MW00845766

12TH EDITION

DIPIRO'S PHARMACOTHERAPY

A PATHOPHYSIOLOGIC APPROACH

Assistant Editors

Angela L. Bingham, PharmD, BCPS, BCNSP, BCCCP
Vice Chair and Clinical Associate Professor
Philadelphia College of Pharmacy
Saint Joseph's University
Philadelphia, Pennsylvania

Scott Bolesta, PharmD, BCPS
Professor
Department of Pharmacy Practice
Nesbitt School of Pharmacy, Wilkes University
Wilkes-Barre, Pennsylvania

Robert J. DiDomenico, PharmD, FCCP, FHFSA, FACC
Associate Professor and Assistant Head
Department of Pharmacy Practice
College of Pharmacy, University of Illinois Chicago
Chicago, Illinois

Rena A. Gosser, PharmD, BCPS
Clinical Ambulatory Pharmacy Manager
Harborview Medical Center
Seattle, Washington

Lisa M. Holle, PharmD, BCOP
Clinical Professor of Pharmacy Practice
Department of Pharmacy Practice
School of Pharmacy, University of Connecticut
Storrs, Connecticut

Amy M. VandenBerg, PharmD, BCPP
Clinical Associate Professor
College of Pharmacy, University of Michigan
Ann Arbor, Michigan

12TH EDITION

DIPIRO'S PHARMACOTHERAPY

A PATHOPHYSIOLOGIC APPROACH

Editors

Joseph T. DiPiro, PharmD
Professor, School of Pharmacy
Associate Vice President for Health Sciences
Virginia Commonwealth University
Richmond, Virginia

Gary C. Yee, PharmD
Professor, College of Pharmacy
Practice
Associate Vice Chancellor for Academic Affairs University of
Nebraska Medical Center
Omaha, Nebraska

Stuart T. Haines, PharmD, BCPS, BCACP
Professor, Department of Pharmacy Practice
Director, Pharmacy Professional Development
School Pharmacy, University of Mississippi
Jackson, Mississippi

Thomas D. Nolin, PharmD, PhD, FCCP, FCP, FASN
Associate Dean for Research and Sponsored Programs
Associate Professor of Pharmacy and Therapeutics
School of Pharmacy, University of Pittsburgh
Pittsburgh, Pennsylvania

Vicki L. Ellingrod, PharmD, FCCP
Dean and John Gideon Searle Professor of Pharmacy
College of Pharmacy
Professor of Psychiatry, Medical School
University of Michigan
Ann Arbor, Michigan

L. Michael Posey, BSPharm, MA
President
PENS Pharmacy Editorial & News Services
Santa Rosa, California

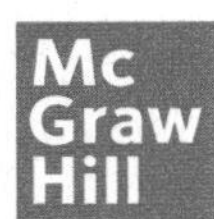

New York Chicago San Francisco Athens London Madrid Mexico City Milan New Delhi Singapore Sydney Toronto

DiPiro's Pharmacotherapy: A Pathophysiologic Approach, Twelfth Edition

1 2 3 4 5 6 7 8 9 LWI 27 26 25 24 23

ISBN 978-1-264-26454-4
MHID 1-264-26454-2

Notice

Medicine is an ever-changing science. As new research and clinical experience broaden our knowledge, changes in treatment and drug therapy are required. The authors and the publisher of this work have checked with sources believed to be reliable in their efforts to provide information that is complete and generally in accord with the standards accepted at the time of publication. However, in view of the possibility of human error or changes in medical sciences, neither the authors nor the publisher nor any other party who has been involved in the preparation or publication of this work warrants that the information contained herein is in every respect accurate or complete, and they disclaim all responsibility for any errors or omissions or for the results obtained from use of the information contained in this work. Readers are encouraged to confirm the information contained herein with other sources. For example and in particular, readers are advised to check the product information sheet included in the package of each drug they plan to administer to be certain that the information contained in this work is accurate and that changes have not been made in the recommended dose or in the contraindications for administration. This recommendation is of particular importance in connection with new or infrequently used drugs.

This book was set in Minion Pro by MPS Limited.
The editors were Michael Weitz and Peter J. Boyle.
The production supervisor was Catherine H. Saggese.
Project management was provided by Poonam Bisht, MPS Limited.
The designer was Alan Barnett.

This book was printed on acid-free paper.

Cataloging-in-publication data for this book is on file at the Library of Congress.

Dedication

To our patients and students, who have challenged and inspired us and given meaning to all our endeavors.

To practitioners who continue to improve patient health outcomes and thereby serve as role models for their colleagues and students while clinging tenaciously to the highest standards of practice.

To our mentors, whose vision provided educational and training programs that encouraged our professional growth and challenged us to be innovators in our patient care, research, and education.

To our faculty colleagues for their efforts and support for our mission to provide a comprehensive and challenging educational foundation for the pharmacists of the future.

And finally to our families for the time that they have sacrificed so that this twelfth edition would become a reality.

—The Editors

PAST EDITORS OF DIPIRO'S *PHARMACOTHERAPY*

Peggy E. Hayes, PharmD
Editions 1 and 2

Gary R. Matzke, PharmD, FCP, FCCP, FASN, FNAP
Editions 2–10

Robert L. Talbert, PharmD, FCCP, BCPS, FAHA
Editions 1–10

Barbara G. Wells, PharmD, FCCP, FASHP
Editions 3–10

Contents

SECTION 4 Cardiovascular Disorders 85

Section Editor: *Stuart T. Haines*

SECTION 5 Respiratory Disorders 355

Section Editor: *Stuart T. Haines*

SECTION 6 Gastrointestinal Disorders 457

Section Editor: *Joseph T. DiPiro*

SECTION 7 Renal Disorders 619

Section Editor: *Thomas D. Nolin*

SECTION 19 Oncologic Disorders 2155

Section Editor: *Gary C. Yee*

SECTION 20 Nutritional Disorders 2455

Section Editor: *Thomas D. Nolin*

SI unit conversions were produced by Ed Randell, PhD, DCC, FCACB, Division Chief and Professor of Laboratory Medicine, Department of Laboratory Medicine, Eastern Health Authority and Faculty of Medicine, Memorial University of Newfoundland, St. John's, Newfoundland, Canada

Conflict of Interest Disclosure and Mitigation

Contributors to *Pharmacotherapy: A Pathophysiologic Approach* must disclose relevant financial and other interests with entities that produce, market, sell, or distribute medications, health products, or services related to the medication use process. All contributors completed, signed, and submitted a conflict of interest (COI) disclosure statement to the Editors. Starting with the 11th edition, the COI disclosure was submitted after an invitation has been extended and before a contributor agreement was signed.

After reviewing the COI disclosure statement submitted by a contributor, the Editors developed and approved a plan to mitigate any and all potential COIs that might be reasonably perceived by the readers of *Pharmacotherapy: A Pathophysiologic Approach* to unduly influence the contributor's favorable or unfavorable portrayal of any product or service. The mitigation plan included, but was not limited to, assigning a coauthor with no COIs to work with the contributor, subjecting the contribution to external peer review, or asking the contributor to divest the interest(s).

No contributor may receive a payment or services from a third party (commercial entity, government agency, professional organization, private foundation, etc.) for any work product submitted to *Pharmacotherapy: A Pathophysiologic Approach.*

Starting with the 11th edition, potential contributors who are employees of a commercial entity that produces, markets, sells, or distributes medications or healthcare products are not invited or re-invited to contribute.

COI disclosures for all contributors to *Pharmacotherapy: A Pathophysiologic Approach* will be made available to readers online. The internet address for the COI disclosure page will be published in the Contributors section of the text.

Contributors

Patrick Aaronson, PharmD, DABAT
Clinical Associate Professor and Emergency Medicine Practitioner
University of Florida Health
Jacksonville, Florida
Chapter 85

Kim G. Adcock, PharmD, CCRC
Professor of Pharmacy Practice and Director of Faculty and Academic Affairs
School of Pharmacy, University of Mississippi
Professor of Pediatrics and Director of the Office of Interprofessional Education
University of Mississippi Medical Center
Jackson, Mississippi
Chapter 47

Bryan T. Alexander, PharmD, BCIDP, AAHIVP
Pharmacy Coordinator, Outpatient Antimicrobial Therapy Program
Nebraska Medicine
Omaha, Nebraska
Chapter 141

Rondall E. Allen, BS, PharmD
Provost and Vice President for Academic Affairs
University of Maryland Eastern Shore
Professor, Pharmacy Practice and Administration
Salisbury, Maryland
Chapter e56

Peter L. Anderson, PharmD
Professor
University of Colorado Anschutz Medical Campus
Aurora, Colorado
Chapter 148

Sarah L. Anderson, PharmD, BCACP, BCPS
Scientific Director
Clinical Care Options
Denver, Colorado
Chapter e35

Rebecca L. Attridge, PharmD, MSc, BCPS, BCCCP
Principal, Pharmacotherapy
The Craneware Group
Colorado Springs, Colorado
Chapter 46

Linda Awdishu, PharmD, MAS
Professor of Clinical Pharmacy, Division Head of Clinical Pharmacy, Director of Simulation and Interprofessional Education
Skaggs School of Pharmacy and Pharmaceutical Sciences, University of California, San Diego
La Jolla, California
Chapter e60

Erin B. Bailey, PharmD, BCOP
Clinical Pharmacist
University of Utah Health, Huntsman Cancer Institute
Salt Lake City, Utah
Chapter e161

Jacquelyn L. Bainbridge, PharmD, MSCS
Professor, Departments of Clinical Pharmacy and Neurology
Skaggs School of Pharmacy and Pharmaceutical Sciences, University of Colorado, Anschutz Medical Campus
Aurora, Colorado
Chapter 74

Gary Bakst, MD
Head, Division of Community Endocrinology
Albany Medical Center
Albany, New York
Chapter 96

Katie E. Barber, PharmD
Associate Professor
School of Pharmacy, University of Mississippi
Jackson, Mississippi
Chapter e126

Jeffrey F. Barletta, BS, PharmD
Professor and Vice Chair of Pharmacy Practice
College of Pharmacy, Midwestern University
Glendale, Arizona
Chapter 41

Kylie N. Barnes, PharmD, BCPS
Clinical Associate Professor
University of Missouri–Kansas City School of Pharmacy
Kansas City, Missouri
Chapter 99

Erin F. Barreto, PharmD, MSc
Associate Professor of Medicine and Pharmacy
Mayo Clinic
Rochester, Minnesota
Chapter e26

Brittany N. Bates, PharmD, BCPS
Assistant Professor of Pharmacy Practice
Ohio Northern University
Ada, Ohio
Chapter 136

Jill S. Bates, PharmD, BCOP
National PHASER Pharmacy Program Manager
Durham VA Health Care System
Associate Professor of Clinical Education
Eshelman School of Pharmacy
Durham VA Health Care System
University of North Carolina
Chapter e160

Seth R. Bauer, PharmD, BCCCP
Critical Care Clinical Specialist
Cleveland Clinic
Clinical Assistant Professor
Cleveland Clinic Lerner College of Medicine
Cleveland, Ohio
Chapter e42

Steven J. Bauer, MD
Medical Director of Certified Community Mental Health Clinic
Human Development Center
Duluth, Minnesota
Chapter e81

Jerry L. Bauman, PharmD
Dean Emeritus and Distinguished Professor Emeritus
College of Pharmacy, University of Illinois at Chicago
Chicago, Illinois
Editor-in-Chief
Journal of the American College of Clinical Pharmacy
Lenexa, Kansas
Chapter 40

Oralia V. Bazaldua, PharmD, BCACP
Professor/Clinical
The University of Texas Health Science Center
Ambulatory Care Clinical Pharmacy Specialist
University Health System San Antonio
San Antonio, Texas
Chapter e2

Scott J. Bergman, PharmD, BCIDP
Nebraska Coordinator Antimicrobial Stewardship, Clinical Professor
College of Pharmacy
University of Nebraska Medical Center
Omaha, Nebraska
Chapter 141

Angela L. Bingham, PharmD, BCPS, BCNSP, BCCCP
Vice Chair and Clinical Associate Professor
Philadelphia College of Pharmacy
Saint Joseph's University
Philadelphia, Pennsylvania
Chapters 69, 164

Jeffrey R. Bishop, PharmD, MS, BCPP
Associate Professor
College of Pharmacy
University of Minnesota
Minneapolis, Minnesota
Chapter e81

Martha G. Blackford, PharmD, BCPS
Clinical Pharmacologist and Toxicologist
Akron Children's Hospital
North Canton, Ohio
Chapter 129

Kathryn V. Blake, PharmD, BCPS
Director, Center for Pharmacogenomics and Translational Research
Nemours Children's Health
Jacksonville, Florida
Chapter 44

Christopher M. Bland, PharmD, BCPS
Clinical Professor
College of Pharmacy, University of Georgia
Antimicrobial Stewardship Pharmacist
St. Joseph's/Candler Health System
Athens, Georgia
Chapter e108

Scott Bolesta, PharmD, BCPS
Professor
Nesbitt College of Pharmacy, Wilkes University
Wilkes-Barre, Pennsylvania
Chapter 57

Jill S. Borchert, PharmD, BCPS, BCACP
Professor and Vice Chair
College of Pharmacy
Midwestern University
Downers Grove, Illinois
Chapter 112

Bonnie Lin Boster, PharmD, BCOP
Clinical Pharmacy Specialist
University of Texas MD Anderson Cancer Center
Houston, Texas
Chapter 151

Jolene R. Bostwick, PharmD
Assistant Dean for Co-curriculum and Professional Development and Clinical Professor of Pharmacy, Department of Clinical Pharmacy, and Clinical Pharmacist, Michigan Medicine
University of Michigan College of Pharmacy
Ann Arbor, Michigan
Chapter 91

Bradley A. Boucher, PharmD, MCCM
Interim Dean and Professor
Department of Clinical Pharmacy and Translational Science
College of Pharmacy
University of Tennessee Health Science Center
Memphis, Tennessee
Chapter 77

Sharya V. Bourdet, PharmD, BCPS
Associate Chief of Pharmacy for Acute Care and Education
San Francisco VA Medical Center
Associate Professor of Clinical Pharmacy
University of California San Francisco School of Pharmacy
San Francisco, California
Chapter 45

Kristina M. Brooks, PharmD
Assistant Professor-Research
University of Colorado Anschutz Medical Campus
Aurora, Colorado
Chapter 148

Caitlin S. Brown, PharmD, BCCCP
Neurocritical and Emergency Medicine Pharmacist
Mayo Clinic
Assistant Professor of Pharmacy & Emergency Medicine
Mayo School of Medicine
Minneapolis, Minnesota
Chapter e27

Jamal Brown, PharmD, BCGP
Associate Professor of Pharmacy Practice
College of Pharmacy, Florida A&M University
Tampa, Florida
Chapter e9

Thomas E. R. Brown, PharmD
Associate Professor
Leslie Dan Faculty of Pharmacy
University of Toronto
Toronto, Ontario
Chapter 143

Peter F. Buckley, MD
Chancellor
University of Tennessee Health Science Center
Memphis, Tennessee
Chapter 87

Yvonne J. Burnett, PharmD, BCIDP
Associate Professor of Pharmacy Practice
University of Health Sciences and Pharmacy in Saint Louis
Clinical Pharmacy Specialist, Infectious Diseases
Missouri Baptist Medical Center
St. Louis, Missouri
Chapter 140

David S. Burgess, PharmD
Professor and Chair, Department of Pharmacy Practice & Science
College of Pharmacy
University of Kentucky
Lexington, Kentucky
Chapter 127

Lakesha M. Butler, PharmD, BCACP, CDFT
Associate Vice President, Inclusion, Diversity and Health Equity and Clinical Professor
College of Pharmacy
University of Florida
Gainesville, Florida
Chapter e3

Morgan A. Butrovich, PharmD
PhD Candidate
University of Pittsburgh School of Pharmacy
Pittsburgh, Pennsylvania
Chapter 67

Lucinda M. Buys, PharmD, BCACP
Clinical Pharmacist and Clinical Services Director
Siouxland Medical Education Foundation
Sioux City, Iowa
Chapter 110

Megan L. Carreon, MHA, RRT, RRT
Assistant Professor, Division of Respiratory Care
UT Health San Antonio
University of Texas Health Science Center
San Antonio, Texas
Chapter e43

Peggy L. Carver, PharmD
Associate Professor
College of Pharmacy
University of Michigan
Clinical pharmacist, Infectious diseases
Ann Arbor, Michigan
Chapter 144

Larisa H. Cavallari, PharmD
Professor of Pharmacotherapy and Translational Research
College of Pharmacy
University of Florida
Gainesville, Florida
Chapter e7

Alexandre Chan, PharmD, MPH, BCPS, BCOP
Founding Chair and Professor of Clinical Pharmacy
University of California, Irvine
Clinical Pharmacist
Chao Family Comprehensive Cancer Center
Irvine, California
Chapter 155

Edward Chang, MD, PhD
Clinical Neurophysiology Fellowship Program Director
Harbor UCLA Medical Center
West Carson, California
Chapter 75

Daniel B. Chastain, PharmD, BCIDP, AAHIVP
Clinical Associate Professor
College of Pharmacy
University of Georgia
Athens, Georgia
Chapter 134

Jack J. Chen, PharmD, BCPS, BCGP
Consultant
Clinical Movement Disorders
Chino Hills, California
Chapter 78

Judy T. Chen, PharmD, BCPS, BCACP, CDCES
Clinical Associate Professor
College of Pharmacy
Purdue University
Clinical Pharmacy Specialist, Women's Health
Indianapolis, Indiana
Chapters 102, 167

Katherine H. Chessman, BS-Pharm, PharmD, BCPS, BCNSP
Professor and Chair, Clinical Pharmacy and Outcome Sciences
College of Pharmacy
Medical University of South Carolina
Clinical Pharmacy Specialist, Pediatrics/Pediatric Surgery/Intestinal Rehabilitation
MUSC Shawn Jenkins Children's Hospital
Charleston, South Carolina
Chapters e21, 68, 164

Mariann D. Churchwell, PharmD, BCPS
Professor
University of Toledo College of Pharmacy and Pharmaceutical Sciences
Clinical Pharmacy Specialist
Toledo, Ohio
Chapter 64

Amber B. Cipriani, PharmD, BCOP
Precision Medicine Pharmacy Coordinator
UNC Health Medical Center
University of North Carolina
Clinical Assistant Professor
UNC Eshelman School of Pharmacy
Chapel Hill, North Carolina
Chapter 154

Nathan P. Clark, PharmD, BCPS
Clinical Pharmacy Cardiovascular Services Manager
Kaiser Permanente Colorado
Denver, Colorado
Chapter 38

Jessica M. Clement, MD
Medical Director of Oncology Research
Hartford HealthCare Cancer Institute
Hartford, Connecticut
Chapter 153

Amber B. Clemmons, PharmD, BCOP
Clinical Professor
College of Pharmacy
University of Georgia
Clinical Pharmacy Specialist - Hematology/Bone Marrow Transplantation
Augusta University (AU) Medical Center
Augusta, Georgia
Chapter 150

Jill M. Comeau, PharmD, BCOP
Associate Professor of Clinical Sciences
College of Pharmacy
University of Louisiana Monroe
Gratis Assistant Professor of Internal Medicine
Feist-Weiller Cancer Center
LSU-Health Shreveport
Monroe, Louisiana
Chapter 158

Kristen M. Cook, PharmD, BCACP
Clinical Associate Professor, College of Pharmacy
University of Nebraska Medical Center
Ambulatory Care Pharmacist
Nebraska Medicine
Omaha, Nebraska
Chapter 122

Lisa M. Cordes, PharmD, BCACP, BCOP
Oncology Clinical Pharmacy Specialist
Office of Clinical Research and National Cancer Institute, National Institutes of Health
Washington, D.C.
Chapter 149

Ryan C. Costantino, PharmD, MS, BCPS, BCGP, CPHIMS
Chief, Data Science Branch
Enterprise Intelligence & Data Solutions Program Management Office
Program Executive Office, Defense Healthcare Management Systems
San Antonio, Texas
Chapter e10

Jason M. Cota, PharmD, MS, BCIDP
Vice Chair and Professor of Pharmacy Practice
Feik School of Pharmacy. University of the Incarnate Word
San Antonio, Texas
Chapter e138

Zachary L. Cox, PharmD
Professor
Lipscomb University College of Pharmacy
Heart Failure Clinical Pharmacy Specialist
Vanderbilt University Medical Center
Nashville, Tennessee
Chapter 37

Elizabeth A. Coyle, PharmD, BCPS
Associate Dean for Academic Affairs, Clinical Professor
College of Pharmacy, University of Houston
Houston, Texas
Chapter 139

Catherine M. Crill, PharmD, FCCP, BCNSP
Associate Professor
Departments of Clinical Pharmacy & Translational Science and Pediatrics
Director of Experiential Learning and International Programs
College of Pharmacy, University of Tennessee Health Science Center
Memphis, Tennessee
Chapter 165

M. Lynn Crismon, PharmD, DABCP, BCPP
Behrens Centennial Professor of Pharmacy
College of Pharmacy
University of Texas at Austin
Professor of Psychiatry
Dell Medical School
University of Texas at Austin
Austin, Texas
Chapter 87

Daniel J. Crona, PharmD, PhD, CPP
Associate Professor
Division of Pharmacotherapy and Experimental Therapeutics
Eshelman School of Pharmacy
Clinical Pharmacist Practitioner
Genitourinary Malignancies, Department of Pharmacy
University of North Carolina Medical Center
Chapel Hill, North Carolina
Chapter 154

Ericka L. Crouse, PharmD, BCPP, BCGP
Associate Professor
Virginia Commonwealth University School of Pharmacy
Clinical Pharmacy Specialist – Psychiatry
VCU Health
Richmond, Virginia
Chapters 73, 91

Sandra Cuellar, PharmD, BCOP
Clinical Associate Professor
College of Pharmacy
University of Illinois
Clinical Oncology Pharmacist
UI Health
Chicago, Illinois
Chapter 149

William Dager, PharmD, BCPS, MCCM
Cardiovascular Pharmacist Specialist
University of California, Davis Medical Center
Clinical Professor of Pharmacy
University of California San Francisco School of Pharmacy
Clinical Professor of Medicine
University of California Davis School of Medicine
Sacramento, California
Chapter 61

Devra K. Dang, CDCES, FNAP
Associate Clinical Professor of Pharmacy Practice
Department of Pharmacy Practice
University of Connecticut College of Pharmacy
Storrs, Connecticut
Chapter 102

Khashayar Dashtipour, MD, PhD
Associate Professor of Neurology and Basic Sciences
Loma Linda University
Loma Linda, California
Chapter 78

Christina M. Davis, PharmD, BCOP
Clinical Oncology Pharmacy Specialist
University of Colorado Hospital
Denver, Colorado
Chapter 162

Lisa E. Davis, PharmD, FCCP, BCPS, BCOP
Clinical Professor
R. Ken Coit College of Pharmacy
University of Arizona
Clinical Pharmacist
University of Arizona Cancer Center
Tucson, Arizona
Chapter 153

Paulina Deming, PharmD
Clinician Educator—Associate Professor
University of New Mexico Health Sciences Center
Albuquerque, New Mexico
Chapter 58

David DeRemer, PharmD, BCOP
Clinical Professor
College of Pharmacy, University of Florida
Assistant Director, Experimental Therapeutics Group
University of Florida Health Cancer Center
Gainesville, Florida
Chapter 157

Sunita Dergalust, PharmD
Neurology Pharmacist
Department of Veterans Affairs
Ventura County, California
Chapter 75

Robert J. DiDomenico, PharmD
Associate Professor and Assistant Head of Pharmacy Practice
University of Illinois Chicago
Chicago, Illinois
Chapters 33, 34

Elizabeth Dimaggio, PharmD, BCOP
Clinical Pharmacy Specialist
Blood and Marrow Transplantation and Cellular Immunotherapy
H. Lee Moffitt Cancer Center
Tampa, Florida
Chapter e163

Dave L. Dixon, PharmD, BCACP, CLS
Nancy L. and Ronald H. McFarlane Professor of Pharmacy
Virginia Commonwealth University School of Pharmacy
Chair
Department of Pharmacotherapy & Outcomes Science
Richmond, Virginia
Chapter 32

Le Hanh Dung Do, MD
Attending Physician
Hiep Loi Cosmetic Surgery Hospital
Ho Chi Minh City, Vietnam
Chapter 120

Paul P. Dobesh, PharmD, BCCP
Professor of Pharmacy Practice and Science
College of Pharmacy
University of Nebraska Medical Center
Cardiology Clinical Pharmacy Specialist
Nebraska Medicine
Omaha, Nebraska
Chapters 33, 34

Krista L. Donohoe, PharmD, BCPS, BCGP
Associate Professor
Virginia Commonwealth University School of Pharmacy
Richmond, Virginia
Chapters e23, 53

Julie A. Dopheide, PharmD, BCPP
Professor of Clinical Pharmacy, Psychiatry and the Behavioral Sciences
University of Southern California School of Pharmacy
Keck School of Medicine
Los Angeles, California
Chapter 82

John M. Dopp, PharmD
Associate Professor
School of Pharmacy
University of Wisconsin
Madison, Wisconsin
Chapter 92

Thomas C. Dowling, PharmD, PhD
Assistant Dean and Professor
Director, Office of Research and Sponsored Programs
College of Pharmacy
Ferris State University
Grand Rapids, Michigan
Chapter e60

Shannon J. Drayton, PharmD, BCPP
Associate Professor
College of Pharmacy
Medical University of South Carolina
Charleston, South Carolina
Chapter 89

Linda D. Dresser, BScPhm, PharmD
Assistant Professor, Teaching Stream
Leslie Dan Faculty of Pharmacy
University of Toronto
Elgin, Ontario
Chapter 143

Lori H. Dupree, PharmD, BCPS
Clinical Assistant Professor
College of Pharmacy
Mercer University
Suwanee, Georgia
Chapter 86

Lauren Duran, PharmD, MBA, BCPPS
Clinical Pharmacist – Hematology/Oncology
Cook Children's Medical Center
Fort Worth, Texas
Chapter 123

Amy L. Dzierba, PharmD, BCCCP
Clinical Pharmacist, Adult Critical Care
NewYork–Presbyterian Hospital
New York, New York
Chapter e26

Deepak P. Edward, MD FACS FARVO
Professor of Ophthalmology
Department of Ophthalmology and Visual Sciences
Chicago, Illinois
Chapter 114

Lea S. Eiland, PharmD, BCPS, BCPPS
Clinical Professor and Associate Department Head
Harrison College of Pharmacy
Auburn University
Auburn, Alabama
Chapter e12

Shareen Y. El-Ibiary, PharmD, BCPS
Professor and Department Chair
College of Pharmacy
Midwestern University
Glendale, Arizona
Chapter 19

Vicki L. Ellingrod, PharmD, FCCP
Dean and John Gideon Searle Professor of Pharmacy,
College of Pharmacy
Professor of Psychiatry, Medical School
University of Michigan
Ann Arbor, Michigan
Chapter e84

Ramy H. Elshaboury, PharmD, BCPS
Director—Clinical Pharmacy Services
Massachusetts General Hospital
Boston, Massachusetts
Chapter 128

Steven R. Erickson, PharmD
Associate Professor
College of Pharmacy
University of Michigan
Ann Arbor, Michigan
Chapter e93

Michael E. Ernst, PharmD
Clinical Professor
College of Pharmacy
University of Iowa
Iowa City, Iowa
Chapter 113

Brian L. Erstad, PharmD, MCCM, BCPS
Professor and Head
R. Ken Coit College of Pharmacy
University of Arizona
Tucson, Arizona
Chapter e42

Alisa K. Escano, PharmD, BCPS
Clinical Assistant Professor
Virginia Commonwealth University, Inova campus
Clinical Pharmacy Specialist, Internal Medicine
Richmond, Virginia
Chapter 115

Gregory A. Eschenauer, PharmD
Clinical Associate Professor
College of Pharmacy
University of Michigan
Clinical Specialist, Infectious Diseases
Michigan Medicine
Ann Arbor, Michigan
Chapter 144

Patricia H. Fabel, PharmD, BCPS
Clinical Associate Professor
University of South Carolina College of Pharmacy
Columbia, South Carolina
Chapter 54

Alireza Fakhriravari, PharmD, BCPS, BCIDP, AAHIVP
Clinical Assistant Professor and Director of Advanced Pharmacy Practice Experiences
School of Pharmacy, Loma Linda University
Loma Linda, California
Chapter e138

Karen M. Fancher, PharmD, BCOP
Associate Professor of Pharmacy Practice
School of Pharmacy, Duquesne University
Clinical Pharmacy Specialist, Oncology
University of Pittsburgh Medical Center Passavant
Pittsburgh, Pennsylvania
Chapter 158

Natalija M. Farrell, PharmD, BCPS, DABAT
Clinical Coordinator—Emergency Medicine & Toxicology
Boston Medical Center
Assistant Professor of Emergency Medicine
Boston University School of Medicine
Boston, Massachusetts
Chapter e8

Joseph P. Fava, PharmD, BCACP
Clinical Assistant Professor
Wayne State University
Detroit, Michigan
Chapter 112

Julianna M. Fernandez, PharmD, BCPS, BCGP
Clinical Associate Professor and Vice Chair of Pharmacy Practice and Translational Research
College of Pharmacy
University of Houston
Houston, Texas
Chapter 139

Shannon W. Finks, PharmD, BCPS, BCCP, ASHCP-CHC
Professor of Clinical Pharmacy and Translational Science
College of Pharmacy, University of Tennessee Health Science Center
Memphis, Tennessee
Chapter 34

Richard Fiscella, PharmD, MPH
Clinical Professor Emeritus
University of Illinois at Chicago
Chicago, Illinois
Chapter 114

Douglas N. Fish, PharmD, BCCCP
Professor and Chair, Department of Clinical Pharmacy
Skaggs School of Pharmacy and Pharmaceutical Sciences
University of Colorado
Aurora, Colorado
Chapters 133, 145

Courtney V. Fletcher, PharmD
Professor
College of Pharmacy
University of Nebraska Medical Center
Omaha, Nebraska
Chapter 148

Rachel W. Flurie, PharmD, BCPS
Assistant Professor
Virginia Commonwealth University School of Pharmacy
Richmond, Virginia
Chapter 70

Alicia B. Forinash, PharmD, BCPS, BCACP
Professor, Pharmacy Practice
Pharmacy Practice
University of Health Science and Pharmacy
St. Louis, Missouri
Chapter 99

Gilles L. Fraser, PharmD, MCCM
Professor of Medicine (ret.)
School of Medicine, Tufts University
Boston, Massachusetts
Clinical Specialist in Critical Care (ret.)
Maine Medical Center
Portland, Maine
Chapter e27

Michelle A. Fravel, PharmD, BCPS
Clinical Associate Professor of Pharmacy Practice and Science
University of Iowa College of Pharmacy
Clinical Pharmacy Specialist
University of Iowa Hospitals and Clinics
Iowa City, Iowa
Chapter 113

Bradi L. Frei, PharmD, MSc, BCPS, BCOP
Professor
Feik School of Pharmacy
University of the Incarnate Word
San Antonio, Texas
Chapter 130

Christopher R. Frei, PharmD, MS, BCPS
Professor and Pharmacotherapy Division Head
University of Texas at Austin College of Pharmacy
Pharmacotherapy Education and Research Center Director
University of Texas Health Science Center at San Antonio Long School of Medicine
Boerne, Texas
Chapter 130

Stormi E. Gale, PharmD, BCCP, BCPS
Clinical Pharmacist, Cardiology
Novant Health Matthews Medical Center
Charlotte, North Carolina
Chapter 37

Roseann S. Gammal, PharmD, BCPS
Associate Professor of Pharmacy Practice
Massachusetts College of Pharmacy and Health Sciences
Boston, Massachusetts
Chapter e7

Kristen N. Gardner, PharmD, BCPP
Clinical Pharmacy Specialist – Behavioral Health
Kaiser Permanente Colorado
Denver, Colorado
Chapter 91

Mandy L. Gatesman, PharmD, BCOP
Clinical Pharmacy Specialist, Hematology & Oncology
VCU Health
Richmond, Virginia
Chapter 53

Jessica E. Geiger, PharmD, MS, BCPS
Pharmacy Coordinator, Palliative Care
OhioHealth
Columbus, Ohio
Chapter e28

Tracey L. Gendron, MS, PhD
Associate Professor and Chair, Department of Gerontology
Virginia Commonwealth University
Executive Director, Virginia Center on Aging
Richmond, Virginia
Chapter e23

James F. Gilmore, PharmD, BCCCP, BCPS
Pharmacy Manager
Adult Critical Care and Emergency Department Medicine
Cedars-Sinai
Los Angeles, California
Chapter e95

Ashley E. Glode, PharmD, BCOP
Associate Professor
Skaggs School of Pharmacy and Pharmaceutical Sciences
University of Colorado
Aurora, Colorado
Chapter 150

Victor R. Gordeuk, MD
Professor of Medicine
Department of Medicine
University of Illinois at Chicago
Chicago, Illinois
Chapter 124

Rena A. Gosser, PharmD, BCPS
Clinical Ambulatory Pharmacy Manager
Harborview Medical Center
Seattle, Washington
Chapter e116

Leigh Anne H. Gravatt, PharmD, BCPS
Associate Professor, Vice-Chair of Education of The Department of Pharmacotherapy and Outcomes Sciences
VCU School of Pharmacy
Clinical Specialist, Internal Medicine
Chesterfield, Virginia
Chapter 53

Shelly L. Gray, PharmD, MS
Professor and Plein Endowed Director
Plein Center for Geriatric Pharmacy Research, Education and Outreach
School of Pharmacy, University of Washington
Seattle, Washington
Chapters e24, e25

Elisa M. Greene, PharmD, BCACP
Associate Professor of Pharmacy Practice
College of Pharmacy
Belmont University
Nashville, Tennessee
Chapter e125

Devon M. Greer, PharmD, BCOP
Clinical Pharmacy Specialist - Medical Oncology
Barnes-Jewish Hospital
St. Louis, Missouri
Chapter 122

Shawn P. Griffin, PharmD, BCOP
Health Sciences Assistant Clinical Professor
School of Pharmacy & Pharmaceutical Sciences
University of California, Irvine
Irvine, California
Chapter 155

Alan E. Gross, PharmD, BCIDP, BCPS
Clinical Associate Professor
Department of Pharmacy Practice, University of Illinois at Chicago College of Pharmacy
Infectious Diseases Pharmacist
University of Illinois Hospital and Health Sciences System
Chicago, Illinois
Chapter 137

Stephanie Gruber, PharmD, BCACP
Clinical Pharmacy Practitioner
William S. Middleton Memorial Veterans Hospital
Madison, Wisconsin
Chapter 111

Wayne P. Gulliver, MD, FRCPC
Professor of Dermatology and Medicine
Memorial University of Newfoundland
Clinical Pharmacy Practitioner
Chapters 118, 119

John G. Gums, PharmD
Associate Dean for Clinical and Administrative Affairs and Professor of Pharmacy and Medicine
College of Pharmacy
St. John's, Newfoundland and Labrador, Canada
Gainesville, Florida
Chapter 97

Tracy M. Hagemann, PharmD
Professor and Associate Dean, Nashville
College of Pharmacy
University of Tennessee Health Science Center
Nashville, Tennessee
Chapter e125

Stuart T. Haines, PharmD, BCPS, BCACP
Professor and Director, Pharmacy Professional Development
Department of Pharmacy Practice
School of Pharmacy, University of Mississippi
Jackson, Mississippi
Chapters 1, 94

Emily R. Hajjar, PharmD, MS, BCPS, BCACP, BCGP
Professor
Jefferson College of Pharmacy
Philadelphia, Pennsylvania
Chapter e24

Elizabeth A. Hall, PharmD, BCPS, BCPPS
Assistant Professor and Director of Assessment
College of Pharmacy, University of Tennessee Health Science Center
Memphis, Tennessee
Chapter 76

Maren Hall, DDS
General Dentist
Elk Plaza Dental
Maple Grove, Minnesota
Chapter e16

Jin Han, PharmD, PhD, BCPS
Clinical Associate Professor and Clinical Pharmacist
College of Pharmacy, University of Illinois at Chicago
Chicago, Illinois
Chapter 124

Jason S. Haney, PharmD, BCPS, BCCCP
Associate Professor
College of Pharmacy, Medical University of South Carolina
Charleston, South Carolina
Chapter 68

Bianca Harris, PharmD
Clinical Pharmacy Practitioner
William S. Middleton Memorial Veteran's Hospital
Madison, Wisconsin
Chapter 111

Delaney E. Hart, PharmD, BCIDP
Clinical Pharmacist
Allina Health
Minneapolis, Minnesota
Chapter 128

Bryan D. Hayes, PharmD, DABAT
Clinical Pharmacy Manager
Massachusetts General Hospital
Associate Professor of Emergency Medicine, Division of Medical Toxicology
Harvard Medical School
Boston, Massachusetts
Chapter e8

Jordan C. Haygood, PharmD, BCPP
Clinical Assistant Professor
University of South Carolina College of Pharmacy
Psychiatric Clinical Pharmacist
Columbia, South Carolina
Chapter 89

Mary S. Hayney, PharmD, MPH, BCPS
Professor
School of Pharmacy
University of Wisconsin
Madison, Wisconsin
Chapter 147

Mojdeh S. Heavner, PharmD, BCPS, BCCCP
Associate Professor and Vice Chair for Clinical Services
School of Pharmacy, University of Maryland
Baltimore, Maryland
Chapter e48

Keith A. Hecht, PharmD, BCOP
Associate Professor, Pharmacy Practice
School of Pharmacy
Southern Illinois University Edwardsville
St Charles, Missouri
Chapter 152

Natalie T. Heinrich, PharmD
Medication Therapy Management (MTM) Pharmacist
M Health Fairview
Minnesota
Chapter 80

Brian A. Hemstreet, PharmD, BCPS
Associate Dean for Student Affairs and Professor
Skaggs School of Pharmacy and Pharmaceutical Sciences
University of Colorado
Aurora, Colorado
Chapter 52

Christopher M. Herndon, PharmD, BCACP
Professor
Southern Illinois University Edwardsville
Edwardsville, Illinois
Chapter 79

Lauren R. Hersh, MD
Associate Professor
Department of Family and Community Medicine, Thomas Jefferson University
Philadelphia, PA
Chapter e24

Tara A. Higgins, PharmD, BCPPS
Assistant Professor
School of Pharmacy
Lake Erie College of Osteopathic Medicine
Bradenton, Florida
Chapter 157

Krista B. Highland, PhD
Research Associate Professor
Uniformed Services University of the Health Sciences
Henry M. Jackson Foundation for the Advancement of Military Medicine
Washington, D.C.
Chapter e10

Yunn-Fang Ho, BPharm, MD, PhD
Associate Professor
Graduate Institute of Clinical Pharmacy, College of Medicine
National Taiwan University
Taipei City, Taiwan
Chapter e5

Sarah E. Hobgood, MD
Associate Professor Internal Medicine and Assistant Dean for Clinical Medical Education
Virginia Commonwealth University
Richmond, Virginia
Chapter 73

Lisa M. Holle, PharmD, BCOP
Clinical Professor
School of Pharmacy, University of Connecticut
UConn Health Carole & Ray Neag Comprehensive Cancer Center
Storrs, Connecticut
Chapter 153

Yen-Ming Huang, BPharm, PhD
Assistant Professor
Graduate Institute of Clinical Pharmacy, College of Medicine
National Taiwan University
Taipei City, Taiwan
Chapter e5

Joanna Q. Hudson, PharmD, BCPS
Professor
College of Pharmacy, University of Tennessee Health Science Center
Clinical Pharmacy Specialist – Nephrology
Memphis, Tennessee
Chapter 63

Humberto R. Jimenez, PharmD, MPH, BCPS, AAHIVP
Clinical Assistant Professor and Director of Diverse Scholar Engagement and Advancement
Ernest Mario School of Pharmacy, Rutgers University
Clinical Pharmacist – HIV / Ambulatory Care
St. Joseph's University Medical Center
Piscataway, New Jersey
Chapter 140

Susan Hylland, MD
Attending Physician—Rheumatology Clinic
William S. Middleton Memorial Veterans Hospital
Madison, Wisconsin
Chapter 111

Kristin M. Janzen, PharmD, BCPS
Clinical Assistant Professor, Pharmacy Practice
College of Pharmacy
University of Texas
Clinical Pharmacy Specialist, Internal Medicine
Dell Seton Medical Center at the University of Texas
Austin, Texas
Chapter e6

Douglas L. Jennings, PharmD, BCPS
Associate Professor of Pharmacy
Clinical Pharmacist, Heart Transplant & LVAD Team
Arnold & Marie Schwartz College of Pharmacy and Health Sciences
Long Island University
New York-Presbyterian Hospital
Columbia University Irving Medical Center
New York, New York
Chapter 109

Brittany N. Johnson, PharmD, CPh
Pain and Palliative Care Stewardship Pharmacist and Clinical Assistant Professor
UF Health Jacksonville
University of Florida
Jacksonville, Florida
Chapter 85

Tami N. Johnson, PharmD, BCPS
Clinical Pharmacy Specialist, Emergency Medicine
University of Texas MD Anderson Cancer Center
Houston, Texas
Chapter 71

Duncan B. Johnstone, MD, PhD
Clinical Associate Professor
School of Medicine, University of Buffalo
Buffalo, New York
Chapter e66

Bruce M. Jones, PharmD, BCPS
Infectious Diseases Clinical Pharmacy Specialist
St. Joseph's/Candler Health System, Inc.
Savannah, Georgia
Chapter e108

Joseph K. Jordan, PharmD, BCPS
Professor of Pharmacy Practice
Butler University
Drug Information Specialist
Indiana University Health
Indianapolis, Indiana
Chapter e98

David Josey Jr., MD
Associate Professor of Pediatrics
University of Mississippi Medical Center
Jackson, Mississippi
Chapter 47

Sul R. Jung, PharmD, BCPS, BCCCP
Associate Director of Pharmacy Services
Ventura County Medical Center
Ventura, California
Chapter 142

Julie Ann Justo, PharmD, MS, BCPS-AQ ID
Clinical Associate Professor
University of South Carolina College of Pharmacy
Infectious Diseases Clinical Pharmacy Specialist
Prisma Health Richland Hospital
Columbia, South Carolina
Chapter e132

Michael P. Kane, PharmD, BCPS, BCACP
Professor, Department of Pharmacy Practice
Albany College of Pharmacy and Health Sciences
Clinical Pharmacy Specialist
Albany Medical Center Division of Community Endocrinology
Albany, New York
Chapter 96

S. Lena Kang-Birken, PharmD, AAHIVP
Associate Professor
Thomas J. Long School of Pharmacy
University of the Pacific
Santa Barbara, California
Chapter 142

Salmaan Kanji, BScPharm, PharmD
Clinical Pharmacy Specialist
The Ottawa Hospital
Associate Scientist
The Ottawa Hospital Research Institute
Ottawa, Ontario
Chapter 146

Jaime Kaushik, PharmD, BCOP
Clinical Pharmacy Specialist
University of Texas MD Anderson Cancer Center
Houston, Texas
Chapter 151

Michael S. Kelly, PharmD, BCACP, CLS
Assistant Professor
School of Pharmacy, Chapman University
Irvine, California
Chapter 32

Scott E. Kincaid, PharmD, BCPS
Assistant Dean for Student Affairs
School of Pharmacy, Presbyterian College
Clinton, South Carolina
Chapter e18

William R. Kirchain, PharmD, CDCES
Clinical Associate Professor and Director Xavier University Health and Wellness Center
Xavier University of Louisiana
New Orleans, Louisiana
Chapter e56

Cynthia K. Kirkwood, PharmD, BCPP
Professor and Executive Associate Dean for Academic Affairs
Virginia Commonwealth University
Richmond, Virginia
Chapter 90

Mary Ann Kliethermes, BS Pharm, PharmD, FAPhA, FCIOM
Director of Medication safety and quality
American Society of Health-System Pharmacists
Bethesda, Maryland
Chapter 1

Jessa M. Koch, PharmD, BCPP
Associate Professor
School of Pharmacy, Loma Linda University
Loma Linda, California
Chapter 78

Courtney M. Kominek, PharmD, BCPS, CPE
Clinical Pharmacy Specialist in Pain Management
Harry S. Truman Memorial Veterans' Hospital
Columbia, Missouri
Chapter 79

Christina Koutsari, PharmD, PhD, BCPS, BCIDP
Antimicrobial Stewardship and Infectious Disease Pharmacist
Children's Minnesota
Minneapolis, Minnesota
Chapter 128

Sum Lam, PharmD, BCPS, BCGP
Clinical Professor
College of Pharmacy and Health Sciences, Saint John's University
Clinical Pharmacotherapy Specialist, Geriatrics
NYU Langone Health
YU Langone Hospital—Long Island
Queens, New York
Chapter 105

Y. W. Francis Lam, PharmD
Professor of Pharmacology
University of Texas Health Science Center at San Antonio, San Antonio, Texas
Clinical Associate Professor of Pharmacy
University of Texas at Austin
Austin, Texas
Chapter e7

Nicholas W. Lange, PharmD, BCTXP
Clinical Pharmacy Manager
NewYork–Presbyterian Hospital
New York, New York
Chapter 109

Devin L. Lavender, PharmD, BCPS, BCACP
Clinical Assistant Professor
College of Pharmacy
University of Georgia
Athens, Georgia
Chapter 50

David T. S. Law, BSc, MD, PhD, CCFP
Assistant Professor
Department of Family and Community Medicine
Temerty Faculty of Medicine, University of Toronto
Staff, Department of Family Practice
The Scarborough Hospital and Rouge Valley Health System
Scarborough, Ontario, Canada
Chapter e121

Rebecca M. Law, PharmD
Associate Professor
Memorial University of Newfoundland
St. John's, Newfoundland
Chapters e17, 118, 119,120, e121

Grace C. Lee, PharmD, PhD, BCPS
Assistant Professor
College of Pharmacy
University of Texas at Austin
Austin, Texas
Chapter 130

Mary Lee, PharmD, BCPS
Vice President and Special Assistant to the President
Midwestern University
Professor of Pharmacy Practice
College of Pharmacy, Midwestern University
Downers Grove, Illinois
Chapters 103, 104

Patrick Leffers, PharmD, DABAT
Emergency Medicine Pharmacist
University of Florida Health Jacksonville
Clinical Assistant Professor
College of Pharmacy, University of Florida
Jacksonville, Florida
Chapters e84, 85

Deborah J. Levine, MD
Professor
Medical Director Lung Transplantation
Director of Pulmonary Hypertension Center
University of Texas Health Science Center at San Antonio
San Antonio, Texas
Chapter 46

Stephanie M. Levine, MD
Professor
Medical Director Lung Transplantation
Director of Pulmonary Hypertension Center
University of Texas Health Science Center
San Antonio, Texas
Chapter e43

Robin Moorman Li, PharmD, BCACP
Clinical Associate Professor
College of Pharmacy, University of Florida
Gainesville, Florida
Chapter 86

Fang-Ju Lin, BPharm, MClinPharm, PhD
Associate Professor
National Taiwan University
Deputy Director, Department of Pharmacy
National Taiwan University Hospital
Taipei City, Taiwan
Chapter e5

Bryan L. Love, PharmD, MPH
Associate Professor
University of South Carolina College of Pharmacy
Columbia, South Carolina
Chapter 51

Amanda M. Loya, PharmD, BCPS
Clinical Associate Professor and Founding Chair of Pharmacy Practice & Clinical Sciences Dept.
College of Pharmacy, University of Texas at El Paso
El Paso, Texas
Chapter e3

Sarah E. Lynch, PharmD, BCACP
Clinical Associate Professor and Director of Skills Education
School of Pharmacy and Pharmaceutical Sciences, Binghamton University
Binghamton, New York
Chapter 101

Robert MacLaren, BSc, PharmD, MPH, MCCM
Professor
Skaggs School of Pharmacy and Pharmaceutical Sciences, University of Colorado
Aurora, Colorado
Chapter e42

Eric J. MacLaughlin, PharmD, BCPS
Professor and Chair, Department of Pharmacy Practice
Texas Tech University Health Sciences Center
Amarillo, Texas
Chapters 30, e31

Howard I. Maibach, MD
Professor
University of California San Francisco
San Francisco, California
Chapters e17, 120, e121

Matthew J. Makelky Sr., PharmD, MSCS
Operations Manager
UCHealth, University of Colorado
Fort Collins, Colorado
Chapter 74

Jenana H. Maker, PharmD, BCPS
Professor
Thomas J. Long School of Pharmacy, University of the Pacific
Santa Barbara, California
Chapter 61

Robert A. Mangione, BPharm, EdD
Provost Emeritus, Professor of Pharmacy (retired)
College of Pharmacy and Health Sciences, Saint John's University
Queens,
New York
Chapter 59

Zachary A. Marcum, PharmD, PhD
Associate Professor
School of Pharmacy, University of Washington
Seattle, Washington
Chapter e25

Ana Elizabeth Markez, MD, LTC, MC, USA
Internal Medicine, Infectious Disease, Fellow ACP and IDSA
Brooke Army Medical Center, United States Army
Chief, Infectious Disease ServiceDeputy Chief of Operations and Administration, Department of Medicine
San Antonio, Texas
Chapter e138

Grace A. Martin, PharmD, BCOP
Clinical Pharmacy Coordinator - Cancer Care
The University of Kansas Cancer Center
Kansas City, Kansas
Chapter 156

Todd W. Mattox, BS, PharmD, BCNSP
Medicine/Surgery Clinical Pharmacist
Moffitt Cancer Center
Tampa, Florida
Chapter 165

Jared E. Matya, PharmD, BCOP
Clinical Pharmacist Practitioner - BMT and Cellular Therapy
Nebraska Medicine
Omaha, Nebraska
Chapter 159

J. Russell May, PharmD
Clinical Professor and Assistant Dean for Extended Campuses
College of Pharmacy, University of Georgia
Athens, Georgia
Chapter e14

Dianne W. May, PharmD, BCPS
Clinical Professor and Campus Director for Pharmacy Practice Experiences
College of Pharmacy
University of Georgia
Athens, Georgia
Chapter 50

Danielle C. Mayer, PharmD, BCACP
Assistant Professor, Department of Pharmacy Practice and Director, Pharmacy Practice Laboratories
Jefferson College of Pharmacy
Philadelphia, Pennsylvania
Chapter 100

Jennifer L. Mazan, PharmD
Professor
Midwestern University
Downers Grove, Illinois
Chapter e15

Timothy L. McCavit, MD, MSCS
Staff Hematologist
Director, Bleeding Disorder Program
Cook Children's Medical Center
Fort Worth, Texas
Chapter 123

Erin K. McCreary, PharmD, BCPS, BCIDP
Director of Infectious Diseases Improvement and Clinical Research Innovation
University of Pittsburgh Medical Center
Clinical Assistant Professor
University of Pittsburgh School of Medicine
Pittsburgh, Pennsylvania
Chapter e132

Mary Lynn McPherson, PharmD, MA, MDE, FAAHPM
Professor and Executive Director, Online Graduate Studies in Palliative Care
University of Maryland, Baltimore
Baltimore, Maryland
Chapter e28

Christopher G. Medlin, PharmD, BCPS
Clinical Assistant Professor
College of Pharmacy, University of Texas at El Paso
El Paso, Texas
Chapter e3

Sarah T. Melton, PharmD, BCPP, BCACP, CGP, FASCP
Professor of Pharmacy Practice
Gatton College of Pharmacy at East Tennessee State University
Clinical Pharmacist
Highpower, PC in Lebanon, Virginia and the Johnson City Community Health Center
Johnson City, Tennessee
Chapter 90

Leigh Ann Mike, PharmD, BCPS, BCGP
Clinical Associate Professor and Assistant Director for Education, Plein Center for Pharmacy Research, Education & Outreach
School of Pharmacy, University of Washington
Seattle, Washington
Chapter e25

Margaret A. Miklich, PharmD, BCACP
Clinical Associate Professor of Pharmacy Practice
School of Pharmacy, Temple University
Philadelphia, Pennsylvania
Chapter e48

Anna S. Milone, PharmD, BCPS
Teaching Specialist and Director of Pharmacy Learning Collaborative
College of Pharmacy, University of Minnesota
Minneapolis, Minnesota
Chapter e16

Augusto Miravelle, MD
Associate Professor of Clinical Neurology University of Colorado, Anschutz Medical Campus
Aurora, Colorado
Chapter 74

Jean Y. Moon, PharmD, BCACP
Associate Professor and Postgraduate Year One Pharmacy Residency Program Director
College of Pharmacy, University of Minnesota
Minneapolis, Minnesota
Chapter 44

Rebecca Moote, PharmD, MSc, BCPS
Clinical Associate Professor and Assistant Division Head
University of Texas at Austin College of Pharmacy
Internal Medicine Clinical Pharmacy Specialist
University Hospital, San Antonio, Texas
Chapter 46

Jessica L. Moreno PharmD, BCPP
Psychiatric Clinical Pharmacist
Integrated Behavioral Health
Detroit Michigan
Chapter e84

Juan Mosley II, PharmD, CPh, AAHIVP
Chair and Associate Professor
College of Pharmacy, Larkin University
Miami, Florida
Chapter e9

Jeffrey J. Mucksavage, PharmD
Clinical Assistant Professor
Department of Pharmacy Practice
University of Illinois at Chicago College of Pharmacy
Chicago, Illinois
Chapter e31

Scott W. Mueller, PharmD, BCCCP
Burn Services and Critical Care Pharmacy Specialist
University of Colorado Hospital
Clinical Associate Professor
University of Colorado Skaggs School of Pharmacy and Pharmaceutical Sciences
Denver, Colorado
Chapter 145

Diana W. Mulherin, PharmD, BCNSP, BCCCP
Clinical Pharmacist Specialist, Nutrition Support
Vanderbilt University Medical Center
Nashville, Tennessee
Chapter 166

Amanda M. Mullins, PharmD, BCPS
Clinical Pharmacist Practitioner
VA St. Louis Healthcare System, St. Louis, Missouri
St. Louis, Missouri
Chapter 79

Kashif M. Munir, MD
Professor of Medicine
School of Medicine, University of Maryland
Baltimore, Maryland
Chapter e98

Milap C. Nahata, PharmD
Director, Institute of Therapeutic Innovations and Outcomes; Professor Emeritus of Pharmacy, Pediatrics and Internal Medicine
Colleges of Pharmacy and Medicine, Ohio State University
Columbus, Ohio
Chapter e20

Rocsanna Namdar, PharmD
PGY1 Residency Director; Strategic Planning and Learning Resources Director
New Mexico Veterans Affairs Health Care System
Clinical Pharmacy Specialist
Albuquerque, New Mexico
Chapter 135

Leigh Anne Nelson, PharmD, BCPP
Professor of Pharmacy Practice and Administration
University of Missouri-Kansas School of Pharmacy
Kansas City, Missouri
Chapter e81

Melissa A. Nestor, PharmD, BCCCP
Clinical Pharmacist, Critical Care/Stroke Neurology
UK HealthCare
Assistant Professor
College of Pharmacy, University of Kentucky
Lexington, Kentucky
Chapter 39

Viet-Huong V. Nguyen, PharmD, MPH, MSc, BCCCP
Associate Professor (Neurology)
School of Pharmacy, Chapman University, Irvine, California
Clinical Pharmacy Specialist, Neurology and Critical Care
Harbor UCLA Medical Center
West Carson, California
Chapter 75

Jessica C. Njoku, PharmD, MPH, BCPS
System Formulary Coordinator
Harris Health System
Pearland, Texas
Chapter 131

Thomas D. Nolin, PharmD, PhD
Associate Dean for Research and Sponsored Programs
University of Pittsburgh School of Pharmacy
Pittsburgh, Pennsylvania
Chapters 65, 67

Cindy L. O'Bryant, PharmD, FCCP, FHOPA, BCOP
Professor of Clinical Pharmacy
Skaggs School of Pharmacy and Pharmaceutical Sciences
University of Colorado Anschutz Medical Campus
Aurora, Colorado
Chapter 162

Mary Beth O'Connell, PharmD, BCPS
Professor
Wayne State University, Eugene Applebaum College of Pharmacy and Health Sciences
Detroit, Michigan
Chapter 112

Kirsten H. Ohler, PharmD, BCPS, BCPPS
Clinical Associate Professor, Pharmacy Practice; Program Director, PGY1 Pharmacy Residency
College of Pharmacy, University of Illinois at Chicago
Clinical Pharmacist, Neonatal Intensive Care Unit
University of Illinois Hospital & Health Sciences System
Chicago, Illinois
Chapter e22

Katie B. Olney, PharmD, BCIDP
Infectious Diseases Clinical Pharmacist
University of Kentucky HealthCare
Lexington, Kentucky
Chapter 127

Keith M. Olsen, Pharm.D
Dean and Professor
College of Pharmacy
University of Nebraska Medical Center
Omaha, Nebraska
Chapters e49, 137

Jared Ostroff, PharmD, MBA, BCACP, BCGP
Ambulatory Pharmacy Supervisor
Baystate Health
Granby, Connecticut
Chapter e11

Ohoud Owaidhah, MD
Senior Consultant, Glaucoma Division
King Khaled Eye Specialist Hospital
Riyadh, Saudi Arabia
Chapter 114

Melissa C. Palmer, PharmD, BCPS, BCPP
Clinical Pharmacist Practitioner
Alaska VA Healthcare System
Eagle River, Alaska
Chapter e83

Lisa M. Palmisano, PharmD, BCACP
Associate Professor and Clinical Pharmacist
College of Pharmacy, Midwestern University
Downers Grove, Illinois
Chapter e15

Robert B. Parker, PharmD
Professor
College of Pharmacy, University of Tennessee Health Science Center
Memphis, Tennessee
Chapter 36

Neelam K. Patel, PharmD, BCOP
Clinical Pharmacy Specialist
The University of Texas MD Anderson Cancer Center
Houston, Texas
Chapter 151

Priti N. Patel, PharmD, BCPS
Clinical Associate Professor and Director of Personal and Professional Development
College of Pharmacy, University of Florida
Gainesville, Florida
Chapter 59

Charles A. Peloquin, PharmD
Professor and Division Head, Translational Research
College of Pharmacy
University of Florida
Gainesville, Florida
Chapter 135

Mark A. Perazella, MD, MS
Professor of Medicine
Yale University School of Medicine
New Haven, Connecticut
Chapter 65

Janelle Perkins, PharmD, BCOP
Professor
Taneja College of Pharmacy
University of South Florida
Tampa, Florida
Chapter e163

Emily P. Peron, PharmD, MS, BCPS, BCGP
Associate Professor
Virginia Commonwealth University School of Pharmacy
Richmond, Virginia
Chapter 73

Jay I. Peters, MD
Professor and Chief (Retired) Division of Pulmonary and Critical Care
UT Health San Antonio
University of Texas Health Science Center
San Antonio, Texas
Chapter e43

Jennifer T. Pham, PharmD, BCPS, BCPPS
Clinical Associate Professor, Department of Pharmacy Practice, College of Pharmacy
Department of Pediatrics, College of Medicine
University of Illinois at Chicago
Clinical Pharmacist, Neonatal Intensive Care Unit
University of Illinois Hospital & Health Sciences System
Chicago, Illinois
Chapter e22

Ha K. Phan, PharmD, CDCES, BCACP
Clinical Assistant Professor
School of Pharmacy, University of Mississippi
Jackson, Mississippi
Chapter 47

Stephanie J. Phelps
Emeritus Professor
University of Tennessee Health Science Center College of Pharmacy
Memphis, Tennessee
Chapter 76

Bradley G. Phillips, PharmD, BCPS, FCCP
Clinical and Administrative Pharmacy
Professor
Director, Biomedical and Translational Sciences Institute
University of Georgia
Augusta, Georgia
Chapter 92

Stephen T. Phillips, MD
Cardiac Electrophysiologist
Advocate Christ Medical Center
Oak Lawn, Illinois
Chapter 40

Amy M. Pick, PharmD, MS, BCOP
Associate Professor
College of Pharmacy
University of Nebraska Medical Center
Omaha, Nebraska
Chapter 159

Christopher R. Piszczatoski, PharmD, BCPS
Clinical Pharmacy Specialist, Ambulatory Care
UF Health Shands Physicians, University of Florida
Gainesville, Florida
Chapter 97

Steven Pliszka, MD
Dielmann Distinguish Professor
Chair of the Department of Psychiatry
University of Texas Health Science Center at San Antonio
San Antonio, Texas
Chapter 82

Jason M. Pogue, PharmD, BCIDP
Clinical Professor of Pharmacy
College of Pharmacy
University of Michigan
Ann Arbor, Michigan
Chapter e132

Samuel M. Poloyac, PharmD, PhD
Dean & James T. Doluisio Regents Chair
University of Texas at Austin College of Pharmacy
Austin, Texas
Chapter e6

Elvin T. Price, PharmD, PhD
Victor A. Yanchick Associate Professor and Director of the Geriatric Pharmacotherapy Program
Virginia Commonwealth University
Richmond, Virginia
Chapter e23

Sarah Rajkovic, PharmD
Senior Clinical Instructor
Skaggs School of Pharmacy and Pharmaceutical Sciences
University of Colorado
Aurora, Colorado
Chapter 74

Gautam Ramani, MD
Associate Professor of Medicine
University of Maryland
Director, Pulmonary Hypertension Program
Baltimore, Maryland
Chapter e29

Satish C. Rao, MD, PhD, ABIM
Professor of Medicine
Augusta University
Augusta, Georgia
Chapter 50

Brent N. Reed, PharmD, MS, BCCP, BCPS
Clinical Associate Professor
School of Pharmacy, University of Maryland
Baltimore, Maryland
Chapters e29, 37

Beth H. Resman-Targoff, PharmD
Clinical Professor
Department of Pharmacy, Clinical and Administrative Sciences
University of Oklahoma College of Pharmacy
Oklahoma City, Oklahoma
Chapter 107

Daniel M. Riche, PharmD, CLS, ASH-CHC
Professor
School of Pharmacy, University of Mississippi
Associate Professor
University of Mississippi Medical Center
Jackson, Mississippi
Chapter 32

Jo E. Rodgers, PharmD, BCPS, BCCP
Professor and Director of Postdoctoral Programs
Eshelman School of Pharmacy
University of North Carolina
Chapel Hill, North Carolina
Chapter 36

Andrew M. Roecker, PharmD, BCPS
Professor and Chair – Department of Pharmacy Practice and Director of Continuing Pharmacy Education
Ohio Northern University
Ada, Ohio
Chapter 136

Kelly C. Rogers, PharmD, BCCP
Professor of Clinical Pharmacy and Translational Science
College of Pharmacy, University of Tennessee Health Science Center
Cardiology Clinical Pharmacy Practitioner
VA Medical Center, Memphis
Lakeland, Tennessee
Chapter 33

Lauren K. Roller, PharmD, BCCCP
Clinical Pharmacist, Critical Care and Addiction Medicine
Alameda Health System, Highland Hospital
Oakland, California
Clinical Associate Professor of Clinical Sciences
Touro University California
Vallejo, California
Chapter 61

Norbert Rosario, PharmD, BCPS
Ambulatory Care Clinical Pharmacist Practitioner
H-E-B Wellness Primary Care Clinics
San Antonio, Texas
Chapter e2

Eric S. Rovner, MD
Professor of Urology
Medical University of South Carolina
Charleston, South Carolina
Chapter 105

Valerie L. Ruehter, PharmD, BCPP
Clinical Associate Professor and Assistant Dean of Experiential Learning
University of Missouri-Kansas City
Kansas City, Missouri
Chapter e83

Melody Ryan, PharmD, MPH, BCPS, BCGP
Professor and Assistant Provost for Global Health
University of Kentucky
Lexington, Kentucky
Chapters 39, e72

Stephen J. Ryan, MD, MA
Professor of Neurology
University of Kentucky
Lexington, Kentucky
Chapter e72

David M. Salerno, PharmD, BCPS, BCTXP
Clinical Pharmacy Manager | Liver Transplantation
NewYork–Presbyterian Hospital/Weill Cornell Medical Center
New York, New York
Chapter 109

Santosh L. Saraf, MD
Associate Professor of Medicine
College of Medicine
University of Illinois at Chicago
Director of Translational Research, Sickle Cell Center
Chicago, Illinois
Chapter 124

Lana J. Sargent, PhD, RN, CRNP, FNP-C, GNP-BC
Assistant Professor
Virginia Commonwealth University
School of Pharmacy
Richmond, Virginia
Chapter 73

Joseph J. Saseen, PharmD, BCPS, BCACP
Professor and Associate Dean for Clinical Affairs
University of Colorado Anschutz Medical Campus
Clinical Pharmacy Specialist, Family Medicine
University of Colorado Health
Aurora, Colorado
Chapter 30

Mark E. Schneiderhan, PharmD, BCPP
Associate Professor
College of Pharmacy
University of Minnesota
Psychiatric Pharmacist
Human Development Center, Department of Psychiatry
Minneapolis, Minnesota
Chapter e81

Julie M. Sease, PharmD, BCPS, CDCES, BCACP
Senior Associate Dean and Clinical Professor
University of South Carolina College of Pharmacy
Columbia, South Carolina
Chapter 55

Eve M. Segal, PharmD, BCOP
Lead Clinical Pharmacist, Hematology/Oncology
Fred Hutchinson Cancer Center/UW Medicine
Seattle, Washington
Chapter 152

Jolynn Knoche Sessions, PharmD, BCOP, CPP
Oncology Program Manager, Clinical Pharmacist Practitioner
Department of Veterans Affairs
Western North Carolina Health Care System
Associate Professor of Clinical Education
Eshelman School of Pharmacy
University of North Carolina
Chapel Hill, North Carolina
Chapter e160

Roohollah Sharifi, MD
Professor
College of Medicine
University of Illinois Chicago
Section Chief of Urology
Jesse Brown Veterans Affairs Medical Center
Chicago, Illinois
Chapters 103, 104

Kayce M. Shealy, PharmD, BCPS, CDCES
Professor of Pharmacy Practice
School of Pharmacy
Presbyterian College
Clinton, South Carolina
Chapter 54

Amy Heck Sheehan, PharmD
Professor of Pharmacy Practice
College of Pharmacy, Purdue University
Indianapolis, Indiana
Chapter e98, 167

Jessica M. Shenberger-Trujillo, PhD
Clinical Assistant Professor
University of Texas at El Paso
El Paso, Texas
Chapter e3

Jeri J. Sias, PharmD, MPH
Clinical Professor
College of Pharmacy
University of Texas at El Paso
El Paso, Texas
Chapter e3

Cathryn Sibbald, MD MSc
Dermatologist
The Hospital for Sick Children
Assistant Professor
University of Toronto
Toronto, Ontario
Chapter 117

Debra Sibbald, BScPhm, ACPR, RPh, MA, PhD
Academic Lead – Admissions, PharmD Program
Associate Professor, Teaching Stream, Division of Pharmacy Practice
Leslie Dan Faculty of Pharmacy
University of Toronto
Education and Competence Assessment/Evaluation Consultant
Mississauga, Ontario
Chapter 117

Douglas Slain, PharmD, BCPS
Professor
West Virginia University
Infectious Diseases Clinical Specialist
Morgantown, West Virginia
Chapter e18

Patricia W. Slattum, PharmD, PhD
Professor and Co-Director, Geriatrics Workforce Enhancement Program
Virginia Center on Aging
Virginia Commonwealth University
Richmond, Virginia
Chapter e23

Erin M. Slazak, PharmD, BCPS, BCACP
Clinical Associate Professor
School of Pharmacy and Pharmaceutical Sciences
University of Buffalo
Buffalo, New York
Chapter 112

Jordan R. Smith, PharmD
Assistant Professor of Clinical Sciences
High Point University
High Point, North Carolina
Chapter e126

Judith A. Smith, BS, PharmD, BCOP, CPHQ
Professor and Director of WHIM Research Program
UT Health McGovern Medical School at Houston
Oncology Clinical Pharmacy Specialist
Memorial Hermann Cancer Center—TMC
Houston, Texas
Chapter 156

Steven M. Smith, PharmD, MPH
Assistant Professor
Department of Pharmaceutical Outcomes and Policy
College of Florida, University of Florida
Gainesville, Florida
Chapter 97

Tawny L. Smith, PharmD, BCPP
Associate Professor of Psychiatry
University of Texas Health Science Center at Austin
Austin, Texas
Chapter 87

Todd D. Sorensen, PharmD, FAPhA, FCCP
Professor and Senior Executive Associate Dean for Strategic Initiatives and Faculty Affairs
University of Minnesota College of Pharmacy
Minneapolis, Minnesota
Chapter 1

Kevin M. Sowinski, PharmD
Professor of Pharmacy Practice and Associate Head for Faculty Affairs
College of Pharmacy, Purdue University
Adjunct Professor of Medicine
Indiana University School of Medicine
Indianapolis, Indiana
Chapter 64

Mary L. Staicu, PharmD, BCIDP
Infectious Diseases Clinical Pharmacy Specialist
Rochester General Hospital
Rochester, New York
Chapter e108

David D. Stenehjem, PharmD, BCOP
Associate Professor and Associate Department Head
Department of Pharmacy Practice and Pharmaceutical Sciences
University of Minnesota
College of Pharmacy
Minneapolis, Minnesota
Chapter e161

Steven C. Stoner, PharmD, BCPP
Clinical Professor and Associate Dean for Student Affairs
School of Pharmacy
University of Missouri Kansas City
Psychiatric Pharmacy Specialist
Kansas City, Missouri
Chapter e83

Danielle L. Stutzman, PharmD, BCPP
Psychiatric Pharmacist
Pediatric Mental Health Institute and Department of Pharmacy
Children's Hospital Colorado
Clinical Assistant Professor
Skaggs School of Pharmacy and Pharmaceutical Sciences, University of Colorado
Denver, Colorado
Chapter 82

Brandon Sucher, Pharm.D., BCACP, CDCES, AE-C
Professor of Pharmacy Practice
Regis University School of Pharmacy
Denver, Colorado
Chapter e13

Paul M. Szumita, PharmD, BCCCP, BCPS
Director, Clinical Pharmacy and Director, PGY2 Critical Care Pharmacy Residency
Brigham and Women's Hospital
Boston, Massachusetts
Chapter e95

Carol K. Taketomo, PharmD
Adjunct Assistant Professor of Pharmacy Practice, School of Pharmacy
University of Southern California
Chief Pharmacy Officer
Children's Hospital Los Angeles
Los Angeles, California
Chapter e20

Kristine M. C. Talley, PhD, CNP, RN
Associate Professor
School of Nursing
University of Minnesota
Minneapolis, Minnesota
Chapter 105

Kimberly B. Tallian, PharmD, APh, BCPP
Advanced Practice Pharmacist—Neuropsychiatry
Adjunct Clinical Professor
UC San Diego—Skaggs School of Pharmacy & Pharmaceutical Sciences
Scripps Mercy Hospital
San Diego, California
Chapter 80

Chia J. Tan, BPharm(Hons), PhD, BCOP
Postdoctoral Research Fellow
University of Utah College of Pharmacy
Salt Lake City, Utah
Chapter 155

Geoffrey M. Thiele, PhD
Umbach Professor of Rheumatology
College of Medicine
University of Nebraska Medical Center
Omaha, Nebraska
Chapter e106

Laura C. Tilley, MD
Assistant Professor
Uniformed Services University of the Health Sciences
Washington, District Columbia
Chapter e10

Jessica J. Tilton, PharmD, BCACP
Clinical Assistant Professor and Clinical Pharmacist
College of Pharmacy, University of Illinois at Chicago
Chicago, Illinois
Chapter 40

Danielle M. Tompkins, PharmD, BCCCP
Clinical Assistant Professor
Ernest Mario School of Pharmacy, Rutgers University
Piscataway, New Jersey
Chapter e31

Erica Torres, PharmD, BCACP
Ambulatory Care Clinical Pharmacy Specialist
University Family Health Center—Southwest
San Antonio, Texas
Chapter e2

Heidi Trinkman, PharmD, BCOP
Clinical Pharmacy Specialist
Pediatric Hematology/Oncology and Stem Cell Transplant
Cook Children's Medical Center
Fort Worth, Texas
Chapter 123

Jennifer M. Trujillo, PharmD, BCPS, CDCES, BC-ADM
Professor
Skaggs School of Pharmacy and Pharmaceutical Sciences, University of Colorado
Aurora, Colorado
Chapters 94, e95

Anne M. Tucker, PharmD, BCNSP
Clinical Pharmacy Specialist - Critical Care / Nutrition Support
University of Texas MD Anderson Cancer Center
Houston, Texas
Chapter 71

Amy M. VandenBerg, PharmD, BCPP
Clinical Associate Professor
College of Pharmacy
University of Michigan
Ann Arbor, Michigan
Chapter 88

Sara R. Vazquez, PharmD, BCPS, CACP
Clinical Pharmacist
University of Utah Health
Adjunct Associate Professor in Pharmacotherapy
University of Utah College of Pharmacy
Salt Lake City, Utah
Chapter 38

Maria I. Velez, MD
Assistant Professor
University of Texas Health Science Center at San Antonio
San Antonio, Texas
Chapter e43

Kathleen M. Vest, PharmD, CDCES, BCACP
Professor of Pharmacy Practice
College of Pharmacy
Midwestern University
Clinical Pharmacist
Northwestern Medicine
Downers Grove, Illinois
Chapters 100, 101

Jamie L. Wagner, PharmD, BCPS
Clinical Associate Professor
Department of Pharmacy Practice
School of Pharmacy, University of Mississippi
Jackson, Mississippi
Chapter 137

Michael A. Wankum, PharmD, BCIDP, BCPS
Clinical Pharmacy Coordinator – Infectious Diseases
Allina Health
Minneapolis, Minnesota
Chapter 128

Casey S. Washington, PharmD, BCPS
Medical Writer
Medscape Education
New York, New York
Chapter 115

Kristin Watson, PharmD, BCCP
Associate Professor
School of Pharmacy, University of Maryland
Baltimore, Maryland
Chapters e29, e35

Lori D. Wazny, BSc(Pharm), PharmD
Clinical Pharmacist
Manitoba Renal Program
Winnipeg, Manitoba, Canada
Chapter 62

Robert J. Weber, PharmD, MS, BCPS, FASHP, FNAP
Administrator, Pharmaceutical Services
The Ohio State University Wexner Medical Center
Assistant Dean for Medical Center Affairs
The Ohio State University College of Pharmacy
Columbus, Ohio
Chapter e4

Brian J. Werth, PharmD
Associate Professor
School of Pharmacy, University of Washington
Seattle, Washington
Chapter e126

James W. Wheless
Professor and Chief, Department of Pediatric Neurology
Director, Le Bonheur Comprehensive Epilepsy Program
The University of Tennessee Health Science Center
Pediatric Neurology
Memphis, Tennessee
Chapter 76

Sara A. Wiedenfeld, PharmD, BCPS, BCACP
Clinical Assistant Professor
College of Pharmacy, University of Iowa
Iowa City, Iowa
Chapter 110

Dennis M. Williams, PharmD, BCPS
Associate Professor
Eshelman School of Pharmacy, University of North Carolina
Clinical Specialist
Chapel Hill, North Carolina
Chapter 45

Kristyn M. Williamson, PharmD, BCACP
Teaching specialist
College of Pharmacy
University of Minnesota
Clinical pharmacist
Minneapolis, Minnesota
Chapter e16

Daniel M. Witt, PharmD, BCPS
Professor and Chair
University of Utah College of Pharmacy, Department of Pharmacotherapy
Salt Lake City, Utah
Chapter 38

Pei Shieen Wong, PharmD, BSPS
Principal Clinical Pharmacist
Singapore General Hospital
Lecturer
National University of Singapore
Singapore
Chapter 74

G. Christopher Wood, PharmD, BCCCP
Professor of Clinical Pharmacy and Translational Science
College of Pharmacy
University of Tennessee Health Science Center
Memphis, Tennessee
Chapter 77

Jack A. Yanovski, MD, PhD
Chief, Section on Growth and Obesity and Associate Scientific Director for Translational Medicine
Eunice Kennedy Shriver National Institute of Child Health and Human Development, NIH
Bethesda, Maryland
Chapter 167

Evan J. Zasowski, PharmD, MPH, BCPS, BCIDP
Associate Professor
College of Pharmacy
Touro University California
Vallejo, California
Chapter 129

Kristin M. Zimmerman, PharmD, BCACP, BCGP
Associate Professor
Virginia Commonwealth University School of Pharmacy
Richmond, Virginia
Chapter 73

Daniel A. Zlott, PharmD, BCOP
Senior Vice President
Education and Business Development
American Pharmacists Association
Washington, D.C.
Chapter e106

Foreword

Thirty-five years have passed since the publication of the first edition of *Pharmacotherapy: A Pathophysiologic Approach*. During those years we have witnessed dramatic changes in healthcare delivery and advances in the prevention and treatment of many diseases and disorders. Also, new diseases such as COVID-19 and monkeypox have become public health emergencies.

As summarized in the Foreword to the 10th edition, major changes in the pharmacy profession have also occurred during our professional journey. We have seen the emphasis on pharmaceutical care, the change to the entry-level doctor of pharmacy degree, and the growing acceptance of credentials (eg, residency and board certification) for pharmacy specialists. Reimbursement for patient care services (through Medicare provider status or other means) has not advanced as quickly.

As the pharmacy profession promoted patient care services to payers and the public, some fundamental questions became evident and still challenge us today. What services do clinical pharmacists provide to improve patient care? Do pharmacists apply a uniform process of care for a given service? What patient care services do payers, providers, and the public need and want? Should some services be performed by pharmacists with specialized training or advanced credentials?

We didn't think about those questions in the early days of the clinical pharmacy movement. The term "clinical pharmacy" described the role of the pharmacist in patient care and "clinical pharmacist" was someone who provided those services. Over time, many healthcare professionals and patients came to value the services provided by clinical pharmacists. However, it was difficult to explain to others the services provided by clinical pharmacists, in part because the process of care and its goals were not uniform. Clinical pharmacy services varied between institutions and could entail a general service such as drug information or a specialized service such as nutrition support or pharmacokinetic dosing. Most clinical pharmacists served primarily as consultants to physicians in the acute care setting and were not ultimately responsible to patients for their care. Whatever you called the service that pharmacists provided, hospitals and healthcare systems wanted more, and clinical pharmacy expanded dramatically over the next few decades. When Medicare Part D benefits were implemented in 2006, the term "medication therapy management" (MTM) became popular to describe a new service for pharmacists. However, the confusion continued because pharmacists and pharmacies offered different services labeled as MTM, delivered using different processes of care.

In the last 10 years, the profession has finally begun to address the important questions about the fundamental role of pharmacists. A Task Force of the Patient-Centered Primary Care Collaborative described the integration of comprehensive medication management (CMM) in the patient-centered medical home. The American College of Clinical Pharmacy (ACCP) published Standards of Practice for Clinical Pharmacists and the Joint Commission of Pharmacy Practitioners approved the Pharmacists' Patient Care Process. These documents described a consistent process for the delivery of pharmacy patient care services. The ACCP Standards of Practice added details to CMM such as the setting (eg, clinical pharmacist working as part of a healthcare team) and qualifications (eg, board certification) of the clinical pharmacist providing CMM. And the 2016 ACPE Standards added new requirements for schools and colleges to teach students about the Pharmacists' Patient Care Process. The ACCP CMM study results and publications have accelerated the growth and adoption of CMM worldwide.

As the profession has recognized the importance of practice standards and practice consistency, implementation science is being applied to clinical pharmacy service delivery. The CMM in Primary Care Study funded by ACCP was the first large-scale study to apply this relatively new science to the delivery of CMM, further defining the CMM patient care process with the degree of specificity required to ensure consistent clinical and economic outcomes (fidelity). As we look into the near future, we can expect that the application of implementation science will accelerate growth and adoption of CMM worldwide to optimize medication use and patient health.

Although pharmacy education and practice has changed dramatically, the importance of pharmacotherapy knowledge has remained the same. In its 2017 update, ACCP listed in-depth pharmacotherapy knowledge as one of the six competencies necessary to provide CMM in team-based, direct patient care environments. Patient-centered pharmacotherapy knowledge represents 65% of the board certification examination for the Pharmacotherapy Specialty. And Pharmacotherapy (or "Therapeutics" or "Pharmacotherapeutics") is a major part of the doctor of pharmacy curriculum, usually a series of courses with the most credit hours. Indeed, it is this in-depth knowledge of pharmacotherapy, combined with the clinical experience gained through postgraduate training in direct patient care practice, that allows the pharmacist to be the "medication therapy expert" on the healthcare team and to proactively address medication-related problems. Some have argued that preventing, identifying, and managing medication-related problems should be at the very core of a pharmacist's professional identity.

Pharmacotherapy: A Pathophysiologic Approach remains as relevant today as it was when originally published 35 years ago. The 12th edition provides students, pharmacists, and other health professionals with the core pharmacotherapy knowledge necessary to prevent, identify, and manage disease and medication-related problems.

Gary C. Yee, PharmD, and Joseph T. DiPiro, PharmD

Preface

Remington's, Stedman's, Goodman & Gilman's, Harrison's, and Koda-Kimble—a few textbooks in the medical and pharmacy fields have become so well known that students often refer to them by the name of a chief editor or author rather than book titles.

This book, *Pharmacotherapy: A Pathophysiologic Approach*, quickly reached that stature in pharmacy education and practice following the publication of the first edition in 1988. By changing our title to *DiPiro's Pharmacotherapy* with this 12th edition, we make permanent the association of this work with the important leadership and vision of our founding editor, Joseph T. DiPiro, PharmD, who had the initial discussions with our original publisher, Elsevier, in 1983. By 1985, a cohesive team of founding editors came together with a unified vision of pharmacotherapy and how it fit into the practice of clinical pharmacy. DiPiro, along with Michael Posey, Robert Talbert, Peggy Hayes, and Gary Yee, took on the difficult chore of identifying more than 200 recognized experts from across the United States who would write, from scratch, 111 chapters. Just two years later, the team began to funnel chapters to the publisher and through to publication.

Gary Matzke, after serving as an author and section editor in the first edition, joined the masthead for the second edition, and Barbara Wells replaced Peggy Hayes beginning with the third edition. That editorial team would remain together through the 10th edition, assuring continuity and cohesiveness for the *Pharmacotherapy* project.

Our founding editors set several lofty goals for *Pharmacotherapy*. The work needed to meet the educational standards of emerging postbaccalaureate doctor of pharmacy programs, serve as an authoritative reference for clinical pharmacists and other clinicians involved in direct patient care, and support the recognition of pharmacotherapy as a board-certified specialty in pharmacy by providing evidence of the field's unique and extensive body of knowledge. Those goals made the book an immediate success and have stood the test of time by guiding the editors for more than 30 years.

Turning to this 12th edition, the current editors met in Atlanta in early January 2020. Nearby, the Centers for Disease Control and Prevention was responding to the emergence of a novel pneumonia of unknown etiology. By the time we departed just two days later, Chinese authorities had identified and isolated a previously unknown coronavirus, then known as Wuhan-Hu-1. Despite the changes, challenges, illnesses, and losses the ensuing pandemic would bring, the editors and more than 300 authors of the 12th edition persevered to complete a record number of chapters (167) on time, online, and in print, including a new chapter regarding the ever-changing topic of COVID-19.

At that 2020 meeting, the editors decided to dive deeper into the digital world. Working with our publisher, we created a process for keeping online chapters updated on a continual basis, so they are current as new drugs are approved, guidelines are issued, and recommendations change on the best use of pharmacotherapeutic agents in prevention, management, and cure of diseases. Also, we published the 12th edition online in AccessPharmacy long before the print version could be released.

To handle this added responsibility, the editors needed help. A group of six assistant editors, each with unique expertise to complement that of the section editors, were recruited. Scott Bolesta (assisting Dr. DiPiro), Lisa Holle (Yee), Robert DiDomenico (Haines), Angela Bingham (Nolin), Amy VandenBerg (Ellingrod), and Rena Gosser (Posey) have provided invaluable assistance to the contributors and editors to produce the final manuscript for this 12th edition. We are pleased to acknowledge their efforts.

For the 12th edition, the editors chose not to make extensive changes in the chapter structure and content. One refinement was to replace the preclass and postclass learning activities that appeared in the 11th edition with a single "Beyond the Book" box placed at the beginning of each chapter. The intent is to prepare and stimulate learners by pointing them to multimedia resources that can deepen their understanding of the material.

Two of our founding editors are retiring from the book after the 12th edition. Drs. DiPiro and Yee have worked on all 12 editions and helped make this work the gold standard textbook in pharmacy and health professions education. The editors are pleased to welcome two new editors to the team: Jennifer Cocohoba, PharmD, MAS, of the University of California, San Francisco, for the chapters managed by Dr. DiPiro, and Lisa M. Holle, PharmD, BCOP, FHOPA, FISOPP, of the University of Connecticut, for Dr. Yee's chapters.

We acknowledge the many hours that numerous authors—including the many contributors since the first edition—have devoted to this labor of love. Without their dedication to the cause of improving pharmacotherapy and maintaining the accuracy, clarity, and relevance of their chapters, this text would unquestionably not be possible.

A special thanks go to Michael Weitz and Juanita Thompson of McGraw Hill and Poonam Bisht of MPS Limited for their input and support and for enhancing the online authoring tools needed to maintain the textbook on the AccessPharmacy website.

Many thanks to Terry Schwinghammer for his insights during our editor meetings and continued devotion to the *Pharmacotherapy Casebook: A Patient-Focused Approach* companion to this work and the tools, chapter updates, and innovations he has shepherded onto the AccessPharmacy website. Finally, we thank James Shanahan, Peter Boyle, and their colleagues at McGraw Hill for their ongoing support of the *Pharmacotherapy* family of resources, insights into publishing and higher education trends, and critical attention to detail.

The Editors, October 2022

1

Patient Care Process

Stuart T. Haines, Mary Ann Kliethermes, and Todd D. Sorensen

KEY CONCEPTS

1. A professional patient care practice is built on three essential elements: a philosophy of practice, a patient care process, and a practice management system.
2. A professional patient care practice is predicated on a patient-practitioner relationship established through respect, trust, and effective communication. Patients, and when appropriate, caregivers and family, are actively engaged in decision making.
3. Adopting a uniform patient care process—a consistently implemented set of methods and procedures—serves as a framework for each patient encounter, increases quality and accountability, and creates shared language and expectations.
4. The patient care process includes five essential steps: collecting subjective and objective information about the patient; assessing the collected data to identify problems and set priorities; creating an individualized care plan that is evidence-based and cost-effective; implementing the care plan; and monitoring the patient over time during follow-up encounters to evaluate the effectiveness of the plan and modify it as needed.
5. The patient care process is supported by three inter-related elements: communication, collaboration, and documentation. Interprofessional teamwork and information technology facilitate the effective and efficient delivery of care.
6. A practice management system includes the infrastructure to deliver care. This includes physical space, documentation systems, payment for services, and qualified support personnel.

BEYOND THE BOOK

For an overview of the importance of applying a consistent process of care in practice, listen to the following Pharmacy Forward podcast episodes:

- PharmacistsPatientCareProcess–EpisodeI(Dr.ToddSorensen) https://pharmacyforward.podbean.com/e/pharmacists-patient-care-process-i/
- Pharmacists Patient Care Process – Episode II (Dr. Mary Ann Kliethermes) https://pharmacyforward.podbean.com/e/pharmacists-patient-care-process-ii/

INTRODUCTION

The *patient care process* is a fundamental series of actions that guide the activities of health professionals. All health professionals who provide direct patient care should use a systematically and consistently applied *process of care* in their practice.[1] Until recently, the language to describe the process for delivering comprehensive medication management services was ill-defined. In 2014, the Joint Commission for Pharmacy Practitioners (JCPP)—representing 11 national pharmacy organizations—endorsed a framework for providing clinically oriented patient care services called the Pharmacist's Patient Care Process.[2] However, the framework and the language to describe the process are not unique to the pharmacy profession. Indeed, medicine, nursing, and dentistry all follow a putatively similar process of care[3] (see Table 1-1). For example, the American

TABLE 1-1 Professional Standards of Patient Care and Their Domains

Primary Care IPC-2[6,7]	Dietician's Nutrition Care Process[8]	Specialty Nursing: Standards of Practice[9]	Physical Therapists[10]
Symptoms, complaints	Nutrition assessment	Assessment	Examination
Diagnostic screening, prevention	Nutrition diagnosis	Diagnosis	Evaluation
Treatment, procedures, medication	Nutrition intervention	Outcome identification	Diagnosis
Test results	Nutrition monitoring and evaluation	Develop plan of care	Prognosis
Administrative		Implement plan	Plan of care
Other		Co-coordination of care	Reexamination
		Health teaching and promotion	
		Prescriptive authority and treatment	
Diagnoses, diseases		Evaluation	Discharge/ Discontinuation summary

Nursing Association (ANA) outlines the nursing process with steps that include assessment, diagnosis, outcomes/planning, implementation, and evaluation.[4] The Academy of Nutrition and Dietetics collapses these general steps into four steps, outlining the nutrition care process to include nutrition assessment, diagnosis, intervention, and monitoring/evaluation.[5] Although the care process is similar across disciplines, each health profession brings a unique set of knowledge, skills, attitudes, and values to the patient encounter.

Health professionals who provide direct patient care are often called *practitioners*. To *practice* is what health professionals do to bring their unique knowledge and skills to patients. A practice is not a physical location or simply a list of activities. Rather, a professional practice requires three essential elements: (1) a philosophy of practice, (2) a process of care, and (3) a practice management system.[3] These three inter-related concepts make the delivery of patient-centered care possible.

Health professionals have an ethical obligation to promote the health and well-being of the patients they serve. Thus, a philosophy—the moral purpose and a commonly held set of values that guides the profession—is the critical foundation on which the practices of pharmacy, medicine, nursing, and dentistry are built.[11] A philosophy of practice is often formally articulated in the professional code of ethics endorsed by professional organizations and an oath that is recited by members of the profession during rituals and ceremonies. In addition to a code of ethics, most professions have an informal set of beliefs and values that inform self-proclaimed and societal expectations. For example, the concept of *pharmaceutical care* is not formally included in the code of ethics for the profession of pharmacy or the oath of a pharmacist.[12,13] However, informally, pharmacists understand they have a unique responsibility for addressing the drug-related needs of patients and should be held accountable for preventing, identifying, and resolving drug therapy problems.[14] Similarly, dentistry, nursing, and medicine have both formal and informal expectations that guide their professional practice.

A process of care that is systematically and consistently applied during each patient encounter increases the likelihood that optimal health outcomes are achieved.[15] The patient care process used throughout this book includes five essential steps: (1) collecting subjective and objective information about the patient; (2) assessing the collected data to identify problems, determine the adequacy of current treatments, and set priorities; (3) creating an individualized care plan that is evidence-based and cost-effective; (4) implementing the care plan; and (5) monitoring the patient over time during follow-up encounters to evaluate the effectiveness of the plan and modify it as needed (see Fig. 1-1). In addition to the five fundamental steps, a patient-centered approach to decision making is essential.[16] To be patient-centered requires effective communication and seeking to understand the patient's needs, preferences, and values. It also requires interprofessional collaboration—working with other health professionals to develop and implement a shared plan of care.[17] Each step of the process must be documented. These steps are interdependent, and completing all five steps is necessary to achieve the greatest impact. While a process of care is common to all, each profession has a unique body of knowledge and skills they bring to bear when assessing the data and formulating plans.[3]

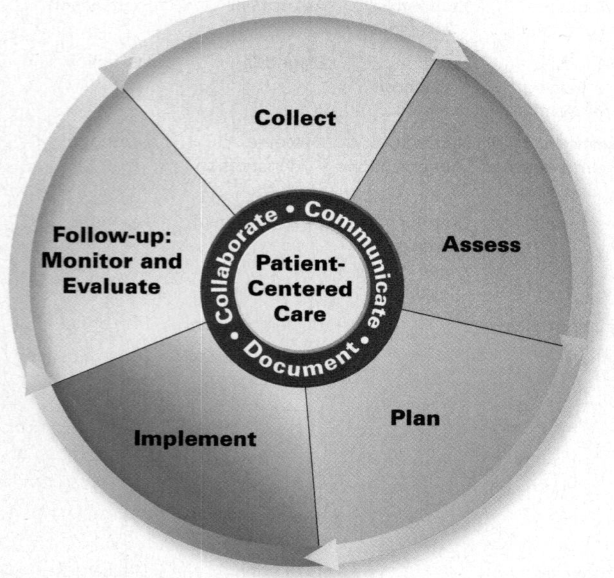

FIGURE 1-1 The Pharmacist's Patient Care Process endorsed by the Joint Commission for Pharmacy Practitioners (2014).

A practice must also have a practice management system that supports the efficient and effective delivery of services.[3] Without a well-defined practice management system, the practice would not be sustainable. This includes the infrastructure—the physical, financial, and human resources—as well as policies and procedures to carry out the patient care work. Successful practices have a clear mission statement that defines who the practice serves, the organizational values, and what they hope to accomplish. Furthermore, to achieve its mission, a practice must implement quality improvement methods that measure, evaluate, and improve the actions of practitioners (individually) and the practice (collectively).

While every practice is built on three essential elements—a philosophy of practice, a well-defined patient care process, and a practice management system—the focus of this chapter is to describe the patient care process applied to drug therapy management and explore some environmental issues that are influencing the adoption and application of this process.

IMPORTANCE OF A CONSISTENT PROCESS OF CARE

It is well understood that healthcare is a complex business. Since the turn of the twenty-first century, much effort has focused on gaining control of a disparate, disjointed, costly health system that is not adequately producing desired patient outcomes despite the healthcare workforce laboring harder than ever. Spurred by the Institute of Medicine's *Crossing the Quality Chasm* report from 2001,[18] which set the framework for redesigning healthcare delivery, healthcare institutions and practitioners have embraced the Triple Aim[19] focusing on patient-centeredness, safety, and quality improvement (see Fig. 1-2). The Triple Aim can only be achieved with significant transformations in the delivery of care and by adopting payment models based on value.

To accelerate the requisite redesign of healthcare delivery, the Institute for Healthcare Improvement has developed guiding principles or "rules" for workforces and healthcare communities. Among these principles is to consistently implement what works in order to reduce unnecessary variation. Standardization is important because healthcare systems are embedded in a network of providers in multiple institutions, settings, and practices.[20] A lack of a consistent process of care creates an environment that leads to unacceptable gaps in care. Thus, a process of care must be sufficiently robust to address the complexity that exists among patients and adaptable to varied settings and different acuity levels. For a specific patient care service to be widely adopted and valued, it is imperative that clarity exists both in the execution of care and the terminology used to describe the care.

The stimulus for developing the patient care process for pharmacy was the wide variation observed as pharmacists provided direct patient care, often using the same terminology to describe diverse services or, conversely, the same service is described using different terminology. As patient care services provided by pharmacists, physicians, nurses, and any healthcare practitioner cannot operate in a silo, the services must be clearly articulated and well understood by patients, their caregivers, payers, and other care team members.

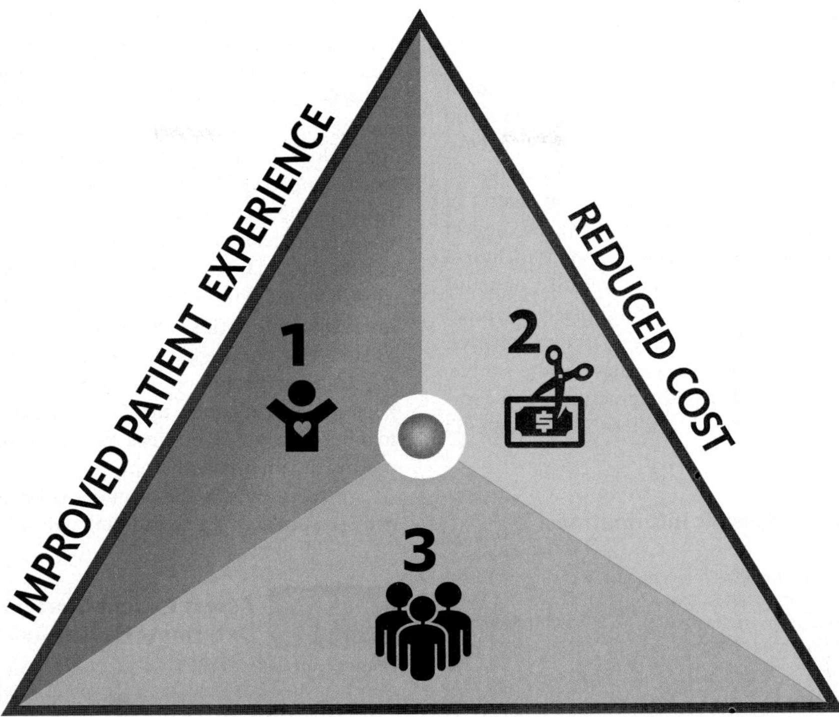

FIGURE 1-2 The Triple Aim in healthcare.

Without a consistent patient care process, it has been challenging for the pharmacy profession to communicate the pharmacist's role to groups external to the profession and establish the distinct value pharmacists bring to an interprofessional care team. Moreover, the patient must know and understand what is to be delivered and to determine how best to receive the care provided. Likewise, other healthcare team members must determine how best to integrate the pharmacist's work into their efforts caring for the patient.

Structure is essential to maintaining consistency. Systematically implementing a framework for care that is consistently applied assures no important step is overlooked and actions that may lead to greater harm than benefit are reduced or eliminated. Defining a standardized process of care enables data collection for quality assurance and research purposes to demonstrate the value of a service. In the hospital setting, care pathways and standard order sets are examples of standardized care processes that have been used for many years. Creating a standardized patient care process is not intended to reinvent "the wheel" but to create a common framework and language. The process of care described throughout this text provides an easily understood approach that is universally recognized.

PATIENT CARE PROCESS TO OPTIMIZE PHARMACOTHERAPY

There are two aspects that typically differentiate a profession-specific process of care. First, the application of the care process is defined within the context of the profession's knowledge and expertise. For pharmacy, the patient care process is focused on a patient's medication-related needs and their experience with medication therapy.[3] Dentists and dental hygienists employ a patient care process focused on a patient's oral health needs.[21] The nursing care process is applied to provide a holistic approach to a patient's health needs and include physical and mental health, sociocultural issues, spirituality, as well as economic and lifestyle factors.[4] The general approach to providing care to an individual patient in each of these disciplines is similar; however, the focus of the process is distinct.

The second way in which each profession uniquely addresses a patient's needs is the manner in which patient-specific information is assessed. When assessing information collected from a patient (eg, history of present illness, physical examination, laboratory data), physicians employ a clinical reasoning process called "differential diagnosis" to weigh the probability of one disease versus other diseases that possibly account for the patient's signs and symptoms. In the case of dental hygienists, the American Dental Hygienists Association notes that an assessment includes not only a health history and clinical assessment but also a "risk assessment" that includes 11 areas of evaluation.[5] For pharmacists providing comprehensive medication management, the assessment step involves a systematic examination of the indication, effectiveness, safety, and adherence for each of the patient's medications. This is a unique way of approaching a patient's health needs. No other discipline applies a systematic assessment process to a patient's medications and their medication experience in this manner.

Several publications and resources have outlined elements of the patient care process to deliver comprehensive medication management services.[2,11,17,22,23] There is relative consistency between these sources regarding the core elements. What varies is the specificity of the operational definition of each of the process components. Detailed operational definitions help to establish consistency across all practitioners applying the patient care process.[23] This care process is not specific to a care setting—the process can be applied in any setting when providing comprehensive medication management. What often varies is the information collected and its source, as well as the duration of time to complete the process. For example, in an ambulatory care clinic, the patient is often the most important source of information, but in a critical care unit of a hospital, there is a greater reliance on laboratory tests and special diagnostic studies. Similarly, the process of care unfolds in hours or days in acute care settings but may extend over weeks or months in chronic care environments.

Collect Information

When initiating the patient care cycle, a practitioner assures the collection of the necessary subjective and objective information about the patient and is responsible for analyzing the data to understand the patient's relevant medical needs, medication-related problems, and clinical status. In some cases, this information is directly collected by interviewing the patient or reviewing a medical record. In other cases, the practitioner may rely on other personnel to collect the information to be used in the assessment. This may include a blood pressure determined by a clinical assistant or a list of active medications recorded by a nurse. However, it is ultimately the practitioner's responsibility to assure that all necessary information is collected and that the data is accurate, regardless of the source. This information is critical to the ability of the practitioner to complete an assessment that will appropriately address all of a patient's medication-related needs (see Table 1-2).

TABLE 1-2 Collect Patient-Specific Information

Functional Definition[23]

The practitioner assures the collection of the relevant and necessary subjective and objective information about the patient and is responsible for analyzing the data to understand the relevant medical/medication history and clinical status of the patient.

Operational Definition

1. Conduct a review of the medical record to gather relevant information (eg, patient demographics, active medical problem list, admission and discharge notes, office visit notes, laboratory values, diagnostic tests, medication lists).
2. Conduct a comprehensive review of medications and associated health and social history with the patient. The practitioner or team member should:
   - Inquire as to whether the patient has any questions or concerns for the visit.
   - Review social history (eg, alcohol, tobacco, caffeine, other substance use).
   - Review social determinants of health relevant to medication use (eg, whether the patient can afford his/her medications, the patient's education level, housing arrangements, or means of transportation affect his/her ability to use medications as intended).
   - Review past medication history, including allergies and adverse medication effects.
   - Obtain and reconcile a complete medication list that includes all current prescription and nonprescription medications as well as complementary and alternative medicine the patient is taking (eg, name, indication, strength and formulation, dose, frequency, duration, and response to medication).
   - Review the indication for each medication.
   - Review the effectiveness of each medication.
   - Review the safety of each medication.
   - Review the patient's medication experience (eg, beliefs, expectations, and cultural considerations related to medications).
   - Review how the patient manages his/her medications at home (eg, independently or with help, pillboxes, calendars, reminders).
   - Gather any additional information that may be needed (eg, physical assessment, review of systems, home-monitored blood glucose, and/or blood pressure readings).
3. Analyze information in preparation for formulating an assessment of medication therapy problems.

Assess Information and Formulate a Medication Therapy Problem List

Once all of the necessary information to conduct a comprehensive assessment of the patient and their medication-related needs has been collected, the assessment is organized into a problem list consisting of the patient's active medical problems and medication therapy problems. Once identified, problems are prioritized to make decisions regarding the patient's medication therapy to offer the best opportunity to achieve the patient's overall health goals. In doing so, the practitioner reviews each medical condition and medication to make sure that each current medication is *indicated* (or necessary) for the condition for which it is being taken and that each condition that requires drug therapy is being appropriately treated. Then the practitioner determines whether each medication the patient is taking is *effective*, achieving the intended outcome. This includes assuring the medication is the most appropriate option for the patient and is at a dose that is expected to achieve the intended effect. Next, the practitioner considers the *safety* of each medication, assuring that the patient is not experiencing or being exposed to an unnecessary risk of adverse effects or an unintended interaction. Finally, the practitioner then evaluates each medication for *adherence*-related concerns. This includes determining if the patient can take the medication as intended, considering issues such as access and affordability, as well as sufficient knowledge and ability to appropriately administer the medication. Throughout the assessment process, practitioners must keep the patient's goals for therapy at the forefront of their decision making. Table 1-3 outlines the assessment process applied when optimizing pharmacotherapy.

It is critical that the practitioner completes their assessment and defines a problem list considering indication, effectiveness, safety, and

TABLE 1-3 Assess Patient-Specific Information to Determine Health-Related Needs

Functional Definition[23]

The practitioner assesses the information collected and formulates a problem list consisting of the patient's active medical problems and medication therapy problems to prioritize medication therapy recommendations to optimize medication use and achieve clinical goals.

Operational Definition

1. Assess and prioritize the patient's active medical conditions taking into account clinical and patient goals of therapy.
2. Assess the **indication** of each medication the patient is taking. When assessing the indication of each medication, consider the following:
   - Does the patient have an indication for the medication?
   - Is the medication appropriate for the medical condition being treated?
   - Does the patient have an untreated medical condition that requires therapy but is not being treated or prevented?
3. Assess the **effectiveness** of each medication the patient is taking. When assessing the effectiveness of each medication, consider the following:
   - Is the patient meeting clinical goals of therapy?
   - Is the patient meeting personal goals of therapy?
   - Is the most appropriate drug product being used for the medical condition?
   - Are the dose and duration appropriate for the patient?
4. Assess the **safety** of each medication the patient is taking. When assessing the safety of each medication, consider the following:
   - Is the patient experiencing an adverse event from a medication?
   - Is the dose too high for the patient? Are the frequency and duration appropriate for the patient?
   - Do safer alternatives exist?
   - Are there any pertinent drug-disease, drug-drug, or drug-food interactions?
   - Do additional labs need to be obtained to monitor the safety of the medication therapy?
5. Assess **adherence** and the patient's ability to take (eg, administration, access, affordability) each medication. When assessing adherence, consider the following:
   - Is the patient receiving the most affordable option to optimize adherence?
   - Is the patient able to obtain the medication(s), and, if not, why?
   - Are the medications taken at times during the day that is appropriate to optimize effectiveness and minimize harm but also convenient for the patient?
   - Is the patient taking the medication as prescribed/instructed, or are doses missed? If doses are missed, why?
   - Are the frequency and formulation appropriate for the patient to optimize adherence?
6. Formulate a medication therapy problem list in accordance with the Pharmacy Quality Alliance Medication Therapy Problem Categories Framework.[26]
7. Prioritize the patient's medication therapy problems.

adherence *in this order*. This order of assessment ensures that the most relevant issue affecting the patient is identified. For example, there is a great deal of emphasis placed on improving patient adherence to medications, with nonadherence rates reported to range from 28% to 65%.[24,25] However, if a patient is prescribed a medication that is not indicated or is causing an adverse effect, focusing time and attention toward improving medication adherence is misguided and does not address the most important medication therapy problem. Selection of the most appropriate medication for the indication is the primary medication-related need that must be resolved.

The output of the assessment is a medication therapy problem list, prioritized in the order of importance from both the patient's and practitioner's perspectives. Typically, the problem list is framed in a categorical system of medication therapy problems. A nationally recognized system for categorizing the output of a practitioner's assessment is now recognized by the Pharmacy Quality Alliance (see Table 1-4). There are 10 medication therapy problem categories, and these align with the four areas of medication use assessment.[26]

TABLE 1-4 Medication Therapy Problem Categories Framework

Medication-Related Needs	Medication Therapy Problem Category
Indication	Unnecessary medication therapy
	Needs additional medication therapy
Effectiveness	Ineffective medication
	Dosage too low
	Needs additional monitoring
Safety	Adverse medication event
	Dosage too high
	Needs additional monitoring
Convenience	Adherence
	Cost

Data from Pharmacy Quality Alliance. *Medication Therapy Problem Categories Framework for PQA Measures*. Alexandria, VA: Pharmacy Quality Alliance, 2017.

When this assessment approach is applied, a relatively consistent pattern of medication therapy problems emerges.[27-29] The categories identified with the greatest frequency are "needs additional therapy" and "dose too low," followed by "adherence." The other categories are observed less frequently. It should be noted that these reported trends all come from the application of this assessment process in ambulatory care settings. The distribution of medication therapy problems would likely differ in acute care settings.

Develop the Care Plan

Upon completing the assessment and establishing a prioritized list of medication therapy problems, an individualized patient-centered care plan that is evidence-based and as affordable as possible for the patient is created. The plan should be developed in collaboration with the patient or caregiver to meet the patient's expectations and priorities. It should also be developed in collaboration with other healthcare professionals to ensure that all healthcare providers involved with the patient's care agree and support the plan.

The care plan will include goals of therapy and outline contingencies to adjust medications, doses, or delivery, as well as monitoring parameters. It will establish time frames for follow-up and clearly state who will be responsible for each component of the care plan. The steps for developing a patient-centered care plan are outlined in Table 1-5.

TABLE 1-5 Develop the Care Plan

Functional Definition[23]

The practitioner develops an individualized, evidence-based care plan in collaboration with other healthcare professionals and the patient or caregiver that is evidence-based and as affordable as possible for the patient.

Operational Definition

1. Develop a care plan in collaboration with the patient and the patient's healthcare providers to address the identified medication therapy problems.
2. Identify the monitoring parameters important to routinely assess indication, effectiveness, safety, and adherence.
3. Review all medication lists to arrive at an accurate and updated medication list.
4. Determine and coordinate who will implement components of the care plan (ie, patient, pharmacist, other healthcare providers).
5. Determine the type of follow-up needed.
6. Determine the appropriate time frame for patient follow-up.
7. Determine the appropriate mode for follow-up (eg, in person, electronically, by phone).

Implement the Care Plan

Once a care plan is established, the practitioner implements the plan designed to prevent and resolve medication therapy problems. The care plan will likely include activities that the patient and other healthcare providers will be responsible for; however, it is the duty of the practitioner to ensure that each of the elements of the plan has been implemented in a time frame that is reasonable and effective (see Table 1-6).

There are many tools and resources that may be used to support a patient and/or their caregivers to successfully implement the care plan. It is in this part of the patient care process where practitioners will employ strategies such as patient education, motivational interviewing techniques, tools that support medication adherence, and patient self-monitoring technologies. These tools and resources are approaches to best meet the needs of the patient and their medication-related goals.

TABLE 1-6 Implement the Care Plan

Functional Definition[23]

The practitioner implements the care plan in collaboration with other healthcare professionals and the patient or caregiver.

Operational Definition

1. Discuss the care plan with the patient.
2. Ensure patient understanding and agreement with the plan and goals of therapy.
3. Provide personalized education to the patient on his/her medications and lifestyle modifications.
4. Provide the patient with an updated, accurate medication list.
5. Implement those recommendations that you have the ability to implement in your scope of practice.
6. Communicate the care plan to the rest of the care team. If you cannot implement a recommendation(s) on your own, reach a consensus on where implementation is required by another team member.
7. Document the encounter in the electronic health record (eg, a summary of relevant patient information, assessment, and plan, including rationale, monitoring, and follow-up).
8. Arrange patient follow-up.
9. Communicate instructions for follow-up to the patient.

Follow-up with the Patient

After the initial implementation of a care plan, ongoing monitoring and follow-up to evaluate the effectiveness and safety of the plan are essential. The plan should be modified as needed in collaboration with other healthcare professionals and the patient or caregiver. This follow-up process is critical and demonstrates the practitioner has assumed responsibility for the patient's medication-related needs. While a practitioner who serves as a consultant may not follow up to determine if the problem has been resolved, this is inconsistent with the expectations of a comprehensive medication management practice or the patient care process. As a healthcare practitioner who has assumed an important role in a patient's care, it is the responsibility of the practitioner to determine the outcome of drug therapy and take additional action if necessary. This follow-up process can occur through a variety of mechanisms, including face-to-face encounters, phone calls, electronic health record messaging, and telehealth technologies (see Table 1-7).

The frequency to which follow-up occurs varies from setting to setting. A practitioner practicing in an acute care environment will possibly transfer responsibility for follow-up to other providers, including another pharmacist, when the patient transitions to another setting. In the ambulatory care setting, a practitioner should ensure that a patient has a comprehensive evaluation of their medications and health status annually, at a minimum. In some cases, the nature of the patient's medication therapy problems may be resolved to the degree to which the patient no longer requires ongoing monitoring. In such cases, the patient should be referred back to the primary care provider for ongoing follow-up and monitoring.

TABLE 1-7 Follow-up with the Patient

Functional Definition[23]

The practitioner provides ongoing follow-up and monitoring to optimize the care plan and identify and resolve mediation therapy problems, with the goal of optimizing medication use and improving care.

Operational Definition

1. Provide targeted follow-up and monitoring (eg, in person, electronically, or via phone), where needed, to monitor response to therapy and/or refine the care plan to achieve patient and clinical goals of therapy. Targeted follow-up includes but is not limited to quick check-ins to monitor blood sugar or blood pressure, adjust insulin, check INRs, and provide education.
2. Repeat comprehensive medication management (CMM) follow-up visits at least annually, whereby all steps of the CMM Patient Care Process are repeated to ensure continuity of care and ongoing medication optimization.
3. If the patient is no longer a candidate for CMM, ensure that a plan for continuity of care with other care team members.

ENVIRONMENTAL ISSUES

The third critical element of practice is a practice management system. The specifics of any practice management system are based on fundamental business principles and the requirements of the particular type of healthcare setting where the practice exists.[30] In today's healthcare environment, there are several aspects of managing a practice that practitioners must consider—the metrics to ensure patient health outcomes are being achieved; efficient workflow; communication and documentation using the power of information technology (IT); and data that accurately attributes and values the work each practitioner brings to patient care.

Quality Metrics

Dr. Avedis Donabedian, considered the father of quality improvement in healthcare, defined standards as the desired and achievable performance related to a specific parameter—an objective, definable, and measurable characteristic of the structure, the process, or the outcome of the care.[31] To determine quality, there must be a standard to measure the level of quality against. The patient care process sets a standard of achievable performance by defining the parameters of the process that can be measured. With the movement toward outcome-based healthcare models and value-based payment systems, it is critical to objectively measure the impact a patient care service has on a patient's health and well-being. This allows the linkage from the standard process, such as what health problems were identified and how they were addressed during the patient encounter, to the desired outcomes. For the process to be measurable, each element must be clearly defined and performed similarly during each patient encounter. The lack of clarity and consistency has been the Achilles heel in the evidence to support the value of pharmacists' patient care services.[32] The standard process gives pharmacists an opportunity to show value on a large scale because the services are comparable and clearly understood across practice settings.

Workflow, Documentation, and Information Systems

The generation and analysis of data regarding the care provided and the resulting health outcomes are becoming increasingly important for organizations and individual providers. Healthcare systems are rapidly embracing the power of technology to analyze information to gain important insights. This technology is only useful if clinical care is robustly documented, collected, and managed. Data is optimally collected as part of the workflow process using IT tools. Creating the requisite tools, however, requires a standard process to build cohesive systems with uniform data sets. Thus, the data elements can be collected using the same collection specifications using different technology systems in different organizations. This allows the reporting of comparable information to providers, payers, and others.

A uniform patient care process sets a standard for the workflow that allows IT systems to capture and extract data for analysis and sharing. Imagine a patient encounter with a practitioner in any setting. The practitioner often has some patient information available before the encounter; however, the practitioner will likely collect new information. This work can now be electronically captured in the collect phase of the workflow. The practitioner will then assess the information and identify new or unresolved medication-related problems. Likewise, this work is captured in the assessment phase of the visit. The practitioner will then update or add to the care plan for the patient, and the information can be electronically captured in the planning phase. During the encounter, the practitioner may implement some or all of the plan, and the tasks or services performed are captured during the implementation phase. During the follow-up and monitoring phase, the resolution of identified problems and the response to treatment are documented. The information collected can now be exchanged, extracted, and analyzed at the provider, population, organizational, and payer levels because it is defined and collected in a uniform manner.

The ability to capture clinical data is available through several coding systems (see Table 1-8). The Pharmacy Health Information

TABLE 1-8 Clinical Coding Systems

System Name	Contents
International Classification of Disease (ICD)	Coding for medical procedures and encounters. The 11th edition was published in 2019.
Systematized Nomenclature of Medicine—Clinical Terms (SNOMED-CT)	A coding system of clinical terminology representing the full scope of clinical information in healthcare.
Logical Observation Identifiers Names and Codes (LOINC)	Vocabulary database of universal identifiers for laboratory and clinical test results.
Healthcare Common Procedural Coding System (HCPCS)	CMS established billing codes for Medicare for medical procedures that include CPT as well as codes not covered by CPT.
Current procedure terminology (CPT)	Coding system for medical procedures developed and maintained by the American Medical Association primarily used for billing services.
RxNorm	Standardized nomenclature for clinical drugs created by the National Library of Medicine.

Technology Collaborative has been at the forefront in assuring pharmacist patient care services are part of the IT systems being developed for the healthcare system in the United States.[33] The collaborative has developed several documents demonstrating how to uniformly document patient-care activities and enables sharing of patient-specific information across technology platforms. These data can be used to improve care coordination, workflows, and quality. Examples include documentation templates that use standard technology coding such as the Systematic Nomenclature of Medicine—Clinical Terms (SNOMED-CT) codes that convert a patient care note into an electronically transferable document (eg, pharmacist e-care plan). The information can then be used to link patient outcomes attributable to the pharmacist-provided care. The documents are easily accessible on the Pharmacy Health Information Technology (HIT) website (http://pharmacyhit.org/). It is unnecessary for practitioners to know the specific codes or technology structure. However, clinicians should understand how IT operates behind the scenes when performing and documenting their clinical activities. This will enable practitioners to assist information technologists in effectively designing systems that accurately and efficiently capture the elements of the patient encounter that can be used for care coordination, quality metrics, and payment in emerging value-based payment models.

Documentation, Attribution, and Payment

Payment to healthcare providers for patient care services in the United States has traditionally been based on the documentation and reporting of standard processes of care. Rules and guidance from Medicare and the Centers for Medicare & Medicaid Services (CMS) are considered the billing and payment standard for healthcare providers, both for governmental and commercial payers. Eligible Medicare Part B providers such as physicians, nurse practitioners, and physician assistants must follow standards outlined in the CMS Documentation Guidelines for Evaluation and Management Services.[34] Pharmacists are familiar with these standards because they often use the Subjective, Objective, Assessment, Plan (SOAP) note format when documenting care, including the patient's chief complaint, history of present illness, past medical history, social history, family history, review of systems, physical examination, assessment, and plan. Built on top of the standard documentation requirement is the reporting of the complexity of the care provided. This added layer of documentation is determined by the number of required elements in each documentation domain. A billing code can then be assigned to that patient care encounter which, in turn, equates to a payment commensurate with the level of care provided. While this process is the basis for the current fee-for-service payment structure, it is likely the general format that will remain in any new payment model. Similarly, other providers such as dieticians and physical therapists have standard processes, workflow, and documentation that enable the payment structures in their practice model.

Pharmacists have traditionally used the SOAP note format when documenting care for patients. This is particularly appropriate when providing services incident to an eligible Medicare Part B provider. It is the standard documentation required in that circumstance. However, some elements for the SOAP note, required when using certain billing codes, are not routinely performed by pharmacists (eg, comprehensive physical examination). The pharmacist patient care process establishes a standard framework that reflects the pharmacist's work. Using a standard care process accompanied with a standard documentation framework will result in efficiencies of practice, enable appropriate and accurate billing, and facilitate the attribution of care to desired patient outcomes needed in value-based payment models.

CONCLUSION

A standard process of care provides the structure that all practitioners should follow and, when implemented correctly and consistently, can improve the quality of care provided to patients. It provides a common language that defines roles, responsibilities, and expectations. Comprehensive medication management involves a five-step process: collect, assess, plan, implement, and follow-up. A standard process of care informs the creation of quality metrics and is the foundation of practitioner workflow, the structure of health information systems, and billing for patient care services.

ABBREVIATIONS

CMS	Centers for Medicare & Medicaid Services
CPT	current procedure terminology
HCPCS	Healthcare Common Procedural Coding System
ICD	International Classification of Disease
IT	information technology
LOINC	Logical Observation Identifiers Names and Codes
SNOMED-CT	CT Systematized Nomenclature of Medicine—Clinical Terms
SOAP	subjective, objective, assessment, plan

REFERENCES

1. Harris IM, Phillips B, Boyce E, et al. Clinical pharmacy should adopt a consistent process of direct patient care. *Pharmacotherapy.* 2014;34(8):e133–e148. doi:10.1002/phar.1459.
2. Joint Commission of Pharmacy Practitioners. *Pharmacists' Patient Care Process.* May 29, 2014. Available at: https://jcpp.net/wp-content/uploads/2016/03/PatientCareProcess-with-supporting-organizations.pdf. Accessed August 19, 2021.
3. Cipolle JR, Strand L, Morley P. Pharmaceutical care as the professional practice for patient-centered medication management services. In: Cipolle JR, Strand L, Morley P, eds. *Pharmaceutical Care Practice: The Patient Centered Approach to Medication Management.* 3rd ed. New York, NY: McGraw-Hill Companies; 2012:37–72.
4. American Nurses Association. The Nursing Process. https://www.nursingworld.org/practice-policy/workforce/what-is-nursing/the-nursing-process/. Accessed August 11, 2021.
5. Writing Group of the Nutrition Care Process/Standardized Language Committee. Nutrition care process and model. Part I: The 2008 update. *J Am Diet Assoc.* 2008;108(7):1113–1117. doi:10.1016/j.jada.2008.04.027.
6. Phillips RLJ, Klinkman M, Green LA. *Conference Report: Harmonizing Primary Care Clinical Classification and Data Standards.* Washington, DC; 2007. http://www.graham-center.org/content/dam/rgc/documents/publications-reports/monographs-books/harmonizing-primary-care.pdf. Accessed August 11, 2021.
7. ICPC Primary Health Care Classification Consortium. International Classification of Primary Care (ICPC-2) Process Codes update 2016. http://www.ph3c.org/4daction/w3_CatVisu/en/icpc.html?wCatIDAdmin=1106. Accessed August 11, 2021.
8. Lacey K, Pritchett E. Nutrition care process and model: ADA adopts road map to quality care and outcomes management. *J Am Diet Assoc.* 2003;103(8):1061–1072. doi:10.1053/jada.2003.50564.
9. Tomajan K, Barker CR, Canariato SV, et al. *Recognition of a Nursing Specialty, Approval of a Speciality Nursing Scope of Practice Statement, and Acknowledgment of Specialty Nursing Standards of Practice.* Silver Spring, MD; 2010. https://www.nursingworld.org/~4989de/globalassets/practiceandpolicy/scope-of-practice/3sc-booklet-final-2017-08-17.pdf. Accessed August 11, 2021.
10. American Physical Therapy Association. *Guidelines: Physical Therapy Documentation of Patient/Client Management.* Alexandria, VA: 2009. https://www.apta.org/uploadedFiles/APTAorg/About_Us/Policies/BOD/Practice/DocumentationPatientClientMgmt.pdf. Accessed August 11, 2021.
11. Cipolle RJ, Strand L, Morley P. Toward a philosophy of pharmaceutical care practice. In: Cipolle RJ, Strand L, Morley P, eds. *Pharmaceutical Care Practice: The Patient-Centered Approach to Medication*

Management Services. 3rd ed. New York, NY: McGraw-Hill Companies; 2012;94–100.

12. American Pharmacists Association. Code of Ethics for Pharmacists. Published 1994. https://portal.pharmacist.com/code-ethics. Accessed August 11, 2021.
13. American Pharmacists Association. Oath of a Pharmacist. Published November 2021. https://www.pharmacist.com/About/Oath-of-a-Pharmacist. Accessed July 29, 2022.
14. American Society of Hospital Pharmacists. ASHP Statement on Pharmaceutical Care. *Am J Hosp Pharm.* 1993;50:1720–1723.
15. Donabedian A. The quality of care: How can it be assessed? *JAMA.* 1988;260(12):1743–1748. doi:10.1001/jama.1988.03410120089033.
16. Epstein RM, Street RL, Jr. The values and value of patient-centered care. *Ann Fam Med.* 2011;9(2):100–103. doi:10.1370/afm.1239.
17. American College of Clinical Pharmacy. Standards of practice for clinical pharmacists. *Pharmacotherapy.* 2014;34(8):794–797. doi:10.1002/phar.1438.
18. Institute of Medicine. *Crossing the Quality Chasm: A New Health System for the 21st Century.* Washington, DC: National Academies Press; 2001. doi:10.17226/12019.
19. Berwick DM, Nolan TW, Whittington J. The triple aim: Care, health, and cost. *Health Aff.* 2008;27(3):759–769. doi:10.1377/hlthaff.27.3.759.
20. Loehrer S, Feeley D, Berwick D. 10 New rules to accelerate healthcare redesign. Bold aspirations to guide healthcare organizations during an era of reform. *Healthc Exec.* 30(6):66, 68–69.
21. American Dental Hygienists' Association. *Standards for Clinical Dental Hygiene Practice.* Chicago, IL: American Dental Hygienists' Association; Revised 2016. https://www.adha.org/resources-docs/2016-Revised-Standards-for-Clinical-Dental-Hygiene-Practice.pdf.
22. McInnis T, Strand L, Webb CE. *Integrating Comprehensive Medication Management to Optimize Patient Outcomes: Resource Guide.* 2nd ed. 2012. https://www.pcpcc.org/sites/default/files/media/medmanagement.pdf.
23. The Patient Care Process for Delivering Comprehensive Medication Management (CMM): Optimizing Medication Use in Patient-Centered, Team-Based Care Settings. CMM in Primary Care Research Team. July 2018. Available at: http://www.accp.com/cmm_care_process.
24. Briesacher BA, Andrade SE, Fouayzi H, Chan KA. Comparison of drug adherence rates among patients with seven different medical conditions. *Pharmacotherapy.* 2008;28(4):437–443. doi:10.1592/phco.28.4.437.
25. Yeaw J, Benner JS, Walt JG, Sian S, Smith DB. Comparing adherence and persistence across 6 chronic medication classes. *J Manag Care Pharm.* 2009;15(9):728–740. doi:10.18553/jmcp.2009.15.9.728.
26. Pharmacy Quality Alliance. *Medication Therapy Problem Categories Framework for PQA Measures.* Alexandria, VA: Pharmacy Quality Alliance; 2017.
27. Sorensen TD, Pestka DL, Brummel AR, Rehrauer DJ, Ekstrand MJ. Seeing the forest through the trees: Improving adherence alone will not optimize medication use. *J Manag Care Spec Pharm.* 2016;22(5):598–604. doi:10.18553/jmcp.2016.22.5.598.
28. Isetts BJ, Schondelmeyer SW, Artz MB, et al. Clinical and economic outcomes of medication therapy management services: The Minnesota experience. *J Am Pharm Assoc.* 2008;48(2):203–214. doi:10.1331/JAPhA.2008.07108.
29. Ramalho de Oliveira D, Brummel AR, Miller DB. Medication therapy management: 10 years of experience in a large integrated health care system. *J Manag Care Pharm.* 2010;16(3):185–195. doi:10.18553/jmcp.2010.16.3.185.
30. Harris IM, Baker E, Berry T, et al. Developing a business-practice model for pharmacy services in ambulatory settings. *Pharmacotherapy.* 2008;28(2):285. doi:10.1592/phco.28.2.285.
31. Donabedian A. Criteria, norms and standards of quality: What do they mean? *Am J Public Health.* 1981;71(4):409–412.
32. Viswanathan M, Kahwati LC, Golin CE, et al. Medication therapy management interventions in outpatient settings. *JAMA Intern Med.* 2015;175(1):76. doi:10.1001/jamainternmed.2014.5841.
33. Pharmacy Health Information Technology Collaborative. http://pharmacyhit.org/. Accessed July 29, 2022.
34. Centers for Medicare and Medicaid Services. *Evaluation and Management Services Guide.* Rockville, MD: Department of Health and Human Services; January 2022. https://www.cms.gov/Outreach-and-Education/Medicare-Learning-Network-MLN/MLNProducts/MLN-Publications-Items/CMS1243514. Accessed July 29, 2022.

Health Literacy and Medication Use

e2

Oralia V. Bazaldua, Norbert Rosario, and Erica Torres

KEY CONCEPTS

1. Limited health literacy is common and must be considered when providing medication management services.
2. Some groups of people are at higher risk for having limited literacy skills, but in general, you cannot tell by looking.
3. Patients with limited health literacy are more likely to misunderstand medication instructions and have difficulty demonstrating the correct dosing regimen.
4. Limited health literacy is associated with increased healthcare costs and worse health outcomes, including increased mortality.
5. Despite numerous efforts to improve safe medication practices, current strategies have been inadequate, and this may have a larger impact in patients with limited literacy.
6. Most printed materials are written at higher comprehension levels than most adults can read.
7. The United States Pharmacopeia has set new standards for prescription medication labeling to minimize patient confusion.
8. Several instruments exist to measure health literacy, but some experts advocate "universal precautions" under which all patients are assumed to benefit from plain language and clear communication.
9. Obtaining a complete medication history and providing medication counseling are vital components in the medication management of patients with limited health literacy.

BEYOND THE BOOK

Watch the YouTube video, "Health and the City" available online (https://youtu.be/ux6c3wYzRJM), and the TEDx Talk, "Are You Confused About Health Information? You're Not Alone (https://www.youtube.com/watch?v=-x6DLqtaK2g)."

Another exercise is useful for translating the material in this chapter to your local area. Working in small groups, make a list of the challenges in health literacy common in the geographic area your educational institution serves. Use resources such as census.gov and cdc.gov to explore the languages spoken in your area, the racial/ethnic background of residents, and cultural practices that can affect patient adherence to medication-related advice and counseling.

INTRODUCTION

Every day, thousands of patients are not taking their medications correctly. Some take too much. Others take too little. Some use a tablespoon instead of a teaspoon. Parents pour an oral antibiotic suspension in their child's ear instead of giving it by mouth because it was prescribed for an ear infection. Others are in the emergency department because they did not know how to use their asthma inhaler. It is not a deliberate revolt against the doctor's orders but rather a likely and an unfortunate result of a hidden risk factor—limited health literacy.

(1) *Literacy*, at the basic level, is simply the ability to read and write. When these skills are applied to a health context, it is called *health literacy*, but health literacy is more than just reading and writing. The definition of health literacy has evolved from that of the Institute of Medicine in 2004 as some have questioned its meaning and point out the lack of consensus on what it represents.[1] To update and address health literacy in Healthy People 2030, Santana and colleagues provide the following definitions that address both personal and organizational health literacy. Among other key points, they incorporate a public health perspective and acknowledge that organizations have a responsibility to address health literacy as well.[2]

- **Personal health literacy** is the degree to which individuals have the ability to find, understand, and use information and services to inform health-related decisions and actions for themselves and others.
- **Organizational health literacy** is the degree to which organizations equitably enable individuals to find, understand, and use information and services to inform health-related decisions and actions for themselves and others.

While some have provided a rigorous definition for medication literacy,[3] we propose that ***medication literacy*** *is simply, the degree to which individuals have the ability to make informed decisions that lead to safe and effective medication use.*

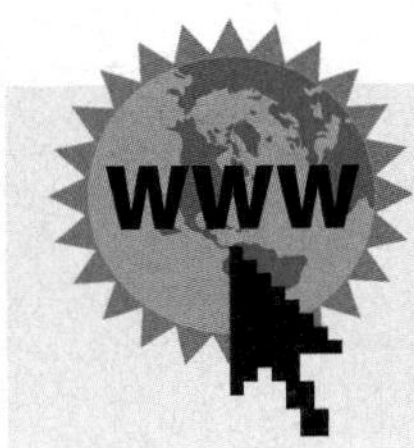

The complete chapter, learning objectives, and other resources can be found at **www.pharmacotherapyonline.com.**

Exploring Cultural Diversity and Equity in Healthcare

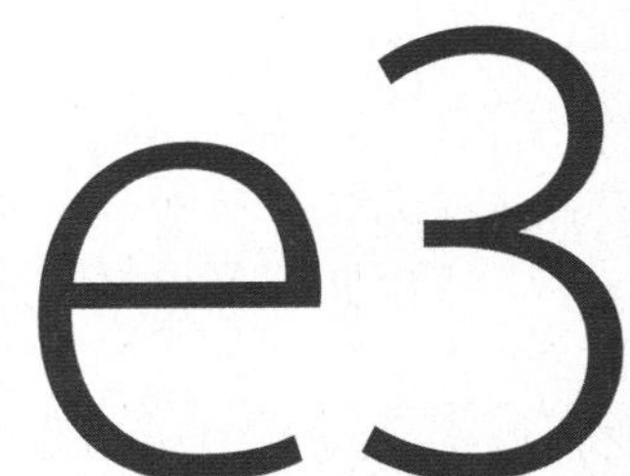

Amanda M. Loya, Jeri J. Sias, Lakesha M. Butler, Christopher G. Medlin, and Jessica M. Shenberger-Trujillo

KEY CONCEPTS

1. Healthcare providers should strive toward cultural competency and equity in the context of social determinants of health and community history to improve care and access unique resources for patients and communities from diverse cultures and backgrounds.
2. Changes in demographics in the United States, health disparities, patient safety, and healthcare workforce shortages are among the reasons for needing cultural and linguistic competency skills and for promoting diversity and equity in healthcare.
3. A variety of models recognize cultural competency as a process, not an achievement.
4. Legal and regulatory issues surrounding cultural competency include understanding and interpreting accreditation standards for healthcare organizations and Title VI of the Civil Rights Act.
5. Patients may enter the healthcare setting with a different explanation of their illnesses than what is found in the Western biomedical model (WBM).
6. Cultural values and beliefs influence decisions and attitudes about healthcare, including race, ethnicity, age, gender, sexual orientation, and religious beliefs.
7. Developing communication skills to interact with diverse populations involves recognizing personal styles and cultural values of communication as well as barriers to patient understanding.
8. Linguistic competency encompasses understanding the capacity of organizations and providers to communicate well with diverse populations such as patients with limited English proficiency (LEP), low literacy, or hearing impairments.
9. Before practitioners can understand other cultures, they should strive to understand the personal and organizational values and beliefs.
10. Skills for working with patients from diverse cultures include being able to listen to the patient's perception of health, acknowledging differences, being respectful, and negotiating treatment options.

BEYOND THE BOOK

Select any one of the patients from diverse backgrounds from the cases introduced in the first section of this chapter. What are the factors that influence their health that are based on genetics? Individual and family choices? Community influences? Larger city and policy structures?

For more in-depth discussions, consider these activities and questions:

1. Use Healthy People 2030 (https://health.gov/healthypeople/objectives-and-data/browse-objectives) to identify Social Determinants of Health found in the cases.
2. Describe what you think would be the acculturation of each patient. What is the host culture? What is the home culture?
3. Explore values and beliefs found in resources provided in the chapter: Based on the information provided, what social identity and acculturation characteristics are involved? Look up information about healthcare beliefs and values based on how the patient self-identifies with religion and race or ethnicity.
4. Discuss what you would describe to be your own "cultural competency" to work with each of the patients. Which models do you prefer?
5. If approached by one of the patients, providers may argue that "we can't solve everything in healthcare. I only have so much time during a visit." How might you respond to those statements? What changes can be made at a provider level, clinic/hospital level, and at a larger system-wide level to improve care across cultures?

CULTURE, COMMUNITY, AND SOCIAL DETERMINANTS OF HEALTH

Culture influences who we are, including our thoughts, behaviors, and beliefs toward healthcare. What is culture? **Culture** can be defined as "the learned and shared beliefs, feelings, and knowledge that individuals and/or groups use to guide their behavior and define their reality as they interact with the world."[1,2]

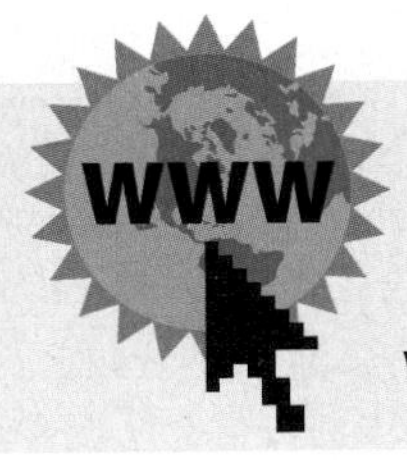

The complete chapter, learning objectives, and other resources can be found at **www.pharmacotherapyonline.com.**

e4

Medication Safety

Robert J. Weber

KEY CONCEPTS

1. Medication errors (MEs) are defined as any mistake at any stage of the medication-use process; adverse drug events (ADEs) are MEs that result in injury.
2. All MEs are preventable, while ADEs can be categorized as preventable and potential.
3. MEs occur at an alarmingly high rate, with some ADEs having fatal outcomes for patients.
4. MEs can occur at any step of the medication-use process: selection and procurement, storage, ordering and transcribing, preparing and dispensing, administration, or monitoring.
5. Determining the actual and potential root causes of MEs helps to correct future errors in the medication-use system.
6. Quality improvement methods that prevent MEs and thereby minimize ADEs include identifying the ME and/or ADE, understanding the reasons for the ME and/or ADE, designing and implementing changes to prevent an ADE or ME, and checking the outcome of that change.
7. Healthcare organizations have implemented various measures to reduce the incidence of MEs and ADEs, such as computerized physician order entry (CPOE), automated drug distribution systems, bar-code scanning, and "smart" infusion pumps with decision support and where information is passed in a bidirectional manner between the pump and the patient's electronic medical record (EMR).
8. Medication reconciliation or comparing a patient's current medication orders to all of the medications that the patient had been taking before any care transition (hospital admission, transfer, or discharge) is a vital process in preventing MEs and ADEs.
9. Promoting a "just culture" of medication safety cultivates trust in the workplace that makes personnel feel comfortable sharing safety information (eg, unsafe situations) and assuming personal responsibility and accountability for complying with safe medication practices.

BEYOND THE BOOK

1. Watch the https://tinyurl.com/tqh8n3k video entitled "CUSP: Understand Just Culture," sponsored by the Agency for Healthcare Research and Quality. This 5.5-minute video describes the fundamental tenets of a "just culture" environment with examples that clarify the concept.
2. Use the above video to think about a patient care situation where a medication error occurred—and how it was managed and resolved. Write down two to four ways the "just culture" concepts were used—or not used—in that situation.

INTRODUCTION

Medical errors are not a new phenomenon. Medical errors causing harm may lead to devastating effects on patients. In 1991, the Harvard Medical Practice Study showed that a significant number of people are victims of medical errors, and a subset experienced MEs. This landmark study reviewed the incidence of adverse events and negligence in hospitalized patients in the state of New York showing that almost 4% of patients experienced an iatrogenic injury (one caused by healthcare practices or procedures), prolonging their hospital stays.[1] Importantly, nearly 14% of those mistakes were fatal. Examples of mistakes noted in the Harvard study included renal failure from angiographic dye and a missed diagnosis of colon cancer. Drug complications were the most common type of outcome attributed to negligence, accounting for 19% of these preventable adverse events.[1]

The goal of medication therapy is achieving defined therapeutic goals to improve a patient's quality of life while minimizing harm.[2] Known and unknown risks are associated with the therapeutic use of prescription and nonprescription drugs and drug administration devices.[3] Mishaps related to medication therapy include both ADEs and MEs.[4]

MEs negatively affect patients' confidence in the healthcare system and increase healthcare costs. Research conducted by the American Society of Health-System Pharmacists (ASHP) showed that 61% of patients surveyed reported that they were "very concerned" about being given the wrong medicine during a hospital stay.[5] MEs are also very costly—to healthcare systems, patients and their families, and healthcare workers. The emotional cost of an ME is also significant, including the burden on the family for grieving loss or stress for the healthcare worker (often referred to as the "second victim") involved in an ME that caused harm.

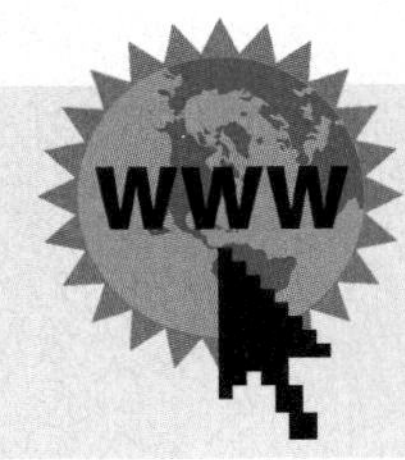

The complete chapter, learning objectives, and other resources can be found at **www.pharmacotherapyonline.com.**

e5

Medication Adherence

Fang-Ju Lin, Yen-Ming Huang, and Yunn-Fang Ho

KEY CONCEPTS

1. Medication adherence is defined as the degree to which an individual takes medications recommended by healthcare providers in terms of the dose, route, frequency, and length of time.
2. Better medication adherence is associated with optimal health outcomes.
3. Approaches to assessing medication adherence are classified as direct and indirect methods with various inherent limitations.
4. Direct methods of assessing medication adherence include bioassays or biomarkers to measure levels of drugs or their metabolites in body fluids.
5. Indirect methods of assessing medication adherence include self-report surveys, pharmacy refill rates, pill counts, clinical response monitoring, and electronic monitoring devices.
6. The World Health Organization suggests five interactive dimensions to describe factors associated with medication adherence: (1) social and economic, (2) healthcare team- and system-related, (3) condition-related, (4) therapy-related, and (5) patient-related factors.
7. To improve and sustain good adherence, healthcare interventions and services must overcome barriers to medication adherence and individualize care by considering multiple factors.

BEYOND THE BOOK

Watch "Medication Adherence," (https://edhub.ama-assn.org/steps-forward/module/2702595) a video from the American Medical Association. This video describes the common reasons for medication nonadherence from patients' perspectives. Then, watch the YouTube video from the FDA Drug Info Rounds (pharmacists), "Taking Medications Correctly—Medication Adherence," (https://www.youtube.com/watch?v=Qh84l557-D0). This video provides a glance at strategies for improving medication adherence.

INTRODUCTION

1 Based on the World Health Organization (WHO) definition, medication adherence refers to the extent to which an individual takes medications corresponding to the agreed recommendations from a healthcare provider.[1] Good medication adherence indicates a person takes medications as prescribed, with the appropriate dose via the suggested route at the right time.[2] Poor medication adherence is associated with suboptimal or adverse health outcomes.[3]

2 Compared with nonadherent patients, adherent patients have lower healthcare costs, including fewer hospitalizations and emergency department visits, reduced costs of acute and outpatient care, and better health outcomes and quality of life.[4] For instance, for every patient with type 2 diabetes in an indigent population in Virginia, every 10% increase in medication adherence is estimated to save US $450 annually in medical care[5] and a decrease in glycosylated hemoglobin (HbA_{1c}) level by 0.16% (0.0016; ~1.8 mmol/mol).[6] As a result, medication adherence is widely used as a proxy measure for evaluating disease management and treatment effects.[7]

The estimated rate of medication adherence for chronic illnesses in developed countries is around 50%, even with patients who have easy access to medications.[8] As such, the WHO further indicated that improving medication adherence may have a far greater influence on public health than any improvement in specific medical treatments.[9]

In this chapter, key aspects of the medication adherence process are presented. These include methods of assessment, barriers, and improvement strategies. When the patient is taking the medication as agreed upon, optimal clinical, economic, and humanistic outcomes can be achieved (Fig. e5-1).

MEASURES OF MEDICATION ADHERENCE

3 The critical first step in improving medication adherence is to appropriately measure how an individual takes medications as prescribed by healthcare providers. Various methods have been proposed to measure medication adherence; however, there is no agreement among clinical practitioners and researchers on the best method for assessing medication adherence.

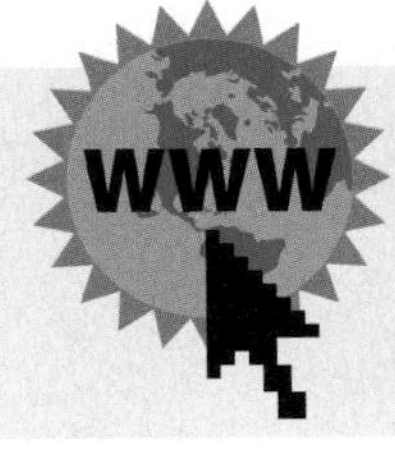

The complete chapter, learning objectives, and other resources can be found at **www.pharmacotherapyonline.com.**

Clinical Pharmacokinetics and Pharmacodynamics

e6

Kristin M. Janzen and Samuel M. Poloyac

KEY CONCEPTS

1 Clinical pharmacokinetics is the discipline that describes the absorption, distribution, and elimination of medications in patients requiring pharmacotherapy.

2 The pharmacokinetic parameter that describes absorption is the bioavailability. Bioavailability refers to the proportion of the dose of a medication that reaches systemic circulation.

3 The pharmacokinetic parameter that describes distribution is the volume of distribution. The volume of distribution is a proportionality constant that relates the amount of medication in the body to the serum concentration.

4 To characterize differences in drug distribution, we can use compartmental models to describe the different behaviors. Compartmental models are mathematical descriptions of the grouped body spaces that the medication penetrates and the overall time it takes to get into each space.

5 The pharmacokinetic parameter that describes elimination is clearance. Clearance describes the volume of plasma cleared of the given drug over time, and it may be either linear or nonlinear.

6 Most drugs follow linear pharmacokinetics, in which serum drug concentrations change proportionally with changes in dose.

7 Some drugs do not follow the rules of linear pharmacokinetics, which leads to a variety of nonlinear pharmacokinetic profiles. Instead of concentration increasing proportionally with dose, serum concentrations change more or less than expected.

8 The pharmacokinetic parameter that describes the time required for serum concentrations to decrease by one-half is half-life. Half-life is dependent on the values of clearance and volume of distribution.

9 Pharmacokinetic models are useful to describe data sets, to predict serum concentrations after several doses or different routes of administration, and to calculate pharmacokinetic constants such as clearance, volume of distribution, and half-life.

10 Many factors should be taken into consideration when deciding on the best drug dose for a patient. These include patient-specific factors, including age, sex, weight, race/ethnic background, genetics, other concurrent disease states, kidney function, and hepatic function, as well as drug-specific factors (drug-drug interactions, drug-food interactions).

11 Cytochrome P450 enzymes are responsible for most drug metabolism oxidation reactions.

12 Membrane transporters are protein molecules that actively transport drugs across cell membranes. Transport proteins are important in the processes of drug bioavailability, elimination, and distribution.

13 When deciding on initial doses for drugs that are renally eliminated, the patient's kidney function should be assessed. A common, useful way to do this is to measure the patient's serum creatinine concentration and convert this value into an estimated creatinine clearance (CL_{cr}).

14 When deciding on initial doses for drugs that are hepatically eliminated, the patient's liver function should be assessed. The Child-Pugh score can be used as an indicator of a patient's ability to metabolize drugs that are eliminated by the liver.

15 For drugs that exhibit linear pharmacokinetics, steady-state drug concentration changes proportionally with dose.

16 Some drugs with narrow therapeutic windows require determination of the pharmacokinetic constants to individualize the patient's dose. In these cases, a small pharmacokinetic evaluation is conducted in the individual.

17 Pharmacodynamics is the study of the relationship between the concentration of a drug and the response obtained in a patient. If pharmacologic effect is plotted against concentration for most drugs, a hyperbola results with an asymptote equal to the maximum attainable effect. The potency of a drug is estimated by the concentration required to achieve 50% of that maximal effect.

BEYOND THE BOOK

Watch the video titled "Introduction to Pharmacokinetics", available at https://www.youtube.com/watch?v=TwSsMHtfQD4. This video provides a brief overview of basic pharmacokinetic concepts. This website is useful to enhance student understanding of basic pharmacokinetic concepts.

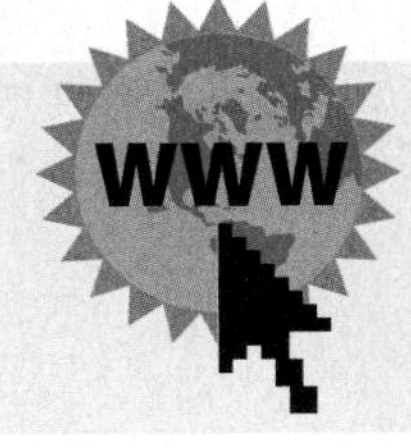

The complete chapter, learning objectives, and other resources can be found at **www.pharmacotherapyonline.com.**

e7

Clinical Pharmacogenomics

Roseann S. Gammal, Larisa H. Cavallari, and Y. W. Francis Lam

KEY CONCEPTS

1. Genetic variation contributes to pharmacokinetic and pharmacodynamic properties of medications.
2. Genetic variation affects drug-metabolizing enzymes, transporters, and target proteins, as well as immune-related proteins that may impact medication response.
3. Genetic polymorphisms may influence medication effectiveness and risk for toxicity.
4. Pharmacogenomics is the study of the impact of genetic polymorphisms on medication response.
5. The goals of pharmacogenomics are to optimize medication efficacy and limit toxicity based on an individual's DNA.
6. Single nucleotide polymorphisms are the most common gene variations associated with medication response.
7. Evidence-based resources, such as US Food and Drug Administration medication labels, Clinical Pharmacogenetics Implementation Consortium Guidelines, and the Pharmacogenomics Knowledgebase, are available to help clinicians select and dose medications based on a patient's genetic profile.
8. The pharmacist plays a key role in advancing pharmacogenomics in clinical practice as part of a multidisciplinary healthcare team.

BEYOND THE BOOK

Visit the CPIC Website: https://cpicpgx.org/. Select and review a gene-drug guideline. Briefly describe how these recommendations may be applied to clinical practice. This activity is intended to build your experience with accessing pharmacogenomic guidelines and how they may be integrated into prescribing decisions.

INTRODUCTION

Great variability exists among individuals in response to medication therapy, and it is difficult to predict how effective or safe a medication will be for a particular patient. For example, when treating a patient with depression, it may be necessary to try several agents or a combination of agents before achieving adequate depressive symptom control with acceptable tolerability. Several clinical factors are known to influence medication response, including age, body size, kidney and liver function, and concomitant medication use. However, considering these factors alone is often insufficient in predicting the likelihood of medication efficacy or safety for a given patient. For example, identical antidepressant therapy in two patients of similar age, sex, race, and with similar medical histories and concomitant medication therapy may produce inadequate control of depressive symptoms in one patient and intolerable adverse effects in the other.

1 2 The observed interpatient variability in medication response may result largely from genetically determined differences in drug metabolism, distribution, and target proteins. The influence of heredity on medication response was demonstrated as early as 1956 with the discovery that an inherited deficiency of glucose-6-phosphate dehydrogenase (G6PD) was responsible for hemolytic reactions to the antimalarial drug primaquine (Fig. e7-1). Variations in genes encoding cytochrome P450 (CYP) and other drug-metabolizing enzymes are now well-recognized as causes of interindividual differences in plasma concentrations of certain medications. These variations may have serious implications for medications with a narrow therapeutic index such as warfarin, phenytoin, and mercaptopurine. Other variations associated with medication response occur in genes for drug transporters such as the solute carrier organic anion transporter (OAT) family member 1B1 (SLCO1B1) as well as drug targets such as receptors and enzymes. Genetic variations for drug-metabolizing enzymes and transporter proteins may influence drug disposition, thus altering pharmacokinetic properties. Drug target genes may alter pharmacodynamic mechanisms by affecting sensitivity to a medication at its target site. Variation in immune-related genes, such as those that encode human leukocyte antigen (HLA) molecules, may affect a patient's predisposition to severe medication hypersensitivity reactions despite having no direct effect on pharmacokinetic or pharmacodynamic mechanisms.

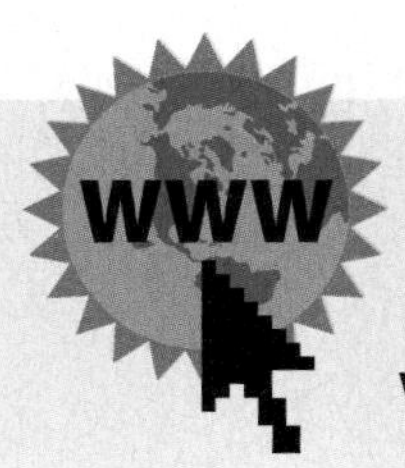

The complete chapter, learning objectives, and other resources can be found at **www.pharmacotherapyonline.com.**

Clinical Toxicology

e8

Bryan D. Hayes and Natalija M. Farrell

KEY CONCEPTS

1. Poisoning can result from exposure to excessive doses of any chemical, with medicines being responsible for most childhood and adult poisonings.
2. The total number and rate of poisonings have been increasing, but preventive measures, such as child-resistant containers, have reduced mortality in young children.
3. Immediate first aid may reduce the development of serious poisoning, and consultation with a poison control center may indicate the need for further therapy.
4. The use of ipecac syrup, gastric lavage, whole bowel irrigation, and cathartics has fallen out of favor as routine therapies, whereas activated charcoal remains useful for gastric decontamination of appropriate patients.
5. Antidotes can prevent or reduce the toxicity of certain poisons, but symptomatic and supportive care is essential for all patients.
6. Acute acetaminophen poisoning produces severe liver injury and occasionally kidney failure. A determination of serum acetaminophen concentration may indicate whether there is risk of hepatotoxicity and the need for acetylcysteine therapy.
7. Anticholinesterase insecticides may produce life-threatening respiratory distress and paralysis by all routes of exposure and can be treated with symptomatic care, atropine, and pralidoxime.
8. An overdose of calcium channel antagonists can produce severe hypotension and bradycardia and should be treated with supportive care, calcium, and insulin with supplemental dextrose.
9. Anticholinergic toxicity is characterized by dry mucous membranes, mydriasis, urinary retention, tachycardia, fever, or agitated delirium with or without hallucinations, which can be treated with physostigmine.
10. Acute opioid poisoning and overdose can produce life-threatening respiratory depression that can be treated with assisted ventilation and naloxone.
11. Chemicals can be used for mass poisonings by acts of terrorism and warfare and typically produce life-threatening effects within minutes to hours, which warrant emergency preparedness at healthcare facilities and communities.

BEYOND THE BOOK

Watch the video entitled "Toxicology—The National Emergency Medicine Board Review Course" <https://www.youtube.com/watch?v=LIfermvH8YU> up to minute 21:00. Dr. William "Billy" Mallon, an emergency medicine physician, provides an overview of basic toxicology principles covered in this chapter including gastrointestinal decontamination, enhanced elimination, and antidotes. The video is useful to enhance student understanding of foundational concepts of clinical toxicology.

Poisoning is an adverse effect from a chemical that has been taken in excessive amounts. The body can tolerate and, in some cases, detoxify a certain dose of a chemical; however, toxicity ensues once a critical exposure threshold is exceeded. Poisoning can produce minor local effects that may be treated readily in the outpatient setting or systemic life-threatening effects that require intensive medical intervention. Virtually any chemical can become a poison when taken in enough quantity, but the potency of some compounds leads to serious toxicity with small quantities (Table e8-1). Poisoning by chemicals includes exposure to drugs, industrial chemicals, household products, plants, venomous animals, agrochemicals, and weapons for warfare and terrorism. This chapter describes some examples of the spectrum of toxicity, outlines means to recognize poisoning risk, and presents principles of treatment.

EPIDEMIOLOGY

Poisonings account for approximately 69,000 deaths, at least 2.3 million emergency department (ED) visits, and over 1.9 million nonfatal poisoning injuries each year in the United States.[1,2] Approximately 0.2% of poisoning deaths involve children younger than 5 years.[1] Of ED visits for drug-related poisoning, typically 1.1 million visits are made each year (3.5 per 100,000 population) with the highest rate observed for patients 20 to 34 years of age. One-fourth of ED visits for drug-related poisonings were hospitalized, which is twice the rate of other types of visits.[2] The age-adjusted death rates from poisonings from all circumstances have been increasing steadily, with a 297% increase from 2000 to 2016, representing 68,995 deaths representing 21.3 deaths per 100,000 population in 2016 of which 92% were drug-related poisonings. This increasing mortality trend has placed poisoning since 2008 as the leading cause of injury-related death in the United States.[1]

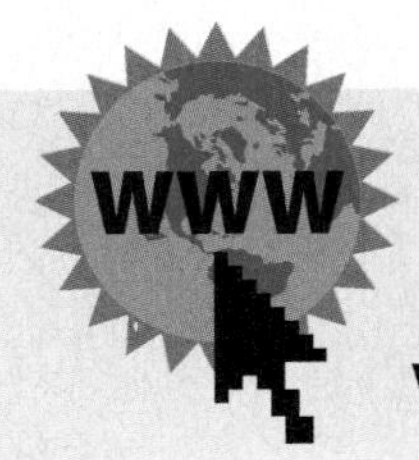

The complete chapter, learning objectives, and other resources can be found at **www.pharmacotherapyonline.com.**

e9 Fever

Jamal Brown and Juan Mosley II

KEY CONCEPTS

1. Fever can be a by-product of various infectious or pathologic processes, vaccinations, medications, and environmental exposure, or of vigorous activity.
2. Normal body temperature fluctuates and is regulated in the thermoregulatory center of the anterior hypothalamus. During a fever, prostaglandins cause an increase in the hypothalamic temperature set point and thereby increase production of heat in the periphery.
3. Healthcare professionals should COLLECT key information on medications, medical history, immunizations, recent travel, social history, barriers of care, and course of fever.
4. Using the gathered data, ASSESS information to differentiate symptoms from surrounding conditions, determine appropriateness for self-care, evaluate history for causes of fever, and consider the most appropriate medication for fever.
5. Goals of therapy include relieving discomfort, reducing body temperature, and when appropriate treating the underlying cause of fever.
6. Nondrug treatments include the use of cooling blankets, which should only be used along with antipyretics. Appropriate hydration and the use of fans also contribute to decreasing body temperature.
7. Nonsteroidal anti-inflammatory drugs (NSAIDs) reduce fever, but they can adversely affect the gastrointestinal tract and platelets. For this reason, acetaminophen is the preferred agent to reduce fever in most patients. Therapy with NSAIDs and acetaminophen combinations can be used in most but not all patients.
8. Medical evaluation should be sought if symptoms of fever do not resolve with over-the-counter treatment within 24 hours in children younger than 2 years, 48 hours in other children and 3 days in adults. Also, a medical evaluation should occur in patients with alarming symptoms regardless of their temperature.

BEYOND THE BOOK

In a small group, create a drug treatment table of OTC products for fever. Consider appropriate age, mechanism of action, dosing schedule, disease interactions, drug interactions, and cost. Compare and contrast these agents based on these factors and create an "optimal" situation to use each medication. Also, create a list of conditions that mimic symptoms of fever. This will assist you during the Assess phase of the Patient Care Process.

INTRODUCTION

Healthcare professionals are often the first point of contact for patients who present with nonspecific symptoms that can be transient and self-limiting or that indicate the presence of serious disease. Collecting the information needed to assess these symptoms and make a recommendation to patients is a common and important activity of health professionals as they provide direct patient care.

1 Elevated body temperature is one of these cardinal manifestations of disease. Fever and elevated temperatures can be associated with many etiologies related to recent travel, illnesses, activity, and environmental factors. Healthcare professionals have an opportunity and responsibility to decipher information to help patients find an appropriate treatment to decrease temperatures and alleviate associated symptoms or to seek more extensive medical evaluations.

A systematic process for assessing elevated temperatures includes asking the patient or caregiver for specific facts about the condition, examining the patient and measuring the body temperature, assessing the collected information, developing and implementing a treatment plan (including referring the patient when red flags to self-treatment are present), and scheduling appropriate follow-up. This chapter reviews the causes of fever in a clinic or pharmacy setting and appropriate evidence-based treatment to alleviate symptoms.

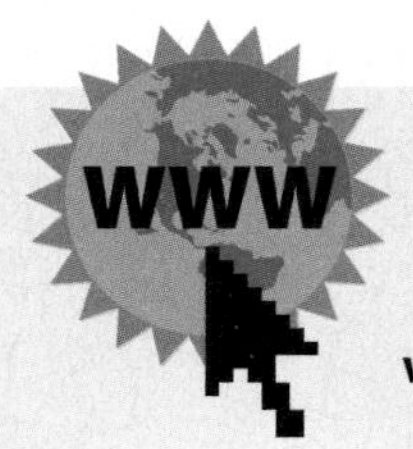

The complete chapter, learning objectives, and other resources can be found at **www.pharmacotherapyonline.com.**

e10

Pain and Headache

Ryan C. Costantino, Krista B. Highland, and Laura C. Tilley

KEY CONCEPTS

1. A comprehensive pain symptom analysis should be performed on each individual reporting pain to determine the type of pain condition.
2. A patient's self-report of pain impact, across a variety of biopsychosocial domains, is important to tailor and monitor treatment.
3. Appropriateness of self-care options to treat pain must be determined after careful review of red flag indicators.
4. The topical route of administration is preferred to oral analgesics whenever feasible.
5. Goals focused on quality of life and function in addition to traditional pain scores are preferred.

BEYOND THE BOOK

Ask a friend or colleague to recall a painful experience from their past. Perform a pain symptom analysis with them using the PQRSTU method described in the chapter. Be sure to analyze each pain report if the pain experience involved multiple sources of pain. The goal of the interview should be to COLLECT information about their painful experience, ASSESS the pain, and classify it appropriately (eg, nociceptive somatic, nociceptive visceral, neuropathic). Ask yourself, could this patient be managed through self-care or is a referral required? This activity is intended to build pain symptom assessment skills and ability to identify pain etiology and pathogenesis.

INTRODUCTION

The International Association for the Study of Pain (IASP) defines pain as: "an unpleasant sensory and emotional experience associated with actual or potential tissue damage or described in terms of such damage."[1] Despite being a top reason patients access the medical system, many patients will attempt to manage their pain with nonprescription medications.[2,3] This gives unique opportunities for health professionals to improve the health, wellness, and medication use among patients experiencing pain.

EPIDEMIOLOGY AND ETIOLOGY

In 2016, approximately one in five people experienced chronic pain, with an estimated 8% of the US population experiencing high-impact chronic pain.[4] While the true incidence and prevalence is difficult to determine, painful disorders have a significant burden on our society. Chronic pain alone is estimated to cost the United States more than US$600 billion each year in medical treatment and lost productivity.[5] Unfortunately, our healthcare system has historically struggled to provide medical professionals with adequate education and training to sufficiently diagnose and treat people with pain.[6,7]

Headache and musculoskeletal disorders are two common etiologies of pain for which there are over-the-counter (OTC) treatment options available for patients. Globally, almost half of people with headache self-treat without a formal diagnosis.[8] This is concerning, as many of the medications commonly used to treat painful conditions carry serious side effects (ie, bleeding with nonsteriodal anti-inflammatory drugs [NSAIDs]). Furthermore, one study demonstrated approximately half of patients may not be aware of the potential side effects of their medication. Many patients are under the impression that OTC medications are safer or carry less risk than their equivalent prescription product.[9]

All healthcare professionals have a role to play in educating and assisting with the care of patients with painful disorders by screening for red flag symptoms (see Table e10-1) and referring patients to a primary care physician or specialist when appropriate. If a patient's presentation is appropriate to self-treat, health professionals can provide guidance on the most appropriate drug based on the patient's symptoms and encourage safe use (eg, dosing, duration of use, and monitoring parameters).

ANATOMY AND MECHANISM OF DISEASE

While pain can create much patient discomfort and disability, it also serves as an essential protective mechanism used to maintain homeostasis in the body. For a detailed review of the pathogenesis of pain, see Chapter 79, Pain Management. For the purposes of self-care, it is helpful to classify pain into subcategories to align treatment modalities.

Pain is often classified as nociceptive, neuropathic, or mixed (see Table e10-2). Nociceptive pain occurs in response to harmful or potentially harmful stimuli when signals are sent to the brain through the process of transduction, conduction, transmission, perception, and modulation. It is typically characterized as either somatic or visceral in nature. Somatic and visceral pain often respond to primary analgesics available OTC (eg, acetaminophen or NSAIDs), whereas neuropathic pain will often require a referral and evaluation for prescription analgesics. However, OTC products containing capsaicin or lidocaine are available and may be beneficial in the initial treatment of patients experiencing neuropathic pain (see Table e10-2).

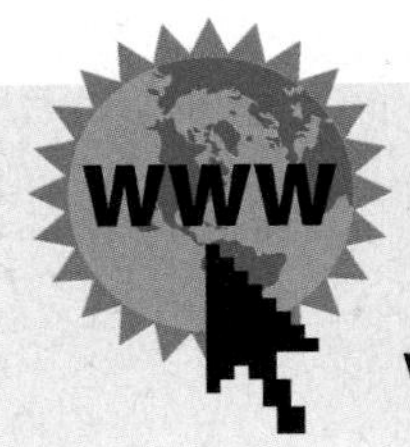

The complete chapter, learning objectives, and other resources can be found at **www.pharmacotherapyonline.com.**

Minor Ophthalmic Disorders

e11

Jared Ostroff

KEY CONCEPTS

1. Pharmacists are often the first healthcare provider that patients will seek with various eye complaints.
2. It is crucial to understand the various products available over-the-counter (OTC) to provide appropriate recommendations.
3. Healthcare professionals should also be familiar with eye conditions that do require referral to a medical provider for further evaluation.

Beyond the Book

Design a list of questions for a patient who is presenting with complaints of dry eyes. Which medications and/or disease states would you screen when reviewing their medication lists? What would be your initial OTC recommendation for symptom relief? This activity will develop your skills with collect, assess, and plan within the Patient Care Process.

INTRODUCTION

1 When it comes to ophthalmic complaints, there are many considerations and other causes to rule out prior to making a pharmacologic recommendation. Patients will sometimes present in the pharmacy or primary care setting with dry eyes, burning eyes, or obstructed vision, or for help selecting appropriate contact lens solutions. While patients may seek a quick cure, the healthcare professional must also realize that a full assessment is encouraged for each patient complaining of symptoms to determine if it is appropriate to use nonpharmacologic or pharmacologic treatments that are available without a prescription or refer to another provider.

This chapter reviews common eye complaints and how to make evidence-based recommendations on management.

DRY EYES

Collect. Dry eye disease, or keratoconjunctivitis sicca, is one of the most common complaints when patients visit the eye doctor, and its prevalence is estimated between 7% and 33%.[1] Risk factors for the development of dry eyes include increasing age and female sex.[2] While onset of dry eyes is often unpredictable, it may correlate with exposure to various changes in environment and current medications.

Patients with dry eyes may present with or without redness of the eyes with various complaints that will need a review of their current medical history and other predisposing factors. Factors such as weather, current medications, recent exposure, and previous experience with the condition are essential in triage and making recommendations for therapy.

Assess. The first step in evaluating a patient with dry eyes is to evaluate the complaints and medical history including any current medications or environmental triggers. Patients may not always recognize that environmental factors could play a role so it is essential to ask for that information. Since dry eyes may be caused by a variety of medications, perform a medication reconciliation with the patient's current medication list. Some of the medications to check for include antihistamines, decongestants, antidepressants, and hormone replacement therapy.[3] While this is not the only mechanism that can cause dry eyes, medications are frequently implicated. If offending medications are identified during reconciliation, advise the patient to stop using if appropriate and recommend an alternative product that would minimize the potential for dry eyes to return.

Plan. Once a thorough medication reconciliation is complete, rule out for any red flags such as complaints of any discharge, blurry vision, or difficulty with vision. Patients with those symptoms should be referred to a medical provider for further evaluation.

Implement. If there are no red flags or urgent symptoms needing further evaluation, the choice of best initial option should be discussed with the patient. A number of factors contribute to selection of an initial treatment option. These may include cost, dosage form (suspension vs solution), administration times, previous experience with a product, and any potential drug or nondrug allergies.

2 When considering OTC treatment for dry eyes, the first-line recommendation is artificial tears, which may include cellulose, polyethylene glycol, and a preservative. Each of these ingredients have a specific role in dry eye treatment and many come in a variety of forms such as liquid, gel, and ointment. Preservative-free forms are also available; these are preferred in patients who wear contact lenses.

Artificial tears are evidence based and have been proven to improve patient symptoms.[4] These products include cellulose ethers, such as hydroxyethylcellulose, carboxymethylcellulose, and hydroxypropyl methylcellulose. Other ingredients used in dry eyes include white petrolatum to assist with lubrication of the eye. There are several randomized trials showing efficacy with artificial tears; anecdotal reports also show that they are effective in keeping the eyes lubricated.[5] A starting dose for artificial tear administration is one drop in each eye, three to four times a day. Many patients experience improvement within 1 to 2 days after administration; however, it may take a week or longer in some cases. Depending on the dosage form, patients may want to consider administration in the evening. Dosage forms such as ointments or gels have specific application instructions and may cause a temporary visual disturbance while the medication is being absorbed.

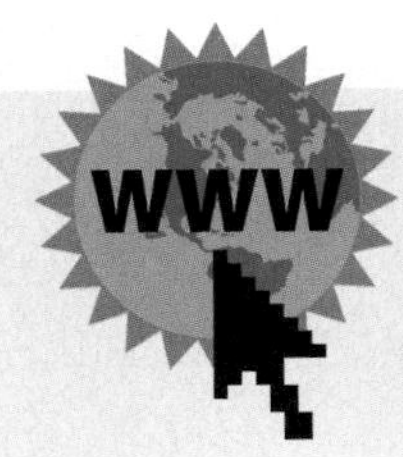

The complete chapter, learning objectives, and other resources can be found at **www.pharmacotherapyonline.com.**

Minor Otic Disorders (Cerumen Impaction, Otitis External)

e12

Lea S. Eiland

KEY CONCEPTS

1. The most common pathogens in acute otitis externa (AOE) are *Pseudomonas aeruginosa* and *Staphylococcus aureus*.
2. Topical antimicrobials are the medication and route of choice for the treatment of AOE.
3. Systemic antimicrobials are not warranted for the initial treatment of diffuse, uncomplicated AOE.
4. Pain should be assessed in all patients and therapy recommended based upon severity.
5. Appropriate counseling points for otic administration of medication should be provided to each patient.
6. Cerumen production is a naturally occurring process of the body.
7. Cerumen impaction may cause discomfort, itching, hearing loss, or tinnitus.
8. Cotton swabs should not be used as they can worsen cerumen impaction or cause trauma to the tympanic membrane.
9. Home-treatment options for cerumen impaction include cerumenolytic agents and/or irrigation.
10. Foreign objects such as pen caps, tweezers, or paper clips should not be inserted in the ear canal.

BEYOND THE BOOK

1. Otic administration of medications: Working individually or in teams, develop a handout or short video for patients and caregivers to teach them how to administer medication into the ear of a child or an adult. Be creative in the education models used for patient education!
2. Cerumenolytics: Which one to recommend first? Working individually or in teams, research the various cerumenolytic agents available for patient use and develop a selection algorithm. The algorithm should clearly state which product (with the respective dosing regimen) would be the first to recommend to a patient, then second, and so forth.

ACUTE OTITIS EXTERNA—INTRODUCTION

Acute otitis externa (AOE) is a diffuse inflammation of the external ear canal secondary to infection.[1] The tympanic membrane or pinna may also be involved in this infectious process. AOE may occur at any age but is uncommon in children younger than 2 years.

The hallmark sign of diffuse AOE is intense tenderness of the pinna when pulled, tragus when pushed, or both, which can be inconsistent with signs observed visually, such as redness or areas of cellulitis. Diagnosis of AOE requires a rapid onset (<48 hours) of signs and symptoms of ear canal inflammation within the past 3 weeks.[1] The signs of inflammation include tenderness of the pinna, tragus, or both or diffuse canal edema, erythema, or both. Signs may also include otorrhea, regional lymphadenitis, erythema of the tympanic membrane, or cellulitis of the pinna and adjacent skin.

Symptoms of inflammation include otalgia (70%), itching (60%), or fullness (22%), with or without jaw pain or hearing loss (32%).[1] Pain best correlates with the severity of the disease.[2]

This chapter focuses on AOE, but patients sometimes present with other types of otitis externa. Chronic otitis externa is defined as otitis externa occurring for 3 months or longer. Necrotizing or malignant otitis externa is defined as the AOE infection extending to the temporal bone causing osteomyelitis. This primarily occurs in patients who are older, have diabetes mellitus, or are immunocompromised.

Epidemiology and Etiology

Patients with AOE commonly seek treatment from healthcare providers in the outpatient setting. In 2007, 2.4 million patients received a diagnosis of AOE in the ambulatory care or emergency department setting (8.1 visits per 1,000 population).[3] In ambulatory care visits in the years 2003 to 2007 for AOE, 18.6% were for children 5 to 9 years of age, 15.8% were for children 10 to 14 years of age, and 53% were for adults 20 years of age or older. One study found a peak incidence of AOE in patients 7 to 12 years of age.[4] Ambulatory care clinicians spend approximately 600,000 hours treating patients with AOE, and annual direct healthcare costs for the nonhospitalized setting in the United States are up to $500 million.[1]

(1) AOE is predominantly of bacterial origin (98%) in North America.[1] The primary organisms are *Pseudomonas aeruginosa* and *Staphylococcus aureus,* with a prevalence of 20% to 60% and 10% to 70%, respectively. A polymicrobial infection occurs in approximately one-third of AOE cases. A study of 173 patients with AOE in the United States from 2014 to 2016 found the most common pathogens were *P. aeruginosa* (42%), methicillin-sensitive *S. aureus* (22%), and methicillin-resistant *S. aureus* (MRSA) (8.7%).[5] This is the first study to have found higher rates of MRSA in AOE than previously reported. Other AOE pathogens found in this study were *Enterococcus faecalis* (5.2%), *Escherichia coli* (2.3%), *Stenotrophomonas maltophilia* (2.3%), *Streptococcus pneumoniae* (2.3%), coagulase-negative *Staphylococcus* species (2.3%), and *Staphylococcus epidermidis* (2.3%).[5]

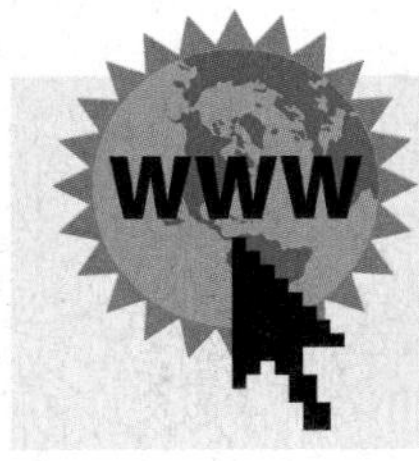

The complete chapter, learning objectives, and other resources can be found at **www.pharmacotherapyonline.com.**

Nonspecific Respiratory Tract Symptoms (with Cough)

e13

Brandon Sucher

KEY CONCEPTS

1. Cough is classified as acute, subacute, or chronic based on duration of symptoms.
2. Cough is an essential component for lung health maintenance, but persistent or excessive cough ceases to be protective, is bothersome, and adversely affects quality of life.
3. Although cough is associated with a variety of diseases, the duration of cough helps narrow the potential etiologies for cough symptoms.
4. The presence of dyspnea, red flag symptoms, and/or symptoms suggestive of acute bacterial rhinosinusitis indicates the need for referral to the patient's primary care physician.
5. Treatment trials (eg, intranasal corticosteroids, first-generation antihistamines, treatments for gastroesophageal reflux disease) can help rule out common causes of chronic cough.

BEYOND THE BOOK

Create a flow chart that outlines the sequence of therapeutic approaches for the four most common causes of chronic cough. Indicate the name of the medication class that may be used for a therapeutic trial when available as an over-the-counter medication. When a therapeutic trial of an over-the-counter medication is not appropriate, indicate referral to the patient's primary care physician for each of the respective causes of chronic cough.

This activity provides an opportunity for students to practice applying the assess, plan, and implement steps of the patient care process.

INTRODUCTION

1 2 Cough is the second most common symptom patients report as the reason for seeking healthcare in ambulatory settings.[1] In addition to occurring as a common symptom associated with respiratory diseases, cough serves as a protective respiratory reflex and also can be initiated voluntarily.[2] Cough is classified as acute, subacute, or chronic based on duration of symptoms (Table e13-1).[3] As a defense mechanism, cough protects the airways from aspiration of foreign substances, expels infectious organisms and harmful environmental insults, and clears excessive mucus secretions.[2,4] However, when cough is excessive or persists, it can be detrimental to patients through adverse consequences such as syncope, urinary incontinence, vomiting, chest pain, rib fractures, sleep disturbances, relationship difficulties, social embarrassment, and depression.[5,6] An increased frequency of cough also adversely affects health-related quality of life.[5]

EPIDEMIOLOGY AND ETIOLOGY

The estimated prevalence of chronic cough varies and depends on the epidemiological study design, duration of symptoms used to define chronic cough, and how the data is obtained (eg, diagnosis codes, patient report, physician diagnosis).[7,8] The global prevalence of chronic cough is approximately 10% and the prevalence of chronic cough in the United States ranges between 10% and 15%.[8] Chronic cough is more common in women and more commonly occurs in patients aged 50 to 70 years old.[7,9] Chronic cough is more common in patients who continue to smoke, which may reflect a protective response to inhaled irritants rather than hypersensitive cough.[10] Results from the ACHOO study revealed the burden associated with acute cough and/or cold symptoms. Fifty-two percent of the survey respondents indicated that their daily lives were affected "a fair amount" or "a lot" when they had a cough and/or cold. Participants also reported a decrease of 26% in their perceived productivity when they were experiencing cough and/or cold symptoms, and 45% of respondents reported missing at least 1 day of work or school.[5]

The etiology of cough may occur anywhere within the realm of the vagus nerve, which is the longest nerve of the autonomic nervous system. Therefore, cough may arise from a variety of systems (eg, respiratory, cardiovascular, gastrointestinal).[4] Viral upper respiratory tract infections are the most common cause of acute cough, followed by exacerbations of underlying diseases (eg, asthma, chronic obstructive pulmonary disease [COPD], upper airway cough syndrome [UACS], bronchiectasis) and pneumonia.[2,3] The most common cause of subacute cough is postinfectious cough followed by exacerbations of underlying diseases.[2,4,8] Asthma (including cough-variant asthma), UACS, nonasthmatic eosinophilic bronchitis (NAEB), and GERD are the most common causes of chronic cough in adult nonsmokers with UACS being the most common cause of chronic cough in the United States.[3,11] Additional causes of chronic cough are included in Table e13-2.[3,12]

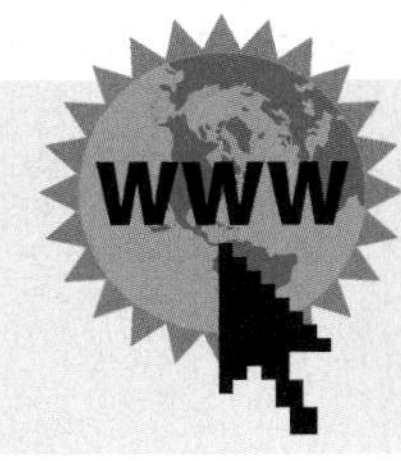

The complete chapter, learning objectives, and other resources can be found at **www.pharmacotherapyonline.com.**

Allergic Rhinitis

J. Russell May

e14

KEY CONCEPTS

1. Allergic rhinitis is a common disease. Prevention measures and treatment are justified in most cases because of the potential for complications.
2. Because an immune response to allergens results in release of inflammatory mediators that cause allergic rhinitis symptoms, patients must understand the rationale for proper timing and administration of prophylactic regimens.
3. Avoidance of allergens is difficult and it may be impractical to expect full success.
4. Antihistamines offer an effective option for treating both seasonal and persistent allergic rhinitis.
5. Intranasal steroids are highly effective in patients who use them properly.
6. While immunotherapy is the only disease-modifying treatment of allergic rhinitis, expense, potential risks, and the major time commitment required make patient selection critical.

BEYOND THE BOOK

Review the patient monitoring recommendations for the most common allergic rhinitis pharmacotherapy options (antihistamines, intranasal steroids, topical and systemic decongestants, mast cell stabilizers, and leukotriene receptor antagonists) in a standard drug information compendium (eg, Facts & Comparisons). This activity is useful to enhance student understanding of the PLAN step in the patient care process.

INTRODUCTION

Allergic rhinitis involves inflammation of the nasal mucous membrane. In a sensitized individual, allergic rhinitis occurs when inhaled allergenic particles contact mucous membranes and elicit a specific response mediated by immunoglobulin E (IgE). This acute response involves the release of inflammatory mediators and is characterized by sneezing, nasal itching, and watery rhinorrhea, often associated with nasal congestion. Itching of the throat, eyes, and ears frequently accompanies allergic rhinitis.

Allergic rhinitis may be regarded as seasonal allergic rhinitis, commonly known as *hay fever*, or persistent allergic rhinitis (formerly known as perennial rhinitis). Seasonal rhinitis occurs in response to specific allergens usually present at predictable times of the year, during plants' pollination (typically the spring or fall). Seasonal allergens include pollen from trees, grasses, and weeds. Persistent allergic rhinitis is a year-round disease caused by nonseasonal allergens, such as house dust mites, animal dander, and molds, or multiple allergic sensitivities. It typically results in less variable, chronic symptoms. Many patients have a combination of these two types of allergic rhinitis, with symptoms year-round and seasonal exacerbations.

EPIDEMIOLOGY AND ETIOLOGY

1 Allergic rhinitis is one of the most common diseases affecting adults and is the most common chronic disease in children in the United States, generating \$2 to \$5 billion in direct healthcare cost each year.[1] Prevalence rates are 14% in adults and 13% in children when using a physician-confirmed diagnosis.[2] Actual sensitization to inhaled allergens is likely higher and is increasing with estimates of 15% to 30% in the United States.[3] Patients may be limited in their ability to carry out normal daily functions; higher levels of general fatigue, mental fatigue, anxiety, depressive disorders, and learning disabilities (secondary to sleep loss and fatigue) are possible.

In addition, the impact of allergic rhinitis goes well beyond these CNS issues. Allergic rhinitis is associated with several other serious medical conditions, including asthma, chronic rhinosinusitis, otitis media, nasal polyposis, respiratory infections, and orthodontic malocclusions.

The development of allergic rhinitis is determined by genetics, allergen exposure, and the presence of other risk factors. A family history of allergic rhinitis, atopic dermatitis, or asthma suggests that rhinitis is allergic. The risk of developing allergic disease appears to increase if one parent is atopic and further increases if two are allergic; however, small sample sizes and the lack of reproducibility prevent generalization.[4]

Allergen exposure is another necessary factor. For allergic rhinitis to occur, an individual must be exposed over time to a protein that elicits the allergic response in that individual. Many potential sufferers never develop symptoms because they do not come into contact with the allergen that would produce symptoms in them.

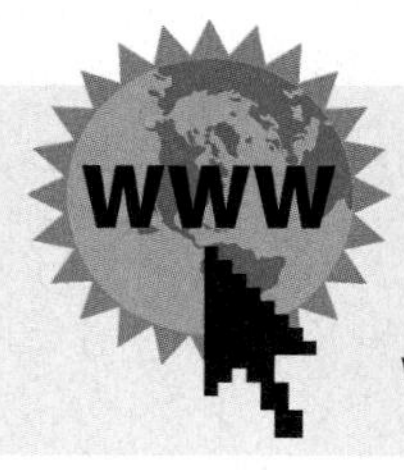

The complete chapter, learning objectives, and other resources can be found at **www.pharmacotherapyonline.com.**

Oral Health and Systemic Conditions

e15

Lisa M. Palmisano and Jennifer L. Mazan

KEY CONCEPTS

1. Oral health is a growing global concern because of its effect on quality of life, morbidity, and mortality.
2. Dental caries in children can significantly impair their overall health status.
3. Periodontal disease in older populations may contribute to progression of noncommunicable diseases (ie, diabetes).
4. Poor oral health conditions are associated with increased mortality risk.
5. Medications taken for various conditions may contribute to significant oral adverse effects that result in worsening oral health outcomes.
6. Diabetes and periodontal disease have a bidirectional relationship on glycemic control and periodontal disease progression.
7. Medications used for various cardiovascular disease conditions have significant oral adverse effects that result in reduced oral health outcomes and patient quality of life.
8. Patients with respiratory conditions and who require inhaler medications are at an increased risk of dental caries, periodontal disease, dental erosion, and oral candidiasis.
9. Poor oral health in patients with psychiatric disorders may result from various contributing factors such as medication-related side effects, existing comorbidities, and barriers to accessing dental care.
10. Tobacco and substance use disorders are significant contributors to poor oral health consequences, particularly in those with other psychiatric conditions.
11. Oral health disparities are noted across patients' lifespans as a result of access to dental coverage, income, education, and race/ethnicity.
12. National and local initiatives have been created to increase awareness, education, and access for oral healthcare for all Americans.
13. Nondental healthcare professionals, including pharmacists, can play an integral role in educating patients on oral health as it pertains to oral health diseases, systemic diseases, and medication-related adverse effects.

BEYOND THE BOOK

Test your baseline knowledge on various oral health topics using the online short quizzes below:

General website (http://www.mouthhealthy.org/en/az-topics/quiz-time)

Specific short oral health quizzes:

1. What causes dry mouth?
2. Is all tobacco bad?
3. Kids' dental health
4. Teen dental health
5. Adults under 40 dental health
6. Adults 40 to 60 dental health
7. Adults over 60 dental health

INTRODUCTION

1 Oral health encompasses the oral tissues, dentition, mastication ability, and tongue movement in the absence of chronic oral-facial pain, cancers, oral lesions, or other oral conditions or diseases that affect the oral, dental, or craniofacial tissues.[1] Poor oral health can result in physical oral dysfunction, malnutrition, sociopsychological impairment, cognitive decline, and a reduced overall quality of life.[2,3] The global concern of oral health is a result of the disparities in accessing providers as well as the growing evidence that it is a modifiable risk factor for chronic systemic conditions and oral disease.[1-4] The manifestation of oral symptoms such as xerostomia, candida infections, and ulcerations are examples of potential indicators of chronic conditions such as diabetes, cardiovascular disease (CVD), autoimmune disease, and others.[3,5] Furthermore, medical condition(s) and medication treatment can negatively affect a person's oral health. The World Health Organization, US Surgeon General, and other healthcare organizations have emphasized the call to action for improvement of oral healthcare.[1,6-8]

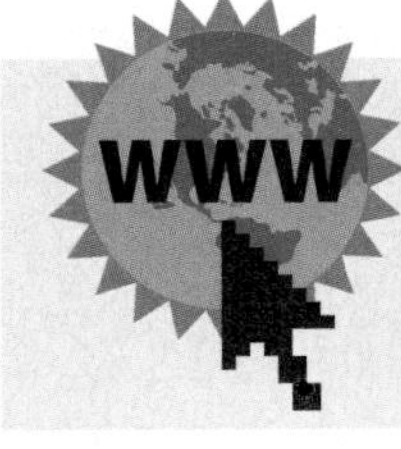

The complete chapter, learning objectives, and other resources can be found at **www.pharmacotherapyonline.com.**

Oral Hygiene and Minor Oral Disorders

e16

Anna S. Milone, Kristyn M. Williamson, and Maren Hall

KEY CONCEPTS

1. Dental caries is one of the most common chronic health conditions in both children and adults. Dental caries stems from an imbalance in saliva defense, microbial load, and lifestyle habits. Modifiable risk factors include oral hygiene practices and lifestyle factors. Dental caries can lead to tooth sensitivity, cause oral pain, and have implications for overall health.
2. For oral health maintenance, teeth should be brushed twice daily with fluoride toothpaste. Patients should floss daily and follow recommended technique for brushing and flossing. Oral health maintenance also includes the use of athletic mouthguards, denture care, and regular dental care by an oral healthcare professional.
3. Toothpaste contains fluoride as its primary active ingredient to prevent tooth decay and gum disease. Other active ingredients, such as potassium salts, may be added for tooth sensitivity, as well as abrasives and carbamide peroxide for tooth whitening.
4. The first-line treatment for dental pain is nonsteroidal anti-inflammatory drugs (NSAIDs), with or without acetaminophen.
5. Benzocaine is available over-the-counter (OTC) in numerous products for adults, children, and infants as a local anesthetic for oral pain. While widely available, benzocaine has significant safety concerns and should not be used for teething pain in children younger than 2 years of age.
6. Canker sores are one of the most common ulcerative conditions of the mouth. Treatment options include pain management with topical agents and eliminating irritating food and drink from the diet.
7. Cold sores are recurrent oral lesions resulting from infection with herpes simplex virus type 1. Referral of patients to their primary care physician is likely warranted, as the most effective treatment options are available as prescription only products.
8. Xerostomia or dry mouth is a common oral condition often caused by medical conditions, medications, or medical treatments. Treatment of xerostomia greatly depends on the cause of the condition, but can be treated symptomatically with a number of OTC products.
9. Dentistry has few true emergencies; however, dental trauma where a permanent tooth is displaced or avulsed constitute a dental emergency, and immediate referral to an oral healthcare provider or urgent care center is warranted.
10. Fluoride is effective in preventing dental caries by inhibiting the demineralization of tooth enamel, enhancing the remineralization of enamel, and inhibiting bacterial enzymes involved in the metabolism of carbohydrates by cariogenic bacteria. Sources of fluoride include toothpaste, fluoridated drinking water, professionally applied topical fluorides, and oral fluoride supplementation.

BEYOND THE BOOK

Explore the oral health section of either the Centers for Disease Control and Prevention (CDC) website: https://www.cdc.gov/OralHealth/index.html), or the oral health portion of http://healthychildren.org by the American Academy of Pediatrics (AAP): https://www.healthychildren.org/English/healthy-living/oral-health/Pages/default.aspx). You can explore overview topics, Question and Answer sections, or topics that stimulate your interest. Find at least one topic that relates directly to community pharmacy practice or the primary care setting, such as the use of OTCs or educating patients. What areas of oral health do you feel knowledgeable in, and in what areas do you have gaps in knowledge? You may wish to reflect on any patient questions you have received on oral health topics. You may also wish to explore (either online or in person) the oral health section of a pharmacy. How large are these sections, and what products are available?

INTRODUCTION

Dentists and other members of the dental community are actively encouraging the involvement of additional health professionals in identification, referral, and in some cases treatment of patients with oral health conditions. Pharmacists, particularly community and health-system pharmacists, are the most accessible health professionals for patients presenting with oral health issues or questions. Furthermore, community pharmacies carry many products for oral health ranging from toothbrushes and mouthguards to rinses and pain relievers.

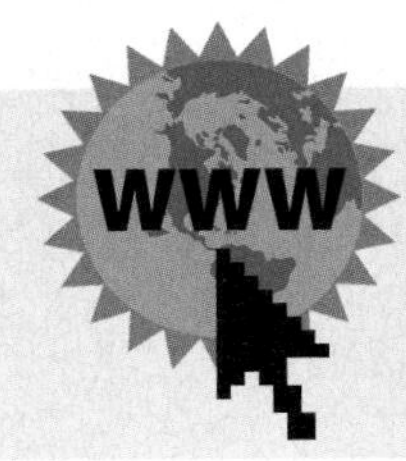

The complete chapter, learning objectives, and other resources can be found at **www.pharmacotherapyonline.com.**

Skin Care and Minor Dermatologic Conditions

e17

Rebecca M. Law and Howard I. Maibach

KEY CONCEPTS

1. The skin is the largest organ of the human body. It performs vital functions such as (a) protecting the body against injury, physical agents, and ultraviolet radiation; (b) regulating body temperature; (c) preventing dehydration, thus helping to maintain fluid balance; (d) acting as a sense organ; and (e) acting as an outpost for immune surveillance. Skin also has a role in vitamin D production and absorption.
2. Age-related factors affect the epidermis, dermis, and subcutis. Pediatric skin is thinner, which enhances topical drug absorption and potential drug toxicities. Neonates, particularly premature neonates, are especially susceptible due to an incomplete skin barrier. Skin of older adults is drier, thinner, and more friable, which may predispose them to external insults and loss of the skin barrier function.
3. Examination of a patient's skin involves assessing skin color (degree of pigmentation, pallor, carotenemia, jaundice), skin temperature (warm, cool, clammy), skin surface characteristics (dryness, seborrhea, turgor, excessive or reduced sweating, texture), and the degree of photoaging.
4. Signs that a mole (nevus) may be dysplastic include: size >5 mm, irregular shape, variable/different pigmentation, indistinct borders; and they may be totally flat or flat with a central elevation.
5. Skin hydration is especially important for people with dry skin conditions. This involves an appropriate daily skin care routine and adequate daily fluid intake.
6. Management of diaper dermatitis includes frequent diaper changes, air drying (removing the diaper for as long as practical), gentle cleansing (preferably with nonsoap cleansers and lukewarm water), and the use of barriers such as zinc oxide 40% ointment. After healing, a barrier such as zinc oxide 10% should be used with each diaper change as prophylaxis.
7. Due to the many negative effects and skin disorders relating to sun damage, sun protection at all times is critical, and this should be emphasized to patients, whether they are on medications with photosensitivity potential or not. Sun protection includes sunscreens, sun avoidance, shading, long sleeve clothing, and wide brim hats or hats with a flap that covers the ears and neck. Sunscreens should always be used except in infants <6 months of age.

BEYOND THE BOOK

Review the anatomy and physiology of the skin as described in this chapter of *Pharmacotherapy*. Audiovisual presentations of this material are available online, including a video on the components of the skin (https://medlineplus.gov/ency/anatomyvideos/000029.htm) from the National Library of Medicine.

INTRODUCTION

The novelist Deen Ferrell has equated skin to life: "Life is too much like skin. It molds to the core of who you are and whether you dress it up, or try to keep busy so you don't have to think about it, it doesn't go away."[1] Too often, we neglect to think about our skin or pay attention to changes on our skin that don't go away. We allow our skin to get so dry it itches, cracks, and hurts. We ignore bumps and lesions on our skin because they are often painless and always present, so we do not notice when slow or subtle changes occur, which may be innocuous—or life threatening. It is easy to grow accustomed to something that is always there. We need to pay attention and teach our patients to pay attention.

1 Although not commonly thought of as such, skin is a vital organ with important functions. In fact, skin is the human body's largest organ, with an average surface area of about 1.8 m^2.[2] The organ system that includes the skin is known as *the integumentary system*.

The human skin consists of an outer epidermis and an inner dermis, with subcutaneous fat. The epidermis (in four layers) primarily provides protection from the environment and performs a critical barrier function—keeping in water and other vital substances and keeping out foreign elements. The dermis is a connective tissue layer that primarily provides resiliency and support for various skin structures and appendages such as sweat glands, sebaceous glands, hair, and nails. It also provides support for nerves and blood vessels. The subcutis (subcutaneous tissue) is a fatty layer below the dermis that helps to maintain the body temperature stable and protect bones and muscles from damage. It also allows nerves and blood vessels from the dermis to pass through and reach the muscles (Fig. e17-1). See the "Structure and Functions of the Skin" section for further discussion.

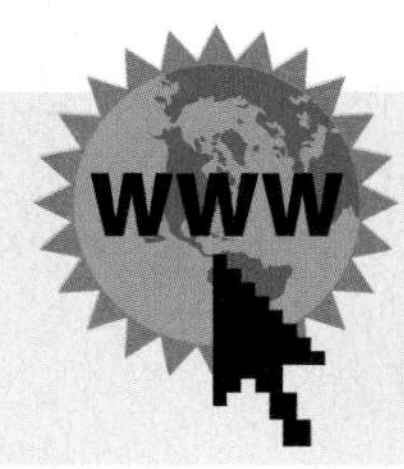

The complete chapter, learning objectives, and other resources can be found at **www.pharmacotherapyonline.com.**

e18

Travel Health

Douglas Slain and Scott E. Kincaid

KEY CONCEPTS

1. Travelers should consult practitioners with travel health expertise when going to tropical or developing countries.
2. For the pretravel consultation recommendations, travelers should be given written material in their language to reinforce and supplement verbal instructions.
3. The pretravel screening appointment should include a discussion of items that should be contained in a travel medical kit.
4. Pregnant travelers should consult obstetric and travel medicine experts prior to traveling to developing countries.
5. Immunocompromised patients may need longer periods of pretravel preparatory time to allow for adequate immunization, given their sometimes blunted antibody responses to vaccines.
6. Travelers to sub-Saharan Africa, Southern Asia, Central and South America, and the Caribbean experience higher rates of infection than those traveling to other parts of the world.
7. Prophylactic antibiotic use may reduce the risk of traveler's diarrhea but is generally not recommended, primarily because of the risk of developing drug resistance or *Clostridioides difficile* infection.
8. Prevention strategies are essential for limiting vector-borne infections during travel.
9. The mainstay of therapy in all altitude-related illnesses is descent to a lower altitude (typically at least a 300-m reduction in altitude).
10. Patients who have previously been diagnosed with depression should continue their prescribed medications and minimize alcohol consumption while traveling.

BEYOND THE BOOK

Design a medication kit for a family of four (two adults and two preteen children) taking a 10-day trip to Aruba.

INTRODUCTION

Global (international) travel has increased dramatically over the past 20 years. A sizable proportion of this increased travel can be explained by individuals traveling from developed countries to developing countries.[1] Reasons for travel to developing countries are variable, but include work-related travel, leisure travel, medical tourism, visiting family, adventure travel, medical mission or outreach, and study abroad programs.

Travel to distant lands has always been associated with risks to mental and physical health. Long-standing estimates of travelers experiencing health problems have been between 22% and 64%, and more recent data tell us that travelers visiting developing and/or tropical nations may experience illness 43% to 79% of the time.[2] Many health problems arising during travel are self-limiting or not bothersome enough for travelers to seek medical care. However, approximately 8% of travelers seek help from physicians either during or soon after traveling.[3] In addition to infectious and noninfectious health problems, global travelers face potential dangers from vehicle and pedestrian traffic accidents, drowning, animal attacks, and assaults. This chapter focuses on health risks and diseases that affect global travelers, with primary emphasis on travel from developed countries to developing or tropical countries. Some travel-related information is included in other chapters, and readers will be referred accordingly.

PRETRAVEL PREPARATION

1 Travelers should review information about their destinations and itinerary and consider potential self-care options for health issues that may arise during travel. Pretravel preparation often involves the assistance of healthcare providers, which is typically more important for patients with chronic health conditions and those traveling internationally, especially to the developing world. About 35% to 50% of travelers from North America and Europe heading to developing countries seek pretravel health advice.[4] Of whom, only about 10% to 20% of travelers consult travel medicine experts or travel clinics. Informed primary care providers without extensive travel health expertise can provide adequate advice to travelers en route to low-risk destinations, but travelers should consult practitioners with travel health expertise when going to tropical or developing countries.[4]

Travel clinics and travel health experts are often underutilized.[4] Two groups of travelers that are less likely to seek expert pretravel health advise are business travelers and immigrants living in developed countries, going back to their home countries to visit friends and relatives (VFR).[5,6] VFR individuals often believe that they are immune to local diseases and do not feel the need to seek advice.[6]

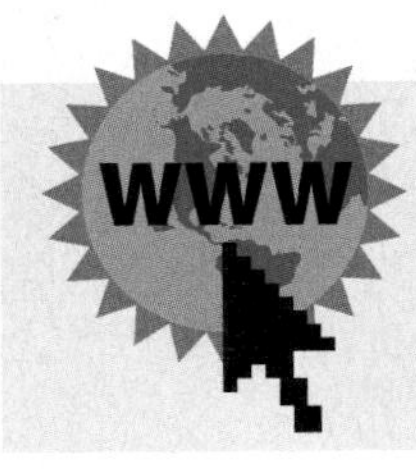

The complete chapter, learning objectives, and other resources can be found at **www.pharmacotherapyonline.com.**

Contraception

19

Shareen Y. El-Ibiary

KEY CONCEPTS

1. Unintended pregnancy is a public health issue. A majority of unintended pregnancies occur due to inconsistent use or nonuse of contraceptives.
2. Contraception implies the prevention of pregnancy; however, some hormonal contraceptives may also provide noncontraceptive benefits.
3. When selecting a contraceptive method consider the following: the effectiveness of the method, its noncontraceptive benefits and adverse medication effects, attitude of the patient and sexual partner toward a contraceptive method, the ability to use it correctly (which may alter its effectiveness), and the ability to pay for the method.
4. Patient-specific factors (eg, frequency of intercourse, age, smoking status, desire for return to fertility, concomitant diseases, medications, contraceptive method preference, and medication interactions) must be evaluated when selecting a contraceptive method.
5. A variety of contraceptive methods are available. Nonhormonal methods include fertility awareness, barriers, spermicides, and the copper intrauterine device. Hormonal methods include progestin-only or combination of estrogen/progestin products.
6. Adverse effects or difficulties in using the selected method should be monitored carefully and managed in regard to patient-specific factors.
7. Some medications may alter the effects of hormonal contraceptives or vice versa; therefore, concomitant medications should be assessed for medication interactions with hormonal contraceptives.
8. Accurate and timely counseling on the management of missed doses is critical for contraceptive effectiveness.
9. Counseling on the optimal use of the contraceptive method and providing strategies for minimizing sexually transmitted infections/diseases (STIs/STDs) must be provided to all patients being initiated on contraceptives and also for those using contraception on an ongoing basis.
10. Emergency contraception (EC) may prevent pregnancy after unprotected intercourse or when regular contraceptive methods have failed.
11. Mifepristone and misoprostol may be used in regimens for medical abortion.

BEYOND THE BOOK

Watch the video entitled "The Menstrual Cycle" (https://www.youtube.com/watch?v=tOluxtc3Cpw) on YouTube from Osmosis. This is a 11-minute video that gives an overview of the menstrual cycle and discusses the cycle phases, ovulation, and the hormones involved. This video is helpful in serving as a quick refresher of the menstrual cycle physiology. Clear understanding of the menstrual cycle is important to understand the mechanisms of action for contraceptive products.

INTRODUCTION

1 Unintended pregnancy is a significant public health issue. In the United States, approximately 6 million individuals become pregnant each year.[1] About 45% of pregnancies are unintended, with the highest rates occurring in individuals aged 20 to 24 years, and in individuals aged 15 to 19 when taking into account only sexually active persons.[2] About half of all unintended pregnancies end in abortion, and 41% occur in sexually active couples who claim they used some method of contraception.[2] Education on the use and effectiveness of contraceptive methods must be improved and provided, if the goal of contraception, for all pregnancies to be planned and desired, is to be realized. While cis-women are the primary users of hormonal contraception, these preparations may also be used by transgender individuals, and thus, this chapter is written with this is mind.

EPIDEMIOLOGY

2 3 Contraception implies the prevention of pregnancy by two methods: first by inhibiting viable sperm from coming into contact with a mature ovum (ie, methods that act as barriers or prevent ovulation) and second, by preventing a fertilized ovum from successfully implanting in the endometrium (ie, mechanisms that create an unfavorable uterine environment). These methods differ in their relative effectiveness, safety, and patient acceptability (Tables 19-1 and 19-2).[3,4]

The actual effectiveness of any contraceptive method is difficult to determine because many factors affect failure (eg, patient had an unintended pregnancy). Failure rates are described as perfect-use failure or typical-use failure. A failure in a patient who used the contraceptive agent properly is considered a method failure or perfect-use failure. User failure or typical-use failure rates take into account the perfect-use failure rate plus the user's ability to follow directions correctly and consistently and is usually higher.[3,4] Because the typical-use rate includes both the method and user failure rates, it is used most often.

TABLE 19-1 Pregnancy and Continuation Rates for Various Pharmacologic Contraceptive Methods

Method	Pregnancy Typical Use	Pregnancy Ideal Use	Continuation After 1 Year
Combined and progestin-oral contraceptive	7%	<1%	67%
• Drospirenone-only contraceptive	4%	–	–
Combined hormonal transdermal contraceptive patch			
• Norelgestromin/Ethinyl estradiol	7%	<1%	–
• Levonorgestrel/Ethinyl estradiol	3%	–	–
Combined hormonal vaginal contraceptive ring			
• Etonogestrel/Ethinyl estradiol	7%	<1%	–
• Segesterone/Ethinyl estradiol	3%	–	–
Depo-medroxyprogesterone acetate	4%	<1%	56%
Copper IUD	<1%	<1%	78%
Levonorgestrel IUD	<1%	<1%	80%
Progestin-only implant	<1%	<1%	89%

Data from References 3 and 5-7.

ETIOLOGY AND PATHOPHYSIOLOGY

Comprehension of the normal menstrual cycle hormonal regulation is essential to understanding contraception (Fig. 19-1). The menstruation cycle begins with menarche, usually around age 12 years, and continues to occur in nonpregnant individuals until menopause, usually around age 50 years. Factors such as race, body weight, medical conditions, and family history can affect the menstrual cycle.[3,4] The cycle concludes in the vaginal discharge of sloughed endometrium called *menses* and is comprised of three phases: (1) follicular (or preovulatory), (2) ovulatory, and (3) luteal (or postovulatory).

The Menstrual Cycle

The first day of menses is referred to as *day 1 of the menstrual cycle* and marks the beginning of the follicular phase[3] which continues until ovulation, which typically occurs on day 14. The time after ovulation is referred to as the *luteal phase,* which lasts until the beginning of the next menstrual cycle. The median menstrual cycle length is 28 days, but can range from 21 to 40 days. Generally, cycle length variation is greatest in the follicular phase, particularly in the years immediately after menarche and before menopause.[3]

The menstrual cycle is influenced by the hormonal relationships among the hypothalamus, anterior pituitary, and ovaries.[3] The hypothalamus secretes gonadotropin-releasing hormone (GnRH) in a pulsatile fashion[3] which stimulates the anterior pituitary to secrete bursts of gonadotropins, follicle-stimulating hormone (FSH), and luteinizing hormone (LH). Secretion of FSH and LH directs events in the ovarian follicles that result in the production of a fertile ovum.

TABLE 19-2 Comparison of Methods of Nonhormonal Contraception

Method	Absolute Contraindications	Advantages	Disadvantages	Percent of with Pregnancy[a] Perfect Use	Typical Use
Condoms, external (traditionally known as male)	Allergy to latex or rubber	Inexpensive STI/STD protection, including HIV (latex only)	High user failure rate Poor acceptance Possibility of breakage Efficacy decreased by oil-based lubricants Possible allergic reactions to latex in either partner	2	13
Condoms, internal (traditionally known as female)	Allergy to polyurethane History of TSS	Can be inserted just before intercourse or ahead of time STI/STD protection, including HIV	High user failure rate Dislike ring hanging outside vagina Cumbersome	5	21
Diaphragm with spermicide	Allergy to latex, rubber, or spermicide Recurrent UTIs History of TSS Abnormal gynecologic anatomy	Low cost Decreased incidence of cervical neoplasia Some protection against STIs/STDs	High user failure rate Decreased efficacy with increased frequency of intercourse Increased incidence of vaginal yeast UTIs, TSS Efficacy decreased by oil-based lubricants Cervical irritation	16	17
Cervical cap (FemCap)	Allergy to spermicide History of TSS Abnormal gynecologic anatomy Abnormal papanicolaou smear	Low cost Latex-free Some protection against STIs/STDs FemCap reusable for up to 2 years	High user failure rate Decreased efficacy with parity Cannot be used during menses	9	16[b]
Spermicides alone (Phexxi)	Allergy to spermicide	Inexpensive	High user failure rate Must be reapplied before each act of intercourse May enhance HIV transmission No protection against STIs/STDs	16	21-28[c]

(Continued)

TABLE 19-2 Comparison of Methods of Nonhormonal Contraception (*Continued*)

Method	Absolute Contraindications	Advantages	Disadvantages	Percent of with Pregnancy[a] Perfect Use	Typical Use
Sponge (Today)	Allergy to spermicide Recurrent UTIs History of TSS Abnormal gynecologic anatomy	Inexpensive	High user failure rate Decreased efficacy with parity Cannot be used during menses No protection against STIs/STDs	9[d]	14[e]

[a]Failure rates in the United States during first year of use.

[b]Failure rate with FemCap reported to be 24% per package insert.

[c]Failure rate with Phexxi reported to be 27.5% per package insert.

[d]Failure rate with Today sponge reported to be 20% in parous individuals.

[e]Failure rate with Today sponge reported to be 27% in parous females.

Data from References 3 and 8-10.

HIV, human immunodeficiency virus; STI/STD, sexually transmitted infection/disease; TSS, toxic shock syndrome; UTI, urinary tract infection.

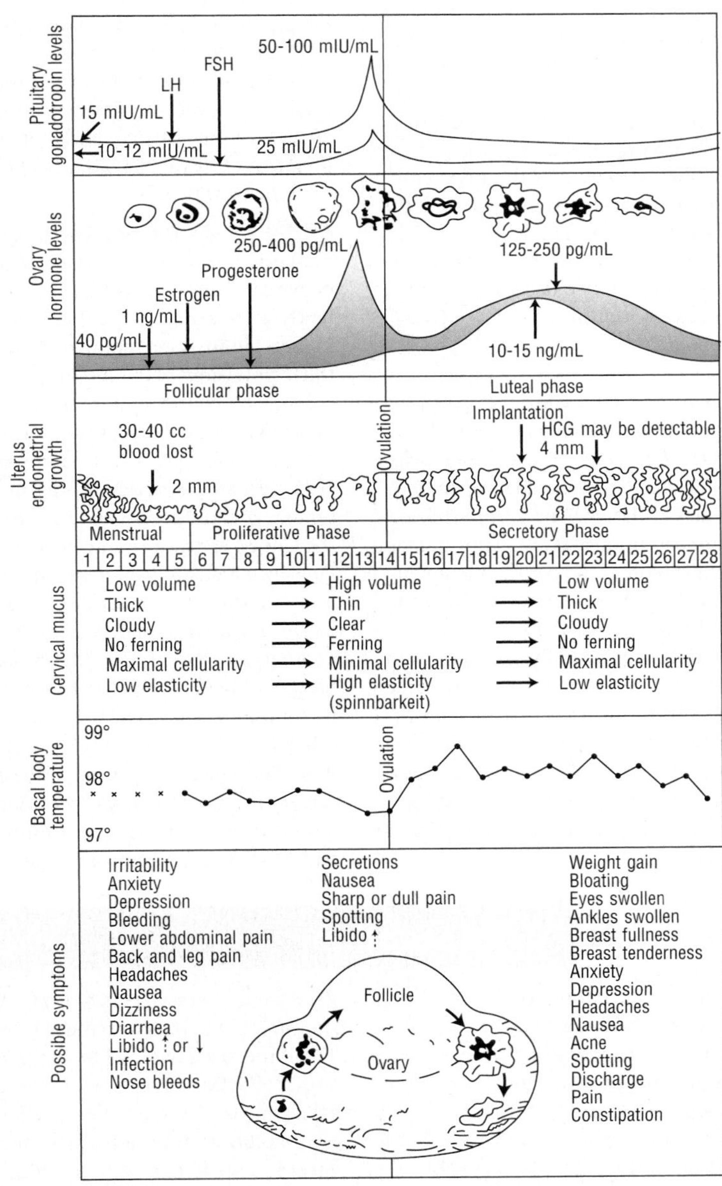

FIGURE 19-1 Menstrual cycle events, idealized 28-day cycle (FSH, follicle-stimulating hormone; HCG, human chorionic gonadotropin; LH, luteinizing hormone).

Follicular Phase

In the first 4 days of the menstrual cycle, FSH levels rise and allow the recruitment of a small group of follicles for continued growth and development (see Fig. 19-1).[3] Between days 5 and 7, one follicle becomes dominant and later ruptures, releasing the oocyte. The dominant follicle develops increasing amounts of estradiol and inhibin, which cause a negative feedback on the hypothalamic secretion of GnRH and pituitary secretion of FSH, causing atresia of the remaining follicles recruited during the cycle.

Once the follicle has received FSH stimulation, it must receive continued FSH stimulation or it will die.[3] FSH allows the follicle to enlarge and synthesize estradiol, progesterone, and androgen. Estradiol stops the menstrual flow from the previous cycle, thickening the endometrial lining of the uterus to prepare it for embryonic implantation. It is responsible for increased production of thin, watery cervical mucus, which will enhance sperm transport during fertilization. FSH regulates the aromatase enzymes that convert androgens to estrogens in the follicle. If a follicle has insufficient aromatase, it will not survive.

Ovulation

When estradiol levels remain elevated for a sustained period of time, the pituitary releases a mid-cycle LH surge (see Fig. 19-1).[3] This LH surge stimulates the final stages of follicular maturation and ovulation (follicular rupture and release of the oocyte). On average, ovulation occurs 24 to 36 hours after the estradiol peak and 10 to 12 hours after the LH peak. The beginning of the LH surge, which occurs about 36 hours before a follicle ruptures, is the most clinically useful predictor of approaching ovulation. After ovulation, the oocyte is released and travels to the fallopian tube, where it can be fertilized and transported to the uterus for embryonic implantation. Conception is most successful when intercourse takes place from 2 days before ovulation to the day of ovulation.

Luteal Phase

After rupture of the follicle and release of the ovum, the remaining luteinized follicles become the corpus luteum, which synthesizes androgen, estrogen, and progesterone (see Fig. 19-1).[3] Progesterone helps maintain the endometrial lining, which sustains the implanted embryo, maintaining pregnancy. It also inhibits GnRH and gonadotropin release, preventing the new follicle development. If pregnancy occurs, human chorionic gonadotropin prevents regression of the corpus luteum and stimulates continued estrogen and progesterone secretion to maintain the pregnancy until the placenta is able to fulfill this role.

If fertilization or implantation does not occur, the corpus luteum degenerates, and progesterone production declines.[3] The life span of the corpus luteum depends on the continuous presence of small amounts of LH, and its average duration of function is 9 to 11 days. As progesterone levels decline, endometrial shedding (menstruation) occurs, and a new menstrual cycle begins. At the end of the luteal phase, when estrogen and progesterone levels are low, FSH levels start to rise, and follicular recruitment for the next cycle begins.

TREATMENT

Desired Outcomes

2 The desired goal of all conceptive methods is to prevent pregnancy. However, other health benefits are associated with various contraceptive methods, including prevention of STIs/STDs (with condoms), improvements in menstrual cycle regularity (with hormonal contraceptives), improvements in certain health conditions (with hormonal contraceptives), and management of perimenopause (with hormonal contraceptives).[3]

General Approach to Treatment

Nonpharmacologic Therapy

3 4 5 **Fertility Awareness-Based Methods** Motivated couples may use fertility awareness-based methods that entail avoiding sexual intercourse during the days of the menstrual cycle when conception is likely to occur. These typically include calendar-based methods such as the standard days or rhythm methods. In addition, there are symptoms-based methods that are based on observed physiologic changes, such as basal body temperature and cervical mucus to determine the fertile period. There are many technology apps available for these methods and the Food and Drug Administration (FDA) approved the first app in this category (Natural Cycles) in 2018.[11] The major drawbacks of these methods are relatively high pregnancy rates and avoidance of intercourse for several days during each menstrual cycle.[3]

3 4 5 9 **Barrier Techniques** The effectiveness of barrier methods (eg, condoms, diaphragms, cervical caps, and sponges) depends almost exclusively on the motivation to use them consistently and correctly (see Table 19-2).[3] Their major disadvantage is higher failure rates compared to most hormonal contraceptives; thus, provision of counseling and an advanced prescription for emergency contraception (EC) are recommended for all patients using barrier methods as their primary contraception means.

External condoms (traditionally known as male condoms) create a mechanical barrier, preventing direct contact of the vagina with semen, genital lesions, and infectious secretions.[3] Most condoms in the United States are made of latex, which is impermeable to viruses. However, a small proportion are made from lamb intestine, which is permeable to viruses and should not be used to prevent STIs/STDs. Synthetic condoms manufactured from polyurethane are another latex-free option that protect against viruses. Condoms are used worldwide for STIs/STDs protection including human immunodeficiency virus (HIV). When used in conjunction with any other barrier method, their effectiveness theoretically approaches 98%. Spillage of semen or perforation and tearing of the condom can occur, but proper use minimizes these problems. Mineral oil-based vaginal medication formulations (eg, Cleocin, Premarin, and Monistat), lotions, or lubricants can decrease the latex barrier

CLINICAL PRESENTATION Contraception

Traditionally, hormonal contraception required breast and pelvic examinations. However, the need for the physical examination may delay contraception access and reinforces the incorrect perception that these methods of contraceptives are harmful. Therefore, in practice, provision of hormonal contraception is followed after a simple medical history, including weight and BP pressure measurement.[5]

3 4 Most annual preventative medicine visits should include an assessment of and counseling about reproductive health, including contraception and STIs/STDs prevention education. Additionally, other preventive measures, such as pelvic and breast examinations, provision of the human papillomavirus vaccine, and screening for cervical neoplasia, can be accomplished during these visits.

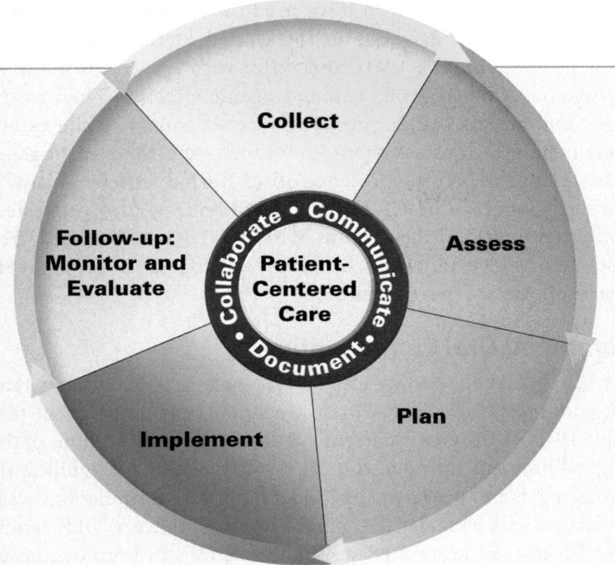

Patient Care Process for Contraception

An illustration shows that patient-centered care includes collaboration, communication, and documentation. The actions associated with the care are collect, assess, plan, implement, and follow-up by monitoring and evaluating.

Collect

- Patient characteristics (eg, age, sex, date of last menstrual period, pregnant, recently postpartum, breastfeeding, desire for pregnancy/return to fertility)
- Patient medical history (personal and family)
- Medication allergies
- Social history (eg, tobacco/ethanol use, relationships, sexual history)
- Current medications including over-the-counter (OTC), herbal products, dietary supplements
- Previous or current use of contraceptives
- Objective data: blood pressure (BP), height, weight

Assess

- Pregnancy status
- Effectiveness of previous contraceptive methods used (Tables 19-1 and 19-2)
- BP
- Weight and optimal method for use
- Precautions and contraindications to various types of contraceptives utilizing the CDC Medical Eligibility for Contraceptive Use, 2016 (see Table 19-6)
- Venous thromboembolism (VTE) risk factors (eg, recent surgery, plaster casting of lower extremity, cancer, prolonged immobility, recent hospitalization, recently postpartum)
- Medication interactions with various forms of contraception (see Table 19-6 for a select listing of medication interactions)
- Patient ability/willingness to use, adhere, or pay for various forms of contraception (Tables 19-1 and 19-2)

Plan*

- Medication therapy regimen including specific contraceptive dosage forms, dose, route, frequency, and duration (see Table 19-3 for select examples)
- Monitoring parameters including effectiveness and safety (eg, ACHES [abdominal pain, chest pain, headaches, eye problems, and severe leg pain]) (Tables 19-4 and 19-5)

Implement*

- Provide patient education regarding all elements of contraceptive plan (eg, adherence, missed doses, adverse medication effects)
- Schedule appropriate follow-up to assess adverse medication effects, adherence issues, access to contraceptive

Follow-up: Monitor and Evaluate

- Presence of adverse effects (Tables 19-3, 19-4, and 19-5)
- For intrauterine devices (IUD), appropriate placement (eg, checking for strings)
- Changes in medical history (eg, increase in BP, migraines, VTE risk, body mass index [BMI], new medications)
- Patient adherence to treatment plan using multiple sources of information

Collaborate with patient, caregivers, and other healthcare professionals.

strength and are not recommended, thus water-soluble lubricants (eg, Astroglide and K-Y Jelly) are the preferred choice. Condoms sold with prelubricated spermicides are no longer recommended as they do not provide additional protection against pregnancy or STIs/STDs and may increase vulnerability to HIV.[3,12]

The internal condom (traditionally referred to as the female condom) is a prelubricated, loose-fitting polyurethane sheath which is closed at one end and has flexible rings at both ends.[3] This method protects against viruses, including HIV. Properly positioned, the ring at the closed end covers the cervix, and the sheath lines the vaginal walls. The outer ring remains outside the vagina, covering the labia. The pregnancy rate of the internal condom is higher compared to external condoms. External and internal condoms should not be used together, as slippage and device displacement may occur.

The diaphragm, a reusable dome-shaped rubber cap with a flexible rim that is inserted vaginally, fits over the cervix to decrease access of sperm to the ovum. The diaphragm must be fitted to the patient for the correct size and requires a prescription.[3] Its efficacy is increased when used in conjunction with a spermicidal cream or jelly. The diaphragm may be inserted up to 6 hours before intercourse and must be left in place for at least 6 hours afterward. However, leaving it in place for more than 24 hours is not recommended due to the potential for toxic shock syndrome (TSS). With subsequent acts of intercourse, the diaphragm should be left in place, and a condom should be used for additional protection.

The cervical cap (FemCap) is a soft, deep cup with a firm round rim that is smaller than a diaphragm and fits over the cervix like a thimble.[3,8] The cervical cap is available in three sizes, is fitted into the patient for the correct size, and requires a prescription. It should be filled with spermicide prior to use. It should be inserted 6 hours prior to intercourse and not be removed for at least 6 hours after intercourse. It can remain in place for multiple episodes of intercourse without adding more spermicide but should not be worn for more than 48 hours at a time to reduce the risk of TSS. Failure rates with the cervical cap are higher than with other methods. Diaphragms and cervical caps do not protect against some STIs/STDs including HIV; thus, condoms should also be used.

Pharmacologic Therapy

Spermicides and Spermicide-Implanted Barrier Techniques

3 4 5 9 Spermicides, most of which contain nonoxynol-9, are chemical surfactants that destroy sperm cell walls and act as barriers to prevent sperm from entering the cervical os.[3] They are available as creams, films, foams, gels, suppositories, sponges, and tablets. Spermicides offer no protection against STIs/STDs. In fact, when used frequently (more than two times per day), nonoxynol-9 may increase the risk of transmission of HIV by causing small disruptions in the vaginal epithelium.[3,12] The World Health Organization (WHO) and the Centers for Disease Control and Prevention (CDC) do not promote products containing nonoxynol-9 for protection against STIs/STDs.

A new prescription spermicide, marketed as Phexxi, is a combination of lactic acid 1.8%, citric acid 1%, and potassium bitartrate 0.4%, and does not contain nonoxynol-9. The product works to lower pH and reduce sperm motility, and should be used within 1 hour before sexual intercourse and with each act of intercourse. Some precautions include avoiding use in individuals with frequent cystitis as this product has been reported to increase risk.[9]

3 4 5 The vaginal contraceptive sponge (Today) contains 1 g of the spermicide nonoxynol-9.[3] It has a concave dimple on one side to fit over the cervix and a loop on the other side to facilitate removal. After being moistened with water, the sponge is inserted into the vagina up to 6 hours before intercourse and provides protection for 24 hours, regardless of the frequency of intercourse during this time. After intercourse, the sponge must be left in place for at least 6 hours but should not be left in place for more than 24 to 30 hours to reduce the risk of TSS. Sponges should not be reused and should be discarded after removal. They come in one size and are available OTC.

The copper IUD (Paragard T380A) contains copper and affects sperm motility to prevent fertilization and implantation (see "Intrauterine Devices" section).

Hormonal Contraception

3 4 5 Hormonal contraceptives contain a combination of estrogen and progestin or a progestin alone. Oral contraceptive (OC) preparations first became available in the 1960s, but options have expanded to include transdermal patches, vaginal rings, a long-acting injection, a subdermal implant, and IUDs.

Combined Hormonal Contraceptives Combined hormonal contraceptives (CHCs) contain both estrogen and progestin and work primarily before fertilization to prevent conception. Progestins provide most of the contraceptive effect by thickening cervical mucus to prevent sperm penetration, slowing tubal motility, delaying sperm transport, and inducing endometrial atrophy. Progestins block the LH surge, to inhibit ovulation, and estrogens suppress FSH release from the pituitary, which may contribute to blocking the LH surge to prevent ovulation. However, the estrogen's primary role in hormonal contraception is to stabilize the endometrial lining and provide cycle control.[3,4]

Estrogens The synthetic estrogens found in hormonal contraceptives available in the United States are ethinyl estradiol (EE), estradiol valerate, and more recently estetrol (E4), with EE being the most commonly used.[3,4,13] Most combined oral contraceptives (COCs), including transdermal patches, and vaginal rings contain EE at doses of 20 to 50 mcg, with a few lower than 20 mcg.[4,13,16]

Progestins Progestin is a term used for a synthetic progesterone and a variety available in the United States. They vary in their progestational activity and differ with respect to inherent estrogenic, antiestrogenic, and androgenic effects.[3,4] Their estrogenic and antiestrogenic properties are secondary to the extent their metabolism to estrogenic substances and their androgenic activity depends on the presence of sex hormone (testosterone)-binding globulin (SHBG-TBG) and the androgen-to-progesterone activity ratio. If the amount of SHBG-TBG is decreased, free testosterone levels increase, and their androgenic adverse medication effects are more prominent.[4]

Combined Oral Contraceptives

3 4 5 With perfect-use, COCs have a 99% efficacy rate, but with typical-use up to 7% of users may become pregnant (see Table 19-1).[3,4] The COCs currently available are modifications of the original products introduced in the 1960s and contain significantly less estrogen and progestin. The older high-dose formulations were associated with vascular and embolic events, cancers, and significant adverse medication effects, but reductions in hormone doses are associated with fewer complications.

Monophasic COCs contain the same amounts of estrogen and progestin for 21 days, followed by a 7-day placebo phase. Multiphasic pills (biphasic, triphasic, or quadriphasic) contain variable amounts of estrogen and progestin for 21 days, also followed by a 7-day placebo phase. Multiphasic and monophasic products are equally effective.[3,14,15] Extended-cycle tablets and continuous combination regimens may offer some benefits for patients in terms of side effects and convenience. With COCs, the types and doses of estrogen and progestin remain constant during the 21 to 24 days that active tablets are taken, though the doses and ratios of estrogens and progestins vary from one preparation to another. The inclusion of three additional days of active pills to shorten the pill-free interval is thought to reduce hormone fluctuation between menstrual cycles. With extended use of COCs, active combination tablets are taken continuously for 84 days or longer followed by 7 days of inactive pills or estrogen-only pills.[4] **Table 19-3** lists the available OC products by brand name and specifies hormonal composition.[3,4,7,13,16]

8 **Initiating a Combined Oral Contraceptive** COCs may be initiated by different methods, including on the first day of bleeding during the menstrual cycle, or on the first Sunday after the menstrual cycle begins, or using the quick start method. The first day method is when the woman starts the COC on the first day of her menstrual cycle. The patient should be instructed to use a second method of contraception (typically recommend condoms) for at least 7 days after initiation for maximum effectiveness, though some sources state that no backup contraceptive method is required for the first day of menses start method.[13] The "Sunday start" method requires taking tablets on the first Sunday after the menstrual cycle begins and may provide weekends free of menstrual periods.[3,4,10,17] Individuals should also be instructed to use a second method of contraception (typically recommend condoms) for at least 7 days after initiation for maximum effectiveness. It may be preferable to have individuals use additional contraception for the entire first cycle, due to user failure in the first month. In the "quick start" method, the patient takes the first tablet on the day of her office visit. Patients should be instructed to use a second method of contraception for at least 7 days and potentially until she begins her next menstrual cycle to ensure optimal effectiveness. Patients should be informed that the menstrual period will be delayed until completion of the active tablets in the current OC pack. This method is more successful in getting individuals to start OCs and to continue using OCs through the third cycle of use.[3] The CDC recommends that individuals start or resume hormonal contraception no sooner than 5 days

TABLE 19-3 Composition of Commonly Prescribed Oral Contraceptives[a]

Common Brand Names	Estrogen	Micrograms[a] (Number of Days)	Progestin	Milligrams[a] (Number of Days)	Spotting and Breakthrough Bleeding by Third Cycle (Up to Tenth Decimal)	Comments
Monophasic Preparations						
Kelnor 1/50	Ethinyl estradiol	50	Ethynodiol diacetate	1	13.9	
Zovia 1/35E, Kelnor 1/35	Ethinyl estradiol	35	Ethynodiol diacetate	1	37.4	
Apri, Cyred, Cyred EQ, Emoquette, Enskyce, Isibloom, Juleber, Kalliga, Reclipsen	Ethinyl estradiol	30	Desogestrel	0.15	13.1	
Azurette, Bekyree, Kariva, Mircette, Pimtrea, Simliya, Viorele, Volnea	Ethinyl estradiol	20 (21) 10 (5)	Desogestrel	0.15	19.7	Contains 2 days of placebo, 5 days of EE 10 mcg only
Nextstellis	Estetrol	14.2 (mg)	Drospirenone	3	N/A	Contains 24 active tablets, 4 days of placebo Contains estetrol (E4), known to have native estrogen selective actions in tissues, acts as nuclear agonist on vascular system, liver, bone, uterus, and vagina; acts as a membrane antagonist on breast, liver, bone, and vascular system.
Ocella, Safyral, Syeda, Tydemy, Yasmin, Zarah, Zumandimine	Ethinyl estradiol	30	Drospirenone	3	14.5	Safyral and Tydemy are FDA-approved for acne, premenstrual dysphoric disorder (PMDD), and provide folate supplementation, 21 active pills with 0.451 mg of levomefolate calcium and 7 days of 0.451 mg of levomefolate calcium instead of placebos.
Beyaz, Gianvi, Jasmiel, Lo-Zumandimine, Loryna, Nikki, Rajani, Vestura, Yaz[b]	Ethinyl estradiol	20	Drospirenone	3	13.8[c]	Extended cycle—24 active hormone tablets, 4 placebo FDA-approved use for treatment of acne and PMDD Beyaz and Rajani provide folate supplementation, 21 active pills with 0.451 mg of levomefolate calcium and 7 days of 0.451 mg of levomefolate calcium instead of placebos
Altavera, Ayuna, Chateal, Chateal EQ, Kurvelo, Levora 0.15/30, Lillow, Marlissa, Portia-28	Ethinyl estradiol	30	Levonorgestrel	0.15	14	
Iclevia, Introvale, Jolessa, Setlakin[d]	Ethinyl estradiol	30	Levonorgestrel	0.15	15.1[c]	Extended cycle—91 tablets (84 active hormone tablets and 7 placebo pills)
Amethia, Ashlyna, Camrese Daysee, Jaimiess, Seasonique, Simpesse	Ethinyl estradiol	30 (84) 10 (7)	Levonorgestrel	0.15	14.3[e]	Extended cycle—91 tablets (84 active hormone tablets and 7 tablets of EE 10 mcg instead of placebos) Considered monophasic since only last 7 days are lower estrogen and act similarly to a placebo
Afirmelle, Aubra, Aubra EQ, Aviane, Balcoltra, Delyla, Falmina, Larissia, Lessina, Lutera, Orsythia, Sronyx, Tyblume, Vienva	Ethinyl estradiol	20	Levonorgestrel	0.1	26.5	Balcoltra contains 7 tables of ferrous bisglycinate instead of placebo

(Continued)

TABLE 19-3 Composition of Commonly Prescribed Oral Contraceptives[a] (*Continued*)

Common Brand Names	Estrogen	Micrograms[a] (Number of Days)	Progestin	Milligrams[a] (Number of Days)	Spotting and Breakthrough Bleeding by Third Cycle (Up to Tenth Decimal)	Comments
Monophasic Preparations						
Camrese Lo, LoJaimiess, LoSeasonique	Ethinyl estradiol	20/10	Levonorgestrel	0.1	21.5[e]	Extended cycle—91 tablets (84 active hormone tablets and 7 tablets of EE 10 mcg instead of placebos)
Amethyst, Dolishale	Ethinyl estradiol	20	Levonorgestrel	0.09	N/A[c]	Extended cycle—intended for 1-year continuous use available in packs of 28 active pills
Estarylla, Femynor, Mili, Mono-Linyah, Mononessa, NymyoPrevifem, Sprintec, VyLibra	Ethinyl estradiol	35	Norgestimate	0.25	14.3	
–	Ethinyl estradiol	50	Norgestrel	0.5	N/A	
Cryselle, Elinest, Low-Ogestrel	Ethinyl estradiol	30	Norgestrel	0.3	9.6	
Balziva, Briellyn, Gildagia, Philith, Vyfemla, Wymzya Fe chewable	Ethinyl estradiol	35	Norethindrone	0.4	11	"Fe" contains 7 days of 75 mg ferrous fumarate instead of placebos "Chewable"—chewable formulation, must drink with 8 oz (~240 mL) of water and rinse mouth
Necon 0.5/35, Nortrel 0.5/35, Norminest Fe, Wera	Ethinyl estradiol	35	Norethindrone	0.5	24.6	
Alyacen 1/35, Cyclafem 1/35, Dasetta 1/35, Nortrel 1/35, Pirmella 1/35	Ethinyl estradiol	35	Norethindrone	1	14.7	
Generess Fe chewable, Kaitlib Fe chewable, Layolis Fe chewable	Ethinyl estradiol	25	Norethindrone	0.8	19.0	Extended cycle—24 active hormone tablets, 4 days of ferrous fumarate 75 mg instead of placebos "Chewable"—chewable formulation, must drink with 8 oz (~240 mL) of water and rinse mouth
Aurovela 1.5/30-21, Aurovela 1.5/30-28, Aurovela Fe 1.5/30, Blisovi Fe 1.5/30, Hailey Fe 1/20, Gildess Fe 1.5/30, Junel 1.5/30, Junel Fe 1.5/30, Larin 1.5/30, LarinFe 1.5/30, Loestrin Fe 1.5/30, Microgestin 1.5/30, Microgestin Fe 1.5/30	Ethinyl estradiol	30	Norethindrone acetate	1.5	25.2	"Fe" contains 7 days of 75 mg ferrous fumarate instead of placebos
Aurovela 1/20, Aurovela Fe 1/20, Blisovi 1/20, Hailey Fe 1/20, Junel Fe 1/20, Junel 1/20, Larin (Fe) 1/20, Loestrin 1/20; Fe 1/20, Microgestin 1/20; Microgestin Fe 1/20, Tarina Fe 1/20, Tarina Fe 1/20 EQ	Ethinyl estradiol	20	Norethindrone acetate	1	29.7	"Fe" contains 7 days of 75 mg ferrous fumarate for 7 days "Chewable"—chewable formulation, must drink with 8 oz (~240 mL) of water and rinse mouth
Aurovela 24 Fe, Blisovi 24 Fe, Gemmily (capsules), Junel Fe 24, Hailey 24 Fe, Larin 24 Fe, Minastrin 24 Fe chewable, Merzee (capsules), Melodetta 24 Fe (chewable), Microgestin 24 Fe, Tarina 24 Fe, Taytulla (capsules)	Ethinyl estradiol	20	Norethindrone acetate	1	23.2[c]	Extended cycle—24 active hormone tablets, 4 placebo "Fe" contains 4 days of 75 mg ferrous fumarate instead of placebos "Chewable"—chewable formulation, must drink with 8 oz (~240 mL) of water and rinse mouth. Gemmily, Merzee, Taytulla—capsule formulations and also contain 75 mg ferrous fumarate for 7 days, instead of placebos

TABLE 19-3 Composition of Commonly Prescribed Oral Contraceptives[a]

Common Brand Names	Estrogen	Micrograms[a] (Number of Days)	Progestin	Milligrams[a] (Number of Days)	Spotting and Breakthrough Bleeding by Third Cycle (Up to Tenth Decimal)	Comments
Monophasic Preparations						
Lo Loestrin-24 Fe[b]	Ethinyl estradiol	10	Norethindrone acetate	1	52.0[c]	Extended cycle—24 active tablets, 2 days of EE 10 mcg only and 2 days of 75 mg ferrous fumarate tablets
Multiphasic Preparations (Biphasic, Triphasic, and Quadriphasic)						
–	Ethinyl estradiol	35 (10)	Norethindrone	0.5 (10)	N/A	Biphasic
		35 (11)		1 (11)		
Caziant, Cyclessa, Velivet	Ethinyl estradiol	25 (7)	Desogestrel	0.1 (7)	11.1	Triphasic
		25 (7)		0.125 (7)		
		25 (7)		0.15 (7)		
Enpresse, Trivora, Levonest Myzilra	Ethinyl estradiol	30 (6)	Levonorgestrel	0.05 (6)	15.1	Triphasic
		40 (5)		0.075 (5)		
		30 (10)		0.125 (10)		
Ortho Tri-Cyclen, Tri-Estarylla, Tri-Femynor, Tri-Linyah, TriNessa, Tri-Previfem, Tri-Sprintec	Ethinyl estradiol	35 (7)	Norgestimate	0.18 (7)	17.7	Triphasic FDA-approved use for treatment of acne
		35 (7)		0.215 (7)		
		35 (7)		0.25 (7)		
Tri-Lo Estarylla, Tri-Lo-Marzia, Tri-Lo-Mili, Tri-Lo-Sprintec, Tri-VyLibra Lo	Ethinyl estradiol	25 (7)	Norgestimate	0.18 (7)	11.5	Triphasic
		25 (7)		0.215 (7)		
		25 (7)		0.25 (7)		
Alyacen 7/7/7, Cyclafem 7/7/7, Dasetta 7/7/7, Nortrel 7/7/7, Nylia 7/7/7, Pirmella 7/7/7	Ethinyl estradiol	35 (7)	Norethindrone	0.5 (7)	14.5	Triphasic
		35 (7)		0.75 (7)		
		35 (7)		1 (7)		
Aranelle, Leena	Ethinyl estradiol	35 (7)	Norethindrone	0.5 (7)	25.5	Triphasic
		35 (9)		1 (9)		
		35 (5)		0.5 (5)		
Estrostep Fe, Tilia Fe, Tri-Legest Fe	Ethinyl estradiol	20 (5)	Norethindrone acetate	1 (5)	21.7	Triphasic Estrophasic (estrogen content changes), FDA-approved use for treatment of acne, "Fe" contains 75 mg ferrous fumarate instead of placebos
		30 (7)		1 (7)		
		35 (9)		1 (9)		
Fayosim, Quartette, Rivelsa	Ethinyl estradiol	20 (42)	Levonorgestrel	0.15	N/A[e]	Quadriphasic, Estrophasic (estrogen content changes), extended cycle—91 tablets (84 active tablets and 7 tablets of EE 10 mcg instead of placebo)
		25 (21)				
		30 (21)				
		10 (7)				

(Continued)

TABLE 19-3 Composition of Commonly Prescribed Oral Contraceptives[a] *(Continued)*

Common Brand Names	Estrogen	Micrograms[a] (Number of Days)	Progestin	Milligrams[a] (Number of Days)	Spotting and Breakthrough Bleeding by Third Cycle (Up to Tenth Decimal)	Comments
Monophasic Preparations						
Natazia	Estradiol valerate	3 (2) 2 (5) 2 (17) 1 (2)	Dienogest	0 (2) 2 (5) 3 (17) 0 (4)	14	Quadriphasic, Estrophasic FDA-approved use for heavy menstrual bleeding
Progestin-Only Oral Contraceptives						
Camila, Deblitane Errin, Heather, Incassia, Jencycla Lyleq, Lyza, Ortho Micronor, Nora-BE, Norlyda, Norlyroc, Orthor Micronor, Sharobel, Tulana	Ethinyl estradiol	–	Norethindrone	0.35 (28)	42.3	Contains 28 days of active tablets, no placebos
Slynd	Ethinyl estradiol	–	Drospirenone	4 (24)	N/A	Contains 24 days of active tablets, 4 days placebo

[a]28-day regimens (21-day active pills, then 7-day pill-free interval) unless otherwise noted.

[b]Number in parentheses refers to the number of days the dose is received in multiphasic oral contraceptives.

[c]28-day regimen (24-day active pills, then 4-day pill-free interval).

[d]91-day regimen (84-day active pills, then 7-day pill-free interval).

[e]Percent reporting after 6 to 12 months of use.

[f]Also contains levomefolate calcium 0.451 mg in all 28 tablets.

Data from References 3, 4, 13 and 16.

N/A—Data not available per references.

after use of the emergency contraceptive ulipristal acetate to maximize the effectiveness of both products (use of the two products together may decrease effectiveness). Long-acting reversible contraception (LARC) methods such as the IUD and implant, however, can be started at the time of ulipristal acetate use.[10,17]

4 5 3 Selecting a Combined Oral Contraceptive Because all COCs are similarly effective in preventing pregnancy (see Table 19-1), the initial choice is based on the hormonal content and dose, preferred formulation, and coexisting medical conditions (see Table 19-6).[4,16,17] In individuals without coexisting medical conditions, an OC containing 35 mcg or less of EE is recommended (see Table 19-3).[4,7,13,16] This strategy is based on evidence that complications and side effects of CHC (ie, VTE, stroke, or myocardial infarction [MI]) result from excessive hormonal content. With nonadherence to OCs, the risk of pregnancy may be greater in individuals taking COCs containing less than 35 mcg of EE. Individuals with oily skin, acne, or hirsutism should be given low androgenic COCs.[4] Choice of an agent based upon coexisting medical conditions can be found in Table 19-6.[17]

It may be easier to identify/manage adverse medication effects and easier to manipulate to alter the timing of the menstrual cycle in patients taking monophasic COCs.[3,4] Continuous COCs either eliminate or reduce the number of menstrual cycles per year, leading to less premenstrual symptoms and dysmenorrhea. Commercially available continuous COCs or monophasic 28-day OCs can be cycled by skipping the 7-day placebo phase. With continued use of extended-cycle or continuous COCs for 1 year, no significant changes in adverse effects have been noted. However, long-term studies have not been performed to assess the risk of cancer, VTE, or changes in fertility. Extended-cycle regimens provide a shortened pill-free interval, from the traditional 7 days to 2 to 4 days. These various extended-cycle and continuous regimens may be beneficial for patients with symptoms such as dysmenorrhea, severe premenstrual syndrome, or menstrual migraines.

TABLE 19-4 Symptoms of a Serious or Potentially Serious Nature Associated with Combined Hormonal Contraception

Symptom	Possible Cause
SERIOUS: Stop immediately	
Loss of vision, proptosis, diplopia, papilledema	Retinal artery thrombosis
Unilateral numbness, weakness, or tingling	Hemorrhagic or thrombotic stroke
Severe pains in chest, left arm, or neck	Myocardial infarction
Hemoptysis	Pulmonary embolism
Severe pains, tenderness or swelling, warmth or palpable cord in legs	Thrombophlebitis or thrombosis
Slurring of speech	Hemorrhagic or thrombotic stroke
Hepatic mass or tenderness	Liver neoplasm
POTENTIALLY SERIOUS: May continue with caution while being evaluated	
Absence of menses	Cervical endometrial or vaginal cancer
Spotting or breakthrough bleeding	Cholecystitis, cholelithiasis, or liver neoplasm
Breast mass, pain, or swelling	Pituitary adenoma
Right upper-quadrant pain	Cholestatic jaundice
Mid-epigastric pain	B6 deficiency
Migraine headache	Leiomyomata, adenomyosis
Severe nonvascular headache	
Galactorrhea	
Jaundice, pruritus	
Depression, sleepiness	
Uterine size increase	

Data from References 3 and 4.

6 Managing Combined Oral Contraceptive Adverse Medication Effects Adverse medication effects occurring with early COC use (eg, nausea, bloating, breakthrough bleeding) may improve spontaneously by the third cycle after adjusting to the altered hormone levels.[3,4,10,17] Patients should be counseled to continue their COC for 2 to 3 months before changing products unless a serious adverse effect is present. Despite the 2- to 3-month adjustment period, a large majority of individuals who discontinue COCs do so because of the adverse medication effects. Therefore, patient education and early reevaluation within 3 to 6 months are necessary to identify and manage adverse effects, and to improve adherence. The most common adverse effect is irregular bleeding. Individuals on extended-cycle regimens should be counseled to expect this during the first 6 months. For those experiencing bleeding irregularities beyond the recommended time frame, the estrogen or progestin content may need to be adjusted.[4,10,17] Early breakthrough bleeding is typically due to insufficient estrogen and late breakthrough bleeding is due to insufficient progestin. Nausea may occur due to the estrogenic effects of these hormonal contraceptives. Skin breakouts occur more often in products with higher androgenic effects. Serious adverse effects that may occur with the use of CHCs are listed in Table 19-4, and common adverse medication effects along with recommended monitoring are reviewed in Table 19-5.[3,4,10] Patients should be instructed to consult with their provider immediately and likely should discontinue CHCs if they experience serious warning signs, described as ACHES.[3,4]

4 6 7 Managing Combined Oral Contraceptive Medication Interactions The effectiveness of a COC is sometimes limited by medication interactions that interfere with GI absorption, increase intestinal motility due to altered gut bacteriologic flora, and alteration of the metabolism, excretion, or binding of the COC.[2] The lower the dose of hormone in the COC, the greater the risk that a medication interaction will compromise effectiveness. Individuals should be instructed to use an additional method of contraception if there is a possible medication interaction altering COC effectiveness.[4] Although less well documented, these recommendations generally apply to patients receiving transdermal and vaginal CHC products.

Rifampin is the one with a true documented COC pharmacokinetic interactions.[3,10] Pharmacokinetic studies of other antibiotics have not shown any consistent interaction, but individual case reports have shown a reduction in EE levels when OCs are taken with tetracyclines and penicillin derivatives, possibly due to the inhibition of enterohepatic recirculation. Individuals receiving concomitant rifampin (or derivatives) and OCs should be counseled on the possibility for decreased efficacy and to use an additional nonhormonal contraception while on the combination and for at least 7 days after the rifampin therapy has been discontinued. Some OC manufacturers recommend to use a backup method for 28 days after the use of any enzyme inducer such as rifampin.[10,17,18] It may be prudent to inform patients of the slight risk of decreased effectiveness with other antimicrobials as well; however, this is not necessarily supported with strong evidence. If a patient is going to be receiving an interacting medication for more than 2 months, switch to depot medroxyprogesterone acetate (DMPA) or an IUD to avoid the interaction and eliminate the need for long-term additional nonhormonal contraception.

7 Individuals receiving certain anticonvulsants for a seizure disorder should be offered another form of contraception such as

TABLE 19-5 Medication Monitoring Table for Hormonal Contraception

Medication (or Medication Class)	Adverse Medication Reactions	Monitoring Parameter	Comments
Combined hormonal contraception	Nausea/vomiting Breast tenderness Weight gain Acne, oily skin Depression, fatigue Breakthrough bleeding/spotting Application site reaction (transdermal) Vaginal irritation (vaginal ring)	Patient symptoms Weight Visual inspection Depression screening Menstrual symptoms Visual inspection Patient symptoms	Typically improves after two to three cycles; consider changing to lower estrogenic. Consider changing to lower androgenic. Data are limited and conflicting. Consider changing to higher estrogenic.
Depo-medroxyprogesterone acetate	Menstrual irregularities[a] Weight gain Acne Hirsutism Depression Decreased bone density	Menstrual symptoms Weight Visual inspection Depression screening bone mineral density (BMD)	Typically improves after 6 months. Data are limited and conflicting. Do not routinely screen with dual-energy X-ray absorptiometry (DXA).
Levonorgestrel IUD	Menstrual irregularities[a] Insertion-related complications Expulsion Pelvic inflammatory disease (PID)	Menstrual symptoms Cramping, pain, spotting, dyspareunia, missing strings Lower abdominal pain, unusual vaginal discharge, fever	Typically spotting, amenorrhea Prophylactic nonsteroidal anti-inflammatory drugs (NSAIDs) or local anesthetic may reduce occurrence. IUD strings should be checked regularly to ensure IUD properly placed. Risk of developing is rare, but counseling on STI/STD prevention is important.
Copper IUD	See levonorgestrel IUD above	See levonorgestrel IUD above	Menstrual irregularities are typically heavier menses with copper IUD.
Progestin-only implant	Menstrual irregularities[a] Insertion-site reactions	Menstrual symptoms Pain, bruising, skin irritation, erythema, pus, fever	Typically well tolerated and resolved without treatment; infection is rare.

[a]Suggested management of irregular bleeding may include use of NSAIDs for 5 to 7 days; hormonal treatment (if medically eligible) with COC or estrogen therapy for 10 to 20 days of treatment.

Data from References 3 and 10.

DMPA or LARC methods rather than OCs (see Table 19-6).[17] Some anticonvulsants (mainly phenobarbital, carbamazepine, phenytoin) induce the metabolism of estrogen and progestin, inducing breakthrough bleeding and potentially reducing contraceptive efficacy. In addition, some antiseizure medications are known as teratogens. Use of COCs with lamotrigine may decrease the effectiveness of lamotrigine and increase the possibility of worsening the seizure disorder.

Other medications that may affect COCs include HIV antiretrovirals such as protease inhibitors which, depending on the HIV medication, may decrease COC effectiveness or the COC may possibly alter the levels of protease inhibitor.[17] In addition, monitoring of potassium levels may be needed in individuals who take medications that increase potassium with drospirenone-containing COCs. Drospirenone is a derivative of spironolactone, a potassium-sparing diuretic, that also has anti-mineralocorticoid activity. Caution may be warranted in patients with a history of hyperkalemia or in patients taking concomitant medications that increase potassium levels or in high-risk patients taking strong inhibitors of CYP3A4.[18] Patients should also be counseled that an OTC herbal product, St. John's wort, may also possibly decrease OC effectiveness. Because there are several possible medication interactions that could affect the levels of COCs, assess all patient medications for possible interactions with COCs.[17]

9 Patient Instructions with Combined Oral Contraceptives Many individuals who take OCs are not educated properly on the appropriate use of these medications. They should be given the package insert that accompanies all products and instructed to read it, as well as supplementing this information with verbal education describing the mechanism of the medication, common and serious adverse medication effects (ie, ACHES symptoms), and their management. Although several transient self-limiting adverse medication effects often occur, the patient should be aware of the danger signals that require immediate medical attention (see Table 19-4). The benefits and risks should be discussed, including the fact that OCs provide no physical barrier to the transmission of STIs/STDs, including HIV. Detailed instructions on when to start taking the OC should be provided. Patients should be told the importance of routine daily administration to ensure consistent plasma concentrations and improve adherence.

8 Missed Doses of Combined Oral Contraceptives Specific instructions should be given regarding what to do if a tablet is missed.[10] For individuals who routinely have difficulty with adhering to daily dosing, counseling regarding other options such as the vaginal ring, transdermal patch, DMPA, implants, or IUDs should be provided. If warranted, suggesting EC may also be necessary.

For COCs, if one tablet is missed or late then it should be taken as soon as remembered, and the rest of the tablets should be continued as prescribed (for most this that means two tablets are taken on the same day). Typically no additional nonhormonal contraception methods are warranted. If two or more consecutive tablets are missed then take one missed tablet as soon as remembered and discard the other missed tablets. Continue taking the OC tablets as scheduled which means two tablets may need to be taken on the same day (ie, one of the missed tablets and one of the regularly scheduled tablets). If tablets were missed in the last week of hormonal tablets, finish the remaining active tablets (tablets with hormone) and then omit the hormone-free interval (skip taking the placebo tablets) and start a new pack of tablets. For both of these scenarios, counsel patients to use additional nonhormonal contraception until active hormone tablets have been taken for seven consecutive days. For all scenarios when two or more consecutive tablets are missed, consider counseling on EC use if warranted.

TABLE 19-6 US Medical Eligibility Criteria for Contraceptive Use: Classifications for Combined Hormonal Contraceptives

Category 4: Unacceptable health risk (method not to be used)
- Breastfeeding or non-breastfeeding <21 days postpartum
- Current breast cancer
- Severe (decompensated) cirrhosis
- Current DVT/PE
- History/higher risk of DVT/PE (not on anticoagulant therapy)
- History/higher risk of DVT/PE (established on anticoagulant therapy for 3 months or greater)
- Thrombogenic mutations
- Major surgery with prolonged immobilization
- Migraines with aura, any age
- Systolic BP ≥160 mm Hg or diastolic ≥100 mm Hg
- Hypertension with vascular disease
- Current and history of ischemic heart disease
- Benign hepatocellular adenoma or malignant liver tumor
- Peripartum cardiomyopathy, moderately or severely impaired cardiac function; normal or mildly impaired cardiac function <6 months
- Smoking ≥15 cigarettes per day and age ≥35
- Complicated solid organ transplantation
- History of cerebrovascular accident
- SLE; positive or unknown antiphospholipid antibodies
- Complicated valvular heart disease

Category 3: Theoretical or proven risks usually outweigh the advantages
- Breastfeeding 21-30 days postpartum with or without risk factors for VTE
- Breastfeeding 30-42 days postpartum with risk factors for VTE
- Non-breastfeeding 21-42 days postpartum with other risk factors for VTE
- Past breast cancer and no evidence of disease for 5 years
- History of DVT/PE (not on anticoagulant therapy or established on anticoagulant therapy for at least 3 months), but lower risk for recurrent DVT/PE
- Current gallbladder disease, symptomatic and medically treated
- History of bariatric surgery; malabsorptive procedures (*COCs only, vaginal ring/transdermal patch category 1*)
- History of cholestasis, past COC-related
- Hypertension; systolic BP 140-159 mm Hg or diastolic 90-99 mm Hg
- Adequately controlled hypertension
- Peripartum cardiomyopathy, normal or mildly impaired cardiac function ≥6 months
- Smoking <15 cigarettes per day and age ≥35
- Use of fosamprenavir
- Use of certain antiseizure medications (phenytoin, carbamazepine, barbiturates, primidone, topiramate, oxcarbazepine, and lamotrigine)
- Use of rifampicin or rifabutin therapy
- Diabetes with vascular disease or >20 years duration (*possibly category 4 depending upon severity*)
- Multiple risk factors for arterial cardiovascular disease (older age, smoking, diabetes, low HDL, high LDL, or high triglycerides and hypertension) (*possibly category 4 depending on category and severity*)
- Acute flare of viral hepatitis (*possibly category 4 depending on severity [initiation]*)
- Multiple sclerosis with prolonged immobility
- Current or history of superficial venous thrombosis

Category 2: Advantages generally outweigh theoretical or proven risks
- Age ≥40 (in the absence of other comorbid conditions that increase CVD risk)
- Sickle cell disease
- Undiagnosed breast mass
- Cervical cancer and awaiting treatment; cervical intraepithelial neoplasia
- Family history (first-degree relatives) of DVT/PE
- Major surgery without prolonged immobilization
- Diabetes mellitus (type 1 or type 2), nonvascular disease
- Gallbladder disease; symptomatic and treated by cholecystectomy or asymptomatic
- Migraines without aura
- History of pregnancy-related cholestasis
- History of high BP during pregnancy
- Benign liver tumors; focal nodular hyperplasia
- Obesity
- Breastfeeding 30-42 days without other VTE risk factors
- Breastfeeding 42 days or more postpartum
- Non-breastfeeding 21-42 days postpartum without risk factors for VTE
- Rheumatoid arthritis on or off immunosuppressive therapy
- Smoking and <35 years old
- Uncomplicated sold organ transplantation
- Stable SLE without antiphospholipid antibodies
- Unexplained vaginal bleeding before evaluation
- Uncomplicated valvular heart disease
- Use of antiretrovirals other than fosamprenavir (*category 1 or 2 depending on agent*)
- Use of St. John's wort
- Inflammatory bowel disease (*possibly category 3 for those with increased risk of VTE*)
- Acute flare of viral hepatitis occurring during use of product (*continuation, category 3 or 4 for initiation of product*)

Category 1: No restriction (method can be used)
- Thalassemia, iron deficiency anemia
- Mild compensated cirrhosis
- Benign ovarian tumors
- Benign breast disease or family history of cancer
- Family history of cancer
- Schistosomiasis
- Cystic fibrosis
- Cervical ectropion
- Viral hepatitis (carrier/chronic)
- Minor surgery without immobilization
- Depression
- Gestational diabetes mellitus
- Endometrial cancer/hyperplasia, endometriosis
- Epilepsy
- Gestational trophoblastic disease
- Nonmigrainous headaches
- History of bariatric surgery; restrictive procedures
- History of pelvic surgery
- HIV infected or high risk
- Malaria
- Multiple sclerosis without prolonged immobility
- Ovarian cancer
- Past ectopic pregnancy
- Parity, parous, or nulliparous
- PID
- Postabortion
- Non-breastfeeding >42 days postpartum
- Severe dysmenorrhea
- STIs
- Varicose veins
- Vaginal bleeding—irregular pattern without heavy bleeding or heavy, prolonged bleeding
- Thyroid disorders
- Tuberculosis
- Uterine fibroids
- Use of SSRIs
- Use of broad-spectrum antibiotics, antifungals, and antiparasitics

CVD, cardiovascular disease; DVT, deep vein thrombosis; HDL, high-density lipoprotein; LDL, low-density lipoprotein; PE, pulmonary embolism; PID, pelvic inflammatory disease; SSRI, selective serotonin reuptake inhibitors.

Data from Reference 17.

6 9 **Vomiting and Severe Diarrhea While on Combined Oral Contraceptives** Efficacy of COCs may be decreased when vomiting or severe diarrhea occurs, and recommendations for dosing in this situation have been developed.[10] These recommendations are based on theoretical concerns and are identical to missed tablet instructions. If vomiting or diarrhea occurs for less than 48 hours, then no redosing of COCs is warranted. If vomiting or diarrhea persists greater than 48 hours then continue taking tablets. If this scenario occurs during the last week of the hormonal tablets, then finish the tablets, skip the hormone-free tablets, and begin a new pack. Patients should be instructed to use additional nonhormonal contraception until hormonal tablets have been taken for seven consecutive days after the vomiting or diarrhea subsides and counsel patients on use of EC if warranted.

3 4 5 **Transdermal Contraceptives** There are two CHCs available as transdermal patches (Xulane, originally marketed as

Ortho Evra, and Twirla). Xulane is a 14-cm^2 square transdermal patch that delivers 35 mcg of EE and 150 mcg of norelgestromin, the active metabolite of norgestimate.[3,4,19] Twirla is a 28 cm^2 circular patch that provides 30 cmg of EE and 120 mcg of levonorgestrel daily.[5] The EE/norelgestromin patch is as effective as COCs in patients weighing less than 90 kg. Of the 15 pregnancies reported in the clinical trials, five were among individuals weighing more than 90 kg; therefore, this product is not recommended as a first-line option for these patients.[3,4,19,20] Similar to the EE/norelgestromin patch, the EE/levonorgestrel patch is recommended for individuals with a BMI of less than 30 kg/m^2, but may also have reduced effectiveness with BMIs ranging from 25 to 30 kg/m^2.[5,19,20] Typical-use failure rates for EE/norelgestromin and EE/levonorgestrel patches are 7% and 3%, respectively (Table 19-1).[3,5]

6 7 ***Managing Transdermal Patch Contraceptive Adverse Medication Effects and Medication Interactions*** Some patients experience application-site reactions, but other adverse medication effects are similar to those experienced with COCs (eg, breast discomfort, headache, breakthrough bleeding, and nausea).[4] A warning from the EE/norelgestromin manufacturer states that individuals using the patch are exposed to approximately 60% more estrogen than from a typical COC containing 35 mcg of EE, which may lead to an increased thromboembolic risk. The labeling for these patches now contains a warning of this risk.[5,17] Medication interactions with the patches are similar to those of COCs. Please see Managing Combined Oral Contraceptive Medication Interactions.

9 **Patient Instructions with Transdermal Patch Contraceptives** The patch is designed to provide estrogen (EE) and progestin (norelgestromin or levonorgestrel) for 7 days. One patch should be worn at a time and applied to the abdomen, buttocks, upper torso, or upper arm. Start applying the patches at the beginning of the menstrual cycle. They should be changed weekly on the same day which is labeled the "Patch Change Day." Apply a new patch weekly for 3 weeks with the fourth week being patch-free for a 4-week cycle.[3,4,5,19]

8 9 **Missed Doses of Transdermal Patch Contraceptives** If the patch detaches and is off less than 24 hours, the detached patch or a new patch can be reapplied, and no additional hormone contraception necessary. If application is delayed for more than 24 hours, start a new 4-week cycle by applying a new patch as soon as possible. An additional nonhormonal contraception should be utilized until the new patch has been worn for 7 consecutive days. This will be the new "Patch Change Day."[15,19] If the delayed application or detachment occurs in the third patch week, the hormone-free week should be omitted and a new patch should be applied immediately.[5,10,19]

If an individual forgets to change the patch at the end of the week, instructions on what to do vary based on where they are in the cycle.[5,19] If they forget to apply a new patch after the hormone-free week, they will need to use a backup method of nonhormonal contraception until they has worn a patch for 7 days. If they forget to apply a new patch in weeks 2 or 3 (left an active hormone patch on and forgot to replace it with a new one) and the delayed application is for only 1 or 2 days (up to 48 hours), a new patch should be applied immediately.[5,19] The next patch should be changed on the same "Patch Change Day," and no backup contraception is needed. If the delayed application of a new patch (old one is still on) is longer than 2 days (more than 48 hours), then they will need to start a new 4-week cycle of patches and use a backup nonhormonal method of contraception until a new patch has been placed for 7 days.[5,19] If the patient forgets to remove the patch for the hormone-free week, they should remove it as soon as they remember and start the next cycle of patches on the regular "Patch Change Day" (day after day 28 of the cycle). No backup contraceptive method is required in this situation. There should not be more than 7 days where a patch is not worn. If this occurs, the individual must use a backup nonhormonal contraceptive method until a new patch has been applied for 7 days.[5,19] Users have greater adherence with the patch than with an COC, but whether this results in reduced pregnancy rates remains to be seen.[3] The benefits of adherence must be weighed against the risk of increased estrogen exposure and possibility of VTE.

Vaginal Rings

3 4 5 There are two marketed vaginal contraceptive rings (NuvaRing and Annovera). NuvaRing is a 54-mm flexible ring, 4 mm in thickness which when vaginally inserted releases approximately 15 mcg/day of EE and 120 mcg/day of etonogestrel.[20] It is formulated to be used for 3 weeks and then discarded.

Annovera is 56 mm in diameter and 8.4 mm in cross-sectional diameter vaginally inserted ring which releases 13 mcg of EE and 150 mcg of segesterone acetate.[6] It is formulated to be used for 3 weeks at a time, but is not discarded. It is used again for a total of 13 cycles.

The vaginal ring is as effective as COCs.

9 **Patient Instructions with Vaginal Ring Contraceptives** On the first cycle of use, the ring should be inserted on or before the fifth day of the menstrual cycle, remain in place for 3 weeks, then removed for 1 week to allow for withdrawal bleeding. The ring should be inserted on the same day of the week as it was during the last cycle, similar to starting a new COC pack or transdermal patch on the same day of the week.

In contrast to diaphragms and cervical caps, precise placement is not an issue because the hormones are absorbed anywhere in the vagina. Individuals should be in a comfortable position, and compress the ring between the thumb and index finger to push it into the vagina. There is no danger of inserting the ring too far because the cervix will prevent it from traveling up the genital tract. Removal of the ring is performed in a similar manner, pulling it out. The NuvaRing should be discarded into the foil patch (the ring should not be flushed down the toilet).[21] The Annovera ring should be removed, washed with warm water, and placed in its original container for later use. After one ring-free week, the Annovera ring can be vaginally inserted again and can be used for a total 13 cycles. Annovera does not require refrigeration, however, NuvaRing may require it if not being used promptly. Individuals should be discouraged from douching, but other vaginal products, including antifungal creams and spermicides, can be used.[3,6,21]

8 9 **Missed Doses of Vaginal Ring Contraceptives** If the NuvaRing has been displaced for less than 3 hours, or less than 2 hours for Annovera, a new ring should be inserted as soon as possible and kept in until the scheduled removal day, with no additional nonhormonal contraception necessary.[6,21] If there is a delay of 3 or more hours, for NuvaRing or 2 or more hours for Annovera, a new ring (for NuvaRing) or current ring (Annovera) should be inserted immediately and either additional nonhormonal contraception should be utilized, or intercourse should be avoided until the ring has been in place for seven consecutive days. If the delayed reinsertion occurs during the third week of ring use, a new ring (for NuvaRing) or current ring (for Annovera) can be reinserted right away to start the next 21-day cycle. There may be some spotting or vaginal bleeding.

If a person forgets to remove the ring after the third week, and there has been prolonged use of the ring for up to one extra week (not more than 4 weeks in place for NuvaRing), they will still be protected and no backup protection will be necessary. Though, the individual should take into account the number of extra weeks the Annovera ring was inserted vaginally and subtract those weeks from the total 13 cycles for use. The ring should be removed for the ring-free week, and a new ring can be inserted after the ring-free week. If NuvaRing has been left in place longer than 4 weeks, the ring should be removed. The individual should then check for possible pregnancy. Once pregnancy has been ruled out, a new cycle of the vaginal ring with 7 days of a nonhormonal contraceptive method may be started.[6,21] With Annovera, a ring-free week should occur and then the regular 3-week ring cycle should be restarted.

6 7 Managing Vaginal Ring Contraceptive Adverse Medication Effects and Medication Interactions Adverse medication effects, precautions, and contraindications for use of the vaginal ring are similar to those for all CHCs. Specific medication interactions with Annovera have been reported that include 1-day or the 3-day oil-based miconazole suppository use increasing exposure up to 67% for EE and 32% for segesterone acetate. These medications and oil-based vaginal suppositories should be avoided with Annovera. Water-based products may be used. Unlike NuvaRing, tampon use with Annovera should be avoided until further studies are completed. The most common reasons for discontinuation of use were device-related issues, such as foreign-body sensation, device expulsion, and vaginal symptoms.[6,21] Cycle control with the vaginal ring appears to be equal or better than with COCs, with a low incidence of breakthrough bleeding and spotting after the second cycle of use. Patient acceptability of the delivery system has been studied, and the majority of patients do not complain of discomfort in general or during intercourse.[4,6,21] A potential concern is the possibility of increased VTE.[6,21]

2 3 4 5 Considerations with Combined Hormonal Contraceptive Use

When selecting a CHC, clinicians are challenged by weighing the benefits and risks associated with the many formulations available. The clinician must determine if the form of contraception is appropriate based upon the patient's lifestyle and potential adherence. A complete medical examination and papanicolaou (Pap) smear are not necessary before a CHC is prescribed. A medical history and BP measurement should be obtained before prescribing a CHC, along with a discussion of the benefits, risks, and adverse effects with each patient.[3,10,17] For example, OCs are associated with noncontraceptive benefits, including relief from menstruation-related problems (eg, decreased menstrual cramps, decreased ovulatory pain [mittelschmerz], and decreased menstrual blood loss), improvement in menstrual regularity, alleviating acne and premenstrual dysphoric disorder, and decreased iron deficiency anemia.[3] Individuals who take COCs have a reduced risk of ovarian and endometrial cancer, which is a 50% reduction after 5 years or more. This protection may persist for more than 10 years post-use.[3] COCs may also reduce the risk of ovarian cysts, ectopic pregnancy, pelvic inflammatory disease (PID), endometriosis, uterine fibroids, and benign breast disease. The CHC transdermal patches and vaginal rings are combined hormonal options that may be more convenient than taking a tablet each day.

3 4 6 9 Adverse effects may hinder adherence and therefore efficacy, so they should be discussed prior to initiating a hormonal contraceptive agent.[10,17] Excessive or deficient amounts of estrogen and progestin are related to the most common adverse effects.[3,10] An important concern regarding the use of CHCs is the lack of protection against STIs/STDs. Because of their high efficacy in preventing pregnancy, patients may choose not to use condoms. In addition to public health awareness, clinicians must encourage patients to use condoms for prevention of STIs/STDs. The health risks associated with pregnancy, the specific health risks associated with CHCs, and the noncontraceptive benefits of CHCs should be factored into risk-to-benefit considerations. To help provide guidance on absolute and relative contraindications to CHC use, the CDC developed a graded list of precautions for clinicians to consider when initiating CHCs (Table 19-6).[10,17]

Individuals Older Than 35 Years Use of a CHC in individuals older than 35 is controversial. Older individuals, especially those in their 40s, retain a level of fertility even in the perimenopausal state and can use hormonal contraception to prevent pregnancy. Formulations with lower doses of estrogen (less than 30 mcg) have increased the use of CHCs in these individuals. In addition to the benefit of pregnancy prevention, they may improve or decrease the chance of developing perimenopausal and menopausal symptoms and increase bone mineral density (BMD). However, the benefits of using CHCs must be weighed against the risks in individuals older than 35. The increased risk of VTE should be considered especially in perimenopausal individuals older than 40. Older data suggest an increased risk of myocardial infarction (MI) is present in older individuals using CHCs, although many of who in these studies were current smokers and used older formulations containing higher doses (greater than 50 mcg) of estrogen. There is no increased risk of cardiovascular disease when low-dose formulations of CHCs are used in healthy, nonobese individuals. Other concerns include the increased risk of ischemic stroke in those with migraines and the increased risk of breast cancer in older individuals.[4,17]

The risks and benefits of using CHCs in individuals greater than 35 must be considered on an individual basis. The use of CHCs (with less than 50 mcg of estrogen) may be considered in healthy nonsmoking individuals. CHCs should not be recommended in individuals older than 35 years with migraine (with aura), uncontrolled hypertension, smoking, or diabetes with vascular disease.[4,17]

Smoking COCs with 50 mcg EE or more were associated with MI in individuals who smoked cigarettes.[3,4] The US case-control studies have found that both nonsmoking and smoking individuals taking OCs with less than 50 mcg EE did not have an increased risk of MI or stroke, regardless of age. However, these studies included few patients older than 35 years who were smokers. European studies, with a higher population of older smoking individuals, demonstrated an increased risk of MI in this population. Therefore, practitioners should prescribe CHC with caution, if at all, to those older than 35 years who smoke. Smoking 15 or more cigarettes per day by those in this age group is a contraindication to CHCs, and the risks generally outweigh the benefits of CHCs in those who smoke fewer than 15 cigarettes per day.[4,17] Progestin-only or nonhormonal contraceptive methods should be considered for individuals in this group.

Hypertension CHCs can cause small increases (ie, 6-8 mm Hg) in BP, regardless of estrogen dosage.[4,17] This is presented in both normotensive and mildly hypertensive individuals when given an OC with 30 mcg EE. OCs have been associated with an increased risk of MI and stroke. Use of low-dose CHC is acceptable in those younger than 35 years with well-controlled and frequently monitored hypertension. If a CHC-related increase in BP occurs, CHC discontinuation usually restores BP to pretreatment values within 3 to 6 months.[4] Systolic BP ≥160 mm Hg or diastolic BP ≥100 mm Hg is considered a contraindication to the use of CHCs. Hypertensive individuals who have a systolic BP of 140 to 159 or diastolic BP of 90 to 99 mm Hg should also avoid CHCs as the risks generally outweigh the benefits. Risks versus benefits should be considered for those who have additional cardiovascular risk factors along with hypertension. Individuals with hypertension who are taking potassium-sparing diuretics, angiotensin-converting enzyme inhibitors, angiotensin-receptor blockers, or aldosterone antagonists may have increased serum potassium concentrations if they are also using an OC-containing drospirenone, which has anti-aldosterone properties.[4,7,18]

Dyslipidemia Generally, synthetic progestins may adversely affect lipid metabolism by decreasing high-density lipoprotein (HDL) and increasing low-density lipoprotein (LDL).[4,17] Estrogens tend to have more beneficial effects by enhancing removal of LDL and increasing HDL levels. They may also moderately increase triglycerides. Today, most low-dose CHCs have no significant impact on HDL,

LDL, triglycerides, or total cholesterol, although historically this was not felt to be true. Although the lipid effects of CHCs theoretically can influence cardiovascular risk, the mechanism of increased cardiovascular disease in CHC users is believed to be due to thromboembolic and thrombotic changes, not atherosclerosis. CHCs use is generally acceptable in individuals with dyslipidemia as the single cardiovascular risk factor. However, careful consideration should be taken in persons with dyslipidemia along with other cardiovascular risk factors and in many cases alternative methods of contraception may be recommended.

Diabetes Any effect of CHCs on carbohydrate metabolism is thought to be due to the progestin component.[4,17] However, most products used today contain low doses of progestins and do not significantly alter insulin, glucose, or glucagon release or daily insulin requirements. CHCs do not appear to alter the hemoglobin A_{1C} values or accelerate the development of microvascular complications in individuals with diabetes. Therefore, nonsmoking patients younger than 35 years with diabetes but no associated vascular disease can safely use CHCs. Diabetic individuals with vascular disease (eg, nephropathy, retinopathy, neuropathy, or other vascular disease) or diabetes of more than 20 years duration should not use CHCs.[4,17]

Migraine Headaches Individuals with migraine headaches may experience a decreased or an increased frequency of migraine headaches when using CHCs.[4,17,22] A higher risk of stroke is seen in patients experiencing migraine with aura compared to those with simple migraine. The risk of stroke in individuals with migraines has been elevated twofold to threefold. However, given the low absolute risk of stroke in those less than 35 years of age, CHCs in healthy, nonsmoking individuals with migraine headaches without aura may still be considered.[17] Likewise, individuals with nonmigrainous headaches may also use CHCs without restriction. However, individuals of any age who have migraine with aura should not use CHC,[1] and those who develop migraines with aura while receiving CHC should discontinue use and consider a progestin-only option.[17] Individuals developing migraines without aura while receiving CHC should have their headaches evaluated to determine severity, evaluate for signs of an aura, and to discuss the risk versus benefit of CHC use.[17]

Breast Cancer Worldwide epidemiologic data from 54 studies in 25 countries (many of which studied high-dose OCs) were collected to assess the relationship between COCs and breast cancer.[3,4] Overall, investigators noted a small increase in the relative risk of having breast cancer diagnosed while COCs are taken and for up to 10 years following discontinuance. There is no increased excess risk of diagnosis 10 years or more after COCs are discontinued. A 2010 analysis of data from the Nurses' Health Study also found that individuals who used OCs had a slight increase in breast cancer risk.[23] In 2017, a large prospective Danish study reported breast cancer risks associated with more recent formulations of COCs.[24] Overall, those who were using or had recently discontinued using hormonal contraception had a modest (20%) increase in the relative risk of breast cancer compared with individuals who had never used hormonal contraception. The risk increased the longer the hormones were used and in individuals over the age of 40. If hormones are discontinued, the breast cancer risk returns to the same levels seen for persons who never used them, although it may take longer for those who had taken for more than 5 to 10 years. For healthy young individuals, the benefits of hormonal contraception in preventing unwanted pregnancies and associated other benefits outweigh any risks. For those over the age of 40 or those who have an elevated risk of breast cancer because of family history or other factors, alternatives may be considered. The choice to use CHCs should not be affected by the presence of benign breast disease or a family history of breast cancer with either mutation. In individuals identified with BRCA1 or BRCA2 mutations, increased risk of breast cancer with COCs has been controversial. The results of two large, case-controlled studies have found conflicting results. Until additional data refutes or affirms these studies, it is important to understand these risks and assure they are discussed with patients as even a small increase in risk may be clinically important.[25,26] Patients with current or past history of breast cancer should not use CHCs.[3,4,17]

Thromboembolism Estrogens increase hepatic production of factor VII, factor X, and fibrinogen in the coagulation cascade, therefore increasing thromboembolic event risk (eg, deep vein thrombosis and pulmonary embolism). These risks are increased in individuals who have underlying hypercoagulable states (eg, deficiencies in antithrombin III, protein C, and protein S; factor V Leiden mutations, prothrombin G2010 A mutations) or who have acquired conditions (eg, obesity, pregnancy, immobility, trauma, surgery, and certain malignancies) that predispose them to coagulation abnormalities.[3,4,17] The incidence of thromboembolism and mortality is increased threefold in current OC users compared to nonusers. However, this risk is still less than the risk of VTE incurred during pregnancy. COCs containing new progestins such as third-generation progestins (eg, desogestrel and norgestimate) and a fourth-generation progestin (eg, drospirenone) have been associated with a slightly higher risk of thromboembolism.[3,4] Although the mechanisms for this increased risk is unclear, this increased risk may be due to: (a) a greater effect on the procoagulant, anticoagulant, and fibrinolytic pathways than earlier generation progestins; (b) an increased resistance to the anticoagulant effect of activated protein C; (c) increased levels of sex hormone-binding globulin; and (d) antiandrogenic effects of drospirenone make the CHC more estrogenic.[2,3,27,28] A continuous, higher exposure to estrogen seen with the transdermal patch or vaginal ring is the reason for an increased thromboembolic risk with these agents as well.[27] An advisory committee to the FDA decided to change the product labeling of the transdermal patch as well as products containing drospirenone to include additional information about the increased risk of thromboembolism.[18,19] In addition, the vaginal ring also has an additional precaution in the product labeling.[21] Therefore, for individuals at an increased risk of thromboembolism (eg, older than 35 years, obesity, smoking, personal or family history of venous thrombosis, prolonged immobilization), it would be prudent to first consider low-dose oral estrogen contraceptives containing older progestins, progestin-only contraceptive methods, or barrier methods. A recent systematic review of progestin-only contraceptives did not suggest an overall significant increase in venous or arterial events.[29] Limited evidence suggests slight increases in thromboembolism in those using these for therapeutic indications or in those with other thromboembolic risk factors. Any slight increase in risk likely translates to a small increase in absolute numbers of thrombotic events at the population level.

Weighing the risks versus benefits of using CHCs containing third- and fourth-generation progestins, transdermal patch, and vaginal ring to determine their place in therapy is controversial. The risk of VTE with CHC use is 3 to 12 per 10,000 person-years, compared with 1 to 5 per 10,000 person-years in non-CHC users and nonpregnant biologically female individuals.[3] The risk increases to about 10 per 10,000 person-years with drospirenone-containing COCs.[30] Risk of VTE is also higher with the transdermal patch and possibly with the vaginal ring.[30] A continuous, higher exposure to estrogen seen with these formulations may be the cause of this increased risk. Regardless of contraceptive product, the risk is still lower than the risk of thromboembolism during pregnancy (5-20 per 10,000 person-years).[27,31]

Obesity The prevalence of obesity continues to rise each year among all age groups including patients of childbearing age. Individuals with increased body weight have increased basal metabolic rates and induction of hepatic enzymes, leading to increased hormonal clearance and decreased serum concentrations of hormonal contraceptives. In addition, patients who are obese have more adipose tissue, increasing hormonal sequestration, and decreased free hormone serum concentrations resulting in lower efficacy.[3,4] There is an additional two to four pregnancies per 100 person-years of use in overweight or obese users.[20,32] Regardless of body weight, IUDs, implants, and DMPA have low failure rates, and progestin-only contraceptives are considered safe in obese indiiduals.[17,20] In addition, the advantages of using an estrogen-containing contraceptive method (pill, patch, ring) generally outweigh the risks.[10,17] DMPA is associated with more weight gain than other methods.[3] With regard to EC, the copper IUD is the most reliable method in obese individuals. Oral EC products may be less effective and the effectiveness of levonorgestrel, in particular, is diminished.[33]

Obese individuals are also at risk of VTE, although studies evaluating the incidence of thromboembolism in obese persons taking hormonal contraceptives have produced conflicting results. With low-dose estrogen containing products, the incidence increases from 5 to 10 cases in nonusers to 15 to 30 cases in users per 10,000 person-years. At baseline, obesity doubles the risk of thromboembolism compared to someone with a normal BMI. Progestin-only hormonal contraception may be more appropriate for obese individuals over the age of 35 years, although the CDC considers the benefits of estrogen-containing contraceptives to outweigh the risks as well.[17,20] Patients should be counseled on any risks and consider alternative contraceptive methods on an individual basis.[20] The risk of thromboembolism during pregnancy and in the peripartum period is significantly greater than the risk with any hormonal contraceptive agent.

Postpartum Use of CHCs In the postpartum phase, there is concern about use of CHCs due to hypercoagulability risks and the effects on lactation. In the first 21 days postpartum (when the risk of thrombosis is higher), estrogen-containing hormonal contraceptives should be avoided (see Table 19-6).[17] If contraception is required during this period, progestin-only contraceptive methods may be acceptable alternatives. Individuals breastfeeding muss avoid CHCs for the first 42 days postpartum if they have risk factors for VTE and for 30 days without risk factors. In those individuals who are not breastfeeding, CHCs should be avoided for up to 42 days postpartum in those with risk factors for VTE.[17] After 42 days postpartum, there is no restriction to the use of CHCs.

Systemic Lupus Erythematosus Contraception is important in biologically female individuals with systemic lupus erythematosus (SLE) because the risks associated with pregnancy are high in this population. CHCs exacerbated the symptoms of SLE,[4] postulating that estrogen may cause cutaneous lupus to progress to systemic lupus by promoting B-cell hyper-responsiveness and inducing or increasing autoimmunity.[4] OCs with less than 50 mcg ethinyl estradiol do not increase the risk of flare in individuals with stable SLE without antiphospholipid/anticardiolipin antibodies. Therefore, CHCs should be avoided in patients with SLE and antiphospholipid antibodies or vascular complications as the risks outweigh the benefits of progestin-only contraceptive use in patient population. The copper IUD may be the best option in this situation.[17] For patients with SLE without antiphospholipid antibodies or vascular complications, progestin-only contraceptives or the copper IUD may be an alternative to CHCs; however, those with SLE and severe thrombocytopenia should avoid the copper IUD and DMPA injection.[17]

Discontinuing Combined Hormonal Contraceptives and Return of Fertility There is no evidence that CHC, transdermal patches, or vaginal ring use decreases subsequent fertility.[3] Return to fertility with CHC use is usually within a few months.[3] However, delayed ovulation is more common in individuals with a history of irregular menses. If amenorrhea does continue beyond 6 months, patients should be counseled to see a physician for further fertility workup.[3,4] Individuals were counseled to allow two to three normal menstrual periods before becoming pregnant to permit the reestablishment of menses and ovulation. However, infants conceived in the first month after discontinuation of an OC had no greater chance of miscarriage or being born with a birth defect than those born in the general population.

Progestin-Only Contraceptives

3 4 5 There are a few hormonal contraceptives that contain only progestin. Formulations include oral tablets, injections, a subdermal implant, and IUDs. Sustained progestin exposure blocks the LH surge, thus inhibiting ovulation. Should ovulation occur, progestins reduce ovum motility in the fallopian tubes. Even if fertilization occurs, progestins thin the endometrium, reducing the chance of implantation. Progestins also thicken the cervical mucus, producing a barrier to sperm penetration. Individuals who may benefit from progestin-only contraceptives are those who are breastfeeding, those who are intolerant to estrogens (ie, have a history of estrogen-related headache, breast tenderness, or nausea), or those with concomitant medical conditions or contraindications in which estrogen is not recommended (see Table 19-6). This method of contraception does not provide any protection from STIs/STDs.[3,4]

8 9 **Oral Progestin-Only Contraceptives and Administration** There are two progestin-only oral products available, norethindrone and drospirenone. Norethindrone tablets are also known as "minipills" and have similar effectiveness to COCs with a perfect-use failure rate of 0.3% and typical-use failure of 7% (Table 19-1).[3] The norethindrone 35-mg product consists of 28 days of active hormone per cycle, which must be taken every day of the menstrual cycle at approximately the same time to maintain contraceptive efficacy. As with other OCs, initiating norethindrone tablets may be done any time during the cycle. If taken within the first 5 days of menstrual bleeding, a backup contraceptive method is not required. Starting any other time in the cycle requires an additional contraceptive method for 2 days.[10] If a norethindrone-only OC is taken more than 3 hours late, patients should use a backup method of contraception for 48 hours.[3]

Drospirenone 4-mg tablets known as the product Slynd contain 24 days of active hormone and 4 days placebo. Drospirenone-only tablets have a typical-use failure rate of 4%.[7] Slynd can be started on day 1 of menses with no additional backup method. If started later in the cycle, a backup contraceptive method is required.[7] There is more flexibility in dose administration with drospirenone compared with norethindrone, a missed dose is considered more than 24 hours after the scheduled administration time. The individual can take the missed tablet as soon as possible and continue with the pill pack as no backup contraception is needed. If two or more active tablets are missed, the individual should take the last missed tablet as soon as possible and continue taking one tablet daily as instructed while using an additional contraceptive method for 7 days.[7]

3 6 7 **Oral Progestin-Only Contraceptives Adverse Effects, and Considerations** Progestin-only pills may not block ovulation, as nearly 40% of patients continue to ovulate normally, so the risk of ectopic pregnancy is higher with their use than with other hormonal contraceptives. Common progestin adverse medication effects may include: irregular menses, acne, headache, nausea, or libido changes. Drospirenone products may have less acne adverse medication effects, but may need monitoring for thromboembolism, hyperkalemia, and bone loss.[7]

Medication interactions are also a consideration for oral progestin-only tablets. In particular, norethindrone formulations are metabolized via the liver through the cytochrome P450 system. Medications that induce the P450 system like phenytoin, carbamazepine, oxcarbazepine, primidone, topiramate, protease inhibitors, and St. John's wort, as examples may affect oral progestin metabolism.[17] With the exception of rifampin, broad spectrum antibiotics do not affect levels of oral progestins.[17] Considerations for drospirenone-only tablets also include medications that may increase potassium levels, such as ACE inhibitors, potassium-sparing diuretics, and high-dose ibuprofen. The concurrent use of these medications with drospirenone should be avoided due to the potential risk of hyperkalemia.

Similar to estrogen containing contraceptives, oral progestin-only contraceptives should be avoided in individuals with a history of breast cancer, unexplained bleeding, and SLE with antiphospholipids. Caution may be needed in patients with a history of current VTE, complicated diabetes, heart or hepatic disease.[17] Starting oral progestin contraceptives postpartum or while breastfeeding may be used though follow-up may be required per the CDC recommendations.[17]

Progestin Injections

Steroid hormones provide longer-term contraception when injected into the skin. In addition, injectable progestins are beneficial for individuals with adherence issues, as they have lower failure rates than CHC methods (see Table 19-1).[3,6,17]

Depo-Provera (DMPA) is similar in structure to naturally occurring progesterone and is administered every 3 months either by deep intramuscular injection in the gluteal or deltoid muscle or subcutaneously in the abdomen or thigh within 5 days of onset of menstrual bleeding.[34,35] With perfect use, the efficacy of DMPA is more than 99%; however, with typical use, 3% of individuals experience unintended pregnancy.[3] The primary mechanism of action is suppression of ovulation. Depo-Provera is available as a 150 mg/mL injection vial or prefilled syringe for IM injection, and Depo-SubQ Provera 104 mg is available as a prefilled syringe.[34,35] The subcutaneous formulation is also FDA-approved for use in treating endometriosis. Administration of both formulations of DMPA requires a medical office visit; however, studies of patient self-administration of subcutaneous DMPA have demonstrated positive results.[36,37]

5 8 9 Progestin Injection Administration Depo-Provera may be administered at any time as long as it is reasonably certain that the patient is not pregnant.[1,34,35] If it is administered between days 1 and 7 of the menstrual cycle in individuals who have not previously used hormonal contraception, then no backup method is needed.[10] If it is administered at any other time of the menstrual cycle, then an additional nonhormonal contraceptive is needed as backup method for 7 days. Additional recommendations on initiating the implant when switching from other methods of contraception are included in the package insert.[34,35] Although these injections may inhibit ovulation for up to 14 weeks, the dose should be repeated every 3 months (12 weeks) to ensure continuous contraception. The patient must be confirmed to not be pregnant if there is a lapse of more than 13 weeks between injections for the intramuscular formulation or 14 or more weeks between injections for the subcutaneous formulation. However, CDC recommendations differ and state for either formulation, and pregnancy should be excluded in individuals with a lapse of 15 or more weeks.[10]

3 4 5 6 Progestin Injection Considerations As with other contraceptive agents, concomitant conditions should be evaluated prior to use of DMPA. Although no adverse effects have been documented in infants exposed to DMPA through breast milk, DMPA must not be initiated until 6 weeks postpartum in breastfeeding patients.[34,35] However, the CDC cites a lack of evidence supporting this claim and classifies DMPA use during this time frame as a category 1 or 2 suggesting that the benefit may outweigh the theoretical risk.[17] Patients who are not breastfeeding but require contraception can receive DMPA immediately postpartum.[17] It is contraindicated in individuals with a current diagnosis of breast cancer due to potential hormonally sensitive tumors, and should be used with precaution in those with a past history of breast cancer, vascular, cardiovascular, or cerebrovascular disease, multiple risk factors for cardiovascular disease, and lupus. There is some concern that the impact of DMPA on lipids (potentially decreased HDL) and the hypoestrogenic pharmacologic effects may increase the risk of a vascular event. However, the risks with DMPA are much lower than with CHCs so risks and benefits should be weighed on an individual basis.[17] Patients with sickle cell disease are good candidates for DMPA, due to a reduction in sickle cell pain crises in those using DMPA.[17] In addition, patients with seizure disorders may experience fewer seizures when taking DMPA for contraception, and there is not a concern with antiseizure medications reducing the contraceptive efficacy of DMPA.[3,17] Because return of fertility may be delayed after discontinuation of DMPA, it should not be recommended to individuals desiring pregnancy in the near future. The median time to conception from the first omitted dose is 10 months and 68% of those are able to conceive within 12 months, 83% within 15 months, and 93% within 18 months of the last injection.[3,34,35]

6 Progestin Injection Adverse Effects Menstrual irregularities are the most frequent adverse effects of both formulations of DMPA and are most common in the first year of use. These irregularities include spotting, prolonged bleeding, and amenorrhea; counseling patients on these possibilities is important before initiation of the method.[10,17] Individuals who cannot tolerate prolonged bleeding may benefit from a short course of NSAIDs (for 5-7 days) during the bleeding, and in addition, a short course of estrogen (if no contraindications are present) for approximately 10 to 20 days.[4] The incidence of irregular bleeding decreases from 30% to 50% in the first 2 years to 10% thereafter, and after 12 months of therapy, 55% of patients report amenorrhea, with the incidence increasing to 68% after 2 years.[34,35]

Other adverse effects, including breast tenderness and depression, occur less commonly. Weight gain is a concern for many patients using DMPA, and the incidence and amount gained vary widely. It has been reported that weight gain averages 1 kg annually and may not resolve until 6 to 8 months after the last injections. In clinical trials 38% of patients reported a weight gain of great than 10 lbs (4.5 kg) at 24 months.[3,4,34,35] However, use of DMPA in obese patients should not be excluded. Appropriate consideration of multiple factors should be evaluated for obese patients and individualized decisions made. For all patients, weight and BMI should be monitored for patients receiving DMPA.[10,17]

DMPA has been associated with short-term bone loss in younger individuals of reproductive age. This potential side effect may be due to lower ovarian estrogen production that occurs when gonadotropin secretion is suppressed.[3,38] Because longitudinal studies demonstrated effects on BMD, the FDA issued a black box warning for DMPA in 2004.[34,35] It states that DMPA should be continued for more than 2 years, only if other contraceptive methods are inadequate. It also states that the loss of BMD seems to be greater with increasing duration of use and may not be completely reversible. However, the majority of clinicians view the effects of DMPA on BMD (which in the majority of cases is reversible) as a surrogate marker and there are no clear data that demonstrate the effects of DMPA on fracture risk.[38,39] The ACOG and CDC continue to recommend that for most patients the benefits of DMPA outweigh the risks even when used beyond 2 years of use.[10,36] It is not routinely recommended to use DMPA in individuals on long-term corticosteroids (eg, patients with rheumatoid arthritis) with a history or high risk of fractures.[17] While the ACOG does not recommend the routine screening of BMD in most patients, a discussion regarding the risks and benefits of this contraceptive option is recommended prior to initiation and with prolonged use.[38]

3 4 5 Subdermal Progestin Implants Nexplanon (similar to the original product Implanon marketed in the United States) is a single 4-cm-long implant, containing 68 mg of etonogestrel, which releases etonogestrel at a rate of 60 mcg daily for the first month, then decreases to an average of 30 mcg daily at the end of the 3 years of recommended use. The etonogestrel implant is placed under the skin of the upper arm using a preloaded inserter,[3,40] and clinicians must receive training from the manufacturer to properly insert or remove of the device. The primary mechanism of action is suppression of ovulation. When ovulation is not suppressed, etonogestrel still is effective as the progestin thickens the cervical mucus and produces an atrophic endometrium. With both perfect and typical use, the efficacy rate is over 99%.[3,40] However, in overweight and obese individuals weighing more than 130% of their ideal body weight, the efficacy is possibly decreased. However, it is noted that overweight individuals were excluded from studies, and recent small studies have not demonstrated any decreased effects.[40]

9 **Progestin Implant Insertion** The etonogestrel implant can be inserted at any time as long as it is reasonably certain the individual is not pregnant.[13,40] If the implant is inserted between days 1 and 5 of the menstrual cycle in those who have not previously used hormonal contraception then no backup method is needed.[13,40] If it is inserted at any other time of the menstrual cycle, then an additional nonhormonal contraceptive is needed as backup method for 7 days. Additional recommendations on initiating the implant when switching from other methods of contraception are included in the package insert.[40] After removal, fertility returns within 30 days.

6 **Progestin Implant Adverse Effects** The major adverse effect associated with Nexplanon is irregular menstrual bleeding, which led to discontinuation of the implant in 11% of patients in clinical trials.[40,41] Patients should be counseled about the risk of irregular bleeding patterns so that patients will not request early removal of Nexplanon. Some individuals (22%) became amenorrheic with continued use, but many continued to have prolonged bleeding and spotting (18% and 34%, respectively) and frequent bleeding (7%).[10,40] Those who cannot tolerate prolonged bleeding may benefit from a short course of NSAIDs (for 5-7 days) during the bleeding and from a short course of estrogen (if no contraindications are present) for approximately 10 to 20 days.[14] Insertion and removal complications are rare (less than 2%).[40] Nexplanon is radio opaque, making it easy to locate for removal by conducting an x-ray if needed.[13] Information from the manufacturer suggests using precaution when there is potential for medication interactions in the presence of potent CYP450 inducers (eg, rifampin, phenytoin, and carbamazepine).[40] This information conflicts with CDC recommendations which classify combining those medications with Nexplanon as a category 2, and suggest that the benefits may outweigh the theoretical risks. However, the CDC does still recommend use of additional nonhormonal contraception or switching to DMPA or an IUD as the preferred methods of managing these potential medication interactions.[17]

Intrauterine Devices

3 4 5 Currently, five IUDs are available, four of them contain levonorgestrel (Mirena, Skyla, Liletta, and Kyleena), one contains copper (ParaGard T 380A, many times referred to as ParaGard). All of the mentioned IUDs are T-shaped and clinicians must receive training from the manufacturer to learn effective insertion or removal of the IUDs. These IUDs have several possible mechanisms of action, including inhibition of sperm migration, damaging ovum or disrupting transport, and possibly damaging the fertilized ovum.[3] Due to the presence of local progestin, the Mirena, Skyla, Liletta, and Kyleena IUDs have additional mechanisms of endometrial suppression and thickening cervical mucus. The most recent evidence regarding the mechanisms of action demonstrates that the contraceptive activity of IUDs occurs before implantation.[3,41] Efficacy rates with IUDs are greater than 99% with both perfect- and typical-use,[3,41] and should not be inserted in the presence of current pregnancy, current PID, current STI/STD, puerperal or postabortion sepsis, purulent cervicitis, undiagnosed abnormal vaginal bleeding, malignancy of genital tract, uterine anomalies or fibroids distorting uterine cavity, allergy to an IUD component, or Wilson's disease (for copper IUD).[42,43] If an IUD is already in place and the patient contracts an STI/STD, the IUD in most cases can remain in place while the STI/STD is being treated.[3,17] The risk of PID among IUD users is low, and there are no long-term effects on fertility, and average time to return of fertility is similar to oral contracpetives.[41] The influence of medication interactions on the efficacy of IUDs is not a primary concern based on manufacturer and CDC recommendations.[42-46]

6 9 ParaGard is a highly effective IUD that contains copper and can be left in place for 10 years.[3,42] A disadvantage of ParaGard is increased menstrual blood flow and dysmenorrhea, as the average monthly blood loss among users increased by 35%. Mirena, Skyla, Liletta, and Kyleena contain the progestin levonorgestrel and are approved for the prevention of pregnancy in the United States.[42-46] Mirena is also approved for up to 5 years of use for the treatment of heavy menstrual bleeding.[43] Liletta and Mirena can be used for up to 6 years and release 20 mcg of levonorgestrel daily, decreasing over time.[43,44] Kyleena can be used for up to 5 years and releases 17.5 mcg of levonorgestrel daily, decreasing over time.[46] Skyla can be used for up to 3 years and releases 14 mcg of levonorgestrel daily, decreasing over time.[45] For all of the levonorgestrel IUDs, the systemic absorption of the progestin is minimal and considerably less than with OCs. There are no direct comparisons of safety or efficacy; when used appropriately all are highly effective and well tolerated.

Intrauterine Device Insertion

9 IUDs can be inserted at any time as long as it is reasonably certain that the user is not pregnant.[10] If the IUD is inserted between days 1 and 7 of the menstrual cycle in those who have not previously used hormonal contraception, then no backup method is needed. If it is inserted at any other time of the menstrual cycle, then it is recommended to use an additional nonhormonal contraceptive backup method for 7 days. Additional recommendations on initiating an IUD when switching from other methods of contraception are included in the package inserts.

Concerns about pain and infection upon insertion of the IUD are common; however, for most patients, insertion-pain is minimal and is not prolonged. If needed, common OTC pain relievers such as NSAIDs or acetaminophen may be helpful. Premedicating with misoprostol or paracervical lidocaine blocks have been studied,[10] but based on the evidence, misoprostol is not recommended for most patients due to lack of efficacy. Paracervical lidocaine blocks may be recommended for pain reduction, but it is not a commonly accepted standard of care. Risk of infection upon IUD insertion is minimal, and it is not recommended to prophylactically treat with antibiotics.[10] Individuals with current PID or STI/STD should delay having their IUD inserted. In contrast, users with an IUD in place that develop PID or an STI/STD should treat the infection, but it is not typically recommended to remove the IUD. Users who have not been screened for STIs/STDs according to CDC guidelines should be screened at the same time as insertion. If results come back positive, then the STI/STD can be treated at that time.[10]

Intrauterine Device Adverse Effects

6 The major adverse effect associated with IUDs is irregular menstrual bleeding. The levonorgestrel IUD produces its effects locally via suppression of the endometrium, causing a reduction in menstrual blood loss over time. In contrast to the copper IUD, menstrual flow in users of the levonorgestrel IUD is decreased, and development of amenorrhea has been observed in 20% of users in the first year and 60% in the fifth year. Mirena specifically has an additional indication for treatment of heavy menstrual bleeding (menorrhagia).[42] A

disadvantage of the levonorgestrel IUD is increased spotting in the first 6 months of use; users should be counseled that the spotting will decline gradually over time.[3,42] Those who cannot tolerate prolonged bleeding may benefit from a short course of NSAIDs (for 5-7 days) during the bleeding. In addition, a short course of estrogen (if no contraindications are present) could be used for approximately 10 to 20 days.[10]

IUD use in nulliparious and adolescent individuals was considered a precaution. However, recent evidence, clinical experience, and expert opinion do not preclude use in these populations. Risks versus benefits should be considered, and the users must be counseled on the efficacy and potential adverse effects.[41,47] Strong consideration of an IUD is appropriate in this population due to high efficacy rates and low complication rates.[47] In addition, Skyla and Liletta included adolescent patients less than 18 years of age in clinical trials.[44,45]

Long-Acting Reversible Contraception

3 5 Long-acting reversible contraception (LARC) refers to a category of hormonal and nonhormonal contraceptives that include IUDs and implants. This type of contraception is highly efficacious in preventing pregnancy, but the effects are quickly reversible upon removal.[41] As LARC does not require effort or adherence by the patient once they are inserted, perfect-use and typical-use efficacy rates do not differ, and the efficacy rate is similar to that of surgical options such as tubal ligation (see Table 19-1).[3,41] When compared to other methods of hormonal contraception, especially OCs, LARC methods are not used as frequently in the United States; however, increased education campaigns are demonstrating effectiveness. The use of LARC has increased to 14% of all individuals biologically female between the ages of 15 and 44,[48] and all patients should be considered potential candidates for this method.[41,47] Due to the high efficacy rates and emerging evidence of LARC methods, increased use may decrease unintended pregnancy rates.[41]

Emergency Contraception

10 EC is used to prevent unintended pregnancy after unprotected or inadequately protected sexual intercourse (eg, no contraception, condom breakage, contraceptive mishap, or nonadherence, sexual assault). Pregnancy occurs when the fertilized egg is implanted into the endometrial lining. After intercourse, implantation of the fertilized egg typically takes approximately 5 days.[49] Progestin-only and progesterone receptor modulator products are approved by the FDA and recommended as first-line EC options.[3,4,49] Insertion of ParaGard (copper IUD) or prescribing higher doses of COCs (Yuzpe method) are other options.

Currently, the progestin-only formulation containing levonorgestrel 1.5 mg tablet × 1 dose (currently marketed in a variety of products, including Aftera, EContra EZ, EContra One-Step, My Way, New Day, Opcicon One-Step, Plan B One Step, Preventeza, React and Take Action) is approved specifically for EC in the United States.[13,16] The primary mechanism of action of progestin-only EC is inhibiting or delaying ovulation.[49] The levonorgestrel-containing EC formulation is the regimen of choice due to availability, improved tolerability, and potentially increased efficacy rates. All formulations are now offered as one-dose options, to be given within 72 hours (3 days) of unprotected intercourse. However, the earlier the medication is given, the greater the efficacy and less chance of a pregnancy. Notably, this regimen may be effective for up to 5 days after unprotected intercourse; but consideration of ulipristal or the copper IUD may be a better option if a patient can get access in time.[49] Levonorgestrel-containing EC products are available without a prescription to patients of all ages in the United States.[49]

10 Ulipristal acetate (ella One) was approved for use as an EC and is a selective progesterone receptor modulator with mixed progesterone agonist and antagonist properties.[49,50] Its mechanism of action depends on the timing of administration relative to the patient's menstrual cycle.[50,51] However, the primary mechanism of action appears to be delay of ovulation. Ulipristal acetate is available by prescription only as a single dose of 30 mg taken within 120 hours (5 days) after unprotected intercourse so that it maintains efficacy for the full 120-hour window.[49,50] Data also exist to support noninferiority of ulipristal acetate compared to levonorgestrel-containing EC.[52]

Ulipristal acetate is not recommended for use in breastfeeding patients. Ulipristal acetate affects progesterone receptors and may interfere with ongoing hormonal contraception. A reliable barrier method is recommended for intercourse that occurs in the same menstrual cycle with ulipristal acetate use, even if the patient is on a regular hormonal contraceptive. In addition, the individual should avoid using a hormonal contraceptive method or initiating a new hormonal contraceptive for at least 5 days after ulipristal acetate administration.[50] Taking hormonal contraception sooner may alter the effect of ulipristal acetate as well as may compromise the effect of the hormonal contraceptive.[50]

10 Determining the exact effectiveness rate of EC is difficult; however, the range has been reported to be between 59% and 94%.[49] EC may prevent an average of 75% of expected pregnancies when taken appropriately. Individuals must have an advanced prescription on hand or access to an OTC formulation to maximize the effectiveness of EC.

Controversy exists regarding the potential for decreased efficacy of oral EC (both levonorgestrel and ulipristal) in overweight or obese individuals. No large-scale studies have been designed to fully resolve the controversy, and data from randomized trials have suggested an association with increased body weight and decreased efficacy of oral EC.[53,54] However, data demonstrate that there may be a decline in efficacy of levonorgestrel in females weighing greater than 75 kg. As oral EC is the most widely used EC method due to its accessibility, this issue is controversial. In 2016, the FDA announced that there was not enough evidence to change levonorgestrel labeling and encouraged further studies.[53] There is no effect of increased body weight on efficacy of a copper IUD.

6 Common adverse effects of EC include nausea, vomiting, and irregular bleeding.[49] Nausea and vomiting occur significantly less when progestin-only and progesterone receptor modulator EC is administered. Many patients will experience irregular bleeding regardless of which EC method is used, with the menstrual period usually occurring 1 week before or after the expected time. Routine screening prior to or after receiving progestin-only and progesterone receptor modulator EC is not recommended. If a pregnancy already exists, the oral EC will not disrupt or harm the embryo. In addition, there are no contraindications to the use of these methods of EC (for the Yuzpe and copper IUD methods clinicians must adhere to their contraindications and precautions). No current data regarding the safety of repeated-use EC are available, but current consensus suggests that the risks are low, and patients can receive multiple regimens if warranted, though use of a regular ongoing contraceptive should be encouraged. Appropriate counseling should be provided regarding timing of the dose, common adverse effects, and use of a regular contraceptive method (additional nonhormonal contraceptive methods should be used after EC for at least 7 days).

Pregnancy Termination

11 For various reasons, medications may be needed for pregnancy termination. There are a variety of protocols and considerations that will not be covered in depth within this chapter. Medications used in early pregnancy (≤70 days) termination supported by most national and international medical organizations include mifepristone and misoprostol typically used in combination or with misoprostol alone.

Mifepristone is a steroid that binds progesterone receptors and causes abortion by blocking progesterone, softening the cervix, increasing uterine contractility, and increasing prostaglandin sensitivity.[3,55] Progesterone is needed to maintain the corpus luteum during pregnancy. Softening of the cervix and increasing prostaglandins also affects the pregnancy by stimulating contractions. Mifepristone is usually administered orally.[3,56] Prescribing of mifepristone is restricted to a prescriber that has met the training and qualifications of the manufacturer, and it is only dispensed out of the prescriber's facility. Although it is only used short term for pregnancy termination, it requires monitoring for medication interactions as it is metabolized by the CYP450 3A4 system. Therefore, caution should be taken when administered with strong inhibitors or inducers of that system.[57]

Boxed warnings for mifepristone include infection and bleeding.[57] Bacterial infections and sepsis may occur without findings upon pelvic examination after the abortion or without signs of infections such as bacteremia and fever. Excessive bleeding may occur and could be a sign of incomplete abortion or other complications and needs prompt medical attention.[57] Prescribers need to inform patients of these risks prior to use and also educate patients on what to do if they feel they experience these events by discussing a patient agreement created by the manufacturer. When used as an abortifacient, mifepristone is contraindicated in patients with bleeding disorders or on anticoagulants.[57]

Misoprostol is a prostaglandin E1 analog, currently marketed as a protective agent in patients at risk for gastric ulcers that also causes softening of the cervix and stimulates uterine contractions. Off-label uses include abortion, labor induction, preventing and treating postpartum hemorrhage, cervical ripening for medical procedures, and treatment of early pregnancy loss.[55] Adverse medication effects of misoprostol may include stomach upset, diarrhea, headache, dizziness, chills, and fever.[3,55,56] There are a variety of dosage forms available, including oral, vaginal, buccal, and sublingual. The oral form is not recommended because of decreased efficacy, as the other formulations have better adsorption. In addition, the vaginal route may cause less gastrointestinal adverse medication effects.[55]

Abortion regimens include mifepristone–misoprostol (most common), or misoprostol used alone. The mifepristone–misoprostol regimen approved for use by the FDA includes mifepristone 200 mg orally on day 1 and then misoprostol 800 mcg administered buccally 24 to 48 hours after the mifepristone dose.[3,4,55] The efficacy of this regimen has been reported as 98% in pregnancies up to 49 days.[55] Efficacy is higher if the regimen is used earlier in the pregnancy. The mifepristone–misoprostol regimen, compared to misoprostol alone, works faster and is more effective in later gestational ages.[3,55]

In all cases, further assessment by the treating provider is required in the days that follow medication administration to ensure complete abortion and to assess for any complications. Abdominal cramps and bleeding are common after medical abortion.[3,55] An individual should be counseled that they will likely have heavy menstrual bleeding, but it is important for them to recognize if there is too much bleeding.[55] Those experiencing bleeding that soaks two maxi pads per hour for 2 consecutive hours should contact their healthcare provider promptly.[55] Acetaminophen or NSAIDs such as ibuprofen may be used to help relieve pain and cramping.[3,55] Use of NSAIDs inhibits new prostaglandins but will not affect the use of misoprostol in pregnancy termination.

EVALUATION OF THERAPEUTIC OUTCOMES

9 Selecting a contraceptive method should involve the patient and clinician using a shared decision-making model. Contraceptive pharmacotherapy should be personalized for each patient, taking into account desired outcomes from a contraceptive and noncontraceptive perspective. Factors to consider include effectiveness, presence of coexisting medical conditions or medications, safety, adverse effects, cost, return to fertility time, and patient preference of the contraceptive method (eg, long-acting, short-acting, hormonal, oral, nonoral, barrier). Patients should receive both verbal and written instructions on the chosen method of contraception. In addition, access to timely contraception is important. In addition, some states have (or are in the process of obtaining) expanded scope of practice to include provision of hormonal contraception by a pharmacist.[57,58] Follow-up appointments can increase adherence and provide opportunities to address other health maintenance issues. The contraceptive outcome of pregnancy prevention can be assessed when needed by obtaining a serum or urine pregnancy test.

Monitoring of the Pharmaceutical Care Plan

3 4 5 8 Contraceptive users should receive an annual preventative medicine exam that may include a cytologic screening (if appropriate) and pelvic and breast examination. Consultation should provide routine health maintenance screening and to assess for clinical problems or adverse effects related to contraception (see Tables 19-4, 19-5, and 19-6). These annual screenings do not have to occur prior to prescribing hormonal contraception.

Annual BP monitoring is recommended for all users of CHC. When a patient with a history of glucose intolerance or diabetes mellitus begins or discontinues the use of hormonal contraception, glucose levels must be monitored. Monitoring for the presence of adverse effects related to hormonal content or the presence of coexisting medical conditions is recommended for individuals using CHCs. Those using the etonogestrel implant should be monitored annually for menstrual cycle disturbances, local inflammation, or infection at the implant site, acne, breast tenderness, headaches, and hair loss. Patients using DMPA should be asked at 3-month follow-up visits about weight gain, menstrual cycle disturbances, and fractures. Those using IUDs should be asked at 1- to 3-month follow-up visits about IUD placement (checking for IUD strings to assure the IUD is still in the proper position), changes in menstrual bleeding patterns, and symptoms and protection against STIs/STDs. Clinicians should check for proper IUD positioning and symptoms of upper genital tract infection.

Finally, clinicians should monitor, and when indicated, screen for HIV and STIs/STDs. All individuals should receive counseling about healthy sexual practices including the use of condoms to prevent the transmission of STIs/STDs when necessary.

CONCLUSION

A variety of contraceptive methods are available. Selection of a contraceptive method depends on many factors. Patient preference, method effectiveness, medical history, contraceptive adverse medication effects, desire for a return to fertility, and available access to products all play a role in choosing the best contraception method for a patient. Clinicians play a critical role in helping patients carefully select an appropriate contraceptive method, monitoring adverse medication effects, and providing education on optimal use, effectiveness, and STI/STD prevention that can help reduce STIs/STDs and unintended pregnancies.

ABBREVIATIONS

ACHES	abdominal pain, chest pain, headaches, eye problems, and severe leg pain
ACOG	American College of Obstetricians and Gynecologists
BMD	bone mineral density
BMI	body mass index

CDC	Centers for Disease Control and Prevention
CHC	combined hormonal contraceptive
COC	combined oral contraceptive
DMPA	depot medroxyprogesterone acetate
DXA	dual-energy x-ray absorptiometry
EC	emergency contraception
EE	ethinyl estradiol
FDA	Food and Drug Administration
FSH	follicle-stimulating hormone
GnRH	gonadotropin-releasing hormone
HDL	high-density lipoprotein
HIV	human immunodeficiency virus
IUD	intrauterine device
LARC	long-acting reversible contraception
LDL	low-density lipoprotein
LH	luteinizing hormone
MI	myocardial infarction
NSAID	nonsteroidal anti-inflammatory drug
OC	oral contraceptive
OTC	over-the-counter
Pap	papanicolaou (smear)
PMDD	premenstrual dysphoric disorder
SHBG-TBG	sex hormone (testosterone)-binding globulin
SLE	systemic lupus erythematosus
STI/STD	sexually transmitted infection/disease
TSS	toxic shock syndrome
VTE	venous thromboembolism

REFERENCES

1. Finer LB, Zolna MR. Declines in unintended pregnancy in the United States, 2008-2011. *N Engl J Med.* 2016;374:843–852. doi:10.1056/NEJMsa1506575
2. Guttmacher Institute. Unintended pregnancy in the United States: Fact sheet. January 2019. Available at: https://www.guttmacher.org/fact-sheet/unintended-pregnancy-united-states. Accessed April 8, 2021.
3. Hatcher RA, Trussell J, Nelson AL, et al. *Contraceptive Technology*. 21st ed. New York, NY: Ardent Median, Inc.; 2018.
4. Dickey RP. *Managing Contraceptive Pill Patients*. 16th ed. Fort Collins, CO: EMIS Inc.; 2020.
5. Twirla [package insert]. Grand Rapids, MI: Corium International, Inc.; February 2020.
6. Annovera [package insert]. Boca Raton, FL: Therapeutics MD, Inc.; January 2020.
7. Slynd [package insert]. Florham Park, NJ: Exeltis USA, Inc.; June 2019.
8. FemCap Website. Available at: https://femcap.com/new/. Accessed May 3, 2021.
9. Phexxi [package insert]. San Diego, CA: Evofem; May 2020.
10. Curtis KM, Jatlaoui TC, Tepper NK, et al. U.S. selected practice recommendations for contraceptive use, 2016. *MMWR Recomm Rep.* 2016;65(No. RR-4):1–66. doi:http://dx.doi.org/10.15585/mmwr.rr6504a1external_icon
11. Natural Cycles App. Available at: https://www.naturalcycles.com/en. Accessed April 8, 2021.
12. Grimes DA, Lopez LM, Raymond EG, et al. Spermicide used alone for contraception. *Cochrane Database Syst Rev.* 2013;(12):CD005218.
13. Oral Contraceptives. Drug Facts and Comparisons. eFacts [online]. Available from Wolters Kluwer Health, Inc. Accessed May 2, 2021.
14. Van Vliet HAAM, Grimes DA, Helmerhorst FM, Schulz KF. Biphasic versus monophasic oral contraceptives for contraception. *Cochrane Database Syst Rev.* 2006;(3):CD002032.
15. Van Vliet HAAM, Grimes DA, Helmerhorst FM, Schulz KF. Triphasic versus monophasic oral contraceptives for contraception. *Cochrane Database Syst Rev.* 2011;3:CD003553.
16. Pharmacist's Letter Detail-Document: Comparison of oral contraceptives and non-oral alternatives. *Pharmacist's Letter/Prescriber's Letter*. February 2021.
17. Curtis KM, Tepper NK, Jatlaoui TC, et al. U.S. medical eligibility criteria for contraceptive use, 2016. *MMWR Recomm Rep.* 2016;65(No. RR-3):1–104. doi:http://dx.doi.org/10.15585/mmwr.rr6503a1
18. Yaz [Package Insert]. Whippany NJ: Bayer HealthCare Pharmaceuticals, Inc. 2012. Available at: https://www.accessdata.fda.gov/drugsatfda_docs/label/2012/021676s012lbl.pdf. Accessed May 3, 2021.
19. Xulane [Package Insert]. Morgantown, WV: Mylan Pharmaceuticals Inc. February 2021.
20. ACOG Practice Bulletin No. 206. Use of hormonal contraception in women with coexisting medical conditions. *Obstet Gynecol.* 2019 Feb;133(2):e128–e150. 10.1097/AOG.0000000000003072. Erratum in: Obstet Gynecol. 2019 Jun;133(6):1288. PMID: 30681544.
21. Nuva Ring [Package Insert] Whitehouse Station, NJ: Merck & Co., Inc. January, 2020. Available at: https://www.nuvaring.com/static/pdf/nuvaring-pi.pdf. Accessed May 4, 2021.
22. MacGregor EA. Contraception and headache. *Headache.* 2013;53:247–276.
23. Bhupathiraju SN, Grodstein F, Stampfer MJ, et al. Exogenous hormone use: Oral contraceptives, postmenopausal hormone therapy, and health outcomes in the nurses' health study. *Am J Public Health.* 2016;106(9):1631–1637. doi:10.2105/AJPH.2016.303349
24. Morch LS, Skovlund CW, Hannaford PC, et al. Contemporary hormonal contraception and the risk of breast cancer. *N Engl J Med.* 2017;377(23):2228–2239. doi:10.1056/NEJMoa1700732
25. Figueiredo JC, Haile RW, Bernstein L, et al. Oral contraceptives and postmenopausal hormones and risk of contralateral breast cancer among BRCA1 and BRCA2 mutation carriers and noncarriers: The WECARE Study. *Breast Cancer Res Treat.* 2010 Feb;120(1):175–183. doi:10.1007/s10549-009-0455-5
26. Kotsopoulos J, Lubinski J, Moller P, et al. Hereditary Breast Cancer Clinical Study Group. Timing of oral contraceptive use and the risk of breast cancer in BRCA1 mutation carriers. *Breast Cancer Res Treat.* 2014 Feb;143(3):579–586. doi:10.1007/s10549-013-2823-4
27. Lidegaard OM, Nielsen LH, Skovlund CW, Lokkegaard E. Venous thromboembolism in users of non-oral hormonal contraception: Follow-up study, Denmark 2001–2010. *BMJ.* 2012;344:e2990. doi:10.1136/bmj.e2990
28. Jick SS, Hernandez RK. Risk of non-fatal thromboembolism in women using oral contraceptives containing drospirenone compared with women using oral contraceptives containing levonorgestrel: Case-control study using United States claims data. *BMJ.* 2011;342:d2151. doi:10.1136/bmj.d2151
29. Tepper NK, Whiteman MK, Marchbanks PA. Progestin-only contraception and thromboembolism: A systematic review. *Contraception.* 2016;94(6):678–700. doi:10.1016/j.contraception.2016.04.014
30. Committee on Gynecologic Practice. ACOG Committee Opinion Number 540: Risk of venous thromboembolism among users of drospirenone-containing oral contraceptive pills. *Obstet Gynecol.* 2012 (Reaffirmed 2020);120(5):1239–1242. doi:10.1097/aog.0b013e318277c93b
31. Practice Committee of the American Society for Reproductive Medicine. Electronic address: ASRM@asrm.org; Practice Committee of the American Society for Reproductive Medicine. Combined hormonal contraception and the risk of venous thromboembolism: a guideline. *Fertil Steril.* 2017;107(1):43–51. doi:10.1016/j.fertnstert.2016.09.027
32. Dinger J, Minh TD, Buttmann N, Bardenheuer K. Effectiveness of oral contraceptive pills in a large U.S. cohort comparing progestogen and regimen. *Obstet Gynecol.* 2011;117:33–40. 10.1097/AOG.0b013e31820095a2
33. Kapp N, Abitbol JL, Mathe H, et al. Effect of body weight and BMI on the efficacy of levonorgestrel emergency contraception. *Contraception.* 2015;91:97–107. doi:10.1016/j.contraception.2014.11.001
34. Depo-Provera [Package Insert]. New York: Pfizer. October 2010. Available at: https://www.accessdata.fda.gov/drugsatfda_docs/label/2010/020246s036lbl.pdf. Accessed May 4, 2021.
35. Depo-SubQ Provera 104 [Package Insert]. New York: Pfizer. December 2020. Available at: http://labeling.pfizer.com/ShowLabeling.aspx?id=549. Accessed May 4, 2021.
36. Beasley A, White K, Cremers S, Westhoff C. Randomized clinical trial of self versus clinical administration of subcutaneous depot medroxyprogesterone acetate. *Contraception.* 2014;89:352–356. doi:10.1016/j.contraception.2014.01.026
37. Kohn JE, Simons HR, Della Badia L, et al. Increased 1-year continuation of DMPA among women randomized to self-administration: Results from a randomized controlled trial at planned parenthood. *Contraception.* 2018;97:198–204. doi:10.1016/j.contraception.2017.11.009
38. American College of Obstetricians and Gynecologists. Committee Opinion No. 602 (reaffirmed 2017). Depot medroxyprogesterone acetate and bone effects. *Obstet Gynecol.* 2014;123:1398–1402. doi:10.1097/01.AOG.0000450758.95422.c8

39. Lopez LM, Chen M, Mullins Long S, et al. Steroidal contraceptives and bone fractures in women: Evidence from observational studies. *Cochrane Database Syst Rev.* 2015;(7):CD009849. doi.10.1002/14651858.CD009849.pub3
40. Nexplanon [Package Insert]. Whitehouse Station, NJ: Merck & Co., Inc. November 2020. Available at: https://www.merck.com/product/usa/pi_circulars/n/nexplanon/nexplanon_pi.pdf. Accessed May 5, 2020.
41. American College of Obstetricians and Gynecologists. Long-acting reversible contraception: Implants and intrauterine devices. Practice Bulletin No. 186. *Obstet Gynecol.* 2017;130:e251–e269. doi:10.1097/AOG.0000000000002400
42. ParaGard T380A [Package Insert]. Trumbull, CT: Cooper Surgical, Inc. February 2020.
43. Mirena [Package Insert]. Whippany, NJ: Bayer HealthCare Pharmaceuticals, Inc. August 2020.
44. Liletta [Package Insert] Parsippany, NJ: Actavis Pharma, Inc. April 2020.
45. Skyla [Package Insert]. Whippany, NJ: Bayer HealthCare Pharmaceuticals, Inc. March 2018.
46. Kyleena [Package Insert]. Whippany, NJ: Bayer HealthCare Pharmaceuticals, Inc. April 2021.
47. American College of Obstetricians and Gynecologists. Adolescents and long-acting reversible contraception: Implants and intrauterine devices. Committee Opinion No. 735. *Obstet Gynecol.* 2018;131:e130–e139. doi:10.1097/AOG.0000000000002632
48. Kavanaugh M, Jerman J. Contraceptive method use in the United States: Trends and characteristics between 2008, 2012, and 2014. *Contraception*. 2018;97:14–21. DOI:10.1016/j.contraception.2017.10.003
49. American College of Obstetricians and Gynecologists. Emergency contraception. Practice Bulletin No. 152. *Obstet Gynecol.* 2015;126:e1–e11. doi:10.1097/AOG.0000000000001047
50. ella [Package Insert]. Charleston, SC: Afaxys Pharma, LLC. March 2015.
51. Brache V, Cochon L, Jesam C, et al. Immediate pre-ovulatory administration of 30 mg ulipristal acetate significantly delays follicular rupture. *Hum Reprod.* 2010;25:2256–2263. doi:10.1093/humrep/deq157
52. Glasier AF, Cameron ST, Fine PM, et al. Ulipristal acetate versus levonorgestrel for emergency contraception: A randomized non-inferiority trial and meta-analysis. *Lancet.* 2010;375:555–579. doi:10.1016/S0140-6736(10)60101-8
53. Trussell J, Raymond EG, Cleland K. Emergency contraception: A last chance to prevent unintended pregnancy. January 2019. Available at: https://ec.princeton.edu/questions/ec-review.pdf. Accessed May 5, 2021.
54. Glasier A, Cameron ST, Blithe D, et al. Can we identify women at risk of pregnancy despite using emergency contraception? Data from randomized trials of ulipristal acetate and levonorgestrel. *Contraception.* 2011;84:363–367. doi:10.1016/j.contraception.2011.02.009
55. Committee on Practice Bulletins—Gynecology; Society of Family Planning. Medication Abortion Up to 70 Days of Gestation: ACOG Practice Bulletin, Number 225. *Obstet Gynecol.* 2020;136(4):e31–e47. doi:10.1097/AOG.0000000000004082
56. Lexicomp. Misoprostol and Methotrexate: Lexi-Drugs. Riverwoods, IL: Wolters Kluwer Clinical Drug Information; 2021. Available at: http//:online.lexi.com. Accessed May 4, 2021.
57. Mifeprex [package insert]. New York: Danco Laboratories, LLC. March 2016. Available at: https://www.accessdata.fda.gov/drugsatfda_docs/label/2016/020687s010-lbl.pdf. Accessed May 5, 2021.
58. National Alliance of State Pharmacy Associations. Pharmacist Prescribing: Hormonal Contraceptives. Available at: https://naspa.us/resource/contraceptives/. Accessed May 5, 2021.

Pediatrics: General Topics in Pediatric Pharmacotherapy

e20

Milap C. Nahata and Carol K. Taketomo

KEY CONCEPTS

1. Children are not just "little adults," and lack of data on important pharmacokinetic and pharmacodynamic differences has led to several disastrous situations in pediatric care.
2. Variations in absorption of medications from the gastrointestinal tract, intramuscular injection sites, and skin are important in pediatric patients, especially in premature and other newborn infants.
3. The rate and extent of organ function development and the distribution, metabolism, and elimination of drugs differ not only between pediatric versus adult patients but also among pediatric age groups.
4. The effectiveness and safety of drugs may vary among age groups and from one drug to another in pediatric versus adult patients.
5. Concomitant diseases may influence dosage requirements to achieve a targeted effect for a specific disease in children.
6. Use of weight-based dosing of medications for obese children may result in suboptimal drug therapy.
7. The myth that neonates and young infants do not experience pain has led to inadequate pain management in this pediatric population.
8. Special methods of drug administration are needed for infants and young children.
9. Many medicines needed for pediatric patients are not available in appropriate dosage forms; thus, the dosage forms of drugs marketed for adults may require modification for use in infants and children, necessitating assurance of potency and safety of drug use.
10. The pediatric medication-use process is complex and error prone because of the multiple steps required in calculating, verifying, preparing, and administering doses.

BEYOND THE BOOK

Visit the US Food and Drug Administration Website and navigate to the New Pediatric Labeling Information Database <https://www.accessdata.fda.gov/scripts/sda/sdNavigation.cfm?sd=labelingdatabase>. The Website provides comprehensive up-to-date information related to pediatric drug labeling changes. Explore available drugs, review recent labeling information for one drug of interest, and summarize the label changes. This Website is useful to enhance student understanding of available resources for pediatric drug dosing information.

INTRODUCTION

Remarkable progress has been made in the clinical management of diseases in pediatric patients. This chapter highlights important principles of pediatric pharmacotherapy that must be considered when the diseases discussed in other chapters of this book occur in pediatric patients, defined as those younger than 18 years. Newborn infants born before 37 weeks of gestational age may experience a variety of health problems and are termed *premature*; those between 1 day and 1 month of age are *neonates*; 1 month to 1 year are *infants*; 1 to 11 years are *children*; and 12 to 16 years are *adolescents*. This chapter covers notable examples of problems in pediatrics, pharmacokinetic differences in pediatric patients, drug efficacy and toxicity in this patient group, and various factors affecting pediatric pharmacotherapy. Specific examples of problems and special considerations in pediatric patients are cited to enhance understanding.

(1) Infant mortality up to 1 year of age has declined from 200 per 1,000 births in the 19th century to 75 per 1,000 births in 1925 and to 5.6 per 1,000 births in 2019.[1] This success has resulted largely from improvements in identification, prevention, and treatment of diseases once common during delivery and the infancy period. Although most marketed drugs are used in pediatric patients, less than one-half of the drugs approved by the US Food and Drug Administration (FDA) are labeled for use in the pediatric population. Data on the pharmacokinetics, pharmacodynamics, efficacy, and safety of drugs in infants and children are scarce. Lack of this type of information led to disasters such as gray baby syndrome from chloramphenicol, phocomelia from thalidomide, and kernicterus from sulfonamide therapy. Gray baby syndrome was first reported in two neonates who died after excessive doses of chloramphenicol (100-300 mg/kg/day); the serum concentrations of chloramphenicol immediately before death were 75 and 100 μg/mL (mg/L; 232 and 309 μmol/L). Patients with gray baby syndrome usually have abdominal distension, vomiting, diarrhea, a characteristic gray color, respiratory distress, hypotension, and progressive shock.

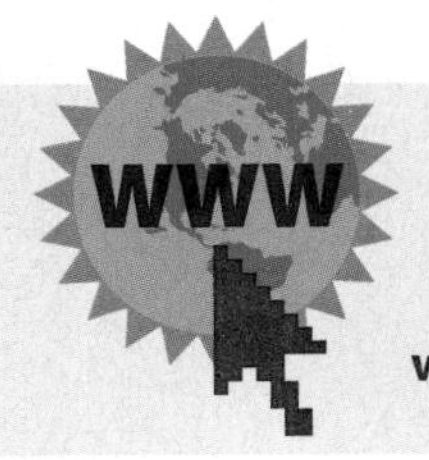

The complete chapter, learning objectives, and other resources can be found at **www.pharmacotherapyonline.com.**

Pediatrics: Oral Nutrition and Rehydration of Infants and Children

e21

Katherine H. Chessman

KEY CONCEPTS

1. Human milk is the preferred source of nutrition for almost all neonates and infants, including those born prematurely.
2. A commercial infant formula is a nutritionally complete substitute if human milk is not available.
3. Cow milk-based formulas are consumed by most US non-breastfeeding infants, although there is increasing usage of other types of infant formulas.
4. When sufficient maternal or donor milk is not available, specific formulas designed for preterm low birth weight infants can be used to meet nutritional needs.
5. Some infants will require specialized formulas with altered macronutrients due to cow milk or soy protein sensitivities or conditions that lead to impaired nutrient digestion, absorption, or utilization.
6. Two nutrients, iron and vitamin D, are of particular importance in infant nutrition.
7. Human milk contains a variety of non-nutritive compounds with specific bioactive characteristics; formula manufacturers continue to modify their products to include these compounds.
8. Enteral formulas are available for children who need supplemental nutrition beyond a regular diet in most of the infant formula categories discussed and are used for similar indications.
9. Expressed human milk and infant formulas must be handled and stored properly.
10. Oral rehydration therapy (ORT) is a mainstay of treatment for mild-to-moderate dehydration; severe dehydration requires intravenous (IV) rehydration.

INTRODUCTION

Nutrition in the first 1,000 days of life can play a pivotal role in infants, especially those born prematurely. Appropriate early nutrition is essential for growth and development to prevent adverse health outcomes later in life and improve cognition in adulthood. Obesity, hypertension, and diabetes mellitus may be programmed by nutrition status during this period.[1] Infancy is a period of rapid growth which is followed by continued but slower growth and development throughout childhood. Healthy term infants will double their birth weight in approximately 4 months and triple it by 12 months. Adequate nutrient intake, absorption, and utilization are vital to ensuring that growth and development progress normally. All practitioners providing health care for infants and children should be knowledgeable about appropriate pediatric nutrition to be able to quickly identify opportunities for intervention. Dietary reference intakes (DRIs)[2] established by the Food and Nutrition Board of the National Academies of Science, Engineering, and Medicine, for energy, protein, fat, trace elements, vitamins, electrolyte, and mineral requirements are discussed in Chapter 164. There are many choices for both standard and specialized formulas for infants and children. This chapter will review human milk and the various available formulas and their appropriate usage. Adolescents requiring nutrition supplementation beyond a regular diet will typically use feeding formulations appropriate for adults (see Chapter 166). Oral rehydration therapy will also be discussed in this chapter.

INFANT NUTRITION

A term newborn's stomach has a capacity of 20-90 mL. Gastric capacity increases to 90 to 180 mL by 1 month of age. Too rapidly advancing oral or enteral nutrition intake can lead to emesis, gastroesophageal reflux (GER), and other gastrointestinal (GI) symptoms. Frequent feedings (every 2-3 hours) are needed early in life due to the stomach's limited capacity and an infant's high metabolic demand (see Table e21-1). Human milk empties from the stomach at a faster rate than formula; thus, breastfed infants fed ad libitum (ad lib) may demand feeding more often than their formula-fed peers. Nutritive sucking ability develops at approximately 34 weeks gestational age; before that time, tube feedings are required. The inability to coordinate sucking, swallowing, and breathing when the respiratory rate is elevated above 60 breaths per minute also may necessitate tube feeding.

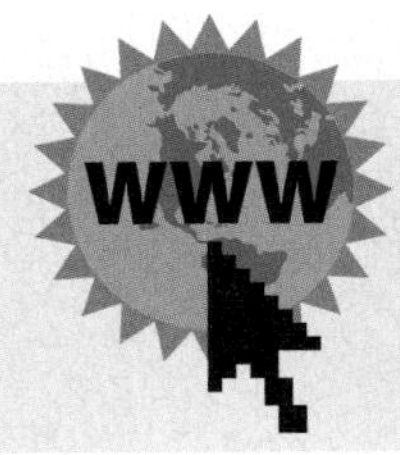

The complete chapter, learning objectives, and other resources can be found at **www.pharmacotherapyonline.com.**

Pediatrics: Neonatal Critical Care

e22

Kirsten H. Ohler and Jennifer T. Pham

KEY CONCEPTS

1. Pharmacokinetic parameters are altered across the age spectrum of the neonatal population (ie, preterm to term) because of developmental maturation and the effect of various disease states on these processes. Therefore, medication selection and monitoring is of utmost importance in this population.
2. Treatment guidelines for neonatal resuscitation have been extrapolated from studies in older children and adults, which may not be optimal because of differences in the pathophysiology of cardiopulmonary arrest among these populations.
3. Neonatal sepsis can be categorized as either early-onset sepsis (EOS) or late-onset sepsis (LOS). Pathogens associated with neonatal sepsis vary depending on the onset of sepsis (EOS vs LOS).
4. Empiric antibiotic therapy should be initiated in infants with suspected sepsis and should target the most common pathogens.
5. Patent ductus arteriosus occurs commonly in preterm neonates and, if hemodynamically significant, requires pharmacologic (with a cyclooxygenase inhibitor) or surgical closure.
6. In certain congenital heart defects (eg, tetralogy of Fallot, hypoplastic left heart syndrome, transposition of the great arteries), it is imperative that the ductus arteriosus remains patent. Prostaglandin E1 (alprostadil) is the drug of choice in these cases.
7. Neonatal hypotension can result in impaired cerebral perfusion and ischemic damage if left untreated. Since there is no clear consensus on the definition of neonatal hypotension, diagnosis and treatment are guided by clinical judgment, and review of the physiological parameters of the infant.
8. Pharmacologic therapy should be selected based on the etiology of hemodynamic instability and may include fluid bolus, vasopressors (eg, dopamine, dobutamine, epinephrine, norepinephrine), hydrocortisone, and vasopressin. Dopamine is the preferred initial vasopressor agent for hemodynamic support in neonates with hypotension.
9. Assessment of the degree of pain and sedation in the preverbal neonatal population is difficult. When using assessment tools, recognize the population and pain type for which each tool has been validated.
10. Opioids and benzodiazepines are commonly used to provide analgesia and sedation for critically ill neonates; however, there are concerns about their effects on long-term neurodevelopment.

BEYOND THE BOOK

Watch the video titled "Healthcare Heroes-NICU episode" at https://www.youtube.com/watch?v=DEheE4rr1GU. This 8-minute video provides a brief overview of the initial assessment and treatment of a critically ill neonate admitted to the neonatal intensive care unit (NICU). The video will enhance the student's understanding of the role of an interprofessional team in the complex care of an NICU patient. After watching the video, the student's reflection should include identification of the roles various healthcare providers (eg, pharmacist, nurse, nurse practitioner, respiratory therapist) can play in the management of an unstable neonate. The ASSESS and PLAN steps of the patient care process will be developed through this exercise.

INTRODUCTION

Healthcare providers working in the neonatal intensive care unit (NICU) care for a wide range of patients—from those born prematurely to term newborns, newly born infants to infants who have spent months to years in the NICU, those with acute illnesses to those with chronic morbidities associated with prematurity. A large proportion of NICU patients are born prematurely. In the United States, almost 1 in 10 births is premature.[1] Preterm birth occurs when a neonate is born before 37 completed weeks of gestation.[2] Prematurity can be further categorized as late preterm (ie, 34-37 weeks), moderate preterm (ie, 32-34 weeks), very preterm (ie, 28-32 weeks), and extremely preterm (ie, less than 28 weeks).[2] Neonates born prematurely can have multiple complications including respiratory distress syndrome, intraventricular hemorrhage (IVH), seizures, necrotizing enterocolitis (NEC), and sepsis, among others. Survivors of preterm birth often have morbidities such as bronchopulmonary dysplasia (BPD), neurodevelopmental delay, and cerebral palsy.[1,3] Despite medical advances, mortality in this population, especially those born extremely premature, remains high (30%-50%).[3]

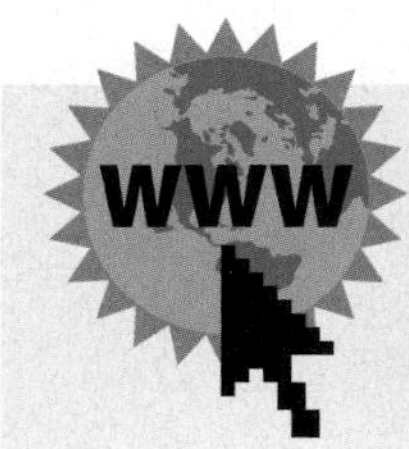

The complete chapter, learning objectives, and other resources can be found at **www.pharmacotherapyonline.com.**

Geriatrics: Physiology of Aging

e23

Krista L. Donohoe, Elvin T. Price, Tracey L. Gendron, and Patricia W. Slattum

KEY CONCEPTS

1. The population of people 65 years and older is increasing.
2. Age-related changes in physiology affect the functions of various organ systems and contribute to the onset of diseases.
3. Age-related changes in physiology can affect the pharmacokinetics (PK) and pharmacodynamics (PD) of numerous medications.
4. Successful aging is determined by individually defined measures of well-being that include maximizing health span and socio-environmental engagement.

BEYOND THE BOOK

Pair up with a classmate and brainstorm a list of age-related changes that occur in the human physiology and the effects they may have on pharmacokinetics (PK)/pharmacodynamics (PD) of medications in older adults.

Interview an older adult and obtain a medication history. Using their medication list, determine the effects that age-related changes in PK/PD will have on the medications and ensure they are appropriately dosed for older adults.

INTRODUCTION

1 Medications can cure or palliate medical conditions in older adults, however, they can also cause a number of drug-related problems. Prevention of drug-related problems requires that health professionals be knowledgeable about the changes that occur with aging and the implications this has on prescribing, monitoring, and evaluating medication regimens in older adults. This chapter will focus on the epidemiology of aging, mechanisms of aging, physiologic changes due to aging with an emphasis on the age-related changes in pharmacokinetics (PK) and pharmacodynamics (PD) of medications, and successful aging to maximize health span and quality of life.

EPIDEMIOLOGY OF AGING

The proportion of persons 65 years and older is increasing worldwide. In 2019, the worldwide number of people aged 65 years or older was 703 million, and this is projected to double to 1.5 billion by 2050.[1] In the United States, the population of older adults has changed from a pyramidal shape to a pillar.[2] The rectangular shape will be top heavy in 2050 because of the large numbers of births in the latter half of the 20th century. In 2018, 16% of the population was considered geriatric in the United States, and in 2050 it is projected to be 22% and 23.4% by 2060.[3] In 2034, the older adult population will outnumber children under 18 years old for the first time in US history.[2]

The population is aging due to people having fewer children and living longer. In the United States, the life expectancy in 2018 at birth is 76.2 years for men and 81.2 years for women.[4] At age 65 and 85 years old, respectively, men are projected to have 18.1 and 6 years of life remaining, compared to 20.7 and 7 years for women.[3] However, based on provisional data for the first half of 2020, US life expectancy has declined due to COVID-19 global pandemic.[5]

Older adults often have multiple chronic conditions and thus need to see a number of specialists and healthcare providers. In 2018, the three most frequently reported chronic health conditions in the United States for adults 65 and older were hypertension, arthritis, and heart disease.[3] Women have a higher prevalence of arthritis (54% vs 46%) and asthma (14% vs 9%), while men have higher rates of heart disease (35% vs 24%), cancer (27% vs 25%), and diabetes (25% vs 19%).[3] In 2018, the six leading causes of death among persons 65 years and older were: heart disease, cancer, chronic lower respiratory diseases, stroke, Alzheimer's disease, unintentional injuries, and influenza and pneumonia. Heart disease and cancer were the top two leading causes of death.[3] COVID-19 has had a significant impact on life expectancy and mortality during the global pandemic.[5]

Older adults have a high prevalence of chronic diseases, and this means they are using numerous medications on a long-term basis. This "polypharmacy" can lead to potential drug-related problems, such as drug-drug interactions.[6–8] To provide the best pharmacotherapy for this diverse and heterogeneous population of older adults, their health care providers need to understand the mechanisms of physiologic changes that occur with aging and resulting pharmacokinetic and pharmacodynamic implications, especially with respect to the common chronic conditions and medications that are used to treat them.

MECHANISMS OF AGING

Aging is associated with alterations in physiologic and homeostatic mechanisms. These alterations affect multiple organ systems and contribute to the presence of common chronic diseases.[9–14]

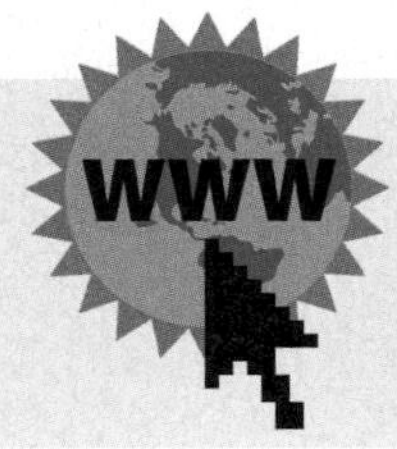

The complete chapter, learning objectives, and other resources can be found at **www.pharmacotherapyonline.com.**

Geriatrics: Medication Use in Older Adults

e24

Emily R. Hajjar, Lauren R. Hersh, and Shelly L. Gray

KEY CONCEPTS

1. Improving and maintaining functional status is a cornerstone of care for older adults.
2. Adverse drug reactions in older adults are common and cause considerable morbidity.
3. Inappropriate prescribing is a major concern and is guided by the Beer's criteria.
4. Polypharmacy can be defined in various ways and is a common occurrence in older adults.
5. Underutilization of medications also occurs and can be improved by using the START criteria.
6. Pharmacists can play a major role in optimizing drug therapy and preventing adverse consequences of medications in older adults.
7. Deprescribing should be considered to reduce medications in older adults.
8. Practitioners may consider targeting high-risk older adults to implement comprehensive management strategies.

BEYOND THE BOOK

Read the current American Geriatrics Society Beers Criteria®[13] and discuss the impact of the recommendations on medication use in older adults.

INTRODUCTION

1 Pharmacotherapy for older adults can cure or palliate disease as well as enhance health-related quality of life (HRQOL). HRQOL considerations for older adults include focusing on improvements in physical functioning (eg, activities of daily living), psychological functioning (eg, cognition, depression), social functioning (eg, social activities, support systems), and overall health (eg, general health perception).[1] Despite the benefits of pharmacotherapy, HRQOL can be compromised by drug-related problems. The clinical response to a medication in an older adult is the result of the interaction of a number of complex processes, including pharmacokinetics, pharmacodynamics, concurrent medications, comorbidities, and frailty. Age-related changes in physiology can affect drug pharmacokinetics and pharmacodynamics.[2] When applying general knowledge of pharmacokinetic and pharmacodynamic alterations in an older adult in the clinical setting, it is necessary to consider the patient's overall condition, age, diseases, frailty status, and concurrent medications. Prevention of drug-related problems in older adults requires that health professionals become knowledgeable about a number of age-specific issues. To address these knowledge needs, this chapter discusses the epidemiology of adverse consequences of medications in older adults and an approach to optimizing medication use through the provision of a comprehensive geriatric assessment.

ADVERSE CONSEQUENCES OF MEDICATION USE

Although medications used by older adults can lead to improvement in HRQOL, adverse outcomes caused by drug-related problems are considerable.[3] Adverse drug reactions (ADRs) and negative consequences of drug therapy are major threats to the HRQOL of outpatient older adults and account for a significant portion of healthcare expenditures.[4] Estimates are that more than $520 billion was spent in 2016 for prescription-associated morbidity and mortality from nonoptimized medications.[4]

ADVERSE DRUG REACTIONS

2 ADRs are a major public health problem for older adults in all settings. ADRs are defined as "a response to a drug that is noxious and unintended and occurs at doses normally used in man for the prophylaxis, diagnosis or therapy of disease, or for modification of physiological function" and exclude therapeutic failure and adverse drug withdrawal events.[5] Approximately 9% of hospitalizations in older adults are caused by ADRs, while 16% of older adults experience a significant ADR while hospitalized.[6,7] Moreover, ADRs occur frequently in community-dwelling older adults (10%-35% yearly). Transitions of care are often high-risk times for adverse drug-related events.[8,9] For example, one study found that 19% of older adults experienced an adverse drug event within 45 days of hospital discharge.[8] Some medication classes, such as anticoagulants, antidiabetic agents, and opioids, are especially problematic for causing serious ADRs in older adults and are high priority targets to improve patient safety.[5,10] The use of potentially inappropriate medications (eg, beers criteria drugs) only cause a small proportion of ADRs.[6,8,10] Number of medications is a consistent risk factor for ADRs.[6]

Inappropriate Prescribing

3 Inappropriate prescribing is defined broadly as prescribing medications outside the bounds of accepted medical standards. However, inappropriate prescribing is challenging to define and operationalize.

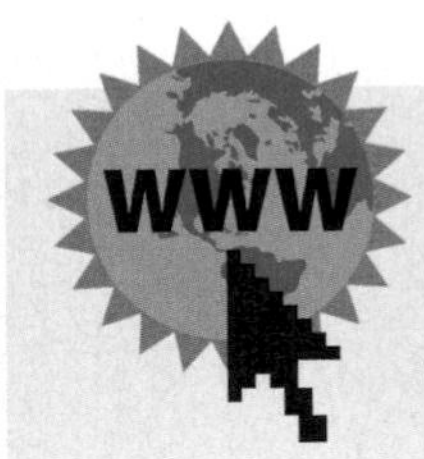

The complete chapter, learning objectives, and other resources can be found at **www.pharmacotherapyonline.com.**

Geriatrics: Assessing Health and Delivering Healthcare to Older Adults

e25

Leigh Ann Mike, Zachary A. Marcum, and Shelly L. Gray

KEY CONCEPTS

1. The population of older adults in the United States is increasing and is expected to become more racially and ethnically diverse.
2. Ageism, or negative ideas about age and aging, can adversely affect health outcomes in older adults.
3. The primary goal of care for older adults is to maximize the amount of time they can live independently.
4. Living arrangements of older adults are tied to health and functional status, presence of disabilities, and caregiver ability, rather than chronological age.
5. Geriatric assessment is a multidisciplinary, multifaceted approach to promote wellness and prolong independence.
6. Geriatric syndromes are multifactorial clinical conditions that are linked with poor health outcomes.
7. Pharmacists can play an important role in identifying medications that may be contributing to geriatric syndromes.
8. Transitions of care are common and risky for older adults.
9. Optimal care transitions require teamwork, and the pharmacist's primary role on the care transitions team is to identify and address current and potential medication-related problems.

BEYOND THE BOOK

As the population of older adults continues to grow, there is a pressing need to reimagine what it means to age, to reframe thoughts about how older people contribute to society, and to combat ageism, which is defined as discrimination based on age. The Reframing Aging Initiative offers important suggestions on how to achieve this goal. Navigate to the Reframing Aging website resource page (https://www.reframingaging.org/Resources/Multimedia). Listen to the two-part podcast "Words Matter: a Podcast with Patricia D'Antonio." As you are listening to the podcast, recognize any implicit bias you may have against older people. Commit to making language choices that are less "othering" of or discriminatory against older people. Start by identifying one or two words that you will either avoid using or start using in your everyday life and future practice. Reframing your thoughts about age and aging can have a positive impact on health outcomes for older adults.

INTRODUCTION

The population of older adults aged 65 years or older is growing both globally and in the United States. This is due to increased life expectancy associated with advances in science and technology in early detection of diseases, therapeutic interventions that increase survival, and overall improved healthcare delivery to the general public such as vaccinations, access to care, and multiple treatment options.[1]

As people are living longer, they are likely to experience multiple chronic medical conditions. The fraction of older adults using healthcare resources will increase, primarily due to the aging of the "Baby Boomer" generation. Despite the development of chronic medical conditions, many older adults lead full, active lives with functional abilities largely preserved. This is contrary to the myth that older age is linked with sickness and disability or poor functional status. Many of these older adults either have few chronic conditions or have them well-controlled. The healthcare needs for an active 65-year-old person are different from an octogenarian living in a skilled-nursing facility. Additionally, with the advances in cancer treatment and the emergence of new therapies that have transformed diseases such as hepatitis C and acquired immunodeficiency syndrome into chronic conditions, it is likely that the healthcare resources used by older adults will include treatment of advanced diseases, life-prolonging measures, and general health maintenance.

The goal of providing optimal healthcare to older adults is to promote and maintain independence, which has a direct effect on quality of life. To achieve and maintain independence, healthcare providers can target interventions and approaches to promote and maintain functional status. The functional status of older adults is impacted by disease, accidents, age-related changes (eg, decreased muscle mass or bone density), and frailty; it is independent of chronological age. Because of this, there has been a shift in focus in older adults from managing health conditions alone to incorporating functional status into the assessment of health and wellness. This requires a holistic, multidisciplinary approach.

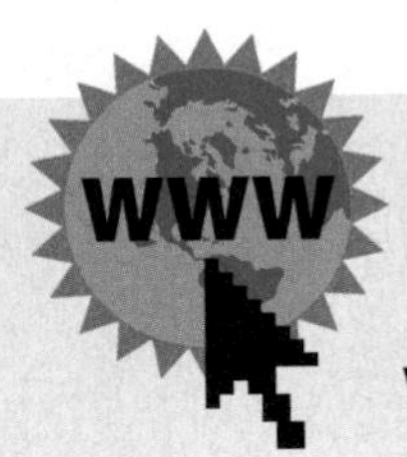

The complete chapter, learning objectives, and other resources can be found at **www.pharmacotherapyonline.com.**

Critical Care: Considerations in Medication Selection, Dosing, Monitoring, and Safety

e26

Erin F. Barreto and Amy L. Dzierba

KEY CONCEPTS

1. Intensive care units (ICU) are designed to support the complex needs of critically ill patients with acute organ dysfunction in need of a higher level of monitoring and treatment.
2. The four phases of critical illness include rescue, optimization, stabilization, and de-escalation, each of which can affect medication selection, dosing, and monitoring.
3. Ideal medications for use in the ICU have predictable bioavailability, fast onset, rapid titratability, and a wide therapeutic window.
4. Critically ill patients exhibit a uniquely complex pharmacokinetic profile and response to therapies that needs to be considered when individualizing drug regimens.
5. Acute changes to end-organ function occur more commonly in the ICU and dynamically affect drugs.
6. Perfusion deficits and iatrogenic exposures can decrease enteral, subcutaneous, and intramuscular drug bioavailability which makes the intravenous route preferred in acutely ill unstable patients in the ICU.
7. The use of advanced organ support devices is common in the ICU and each device differentially affects the pharmacokinetics and pharmacodynamics of medications.
8. Key properties of drugs susceptible to sequestration in the extracorporeal membrane oxygenation (ECMO) circuit include high percentage of protein binding and high degree of lipophilicity.
9. Highly protein-bound medications are readily cleared by molecular adsorbent recirculating system (MARS) and therapeutic plasma exchange (TPE), but not efficiently cleared by renal replacement therapies.
10. Many patient, provider, and environmental factors increase an ICU patient's vulnerability to medical errors, adverse medication reactions, and their related consequences, relative to their noncritically ill counterparts.

BEYOND THE BOOK

Watch the first 12 minutes of the video "Right dose, right now: customizing drug dosing for the critically ill patient" available at https://youtu.be/mG9BdYFocQk. This video briefly overviews some of the key pharmacokinetic and pharmacodynamic changes present in critically ill patients and the potential impact on anti-infective effectiveness and safety in the ICU.

INTRODUCTION

Epidemiology of Critical Illness

Since the poliomyelitis epidemic of the 1950s when mechanical ventilation was first introduced, significant advancements have been made in our understanding of the pathophysiology of syndromes of critical illness and the interventions needed to improve patient outcomes.[1] Only recently, however, have we begun to quantify the true global burden of critical illness. In the United States, 27% of all hospitalizations or 4.6 million stays annually include an intensive care unit (ICU) admission.[2] Short-term mortality for ICU patients is 8% to 22%, but can be much higher in patients with sepsis, acute respiratory distress syndrome, shock, or those in the developing world, where mortality may reach 50% to 60%.[3] Although surviving critical illness is a short-term goal, survivors can experience long-term physical, psychological, and cognitive consequences, collectively termed "post-intensive care syndrome." When considering these sequelae, care of critically ill patients is estimated to cost $121 to $263 billion annually in the United States, on par with the financial burden of cancer care or cardiovascular disease.[4] Clinicians and scientists seek new ways to more effectively prevent and treat critical illness to improve patient outcomes and limit the global health burden.

The Dynamic Trajectory of Critical Illness

1 Critical care medicine is a diverse discipline that integrates aspects of medicine, surgery, and anesthesia. Broadly, contemporary ICU patients include those with acute organ dysfunction in need of resuscitation or organ support and those in need of monitoring after a major event or intervention who are at high risk for complications (eg, surgical procedure, trauma, bleed).[5]

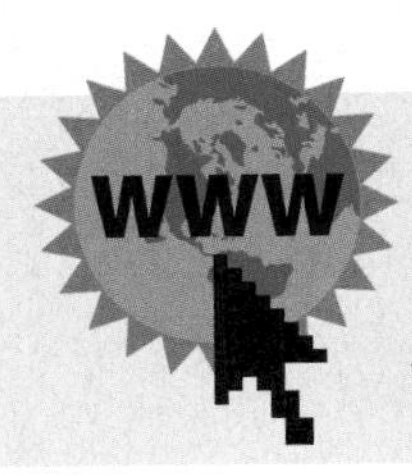

The complete chapter, learning objectives, and other resources can be found at **www.pharmacotherapyonline.com.**

Critical Care: Pain, Agitation, and Delirium

e27

Caitlin S. Brown and Gilles L. Fraser

KEY CONCEPTS

1. The primary goal of pain, agitation, and delirium (PAD) management is to provide patient comfort and safety with secondary goals to prevent immediate and long-term adverse physical and psychological outcomes.
2. PAD are interrelated and can confound efforts to provide intensive care including mobility, sleep, participation in care, and in shared patient/caregiver decisions about appropriate levels of care.
3. It is important to systematically evaluate PAD with validated tools for timely identification and correction of inciting clinical issues.
4. Preventative measures and nonpharmacologic strategies for PAD management should be initiated as early as possible.
5. A multifaceted, interprofessional approach to PAD management impacts care and clinical outcomes.
6. Pain is an important cause of agitation in the intensive care unit (ICU) and should be assessed and treated before administration of sedatives.
7. No proven pharmacologic strategies limit the severity and duration of ICU delirium.
8. Sedative choice (dexmedetomidine or propofol) and depth of sedation may have an important impact on patient assessments and outcomes.

BEYOND THE BOOK

Watch the video entitled "CAM-ICU Delirium Test" at the following link: <https://www.youtube.com/watch?v=6WyJ0zL7VkI>. This brief 3-minute video is an overview of a common and valid method of screening for delirium in critically ill adults who are unable to verbalize. This activity is useful to enhance student understanding of the COLLECT and ASSESS steps in the patient care process.

INTRODUCTION

Pain, agitation, and delirium are considered the most common clinical conditions confronting critically ill patients and their caregivers. These issues are stressful for patients as well as families and are often precipitated by factors that are frequently seen in the critically ill such as hemodynamic instability, inadequate oxygenation, metabolic derangements, pain, the inability to communicate, immobility, sleep deprivation, the need for invasive instrumentation, and loss of autonomy all occurring in an unfamiliar and threatening environment.

1 Short-term patient goals for PAD management include the provision of comfort and safety. It is also important to consider newly recognized long-term outcomes in critical care survivors that affect their quality of life such as the inability to return to baseline physiologic and cognitive function and a high frequency (50%) of unemployment for a year or longer after discharge from the hospital.[1-3] In addition, post-discharge post-traumatic stress disorder (PTSD) and depression are experienced by 7% and 20% to 30% of ICU survivors respectively at 1 year.[4,5]

All of these outcomes are impacted by our choice of therapeutics for PAD management. For example, the provision of inadequate pain relief can be regarded as inhumane, but conversely, overaggressive opioid therapy continued in the outpatient setting represents an obvious and avoidable risk factor in this era of opioid misuse.[6] The complexity of the pharmacologic and nonpharmacologic management of PAD requires knowledge of the risks and benefits of each option and necessitates a standardized, but flexible evidence-based approach[7] (Table e27-1).

Although we will be discussing PAD in this chapter as discrete clinical issues, the reader should appreciate that they are inter-related.[9] The interwoven nature of PAD is well demonstrated by a patient with unrelieved pain (a risk factor for delirium) who develops agitation. Dangerous agitation can result in patient harm or injury, but attempts to control these behaviors with sedatives can inadvertently precipitate delirium without addressing the inciting problem of pain.

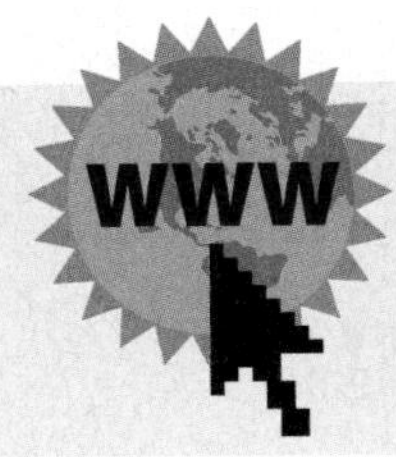

The complete chapter, learning objectives, and other resources can be found at **www.pharmacotherapyonline.com.**

Palliative and End-of-Life Care e28

Mary Lynn McPherson and Jessica E. Geiger

KEY CONCEPTS

1. Palliative care may be provided to any patient with a serious illness, at any point in the course of the illness, including while a patient receives curative or disease-focused therapy.
2. Hospice is a form of palliative care, which has been defined by Medicare to encompass care solely focused on comfort and quality of life for patients with a likely prognosis of 6 months or less.
3. Pain is a common symptom among patients receiving palliative care and may be managed safely and effectively using nonopioid, adjuvant, and/or opioid therapies.
4. Opioids are the drug of choice for the management of dyspnea.
5. Constipation, nausea, vomiting, anxiety, and delirium are common symptoms among patients receiving palliative care and may be managed effectively with drug and nondrug therapies.
6. End-of-life care can be provided to patients in the last days of their lives through palliative or hospice care and provides the management of common terminal symptoms.
7. Identifying a patient's goals and structuring care to achieve these goals is a key component of palliative care. Identifying a patient's goals of care involves communication with patients, their families and/or caregivers, as well as other healthcare professionals.
8. Addressing nonphysical needs—including spiritual, faith, and psychosocial—is a key component of providing quality palliative care.

BEYOND THE BOOK

Navigate to the website http://www.graduate.umaryland.edu/palliative, then click on "Palliative Care Chat Podcast" on the left-hand side. Scroll down to Episode 15: "Ten Tips Palliative Care Pharmacists Want the Palliative Care Team to Know When Caring for Patients." Select any two tips discussed in the podcast and critically think through why the tip is an important one for the rest of the hospice or palliative care team. This podcast is useful to enhance your understanding regarding the PLAN and MONITORING and FOLLOW-UP steps in the patient care process.

INTRODUCTION

1 Palliative care, or palliative medicine, is specialized care provided to patients with serious illness with a goal of managing symptoms and helping patients to cope with their illnesses.[1] It is provided by an interdisciplinary team of healthcare professionals, including physicians, pharmacists, nurses, nurse practitioners, social workers, chaplains, and others.[2] Palliative care is appropriate for any patient with a serious or potentially life-limiting illness, at any point during the time course of that illness. Common diseases for which palliative care is appropriate include cancer, heart failure, advanced lung disease such as chronic obstructive pulmonary disease (COPD), organ failure such as liver or renal failure, and neurologic diseases such as dementia and Parkinson disease.[2] Patients may receive palliative care throughout the course of a serious illness, including while the patient receives treatment aimed at managing or curing the disease. If or when the serious illness progresses and disease-focused therapies are no longer helpful or desired, palliative care continues to be provided to manage symptoms and maximize quality of life.

Provision of palliative and end-of-life care to patients with limited prognoses has been shown to improve patient and caregiver satisfaction,[3-5] reduce healthcare utilization,[3,4] and decrease healthcare costs.[3,4,6] In addition to providing symptom management, improving patient and caregiver satisfaction, and reducing healthcare costs, early integration of palliative care has been shown to increase survival among patients with advanced cancer.[7,8]

Because of the evidence supporting the benefits of palliative care, clinical practice guidelines for serious illnesses incorporate palliative care into treatment recommendations. Both the American Society of Clinical Oncology and National Comprehensive Cancer Network recommend palliative care as a component of oncology management.[9,10] In addition, the American College of Cardiology Foundation/American Heart Association practice guideline for the management of heart failure supports the incorporation of palliative care into the management of patients with advanced heart failure due to its effectiveness in increasing quality of life.[11]

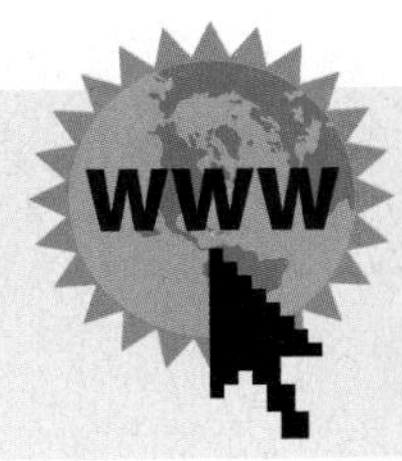

The complete chapter, learning objectives, and other resources can be found at **www.pharmacotherapyonline.com.**

Evaluation of Cardiovascular Function

e29

Brent N. Reed, Kristin Watson, and Gautam Ramani

KEY CONCEPTS

1. Many cardiovascular disorders develop over years to decades. Evaluation of the patient with or at risk for cardiovascular disease (CVD) must therefore include a comprehensive patient (or caregiver) interview to identify traditional risk factors and risk-enhancing factors for CVD. Along with other key information (eg, vital signs, laboratory values), these data can be used to determine a patient's risk for future cardiovascular events.
2. Changes in the frequency, duration, and severity of cardiac-related symptoms (eg, ischemic chest pain, dyspnea) are essential to the assessment of CVD and often guide the urgency of intervention as well as the specific pharmacologic strategies selected. A comprehensive patient interview can also be useful for discerning CVD from noncardiac disorders that share similar symptomology.
3. Obtaining an accurate blood pressure measurement is paramount to the evaluation and treatment of several cardiovascular disorders. Guidelines for appropriate measurement techniques include recommendations on patient preparation and position, cuff size, and blood pressure documentation.
4. Several cardiovascular disorders, such as heart failure (HF) and peripheral arterial disease, warrant physical examination of areas that are more distal from the heart, including the neck (eg, carotid arteries, jugular venous pressure, abdominojugular reflux) and lower extremities (eg, peripheral pulses, edema). Abnormal findings can prompt further evaluation or alterations in pharmacologic therapy.
5. Auscultation of the chest provides key information on valvular structure and function. Abnormal heart sounds can be used to guide the need for further evaluation.
6. Two key cardiac-specific laboratory tests are cardiac troponin and brain natriuretic peptide (BNP). Elevations in cardiac troponin may indicate the presence of myocardial infarction and can be used to guide both pharmacologic and nonpharmacologic interventions. A normal BNP concentration in a patient with dyspnea excludes the presence of HF whereas elevations are correlated with disease severity as well as long-term morbidity and mortality.
7. An electrocardiogram (ECG) records the pattern of electrical activity across the heart and each segment corresponds to an event in the cardiac cycle. The ECG provides an electrical map of the heart, which can be used to locate areas of ischemia or other pathology and identify arrhythmias. Alterations in the ECG such as QT-interval prolongation can be drug-related and may place patients at risk of potentially life-threatening arrhythmias.
8. Stress testing remains the most common initial strategy for evaluating chest pain suspicious for myocardial ischemia. The two main modalities for testing are inducing stress via exercise or the administration of a pharmacologic agent such as dobutamine or adenosine. The information provided by a stress test is often combined with echocardiography and radionuclide myocardial perfusion imaging.
9. Echocardiography uses sound waves to create an image of the heart, providing important information on the structure and function of heart valves and chambers. Although a transthoracic echocardiogram (TTE) is less invasive and provides the key information necessary for most clinical decisions, a transesophageal echocardiogram (TEE) may be required to visualize structures located in posterior areas of the heart (eg, mitral valve, left atrial appendage) and to guide surgical planning.
10. Left heart catheterization (LHC) is an invasive procedure in which a catheter is inserted into a large artery and advanced to the left side of the heart. The most common indication for LHC is coronary angiography, in which radiocontrast dye is used to visualize the coronary anatomy, most often for evaluation of chest pain, concern for myocardial infarction, and abnormal stress testing, and to guide decision-making regarding medical therapy, percutaneous coronary intervention, or coronary artery bypass grafting.
11. Right heart catheterization (RHC) involves advancing a catheter through a large vein and into the right side of the heart, where information on pulmonary and intracardiac hemodynamics can be obtained. Key parameters obtained during RHC include pulmonary artery pressures (including pulmonary capillary wedge pressure), cardiac output, and systemic and pulmonary vascular resistance, and these can be used to guide pharmacologic therapies in patients with HF or pulmonary hypertension.

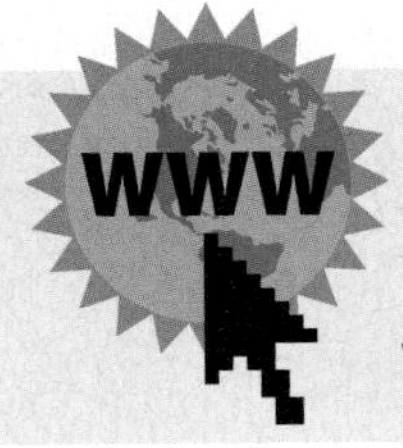

The complete chapter, learning objectives, and other resources can be found at **www.pharmacotherapyonline.com.**

Hypertension

30

Eric J. MacLaughlin and Joseph J. Saseen

KEY CONCEPTS

1. The risk of cardiovascular (CV) morbidity and mortality is directly correlated with blood pressure (BP).
2. Evidence definitively demonstrates that antihypertensive drug therapy substantially reduces the risks of CV events and death in patients with high BP.
3. Essential hypertension is usually an asymptomatic disease. A diagnosis cannot be made based on one elevated BP measurement. An elevated BP value from the average of two or more BP measurements, present during two or more clinical encounters, is required to establish a diagnosis of hypertension.
4. The overall goal of treating hypertension is to reduce associated morbidity and mortality from CV events. Antihypertensive drug therapy should be selected based on evidence demonstrating CV event reduction.
5. A goal BP of <130/80 mm Hg is appropriate for nearly all patients with hypertension.
6. The magnitude of BP elevation should be used to guide the number of antihypertensive agents to start when implementing drug therapy. Most patients with stage 1 hypertension should start on one medication as initial therapy. Most patients presenting with stage 2 hypertension should be started on two medications as initial therapy.
7. Lifestyle modifications should be prescribed to all patients, especially those with elevated BP and hypertension.
8. Angiotensin-converting enzyme inhibitors (ACEi), angiotensin II receptor blockers (ARBs), calcium channel blockers (CCBs), and thiazides are preferred first-line antihypertensive agents for most patients with hypertension. These first-line options are for patients with hypertension who do not have a compelling indication for a specific antihypertensive drug class.
9. For most patients with hypertension, β-blocker is not an appropriate first-line treatment. While β-blocker will reduce CV events in hypertension compared to no treatment, it will not reduce CV events as much as has been demonstrated with an ACEi, ARB, CCB, or thiazide.
10. Compelling indications are comorbid conditions where specific antihypertensive drug classes have been shown in clinical trials to reduce CV events in patients with these specific comorbidities.
11. Older patients are often at higher risk for adverse reactions related to antihypertensive medications. Antihypertensive drug therapy selection should be the same as in younger patients, but lower initial doses should be used to minimize the risk of side effects in older patients.
12. Patients are categorized as having resistant hypertension when they fail to achieve goal BP while adherent to a regimen that includes three antihypertensive agents (one of which includes a diuretic) at full doses, or when four or more antihypertensive agents are needed to treat hypertension regardless of goal BP achievement.
13. Alternative antihypertensive agents should only be used in combination with first-line antihypertensive agents to provide additional BP lowering because they do not have sufficient evidence demonstrating CV event reduction.

BEYOND THE BOOK

Clinical Interaction: Patient with Hypertension

Prepare for this activity by completing the following tasks:

- View the instructional video "How to Use Your Home Blood Pressure Monitor" at: https://www.youtube.com/watch?v=K9HU2F3TOal.
- Read the iForumRx.org commentary and listen to the podcast episode "Ten Things Every Clinician Should Know About the 2017 Hypertension Guidelines" available at: https://iforumrx.org/commentary/ten-things-every-clinician-should-know-about-the-2017-hypertension-guidelines/.

Complete the activity by doing the following:

- Identify a patient with hypertension that has been prescribed two or more antihypertensive agents.
- Measure a patient's BP using the technique demonstrated in the video.
- Engage in a brief discussion with your patient and address the following topics related to hypertension:
  - How long has the patient had hypertension?
  - What strategies does the patient use to take their antihypertensive medications regularly?
  - What does the patient believe are the benefits of the current antihypertensive drug regimen?
  - What does the patient identify as some of the risks of their current antihypertensive drug regimen?
  - How well does the patient think the drug therapy regimen is working?
  - What is the patient's goal BP?
  - Has the patient taken any other antihypertensive medications in the past and how did he/she respond to them?
  - What lifestyle modifications does the patient engage in to help control BP?
- At the end of this interview, write some brief notes about this patient encounter.

INTRODUCTION

Hypertension is a common disease that is defined as persistently elevated arterial blood pressure (BP). Although elevated BP was perceived to be "essential" for adequate perfusion of vital organs during the early and middle 1900s, it is one of the most significant risk factors for cardiovascular (CV) disease for decades. Therefore, increasing awareness and diagnosis of hypertension and improving BP control with appropriate treatment are considered critical public health initiatives to reduce CV morbidity and mortality.

The 2017 American College of Cardiology/American Heart Association (ACC/AHA) guideline for the Prevention, Detection, Evaluation, and Management of High Blood Pressure in Adults is the evidence-based clinical guideline in the United States to manage hypertension.[1] The 2017 ACC/AHA guideline provides recommendations on the definition of high BP, the diagnosis, patient evaluation, treatment goals, and management in various patient populations and provides additional strategies to improve BP control. This chapter incorporates relevant components of the 2017 ACC/AHA high BP guideline and additional evidence from clinical trials and meta-analyses, focusing on the pharmacotherapy for hypertension.

Pooled data from 2011 to 2014 indicate that approximately 103.3 million Americans aged 20 years and above met the definition of hypertension according to the 2017 ACC/AHA guideline.[2] More than half (53.4%) of the US adults taking antihypertensive medications had a BP above treatment goal. Considering the health consequences associated with high BP, there remain many opportunities for clinicians to improve the care of patients with hypertension.

EPIDEMIOLOGY

The definition of hypertension changed with the 2017 ACC/AHA guideline from a BP of ≥140/90 to ≥130/80 mm Hg. Hence, the prevalence of hypertension has increased considerably. According to the ACC/AHA definition, almost half (46%) of American adults aged 20 years and older have hypertension.[2] Although the overall prevalence has increased, only 1.9% would require additional drug therapy as the majority of newly diagnosed patients would require nonpharmacologic treatment only.[2]

The overall incidence of hypertension is similar between men and women but varies depending on age. The prevalence of high BP is higher in men than women before the age of 65 and is similar between the ages 65 and 74. However, after the age of 74, more women have high BP than men.[1] Prevalence rates are highest in non-Hispanic Blacks (59% in men, 56% in women), followed by non-Hispanic Whites (47% in men, 41% in women), non-Hispanic Asians (45% in men, 36% in women), and Hispanics (45% in men, 42% in women).[1]

BP values increase with age, and hypertension (persistently elevated BP values) is prevalent in older patients. The lifetime risk of developing hypertension among those 55 years of age and older who are normotensive is higher than 90%.[1] Most patients have elevated BP before being diagnosed with hypertension, with most diagnoses occurring between the third and fifth decades of life.

ETIOLOGY

Hypertension usually results from unknown pathophysiologic etiology (*essential* or *primary hypertension*). While this form of hypertension cannot be cured, it can be controlled. A smaller percentage of patients have a specific cause of their hypertension (*secondary hypertension*). There are many potential secondary causes of hypertension. If identified, hypertension in these patients can be mitigated or potentially be cured.

Primary Hypertension

Over 90% of individuals with high BP have essential or primary hypertension.[1] Numerous potential mechanisms have been identified that contribute to the pathogenesis of essential hypertension, so identifying the exact underlying abnormality is not possible. Genetic factors may play a role in developing essential hypertension by affecting sodium balance or other BP regulating pathways.

Secondary Hypertension

Secondary hypertension, where either a comorbid disease or a drug (or other product) is responsible for elevating BP (see Table 30-1), is much less common than primary hypertension (up to 10%).[1] In most cases, renal dysfunction resulting from severe chronic kidney disease (CKD) or renovascular disease is the most common secondary cause. Certain drugs (or other products) can directly or indirectly increase BP. The most common agents are listed in Table 30-1. When a secondary cause is identified, removing the offending agent (when feasible) or treating/correcting the underlying comorbid condition should be the first step in management.[1]

TABLE 30-1 Secondary Causes of Hypertension[a]

Diseases
- Chronic kidney disease
- Cushing's syndrome
- Coarctation of the aorta
- Obstructive sleep apnea
- Parathyroid disease
- Pheochromocytoma
- Primary aldosteronism
- Renovascular disease
- Thyroid disease

Medications
- Amphetamines (eg, amphetamine, dexmethylphenidate, dextroamphetamine, lisdexamfetamine, methylphenidate, phendimetrazine, phentermine)
- Antivascular endothelin growth factor agents (bevacizumab, sorafenib, sunitinib)
- Corticosteroids (cortisone, dexamethasone, fludrocortisone, hydrocortisone, methylprednisolone, prednisolone, prednisone, triamcinolone)
- Calcineurin inhibitors (cyclosporine, tacrolimus)
- Decongestants (pseudoephedrine, ocular phenylephrine)
- Ergot alkaloids (ergonovine, dihydroergotamine, methysergide)
- Erythropoiesis-stimulating agents (erythropoietin, darbepoetin)
- Estrogen-containing oral contraceptives
- Nonsteroidal anti-inflammatory drugs—cyclooxygenase-2 selective (celecoxib) and nonselective (aspirin [at higher doses], choline magnesium trisalicylate, diclofenac, diflunisal, etodolac, fenoprofen, flurbiprofen, ibuprofen, indomethacin, ketoprofen, ketorolac, meclofenamate, mefenamic acid, meloxicam, nabumetone, naproxen, naproxen sodium, oxaprozin, piroxicam, salsalate, sulindac, tolmetin)
- Testosterone
- Others: desvenlafaxine, venlafaxine, bupropion

Special situations with medications
- β-Blocker or centrally acting α-agonists (when abruptly discontinued)
- β-Blocker without α-blocker first when treating pheochromocytoma
- Use of a monoamine oxidase inhibitor (isocarboxazid, phenelzine, tranylcypromine) with tyramine-containing foods or certain drugs

Street drugs and other products
- Cocaine and cocaine withdrawal
- Methamphetamine
- Ephedra alkaloids (eg, Ma huang), "herbal ecstasy," other analogs
- Anabolic steroids
- Ergot-containing herbal products
- St. John's wort

Excessive consumption of food substances
- Sodium
- Ethanol
- Licorice

[a]Agents of most clinical importance.

PATHOPHYSIOLOGY

Multiple physiologic factors control BP, and abnormalities of these factors are potential contributing components in developing essential hypertension. These include malfunctions in either humoral (ie, the renin–angiotensin–aldosterone system [RAAS]) or vasodepressor mechanisms, abnormal neuronal mechanisms, defects in peripheral autoregulation, and disturbances in sodium, calcium, and natriuretic hormones. Many of these factors are cumulatively affected by the multifaceted RAAS, which ultimately regulates arterial BP. No one factor is probably solely responsible for essential hypertension.

Arterial BP

Arterial BP is the pressure in the arterial wall measured in millimeters of mercury (mm Hg). The two arterial BP values are *systolic BP* (SBP) and *diastolic BP* (DBP). SBP represents the peak pressure achieved during cardiac contraction. DBP is achieved after contraction when the cardiac chambers are filling and represents the nadir pressure. The absolute difference between SBP and DBP is called the pulse pressure and measures arterial wall tension. Mean arterial pressure (MAP) is the average pressure throughout the cardiac contraction cycle. It can be used clinically to represent overall arterial BP, especially in a hypertensive emergency. During a cardiac cycle, two-thirds of the time is spent in diastole and one-third in systole. Therefore, the MAP is calculated by using the following equation:

$$\text{MAP} = \left(\text{SBP} \times \frac{1}{3}\right) + \left(\text{DBP} \times \frac{2}{3}\right)$$

Arterial BP is hemodynamically generated by the interplay between blood flow and the resistance to blood flow. It is mathematically defined as the product of cardiac output (CO) and total peripheral resistance (TPR) according to the following equation:

$$\text{BP} = \text{CO} \times \text{TPR}$$

CO is the primary determinant of SBP, whereas TPR largely determines DBP. In turn, CO is a function of stroke volume, heart rate, and venous capacitance. Table 30-2 lists physiologic causes of increased CO and TPR and correlates them to potential mechanisms of pathogenesis.

Under normal physiologic conditions, arterial BP fluctuates throughout the day following a circadian rhythm. BP decreases to its lowest values during sleep, followed by a sharp rise starting a few hours before awakening, with the highest values occurring midmorning. BP also increases acutely during physical activity or emotional stress.

Classification

The classification of BP in adults (aged 18 years and older) is based on the average of two or more properly measured BP values from two or more clinical encounters (Table 30-3).[1] According to the ACC/AHA, there are four BP categories: normal, elevated, stage 1 hypertension, and stage 2 hypertension. Elevated BP is not a disease category but is associated with increased adverse CV risks compared to patients with normal BP.[3] It identifies patients whose BP is likely to progress to hypertension in the future, and thus for whom lifestyle modifications should be enacted to attenuate this progression.

Hypertensive crises are clinical situations where patients have extreme BP elevations, typically >180/120 mm Hg. They are categorized as either *hypertensive emergency* or *hypertensive urgency*. Hypertensive emergencies are extreme BP elevations that are accompanied by acute or progressing end-organ damage. Hypertensive urgencies are extreme BP elevations without acute or progressing end-organ injury.

TABLE 30-2 Potential Mechanisms of Pathogenesis

Blood pressure (BP) is the mathematical product of cardiac output and peripheral resistance. Elevated BP can result from increased cardiac output and/or increased total peripheral resistance.

Increased cardiac output	*Increased cardiac preload:* • Increased fluid volume from excess sodium intake or renal sodium retention *Venous constriction:* • Excess stimulation of the renin–angiotensin–aldosterone system (RAAS) • Sympathetic nervous system overactivity
Increased peripheral resistance	*Functional vascular constriction:* • Excess stimulation of the RAAS • Sympathetic nervous system overactivity • Genetic alterations of cell membranes • Endothelial-derived factors *Structural vascular hypertrophy:* • Excess stimulation of the RAAS • Sympathetic nervous system overactivity • Genetic alterations of cell membranes • Endothelial-derived factors • Hyperinsulinemia

TABLE 30-3 Classification of Blood Pressure in Adults (Age ≥18 Years)[a]

Classification	Systolic Blood Pressure (mm Hg)		Diastolic Blood Pressure (mm Hg)
Normal	<120	and	<80
Elevated	120-129	and	<80
Stage 1 hypertension	130-139	or	80-89
Stage 2 hypertension	≥140	or	≥90

[a]Classification is determined based on the average of two or more properly measured seated BP values from two or more clinical encounters. Out-of-office measurements should be used to confirm the diagnosis. If systolic and diastolic BP values yield different classifications, the highest category is used for the purpose of determining a classification.

Cardiovascular Risk and Blood Pressure

1 Epidemiologic data demonstrate a strong correlation between BP and CV morbidity and mortality.[4] Risk of hypertension-associated complications (eg, stroke, myocardial infarction [MI], angina, heart failure [HF], kidney failure, early death from CV causes) is directly correlated with BP. Starting at a BP of 115/75 mm Hg, the risk of CV disease doubles with every 20/10 mm Hg increase.[1] Therefore, patients with elevated BP have an increased risk of CV disease.

2 Treating patients with hypertension with antihypertensive drug therapy reduces the risk of CV events. Evidence from large-scale placebo-controlled clinical trials has repeatedly shown that the increased risks of CV events and death associated with elevated BP are reduced substantially by antihypertensive drug therapy (see Treatment section).[5-8]

SBP is a stronger predictor of CV disease than DBP in adults aged 50 years and older; it is the most important BP parameter for most patients.[1] Patients are considered to have *isolated systolic hypertension* when their SBP values are elevated (ie, ≥130 mm Hg) and DBP values are normal (ie, <80 mm Hg). Isolated systolic hypertension is believed to result from pathophysiologic changes in the arterial vasculature, consistent with aging, that result in decreased compliance of the arterial wall and portend an increased risk of CV morbidity and mortality. A higher than normal pulse pressure (SBP minus DBP) is believed to reflect the extent of atherosclerotic disease in older patients and is a measure of increased arterial stiffness. Higher pulse pressure values are directly correlated with the risk of CV mortality.

Humoral Mechanisms

Several humoral abnormalities involving the RAAS, natriuretic hormone, and hyperinsulinemia may be involved in developing essential hypertension.

The Renin–Angiotensin–Aldosterone System

The RAAS is a complex endogenous system that is involved with most regulatory components of arterial BP. Activation and regulation are primarily governed by the kidney (see Fig. 30-1). The RAAS regulates sodium, potassium, and blood volume. Therefore, this system significantly influences the vascular tone and sympathetic nervous system activity and is the most influential contributor to the homeostatic regulation of BP.

Renin is an enzyme stored in the juxtaglomerular cells within the afferent arterioles of the kidney. The release of renin is modulated by several factors: intrarenal factors (eg, renal perfusion pressure, catecholamines, angiotensin II) and extrarenal factors (eg, sodium, chloride, potassium).

Juxtaglomerular cells function as a baroreceptor-sensing device. Decreased renal artery pressure and kidney blood flow are sensed by these cells and stimulate renin secretion. A decrease in sodium and chloride delivered to the distal tubule stimulates renin release. Catecholamines increase renin release, most likely by directly stimulating sympathetic nerves on the afferent arterioles that, in turn, activate the juxtaglomerular cells.

Renin catalyzes the conversion of angiotensinogen to angiotensin I in the blood. Angiotensin I is then converted to angiotensin II by angiotensin-converting enzyme (ACE). After binding to specific receptors (classified as either angiotensin II type 1 [AT_1] or angiotensin II type 2 [AT_2] subtypes), angiotensin II exerts biologic effects in several tissues. AT_1 receptors are located in the brain, kidneys, myocardium, peripheral vasculature, and adrenal glands. These receptors mediate most responses that are critical to CV and kidney function. AT_2 receptors are located in the adrenal medullary tissue, uterus, and brain. Stimulation of the AT_2 receptor does not influence BP regulation.

Circulating angiotensin II can elevate BP through pressor and volume effects. Pressor effects include direct vasoconstriction, stimulation of catecholamine release from the adrenal medulla, and centrally mediated increases in sympathetic nervous system activity. Angiotensin II also stimulates aldosterone synthesis from the adrenal cortex, leading to sodium and water reabsorption, increasing plasma volume, TPR, and ultimately BP. Aldosterone also has a deleterious role in the pathophysiology of other CV diseases (eg, HF, MI, kidney disease) by promoting tissue remodeling leading to myocardial fibrosis and vascular dysfunction. Clearly, any disturbance that leads to activation of the RAAS could explain chronic hypertension.

Natriuretic Hormone

Natriuretic hormone inhibits sodium and potassium-ATPase and thus interferes with sodium transport across cell membranes.

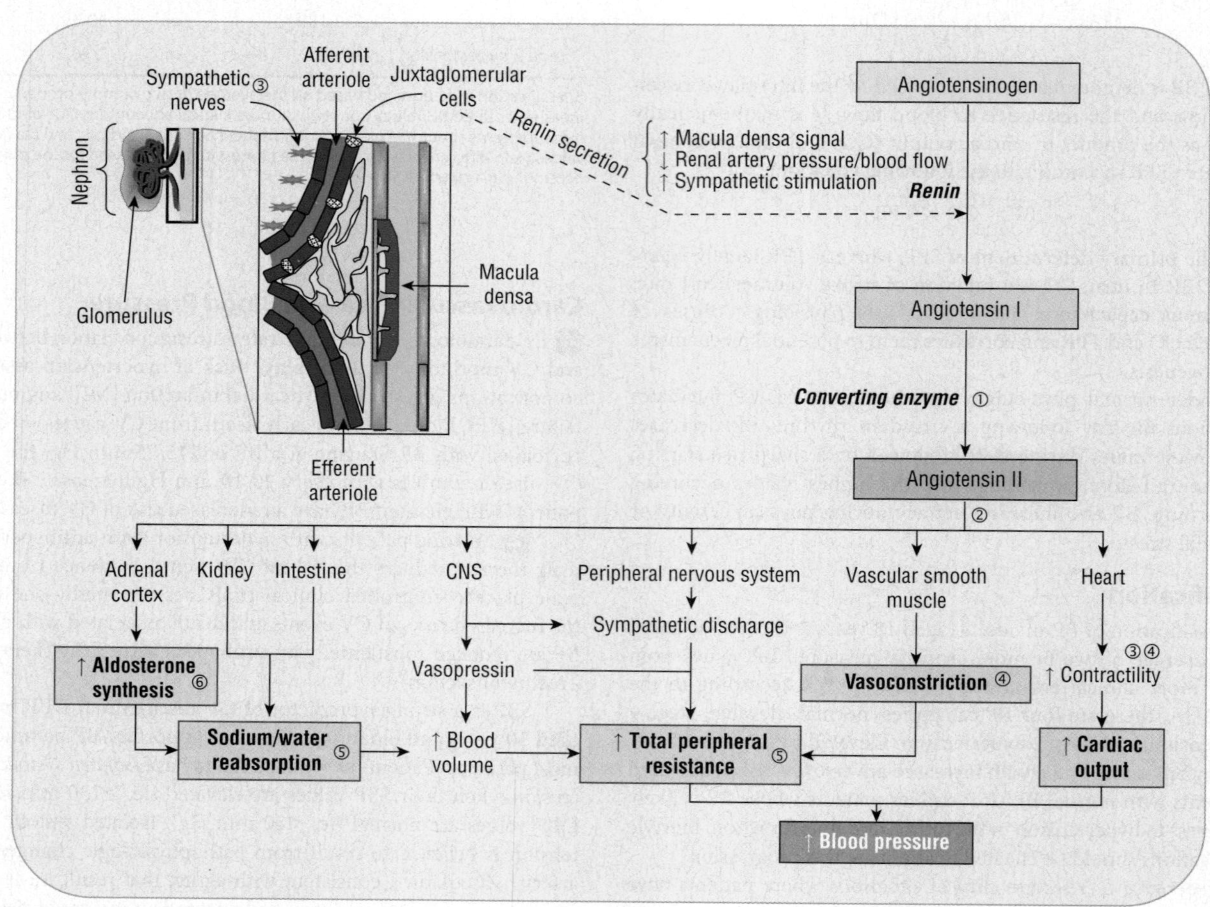

FIGURE 30-1 Diagram representing the renin–angiotensin–aldosterone system. The interrelationship between the kidney, angiotensin II, and regulation of blood pressure is depicted. Renin secretion from the juxtaglomerular cells in the afferent arterioles is regulated by three major factors that trigger the conversion of angiotensinogen to angiotensin 1. The primary sites of action for major antihypertensive agents are included: ① ACE inhibitor; ② angiotensin II receptor blocker; ③ β-blocker; ④ calcium channel blocker; ⑤ thiazide; ⑥ mineralocorticoid receptor antagonist.

Inherited defects in the kidney's ability to eliminate sodium can cause increased blood volume. A compensatory increase in the concentration of circulating natriuretic hormone theoretically could increase urinary excretion of sodium and water.

Neuronal Regulation

Central and autonomic nervous systems are intricately involved in the regulation of arterial BP. Many receptors that either enhance or inhibit norepinephrine release are located on the presynaptic surface of sympathetic terminals. The α and β presynaptic receptors play a role in negative and positive feedback to the norepinephrine-containing vesicles. Stimulation of presynaptic α-receptors (α_2) exerts a negative inhibition on norepinephrine release. Conversely, stimulation of presynaptic β-receptors facilitates norepinephrine release.

Sympathetic neuronal fibers located on the surface of effector cells innervate the α- and β-receptors. Stimulation of postsynaptic α-receptors (α_1) on arterioles and venules results in vasoconstriction. There are two types of postsynaptic β-receptors, β_1 and β_2. Both are present in all tissues innervated by the sympathetic nervous system. However, in some tissues, β_1-receptors predominate (eg, heart), and in other tissues, β_2-receptors predominate (eg, bronchioles). Stimulation of β_1-receptors in the heart increases heart rate (chronotropy) and force of contraction (inotropy), whereas stimulation of β_2-receptors causes vasodilation in arteries and veins.

The baroreceptor reflex system is the primary negative feedback mechanism that controls sympathetic activity. Baroreceptors are nerve endings lying in the walls of large arteries, especially in the carotid arteries and aortic arch. Changes in arterial BP rapidly activate baroreceptors that then transmit impulses to the brain stem through the ninth cranial nerve and vagus nerve. In this reflex system, a decrease in arterial BP stimulates baroreceptors, causing reflex vasoconstriction, increased heart rate, and increased force of cardiac contraction. However, baroreceptor reflex mechanisms may be less responsive in older patients and those with diabetes.

Stimulation of specific areas within the central nervous system (eg, nucleus tractus solitarius, vagal nuclei, vasomotor center, area postrema) can either increase or decrease BP. For example, α_2-adrenergic stimulation within the central nervous system decreases BP through inhibitory effects on the vasomotor center. However, angiotensin II increases sympathetic outflow from the vasomotor center, which increases BP.

Neuronal mechanisms regulate BP and maintain homeostasis. Pathologic disturbances in any of the four major components (autonomic nerve fibers, adrenergic receptors, baroreceptors, and central nervous system) could chronically elevate BP. These systems are physiologically interrelated. A defect in one component may alter normal function in another. Therefore, cumulative abnormalities may explain the development of essential hypertension.

Peripheral Autoregulatory Components

Abnormalities in renal or tissue autoregulatory systems could cause hypertension. For example, renal defects in sodium excretion may develop, which can then cause resetting of tissue autoregulatory processes resulting in a higher BP. The kidney usually maintains a normal BP through a volume-pressure adaptive mechanism. When BP drops, the kidneys respond by increasing retention of sodium and water, which leads to plasma volume expansion that increases BP. Conversely, when BP rises above normal, renal sodium and water excretion increase to reduce plasma volume and CO.

Local autoregulatory processes maintain adequate tissue oxygenation. When tissue oxygen demand is normal to low, the local arteriolar bed remains relatively vasoconstricted. However, increased metabolic demand triggers arteriolar vasodilation that lowers peripheral vascular resistance (PVR) and increases blood flow and oxygen delivery.

Defects in renal adaptive mechanisms could lead to plasma volume expansion and increased blood flow to peripheral tissues, even when BP is normal. Local tissue autoregulatory processes that vasoconstrict would then be activated to offset the increased blood flow. This effect would result in increased PVR and, if sustained, would also thicken the arteriolar walls. This pathophysiologic component is plausible because increased TPR is a common underlying finding in essential hypertension.

Vascular Endothelial Mechanisms

Vascular endothelium and smooth muscle play essential roles in regulating blood vessel tone and BP. Regulating functions are mediated by vasoactive substances that are synthesized by endothelial cells. It has been postulated that a deficiency in local synthesis of vasodilating substances (eg, prostacyclin and bradykinin) or excess vasoconstricting substances (eg, angiotensin II and endothelin I) contributes to essential hypertension.

Nitric oxide is produced in the endothelium, relaxes the vascular epithelium, and is a potent vasodilator. The nitric oxide system is an important regulator of arterial BP. Patients with hypertension may have an intrinsic nitric oxide deficiency, resulting in impaired vasodilation.

Electrolytes

Population-based studies demonstrate that high-sodium diets are associated with a high prevalence of stroke and hypertension. Conversely, low-sodium diets are associated with a lower prevalence of hypertension. Clinical studies have shown that dietary sodium restriction lowers BP in many (but not all) patients with elevated BP. The exact mechanisms by which excess sodium leads to hypertension are not known.

Alterations in calcium and potassium may also play an important role in the pathogenesis of hypertension. A lack of dietary calcium hypothetically can disturb the balance between intracellular and extracellular calcium, resulting in an increased intracellular calcium concentration and alterations in vascular smooth muscle function. Dietary potassium intake is inversely related to BP and may blunt the effect of sodium on BP.[1] Potassium depletion may also increase PVR, but the clinical significance of small serum potassium concentration changes in relation to BP is unclear. While altered calcium and potassium may play a role in the development of hypertension, data demonstrating reduced CV risk with supplementation are limited.

CLINICAL PRESENTATION

Diagnostic Considerations

3 Hypertension is called the *silent killer* because most patients do not have symptoms. The primary physical finding is persistently increased BP. The diagnosis of hypertension cannot be made based on one elevated BP measurement. The average of two or more BP measurements taken during two or more clinical encounters is required to diagnose hypertension.[1] This BP average should be used to establish a diagnosis and then classify the initial stage of hypertension using Table 30-3. Out-of-office measurements should be used to confirm elevated readings.

Measuring BP

The measurement of BP is a medical screening tool and should be conducted at every healthcare encounter.[1]

Cuff Measurement The most common method to measure BP in clinical practice is the indirect measurement of BP using an oscillometric device or sphygmomanometry. The AHA describes the appropriate procedure to measure BP indirectly.[9] The measurement equipment (ie, inflation cuff, stethoscope, and manometer) must meet national standards to ensure maximum quality and precision with measurement.

The AHA stepwise technique is recommended:

1. Patients should ideally refrain from nicotine and caffeine ingestion for 30 minutes, have emptied his/her bladder, and sit with lower back supported in a chair. Their bare arm should be supported and rest near heart level. The feet should be flat on the floor (with legs not crossed). The measurement environment should be relatively quiet and ideally provide privacy. Measuring BP in a position other than seated (supine or standing position) may be required under special circumstances (eg, suspected orthostatic hypotension, dehydration).
2. Measurement should begin only after a 5-minute period of rest in the seated position.
3. Neither the patient nor the clinician measuring the BP should talk during measurement.
4. A properly sized cuff (pediatric, small, regular, large, or extra-large) should be used. The inflatable rubber bladder should cover at least 80% of arm circumference and a width that is at least 40% of arm circumference.
5. The palpatory method should be used to estimate the SBP:
   a. Place the cuff on the upper arm with the bottom resting 2 to 3 cm above the antecubital fossa and attach it to the manometer.
   b. Close the inflation valve and inflate the cuff to 70 mm Hg. Palpate the radial pulse with the index and middle fingers of the opposite hand.
   c. Inflate further in increments of 10 mm Hg until the radial pulse can no longer be palpated.
   d. Note the pressure at which the radial pulse is no longer palpated. This is the estimated SBP.
   e. Rapidly release the pressure in the cuff by opening the valve.
6. The stethoscope (either diaphragm or bell) should be placed on the bare skin of the antecubital fossa, directly over where the brachial artery is palpated. The stethoscope earpieces should be inserted appropriately. The valve should be closed and then the cuff inflated to 30 mm Hg above the estimated SBP from the palpatory method. The valve should then be slightly opened to slowly release pressure at a rate of approximately 2 mm Hg/s.
7. The clinician should listen for Korotkoff sounds with the stethoscope. The first phase of Korotkoff sounds is the initial presence of clear tapping sounds indicating cardiac contraction. Note the pressure at the first recognition of these sounds. This is the SBP. As pressure deflates, note the pressure when all sounds disappear, right at the last sound. This is the DBP.
8. Record the SBP and DBP to the nearest even number (eg, 145 mm Hg rounded up to 146 mm Hg).
9. A second measurement should be obtained after 1 to 2 minutes. If the two measurements (SBP and/or DBP) differ by more than 5 mm Hg, additional measurement(s) should be obtained.
10. When first establishing care with a patient, BP should be measured in both arms. If consistent inter-arm differences exist, the arm with the higher value should be used.

Inaccuracies with indirect measurements result from inherent biologic variability of BP, errors related to incorrect technique, and the white coat effect.[9] Variations in BP occur with environmental temperature, the time of day, meals, physical activity, posture, alcohol, nicotine, and emotions. In the clinical setting, standard BP measurement procedures (eg, appropriate rest period, correct technique, wrong cuff size) are often not followed, which results in incorrect estimation of true BP. In addition, variations may occur between individuals measuring BP. Due to these factors, the use of oscillometric devices is generally preferred.

Approximately 15% to 20% of patients have *white coat hypertension*, where BP values rise in a clinical setting but are normal in nonclinical environments as measured with home or ambulatory BP (ABP) monitors.[1] Interestingly, the rise in BP dissipates gradually after leaving the clinical setting. This is in contrast to *masked hypertension*, where a decrease in BP occurs in the clinical setting.[1] With masked hypertension, home BP is much higher than the in-office BP measurement. This situation may lead to undertreatment or lack of treatment for hypertension. While white coat hypertension is associated with a minimal increase in CV events, masked hypertension increases the risk similar to those with sustained hypertension. Moreover, patients with either white coat or masked hypertension are at higher risk of progressing to sustained hypertension.[10]

Pseudohypertension is a falsely elevated BP measurement. It may be seen in older patients, those with long-standing diabetes, or those with CKD due to rigid, calcified brachial arteries.[9] In these patients, the true arterial BP, when measured directly with intraarterial measurement (the most accurate BP measurement), is much lower than that measured using the indirect cuff method.

Ambulatory and Home BP Monitoring ABP monitoring using an automated device records BP at frequent time intervals (eg, every 15-30 minutes) throughout a 24-hour period.[9] Home BP monitoring is performed by patients or a caregiver, preferably in the morning. Upper arm devices are preferred over wrist monitors because of concerns regarding the precision of readings. Many wrist monitors are not validated, and positioning of the device (directly over the radial artery) is essential, and the wrist must be placed directly over the heart. However, a validated wrist monitor may be an option for patients whose arm measurements with home devices are difficult or not possible (eg, manual dexterity, extreme obesity). Patients should be counseled to obtain BP monitors that have been validated (see https://www.validatebp.org).

Home BP monitoring values and ABP values are often lower than clinic-measured values, particularly as BP increases beyond elevated to stage 1 and stage 2 hypertension.[1] For example, a clinic BP of 130/80 mm Hg corresponds to a home BP reading of 130/80 mm Hg and a 24-hr ABP of 125/75 mm Hg. However, a clinic BP of 140/90 mm Hg corresponds to a home BP monitoring value of 135/85 mm Hg and a 24-hours ABP value of 130/80 mm Hg.

Neither ABP nor home BP monitoring is needed for the diagnosis of hypertension, but they are recommended. These modalities are needed to identify patients with white coat or masked hypertension.[1] In addition, ABP monitoring may be a stronger predictor of all-cause and CV mortality than clinic measurements.[11] The 2017 ACC/AHA guideline recommends out-of-office measurements for diagnostic confirmation and to assist in titrating antihypertensive medication.[1] ABP monitoring may be helpful for patients with apparent drug resistance, hypotensive symptoms while on antihypertensive therapy, episodic hypertension (eg, white coat hypertension), and autonomic dysfunction, and in identifying "nondippers" whose BP does not decrease by >10% during sleep and who may portend an increased risk of hypertension-associated complications.

Limitations of ABP and home BP measurements include the complexity of use and costs. Although home BP monitoring is less complicated and less costly than ambulatory monitoring, patients may omit or fabricate readings or have a poor technique (eg, not resting for an adequate period, improper placement, wrong cuff size). Therefore, patients should be educated on the appropriate

CLINICAL PRESENTATION Hypertension

General: May appear healthy or may have additional CV risk factors:

- Age (≥55 years for men, ≥65 years for women)
- Diabetes (type 1 or type 2)
- Dyslipidemia
- Albuminuria
- Family history of premature CV disease
- Overweight (body mass index [BMI] 25-29.9 kg/m^2) or obesity (BMI ≥ 30 kg/m^2)
- Physical inactivity
- Tobacco use

Symptoms: Usually none related to elevated BP

Signs: Previous BP (SBP or DBP) values in the elevated or the hypertension category.

Routine laboratory tests: Blood urea nitrogen (BUN)/serum creatinine with estimated glomerular filtration rate (using CKD-EPI Creatinine Equation [2021]; available at https://https://www.kidney.org/professionals/kdoqi/gfr_calculator), lipid panel, fasting blood glucose, serum electrolytes (sodium, potassium, calcium), hemoglobin and hematocrit, and electrocardiogram. May have normal values and still have hypertension. However, some may have abnormal values consistent with either additional CV risk factors or hypertension-related damage.

Other tests: Echocardiogram, spot urine albumin-to-creatinine ratio, uric acid

Hypertension-related complications: The patient may have a previous medical history or diagnostic findings that indicate the presence of hypertension-associated complications:

- Brain (stroke, transient ischemic attack, dementia)
- Eyes (retinopathy)
- Heart (left ventricular hypertrophy [LVH], angina, prior MI, prior coronary revascularization, HF)
- Kidney (chronic kidney disease [CKD])
- Peripheral vasculature (peripheral arterial disease [PAD])

selection of a home BP device (eg, validated machine, ideally has a memory feature, right cuff size) and how to use it correctly.

Clinical Evaluation

The most common sign of essential hypertension is increased BP. The rest of the physical examination may be completely normal. However, a complete medical evaluation is recommended after diagnosis to (a) identify secondary causes, (b) identify other CV risk factors or comorbid conditions that may define prognosis and/or guide therapy, and (c) assess for the presence or absence of hypertension-associated complications. All patients with hypertension should have the tests described in the Clinical Presentation box before initiating antihypertensive drug therapy.[1] For patients *without* a history of atherosclerotic cardiovascular disease (ASCVD), CKD or diabetes, it is also important to estimate future risk of ASCVD using the Pooled Cohort Equations calculator. This calculator estimates the 10-year risk of clinical ASCVD (defined as coronary death or nonfatal myocardial infarction, or fatal or nonfatal stroke) and lifetime risk in certain patients (found at http://tools.acc.org/ASCVD-Risk-Estimator-Plus/#!/calculate/estimate/).

Secondary Causes

The most common secondary causes of hypertension are listed in Table 30-1. A complete medical evaluation should provide clues for identifying secondary hypertension. Patients with secondary hypertension might have signs or symptoms suggestive of the underlying disorder. Patients with pheochromocytoma may have a history of paroxysmal headaches, sweating, tachycardia, and palpitations. Over half of these patients suffer from episodes of orthostatic hypotension. In primary hyperaldosteronism, symptoms related to hypokalemia usually include muscle cramps and muscle weakness. Patients with Cushing's syndrome may complain of weight gain, polyuria, edema, menstrual irregularities, recurrent acne, or muscular weakness and have several classic physical features (eg, moon face, buffalo hump, hirsutism). Patients with coarctation of the aorta may have higher BP in the arms than in the legs and diminished or even absent femoral pulses. Patients with renal artery stenosis may have an abdominal systolic-diastolic bruit.

Laboratory tests may also help identify secondary hypertension. Baseline hypokalemia may suggest mineralocorticoid-induced hypertension. Protein, red blood cells, and casts in the urine may indicate renovascular disease. Some laboratory tests are used specifically to diagnose secondary hypertension. These include plasma norepinephrine and urinary metanephrine for pheochromocytoma, plasma and urinary aldosterone concentrations for primary hyperaldosteronism, and plasma renin activity, captopril stimulation test, renal vein renin, and renal artery angiography for renovascular disease.

Certain drugs and other products can increase BP (see Table 30-1). For some patients, the addition of these agents can be the cause of hypertension or can exacerbate underlying hypertension. Identifying a temporal relationship between starting the suspected agent and developing elevated BP suggests drug-induced BP elevation.

Natural Course of Disease

The onset of hypertension is usually preceded by increased BP values that are in the elevated BP category. BP values may fluctuate between elevated and normal levels for a period of time. As the disease progresses, PVR increases, and BP elevation becomes chronic.

Hypertension-Associated Complications

Several complications can result from high BP in patients with hypertension (see Clinical Presentation box). CV events (eg, MI, cerebrovascular events, kidney failure) are the primary causes of CV morbidity and mortality in patients with hypertension. The probability of CV events and CV morbidity and mortality in patients with hypertension is directly correlated with the severity of BP elevation.

Hypertension accelerates the development of atherosclerosis and stimulates left ventricular and vascular dysfunction. These pathologic changes are thought to be secondary to both a chronic pressure overload and a variety of nonhemodynamic stimuli. Atherosclerosis in hypertension is accompanied by the proliferation of smooth muscle cells, lipid infiltration into the vascular endothelium, and enhancement of vascular calcium accumulation.

Cerebrovascular disease is a consequence of hypertension. Either gross neurologic deficits or a slight hemiparesis with some incoordination and hyperreflexia is indicative of cerebrovascular disease. Stroke can result from lacunar infarcts caused by thrombotic occlusion of small vessels or intracerebral hemorrhage resulting from ruptured microaneurysms. Transient ischemic attacks (TIAs) secondary to atherosclerosis in the carotid arteries can also develop in patients with hypertension.

Retinopathies can occur in hypertension and may manifest as a variety of different findings. A funduscopic examination can detect hypertensive retinopathy, which manifests as arteriolar narrowing, focal arteriolar constrictions, arteriovenous crossing changes (nicking), retinal hemorrhages and exudates, and disk edema. Focal arteriolar narrowing, retinal infarcts, and flame-shaped hemorrhages usually suggest an accelerated or malignant phase of hypertension (seen in some hypertensive emergencies). Papilledema (swelling of the optic disk) is usually only present in hypertensive emergencies.

Heart disease is a commonly identified complication of hypertension. A thorough cardiac and pulmonary examination can identify cardiopulmonary abnormalities. Clinical manifestations include stable ischemic heart disease (angina, prior MI, prior coronary revascularization), acute coronary syndromes (aka, acute MI), and HF. These complications may lead to cardiac arrhythmias, angina, MI, and sudden death. Stable ischemic heart disease (also called *coronary artery disease* or *coronary heart disease*) and associated acute coronary syndromes (also called *CV events*) are the most common causes of death in patients with hypertension.

The kidney damage caused by hypertension is characterized pathologically by hyaline arteriosclerosis, hyperplastic arteriosclerosis, arteriolar hypertrophy, fibrinoid necrosis, and atheroma of the major renal arteries. Glomerular hyperfiltration and intraglomerular hypertension are early stages of hypertensive nephropathy, followed by persistent albuminuria and then a gradual decline in kidney function. The primary renal complication in hypertension is nephrosclerosis, which is secondary to arteriosclerosis. Atheromatous disease of a major renal artery may give rise to renal artery stenosis. Overt kidney failure is an important cause of end-stage kidney disease, especially in Black patients, Hispanic persons, and Native Americans.

The peripheral vasculature is a target organ affected by hypertension. Physical examination of the vascular system can detect evidence of atherosclerosis, which may present as arterial bruits (aortic, abdominal, or peripheral), distended veins, diminished or absent peripheral arterial pulses, or lower extremity edema. Peripheral arterial disease (PAD) is a clinical condition that can result from atherosclerosis.

TREATMENT

Overall Goal of Treatment

4 The overall goal of treating hypertension is to reduce morbidity and mortality from CV events (eg, acute coronary syndromes, cerebrovascular events, HF) and kidney disease. Therefore, the specific selection of antihypertensive drug therapy should be based on evidence demonstrating a reduction in morbidity and mortality, not merely a reduction in BP.

Blood Pressure Goals

5 Treating patients with hypertension to achieve a desired goal BP is a surrogate goal of therapy. Reducing BP to a goal does not guarantee the prevention of hypertension-associated complications but significantly lowers risk. Targeting a goal BP is the standard of care for how clinicians evaluate response to therapy. It is the primary method used to determine the need for titration and regimen modification.

The 2017 ACC/AHA guideline recommends a goal BP of <130/80 mm Hg for the management of hypertension in most patients (Box A), including those with ASCVD, diabetes, or chronic kidney disease.[1] The American Diabetes Association recommends a minimum goal of <140/90 mm Hg for patients with diabetes and lowers CV risk, with a lower goal of <130/80 mm Hg for certain individuals (eg, those at higher risk of ASCVD) if achieved without undue treatment burden.[12] The Kidney Disease Improving Global Outcomes (KDIGO) guidelines recommend an SBP goal of <120 mm Hg for patients with CKD (not receiving dialysis) when tolerated.[13]

BOX A DESIRED OUTCOMES: GOAL BP FOR CHRONIC TREATMENT

Most patients (includes patients with clinical ASCVD [secondary prevention], diabetes, or CKD; primary prevention patients regardless of 10-year ASCVD risk score)

- <130/80 mm Hg

Older ambulatory, community-dwelling patients

- SBP <130 mm Hg

Institutionalized older patients, those with high disease burden and comorbidities, or limited life-expectancy:

- Consider a relaxed SBP goal of at least <150 mm Hg; <140 mm Hg in some patients if tolerated
- Use a team-based decision process weighing patient preferences, risks, and benefits

Historically, most patients with hypertension were treated to a goal BP of <140/90 mm Hg, with <130/80 mm Hg recommended for higher-risk patients. However, evidence demonstrates a significantly lower risk of CV events with lower BP goals. Some of the strongest data supporting the lower BP goals comes from the Systolic Blood Pressure Intervention Trial (SPRINT). SPRINT evaluated a systolic BP goal of <120 mm Hg versus <140 mm Hg in patients with hypertension at high CV risk but without diabetes.[14] The study was stopped early after a median follow-up of 3.3 years due to a significantly lower risk of the primary composite outcome (MI, other acute coronary syndromes, stroke, HF, or death from CV causes) and all-cause mortality in patients treated to the lower BP goals. The final results when the trial was fully adjudicated were consistent with the initially published report.[15] Despite an increased risk of adverse events in the intensive treatment group (eg, hypotension, syncope, electrolyte abnormalities, and acute kidney injury or failure), the significant benefits outweighed these risks, with intensive BP control improving survival by 6 months to 3 years in middle-aged and older adults with high CV risk.[16]

In addition to SPRINT, several other systematic reviews and meta-analyses demonstrate that lower BP goals improve clinical outcomes better than higher BP goals.[17-21] In a systematic review and meta-analysis of 19 trials involving 44,989 patients, intensive treatment (mean BP 133/76 mm Hg) was associated with a reduced risk of major CV events, MI, stroke, albuminuria, and retinopathy progression compared to less intensive BP-lowering (mean BP 140/81 mm Hg).[18] The risk of serious adverse events with intensive therapy was low and did not differ significantly compared to less-intensive treatment, though severe hypotension was more frequent.

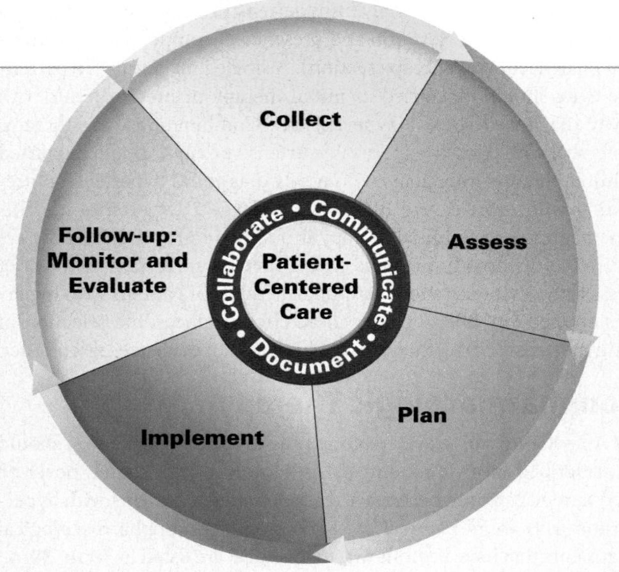

Patient Care Process for the Management of Hypertension

Collect

- Patient characteristics (eg, age, race, sex, pregnant)
- Patient history (past medical, family, social—dietary habits, tobacco use)
- Home blood pressure (BP) readings
- Current medications and prior antihypertensive medication use
- Objective data (see Box 30-1.)
  - BP, heart rate (HR), height, weight, and body mass index (BMI)
  - Labs (eg, serum electrolytes, Scr, BUN)
  - Other diagnostic tests when indicated (eg, electrocardiogram [ECG])

Assess

- Presence of compelling indications (eg, stable ischemic heart disease, chronic kidney disease; see Fig. 30-3)
- Hypertension-related complications (eg, albuminuria, retinopathy; see Box 30-1.)
- 10-year atherosclerotic cardiovascular disease (ASCVD) risk when indicated
- Current medications that may contribute to or worsen hypertension
- BP goal and whether the goal has been achieved (see Box 30-2.)
- Appropriateness and effectiveness of the current antihypertensive regimen
- For resistant hypertension if taking three or more antihypertensive medications (see Table 30-8)

Plan*

- Tailored lifestyle modifications (eg, diet, exercise, weight management; see Table 30-4)
- Drug therapy regimen including specific antihypertensive(s), dose, route, frequency, and duration; specify the continuation and discontinuation of existing therapies (see Tables 30-5, 30-6, 30-7, and 30-9)
- Monitoring parameters including efficacy (eg, BP, CV events, kidney health), safety (medication-specific adverse effects), and timeframe (see Table 30-10)
- Patient education (eg, purpose of treatment, dietary and lifestyle modification, drug therapy)
- Self-monitoring of BP, HR, and weight—where and how to record results
- Referrals to other providers when appropriate (eg, physician, dietician)

Implement*

- Provide patient education regarding all elements of the treatment plan
- Use motivational interviewing and coaching strategies to maximize adherence
- Schedule follow-up

Follow-up: Monitor and Evaluate

- Determine BP goal attainment
- Presence of adverse effects
- Occurrence of CV events and development/progression of kidney impairment
- Patient adherence to treatment plan using multiple sources of information

**Collaborate with patient, caregivers, and other healthcare professionals.*

BP goal values for patients with diabetes have been a subject of debate for a number of years. A BP goal of <130/80 mm Hg was historically recommended for patients with diabetes by multiple organizations. The primary evidence supporting this recommendation was from the Hypertension Optimal Treatment (HOT) study, which compared diastolic BP goals of <90, <85, or <80 mm Hg on CV outcomes.[22] Only the subgroup of patients with diabetes ($n = 1{,}501$) had a lower risk of major CV events in the <80 mm Hg group versus the <90 mm Hg group.

However, the NHLBI-sponsored Action to Control Cardiovascular Risk in Diabetes Blood Pressure (ACCORD-BP) study questioned the benefit of lower BP goals for patients with diabetes.[23] The ACCORD-BP was an open-label, factorial study that randomized 4,733 patients with type 2 diabetes to an SBP of <120 or <140 mm Hg. After a mean follow-up of 4.7 years, there was no significant difference in the annual rate of the primary endpoint (nonfatal MI, nonfatal stroke, or CV death) between the two groups. However, the annual incidence of the secondary endpoint of stroke was significantly lower with the <120 mm Hg goal. Also, there are significant limitations to ACCORD-BP. First, ACCORD-BP was underpowered, as only half of the expected primary composite endpoint events occurred during the study. It was also a factorial study design. A posthoc analysis of ACCORD-BP that examined CV outcomes for participants with CVD risk factors that would have been eligible for SPRINT found similar CV event rates and adverse effect rates as seen in SPRINT.[24] Also, the evidence-based review performed for the 2017 ACC/AHA guideline found a lower risk of fatal or nonfatal stroke with lower BP goals in patients with diabetes.[17]

Therefore, most patients with diabetes should be treated to a BP of <130/80 mm Hg.

Avoiding Clinical Inertia

Although hypertension is one of the most common medical conditions, BP control rates are poor. *Clinical inertia* in hypertension is defined as an office visit for which no therapeutic move was made to lower BP in a patient with uncontrolled hypertension.[25] Clinical inertia is not the entire reason why many patients with hypertension do not achieve goal BP values. However, it is a major reason that can be remedied simply through more aggressive antihypertensive drug therapy. This strategy can include initiating, titrating, or changing drug therapy.

General Approach to Treatment

All patients with elevated blood pressure, stage 1 hypertension, and stage 2 hypertension should be engaged in lifestyle modifications. For patients with elevated blood pressure and those with stage 1 hypertension who are at low risk of ASCVD (ie, primary prevention, without CKD, without diabetes but with a 10-year ASCVD risk <10%), lifestyle modification alone is an appropriate initial treatment. The *threshold* for when these low-risk patients should start drug therapy is when the BP is ≥140/90 mm Hg with a *goal* BP of <130/80 mm Hg. For patients with stage 1 or 2 hypertension who already have ASCVD (secondary prevention) or who have an elevated 10-year ASCVD risk ≥10% (including patients with diabetes and patients with CKD), the *threshold* for starting drug therapy is ≥130/80 mm Hg with a *goal* BP of <130/80 mm Hg.

6 The choice of initial antihypertensive drug therapy depends on the degree of BP elevation and presence of compelling indications (see Pharmacologic Therapy section). A single first-line antihypertensive drug should be started as initial therapy in most patients with newly diagnosed stage 1 hypertension. Combination drug therapy, preferably with two first-line antihypertensive drugs, should be started as initial therapy in patients with newly diagnosed hypertension presenting with more severe BP elevation (stage 2 hypertension). This general approach to initial therapy is outlined in Fig. 30-2. There are several compelling indications where specific antihypertensive drug classes have evidence showing unique benefits in patients with hypertension (see Fig. 30-3). Under these circumstances, the selection of antihypertensive drug therapy should follow an evidence-based order.

Nonpharmacologic Therapy

7 All patients with elevated blood pressure and hypertension should be prescribed lifestyle modifications. However, they should never be used to replace antihypertensive drug therapy for patients with hypertension who are not at goal BP. Recommended nonpharmacological treatments that have been shown to lower BP are listed in Table 30-4.[1] Lifestyle modifications can provide small to moderate reductions in SBP. Aside from reducing BP in patients with known hypertension, strict adherence to lifestyle modification can decrease the progression to hypertension in patients with elevated BP values, and improve other aspects of CV health (eg, cholesterol, weight).

A sensible dietary program is designed to reduce weight gradually for overweight and obese patients and restricts sodium intake with limited alcohol consumption (for patients who consume alcohol). Patients' successful implementation of dietary and lifestyle

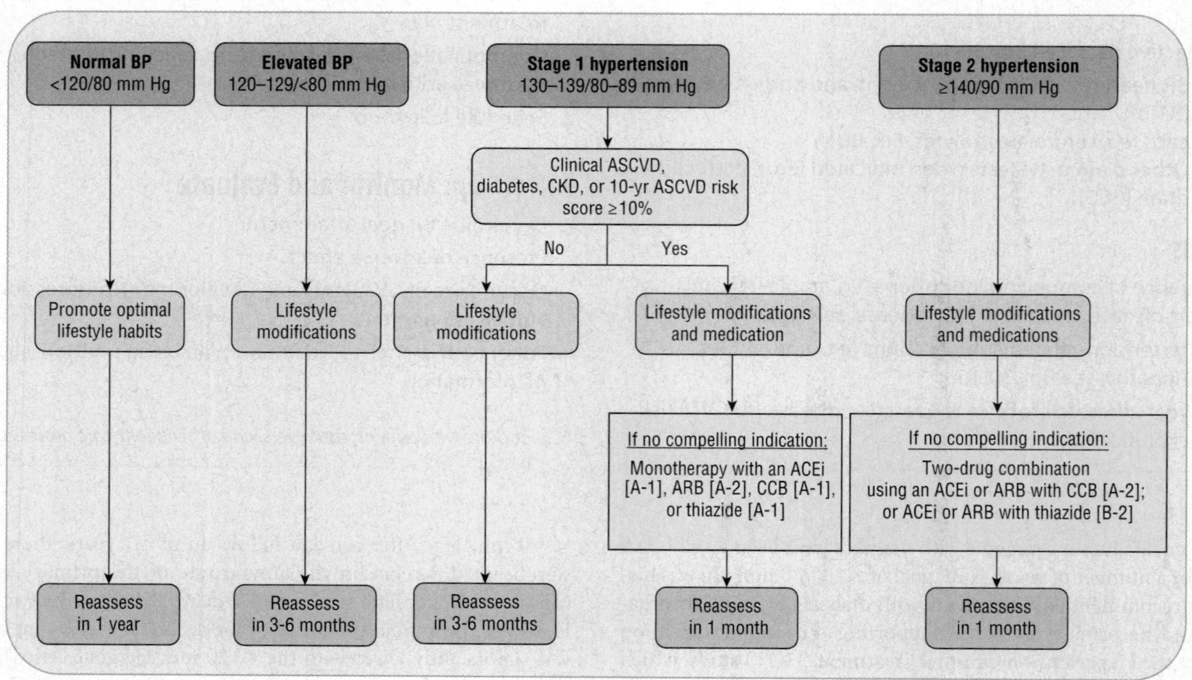

FIGURE 30-2 Algorithm for treatment of elevated BP and hypertension based on BP category at initial diagnosis. Drug therapy recommendations are graded with the strength of recommendation and quality of evidence in brackets. Strength of recommendations: A, B, and C are good, moderate, and poor evidence to support recommendations, respectively. Quality of evidence: (1) evidence from more than one properly randomized controlled trial; (2) evidence from at least one well-designed clinical trial with randomization, from cohort or case-controlled studies, or dramatic results from uncontrolled experiments or subgroup analyses; (3) evidence from opinions of respected authorities, based on clinical experience, descriptive studies, or reports of expert communities. *Monotherapy with an ACEi, ARB, CCB, or thiazide is appropriate in patients presenting in Stage 2 hypertension if they are at high risk for orthostatic hypertension or are very elderly.

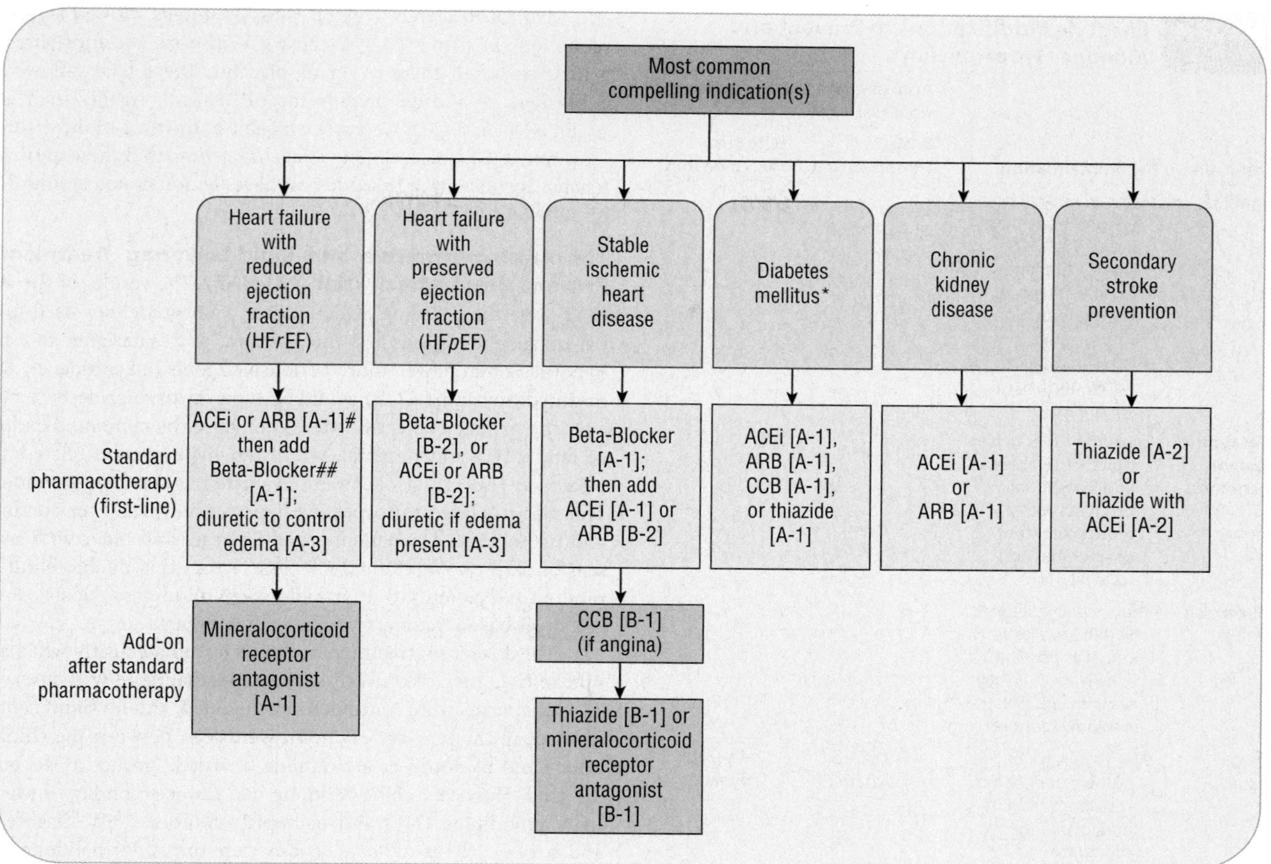

FIGURE 30-3 The most common compelling indications for individual drug classes. Compelling indications for specific drugs are evidenced-based recommendations from outcome studies or existing clinical guidelines. The order of drug therapies serves as a general guidance that should be balanced with clinical judgment and patient response. Add-on pharmacotherapy recommendations are when additional medications are needed to lower blood pressure to goal. Blood pressure control should be managed concurrently with the compelling indication. Drug therapy recommendations are graded with the strength of recommendation and quality of evidence in brackets. Strength of recommendations: A, B, and C are good, moderate, and poor evidence to support recommendations, respectively. Quality of evidence: (1) evidence from more than one properly randomized controlled trial; (2) evidence from at least one well-designed clinical trial with randomization, from cohort or case-controlled analytic studies or multiple time series, or dramatic results from uncontrolled experiments or subgroup analyses; (3) evidence from opinions of respected authorities, based on clinical experience, descriptive studies, or reports of expert communities.
#An ARB with an angiotensin receptor neprilysn inhibitor preferred ahead of an ACEi or ARB for the treatment of HFrEF.
##In HFrEF only, use bisprolol, carvedilol, or metoprolol succinate, titrated to the evidence-based dose.
*If albuminuria is present in diabetes, treat like chronic kidney disease and use an ACEi or ARB titrated to the maximum tolerated dose.

modifications requires aggressive promotion by clinicians through patient education, encouragement, and continued reinforcement. Weight loss, as little as 5% of body weight, can decrease BP significantly in overweight or obese patients. Diets rich in fruits and vegetables and low in saturated fat have been shown to lower BP in patients with hypertension.

The Dietary Approaches to Stop Hypertension (DASH) eating plan is a diet rich in fruits, vegetables, and low-fat dairy products with a reduced content of saturated and total fat. It is an evidence-based diet that lowers BP. Intake of sodium should be minimized as much as possible, ideally to 1.5 g/day, although an interim goal of a 1 g/day reduction may be reasonable considering the challenges in achieving low sodium intake. Patients should be aware of the multiple sources of dietary sodium (eg, processed foods, soups, table salt) so that they may implement the restriction. Potassium intake should be encouraged through fruits and vegetables with a high content (ideally 3,500-5,000 g/day) in those with normal kidney function or without impaired potassium excretion. Excessive alcohol use can either cause or worsen hypertension. Patients with hypertension who drink alcoholic beverages should restrict their daily intake.

Physical activity consisting of aerobic or dynamic resistance training of 90 to 150 min/week (eg, 3-4 sessions/week, lasting on average 40 min/session) and involving moderate-to-vigorous intensity should be encouraged when possible. Studies have shown that physical activity, and in particular aerobic activity, can reduce BP, even in the absence of weight loss. Patients should consult their physicians before starting an exercise program, especially those with hypertension-associated complications.

Smoking (tobacco or other products) is not a secondary cause of essential hypertension. However, smoking is a major, independent, modifiable risk factor for CV disease. Therefore, while smoking cessation is not a recommended strategy to control BP, patients with hypertension who smoke should be counseled regarding the additional health risks that result from smoking and be encouraged to quit.

TABLE 30-4 Lifestyle Modifications to Prevent and Manage Hypertension[a]

Modification	Recommendation	Approximate SBP Reduction (mm Hg) With Hypertension	Approximate SBP Reduction (mm Hg) Without Hypertension
Weight loss	Maintain normal body weight (body mass index, 18.5-24.9 kg/m^2), but aim for at least ≥1 kg weight reduction. Approximate 1 mm Hg BP reduction noted per 1 kg weight loss	5	2-3
DASH-type dietary patterns	Consume a diet rich in fruits, vegetables, and low-fat dairy products with a reduced content of saturated and total fat	11	3
Reduced salt intake	Reduce daily dietary sodium intake as much as possible, ideally to 1.5 g/day sodium (3.8 g/day sodium chloride)	5-6	2-3
Physical activity	90-150 min/wk of aerobic or dynamic resistance training, and involving moderate-to-vigorous intensity[b]	• 5-8 aerobic • 4 dynamic	• 2-4 aerobic • 2 dynamic
Moderation of alcohol intake	Limit consumption to ≤2 drink equivalents per day in men and ≤1 drink equivalent per day in women and lighter-weight persons[c]	4	3

[a]Effects of implementing these modifications are time- and dose-dependent and could be greater for some patients.

[b]Aerobic exercise at 65%-75% heart rate reserve; dynamic resistance consisting of 6 exercises, 3 sets/exercise, 10 repetitions/set at 50%-80% of 1 rep maximum.

[c]One drink equivalent is equal to 1.5 oz (~45 mL) of 80-proof distilled spirits (eg, whiskey), a 5 oz (~150 mL) glass of wine (12%), or 12 oz (~350 mL) of beer.

Pharmacologic Therapy

8 An ACEi, ARB, CCB, or thiazide are preferred first-line antihypertensive agents for most patients (Table 30-5).[1] These agents should be used to treat the majority of patients with hypertension because of evidence demonstrating CV event reduction. Several of these medications have subclasses where significant differences in the mechanism of action, clinical use, side effects, or evidence from outcome studies exist. β-Blocker therapy should be reserved to treat a specific, compelling indication or may be used in combination with one or more first-line antihypertensive agents for patients without a compelling indication. Other antihypertensive drug classes are considered alternative drug classes that should be limited for use in select patients after implementing first-line agents (Table 30-6).

Historical Evidence Supporting Thiazide Therapy

Landmark placebo-controlled clinical trials demonstrate that thiazide therapy irrefutably reduces the risk of CV morbidity and mortality. The Systolic Hypertension in the Elderly Program (SHEP),[6] Swedish Trial in Old Patients with Hypertension (STOP-Hypertension),[5] and Medical Research Council (MRC)[7] studies showed significant reductions in stroke, MI, all-cause CV disease, and mortality with a thiazide-based therapy versus placebo. These trials allowed for β-blockers as add-on therapy for BP control. Agents such as an ACEi, ARB, and CCB were not available at the time of these studies. However, subsequent clinical trials have compared these antihypertensive agents with a thiazide and have demonstrated similar long-term benefits.[26-32]

The Antihypertensive and Lipid-Lowering Treatment to Prevent Heart Attack Trial (ALLHAT) The results of the ALLHAT were the deciding evidence that prior guidelines used to justify thiazide therapy as first-line therapy.[26] It was designed to test the hypothesis that newer antihypertensive agents (an α-blocker, ACEi, or dihydropyridine CCB) would be superior to thiazide-based therapy. The primary objective was to compare the combined endpoint of fatal CHD and nonfatal MI. Other hypertension-related complications (eg, HF, stroke) were evaluated as secondary endpoints. This was the largest prospective hypertension trial ever conducted and included 42,418 patients aged 55 years and older with hypertension and one additional CV risk factor. This double-blind trial randomized patients to chlorthalidone-, amlodipine-, doxazosin-, or lisinopril-based therapy for a mean of 4.9 years.

The doxazosin treatment arm was terminated early when a significantly higher risk of HF versus chlorthalidone was observed.[33] The other arms were continued as scheduled, and no significant differences in the primary endpoint were seen between the chlorthalidone and lisinopril or amlodipine treatment groups at the end of the trial. However, chlorthalidone had fewer secondary endpoints than amlodipine (HF) and lisinopril (combined CV disease, HF, and stroke). The study conclusions were that chlorthalidone-based therapy was superior in preventing one or more major forms of CV disease and was less expensive than amlodipine- or lisinopril-based therapy.

ALLHAT was designed as a superiority study with the hypothesis that amlodipine, doxazosin, and lisinopril would be better than chlorthalidone.[34] It did not prove this hypothesis. Several subgroup analyses of specific populations (eg, Black patients, CKD, diabetes) from the ALLHAT have been conducted to assess response in certain unique patient populations.[35-37] Surprisingly, none of these analyses demonstrated superior CV event reductions with lisinopril or amlodipine versus chlorthalidone. Overall, thiazides remain unsurpassed in their ability to reduce CV morbidity and mortality in most patients.

The 2017 ACC/AHA high BP guideline recommends a thiazide as first-line therapy for most patients.[1] However, an ACEi, ARB, or CCB are also comparable first-line options. Contrary to the historical preference to use a thiazide as preferred for treating most patients with hypertension, they are simply one of the four first-line drug therapy options. Figure 30-2 displays the algorithm for treating hypertension and highlights the four first-line antihypertensive options for patients without a compelling indication for a specific drug class.

ACEi, ARB, and CCB as First-Line Agents

Clinical trial data cumulatively demonstrate that ACEi-, CCB-, or ARB-based antihypertensive therapy reduces CV events. These agents are first-line options for patients without a compelling indication. The Blood Pressure Lowering Treatment Trialists' Collaboration has evaluated the incidence of major CV events and death among different antihypertensive drug classes from 29 major randomized trials in 162,341 patients.[38] In placebo-controlled trials, major CV events were significantly lower with ACEi- and CCB-based regimens versus placebo. Although there were minor differences in the incidence of certain CV events in some comparisons, there were no differences in total major CV events when an ACEi, CCB, or thiazide

TABLE 30-5 Most Common First-Line and Other Antihypertensive Agents

Class	Subclass	Medication (Brand Name)	Usual Dose Range (mg/day)	Daily Frequency	Comments
ACEi		Benazepril (Lotensin) Captopril (Capoten) Enalapril (Vasotec) Fosinopril (Monopril) Lisinopril (Prinivil, Zestril) Moexipril (Univasc) Perindopril (Aceon) Quinapril (Accupril) Ramipril (Altace) Trandolapril (Mavik)	10-40 12.5-150 5-40 10-40 10-40 7.5-30 4-16 10-80 2.5-10 1-4	1 or 2 2 or 3 1 or 2 1 1 1 or 2 1 1 or 2 1 or 2 1	May cause hyperkalemia in patients with chronic kidney disease or in those receiving a potassium-sparing diuretic, or MRA; should not be used in combination with an ARB, or direct renin inhibitor; can cause acute kidney injury in patients with severe bilateral renal artery stenosis or severe stenosis in artery to solitary kidney; contraindicated in pregnancy or in patients with a history of angioedema; starting dose should be reduced 50% in patients who are on a thiazide, are volume depleted, or are very elderly due to risks of hypotension.
ARB		Azilsartan (Edarbi) Candesartan (Atacand) Eprosartan (Teveten) Irbesartan (Avapro) Losartan (Cozaar) Telmisartan (Micardis) Olmesartan (Benicar) Valsartan (Diovan)	40-80 8-32 600-800 150-300 50-100 20-40 20-80 80-320	1 1 or 2 1 or 2 1 1 or 2 1 1 1	May cause hyperkalemia in patients with chronic kidney disease or in those receiving a potassium-sparing diuretic, or MRA; should not be used in combination with an ACEi or direct renin inhibitor; can cause acute kidney injury in patients with severe bilateral renal artery stenosis or severe stenosis in artery to solitary kidney; do not cause a dry cough like an ACEi may; contraindicated in pregnancy; starting dose should be reduced 50% in patients who are on a thiazide, are volume depleted, or are very elderly due to risks of hypotension.
Calcium channel blocker	Dihydropyridine	Amlodipine (Norvasc) Felodipine (Plendil) Nifedipine long-acting (Afeditab CR Adalat CC, Nifediac CC, Nifedical XL, Procardia XL) Nisoldipine (Sular)	2.5-10 5-20 30-90 10-40	1 1 1 1	Do not use immediate-release nifedipine or immediate-release nicardipine; dihydropyridines are more potent arterial vasodilators than nondihydropyridines and may cause more peripheral edema; have additional benefits in Raynaud's syndrome.
	Nondihydropyridine	Diltiazem sustained release (Cardizem CD, Cartia XT, Dilacor XR, Diltia XT, Tiazac, Taztia XT) Diltiazem extended release (Cardizem LA, Matzim LA) Verapamil sustained release (Calan SR, Isoptin SR, Verelan) Verapamil chronotherapeutic oral drug absorption system (Verelan PM)	120-480 180-480 180-420 100-400	1 1 (morning or evening) 1 or 2 1 (in the evening)	Use extended-release products for hypertension; these agents block the A-V node, reduce heart rate, and may produce heart block, especially in combination with β-blockers; not all products are not AB rated as interchangeable on an equipotent milligram-per-milligram basis due to different release mechanisms and bioavailability; Cardizem LA, Matzim LA, and Verelan PM have delayed drug release for several hours after dosing and can provide chronotherapeutic drug delivery, but this does not have any clinical advantages; have additional benefits in patients with atrial tachyarrhythmia.
Diuretic	Thiazide	Chlorthalidone (Thalitone) Hydrochlorothiazide (Microzide) Indapamide (Lozol) Metolazone (Zaroxolyn)	12.5-25 12.5-50 1.25-2.5 2.5-10	1 1 1 1	Hydrochlorothiazide is a "thiazide-type" while chlorthalidone, indapamide, and metolazone are "thiazide-like." Dose in the morning to avoid nocturnal diuresis; thiazides are more effective antihypertensives than loop diuretics in most patients; use usual doses to avoid adverse metabolic effects; hydrochlorothiazide, chlorthalidone, and indapamide are preferred; chlorthalidone is approximately 1.5 times as potent as hydrochlorothiazide; have additional benefits in osteoporosis; use with caution in patients with a history of gout.
	Loop	Bumetanide (Bumex) Furosemide (Lasix) Torsemide (Demadex)	0.5-4 20-80 5-10	2 2 1	Dose in the morning and late afternoon (when twice daily) to avoid nocturnal diuresis; higher doses may be needed for patients with severely decreased glomerular filtration rate or HF; preferred over thiazides in patient with severe kidney dysfunction and resistant hypertension.
	Potassium-sparing	Amiloride (Midamor) Amiloride/hydrochlorothiazide (Moduretic) Triamterene (Dyrenium) Triamterene/hydrochlorothiazide (Dyazide, Maxide)	5-10 5/50 50-100 37.5-75/25-50	1 or 2 1 1 or 2 1	Weak diuretics that are used in combination with a thiazide to minimize hypokalemia; do not significantly lower BP unless used with a thiazide; should be reserved for patients experiencing diuretic-induced hypokalemia; avoid in patients with severe chronic kidney disease (estimated glomerular filtration rate <30 mL/min/1.73m^2); may cause hyperkalemia, especially in combination with an MRA, ACEi, ARB, direct renin inhibitor, or potassium supplements.
	MRA	Eplerenone (Inspra) Spironolactone (Aldactone, CaroSpir)	50-100 25-50	1 or 2 1 or 2	Dose in the morning and late afternoon (when twice daily) to avoid nocturnal diuresis; eplerenone contraindicated in patients with an estimated creatinine clearance <50 mL/min (0.83 mL/s), elevated serum creatinine (>1.8 mg/dL [115 µmol/L] in women, >2 mg/dL [177 µmol/L]) in men), and type 2 diabetes with albuminuria; often used as add-on therapy in resistant hypertension; avoid in patients with severe chronic kidney disease (estimated glomerular filtration rate <30 mL/min/1.73m^2); may cause hyperkalemia, especially in combination with an ACEi, ARB, direct renin inhibitor, or potassium supplements.

(continued)

TABLE 30-5 Most Common First-Line and Other Antihypertensive Agents (*Continued*)

Class	Subclass	Medication (Brand Name)	Usual Dose Range (mg/day)	Daily Frequency	Comments
β-Blocker	Cardio-selective	Atenolol (Tenormin)	25-100	1 or 2	Abrupt discontinuation may cause rebound hypertension; have additional benefits in patients with atrial tachyarrhythmia or preoperative hypertension; in general, cardioselective agents inhibit β_1-receptors at low to moderate dose, higher doses may also block β_2-receptors (especially metoprolol); additional vasodilation with nebivolol does not result in more orthostatic hypotension; nonselective agents inhibit β_1- and β_2-receptors at all doses, can exacerbate asthma, and have additional benefits in patients with essential tremor, migraine headache, portal hypertension, and thyrotoxicosis. Agents with intrinsic sympathomimetic activity (acebutolol and pindolol) partially stimulate β-receptors while blocking against additional stimulation; no role in the management of hypertension and are contraindicated in patients with stable ischemic heart disease. Mixed α- and β-blockers produce vasodilation and have more orthostatic hypotension.
		Betaxolol (Kerlone)	5-20	1	
		Bisoprolol (Zebeta)	2.5-10	1	
		Metoprolol tartrate (Lopressor)	100-200	2	
		Metoprolol succinate extended release (Toprol XL)	50-200	1	
		Nebivolol (Bystolic)	5-20	1	
	Nonselective	Nadolol (Corgard)	40-120	1	
		Propranolol (Inderal)	160-480	2	
		Propranolol long acting (Inderal LA, Inderal XL, InnoPran XL)	80-320	1	
		Timolol (Blocadren)	10-40	1	
	Mixed α- and β-blockers	Carvedilol (Coreg)	12.5-50	2	
		Carvedilol phosphate (Coreg CR)	20-80	1	
		Labetalol (Normodyne, Trandate)	200-800	2	

TABLE 30-6 Alternative Antihypertensive Agents

Class	Medication (Brand Name)	Usual Dose Range (mg/day)	Daily Frequency	Comments
α_1-Blocker	Doxazosin (Cardura)	1-8	1	Give first dose at bedtime; patients should rise from sitting or lying down slowly to minimize risk of orthostatic hypotension; additional benefits in men with benign prostatic hyperplasia
	Prazosin (Minipress)	2-20	2 or 3	
	Terazosin (Hytrin)	1-20	1 or 2	
Direct renin inhibitor	Aliskiren (Tekturna)	150-300	1	May cause hyperkalemia in patients with chronic kidney disease and diabetes or in those receiving a potassium-sparing diuretic, MRA; do not use in combination with an ACEi or ARB; may cause acute kidney failure in patients with severe bilateral renal artery stenosis or severe stenosis in artery to solitary kidney; do not use in pregnancy
Central α_2-agonist	Clonidine (Catapres)	0.1-0.8	2	Oral form should be avoided due to need for frequent administration and potential rebound HTN with abrupt discontinuation or nonadherence; most effective if used with a thiazide to diminish fluid retention; clonidine patch is replaced once per week
	Clonidine patch (Catapres-TTS)	0.1-0.3	1 weekly	
	Methyldopa (Aldomet)	250-1,000	2	
Direct arterial vasodilator	Minoxidil (Loniten)	10-40	1 or 2	Should be used with thiazide and β-blocker to diminish fluid retention and reflex tachycardia
	Hydralazine (Apresoline)	20-100	2 to 4	

was compared with each other. In studies evaluating ARB-based therapy to control regimens, the incidence of major CV events was lower with ARB-based therapy. However, the control regimens used in these comparisons included both antihypertensive drug therapies and placebo. These results were largely consistent with the network meta-analysis conducted for the 2017 ACC/AHA guideline, which found that an ACEI, ARB, CCB, or thiazide were all similar as first-line treatment for hypertension.[17]

Data from meta-analyses that incorporate high-quality randomized controlled trials provide more robust data than any single trial alone. High-quality meta-analyses are considered the highest level of evidence by the ACC/AHA guidelines and provide clinically useful data that support using ACEi-, CCB-, or ARB-based treatment for hypertension as first-line antihypertensive agents. Clinicians should use meta-analyses data as supporting evidence when selecting a first-line antihypertensive regimen for hypertension in most patients.

β-Blocker Versus First-Line Agents 9 Clinical trial data and meta-analyses cumulatively suggest that treatment with a β-blocker may reduce CV events better than placebo but not to the extent that an ACEi, ARB, CCB, or particularly thiazide diuretics do.[1] In the systematic review and network analysis conducted for the 2017 ACC/AHA guideline, β-blockers were less effective for preventing stroke and CV events than diuretics.[17]

Meta-analyses data evaluating β-blockers and their ability to reduce CV events have limitations. Most studies that were included in these analyses used atenolol as the β-blocker studied. Therefore, it is possible that atenolol is inferior and is the only β-blocker that does not reduce CV events as much as other first-line antihypertensive drug classes. A network meta-analysis comparing the effects of different β-blockers found a decreased risk of mortality and CV events with lipophilic agents (metoprolol, propranolol, and oxprenolol) compared to hydrophilic agents (atenolol).[39] However, due to challenges in the interpretation of meta-analyses of β-blockers compared to other first-line agents (eg, trials conducted at different times, use of different beta-blockers, changes in the efficacy of agents), most guideline recommendations do not differentiate between the β-blocker drug class. In the absence of a compelling indication, a β-blocker can be considered only after other first-line antihypertensive agents (ACEi or ARB, CCB, thiazide) have been used.[1,40] These findings also call into question the validity of results from prominent prospective, controlled clinical trials evaluating antihypertensive drug therapy that used β-blocker–based therapy, especially atenolol, as the primary comparator.[28,30] These studies used once-daily atenolol, which in addition to being hydrophilic, may have been inadequately dosed based on the short half-life of this agent.

β-Blocker–based antihypertensive therapy does not increase the risk of CV events; β-blocker–based therapy reduces the risk of CV events compared with no antihypertensive therapy. Using a β-blocker as a first-line antihypertensive agent is an option when an ACEi, ARB, CCB, or thiazide cannot be used. β-Blockers also have an important role as add-on therapy to first-line agents to reduce BP in patients with hypertension but without compelling indications.

Many of the clinical trials included in the meta-analyses suggest that β-blocker–based therapy may not reduce CV events as well as these other agents, used atenolol dosed once daily.[41] Atenolol has a half-life of 6 to 7 hours and is nearly always dosed once daily, while immediate-release forms of carvedilol and metoprolol have half-lives of 6 to 10 and 3 to 7 hours, respectively, and are dosed at least twice daily.[41] It is also hydrophilic, which may not penetrate the brain and cell membrane as easily as lipophilic agents, and is inferior to lipophilic agents (metoprolol, propranolol, and oxprenolol).[39] Therefore, it is possible that these findings might only apply to atenolol, particularly dosed once daily instead of twice daily. Based on available evidence, metoprolol succinate or carvedilol are the preferred β-blockers if a β-blocker is to be used.

Patients with Compelling Indications

10 Compelling indications represent specific comorbid conditions where evidence from clinical trials supports using specific antihypertensive classes to treat both the compelling indication and hypertension. Antihypertensive medication recommendations typically consist of combination drug therapy (see Fig. 30-3). Data from clinical trials have demonstrated a reduction in CV morbidity and/or mortality that justifies use for patients with hypertension and with such a compelling indication.

Heart Failure with Reduced Ejection Fraction Five drug classes have compelling indications for HF with reduced ejection fraction (HFrEF), also known as systolic HF or left ventricular dysfunction.[42] The primary physiologic abnormality in HFrEF is decreased CO resulting from a decreased left ventricular ejection fraction. An evidence-based pharmacotherapy regimen for HFrEF, called *guideline-directed medical therapy*, consists of three to four drugs: an ACEi or ARB (although ARB with a neprilysin inhibitor [aka angiotensin receptor neprilysin inhibitor; ARNI] is preferred ahead of an ACEi or ARB alone according to HFrEF recommendations), an evidence-based β-blocker (ie, bisoprolol, carvedilol, metoprolol succinate) titrated to the maximum dose, and then possibly an MRA.[43] Diuretics are often needed in patients with HFrEF primarily to provide symptomatic relief of edema by inducing diuresis. Loop diuretics are often needed, especially for patients with more advanced HF and/or advanced stages of CKD. However, some patients with well-controlled HF and without significant CKD may be managed with a thiazide.

For patients with hypertension and HFrEF full implementation for guideline-directed medical therapy to treat HFrEF using multiple pharmacologic therapies should be the primary driver of pharmacotherapy. When done correctly and completely, not only are benefits related to HFrEF realized but lowering of BP to goal is usually achieved.

β-Blocker therapy modifies disease in HFrEF and is a component of standard treatment for these patients. For patients on an initial regimen of a diuretic with an ACEi or ARB (or ARNI), add-on β-blocker therapy has been shown to reduce CV morbidity and mortality.[42,44] It is of paramount importance that β-blockers be dosed appropriately due to the risk of inducing an acute exacerbation of HF. They must be started in low doses (much lower than that used to treat hypertension) and titrated slowly to high doses based on tolerability. Bisoprolol, carvedilol, and metoprolol succinate are the only β-blockers that are proved to be beneficial in HFrEF.

After implementing a standard HFrEF regimen (diuretic, ACEi or ARB alone [or ARNI], and evidence-based β-blocker), other agents may be added to reduce CV morbidity and mortality further and reduce BP if needed. The addition of a mineralocorticoid receptor antagonist (spironolactone or eplerenone) can reduce CV morbidity and mortality in HFrEF.[44]

Heart Failure with Preserved Ejection Fraction Approximately 50% of patients with HF have a preserved ejection fraction (HFpEF). In HFpEF, patients have signs and symptoms of HF such as dyspnea, fatigue, and possibly edema, but they have a preserved left ventricular ejection fraction (≥50%).

Unlike interventions using GDMT in HFrEF, which have been shown to decrease morbidity and mortality in HF, trials using the same antihypertensive medications in HFpEF have not shown similar benefits.[44] Therefore, treatment should be targeted at any underline symptoms, appropriate management of any underlying coronary artery disease, and attainment of goal BP to prevent progression of HF. Patients should use a β-blocker or an ACEi or ARB to treat hypertension, but if signs and symptoms of edema are present, they should receive a diuretic.[1] A mineralocorticoid receptor antagonist may be considered in patients with elevated brain natriuretic peptide concentrations or heart failure admission within one year and adequate kidney function to reduce the risk of hospitalizations.[42]

Stable Ischemic Heart Disease Chronic stable angina and a history of acute coronary syndrome (unstable angina or acute MI) are forms of stable ischemic heart disease (aka, coronary artery disease, or coronary heart disease).[1] These are the most common forms of hypertension-associated complications. Patients with stable ischemic heart disease are at high risk for a CV event.

β-Blocker therapy has been a standard of care for treating patients with stable ischemic heart disease and hypertension for decades because they can reduce BP and improve angina symptoms by decreasing myocardial oxygen consumption and demand.[1] They also decrease cardiac adrenergic stimulation and have been shown in clinical trials to reduce the risk of a subsequent MI and sudden cardiac death. β-Blocker therapy seems to be most effective in reducing the risk of CV events in patients with recent MI and/or ischemic symptoms. While data indicate that the long-term risk of CV events and mortality may not be reduced with β-blocker therapy in patients with stable coronary artery disease (ie, do not have ischemic symptoms or have a distant history of MI),[45] β-blockers should be used for the treatment of hypertension in patients with stable ischemic heart disease.[1] An ACEi (or ARB as an alternative) has been shown to improve cardiac remodeling and cardiac function and reduce CV events in stable ischemic heart disease as an add-on to a β-blocker.

A long-acting nondihydropyridine CCB is an alternative to a β-blocker (diltiazem and verapamil) in stable ischemic heart disease.[46] The International Verapamil–Trandolapril Study (INVEST) demonstrated no difference in CV risk reduction when β-blocker-based therapy was compared with nondihydropyridine CCB-based treatment in this population.[47] Nonetheless, the preponderance of data is with β-blockers, and they remain the therapy of choice.[1,46] Importantly, the combined use of a nondihydropyridine CCB with a β-blocker should be avoided in general due to the increased risk of bradycardia.

A dihydropyridine CCB (eg, amlodipine, felodipine) is recommended as add-on therapy in stable ischemic heart disease patients who have ongoing ischemic symptoms (aka, angina or chest pain).[46] CCBs (especially nondihydropyridine CCBs) and β-blockers provide anti-ischemic effects; they lower BP and reduce myocardial oxygen demand in patients with hypertension and stable (and unstable) ischemic heart disease. Moreover, a dihydropyridine CCB can be used in combination with a β-blocker because there is not an increased risk of bradycardia. However, cardiac stimulation may occur with dihydropyridine CCBs (particularly immediate-release formulations) or β-blockers with intrinsic sympathomimetic activity (ISA), making these agents less desirable. Moreover, β-blockers with ISA should be avoided due to these deleterious effects.

Once ischemic symptoms are controlled with β-blocker and/or CCB therapy, other antihypertensive drugs can be added to provide additional CV risk reduction. Clinical trials have demonstrated that the addition of an ACEi further reduces CV events in patients with stable ischemic heart disease.[46] ARBs may provide similar benefits but have not been as extensively studied as ACEi therapy. Therefore, in stable ischemic heart disease, an ARB is generally considered an alternative to an ACEi. Thiazides can be added after that to provide additional BP lowering and to reduce CV risk further. However, thiazides do not provide anti-ischemic effects.

Diabetes Mellitus The primary cause of mortality in patients with diabetes is CV disease, and hypertension management is an important risk reduction strategy.[1] All four first-line antihypertensive agents (ACEi, ARB, CCB, and thiazides) have been shown to reduce CV events in patients with diabetes (see Fig. 30-3).[1] The evidence-based review performed for the 2017 ACC/AHA guideline found no difference in all-cause mortality, CV mortality, HF, or stroke between ACEi-, ARB-, CCB-, or thiazide-based regimen in patients with diabetes.[17]

Traditionally, an ACEi or ARB was considered as a preferred antihypertensive agent for patients with diabetes. The reasons for this were that pharmacologically, ACEis and ARBs should provide nephroprotection due to vasodilation in the efferent arteriole of the kidney. Evidence from clinical studies has shown reductions in both CV risk (mostly with an ACEi) and reduction in risk of progressive kidney dysfunction (mainly with ARBs) in patients with diabetes.[13,48] However, data indicate that an ACEi or ARB does not confer significantly better CV risk reduction compared to CCBs, thiazides, or β-blockers in patients with diabetes.[48,49] In addition, the risk of kidney disease progression is low in the absence of albuminuria (urine albumin-to-creatinine ratio ≥30 mg/g [3.4 mg/mmol]),[13,48] and many of the studies evaluating the ability of an ACEi or ARB to slow the progression of kidney dysfunction were placebo-controlled.[49] Therefore, an ACEi or ARB is recommended similarly to a CCB or thiazide in patients with diabetes and hypertension that do not have persistent albuminuria.[1]

After first-line antihypertensives (ACEi, ARB, CCB, and thiazide), a β-blocker is useful add-on therapy for BP control for patients with diabetes or to treat another compelling indication (eg, stable ischemic heart disease). A β-blocker (especially nonselective agents) can mask the signs and symptoms of hypoglycemia in patients with tightly controlled diabetes because most of the symptoms of hypoglycemia (eg, tremor, tachycardia, and palpitations) are mediated through the sympathetic nervous system. In addition, sweating, a cholinergically mediated symptom of hypoglycemia, still occurs during a hypoglycemic episode despite β-blocker therapy. Patients may also have a delay in hypoglycemia recovery time because compensatory recovery mechanisms need the catecholamine inputs that are antagonized by β-blocker therapy. Finally, unopposed α-receptor stimulation during the acute hypoglycemic recovery phase (due to endogenous epinephrine release intended to reverse hypoglycemia) may result in acutely elevated BP due to vasoconstriction. Despite these potential concerns, β-blockers can be safely used for patients with diabetes, and are recommended in patients with diabetes that also have a compelling indication (eg, stable ischemic heart disease, HF).

Based on the weight of all evidence, any first-line agent can be used for controlling hypertension for patients with diabetes in the absence of albuminuria. However, regardless of what agent is initially chosen, most patients will require combination therapy (discussed later), typically involving and ACEi or ARB with a CCB or thiazide.

Chronic Kidney Disease Hypertension, especially uncontrolled BP, can damage the renal tissue (parenchyma) and/or the renal arteries that lead to CKD.[13] CKD in patients with hypertension initially presents as moderately increased albuminuria (urine albumin-to-creatinine ratio 30-299 mg/g [3.4-33.8 mg/mmol] on a spot urine sample or ≥30 mg albumin in a 24-hour urine collection) that can progress to overt kidney failure. The rate of kidney function deterioration is accelerated when both hypertension and diabetes are present. Patients with significant CKD (eg, GFR <60 mL/min/1.73 m^2 and/or albuminuria) have an increased risk of CV disease, and further progression to severe CKD.[1] BP control can slow the decline in kidney function and reduce the risk of a CV event in patients with CKD.

In addition to lowering BP, ACEi and ARB therapy can reduce intraglomerular pressure, which can theoretically provide additional benefits by slowing CKD progression in patients with diabetes[48] and those without diabetes.[13] It is difficult to differentiate whether the kidney protection benefits are from RAAS blockade versus BP lowering. A meta-analysis failed to demonstrate any unique long-term kidney protective effects of RAAS-blocking drugs compared with other antihypertensive drugs, suggesting that benefits may be attributed to BP lowering.[50] Moreover, a subgroup analysis of patients from the ALLHAT stratified by different baseline GFR values also did not show a difference in long-term outcomes with chlorthalidone versus lisinopril among patients with significant CKD.[35]

Patients may experience a rapid and profound drop in BP or acute kidney injury when initially starting an ACEi or ARB. The potential to produce acute kidney injury is particularly problematic in patients with significant bilateral renal artery stenosis or a solitary functioning kidney with stenosis. Patients with renal artery stenosis are usually older, and this condition is more common in patients with diabetes or those who smoke. Patients with renal artery stenosis do not always have evidence of kidney disease unless specific tests are performed. Starting with low dosages and evaluating serum creatinine soon after starting either an ACEi or ARB can minimize this risk.

Secondary Stroke Prevention Ischemic stroke (not hemorrhagic stroke) and TIA are considered hypertension-associated complications. More than two-thirds of patients who have had an ischemic stroke or TIA have hypertension.[1] Achieving goal BP values in patients who have experienced an ischemic stroke is considered a primary modality to reduce the risk of recurrent stroke or TIA. A thiazide, either in combination with an ACEi or as monotherapy, is an evidence-based antihypertensive regimen for patients with a history of stroke or TIA.[1,51,52] ARB-based therapy has also been studied in this population.[53,54] Antihypertensive drug therapy should only be implemented after patients have stabilized following an acute cerebrovascular event, typically a few days after the event.[1] Moreover, the threshold for starting antihypertensive drug therapy in patients with a history of stroke is when BP is above 140/90 mm Hg.[1] Once antihypertensive therapy is initiated, these patients should be treated to a goal of <130/80 mm Hg.

Alternative Drug Treatments

It is sometimes necessary to use other antihypertensive agents such as a mineralocorticoid receptor antagonist, α-blocker, central α_2-agonist, adrenergic inhibitor, or arterial vasodilator. Although these agents effectively lower BP, they either do not have convincing evidence showing reduced morbidity and mortality in hypertension or have a high incidence of adverse effects that significantly hinder tolerability. Alternative agents are generally reserved for patients with resistant hypertension or as add-on therapy with multiple other first-line antihypertensive agents.

Special Populations

Drug therapy selection should always follow the recommendations provided by evidence-based guidelines, summarized in Figs. 30-2 and 30-3.[1] These should be maintained as the guiding principles of drug therapy. However, there are some patient populations where the approach to drug therapy may be slightly altered. In some cases, this is because other agents have unique properties that benefit a coexisting condition but may not be based on evidence from outcome studies in hypertension.

Hypertension in Older People Hypertension often presents as isolated systolic hypertension in older patients.[1] Epidemiologic data indicate that CV morbidity and mortality are more directly correlated to SBP than to DBP for patients aged 50 years and older. This population is also at high risk for hypertension-associated complications.[1] Although several placebo-controlled trials have specifically demonstrated risk reduction in this population, many older people with hypertension are either not treated or are treated but not at goal BP.

The SHEP was a landmark double-blind, placebo-controlled trial that evaluated chlorthalidone-based treatment for isolated systolic hypertension.[6] A 36% reduction in total stroke, a 27% reduction in coronary artery disease, and 55% reduction in HF were demonstrated versus placebo. The Systolic Hypertension in Europe (Syst-Eur) trial was another placebo-controlled trial that evaluated treatment with a long-acting dihydropyridine CCB.[8] Treatment resulted in a 42% reduction in stroke, 26% reduction in coronary artery disease, and 29% reduction in HF. These data demonstrate reductions in CV morbidity and mortality in older patients with isolated systolic hypertension, especially with thiazides and long-acting dihydropyridine CCBs.

The "very elderly" population (80 years of age and older) were underrepresented in the SHEP and Syst-Eur studies. Historically, this population was often not treated to goal either due to fear of side effects or limited evidence demonstrating benefit. However, the Hypertension in the Very Elderly Trial (HYVET) provided definitive evidence that antihypertensive drug therapy offers significant clinical benefits in these patients.[55] The HYVET was a prospective controlled clinical trial that randomized patients 80 years and older with hypertension to placebo or antihypertensive drug therapy. It was stopped early after a median of only 1.8 years because the incidence of death was 21% higher in placebo-treated patients. Based on these results, hypertension should be treated with antihypertensive drug therapy in patients age 80 years and older.

Thiazide or β-blocker therapy has been compared with either an ACEi or CCB in older patients with systolic hypertension, diastolic hypertension, or both in the Swedish Trial in Old Patients with Hypertension-2 (STOP-2) study.[56] In this trial, no significant differences in the primary CV event endpoint were seen between the thiazide-based treatment and either an ACEi or CCB. Overall, selecting a treatment that is well-tolerated and affordable may be more important than using specific antihypertensive agents in this population.

Older patients are more sensitive to volume depletion and sympathetic inhibition than younger patients. This may lead to orthostatic hypotension (see Patients at Risk for Orthostatic Hypotension). In older patients, this can increase the risk of falls due to the associated dizziness. Therefore, centrally acting agents and α_1-blockers should generally be avoided or used with caution in older patients because they are frequently associated with dizziness and orthostatic hypotension. First-line antihypertensives provide significant benefits and can safely be used in older patients, especially those age 80 years and older, but smaller-than-usual initial doses must be used for initial therapy.

The best evidence for lower BP goals in older patients comes from the SPRINT-Senior trial, a prespecified subanalysis of patients aged 75 years and older enrolled in the SPRINT study.[57] In this cohort, older (mean age 79.9 years), community-dwelling patients without dementia and an expected life expectancy of 3 or more years who were treated to an SBP of <120 mm Hg compared an SBP of <140 mm Hg experienced a 34% reduced risk of the primary composite outcome of CVD and 33% reduced risk of all-cause mortality. While the lower SBP goal was associated with an increased risk of hypotension and electrolyte abnormalities, there was no difference in serious adverse events. The benefits of lower BP goals in older patients significantly outweighed the risk, though careful monitoring is essential to ensure safe medication use. A subsequent meta-analysis examining the risks and benefits of lower BP compared to a "relaxed" goal of <150 mm Hg found similar results.[58] Therefore, based on the totality of the evidence, older ambulatory patients should be treated to an SBP goal of <130 mm Hg.[1]

The treatment of hypertension in older patients should follow the same principles outlined for general care of hypertension. However, in patients with multiple comorbidities or disease states, or in whom the benefit of therapy may be less established (eg, nursing home resident, dementia), the risks and benefits of using a lower BP goal should be considered, taking into account patient preference and using a team-based approach. A relaxed SBP goal of <150 mm Hg (<140 mm Hg if tolerated) may be considered appropriate in these patients. Also, while the general approach to treatment is similar to younger patients, initial drug doses may be lower, and dosage titrations over a more extended period are usually needed to minimize the risk of hypotension.

Patients at Risk for Orthostatic Hypotension 11 Orthostatic hypotension is a significant drop in BP when standing and can be associated with dizziness and/or fainting. It is defined as an SBP decrease of >20 mm Hg or DBP decrease of >10 mm Hg when changing from supine to standing.[1] The risk of orthostatic hypotension is increased in older patients (especially those with isolated systolic hypotension, or those aged 80 years or older) and those with long-standing diabetes, severe volume depletion, baroreflex dysfunction, autonomic insufficiency, and concomitant use of medications that cause venodilation (α-blockers, mixed α-/β-blockers, nitrates, and phosphodiesterase inhibitors). Interestingly, in a meta-analysis of 18,466 adults enrolled in randomized trials, intensive BP-lowering treatment was associated with a lower risk of orthostatic hypotension, possibly through improvement in long-term maladaptive mechanisms associated with high blood pressure.[59] For patients with risk factors for orthostatic hypotension, antihypertensive agents, especially a thiazide, ACEi, or ARB, should be started in low doses.

Hypertension in Children and Adolescents Detecting hypertension in children requires customized evaluation. Hypertension is defined as SBP or DBP that is >95th percentile for sex, age, and height on at least three occasions for children.[60] BP values between the 90th and 95th percentile, or >120/80 mm Hg in adolescents, is considered elevated BP. Hypertensive children often have a family history of high BP, and many are overweight or obese, predisposing them to insulin resistance and associated CV risk. Unlike hypertension in adults, secondary hypertension is more common in children and adolescents. Therefore, an appropriate workup for secondary causes is required if elevated BP is identified. Kidney disease (eg, pyelonephritis, glomerulonephritis) is the most common cause of secondary hypertension in children.

Nonpharmacologic treatment (eg, weight loss if overweight or obese, healthy diet, sleep, physical activity) is the cornerstone of therapy for essential hypertension in children.[60] The goal is to reduce the BP to <90th percentile for sex, age, and height and <130/80 mm Hg in adolescents aged 13 years and older.[60] An ACEi, ARB, β-blocker, CCB, and thiazide are all acceptable choices in children and have data supporting their use.[60] If an ACEi or ARB is to be used in adolescent girls of childbearing age, it is important to counsel regarding the risk of fetal injury and death since these agents are teratogenic, and an alternative antihypertensive may be considered. As with adults, the selection of initial agents should be based on the presence of compelling indications or concurrent conditions that may warrant their use.

Pregnancy Hypertension during pregnancy is a major cause of maternal and neonatal morbidity and mortality.[1] Hypertension during pregnancy can be categorized as preeclampsia, eclampsia, chronic hypertension, preeclampsia superimposed on chronic hypertension, and gestational hypertension.[61] *Preeclampsia* is defined as hypertension (elevated BP ≥140/90 mm Hg on >2 occasions at least 4 hours apart after 20 weeks of gestation or ≥160/110 mm Hg confirmed within a short interval) and either proteinuria or new-onset hypertension with the onset of thrombocytopenia, impaired liver function, new-onset renal insufficiency, pulmonary edema, or new-onset cerebral or visual disturbances. It can lead to life-threatening complications for both mother and fetus. *Eclampsia*, the onset of convulsions in preeclampsia, is a medical emergency. Chronic hypertension is hypertension that predates pregnancy; superimposed preeclampsia is chronic hypertension associated with preeclampsia. *Gestational hypertension* is defined as new-onset hypertension arising after 20 weeks of gestation in a patient with normal BP before pregnancy that is not in the severe range (≥160/110 mm Hg), without proteinuria or other systemic findings (eg, thrombocytopenia, renal insufficiency, pulmonary edema, cerebral or visual disturbances).

It is controversial whether treating mild-to-moderate hypertension in pregnancy is beneficial. However, women with chronic hypertension before pregnancy are at increased risk of several complications, including superimposed preeclampsia, preterm delivery, fetal growth restriction or demise, placental abruption, HF, and acute kidney failure.[61,62] In an open, international, multicenter study of patients with nonproteinuric preexisting or gestational hypertension, tighter DBP goals (<85 mm Hg) was not associated with decreased rates of the primary composite outcome of pregnancy loss or high-level neonatal care compared to less-tight control (DBP <100 mm Hg).[63] However, severe hypertension (≥160/110 mm Hg) developed less often in patients randomized to the tight control group compared to less-tight control (40.6% vs 27.5%).

The treatment of severe hypertension, pre-eclampsia, and eclampsia is discussed in Chapter e31. For chronic hypertension in pregnancy, several agents may be considered (Table 30-7). Unfortunately, there are few data regarding the most appropriate therapy in pregnancy. Labetalol, long-acting nifedipine, or methyldopa are recommended as first-line agents due to their favorable safety profile.[62] Other β-blockers (not atenolol) and CCBs are also reasonable alternatives. An ACEi, ARB, and direct renin inhibitor are known teratogens and are absolutely contraindicated.

TABLE 30-7 Treatment of Chronic Hypertension in Pregnancy

Medication/Class	Comments
Methyldopa	Long-term follow-up data supports safety; considered a preferred agent
β-Blockers	Generally safe, but intrauterine growth retardation reported (mostly with atenolol)
Labetalol	Increasingly used over methyldopa because of fewer side effects; considered a first-line agent
Clonidine	Limited data available; mainly an option in the third trimester
CCB	Limited data available; no increase in major teratogenicity with exposure (except immediate-release oral nifedipine should not be used); long-acting nifedipine considered a preferred agent
Thiazide	Not first-line agents but probably safe in low doses if started prior to conception when treating essential hypertension
ACEi, ARB, direct renin inhibitor	Contraindicated; major teratogenicity reported with exposure (fetal toxicity and death)

Black Patients Hypertension affects Black patients at a disproportionately higher rate, and hypertension-associated complications are more prevalent than in other populations.[1] Reasons for these differences are not fully understood. Hypertension is also more challenging to control in Black patients and usually requires two or more antihypertensives to reach a goal of <130/80 mm Hg.[1]

BP-lowering effects of antihypertensive medication classes vary in Black patients but individual treatment response should always guide therapy, not race. CCBs and thiazides, as monotherapy, are more effective at lowering BP in Black patients and should be used first-line in the absence of a compelling indication.[1] When either of these two classes (especially thiazides) are used in combination with a β-blocker, ACEi, or ARB (which are three classes known to be less effective, on average, at lowering BP in Black patients), the antihypertensive response is increased. This may be due to the low-renin pattern of hypertension in Black patients, resulting in less BP lowering with a β-blocker, ACEi, or ARB when used as monotherapy when compared with other patient populations. Importantly, Black patients have a higher risk of angioedema from an ACEi compared with White patients, though this is not a common adverse effect.[1]

Despite potential differences in antihypertensive effects with monotherapy treatment, drug therapy selection is no different from what is recommended for the hypertensive population in general, and individual treatment response should always guide therapy, not race. Medications recommended for specific compelling indications should be used when such compelling indications are present, even if the antihypertensive effect may not be as great as with another drug class (eg, use a β-blocker first-line for hypertension in a Black patient with stable ischemic heart disease or an ACE or ARB in a Black patient with CKD).

Other Conditions

Most patients with hypertension have other coexisting conditions that may influence the selection of drug therapy. The influence of comorbid conditions should only be complementary to, and never replace, drug therapy choices recommended to treat a compelling indication. Under some circumstances, these considerations help decide on a particular antihypertensive agent when more than one antihypertensive class is recommended. In some cases, an agent should be avoided because it may aggravate a concomitant disorder. In other cases, an antihypertensive can be used to treat hypertension and another concomitant condition. These are briefly summarized in Table 30-5.

Pulmonary Disease and Peripheral Arterial Disease β-Blockers, especially nonselective agents, have generally been avoided for patients with hypertension and reactive airway disease (asthma or chronic obstructive pulmonary disease [COPD] with a reversible obstructive component) due to a fear of inducing bronchospasm. However, cardioselective β-blockers can safely be used in patients with asthma or COPD.[1] Therefore, cardioselective β-blockers should be used to treat a compelling indication (ie, stable ischemic heart disease or HF) for patients with reactive airway disease.

PAD is a non-coronary form of ASCVD. Patients with PAD are at an increased risk of stroke and CV events.[1,64] While β-blockers can theoretically be problematic for patients with PAD due to possible decreased peripheral blood flow secondary to unopposed stimulation of α_1-receptors that results in vasoconstriction, available data indicate that β-blockers do not worsen claudication symptoms or cause functional impairment.[64] Antihypertensive treatment for patients with PAD should follow the same general principles as patients without PAD.[1]

Metabolic Syndrome Metabolic syndrome is a cluster of multiple cardiometabolic risk factors.[1] It has been defined as the presence of three of the following five criteria: abdominal obesity, elevated triglycerides, low HDL cholesterol, elevated BP (or receiving drug treatment for high BP), and elevated fasting blood glucose.[65] It is widely accepted that patients with metabolic syndrome are at increased risk of developing CV disease and/or type 2 diabetes. The cornerstone of treatment involves lifestyle modification (eg, weight loss if overweight or obese, exercise, dietary modifications). There is no definitive evidence that any first-line antihypertensive medication class is better or worse than another in reducing CV events in patients with metabolic syndrome.[1] While thiazides have been associated with a slight increase in blood glucose and faster progression to diabetes, a subgroup analysis of ALLHAT found that CV events were reduced more with chlorthalidone when compared to lisinopril in patients with impaired fasting glucose.[36] Therefore, any first-line antihypertensive can be used for patients with metabolic syndrome.

Erectile Dysfunction Most antihypertensive agents, particularly β-blockers and mineralocorticoid receptor antagonists, have been associated with erectile dysfunction in men. However, it is not clear if erectile dysfunction associated with antihypertensive treatment is solely a result of drug therapy or rather a symptom of underlying vascular disease. β-Blockers have historically been labeled as agents that cause significant sexual dysfunction. However, evidence supporting this notion is limited. A systematic review of 15 studies involving 35,000 patients assessing β-blocker use for MI, HF, and hypertension found only a slight increased risk for erectile dysfunction.[66] In addition, prospective long-term data from the Treatment of Mild Hypertension Study (TOMHS) and the Veterans Administration Cooperative trial show no difference in the incidence of erectile dysfunction between thiazide and β-blocker versus an ACEi and CCB.[67,68] Centrally acting agents are associated with higher rates of sexual dysfunction and should be avoided in men with erectile dysfunction.

Hypertensive men frequently have ASCVD, which frequently results in erectile dysfunction. Therefore, erectile dysfunction is associated with chronic arterial changes resulting from elevated BP, and lack of control may increase the risk of erectile dysfunction. These changes are even more pronounced in hypertensive men with diabetes.

Resistant Hypertension

12 Resistant hypertension is defined as failure to achieve goal BP using three or more antihypertensive drugs with complementary mechanisms of action (ideally using optimal doses, one of which is a diuretic) or when four or more antihypertensive drugs are needed to achieve BP control.[1,69] Approximately 12% to 15% of patients with hypertension have apparent treatment-resistant hypertension.[69] Patients with newly diagnosed hypertension or who are not receiving drug therapy should not be considered to have resistant hypertension. Difficult-to-control hypertension is persistently elevated BP despite treatment with two or three drugs, which fails to meet the criteria for resistant hypertension.

Several causes of resistant hypertension are listed in Table 30-8. Volume overload is a common cause, thus highlighting the importance of diuretic therapy in managing hypertension. Pseudoresistance should also be ruled out by assuring adherence to prescribed therapy and possibly using home BP measurements (using a self-monitoring device or 24-hour ABP monitor).[1] Patients should be closely evaluated to see if any of these causes can be reversed.

Treatment of patients with resistant hypertension should ultimately follow the principle of drug therapy selection from the 2017 ACC/AHA guideline. Compelling indications, if present, should guide selection assuming that these patients are on a thiazide or other type of diuretic. However, there are treatment philosophies that are germane to the management of resistant hypertension: (a) assuring adequate diuretic therapy, (b) appropriate use of combination therapy, and (c) using alternative antihypertensive agents when needed.

Assuring Appropriate Diuretic Therapy

Diuretics have a prominent role in the pharmacotherapy of resistant hypertension. Thiazides are first-line antihypertensive agents, but chlorthalidone (thiazide-like) is recommended ahead of hydrochlorothiazide for patients with resistant hypertension because it is more potent on a milligram-per-milligram basis.[69] Though less commonly used, indapamide (similar to chlorthalidone as "thiazide-like") is also a more potent antihypertensive agent than hydrochlorothiazide at commonly prescribed doses, and the evidence does not demonstrate a higher risk of metabolic side effects.[70]

A mineralocorticoid receptor antagonist (eg, spironolactone) is a highly effective add-on agent.[1,69] Data indicate that many patients with resistant hypertension have some degree of underlying hyperaldosteronism, justifying the role of adding a mineralocorticoid receptor antagonist. Spironolactone has been compared to an α-blocker and a β-blocker as add-on therapy for resistant hypertension in the PATHWAY-2 study.[71] The BP-lowering effect of spironolactone was approximately double that of doxazosin and bisoprolol, reinforcing the benefits of blocking aldosterone by using a mineralocorticoid receptor antagonist in managing resistant hypertension.

TABLE 30-8 Causes of Resistant Hypertension

Improper BP measurement
Volume overload:
– Excess sodium intake
– Volume retention from kidney disease
– Inadequate diuretic therapy
Drug-induced or other causes:
– Nonadherence
– Inadequate doses
– Agents listed in Table 30-1
Associated conditions:
– Obesity
– Excess alcohol intake
– Obstructive sleep apnea
Secondary hypertension

Clinicians may consider using a loop diuretic, even in place of a thiazide, for patients with resistant hypertension who have compromised kidney function (eg, estimated GFR <15 mL/min/1.73 m^2).[1,69] When a loop diuretic is used, a long-acting agent such as torsemide, which can be dosed once daily, should be used over shorter-acting agents such as furosemide and bumetanide, which may need to be dosed multiple times a day.[69]

First-Line Antihypertensive Agents

Angiotensin-Converting Enzyme Inhibitors (ACEi) An ACEi is a first-line therapy option in most patients with hypertension.[1] The ALLHAT demonstrated less HF and stroke with chlorthalidone versus lisinopril,[26] while another outcome study showed similar, if not better, outcomes with an ACEi versus hydrochlorothiazide.[32] It is possible that the different thiazides have different abilities to reduce CV events. Nonetheless, strong evidence demonstrates that ACEi therapy overall reduces CV events comparably to other first-line antihypertensive agents.

ACE facilitates the production of angiotensin II that has a major role in arterial BP regulation, as depicted in Fig. 30-1. ACE is distributed in many tissues and is present in several different cell types, but its main location is endothelial cells. Therefore, the primary site for angiotensin II production is in the blood vessels, not the kidney. An ACEi blocks the ACE, thus inhibiting the conversion of angiotensin I to angiotensin II. Angiotensin II is a potent vasoconstrictor that stimulates aldosterone secretion, causing an increase in sodium and water reabsorption with accompanying potassium loss. By blocking the ACE, vasodilation and a decrease in aldosterone occur.

An ACEi also blocks the degradation of bradykinin and stimulates the synthesis of other vasodilating substances (prostaglandin E_2 and prostacyclin). Because an ACEi lowers BP in patients with normal plasma renin activity, bradykinin and perhaps tissue production of ACE are important in hypertension. Increased bradykinin enhances the BP-lowering effects of an ACEi, and is also responsible for the side effect of a dry cough. An ACEi may effectively prevent or regress LVH by reducing direct stimulation of angiotensin II on myocardial cells.

There are many evidence-based indications for an ACEi (see Fig. 30-3). An ACEi reduces CV morbidity and mortality in patients with HFrEF and decreases the progression of CKD. An ACEi is a first-line option for patients with diabetes and hypertension because of demonstrated CV disease and kidney benefits. A two-drug regimen of an ACEi with a thiazide is first-line in recurrent stroke prevention based on benefits demonstrated from the PROGRESS trial showing a reduced risk of secondary stroke.[31] As an add-on to β-blocker therapy, evidence indicates that an ACEi further reduces CV risk in patients with stable ischemic heart disease.[46,72-74]

Most ACEi medications can be dosed once daily for hypertension (Table 30-5). In some patients, especially when higher doses are used, twice-daily dosing is needed to maintain 24-hour effects with enalapril, benazepril, moexipril, quinapril, and ramipril.

ACEi therapy is generally well tolerated. Because they decrease aldosterone, an increase in potassium serum concentrations can occur. While this increase is usually small, hyperkalemia is possible. Patients with CKD or taking other agents which may increase potassium (eg, potassium supplements, potassium-sparing diuretics, mineralocorticoid receptor antagonists) are at the highest risk for hyperkalemia. Judicious monitoring of serum potassium and creatinine values within 4 weeks of starting or increasing the dose of an ACEi can often identify abnormalities early before they evolve into serious adverse events.

The most worrisome adverse effect of ACEi therapy is acute kidney injury. This serious adverse effect is uncommon, and the development of severe acute kidney failure is rare, occurring in less than 1% of patients. Preexisting kidney disease increases the risk of this side effect. Severe bilateral renal artery stenosis or unilateral stenosis of a solitary functioning kidney renders patients dependent on the vasoconstrictive effect of angiotensin II on the efferent arteriole of the kidney, thus explaining why these patients are particularly susceptible to acute kidney injury from an ACEi. Slow titration of the ACEi dose and judicious kidney function monitoring can minimize risk and allow early detection of patients with renal artery stenosis.

GFR does decrease somewhat in patients when started on an ACEi.[1] This is attributed to the inhibition of angiotensin II vasoconstriction on the efferent arteriole. This decrease in GFR often increases serum creatinine, and small increases should be anticipated when monitoring patients newly started on an ACEi. Either modest elevations of ≤35% (for baseline creatinine values ≤3 mg/dL [265 μmol/L]) or absolute increases <1 mg/dL (88 μmol/L) do not warrant changes. If larger increases occur, ACEi therapy should be stopped or the dose reduced.

Angioedema is a serious potential complication of ACEi therapy. It occurs in <1% of the population and is more likely in Black patients and smokers. Symptoms include lip and tongue swelling and possibly difficulty breathing. All patients with ACEi-induced angioedema should have ACEi therapy stopped. However, angioedema associated with laryngeal edema and/or pulmonary symptoms occasionally occurs and requires additional treatment with a bradykinin-2 receptor antagonist (eg, icatibant), fresh frozen plasma, and/or emergent intubations to support respiration. Even if not from an ACEi, a history of angioedema precludes the use of an ACEi (it is a contraindication). Cross-reactivity between an ACEi and an ARB does not appear to be a significant concern. The Telmisartan Randomized Assessment Study in ACE-Intolerant Subjects with Cardiovascular Disease (TRANSCEND) trial enrolled 75 patients with a history of ACEi-induced angioedema and randomized these patients to either placebo or ARB therapy.[75] There were no cases of repeat angioedema among these patients. These data suggest that the cross-reactivity is low. Hence, an ARB can be used in a patient with a history of ACEi-induced angioedema when needed. However, clinicians should monitor for repeat occurrences since idiopathic angioedema may still occur.

A persistent dry cough may develop in up to 20% of patients treated with an ACEi. The inhibition of bradykinin breakdown pharmacologically explains it. This cough does not cause pulmonary disease but is annoying and can compromise adherence. It should be differentiated from a "wet" cough due to pulmonary edema, which may be a sign of uncontrolled HF and not an ACEi-induced cough.

An ACEi (and ARB or direct renin inhibitor) is absolutely contraindicated in pregnancy. Female patients of childbearing age should be counseled regarding effective birth control as ACEi therapy are fetotoxic.[1] Fetopathy (group of conditions that includes renal failure, renal dysplasia, hypotension, oligohydramnios, pulmonary hypotension, hypocalvaria, and death) has occurred with ACEi exposure in the second and third trimesters. Similar to a thiazide, an ACEi can increase lithium serum concentrations in patients on lithium therapy. Concurrent use of an ACEi with a potassium-sparing diuretic, potassium supplements, or mineralocorticoid receptor antagonist may result in hyperkalemia. An ACEi should not be used with an ARB or direct renin inhibitor to avoid possible hyperkalemia.

Lower than normal starting doses of an ACEi should be used for patients at risk for orthostatic hypotension or severe renal dysfunction (eg, elderly patients, those with CKD). Acute hypotension may occur at the onset of ACEi therapy. Patients who are sodium or volume-depleted, in an HF exacerbation, very elderly, or on concurrent vasodilators or thiazide therapy are at high risk for this effect. It is important to start with half the usual dose of an ACEi for all patients with these risk factors and use slow dose titration.

Angiotensin Receptor Blockers (ARBs) Two enzymatic pathways generate angiotensin II: the RAAS, which involves ACE, and an alternative path that uses other enzymes such as chymase (aka "tissue ACE"). An ACEi inhibits only the effects of angiotensin II produced through the RAAS, whereas ARBs inhibit angiotensin II from all pathways. It is unclear how these differences affect tissue concentrations of ACE.

ARB therapy directly blocks the AT_1 receptor, which mediates the known effects of angiotensin II in humans: vasoconstriction, aldosterone release, sympathetic activation, antidiuretic hormone release, and constriction of the efferent arterioles of the glomerulus. They do not block the AT_2 receptor. Therefore, the beneficial effects of AT_2 receptor stimulation (vasodilation, tissue repair, and inhibition of cell growth) remain intact with ARB use. Unlike an ACEi, an ARB does not block the breakdown of bradykinin. Therefore, some of the beneficial effects of bradykinin (eg, vasodilation) are not present with ARB therapy.

An ARB is a first-line therapy option in most patients with hypertension.[1] ARB therapy has been directly compared with ACEi therapy in patients with high CV risk.[76] The Ongoing Telmisartan Alone and in Combination with Ramipril Global End Point Trial (ON-TARGET) was a double-blind trial that randomized 25,620 patients (69% with a history of hypertension-based historical standards, mean BP of 142/82 mm Hg) to ACEi-based therapy, ARB-based therapy, or the combination of an ACEi with an ARB. After a median follow-up of 56 months, there was no difference in the primary endpoint (CV death or hospitalization for HF) between any of the three treatment groups. Therefore, these data establish that the CV event–lowering benefits of ARB therapy is similar to ACEi therapy. Moreover, the combination of an ACEi with an ARB had no additional benefits on CV events and was associated with a higher risk of side effects (renal dysfunction, hypotension, hyperkalemia). Therefore, concurrent use of an ACEi with an ARB for the management of hypertension is not recommended.[1]

For patients with type 2 diabetes and CKD, the progression of kidney disease is significantly reduced with ARB therapy.[48] Some benefits are independent of BP lowering, suggesting that the pharmacologic effects of ARBs on the efferent arteriole may result in attenuated progression of kidney disease. For patients with HFrEF, ARB therapy has been shown to reduce the risk of hospitalization for HF when used as an alternative therapy in ACEi-intolerant patients.[44]

ARBs have been compared head-to-head with CCBs. The Morbidity and Mortality After Stroke: Eprosartan Versus Nitrendipine in Secondary Prevention (MOSES) trial demonstrated that eprosartan reduced the risk of recurrent stroke greater than nitrendipine in patients with a past medical history of cerebrovascular disease.[53] These data support the common notion that ARBs may have cerebroprotective effects that may explain CV event reductions. Another outcome study, the Valsartan Antihypertensive Long-Term Use Evaluation (VALUE) trial, showed that valsartan-based therapy is equivalent to amlodipine-based therapy for the primary composite outcome of first CV event in patients with hypertension and additional CV risk factors.[30] However, the occurrence of certain components of the primary endpoint (stroke and MI) was lower in the valsartan group. Although patients treated with amlodipine had slightly lower mean BP values than valsartan-treated patients, there was no difference in the primary endpoint.

The addition of a CCB or thiazide to an ARB significantly increases antihypertensive efficacy. Similar to an ACEi, most ARBs have long enough half-lives to allow for once-daily dosing. However, candesartan, eprosartan, losartan, and valsartan have the shortest half-lives and may require twice-daily dosing for sustained BP lowering.

ARB therapy has the lowest incidence of side effects compared with other antihypertensive agents.[77] ARBs do not affect bradykinin and do not elicit a dry cough like an ACEi. While referred to as an "ACEi without a cough," pharmacologic differences between an ARB and ACEi highlight that they could have different effects on vascular smooth muscle and myocardial tissue that can correlate to different effects. Regardless, they are first-line options for hypertension, and they are reasonable alternatives for patients who do not tolerate ACEi therapy because of a cough. Due to their excellent tolerability, safety profile, and generic availability, ARBs are increasingly preferred by clinicians over an ACEi for hypertension.

An ARB may cause renal insufficiency, hyperkalemia, and orthostatic hypotension in a manner identical to that of an ACEi. The same precautions that apply to ACEi therapy regarding suspected bilateral renal artery stenosis, concomitant medications that can raise potassium, and/or increase the risk of hypotension apply to ARBs. As previously discussed, patients with a history of ACEi angioedema can be treated with an ARB when needed.[78] An ARB should never be used in pregnancy. An ARB should not be used with an ACEi or direct renin inhibitor.

Calcium Channel Blockers (CCB) Both dihydropyridine CCBs and nondihydropyridine CCBs are first-line therapies for hypertension.[1] CCBs also have compelling indications in stable ischemic heart disease as an add-on to a β-blocker, while a nondihydropyridine CCB should be used as an alternative to a β-blocker. However, they are primarily used as add-on therapy to other antihypertensive drug classes with this compelling indication.

Contraction of cardiac and smooth muscle cells requires increased free intracellular calcium concentrations from the extracellular fluid. When the cardiac or vascular smooth muscle is stimulated, voltage-sensitive channels in the cell membrane are opened, allowing calcium to enter the cells. The influx of extracellular calcium into the cell releases stored calcium from the sarcoplasmic reticulum. As intracellular free calcium concentration increases, it binds to a protein, calmodulin, which then activates myosin kinase enabling myosin to interact with actin to induce contraction. CCBs work by inhibiting the influx of calcium across the cell membrane. There are two types of voltage-gated calcium channels: a high-voltage channel (L-type) and a low-voltage channel (T-type). Available CCBs only block the L-type channel, which leads to coronary and peripheral vasodilation.

The two subclasses, dihydropyridines and nondihydropyridines (see Table 30-5), are pharmacologically different from each other. While their antihypertensive effectiveness is similar, they differ somewhat in other pharmacodynamic effects. Nondihydropyridines (verapamil and diltiazem) decrease heart rate and slow atrioventricular nodal conduction. Similar to a β-blocker, these drugs may also treat supraventricular tachyarrhythmias (eg, atrial fibrillation). Verapamil (and diltiazem to a lesser extent) produces negative inotropic and chronotropic effects that are responsible for its propensity to precipitate or cause systolic HF in high-risk patients. All CCBs (except amlodipine and felodipine) have negative inotropic effects. Dihydropyridines may cause a baroreceptor-mediated reflex tachycardia because of their potent peripheral vasodilating effects. This effect is more pronounced with the first-generation dihydropyridines (eg, nifedipine) and is significantly diminished with the newer agents (eg, amlodipine) and when given in sustained-release dosage forms. Dihydropyridines do not alter conduction through the atrioventricular node and thus are not effective agents in supraventricular tachyarrhythmias.

Dihydropyridine CCBs have been extensively studied in hypertension and are the primary agents used for this indication. In ALLHAT, there was no difference in the primary outcome between chlorthalidone and amlodipine, and only the secondary outcome of HF was higher with amlodipine.[26] A subgroup analysis of ALLHAT directly compared amlodipine with lisinopril and demonstrated that there was no difference in the primary outcome.[79] However, amlodipine was superior to lisinopril for BP control in Black patients, and for stroke reduction in Black patients and women. As discussed previously, the VALUE study also showed no difference between valsartan and amlodipine in the primary outcome of the first CV event in high-risk patients.[30]

Dihydropyridine CCBs are effective in older patients with isolated systolic hypertension. The placebo-controlled Syst-Eur trial demonstrated that a long-acting dihydropyridine CCB reduced the risk of CV events markedly in isolated systolic hypertension.[8] A long-acting dihydropyridine CCB, similar to a thiazide, should be strongly considered as preferred therapy in a patient with isolated systolic hypertension and no other compelling indications.

Among dihydropyridine CCBs, short-acting nifedipine may rarely cause an increase in the frequency, intensity, and duration of angina in association with acute hypotension. This effect is most likely due to reflex sympathetic stimulation and is likely avoided by using sustained-release formulations of nifedipine. For this reason, all other dihydropyridines have an intrinsically long half-life or are sustained-release formulations. Immediate-release nifedipine has been associated with an increased incidence of adverse CV effects, is not approved for the treatment of hypertension, and should never be used to treat hypertension. Other side effects of dihydropyridine CCBs include dizziness, flushing, headache, gingival hyperplasia, peripheral edema, mood changes, and various GI complaints. Side effects due to vasodilation such as dizziness, flushing, headache, and peripheral edema occur more frequently with all dihydropyridine CCBs than with the nondihydropyridine CCBs because they are less potent vasodilators.

Diltiazem and verapamil are nondihydropyridine CCBs that can cause cardiac conduction abnormalities such as bradycardia or atrioventricular block. These problems occur mainly with high doses or when used for patients with preexisting cardiac conduction abnormalities. HF has been reported in otherwise healthy patients due to negative inotropic effects. Both drugs can cause peripheral edema and hypotension. Verapamil causes constipation in some patients. This side effect also occurs with diltiazem, but to a lesser extent.

Verapamil and diltiazem are moderate cytochrome P450 3A4 isoenzyme system inhibitors and can cause drug-drug interactions that result in increased serum concentrations of other drugs metabolized by this isoenzyme system (eg, cyclosporine, digoxin, lovastatin, simvastatin, tacrolimus, theophylline). The use of verapamil or diltiazem with a β-blocker should be avoided for the treatment of hypertension because there is an increased risk of heart block with these combinations. When a CCB is needed in combination with a β-blocker for BP lowering, a dihydropyridine should be selected because it will not increase the risk of heart block. The hepatic metabolism of CCBs, especially felodipine, nicardipine, nifedipine, and nisoldipine, may be inhibited by ingesting large quantities of grapefruit juice (eg, ≥1 quart daily).

Many different formulations of verapamil and diltiazem are currently available (see Table 30-5). Although certain individual sustained-release verapamil and diltiazem products contain the same active drug, they are usually not AB-rated by the FDA as interchangeable on a milligram-per-milligram basis due to different biopharmaceutical release mechanisms. However, the clinical significance of these differences is likely negligible.

Thiazides and Other Diuretics There are four subclasses of diuretics: thiazides, loops, potassium-sparing agents, and mineralocorticoid receptor antagonists (see Table 30-5).[1,80] A thiazide is the preferred diuretic for hypertension and is considered a first-line therapy option in most patients.[1] The best available evidence justifying this recommendation is from the ALLHAT.[26] Moreover, when combination therapy is needed in hypertension to control BP, a thiazide as an add-on agent, but not necessarily the second agent, is effective in augmenting BP lowering.

Loop diuretics are more potent agents for inducing diuresis but are not ideal antihypertensives unless treating edema is also needed. In general, loop diuretics are sometimes required over a thiazide for hypertension in patients with severe CKD when estimated GFR is <30 mL/min/1.73m^2, especially in the case of hydrochlorothiazide or when edema is present.[69] However, many patients with an estimated GFR between 25 and 30 mL/min/1.73m^2, but not on dialysis, will still have antihypertensive effects with thiazides. This is especially true with chlorthalidone.[69]

Potassium-sparing diuretics are weak antihypertensive agents when used alone and do not enhance antihypertensive effects when combined with a thiazide or loop diuretic. Their use in hypertension is in combination with another diuretic to counteract the potassium-wasting properties of the other diuretic agent.

Mineralocorticoid receptor antagonists (MRAs; spironolactone and eplerenone) inhibit aldosterone activity and are sometimes considered potassium-sparing diuretics. However, they are more potent as antihypertensives and should be viewed as an independent class due to evidence supporting different compelling indications. Mineralocorticoid receptor antagonists are most commonly used to treat resistant hypertension, as elevated aldosterone concentrations are prevalent in this setting. They are also used as an add-on agent in patients with HF, with or without concomitant hypertension.

The exact antihypertensive mechanism of action of non-MRA diuretics is not completely known but has been well hypothesized. The drop in BP seen when they are first started is caused by an initial diuresis. Diuresis causes reductions in plasma and stroke volume, which decreases CO and BP. This initial drop in CO causes a compensatory increase in PVR. With chronic diuretic therapy, extracellular fluid and plasma volume return to near pretreatment values. However, PVR decreases to values that are lower than the pretreatment baseline. This reduction in PVR is responsible for persistent antihypertensive effects.

With thiazides, additional actions may further explain their antihypertensive effects. They mobilize sodium and water from arteriolar walls. This effect would lessen the amount of physical encroachment on the lumen of the vessel created by the excessive accumulation of intracellular fluid. As the diameter of the lumen relaxes and increases, there is less resistance to the flow of blood, and PVR further drops. High dietary sodium intake can blunt this effect, and a low salt intake can enhance this effect. Thiazides are also postulated to cause direct relaxation of vascular smooth muscle.

Diuretics should be dosed in the morning when given once daily and in the morning and late afternoon when dosed twice daily to minimize nocturnal diuresis. However, with chronic use, thiazides, potassium-sparing diuretics, and MRAs rarely cause a pronounced diuresis.

The major pharmacokinetic differences between the different thiazide medications are serum half-life and duration of diuretic effect. The clinical relevance of these differences is unknown because the serum half-life of most antihypertensive agents does not correlate with the hypotensive duration of action. Moreover, diuretics lower BP primarily through extrarenal mechanisms. Hydrochlorothiazide and, to a greater extent, chlorthalidone are the two most frequently used thiazides in landmark clinical trials that have demonstrated reduced morbidity and mortality. Hydrochlorothiazide is considered a "thiazide-type" agent, while chlorthalidone is a "thiazide-like" agent. These agents are not equipotent on a milligram-per-milligram basis; chlorthalidone is 1.5 to 2 times more potent than hydrochlorothiazide.[80] This is likely attributed to a longer half-life (45-60 hours vs 8-15 hours) and a longer duration of effect (48-72 hours vs 16-24 hours) with chlorthalidone.

Thiazides are effective in lowering BP, especially when used in combination with most other antihypertensives. Two independent pharmacodynamic effects explain this additive response. First, when two drugs cause the same overall pharmacologic effect (BP lowering) through different mechanisms of action, their combination usually results in an additive or synergistic effect. This is especially relevant when a β-blocker, ACEi, or ARB is indicated in a Black patient but does not elicit sufficient antihypertensive effect. Adding a thiazide, similar to a CCB, in this situation can often significantly lower BP. Second, a compensatory increase in sodium and fluid retention may be seen with antihypertensive agents. This problem is counteracted with the concurrent use of a thiazide.

Side effects of a thiazide include hypokalemia, hypomagnesemia, hypercalcemia, hyperuricemia, hyperglycemia, dyslipidemia, and sexual dysfunction. Many of these side effects were identified when high doses of thiazides were used in the past (eg, hydrochlorothiazide up to 200 mg/day). Current guidelines recommend dosing hydrochlorothiazide up to 50 mg/day or chlorthalidone up to 25 mg/day, which markedly reduces the risk for most metabolic side effects. Loop diuretics may cause the same side effects. Although the effect on serum lipids and glucose is even less significant, hypokalemia is more pronounced, and hypocalcemia may occur.

Hypokalemia and hypomagnesemia may cause muscle fatigue or cramps. However, serious cardiac arrhythmias can occur in patients with severe hypokalemia and hypomagnesemia. Low-dose therapy (ie, 25 mg hydrochlorothiazide or 12.5 mg chlorthalidone daily) causes less electrolyte disturbances than higher doses. However, because the most effective doses of these two thiazides are hydrochlorothiazide 50 mg daily and chlorthalidone 25 mg daily, efforts should be made to keep potassium in the therapeutic range by careful monitoring, especially when higher doses are used.

Thiazide-induced hyperuricemia can precipitate gout. This side effect may be especially problematic for patients with a previous history of gout and is more common with thiazides. However, acute gout is unlikely in patients with no prior history of gout. If gout occurs in a patient who requires thiazide therapy, allopurinol can be given to prevent gout and not compromise thiazide's antihypertensive effects. High doses of thiazide and loop diuretics may increase fasting glucose and serum cholesterol values. These effects, however, usually are transient and often inconsequential.[80]

Potassium-sparing diuretics can cause hyperkalemia, especially in patients with CKD or diabetes and in patients receiving concurrent treatment with an MRA, ACEi, ARB, direct renin inhibitor, or potassium supplements. Hyperkalemia is especially problematic for the MRA eplerenone, a selective antagonist of aldosterone. Due to this increased risk of hyperkalemia, eplerenone is contraindicated for patients with impaired kidney function or type 2 diabetes with proteinuria (see Table 30-5). While spironolactone may cause gynecomastia in up to 10% of patients, this rarely occurs with eplerenone.

A thiazide can be used safely with most other agents. However, concurrent administration with lithium may increase lithium serum concentrations and predispose patients to lithium toxicity.

β-Blockers β-blockers have been used in several large outcome trials in hypertension. However, in most of these trials, a thiazide was the first-line agent with a β-blocker added for additional BP lowering. For patients with hypertension but without compelling indications, a β-blocker should not be used as the initial first-line agent. This recommendation is based on meta-analyses that suggest β-blocker-based therapy may not reduce CV events as well as these other agents when used as the initial drug to treat patients with hypertension who do not have a compelling indication for a β-blocker.[1]

A β-blocker is only an appropriate first-line agent in hypertension when treating specific, compelling indications (eg, stable ischemic heart disease, HF). Numerous trials have shown a reduced risk of CV events when β-blockers are used following an MI, during an acute coronary syndrome, or in patients with chronic stable angina with ischemic symptoms. Although once contraindicated in HF, studies have shown that bisoprolol, carvedilol, and metoprolol succinate reduce mortality in patients with HFrEF who are treated with a diuretic and ACEi.

Several mechanisms of action have been proposed for β-blockers, but none alone has been consistently associated with reducing arterial BP. β-Blocker therapy has negative chronotropic and inotropic effects that reduce CO, which explains some of the antihypertensive effects. However, CO falls equally for patients treated with a β-blocker regardless of BP lowering. Additionally, β-blockers with ISA do not reduce CO, yet they lower BP and decrease peripheral resistance. However, β-blockers with ISA are contraindicated in stable ischemic heart disease because they stimulate β-receptors.

β-adrenoceptors are also located on the surface membranes of juxtaglomerular cells, and a β-blocker inhibits these receptors and thus the release of renin. However, there is a weak association between plasma renin and the antihypertensive efficacy of β-blocker therapy. Some patients with low plasma renin concentrations do respond to β-blocker treatment. Therefore, additional mechanisms likely also account for the antihypertensive effect of a β-blocker.

There are important pharmacodynamic and pharmacokinetic differences among β-blockers, but all agents provide a similar degree of BP lowering. There are three pharmacodynamic properties of β-blocker therapy that differentiate this class: cardioselectivity, ISA, and membrane-stabilizing effects. β-Blocker agents that possess a greater affinity for β_1-receptors than for β_2-receptors are *cardioselective*.

β_1-adrenoceptors and β_2-adrenoceptors are distributed throughout the body, but they concentrate differently in specific organs and tissues. There is a preponderance of β_1-receptors in the heart and kidney and a preponderance of β_2-receptors in the lungs, liver, pancreas, and arteriolar smooth muscle. β_1-Receptor stimulation increases heart rate, contractility, and renin release. β_2-Receptor stimulation results in bronchodilation and vasodilation. A cardioselective β-blocker is not likely to provoke bronchospasm and vasoconstriction. β_2-Receptors mediate insulin secretion and glycogenolysis. Blocking β_2-receptors may reduce these processes and increase blood glucose or blunt recovery from hypoglycemia.

Cardioselective β-blockers (eg, bisoprolol, metoprolol, nebivolol) have clinically significant advantages over nonselective agents (eg, propranolol, nadolol) and are preferred when using a β-blocker to treat hypertension. Cardioselective agents are safer than nonselective agents for patients with asthma or diabetes who have a compelling indication for a β-blocker. However, cardioselectivity is a dose-dependent phenomenon; at higher doses, some cardioselective agents lose their relative selectivity for β_1-receptors and block β_2-receptors as effectively as they block β_1-receptors. The dose at which cardioselectivity is lost varies from patient to patient and may not occur with highly selective β-blockers (eg, bisoprolol).

Some β-blockers (eg, acebutolol, pindolol) have ISA and act as partial β-receptor agonists. When they bind to the β-receptor, they stimulate it, but far less than a pure β-agonist. If the sympathetic tone is low, as it is during resting states, β-receptors are partially stimulated by ISA β-blockers. Therefore, resting heart rate, CO, and peripheral blood flow are not reduced when these types of β-blockers are used. Theoretically, ISA agents have advantages over non-ISA β-blockers in certain patients with HF or sinus bradycardia. Unfortunately, they do not reduce CV events as well as other β-blockers. In fact, they may increase CV risk in patients with stable ischemic heart disease. Thus, agents with ISA are rarely needed and have no role in the management of hypertension.

Pharmacokinetic differences among β-blockers relate to first-pass metabolism, route of elimination, the degree of lipophilicity, and serum half-lives. Propranolol and metoprolol undergo extensive first-pass metabolism, so the dose needed to attain β-blockade with either drug varies from patient to patient. Atenolol and nadolol are renally excreted. The dose of these agents may need to be reduced for patients with moderate-to-severe CKD.

β-blockers, especially those with high lipophilic properties, penetrate the central nervous system and may cause other effects.

Propranolol is the most lipophilic. It is thought that higher lipophilicity is associated with more central nervous system side effects (dizziness, drowsiness). However, the lipophilic properties provide better effects for non-CV conditions such as migraine headache prevention, essential tremor, and thyrotoxicosis. BP lowering is equal among β-blockers regardless of lipophilicity.

Most side effects of β-blockers are extensions of their ability to antagonize β-adrenoceptors. β-blockade in the myocardium can be associated with bradycardia, atrioventricular conduction abnormalities (eg, second- or third-degree heart block), and the development of acute HF. The decrease in heart rate may benefit certain patients with atrial arrhythmias (atrial fibrillation, atrial flutter) and hypertension by both providing rate control and BP lowering. β-blocker therapy usually only produces HF if used in high initial doses for patients with preexisting left ventricular dysfunction or if started in these patients during an acute HF exacerbation. Blocking β_2-receptors in arteriolar smooth muscle may cause cold extremities and may aggravate intermittent claudication or Raynaud's phenomenon due to decreased peripheral blood flow. Also, there is an increase of sympathetic tone during periods of hypoglycemia in patients with diabetes that may result in a significant increase in BP because of unopposed α-receptor-mediated vasoconstriction.

Abrupt cessation of β-blocker therapy can cause harm. Abrupt cessation may lead to rebound hypertension (a sudden increase in BP to or above pretreatment values). Cardiac ischemia (aka, angina, or chest pain), a CV event, or even death in patients with coronary artery disease can also result from abrupt cessation. To avoid this, β-blockers should always be tapered gradually over 1 to 2 weeks before eventually discontinuing the drug. This acute withdrawal syndrome is believed to be secondary to the progression of underlying coronary disease, hypersensitivity of β-adrenergic receptors due to upregulation, and increased physical activity after withdrawal of a drug that decreases myocardial oxygen requirements. For patients without coronary disease, abrupt discontinuation may present as tachycardia, sweating, and generalized malaise in addition to increased BP.

Like a thiazide, β-blocker therapy has been shown to increase serum cholesterol and glucose values, but these effects are transient and of little-to-no clinical significance. For patients with diabetes, the reduction in CV events was as great with β-blocker therapy as with an ACEi in the United Kingdom Prospective Diabetes Study (UKPDS)[81] and far superior to placebo in the SHEP trial.[6] In the Glycemic Effects in Diabetes Mellitus: Carvedilol-Metoprolol Comparison in Hypertensives (GEMINI) trial, patients with diabetes and hypertension who were randomized to metoprolol tartrate had a small increase in hemoglobin A1C values, while patients randomized to carvedilol did not.[82] This suggests that mixed α- and β-blocking effects of carvedilol may be preferential to metoprolol for patients with uncontrolled diabetes.

Nebivolol is a third-generation β-blocker. Similar to carvedilol and labetalol, this β-blocker results in vasodilation. However, carvedilol and labetalol cause vasodilation because of their ability to block α_1-receptors, while nebivolol causes vasodilation through the release of nitric oxide. There are no proven long-term clinical benefits of the nitric oxide effects seen with nebivolol, but this might explain a lower risk of β-blocker–associated fatigue, erectile dysfunction, and metabolic side effects (eg, hyperglycemia) with this agent.

Alternative Agents 13 Alternative antihypertensive agents may be used as add-on therapy to provide additional BP lowering in patients who are already treated with combination therapy consisting of first-line antihypertensives.

α_1-Blocker Selective α_1-receptor blockers (doxazosin, prazosin, and doxazosin) work in the peripheral vasculature and inhibit the uptake of catecholamines in smooth muscle cells resulting in vasodilation and BP lowering.

Doxazosin was one of the original treatment arms of the ALLHAT. However, it was stopped prematurely when more secondary endpoints of stroke, HF, and CV events were seen with doxazosin than chlorthalidone.[33] These data demonstrated that thiazides are superior to α_1-blockers in preventing CV events in patients with hypertension. Therefore, α_1-blockers should only be used in combination with first-line antihypertensive agents.

An α_1-blocker can provide symptomatic benefits in men with benign prostatic hypertrophy. These agents block postsynaptic α_1-adrenergic receptors located on the prostate capsule, causing relaxation and decreased resistance to urinary outflow. However, when used to lower BP, they should only be in addition to first-line antihypertensive agents.

A potentially severe side effect of an α_1-blocker is a "first-dose" phenomenon characterized by transient dizziness or faintness, palpitations, and even syncope within 1 to 3 hours of the first dose. This adverse reaction can also happen after a dose increase. These episodes are accompanied by orthostatic hypotension and can be mitigated by taking the first dose and subsequent first increased doses at bedtime. Because orthostatic hypotension and dizziness often persist with chronic administration, these agents should be used cautiously in older patients that are at an increased risk of falls. Sodium and water retention can occur with higher doses and sometimes even with chronic administration of low doses. Therefore, these agents are most effective when given in combination with a thiazide to maintain antihypertensive efficacy and minimize potential edema.

Aliskiren Aliskiren is the only direct renin inhibitor. This drug blocks the RAAS at its point of activation, which results in reduced plasma renin activity and BP lowering.

The role of this drug class in the management of hypertension is limited. Since aliskiren is a RAAS blocker, it should not be used in combination with an ACEi or an ARB because of a higher risk of serious adverse effects without providing any additional reduction in CV events.[1]

Many of the cautions and adverse effects observed with an ACEi or ARB apply to aliskiren. Aliskiren should never be used in pregnancy due to the known teratogenic effects of using other drugs that block the RAAS system. Angioedema has also been reported in patients treated with aliskiren, as well as increases in serum creatinine and serum potassium values. The mechanisms of these adverse effects are likely similar to those with an ACEi or ARB. It is reasonable to utilize similar monitoring strategies by measuring serum creatinine and serum potassium in patients treated with aliskiren.

Central α_2-Agonist Clonidine, guanfacine, and methyldopa lower BP primarily by stimulating α_2-adrenergic receptors in the brain. This stimulation reduces sympathetic outflow from the vasomotor center in the brain and increases vagal tone. It is also believed that peripheral stimulation of presynaptic α_2-receptors may further reduce sympathetic tone. Reduced sympathetic activity together, with enhanced parasympathetic activity, can decrease heart rate, CO, TPR, plasma renin activity, and baroreceptor reflexes. Clonidine is usually reserved for resistant hypertension, and methyldopa, when used, is primarily for pregnancy-induced hypertension.

Chronic use of centrally acting α_2-agonist results in sodium and water retention, which is most prominent with methyldopa. Low doses of clonidine and guanfacine can be used to treat hypertension without the addition of a thiazide. However, methyldopa should be given in combination with a thiazide to avoid blunting the antihypertensive effect that happens with prolonged use when treating chronic hypertension (but not in pregnancy). Sedation and dry mouth are common anticholinergic side effects that typically improve with chronic use of low doses, but they are more troublesome in older patients. As with other centrally acting antihypertensives, depression can occur, especially with high doses. The incidence of orthostatic hypotension and dizziness is higher than with other antihypertensive agents, so they should be used cautiously in the elderly. Lastly, clonidine has a relatively high incidence of anticholinergic side effects (sedation, dry mouth, constipation, urinary retention, and blurred vision). Thus, it should generally be avoided for chronic antihypertensive therapy in older patients.

Abrupt cessation of a central α_2-agonist may lead to rebound hypertension. This effect is thought to be secondary to a compensatory increase in norepinephrine release after abrupt discontinuation. In addition, other effects such as nervousness, agitation, headache, and tremor can also occur, which may be exacerbated by concomitant β-blocker use, particularly with clonidine. Thus, if clonidine is to be discontinued, it should be tapered. For patients who are receiving concomitant β-blocker therapy, the β-blocker should be gradually discontinued first several days before gradual discontinuation of clonidine. Considering the increased risk of adverse effects and the need for frequent administration with the oral dosage formulation, which increases the risk of rebound hypertension during periods of nonadherence, the transdermal form rather than tablets should be used when clonidine therapy is needed.[69]

Methyldopa can cause hepatitis or hemolytic anemia, although this is rare. Methyldopa should be quickly discontinued if persistent increases in serum hepatic transaminases or alkaline phosphatase are detected because this may indicate the onset of fulminant life-threatening hepatitis. Coombs-positive hemolytic anemia occurs in <1% of patients receiving methyldopa, although 20% exhibit a positive direct Coombs test without anemia. For these reasons, methyldopa has limited use in the routine management of hypertension, except in pregnancy.

Direct Arterial Vasodilator Hydralazine and minoxidil directly relax arteriolar smooth muscle resulting in vasodilation and BP lowering. They exert little to no venous vasodilation. Both agents cause potent reductions in perfusion pressure that activate baroreceptor reflexes. Activation of baroreceptors results in a compensatory increase in sympathetic outflow, which leads to an increase in heart rate, CO, and renin release. Consequently, tachyphylaxis (loss of antihypertensive effect) can develop with continued use. This compensatory baroreceptor response can be counteracted by concurrent use of a β-blocker.

All patients receiving hydralazine or minoxidil for chronic therapy should first receive both a thiazide and a β-blocker. Direct arterial vasodilators can precipitate angina in patients with stable ischemic heart disease unless the baroreceptor reflex mechanism is blocked with a β-blocker (diltiazem or verapamil can be used as an alternative to β-blockers for this purpose). The side effect of sodium and water retention is significant but is minimized by using a thiazide concomitantly.

One side effect unique to hydralazine is a dose-dependent drug-induced lupus-like syndrome. Hepatic *N*-acetyltransferase eliminates hydralazine. This enzyme displays genetic polymorphism, and "slow acetylators" are especially prone to develop drug-induced lupus with hydralazine. This syndrome is more common in women and is reversible on discontinuation. Drug-induced lupus may be avoided by using less than 200 mg of hydralazine daily. Because of side effects, hydralazine has limited clinical use for chronic management of hypertension. However, it is especially useful for patients with severe CKD and kidney failure. When used in combination with isosorbide dinitrate, hydralazine has been shown to reduce the risk of CV events in Black patients with HFrEF when added to a standard regimen of a diuretic, ACEi, or ARB, and evidence-based β-blocker therapy.[44]

Minoxidil is a more potent vasodilator than hydralazine. Therefore, the compensatory increases in heart rate, CO, renin release, and sodium retention are even more dramatic. Due to significant water retention, a loop diuretic is often more effective than a thiazide in patients treated with minoxidil. A troublesome side effect of minoxidil is hypertrichosis (hirsutism), presenting as increased hair growth on the face, arms, back, and chest. Hypertrichosis usually ceases when the drug is discontinued. Other minoxidil side effects include pericardial effusion and a nonspecific T-wave change on the electrocardiogram. Minoxidil is reserved for resistant hypertension as an alternative to hydralazine.

Combination Therapy

13 A combination of two antihypertensive drugs is recommended for patients initially presenting with stage 2 hypertension.[1] Using a fixed-dose combination product is an option for these types of patients and has been shown to improve adherence. Initial two-drug combination therapy may also be appropriate for patients with multiple compelling indications for different antihypertensive agents. Moreover, combination therapy is often needed to control BP in patients who are already treated with drug therapy.[1]

The long-term safety and efficacy of initial two-drug therapy for hypertension were evaluated in the ACCOMPLISH trial.[83] This was a prospective, randomized, double-blind trial in 11,506 patients with hypertension and other CV risk factors. All these patients either had stage 2 hypertension or were on antihypertensive drug therapy at enrollment. Patients were randomized to receive either benazepril-with-hydrochlorothiazide or benazepril-with-amlodipine as initial drug therapy. Treatment was titrated to a goal BP of <140/90 mm Hg for most patients and <130/80 mm Hg for patients with diabetes or CKD.

The trial was terminated early after a mean of 36 months because the incidence of CV events was 20% lower in the benazepril-with-amlodipine group compared with the benazepril-with-hydrochlorothiazide group. What is most important for clinical practice is that this trial established that initial two-drug therapy for stage 2 hypertension was safe and effective. Mean BP measurements were 132/73 and 133/74 mm Hg in the benazepril-with-amlodipine and benazepril-with-hydrochlorothiazide groups.

The ACCOMPLISH trial established initial two-drug antihypertensive therapy as an evidence-based strategy to treat hypertension. Clinicians should consider this study as justification for implementing initial two-drug therapy antihypertensive regimens in appropriate patients. Moreover, the ACCOMPLISH trial demonstrated that the combination of an ACEi with a dihydropyridine CCB was more effective in reducing CV events than the combination of an ACEi with hydrochlorothiazide. However, thiazides are effective at lowering BP, particularly chlorthalidone and indapamide, especially when combined with other agents, and hydrochlorothiazide is available in many fixed-dose combination products.

Optimal Use of Combination Therapy

Clinicians should anticipate the need for combination therapy to control BP in most patients. Using low-dose combinations also provides greater BP reductions than high doses of single agents, with fewer drug-related side effects.[71] Contrary to popular myth, appropriately increasing the number of antihypertensive medications to attain goal BP values does not increase the risk of adverse effects. The American Society of Hypertension has recommended three categories of combination therapy (see Box B).[84] Preferred combinations are ideal for lowering BP, have complementary mechanisms of action, and use evidence-based first-line agents. Acceptable combinations may not provide all of the benefits that preferred combinations do and may have additive side effect profiles. Less-effective combinations are limited in their overall benefits and should only be used when necessary, except when treating compelling indications.

BOX B AMERICAN SOCIETY OF HYPERTENSION RECOMMENDATIONS FOR COMBINATION THERAPY

Preferred	Acceptable	Less Effective
• ACEi/CCB • ARB/CCB • ACEi/thiazide • ARB/thiazide	• β-Blocker/thiazide • CCB (dihydropyridine)/β-blocker • CCB/thiazide • Thiazide/potassium-sparing diuretic	• ACEi/β-blocker • ARB/β-blocker • CCB (nondihydropyridine)/β-blocker • Centrally acting agent/β-blocker

Data from Reference 85.

Some combinations should be avoided when treating hypertension. As previously discussed, the ON-TARGET demonstrated that using an ACEi with an ARB in the management of hypertension resulted in no additional reduction in the incidence of CV events.[85] Moreover, this combination resulted in a higher risk of adverse events, which was also demonstrated in other trials. These same negative effects are seen when aliskiren is used in combination with an ARB.[86] These combinations (using two RAAS blockers together) should be avoided in the management of hypertension.[1] Other combinations, such as a thiazide with a potassium-sparing diuretic, both of which have overlapping mechanisms of action, should be implemented only to minimize hypokalemia; not for additional BP lowering. Combining two CCBs, a dihydropyridine with a nondihydropyridine, can provide additional BP lowering but has limited use in the routine management of most patients. Under no circumstance should two drugs from the exactly same class of medications be used to treat hypertension.

Fixed-Dose Combination Products Many fixed-dose combination products are available, and nearly all are generic (see Table 30-9). Most combination products contain a thiazide and have multiple dose strengths. Individual dose titration is more complicated with fixed-dose combination products, but this strategy can reduce the number of daily tablets/capsules and simplify regimens to improve adherence by decreasing pill burden. This alone may increase the likelihood of achieving or maintaining goal BP values and is recommended to improve adherence.[1,87] Most generic combination products are less expensive to patients and health systems. Nonadherence rates are lower when fixed-dose combination products are used to treat hypertension compared with using free drug components (separate pills) to treat hypertension and therefore is recommended preferentially.[1]

Chronotherapy

Chronotherapy refers to targeting medication release and its effects at specific times of the day. The rationale behind chronotherapy in hypertension is that blunting the early morning BP surge may result in more significant reductions in CV events than dosing conventional antihypertensive products in the morning.

Two nondihydropyridine CCBs, sustained-release verapamil (Verelan PM) and long-acting diltiazem (Cardizem LA), are designed to target the circadian BP rhythm. When dosed in the evening, the drug is released during the early morning hours when BP first increases. However, evidence from the Controlled Onset Verapamil Investigation of Cardiovascular End-Points (CONVINCE) trial showed that chronotherapeutic verapamil was similar to, but not better than, a thiazide–β-blocker–based regimen for CV events.[27]

TABLE 30-9 Fixed-Dose Combination Products

Combination	Medication (Brand Name)
ACEi with CCB	• Amlodipine/benazepril (Lotrel) • Perindopril/amlodipine (Prestalia) • Trandolapril/verapamil (Tarka)
ARB with CCB	• Amlodipine/olmesartan (Azor) • Telmisartan/amlodipine (Twynsta) • Valsartan/amlodipine (Exforge)
ACEi with a thiazide	• Benazepril/hydrochlorothiazide (Lotensin HCT) • Captopril/hydrochlorothiazide (Capozide) • Enalapril/hydrochlorothiazide (Vaseretic) • Fosinopril/hydrochlorothiazide (Monopril HCT) • Lisinopril/hydrochlorothiazide (Prinizide, Zestoretic) • Moexipril/hydrochlorothiazide (Uniretic) • Quinapril/hydrochlorothiazide (Accuretic)
ARB with a thiazide	• Azilsartan/chlorthalidone (Edarbyclor) • Candesartan/hydrochlorothiazide (Atacand HCT) • Eprosartan/hydrochlorothiazide (Teveten HCT) • Irbesartan/hydrochlorothiazide (Avalide) • Losartan/hydrochlorothiazide (Hyzaar) • Olmesartan/hydrochlorothiazide (Benicar HCT) • Telmisartan/hydrochlorothiazide (Micardis HCT) • Valsartan/hydrochlorothiazide (Diovan HCT)
β-Blocker with a thiazide	• Atenolol/chlorthalidone (Tenoretic) • Bisoprolol/hydrochlorothiazide (Ziac) • Metoprolol succinate/hydrochlorothiazide (Dutoprol) • Metoprolol tartrate/hydrochlorothiazide (Lopressor HCT) • Nadolol/Bendroflumethiazide (Corzide) • Propranolol/hydrochlorothiazide (Inderide)
Direct renin inhibitor with thiazide	Aliskiren/hydrochlorothiazide (Tekturna HCT)
Mineralocorticoid receptor antagonist with thiazide	Spironolactone/hydrochlorothiazide (Aldactazide)
ARB with CCB with a thiazide	• Amlodipine/valsartan/hydrochlorothiazide (Exforge HCT) • Olmesartan/amlodipine/hydrochlorothiazide (Tribenzor)

The Hygia Chronotherapy Trial sought to assess whether dosing one or more antihypertensives at bedtime reduced CVD events more than upon waking.[88] The trial reported that evening dosing dramatically reduced CV events and CV death. However, results of the Hygia trial should be viewed cautiously due to several issues, including the methods (eg, open-label design, statistics used), and the magnitude of benefit on CV outcomes was inconsistent with the minimal BP difference between groups (1 mm Hg). Therefore, data are lacking based on the current evidence, demonstrating an advantage for chronotherapy in treating hypertension.

Pharmacoeconomic Considerations

The cost of effectively treating hypertension based on estimated annual healthcare expenditures is approximately $2,000 more for patients with hypertension than without hypertension.[89] The average yearly direct and indirect cost of hypertension from 2016 to 2017 was $52.4 billion.[90,91] However, costs of care are offset by savings that would be realized by reducing CV morbidity and mortality. Costs related to treating CV events (eg, MI, end-stage kidney failure) can drastically increase healthcare costs.

Antihypertensive drug costs are generally inexpensive and are not a significant portion of the total cost of hypertensive care. Nearly all antihypertensive agents, including first-line antihypertensive drug classes (ACEis, ARBs, CCBs, and thiazides), are generic. Many are available on discount formularies, including many generic fixed-dose combinations.

It is crucial to identify ways to control the cost of care without increasing the morbidity and mortality associated with uncontrolled hypertension. Using evidence-based pharmacotherapy will save costs. An ACEi, ARB, CCB, and thiazide are all first-line treatment options in most patients without compelling indications, and with few exceptions, are inexpensive. Utilizing generic agents, either as monotherapy or combined, is appropriate under nearly all circumstances in hypertension management. Use of once-daily and fixed-dose generic combination antihypertensives that are economical is preferred.[1]

Team-Based Collaborative Care

Team-based care for patients with cardiovascular disease is optimal for the comprehensive care of patients.[1] A collaborative approach to the management of hypertension is a proven strategy that improves goal BP attainment rates.[1] Ideal patient care models are interprofessional and utilize physicians, pharmacists, nurses, and other healthcare professionals.

With the advent of healthcare reform, collaborative team-based approaches to chronic diseases are viewed as high-quality and cost-effective improvement modalities. Within these models, pharmacists have been proven to be an effective component of team-based models not only in a community pharmacy or ambulatory clinic settings[92] but also in community outreach sites such as barbershops.[93] In addition to optimizing the selection and implementation of antihypertensive drug therapy and increased attainment of goal BP, clinical interventions by pharmacists have been proven to reduce the risk of adverse drug events and medication errors in ambulatory patients with CV disease.[94] Pharmacists have a substantial effect in various roles in clinical settings, through comprehensive medication management, optimization of drug use, avoidance of adverse drug events, and patient education.

EVALUATION OF THERAPEUTIC OUTCOMES

Monitoring the Pharmacotherapy Plan

Routine, ongoing monitoring to assess the desired effects of antihypertensive therapy (efficacy, including BP goal attainment), undesired adverse effects (side effects and toxicity), and disease progression is needed in all patients treated with antihypertensive drug therapy.

Efficacy

The most important strategy to prevent CV morbidity and mortality from CV events in hypertension is BP control to a goal (see Box A). Treating to a goal BP of <130/80 mm Hg should be attained in older patients and those with isolated systolic hypertension. For older patients, actual BP lowering can occur at a more gradual pace to avoid orthostatic hypotension. Modifying other CV risk factors (eg, smoking, dyslipidemia, diabetes) is also essential.

Both clinic-based and self-measurement home BP monitoring are important components for monitoring and managing hypertension. Patients should be encouraged to obtain a validated home BP monitor, record the results, and send or bring them to follow-up clinic visits. BP response should be evaluated in the clinic 4 weeks after initiating or making changes in therapy and results compared to home BP readings. Once goal BP is attained, clinic BP monitoring can be done every 3 to 6 months. More frequent evaluations are required for patients with a history of poor control, nonadherence, other significant comorbidities, or symptoms of adverse drug effects.

Automated ABP monitoring can be useful clinically to establish effective 24-hour control. This type of monitoring may become the standard of care in the future because evolving data have demonstrated significant benefits of using these types of measurements to diagnose hypertension, confirm white coat or masked uncontrolled hypertension, and could be a stronger predictor of CVD.[1]

For patients self-measuring their BP at home, it is important that they measure during the early morning hours, taking at least two measurements 1 minute apart before taking antihypertensive medications, for most days and then in the evening on alternate days of the week using appropriate technique.[1] BP measurements should be recorded daily, or ideally, a monitor with a built-in memory should be used. Patients should be instructed to bring their actual measurements and/or BP monitor with built-in memory to follow-up clinic appointments, and any changes to drug therapy should be based on an average BP reading from two or more occasions.[1]

Side Effects and Toxicity

The most common side effects associated with each class of antihypertensive agents were discussed in the "First-Line Antihypertensive Agents" and "Alternative Agents" sections, and laboratory parameters for first-line agents are listed in Table 30-10. Laboratory monitoring should typically occur 4 weeks after starting a new agent or dose increase, and then every 6 to 12 months in stable patients. Additional disease-specific monitoring might be needed (eg, diabetes, dyslipidemia, gout) depending on which agents are used. Moreover, patients treated with a mineralocorticoid receptor antagonist (eplerenone or spironolactone) should ideally have potassium concentrations and kidney function assessed within 3 days of initiation and again at 1 week to detect potential hyperkalemia, especially for patients at high risk for hyperkalemia. The occurrence of an adverse drug event may require dosage reduction or substitution with an alternative antihypertensive agent.

Disease Progression

Patients should be monitored for signs and symptoms of hypertension-associated complications. A careful history for ischemic chest pain (or pressure), palpitations, dizziness, dyspnea, orthopnea, headache, sudden change in vision, one-sided weakness, slurred speech, and loss of balance should be taken to determine the presence of CV and cerebrovascular disease. Other monitoring parameters that may be used include funduscopic changes on an eye examination, LVH on electrocardiogram, albuminuria, and changes in kidney function by calculating estimated GFR. These parameters should be monitored periodically because any sign of deterioration requires additional assessment and follow-up.

Adherence and Persistence

Poor medication use behaviors and lack of persistence with antihypertensive pharmacotherapy is a major problem and associated with

TABLE 30-10 Routine Monitoring for Select Antihypertensive Agents

Class	Parameters
ACEi	BP; BUN/serum creatinine; serum potassium
ARB	BP; BUN/serum creatinine; serum potassium
β-Blocker	BP; heart rate
Calcium channel blocker	BP; heart rate
Mineralocorticoid receptor antagonist	BP; BUN/serum creatinine; serum potassium
Thiazide	BP; BUN/serum creatinine; serum electrolytes (potassium, magnesium, sodium); uric acid (for thiazides)

significant increases in costs due to the development of complications. Since hypertension is nearly always an asymptomatic disease, poor adherence is frequent, particularly in newly treated patients. Up to 25% of patients do not fill their initial prescription for antihypertensive medication, and during the first year of treatment, an average patient possesses their BP medication only half of the time.[1] Long-term risk of CV events can be significantly reduced when patients adhere to their antihypertensive drug therapy. Therefore, it is imperative to assess patient adherence and medication-taking behavior on a regular basis.

Improving adherence to antihypertensive treatment and hypertension control requires a multifactorial approach.[1] These include interventions aimed at the patient, provider, and health-system level. Examples can include (a) focusing on clinical outcomes (eg, following national guidelines, use of once-daily antihypertensives and combination rather than free individual components, encouraging self-monitoring of BP), (b) empowering informed activated patients (eg, behavioral and motivational strategies, use of pillboxes, systems to prompt patients to refill prescriptions), (c) implementing a team approach (eg, collaborative interprofessional models of care), (d) use of telehealth strategies, and (e) advocating for health policy reform (eg, use of performance measures, reimbursement for telehealth strategies).

After identifying less than optimal adherence in a patient with hypertension, appropriate patient education, counseling, and intervention should occur. Once-daily regimens are recommended in most patients to improve adherence. Some patients may incorrectly believe that aggressive treatment may negatively impact the quality of life and thus result in nonadherence. However, several studies have found that most patients feel better once their BP is controlled, and patients should be aware of this. Patients on antihypertensive therapy should be questioned periodically about changes in their general health perception, physical functioning, and overall satisfaction with treatment. Lifestyle modifications should always be recommended to augment antihypertensive drug therapy and provide other potential health benefits. Persistence with lifestyle modifications should also be continually encouraged.

Hypertensive Urgencies and Emergencies

Both hypertensive urgencies and emergencies (aka hypertensive crisis) are characterized by elevated BP, typically >180/120 mm Hg.[1] However, the need for urgent or emergent antihypertensive therapy must be determined based on the presence of acute or immediately progressing end-organ injury, not elevated BP alone. Urgencies are not associated with acute or immediately progressing end-organ injury, while emergencies are. Examples of acute end-organ injury include encephalopathy, intracranial hemorrhage, acute left ventricular failure with pulmonary edema, dissecting aortic aneurysm, unstable angina, acute renal failure, and eclampsia.

Hypertensive urgencies are ideally managed by adjusting maintenance therapy, whereas hypertensive emergencies require immediate BP reduction parenteral agents to limit new or progressing end-organ damage. The Acute Hypertensive Crisis Chapter (Chapter e31) discusses the pathophysiology and pharmacotherapeutic treatment of hypertensive urgencies and emergencies.

CONCLUSIONS

Hypertension is a common medical condition in the United States with significant health consequences if not controlled. Treatment of patients with hypertension should include both lifestyle modifications and pharmacotherapy. Evidence from outcome-based clinical trials has definitively demonstrated that treating hypertension reduces the risk of CV events and subsequently reduces morbidity and mortality. Moreover, evidence evaluating individual drug classes has resulted in an evidence-based approach to selecting pharmacotherapy in an individual patient. An ACEi, ARB, CCB, and thiazide are all first-line agents. Data suggest that using a β-blocker first-line to treat patients with hypertension, without the presence of a compelling indication, is better than not treating hypertension. However, β-blocker therapy is not as beneficial in reducing the risk of CV events compared with ACEi-, ARB-, CCB-, or thiazide-based therapy and is not a first-line therapy option without an appropriate compelling indication.

Patients should be treated to a goal BP value. In addition to selecting an appropriate antihypertensive regimen, attaining a goal BP is also of paramount importance to ensure a maximum reduction in risk for CV events is provided. A BP goal of <130/80 mm Hg is recommended for most patients with hypertension. Most patients with hypertension require more than one drug to attain goal BP values; therefore, combination therapy should be anticipated.

Optimizing hypertension management can be achieved in many ways. Team-based approaches to implementing care and attaining goal BP values are preferred. Judicious use of cost-effective medications and fixed-dose combination products should always be considered to improve the sustainability of treatment. Lastly, interventions to reinforce adherence and lifestyle modifications are needed for the comprehensive management of hypertension.

ABBREVIATIONS

ABP	ambulatory blood pressure
ACC	American College of Cardiology
ACCOMPLISH	Avoiding Cardiovascular Events Through Combination Therapy in Patients Living with Systolic Hypertension
ACCORD-BP	Action to Control Cardiovascular Risk in Diabetes Blood Pressure
ACE	angiotensin-converting enzyme
AHA	American Heart Association
ALLHAT	Antihypertensive and Lipid Lowering Treatment to Prevent Heart Attack Trial
ARB	angiotensin II receptor blocker
ASCVD	atherosclerotic cardiovascular disease
AT_1	angiotensin II type 1
AT_2	angiotensin II type 2
BP	blood pressure
BUN	blood urea nitrogen
CCB	calcium channel blocker
CKD	chronic kidney disease
CO	cardiac output
CONVINCE	Controlled Onset Verapamil Investigation of Cardiovascular End-Points
COPD	chronic obstructive pulmonary disease
CV	cardiovascular
DASH	Dietary Approaches to Stop Hypertension
DBP	diastolic blood pressure
GEMINI	Glycemic Effects in Diabetes Mellitus: Carvedilol–Metoprolol Comparison in Hypertensives
GFR	glomerular filtration rate
HOT	Hypertension Optimal Treatment
HF	heart failure
HFpEF	heart failure with preserved ejection fraction
HFrEF	heart failure with reduced ejection fraction
HYVET	Hypertension in the Very Elderly Trial
INVEST	International Verapamil–Trandolapril Study
ISA	intrinsic sympathomimetic activity
KDIGO	Kidney Disease Improving Global Outcomes
LVH	left ventricular hypertrophy
MAP	mean arterial pressure

MI	myocardial infarction
MOSES	Morbidity and Mortality After Stroke: Eprosartan Versus Nitrendipine in Secondary Prevention
MRA	mineralocorticoid receptor antagonists
MRC	Medical Research Council
NHLBI	National Heart, Lung, and Blood Institute
ON-TARGET	Ongoing Telmisartan Alone and in Combination with Ramipril Global End Point Trial
PAD	peripheral arterial disease
PATHWAY-2	Prevention And Treatment of Hypertension With Algorithm based therapY-2
PVR	peripheral vascular resistance
RAAS	renin–angiotensin–aldosterone system
SBP	systolic blood pressure
SHEP	Systolic Hypertension in the Elderly Program
SPRINT	Systolic Pressure Intervention Trial
STOP-2	Swedish Trial in Old Patients with Hypertension-2
STOP-Hypertension	Swedish Trial in Old Patients with Hypertension
Syst-Eur	Systolic Hypertension in Europe
TOMHS	Treatment of Mild Hypertension Study
TPR	total peripheral resistance
TRANSCEND	Telmisartan Randomized Assessment Study in ACE-Intolerant Subjects with Cardiovascular Disease
UKPDS	United Kingdom Prospective Diabetes Study
VALUE	Valsartan Antihypertensive Long-Term Use Evaluation

REFERENCES

1. Whelton PK, Carey RM, Aronow WS, et al. 2017 ACC/AHA/AAPA/ABC/ACPM/AGS/APhA/ASH/ASPC/NMA/PCNA Guideline for the prevention, detection, evaluation, and management of high blood pressure in adults: A report of the American College of Cardiology/American Heart Association Task Force on Clinical Practice Guidelines. *Hypertension*. 2018;71(6):e13–e115. doi:10.1161/HYP.0000000000000065.
2. Muntner P, Carey RM, Gidding S, et al. Potential U.S. population impact of the 2017 ACC/AHA High Blood Pressure Guideline. *J Am Coll Cardiol*. 2018;71(2):109–118. doi:10.1016/j.jacc.2017.10.073.
3. Guo X, Zhang X, Guo L, et al. Association between pre-hypertension and cardiovascular outcomes: A systematic review and meta-analysis of prospective studies. *Curr Hypertens Rep*. 2013;15(6):703–716. doi:10.1007/s11906-013-0403-y.
4. Lewington S, Clarke R, Qizilbash N, Peto R, Collins R, Prospective Studies Collaboration. Age-specific relevance of usual blood pressure to vascular mortality: A meta-analysis of individual data for one million adults in 61 prospective studies. *Lancet*. 2002;360(9349):1903–1913.
5. Dahlof B, Lindholm LH, Hansson L, Schersten B, Ekbom T, Wester PO. Morbidity and mortality in the Swedish Trial in Old Patients with Hypertension (STOP-Hypertension). *Lancet*. 1991;338(8778):1281–1285.
6. SHEP Cooperative Research Group. Prevention of stroke by antihypertensive drug treatment in older persons with isolated systolic hypertension. Final results of the Systolic Hypertension in the Elderly Program (SHEP). *JAMA*. 1991;265(24):3255–3264.
7. MRC Working Party. Medical Research Council trial of treatment of hypertension in older adults: Principal results. *BMJ*. 1992;304(6824):405–412.
8. Staessen JA, Fagard R, Thijs L, et al. Randomised double-blind comparison of placebo and active treatment for older patients with isolated systolic hypertension. The Systolic Hypertension in Europe (Syst-Eur) Trial Investigators. *Lancet*. 1997;350(9080):757–764.
9. Muntner P, Shimbo D, Carey RM, et al. Measurement of blood pressure in humans: A scientific statement from the American Heart Association. *Hypertension*. 2019;73(5):e35–e66. doi:10.1161/HYP.0000000000000087.
10. Mancia G, Bombelli M, Facchetti R, et al. Long-term risk of sustained hypertension in white-coat or masked hypertension. *Hypertension*. 2009;54(2):226–232. doi:10.1161/HYPERTENSIONAHA.109.129882.
11. Banegas JR, Ruilope LM, de la Sierra A, et al. Relationship between clinic and ambulatory blood-pressure measurements and mortality. *N Engl J Med*. 2018;378(16):1509–1520. doi:10.1056/NEJMoa1712231.
12. American Diabetes Association. 10. Cardiovascular disease and risk management: Standards of medical care in diabetes—2021. *Diabetes Care*. 2021;44(Suppl 1):S125–S150. doi:10.2337/dc21-S010.
13. Kidney Disease: Improving Global Outcomes Blood Pressure Work Group. KDIGO 2021 clinical practice guideline for the management of blood pressure in chronic kidney disease. *Kidney Int*. 2021;99(3S):S1–S87. doi:10.1016/j.kint.2020.11.003.
14. The SPRINT Research Group. A randomized trial of intensive versus standard blood-pressure control. *N Engl J Med*. 2015;373(22):2103–2116. doi:10.1056/NEJMoa1511939.
15. The Sprint Research Group. Final report of a trial of intensive versus standard blood-pressure control. *N Engl J Med*. 2021;384(20):1921–1930. doi:10.1056/NEJMoa1901281.
16. Vaduganathan M, Claggett BL, Juraschek SP, Solomon SD. Assessment of long-term benefit of intensive blood pressure control on residual life span: Secondary analysis of the Systolic Blood Pressure Intervention Trial (SPRINT). *JAMA Cardiol*. 2020;5(5):576–581. doi:10.1001/jamacardio.2019.6192.
17. Reboussin DM, Allen NB, Griswold ME, et al. Systematic review for the 2017 ACC/AHA/AAPA/ABC/ACPM/AGS/APhA/ASH/ASPC/NMA/PCNA Guideline for the Prevention, Detection, Evaluation, and Management of High Blood Pressure in Adults: A Report of the American College of Cardiology/American Heart Association Task Force on Clinical Practice Guidelines. *Hypertension*. 2017. doi:10.1161/hyp.0000000000000067.
18. Xie X, Atkins E, Lv J, et al. Effects of intensive blood pressure lowering on cardiovascular and renal outcomes: Updated systematic review and meta-analysis. *Lancet*. 2016;387(10017):435–443. doi:10.1016/s0140-6736(15)00805-3.
19. Bundy JD, Li C, Stuchlik P, et al. Systolic blood pressure reduction and risk of cardiovascular disease and mortality: A systematic review and network meta-analysis. *JAMA Cardiol*. 2017;2(7):775–781. 10.1001/jamacardio.2017.1421.
20. The Blood Pressure Lowering Treatment Trialists' Collaboration. Blood pressure-lowering treatment based on cardiovascular risk: A meta-analysis of individual patient data. *Lancet*. 2014;384(9943):591–598. doi:10.1016/s0140-6736(14)61212-5.
21. Thomopoulos C, Parati G, Zanchetti A. Effects of blood pressure lowering on outcome incidence in hypertension: 7. Effects of more vs less intensive blood pressure lowering and different achieved blood pressure levels: updated overview and meta-analyses of randomized trials. *J Hypertens*. 2016;34(4):613–622. doi:10.1097/hjh.0000000000000881.
22. Hansson L, Zanchetti A, Carruthers SG, et al. Effects of intensive blood-pressure lowering and low-dose aspirin in patients with hypertension: Principal results of the Hypertension Optimal Treatment (HOT) randomised trial. HOT Study Group. *Lancet*. 1998;351(9118):1755–1762.
23. The ACCORD Study Group. Effects of intensive blood-pressure control in type 2 diabetes mellitus. *N Engl J Med*. 2010;362(17):1575–1585. doi:10.1056/NEJMoa1001286.
24. Buckley LF, Dixon DL, Wohlford GFt, Wijesinghe DS, Baker WL, Van Tassell BW. Intensive versus standard blood pressure control in SPRINT-eligible participants of ACCORD-BP. *Diabetes Care*. 2017;40(12):1733–1738. doi:10.2337/dc17-1366.
25. O'Connor PJ. Overcome clinical inertia to control systolic blood pressure. *Arch Intern Med*. 2003;163(22):2677–2678.
26. ALLHAT Officers and Coordinators for the ALLHAT Collaborative Research Group. Major outcomes in high-risk hypertensive patients randomized to angiotensin-converting enzyme inhibitor or calcium channel blocker vs diuretic: The Antihypertensive and Lipid-Lowering Treatment to Prevent Heart Attack Trial (ALLHAT). *JAMA*. 2002;288(23):2981–2997.
27. Black HR, Elliott WJ, Grandits G, et al. Principal results of the Controlled Onset Verapamil Investigation of Cardiovascular End Points (CONVINCE) trial. *JAMA*. 2003;289(16):2073–2082.
28. Dahlof B, Devereux RB, Kjeldsen SE, et al. Cardiovascular morbidity and mortality in the Losartan Intervention For Endpoint reduction in hypertension study (LIFE): A randomised trial against atenolol. *Lancet*. 2002;359(9311):995–1003.
29. Dahlof B, Sever PS, Poulter NR, et al. Prevention of cardiovascular events with an antihypertensive regimen of amlodipine adding

perindopril as required versus atenolol adding bendroflumethiazide as required, in the Anglo-Scandinavian Cardiac Outcomes Trial-Blood Pressure Lowering Arm (ASCOT-BPLA): A multicentre randomised controlled trial. *Lancet*. 2005;366(9489):895–906.

30. Julius S, Kjeldsen SE, Weber M, et al. Outcomes in hypertensive patients at high cardiovascular risk treated with regimens based on valsartan or amlodipine: The VALUE randomised trial. *Lancet*. 2004;363(9426):2022–2031.
31. PROGRESS Collaborative Group. Randomised trial of a perindopril-based blood-pressure-lowering regimen among 6,105 individuals with previous stroke or transient ischaemic attack. *Lancet*. 2001;358(9287):1033–1041.
32. Wing LM, Reid CM, Ryan P, et al. A comparison of outcomes with angiotensin-converting-enzyme inhibitors and diuretics for hypertension in the elderly. *N Engl J Med*. 2003;348(7):583–592.
33. Antihypertensive and Lipid-Lowering Treatment to Prevent Heart Attack Trial Collaborative Research Group. Diuretic versus alpha-blocker as first-step antihypertensive therapy: Final results from the Antihypertensive and Lipid-Lowering Treatment to Prevent Heart Attack Trial (ALLHAT). *Hypertension*. 2003;42(3):239–246.
34. Davis BR, Cutler JA, Gordon DJ, et al. Rationale and design for the Antihypertensive and Lipid Lowering Treatment to Prevent Heart Attack Trial (ALLHAT). ALLHAT Research Group. *Am J Hypertens*. 1996;9(4 Pt 1):342–360.
35. Rahman M, Pressel S, Davis BR, et al. Renal outcomes in high-risk hypertensive patients treated with an angiotensin-converting enzyme inhibitor or a calcium channel blocker vs a diuretic: A report from the Antihypertensive and Lipid-Lowering Treatment to Prevent Heart Attack Trial (ALLHAT). *Arch Intern Med*. 2005;165(8):936–946.
36. Whelton PK, Barzilay J, Cushman WC, et al. Clinical outcomes in antihypertensive treatment of type 2 diabetes, impaired fasting glucose concentration, and normoglycemia: Antihypertensive and Lipid-Lowering Treatment to Prevent Heart Attack Trial (ALLHAT). *Arch Intern Med*. 2005;165(12):1401–1409.
37. Wright JTJ, Dunn JK, Cutler JA, et al. Outcomes in hypertensive black and nonblack patients treated with chlorthalidone, amlodipine, and lisinopril. *JAMA*. 2005;293(13):1595–1608.
38. Turnbull F. Effects of different blood-pressure-lowering regimens on major cardiovascular events: Results of prospectively-designed overviews of randomised trials. *Lancet*. 2003;362(9395):1527–1535.
39. Zhang Y, Sun N, Jiang X, Xi Y. Comparative efficacy of beta-blockers on mortality and cardiovascular outcomes in patients with hypertension: A systematic review and network meta-analysis. *J Am Soc Hypertens*. 2017;11(7):394–401. doi:10.1016/j.jash.2017.05.001.
40. National Institute for Health and Clinical Excellence (NICE) Clinical Guideline. Hypertension in adults: Diagnosis and management. https://www.nice.org.uk/guidance/cg127. Accessed May 29, 2018.
41. Ripley TL, Saseen JJ. Beta-blockers: A review of their pharmacological and physiological diversity in hypertension. *Ann Pharmacother*. 2014;48(6):723–733. doi:10.1177/1060028013519591.
42. Yancy CW, Jessup M, Bozkurt B, et al. 2017 ACC/AHA/HFSA focused update of the 2013 ACCF/AHA guideline for the management of heart failure: A report of the American College of Cardiology/American Heart Association Task Force on Clinical Practice Guidelines and the Heart Failure Society of America. *Circulation*. 2017;136(6):e137–e161. doi:10.1161/CIR.0000000000000509.
43. Writing Committee, Maddox TM, Januzzi JL Jr, et al. 2021 update to the 2017 ACC expert consensus decision pathway for optimization of heart failure treatment: Answers to 10 pivotal issues about heart failure with reduced ejection fraction: A report of the American College of Cardiology Solution Set Oversight Committee. *J Am Coll Cardiol*. 2021;77(6):772–810. doi:10.1016/j.jacc.2020.11.022.
44. Yancy CW, Jessup M, Bozkurt B, et al. 2013 ACCF/AHA guideline for the management of heart failure: executive summary: A report of the American College of Cardiology Foundation/American Heart Association Task Force on practice guidelines. *Circulation*. 2013;128(16):1810–1852. doi:10.1161/CIR.0b013e31829e8807.
45. Bangalore S, Steg G, Deedwania P, et al. Beta-blocker use and clinical outcomes in stable outpatients with and without coronary artery disease. *JAMA*. 2012;308(13):1340–1349. doi:10.1001/jama.2012.12559.
46. Fihn SD, Blankenship JC, Alexander KP, et al. 2014 ACC/AHA/AATS/PCNA/SCAI/STS focused update of the guideline for the diagnosis and management of patients with stable ischemic heart disease: A report of the American College of Cardiology/American Heart Association Task Force on Practice Guidelines, and the American Association for Thoracic Surgery, Preventive Cardiovascular Nurses Association, Society for Cardiovascular Angiography and Interventions, and Society of Thoracic Surgeons. *Circulation*. 2014;130(19):1749–1767. doi:10.1161/CIR.0000000000000095.
47. Pepine CJ, Handberg EM, Cooper-DeHoff RM, et al. A calcium antagonist vs a non-calcium antagonist hypertension treatment strategy for patients with coronary artery disease. The International Verapamil-Trandolapril Study (INVEST): A randomized controlled trial. *JAMA*. 2003;290(21):2805–2816.
48. American Diabetes Association. 11. Microvascular complications and foot care: Standards of medical care in diabetes—2021. *Diabetes Care*. 2021;44(Suppl 1):S151–S167. doi:10.2337/dc21-S011.
49. Bangalore S, Fakheri R, Toklu B, Messerli FH. Diabetes mellitus as a compelling indication for use of renin angiotensin system blockers: Systematic review and meta-analysis of randomized trials. *BMJ*. 2016;352:i438. doi:10.1136/bmj.i438.
50. Casas JP, Chua W, Loukogeorgakis S, et al. Effect of inhibitors of the renin-angiotensin system and other antihypertensive drugs on renal outcomes: Systematic review and meta-analysis. *Lancet*. 2005;366(9502):2026–2033.
51. Kernan WN, Ovbiagele B, Black HR, et al. Guidelines for the prevention of stroke in patients with stroke and transient ischemic attack: A guideline for healthcare professionals from the American Heart Association/American Stroke Association. *Stroke*. 2014;45(7):2160–2236. doi:10.1161/STR.0000000000000024.
52. Rashid P, Leonardi-Bee J, Bath P. Blood pressure reduction and secondary prevention of stroke and other vascular events: A systematic review. *Stroke*. 2003;34(11):2741–2748. doi:10.1161/01.STR.0000092488.40085.15.
53. Schrader J, Luders S, Kulschewski A, et al. Morbidity and mortality after stroke, eprosartan compared with nitrendipine for secondary prevention: Principal results of a prospective randomized controlled study (MOSES). *Stroke*. 2005;36(6):1218–1226.
54. Yusuf S, Diener HC, Sacco RL, et al. Telmisartan to prevent recurrent stroke and cardiovascular events. *N Engl J Med*. 2008;359(12):1225–1237. doi:10.1056/NEJMoa0804593.
55. Beckett NS, Peters R, Fletcher AE, et al. Treatment of hypertension in patients 80 years of age or older. *N Engl J Med*. 2008;358(18):1887–1898. doi:10.1056/NEJMoa0801369.
56. Hansson L, Lindholm LH, Ekbom T, et al. Randomised trial of old and new antihypertensive drugs in elderly patients: Cardiovascular mortality and morbidity the Swedish Trial in Old Patients with Hypertension-2 study. *Lancet*. 1999;354(9192):1751–1756.
57. Williamson JD, Supiano MA, Applegate WB, et al. Intensive vs standard blood pressure control and cardiovascular disease outcomes in adults aged ≥75 years: A randomized clinical trial. *JAMA*. 2016;315(24):2673–2682. doi:10.1001/jama.2016.7050.
58. Bavishi C, Bangalore S, Messerli FH. Outcomes of intensive blood pressure lowering in older hypertensive patients. *J Am Coll Cardiol*. 2017;69(5):486–493. doi:10.1016/j.jacc.2016.10.077.
59. Juraschek SP, Hu JR, Cluett JL, et al. Effects of intensive blood pressure treatment on orthostatic hypotension: A systematic review and individual participant-based meta-analysis. *Ann Intern Med*. 2021;174(1):58–68. doi:10.7326/M20-4298.
60. Flynn JT, Kaelber DC, Baker-Smith CM, et al. Clinical practice guideline for screening and management of high blood pressure in children and adolescents. *Pediatrics*. 2017;140(3). doi:10.1542/peds.2017-1904.
61. Gestational hypertension and preeclampsia: ACOG practice bulletin, number 222. *Obstet Gynecol*. 2020;135(6):e237–e260. doi:10.1097/AOG.0000000000003891.
62. American College of Obstetricians and Gynecologists Task Force on Hypertension in Pregnancy. Hypertension in pregnancy. Report of the American College of Obstetricians and Gynecologists' Task Force on Hypertension in Pregnancy. *Obstet Gynecol*. 2013;122(5):1122–1131. doi:10.1097/01.AOG.0000437382.03963.88.
63. Magee LA, von Dadelszen P, Rey E, et al. Less-tight versus tight control of hypertension in pregnancy. *N Engl J Med*. 2015;372(5):407–417. doi:10.1056/NEJMoa1404595.
64. Gerhard-Herman MD, Gornik HL, Barrett C, et al. 2016 AHA/ACC guideline on the management of patients with lower extremity peripheral artery disease: A report of the American College of Cardiology/American Heart Association Task Force on Clinical Practice Guidelines. *J Am Coll Cardiol*. 2017;69(11):e71–e126. doi:10.1016/j.jacc.2016.11.007.
65. Alberti KG, Eckel RH, Grundy SM, et al. Harmonizing the metabolic syndrome: A joint interim statement of the International Diabetes Federation Task Force on Epidemiology and Prevention; National Heart, Lung, and Blood Institute;

American Heart Association; World Heart Federation; International Atherosclerosis Society; and international association for the Study of Obesity. *Circulation*. 2009;120(16):1640–1645. doi:10.1161/CIRCULATIONAHA.109.192644.

66. Ko DT, Hebert PR, Coffey CS, Sedrakyan A, Curtis JP, Krumholz HM. Beta-blocker therapy and symptoms of depression, fatigue, and sexual dysfunction. *JAMA*. 2002;288(3):351–357.
67. Grimm RH Jr, Grandits GA, Prineas RJ, et al. Long-term effects on sexual function of five antihypertensive drugs and nutritional hygienic treatment in hypertensive men and women. Treatment of Mild Hypertension Study (TOMHS). *Hypertension*. 1997;29(1 Pt 1):8–14.
68. Materson BJ, Reda DJ, Cushman WC, et al. Single-drug therapy for hypertension in men. A comparison of six antihypertensive agents with placebo. The Department of Veterans Affairs Cooperative Study Group on Antihypertensive Agents. *N Engl J Med*. 1993;328(13):914–921. doi:10.1056/NEJM199304013281303.
69. Carey RM, Calhoun DA, Bakris GL, et al. Resistant hypertension: Detection, evaluation, and management: A scientific statement from the American Heart Association. *Hypertension*. 2018;72(5):e53–e90. doi:10.1161/HYP.0000000000000084.
70. Roush GC, Ernst ME, Kostis JB, Tandon S, Sica DA. Head-to-head comparisons of hydrochlorothiazide with indapamide and chlorthalidone: Antihypertensive and metabolic effects. *Hypertension*. 2015;65(5):1041–1046. doi:10.1161/HYPERTENSIONAHA.114.05021.
71. Williams B, MacDonald TM, Morant S, et al. Spironolactone versus placebo, bisoprolol, and doxazosin to determine the optimal treatment for drug-resistant hypertension (PATHWAY-2): A randomised, double-blind, crossover trial. *Lancet*. 2015;386(10008):2059–2068. doi:10.1016/S0140-6736(15)00257-3.
72. Smith SCJ, Benjamin EJ, Bonow RO, et al. AHA/ACCF secondary prevention and risk reduction therapy for patients with coronary and other atherosclerotic vascular disease: 2011 update: A guideline from the American Heart Association and American College of Cardiology Foundation. *Circulation*. 2011;124(22):2458–2473. doi:10.1161/CIR.0b013e318235eb4d.
73. Amsterdam EA, Wenger NK, Brindis RG, et al. 2014 AHA/ACC Guideline for the management of patients with non-ST-elevation acute coronary syndromes: A report of the American College of Cardiology/American Heart Association Task Force on Practice Guidelines. *J Am Coll Cardiol*. 2014;64(24):e139–e228. doi:10.1016/j.jacc.2014.09.017.
74. American College of Emergency Physicians, Society for Cardiovascular Angiography Interventions, O'Gara PT, et al. 2013 ACCF/AHA guideline for the management of ST-elevation myocardial infarction: Areport of the American College of Cardiology Foundation/American Heart Association Task Force on Practice Guidelines. *J Am Coll Cardiol*. 2013;61(4):e78–e140. doi:10.1016/j.jacc.2012.11.019.
75. Telmisartan Randomised AssessmeNt Study in ACE iNtolerant subjects with cardiovascular Disease (TRANSCEND) Investigators, Yusuf S, Teo K, et al. Effects of the angiotensin-receptor blocker telmisartan on cardiovascular events in high-risk patients intolerant to angiotensin-converting enzyme inhibitors: A randomised controlled trial. *Lancet*. 2008;372(9644):1174–1183. doi:10.1016/S0140-6736(08)61242-8.
76. Yusuf S, Teo KK, Pogue J, et al. Telmisartan, ramipril, or both in patients at high risk for vascular events. *N Engl J Med*. 2008;358(15):1547–1559. doi:10.1056/NEJMoa0801317.
77. Abraham HM, White CM, White WB. The comparative efficacy and safety of the angiotensin receptor blockers in the management of hypertension and other cardiovascular diseases. *Drug Saf*. 2015;38(1):33–54. doi:10.1007/s40264-014-0239-7.
78. Yusuf S, Teo K, Anderson C, et al. Effects of the angiotensin-receptor blocker telmisartan on cardiovascular events in high-risk patients intolerant to angiotensin-converting enzyme inhibitors: A randomised controlled trial. *Lancet*. 2008;372(9644):1174–1183. doi:10.1016/S0140-6736(08)61242-8.
79. Leenen FH, Nwachuku CE, Black HR, et al. Clinical events in high-risk hypertensive patients randomly assigned to calcium channel blocker versus angiotensin-converting enzyme inhibitor in the antihypertensive and lipid-lowering treatment to prevent heart attack trial. *Hypertension*. 2006;48(3):374–384.
80. Ernst ME, Moser M. Use of diuretics in patients with hypertension. *N Engl J Med*. 2009;361(22):2153–2164. doi:10.1056/NEJMra0907219.
81. UK Prospective Diabetes Study Group. Efficacy of atenolol and captopril in reducing risk of macrovascular and microvascular complications in type 2 diabetes: UKPDS 39. *BMJ*. 1998;317(7160):713–720.
82. Bakris GL, Fonseca V, Katholi RE, et al. Metabolic effects of carvedilol vs metoprolol in patients with type 2 diabetes mellitus and hypertension: A randomized controlled trial. *JAMA*. 2004;292(18):2227–2236.
83. Jamerson K, Weber MA, Bakris GL, et al. Benazepril plus amlodipine or hydrochlorothiazide for hypertension in high-risk patients. *N Engl J Med*. 2008;359(23):2417–2428. doi:10.1056/NEJMoa0806182.
84. Gradman AH, Basile JN, Carter BL, Bakris GL. Combination therapy in hypertension. *J Am Soc Hypertens*. 2010;4(1):42–50. doi:10.1016/j.jash.2010.02.005.
85. ONTARGET Investigators, Yusuf S, Teo KK, et al. Telmisartan, ramipril, or both in patients at high risk for vascular events. *N Engl J Med*. 2008;358(15):1547–1559. doi:10.1056/NEJMoa0801317.
86. Parving HH, Brenner BM, McMurray JJ, et al. Cardiorenal end points in a trial of aliskiren for type 2 diabetes. *N Engl J Med*. 2012;367(23):2204–2213. doi:10.1056/NEJMoa1208799.
87. Bangalore S, Kamalakkannan G, Parkar S, Messerli FH. Fixed-dose combinations improve medication compliance: A meta-analysis. *Am J Med*. 2007;120(8):713–719. doi:10.1016/j.amjmed.2006.08.033.
88. Hermida RC, Crespo JJ, Dominguez-Sardina M, et al. Bedtime hypertension treatment improves cardiovascular risk reduction: The Hygia Chronotherapy Trial. *Eur Heart J*. 2020;41(48):4565–4576. doi:10.1093/eurheartj/ehz754.
89. Kirkland EB, Heincelman M, Bishu KG, et al. Trends in healthcare expenditures among US adults with hypertension: National estimates, 2003-2014. *J Am Heart Assoc*. 2018;7(11). doi:10.1161/JAHA.118.008731.
90. Virani SS, Alonso A, Aparicio HJ, et al. Heart disease and stroke statistics—2021 update: A report from the American Heart Association. *Circulation*. 2021;143(8):e254–e743. doi:10.1161/CIR.0000000000000950.
91. Benjamin EJ, Virani SS, Callaway CW, et al. Heart disease and stroke statistics—2018 update: A report from the American Heart Association. *Circulation*. 2018;137(12):e67–e492. doi:10.1161/CIR.0000000000000558.
92. Santschi V, Chiolero A, Colosimo AL, et al. Improving blood pressure control through pharmacist interventions: A meta-analysis of randomized controlled trials. *J Am Heart Assoc*. 2014;3(2):e000718. doi:10.1161/JAHA.113.000718.
93. Victor RG, Lynch K, Li N, et al. A cluster-randomized trial of blood-pressure reduction in black barbershops. *N Engl J Med*. 2018;378(14):1291–1301. doi:10.1056/NEJMoa1717250.
94. Murray MD, Ritchey ME, Wu J, Tu W. Effect of a pharmacist on adverse drug events and medication errors in outpatients with cardiovascular disease. *Arch Intern Med*. 2009;169(8):757–763. doi:10.1001/archinternmed.2009.59.

e31

Acute Hypertensive Crisis

Jeffrey J. Mucksavage, Danielle M. Tompkins, and Eric J. MacLaughlin

KEY CONCEPTS

1. Hypertensive crisis is an acute condition of very high blood pressure (BP), with either a systolic BP (SBP) > 180 mm Hg, diastolic (DBP) > 120 mm Hg, or both.
2. The presence of new or worsening target end-organ damage differentiates hypertensive emergency from hypertensive urgency.
3. Autoregulation of perfusion is a key physiological concept that explains the pathophysiology of hypertensive crisis.
4. The affected organs during a hypertensive emergency commonly include the heart, lungs, brain, vasculature, kidneys, and eyes.
5. Hypertensive urgency does not require rapid (ie, immediate) BP reduction because the benefit does not outweigh the risk. A more gradual BP reduction over several hours to days is optimal. Hypertensive urgency is managed by resuming omitted antihypertensive therapy, increasing current doses of antihypertensives, or adding additional agents to achieve control.
6. Hypertensive emergency is a medical emergency that requires acute hospitalization, frequent monitoring, and, in most cases, intravenous (IV) antihypertensive therapy to control BP.
7. The goal for managing hypertensive emergencies is to prevent additional organ damage. Target BP goals are different than those for chronic treatment of high BP, and the timeframe for achieving goals is determined by the organ systems affected and comorbities.
8. Despite no clear mortality benefit with the use of IV antihypertensive agents, their use is still the standard of care intended to reduce further organ damage. There are multiple IV antihypertensive infusions to choose from. The type of organ damage present, clinical characteristics of the patient, and pharmacological properties of the medication should guide therapy selection.
9. Medication nonadherence is a modifiable risk factor that commonly leads to hypertensive crises. Interventions aimed at improving adherence (eg, patient education regarding the importance of medication adherence, simplification of medication regimens, use of fixed-dose combination antihypertensives products, use of low-cost generic agents) and periodic, scheduled follow-up are essential.

BEYOND THE BOOK

To improve your ability to identify the clinical nuances encountered when treating patients with hypertensive crises and also aid in your understanding of the concept of autoregulation, please listen to the podcast and watch the video below.

1. Hypertensive Emergencies Demystified: A Brief Clinical Review on the management of hypertensive crisis—HelixTalk: https://www.rosalindfranklin.edu/academics/college-of-pharmacy/helixtalk/helixtalk-episode-134-hypertensive-emergencies-demystified-a-brief-clinical-review/
    - The discussion of hypertensive emergency uses an illustrative case in which a patient presents with acute ischemic stroke to highlight the complexities in care with which these patients present.
2. Autoregulation—Baroreceptors—Rishi Desai (Khan Academy): https://www.youtube.com/watch?v=R07V4NOwfsk&t=602s

INTRODUCTION

As implied by its nomenclature, an acute hypertensive crisis is both a temporal and numerical characterization of dangerously elevated blood pressure (BP) that requires prompt assessment and clinical intervention. However, this broad terminology does not distinguish between patients who require chronic versus emergent interventions to control BP and prevent or minimize complications. For example, some patients with acute hypertensive crisis require emergent escalation to intensive care and intravenous (IV) antihypertensive therapy while others can be managed less aggressively by resuming or adjusting chronic antihypertensive treatment and monitoring.

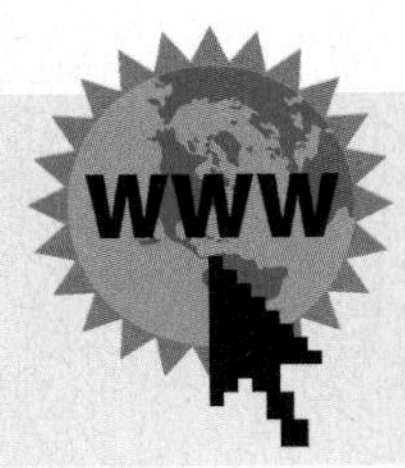

The complete chapter, learning objectives, and other resources can be found at **www.pharmacotherapyonline.com.**

32

Dyslipidemia

Dave L. Dixon, Daniel M. Riche, and Michael S. Kelly

KEY CONCEPTS

1. Lipid abnormalities increase the risk of atherosclerotic cardiovascular disease (ASCVD) which includes ischemic coronary heart disease, ischemic stroke, and peripheral arterial disease.
2. Low-density-lipoprotein cholesterol (LDL-C) is the primary target to reduce the risk of ASCVD events.
3. Genetic abnormalities and environmental factors are involved in the development of dyslipidemia.
4. Therapeutic lifestyle change is the first-line therapy for any lipoprotein disorder.
5. If therapeutic lifestyle changes are insufficient, lipid-lowering agents should be chosen based on which lipid is at an undesirable level and the degree to which it is expected to increase the risk of ASCVD.
6. Statins are the drug of choice for dyslipidemia because they significantly lower LDL-C and the risk of ASCVD events, and are generally well tolerated.
7. If statin monotherapy is insufficient, patients may be treated with evidence-based combination therapy but should be monitored closely for drug-drug interactions.
8. Reducing total cholesterol and LDL-C reduces CHD and total mortality.
9. Lipid-lowering therapies that reduce ASCVD event rates are cost-effective.
10. Several novel medications including antisense oligonucleotide inhibitors of apoB, microsomal triglyceride transport protein inhibitors, adenosine triphosphate-citrate lyase (ACL) inhibitors, and proprotein convertase subtilisin/kexin type 9 (PCSK9) modulating therapies can be used as add-on therapy or in lieu of statin therapy in select high-risk patients.

BEYOND THE BOOK

Watch these YouTube videos to learn about cholesterol basics as well as the physiology of lipoprotein cholesterol and metabolism:

- Cholesterol Good and Bad (https://tinyurl.com/yx6a5ufj) by the US National Library of Medicine
- Physiology of Lipoprotein Cholesterol (https://tinyurl.com/hcy239y) by Armando Hasudungan
- Physiology of Lipoprotein Metabolism (https://tinyurl.com/pwo856o) by National Heart, Lung, and Blood Institute

INTRODUCTION

Cholesterol, triglycerides, and phospholipids are the major lipids that combine with proteins to be transported as complexes of lipid and proteins known as lipoproteins. Lipids, such as cholesterol and triglycerides, are insoluble in plasma, which is why the lipoproteins are required for transportation (Fig. 32-1).[1,2]

There are three major classes of lipoproteins in the serum. These include low-density lipoproteins (LDL), high-density lipoproteins (HDL), and very-low-density lipoproteins (VLDL). VLDL is the primary carrier of triglycerides (TG) in the circulation. Intermediate-density lipoprotein (IDL) is between VLDL and LDL and is included in LDL-C measurement (Fig. 32-2).[3]

1 2 Lipid abnormalities increase the risk of coronary, cerebrovascular, and peripheral vascular arterial disease collectively known as atherosclerotic cardiovascular disease (ASCVD). The ASCVD-risk assessment evaluates a 10-year ASCVD incident. Developing a first ASCVD event is defined as nonfatal myocardial infarction or coronary heart disease (CHD) death, or fatal or nonfatal stroke, over a 10-year period. Premature coronary atherosclerosis is the most common and significant consequence of dyslipidemia. The 2013 guidelines from the American Heart Association (AHA) and American College of Cardiology (ACC) state that there is not sufficient evidence to recommend treating to specific lipid targets but suggests four statin benefit patient populations.[5] Low-density lipoprotein cholesterol (LDL-C) is the primary target of lipid-lowering therapy. Methods for risk assessment were also updated, which increases the number of patients who would qualify for therapy. Primary and secondary CHD prevention measures are provided as well.[4-7]

There are several subtypes of dyslipidemias, including hypertriglyceridemia, low HDL cholesterol (HDL-C), and diabetic dyslipidemia. Hypertriglyceridemia can lead to pancreatitis when very high TG levels (>500 mg/dL [5.65 mmol/L]) are seen. High serum triglycerides should primarily be treated by achieving desirable body weight, consumption of low saturated fat and cholesterol diet, regular exercise, smoking cessation, and restriction of alcohol.[3,4] In patients with borderline-high TG but with accompanying risk factors of established congenital heart disease, family history of premature CHD, concomitant LDL-C elevation or low HDL-C, and genetic forms of hypertriglyceridemia associated with CHD, lipid-lowering therapy should be considered.[8-10]

Low HDL-C is another dyslipidemia subtype that can occur due to insulin resistance, physical inactivity, diabetes, cigarette smoking, high carbohydrate intake, and some medications. In

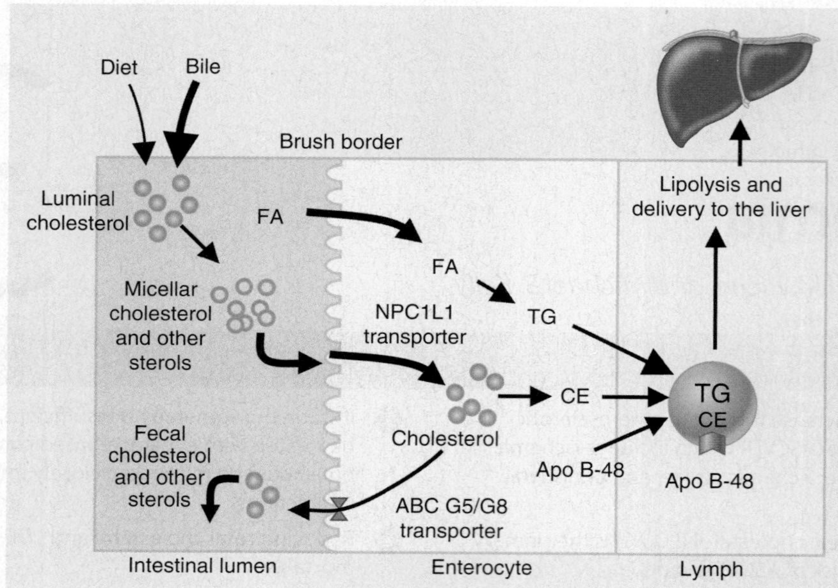

FIGURE 32-1 Intestinal cholesterol absorption and transportation. Cholesterol from food and bile enters the gut lumen and is emulsified by bile acids into micelles. Micelles bind to intestinal enterocytes and cholesterol, and other sterols are transported from the micelles to the enterocytes by sterol transporters. Triglycerides (TG) synthesized by absorbed fatty acids (FA) are incorporated into chylomicrons. Chylomicrons are released into lymphatic circulation and converted to chylomicron remnants (by losing triglyceride), and are then taken up by hepatic LDL-receptor–related protein. (Apo, apolipoprotein; ABC, ATP-binding cassette; CE, cholesterol ester; FA, fatty acid; NPC1L1, Niemann-Pick C1-Like1 protein; TG, triglyceride.) *(Reproduced, with permission, from Chisholm-Burns MA, Schwinghammer TL, Malone PM, Kolesar JM, Bookstaver PB, Lee KC, eds. Pharmacotherapy Principles & Practice. 5th ed. New York: McGraw Hill; 2019.)*

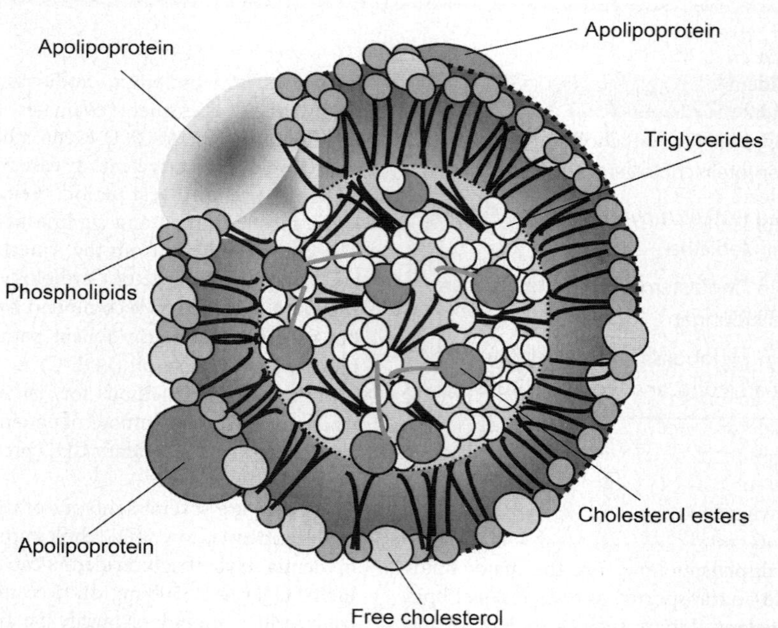

FIGURE 32-2 Lipoprotein structure, which contains variable amounts of core cholesterol esters and triglycerides and have varying numbers and types of surface apolipoproteins.

patients with low HDL-C, the primary target remains LDL-C, but an emphasis on weight loss, increased physical activity, and smoking cessation are recommended. No randomized controlled trials (RCT) have shown a reduction in ASCVD risk by raising HDL-C levels.[3,11]

Hypertriglyceridemia, low HDL-C, and minimally elevated LDL-C characterize diabetic dyslipidemia. Because the primary target is LDL-C in diabetic dyslipidemia, statins are considered the drugs of choice.[3,4,12,13]

EPIDEMIOLOGY

Total cholesterol and LDL-C increase throughout life in both men and women. According to AHA estimates, approximately 49% of American adults aged 20 years or older have total cholesterol levels exceeding 200 mg/dL (5.17 mmol/L).[14] The prevalence of elevated LDL cholesterol as a risk factor for death in adults has increased from 15th in 1990 to 8th in 2019.[15] Westernized societal diets high in cholesterol are a strong contributor to the increase in total and LDL-C cholesterol. In 2011, CHD caused one in every seven deaths in the United States. About one-third of treated patients are achieving their LDL-C goal; fewer than 20% of CHD patients are at their LDL-C goal. Estimates from the National Cholesterol Education Program (NCEP) state that only 26% of patients have an optimal LDL-C (<100 mg/dL [2.59 mmol/L]), and that large numbers of patients are either untreated or undertreated. Patients at the highest risk are less likely to be treated to desirable LDL-C values.[15-17] When patients who are at risk but who have not yet experienced initial cardiovascular (eg, myocardial infarction [MI]) or cerebrovascular (eg, ischemic stroke) events are treated, it is termed primary prevention. Treatment for those with manifest ASCVD is termed secondary prevention.[17] Studies, such as the Framingham Heart Study, show that risk for developing cardiovascular disease is related to the degree of LDL-C elevation in a continuous fashion.[3] Hypercholesterolemia, cigarette smoking, hypertension, diabetes, and low HDL-C levels are all additive risk factors for CHD. The risk of MI increases five to seven times with any preexisting CHD or previous MI compared to patients with no history of these. Patients with a history of CHD or MI should be screened, identified, and treated for dyslipidemias. Fifty percent of all MIs and 70% of all deaths due to CHD occur in patients with known CHD.

ETIOLOGY

3 Genetic abnormalities and environmental factors are involved in the development of dyslipidemia. The underlying causes of dyslipidemias can be categorized into two types: primary or secondary. Genetic factors that increase lipid levels can be inherited and cause primary or familial dyslipidemia. By contrast, lifestyles, diseases, medications, and diet can all lead to abnormal lipid levels and cause secondary or "acquired" dyslipidemia.

Primary or Familial Dyslipidemias

Primary or familial dyslipidemias account for a large number of cases of increased total cholesterol, LDL-C, TGs, or decreased HDL-C. There are certain familial or genetic defects that can contribute. Genetic disorders can cause an increase or decrease in different lipoproteins. Primary dyslipidemias result in an increased risk of premature ASCVD due to significant elevations in cholesterol levels. There are different types of familial dyslipidemias, including hypercholesterolemia, hypertriglyceridemia, combined hyperlipidemia, and disorders of HDL-C metabolism, and an excess of lipoproteins. Two other primary disorders include homozygous familial hypercholesterolemia (HoFH) and heterozygous familial hypercholesterolemia (HeFH). HeFH is more common with one case per 250 people versus HoFH with one case per one million people. Heterozygous gene dysfunction usually causes elevations in LDL-C between 250 and 450 mg/dL (6.47-11.64 mmol/L), and homozygous patients may present with LDL-C concentrations above 500 mg/dL (12.93 mmol/L). Tendon xanthomas are thick cholesterol deposits. Xanthelasmas and arcus cornea can also occur, and these are cholesterol deposits in the eyelids and around the corneal rim.[18-20] In familial hypertriglyceridemia, TGs are elevated in the range of 200 to 500 mg/dL (2.26-5.65 mmol/L), but at times can be greater than 1,000 mg/dL (11.3 mmol/L). Patients presenting with TG concentrations greater than or equal to 500 mg/dL (5.65 mmol/L) can have eruptive xanthomas and/or acute pancreatitis.

Secondary or Acquired Dyslipidemias

Secondary or acquired dyslipidemias can accompany genetic disorders or cause lipid imbalances. "The 4D classification" of secondary causes of dyslipidemia include diet, drugs, disorder, and diseases.[19] Regarding diet, an increase in cholesterol can be caused by excessive alcohol use, anorexia, weight gain, excessive carbohydrate intake, and high saturated fat intake. Certain medications can also contribute. For example, some medications that can increase both LDL-C and TGs include atypical antipsychotics, diuretics, beta-blockers, glucocorticoids, oral estrogen and progestin, tacrolimus, and cyclosporine.

Certain metabolism disorders can contribute to cholesterol imbalances. Nephrotic syndrome, renal failure, biliary obstruction, hypothyroidism, and pregnancy can all potentially contribute. Comorbid conditions or diseases such as hypothyroidism, pregnancy, obesity, polycystic ovarian syndrome (PCOS), uncontrolled diabetes, liver disease, and chronic kidney disease can also play a role.

Although we classify the lipid disorders into primary and secondary dyslipidemias based on etiologies, most dyslipidemias are a result of a combination of both.[4,19]

PATHOPHYSIOLOGY

Lipoproteins and Cholesterol Synthesis

There are four types of lipoproteins: chylomicrons, VLDL, LDL, and HDL. These lipoproteins vary in the content of lipid and protein. The ratio of protein and lipid in these lipoproteins contributes to the function of each. Chylomicrons contain the most lipid and little protein. HDL contains the most protein and a small amount of lipids. The small amount of lipid, and in turn cholesterol, in HDL lipoproteins gives HDL the role of picking up extra cholesterol from the tissue. LDL is not necessarily "bad" cholesterol, but in excess, this generates the problem. We need cholesterol for the transportation of fats that are absorbed in our diet and delivered to our tissues. Chylomicrons are not normally in plasma during periods of fasting. In the small intestine, fats are digested and emulsified into micelles. Cholesterol is also absorbed. Fatty acids, cholesterol, and proteins or apoproteins are packaged and form chylomicrons. The chylomicrons circulate around the body and deliver lipids and TGs to tissues in need. The remaining chylomicrons are transported to the liver and bind to LDL receptors. Glucose that has also been absorbed from our diet is delivered to the liver. In the liver, glucose is converted to pyruvate and then to acetyl-CoA. Acetyl-CoA is eventually converted to cholesterol through 3-hydroxy-3-methylglutaryl-coenzyme A (HMG-CoA) reductase. HMG-CoA reductase is a target for statins, thus stopping cholesterol synthesis. Glycolysis also synthesizes glycerol. Combining glycerol and one fatty acid forms monoacylglycerol, and two more fatty acids form triglycerides. Triglycerides and apoproteins are packed through the Golgi apparatus and form lipoproteins. Lipoproteins contain proteins, apoproteins, TGs, phospholipids, and cholesterol. The liver does not make all lipoproteins. In fact, only empty HDL and VLDL are made in the liver. VLDL has more TGs and lipids than HDL. VLDL transports these lipids and TGs to tissues in need of energy or storage. Adipose tissue stores fat, and many tissues use fatty acids for energy. VLDL is transported across lipase, which changes the VLDL to IDL or intermediate-density lipoproteins. IDL can then be converted to LDL. LDL mainly transports cholesterol to body tissues, which is why LDL contains the most cholesterol. Tissues need cholesterol to make hormones and maintain cell membrane integrity. Once LDL gives these tissues cholesterol, it returns to the liver. LDL binds to LDL receptors and is then either recycled to make more lipoproteins or excreted into the bile. Any excess cholesterol is excreted into the bile, so the body maintains cholesterol balance. HDL or empty HDL plays a role in picking up any or excess cholesterol and returning it to the liver. The full HDL containing the picked up cholesterol binds to scavenger receptors. They are then either recycled or excreted depending on how much cholesterol is needed.[1]

Lipid Metabolism and Transport

Cholesterol is water-insoluble so it cannot circulate through blood without help. Lipoproteins are large carrier proteins to help with transport because they are water-soluble. This allows major lipids to be circulated through the blood. Lipoproteins vary in characteristics depending on the amount of cholesterol, TG, and apolipoproteins. All lipoproteins also have something called apolipoproteins on its surface. Apolipoproteins are necessary for the assembly and secretion of lipoproteins. They are also major structural components of lipoproteins that have ligands for binding to receptors or cell surfaces. These are the cofactors for the activation of enzymes. Apolipoproteins have various functions that transport lipids from sites of absorption to sites where they are used. Apolipoprotein B containing lipoproteins, known as non-HDL, make up the lipid-delivery pathway. Apolipoprotein A-1 or HDL participates in reverse cholesterol transport. ApoB containing lipoproteins arise from two sources, one being intestinal ApoB-48 and the other hepatic ApoB-100 lineage. ApoB containing lipoproteins are secreted from the intestine or liver into the plasma. Apolipoproteins E, C-II, and C-III are secreted with them. These may also be acquired from HDL. Apolipoprotein remodeling begins, and ApoC-II activates lipoprotein lipase (LPL), which hydrolyzes the lipoprotein core TGs into free fatty acids. The fatty acids exit and the lipoproteins become smaller and smaller. Remodeling of the ApoB-100 hepatic lipoprotein, another step by hepatic lipase (HL) is needed to convert IDL to LDL. Most ApoB remnants are recycled to the liver by the LDL-receptor–related protein (LRP). They can have other metabolic requirements, too. Excess ApoB particles can invade arterial walls and become oxidized. Once oxidized, they are taken up by macrophage scavenger receptors creating foam cells that lead to atheroma.

ApoA-1 or HDL pathways are believed to protect our bodies from atherogenesis. HDL has two major protective roles in preventing atherogenesis. Reverse cholesterol transport is the transfer of excess cholesterol from peripheral tissues by HDL. ApoA-1 is secreted from the liver or intestine and is transported to the cells to remove excess cholesterol. HDL has several cholesterol removing mechanisms. Upregulation of the ATP-binding cassette transporter or ABCA-1 transporter is triggered by excess cholesterol in the macrophages. ABCA-1 harvests free cholesterol and delivers it to the cell membrane. The free cholesterol is esterified by lecithin-cholesterol acyltransferase (LCAT). The cholesterol ester moves to the core of the lipoprotein forming the mature HDL3. Further removal of cholesterol by HDL3 occurs through scavenger receptor class B type 1, or SR-B1 receptors and is acted on by LCAT, which expands to HDL2. ABCA-1 and SR-B1 are key for cholesterol efflux. HDL2 cholesterol is transferred to ApoB containing lipoproteins. HDL now has one of three options: HDL triglycerides may be hydrolyzed by HL back into HDL3; HDL2 can return to the liver and through SR-B1 converted back to HDL3; or HDL2 may be catabolized by the liver. All of these systems work together to maintain cholesterol homeostasis (Figs. 32-3 and 32-4).[1]

Familial Hypercholesterolemia

Familial hypercholesterolemia is characterized by (a) a selective elevation in the plasma level of LDL; (b) deposition of LDL-derived cholesterol in tendons (xanthomas) and arteries (atheromas); and (c) inheritance as an autosomal dominant trait with homozygotes more severely affected than heterozygotes. The primary defect in familial hypercholesterolemia is the inability to bind LDL to the LDL receptor (LDL-R) or, rarely, a defect of internalizing the LDL-R complex into the cell after normal binding. This leads to a lack of LDL degradation by cells and unregulated biosynthesis of cholesterol, with total cholesterol and LDL-C being inversely proportional to the deficit in LDL receptors. Homozygotes (prevalence 1 in 1,000,000) have severe hypercholesterolemia (650-1,000 mg/dL [16.8-25.9 mmol/L]), with the early appearance of cutaneous xanthomas and fatal CHD generally before the age of 20 and have essentially no functional LDL receptors. Heterozygotes have only about one-half of the normal number of LDL receptors, total cholesterol levels in the range of 300 to 600 mg/dL (7.76-15.52 mmol/L), and cardiovascular events beginning in the third and fourth decades of life.

Secondary causes of dyslipidemia exist and that several drugs and conditions may contribute to abnormal lipid levels (Table 32-1). These secondary forms of dyslipidemia should be managed by addressing the underlying abnormality, including the modification of drug therapy when appropriate.

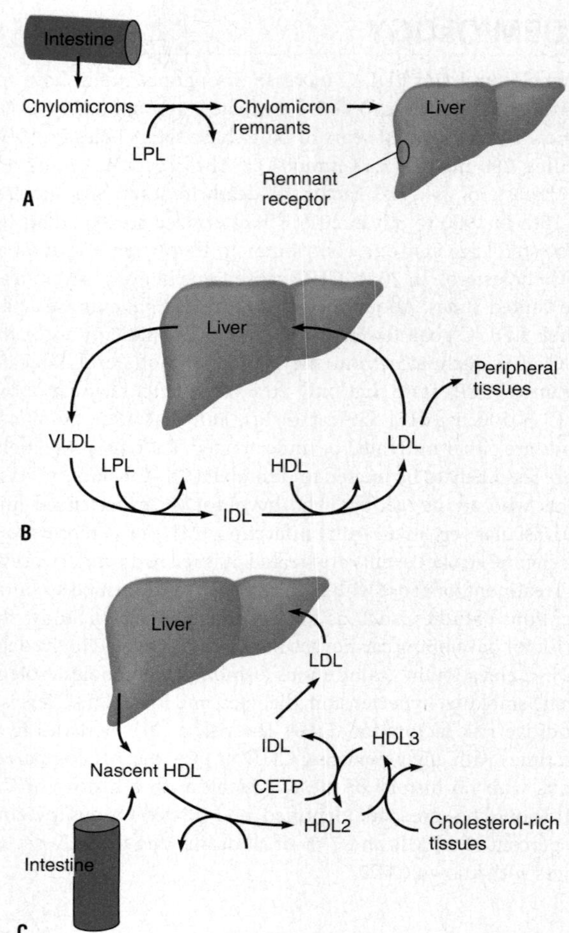

FIGURE 32-3 Biosynthetic pathway for cholesterol. The rate-limiting enzyme in this pathway is 3-hydroxy- 3-methylglutaryl-coenzyme A reductase (HMG-CoA reductase). (CETP, cholesterol ester transfer protein; HDL, high-density lipoprotein; IDL, intermediate-density lipoprotein; LDL, low-density lipoprotein; LPL, lipoprotein lipase; VLDL, very-low-density lipoprotein.) (*A*) Exogenous pathway; (*B*) Endogenous pathway; (*C*) Reverse cholesterol transport. *(Adapted from Breslow JL. Genetic basis of lipoprotein disorders. J Clin Invest. 1989;84:373.)*

Pathogenesis of Atherosclerotic Cardiovascular Disease

The "response-to-injury" hypothesis states that risk factors such as oxidized LDL, mechanical injury to the endothelium, excessive

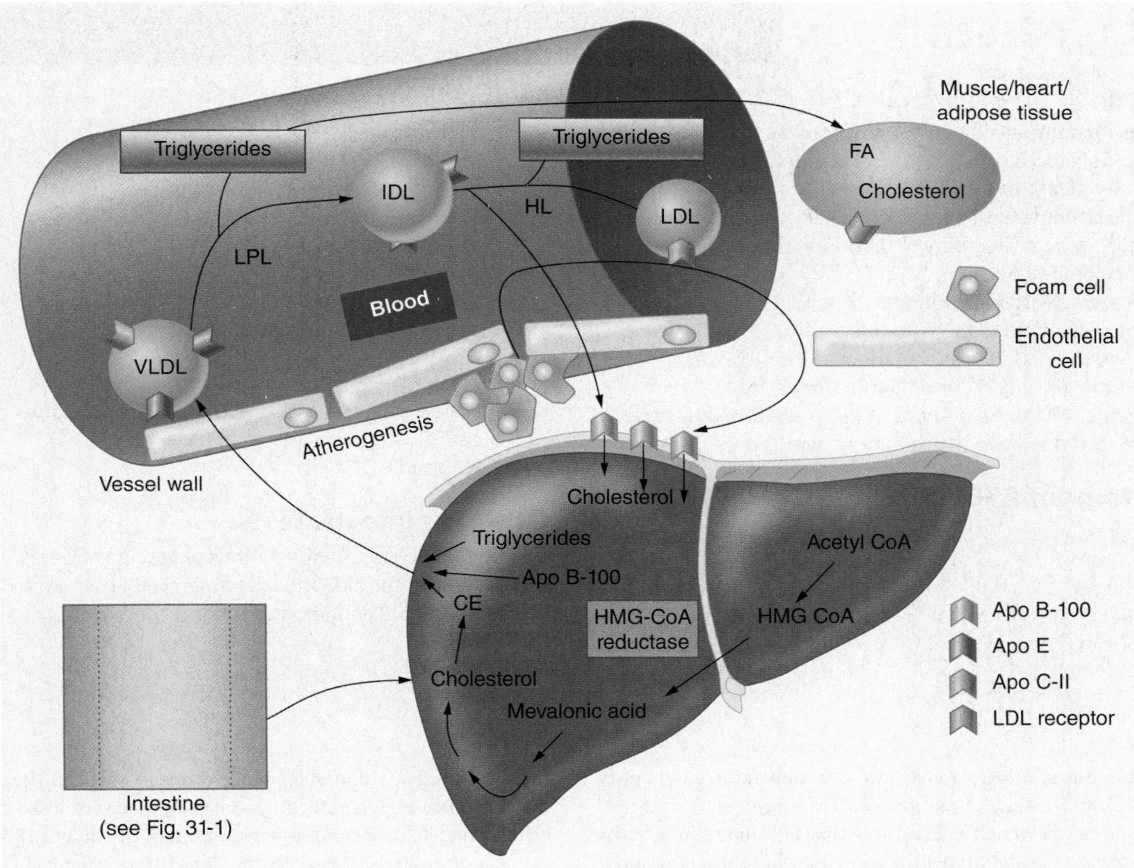

FIGURE 32-4 Endogenous lipoprotein metabolism. In the liver, the cholesterol and triglycerides are packed into VLDL particles and sent into the blood. They are then converted into IDL, which can be cleared by hepatic IDL receptors or metabolized into LDL. LDL can be cleared by LDL receptors or it can enter the arterial walls and contribute to the development of atherosclerotic plaques and cardiovascular disease.

TABLE 32-1 Secondary Causes of Lipoprotein Abnormalities

Hypercholesterolemia	• Hypothyroidism • Obstructive liver disease • Nephrotic syndrome • Anorexia nervosa • Acute intermittent porphyria • Drugs: progestins, thiazide diuretics, glucocorticoids, beta-blockers, isotretinoin, protease inhibitors, cyclosporine, mirtazapine, sirolimus
Hypertriglyceridemia	• Obesity • Diabetes mellitus • Lipodystrophy • Glycogen storage disease • Ileal bypass surgery • Sepsis • Pregnancy • Acute hepatitis • Systemic lupus erythematosus • Monoclonal gammopathy: multiple myeloma, lymphoma • Drugs: alcohol, estrogens, isotretinoin, beta-blockers, glucocorticoids, bile-acid resins, thiazides, asparaginase, interferons, azole antifungals, mirtazapine, anabolic steroids, sirolimus, bexarotene
Hypocholesterolemia	• Malnutrition • Malabsorption • Myeloproliferative diseases • Chronic infectious diseases: tuberculosis • Monoclonal gammopathy
Low HDL	• Malnutrition • Obesity • Drugs: non-ISA beta-blockers, anabolic steroids, probucol, isotretinoin, progestins

CLINICAL PRESENTATION Dyslipidemias

General

- Most patients are asymptomatic for years before they develop ASCVD; the initial presentation may be sudden death due to a CHD event.
- Many patients with dyslipidemia also present with one or more of the following abnormalities:
  - Abdominal obesity
  - Atherogenic dyslipidemia
  - Increased blood pressure
  - Insulin resistance and/or glucose intolerance
  - Prothrombotic or proinflammatory state
- Patients with three or more of these abnormalities are considered to have the metabolic syndrome

Symptoms of ASCVD

- Chest pain
- Palpitations
- Sweating
- Anxiety
- Shortness of breath
- Loss of consciousness
- Difficulty with speech or movement
- Abdominal pain

Signs

- Abdominal pain
- Pancreatitis
- Eruptive xanthomas
- Peripheral polyneuropathy

Laboratory Tests

- Elevated total cholesterol, LDL-C, TGs, apolipoprotein B, hsCRP
- Decreased HDL-C

Other Diagnostic Tests

- Screenings for manifestations of vascular disease, including carotid ultrasound, coronary calcium score, ankle-brachial index, and heart catheterization

homocysteine, immunologic attacks, or infection-induced changes in endothelial and intimal function lead to endothelial dysfunction and a series of cellular interactions that culminate in atherosclerosis. C-reactive protein (CRP) is an acute-phase reactant and a marker for inflammation. Measuring one's CRP levels by means of a high-sensitivity CRP may be useful in identifying patients at risk for developing CAD. Lipid abnormalities increase the risk for CHD and cerebrovascular morbidity and mortality. The eventual outcomes of this atherogenic cascade are clinical events such as angina, MI, arrhythmias, stroke, peripheral arterial disease, abdominal aortic aneurysm, and sudden death. Atherosclerotic lesions are thought to arise from transport and retention of plasma LDL-C through the endothelial cell layer into the extracellular matrix of the subendothelial space. Once in the artery wall, LDL-C is chemically modified through oxidation and nonenzymatic glycation. Mildly oxidized LDL-C then recruits monocytes which transforms into macrophages in the artery wall. Macrophages accelerate LDL-C oxidation and apolipoprotein B accumulation and alter the receptor-mediated uptake of LDL-C into the artery wall from the usual LDL-R to a "scavenger receptor" not regulated by the cell content of cholesterol. Oxidized LDL-C increases plasminogen inhibitor levels (promotion of coagulation), induces the expression of endothelin (vasoconstrictive substance), inhibits the expression of nitric oxide (a vasodilator and platelet inhibitor), and is toxic to macrophages if highly oxidized. As oxidation of biologically active lipids proceeds, other lipids breakdown products of fatty acids and oxysterol are formed, which continue the reaction within the tissue. These events lead to a massive accumulation of cholesterol. The cholesterol-laden macrophages become foam cells; foam cells are the earliest recognized cells of the arterial fatty streak. Oxidized LDL-C provokes an inflammatory response, which is mediated by a number of chemoattractants and cytokines. The process of aging may lead to lipoproteins that are more susceptible to oxidation and have longer resident time in the vascular compartment. Repeated injury and repair within an atherosclerotic plaque eventually leads to fibrous caps protecting the underlying core of lipids, collagen, calcium, and inflammatory cells such as T-lymphocytes. Maintenance of the fibrous plaque is critical to prevent plaque rupture and subsequent coronary thrombosis.[21] An imbalance between plaque synthesis and degradation may lead to a weakened or vulnerable plaque prone to rupture. The fibrous cap may become weakened through the decreased synthesis of the extracellular matrix or increased degradation of the matrix (Fig. 32-5).

Lipoprotein(a) (Lp[a]), a low-density lipoprotein (LDL) variant, containing both apolipoprotein(a) (apo[a]) and apolipoprotein(b) (apo[b]) covalently bound via a disulfide bridge. Lp(a) is an independent risk factor for ASCVD.[22,23] Thought to be elevated in about 20% of the population, the significance of Lp(a) has been utilized to improve ASCVD risk assessment strategies.[22,23] Most recent evidence supports a relationship between elevated Lp(a) levels and both ASCVD and valvular aortic stenosis (VAS) risks, yet the precise pathophysiological mechanism(s) is not completely understood.[22,23]

Theoretically, the pathophysiological mechanisms of Lp(a)-induced ASCVD events include the interaction between oxidized phospholipids and the apo(a) component of Lp(a), resulting in endothelial disruption, lipid deposition, inflammation, and calcification of the vasculature.[22] Apo(a) has structural similarity with plasminogen which may account for its atherogenic properties because it competitively inhibits fibrinolysis and release of plasminogen activator inhibitor-1.[23] This process could further lead to thrombus formation within arterial plaques or turbulent blood flow within stenosis, therefore, causing blockage(s) or embolism in VAS.[22]

While recommendations are still being considered and developed regarding how Lp(a) alters therapy in patients with dyslipidemia, the National Lipid Association (NLA) released a scientific statement in May 2019 detailing recommendations for testing and identifying those at high risk of ASCVD due to Lp(a) elevations.[23] These recommendations describe screening considerations, potential Lp(a) cut-points when to initiate treatment as well as primary and secondary prevention strategies.[23]

TREATMENT

Desired Outcomes

Desired levels of TC, LDL-C, HDL-C, and TG for adults are provided in Table 32-2. While abnormalities in these surrogate markers may impart an increased risk for ASCVD events, the goal of

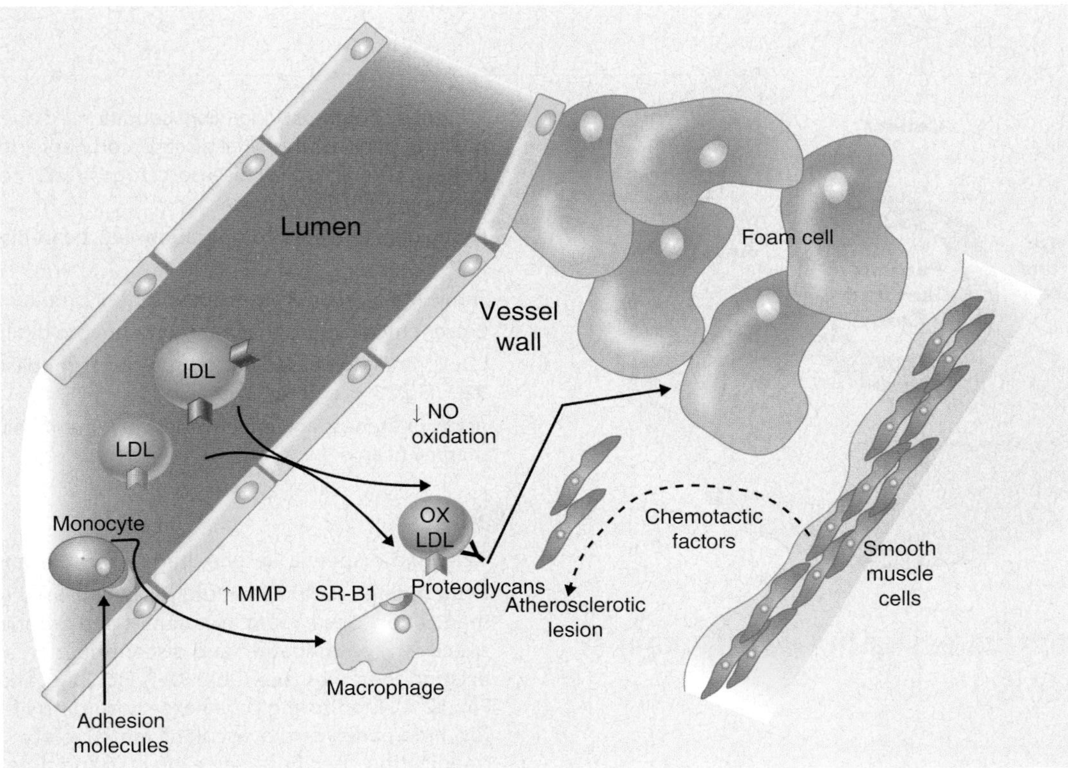

FIGURE 32-5 Atherogenesis is initiated by the migration of LDL and remnant lipoprotein particles into the vessel walls. These particles undergo oxidation and are taken up by macrophages in an unregulated fashion, which induces endothelial cell dysfunction. This, in turn, reduces the ability of the endothelium to dilate the artery and cause a prothrombotic state. Unregulated uptake of cholesterol by macrophages leads to foam cell formation, and thus the development of atherosclerotic plaques. Macrophages eventually produce and secrete matric metalloproteinases, which degrade the collagen matrix of the plaques and cause them to be unstable. This can potentially lead to a myocardial infarction. This is a progressive process. (IDL, intermediate-density lipoprotein; LDL, low-density lipoprotein; MMP, matrix metalloproteinase; NO, nitric oxide; SR-B1, scavenger receptor class B type 1.) *(Reproduced, with permission, from Chisholm-Burns MA, Schwinghammer TL, Malone PM, Kolesar JM, Bookstaver PB, Lee KC, eds. Pharmacotherapy Principles & Practice. 5th ed. New York: McGraw Hill; 2019.)*

TABLE 32-2 Classification of Total-, LDL-, HDL-Cholesterol, and Triglycerides in Adults

Total Cholesterol	
<200 mg/dL (5.17 mmol/L)	Desirable
200-239 mg/dL (5.17-6.20 mmol/L)	Borderline high
≥240 mg/dL (6.21 mmol/L)	High
Low-Density Lipoprotein Cholesterol	
<100 mg/dL (2.59 mmol/L)	Optimal
100-129 mg/dL (2.59-3.35 mmol/L)	Near or above optimal
130-159 mg/dL (3.36-4.13 mmol/L)	Borderline high
160-189 mg/dL (4.14-4.90 mmol/L)	High
≥190 mg/dL (4.91 mmol/L)	Very high
High-Density Lipoprotein Cholesterol	
<40 mg/dL (1.03 mmol/L)	Low (Men)
<50 mg/dL (1.29 mmol/L)	Low (Women)
Triglycerides	
<150 mg/dL (1.70 mmol/L)	Normal
150-199 mg/dL (1.70-2.25 mmol/L)	Borderline high
200-499 mg/dL (2.26-5.64 mmol/L)	High
≥500 mg/dL (5.65 mmol/L)	Very high

treatment is to not merely correct lab abnormalities but prevent the development and progression of ASCVD. Thus, the desired outcome is to prevent ASCVD-related morbidity and mortality, including revascularization procedures, MI, and ischemic stroke. Initiation of lipid-lowering therapies primarily involves the use of those agents shown in RCT to reduce ASCVD risk.[17,24]

General Approach

6 A comprehensive approach to treating dyslipidemia and all modifiable ASCVD risk factors is required to significantly reduce the risk of first and recurrent CV events. Therapeutic lifestyle change is the first-line therapy for any lipoprotein disorder. A healthy lifestyle should be implemented in all patients with the general components including a reduction in the percent of calories from saturated and *trans* fats, increased intake of soluble fiber, weight reduction if overweight or obese, increased physical activity, and avoiding or quitting tobacco use.[24] Additionally, patients with a diagnosis of hypertension should achieve optimal blood pressure control based on the 2017 ACC/AHA Guidelines for control of hypertension (see Chapter 30, "Hypertension").[25] Persons with diabetes mellitus, especially those with established ASCVD, should receive glucose-lowering therapies that reduce ASCVD risk (see Chapter 94, "Diabetes Mellitus").[26]

5 If therapeutic lifestyle changes are insufficient, lipid-lowering agents should be chosen based on which lipid is at an undesirable level and the degree to which it is expected to increase the risk of ASCVD. The decision to initiate lipid-lowering therapy in the management of dyslipidemia should be based on an individual's ASCVD risk and not merely plasma levels of atherogenic lipoproteins

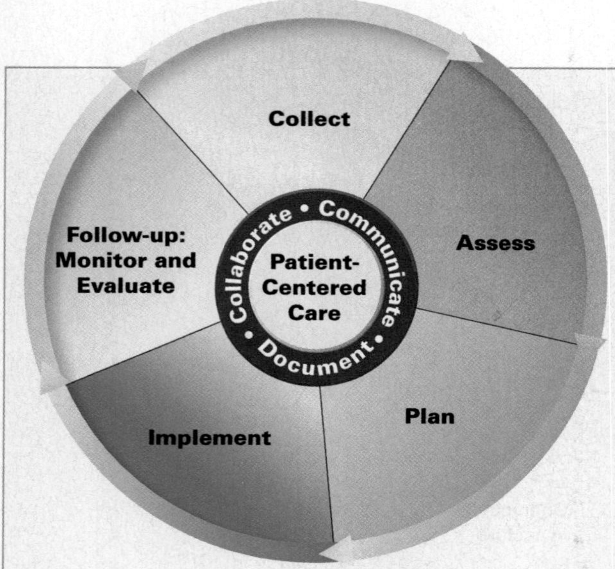

Patient Care Process for the Management of Dyslipidemias

Collect

- Patient characteristics (eg, age, race, gender, pregnant)
- Patients history: Past medical (eg, HTN), family (eg, early-onset coronary heart disease), social
- Current medications (including over-the-counter [OTC]) and prior lipid-lowering medication use
- Socioeconomic factors that may affect access to treatment or other aspects of care
- Lifestyle assessment: smoking status, exercise, diet, and alcohol intake
- Symptoms indicative of ischemic injury (eg, chest pain)
- Objective data
  - Height, weight, BMI, and blood pressure
  - Lipoprotein concentrations (eg, total cholesterol/LDL-C/HDL-C/triglycerides)
  - Laboratory findings (eg, AST/ALT, urinalysis, TSH, glucose, serum creatinine, and BUN at baseline)

Assess

- Potential secondary causes (eg, diabetes mellitus, alcohol abuse, kidney dysfunction, liver disease, drug-induced, thyroid disorder)
- Special needs of specific patient populations such as children/adolescents, pregnant or menopausal women, older adults, ethnic/racial groups, or high-risk conditions/residual risks (eg, patients with rheumatoid arthritis or residual risk despite statin and lifestyle therapy)
- Presence of high-risk comorbid conditions: diabetes mellitus, peripheral arterial disease, coronary artery disease, chronic kidney disease, carotid artery stenosis, and abdominal aortic aneurysm
- Dyslipidemia-related complications (eg, heart disease, stroke)
- Ten-year ASCVD-risk assessment (only if primary prevention)
- Current medications that may contribute to dyslipidemia
- LDL-C reduction based on statin benefit group (see Table 32-5, Fig. 32-6, and Fig. 32-7)
- Appropriateness and effectiveness of current lipid-lowering therapy (if any)

Plan

- Tailored therapeutic lifestyle changes (eg, diet and nutrition)
- Drug therapy regimen including specific lipid-lowering medication, dose, route, frequency, and duration; specify the continuation and discontinuation of existing therapies (see Table 32-5, Fig. 32-6, and Fig. 32-7). Monitoring parameters including efficacy (eg, lipid panel, cardiovascular events), safety (medication-specific adverse effects), and time frame (3-month initial follow-up intervals, followed by 6 to 12 month intervals once at goal)
- Patient education (eg, purpose of treatment, dietary and lifestyle modification, drug therapy). Self-monitoring of weight, exercise, diet, drug adherence/adverse effects
- Referrals to other providers when appropriate for coordination of care (eg, physician, dietician)

Implement*

- Provide patient education regarding all elements of the treatment plan, including self-management training
- Use motivational interviewing and coaching strategies to maximize adherence
- Schedule follow-up; consider the time frame to achieve goals of therapy

Follow-up: Monitor and Evaluate

- The occurrence of cardiovascular (CV) events
- Determine patient adherence to treatment plan using multiple sources of information
- Determine response to lipid-lowering therapy and weight-loss goals
- Presence of medication-induced adverse effects (eg, elevated transaminases or myalgia on statins)

**Collaborate with patient, caregivers, and other healthcare professionals.*

(such as LDL-C) alone.[27] Patients with established ASCVD are at the highest risk and most likely to benefit from select lipid-lowering therapies (such as statins). Risk assessment in patients without established ASCVD is more of an art that requires careful consideration of traditional (eg, age, hypertension) and nontraditional (eg, autoimmune diseases, socioeconomic status) risk factors, the risks of lipid-lowering therapy, and patient preference. For patients between 40 and 79 years of age and no history of ASCVD, the ASCVD Risk Estimator Plus (available at: www.tools.acc.org/ascvd-risk-estimator-plus) should be used to facilitate a clinician-patient discussion regarding the benefit and risks of lipid-lowering therapy, especially in patients whose 10-year risk is 7.5% or greater (see Figure 32-6). The Risk Estimator is comprised of the patient's age, gender, race, TC, HDL-C, blood pressure, diabetes status, smoking status, and use of antihypertensives, statins, and aspirin. Importantly, the Risk Estimator is based on data from large population studies of mostly African American and non-Hispanic white men and women. The Risk Estimator can be used for other ethnic groups if they are designated as non-Hispanic white; however, the Risk Estimator will underestimate the risk of American Indians and Asian Americans of South Asian ancestry, while overestimating the risk of Asian Americans of East Asian ancestry and some Hispanics (eg, Mexican Americans).[27] An estimated lifetime risk for ASCVD can also be performed for patients between age 20 and 39, but results should only be used to justify the need for lifestyle changes and not the initiation of lipid-lowering therapy. Additional tools for ASCVD-risk assessment include high-sensitivity C-reactive protein (hsCRP), apolipoprotein B, and Lp(a) levels that may be obtained to inform decision making in low-intermediate risk patients or those with recurrent ASCVD events despite appropriate lipid-lowering therapy.[27]

6 7 The HMG-CoA reductase inhibitors or "statins" are the drugs of choice for most patients with dyslipidemia.[17] A large body of evidence from randomized, double-blind, placebo-controlled trials has demonstrated the effectiveness of statins on reducing first and recurrent cardiovascular events, cardiovascular mortality, and all-cause mortality.[28] The 2018 ACC/AHA Blood Cholesterol Guideline identified four statin benefit groups where the data from RCT demonstrate clear evidence that the benefit of statin therapy outweighs the potential risks (Figs. 32-6 and 32-7).[17] Nonstatin lipid-lowering therapies (ie, ezetimibe, bempedoic acid, and PCSK9 inhibitors) play a supportive role in the management of dyslipidemia and are primarily used in combination with statins when adequate LDL-C lowering cannot be achieved with statins alone, or in patients unable to tolerate the recommended dose of a statin (Table 32-5).[17]

8 Numerous clinical outcome trials have been performed to determine whether lipid-lowering therapies reduce ASCVD risk in primary and secondary prevention populations. It is beyond the scope of this chapter, however, to discuss each of these trials in detail. Table 32-3 summarizes select trials supporting the use of statins and select nonstatins (ezetimibe and PCSK9 inhibitors) to reduce ASCVD risk. Most of the primary and secondary prevention studies were double-blinded, randomized, and placebo-controlled, lasting 2 to 7 years, and had sufficient patient numbers to be meaningful. The body of evidence supporting the role of statin therapy to reduce ASCVD is substantial and meta-analysis confirms the first-line role this class of drugs should play in dyslipidemia management.[29] As mentioned previously in this chapter, not all lipid-lowering therapies have translated to reducing ASCVD risk, despite having favorable effects on the lipid profile.

Nonpharmacologic Therapy

Lifestyle modification is the cornerstone of ASCVD-risk reduction and is recommended in all patients, including those receiving lipid-lowering therapy. Weight and body mass index (BMI) should be determined at each visit and lifestyle patterns to induce a weight loss of 5% to 10% should be discussed in persons who are overweight or obese (Table 32-4). Moderate-to-vigorous intensity physical activity

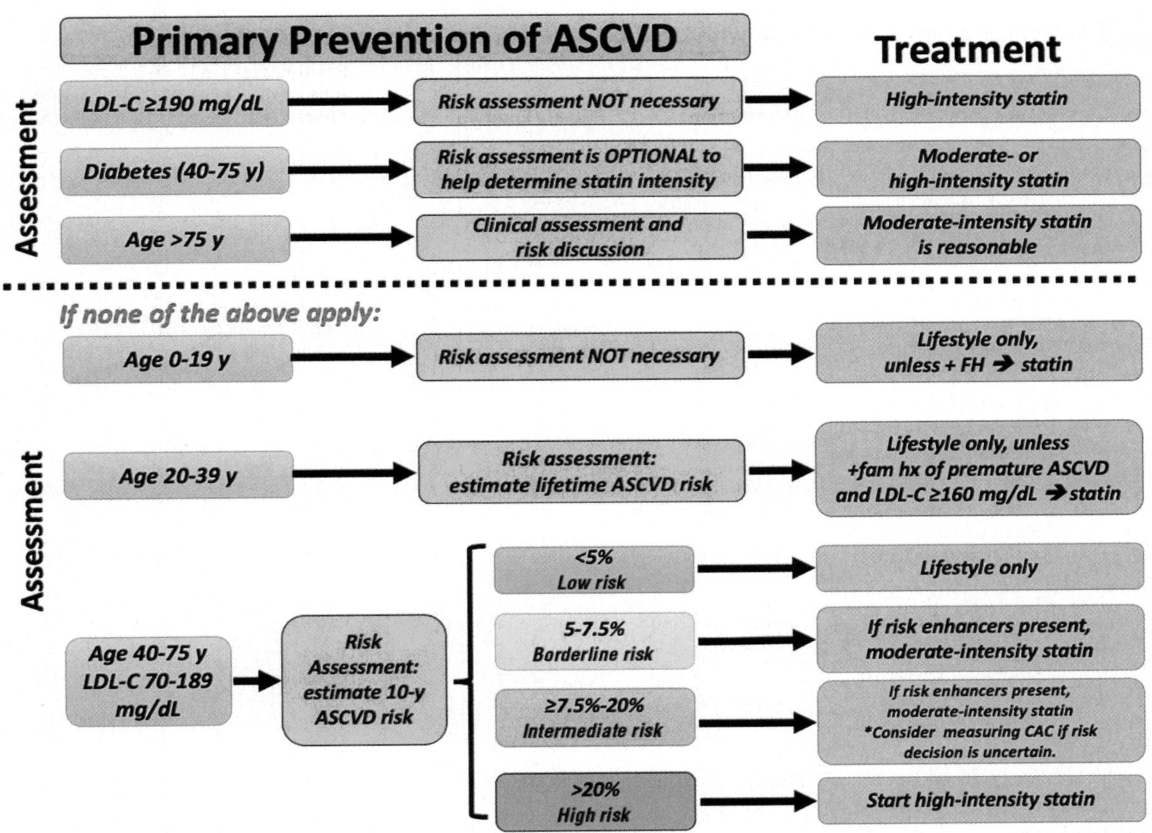

FIGURE 32-6 The assessment and treatment decision regarding the use of statin therapy for primary prevention is complex and must consider multiple factors. Patient groups with an untreated LDL-C ≥190 mg/dL (4.91 mmol/L) or type 1 or 2 diabetes (age 40-75 years) are eligible for statin therapy without estimating ASCVD risk using the Pooled Cohorts Equation. Given the limited data in adults over age 75, a patient-clinician discussion regarding the benefits and risks of statin therapy for primary prevention is warranted. For all other individuals, age is a primary consideration to determine the appropriate method of risk assessment and treatment recommendations. For conversion of LDL-C levels from units of mg/dL to SI units of mmol/L multiply by 0.02586.

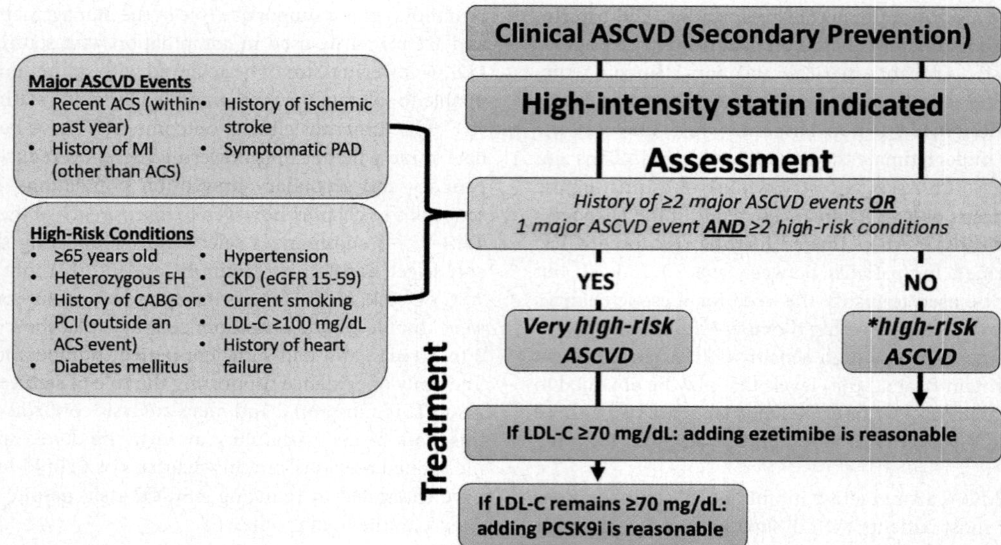

FIGURE 32-7 Patients with established clinical ASCVD are considered secondary prevention and high-intensity statin therapy is automatically indicated. Moderate-intensity statin should only be considered in adults >75 years of age and those unable to tolerate high-intensity statin therapy. After high-intensity statin therapy is initiated, ezetimibe may be added if the LDL-C remains ≥70 mg/dL (1.81 mmol/L). In select, very high-risk patients, adding a PCSK9i is reasonable if the LDL-C remains ≥70 mg/dL (1.81 mmol/L) after adding ezetimibe. For conversion of LDL-C levels from units of mg/dL to SI units of mmol/L multiply by 0.02586.

TABLE 32-3 Select Landmark Clinical Trials with Lipid-Lowering Drugs Targeting LDL Cholesterol

Trial	Patient Population (*n*)	Intervention	Primary Endpoint	Event Rates, Intervention vs Control (%)	RRR (%)	ARR (%)	NNT
Statin Landmark Trials—*Primary prevention*							
AFCAPS/TexCAPS	LDL-C 130-190 mg/dL (3.36-4.91 mmol/L) and HDL-C <47 mg/dL (1.22 mmol/L) (*n* = 6,605)	Lovastatin 20-40 mg vs placebo	Acute major coronary events	3.5 vs 5.5	36.4	2.0	50
CARDS	Age 40-75 years with T2DM and LDL-C <160 mg/dL (4.14 mmol/L) plus additional risk factor (*n* = 2,383)	Atorvastatin 10 mg vs placebo	Coronary heart disease events, coronary revascularization, or stroke	5.8 vs 9.0	37	3.2	32
JUPITER	LDL-C <130 mg/dL (3.36 mmol/L) and hsCRP ≥2.0 mg/L (*n* = 17,802)	Rosuvastatin 20 mg vs placebo	5-point MACE	1.6 vs 2.8	44	1.2	82
HOPE-3	Men and women (age 55 years and older) with at least one cardiovascular risk factor (*n* = 12,705)	Rosuvastatin 10 mg vs placebo	3-point MACE	3.7 vs 4.8	24	1.1	91
Statin Landmark Trials—*Secondary prevention*							
HPS	Previous ASCVD or high risk (*n* = 20,536)	Simvastatin 40 mg vs placebo	All-cause mortality	12.9 vs 14.7	13	1.8	56
PROSPER	Elderly (age 70-82 years) with previous vascular disease or elevated risk (*n* = 5,804)	Pravastatin 40 mg vs placebo	3-point MACE	14.1 vs 16.2	15	2.1	48
TNT	Clinical coronary heart disease (*n* = 10,001)	Atorvastatin 80 mg vs 10 mg	4-point MACE	8.7 vs 10.9	22	2.2	45
Nonstatin Landmark Trials							
IMPROVE-IT	Recent ACS (*n* = 18,144)	Ezetimibe + simvastatin vs simvastatin	5-point MACE	32.7 vs 34.7	6	2	50
FOURIER	Previous ASCVD (*n* = 27,564)	Evolocumab + statin vs statin	5-point MACE	9.8 vs 11.3	15	1.5	67

(*continued*)

TABLE 32-3 Select Landmark Clinical Trials with Lipid-Lowering Drugs Targeting LDL Cholesterol (*Continued*)

Trial	Patient Population (*n*)	Intervention	Primary Endpoint	Event Rates, Intervention vs Control (%)	RRR (%)	ARR (%)	NNT
ODYSSEY-OUTCOMES	Recent ACS ($n = 18{,}924$)	Alirocumab + statin vs statin	4-point MACE	9.5 vs 11.1	15	1.6	63

ACS, acute coronary syndrome; ARR, absolute risk reduction; AFCAPS/TexCAPS, Air Force/Texas Coronary Atherosclerosis Prevention Study[30]; ASCVD, atherosclerotic cardiovascular disease; CARDS, Collaborative Atorvastatin Diabetes Study[12]; FOURIER, Further Cardiovascular Outcomes Research with PCSK9 Inhibition in Patients with Elevated Risk[31]; HOPE-3, Heart Outcomes Prevention Evaluation 3[32]; HPS, Heart Protection Study[34]; hsCRP, high-sensitivity C-reactive protein; IMPROVE-IT, Improved Reduction of Outcomes: Vytorin Efficacy International Trail[35]; JUPITER, Justification for the Use of Statins in Prevention[36]; LDL-C, Low-Density Lipoprotein Cholesterol; MACE, Major Adverse Cardiovascular Events; MI, myocardial infarction; NNT, Number Needed to Treat; ODYSSEY-OUTCOMES, Evaluation of Cardiovascular Outcomes After an Acute Coronary Syndrome During Treatment with Alirocumab[73]; PROSPER, Pravastatin in elderly individuals at risk of vascular disease[37]; RRR, relative risk reduction; T2DM = Type 2 Diabetes Mellitus; TNT, Treat to New Targets Trial[38]; 3-point MACE = cardiovascular death, nonfatal myocardial infarctions, nonfatal stroke. 4-point MACE = death from coronary heart disease, nonfatal MI, fatal or nonfatal stroke, hospitalization for unstable angina. 5-point MACE = cardiovascular death, nonfatal myocardial infarctions, nonfatal stroke, arterial revascularization, hospitalization for unstable angina.

TABLE 32-4 Nonpharmacologic Therapy to Improve Lipid Levels and ASCVD Risk

Recommendations to Modify Select Lipid Parameters	
Lower LDL cholesterol	• Increase soluble fiber intake • Phytosterol (2 g/day) supplementation
Increase HDL cholesterol	• Increase physical activity • Smoking cessation
Lower triglycerides	• Lose weight (5%-10% body weight loss) • Increase physical activity • Abstain from alcohol • Reduce intake of refined carbohydrates and sugars
Recommendations to Reduce ASCVD Risk	
Nutrition and diet	• Avoid eating trans fats • Increase intake of vegetables, fruits, legumes, nuts, whole grains, and fish • Replace foods containing saturated fats with unsaturated (monounsaturated and polyunsaturated) fats • Minimize intake of processed meat products, refined carbohydrate foods, and sweetened beverages • Reduce intake of cholesterol and sodium-containing foods • For patients who are overweight or obese, reduce daily calories to achieve and maintain weight loss of 5%-10%
Physical activity	• Obtain at least 150 min/week of moderate-intensity or 75 minutes of vigorous-intensity physical activity • Decrease sedentary behaviors
Other lifestyle factors	• Smoking cessation and avoiding tobacco products • Avoid secondhand smoke exposure

ASCVD, atherosclerotic cardiovascular disease.

is recommended three to four times per week with each session lasting 40 minutes on average. All patients should also be counseled to stop smoking and avoid tobacco products altogether.[24]

It is important to recognize that there is no single diet suitable for every patient. Instead, advise patients to reduce the percent of calories from saturated and *trans* fats by following a dietary pattern that emphasizes vegetables, fruits, whole grains, low-fat dairy, poultry, fish, legumes, and nuts, while limiting the intake of sweets, sugary beverages, and red meat. Plans that closely mirror this dietary pattern and effectively lower LDL-C include DASH, the USDA Food Pattern, and AHA Diet. Although the Mediterranean-style diet has no consistent effect on LDL-C levels, it reduces major cardiovascular events among persons at high cardiovascular risk when compared to a control diet. Any recommended dietary pattern should be adapted to a patient's caloric requirements, cultural food preferences, and other medical conditions (eg, diabetes mellitus). Individualized diet counseling that provides acceptable substitutions for unhealthy foods and ongoing reinforcement by a registered dietitian are necessary for maximal effect. It is also important to involve all family members, especially if the patient is not the primary person preparing food.[24]

Less than one-third of Americans meet the 2015-2020 Dietary Guidelines for Americans limit of less than 10% of calories from saturated fats.[39] In patients with lipid disorders, the 2013 AHA/ACC Lifestyle Management Guideline recommended only 5% to 6% of total calories from saturated fat.[24] This can be achieved by recommending patients limit or avoid fast food, high-fat dairy products, and sweets. Previous dietary guideline recommendations to limit dietary cholesterol to 300 mg/day was omitted in 2015. However, it is still recommended that individuals limit their daily dietary cholesterol intake. A dietary pattern low in saturated and *trans* fats will typically result in a reduction in dietary cholesterol since foods high in saturated and *trans* fats are often high in cholesterol. A 12-week trial of lifestyle modification is generally recommended before considering lipid-lowering therapy in patients without evidence of ASCVD, diabetes, or other high-risk features. Importantly, lifestyle modification alone is inappropriate for patients with established ASCVD or diabetes given the benefit of statins in these high-risk patients.

Dietary Supplements

Select dietary supplements may be useful to augment diet and lipid-lowering therapy. Increased intake of soluble fiber in the form of oat bran, pectins, certain gums, and psyllium products can reduce total and LDL-C, but have little or no effect on HDL-C or TG levels. Soluble fiber binds cholesterol and bile acids in the small intestine, which decreases absorption and reabsorption. Total daily fiber intake should be about 25 g/day, yet most Americans average only half of the recommended amount.[40] Dietary supplements containing fiber may be used to supplement the diet and achieve the recommended daily intake. An intake of 3 to 12 g/day show reductions in total and LDL-C of 10 mg/dL (0.26 mmol/L) and 12 mg/dL (0.31 mmol/L), respectively, compared to control.[27] It remains unknown if soluble fiber supplements have any impact on cardiovascular morbidity and mortality. Although seemingly safe, patients should be advised to stay well hydrated to avoid gastrointestinal distress. These products may also be useful in managing constipation associated with the bile acid sequestrants (BASs).

In epidemiologic studies, ingestion of large amounts of oily, cold-water fish (such as salmon) is associated with a reduction in ASCVD risk. Modest consumption (1-2 servings per week) reduces the risk of cardiovascular death and total mortality.[41] The American Heart Association recommends eating oily fish at least twice a week; however, there are concerns with some types of fish (such as tuna) that often have high levels of environmental contaminants. There are also concerns about environmental sustainability. Fish oil supplementation is an alternative option that provides a consistent daily intake of omega-3 PUFA such as eicosapentaenoic acid (EPA) and docosahexaenoic acid (DHA). Fish oil supplementation significantly reduces TG levels and VLDL-C but may increase total cholesterol and LDL-C. Other potentially favorable cardiovascular effects of fish oil supplementation include antiarrhythmic, antiplatelet, and anti-inflammatory properties. Despite this, a meta-analysis of 10 RCTs found low doses (less than 2 g/day) of omega-3 PUFA supplementation did not reduce the risk of ASCVD events.[42] Low-dose omega-3 PUFA supplementation is not recommended in primary prevention patients, especially those with diabetes who do not have established ASCVD.[43,44] Additional details regarding prescription omega-3 PUFA products are further discussed under drug therapy.

Phytosterols, including plant sterols and stanols isolated from vegetable oils, also reduce LDL-C levels. Ingestion of 2 g/day will reduce LDL-C by 5% to 15%, while doses above 3 g/day confer no additional LDL-C lowering.[27] The efficacy of plant sterols and plant stanols is comparable. The mechanism by which phytosterols reduce LDL-C remains unclear but may decrease the transport of cholesterol in the intestinal brush border membrane and affect cholesterol uptake via Niemann-Pick C1-Like 1 (NPC1L1) and other transporters. Because lipids are needed to solubilize stanol/sterol esters, they are usually available in commercial butter-like spreads (such as Benecol®). The presence of plant stanols/sterols is listed on the food label. Phytosterols should be administered 2 to 4 hours before or after BASs to avoid the binding of phytosterols in the gut. Although phytosterols are generally recognized as safe (GRAS) in the United States, they can cause gastrointestinal distress and should be avoided in patients with sitosterolemia, a rare genetic disorder characterized by a 50- to 100-fold increase in plant sterol levels and rapid onset of atherosclerosis.[45] The effects of long-term phytosterol supplementation on ASCVD risk remains unknown.

Red yeast rice is a commonly used dietary supplement in the United States that originates from Chinese medicine. The active ingredient of red yeast rice is monacolin K, which is chemically identical to lovastatin. This leads some patients to believe red yeast rice is a "natural" statin and, therefore, safer than statins available only by prescription; however, the active ingredient in over-the-counter (OTC) red yeast rice products vary by over 120-fold. Many products contain little to no monacolin.[46] Conversely, case reports of rhabdomyolysis, liver toxicity, and renal failure have raised concerns about some red yeast rice formulations containing significantly higher levels of monacolin K than described on the label.[47] Red yeast rice is not recommended as a suitable alternative to statins. However, if patients choose to take red yeast rice, it is recommended that they purchase it from a reputable supplier and avoid concurrent use with prescription statins.

Pharmacologic Therapy

9 There are numerous randomized, double-blinded clinical trials demonstrating that reduction of LDL-C reduces ASCVD-event rates in the setting of primary and secondary prevention.[29] Epidemiological studies suggest that every 38 mg/dL (0.98 mmol/L) reduction in LDL-C produces a 21% reduction in ASCVD event rates over 5 years.[48] Additional findings from large prospective cohort studies and Mendelian randomization studies have also demonstrated a dose-dependent log-linear association between LDL-C and ASCVD risk[49] and that lower levels of LDL-C achieve significant reductions in ASCVD risk. These studies provide a strong rationale for attempting to lower plasma cholesterol and LDL-C in patients at risk for ASCVD.[49] It should be noted, however, that not all lipid-lowering agents that reduce LDL-C have resulted in a reduction in ASCVD events (eg, CETP inhibitors). Thus, LDL-C lowering alone should not be the sole basis for selecting an appropriate agent.[17,27]

Lipid-lowering drugs can be broadly divided into agents that primarily decrease atherogenic cholesterol-containing lipoprotein particles (such as statins) and those that primarily decrease TG levels (such as fibrates).

Treatment of Specific Dyslipidemia Subtypes

Familial Hypercholesterolemia

Individuals with familial hypercholesterolemia (FH) have a high lifetime risk of developing ASCVD. Compared to the general population, FH is associated with a 24-fold higher risk of developing acute MI before the age of 40 years.[50] FH should be suspected in adults with untreated LDL-C levels of 190 mg/dL (4.91 mmol/L) or greater or non-HDL cholesterol levels of 220 mg/dL (5.69 mmol/L) or greater who have a family history of high cholesterol or ASCVD in first-degree relatives. Physical findings (such as xanthomas or corneal arcus) may be present in some patients with FH, but their absence does not rule out a diagnosis of FH. In clinical practice, one of several validated tools, including the Dutch Lipid Clinic Network, US Make Early Diagnosis Prevent Early Death (MEDPED), and Simon-Broome Registry, are used to make a formal diagnosis of FH. Genetic testing is available, however, approximately 20% of patients with clinically definite FH will not have an identifiable mutation; therefore, a negative genetic test does not exclude FH.[51] Importantly, cascade screening of all first-degree relatives of diagnosed FH patients is highly recommended as an effective strategy to identify previously undiagnosed FH patients.

Intensive lifestyle and pharmacological therapy are often necessary for adults with FH. In patients with FH who have not had an ASCVD event, a high-intensity statin is warranted and those with an LDL-C ≥100 mg/dL (2.59 mmol/L) despite max-tolerated statin should receive ezetimibe, bempedoic acid, and/or a PCSK9 inhibitor. The LDL-C threshold to consider nonstatin therapies in patients with FH and a history of ASCVD, however, is ≥70 mg/dL (1.81 mmol/L).

10 Mipomersen and lomitapide are orphan drugs indicated for use in patients with HoFH and reduce LDL-C levels by ~25% and ~40%, respectively.[52] Mipomersen is an oligonucleotide inhibitor of apolipoprotein B-100 synthesis administered via subcutaneous injection, while the orally administered lomitapide is a microsomal triglyceride transfer protein, or microsomal TG transfer protein inhibitor, which reduces the level of cholesterol that the liver and intestines assemble and secrete into the circulation. Mipomersen is associated with injection site pain and reactions, while both mipomersen and lomitapide have a black box warning for severe hepatotoxicity and are only available through restricted Risk Evaluation and Mitigation Strategy (REMS) programs.[52] Other treatment options for HoFH patients include LDL apheresis (a process similar to dialysis that removes LDL from the blood) and liver transplant.[50]

Evinacumab was approved to lower LDL-C in patients with HoFH at the age of 12 years and older. Evanicumab is a humanized monoclonal antibody that inhibits angiopoietin-like 3 (ANGPTL3) protein and is administered as an IV infusion every 4 weeks. The ANGPTL3 protein regulates lipid metabolism by inhibiting LPL and endothelial lipase enzymes. Inhibition of ANGPTL3 with Evinacumab reduces LDL-C by ~50% and also reduces TG by ~55% in patients with HoFH.[53] Adverse effects of Evinacumab include infusion-site reactions, influenza-like illness, and rhinorrhea. It is unknown whether evinacumab reduces ASCVD events.

Hypertriglyceridemia

10 Elevated TG levels are strongly associated with an increased risk of ASCVD; however, the direct role of TG in the development of ASCVD is debated.[54] All patients with elevated TG levels (see Table 32-2)

should be advised to implement lifestyle interventions that reduce TG levels, including a 5% to 10% reduction in body weight, reducing consumption of sugar and refined carbohydrates, increasing physical activity, smoking cessation, and restricting alcohol. Secondary causes of hypertriglyceridemia should also be identified and addressed. Uncontrolled diabetes and chronic kidney disease are common causes of elevated TG levels, along with certain medications (such as protease inhibitors and atypical antipsychotics). The best approach to managing patients whose TG levels remain elevated after optimizing lifestyle interventions and addressing secondary causes remains unclear, but statins are generally considered first-line given they can reduce TG levels by up to 30% at higher doses and help achieve desired levels of LDL-C.[55] Fibrates effectively lower TG levels but are not routinely used for borderline-high TG levels as there is no evidence supporting their use to reduce ASCVD risk. Omega-3 PUFA also significantly lower TG levels at higher doses (2-4 g/d) but only icosapent ethyl (EPA-only) prescription product is indicated for borderline-high TG levels and to reduce ASCVD risk.[56]

Fasting TG levels exceeding 500 mg/dL (5.65 mmol/L) are more commonly associated with pancreatitis and other consequences of hyperchylomicronemia (such as eruptive xanthomas). At this level of elevated TG, a genetic form of hypertriglyceridemia often coexists with other causes of elevated triglycerides such as diabetes. Dietary fat restriction is a basic element of treatment as this reduces the synthesis and entry of additional chylomicrons into the circulation. Lipid-lowering therapies that primarily lower TG levels (ie, fibrates and omega-3 PUFA) are recommended as first-line agents.[56] Statins may be reasonable first-line options in those patients with an ASCVD risk of 7.5% or greater. If TG levels are persistently over 500 mg/dL (5.65 mmol/L), it is reasonable to consider adding omega-3 PUFA or fibrate therapy. Success in treatment is defined as a reduction in triglycerides below 500 mg/dL (5.65 mmol/L) and preventing pancreatitis.

Low HDL Cholesterol

Low HDL-C is a strong independent risk predictor of ASCVD5.[7] Low HDL-C is defined as less than 40 mg/dL (1.03 mmol/L) for men and less than 50 mg/dL (1.29 mmol/L) for women, but there is no specified goal for HDL-C raising. Low HDL-C may be a consequence of insulin resistance, physical inactivity, diabetes, cigarette smoking, high carbohydrate intake, and certain drugs. In patients with low HDL-C levels, the primary target remains LDL-C. Niacin has the potential for the greatest increase in HDL-C compared to other lipid-lowering therapies and the effect is more pronounced with regular or immediate-release forms than with sustained-release forms. However, no RCT has resulted in a reduction in ASCVD risk by increasing HDL-C5.[8,59] Additionally, several CETP inhibitors capable of raising HDL-C levels as much as 135% were evaluated in randomized, placebo-controlled trials but no additional benefit was found when these drugs were added to background statin therapy.[57] Due to the lack of pharmacological agents demonstrating an improvement in clinical outcomes by focusing on raising HDL-C, lifestyle modification (such as smoking cessation and increasing physical activity) remains the preferred approach. Although alcohol consumption increases HDL-C, it is not acceptable to recommend this to patients who do not already consume alcohol.

Medications That Primarily Lower Atherogenic Cholesterol

HMG-CoA Reductase Inhibitors (Statins)

Statins (such as atorvastatin) are considered the first-line lipid-lowering therapies for managing dyslipidemia due to robust evidence from multiple RCTs demonstrating that statins significantly decrease the risk of first (primary prevention) and recurrent (secondary prevention) cardiovascular events.[17,48] Statins significantly

TABLE 32-5 Intensity of Statin Therapy by Drug and Daily Dose

High-Intensity Statin Therapy	Moderate-Intensity Statin Therapy	Low-Intensity Statin Therapy
Lowers LDL-C on average by ≥50%	Lowers LDL-C on average by 30% to <50%	Lowers LDL-C on average by <30%
Atorvastatin 40-80 mg **Rosuvastatin 20-40 mg**	**Atorvastatin 10-20 mg** **Rosuvastatin 5-10 mg** **Simvastatin 20-40 mg**[a] Pravastatin 40-80 mg **Lovastatin 40 mg** Fluvastatin XL 80 mg **Fluvastatin 40 mg BID** Pitavastatin 2-4 mg	Simvastatin 10 mg **Pravastatin 10-20 mg** **Lovastatin 20 mg** Fluvastatin 20-40 mg Pitavastatin 1 mg

[a]Simvastatin is not recommended by the FDA to be initiated at 80 mg/day due to increased risk of myopathy and rarely rhabdomyolysis.

FDA, Food and Drug Administration; RCT, randomized clinical trials.

Boldface type indicates medications that have cardiovascular outcome data from RCTs when given in the specified dose.

reduce LDL-C levels (20%-60%), modestly increase HDL-C (6%-12%), and decrease TG levels (10%-29%).[60] Statins interrupt the conversion of HMG-CoA to mevalonate, the rate-limiting step in de novo cholesterol biosynthesis, by inhibiting HMG-CoA reductase (see Fig. 32-4). Metabolic studies with statins in normal volunteers and patients with hypercholesterolemia suggest a reduced synthesis of LDL-C, as well as enhanced catabolism of LDL mediated through LDL receptors, as the principal mechanisms for lipid-lowering effects. Statin selection is primarily based on the patient's individual ASCVD risk and indicated intensity (see Table 32-5). Currently available products in order of decreasing LDL-C lowering potency include rosuvastatin, atorvastatin, pitavastatin, simvastatin, lovastatin, pravastatin, and fluvastatin.[60] The plasma half-lives for all the statins are relatively short (1-3 hours) except for atorvastatin, pitavastatin, and rosuvastatin, which may account for their potency.[60] Statins are generally well tolerated but are not without adverse effects. However, discontinuation rates due to adverse effects in randomized, double-blind, placebo-controlled trials have often been similar between statin and placebo.[61]

Statin-associated muscle symptoms (SAMS) are reported by 10% to 25% of statin users and are frequently reported by patients as a reason for statin discontinuation.[62] While various definitions of SAMS exist, the clinical diagnosis of SAMS is based on a subjective clinical assessment. Myalgia is the most reported muscle-related adverse effect with statin therapy and refers to bilateral muscle achiness, weakness, or cramps affecting larger muscle groups (such as thighs and back). Myopathy is often used interchangeably with myalgia, but myopathy is a general term used for any muscle-related symptoms. The most concerning of SAMS is rhabdomyolysis, which is a rapid breakdown of skeletal muscle resulting in creatine kinase (CK) elevations greater than 10 times the upper limit of normal. The release of myoglobin from damaged muscle tissue may also compromise renal function and lead to acute kidney injury. Patients presenting with rhabdomyolysis will often describe their urine as dark or "tea-colored" and present with nausea, vomiting, confusion, coma, cardiac arrhythmias, electrolyte disturbances, and even death. Fortunately, rhabdomyolysis in statin-treated patients is exceedingly rare occurring in only 0.1% of patients in RCT compared to 0.04% of patients receiving placebo. Rhabdomyolysis is not only caused by statins but can also be induced by extreme physical exercise, certain metabolism disorders (eg, diabetic ketoacidosis), other drugs (eg, colchicine), toxins, and infection.

Certain risk factors are known to increase the risk of developing SAMS and recognition of these risk factors at the time of statin initiation may minimize the risk of SAMS. Known risk factors include advanced age, female gender, low body mass index, frequent heavy exercisers, comorbidities (eg, kidney disease, hypothyroidism), and increased serum statin concentrations due to drug-drug interactions.[62] A lower dose might be necessary for patients with multiple risk factors for SAMS, and once the starting dose is tolerated, the dose can be titrated to the desired potency. Avoiding major drug-drug interactions is a significant modifiable risk factor for SAMS that pharmacists can directly impact. Nearly 80% of all medications are metabolized in the liver by the cytochrome P450 system (CYP) with CYP3A4 being the most predominant.[63] Statins are no different as nearly all statins, except pravastatin, are metabolized to some degree by CYP isoenzymes. Lovastatin, simvastatin, and atorvastatin are associated with more significant drug-drug interactions since they are predominantly metabolized by CYP3A4, while fluvastatin, pitavastatin, and rosuvastatin rely on other CYP isoenzymes (eg, CYP2C9, CYP2C8, CYP2C19).[64]

The co-prescribing of medications that compete with or inhibit the same CYP isoenzyme (ie, verapamil) can increase serum statin concentrations and the risk for SAMS. The concurrent use of medications such as gemfibrozil that interfere with statin glucuronidation, which is responsible for statin clearance, increases the risk of SAMS.

The management of SAMS requires a multifaceted approach. Documentation of the patients' reported symptoms and determining the probability of SAMS is an important first step. A Statin Intolerance App (available at: http://www.acc.org/statinintolerance-app) created by the ACC is a helpful resource that can be used to determine the possibility of SAMS and provide guidance on managing patients with possible SAMS. Statin therapy should be generally discontinued in patients with intolerable symptoms. If symptoms resolve, initiate a different statin at a lower dose.[62,65] Additionally, hydrophilic statins (such as rosuvastatin) may be better tolerated than lipophilic statins (such as simvastatin). In patients where symptoms do not improve, other potential causes of muscle pain should be excluded, including hypothyroidism and vitamin D deficiency, before a statin rechallenge.[65] Alternative dosing strategies (eg, every other day) using statins with long half-lives (atorvastatin, rosuvastatin, and likely pitavastatin) may also be considered. Nonstatin therapies may be considered in patients who fail multiple statins. While routine CK monitoring is not recommended, a CK measurement prompted by patient symptoms can be used to exclude rhabdomyolysis and can assist with identifying those with definite myalgia. Importantly, patients should be reassured that statins are effective and safe, and SAMS is reversible with statin discontinuation.

Other notable adverse effects of statins include mild elevations in serum transaminase levels (primarily alanine aminotransferase [ALT]). Liver enzymes are not, however, an accurate measure of liver function and there is no causal relationship between statin use and liver failure. Therefore, routine periodic monitoring of liver enzymes is not required, but liver enzyme tests should be obtained before starting statin therapy to have a baseline value for comparison if liver enzymes are later discovered to be elevated. Other potential causes for elevated liver enzymes, including excessive alcohol intake, infection, and select medications should also be evaluated. Statins may be initiated in patients with chronic liver disease, compensated cirrhosis, and nonalcoholic fatty liver disease; however, statins are contraindicated in patients with decompensated cirrhosis or acute liver failure.[65]

Statin use is also associated with a small increased risk of new-onset diabetes.[62] This was first observed in the JUPITER (Justification for the Use of Statins in Prevention: an Intervention Trial Evaluating Rosuvastatin) trial, where the number of new-onset diabetes cases was 0.6% higher in those receiving rosuvastatin 20 mg/day compared to placebo.[36] Subsequent meta-analyses of statin trials have also found a modest increase in the number of new-onset diabetes cases among statin-treated patients compared to placebo, but the absolute risk increase is <1%.[66,67] Common attributes of statin users who develop new-onset diabetes include receiving higher doses of statins and having other risk factors for diabetes, including obesity, impaired fasting glucose, HbA1c >6% (0.06; 42 mmol/mol), or metabolic syndrome.[68] Mechanisms to explain the association between statin use and new-onset diabetes remain unclear. However, observational data suggest that higher cholesterol levels are protective against developing diabetes. This may be attributable to changes at the cellular level involving disruption of cholesterol-sensitive cellular functions that affect insulin secretion and insulin sensitivity.[62] Ultimately, the benefit of statin therapy greatly outweighs the risk of new-onset diabetes as statin use in patients at high ASCVD risk will prevent approximately three ASCVD events for every new case of diabetes. Table 32-6 lists common adverse effects of available lipid-lowering therapies.

Cholesterol Absorption Inhibitors

Ezetimibe is a preferred adjunct therapy given, it modestly reduces the risk of recurrent cardiovascular events in a secondary prevention population when used in combination with statin therapy.[35] The primary lipid-lowering effect of ezetimibe is a modest reduction in LDL-C of 15% to 24%; with higher reductions achievable when used in combination with statin therapy.[35,69] Ezetimibe reduces LDL-C by inhibiting the NPC1L1 protein, an important transporter of cholesterol absorption in the small intestine and hepatocytes.[69] Known polymorphisms of *NPC1L1* are associated with lower LDL-C levels and decreased ASCVD risk, thus providing a rationale why ezetimibe reduces ASCVD risk.[70] Other than mild gastrointestinal complaints (ie, diarrhea) and post-marketing reports of myalgia and mild ALT elevations when used in combination with statins, ezetimibe is generally well tolerated. Previous concerns over a potential increased risk of cancer have been nullified given recent prospective clinical trial data showing there is no increased risk of cancer with ezetimibe use.[35] Ezetimibe has no effects on the CYP450 enzyme system; however, concomitant use with cyclosporine can lead to increased exposure to both ezetimibe and cyclosporine.[69]

The BASs, such as colesevelam, modestly reduce LDL-C (13%-20%) and reduce cardiovascular events when used as monotherapy.[71] There is no data to determine if the benefits observed with BAS monotherapy translates to its use in combination with statin therapy. As such, BAS are generally used as adjunct therapy with statins when desired LDL-C levels are not achieved with statins alone. Importantly, BAS are considered first line during pregnancy since they are not systemically absorbed and pose no risk to the fetus. The primary action of BAS is to bind bile acids in the intestinal lumen, with a concurrent interruption of enterohepatic circulation of bile acids and a markedly increased excretion of acidic steroids in the feces. This decreases the bile acid pool size and stimulates the hepatic synthesis of bile acids from cholesterol. Depletion of the hepatic pool of cholesterol results in an increase in cholesterol biosynthesis and an increase in the number of LDL-R on the hepatocyte membrane. The increased number of receptors stimulates an enhanced rate of catabolism from plasma and lowers LDL-C levels. The increase in hepatic cholesterol biosynthesis may be paralleled by increased hepatic VLDL production and, consequently, BAS may aggravate hypertriglyceridemia and should be avoided in those with TG levels exceeding 300 mg/dL (3.39 mmol/L).[33]

One of the main barriers to BAS is their poor tolerability profile. Early BAS (such as cholestyramine) were developed as powders that require mixing with water or juice to create a slurry for oral administration. Gastrointestinal complaints of constipation, bloating, epigastric fullness, nausea, and flatulence are commonly reported with these formulations.[33] These adverse effects can be minimized by increasing fluid intake, modifying the diet to increase bulk, and using stool softeners. Tablet forms of BAS (ie, colesevelam) are generally better tolerated than resin powders and associated with

TABLE 32-6 Safety of Lipid-Lowering Therapies

Lipid-Lowering Drug Class	Adverse Effects: Common/Possible (1%-10%)	Adverse Effects: Rare/unlikely (<1%)	Contraindications
Statins	• Statin associated muscle symptoms (myalgia/myopathy) • New-onset diabetes mellitus • Transient, mild elevation in transaminase levels	• Rhabdomyolysis • Severe hepatotoxicity	• Pregnancy/breastfeeding • Decompensated cirrhosis • Acute liver failure
Cholesterol absorption inhibitors	• GI adverse effects • Myalgias (when used with statin) • Elevated transaminase levels (when used with statin)	• Thrombocytopenia	• Pregnancy/breastfeeding • Acute liver failure
Bile acid sequestrants	• GI adverse effects and/or obstruction • Impaired absorption of fat-soluble vitamins • Reduced bioavailability of select drugs	• Ileus • Cholecystitis • Severe hypertriglyceridemia	• History of bowel obstruction • Fasting TG are 300 mg/dL or higher
ACL inhibitors	• Hyperuricemia	• Increased risk of tendon rupture • Increased risk of benign prostate hyperplasia	
PCSK9 mAbs	• Injection-site reactions • Flu-like symptoms post-injection		• Hypersensitivity reaction to alirocumab or evolocumab
Fibrates	• GI adverse effects • Transient elevation in transaminases • Myalgias (especially when used with statin) • Mild increase in serum creatinine	• Increased risk of gallstones	• Pre-existing gallbladder disease • CrCl of 30 mL/min (0.5 mL/s) or lower
Omega-3 PUFA	• GI adverse effects • Eructation • Increased risk of bleeding when used with antiplatelets or anticoagulants • Increased risk of atrial fibrillation or flutter		• Caution in patients with allergy or sensitivity to fish and/or shellfish
Niacin	• Dermatologic effects (flushing/itching) • Increased transaminases • Hyperuricemia • Hyperglycemia	• Increased risk of atrial fibrillation or flutter • Rhabdomyolysis (with statin) • Hepatotoxicity (with statin)	• Active peptic ulcer • Arterial hemorrhage • Persistently elevated transaminase levels
Inclisiran	• Injection-site reactions		• Pregnancy/breastfeeding
Evinacumab	• Infusion-site pruritus • Influenza-like reactions • Rhinorrhea		• Pregnancy/breastfeeding

ACL, Adenosine Triphosphate-citrate Lyase; CrCl, Creatinine Clearance; mAbs, monoclonal antibodies; PUFA, Polyunsaturated Fatty Acids; SAMS, Statin-associated Muscle Symptoms.

lower overall discontinuation rates.[72] Other potential adverse effects include impaired absorption of fat-soluble vitamins A, D, E, and K; gastrointestinal obstruction; and reduced bioavailability of other drugs such as warfarin, levothyroxine, and phenytoin.[33] Drug-drug interactions may be avoided by taking other medications 1 hour before or 4 hours after the BAS.[33] Colesevelam is not only approved as a lipid-lowering agent but also as an antihyperglycemic that modestly lowers glucose levels in patients with type 2 diabetes mellitus.[73] Given the better safety and tolerability profile of ezetimibe, BAS should be reserved only for those patients unable to tolerate ezetimibe who need additional LDL-C lowering despite maximally tolerated statin therapy.[33]

Proprotein Convertase Subtilisin/Kexin Type 9 (PCSK9) Modulating Therapies

Inhibition of PCSK9 reduces LDL-C by as much as 60% when added to background statin therapy. Reducing PCSK9 levels promotes LDL-R recycling to the cell surface, which increases LDL-C clearance from the circulation. Both alirocumab and evolocumab are fully human monoclonal antibodies to PCSK9 and were approved by the FDA in 2015.[31] Randomized, double-blind clinical trials have also shown that these agents effectively reduce recurrent cardiovascular events in patients following an acute coronary event and secondary prevention populations when added to background statin therapy.[31,74] Alirocumab and evolocumab are both administered by subcutaneous injection. Although this may be a barrier for some patients, PCSK9 inhibitors can be administered bi-weekly or once monthly. The most common adverse effect reported are injection site reactions, which can be minimized by allowing the injection to come to room temperature before use and icing the site before injecting. Some patients may also report "flu-like" symptoms after the injection. There were initial concerns over a potential increased risk for neurocognitive adverse effects; however, a randomized trial found no difference in cognitive function between those randomized to evolocumab *versus* placebo over 19 months of follow-up.[75] Furthermore, those patients who reach low levels of LDL-C (less than 20 mg/dL [0.52 mmol/L]) do not appear to be an increased risk of adverse events.[76] Despite this favorable data, the long-term effects of achieving low levels of LDL-C with PCSK9 inhibitors remain unknown. Despite their LDL-C lowering potency and favorable safety profile, PCSK9 inhibitors frequently require a prior authorization due to their higher cost compared to other LDL-C lowering therapies. Although PCSK9 inhibitors should primarily be used in combination with maximally tolerated statins in high-risk patients unable to achieve desired LDL-C levels with a statin alone, alirocumab and evolocumab are FDA-approved for use as monotherapy in patients with primary hyperlipidemia (ie, heterozygous familial hypercholesterolemia).[31,74]

Inclisiran is a small interfering RNA (siRNA) molecule that reduces the production of PCSK9 by inhibiting messenger RNA.[77] This novel biological agent has a sustained effect on LDL-lowering and is given subcutaneously every 6 months. In Phase 3 clinical trials, inclisiran reduced LDL-C by an average of 50% when given as add-on therapy in patients who were treated with a high-intensity statin but had not achieved their LDL-C goal. Inclisiran is approved as an additional treatment to maximally tolerated statin therapy to further lower LDL-C in adults with HeFH or ASCVD. The most common adverse effects reported are injection-site reactions, which are generally transient and mild. Whether inclisiran lowers cardiovascular event rates is currently being investigated in the ORION-4 trial (NCT03705234).

Adenosine Triphosphate-Citrate Lyase Inhibitors

Adenosine triphosphate-citrate lyase (ACL) is a cytoplasmic enzyme responsible for generating acetyl coenzyme A which is needed during the de novo synthesis of fatty acids and cholesterol. ACL inhibitors prevent cholesterol production upstream from HMG CoA reductase inhibitors (ie, statins) and the two therapeutic strategies can be used in combination. Bempedoic acid is an orally administered ACL inhibitor that provides additional LDL-C lowering. In Phase 3 clinical trials, bempedoic acid produced modest reductions in LDL-C (15%-20%) when combined with statin therapy or used as monotherapy in patients who are unable to tolerate statins.[77] Bempedoic acid is also available in a combination product that contains ezetimide. Bempedoic acid plus ezetimibe resulted in a 36% reduction in LDL-C from baseline in a Phase 3 clinical trial.[78] Bempedoic acid is generally well tolerated and associated with fewer muscle symptoms when compared to statins. However, bempedoic acid may cause hyperuricemia and tendon rupture. Increased blood concentrations of uric acid were seen in some patients treated with bempedoic acid and this may increase the risk of acute gout in those with a history of gouty arthritis. Mechanistically, bempedoic acid inhibits the renal tubular organic anion transporter 2 (OAT2), which plays a role in the renal uptake of uric acid from the blood. Though rare, bempedoic acid was associated with an increased risk of tendon rupture or injury (0.5%) in clinical trials. This uncommon but potentially debilitating adverse effect was not reported in patients who received a placebo. Risk factors for tendon rupture are age greater than 60 years, concurrent use of corticosteroids or fluoroquinolones, renal failure, and history of tendon disorders. Until the results of the long-term cardiovascular outcome trial are published, the role of bempedoic acid in the management of dyslipidemia should be limited to patients unable to achieve desired treatment goals on maximally tolerated statin plus ezetimibe who prefer a non-injectable therapeutic option.

Drug That Primarily Lower Triglycerides

Fibric Acid Derivatives (Fibrates)

Although fibrates, such as gemfibrozil, reduce cardiovascular events when used as monotherapy, there is less evidence to support their use in combination with statin therapy.[54,55] Fibrates are primarily used in patients with TG levels that exceed 500 mg/dL (5.65 mmol/L) to reduce the risk of acute pancreatitis. The two available fibrates, gemfibrozil and fenofibrate, are potent TG-lowering therapies (20%-50%), but may cause a modest reciprocal rise in LDL-C in patients with severely elevated TG levels.[55] Plasma HDL-C concentrations may rise 10% to 15% or more with fibrates. Gemfibrozil increases the activity of LPL and reduces to a lesser extent the synthesis or secretion of VLDL from the liver into the plasma. Fenofibrate increases LPL activity and reduces apoprotein C-III (an inhibitor of LPL) by activating peroxisome proliferator-activated receptor α (PPARα), which regulates the expression of genes involved in the regulation of lipids and other metabolic processes.

Fibrates are generally well tolerated, but gastrointestinal complaints and transient elevations in transaminase levels have been reported.[79] Both gemfibrozil and fenofibrate require dose adjustments for significant renal impairment and fenofibrate has been reported to worsen renal function, although this is usually transient and self-limiting.[17,80] Muscle-related adverse effects can occur with both gemfibrozil and fenofibrate alone but is more common when used in combination with statins to manage complex dyslipidemia or elevated TG levels. Gemfibrozil, and its glucuronide metabolite, has potent effects on CYP450 enzymes (ie, CYP3A4), intestinal, hepatic, and renal transporters making it highly prone to significantly increasing serum statin concentrations and the risk of SAMS.[64] For this reason, current guidelines do not recommend gemfibrozil to be initiated in patients receiving statin therapy; fenofibrate is favored instead.[17] Fenofibrate and gemfibrozil and may enhance the formation of gallstones, but this occurs rarely.[81] Fibrates may potentiate the effects of warfarin and the international normalized ratio (INR) should be monitored closely with this combination.[82]

Omega-3 Polyunsaturated Fatty Acids (PUFA)

High doses of omega-3 PUFA (2-4 g/day of EPA/DHA) significantly reduce TG and VLDL cholesterol levels (20%-50%) with lesser effects on other lipoproteins.[54] The mechanisms by which omega-3 PUFA reduce TG levels include increasing hepatic oxidation of free fatty acids, increasing LDL hydrolysis by activating PPARα, and inhibiting apolipoprotein C-III. The omega-3 PUFA formulations approved by the FDA for treating TG levels of 500 mg/dL (5.65 mmol/L) or greater include an omega-3-acid ethyl ester of EPA/DHA (Lovaza®), omega-3-carboxylic acid of EPA/DHA (Epanova®), and ethyl ester of EPA only (Vascepa®). DHA and EPA have different effects on LDL-C as EPA prevents LDL oxidation and promotes LDL clearance, whereas DHA does not; however, the clinical significance of this remains unclear.[83] Prescription omega-3 PUFA products contain approximately 1 g of EPA/DHA per capsule, whereas the EPA/DHA content of OTC "fish oil" supplements is often less than 300 mg/capsule and are not regulated by the FDA. Unless patient affordability is an issue, prescription omega-3 PUFA is preferred to minimize pill burden and ensure product quality.

Randomized clinical trials of omega-3 PUFA have shown mixed results due to the lack of generalizability due to the population studied, the background lipid-lowering therapy used, and the dose taken.[83] Table 32-7 lists select TG-lowering and cardiovascular trials of available omega-3 PUFA products. The REDUCE-IT study evaluated the effects of icosapent ethyl (4 g/day), a high-potency EPA derivative, used as add-on therapy to statins compared to mineral oil placebo.[84] At baseline, patients enrolled in the REDUCE-IT study had a median TG level of 216 mg/dL (2.44 mmol/L) and the majority had a history of ASCVD. Icosapent ethyl reduced the rate of ischemic events by 25% and significantly reduced the risk of cardiovascular death when compared to placebo. This benefit is not related to TG reduction, however, and may be due to increases in EPA levels. In contrast, the STRENGTH trial evaluated the omega-3-carboxylic acid of EPA/DHA in a randomized controlled trial using corn oil placebo in a population similar to that of REDUCE-IT; however, there was no observed benefit with the intervention.[85] The debate is ongoing as to why these trials produced completely different results, including differences in the omega-3 PUFA product used (EPA only vs EPA/DHA) and type of placebo used (mineral oil vs corn oil).

Gastrointestinal complaints (ie, abdominal pain and "fishy burps") are common with omega-3 PUFA products but may be minimized by refrigerating the capsules. However, they should not be kept frozen in the freezer. Caution is advised in patients with known sensitivities or allergies to fish or shellfish. Drug-drug interactions are minimal with omega-3 PUFA, although caution is advised when used concomitantly with antiplatelet agents or anticoagulants since omega-3 PUFA may prolong bleeding time. Both low- and high-dose omega-3 PUFA supplementation has been observed to increase the risk of incident atrial flutter or fibrillation.[86]

Niacin

Niacin (nicotinic acid) increases HDL-C (5%-30%), and lowers TG (20%-50%) and LDL-C (5%-20%). Despite these favorable changes

TABLE 32-7 Select Clinical Trials of Omega-3 PUFA Effects on TG Lowering and Cardiovascular Events

Product	Omega-3 Acid Ethyl Esters (Lovaza)	Icosapent Ethyl (Vascepa)	Omega-3 Carboxylic Acids (Epanova)
Indicated uses	To reduce TG in adults with severe hypertriglyceridemia (TG ≥500 mg/dL [5.65 mmol/L])	Reduce major vascular events in adults with elevated TG (150-499 mg/dL [1.70-5.64 mmol/L]) and elevated cardiovascular risk while taking statin therapy	
Omega-3 fatty acid contents (per 1 g)	465 mg EPA 375 mg DHA	1 g EPA	550 mg EPA 200 mg DHA
TG-lowering efficacy in patients w/TG ≥ 500 mg/dL	**Harris et al.**[90] Patients with TG 500-2,000 mg/dL (5.65-22.6 mmol/L) Intervention: 4 g/d EPA + DHA ethyl esters vs placebo TG-lowering from baseline: −45% vs +16%	**MARINE** Patients with TG 500-2,000 mg/dL (5.65-22.6 mmol/L) Intervention: 4 g/d EPA vs placebo TG-lowering from baseline: −26.6% vs +9.7%	**EVOLVE** Patients with TG 500-2,000 mg/dL (5.65-22.6 mmol/L) Intervention: 4g/d EPA + DHA carboxylic acids vs 4 g/d olive oil TG-lowering from baseline: −30.9% vs −4.3%
Cardiovascular event reduction in patients at high risk of cardiovascular events	**VITAL** US patients without ASCVD (*n* = 25,871) **Intervention:** 1 g EPA + DHA ethyl esters vs placebo **Event rates:** 3.0% vs 3.2% HR 0.92 (0.80-1.06)	**REDUCE-IT** Patients with increased CV risk and elevated TG while receiving max-tolerated statin (*n* = 8,179) **Intervention:** 4 g/day EPA vs mineral oil **Event rates:** 17.2% vs 22.2% HR 0.75 (0.68-0.83)	**STRENGTH** Patients with increased CV risk and elevated TG and low HDL-C while receiving max-tolerated statin (*n* = 13,078) **Intervention:** 4 g/day EPA + DHA carboxylic acids vs corn oil **Event rates:** 12.0% vs 12.2% HR 0.99 (0.9-1.09)

DHA, docosahexaenoic acid; EPA, eicosapentaenoic acid; EVOLVE, epanova for lowering very high triglycerides[87]; MARINE, multi-center, placebo-controlled, randomized, double-blind, 12-week study with an open-label extension[88]; REDUCE-IT, reduction of cardiovascular events with icosapent ethyl–intervention trial[84]; STRENGTH, effect of high-dose omega-3 fatty acids vs corn oil on major adverse cardiovascular events in patients at high cardiovascular risk[85]; TG, triglycerides; VITAL, marine n–3 fatty acids and prevention of cardiovascular disease and cancer.[89]

in the lipid profile, niacin has not been shown to improve cardiovascular outcomes in patients on background statin therapy with relatively well-controlled lipids at baseline.[58,59] Niacin primarily lowers TG levels by inhibiting lipolysis with a decrease in free fatty acids in plasma and decreased hepatic esterification of TG. It also significantly raises HDL-C by reducing its catabolism and selectively decreasing hepatic removal of HDL apoA-I but not the removal of cholesterol esters, thereby increasing the capacity of retained apoA-I to augment reverse cholesterol transport in isolated hepatic cells. Niacin also reduces the hepatic synthesis of VLDL, which, in turn, leads to a reduction in the synthesis of LDL. However, the modest decrease in serum LDL-C levels is dose dependent.

Niacin has many adverse drug reactions that frequently limit its use. Cutaneous flushing and itching are prostaglandin mediated and can be reduced by administering aspirin 325 mg given shortly before niacin ingestion.[91] Flushing seems to be related to rising plasma concentrations of niacin and the use of immediate-release formulations; taking the dose with meals and slowly titrating the dose upward may also minimize these effects. Extended- or sustained-release products may minimize these complaints in some patients. The only legend form of niacin, Niaspan® (Abbott), is an extended-release form of niacin with pharmacokinetics intermediate between immediate- and sustained-release products that are sold as food supplements rather than legend products. In controlled trials, Niaspan® is reported to have fewer dermatologic reactions and has a lower risk for hepatoxicity.[91] Potentially important laboratory abnormalities occurring with niacin therapy include elevated liver function tests, hyperuricemia, and hyperglycemia. With less than 3 g/day, the degree of liver function test elevation is generally not marked and often transient, and a temporary reduction in dosage frequently corrects the problem. Pre-existing gout and diabetes may be exacerbated by niacin; these patients should be monitored more closely and their medication titrated appropriately.[92,93] Niacin is contraindicated in patients with active liver disease and active peptic ulcer disease. Concomitant alcohol and hot beverages may magnify flushing and pruritus with niacin and they should be avoided at the time of ingestion. Nicotinamide should not be used in the treatment of hyperlipidemia, as it does not effectively lower cholesterol or TG levels.

Special Populations

Older Adults

Dyslipidemia is an independent risk factor for ASCVD in older adults (older than 65 years), as it is in younger patients.[94] The attributable risk, which is the difference in absolute rates of cardiovascular events between segments of the population with higher or lower serum cholesterol levels, increases with age. Drug therapy in principle differs little from younger patients, and older patients respond to lipid-lowering therapies as well as younger patients. Primary prevention in younger patients requires about 2 years before reduction in ASCVD risk is apparent, and this lag time should be taken into consideration, along with life expectancy, when determining if statin therapy is appropriate in older adults. The gain in life expectancy may be small depending on the age at the start of treatment and the magnitude of LDL-C reduction. The benefits of moderate-to-high intensity statin therapy in older adults for secondary prevention is quite clear, while the benefit of statins in older adults for primary prevention is more controversial.[94] This is especially true in individuals older than 75 years since this age group is poorly represented in RCTs.[17] One observational cohort study assessed cardiovascular events among a cohort of patients aged 75 years with no previous ASCVD who either continued or discontinued statin therapy prior to their 75th birthday.[95] Compared to patients who continued, patients who discontinued statin therapy had a 33% increased risk of being admitted for a cardiovascular event. A posthoc meta-analysis of the

JUPITER and HOPE-3 primary prevention trials assessed major cardiovascular events by age (<65 years, 65-69 years, and 70 years or older).[96] Combined results of both trials reported that statin treatment was associated with a 26% lower risk of major cardiovascular events among patients aged 70 years or older, but was only significant within the JUPITER population. The ongoing Statin Therapy for Reducing Events in the Elderly (STAREE) trial (NCT02099123) is evaluating the efficacy of atorvastatin 40 mg/day for primary prevention in those 70 years or older without diabetes and will provide additional information as to the benefits of statin for primary ASCVD prevention in the elderly.

The risks of statin therapy in older adults must also be considered. Changes in body composition, renal function, and other physiologic changes of aging may make older patients more susceptible to the adverse effects of lipid-lowering drug therapy.[94] Older adults are more prone to developing SAMS and the effects of SAMS on the risk of falls and functional status remains unclear.[83] There is also concern regarding the potential negative effects of statins on cognitive function; however, data from meta-analyses have suggested statins are not associated with adverse cognitive effects.[97,98] Statin use has also been associated with increased risk of cataracts, which is highly prevalent among older adults, yet a meta-analysis found no clear evidence showing statins increase the risk of cataracts.[99] Older adults are also more likely to develop type 2 diabetes and the impact of statin therapy on new-onset diabetes in older adults is a concern warranting further study. Several factors including worsening physical or cognitive function, multi- or worsening comorbidities, advancing frailty, and/or reduced life expectancy may favor discontinuing statin therapy in adults 75 years and older taking statins for primary prevention.[17] Clinician-patient discussion regarding potential benefits and risks of discontinuing statin therapy is recommended to ensure individualized treatment decisions.

Children

While cardiovascular events rarely occur in those under 18 years of age, the process of atherosclerosis often begins during childhood.[100] Early identification and management of risk factors is critical for primordial prevention of ASCVD. Dyslipidemia in children can develop from secondary causes, similar to adults, or may present as primary dyslipidemia (ie, FH). Universal lipid screening is recommended between age 9 and 11 years as this is a stable time for lipid assessment before the onset of puberty, which decreases cholesterol levels 10% to 20%.[100] Lipid screening before age 9 is only recommended in children with a significant family history of premature ASCVD, known first-degree relatives with dyslipidemia, or other cardiovascular risk factors (ie, diabetes, obesity, or hypertension).[100]

Drug therapy in children is not recommended until the age of 10 years or older and the guidelines for initiation of therapy and acceptable levels of cholesterol and lipoproteins are quite different than adults.[100] Children younger than 10 years should only receive drug therapy if they have a genetic lipid disorder (ie, FH) or high-risk ASCVD condition (ie, diabetes); these children should be referred to a pediatric lipid specialist.[100] Lifestyle interventions are generally the mainstay of therapy, yet children with FH will often require drug therapy. Rosuvastatin may be used in children with HoFH at age 7. Pravastatin, pitavastatin, and rosuvastatin may be used in children as young as 8 years, while all other statins are indicated for use in children 10 years of age and older.[100] Start with the lowest available statin dose and titrate every 3 months as necessary to achieve treatment goals. Appropriate contraception strategies are recommended in females taking statins who are sexually active. Ezetimibe and BAS also have data suggesting that they are safe and effective to use in children aged 10 years or older. Now, evolocumab is the only PCSK9 inhibitor with safety and efficacy data in children aged 13 years or older with HoFH.[101] The safety and efficacy of fibrates and omega-3 PUFA have not been established.

Women

The leading cause of death in women is ASCVD and as many women as men die of ASCVD annually. This is mostly due to a longer average life expectancy and a higher lifetime risk of ischemic stroke than men.[102] Age is an important factor when estimating cardiovascular risk in women as most ASCVD events occur in postmenopausal women. The decline in estrogen levels that occurs during menopause is associated with increased cardiovascular risk, yet hormone replacement therapy is not recommended as studies have shown it does not reduce cardiovascular risk.[103,104] Other age-related changes, including increases in blood pressure and LDL-C, play a significant role as well in both women and men. Women have been underrepresented in RCT of lipid-lowering therapies; however, a meta-analysis of 27 RCTs found that statin therapy is equally effective in men and women.[105] Nonstatin therapies also appear to be equally effective except for fenofibrate, which is associated with an increased ASCVD risk in women when combined with simvastatin.[106] This finding was not, however, observed in another RCT comparing fenofibrate to placebo.[107] The clinical significance of this subgroup finding remains unknown.

Pregnancy is associated with a progressive rise in cholesterol and TG levels, yet dietary therapy is the mainstay of treatment, with emphasis on maintaining a nutritionally balanced diet as per the needs of pregnancy.[108] If the patient is at high risk or has FH, a BAS may be considered during pregnancy since there is no systemic drug exposure.[108] In July 2021, the FDA recommended that statins no longer be considered contraindicated in pregnant patients, but may be used in select pregnant patients with a high risk of cardiovascular events. Most pregnant patients should still be advised to discontinue statin treatment; statin use while breast feedings is not recommended. Women of childbearing age who are on statin therapy and are sexually active should use a reliable form of contraception to prevent pregnancy. Women who plan to become pregnant should discontinue the statin 1 to 2 months before pregnancy is attempted. Ezetimibe and niacin are pregnancy category C drugs but no data are available in humans. Increased intake of omega-3 PUFA, particularly DHA, during pregnancy is important for fetal brain development; however, prescription omega-3 PUFA products are pregnancy category C.[109] There is no information on the safety of PCSK9 inhibitors in pregnant women.

Patients with Diabetes

Diabetes is a major risk factor for ASCVD and persons with type 1 or type 2 diabetes are at greater risk of morbidity and mortality following an ASCVD event.[17] The dyslipidemia commonly found in persons with diabetes is often characterized by hypertriglyceridemia, low HDL-C, and modestly elevated, but dense, LDL-C that are highly atherogenic.[110] Despite the modest elevation in LDL-C observed in these patients, statins are the first-line therapy given the significant body of evidence from RCT demonstrating that statins reduce ASCVD events and mortality in persons with diabetes.[17] However, the risk among those with diabetes who have no history of ASCVD is not homogenous, so the 10-year ASCVD-risk score may be used to determine the appropriate statin intensity (see Table 32-5 and Fig. 32-6).[17] High-intensity statin therapy is preferred in those with diabetes and a history of ASCVD (secondary prevention) given these patients are at high risk of recurrent ASCVD events.

The role of nonstatin therapies in persons with diabetes is complex but has become clearer in recent years. In the Improved Reduction of Outcomes: Vytorin Efficacy International Trial (IMPROVE-IT) the benefit of adding ezetimibe to simvastatin was significantly enhanced in those with diabetes compared to patients without diabetes.[111] The addition of evolocumab to background statin therapy in the Further Cardiovascular Outcomes Research with PCSK9 Inhibition in Subjects with Elevated Risk (FOURIER) trial was equally effective in those with, and without, diabetes.[112] Given the mixed dyslipidemia associated with diabetes, there has been considerable interest in the potential of fibrates to reduce ASCVD risk. However, in the Action to Control Cardiovascular Risk in Diabetes (ACCORD), the combination of fenofibrate and a statin in patients with type 2 diabetes did not reduce the rate of fatal cardiovascular events, nonfatal myocardial infarction, or nonfatal stroke compared to simvastatin alone.[106] Subgroup analyses from two RCTs have suggested a potential benefit with fenofibrate in those with TG levels >204 mg/dL (2.31 mmol/L) and HDL-C <34 mg/dL (0.88 mmol/L), but this has not been evaluated in a prospective RCT.[106,107] Additionally, fenofibrate reduces the progression of diabetic retinopathy, as well as the need for laser treatment.[113] The BAS colesevelam is FDA-approved to improve both glycemic and lipid control, but it can exacerbate hypertriglyceridemia, which is commonly observed in those with diabetes.[55] Niacin modestly increases fasting plasma glucose (~4%-5%) and HbA1c levels (~0.25%).[92] As such, niacin should not be routinely used in persons with diabetes especially given the lack of evidence to support its use.

Patients with Kidney Disease

Dyslipidemia is highly prevalent among patients with kidney disease.[114] The dyslipidemia pattern in patients with kidney disease includes hypertriglyceridemia, slightly elevated total cholesterol, and LDL-C and low HDL-C levels.[114] These abnormalities are thought to be caused by a deficiency in apolipoprotein C-II, perhaps as a result of sustained use of heparin during hemodialysis and depletion of LPL, carbohydrate-induced obesity and hypertriglyceridemia, loss of carnitine during hemodialysis, use of acetate buffer (acetate is a precursor to fatty acid synthesis) during hemodialysis, and decreased LCAT activity during hemodialysis.[115] Dialysis does not correct the lipid abnormalities. Renal transplantation may correct lipid abnormalities in some patients; however, in others, the use of transplantation-related medications such as corticosteroids and cyclosporine may aggravate lipid abnormalities.[115]

Statins effectively reduce LDL-C in patients with kidney disease, yet the cardiovascular event reduction is less robust in patients with kidney disease.[114] Notably, rosuvastatin failed to prevent cardiovascular events in an RCT of patients undergoing hemodialysis suggesting statins should not be initiated in this population.[116] Statins are generally continued, however, in patients who are on statins before progressing to end-stage renal disease and requiring dialysis.[114] Moderate-intensity statins are generally preferred in patients with kidney disease to minimize the risk of adverse effects (ie, SAMS).[114] Kidney transplant recipients are at considerably high risk of future cardiovascular events and should receive statin therapy; however, appropriate statin selection is important given the potential for drug-drug interactions with antirejection therapies (ie, cyclosporine).[114] Ezetimibe may also be used in combination with statin therapy based on RCT evidence showing that this combination reduces cardiovascular events compared to placebo in patients at various stages of advanced kidney disease.[117] Current guidelines do not advocate for routine use of other nonstatin therapies, given the paucity of efficacy data and safety concerns.[114]

Patients with Chronic Inflammatory Disorders and HIV

It is well established that chronic inflammation and immune activation occur with chronic inflammatory disorders (eg, rheumatoid arthritis, lupus) and human immunodeficiency virus (HIV) and this accelerates the development and progression of atherosclerosis. These nontraditional risk factors are not included in the ASCVD-risk estimator, but they should be considered when assessing individual ASCVD risk. After a 3- to 6-month trial of lifestyle interventions, these patients should have their 10-year ASCVD risk estimated. In those with a 10-year ASCVD risk of 5% or greater, it is reasonable to initiate moderate-intensity statin therapy.

In addition to considering statin therapy, there are additional considerations with the treatments used for chronic inflammatory disorders and HIV. Long-term use of antiretroviral therapy, for example, mediates atherosclerosis progression and development in patients with HIV. Many antiretrovirals (eg, protease inhibitors) can significantly increase TG levels. Anti-inflammatory therapies (eg, tociluzimab, methotrexate) used in the management of rheumatoid arthritis have produced mixed results in terms of their effects on lipid levels and ASCVD risk.

EVALUATION OF THERAPEUTIC OUTCOMES

Short-term evaluation of therapy for dyslipidemia is based on a complete lipid panel obtained 4 to 12 weeks after initiation or following a dose adjustment of lipid-lowering therapy to evaluate therapeutic response.[17] This is especially important with statin therapy given there are numerous pharmacokinetic and pharmacodynamic differences among statins that give rise to variable response to therapy.[118] Long-term evaluation is based on a repeat lipid panel obtained every 3 to 12 months to ensure adherence to lipid-lowering therapy and maintenance of desired levels of LDL-C.[17] It should be noted that although total cholesterol (TC) HDL-C, and TG levels are directly measured, LDL-C is typically estimated using the Friedewald equation, LDL-C = TC – HDL-C – (TG/5) (or LDL-C = TC – HDL-C – [TG/2.2] when lipid levels are all expressed in mmol/L), which does not provide an accurate estimate of VLDL-C.[119] As such, the Friedewald equation can underestimate LDL-C in patients with high TG levels as well as those with very low LDL-C levels. Given VLDL-C concentrations are typically small in comparison to LDL-C, the inaccuracy of VLDL-C has previously been accepted. However, given the increased prevalence of obesity, metabolic syndrome, and diabetes, more patients have elevated levels of VLDL-C. Useful alternatives in these patients include apoB, non-HDL-C (TC minus HDL-C), and direct LDL-C measurements, which are more accurate than estimated LDL-C using the Friedewald equation.[119] A nonfasting lipid panel is generally acceptable, except in patients with hypertriglyceridemia, where a fasting lipid panel is preferred to minimize interference from chylomicrons.[120] Routine safety monitoring of hepatic function and CK levels is not recommended in statin-treated patients, but these may be obtained if the patient has signs or symptoms suggestive of liver or muscle injury.[17] Patients taking niacin, on the other hand, should have hepatic function tests performed at baseline, after each dosage increase, and every 6 months thereafter while taking a stable dose.[17] Periodic monitoring of A1c is warranted in persons with diabetes receiving niacin and patients treated with statins who are at high risk for developing diabetes.[17]

In patients treated with lipid-lowering therapy for secondary prevention, symptoms such as angina or intermittent claudication may improve over months to years. If patients have xanthomas or other external manifestations of dyslipidemia, these lesions should regress with therapy.[50] Modifiable risk factors such as hypertension, smoking, exercise and weight control, and glycemic control in persons with diabetes should also be monitored and evaluated.[17,27] Dietary therapy is an important part of treating dyslipidemia and a dietitian should be consulted to perform an initial evaluation with periodic follow-up thereafter if the goals of therapy are not achieved.[24] Use of food diaries and recall surveys enable the collection of information about diet in a systematic manner and may improve patient adherence to dietary recommendations.

ABBREVIATIONS

ACL	adenosine triphosphate-citrate lyase
Apo	apolipoprotein
ASCVD	atherosclerotic cardiovascular disease
ALT	alanine transaminase
ANGPTL3	angiopoietin-like 3
AST	aspartate transaminase
ATP	adenosine triphosphate
BASs	bile acid sequestrants
BMI	body mass index
BUN	blood urea nitrogen
CE	cholesterol ester
CETP	cholesterol ester transfer protein
CHD	coronary heart disease
CKD	chronic kidney disease
CVD	cardiovascular disease
DHA	docosahexaenoic acid
EPA	eicosapentaenoic acid
HbA1c	glycosylated hemoglobin A1c
HDL-C	high-density lipoprotein-cholesterol
HIV	human immunodeficiency virus
HMG-CoA	β-hydroxy β-methylglutaryl coenzyme A
HTN	hypertension
IDL-C	intermediate-density lipoprotein-cholesterol
LCAT	lecithin-cholesterol acyltransferase
LDL-C	low-density lipoprotein-cholesterol
LPL	lipoprotein lipase
LRP	LDL-receptor-related protein
NPC1L1	Niemann-Pick C1-like1
OTC	over-the-counter
PCOS	polycystic ovarian syndrome
PSCK9	proprotein convertase subtilisin/kexin type 9
PUFA	polyunsaturated fatty acid
RCT	randomized controlled trial
SAMS	statin-associated muscle symptoms
T2DM	type 2 diabetes mellitus
TC	total cholesterol
TG	triglyceride
TSH	thyroid-stimulating hormone
UA	urinalysis
VLDL-C	very-low-density lipoprotein-cholesterol

REFERENCES

1. Wiggins BS, Saseen JJ. *Pharmacist's Guide to Lipid Management*. 2nd ed. Lenexa, KS: American College of Clinical Pharmacy; 2014.
2. Expert Panel on Detection, Evaluation, and Treatment of High Blood Cholesterol in Adults. Executive Summary of the Third Report of the National Cholesterol Education Program (NCEP). (Adult Treatment Panel III). *JAMA*. 2001;285:2486–2497.
3. Grundy SM, Cleeman JI, Merz CN, et al. Implications of recent clinical trials for the national cholesterol education program adult treatment panel III guidelines. *Circulation*. 2004;110:227–239.
4. Smith SC Jr, Allen J, Blair SN, et al. AHA/ACC guidelines for secondary prevention for patients with coronary and other atherosclerotic vascular disease: 2006 Update: Endorsed by the National Heart, Lung, and Blood Institute. *Circulation*. 2006;113:2363–2372.
5. Stone NJ, Robinson JG, Lichtenstein AH, et al. 2013 ACC/AHA guideline on the treatment of blood cholesterol to reduce atherosclerotic cardiovascular risk in adults: A report of the American College of Cardiology/American Heart Association Task Force on Practice Guidelines. *J Am Coll Cardiol*. 2014;63(25 Pt B):2889–2934.
6. Mosca L, Banka CL, Benjamin EJ, et al. Evidence-based guidelines for cardiovascular disease prevention in women: 2007 Update. *Circulation*. 2007;115:1481–1501.
7. Fletcher B, Berra K, Ades P, et al. Managing abnormal blood lipids: A collaborative approach. *Circulation*. 2005;112:3184–3209.
8. Yuan G, Al-Shali KZ, Hegele RA. Hypertriglyceridemia: Its etiology, effects, and treatment. *CMAJ Can Med Assoc J*. 2007;176:1113–1120.
9. Mckenney JM, Sica D. Prescription omega-3 fatty acids for the treatment of hypertriglyceridemia. *Am J Health Syst Pharm*. 2007;64:595–605.
10. Oh RC, Lanier JB. Management of hypertriglyceridemia. *Am Fam Physician*. 2007;75:1365–1371.
11. Mckenney J. New perspectives on the use of niacin in the treatment of lipid disorders. *Arch Intern Med*. 2004;164:697–705.
12. Colhoun HM, Betteridge DJ, Durrington PN, et al. Primary prevention of cardiovascular disease with atorvastatin in type 2 diabetes in the Collaborative Atorvastatin Diabetes Study (CARDS): Multicentre randomised placebo-controlled trial. *Lancet*. 2004;364:685–696.
13. Collins R, Armitage J, Parish S, et al. Heart protection study collaborative G. effects of cholesterol-lowering with simvastatin on stroke and other major vascular events in 20536 people with cerebrovascular disease or other high-risk conditions. *Lancet*. 2004;363:757–767.
14. Ford ES, Mokdad AH, Giles WH, Mensah GA. Serum total cholesterol concentrations and awareness, treatment, and control of hypercholesterolemia among US adults: Findings from the National Health and Nutrition Examination Survey, 1999 to 2000. *Circulation*. 2003;107(17):2185–2189.
15. Pirillo A, Casula M, Olmastroni E, Norata GD, Catapano AL. Global epidemiology of dyslipidaemias. *Nat Rev Cardiol*. 2021;18(10):689–700.
16. Foley Ka, Denke MA, Kama-Bahl S, et al. The impact of physician attitudes and beliefs on treatment decisions: Lipid therapy in high-risk patients. *Med Care*. 2006;44:421–428.
17. Grundy SM, Stone NJ, Bailey AL, et al. 2018 AHA/ACC/AACVPR/AAPA/ABC/ACPM/ADA/AGS/APhA/ASPC/NLA/PCNA guideline on the management of blood cholesterol: A report of the American College of Cardiology/American Heart Association Task Force on Clinical Practice Guidelines. *J Am Coll Cardiol*. Nov 2018;1097:S1. doi:10.1016/j.jacc.2018.11.003.
18. Menotti A, Lanti M, Nedeljkovic S, et al. The relationship of age, blood pressure, serum cholesterol, and smoking habits with the risk of typical and atypical coronary heart disease death in the European Cohorts of seven countries study. *Int J Cardiol*. 2006;106:157–163.
19. Stone NJ. Secondary causes of hyperlipidemia. *Med Clin North Am*. 1994;78:117–141.
20. Yuan F, Wang J, Hegele RA. Heterozygous familial hypercholesterolemia: An underrecognized cause of early cardiovascular disease. *CMAJ*. 2006;174:1124–1129.
21. Libby P. How our growing understanding of inflammation has reshaped the way we think of disease and drug development. *Clin Pharmacol Ther*. 2010;87:389–391.
22. Scheel P, Meyer J, Blumenthal RS, Martin SS. Lipoprotein(a) in Clinical Practice—American College of Cardiology. Published 2019. Available at https://www.acc.org/Latest-in-Cardiology/Articles/2019/07/02/08/05/Lipoproteina-in-Clinical-Practice. Accessed October 11, 2021.
23. Wilson DP, Jacobson TA, Jones PH, et al. Use of Lipoprotein(a) in clinical practice: A biomarker whose time has come. A scientific statement from the National Lipid Association. *J Clin Lipidol*. 2019;13(3):374–392. doi:10.1016/j.jacl.2019.04.010.
24. Eckel RH, Jakicic JM, Ard JD, et al. 2013 AHA/ACC guideline on lifestyle management to reduce cardiovascular risk. *J Am Coll Cardiol*. 2014;53(25):2960–2984.
25. Whelton PK, Carey RM, Aronow WS. 2017 ACC/AHA/AAPA/ABC/ACPM/AGS/APhA/ASPC/NMA/PCNA guideline for the prevention, detection, evaluation, and management of high blood pressure in adults. *J Am Coll Cardiol*. 71(19):e127–e248. doi:10.1016/j.jacc.2017.11.006.
26. American Diabetes Association. 2018 Standards of Medical Care in Diabetes. *Diabetes Care*. 2018.
27. Goff DC, Lloyd-Jones DM, Bennett G, et al. 2013 ACC/AHA guideline on the assessment of cardiovascular risk: A report of the American College of Cardiology/American Heart Association Task Force on Practice Guidelines. *J Am Coll Cardiol*. 2014;63(25):2935–2959.
28. Navarese EP, Robinson JG, Kowalewski M, et al. Association between baseline LDL-C level and total and cardiovascular mortality after LDL-C lowering: A systematic review and meta-analysis. *JAMA*. 2018;319(15):1566–1579.
29. Cholesterol Treatment Trialists Collaboration. Efficacy and safety of more intensive lowering of LDL cholesterol: A meta-analysis of data from 170,000 participants in 26 randomised trials. *Lancet*. 2010;376:1670–1681.
30. Downs JR, Clearfield M, Weis S, et al. Primary prevention of acute coronary events with lovastatin in men and women with

average cholesterol levels: Results of AFCAPS/TexCAPS. Air Force/Texas Coronary Atherosclerosis Prevention Study. *JAMA.* 1998;279(20):1615–1622.

31. Sabatine MS, Giugliano RP, Keech AC, et al. Evolocumab and clinical outcomes in patients with cardiovascular disease. *N Engl J Med.* 2017;376(18):1713–1722.
32. Yusuf S, Bosch J, Dagenais G, et al. Cholesterol lowering in intermediate-risk persons without cardiovascular disease. *N Engl J Med.* 2016;374(21):2021–2031.
33. Lloyd-Jones DM, Morris PB, Ballantyne CM, et al. 2017 Focused update on the 2016 ACC expert consensus decision pathway on the role of non-statin therapies for LDL-Cholesterol lowering in the management of atherosclerotic cardiovascular disease risk. *J Am Coll Cardiol.* 2017;70(14):1785–1822.
34. MRC/BHF Heart Protection Study of cholesterol lowering with simvastatin in 20,536 high-risk individuals: A randomised placebo-controlled trial. *Lancet.* 2002;360(9326):7–22. 12114036.
35. Cannon CP, Blazing MA, Giugliano RP, et al. Ezetimibe added to statin therapy after acute coronary syndromes. *N Engl J Med.* 2015;372:2387–2397.
36. Ridker PM, Danielson E, Fonseca FAH, et al. Rosuvastatin to prevent vascular events in men and women with elevated C-reactive protein. *N Engl J Med.* 2008;359(21):2195–2207.
37. Shepherd J, Blauw GJ, Murphy MB, et al. Pravastatin in elderly individuals at risk of vascular disease (PROSPER): A randomised controlled trial. *Lancet (London, England).* 2002;360(9346):1623–1630.
38. LaRosa JC, Grundy SM, Waters DD, et al. Intensive lipid lowering with atorvastatin in patients with stable coronary disease. *N Engl J Med.* 2005;352(14):1425–1435.
39. U.S. Department of Health and Human Services and U.S. Department of Agriculture. *2015–2020 Dietary Guidelines for Americans.* 8th ed. December 2015. Available at:http://health.gov/dietaryguidelines/2015/guidelines.
40. Hoy MK, Goldman JD. Fiber intake of the U.S. population: What we eat in America, NHANGES 2009–2010. Food Surveys Research Group Dietary Data Brief No. 12. September 2014.
41. Mozaffarian D, Rimm EB. Fish intake, contaminants and human health: Evaluating the risks and benefits. *JAMA.* 2006;296(15):1885–1899.
42. Aung T, Halsey J, Kromhout D, et al. Associations of omega-3 fatty acid supplement use with cardiovascular disease risks: Meta-analysis of 10 trials involving 77,917 individuals. *JAMA Cardiol.* 2018;3(3):225–234.
43. Siscovick DS, Barringer TA, Fretts AM, et al. Omega-3 polyunsaturated fatty acid (Fish Oil) supplementation and the prevention of clinical cardiovascular disease: A science advisory from the American Heart Association. *Circulation.* 2017;135:e867–e884.
44. Bowman L, Mafham M, Wallendszus K, et al. ASCEND Study Collaborative Group. Effects of n-3 fatty acid supplements in diabetes mellitus. *N Engl J Med.* 2018;379(16):1540–1550.
45. Yoo EG. Sitosterolemia: A review and update of pathophysiology, clinical spectrum, diagnosis, and management. *Ann Pediatr Endocrinol Metab.* 2016;21(1):7–14.
46. Cohen PA, Avula B, Khan IA. Variability in strength of red yeast rice supplements purchased from mainstream retailers. *Eur J Prev Cardiol.* 2017;24(13):1431–1434.
47. Dujovne CA. Red yeast rice preparations: Are they suitable substitutions for statins? *Am J Med.* 2017;130(10):1148–1150.
48. Baigent C, Keech A, Kearney PM, et al. Efficacy and safety of cholesterol-lowering treatment: Prospective meta-analysis of data from 90,056 participants in 14 randomized trials of statins. *Lancet.* 2005;366:1267–1278.
49. Ference BA, Ginsberg HN, Graham I, et al. Low-density lipoproteins cause atherosclerotic cardiovascular disease. 1. Evidence from genetic, epidemiologic, and clinical studies. A consensus statement from the European Atherosclerosis Society Consensus Panel. *Eur Heart J.* 2017;38(32):2459–2472.
50. Robinson JG, Goldberg AC. Treatment of adults with familial hypercholesterolemia and evidence for treatment: Recommendations from the National Lipid Association Expert Panel on Familial Hypercholesterolemia. *J Clin Lipidol.* 2011;5:S18–S29.
51. Hopkins PN, Toth PP, Ballantyne CM. Rader DJ national lipid association expert panel on familial hypercholesterolemia. Familial hypercholesterolemias: Prevalence, genetics, diagnosis and screening recommendations from the National Lipid Association Expert Panel on Familial Hypercholesterolemia. *J Clin Lipidol.* 2011;5(3 Suppl):S9–S17.
52. Dixon DL, Sisson EM, Butler M, et al. Lomitapide and mipomersen: Novel lipid-lowering therapies for the management of familial hypercholesterolemia. *J Cardiovasc Nurs.* 2014;29(5):E7–E12.
53. Raal FJ, Rosenson RS, Reeskamp LF, et al. Evinacumab for homozygous familial hypercholesterolemia. *N Engl J Med.* 2020;383(8):711–720.
54. Miller M, Stone NJ, Ballantyne C, et al. Triglycerides and cardiovascular disease: A scientific statement from the American Heart Association. *Circulation.* 2011;123(20):2292–2333.
55. Jacobson TA, Ito MK, Maki KC, et al. National lipid association recommendations for patient-centered management of dyslipidemia: Part 1—full report. *J Clin Lipidol.* 2015;9:129–169.
56. Virani SS, Morris PB, Agarwala A, et al. 2021 ACC expert consensus decision pathway on the management of ASCVD risk reduction in patients with persistent hypertriglyceridemia: A report of the American College of Cardiology solution set oversight committee. elevated triglycerides (150–499 mg/dL). *J Am Coll Cardiol.* 2021;78(9):960–993.
57. Toth PP, Barter PJ, Rosenson RS, et al. High-density lipoproteins: A consensus statement from the National Lipid Association. *J Clin Lipidol.* 2013;7(5):484–525.
58. Landray MJ, Haynes R, Hopewell JC, et al. HPS2-THRIVE Collaborative Group. Effects of extended-release niacin with laropiprant in high-risk patients. *N Engl J Med.* 2014;371(3):203–212.
59. Boden WE, Probstfield JL, Anderson T, et al. AIM-HIGH Investigators. Niacin in patients with low HDL cholesterol levels receiving intensive statin therapy. *N Engl J Med.* 2012;365(24):2255–2267.
60. Schachter M. Chemical, pharmacokinetics and pharmacodynamic properties of statins: An update. *Fundam Clin Pharmacol.* 2005;19(1):117–125.
61. Tobert JA, Newman CB. Statin tolerability: In defense of placebo-controlled trials. *Eur J Prev Cardiol.* 2016;23:891–896.
62. Thompson PD, Panza G, Zaleski A, Taylor B. Statin-associated side effects. *J Am Coll Cardiol.* 2016;67(20):2396–2410.
63. Zanger UM, Schwab M. Cytochrome P450 enzymes in drug metabolism: Regulation of gene expression, enzyme activities, and impact of genetic variation. *Pharmacol Ther.* 2013;138(1):103–141.
64. Wiggins BS, Saseen JJ, Page RL, et al. Recommendations for management of clinically significant drug-drug interactions with statins and select agents used in patients with cardiovascular disease. *Circulation.* 2016;134(21):e468–e495.
65. Rosenson RS, Baker SK, Jacobson TA, et al. An assessment by the statin muscle safety task force: 2014 Update. *J Clin Lipidol.* 2014;8(3):S58–S71.
66. Preiss D, Seshasai SR, Welsh P, et al. Risk of incident diabetes with intensive-dose compared with moderate-dose statin therapy: A meta-analysis. *JAMA.* 2011;305:2556–2564.
67. Sattar N, Preiss D, Murray HM, et al. Statins and risk of incident diabetes: A collaborative meta-analysis of randomised statin trials. *Lancet.* 2010;375:735–742.
68. Ridker PM, Pradhan A, MacFadyen JG, et al. Cardiovascular benefits and diabetes risks of statin therapy in primary prevention: An analysis from the JUPITER trial. *Lancet.* 2012;380(9841):565–571.
69. Ezetimibe (Zetia®) [package insert]. Whitehouse Station, NJ: Merck & Co., Inc; 2007.
70. The Myocardial Infarction Genetics Consortium Investigators. Inactivating mutations in NPC1L1 and protection from coronary heart disease. *N Engl J Med.* 2014;371:2072–2082.
71. The lipid research clinics coronary primary prevention trial results. I. Reduction in incidence of coronary heart disease. *JAMA.* 1984;251(3):351–364.
72. Brunetti L, DeSantis EH. Patient tolerance and acceptance of colesevelam hydrochloride: Focus on type-2 diabetes mellitus. *Pharmacy and Therapeutics.* 2015;40(1):62–67.
73. Fonseca VA, Handelsman Y, Staels B. Coleseveal lowers glucose and lipid levels in type 2 diabetes: The clinical evidence. *Diabetes Obes Metab.* 2010;12(5):384–392.
74. Schwartz GG, Steg PG, Szarek M, et al. Alirocumab and cardiovascular outcomes after acute coronary syndrome. *N Engl J Med.* November 29, 2018;379(22):2097–2107.
75. Giugliano RP, Mach F, Zavitz K, et al. Cognitive function in a randomized trial of evolocumab. *N Engl J Med.* 2017;377:633–643.
76. Giugliano RP, Pedersen TR, Park JG, et al. Clinical efficacy and safety of achieving very low LDL-cholesterol concentrations with the PCSK9 inhibitor evolocumab: A prespecified secondary analysis of the FOURIER trial. *Lancet.* 2017;390:1692–1671.
77. Markham A Bempedoic acid: First approval. *Drugs.* 2020;80(7):747–753. doi:10.1007/s40265-020-01308-w32314225.
78. Ballantyne CM, Banach M, Mancini GBJ. Efficacy and safety of bempedoic acid added to ezetimibe in statin-intolerant patients with hypercholesterolemia: A randomized, placebo-controlled study. *Atherosclerosis.* 2018;277:195–203. doi:10.1016/j.atherosclerosis.2018.06.00229910030.

79. Fenofibrate (Tricor®) [package insert]. North Chicago, IL: Abbott Laboratories; 2010.
80. Mychaleckyj JC, Craven T, Nayak U, et al. Reversibility of fenofibrate therapy-induced renal function impairment in ACCORD type 2 diabetic participants. *Diabetes Care.* 2012;35(5):1008–1014.
81. Caroli-Bosc FX, Le Gall P, Pugliese P, et al. Role of fibrates and HMG-CoA reductase inhibitors in gallstone formation. *Digestive Diseases and Sciences*. 2001;46(3):540–544.
82. Dixon DL, Williams VG. Interaction between gemfibrozil and warfarin: Case report and review of the literature. *Pharmacotherapy.* 2009;29(6):744–748.
83. Bradberry JC, Hilleman DE. Overview of omega-3 fatty acid therapies. *Pharmacy and Therapeutics*. 2013;38(11):681–691.
84. Bhatt DL, Steg PG, Miller M, et al. Cardiovascular risk reduction with icosapent ethyl for hypertriglyceridemia. *N Engl J Med.* 2019;380(1):11–22. doi:10.1056/NEJMoa1812792.
85. Nicholls SJ, Lincoff AM, Garcia M, et al. Effect of high-dose omega-3 fatty acids vs corn oil on major adverse cardiovascular events in patients at high cardiovascular risk: The STRENGTH randomized clinical trial. *JAMA.* 2020;324(22):2268–2280.
86. Lombardi M, Carbone S, Del Buono MG, et al. Omega-3 fatty acids supplementation and risk of atrial fibrillation: An updated meta-analysis of randomized controlled trials. *Eur Hear Journal Cardiovasc Pharmacother.* 2021;7(4):e69–e70.
87. Kastelein JJP, Maki KC, Susekov A, et al. Omega-3 free fatty acids for the treatment of severe hypertriglyceridemia: The EpanoVa fOr Lowering Very high triglyceridEs (EVOLVE) trial. *J Clin Lipidol.* 2014;8(1):94–106.
88. Bays HE, Ballantyne CM, Kastelein JJ, Isaacsohn JL, Braeckman RA, Soni PN. Eicosapentaenoic acid ethyl ester (AMR101) therapy in patients with very high triglyceride levels (from the Multi-center, plAcebo-controlled, randomized, double-blINd, 12-week study with an open-label extension [MARINE] trial). *Am J Cardiol.* 2011;108(5):682–690.
89. Manson JE, Cook NR, Lee I-M, et al. Marine n−3 fatty acids and prevention of cardiovascular disease and cancer. *N Engl J Med.* 2018;380(1):23–32.
90. Harris WS, Ginsberg HN, Arunakul N, et al. Safety and efficacy of Omacor in severe hypertriglyceridemia. *J Cardiovasc Risk.* 1997;4(5-6):385–391.
91. Jacobson TA. A "Hot" topic in dyslipidemia management—"How to Beat a Flush": Optimizing niacin tolerability to promote long-term treatment adherence and coronary disease prevention. *Mayo Clin Proc.* 2010;85(4):365–379.
92. Goldberg RB, Jacobson TA. Effects of niacin on glucose control in patients with dyslipidemia. *Mayo Clin Proc.* 2008 Apr;83(4):470–478.
93. Salem CB, Slim R, Fathallah N, Hmouda H. Drug-induced hyperuricemia and gout. *Rheumatology.* 2017;56(5):679–688.
94. Dixon DL, Donohoe KL, Ogbonna KC, Barden SM. Current drug treatment of hyperlipidemia in older adults. *Drugs Aging.* 2015;32:127–138.
95. Giral P, Neumann A, Weill A, Coste J. Cardiovascular effect of discontinuing statins for primary prevention at the age of 75 years: A nationwide population-based cohort study in France. *Eur Heart J.* 2019;40(43):3516–3525.
96. Ridker PM, Lonn E, Paynter NP, et al. Primary prevention with statin therapy in the elderly: New meta-analyses from the contemporary JUPITER and HOPE-3 randomized trials. *Circulation.* 2017;135(20):1979–1981.
97. Swiger KJ, Manalac RJ, Blumenthal RS, et al. Statins and cognition: A systematic review and meta-analysis of short- and long-term cognitive effects. *Mayo Clin Proc.* 2013;88(11):1213–1221.
98. Ott BR, Daiella LA, Dahabreh IJ, et al. Do statins impair cognition? A systematic review and meta-analysis of randomized controlled trials. *J Gen Intern Med.* 2015;30(3):348–358.
99. Yu S, Chu Y, Li G, et al. Statin use and the risk of cataracts: A systematic review and meta-analysis. *J Am Heart Assoc.* 2017;6(3):pii: e004180. doi:10.1161/JAHA.116.004180.
100. Expert Panel on Integrated Guidelines for Cardiovascular Health and Risk Reduction in Children and Adolescents, National Heart, Lung, and Blood Institute. Expert panel on integrated guidelines for cardiovascular health and risk reduction in children and adolescents: Summary report. *Pediatrics.* 2011;128(suppl 5):S213–S256.
101. Evolocumab (Repatha®) [package insert]. Thousand Oaks, CA: Amgen; 2015.
102. Benjamin EJ, Virani SS, Callaway CW, et al. Heart disease and stroke statistics—2018 update: A report from the American Heart Association. *Circulation.* 2018;137(12):e67–e492.
103. Manson JE, Hsia J, Johnson KC, et al. Estrogen plus progestin and the risk of coronary heart disease. *N Engl J Med.* 2003;349:523–534.
104. Hulley S, Grady D, Bush T, et al. For the heart and estrogen/progestin replacement study (HERS) research group. Randomized trial of estrogen plus progestin for secondary prevention of coronary heart disease in postmenopausal women. *JAMA.* 1998;280:605–613.
105. Cholesterol Treatment Trialists Collaboration. Efficacy and safety of LDL-lowering therapy among men and women: Meta-analysis of individual data from 174 000 participants in 27 randomised trials. *Lancet.* 2015;385:1397–1405.
106. Ginsberg HN, Elam MB, Lovato LC, et al. Effects of combination lipid therapy in type 2 diabetes mellitus. *N Engl J Med.* 2010;362:1563–1574.
107. Keech A, Simes RJ, Barter P, et al. Effects of long-term fenofibrate therapy on cardiovascular events in 9795 people with type 2 diabetes mellitus (the FIELD study): Randomised controlled trial. *Lancet.* 2005;366(9500):1849–1861.
108. Wild R, Weedin EA, Wilson D. Dyslipidemia in pregnancy. *Cardiol Clin.* 2015;33:209–215.
109. Coletta JM, Bell SJ, Roman AS. Omega-3 fatty acids and pregnancy. *Rev Obstet Gynecol.* 2010;3(4):163–171.
110. Goldberg IJ. Diabetic dyslipidemia: Causes and consequences. *J Clin Endocrinol Metab.* 2001;86(3):965–971.
111. Giugliano RP, Cannon CP, Blazing MA, et al. Benefit of adding ezetimibe to statin therapy on cardiovascular outcomes and safety in patients with versus without diabetes mellitus: Results from IMPROVE-IT (Improved Reduction of Outcomes: Vytorin Efficacy International Trial). *Circulation.* 2018;137(151):1571–1582.
112. Sabatine MS, Leiter LA, Wiviott SD, et al. Cardiovascular safety and efficacy of the PCSK9 inhibitor evolocumab in patients with and without diabetes and the effect of evolocumab on glycaemia and risk of new-onset diabetes: A prespecified analysis of the FOURIER randomised controlled trial. *Lancet Diabetes Endocrinol.* 2017;5(12):941–950.
113. Chew EY, Ambrosius WT, Davis MD, et al. Effects of medical therapies on retinopathy progression in type 2 diabetes. *N Engl J Med.* 2010;363(3):233–244.
114. Kidney Disease: Improving Global Outcomes (KDIGO) Lipid Work Group. Clinical practice guidelines for lipid management in CKD: Summary of recommendation statements and clinical approach to the patient. *Kindey Int Suppl.* 2013;3(3):259–305.
115. Vaziri ND. Dyslipidemia of chronic renal failure: The nature, mechanisms, and potential consequences. *Am J Physiol Renal Physiol.* 2006;290(2):F262–F272.
116. Fellstrom BC, Jardine AG, Schmieder RE, et al. Rosuvastatin and cardiovascular events in patients undergoing hemodialysis. *N Engl J Med.* 2009;360:1395–1407.
117. Baigent C, Landray MJ, Reith C, et al. The effects of lowering LDL cholesterol with simvastatin plus ezetimibe in patients with chronic kidney disease (study of heart and renal protection): A randomized placebo-controlled trial. *Lancet.* 2011;377(9784):2181–2192.
118. Karlson BW, Wiklund O, Palmer MK, et al. Variability of low-density lipoprotein cholesterol response with different doses of atorvastatin, rosuvastatin, and simvastatin: Results from VOYAGER. *Eur Heart J Cardiovasc Pharmacother.* 2016;2(4):212–217.
119. Martin SS, Blaha MJ, Elshazly MB, et al. Friedewald-estimated versus directly measured low-density lipoprotein cholesterol and treatment implications. *J Am Coll Cardiol.* 2013;62(8):732–739.
120. Nordestgaard BG, Langsted A, Mora S, et al. Fasting is not routinely required for determination of a lipid profile: Clinical and laboratory implications including flagging at desirable concentration cut-points—a joint consensus statement from the European Atherosclerosis Society and European Federation of Clinical Chemistry and Laboratory Medicine. *Eur Heart J.* 2016;37(25):1944–1958.

Stable Ischemic Heart Disease

33

Paul P. Dobesh, Robert J. DiDomenico, and Kelly C. Rogers

KEY CONCEPTS

1. Stable ischemic heart disease (SIHD) is caused by an obstructive atherosclerotic plaque in one or more epicardial coronary arteries. Increases in myocardial oxygen demand in the setting of a fixed decrease in myocardial oxygen supply result in myocardial ischemia. Some patients with SIHD may have a component of vasospasm that requires a slightly different pharmacologic approach.
2. Chest pain (angina) from exertion is the cardinal symptom of myocardial ischemia in patients with SIHD.
3. Assessment of successful treatment of angina includes reducing the number of episodes, enabling patients to participate in activities that provide a high-level quality of life, and decreasing mortality by using guideline-directed medical therapy (GDMT).
4. Management of modifiable atherosclerotic risk factors is key to improving the quantity of life in patients with SIHD.
5. Aspirin, angiotensin-converting enzyme inhibitors, and statins play an important role in preventing adverse cardiovascular events in patients with SIHD.
6. β-Blockers are typically regarded as first-line therapy in the management and control of episodes of angina in patients with SIHD.
7. Calcium channel blockers, long-acting nitrates, and ranolazine are often used as additional therapies for angina. Calcium channel blockers and nitrates are first-line therapies in vasospastic disease.
8. All patients with SHID should receive sublingual nitroglycerin for acute treatment and should receive education regarding its proper use.
9. Revascularization procedures may provide a survival advantage over GDMT in SIHD patients with more extensive atherosclerotic disease but have not demonstrated a clear advantage over GDMT in those with less extensive disease. Antithrombotic therapy is necessary after revascularization for a variable duration of time.

BEYOND THE BOX

To better understand the normal physiology of the heart and the pathophysiology of coronary artery disease (CAD), please watch the following videos. These videos are useful to enhance learner's understanding regarding the COLLECT and ASSESS steps in the Patient Care Process.

1. Pathophysiology of CAD—What is Coronary Artery Disease? Khan Academy: https://tinyurl.com/y3cjyb8v (Duration: 13:38 minutes)
2. Myocardial oxygen supply—University of British Columbia, UBC Anesthesiology: https://tinyurl.com/yxjouoh3 (Duration: 4:59 minutes)
3. Myocardial oxygen demand—University of British Columbia, UBC Anesthesiology: https://tinyurl.com/y5488brm (Duration: 4:37 minutes)

INTRODUCTION

Coronary artery disease (CAD) is the leading cause of ischemic heart disease and is typically the result of atherosclerotic plaques in the epicardial vessels. The process of atherosclerosis begins early in life, with fatty steaks developing in many people in their teenage years or early twenties. These plaques grow over decades and start to become pathologic in a person's fifth decade of life and beyond. In addition to CAD, atherosclerosis also manifests in other vascular beds leading to cerebrovascular disease (Stroke, Chapter 39) and peripheral arterial disease (Chapter e35). Ischemic heart disease may present as an acute coronary syndrome (ACS) (Chapter 34), which includes unstable angina, non-ST-segment myocardial infarction (MI), or ST-segment elevation MI. While the pathophysiology is similar, stable ischemic heart disease (SIHD) is not an acute event but rather manifests as either chronic stable exertional angina or ischemia without clinical symptoms (silent ischemia). Less common causes of SIHD include microvascular angina, which is due to atherosclerosis in endocardial instead of epicardial vessels. Microvascular angina is more common in women and those with metabolic syndrome. Coronary vasospasm represents a form of angina that results from an increase in coronary vascular tone that can occur in either normal or diseased vessels. Prinzmetal's angina is a form of vasospastic angina that does not involve atherosclerotic plaque. Inappropriate, insufficient, or untreated SIHD can lead not only to MI and cardiac death, but also to the development of heart failure (HF), arrhythmias, and valvular disease. The American College of Cardiology (ACC) and American Heart Association (AHA) have published guidelines for the diagnosis and management of SIHD.[1]

EPIDEMIOLOGY

According to AHA statistics, in 2018, an estimated 126.9 million (49%) adult Americans had at least one form of cardiovascular disease (CVD), which includes CAD, HF, stroke, and hypertension (HTN).[2] Among patients with CVD, approximately 20.1 million adult Americans had CAD, corresponding to an estimated prevalence of 7.2%. The prevalence of CAD increases with age and is higher in men. Among patients with CAD, the total number of patients with SIHD is difficult to determine. Statistics from the AHA estimate that approximately 11 million Americans have angina pectoris while the prevalence of MI among adult Americans is approximately 8.8 million, together approximating the prevalence of CAD.[2] Stable angina is the initial manifestation of ischemic heart disease in approximately one-half of all patients who eventually have an MI.

The mortality and costs associated with CAD are enormous. In 2018, CVD was the number one cause of death in the United States with CAD being the most common cause of CVD death, accounting for almost 400,000 deaths—42% of all CVD-related mortality.[2] Adjusting for age, death rates per 100,000 are highest among black patients compared to those of white and Hispanic ancestry and among men compared to women within each racial demographic. The estimated direct and indirect cost of CAD was $220 billion in 2016-2017, with direct healthcare spending of $89 billion.[2]

The prognosis of patients with SIHD is related to the extent of atherosclerotic disease, the presence of left ventricular (LV) dysfunction, and the presence of other comorbidities. The severity of angina symptoms may also be useful in determining the prognosis.[3] In a study of veterans with CAD, the risk of death increased with the degree of self-reported physical limitation due to angina.[4] It is thought that the degree of physical limitation reflects the extent of underlying atherosclerotic disease. In addition to mortality, SIHD leads to significant morbidity. Most patients will eventually need to be hospitalized for ACS. Patients often have a reduced quality of life due to their inability to perform activities of daily living without chest pain.[5,6] Time lost from work and lost productivity have a large indirect cost to patients and society. Approximately 15% to 20% of patients rate their health as fair or poor despite revascularization, and 30% of patients are never able to return to work.[7]

ETIOLOGY AND PATHOPHYSIOLOGY

1 Angina pectoris is most often the result of an imbalance between myocardial oxygen supply and myocardial oxygen demand (MVO_2). The process of maintaining adequate coronary blood flow to meet the metabolic demands of the myocytes is complex. Multiple factors influence the supply/demand equation.

The pathophysiology of SIHD is driven by an increase in MVO_2 in the setting of a fixed decrease in myocardial oxygen supply.[8] The etiology of the fixed decrease in supply is long-standing, well-developed atherosclerotic plaque. These plaques grow over several decades. The extent and rate of growth are related to risk factors such as smoking, dyslipidemia, HTN, diabetes mellitus (DM), and genetics. The process and development of atherosclerosis are detailed in Chapter 32 (Dyslipidemia). Unlike ACS, the episodes of angina in patients with SIHD are not caused by ruptured atherosclerotic plaque, which leads to thrombus formation and a rapid reduction in coronary blood flow.[9,10] Rather, the atherosclerotic plaques are stable, have a reduced lipid core, and a firm calcified covering. Since the vessel lumen size does not acutely change, the atherosclerotic plaque produces a relatively fixed decrease in myocardial oxygen supply.

Determinants of Myocardial Oxygen Demand

The major determinants of MVO_2 include heart rate (HR), myocardial contractility, and intramyocardial wall tension. A twofold increase in any of these determinants requires an approximate 50% increase of coronary flow to maintain the myocardial oxygen supply. Intramyocardial wall tension is the leading contributor to increased MVO_2 and is directly related to the radius or size of the ventricular cavity and blood pressure (BP), and indirectly related to the ventricular muscle mass. The larger the size of the ventricular cavity, the more energy or myocardial work is needed for myocardial contraction (systole). During early systole, myocardial work peaks when the pressure in the LV overcomes the pressure outside the aortic valve. The aortic valve is then pushed open and blood is ejected into the systemic circulation. The higher the blood pressure outside the aortic valve, the more MVO_2 needed. Increased ventricular muscle mass should make myocardial work easier and reduce MVO_2. For example, some athletes have increased ventricular muscle mass and their heart works more efficiently. Unfortunately, left ventricular hypertrophy results in dysfunctional myocytes that do not improve MVO_2. Left ventricular hypertrophy can worsen the supply/demand balance because the blood vessel development (supply) is less than the native myocardium.

The rate-pressure product, or double product, is a common non-invasive measure of MVO_2. To determine the rate-pressure product, multiply the HR and systolic BP. However, changes in contractility or volume loading of the LV are not accounted for in this calculation. An increase in MVO_2 requirements commonly stems from the release of norepinephrine by adrenergic nerve endings in the myocardium and vascular bed as part of the physiologic response to exertion, emotion, or mental stress. The rate of increase of MVO_2, which correlates to the speed at which a physical task is carried out, can be as important as the total amount of MVO_2. A rapid increase in physical exertion is particularly likely to precipitate angina. Tasks involving motion of the hands over the head can also provoke chest pain. Mental and emotional stress may precipitate angina, presumably by increasing adrenergic tone and reducing vagal activity. Sexual activity may precipitate angina due to the combination of physical exertion and emotional stimulation. Similarly, anger can produce constriction of coronary arteries. Other precipitates of angina include physical exertion after a heavy meal and excessive metabolic demands imposed by chills, fever, exposure to cold, thyrotoxicosis, hypoglycemia, and other causes of tachycardia.

Determinants of Myocardial Oxygen Supply

Coronary Blood Flow

Meeting the metabolic demands of the myocardium is centered on the ability to maintain adequate coronary blood flow and coronary arterial pressure. The coronary vasculature is made up of larger epicardial vessels, also referred to as R_1 or conductance vessels, and smaller endocardial vessels called R_2 or resistance vessels (Fig. 33-1).[11] Resistance to coronary blood flow is the sum of the resistance in the R_1 and R_2 vessels. The larger epicardial vessels typically offer little resistance to blood flow and can accommodate large increases in coronary blood flow without producing a significant change in pressure. These vessels primarily serve a conduit function. In healthy coronary arteries, resistance to flow is controlled by smaller endocardial (R_2) vessels. These vessels will contract and dilate to maintain blood flow based on the metabolic demands of the myocardium. When a person is at rest or not engaged in physical activity, MVO_2 is low and endocardial vessels constrict. The need for blood flow is low. When there is physical exertion or emotional stress, MVO_2 increases and the endocardial vessels dilate to increase myocardial oxygen supply in proportion to the increase in MVO_2 (Fig. 33-1). The process of constricting and dilating the resistance vessels based on MVO_2 is called autoregulation.[8,11] In response to increased MVO_2, several vasodilatory substances (eg, nitric oxide, prostacyclin, and bradykinin) are secreted and this can increase coronary blood flow four- to fivefold over normal resting conditions.[8] The increase in coronary flow above resting conditions is the coronary flow reserve.

Coronary atherosclerotic plaques typically develop in the larger epicardial vessels. As plaques grow and cause luminal narrowing,

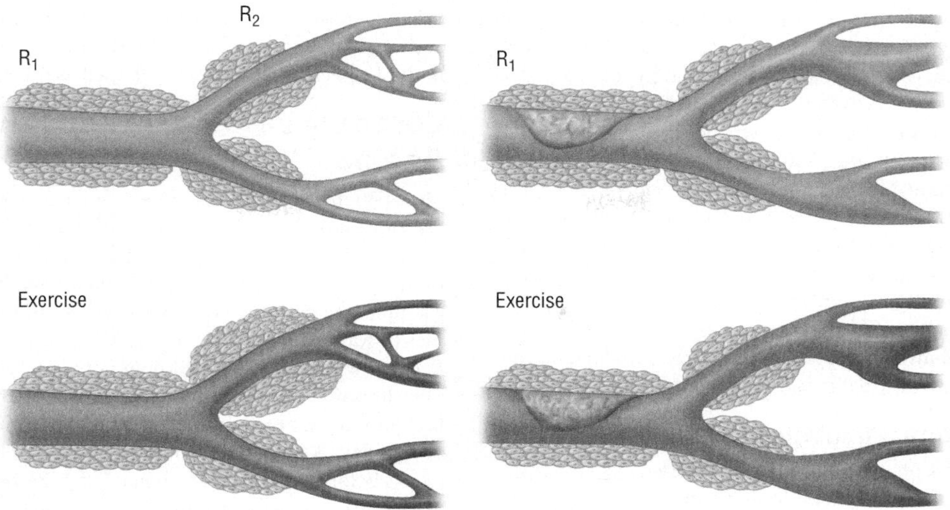

FIGURE 33-1 The coronary circulation with large epicardial conductance vessels (R_1) and intramyocardial resistance arterioles (R_2). Resistance to flow equals $R_1 + R_2$. R_2 resistance is normally much greater than R_1; hence, flow is equal to the driving pressure across the coronary bed divided by the resistance in R_2. Dilation in R_2 normally occurs in response to exercise or increased myocardial oxygen demand. When an atherosclerotic lesion narrows the conductance vessel, the arterioles dilate under resting conditions to prevent ischemia. However, during the period of exertion, the vasodilator reserve is limited. *(Reproduced from Epstein SE, O'Cannon R, Talbot TL. Hemodynamic principles in the control of coronary blood flow. Am J Cardiol. 1985;56:4E-10E.)*

resistance to blood flow in epicardial vessels transforms from minimal to considerable. This continues to a point where the resistance from the epicardial vessels becomes dominant. Through autoregulation, the increase in resistance from the R_1 or conductance vessels is offset by vasodilation in the R_2 or resistance vessels to maintain flow.[11]

The luminal diameter occupied by the atherosclerotic plaque determines the drop in pressure and blood flow distal to the stenosis. The most important determinant of resistance for any given level of flow is the minimum stenosis cross-sectional area.[8] Because resistance is inversely proportional to the square of the cross-sectional area, small dynamic changes in the luminal area caused by atherosclerotic plaque size, thrombus creation, or vasospasm can lead to large changes in the stenosis pressure-flow relationship and reduce maximal perfusion during vasodilation.[8]

Coronary plaques that occupy less than 50% to 70% of the vessel luminal diameter are often referred to as "non-obstructive". They rarely produce ischemia or angina.[11] These smaller plaques do not produce symptoms, and therefore, the patient and clinician typically have no idea they exist. Small plaques have a rich lipid core and thin fibrous cap, they are more prone to rupture and provoke acute thrombus formation, making them potentially lethal (see Chapter 34 "Acute Coronary Syndrome").[9,10]

Once the epicardial vessel is narrowed by 70% or more of the luminal diameter, the endocardial vessels must fully dilate in order to maintain normal coronary flow. These larger plaques are considered "obstructive."[8,11] At this point, much of the coronary flow reserve has been used to preserve resting coronary blood flow and minimal physical exertion exhausts any remaining capacity. Further increases in exercise intensity are no longer accompanied by decreases in endocardial (R_2) resistance. Blood flow cannot increase to accommodate the demand and autoregulation has reached its ceiling. The resulting flow deficit causes myocardial ischemia and, frequently, angina. The amount of exertion a patient can endure is largely based on the extent of vessel stenosis and the remaining coronary flow reserve. The endocardial flow reserve is exhausted when the epicardial stenosis severity exceeds 90%. Narrowing of the luminal diameter by 90% or more is called a critical stenosis.

Heart Rate and Systole

Increasing HR not only increases MVO_2 but also reduces myocardial oxygen supply. While most tissues and organs are perfused during systole, the heart is the only organ that is perfused during diastole, the phase of myocardial relaxation. There are two physiologic explanations.[8] First, the pressure created in the ventricles during systole creates an increase in pressure in the coronary circulation well above the pressure for coronary perfusion (50-60 mm Hg). Only during diastole do the pressures drop sufficiently to allow coronary flow. Second, the physical compression force of the myocardium that occurs during systole squeezes the coronary vessels closed, preventing blood flow. During a typical cardiac cycle with a normal resting HR, the myocardium spends twice as much time in diastole compared to systole. When the HR increases, time spent in diastole is reduced while time in systole remains relatively unchanged. During times of exertion and increased HR, the ratio of time spent in diastole to systole is reduced from 2:1 to as little as 1:1. This reduces the time for myocardial perfusion, and thus, myocardial oxygen supply is significantly diminished.[8]

Oxygen Extraction and Oxygen Carrying Capacity

Two additional determinants of myocardial oxygen supply are myocardial oxygen extraction and oxygen-carrying capacity. The oxygen-carrying capacity of the coronary arteries is relatively fixed under normal circumstances and not capable of changing in response to increased MVO_2. Therefore, during exertion, the ability to increase oxygen delivery to myocytes is limited mainly through increasing oxygen extraction from the arterial blood. However, this compensatory mechanism provides little additional oxygen as myocardial arterial oxygen extraction is already approximately 75% under normal circumstances.[12]

Arterial oxygen content is related to hemoglobin concentration and oxygen saturation. Consequently, patients with anemia (low hemoglobin) or hypoxia (low oxygen saturation) have lower than normal oxygen-carrying capacity. Anemia is thought to impact total oxygen-carrying capacity to a greater degree than hypoxia until the oxygen saturation falls below 50% (0.50). This explains why patients with SIHD often require transfusions when hemoglobin concentrations fall below 9 to 10 g/dL (90-100 g/L; 5.59-6.21 mmol/L), whereas patients without SIHD can tolerate hemoglobin concentrations as low as 6 g/dL (60 g/L; 3.72 mmol/L). Most patients have arterial oxygen saturation between 95% and 100% (0.95 and 1.0) so oxygen therapy would not improve oxygen delivery. Therefore, there is little opportunity to improve myocardial oxygen supply by improving myocardial oxygen extraction or oxygen-carrying capacity, leaving increased myocardial blood flow as the principal mechanism for increasing myocardial oxygen supply.

Coronary Collateral Circulation

In the setting of SIHD, preexisting collateral vessels develop in a process termed arteriogenesis. When coronary stenosis exceeds 70%, endocardial vessel pressure falls due to maximized autoregulation. This extent of stenosis also contributes to the severity and duration of the episodes of exertion-induced ischemia. The ischemic episodes stimulate nitric oxide synthase and lead to the production of vascular endothelial growth factor and basic fibroblast growth factor. The combination of altered coronary pressure, growth factors, and endogenous vasodilators (eg, nitrous oxide and prostacyclin) change native collateral vessels in existing epicardial anastomoses into mature vessels.[13] While most functional collateral flow develops from the process of arteriogenesis, collateral perfusion can also occur from the development of new collateral vessels in a process called angiogenesis. The process of angiogenesis is also driven by physical forces and growth factors but produces smaller, capillary-like vessels. These vessels can provide collateral flow in the border between ischemic and nonischemic regions of the myocardium.[13] Capillary angiogenesis may also occur within the ischemic region and can reduce the intercapillary distance for oxygen delivery.

Other Factors

While atherosclerotic coronary stenosis is the leading etiology in the development of SIHD and angina, there are additional pathophysiologic mechanisms that also contribute to disease onset and progression. These mechanisms include endothelial dysfunction, microvascular dysfunction, vasospasm, platelet activation, and coagulation, as well as inflammation.[13] A reduction in nitric oxide-mediated vasodilation leads to endothelial dysfunction. This can be due to impaired nitric oxide synthesis or availability. Reduced vasodilator response may lead to ischemia at lower levels of exertion. There can also be impairments that reduce microvascular response to endogenous vasodilators or exaggerate the response to vasoconstrictors.[13]

Patients with an ACS event have ruptured atherosclerotic plaque with platelet accumulation and coagulation response producing an acute reduction in myocardial oxygen supply.[9,10] While this is not the pathophysiology of ischemia in patients with SIHD, there can be smaller plaques (30%-50% stenosis) that rupture and produce a limited platelet and coagulation response that does not produce an acute compromise in myocardial oxygen supply. Instead, the thrombotic process is arrested and the thrombus undergoes re-endothelialization.[9] This greatly accelerates plaque accumulation. Finally, inflammation plays a role in the pathophysiology of SIHD. Macrophages and T lymphocytes produce and secrete cytokines, chemokines, and growth factors that activate endothelial cells, increase vasoreactivity, and proliferation of vascular smooth muscle cells.[13,14] C-reactive protein, a marker of inflammation, has been shown to be elevated in patients with SIHD and correlates to adverse CV events. Statin therapy in patients with elevated C-reactive protein and normal cholesterol levels reduces the risk of CV events.[15]

While an obstructive atherosclerotic plaque contributes to ischemia and angina in patients with SIHD, the pathophysiology involves multiple mechanisms that can be used as therapeutic targets.

Coronary Vasospasm and Prinzmetal's Angina

Most patients with SIHD have an obstructive coronary stenosis and exertion-induced ischemia. Since the size of the obstructive lesion does not change acutely, the amount of exertion needed to induce ischemia and angina is often predictable in an individual patient. For example, the patient knows that working in the garden for 20 minutes or walking five blocks at a certain pace will produce chest pain. Patients with this pattern of angina have a fixed angina threshold. The threshold of angina varies in some patients. In these patients, the amount of exertion needed to provoke chest pain differs from day-to-day. An example would be the patient who could walk six blocks before experiencing angina yesterday, but today they can only walk one block before becoming symptomatic. These patients have an obstructing atherosclerotic plaque leading to a fixed decrease in myocardial oxygen supply, but also have transient vasospasm superimposed at the site of the obstructing plaque.[11,13] The vasospasm at or distal to the location of atherosclerotic plaque is typically induced by endothelial damage. Damaged endothelial cells produce less than normal amounts of vasodilator substances such as endothelium-derived relaxing factor (EDRF) and often have an exaggerated response to vasoconstrictors during exercise.[13] Symptoms will differ based on the extent of the underlying fixed obstruction and the degree of dynamic change in coronary arterial tone. The changing pattern of ischemia in these patients reflects varying amounts of vasospasm. Angina episodes are typically more common in the morning hours due to the circadian release of vasoconstrictors. Exposure to cold temperature, emotion, and mental stress may also lower the angina threshold in patients with variable threshold angina.

Some patients have variant angina, also known as Prinzmetal's angina. Patients with variant angina usually do not have flow-obstructing atherosclerotic plaques in their coronary arteries, but instead, have vasospasm in epicardial vessels.[8,13] The vasospasm is due to the reduced production of vasodilators and an exaggerated response to endogenous vasoconstrictors. Patients with Prinzmetal's angina also have a different clinical presentation when compared to patients with SIHD due to an obstructive coronary plaque. Patients with Prinzmetal's angina are typically younger, may experience chest pain at rest, often in the early morning, and have transient ST-segment elevation on the electrocardiogram (ECG).

CLINICAL PRESENTATION

2 A thorough patient history is key to the clinical assessment of a patient with SIHD. Exertional chest pain is the classic presenting symptom of patients with SIHD. The differential diagnosis of "chest pain" is broad (Table 33-1). Therefore, it is important to determine if symptoms are due to cardiac or noncardiac pathology. The patient's description of chest pain can be helpful in determining if the pain is more likely SIHD or ACS. The PQRST pneumonic is commonly used when conducting the patient interview to gather important aspects of the chest pain story (Table 33-2).

The chest pain in a patient with SIHD is often precipitated by exertion, such as walking, gardening, sexual activity, or activities of daily living such as showering, cleaning the house, or doing laundry. In this setting, the exertion produces an increase in MVO_2 that exceeds what can be provided by the fixed decrease in myocardial oxygen supply from the obstructive atherosclerotic plaque. Typically, rest or the use of sublingual (SL) nitroglycerin relieves the symptoms. As the patient rests for a few minutes, the HR and

CLINICAL PRESENTATION Stable Ischemic Heart Disease (SIHD)

General

- The patient is not typically in acute distress; however, careful assessment to identify features consistent with ACS is important.

Symptoms

- The classic symptom of ACS is abrupt-onset substernal chest pain or discomfort often described as a squeezing, heaviness, or tightness (Table 33-1). Symptoms may radiate to the arms, shoulders, back, abdomen, or jaw. Nausea, vomiting, diaphoresis, or shortness of breath may also be present.
- The PQRST pneumonic (Table 33-2) is useful for structuring the patient interview to assess the history of chest pain.
- Evaluation of symptoms should include an evaluation of the limitations in daily activities due to angina (eg, CCS classification, see Table 33-3).

Signs

- BP may be elevated in patients with SIHD
- No physical findings are specific for SIHD. Nonspecific findings include S4 or paradoxical splitting of S2 on auscultation.
- Patients with SIHD may present with signs of HF, including jugular venous distention, pulmonary edema, and an S3 on auscultation.

Laboratory Tests

- Cardiac troponin (cTn, either cTnI or cTnT) are not typically elevated in patients with SIHD.
- Fasting lipid panel should be evaluated to assess for the presence of dyslipidemia.
- C-reactive protein may be obtained but is more valuable as a screening tool to detect CAD rather than guide treatment decisions.

Other Diagnostic Tests

- A 12-lead ECG should be obtained in a patient with symptoms of SIHD. However, it is often normal in patients with SIHD.
- Exercise stress testing is a noninvasive test to detect CAD in patients presenting with symptoms of SIHD.
- Coronary angiography is often performed in patients with a high likelihood of SIHD (eg, "positive" exercise stress test) to detect the presence and extent of CAD.
- Other diagnostic tests may be used in select patients to detect CAD or assess for progression of disease and include myocardial perfusion imaging, cardiac magnetic resonance, "ultra-fast computed tomography (CT)," and CT angiography.

TABLE 33-1 Differential Diagnosis of Episodic Chest Pain Resembling Angina Pectoris

	Duration	Quality	Provocation	Relief	Location	Comment
Effort angina	5-15 minutes	Visceral (pressure)	During effort or emotion	Rest, nitroglycerin	Substernal, radiates	First episode vivid
Rest angina	5-15 minutes	Visceral (pressure)	Spontaneous	Nitroglycerin	Substernal, radiates	Often nocturnal
Mitral prolapse	Minutes to hours	Superficial (rarely visceral)	Spontaneous (no pattern)	Time	Left anterior	No pattern, variable
Esophageal reflux	10 minutes to 1 hour	Visceral	Spontaneous, cold liquids, exercise, lying down	Foods, antacids, H_2 blockers, proton pump inhibitors, nitroglycerin	Substernal, radiates	Mimics angina
Peptic ulcer	Hours	Visceral, burning	Lack of food, "acid" foods	Foods, antacids, H_2 blockers, proton pump inhibitors	Epigastric, substernal	
Biliary disease	Hours	Visceral (wax and wane)	Spontaneous, food	Time, analgesia	Epigastric, radiates	Colic
Cervical disk	Variable (gradually subsides)	Superficial	Spontaneous, food	Time, analgesia	Arm, neck	Not relieved by rest
Hyperventilation	2-3 minutes	Visceral	Emotion, tachypnea	Stimulus removed	Substernal	Facial paresthesia
Musculoskeletal	Variable	Superficial	Movement, palpation	Time, analgesia	Multiple	Tenderness
Pulmonary	Minutes to hours	Visceral (pressure)	Often spontaneous	Rest, time bronchodilator	Substernal	Dyspneic

BP come down, re-establishing a balance between myocardial oxygen supply and demand, relieving their chest pain. The use of SL nitroglycerin provides acute relief by increasing myocardial oxygen supply through vasodilation of epicardial vessels and a reduction in preload.

Cardiac chest pain is often described as squeezing, crushing, heaviness, or tightness in the chest. It can also be described as numbness or burning in the chest. Chest pain that is described as sharp, increases with inspiration or expiration, or is reproducible with palpation is less likely to be cardiac in origin. The pain is often substernal

TABLE 33-2 PQRST Approach to Assessment of a Patient's Chest Pain

Factor	Presentation in Stable Ischemic Heart Disease	Questions to Ask
Precipitating factors	Typically brought on by some level of exercise or exertion	What were you doing when the pain started? What brought on this chest pain?
Palliative measures	Relieved by rest with or without sublingual nitroglycerin in 5-10 minutes	Is there anything that helps the pain go away? If you rest, does the pain get better? Does your sublingual nitroglycerin help?
Quality of the pain	Described as a continuous squeezing, heaviness, or tightness	How would you describe the pain? Does the pain change when you breathe in and out?
Region	Substernal	Where is the pain located? Can you point to where the pain seems to originate?
Radiation	Left or right arm, back, down into the abdomen, up into the neck	Does the pain seem to radiate or go to other locations?
Severity	While pain is subjective, those who have pain report a 5 or higher on a 10-point scale	On a scale from 1 to 10, with 1 being no pain, and 10 being the worst pain you have ever had, how would you rate this pain?
Temporal pattern (timing)	Pain lasts less than 20 minutes and is usually relieved in 5-10 minutes	How long did the pain last? How long before the pain went away? After you started to rest, how long before the pain went away?

and may radiate to the right or left shoulder, right or left arm (left more commonly than right), neck, back, or abdomen. Cardiac chest pain rarely radiates above the mandible (jaw) or below the umbilicus (belly button). The severity of cardiac chest pain can be difficult to quantify since pain is subjective, but most patients will state the pain is severe and rate it five or higher on a 10-point scale. The duration of chest pain in patients with SIHD is less than 20 minutes, usually only 5 to 10 minutes. Other symptoms that may be present during times of ischemia include diaphoresis, nausea, vomiting, and dyspnea.

1 It is helpful to connect the pathophysiology with the clinical presentation. In SIHD, ischemia is produced by an increase in MVO_2 in the setting of a fixed decrease in supply. The exertion exhausts autoregulation and coronary flow reserve. The patient experiences chest pain. When the patient rests for 5 to 10 minutes or uses an SL nitroglycerin, the MVO_2 decreases to a point in which myocardial supply and demand are back in balance—the pain and other symptoms go away. The major differences between the pain with SIHD compared to ACS would be the precipitating factors and the duration of the chest pain. The patient with an ACS typically has angina at rest that lasts longer than 20 minutes. The pathophysiology in a patient with an ACS is an abrupt decrease in myocardial oxygen supply precipitated by a plaque rupture.

The severity of chest pain and the impact of SIHD on daily activities are often evaluated using the Canadian Cardiovascular Society (CCS) classification system (Table 33-3).[16] The CSS system evaluates the level of activity needed to produce angina. All the current severity scores are limited by the subjective nature of a patient's pain as well as the reliability and reproducibility of patient observations.

TABLE 33-3 Grading of Angina Pectoris by the Canadian Cardiovascular Society Classification System

Class	Description of Stage
Class I	Ordinary physical activity does not cause angina, such as walking and climbing stairs. Angina occurs with strenuous, rapid, or prolonged exertion at work or recreation
Class II	Slight limitation or ordinary activity. Angina occurs on walking or climbing stairs rapidly, on walking uphill, on walking or stair climbing after meals, in cold, in wind, under emotional stress, or only during the few hours after awakening. Walking more than two blocks on the level and climbing more than one flight of ordinary stairs at a normal pace and in normal condition
Class III	Marked limitations of ordinary physical activity. Angina occurs on walking one to two blocks on the level and climbing one flight of stairs in normal conditions and at a normal pace
Class IV	Inability to carry on any physical activity without discomfort—anginal symptoms may be present at rest

Reproduced from Campeau L. Grading of angina pectoris. *Circulation* 1976;54:522-523.

Not all patients have a typical chest pain presentation.[1] "Typical" angina is comprised of three components: (1) substernal chest discomfort with a characteristic quality and duration, which is (2) provoked by exertion or emotional stress, and (3) relieved by rest or nitroglycerin. Patients with "atypical" angina meet two of the three criteria. Patients meeting one or none of the typical angina characteristics likely have non-cardiac causes of chest pain. Patient groups more likely to present with atypical angina include women and older patients. Patients with DM may also have decreased sensation of pain due to neuropathy.[13] Features of atypical angina or angina equivalents include symptoms such as midepigastric discomfort, effort intolerance, dyspnea, and excessive fatigue. One study found that 65% of women with ischemia present with atypical symptoms.[17]

After a description of the chest pain has been obtained, a review of the patient's CAD risk factors should be performed. Nonmodifiable risk factors include the patient's age, sex, and a family history of premature atherosclerotic cardiovascular disease (ASCVD) in first-degree relatives (onset in a male before the age of 55 years or a female before the age of 65 years). Modifiable risk factors including HTN, DM, dyslipidemia, and cigarette smoking should also be explored. In addition to considering traditional risk factors, markers of inflammation, such as high sensitive C-reactive protein, may also be obtained. The evidence regarding the utility of C-reactive protein in the setting of primary prevention is growing but its value in guiding therapy in the setting of established CAD (secondary prevention) is less certain. Due to the systemic nature of atherosclerotic cardiovascular disease (ASCVD), patients with a history of cerebrovascular or peripheral arterial disease are also at high risk for CAD. It is likely that patients who have atherosclerosis in cerebral or peripheral arteries also have atherosclerosis in their coronary arteries even if it has not yet led to episodes of angina.

The physical examination of a patient with SIHD usually produces nonspecific findings. At the time of an angina episode, patients may have tachycardia, diaphoresis, and shortness of breath. Patients may also have symptoms of nausea, vomiting, and lightheadedness. Other physical findings may relate to cardiovascular risk factors including an increased BP or a fourth heart sound reflecting long-standing HTN. Other findings may include pulmonary crackles, a displaced point of maximal impulse, or a third heart sound in patients with HF with reduced ejection fraction (HFrEF).

Diagnostic and Prognostic Testing

Several noninvasive and invasive testing can be done to assist in the diagnosis and evaluation of patients with SIHD. A detailed

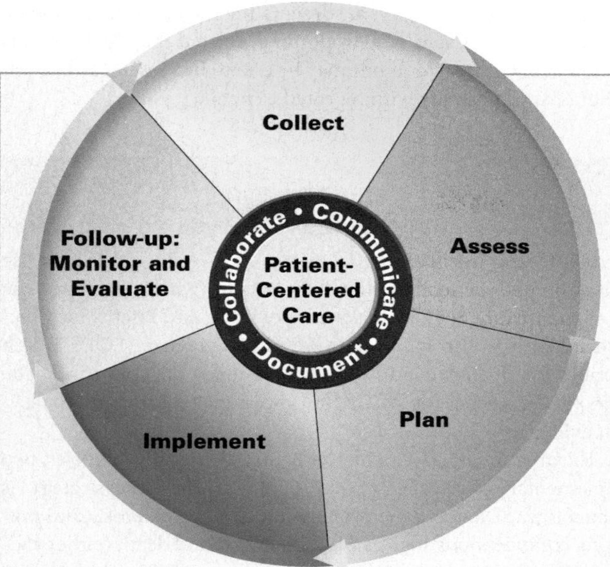

Patient Care Process for Stable Ischemic Heart Disease (SIHD)

The image shows the five fundamental steps included in The Pharmacist's Care Process endorsed by the Joint Commission for Pharmacy Practitioners (2014). The tagline of this process reads collaborate, communicate, and document. The five fundamental steps listed here are collect, assess, plan, implement, and follow-up: monitor and evaluate. All these steps are listed in a circular block diagram.

Collect

- Patient characteristics (eg, age, sex, pregnant)
- Description of chest discomfort and/or related symptoms (eg, precipitating factors, palliative measures, quality, location, radiation, and severity)
- Patient medical (personal and family) and social histories (eg, tobacco/ethanol use), dietary habits (eg, intake of foods high in sodium, cholesterol, and/or saturated fat), and physical activity (eg, frequency and duration of moderate-intensity aerobic activity)
- Current medications including over-the-counter (OTC) medications (eg, aspirin-containing medications), herbals/dietary supplements
- History of allergy or intolerance to previous medications
- Objective data
- Blood pressure (BP), heart rate (HR), respiratory rate (RR), height, weight, O_2-saturation
    - Labs: serum creatinine (SCr), potassium (K^+), hemoglobin (Hgb), platelets, liver function tests (LFTs), lipid profile, blood glucose, A1c
    - Diagnostic testing results

Assess

- Description of chest discomfort to determine differential diagnosis and classification of angina symptoms
- Presence of provoking factors (eg, exertion, mental/emotional stress, tachyarrhythmia, high adrenergic state including the use of stimulant medications, and exposure to cold)
- Presence/control of risk factors for SIHD (eg, hypertension, dyslipidemia, diabetes, smoking, and obesity)
- Presence/control of SIHD-related complications (eg, myocardial infarction [MI], heart failure [HF], and stroke)
- Adverse drug reactions from current/previous medications used to treat/prevent angina symptoms or major adverse cardiac events (MACE)
- Previous/recent revascularization procedures (eg, percutaneous coronary intervention [PCI] with/without stenting, and coronary artery bypass graft [CABG] surgery)
- Contraindications to medications to treat/prevent angina symptoms and/or prevent MACE
- Barriers that may impair adherence to the care plan

Plan*

- Initiate/modify drug therapy to treat and prevent angina symptoms, prevent MACE, and address risk factors for SIHD including specific drug(s), dose, route, frequency, and duration (see Fig. 33-2, Tables 32-6 and 32-7)
- Monitoring parameters: efficacy (eg, signs and symptoms of angina and SIHD-related complications) and adverse drug reactions; frequency and timing of follow-up
- Patient education: the purpose of treatment, lifestyle modifications, planned procedures, and drug-specific information (eg, indication, dose, route, frequency, adverse drug reactions; see Table 33-8)
- Self-monitoring for worsening angina symptoms, signs and symptoms of SIHD-related complications, adverse drug reactions, when to seek emergency medical attention
- Address barriers to adherence to medications and lifestyle modification
- Referrals to other providers (eg, primary care provider, endocrinologist, dietician, and smoking cessation)

Implement*

- Provide patient education regarding all elements of the treatment plan as described above
- Use motivational interviewing and coaching strategies to maximize adherence
- Schedule follow-up (eg, every 1-2 months until goals achieved, then every 6-12 months)

Follow-up: Monitor and Evaluate

- Frequency and severity of chest discomfort, sublingual nitroglycerin use, exercise tolerance, presence/control of SIHD risk factors, and presence/control of SIHD-related complications
- Presence of adverse drug reactions and drug-drug interactions
- Patient adherence to treatment plan using multiple sources of information

**Collaborate with the patient, caregivers, and other healthcare professionals.*

discussion of these tests and when they should be used can be found in the ACC/AHA SIHD guidelines.[1] More information on how each test is performed is available in Chapter e29, "Evaluation of Cardiovascular Function."

The results of cardiac testing can provide prognostic information, may help guide pharmacotherapy, and identify patients who need revascularization. All patients with angina symptoms should receive a 12-lead electrocardiogram (ECG). In the resting state, the ECG will be normal in ≥50% of patients with SIHD. In SIHD patients with a normal ECG at rest, about 50% will develop ischemic ST-T wave changes during an episode of angina. These changes can be observed on the ECG conducted during an exercise stress test. Exercise stress testing is a relatively easy and inexpensive method for detecting CAD. Since many patients cannot physically endure an exercise stress test, the myocardium can also be stressed pharmacologically with adenosine, regadenoson, dipyridamole, or dobutamine. Stress testing can provide important diagnostic and prognostic information, especially when conducted with a nuclear imaging study to evaluate myocardial perfusion.

Coronary angiography is the most accurate test for the diagnosis and assessment of patients with CAD and is considered the "gold standard." Unfortunately, coronary angiography is an invasive technique that requires arterial access. Coronary angiography in patients with SIHD routinely reveals that approximately 25% of patients have a single-vessel disease, 25% have double-vessel disease, and 25% have triple-vessel disease, with 5% to 10% presenting with left main coronary disease and another 15% with no detectable critical vessel obstruction.

Coronary angiography is also useful in determining the fractional flow reserve (FFR) in patients with obstructive coronary stenosis. FFR is an indirect index determined by measuring the driving pressure of microcirculatory flow distal to the area of stenosis relative to the coronary driving pressure available in the absence of stenosis.[18] The FFR is attractive for clinical use in that it can immediately assess the physiologic significance of intermediate stenosis to help guide decisions regarding coronary intervention. Moreover, the FFR is unaffected by alterations in resting flow. Data suggest that patients with an FFR of less than or equal to 0.80 may have a better outcome with a revascularization procedure compared to medical therapy, but more studies are needed to determine the best use of this index.[18,19]

Additional noninvasive diagnostic tests may be used to establish the diagnosis of CAD or follow the progression of disease in patients with SIHD. Myocardial perfusion imaging (eg, nuclear imaging studies) involves the administration of an intravenous radioactive tracer before and after a stressor (exercise or pharmacologic). The uptake of the radioactive tracer is proportional to coronary blood flow in normal myocytes and the resulting images can detect perfusion defects. Cardiac magnetic resonance combined with physiologic or pharmacologic stressors can also detect the presence of perfusion defects as well as wall motion abnormalities. Coronary artery calcium scoring using computed tomography (CT), often called "ultra-fast CT" or electron beam CT, multislice or multidetector CT, and CT angiography can also be used to detect the presence of CAD.

Biomarkers

Cardiac troponin concentrations are released with myocyte death (infarction) and hence are not typically elevated in patients with SIHD. A study of patients undergoing percutaneous coronary intervention (PCI) for the treatment of SIHD found that 6% of patients had an elevated troponin before PCI and these patients were more likely to have an MI or die in-hospital when compared to patients without an elevated troponin (13.4% vs 5.6%).[20] The differences in these outcomes were significant even after 1 year.[20] The study was conducted at multiple sites and, given the lack of a single reference range, no specific troponin value designating increased risk could be determined. The reasons why troponin predicted these outcomes is not completely understood but may be due to increased cardiac cell membrane permeability with repeated ischemia.

TREATMENT

Treatment recommendations from the ACC/AHA guidelines use a Class of Recommendation (COR) system, which estimates the size of the treatment effect, balancing efficacy, and safety. Each recommendation is also based on a Level of Evidence (LOE), which describes the quality, quantity, and consistency of supporting data. Table 33-4 describes the ACC/AHA recommendations and the levels of evidence.[1]

The treatment of patients with SIHD typically involves two complementary strategies.[1] See Fig. 33-2. The first strategy is directed toward slowing the progression of atherosclerosis and preventing complications such as MI, HF, stroke, and death (either sudden cardiac death or progression of underlying CVD). This strategy focuses on risk-factor modification and providing vasculoprotection therapies (see Table 33-5). While vasculoprotective therapies have demonstrated the ability to reduce mortality, and therefore, the quantity of life, they have minimal impact on improving symptoms and the functional limitations caused by angina, or the quality of life. The second strategy is focused on reducing the number of ischemic episodes as well as increasing the amount of exertion or exercise a patient can accomplish before chest pain occurs (see Table 33-6). Antianginal therapies used to prevent or decrease ischemic episodes rarely have demonstrated a survival benefit but improve quality of life through symptom reduction. Each of the antianginal therapies is relatively equivalent in its ability to reduce ischemic episodes.[21]

Desired Outcomes

4 In addition to reducing the risk of CV events and mortality, the ACC/AHA SIHD guidelines state that a goal of therapy should be the complete, or nearly complete, elimination of chest pain and return to normal activities with a functional capacity of CCS class I angina.[1]

Pharmacologic Therapy

Providing guideline-directed medical therapy (GDMT), also referred to as optimal medical therapy, reduces the risk of mortality

TABLE 33-4 The American College of Cardiology and American Heart Association Evidence Grading System

Recommendation Class	Level of Evidence
I. Conditions for which there is evidence or general agreement that a given procedure or treatment is useful and effective	A. Data derived from multiple randomized clinical trials with large numbers of patients
II. Conditions for which there is conflicting evidence or a divergence of opinion that the usefulness/efficacy of a given procedure or treatment is useful and effective a. The weight of evidence/opinion is in favor or usefulness/efficacy b. Usefulness/efficacy is less well established by evidence/opinion	B. Data derived from a limited number of randomized trials with small numbers of patients, careful analyses of nonrandomized studies, or observational registries C. Expert consensus was the primary basis for the recommendation
III. Conditions for which there is evidence or general agreement that a given procedure or treatment is not useful/effective and in some cases may be harmful	

Data from Reference 1.

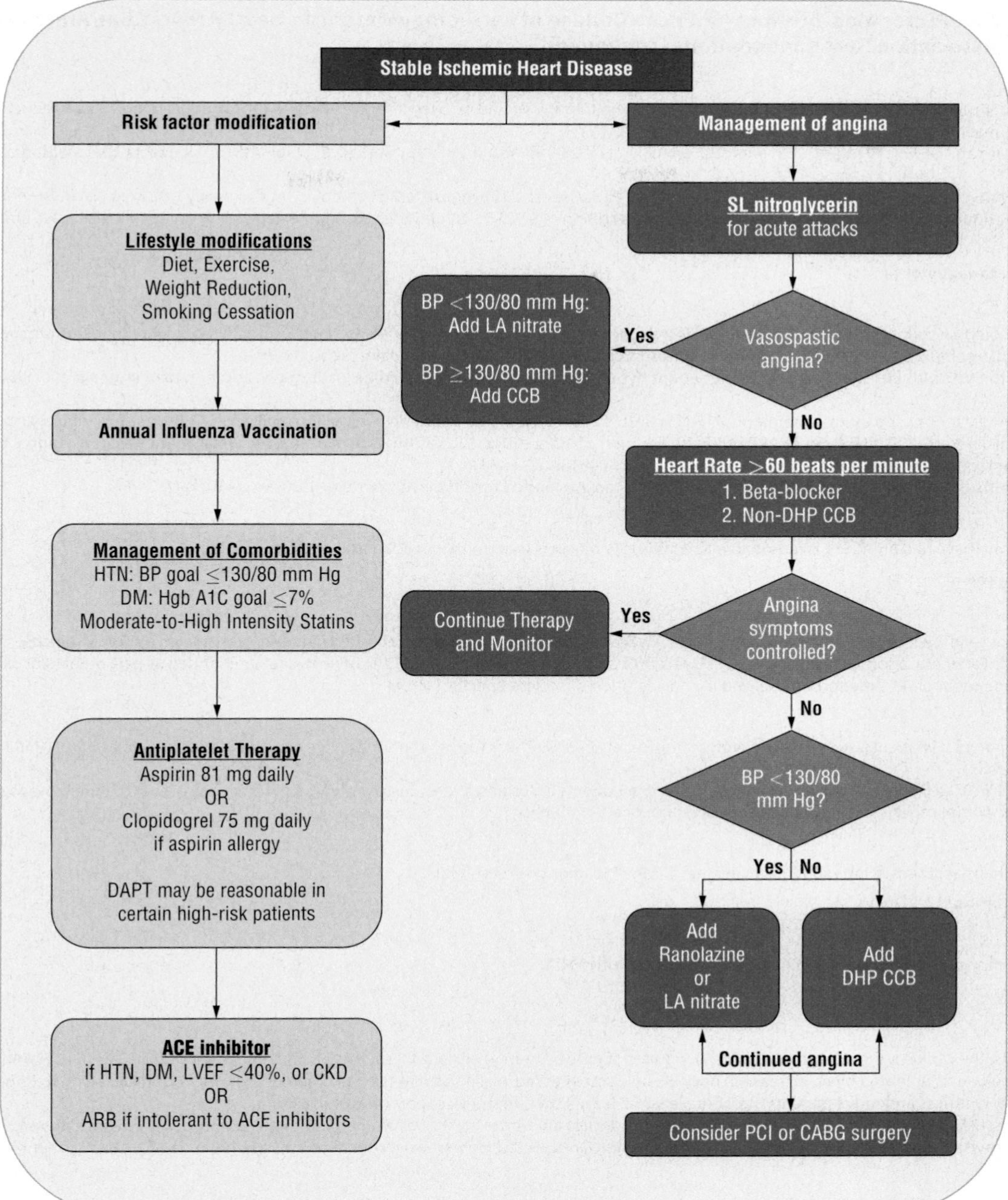

FIGURE 33-2 Treatment algorithm for stable ischemic heart disease (guideline-directed medical therapy). The Hgb A1c goal of ≤7% (0.07) is equivalent to 53 mmol/mol. (ACE, angiotensin-converting enzyme; ARB, angiotensin receptor blocker; BP, blood pressure; CCB, calcium channel blocker; CKD, chronic kidney disease; DAPT, dual antiplatelet therapy; DHP, dihydropyridine; DM, diabetes mellitus; HTN, hypertension; LA, long-acting; LVEF, left ventricular ejection fraction.)

TABLE 33-5 Risk Factor Modification: American College of Cardiology/American Heart Association/American Diabetes Association Recommendations

Lipid Management

Class I

1. Lifestyle modifications, including daily physical activity and weight management, are strongly recommended for all patients with SIHD.
2. Dietary therapy for all patients should include reduced intake of saturated fats (to <7% of total calories), *trans*-fatty acids (to <1% of total calories), and cholesterol (to <200 mg/day).
3. In addition to therapeutic lifestyle changes, a high-intensity statin should be prescribed with a goal of achieving a ≥50% decrease in LDL-C, in the absence of contraindications or documented adverse drug reactions.
4. In patients with contraindications or intolerant to high-intensity statin therapy, moderate-intensity statins should be used, if tolerated, with a goal of achieving a 30%-49% decrease in LDL-C.

(continued)

TABLE 33-5 Risk Factor Modification: American College of Cardiology/American Heart Association/American Diabetes Association Recommendations (*continued*)

Class IIa

1. In patients older than 75 years, moderate- or high-intensity statin therapy should be used after considering the potential benefits (risk reduction) and risks (adverse drug reactions, drug-drug interactions, patient frailty).
2. For patients with an LDL-C >70 mg/dL (1.81 mmol/L) on maximally tolerated statin therapy and at very high risk for CV events, the addition of ezetimibe is reasonable.
3. For patients with an LDL-C >70 mg/dL (1.81 mmol/L) or a non-HDL-C level ≥100 mg/dL (≥2.59 mmol/L) on maximally tolerated LDL-C lowering therapy (statin plus ezetimibe) and at very high risk for CV events, the addition of a PCSK-9 inhibitor is reasonable depending on benefit, risk, cost, and patient preference.

Blood Pressure Management

Class I

1. All patients should be counseled about the need for lifestyle modification: weight control; increased physical activity; alcohol moderation; sodium reduction; and emphasis on increased consumption of fresh fruits, vegetables, and low-fat dairy products.
2. In patients with SIHD with BP 130/80 mm Hg or higher, antihypertensive drug therapy should be instituted in addition to or after a trial of lifestyle modifications.
3. The specific medications used for the treatment of HTN in SIHD patients should be based on compelling indications (eg, prior MI, angina, and HFrEF) and may include β-blockers, ACE inhibitors, or ARBs with the addition of other drugs, such as thiazide diuretics, dihydropyridine calcium channel blockers, or aldosterone antagonists, if needed to achieve a goal of BP less than 130/80 mm Hg.
4. For patients with angina and persistent uncontrolled HTN, it is recommended to add dihydropyridine CCBs to β-blockers.

Class IIa

1. For patients who have had an ACS, it is reasonable to continue β-blockers long-term if needed for treatment of HTN.

Diabetes Management

Class I*

1. Among patients with type 2 DM who have established ASCVD or indicators of high-risk, established kidney disease, or HF, a sodium-glucose cotransporter 2 (SGLT2) inhibitor or glucagon-like peptide 1 (GLP-1) receptor agonist with demonstrated CVD benefit is recommended as part of the glucose-lowering regimen independent of A1c, metformin use, and in consideration of patient-specific factors.

Class IIa

1. For selected individual patients, such as those with a short duration of diabetes mellitus and a long life expectancy, a goal A1c of 7% (0.07; 53 mmol/mol) or less is reasonable.
2. A goal A1c <8% (0.08; 64 mmol/mol) is reasonable for certain patients according to age, history of hypoglycemia, the presence of microvascular or macrovascular complications, or presence of coexisting medical conditions.

Class IIb

1. Initiation of pharmacotherapy interventions to achieve target A1c might be reasonable.

Influenza Vaccination

Class I

1. Annual influenza vaccinations are recommended for patients with SIHD.

Physical Activity

Class I

1. For all patients, the clinician should encourage 30-60 minutes of moderate-intensity aerobic activity, such as brisk walking, at least 5 days and preferably 7 days per week, supplemented by an increase in daily lifestyle activities (eg, walking breaks at work, gardening, and household work) to improve cardiorespiratory fitness and move patients out of the least-fit, least-active, high-risk cohort (bottom 20%).
2. For all patients, risk assessment with a physical activity history and/or an exercise test is recommended to guide prognosis and prescription.
3. Medically supervised programs (cardiac rehabilitation) and physician-directed, home-based programs are recommended for at-risk patients at first diagnosis.

Class IIa

1. It is reasonable for the clinician to recommend complementary resistance training at least 2 days per week.

Weight Management

Class I

1. BMI and/or waist circumference should be assessed at every visit, and the clinician should consistently encourage weight maintenance or reduction through an appropriate balance of lifestyle, physical activity, structured exercise, caloric intake, and formal behavioral programs when indicated to maintain or achieve a BMI between 18.5 and 24.9 kg/m^2 and a waist circumference less than 102 cm (40 in.) in men and less than 88 cm (35 in.) in women (less for certain racial groups).
2. The initial goal of weight loss therapy should be to reduce body weight by approximately 5%-10% from baseline. With success, further weight loss can be attempted if indicated.

Smoking Cessation Counseling

Class I

1. Smoking cessation and avoidance of exposure to environmental tobacco smoke at work and home should be encouraged for all patients with SIHD. Follow-up, referral to special programs, and pharmacotherapy are recommended along with a systematic strategy for smoking cessation (Ask, Advise, Assess, Assist, Arrange, Avoid).

Management of Psychological Factors

Class IIa

1. It is reasonable to consider screening SIHD patients for depression and to refer or treat when indicated.

Class IIb

1. Treatment of depression has not been shown to improve cardiovascular disease outcomes but might be reasonable for its other clinical benefits.

(*continued*)

TABLE 33-5 Risk Factor Modification: American College of Cardiology/American Heart Association/American Diabetes Association Recommendations (*continued*)

Alcohol Consumption

Class IIb

1. In patients with SIHD who use alcohol, it might be reasonable for nonpregnant women to have one drink (4 ounces [~120 mL] of wine, 12 ounces [355 mL] of beer, or 1 ounce [30 mL] of spirits) a day and for men to have one or two drinks per day unless alcohol is contraindicated (such as in patients with a history of alcohol abuse or dependence or with liver disease).

Avoiding Exposure to Air Pollution

Class IIa

1. It is reasonable for patients with SIHD to avoid exposure to increased air pollution to reduce the risk of cardiovascular events.

*American Diabetes Association Standards of Medical Care in Diabetes recommendation is A: clear evidence from well-conducted, generalizable randomized controlled trials that are adequately powered.[24] This recommendation was considered equivalent to a Class I recommendation by the American College of Cardiology/American Heart Association.

Data from References 1 and 22-24.

TABLE 33-6 American College of Cardiology/American Heart Association Class of Recommendations for Pharmacotherapy to Relieve Symptoms

Class I

1. β-Blockers should be prescribed as initial therapy for the relief of symptoms in patients with SIHD (LOE B).
2. Calcium channel blockers or long-acting nitrates should be prescribed for the relief of symptoms when β-blockers are contraindicated or cause unacceptable adverse drug reactions in patients with SIHD (LOE B).
3. Calcium channel blockers or long-acting nitrates, in combination with β-blockers, should be prescribed for the relief of symptoms when initial treatment with β-blockers is unsuccessful in patients with SIHD (LOE B).
4. Sublingual nitroglycerin or nitroglycerin spray is recommended for the immediate relief of angina in patients with SIHD (LOE B).

Class IIa

1. Treatment with a long-acting nòn-dihydropyridine calcium channel blocker (verapamil or diltiazem) instead of a β-blocker as initial therapy for relief of symptoms is reasonable in patients with SIHD (LOE B).
2. Ranolazine can be useful when prescribed as a substitute for β-blockers for the relief of symptoms in patients with SIHD if initial treatment with β-blockers leads to unacceptable adverse drug reactions or is ineffective or if initial treatment with β-blockers is contraindicated (LOE B).
3. Ranolazine in combination with β-blockers can be useful when prescribed for relief of symptoms when initial treatment with β-blockers is not successful in patients with SIHD (LOE A).

Data from Reference 1.

in patients with SIHD.[1] In the absence of proximal CAD, multivessel CAD, or acute ischemia, GDMT reduces the rate of death and MI similar to revascularization therapy for most patients with SIHD. Most of the evidence-based GDMT target risk-factor modification (Table 33-5), but also include aspirin and angiotensin-converting enzyme (ACE) inhibition.

Antithrombotic Therapy

5 Aspirin produces an antiplatelet effect by irreversibly blocking cyclooxygenase-1 (COX-1) activity (~95%) for the life of the platelet, thereby inhibiting thromboxane A_2 production. The reduction in thromboxane A_2 leads to reduced platelet activation and aggregation. Aspirin doses as small as 30 mg daily effectively inhibit COX-1. Aspirin doses above 75 to 100 mg provide little additional antiplatelet activity.[25] Aspirin may also provide benefits through some non-platelet-mediated effects. Higher doses of aspirin (≥325 mg daily) significantly impair endothelial secretion of prostacyclin, which is a natural vasodilator. Low-dose aspirin does not have this deleterious effect. Although aspirin may inhibit prostacyclin secretion, the effects on the endothelium are reversible, unlike its effect on platelets.[26] After unbound aspirin has been removed from the circulation (half-life is about 30 minutes), prostacyclin secretion and its vasodilation effects are restored. Aspirin may also attenuate the synthesis of cytokines such as interleukin-2, interleukin-6, and interferon in leukocytes as well as prevent leukocyte rolling and macrophage-induced endothelial activation.[26] The extent to which these pharmacologic properties contribute to the clinical benefits of aspirin is unknown.

Evidence supporting the effectiveness of aspirin in patients with SIHD first came from a subgroup analysis of the Physicians Health Study.[27] Patients with SIHD who took aspirin (325 mg every other day) had an 87% reduction in first MI compared to placebo. This benefit came with a significant increase in hemorrhagic stroke, although none of the strokes were fatal. These beneficial effects were confirmed in the more robust Swedish Angina Pectoris Aspirin Trial.[28] Patients with controlled angina on sotalol treated with 75 mg of aspirin daily had a 34% reduction in first MI or sudden death compared to placebo. There was no difference in major bleeding or stroke between the groups.

Some patients are nonresponsive to the antiplatelet effects of aspirin, and therefore, do not receive a clinical benefit. In patients with CAD, the risk of recurrent CV events was more than threefold higher in patients with aspirin non-responsiveness.[29] The rate of aspirin non-responsiveness was estimated to be 24% in one meta-analysis, but the range reported in the included studies was wide (0%-57%).[30] In studies that used light transmission aggregotomy induced with arachidonic acid (the gold standard test) or measured serum thromboxane B_2, the rate of aspirin non-responsiveness was only 6%.[30] These results are similar to the findings of the Aspirin-Induced Platelet Effects (ASPECT) trial, in which aspirin non-responsiveness defined by COX-1-nonspecific methods was 27%, compared to only 6% when COX-1-specific methods were used.[31] The ASPECT investigators also reported no difference in aspirin non-responsiveness between patients receiving 81, 162, or 325 mg daily.[31] A lack of dose-response is consistent with the findings of the Antithrombotic Trialists' Collaboration meta-analysis which demonstrated a similar reduction in vascular events regardless if patients were receiving low dose (75-150 mg daily), moderate dose (160-325 mg daily), or high dose (500-1,500 mg daily) aspirin.[25]

Aspirin non-responsiveness may occur because of changes to the COX-1 enzyme, such as changes to the enzyme structure, or temporary blockade of the active site on the enzyme. Of particular concern is the potential for nonsteroidal anti-inflammatory drug (NSAID) therapy to block the COX-1 enzyme. Naproxen and ibuprofen have been shown to interfere with aspirin's antiplatelet effect when coadministered by competing for the site of action.[26] The timing of coadministration appears to be an important factor. The effect of aspirin on platelet aggregation is impaired when ibuprofen is given 2 hours before aspirin, but when aspirin is given first, antiplatelet activity is retained.

While aspirin non-responsiveness does exist, the incidence is probably not as high as once believed. Although patients with aspirin non-responsiveness are more likely to have ischemic events, routinely testing patients is not recommended. Given that increasing the dose of aspirin does not impact responsiveness or improve clinical outcomes, the only effective strategy would be to change to or add an alternative antiplatelet agent.

For patients unable to take aspirin due to allergy or intolerance, clopidogrel represents a suitable alternative antiplatelet agent to prevent MI and death in patients with CAD.[1] While clopidogrel significantly reduced the incidence of stroke, MI, or vascular death in patients with ASCVD compared to aspirin in the The Clopidogrel versus Aspirin in Patients at Risk of Ischemic Events trial, the absolute difference between the two strategies was small (0.5%; number needed to treat = 200).[26] Given the small magnitude of benefit and potential for non-responsiveness to clopidogrel, it remains a second-line choice in patients with CAD. When used in patients with SIHD, clopidogrel should be given 75 mg daily.

Dual antiplatelet therapy (DAPT) with aspirin plus a $P2Y_{12}$ inhibitor, such as clopidogrel, has a clear benefit in patients after a PCI with coronary stent placement and following treatment for ACS. The combination of aspirin plus clopidogrel for 28 months did not reduce the risk of death, MI, stroke, or coronary revascularization when compared to aspirin alone but increased the risk of moderate bleeding.[32] However, in those patients with established vascular disease at study entry receiving aspirin plus clopidogrel, there was a significant reduction in the risk of death, MI, and stroke compared to aspirin alone (7.3% vs 8.8%).[32] In patients with a history of MI at least 1 year prior, the combination of ticagrelor 60 mg twice daily plus aspirin reduced the risk of cardiac events compared to aspirin alone but more than doubled the risk of major bleeding complications.[32] This dose of ticagrelor plus aspirin was evaluated in patients with both SIHD and type 2 DM. Although a significant reduction in CV death, MI, and stroke was observed with a similar increase in major bleeding in the overall study population, the benefit was greatest in patients with a previous PCI and may be considered in this setting.[32]

Patient responsiveness to clopidogrel is highly variable and the antiplatelet activity follows a bell-shaped curve.[33] Several tests have been used to evaluate clopidogrel's antiplatelet activity and there are different definitions of non-responsiveness. Thus, estimates of non-responsiveness to clopidogrel range from 5% to 44%.[34,35] Several trials have correlated clopidogrel non-responsiveness with poor clinical outcomes.

It is unclear what to do if a patient is found to have a lack of appropriate response to clopidogrel. The most common cause of non-responsiveness is poor adherence. Even a small number of missed doses will result in an inadequate response to clopidogrel. Data from a large registry provides evidence that poor adherence is associated with increased ischemic events, as well as important insight into patient predictors of poor adherence.[36] Lack of response may also be due to polymorphisms in cytochrome P450 2C19, which is responsible for the conversion of clopidogrel into its active compound.[37] There may also be drug interactions with the cytochrome P450 2C19, such as proton pump inhibitors, that may alter clopidogrel's effectiveness. A more detailed discussion on the clinical impact of these polymorphisms and drug interactions can be found in Chapter 34 (Acute Coronary Syndrome).

Rivaroxaban, a direct factor Xa anticoagulant, has demonstrated benefit in patients with CAD when added to aspirin therapy. In a large, randomized trial, rivaroxaban 2.5 mg twice daily added to low-dose aspirin provided a 24% relative reduction in CV death, MI, and stroke compared to low-dose aspirin alone.[38] Although there was also a significant increase in major bleeding with patients receiving rivaroxaban, 75% of the major bleeding events would not have been considered a major bleed by standard bleeding definitions. Patients with polyvascular disease, heart failure, diabetes mellitus, or at least moderate renal insufficiency seemed to obtain the most benefit from the addition of rivaroxaban to aspirin therapy.[39]

Recommendations from the ACC/AHA for the use of antiplatelet agents in the management of SIHD include a Class I recommendation for the use of aspirin 75 to 162 mg daily.[1] Aspirin should be continued indefinitely in the absence of contraindications (LOE A). Clopidogrel is considered an appropriate alternative when aspirin is contraindicated (LOE B). The guidelines state that treatment with aspirin (75-162 mg daily) and clopidogrel 75 mg daily might be reasonable in certain high-risk patients with SIHD (Class IIb, LOE B recommendation). Data supporting the combination of rivaroxaban and aspirin in patients with SIHD were not available when the ACC/AHA guidelines were published. However, this combination is recommended by the American Diabetes Association.[24]

ACE Inhibitors

6 In the setting of ASCVD, ACE inhibitors stabilize coronary plaque, provide restoration or improvement in endothelial function, inhibit vascular smooth muscle cell growth, decrease macrophage migration, and possibly prevent oxidative stress. They may also possess some antithrombotic properties by inhibiting platelet aggregation and augmenting the endogenous fibrinolytic system. However, ACE inhibitors have not been shown to improve symptomatic ischemia or chest pain episodes.[40]

The role of ACE inhibitors in patients at high risk for CV events was evaluated in the HOPE (Heart Outcomes Prevention Evaluation) trial.[41] Patients with normal LV function and either ASCVD (history of CAD [~80% of patients, including 55% with SIHD], stroke, peripheral arterial disease) or its equivalent (eg, DM with at least one additional risk factor) treated with ramipril 10 mg daily were significantly less likely to experience one of the primary endpoints (CV death, MI, or stroke) compared to placebo. These impressive benefits were seen despite a minimal reduction in BP with the use of ramipril. Benefits were consistent across all groups of patients enrolled, regardless of the location of ASCVD.

Subsequent trials have produced conflicting results. One trial using perindopril 8 mg daily significantly reduced the incidence of CV death, MI, or cardiac arrest compared to placebo in patients with SIHD.[42] In contrast, the addition of trandolapril 4 mg daily to standard therapy in patients with documented CAD did not significantly reduce the incidence of CV death, MI, or coronary revascularization in another trial.[43] A meta-analysis of seven trials with 33,960 patients demonstrated a significant 14% reduction in mortality in patients with CAD treated with an ACE inhibitor.[44] Based on the well-established benefits, it is appropriate to use ACE inhibitors in patients with SIHD who have HTN, DM, HFrEF, or following an MI.[1]

Trials have evaluated the role of angiotensin receptor blockers (ARB) to determine if they provide a similar benefit as ACE inhibitors in the setting of CAD. A trial in patients with preexisting CVD or DM with end-organ damage treated with either the ACE inhibitor ramipril 10 mg daily or the ARB telmisartan 80 mg daily appeared to have a similar benefit.[45] However, there was no added benefit from combining the two agents. There were significantly more episodes of hypotension, syncope, and renal dysfunction in patients treated with combination therapy. In a second trial, telmisartan failed to demonstrate a CV benefit over placebo in patients who were intolerant to ACE inhibitors.[46] Based on these conflicting data, an ARB may be considered if the patient cannot tolerate ACE inhibitor therapy, and combination therapy should be avoided.

Recommendations from the ACC/AHA include a Class I recommendation to use ACE inhibitors in all patients with SIHD who also have HTN, DM, HFrEF, or chronic kidney disease, unless contraindicated (LOE A).[1] ARBs are recommended for the same patient populations if they are intolerant to ACE inhibitors (LOE A). It is a Class IIa recommendation to use ACE inhibitors in patients with both SIHD and other vascular diseases (LOE B), and ARBs in these patients if intolerant to ACE inhibitors (LOE B).

Lipid Management

7 Multiple studies have demonstrated a continuous increase in coronary events with increasing low-density lipoprotein cholesterol (LDL-C) in men and women with and without SIHD. Statin therapy significantly lowers LDL-C and reduces CV event rates. The Cholesterol Treatment Trialist Collaborators found a 10% reduction in all-cause mortality and a 20% reduction in cardiac mortality for every 40 mg/dL (1.03 mmol/L) reduction in LDL-C.[47] Statin therapy also reduces the risk of MI, stroke, and the need for coronary revascularization. Higher dose and high potency statin regimens are more effective than lower dose, low-potency regimens.[47]

Current guidelines recommend that all patients with known ASCVD, such as SIHD, should receive high-intensity statin therapy to achieve a 50% or more reduction in LDL-C.[23] Patients over the age of 75 years and those who cannot tolerate high-intensity statin therapy should receive moderate-intensity statin therapy to achieve a 30% to 49% reduction in LDL-C. In patients with clinical ASCVD who do not achieve a 50% reduction in LDL-C or who have an LDL ≥70 mg/dL (1.81 mmol/L) on maximally tolerated high-intensity statin therapy, the additional non-statin therapies such as ezetimibe, PCSK9-inhibitors, or bile-acid sequestrates may be considered.[23] In patients with clinical ASCVD with DM, a recent ASCVD event, CKD, or poorly controlled risk factors, targeting an LDL-C less than 70 mg/dL (1.81 mmol/L) or non–HDL-C less than 100 mg/dL (2.59 mmol/L) may be considered.[23]

High-intensity statin options include atorvastatin 40 or 80 mg daily or rosuvastatin 20 or 40 mg daily. Atorvastatin 80 mg is the preferred dose. The 40 mg dose of atorvastatin was only used in one trial in patients who could not tolerate the 80 mg dose.[48] Also, rosuvastatin 20 mg daily is the preferred regimen based on the trial evidence, with the 40 mg daily dose being recommended because it is also an approved dose.[23] Moderate-intensity statin regimens include once-daily atorvastatin 10 to 20 mg, rosuvastatin 5 to 10 mg, simvastatin 20 to 40 mg, pravastatin 40 to 80 mg, lovastatin 40 to 80 mg, pitavastatin 1 to 4 mg, fluvastatin extended-release 80 mg, or twice daily fluvastatin 40 mg.[23]

Regular physical activity, dietary changes, and weight management should also be implemented (Table 33-8). Dietary approaches to lowering LDL-C include replacing saturated and *trans* fatty acids with dietary carbohydrates or unsaturated fatty acids and reducing dietary cholesterol. A diet low in saturated fat and cholesterol typically lowers LDL-C by 10% to 15%. The addition of plant stanols/sterols (2 g/d) can lower LDL-C by 5% to 15%. Viscous fiber (>10 g/d) reduces LDL-C by 3% to 5%. A 10 lb (4.5 kg) weight loss reduces LDL-C by 5% to 8%. Regular physical exercise improves cardiac fitness and facilitates weight loss but does not reliably lower LDL-C.

Blood Pressure Management

A number of observational trials have demonstrated a continuous relationship between BP and the risk of CV events. The risk of vascular death increases linearly over the BP range of 115/75 mm Hg to 185/115 mm Hg. The risk doubles for every 20 mm Hg increase in systolic BP or 10 mm Hg increase in diastolic BP.[22] Clinical trials have evaluated when to initiate therapy and attempted to define the target BP goal for patients with HTN. However, the specific BP target for patients with and without SIHD has been debated. Clinical trials and meta-analyses support the current guidelines which recommend initiating pharmacotherapy in patients with SIHD with a BP of 130/80 mm Hg or higher and treating to a BP goal of less than 130/80 mm Hg.[22,49,50]

Optimal BP should be achieved using lifestyle modifications as well as pharmacotherapy (Table 33-5). This includes a diet rich in fruits, vegetables, and low-fat dairy products, regular physical exercise, a reduction in dietary sodium, and limited alcohol consumption. Lifestyle modifications can also contribute to weight loss. A 10 kg weight loss can reduce systolic BP by 5 to 20 mm Hg.

Drugs used to treat HTN in patients with SIHD commonly include agents that can be used to treat the symptoms of the disease. β-Blockers are often used to control angina symptoms and they also lower BP. Patients may also be on ACE inhibitors to reduce CV risk. Therefore, most patients with SIHD will receive these two classes of agents for the treatment of HTN. If additional therapy is needed, dihydropyridine (DHP) calcium channel blockers (CCBs) are often added because they treat both HTN and reduce angina symptoms. If the patient's angina symptoms are well controlled, thiazide diuretics may be considered as add-on therapy for HTN. They are considered a first-line treatment in most populations and do not appear to be detrimental when used by patients with SIHD.[22]

Smoking Cessation

The relationship between tobacco use and increased risk of CVD is well documented.[51] Cigarette smoking promotes and accelerates ASCVD through a number of mechanisms including increased platelet adhesion, elevated fibrinogen concentrations, endothelial dysfunction, altered serum lipids, and vasoconstriction.[52] Smoking is perhaps the most important cause of preventable CVD and death.[51] Compared to those who never smoked, smokers lose approximately 10 years of life expectancy and early cessation is associated with an approximately 90% reduction in mortality and improved quality of life.[53] Therefore, abstinence and smoking cessation are key components of lifestyle modifications for patients with SIHD.

Advice from a clinician recommending and discussing the importance of smoking cessation significantly increases the likelihood that a patient will quit. Clinicians should approach smoking cessation by using the 6 A's framework[1]:

1. Ask each patient about tobacco use at every visit
2. Advise each smoker to quit
3. Assess each smoker's willingness to make a quit attempt
4. Assist each smoker in making a quit attempt by offering medication and referral for counseling
5. Arrange for follow-up
6. Avoid exposure to environmental tobacco smoke

Several pharmacologic agents are available over the counter or with a prescription and are all more effective than placebo.[54] Nicotine replacement therapy is available in a number of dosage forms without a prescription to fit the patient's lifestyle including patches, tablets, gum, lozenges, and nasal spray. Sustained-release bupropion and the partial agonist of the $\alpha_4\beta_2$ nicotinic receptor, varenicline, are also first-line medications to treat tobacco dependence in adults. In one study, no evidence of serious CVD or CV adverse events occurred in patients receiving smoking cessation medications, demonstrating all three pharmacotherapies are safe from a cardiovascular standpoint.[55] Nonpharmacologic methods for smoking cessation are just as important as pharmacotherapy. Self-help programs, telephone counseling, behavioral therapy, and exercise all can be used to help patients quit smoking.

Diabetes Management

8 DM is a strong risk factor for the development of CVD. Patients with type 1 DM have a 10-fold increased risk of having a CV event and patients with type 2 DM have a two- to sixfold risk of CV death compared to those without DM.

Like HTN, the glycemic target for patients with DM, including those with SIHD, is the subject of considerable debate. Studies have found that achieving an A1c of less than 7% (0.07; 53 mmol/mol) reduces microvascular complications from DM such as retinopathy, nephropathy, and neuropathy.[56] While subgroup analyses of larger trials have suggested lower rates of ischemic events in patients randomized to intensive glycemic control (A1c less than 7% [0.07; 53 mmol/mol]), macrovascular events were not significantly reduced in trials comparing intensive to more lenient glycemic control in high-risk patients with DM, including those with preexisting CVD.[56] In these trials, patients in the intensive glycemic control groups had higher rates of adverse events including severe hypoglycemia, CVD death, and overall mortality.[56] In patients with SIHD, current AHA/ACC recommendations target an A1c of less than 7% (0.07; 53 mmol/mol) for patients with DM of short duration and a long life expectancy (Class IIa, LOE B) but a more lenient goal (A1c $<$8% [0.08; 64 mmol/mol]) for frail or high-risk patients (Class IIa, LOE C Table 33-5).[1]

Metformin is the drug of first choice for the treatment of type 2 DM, including patients with SIHD. While sulfonylureas provide a similar reduction in A1c, their potential to induce hypoglycemia and weight gain make metformin a more attractive option. Although debate remains regarding the effect of metformin and sulfonylureas on CV events, a recent meta-analysis did not find a significant association between the use of either therapy and CV outcomes.[56] Some newer therapies for the treatment of type 2 DM significantly reduce the risk of CV events, including all-cause mortality.[57] In a recent meta-analysis, the risk of death was reduced by 20% (hazard ratio [HR] 0.80, 95% credible interval [CrI] 0.71-0.89) in patients treated with sodium-glucose-cotransporter 2 (SGLT-2) inhibitors and by 12% (HR 0.88, 95% CrI 0.81-0.94) in patients treated with glucagon-like peptide 1 (GLP-1) agonists compared to patients treated with standard therapies in the control groups.[58] Cardiovascular mortality was also lower in patients treated with either SGLT-2 inhibitors or GLP-1 agonists compared to control subjects.[58] The risk of adverse event rates leading to discontinuation was higher with GLP-1 agonists compared to SGLT-2 inhibitors and dipeptidyl peptidase 4 inhibitors.[58] Consequently, updated guidelines for the treatment of DM now recommend using agents that have been shown to reduce CV events (eg, empagliflozin, canagliflozin, and liraglutide) as part of the glucose-lowering regimen, regardless of the patient's current glycemic control and should be added to metformin therapy in patients with DM type 2 and ASCVD.[24]

Influenza Vaccination

Patients with cardiac disease who develop seasonal influenza are at high risk for complications and more likely to die. In patients with CAD, influenza vaccination has been associated with lower rates of ischemic events, although the benefit may be greatest in those with a recent ACS prior to vaccination.[59,60] Current guidelines recommend that all patients with SIHD should receive an annual influenza vaccination to prevent morbidity and mortality.[1]

Pharmacotherapy to Reduce Symptoms

β-Blockers

9 β-Adrenergic blocking agents are commonly used in the management of patients with SIHD and reduce both symptomatic and silent episodes of myocardial ischemia. β-Adrenergic blocking agents competitively inhibit the effects of circulating catecholamines on β-adrenoceptors. The predominant adrenergic receptor type in the heart is the β_1-receptor, and competitive blockade minimizes the influence of endogenous catecholamines on the chronotropic and inotropic state of the myocardium. β-Blockers also produce a reduction in BP through competitive inhibition of β_1-receptors in the kidney, leading to a reduction in renin release. By reducing HR, myocardial contractility, and intramyocardial wall tension through BP reduction, β-blockers impact all major contributing factors to MVO_2.[61] Reductions in HR may also improve myocardial oxygen delivery by prolonging diastole filling time and increasing myocardial perfusion.

β_1-Selectivity does not improve the efficacy of β-blockers for the treatment of SIHD and all agents appear equally effective. β_1-Selective agents would be preferred in patients with chronic obstructive pulmonary disease, peripheral arterial disease, DM, dyslipidemias, and sexual dysfunction, where blocking β_2-adrenergic receptors may be problematic. It should be noted that even β_1-selective agents lose their selectivity at higher doses. β-Blockers with combined α_1 and β-blockade are also effective in the management of angina. β-Blockers with intrinsic sympathomimetic activity cause a slight-to-moderate activation of the β-receptor, in addition to competing with endogenous catecholamines. Due to this unique pharmacologic property, they do not affect resting HR but do modestly lower HR when catecholamine concentrations are increased during exercise. While agents with intrinsic sympathomimetic activity may be useful for patients with peripheral arterial disease and dyslipidemia, they are not preferred in patients with CAD. The selection of a β-blocker in patients with SIHD should be guided by the presence of comorbid diseases, preferred dosing frequency, and cost.

Most adverse drug reactions experienced with the use of β-blockers are an extension of their pharmacologic activity. Patients receiving β-blockers may experience bradycardia, hypotension, heart block, impaired glucose metabolism, and altered serum lipids. β-Blockers may alter the lipid profile by increasing triglycerides and decreasing HDL-C. They have no impact on LDL-C. Changes in the lipid profile are greater with non-selective β-blockers and are usually transient. Central nervous system adverse drug reactions such as fatigue, depression, insomnia, and general malaise are usually mild but among the most common reasons for treatment discontinuation. Impotence has been reported in approximately 1% of men receiving β-blockers. Patients with a history of airway disease may suffer from bronchospasm and patients with HFrEF may become fluid overloaded. Patients without these preexisting disease states usually do not suffer from these adverse drug reactions and it is important to note that even patients at risk for adverse drug reactions receive significant benefit from the use of β-blockers. β-Blockers are absolutely contraindicated in patients with preexisting bradycardia, second or third-degree atrioventricular block, a history of uncontrolled reactive airway disease (asthma), severe peripheral arterial disease (critical limb ischemia), hypotension, HFrEF with unstable fluid status, and patients with DM who have frequent episodes of hypoglycemia. All patients should receive a β-blocker following an MI unless there is an absolute contraindication. A patient with SIHD who has never had an ACS, especially acute MI, and who has concurrent chronic obstructive pulmonary disease (COPD) may be treated with a cardioselective β-blocker if there are compelling reasons to use a β-blocker over another antianginal medication. However, in patients with moderate to severe COPD, β-blockers may increase the risk COPD-related hospitalizations.[62]

If β-blocker therapy needs to be discontinued, doses need to be tapered over 2 to 3 weeks to prevent abrupt withdrawal. During β-blocker therapy, β-receptors become up-regulated in the myocardium. After an abrupt withdrawal of β-blocker therapy, these new receptors, along with all of the blocked receptors, are now stimulated by endogenous catecholamines. This can produce a significant increase in MVO_2, induce ischemia, and even MI. If for some reason β-blockers cannot be tapered, patients should be instructed to avoid exertion as much as possible and manage angina episodes with SL nitroglycerin. Using a non-DHP CCB would be the preferred second-line choice if β-blockers are contraindicated or must be discontinued.

Calcium Channel Blockers

7 CCBs effectively reduce the frequency and duration of angina episodes in patients with SIHD. All CCBs reduce MVO_2, as well as provide some increase in supply by inducing coronary vasodilation and preventing vasospasm. CCBs modulate calcium entry into the myocardium and vascular smooth muscle, as well as other tissues. This leads to a reduction in the cytosolic concentration of calcium responsible for activation of the actin-myosin complex leading to the contraction of vascular smooth muscle and myocardium.

CCBs should be considered as two separate classes of drugs. While all CCBs inhibit the influx of calcium ions, the location of the inhibition differs based on the chemical structure of the agents. The DHP CCBs, such as nifedipine, amlodipine, isradipine, and felodipine, primarily block calcium receptors in vascular smooth muscle cells, such as arterioles, with minimal effect on the myocardium. In contrast, the phenylalkylamine (verapamil) and benzothiazepine (diltiazem) agents, commonly referred to as non-DHP CCBs, block calcium ion entry mostly in the myocardium, with minimal effect on vascular smooth muscle. Verapamil has the greatest impact on myocardial calcium channels with diltiazem having an intermediate effect.

All CCBs reduce MVO_2 by reducing wall tension by lowering arterial blood pressure, and to a minor extent, depressing cardiac contractility. Like β-blockers, non-DHP CCBs also reduce HR and contractility through blockade of myocardial calcium channels. The DHP CCBs slightly reduce cardiac contractility and produce either a neutral or increase in HR due to potential reflex tachycardia from direct arterial dilation. The effect on contractility and reflex tachycardia is not uniform across the class of DHP CCBs. Agents such as nifedipine produce more impairment of LV function than amlodipine and felodipine. Due to their potential to cause reflex tachycardia, short-acting DHP CCBs should be avoided when treating SIHD, chronic HTN, hypertensive crisis, or during an ACS event. Reflex tachycardia from longer-acting DHP CCBs can be prevented with concurrent β-blocker therapy.

Common adverse drug reactions of CCBs vary between the two classes. Patients taking non-DHP CCBs may experience bradycardia, hypotension, atrioventricular block, and symptoms of LV depression. Non-DHP CCBs should not be used in patients who have contraindications or cannot tolerate the rate-slowing effects of β-blockers due to their similar pharmacodynamic effects. Non-DHP CCBs should be avoided in patients with concomitant HFrEF due to their negative inotropic effects but can provide benefit to patients in atrial fibrillation with a rapid ventricular response due to their negative dromotropic effects. Verapamil has also been reported to cause constipation in up to 8% of patients. Patients taking DHP CCBs may experience reflex tachycardia, hypotension, headache, gingival hyperplasia, and peripheral edema. While most DHP CCBs are contraindicated in patients with HFrEF, amlodipine, and felodipine are considered safe options in patients with HFrEF and concomitant SIHD or HTN.

CCBs undergo hepatic oxidative biotransformation via the cytochrome P450 isoenzyme 3A4 and other isoenzymes. Verapamil and diltiazem inhibit the clearance of other substrates for the 3A4 isoenzyme such as carbamazepine, cyclosporine, lovastatin, simvastatin, and benzodiazepines. The DHP CCBs do not produce a clinically meaningful interaction with these medications. Verapamil, and to a lesser extent diltiazem, also inhibit P-glycoprotein mediated drug transport. This interaction is partially responsible for increases in serum concentrations of agents such as digoxin and cyclosporine. Because verapamil decreases digoxin clearance, digoxin levels must be closely monitored if these agents are used together. Agents that induce the P450 3A4 isoenzyme can reduce the effectiveness of all CCBs. Potential pharmacodynamic interactions also need to be monitored in patients taking CCBs. Patients receiving verapamil or diltiazem concurrently with other agents that reduce HR and atrioventricular nodal conduction (β-blockers, digoxin, and amiodarone) should be monitored for the development of bradycardia or heart block.

Nitrates

7 Organic nitrates were found to have antianginal properties over 100 years ago when Murrell first reported in 1879, the ability of a 1% nitroglycerin solution administered orally to relieve and prevent angina attacks. Organic nitrates are prodrugs that require biotransformation into the active compounds. This process leads to denitration of the nitrate and the release of nitric oxide, also known as EDRF. Nitric oxide increases concentrations of cyclic guanosine monophosphate in the vascular endothelium leading to a reduction in cytoplasmic calcium and subsequent vasodilation. Vasodilation occurs predominantly in the venous vasculature thereby reducing preload, myocardial wall tension, and MVO_2. As doses are increased, arterial vasodilation also occurs. Arterial vasodilation can produce reflex tachycardia that can negate some of the antianginal benefits. Patients on adequate doses of β-blockers will not have reflex tachycardia, making this an effective combination for controlling a patient's acute and chronic angina symptoms.

Nitrates also vasodilate stenotic vessels as well as the intracoronary collaterals. Given that blood flow is exponentially related to the degree of stenosis, small increases in vasodilation in these narrowed vessels can produce significant increases in myocardial oxygen supply to ischemic areas of the myocardium. Nitrate-induced coronary vasodilation occurs predominately in epicardial vessels, with minimal effect on coronary microcirculation. This explains why nitrates do not cause coronary steal similar to other vasodilators like dipyridamole or sodium nitroprusside. In coronary steal, there is vasodilation in coronary vessels without atherosclerotic disease but coronary vessels with disease are not dilated. Therefore, more blood flow is shifted, or "stolen," to non-diseased vessels away from atherosclerotic vessels that have reduced blood flow. Nitrates may also have anti-aggregant effects on platelets, but the clinical impact is negligible.

Common adverse drug reactions from nitrate therapy include headache, flushing, nausea, postural hypotension, and syncope. While the hypotension is usually not severe, patients who are volume-depleted may experience paradoxical bradycardia if they attempt to rapidly stand. The headache will usually resolve after about 2 weeks when nitrates are used for chronic therapy. It is important to note that this does not represent tolerance or loss of antianginal effectiveness. Acetaminophen is effective in managing nitrate-induced headaches during the initial weeks of therapy. Patients using transdermal nitroglycerin may experience skin erythema and inflammation. Initiating therapy with smaller doses and rotating the application site can mitigate some of the adverse drug reactions of transdermal nitroglycerin.

8 Several formulations of nitrates are available for acute and chronic use (Table 33-7). All patients with CAD should have access to SL nitroglycerin tablets or spray for the treatment of acute episodes of angina. Patient education is critical to ensure appropriate SL nitroglycerin use (Table 33-8). The SL route of administration avoids gastrointestinal absorption and hepatic first-pass metabolism. SL nitroglycerin 300 to 400 μg typically provides relief of angina within 5 minutes of administration. SL nitroglycerin can also relieve symptoms even if the patient is chronically taking long-acting nitrates. The adverse drug reactions of flushing, headache, and postural hypotension can appear rapidly and the patient should be aware of this potential. SL nitroglycerin can also be used to prevent acute episodes of angina. When patients want to participate in activities that they know lead to angina, they can take a dose of SL nitroglycerin 2 to 5 minutes in advance. This prophylactic dose provides up to 30 minutes of protection and allows patients to participate in activities that they might otherwise be unable.

TABLE 33-7 Nitrate Products

Product	Onset (minutes)	Duration	Initial Dose
Nitroglycerin			
IV	1-2	3-5 minutes	5-10 μg/min
Sublingual[*]	1-3	30-60 minutes	0.3-0.4 mg
Oral	40	3-6 hours	2.5-6.5 mg three times a day
Ointment	20-60	2-8 hours	0.5-1 in. (1.3-2.5 cm)
Patch	40-60	>8 hours	0.2-0.4 mg/hour (1 patch)
Isosorbide dinitrate			
Immediate release	20-40	4-6 hours	5-20 mg three times a day
Sustained release	60	8 hours	40 mg once daily
Isosorbide mononitrate			
Immediate release	30-60	6-8 hours	20 mg twice a day
Extended release	30-60	12-24 hours	30-60 mg daily

[*]Sublingual nitroglycerin exists in three different formulations: tablets, spray, and powder packets.

TABLE 33-8 Appropriate Use of Sublingual Nitroglycerin

Education Point	Rationale
Keep in original dark glass container	SL nitroglycerin will interact with plastic and can lose potency when exposed to light. This is why it is packaged in a dark glass container.
Do not store in a larger plastic vial with a child-resistant safety cap	During an episode of angina, you do not want the patient struggling to figure out how to open the safety cap.
Do not store in the bathroom	SL nitroglycerin will degrade in moisture and tablets will lose their integrity and potency.
Keep SL nitroglycerin close by at all times; may need multiple vials	SL nitroglycerin does not do any good to the patient if they do not have it with them at the time of an episode of angina. The patient should consider having one at home, at work, in the garage, etc.
The patient should be sitting down and resting while taking the tablet	While the SL nitroglycerin tablets are small, the dose is not. It is likely the patient will have some flushing, may get a headache, and even become a little light-headed. They need to know this can happen.
Describe how to use a sublingual tablet	The SL nitroglycerin is administered under the tongue in order to provide rapid absorption and avoid first-pass metabolism. The patient needs to keep the tablet under the tongue until dissolved. Avoid swallowing the tablet.
Once opened, tablets need to be refilled every 6 months and spray every 3 years	Due to the instability of SL nitroglycerin tablets, they are typically only good for 6 months after the bottle is opened.[a] Shelf-life of the spray is longer. Patients need to be advised to refill SL nitroglycerin even if all doses have not been taken.
Remove the cotton plug from the bottle	Larger quantity bottles commonly have a cotton plug. During an episode of angina, you do not want the patient to be struggling with trying to get the cotton plug out of the bottle.
May be taken in advance of events known to cause chest pain	SL nitroglycerin can be used to prevent episodes of angina if taken before partaking in an exertional event known to precipitate angina/chest discomfort.
Contact 911 if first SL nitroglycerin does not relieve angina[b]	Most episodes of angina are relieved within 5-10 minutes of rest and a single SL nitroglycerin. If pain persists, the episode may be an acute coronary syndrome, not stable ischemic heart disease. This requires rapid medical attention.

[a]Product-specific.

[b]May be patient-specific based on their experience with SL nitroglycerin and angina episodes.

The development of nitrate tolerance must be considered when chronically using long-acting nitrate therapy for SIHD. Several trials have shown that continuous nitrate therapy for more than 24 hours leads to a reduction or loss of the hemodynamic and antianginal effects of nitrates. In a large study in patients receiving 24 hours of transdermal nitroglycerin, almost all patients lost control of their angina symptoms within 24 hours to 1 week, which cannot be overcome with higher doses.[63]

Nitrate tolerance is not an "all or none" phenomenon. Responsiveness is reduced in some patients while others experience a total loss of efficacy. Despite the continued use of nitrates and a loss of antianginal effect, plasma volume remains expanded and some hemodynamic effects are maintained. Chronic administration of nitrates produces a state of oxidative stress leading to dysfunction of mitochondrial aldehyde dehydrogenase, the enzyme responsible for converting nitrates to the active agent NO.[64,65] Consequentially, the dysfunctional enzyme is unable to produce active NO and the angina relieving effect of nitrate agents is reduced or lost.

Why nitrate tolerance develops remains unknown, but several pharmacologic approaches have been developed to manage and prevent it. One thought is that tolerance is due to an exhausting of sulfhydryl groups needed to use organic nitrates.[64] Based on this hypothesis, acetylcysteine and ACE inhibitors such as captopril, which supply sulfhydryl groups, have been investigated as a potential strategy for preventing nitrate tolerance. Unfortunately, both agents have provided inconsistent results. ACE inhibitors may prevent nitrate tolerance through other mechanisms. The inhibition of angiotensin II production can reduce superoxide anion production, leading to reduced nitrate degradation, as well as a reduction in protein kinase C and endothelin leading to a reduction in vasoconstriction. Unfortunately, none of these approaches have shown to be effective in maintaining the antianginal effects of continuous nitrate therapy.

The preferred management of nitrate tolerance for patients with CAD is to ensure a 10- to 14-hour nitrate-free interval every day. This approach has been shown to maintain antianginal efficacy with the use of chronic nitrates. The rationale for this approach is based on the observation that although nitrate tolerance develops rapidly, it is also reversed rapidly. Unfortunately, this approach does not provide the patient with anti-ischemic coverage for a full 24 hours and places the patient at risk for angina episodes. Typically, the nitrate-free interval is provided during the nighttime hours when the patient is sleeping and, in most cases, has lower MVO_2. Several trials have used chronic nitrates with a daily nitrate-free interval and demonstrated increased exercise time, reduced exercise-induced ischemic events, and reduced need for SL nitroglycerin. Despite these benefits, a nitrate-free interval would not provide protection to the 20% to 30% of patients with SIHD who experience nocturnal episodes of angina. Moreover, it is well documented that angina episodes and MI commonly occur in the morning hours, immediately before or after awakening. Patients using chronic nitrate therapy are unlikely to have taken or applied their nitrate therapy for the day during this critical time period. Therefore, nitrates should not be routinely used as monotherapy in patients with SIHD due to the lack of 24-hour coverage, lack of protection against circadian-related ischemic events, and potential for reflex tachycardia. Trials have demonstrated that patients taking intermittent transdermal nitroglycerin did not experience rebound ischemia during the nitrate-free interval when β-blockers or diltiazem were concurrently used.

7 Several nitrate preparations can be used for chronic long-term prevention of angina episodes. Transdermal patches and isosorbide mononitrate are the most commonly prescribed chronic nitrates. Although isosorbide dinitrate is effective, the three times daily dosing regimen requires patients to take a dose every 4 to 5 hours in order to provide an adequate nitrate-free interval. Two of the isosorbide mononitrate preparations are dosed twice daily. The twice-daily preparations should be dosed 7 hours apart, such as 7 am and 2 pm. It is critical to be specific about the times each dose should be taken so that patients do not take the doses 12 hours apart, thus compromising the nitrate-free interval. One isosorbide mononitrate preparation is dosed once daily. It is an extended-release preparation that provides 12 hours of nitrate exposure. This should be followed by a 12-hour nitrate-free interval. Transdermal nitroglycerin patches are typically prescribed as "on in the am and off in the pm." It is best to provide specific times for application and remove (eg, apply at 8 am and remove at 8 pm). Patients who work evening or night shifts need to have the timing of their nitrate doses adjusted to coincide with when they are active during the day.

Ranolazine

Unlike other agents used for angina, ranolazine does not impact HR, BP, the inotropic state, or coronary blood flow. Animal studies have demonstrated that ranolazine has little affinity for α_1, β_1, and β_2 adrenoreceptors and has minimal calcium channel blocking activity. Ranolazine reduces ischemic episodes by selective inhibition of late sodium current (I_{Na}). Total sodium entry during an action potential is comprised of an early (fast) and late (slow) component. Under normal conditions, late I_{Na} constitutes only 1% of total I_{Na}. Several preclinical studies have observed an increase in late I_{Na} in ischemic and failing hearts.[66] It is not fully appreciated if this increase in late I_{Na} is due to an increase in the density of the late Na^+ channels or dysfunction of these channels. The increase in intracellular Na^+ triggers an increase in the influx of Ca^{2+} through the reverse mode of the Na^+/Ca^{2+} exchanger, resulting in intracellular Ca^{2+} overload and eventually myocardial stunning.[66] Therefore, it is not the intracellular Na^+ concentration that produces ischemic damage, but its recognized role in Ca^{2+} accumulation via Na^+/Ca^{2+} exchange.[66] By inhibiting late I_{Na}, ranolazine produces a reduction in intracellular Na^+. The reduction in intracellular Na^+ contributes to a reduction in the magnitude of ischemia-induced Ca^{2+} overload and improves myocardial function as well as myocardial perfusion.[66]

Ranolazine is available as a sustained-release preparation dosed twice daily. With a half-life of approximately 7 hours, ranolazine achieves a steady-state within 3 days. Since ranolazine 1,000 mg twice daily significantly improves exercise tolerance more than 500 mg twice daily, titration to 1,000 mg twice daily should be attempted. When ranolazine was added to atenolol (50 mg daily), diltiazem (180 mg daily), or amlodipine (5 mg or 10 mg daily), there was an increase in exercise duration, time to angina, time to 1 mm ST-depression, and a reduction in the number of angina episodes and SL nitroglycerin tablets used per week compared to placebo.[67,68] In these trials, the magnitude of increase in exercise duration during testing was associated with a 25% reduction in the weekly number of angina episodes and SL nitroglycerin use over placebo and almost a 50% reduction from baseline.[68,69] The improvement in exercise duration demonstrated with ranolazine is consistent with results produced with β-blockers, CCBs, and chronic nitrates.[8,70]

Patients should be initiated on ranolazine 500 mg twice daily, with the dose increased to 1,000 mg twice daily within the next 1 to 2 weeks if tolerated. Ranolazine is primarily metabolized by CYP3A4 (70%-85%) and CYP2D6 (10%-15%) in the liver and is a substrate for *P*-glycoprotein, making it prone to several clinically important drug interactions. Potent inhibitors of CYP3A4 and *P*-glycoprotein such as ketoconazole, itraconazole, protease inhibitors, and clarithromycin will significantly increase ranolazine drug concentrations. Conversely, potent CYP3A4 inducers such as phenytoin, phenobarbital, carbamazepine, rifampin, rifabutin, rifapentine, and St. John's wort significantly decrease ranolazine drug concentrations. Concurrent use of these strong inhibitors and inducers with ranolazine is contraindicated. Moderate inhibitors of CYP3A4, such as diltiazem, verapamil, erythromycin, and fluconazole, can be used with ranolazine, but the dose should not exceed 500 mg twice daily. Due to inhibition of CYP3A4 by ranolazine, doses of simvastatin should not exceed 20 mg daily. Ranolazine increases digoxin 1.4- to 1.6-fold at trough and 2-fold at peak plasma concentrations, likely through competition for intestinal and renal *P*-glycoprotein. Digoxin doses may need to be reduced to avoid toxicity. Agents that are potent inhibitors of *P*-glycoprotein, such as cyclosporine, may increase ranolazine concentrations and adverse drug reactions. The dose of ranolazine should be reduced.

Ranolazine and metformin compete for renal clearance through the organic cation transporter 2, which has the potential to increase metformin drug concentrations and increase the risk of lactic acidosis. This interaction is only clinically meaningful when both full-dose ranolazine (1,000 mg twice daily) and full-dose metformin (1,000 mg twice daily) are used together. In this setting, the metformin dose should be reduced to 850 mg twice daily. Patients on ranolazine 500 mg twice daily do not need to alter their metformin doses. Ranolazine produces reductions in A1c by 0.6% to 0.7% (0.006-0.007; 7-8 mmol/mol).[68,71] Reductions in blood glucose were observed in patients with or without diabetes, without causing hypoglycemia. While ranolazine is not a treatment for DM, clinicians may find this property useful.

The most common adverse drug reactions from ranolazine use are constipation, nausea, dizziness, and headache. At therapeutic doses, ranolazine produces a modest prolongation of QTc (15 msec or less). A linear relationship exists between ranolazine plasma concentration and the QTc interval, but the effect is modest when used at recommended doses. Patients should not receive doses of more than 1,000 mg twice daily and caution should be used in patients receiving concomitant QTc-prolonging agents.

While ranolazine is safe and effective for treating angina episodes, it would only be an option as monotherapy in patients with SIHD who cannot tolerate traditional antianginal agents due to hemodynamic or other adverse drug reactions. Ranolazine is recommended as an add-on therapy to traditional antianginal agents. In patients who have achieved HR and BP targets on maximally tolerated doses of traditional agents but continue to have exertional angina symptoms, ranolazine is a reasonable choice because it does not impact these hemodynamic parameters.

Nonpharmacologic Therapy (Revascularization)

Surgical revascularization plays a role in the treatment of SIHD. The most common revascularization procedures are coronary artery bypass grafting (CABG) surgery or PCI with or without stent placement. In 2017, more than 600,000 PCI procedures were performed in the United States and approximately a third of these were done electively (eg, in patients with SIHD).[72] Stents are placed in over 90% of patients undergoing PCI, with drug-eluting stents (DES) accounting for 82% of all stents. Bare metal stents (BMS) are placed less commonly (18%). Approximately 371,000 CABG surgeries are performed annually.[2] Other revascularization options are under development.

9 The primary goal of revascularization is to prolong life and, secondarily, to eliminate or reduce symptoms. Revascularization is recommended over medical therapy as initial management of SIHD in select patients, such as those with significant stenosis of the left main coronary artery, multivessel disease and LV dysfunction, or refractory angina. Whereas most of the pharmacologic approaches reduce MVO_2, revascularization increases myocardial oxygen supply in vessels with critical stenosis. This is accomplished by opening the vessel (PCI) or using alternative transplanted vessels to bypass a critical stenosis (CABG). While both procedures are highly effective and have advantages in certain groups of patients over pharmacologic approaches, both have limitations.

Percutaneous Coronary Intervention

The term PCI encompasses the use of balloon angioplasty with stent placement as well as other less commonly performed intracoronary procedures such as rotational atherectomy and aspiration thrombectomy. During a PCI, a catheter is guided into coronary arteries through either femoral or radial access. A sheath is placed in either the femoral or radial artery to maintain access during the procedure. A guide catheter is then introduced through the sheath and advanced to the ostium of the coronary arteries. A guidewire is then advanced through the guide catheter and across the stenosis in the coronary vessel. The deflated balloon is then slid along the guidewire and to the site of the coronary stenosis. The balloon is then inflated. The inflated balloon expands the coronary lumen by stretching and tearing the atherosclerotic plaque (see Acute Coronary Syndromes, Chapter 34 for detailed review). Most elective PCI procedures are completed in 30 to 60 minutes.

Abrupt vessel closure is a potential complication of balloon angioplasty. Abrupt vessel closure is provoked by physical disruption of the plaque on the vessel walls during the procedure. In the past, this complication occurred in 5% to 8% of cases and required emergency CABG surgery in 3% to 5% of patients. A second complication from PCI is restenosis, which can lead to recurrent symptoms and the need for another revascularization procedure in approximately 30% to 50% of patients within a year.[73] These complications have now been dramatically reduced with the use of antithrombotic therapy and intracoronary stents.

Stents are scaffolds made from stainless steel or other metal alloys placed within coronary arteries that can prevent acute vessel closure and restenosis. The stent is placed over the deflated balloon and advanced to the area of coronary stenosis. When the balloon is inflated, the stent expands into the coronary vascular wall. The balloon is then deflated, leaving the expanded stent permanently in the diseased coronary vessel. While stents have had a dramatic effect of reducing restenosis, and therefore repeat revascularization procedures, they do not prevent death or MI more effectively than balloon angioplasty alone.

Restenosis is a phenomenon characterized by a greater than 50% diameter loss in the vessel lumen at the site of the intervention. Restenosis most often occurs within the first 3 to 6 months following the procedure. The pathophysiology of restenosis involves a complex cascade of various growth factors and cytokines that promote smooth muscle cell proliferation and result in a progressive loss of luminal diameter.[73] Restenosis typically occurs through the following mechanisms: early vessel recoil, late constrictive remodeling, and neointimal proliferation.[73]

Elastic recoil is a nearly instantaneous phenomenon, occurring during the first hour after the successful dilation of the vessel. As the vessel is stretched during balloon angioplasty, the endothelium lining the vessel becomes damaged. In response to the stretching, the fibers begin to recoil back to their previous size.[73] Late constrictive remodeling, also referred to as negative remodeling, is mediated by myofibroblasts of the adventitia layer of the coronary vessel. Balloon-induced injury often results in exposure of the adventitia to the lumen. Cell proliferation begins as activated fibroblasts contribute to the enlargement of the adventitia. These activated fibroblasts differentiate into myofibroblasts that are involved in the profibrotic and remodeling effects of the vessel.[73] As the adventitia becomes thick and fibrotic, a decrease in arterial cross-sectional area results.

The scaffold-like properties of a BMS prevent restenosis by controlling elastic recoil and negative remodeling. Restenosis rates dropped from 30% to 50% with balloon angioplasty alone to 15% to 30% with the use of BMS. However, stent-induced vessel injury and inflammatory reactions around the stent struts trigger a set of events that promote neointimal hyperplasia, a normal response to vascular damage.[73] The anti-proliferative drugs used in DES target neointimal hyperplasia. DES are coated with sirolimus, paclitaxel, zotarolimus, or everolimus. These agents interrupt the cell cycle to prevent neointimal proliferation and reduce restenosis rates to 5% to 10%.[73]

Although stents can effectively reduce restenosis, the exposed stent struts can provoke thrombosis. Stent thrombosis is driven by the implantation of the stent into an atherosclerotic plaque, exposing platelet adhering proteins to the stent surface. Patients remain at risk for stent thrombosis until a thin layer of endothelial tissue can grow around the stent struts. This process is called re-endothelialization and typically occurs in 2 to 4 weeks after BMS deployment, with most adverse events occurring within the first 2 weeks. The process of re-endothelialization is significantly prolonged with the use of DES. The drugs in a DES prevent smooth muscle, neointimal, and endothelial cell growth. Therefore, while DES effectively reduces neointimal proliferation and the risk of restenosis, they also increase the period of risk for stent thrombosis.

Stent thrombosis is uncommon (<5% of cases) but catastrophic when it occurs. Stent thrombosis results in a large MI or death in two-thirds of cases. The mortality rate from stent thrombosis ranges from 20% to 45%. Stent thrombosis can be largely prevented by using DAPT.

Pharmacotherapy with PCI

The physical damage imposed on the atherosclerotic plaque during PCI with stent placement induces platelet recruitment and activation, leading to the potential for thrombus formation. Therefore, antithrombotic therapy with antiplatelet and anticoagulant agents are necessary to produce a successful outcome. Antiplatelet therapy is also used after the procedure to reduce the risk of stent thrombosis.

All patients without a contraindication should receive aspirin before PCI. Patients already on chronic aspirin therapy should take an additional 75 to 325 mg before PCI. Aspirin-naïve patients should be given a dose of 325 mg, preferably at least 2 but up to 24 hours before PCI. Chronic treatment with aspirin 81 mg daily is recommended after PCI. Patients receiving a stent should also receive a $P2Y_{12}$ inhibitor (eg, clopidogrel) before PCI. The ACC/AHA guidelines recommend against stent placement if it is believed the patient will not tolerate or comply with the recommended duration of DAPT.[1]

After elective PCI, DAPT should be continued to reduce the risk of stent thrombosis. For patients who receive a BMS, a minimum of 1 month of DAPT is sufficient.[74] In patients at high risk of bleeding, a minimum of 2 weeks can be given, as most re-endothelialization of the stent surface occurs within 2 weeks. Patients receiving a DES should receive at least 6 months of DAPT due to the delayed and somewhat unknown duration of the re-endothelialization process.[73,74] However, it is reasonable for those patients who receive a DES and are at high risk of bleeding or develop significant bleeding to stop the $P2Y_{12}$ inhibitor after only 3 months of therapy.[74] An alternative approach in patients undergoing PCI for SIHD, continuing the P2Y12 inhibitor but discontinuing aspirin 1-3 months after PCI, reduces the risk of bleeding and may be considered.[75]

The results of the DAPT (Dual Antiplatelet Therapy Trial) found that a longer duration of DAPT (up to 30 months) provides a greater reduction in CV adverse events when compared to 12 months of treatment, but also a significant increase in major bleeding.[76] Therefore, the guidelines state that a longer treatment regimen for both BMS and DES can be considered in patients who have tolerated therapy, are not at high risk of bleeding, nor have experienced any bleeding complications. This longer duration of DAPT for patients receiving a DES is a Class IIb recommendation.[74]

PCI Versus Medical Management

Despite advancements in PCI technique and stent technology, no study to date has demonstrated that PCI in patients with SIHD improves survival. This is most likely due to the advancements in pharmacotherapy and the use of GDMT. PCI resulted in fewer angina episodes when compared to medical therapy, but in these trials PCI rarely included the use of stents and medical therapy did not include the use of high-intensity statins or ACE inhibitors.[77]

Contemporary PCI and GDMT have been compared in recent clinical trials. In the COURAGE (Clinical Outcomes Utilizing Revascularization and Aggressive Drug Evaluation) trial, the rate of death and MI were not different between patients who were randomized to GDMT alone compared to PCI with GDMT (19.0% in PCI group vs 18.5% in GDMT group).[78] While more patients were angina-free in the PCI group compared to the GDMT group at 1 year (66% vs 58%), there was no difference at the 5-year follow-up time point (74% vs 72%). The need for revascularization after 5 years was lower in the PCI group (21.1% vs 32.6%). This trial confirms that PCI with GDMT does not lower the risk of death and MI compared to GDMT alone, and PCI should be reserved for patients with SIHD refractory angina after receiving optimal GDMT. These data underscore the importance of aggressive, goal-oriented, pharmacotherapy in patients with SIHD. While one-third of patients in the COURAGE study randomized to the GDMT group did need to receive PCI during the 5-year study, two-thirds did not. Similar to the COURAGE trial, the incidence of CV death, MI, and CV hospitalizations (unstable angina, HF, or resuscitated cardiac arrest) was not significantly different between patients with SIHD treated with an initial invasive strategy consisting of coronary angiography, revascularization, and GDMT compared to an initial conservative strategy in, the more recent ISCHEMIA (International Study of Comparative Health Effectiveness with Medical and Invasive Approaches) trial.[79]

Thus, based on the available evidence, PCI cannot be supported as the initial management strategy in most patients with SIHD. Existing evidence suggests that PCI in SIHD should be reserved for patients with chest pain despite optimal GDMT often referred to as refractory angina.

Coronary Artery Bypass Graft Surgery

9 While PCI is the most common form of revascularization, CABG surgery is recommended to prolong survival or relieve refractory symptoms of angina in select patients.[1,80,84] In the majority of CABG surgeries, a sternotomy, and division of the sternum is done to provide the surgeons with direct access to the heart. Thus, it is often referred to as "open-heart surgery." Once the heart is exposed, vascular conduits surgically harvested from other areas of the body are used to "bypass" the atherosclerotic plaque. The most commonly used vascular conduits are the saphenous vein grafts (SVG) from the leg and the left internal mammary artery (LIMA) from the chest wall. The radial and gastroepiploic arteries are also occasionally used. When a LIMA graft is performed, the distal portion is detached from its insertion point behind the sternum and an anastomosis is made distal to the atherosclerotic plaque of the diseased coronary artery to restore blood flow beyond the blockage. The other vascular conduits (eg, SVG) are considered "free grafts" and are anastomosed distally to atherosclerotic plaques of the other diseased coronary arteries. The proximal ends of the free grafts are then anastomosed to the aorta restoring blood flow distal to the blockage. Prior to and during the anastomoses of the bypass grafts, patients are often placed on cardiopulmonary bypass which redirects blood from the heart to a bypass machine. In the bypass machine, venous blood is oxygenated and then returned to the systemic circulation to maintain myocardial and systemic perfusion during the surgery. The heart is then arrested allowing the surgeon to perform the surgery without the heart actively beating. After the bypass grafts have been installed, the patient is weaned from the cardiopulmonary bypass machine, the heart and lung resume their normal functioning, the cannulas are removed, and the sternum and incisions are closed.

While a critical obstruction of a native coronary vessel due to atherosclerosis usually takes five or more decades, the lifespan of an SVG is significantly shorter. This is due to the higher BP in arterial circulation compared to venous pressures. Endothelial damage and LDL-C accumulation significantly accelerate the atherosclerotic process. The use of arterial grafts provides greater long-term graft patency compared to SVG. Arterial grafts are more prone to vasospasm and require longer surgical times to harvest.

Despite the advancements in technique and patient care, CABG surgery is associated with several complications. Death, neurological impairment, MI, major bleeding, acute kidney injury, atrial fibrillation, and surgical wound infections are all potential complications following CABG surgery. Early mortality within 30 days is generally low (1%-2%) but is higher in emergent or high-risk cases (eg, multiple comorbidities, older patients).[82] Neurological complications such as stroke (1%-3%), delirium (8%-50%), and cognitive deficits can occur due to hypoxia, emboli, hemorrhage, or a metabolic abnormality during or shortly after the surgery.[82] Patients with advanced age, previous stroke or transient ischemic attack, HTN, ASCVD, atrial fibrillation, and prolonged cardiopulmonary bypass duration are at higher risk of neurological complications. Atrial fibrillation occurs in as many as 30% of patients undergoing CABG surgery but is often transient. An infection of the sternum, known as mediastinitis, occurs in 0.5%-3% of patients and may prolong hospital stays, increase recovery time, and result in repeat surgical intervention.[82] MI, major bleeding requiring surgical re-exploration, and acute kidney injury requiring hemodialysis each occur in 1% to 4% of patients following CABG surgery.[82]

New approaches to CABG surgery have been developed in an attempt to minimize complications. One of these approaches is the off-pump bypass coronary surgery that is performed while the heart is beating. By reducing the need for cardiopulmonary bypass and aortic clamping, rates of adverse neurologic and renal events are significantly lower.[82] Another approach to surgical revascularization is the use of minimally invasive direct coronary artery bypass during which a small left anterior thoracotomy is done in lieu of a sternotomy. Due to the small incision and technical difficulty of the surgery, only patients with single-vessel disease in either the left anterior descending or right coronary artery currently are candidates for the procedure. Although postoperative pain is often increased, clinical outcomes of minimally invasive direct coronary artery bypass are similar to conventional CABG but recovery time is quicker.[82]

In suitable surgical candidates, CABG surgery is the preferred revascularization strategy in several clinical scenarios. Examples include patients with left main CAD (≥50% stenosis) "unprotected" by collateral coronary blood flow or patent bypass grafts, 2-vessel CAD (≥70% stenosis in the proximal left anterior descending coronary artery and one additional major coronary artery), and multivessel CAD (≥70% stenosis in three or more major coronary arteries). CABG surgery is preferred to PCI and medical management because it is associated with prolonged survival.[84] CABG surgery is also recommended to decrease mortality in patients who survived an episode of sudden cardiac death due to ischemia from significant (≥70% stenosis) CAD in one or more arteries. In patients with SIHD whose symptoms are refractory to GDMT, CABG surgery may be considered.[1,84] However, because it is less invasive than CABG surgery, PCI is often the preferred strategy in this setting.

Pharmacotherapy with CABG

Prior to CABG surgery, attention to pharmacotherapeutic needs is important to minimize postoperative complications. Patients taking aspirin 81 to 325 mg daily preoperatively should continue taking aspirin until the time of surgery to reduce ischemic events. Although patients undergoing elective CABG who were not taking aspirin preoperatively have commonly been initiated on aspirin within 24 hours of surgery, this approach offers no benefit and is no longer recommended.[84] To reduce the risk of CABG-related major bleeding, $P2Y_{12}$ inhibitors should be discontinued well in advance of an elective CABG surgery (5 days for clopidogrel and ticagrelor; 7 days for prasugrel) and at least 24 hours prior to urgent CABG surgery, if possible. Initiation of β-blockers or amiodarone prior to CABG surgery may be considered to reduce the risk of postoperative atrial fibrillation.[84]

Pharmacotherapy after CABG surgery includes aspirin, high-intensity statins, β-blockers, and the continuation of ACE inhibitors (ACC/AHA Class I recommendations).[1,84] Aspirin 81 to 325 mg daily should be resumed or initiated within 6 hours of CABG surgery and continued indefinitely to reduce the risk of graft closure and acute MI. If patients are truly aspirin allergic, clopidogrel is an acceptable alternative. For patients treated with DAPT following PCI who subsequently undergo CABG surgery, DAPT should be resumed postoperatively and continued for the initially recommended duration of therapy is completed.[74] Due to the accelerated atherosclerotic process in the bypass grafts, high-intensity statin therapy should be resumed or initiated in all patients following CABG surgery. β-Blockers should be initiated after CABG surgery to reduce the incidence of postoperative atrial fibrillation.[84] The safety and efficacy of initiating ACE inhibitors following CABG surgery are uncertain and may increase the risk of hypotension and acute kidney injury, particularly if administered during the early postoperative period.[81] However, the continuation of previous ACE inhibitor therapy following CABG surgery is associated with a significant reduction in nonfatal cardiac, cerebral, and renal events, whereas ACE inhibitor withdrawal following CABG surgery is associated with increased event rates.[83] Therefore, for patients taking ACE inhibitors or ARBs prior to CABG surgery, these therapies should be resumed following surgery once patients have demonstrated stable hemodynamics and renal function.[81] For ACE inhibitor-naïve patients, initiation of an ACE inhibitor should be considered in stable patients with compelling indications (eg, HFrEF, HTN, DM, and chronic kidney disease).[81] For symptomatic relief of chest pain episodes, patients need access to SL nitroglycerin after surgery. Smoking cessation and cardiac rehabilitation are also critical to successful postoperative outcomes.

Management of Angina

8 Medical management of angina episodes follows a stepwise approach (see Fig. 33-2 and Table 33-6). All patients should have access to SL nitroglycerin for the treatment of an acute episode of angina. Patients need to be adequately educated on appropriate use and storage, assuring consistent access to the tablets or spray (Table 33-8). This may require patients to have multiple vials or canisters that are in areas that they spend time (eg, home, work, car). While some patients may only need SL nitroglycerin for infrequent attacks, many patients with SIHD will need chronic therapy to prevent angina episodes. Patients experiencing frequent angina episodes or in whom angina is impacting the quality of life should receive chronic therapy. The goal of chronic therapy is to provide complete or nearly complete elimination of angina episodes while having the patient take part in normal activities.

Since increased heart rate can increase MVO_2 and precipitate angina, either a β-blocker or a non-DHP CCB (verapamil or diltiazem) can be used for the initial chronic management of angina. The goal is to lower the patient's resting HR to 50 to 60 beats per minute and an exercise HR of less than 100 beats per minute. Not all patients, especially older adults, can tolerate an HR in this range; the goal HR would be as low as the patient can tolerate above 50 beats per minute. Both β-blockers and CCBs can improve exercise duration and reduce the number of weekly angina episodes.[70]

6 β-Blockers are recommended over CCBs as initial therapy for control of angina episodes in patients with SIHD.[1] This recommendation is based on improved survival demonstrated with the use of β-blockers in patients after MI and with HFrEF. Only carvedilol, metoprolol succinate, and bisoprolol should be used in patients with HFrEF, starting with low doses and titrating up in a slow and set regimen. CCBs have not demonstrated similar benefits in patients following an MI or with HFrEF. Patients with contraindications or intolerable adverse drug reactions to β-blocker therapy may be treated with a CCB, with verapamil or diltiazem preferred in patients needing HR reduction. In patients without a history of MI or HF, the use of β-blocker therapy does not provide a survival advantage and is used purely for the control of ischemic episodes and symptoms of angina.[70]

5 If angina symptoms are controlled once the HR goal is achieved, no additional antianginal therapy is necessary and patients are monitored for continued efficacy and adverse drug reactions. Regardless of whether a β-blocker or non DHP CCB are selected as initial therapy for HR reduction, many patients will require combination therapy to attain adequate control of their symptoms. If additional therapy is required, the need for additional antihypertensive agents should be considered in the next step. Patients with angina symptoms refractory to β-blockers who continue to have elevated BP above the goal of 130/80 mm Hg should be prescribed a DHP CCB. Unlike long-acting nitrates and ranolazine, DHP CCBs decrease both MVO_2 and BP. While not commonly combined, DHP CCB and non-DHP CCB target different calcium channels and are a rational regimen for patients with SIHD with contraindications or intolerance to β-blockers. It is important to monitor the patient for peripheral edema and signs and symptoms of reduced cardiac output.

7 In patients with continued angina episodes despite achieving BP and HR goals, a long-acting nitrate or ranolazine should be added to the regimen. Both agents have demonstrated efficacy when used in combination with SL nitroglycerin and medications to control HR and BP. While long-acting nitrates are not optimal agents when used as monotherapy due to reflex tachycardia, this is attenuated in patients who are taking a β-blocker or non-DHP CCB. Ranolazine does not reduce HR or BP, making it an option in patients who have already achieved their HR and BP goals, but still have exertional angina. The selection of a long-acting nitrate or ranolazine should be based on patient preferences, tolerability, and cost. Long-acting nitrates do not provide 24-hour angina protection, but this may not be an issue for all patients. While ranolazine provides 24 hours protection and has a more attractive adverse drug reaction profile compared to long-acting nitrates, it is more expensive and associated with numerous drug interactions.

Patients who are unable to fully participate in the activities that bring them joy in life because of inadequate control of chest pain symptoms, despite the use of maximally tolerated therapies, have refractory angina. Some patients may have refractory angina while taking relatively fewer antianginal medications or lower doses due to intolerances or contraindications. Patients with refractory angina should be referred for revascularization therapy.

Management of Vasospastic Angina

In patients where the onset of angina varies, pharmacotherapy that targets vasospasm is needed. While β-blockers are typically the agents of first choice in patients with a consistent angina threshold, they are less useful in patients with vasospasm. Although not all studies report increased chest pain episodes with β-blockers in patients with vasospasm, they can induce coronary vasoconstriction and prolong ischemia. Worsening angina is most likely due to unopposed α1-adrenergic receptor stimulation during β-blockade. A similar phenomenon may occur in patients with SIHD treated with β-blockers who also abuse cocaine or methamphetamines.

Both nitrates and CCBs reduce vasospasm. Most patients respond well to SL nitroglycerin for acute attacks. While long-acting nitrates can be used in the treatment of vasospasm, the high doses typically needed for adequate symptom control are not well tolerated. Therefore, CCBs are often used. There is no preference to which agent is selected first, but CCBs are dosed less frequently and a single agent may be sufficient to manage symptoms. Nifedipine, verapamil, and diltiazem are all equally effective for the initial management of coronary vasospasm. Dose titration is important to maximize the response with CCBs. Patients unresponsive to calcium antagonists alone may add long-acting nitrates.

EVALUATION OF THERAPEUTIC OUTCOMES

The therapeutic goals in the management of patients with SIHD are to prolong life, reduce symptoms of angina, and improve quality of life. Improving the patient's quality of life requires careful attention to the potential adverse drug reactions from medications. Surrogate endpoints such as BP goal attainment, use of high-intensity statin, A1c goal attainment, smoking cessation, and achieving a healthy weight should be used to determine progress toward the ultimate goal—reduced risk of mortality and major cardiovascular events. Patients should be evaluated every 1 to 2 months until goals are achieved. Follow-up every 6 to 12 months thereafter is appropriate.

3 Monitoring for improvements in symptoms related to angina should include asking the patients about the number and severity of angina episodes and weekly SL nitroglycerin use as well as inquiring about exercise capacity or duration of exertion needed to induce angina. It is important to ask the patient about their ability to engage in activities they want to do. It is not uncommon for patients to report reduced or no episodes of angina because they have stopped engaging in activities that bring on angina. Patients experiencing worsening angina may complain of increasing frequency and severity of symptoms, increased SL nitroglycerin use, decreased exercise capacity, or a combination of these. Once patients have received optimal medical therapy, symptoms should improve in 2 to 4 weeks and remain stable until the disease progresses. Instruments such as the Seattle Angina Questionnaire and CCS Angina Grading Scale can be used to improve the assessment of symptoms.[1] While objective tests such as an exercise tolerance test with or without cardiac imaging can be obtained to assess the adequacy of treatment, they are primarily performed in patients who do not achieve adequate symptom control. Following a revascularization procedure, the patients' symptoms should be assessed every 6 to 12 months.

ABBREVIATIONS

ACC American College of Cardiology
ACE angiotensin-converting enzyme
ACS acute coronary syndrome
AHA American Heart Association
ARB angiotensin receptor blocker
ASCVD atherosclerotic cardiovascular disease
BMS bare-metal stent
BP blood pressure
CABG coronary artery bypass grafting
CAD coronary artery disease
CCS Canadian Cardiovascular Society
CCB calcium channel blocker
COR class of recommendation
COX cyclooxygenase
COPD chronic obstructive pulmonary disease
CT computer topography
CVD cardiovascular disease
DES drug-eluting stent
DHP dihydropyridine
DM diabetes mellitus
ECG electrocardiogram
EDRF endothelium-derived relaxing factor
FFR fractional flow reserve
GDMT guideline-directed medical therapy
HDL-C high-density lipoprotein cholesterol
HF heart failure
HFrEF heart failure with reduced ejection fraction
HR heart rate
HTN hypertension
LDL-C low-density lipoprotein cholesterol
LIMA left internal mammary artery
LOE level of evidence
LV left ventricle
MI myocardial infarction
MVO_2 myocardial oxygen demand
PCI percutaneous coronary intervention
SIHD stable ischemic heart disease
SVG saphenous vein graft

REFERENCES

1. Fihn SD, Gardin JM, Abrams J, et al. 2012 ACCF/AHA/AATS/PCNA/SCAI/STS Guideline for the diagnosis and management of patients with stable ischemic heart disease: A report of the American College of Cardiology Foundation/American Heart Association task force on practice guidelines, and the American College of Physicians, American Association of Thoracic Surgery, Preventive Cardiovascular Nurses Association, Society for Cardiovascular Angiography and Interventions, and Society of Thoracic Surgeons. *J Am Coll Cardiol.* 2012;60:e44–e164.
2. Virani SS, Alonso A, Aparicio HJ, et al. Heart disease and stroke statistics—2021 update. *Circulation.* 2021;143:e254–e743. 10.1161/cir.0000000000000950.
3. Steg PG, Greenlaw N, Tendera M, et al. Prevalence of angina symptoms and myocardial ischemia and their effect on clinical outcomes in outpatients with stable coronary artery disease: Data from the International Observational CLARIFY Registry. *JAMA Intern Med.* 2014;174:1651–1659.
4. Mozaffarian D, Bryson CL, Spertus JA, et al. Anginal symptoms consistently predict total mortality among outpatients with coronary artery disease. *Am Heart J.* 2003;146:1015–1022.
5. Five-year clinical and functional outcome comparing bypass surgery and angioplasty in patients with multivessel coronary disease: A multicenter randomized trial. Writing Group for the Bypass Angioplasty Revascularization Investigation (BARI) Investigators. *JAMA.* 1997;277:715–721.
6. Boini S, Briancon S, Guillemin F, Galan P, Hercberg S. Occurrence of coronary artery disease has an adverse impact on health-related quality of life: A longitudinal controlled study. *Int J Cardiol.* 2006;113:215–222.
7. Hlatky MA, Rogers WJ, Johnstone I, et al. Medical care costs and quality of life after randomization to coronary angioplasty or coronary bypass surgery. Bypass Angioplasy Revascularization Investigation (BARI) Investigators. *N Engl J Med.* 1997;336:92–99.
8. Tarkin JM, Kaski JC. Pharmacological treatment of chronic stable angina pectoris. *Clin Med.* 2013;13:63–70.
9. Fuster V, Badimon L, Badimon JJ, Chesebro JH. The pathogenesis of coronary heart disease and the acute coronary syndrome (first of two parts). *N Engl J Med.* 1992;326:242–250.
10. Fuster V, Badimon L, Badimon JJ, Chesebro JH. The pathogenesis of coronary heart disease and the acute coronary syndrome (second of two parts). *N Engl J Med.* 1992;326:310–318.

11. Epstein SE, Cannon RO III, Talbot TL. Hemodynamic principles in the control of coronary blood flow. *Am J Cardiol.* 1985;56:4E–10E.
12. Laughlin MH, Davis MJ, Secher NH, et al. Peripheral circulation. *Compr Physiol.* 2012;2:321–447.
13. Marzilli M, Merz CNB, Boden WE, et al. Obstructive coronary atherosclerosis and ischemic heart disease: An elusive link! *J Am Coll Cardiol.* 2012;60:951–956.
14. Pepine CJ, Douglas PS. Rethinking stable ischemic heart disease: Is this the beginning of a new era? *J Am Coll Cardiol.* 2012;60:957–959.
15. Ridker PM, Danielson E, Fonseca FAH, et al. JUPITER Study Group. Rosuvastatin to prevent vascular events in men and women with elevated C-reactive protein. *N Engl J Med.* 2008;359:2195–2207.
16. Campeau L. Grading of angina pectoris (letter). *Circulation.* 1976;54:522–523.
17. Pepine CJ, Balaban RS, Bonow RO, et al. Women's ischemic syndrome evaluation: Current status and future research directions: Report of the National Heart, Lung and Blood Institute workshop. October 2–4, 2002; Section 1: diagnosis of stable ischemia and ischemic heart disease. *Circulation.* 2004;109:e44–e46.
18. Gould KL, Johnson NP, Bateman TM, et al. Anatomic versus physiologic assessment of coronary artery disease: Role of coronary flow reserve, fractional flow reserve, and positron emission tomography imaging in revascularization decision-making. *J Am Coll Cardiol.* 2013;62:1639–1653.
19. van de Hoef TP, Echavarría-Pinto M, van Lavieren MA, et al. Diagnostic and prognostic implications of coronary flow capacity: A comprehensive cross-modality physiological concept in ischemic heart disease. *J Am Coll Cardiol Intv.* 2015;8:1670–1680.
20. Jeremias A, Kleiman NS, Nassif D, et al. EVENT Registry Investigators. Prevalence and prognostic significance of preprocedural cardiac troponin elevation among patients with stable coronary artery disease undergoing percutaneous coronary intervention: Results from the Evaluation of Drug Eluting Stents and Ischemic Events Registry. *Circulation.* 2008;118:632–638.
21. Ferrari R, Pavasini R, Camici PG, et al. Anti-anginal drugs–beliefs and evidence: Systematic review covering 50 years of medical treatment. *European Heart Journal.* 2018;40:190–194. 10.1093/eurheartj/ehy504.
22. Whelton PK, Carey RM, Aronow WS, et al. 2017 ACC/AHA/AAPA/ABC/ACPM/AGS/APhA/ASH/ASPC/NMA/PCNA guideline for the prevention, detection, evaluation, and management of high blood pressure in adults—a report of the American College of Cardiology/American Heart Association Task Force on Clinical Practice Guidelines. *J Am Coll Cardiol.* 2018;71:e127–e248.
23. Grundy SM, Stone NJ, Bailey AL, et al. 2018 AHA/ACC/AACVPR/AAPA/ABC/ACPM/ADA/AGS/APhA/ASPC/NLA/PCNA guideline on the management of blood cholesterol. *J Amer Coll Cardiol.* 2019;73:e285–e350.
24. American Diabetes Association. Pharmacologic approaches to glycemic treatment: standards of medical care in diabetes—2022. *Diabetes Care.* 2022;45:S125–S143. 10.2337/dc22-S009.
25. Antithrombotic Trialists' Collaboration. Collaborative meta-analysis of randomised trials of antiplatelet therapy for prevention of death, myocardial infarction, and stroke in high risk patients. *BMJ.* 2002;324:71–86.
26. Dobesh PP, Varnado S, Doyle M. Antiplatelet agents in cardiology: A report on aspirin, clopidogrel, prasugrel, and ticagrelor. *Cur Pharm Des.* 2016;22:1918–1932.
27. Ridker PM, Manson JE, Gaziano JM, et al. Low-dose aspirin therapy for chronic stable angina. A randomized, placebo-controlled clinical trial. *Ann Intern Med.* 1991;114:835–839. doi: 10.7326/0003-4819-114-10-835.
28. Juul-Möller S, Edvardsson N, Jahnmatz B, et al. Double-blind trial of aspirin in primary prevention of myocardial infarction in patients with stable chronic angina pectoris. The Swedish Angina Pectoris Aspirin Trial (SAPAT) Group. *Lancet.* 1992;340:1421–1425. doi: 10.1016/0140-6736(92)92619-q.
29. Sofi F, Marcucci R, Gori AM, Abbate R, Gensini GF. Residual platelet reactivity on aspirin therapy and recurrent cardiovascular events—at meta-analysis. *Int J Cardiol.* 2008;128:166–171.
30. Hovens MMC, Snoep JD, Eikenboom JCJ, van der Bom JG, Mertens BJA, Huisman MV. Prevalence of persistent platelet reactivity despite use of aspirin: A systematic review. *Am Heart J.* 2007;153:175–181.
31. Gurbel PA, Bliden KP, DiChiara J, et al. Evaluation of dose-related effects of aspirin on platelet function: Results from the Aspirin-Induced Platelet Effect (ASPECT) study. *Circulation.* 2007;115:3156–3164.
32. Dobesh PP, Finks SW, Trujillo TC. Dual antiplatelet therapy for long-term secondary prevention of atherosclerotic cardiovascular events. *Clin Ther.* 2020;42:2084–2097. 10.1016/j.clinthera.2020.08.003.
33. Serebruany VL, Steinhubl SR, Berger PB, et al. Variability in platelet responsiveness to clopidogrel among 544 individuals. *J Am Coll Cardiol.* 2005;45:246–251.
34. Wismann PP, Roest M, Asselbergs FW. Platelet-reactivity tests identify patients at secondary risk of secondary cardiovascular events: A systematic review and meta-analysis. *J Thromb Haemost.* 2014;12:736–747.
35. Bonello L, Tantry US, Marcucci R, et al. Consensus and future directions on the definition of high on-treatment platelet reactivity to adenosine diphosphate. *J Am Coll Cardiol.* 2010;56:919–933.
36. Spertus JA, Kettelkamp R, Vance C, et al. Prevalence, predictors, and outcomes of premature discontinuation of thienopyridine therapy after drug-eluting stent placement: Results from the PREMIER registry. *Circulation.* 2006;113:2803–2809.
37. Scott SA, Sangkuhl K, Stein CM, et al. Clinical pharmacogenetics implementation consortium guidelines for cytochrome P450-2C19 (CYP2C19) genotype and clopidogrel therapy: 2013 update. *Clin Pharmacol Ther.* 2013;94:317–323.
38. Eikelboom JW, Connolly SJ, Bosch J, et al. Rivaroxaban with or without aspirin in stable cardiovascular disease. *N Engl J Med.* 2017;377(14):1319–1330. 10.1056/NEJMoa1709118 28844192.
39. Anand SS, Eikelboom JW, Dyal L, et al. Rivaroxaban plus aspirin versus aspirin in relation to vascular risk in the COMPASS Trial. *J Am Coll Cardiol.* 2019;73:3271–3280. 10.1016/j.jacc.2019.02.079.
40. Rousan TA, Mathew ST, Thadani U. Drug therapy for stable angina pectoris. *Drugs.* 2017;77:265–284.
41. HOPE Investigators. Effects of an angiotensin-converting enzyme inhibitor, ramipril, on cardiovascular events in high risk patients. *N Engl J Med.* 2000;342:145–153.
42. The European trial on reduction of cardiac events with perindopril in stable coronary artery disease investigators. Efficacy of perindopril in reduction of cardiovascular events among patients with stable coronary artery disease: Randomised, double-blind, placebo-controlled, multicenter trial (the EUROPA study). *Lancet.* 2003;362:782–788.
43. PEACE Trial Investigators. Angiotensin-converting-enzyme inhibition in stable coronary artery disease. *N Engl J Med.* 2004;351:2058–2068.
44. Danchin N, Cucherat M, Thuillez C, Durand E, Kadri Z, Steg PG. Angiotensin-converting enzyme inhibitors in patients with coronary artery disease and absence of heart failure or left ventricular systolic dysfunction: An overview of long-term randomized controlled trials. *Arch Intern Med.* 2006;166:787–796.
45. The ONTARGET Investigators. Telmisartan, ramipril, or both in patients at high risk for vascular events. *N Engl J Med.* 2008;358:1547–1559.
46. The TRANSCEND Investigators. Effects of angiotensin-receptor blocker telmisartan on cardiovascular events in high-risk patients intolerant to angiotensin-converting enzyme inhibitors: A randomised controlled trial. *Lancet.* 2008;372:1174–1183.
47. Baigent C, Blackwell L, Emberson J, et al. Efficacy and safety of more intensive lowering of LDL cholesterol: A meta-analysis of data from 170,000 participants in 26 randomised trials. *Lancet.* 2010;376:1670–1681.
48. Pedersen TR, Faergeman O, Kastelein JJP, et al. High-dose atorvastatin vs usual-dose simvastatin for secondary prevention after myocardial infarction: The IDEAL study: A randomized controlled trial. *JAMA.* 2005;294:2445.
49. The SPRINT Research Group. A randomized trial of intensive versus standard blood pressure control. *N Engl J Med.* 2015;373:2103–2116.
50. Reboussin DM, Allen NB, Griswold ME, et al. Systematic review for the 2017 ACC/AHA/AAPA/ABC/ACPM/AGS/APhA/ASH/ASPC/NMA/PCNA guideline for the prevention, detection, evaluation, and management of high blood pressure in adults—a report of the American College of Cardiology/American Heart Association Task Force on Clinical Practice Guidelines. *J Am Coll Cardiol.* 2018;71:2176–2198.
51. National Center for Chronic Disease Prevention and Health Promotion (US) Office on Smoking and Health. The health consequences of smoking-50 years of progress: A report of the Surgeon General. http://www.ncbi.nlm.nih.gov/pubmed/24455788. Published 2014; accessed June 13, 2018.
52. Ambrose JA, Barua RS. The pathophysiology of cigarette smoking and cardiovascular disease: An update. *J Am Coll Cardiol.* 2004;43:1731–1737.
53. Jha P, Ramasundarahettige C, Landsman V, et al. 21st-century hazards of smoking and benefits of cessation in the United States. *N Engl J Med.* 2013;368:341–350.
54. Anthenelli RM, Benowitz NL, West R, et al. Neuropsychiatric safety and efficacy of varenicline, bupropion, and nicotine patch

in smokers with and without psychiatric disorders (EAGLES): A double-blind, randomised, placebo-controlled clinical trial. *Lancet.* 2016;387(10037):2507.

55. Benowitz NL, Pipe A, West R, et al. Cardiovascular safety of varenicline, buproprion, and nicotine patch in smokers: A randomized clinical trial. *JAMA Intern Med.* 2018;178:622–631.
56. Hong KN, Fuster V, Rosenson RS, Rosendorff C, Bhatt DL. How low to go with glucose, cholesterol, and blood pressure in primary prevention of CVD. *J Am Coll Cardiol.* 2017;70:2171–2185.
57. Lee G, Oh S-W, Hwang S-S, et al. Comparative effectiveness of oral antidiabetic drugs in preventing cardiovascular mortality and morbidity: A network meta-analysis. *PLoS ONE.* 2017;12:e0177646. https://doi.org/10.1371/journal.pone.0177646.
58. Zheng SL, Roddick AJ, Aghar-Jaffar R, et al. Association between use of sodium-glucose-cotransporter 2 inhibitors, glucagon-like peptide 1 agonists, and dipeptidyl peptidase 4 inhibitors with all-cause mortality in patients with type 2 diabetes: A systematic review and meta-analysis. *JAMA.* 2018;319:1580–1591.
59. Udell JA, Zawi R, Bhatt DL, et al. Association between influenza vaccination and cardiovascular outcomes in high-risk patients. *JAMA.* 2013;310:1711–1720. 10.1001/jama.2013.279206.
60. Frøbert O, Götberg M, Erlinge D, et al. Influenza vaccination after myocardial infarction: a randomized, double-blind, placebo-controlled, multicenter trial. *Circulation.* 2021;144. 10.1161/circulationaha.121.057042.
61. Messerli FH, Bangalore S, Yao SS, Steinberg JS. Cardioprotection with beta-blockers: Myths, facts and Pascal's wager. *J Intern Med.* 2009;266:232–241.
62. Dransfield MT, Voelker H, Bhatt SP, et al. Metoprolol for the Prevention of Acute Exacerbations of COPD. *New England Journal of Medicine.* 2019;381:2304–2314. 10.1056/nejmoa1908142.
63. Steering Committee Transdermal Nitroglycerin Cooperative Study. Acute and chronic antianginal efficacy of continuous twenty-four-hour application of transdermal nitroglycerin. *Am J Cardiol.* 1991;68:1263–1273.
64. Munzel T, Daiber A, Mulsch A. Explaining the phenomenon of nitrate tolerance. *Circ Res.* 2005;97:618–628.
65. Daiber A, Oelze M, Wenzel P, et al. Nitrate tolerance as a model of vascular dysfunction: Roles for mitochondrial aldehyde dehydrogenase and mitochondrial oxidative stress. *Pharmacol Rep.* 2009;61:33–48.
66. Dobesh PP, Trujillo TC. Ranolazine: A new option in the management of chronic stable angina. *Pharmacotherapy.* 2007;27:1659–1676.
67. Chaitman BR, Skettino SL, Parker JO, et al., for the MARISA Investigators. Anti-ischemic effects and long-term survival during ranolazine monotherapy in patients with chronic severe angina. *J Am Coll Cardiol.* 2004;43:1375–1382.
68. Chaitman BR, Pepine CJ, Parker JO, et al. CARISA Investigators. Effects of ranolazine with atenolol, amlodipine, or diltiazem on exercise tolerance and angina frequency in patients with severe chronic angina. A randomized controlled trial. *JAMA.* 2004;291:309–316.
69. Stone PH, Gratsiansky NA, Blokhin A, Huang I-Z, Meng L. Antianginal efficacy of ranolazine when added to treatment with amlodipine. The ERICA (Efficacy of Ranolizine in Chronic Angina) Trial. *J Am Coll Cardiol.* 2006;48:566–575.
70. Mody P, Sidhu MS, Brilakis ES, Sacco JD, Banerjee S, Boden WE. Antianginal agents for the management for stable ischemic heart disease: A review. *Card Rev.* 2016;24:177–189.
71. Morrow DA, Scirica BM, Karwatowska-Prokopczuk E, et al. , for the MERLIN-TIMI 36 Trial Investigators. Effects of Ranolazine on recurrent cardiovascular events in patients with non-ST-elevation acute coronary syndromes: The MERLIN-TIMI 36 randomized trial. *JAMA.* 2007;297:1775–1783.
72. Inohara T, Kohsaka S, Spertus JA, et al. Comparative trends in percutaneous Coronary Intervention in Japan and the United States, 2013 to 2017. *Journal of the American College of Cardiology.* 2020;76:1328–1340. 10.1016/j.jacc.2020.07.037.
73. Dobesh PP, Stacy ZA, Ansara AJ, Enders JM. Drug-eluting stents: A mechanical and pharmacologic approach to coronary artery disease. *Pharmacotherapy.* 2004;24:1554–1577.
74. Levine GN, Bates ER, Bittl JA, et al. 2016 ACC/AHA guideline focused update on duration of dual antiplatelet therapy in patients with coronary artery disease. A report of the American College of Cardiology/American Heart Association Task Force on Clinical Practice Guidelines. *J Am Coll Cardiol.* 2016;68:1082–1115.
75. O'Donoghue ML, Murphy SA, Sabatine MS The Safety and Efficacy of Aspirin Discontinuation on a Background of a P2Y 12 Inhibitor in Patients After Percutaneous Coronary Intervention. *Circulation.* 2020;142:538–545. 10.1161/circulationaha.120.046251.
76. Mauri L, Kereiakes DJ, Yeh RW, et al., for the DAPT Study Investigators. Twelve or 30 months of dual antiplatelet therapy after drug-eluting stents. *N Engl J Med.* 2014;371:2155–2166.
77. Stergiopoulos K, Boden WE, Hartigan P, et al. Percutaneous coronary intervention outcomes in patients with stable obstructive coronary artery disease and myocardial ischemia: A collaborative meta-analysis of contemporary randomized clinical trials. *JAMA Intern Med.* 2014;174:232–240.
78. Boden WE, O'Rourke RA, Teo KK, et al. COURAGE Trial Research Group.Optimal medical therapy with or without PCI for stable coronary disease. *N Engl J Med.* 2007;356:1503–1516.
79 Maron DJ, Hochman JS, Reynolds HR, et al. Initial invasive or conservative strategy for stable coronary disease. *N Engl J Med.* 2020;382:1395–1407.
80. Fihn SD, Blankenship JC, Alexander KP, et al. 2014 ACC/AHA/AATS/PCNA/SCAI/STS focused update of the guidelines for the diagnosis and management of patients with stable ischemic heart disease. *J Am Coll Cardiol.* 2014;64:1929–1949.
81. Hillis LD, Smith PK, Anderson JL, et al. 2011 ACCF/AHA guideline for coronary artery bypass graft surgery. *J Am Coll Cardiol.* 2011;58:e123–e210.
82. Head SJ, Milojevic M, Taggart DP, Puskas JD. Current practice of state-of-the-art surgical coronary revascularization. *Circulation.* 2017;136:1331–1345.
83. Drenger B, Fontes ML, Miao Y, et al. Patterns of use of perioperative angiotensin-converting enzyme inhibitors in coronary artery bypass graft surgery with cardiopulmonary bypass—effects on in-hospital morbidity and mortality. *Circulation.* 2012;126:261–269.
84. Lawton JS, Tamis-Holland JE, Bangalore S, et al. 2021 ACC/AHA/SCAI Guideline for Coronary Artery Revascularization: A Report of the American College of Cardiology/American Heart Association Joint Committee on Clinical Practice Guidelines. *Circulation.* 2022;14510.1161/cir.0000000000001038.

34

Acute Coronary Syndrome

Robert J. DiDomenico, Paul P. Dobesh, and Shannon W. Finks

KEY CONCEPTS

1. The cause of acute coronary syndrome (ACS) in more than 90% of patients is the acute rupture, fissure, or erosion of an unstable atherosclerotic plaque followed by subsequent thrombus formation that impairs distal blood flow resulting in acute myocardial ischemia.
2. Patients with symptoms of myocardial ischemia suspected of having ACS should undergo risk stratification that incorporates their past medical history, presenting signs and symptoms, 12-lead electrocardiogram (ECG), and cardiac troponin (cTn); dynamic elevation in serial cTn values confirms the diagnosis of myocardial infarction (MI).
3. Intravenous (IV) nitroglycerin should be considered to alleviate anginal pain and/or treat acute comorbidities such as uncontrolled hypertension (HTN) or heart failure (HF), oxygen should be administered to patients with hypoxia (oxygen saturation less than 90% [0.90]), and IV morphine may be considered in patients with refractory anginal pain.
4. In the absence of contraindications, an oral β-blocker should be initiated for all patients with ACS and continued for 3 years or more to reduce the risk of major adverse cardiac events (MACE); calcium channel blockers (CCBs) may be considered in patients with vasospasm and those refractory to or with contraindications or intolerance to β-blockers.
5. Reperfusion of the infarct-related artery in ST-segment elevation myocardial infarction (STEMI) with primary percutaneous coronary intervention (PCI) within 90 minutes of first medical contact is preferred to fibrinolytic therapy unless primary PCI cannot be performed within 120 minutes of presentation.
6. Antiplatelet therapy is a central component to the acute and chronic management of patients with ACS to reduce MACE, frequently includes aspirin plus a $P2Y_{12}$ inhibitor, and requires careful attention paid to the clinical scenario to select the regimen that optimizes efficacy and safety.
7. Use of parenteral anticoagulant agents (unfractionated heparin, low-molecular-weight heparin [LMWH], fondaparinux, bivalirudin) during hospitalization have the ability to reduce MACE in patients with ACS and requires knowledge of the diagnosis, selected management strategy, and other factors to select the drug and dosing regimen that optimize efficacy and safety.
8. Dual antiplatelet therapy (DAPT) with aspirin plus a $P2Y_{12}$ receptor inhibitor is indicated for all patients post-ACS for a minimum of 12 months regardless of whether the patient is managed with an ischemia-driven approach or if the patient undergoes revascularization.
9. All patients post-ACS should receive maximally tolerated high-intensity statin therapy to reduce the risk of MACE; patients with low-density lipoprotein cholesterol (LDL-C) of 70 mg/dL (1.81 mmol/L) or greater on maximally tolerated high-intensity statin therapy should be considered for the addition of nonstatin therapies (eg, ezetimibe, proprotein convertase subtilisin kexin 9 [PCSK9] inhibitor).
10. To reduce the risk of MACE, all post-MI patients should receive oral treatment with an angiotensin-converting enzyme inhibitor (ACEI) or angiotensin receptor blocker (ARB) unless contraindicated and a mineralocorticoid receptor antagonist if the left ventricular ejection fraction (LVEF) is 40% (0.40) or less and HF symptoms or diabetes mellitus (DM) are also present.

BEYOND THE BOOK

To better understand the pathophysiology of acute coronary syndrome (ACS), clinical presentation, and the rationale for pharmacotherapy to treat ACS, please watch the videos below. These videos should enhance learner understanding regarding the COLLECT, ASSESS, and PLAN steps in the Patient Care Process.

1. Thrombotic cascade in ACS—Acute coronary syndrome (ACS) pathology—Thrombosis Advisor https://www.youtube.com/watch?v=VIYAAdkOOrk (Duration 1:48 minutes)
2. Acute Coronary Syndrome DETAILED Overview (MI, STEMI, NSTEMI)—Armando Hasudungan https://www.youtube.com/watch?v=TBG9Jw3yd9I (Duration: 24:10)

Learners are encouraged to review Chapter 16: Acute coronary syndrome "ST-elevation myocardial infarction: I can't handle the pressure level III" in the *Pharmacotherapy Casebook: A Patient-Focused Approach* to practice applying their knowledge to develop a patient-centered care plan for a patient with ACS.

INTRODUCTION

Acute coronary syndrome (ACS) is an acute manifestation of coronary artery disease (CAD) and, for many patients, is the first indication they have CAD. Patients with ACS typically experience an acute reduction in coronary blood flow most often due to a ruptured atherosclerotic plaque and subsequent formation of an intracoronary thrombus. The reduction in coronary blood flow produces myocardial ischemia and, if left untreated, may lead to myocardial infarction (MI).

Patients with ACS typically experience acute chest discomfort similar to those with stable ischemic heart disease (SIHD) but the symptoms are often more severe, prolonged, or refractory despite medical interventions. Like patients with SIHD, those experiencing ACS are at risk for complications such as MI, heart failure (HF), ventricular arrhythmias, and death. The spectrum of ACS includes ST-segment elevation myocardial infarction (STEMI), non-ST-segment elevation myocardial infarction (NSTEMI), and unstable angina (UA). The American College of Cardiology (ACC) and the American Heart Association (AHA) have published guidelines for the diagnosis and management of patients with STEMI and non-ST-segment elevation acute coronary syndrome (NSTE-ACS), which includes NSTEMI and UA.[1,2]

EPIDEMIOLOGY

The AHA estimates that every 40 seconds an American will experience an MI.[3] There is a direct relationship between age and the prevalence of both CAD and CAD-related events such as MI. More than 1 million persons are discharged from the hospital annually with a primary or secondary diagnosis of an ACS.[3] MI accounts for more than 70% of these hospitalizations, the majority of cases are the first occurrence of a coronary event.[3] The presentation of MI has changed over the last two decades. Since 2000, the proportion of all patients with MI experiencing STEMI has declined while the proportion experiencing an NSTEMI has increased, the latter representing 74% of patients with MI between 2010 and 2014 in one study.[4] While many patients who experience an MI have symptoms prompting emergent care, an estimated 170,000 Americans will suffer an MI with minimal or no symptoms (eg, "silent MI") that may go undetected, placing them at high risk for major adverse cardiovascular events (MACE).[3]

Patients who experience ACS are at high risk for developing complications. The 1-year and 5-year mortality rates for patients experiencing MI are estimated at 18% to 23% and 36% to 47% for males and females, respectively.[3] Patients experiencing STEMI have a greater short-term (eg, 30 days) risk of complications, including death, compared to patients experiencing NSTEMI, whereas NSTEMI is associated with a greater long-term (eg, 2 years) risk.[3] In addition to death, patients experiencing ACS are also at risk for developing HF, cardiogenic shock, and ventricular arrhythmias, each of which contributes to the mortality associated with this disease state. Fortunately, declines in STEMI prevalence and overall severity of MI coupled with therapeutic advances have contributed to a reduction in complications associated with ACS globally. For instance, the rate of HF hospitalizations following MI declined more than 60% between 2000 and 2015 and the risk of death has similarly declined.[5] Lower rates of in-hospital death and MACE have been associated with increased utilization of percutaneous coronary intervention (PCI) and optimal medical therapy in patients treated for MI.[6] Therefore, the use of evidence-based therapies to treat ACS, the focus of this chapter, improves outcomes in these patients and should be prioritized in care plans.

The treatment of ACS is associated with significant healthcare resource utilization and related costs. For patients hospitalized for ACS, the mean and median length of stay were 5.5 and 4 days, respectively, in a recent analysis.[7,8] Frequent hospitalizations and utilization of revascularization therapies (eg, PCI, coronary artery bypass grafting [CABG]) lead to high costs associated with treating patients with ACS. In the United States, the mean cost of treating patients hospitalized for UA was $7,916 (median cost $7,841) while the average cost of hospitalization for MI was $24,695 (median cost $26,749).[9] In fact, MI ranks among the top 10 most expensive conditions treated in the United States.[3] While the adjusted hospitalization cost of treating MI remained relatively unchanged between 2001 and 2011 in one analysis, hospital costs increased by 10% if MI was treated with PCI and approximately 20% if CABG surgery was performed.[8]

ETIOLOGY

1 Endothelial dysfunction, inflammation, and the formation of fatty streaks contribute to the formation of atherosclerotic coronary artery plaques, the underlying cause of CAD.[9] The predominant cause of ACS in more than 90% of patients is the acute rupture, fissure, or erosion of an unstable atherosclerotic plaque followed by subsequent thrombus formation that impairs distal blood flow resulting in acute myocardial ischemia. If myocardial ischemia persists sufficiently long, MI can occur. This presentation of MI is classified as a type 1 MI.[10] Less commonly, ACS may occur due to an acute mismatch between oxygen supply and demand (eg, coronary vasospasm, coronary embolism, coronary artery dissection, a concomitant condition that acutely increases oxygen demand). When the latter results in myocardial injury, it is classified as a type 2 MI.[10] Other classifications of MI include patients who suffer cardiac death with symptoms suggestive of myocardial ischemia for whom biomarker detection is not possible (type 3), MI associated with PCI-related myocardial injury (type 4), and MI associated with CABG surgery (type 5).[10]

PATHOPHYSIOLOGY

The "Vulnerable Plaque"

1 The basic pathophysiologic process leading to an ACS event typically involves the rupture of an atherosclerotic plaque and subsequent thrombus formation. This thrombus formation produces an abrupt decrease in myocardial blood flow and oxygen supply leading to ischemia and potentially the death of myocytes and infarction.[11] The development of atherosclerotic plaques is complex and discussed in detail in Chapter 32, "Dyslipidemia." The atherosclerotic plaques that produce demand-driven angina in patients with SIHD are different from those that produce an ACS. The atherosclerotic plaques in patients with SIHD typically have thicker fibrous caps, and rarely rupture. The atherosclerotic plaques that rupture in patients with ACS typically have thin fibrous caps and are "vulnerable" to rupture.[12] The plaques in patients with ACS also have a larger cholesterol necrotic core while those in patients with SIHD are more likely to be solidified with calcium deposits. Atherosclerotic plaques that rupture in patients with ACS tend to be "nonobstructive," occluding less than 70% of the luminal diameter. Thus, patients with nonobstructive plaques may not experience angina symptoms prior to plaque rupture due to adequate autoregulation to maintain blood flow and oxygen supply in times of increased myocardial oxygen demand (coronary autoregulation is discussed in Chapter 33, "Stable Ischemic Heart Disease"). Therefore, patients are often unaware they have atherosclerotic plaques until the ACS event occurs.

The fibrous cap of an atherosclerotic plaque is what separates its lipid core from circulating platelets and coagulation factors in the blood. The cap initially is normal arterial intima or thickened intima tissue. As the atherosclerotic plaque grows this is replaced and expanded by fibrous tissue with high amounts of type 1 collagen.[13] In "vulnerable plaques," increased breakdown of collagen in the fibrous matrix and a reduction in collagen production cause the fibrous cap to become thinned and prone to rupture. Inflammatory processes are involved with both mechanisms.

The reduction in collagen production originates from a reduction in the number of secretory smooth muscle cells within the plaque, and a reduction in the synthesis within these cells.[13,14] Alteration of collagen synthesis and breakdown by macrophages and T cells demonstrates the significant role inflammation plays in thinning and weakening of the fibrous cap and increasing the potential for plaque rupture triggering an ACS event.[13-15] Altering the role of these inflammatory processes continues to be an active area of investigation to prevent and treat patients with atherosclerosis and ACS.

A thinning fibrous cap by itself does not usually produce plaque rupture. There is typically a connection to physiological or psychological stress which enhances the likelihood of an acute event.[16,17] Approximately two-thirds of ACS events occur in the morning. This is likely related to circadian rhythm activation of the sympathetic nervous system (SNS) and catecholamine release that produces an increase in heart rate, blood pressure, and vasoconstriction. An increase in catecholamines may occur due to physical and emotional stress. These changes in conjunction with a thin fibrous cap place patients at risk for ruptured atherosclerotic plaque and subsequent ACS.

Plaque Rupture and Clot Formation

1 The process of thrombus formation at the site of the ruptured atherosclerotic plaque is complex. Thrombus formation involves platelets and the coagulation cascade. While these two components of thrombus formation are often described separately, they are intertwined and each depends on the other.[18] These components do not contribute equally to thrombus formation in all vascular types. In venous thrombosis, the coagulation cascade dominates thrombus formation and platelets play a more minor role. In arterial thrombosis, such as ACS, platelets dominate, with the coagulation process having less contribution. This is evident by the use of pharmacotherapy to manage thrombosis in each vascular type. While the prevention and treatment of venous thrombosis are managed with anticoagulant agents almost exclusively, patients with arterial thrombosis are treated with two, and sometimes three, antiplatelet agents and typically receive a single anticoagulant agent for a short duration.

Upon plaque rupture, the barrier between the necrotic core of the plaque and blood components is breached.[18] Circulating platelets are initially attracted and adhere to the area of injury. The adhesion of these initial platelets occurs via platelet glycoprotein (GP) VI receptors binding to collagen within the damaged fibrotic cap, as well as platelet GP Ib-IX receptors and von Willebrand factor. Platelets may then be activated by numerous substances including collagen, thrombin, thromboxane A_2, adenosine diphosphate (ADP), epinephrine, and serotonin. These substances have different potency in their ability to activate platelets, with thrombin (from the clotting cascade) and collagen being the strongest activators. Each of these activators has individual receptors found on the platelet surface (eg, $P2Y_{12}$ receptor for ADP, protease-activated receptor [PAR]-1 for thrombin).

Once an activator binds to its specific receptor a chain reaction is initiated within the platelet with an influx of calcium leading to multiple changes in the platelet.[18] During platelet activation, the platelet changes shape from a disc-like structure to a polymorphic structure with protruding arms that significantly increases the surface area of the platelet. Granules with high concentrations of platelet activators (eg, thromboxane A_2, ADP, serotonin) make their way to the surface of the platelet and release their contents into the circulation. This leads to additional localized activation of platelets that have not adhered to the area of vascular injury. The activated platelet is also the location of the assembly of the tenase and prothrombinase complex that produces most of the activated factors Xa and IIa (thrombin) in the coagulation cascade. Therefore, this represents the interface between platelets and the clotting cascade in thrombosis. Finally, platelet activation leads to the expression of active GP IIb/IIIa receptors.[18] Upon platelet activation, there are approximately 90,000 to 100,000 GP IIb/IIIa receptors, making it the most abundant receptor found on any cell in the body.[18] Through activation, the GP IIb/IIIa receptors undergo a conformational change that exposes the binding site. The main ligand that binds to this receptor is fibrinogen, a linear molecule with a binding site for GP IIb/IIIa on each side. Therefore, each fibrinogen molecule can bind to a GP IIb/IIIa receptor on different platelets, linking those platelets together. The linking of platelets together via the GP IIb/IIIa receptors and fibrinogen is the process of platelet aggregation. Hence, the process of platelet adhesion, activation, and aggregation produces a platelet plug in the area of atherosclerotic plaque rupture.

The platelet plug by itself is rarely enough to significantly occlude myocardial blood flow and oxygen supply.[16] A fibrin meshwork then forms within and on top of the platelet plug that more completely traps cellular components such as red blood cells and produces the abrupt reduction in myocardial blood flow. The formation of this fibrin meshwork involves activation of the clotting cascade.

The initiation of the clotting cascade begins with the interaction and activation of factor VII and tissue factor.[18] Tissue factor is found in endothelial cells, as well as on macrophages at the site of the ruptured fibrous cap. This tissue factor–factor VIIa complex is able to activate small amounts of factor X, which then can activate small amounts of thrombin (factor IIa). The amount of thrombin produced during this initiation phase of coagulation is not enough to promote thrombosis. However, this initial amount of thrombin activates factor VIII. Activated factor VIII (factor VIIIa), with factor IXa (produced from the tissue factor–factor VIIa complex as well as factor XIa), creates the tenase complex on the platelet surface which activates large amounts of factor X. The initial thrombin produced also activates factor V. Activated factor V (factor Va) and activated factor X (factor Xa produced from the tenase complex) create the prothrombinase complex on the surface of the activated platelet where the majority of the thrombin involved in thrombosis is produced. Thrombin is now able to convert fibrinogen into fibrin, which creates the meshwork in the thrombosis and solidifies the clot. Thrombin also activates factor XIII, which provides additional clot stability, continues the positive feedback with the creation of factors VIIIa and Va, as well as provides significant platelet activation via PAR-1 receptors. The contributions of platelets and the coagulation cascade in thrombus formation in ACS are depicted in Fig. 34-1.

Thrombus formation in the area of atherosclerotic plaque rupture produces an abrupt reduction in myocardial blood flow and oxygen supply. This abrupt blockage produces ischemia and, if untreated, potentially infarction which results in myocyte necrosis and cell death.[12,16,17] Therefore, early recognition and prompt initiation of treatment can limit ACS-related sequelae. The progression to infarction and the extent of infarction depends on a number of factors. These may include both the location and size of the thrombus, activity of the endogenous fibrinolytic system, as well as the extent of collateral circulation.[16,17]

Ventricular Remodeling After MI

In the setting of MI, acute and chronic adaptations occur to prevent hemodynamic collapse that may also lead to ventricular remodeling and the development of post-MI complications. Similar to what occurs locally within the infarct-related artery, inflammation at the site of myocardial injury plays a key role in ventricular remodeling. In addition, stimulation of the neurohormonal system occurs and contributes to this process.

In patients who experience a decrease in cardiac output following MI, stimulation of both the SNS and renin–angiotensin–aldosterone system (RAAS) occurs to compensate for the decrease in cardiac output similar to what is observed in patients with acute and chronic HF (see Chapter 36, "Chronic Heart Failure" and Chapter 37, "Acutely Decompensated Heart Failure"). Activation of the SNS is immediate, resulting in increased contractility, heart rate, and peripheral resistance.[20] However, because the synthesis of components of the RAAS is

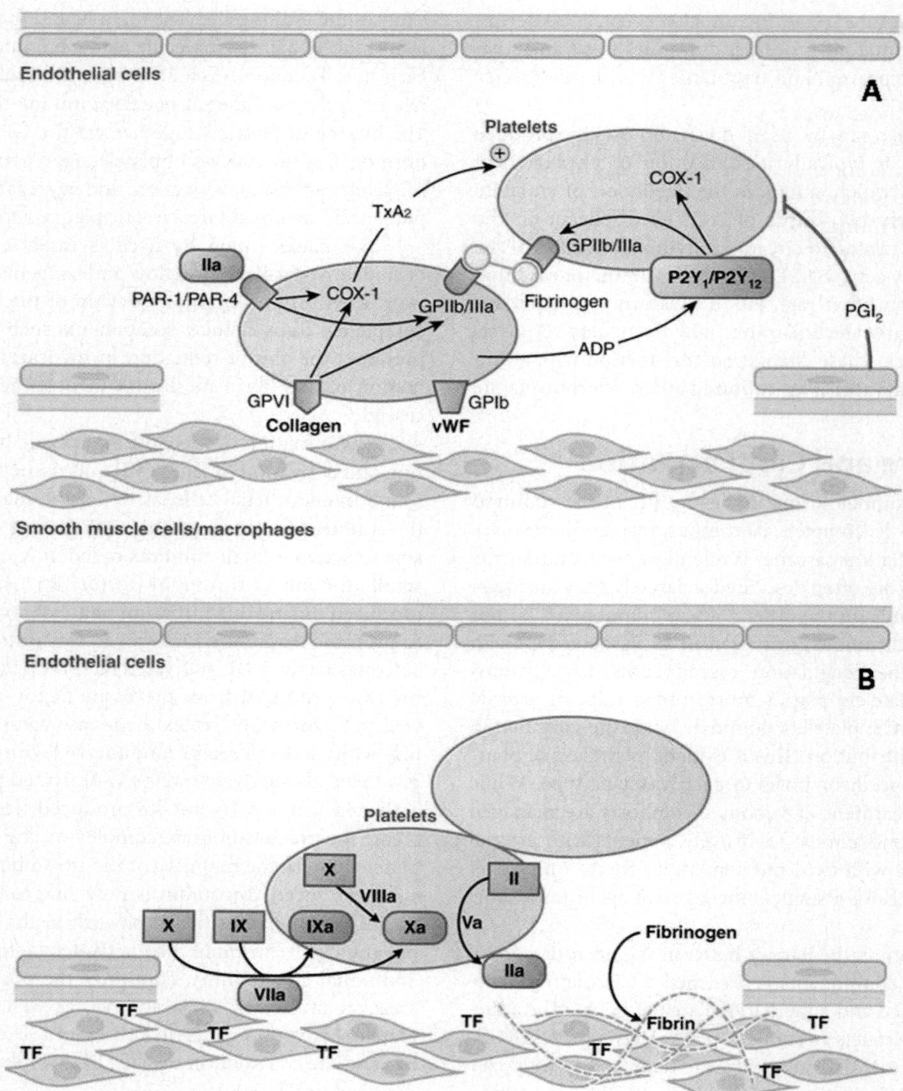

FIGURE 34-1 Role of platelets and coagulation cascade in thrombus formation in ACS. Panel A depicts receptors and mediators of platelet adhesion, activation, and aggregation during acute coronary syndrome (ACS). Panel B depicts components of the coagulation cascade during thrombus formation in ACS. Boxes enclose the coagulation factor zymogens (indicated by Roman numerals); the rounded boxes represent the active proteases. Activated coagulation factors are followed by the letter a: II, prothrombin; IIa, thrombin. (TxA2, thromboxane; PAR, protease-activated receptor; GP, glycoprotein; ADP, adenosine diphosphate; COX, cyclooxygenase; PG, prostaglandin; vWF, von Willebrand factor; TF, tissue factor.) (*From Reference 19.*)

dependent on an increase in mRNA and protein levels, the response is slower.[20] Stimulation of the RAAS results in sodium and water retention as well as peripheral vasoconstriction in an attempt to maintain adequate hemodynamics and perfusion. Vasopressin and endothelin are also released following MI but play a lesser role.[20]

Following MI, some patients experience chronic hyperactivity of either or both the SNS and RAAS, both of which contribute to adverse cardiac remodeling.[20] Chronic hyperactivation of the SNS leads to desensitization and downregulation of β_1-adrenergic receptors, modification of the excitation-contraction coupling mechanism, ventricular hypertrophy, and further impairment of contractility and cardiac output. Likewise, increased production of both angiotensin II and aldosterone via chronic hyperactivation of the RAAS leads to ventricular hypertrophy. Angiotensin II also increases oxidative stress, the release of inflammatory mediators, and collagen deposition, each of which contributes to myocardial fibrosis, or scarring. While myocardial fibrosis is essential for tissue repair following MI, its development impairs ventricular contraction and elasticity. This can lead to the thinning of the left ventricular wall and eventually to the development of dilated cardiomyopathy.

Complications

Depending on the extent and area of ischemia, various complications are possible in patients with ACS, particularly those with MI, which can manifest hours to weeks after the index event.[21] Electrophysiologic disturbances including ventricular arrhythmias, bradyarrhythmias, and heart block are possible and may occur either in the acute phase of the ischemic event due to electrical instability generated during myocyte destruction or in the recovery phase due to ventricular remodeling. HF is possible depending on the extent of myocardial necrosis and subsequent impairment of ventricular contractility. In fact, approximately 5% to 6% of patients with STEMI develop cardiogenic shock, an acute, severe form of HF associated with hypotension, systemic hypoperfusion, and poor outcomes.[21] Myocardial rupture of the papillary muscle, ventricular septum, or free wall of the ventricle is possible within the first 10 days of infarction due to extensive myocyte necrosis in those areas.[21] Thromboembolism, including stroke, is also possible due to the embolization of left ventricular thrombi that can form due to infarct-related ventricular aneurysm or left ventricular dysfunction. Pericarditis, an autoimmune-mediated inflammation of the pericardium, can occur weeks after an MI, particularly after a large infarct.[21] Mental health can also be impacted as many patients with ACS develop depression during the convalescent period.

CLINICAL PRESENTATION

Signs and Symptoms

2 The symptoms and clinical presentation of ACS are similar to those of stable angina (see Chapter 33, "Stable Ischemic Heart

CLINICAL PRESENTATION Acute Coronary Syndrome

General

- The patient is typically in acute distress and may develop or present with hypertensive crisis, acute HF, cardiogenic shock, or cardiac arrest.

Symptoms

- The classic symptom of ACS is abrupt-onset substernal chest pain or discomfort often described as a squeezing, heaviness, or tightness that persists for 10 minutes or longer. Symptoms may radiate to the arms, shoulders, back, abdomen, or jaw. Nausea, vomiting, diaphoresis, or shortness of breath may also be present.
- Patients likely to present with atypical symptoms include those aged 75 years or greater, women, and patients with diabetes mellitus (DM), impaired renal function, and dementia.

Signs

- No physical findings are specific for ACS. Nonspecific findings include S_4 or paradoxical splitting of S_2 on auscultation.
- Patients with ACS may present with signs of acute decompensated HF including jugular venous distention, pulmonary edema, and an S_3 on auscultation.
- Patients with ischemia-related papillary muscle dysfunction may present with a new murmur of mitral regurgitation.
- Patients may also present with arrhythmias, including tachycardia or bradycardia, as well as heart block.
- Hemodynamic abnormalities may include hypertension (HTN) and hypotension or shock.

Laboratory Tests

- Cardiac troponin (cTn, either cTnI or cTnT) is measured at the time of presentation and repeated 3 to 6 hours later (1 to 3 hours later if high-sensitivity cTn assays used) to detect myocardial injury; elevated levels in a patient with ACS symptoms, ischemic changes on ECG, or other diagnostic evidence of ischemia confirm the diagnosis of MI. Additional cTn levels should be obtained beyond 6 hours after symptom onset in patients with intermediate to high-risk features of ACS but normal cTn levels during serial measurements.
- For patients with ACS symptoms who do not have ST-segment elevation on ECG but an elevated cTn, NSTEMI is the appropriate diagnosis. Patients with ACS symptoms but normal cTn may have unstable angina (UA) or an alternative diagnosis.
- Blood chemistry tests are performed with particular attention given to potassium and magnesium, which may affect heart rhythm.
- Serum creatinine (SCr) is measured and creatinine clearance (CrCl) is used to identify patients who are at high risk of morbidity and mortality—dosage adjustments for renally cleared medications may be necessary.
- Baseline complete blood count and coagulation tests (activated partial thromboplastin time [aPTT] or anti-Xa levels, international normalized ratio [INR]) should be obtained; most patients will receive antithrombotic therapy and these tests are useful in monitoring for complications related to antithrombotic therapy, including bleeding.
- Fasting lipid panel.

Other Diagnostic Tests

- The 12-lead ECG is the first step in evaluating a patient with ACS. Patients are risk-stratified into two groups: those with STEMI and those without (NSTE-ACS). Patients with NSTE-ACS may have other ischemic ECG changes including ST-segment depression or T-wave inversion.
- Patients with STEMI and intermediate- to high-risk NSTE-ACS are likely to undergo coronary angiography via a left heart catheterization to diagnose CAD and may be treated with PCI during the procedure.
- An assessment of left ventricular (LV) function via echocardiography or equivalent modality should be performed to identify patients with LV dysfunction (LV ejection fraction [LVEF] less than 40% [0.40]) who are at high risk of death and candidates for guideline-directed medical therapy and device therapy.
- Selected intermediate-risk patients may undergo coronary computed tomography angiography or stress testing in lieu of invasive coronary angiography.
- Selected low-risk patients may undergo early stress testing or coronary artery calcium scanning.

Risk Stratification

- A risk assessment that incorporates the clinical presentation, past medical history, ECG, and cTn should be performed to identify high-risk patients and guide therapeutic interventions. One or more of the validated risk estimators (see Table 34-1) should be used for this purpose and incorporated into clinical decision pathways.

Disease"). The "classic" presentation of ACS is an abrupt onset of substernal chest pain often described as a sensation of squeezing, heaviness, or tightness in the chest that radiates to either or both arms or shoulders (radiation to the left side is more common), the neck, or the jaw. Patients with ACS may also experience diaphoresis, nausea, vomiting, and dyspnea. Many patients—as many as one-third—with ACS may present with atypical symptoms that do not include substernal chest pain.[1] Atypical symptoms include epigastric pain, indigestion, stabbing, or pleuritic chest pain, and increasing exertional dyspnea, the latter representing the most common "angina equivalent."[2] Older adults (75 years of age or older), women, and patients with diabetes mellitus (DM), impaired renal function, and dementia are more likely to present with atypical features.[2]

2 Features that differentiate ACS from stable angina include symptom severity and duration. Unlike SIHD, patients with ACS often experience symptom durations lasting 10 minutes or longer.[2] New or worsening symptoms or a change in symptom pattern (eg, acute increase in frequency or severity, occurring at rest or minimal exertion, longer duration) may be indicative of ACS.[1,2]

On physical examination, there are no specific findings indicative of ACS. In fact, the physical examination may be normal in many patients. Acute myocardial ischemia can cause an S_4 or paradoxical splitting of S_2 on auscultation, but these are nonspecific findings. Rather, clinicians should evaluate for the presence of complications of MI (eg, HF, new murmur of mitral regurgitation due to papillary muscle dysfunction) which, if present, should expedite the evaluation and therapeutic interventions.[2]

12-Lead Electrocardiogram

2 The presenting electrocardiogram (ECG) is critical for expeditious risk stratification and triage of patients presenting with ACS. Patients with possible ACS should have a 12-lead ECG performed and interpreted within 10 minutes of presentation to an emergency department (ED).[2] Ideally, a 12-lead ECG should be performed by emergency medical services (EMS) providers and communicated to the ED staff prior to hospital arrival in order to expedite reperfusion, if necessary.[1] Electrocardiographic changes suggestive of acute ischemia include ST-segment elevation or ST-segment depression of 0.05 mm or greater and T-wave inversion of at least 1 mm in at least two contiguous leads (Fig. 34-2).[2,10] Except for leads V_2-V_3 where greater ST-segment elevation is required, when ST-segment elevation of at least 1 mm is present in patients suspected of having ACS, the presumptive diagnosis of STEMI is made and the patient should be considered for emergent reperfusion therapy (Fig. 34-2).[1,10] In addition, the presence of a new left bundle–branch block (LBBB) in patients suspected of having ACS is strongly suggestive of acute MI and has been considered a STEMI equivalent.[1] However, because new LBBB occurs infrequently, a prior 12-lead ECG should be reviewed, if available, to determine if the LBBB is new or old. Patients with a high suspicion of ACS but with a normal ECG on presentation should have serial ECGs performed (eg, every 15-30 minutes for the first hour) to detect ischemic changes.[2] In approximately 1% to 6% of patients with ACS, often those with occlusions of the left circumflex or right coronary arteries, the 12-lead ECG may be normal or "electrically silent." Therefore, appropriate evaluation and risk stratification for patients with ACS must incorporate the evaluation of the patient's medical history, presenting symptoms, ECG findings, and biomarkers.

Cardiac Troponin

The cardiac troponins (cTn) are part of the contractile apparatus of myocardial cells and are the most sensitive and specific biomarkers for detecting myocardial injury.[2,10] Within 2 to 4 hours of myocyte injury or necrosis, these proteins are released into the bloodstream resulting in elevated blood levels (exceeding the 99th percentile of the upper reference limit).[2,10] The emerging high-sensitivity cTn assays are capable of measuring relatively low concentrations much earlier in the clinical course of myocardial injury that could not be detected with traditional cTn assays. The use of high-sensitivity cTn assays likely increases the frequency of NSTEMI diagnosis. Elevations in cTn may persist for several days, and as long as 2 weeks.[2]

2 There are several nonischemic causes of myocardial injury (eg, HF, myocarditis, Takotsubo syndrome, chronic kidney disease) that result in elevated cTn, particularly if high-sensitivity cTn assays are used.[2,10] Therefore, clinical context is required to establish the diagnosis of ACS. Myocardial injury is considered acute if there is a dynamic rise and/or fall by 20% or more in serial cTn values.[10] In contrast, when using a high-sensitivity cTn assay, the absolute change (in ng/L), rather than a relative change, increases diagnostic accuracy and may be useful in distinguishing an MI from other causes of cTn elevation.[10] Attention must be paid to the units of measure between traditional and high-sensitivity cTn; they are not interchangeable. When an acute myocardial injury is detected (eg, the dynamic elevation of cTn) in a patient presenting with ACS symptoms, ischemic changes on ECG, or other diagnostic evidence of ischemia (eg, imaging that demonstrates loss of myocardium or new regional wall motion abnormality, coronary thrombus detected during angiography or autopsy), the diagnosis of MI is appropriate.[10] Classification of MI is made based on the presenting ECG findings. For patients with dynamic cTn elevations whose presenting ECG demonstrated ST-segment elevation of at least 1 mm in two contiguous leads or new LBBB, the diagnosis of STEMI is confirmed.[10] In contrast, for patients with symptoms of ACS without at least 1 mm ST-segment elevation on the ECG at presentation but with a dynamic elevation of cTn, the diagnosis of NSTEMI is appropriate.[2,10] Patients with symptoms consistent with ACS but in whom the cTn is not elevated may have UA or an alternative diagnosis.[10]

Given that dynamic changes in cTn are needed to establish the diagnosis of MI, serial cTn levels should be obtained when the patient presents to the ED and again 3 to 6 hours after symptom onset (1-3 hours later if using high-sensitivity cTn).[2,26] If the time of symptom onset is unclear from the patient's history, the time of presentation to the ED should be considered the time of symptom onset.[2] For patients with intermediate- to high-risk features of ACS (eg, ECG changes, clinical presentation) but normal cTn values during serial measurements, an additional measurement of cTn after the 6 hours (3 hours if using high-sensitivity cTn) may be warranted.[2,26]

Risk Stratification

2 For patients with ACS, acute risk stratification is essential to determine which patients may benefit from reperfusion therapy, an early invasive approach, or medical management (Fig. 34-2).[1,2] Initial evaluation of risk should include the clinical presentation, past medical history, and both ECG and cTn upon presentation. For example, because STEMI has the highest short-term risk of death, patients with ACS who present with significant ST-segment elevation on ECG should be considered for emergent reperfusion therapy; confirmation of elevated cTn should not delay treatment.

Several risk scoring tools have been developed that predict both short-term and long-term event rates, such as mortality, in patients with ACS (Table 34-1).[22-25] These tools have been well-studied and can be easily applied in the clinical setting. Each of the risk assessment tools incorporates the patient's symptoms, past medical history, ECG, and cTn, while the Global Registry of Acute Coronary Events (GRACE) score also includes additional clinical indicators. For each risk estimator, there is a linear relationship between increasing score and the risk of MACE. For example, in patients with NSTE-ACS, the incidence of MACE through 14 days was 4.7% to 8.3%, 13.2% to 19.9%, and 26.2% to 40.9% in the low (Thrombolysis in Myocardial Infarction [TIMI] risk score 0-2), intermediate (TIMI risk score 3-4), and high (TIMI risk score 5-7) risk groups, respectively.[23] Compared to both the TIMI and GRACE risk estimators,

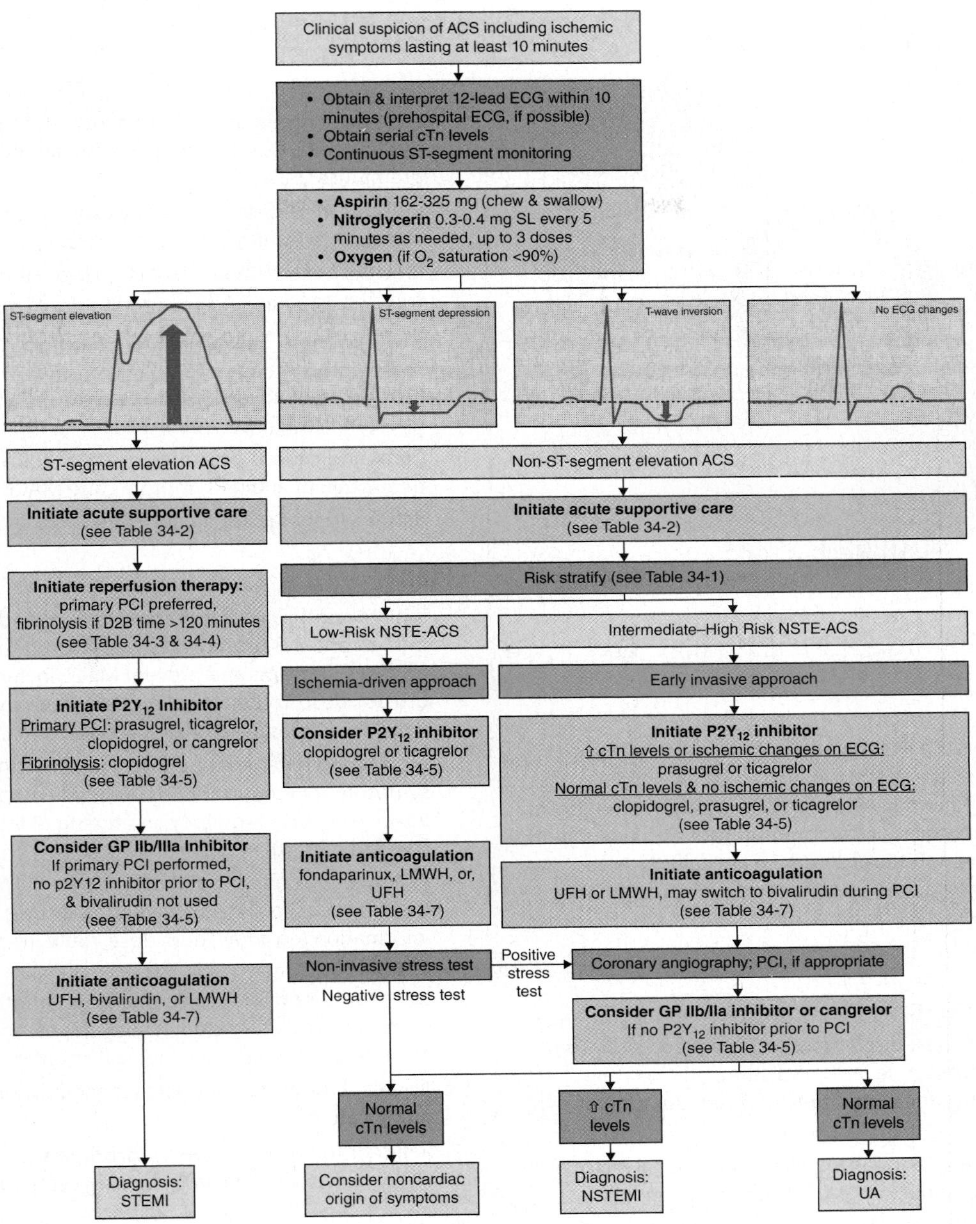

FIGURE 34-2 Evaluation and initial management of patients with suspected acute coronary syndrome (ACS). O_2, oxygen saturation; D2B, door-to-balloon; UFH, unfractionated heparin; LMWH, low-molecular-weight heparin.

the History, ECG, Age, Risk factors, and Troponin (HEART) score is better at identifying patients who present to the hospital with suspected ACS at low risk of MACE.[27] While this prognostic information is useful, the ability of the risk scoring tools to identify patients with ACS who may benefit from specific therapeutic interventions described below makes them particularly useful in the development of the treatment plan.

TREATMENT

Treatment decisions for patients with ACS are made based on the initial and ongoing risk stratification (Fig. 34-2). Rapid identification and delineation of ACS subtype (STEMI, NSTE-ACS) are imperative as treatment goals and timeframes for intervention differ slightly based on the clinical presentation and subsequent risk of death or complications from the index event (eg, patient with STEMI). When ACS is suspected, the patient should be immediately referred to an ED, chest pain unit, or equivalent facility for evaluation which should include 12-lead ECG and cTn such that expeditious treatment can be initiated.[1,2] Patients with possible ischemic symptoms, particularly if high-risk features (persistent chest pain, severe dyspnea, syncope or presyncope, or palpitations) are present, should be educated to activate the EMS system (eg, call 9-1-1) and seek transport via ambulance. EMS personnel are equipped to treat cardiac arrest should it occur; this approach is associated with earlier initiation of reperfusion therapy.

Desired Outcomes

In patients with ACS, treatment is aimed at achieving both short-term and long-term outcomes. Desired short-term outcomes in a patient with ACS are as follows: (a) early restoration of blood flow to the infarct-related artery to prevent infarct expansion (in the case of MI) or prevent complete occlusion and MI (in UA); (b) prevention of death and other MI complications; (c) prevention of coronary artery reocclusion; and (d) relief of ischemic chest discomfort. Long-term goals are control of atherosclerosis risk factors, prevention

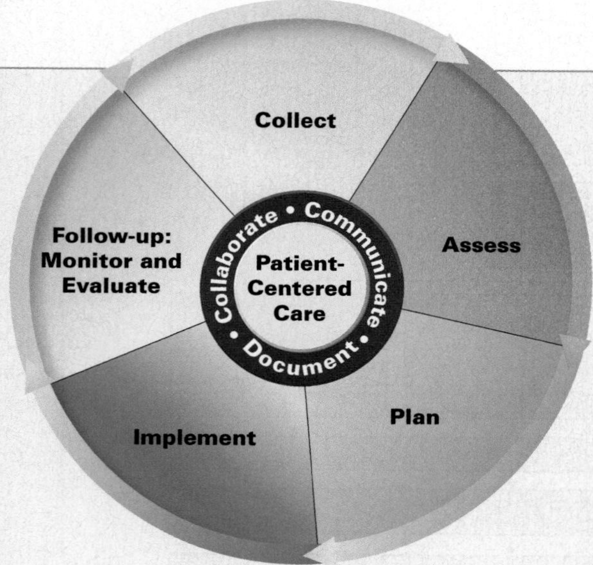

Patient Care Process for Acute Coronary Syndrome

The image shows the five fundamental steps included in The Pharmacist's Care Process endorsed by the Joint Commission for Pharmacy Practitioners (2014). The tagline of this process reads collaborate, communicate, and document. The five fundamental steps listed here are collect, assess, plan, implement, and follow-up: monitor and evaluate. All these steps are listed in a circular block diagram.

Collect

- Patient characteristics (eg, age, sex, pregnant)
- Description of chest discomfort and/or related symptoms (eg, quality, location, severity, radiation, precipitating factors, palliative measures, time of onset, duration of symptoms)
- Patient medical (personal and family) and social histories (eg, tobacco/ethanol, drugs of abuse [eg, cocaine])
- Current medications with particular attention to phosphodiesterase-5 inhibitors, over-the-counter medications (eg, aspirin-containing medications, nonsteroidal anti-inflammatory drugs), and herbals/dietary supplement use
- History of allergy or intolerance to medications
- Objective data
    - Blood pressure, heart rate, respiratory rate, height, weight, O_2-saturation, physical exam
    - Labs: cTn, Scr, potassium, hemoglobin, platelets, lipid profile
    - Diagnostic tests: 12-lead ECG; coronary angiogram and stress testing as necessary

Assess

- Description of chest discomfort to determine differential diagnosis and classification of ACS
- Presence of provoking factors (eg, exertion, mental/emotional stress, tachyarrhythmia, high adrenergic state including the use of stimulant medications, exposure to cold)
- Presence/control of risk factors for CAD (eg, HTN, dyslipidemia, DM, smoking, obesity, family history of premature CAD)
- Presence of ACS-related complications (eg, HF, cardiogenic shock, arrhythmias, heart block, stroke)
- Previous/recent revascularization procedures (eg, PCI with/without stenting, CABG surgery)
- Presence of ST-segment elevation or equivalent on 12-lead ECG
- Risk for major adverse cardiac events (MACE) (eg, perform risk stratification [see Table 34-1])
- Contraindications or intolerance to medications used to treat/prevent angina symptoms and MACE
- Barriers that may impair adherence to the care plan

Plan*

- Initiate antithrombotic therapy to treat and prevent intracoronary thrombosis as well as drug therapy to alleviate angina symptoms and prevent MACE including specific drug(s), dose, route, frequency, and duration (see Figs. 34-2 and 34-3; Tables 34-2–34-5, 34-7, and 34-8).
- Monitoring parameters: efficacy (eg, resolution of signs and symptoms of angina and ACS-related complications) and adverse effects; frequency and timing of follow-up (see Table 34-10)
- Patient education: purpose of treatment, lifestyle modifications, planned procedures, drug-specific information (eg, indication, dose, route, frequency, adverse effects)
- Self-monitoring for recurrent angina symptoms, signs and symptoms of ACS-related complications, adverse effects, when to seek emergency medical attention
- Address barriers to adherence to medications and lifestyle modification
- Referrals to other providers (eg, primary care provider, endocrinologist, dietician, smoking cessation)

Implement*

- Provide patient education regarding all elements of the treatment plan as described above.
- Use motivational interviewing and coaching strategies to maximize adherence.
- Schedule follow-up (eg, usually within 1-2 weeks but no later than 6 weeks after discharge).

Follow-up: Monitor and Evaluate

- Presence of angina symptoms, exercise tolerance, presence/control of CAD risk factors, presence/control of ACS-related complications
- Appropriate use and doses of evidence-based pharmacotherapy for ACS
- Presence of adverse effects and drug-drug interactions
- Patient adherence to treatment plan using multiple sources of information

Collaborate with patients, caregivers, and other healthcare professionals.

TABLE 34-1 Tools to Assess Risk of Major Adverse Cardiac Events in Patients with Acute Coronary Syndrome

TIMI Risk Score (STEMI)[22]	TIMI Risk Score (NSTE-ACS)[23]	GRACE Risk Score[24]	HEART Score[25]
Component (points)	**Each component worth 1 point**	**Points for each component vary based on value**	**Component (points)**
Age <65 years (0)	Age ≥65 years	Age	History highly suspicious (2)
Age 65-74 years (2)	≥3 CAD risk factors[a]	Killip class	Moderately suspicious (1)
Age ≥75 years (3)	Known CAD[b]	Systolic BP	Slightly suspicious (0)
HTN, DM, or angina[c] (1)	Aspirin use within 7 days	Heart rate	ECG: significant ST
Systolic BP <100 mm Hg (3)	≥2 angina episodes within 24 hours	Serum creatinine	Depression (2), nonspecific
Heart rate >100 bpm (2)	Transient STE or ST depression	Cardiac arrest on admission	Repolarization disturbance (1)
Killip class II–IV (2)	Elevated biomarkers (eg, cTn)	Elevated biomarkers (eg, cTn)	Normal (0)
Weight <67 kg (1)		ST deviation[d]	Age: ≤65 years (2), 45-65 years (1),
Anterior STE or LBBB (1)			<45 years (0)
Time to treatment >4 hours (1)			Risk factors for CAD: ≥3 (2),
			1-2 (1), no risk factors (0)
			cTn: ≥2 × ULN (2),
			1-2 × ULN (1), ≤ULN (0)
Calculate point total and determine risk for major adverse cardiac events			
Low risk: 0-3 points	Low risk: 0-2 points	Low risk: <109 points	Low risk: 0-3 points
Intermediate risk: 4-5 points	Intermediate risk: 3-4 points	Intermediate risk: 109-140 points	Intermediate risk: 4-6 points
High risk: ≥6 points	High risk: ≥5 points	High risk: >140 points	High risk: ≥7 points

BP, blood pressure; DM, history of diabetes; cTn, cardiac troponin; ECG, electrocardiogram; GRACE, Global Registry of Acute Coronary Events; HEART, History, Electrocardiogram (ECG), Age, Risk factors, Troponin; LBBB, left bundle branch block; ST, ST-segment; STE, ST-segment elevation; STEMI, ST-segment elevation myocardial infarction; TIMI, thrombolysis in myocardial infarction; ULN, upper limit of normal.

Online calculator available for TIMI Risk Score (STEMI) at: https://www.mdcalc.com/timi-risk-score-stemi

Online calculator available for TIMI Risk Score (NSTE-ACS) at: https://timi.org/calculators/timi-risk-score-calculator-for-ua-nstemi/

Online calculator available for GRACE score at: https://www.outcomes-umassmed.org/grace/acs_risk2/index.html

[a]Risk factors include a family history of coronary artery disease, hypertension, hypercholesterolemia, diabetes, and current smoker.

[b]Prior coronary stenosis ≥50%.

[c]History of angina.

[d]Includes transient ST-segment elevation ≥1 mm, ST-segment depression ≥1 mm, new T wave inversions ≥1 mm, pseudo-normalization of previously inverted T waves, new Q waves, new R wave >S wave in lead V_1, new left bundle branch block.

of additional MACE, including reinfarction, stroke, and HF, and improvement in quality of life.

General Approach to Treatment

The general treatment approach to ACS includes rapid diagnostic triage to determine an appropriate management strategy (Fig. 34-2). Patients with STEMI are of the highest priority and should be emergently referred to the cardiac catheterization lab for primary PCI with the goal of mechanically restoring blood flow to the infarct-related artery as quickly as possible. Patients with NSTE-ACS will undergo additional risk stratification to determine the best approach, which is usually an early invasive approach (eg, PCI) for intermediate- and high-risk patients or a more conservative, ischemia-guided management plan without planned PCI for those with either the lowest risk for coronary event or contraindications to the invasive procedure itself (Fig. 34-2). Regardless of treatment strategy planned (early invasive approach or ischemia-guided approach), general treatment measures for intermediate- and high-risk patients include admission to the hospital, oxygen administration (if oxygen saturation is <90% [0.90]), bed rest with continuous multi-lead ECG monitoring for arrhythmias and ischemia, frequent measurement of vital signs, ischemic pain relief, and prompt initiation of antithrombotic therapy.

Acute Supportive Care

Historically, clinicians and educators have used the mnemonic MONA (Morphine, Oxygen, Nitroglycerin, Aspirin) as a reminder for acute supportive care interventions to be considered in patients with ACS. However, in recent years, recommendations for the routine use of some of these therapies (eg, morphine, oxygen) have been tempered. Further, MONA ignores other potentially useful interventions to consider in the early phase of ACS treatment. Thus, the mnemonic $THROMBINS_2$ (Thienopyridine, Heparin, Renin-angiotensin-aldosterone system, Oxygen, Morphine, β-blocker, Intervention [eg, PCI], Nitroglycerin, Statin/Salicylate [eg, aspirin]) has been developed as a more contemporary reminder for early interventions to consider in patients with ACS.[28] Acute supportive therapies used to treat patients with ACS are summarized in Table 34-2.

Nitroglycerin

Nitrates, including nitroglycerin, are effective anti-ischemic medications and are routinely recommended as part of the initial management of patients with ACS.[1,2] Nitrates promote the release of nitric oxide from the endothelium, which results in venous and arterial vasodilation. Venodilation, the predominant effect, decreases preload, reducing ventricular wall tension, and myocardial oxygen demand. The effects on arterial vasodilation are less prominent but may lower systemic vascular resistance and blood pressure at higher doses, thus reducing myocardial oxygen demand. Nitrates also dilate coronary arteries and increase collateral blood flow.

However, the rationale for treating ACS patients with nitrates is extrapolated from an understanding of the pathophysiology of ACS, pharmacology of nitrates, numerous uncontrolled studies, and clinical experience—not their ability to reduce MACE.[2] In the reperfusion era, there is a paucity of data demonstrating that nitrate administration to patients with ACS is effective in providing symptom relief

TABLE 34-2 Acute Supportive Care Medications Initiated During the Initial 24 Hours of ACS Treatment

Drug	Indication (Class of Recommendation)[a]	Contraindication/Caution	Dose/Administration	Adverse Effects
Morphine	Refractory pain (IIb)	Known hypersensitivity Hypotension Bradycardia Lethargic or moribund patient	STEMI: 4-8 mg IV × 1 (lower dose in older patients), then 2-8 mg IV every 5-15 minutes PRN NSTE-ACS: 1-5 mg IV every 5-30 minutes PRN	Constipation, nausea, vomiting, hypotension, respiratory depression
Oxygen	Oxygen saturation <90% [0.90] (I)	Chronic obstructive pulmonary disease Carbon dioxide retention	2-4 L/min, increasing rate and/or changing to face mask PRN	Increased coronary vascular resistance, decreased coronary blood flow, increased mortality
Nitroglycerin	Angina (I) Uncontrolled hypertension (I) Acute heart failure (I)	SBP less than 90 mm Hg or greater than 30 mm Hg below baseline Avoid if recent PDE_5 inhibitor use: • Avanafil: within 12 hours • Sildenafil: within 24 hours • Vardenafil: within 24 hours • Tadalafil: within 48 hours Use with caution if RV infarct suspected Avoid abrupt cessation of IV nitroglycerin; wean gradually	SL: 0.3-0.4 mg every 5 minutes, up to 3 doses PRN IV: 10 mcg/min titrated to symptom relief and desired blood pressure	Flushing, headache, hypotension, tachycardia
β-Blockers	All patients without contraindications (I) *Associated with mortality reduction, especially in patients with HFrEF*	Signs of heart failure Low cardiac output state Risk factors for cardiogenic shock: • Age 70 years or greater • SBP less than 120 mm Hg • Sinus tachycardia (HR greater than 110 bpm) • Sinus bradycardia (HR less than 60 bpm) • Killip class III • Prolonged time from symptom onset High-grade AV block Active asthma or reactive airway disease	Carvedilol 6.25 mg twice daily; target dose is 25 mg twice daily as tolerated Metoprolol • Oral: 25-50 mg every 6-12 hours for 2-3 days, then once (metoprolol succinate) or twice daily (metoprolol tartrate); target dose is 200 mg daily • IV: 5 mg every 5 min as tolerated up to 3 doses, titrated to BP and HR; should only be considered if BP is uncontrolled or refractory symptoms Continue indefinitely in patients with concomitant HFrEF Other β-blockers may be considered; in patients with HFrEF, use either metoprolol succinate, carvedilol, or bisoprolol	Hypotension, heart failure, bradycardia, cardiogenic shock, AV block, exacerbation of asthma or reactive airway disease
Calcium channel blockers	Angina, normal LVEF, and contraindication or intolerance to β-blocker (I) Angina refractory to β-blocker and normal LVEF (I) Coronary vasospasm (I)	Signs of heart failure Low cardiac output state Risk factors for cardiogenic shock: • Age 70 years or greater • SBP less than 120 mm Hg, sinus tachycardia (HR greater than 110 bpm) • Sinus bradycardia (HR less than 60 bpm) • Killip class III • Prolonged time from symptom onset High-grade AV block	Diltiazem 120-360 mg/day orally[b] Verapamil 240-480 mg/day orally[b] Amlodipine 5-10 mg orally once daily Nicardipine 60-120 mg/day orally[b] Nifedipine ER 30-120 mg orally once daily	Hypotension, diltiazem and verapamil: heart failure, cardiogenic shock, bradycardia, AV block

[a]Dose and frequency may differ based on formulation.

[b]AHA/ACC class of recommendations: I, benefit far outweighs the risk, treatment should be administered; IIb, the benefit is equal to or exceeds the risk, additional studies with broad objectives are needed, treatment may be considered.

AV, atrioventricular; BP, blood pressure; ER, extended-release; HFrEF, heart failure with reduced ejection fraction; HR, heart rate; IV, intravenous; PDE5, phosphodiesterase-5; PRN, as needed; RV, right ventricular; SBP, systolic blood pressure.

Data from References 1, 2, and 29.

or reducing the incidence of MACE. In two large studies of patients with suspected MI, neither IV nitroglycerin (for 24 hours) followed by daily transdermal nitroglycerin nor daily isosorbide mononitrate reduced the incidence of MACE.[30,31] Postinfarction angina and cardiogenic shock were lower with the IV followed by transdermal nitroglycerin approach but not with the isosorbide mononitrate strategy. The use of IV sodium nitrite in 229 patients with STEMI treated with primary PCI had no effect on infarct size.[32]

3 Because nitroglycerin is effective in relieving angina symptoms, it is often utilized in patients with ACS with ongoing angina who are not hypotensive.[1,2] The recommended use for nitroglycerin in patients with ACS is provided in Table 34-2. Initially, SL nitroglycerin

should be administered every 5 minutes for up to three doses as needed for angina. For patients with persistent angina despite SL nitroglycerin, IV nitroglycerin should be considered, particularly in patients with uncontrolled HTN or evidence of HF on presentation. Because nitroglycerin dilates coronary arteries, it is useful in treating ACS related to vasospasm, particularly if cocaine intoxication is thought to be contributory. In fact, in patients with cocaine-induced chest pain, IV nitroglycerin is often the initial anti-ischemic medication recommended, especially if uncontrolled HTN is present.[33] Intravenous nitroglycerin should be continued until symptoms have resolved, blood pressure is controlled, and HF symptoms (if present) have subsided. Hemodynamic tolerance to IV nitroglycerin can occur within 8 to 12 hours, requiring higher doses with prolonged therapy. The most significant adverse effects of nitrates are flushing, headache, hypotension, and tachycardia. Because a synergistic reduction in blood pressure can occur leading to hypotension, nitrate administration is contraindicated in patients who have recently taken oral phosphodiesterase-5 inhibitors (Table 34-2).[1,2,34]

Morphine

Intravenous morphine is a potent analgesic and anxiolytic agent that also causes venodilation and increases vagal tone which reduces heart rate.[1,2] The analgesic and anxiolytic effects may improve patient comfort while the hemodynamic effects may reduce oxygen demand, thereby making IV morphine an attractive treatment option in patients with ACS. However, randomized clinical trials have not been conducted to determine the optimal dose nor evaluate the safety and efficacy of IV morphine in patients with ACS.

The safety of routinely using IV morphine to treat ACS has been recently questioned. Patients treated for ACS with IV morphine had higher rates of in-hospital death, MACE, and bleeding.[35] Studies evaluating IV morphine to treat ACS have high risk of bias, contributing to low confidence in the observed outcomes.

A proposed mechanism for the adverse outcomes associated with IV morphine in patients with ACS is the presence of a drug-drug interaction with $P2Y_{12}$ inhibitors. Morphine stimulates opioid receptors in the GI tract leading to inhibition of gastric emptying, which may slow the absorption of the antiplatelet agent.[36] Additionally, common side effects of morphine include nausea and vomiting. The coadministration of IV morphine and $P2Y_{12}$ inhibitors prolongs the time to peak concentrations, decreases total drug exposure, and produces less platelet inhibition.[36]

3 There is uncertainty regarding the role of IV morphine in patients with ACS. In patients with STEMI, current guidelines state that IV morphine is the drug of choice for pain relief but do not provide a class recommendation.[1] In NSTE-ACS, the use of IV morphine is recommended only in patients refractory to treatment with other anti-ischemic medications (Class IIb recommendation).[2] If IV morphine is used to treat patients with ACS, doses between 1 and 5 mg every 5 to 30 minutes are recommended (Table 34-2).[1,2] While nausea and vomiting are common, the most serious adverse effects to monitor are hypotension and respiratory depression.

Oxygen

3 Although routine oxygen is often administered to patients with ACS, it should be reserved for a minority of patients, particularly those with oxygen saturation less than 90% [0.90].[1,2] The routine use of oxygen may adversely affect patients with ACS by increasing coronary vascular resistance and reducing coronary blood flow.[1,2] The routine use of supplemental oxygen to patients treated for MI was of no benefit with signals suggesting infarct size may be increased.[37]

β-Blockers

Because β-blockers not only possess beneficial anti-ischemic effects but also lower the risk of MACE, their use is recommended for all patients with ACS without contraindications.[1,2] β-Blockers antagonize the β_1-adrenergic receptors causing a decrease in heart rate, contractility, blood pressure, and, subsequently, myocardial oxygen demand. Additionally, the reduction in heart rate increases diastole, prolonging myocardial perfusion and filling time. β-Blockers increase coronary blood flow to the ischemic myocardium by increasing coronary collateral resistance, preventing the shunting of blood away from ischemic areas.[19] The reduction in myocardial oxygen demand coupled with improved coronary blood flow to ischemic areas make β-blockers effective anti-ischemic medications in patients with ACS.

The anti-ischemic effects described above also contribute to the reduction in risk of MACE observed in patients with ACS treated with β-blockers. The risk of reinfarction and post-infarction angina is reduced in patients with MI treated with β-blockers.[38,39] Additionally, β-blockers improve survival in patients with MI, although this benefit has been questioned in recent years. Many β-blocker trials in MI that demonstrated a mortality benefit were conducted in the pre-reperfusion era. In a contemporary trial conducted in patients with MI during the reperfusion era, the use of early IV followed by oral metoprolol was associated with reductions in reinfarction, ventricular fibrillation, and arrhythmic death.[40] However, the primary composite endpoint (death, reinfarction, ventricular fibrillation, or cardiac arrest) was not significantly different from placebo and the risk of developing shock, including cardiogenic shock, was significantly increased. Consistent with this theme, the evaluation of β-blockers in MI had a modest mortality benefit for studies conducted during the pre-reperfusion era but no benefit was observed in studies completed during the reperfusion era.[38] Some of the uncertainty regarding mortality stems from variations in the duration of therapy and follow-up duration in many of the trials. β-Blockers had no influence on the odds of death in short-term trials (up to 6 weeks of treatment) but were associated with a 23% lower risk in long-term trials (treatment durations of 6-48 months).[39] In a recent observational study of patients with MI, 5-year mortality was approximately 30% lower for patients treated with β-blockers at hospital discharge; however, the benefits were no longer significant for those continuing therapy beyond 1 year.[41,42] Consequently, at least one international guideline recommends initiating a discussion with patients who are post-MI with normal left ventricular ejection fraction (LVEF greater than 40% [0.40]) regarding the risks and benefits of continuation beyond 12 months based on recent evidence.

4 Although the mortality benefit of β-blockers in the reperfusion era is uncertain, because they reduce the risk of MI, angina, and arrhythmias, in the absence of contraindications, current ACC/AHA guidelines recommend the initiation of oral β-blockers within the first 24 hours of presentation and continuation of therapy for at least 3 years (Table 34-2).[1,2,29] For patients with ACS and concomitant left ventricular dysfunction (LVEF less than 40% [0.40]), β-blocker therapy is often lifelong.[1,29] Although several β-blockers have been studied in the setting of ACS, the most commonly used agents are metoprolol and carvedilol largely due to the mortality benefit associated with their use in the treatment of HF, a common complication of ACS.

The most serious adverse effects observed in patients with ACS treated with β-blockers include HF, hypotension, bradycardia, and cardiogenic shock.[40] Therefore, in patients with evidence of or risk of developing these complications, β-blocker therapy should be withheld and initiation reassessed later during hospitalization.[1,2] Advanced age (70 years or older), presenting systolic blood pressure less than 120 mm Hg, sinus tachycardia (heart rate greater than 110 bpm) or bradycardia (heart rate less than 60 bpm) upon presentation, Killip class III (eg, pulmonary edema), and a prolonged time from symptom onset are patient characteristics associated with an increased risk of cardiogenic shock for whom β-blocker initiation should be postponed.[1,2,40] While β-blocker initiation should be avoided in patients with ACS and decompensated HF due to left ventricular dysfunction, the initiation of β-blocker therapy once HF symptoms have been stabilized and prior to discharge is safe, has been associated with lower mortality, and should be considered for all patients with ACS and compensated HF with reduced ejection fraction (HFrEF).[2,43] For patients with ACS and acute intoxication with cocaine or methamphetamine, β-blockers should be avoided unless a concomitant coronary vasodilator is also used to minimize the risk of causing or potentiating coronary vasospasm via unopposed α_1-adrenergic stimulation.[2,33,44] Because early initiation of IV β-blockers has been associated with an increased risk of HF and cardiogenic shock, parenteral therapy should be reserved for patients with STEMI who have acute, uncontrolled HTN or refractory symptoms and no contraindications.[1,29]

Calcium Channel Blockers

Calcium channel blockers (CCBs) possess beneficial anti-ischemic effects and are recommended for some patients with ACS, particularly those who are unable to take β-blockers.[1,2] CCBs cause arterial vasodilation, including coronary vasodilation, decreasing peripheral resistance, afterload, blood pressure, and myocardial oxygen demand.[19] All CCBs are also negative inotropes. However, because dihydropyridine (DHP) CCBs are potent peripheral vasodilators, they cause a baroreceptor-mediated increase in sympathetic activity that negates their negative inotropic effect.[19] Non-DHP CCBs decrease sinoatrial node activity and slow atrioventricular node conduction resulting in a decreased heart rate.[19]

4 Although CCBs are effective as anti-ischemic agents, reports of harm, lack of consistent benefit in clinical trials, and the data supporting β-blockers have narrowed the indications for CCBs in patients with ACS. In a systematic review, CCBs had no effect on mortality, MI, or recurrent MI in patients treated for ACS.[42] Consequently, current guidelines recommend non-DHP CCBs (eg, diltiazem, verapamil) to treat angina symptoms in patients with ACS who have a contraindication, have an intolerance, or are refractory to β-blockers in the absence of left ventricular dysfunction, risk factors for cardiogenic shock, and atrioventricular conduction defects (Table 34-2).[1,2] Because of their ability to dilate coronary arteries, long-acting CCBs are recommended in patients with ACS with known or suspected vasospasm.[2] However, if vasospasm is secondary to cocaine intoxication, the use of CCBs should be considered only after treatment with IV nitroglycerin and benzodiazepines.[33,44] Although long-acting formulations may be reasonable, immediate-release nifedipine should be avoided as it has been associated with increased mortality risk in patients with CAD, including those with ACS.[2,45] The most common adverse effects associated with the use of non-DHP CCBs in patients with ACS include heart block, bradycardia, hypotension, and GI disturbances.

Treatment Strategies in STEMI

The widespread use of reperfusion during ACS is responsible for the dramatic decrease in MI-related mortality over the past three decades in the United States.[46] Reperfusion strategies include fibrinolysis and mechanical intervention via PCI with or without stenting, both with the aim of restoring blood flow to the infarct-related artery. Appropriate choice and timing of reperfusion in ACS to facilitate revascularization are critical in STEMI to improve outcomes. Strategies to reduce delays in reperfusion include prehospital assessment of the initial ECG by EMS, early anti-ischemic medication administration, and transport to a hospital with PCI-capable facilities.

Primary PCI

5 In STEMI, the degree of myonecrosis is curvilinear, with the maximum amount of damage occurring in the first few hours of infarction.[47] Therefore, prompt efforts to restore blood flow to the infarct-related artery are paramount. During PCI, mechanical reperfusion is performed using intracoronary balloons, stents, and other devices. The reader is referred to Chapter 33, "Stable Ischemic Heart Disease," for a more detailed description of both coronary angiography and PCI. Compared to reperfusion with fibrinolysis, primary PCI improves survival, establishes consistent revascularization to the infarct-related artery, significantly reduces the risk of stroke and intracranial hemorrhage, and reduces reinfarction and recurrent ischemia. However, the mortality benefit of primary PCI over fibrinolysis is lost when door-to-balloon time exceeds 120 minutes.[48] More rapid performance of primary PCI can result in superior clinical outcomes for patients with STEMI.[1,49,50] In patients with STEMI treated with primary PCI, the risk of in-hospital death was increased by more than 40% when the door-to-balloon time was more than 90 minutes compared to 90 minutes or less.[51] In the United States, quality improvement programs have reduced mean door-to-balloon times from 120 minutes to 87 minutes, decreasing the in-hospital mortality rate from 8.3% to 6.6%.[52] Therefore, early reperfusion with primary PCI is of utmost importance and is preferred by guidelines for patients presenting with STEMI, with the goal of reperfusion within 90 minutes from the time of first medical contact.[1] However, in the United States, only 39% of all hospitals can perform PCI.[53] Given the benefits of primary PCI, patients presenting with STEMI to a hospital unable to perform PCI should be transferred to a PCI-capable hospital to achieve reperfusion within 120 minutes of the first medical contact.[1] Every minute delay results in additional myocardial cell damage that may be irreversible. Patients with STEMI undergoing primary PCI also require adjunctive antiplatelet and anticoagulant therapy which is discussed in greater detail later in this chapter.[1]

Fibrinolysis

5 When primary PCI for patients with STEMI is not possible within a timely fashion, pharmacological reperfusion, or fibrinolysis, is an alternative to primary PCI. The available fibrinolytic agents are plasminogen activators that increase the conversion of plasminogen to plasmin. Plasmin binds to the fibrin strands within the thrombus, breaking them down and allowing blood flow to be restored.

Fibrinolysis is an important means of reperfusion and prevents 30 early deaths per 1,000 patients treated within 6 hours of symptom onset.[54] The mortality advantage of primary PCI over fibrinolysis in patients with STEMI is lost when primary PCI is delayed more than 120 minutes.[48] Therefore, guidelines recommend fibrinolysis when primary PCI cannot be performed within 120 minutes.[1] This may apply when patients have immediate contraindications to receiving contrast dye, the facility to which patients present is unable to perform PCI and transfer time would exceed 120 minutes, or when patients present at off-peak hours when the catheterization laboratory cannot be adequately staffed within 120 minutes. Non-PCI-capable hospitals should aspire to transfer patients with STEMI to a PCI-capable hospital within 30 minutes of arrival (door-in-door-out goal).[1] Yet, when the anticipated time to PCI is expected to exceed 120 minutes, fibrinolytic therapy should be given within 30 minutes of hospital arrival provided no contraindications are present.[1] In fact, for patients with STEMI, the time from hospital presentation until the start of fibrinolytic therapy (door-to-needle time) is a quality performance measure of timely and effective care.[55] In a recent analysis evaluating the timeliness of reperfusion for patients with STEMI, the median door-to-needle time for patients treated with fibrinolytics was approximately 24 minutes with approximately 60% meeting the goal of less than 30 minutes.[56] A coordinated approach among EMS, ED, cardiology, and pharmacy personnel is needed in order to improve this further.

Indications and contraindications to fibrinolytic therapy are outlined in Table 34-3. Fibrinolytic therapy is associated with a slight but significant risk for stroke, largely attributed to intracranial hemorrhage (ICH), which occurs in 0.9% to 1.0% of patients.[57]

TABLE 34-3 Indications and Contraindications to Fibrinolytic Therapy for STEMI

Indications	Absolute Contraindications	Relative Contraindications
• Symptoms of acute coronary syndrome with an onset within 12 hours of first medical contact • ST-segment elevation of 1 mm or greater in two contiguous leads or new left bundle branch block on a 12-lead ECG • Anticipated that primary PCI cannot be performed within 120 minutes of first medical contact	• Any prior hemorrhagic stroke • Ischemic stroke within 3 months (except in past 4.5 hours) • Intracranial neoplasm or arteriovenous malformation • Active internal bleeding • Aortic dissection • Considerable facial trauma or closed-head trauma in the past 3 months • Intracranial or intraspinal surgery within 2 months • Severe, uncontrolled hypertension (unresponsive to emergency therapy) • For streptokinase,[a] treatment within the previous 6 months (if considering streptokinase again)	• BP >180/110 mm Hg on presentation or history of chronic poorly controlled hypertension • History of ischemic stroke greater than 3 months before • Recent major surgery (less than 3 weeks before) • Traumatic or prolonged CPR (greater than 10 minutes) • Recent internal bleeding (within 2-4 weeks) • Active peptic ulcer • Noncompressible vascular punctures • Pregnancy • Known intracranial pathology (dementia) • Oral anticoagulant therapy

[a]Streptokinase is no longer marketed in the United States but is available in other countries.

BP, blood pressure; CPR, cardiopulmonary resuscitation.

Data from Reference 1.

Significant predictors for ICH include advanced age, lower total body weight, female sex, preexisting cerebrovascular disease, and systolic and diastolic HTN at time of presentation.[57]

Relative contraindications to fibrinolytic therapy should be mitigated where possible (eg, giving antihypertensive medications to reduce blood pressure to less than 185/110 mm Hg) to reduce the risk for ICH, prior to administration. Patients at high risk for major bleeding (including a history of ICH) presenting with an absolute contraindication should not receive fibrinolytic therapy and should be transferred to a hospital capable of performing PCI. It is important to weigh the potentially life-saving effect against the life-threatening potential for an adverse event in those with contraindications to fibrinolytic therapy, taking into consideration alternative options such as delayed PCI. The mortality benefit of fibrinolysis is highest when administered early after symptom onset but is negligible if administered to patients with symptom durations exceeding 12 hours. The use of fibrinolytics between 12 and 24 hours after symptom onset should be limited to patients with clinical and/or electrocardiographic evidence of ongoing ischemia.[1] Noncerebral bleeding from fibrinolysis has been reported to be as high as 13%.[57]

When fibrinolytic therapy is indicated, a fibrin-specific agent (alteplase, reteplase, or tenecteplase) is recommended over a non-fibrin-specific agent (eg, streptokinase) because of greater reperfusion success and less systemic bleeding with fibrin-specific agents.[1] Any fibrin-specific agent is acceptable as no drug has demonstrated superiority over the others with regard to the mortality benefit.[58] However, in a systematic review, there was a trend toward a lower risk of major bleeding with tenecteplase compared to other fibrin-specific agents.[58] Therefore, safety considerations along with ease of administration or formulary restrictions may dictate the institutional preference of one agent over another. All hospitals should have protocols addressing fibrinolysis eligibility, dosing, and monitoring. Dosing considerations for the use of fibrinolytics in STEMI are provided in Table 34-4.

TABLE 34-4 Fibrinolytic Therapy Dosing in Patients with STEMI

Drug	Dosing Considerations
Alteplase (tPA)	15 mg IVP over 1-2 minutes, then 0.75 mg/kg (maximum 50 mg) IV over 30 minutes, then 0.5 mg/kg (maximum 35 mg) IV over 60 minutes; total dose not to exceed 100 mg
Reteplase (rPA)	10 units IVP over 2 minutes × 2 doses given 30 minutes apart
Tenecteplase (TNK-tPA)	<60 kg: 30 mg IVP[a]; 60-69 kg: 35 mg IVP[a]; 70-79 kg: 40 mg IVP[a]; 80-89 kg: 45 mg IVP[a]; >90 kg: 50 mg IVP[a];

[a]In patients 75 years or older, the dose may be reduced by 50% to decrease the risk of intracranial hemorrhage.[59]

IVP, intravenous push. Please refer to Tables 34-5 and 34-7 for appropriate adjunctive antiplatelet and anticoagulant therapy for patients with STEMI treated with fibrinolytics.

Data from Reference 1.

As with primary PCI, antiplatelet therapy and parenteral anticoagulation should be given concomitantly in patients treated with fibrinolytic therapy to improve vessel patency and to prevent reocclusion.[1] Adjunctive antiplatelet and anticoagulant therapies are discussed later in this chapter.

Despite data suggesting a benefit and the feasibility of prehospital fibrinolysis, the administration of fibrinolytic therapy by EMS personnel to patients during transport to the hospital is not routine practice in the United States. Early angiography after fibrinolytic therapy, a practice referred to as a pharmacoinvasive approach, may reduce cardiovascular events compared to patients transferred for immediate PCI, yet increased rates of ICH have been implicated with this approach.[46,59] Transfer to a PCI-capable facility for possible "rescue PCI" after fibrinolysis is appropriate for those who fail fibrinolytic therapy and those patients with acute, severe HF or cardiogenic shock.[1]

Treatment Strategies in NSTE-ACS

Early Invasive Approach

While patients presenting with STEMI benefit from immediate reperfusion of the infarct-related artery due to complete arterial occlusion, patients presenting with NSTE-ACS typically have a partially occluded coronary artery with some residual perfusion and, therefore, the need for and urgency to perform PCI is not as critical. With an early invasive approach, the patient has a diagnostic angiography performed early in the hospital course, typically within the first 24 hours, with the intent to perform revascularization if appropriate, depending on the coronary anatomy.[2] An early invasive strategy improves cardiovascular outcomes in patients presenting with NSTE-ACS with the greatest benefits achieved in those patients with the highest risk for MACE. Risk stratification is, therefore, essential in NSTE-ACS to determine which patients will derive the most benefit from an early invasive approach. The benefit of routine invasive therapy is superior to an ischemia-guided approach (a more conservative watch and wait approach) usually in patients with advanced age (older than age 70), previous MI or revascularization, ST-segment changes, HF (especially with left ventricular dysfunction), elevated cTn, DM, and in those with positive results from noninvasive stress tests. Practice guidelines recommend an early invasive strategy in those with an elevated risk for death or MI (eg, high-risk and select intermediate-risk patients [see Table 34-1]), those with refractory angina, acute HF, other symptoms of cardiogenic shock, or arrhythmias.[2,26,60]

Ischemia-Guided Approach ("Medical Management")

In contrast to an early invasive approach, a more conservative management strategy for those with the lowest risk is referred to as an ischemia-guided approach, or "medical management," where anti-ischemic, antiplatelet, and anticoagulant medications are administered and PCI is not initially planned. The patient is evaluated for signs and symptoms of recurrent ischemia or hemodynamic instability and taken for invasive coronary angiography and possible PCI only if recurrent symptoms develop or noninvasive diagnostic testing (eg, coronary computed tomography angiography, stress testing) suggest obstructive CAD. This strategy is appropriate for select low- and intermediate-risk patients, for those with serious comorbidities or contraindications to angiography/PCI (eg, renal failure), or when the risks of the procedure outweigh the benefits of revascularization.[2] The ischemia-driven approach is also preferred by guidelines for those with a low likelihood of ACS, in women without troponin elevation, and in those who do not consent for revascularization.[2]

Antithrombotic Therapy

Due to the role of thrombus formation in the setting of ACS, timely and appropriate antithrombotic therapy is an important component of optimal pharmacotherapy. Antithrombotic therapy consists of antiplatelet and anticoagulant therapy. While platelets dominate the pathophysiologic process in arterial thrombosis, the central role of thrombin in both platelet activation and coagulation makes both types of therapy necessary in the acute phase of treatment in a patient with ACS. After hospital discharge, most patients are typically continued on long-term antiplatelet therapy only, although evidence for use of long-term anticoagulant therapy after ACS is emerging for some high-risk groups.

One of the most challenging aspects of the use of antithrombotic therapy in patients with ACS is that not all agents have been studied across the spectrum of ACS and its different management strategies. While some agents may have data in the setting of NSTE-ACS, they may not have data in STEMI. For patients with NSTE-ACS, data are different for patients being managed with an ischemia-driven approach compared to those receiving PCI.[2] Some agents may have data in the setting of primary PCI in STEMI, but not with the use of fibrinolytics in STEMI.[1] Lastly, agents may have data in these different settings, but the doses may differ depending on the diagnosis or management strategy. Therefore, clinicians must know the evidence on appropriate antithrombotic drug use, dose, and duration based on the patient's diagnosis and management strategy to optimize patient outcomes and prevent adverse events.

Antiplatelet Therapy

The use and dosing of antiplatelet therapies for the treatment of ACS are summarized in Table 34-5.

Aspirin Aspirin, or acetylsalicylic acid, has been a standard part of the treatment for ACS for several decades. Aspirin provides its antiplatelet effect by acetylating a hydroxyl group of serine 530 on the cyclooxygenase (COX)-1 enzyme on platelets and thereby preventing the conversion of arachidonic acid into a number of prostaglandins, and eventually thromboxane A_2.[61] Thromboxane A_2 produces platelet activation as well as vasoconstriction. While unbound aspirin has a half-life of only about 15 to 20 minutes, the irreversible binding of aspirin to the platelet COX-1 enzyme inhibits thromboxane A_2–induced platelet activation for the life of the platelet (7-10 days).

6 Aspirin is recommended for all patients with ACS without contraindications, regardless of the type of ACS or the management strategy. The initial dose of aspirin should be 162 to 325 mg (non-enteric coated) given as soon as possible.[1,2] Typically, this is given as 2 to 4 "baby" aspirin (81 mg in the United States) to be chewed and swallowed. The process of chewing allows for faster dissolution time and platelet inhibition in less than 30 minutes compared to about 60 minutes when tablets are consumed whole.[61] Patients undergoing PCI for NSTE-ACS or STEMI already receiving chronic aspirin doses of 81 mg daily should be given an additional dose of 81 to 325 mg before the procedure.[1,2]

After the initial dose of aspirin, daily doses of aspirin should be 81 mg daily and continued indefinitely.[1,2] Higher daily maintenance doses of aspirin (300-325 mg) do not reduce CV death, MI, or stroke compared to lower daily maintenance doses (75-100 mg), but significantly increase the incidence of gastrointestinal (GI) bleeding.[62]

Contraindications to aspirin include hypersensitivity to aspirin and major GI intolerance. In these rare cases, clopidogrel with a loading dose followed by a maintenance dose should be used as an alternative.[1,2] While ticagrelor may also be considered, there are no direct comparative data to aspirin available. The main adverse effects of aspirin include dyspepsia and GI bleeding, which is an extension of its inhibition of prostaglandins responsible for GI protection.[61] The use of low-dose and/or enteric-coated aspirin can provide a reduction in these adverse effects. Aspirin with an antacid, known as "buffered aspirin," does not provide GI protection. Although most surgical procedures can be conducted with patients on aspirin, it should be discontinued approximately 5 days before the procedure if desired.

$P2Y_{12}$ Inhibitors 6 Aspirin is rarely used as the sole antiplatelet agent in patients with ACS and is typically combined with an oral $P2Y_{12}$ inhibitor as part of dual antiplatelet therapy (DAPT). There are three orally administered $P2Y_{12}$ inhibitors (clopidogrel, prasugrel, and ticagrelor) and one IV agent (cangrelor) available in the United States, and their pharmacology is summarized in Table 34-6. Clopidogrel and prasugrel both belong to the chemical class of thienopyridines that are prodrugs requiring hepatic activation. Both agents have a thiol ring that must be opened to expose the sulfur atom. This sulfur then interacts with the sulfur within the $P2Y_{12}$ receptor creating an irreversible disulfide bond. The binding of the thienopyridine agent to the receptor prevents the receptor's ability to be activated by adenosine diphosphate and subsequent platelet activation and aggregation.

Ticagrelor and cangrelor are not thienopyridines, and therefore do not require hepatic activation to provide their antiplatelet effect. Cangrelor is an adenosine triphosphate analog and ticagrelor belongs to the chemical class of a cyclopentyltriazolopyrimidine that has structural components similar to adenosine triphosphate. While adenosine diphosphate is a known activator of platelets through the $P2Y_{12}$ receptor, adenosine triphosphate is a known inhibitor of this receptor. Ticagrelor and cangrelor do not form an irreversible bond with the $P2Y_{12}$ receptor as thienopyridines but instead, bind reversibly in a different location. With ticagrelor and cangrelor, adenosine diphosphate is allowed to bind to the $P2Y_{12}$ receptor, but the signal

TABLE 34-5 Antiplatelet Drug Use and Dosing Across the Spectrum of ACS and Management Strategy

	STEMI		NSTE-ACS	
Drug	**Primary PCI**	**Fibrinolytic Reperfusion**	**Early Invasive Strategy**	**Ischemia-Driven Strategy**
Aspirin				
Loading dose	162-325 mg	162-325 mg	162-325 mg	162-325 mg
Maintenance dose	81 mg daily	81 mg daily	81 mg daily	81 mg daily
$P2Y_{12}$ inhibitors				
Clopidogrel				
Loading dose	600 mg	300 mg Age greater than 75 years: No loading dose given	600 mg	300 mg
Maintenance dose	75 mg daily	75 mg daily	75 mg daily	75 mg daily
Prasugrel		No recommendation		No recommendation[a]
Loading dose	60 mg		60 mg	
Maintenance dose	10 mg daily Weight less than 60 kg: 5 mg daily		10 mg daily Weight less than 60 kg: 5 mg daily	
Ticagrelor		No recommendation		
Loading dose	180 mg		180 mg	180 mg
Maintenance dose	90 mg twice daily		90 mg twice daily	90 mg twice daily
Cangrelor	30 mcg/kg IV bolus, followed by 4 mcg/kg/min IV infusion for at least 2 hours or duration of PCI	No recommendation	30 mcg/kg IV bolus, followed by 4 mcg/kg/min IV infusion for at least 2 hours or duration of PCI	No recommendation
GP IIb/IIIa inhibitor				
Eptifibatide	180 mcg/kg IV bolus × 2 given 10 minutes apart, followed by 2 mcg/kg/min IV infusion started after first bolus and continued for 18-24 hours after PCI CrCl less than 50 mL/min (0.83 mL/s): Reduce infusion by 50% Hemodialysis: Avoid use	No recommendation	180 mcg/kg IV bolus × 2 given 10 minutes apart, followed by 2 mcg/kg/min IV infusion started after first bolus and continued for 18-24 hours after PCI CrCl less than 50 mL/min (0.83 mL/s): Reduce infusion by 50% Hemodialysis: Avoid use	No recommendation
Tirofiban	25 mcg/kg IV bolus, followed by 0.15 mcg/kg/min CrCl less than 60 mL/min (1.0 mL/s): Reduce infusion by 50%	No recommendation	25 mcg/kg IV bolus, followed by 0.15 mcg/kg/min CrCl less than 60 mL/min (1.0 mL/s): Reduce infusion by 50%	No recommendation

CrCl, creatinine clearance; IC, intracoronary; IV, intravenous.

[a]Not mentioned in the ACC/AHA guidelines, but evidence of noninferiority compared to clopidogrel exists. Prasugrel dosing was a 30 mg loading dose followed by 10 mg daily. Patients weighing less than 60 kg or age 75 years or more received a maintenance dose of 5 mg daily.

Data from References 1 and 2.

TABLE 34-6 $P2Y_{12}$ Inhibitor Pharmacology Comparisons

Property	Clopidogrel	Prasugrel	Ticagrelor	Cangrelor
Drug class	Thienopyridine	Thienopyridine	Cyclopentyltriazolopyrimidine	ATP analogue
Absorption	≥50%	80%	36%	100%
Tmax	2 hours	30 minutes	60 minutes	2 minutes
Onset of action	75 mg: 3-5 days 300 mg: 6-8 hours 600 mg: 2-4 hours	10 mg: 3 days 60 mg: 30-60 minutes	90 mg: 2-3 days 180 mg: 60 minutes	2 minutes
Metabolism	Hepatic	Hepatic	Hepatic	ATPases in vascular endothelium
(CYP isoenzymes)	(2C19, 3A4, 1A2, 2B6)	(2B6, 3A4, 2C9, 2C19)	(3A4, 2C9)	
Prodrug	Yes	Yes	No	No
$P2Y_{12}$ Binding	Irreversible	Irreversible	Reversible	Reversible
Half-life	6 hours	7 hours	12 hours	3-5 minutes
Platelet recovery after cessation of therapy	~5 days	~7 days	~3 days	1-2 hours

ATP, adenosine triphosphate; CYP, cytochrome p450.

Data from References 61 and 63.

is blocked and does not lead to platelet activation and aggregation. Hence, ticagrelor and cangrelor are $P2Y_{12}$ receptor inhibitors, just by a different mechanism than thienopyridines. Because they reversibly bind to the $P2Y_{12}$ receptor, more frequent dosing of ticagrelor (twice-daily dosing) and cangrelor (continuous infusion) is required.

6 Bleeding risk in patients treated with $P2Y_{12}$ inhibitors undergoing major surgery is of concern. In patients with ACS treated with a clopidogrel-based DAPT regimen, the risk of CABG-related major bleeding was approximately 50% higher in clopidogrel-treated patients when surgery was performed within 5 days of clopidogrel cessation compared to patients treated with aspirin alone.[64] The risk of CABG-related major bleeding in ACS patients treated with DAPT is more than four times higher with prasugrel than clopidogrel.[65] Consequently, clopidogrel and ticagrelor should be held for at least 5 days and prasugrel should be held for 7 days prior to elective surgery (eg, CABG surgery).[1,2] Because of its short duration of action, cangrelor can be continued until just a few hours before surgery, which is a favorable property of this agent.[63] Given the known bleeding risk associated with $P2Y_{12}$ inhibitor use and CABG, preloading patients with NSTE-ACS with a $P2Y_{12}$ inhibitor prior to PCI is controversial given that some may require CABG surgery. Administration of an oral $P2Y_{12}$ inhibitor prior to PCI does not offer a reduction in thrombotic outcomes compared to administration immediately following PCI.[66,67] It would still be prudent to preload the oral $P2Y_{12}$ inhibitor in patients with STEMI undergoing primary PCI, especially since CABG surgery is uncommon in these patients.

Clopidogrel Conversion of clopidogrel to its active compound takes two cytochrome P450 (CYP) enzyme steps.[61] While multiple CYP enzymes take part in this conversion, CYP2C19 is responsible for at least 50% of this conversion. Patients with loss of function alleles (*2 or *3) have demonstrated a reduced ability to convert clopidogrel to its active form and have less platelet inhibition compared to patients with wild-type CYP2C19 (*1). It has also been demonstrated that up to 40% of patients receiving clopidogrel fail to achieve an optimal antiplatelet effect.[68] While there is a fair amount of variability in how the antiplatelet effect is determined, patients who fail to respond adequately to clopidogrel have a greater risk for MACE compared to patients with an adequate antiplatelet response. Clopidogrel is less effective than prasugrel or ticagrelor in patients with loss-of-function alleles, but has comparable efficacy to other oral $P2Y_{12}$ inhibitors in patients wild-type CYP2C19.[1,2,69,70] Although genetic polymorphisms of CYP2C19 contribute to the inadequate response to clopidogrel, CYP2C19 status only explains 12% to 15% of the variability demonstrated with clopidogrel.[68] Consequentially, lack of response to clopidogrel is multifaceted and can occur in patients with wild-type CYP2C19. Patients treated for ACS in whom de-escalation of DAPT is being considered (discussed below), platelet function testing to screen for high platelet reactivity may be considered 1 week after switching to clopidogrel in special circumstances (bleeding event, high bleeding risk, financial barriers).[70] Since proton pump inhibitors are known inhibitors of CYP2C19, concern has been raised about an increased risk for MACE in patients receiving these agents with clopidogrel. While the clopidogrel labeling information lists omeprazole and esomeprazole as being contraindicated, clinical evidence supporting this interaction is inconsistent.[68]

Clopidogrel has been extensively evaluated in patients with ACS. The CURE trial (Clopidogrel in Unstable Angina to Prevent Recurrent Events) compared aspirin alone to clopidogrel given as a 300 mg loading dose, followed by 75 mg daily for up to 12 months.[64] Patients receiving DAPT demonstrated a significant reduction in CV death, MI, and stroke compared to aspirin alone. This trial not only demonstrated the efficacy of clopidogrel but also established DAPT as the standard of care for patients presenting with ACS. Since 80% of the patients in this trial were medically managed, this dosing regimen is used in patients undergoing an ischemia-driven approach for NSTE-ACS.

A 600-mg loading dose provides a more potent and faster onset of antiplatelet activity and has demonstrated better efficacy in patients undergoing PCI compared to initially receiving a 300-mg loading dose of clopidogrel.[62] Patients who received an ischemia-driven approach did best with a 300-mg loading dose as in the CURE trial in regards to efficacy and safety outcomes. These data support the 600-mg clopidogrel loading dose in patients undergoing PCI for NSTE-ACS and STEMI.

Finally, clopidogrel is the only $P2Y_{12}$ inhibitor to be evaluated in large clinical trials in patients with STEMI receiving reperfusion with fibrinolytic therapy. Two trials have demonstrated the efficacy and safety of clopidogrel as part of DAPT in these patients.[71,72] Due to the increased concern of ICH in patients receiving fibrinolytics, only a 300 mg loading dose is used except for patients aged 75 or older who should not receive any loading dose.

Prasugrel Prasugrel must also be converted to an active compound through hepatic conversion, but the conversion of prasugrel is more efficient, requiring a single CYP enzyme step, and multiple enzymes are capable of making the conversion.[19] Consequentially, the ability of prasugrel to be converted to its active compound is not limited and leads to faster and more potent platelet inhibition compared to clopidogrel. In patients undergoing PCI for NSTE-ACS or STEMI, prasugrel (as part of DAPT with aspirin) provided a significant reduction in CV death, MI, or stroke compared to clopidogrel.[65] The benefit of prasugrel was similar in the first few days of therapy, and after the first few days out to 1 year. Therefore, the reduction in MACE was due to not only more potent early antiplatelet therapy but also sustained potent antiplatelet therapy.

6 Greater efficacy, however, came at a cost of more non-CABG major bleeding and fatal bleeding. Upon further evaluation of the net clinical benefit (CV death, MI, stroke, and major bleeding), patients entering the trial with a history of stroke or transient ischemic attack were at greater risk for harm from prasugrel.[65] Therefore, these patients have an absolute contraindication to receiving prasugrel. Patients over the age of 75 years and those weighing less than 60 kg also had more bleeding with prasugrel compared to clopidogrel, but the overall net clinical benefit was neutral. Prasugrel should generally be avoided in patients over the age of 75 years. Exceptions may be made for patients who present with prior MI or DM, as the benefit in these patients outweighed the harm. Finally, in patients weighing less than 60 kg, the 60 mg loading dose of prasugrel is still given, but a 5 mg maintenance dose is recommended instead of the typical 10 mg dose.

Prasugrel has been compared to clopidogrel in patients undergoing an ischemia-driven approach.[73] Although there was no increased risk of bleeding with prasugrel in this trial, there was also no difference in efficacy. The use of prasugrel in these patients is not mentioned in the current guidelines.[2] Prasugrel has also not been evaluated in patients with STEMI receiving reperfusion therapy with fibrinolytics.

Ticagrelor 6 As with prasugrel, ticagrelor provides faster and more potent inhibition of platelets compared to clopidogrel.[74] Although ticagrelor does not require hepatic activation, it is metabolized by CYP3A4. Therefore, ticagrelor is contraindicated in patients receiving strong CYP3A4 inhibitors such as azole antifungals and protease inhibitors, as well as strong inducers of this enzyme such as carbamazepine, phenytoin, rifamycins, and St. John's Wort. Patients on ticagrelor should not receive doses of simvastatin or lovastatin higher than 40 mg daily. Due to competition for P-glycoprotein, ticagrelor can increase digoxin concentrations by 30% to 50%.

Ticagrelor has been compared to clopidogrel as part of DAPT with aspirin in patients undergoing PCI (NSTE-ACS or STEMI) or undergoing an ischemia-driven approach for NSTE-ACS in a large clinical trial.[75] Patients receiving ticagrelor had a significant reduction in CV death, MI, or stroke compared to clopidogrel. While this reduction was evident within the first 30 days of therapy, two-thirds of the benefit was after the first 30 days out to 1 year. As with prasugrel, the benefit of ticagrelor was not simply due to more potent antiplatelet therapy early but also sustained potent antiplatelet therapy. The magnitude of benefit was similar in patients receiving an ischemia-driven approach to those receiving PCI. There was also a significant 21% reduction in CV mortality with the use of ticagrelor over clopidogrel, which has not been seen in other trials of $P2Y_{12}$ inhibitors. In the trial, higher doses of aspirin attenuated the benefit of ticagrelor compared to clopidogrel; only patients receiving low-dose aspirin (daily dose of 100 mg or less) received a benefit.[76] Based on these data, ticagrelor is contraindicated in patients receiving chronic aspirin daily doses of more than 100 mg. The mechanism of this interaction remains unknown. Although non-CABG major bleeding was significantly increased, there was no increase in fatal bleeding. Due to the increased risk of bleeding in older patients, clopidogrel may be a safer option based on data from trials evaluating patients aged 70 or 80 years or older.[77,78]

Ticagrelor has been compared to prasugrel as part of DAPT with aspirin in patients with ACS (NSTE-ACS or STEMI) for whom an early invasive treatment strategy was planned.[79] Prasugrel-treated patients had significantly lower rates of death, MI, or stroke compared to ticagrelor with similar rates of major bleeding. While ticagrelor is noninferior to clopidogrel for major bleeding risk in patients with STEMI receiving reperfusion with fibrinolytics, clopidogrel is the only $P2Y_{12}$ inhibitor with specific recommendations as an adjunct to fibrinolytic therapy in patients with STEMI.[80]

While all antiplatelet agents have the adverse effect of bleeding, the unique structure of ticagrelor produces additional adverse effects. Ticagrelor can interfere with adenosine degradation and increase adenosine concentrations via inhibition of adenosine uptake by erythrocytes.[1,74] This interaction most likely occurs through inhibition of the sodium-independent equilibrative nucleoside transporter (ENT)-1. Erythrocyte ENT-1 is responsible for the uptake of adenosine into the cell where it is metabolized by multiple mechanisms. The ability of ticagrelor to inhibit adenosine's uptake via ENT-1 is likely due to the adenosine core of the ticagrelor chemical structure.[74,77] This interaction produces an increase in adenosine exposure that likely explains these unique adverse effects. Significantly more patients receiving ticagrelor complained of dyspnea (13.8%) compared to those receiving clopidogrel (7.8%).[75] Symptoms of dyspnea are typically mild to moderate, require no specific therapy or workup, and usually dissipate within 2 to 4 weeks. Coaching of the patient through these episodes is often successful as ticagrelor was discontinued due to dyspnea in less than 1% of patients in the clinical trial. The use of ticagrelor has also been associated with an increase in asymptomatic ventricular pauses, increases in uric acid, and small increases in serum creatinine.[1,74]

Cangrelor Cangrelor is the only available intravenously administered $P2Y_{12}$ inhibitor. Similar to ticagrelor, cangrelor is a reversible inhibitor of the $P2Y_{12}$ receptor and binds to the receptor at a different location than adenosine diphosphate. Despite the recommended loading doses, oral $P2Y_{12}$ inhibitors take a minimum of 1 to 2 hours to obtain maximum platelet inhibition and 3 to 7 days for platelet recovery after discontinuation.[63] Cangrelor achieves maximum platelet inhibition within approximately 2 minutes of an IV bolus dose, with the restoration of normal platelet reactivity within 1 to 2 hours of cessation of the infusion.[63] Cangrelor has an elimination half-life of less than 9 minutes and is metabolized by ATPases in the blood. Therefore, hepatic or renal dysfunction are not likely to impact the pharmacokinetics of cangrelor.[63] The fast return to normal platelet function may provide safety advantages for cangrelor over other $P2Y_{12}$ inhibitors in the context of bleeding or transition to CABG surgery.

The use of cangrelor in patients with ACS is not well defined. In a clinical trial evaluating the efficacy and safety of cangrelor for patients undergoing PCI (44% of whom had ACS), cangrelor provided a significant reduction in MACE with an increase in minor bleeding, but not major bleeding.[81] When used in this setting, cangrelor (bolus dose followed by an infusion) should be initiated before PCI. After PCI, an oral P2Y12 inhibitor (loading dose followed by maintenance dose) should be initiated; the overall duration of cangrelor infusion should be at least 2 hours. Since the chemical structure is similar to ticagrelor, dyspnea may occur with the use of cangrelor, but the shorter drug exposure time likely contributes to a lower incidence (1.2%) and discontinuation rate (0.1%) compared to ticagrelor (13.8% and 0.9%, respectively).[81,82]

Cangrelor may interfere with the binding of the active metabolites of clopidogrel and prasugrel. When clopidogrel is given with cangrelor, the ability of the thienopyridines to irreversibly inhibit platelet function was reduced.[82,83] Cangrelor directly prevents binding of the short-lived but irreversible active metabolite of clopidogrel. Once the infusion is discontinued, no impact on the pharmacodynamic effect of clopidogrel was seen. This same interaction would be expected with prasugrel. Therefore, if cangrelor is used, the loading dose of the thienopyridine should not be given until the cangrelor infusion has been discontinued. This interaction does not exist with ticagrelor.

Switching Antiplatelet Agents Situations may occur after initial DAPT is chosen whereby therapy needs to change based upon some unique clinical scenario. Switching of therapy can be described as an escalation of therapy whereby clopidogrel is switched to a more potent $P2Y_{12}$ inhibitor such as ticagrelor or prasugrel. Reasons for escalation include cases of heightened risk for a coronary event or stent thrombosis, development of drug interaction, intolerance or nonadherence, identification of a genetic polymorphism to clopidogrel, or confirmation of inadequate platelet inhibition. In contrast, de-escalation typically refers to switching from a more potent $P2Y_{12}$ inhibitor to clopidogrel. Need for a de-escalation of $P2Y_{12}$ inhibitor therapy may be needed in response to bleeding, when there is a new indication to concurrently use an oral anticoagulant, or in cases when the cost is limiting medication access or leading to suboptimal adherence. Data on switching antiplatelet therapies is limited and is primarily based on pharmacodynamic studies. The efficacy and safety of switching agents during the first 12 months following ACS, therefore, is not fully known. But clinical decisions based on the reason for switching (ie, escalation versus de-escalation) and the timing from index event (ie, acute/early phase within the first 30 days versus later) must be weighed. One international consensus panel recommends that no loading dose be given when de-escalating therapy due to bleeding.[84] Loading doses are generally not needed when de-escalating therapy except when being when switching from ticagrelor to another $P2Y_{12}$ inhibitor.[84] Any escalation in therapy should be accompanied by a loading dose of the new agent regardless of the time of last $P2Y_{12}$ inhibitor dose, followed by maintenance therapy 24 hours after the last $P2Y_{12}$ inhibitor dose.[84] Finally, when switching between $P2Y_{12}$ inhibitors within 30 days of the index event, loading doses are recommended in most cases, except when the reason for switching is because of bleeding.[84] In general, the switch should occur 24 hours after the last dose of previous $P2Y_{12}$ inhibitor.[84]

Glycoprotein IIb/IIIa Inhibitors The binding of fibrinogen to activated GP IIb/IIIa receptors represents the final step in platelet aggregation, making inhibition of this receptor an ideal target in patients with ACS. Each of the agents is only available as an IV infusion.

Eptifibatide and tirofiban are peptide and nonpeptide inhibitors of the GP IIb/IIIa receptor, respectively. These agents have a reversible binding of the GP IIb/IIIa receptor. Therefore, platelet function recovery occurs in 2 to 4 hours after discontinuation of the infusion.

The reversible binding of these agents requires that they overwhelm the ability of fibrinogen to bind to the GP IIb/IIIa receptor with high concentrations. Consequently, platelet transfusion would not be able to absorb the excess drug and would not be helpful in the management of bleeding with eptifibatide or tirofiban.

Besides bleeding, GP IIb/IIIa inhibitors can also cause significant thrombocytopenia in about 0.5% of patients.[19] Given that GP IIb/IIIa inhibitors should be administered with a heparin, it is important to differentiate GP IIb/IIIa inhibitor-induced thrombocytopenia from heparin-induced thrombocytopenia (HIT).[85] Thrombocytopenia from a GP IIb/IIIa inhibitor occurs more rapidly (within hours) and the platelet count nadir is typically lower (about 20,000/μL [20×10^9/L]) compared to HIT. While the efficacy of platelet transfusion for thrombocytopenia from eptifibatide or tirofiban is limited, it would unlikely be harmful as in HIT.[85]

Although GP IIb/IIIa inhibitors significantly reduce MACE, the majority of trials were conducted before DAPT became standard-of-care and before the more potent $P2Y_{12}$ inhibitors prasugrel and ticagrelor were available. In a study comparing the combination of a GP IIb/IIIa inhibitor and unfractionated heparin to unfractionated heparin alone in patients with NSTE-ACS receiving PCI and a 600 mg loading dose of clopidogrel, patients treated with the GP IIb/IIIa inhibitor had a significant reduction in MACE but the benefit was only in patients who had an elevated cTn.[86] Therefore, GP IIb/IIIa inhibitors provide added benefit in the setting of early DAPT but should be reserved for high-risk patients with elevated cTn. The ability of GP IIb/IIIa inhibitors to reduce MACE in patients receiving prasugrel or ticagrelor remains unknown. In trials comparing a strategy of GP IIb/IIIa inhibitors plus unfractionated heparin to bivalirudin alone in patients with ACS undergoing PCI, no differences in MACE were observed, but there was significantly less major bleeding with bivalirudin alone.[87,88] While these trials have many limitations, clinicians have consistently used less GP IIb/IIIa inhibitors over the last decade.

Patients with NSTE-ACS undergoing an ischemia-driven approach do not derive benefit from GP IIb/IIIa inhibitors and should not be used in these patients.[2] Patients with STEMI receiving reperfusion with fibrinolytics have significant increases in major bleeding and ICH when GP IIb/IIIa inhibitors are used concomitantly and they should be avoided in these patients as well.[1]

6 While the use of GP IIb/IIIa inhibitors has been diminishing over the years, the patient for whom GP IIb/IIIa inhibitors may provide the most benefit is one receiving PCI for NSTE-ACS with elevated cTn, (eg, suffering MI) or STEMI who has not been preloaded with a $P2Y_{12}$ inhibitor and is not being treated with bivalirudin. Guidelines also state that it is reasonable to use a GP IIb/IIIa inhibitor in patients who are preloaded with clopidogrel.[1,2,60,86] In this setting, consensus guidelines recommend the use of an 18- to 24-hour infusion (eptifibatide and tirofiban) but the contemporary use of these drugs continues to evolve. These agents should always be given concurrently with unfractionated heparin or a low-molecular-weight heparin (LMWH) but the anticoagulant should be discontinued immediately following the PCI procedure to reduce the risk of major bleeding.

Anticoagulants

Although patients with ACS are typically treated with two antiplatelet agents for at least a year, usually a single anticoagulant is used in these patients and the duration is abbreviated (typically the initial few days of hospitalization).[1,2] Currently available anticoagulants inhibit the production of thrombin by inhibiting factor Xa, inhibiting thrombin itself, or a combination of these. While the use of oral anticoagulants may be common for other thromboembolic disease states, all of the current evidence in the acute management of ACS is with injectable agents. The use and dosing of anticoagulant therapies for the treatment of ACS are summarized in Table 34-7.

Unfractionated Heparin Unfractionated heparin has been widely used in the management of patients with ACS for several decades. The unfractionated heparin molecule is a highly sulfated polysaccharide. Unfractionated heparin provides its anticoagulant activity by binding to the endogenous anticoagulant antithrombin (AT) via a unique pentasaccharide sequence, substantially increasing its affinity for clotting factor inhibition.[89] These unfractionated heparin–AT complexes can then inhibit clotting factors IXa, Xa, XIa, XIIa, and thrombin, with most of the impact provided through inhibition of factor Xa and thrombin. Inhibition of thrombin requires a tertiary binding between the unfractionated heparin–AT and thrombin molecules. This requires that the chain length of the inhibitory molecule be at least 18 saccharides long.[89] This additional binding is not necessary for inhibition of factor Xa. Since most unfractionated heparin molecules are approximately 45 to 50 saccharides long, unfractionated heparin can inhibit factor Xa and thrombin in an equal 1:1 ratio.[89]

The anticoagulant effect of unfractionated heparin has significant interpatient variability.[89] This is due to the additional binding of unfractionated heparin with endothelial cells, plasma protein, and ingestion by macrophages. As a result of the unpredictable anticoagulant response of unfractionated heparin, therapy needs to be monitored with an activated partial thromboplastin time (aPTT). The aPTT should be measured every 6 hours until two consecutive readings are within the therapeutic range, as determined by the individual institutional protocols, then every 24 hours for the duration of unfractionated heparin therapy. Although goal ranges for aPTT vary by institution based on the assays used, an aPTT goal of 1.5 to 2 times the institution's control value is recommended.[1] If a dose adjustment is made, the same monitoring schedule should be restarted. While some institutions have adopted the use of anti-Xa levels instead of aPTT to monitor heparin therapy, guideline recommendations are specific to aPTT. Due to the short duration of anticoagulant therapy in patients with ACS, it is not uncommon for unfractionated heparin to be discontinued before the patient ever achieves two consecutive therapeutic aPTT measurements. Platelet counts should also be monitored daily or every other day to monitor for HIT. While HIT typically presents 5 days or more after unfractionated heparin exposure, it can occur within hours if the patient has been exposed to heparin in the last 3 months.[85] If HIT is suspected, unfractionated heparin should be discontinued and anticoagulation with an IV direct thrombin inhibitor should be provided.

7 Based on experience, unfractionated heparin can be used across the spectrum of ACS, and regardless of the management strategy.[1,2] The recommended dosing of unfractionated heparin has changed several times over the past decades in an attempt to maximize efficacy and minimize bleeding. The recommended dose of unfractionated heparin is an IV bolus of 60 units/kg (initial maximum total dose of 4,000 units) and an initial infusion rate of 12 units/kg/hr (initial maximum 1,000 units/hr). This is the recommended dose regardless of the ACS diagnosis or management strategy.[1,2] After initiation of heparin, dosage adjustments can exceed the recommended maximums as necessary to achieve the aPTT goal. Bolus doses of 2,000 to 5,000 units can also be given in the cardiac catheterization laboratory at the time of PCI to maintain an adequate activated clotting time (ACT). In a meta-analysis comparing the use of heparin plus aspirin to aspirin alone in patients with NSTE-ACS, the risk of death or MI was reduced by 33% in heparin-treated patients.[90] Because of the long-standing experience and use of unfractionated heparin in patients with ACS, it is the standard-of-care comparison in clinical trials.

Low-Molecular-Weight Heparins Similar to unfractionated heparin, LMWHs must first bind to AT to provide their anticoagulant activity. LMWHs are created through chemical or enzymatic depolymerization of unfractionated heparin molecules.[89] This

TABLE 34-7 Anticoagulant Drug Use and Dosing Across the Spectrum of ACS and Management Strategy

	STEMI		NSTE-ACS	
Drug	**Primary PCI**	**Fibrinolytic reperfusion**	**Early invasive strategy**	**Ischemia-driven strategy**
Bivalirudin	0.75 mg/kg IV bolus, followed by 1.75 mg/kg/hr IV infusion until completion of PCI CrCl less than 30 mL/min (0.5 mL/s): Reduce infusion to 1 mg/kg/hr	No recommendation	0.10 mg/kg IV bolus, followed by 0.25 mg/kg/hr IV infusion continued until completion of PCI	No recommendation
Enoxaparin	0.5 mg/kg one time IV bolus[a]	30 mg IV bolus, followed by 1 mg/kg SC every 12 hours for up to 8 days or hospital discharge SC doses should be initiated within 15 minutes of the IV bolus. The first two SC doses should be capped at 100 mg CrCl less than 30 mL/min (0.5 mL/s): 30 mg IV bolus, followed by 1 mg/kg SC every 24 hours The first SC dose should be capped at 100 mg Age 75 years or more: No IV bolus. Initiate at 0.75 mg/kg SC every 12 hours The first two SC doses should be capped at 75 mg CrCl less than 30 mL/min (0.5 mL/s) AND age 75 years or more: No IV bolus. Initiate at 1 mg/kg every 24 hours The first dose should be capped at 100 mg	1 mg/kg SC every 12 hours until PCI A 0.3 mg/kg IV bolus should be given if PCI occurs before two SC doses have been given, or if the last dose was given 8 hours or more prior to PCI CrCl less than 30 mL/min (0.5 mL/s): 1 mg/kg SC every 24 hours An initial 30 mg IV bolus can be given	1 mg/kg SC every 12 hours for the duration of hospitalization An initial 30 mg IV bolus can be given CrCl less than 30 mL/min (0.5 mL/s): 1 mg/kg SC every 24 hours
Fondaparinux	No recommendation	2.5 mg IV first dose, followed by 2.5 mg SC daily for up to 8 days or hospital discharge	2.5 mg SC daily until PCI At the time of PCI: No GP IIb/IIIa: IV UFH 85 units/kg[b] With GP IIb/IIIa: IV UFH 60 units/kg[b]	2.5 mg SC daily for up to 8 days or duration of hospitalization
Unfractionated heparin	No GP IIb/IIIa: 70-100 units/kg IV bolus to achieve a therapeutic ACT[b] GP IIb/IIIa: 50-70 units/kg IV bolus to achieve a therapeutic ACT[b]	60 units/kg (maximum initial bolus: 4,000 units) IV bolus, followed by 12 units/kg/hr (maximum initial infusion rate: 1,000 units/hr)	60 units/kg (maximum initial bolus: 4,000 units) IV bolus, followed by 12 units/kg/hr (maximum initial infusion rate: 1,000 units/hr)[b]	60 units/kg (maximum initial bolus: 4,000 units) IV bolus, followed by 12 units/kg/hr (maximum initial infusion rate: 1,000 units/hr)

[a]Not mentioned in the ACC/AHA guidelines, but evidence exists.

[b]Additional IV boluses of unfractionated heparin may be needed to maintain a therapeutic ACT.

ACT, activated clotting time; CrCl, creatinine clearance; IV, intravenous; SC, subcutaneous; UFH, unfractionated heparin.

Data from References 1 and 2.

creates a mixture of lower molecular weight fragments compared to the larger intact unfractionated heparin molecule. Most of these fragments are less than 18 saccharides long. Consequently, LMWH's anticoagulants primarily inhibit factor Xa due to the fewer number of larger fragments able to inhibit thrombin. The ratio of factor Xa to thrombin inhibition for a LMWH is typically 3:1 or 4:1, depending on the process of depolymerization.[89]

Compared to unfractionated heparin, LMWHs provide a predicable anticoagulant dose-response with no need for routine therapeutic monitoring. While most patients receiving a LMWH do not require therapeutic monitoring, an anti-Xa level may be desired in certain patient populations.[89] Patient groups where anti-Xa monitoring may be helpful would be pediatrics, pregnancy, obesity (greater than 190 kg), and patients with severe renal insufficiency (eg, creatinine clearance [CrCl] less than 30 mL/min [0.5 mL/s]). While pediatric and pregnant patients rarely have ACS, obesity and severe renal insufficiency are more common in patients with ACS. The target peak anti-Xa level is 0.3 to 0.7 IU/mL (kIU/L) drawn 4 hours after the third dose. Since patients with ACS typically receive anticoagulant therapy for only a few days, the utility of anti-Xa monitoring in these patients is limited. There is also a lower incidence of HIT with the use of LMWHs (less than 2%) compared to unfractionated heparin (2%-5%).[85] Even though the risk of HIT is lower with LMWH, the monitoring of platelet counts is still warranted. Due to the 90% cross-reactivity between HIT antibodies from LMWH and unfractionated heparin, LMWH is not considered a safe alternative in patients who develop HIT from unfractionated heparin and vice versa.[85]

While other LMWHs are available, enoxaparin is the most widely studied agent in patients with ACS and is the only LMWH recommended in the ACC/AHA guidelines.[1,2] Data supporting the use of enoxaparin exist in patients with NSTE-ACS and STEMI regardless of the management or reperfusion strategy used. Unfortunately, the dosing of enoxaparin varies across these different settings, requiring careful attention to assure the right dose is used in the right patient to maximize efficacy and safety (Table 34-7).

7 In patients with NSTE-ACS undergoing an ischemia-driven approach, the use of subcutaneous (SC) enoxaparin 1 mg/kg every 12 hours for up to 3 days significantly reduces the risk of MACE without increasing major bleeding compared to IV unfractionated

heparin.[91] In patients with NSTE-ACS treated with an early invasive strategy, SC enoxaparin (1 mg/kg every 12 hours) has similar efficacy but more major bleeding compared to unfractionated heparin.[92] This trial was complicated by a large number of patients receiving both anticoagulants during the trial. Interestingly, in patients who were treated with either enoxaparin or IV unfractionated heparin alone, those randomized to enoxaparin had a 17% reduction in the risk of death or MI at 30 days and at 6 months without a significant increase in major bleeding compared to IV unfractionated heparin. Based on these data, either unfractionated heparin or enoxaparin is recommended in patients with NSTE-ACS. Patients who have received less than two SC doses prior to PCI should receive a supplemental IV enoxaparin bolus dose of 0.3 mg/kg to provide sufficient anticoagulation during the procedure.[2] Patients who have received at least two SC doses and arrive at PCI within 8 hours of their last dose do not require any additional anticoagulation for PCI.[2,92] Patients having PCI performed within 8 to 12 hours of their last dose should also receive the supplemental IV enoxaparin bolus dose.[2,92] Patients with a CrCl less than 30 mL/min (0.5 mL/s) should receive enoxaparin 1 mg/kg every 24 hours instead of every 12 hours.

7 In patients with STEMI receiving reperfusion with fibrinolytics, enoxaparin significantly reduced death and MI when compared to unfractionated heparin.[93] Major bleeding was increased, but there was no increase in ICH which occurred in less than 1% of patients. Dosing of enoxaparin in this trial used a 30 mg IV bolus followed immediately by 1 mg/kg SC every 12 hours. The bolus dose is necessary in the setting of STEMI due to the rapid need for reperfusion therapy. Patients aged 75 years or greater and those with a CrCl less than 30 mL/min (0.5 mL/s) need to receive altered dosing to reduce the risk of bleeding in these higher-risk patients (Table 34-7). Trials in patients receiving primary PCI for STEMI have used a single IV dose of 0.5 mg/kg of enoxaparin. In a meta-analysis of trials evaluating this dose of enoxaparin in primary PCI, there is a reduction in mortality and significantly less major bleeding compared to unfractionated heparin.[94] Despite these data, a definitive clinical trial has not been conducted with enoxaparin in this setting.

Fondaparinux Fondaparinux is a synthetic molecule existing of only the five saccharides needed to bind to and potentiate the activity of AT.[89] While others have been investigated, fondaparinux is the only available pentasaccharide worldwide. Due to the small size of the molecule, once it binds to AT it can only inhibit factor Xa and has no activity against thrombin. Similar to LMWH, fondaparinux also provides a predictable anticoagulant dose-response and no need for therapeutic monitoring.[89] While case reports of fondaparinux-induced thrombocytopenia have been reported, the incidence is thought to be extremely rare.[85] Based on the lack of antibody cross-reactivity, it is reasonable to consider the use of fondaparinux in patients with a history of HIT.[85] Based on the long half-life of fondaparinux, the SC dose (2.5 mg) is only given once daily. Fondaparinux is contraindicated in patients with a CrCl of less than 30 mL/min (0.5 mL/s) due to the significant degree of renal elimination. There can also be accumulation in patients with a CrCl between 30 and 60 mL/min (0.5 and 1.0 mL/s), but this is typically not a factor with the short duration of therapy in patients with ACS.[95]

7 The use of fondaparinux in patients with ACS has been evaluated in two large trials.[96,97] The trial in NSTE-ACS evaluated patients receiving either an ischemia-driven or invasive management strategy and found similar efficacy between fondaparinux and enoxaparin, with significantly less major bleeding in patients receiving fondaparinux.[97] Although a number of issues in the trial may have explained the observed difference in bleeding, fondaparinux can be considered in patients undergoing an ischemia-driven approach who are at a high risk of bleeding.[2] Patients undergoing PCI experienced an increase in catheter-related thrombosis if they received fondaparinux compared to enoxaparin.[97] Due to this concern, supplemental doses of IV unfractionated heparin must be given if a patient receiving fondaparinux requires PCI.[2] Consequently, fondaparinux is rarely used and not recommended in the United States for patients with NSTE-ACS receiving an invasive management approach.[60]

7 The trial utilizing fondaparinux in STEMI evaluated patients receiving reperfusion with either fibrinolytics or primary PCI.[96] In this trial, fondaparinux was compared to unfractionated heparin. Similar to the NSTE-ACS trial, patients receiving primary PCI had significantly higher rates of catheter-related thrombosis if they received fondaparinux compared to unfractionated heparin.[1,96] As in NSTE-ACS, fondaparinux use has been constrained by this limitation and is not recommended in patients receiving primary PCI.[60] In patients receiving fibrinolytics, the use of fondaparinux has similar efficacy and safety compared to unfractionated heparin.[96] Based on the lack of benefit over unfractionated heparin, and the benefit with enoxaparin over unfractionated heparin in this population, fondaparinux is rarely used in patients with STEMI.

Bivalirudin Bivalirudin is an intravenously administered direct thrombin inhibitor. Being a "direct" inhibitor means bivalirudin does not have to first bind to AT to provide its anticoagulant effect.[89] Because of the lack of AT binding, bivalirudin can inhibit not only free or soluble thrombin, similar to unfractionated heparin and LMWH but also fibrin-bound thrombin. Fibrin-bound thrombin is still enzymatically active, but the large AT–anticoagulant complexes are unable to gain access and, therefore, exert anticoagulant activity.[89] The clinical benefit of bivalirudin's inhibition of this larger pool of thrombin is difficult to quantify.

7 Bivalirudin has not been evaluated in patients with NSTE-ACS undergoing an ischemia-driven approach or in patients with STEMI receiving reperfusion with fibrinolytics. Therefore, bivalirudin is only used in patients with ACS who receive PCI and can be monitored with an ACT in the catheterization laboratory.[1,2,89] In one NSTE-ACS trial evaluating anticoagulation as part of an early invasive approach, patients received a heparin derivative (unfractionated heparin or enoxaparin) with a GP IIb/IIIa inhibitor, bivalirudin with a GP IIb/IIIa inhibitor, or bivalirudin alone.[87] There was no difference in efficacy or safety in patients receiving heparin or LMWH with a GP IIb/IIIa inhibitor compared to bivalirudin with a GPII/IIIa inhibitor. Consequently, because of the lack of benefit and increased cost associated with the combination of bivalirudin and a GP IIb/IIIa inhibitor, this regimen is not recommended in patients with NSTE-ACS undergoing PCI. Patients receiving bivalirudin alone had similar efficacy but significantly less major bleeding compared to heparin or LMWH with a GP IIb/IIIa inhibitor. The patients who were not preloaded with clopidogrel in the trial had significantly more MACE if they received bivalirudin alone.[2,87] Therefore, bivalirudin may not be as protective in patients who do not receive a $P2Y_{12}$ inhibitor prior to PCI. Similar to the study in NSTE-ACS, bivalirudin alone had similar efficacy with significantly less major bleeding compared to unfractionated heparin with a GP IIb/IIIa in patients undergoing primary PCI for STEMI.[88] These data led to a significant reduction in the use of GP IIb/IIIa inhibitors. Bivalirudin does not offer efficacy or safety benefit over unfractionated heparin alone in the setting of primary PCI for STEMI, particularly as vascular access to perform PCI has moved from a predominantly femoral arterial approach associated with higher rates of bleeding to a radial artery approach associated with less bleeding.[98-100] While the role of bivalirudin in these patients is recommended in the guidelines, many cardiologists have come full circle and often use unfractionated heparin for primary PCI for patients with STEMI instead of bivalirudin.

Secondary Prevention of Ischemic Events

For most patients, the initial 24 hours of ACS care are focused on reperfusion (if appropriate), antithrombotic therapy, and acute supportive measures. After a diagnosis of ACS, patients are considered to have atherosclerotic cardiovascular disease (ASCVD) and should be treated aggressively because they are at the highest risk of recurrent MACE. Secondary prevention strategies proved to accomplish these goals typically include anti-ischemic, antiplatelet, lipid-lowering, and antihypertensive therapies (Table 34-8).[1,2,29] Specific pharmacotherapy proved to decrease mortality, HF, reinfarction or stroke, and stent thrombosis should be initiated prior

TABLE 34-8 Chronic Medications to Reduce Risk of MACE and Control Symptoms Following ACS

Drug	Indication in ACS Patients (Class of Recommendation)[a]	Contraindication/Caution	Dose (All doses are oral unless indicated)	Adverse Effects
Aspirin	All patients without contraindications	• Hypersensitivity to aspirin or NSAID • History of asthma, rhinitis, and nasal polyps • History of upper GI bleeding • Bleeding disorder/active bleeding	• 81 mg once daily	Dyspepsia, GI bleeding
$P2Y_{12}$ inhibitors	All patients without contraindications	• Thienopyridine hypersensitivity • Bleeding disorder/active bleeding • Previous intracranial hemorrhage • Prasugrel: prior TIA or stroke • Ticagrelor: aspirin doses greater than 100 mg daily; strong CYP3A4 inhibitors or inducers	• Clopidogrel 75 mg once daily • Prasugrel 10 mg once daily; weight less than 60 kg: 5 mg daily • Ticagrelor 90 mg twice daily	Bleeding, rash; Ticagrelor: dyspnea, ventricular pauses, bradycardia
β-Blockers	All patients without contraindications	• Signs of heart failure • Low cardiac output state • High-grade AV block • Active asthma or reactive airway disease	• Carvedilol 6.25 mg twice daily; target dose (in patients with HFrEF): 25 mg twice daily as tolerated • Metoprolol 25-50 mg every 6-12 hours for 2-3 days, then once (metoprolol succinate) or twice daily (metoprolol tartrate); target dose (in patients with HFrEF): 200 mg daily • Continue therapy for at least 3 years, indefinitely in patients with concomitant HFrEF • Other β-blockers may be considered; in patients with HFrEF, use either metoprolol succinate, carvedilol, or bisoprolol	Hypotension, heart failure, bradycardia, cardiogenic shock, AV block, exacerbation of asthma or reactive airway disease
Statins	All patients without contraindications	• Active liver disease • Pregnancy • Breastfeeding • Concomitant use of fibrate	• Atorvastatin 80 mg daily • Rosuvastatin 20-40 mg daily	GI discomfort, arthralgia, myalgia, musculoskeletal pain, hepatotoxicity
Nonstatin therapies	Patients with very high-risk ASCVD (eg, post-ACS) with LDL-C greater than 70 mg/dL (1.81 mmol/L) on maximally tolerated statin therapy	• Hypersensitivity • Simvastatin/ezetimibe: strong CYP3A4 inhibitors	• Ezetimibe 10 mg daily • Simvastatin 40 mg/ezetimibe 10 mg • Alirocumab 75 mg SC every 2 weeks or 300 mg SC every 4 weeks • Evolocumab 140 mg SC every 2 weeks or 420 mg SC monthly	Ezetimibe and combination: GI discomfort, arthralgia, myalgia, musculoskeletal pain Alirocumab: injection site pain, hypersensitivity Evolocumab: nasopharyngitis, injection site pain
ACE inhibitors	All patients without contraindications	• Hypotension • Renal failure • Hyperkalemia	• Lisinopril 2.5-5 mg daily; target dose: 10-40 mg daily • Enalapril 2.5-5 mg twice daily; target dose: 10-20 mg twice daily • Captopril 6.25-12.5 mg three times daily; target dose: 25-50 mg three times daily • Ramipril 2.5 mg twice daily; target dose: 5 mg twice daily • Trandolapril 0.5-1 mg daily; target dose: 4 mg daily	Hypotension, hyperuricemia, hyperkalemia, worsening renal function, chronic cough, angioedema
ARBs	Patients intolerant to ACE inhibitors	• Hypotension • Renal failure • Hyperkalemia	• Valsartan 20 mg twice daily; target dose: 160 mg twice daily	Hypotension, hyperuricemia, hyperkalemia, worsening renal function

(continued)

TABLE 34-8 Chronic Medications to Reduce Risk of MACE and Control Symptoms Following ACS (*Continued*)

Drug	Indication in ACS Patients (Class of Recommendation)[a]	Contraindication/Caution	Dose (All doses are oral unless indicated)	Adverse Effects
Aldosterone antagonist	Patients with LVEF 40% (0.40) or less and either DM or symptoms of HF	• Elevated serum creatinine • Men: 2.5 mg/dL (221 μmol/L) or greater • Women: 2.0 mg/dL (177 μmol/L) or greater • CrCl 30 mL/min (0.5 mL/s) or less • Serum potassium 5.0 mEq/L (mmol/L) or greater	• Eplerenone 25 mg daily; target dose: 50 mg daily • Spironolactone 12.5-25 mg daily; target dose: 25-50 mg daily	Hyperkalemia, worsening renal function
Nitroglycerin	All patients without contraindications	• Hypotension • Avoid if recent PDE_5 inhibitor use • Avanafil: within 12 hours • Sildenafil: within 24 hours • Vardenafil: within 24 hours • Tadalafil: within 48 hours	• SL: 0.3-0.4 mg every 5 minutes, up to 3 doses PRN	Flushing, headache, hypotension, tachycardia

[a]AHA/ACC class of recommendations: I, benefit far outweighs the risk, treatment should be administered; IIb, the benefit is equal to or exceeds the risk, additional studies with broad objectives are needed, treatment may be considered.

AV, atrioventricular; CrCl, creatinine clearance; CYP3A4, cytochrome p450 isoenzyme 3A4; GI, gastrointestinal; HF, heart failure; NSAID, nonsteroidal anti-inflammatory drug; PDE5, phosphodiesterase-5; PRN, as needed; SC, subcutaneously; TIA, transient ischemic attack.

Data from References 1, 2, and 101-103.

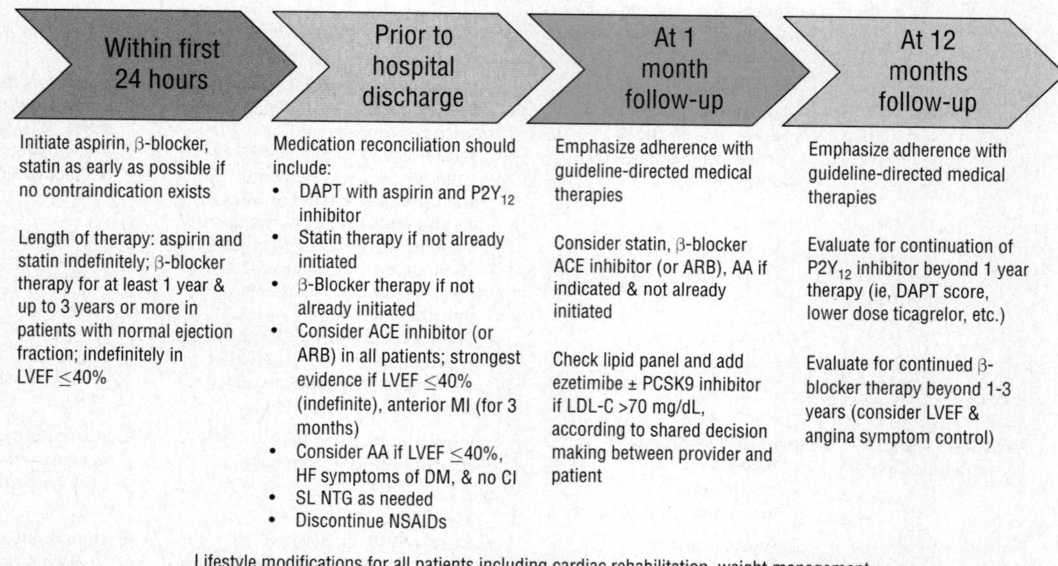

FIGURE 34-3 Secondary prevention of ischemic events over time. (AA, aldosterone antagonist; CI, contraindications; DM, diabetes mellitus; LDL-C, low-density lipoprotein cholesterol [70 mg/dL is expressed in SI units as 1.81 mmol/L]; NSAID, nonsteroidal anti-inflammatory drug; SL NTG, sublingual nitroglycerin.)

to hospital discharge in all patients without contraindications. Medication reconciliation at discharge should include assessment for DAPT, β-blocker, angiotensin-converting enzyme (ACE) inhibitor or angiotensin receptor blocker (ARB), and statin therapy unless a contraindication exists (Fig. 34-3). In addition, short-acting nitroglycerin should be prescribed as needed for any subsequent episode of acute angina for patients not taking phosphodiesterase-5 inhibitors. Select patients may also meet the criteria for aldosterone antagonist use.

In addition to evaluating patients for the use of medications proved to reduce the risk of MACE or recurrent symptoms of angina, additional interventions may be appropriate to optimize outcomes and improve safety. Aggressive risk factor modification strategies such as increased physical activity, dietary modification, weight loss, blood pressure modification, and smoking cessation should be communicated to all patients, initiated, and continued indefinitely.[104] Proton pump inhibitors provide a protective benefit in patients at the highest risk for GI bleeding from DAPT and may be considered for select patients (eg, history of GI bleeding, triple therapy with DAPT, and an oral anticoagulant with or without a history of GI bleeding).[2] All patients should refrain from chronic use of nonsteroidal anti-inflammatory drugs with a high degree of cyclo-oxygenase-2 selectivity as they are associated with increased cerebrovascular and cardiovascular events.[1,2] Finally, for patients with cardiovascular disease, including those hospitalized for ACS, an annual influenza vaccination lowers the risk of MACE and is recommended as part of the care plan.[1,2,105,106]

Duration of Dual Antiplatelet Therapy (DAPT)

8 The ACC/AHA has published guidelines specifically related to dosing, initiation, and duration of DAPT after ACS, including situations when therapy should be discontinued.[1,2,107,120] In general, shorter durations of DAPT are appropriate for those patients with a lower ischemic risk who are at high-risk for bleeding. Conversely, longer durations of DAPT may be reasonable in patients at higher ischemic risk if bleeding risk is low. No randomized trials have compared different durations of DAPT specifically in the ACS setting. Yet, because the ischemic risk following ACS is considered high, DAPT with aspirin plus a $P2Y_{12}$ receptor inhibitor is indicated for most patients treated for ACS for a minimum of 12 months regardless of whether the patient was medically managed or if the patient undergoes some type of revascularization.[1,2,107,120] For patients with STEMI treated with fibrinolysis, the minimum recommended duration of DAPT is 14 days.[1,107] Every patient receiving DAPT should understand the benefit as well as risks associated with the therapy and the importance of maintaining adherence with therapy for the appropriate duration of therapy. For patients at high risk of bleeding, a shorter duration of DAPT may be warranted. In these patients, a brief (1 to 3 months) duration of DAPT followed by $P2Y_{12}$ monotherapy or 6-month duration of DAPT followed by aspirin monotherapy may lower the risk of bleeding.

Continuation of DAPT beyond 12 months may be reasonable for patients at higher ischemic risk provided they also have a lower bleeding risk. This should be an individualized decision, considering both ischemic and bleeding risks. The DAPT risk score has been derived from the DAPT study and is supported by guidelines to aid in making decisions regarding prolonging DAPT beyond 12 months (Table 34-9).[107,108] A risk score of 2 or more suggests that prolonging therapy is favorable and would reduce ischemic events with perhaps only a modest increase in bleeding risk. Conversely, for those with a DAPT risk score less than 2, the risk for bleeding is anticipated to be greater than an ischemic benefit and the $P2Y_{12}$ inhibitor should be discontinued. The DAPT score was developed from a study comparing standard DAPT (12 months) to an extended duration of 30 months of therapy in patients who had PCI with intracoronary stenting for either SIHD or ACS and is not appropriate for determining DAPT duration shorter than 12 months. Further, 65% of patients enrolled in this study were administered clopidogrel and 35% were treated with prasugrel; ticagrelor was not used. Other risk prediction models are being developed and evaluated.

TABLE 34-9 Factors Used to Calculate DAPT Score and Predict Ischemic and Bleeding Events

Points	+2	+1	−1	−2
Clinical variables	CHF or LVEF less than 30% (0.30) Saphenous vein graft PCI	Current tobacco user DM NSTEMI or STEMI at presentation Prior MI or PCI Stent diameter less than 3 mm Paclitaxel-eluting stent	Age 65-74	Age ≥75 years

Risk factors ordered from left to right include those with highest ischemic risk and highest point accrual to those with the highest bleeding risk and negative point accrual. A score of ≥2 favors prolonged DAPT; a score of <2 is of unfavorable risk/benefit. Total score ranges from −2 to 10.

Data from References 107 and 108.

Continued use of DAPT with ticagrelor beyond 12 months after ACS can be considered. One trial compared standard-dose ticagrelor to a reduced dose of 60 mg twice daily in combination with low-dose aspirin to aspirin alone in patients who had suffered an MI 1 to 3 years prior.[109] Continuation of DAPT with either dose of ticagrelor decreased the composite of CV death, MI, or stroke compared to aspirin alone. While major bleeding was increased in patients treated with ticagrelor compared to aspirin alone, there were fewer bleeds in the low-dose ticagrelor group compared to the standard dose. The lower dose of ticagrelor (60 mg twice daily) has not been studied in the first 12 months after ACS; therefore, only the 90 mg twice daily is appropriate for the first year after the index event.

Cholesterol Management

Statins 9 Following ACS, statins reduce total mortality, CV mortality, MI, and stroke. Results from landmark clinical trials have unequivocally demonstrated the value of statins in secondary prevention following MI and provide an approximate 1% reduction in risk of ASCVD event per 1% reduction in low-density lipoprotein cholesterol (LDL-C) over time.[101] Further, clinical trial results confirm the benefit of high-intensity statins initiated 1 to 10 days after ACS presentation. In a meta-analysis of randomized controlled clinical trials of patients with recent ACS (less than 14 days), statin therapy reduces mortality by 19%, with benefits observed after approximately 4 months of treatment.[110] Therefore, high-intensity statin therapy should be initiated during the index hospitalization once the patient has been stabilized and continued indefinitely. Risk reductions from high-intensity statin therapy occur regardless of cholesterol concentrations at presentation. Therefore, all patients with ACS should receive the highest dose of maximally tolerated statin, even those with "normal" LDL-C at baseline.[1,2,101]

In those patients who are already taking low- or moderate-intensity statin therapy at the time of ACS presentation, consideration should be given to switching to a high-intensity statin. For ACS patients with a history of statin intolerance or those at high risk for statin-related adverse effects (older patients, drug interaction, etc.), the use of moderate-intensity statins or lower doses of high-intensity statins may be considered.[101] Patients aged greater than 75 years may be prescribed a moderate-intensity statin as initial therapy because they are at higher risk of adverse drug effects and the data using high-dose statins in this patient subgroup are less robust.[101]

A lipid panel should be reassessed 4 to 6 weeks after initiation of therapy with the goal of a 50% reduction in LDL-C from baseline. Baseline lipid concentrations should be drawn as early as possible, ideally within the first 24 hours of ACS presentation, as phasic changes may occur that falsely lower total cholesterol, LDL-C, and high-density lipoprotein cholesterol. Triglycerides may be falsely elevated during this immediate period of ACS. See Chapter 32, "Dyslipidemia," for a more detailed discussion on the management of patients with dyslipidemia.

Other Cholesterol-Lowering Therapies Nonstatin therapies lower the risk of MACE in patients with ACS already receiving statin therapy and may be considered as add-on therapy in select patients. The combination of moderate-dose simvastatin and ezetimibe, a nonstatin, in patients with recent (within 10 days) ACS and an LDL-C level between 50 and 100 mg/dL (1.29 and 2.59 mmol/L) resulted in a modest reduction (6.4% relative risk reduction) in the rate of MACE compared to moderate-dose simvastatin alone.[111] Event rates were lower in patients who achieved lower LDL-C, suggesting a direct relationship between LDL-C and benefit. A new class of potent, injectable cholesterol-lowering drugs, the proprotein convertase subtilisin-kexin type 9 (PCSK9) inhibitors, lower the risk of MACE when added to high-intensity statin therapy in patients with recent ACS (within 1 to 12 months). Alirocumab reduced LDL-C by approximately 60% and the risk of MACE at 4 years by

15% compared to high-intensity statin therapy alone.[102] Another PCSK9 inhibitor, evolocumab, yielded similar reductions in LDL-C and MACE in patients with ASCVD, most of whom had a distant history of MI.[103] However, at the current cost of approximately $6,000 to $7,000 annually, the cost-effectiveness of PCSK9 inhibitors in this setting remains uncertain and may be dependent on baseline LDL-C.[101,112] Nevertheless, for patients with clinical ASCVD treated with maximally tolerated statin therapy at very high risk (eg, recent ACS event) and persistently elevated LDL-C (70 mg/dL [1.81 mmol/L]or greater), current guidelines suggest adding ezetimibe.[101] If LDL-C remains elevated despite maximally tolerated statin therapy and ezetimibe, the addition of a PCSK9 inhibitor is reasonable.[101]

ACE Inhibitors or Angiotensin Receptor Blockers

10 Following MI, ACE inhibitors lower mortality, reinfarction rates, and HF, most likely through the prevention of adverse cardiac remodeling.[1,2,113,114] While the use of IV enalaprilat within 24 hours of MI should be avoided due to increased risk of adverse events, early administration (within 48 hours of presentation) of ACE inhibitors is associated with lower mortality within the first month of therapy with additional benefit observed during longer treatment durations.[113,114] Data supporting the use of ACE inhibitors is strongest for those with left ventricular dysfunction (LVEF 40% [0.40] or less) or in those who developed HF symptoms in the early phase of ACS.[113] Therefore, treatment with ACE inhibitor is recommended in all patients with MI and concomitant HFrEF, HTN, DM, or stable chronic kidney disease.[1,2,29] For patients without those comorbidities who suffer an MI, treatment with an ACE inhibitor is also reasonable.[1,29] Because they have a comparable benefit to ACE inhibitors in patients with MI, an ARB may be prescribed for those who cannot tolerate an ACE inhibitor.[1,2,29,115]

Although ACE inhibitors and ARBs are generally well-tolerated, it is important to monitor closely for the development of noteworthy adverse effects. The most common adverse effects associated with ACE inhibitors and ARBs are worsening renal function and hypotension. Hyperkalemia is also possible and is more likely in patients who develop acute kidney injury. Therefore, close monitoring of renal function, potassium levels, and blood pressure are warranted 1 to 2 weeks following initiation and dose adjustments. Although angioedema and chronic cough are possible with each of these therapies, both adverse effects are more common with ACE inhibitors and occur infrequently with ARBs.

Aldosterone Antagonists

10 To reduce mortality, administration of an aldosterone antagonist, either eplerenone or spironolactone, should be considered within the first 14 days following MI in all patients with left ventricular dysfunction (LVEF of 40% [0.40] or less) and either HF symptoms or DM treated with both an ACE inhibitor (or ARB) and β-blocker.[1,2,29] Aldosterone antagonists attenuate the adverse hemodynamic and metabolic effects from chronic excessive aldosterone production as well as the cardiac remodeling that occurs in patients with MI.[116] In patients who suffered MI, aldosterone antagonists improved LVEF, lowered the risk for new or worsening HF by 26%, and reduced the risk of both all-cause mortality and CV mortality by 18%.[116] Although mortality was lower in patients with and without HF treated with aldosterone antagonists, the difference was only significant in patients with HF.

Both eplerenone and spironolactone block the mineralocorticoid receptor to which aldosterone binds contributing to some of the observed adverse effects. Spironolactone is a nonspecific steroid hormone receptor antagonist that also binds progesterone and androgen receptors and can cause gynecomastia in men and menstrual irregularities in women.[19] In contrast, eplerenone is selective for the mineralocorticoid receptor, thereby minimizing the risk of gynecomastia, sexual dysfunction, and menstrual irregularities.[19]

In post-MI clinical trials, aldosterone antagonists have been associated with a more than twofold increase in the risk of hyperkalemia with an overall incidence of 11.6%.[116] Therefore, patients who are post-MI with serum potassium concentrations greater than 5 mmol/L (mEq/L) should not receive an aldosterone antagonist.[2] Additional contraindications for aldosterone antagonists include a serum creatinine greater than 2.5 mg/dL (221 μmol/L) for men or 2 mg/dL (177 μmol/L) for women, or CrCl less than 30 mL/min (0.5 mL/s).[2] Because of the increased risk of hyperkalemia, especially in patients with chronic kidney disease, both serum potassium and renal function should be monitored diligently: 3 days and 1 week after initiation or dose titration, then monthly for the first 3 months, and every 3 months thereafter. There are no data to support the use of the more selective but more expensive eplerenone over the generically available spironolactone unless a patient experiences gynecomastia, breast pain, or impotence while receiving spironolactone.

Nitroglycerin

All patients should be prescribed and instructed on the appropriate use of short-acting nitroglycerin, typically either sublingual tablets or lingual spray, to relieve acute anginal symptoms on an as-needed basis.[1,2] Appropriate patient education for patients prescribed short-acting nitroglycerin is provided in Chapter 33, "Stable Ischemic Heart Disease." Chronic long-acting nitrate therapy does not reduce MACE following ACS and its role is typically limited to the prevention of recurrent symptoms of angina for patients treated for ACS with significant coronary stenoses not amenable to revascularization who experience symptomatic SIHD. For patients with ACS for whom vasospasm is believed to be contributory, long-acting nitrates are recommended to treat and reduce the frequency of anginal episodes.[2]

EVALUATION OF THERAPEUTIC OUTCOMES

Evaluation of short-term efficacy focuses on the restoration or preservation of coronary blood flow, symptom relief, and prevention of MACE. Restoration of blood flow and relief of ischemia can be detected by resolution of the ischemic changes on ECG at the time of presentation, which should occur soon after revascularization. Although cTn levels may remain elevated for several days, for patients with MI, cTn levels should peak within 12 to 24 hours and should decline steadily thereafter once ischemia is relieved. More importantly, if blood flow is restored or preserved and the angina is managed effectively, the patients should have a resolution of symptoms rather quickly. In terms of MACE, monitoring for the development of complications from ACS (eg, HF, arrhythmias) should occur frequently. Lastly, assuring that evidence-based therapies that reduce the risk of MACE following ACS have been initiated in appropriate patients is critical.

Long-term evaluation of outcomes is directed largely at functional capacity and continued focus on risk reduction. Returning to and maintaining a high quality of life is an important goal following an ACS hospitalization. Patients should eventually be able to return to their activities of daily living, perhaps following a cardiac rehabilitation program to assist them with this goal. Additionally, patients should be monitored at every healthcare encounter for the development of adverse effects from ACS pharmacotherapy (Table 34-10). If patients show signs of adverse effects or intolerance, particularly serious adverse events such as bleeding or hypotension, the offending agent(s) may need to be discontinued until the symptoms have resolved. Clinical signs of bleeding include bloody stools, melena, hematuria, hematemesis, bruising, and oozing from arterial or venous puncture sites. Oral antiplatelet agents are a leading cause of hospitalizations and ED visits for adverse drug reactions among

TABLE 34-10 Therapeutic Drug Monitoring of Pharmacotherapy for ACS

Drug	Adverse Effects	Monitoring
Fibrinolytics	Bleeding (ICH)	Clinical signs of bleeding[a]; baseline aPTT, INR; Hgb, Hct, platelet count at baseline then daily; mental status every 2 hours for signs of ICH
Aspirin	Dyspepsia, GI bleeding	Clinical signs of bleeding[a]; GI upset; Hgb, Hct, and platelet count at baseline & every 6 months
$P2Y_{12}$ inhibitors	Bleeding, rash	Clinical signs of bleeding[a]; evidence of rash; Hgb, Hct, platelet count at baseline and every 6 months
	Ticagrelor: dyspnea, ventricular pauses, bradycardia	Ticagrelor: dyspnea, heart rate, telemetry during hospitalization
Glycoprotein IIb/IIIa inhibitors	Bleeding, thrombocytopenia (can be profound with abciximab)	Clinical signs of bleeding[a]; Hgb, Hct, and platelet count at baseline, 2 hours, then daily
		Eptifibatide and tirofiban: serum creatinine at baseline then daily
Anticoagulants	Bleeding	Clinical signs of bleeding[a]; baseline aPTT, INR; Hgb, Hct, platelet count at baseline then daily
	Unfractionated heparin and LMWH: heparin-induced thrombocytopenia	Unfractionated heparin: aPTT every 6 hours until two consecutive aPTT values are at goal, then every 24 hours; ACT during PCI
		Enoxaparin, bivalirudin, and fondaparinux: serum creatinine at baseline then daily
		Enoxaparin: may consider steady-state anti-Xa levels in special populations
β-Blockers	Hypotension, heart failure, bradycardia, cardiogenic shock, AV block, exacerbation of asthma or reactive airway disease	Continuous telemetry (while hospitalized); blood pressure, heart rate, signs and symptoms of heart failure; monitor every 5 minutes before each IV bolus dose; monitor every shift while hospitalized then at each healthcare encounter after discharge
Nitroglycerin	Flushing, headache, hypotension, tachycardia	Blood pressure and heart rate; monitor every 5-15 minutes following dosage adjustment of intravenous nitroglycerin then every 1-2 hours; monitor every 5 minutes following administration of short-acting nitroglycerin
Morphine	Hypotension, respiratory depression, sedation, hypersensitivity	Blood pressure, heart rate, respiratory rate, sedation level 5 minutes after administration then every 1-2 hours for 4 hours after the last dose
Calcium channel blockers	Hypotension	Blood pressure, heart rate, every shift while hospitalized then at each healthcare encounter after discharge
	Verapamil and diltiazem: heart failure, cardiogenic shock, bradycardia, AV block	Verapamil and diltiazem: continuous telemetry (while hospitalized); signs and symptoms of heart failure every shift while hospitalized then at each healthcare encounter after discharge
Statins	GI discomfort, arthralgia, myalgia, musculoskeletal pain, hepatotoxicity	Liver function tests at baseline (prior to discharge) and if signs or symptoms of hepatotoxicity develop; creatinine kinase if severe myalgia or musculoskeletal symptoms occur; LDL-C at baseline, 4-12 weeks after initiation or dose adjustment, then every 3-12 months
Nonstatin therapies	Ezetimibe and combination: GI discomfort, arthralgia, myalgia, musculoskeletal pain	Simvastatin/ezetimibe: liver function tests at baseline (prior to discharge) and if signs or symptoms of hepatotoxicity develop; creatinine kinase if severe myalgia or musculoskeletal symptoms occur; LDL-C at baseline, 4-12 weeks after initiation or dose adjustment, then every 3-12 months
	PCSK9 inhibitors: injection site pain, hypersensitivity, nasopharyngitis	PCSK9 inhibitors: LDL-C at baseline and 4-8 weeks after initiation or dose adjustment; evaluation of injection site if injection site pain develops, signs and symptoms of hypersensitivity with each healthcare encounter
ACE inhibitors	Hypotension, hyperuricemia, hyperkalemia, worsening renal function, chronic cough, angioedema	Blood pressure every shift while hospitalized, 1-2 weeks after initiation or dose adjustment, then with each healthcare encounter; serum creatinine and potassium at baseline, 1-2 weeks after initiation, then every 6-12 months; signs and symptoms of angioedema or cough with each healthcare encounter
ARBs	Hypotension, hyperuricemia, hyperkalemia, worsening renal function	Blood pressure every shift while hospitalized, 1-2 weeks after initiation or dose adjustment, then with each healthcare encounter; serum creatinine and potassium at baseline, 1-2 weeks after initiation, then every 6-12 months
Aldosterone antagonist	Hyperkalemia, worsening renal function	Blood pressure every shift while hospitalized, 1-2 weeks after initiation or dose adjustment, then with each healthcare encounter; serum creatinine and potassium at baseline, after initiation or dose adjustment: at 3 days, 1 week, monthly for 3 months, then every 3 months

GI, gastrointestinal; Hct, hematocrit; Hgb, hemoglobin; ICH, intracranial hemorrhage; INR, international normalized ratio; LDL-C, low-density lipoprotein cholesterol; PCI, percutaneous coronary intervention; PCSK9, proprotein convertase subtilisin-kexin type 9.

[a]Clinical signs of bleeding include bloody stools, melena, hematuria, hematemesis, bruising, and oozing from arterial or venous puncture sites.

senior citizens.[117] Patients should be counseled on the risks and sites of potential bleeding and should be told to seek medical care immediately if significant bleeding is noticed. If bleeding occurs while on chronic therapy, the patient should be referred to the prescribing physician as the severity of the bleed and the timing since index event (and presence of stent placement) may influence supportive measures and cessation of therapy.

For long-term risk reduction, the focus centers on control of CAD risk factors and the appropriate use of and adherence to an evidence-based medication regimen known to reduce the risk of MACE. Lifestyle modifications should be reinforced during each healthcare encounter. Similarly, control of CAD risk factors should be assessed and interventions made to improve risk factor control, if necessary. Finally, it is important to reassess the evidence-based regimen to determine the need to either escalate (eg, add additional evidence-based ACS therapies or increase their doses) or de-escalate therapy (eg, consider discontinuation of $P2Y_{12}$ inhibitor after 12 months or β-blocker after 3 years in a post-MI patient with a normal LVEF).

Medication adherence must also be assessed during each healthcare encounter. Despite evidence to support mortality reduction with secondary prevention strategies, typically less than 50% of patients remain adherent at 1 year.[118] Because nonadherence with secondary prevention medications following ACS leads to poor CV outcomes, patients must receive thorough medication counseling (including counseling prior to hospital discharge) and be monitored for medication persistence.[1,2,104] Counseling should include assessments of health literacy level, barriers to adherence, access to medications, and understanding of instructions.[104] Additionally, patients and their caregivers should be provided written and verbal instructions about the purpose of each medication, changes to previous medication regimen, the optimal time to take each medication, new allergies or medication intolerances, need for a timely prescription fill after discharge, anticipated duration of therapy, consequences of nonadherence, common and/or serious adverse reactions that may develop, and drug-drug and drug-food interactions.[104] Early follow-up (within 6 weeks) after discharge has been associated with improved medication adherence and, for this reason, post-discharge follow-up is often scheduled within 1 to 2 weeks.[119]

CONCLUSION

For the majority of patients, the pathophysiology of ACS involves an acute disruption of an atherosclerotic plaque followed by platelet activation and aggregation leading to intracoronary thrombus formation. Myocardial ischemia ensues due to an acute imbalance between myocardial oxygen supply and demand and may lead to infarction depending on the severity and duration of thrombotic occlusion. Therefore, the acute pharmacotherapeutic management of ACS is focused on antiplatelet, anticoagulation, and anti-ischemic therapies. Appropriate selection of these agents depends upon patient presentation (eg, STEMI or NSTE-ACS), the decision for reperfusion (eg, PCI, fibrinolysis, or no reperfusion), and individual considerations for efficacy and safety associated with individual agents (eg, pharmacokinetic alterations, drug-drug interactions, contraindications). High-intensity statins should be initiated early and continued indefinitely for all patients with ACS without contraindications to lower LDL-C and stabilize atherosclerotic plaques. Long-term use of DAPT lowers the risk of MACE after ACS and maintains stent patency in patients who had intracoronary stent implantation during PCI. Neurohormonal blocking drugs such as β-blockers and inhibitors of the RAAS system are also associated with a lower risk of MACE and should be initiated prior to hospital discharge in appropriate patients. Each member of the healthcare team plays an important role in the patient care process for ACS, collecting and analyzing clinical information, collaborating in the development and implementation of the care plan, and evaluating therapeutic outcomes.

ABBREVIATIONS

ACC	American College of Cardiology
ACE	angiotensin-converting enzyme
ACS	acute coronary syndrome
ACT	activated clotting time
ADP	adenosine diphosphate
AHA	American Heart Association
aPTT	activated partial thromboplastin time
ARB	angiotensin receptor blocker
ASCVD	atherosclerotic cardiovascular disease
AT	antithrombin
CABG	coronary artery bypass grafting
CAD	coronary artery disease
CCB	calcium channel blocker
COX	cyclooxygenase
CrCl	creatinine clearance
cTn	cardiac troponin
CV	cardiovascular
CYP	cytochrome P450
DAPT	dual antiplatelet therapy
DHP	dihydropyridine
DM	diabetes mellitus
ECG	electrocardiogram
ED	emergency department
EMS	emergency medical services
ENT	equilibrative nucleoside transporter
GI	gastrointestinal
GP	glycoprotein
GRACE	Global Registry of Acute Coronary Events
HEART	History, ECG, age, risk factors, and troponin
HF	heart failure
HFrEF	heart failure with reduced ejection fraction
HIT	heparin-induced thrombocytopenia
HTN	hypertension
ICH	intracranial hemorrhage
IV	intravenous
LBBB	left bundle branch block
LDL-C	low-density lipoprotein cholesterol
LMWH	low-molecular-weight heparin
LVEF	left ventricular ejection fraction
MACE	major adverse cardiovascular events
MI	myocardial infarction
MONA	morphine, oxygen, nitroglycerin, aspirin
NSTE-ACS	non-ST-segment elevation acute coronary syndromes
NSTEMI	non-ST-segment elevation myocardial infarction
PAR	protease-activated receptor
PCI	percutaneous coronary intervention
PCSK9	proprotein convertase subtilisin-kexin type 9
RAAS	renin–angiotensin–aldosterone system
SCr	serum creatinine
SIHD	stable ischemic heart disease
SNS	sympathetic nervous system
STEMI	ST-segment-elevation myocardial infarction
SC	subcutaneous
TIMI	thrombolysis in myocardial infarction
UA	unstable angina

REFERENCES

1. O'Gara PT, Kushner FG, Ascheim DD, et al. 2013 ACCF/AHA guideline for the management of ST-elevation myocardial infarction: A report of the American College of Cardiology Foundation/American Heart Association Task Force on Practice Guidelines. *J Am Coll Cardiol.* 2013;61:e78–e140.
2. Amsterdam EA, Wenger NK, Brindis RG, et al. 2014 AHA/ACC guideline for the management of patients with non-ST-elevation acute coronary syndromes: A report of the American College of Cardiology/American Heart Association Task Force on Practice Guidelines. *J Am Coll Cardiol.* 2014;64:e139–e228.
3. Virani SS, Alonso A, Aparicio HJ, et al. Heart disease and stroke statistics—2021 update. *Circulation.* 2021;143:e254–e743. doi: 10.1161/cir.0000000000000950.
4. Chi GC, Kanter MH, Li BH, et al. Trends in acute myocardial infarction by race and ethnicity. *J Am Heart Assoc.* 2020;9:e013542. doi: 10.1161/jaha.119.013542.

5. Wellings J, Kostis JB, Sargsyan D, et al. Risk factors and trends in incidence of heart failure following acute myocardial infarction. *Am J Cardiol.* 2018;122:1–5. doi: 10.1016/j.amjcard.2018.03.005.
6. Jernberg T, Johanson P, Held C, et al. Association between adoption of evidence-based treatment and survival for patients with ST-elevation myocardial infarction. *JAMA.* 2011;305:1677–1684. doi: 10.1001/jama.2011.522.
7. Tickoo S, Bhardwaj A, Fonarow GC, Liang L, Bhatt DL, Cannon CP. Relation between hospital length of stay and quality of care in patients with acute coronary syndromes (from the American Heart Association's Get with the Guidelines—coronary artery disease data set). *Am J Cardiol.* 2016;117:201–205.
8. Sugiyama T, Hasegawa K, Kobayashi Y, Takahashi O, Fukui T, Tsugawa Y. Differential time trends of outcomes and costs of care for acute myocardial infarction hospitalizations by ST elevation and type of intervention in the United States, 2001–2011. *J Am Heart Assoc.* 2015;4:e001445.
9. Nicholson G, Gandra SR, Halbert RJ, Richhariya A, Nordyke RJ. Patient-level costs of major cardiovascular conditions: A review of the international literature. *Clinicoecon Outcomes Res.* 2016;8:495–506.
10. Thygesen K, Alpert JS, Jaffe AS, et al. Fourth universal definition of myocardial infarction (2018). *J Am Coll Cardiol.* 2018. doi: 10.1016/j.jacc.2018.08.1038.
11. Ford TJ, Berry C, De Bruyne B, et al. Physiological predictors of acute coronary syndromes: Emerging insights from the plaque to the vulnerable patient. *JACC Cardiovasc Interv.* 2017;10:2539–2547.
12. Crea F, Liuzzo G. Pathogenesis of acute coronary syndromes. *J Am Coll Cardiol.* 2013;61:1–11.
13. Libby P. Mechanisms of acute coronary syndromes and their implications for therapy. *N Engl J Med.* 2013;368:2004–2013.
14. Bentzon JF, Otsuka F, Virmani R, Falk E. Mechanisms of plaque formation and rupture. *Circ Res.* 2014;114:1852–1866.
15. Libby P, Tabas I, Fredman G, Fisher EA. Inflammation and its resolution as determinants of acute coronary syndromes. *Circ Res.* 2014;114:1867–1879.
16. Crea F, Libby P. Acute coronary syndromes: The way forward from mechanisms to precision treatment. *Circulation.* 2017;136:1155–1166.
17. Fuster V, Kovacic JC. Acute coronary syndromes: Pathology, diagnosis, genetics, prevention, and treatment. *Circ Res.* 2014;114:1847–1851.
18. Furie B, Furie BC. Mechanisms of thrombus formation. *N Engl J Med.* 2008;359:938–949.
19. Brunton LL, Hilal-Dandan R, Knollmann BC. *Goodman & Gilman's: The Pharmacological Basis of Therapeutics.* 13th ed. New York, NY: McGraw Hill; 2018.
20. Gabriel-Costa D. The pathophysiology of myocardial infarction-induced heart failure. *Pathophysiology.* 2018;25:277–284.
21. Reed GW, Rossi JE, Cannon CP. Acute myocardial infarction. *Lancet.* 2017;389:197–210.
22. Morrow DA, Antman EM, Charlesworth A, et al. TIMI risk score for ST-elevation myocardial infarction: A convenient, bedside, clinical score for risk assessment at presentation: An intravenous nPA for treatment of infarcting myocardium early II trial substudy. *Circulation.* 2000;102:2031–2037.
23. Antman EM, Cohen M, Bernink PJ, et al. The TIMI risk score for unstable angina/non-ST elevation MI: A method for prognostication and therapeutic decision making. *JAMA.* 2000;284:835–842.
24. Granger CB, Goldberg RJ, Dabbous O, et al. Predictors of hospital mortality in the global registry of acute coronary events. *Arch Intern Med.* 2003;163:2345–2353.
25. Six AJ, Backus BE, Kelder JC. Chest pain in the emergency room: Value of the HEART score. *Neth Heart J.* 2008;16:191–196.
26. Gulati Martha, Levy Phillip D, Mukherjee Debabrata, et al. 2021 AHA/ACC/ASE/CHEST/SAEM/SCCT/SCMR Guideline for the evaluation and diagnosis of chest pain: A report of the American College of Cardiology/American Heart Association Joint Committee on Clinical Practice Guidelines. *Circulation.* 2021;144:e368–e454. 10.1161/cir.0000000000001029.
27. Poldervaart JM, Langedijk M, Backus BE, et al. Comparison of the GRACE, HEART and TIMI score to predict major adverse cardiac events in chest pain patients at the emergency department. *Int J Cardiol.* 2017;227:656–661.
28. Kline KP, Conti CR, Winchester DE. Historical perspective and contemporary management of acute coronary syndromes: From MONA to THROMBINS2. *Postgrad Med.* 2015;127:855–862.
29. Smith SC Jr, Benjamin EJ, Bonow RO, et al. AHA/ACCF secondary prevention and risk reduction therapy for patients with coronary and other atherosclerotic vascular disease: 2011 update: A guideline from the American Heart Association and American College of Cardiology Foundation endorsed by the World Heart Federation and the Preventive Cardiovascular Nurses Association. *J Am Coll Cardiol.* 2011;58:2432–2446.
30. GISSI-3: Effects of lisinopril and transdermal glyceryl trinitrate singly and together on 6-week mortality and ventricular function after acute myocardial infarction. Gruppo Italiano per lo Studio della Sopravvivenza nell'infarto Miocardico. *Lancet.* 1994;343:1115–1122.
31. ISIS-4: A randomised factorial trial assessing early oral captopril, oral mononitrate, and intravenous magnesium sulphate in 58,050 patients with suspected acute myocardial infarction. ISIS-4 (Fourth International Study of Infarct Survival) Collaborative Group. *Lancet.* 1995;345:669–685.
32. Siddiqi N, Neil C, Bruce M, et al. Intravenous sodium nitrite in acute ST-elevation myocardial infarction: A randomized controlled trial (NIAMI). *Eur Heart J.* 2014;35:1255–1262.
33. McCord J, Jneid H, Hollander JE, et al. Management of cocaine-associated chest pain and myocardial infarction: A scientific statement from the American Heart Association Acute Cardiac Care Committee of the Council on Clinical Cardiology. *Circulation.* 2008;117:1897–1907.
34. Ventimiglia E, Capogrosso P, Montorsi F, Salonia A. The safety of phosphodiesterase type 5 inhibitors for erectile dysfunction. *Expert Opin Drug Saf.* 2016;15:141–152.
35. Duarte GS, Nunes-Ferreira A, Rodrigues FB, et al. Morphine in acute coronary syndrome: Systematic review and meta-analysis. *BMJ Open* 2019;9(3):e025232. 10.1136/bmjopen-2018-025232.
36. Kubica J, Kubica A, Jilma B, et al. Impact of morphine on antiplatelet effects of oral P2Y12 receptor inhibitors. *Int J Cardiol.* 2016;215:201–208.
37. Cabello JB, Burls A, Emparanza JI, Bayliss SE, Quinn T. Oxygen therapy for acute myocardial infarction. *Cochrane Database Syst Rev.* 2016;12:CD007160.
38. Bangalore S, Makani H, Radford M, et al. Clinical outcomes with beta-blockers for myocardial infarction: A meta-analysis of randomized trials. *Am J Med.* 2014;127:939–953.
39. Freemantle N, Cleland J, Young P, Mason J, Harrison J. Beta blockade after myocardial infarction: Systematic review and meta regression analysis. *BMJ.* 1999;318:1730–1737.
40. Chen ZM, Pan HC, Chen YP, et al. Early intravenous then oral metoprolol in 45,852 patients with acute myocardial infarction: Randomised placebo-controlled trial. *Lancet.* 2005;366:1622–1632.
41. Park JJ, Kim SH, Kang SH, et al. Effect of beta-blockers beyond 3 years after acute myocardial infarction. *J Am Heart Assoc.* 2018;(7):e007567.
42. Held PH, Yusuf S, Furberg CD. Calcium channel blockers in acute myocardial infarction and unstable angina: An overview. *BMJ.* 1989;299:1187–1192.
43. Dargie HJ. Effect of carvedilol on outcome after myocardial infarction in patients with left-ventricular dysfunction: The CAPRICORN randomised trial. *Lancet.* 2001;357:1385–1390.
44. Agrawal PR, Scarabelli TM, Saravolatz L, et al. Current strategies in the evaluation and management of cocaine-induced chest pain. *Cardiol Rev.* 2015;23:303–311.
45. Furberg CD, Psaty BM, Meyer JV. Nifedipine. Dose-related increase in mortality in patients with coronary heart disease. *Circulation.* 1995;92:1326–1331.
46. Bagai A, Dangas GD, Stone GW, Granger CB. Reperfusion strategies in acute coronary syndromes. *Circ Res.* 2014;114:1918–1928.
47. Gersh BJ, Stone GW, White HD, Holmes DR Jr. Pharmacological facilitation of primary percutaneous coronary intervention for acute myocardial infarction: Is the slope of the curve the shape of the future? *JAMA.* 2005;293:979–986.
48. Pinto DS, Frederick PD, Chakrabarti AK, et al. Benefit of transferring ST-segment-elevation myocardial infarction patients for percutaneous coronary intervention compared with administration of onsite fibrinolytic declines as delays increase. *Circulation.* 2011;124:2512–2521.
49. Bagai A, Jollis JG, Dauerman HL, et al. Emergency department bypass for ST-segment-elevation myocardial infarction patients identified with a prehospital electrocardiogram: A report from the American Heart Association Mission: Lifeline program. *Circulation.* 2013;128:352–359.
50. Ting HH, Krumholz HM, Bradley EH, et al. Implementation and integration of prehospital ECGs into systems of care for acute coronary syndrome: A scientific statement from the American Heart Association Interdisciplinary Council on Quality of Care and Outcomes Research, Emergency Cardiovascular Care Committee, Council on Cardiovascular Nursing, and Council on Clinical Cardiology. *Circulation.* 2008;118:1066–1079.

51. McNamara RL, Wang Y, Herrin J, et al. Effect of door-to-balloon time on mortality in patients with ST-segment elevation myocardial infarction. *J Am Coll Cardiol.* 2006;47:2180–2186.
52. Gibson CM, Pride YB, Frederick PD, et al. Trends in reperfusion strategies, door-to-needle and door-to-balloon times, and in-hospital mortality among patients with ST-segment elevation myocardial infarction enrolled in the National Registry of Myocardial Infarction from 1990 to 2006. *Am Heart J.* 2008;156:1035–1044.
53. Langabeer JR, Henry TD, Kereiakes DJ, et al Growth in percutaneous coronary intervention capacity relative to population and disease prevalence. *J Am Heart Assoc.* 2013;2:e000370.
54. Bonnefoy E, Lapostolle F, Leizorovicz A, et al. Primary angioplasty versus prehospital fibrinolysis in acute myocardial infarction: A randomised study. *Lancet.* 2002;360:825–829.
55. Jneid H, Addison D, Bhatt DL, et al. 2017 AHA/ACC clinical performance and quality measures for adults with ST-elevation and non-ST-elevation myocardial infarction: A report of the American College of Cardiology/American Heart Association Task Force on Performance Measures. *Circ Cardiovasc Qual Outcomes.* 2017;70(16):2048–2090.
56. Dasari TW, Roe MT, Chen AY, et al. Impact of time of presentation on process performance and outcomes in ST-segment-elevation myocardial infarction: A report from the American Heart Association: Mission Lifeline program. *Circ Cardiovasc Qual Outcomes.* 2014;7:656–663.
57. Ibanez B, James S, Agewall S, et al. 2017 ESC Guidelines for the management of acute myocardial infarction in patients presenting with ST-segment elevation: The Task Force for the management of acute myocardial infarction in patients presenting with ST-segment elevation of the European Society of Cardiology (ESC). *Eur Heart J.* 2018;39:119–177.
58. Jinatongthai P, Kongwatcharapong J, Foo CY, et al. Comparative efficacy and safety of reperfusion therapy with fibrinolytic agents in patients with ST-segment elevation myocardial infarction: A systematic review and network meta-analysis. *Lancet.* 2017;390:747–759.
59. Armstrong PW, Gershlick AH, Goldstein P, et al. Fibrinolysis or primary PCI in ST-segment elevation myocardial infarction. *N Engl J Med.* 2013;368:1379–1387.
60. Levine GN, Bates ER, Blankenship JC, et al. 2011 ACCF/AHA/SCAI guideline for percutaneous coronary intervention. A report of the American College of Cardiology Foundation/American Heart Association Task Force on Practice Guidelines and the Society for Cardiovascular Angiography and Interventions. *J Am Coll Cardiol.* 2011;58:e44–e122.
61. Dobesh PP, Varnado S, Doyle M. Antiplatelet agents in cardiology: A report on aspirin, clopidogrel, prasugrel, and ticagrelor. *Curr Pharm Des.* 2016;22:1918–1932.
62. Current-Oasis Investigators. Dose comparisons of clopidogrel and aspirin in acute coronary syndromes. *N Engl J Med.* 2010;363:930–942.
63. Akers WS, Oh JJ, Oestreich JH, Ferraris S, Wethington M, Steinhubl SR. Pharmacokinetics and pharmacodynamics of a bolus and infusion of cangrelor: A direct, parenteral P2Y12 receptor antagonist. *J Clin Pharmacol.* 2010;50:27–35.
64. Yusuf S, Zhao F, Mehta SR, et al. Effects of clopidogrel in addition to aspirin in patients with acute coronary syndromes without ST-segment elevation. *N Engl J Med.* 2001;345:494–502.
65. Wiviott SD, Braunwald E, McCabe CH, et al. Prasugrel versus clopidogrel in patients with acute coronary syndromes. *N Engl J Med.* 2007;357:2001–2015.
66. Montalescot G, Bolognese L, Dudek D, et al. Pretreatment with prasugrel in non–ST-segment elevation acute coronary syndromes. *N Engl J Med.* 2013;369:999–1010. doi: 10.1056/nejmoa1308075.
67. Tarantini G, Mojoli M, Varbella F, et al. Timing of oral P2Y12 inhibitor administration in patients with non-ST-segment elevation acute coronary syndrome. *J Am Coll Cardiol.* 2020;76:2450–2459. doi: 10.1016/j.jacc.2020.08.053.
68. Tantry US, Bonello L, Aradi D, et al. Consensus and update on the definition of on-treatment platelet reactivity to adenosine diphosphate associated with ischemia and bleeding. *J Am Coll Cardiol.* 2013;62:2261–2273.
69. Pereira NL, Rihal C, Lennon R, et al. Effect of CYP2C19 genotype on ischemic outcomes during oral P2Y12 inhibitor therapy. *J Am Coll Cardiol Intv.* 2021;14:739–750. doi: 10.1016/j.jcin.2021.01.024.
70. Sibbing D, Aradi D, Alexopoulos D, et al. Updated expert consensus statement on platelet function and genetic testing for guiding $P2Y_{12}$ receptor inhibitor treatment percutaneous coronary intervention. *JACC Cardiovasc Interv.* 2019;12:1521–1537.
71. Chen ZM, Jiang LX, Chen YP, et al. Addition of clopidogrel to aspirin in 45,852 patients with acute myocardial infarction: Randomised placebo-controlled trial. *Lancet.* 2005;366:1607–1621.
72. Sabatine MS, Cannon CP, Gibson CM, et al. Addition of clopidogrel to aspirin and fibrinolytic therapy for myocardial infarction with ST-segment elevation. *N Engl J Med.* 2005;352:1179–1189.
73. Roe MT, Armstrong PW, Fox KA, et al. Prasugrel versus clopidogrel for acute coronary syndromes without revascularization. *N Engl J Med.* 2012;367:1297–1309.
74. Dobesh PP, Oestreich JH. Ticagrelor: Pharmacokinetics, pharmacodynamics, clinical efficacy, and safety. *Pharmacotherapy.* 2014;34:1077–1090.
75. Wallentin L, Becker RC, Budaj A, et al. Ticagrelor versus clopidogrel in patients with acute coronary syndromes. *N Engl J Med.* 2009;361:1045–1057.
76. Mahaffey KW, Wojdyla DM, Carroll K, et al. Ticagrelor compared with clopidogrel by geographic region in the Platelet Inhibition and Patient Outcomes (PLATO) trial. *Circulation.* 2011;124:544–554.
77. Gimbel M, Qaderdan K, Willemsen L, et al. Clopidogrel versus ticagrelor or prasugrel in patients aged 70 years or older with non-ST-elevation acute coronary syndrome (POPular AGE): The randomised, open-label, non-inferiority trial. *Lancet.* 2020;395:1374–1381. doi: 10.1016/s0140-6736(20)30325-1.
78. Szummer K, Montez-Rath ME, Alfredsson J, et al. Comparison between ticagrelor and clopidogrel in elderly patients with an acute coronary syndrome. *Circulation.* 2020;142:1700–1708. doi: 10.1161/circulationaha.120.050645.
79. Schüpke S, Neumann FJ, Menichelli M, et al. Ticagrelor or prasugrel in patients with acute coronary syndromes. *N Engl J Med.* 2019;381:1524–1534.
80. Berwanger O, Nicolau JC, Carvalho AC, et al. Ticagrelor vs clopidogrel after fibrinolytic therapy in patients with ST-elevation myocardial infarction: A randomized clinical trial. *JAMA Cardiol.* 2018;3:391–399.
81. Bhatt DL, Stone GW, Mahaffey KW, et al. Effect of platelet inhibition with cangrelor during PCI on ischemic events. *N Engl J Med.* 2013;368:1303–1313.
82. Steinhubl SR, Oh JJ, Oestreich JH, Ferraris S, Charnigo R, Akers WS. Transitioning patients from cangrelor to clopidogrel: Pharmacodynamic evidence of a competitive effect. *Thromb Res.* 2008;121:527–534.
83. Dovlatova NL, Jakubowski JA, Sugidachi A, Heptinstall S. The reversible P2Y antagonist cangrelor influences the ability of the active metabolites of clopidogrel and prasugrel to produce irreversible inhibition of platelet function. *J Thromb Haemost.* 2008;6:1153–1159.
84. Angiolillo DJ, Rollini F, Storey RF, et al. International expert consensus on switching platelet P2Y12 receptor-inhibiting therapies. *Circulation.* 2017;136:1955–1975.
85. Linkins LA, Dans AL, Moores LK, et al. Treatment and prevention of heparin-induced thrombocytopenia: Antithrombotic Therapy and Prevention of Thrombosis, 9th ed: American College of Chest Physicians Evidence-Based Clinical Practice Guidelines. *Chest.* 2012;141:e495S–e530S.
86. Kastrati A, Mehilli J, Neumann FJ, et al. Abciximab in patients with acute coronary syndromes undergoing percutaneous coronary intervention after clopidogrel pretreatment: The ISAR-REACT 2 randomized trial. *JAMA.* 2006;295:1531–1538.
87. Stone GW, McLaurin BT, Cox DA, et al. Bivalirudin for patients with acute coronary syndromes. *N Engl J Med.* 2006;355:2203–2216.
88. Stone GW, Witzenbichler B, Guagliumi G, et al. Bivalirudin during primary PCI in acute myocardial infarction. *N Engl J Med.* 2008;358:2218–2230.
89. Garcia DA, Baglin TP, Weitz JI, Samama MM. Parenteral anticoagulants: Antithrombotic Therapy and Prevention of Thrombosis, 9th ed: American College of Chest Physicians Evidence-Based Clinical Practice Guidelines. *Chest.* 2012;141:e24S–e43S.
90. Oler A, Whooley MA, Oler J, Grady D. Adding heparin to aspirin reduces the incidence of myocardial infarction and death in patients with unstable angina. A meta-analysis. *JAMA.* 1996;276:811–815.
91. Antman EM, Cohen M, Radley D, et al. Assessment of the treatment effect of enoxaparin for unstable angina/non-Q-wave myocardial infarction. TIMI 11B-ESSENCE meta-analysis. *Circulation.* 1999;100:1602–1608.
92. Ferguson JJ, Califf RM, Antman EM, et al. Enoxaparin vs unfractionated heparin in high-risk patients with non-ST-segment elevation acute coronary syndromes managed with an intended early invasive strategy: Primary results of the SYNERGY randomized trial. *JAMA.* 2004;292:45–54.

93. Antman EM, Morrow DA, McCabe CH, et al. Enoxaparin versus unfractionated heparin with fibrinolysis for ST-elevation myocardial infarction. *N Engl J Med.* 2006;354:1477–1488.
94. Navarese EP, De Luca G, Castriota F, et al. Low-molecular-weight heparins vs. unfractionated heparin in the setting of percutaneous coronary intervention for ST-elevation myocardial infarction: A meta-analysis. *J Thromb Haemost.* 2011;9:1902–1915.
95. Turpie AG, Lensing AW, Fuji T, Boyle DA. Pharmacokinetic and clinical data supporting the use of fondaparinux 1.5 mg once daily in the prevention of venous thromboembolism in renally impaired patients. *Blood Coagul Fibrinolysis.* 2009;20:114–121.
96. Yusuf S, Mehta SR, Chrolavicius S, et al. Effects of fondaparinux on mortality and reinfarction in patients with acute ST-segment elevation myocardial infarction: The OASIS-6 randomized trial. *JAMA.* 2006;295:1519–1530.
97. Fifth Organization to Assess Strategies in Acute Ischemic Syndromes I, Yusuf S, Mehta SR, et al. Comparison of fondaparinux and enoxaparin in acute coronary syndromes. *N Engl J Med.* 2006;354:1464–1476.
98. Kastrati A, Neumann FJ, Mehilli J, et al. Bivalirudin versus unfractionated heparin during percutaneous coronary intervention. *N Engl J Med.* 2008;359:688–696.
99. Schulz S, Richardt G, Laugwitz KL, et al. Prasugrel plus bivalirudin vs. clopidogrel plus heparin in patients with ST-segment elevation myocardial infarction. *Eur Heart J.* 2014;35:2285–2294.
100. Shahzad A, Kemp I, Mars C, et al. Unfractionated heparin versus bivalirudin in primary percutaneous coronary intervention (HEAT-PPCI): An open-label, single centre, randomised controlled trial. *Lancet.* 2014;384:1849–1858.
101. Grundy SM, Stone NJ, Bailey AL, et al. 2018 AHA/ACC/AACVPR/AAPA/ABC/ACPM/ADA/AGS/APhA/ASPC/NLA/PCNA Guideline on the management of blood cholesterol: A report of the American College of Cardiology/American Heart Association Task Force on Clinical Practice Guidelines. *J Am Coll Cardiol.* 2018. https://doi.org/10.1016/j.jacc.2018.11.003.
102. Schwartz GG, Steg PG, Szarek M, et al. Alirocumab and cardiovascular outcomes after acute coronary syndrome. *N Engl J Med.* 2018;379:2097–2107.
103. Sabatine MS, Giugliano RP, Keech AC, et al. Evolocumab and clinical outcomes in patients with cardiovascular disease. *N Engl J Med.* 2017;376:1713–1722. doi: 10.1056/nejmoa1615664.
104. Wiggins BS, Rodgers JE, DiDomenico RJ, Cook AM, Page RL II. Discharge counseling for patients with heart failure or myocardial infarction: A best practices model developed by members of the American College of Clinical Pharmacy's Cardiology Practice and Research Network based on the Hospital to Home (H2H) Initiative. *Pharmacotherapy.* 2013;33:558–580.
105. Frøbert O, Götberg M, Erlinge D, et al. Influenza vaccination after myocardial infarction: A randomized, double-blind, placebo-controlled, multicenter trial. *Circulation.* 2021;144(18):1476–1484. doi: 10.1161/circulationaha.121.057042.
106. Udell JA, Zawi R, Bhatt DL, et al. Association between influenza vaccination and cardiovascular outcomes in high-risk patients. *JAMA.* 2013;310:1711–1720. doi: 10.1001/jama.2013.279206.
107. Levine GN, Bates ER, Bittl JA, et al. 2016 ACC/AHA Guideline focused update on duration of dual antiplatelet therapy in patients with coronary artery disease: A report of the American College of Cardiology/American Heart Association Task Force on Clinical Practice Guidelines. *J Am Coll Cardiol.* 2016;68:1082–1115.
108. Yeh RW, Secemsky EA, Kereiakes DJ, et al. Development and validation of a prediction rule for benefit and harm of dual antiplatelet therapy beyond 1 year after percutaneous coronary intervention. *JAMA.* 2016;315:1735–1749.
109. Bonaca MP, Bhatt DL, Cohen M, et al. Long-term use of ticagrelor in patients with prior myocardial infarction. *N Engl J Med.* 2015;372:1791–1800.
110. Hulten E, Jackson JL, Douglas K, George S, Villines TC. The effect of early, intensive statin therapy on acute coronary syndrome: A meta-analysis of randomized controlled trials. *Arch Intern Med.* 2006;166:1814–1821.
111. Cannon CP, Blazing MA, Giugliano RP, et al. Ezetimibe added to statin therapy after acute coronary syndromes. *N Engl J Med.* 2015;372:2387–2397.
112. Bhatt DL, Briggs AH, Reed SD, et al. Cost-effectiveness of alirocumab in patients with acute coronary syndromes. *J Am Coll Cardiol.* 2020;75:2297–2308. doi:10.1016/j.jacc.2020.03.029.
113. Garg R, Yusuf S. Overview of randomized trials of angiotensin-converting enzyme inhibitors on mortality and morbidity in patients with heart failure. Collaborative Group on ACE Inhibitor Trials. *JAMA.* 1995;273:1450–1456.
114. Rodrigues EJ, Eisenberg MJ, Pilote L. Effects of early and late administration of angiotensin-converting enzyme inhibitors on mortality after myocardial infarction. *Am J Med.* 2003;115:473–479.
115. Lee VC, Rhew DC, Dylan M, Badamgarav E, Braunstein GD, Weingarten SR. Meta-analysis: Angiotensin-receptor blockers in chronic heart failure and high-risk acute myocardial infarction. *Ann Intern Med.* 2004;141:693–704.
116. Bossard M, Binbraik Y, Beygui F, et al. Mineralocorticoid receptor antagonists in patients with acute myocardial infarction: A systematic review and meta-analysis of randomized trials. *Am Heart J.* 2018;195:60–69.
117. Budnitz DS, Lovegrove MC, Shehab N, Richards CL. Emergency hospitalizations for adverse drug events in older Americans. *N Engl J Med.* 2011;365:2002–2012.
118. Kumbhani DJ, Steg PG, Cannon CP, et al. Adherence to secondary prevention medications and four-year outcomes in outpatients with atherosclerosis. *Am J Med.* 2013;126:693–700e1.
119. Faridi KF, Peterson ED, McCoy LA, Thomas L, Enriquez J, Wang TY. Timing of first postdischarge follow-up and medication adherence after acute myocardial infarction. *JAMA Cardiol.* 2016;1:147–155.
120. Lawton JS, Tamis-Holland JE, Bangalore S, et al. 2021 ACC/AHA/SCAI Guideline for Coronary Artery Revascularization: A Report of the American College of Cardiology/American Heart Association Joint Committee on Clinical Practice Guidelines. *Circulation.* 2022;145:e18–e114. doi: 10.1161/CIR.0000000000001038.

e35

Peripheral Arterial Disease

Kristin Watson and Sarah L. Anderson

KEY CONCEPTS

1 Peripheral arterial disease (PAD) is a form of atherosclerotic cardiovascular disease (ASCVD) that occurs in the peripheral arteries. Lower extremity PAD is the most common form of PAD.

2 Lower extremity PAD is associated with an increased risk of limb loss and death.

3 The most prevalent PAD risk factors are tobacco smoking, diabetes mellitus (DM), hypertension, and dyslipidemia. The risk of developing PAD increases with age.

4 Symptoms of lower extremity PAD may include cramping or discomfort in the affected lower extremity(ies). A significant portion of those with PAD will be asymptomatic. Signs of lower extremity PAD include, but are not limited to, diminished or absent pedal pulses, nonhealing wounds, brittle and hypertrophic toenails, and/or cool skin. The presence of signs and/or symptoms in those at risk for PAD should prompt further evaluation.

5 The ankle-brachial index (ABI) is the most common test used to diagnose lower extremity PAD. PAD is defined by an ABI score ≤0.9 for one or more of the pedal pulses (ie, dorsalis pedis, posterior tibial). A score >1.4 is indicative of noncompressible arteries which may be present in those with DM and/or chronic kidney disease (CKD).

6 ASCVD risk reduction is prudent to lower the risk of cardiovascular (CV) complications associated with PAD. This includes acheiving good glycemic and blood pressure (BP) control. A high-intensity statin is recommended to reduce the risk of CV and limb-related events. Smoking cessation has been shown to reduce the risk of limb loss and death.

7 Participation in a structured exercise training program has been shown to improve functional status and quality of life and to decrease lower extremity symptoms.

8 Revascularization surgery is a potential therapeutic option for patients who have persistent lower extremity PAD symptoms despite pharmacological therapy, exercise, and smoking cessation.

9 Low-dose aspirin or clopidogrel is recommended for patients with symptomatic lower extremity PAD to lower the risk of CV events and death.

10 An antithrombotic regimen should be prescribed after revascularization surgery to lower the risk of CV events and limb-related events. Options include aspirin or clopidogrel monotherapy, dual antiplatelet therapy with aspirin and clopidogrel, or rivaroxaban 2.5 mg twice daily combined with low-dose aspirin.

11 Cilostazol can be considered in those with lower extremity PAD symptoms despite other pharmacological therapy, exercise, and smoking cessation. This agent is not to be used in those with heart failure due to an increased risk of death.

BEYOND THE BOOK

Readers are encouraged to watch the following videos:

- Overview of the physical examination for peripheral arterial disease (PAD): https://youtu.be/sJ6YkxQeAbo (Duration: 10:08 minutes)
- Overview of Surgical Approaches for Peripheral Arterial Disease (PAD) https://www.youtube.com/watch?v=Y1WK6p0l80A&ab_channel=ColumbiaUniversityDepartmentofSurgery (Duration: 5:38 minutes)

INTRODUCTION

1 Peripheral arterial disease (PAD) is characterized by atherosclerosis of the peripheral arteries. Lower extremity PAD specifically refers to atherosclerotic disease from the aortoiliac segments to the pedal arteries.[1] While PAD can occur in several peripheral arteries, this chapter will focus predominantly on the treatment of lower extremity PAD because it is most common. The atherosclerotic process leads to the accumulation of plaque material within the arterial wall, narrowing the lumen and reducing blood flow to the lower extremities. Risk factors for PAD are similar to those for atherosclerosis in other parts of the body and include age ≥65 years old, tobacco smoking, diabetes mellitus (DM), hypertension (HTN), and dyslipidemia.[2,3] Presence of PAD is associated with a high risk of morbidity and mortality; those with PAD have a threefold increased risk of all-cause mortality compared to those without the disease.[2,3] PAD is a marker for atherosclerotic cardiovascular disease (ASCVD) that requires multiple interventions aimed at lowering risk.[4] The treatment of lower extremity PAD focuses on minimizing and managing risk factors, alleviating symptoms, and reducing cardiovascular disease (CVD) progression through nonpharmacologic and pharmacologic therapy.[3,4]

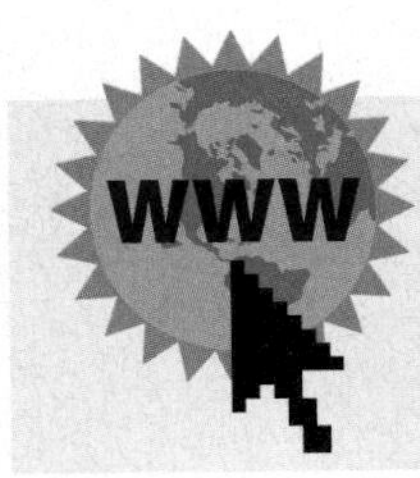

The complete chapter, learning objectives, and other resources can be found at **www.pharmacotherapyonline.com.**

36

Chronic Heart Failure

Robert B. Parker and Jo E. Rodgers

KEY CONCEPTS

1 Heart failure (HF) is a clinical syndrome associated with symptoms signs due to abnormalities in cardiac structure and/or function substantiated by the presence of increased natriuretic peptide plasma concentrations or objective evidence of pulmonary or systemic congestion of cardiogenic origin. The left ventricular ejection fraction (LVEF) is used to classify patients into four different types of HF, the two primary classifications being heart failure with reduced ejection fraction (HFrEF) or heart failure with preserved ejection fraction (HFpEF). Patients with HFrEF or HFpEF commonly present with signs and symptoms of fluid overload.

2 With HFpEF, systolic function is preserved, but the heart does not relax nor fill sufficiently resulting in compromised diastolic function. Despite the activation of similar neurohormonal systems as HFrEF, patients with HFpEF are often treated differently than those with HFrEF. Most of the pharmacotherapies known to benefit patients with HFrEF have been less beneficial in HFpEF. Targeting the underlying cause, most commonly uncontrolled hypertension, has been the primary strategy for managing patient with HFpEF. However, recent trials have identified new therapies that benefit patients with HFpEF.

3 In HFrEF, systolic dysfunction results in a decline in cardiac output leading to the activation of a number of neurohormonal compensatory responses that attempt to maintain adequate cardiac output. These responses include activation of the sympathetic nervous system (SNS) and the renin-angiotensin-aldosterone system (RAAS) and other systems. These compensatory mechanisms play an important role in ventricular remodeling and contribute to the progression of HF. Importantly, pharmacotherapy targeted at antagonizing this neurohormonal activation slows the progression of HFrEF and improves survival.

4 Most patients with HFrEF should be routinely treated with guideline-directed medical therapy (GDMT)—medications known to reduce mortality in these patients. GDMT includes four medication classes: an angiotensin receptor II receptor blocker/neprilysin inhibitor (ARNI) or angiotensin-converting enzyme (ACE) inhibitor or angiotensin II receptor blocker (ARB), an evidence-based β-blocker, an aldosterone antagonist, and a sodium-glucose cotransporter-2 (SGLT2) inhibitor. In patients with HFrEF, GDMT dosing should be titrated to achieve target doses known to be effective in randomized clinical trials. Patients with HFpEF may benefit from an ARNI and SGLT2 inhibitor.

5 The ARNI, sacubitril/valsartan, is approved to treat patients with HFrEF and many with HFpEF. In patients with HFrEF, ARNI is preferred over either ACE inhibitors or ARBs to improve survival, slow disease progression, reduce hospitalizations, and improve quality of life. Patients receiving ACE inhibitors or ARBs can be switched to ARNI or ARNI can be used as initial treatment in patients with newly detected HFrEF without previous exposure to ACE inhibitors or ARBs. The doses for these agents should be targeted at those shown in clinical trials to improve survival.

6 The β-blockers carvedilol, metoprolol succinate, and bisoprolol prolong survival, decrease hospitalizations, reduce the need for transplantation, and promote "reverse remodeling" of the left ventricle. These agents are recommended for all patients with HFrEF unless contraindicated. Therapy must be instituted at low doses, with slow upward titration to the target dose.

7 The aldosterone antagonists prolong survival and decrease hospitalizations in patients with HFrEF. These agents may be used provided that potassium and renal function can be carefully monitored. The aldosterone antagonists may be considered to reduce the risk of hospitalization in patients with HFpEF.

8 The SGLT2 inhibitors dapagliflozin or empagliflozin reduce the risk of cardiovascular death, hospitalization, and worsening HF in patients with HFrEF. In addition, empagliflozin reduces the composite outcome of cardiovascular death or HF hospitalization in patients with HFpEF. In both HFrEF and HFpEF, these benefits were demonstrated in patients with and without type 2 diabetes. SGLT2 inhibitors require assessment of renal function prior to initiation.

9 Although chronic loop diuretic therapy frequently is used in patients with HFrEF or HFpEF, it is not mandatory. Diuretic therapy is required only in those patients with peripheral edema and/or pulmonary congestion. Many patients will need continued diuretic therapy to maintain euvolemia after fluid overload is resolved.

10 The combination of hydralazine and nitrates improves the composite endpoint of mortality, hospitalizations for HF, and quality of life in Black patients receiving GDMT for HFrEF. Hydralazine and nitrates should be used in Black patients with persistent symptoms despite GDMT. Hydralazine and a nitrate might be reasonable in patients unable to tolerate either an ACE inhibitor or ARB because of renal insufficiency, hyperkalemia, or possibly hypotension.

11 Other therapies including digoxin, ivabradine, and vericiguat may be used in select patients with HFrEF to improve symptoms or reduce the risk of hospitalization.

BEYOND THE BOOK

Watch the video by Osmosis regarding congestive heart failure (CHF)—systolic, diastolic, left side, right side, and symptoms. This video provides an overview of the pathophysiology of heart failure due to both systolic and diastolic dysfunction. It also explains how heart failure symptoms relate to the underlying pathophysiology. A thorough understanding of heart failure pathophysiology and symptoms is key for students to learn how pharmacotherapy affects symptoms and improves overall outcomes. This will assist students in understanding the COLLECT and ASSESS steps in the patient care process.

INTRODUCTION

1 Heart failure (HF) is a clinical syndrome associated with symptoms and/or signs due to abnormalities in cardiac structure and/or function substantiated by the presence of increased natriuretic peptide plasma concentrations or objective evidence of pulmonary or systemic congestion of cardiogenic origin.[1] HF is the final common pathway for numerous cardiac disorders including those affecting the pericardium, heart valves, and myocardium. HF may be caused by an abnormality that affects cardiac systolic function, diastolic function, or both. Making the distinction is important because the treatment of HF may be quite different depending on whether the predominant mechanism of the disorder is systolic (ie, reduced left ventricular ejection fraction [LVEF]), now referred to as heart failure with reduced ejection fraction (HFrEF) or diastolic dysfunction (HF with normal LVEF, termed heart failure with preserved ejection fraction, HFpEF). Approximately 50% of patients with HF have HFpEF with disturbances in relaxation (lusitropic) properties of the heart or diastolic dysfunction.[2] However, regardless of the etiology of HF, the principal clinical manifestations (fatigue, dyspnea, and often volume overload) are similar and appear to be independent of the initial cause. This chapter focuses on the treatment of patients with chronic HFrEF and HFpEF. Chapter 37, "Acute Decompensated Heart Failure," discusses the treatment of acute decompensated HF.

EPIDEMIOLOGY

HF is an epidemic public health problem in the United States.[2] Approximately 6 million Americans have HF with 1,000,000 new cases diagnosed each year.[2] Unlike most other cardiovascular diseases, the incidence and prevalence of HF are increasing and are expected to continue to increase over the next few decades as the population ages. A large majority of patients with HF are elderly, with multiple comorbid conditions that influence morbidity and mortality.[2] Improved survival from the treatment of comorbidities such as hypertension and coronary artery disease as well as the more widespread use of device therapy including implantable cardioverter-defibrillators and cardiac resynchronization therapy are likely contributors to the increased incidence and prevalence of HF.[2,3] Annual hospital discharges for HF are approximately 800,000, and HF is a common hospital discharge diagnosis in individuals over age 65 years.[2] The disorder also has a tremendous economic impact, with this expected to increase markedly as the baby-boom generation ages. The annual expenditures for HF were over $30 billion, with estimates approaching $70 billion by 2030.[2] Thus, HF is a major medical problem, with a substantial economic impact that is expected to become even more significant as the population ages.

Marked racial and ethnic disparities in the epidemiology and clinical outcomes of HF exist.[2,4] Black patients are at the highest risk of developing and dying from HF (HFrEF or HFpEF) and are hospitalized at higher rates than White patients.[2,4] The reasons for these differences are multifactorial and represent a complex mix of higher prevalence of cardiovascular risk factors (hypertension, diabetes, obesity, chronic kidney disease), genetic susceptibility, access to care, socioeconomic factors and other social determinants of health, and implicit biases in healthcare providers and systems.[4]

Despite prodigious advances in our understanding of the etiology, pathophysiology, and pharmacotherapy of HF, the prognosis for patients with this disorder remains grim. Although the mortality rates have declined over the last 50 years, the overall 5-year survival remains approximately 42% for all patients with a diagnosis of HF, with mortality increasing with symptom severity.[2] Death is classified as sudden in about 40% of patients, implicating serious ventricular arrhythmias as the underlying cause. Factors affecting the prognosis of patients with HF include, but are not limited to, age, gender, LVEF, renal function, natriuretic peptide plasma concentrations, diabetes, metabolic syndrome, the extent of underlying coronary artery disease, blood pressure (BP), HF etiology, and medical or device therapies.[2] Models incorporating these and other factors enable clinicians to develop reliable estimates of an individual patient's prognosis.[5-7]

CLASSIFICATION AND ETIOLOGY

1 The LVEF is used to classify patients with HF as it identifies specific groups in which guideline-directed medical therapy (GDMT) improves key clinical outcomes such as mortality, hospitalization, and symptoms. Four classifications of HF are proposed: (1) HFrEF; (2) HF with mildly reduced ejection fraction (HFmrEF); (3) HFpEF; and (4) HF with improved EF (HFimpEF) (Table 36-1).[1]

HF can result from any disorder that affects the ability of the heart to contract (systolic function) and/or relax (diastolic dysfunction); common causes of HF are shown in Table 36-2.[8] HFrEF is

TABLE 36-1 Classification of Heart Failure According to Left Ventricular Ejection Fraction

HF with reduced EF (HFrEF)	HF with LVEF <40% (0.4)
HF with mildly reduced EF (HFmrEF)	HF with LVEF 41%-49% (0.41-0.49)
HF with preserved EF (HFpEF)	HF with LVEF ≥50% (0.5)
HF with improved EF (HFimpEF)	HF with baseline LVEF <40% (0.4), a >10 point increase from baseline LVEF, and a second measurement of LVEF >40% (0.4)

HF, heart failure; LVEF, left ventricular ejection fraction.

Data from Reference 1.

TABLE 36-2 Common Causes of Chronic Heart Failure

Heart failure with reduced ejection fraction (HFrEF)

- Coronary artery disease (eg, myocardial infarction or ischemia)
- Dilated cardiomyopathies (eg, drug-induced, viral infections, postpartum)
- Pressure overload (eg, systemic or pulmonary hypertension, or aortic valve or pulmonic valve stenosis)
- Volume overload (eg, valvular regurgitation, shunts, high-output states)

Heart failure with preserved ejection fraction (HFpEF)

- Increased ventricular stiffness
  - Ventricular hypertrophy (eg, hypertrophic cardiomyopathy, hypertension)
  - Infiltrative myocardial diseases (eg, amyloidosis, sarcoidosis, endomyocardial fibrosis)
  - Myocardial infarction or ischemia
- Mitral or tricuspid valve stenosis
- Pericardial disease (eg, pericarditis, pericardial tamponade)

Data from Reference 8.

the classic, more familiar form of the disorder although up to 50% of patients with HF have preserved left ventricular systolic function with presumed diastolic dysfunction, now termed HFpEF.[9] Patients with HFpEF typically are elderly, female, and obese, and have hypertension (HTN), atrial fibrillation, or diabetes.[2,10] Mortality is lower in patients with HFpEF compared to patients with HFrEF, despite HFpEF patients being older.[10]

Patients with LVEF between the HFrEF and HFpEF range are considered as "HF with mid-range EF" or "HF with mildly-reduced EF" (HFmrEF).[1] HFmrEF may represent patients with prior HFrEF but with improved LVEF or patients with deterioration in LVEF possibly progressing to HFrEF. To improve the specificity of diagnosing HFmrEF and HFpEF, the clinical diagnosis of HF in these EF categories should be further supported by objective measures. In addition, patients with HF with baseline LVEF <40% (0.4) who experience a greater than 10 point increase from baseline LVEF and a subsequent measurement of LVEF >40% (0.4) may be classified as HFimpEF. Both characteristics of and optimal management of patients with HFmrEF and HFimpEF are areas of ongoing investigations.

Coronary artery disease is the most common cause of HFrEF, accounting for up to 75% of cases.[8] Myocardial infarction (MI) leads to a reduction in muscle mass due to the death of affected myocardial cells. The degree to which contractility is impaired depends on the size of the infarction. To attempt to maintain cardiac output (CO), the surviving myocardium undergoes a compensatory remodeling, thus beginning the maladaptive process that initiates the HF syndrome and leads to further injury to the heart. This is discussed in greater detail in the "Pathophysiology" section. Myocardial ischemia and infarction also affect the diastolic properties of the heart by increasing ventricular stiffness and slowing ventricular relaxation. Thus, MI frequently results in systolic and diastolic dysfunctions.

Impaired systolic function is a cardinal feature of dilated cardiomyopathies. Although the cause of reduced contractility frequently is unknown, abnormalities such as interstitial fibrosis, cellular infiltrates, cellular hypertrophy, and myocardial cell degeneration are seen commonly on histologic examination. Inherited forms of dilated as well as hypertrophic cardiomyopathies may also occur.[8]

Pressure or volume overload causes ventricular hypertrophy, which attempts to return contractility to a near-normal state. If the pressure or volume overload persists, the remodeling process results in alterations in the geometry of the hypertrophied myocardial cells and is accompanied by increased collagen deposition in the extracellular matrix. Thus, both systolic and diastolic functions may be impaired.[11] Examples of pressure overload include systemic or pulmonary HTN and valvular heart disease.

HTN remains an important cause and/or contributor to both HFrEF and HFpEF in many patients, particularly women, the elderly, and African Americans.[2,4,8] The role of HTN should not be underestimated because it is an important risk factor for ischemic heart disease and is present in a high percentage of patients with coronary artery disease. HF is a largely preventable disorder; control of lifestyle risk factors (eg, HTN, coronary heart disease, smoking, obesity, physical inactivity, diabetes) is key to minimizing the risk of HF development. Two causes of HF that have been increasingly recognized include amyloidosis and cardiotoxicity with cancer therapies.

PATHOPHYSIOLOGY

Normal Cardiac Function

To understand the pathophysiologic processes in HF, a basic understanding of normal cardiac function is necessary. CO is defined as the volume of blood ejected per unit time (L/min) and is the product of heart rate (HR) and stroke volume (SV):

$$CO = HR \times SV$$

The relationship between CO and mean arterial pressure (MAP) is as follows:

$$MAP = CO \times \text{systemic vascular resistance (SVR)}$$

HR is controlled by the autonomic nervous system. The volume of blood ejected during systole, or stroke volume, depends on preload, afterload, and contractility.[11] As defined by the Frank-Starling mechanism, the ability of the heart to alter the force of contraction depends on changes in preload. As myocardial sarcomere length is stretched, the number of cross-bridges between thick and thin myofilaments increases, resulting in an increase in the force of contraction. The length of the sarcomere is determined primarily by the volume of blood in the ventricle; therefore, left ventricular end-diastolic volume (LVEDV) is the primary determinant of preload. In normal hearts, the preload response is the primary compensatory mechanism such that a small increase in end-diastolic volume results in a large increase in CO. Because of the relationship between pressure and volume in the heart, left ventricular end-diastolic pressure (LVEDP) is often used in the clinical setting to estimate preload. The hemodynamic measurement used to clinically estimate LVEDP is the pulmonary capillary wedge pressure (PCWP) also known as the pulmonary artery occlusion pressure (PAOP). Afterload is a more complex physiologic concept that can be viewed pragmatically as the sum of forces preventing the active forward ejection of blood by the ventricle. Major components of afterload are ejection impedance, wall tension, and regional wall geometry. In patients with left ventricular systolic dysfunction, an inverse relationship exists between afterload (estimated clinically by SVR) and SV such that increasing afterload causes a decrease in SV (Fig. 36-1). Contractility is the intrinsic property of cardiac muscle describing fiber shortening and tension development.

Heart Failure with Preserved Ejection Fraction

2 This disorder can be defined as a condition in which myocardial relaxation and filling are impaired and incomplete. The ventricle is unable to accept an adequate volume of blood from the venous system, does not fill at low pressure, and/or is unable to maintain normal SV. In its most severe form, HFpEF results in overt symptoms of HF. In modest HFpEF, symptoms of dyspnea and fatigue occur only during stress or activity, when HR and end-diastolic volume

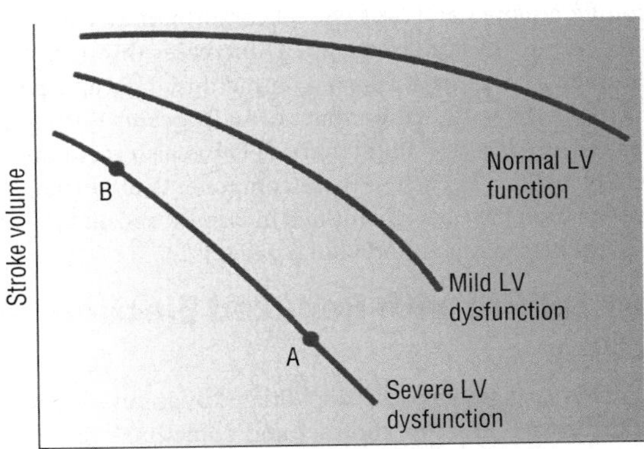

FIGURE 36-1 Relationship between stroke volume and systemic vascular resistance. In an individual with normal left ventricular (LV) function, increasing systemic vascular resistance has little effect on stroke volume. As the extent of LV dysfunction increases, the negative, inverse relationship between stroke volume and systemic vascular resistance becomes more important (B to A).

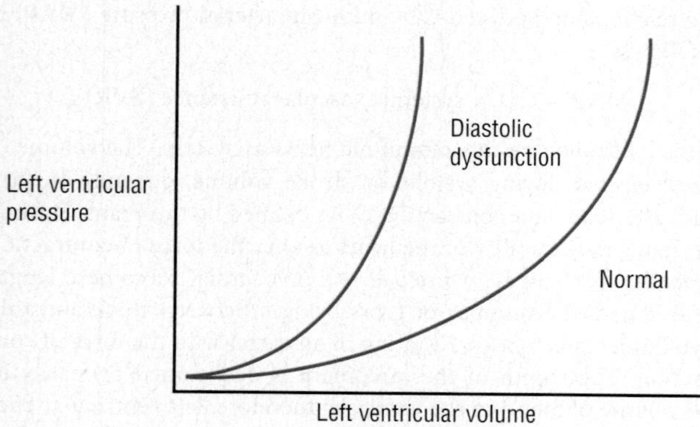

FIGURE 36-2 Diastolic pressure-volume relationship in a normal patient (right trace) and a patient with diastolic dysfunction (left trace).

increase. In its mildest form, HFpEF can be manifested as a slow or delayed pattern of relaxation and filling with little or no elevation in diastolic pressure and few or no cardiac symptoms. The congestive symptoms that occur with HFpEF are a manifestation of increased pulmonary venous pressures. HFpEF is caused by impaired myocardial relaxation and/or increased diastolic stiffness. When HF is caused by a predominant abnormality in diastolic function, the ventricular chamber is not enlarged, and EF may be normal or even elevated.[12] Figure 36-2 shows the pressure-volume relationship in a patient with normal versus abnormal diastolic function. The changes in the myocardium are associated with a shift upward and to the left of the pressure-volume curve so that for any increase in LV volume, diastolic pressure rises to a much greater level than normally would occur. Clinically, patients present with reduced exercise tolerance and dyspnea when they have elevated LV diastolic pressures. Patients with HFpEF have a predominant abnormality in diastolic function, whereas patients with HFrEF have a predominant abnormality in the systolic function of the LV.

HFpEF may represent a collection of syndromes because there is significant variability in morphology and functional presentation.[13] Some feel that a systemic inflammatory state and microvascular endothelial dysfunction play a role.[9] Although CAD is a common comorbidity, HF symptoms are often disproportionate to the severity of coronary artery disease. Obesity, HTN, and diabetes are proinflammatory and are frequent comorbidities in patients with HFpEF. During physical exertion, CO increases through integrated enhancements in venous return, contractility, HR, and peripheral vasodilation. The vasodilation that normally occurs during exercise is impaired in HFpEF.[13] Pulmonary HTN is also a common finding. Abnormalities in each of these components of normal exercise reserve function have been identified in HFpEF and all may contribute to pathophysiology in individual patients.[9,12]

Heart Failure with Reduced Ejection Fraction

3 HFrEF is a progressive disorder initiated by any event that impairs the ability of the heart to contract and sometimes relax resulting in a decrease in CO. The index event may have an acute onset, as with MI, or the onset may be slow, as with long-standing HTN. Regardless of the index event, a decrease in CO results in the activation of compensatory responses to maintain circulation.[11,14] These compensatory responses include: (a) tachycardia and increased contractility through sympathetic nervous system (SNS) activation, (b) the Frank-Starling mechanism, whereby an increase in preload results in an increase in SV, (c) vasoconstriction, and (d) ventricular hypertrophy and remodeling. Compensatory responses evolved to provide short-term support to maintain circulatory homeostasis after acute reductions in BP or renal perfusion. However, the persistent decline in CO in HF triggers long-term activation of these compensatory responses resulting in the complex functional, structural, biochemical, and molecular changes important for the development and progression of HF. The beneficial and detrimental effects of these compensatory responses are described below and are summarized in Table 36-3.

TABLE 36-3 Beneficial and Detrimental Effects of the Compensatory Responses in Heart

Compensatory Response	Beneficial Effects of Compensation	Detrimental Effects of Compensation
Increased preload due to sodium and water retention)	Optimizes stroke volume via Frank-Starling mechanism	Pulmonary and systemic congestion and edema formation Increased MVO_2
Vasoconstriction	Maintains BP despite reduced CO Shunts blood from nonessential organs to brain and heart	Increased MVO_2 Increased afterload decreases stroke volume and further activates the compensatory responses
Tachycardia and increased contractility (due to SNS activation)	Helps maintain CO	Increased MVO_2 Shortened diastolic filling time β_1-Receptor downregulation, decreased receptor sensitivity Precipitation of ventricular arrhythmias Increased risk of myocardial cell death
Ventricular hypertrophy and remodeling	Helps maintain CO Reduces myocardial wall stress Decreases MVO_2	Diastolic dysfunction Systolic dysfunction Increased risk of myocardial cell death Increased risk of myocardial ischemia Increased arrhythmia risk Fibrosis

BP, blood pressure; CO, cardiac output; MVO_2, myocardial oxygen demand; SNS, sympathetic nervous system.

Tachycardia and Increased Contractility

The increase in HR and contractility that rapidly occurs in response to a drop in CO is primarily due to the release of norepinephrine (NE) from adrenergic nerve terminals, although parasympathetic nervous system activity is also diminished.[14] Loss of atrial contribution to ventricular filling also can occur (atrial fibrillation, ventricular tachycardia), reducing ventricular performance even more. Because ionized calcium is sequestered into the sarcoplasmic reticulum and pumped out of the cell during diastole, the shortened diastolic time with increases in HR also results in a higher average intracellular calcium concentration during diastole, increasing actin-myosin interaction, augmenting the active resistance to fibril stretch, and reducing lusitropy. Conversely, the higher average calcium concentration translates into greater filament interaction during systole, generating more tension.[11] Increasing HR also increases myocardial oxygen demand. If ischemia is induced or worsened, both diastolic and systolic functions may become impaired, and SV can drop precipitously.

Fluid Retention and Increased Preload

Augmentation of preload is another compensatory response that is rapidly activated in response to decreased CO. Renal perfusion in HF is reduced due to both depressed CO and redistribution of blood away from nonvital organs. The kidney interprets the reduced

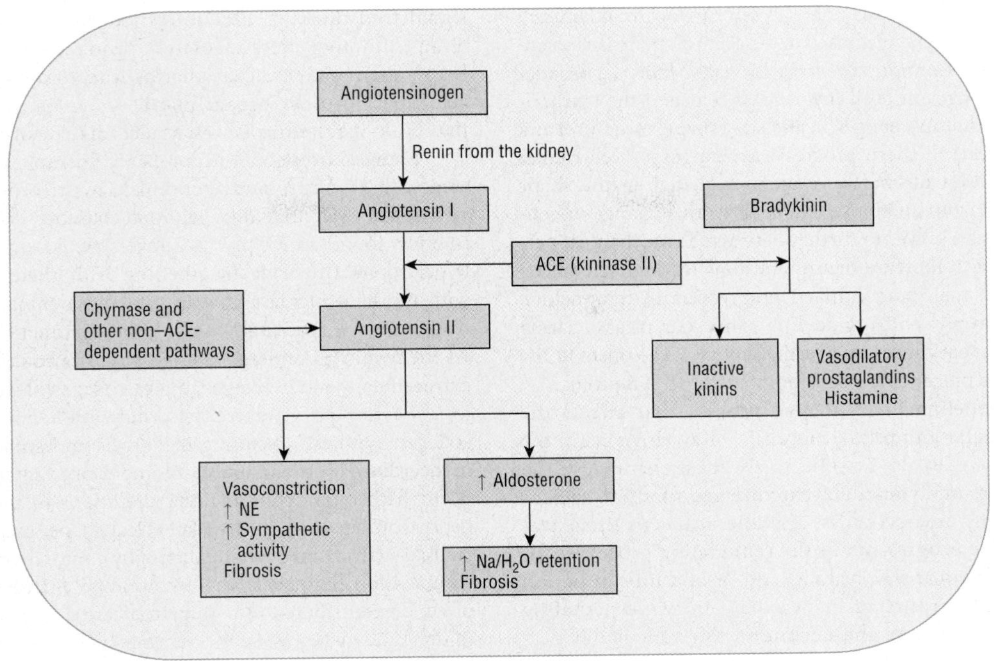

FIGURE 36-3 Physiology of the renin-angiotensin-aldosterone system. converts angiotensinogen to angiotensin I. Angiotensin I is cleaved to angiotensin II by the angiotensin-converting enzyme (ACE). Angiotensin II has a number of physiologic actions that are detrimental in HF. Note that angiotensin II can be produced in a number of tissues, including the heart, independent of ACE activity. ACE is also responsible for the breakdown of bradykinin. Inhibition of ACE results in the accumulation of bradykinin that, in turn, enhances the production of vasodilatory prostaglandins.

perfusion as an ineffective blood volume, resulting in activation of the renin-angiotensin-aldosterone system (RAAS) in an attempt to maintain BP and increase renal sodium and water retention. Reduced renal perfusion and increased sympathetic tone also stimulate renin release from juxtaglomerular cells in the kidney. As shown in Fig. 36-3, renin is responsible for the conversion of angiotensinogen to angiotensin I. Angiotensin I is converted to angiotensin II by angiotensin-converting enzyme (ACE). Angiotensin II may also be generated via non–ACE-dependent pathways. Angiotensin II stimulates aldosterone release from the adrenal gland, thereby providing an additional mechanism for renal sodium and water retention. As intravascular volume increases secondary to sodium and water retention, left ventricular volume and pressure (preload) increase, sarcomeres are stretched, and the force of contraction is enhanced.[11] While the preload response is the primary compensatory mechanism in normal hearts, the chronically failing heart usually has exhausted its preload response.[11] As shown in Fig. 36-4, increases in preload will increase SV only to a certain point. Once the flat portion of the curve is reached, further increases in preload will only lead to pulmonary or systemic congestion, a detrimental result.[11] Figure 36-4 also shows that the curve is flatter in patients with left ventricular dysfunction. Consequently, a given increase in preload in a patient with HF will produce a smaller incremental increase in SV than in an individual with normal ventricular function.

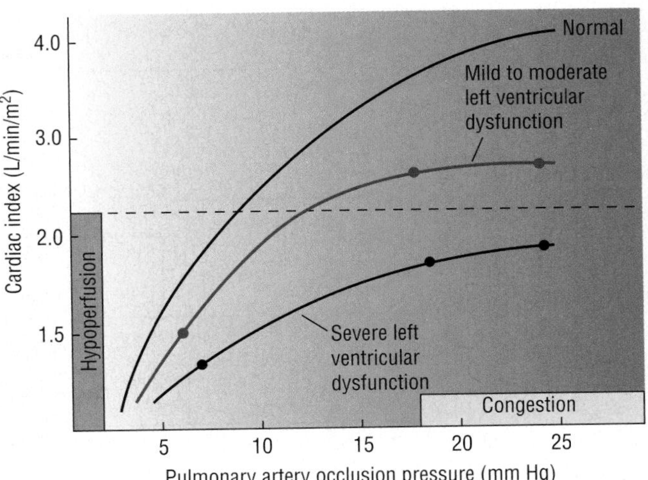

FIGURE 36-4 Relationship between cardiac output (shown as cardiac index which is CO/BSA) and preload (shown as pulmonary artery occlusion pressure).

Vasoconstriction and Increased Afterload

Vasoconstriction occurs in patients with HFrEF to help redistribute blood flow away from nonessential organs to coronary and cerebral circulations which may be reduced secondary to a decrease in CO (MAP = CO × SVR).[11] A number of neurohormones likely contribute to the vasoconstriction, including NE, angiotensin II, endothelin-1 (ET-1), neuropeptide Y, urotensin II, and arginine vasopressin (AVP).[11,14] Vasoconstriction impedes forward ejection of blood from the ventricle, further depressing CO and heightening the compensatory responses. The failing ventricle is exquisitely sensitive to changes in afterload (Fig. 36-1). Thus, increases in afterload often potentiate a vicious cycle of continued worsening and downward spiraling of the HF state.

Ventricular Hypertrophy and Remodeling

3 While the signs and symptoms of HF are closely associated with the items described above, the progression of HF appears to be independent of the patient's hemodynamic status. It is now recognized that left ventricular hypertrophy and remodeling are key

components in the pathogenesis of progressive myocardial failure.[11] *Ventricular hypertrophy* is a term used to describe an increase in ventricular muscle mass. *Cardiac or ventricular remodeling* is a broader term describing changes in both myocardial cells and the extracellular matrix that result in changes in the size, shape, structure, and function of the heart.[15] These progressive changes in ventricular structure and function ultimately result in a change in the shape of the left ventricle from an ellipse to a sphere. This change in ventricular size and shape serves to further depress the mechanical performance of the heart, increase regurgitant flow through the mitral valve, and, in turn, fuel the continued progression of remodeling. Ventricular hypertrophy and remodeling can occur in association with any condition that causes myocardial injury.[15] The onset of the remodeling process precedes the development of HF symptoms.

Cardiac remodeling is a complex process that affects the heart at the molecular and cellular levels.[11,15] Key elements in the process are shown in Fig. 36-5. Collectively, these events result in progressive changes in myocardial structure and function such as cardiac hypertrophy, myocyte loss, and alterations in the extracellular matrix. The progression of the remodeling process leads to reductions in myocardial systolic and/or diastolic function that, in turn, results in further myocardial injury, perpetuating the remodeling process and the decline in left ventricular performance. Angiotensin II, NE, ET, aldosterone, vasopressin, and numerous inflammatory cytokines, as well as substances under investigation, are active both systemically and locally in the heart. These substances play an important role in initiating the signal transduction cascade responsible for ventricular remodeling. Although these mediators produce harmful effects on the heart, their increased circulating and tissue concentrations are also toxic to other organs and serve as an important reminder that HF is a systemic as well as a cardiac disorder.[11,14,15]

Pressure overload (and probably hormonal activation) associated with HTN produces concentric hypertrophy (increase in the ventricular wall thickness without chamber enlargement), which is often found in HFpEF.[12] Conversely, eccentric left ventricular hypertrophy (myocyte lengthening with increased chamber size with minimal increase in wall thickness) characterizes the hypertrophy seen in patients with systolic dysfunction or previous MI. As the myocytes undergo change, so do various components of the extracellular matrix. For example, collagen degradation may lead to myocyte slippage, fibroblast proliferation, and increased fibrillar collagen synthesis, resulting in fibrosis and stiffening of the entire myocardium. Thus, a number of important ventricular changes that occur with remodeling include alterations in the geometry of the heart from an elliptical to a spherical shape, increases in ventricular mass (from myocyte hypertrophy), and changes in ventricular composition (especially the extracellular matrix) and volumes, all of which contribute to the impaired cardiac function. If the cardiac injury is acute (eg, MI), the ventricular remodeling process begins immediately. However, it is the progressive nature of this process that results in the continual worsening of the HF state, and thus is now the major focus for the identification of new therapeutic targets. In fact, HF pharmacotherapy associated with decreased mortality,

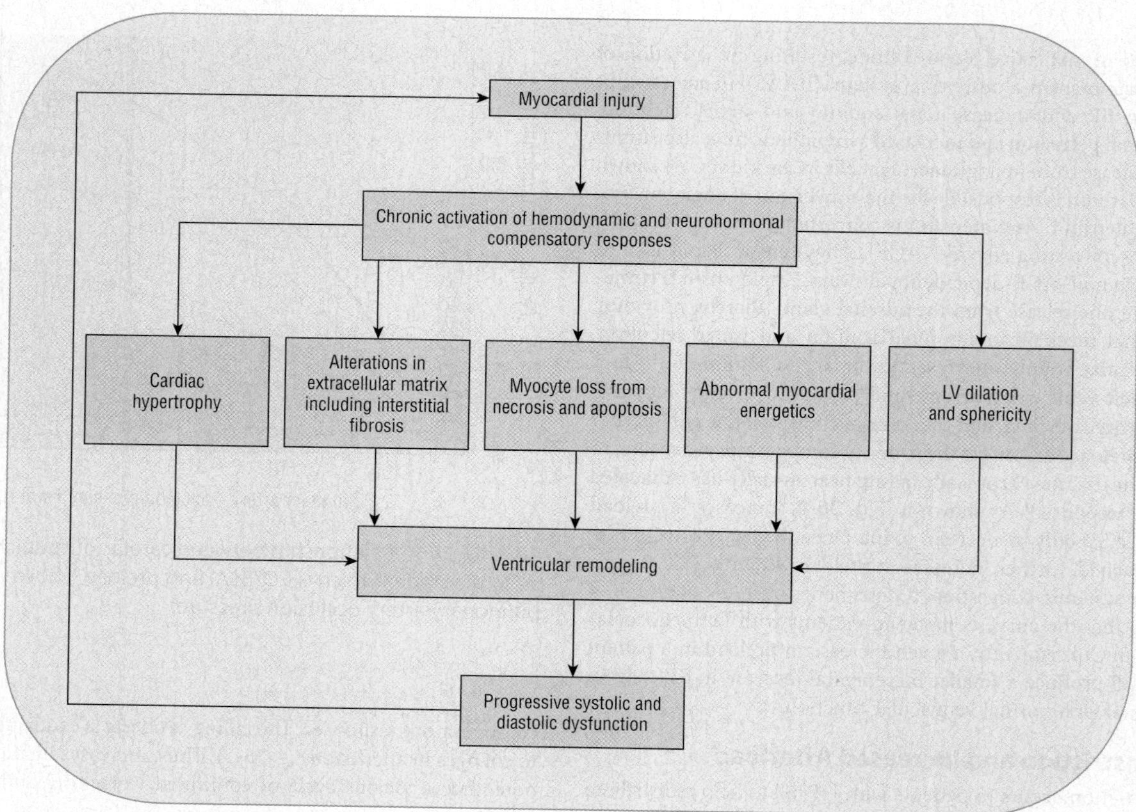

FIGURE 36-5 Key components of the pathophysiology of cardiac remodeling. Myocardial injury (eg, myocardial infarction) results in the activation of a number of hemodynamic and neurohormonal compensatory responses in an attempt to maintain circulatory homeostasis. Chronic activation of the neurohormonal systems results in a cascade of events that affect the myocardium at the molecular and cellular levels. These events lead to the changes in ventricular size, shape, structure, and function known as ventricular remodeling. The alterations in ventricular function result in further deterioration in cardiac systolic and diastolic functions that further promotes the remodeling process.

and/or slowing the progression of the disease, produce these effects largely by slowing or reversing ventricular remodeling, a process often referred to as *reverse remodeling*.

Amyloid Cardiomyopathy

Amyloidosis is an multisystem disorder in which protein-based infiltrates deposit in tissues including the heart, kidneys, nerves, liver, lungs, and bowel leading to organ dysfunction and death. The vast majority of cardiac amyloidosis is caused by one of two proteins, light chains or transthyretin, resulting in distinct pathophysiology. While the two primary types of amyloidosis, immunoglobulin light chain (AL) and transthyretin (ATTR) are considered rare, ATTR amyloidosis is found in as many as 25% of adults older than 85 years on autopsy. Both forms of amyloidosis are underdiagnosed. Overall, 25% of patients with AL amyloidosis die within 6 months of diagnosis and 25% of patients with ATTR amyloidosis die within 24 months of diagnosis.

Cardiac amyloidosis occurs with the deposition of abnormal proteins into the extracellular space in the myocardium. Heart involvement may result in HF, more commonly HFpEF. Approximately 30 proteins are associated with amyloid cardiomyopathy; however, the most common is transthyretin. The DNA coding sequence for misfolded transthyretin can be inherited, causing the proteins to easily disassociate (hereditary type). ATTR cardiomyopathy is under-recognized and may be present in up to 15% of older adults with HF. Most cases of cardiac amyloidosis are not inherited but rather related to the aging process. The non-hereditary type (wild-type) is mostly observed in patients older than 60 years. Progressive HF, complicated by arrhythmias and conduction disturbances, may be part of the natural history of the disorder.[16]

Recent advances in standard chemotherapy to treat AL amyloidosis have markedly improved patient outcomes such that auto-stem-cell transplant is now only rarely indicated. ATTR cardiomyopathy was treated only by cardiac transplantation. However, there are now three therapies approved for managing ATTR amyloidosis, depending on the clinical phenotype.[17-19]

Hypertrophic Cardiomyopathy

Hypertrophic cardiomyopathy (HCM) is the most common genetic disorder of the heart, occurring in one of every 200 to 500 persons. It is characterized by the presence of increased left ventricular (LV) wall thickness that is typically severe, asymmetric, and primarily affects the interventricular septum often resulting in obstruction of the left ventricular outflow tract. In up to 60% of adults with HCM, this disease is inherited in an autosomal dominant pattern, associated with mutations in genes encoding proteins of thick and thin myofilament contractile components of the cardiac sarcomere. HCM often remains clinically silent and is the most common cause of sudden death in athletes. Fortunately, pharmacologic, electrical, and surgical interventions have reduced mortality to 0.5% per year. Assessment of the risk of sudden cardiac death (SCD) is of paramount importance since sudden death is considered the main cause of death in younger patients with HCM. Genetic testing is increasingly being applied to patients who meet diagnostic criteria for HCM in order to identify the causative mutation for the disease and to determine the genetic predisposition of asymptomatic relatives. Typical symptoms of HCM include dyspnea, chest pain, palpitations, and syncope. Treatment is aimed at the improvement of symptoms, exercise capacity, and functional status. While pharmacological therapy is first-line, patients may experience symptoms refractory to medications, primarily related to left ventricular outflow obstruction, and surgical or other interventions may be needed.[20]

Neurohormonal Model of Heart Failure

2 3 The current paradigm used to describe HF pathogenesis is the *neurohormonal model*.[11] This model recognizes an initiating event (eg, MI, long-standing HTN) that leads to decreased CO and begins the "HF state." The problem then moves beyond the heart, and it becomes a systemic disease whose progression is mediated largely by neurohormones and autocrine/paracrine factors that drive myocyte injury, oxidative stress, inflammation, and extracellular matrix remodeling. While the former paradigms still guide us to some extent in the symptomatic management of the disease (eg, diuretics), it is this latter paradigm that helps us understand disease progression and, more importantly, the ways to slow disease progression. In the sections that follow, key neurohormones and autocrine/paracrine factors, collectively termed biomarkers, are described with respect to their role in HF and its progression. The benefits of current and investigational drug therapies can be better understood through a solid understanding of the neurohormones they regulate. Although the neurohormonal model provides a logical framework for our current understanding of HF progression and the role of various medications in attenuating this progression, it must be emphasized that this model does not completely explain HF progression.

Angiotensin II

Of the neurohormones and autocrine/paracrine factors that play an important role in HFrEF pathophysiology, angiotensin II is probably the best understood.[11,21] Angiotensin II has multiple actions that contribute to its detrimental effects. It is a potent vasoconstrictor mediated by binding to the angiotensin type 1 (AT1) receptor in the vasculature, and it also causes a release of AVP and ET-1. Angiotensin II facilitates the release of NE from adrenergic nerve terminals, heightening SNS activation. It promotes sodium retention through direct effects on the renal tubules and by stimulating aldosterone release. Its vasoconstriction of the efferent glomerular arteriole helps to maintain renal perfusion pressure in patients with severe HF or impaired renal function. Finally, angiotensin II and many of the neurohormones released in response to angiotensin II play central roles in stimulating ventricular hypertrophy, remodeling, myocyte apoptosis, oxidative stress, inflammation, and alterations in the myocardial extracellular matrix. Clinical trials showing that attenuating angiotensin II-mediated effects with ACE inhibitors or ARBs improve hemodynamics, symptoms, hospitalizations, and survival highlight the importance of angiotensin II in HF pathophysiology.[22]

Norepinephrine

NE plays a central role in tachycardia, vasoconstriction, and increased contractility and plasma renin activity in HFrEF.[14] Plasma NE concentrations are elevated in correlation with the degree of HF, and patients with the highest plasma NE concentrations have the poorest prognosis.[11] Excessive SNS activation causes β_1-receptor downregulation with a subsequent loss of sensitivity to receptor stimulation. Excess catecholamines increase the risk of arrhythmias and can cause myocardial cell loss by stimulating both necrosis and apoptosis. Finally, NE contributes to ventricular hypertrophy and remodeling. The beneficial effects of β-blockers on outcomes in patients with HFrEF support the critical role of sympathetic nervous system activation and NE in the pathophysiology of the HF state.[8,22]

Aldosterone

Aldosterone-mediated sodium retention and its key role in volume overload and edema have long been recognized as important components of the HF syndrome.[11] Circulating aldosterone is increased in HF due to angiotensin II-stimulated synthesis, release of aldosterone from the adrenal cortex, and reduced hepatic clearance of aldosterone due to reduce hepatic perfusion. The direct effects of aldosterone on the heart may be even more important than sodium retention in HF pathophysiology. Aldosterone produces interstitial cardiac fibrosis through increased collagen deposition in the extracellular matrix of the heart. By increasing the stiffness of the myocardium, cardiac fibrosis may decrease systolic function and impair diastolic function. Extra-adrenal production of aldosterone in the heart, kidneys, and vascular smooth muscle also contributes to the progressive nature of HF through target organ fibrosis and vascular remodeling. Induction of a systemic proinflammatory state, increased oxidative stress, wasting of soft tissues and bone, secondary hyperparathyroidism, and mineral/micronutrient dyshomeostasis are other important pathologic actions of aldosterone that directly contribute to ventricular remodeling and HF progression.[11,21] Clinical trials with the aldosterone antagonists spironolactone[23] and eplerenone[24,25] showing significant reductions in morbidity and mortality in patients with HFrEF provide compelling evidence of the important role of aldosterone in HFrEF initiation and progression. Although not studied as extensively as in HFrEF, aldosterone antagonists also show benefit in select patients with HFpEF.[26,27]

Natriuretic Peptides

The natriuretic peptide family has three members, atrial natriuretic peptide, B-type natriuretic peptide (BNP), and C-type natriuretic peptide. Of these, BNP and its biologically related inactive peptide NT-proBNP are the most useful in the diagnosis and management of HF.[22,28] BNP and NT-proBNP are synthesized and released from the ventricle in response to pressure or volume overload. BNP or NT-proBNP plasma concentrations are elevated in patients with HF, increasing natriuresis and diuresis and attenuating activation of the RAAS and SNS. A recent clinical trial showing that neprilysin-mediated inhibition of natriuretic peptide breakdown improves outcomes in patients with HFrEF supports the importance of these peptides in HF pathophysiology.[29]

The development of easily performed commercial assays for BNP and NT-proBNP resulted in widespread interest in the role of these peptides as a biomarker for prognostic, diagnostic, and therapeutic use. In patients with chronic HFrEF, the degree of elevation in BNP concentrations is closely associated with poor outcomes.[28] Elevation of natriuretic peptide plasma concentrations now plays a key role in establishing the diagnosis of HF.[22] Clinicians should be aware that many cardiovascular and non-cardiovascular comorbidities (eg, pulmonary embolism, pulmonary hypertension) as well as sex, race/ethnicity, and age may also affect natriuretic peptide levels.[22] In addition, obesity is associated with lower levels of BNP and NT-proBNP, and thus, diagnostic sensitivity in morbidly obese patients is reduced. The most well-established clinical application of BNP testing is in the urgent care setting where the BNP or NT-proBNP assay is useful when combined with clinical evaluation for differentiating dyspnea secondary to either HFrEF or HFpEF from other causes. In patients with either chronic or acute/hospitalized HF, measurements of BNP or NT-proBNP also have utility for risk stratification and prognosis.[28]

Studies evaluating the role of serial BNP measurement to guide drug therapy have not shown consistent improvement in long-term outcomes compared with standard medical therapy, particularly in patients with HFpEF.[28] Guidelines reflect this uncertainty and do not support the routine use of serial BNP measurement in chronic HF management.[28,30] Measurement of BNP should not preclude good clinical judgment and an individualized approach to each patient is imperative.

Other Factors

AVP is a pituitary peptide hormone that regulates renal water excretion and plasma osmolality.[11] Plasma concentrations of AVP are elevated in patients with HF, supporting its role in the pathophysiology of this disorder. The physiologic effects of AVP are mediated through the V_{1a}, V_{1b}, and V_2 receptors. Stimulation of these receptors by increased circulating AVP results in several maladaptive responses including: (a) increased renal free water reabsorption in the face of plasma hypoosmolality resulting in volume overload and hyponatremia; (b) increased arterial vasoconstriction that contributes to reduced CO; and (c) stimulation of remodeling by cardiac hypertrophy and extracellular matrix collagen deposition. Although the AVP antagonists tolvaptan and conivaptan improve acute symptoms and increase serum sodium and urine output without affecting HR, BP, renal function, or other electrolytes, no improvements in morbidity and mortality were seen in clinical trials.[31]

The sodium-glucose-cotransporter-2 (SGLT2) is highly expressed in the renal proximal tubule and is responsible for reabsorbing more than 90% of filtered glucose that is coupled with Na^+ ions.[32] The SGLT2 inhibitors (eg, empagliflozin, dapagliflozin) lower blood glucose by increasing urinary glucose (and sodium) excretion resulting in diuresis and natriuresis. Clinical trials reported that these agents also reduce the risk of cardiovascular events in patients with HF, including hospitalizations, even in patients without diabetes, suggesting that mechanism(s) other than simply lowering blood glucose are important.[33] Although the exact beneficial mechanisms remain uncertain, these agents reduce inflammation, oxidative stress, and sympathetic nervous system activity as well as improve cardiac remodeling and myocardial energetics.[32,33] The impressive outcomes with these medications in patients with HF further support the notion of HF as a disorder driven by multiple systemic mechanisms.

Factors Precipitating/Exacerbating Heart Failure

Although significant advances have been made in treatment, symptom exacerbation, to the point that hospitalization is required, is a common and growing problem in patients with chronic HF. Hospitalization for HF exacerbation consumes large amounts of healthcare dollars and significantly impairs the patient's quality of life. Thus, there is great interest in identifying and then remedying factors that increase the risk of decompensation. Appropriate therapy can often maintain patients in a "compensated" state, indicating that they are relatively symptom-free. However, there are many aggravating or precipitating factors that may cause a previously compensated patient to develop worsened symptoms necessitating hospitalization. Often, these precipitating factors are reversible or treatable, thus thorough evaluation for their presence is imperative.

Cardiac events are a frequent cause of worsening HF.[34] Myocardial ischemia and infarction are potentially reversible causes that must be carefully considered since nearly 70% of patients with HF have coronary artery disease. Revascularization should be considered in eligible patients. Atrial fibrillation is a common comorbidity in patients with HF and is associated with increased morbidity and mortality.[35] Control of ventricular response, maintenance of sinus rhythm in appropriate patients, and prevention of thromboembolism are important elements in the treatment of patients with concomitant HF and atrial fibrillation. Uncontrolled HTN is also an important contributing factor and should be treated according to current guidelines.[36]

Noncardiac events are also associated with HF decompensation. Pulmonary infections frequently cause worsening HF. Many of these events would be preventable with the more widespread use of the pneumococcal and influenza vaccines. Pulmonary embolus, diabetes, chronic kidney disease, hypothyroidism, and hyperthyroidism should also be considered.

Nonadherence with prescribed HF medications or with dietary recommendations (eg, sodium intake and fluid restriction) is also a common cause of HF exacerbation.[34] Polypharmacy is common in patients with HF.[37] Thus, nonadherence is an important contributor to poor outcomes and socioeconomically disadvantaged patients appear to be disproportionately affected.

Many medications can precipitate or exacerbate HF by one or more mechanisms: (a) negative inotropic effects; (b) direct cardiotoxicity; or (c) increased sodium and/or water retention (Table 36-4).[38]

TABLE 36-4 Selected Drugs That May Precipitate or Exacerbate Heart Failure

Negative inotropic effect
Antiarrhythmics (disopyramide, dronedarone, flecainide, propafenone, sotalol)
β-Blockers (eg, propranolol, metoprolol, carvedilol)
Calcium channel blockers—nondihydropyridine type (verapamil, diltiazem)
Itraconazole
Cardiotoxic
Alkylating agents (eg, cyclophosphamide, ifosfamide, melphalan)
Amphetamines (eg, cocaine, methamphetamine)
Anthracyclines (eg, doxorubicin, daunorubicin, epirubicin, idarubicin)
Antiarrhythmics (eg, disopyramide, dronedarone, flecainide, propafenone, sotalol)
Antimetabolites (eg, fluorouracil, capecitabine, fludarabine, decitabine)
Antimicrotubules (eg, docetaxel, paclitaxel)
BCR-ABL inhibitors (eg, bosutinib, dastinib, imatinib, ponatinib)
BRAF inhibitors (eg, dabrafenib)
Carbamazepine
Chimeric antigen receptor (CAR) T-cell therapy (eg, tisagenlecleucel, axicabtageneciloleucel)
Daunomycin
Ethanol
Hormonal therapy (eg, aplalutamide, bicalutamide, darolutamide, nilutamide)
Human epidermal growth factor receptor (HER/EGFR) inhibitors (eg, lapatinib, osimertinib)
Human epidermal growth factor receptor 2 (HER2) inhibitors (eg, pertuzamab, trastuzumab)
Immune checkpoint inhibitors (eg, nivolumab, ipilimumab, pembrolizumab)
Immunomodulators (eg, lenalidomide, pomalidomide, thalidomide)
MEK inhibitors (eg, binimetinib, cobimetinib, trametinib)
Mitomycin
Mitoxantrone
Mitomycin
Vascular endothelial growth factor (VEGF) inhibitors (eg, axitinib. bevacizumab, cabazantobinib, lenvatinib, pazopanib, sorafenib, sunitinib, vandetanib)
Miscellaneous (eg, entrectinib, fedratinib, ripretinib, tretinoin)
Sodium and water retention
Androgens and estrogens
Cyclooxygenase-2 (COX-2) inhibitors
Rosiglitazone and pioglitazone
Glucocorticoids
Nonsteroidal anti-inflammatory drugs (NSAIDs)
Pioglitazone and rosiglitazone
Salicylates (high dose)
Sodium-containing drugs (eg, carbenicillin disodium, ticarcillin disodium)
Uncertain mechanism
Dipeptidyl peptidase-4 (DPP-4) inhibitors (eg, saxagliptin)
TNF-α inhibitors (eg, adalimumab, infliximab, etanercept)

Agents with negative inotropic effects are primarily a concern in patients with HFrEF. Nonsteroidal anti-inflammatory drugs (NSAIDs) are increasingly recognized for their ability to exacerbate HF and increase the risk of hospitalization and mortality through volume retention, decreased renal function, and increased BP.[38] The ability of numerous antineoplastic agents to cause or worsen HF is increasingly recognized.[39,40]

Many of the precipitating factors for HF are preventable, particularly through appropriate healthcare professional intervention. First and foremost, multidisciplinary teams should work collaboratively to identify and address such factors. Given medications are often a precipitating factor, engaging a pharmacist in HF care is recommended to assist with identifying inadequate HF therapy, detecting medication nonadherence, and avoiding drug-drug interactions or other medication-related causes of HF.[41,42] A careful medication history is an important aspect of evaluating the cause(s) of HF exacerbation as many are amenable to pharmacist intervention. Attention to these factors can contribute to reducing the risk of adverse cardiovascular outcomes and improving the patient's quality of life.

CLINICAL PRESENTATION

Signs and Symptoms

1 The primary manifestations of both HFrEF and HFpEF are dyspnea and fatigue, which lead to exercise intolerance, and fluid overload, which can result in peripheral edema and pulmonary congestion.[34,43] The presence of these signs and symptoms may vary considerably from patient to patient such that some patients have dyspnea but no signs of fluid retention, whereas others may have marked volume overload with few complaints of dyspnea or fatigue. However, many patients have both dyspnea and volume overload. Clinicians should remember that symptom severity often does not correlate with the degree of LV dysfunction. Patients with a low LVEF (less than 20%-25% [0.20-0.25]) may be asymptomatic, whereas those with preserved LVEF may have significant symptoms. Symptoms can vary considerably over time in a given patient, even in the absence of changes in ventricular function or medications.

Systemic congestion is associated with a number of signs and symptoms. Jugular venous distension (JVD) is the simplest and most reliable sign of fluid overload. Examination of the right internal jugular vein with the patient at a 45° angle is the preferred method for assessing JVD. The presence of JVD more than 4 cm above the sternal angle suggests systemic venous congestion. In patients with mild systemic congestion, JVD may be absent at rest, but the application of pressure to the abdomen will cause an elevation of JVD (hepatojugular reflux).

Peripheral edema is a cardinal finding in HF. Edema usually occurs in dependent parts of the body and is often seen as ankle or pedal edema in ambulatory patients, although it may be manifested as sacral edema in bedridden patients. Adults typically have a 10-lb (4.5-kg) fluid weight gain before trace peripheral edema is evident; therefore, patients with acute decompensated HF may have no clinical evidence of systemic congestion except weight gain. Body weight is thus an excellent short-term endpoint for evaluating fluid status. Nonfluid weight gain and loss of muscle mass due to cardiac cachexia are potential confounders for long-term use of weight as a marker for fluid status. Hepatomegaly and ascites are other signs of systemic congestion.

Patients with HFrEF may exhibit signs and symptoms of low CO alone or in addition to volume overload. The primary complaint associated with hypoperfusion is fatigue. Objective indicators of low CO include worsening renal function, cool extremities, altered mental status, resting tachycardia, low systolic blood pressure, and narrow pulse pressure.

Diagnosis

No single test is available to confirm the diagnosis of HF—it is a clinical syndrome with current or prior signs and symptoms due to any cardiac structural and/or functional disorder corroborated by elevated plasma natriuretic peptide concentrations or objective evidence of pulmonary or systemic congestion from a cardiogenic cause.[1,43] Because HF can be caused or worsened by multiple cardiac and noncardiac disorders, some of which may be treatable or reversible, accurate diagnosis is essential for the development of therapeutic strategies. HF is often initially suspected in a patient based on symptoms. However, signs and symptoms lack sensitivity for diagnosing HF since they are frequently found with many other disorders. Even in patients with known HF, there is a poor correlation between the presence or severity of symptoms and the hemodynamic abnormality. With few exceptions, HFpEF cannot be distinguished from HFrEF on the basis of the history, physical examination, chest x-ray, and ECG alone.[9] Patients with HFpEF are often elderly, with multiple comorbidities.[9]

CLINICAL PRESENTATION Heart Failure

Symptoms

Common

- Dyspnea, particularly on exertion
- Orthopnea
- Paroxysmal nocturnal dyspnea
- Exercise intolerance
- Fatigue
- Swollen ankles or other parts of the body
- Bendopnea

Less Common

- Cough
- Wheezing
- Nocturia
- Anorexia, poor appetite, early satiety
- Nausea
- Bloating
- Weight gain or loss
- Dizziness or syncope
- Depression
- Reduced cognitive function (especially in the elderly)

Signs

Specific for Heart Failure

- Jugular venous distention
- Cardiomegaly, lateral displacement of the apical impulse
- Hepatojugular reflux
- S_3 gallop
- Cheyne-Stokes respiration (advanced HF)

Less Specific for Heart Failure

- Peripheral edema (lower extremities, sacral, scrotal)
- Pulmonary rales
- Pulmonary edema
- Weight gain (>2 kg/week)
- Weight loss with muscle wasting/cachexia (advanced HF)
- Pleural effusion
- Tachycardia/irregular pulse
- Tachypnea
- Hepatomegaly/ascites
- Cool extremities
- Oliguria
- Narrow pulse pressure
- Cardiomegaly
- Peripheral edema
- Hepatomegaly
- Venous stasis changes

Laboratory tests

- BNP >35 pg/mL (ng/L; 10 pmol/L) for ambulatory patients or >100 pg/mL (ng/L; 29 pmol/L) for patients hospitalized or with decompensated HF
- NT-proBNP >125 pg/mL (ng/L; 15 pmol/L) for ambulatory patients or >300 pg/mL (ng/L; 35 pmol/L) for patients hospitalized or with decompensated HF
- An electrocardiogram may be normal or it could show numerous abnormalities including acute ST-T wave changes from myocardial ischemia, atrial fibrillation, bradycardia, left ventricular hypertrophy
- Serum creatinine: It may be increased due to hypoperfusion. Preexisting renal dysfunction can contribute to volume overload
- Complete blood count is useful to determine if HF is due to reduced oxygen-carrying capacity
- Chest x-ray: Useful for detection of cardiac enlargement, pulmonary edema, and pleural effusions
- Echocardiogram: Used to assess LV size, valve function, pericardial effusion, wall motion abnormalities, and ejection fraction
- Hyponatremia: Serum sodium <130 mEq/L (mmol/L) is associated with reduced survival and may indicate worsening volume overload and/or disease progression

Data from Reference 1.

A complete history and physical examination targeted at identifying cardiac or noncardiac disorders or behaviors that may cause or hasten HF development or progression are essential in the initial patient evaluation. Careful medication history should also be obtained with a focus on the use of medications that can precipitate or exacerbate HF (Table 36-4).[38]

Particular attention should be paid to cardiovascular risk factors and to other disorders that can cause or exacerbate HF such as HTN, diabetes, atrial fibrillation, dyslipidemia, tobacco use, sleep-disordered breathing, iron deficiency, and thyroid disease. Since coronary artery disease is the cause of HF in many patients, evaluation of the possibility of coronary disease is essential, especially in men. If coronary artery disease is detected, appropriate revascularization procedures may then be considered. The patient's volume status should be documented by assessing the body weight, JVD, and presence or absence of pulmonary congestion and peripheral edema. The biomarkers BNP or NT-proBNP are increased in most patients and their measurement is a key component of establishing the diagnosis of HF, particularly for differentiating dyspnea caused by HF from other causes.[1,30] The initial evaluation should include a complete blood count, serum electrolytes (including calcium and magnesium), assessment of renal and hepatic function, urinalysis, lipid profile, hemoglobin A1C, thyroid function tests, iron studies, chest x-ray, and 12-lead ECG.

Although the history, physical examination, and laboratory tests provide important insight into the underlying cause of HF, the echocardiogram is a standard test routinely used in the evaluation of the patient with HF. The echocardiogram is used to assess abnormalities in cardiac structure and function and should include evaluation of the pericardium, myocardium, and heart valves, and quantification of the LVEF to determine if systolic or diastolic dysfunction is present. Other imaging modalities may occasionally be used in conjunction with the echocardiogram including radionucleotide ventriculography, cardiac, computed tomography, and cardiac magnetic resonance.

TREATMENT

Desired Outcomes

The goals of therapy in the management of chronic HF are to improve the patient's quality of life, relieve or reduce symptoms, prevent or minimize hospitalizations, slow progression of the disease, and prolong survival. Pharmacotherapy plays a key role in achieving these goals.[22,30] In addition, identification of risk factors for HF development and recognition of its progressive nature has led to increased emphasis on preventing the development of this disorder. In an attempt to standardize the definition of HF and provide clarity to clinicians and patients on optimal preventive and treatment approaches, an international group that included the Heart Failure Society of America developed a staging system to emphasize that HF is a continuum and that not only recognizes the evolution and progression of the disorder but also emphasizes risk factor modification and preventive treatment strategies (Table 36-5).[1]

The four stages of this system differ from the NYHA functional classification that classifies symptoms according to the clinician's subjective evaluation and does not recognize preventive measures or the progression of the disorder (Table 36-6). For patients with symptomatic HF (Stage C or D), symptoms can change frequently over a short period of time due to changes in medications, diet, intercurrent illnesses, or other causes. For example, a patient with Stage C HF with NYHA class IV symptoms such as marked volume overload could improve to class I or II with appropriate GDMT, yet they will remain categorized as Stage C.

The general principles used to guide the treatment of HFrEF are based on numerous large, randomized, double-blind, multicenter trials. No such randomized trials had been performed in patients with HFpEF. Consequently, the guidelines for the management of HFpEF are based primarily on clinical investigations in relatively small groups of patients, clinical experience, and concepts based on the knowledge and understanding of the pathophysiology of the disease process. Treatment of HFpEF has been directed primarily at alleviation of congestion with diuretics, managing precipitating factors and comorbid conditions (eg, ischemia, HTN, atrial fibrillation), and addressing underlying microvascular inflammation.[10] Previously, the typical therapies used for HFrEF have not shown a significant benefit for patients with HFpEF. However, more recent studies identified several agents that are also beneficial for HFpEF.

TABLE 36-6 New York Heart Association Functional Classification

Functional Class	Physical Limitations and Symptoms
Class I	Patients with cardiac disease but without limitations of physical activity. Ordinary physical activity does not cause undue fatigue, dyspnea, or palpitation.
Class II	Patients with cardiac disease that results in slight limitations of physical activity. Ordinary physical activity results in fatigue, palpitation, dyspnea, or angina.
Class III	Patients with cardiac disease that results in marked limitation of physical activity. Although patients are comfortable at rest, less than ordinary activity will lead to symptoms.
Class IV	Patients with cardiac disease that results in an inability to carry on physical activity without discomfort. Symptoms of congestive HF are present even at rest. With any physical activity, increased discomfort is experienced.

TABLE 36-5 Stages of Heart Failure

Stages	Definition
Stage A At-risk for heart failure	Patients at risk for HF but without current or prior symptoms or signs of HF and without structural, biomarker, or genetic markers of heart disease • Patients with HTN, CVD, DM, obesity, known exposure to cardiotoxins, family history of cardiomyopathy
Stage B Pre-heart failure	Patients without current or prior symptoms or signs of HF but evidence of *one* of the following: • Structural heart disease: eg, LVH, chamber enlargement, wall motion abnormality, myocardial tissue abnormality, valvular heart disease • Abnormal cardiac function: eg, reduced LV or RV systolic function, evidence of increased filling pressures or abnormal diastolic dysfunction • Elevated natriuretic peptide levels or elevated cardiac troponin levels in the setting of exposure to cardiotoxins
Stage C Heart failure	Patients with current or prior symptoms and/or signs of HF caused by structural and/or cardiac abnormality • HF in remission *or* persistent HF
Stage D Advanced heart failure	Severe symptoms and/or signs of HF at rest, recurrent hospitalizations despite GDMT, refractory or intolerant to GDMT • Requiring advanced therapies such as consideration for transplant, mechanical circulatory support, or palliative care

CVD, cardiovascular disease; DM, diabetes; GDMT, guideline-directed medical therapy; HF, heart failure; HTN, hypertension; LV, left ventricle; LVH, left ventricular hypertrophy; RV, right ventricle.

Data from Reference 1.

General Approach to Treatment

The complexity of the HF syndrome necessitates a comprehensive approach to management that includes accurate diagnosis, identification, and treatment of risk factors, elimination or minimization of precipitating factors, appropriate pharmacologic and nonpharmacologic therapy, and close monitoring and follow-up.

The first step in the management of chronic HF is to determine the classification of HF based upon LVEF and symptoms based upon NYHA functional class (see Tables 36-1 and 36-6) and/or any precipitating factors. Appropriate treatment of underlying disorders (eg, hyperthyroidism, valvular heart disease) may obviate the need for specific HF treatment. Revascularization or anti-ischemic therapy in patients with coronary disease may reduce HF symptoms. Drugs that aggravate HF (see Table 36-4) should be discontinued if possible.

Restriction of dietary sodium and fluid intake is an important lifestyle intervention for both HFrEF and HFpEF. Mild (<3 g/day) to moderate (<2 g/day) sodium restriction, in conjunction with daily measurement of weight, should be implemented to minimize volume retention and allow the use of lower and safer diuretic doses. Patients should avoid adding salt to prepared foods and eliminate foods high in sodium (eg, salt-cured meats, salted snack foods, pickles, soups, delicatessen meats, and processed foods). In patients with hyponatremia (serum Na <130 mEq/L [mmol/L]) or those with persistent volume retention despite high diuretic doses and sodium restriction, daily fluid intake should be limited to 2 L/day from all sources. However, both sodium and fluid restriction must be done with care in patients with HFpEF. Excessive restriction can lead to hypotension, a low-output state, and/or renal insufficiency. Daily weights may help assess volume status. Dietary and lifestyle factors that decrease the risk of development of CAD, HTN, diabetes, and obesity should be encouraged. Although guidelines indicate sodium restriction is reasonable to minimize congestion, proven benefits on clinical outcomes are lacking.

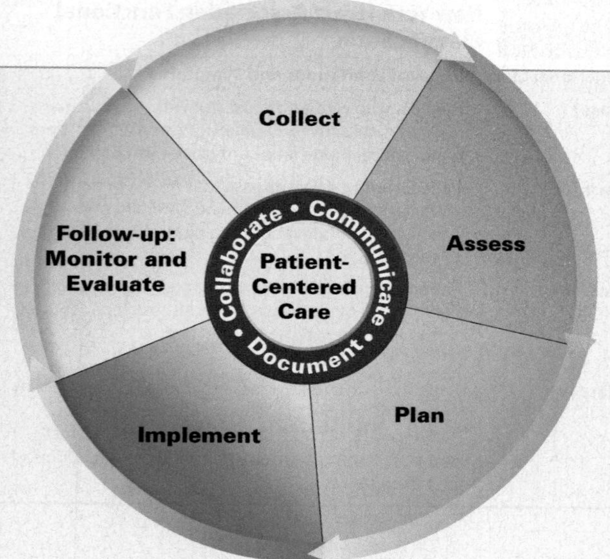

Patient Care Process for Heart Failure

An illustration shows that patient-centered care includes collaboration, communication, and documentation. The actions associated with the care are collect, assess, plan, implement, and follow-up by monitoring and evaluating.

The processes of Collect and Assess are similar for patients with heart failure with reduced ejection fraction (HFrEF) and heart failure with preserved ejection fraction (HFpEF) as are the processes of Implement and Follow-up: Monitor and Evaluate. In contrast, while the Plan process has many similarities between HFrEF and HFpEF, some important differences in the Plan are described below.

Collect

- Patient characteristics (eg, age, sex)
- Patient medical history (personal and family)
- Social history (eg, tobacco/ethanol use) and dietary habits including intake of sodium-containing foods and fluid
- Current medications including over-the-counter (OTC), herbal products, dietary supplements
- Etiology of heart failure (Table 36-1)
- Objective data
  - Blood pressure (BP), heart rate (HR), respiratory rate (RR), height, weight, left ventricular ejection fraction, echocardiogram, chest x-ray
  - Labs including complete blood count, comprehensive metabolic panel (eg, serum Na, K, BUN, creatinine), urinalysis, liver function tests, thyroid-stimulating hormone, iron studies (serum ferritin and transferrin saturation), brain natriuretic peptide (BNP) or NT-pro-BNP, electrocardiogram (ECG)
  - Physical examination (eg, signs/symptoms of volume overload [see the "Clinical Presentation" box])

Assess

- Hemodynamic stability (eg, systolic BP <90 mm Hg, signs/symptoms of hypotension or poor perfusion)
- Presence of comorbidities (eg, coronary artery disease, hypertension, diabetes, atrial fibrillation)
- Presence of volume overload (eg, weight gain, rales, jugular vein distension, peripheral edema)
- Presence of exertional dyspnea, orthopnea, fatigue
- Emotional status (eg, presence of anxiety, depression)

Plan*

- HFrEF
  - Initiate and titrate guideline-directed medical therapy (GDMT) with ARNI/ACEI/ARB (ARNI preferred) + β-blocker + aldosterone antagonist + SGLT2 inhibitor (Fig. 36-6, Tables 36-7 and 36-9). Add diuretics if the patient is volume overloaded
  - Add additional drug therapy as indicated based on patient characteristics (eg, isosorbide/hydralazine, ivabradine, digoxin, vericiguat [Figs. 36-6 and 36-7, Tables 36-7 and 36-9])
- HFpEF
  - Initiate and titrate GDMT with ARNI + aldosterone antagonist + SGLT2 inhibitor in select patients (Tables 36-7 to 36-9). Add diuretics if the patient is volume overloaded.
- Monitoring parameters including efficacy (eg, shortness of breath, lower extremity edema, pulmonary congestion) and safety (eg, worsening renal function, hypotension, bradycardia [if prescribed β-blocker, ivabradine, or digoxin], hyperkalemia); follow-up frequency and timing
- Patient education (eg, the purpose of treatment, dietary and lifestyle modification, invasive procedures, drug-specific information, medication administration)
- Self-monitoring for HF symptoms (eg, daily weights, sodium and fluid intake)
- Referrals to other providers when appropriate (eg, HF specialist for consideration of advanced therapies [HFrEF], electrophysiologist for placement of ICD [HFrEF, secondary prevention of sudden cardiac death in select patients with HFpEF] and/or CRT [HFrEF], dietician)

Implement*

- Provide patient education regarding all elements of the treatment plan
- Use motivational interviewing and coaching strategies to maximize adherence
- Schedule follow-up (eg, serum creatinine, electrolytes, vital signs, adherence assessment)

Follow-up: Monitor and Evaluate

- Resolution of HF signs and symptoms (eg, JVD, weight, shortness of breath)
- Evaluate the need for dose titration of GDMT and/or the initiation of additional therapies
- Presence of adverse effects (eg, serum creatinine, electrolytes, BP, HR)
- Patient adherence to treatment plan using multiple sources of information

**Collaborate with the patient, caregivers, and other healthcare professionals.*

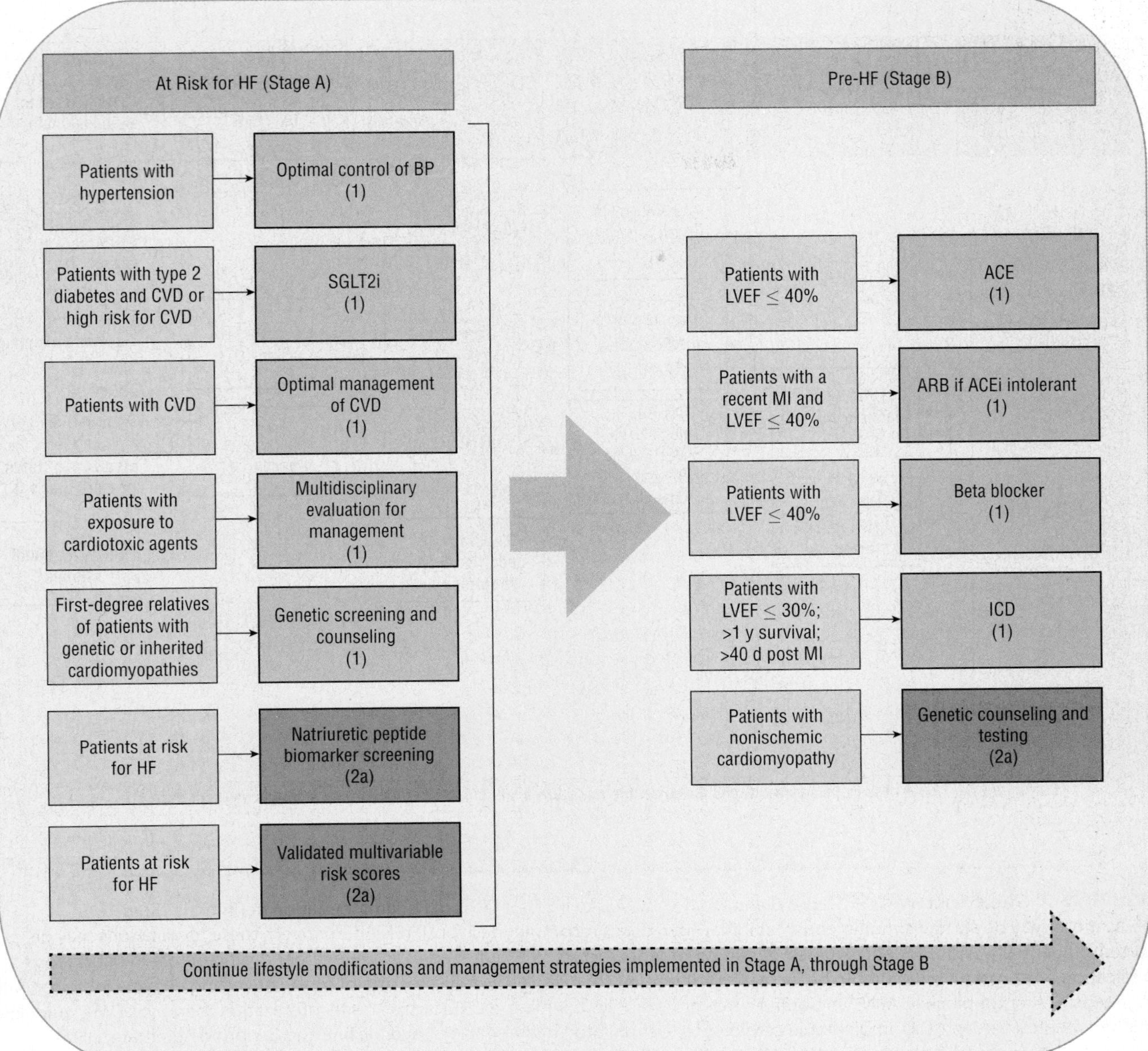

FIGURE 36-6 Recommendations (Class 1 and 2a) for Patients at Risk of HF (stage A) and those with Pre-HF (stage B). See ACC/AHA/HFSA for Class of Recommendation definitions provided under each recommendation (e.g., 1, 2a). ACEi, angiotensin converting enzyme inhibitor; ARB, angiotensin receptor blocker; BP, blood pressure; CVD, cardiovascular disease; HF, heart failure; ICD, implantable cardioverter-defiibrillator; LVEF, left ventricular ejection fraction; MI, myocardial infarction; SGLT2i, sodium glucose cotransporter 2 inhibitor *(Data from Reference 22.)*

Other important general measures include patient and family counseling on the signs and symptoms of HF, detailed written instructions on the importance of appropriate medication use and compliance, activity level, diet, discharge medications, weight monitoring, continuity of care, and the need for close monitoring and follow-up to reinforce compliance and minimize the risk of HF exacerbations and subsequent hospitalization.[22]

4 Treatment guidelines are organized around the four identified stages of HFrEF, and the recommendations are summarized in Fig. 36-6 and Fig. 36-7.[22,34] These figures address stages A-D with stage D discussed in greater detail in "Acute Decompensated Heart Failure," Chapter 37. While the guidelines primarily focus on HFrEF, discussions of HFpEF, acute decompensated HF, and management of patients with comorbid diseases often encountered in this population are included. Dosing recommendations for GDMT used to treat patients with HFrEF and HFpEF are provided in Table 36-7.

Less information guiding the treatment of HFpEF is available. This relative paucity of evidence is reflected in guidelines for the diagnosis and management of HFpEF; however, the most recent ACC/AHA/HFSA guidelines provided greater clarity.[22,30,44] In general, all three guidelines recommend treating comorbid conditions by controlling HR and BP, alleviating causes of myocardial ischemia, reducing volume, and restoring and maintaining sinus rhythm in

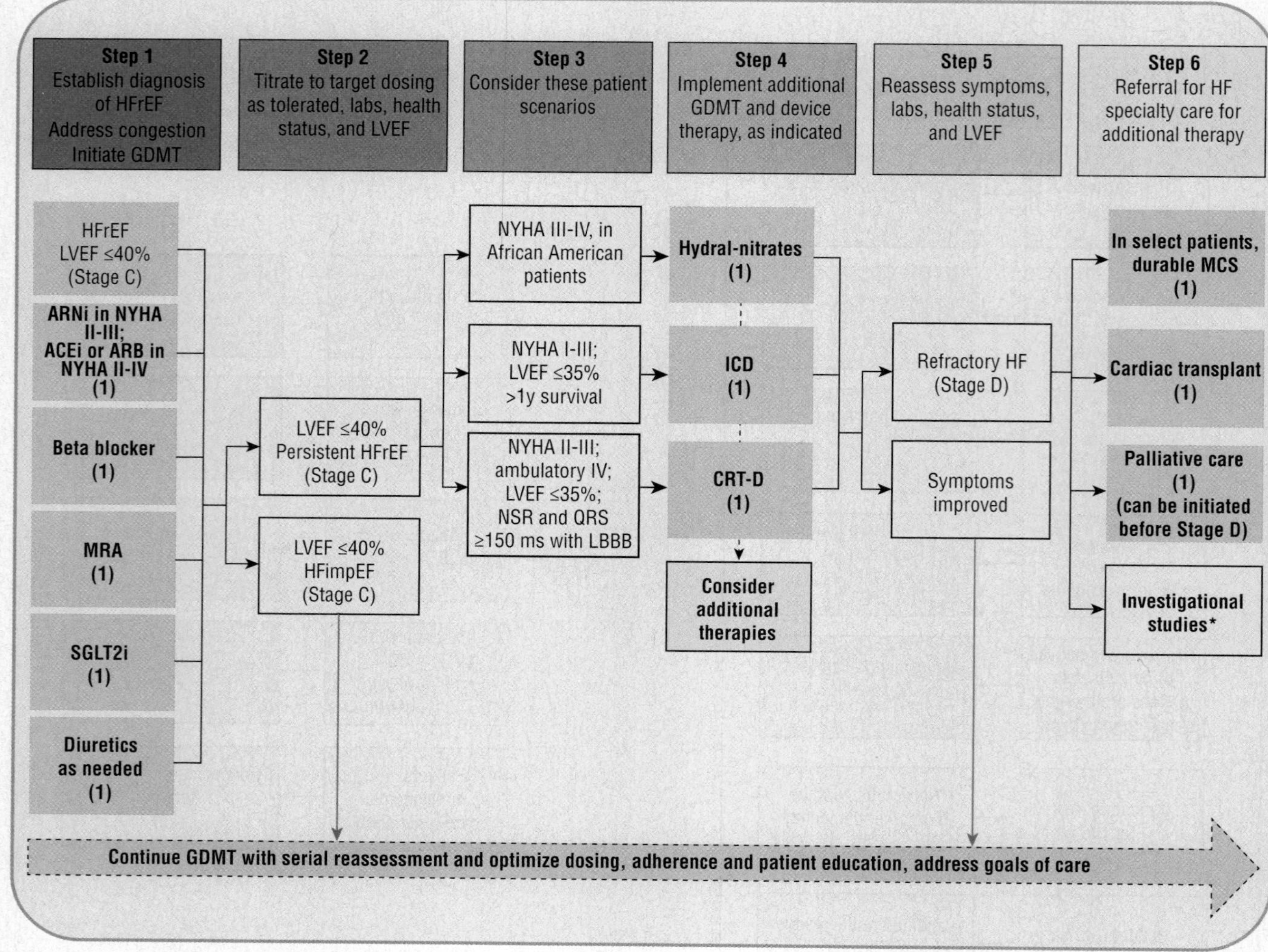

FIGURE 36-7 GTreatment of HFrEF Stages C and D. See ACC/AHA/HFSA for Class of Recommendation definitions. Step 1 medications may be started simultaneously at initial (low) doses recommended for HFrEF. Alternatively, these medications may be started sequentially, with sequence guided by clinical or other factors, without need to achieve target dosing before initiating next medication. Medication doses should be increased to target as tolerated. ACEi indicates angiotensin-converting enzyme inhibitor; ARB, angiotensin receptor blocker; ARNi, angiotensin receptor-neprilysin inhibitor; CRT, cardiac resynchronization therapy; GDMT, guideline-directed medical therapy; ICD, implantable cardioverter-defibrillator; hydral-nitrates, hydralazine and isosorbide dinitrate; HFrEF, heart failure with reduced ejection fraction; LBBB, left bundle branch block; MCS, mechanical circulatory support; LVEF, left ventricular ejection fraction; MRA, mineralocorticoid receptor antagonist; NSR, normal sinus rhythm; NYHA, New York Heart Association; and SGLT2i, sodium-glucose cotransporter 2 inhibitor.
*Participation in investigational studies is appropriate for stage C, NYHA class II and III HF. *(Data from Reference 22.)*

patients with atrial fibrillation. Table 36-8 summarizes the therapeutic recommendations for HFpEF.

As the management of HF has become increasingly complex, disease management programs that include HF specialty clinics, home-based interventions, structured telephone support, and close patient follow-up are frequently used. Most are multidisciplinary and may include physicians, advanced practice nurses, dieticians, and pharmacists. In general, the programs focus on optimization of drug and non-drug therapy, patient and family education and counseling, exercise and dietary advice, intense follow-up by telephone or home visits, improving adherence to medications and lifestyle recommendations, encouragement of self-care, early recognition of and management of volume overload, and referral to palliative care when appropriate.[22] Such programs typically focus on patients with more severe HF who are at high risk for hospital admission. In general, multidisciplinary disease management programs improve quality of life and reduce HF and all-cause hospitalizations and costs, although these benefits are not consistently demonstrated in all studies.

Treatment of Stage A Heart Failure

Patients who are at risk for HF are classified as Stage A.[1] These patients have no HF signs and symptoms or structural or biomarker evidence of heart disease but are at risk for developing HF because of the presence of risk factors (Fig. 36-6). The emphasis in these patients is on risk factor identification and modification to prevent the development of structural heart disease and subsequent HF. Commonly encountered risk factors

TABLE 36-7 Guideline Recommended Drug Therapies and Doses for HFrEF and HFpEF

Drug	Brand Name	Initial Dose	Usual Range	Special Population Dose	Comments
Loop Diuretics					
Furosemide	Lasix®	20-40 mg once or twice daily	20-160 mg once or twice daily	Cl_{cr} 20-50 mL/min (0.33-0.83 mL/s): 160 mg once or twice daily Cl_{cr} <20 mL/min (0.33 mL/s): 400 mg daily	Single doses exceeding those listed are unlikely to elicit additional response
Bumetanide	Bumex®	0.5-1.0 mg once or twice daily	1-2 mg once or twice daily	Cl_{cr} 20-50 mL/min (0.33-0.83 mL/s): 2 mg once or twice daily Cl_{cr} <20 mL/min (0.33 mL/s): 8-10 mg daily	Single doses exceeding those listed are unlikely to elicit additional response
Torsemide	Demadex®	10-20 mg once daily	10-80 mg once daily	Cl_{cr} 20-50 mL/min (0.33-0.83 mL/s): 40 mg once daily Cl_{cr} <20 mL/min (0.33 mL/s): 200 mg daily	Single doses exceeding those listed are unlikely to elicit additional response
ACE Inhibitors					
Captopril	Capoten®	6.25 mg three times daily	50 mg three times daily[a]		
Enalapril	Vasotec®	2.5 mg twice daily	10-20 mg twice daily[a]		
Lisinopril	Zestril®, Prinivil®	2.5-5.0 mg once daily	20-40 mg once daily[a]		
Quinapril	Accupril®	5 mg twice daily	20-40 mg twice daily		
Ramipril	Altace®	1.25-2.5 mg once daily	10 mg once daily[a]		
Fosinopril	Monopril®	5-10 mg once daily	40 mg once daily		Undergoes both hepatic and renal elimination
Trandolapril	Mavik®	1.0 mg once daily	4 mg once daily[a]		Undergoes both hepatic and renal elimination
Perindopril	Aceon®	2 mg once daily	8-16 mg once daily		Undergoes both hepatic and renal elimination
Angiotensin Receptor Blockers					
Candesartan	Atacand®	4-8 mg once daily	32 mg once daily[a]		
Valsartan	Diovan®	20-40 mg twice daily	160 mg twice daily[a]		
Losartan	Cozaar®	25-50 mg once daily	150 mg once daily[a]		
Angiotensin Receptor Blocker/Neprilysin Inhibitor					
Sacubitril/valsartan	Entresto®	49/51 mg sacubitril/valsartan twice daily	97/103 mg sacubitril/valsartan twice daily[a]		For patients taking a low dose of or not taking an ACE inhibitor or ARB or if eGFR is <30 mL/min/1.73 m², the starting dose is 24/26-mg sacubitril/valsartan twice daily
Beta-blockers					
Bisoprolol	Zebeta®	1.25 mg once daily	10 mg once daily[a]		
Carvedilol	Coreg®	3.125 mg twice daily	25 mg twice daily[a]	Target dose for patients weighing >85 kg is 50 mg twice daily	Should be taken with food
Carvedilol phosphate	Coreg CR®	10 mg once daily	80 mg once daily		Should be taken with food
Metoprolol succinate CR/XL	Toprol-XL®	12.5-25 mg once daily	200 mg once daily[a]		
Aldosterone Antagonists					
Spironolactone	Aldactone®	eGFR >50 mL/min/1.73 m²: 12.5-25 mg once daily	25-50 mg once daily[a]	eGFR 30-49 mL/min/1.73 m²: 12.5 mg once daily or every other day	The risk of hyperkalemia increases if serum creatinine is >1.6 mg/dL (141 µmol/L). Avoid if baseline potassium is >5 mEq/L (mmol/L)
Eplerenone	Inspra®	eGFR >50 mL/min/1.73 m²: 25 mg once daily	50 mg once daily[a]	eGFR 30-49 mL/min/1.73 m²: 25 mg every other day	The risk of hyperkalemia increases if serum creatinine is >1.6 mg/dL (141 µmol/L). Avoid if baseline potassium is >5 mEq/L (mmol/L)

(continued)

TABLE 36-7 Guideline Recommended Drug Therapies and Doses for HFrEF and HFpEF (*Continued*)

Drug	Brand Name	Initial Dose	Usual Range	Special Population Dose	Comments
SGLT2 Inhibitors					
Dapagliflozin	Farxiga®	10 mg daily	10 mg daily	eGFR ≥30 mL/min/1.73 m²	
Empagliflozin	Jardiance®	10 mg daily	10 mg daily	eGFR ≥20 mL/min/1.73 m²	
Others					
Hydralazine-Isosorbide Dinitrate	Bidil®	Hydralazine 37.5 mg three times daily	Hydralazine 75 mg three times daily[a]		Indicated in conjunction with standard heart failure therapy in patients with HFrEF to improve survival and reduce hospitalizations in Black patients. Also an alternative if intolerance to ACEI/ARB/ARNI (eg, angioedema)
Digoxin	Lanoxin®	Isosorbide dinitrate 20 mg three times daily 0.125-0.25 mg once daily	Isosorbide dinitrate 40 mg three times daily[a] 0.125-0.25 mg once daily	Reduce dose in elderly, patients with low lean body mass, and patients with impaired renal function	Indicated in conjunction with standard HF therapy in patients with HFrEF to improve symptoms and reduce hospitalizations. Target plasma concentration range is 0.5-0.9 ng/mL (μg/L; 0.6-1.2 nmol/L). Does not improve survival in patients with HFrEF
Ivabradine	Corlanor®	5 mg twice daily	5-7.5 mg twice daily	Avoid if resting heart rate <60 BPM before treatment	Indicated in conjunction with standard HF therapy in patients with HFrEF to reduce the risk of hospitalization in patients with HFrEF with a resting heart rate >70 BPM receiving maximally tolerated beta-blocker doses. Take with meals
Vericiguat	Verquvo®	2.5 mg once daily	10 mg once daily		Indicated in conjunction with standard HF therapy in patients with HFrEF to improve CV survival and reduce HF hospitalization. Take with food

[a]Regimens proven in large clinical trials to reduce mortality.

BPM, beats per minute; Cl_{cr}, creatinine clearance; CV, cardiovascular; eGFR, estimated glomerular filtration rate; HF, heart failure; HFrEF, heart failure with reduced ejection fraction.

Data from References 22 and 86.

TABLE 36-8 Pharmacotherapy for Heart Failure with Preserved Ejection Fraction

Recommendations

- Patients with HFpEF and hypertension should have medication titrated to attain blood pressure targets in accordance with published clinical practice guidelines to prevent morbidity. (a)
- In patients with HFpEF, SGLT2i can be beneficial in decreasing HF hospitalizations and cardiovascular mortality. (2a)
- In patients with HFpEF, management of AF can be useful to improve symptoms. (2a)
- In selected patients with HFpEF, MRAs may be considered to decrease hospitalizations, particularly among patients with LVEF on the lower end of this spectrum. (2b)
- In selected patients with HFpEF, the use of ARBs may be considered to decrease hospitalizations, particularly among patients with LVEF on the lower end of this spectrum. (2b)
- In selected patients with HFpEF, ARNI may be considered to decrease hospitalizations, particularly among patients with LVEF on the lower end of this spectrum (2b).

See ACC/AHA/HFSA for Class of Recommendation definitions provided under each recommendation (e.g., 1, 2a, 2b).

AF, atrial fibrillation; ARB, angiotensin receptor blocker; ARNI, angiotensin II receptor-neprilysin inhibitor; HFpEF, heart failure with preserved ejection fraction; LVEF, left ventricular ejection fraction; MRA mineralcorticoid receptor antagonist; SGLT2i, sodium glucose cotransporter 2 inhibitor

Data from Reference 22 and 30.

include HTN, dyslipidemia, diabetes, obesity, metabolic syndrome, smoking, exposure to cardiotoxins, and coronary artery disease, among others. Although each of these disorders individually increases risk, they frequently coexist in many patients and act synergistically to foster the development of both HFrEF and HFpEF.[3] Effective blood pressure control reduces the risk of developing HF by approximately 50%; thus, current HTN-treatment guidelines should be followed.[3,22,36] Obesity, diabetes, and metabolic syndrome also importantly contribute to the risk of developing HF.[3,45] Appropriate management of coronary disease and its associated risk factors are also important. Although treatment must be individualized, ACE inhibitors or ARBs and statins are recommended for HF prevention in select patients with atherosclerotic vascular disease or diabetes.[34] New to the into guidelines addressing Stage A HF, sodium-glucose cotransporter type 2 (SGLT2) inhibitors should be strongly considered in patients with with type 2 diabetes and CVD or high risk for CVD as these agents reduce the risks of adverse cardiovascular events and hospitalization for HF.[45,46]

Treatment of Stage B Heart Failure

Patients in Stage B, or pre-HF, have structural heart disease, abnormal cardiac function (eg, systolic and/or diastolic dysfunction), or increased natriuretic peptide plasma concentrations, but do not have current or prior HF symptoms.[1] This group includes patients with left ventricular hypertrophy, recent or remote MI, valvular disease, or LVEF <40% (0.4). Treatment is targeted at minimizing additional injury and preventing or slowing the remodeling process. In addition to the treatment measures outlined in Stage A, all patients with an LVEF <40% (0.4) should receive an ACE inhibitor or ARB and a β-blocker, especially if there is a history of MI.[22] Management strategies implemented in patients at risk for HF (stage A) should be continued through stage B.[22]

Treatment of Stage C Heart Failure

Patients with structural heart disease and previous or current symptoms are classified in Stage C. Most patients with HFrEF in Stage C should be routinely treated with GDMT proven to improve morbidity and mortality (Fig. 36-7).[22] In select patients, hydralazine-isosorbide dinitrate (ISDN), loop diuretics, digoxin, ivabradine, and vericiguat may also be considered.[22] Nonpharmacologic therapy with devices such as an implantable cardioverter-defibrillator (ICD) or cardiac resynchronization therapy (CRT) with a biventricular pacemaker is also indicated in certain patients with HFrEF in Stage C (see the "Nonpharmacologic Therapy" section).[22]

Treatment of Stage D Heart Failure

Patients with advanced HF are classified as Stage D.[1] These patients experience persistent symptoms despite receiving maximally tolerated GDMT. This stage is often also referred to as refractory or end-stage HF. These patients often undergo recurrent hospitalizations or cannot be discharged from the hospital without special interventions, have a poor quality of life, and are at high risk for morbidity and mortality. Patients with advanced HFrEF should be considered for referral to HF management programs so that specialized therapies including mechanical circulatory support, cardiac transplantation, and palliative care may be considered in addition to standard treatments outlined in Stages A to C.[34,49] Unfortunately, these same advanced therapies are not beneficial for patients with HFpEF. For all patients with advanced HFrEF or HFpEF, discussions with the patient and family members regarding prognosis, patient priorities for minimizing symptoms versus prolonging survival, options for additional treatments, and end-of-life and hospice care should be initiated.[22] The approach to the treatment of patients with Stage D HF is discussed in more detail in Chapter 37.

Nonpharmacologic Therapy

Sudden cardiac death, primarily due to ventricular tachycardia and fibrillation, is responsible for 40% to 50% of the mortality in patients with HFrEF. Implantation of an ICD prevents sudden cardiac death and is an effective primary prevention strategy to reduce the risk of mortality in selected patients with HFrEF.[50] Current guidelines recommend the use of an ICD for primary prevention in patients receiving GDMT with NYHA class II-III symptoms and an LVEF <35% (0.35) that are expected to live for at least 1 year.[50] In patients with NYHA class I symptoms and an LVEF <30% (0.30), an ICD is also recommended for primary prevention if life expectancy exceeds 1 year.[50]

Delayed electrical activation of the left ventricle, characterized on the ECG by a QRS duration that exceeds 120 ms, occurs in approximately one-third of patients with moderate-to-severe HFrEF. Since the left and right ventricles normally activate simultaneously, this delay results in asynchronous contraction of the ventricles and contributes to the hemodynamic abnormalities of HF. Implantation of a specialized biventricular pacemaker, cardiac resynchronization therapy (CRT), to restore synchronous activation of the ventricles improves ventricular function and hemodynamics and is associated with reverse remodeling and increased LVEF. The use of CRT improves exercise capacity, symptoms, quality of life, hospitalizations, and mortality in patients with HRrEF.[22] Guidelines recommend CRT in patients receiving GDMT that have NYHA class II-III or ambulatory class IV symptoms and with a QRS duration >150 ms and LVEF <35% (0.35).[22] CRT can also be considered in selected patients with a QRS duration between 120 and 149 ms. Combined CRT and ICD devices are used if the patient meets the indications for both devices.

Wireless hemodynamic monitoring of pulmonary artery pressures remotely as a supplemental measurement of fluid status in patients at high risk for HF-related hospitalization is now possible.[51] The CardioMEMS™ implantable pulmonary artery sensor reduces the risk of HF hospitalization in selected patients.[52] In contrast, the usefulness of noninvasive telemonitoring or remote monitoring of physiological parameters (eg, patient activity, impedance, HR) via implanted electrical devices (ICDs or CRT-Ds) to improve clinical outcomes remains uncertain.

In patients with stage D HFrEF receiving GDMT, the use of mechanical circulatory support with a left ventricular assist device (LVAD) can be considered in certain patients.[22] Although the criteria for use of these devices continue to rapidly evolve, they are frequently used to bridge patients to cardiac transplant or as destination therapy in patients ineligible for transplant, and their use in these settings is associated with better survival and improved functional capacity.[22,53] Their use is covered in more detail in Chapter 37 (Acute Decompensated Heart Failure).

Pharmacologic Therapy

Pharmacologic Therapy for Stages B-D HFrEF

A treatment algorithm for the management of patients with Stages A or B HFrEF is shown in Fig. 36-6 and for Stages C and D HFrEF in Fig. 36-7. In general, patients with Stage B HFrEF should receive an ACE inhibitor or ARB and β-blocker and, in select patients, an SGLT2 inhibitor.[22] Patients with Stage C HFrEF should receive combined therapy with an ARNI (preferred) or ACE inhibitor or ARB, β-blocker, aldosterone antagonist, and SGLT2 inhibitor.[22] The optimal sequence for initiating these four medication classes remains uncertain. However, there is growing interest in simultaneous initiation of low doses of each drug class due to the incremental and early benefits of these different medications on morbidity and mortality.[54,55] Given the demonstrated benefits of optimal GDMT on crucial outcomes and that large numbers of patients receive inadequate GDMT, strategies to improve the initiation and dose titration of these life-saving treatments are clearly needed.[56,57]

A diuretic should be administered if there is evidence of fluid retention. Other therapies including the combination of hydralazine-nitrates, digoxin, ivabradine, or vericiguat can be considered in selected patients.[22] Drug dosing and monitoring are summarized in Tables 36-7 and 36-9.

Pharmacologic Therapy for HFpEF

With a few notable exceptions, the drugs used to treat HFpEF are the same as those used to treat HFrEF. However, the rationale for their use, the pathophysiologic process that is being addressed by the drug, and the dosing regimen may be different. For example, β-blockers are recommended for the treatment of both HFrEF and HFpEF. However, in HFpEF, β-blockers should only be prescribed to those patients who have a comorbid condition that have an indication for β-blocker therapy. In HFpEF, ACE inhibitors, ARBs, and β-blockers have not demonstrated efficacy in the absence of other comorbid conditions such as HTN or myocardial infarction. Diuretics also are used in the treatment of both HFrEF and HFpEF. However, the doses of diuretics used to treat HFpEF are, in general, much lower than those used to treat HFrEF. Some drugs, however, are used to treat HFpEF, but not HFrEF. Calcium channel blockers such as diltiazem, amlodipine, and verapamil have little utility in the treatment of HFrEF and are often contraindicated as described in Table 36-4. In contrast, each of these drugs may be useful in the treatment of HFpEF when used for the treatment of HTN. ARNIs and SGLT2 inhibitors are beneficial in select patients with HFpEF. Drug dosing and monitoring for these agents is similar in HFrEF and HFpEF and are summarized in Tables 36-7 and 36-9.

While dozens of trials demonstrated the benefit of pharmacotherapy in patients with HFrEF, only a few recent studies

TABLE 36-9 Drug Monitoring

Drug Class	Adverse Effect	Monitoring Parameters	Comments
Diuretics	Hypovolemia, hypotension, hyponatremia, hypokalemia, hypomagnesemia, hyperuricemia, renal dysfunction, thirst	BP, electrolytes, BUN, creatinine, glucose, uric acid, changes in weight, JVD	Dose should be adjusted based on volume status, renal function, electrolytes, and BP. Reassess these parameters 1-2 weeks after dose changes. Goal is lowest dose that maintains euvolemia.
ACE inhibitors	Angioedema, cough, hyperkalemia, hypotension, renal dysfunction	BP, electrolytes, BUN, and creatinine	Contraindicated in patients with bilateral renal artery stenosis, history of angioedema, or pregnancy. Assess BP, BUN, creatinine, and electrolytes at baseline and 1-2 weeks after initiation or increase in dose. Goal is target dose from clinical trials or highest tolerated.
ARBs	Hyperkalemia, hypotension, renal dysfunction	BP, electrolytes, BUN, and creatinine	Contraindicated in patients with bilateral renal artery stenosis or pregnancy. Assess BP, BUN, creatinine, and electrolytes at baseline and 1-2 weeks after initiation or increase in dose. Use with caution in patients with a history of ACE inhibitor-associated angioedema. Goal is target dose from clinical trials or highest tolerated.
ARNI	Angioedema, hyperkalemia, hypotension, dizziness, renal dysfunction	BP, electrolytes, BUN, and creatinine	Contraindicated in patients with a history of angioedema associated with ACE inhibitor or ARB therapy or in pregnancy. ACE inhibitors should be discontinued at least 36 hours before ARNI initiation. Assess BP, BUN, creatinine, and electrolytes at baseline and 1-2 weeks after initiation or dose increase. Start with a low dose and double the dose every 2-4 weeks as tolerated based on BP, serum potassium, and renal function. Goal is target dose from clinical trials or highest tolerated.
β-Blockers	Bradycardia, heart block, bronchospasm, hypotension, worsening HF	BP, HR, ECG, signs and symptoms of worsening HF, blood glucose	Start with low dose and titrate upward no more often than every 2 weeks as tolerated based on BP, HR, and symptoms. Goal is target dose from clinical trials or highest tolerated. Patients may feel worse before they feel better.
Aldosterone antagonists	Gynecomastia/breast tenderness/ menstrual irregularities (spironolactone), hyperkalemia, worsening renal function	BP, electrolytes, BUN, and creatinine	Assess BP, BUN, creatinine, and electrolytes at baseline. Check potassium 3 days and 1 week after initiation and then monthly for the first 3 months. Change to eplerenone if gynecomastia develops with spironolactone.
SGLT2 inhibitors	Mycotic genital infections, volume depletion, acute kidney injury, or impairment of renal function, necrotizing fasciitis of the perineum (Fournier's gangrene), urosepsis or pyelonephritis, diabetic ketoacidosis	Volume status (weight, BP, hematocrit, electrolytes), BUN, and creatinine, blood glucose and HbA1c if diabetic	Contraindicated for patients on dialysis (per package insert), lactating (no data), or with type 1 diabetes (risk of euglycemic acidosis). Monitor volume status, especially if receiving concomitant diuretics. Benefit for HFrEF is regardless of presence of diabetes.
Hydralazine	Hypotension, headache, rash, arthralgia, lupus, tachycardia	BP, HR	
Nitrates	Hypotension, headache, lightheadedness	BP, HR	
Digoxin	GI and CNS adverse effects, brady- and tachyarrhythmias	Electrolytes, BUN, creatinine, ECG, serum digoxin concentration	Target serum digoxin concentration 0.5-0.9 ng/mL (μg/L; 0.6-1.2 nmol/L)
Ivabradine	Bradycardia, hypertension, atrial fibrillation, luminous phenomena (phosphenes, transiently enhanced brightness in a portion of the visual field)	BP, HR, ECG	Start with 5 mg twice daily and after 2 weeks adjust dose to achieve a resting HR 50-60 BPM. Only use in patients in sinus rhythm.
Vericiguat	Hypotension, anemia	BP, Hgb, Hct	

demonstrated benefit in patients with HFpEF. Early trials led to ARBs and spironolactone being recommended in HFpEF patients to reduce hospitalization.[27,58] While most studies targeting the renin-angiotensin-aldosterone system have been disappointing, the PARAGON-HF trial led to sacubitril/valsartan being the first therapy approved in the United States to reduce cardiovascular mortality and hospitalizations in patients diagnosed with HF regardless of LVEF, with the greatest benefit evident in patients with LVEF below normal.[48] Shortly afterward, the EMPEROR-Preserved Trial also demonstrated benefit with the SGLT2 inhibitor empagliflozin.[47] The results of these two pivotal HFpEF clinical trials are summarized in Table 36-10.

ACE Inhibitors

5 For decades, ACE inhibitors have been a key component of the pharmacotherapy of patients with HFrEF.[22] By blocking the conversion of angiotensin I to angiotensin II by ACE, the production of angiotensin II and, in turn, aldosterone is decreased. This decrease in angiotensin II and aldosterone attenuates many of the deleterious effects of these neurohormones that drive HF initiation and progression. ACE inhibitors also inhibit the breakdown of bradykinin, which increases vasodilation and also leads to cough. The evidence that ACE inhibitors improve symptoms, slow disease progression, and decrease mortality in patients with HFrEF is unequivocal. As a result, prior and current guidelines recommend that all patients

TABLE 36-10 Key Clinical Trials for HFpEF

Trial (No. of Patients)	Treatment	Inclusion Criteria	Primary Endpoint	Results
EMPEROR-Preserved (n = 5,988)[47]	Empagliflozin vs placebo daily for a median follow-up of 26.2 months, in addition to usual therapy	NYHA II-IV, EF >40% (0.40), NT-proBNP >300 pg/mL (ng/L; 35 pmol/L) (>900 pg/mL [ng/L; 106 pmol/L] for patients with atrial fibrillation at baseline)	Composite of adjudicated CV death or hospitalization for HF	The primary outcome occurred in 13.8% of the empagliflozin group and 17.1% of the placebo group (HR 0.79, $P < 0.001$). Of the two composite endpoints, there was only a significant reduction, in the risk of hospitalization for heart failure.
PARAGON-HF[48] (n = 4,822)	Sacubitril/valsartan vs valsartan	NYHA class II-IV with EF >45% (0.45)	Composite of CV death and total HF hospitalization	No significant difference was found in the primary endpoint between treatment groups (rate ratio 0.87; 95% CI 0.75-1.01, $P = 0.06$). A prespecified subgroup demonstrated benefit in patients with an EF in the lower part (45%-57% [0.45-0.57]) of the range.

NYHA, New York Heart Association; EF, ejection fraction; CV, cardiovascular; HF, heart failure; HR, hazard ratio; CI, confidence interval.

with HFrEF, regardless of whether or not symptoms are present, should receive ACE inhibitors to reduce morbidity and mortality, unless there are contraindications.[22,30,34] As described above, more recent evidence suggests that sacubitril/valsartan is preferred over ACE inhibitors (or ARBs) for HFrEF unless other circumstances (eg, affordability) are present in individual patients.

Numerous placebo-controlled clinical trials in both symptomatic and asymptomatic patients with reduced LVEF have documented the favorable effects of ACE inhibitor therapy on symptoms, HF progression, hospitalizations, and quality of life.[22] ACE inhibitors improve survival compared with placebo, and these benefits are maintained with continued therapy.[22] The benefits of ACE inhibitor therapy are independent of the etiology of HF (ischemic vs nonischemic) and are greatest in patients with the most severe symptoms. As efficacy has been demonstrated with numerous agents, the improved outcomes are a "class effect" of ACE inhibitors.

ACE inhibitor therapy should be started with low doses followed by gradual titration as tolerated to the target or maximally tolerated doses.[34,59] Dose titration is usually accomplished by doubling the dose every 2 weeks. Higher doses further reduce the risk of hospitalization, but not mortality, compared to lower doses.[34] Blood pressure, renal function, and serum potassium should be evaluated at baseline and within 1 to 2 weeks after therapy is started and after each dose increase. Although symptoms may improve within a few days of initiating therapy, it may take weeks to months before the full benefits are apparent. Even if symptoms do not improve, long-term ACE inhibitor therapy should be continued to reduce the risk of mortality and hospitalization.

A number of ACE inhibitors are available; those commonly used in the treatment of patients with HF are summarized in Table 36-7. Although ACE inhibitors vary in their chemical structure (eg, sulfhydryl vs non–sulfhydryl-containing agents) and tissue affinity, all ACE inhibitors studied improve symptoms and mortality in patients with HFrEF.[22] However, it seems most prudent to use those agents documented to reduce morbidity and mortality because the dose required for these endpoints has been determined.

Similar to sacubitril/valsartan and ARBs, the primary adverse effects of ACE inhibitors are secondary to their major pharmacologic action of suppressing angiotensin II and increasing bradykinin. Hence, common adverse effects of ACE inhibitors are hypotension, renal dysfunction, and hyperkalemia.

A dry, nonproductive cough is the most common reason for discontinuation of ACE inhibitors, occurring in up to 15% to 20% of patients with a similar frequency with all the agents.[34] The cough usually occurs within the first few months of therapy, resolves within 1 to 2 weeks of drug discontinuation, and reappears with rechallenge. Because cough is a bradykinin-mediated effect, the replacement of ACE inhibitor therapy with sacubitril/valsartan (preferred) or an ARB is reasonable. Angioedema is a potentially life-threatening complication that is also due to bradykinin accumulation and occurs in approximately 1% of patients receiving an ACE inhibitor. It occurs more frequently in patients older than 65 years, Black patients, women, and patients with histories of drug rashes or seasonal allergies.[60] The use of ACE inhibitors is contraindicated in patients with a history of angioedema. Caution should be exercised if ARBs are used as an alternative therapy in patients with ACE inhibitor-induced angioedema, as cross-reactivity is reported.[34] ACE inhibitors are contraindicated in pregnancy due to the increased risk of fetal renal failure, intrauterine growth retardation, and other congenital defects.

Angiotensin II Receptor Blockers

5 The crucial role of the RAAS in the HF development and progression is well established as are the benefits of inhibiting this system with ACE inhibitors. However, angiotensin II can be formed in a number of tissues, including the heart, through non–ACE-dependent pathways (eg, chymase, cathepsin, and kallikrein).[11] By blocking the angiotensin II receptor subtype, AT1, ARBs attenuate the deleterious effects of angiotensin II on ventricular remodeling, regardless of the site of origin of the hormone. Since ARBs do not inhibit the ACE enzyme, these agents do not affect bradykinin, which is linked to ACE inhibitor cough and angioedema.

While ARBs are a guideline-recommended alternative in patients who are unable to tolerate an ACE inhibitor due to cough or angioedema, sacubitril/valsartan is preferred for patients with cough associated with an ACE inhibitor.[22] Numerous ARBs are available but only three agents, candesartan, valsartan, and losartan, are recommended in the treatment guidelines.[22] The efficacy of these agents is supported by the clinical trial data that document a target dose associated with improved survival and other important outcomes in patients with decreased EF.[34] The specific drugs and doses proven to be effective in clinical trials should be used (Table 36-7). The clinical use of ARBs is similar to that of sacubitril/valsartan and ACE inhibitors. Therapy should be initiated at low doses and then titrated to target doses (Table 36-7). Blood pressure, renal function, and serum potassium should be evaluated within 1 to 2 weeks after initiation of therapy and after increases in the dose, and these monitoring, parameters should be used to guide subsequent dose changes.

The role of ARBs in the treatment of HFpEF is less clear. The CHARM-Preserved trial was the first large prospective study to demonstrate some benefit (reduction in hospitalizations for HF) of an ARB in patients with HFpEF receiving standard background treatment, although no improvement in cardiovascular death was observed.[58] Adverse effects of candesartan in this study were frequent with candesartan-treated patients discontinuing therapy because of hypotension, increased serum creatinine, or hyperkalemia.

Similar to ARNI and ACE inhibitors, the major adverse effects of ARBs are related to the suppression of the RAAS. The incidence of and risk factors for developing hypotension, impaired renal function, and hyperkalemia with the ARBs are similar to those with ARNI and ACE inhibitors.[22] Thus, ARBs are not alternatives in patients who develop these complications from ACE inhibitors. Similar to ACE inhibitors, careful monitoring is required when an ARB is used with an aldosterone antagonist as this combination increases the risk of these adverse effects. Since ARBs do not affect bradykinin, they are not associated with cough and have a lower risk of angioedema than ACE inhibitors.[60] However, because of reports of recurrences of angioedema after ARB use in patients with a history of ACE inhibitor-related angioedema, ARBs should be used with caution in any patient with a history of angioedema as cross-reactivity may occur.[60] Like ARNI and ACE inhibitors, ARBs are contraindicated in pregnancy.

Angiotensin II Receptor Blocker/Neprilysin Inhibitor (ARNI)

5 The first and only angiotensin receptor/neprilysin inhibitor approved for the treatment of patients with HFrEF is sacubitril/valsartan. It is a crystalline complex composed of the ARB valsartan and sacubitril, a neprilysin inhibitor prodrug. After ingestion, sacubitril dissociates from the complex and is cleaved into its active form LBQ657, which inhibits the action of neprilysin that degrades natriuretic peptides, bradykinin, and other endogenous vasodilator and natriuretic peptides.[61] By reducing the neprilysin-mediated breakdown of these compounds, vasodilation, diuresis, and natriuresis are enhanced and renin and aldosterone secretion is inhibited.

The PARADIGM-HF study compared sacubitril/valsartan to enalapril in patients with NYHA Class II-IV HFrEF.[29] There was a statistically significant reduction in the primary outcome of combined death from cardiovascular causes or first hospitalization for HF in patients receiving sacubitril/valsartan compared to enalapril. A similar reduction was seen in each component of the primary endpoint and death from any cause was also significantly reduced. Hypotension occurred more frequently in patients randomized to sacubitril/valsartan compared to enalapril. However, more patients receiving enalapril experienced cough and hyperkalemia greater than 6.0 mEq/L (mmol/L). Angioedema was rare in either treatment group.

In the PARAGON-HF study, patients with HFpEF (LVEF of at least 45% [0.45] and NYHA class II-IV symptoms) were randomized to either sacubitril/valsartan or placebo (Table 36-10).[48] The primary endpoint, a composite of total hospitalizations for HF and death from cardiovascular causes, was not significantly different between the sacubitril/valsartan and placebo groups. A prespecified subgroup in patients with an LVEF in the lower part (45%-57% [0.45-0.57]) of the range suggested benefit. Based upon this subgroup analysis, the current guidelines for sacubitril/valsartan have been expanded to include those with HFpEF, particularly those with an LVEF on the lower end of this spectrum.[22]

In patients with HFrEF, ARNI is preferred over either ACE inhibitors or ARBs to improve survival, slow disease progression, reduce hospitalizations, and improve quality of life.[22] Patients receiving ACE inhibitors or ARBs can be switched to ARNI or ARNI can be used as initial treatment in patients with newly detected HFrEF without previous exposure to ACE inhibitors or ARBs.[22] ACE inhibitors should be discontinued 36 hours prior to initiating ARNI; no waiting period is needed in patients receiving an ARB. The rationale for avoiding overlap is due to an increased risk of angioedema given the neprilysin inhibitor, like an ACE inhibitor, prevents the breakdown of bradykinin. The initial starting dose for most patients being treated for HFrEF is 49/51 mg sacubitril/valsartan twice daily and titrated to the target dose of 97/103 mg sacubitril/valsartan twice daily after 2 to 4 weeks. A reduced dose of 24/26 mg sacubitril/valsartan is available for patients taking a low dose of either an ACE inhibitor or an ARB prior to initiation or those with severe renal dysfunction (eGFR <30 mL/min/1.73 m^2). Blood pressure, serum potassium, and renal function should be closely monitored after the start of therapy and after each titration step. The valsartan component of the combination product is 40% to 60% more bioavailable than conventional valsartan tablets. Thus, the 24-mg sacubitril/26-mg valsartan tablet is equivalent to 40 mg of valsartan.[62]

The primary adverse effects of ARNIs are secondary to their major pharmacologic action of suppressing angiotensin II, increasing bradykinin, and increasing BNP. The most common adverse effects of this agent are hypotension, renal dysfunction, and hyperkalemia. Given similar pharmacologic effects of ACE inhibitors and ARBs, specifically on angiotensin II (ACE inhibitors and ARBs) and bradykinin (primarily ACEIs), a similar side effect profile is generally observed. ARNIs, ACE inhibitors, and ARBs reduce BP in nearly all patients. Hypotension occurs most frequently soon after therapy is started, after an increase in dose, or in patients who are volume-depleted as may occur with diuretics. An often overlooked solution to hypotension is to space the administration times of vasoactive medications (eg, diuretics and β-blockers) throughout the day so that these medications are not all administered at or near the same time.

Functional renal insufficiency causes an increase in serum creatinine and blood urea nitrogen (BUN). As CO and renal blood flow decline, renal perfusion is maintained by the vasoconstrictor effect of angiotensin II on the efferent arteriole. Patients most dependent on this system for maintenance of renal perfusion (and therefore most likely to develop renal insufficiency with an ARNI, ACE inhibitor, or ARB) are those with severe HF, hypotension, hyponatremia, volume depletion, bilateral renal artery stenosis, and concomitant use of NSAIDs.[34,59] Increases in serum creatinine of >0.5 mg/dL (44 μmol/L) if the baseline creatinine is <2 mg/dl (177) or >1 mg/dl (88 umol/L) if the baseline creatinine is >2 mg/dL (177 μmol/L) should prompt clinicians to dose reduce or discontinue therapy and evaluate potential causes for the abrupt decline in the renal function. Since renal dysfunction with these agents is secondary to alterations in renal hemodynamics, it is almost always reversible on discontinuation of the drug.

Hyperkalemia with ARNI, ACE inhibitors, or ARBs is most likely to occur in patients with renal insufficiency, in elderly patients, and in those taking concomitant potassium supplements, potassium-containing salt substitutes, or potassium-sparing diuretic therapy (including an aldosterone antagonist), especially if they have diabetes.[63] Patiromer or sodium zirconium cyclosilicate can be used to treat or prevent hyperkalemia in these patients.[63]

In contrast to ACE inhibitors, bradykinin side effects of cough and angioedema are rare with both ARNI and ARBs (the latter by virtue of combining sacubitril with the ARB, valsartan, rather than an ACE inhibitor). In fact, ACE inhibitor cough is a common reason to switch to sacubitril/valsartan or an ARB. While extremely rare, angioedema occurred more frequently with sacubitril/valsartan compared to enalapril (0.5% vs 0.2%, respectively).[29] The risk of angioedema is fourfold higher in Black patients.[63] Unlike ACE inhibitor cough, sacubitril/valsartan is contraindicated in patients with a history of angioedema associated with an ACE inhibitor or ARB. Sacubitril/valsartan is also contraindicated in pregnancy and should not be used concurrently with ACE inhibitors or other ARBs. As previously stated, ARNIs, ACE inhibitors, and ARBs are contraindicated in pregnancy.

β-Blockers

6 β-Blockers antagonize the detrimental effects of the SNS in HF and slow disease progression. Favorable effects of β-blockers in HF include antiarrhythmic effects, attenuation or reversal of ventricular remodeling, reduction in myocyte death from catecholamine-induced necrosis or apoptosis, improvement in left

ventricular systolic function, reductions in HR and ventricular wall stress thereby reducing myocardial oxygen demand, and inhibition of plasma renin release.[34] There is overwhelming clinical trial evidence that β-blockers reduce morbidity and mortality in patients with HFrEF. As such, the ACC/AHA guidelines on the management of HF recommend that evidence-based β-blockers should be used in all stable patients with Stages B-D HFrEF (Figure 36-7) in the absence of contraindications or a clear history of β-blocker intolerance.[22] Patients should receive a β-blocker even if their symptoms are mild or well-controlled with other GDMT. Importantly, it is not essential that doses of other agents (eg, RAAS inhibitors) be optimized before a β-blocker is started because the addition of a β-blocker is likely to be of greater benefit than an increase in the dose of other medications.[30,34] β-Blockers are also recommended for patients with a reduced left ventricular EF (Stage B) to decrease the risk of progression to HF.[22,64]

Three β-blockers, in particular, reduced morbidity and mortality compared with placebo in randomized, controlled trials: carvedilol, metoprolol succinate (CR/XL), and bisoprolol. Each was studied in a large population with the primary endpoint of mortality, and in each case, the trial was stopped early because of significant survival benefit with the β-blocker. The US Carvedilol Heart Failure Study, the MERIT-HF trial with metoprolol succinate (Toprol-XL®), and the CIBIS II trial with bisoprolol each demonstrated a reduction in mortality; the latter two trials also showed a reduction in sudden death and death due to worsening HF compared with placebo.[65-67] Multiple post hoc subgroup analyses of the MERIT-HF and CIBIS II trials suggest that the benefits of β-blockade occur regardless of HF etiology or disease severity.

In contrast to earlier trials in which the majority of participants had either NYHA class II or class III HFrEF, the COPERNICUS trial examined the efficacy and safety of β-blockers in clinically stable patients with class IV HF who had symptoms at rest or with minimal exertion.[68] Like the other studies, COPERNICUS was stopped early after carvedilol demonstrated a significant reduction in mortality. Carvedilol was well tolerated in this population, with fewer participants receiving carvedilol compared with placebo requiring discontinuation of study medication.

In addition to improving survival, β-blockers improve multiple other endpoints. Clinical trials demonstrate reductions in all-cause hospitalization and hospitalizations for worsening HF with the β-blocker therapy.[67,69,70] Increases in LVEF of 5 to 10 units occur after several weeks to months of therapy. β-Blockers decrease ventricular mass, improve the sphericity of the ventricle, and reduce systolic and diastolic volumes (left ventricular end-systolic volume and LVEDV).[8,34] These effects are often collectively called reverse remodeling, referring to the fact that they return the heart toward a more normal size, shape, and function. β-Blockers are also associated with improvements in NYHA functional class, patient symptom scores or quality-of-life assessments, and exercise performance, as assessed by the 6-minute walk test.

6 The benefits of β-blockers in HFrEF are not a class effect; therefore, one of the three agents with proven survival benefits (carvedilol, metoprolol succinate, or bisoprolol) should be used.[22] Metoprolol and bisoprolol selectively block the β1-receptor, while carvedilol blocks the β1-, β2-, and α1-receptors and also possesses antioxidant effects. The smallest commercially available tablet of bisoprolol is a scored 5-mg tablet. Since the recommended starting dose of 1.25 mg/day is not readily available, bisoprolol is the least commonly used of the three agents and, in fact, is not approved for use in HFrEF. Thus, therapy is generally limited to either carvedilol or metoprolol succinate, and there is no compelling evidence that one drug is superior to the other. While one trial found a lower mortality rate in patients treated with carvedilol 25 mg twice daily compared to immediate-release metoprolol 50 mg twice daily,[71] concerns regarding the formulation (immediate-release vs sustained-release) and dose (100 vs 200 mg/day) of metoprolol used limit the conclusions that can be drawn from the trial. The efficacy of the immediate-release formulation in reducing mortality in HF has not been proven. Metoprolol succinate provides more consistent plasma concentrations over a 24-hour period and appears to provide more favorable effects on HR variability, autonomic balance, and BP, suggesting that this formulation might be superior to immediate-release metoprolol. Data from HF registries suggest that metoprolol succinate and carvedilol are similarly effective.[72,73]

Pharmacologic differences between β-blockers may aid in the selection of a specific agent. Carvedilol is expected to have greater antihypertensive effects than the other agents because of its α-receptor blocking properties and may be preferred in patients with poorly controlled BP. Conversely, metoprolol or bisoprolol may be preferred in patients with low BP or dizziness and in patients with significant airway disease given their β-1 selectivity.

Most participants in β-blocker trials were on ACE inhibitors at baseline since the benefits of these agents were proven prior to β-blocker trials. The risk for decompensation during β-blocker initiation may be greater in the absence of preexisting ACE inhibitor, ARB, or ARNI therapy. Thus, ACE inhibitors, ARBs, or ARNIs are generally started first in most patients, especially if there is evidence of volume overload. Initiating a β-blocker first may be advantageous for patients with evidence of excessive SNS activity (eg, tachycardia) and may also be appropriate for patients whose renal function or potassium concentrations preclude starting an ACE inhibitor, ARB, or ARNI at that time.

Components that are critical for successful β-blocker therapy include appropriate patient selection, drug initiation and titration, and patient education. β-Blockers should be initiated in stable patients who have no or minimal evidence of fluid overload.[34] While β-blockers are typically started in the outpatient setting, initiation of a β-blocker prior to discharge in patients who are hospitalized for decompensated HF increases β-blocker usage compared with outpatient initiation without increasing the risk of serious adverse effects.[74,75] However, β-blockers should not be started in patients who are hospitalized in the intensive care unit or required intravenous inotropic support. In unstable patients, other HF therapy should be optimized, and then β-blocker therapy reevaluated once stability is achieved.

Initiation of a β-blocker at normal doses in patients with HF may lead to symptomatic worsening or acute decompensation owing to the drug's negative inotropic effect. For this reason, β-blockers are listed as drugs that may exacerbate or worsen HF (see Table 36-4). To minimize the likelihood of acute decompensation, β-blockers should be started in low doses with slow upward dose titration and close monitoring. β-Blocker doses should be doubled no more often than every 2 weeks, as tolerated, until the target or maximally tolerated dose is reached. Uptitration should be avoided if the patient experiences signs of worsening HF, including volume overload and poor perfusion. Fluid overload may be asymptomatic and manifest solely as an increase in body weight. Mild fluid overload may be managed by intensifying the diuretic therapy. Once the patient has been stabilized, dose titration may continue as tolerated until the target or highest tolerated dose is reached.[34] According to current guidelines, target doses are those associated with reductions in mortality in placebo-controlled clinical trials.[22] The starting and target doses achieved in clinical trials are described in Table 36-7. Data with both metoprolol and carvedilol suggest that HR may serve as a guide to the degree of β-blockade, with a greater magnitude of HR reduction associated with greater improvement in survival. Thus, lower β-blocker doses might be considered reasonable if the reduction in HR indicates a good response to β-blocker therapy.[76] Chapter 37, "Acute Decompensated Heart Failure," will discuss optimal management of β-blocker therapy during hospitalization, addressing appropriate scenarios for continuation and withdrawal of β-blocker therapy.

Good communication between the patient and the healthcare provider(s) is particularly important for successful therapy. It is important to educate patients that β-blocker therapy is expected to positively influence disease progression and survival even if there is little to no symptomatic improvement. Patients should understand that dose titration is a long, gradual process. Patients should also be aware that response to therapy may be delayed and that HF symptoms may actually worsen during the initiation period. In the event of worsening symptoms, patients who understand the potential benefits of long-term β-blocker therapy may be more likely to continue treatment.

As previously discussed, the primary utility of beta-blockers in HFpEF is treating comorbid conditions such as HTN, angina, and myocardial infarction. In patients with HFpEF, β-blockers may help to lower and maintain low pulmonary venous pressures by decreasing HR and increasing the duration of diastole. Tachycardia is poorly tolerated in patients with HFpEF for a variety of reasons. However, excessive bradycardia can result in a fall of CO despite an increase in LV filling. Such considerations underscore the need for individualizing therapeutic interventions that affect HR. In general, it is not necessary to start at an extremely low dose and titrate the β-blocker in a slow, progressive fashion in HFpEF as it is in HFrEF. However, because patients tend to be older, have numerous comorbidities, and take many concomitant medications, it is prudent to start with a moderate dose of β-blockers in HFpEF. A meta-analysis examining the effects of β-blocker therapy on clinical outcomes in patients with HFpEF found lower all-cause mortality but no significant reduction for HF hospitalizations in observational studies.[77] In contrast, an individual patient-level meta-analysis found no benefit of β-blocker therapy in patients with HFpEF (EF >50% [0.5]) in normal sinus rhythm as compared to patients with reduced (EF <40% [0.4]) or mid-range EF (40%-49% [0.4-0.49]).[78]

Possible adverse effects with β-blocker use in HF include bradycardia or heart block, hypotension, fatigue, impaired glycemic control in diabetic patients, bronchospasm in patients with asthma, and worsening HF. Clinicians should monitor vital signs and carefully assess for signs and symptoms of worsening HF during β-blocker initiation and titration. Hypotension is more common with carvedilol due to its α1-receptor blocking properties. Bradycardia and hypotension generally are asymptomatic and require no intervention; however, β-blocker dose reduction is warranted in symptomatic patients. Fatigue usually resolves after several weeks of therapy, but sometimes requires dose reduction. In diabetic patients, β-blockers may worsen glucose tolerance and can mask the tachycardia and tremor (but not sweating) that accompany hypoglycemia. In addition, nonselective agents such as carvedilol may prolong insulin-induced hypoglycemia and slow recovery from a hypoglycemic episode. Despite this, there is evidence that carvedilol may improve insulin sensitivity and that β-blockers are well tolerated and significantly reduce morbidity and mortality in patients with diabetes and HFrEF. Thus, while β-blockers should be used cautiously in patients with recurrent hypoglycemia, concerns of masking symptoms of hypoglycemia or worsening glycemic control should not preclude β-blocker use in patients with diabetes. Patients with diabetes should be warned of these potential adverse effects and blood glucose should be monitored when initiating, adjusting, and discontinuing β-blocker therapy. Adjustment of hypoglycemic therapy may be necessary with concomitant β-blocker use in diabetics.

Absolute contraindications to β-blocker use include uncontrolled bronchospastic disease, symptomatic bradycardia, advanced heart block without a pacemaker, and acute decompensated HF. However, β-blockers may be tried with caution in patients with asymptomatic bradycardia, COPD, or well-controlled asthma. Particular caution is warranted in patients with marked bradycardia (HR <55 BPM) or hypotension (systolic BP <80 mm Hg).

Aldosterone Antagonists

7 Spironolactone and eplerenone are aldosterone antagonists that work by blocking the mineralocorticoid receptor, the target site for aldosterone, and, thus, they are also referred to as mineralocorticoid receptor antagonists. In the kidney, aldosterone antagonists inhibit sodium reabsorption and potassium excretion. While the diuretic effects with low doses of aldosterone antagonists are minimal, the potassium-sparing effects can have significant consequences as discussed below. In the heart, aldosterone antagonists inhibit cardiac extracellular matrix and collagen deposition, thereby attenuating cardiac fibrosis and ventricular remodeling.[79] Aldosterone antagonists also attenuate the systemic pro-inflammatory state, atherogenesis, and oxidative stress caused by aldosterone. Thus, as with ACE inhibitors and β-blockers, the data on aldosterone antagonists also support the neurohormonal model of HF. In addition, there is evidence that aldosterone antagonists may attenuate aldosterone-induced calcium excretion and reductions in bone mineral density and protect against fractures in HF.[79]

Three randomized, placebo-controlled trials have evaluated low-dose aldosterone antagonism in patients with HFrEF or post-MI and left ventricular dysfunction. In each trial, the aldosterone antagonist was added to the standard therapy, which included an ACE inhibitor and diuretic. While the initial trial was conducted before the benefits of β-blockers were fully appreciated, participants in the latter two trials received β-blockers. All three trials excluded patients with significant renal dysfunction (eg, serum creatinine above 2.5 mg/dL [221 μmol/L]) and elevated serum potassium (eg, above 5 mEq/L [mmol/L]) at baseline.

The RALES trial was the first to examine the efficacy of aldosterone antagonism in HFrEF. Patients with current or recent NYHA class IV HFrEF were randomized to spironolactone 25 mg/day or placebo.[23] The study was stopped prematurely because of a significant reduction in the primary endpoint of total mortality with spironolactone. Spironolactone also significantly reduced hospitalizations for worsening HF and improved symptoms. The EPHESUS trial evaluated eplerenone in patients with left ventricular dysfunction after MI.[24] Treatment with eplerenone titrated to 50 mg/day was associated with significant reductions in mortality and hospitalizations from HF compared to placebo. The EMPHASIS-HF trial demonstrated significant improvements in clinical outcomes with eplerenone, titrated to 50 mg/day (mean dose of 39 mg/day), in patients with NYHA class II HF and an LVEF of 35% [0.35] or less.[25] Eplerenone treatment reduced the primary endpoint of cardiovascular death or HF hospitalization as well as all-cause and cardiovascular mortality and hospitalization for HF.

The TOPCAT trial examined the effect of spironolactone (mean dose 25 mg/day) in patients with HFpEF (EF >45% [0.45]).[27] There was no difference in the primary outcome composite of death from cardiovascular causes, aborted cardiac arrest, or hospitalization for HF between the spironolactone and placebo groups; however, there was a significant reduction in the risk for hospitalization for HF. There appeared to be a difference in outcomes by region of enrollment. Post hoc analysis showed a greater reduction in the primary outcome with spironolactone among patients from the Americas, but not in those from Eastern Europe.[26] While the prespecified test for an interaction between region and study arm was not significant, differences in baseline characteristics by region and the lower event rate overall in patients from Eastern Europe confound the interpretation of the study results.

For optimal GDMT in patients with HFrEF and NYHA class II-IV symptoms, a low-dose aldosterone antagonist should be used to improve symptoms, reduce the risk of HF hospitalization, and increase survival provided that serum potassium and renal function can be carefully monitored.[22] Current guidelines recommend adding an aldosterone antagonist to decrease the risk for hospitalization for HF in patients with HFpEF, especially if LVEF is on the lower end of this spectrum.[30]

TABLE 36-11 Recommended Strategies for Reducing the Risk for Hyperkalemia with Aldosterone Antagonists

- Avoid starting aldosterone antagonists in patients with any of the following:
  - Serum creatinine concentration >2.0 mg/dL (177 μmol/L) in women or >2.5 mg/dL (221 μmol/L) in men or a creatinine clearance <30 mL/min/1.73 m² (0.29 mL/s/m²)
  - Recent worsening of renal function
  - Serum potassium concentration >5.0 mEq/L (mmol/L)
  - History of severe hyperkalemia
- Start with low doses (12.5 mg/day for spironolactone and 25 mg/day for eplerenone) especially in the elderly and in those with diabetes or a creatinine clearance <50 mL/min/1.73 m² (0.48 mL/s/m²).
- Decrease or discontinue potassium supplements when starting an aldosterone antagonist.
- Avoid concomitant use of NSAIDs or COX-2 inhibitors.
- Avoid concomitant use of high-dose ACE inhibitors or ARBs.
- Avoid triple therapy with an ACE inhibitor, ARB, and aldosterone antagonist.
- Monitor serum potassium concentrations and renal function within 3 days and 1 week after the initiation or dose titration of an aldosterone antagonist or any other medication that could affect potassium homeostasis. Thereafter, potassium concentrations and renal function should be monitored monthly for the first 3 months, and then every 3 months.
- If potassium exceeds 5.5 mEq/L (mmol/L) at any point during therapy, discontinue any potassium supplementation or, in the absence of potassium supplements, reduce or stop aldosterone antagonist therapy.
- Counsel patients to:
  - limit intake of high potassium-containing foods and salt substitutes.
  - avoid the use of over-the-counter NSAIDs.
  - temporarily discontinue aldosterone antagonist therapy if diarrhea develops or diuretic therapy is interrupted.

Data from Reference 34.

Aldosterone antagonist use in clinical trials was associated with significant increases in serum potassium and creatinine. Most trials demonstrated a higher rate of hyperkalemia (serum potassium ≥5.5 mEq/L [mmol/L] or ≥6.0 mEq/L [mmol/L]) with the aldosterone antagonist compared to placebo.[24,25,27] However, hyperkalemia occurs more commonly in clinical practice than in clinical trials.[80] Risk factors for hyperkalemia include impaired renal function, high potassium concentrations, failure to decrease or stop potassium supplements when starting aldosterone antagonists, diabetes, inadequate laboratory monitoring, high potassium intake, and concomitant use of both ACE inhibitors and ARBs or NSAIDs.[81] The ACC/AHA recommended strategies to minimize the risk for hyperkalemia with aldosterone antagonists in HF and are summarized in Table 36-11.[34] Chief among these recommendations is to avoid aldosterone antagonists in patients with renal dysfunction or elevated serum potassium. Serum creatinine may overestimate renal function in the elderly and in patients with decreased muscle mass, in whom creatinine clearance should serve as a guide for the appropriateness of aldosterone antagonist therapy. The risk for hyperkalemia is dose-dependent, and the morbidity and mortality reductions with aldosterone antagonists in clinical trials occurred at low doses (ie, spironolactone 25 mg/day and eplerenone 50 mg/day). Therefore, the doses of aldosterone antagonists should be limited to those associated with beneficial effects in order to decrease the risk for hyperkalemia. Initiation of every other-day dosing is appropriate for patients with marginal renal function or who are otherwise at high risk for hyperkalemia. Notably, both ARNI and SGLT2 inhibitors may reduce the risk of hyperkalemia with aldosterone antagonists.[82] Spironolactone also interacts with androgen and progesterone receptors, which may lead to gynecomastia, impotence, and menstrual irregularities in some patients. Such adverse effects are less frequent with eplerenone owing to its low affinity for the progesterone and androgen receptors.

Sodium-Glucose Cotransporter Type 2 (SGLT2) Inhibitors

8 Initially developed for diabetes given their glucose-lowering potential by blocking renal tubular glucose reabsorption, SGLT2 inhibitors are also benefical in HF. These agents inhibit glucose and sodium reabsorption in the proximal renal tubule which promotes urinary glucose excretion and causes a modest diuresis.[83] Under normoglycemic conditions, the kidneys contribute to blood glucose homeostasis by nearly complete reabsorption of filtered glucose. The majority (>90%) of glucose reabsorption occurs early in the proximal tubule via SGLT2, while the remainder is reabsorbed by SGLT1 in the late proximal tubule. Although the mechanism of benefit from these agents in HF remains uncertain, treatment with SGLT2 inhibitors leads to osmotic diuresis and natriuresis, reduction in arterial pressure and stiffness, and a shift to ketone-based myocardial metabolism. Additional benefit may be related to the reduction of preload and afterload, thereby reducing cardiac stress and injury and ultimately leading to reduced myocardial hypertrophy, fibrosis, and remodeling.[32,83]

Cardiovascular outcome trials in patients with type 2 diabetes demonstrated that SGLT2 inhibitors improved both CV and renal outcomes as well as a reduction in hospitalizations for HF. Thus, outcome trials in patients with HF with and without diabetes were designed. In the DAPA-HF and EMPEROR-Reduced trials, patients with HFrEF and NYHA class II-IV symptoms, both dapagliflozin and empagliflozin reduced the risk of worsening HF and cardiovascular death compared to placebo. In addition, both agents demonstrated a significant reduction in each of the individual components of the composite endpoint.[84,85] Importantly, these benefits were observed both in patients with and without diabetes. As a result, both agents are now foundational components of optimal GDMT for patients with HFrEF (with or without diabetes) and are recommended by current guidelines for use in this population.[22] In the EMPEROR-Preserved trial, empagliflozin (fixed dose of 10 mg daily) also reduced the primary outcome of cardiovascular death or HF hospitalization in patients with HFpEF.[47]

Dosing, monitoring, and related recommendations for SGLT2 inhibitors are detailed in Tables 36-7 and 36-9. The DAPA-HF trial did not enroll patients with an eGFR <30 mL/min/1.73 m² and the limit of eGFR for inclusion in the EMPEROR-Reduced trial was 20 mL/min/1.73 m². These agents are indicated in patients with renal function above or very near these eGFR thresholds. Renal function (eGFR) may initially decrease with SGLT2 inhibitor initiation but improve over time. Patient counseling is imperative with the use of SGLT2 inhibitors, especially in the HF population. It is unclear if SGLT2 inhibitors will contribute to volume depletion and the potential need for diuretic dose adjustment. And thus, patients should be counseled to weigh daily and contact their healthcare provider should their weight start to decline and to avoid abrupt changes in position as orthostasis may occur in the setting of over diuresis. Patients should be monitored for acute kidney injury and renal function impairment; temporary discontinuation of diuretic may be required in settings of reduced oral intake or fluid losses. Patients should also be advised to monitor for and report mycotic genital infections and urinary tract infections. Urosepsis and pyelonephritis are also potential risks with SGLT2 inhibitors. Necrotizing fasciitis of the perineum, also known as Fournier's gangrene, is a rare but serious and potentially life-threatening adverse effect that may occur in either females or males. Patients presenting with pain or tenderness, erythema, or swelling in the genital or perineal area should also be assessed for fever or malaise. Patients with diabetes may be at increased risk for ketoacidosis and temporary discontinuation before scheduled surgery is recommended to avoid this potential risk. Patients who present with signs and symptoms of metabolic acidosis should be assessed for ketoacidosis, regardless of blood glucose level.

Diuretics

9 The compensatory mechanisms in HF stimulate excessive sodium and water retention, often leading to pulmonary and systemic congestion.[86,87] Diuretic therapy, in addition to sodium restriction, is recommended in all patients with clinical evidence of fluid retention. Once fluid overload has been resolved, many patients require chronic diuretic therapy to maintain euvolemia. Among the drugs used to manage HF, diuretics are the most rapid in producing symptomatic benefits. However, diuretics do not prolong survival or alter disease progression, and therefore are not considered mandatory therapy. Thus, patients who do not have fluid retention would not require diuretic therapy.

The primary goals of diuretic therapy are to reduce symptoms associated with fluid retention, improve exercise tolerance and quality of life, and reduce hospitalizations from HF. Diuretics accomplish this by decreasing pulmonary and peripheral edema through the reduction of preload. Although preload is a determinant of CO, the Frank-Starling curve (see Fig. 36-4) shows that patients with congestive symptoms have reached the flat portion of the curve. A reduction in preload improves symptoms but has little effect on the patient's SV or CO until the steep portion of the curve is reached. However, diuretic therapy must be used judiciously because over-diuresis can lead to a reduction in CO, renal perfusion, and symptoms of volume depletion.

Diuretic therapy is usually initiated in low doses in the outpatient setting, with dosage adjustments based on symptom assessment and daily body weight. Change in body weight is a sensitive marker of fluid retention or loss, and it is recommended that patients monitor their status by taking daily morning body weights. Patients who gain 1 lb/day (~0.5 kg/day) for several consecutive days or 3 to 5 lb (1.4-2.3 kg) in a week should contact their healthcare provider for instructions (which often will be to increase the diuretic dose temporarily). Such action often will allow patients to prevent a decompensation that requires hospitalization. Patients may be directed to self-adjust their diuretic dose based on changes in HF symptoms and daily body weight. Hypotension or worsening renal function (eg, increases in serum creatinine) may be indicative of volume depletion and necessitates a reduction in the diuretic dose. Assessing volume status is particularly important before ACE inhibitor/ARB/ARNI initiation or dose titration as over-diuresis may predispose patients to hypotension and other adverse effects with these agents.

In patients with HFpEF, diuretic treatment should be initiated at low doses in order to avoid hypotension and fatigue. Hypotension can be a significant problem in the treatment of HFpEF because patients have a steep LV diastolic pressure-volume curve such that a small change in volume causes a large change in filling pressure and CO. Hence, diuretic dosing should be tailored to individual patient needs.

Loop Diuretics Loop diuretics are usually necessary to restore and maintain euvolemia in HF. They act by inhibiting a Na–K–2Cl transporter in the thick ascending limb of the loop of Henle, where 20% to 25% of filtered sodium normally is reabsorbed. Loop diuretics also induce a prostaglandin-mediated increase in renal blood flow, which contributes to their natriuretic effect. Coadministration of NSAIDs, including cyclooxygenase-2 inhibitors, blocks this prostaglandin-mediated effect and can diminish diuretic efficacy. Excessive dietary sodium intake may also reduce the efficacy of loop diuretics. Unlike thiazides, loop diuretics maintain their effectiveness in the presence of impaired renal function, although higher doses may be necessary to obtain adequate delivery of the drug to the site of action.

There are three loop diuretics available that are routinely used: furosemide, bumetanide, and torsemide.[86,87] They share many similarities in their pharmacodynamics, with their differences being largely pharmacokinetic in nature. Relevant information on the loop diuretics is listed in Tables 36-7 and 36-9. Following oral administration, the peak effect with all the agents occurs in 30 to 90 minutes, with a duration of 4 to 8 hours (longer for torsemide). Following IV administration, the diuretic effect begins within minutes. All three drugs are highly (>95%) bound to plasma proteins, and reach the tubular lumen by active transport via the organic acid transport pathway. The magnitude of the effect is determined by the peak concentration achieved in the nephron, and there is a threshold concentration that must be achieved before any diuresis occurs. Competitors for the organic acid transport pathway (probenecid or organic by-products of uremia) can inhibit the delivery of loop diuretics to their site of action and decrease effectiveness.

The greatest difference between the agents is bioavailability. The bioavailability of bumetanide and torsemide is essentially complete (80%-100%), whereas furosemide bioavailability exhibits marked intra- and inter-patient variability.[86,87] Furosemide bioavailability ranges from 10% to 100%, with an average of 50%. Thus, if bioequivalent IV and oral doses are desired, oral furosemide doses should be approximately double that of the IV dose, whereas IV and oral doses are the same for torsemide and bumetanide. Coadministration of furosemide and bumetanide with food can decrease bioavailability significantly, whereas food has no effect on the bioavailability of torsemide. The intra-abdominal congestion that can occur in HF also may slow the rate (and thus decrease the peak concentration) of furosemide, which can reduce its efficacy. Thus, furosemide is most problematic with respect to the rate and extent of absorption and the factors that influence it, whereas torsemide has the least variable bioavailability.

These differences in bioavailability and variability may have clinical implications. For example, several studies suggest that torsemide is absorbed reliably and may be associated with better outcomes than the more variably absorbed furosemide.[86] Torsemide may modulate neurohormonal levels resulting in attenuation of cardiac remodeling. Torsemide is preferred in patients with persistent fluid retention despite high doses of other loop diuretics. While the costs of torsemide exceed those of furosemide, pharmacoeconomic analyses suggest that the costs of care are similar or less with torsemide.

Heart failure is one of the disease states in which the maximal response to loop diuretics is reduced. This is believed to result from a decrease in the rate of diuretic absorption and/or increased proximal or distal tubule reabsorption of sodium, possibly due to increased activity of the Na–K–2Cl transporter.[86,87] As a consequence, loop diuretics exhibit a ceiling effect in HF, meaning that once the ceiling dose is reached, no additional diuretic response is achieved by increasing the dose. Thus, when this dose is reached, additional diuresis can be achieved by giving the drug more often (twice daily or occasionally three times daily) or by giving combination diuretic therapy. Multiple daily dosing achieves a more sustained diuresis throughout the day. When dosed two or three times daily, the first dose is usually given first thing in the morning and the final dose in the late afternoon/early evening. The appropriate chronic dose of a loop diuretic is that which maintains the patient at a stable dry weight without symptoms of dyspnea. Loop diuretic dose ranges and recommended ceiling doses are listed in Table 36-7.

Diuretics cause a variety of metabolic abnormalities, with severity related to the potency of the diuretic.[86,87] The reader is referred to Chapter 37, "Acute Decompensated Heart Failure" for a detailed discussion on the adverse effects of diuretic therapy. Hypokalemia is the most common metabolic disturbance with thiazide and loop diuretics, which in HF patients may be exacerbated by hyperaldosteronism. Hypokalemia increases the risk for ventricular arrhythmias in HF and is especially worrisome in patients receiving digoxin. It is often accompanied by hypomagnesemia. Since adequate magnesium is necessary for the entry of potassium into the cell, co-supplementation with both magnesium and potassium may be necessary to correct the hypokalemia. Concomitant ARNI, ACE inhibitor/ARB and/or aldosterone antagonist therapy may help minimize diuretic-induced hypokalemia because these drugs tend to increase serum potassium concentration through their inhibitory effect on aldosterone secretion. Nonetheless, the serum potassium concentration should be monitored closely in patients with HF and supplemented appropriately when needed.

Thiazide Diuretics Thiazide diuretics such as hydrochlorothiazide block sodium reabsorption in the distal convoluted tubule (~5%-8% of filtered sodium). The thiazides, therefore, are relatively weak diuretics and infrequently used alone in HF. However, thiazides or the thiazide-like diuretic, metolazone, can be used in combination with loop diuretics to promote an effective diuresis. In addition, thiazide diuretics may be preferred in patients with only mild fluid retention and elevated BP because of their more persistent antihypertensive effects compared with loop diuretics. Given patients with HFpEF often have ongoing uncontrolled HTN, thiazide diuretics may be used to manage this disorder.

Other Treatments for Heart Failure in Select Patients

Nitrates and Hydralazine

11 Nitrates and hydralazine were originally combined in the treatment of HFrEF because of their complementary hemodynamic actions. Nitrates, by serving as nitric oxide donors, activate guanylate cyclase to increase cyclic guanosine monophosphate (cGMP) in vascular smooth muscle resulting in venodilation and decreased preload. Hydralazine is a direct-acting arterial vasodilator causing a decrease in SVR and resultant increases in SV and CO (Fig. 36-1). However, the beneficial effects of hydralazine and nitrates extend beyond their hemodynamic actions and are likely related to attenuating the biochemical processes driving HF progression.

Based on the results of initial clinical trials showing ISDN and hydralazine were more effective in African Americans, the African-American Heart Failure Trial (A-HeFT) enrolled self-identified African Americans with NYHA class III or IV HFrEF receiving standard HF therapy and compared outcomes in patients randomized to the fixed-dose combination of hydralazine/Isosorbide dinitrate (BiDil®) or placebo.[88] The trial was terminated early because of a significant reduction in all-cause mortality in patients receiving hydralazine/isosorbide compared with placebo. Based on these results, BiDil® was approved by the FDA to treat HFrEF in African Americans.

Guidelines recommend the addition of hydralazine/ISDN to African American patients with HFrEF with persistent symptoms despite ARNI, β-blocker, aldosterone antagonist, and SGLT2 inhibitor therapy.[22] Hydralazine/ISDN can also be useful in patients unable to tolerate either an ACE inhibitor or ARB because of renal insufficiency, hyperkalemia, or possibly hypotension.

Despite its efficacy, the use of hydralazine/ISDN is limited by the need for three times daily dosing and frequent adverse effects including dizziness, headache, and GI distress. Because of cost, some clinicians use generic hydralazine and ISDN as separate agents, rather than BiDil®. Although the generic and brand name products are not bioequivalent as determined in healthy volunteer studies, it is unknown if these pharmacokinetic differences impact clinical outcomes.

In contrast to the beneficial effects of hydralazine/ISDN in patients with HFrEF, in patients with HFpEF nitrates reduce exercise capacity and do not improve quality of life or plasma NT-proBNP concentrations.[89] Adverse events, including worsening HF and presyncope/syncope, were more frequent with nitrate treatment. These findings suggest that in the absence of another indication for nitrate therapy (eg, angina), nitrates provide no benefits to patients with HFpEF.

Ivabradine

11 Ivabradine reduces HR and is used in the treatment of HFrEF.[90] Ivabradine selectively inhibits the I_f current responsible for controlling the depolarization rate of the sinus node.[90] By blocking this current, ivabradine slows the spontaneous depolarization of the sinus node resulting in a dose-dependent slowing of the HR. Ivabradine does not affect AV conduction, blood pressure, or myocardial contractility.[90]

Elevated resting HR (>70-80 BPM) is emerging as an important independent risk factor for adverse outcomes in patients with HFrEF and is associated with increased hospital admissions, disease progression, and mortality.[91] New approaches to address increased HR in these patients are needed because, for a variety of reasons, β-blockers are frequently underdosed in clinical practice and the benefits of β-blockers are associated with the degree of HR reduction and the dose administered.[91,92] In the SHIFT trial, ivabradine reduced the risk of hospitalization for worsening HF in patients with HFrEF in sinus rhythm.[93] As a result, guidelines recommend the use of ivabradine after GDMT is optimized in patients with HFrEF in sinus rhythm who have a resting HR >70 BPM and are receiving maximally tolerated β-blocker doses.[22]

The starting dose of ivabradine in most patients is 5 mg twice daily with meals. After 2 weeks of treatment, the resting HR should be evaluated, and if between 50 and 60 BPM, the dose should be continued. If the heart rate is >60 BPM, the dose can be increased to a maximum of 7.5 mg twice daily. If at any point, the HR is <50 BPM or if the patient has symptomatic bradycardia, the dose should be reduced by 2.5 mg twice daily. In this case, if the patient is receiving only 2.5 mg twice daily, then ivabradine should be discontinued. Because of the clear benefits of β-blockers on mortality and that many patients treated with β-blockers are under-dosed, clinicians should remember to titrate to the maximum tolerated doses before determining the need for ivabradine. The most common adverse effects associated with ivabradine were bradycardia, atrial fibrillation, and visual disturbances.

Digoxin

11 The benefits of digoxin in HF are related to its neurohormonal modulating activity.[94] These benefits occur at low plasma concentrations and little inotropic effect is produced. Digoxin attenuates the excessive SNS activation present in HF patients. Chronic HF is also marked by autonomic dysfunction, most notably suppression of the parasympathetic (vagal) system. Digoxin increases parasympathetic activity in HF patients and leads to a decrease in HR, thus enhancing diastolic filling. The vagal effects also result in slowed conduction and prolongation of AV node refractoriness, thus slowing the ventricular response in patients with atrial fibrillation. This leads to a decrease in HR, which enhances diastolic filling. Because atrial fibrillation is a common complication of HF, the combined neurohormonal and negative chronotropic effects of digoxin may be beneficial for such patients.

The Digitalis Investigation Group (DIG) trial examined the effects of digoxin on survival and hospitalization in patients with HF symptoms, an LVEF of <45% (0.45), and in sinus rhythm.[95] No significant differences in all-cause mortality were found between patients receiving digoxin and placebo. Digoxin reduced hospitalizations for worsening HF compared with placebo. Among patients with an LVEF greater than 45% (0.45) (HFpEF) who were enrolled in an ancillary DIG trial, there was no apparent benefit of digoxin on hospitalizations or mortality.[96] Therefore, digoxin is recommended in HFrEF after GDMT is optimized.[22] An analysis of the trial database found that lower serum digoxin concentrations (SDCs) were associated with decreased mortality, whereas higher concentrations were not.[97] Specifically, compared with placebo, SDCs of 0.5 to 0.9 ng/mL (μg/L; 0.6-1.2 nmol/L) were associated with lower mortality, all-cause hospitalizations, and HF hospitalizations. Based on these data, for most patients, the target SDC should be 0.5 to 0.9 ng/mL (μg/L; 0.6-1.2 nmol/L).[34] In most patients with normal renal function, this serum concentration range can be achieved with a daily dose of 0.125 mg. Patients with decreased renal function or low body weight, the elderly, or those receiving interacting drugs (eg, amiodarone) should receive 0.125 mg daily or every other day. Routinely measuring SDCs is not necessary unless digoxin toxicity is suspected or there are other conditions that may significantly affect SDC such as worsening renal function or the initiation of an interacting drug. Digoxin combined with a β-blocker or amiodarone is superior to either agent alone for controlling ventricular response in patients with concomitant atrial fibrillation and HF.[34] Target SDCs are the same regardless of whether the patient is in sinus rhythm or atrial fibrillation. Several equations and nomograms have been proposed to estimate digoxin maintenance doses based on estimated renal function for a particular patient and population pharmacokinetic parameters. These methods are extensively reviewed elsewhere.[98]

The DIG trial was conducted prior to the proven benefits and widespread use of β-blockers in HF. Observational studies have reexamined digoxin in the context of contemporary HF therapy and shown variable results.[99-101] In patients with HFrEF receiving more contemporary GDMT, digoxin withdrawal is associated with an increased risk of hospital readmissions for HF and the combined endpoint of HF readmission and mortality.[102] Based on the totality of data, digoxin is not considered a first-line agent in HF but a trial may be considered in conjunction with GDMT in patients with symptomatic HFrEF to improve symptoms and reduce hospitalizations.[22] Digoxin may also be considered to help control ventricular response rate in patients with HFrEF and supraventricular arrhythmias.

There is no established role for digoxin in HFpEF when patients are in normal sinus rhythm. Digoxin may be of benefit in patients with concomitant HFpEF and atrial fibrillation.[103]

Digoxin pharmacokinetics are well described.[98] There is a long "distribution phase" after administration of oral or IV digoxin, resulting in a lag time before a maximum pharmacologic response is observed. Blood samples for measurement of SDCs should be collected at least 6 hours and preferably 12 hours or more after the last dose. The drug efflux transporter P-glycoprotein (P-gp) plays an important role in the bioavailability, renal and nonrenal clearance, and drug interactions with digoxin. Clinically important pharmacokinetic/pharmacodynamic drug interactions exist with a range of mechanisms including reduced bioavailability through various processes (eg, antacids, cholestyramine, kaolin-pectin, metoclopramide), altered gut bacteria (eg, clarithromycin, tetracycline), reduced clearance through P-glycoprotein inhibition (e.g, cyclosporine, ranolazine, ritonavir) and hypokalemia/hypomagnesemia increasing risk of digoxin toxicity (eg, thiazide or loop diuretics). Select interactions occur through multiple mechanisms such as increased bioavailability and reduced renal and nonrenal clearance through P-glycoprotein inhibition resulting in 50% to 100% or greater increases in serum digoxin concentrations (eg, amiodarone, verapamil, quinidine, ketoconazole, macrolide antibiotics) requiring up to a 50% reduction in dose. One standard GDMT, spironolactone, may alter the clearance of digoxin, and thus close monitoring of serum concentrations is warranted. In addition, spironolactone may interfere with some digoxin assays, thus, increasing apparent digoxin concentrations.

Digoxin can produce a variety of cardiac and noncardiac adverse effects, but it is usually well tolerated by most patients.[94] Noncardiac adverse effects frequently involve the GI (nausea/vomiting) or CNS (halos, photophobia, problems with color perception including red-green or yellow-green vision) systems but also may be nonspecific (eg, fatigue, weakness, confusion). Cardiac manifestations include numerous different arrhythmias caused by the drug's multiple electrophysiologic effects including both various tachy- and bradyarrhythmias ranging from sinus bradycardia to third-degree heart block and premature ventricular contractions to ventricular arrhythmias. Rhythm disturbances are of particular concern because patients with chronic HF are already at increased risk for sudden cardiac death, presumably due to ventricular arrhythmias. Patients at increased risk of toxicity include those with impaired renal function, decreased lean body mass, the elderly, and those taking interacting drugs. Hypokalemia, hypomagnesemia, and hypercalcemia will predispose patients to cardiac manifestations of digoxin toxicity. Thus, concomitant therapy with diuretics may lead to electrolyte abnormalities and increase the likelihood of cardiac arrhythmias. Similarly, hypothyroidism, myocardial ischemia, and acidosis will also increase the risk of cardiac adverse effects. Although digoxin toxicity is commonly associated with plasma concentrations greater than 2 ng/mL (μg/L; 2.6 nmol/L), toxicity may occur at lower concentrations, and clinicians should remember that digoxin toxicity is based on the presence of symptoms rather than a specific plasma concentration.[98] Usual treatment of digoxin toxicity includes drug withdrawal or dose reduction and treatment of cardiac arrhythmias and electrolyte abnormalities. In patients with life-threatening digoxin toxicity, purified digoxin-specific Fab antibody fragments should be administered.

Vericiguat

11 One of the detrimental consequences of HF is endothelial dysfunction and reactive oxygen species generation.[104] Vericiguat is a novel pharmacotherapy that modulates endothelial dysfunction.[105] Under normal conditions, the vascular endothelium generates nitric oxide (NO) which stimulates soluble guanylate cyclase (sGC) mediated cyclic guanosine monophosphate (cGMP) production. The endocardial endothelium is also sensitive to NO and relies upon increasing intracellular cGMP to regulate contractility and diastolic function. In HF, this process becomes dysregulated, leading to insufficiency of NO, sGC and cGMP, resulting in impaired diastolic relaxation and microvascular dysfunction. While administration of nitrates, in combination with hydralazine, reduce mortality in HFrEF, this benefit has only been demonstrated in self-identified African American patients.[88] Vericiguat is an sGC activator that binds to sGC and enhances the effect of NO to increase cGMP activity.[105]

In the VICTORIA trial, patients with HFrEF (LVEF <45% [0.45]), recent ADHF requiring hospitalization or outpatient intravenous diuretics, and elevated BNP levels were randomized to vericiguat or placebo.[106] Patients receiving vericiguat demonstrated a significant, but modest, reduction in the primary endpoint of cardiovascular death or HF hospitalization. Vericiguat was well tolerated with no differences in symptomatic hypotension or syncope between groups. While renal function and electrolytes were unaffected, there was a concerning and as yet unexplained greater incidence of anemia found in patients receiving vericiguat. The place in therapy for verciguat is unclear given the limited benefit but it may lie in the lack of significant hemodynamic, renal, and electrolyte effects in the setting of a high-risk population that often does not tolerate GDMT. Similar to digoxin, it is[22] Vericiguat is not indicated in HFpEF given the lack of benefit and potential lack of safety (hypotension, syncope) demonstrated in the VITALITY-HFpEF Trial.[107]

Calcium Channel Blockers

Calcium channel blockers have a limited role in HFrEF. While dihydropyridine type agents (eg, amlodipine, felodipine) are safe to use in patients with HFrEF, these agents have a neutral effect on morbidity or mortality. Hence, they can be safely used to manage HTN or angina in patients with HFrEF but they should only be considered after other doses of GDMT with blood pressure–lowering effects are optimized. In contrast, the nondihydropyridine calcium channel blockers, verapamil and diltiazem, are contraindicated in HFrEF due to their negative inotropic effects. As such, nondihydropyridines are listed as medications that can exacerbate HF in Table 36-4.

Calcium channel blockers can provide symptom-targeted treatment in patients with HFpEF by decreasing HR and increasing exercise tolerance. They can also provide disease-targeted therapy by treating HTN and coronary artery disease. However, the beneficial effect of these agents on exercise tolerance is not always paralleled by improved LV diastolic function or increased relaxation rate. Of the calcium channel blockers, the nondihydropyridines are the most effective because they lower heart rate in addition to lowering BP. Nondihydropyridines are also frequently used to treat the comorbidities of HTN and atrial fibrillation in patients with HFpEF. Sustained-release nifedipine, because of its strong vasodilator properties, tends to cause hypotension, reflex tachycardia, and peripheral edema. These characteristics make it less useful in HFpEF. Amlodipine may be effective because it reduces BP. Initial daily doses are verapamil 120 to 240 mg, diltiazem 90 to 120 mg, and amlodipine 2.5 mg.

Heart block is a contraindication for nondihydropyridines. The most common adverse effects are bradycardia and heart block (for the nondihydropyridines). Peripheral edema and headache also are common. Nondihydropyridines exacerbate the bradycardic effects of β-blockers, and verapamil raises digoxin serum concentrations by 70%. Generic formulations, but not necessarily generic equivalents to the original brand names, are available for some of the calcium channel blockers.

Tafamidis

Tafamidis stabilizes the TTR tetramer by binding to the thyroxine-binding sites and thereby slowing its disassociation into monomers and halting the amyloid deposition process. The Transthyretin Amyloidosis Cardiomyopathy Clinical Trial (ATTR-ACT) included 441 patients with either hereditary (24%) or wild type (76%) ATTR cardiomyopathy.[17] The trial results showed the superiority of tafamidis meglumine to placebo in reducing all-cause mortality and reducing the rate of hospitalizations due to cardiovascular complications. No differences in the primary outcome were observed between hereditary and wild-type ATTR patients. Approved in the United States in 2019, tafamidis is dosed once daily as either a single 61 mg capsule or four 20 mg capsules (80 mg total) of tafamidis meglumine. Recent guidelines recommended tafamadis in select patients with ATTR cardiac amyloidosis to reduce cardiovascular morbidity and mortality.[22]

Special Populations

HF is often accompanied by other cardiovascular and non-cardiovascular disorders whose natural history or therapy may affect morbidity, mortality, and treatment approach.[3,33] Optimal management of these concomitant disorders in the context of the patient's HF is an important consideration in the overall care of the patient.

Although HTN has been replaced by ischemic heart disease as the most common cause of HF, up to 90% of patients with HF have a current or a previous history of HTN.[3] HTN directly contributes to the development of both HFrEF and HFpEF as well as indirectly by increasing the risk of coronary artery disease. Effective treatment of HTN markedly reduces the risk of developing HF.[3] Pharmacotherapy of HTN in patients with HFrEF should initially involve GDMT with blood pressure reducing effects (eg, ARNI, β-blockers, aldosterone antagonists). If control of HTN is not achieved after optimizing treatment with these agents, the addition of ISDN/hydralazine or a dihydropyridine calcium channel blocker such as amlodipine may be considered. In patients with HFpEF, both verapamil and diltiazem can be safely used in conjunction with other therapies known to benefit select patients with HFpEF, specifically ARNI or ARBs. In patients with either HFrEF or HFpEF, target levels of BP should be less than 130/80 mm Hg, consistent with current guidelines (see Chapter 30, "Hypertension").[30,36]

Coronary artery disease is the most common cause of HFrEF and a less common cause of HFpEF. Appropriate management of coronary disease and its risk factors is thus an important strategy for the prevention and treatment of HF (see Chapter 32, "Stable Ischemic Heart Disease"). Coronary revascularization should be strongly considered in patients with both HF and angina.[34] Pharmacotherapy of angina in patients with HF should utilize drugs that can effectively treat both disorders. In HFrEF, nitrates and β-blockers are effective antianginals and are the preferred agents for patients with both disorders since they may improve clinical outcomes. In HFrEF, both amlodipine and felodipine are safe to use in this setting while nondihydropyrindines should be avoided. In HFpEF, given nitrates, β-blockers and verapamil have neutral effects on HF outcomes, they can also be safely used. Optimization of treatments for secondary prevention of coronary and atherosclerotic vascular disease should also be considered.[3]

Atrial fibrillation is the most frequently encountered arrhythmia and it is commonly found in both HFrEF and HFpEF, with the prevalence increasing in parallel to the severity of HF and an association with worse long-term prognosis.[34,35] Moreover, HF exacerbations and atrial fibrillation are closely linked causes of hospitalization and it is often difficult to determine which disorder caused the other. Thus, optimal management according to established guidelines is required with careful attention paid to control of ventricular response, symptoms, and anticoagulation for stroke prevention (see Chapter 40, "Arrhythmias").[35,108]

Digoxin is frequently used to slow ventricular response in patients with HF and atrial fibrillation. However, it is more effective at rest than with exercise and it does not affect the progression of HF. In addition, the potential for digoxin to increase mortality in patients with atrial fibrillation is a growing concern.[109] β-Blockers are more effective than digoxin and have the added benefits of improving morbidity and mortality in patients with HFrEF. Combination therapy with digoxin and a β-blocker may be more effective for rate control than either agent used alone. Calcium channel blockers with negative inotropic effects such as verapamil or diltiazem should be avoided in patients with HFrEF but are effective in patients with HFpEF.

There appear to be no differences in outcomes between the rhythm- (restoration and maintenance of sinus rhythm) and rate-control approaches to atrial fibrillation in patients with HF.[35,103] In general, amiodarone and dofetilide are the preferred agents if rhythm control is needed in HFrEF.[103] Class I antiarrhythmics and dronedarone should be avoided in HFrEF. Because of the limited efficacy and potential for serious adverse effects with antiarrhythmic drugs, there is a growing interest in the use of catheter ablation for restoring sinus rhythm in HF.[108,110] Several recent studies have shown an improvement in clinical outcomes after AF ablation in HF patients highlighting the emerging role of the invasive approach in this subset of patients.[110,22]

Several noncardiovascular diseases warrant special consideration in HF including diabetes, COPD, depression, gout, chronic kidney disease (CKD), and iron deficiency.[33]

Type 2 diabetes is a common comorbid condition in patients with HF with each disorder independently enhancing the risk of the other.[111] Patients with diabetes are at two- to fourfold increased risk of developing HF compared to those without diabetes through increased risk of coronary artery disease and multiple other mechanisms.[111] Adequate glycemic control is critical to reducing the risk of HF development and progression.[111] For most patients with diabetes and HF, a more lenient HbA1c goal of 7% to 8% (53-64 mmol/mol) is suggested and should be individualized based on numerous patient characteristics.[111] Metformin remains a first-line therapy in patients at risk for or with established HF unless contraindications are present.[111] As previously discussed, SGLT2 inhibitors are now standard GDMT for HFrEF.[22] If additional glucose-lowering is needed, a glucagon-like peptide-1 (GLP-1) receptor agonist demonstrating CV benefits (dulaglutide, liraglutide, or semaglutide) should be considered.[111] The dipeptidyl peptidase-4 (DPP-4) inhibitors should be avoided due to the increased risk of HF. The thiazolidinediones and sulfonylureas should be avoided. Insulin therapy may be necessary for some patients to achieve glycemic control. Readers are referred to Chapter 94 ("Diabetes Mellitus") for more in-depth treatment recommendations.

Given COPD (see Chapter 45, "Chronic Obstructive Pulmonary Disease") co-presents in many patients with HF, concern about the safe use of β-blockers exists.[33] Overall, the benefit of β-blockers in HFrEF outweighs the risk of worsening pulmonary disease with the exception of those with acute bronchospasm. Use of β1-selective agents (eg, bisoprolol, metoprolol succinate) over nonselective agents are preferred and patients should be counseled to monitor for and report worsening pulmonary symptoms.[33] Limited retrospective data suggest preference may be given to the use of ARBs over ACE inhibitors.[33]

While there have been several studies assessing the role of interventions addressing depression in HF patients, it remains unclear if antidepressants have any benefit. Still, antidepressants should still be considered in patients voicing depressive symptoms (see Chapter 88, "Depressive Disorders"). The selective serotonin receptor inhibitors have been safe in HF, and thus, these agents are preferred over serotonin-norepinephrine receptor inhibitors and TCAs.[33]

Gout (see Chapter 113, "Gout and Hyperuricemia") is common in HF patients receiving diuretic therapy. Colchicine is safe and effective in patients with HF experiencing an acute gout flare.[33] Close monitoring for gastrointestinal symptoms and myelosuppression is warranted in the setting of renal dysfunction or concomitant use of CYP3A4 or P-glycoprotein inhibitors. If patients do not tolerate or fail colchicine, corticosteroids are an alternative; however, dose and duration should be limited. NSAIDs are contraindicated in patients with HF as is febuxostat. Allopurinol is the preferred urate-lowering therapy.

Present in over 50% of patients with HFrEF, the effect of CKD on serum potassium and creatinine can substantially impact GDMT use, particularly ACE inhibitors, ARBs, ARNI, and aldosterone antagonists.[33] These agents, along with the SGLT2 inhibitors, are also renoprotective and should be used if at all possible in patients with HFrEF and CKD. Potassium binders may be necessary if hyperkalemia develops. Erythrocyte stimulating agents should not be used to correct anemia in patients with HF alone but may be considered in those with concomitant CKD, low hemoglobin concentrations (ie, <10 g/dL [100 g/L; 6.21 mmol/L]), and adequate or repleted iron stores.

Iron deficiency, defined as ferritin <100 ng/mL (mcg/L) or 100 to 299 ng/mL (mcg/L) with a transferrin saturation (TSAT) <20% [0.2]), is present in approximately 50% of patients with chronic HFrEF and 80% of individuals admitted to the hospital for ADHF.[112] Thus, iron studies should be routinely assessed in patients with symptomatic HFrEF, regardless of the presence or absence of anemia. If iron deficiency is present, the total iron deficit should be calculated using the Ganzoni equation and intravenous repletion should occur with iron product selection taking into consideration cost and feasibility (eg, inpatient versus outpatient) to improve symptoms, functional status and reduce HF hospitalizations.[30,33,113]

EVALUATION OF THERAPEUTIC OUTCOMES

Although mortality is an important endpoint, it does not give a complete measure of the overall impact of HF because many patients are repeatedly hospitalized for HF exacerbations and continue to survive, albeit with a significantly reduced quality of life. Thus, some of the more important therapeutic outcomes in HF management, such as prolonged survival or prevention or slowing of the progression of HF, are difficult to quantify in an individual patient. However, after appropriate diagnostic evaluation to determine the etiology of HF, ongoing clinical assessment of patients typically focuses on the evaluation of three general areas: (a) functional capacity, (b) volume status, and (c) laboratory monitoring.

The evaluation of functional capacity should focus on the presence and severity of symptoms the patient experiences during activities of daily living and how their symptoms affect these activities. Questions directed toward the patient's ability to perform specific activities may be more informative than general questions about what symptoms the patient may be experiencing. For example, patients should be asked if they could exercise, climb stairs, get dressed without stopping, check the mail, go shopping, or clean the house. Another important component of the assessment of functional capacity is to ask patients what activities they would like to do but are now unable to perform.

Assessment of volume status is a vital component of the ongoing care of patients with HF. This evaluation provides the clinician with important information about the adequacy of diuretic therapy. Since the cardinal signs and symptoms of HF are caused by excess fluid retention, the efficacy of diuretic treatment is readily evaluated by the disappearance of these signs and symptoms. The physical examination is the primary method for the evaluation of fluid retention, and specific attention should be focused on the patient's body weight, the extent of JVD, the presence of hepatojugular reflux, presence, and the severity of pulmonary congestion, and peripheral edema. Specifically, in a patient with pulmonary congestion, monitoring is indicated for resolution of rales and pulmonary edema and improvement or the resolution of DOE, orthopnea, and PND. For patients with systemic congestion, a decrease or disappearance of peripheral edema, JVD, and hepatojugular reflux is sought. Other therapeutic outcomes include an improvement in exercise tolerance and fatigue, decreased nocturia, and a decrease in HR. Clinicians also will want to monitor BP and ensure that the patient does not develop symptomatic hypotension as a result of drug therapy. Body weight is a sensitive short-term marker of fluid loss or retention, and patients should be counseled to weigh themselves daily, reporting changes of 3 to 5 lb (1.4-2.3 kg) to their healthcare provider so that adjustments can be made in diuretic doses. Patients and healthcare providers should be aware that HF progression may be slowed even though symptoms have not been resolved.

Routine monitoring of serum electrolytes and renal function is required in patients with HF. Assessment of serum potassium and magnesium is especially important because hypokalemia and hypomagnesemia are common adverse effects of diuretic therapy and are associated with an increased risk of arrhythmias and digox in toxicity (hypokalemia). The risk of hyperkalemia is also high as expected with the use of ACE inhibitors, ARBs, ARNI, and aldosterone antagonists and is associated with adverse outcomes.[80,114] A serum potassium ≥4 mEq/L (mmol/L) should be maintained with some evidence suggesting it should be ≥4.5 mEq/L (mmol/L).[115] Assessment of renal function (BUN and serum creatinine) is also an important endpoint for monitoring diuretic and RAAS inhibitor therapy. Common causes of worsening renal function in patients with HF include over-diuresis, adverse effects of RAAS inhibition, and hypoperfusion.

Excellent overviews on approaches to initiating and titrating evidence-based therapies, care coordination, monitoring parameters, therapeutic endpoints, improving adherence, care of common comorbidities that impact treatment, and solutions to frequently encountered problems when evaluating and treating patients with HF are available.[22,59]

ABBREVIATIONS

ACC	American College of Cardiology
ACE	angiotensin-converting enzyme
AHA	American Heart Association
ARB	angiotensin receptor blocker
ARNI	angiotensin-receptor blocker/neprilysin inhibitor
AVP	arginine vasopressin
BNP	B-type natriuretic peptide
BP	blood pressure
BPM	beats per minute
BUN	blood urea nitrogen
cAMP	cyclic adenosine monophosphate
CKD	chronic kidney disease
CO	cardiac output
COX-2	cyclooxygenase-2
CRT	cardiac resynchronization therapy
ESC	European Society of Cardiology
ET	endothelin
GDMT	guideline-directed medical therapy
HF	heart failure
HFpEF	heart failure with preserved ejection fraction
HFrEF	heart failure with reduced ejection fraction
HFSA	Heart Failure Society of America
HR	heart rate
HTN	hypertension
IABP	intra-aortic balloon pump
ICD	implantable cardioverter-defibrillator
JVD	jugular venous distension
LVAD	left ventricular assist device
LVEDV	left ventricular end-diastolic volume
LVEDP	left ventricular end-diastolic pressure
LVEF	left ventricular ejection fraction
MI	myocardial infarction
NE	norepinephrine
NSAID	nonsteroidal anti-inflammatory drug
NYHA	New York Heart Association
PCWP	pulmonary capillary wedge pressure
P-gp	P-glycoprotein
RAAS	renin–angiotensin–aldosterone system
SDC	serum digoxin concentration
SNS	sympathetic nervous system
SVR	systemic vascular resistance
TNF-α	tumor necrosis factor-α
TZD	thiazolidinedione

REFERENCES

1. Bozkurt B, Coats AJ, Tsutsui H, et al. Universal Definition and Classification of Heart Failure: A Report of the Heart Failure Society of America, Heart Failure Association of the European Society of Cardiology, Japanese Heart Failure Society and Writing Committee of the Universal Definition of Heart Failure. *J Card Fail.* 2021.
2. Virani SS, Alonso A, Aparicio HJ, et al. Heart disease and stroke Statistics—2021 Update: A report from the American Heart Association. *Circulation.* 2021;143(8):e254–e743.
3. Bozkurt B, Aguilar D, Deswal A, et al. Contributory risk and management of comorbidities of hypertension, obesity, diabetes mellitus, hyperlipidemia, and metabolic syndrome in chronic heart failure: A scientific statement from the American Heart Association. *Circulation.* 2016;134:e535–e578.
4. Nayak A, Hicks AJ, Morris AA. Understanding the complexity of heart failure risk and treatment in Black patients. *Circ Heart Fail.* 2020;13(8): e007264.
5. Reddy YNV, Carter RE, Obokata M, Redfield MM, Borlaug BA. A simple, evidence-based approach to help guide diagnosis of heart failure with preserved ejection fraction. *Circulation.* 2018;(9):861–870.
6. Levy WC, Mozaffarian D, Linker DT, et al. The Seattle heart failure model: Prediction of survival in heart failure. *Circulation.* 2006;113(11):1424–1433.
7. Rich JD, Burns J, Freed BH, Maurer MS, Burkhoff D, Shah SJ. Meta-Analysis Global Group in Chronic (MAGGIC) Heart Failure Risk Score: Validation of a Simple Tool for the Prediction of Morbidity and Mortality in Heart Failure with Preserved Ejection Fraction. *J Am Heart Assoc.* 2018;7(20):e009594.
8. Mann DL. Management of patients with heart failure with reduced ejection fraction. In: Zipes DP, Libby P, Bonow RO, Mann DL, Tomaselli GF, Braunwald E, eds. *Braunwald's Heart Disease: A Textbook of Cardiovascular Medicine.* 11th ed. Philadelphia, PA: Elsevier; 2019:490–522.
9. Zakeri R, Cowie MR. Heart failure with preserved ejection fraction: Controversies, challenges and future directions. *Heart.* 2018;104:377–384.
10. Lam CSP, Voors AA, de Boer RA, Solomon SD, van Veldhuisen DJ. Heart failure with preserved ejection fraction: From mechanisms to therapies. *Eur Heart J.* 2018;39:2780–2792.
11. Hasenfuss G, Mann DL. Pathophysiology of heart failure. In: Zipes DP, Libby P, Bonow RO, Mann DL, Tomaselli GF, Braunwald E, eds. *Braunwald's Heart Disease: A Textbook of Cardiovascular Medicine.* 11th ed. Philadelphia, PA: Elsevier; 2019:442–461.
12. Borlaug BA. The pathophysiology of heart failure with preserved ejection fraction. *Nature Reviews Cardiology.* 2014;11:507–515.
13. Lewis GA, Schelbert EB, Williams SG, et al. Biological phenotypes of heart failure with preserved ejection fraction. *J Am Coll Cardiol.* 2017;70:2186–2200.
14. Lymperopoulos A, Rengo G, Koch WJ. Adrenergic nervous system in heart failure: Pathophysiology and therapy. *Circ Res.* 2013;113:739–753.
15. Aimo A, Gaggin HK, Barison A, Emdin M, Januzzi JL Jr. Imaging, biomarker, and clinical predictors of cardiac remodeling in heart failure with reduced ejection fraction. *JACC Heart Fail.* 2019;7(9):782–794.
16. Ruberg FL, Grogan M, Hanna M, Kelly JW, Maurer MS. Transthyretin amyloid cardiomyopathy: JACC state-of-the-art review. *J Am Coll Cardiol.* 2019;73:2872–2891.
17. Maurer MS, Schwartz JH, Gundapaneni B, et al. Tafamidis treatment for patients with transthyretin amyloid cardiomyopathy. *N Engl J Med.* 2018;379:1007–1016.
18. Gertz MA, Dispenzieri A. Systemic amyloidosis recognition, prognosis, and therapy: A systematic review. *JAMA.* 2020;324(1):79–89.
19. Kittleson MM, Maurer MS, Ambardekar AV, et al. Cardiac amyloidosis: Evolving diagnosis and management: A scientific statement from the American Heart Association. *Circulation.* 2020;142(1):e7–e22.
20. Ommen SR, Mital S, Burke MA, et al. 2020 AHA/ACC Guideline for the Diagnosis and Treatment of Patients with Hypertrophic Cardiomyopathy: A Report of the American College of Cardiology/American Heart Association Joint Committee on Clinical Practice Guidelines. *J Am Coll Cardiol.* 2020;76(25):e159–e240.
21. Hartupee J, Mann DL. Neurohormonal activation in heart failure with reduced ejection fraction. *Nature Reviews Cardiology.* 2017;14:30–38.
22. Heidenreich PA, Bozkurt B , Aguilar D, et al. 2022 AHA/ACC/HFSA guideline for the management of heart failure: a report of the American College of Cardiology/American Heart Association Joint Committee on Clinical Practice Guidelines. *J Am Coll Cardiol.* 2022;79:e263–e421.
23. Pitt B, Zannad F, Remme WJ, et al. The effect of spironolactone on morbidity and mortality in patients with severe heart failure. Randomized Aldactone Evaluation Study Investigators. *N Engl J Med.* 1999;341:709–717.
24. Pitt B, Remme W, Zannad F, et al. Eplerenone, a selective aldosterone blocker, in patients with left ventricular dysfunction after myocardial infarction. *N Engl J Med.* 2003;348:1309–1321.
25. Zannad F, McMurray JJ, Krum H, et al. Eplerenone in patients with systolic heart failure and mild symptoms. *N Engl J Med.* 2011;364:11–21.
26. Pfeffer MA, Claggett B, Assmann SF, et al. Regional variation in patients and outcomes in the treatment of preserved cardiac function heart failure with an aldosterone antagonist (TOPCAT) trial. *Circulation.* 2015;131:34–42.
27. Pitt B, Pfeffer MA, Assmann SF, et al. Spironolactone for heart failure with preserved ejection fraction. *N Engl J Med.* 2014;370:1383–1392.
28. Chow SL, Maisel AS, Anand I, et al. Role of biomarkers for the prevention, assessment, and management of heart failure: A scientific statement from the American Heart Association. *Circulation.* 2017;135:e1054–e1091.
29. McMurray JJ, Packer M, Desai AS, et al. Angiotensin-neprilysin inhibition versus enalapril in heart failure. *N Engl J Med.* 2014;371:993–1004.
30. Yancy CW, Jessup M, Bozkurt B, et al. 2017 ACC/AHA/HFSA focused update of the 2013 ACCF/AHA guideline for the management of heart failure: A report of the American College of Cardiology/American

Heart Association Task Force on Clinical Practice Guidelines and the Heart Failure Society of America. *Circulation*. 2017;136:e137–e161.
31. Houston BA, Kalathiya RJ, Kim DA, Zakaria S. Volume overload in heart failure: An evidence-based review of strategies for treatment and prevention. *Mayo Clin Proc*. 2015;90:1247–1261.
32. Zelniker Thomas A. Braunwald Eugene Mechanisms of cardiorenal rffects of sodium-glucose cotransporter 2 inhibitors. *J Am Coll Cardiol*. 2020;75:422-434.
33. Gale SE, Mardis A, Plazak ME, Kukin A, Reed BN. Management of noncardiovascular comorbidities in patients with heart failure with reduced ejection fraction. *Pharmacotherapy*. 2021;41(6):537–545.
34. Yancy CW, Jessup M, Bozkurt B, et al. 2013 ACCF/AHA guideline for the management of heart failure: A report of the American College of Cardiology Foundation/American Heart Association Task Force on Practice Guidelines. *J Am Coll Cardiol*. 2013;62:e147–e239.
35. Verma A, Kalman JM, Callans DJ. Treatment of patients with atrial fibrillation and heart failure with reduced ejection fraction. *Circulation*. 2017;135:1547–1563.
36. Whelton PK, Carey RM, Aronow WS, et al. 2017 ACC/AHA/AAPA/ABC/ACPM/AGS/APhA/ASH/ASPC/NMA/PCNA guideline for the prevention, detection, evaluation, and management of high blood pressure in adults: Executive summary: A report of the American College of Cardiology/American Heart Association Task Force on Clinical Practice Guidelines. *J Am Coll Cardiol*. 2018;71:2199–2269.
37. Unlu O, Levitan EB, Reshetnyak E, et al. Polypharmacy in older adults hospitalized for heart failure. *Circ Heart Fail*. 2020;13(11):e006977.
38. Page RL 2nd, O'Bryant CL, Cheng D, et al. Drugs that may cause or exacerbate heart failure: A scientific statement from the American Heart Association. *Circulation*. 2016;134:e32–e69.
39. Rao VU, Reeves DJ, Chugh AR, et al. Clinical approach to cardiovascular toxicity of oral antineoplastic agents: JACC state-of-the-art review. *J Am Coll Cardiol*. 2021;77(21):2693–2716.
40. Witteles RM, Bosch X. Myocardial protection during cardiotoxic chemotherapy. *Circulation*. 2015;132(19):1835–1845.
41. Milfred-LaForest SK, Chow SL, DiDomenico RJ, et al. Clinical pharmacy services in heart failure: An opinion paper from the Heart Failure Society of America and American College of Clinical Pharmacy Cardiology Practice and Research Network. *Pharmacotherapy*. 2013;33:529–548.
42. Stough WG, Patterson JH. Role and value of clinical pharmacy in heart failure management. *Clin Pharmacol Ther*. 2017;102:209–212.
43. Januzzi JL, Mann DL. Approach to the patient with heart failure. In: Zipes DP, Libby P, Bonow RO, Mann DL, Tomaselli GF, Braunwald E, eds. *Braunwald's Heart Disease: A Textbook of Cardiovascular Medicine*. 11th ed. Philadelphia, PA: Elsevier; 2019:403–417.
44. Ponikowski P, Voors AA, Anker SD, et al. 2016 ESC Guidelines for the diagnosis and treatment of acute and chronic heart failure: The task force for the diagnosis and treatment of acute and chronic heart failure of the European Society of Cardiology (ESC) developed with the special contribution of the Heart Failure Association (HFA) of the ESC. *Eur Heart J*. 2016;37:2129–2200.
45. Kalyani RR. Glucose-lowering drugs to reduce cardiovascular risk in type 2 diabetes. *N Engl J Med*. 2021;384(13):1248–1260.
46. Das SR, Everett BM, Birtcher KK, et al. 2020 Expert Consensus Decision Pathway on Novel Therapies for Cardiovascular Risk Reduction in Patients with Type 2 Diabetes: A Report of the American College of Cardiology Solution Set Oversight Committee. *J Am Coll Cardiol*. 2020;76(9):1117–1145.
47. Anker SD, Butler J, Filippatos G, et al. Empagliflozin in heart failure with a preserved ejection fraction. *N Engl J Med*. 2021;385(16):1451–1461.
48. Solomon SD, McMurray JJV, Anand IS, et al. Angiotensin-neprilysin inhibition in heart failure with preserved ejection fraction. *N Engl J Med*. 2019;381:1609–1620.
49. Fang JC, Ewald GA, Allen LA, et al. Advanced (stage D) heart failure: A statement from the Heart Failure Society of America Guidelines Committee. *J Card Fail*. 2015;21:519–534.
50. Al-Khatib SM, Stevenson WG, Ackerman MJ, et al. 2017 AHA/ACC/HRS Guideline for Management of Patients with Ventricular Arrhythmias and the Prevention of Sudden Cardiac Death: A Report of the American College of Cardiology/American Heart Association Task Force on Clinical Practice Guidelines and the Heart Rhythm Society. *Circulation*. 2018;138(13):e272–e391.
51. Lander MM, Aldweib N, Abraham WT. Wireless hemodynamic monitoring in patients with heart failure. *Curr Heart Fail Rep*. 2021;18(1): 12–22.
52. Abraham WT, Adamson PB, Bourge RC, et al. Wireless pulmonary artery haemodynamic monitoring in chronic heart failure: A randomised controlled trial. *Lancet*. 2011;377(9766): 658–666.
53. Sajgalik P, Grupper A, Edwards BS, et al. Current status of left ventricular assist device therapy. *Mayo Clin Proc*. 2016;91:927–940.
54. Greene SJ, Butler J, Fonarow GC. Simultaneous or rapid sequence initiation of quadruple medical therapy for heart failure-optimizing therapy with the need for speed. *JAMA Cardiol*. 2021.
55. McMurray JJV, Packer M. How should we sequence the treatments for heart failure and a reduced ejection fraction? A redefinition of evidence-based medicine. *Circulation*. 2021;143(9): 875–877.
56. Greene SJ, Fonarow GC, DeVore AD, et al. Titration of medical therapy for heart failure with reduced ejection fraction. *J Am Coll Cardiol*. 2019;73(19):2365–2383.
57. Srivastava PK, DeVore AD, Hellkamp AS, et al. Heart failure hospitalization and guideline-directed prescribing patterns among heart failure with reduced ejection fraction patients. *JACC Heart Fail*. 2021;9(1):28–38.
58. Yusuf S, Pfeffer MA, Swedberg K, et al. Effects of candesartan in patients with chronic heart failure and preserved left-ventricular ejection fraction: The CHARM-Preserved trial. *Lancet*. 2003;362:777–781.
59. Yancy CW, Januzzi JL Jr, Allen LA, et al. 2017 ACC expert consensus decision pathway for optimization of heart failure treatment: Answers to 10 pivotal issues about heart failure with reduced ejection fraction: A report of the American College of Cardiology Task Force on expert consensus decision pathways. *J Am Coll Cardiol*. 2018;71:201–230.
60. Kostis WJ, Shetty M, Chowdhury YS, Kostis JB. ACE inhibitor-induced angioedema: A review. *Curr Hypertens Rep*. 2018;20:55.
61. Vardeny O, Miller R, Solomon SD. Combined neprilysin and renin-angiotensin system inhibition for the treatment of heart failure. *JACC Heart Fail*. 2014;2:663–670.
62. King JB, Bress AP, Reese AD, Munger MA. Neprilysin inhibition in heart failure with reduced ejection fraction: A clinical review. *Pharmacotherapy*. 2015;35:823–837.
63. Sarwar CM, Papadimitriou L, Pitt B, et al. Hyperkalemia in heart failure. *J Am Coll Cardiol*. 2016;68:1575–1589.
64. Dargie HJ. Effect of carvedilol on outcome after myocardial infarction in patients with left-ventricular dysfunction: The CAPRICORN randomised trial. *Lancet*. 2001;357:1385–1390.
65. Packer M, Bristow MR, Cohn JN, et al. The effect of carvedilol on morbidity and mortality in patients with chronic heart failure. U.S. Carvedilol Heart Failure Study Group. *N Engl J Med*. 1996;334:1349–1355.
66. Effect of metoprolol CR/XL in chronic heart failure: Metoprolol CR/XL randomised intervention trial in congestive heart failure (MERIT-HF). *Lancet*. 1999;353(9169):2001–2007.
67. The cardiac insufficiency bisoprolol study II (CIBIS-II): A randomised trial. *Lancet*. 1999;353:9–13.
68. Packer M, Coats AJ, Fowler MB, et al. Effect of carvedilol on survival in severe chronic heart failure. *N Engl J Med*. 2001;344:1651–1658.
69. Hjalmarson A, Goldstein S, Fagerberg B, et al. Effects of controlled-release metoprolol on total mortality, hospitalizations, and well-being in patients with heart failure: The Metoprolol CR/XL randomized intervention trial in congestive heart failure (MERIT-HF). MERIT-HF Study Group. *JAMA*. 2000;283:1295–1302.
70. Packer M, Fowler MB, Roecker EB, et al. Effect of carvedilol on the morbidity of patients with severe chronic heart failure: Results of the carvedilol prospective randomized cumulative survival (COPERNICUS) study. *Circulation*. 2002;106:2194–2199.
71. Poole-Wilson PA, Swedberg K, Cleland JG, et al. Comparison of carvedilol and metoprolol on clinical outcomes in patients with chronic heart failure in the Carvedilol or Metoprolol European Trial (COMET): Randomised controlled trial. *Lancet*. 2003;362:7–13.
72. Frohlich H, Zhao J, Tager T, et al. Carvedilol compared with metoprolol succinate in the treatment and prognosis of patients with stable chronic heart failure: Carvedilol or metoprolol evaluation study. *Circulation Heart failure*. 2015;8:887–896.
73. Pasternak B, Svanstrom H, Melbye M, Hviid A. Association of treatment with carvedilol vs metoprolol succinate and mortality in patients with heart failure. *JAMA Intern Med*. 2014;174:1597–1604.
74. Willenheimer R, van Veldhuisen DJ, Silke B, et al. Effect on survival and hospitalization of initiating treatment for chronic heart failure with bisoprolol followed by enalapril, as compared with the opposite sequence: Results of the randomized Cardiac Insufficiency Bisoprolol Study (CIBIS) III. *Circulation*. 2005;112:2426–2435.
75. Gattis WA, O'Connor CM, Gallup DS, Hasselblad V, Gheorghiade M. Predischarge initiation of carvedilol in patients hospitalized for decompensated heart failure: Results of the Initiation Management Predischarge: Process for Assessment of Carvedilol Therapy in Heart Failure (IMPACT-HF) trial. *J Am Coll Cardiol*. 2004;43:1534–1541.

76. McAlister FA, Wiebe N, Ezekowitz JA, Leung AA, Armstrong PW. Meta-analysis: Beta-blocker dose, heart rate reduction, and death in patients with heart failure. *Ann Intern Med.* 2009;150:784–794.
77. Bavishi C, Chatterjee S, Ather S, Patel D, Messerli FH. Beta-blockers in heart failure with preserved ejection fraction: A meta-analysis. *Heart Fail Rev.* 2015;20:193–201.
78. Cleland JGF, Bunting KV, Flather MD, et al. Beta-blockers for heart failure with reduced, mid-range, and preserved ejection fraction: An individual patient-level analysis of double-blind randomized trials. *Eur Heart J.* 2018;39:26–35.
79. Flatt DM, Brown MC, Mizeracki AM, King BJ, Weber KT. Mineralocorticoid receptor antagonists in the management of heart failure and resistant hypertension: A review. *JAMA Cardiol.* 2016;1:607–612.
80. Trevisan M, de Deco P, Xu H, et al. Incidence, predictors and clinical management of hyperkalaemia in new users of mineralocorticoid receptor antagonists. *Eur J Heart Fail.* 2018;20:1217–1226.
81. Ferreira JP, Butler J, Rossignol P, et al. Abnormalities of potassium in heart failure: JACC State-of-the-Art Review. *J Am Coll Cardiol.* 2020;75(22):2836–2850.
82. Desai AS, Vardeny O, Claggett B, et al. Reduced risk of hyperkalemia during treatment of heart failure with mineralocorticoid receptor antagonists by use of sacubitril/valsartan compared with enalapril: A secondary analysis of the PARADIGM-HF Trial. *JAMA Cardiol.* 2017;2(1):79–85.
83. Vallon V, Verma S. Effects of SGLT2 inhibitors on kidney and cardiovascular function. *Annu Rev Physiol.* 2021;83:503–528.
84. McMurray JJV, Solomon SD, Inzucchi SE, et al. Dapagliflozin in patients with heart failure and reduced ejection fraction. *N Engl J Med.* 2019;381:1995–2008.
85. Packer M, Anker SD, Butler J, et al. Cardiovascular and renal outcomes with empagliflozin in heart failure. *New Engl J Med.* 2020;Aug 29. Online ahead of print. doi:10.1056/nejmoa2022190.
86. Ellison DH, Felker GM. Diuretic treatment in heart failure. *N Engl J Med.* 2017;377:1964–1975.
87. Mullens W, Damman K, Harjola VP, et al. The use of diuretics in heart failure with congestion: A position statement from the Heart Failure Association of the European Society of Cardiology. *Eur J Heart Fail.* 2019;21(2):137–155.
88. Taylor AL, Ziesche S, Yancy C, et al. Combination of isosorbide dinitrate and hydralazine in blacks with heart failure. *N Engl J Med.* 2004;351(20):2049–2057.
89. Redfield MM, Anstrom KJ, Levine JA, et al. Isosorbide mononitrate in heart failure with preserved ejection fraction. *N Engl J Med.* 2015;373:2314–2324.
90. Koruth JS, Lala A, Pinney S, Reddy VY, Dukkipati SR. The clinical use of Ivabradine. *J Am Coll Cardiol.* 2017;70:1777–1784.
91. Bhatt AS, DeVore AD, DeWald TA, Swedberg K, Mentz RJ. Achieving a maximally tolerated beta-blocker dose in heart failure patients: Is there room for improvement? *J Am Coll Cardiol.* 2017;69:2542–2550.
92. Greene SJ, Butler J, Albert NM, et al. Medical therapy for heart failure with reduced ejection fraction: The CHAMP-HF registry. *J Am Coll Cardiol.* 2018;72:351–366.
93. Swedberg K, Komajda M, Bohm M, et al. Ivabradine and outcomes in chronic heart failure (SHIFT): A randomised placebo-controlled study. *Lancet.* 2010;376:875–885.
94. Ambrosy AP, Butler J, Ahmed A, et al. The use of digoxin in patients with worsening chronic heart failure: Reconsidering an old drug to reduce hospital admissions. *J Am Coll Cardiol.* 2014;63:1823–1832.
95. The Digitalis Investigation Group. The effect of digoxin on mortality and morbidity in patients with heart failure. *N Engl J Med.* 1997;336:525–533.
96. Ahmed A, Rich MW, Fleg JL, et al. Effects of digoxin on morbidity and mortality in diastolic heart failure: The ancillary digitalis investigation group trial. *Circulation.* 2006;114:397–403.
97. Ahmed A, Rich MW, Love TE, et al. Digoxin and reduction in mortality and hospitalization in heart failure: A comprehensive post hoc analysis of the DIG trial. *Eur Heart J.* 2006;27:178–186.
98. DiDomenico RJ, Page RL. Digoxin. *Clinical Pharmacokinetics.* J. E. Murphy. Bethesda, MD, American Society of Health-System Pharmacists: 2017;239–248.
99. Allen LA, Fonarow GC, Simon DN, et al. Digoxin use and subsequent outcomes among patients in a contemporary atrial fibrillation cohort. *J Am Coll Cardiol.* 2015;65:2691–2698.
100. Lam PH, Bhyan P, Arundel C, et al. Digoxin use and lower risk of 30-day all-cause readmission in older patients with heart failure and reduced ejection fraction receiving beta-blockers. *Clin Cardiol.* 2018;41:406–412.
101. Freeman JV, Yang J, Sung SH, Hlatky MA, Go AS. Effectiveness and safety of digoxin among contemporary adults with incident systolic heart failure. *Circ Cardiovasc Qual Outcomes.* 2013;6:525–533.
102. Malik A, Masson R, Singh S, et al. Digoxin discontinuation and outcomes in patients with heart failure with reduced ejection fraction. *J Am Coll Cardiol.* 2019;74(5):617–627.
103. January CT, Wann LS, Alpert JS, et al. 2014 AHA/ACC/HRS guideline for the management of patients with atrial fibrillation: A report of the American College of Cardiology/American Heart Association Task Force on practice guidelines and the Heart Rhythm Society. *Circulation.* 2014;130:e199–e267.
104. Emdin M, Aimo A, Castiglione V, et al. Targeting cyclic guanosine monophosphate to treat heart failure: JACC review topic of the week. *J Am Coll Cardiol.* 2020;76(15):1795–1807.
105. Markham A, Duggan S. Vericiguat: First approval. *Drugs.* 2021;81(6):721–726.
106. Armstrong PW, Pieske B, Anstrom KJ, et al. Vericiguat in patients with heart failure and reduced ejection fraction. *N Engl J Med.* 2020;382(20):1883–1893.
107. Armstrong PW, Lam CSP, Anstrom KJ, et al. Effect of vericiguat vs placebo on quality of life in patients with heart failure and preserved ejection fraction: The VITALITY-HFpEF Randomized Clinical Trial. *JAMA.* 2020;324(15):1512–1521.
108. January CT, Wann LS, Calkins H, et al. 2019 AHA/ACC/HRS Focused Update of the 2014 AHA/ACC/HRS Guideline for the Management of Patients with Atrial Fibrillation: A Report of the American College of Cardiology/American Heart Association Task Force on Clinical Practice Guidelines and the Heart Rhythm Society. *J Am Coll Cardiol.* 2019;74(1):104–132.
109. Vamos M, Erath JW, Hohnloser SH. Digoxin-associated mortality: A systematic review and meta-analysis of the literature. *Eur Heart J.* 2015;36:1831–1838.
110. Balla C, Cappato R. Atrial fibrillation ablation in heart failure. *Eur Heart J.* 2020;Suppl 22(Suppl E):E50–E53.
111. Dunlay SM, Givertz MM, Aguilar D, et al. Type 2 diabetes mellitus and heart failure: A scientific statement from the American Heart Association and the Heart Failure Society of America: This statement does not represent an update of the 2017 ACC/AHA/HFSA heart failure guideline update. *Circulation.* 2019;14010.1161/cir.0000000000000691.
112. Rocha BML, Cunha GJL, Menezes Falcao LF. The burden of iron deficiency in heart failure: Therapeutic approach. *J Am Coll Cardiol.* 2018;71(7):782–793.
113. Ponikowski P, Kirwan BA, Anker SD, et al. Ferric carboxymaltose for iron deficiency at discharge after acute heart failure: A multicentre, double-blind, randomised, controlled trial. *Lancet.* 2020;396(10266):1895–1904.
114. Thomsen RW, Nicolaisen SK, Hasvold P, et al. Elevated potassium levels in patients with congestive heart failure: Occurrence, risk factors, and clinical outcomes: A Danish population-based cohort study. *J Am Heart Assoc.* 2018;7(11).
115. Weiss JN, Qu Z, Shivkumar K. Electrophysiology of hypokalemia and hyperkalemia. *Circ Arrhythm Electrophysiol.* 2017;10(3):pii: e004667.

Acute Decompensated Heart Failure

37

Brent N. Reed, Stormi E. Gale, and Zachary L. Cox

KEY CONCEPTS

1. Patients presenting to the hospital with acute decompensated heart failure (ADHF) can be categorized into four hemodynamic subsets based on volume status (euvolemic or "dry" vs volume overloaded or "wet") and cardiac output (adequate cardiac output or "warm" vs hypoperfusion or "cold"). Patients may be warm and dry, warm and wet, cold and dry, or cold and wet.
2. While invasive hemodynamic monitoring using a pulmonary artery (PA) catheter does not alter outcomes in a broad population of ADHF patients, it may be considered in those who are refractory to initial therapy, in those whose hemodynamic status is unclear, or in those with clinically significant hypotension (ie, systolic blood pressure <80 mm Hg) or worsening renal function despite standard therapy.
3. Key hemodynamic parameters monitored with a PA catheter include pulmonary capillary wedge pressure (PCWP; reflecting fluid status or "preload"), cardiac output or cardiac index (CI; often used to reflect the innate contractility of the heart), and systemic vascular resistance (SVR; reflecting vascular tone or "afterload"). Although a normal PCWP (6-12 mm Hg) is desirable in healthy patients, higher ventricular filling pressures (15-18 mm Hg) are often necessary for patients with heart failure (HF).
4. Treatment goals for ADHF include relief of congestive symptoms, restoration of systemic tissue perfusion via improved cardiac output, and minimization of further cardiac damage and other adverse drug reactions.
5. Optimizing oral chronic HF therapy in the setting of ADHF may assist with improving cardiac output, relieving congestion, and preventing hospital readmission.
6. Pharmacologic therapies used in the management of ADHF can be broadly classified according to whether they improve volume overload and/or low cardiac output. No therapy studied to date has conclusively been shown to reduce mortality, and some may worsen outcomes.
7. Intravenous (IV) loop diuretics are considered first-line therapy for the management of ADHF associated with volume overload. Administration as a bolus or continuous infusion appears to be equally effective and safe when selected as initial therapy, although high-dose loop diuretic therapy (ie, 2.5 times the oral regimen prior to admission) is associated with greater volume removal. The addition of a thiazide-type diuretic may be considered in patients with diuretic resistance. If patients continue to be refractory to, or experience worsening of renal function with, diuretic therapy, placement of a PA catheter may help guide therapies such as IV vasodilators and/or inotropes.
8. Ultrafiltration may be considered in patients with diuretic resistance or those with worsening renal impairment despite IV vasodilator and/or inotrope therapy.
9. Intravenous vasodilators may be added to diuretics for rapid resolution of congestive symptoms, especially in patients with acute pulmonary edema or severe hypertension. Such therapy may also be considered in patients who fail to respond to aggressive treatment with diuretics. In the absence of hypotension (systolic blood pressure <90 mm Hg or symptomatic hypotension) or reduced left ventricular filling pressures, IV vasodilators should also be considered prior to IV inotropes in patients with ADHF and evidence of low cardiac output. Frequent blood pressure monitoring is necessary to ensure their safe use.
10. Intravenous inotropes are recommended for maintaining systemic perfusion and end-organ function in hypotensive patients with evidence of severe left ventricular dysfunction and low cardiac output. Inotropic therapy may also be considered in patients who do not tolerate or respond to IV vasodilators or in patients with worsening renal function despite standard therapy. Patients receiving IV inotropes should be monitored continuously for arrhythmias.
11. Temporary mechanical circulatory support (MCS) is indicated in select patients with severe ADHF or those with advanced HF who are refractory to pharmacologic therapy. The intra-aortic balloon pump (IABP) is the most common type of temporary MCS but provides the least amount of hemodynamic support. Other types of temporary MCS include temporary ventricular assist devices (VADs) and extracorporeal membrane oxygenation (ECMO).
12. Cardiac transplantation remains the only definitive therapy for advanced HF. Given the extended wait time for identifying suitable donors, implantation of a durable VAD may be considered for patients who are eligible for cardiac transplantation (ie, "bridge to transplant") or in whom transplantation is not an option (ie, "destination therapy").

BEYOND THE BOOK

Pair up with a classmate and create a series of flashcards, in which you describe and list several characteristics of a patient in one of the four hemodynamic subsets on one side (ie, signs, symptoms, physical examination findings, laboratory values) and the appropriate classification and treatment approach on the other side. Present your partner with the case, and ask them to recommend an initial treatment and monitoring plan. Ensure that at least one of each of the four hemodynamic subsets is represented in your stack of cards, but also try varying the complexity and severity of each case/list. For example, start with a simple case/list of characteristics consistent with fluid overload (ie, subset II or "warm and wet"), and ask your partner to recommend an intravenous diuretic regimen based on the patient's home diuretic dose. Later, progress to patient scenarios/cards representing subset III ("cold and dry") and IV ("cold and wet"). For each case/card, ask your partner to list patient-specific factors that might influence the treatment approach (eg, hypotension when deciding between a vasodilator and inotrope) as well as monitoring parameters for the therapies selected. For an extra challenge, add in some cases/cards where you provide values from a pulmonary artery catheter or include a patient who develops diuretic resistance. Compare and contrast your partner's recommendations with those you wrote on the back of the card.

INTRODUCTION

The clinical course of heart failure (HF) manifests as periods of relative stability with increasingly frequent episodes of decompensation as the disease progresses.[1] Several terms have been used to characterize worsening HF requiring hospitalization. Patients with persistent symptoms requiring specialized interventions despite guideline-directed medical therapy (GDMT) are classified as having advanced HF or Stage D, according to the American College of Cardiology Foundation/American Heart Association (ACCF/AHA) system.[2] Due to the presence of HF symptoms with minimal activity or at rest, these patients are also typically classified as New York Heart Association (NYHA) class III or IV, respectively. The terms *acute decompensated heart failure* (ADHF) and *exacerbation of heart failure* refer to those patients with new or worsening signs or symptoms of HF (often as a result of volume overload and/or low cardiac output [CO]) requiring medical intervention such as an emergency department visit or hospitalization. The term *acute heart failure* may be misleading as it more often refers to patients with a sudden onset of HF signs or symptoms following previously normal cardiac function (eg, following myocardial infarction [MI]). This chapter focuses on the management of patients with ADHF, which may include those with heart failure with reduced ejection fraction (HFrEF) or heart failure with preserved ejection fraction (HFpEF).

Despite the considerable morbidity and mortality associated with ADHF, few randomized controlled trials have been conducted in this patient population. For those studies that have been published, the heterogeneity of patients enrolled often limits clinical application. Nonetheless, clinical practice guidelines for HF issued by ACCF/AHA include sections specifically focused on the management of advanced HF and ADHF; these and other consensus-based recommendations will be referenced where relevant throughout this chapter.[2,3]

EPIDEMIOLOGY

An estimated 6 million American adults have HF, and projections indicate that prevalence is likely to increase nearly 50% by 2030.[4] The growing number of patients living with HF has led to substantial increases in hospitalization rates for ADHF. Recent data indicate that over 1 million patients are hospitalized for HF annually, contributing to significant increases in morbidity and mortality and adding substantial burden to the healthcare system.[4,5] Hospitalization for HF has been independently associated with increases in subsequent hospitalization as well as decreased survival, which may explain why the mortality rate at 5 years remains high (42.3%).[4,6] The cost of HF is projected to approach $70 billion by 2030, an increase thought to be driven primarily by the costs of acute care.[4]

ETIOLOGY AND PATHOPHYSIOLOGY

The underlying etiology of ADHF varies and is often multifactorial. De novo HF may occur due to left ventricular dysfunction following a large MI or sudden elevation in blood pressure; such cases represent approximately 25% of admissions.[6] However, most hospitalizations for ADHF (70%) comprise patients experiencing an acute worsening of chronic HF[7]; readers are referred to Chapter 36, "Chronic Heart Failure," for a more detailed discussion of the etiology and pathophysiology of chronic HF including precipitating factors. Patients can become refractory to oral therapies and decompensate after even a relatively mild insult (eg, dietary indiscretion, nonsteroidal anti-inflammatory drug use), medication nonadherence, or concurrent noncardiac illness (eg, infection). New or worsening cardiac processes, such as MI, atrial or ventricular arrhythmias, hypertensive crises, myocarditis, or acute valvular insufficiency, may also produce ADHF in an otherwise stable patient. Exacerbations of chronic HFrEF and HFpEF occur in approximately equal numbers.[2] A minority of patients (5%) present with gradual, progressive worsening of CO and refractoriness to therapy due to advanced left ventricular systolic dysfunction.[7]

Several studies have provided a better understanding of the prognostic factors associated with ADHF. Blood urea nitrogen (BUN) is the best individual predictor of in-hospital mortality, followed by low systolic blood pressure and elevated serum creatinine.[7] Hyponatremia, elevations in troponin I, ischemic etiology, and poor functional capacity are also negative prognostic factors.[6,9] Use of GDMT at discharge and coronary angiography or implantable cardioverter-defibrillator placement during hospitalization are associated with improved prognosis, suggesting that optimal management during hospitalization can yield beneficial effects on subsequent prognosis.[9]

CLINICAL PRESENTATION

1 A careful history and physical examination are key components of an ADHF diagnosis. The history should focus on potential etiologies of ADHF; the presence of precipitating factors; the onset, duration, and severity of symptoms; and a careful medication history. Hemodynamic status should also be ascertained to guide initial therapy. Patients presenting with ADHF may be categorized into one of four hemodynamic subsets based on volume status (euvolemic or "dry" vs volume overloaded or "wet") and CO (adequate CO or "warm" vs hypoperfusion or "cold"). The corresponding subsets are warm and dry (subset I), warm and wet (subset II), cold and dry (subset III), or cold and wet (subset IV; Fig. 37-1). The term *cardiogenic shock* may also be used to describe patients in subsets III and IV who present with low blood pressure and evidence of tissue hypoperfusion. In addition to guiding therapeutic decision making, these four hemodynamic profiles are also predictive of clinical outcomes. Compared to dry-warm patients, patients in the wet-warm

CLINICAL PRESENTATION Acute Decompensated Heart Failure

General

- Patients with ADHF typically present in one of four hemodynamic subsets (Fig. 37-1) based on the presence of volume overload (ie, congestion) and/or low cardiac output (ie, tissue hypoperfusion).
- Hemodynamic status can be ascertained in most patients based on their history and physical examination; some may require invasive hemodynamic monitoring.

Symptoms

- Volume overload: dyspnea, orthopnea, paroxysmal nocturnal dyspnea, ascites, gastrointestinal symptoms (poor appetite, nausea, early satiety), peripheral edema, weight gain.
- Low output: altered mental status, fatigue, gastrointestinal symptoms (similar to volume overload), decreased urine output.

Signs

- Volume overload: pulmonary crackles (or rales), elevated jugular venous pressure, abdominojugular reflux, S3 gallop, peripheral edema.
- Low output: tachycardia, hypotension (more commonly) or hypertension, narrow pulse pressure, cool extremities, pallor, cachexia.

Laboratory Values

- Volume overload: B-type natriuretic peptide <100 pg/mL (ng/L; 29 pmol/L) and N-terminal B-type natriuretic peptide <300 pg/mL (ng/L; 35 pmol/L) are negatively predictive for congestive ADHF; serum sodium concentration <130 mEq/L (mmol/L); elevated alkaline phosphatase; elevated gamma-glutamyl transferase.
- Low cardiac output: evidence of end-organ injury due to impaired perfusion, such as elevated liver transaminases and serum creatinine; mixed venous oxygen concentration <60% (0.60); elevated serum lactate.

Hemodynamic Monitoring

- Volume overload: pulmonary capillary wedge pressure >18 mm Hg; other volumetric pressures (eg, right atrial pressure, pulmonary artery diastolic pressure) are also commonly elevated.
- Low cardiac output: cardiac index <2.2 L/min/m^2 (0.037 L/s/m^2), with or without systemic vascular resistance >1,400 dyne·sec·cm^{-5} (18 Wood units; 140 MPa·s/m^3).

and wet-cold subsets have a 2-fold and 2.5-fold greater risk of death at 1 year, respectively.[7]

Although hemodynamic status can be determined in most patients based on signs and symptoms, a small subset of patients may require invasive hemodynamic monitoring to guide therapy. In this latter population, measurement of the pulmonary capillary wedge pressure (PCWP) and cardiac index (CI) may be used to categorize patients by volume status and CO, respectively. A PCWP greater than 18 mm Hg often reflects volume overload and is generally used to distinguish "wet" from "dry" subsets, whereas a CI less than 2.2 L/min/m^2 (0.037 L/s/m^2) is often used to distinguish "cold" from "warm" subsets; use of these invasive hemodynamic parameters will be discussed in further detail later in this chapter.

Hospitalization for ADHF should be considered based on the clinical findings listed in Table 37-1. Most patients do not require admission to an intensive care unit and may be admitted to a monitored unit or general medical floor. If a patient experiences hemodynamic instability necessitating frequent monitoring of vital signs, invasive hemodynamic monitoring, or rapid titration of IV medications (with concurrent monitoring), admission to an intensive care unit may be required to ensure optimal outcomes.

Signs and Symptoms

Important elements of the physical examination include assessment of vital signs and weight, cardiac auscultation for heart sounds and murmurs, pulmonary auscultation for crackles, presence and severity of peripheral edema, and evidence of end-organ dysfunction. The most common presentation of ADHF is severe volume overload. Symptoms consistent with pulmonary congestion include orthopnea and dyspnea with minimal exertion, and those associated with systemic congestion include gastrointestinal (GI) discomfort, ascites, and peripheral edema. Orthopnea is the symptom that best correlates with elevated pulmonary pressure, whereas jugular venous pressure is the most reliable sign of volume status, warranting evaluation at admission as well as throughout hospitalization as an indicator of diuretic efficacy.[7] An S3 gallop, suggestive of increased volume in the left ventricle, has high diagnostic specificity for ADHF.[7] Other physical findings, such as pulmonary crackles and lower extremity edema, have low specificity and sensitivity for the diagnosis of ADHF.

Signs and symptoms of low CO are often nonspecific and may include generalized fatigue, cool extremities, and pallor. Manifestations of impaired end-organ perfusion may also be present, such as altered mental status (decreased perfusion to the central nervous system) or decreased urine output (decreased renal perfusion). Hypotension and narrow pulse pressure may also suggest low CO. Gastrointestinal symptoms such as poor appetite, nausea, and early satiety may be a sign of poor perfusion to the GI tract, abdominal congestion, or both. Many patients will present with signs and symptoms of both wet and cold subsets; in these patients, symptoms of low CO may not be obvious until the congestion has been optimally treated.

Laboratory Findings

Plasma B-type natriuretic peptide (BNP) and N-terminal pro-BNP (NT-proBNP) concentrations are positively correlated with the degree of left ventricular dysfunction and HF, and are now frequently used to assist in the differential diagnosis of dyspnea (HF vs pulmonary disorders). A low BNP concentration, often defined as less than 100 pg/mL (ng/L; 29 pmol/L), is highly predictive for excluding HF as an underlying etiology for dyspnea.[7] An NT-proBNP concentration of less than 300 pg/mL (ng/L; 35 pmol/L) is similarly predictive for excluding HF. In addition, an elevated BNP concentration prior to discharge is associated with an increased risk of poor long-term outcomes. However, some limitations exist. For example, any

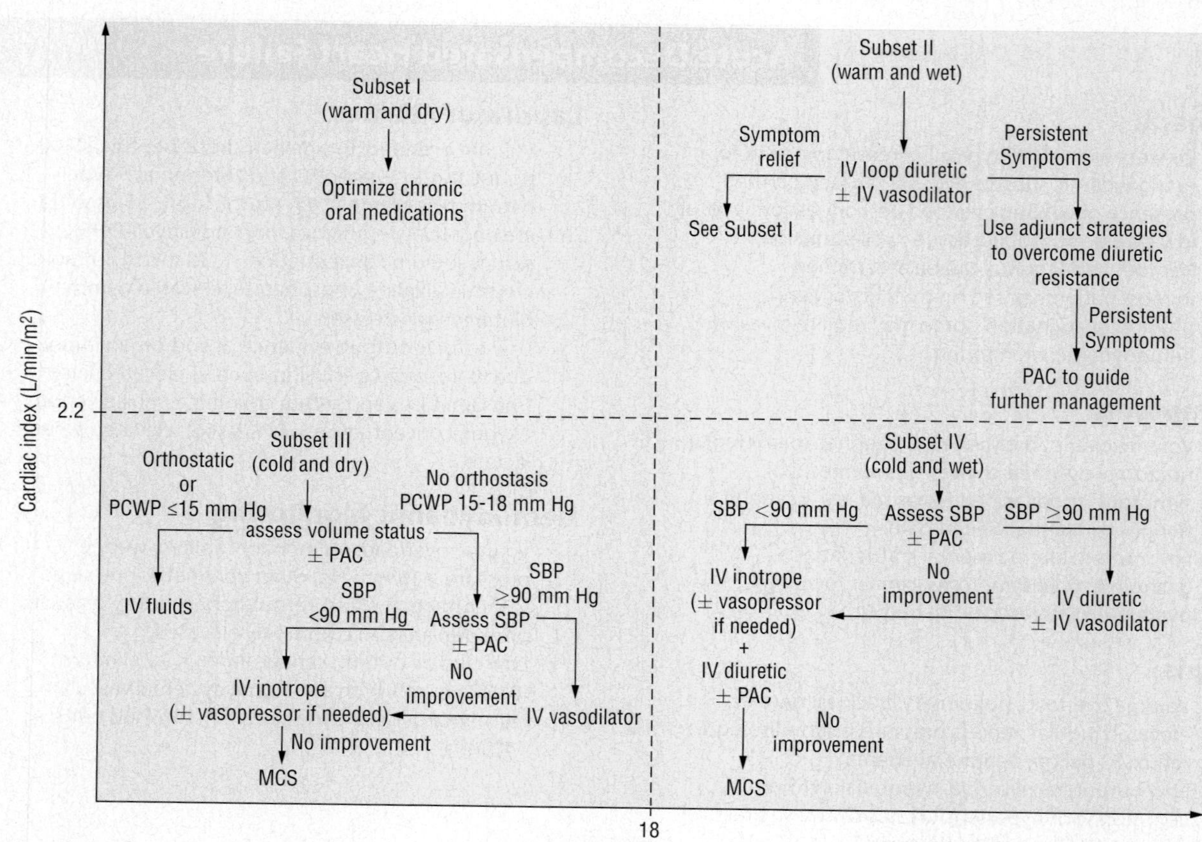

FIGURE 37-1 General management algorithm for ADHF based on clinical presentation. Patients may be categorized into a hemodynamic subset based on signs and symptoms or invasive hemodynamic monitoring. Adjunct strategies for overcoming diuretic resistance include increasing the dose of loop diuretic; switching to a continuous infusion; adding a diuretic with an alternative mechanism of action, an IV vasodilator, or an IV inotrope; and in select patients, adding MCS. (IV, intravenous; MCS, mechanical circulatory support; PAC, pulmonary artery catheter; PCWP, pulmonary capillary wedge pressure; SBP, systolic blood pressure.)

TABLE 37-1 Indications for Hospitalization in Patients Presenting with ADHF

Presenting Features	Clinical Findings
Evidence of fluid overload	• Weight gain >10 kg (consider if >5 kg) • Symptoms of congestion (eg, dyspnea on exertion or at rest, orthopnea, PND, and early satiety[a]) • Signs of congestion (eg, tachypnea with oxygen saturation <90% [0.90], JVD, crackles, hepatomegaly, and lower extremity edema)
Evidence of low cardiac output	• Extreme fatigue • Hypotension, narrow pulse pressure • Cool extremities
Evidence of organ hypoperfusion	• Worsening renal or hepatic function • Altered mental status
Concomitant cardiovascular diseases that could compromise hemodynamic status	• Uncontrolled hypertension • Myocardial ischemia or infarction • Valvular disease • Arrhythmia (eg, atrial fibrillation with rapid ventricular response, ventricular tachycardia, and repeated ICD shocks)
Other conditions that could compromise hemodynamic status	• Severe electrolyte deficiency (potassium and magnesium) • Acute exacerbation of pulmonary disease (eg, asthma, COPD, or pulmonary embolus) • Infection such as pneumonia or urosepsis • Symptomatic hypothyroidism or hyperthyroidism • Use of medications with negative inotropic effects (eg, nondihydropyridine calcium antagonists)

COPD, chronic obstructive pulmonary disease; ICD, implantable cardioverter defibrillator; JVD, jugular venous distension; PND, paroxysmal nocturnal dyspnea.

[a]Early satiety may also be a symptom of low cardiac output.

disease process that increases right heart pressures will elevate BNP, such as pulmonary emboli, chronic obstructive lung disease, and pulmonary arterial hypertension. In addition, BNP concentrations may be mildly increased with advanced age, female gender, renal dysfunction, and use of sacubitril/valsartan, and may be lower in the setting of obesity. Although the role of BNP in HF remains an area of ongoing research, guidelines recommend obtaining a BNP or NT-proBNP in order to assist with clinical decision making when the diagnosis of ADHF is uncertain and for determining the prognosis or severity of disease.[2]

A number of other laboratory tests should also be obtained to identify precipitating factors for ADHF (eg, thyroid function tests, complete blood count to assess for infection). In particular, cardiac enzymes (eg, troponin) should be obtained to exclude the presence of myocardial ischemia. Routine serum chemistries (eg, serum creatinine, liver function tests) should also be obtained to assess end-organ perfusion. Ferritin, serum iron, and transferrin iron-binding capacity should be obtained to screen for iron deficiency, even in patients without anemia. Profound volume overload may also contribute to aberrations in serum markers of end-organ function due to venous congestion. Other helpful laboratory tests include markers of peripheral tissue perfusion, such as venous oxygenation saturation and serum lactate concentrations.

Invasive Hemodynamic Monitoring

2 Invasive hemodynamic monitoring is usually performed with a flow-directed pulmonary artery (PA) catheter (also known as Swan-Ganz catheter) placed percutaneously into a central vein and advanced through the right side of the heart and into the PA. This process may also be referred to as right heart catheterization (in contrast to left heart catheterization, which is often used to visualize the coronary arteries). Because routine use of a PA catheter in patients with ADHF does not improve survival, invasive hemodynamic monitoring should be reserved for select patients with ADHF.[10] For example, it often provides important information in patients whose clinical status is unclear or complicated (eg, cardiogenic shock), or as a guide for titrating rapidly acting medications (eg, IV vasodilators).[3] As a consequence, invasive hemodynamic monitoring should be considered in patients who are refractory to initial therapy, whose volume status is unclear, or who have clinically significant hypotension (eg, systolic blood pressure <80 mm Hg) or worsening renal function (WRF) despite appropriate initial therapy.[11] Hemodynamic assessment is also required in patients being evaluated for mechanical circulatory support (MCS) or cardiac transplantation. Finally, documentation of an adequate hemodynamic response to IV inotropic therapy is often necessary in order to obtain approval for reimbursement for chronic outpatient inotropic therapy.[2]

3 Several important hemodynamic parameters can be obtained from a PA catheter. Inflation of a balloon proximal to the end port allows the catheter to be "wedged" inside a pulmonary capillary, yielding the PCWP. In the absence of an intracardiac shunt, mitral valve disease, or severe pulmonary disease, the PCWP may be used to estimate left ventricular end-diastolic pressure, or "preload." Preload refers to the stretch incurred by cardiac myocytes in response to increased volumetric pressure. Thus, PCWP can be a useful marker of volume status; elevated PCWP is often indicative of volume overload, whereas reduced PCWP indicates dehydration or inadequate ventricular filling pressure. The relationship between preload (or PCWP) and CO is described by the Frank-Starling mechanism, which is depicted in Fig. 37-2. Due to the much flatter curve observed in patients with HF, increases in preload do not confer the same improvements in CO observed in patients with normal cardiac function. Consequently, higher pressures (ie, 15-18 mm Hg, compared to a normal range of 6-12 mm Hg) are often required in patients with HF in order to optimize CO. Excess preload (PCWP >18 mm Hg) manifests as signs and symptoms of congestion. Fortunately, PCWP can be lowered to 15 to 18 mm Hg with relatively little decrease in CO due to the flatter shape of the Frank–Starling curve in HF. Extreme elevations in PCWP (representing profound volume overload) are also thought to worsen cardiac function, although a precise mechanism for this phenomenon is unknown. Of the parameters that can be obtained via PA catheterization, an elevated PCWP is most consistently associated with a worse prognosis.[12]

A PA catheter may also be used to determine CO or the volume of blood being pumped by the heart (particularly by the left ventricle) over a unit of time. CO is often normalized for body surface area to yield CI, which allows measurements to be made without considering the body size. Using parameters derived from the PA catheter, CO is calculated based on one of two methods. The thermodilution method for determining CO is performed by releasing cooled fluid from a proximal port on the PA catheter and measuring the resulting change in temperature at a downstream thermistor over a period of time. In the Fick method, blood flow is calculated using the difference between arterial and venous oxygen concentration, the oxygen-carrying capacity of hemoglobin, and a population constant for oxygen consumption over time. The preferred method for determining CO varies by clinician, although the presence of certain comorbid conditions (eg, valvular abnormalities and pulmonary disease) may make one method more or less accurate in an individual patient. However, because the determination of CO by the Fick method depends on a set of assumptions (eg, rate of oxygen consumption according to gender and body size), the thermodilution method is generally thought to be a more reliable predictor of outcomes in critically ill patients.[13]

The systemic vascular resistance (SVR) can also be calculated using parameters measured by the PA catheter, including CO, mean arterial pressure (MAP), and central venous pressure (CVP). Also referred to as total peripheral resistance or arterial impedance, SVR reflects "afterload," or the total sum of forces impeding the ejection of blood from the left ventricle. Vasoconstriction (ie, decreased diameter of arterial vessel lumen) increases vascular resistance, whereas vasodilation decreases it. Although SVR is inversely related to CO, patients with normal left ventricular function can often withstand relatively high elevations in SVR, as shown in Fig. 37-2. However, in patients with HF, even a moderately elevated SVR can compromise left ventricular performance. Elevated SVR is common in untreated HF and generally responsive to oral or IV vasodilators. Conversely, a reduction in resistance is consistent with vasodilatory shock (eg, sepsis) and is routinely managed with IV vasopressor therapy (see Chapter e42, "Shock Syndromes").

When the heart rate is held constant, CO reflects stroke volume, or the volume of blood being pumped by the heart (particularly by the left ventricle) with each beat. Although stroke volume is in part determined by cardiac contractility, it is also influenced by preload and afterload, and alterations in CO (or CI) should therefore be interpreted in the context of PCWP and SVR. For example, a low CI (<2.2 L/min/m^2[0.037 L/s/m^2]) in the setting of a low PCWP (<6 mm Hg) may represent decreased preload due to hypovolemia rather than impaired contractility (Fig. 37-2). Similarly, a low CI in the setting of high SVR (>1,400 dyne·sec·cm^{-5} [18 Wood units; 140 MPa·s/m^3]) may represent impaired left ventricular performance due to excess afterload (Fig. 37-2). In both of these cases, CI could be increased directly (via inotropic therapy, for example), but a more optimal strategy would be to first address the aberrations in PCWP or SVR contributing to low CI.

A PA catheter can also be used to measure pulmonary vascular resistance (PVR), which represents the impedance of blood flow from the right ventricle to the pulmonary circulation. Pulmonary hypertension and pulmonary edema are two common causes of elevated PVR. Just as SVR is calculated using MAP, PVR is calculated using the mean PA pressure, which incorporates the PA systolic and diastolic pressures. The PA diastolic pressure may also be useful if the PA catheter fails to wedge (making it impossible to obtain PCWP). If the PCWP and PA diastolic pressure have been correlated

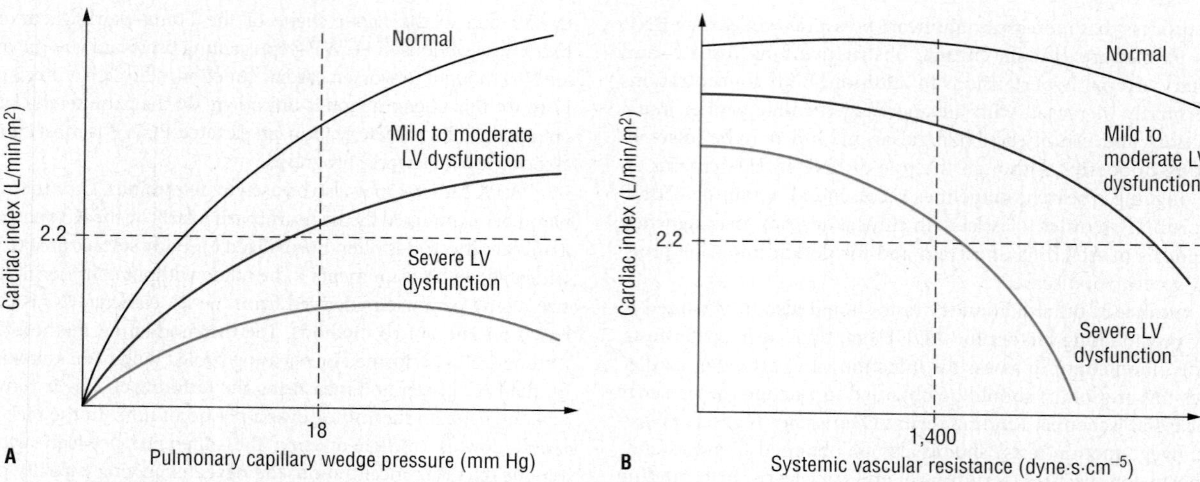

FIGURE 37-2 Hemodynamic alterations in HF. (A) An illustration of the relationship between cardiac output (displayed as cardiac index, which is cardiac output normalized for body surface area) and preload (displayed as pulmonary capillary wedge pressure) according to the severity of left ventricular function. (B) An illustration of the corresponding relationship between cardiac output and afterload (displayed as systemic vascular resistance). (LV, left ventricular.)

TABLE 37-2 Normal Hemodynamic Values

Central Venous (Right Atrial) Pressure, mean, CVP	<5 mm Hg
Right Ventricular Pressure (Systolic/Diastolic)	25/0 mm Hg
Pulmonary Artery Pressure (Systolic/Diastolic), PAS/PAD	25/10 mm Hg
Pulmonary Arterial Pressure, mean, PAP	<18 mm Hg
Pulmonary Capillary Wedge Pressure, PCWP	<12 mm Hg[a]
Systemic Arterial Pressure (Systolic/Diastolic), SBP/DBP	120/80 mm Hg
Mean Arterial Pressure, MAP = (DBP+[1/3 (SBP-DBP])	70-110 mm Hg
Cardiac Output, CO	4-6 L/min
Cardiac Index, CI = CO/BSA	2.8-4.2 L/min/m² (0.047-0.070 L/s/m²)
Systemic Vascular Resistance, SVR = ([MAP–CVP]*80)/(CO)	800-1,400 dyne·sec·cm^{-5} (10-18 Wood units; 80 - 140 MPa·s/m³)
Pulmonary Vascular Resistance, PVR = ([PAP–CVP]*80)/(CO)	100-200 dyne·sec·cm^{-5} (1.25-2.5 Wood units; 10 - 20 MPa·s/m³)
Arterial Oxygen Saturation	90%-94% (0.90-0.94)
Mixed Venous Oxygen Saturation	60%-80% (0.60-0.80)

BSA, body surface area.

[a]A higher than normal pulmonary capillary wedge pressure (ie, 15-18 mm Hg) is often accepted in patients with HF. See text for details.

prior to the failure to wedge, then the PA diastolic pressure may be followed as a surrogate marker of volume status. Normal values for these hemodynamic parameters are listed in Table 37-2.

TREATMENT

Desired Outcomes

4 The overall goals of therapy in ADHF evolve over the course of a hospitalization (Fig. 37-3).[3] During the acute phase, the goals are to relieve symptoms, improve hemodynamic stability (ie, restore end-organ perfusion if compromised), and reduce short-term mortality, and address precipitating factors (eg, arrhythmias, hypertension, myocardial ischemia, medication or dietary nonadherence). Other key considerations include evaluating medications (including noncardiac medications) that may worsen cardiac function. Although IV diuretic, vasodilator, and inotropic therapy can be very effective at achieving these short-term goals, their efficacy must be balanced against the potential for serious adverse drug reactions. Decongestion should be prioritized even if it is accompanied by mild to moderate WRF, as failure to relieve congestion prior to discharge increases the risk of rehospitalization and mortality.[14-16] Patients should be routinely evaluated for their progress toward these goals as care may need to be escalated for those whose progress stalls or worsens despite routine therapy. For patients whose course improves with therapy, the focus of care shifts to the optimization of GDMT, patient education, and coordination of care, all of which are critical to preventing rehospitalization and improving survival. When available and appropriate, patients should be referred to an HF disease management program.[2]

General Approach to Treatment

5 An important step in the management of ADHF is to assess medications being taken prior to admission and determine whether adjustment or discontinuation is required. Medications that may cause or contribute to ADHF due to negative inotropic effects (eg, nondihydropyridine calcium channel blockers) or by promoting fluid retention (eg, NSAIDs, mineralocorticoids, thiazolidinediones) should be discontinued. If fluid retention is evident on physical examination, aggressive diuresis should be pursued. The use of IV diuretics is recommended over increased doses of oral diuretics, and the regimen being taken prior to admission should be used to guide initial IV diuretic dosing.[2] In the absence of cardiogenic shock or symptomatic hypotension, every effort should be made to continue all GDMT for HF. β-Blocker therapy may be temporarily held or dose-reduced if recent initiation or up-titration is responsible for acute decompensation. Otherwise, β-blocker discontinuation is discouraged as it worsens outcomes in patients with ADHF.[17,18] Appropriateness of initiating β-blockers prior to discharge will be discussed later in this chapter.

Select GDMT may also need to be temporarily held in the setting of renal dysfunction, especially if oliguria or hyperkalemia is present (eg, ACE inhibitors, angiotensin receptor blockers,

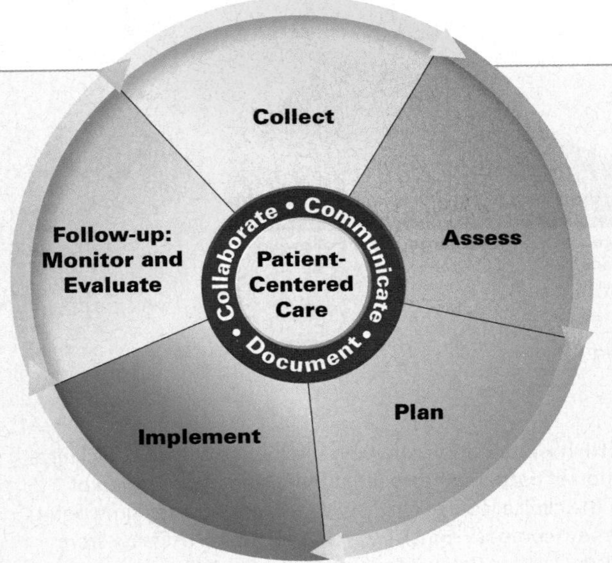

Patient Care Process for Acute Decompensated Heart Failure (ADHF)

Collect (see Tables 37-1 and 37-6)

- Patient characteristics (eg, age, sex, genetic ancestry, pregnancy status)
- Patient medical history (personal and family)
- Social history (eg, tobacco, ethanol, illicit drug use) and dietary habits, including fluid intake and sodium intake
- Current medications, including over-the-counter (OTC) medications (especially nonsteroidal anti-inflammatory drug [NSAID] and decongestant use), herbal products, and dietary supplements
- Subjective data
  - Signs/symptoms of fluid overload (eg, weight changes, dyspnea on exertion or at rest, orthopnea, paroxysmal nocturnal dyspnea, abdominal fullness, lower extremity edema, early satiety)
  - Signs/symptoms of low cardiac output (eg, fatigue, dyspnea on exertion, early satiety)
  - Signs/symptoms associated with precipitating factors (eg, chest pain, palpitations, presyncope, and syncope)
  - Ability to complete activities of daily living
  - Adherence to medications and dietary restrictions
- Objective data
  - Weight on admission and daily throughout hospital stay (standing weight preferred if not bedridden)
  - Blood pressure (BP), heart rate (HR), respiratory rate (RR), and arterial oxygen saturation every 1 to 6 hours depending on the severity of illness
  - Continuous telemetry monitoring, especially if administering intravenous inotropes or if concerned for arrhythmias
  - Pertinent laboratory values, especially sodium, potassium, serum creatinine, blood urea nitrogen (BUN), liver function tests, B-type natriuretic peptide
  - Various diagnostic tests depending on presumed etiology of acute decompensation, the severity of illness, and drug therapy selection

Assess (see Table 37-1; Figs. 37-1 and 37-2)

- Potential etiologies of decompensation
- Volume status (eg, increase in weight, signs/symptoms of fluid overload)
- Perfusion status (eg, complaints of fatigue, objective data consistent with low cardiac output)
- Ability/willingness to pay for newer guideline-directed medical therapies for heart failure (eg, sacubitril/valsartan, sodium-glucose co-transporter-2 inhibitors)
- Ability/willingness to obtain laboratory monitoring tests
- Emotional status (eg, presence of anxiety, depression)

Plan (see Tables 37-3 to 37-6; Figs. 37-1, 37-3, and 37-4)

- Drug therapy regimen, including guideline-directed medical therapies for heart failure as well as dose, route, frequency, and duration
- Monitoring parameters for efficacy (eg, weight to maintain euvolemia, surrogate markers of end-organ function) and safety (eg, orthostasis); frequency and timing of follow-up
- Patient education (eg, purpose of treatment, dietary and lifestyle modification, drug-specific information
- Referrals to other providers when appropriate

Implement (see Table 37-6)*

- Provide patient education regarding all elements of the treatment plan (eg, self-monitoring of weight, sodium and fluid dietary restriction, self-titration of diuretic dose in select patients)
- Use motivational interviewing and coaching strategies to maximize adherence
- Schedule follow-up in 3 to 8 days following hospital discharge

Follow-up: Monitor and Evaluate (see Tables 37-1 and 37-6)

- Resolution of symptoms of fluid overload or low cardiac output
- Presence of adverse drug reactions (eg, orthostasis due to over-diuresis or excess vasodilation)
- Obtain relevant laboratory monitoring data (eg, potassium, magnesium, BUN/serum creatinine [diuretics]; BP [eg, sacubitril/valsartan, ACE inhibitor, ARB, β-blocker]; and HR [eg, β-blocker])
- Patient adherence to treatment plan
- Reevaluate need for escalation of guideline-directed medical therapy (up-titration or initiation of additional therapies) or referral for nonpharmacologic therapies (eg, ICD, CRT, mitral valve repair) or advanced therapies (eg, ventricular assist device, transplant)

In collaboration with the patient, caregivers, and other healthcare professionals.

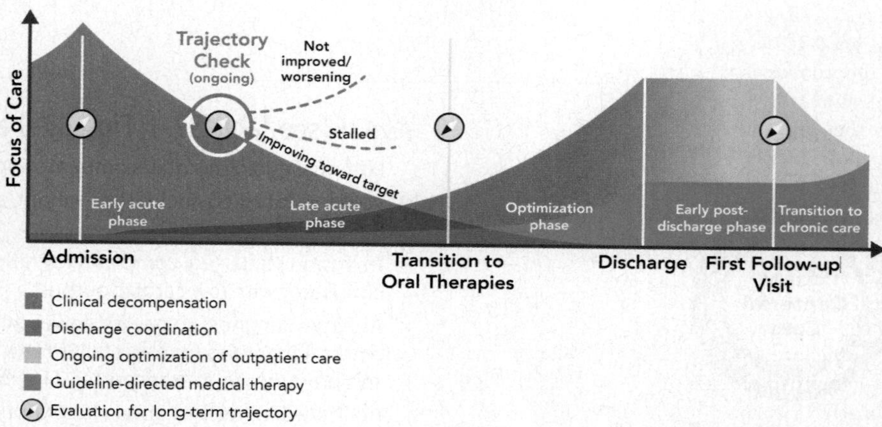

FIGURE 37-3 Clinical course of HF hospitalization. Graphic depiction of HF hospitalization, showing the degree of focus on clinical decompensation (red), discharge coordination (blue), ongoing coordination of outpatient care (light blue), and optimization of guideline-directed medical therapy (green), with ongoing assessment of the clinical course (circle with arrows), and key time points for review and revision of the long-term disease trajectory for the HF journey (compass signs). *(Reproduced, with permission, from Hollenberg SM, Warner Stevenson L, Ahmad T, et al. 2019 ACC Expert Consensus Decision Pathway on Risk Assessment, Management, and Clinical Trajectory of Patients Hospitalized With Heart Failure: A Report of the American College of Cardiology Solution Set Oversight Committee. J Am Coll Cardiol. 2019;74(15):1966-2011.)*

angiotensin receptor-neprilysin inhibitors, aldosterone antagonists). Therapies that may cause WRF (eg, ACE inhibitors, angiotensin receptor blockers, angiotensin receptor-neprilysin inhibitors) should only be initiated or up-titrated cautiously during aggressive volume removal with IV diuretic therapy. In addition, serum potassium concentrations should be monitored closely as IV diuretic therapy is transitioned to oral diuretic therapy, especially if an aldosterone antagonist has been initiated during the hospital stay; this ensures therapy can be tolerated on the intended oral diuretic dose prescribed at discharge. Most patients may continue to receive digoxin at doses targeting a trough serum concentration of 0.5 to 0.9 ng/mL (mcg/L; 0.6-1.2 nmol/L).[2] Discontinuation of digoxin is generally discouraged as withdrawal of therapy can worsen HF.[19,20] Digoxin should only be discontinued if serum concentrations cannot be safely maintained within the desirable range (eg, fluctuating renal function) or if patients demonstrate evidence of toxicity.

6 The acute management of ADHF is based primarily on hemodynamic status.[2] Patients with underlying HFrEF may present in any of the four hemodynamic subsets, whereas those with HFpEF usually present in subset II. Two general approaches exist for determining hemodynamic status. One is to use simple clinical parameters (eg, signs and symptoms, blood pressure, and organ function), and the other is to use these in conjunction with invasive hemodynamic monitoring. A management algorithm based on the hemodynamic subset is depicted in Fig. 37-1. The hemodynamic effects exerted by pharmacologic therapies used in the management of ADHF are illustrated in Fig. 37-4.

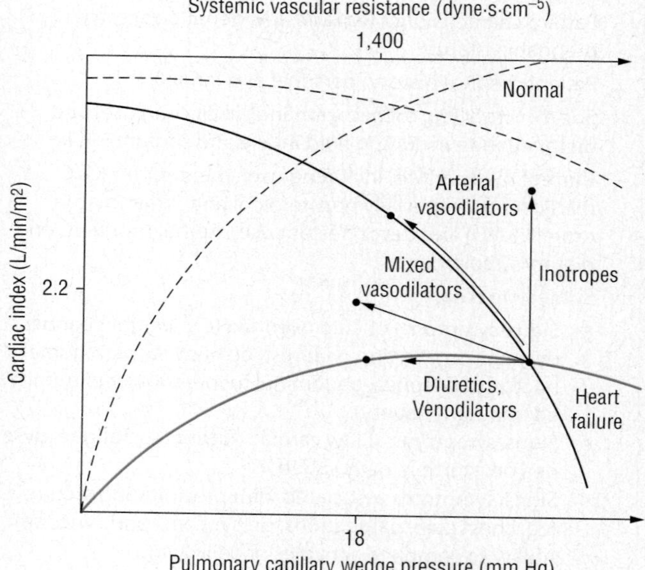

FIGURE 37-4 Hemodynamic effects of pharmacologic therapy in ADHF. Pharmacologic agents used in the management of ADHF exert important effects on cardiovascular hemodynamics. Although diuretics and venodilators reduce preload, this does not substantially reduce cardiac output in patients with heart failure and adequate filling pressures due to a flatter Frank–Starling curve. Arterial vasodilators reduce afterload, producing an increase in cardiac output as a consequence of improved left ventricular performance in patients with reduced ejection fraction. Vasodilators with effects on both venous and arterial tissue may reduce both preload and afterload. Inotropes improve contractility directly, although some agents (eg, milrinone) may exert salutary effects on afterload via vasodilation.

Subset I (Warm and Dry)

Patients in subset I generally do not have signs and symptoms of volume overload or hypoperfusion and usually have CI and PCWP values within appropriate ranges. Patients in this subset have the lowest risk of mortality and do not require immediate intervention other than optimization of GDMT for HF.

Subset II (Warm and Wet)

Patients in subset II are likely to present with signs and symptoms of congestion (eg, orthopnea and peripheral edema) due to increased hydrostatic pressure in the pulmonary and systemic circulation, but without evidence of peripheral hypoperfusion. As a consequence, they often have adequate CO but a PCWP greater than 18 mm Hg. The primary goal of therapy in these patients is to relieve symptoms of congestion by lowering PCWP to an acceptable range (ie, 15-18 mm Hg). Considerably greater reductions should generally be avoided, as these could compromise CO, increase heart rate, or provoke neurohormonal activation.

Intravenous agents that reduce preload via diuresis and/or direct venodilation (eg, loop diuretics) are the most appropriate initial therapy for patients presenting in subset II. Although symptomatic improvement may occur within minutes of IV loop diuretic administration, significant relief of congestive symptoms may require several hours in select patients. Resistance to loop diuretics may occur, requiring dose escalation or addition of thiazide-type diuretics. IV vasodilators with effects on primarily the venous vasculature (eg, nitroglycerin) may be used for rapid venodilation (see Fig. 37-4), which can aid in acutely improving dyspnea. IV vasodilators do not improve outcomes in ADHF beyond dyspnea relief and should therefore be reserved for patients with acute pulmonary edema with respiratory distress or severe hypertension and avoided in patients with low blood pressure. Failure to respond to these therapies may indicate the presence of impaired CO and should prompt a reevaluation of perfusion status (with or without PA catheter insertion).

Patients in subset II should also be placed on a sodium restriction (2-3 g daily). In patients with moderate hyponatremia (<130 mEq/L [mmol/L]) or excess fluid intake that limits effective decongestion, fluid restriction (<2 L daily) should be considered. In patients with worsening or severe hyponatremia (<125 mEq/L [mmol/L]), a stricter fluid restriction may be necessary and an arginine vasopressin (AVP) antagonist may be considered in patients who develop neurologic symptoms.[2] Finally, supplemental oxygen should be administered as needed for hypoxemia (arterial oxygen saturation <90% [0.90]).

Subset III (Cold and Dry)

Patients in subset III present with evidence of peripheral hypoperfusion (eg, weakness, decreased urine output, and weak pulses) but no signs or symptoms of congestion. They often present with a CI of less than 2.2 L/min/m^2 (0.037 L/s/m^2) but no abnormal elevation in PCWP. The mortality rate of patients in subset III is higher than that of patients with adequate perfusion.[21] Although the treatment goal is to alleviate signs and symptoms of hypoperfusion by increasing CI and perfusion to essential organs, therapy may differ based on initial presentation. If evidence of hypovolemia exists (eg, orthostatic hypotension) or PCWP is below 15 mm Hg, IV fluids should be cautiously administered to provide a more optimal left ventricular filling pressure (ie, 15-18 mm Hg), consequently improving CI (see Fig. 37-1). As this presentation most often occurs in the setting of overly aggressive diuresis, diuretic therapy should be withheld and fluid restriction liberalized; these interventions alone may obviate the need for IV fluids.

In patients whose CI remains low despite restoration of optimal left ventricular filling pressures, IV positive inotropic agents (eg, dobutamine and milrinone) and/or IV arterial vasodilators (eg, nitroprusside) may be necessary to achieve adequate CI (see Fig. 37-4). IV inotropes should also be avoided in patients with low left ventricular filling pressure and generally reserved for patients with evidence of severely low CO who are not candidates for IV vasodilators (ie, hypotension). They may also be used to "bridge" patients to MCS or heart transplantation, or as palliative therapy to improve functional status and quality of life in patients who are ineligible for definitive therapies.

Subset IV (Cold and Wet)

Patients in subset IV present with signs and symptoms of both volume overload and peripheral hypoperfusion, and often have a PCWP exceeding 18 mm Hg and a CI of less than 2.2 L/min/m^2 (0.037 L/s/m^2). This subset is characterized by the worst prognosis of all four and represents the most common hemodynamic profile for patients with end-stage HF. Given the severity of HF, patients in subset IV cannot maintain adequate CI despite elevated left ventricular filling pressure and increased myocardial fiber stretch. Treatment goals for these patients include alleviation of signs and symptoms of congestion and hypoperfusion by increasing CI to above 2.2 L/min/m^2 (0.037 L/s/m^2) and reducing PCWP to 15 to 18 mm Hg while maintaining adequate MAP. Therapy often involves a combination of agents used in subsets II and III (ie, a combination of IV diuretic plus vasodilator or inotrope). These targets may be difficult to achieve and often necessitate careful monitoring and individualization of drug therapy. In the presence of significant hypotension and low MAP (and SVR is low to normal or unknown), vasodilators should be avoided. In some cases, even the vasodilating effects of inotropic therapy may compromise MAP, requiring that combined inotrope and vasopressor therapy (eg, dobutamine plus norepinephrine) or an inotrope with vasopressor activity (eg, dopamine) be used to achieve adequate end-organ perfusion. Once end-organ perfusion and hemodynamic stability have been restored, therapy can then be adjusted to obtain the desired clinical response (see Fig. 37-1).

Pharmacologic Therapy

Despite advances in the care of patients with HF, none of the therapies used in the treatment of ADHF confer long-term improvements in morbidity and mortality, and some may cause harm when used indiscriminately (eg, IV inotropes). Therefore, the primary role of pharmacologic therapy in ADHF is to relieve acute symptoms and stabilize patients so that GDMT may be safely initiated or titrated.

Loop Diuretics

7 The IV loop diuretics furosemide and bumetanide are the mainstay of therapy for relieving congestion in the setting of ADHF (Table 37-3); furosemide remains the most widely studied and used in this setting.[22] Bolus administration reduces preload within 5 to 15 minutes by functional venodilation and later (>20 minutes) via sodium and water excretion, thereby improving pulmonary congestion. Although patients with HFrEF can tolerate significant reductions in preload without compromising stroke volume, excessive diuresis (ie, PCWP <12 mm Hg or CVP <3 mm Hg) can lead to a decline in CO (see Fig. 37-4). Excessive or rapid reductions in preload may also compromise CO in patients with preload-dependent conditions (eg, aortic stenosis, hypertrophic obstructive cardiomyopathy, restrictive or constrictive cardiomyopathies, right ventricular failure, or severe diastolic dysfunction) or if diuresis exceeds the rate at which fluid can migrate from the interstitial space back into the systemic vasculature (ie, transcapillary refill rate). One scenario in which the latter may occur is with reduced oncotic pressure resulting from hypoalbuminemia, which is common in patients with advanced HF who become malnourished due to early satiety (as a consequence of abdominal edema and/or reduced perfusion to the GI tract). Patients with these conditions often require less aggressive decongestion goals (eg, net negative 1 L per day, or an amount of urine output that is approximately 1 L more than all of the fluid taken in over the course of a day).

Unlike arterial vasodilators and positive inotropic agents, diuretics do not cause an upward shift in the Frank–Starling curve or significantly increase CO in most patients (see Fig. 37-4). In some cases, patients with severe congestion may experience improvements in CO as PCWP approaches the normal range (see Fig. 37-4), which may explain why renal function occasionally improves in the setting of diuresis. Alternatively, improvements in renal function may reflect the relief of congestive nephropathy.

IV loop diuretics are recommended as first-line therapy for patients with ADHF and volume overload.[2] Although the oral bioavailability of loop diuretics is relatively unchanged in patients with HF who have adequate GI perfusion, the rate of absorption is prolonged by approximately twofold and peak concentrations are

TABLE 37-3 Diuretics Commonly Used for the Management of ADHF

Loop Diuretics

Characteristic	Furosemide	Bumetanide
Oral bioavailability	10-100% (mean 50%)	80-90%
Dose equivalence (IV)[a]	20-40 mg	1 mg
Usual intermittent bolus dose (maximum)[b]	40-160 mg (200-300 mg)	1-4 mg (6-8 mg)
Usual infusion rate (maximum)[b]	10-20 mg/hr (40-80 mg/hr)	0.5 mg/hr (2-4 mg/hr)
Duration of action	4-6 hours	4-6 hours

Thiazide-Type Diuretics

Characteristic	Metolazone	Chlorothiazide	Hydrochlorothiazide
Usual dose (maximum)[b]	2.5-5 mg orally once daily (20 mg/day)	500 mg IV twice daily (2,000 mg/day)	50 mg orally once daily (200 mg/day)
Duration of action	12-24 hours	6-12 hours	5-15 hours
Other considerations	Oral absorption is erratic and delayed. No evidence of superiority to other thiazides but is most commonly used.	Oral formulations have poor absorption and should not be used. More costly but no evidence of superiority over other thiazides.	Higher doses than those used for hypertension are typically required to facilitate diuresis.

IV, intravenous.

[a]Torsemide is currently unavailable in an intravenous formulation, but its IV dose equivalence is 20 mg.

[b]Some institutions have published experience with higher doses; the ranges and maximum doses listed may be exceeded if the benefits justify the risks.

reduced by approximately half. Because loop diuretics have a sigmoidal-shaped concentration–response curve, prolonged absorption may result in concentrations that fail to reach the threshold necessary for producing diuresis, necessitating the use of IV therapy.

Low doses (ie, doses equivalent to IV furosemide 20-40 mg) once to twice daily should initially be selected in patients with ADHF who are naïve to loop diuretics. For patients taking loop diuretics prior to admission, a total daily dose of 1 to 2.5 times their home dose is recommended.[2,22] Higher doses are associated with more rapid relief of congestive symptoms but may also mildly increase the risk of transient worsening of renal function (WRF).[22,23]

Once an initial total daily dose is determined from the home diuretic regimen, doses may be administered as either an IV bolus (ie, divided every 12 hours) or continuous IV infusion.[2] Although major differences in relief of congestive symptoms, weight loss, or long-term outcomes have not been observed between these two methods of administration, a greater natriuretic effect may occur when the same total daily dose is administered as a continuous infusion rather than an IV bolus.[22-24] Given limitations in the designs of published trials, the appropriate method of administration for loop diuretic therapy in ADHF remains an area of controversy.[25,26]

Subsequent doses of loop diuretic therapy should be adjusted to patient response, as determined by urine output, weight loss, or urine sodium concentrations (goal >70 mEq/L [mmol/L]). Most patients tolerate at least a 2-L per day net negative diuresis (or a 2-kg weight loss), but diuretic therapy must be highly individualized in order to obtain the desired improvement in congestive symptoms while avoiding a reduction in CO, symptomatic hypotension, or WRF. Importantly, WRF alone should not be interpreted as evidence of euvolemia or as a reason to discontinue diuretics, as at least mild to moderate WRF occurs in approximately half of patients with ADHF.[22,27] The prognostic significance of WRF is strongly associated with the etiology of injury and among patients achieving decongestion with diuresis, WRF is not indicative of renal tubular injury or a worsened prognosis.[16,27,28] Therefore, careful evaluation of the patient's volume status and clinical context should guide decisions about diuretic therapy and GDMT (eg, ACE inhibitors, angiotensin receptor blockers, sacubitril/valsartan). Invasive hemodynamic monitoring can also be used to confirm volume status when the appropriate next steps are unclear based on changes to physical examination or laboratory findings. Finally, electrolyte depletion (eg, potassium, magnesium) should also be monitored daily at minimum and more frequently when high doses or combination diuretic therapy is used.

Strategies to Overcome Diuretic Resistance

Occasionally, patients respond inadequately to appropriate doses of loop diuretics, a phenomenon subjectively referred to as diuretic resistance. Unfortunately, attempts to define diuretic resistance in quantitative terms have not resulted in clinically applicable measures, and the mechanisms responsible for diuretic resistance are diverse.[29] However, the predominant mechanisms of diuretic resistance are intra-renal, specifically diminished diuretic response in the loop of Henle, and compensatory sodium reabsorption in the distal convoluted tubule.[29] Over time, the distal tubule may also undergo hypertrophy, thereby enhancing its ability to reabsorb sodium. Impaired CO resulting in reduced renal perfusion is an infrequent contributor to diuretic resistance, thus IV inotropic therapy should only be used to treat diuretic resistance if patients are in hemodynamic subset IV (ie, cold and wet).

Diuretic resistance is primarily treated by increasing the doses of loop diuretics or augmenting them by adding a diuretic with an alternative mechanism of action (eg, thiazide-type diuretics).[2] Although an escalation of loop diuretics should be prioritized due to an increased risk of adverse events with combination diuretic therapy, no consensus exists regarding the dose at which alternative diuretics should be added.[29,30] Given the sigmoidal dose–response curve of loop diuretics, a doubling of the dose is required to improve diuresis. Bolus doses should be increased if an inadequate response is not observed within six hours and the frequency of dosing should be increased if a response is observed but patients still fail to meet overall diuresis goals. Transitioning to continuous infusion loop diuretics may also be considered provided it is accompanied by a substantial increase in the total daily dose, although studies comparing this approach to IV bolus administration in patients with diuretic resistance have not been performed.

For patients with refractory congestion despite increased doses of loop diuretics, adding a distal tubule blocker such as oral metolazone, oral hydrochlorothiazide, or IV chlorothiazide (Table 37-3) can produce a synergistic diuretic effect.[2] Inhibition of sodium reabsorption in the loop of Henle increases sodium delivery to (and reabsorption in) the distal convoluted tubule, which can be subsequently blocked by a thiazide-type diuretic. When added to loop diuretics, IV chlorothiazide and oral metolazone are similarly efficacious and safe, as the higher potency and longer duration of metolazone likely compensate for its erratic absorption and delayed onset of action.[31] Sequential nephron blockade with a loop and thiazide-type diuretic should generally be reserved for hospitalized patients, as profound diuresis with severe electrolyte and intravascular volume depletion may occur. Patients should also receive close follow-up (eg, weight, vital signs, serum potassium, and assessment for orthostatic hypotension) to avoid serious adverse events.

Several other pharmacologic strategies have been investigated for relieving congestion or overcoming diuretic resistance in ADHF.[32] Studies are currently underway to investigate the addition of acetazolamide, a carbonic anhydrase inhibitor, to loop diuretics in patients with ADHF. On the basis of their benefits in patients with chronic HFrEF, sodium-glucose cotransporter-2 (SGLT2) inhibitors are also being explored for their diuretic and natriuretic effects in patients with ADHF. One strategy for enhancing diuresis that has fallen out of favor is the administration of low doses of dopamine (ie, 2-5 mcg/kg/min), as this approach does not consistently improve congestive symptoms or diuresis and it increases the risk of tachyarrhythmias.[33,34] Given the evidence of β-mediated effects at lower infusion rates, dopamine likely does not provide any advantages over a traditional inotrope when used in this setting.

Vasopressin Antagonists

Vasopressin receptor antagonists have been extensively studied in ADHF, particularly when complicated by severe hyponatremia, which is commonly defined as a serum sodium concentration of less than 125 mEq/L (mmol/L). Heart failure is most commonly associated with hypervolemic hyponatremia and is often characterized by inappropriately elevated concentrations of AVP or antidiuretic hormone. In the setting of HF, reduced CO leads to excess stimulation of arterial baroreceptors, which in turn enhances AVP secretion and consequently, stimulation of vasopressin receptors. Of particular importance in ADHF are V_2 receptors, which are located in the renal tubules, where stimulation by AVP results in net water reabsorption.

Although the prevalence of hyponatremia in patients with HF varies by the serum sodium threshold used, as many as one in five patients hospitalized with ADHF present with serum sodium concentrations less than 136 mEq/L (mmol/L).[35] Furthermore, the presence of hyponatremia has been associated with increased mortality in this population.[36]

Most cases of hyponatremia are mild, asymptomatic, and self-limited, but prompt diagnosis and management is critical for the less common but life-threatening presentation, which may include lethargy, confusion, respiratory arrest, cerebral edema, seizures, coma, or death. Because vasopressin antagonists have failed to improve outcomes in ADHF beyond increases in serum sodium concentrations and marginal improvements in urine output and congestive symptoms, their role is limited to the treatment of severe hyponatremia.[2,37,38]

The two currently available vasopressin receptor antagonists are tolvaptan and conivaptan. Tolvaptan selectively binds to and inhibits the V_2 receptor, whereas conivaptan nonselectively inhibits both V_{1A} and V_2 receptors. Stimulation of V_{1A} receptors in vascular smooth muscle and myocardium results in vasoconstriction, myocyte hypertrophy, and positive inotropic effects, but the clinical consequences of inhibiting these effects with conivaptan are unknown. Conivaptan is an IV agent indicated for hypervolemic and euvolemic hyponatremia resulting from a variety of causes, but because it is not indicated in patients with ADHF, its use will not be discussed in further detail here.

Tolvaptan is orally bioavailable and indicated for the management of hypervolemic and euvolemic hyponatremia in patients with SIADH, cirrhosis, or HF. It is typically initiated at 15 mg daily and then titrated to 30 mg or 60 mg as needed for resolution of hyponatremia (ie, typically no longer than several days to a week). Importantly, tolvaptan is a substrate of cytochrome P450 3A4 and is contraindicated with potent inhibitors of this enzyme. Patients receiving vasopressin antagonists must be monitored closely to avoid an overly rapid rise in serum sodium (>12 mEq/L [mmol/L] per 24 hours); fluid restrictions should be liberalized to reduce this risk.

Vasodilators

9 Current guidelines focus on the role of IV vasodilators as an adjunct treatment for refractory congestive symptoms,[2] but they may also be helpful for restoring tissue perfusion in select patients with low CO. Vasodilators are commonly classified according to their most prominent site of action (ie, arterial or venous circulation). As described in the section on patients in subset II, venodilators act as preload reducers by increasing venous capacitance, thus reducing symptoms of pulmonary congestion in patients with high ventricular filling pressures. Arterial vasodilators exert their beneficial effects by counteracting the peripheral vasoconstriction and impaired CO that can result from the activation of the sympathetic nervous system, renin–angiotensin–aldosterone system, and other neurohormonal mediators in both acute and chronic HF. In these patients, arterial vasodilators act as impedance-reducing agents, reducing afterload and causing a reflexive improvement in left ventricular performance and thus an increase in CO. Mixed vasodilators act on both resistance and capacitance vessels, reducing congestive symptoms while increasing CO.

Intravenous vasodilators should, therefore, be considered prior to positive inotropic therapy in patients with low CO and elevated SVR (or elevated blood pressure in those without a PA catheter). For patients in whom blood pressure or SVR is already low, including those receiving GDMT with vasodilating effects (eg, ACE inhibitors) or those with advanced HF, hypotension may preclude the use of IV vasodilators. In patients with advanced HF and limited contractile reserve, increases in left ventricular performance may not fully compensate for reductions in afterload, leading to worsening hypotension. In addition, IV vasodilators have not been extensively studied in patients with HFpEF, where a sudden drop in preload may compromise existing defects in ventricular filling, leading to decreased CO.[39]

The most commonly used IV vasodilators in ADHF are nitroglycerin and sodium nitroprusside, which differ according to their effects on arterial and venous circulation (Table 37-4). Nitroglycerin is primarily a venodilator (except at high doses), whereas sodium nitroprusside is a mixed venous and arterial vasodilator. Once stabilized on IV therapies, transitioning to oral vasodilators (eg, nitrates/hydralazine, ACE inhibitors) should be considered.

Nitroglycerin Intravenous nitroglycerin is often preferred for preload reduction in patients with ADHF, especially those requiring urgent relief of dyspnea (ie, acute pulmonary congestion). Because of its short half-life (1-3 minutes), IV nitroglycerin is administered by continuous infusion. Its major hemodynamic effects are reductions in preload and PCWP via functional venodilation and mild arterial vasodilation that is particularly evident in patients with HF and elevated SVR or when given in doses exceeding 100 mcg/min (see Table 37-4).[40] At higher doses, nitroglycerin displays potent coronary vasodilating properties, exerting beneficial effects on myocardial oxygen demand and supply and making it the vasodilator of choice for patients with severe HF and ischemic heart disease.

Nitroglycerin should be initiated at a dose of 5 to 10 mcg/min (0.1 mcg/kg/min) and increased every 5 to 10 minutes as tolerated. Hypotension and an excessive decrease in PCWP are important

TABLE 37-4 Vasodilators Commonly Utilized for the Management of ADHF[a]

Drug (Vasodilatory Effect)	Onset, Half-life	Elimination	Dose	HR	MAP	PCWP	CO[b]	SVR
Nitroglycerin (venous > arterial)	Immediate, <4 mins	Inactive metabolites in urine	10-20 mcg/min and titrate 10-20 mcg/min q10–20 mins, max 200 mcg/kg/min	0/↑	0/↓	↓	0/↑	0/↓
Nitroprusside (venous = arterial)	Immediate, 2 mins	Cyanide (hepatic), thiocyanate (renal)	0.1-0.2 mcg/kg/min, titrate 0.1-0.2 mcg/kg/min q10-20 mins, max 3 mcg/kg/min	0/↑	0/↓	↓	↑	↓
Furosemide (venous only)	1 hr (PO)/5 mins (IV), 2 hrs	Urine	Variable[c]	0	0/↓	↓	0	0
Isosorbide dinitrate (venous only)	1 hr, 2-5 hrs for active metabolites	Hepatic	10-60 mg q8h	0/↑	0	↓	0	0
Hydralazine (arterial only)	1-2 hrs (PO), 3-7 hrs	Hepatic	12.5-100 mg q6–8h	0/↑	0/↓	0	↑	↓
Captopril (arterial > venous)	<15 mins, 2-4 hrs	Urine	6.25-50 mg q8h	0	0/↓	↓	↑	↓

[a]See text for a more detailed description of the interpatient variability in response.

[b]Indirect effects due to decreased arterial impedance.

[c]Intravenous bolus administered <0.4 mg/min.

↑, increase; ↓, decrease; 0, no change; HR, heart rate; MAP, mean arterial pressure; PCWP, pulmonary capillary wedge pressure; CI, continuous infusion; CO, cardiac output; IVB, intravenous bolus; SVR, systemic vascular resistance.

dose-limiting adverse drug reactions. Maintenance doses usually vary from 35 to 200 mcg/min (0.5-3 mcg/kg/min). While tolerance to the hemodynamic effects of nitroglycerin may develop within hours of continuous administration, some patients experience a sustained response; this variability in response to nitroglycerin requires that patients be continuously monitored (eg, symptoms, hemodynamic parameters) to guide adjustments to therapy. Nitroglycerin should not be used in the presence of elevated intracranial pressure because it may worsen cerebral edema in this setting.

Sodium Nitroprusside As a result of its balanced effects in arterial and venous tissue, sodium nitroprusside increases CI to a similar degree as dobutamine and milrinone despite having no direct inotropic activity; however, greater decreases in PCWP, SVR, and blood pressure are generally observed. MAP may remain fairly constant due to reflexive improvements in stroke volume and CO but can decrease based on the extent of arterial smooth muscle relaxation. Patients with normal left ventricular function do not experience an increase in stroke volume when SVR falls because the normal ventricle is fairly insensitive to changes in afterload. Consequently, these patients may experience a significant decrease in blood pressure in response to arterial vasodilators. These differences explain why sodium nitroprusside is a potent antihypertensive agent in patients without HF but causes less hypotension and reflex tachycardia in the presence of left ventricular dysfunction (see Fig. 37-2). Nonetheless, hypotension remains an important dose-limiting effect of sodium nitroprusside, and its use should be primarily reserved for patients with elevated SVR. Close monitoring of therapy is warranted, as even modest increases in heart rate can have adverse consequences in patients with underlying ischemic heart disease and/or resting tachycardia.

Sodium nitroprusside is an effective strategy for the short-term management of patients with acute HF across a variety of settings (eg, acute MI, valvular regurgitation, postcoronary bypass surgery, and ADHF). Generally, sodium nitroprusside does not worsen, and may even improve, the balance between myocardial oxygen demand and supply by lowering both left ventricular wall tension (thus reducing oxygen demand) and end-diastolic pressure (thereby increasing subendocardial blood flow). However, an excessive decrease in systemic arterial pressure may reduce coronary perfusion and worsen ischemia due to coronary steal. Consequently, therapy should be avoided in patients with recent MI in the absence of persistent congestive symptoms or elevated ventricular filling pressures.[41] In ADHF specifically, sodium nitroprusside improves low CO and may support the initiation and titration of GDMT, even among patients with lower MAP (<85 mm Hg).[42]

Sodium nitroprusside has a rapid onset of action, but its effects last less than 10 minutes, necessitating administration by continuous IV infusion. Its short duration of action also allows precise dose-titration based on clinical and hemodynamic response. As with nitroglycerin, sodium nitroprusside should be initiated at low doses (0.1-0.2 mcg/kg/min) to avoid excessive hypotension and increased by small increments (0.1-0.2 mcg/kg/min) every 5 to 10 minutes as tolerated. Effective doses usually range from 0.5 to 3 mcg/kg/min. A rebound phenomenon, which may be due to reflex neurohormonal activation during sodium nitroprusside therapy, has been reported following abrupt withdrawal in patients with HF. Therefore, therapy should be tapered slowly when transitioning patients to oral medications. As with nitroglycerin, sodium nitroprusside should be avoided in the presence of elevated intracranial pressure as it may worsen cerebral edema in this setting.

Following IV administration, sodium nitroprusside interacts with hemoglobin to release cyanide, which undergoes hepatic conversion to thiocyanate before it is eliminated renally. As a consequence, sodium nitroprusside can cause cyanide and thiocyanate toxicity, but these effects are unlikely when doses less than 3 mcg/kg/min are administered for less than 3 days, except in patients with significant renal impairment (ie, serum creatinine concentration >3 mg/dL (265 μmol/L). Closer monitoring for signs and symptoms of toxicity (eg, altered mental status, nausea or vomiting, metabolic acidosis) should be considered in patients with renal impairment or when higher doses or prolonged durations of sodium nitroprusside must be used.

Inotropes

10 Patients in subsets III and IV ("cold" subsets) require prompt correction of low CO in order to restore peripheral tissue perfusion and

preserve end-organ function. Although IV inotropes can improve peripheral hypoperfusion by directly enhancing cardiac contractility, their association with adverse outcomes (eg, arrhythmias, in-hospital mortality) necessitates that they are reserved for select patients with refractory ADHF, particularly those unable to tolerate vasodilators due to hypotension.[43] Inotrope therapy should be considered only as a temporizing measure for maintaining end-organ perfusion in patients with cardiogenic shock or evidence of severely depressed CO and low systolic blood pressure (ie, ineligible for IV vasodilators) until definitive therapy can be initiated, as a "bridge" for those with advanced HF who are eligible for MCS or cardiac transplantation, or for palliation of symptoms in patients with advanced HF who are not eligible for MCS or cardiac transplantation.[2]

Patients in these latter two groups may require placement of an indwelling IV catheter for continuous outpatient administration of inotropic therapy. Palliative use of IV inotropes should only be considered after multiple unsuccessful attempts have been made to wean therapy and maximize GDMT, as the risk of mortality is likely increased with IV inotrope use.

Importantly, IV inotropes rarely, if ever, produce a single cardiovascular action. Even when intended for a specific purpose (eg, positive inotropic effects), other cardiovascular effects (tachycardia, vasodilation, or vasoconstriction) may either add to the therapeutic effect of the drug or cause adverse drug reactions that negate or even outweigh its intended therapeutic benefit. How an individual patient will respond to an intervention is often difficult to anticipate. For this reason, hemodynamic monitoring with a PA catheter may be useful.

The two IV inotropic agents most commonly used for the management of ADHF are dobutamine and milrinone. Although both drugs increase intracellular concentrations of cAMP, they do so by different mechanisms. Dobutamine activates adenylate cyclase through direct stimulation of β-adrenergic receptors, thus catalyzing the conversion of adenosine triphosphate to cAMP, whereas milrinone reduces degradation of cAMP by inhibiting phosphodiesterase type 3. Increased intracellular cAMP enhances phospholipase (and subsequently phosphorylase) activity, increasing the rate and extent of calcium influx during systole and thus enhancing contractility. In addition, cAMP enhances the reuptake of calcium by the sarcoplasmic reticulum during diastole, improving active relaxation (ie, positive lusitropic effects). Comparisons between dobutamine and milrinone indicate that the two agents generally produce similar hemodynamic effects, although dobutamine is usually associated with more pronounced increases in heart rate and milrinone is associated with greater relaxation in arterial smooth muscle. Differences in the pharmacologic effects of the two agents may confer advantages or disadvantages in an individual patient; these and other clinical considerations for their use in the management of ADHF will be reviewed in the sections to follow.

Digoxin rarely has a role in hemodynamically unstable patients due to its limited inotropic effects. In patients who take digoxin as chronic therapy, discontinuation or dose-adjustment during an acute decompensation is generally unnecessary unless changes in renal function increase the risk of toxicity. As discussed previously in this chapter, discontinuation should be discouraged in the absence of toxicity, given the potential for digoxin withdrawal.[19,20]

Dobutamine The receptor activities of dobutamine and other adrenergic agonists are summarized in Table 37-5. Dobutamine, a synthetic catecholamine, is a β_1- and β_2-receptor agonist with some α_1-agonist effects. Because dobutamine does not cause the release of norepinephrine from nerve terminals, its positive inotropic effects are attributed to its action on β_1-receptors. Stimulation of cardiac β_1-receptors by dobutamine does not generally produce a significant change in heart rate, thus explaining its modest chronotropic effects. Modest peripheral β_2-receptor-mediated vasodilation tends to offset minor α_1-receptor-mediated vasoconstriction. In addition, the increase in CO often results in a reflexive decline in SVR. As a consequence, the net hemodynamic effect of dobutamine, particularly at low doses, is usually vasodilation.

The effects of dobutamine are observed within minutes, but its peak effects may take up to 10 minutes to occur. Initial doses of 2.5 to 5 mcg/kg/min may be adjusted based on clinical and hemodynamic responses. Although doses of up to 20 mcg/kg/min are occasionally used, most patients are maintained at doses of 7.5 mcg/kg/min or less. The cardiac index is increased due to inotropic stimulation, arterial vasodilation, and a variable increase in heart rate. Because of offsetting changes in arteriolar resistance and CI, dobutamine usually causes relatively little change in MAP, unlike the more consistent increases observed with vasopressors. Although its impact on heart rate is variable, the major adverse drug reactions of dobutamine are tachycardia and ventricular arrhythmias. Potentially detrimental increases in oxygen consumption have also been observed. While concerns exist regarding the attenuation of its effects during prolonged administration, changes in receptor expression require that dobutamine be slowly tapered rather than abruptly discontinued.

Milrinone Milrinone is a bipyridine derivative that inhibits phosphodiesterase 3, an enzyme responsible for the breakdown of cAMP to adenosine monophosphate (AMP). Because both inotropic and vasodilating effects contribute to its therapeutic effects in ADHF, milrinone is often referred to as an inodilator. The relative balance of these pharmacologic effects may vary with dose and underlying cardiovascular pathology.

During IV administration, milrinone produces an increase in stroke volume (and therefore CO) with minimal change in heart rate (see Table 37-5). Despite an increase in CI, MAP may remain constant due to a concomitant decrease in arteriolar resistance. However, the vasodilating effects of milrinone may predominate, leading to a decrease in blood pressure and reflex tachycardia. As such, milrinone should be used cautiously in severely hypotensive patients because it does not increase, and may even decrease, arterial blood pressure.

TABLE 37-5 Inotropes Commonly Used for the Management of ADHF[a]

Drug	Onset, Half-life	Dose	Receptor Affinity (α_1/β_1/β_2)	HR	MAP	PCWP	CO	SVR
Dobutamine	<10 mins, 2 mins	1-2 mcg/kg/min, titrate 1-2 mcg/kg/min q10–20 mins, max 20 mcg/kg/min	↑/↑↑↑↑/↑↑	0/↑	0	↓	↑	0/↓
Milrinone	5-15 mins, 1-4 hrs, (prolonged if renal dysfunction)	0.1-0.2 mcg/kg/min, titrate 0.1 mcg/kg/min q4–16 hrs (titrate slowly in renal dysfunction), max 0.75 mcg/kg/min (IVB dose generally avoided)	Phosphodiesterase inhibition	0/↑	0/↓	↓	↑	↓

[a]See text for a more detailed description of the dose-dependent hemodynamic effects.

The half-life of milrinone is about one hour but may be as long as 3 to 6 hours in patients with renal dysfunction. The longer elimination half-life of milrinone presents several disadvantages in patients with ADHF, including the inability to perform minute-to-minute titrations based on hemodynamic changes and persistence of adverse drug reactions (eg, arrhythmias or hypotension) following drug discontinuation. Although a loading dose is still listed in the product labeling for milrinone (50 mcg/kg administered over 10 minutes), this practice is uncommon due to an increased risk of hypotension.[44] Most patients are started on a maintenance infusion of 0.1 to 0.3 mcg/kg/min (up to 0.75 mcg/kg/min). Milrinone is excreted unchanged in the urine, and thus its infusion rate should be decreased by 50% to 70% in patients with significant renal impairment.

The most notable adverse drug reactions associated with milrinone are arrhythmia, hypotension, and thrombocytopenia. Although the incidence of thrombocytopenia is rare, patients should still have platelet counts measured before and during therapy.

Inotrope Selection Although outcomes are similar between dobutamine and milrinone in patients with cardiogenic shock, certain characteristics may make one agent more ideal in an individual patient.[45] Dobutamine should be considered when a significant decrease in MAP might further compromise hemodynamic function, as this is more common with the initiation of milrinone. The selection of an inotropic drug should also consider whether patients are receiving chronic β-blocker therapy and whether a β_1-selective agent (eg, metoprolol succinate) or mixed α, β-blocking agent (eg, carvedilol) is used. Traditionally, milrinone has been advocated in patients who are receiving chronic β-blocker therapy because its inotropic effects do not involve β-receptor stimulation. However, the hemodynamic effects of dobutamine may persist in the presence of β-blocker therapy, particularly with β_1-selective agents as a result of β-receptor upregulation or selective activation of β_2-receptors by dobutamine.[46] Similar effects are not observed in the presence of carvedilol, which may inhibit the hemodynamic benefits of dobutamine entirely. Concomitant carvedilol therapy may augment the hemodynamic effects of milrinone based on studies with a structurally similar phosphodiesterase inhibitor, enoximone.[46]

The combination of dobutamine and milrinone is likely to produce additive effects on CO and PCWP, suggesting that this regimen may be considered in patients who have dose-limiting adverse drug reactions with either drug class. However, whether this combination provides a therapeutic advantage over the combined use of a positive inotrope and a traditional vasodilator (eg, sodium nitroprusside) is unclear.

Agents with Combined Inotropic and Vasopressor Activity

Although therapies that can increase SVR are generally avoided in ADHF, agents with combined inotropic and vasopressor activity, such as norepinephrine or dopamine, may be required in select scenarios where marked systemic hypotension may preclude the use of traditional IV inotropes (eg, mixed shock, refractory cardiogenic shock). Alternatively, these agents may be used in combination with traditional inotropes so that adjustments can be made to each agent independently to achieve the desired hemodynamic response. Although these strategies are common in clinical practice, minimal data exist to support their use.

Norepinephrine is an endogenous catecholamine that exerts its hemodynamic effects via direct stimulation of α_1- and β_1-adrenergic receptors. Its effects on β_1-adrenergic receptors in myocardial tissue are thought to confer improvements in CO because of increases in heart rate and cardiac contractility. However, despite having a similar affinity for α_1- and β_1-adrenergic receptors, enhanced vasoconstriction via activation of peripheral α_1-receptors appears to be the predominant hemodynamic effect observed clinically. The limited impact of norepinephrine on CO may be due to its lack of affinity for β_2-receptors, which would both enhance cardiac contractility and balance its effects on α_1-receptors in vascular smooth muscle. The affinity of norepinephrine for adrenergic receptors does not appreciably differ based on dose.

Dopamine is an endogenous precursor of norepinephrine and exerts its effects by directly stimulating adrenergic receptors as well as causing the release of norepinephrine from adrenergic nerve terminals. In contrast with norepinephrine, dopamine produces dose-dependent hemodynamic effects because of its relative affinity for α_1-, β_1-, β_2-, and D_1- (vascular dopaminergic) receptors (see Table 37-5). The positive inotropic effects of dopamine are mediated primarily by β_1-receptors and become more prominent at doses of 2 to 5 mcg/kg/min. The cardiac index is increased because of an increase in stroke volume and a variable increase in heart rate, which is also partially dose-dependent. Minimal changes in SVR occur, presumably because neither vasodilation (D_1- and β_2-receptor-mediated) nor vasoconstriction (α_1-receptor-mediated) predominates. However, at doses between 5 and 10 mcg/kg/min, chronotropy and α1-receptor-mediated vasoconstriction become more prominent. MAP is usually raised because of increases in both CI and SVR (see Table 37-5).

Epinephrine is also an endogenous catecholamine that exerts its hemodynamic effects via direct stimulation of α_1-, α_2-, and β_1-adrenergic receptors. Similar to dopamine, epinephrine exerts dose-dependent hemodynamic effects, including increased selectivity for β_1-adrenergic receptors at lower doses (ie, 0.01-0.05 mcg/kg/min) whereas increased α-adrenergic activity is seen at higher doses (ie, >0.5 mcg/kg/min).

The vasoconstriction observed with higher doses of norepinephrine and dopamine may limit improvements in CI by concomitantly increasing afterload and preload. Consequently, they should generally be reserved for patients with low CO and low systolic blood pressure despite adequate ventricular filling pressures, or as an adjunct to inotrope therapy when hypotension precludes the use of inotrope therapy alone. At higher doses, agents with vasopressor activity may alter several parameters that increase myocardial oxygen demand (eg, increased heart rate, contractility, and systolic pressure) and potentially decrease myocardial blood flow (eg, coronary vasoconstriction and increased wall tension), which may worsen ischemia in patients with coronary artery disease. As with dobutamine and milrinone, arrhythmogenesis is also more common at higher doses, although this risk appears to be greater with dopamine than with norepinephrine.[47]

Nonpharmacologic Therapy

Several nonpharmacologic therapies are routinely used in ADHF. All patients with congestive symptoms should be placed on a sodium restriction. Given a complex relationship between sodium restriction and ADHF outcomes, no consensus exists on an appropriate sodium limit. For example, intense targets (<0.8 g/day) do not improve outcomes in ADHF, and higher levels of sodium intake (including the administration of hypertonic saline) may counterintuitively improve diuresis in select patients.[48,49] Based on these uncertainties, a general range of <2-3 g daily is recommended for most patients with ADHF.[2] Fluid restriction should also be considered for those with refractory symptoms. Noninvasive ventilation may be considered in patients with respiratory distress due to acute pulmonary edema, particularly those at risk for intubation. Although most patients with limited mobility should receive pharmacologic thromboprophylaxis with unfractionated heparin or low-molecular-weight heparin, mechanical thromboprophylaxis with intermittent pneumatic compression devices may be considered in patients at high risk for bleeding complications.

Most of the nonpharmacologic therapies used in ADHF are primarily reserved for patients who have failed pharmacologic therapy. Ultrafiltration and wireless invasive hemodynamic monitoring

(W-IHM) may be used in the management of congestive symptoms, whereas MCS (temporary or durable devices) and cardiac transplantation may be considered in those with advanced disease.[2]

Ultrafiltration

8 Renal impairment is common among patients with ADHF, and advanced forms may warrant the use of renal replacement therapy (eg, hemodialysis, ultrafiltration). Ultrafiltration involves the circulation of blood through a high-pressure circuit, where plasma water is removed from whole blood via a semipermeable membrane. Hemodialysis also involves the use of a semipermeable membrane, but water and solutes (eg, electrolytes, toxins) are removed via diffusion as a result of concentration differences between blood and dialysate (a fluid mixture that runs countercurrent to blood flow on the other side of the membrane). As a result of its mechanism of action, ultrafiltration reduces PCWP without adversely affecting hemodynamics or serum electrolyte concentrations.

Ultrafiltration has emerged as an effective strategy for fluid removal in patients with ADHF (up to 500 mL/h), but it is not superior to adequate doses of diuretic therapy and also increases the risk of adverse events.[50-52] Complications of ultrafiltration include those associated with central venous access (eg, infection), adverse effects from the use of IV heparin (to prevent thrombosis of the access line), and intravascular volume depletion, which increases the risk of WRF. Taken altogether, ultrafiltration should generally be reserved for patients demonstrating diuretic resistance despite optimal diuretic therapy, severe renal impairment following diuretic administration, or continued renal impairment despite inotropic therapy.

Wireless Implantable Hemodynamic Monitoring

Increases in cardiac filling pressures often precede the development of congestive symptoms, and W-IHM has recently emerged as a strategy for using early hemodynamic changes to adjust therapy and thus prevent ADHF in high-risk patients.[53] The CardioMEMS Heart Failure System (Abbott; Lake Bluff, IL) consists of a wireless sensor implanted into the PA during a right heart catheterization and an electronic capturing system that collects information on PA systolic, diastolic, and mean pressures. In addition to guiding therapy adjustments during acute hospitalization, W-IHM can also be telemonitored after patients are discharged from the hospital, permitting further titration of diuretic therapy and GDMT. Despite decreasing the risk of HF hospitalization, widespread use of W-IHM has been limited due to concerns regarding the long-term durability and cost-effectiveness of the device.

Temporary MCS

11 For patients with refractory ADHF, temporary MCS may be considered for hemodynamic stabilization until the underlying etiology of cardiac dysfunction resolves or has been corrected ("bridge to recovery") or until evaluation for definitive therapy (eg, durable MCS or cardiac transplantation) can be completed ("bridge to decision").[2] Due to the invasive nature of MCS and its potential complications, therapy should be reserved for patients who are refractory to maximally tolerated pharmacologic therapy. Intravenous vasodilators and inotropic agents may also be used in conjunction with temporary MCS to maximize hemodynamic and clinical benefits or to facilitate device removal. Regardless of the modality selected, systemic anticoagulation with intravenous therapies (eg, unfractionated heparin) is required to prevent device thrombosis. Temporary MCS should generally be avoided in patients with irreversible advanced HF and no plan for definitive management, those with contraindications to anticoagulation therapy, and those with comorbid conditions or anatomical abnormalities that preclude device implantation. The three most common modalities of temporary MCS are the IABP, VAD, and extracorporeal membrane oxygenation (ECMO) (Fig. 37-5). Unique features, contraindications, and complications of each type of device will be discussed in the sections to follow.

Intra-aortic Balloon Pump An IABP consists of a polyethylene balloon mounted on a catheter that is inserted percutaneously into the femoral artery and advanced into the descending thoracic aorta (see Fig. 37-5). During counterpulsation, the balloon is synchronized with the electrocardiogram (or alternatively, changes in pressure) so that it inflates during diastole and displaces blood to the proximal aorta, thus increasing diastolic pressure and coronary perfusion. The balloon deflates just prior to the opening of the aortic valve during systole, which causes a sudden "vacuum-like" decrease in aortic pressure, allowing the left ventricle to pump against reduced arterial impedance. Although the IABP is the most commonly employed modality of temporary MCS due to its ease of use, it only provides an estimated 1.0 L/min of CO. As a consequence, the primary benefits of an IABP are enhanced coronary perfusion, increased myocardial oxygen supply, and reduced myocardial oxygen demand. It may be particularly useful for patients with myocardial ischemia complicated by cardiogenic shock, although it has not been shown to improve mortality in this setting.[54] Systemic anticoagulation is generally recommended, although cases of IABP use without anticoagulation have been reported and practices vary across institutions.[55] Complications of the IABP include vascular injury, thrombocytopenia, and renal impairment due to obstruction of the splanchnic circulation by balloon malposition. Use should be avoided in patients with severe peripheral vascular disease or significant aortic regurgitation (eg, aortic insufficiency).

Ventricular Assist Devices A VAD provides hemodynamic support by assisting and, in some cases, replacing the pumping functions of the right and/or left ventricles. Compared to an IABP, temporary VADs confer greater hemodynamic improvements but no differences in long-term survival.[56] A left ventricular assist device (LVAD) propels blood from the left ventricle or left atrium to the ascending aorta, whereas a right VAD propels blood from the right ventricle or right atrium to the PA. A right VAD may be used alone or in conjunction with an LVAD; this latter configuration is known as a biventricular assist device. All VADs are preload-dependent, meaning that adequate intra-ventricular filling pressure (ie, volume) is required to optimize blood flow. As with the native ventricle in HF, VADs are also afterload-sensitive, meaning that excess peripheral resistance can impair blood flow. Complications of VAD implantation include bleeding, infections, stroke, and risks associated with the specific implantation technique. In addition, the devices can cause thrombosis, renal and hepatic dysfunction, and arrhythmias. Right ventricular failure is a unique complication of LVAD implantation as a result of increased venous return, persistently elevated pulmonary pressures, and changes in right ventricular geometry.

Percutaneous VADs include the Impella series (Abiomed, Danvers, MA) and TandemHeart (CardiacAssist, Pittsburgh, PA). Most Impella devices are inserted percutaneously into a large peripheral artery and advanced in a retrograde fashion across the aortic valve, where blood is advanced from the left ventricle to the ascending aorta via axial flow (see Fig. 37-5). The amount of CO augmented by the Impella device depends on the model used; for example, the Impella 2.5 and 5.0 models supply 2.5 L and 5.0 L/min of flow, respectively. Hemolysis is a common complication of Impella use due to the axial flow facilitated by the device. The TandemHeart device consists of an inflow cannula placed percutaneously into a large peripheral vein and advanced transseptally into the left atrium (see Fig. 37-5). Blood is withdrawn from the left atrium by an extracorporeal pump and propelled via an outflow cannula placed percutaneously into a large artery. Up to 5.0 L/min of flow can be provided by the TandemHeart. Due to its placement across the intra-atrial septum, perforation and shunt formation are potential complications with this device.

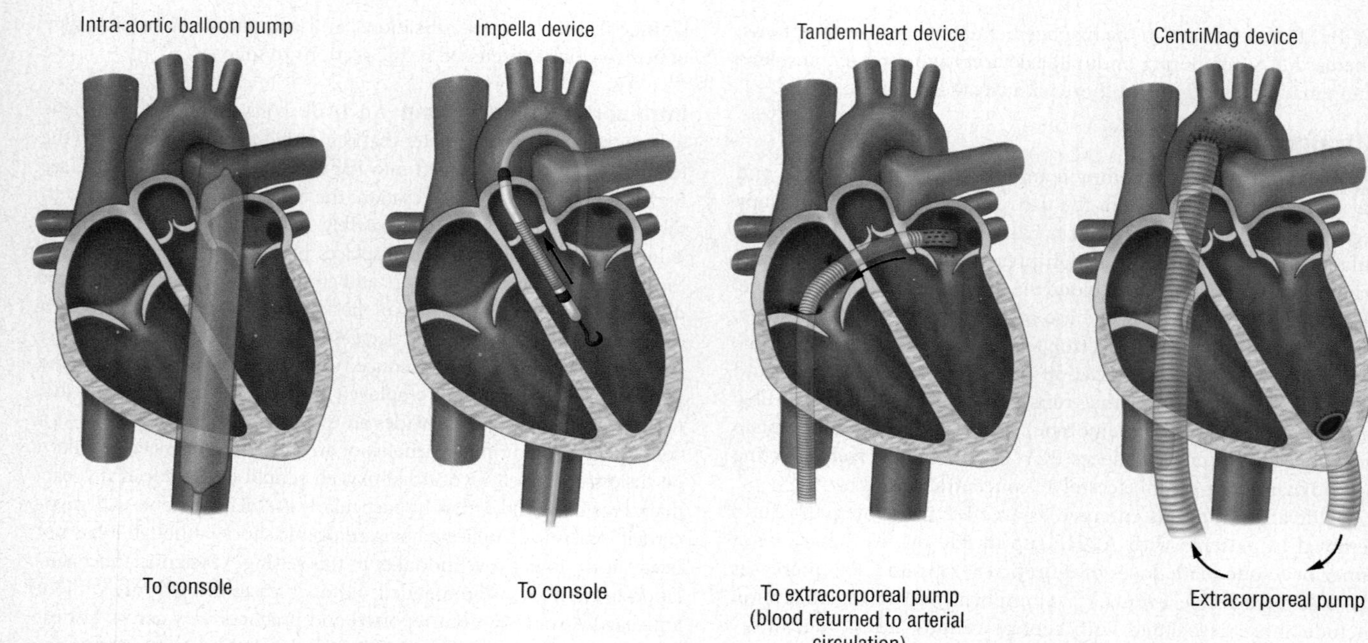

FIGURE 37-5 Common types of temporary MCS. An intra-aortic balloon pump (IABP) is advanced into the descending aorta where it inflates during diastole (shown), displacing blood and improving coronary filling. During systole (not shown), the IABP deflates, producing a vacuum-like effect that reduces peripheral resistance. An example of a percutaneous VAD is the Impella device, which is advanced through the aortic valve, where blood is transferred from the left ventricle to the aorta by an axial flow pump. The TandemHeart VAD is also a device inserted percutaneously into a large peripheral vein and advanced across the intra-atrial septum. Blood is removed from the left atrium and propelled by an extracorporeal centrifugal flow pump back into the systemic circulation (not shown). The CentriMag VAD uses an inflow cannula that is surgically inserted into the apex of the left ventricle, where blood is transferred to an extracorporeal centrifugal flow pump (not shown), where it is returned to the systemic circulation via an outflow cannula surgically inserted into the aorta. In extracorporeal membrane oxygenation (ECMO) (not shown), the inflow and outflow cannula are inserted into peripheral vessels.

The most common surgically implanted temporary VAD is the CentriMag (Thoractec Corp., Pleasanton, CA), which can provide right, left, or biventricular support and up to 10 L/min of CO. The CentriMag device consists of a centrifugal flow extracorporeal pump and surgically placed inflow and outflow cannula supporting the affected ventricle (see Fig. 37-5). Given the surgical technique required for placement of the CentriMag device, tissue injury is its most common complication.

Extracorporeal Membrane Oxygenation Extracorporeal membrane oxygenation may be venoarterial or venovenous in nature. In venoarterial ECMO, deoxygenated blood is transported from the venous circulation to an extracorporeal oxygenator and centrifugal flow pump and returned as oxygenated blood to the arterial circulation. In contrast, venovenous ECMO consists of only extracorporeal oxygenation; hemodynamic support is provided by native cardiac function. As a consequence, venoarterial ECMO is more common in the management of refractory ADHF, where up to 8 L/min of cardiac support can be provided. Complications of ECMO include bleeding, infections, and organ dysfunction. Serum drug concentrations can also be significantly impacted as a result of an increased volume of distribution, decreased elimination due to hepatic and/or renal impairment, and sequestration of drugs in the ECMO circuit.

Advanced Therapies

No consensus definition exists for advanced HF or the stage at which patients should be considered for definitive therapies such as durable MCS and heart transplantation. Nonetheless, evaluation for these advanced therapies is commonly initiated during an admission for ADHF, particularly if hospitalization is accompanied by severe symptoms at rest, intolerance of GDMT, decline in organ function, refractory arrhythmias, or an inability to be successfully weaned from inotropic or temporary MCS support. Because of the complexity of care, potential risks, and resource implications of durable MCS and heart transplantation, patients with advanced HF must undergo a rigorous interdisciplinary evaluation before becoming eligible candidates. Components of this evaluation commonly include past medical, surgical, and psychosocial history, medication and adverse event history, adherence to medications and medical care, comorbid conditions, risks for postoperative complications, and health insurance coverage. Relative contraindications to the use of advanced therapies include excess perioperative risk, irreversible pulmonary hypertension, inability to manage postoperative care (eg, medication therapy, monitoring), and concurrent survival-limiting diseases (eg, malignancy).

Durable MCS The most common indications for durable MCS are temporary device implantation in patients awaiting heart transplantation who are unlikely to survive the duration of time required for identifying a suitable donor ("bridge to transplantation") and permanent device implantation in patients who are ineligible for heart transplantation due to advanced age or comorbid conditions ("destination therapy"). Although far less common than with temporary MCS, durable VADs may be implanted in patients who are likely to become eligible transplant candidates ("bridge to decision") but the evaluation is incomplete or has been delayed until certain requirements can be satisfied (eg, smoking cessation). Durable MCS is almost exclusively comprised of LVAD implantation, although select patients may remain hospitalized with right VAD or biventricular support while awaiting transplantation.

Durable LVADs are implanted by inserting an inflow cannula into the apex of the left ventricle, which is connected to an intracorporeal pumping unit; blood is returned to the systemic circulation via an outflow cannula inserted into the aorta. Whereas previous devices provided hemodynamic support via pulsatile flow, newer-generation devices utilize a continuous flow mechanism, allowing them to be smaller in size, less subject to deterioration over time, and conferring an improvement in event-free survival.[57] Prolonged unloading of the left ventricle with an LVAD in combination with drug therapy can produce sustained recovery in LV function, amelioration of symptoms, and in some cases, device explantation.[58] The three continuous flow LVADs currently approved for use in the United States are the axial flow HeartMate II LVAD (Abbott; Lake Bluff, IL) and centrifugal flow HeartMate 3 LVAD (Abbott) and HeartWare Ventricular Assist Device (HVAD) (HeartWare, Inc; Framingham, MA). All three devices are capable of providing up to 10 L/min of CO. For complete heart replacement therapy, total artificial heart systems continue to be investigated, although their size and embolic complications limit widespread use.

Complications following durable LVAD placement are similar to those described for temporary devices. Device malfunction may occur with long-term use but has become rare with advances in technology. The most perplexing challenge in the care of LVAD patients remains identifying a chronic antithrombotic regimen that balances the risk of device thrombosis and bleeding. Antithrombotic regimens most often include a vitamin K antagonist and antiplatelet agent, although the goal international normalized ratio (INR) range and antiplatelet agents selected (eg, aspirin, dipyridamole, clopidogrel) may vary significantly by the center. The efficacy and safety of direct oral anticoagulants in LVAD recipients have yet to be established. Suspected pump thrombosis should be promptly evaluated, although no consensus exists on an appropriate treatment strategy (eg, enhanced antiplatelet or anticoagulant therapy, thrombolysis, or pump exchange).[59]

Heart Transplantation 12 Orthotopic heart transplantation remains the optimal management strategy for patients with irreversible advanced HF, as 10-year survival rates approach 60% among patients transplanted after 2001.[60] Unfortunately, the shortage of acceptable donor hearts has prolonged waiting times and many patients succumb to their disease prior to transplantation. Another significant percentage of patients are deemed ineligible for heart transplantation because of age, concurrent illnesses, psychosocial factors, or other reasons. The shortage of donor hearts has prompted the development of new surgical strategies, including ventricular aneurysm resection, mitral valve repair, and myocardial cell transplantation, which have resulted in variable degrees of improvement. Further development of these and other techniques may offer additional options in patients who are not eligible for VAD implantation or heart transplantation. For a more detailed discussion of heart transplantation, see Chapter 109 "Solid Organ Transplantation."

EVALUATION OF THERAPEUTIC OUTCOMES

Daily monitoring to assess the efficacy of drug therapy is critical to assuring optimal outcomes and should include weight, strict measurement of fluid intake and output, and HF signs and symptoms (Table 37-6). Foley catheter placement is not recommended unless close monitoring of urine output is not otherwise possible. Safety endpoints such as monitoring for electrolyte depletion, symptomatic hypotension, and renal dysfunction should be assessed frequently. While many safety parameters can be monitored daily, some will need to be monitored more frequently based on the patient's clinical status. Vital signs should be assessed multiple times throughout the day at a frequency that is appropriate for the patient's degree of stability. Orthostatic blood pressure should be assessed at least once daily.

TABLE 37-6 Monitoring Recommendations for Patients Hospitalized with ADHF

Parameter	Frequency	Notes
Weight	Daily	Assess after voiding in the morning
		Use the same scale each day, standing weight if possible
		Account for increase or decrease in food intake
Fluid balance	Daily[a]	Strict intake and output
Vital signs	More than daily	Blood pressure and heart rate, including signs/symptoms of orthostatic hypotension, rhythm (continuous)
Signs of congestion and/or low output	Daily[a]	Jugular venous distension, crackles, hepatomegaly, splenomegaly, hepatojugular reflux, ascites, lower extremity edema, hypotension, narrow pulse pressures, cool extremities, altered mental status, worsening renal or hepatic function
Symptoms of congestion and/or low output	Daily[a]	Dyspnea on exertion or at rest, orthopnea, paroxysmal nocturnal dyspnea, nausea/vomiting, early satiety, fatigue, lightheadedness, chest pain, palpitations
Electrolytes	Daily[a]	Potassium, magnesium, sodium
Renal function	Daily[a]	Blood urea nitrogen and serum creatinine including ratio to assess volume status (ie, over-diuresis)
Hepatic function	Variable[a]	Alk Phos and GGT primarily for fluid overload, AST and ALT primarily for hypoperfusion
BNP, NT-proBNP	Admission, discharge	Admission for diagnosis, discharge for prognosis
Other	Variable	Troponin and other cardiac enzymes if myocardial strain
		Arterial blood gas if hypoxic
		Lactate, if hypoperfusion present
		Iron panel, regardless of hemoglobin concentrations

Alk Phos, alkaline phosphatase; AST, aspartate aminotransferase; ALT, alanine aminotransferase; BNP, B-type natriuretic peptide; GGT, gamma-glutamyltransferase; NT-proBNP, N-terminal pro-B-type natriuretic peptide.

[a]Daily unless a change in clinical status warrants more frequent assessment (eg, high-dose, continuous infusion, and/or combination diuretic therapy; rapidly changing clinical status).

Patients with ADHF may have critically reduced CO, usually with low arterial blood pressure and systemic hypoperfusion resulting in organ system dysfunction (ie, cardiogenic shock). They may also have pulmonary edema with hypoxemia, respiratory acidosis, and markedly increased work of breathing. With cardiopulmonary support, response to interventions should be assessed promptly to allow for timely adjustments in treatment. Continuous telemetry monitoring, continuous pulse oximetry, urine flow, and automated blood pressure recordings are standards of care for critically ill patients with cardiopulmonary decompensation. Peripheral or femoral arterial catheters may be used for continuous and accurate assessment of arterial pressure.

Preparing for Discharge

Patients should not be discharged until optimal volume status is achieved and they have been successfully transitioned from an IV to an oral diuretic regimen and IV inotropes and vasodilators have been discontinued for at least 24 hours. Given the known benefits of discharging patients on GDMT, hospitalization for ADHF represents an ideal opportunity to optimize these therapies. As such, efforts should be made to initiate (or reinitiate if held earlier in the admission) GDMT in hemodynamically stable patients without contraindications.[3] For example, low-dose β-blocker therapy may be safely initiated at discharge without increasing the risk of readmission,[61] and transitioning eligible patients to the angiotensin receptor neprilysin inhibitor (ARNI) sacubitril/valsartan should also be considered.[62] Patients who are hemodynamically stable and have been successfully transitioned to oral diuretics should be considered for SGTL2 inhibitor therapy given reductions in the risk of cardiovascular death and rehospitalization when these therapies are initiated prior to or shortly after discharge.[63] In patients with iron deficiency (ie, serum ferritin <100 ng/mL [mcg/L] or 100 to 299 ng/mL [mcg/L] with transferrin saturation <20%), IV iron repletion should be considered prior to or shortly after discharge to improve symptoms and quality of life and potentially reduce the risk of HF rehospitalization.[64] If relevant, smoking cessation must be addressed to avoid delay in consideration for advanced therapies. In patients with reduced LVEF, use of GDMT or intolerance to such should be documented in the medical record.[65]

Prior to discharge, patients and caregivers should be counseled on dietary sodium restriction as well as monitoring body weight daily and parameters for when to titrate diuretics or call a healthcare provider for further instruction (eg, 3-lb [1.4 kg] weight gain in 24 hours). Medication changes (initiation, discontinuation, dose change) should be clearly conveyed verbally and in writing and financial coverage for all medication assured. The importance of dietary and medication adherence should be emphasized. Appropriate follow-up should be scheduled, including an appointment within 7 days post-discharge and a nurse visit or phone call at 3 days for select patients. Pertinent follow-up labs (eg, potassium, serum creatinine) should also be scheduled, including other medication-related labs (eg, INR for warfarin, serum digoxin concentration). All patients should be considered for referral to a multidisciplinary disease management program.[66,67]

CONCLUSION

Several recent clinical trials have addressed many controversies in the management of ADHF, including the appropriate dosing of diuretics and the use of vasoactive therapies in patients with volume overload. Still, many unanswered questions remain, including optimal use of GDMT in the setting of ADHF. Many advances in MCS have extended the lives of patients awaiting a transplant; however, limited evidence exists to guide the management of this patient population, including how to avoid and manage complications associated with these devices. Finally, ideal management of patients with ADHF includes optimization of GDMT, optimal communication with patients, caregivers, and other healthcare providers with each care transition, and outpatient follow-up with a collaborative, multidisciplinary team.

ABBREVIATIONS

ACCF	American College of Cardiology Foundation
ACE	angiotensin-converting enzyme
ADHF	acute decompensated heart failure
AHA	American Heart Association
AMP	adenosine monophosphate
AVP	arginine vasopressin
BNP	B-type natriuretic peptide
BUN	blood urea nitrogen
cAMP	cyclic adenosine monophosphate
cGMP	cyclic guanosine monophosphate
CI	cardiac index
CO	cardiac output
CVP	central venous pressure
DT	destination therapy
ECMO	extracorporeal membrane oxygenation
GDMT	guideline-directed medical therapy
GI	gastrointestinal
HF	heart failure
HFpEF	heart failure with preserved ejection fraction
HFrEF	heart failure with reduced ejection fraction
HVAD	HeartWare Ventricular Assist Device
IABP	intra-aortic balloon pump
INR	international normalized ratio
IV	intravenous
JVD	jugular venous distension
LVAD	left ventricular assist device
MAP	mean arterial pressure
MCS	mechanical circulatory support
MI	myocardial infarction
NYHA	New York Heart Association
PA	pulmonary artery
PCWP	pulmonary capillary wedge pressure
PVR	pulmonary vascular resistance
SIADH	syndrome of inappropriate diuretic hormone
SVR	systemic vascular resistance
VAD	ventricular assist device
W-IHM	wireless invasive hemodynamic monitoring
WRF	worsening renal function

REFERENCES

1. McIlvennan Colleen K, Allen Larry A. Palliative care in patients with heart failure. *BMJ.* 2016;353:i1010. 10.1136/bmj.i1010.
2. Yancy CW, Jessup M, Bozkurt B, et al. 2013 ACCF/AHA guideline for the management of heart failure: A report of the American College of Cardiology Foundation/American Heart Association Task Force on Practice Guidelines. *J Am Coll Cardiol.* 2013;62(16):e147–e239.
3. Hollenberg SM, Warner Stevenson L, Ahmad T, et al. 2019 ACC expert consensus decision pathway on risk assessment, management, and clinical trajectory of patients hospitalized with heart failure: A report of the American College of Cardiology solution set oversight committee. *J Am Coll Cardiol.* 2019;74(15):1966–2011. 10.1016/j.jacc.2019.08.001 31526538.
4. Virani SS, Alonso A, Aparicio HJ, et al. Heart disease and stroke statistics-2021 update: A report from the American Heart Association. *Circulation.* 2021;143(8):e254–e743. 10.1161/CIR.0000000000000950 33501848.
5. Ambrosy AP, Fonarow GC, Butler J, et al. The global health and economic burden of hospitalizations for heart failure: Lessons learned from hospitalized heart failure registries. *J Am Coll Cardiol.* 2014;63(12):1123–1133.

6. Kurmani S, Squire I. Acute heart failure: Definition, classification and epidemiology. *Curr Heart Fail Rep.* 2017;14(5):385–392. 10.1007/s11897-017-0351-y 28785969.
7. Fonarow GC, Adams KF, Abraham WT, et al. Risk stratification for in-hospital mortality in acutely decompensated heart failure: Classification and regression tree analysis. *JAMA.* 2005;293(5):572–580.
8. O'Connor CM, Abraham WT, Albert NM, et al. Predictors of mortality after discharge in patients hospitalized with heart failure: An analysis from the Organized Program to Initiate Lifesaving Treatment in Hospitalized Patients with Heart Failure (OPTIMIZE-HF). *Am Heart J.* 2008;156(4):662–673.
9. Binanay C, Califf RM, Hasselblad V, et al. Evaluation study of congestive heart failure and pulmonary artery catheterization effectiveness: The ESCAPE trial. *JAMA.* 2005;294(13):1625–1633.
10. Garan AR, Kanwar M, Thayer KL, et al. Complete hemodynamic profiling with pulmonary artery catheters in cardiogenic shock is associated with lower in-hospital mortality. *J Am Coll Cardiol Heart Fail.* 2020;8(11):903–913. 10.1016/j.jchf.2020.08.012 33121702.
11. Opotowsky AR, Hess E, Maron BA, et al. Thermodilution vs estimated fick cardiac output measurement in clinical practice: An analysis of mortality from the veterans affairs clinical assessment, reporting, and tracking (VA CART) program and vanderbilt university. *JAMA Cardiol.* 2017;2(10):1090–1099. 10.1001/jamacardio.2017.2945 28877293.
12. Aalders M, Kok W. Comparison of hemodynamic factors predicting prognosis in heart failure: A systematic review. *J Clin Med.* 2019;8(10):1757. 10.3390/jcm8101757 31652650.
13. Chioncel O, Mebazaa A, Maggioni AP, et al. Acute heart failure congestion and perfusion status: Impact of the clinical classification on in-hospital and long-term outcomes; insights from the ESC-EORP-HFA Heart Failure Long-Term Registry. *Eur J Heart Fail.* 2019;21(11):1338–1352. 10.1002/ejhf.1492 31127678.
14. Testani JM, Chen J, McCauley BD, et al. Potential effects of aggressive decongestion during the treatment of decompensated heart failure on renal function and survival. *Circulation.* 2010;122(3):265–72. 10.1161/CIRCULATIONAHA.109.933275 20606118.
15. Damman K, Testani JM. The kidney in heart failure: An update. *Eur Heart J.* 2015;36(23):1437–1444. 10.1093/eurheartj/ehv010 25838436.
16. Fonarow GC, Abraham WT, Albert NM, et al. Influence of beta-blocker continuation or withdrawal on outcomes in patients hospitalized with heart failure: Findings from the OPTIMIZE-HF program. *J Am Coll Cardiol.* 2008;52(3):90–199.
17. Jondeau G, Neuder Y, Eicher J-C, et al. B-CONVINCED: Beta-blocker CONtinuation Vs. INterruption in patients with Congestive heart failure hospitalizED for a decompensation episode. *Eur Heart J.* 2009;30(18):2186–2192.
18. Packer M, Gheorghiade M, Young JB, et al. Withdrawal of digoxin from patients with chronic heart failure treated with angiotensin-converting-enzyme inhibitors. RADIANCE Study. *N Engl J Med.* 1993;329(1):1–7.
19. Uretsky BF, Young JB, Shahidi FE, Yellen LG, Harrison MC, Jolly MK. Randomized study assessing the effect of digoxin withdrawal in patients with mild to moderate chronic congestive heart failure: Results of the PROVED trial. PROVED Investigative Group. *J Am Coll Cardiol.* 1993;22(4):955–962.
20. Forrester JS, Diamond G, Chatterjee K, Swan HJ. Medical therapy of acute myocardial infarction by application of hemodynamic subsets (first of two parts). *N Engl J Med.* 1976;295(24):1356–1362.
21. Felker GM, Lee KL, Bull DA, et al. Diuretic strategies in patients with acute decompensated heart failure. *N Engl J Med.* 2011;364(9):797–805.
22. Dormans TP, van Meyel JJ, Gerlag PG, Tan Y, Russel FG, Smits P. Diuretic efficacy of high dose furosemide in severe heart failure: Bolus injection versus continuous infusion. *J Am Coll Cardiol.* 1996;28(2):376–382.
23. Thomson MR, Nappi JM, Dunn SP, Hollis IB, Rodgers JE, Van Bakel AB. Continuous versus intermittent infusion of furosemide in acute decompensated heart failure. *J Card Fail.* 2010;16(3):88–193.
24. Sharma K, Vasihnav J, Kalathiya R, et al. Randomized evaluation of heart failure with preserved ejection fraction patients with acute heart failure and dopamine: The ROPA-DOP trial. *JACC Heart Fail.* 2018;6(10):859–870.
25. Reed BN, Gottlieb SS. Diuretic strategies and renal dysfunction in heart failure with preserved ejection fraction. *JACC Heart Fail.* 2018;6(12):1049–1050.
26. Mullens W, Damman K, Testani JM, et al. Evaluation of kidney function throughout the heart failure trajectory: A position statement from the Heart Failure Association of the European Society of Cardiology. *Eur J Heart Fail.* 2020;22(4):584–603. 10.1002/ejhf.1697 31908120.
27. Ahmad T, Jackson K, Rao VS, et al. Worsening renal function in patients with acute heart failure undergoing aggressive diuresis is not associated with tubular injury. *Circulation.* 2018;137(19):2016–2028. 10.1161/CIRCULATIONAHA.117.030112 29352071.
28. Felker GM, Ellison DH, Mullens W, et al. Diuretic therapy for patients with heart failure: JACC state-of-the-art review. *J Am Coll Cardiol.* 2020;75(10):1178–1195. 10.1016/j.jacc.2019.12.059 32164892.
29. Mullens W, Damman K, Harjola VP, et al. The use of diuretics in heart failure with congestion: A position statement from the Heart Failure Association of the European Society of Cardiology. *Eur J Heart Fail.* 2019;21(2):137–155. 10.1002/ejhf.1369 30600580.
30. Cox ZL, Hung R, Lenihan DJ, et al. Diuretic strategies for loop diuretic resistance in acute heart failure: The 3T trial. *J Am Coll Cardiol Heart Fail.* 2020;8(3):157–168. 10.1016/j.jchf.2019.09.012 31838029.
31. Butler J, Anstrom KJ, Felker GM, et al. Efficacy and safety of spironolactone in acute heart failure: The ATHENA-HF randomized clinical trial. *JAMA Cardiol.* 2017;2(9):950–958. 10.1001/jamacardio.2017.2198 28700781.
32. Giamouzis G, Butler J, Starling RC, et al. Impact of dopamine infusion on renal function in hospitalized heart failure patients: Results of the Dopamine in Acute Decompensated Heart Failure (DAD-HF) Trial. *J Card Fail.* 2010;16(12):922–930.
33. Chen HH, Anstrom KJ, Givertz MM, et al. Low-dose dopamine or low-dose nesiritide in acute heart failure with renal dysfunction: The ROSE acute heart failure randomized trial. *JAMA.* 2013;310(23):2533–2543.
34. Gheorghiade M, Gattis WA, O'Connor CM, et al. Effects of tolvaptan, a vasopressin antagonist, in patients hospitalized with worsening heart failure: A randomized controlled trial. *JAMA.* 2004;291(16):1963–1971.
35. Lee WH, Packer M. Prognostic importance of serum sodium concentration and its modification by converting-enzyme inhibition in patients with severe chronic heart failure. *Circulation.* 1986;73(2):257–267.
36. Gheorghiade M, Konstam MA, Burnett JC, et al. Short-term clinical effects of tolvaptan, an oral vasopressin antagonist, in patients hospitalized for heart failure: The EVEREST Clinical Status Trials. *JAMA.* 2007;297(12):1332–1343.
37. Felker GM, Mentz RJ, Cole RT, et al. Efficacy and safety of tolvaptan in patients hospitalized with acute heart failure. *J Am Coll Cardiol.* 2017;69(11):1399–1406.
38. Schwartzenberg S, Redfield MM, From AM, Sorajja P, Nishimura RA, Borlaug BA. Effects of vasodilation in heart failure with preserved or reduced ejection fraction implications of distinct pathophysiologies on response to therapy. *J Am Coll Cardiol.* 2012;59(5):442–451.
39. Publication Committee for the VMAC Investigators (Vasodilatation in the Management of Acute CHF). Intravenous nesiritide vs nitroglycerin for treatment of decompensated congestive heart failure: A randomized controlled trial. *JAMA.* 2002;287(12):1531–1540.
40. Cohn JN, Franciosa JA, Francis GS, et al. Effect of short-term infusion of sodium nitroprusside on mortality rate in acute myocardial infarction complicated by left ventricular failure: results of a Veterans Administration cooperative study. *N Engl J Med.* 1982;306:1129–1135. doi: 10.1056/NEJM198205133061902.
41. Mullens W, Abrahams Z, Francis GS, et al. Sodium nitroprusside for advanced low-output heart failure. *J Am Coll Cardiol.* 2008;52(3):200–207.
42. Abraham WT, Adams KF, Fonarow GC, et al. In-hospital mortality in patients with acute decompensated heart failure requiring intravenous vasoactive medications: An analysis from the Acute Decompensated Heart Failure National Registry (ADHERE). *J Am Coll Cardiol.* 2005;46(1):57–64.
43. Cuffe MS, Califf RM, Adams KF, et al. Short-term intravenous milrinone for acute exacerbation of chronic heart failure: A randomized controlled trial. *JAMA.* 2002;287(12):1541–1547.
44. Mathew R, Di Santo P, Jung RG, et al. Milrinone as compared with dobutamine in the treatment of cardiogenic shock. *N Engl J Med.* 2021;385(6):516–525. 10.1056/NEJMoa2026845 34347952.
45. Metra M, Nodari S, D'Aloia A, et al. Beta-blocker therapy influences the hemodynamic response to inotropic agents in patients with heart failure: A randomized comparison of dobutamine and enoximone before and after chronic treatment with metoprolol or carvedilol. *J Am Coll Cardiol.* 2002;40(7):1248–1258.
46. De Backer D, Biston P, Devriendt J, et al. Comparison of dopamine and norepinephrine in the treatment of shock. *N Engl J Med.* 2010;362(9):779–789.
47. Aliti GB, Rabelo ER, Clausell N, et al. Aggressive fluid and sodium restriction in acute decompensated heart failure: A randomized clinical trial. *JAMA Intern Med.* 2013;173(12):1058–1064. 10.1001/jamainternmed.2013.552 23689381.

48. Griffin M, Soufer A, Goljo E, et al. Real world use of hypertonic saline in refractory acute decompensated heart failure: A U.S. center's 2xperience. *J Am Coll Cardiol Heart Fail.* 2020;8(3):199–208. 10.1016/j.jchf.2019.10.012 32035891.
49. Costanzo MR, Guglin ME, Saltzberg MT, et al. Ultrafiltration versus intravenous diuretics for patients hospitalized for acute decompensated heart failure. *J Am Coll Cardiol.* 2007;49(6):675–683.
50. Bart BA, Goldsmith SR, Lee KL, et al. Ultrafiltration in decompensated heart failure with cardiorenal syndrome. *N Engl J Med.* 2012;367(24):2296–2304.
51. Costanzo MR, Negoianu D, Jaski BE, et al. Aquapheresis versus intravenous diuretics and hospitalizations for heart failure. *J Am Coll Cardiol Heart Fail.* 2016;4(2):95–105. 10.1016/j.jchf.2015.08.005 26519995.
52. Abraham WT, Adamson PB, Bourge RC, et al. Wireless pulmonary artery haemodynamic monitoring in chronic heart failure: A randomised controlled trial. *Lancet.* 2011;377(9766):658–696.
53. Thiele H, Zeymer U, Neumann F-J, et al. Intraaortic balloon support for myocardial infarction with cardiogenic shock. *N Engl J Med.* 2012;367(14):1287–1296.
54. Pucher PH, Cummings IG, Shipolini AR, McCormack DJ. Is heparin needed for patients with an intra-aortic balloon pump? *Interact Cardiovasc Thorac Surg.* 2012;15(1):36–139.
55. Cheng JM, den Uil CA, Hoeks SE, et al. Percutaneous left ventricular assist devices vs. intra-aortic balloon pump counterpulsation for treatment of cardiogenic shock: A meta-analysis of controlled trials. *Eur Heart J.* 2009;30(17):2102–2108.
56. Slaughter MS, Rogers JG, Milano CA, et al. Advanced heart failure treated with continuous-flow left ventricular assist device. *N Engl J Med.* 2009;361(23):2241–2251.
57. Birks EJ, Tansley PD, Hardy J, et al. Left ventricular assist device and drug therapy for the reversal of heart failure. *N Engl J Med.* 2006;355(18):1873–1884.
58. Goldstein DJ, John R, Salerno C, et al. Algorithm for the diagnosis and management of suspected pump thrombus. *J Heart Lung Transplant.* 2013;32(7):667–670.
59. Khush KK, Cherikh WS, Chambers DC, et al. The international thoracic organ transplant registry of the International Society for Heart and Lung Transplantation: Thirty-sixth adult heart transplantation report - 2019; focus theme: donor and recipient size match. *J Heart Lung Transplant.* 2019;38(10):1056–1066. 10.1016/j.healun.2019.08.004 31548031.
60. Gattis WA1, O'Connor CM, Gallup DS, Hasselblad V, Gheorghiade M; IMPACT-HF Investigators and Coordinators. Predischarge initiation of carvedilol in patients hospitalized for decompensated heart failure: Results of the Initiation Management Predischarge: Process for Assessment of Carvedilol Therapy in Heart Failure (IMPACT-HF) trial. *J Am Coll Cardiol.* 2004;43(9):1534–1541.
61. Velazquez Eric J, Morrow David A, DeVore Adam D, et al. Angiotensin–neprilysin inhibition in acute decompensated heart failure. *N Engl J Med.* 2019;380:539–548. 10.1056/nejmoa1812851.
62. Bhatt DL, Szarek M, Steg PG, et al. Sotagliflozin in patients with diabetes and recent worsening heart failure. *N Engl J Med.* 2021;384(2):117–128. 10.1056/NEJMoa2030183 33200892.
63. Ponikowski P, Kirwan BA, Anker SD, et al. Ferric carboxymaltose for iron deficiency at discharge after acute heart failure: A multicentre, double-blind, randomised, controlled trial. *Lancet.* 2020;396(10266):1895–1904. 10.1016/S0140-6736(20)32339-4 33197395.
64. Heidenreich PA, Fonarow GC, Breathett K, et al. 2020 ACC/AHA clinical performance and quality measures for adults with heart failure: A report of the American College of Cardiology/American Heart Association task force on performance measures. *J Am Coll Cardiol.* 2020;76:2527–2564. doi: 10.1016/j.jacc.2020.07.023
65. Milfred-LaForest SK, Chow SL, DiDomenico RJ, et al. Clinical pharmacy services in heart failure: An opinion paper from the Heart Failure Society of America and American College of Clinical Pharmacy Cardiology Practice and Research Network. *Pharmacotherapy.* 2013;33(5):529–548.
66. Albert NM, Barnason S, Deswal A, et al. Transitions of care in heart failure: A scientific statement from the American Heart Association. *Circ Heart Fail.* 2015;8(2):384–409.

38

Venous Thromboembolism

Daniel M. Witt, Nathan P. Clark, and Sara R. Vazquez

KEY CONCEPTS

1. Venous thromboembolism (VTE) is often associated with identifiable risk factors.
2. The diagnosis of suspected VTE should be confirmed by objective testing.
3. During hospitalization, patients should receive VTE prophylaxis based on the VTE risk factors present and the anticipated duration of risk.
4. Initial VTE treatment should include a rapid-acting anticoagulant.
5. For VTE treatment, injectable anticoagulants should be overlapped with warfarin for at least 5 days and until the patient's international normalized ratio is ≥2.0 for at least 24 hours.
6. Direct oral anticoagulants (DOACs) such as apixaban, dabigatran, edoxaban, and rivaroxaban are significant advancements in VTE prevention and treatment.
7. Most patients with uncomplicated deep vein thrombosis (DVT) or pulmonary embolism (PE) can be safely treated as outpatients.
8. Most patients with VTE should receive 3 months of anticoagulation therapy; treatment beyond 3 months should be based on the risk of VTE recurrence and bleeding as well as patient preferences.
9. Optimal anticoagulant therapy management requires knowledge of pharmacologic and pharmacokinetic characteristics as well as a systematic management approach with ongoing patient education.

BEYOND THE BOOK

Visit the **National Blood Clot Alliance: Stop The Clot** website and read the stories of at least five different patients (https://www.stoptheclot.org/patient-stories/). These stories are useful to enhance student understanding regarding the impact of VTE and its treatment on the lives of patients and their families.

INTRODUCTION

Venous thromboembolism (VTE) is a potentially fatal disorder and a significant health problem in our aging society.[1] VTE results from clot formation within the venous circulation and manifests as deep vein thrombosis (DVT) and/or pulmonary embolism (PE) (Fig. 38-1).[1] DVT is rarely fatal, but PE can result in death within minutes of symptom onset before effective treatment can be given. Late VTE complications, such as the postthrombotic syndrome and chronic thromboembolic pulmonary hypertension (CTPH), also cause substantial morbidity.[1] Identifying VTE risk factors is important for targeting patients at high risk for VTE who would most benefit from VTE prevention strategies.[2,3]

Rapid and accurate diagnosis is critical to making appropriate treatment decisions when VTE is suspected.[4] Optimal prevention and treatment of VTE using anticoagulant drugs requires an in-depth knowledge of their pharmacology and pharmacokinetic properties, and a comprehensive approach to patient management.[5] Bleeding is a common and serious complication of anticoagulant therapy.[5]

EPIDEMIOLOGY

VTE is associated with a significant global disease burden.[6] The incidence rate of symptomatic first VTE is estimated at 132 per 100,000 patient-years and occurs more frequently in women (55.6%).[7] When standardized by age, Asian patients appear to have the lowest VTE incidence (122 per 100,000 patient-years) followed by White (191) and Black (203) patients.[7] Recurrent VTE rates are highest in the 180 days following the initial event and decline slowly over the next 4 to 10 years. In the absence of secondary prevention, the 10-year cumulative recurrent VTE risk is approximately 25.0%.[7]

ETIOLOGY

(1) A number of identifiable factors increase VTE risk (Table 38-1). Many risk factors fall into categories constituting what is known as Virchow's triad: blood stasis, vascular injury, and hypercoagulability.

Blood Stasis

Blood stasis favors clotting in part through concentrating the elements responsible for blood clot formation.[11] Contraction of the calf and thigh muscles coupled with one-way valves in leg veins facilitate blood flow back to the heart and lungs. Thus, damage to venous valves and prolonged immobility result in venous stasis, which partly explains why numerous medical conditions and surgical procedures are associated with increased VTE risk (Table 38-1).[12]

Vascular Injury

An intact vascular endothelium separates flowing blood from subendothelial vessel wall components responsible for preventing blood loss through clot formation (see detailed description in section "Pathophysiology"). Vascular injury (eg, surgery, trauma) disrupts this protective barrier initiating blood clot formation.[13]

Hypercoagulability

Several inherited and acquired disorders as well as drugs have been linked to blood hypercoagulability (Table 38-1). Estrogen-containing

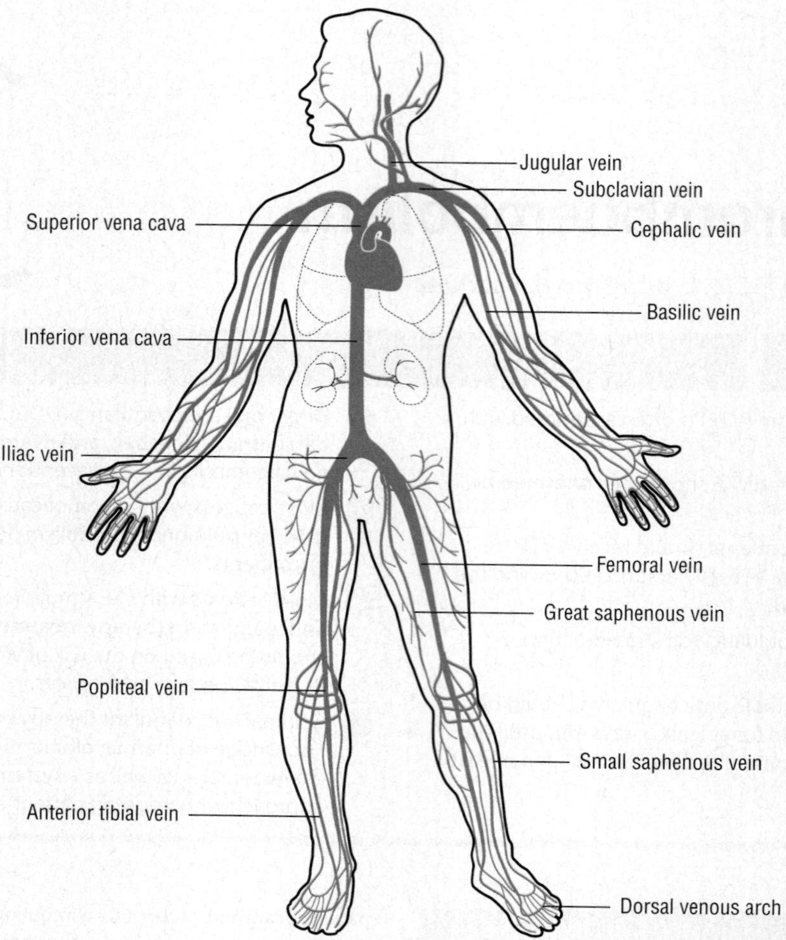

FIGURE 38-1 Venous circulation.

TABLE 38-1 Risk Factors for VTE

Risk Factor	Comments/Examples
Age	Incidence of VTE in adults age 75 and older is seven to ten times higher than adults younger than 55 years, with risk increasing even more over age 85
Prior VTE History	Potent risk factor for recurrence; risk is highest during the first 180 days after VTE
Blood stasis	Acute medical illness requiring hospitalization Surgery (especially general anesthesia >30 minutes) Paralysis (eg, status post-stroke, spinal cord injury) Immobility (eg, plaster casts, status post-stroke, or spinal cord injury) Polycythemia vera Obesity
Vascular injury	Major orthopedic surgery (eg, knee or hip replacement) Trauma (especially fractures of the pelvis, hip, or leg) Indwelling venous catheters
Hypercoagulability	Malignancy Factor V Leiden (homozygous >>heterozygous) Prothrombin (G20210A) gene mutation Protein C deficiency Protein S deficiency Antithrombin deficiency Factor VIII excess (>90th percentile) Factor XI excess (>90th percentile) Antiphospholipid antibodies Lupus anticoagulant Anticardiolipin antibodies (IgG and/or IgM >99th percentile) Anti–β_2-glycoprotein I antibodies (IgG and/or IgM >99th percentile) Inflammatory bowel disease Nephrotic syndrome Paroxysmal nocturnal hemoglobinuria Pregnancy or up to 6 weeks postpartum Drug therapy (eg, estrogen-containing contraceptives, estrogen replacement therapy, tamoxifen, raloxifene, cancer therapy, heparin-induced thrombocytopenia)

Data from References 2, 3, and 8-10.

contraception, estrogen replacement therapy, and selective estrogen receptor modulators are all linked to VTE risk.[8] Women with inherited hypercoagulability disorders are at particularly high risk of developing VTE during pregnancy and while taking estrogen.[8]

In many cases, VTE results from combinations of inherited and acquired thrombotic risk factors. Thus, an individual with inherited hypercoagulability may experience VTE only after being placed in high-risk situations such as surgery, immobilization, the use of estrogen-containing oral contraceptives, or pregnancy. Approximately a third of VTEs are provoked by identifiable risk factors.[7]

PATHOPHYSIOLOGY

Hemostasis is the process responsible for maintaining circulatory system integrity following blood vessel damage (Fig. 38-2).[13] Hemostatic clots are formed rapidly and remain localized to the vessel wall without significantly impairing blood flow. In contrast, pathologic clots like those causing VTE form slowly, impair blood flow, and often cause complete vessel occlusion.[13]

Collagen and tissue factor (TF) form a subendothelial hemostatic barrier around blood vessels and organs. Under normal circumstances, endothelial cells lining the vessel wall physically separate collagen and TF from circulating platelets and clotting factors (namely, activated factor VII [VIIa]). Vessel injury results in platelet activation and TF-mediated clotting factor cascade initiation that culminates in thrombin formation. Ultimately, a fibrin clot forms and seals the breach (Fig. 38-2).[13] In contrast to physiologic hemostasis, pathologic VTE often occurs without gross vessel wall damage and may be triggered by TF brought to the growing thrombus by circulating microparticles. Venous clots are mainly composed of fibrin, platelets, and trapped red blood cells and often occur in areas of disturbed blood flow, like deep leg vein valve cusps.[13]

Platelet and coagulation cascade activation occur nearly simultaneously. Platelets become actively involved in thrombus formation after binding to adhesion proteins like von Willebrand factor and collagen when blood is exposed to damaged vessel endothelium.[13] A platelet thrombus grows as activated platelets recruit and activate additional platelets. Activated platelets change shape and release components critical for sustaining further thrombus formation into the environment surrounding the developing clot.[13] Activated platelets accumulating in the thrombus also express P-selectin, an adhesion molecule that facilitates the capture of blood-borne TF bearing microparticles resulting in fibrin clot formation via the coagulation cascade (Fig. 38-3).[13] Activated platelets provide phospholipid-rich surfaces necessary for coagulation cascade reactions.[13]

The conceptual coagulation cascade model has evolved from the classic depiction of extrinsic, intrinsic, and common pathways (Fig. 38-4) to one in which highly regulated reactions take place on cell surfaces in three overlapping phases: initiation, amplification,

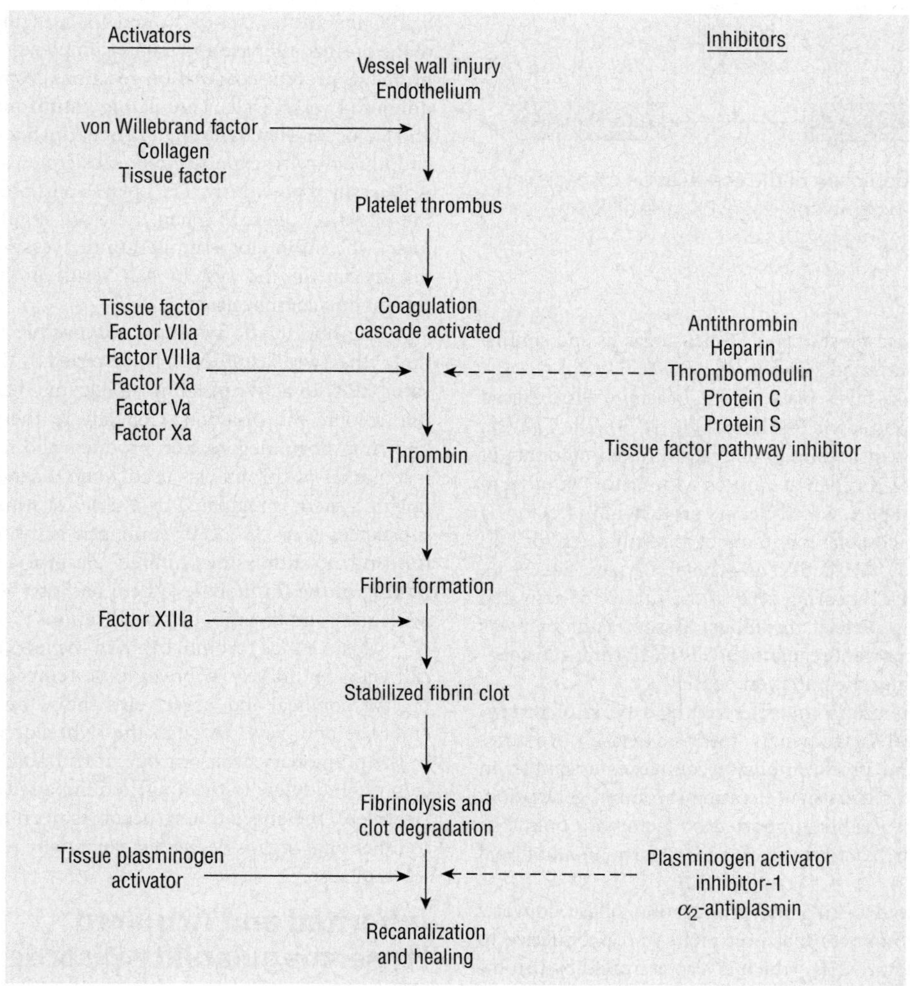

FIGURE 38-2 Overview of hemostasis.

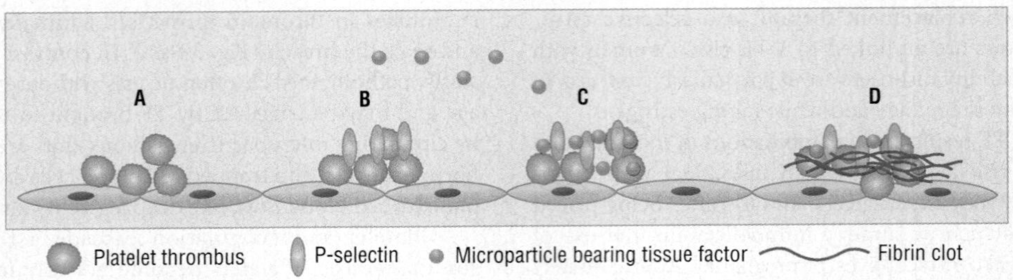

FIGURE 38-3 Model of pathologic thrombus formation: (A) activated platelets adhere to vascular endothelium; (B) activated platelets express P-selectin; (C) pathologic microparticles express active tissue factor and are present at a high concentration in the circulation—these microparticles accumulate, perhaps by binding to activated platelets expressing P-selectin; (D) tissue factor can lead to thrombin and fibrin generation. *(Adapted from De Caterina R, et al. General mechanisms of coagulation and targets of anticoagulants (Section I). Position Paper of the ESC Working Group on Thrombosis—Task Force on Anticoagulants in Heart Disease. Thromb Haemost. 2013;109:569–579.)*

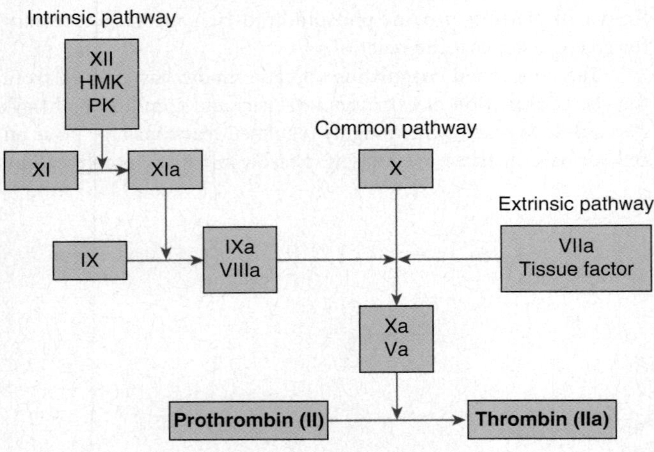

FIGURE 38-4 Classic depiction of the coagulation cascade. (HMK, high-molecular-weight kininogen; PK, prekallikrein.)

and propagation. The cascade starts on TF-bearing cells and continues on the surfaces of activated platelets (Fig. 38-5).[13]

The initiation phase takes place on TF-bearing cells exposed after vessel injury or captured via P-selectin (Fig. 38-3). The TF/VIIa complex (known as extrinsic tenase) activates limited amounts of factors IX and X. Factor Xa then associates with factor Va to form the prothrombinase complex, which cleaves prothrombin (factor II) to generate a small (picomolar) amount of thrombin (factor IIa) which activates factors V, VIII, and XI on platelet surfaces (Fig. 38-5). Factor IXa moves from TF-bearing cells to the surface of activated platelets in the growing platelet thrombus. Tissue factor pathway inhibitor (TFPI), an important regulator of TF/FVIIa-induced coagulation, rapidly terminates the initiation phase.[13]

The propagation phase is characterized by a burst of thrombin generation as VIIIa/IXa (known as "intrinsic tenase") promotes factor Xa formation and prothrombinase complexes assemble on the surface of activated platelets accelerating thrombin generation. Thrombin generation is further supported by factor XIa bound to the platelet surface, which activates factor IX to form an additional intrinsic tenase.[13]

Thrombin generated during the propagation phase converts fibrinogen to fibrin monomers that precipitate and polymerize to form fibrin strands. Factor XIIIa, which is also activated by thrombin, covalently bonds these strands together (Fig. 38-5) to form an extensive meshwork that surrounds and encases the aggregating platelet thrombus and red blood cells to form a stabilized fibrin clot.[13] Clot formation eventually terminates when the expanding meshwork of platelets and fibrin "paves over" the initiation site preventing activated factors from diffusing through the overlying clot layer.

A number of tempering mechanisms control coagulation (Fig. 38-2). Without effective self-regulation, thrombus formation results in vascular occlusion. Intact endothelium adjacent to the growing thrombus actively produces several antithrombotic substances.[11] Thrombomodulin modulates thrombin activity by converting protein C to its active form (aPC). With its cofactor protein S, aPC inactivates factors Va and VIIIa regulating the functionality of the prothrombinase and tenase complexes, respectively.[11] aPC and protein S prevent coagulation reactions from spreading to healthy, uninjured vessel walls. Circulating antithrombin inhibits thrombin and factor Xa. Heparan sulfate, a heparin-like compound secreted by endothelial cells, exponentially accelerates antithrombin activity.[11] As described previously, TFPI plays an important role by regulating the initiation phase.[13] When these self-regulatory mechanisms are intact, the fibrin clot is limited to the vessel injury zone. However, disruptions in the system can result in hypercoagulability and thrombotic complications.[14]

The fibrinolytic system is responsible for blood clot dissolution.[15] Inactive plasminogen is converted by tissue plasminogen activator (tPA) to active plasmin, an enzyme that degrades fibrin mesh into soluble end products. Collectively, these soluble products are known as fibrin degradation products and include D-dimer, which is a marker of thrombosis used when diagnosing VTE.[15] The fibrinolytic system is regulated by a series of stimulatory and inhibitory substances (Fig. 38-2). Plasminogen activator inhibitor-1 inhibits tPA and α_2-antiplasmin inhibits plasmin activity. Impaired functioning of the fibrinolytic system has also been linked to hypercoagulability and thrombotic complications.[15]

Most venous thrombi begin in the leg(s). Thrombus isolated in calf veins is unlikely to break loose (embolize). Thrombus involving the popliteal and larger veins above the knee is more likely to embolize and travel through the right side of the heart and lodge in the pulmonary artery or one of its branches, causing PE, occlusion of blood flow to the lung, and impaired gas exchange. Without treatment, the affected lung becomes necrotic and oxygen delivery to other vital organs decreases, potentially resulting in fatal circulatory collapse.[1]

Inherited and Acquired Hypercoagulability Disorders

Disturbances in hemostatic regulation may result in inherited or acquired hypercoagulability.[14] aPC resistance increases the risk of

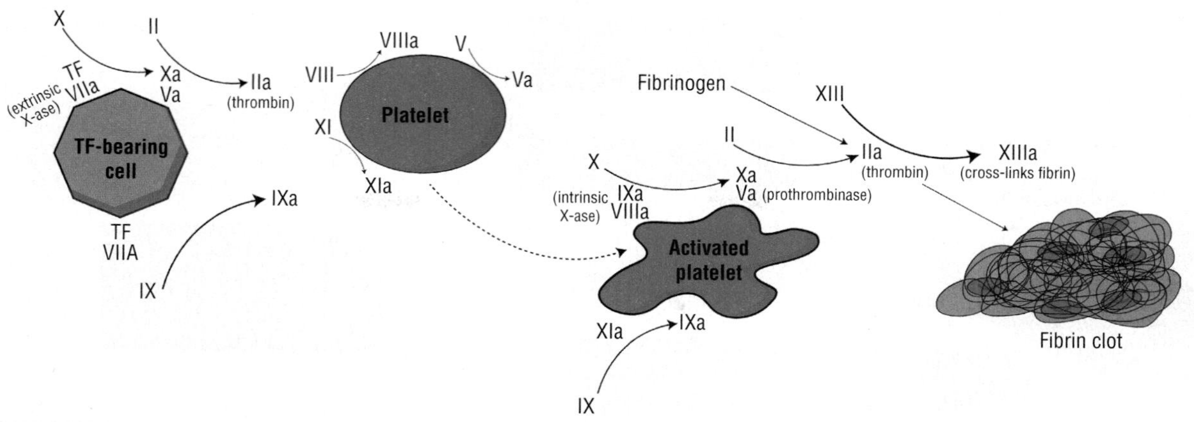

FIGURE 38-5 Cellular coagulation cascade model. *(Adapted from De Caterina R, et al. General mechanisms of coagulation and targets of anticoagulants (Section I). Position Paper of the ESC Working Group on Thrombosis—Task Force on Anticoagulants in Heart Disease. Thromb Haemost. 2013;109:569-579.)*

VTE approximately threefold and is the most common inherited hypercoagulability disorder with a prevalence rate of 2.0% to 7.0% in White individuals.[14] aPC resistance most often results from a gene mutation that renders factor V resistant to degradation by aPC. This mutation is known as factor V Leiden.[14]

The prothrombin G20210A mutation also imparts about a threefold increased VTE risk and is the second most frequent inherited hypercoagulability disorder, occurring in about 2.0% to 4.0% of White individuals.[14] This mutation increases circulating prothrombin, enhancing thrombin generation potential.[10] Some patients inherit both factor V Leiden and prothrombin G20210A mutations, significantly increasing their lifetime VTE risk.[14]

Experts believe the lifetime risk associated with inherited protein C, protein S, and antithrombin deficiencies (present in <1% of the population) is high, perhaps sevenfold higher than patients without such disorders. Many patients with protein C, protein S, or antithrombin deficiency suffer VTE prior to age 60.[10]

Acquired disorders of hypercoagulability may result from cancer, the presence of antiphospholipid antibodies, or estrogen use. A strong link between cancer and thrombosis has long been recognized.[16] Tumor cells secrete procoagulant substances that activate the coagulation cascade, and patients with cancer often have suppressed protein C, protein S, and antithrombin levels. Cancer cells use thrombotic mechanisms to recruit a blood supply, metastasize, and create barriers against host defense mechanisms.[16]

Antiphospholipid antibodies are a heterogeneous group of antibodies targeting proteins that bind phospholipids.[10] These include antibodies that prolong phospholipid-based clotting assays, known as lupus anticoagulants, as well as anticardiolipin and β_2-glycoprotein (β_2-gp) I antibodies. Antiphospholipid antibodies are more common among patients with autoimmune disorders (eg, systemic lupus erythematosus and inflammatory bowel disease) compared to healthy individuals. The precise mechanism by which antiphospholipid antibodies provoke thrombosis remains uncertain. Contributing factors include complement activation, protein C and fibrinolysis inhibition, platelet activation, and increased TF expression.[10]

CLINICAL PRESENTATION (INCLUDING DIAGNOSTIC CONSIDERATIONS)

2 The symptoms of DVT or PE are nonspecific and objective tests are required to confirm or exclude the diagnosis. Patients with DVT frequently present with unilateral leg pain and swelling. Postthrombotic syndrome, a long-term complication of DVT caused by damage to the venous valves, may also result in chronic lower extremity swelling, pain, tenderness, skin discoloration, and, in the most severe cases, ulceration. PE typically presents with chest pain, shortness of breath, tachypnea, and tachycardia, which in some cases may result in cardiopulmonary collapse.[17,18]

Because VTE can be debilitating or fatal, it is important to treat it quickly and aggressively. Conversely, because major bleeding induced by anticoagulant drugs can be equally harmful, it is important to avoid treatment when the diagnosis is not a reasonable certainty. Assessment of the patient's status should focus on the search for risk factors in the patient's medical history (Table 38-1). Even in the presence of mild, seemingly inconsequential symptoms, VTE should be strongly suspected in those with multiple risk factors.[17]

Clinical assessment significantly improves the diagnostic accuracy of noninvasive tests such as compression ultrasound (CUS), computed tomography pulmonary angiography (CTPA), and D-dimer. Simple clinical assessment checklists such as the Wells score for DVT or PE or the revised Geneva score for PE can be used to determine if a patient is "likely" or "unlikely" to have DVT or PE (Figs. 38-6 and 38-7).[19] Patients with a likely probability of VTE have a >60% chance of VTE, compared with a <10% chance for patients with an unlikely probability.[20] In general, patients with an unlikely probability of VTE should first have their D-dimer tested. If the D-dimer result is below the defined cutoff point or reported as "negative," VTE is ruled out. D-dimer results above the cutoff point warrant appropriate diagnostic imaging (CUS for suspected DVT, or CTPA or ventilation/perfusion [V/Q] scanning for suspected PE).

D-dimer is a fibrin clot degradation product and levels are significantly elevated in patients with acute thrombosis. A variety of conditions other than VTE are associated with D-dimer elevations, including recent surgery or trauma, pregnancy, advanced age, and cancer; therefore, a positive D-dimer test is not conclusive evidence of VTE diagnosis. However, a *negative* D-dimer, for most assays defined as <500 ng/mL (mcg/L), can be useful in ruling out the diagnosis of VTE.[20] Appropriate use of D-dimer should include initial risk stratification using a validated clinical assessment tool.[20]

All patients with a likely probability of DVT should receive either proximal (popliteal, femoral, and iliac veins) or whole leg CUS. A normal whole leg ultrasound rules out DVT, whereas a normal proximal ultrasound requires whole leg ultrasound or repeat proximal ultrasound surveillance in 1 week. Patients with CUS indicating proximal DVT should receive anticoagulant treatment. Evidence of

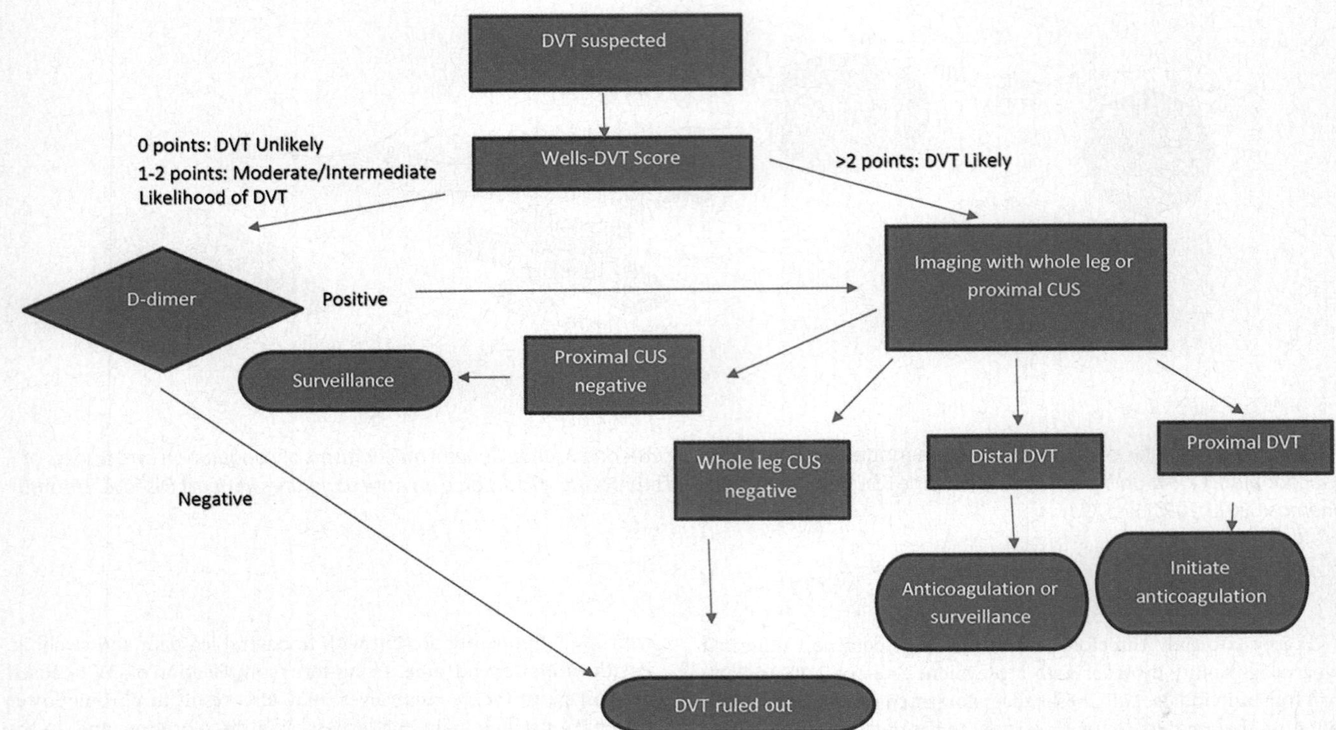

FIGURE 38-6 Deep vein thrombosis diagnostic algorithm. Wells score: 1 pt each for: active cancer, paralysis, or recent plaster cast, immobilization >3 days or surgery in previous 12 weeks, tenderness along the venous system, entire leg swollen, calf swelling >3 cm, pitting edema, collateral superficial veins, history of DVT. Alternate diagnosis as likely as DVT, subtract 2 pts. Surveillance, follow-up CUS in 7-14 days to assess for proximal DVT. *(Data from References 19-21.)*

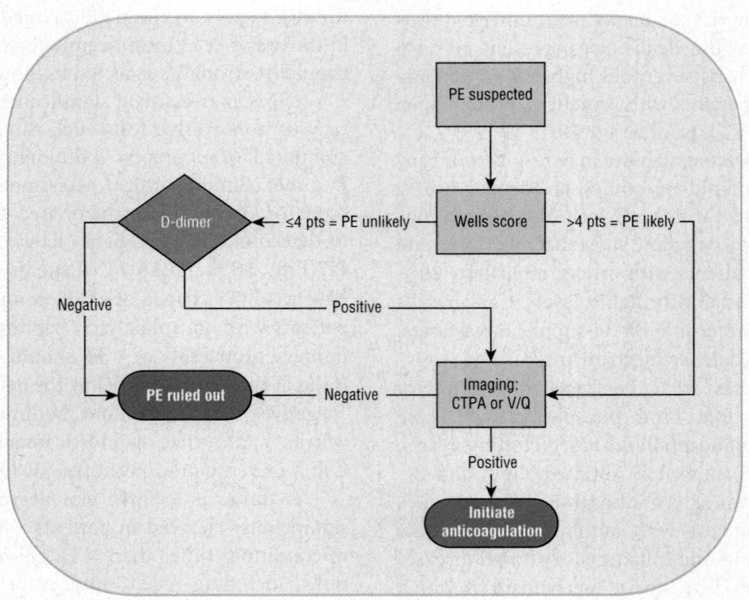

FIGURE 38-7 Pulmonary embolism diagnostic algorithm. (Simplified Wells PE Score, signs/symptoms of DVT, alternative diagnosis less likely than PE [3 pts each], HR >100 bpm, immobile >3 days in past 4 weeks, history of DVT/PE [1.5 pts each], hemoptysis or malignancy [1 pt each]). *(Data from References 17 and 22.)*

distal DVT (anterior and posterior tibial, peroneal, gastrocnemius veins) after whole leg ultrasound may be managed with anticoagulants or repeated ultrasound surveillance in 1 to 2 weeks to assess for propagation into the proximal deep veins of the leg (Fig. 38-6).

Patients with a likely probability of PE should receive imaging with either CTPA or V/Q scan. A negative imaging result rules out PE, whereas a positive imaging result indicates need for anticoagulant treatment (Fig. 38-7).[17,19,20]

CLINICAL PRESENTATION Deep Vein Thrombosis

General

DVT most commonly develops in patients with identifiable risk factors (see Table 38-1). Some may have asymptomatic disease.

Symptoms

The patient may complain of leg swelling, pain, or warmth. Symptoms are nonspecific and objective testing must be performed to establish the diagnosis

Signs

The patient's superficial veins may be dilated and a "palpable cord" may be felt in the affected leg. The patient may experience pain in the back of the knee when the examiner dorsiflexes the foot of the affected leg (Homan's sign).

Laboratory Tests

Serum concentration of D-dimer, a by-product of fibrin degradation, is nearly always elevated. A negative D-dimer (values <500 ng/mL [mcg/L]) combined with clinical decision rules are useful in ruling out the diagnosis of DVT.

Diagnostic Tests

Compression ultrasound is the most commonly used test to diagnose DVT. It is a noninvasive test that can visualize clot formation in veins of the legs. Coupled with a careful clinical assessment, it can rule in or out the diagnosis in the majority of cases. Venography is the gold standard for the diagnosis of DVT. However, it is an invasive test that involves the injection of radiopaque contrast dye into a foot vein. It is expensive and can cause anaphylaxis and nephrotoxicity.

CLINICAL PRESENTATION Pulmonary Embolism

General

PE most commonly develops in patients with risk factors for VTE (see Table 38-1). Although many patients develop a symptomatic DVT prior to developing a PE, some do not. Patients may die suddenly from cardiogenic shock and circulatory collapse before effective treatment can be initiated.

Symptoms

The patient may complain of cough, chest pain, chest tightness, shortness of breath, or palpitation. The patient may spit or cough up blood (hemoptysis). When PE is massive, the patient may complain of dizziness or light-headedness. Symptoms may be confused with myocardial infarction, requiring objective testing to establish the diagnosis.

Signs

The patient may have tachypnea, tachycardia, and appear diaphoretic. The patient's neck veins may be distended. In massive PE, the patient may appear cyanotic and become hypotensive. In such cases, oxygen saturation by pulse oximetry or arterial blood gas will likely indicate that the patient is hypoxic. In the worse cases, the patient may go into cardiogenic shock and die within minutes.

Laboratory Tests

Serum concentration of D-dimer, a by-product of fibrin degradation, is nearly always elevated. D-dimer values <500 ng/mL (mcg/L) combined with clinical decision rules are useful in ruling out the diagnosis of PE.

Diagnostic Tests

Computerized tomography pulmonary angiography (CTPA) is the most commonly used test to diagnose PE, but some centers still use the V/Q scan. A V/Q scan measures the distribution of blood and airflow in the lungs. When there is a large mismatch between blood and airflow in one area of the lung, there is a PE.

Pulmonary angiography is the gold standard for the diagnosis of PE. However, it is an invasive test that involves the injection of radiopaque contrast dye into the pulmonary artery. The test is expensive and associated with a significant risk of mortality.

PREVENTION OF VENOUS THROMBOEMBOLISM

Unfortunately, public awareness of the life-threatening nature of DVT and PE is lacking with many patients having little or no awareness of VTE symptoms or risk factors.[23] VTE awareness is substantially lower than for other disease states like stroke, heart attack, and breast cancer and there is a need to increase knowledge of the risks, signs, and symptoms of VTE.

Desired Outcomes

Prevention strategies in at-risk populations positively impact patient outcomes because VTE is potentially fatal and costly to treat.[26] Treatment of VTE is aimed at preventing thrombus extension and embolization, reducing recurrence risk, and preventing long-term complications such as the postthrombotic syndrome and CTPH. Carefully managed anticoagulant drug use is important to reduce the risk of bleeding associated with these agents.

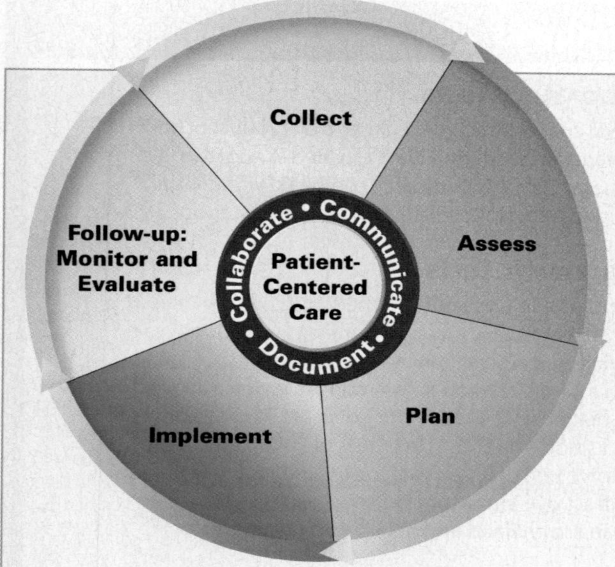

Patient Care Process for the Prevention of VTE

The image shows the five fundamental steps included in The Pharmacist's Care Process endorsed by the Joint Commission for Pharmacy Practitioners (2014). The tagline of this process reads collaborate, communicate, and document. The five fundamental steps listed here are collect, assess, plan, implement, and follow-up: monitor and evaluate. All these steps are listed in a circular block diagram.

Collect

- Patient characteristics (eg, age, sex, active cancer, pregnant)
- Patient history (past medical [eg, bleeding history], family, social—dietary habits including intake of vitamin K-containing foods [see Table 38-12], tobacco/ethanol use)
- Current medications including over-the-counter aspirin and NSAID use; prior anticoagulant medication use
- Objective data
  - Blood pressure (BP), heart rate (HR), respiratory rate (RR), O_2-saturation, height, weight
  - Labs (eg, hemoglobin [Hgb], serum creatinine [Scr], platelets, activated partial thromboplastin time [aPTT], prothrombin time [PT])

Assess

- Presence of VTE risk factors (see Table 38-1); consider using risk stratification tools appropriate for medical or surgical patients (see Table 38-2)
- Presence of active bleeding and/or bleeding risk factors (see Table 38-10)
- Presence of medications that increase VTE risk (eg, estrogen)
- Presence of contraindications to anticoagulation therapy
- Ability/willingness to self-inject LMWH or fondaparinux if extended parenteral therapy is being considered
- Ability/willingness to pay for various anticoagulation therapy options if extended therapy is being considered
- Ability/willingness to obtain appropriate laboratory monitoring if extended therapy is being considered (eg, INR [international normalized ratio] for warfarin)

Plan*

- Drug therapy regimen including specific anticoagulant(s) or reversal agent(s), dose, route, frequency, and duration (see Fig. 38-9)
- Monitoring parameters including effectiveness (eg, INR results, signs and symptoms of VTE), safety (bleeding, platelet count [heparin]), and timing of assessments
- Patient education (eg, purpose of treatment, dietary and lifestyle modification, drug therapy; see Table 38-5)
- Self-monitoring for VTE symptoms, occurrence of bleeding, when to seek emergency medical attention

Implement

- Ensure appropriate VTE prevention is initiated based on patient-specific VTE/bleeding risk
- Provide patient education regarding all elements of the treatment plan
- Use motivational interviewing and coaching strategies to maximize adherence if extended therapy being considered
- Schedule follow-up (eg, INR tests [warfarin], bleeding assessment, duration of therapy assessment)

Follow-up: Monitor and Evaluate

- Occurrence of VTE symptoms (eg, shortness of breath, chest pain, leg or arm swelling, redness, pain)
- Presence of adverse drug reactions (eg, bleeding, gastrointestinal upset [dabigatran only], HIT [heparin-induced thrombocytopenia])
- INR results (adjust warfarin dose as needed to keep within target range)
- Patient adherence to the treatment plan if extended therapy
- Inquire whether the patient is ambulatory and/or weight-bearing (following orthopedic surgery)

**Collaborate with patient, caregivers, and other healthcare professionals.*

General Approach to the Prevention of Venous Thromboembolism

Effective prophylaxis can reduce the risk of fatal PE in high-risk medical and surgical populations. Early ambulation is often sufficient for those at low risk of VTE.[27] Educational programs and clinical decision support systems have been shown to improve the appropriate use of VTE prevention methods.[28]

3 VTE continues to be a major risk for patient morbidity and mortality in hospitalized patients. Approximately half of all VTE occurs secondary to hospital admission or surgery, often occurring after hospital discharge. Effective VTE prophylaxis can prevent as much as 70% of VTE events related to hospitalization or surgery.[29-31] Safe and effective prophylaxis strategies must balance the risks for thromboembolism and bleeding. There is evidence that VTE prophylaxis is both underused in patients at high risk for VTE and

overused in low-risk populations.[32] It is essential that patients are assessed for risks of VTE and bleeding (Table 38-2) prior to deciding whether VTE prophylaxis is appropriate. Distinct populations to consider for VTE prophylaxis include the medically ill and those undergoing surgery (Table 38-3). Each group has unique risk factors for VTE and bleeding to consider in determining an approach to VTE prophylaxis (Fig. 38-8).

Nonpharmacologic Therapy

Graduated compression stockings and intermittent pneumatic compression (IPC) devices prevent VTE by increasing the velocity of lower extremity venous blood flow through graded pressure application. IPC devices utilize a series of cuffs wrapped around the patient's legs that inflate in continuous 1- to 2-minute cycles from the ankles to the knees or thighs. IPC devices should be worn at least 18 hr/day for optimal effectiveness.

Graduated compression stockings do not reliably reduce VTE in medically ill patients.[33] However, they reduce the incidence of VTE (including asymptomatic and distal DVT) by approximately 65% when used after orthopedic surgery, cardiac surgery, gynecologic surgery, or neurosurgery.[34] IPC reduces the risk of VTE by more than 60% following general surgery, neurosurgery, and orthopedic surgery.[34] Both modalities can be used in combination with anticoagulation in appropriate settings (see below) to maximize VTE prevention.[35]

Mechanical methods do not increase bleeding risk, which makes them attractive for VTE prophylaxis following surgery, especially in patients with contraindications to anticoagulation. However, they are not risk-free, as discomfort, skin breakdown, and ulceration can occur.[33]

Inferior vena cava (IVC) filters can provide short-term protection against PE in very high-risk patients by blocking embolization of thrombus formed below the filter.[36] Percutaneous insertion of an IVC filter is a minimally invasive procedure performed using fluoroscopic imaging to verify placement. Frequently "retrievable" IVC filters are never retrieved, increasing the risk for long-term complications such as DVT, filter migration, IVC occlusion, and insertion site thrombosis.[34] Therefore, IVC filters should be reserved for patients

TABLE 38-2 VTE and Bleeding Risk Assessment for Medically Ill Patients

VTE Risk Assessment		Bleeding Risk Assessment	
Characteristic	Points	Characteristic	Points
Reduced mobility	3	Renal failure (GFR 30-59 mL/min/1.73 m^2)	1
Active cancer	3	Male	1
Previous VTE (excluding superficial thrombophlebitis)	3	Age 40-80	1.5
Known thrombophelia	3	Current cancer	2
Recent trauma or surgery (within 1 month)	2	Rheumatic disease	2
Age >70 years	1	Central venous catheter	2
Heart or respiratory failure	1	Intensive or critical care unit stay	2.5
Acute myocardial infarction or ischemic stroke	1	Renal failure (GFR <30 mL/min/1.73 m^2)	2.5
Ongoing hormonal treatment	1	Hepatic failure (INR >1.5)	2.5
Obesity (BMI >30 kg/m^2)	1	Age ≥85	3.5
Active infection or rheumatologic disorder	1	Platelet count <50,000/mm^3 (50 × 10^9/L)	4
		Bleeding in previous 3 months	4
		Active gastroduodenal ulcer	4.5
4 points or greater is high risk for VTE		7 points or greater is high risk for major bleeding	

BMI, body mass index; GFR, glomerular filtration rate; INR, international normalized ratio. GFR expressed in units of mL/min/1.73 m^2 is converted to SI units of mL/s/m^2 by multiplying by 0.0096. *Data from References 39 and 40.*

TABLE 38-3 Summary of Guideline Recommended Therapies Indicated for VTE Prophylaxis

		Orthopedic Surgery		
Indication	**Medically ill**	**TKA/THA**	**Hip fracture repair**	**Other major surgeries[a]**
Preferred agents	LMWH or fondaparinux	Aspirin or anticoagulants (DOACs favored; LMWH also supported)	LMWH or UFH	LMWH or UFH
Combined pharmacological and mechanical prophylaxis[b]	No	Yes	Yes	Yes
Extended duration pharmacological prophylaxis	No	Yes	Yes	Yes
Alternative pharmacologic agents	UFH or rivaroxaban	Fondaparinux, low-dose UFH, or warfarin	Fondaparinux or warfarin	n/a
Alternative mechanical prophylaxis in high bleeding risk	IPC	IPC and/or compression stockings	IPC and/or compression stockings	IPC and/or compression stockings

THA, total hip arthroplasty; TKA, total knee arthroplasty; LMWH, low-molecular weight heparin; DOACs, direct-acting oral anticoagulants; UFH, unfractionated heparin; IPC, intermittent pneumatic compression.

[a]Excludes prostate resection, prostatectomy, and neurosurgery.

[b]Combination of aspirin or anticoagulation plus IPC or graduated compression stockings.

Data from References 2, 3, 34, and 37.

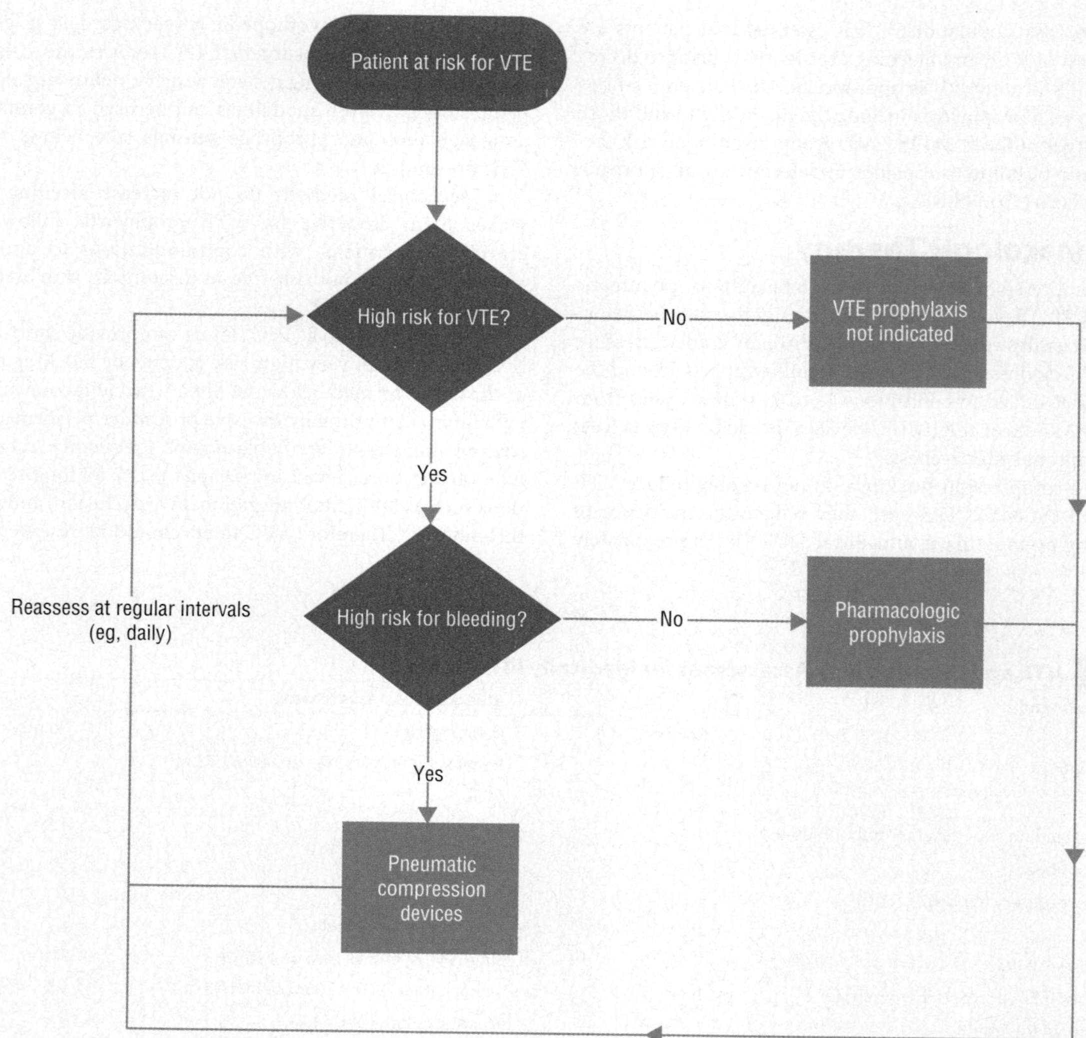

FIGURE 38-8 General approach to VTE prophylaxis. *(Data from References 2 and 3.)*

at the highest VTE risk in whom other prophylactic strategies cannot be used. The data supporting the use of IVC filters for primary VTE prophylaxis in patients at high risk of bleeding is very weak.[2] Routine use of IVC filters is not recommended and their potential role in high bleeding risk patients remains to be determined.[2] IVC filters should be removed when VTE risk has passed or when anticoagulation is no longer contraindicated.[36]

Pharmacologic Therapy

Pharmacologic options for preventing VTE have been extensively evaluated in randomized clinical trials and significantly reduce the risk of VTE following hip and knee replacement, hip fracture repair, general surgery, myocardial infarction, ischemic stroke, and in selected hospitalized medical patients.[33,34,37] The optimal agent and dose for VTE prevention must be based on an assessment of VTE and bleeding risk, as well as cost and availability. In general, pharmacologic therapy is preferred over mechanical interventions in patients without active bleeding or high risk for bleeding. Pharmacologic prophylaxis options include UFH, LMWH, DOACs, aspirin, and warfarin. Each can be used safely and effectively given the appropriate clinical scenario.

Medical Patients

Low-dose UFH, LMWH, and fondaparinux all reduce symptomatic VTE and fatal PE among high-risk medical patients.[2] Rivaroxaban is as effective as enoxaparin for VTE prophylaxis during hospitalization and is approved for VTE prophylaxis in medically ill patients including after hospital discharge for a total duration of 39 days.[38] However, routine use of extended duration prophylaxis beyond hospital discharge is not supported by guidelines.[3]

Hospitalized and acutely ill medical patients at high VTE risk and low bleeding risk should receive pharmacologic prophylaxis with low-dose UFH, LMWH, fondaparinux, or rivaroxaban during hospitalization or until fully ambulatory. The use of extended prophylaxis beyond hospital discharge reduces the risk of VTE but with a comparable increase in bleeding and is not recommended in the medically ill population.[3] LMWH or fondaparinux are preferred to low-dose UFH or DOACs for VTE prophylaxis in medically ill inpatients. Routine pharmacologic prophylaxis is not warranted in low-VTE-risk medical patients.

Several risk assessment models have been developed to identify hospitalized and critically ill patients at high VTE risk likely to benefit from thromboprophylaxis. The Padua Prediction Score is a prospectively validated VTE risk assessment tool for hospitalized medical patients.[39] Among high-risk patients (score ≥4 points) not receiving prophylaxis, VTE occurred in 11.0% within 90 days compared with just 0.3% of low-risk patients. Bleeding risk can be estimated using various risk stratification tools such as the IMPROVE bleeding score.[40] An IMPROVE score of ≥7 points was associated with a major bleeding risk of 4.1%. Mechanical prophylaxis is preferred over anticoagulation therapy in medical patients at high bleeding risk.[2] Patients with severe hepatic insufficiency are not adequately protected from VTE even if baseline INR is elevated. This population is particularly challenging as they are at risk for VTE without prophylaxis and bleeding with pharmacologic prophylaxis.[41,42]

Table 38-2 summarizes a scoring system for VTE risk and bleeding assessment in medically ill patients. Figure 38-8 outlines a general approach to deciding on VTE prophylaxis once VTE and bleeding risk scores have been estimated.

Surgical Patients

General recommendations for reducing perioperative VTE risk include using regional rather than general anesthesia, whenever possible, and having patients ambulate as soon as it is safe to do so.[17]

Risk stratification tools (eg, Caprini score) also exist for estimating VTE risk in surgical populations. However, current guidelines provide recommendations according to the type of surgery rather than based on specific risk assessment models.[2] Most patients having general, gynecologic, cardiac, and vascular surgery should receive pharmacologic prophylaxis with LMWH or low-dose UFH to prevent VTE. Patients unable to receive pharmacologic prophylaxis should use IPCs or compression stockings.[2] Combination of pharmacologic and mechanical VTE prevention methods have the potential to reduce the risk for VTE as well as mortality compared to pharmacologic prophylaxis alone. The addition of mechanical prophylaxis is generally well tolerated and should be particularly advantageous to patients with additional risk factors for VTE.[2]

There are a few surgery types excluded from the general recommendations above. Uncomplicated laparoscopic cholecystectomy does not routinely require VTE prophylaxis unless the patient has additional VTE risk factors, such as a history of VTE, hypercoagulability, or active cancer. Patients undergoing surgery that involves high bleeding risk (eg, urologic procedures) or where small amounts of bleeding can result is substantial morbidity (eg, intracranial or spinal surgery) are typically managed with IPCs rather than pharmacologic prophylaxis.[2]

Total joint arthroplasty has historically been associated with very high postoperative VTE risk.[37] Pharmacologic agents for VTE prevention following joint replacement surgery include aspirin, adjusted-dose warfarin, low-dose UFH, LMWH, fondaparinux, dabigatran, apixaban, and rivaroxaban for a minimum of 10 days postsurgery.[37] Optimal timing of anticoagulation initiation is between 6 and 12 hours postop. Earlier initiation increases bleeding risk up to fivefold.[37] Extended duration prophylaxis is also recommended to prevent delayed VTE up to 35 days postoperatively.

Warfarin remains a commonly prescribed agent for VTE prevention after total joint arthroplasty due to low acquisition cost, oral administration, and delayed onset, potentially reducing the risk of early postoperative bleeding (see Fig. 38-9).[43] The optimal target INR during warfarin prophylaxis is not clear. It is common for INR targets lower than the standard range of 2 to 3 to be employed as the American Academy of Orthopaedic Surgery guidelines do not recommend a specific INR target.[37,44]

DOACs offer convenient oral administration and fixed dosing without the need for routine coagulation testing. The safety and efficacy of DOACs are similar to enoxaparin after total joint replacement, but studies after hip fracture surgery are lacking.[37] The American Society of Hematology recommends DOACs over other anticoagulants for VTE prophylaxis after total joint replacement.[2] If a DOAC is not available or contraindicated, LMWHs are generally preferred over UFH or warfarin (see Table 38-3 for VTE prophylaxis summary). If aspirin is used, a two-tiered approach might be considered where aspirin is the default option for patients who have no additional VTE risk factors and DOACs, warfarin, or LMWH reserved for patients with additional VTE risk factors (eg, obesity, active cancer, history of VTE). Finally, a short course (eg, 5 days) of DOAC therapy followed by aspirin provides an early anticoagulant effect and may optimally balance the use of an anticoagulant to prevent early postoperative thrombosis when the risk is highest, and a low-cost oral option (aspirin) that can be easily administered after hospital discharge.[45]

Duration of Therapy

VTE incidence is relatively high in the month following hospital discharge among patients undergoing lower extremity orthopedic procedures; therefore, extended prophylaxis appears to be beneficial.[2] Most clinical trials support the use of antithrombotic prophylaxis for 15 to 42 days following total knee or hip replacement surgery.[2] Optimal VTE prophylaxis duration following other major surgeries is not well established. Prophylaxis should be given throughout the period of increased VTE risk. Guidelines support extended VTE prophylaxis for up to 42 days after major surgery.[2] However, it may be reasonable to forego extended prophylaxis after less extensive procedures where patients are ambulatory and other risk factors are no longer present.

TREATMENT OF VENOUS THROMBOEMBOLISM

General Approach to the Treatment of Venous Thromboembolism

Anticoagulation therapies remain the mainstay of VTE treatment. DVT and PE are manifestations of the same disease process and are treated similarly (Figs. 38-10 and 38-11). Before prescribing anticoagulation therapy for VTE treatment, establishing an accurate diagnosis is imperative to prevent unnecessary bleeding risk and expense to the patient.[18] Patients with a likely VTE probability (Figs. 38-6 and 38-7) may need rapid-onset anticoagulation therapy while awaiting diagnostic testing results. However, patients with unlikely VTE probability may only need rapid-onset anticoagulation in the setting of a positive D-dimer with anticipated delays in diagnostic testing exceeding 4 hours.[17]

Strict bed rest was traditionally recommended following acute DVT based on the assumption that leg movement would dislodge the clot, resulting in PE. However, ambulation in conjunction with graduated compression stockings results in a faster reduction of pain and swelling with no apparent increase in embolization rate. Patients should be encouraged to ambulate as much as symptoms permit. If ambulation increases pain and swelling, the patient should be instructed to lie down and elevate the affected leg until symptoms subside.

IVC filters have a limited role in the management of acute VTE and should only be used when anticoagulants are contraindicated due to active bleeding.[21] As soon as the bleeding resolves, patients should receive a conventional course of anticoagulant therapy and have the filter removed within 90 to 120 days of implantation.[17,18,36] In life- or limb-threatening circumstances, elimination of the obstructing thrombus may be warranted and the use of thrombolysis or thrombectomy considered.[18,46]

4 7 Once the diagnosis of VTE has been objectively confirmed (see details regarding Clinical Presentation and Diagnosis above), anticoagulant therapy with a rapid-acting anticoagulant should be instituted as soon as possible. Available anticoagulants can be administered in the outpatient setting in most patients with DVT and in carefully selected hemodynamically stable patients with PE. Given the predictable response and reduced need for laboratory monitoring with LMWH and DOACs, stable patients with DVT or PE who have normal vital signs, low bleeding risk, and no other uncontrolled comorbid conditions requiring hospitalization can be discharged early or treated entirely on an outpatient

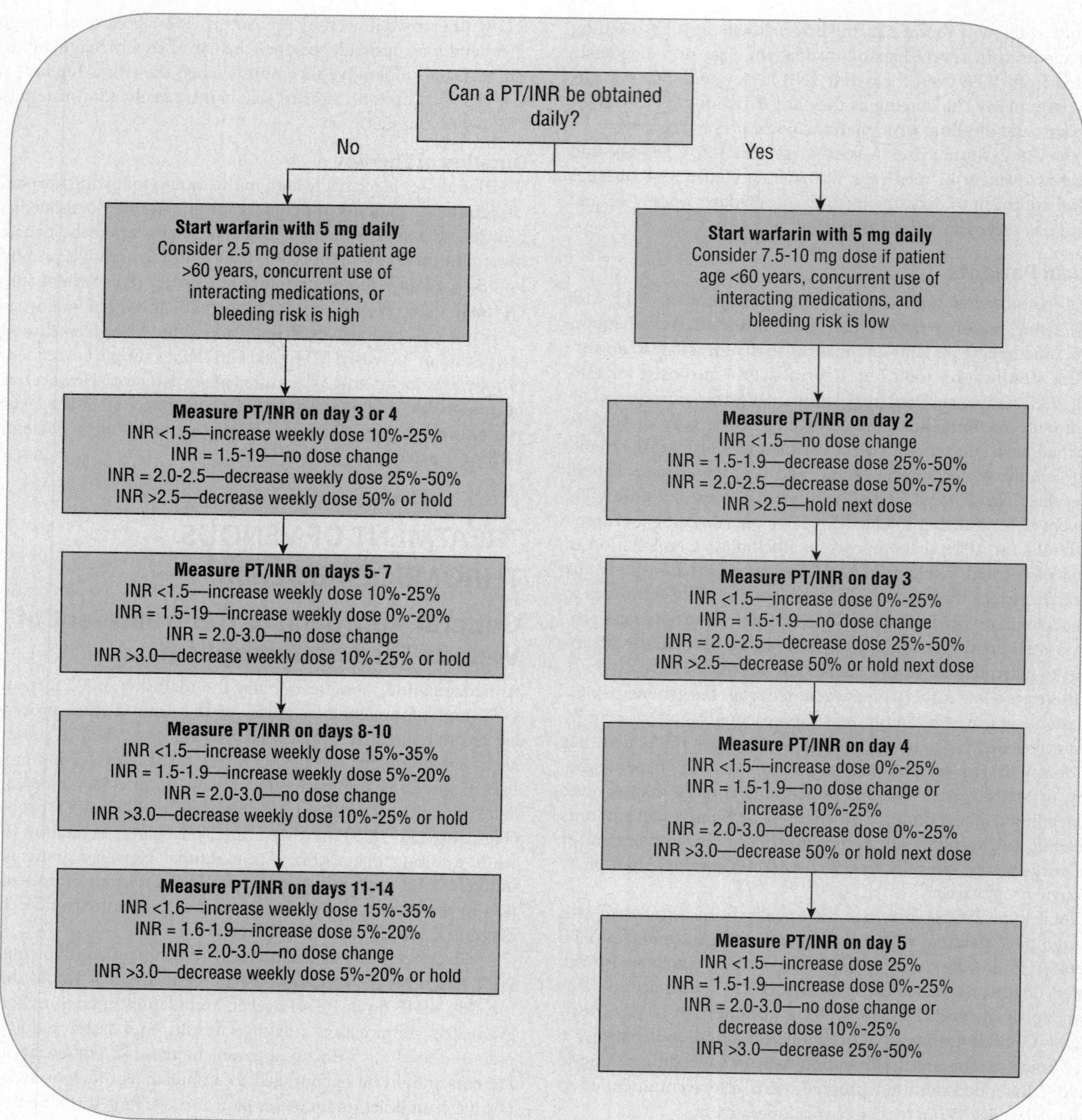

FIGURE 38-9 Initiation of warfarin therapy.

basis (Table 38-4).[47] Not all patients are appropriate candidates for outpatient VTE treatment. At a minimum, patients must be reliable or have adequate caregiver support and be willing and active participants in outpatient VTE management. Important patient education aspects for outpatient VTE treatment are summarized in Table 38-5. Hemodynamically unstable patients with PE should be admitted for anticoagulation therapy initiation. The decision to initiate outpatient therapy should be based on institutional resources and patient-specific variables.[46,48]

8 The appropriate initial duration of anticoagulation therapy to effectively treat an acute first episode of VTE for all patients is 3 months.[47] To prevent new VTE episodes not directly related to the preceding episode, continuing anticoagulation therapy may be required.[1] Individually tailoring anticoagulation therapy duration therapy beyond 3 months requires careful consideration of the circumstances surrounding the initial thromboembolic event, the presence of ongoing thromboembolic risk factors, bleeding risk, and patient preference.[47]

The most important considerations in determining recurrent VTE risk are whether the initial thrombotic event was associated with a major transient or reversible risk factor (eg, surgery, plaster cast leg immobilization, or hospitalization in the month prior to VTE) and the presence of active cancer.[47] The estimated cumulative risk of recurrent VTE after stopping anticoagulant therapy for VTE provoked by surgery is 1% after 1 year and 3% after 5 years. The cumulative risk of recurrent VTE provoked by a nonsurgical reversible risk factor is higher, 5% and 15% after 1 and 5 years, respectively. Three months of anticoagulation therapy is recommended in these situations.[18] Patients with a first unprovoked (idiopathic) VTE have approximately 10% recurrence risk in the first year and

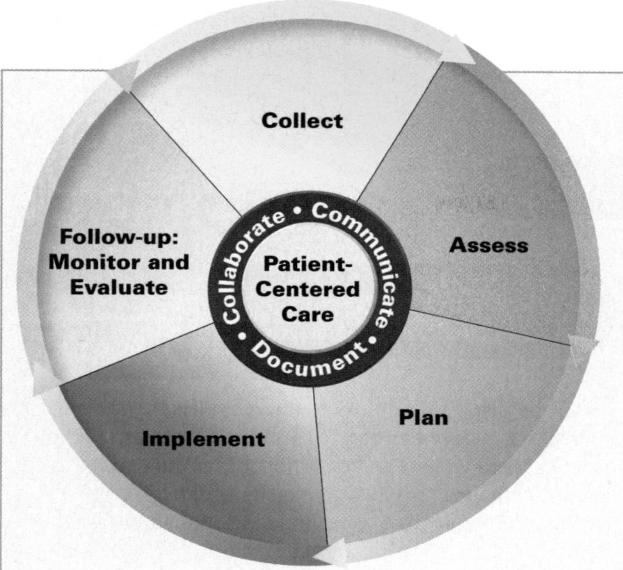

Patient Care Process for the Treatment of VTE

The image shows the five fundamental steps included in The Pharmacist's Care Process endorsed by the Joint Commission for Pharmacy Practitioners (2014). The tagline of this process reads collaborate, communicate, and document. The five fundamental steps listed here are collect, assess, plan, implement, and follow-up: monitor and evaluate. All these steps are listed in a circular block diagram.

Collect

- Patient characteristics (eg, age, sex, pregnant)
- Patient history (past medical, family, social—dietary habits including intake of vitamin K-containing foods (see Table 38-12), tobacco/ethanol use
- Current medications including over-the-counter aspirin/NSAID use; prior anticoagulant medication use
- Objective data
  - BP, HR, RR, O_2-saturation, height, weight
  - Labs (eg, Hgb, Scr, platelets, aPTT, PT)
  - Do NOT order hypercoagulability tests
  - Objective confirmation of VTE (see Figs. 38-6 and 38-7)

Assess

- For PE, hemodynamic instability (eg, SBP <90 mm Hg, HR >110 bpm, O_2-sat <90% [0.90])
- Presence of active bleeding and/or bleeding risk factors (see Table 38-10)
- Presence of VTE provoking factors (eg, recent surgery, plaster casting of lower extremity, indwelling catheter, cancer, pregnancy, estrogen use, prolonged immobility, recent hospitalization)
- Ability/willingness to self-inject LMWH/fondaparinux
- Ability/willingness to pay for various anticoagulation therapy options
- Ability/willingness to obtain appropriate laboratory monitoring (eg, INR for warfarin)
- Emotional status (eg, presence of anxiety, depression)

Plan*

- Drug therapy regimen including specific anticoagulant(s), dose, route, frequency, and duration (see Figs. 38-8 to 38-11, Tables 38-4–38-6)
- Monitoring parameters including effectiveness (eg, INR results, pain control, limb swelling, shortness of breath), safety (bleeding, VTE recurrence), and timing of assessments
- Patient education (eg, purpose of treatment, dietary and lifestyle modification, invasive procedures, drug therapy; see Table 38-5)
- Self-monitoring for resolution of VTE symptoms, the occurrence of bleeding, when to seek emergency medical attention
- Referrals to other providers when appropriate (eg, thrombosis specialist, behavioral health, dietician)

Implement

- Provide patient education regarding all elements of the treatment plan
- Use motivational interviewing and coaching strategies to maximize adherence
- Schedule follow-up (eg, INR tests [warfarin], Scr [DOACs], adherence assessment, bleeding risk assessment, duration of therapy assessment)

Follow-up: Monitor and Evaluate

- Resolution of VTE symptoms (eg, shortness of breath, chest pain, swelling, redness, pain)
- Presence of adverse drug reactions (eg, bleeding, GI upset [dabigatran])
- INR results (adjust warfarin dose as needed to keep between 2 and 3)
- Patient adherence to treatment plan using multiple sources of information
- Duration of therapy after 90 days

Collaborate with patient, caregivers, and other healthcare professionals.

approximately 30% and 50% over 5 and 10 years, respectively. These patients should be considered for extended anticoagulation therapy when feasible.[47] With extended therapy, anticoagulation continues beyond 3 months, stopping only if bleeding risk increases substantially or change in patient preference for anticoagulation changes.[47] For patients with a second idiopathic VTE episode, extended anticoagulation is recommended.[47] Anticoagulation is rarely stopped in patients with VTE and active cancer because of the high recurrence risk.[47] Factors that may lead to the decision to stop anticoagulation therapy after 3 months include nonadherence with therapy, initial clot isolated in calf veins (even if idiopathic), moderate-to-high bleeding risk, or patient preference.[47]

Important risk factors for bleeding include age >75 years, previous noncardioembolic stroke, history of gastrointestinal bleeding, renal or hepatic impairment, anemia, thrombocytopenia, concurrent antiplatelet use (avoid if possible), nonadherence, poor

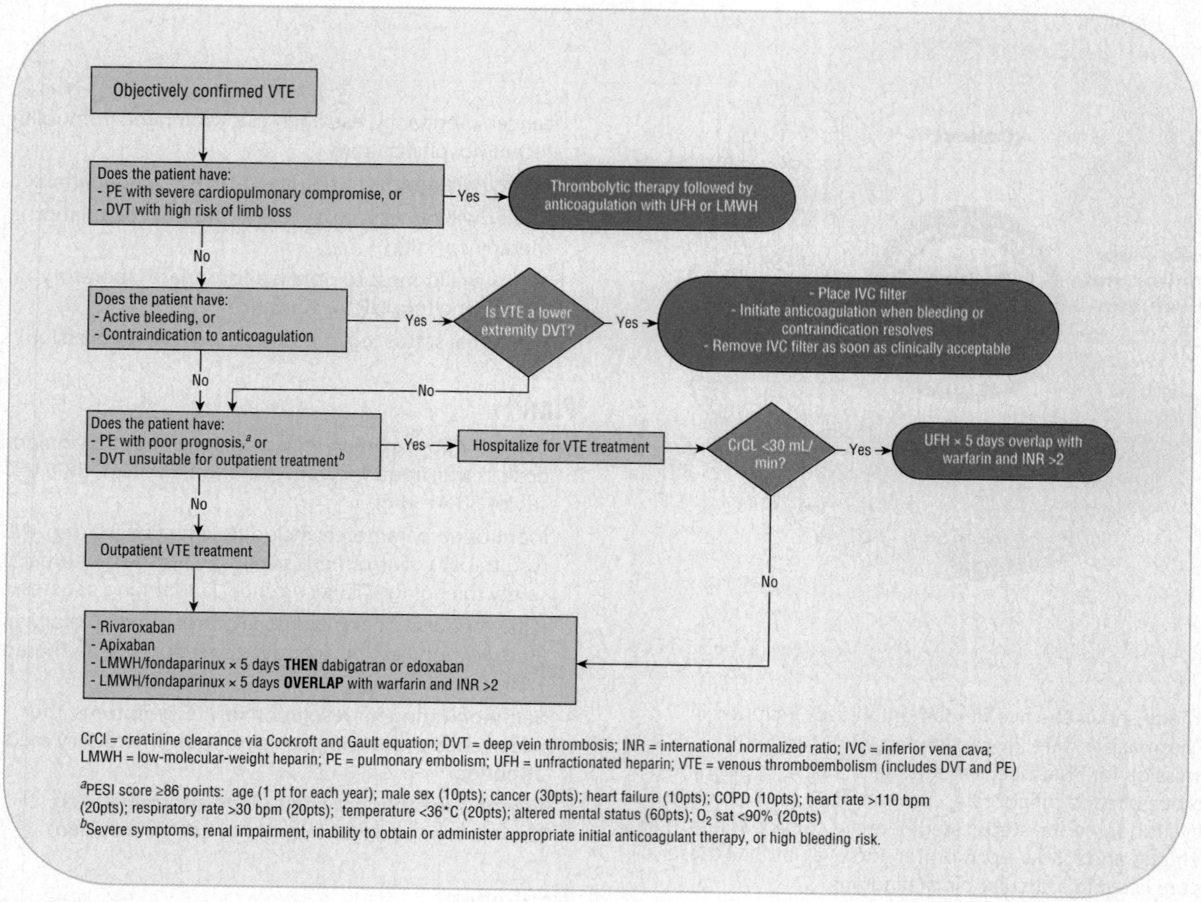

Objectively confirmed VTE
Does the patient have:
- PE with severe cardiopulmonary compromise, or
- DVT with high risk of limb loss
Yes
Thrombolytic therapy followed by anticoagulation with UFH or LMWH
No
Does the patient have:
- Active bleeding, or
- Contraindication to anticoagulation
Yes
Is VTE a lower extremity DVT?
Yes
- Place IVC filter
- Initiate anticoagulation when bleeding or contraindication resolves
- Remove IVC filter as soon as clinically acceptable
No
No
Does the patient have:
- PE with poor prognosis,[a] or
- DVT unsuitable for outpatient treatment[b]
Yes
Hospitalize for VTE treatment
CrCL <30 mL/min?
Yes
UFH × 5 days overlap with warfarin and INR >2
No
No
Outpatient VTE treatment
- Rivaroxaban
- Apixaban
- LMWH/fondaparinux × 5 days THEN dabigatran or edoxaban
- LMWH/fondaparinux × 5 days OVERLAP with warfarin and INR >2
CrCl = creatinine clearance via Cockroft and Gault equation; DVT = deep vein thrombosis; INR = international normalized ratio; IVC = inferior vena cava; LMWH = low-molecular-weight heparin; PE = pulmonary embolism; UFH = unfractionated heparin; VTE = venous thromboembolism (includes DVT and PE)
[a]PESI score ≥86 points: age (1 pt for each year); male sex (10pts); cancer (30pts); heart failure (10pts); COPD (10pts); heart rate >110 bpm (20pts); respiratory rate >30 bpm (20pts); temperature <36°C (20pts); altered mental status (60pts); O2 sat <90% (20pts)
[b]Severe symptoms, renal impairment, inability to obtain or administer appropriate initial anticoagulant therapy, or high bleeding risk.

FIGURE 38-10 Decision algorithm: Acute treatment of VTE. (CrCl, creatinine clearance via Cockroft and Gault equation; VTE, venous thromboembolism [includes DVT and PE].) *(Data from References 37 and 39.)*

Treatment
Prevention
Acute phase Day 0-7
Early maintenance Day 8-90
Extended Day 91+
Oral only
Apixaban 10 mg PO BID × first 7 days
Apixaban 5 mg PO BID
Optional: Reduce to Apixaban 2.5 mg PO BID after first 6 months
Rivaroxaban 15 mg PO BID × first 21 days
Rivaroxaban 20 mg PO daily
Optional: Reduce to Rivaroxaban 10 mg PO daily after first 6 months
Switch
UFH, LMWH, or fondaparinux (all SC) × first 5 days
Dabigatran 150 mg PO BID or Edoxaban 60 mg PO daily
Overlap
UFH, LMWH, or fondaparinux (all SC)
Warfarin PO daily, overlapped with parenteral anticoagulant for at least 5 days AND the INR ≥2.0, then dose adjusted to INR target 2.5 (range 2.0-3.0)

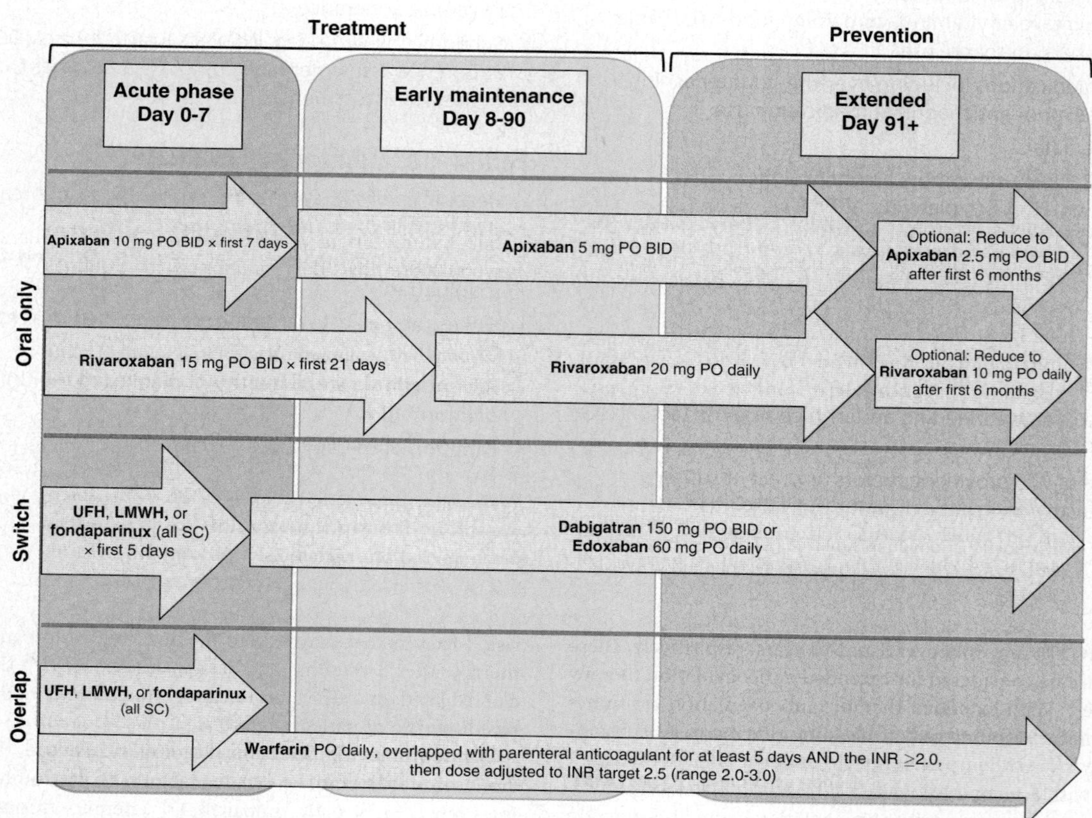

FIGURE 38-11 Overview of VTE treatment strategies: Acute, early maintenance, and extended treatment phases.

TABLE 38-4 Outpatient Treatment Suggestions for DVT and PE

Inclusion: Patients with objectively diagnosed VTE
Exclusion: Hemodynamically unstable, arterial thromboembolism or patients currently receiving dialysis, actively bleeding, recent (within 2 weeks) major surgery/trauma, or other severe uncompensated comorbid conditions
Suggested procedure may vary depending on the patient's clinical condition
Confirm diagnosis of VTE by objective testing

Day 1

Baseline laboratory evaluation
- INR—if use of warfarin anticipated
- SCr
- Complete blood count (CBC) with platelets

Medication—see Fig. 38-11
Patient education
- Clinical pharmacy/nursing
  - Educate patient regarding the importance of proper monitoring of anticoagulation therapy (if applicable) and warning signs that should prompt additional medical evaluation; document activities in the medical record
  - If applicable, teach patient how to self-administer LMWH/fondaparinux (if patient or family member unwilling or unable to self-administer injection, visiting nurse services should be arranged or consider single oral anticoagulant approach); initial injection should be administered in the medical office or hospital
  - Instruct patient regarding local therapy: elevation of affected extremity, localized heat, anti-embolic exercises (flexion–extension of ankle for lower extremity VTE, or hand squeezing–relaxation for upper extremity VTE)
- Dispensing pharmacy
  - Reinforce patient education regarding indication, use, monitoring, adverse drug reactions, and drug interactions with antithrombotic therapy
  - Screen patient's pharmacy profile for potential drug-drug interactions with anticoagulation therapy
  - Dispense anticoagulant therapy
  - Verify anticoagulation service enrollment

Days 3-4

Laboratory evaluation if on warfarin: check INR
Assess for symptoms of pulmonary embolism or bleeding
Medications: continue anticoagulant medication(s) as directed
Anticoagulation service
- If on warfarin interpret results of INR and adjust dose of warfarin to achieve an INR of 2 to 3
- Patient activity: continue reduced activity as long as pain persists (when possible, elevate extremity); increase activity as tolerated
- Document activities in medical record

Day 5

Laboratory evaluation if on warfarin: check INR
Assess for symptoms of bleeding or pulmonary embolism
Medications: continue anticoagulant medication(s) as directed
Anticoagulation service
- If on warfarin interpret results of INR and adjust dose of warfarin to achieve an INR of 2 to 3 (stop LMWH if INR ≥2.0)
- Patient activity: no restriction; if pain increases, contact primary care provider
- Document activities in medical record

Day 6 (Dabigatran or Edoxaban)

Medications: transition from parenteral to oral medication
Assess for symptoms of bleeding or pulmonary embolism
Anticoagulation service
- Verify adherence, affordability, and tolerability of oral medication
- Patient activity: no restriction; if pain increases, contact primary care provider
- Review key education points (eg, keep in original container [dabigatran])
- Document activities in medical record

Day 8 (Apixaban)

Medications: decrease apixaban dose
Anticoagulation service
- Patient activity: no restrictions; if pain increases contact primary care provider
- Verify adherence, affordability, and tolerability of oral medication
- Document activities in medical record

Day 22 (Rivaroxaban)

Medications: decrease rivaroxaban dose
Anticoagulation service
- Verify adherence, affordability, and tolerability of oral medication
- Patient activity: no restriction; if pain increases, contact primary care provider
- Review key education points (eg, take with food [rivaroxaban])
- Document activities in medical record

anticoagulant control (for patients on warfarin), serious acute or chronic illness, and the presence of structural lesions (eg, tumor, recent surgery) that could bleed. One to two bleeding risk factors suggest moderate bleeding risk while three or more suggest high bleeding risk.[18]

Various risk prediction rules aimed at identifying patients with very low recurrence risk after a first idiopathic VTE have evaluated whether the safe withdrawal of anticoagulation therapy may be possible after 3 months. Some factors that may predict lower recurrence risk include female sex, low D-dimer levels 1 month after stopping

TABLE 38-5 Patient Education for Outpatient VTE Therapy

General Information Regarding VTE and the Goals of Treatment

- Anticoagulant medications (injections and warfarin tablets, injections and dabigatran or edoxaban, or rivaroxaban or apixaban) have been prescribed to prevent your blood clot from growing larger so that the body can begin to dissolve the clot.
- Your body may be able to completely dissolve the clot, but in some cases, the clot never goes completely away; even with adequate anticoagulation therapy, some people will have chronic pain and swelling in the affected limb; people who have had one clot are at increased risk of having future clots.
- Warfarin tablets take several days to begin to work, so at first, LMWH or fondaparinux injections and warfarin tablets are used together.
- When the warfarin has become effective, you will be able to stop the LMWH or fondaparinux injections; you will continue to take warfarin tablets for 3 months or longer to prevent blood clots from returning.
- It is important for you to administer your LMWH or fondaparinux and warfarin exactly as directed.
- It is important not to use LMWH at the same time as dabigatran or edoxaban—first use LMWH then switch to dabigatran or edoxaban.

Subcutaneous Injection Technique (If Needed)

- You must learn to give yourself an injection of LMWH or fondaparinux under the skin; alternatively, you may have a family member or visiting nurse give it to you.
- If your LMWH or fondaparinux syringes were filled by the manufacturer, they can be stored at room temperature; if your syringes were filled by the pharmacy, they should be stored in the refrigerator; if you were instructed to fill your own syringes, you should prepare the syringe immediately prior to injecting its contents.
- If you see a bubble in the syringe, do not try to get it out; you may accidentally squirt out part of your dose.
- Choose an injection site on your abdomen; clean the area with alcohol, and then position an uncapped syringe at a 90° angle; pinch the skin, stick the needle in as far as it will go, and gently but firmly push the plunger down; this will inject the medicine into the skin; when all the medication has been injected, remove the needle and dispose of it in an appropriate container.
- You will likely experience a burning sensation when the medication is injected; this will go away after a few minutes.
- Rotate injection sites from side to side; do not inject into the same site more than once; avoid the area around your navel; do not inject into any bruises.

Blood Test Monitoring

- If you are taking warfarin, regular blood tests are required to make sure your medication is working properly.
- The PT tells how quickly your blood forms a clot; it is used to tell how well warfarin is working.
- The INR is a way to standardize the PT between laboratories; your goal INR range is between 2 and 3; if your INR is less than 2, you are at higher risk for clotting; if your INR is greater than 3, you are at higher risk for bleeding; your dose of warfarin will be adjusted based on the results of this test.
- If you are taking LMWH, fondaparinux, dabigatran, edoxaban, rivaroxaban, or apixaban, you need to have a blood test to determine how well your kidneys are working.

Warfarin Information

- Each strength of warfarin has a unique color; each time you refill your prescription, make sure your new tablets are the same color as the ones you have been taking; if not, ask your pharmacist why.
- Warfarin should be taken at approximately the same time each day.
- The most common and serious adverse drug reaction of warfarin is bleeding; you should be careful to avoid situations or activities that increase your risk of injury; apply direct pressure to control bleeding from superficial cuts.
- Warfarin has many drug interactions; always check with your provider before taking any new medications (including nonprescription medications and dietary supplements).
- Foods rich in vitamin K (dark green leafy vegetables, etc.) may interfere with warfarin; do not avoid foods rich in vitamin K, but try to maintain consistent dietary habits.
- Alcohol can increase your risk for bleeding and interfere with warfarin therapy; drink alcohol in moderation (one to two drinks per day); avoid binge drinking.
- If you need to have a surgery or diagnostic procedure, talk to your provider to make a plan for how to take your anticoagulant medication before and after the procedure. Do not stop taking your anticoagulant medication without first talking to your provider.

Dabigatran, Edoxaban, Rivaroxaban, and Apixaban Information

- Take rivaroxaban 15- or 20-mg doses with food to make sure the medication is well absorbed from your stomach.
- It is very important that you take each dose of your medication. These medications leave your body within hours; so missing a dose of medication may place you at a higher risk of blood clots.
- If you need to have a surgery or procedure, talk to your provider to make a plan for how to take your anticoagulant medication before and after the procedure. Do not stop taking your anticoagulant medication without first talking to your provider.
- There are a few drug interactions with dabigatran, edoxaban, rivaroxaban, and apixaban; always check with your provider before taking any new medications (including nonprescription medications and dietary supplements).

Contact Your Provider If You Experience

- Prolonged bleeding from a cut or scrape
- Blood in your urine
- Blood in your stool
- Prolonged nose bleeding (longer than 30 minutes)
- Increased swelling or pain where the blood clot was

Go to the Emergency Department If You Experience

- Sudden onset of shortness of breath
- Chest pain
- Coughing up blood
- Black tarry-appearing stool
- Severe headache of sudden onset
- Drooping of one side of your face
- Weakness in one of your arms
- Slurred speech

anticoagulation therapy, absence of residual clot on ultrasound, absence of hereditary and acquired thrombophilia, and absence of the postthrombotic syndrome. Risk assessment derived from combining several independent recurrence risk factors has also been investigated.[18] Further validation is needed before any one factor or prediction rule using a combination of factors can justify stopping anticoagulation. The decision to continue extended anticoagulation therapy should be reassessed periodically. Patients should be involved in any decision to continue therapy with consideration given to long-term prognosis, risk of bleeding, ability to adhere to anticoagulation therapy instructions, financial resources, lifestyle, and quality of life.[18] When anticoagulation therapy is stopped, there is a similar risk of recurrence whether patients have been treated for 3 months or longer.[47]

Patients with VTE are often tested for hereditary and acquired hypercoagulable states (thrombophilia). The available evidence does not support a strong association between genetically transmitted thrombophilia (especially factor V Leiden and prothrombin G20210A) and higher recurrent VTE rates.[10] For this reason, routine testing for thrombophilia is not recommended.[17]

For patients with proximal DVT, wearing graduated compression stockings does not reduce the risk of developing the postthrombotic syndrome.[49] However, for patients with persistent leg pain and swelling, graduated compression stockings can be suggested for symptomatic relief.

Pharmacologic Therapy

The anticoagulant drugs used to treat VTE are the same as those used for VTE prevention. However, there are important differences in the approach to VTE treatment regarding the doses used and duration of therapy.

Direct Oral Anticoagulants

Clinical trials have demonstrated that single-drug therapy with rivaroxaban or apixaban produces similar rates of recurrent VTE when compared to the traditional approach of initiating warfarin overlapped with enoxaparin for both acute DVT and PE.[50-52] The rate of major bleeding was lower with rivaroxaban in the PE trial,[51] but not in the DVT trial.[52] Apixaban was associated with significantly fewer major bleeding episodes than traditional therapy.[50] Both drugs are initiated with a higher dose and subsequently reduced to a maintenance dose (Fig. 38-11). Patients with CrCl <25 to 30 mL/min (0.42-0.5 mL/s), active cancer, and those requiring thrombolytic therapy were excluded from these clinical trials.[50-52] Subsequent studies have shown that edoxaban and rivaroxaban can be used in cancer patients with VTE and prescribing information for apixaban contains no restrictions based on creatinine clearance.[53,54] Replacing the effective but cumbersome combination warfarin overlapped with an injectable anticoagulant with a single-drug regimen simplifies VTE treatment. However, the higher acquisition cost of rivaroxaban and apixaban may be a barrier for some patients.

6 Oral dabigatran 150 mg twice daily and oral edoxaban 60 mg once daily have each been compared with traditional therapy in randomized, double-blind, noninferiority trials involving patients with acute VTE.[55,56] In these trials, all patients were initially given at least 5 days of parenteral anticoagulation therapy (UFH or LMWH) and then randomized to study treatment. Both dabigatran and edoxaban were noninferior to warfarin following the use of a parenteral anticoagulant. Dabigatran caused similar rate of major bleeding[55] and edoxaban significantly fewer major bleeding events when compared to warfarin.[56] The requirement for parenteral anticoagulation prior to initiation of dabigatran or edoxaban therapy is a disadvantage compared with single-drug approaches to VTE treatment. DOACs are preferred over traditional anticoagulation therapy approaches for the treatment of VTE in consensus guidelines.[57,58] Edoxaban and rivaroxaban may be reasonable alternatives to LMWH monotherapy for patients with cancer-associated VTE.[47,59]

Low-Molecular-Weight Heparin

LMWH given subcutaneously in fixed, weight-based doses (enoxaparin 1 mg/kg twice daily or 1.5 mg/kg once daily) is at least as effective as UFH given intravenously for the treatment of VTE.[60] UFH is preferred as the initial anticoagulant for unstable patients in case thrombolytic therapy or embolectomy is needed.[61] Among patients without cancer treated initially with LMWH, acute treatment with LMWH is generally transitioned to long-term warfarin therapy after at least 5 days of overlap with warfarin and an INR of 2.0 or greater.

Fondaparinux

Fondaparinux is a safe and effective option for acute VTE treatment.[18] Compared with weight-based LMWH dosing, fondaparinux's more flexible dosing scheme may be particularly useful with obese patients and those whose weight falls between commercially available prefilled LMWH syringes. Fondaparinux may be used to overlap with warfarin during initiation or for at least 5 days of parenteral anticoagulation prior to edoxaban or dabigatran initiation for acute VTE. Careful attention should be paid to renal function as fondaparinux is contraindicated if CrCl is <30 mL/min (0.5 mL/s).[62]

Unfractionated Heparin

UFH may be administered subcutaneously (SQ) or by continuous intravenous (IV) infusion (Table 38-6). The anticoagulant response to UFH is highly variable when given intravenously and it is standard practice to adjust the dose according to coagulation test results. The aPTT and antifactor Xa concentration are the two most commonly used tests to monitor the UFH anticoagulant effect. The therapeutic aPTT range at each institution should be adapted to the responsiveness of the reagent and instrument used.[60] Weight-based UFH dosing by IV infusion is preferred. However, failure to give a sufficient IV UFH dose increases VTE recurrence risk.[60] IV UFH requires hospitalization with frequent aPTT monitoring and dose adjustment. Failure to achieve an adequate response to UFH therapy is common despite close monitoring.[60] Consequently, UFH has largely been replaced by LMWH, fondaparinux, and DOACs for the management of acute VTE. However, because the clearance of LMWH, fondaparinux, and DOACs is dependent on renal function, UFH continues to have a role in acute VTE treatment in patients with CrCl <30 mL/min (0.5 mL/s).[18,63] UFH should also be used in unstable patients potentially requiring invasive interventions or thrombolytic therapy.[18,63]

Warfarin

5 Warfarin monotherapy is unacceptable for acute VTE treatment because of the slow onset of effect. However, warfarin is effective for long-term VTE management provided it is started concurrently

TABLE 38-6 Weight-Based[a] Dosing for UFH Administered by Continuous IV Infusion for Acute VTE

Initial Bolus Dose	Initial Infusion Rate
80 units/kg (maximum = 10,000 units)	18 units/kg/hr (maximum = 2,300 units/hr)
Maintenance Infusion Rate	
Activated Partial Thromboplastin Time (seconds)	**Dose Adjustment**
<37 (or antifactor Xa <0.20 unit/mL [kU/L])	80 units/kg bolus, and then increase infusion by 4 units/kg/hr
37-47 (or antifactor Xa 0.20-0.29 unit/mL [kU/L])	40 units/kg bolus, and then increase infusion by 2 units/kg/hr
48-71 (or antifactor Xa 0.30-0.70 unit/mL [kU/L])	No change
72-93 (or antifactor Xa 0.71-1 unit/mL [kU/L])	Decrease infusion by 1-2 units/kg/hr
>93 (or antifactor Xa >1 unit/mL [kU/L])	Hold infusion for 1 hr, and then decrease by 3 units/kg/hr

[a]Use actual body weight for all calculations. Adjusted body weight may be used for obese patients (>130% of ideal body weight).

Data from Reference 60.

with rapid-acting injectable anticoagulant therapy.[58] Injectable anticoagulation should overlap with warfarin therapy for at least 5 days and until an INR ≥2 has been achieved for at least 24 hours.[58] The initial dose of warfarin should be 5 to 10 mg for most patients with subsequent adjustments to achieve and maintain an INR between 2 and 3 (Fig. 38-9).

Thrombolysis and Thrombectomy

Most VTE cases require only anticoagulation therapy. In select cases, removing the occluding thrombus by pharmacologic or surgical means may be warranted.[58] Thrombolytic agents are proteolytic enzymes that enhance the conversion of plasminogen to plasmin. Thrombolytic therapy for DVT improves early venous patency, but this does not necessarily translate into improved long-term outcomes.[58] If thrombolytic therapy is pursued, catheter-directed thrombolysis is suggested over systemic thrombolysis as the latter is not considered appropriate for DVT treatment in the United States.[58] Patients with extensive proximal DVT presenting within 14 days of symptom onset, with good functional status, low bleeding risk, and a life expectancy of a year or more are thrombolysis candidates (Table 38-7). Patients with DVT involving the iliac and common femoral veins are at the highest risk for postthrombotic syndrome and may derive the most benefit from thrombus removal strategies.

In acute PE, successful clot dissolution with thrombolytic therapy reduces elevated pulmonary artery pressure and normalizes right ventricular dysfunction. However, the risk of death from PE should outweigh the risk of serious bleeding associated with thrombolytic therapy. Therefore, patients being considered for thrombolytic therapy should be screened carefully for contraindications relating to bleeding risk (Table 38-7).[58,64] Thrombolytic therapy is considered necessary in addition to aggressive interventions such as volume expansion, vasopressor therapy, intubation, and mechanical ventilation for patients with massive PE accompanied by shock and cardiovascular collapse (about 5% of patients with PE).[58,64] Thrombolytic therapy in these patients should be administered without delay to reduce risk of progression to multisystem organ failure and death.

The benefit of thrombolytic therapy in patients with PE without hemodynamic compromise is less clear and requires rapid risk stratification to determine the initial treatment intensity.[61] Low-risk patients can be discharged early or managed as outpatients, and high-risk patients should be admitted to an intensive care unit for surveillance and/or advanced therapies such as thrombolysis.[65] The Pulmonary Embolism Severity Index (PESI) is a prognostic tool utilizing 11 routinely available clinical parameters: demographics (age and gender), comorbid illnesses (cancer, heart failure, and chronic lung disease), and clinical findings (pulse, systolic blood pressure, respiratory rate, temperature, mental status, and arterial oxygen saturation). PESI stratifies patients into five risk classes with classes I and II considered low risk.[65] Patients with acute PE and evidence of hemodynamic compromise, right ventricular strain by echocardiography, or elevated cardiac biomarker levels have higher mortality risk than patients without these findings, but the risk of death is much less than patients with hemodynamic compromise. Therefore, routine use of thrombolytic therapy is not recommended in these patients, but this decision needs to be individualized (Table 38-7).[58]

In rare circumstances, surgical thrombectomy for extensive ileofemoral DVT may be necessary, but catheter-directed thrombolysis is preferred if bleeding risk is acceptable.[21] For acute PE treatment, catheter-based embolectomy might be suitable in settings where the necessary expertise and resources are available for patients who have contraindications to thrombolytic therapy, have failed thrombolytic therapy, or in whom death is likely before thrombolytic onset.[21] Surgical embolectomy is reserved for patients experiencing massive PE with hemodynamic instability when thrombolysis is either contraindicated or failed, or when insufficient time exists for thrombolysis to take effect.[18] In chronic PE cases—where persistent emboli produce CTPH, hypoxemia, and right-sided heart failure—surgical pulmonary thromboendarterectomy offers greater benefit than anticoagulants and may be the treatment of choice if performed by an experienced surgical team.[21] A permanent IVC filter is usually inserted before or during the procedure and long-term anticoagulation therapy is needed.[18]

Special Populations

Some patient populations with VTE require special consideration due to increased risk for recurrence, adverse events, or altered anticoagulant pharmacokinetics.

TABLE 38-7 Thrombolysis for the Treatment of VTE

- The majority of patients with VTE do not require thrombolytic therapy
- Thrombolytic therapy for DVT should be reserved for patients who present with extensive proximal DVT (eg, ileofemoral) within 14 days of symptom onset, have good functional status, and are at low risk of bleeding
- Thrombolytic therapy should be administered to patients with massive PE with evidence of hemodynamic compromise (hypotension or shock) unless contraindicated by bleeding risk
- Routine use of thrombolytic therapy is not recommended for PE without hypotension or shock but might be appropriate for selected high-risk patients (see below) provided the risk of bleeding is acceptable
- Factors associated with high risk for adverse PE outcomes include:
  - Ill-appearing patients with marked dyspnea, anxiety, and low oxygen saturation
  - Elevated troponin levels
  - Right ventricular dysfunction on echocardiography
  - Right ventricular enlargement on chest CT
- Factors that increase the risk of bleeding must be evaluated before thrombolytic therapy is initiated (ie, recent surgery, trauma or internal bleeding, uncontrolled hypertension, recent stroke or intracranial hemorrhage)
- Baseline labs should include CBC and blood typing in case transfusion is needed
- Alteplase 100 mg infused via peripheral vein over 2 hours is the most commonly used thrombolytic for patients with PE
- Before thrombolytic therapy for PE, IV UFH should be administered in full therapeutic doses
- During thrombolytic therapy, it is acceptable to either continue or suspend IV UFH (suspending UFH is the most common practice in the United States)
- aPTT should be measured following the completion of thrombolytic therapy
  - If aPTT is <80 seconds, UFH infusion should be started and adjusted to maintain aPTT in the therapeutic range
  - If aPTT is >80 seconds, measure every 2-4 hours and start UFH infusion when aPTT is <80 seconds
- Avoid phlebotomy, arterial puncture, and other invasive procedures during thrombolytic therapy to minimize the risk of bleeding

CBC, complete blood cell count; CT, computed tomography.

Data from References 1 and 58.

Pregnancy

Anticoagulation therapy is commonly used for the prevention and treatment of VTE during pregnancy.[8] UFH and LMWH do not cross the placenta and are preferred during pregnancy (Table 38-8).[8] Warfarin crosses the placenta and can result in fetal bleeding, central nervous system abnormalities, and embryopathy and should not be used for VTE treatment during pregnancy.[8] Women of childbearing age taking warfarin must be counseled regarding fetal risks and the need for effective contraception. DOACs should be avoided in pregnancy until more information regarding their safety is available.[66-69] Fondaparinux has not been extensively studied in pregnancy and may cross the placenta.[62] However, fondaparinux may be considered in pregnant patients intolerant to LMWH or those with a history of HIT.[70]

Pregnant women with a history of VTE should receive VTE prophylaxis for 6 weeks after delivery.[71] Antenatal prophylaxis may also be indicated in women with a history of multiple VTE, VTE associated with pregnancy or estrogen therapy, or known thrombophilia. Anticoagulation for acute VTE during pregnancy should continue for at least 6 weeks postpartum and a minimum total duration of 3 months.[8] Warfarin, UFH, and LMWH are safe during breastfeeding.[60,72] It is not known if DOACs are excreted in human milk and breastfeeding is not recommended.[66-69]

Pediatric Patients

VTE in pediatric patients is increasing secondary to prematurity, cancer, trauma, surgery, congenital heart disease, and systemic lupus erythematosus. Pediatric patients rarely experience unprovoked VTE, but often develop DVTs associated with indwelling central venous catheters.[73] In many cases, recommendations for anticoagulant therapy in pediatric patients are largely extrapolated from data from clinical trials in adults. However, in recent years, the available information, knowledge, and expertise in relation to appropriate diagnosis, prevention, and clinical management of VTE in neonates and children have increased dramatically.[73] When possible, a pediatric hematologist with experience treating VTE should manage pediatric patients.[74]

Anticoagulation with LMWH and warfarin remains the most frequently used approach for VTE treatment in pediatric patients. The decision between LMWH and warfarin should depend on patient values and preferences, health services resources, infrastructure and support, indication for anticoagulation, comorbidities, and other medications. The recommended target INR range, as well as the duration of therapy, is the same as for adults.[73] Frequent INR monitoring and warfarin dose adjustments are typically required. Obtaining blood for coagulation monitoring tests in pediatric patients is challenging because many have poor venous access. Using finger-stick blood samples with point-of-care INR monitors is an option in this situation. Despite the need for daily injections, LMWH is an attractive alternative for pediatric patients due to the low potential for drug-drug interactions and less frequent laboratory testing. Most experts recommend anti-Xa activity monitoring with goal antifactor Xa levels between 0.5 and 1.0 unit/mL (kU/L) 4 to 6 hours following subcutaneous injection. Warfarin should be initiated concurrently with UFH or LMWH therapy. Similar to adults, therapy should be overlapped for a minimum of 5 days and until the INR is therapeutic. Anticoagulation should be continued for up to 3 months for provoked VTE and 6 to 12 months for unprovoked VTE.[73] DOACs are attractive alternatives in pediatric patients due to oral administration and no need for routine coagulation monitoring; however, safety, effectiveness, and dosing in this population have

TABLE 38-8 Anticoagulant Use During Pregnancy and Delivery

Acute treatment[a]	LMWH • Enoxaparin 1 mg/kg SC q 12 hr or 1.5 mg/kg q 24 hr *Or* • Dalteparin 100 units/kg SC q 12 hr *Or* UFH • Initiate using weight-based IV therapy and adjust dose to achieve therapeutic anti-Xa level for at least 5 days • Transition to SC adjusted-dose UFH administered q 8-12 hr with mid-interval anti-Xa activity adjusted to achieve an anti-Xa level of 0.3-0.7 unit/mL [kU/L][b]
Long-term treatment[c]	LMWH • Maintain initial LMWH dose regimen throughout pregnancy *Or* • Alter LMWH dose in proportion to any weight change (usually gain) *Or* UFH • Obtain anti-Xa level at the midpoint of the dosing interval and adjust UFH dose to achieve an anti-Xa level of 0.3-0.7 unit/mL (kU/L)
Issues at the time of delivery	Elective induction of labor • Discontinue UFH or LMWH 24 hr prior to induction • Initiate therapeutic doses of UFH by IV infusion and discontinue 4-6 hr prior to the expected time of delivery if the risk of recurrent VTE is deemed high Spontaneous labor • For LMWH, if there is a reasonable expectation that significant anticoagulant effect will be present at the time of delivery: (a) epidural should be avoided and (b) reversal with protamine sulfate may be considered • For UFH, monitor the aPTT and reverse with protamine sulfate if aPTT is prolonged near the time of delivery Postpartum • Commence UFH or LMWH as soon as safely possible (usually 12 hr following delivery) • Concurrently initiate warfarin therapy and discontinue UFH or LMWH when the INR is 2 or greater • Continue anticoagulants for at least 6 weeks following delivery • Warfarin can be safely used by women who are breast-feeding

[a]Twice-daily LMWH preferred during pregnancy due to increased clearance.

[b]Anti-Xa monitoring preferred as the relationship between aPTT and heparin levels differs in pregnant compared with nonpregnant patients.

[c]As pregnancy progresses the volume of distribution of LMWH changes, glomerular filtration rate increases, and most women gain weight.

SC, subcutaneously.

Data from Reference 8.

not been established.[66-69] Thrombolysis has been used in pediatric patients, but published data are very limited—routine use is not recommended with the exception of PE associated with hemodynamic compromise.[73]

Patients with Cancer

Cancer-related VTE is associated with threefold higher rates of recurrent VTE and up to sixfold higher rates of bleeding. In addition, increased rates of recurrent VTE have been associated with warfarin-based approaches to VTE treatment in patients with active cancer.[75] Warfarin therapy in cancer patients is often complicated by drug interactions (eg, chemotherapy and antibiotics) and the need to interrupt therapy for invasive procedures. Maintaining stable INR control is also more difficult in this patient population because of nausea, anorexia, and vomiting.[18]

Long-term LMWH monotherapy (dalteparin 200 units/kg every 24 hr for 30 days, followed by 150 units every 24 hr, or enoxaparin as described above) is a preferred option for patients with cancer-associated VTE. Treatment of cancer-related VTE with LMWH monotherapy rather than traditional warfarin-based therapy decreases recurrent VTE rates without increasing bleeding risk but does not affect overall mortality.[16,18,76,77] Advantages of LMWH over warfarin for VTE treatment in cancer are expected to be greatest in those with one or more of the following: metastatic disease, treatment with aggressive chemotherapy, extensive VTE at presentation, liver dysfunction, poor or unstable nutritional status, or desire to avoid frequent blood draws for coagulation monitoring.[18]

For patients with cancer and VTE receiving LMWH, therapy should continue for 3 to 6 months after which the LMWH can be continued or warfarin or DOAC therapy substituted. Anticoagulation therapy should continue for as long as the cancer is "active" and while the patient is receiving antitumor therapy.[18] A risk-to-benefit assessment should be performed on a regular basis considering overall clinical status, bleeding risk, quality of life, and life expectancy.[18] For patients with cancer who experience a VTE recurrence despite receiving anticoagulant therapy, LMWH appears to be more effective than warfarin-based therapy in preventing further recurrences, and increasing the anticoagulant intensity may not be necessary for this situation.[75]

Edoxaban and rivaroxaban have been compared to dalteparin monotherapy for the treatment of cancer-related VTE and were as effective as dalteparin for preventing VTE recurrence but caused more bleeding.[53,54] Excess DOAC-related bleeding often occurred in the gastrointestinal tract in patients with gastrointestinal malignancy.[53] Thus, DOACs may be an important alternative to LMWH for cancer-related VTE given the limited tolerability of long-term LMWH but should be used with caution in patients with tumors involving the gastrointestinal lumen.

Patients with Renal Insufficiency

Patients with acute or chronic kidney disease often require anticoagulation for VTE prevention or treatment. With the exception of warfarin and UFH, most anticoagulants require adequate renal function for their elimination. Accumulation of drug is possible during treatment with LMWH, fondaparinux, and most DOACs.[60,72] In addition, patients with chronic kidney disease are at increased risk of bleeding, regardless of anticoagulant choice.[25]

LMWHs are renally eliminated and should be used with caution in patients with severe renal impairment.[78] Enoxaparin has specific labeling for patients with CrCl <30 mL/min (0.5 mL/s), but supporting evidence is limited to pharmacokinetic modeling analyses.[79] Bleeding and recurrent VTE outcomes for patients with CrCl <30 mL/min (0.5 mL/s) receiving enoxaparin 1 mg/kg once daily for acute VTE treatment was comparable to patients with normal renal function in one retrospective study.[63] However, UFH remains preferred for acute VTE treatment in this setting until further evidence becomes available.[18] Fondaparinux is contraindicated in patients with CrCl <30 mL/min (0.5 mL/s).

DOACs are eliminated to varying[80] degrees through the kidney and require dose adjustment for renal impairment.[66-69] Periodic renal function assessment is important during long-term DOAC therapy, especially for patients with CrCl <50 mL/min (0.83 mL/s). The use of dabigatran and rivaroxaban in patients with CrCl <30 mL/min (0.5 mL/s) should be avoided.[67,68] Edoxaban dosing is reduced to 30 mg once daily in patients with CrCl 15 to 50 mL/min (0.25-0.83 mL/s).[69] Product labeling for apixaban permits its use in patients with end-stage kidney disease and emerging data suggest that apixaban may be an option for these patients.[66,80]

Patients Undergoing Invasive Procedures

Patients scheduled to undergo invasive procedures often require temporary discontinuation of anticoagulation therapy.[81] The decision to withhold anticoagulation therapy should be based on the bleeding risk associated with the procedure and the patient's underlying thromboembolic risk. Anticoagulation therapy is typically continued in patients undergoing minimally invasive procedures such as dental work, cataract surgery, or minor dermatologic procedures.[82] If the bleeding risk from the procedure is considerable, near-normal hemostasis should be achieved prior to the procedure. For DOACs the time required for the restoration of normal hemostasis after interrupting therapy is dependent on renal function and medication half-life. Stopping DOACs 2 days prior to invasive procedures is usually sufficient to restore near-normal hemostasis for patients with normal renal function. Additional days off therapy may be required for patients with impaired renal function.[66-69] The anticoagulant effect of dabigatran can be rapidly reversed with idarucizumab and andexanet can be used to reverse the effect of rivaroxaban and apixaban for patients requiring urgent surgical interventions.[83,84] Up to 5 days may be required for the restoration of normal hemostasis after warfarin discontinuation. Patients at high thromboembolic risk (ie, DVT or PE in the previous month) may be considered for so-called "bridge therapy" with UFH or an LMWH given before and after the procedure.[82] Bridge therapy has been associated with increased major bleeding without offering additional recurrent VTE risk reduction in low-to-moderate risk patients. Therefore, most patients with VTE can safely interrupt warfarin for invasive procedures without using bridge therapy.[81] Resumption of anticoagulation following an invasive procedure is based on post-procedure bleeding risk and drug-specific time to onset of the anticoagulant effect (Table 38-9).

DRUG CLASS INFORMATION

9 Optimal use of anticoagulant therapies requires knowledge of pharmacologic and pharmacokinetic characteristics as well as systematic management and ongoing patient education (Table 38-5) to reduce the risks of bleeding and therapeutic failure (Table 38-10).

Direct Oral Anticoagulants

Shortcomings with warfarin, LMWH, fondaparinux, and UFH have driven the search for replacements with rapid anticoagulant onset and oral administration without the need for monitoring. The DOACs have provided a major advance in VTE prevention and treatment.

Pharmacology/Mechanism of Action

Rivaroxaban, apixaban, and edoxaban are potent and selective inhibitors of both free and clot-bound factor Xa that do not require antithrombin to exert their anticoagulant effect.[58] Dabigatran is a selective, reversible, direct factor IIa (thrombin) inhibitor.[67]

TABLE 38-9 Anticoagulant Interruption and Resumption Around High Bleeding-Risk Invasive Procedures

Anticoagulant	Timing of Anticoagulant Interruption Prior to Procedure	Day of Procedure	Timing of Anticoagulant Resumption After Procedure[a]
UFH	IV: hold infusion 6-8 hours prior to the procedure SC: last dose 12 hours prior to the procedure	No anticoagulation	24-48 hours after the procedure
LMWH	Last dose 24 hours prior to the procedure		
Fondaparinux	Last dose 2 days prior to the procedure		
Apixaban	Last dose 2 days prior to the procedure		
Dabigatran • CrCl <50 mL/min (0.83 mL/s) • CrCl ≥50 mL/min (0.83 mL/s)	 Last dose 3-4 days prior to the procedure Last dose 2 days prior to the procedure		
Edoxaban	Last dose 2 days prior to the procedure		
Rivaroxaban	Last dose 2 days prior to the procedure		
Warfarin[b]	Last dose 4-5 days prior to the procedure		Day of or 1 day after the procedure

[a]Assumes hemostasis has been achieved.

[b]Warfarin hold time is dependent on the INR prior to beginning the interruption and the target INR for the day of the procedure (eg, patients beginning with elevated INR may require a longer holding period to achieve target INR for the day of procedure)

TABLE 38-10 Risk Factors for Major Bleeding While Taking Anticoagulation Therapy

Higher anticoagulation intensity
Initiation of therapy (first few days and weeks)
Unstable anticoagulation response
Age >65 years
Concurrent aspirin or other antiplatelet therapy
Concurrent nonsteroidal anti-inflammatory drug use
History of gastrointestinal tract bleeding
Recent surgery or trauma
High risk for fall/trauma
Heavy alcohol use
Renal failure
Cerebrovascular disease
Malignancy

Data from Reference 25.

Pharmacokinetics

Rivaroxaban, apixaban, and edoxaban have good oral bioavailability (greater than 60%), whereas dabigatran is formulated as a prodrug (dabigatran etexilate) to overcome poor oral bioavailability.[66-69] All DOACs reach peak plasma concentrations in less than 4 hours. Each drug is renally eliminated to a variable extent, as low as 27% for apixaban and as high as 80% for dabigatran.[66-69] Terminal half-lives range from 9 to 12 hours for rivaroxaban, apixaban, and edoxaban, and 14 to 17 hours for dabigatran.[66-69] DOACs should be used with caution in patients with renal dysfunction.[85] Rivaroxaban and apixaban are substrates of cytochrome p450 (CYP) 3A4 and the P-glycoprotein (P-gp) transporter.[66] Edoxaban and dabigatran do not undergo significant CYP 3A4 metabolism, but all are P-gp substrates. Strong inhibitors and inducers of CYP 3A4 enzymes or P-gp may cause changes in DOAC exposure and increase the risk of bleeding or VTE events.[66-69]

Efficacy

DOACs are noninferior to warfarin therapy overlapped with LMWH for VTE treatment.[66-69] For patients who are at high risk of VTE recurrence who require extended anticoagulant therapy beyond 6 months, rivaroxaban and apixaban at either the treatment or prophylactic doses were superior to low-dose aspirin or placebo, respectively.[86,87] Similarly, when compared to LMWH, rivaroxaban and apixaban are noninferior for preventing VTE following hip or knee replacement surgery.[66-68,88]

Adverse Drug Reactions

The most common adverse drug reaction associated with DOAC therapy is bleeding.[66-69] The International Society for Thrombosis and Haemostasis defines major bleeding as fatal bleeding, any bleeding into a critical anatomic space (eg, intracranial bleeding, hemarthrosis, pericardial bleeding, or intraocular bleeding), bleeding that requires transfusion of two or more units of whole blood or red cells, or bleeding that leads to a greater than 2 g/dL (20 g/L; 1.24 mmol/L) drop in hemoglobin concentration. Bleeding that does not meet the major bleeding criteria but requires medical intervention or alteration of therapy is sometimes termed clinically relevant nonmajor bleeding. All other bleeding is considered minor and is common during anticoagulation therapy even in the most expertly managed patients. The most frequent nonbleeding adverse events in clinical trials of DOACs were gastrointestinal complaints.[66-69]

Patients presenting with significant bleeding during DOAC therapy should receive routine supportive care (fluid resuscitation, blood transfusion, maintenance of renal function, bleeding source identification, and surgical intervention if needed), and discontinuation of anticoagulation therapy.[89] Because DOACs have relatively short half-lives, these measures may control bleeding in many patients, especially those with normal renal function.[89] Activated charcoal may provide some benefit if drug intake occurred within the previous 2 hours.[89]

Idarucizumab is a humanized monoclonal antibody fragment that rapidly reverses dabigatran's anticoagulant effect following IV administration.[83] Idarucizumab can be used during emergency situations such as life-threatening bleeding and when there is a need for urgent surgical intervention. Andexanet is a recombinant Factor Xa molecule that binds the Factor Xa inhibitors rivaroxaban and apixaban without having intrinsic antithrombotic activity. It can be used for the reversal of life-threatening bleeding in patients taking rivaroxaban or apixaban (Table 38-11). If traditional hemostatic measures fail or drug-specific reversal agents are not available in a life-threatening bleeding situation, it may be reasonable to consider the use of 4-factor prothrombin complex concentrates (PCCs) while weighing the associated risk for thrombotic events. Animal, in vitro,

TABLE 38-11 Reversal Agents for the DOACs

Reversal Agent	Target	Outcomes and Current Status
Idarucizumab (monoclonal antibody fragment)	Dabigatran	Reversed anticoagulant effect of dabigatran in patients with serious bleeding or needing urgent reversal for a procedure Approved by the FDA in October 2015
Andexanet (modified recombinant Factor Xa)	Rivaroxaban, Apixaban	Reversed anticoagulant effect of rivaroxaban and apixaban in patients with intracranial hemorrhage Approved by the FDA in May 2018

Data from References 83 and 90-92.

and healthy volunteer studies have shown that these agents reverse coagulation laboratory parameters, but controlled studies of these agents in bleeding patients taking DOACs are not available. Fresh-frozen plasma (FFP) is unlikely to provide clinical benefit.[89]

Drug-Drug and Drug-Food Interactions

Adding aspirin to DOAC therapy nearly doubles bleeding rates and should be avoided in most patients with VTE. Although the DOACs have far fewer drug interactions than warfarin, all DOACs are P-gp substrates and subject to changes in anticoagulant effect when coadministered with strong P-gp inhibitors or inducers. Rivaroxaban and apixaban are subject to interactions involving inhibitors or inducers of CYP 3A4.[66-69] Which drug interactions must be avoided is a matter of debate. Strong inducers of P-gp and CYP 3A4 enzymes such as carbamazepine and rifampin should be avoided. Caution should be used with concurrent use of strong P-gp or combination P-gp/CYP 3A4 inhibitors with a DOAC, particularly in the setting of renal insufficiency.[66-69] When interacting drugs cannot be avoided it may be best to switch to warfarin for dose adjustment guided by INR monitoring.

Dosing and Administration

Rivaroxaban and apixaban can be used in a single-drug approach for acute VTE treatment, whereas at least 5 days of parenteral anticoagulant therapy is required prior to initiating edoxaban or dabigatran for acute VTE (Fig. 38-11). The 15- and 20-mg doses of rivaroxaban should be taken with food to enhance oral absorption, but all other DOACs can be taken irrespective of food.[66-69]

Low-Molecular-Weight Heparin

LMWH fragments produced by either chemical or enzymatic depolymerization of UFH are heterogeneous mixtures of sulfated glycosaminoglycans with approximately one-third the mean molecular weight of UFH.[60] Advantages of LMWH over UFH include predictable anticoagulation dose-response, improved subcutaneous bioavailability, dose-independent clearance, longer biologic half-life, lower incidence of thrombocytopenia, and reduced need for routine laboratory monitoring.[60]

Pharmacology/Mechanism of Action

LMWH prevents thrombus growth and propagation by enhancing and accelerating the activity of antithrombin.[60] The anticoagulant effect of LMWH (and UFH) is mediated through a specific pentasaccharide sequence that binds to antithrombin, provoking a conformational change (Fig. 38-12). To inactivate thrombin, the heparin molecule must form a ternary complex bridging between antithrombin and thrombin.[60] Only molecules containing more than 18 saccharides are able to bind to both antithrombin and thrombin simultaneously. Smaller heparin molecules cannot facilitate the interaction between antithrombin and thrombin. In contrast, the inactivation of factor Xa does not require the formation of a bridge with antithrombin but requires only heparin binding to antithrombin via the specific pentasaccharide sequence. Heparin molecules with as few as five saccharide units are able to catalyze the inhibition of factor Xa. The principal difference in the pharmacologic activity of LMWH and UFH is their relative inhibition of factor Xa and thrombin. Because of smaller chain lengths, LMWH has limited activity against thrombin (Fig. 38-12). The ratio of antifactor Xa:IIa activity varies between 4:1 and 2:1.

Pharmacokinetics

Compared with UFH, LMWH has a more predictable anticoagulation response. The improved pharmacokinetic profile of LMWH is the result of reduced binding to proteins and cells.[60] The bioavailability of LMWH is about 90% when administered subcutaneously. The peak anticoagulation effect is seen within 3 to 5 hours of subcutaneous LMWH injection and the predominant mode of elimination for LMWH is renal. Consequently, the biologic half-life may be prolonged in patients with renal impairment.[60] The plasma half-life of LMWH preparations is 3 to 6 hours. Unlike UFH, the clearance of LMWH is independent of dose.[60]

Efficacy

The efficacy of LMWH for the prevention of VTE was established in clinical trials in comparison to low-dose UFH and placebo. For the

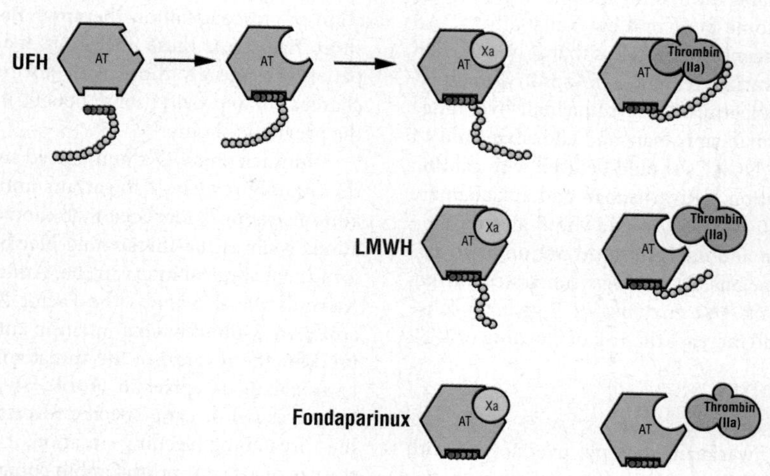

FIGURE 38-12 Pharmacologic activity of UFH, LMWHs, and fondaparinux. (AT, antithrombin.)

treatment of VTE, the efficacy of fixed weight-based LMWH was compared to aPTT-adjusted IV UFH; all patients were transitioned to warfarin for long-term therapy.[79,93]

Adverse Drug Reactions

As with other anticoagulants, bleeding is the most common LMWH adverse drug reaction.[25] The frequency of major bleeding may be less with LMWH than with UFH, but this has not been consistently demonstrated in clinical trials.[25] Although there is no proven method for reversing LMWH anticoagulation if major bleeding occurs, IV protamine sulfate can be administered. However, because of limited binding to the shorter LMWH chains, protamine sulfate neutralizes only around 60% to 75% of LMWH anticoagulant activity.[60] The recommended dose of protamine sulfate is 1 mg/1 mg of enoxaparin or 1 mg/100 antifactor Xa units of dalteparin administered in the previous 8 hours. A second protamine sulfate dose of 0.5 mg/1 mg or 100 antifactor Xa units can be given if bleeding continues. Smaller doses of protamine sulfate can be used if the LMWH dose was given in the previous 8 to 12 hours. The use of protamine sulfate is not recommended if LMWH was administered more than 12 hours earlier.[60]

Although thrombocytopenia can occur with LMWH use, the incidence of HIT is one-third of that observed with UFH, perhaps due to the reduced propensity of LMWH to bind to platelets.[60] However, LMWH exhibits nearly 100% cross-reactivity with UFH antibodies in vitro, and thus LHWH should be avoided in patients with an established diagnosis or history of HIT.[60] The risk of osteoporosis appears to be lower with LMWH than with UFH.[60]

Drug-Drug Interactions

The concurrent use of drugs that enhance bleeding risk should be avoided during LMWH therapy if possible. This includes aspirin or other antiplatelet agents, nonsteroidal anti-inflammatory drugs, dipyridamole, or sulfinpyrazone.[79,93]

Dosing and Administration

LMWH is given in fixed or weight-based doses based on the product and indication. Doses should be based on actual body weight and dose capping (ie, a fixed, maximum daily dose) is not recommended.[78] The dose for enoxaparin is expressed in milligrams, whereas dalteparin doses are expressed in units of antifactor Xa activity. LMWH is given by subcutaneous injection.

Significant LMWH accumulation is possible in patients with severe renal impairment.[60] The enoxaparin dose should be reduced or the dosing interval extended to once daily in patients with CrCl <30 mL/min (0.5 mL/s).[79] Dalteparin is less reliant upon renal elimination than enoxaparin; however, its pharmacokinetics are insufficiently characterized in renal insufficiency.[94] LMWH use in patients with end-stage renal disease receiving hemodialysis is poorly understood; thus, UFH is preferred for these patients.[60] Some experts recommend measuring antifactor Xa activity if LMWH therapy is continued for more than a few days in patients with severe renal disease.[60] For patients with CrCl <30 mL/min (0.5 mL/s) who require VTE prophylaxis, enoxaparin 30 mg once daily is recommended.[60]

Fondaparinux

Fondaparinux is a synthetic molecule consisting of the five critical saccharide units that bind specifically, but reversibly, to antithrombin. Unlike UFH or LMWH, fondaparinux inhibits only factor Xa activity.[60]

Pharmacology/Mechanism of Action

Fondaparinux prevents thrombus generation and clot formation by indirectly inhibiting factor Xa activity through its interaction with antithrombin (Fig. 38-12). Fondaparinux is not destroyed during this process and is released to bind to other antithrombin molecules.[60]

Pharmacokinetics

Fondaparinux is rapidly and completely absorbed following subcutaneous administration achieving peak plasma concentrations approximately 2 hours after a single dose and 3 hours with repeated once-daily dosing. At therapeutic concentrations, fondaparinux does not bind to red blood cells or other plasma proteins.[60] Fondaparinux is primarily eliminated unchanged in the urine and its terminal elimination half-life is 17 to 21 hours.[60] The anticoagulant effect of fondaparinux persists for 2 to 4 days following discontinuation of the drug in patients with normal renal function.

Efficacy

The efficacy of fondaparinux for the prevention of VTE was established in several clinical trials in comparison to LMWH. For the treatment of VTE, the efficacy of fixed weight-based dosing of fondaparinux was compared to weight-based dosing of LMWH; all patients were transitioned to warfarin for long-term therapy.[62]

Adverse Drug Reactions

The primary adverse drug reaction associated with fondaparinux therapy is bleeding.[62] Fondaparinux should be used with extreme caution with neuraxial anesthesia or following spinal puncture because of the risk for spinal or epidural hematoma formation.[62] Some case reports have implicated fondaparinux as a cause of HIT, while others have documented successful HIT treatment with fondaparinux.[95] A specific antidote to reverse the antithrombotic activity of fondaparinux is not currently available.[60]

Drug-Drug Interactions

Fondaparinux has no known pharmacokinetic drug interactions; other drugs with anticoagulant, fibrinolytic, or antiplatelet activity increase the risk of bleeding.[62]

Dosing and Administration

The dose of fondaparinux for VTE prevention is 2.5 mg injected subcutaneously once daily following surgery if hemostasis has been established. It is important to avoid initiating fondaparinux too soon because there is a significant relationship between first dose timing and major bleeding risk.[60] Patients weighing less than 50 kg should not receive VTE prophylaxis with fondaparinux.[62] The usual duration of prophylaxis is 5 to 9 days, but extended prophylaxis for up to 35 days following a lower extremity orthopedic procedure may be used.[37] For the treatment of DVT or PE, the dose of fondaparinux is 5 mg for patients up to 50 kg, 7.5 mg for 50 to 100 kg, and 10 mg for >100 kg.[62]

Unfractionated Heparin

UFH has been used for VTE prevention and treatment for decades. Commercially available UFH preparations are derived from bovine lung or porcine intestinal mucosa. Although some differences exist between the two sources, no differences in antithrombotic activity have been demonstrated.[60]

Pharmacology/Mechanism of Action

UFH is a heterogeneous mixture of sulfated mucopolysaccharides of variable lengths and pharmacologic properties.[60]

Only one-third of the UFH molecules possess the unique pentasaccharide sequence with an affinity for antithrombin. Antithrombin inhibits factor IXa, Xa, XIIa, and IIa activity. Thrombin and Xa are most sensitive to UFH–antithrombin complex inhibition. UFH has an antifactor Xa:IIa activity ratio of 1:1 (Fig. 38-12).[60] UFH prevents thrombus growth and propagation allowing endogenous thrombolytic systems to lyse the clot.[60]

After it has produced its effect UFH uncouples from antithrombin and quickly recouples with another antithrombin molecule.[60]

Pharmacokinetics

UFH is not reliably orally absorbed because of its large molecular size and anionic structure. The bioavailability and biologic activity of UFH are limited by a propensity to bind plasma proteins, platelet factor-4, macrophages, fibrinogen, lipoproteins, and endothelial cells. This may explain the substantial interpatient and intrapatient variability observed in the anticoagulation response to UFH.[60]

The onset of anticoagulant effect after subcutaneous injection is 1 to 2 hours, peaking at 3 hours.[60] Continuous infusion is preferred for IV UFH administration.[18] Intramuscular administration is discouraged because of the risk of large hematoma formation.

UFH has a dose-dependent half-life of approximately 30 to 90 minutes.[60] There are two primary mechanisms for UFH elimination, a rapid, but saturable zero-order process involving enzymatic inactivation of heparin molecules bound to endothelial cells and macrophages, and renal elimination via a slower, nonsaturable first-order process. With typical therapeutic UFH regimens, the zero-order process predominates.[60]

Efficacy

UFH has demonstrated clinical effectiveness for the prevention and treatment of VTE over many years of clinical use.

Adverse Drug Reactions

Low-dose subcutaneous UFH is associated with a minimal risk of major bleeding. Bleeding rates for patients receiving therapeutic UFH doses range from 0% to 2%.[25] Close monitoring for bleeding signs and symptoms during UFH therapy is crucial.[25,60] When major bleeding occurs, UFH should be discontinued and the underlying bleeding source should be identified and treated. Protamine sulfate in a dose of 1 mg per 100 units of UFH (maximum of 50 mg) can be administered via slow IV infusion to reverse the anticoagulant effects of UFH.[60] Protamine sulfate neutralizes UFH in 5 minutes and persists for 2 hours. Multiple doses or prolonged infusion of protamine sulfate may be necessary if bleeding continues.[60]

HIT is a rare drug-induced immunologic reaction requiring immediate intervention.[96] The most common complication of HIT is VTE; arterial thromboembolic events occur less frequently. Approximately 5% to 10% of patients with HIT die, usually from thrombotic complications.[96] Thrombocytopenia (defined as a platelet count $<150 \times 10^3/\text{mm}^3$ [$150 \times 10^9/\text{L}$]) is the most common clinical HIT manifestation. HIT should be suspected if platelet counts decrease by 30% to 50% but remain above $150 \times 10^3/\text{mm}^3$ ($150 \times 10^9/\text{L}$).[96] The characteristic onset of falling platelet count occurs in the first 5 to 10 days after initiation of UFH (Day 0 being the first day of UFH), particularly when administered perioperatively.[96] Thrombocytopenia alone is not sufficient for diagnosing HIT; serologic confirmation of heparin antibodies using an assay available only in a few specialty laboratories is required.[96] Falsely diagnosing HIT can have serious consequences including unnecessary anxiety, unnecessary UFH withdrawal, and the use of alternative anticoagulants with higher bleeding risk. The use of a clinical prediction rule, such as the 4Ts score (thrombocytopenia, timing of platelet count fall or thrombosis, thrombosis, other explanations for thrombocytopenia) can improve the predictive value of platelet count monitoring and heparin antibody testing.[96,97] A 4Ts score should be calculated when HIT is suspected in patients receiving heparin (UFH or LMWH). If the 4Ts score is low (3 or less), no further workup is needed, whereas a moderate (4 to 5) or high (6 to 8) 4Ts score requires further HIT workup including serologic testing.[98] In the setting of new thrombosis occurring in conjunction with falling platelets and a moderate or high 4Ts score, all sources of heparin should be discontinued. Alternative anticoagulation with a direct thrombin inhibitor or fondaparinux should then be initiated. If warfarin therapy is being used, it should be discontinued and reversed with vitamin K. Once platelet counts have recovered, warfarin can be resumed so long as it is overlapped with a direct thrombin inhibitor or fondaparinux until the INR is ≥2.0.[96]

Using UFH in doses ≥20,000 units/day for more than 6 months, especially during pregnancy, is associated with significant bone loss and may lead to osteoporosis.[60]

Drug-Drug and Drug-Food Interactions

Few drug interactions are reported with UFH, but concurrent use with other anticoagulants, thrombolytics, and antiplatelet agents increases bleeding risk.[60]

Dosing and Administration

UFH dose is expressed in units of activity. For VTE prevention, UFH is given by subcutaneous injection in the abdominal fat layer. The typical prophylaxis dose is 5,000 units every 8 to 12 hours. When immediate and full anticoagulation is required, an IV bolus dose followed by a continuous infusion is preferred (Table 38-6).[60] Subcutaneous UFH (initial dose of 333 units/kg followed by 250 units/kg every 12 hours) also provides adequate therapeutic anticoagulation for the treatment of acute VTE and does not require aPTT or anti-Xa monitoring.[60]

Warfarin

Because of its narrow therapeutic index, predisposition to drug and food interactions, and propensity to exacerbate bleeding, warfarin requires frequent monitoring and extensive patient education to achieve optimal outcomes.[72]

Pharmacology/Mechanism of Action

Warfarin exerts its anticoagulation effect by inhibiting the enzymes responsible for the cyclic vitamin K interconversion in the liver.[72] Vitamin K in its reduced form is a required cofactor for vitamin K-dependent carboxylation of factors II, VII, IX, and X, as well as the endogenous anticoagulant proteins C and S. Hepatic carboxylation of the N-terminal region of these proteins is required for biologic activity. By inhibiting the reduced vitamin K supply used in the production of these proteins, warfarin therapy produces partially carboxylated and decarboxylated coagulation proteins with reduced activity.[72] Warfarin has no direct effect on previously circulating clotting factors or previously formed thrombus. The time required for warfarin to achieve its pharmacologic effect is dependent on coagulation protein elimination half-lives (6 hours for factor VII and 72 hours for prothrombin).[72] Full antithrombotic effect is not achieved for at least 6 days after warfarin therapy initiation. By suppressing fully functional clotting factor production, warfarin prevents initial thrombus formation and propagation.[72]

Pharmacokinetics

Warfarin is a racemic mixture of *R* and *S* isomers, with *S*-warfarin being 2.7 to 3.8 times more potent than *R*-warfarin.[72] Warfarin is rapidly and extensively absorbed from the gastrointestinal tract (bioavailability >90%) and reaches peak plasma concentration within 4 hours of oral administration. Warfarin is 99% bound to plasma proteins and undergoes stereoselective metabolism via CYP 1A2, 2C9, 2C19, 2C8, 2C18, and 3A4 isoenzymes in the liver, with 2C9 being the main enzyme to modulate the elimination of *S*-warfarin.[99] Warfarin pharmacokinetics varies substantially between individuals leading to large interpatient differences in dose requirements. Genetic variations in the 2C9 isoenzyme and vitamin K epoxide reductase (VKOR) have been shown to correlate with warfarin dose requirements.[72] Given the greater potency of *S*-warfarin, coadministration of drugs that induce or inhibit the CYP 2C9 isoenzyme is more likely to cause clinically significant interactions.[72]

Efficacy

Warfarin has demonstrated clinical effectiveness for the prevention and treatment of VTE over many years of clinical use.

Adverse Drug Reactions

Warfarin's primary adverse drug reaction is bleeding that can range from mild to life-threatening.[72] Although warfarin does not cause bleeding per se, it exacerbates bleeding from existing lesions and can enable massive bleeding from ordinarily minor sources.[72] Anticoagulation therapy intensity is an important bleeding risk factor; the likelihood of bleeding rises with increasing INR values.[72] Therefore, maintaining the INR within the target range is important to reduce bleeding risk. Most patients with asymptomatic INR elevations between 4.5 and 10 can be safely managed by withholding warfarin alone.[5] For an INR >10 without evidence of bleeding, oral vitamin K 2.5 mg is recommended but does not improve clinical outcomes compared to withholding warfarin alone.[100] Vitamin K can be administered subcutaneously, IV, or orally; the oral route is preferred in the absence of serious bleeding. Vitamin K should be used cautiously in patients at high thromboembolism risk due to the possibility of INR overcorrection. Conversely, simply withholding warfarin therapy may not lower high INRs quickly enough in patients at high bleeding risk or in situations associated with prolonged INR elevations such as drug interactions and intentional overdoses.

Patients with warfarin-associated life-threatening bleeding require supportive care and rapid reversal of anticoagulation with both 4-factor PCC (rather than FFP) and 5 to 10 mg of vitamin K (administered via slow IV injection).[5]

Other adverse drug reactions associated with warfarin are uncommon but can be serious.[72] The etiology of the "purple toe syndrome" is unknown, but is thought to be the result of cholesterol microembolization into the arterial circulation of the toes.[72] If recognized early, complete resolution can be achieved by simply substituting a different anticoagulant for warfarin.[101] Warfarin-induced skin necrosis is a serious dermatologic reaction usually manifesting in the first week of therapy as a painful maculopapular rash and ecchymosis or purpura that subsequently progresses to necrotic gangrene. Areas of the body rich in subcutaneous fat, such as the breasts, thighs, buttocks, and abdomen are most commonly affected.[72] If skin necrosis is suspected, warfarin therapy should be discontinued immediately, reversed with vitamin K and either FFP or PCC, and full-dose UFH or LMWH therapy initiated. Patients with a history of skin necrosis should restart warfarin with extreme caution, if at all, using small doses and gradual titration under full-dose unfractionated heparin or LMWH coverage until a therapeutic INR is achieved.[72]

Drug-Food and Drug-Drug Interactions

The pharmacokinetic and pharmacodynamic properties of warfarin predispose patients to numerous clinically important food and drug interactions.[102] Vitamin K can reverse warfarin's pharmacologic activity; many foods contain sufficient vitamin K to reduce the anticoagulation effect if consumed in large portions or repetitively within a short period of time.[72] Patients should be instructed to maintain a relatively consistent intake of vitamin K–rich foods (Table 38-12). It is important to stress consistency rather than abstinence.

Pharmacokinetic drug interactions with warfarin primarily result from alterations in hepatic metabolism. Drugs inhibiting or inducing CYP 2C9, 1A2, and 3A4 isoenzymes have the greatest potential to significantly alter warfarin therapy response.[72] Drugs altering hemostasis or platelet function (eg, aspirin, clopidogrel) can increase bleeding risk without altering warfarin pharmacokinetics or impacting the INR.[72] Clinicians should advise patients on warfarin to report potential interactions to their anticoagulation provider whenever a drug product, dietary supplement, or herbal product is initiated or stopped, whether prescribed or available over the counter. If there is a known drug interaction or doubt about the potential to alter the warfarin response, more frequent INR testing

TABLE 38-12 Vitamin K Content of Select Foods[a]

Very High (>200 mcg)	High (100-200 mcg)	Medium (50-100 mcg)	Low (<50 mcg)
Brussel sprouts	Basil	Apple, green	Apple, red
Chickpeas	Broccoli	Asparagus	Avocado
Collard greens	Chive	Cabbage	Beans
Coriander	Coleslaw	Cauliflower	Breads, grains
Endive	Cucumber (with peel)	Mayonnaise	Carrot
Kale	Canola oil	Nuts, pistachio	Cereal
Lettuce, red leaf	Green onion/scallion	Squash, summer	Celery
Parsley	Lettuce, butterhead		Coffee
Spinach	Mustard greens		Corn
Swiss chard	Soybean oil		Cucumber (without peel)
Tea, green			Dairy products
Tea, black			Eggs
Turnip greens			Fruit (varies)
Watercress			Lettuce, iceberg
			Meats, fish, poultry
			Pasta
			Peanuts
			Peas
			Potato
			Rice
			Tomato

[a]Approximate amount of vitamin K per 100 g (3.5 oz) serving.

Data from Reference 24.

is recommended with warfarin dose adjustments as needed to maintain INRs in the target range.[102]

Dosing and Administration

The dose of warfarin is individualized based on the desired target INR range and anticoagulant response by periodically measuring the PT and calculating the INR.[72] The pharmacodynamic response and pharmacokinetic disposition of warfarin between and within patients are highly variable. Therefore, the dose of warfarin must be individualized based on frequent clinical and laboratory monitoring.[72] The average weekly warfarin dose is between 25 and 55 mg. Some patients require lower than usual dose requirements, including patients who are of advanced age (>65 years), have an elevated baseline INR, poor nutritional status, liver disease, genetic polymorphisms in CYP 2C9 and VKOR, and concurrent use of medications known to enhance the effect of warfarin.[72] Higher than usual dose requirements are also necessary in some patients, including concurrent use of medications known to induce the metabolism of warfarin such as rifampin and carbamazepine, high dietary vitamin K intake, and genetic polymorphisms in CYP 2C9. It is important to collect a complete medication history, including the use of herbal and nutritional products as these can influence warfarin's metabolism, dose requirements, and the risk of bleeding.[72]

Initiating warfarin therapy with 5 to 10 mg daily and adjusting the dose based on the INR response will produce therapeutic INRs in 5 to 7 days for most patients (Fig. 38-9). Lower starting doses may be acceptable based on patient-related factors such as advanced age, malnutrition, liver disease, or heart failure. Starting doses >10 mg should be avoided.[72] When warfarin therapy is initiated in the outpatient setting, the INR should be measured every 3 to 4 days until stabilized. For patients with acute VTE, a parenteral, rapid-acting anticoagulant such as UFH, LMWH, or fondaparinux should be overlapped with warfarin therapy for at least 5 days regardless of whether the target INR has been achieved earlier.[18,72]

It is important to allow sufficient time for changes in the INR to occur when adjusting warfarin doses. In general, maintenance dose changes should not be made more frequently than every 3 days. When adjusting maintenance warfarin doses, the weekly dosage should be reduced or increased by 5% to 25%; the full effect of dose changes may not become evident for 5 to 7 days or longer.[72] Patients demonstrating a stable response to warfarin as evidenced by consistently therapeutic INR results on the same warfarin dose can have INRs checked as infrequently as every 8 to 12 weeks, although most stable patients are tested approximately every 4 to 6 weeks.[5]

Therapeutic Considerations

Prevention Versus Treatment of Venous Thromboembolism

Lower doses of LMWH and DOACs are used for VTE prevention than during VTE treatment. Warfarin may be targeted to a traditional INR range (2.0 to 3.0) or reduced-intensity (1.5 to 2.5) for VTE prophylaxis. Orthopedic surgeons frequently prefer the lower INR range due to perceived lower bleeding risk. VTE prophylaxis in high-risk hospitalized patients is typically discontinued at discharge. In contrast, after certain surgeries (eg, major orthopedic surgery), VTE prophylaxis continues following hospital discharge for up to 35 days.

VTE treatment requires full therapeutic anticoagulant doses for at least 3 months. Patients unwilling to self-administer LMWH or fondaparinux injections may prefer apixaban or rivaroxaban. The duration of anticoagulant therapy after acute VTE is principally determined by whether the clot was provoked, unprovoked, or recurrent. Three months of therapeutic anticoagulation is sufficient following a first episode of VTE provoked by major transient risk factors such as surgery, pregnancy, or trauma. Most patients with unprovoked or recurrent VTE should receive long-term anticoagulation for secondary VTE prevention. Patients selected for long-term secondary anticoagulation traditionally receive standard therapeutic doses. In patients for whom there is clinical equipoise regarding anticoagulation continuation, prophylactic doses of apixaban and rivaroxaban are as effective as full therapeutic doses after 6 months of treatment has been completed.[86,87] However, prophylactic doses were not safer than therapeutic doses as the risk of major bleeding was low for both options. Switching to aspirin for long-term secondary VTE prevention is also an option but is less effective than continuing anticoagulation therapy.[103,104]

Weight

Patients at extremes of body weight were underrepresented in DOAC VTE treatment trials. There is speculation regarding whether very obese or very small patients receive equivalent anticoagulant effects with DOAC when compared to other patients. The International Society of Thrombosis and Haemostasis suggests that standard doses of rivaroxaban or apixaban, without monitoring of peak and trough concentrations, are among the appropriate anticoagulant options for VTE treatment or prevention regardless of high BMI and weight.[105] They suggest avoiding dabigatran and edoxaban for VTE treatment and prevention in patients with BMI >40 kg/m^2 or weight >120 kg, given that data are either unconvincing (dabigatran) or lacking (edoxaban). DOACs should be avoided for both prevention and treatment of VTE in the acute setting following bariatric surgery because of concerns of decreased absorption.[105] Switching to a DOAC after at least 4 weeks following surgery may be reasonable but obtaining a DOAC trough level to check for drug absorption and bioavailability is suggested (see Evaluation of Therapeutic Outcomes section).[105]

LMWH dosing in obesity frequently causes concern. Patients weighing more than 90 kg would exceed the maximum dose specified in the approved labeling for dalteparin (18,000 units).[93] However, evidence supports similar anti-Xa exposure to LMWH and no increase in bleeding risk compared to nonobese patients when doses based on actual body weight without capping are administered.[106] Fondaparinux is a convenient option for obese patients as the 10 mg dose is suitable for acute VTE treatment in patients >100 kg.[62] Obese patients requiring VTE prophylaxis may need higher than normal LMWH doses. For example, enoxaparin 40 mg subcutaneously twice daily may be more effective than usual VTE prophylaxis doses for patients undergoing bariatric surgery.[107]

Response to Previous Therapy

Other than bleeding, anticoagulants are generally well tolerated. However, adverse reactions, treatment failure, or allergies during previous therapy may necessitate preferential use of one anticoagulant over another.

Warfarin allergy is rare and often related to dyes or tablet excipients rather than the active ingredient. Warfarin 10 mg tablets contain no dye and can be considered when an allergy is suspected. Patients experiencing dabigatran-related dyspepsia can try taking the dose with a full glass of water or food. Transitioning to another DOAC or warfarin may be necessary.

Cost is an important aspect of personalizing anticoagulant therapy for VTE prevention and treatment. For patients unable to afford DOACs, warfarin remains a cost-effective option.

Patients suspected of having a recurrent VTE during anticoagulant therapy should have their adherence to therapy assessed and imaging compared to historical data to ensure the clot is new. Determining and correcting the causes of poor medication adherence to anticoagulation therapy should occur before switching anticoagulants. Malignancy should be considered when anticoagulant adherence is verified. Switching to an LMWH is recommended for breakthrough VTE occurring during oral anticoagulation therapy.[21]

Patients having breakthrough VTE during LMWH should be switched to twice daily injections (if receiving once-daily LMWH) and considered for dose escalation of 25% to 33%.[21] Switching to an oral factor Xa inhibitor may also be an option given the comparable efficacy of edoxaban and dalteparin for the treatment of cancer-related VTE; however, less is known regarding their use in breakthrough VTE.

Pharmacogenomics

CYP2C9 is the hepatic microsomal enzyme responsible for the metabolism of the more potent S-enantiomer of warfarin. Polymorphisms in CYP 2C9 and the gene coding for VKOR (known as vitamin K epoxide reductase complex 1) explain a substantial proportion of warfarin dose variability between patients. Dosing algorithms using CYP 2C9 and VKOR pharmacogenomics, as well as clinical and drug interaction information, have been developed to assist providers more accurately select initial warfarin doses based upon a predicted maintenance warfarin dose for an individual patient (see www.warfarindosing.org). The Food and Drug Administration (FDA) updated the warfarin package label to include the use of pharmacogenetic testing in 2007.[99]

There are several barriers to the widespread application of pharmacogenomic testing for warfarin. First, and most important, is the INR. The ability to rapidly assess a patient's physiologic response to warfarin using an inexpensive and widely available test limits the need for pharmacogenomic information. Second is the timeliness of receiving pharmacogenomic test results. Pharmacogenomic information is most valuable when selecting the first 3 or 4 warfarin doses. However, pharmacogenomic testing outside of clinical trials may require several days or longer before results become available. Delaying warfarin initiation is rarely safe, thus pharmacogenomic test results are only meaningful if they are available in the first 2 to 3 days after treatment initiation. Although poor metabolizing CYP2C9 subtypes have been associated with increased risk of bleeding compared to the wild-type, clinical trials have not demonstrated improved bleeding or thromboembolic outcomes with the routine use of pharmacogenomic information to guide warfarin dosing when compared to usual care.[108,109] As a result, the clinical utility and cost-effectiveness of warfarin pharmacogenomics remains ill-defined and the American College of Chest Physicians guidelines does not recommend routine use.[110]

EVALUATION OF THERAPEUTIC OUTCOMES

Warfarin dose titration based on INR monitoring and UFH dose titration based on aPTT or anti-Xa monitoring allows a degree of personalized therapy not available with other anticoagulants. The intensity of warfarin or UFH therapy can be easily titrated in high-risk situations such as invasive procedures, accidental or intentional overdose, suspected nonadherence, or concomitant therapy with interacting drugs. Titrating DOAC therapy cannot be accomplished due to lack of readily available quantitative coagulation assays and dosing guidelines in these clinical scenarios.[111] In rare circumstances, such as patients who have previously had bariatric surgery, measuring trough levels of rivaroxaban or apixaban has been suggested.[105] This should be accomplished using an anti-Xa level specific to rivaroxaban or apixaban.

While laboratory coagulation monitoring is unnecessary during DOAC therapy, clinical surveillance is likely beneficial. In clinical trials comparing DOACs to warfarin, patients receiving DOAC therapy had regular contact with healthcare providers who screened for bleeding, changes in renal or hepatic function, drug adherence, potential drug interactions, and plans for invasive procedures.

Adherence is essential to preventing recurrent VTE during DOAC therapy due to their short half-lives. A study performed in patients with atrial fibrillation taking dabigatran found that pharmacist involvement during initial drug selection, patient education, and follow-up contacts improved drug adherence.[112] Pharmacist involvement during DOAC initiation may be especially important to ensure proper transitions from LMWH to dabigatran or edoxaban or from initiation to maintenance dosing with rivaroxaban or apixaban. An ABCDEF checklist may be helpful when monitoring patients on DOACs: A—Adherence with therapy, B—Bleeding risk assessment, C—Creatinine clearance/renal function monitoring, D—Drug interaction evaluation, E—Examination for adverse events and therapeutic effectiveness, and F—Final assessment and recommendations regarding the need for ongoing DOAC therapy.[113] What remains unclear is how frequently patient monitoring should be performed for patients on DOACs and whether it should be performed for all patients taking DOACs or only those at highest risk.

Because LMWH anticoagulant response is predictable when given subcutaneously, routine laboratory monitoring is unnecessary.[60] Prior to LMWH initiation, baseline complete blood cell counts with platelets and SCr should be obtained. If neuraxial anesthesia has been used, patients should be closely monitored for signs and symptoms of neurologic impairment.[79]

Antifactor Xa activity is the most widely used test to monitor the anticoagulant effect of LMWH in clinical practice. Routine antifactor Xa activity measurement is unnecessary in uncomplicated patients who are stable.[60] Measuring antifactor Xa activity may be considered in patients who are morbidly obese, pregnant, or have a significant renal impairment (eg, CrCl <30 mL/min [0.5 mL/s]).[60] However, many laboratories do not standardize the measurement of anti-factor Xa levels for specific LMWH products. For this reason and because the correlation between antifactor Xa levels and adverse outcomes is uncertain, guidelines recommend against measuring antifactor Xa activity in these situations.[5,114]

When antifactor Xa activity is used to monitor LMWH therapy, the sample should be drawn during the peak antifactor Xa activity—once a steady state has been achieved (after the second or third dose) and approximately 4 hours after the subcutaneous injection.[60] The antifactor Xa activity therapeutic range is not well-defined and has not been clearly correlated with efficacy or the risk of bleeding. For the treatment of VTE, an acceptable target range for the peak anti-Xa level for twice-daily enoxaparin dosing is 0.6 to 1 unit/mL (kU/L). For once-daily dosing, peak targets >1 unit/mL (kU/L) for enoxaparin and 1.05 units/mL (kU/L) for dalteparin have been suggested.[60] The target range for peak anti-Xa concentrations during cancer-associated VTE treatment with dalteparin is 0.5 to 1.5 units/mL (kU/L).[93]

Prior to initiating fondaparinux, baseline kidney function should be determined as fondaparinux is contraindicated when CrCL is <30 mL/min (0.5 mL/s).[62] Signs and symptoms of bleeding should be monitored daily, particularly in patients with a baseline CrCl between 30 and 50 mL/min (0.5 and 0.83 mL/s). If neuraxial anesthesia has been used, patients should be closely monitored for signs and symptoms of neurologic impairment.[62] The role of antifactor Xa monitoring during fondaparinux is not well-defined, but routine coagulation testing is not required.[62]

Administration of UFH requires close monitoring because each patient's anticoagulant response is unpredictable.[60] Although the aPTT has several limitations, most experts advocate using the aPTT to monitor UFH provided that institution-specific therapeutic ranges are defined.[60] The aPTT should be measured prior to the initiation of therapy to determine the patient's baseline. With IV infusion, the aPTT response to UFH therapy should be measured 6 hours after initiation or dose changes. UFH doses should be adjusted based on patient response and the institution-specific aPTT therapeutic range (Table 38-6).[60]

The PT measures the biologic activity of factors II, VII, and X and has been used for decades to monitor the anticoagulation effects of warfarin. The PT is performed by measuring the time required for clot formation after adding calcium and thromboplastin to citrated plasma.[72] Interpreting the PT is problematic because thromboplastins of differing sensitivity produce substantially different results, some of which could lead to inappropriate dosing decisions. The World Health Organization (WHO) addressed the need for standardization in the late 1970s by developing a reference thromboplastin and recommending the use of the INR to monitor warfarin therapy.[72] The INR attempts to correct for differences in thromboplastin reagents through the following formula:

$$\text{INR} = \left(\frac{\text{PT}^{\text{patient}}}{\text{PT}^{\text{control}}}\right)^{\text{ISI}}$$

The International Sensitivity Index (ISI) is a measure of thromboplastin responsiveness compared with the WHO reference standard.[72] Although the INR system has a number of limitations, it remains the preferred method for monitoring warfarin therapy.[72]

Referring patients with VTE to anticoagulation therapy management services is recommended to optimize the care of patients who take warfarin therapy by providing structured care, comprehensive patient education, and evaluation of outcomes.[5] When anticoagulation management services are not available, individual clinicians should strive to implement similar structured care processes.[110]

Portable finger-stick INR devices are available for monitoring warfarin therapy. These devices permit clinicians to do "real-time" therapeutic INR monitoring and enable patients to engage in self-testing at home.[5] Patients who engage in INR self-testing and warfarin self-management have fewer thromboembolic complications, report high levels of satisfaction with care, and maintain INRs within the therapeutic range slightly more frequently than those managed by "usual care." However, home INR testing and self-management is not for everyone and requires careful patient selection and considerable patient education.[110] Finger-stick INR devices are relatively expensive, but some patients qualify for insurance coverage for the monitor and testing supplies.

CONCLUSION

VTE is a significant public health issue, yet there is little public awareness of the life-threatening nature of this commonly occurring condition. Given the number and variety of clinical circumstances that place individuals at risk for VTE, improvements in VTE prevention and care have the potential to benefit many patients. Over the past decade, the focus on quality healthcare has included systematic measures to improve the use of effective VTE prophylaxis and evidence-based VTE treatments. The concerted efforts of government and accrediting agencies working with hospitals and other healthcare institutions will hopefully reduce VTE rates. Systematic approaches to this problem are needed at every level, starting with increased public and health practitioner awareness, continuing with the uniform use of effective prophylactic strategies in patients at risk, and concluding with the application of high-quality VTE treatment strategies.

ABBREVIATIONS

aPC	activated protein C
aPTT	activated partial thromboplastin time
β_2-gp	β_2-glycoprotein
BMI	body mass index
CrCl	creatinine clearance
CTPA	computed tomography pulmonary angiography
CTPH	chronic thromboembolic pulmonary hypertension
CUS	compression ultrasound
CYP	cytochrome P450
DOAC	direct-acting oral anticoagulant
DVT	deep vein thrombosis
FFP	fresh-frozen plasma
HIT	heparin-induced thrombocytopenia
INR	international normalized ratio
IPC	intermittent pneumatic compression
ISI	International Sensitivity Index
IVC	inferior vena cava
LMWH	low-molecular-weight heparin
NICE	National Institute for Health and Care Excellence
PCCs	prothrombin complex concentrates
PE	pulmonary embolism
PESI	Pulmonary Embolism Severity Index
P-gp	P-glycoprotein
PT	prothrombin time
SBP	systolic blood pressure
TF	tissue factor
TFPI	tissue factor pathway inhibitor
tPA	tissue plasminogen activator
UFH	unfractionated heparin
V/Q	ventilation/perfusion
VKOR	vitamin K epoxide reductase
VTE	venous thromboembolism
WHO	World Health Organization

REFERENCES

1. Goldhaber SZ, Bounameaux H. Pulmonary embolism and deep vein thrombosis. *Lancet*. 2012;379:1835–1846.
2. Anderson DR, Morgano GP, Bennett C, et al. American Society of Hematology 2019 guidelines for management of venous thromboembolism: Prevention of venous thromboembolism in surgical hospitalized patients. *Blood Adv.* 2019;3:3898–3944. doi:10.1182/bloodadvances.2019000975.
3. Schünemann HJ, Cushman M, Burnett AE, et al. American Society of Hematology 2018 guidelines for management of venous thromboembolism: Prophylaxis for hospitalized and nonhospitalized medical patients. *Blood Adv.* 2018;2:3198–3225. doi:10.1182/bloodadvances.2018022954.
4. Lim W, Le Gal G, Bates SM, et al. American Society of Hematology 2018 guidelines for management of venous thromboembolism: Diagnosis of venous thromboembolism. *Blood Adv.* 2018;2:3226–3256. doi:10.1182/bloodadvances.2018024828.
5. Witt DM, Nieuwlaat R, Clark NP, et al. American Society of Hematology 2018 guidelines for management of venous thromboembolism: Optimal management of anticoagulation therapy. *Blood Adv.* 2018;2:3257–3291. doi:10.1182/bloodadvances.2018024893.
6. ISTH Steering Committee for World Thrombosis Day. Thrombosis: A major contributor to the global disease burden. *J Thromb Haemost.* 2014;12:1580–1590.
7. Martinez C, Cohen AT, Bamber L, Rietbrock S. Epidemiology of first and recurrent venous thromboembolism: A population-based cohort study in patients without active cancer. *Thromb Haemost.* 2014;112:255–263.
8. Bates SM, Rajasekhar A, Middeldorp S, et al. American Society of Hematology 2018 guidelines for management of venous thromboembolism: Venous thromboembolism in the context of pregnancy. *Blood Adv.* 2018;2:3317–3359. doi:10.1182/bloodadvances.2018024802.
9. Johnson SA, Eleazer GP, Rondina MT. Pathogenesis, diagnosis, and treatment of venous thromboembolism in older adults. *J Am Geriatr Soc.* 2016;64:1869–1878.
10. Anderson JA, Weitz JI. Hypercoagulable states. *Crit Care Clin.* 2011;27:933–952,vii.
11. Turpie AG, Esmon C. Venous and arterial thrombosis: Pathogenesis and the rationale for anticoagulation. *Thromb Haemost.* 2011;105:586–596.

12. Reitsma PH, Versteeg HH, Middeldorp S. Mechanistic view of risk factors for venous thromboembolism. *Arterioscler Thromb Vasc Biol.* 2012;32:563–568.
13. De Caterina R, Husted S, Wallentin L, et al. General mechanisms of coagulation and targets of anticoagulants (Section I). Position Paper of the ESC Working Group on Thrombosis: Task Force on Anticoagulants in Heart Disease. *Thromb Haemost.* 2013;109:569–579.
14. Margaglione M, Grandone E. Population genetics of venous thromboembolism. A narrative review. *Thromb Haemost.* 2011;105:221–231.
15. Rijken DC, Lijnen HR. New insights into the molecular mechanisms of the fibrinolytic system. *J Thromb Haemost.* 2009;7:4–13.
16. Khorana AA. Cancer and coagulation. *Am J Hematol.* 2012;87(Suppl 1):S82–S87.
17. Chong LY, Fenu E, Stansby G, Hodgkinson S, Guideline Development G. Management of venous thromboembolic diseases and the role of thrombophilia testing: Summary of NICE guidance. *BMJ.* 2012;344:e3979.
18. Kearon C, Akl EA, Comerota AJ, et al. Antithrombotic therapy for VTE disease: Antithrombotic Therapy and Prevention of Thrombosis, 9th ed: American College of Chest Physicians Evidence-Based Clinical Practice Guidelines. *Chest.* 2012;141:e419S–e494S.
19. Bates SM, Jaeschke R, Stevens SM, et al. Diagnosis of DVT: Antithrombotic Therapy and Prevention of Thrombosis, 9th ed: American College of Chest Physicians Evidence-Based Clinical Practice Guidelines. *Chest.* 2012;141:e351S–e418S.
20. Le Gal G, Righini M. Controversies in the diagnosis of venous thromboembolism. *J Thromb Haemost.* 2015;13(Suppl 1):S259–S265.
21. Kearon C, Akl EA, Ornelas J, et al. Antithrombotic Therapy for VTE Disease: CHEST Guideline and Expert Panel Report. *Chest.* 2016;149:315–352.
22. Wells PS, Anderson DR, Rodger M, et al. Derivation of a simple clinical model to categorize patients probability of pulmonary embolism: Increasing the models utility with the SimpliRED D-dimer. *Thromb Haemost.* 2000;83:416–420.
23. Wendelboe AM, McCumber M, Hylek EM, et al. Global public awareness of venous thromboembolism. *J Thromb Haemost.* 2015;13:1365–1371.
24. Booth SL, Centurelli MA. Vitamin K: A practical guide to the dietary management of patients on warfarin. *Nutr Rev.* 1999;57:288–296.
25. Schulman S, Beyth RJ, Kearon C, Levine MN. Hemorrhagic complications of anticoagulant and thrombolytic treatment: American College of Chest Physicians Evidence-Based Clinical Practice Guidelines (8th Edition). *Chest.* 2008;133:257S–298S.
26. Mahan CE, Holdsworth MT, Welch SM, Borrego M, Spyropoulos AC. Deep-vein thrombosis: A United States cost model for a preventable and costly adverse event. *Thromb Haemost.* 2011;106:405–415.
27. Guyatt GH, Eikelboom JW, Gould MK, et al. Approach to outcome measurement in the prevention of thrombosis in surgical and medical patients: Antithrombotic Therapy and Prevention of Thrombosis, 9th ed: American College of Chest Physicians Evidence-Based Clinical Practice Guidelines. *Chest.* 2012;141:e185S–e194S.
28. Gray J, Razmus I. Improving venous thromboembolism prevention processes and outcomes at a community hospital. *Jt Comm J Qual Patient Saf.* 2012;38:61–66.
29. Zeidan AM, Streiff MB, Lau BD, et al. Impact of a venous thromboembolism prophylaxis "smart order set": Improved compliance, fewer events. *Am J Hemat.* 2013;88:545–549. doi:10.1002/ajh.23450.
30. Streiff MB, Agnelli G, Connors JM, et al. Guidance for the treatment of deep vein thrombosis and pulmonary embolism. *J Thromb Thrombolysis.* 2016;41:32–67. doi:10.1007/s11239-015-1317-0.
31. Streiff MB, Brady JP, Grant AM, et al. CDC Grand Rounds: Preventing hospital-associated venous thromboembolism. *MMWR Morb Mortal Wkly Rep.* 2014;63(9):190–3. 24598595.
32. Grant PJ, Conlon A, Chopra V, et al. Use of venous thromboembolism prophylaxis in hospitalized patients. *JAMA Intern Med.* 2018;178:1122. doi:10.1001/jamainternmed.2018.2022.
33. Kahn SR, Lim W, Dunn AS, et al. Prevention of VTE in nonsurgical patients: Antithrombotic Therapy and Prevention of Thrombosis, 9th ed: American College of Chest Physicians Evidence-Based Clinical Practice Guidelines. *Chest.* 2012;141:e195S–e226S.
34. Gould MK, Garcia DA, Wren SM, et al. Prevention of VTE in nonorthopedic surgical patients: Antithrombotic Therapy and Prevention of Thrombosis, 9th ed: American College of Chest Physicians Evidence-Based Clinical Practice Guidelines. *Chest.* 2012;141:e227S–e277S.
35. Zareba P, Wu C, Agzarian J, Rodriguez D, Kearon C. Meta-analysis of randomized trials comparing combined compression and anticoagulation with either modality alone for prevention of venous thromboembolism after surgery. *Br J Surg.* 2014;101:1053–1062.
36. Rajasekhar A, Streiff MB. Vena cava filters for management of venous thromboembolism: A clinical review. *Blood Rev.* 2013;27:225–241.
37. Falck-Ytter Y, Francis CW, Johanson NA, et al. Prevention of VTE in orthopedic surgery patients: Antithrombotic Therapy and Prevention of Thrombosis, 9th ed: American College of Chest Physicians Evidence-Based Clinical Practice Guidelines. *Chest.* 2012;141:e278S–e325S.
38. Cohen AT, Spiro TE, Büller HR, et al. Rivaroxaban for thromboprophylaxis in acutely ill medical patients. *N Engl J Med.* 2013;368:513–523. doi:10.1056/nejmoa1111096.
39. Barbar S, Noventa F, Rossetto V, et al. A risk assessment model for the identification of hospitalized medical patients at risk for venous thromboembolism: The Padua Prediction Score. *J Thromb Haemost.* 2010;8:2450–2457. doi:10.1111/j.1538-7836.2010.04044.x.
40. Decousus H, Tapson VF, Bergmann JF, et al. Factors at admission associated with bleeding risk in medical patients. *Chest.* 2011;139:69–79. doi:10.1378/chest.09-3081.
41. Reichert JA, Hlavinka PF, Stolzfus JC. Risk of hemorrhage in patients with chronic liver disease and coagulopathy receiving pharmacologic venous thromboembolism prophylaxis. *Pharmacotherapy.* 2014;34:1043–1049.
42. Ali M, Ananthakrishnan AN, McGinley EL, Saeian K. Deep vein thrombosis and pulmonary embolism in hospitalized patients with cirrhosis: A nationwide analysis. *Dig Dis Sci.* 2011;56:2152–2159.
43. Anderson FA Jr., Huang W, Friedman RJ, et al. Prevention of venous thromboembolism after hip or knee arthroplasty: Findings from a 2008 survey of US orthopedic surgeons. *J Arthroplasty.* 2012;27:659–666. e5.
44. Mont MA, Jacobs JJ, Boggio LN, et al. Preventing venous thromboembolic disease in patients undergoing elective hip and knee arthroplasty. *J Am Acad Orthop Surg.* 2011;19:768–776.
45. Anderson DR, Dunbar M, Murnaghan J, et al. Aspirin or Rivaroxaban for VTE prophylaxis after hip or knee arthroplasty. *N Engl J Med.* 2018;378:699–707.
46. Wells PS, Forgie MA, Rodger MA. Treatment of venous thromboembolism. *JAMA.* 2014;311:717–728.
47. Young AM, Marshall A, Thirlwall J, et al. Comparison of an oral factor Xa inhibitor with low molecular weight heparin in patients with cancer with venous thromboembolism: Results of a randomized trial (SELECT-D). *J Clin Oncol.* 10, 2018;36(20):2017–2023. doi:10.1200/JCO.2018.78.8034.
48. Meyer G, Planquette B, Sanchez O. Pulmonary embolism: Whom to discharge and whom to thrombolyze? *J Thromb Haemost.* 2015;13(Suppl 1):S252–S258.
49. Kahn SR, Shapiro S, Wells PS, et al. Compression stockings to prevent post-thrombotic syndrome: A randomised placebo-controlled trial. *Lancet.* 2014;383:880–888.
50. Agnelli G, Buller HR, Cohen A, et al. Oral apixaban for the treatment of acute venous thromboembolism. *N Engl J Med.* 2013;369:799–808.
51. Investigators E-P, Buller HR, Prins MH, et al. Oral rivaroxaban for the treatment of symptomatic pulmonary embolism. *N Engl J Med.* 2012;366:1287–1297.
52. Investigators E, Bauersachs R, Berkowitz SD, et al. Oral rivaroxaban for symptomatic venous thromboembolism. *N Engl J Med.* 2010;363:2499–2510.
53. Raskob GE, van Es N, Verhamme P, et al. Edoxaban for the treatment of cancer-associated venous thromboembolism. *N Engl J Med.* 2018;378:615–624.
54. Young AM, Marshall A, Thirlwall J, et al. Comparison of an oral factor Xa inhibitor with low molecular weight heparin in patients with cancer with venous thromboembolism: Results of a randomized trial (SELECT-D). *J Clin Oncol.* 2018;36(20):2017–2023.
55. Schulman S, Kakkar AK, Goldhaber SZ, et al. Treatment of acute venous thromboembolism with dabigatran or warfarin and pooled analysis. *Circulation.* 2014;129:764–772.
56. Hokusai VTEI, Buller HR, Decousus H, et al. Edoxaban versus warfarin for the treatment of symptomatic venous thromboembolism. *N Engl J Med.* 2013;369:1406–1415.
57. Kearon C, Akl EA, Ornelas J, et al. Antithrombotic therapy for VTE disease: CHEST guideline and expert panel report. *Chest.* 2016;149(2):315–352. doi:10.1016/j.chest.2015.11.026 26867832.
58. Ortel TL, Neumann I, Ageno W, et al. American Society of Hematology 2020 guidelines for management of venous thromboembolism: Treatment of deep vein thrombosis and pulmonary embolism. *Blood Adv.* 2020;4:4693–4738. doi:10.1182/bloodadvances.2020001830.
59. Raskob GE, van Es N, Verhamme P, et al. Edoxaban for the treatment of cancer-associated venous thromboembolism. *N Engl J Med.* 15, 2018;378(7):615–624. doi: 10.1056/NEJMoa1711948.

60. Garcia DA, Baglin TP, Weitz JI, Samama MM, American College of Chest P. Parenteral anticoagulants: Antithrombotic Therapy and Prevention of Thrombosis, 9th ed: American College of Chest Physicians Evidence-Based Clinical Practice Guidelines. *Chest.* 2012;141:e24S–e43S.
61. Goldhaber SZ. Advanced treatment strategies for acute pulmonary embolism, including thrombolysis and embolectomy. *J Thromb Haemost.* 2009;7(Suppl 1):322–327.
62. GlaxoSmithKline. Arixtra Prescribing Information 2018.
63. Martinez K, Kosirog E, Billups SJ, Clark NP, Delate T, Witt DM. Clinical outcomes and adherence to guideline recommendations during the initial treatment of acute venous thromboembolism. *Ann Pharmacother.* 2015;49:869–875.
64. Wang TF, Squizzato A, Dentali F, Ageno W. The role of thrombolytic therapy in pulmonary embolism. *Blood.* 2015;125:2191–2199.
65. Aujesky D, Hughes R, Jimenez D. Short-term prognosis of pulmonary embolism. *J Thromb Haemost.* 2009;7(Suppl 1):318–321.
66. Bristol Myers Squibb C. Eliquis Prescribing Information. 2021. Available at: https://packageinserts.bms.com/pi/pi_eliquis.pdf. Accessed October 20, 2021.
67. Boehringer-Ingelheim. Pradaxa Prescribing Information. 2021. Available at: https://docs.boehringer-ingelheim.com/Prescribing%20Information/PIs/Pradaxa/Pradaxa.pdf. Accessed October 30, 2021.
68. Janssen Pharmaceuticals I. Xarelto Prescribing Information. 2021. Available at: https://www.janssenlabels.com/package-insert/product-monograph/prescribing-information/XARELTO-pi.pdf. Accessed October 30, 2021.
69. Daiichi Sankyo I. Savaysa Prescribing Information. 2021. Available at: https://daiichisankyo.us/prescribing-information-portlet/getPIContent?productName=Savaysa&inline=true. Accessed October 30, 2021.
70. Knol HM, Schultinge L, Erwich JJ, Meijer K. Fondaparinux as an alternative anticoagulant therapy during pregnancy. *J Thromb Haemost.* 2010;8:1876–1879.
71. Kamel H, Navi BB, Sriram N, Hovsepian DA, Devereux RB, Elkind MS. Risk of a thrombotic event after the 6-week postpartum period. *N Engl J Med.* 2014;370:1307–1315.
72. Ageno W, Gallus AS, Wittkowsky A, et al. Oral anticoagulant therapy: Antithrombotic Therapy and Prevention of Thrombosis, 9th ed: American College of Chest Physicians Evidence-Based Clinical Practice Guidelines. *Chest.* 2012;141:e44S–e88S.
73. Monagle P, Cuello CA, Augustine C, et al. American Society of Hematology 2018 guidelines for management of venous thromboembolism: Treatment of pediatric venous thromboembolism. *Blood Adv.* 2018;2:3292–3316. doi:10.1182/bloodadvances.2018024786.
74. Monagle P, Chan AK, Goldenberg NA, et al. Antithrombotic therapy in neonates and children: Antithrombotic Therapy and Prevention of Thrombosis, 9th ed: American College of Chest Physicians Evidence-Based Clinical Practice Guidelines. *Chest.* 2012;141:e737S–e801S.
75. Schulman S, Zondag M, Linkins L, et al. Recurrent venous thromboembolism in anticoagulated patients with cancer: Management and short-term prognosis. *J Thromb Haemost.* 2015;13:1010–1018.
76. Easaw JC, Shea-Budgell MA, Wu CM, et al. Canadian consensus recommendations on the management of venous thromboembolism in patients with cancer. Part 2: Treatment. *Curr Oncol.* 2015;22:144–155.
77. Farge D, Debourdeau P, Beckers M, et al. International clinical practice guidelines for the treatment and prophylaxis of venous thromboembolism in patients with cancer. *J Thromb Haemost.* 2013;11:56–70.
78. Clark NP. Low-molecular-weight heparin use in the obese, elderly, and in renal insufficiency. *Thromb Res.* 2008;123(Suppl 1):S58–S61.
79. Sanofi-Aventis. Lovenox Prescribing Information. 2018. Available at: http://products.sanofi.us/lovenox/lovenox.html. Accessed May 29, 2018.
80. Hanni Claudia, Petrovitch Elizabeth, Ali Mona, et al. Outcomes associated with apixaban vs warfarin in patients with renal dysfunction. *Blood Adv.* 2020;4:2366–2371. doi:10.1182/bloodadvances.2019000972.
81. Clark NP, Witt DM, Davies LE, et al. Bleeding, recurrent venous thromboembolism, and mortality risks during warfarin interruption for invasive procedures. *JAMA Intern Med.* 2015;175:1163–1168.
82. Douketis JD, Spyropoulos AC, Spencer FA, et al. Perioperative management of antithrombotic therapy: Antithrombotic Therapy and Prevention of Thrombosis, 9th ed: American College of Chest Physicians Evidence-Based Clinical Practice Guidelines. *Chest.* 2012;141:e326S–e350S.
83. Pollack CV Jr., Reilly PA, Eikelboom J, et al. Idarucizumab for dabigatran reversal. *N Engl J Med.* 2015;373:511–520.
84. Alexion Pharmaceuticals, Inc. Andexxa (coagulation factor Xa (recombinant), inactivated-zhzo) prescribing information. 2021. Available at: https://alexion.com/Documents/andexxa_uspi.pdf. Accessed October 30, 2021.
85. Yeh CH, Gross PL, Weitz JI. Evolving use of new oral anticoagulants for treatment of venous thromboembolism. *Blood.* 2014;124:1020–1028.
86. Agnelli G, Buller HR, Cohen A, et al. Apixaban for extended treatment of venous thromboembolism. *N Engl J Med.* 2013;368:699–708.
87. Weitz JI, Lensing AWA, Prins MH, et al. Rivaroxaban or aspirin for extended treatment of venous thromboembolism. *N Engl J Med.* 2017;376:1211–1222.
88. Portola Pharmaceuticals I. Betrixaban prescribing information. 2018. Available at: https://www.accessdata.fda.gov/drugsatfda_docs/label/2017/208383s000lbl.pdf. Accessed May 19, 2018.
89. Weitz JI, Pollack CV Jr. Practical management of bleeding in patients receiving non-vitamin K antagonist oral anticoagulants. *Thromb Haemost.* 2015;114.
90. Greinacher A, Thiele T, Selleng K. Reversal of anticoagulants: An overview of current developments. *Thromb Haemost.* 2015;113:931–942.
91. Tornkvist M, Smith JG, Labaf A. Current evidence of oral anticoagulant reversal: A systematic review. *Thromb Res.* 2018;162:22–31.
92. Ansell JE, Bakhru SH, Laulicht BE, et al. Use of PER977 to reverse the anticoagulant effect of edoxaban. *N Engl J Med.* 2014;371:2141–2142.
93. PfizerLabs. Fragmin Prescribing Information. 2018. Available at: http://labeling.pfizer.com/ShowLabeling.aspx?id=2293. Accessed May 19, 2018.
94. Park D, Southern W, Calvo M, et al. Treatment with dalteparin is associated with a lower risk of bleeding compared to treatment with unfractionated heparin in patients with renal insufficiency. *J Gen Intern Med.* 2016;31(12):182–187.
95. Blackmer AB, Oertel MD, Valgus JM. Fondaparinux and the management of heparin-induced thrombocytopenia: The journey continues. *Ann Pharmacother.* 2009;43:1636–1646.
96. Linkins LA, Dans AL, Moores LK, et al. Treatment and prevention of heparin-induced thrombocytopenia: Antithrombotic Therapy and Prevention of Thrombosis, 9th ed: American College of Chest Physicians Evidence-Based Clinical Practice Guidelines. *Chest.* 2012;141:e495S–e530S.
97. Crowther MA, Cook DJ, Albert M, et al. The 4Ts scoring system for heparin-induced thrombocytopenia in medical-surgical intensive care unit patients. *J Crit Care.* 2010;25:287–293.
98. Cuker A, Gimotty PA, Crowther MA, Warkentin TE. Predictive value of the 4Ts scoring system for heparin-induced thrombocytopenia: A systematic review and meta-analysis. *Blood.* 2012;120:4160–4167.
99. Bristol Myers Squibb C. Coumadin Prescribing Information. 2018. Available at: http://packageinserts.bms.com/pi/pi_coumadin.pdf. Accessed May 19, 2018.
100. Farrow GS, Delate T, McNeil K, et al. Vitamin K versus warfarin interruption alone in patients without bleeding and an international normalized ratio >10. *J Thromb Haemost.* 2020;18(5):1133–1140. doi:10.1111/jth.14772 32073738.
101. Cakebread HE, Knight HM, Gajendragadkar PR, Cooper JP. Warfarin-induced purple toe syndrome successfully treated with apixaban. *BMJ Case Rep.* 2014;2014doi:10.1136/bcr-2014-205320.
102. Clark NP, Delate T, Riggs CS, et al. Warfarin interactions with antibiotics in the ambulatory care setting. *JAMA Inter Med.* 2014;174:409–416.
103. Brighton TA, Eikelboom JW, Mann K, et al. Low-dose aspirin for preventing recurrent venous thromboembolism. *N Engl J Med.* 2012;367:1979–1987.
104. Becattini C, Agnelli G, Schenone A, et al. Aspirin for preventing the recurrence of venous thromboembolism. *N Engl J Med.* 2012;366:1959–1967.
105. Martin KA, Beyer-Westendorf J, Davidson BL, et al. Use of direct oral anticoagulants in patients with obesity for treatment and prevention of venous thromboembolism: Updated communication from the ISTH SSC Subcommittee on Control of Anticoagulation. *J Thromb Haemost.* 2021;19:1874–1882. 10.1111/jth.15358.
106. Al-Yaseen E, Wells PS, Anderson J, Martin J, Kovacs MJ. The safety of dosing dalteparin based on actual body weight for the treatment of acute venous thromboembolism in obese patients. *J Thromb Haemost.* 2005;3:100–102.
107. Parker SG, McGlone ER, Knight WR, Sufi P, Khan OA. Enoxaparin venous thromboembolism prophylaxis in bariatric surgery: A best evidence topic. *Int J Surg.* 2015;23:52–56.
108. Pirmohamed M, Burnside G, Eriksson N, et al. A randomized trial of genotype-guided dosing of warfarin. *N Engl J Med.* 2013;369:2294–2303.

109. Kimmel SE, French B, Kasner SE, et al. A pharmacogenetic versus a clinical algorithm for warfarin dosing. *N Engl J Med.* 2013;369:2283–2293.
110. Holbrook A, Schulman S, Witt DM, et al. Evidence-based management of anticoagulant therapy: Antithrombotic therapy and prevention of thrombosis, 9th ed: American College of Chest Physicians Evidence-Based Clinical Practice Guidelines. *Chest.* 2012;141:e152S–e184S.
111. Cuker A, Siegal DM, Crowther MA, Garcia DA. Laboratory measurement of the anticoagulant activity of the non-vitamin K oral anticoagulants. *J Am Coll Cardiol.* 2014;64:1128–1139.
112. Shore S, Ho PM, Lambert-Kerzner A, et al. Site-level variation in and practices associated with dabigatran adherence. *JAMA.* 2015;313:1443–1450.
113. Gladstone DJ, Geerts WH, Douketis J, Ivers N, Healey JS, Leblanc K. How to Monitor Patients Receiving Direct Oral Anticoagulants for Stroke Prevention in Atrial Fibrillation: A Practice Tool Endorsed by Thrombosis Canada, the Canadian Stroke Consortium, the Canadian Cardiovascular Pharmacists Network, and the Canadian Cardiovascular Society. *Ann Intern Med.* 2015;163:382–385.
114. Baglin T. What happens after venous thromboembolism? *J Thromb Haemost.* 2009;7(Suppl 1):287–290.

39

Stroke

Melody Ryan and Melissa A. Nestor

KEY CONCEPTS

1. Stroke can be either ischemic (87%) or hemorrhagic (13%) and the two types are treated differently.
2. Transient ischemic attacks (TIAs) require urgent intervention to reduce the risk of stroke, which is known to be highest in the first few days after TIA.
3. In patients with an ischemic stroke and a blood pressure (BP) <220/120 mm Hg without comorbid conditions requiring acute hypertensive treatment, the acute lowering of BP in the first 48 to 72 hours after stroke onset does not improve survival or the level of dependency; "permissive hypertension" (BP up to 220/120 mm Hg) is often allowed. In patients with intracranial hemorrhage and elevated systolic blood pressure (SBP) between 150 and 220 mm Hg, the acute lowering of SBP to lower than 140 mm Hg is safe and may improve functional outcomes.
4. Thrombectomy is strongly recommended for patients with anterior circulation arterial occlusion in the internal carotid artery (ICA) or the M1 segment of the middle cerebral artery (MCA) who are within 6 hours of symptom onset and may be considered in select patients within 6 to 24 hours of symptom onset.
5. In patients with ischemic stroke and 70% to 99% stenosis of the carotid artery, carotid endarterectomy or carotid stenting should be performed.
6. Early pharmacologic reperfusion (initiated less than 4.5 hours from symptom onset) with intravenous alteplase has been shown to improve functional ability after ischemic stroke.
7. Antiplatelet therapy is the cornerstone of antithrombotic therapy for the secondary prevention of noncardioembolic ischemic stroke.
8. Oral anticoagulation is recommended for the secondary prevention of cardioembolic stroke in moderate- to high-risk patients.
9. Elevated blood pressure is very common in ischemic stroke patients and treatment of hypertension in these patients is associated with a decreased risk of stroke recurrence.
10. Statin therapy is recommended for all ischemic stroke patients, regardless of baseline cholesterol, to reduce stroke recurrence.

BEYOND THE BOOK

Watch the video entitled "What is a stroke?" (https://youtu.be/QIAI6KOwKII">) in Khan Academy. This 11-minute video provides an overview of stroke and is useful to enhance understanding of stroke pathophysiology.

INTRODUCTION

Stroke is the leading cause of disability among adults and the fifth leading cause of death in the United States, behind cardiovascular disease, cancer, unintentional injuries, and chronic lower respiratory diseases.[1] Although the incidence of stroke has been trending downward, approximately 795,000 strokes occur annually, contributing to nearly 148,000 deaths each year.[2] Aggressive efforts to organize stroke care at the local and regional levels and increased utilization of evidence-based recommendations and national guidelines may have contributed to the improved outcomes.

EPIDEMIOLOGY

There are about 7.6 million stroke survivors in the United States and stroke is the leading cause of adult disability, with women having worse outcomes than men.[2] Owing in part to the need for expensive posthospitalization rehabilitation and nursing home care, the annual cost of stroke in the United States is estimated to be nearly $50 billion.[2]

Not all groups have benefitted equally from advances in care and prevention of stroke. Black Americans have stroke rates that are 1.5 times higher than White Americans; rates are up to four times higher at younger ages.[2] Genome-wide studies provide some evidence that part of this racial disparity is genetic. However, age-adjusted death rates for stroke are still 1.6 times higher for Black men compared to White men and 1.3 times higher for Black women compared to White women.[2] In addition, geographic disparity in stroke incidence exists, such that many southeastern states in the United States have stroke mortality rates 30% to 40% higher than the national average.[2] Lastly, case fatality due to hemorrhagic stroke has not declined in the past decade, with 30-day rates remaining around 46%.[2]

ETIOLOGY

1 Stroke is subdivided into either ischemic or hemorrhagic types (87% and 13%, respectively).[2] Hemorrhagic stroke includes subarachnoid hemorrhage (SAH) and intracerebral hemorrhage (ICH). SAH occurs when blood enters the subarachnoid space, which can occur due to trauma, rupture of an intracerebral aneurysm, or rupture of an arteriovenous malformation (AVM). ICH, however, occurs when bleeding occurs in the brain parenchyma itself, with

the formation of a hematoma within the brain. Uncontrolled hypertension is the most common cause for ICH, but antithrombotic therapy, cerebral amyloid angiopathy, and some drugs of abuse are also associated with ICH.[3] Hemorrhagic stroke, though less frequent in occurrence, has significantly higher mortality than ischemic stroke and is dependent on the quality and availability of critical care. In high-income countries, the mortality rate is 25% to 30%, but it is 30% to 48% in low- and middle-income countries.[3]

Ischemic stroke is caused by occlusion within a cerebral artery or emboli from a more proximal source resulting in occlusion of a cerebral artery. Atherosclerosis of large arteries, either intracranial or extracranial, as well as small artery damage, can give rise to ischemic stroke. Emboli can also arise centrally from the heart in patients with atrial fibrillation, valvular heart disease, or other prothrombogenic heart problems and are responsible for approximately 25% of ischemic stroke. While large artery atherosclerosis, small artery disease, and cardioembolism comprise the majority of ischemic stroke mechanisms, the cause of stroke is undetermined in some cases.[2] Determining the stroke mechanism (eg, cardiogenic mechanism vs other causes) is important when selecting the most appropriate long-term pharmacotherapy in stroke patients.

Risk Factors

Risk factors for ischemic stroke can be described as nonmodifiable or modifiable, with some risk factors more well-documented than others. The main risk factors of ischemic stroke are listed in Table 39-1.[4] The risk of stroke doubles for each decade older than 55 years. Men are at a higher risk of ischemic stroke than women at a younger age, but women have higher mortality and lifetime risk of ischemic stroke overall. Individuals who identify as Black, Asian-Pacific Islanders, or Hispanic have higher rates of death from ischemic stroke compared to those who identify as White.[4] Recommendations for ischemic stroke prevention focus on aggressive management of modifiable, well-documented risk factors.

The most common modifiable, well-documented risk factors for ischemic stroke include hypertension, cigarette smoking, diabetes, atrial fibrillation, and dyslipidemia. Hypertension is the most common risk factor, affecting up to one in three adults in the United States. Cardiac disease, including coronary artery disease, heart failure, left ventricular hypertrophy, and particularly atrial fibrillation, is also a very important risk factor. Atrial fibrillation increases an individual's risk of ischemic stroke to 5% to 20% per year, depending on concomitant comorbidities. Diabetes mellitus, dyslipidemia, and cigarette smoking contribute to atherogenic disease and increase the risk of ischemic stroke.[4]

TABLE 39-1 Risk Factors for Ischemic Stroke

Nonmodifiable Risk Factors
Age
Race
Sex
Low birth weight
Genetic factors
Modifiable, Well Documented
Cigarette smoking
Hypertension
Diabetes
Asymptomatic carotid stenosis
Dyslipidemia
Atrial fibrillation
Sickle cell disease
Poor diet
Obesity
Physical inactivity
Other cardiac diseases (coronary heart disease, heart failure, peripheral arterial disease)
Potentially Modifiable, Less Well Documented
Migraine
Metabolic syndrome
Drug and alcohol abuse
Inflammation and infection
Elevated lipoprotein (a)
Homocysteinemia
Patent foramen ovale
Sleep-disordered breathing

Data from Reference 4.

PATHOPHYSIOLOGY

Ischemic Stroke

Ischemic stroke is the manifestation of neurologic deficit due to occlusion of a cerebral artery, causing a reduction in cerebral blood flow and neuronal ischemia. The pathophysiologic mechanisms of ischemic stroke are depicted in Fig. 39-1. These arterial occlusions are most commonly due to artery-to-artery emboli, cardiac sources of emboli, or by vascular changes leading to occlusion of the cerebral artery itself. Cerebral blood flow is maintained at an average rate of 50 mL/100 g per minute over a wide range of blood pressure (mean arterial pressures of 50-150 mm Hg) by a process called cerebral autoregulation. Cerebral blood vessels dilate and constrict in response to changes in blood pressure, but this process can be impaired by atherosclerosis, chronic hypertension, and acute injury, such as stroke. Decreased cerebral blood flow due to arterial occlusion can lead to infarction of cerebral tissue. Surrounding a core area of infarct is tissue that is ischemic

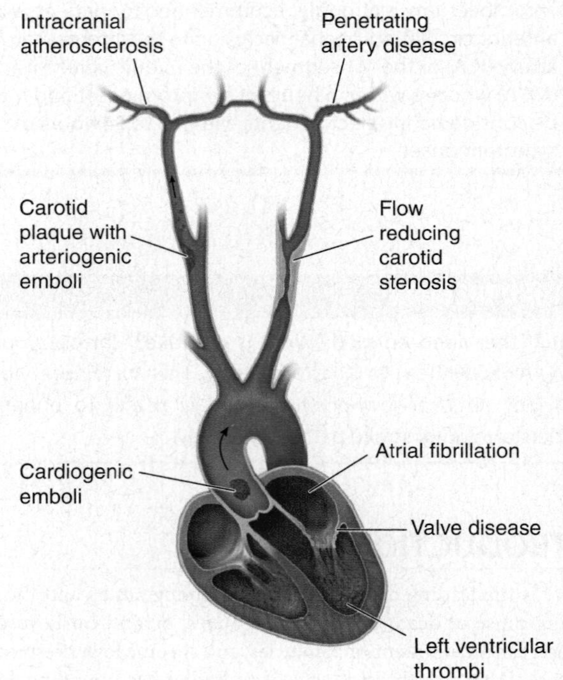

FIGURE 39-1 Pathophysiology of ischemic stroke. Diagram illustrating the three major mechanisms underlying ischemic stroke including occlusion of an intracranial vessel by an embolus that arises from a distant site (eg, cardiogenic embolus), in situ thrombosis of an intracranial vessel, typically affecting the small penetrating arteries, and hypoperfusion caused by flow-limiting stenosis of a major extracranial artery. *(Reproduced, with permission, from Smith WS, Johnston S, Hemphill J III. Ischemic stroke. In: Jameson J, Fauci AS, Kasper DL, et al., eds. Harrison's Principles of Internal Medicine. 20th ed. New York, NY: McGraw Hill; 2018.)*

CLINICAL PRESENTATION Stroke

General

- The patient may not be able to reliably report the history due to cognitive or language deficits. A reliable history may have to come from a family member or witness.

Symptoms

- The patient may complain of weakness on one side of the body, inability to speak, loss of vision, vertigo, and/or falling. Ischemic stroke is not usually painful, but some patients may complain of headache. Pain and headache, often severe, are more common with hemorrhagic stroke.

Signs

- The specific areas of neurologic deficit are determined by the area of the brain involved.
- Hemiparesis or monoparesis occurs commonly, as does a hemisensory deficit.
- Patients with vertigo and double vision are likely to have posterior circulation involvement.
- Aphasia is seen commonly in patients with anterior circulation strokes.
- Patients may also suffer from dysarthria, visual field deficits, and altered levels of consciousness.

Laboratory Tests

- In acute stroke, assessment of blood glucose, platelet count, and coagulation parameters (eg, prothrombin time, aPTT) are used to determine treatment eligibility.
- Tests for hypercoagulable states (protein C/S deficiency, antiphospholipid antibody) should be done only when the cause of the stroke cannot be determined based on the presence of well-known risk factors.

Other Diagnostic Tests

- CT scan of the head will reveal an area of hyperdensity (bright) in patients with hemorrhage and will be normal or hypodense (dark) in patients with infarction. It may take 24 hours before the CT scan will reveal the area of infarction.
- MRI of the head will reveal areas of ischemia with higher resolution and an MRI with diffusion-weighted imaging (DWI) will reveal an evolving infarct within minutes of stroke onset.
- Vascular imaging with CTA is recommended in patients with endovascular treatment indications. CTA can identify both acute treatment candidacy as well as identify intracranial and extracranial arterial stenosis.
- An ECG can help determine whether the patient is presenting in atrial fibrillation.
- TTE can identify cardiac valve abnormalities or wall-motion abnormalities as sources of emboli to the brain. A "bubble study" in which a solution with tiny bubbles is injected intravenously can be done to look for an intra-arterial shunt indicating an atrial-septal defect or a patent foramen ovale. The bubbles can be seen moving through the heart chambers during the TTE.
- In patients unable to undergo CTA, carotid Doppler (CD) and transcranial Doppler (TCD) can be used to determine extracranial carotid artery stenosis and intracranial artery stenosis.

but may maintain membrane integrity and is referred to as the *ischemic* penumbra.[5] This penumbra is the area of brain tissue that is potentially salvageable with urgent pharmacologic and endovascular interventions in acute ischemic stroke.

Insufficient oxygen supply in ischemic tissue leads to adenosine triphosphate (ATP) depletion and anaerobic metabolism. This results in an accumulation of intracellular lactate, sodium, and water, which may cause cytotoxic edema and eventual cell lysis. There is also an influx of intracellular calcium leading to activation of lipases and proteases that degrade proteins and release free fatty acids from cellular membranes. Additionally, excitatory amino acids, such as glutamate and aspartate, are released in ischemic tissue that perpetuate neuronal damage and production of damaging prostaglandins, leukotrienes, and reactive oxygen species. These processes occur within 2 to 3 hours from the onset of ischemia and, ultimately, lead to cellular apoptosis and necrosis.[5]

Hemorrhagic Stroke

Hemorrhagic stroke causes neuronal damage by a variety of mechanisms and timelines. In patients with ICH, the hematoma causes primary injury and mechanical compression of the brain parenchyma itself. Early hematoma expansion, which may occur in up to 38% of patients within 3 hours of ICH onset, is associated with worsened functional outcome and increased mortality. The highest rates of mortality are associated with a low Glasgow Coma Score (GCS) on presentation (GCS 3-4), ICH volume greater than 30 cc (mL), intraventricular extension, brain stem location, and age greater than 80.[6] Secondary mechanisms of injury in ICH patients are mediated by subsequent inflammatory response, cerebral edema, and damage from blood product degradation.[3]

CLINICAL PRESENTATION

The term stroke describes patients with an episode of neurologic dysfunction caused by focal cerebral, spinal, or retinal infarction. The syndrome of arterial ischemia with transient symptoms (<24 hours) and without evidence of infarction is a transient ischemic attack (TIA). Appropriate patient history obtainment helps determine the nature of symptom onset and duration of neurologic dysfunction. The location of the central nervous system (CNS) injury and its reference to a specific arterial distribution in the brain are determined through neurologic examination and confirmed by imaging studies such as computed tomography (CT) and magnetic resonance imaging (MRI). The main arterial supply to the cerebral hemispheres is illustrated in Figs. 39-2 and 39-3. Vascular imaging with computed tomography angiography (CTA) can aid clinicians in determining the cause of stroke and whether urgent mechanical intervention is necessary.

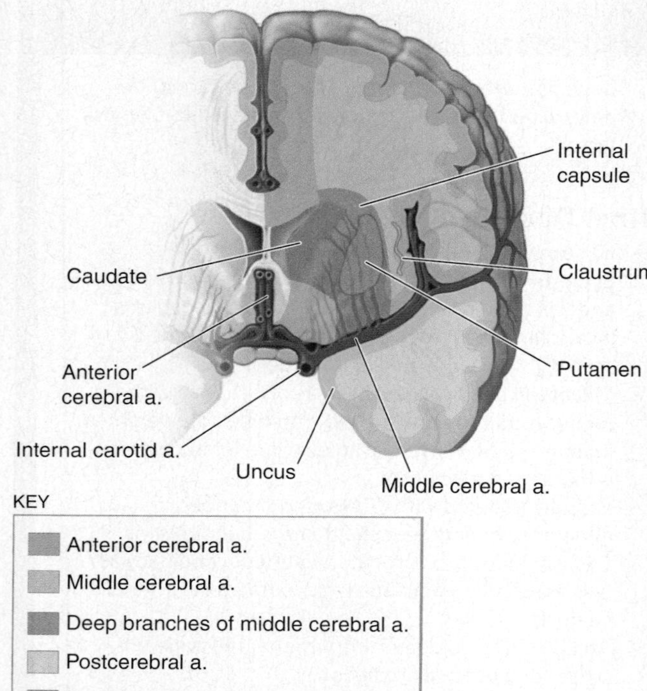

FIGURE 39-2 Diagram of a cerebral hemisphere in coronal section showing the territories of the major cerebral vessels branching from the internal carotid arteries. *(Reproduced, with permission, from Smith WS, Johnston S, Hemphill J III. Cerebrovascular Diseases. In: Jameson J, Fauci AS, Kasper DL, et al., eds. Harrison's Principles of Internal Medicine. 20th ed. New York, NY: McGraw Hill; 2018.)*

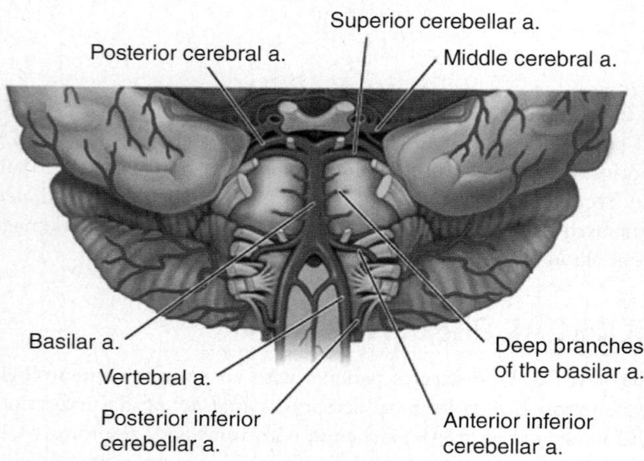

FIGURE 39-3 Diagram of the posterior circulation, showing the intracranial vertebral arteries forming the basilar artery that gives off the anterior inferior cerebellar, superior cerebellar, and posterior cerebral arteries. The posterior inferior cerebellar artery arises from each of the vertebral segments. The majority of brainstem blood flow arises from numerous deep branches of the basilar artery that penetrate directly into the brainstem. *(Reproduced, with permission, from Smith WS, Johnston S, Hemphill J III. Cerebrovascular diseases. In: Jameson J, Fauci AS, Kasper DL, et al., eds. Harrison's Principles of Internal Medicine. 20th ed. New York, NY: McGraw Hill; 2018.)*

TREATMENT

Desired Outcomes

The goals of treatment of acute stroke are to (a) minimize the ongoing neurologic injury in the acute setting to reduce mortality and long-term disability, (b) prevent complications secondary to immobility and neurologic dysfunction, and (c) prevent stroke recurrence. Primary prevention of stroke is described in the Chapter 30 (Hypertension), Chapter e31 (Acute Hypertensive Crisis), and Chapter 32 (Dyslipidemia).[4]

General Approach to Treatment

2 3 Patients with presumed acute stroke should have a CT scan performed urgently to identify the type of injury (eg, ischemic or hemorrhagic), provided respiratory and cardiac indices are stable. Ischemic stroke patients presenting within hours of symptom onset should be evaluated for pharmacologic and mechanical reperfusion therapy. Patients with TIA require urgent assessment and intervention to reduce the risk of stroke, which is highest in the first few days after TIA.[4]

In the absence of comorbid conditions, in patients with an acute ischemic stroke and uncontrolled hypertension with a BP <220/120 mm Hg, acutely lowering BP in the first 48 to 72 hours does not prevent death or improve the level of dependency. Therefore, "permissive hypertension" is often part of routine care in these patients. However, for patients who are candidates for alteplase or those with comorbid conditions, such as aortic dissection, acute myocardial infarction, pulmonary edema, or hypertensive encephalopathy, treatment of acute hypertension may be required. If BP is treated, the use of short-acting and easily titrated agents, such as labetalol or nicardipine/clevidipine, is preferred. See Chapter e31, Acute Hypertensive Crisis. Table 39-2 outlines current recommendations regarding the management of arterial hypertension in patients with acute ischemic stroke. In patients with ICH and elevated BP, the acute lowering of SBP to 140 mm Hg has been shown to be safe and may improve functional outcome.[6]

Once the patient is out of the hyperacute phase (eg, first 24 hours), management is focused on preventing worsening of stroke, minimizing complications, and secondary prevention. The acute phase of the stroke includes the first week after the event.[4]

Nonpharmacologic Therapy

Ischemic Stroke

4 To reperfuse ischemic brain tissue, endovascular intervention and thrombectomy is recommended by the American Heart Association (AHA)/American Stroke Association (ASA) since 2015 based on data from several clinical trials.[7] Thrombectomy is strongly recommended for patients with anterior circulation arterial occlusion in the ICA or the M1 segment of the MCA who are within 6 hours of symptom onset and may be considered in select patients within 6 to 24 hours of symptom onset. Patients with ICA and M1 MCA arterial occlusions and symptom onset within 24 hours may be candidates for endovascular intervention if imaging studies suggest a significant area of salvageable penumbra is present. The benefit of mechanical thrombectomy is less clear in patients with posterior circulation occlusions and should be considered in a case-by-case basis.[7] The availability of this mechanical intervention for stroke has greatly increased the importance of early vascular diagnostic imaging followed by rapid transfer to centiers with interventional capabilities and escalation of care in patients with these emergent large vessel occlusions.

Large infarcts of the MCA are often devastating and, in patients without recanalization via pharmacologic or mechanical intervention, are associated with high rates of morbidity and

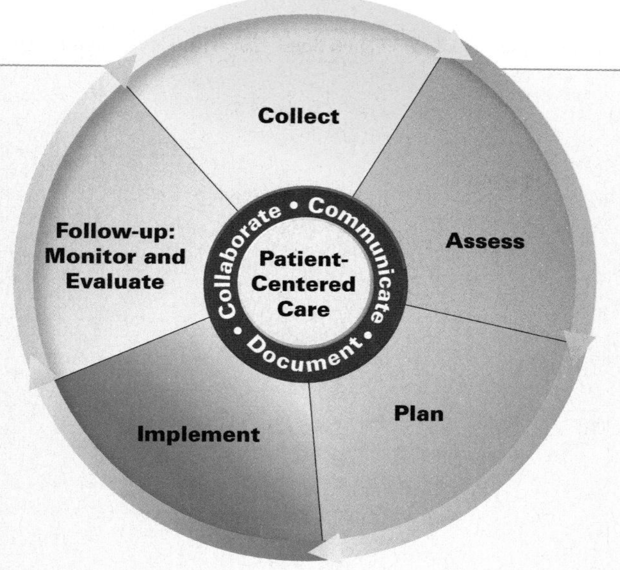

Patient Care Process for Acute Ischemic Stroke

Collect

- Patient characteristics (eg, age, sex, race)
- Patient medical history (personal and family)
- Social history (eg, tobacco/ethanol use)
- Current medications including nonprescription aspirin/nonsteroidal anti-inflammatory drug (NSAID) use, herbal products, dietary supplements, and prior antiplatelet and anticoagulant medication use
- Medication allergies
- Symptoms (time of onset, duration)
- Objective data
    - Blood pressure (BP), heart rate, respiratory rate, height, weight
    - Labs including hemoglobin, platelets, serum creatinine, activated partial thromboplastin time (aPTT), prothrombin time, blood glucose, troponin
    - Noncontrast computed tomography (CT) scan, magnetic resonance imaging (MRI), and/or computed tomography angiography (CTA) may be needed
    - Neurologic examination (eg, National Institutes of Health Stroke Scale [NIHSS] score)
    - Electrocardiogram (ECG) and, in some patients, transthoracic echocardiogram (TTE)

Assess

- Hemodynamic stability (eg, systolic blood pressure [SBP] <110 mm Hg, diastolic blood pressure [DBP] <185 mm Hg, if candidate for tissue plasminogen activator candidate; otherwise, BP less than 220/120 mm Hg; O_2-sat >94% [0.94]; temperature <38°C [100.4°F])
- Blood glucose (<60 mg/dL [3.7 mmol/L] or >180 mg/dL [10.0 mmol/L] should be treated)
- Presence of active bleeding and/or bleeding risk factors (Table 39-6)
- Patient's candidacy for tissue plasminogen activator treatment (Table 39-2) or thrombectomy
- Presence of dysphagia (swallowing disorder)

Plan

- Aspirin within 24 to 48 hours unless contraindicated; delay for 24 hours if the patient has been given tissue plasminogen activator
- Antiplatelet drug therapy regimen including specific medication(s), dose, frequency, and duration OR oral anticoagulant, if the patient has atrial fibrillation (see Table 39-2)
- Evaluation for carotid endarterectomy or carotid stenting
- Prophylaxis for venous thromboembolism, if immobile
- Nutritional plan; if the patient has dysphagia, nutrition via nasogastric tube or percutaneous gastrostomy tube
- Treat and manage stroke risk factors (Table 39-2) (eg, BP control, dyslipidemia, diabetes)
- Monitoring parameters including efficacy (eg, stroke symptoms) and safety (eg, signs and symptoms of bleeding [all antiplatelets and oral anticoagulants], headache [dipyridamole]); frequency and timing of follow-up
- Patient education (eg, the purpose of treatment, dietary and lifestyle modification, invasive procedures, drug-specific information, medication administration)
- Self-monitoring for stroke recurrence, the occurrence of bleeding, and when to seek emergency medical attention
- Referrals to other providers when appropriate (eg, physical therapist, occupational therapist, behavioral health, dietician)

Implement*

- Provide patient education regarding all elements of the treatment plan
- Use motivational interviewing and coaching strategies to maximize adherence
- Schedule follow-up

Follow-up: Monitor and Evaluate

- Improvement of stroke symptoms; neurological examination
- Presence of adverse drug reactions (eg, bleeding [all medications], gastrointestinal upset [aspirin], headache [dipyridamole], cerebral edema, seizures)
- Patient adherence to treatment plan using multiple sources of information
- Adherence to recommended follow-up appointments (eg, neurology, physical therapy)
- Assess for poststroke depression

**Collaborate with patient, caregivers, and other healthcare professionals.*

TABLE 39-2 Blood Pressure Treatment Guidelines in Stroke

Recommendation	Class (Strength) of Recommendation[a]	Level (Quality) of Evidence[b]
Ischemic Stroke with Alteplase Treatment		
• Pre-alteplase: lower BP to SBP <185 mm Hg and DBP <110 mm Hg • Post-alteplase: maintain SBP <180 mm Hg and DBP <105 mm Hg for 24 hours	I	B-NR
Ischemic Stroke Without Alteplase Treatment		
• Treatment benefit uncertain/not recommended unless BP >220/120 mm Hg	IIb	C-EO
• If comorbid conditions (eg, acute coronary event, acute heart failure, aortic dissection, symptomatic intracranial hemorrhage, preeclampsia/eclampsia) are present that require acute lowering of BP, lowering BP by 15% is probably safe)	I	C-EO
Ischemic Stroke with Mechanical Thrombectomy Without Fibrinolytic Treatment		
• It is reasonable to maintain BP ≤185/110 mm Hg before the procedure	IIb	C-EO
Intracranial Hemorrhage		
• Treatment is reasonable for ICH patients with SBP >220 mm Hg	IIb	C
• For ICH patients with SBP 150-220 mm Hg, acute lowering of SBP to 140 mm Hg is safe	I	A
Pharmacologic Options for Blood Pressure Lowering in Acute Stroke		
• Labetalol 10-20 mg IV over 1-2 minutes, may repeat • Nicardipine 5 mg/hr IV, titrate up by 2.5 mg/hr every 5-15 minutes, maximum 15 mg/hr • Clevidipine 1-2 mg/hr IV, titrate by doubling the dose every 2-5 minutes, maximum 21 mg/hr • Other agents to consider: hydralazine, enalaprilat, nitroprusside IV infusion, labetalol IV infusion	IIb	C-EO

ASCVD, atherosclerotic cardiovascular disease; BMI, body mass index; GLP1, glucagon-like peptide 1; HbA1c, hemoglobin A1c; ICH, intracerebral hemorrhage; INR, international normalized ratio; IV, intravenous; LDL, low-density lipoprotein; NIHSS, National Institutes of Health Stroke Scale.

Data from References 6 and 7.

[a]Class (strength) of recommendation : I, strong; IIa, moderate; IIb, weak; III, no benefit (moderate); 3, harm (strong).

[b]Level (quality) of evidence: A, high-quality evidence from more than 1 randomized clinical trial, meta-analyses of high-quality randomized clinical trials, or one or more randomized clinical trials corroborated by high-quality registry studies; B-R (randomized), moderate-quality evidence from one or more randomized clinical trials or meta-analyses of moderate-quality randomized clinical trials; B-NR (nonrandomized), moderate-quality evidence from one or more well-designed, well-executed nonrandomized studies, observational studies, or registry studies or meta-analyses of such studies; C-LD (limited data), randomized or nonrandomized observational or registry studies with limitations or design or execution, meta-analyses of such studies, or physiological or mechanistic studies in human subjects; C-EO (expert opinion), consensus of expert opinion based on clinical experience.

mortality. Decompressive hemicraniectomy is a surgical procedure that can be done to reduce intracranial pressure, typically due to cerebral edema, and can reduce mortality and improve functional outcome. In patients under 60 years of age with unilateral MCA infarcts and significant cerebral edema, surgical intervention with decompressive craniectomy has been shown to reduce mortality by almost 50% and improve favorable neurologic outcomes at 1 year. This surgical intervention can be considered for patients over the age of 60 but the likelihood of favorable neurologic outcome is less robust. In patients with cerebellar infarction and significant swelling, surgical decompression can be lifesaving. For all ischemic stroke patients coordinated care with a multidisciplinary approach to assessment and early rehabilitation is effective in reducing overall disability due to stroke.[7]

5 For the secondary prevention of ischemic stroke, carotid endarterectomy of an ulcerated and/or stenotic carotid artery is a very effective way to reduce stroke incidence and recurrence in patients with 70% to 99% stenosis if performed in centers with low operative morbidity and mortality.[8] Carotid stenting is a less invasive alternative that can be effective in reducing recurrent stroke risk when combined with aspirin and clopidogrel therapy.[8] However, it is associated with a higher periprocedural stroke rate.[8]

A patent foramen ovale (PFO) occurs when the septum between the right and left atria fails to close after birth. A PFO is present in 20% to 25% of adults; but in patients with stroke from unknown causes, 40% to 50% have a PFO.[9] The PFO can be closed surgically. People who benefit most from this surgery are 18 to 60 years of age with nonlacunar ischemic strokes of undetermined cause.[8]

Other nonpharmacological approaches for secondary stroke prevention include diet modification, exercise, smoking cessation, avoidance of environmental tobacco smoke, moderation of alcohol consumption, and avoidance of stimulants such as amphetamines and cocaine. A Mediterranean-type diet and, in patients with hypertension, reducing sodium intake is recommended. Exercise plans should take any mobility considerations into account. Alcohol consumption should be no greater than two drinks per day for men or one drink per day for women.[8]

Hemorrhagic Stroke

SAH often arises from a ruptured intracranial aneurysm or AVM and intervention as early as possible with either surgical clipping or endovascular coiling of the vascular anomaly reduces the risk of rebleeding and improves mortality.[6] For patients with cerebellar ICH and neurologic deterioration, brainstem compression, and/or hydrocephalus from ventricular obstruction, early surgical intervention and hematoma removal is recommended. For patients with cerebral ICH, the usefulness of surgical hematoma evacuation or use of minimally invasive clot evacuation is not well established. Ventricular drainage with an extraventricular drain (EVD) is reasonable in patients with hydrocephalus causing decreased consciousness.[6]

Temperature Management

Fever worsens outcomes in patients with both hemorrhagic and ischemic stroke types. Identification of the source of fever and management is recommended to maintain patients within normothermia ranges. Pharmacologic and nonpharmacologic interventions can be considered and applied. Data are limited to support induced hypothermia; it should be done only in a controlled, clinical trial setting.[6,7]

Pharmacologic Therapy

Ischemic Stroke

Acute Treatment The stroke council of the ASA has created and published guidelines that address the management of acute ischemic stroke.[7] For acute treatment, the only two pharmacologic agents with class I recommendations are alteplase initiated within 4.5 hours of stroke onset and aspirin started within 24 to 48 hours of stroke onset (Table 39-3).[7]

Alteplase 6 Early pharmacologic reperfusion (initiated less than 4.5 hours from symptom onset) with IV alteplase has been a mainstay of acute pharmacologic treatment to improve functional ability after ischemic stroke as compared to no intervention.[7] Alteplase, or recombinant

TABLE 39-3 Recommendations for Pharmacotherapy of Ischemic Stroke

Acute Treatment of Ischemic Stroke[7]		
Recommendation	**Class (Strength) of Recommendation[a]**	**Level (Quality) of Evidence[b]**
Alteplase 0.9 mg/kg IV (maximum 90 mg), 10% as a bolus with the remainder given over 1 hour in selected patients		
• Within 3 hours of onset	I	A
• Between 3 and 4.5 hours of onset	I	B-R
Tenecteplase 0.25 mg/kg IV bolus (maximum 25 mg) may be a reasonable alternative to alteplase for patients who are also eligible to undergo mechanical thrombectomy	IIb	B-R
Tenecteplase 0.4 mg/kg IV bolus (maximum 40 mg) has not been proved to be superior or non-inferior to alteplase but may be considered as an alternative to alteplase in patients with minor neurological impairment and no major intracranial occlusion	IIb	B-R
Aspirin 160-325 mg daily started within 48 hours of onset	I	A
Aspirin 81 mg daily and clopidogrel 75 mg daily for 21 days may be effective in reducing recurrent stroke in patients who do not receive IV alteplase and present with minor, non-cardioembolic stroke (NIHSS ≤ 3)	I	A
Ticagrelor is not recommended over aspirin for treatment of patients with minor acute stroke	III	B-R
Acute Treatment of Spontaneous Intracerebral Hemorrhage[6]		
Patients with a severe coagulation factor deficiency or severe thrombocytopenia should receive appropriate factor replacement therapy or platelets	I	C
Prophylactic antiseizure medication is not recommended	III	B

Secondary Prevention of Ischemic Stroke			
Stroke Etiology	**Recommendation**	**Class (Strength) of Recommendation[a]**	**Level (Quality) of Evidence[b]**
Noncardioembolic	Antiplatelet therapy[7]		
	• Aspirin 50-325 mg daily	I	A
	• Aspirin 25 mg + extended-release dipyridamole 200 mg twice daily	I	A
	• Clopidogrel 75 mg daily	I	A
Cardioembolic (especially atrial fibrillation)	Anticoagulant therapy[7]		
	• Vitamin K antagonist (warfarin) (INR = 2-3)	I	A
	• Apixaban 5 mg twice daily	I	A
	• Dabigatran 150 mg twice daily	I	A
	• Edoxaban 60 mg daily	I	A
	• Rivaroxaban 20 mg daily	I	A
Atrial fibrillation without moderate to severe mitral stenosis or a mechanical heart valve	Apixaban, dabigatran, endoxaban, or rivaroxaban is preferred over warfarin	I	B-R
Risk Factor	**Recommendation[10]**	**Class (Strength) of Recommendation[a]**	**Level (Quality) of Evidence[b]**
LDL cholesterol >100 mg/dL (2.59 mmol/L) with no known coronary heart disease, and no major cardiac sources of embolism	Atorvastatin 80 mg daily	I	A
Patients with atherosclerotic disease	Statins and ezetimibe, if needed; goal LDL cholesterol <70 mg/dL (1.81 mmol/L)	I	A
Very high risk (stroke + another major ASCVD or stroke + multiple high-risk conditions)[c] already taking statins at maximally tolerated dose and ezetimibe, but who still have LDL-cholesterol >70 mg/dL (1.81 mmol/L)	Proprotein convertase subtilisin/kexin type 9 inhibitor therapy	IIa	B-NR

(continued)

TABLE 39-3 Recommendations for Pharmacotherapy of Ischemic Stroke *(Continued)*

Acute Treatment of Ischemic Stroke[7]

Recommendation		Class (Strength) of Recommendation[a]	Level (Quality) of Evidence[b]
Fasting triglycerides 135-499 mg/dL (1.53-5.64 mmol/L) and LDL cholesterol 41-100 mg/dL (1.06-2.59 mmol/L) who are on moderate- or high-intensity statin therapy, with HbA1c <10% (86 mmol/mol), and no history of pancreatitis, atrial fibrillation, or severe heart failure	Icoaspent ethyl 2 g twice daily	IIa	B-R
Fasting triglycerides ≥500 mg/dL (5.65 mmol/L)	Identify and address causes of hypertriglyceridemia; implement a very low-fat diet, avoid refined carbohydrates and alcohol; omega-3 fatty acids; fibrate therapy, if needed to prevent acute pancreatitis	IIa	B-NR
BP >130/80	BP reduction, goal <130/80 mm Hg	I	B-R
Patients who smoke	Smoking cessation with or without drug therapy	I	A
Men who drink >2 alcoholic drinks per day or women who drink >1 alcoholic drink per day	Reduce or eliminate alcohol consumption	I	B-NR
Patients who use stimulants and patients with infective endocarditis in the context of intravenous drug use	Cessation of use of substance	I	C-EO
Diabetes - treatment goal	Goal HbA1c ≤7% (53 mmol/mol)	I	A
Diabetes - drug therapy selection	Treatment with glucose-lowering agents with proven cardiovascular benefit (metformin + GLP1 receptor agonist therapy or sodium-glucose cotransporter 2 inhibitor) regardless of baseline HbA1C	I	B-R
Prediabetes, particularly with BMI ≥35 kg/m², <60 years, women with a history of gestational diabetes	Metformin 850 mg twice daily	IIb	B-R

[a]Class (strength) of recommendation: I, strong; IIa, moderate; IIb, weak; III, no benefit (moderate); 3, harm (strong).

[b]Level (quality) of evidence: A, high-quality evidence from more than 1 randomized clinical trial, meta-analyses of high-quality randomized clinical trials, or one or more randomized clinical trials corroborated by high-quality registry studies; B-R (randomized), moderate-quality evidence from one or more randomized clinical trials or meta-analyses of moderate-quality randomized clinical trials; B-NR (nonrandomized), moderate-quality evidence from one or more well-designed, well-executed nonrandomized studies, observational studies, or registry studies or meta-analyses of such studies; C-LD (limited data), randomized or nonrandomized observational or registry studies with limitations or design or execution, meta-analyses of such studies, or physiological or mechanistic studies in human subjects; C-EO (expert opinion), consensus of expert opinion based on clinical experience.

[c]Very high risk of future ASCVD events includes a history of multiple major ASCVD events or 1 major ASCVD event and multiple high-risk conditions. Major ASCVD events are history of ischemic stroke, acute coronary syndrome within the past 12 months, history of myocardial infarction, symptomatic peripheral arterial disease. High-risk conditions include: age ≥65 years; heterozygous familial hypercholesterolemia; history of coronary artery bypass surgery or percutaneous coronary intervention outside of the major ASCVD events; diabetes; hypertension; chronic kidney disease; current smoking.

ASCVD, atherosclerotic cardiovascular disease; BMI, body mass index; GLP1, glucagon-like peptide 1; HbA1c, hemoglobin A1c; ICH, intracerebral hemorrhage; INR, international normalized ratio; IV, intravenous; LDL, low-density lipoprotein; NIHSS, National Institutes of Health Stroke Scale.

tissue plasminogen activator (rt-PA), is a fibrinolytic agent that exhibits a moderate binding preference for fibrin and facilitates the conversion of plasminogen to plasmin, leading to degradation of fibrin clots. Alteplase has a short half-life (approximately 4 minutes). The total dose for acute ischemic stroke is 0.9 mg/kg (maximum 90 mg), 10% administered as an intravenous (IV) bolus over 1 minute, and the remaining 90% given as an IV infusion over 60 minutes.[7]

The first large trial demonstrating the effectiveness of IV alteplase in the treatment of ischemic stroke was published in 1995. A subsequent study demonstrated improved functional outcome at 3 months in patients with acute ischemic stroke treated with alteplase between 3 and 4.5 hours of stroke symptom onset when compared with placebo (52.4% vs 45.2%).[7] Based on these data, the AHA/ASA guidelines extended the window for alteplase from 3 hours to up to 4.5 hours from symptom onset. However, there may be diminished benefit of alteplase in patients presenting within 3 to 4.5 hours from symptom onset and severe stroke (NIHSS>25 or evidence of more than one-third of MCA territory infarct on initial imaging).[7] Consequently, delays in alteplase therapy should be minimized and early administration prioritized since this approach is associated with improved outcomes.

Alteplase use is associated with a high risk for bleeding, including ICH. Therefore, adherence to the guideline-recommended protocol is essential for achieving a positive outcome and minimizing the risk. This protocol can be summarized as (a) stroke team activation, (b) brain imaging study (eg, CT scan), (c) treatment as early as possible within 4.5 hours of symptom onset, (d) meeting inclusion and exclusion criteria (Table 39-4), (e) administration of alteplase 0.9 mg/kg total dose (maximum dose of 90 mg), 10% given as a bolus over 1 minute and the remaining 90% given as an IV infusion over 1 hour, (f) avoidance of antithrombotic therapy (anticoagulant or antiplatelet) for 24 hours after alteplase, and (g) close patient monitoring for BP, neurologic status, and hemorrhage. Endovascular intervention is not a contraindication to alteplase and patients eligible for alteplase should receive pharmacologic treatment in addition to mechanical thrombectomy.[7]

Tenecteplase Tenecteplase is a modified form of tissue plasminogen activator with protein substitutions that yield a higher degree of fibrin specificity and a longer half-life than alteplase. Unlike alteplase, tenecteplase can be administered as a single, rapid IV bolus dose. While tenecteplase is FDA-approved for the management of

TABLE 39-4 Inclusion and Exclusion Criteria for Alteplase Use in Acute Ischemic Stroke

Inclusion Criteria
Age ≥18 years
Clinical diagnosis of ischemic stroke with neurologic deficit
Time of symptom onset well established to be <4.5 hours from treatment initiation
Contraindications
History of intracranial hemorrhage
History of ischemic stroke within prior 3 months
Symptoms/imaging consistent with subarachnoid hemorrhage or acute intracerebral hemorrhage
Current use of direct thrombin inhibitors or direct factor Xa inhibitors in prior 48 hours
Use of treatment-dose low molecular weight heparin in prior 24 hours
Infective endocarditis
Intra-axial, intracranial neoplasm
Aortic arch dissection
Active internal bleeding or coagulopathy (platelets <100,000/mm³ [100 × 10⁹/L], INR>1.7, aPTT>40s, PT>15s)
Severe head trauma in prior 3 months
Gastrointestinal malignancy or bleeding within prior 21 days
Warnings/Use Clinical Judgment
Unruptured/unsecured AVM or aneurysm >10 mm
Major surgery or nonhead trauma
History of bleeding diathesis
Extensive regions of clear hypoattenuation on initial CT scan

aPTT, activated partial thromboplastin time; AVM, arteriovenous malformation; CT, computed tomography; INR, international normalized ratio; PT; prothrombin time.

Data from Reference 7.

patients with acute ST-elevation myocardial infarction, use for ischemic stroke remains off-label. Tenecteplase has been studied in a variety of acute ischemic stroke populations and is specifically mentioned in the 2019 update to the AHA/ASA guidelines. Tenecteplase 0.4 mg/kg (maximum 40 mg), given as an IV bolus, may be considered as an alternative to alteplase for patients with ischemic stroke and mild neurologic impairment (class IIb recommendation).[7] It may also be reasonable to choose an IV bolus of tenecteplase 0.25 mg/kg (maximum 25 mg) over alteplase for patients who are also eligible to undergo mechanical thrombectomy (class IIb recommendation).[7] Ongoing studies may further define the role of tenecteplase in patients with acute ischemic, identify the optimal dose, and support stronger recommendations in the future.

Aspirin Early aspirin therapy, within 24 to 48 hours from symptom onset, should be given to patients with acute ischemic stroke in the absence of aspirin allergy or other contraindications. For patients receiving alteplase, aspirin and other antithrombotics are generally held for 24 hours after alteplase administration to reduce the risk of hemorrhage.[7]

Early use of aspirin in ischemic stroke patients is recommended by the AHA/ASA guidelines to reduce the long-term risk of death and disability.[7] Data are limited to describe acute use of non-aspirin antiplatelet agents in the acute stroke phase, apart from combination therapy regimens described below. However, using an alternative antiplatelet agent in patients with acute ischemic stroke who have a severe allergy or contraindication to aspirin may be reasonable.[7]

Aspirin exerts its antiplatelet effect by irreversibly inhibiting cyclooxygenase (COX)-1, which, in platelets, prevents the conversion of arachidonic acid to thromboxane A2 (TXA2), a powerful vasoconstrictor and stimulator of platelet aggregation. The onset of the antiplatelet effect of aspirin is less than 60 minutes, and platelets remain impaired for their life span (5-7 days) after exposure to aspirin.[11] Aspirin also inhibits COX-2 in a dose-dependent manner, leading to decreased prostacyclin (PGI2) activity in vascular smooth muscle.[12] There is probably a point at which lower doses of aspirin do not completely block TXA2, and studies indicate that the lowest effective dose may be in the range of 75 mg/day.[12] Upper gastrointestinal (GI) discomfort and bleeding are the most common adverse effects of aspirin and have been shown to be dose-related. The risk of major bleeding is 43% higher in patients treated with aspirin compared to patients not receiving aspirin. The risk of bleeding is dose-dependent and increases with increasing age; therefore, the upper limit of the aspirin dose is between 300 mg and 325 mg.[7]

Some patients either have or develop high on-treatment platelet reactivity ("aspirin resistance") and can require higher doses or twice daily dosing to achieve the desired antiplatelet effect.[13] Several factors contribute to this effect, including aging, diabetes, hyperlipidemia, smoking, chronic kidney disease, and drug-drug interactions (eg, nonsteroidal anti-inflammatory drugs).[14] Genetic polymorphisms, including those influencing activity of COX-1, COX-2, glycoprotein IIb/IIIa receptors, and adenosine diphosphate (ADP) receptors, may contribute to aspirin resistance.[15] Despite the growing evidence linking aspirin resistance to worse outcomes in patients with stroke, routine testing for aspirin resistance is not recommended.

Blood Pressure Management In general, patients with acute ischemic stroke commonly present with elevated or normal BP. However, hypotension and hypovolemia, if present, should be corrected to maintain systemic perfusion and end organ function. For patients with elevated BP who are otherwise eligible for alteplase, the treatment of hypertension to a goal SBP of less than 185 mm Hg and diastolic BP of less than 110 mm Hg is recommended before thrombolytic administration. While data are limited, it is also reasonable to maintain blood pressure less than 185/110 mm Hg for patients undergoing mechanical thrombectomy. For patients not requiring IV thrombolytic therapy or endovascular intervention, "permissive hypertension," allowing BP to rise as high as 220/120 mm Hg for the first 48 to 72 hours, is often implemented as early initiation of antihypertensive therapy does not prevent death or dependency. For patients with comorbid conditions requiring BP lowering, a reduction of 15% is reasonable. See Table 39-3 for a summary of these recommendations and pharmacotherapeutic options.[7] When treating hypertension in acute ischemic stroke, it is typical to use IV drugs with a faster time to onset and ability to titrate to patient response. Calcium channel blocker infusions, such as nicardipine and clevidipine, are often preferred. Labetalol can be administered as an IV bolus dose or as a continuous infusion. In patients with refractory hypertension, there may be a role for last-line agents such as sodium nitroprusside to achieve BP goals.

Therapeutic Anticoagulation Use of therapeutic anticoagulation (eg, unfractionated heparin or low-molecular-weight heparin) is not routinely recommended in the early phase of acute ischemic stroke treatment. The clinical benefit of therapeutic anticoagulation in the setting of nonocclusive intraluminal thrombus in acute stroke is limited. Restricted use on a case-by-case basis or in a clinical trial setting may be considered. Anticoagulation for non-stroke indications (eg, venous thromboembolism prophylaxis or treatment) must be weighed against the risk of hemorrhagic conversion in patients with acute ischemic stroke.[7] Patients with immobility after stroke should be receive either mechanical or pharmacologic venous thromboembolism prophylaxis. Drug selection, dosing, and timing of pharmacologic venous thromboembolism prophylaxis will depend on patient factors and conconimitant treatment for stroke.

Secondary Prevention (7) Antiplatelet therapy is the cornerstone of antithrombotic therapy for the secondary prevention of ischemic stroke and should be used in noncardioembolic strokes. Aspirin, extended-release dipyridamole plus aspirin, clopidogrel, and ticagrelor are all recommended for secondary stroke prevention.[4] In patients with atrial fibrillation, oral anticoagulation with apixaban, dabigatran, edoxaban, rivaroxaban, or warfarin is recommended for secondary stroke prevention.[4] Other pharmacotherapy recommended for secondary prevention of stroke includes treatment of hypertension and statin therapy. Current recommendations regarding the acute treatment and secondary prevention of stroke are given in Table 39-2.

Antiplatelet Agents All patients who have had an acute ischemic stroke or TIA should receive long-term antithrombotic therapy for secondary prevention.[4] In patients with noncardioembolic stroke, this will be some form of antiplatelet therapy. In a comprehensive meta-analysis, antiplatelet therapy reduced the odds of a second stroke by 16% to 41% in patients with previous stroke.[16] While aspirin is the antiplatelet agent with the most data supporting its use, there is also evidence to support using clopidogrel and the combination product extended-release dipyridamole plus aspirin as alternative first-line agents for secondary stroke prevention.[8] For patients already taking aspirin at the time of a noncardioemoblic ischemic stroke or TIA, there is no evidence that increasing the dose of aspirin is more effective at preventing additional strokes.[8]

Clopidogrel Clopidogrel exerts its antiplatelet effect by inhibiting the ADP pathway of platelet aggregation through antagonism of the purinergic receptor P2Y, G-protein coupled 12 ($P2Y_{12}$) receptor.[12,17] This effect causes an alteration of the platelet membrane and interference with the membrane–fibrinogenic interaction leading to a blocking of the platelet glycoprotein IIb/IIIa receptor. In the absence of a loading dose, the maximal antiplatelet effect is delayed for 3 to 7 days.

Clopidogrel is a prodrug and requires activation by the cytochrome P450 isoenzyme 2C19 (CYP2C19) to achieve its antiplatelet effect. There are polymorphisms of various alleles encoding for this enzyme, with *1 being the wild type, *17 leading to increased metabolism, and *2 and *3 causing decreased metabolism. Thus, individuals with one copy of *2 or *3 are classified as intermediate metabolizers and those with two copies of *2 or *3 or one copy of each (*2/*3) are termed poor metabolizers, leading to diminished antiplatelet activity.[18] Poor metabolizers are found in about 2% of Caucasians, 4% of African Americans, and 14% of Chinese.[18] Consequently, the Clinical Pharmacogenetics Implementation Consortium and the Dutch Pharmacogenetics Working Group of the Royal Dutch Association for the Advancement of Pharmacy both suggest pharmacogenetic testing prior to using clopidogrel.[18] However, current AHA/ASA guidelines for acute treatment of stroke do not suggest doing so.[8] Medications that inhibit CYP2C19 may also reduce the antiplatelet activity of clopidogrel. Omeprazole and esomeprazole both inhibit CYP2C19 and their use should be avoided in patients taking clopidogrel. Opioids slow gastric emptying, delaying and decreasing absorption, leading to reduced antiplatelet activity and, potentially, decreased efficacy.[19]

In a study of patients with atherothrombotic disorders (eg, ischemic stroke, myocardial infarction, or peripheral arterial disease), clopidogrel was slightly more effective than aspirin in preventing vascular events and had a similar incidence of adverse effects.[20] The tolerability of clopidogrel 75 mg/day is at least as good as medium-dose (325 mg/day) aspirin and there is less GI bleeding.[20] Clopidogrel is associated with an increased risk of diarrhea and rash, but discontinuation rates due to adverse effects are similar to those with aspirin 325 mg/day (5.3% and 6%, respectively).[20]

Extended-Release Dipyridamole Plus Aspirin Dipyridamole, in high doses, is thought to inhibit phosphodiesterase, increasing intracellular cyclic adenosine monophosphate (cAMP) and cyclic guanosine monophosphate (cGMP), leading to inhibition of platelet activation.[12] Early studies of the role of dipyridamole in stroke prevention failed to show a benefit over aspirin alone. However, 25% of the patients who received combination dipyridamole and aspirin discontinued the therapy early, many due to adverse drug reactions. The discontinuation due to headache was more than threefold higher (10%) than the aspirin-alone group (3%).[21] Another study demonstrated similar efficacy in preventing recurrent stroke between the combination of extended-release dipyridamole and aspirin and clopidogrel.[22] However, clopidogrel was better tolerated with less bleeding and headache. Despite carefully educating and coaching patients on managing headache, discontinuation due to headache was six times higher in the extended-release dipyridamole plus aspirin group (5.9% vs 0.9%) compared to clopidogrel.[22] The extended-release formulation of dipyridamole is important in that it allows twice-daily administration. The use of immediate-release dipyridamole in combination with regular aspirin, in order to reduce costs, is unproven and should be discouraged.

Ticagrelor Ticagrelor is a direct-acting $P2Y_{12}$ receptor inhibitor.[17] Ticagrelor (loading dose of 180 mg then 90 mg twice daily for 90 days) was compared to aspirin (300 mg loading dose then 100 mg daily 90 days) in a large clinical trial of patients with noncardioembolic stroke not treated with alteplase.[23] Ticagrelor did not demonstrate superiority to aspirin in this trial.[23] However, in a subgroup analysis of patients with an atherosclerotic cause of stroke, there was a 32% lower risk of secondary stroke within 90 days in patients treated with ticagrelor.[24] Despite this subgroup analysis, ticagrelor is not FDA-approved for secondary stroke prevention.

Dual Antiplatelet Therapy The combination of two or more antiplatelet medications for secondary stroke prevention may be an option for select patients (Table 39-5). The combination of clopidogrel and aspirin has been the most studied dual antiplatelet strategy. A systematic review determined that short-term use of dual antiplatelet therapy (≤90 days) was associated with a significantly lower risk of recurrent stroke without an accompanying risk of major bleeding.[25] However, in longer-term studies (>90 days), the dual therapy was not associated with a reduced number of strokes but did increase the risk of major bleeding. Therefore, use of dual antiplatelet therapy with aspirin and clopidogrel for longer than 90 days is not recommended.[8]

Ticagrelor (180 mg loading dose then 90 mg twice daily for 30 days) in combination with aspirin (300-325 mg loading dose then 75-100 mg daily) has been compared to aspirin alone in patients with mild-moderate noncardioembolic stroke.[26] Fewer patients in the dual therapy group had stroke or death in the first 30 days compared to the aspirin-only group. However, the overall level of disability was not different between the groups, and the incidence of severe bleeding, including ICH, was increased in the dual therapy group. A subgroup analysis of patients at higher risk for recurrent stroke found rates of stroke and death were lower in the combination therapy group compared to aspirin alone while no difference in severe bleeding was observed between the groups.[27] Consequently, that the use of ticagrelor and aspirin together for secondary stroke prevention is only recommended for patients with minor stroke or TIA with more than 30% stenosis of an ipsilateral major intercranial artery; combination therapy should be limited to a duration of 30 days.[8]

The positive results of dual antiplatelet therapy led researchers to investigate triple antiplatelet therapy. One trial compared the combination of aspirin, sustained-release dipyridamole, and clopidogrel to a "guideline group" which received either clopidogrel or aspirin and sustained-release dipyridamole. This trial was stopped early because of a doubling of the risk of major bleeding in the triple therapy group. There was no difference in risk of recurrent stroke between the groups.[28] Therefore, the use of triple antiplatelet therapy is not recommended.[8]

Oral Anticoagulants 8 Oral anticoagulation is the treatment of choice for the prevention of stroke in patients with atrial fibrillation and atrial flutter.[4,29] Patients with atrial fibrillation and a recent history of stroke or TIA are among the highest risk groups for stroke recurrence. However, there is a significant risk of bleeding

TABLE 39-5 Dual Antiplatelet Recommendations for Patients with Noncardioembolic Ischemic Stroke or TIA

Patient Sub-type	Recommendation	Class (Strength) of Recommendation[a]	Level (Quality) of Evidence[b]
Minor stroke (NIHSS score ≤3)or high-risk TIA (ABCD2 score ≥4)[c]	Aspirin and clopidogrel should be initiated within 7 days (ideally within 12-24 hours). Continue for 21-90 days followed by single agent antiplatelet therapy	I	A
Recent (<30 days) minor stroke or TIA attributable to 70-99% stenosis of a major intracranial artery	Aspirin and clopidogrel 75 mg daily for up to 90 days followed by single agent antiplatelet therapy	IIa	B-NR
Recent (within 24 hours) minor stroke or high-risk TIA and concomitant ipsilateral >30% stenosis of a major intracranial artery	Ticagrelor 90 mg twice a day may be added to aspirin for up to 30 days	IIb	B-NR

[a]Class (strength) of recommendation: I, strong; IIa, moderate; IIb, weak; III, no benefit (moderate); III, harm (strong).

[b]Level (quality) of evidence: A, high-quality evidence from more than 1 randomized clinical trial, meta-analyses of high-quality randomized clinical trials, or one or more randomized clinical trials corroborated by high-quality registry studies; B-R (randomized), moderate-quality evidence from one or more randomized clinical trials or meta-analyses of moderate-quality randomized clinical trials; B-NR (nonrandomized), moderate-quality evidence from one or more well-designed, well-executed nonrandomized studies, observational studies, or registry studies or meta-analyses of such studies; C-LD (limited data), randomized or nonrandomized observational or registry studies with limitations or design or execution, meta-analyses of such studies, or physiological or mechanistic studies in human subjects; C-EO (expert opinion), consensus of expert opinion based on clinical experience.

[c]The ABCD2 score is a clinical prediction rule used to determine the risk for stroke soon after a TIA. Score 1 point each for age ≥60 years, blood pressure ≥140/90 mm Hg, speech disturbance, unilateral weakness, 10-59 minute duration, diabetes and 2 points for duration ≥60 minutes.

NIHSS, National Institutes of Health Stroke Scale; TIA, transient ischemic attack.

Data from Reference 8.

TABLE 39-6 HAS-BLED Score for Assessing Bleeding Risk with Oral Anticoagulants

HAS-BLED Symbol	Risk Factor	Score
H	**H**ypertension (SBP >160 mm Hg)	1
A	**A**bnormal renal or liver function	1
S	Prior **S**troke	1
B	Prior major **B**leeding or **B**leeding predisposition	1
L	**L**abile INRs (in therapeutic range <60% of time)	1
E	**E**lderly (age >65 years)	1
D	**D**rugs of abuse or excessive alcohol use	1

HAS-BLED score >2 associated with clinically relevant and major bleeding.

SBP, systolic blood pressure, INR, international normalized ratio.

Data from References 4 and 30.

with anticoagulation. Thus, a stroke risk stratification tool known as CHA_2DS_2-VASc has been developed to determine the patient's risk of stroke (see Chapter 40 "The Arrhythmias"). CHA_2DS_2-VASc scores greater than zero should receive oral anticoagulation therapy.[4] Several risk stratification tools have been developed to evaluate bleeding and determine bleeding risk. HAS-BLED is a simple tool that is widely used.[30] A HAS-BLED score >2 indicates a high risk for bleeding and should be accompanied by more intensive patient monitoring (Table 39-6).

In patients with atrial fibrillation, adjusted-dose warfarin reduces stroke risk by 62% when compared to placebo and by 36% when compared to aspirin.[31] When using warfarin, targeting an international normalized ratio (INR) of 2 to 3 prevents stroke with the lowest bleeding risk; therefore, a target INR of 2 to 3 is recommended for the secondary prevention of stroke.[4,7,29] In settings of atrial fibrillation with mechanical heart valves or moderate to severe mitral stenosis, warfarin should be used.[8]

Direct-acting oral anticoagulants (DOAC), including direct thrombin inhibitors (dabigatran) and direct factor Xa inhibitors (rivaroxaban, edoxaban, and apixaban), have significant advantages over warfarin in terms of ease of dosing and less food and drug interactions. In addition, all four agents have been shown to be as effective, and in some cases, superior to warfarin in reducing stroke risk with reduced rates of serious hemorrhage.[29]

TABLE 39-7 Direct-acting Oral Anticoagulant Dosing Adjustments Required for Renal Impairment

Direct-acting Oral Anticoagulant	Usual Oral Dosing for Stroke Prevention in Atrial Fibrillation	Dosing Adjustments
Apixaban	5 mg twice daily	2.5 mg twice daily in patients with at least two high-risk characteristics below: Age ≥80 years Body weight ≤60 kg Serum creatinine ≥1.5 mg/dL (133 μmol/L)
Dabigatran	150 mg twice daily	75 mg orally twice daily if creatinine clearance 15-30 mL/min (0.25-0.50 mL/s)
Edoxaban	60 mg daily	30 mg orally daily if creatinine clearance is 15-50 mL/min (0.25-0.83 mL/s)
Rivaroxaban	20 mg daily with food	15 mg orally daily with evening meal if creatinine clearance is ≤50 mL/min (0.83 mL/s)

Before using a DOAC, the patient's renal function must be evaluated and the dose adjusted if significant renal impairment is present (Table 39-7). Patients with creatinine clearance less than 15 mL/min (0.25 mL/s) or who require hemodialysis, either warfarin or apixaban, are preferred.[29] Additionally, edoxaban should not be given to patients with creatinine clearances above 95 mL/min because the risk of stroke is increased compared to warfarin.[29] There is limited information on the use of these agents in patients with a body mass index over 40 kg/m^2.[32] However, emerging data suggest that apixaban and rivaroxaban may be the best options for patients with a body weight over 120 kg or body mass index over 40 kg/m^2.[33]

The timing of oral anticoagulant initiation has been in question due to the risk of hemorrhagic conversion of the infarcted area. Guidelines suggest for patients with a low risk of hemorrhagic conversion, anticoagulation can begin 2 to 14 days after the stroke. However, in patients with a high risk of hemorrhagic conversion, waiting at least 14 days is recommended.[8]

Blood Pressure Management 9 Elevated BP is very common in ischemic stroke patients, and treatment of hypertension in these patients is associated with a decreased risk of stroke recurrence.[8] Current guidelines have the following recommendations for BP control after ischemic stroke to prevent future strokes:

- Adults with previously treated hypertension who experience a stroke or TIA should be restarted on antihypertensive treatment after the first few days of the index event to reduce the risk of recurrent stroke and other vascular events.
- For adults with hypertension who experience a stroke or TIA, treatment with a thiazide diuretic, angiotensin-converting enzyme (ACE) inhibitor, or angiotensin II receptor blocker is useful.
- Adults not previously treated for hypertension who experience a stroke or TIA and have an average BP of 130/80 mm Hg or higher should be prescribed antihypertensive treatment a few days after the index event to reduce the risk of recurrent stroke and other vascular events.
- For adults who experience a stroke or TIA, a BP goal of less than 130/80 mm Hg is recommended.[8,34]

Cholesterol Management 10 The statins have been shown to reduce the risk of stroke by approximately 30% in patients with coronary artery disease and elevated plasma lipids.[8] Patients with ischemic stroke without known heart disease but who have LDL cholesterol over 100 mg/dL (2.59 mmol/L) should be given atorvastatin 80 mg daily to reduce the risk of stroke recurrence.[8] Patients with ischemic stroke or TIA who have atherosclerotic cardiovascular disease (ASCVD) should be given lipid-lowering therapy with a high-intensity statin (and ezetimibe, if necessary) to reach a goal of LDL cholesterol of less than 70 mg/dL (1.81 mmol/L).[8] In very high-risk patients (multiple major atherosclerotic cardiovascular events or one major atherosclerotic cardiovascular event and multiple high-risk conditions) who are taking maximally tolerated statins and ezetimibe with LDL cholesterol ≥70 mg/dL (1.81 mmol/L), a proprotein convertase subtilisin/kexin type 9 (PCSK9) inhibitor may be considered.[8]

Hypertriglyceridemia has recently been recognized as a risk factor for ASCVD but lowering triglycerides with extended-release niacin or fibrates has not been shown to change cardiovascular outcomes. In contrast, adding icosapent ethyl 2 g twice daily to statin therapy has been shown to reduce major adverse cardiovascular events, including stroke, in patients with fasting triglycerides of 135 to 499 mg/dL (1.53 to 5.64 mmol/L) and LDL cholesterol of 41 to 100 mg/dL (1.06 to 2.59 mmol/L).[35] Therefore, icosapent ethyl is recommended for these patients with provided they have HbA1c <10% (86 mmol/mol) and no history of pancreatitis, atrial fibrillation, or severe heart failure.[8] When patients have fasting triglycerides of 500 mg/dL (5.65 mmol/L) or more, non-pharmacologic efforts to reduce them should be initiated along with fibrate therapy, if needed.[8]

Hemorrhagic Stroke

Acute Treatment The stroke council of the AHA/ASA has published guidelines on the management of spontaneous ICH in 2015.[6] While the usefulness of pharmacologic interventions is limited in this stroke type, the management of hypertension and reversal of coagulopathy in anticoagulant-associated ICH should be considered.

Blood Pressure Management Hypertension in patients with hemorrhagic stroke increases the risk of hematoma expansion. For patients with ICH presenting with a SBP above 220 mm Hg, aggressive lowering of BP with continuous IV infusion medications is reasonable. Clinical trials have demonstrated that acute lowering of SBP to a goal of 140 mm Hg is safe and may be effective at improving functional outcomes.[6] For patients with SAH due to aneurysm rupture, targeting an SBP less than 160 mm Hg is reasonable in the time period from symptom onset to aneurysm obliteration.[6] Refer to Table 39-3 for a summary of these recommendations and pharmacologic treatment options.

Anticoagulation Reversal When ICH occurs in a patient on anticoagulants, the use of reversal agents to correct the medication-induced coagulopathy should be considered. For patients on warfarin with elevated INR, reversal with vitamin K, typically IV, in combination with a four-factor prothrombin complex concentrate is recommended. Fresh frozen plasma can be used in place of a prothrombin complex concentrate, if necessary, but is not preferred.[6] Idarucizumab may be considered for reversing the effect of dabigatran specifically.[36] Factor Xa inhibitors, such as rivaroxaban and apixaban, may be reversed with andexanet alfa[37] (Table 39-8).

TABLE 39-8 Selected Anticoagulant Reversal

Drug	First-Line Reversal Recommendation	Alternate Treatment
Warfarin	Vitamin K 10 mg IV ×1 -and- 4-Factor Prothrombin Complex Concentrate (4PCC) INR 2 to <4: 25 units/kg, max 2,500 units INR 4-6: 35 units/kg, max 3,500 units INR >6: 50 units/kg, max 5,000 units	Vitamin K 10 mg IV ×1 -and- Fresh Frozen Plasma (FFP) 10-15 mL/kg
Dabigatran	Idarucizumab 5 gm IV ×1	Hemodialysis 4PCC 50 units/kg
Rivaroxaban ≤10 mg	Andexanet alfa 400 mg IV Bolus at rate of 30 mg/min, followed by 4 mg/min IV infusion up to 120 minutes	4PCC 50 units/kg
Rivaroxaban >10 mg or unknown dose	If <8 hours since last dose or unknown time andexanet alfa 800 mg IV bolus at rate of 30 mg/min, followed by 8 mg/min IV infusion up to 120 minutes If ≥8 hours since last dose Andexanet alfa 400 mg IV Bolus at rate of 30 mg/min, followed by 4 mg/min IV infusion up to 120 minutes	4PCC 50 units/kg
Apixaban ≤5 mg	Andexanet alfa 400 mg IV Bolus at rate of 30 mg/min, followed by 4 mg/min IV infusion up to 120 minutes	4PCC 50 units/kg

(continued)

TABLE 39-8 Selected Anticoagulant Reversal (*Continued*)

Drug	First-Line Reversal Recommendation	Alternate Treatment
Apixaban >5 mg or unknown dose	If <8 hours since last dose or unknown time Andexanet alfa 800 mg IV bolus at rate of 30 mg/min, followed by 8 mg/min IV infusion up to 120 minutes If ≥8 hours since last dose Andexanet alfa 400 mg IV Bolus at rate of 30 mg/min, followed by 4 mg/min IV infusion up to 120 minutes	4PCC 50 units/kg
Edoxaban	Andexanet alfa not studied	4PCC 50 units/kg

FFP, fresh frozen plasma; IV, intravenous; 4PCC, 4-factor prothrombin complex concentrate; INR, international normalized ratio.

TABLE 39-9 Monitoring Stroke Therapy in Hospitalized Patients

Drug	Adverse Effect	Monitoring Parameters	Comments
Alteplase and tenecteplase	Bleeding	Neurologic examination, blood pressure	Every 15 minutes × 1 hour; every 30 minutes × 6 hours; every 1 hour × 17 hours; every shift after
Aspirin	Bleeding		Daily
Clopidogrel	Bleeding		Daily
Extended-release dipyridamole plus aspirin	Headache, bleeding		Daily
Ticagrelor	Bleeding, bradycardia, dyspnea	Heart rate, respiratory rate	Bleeding daily, heart rate and respiratory rate as clinically indicated
Direct-acting oral anticoagulants	Bleeding		Daily
Warfarin	Bleeding	PT/INR, hemoglobin, hematocrit	Daily

INR, international normalized ratio; PT, prothrombin time.

EVALUATION OF THERAPEUTIC OUTCOMES

Patients with acute stroke should be monitored intensely for the development of neurologic worsening (recurrence or extension of stroke), complications (venous thromboembolism or infection), and adverse effects from pharmacologic or nonpharmacologic interventions. The most common reasons for deterioration in a stroke patient are (a) extension of the original lesion—ischemic or hemorrhagic—in the brain, (b) development of cerebral edema and elevated intracranial pressure, (c) hypertensive emergency, (d) infection (urinary and respiratory most common), (e) venous thromboembolism (deep vein thrombosis and pulmonary embolism), (f) electrolyte abnormalities and cardiac rhythm disturbances (can be associated with brain injury), and (g) recurrent stroke.

The approach to monitoring drug therapy in the hospitalized stroke patient is summarized in Table 39-9. The plan should be customized for individual patients based on the etiology of the stroke, their comorbidities, and ongoing disease processes.

For survivors of noncardioembolic strokes, approximately 3% to 4% per year will experience another stroke. One-third to one-half of these strokes occur while patients are on antiplatelet therapy to prevent stroke.[38] None of these agents reduces stroke risk to zero; some of the most important causes of breakthrough strokes are nonadherence, inappropriate dosing, reduced absorption, increased metabolism, drug-drug interactions, and genetic polymorphisms.[38] The healthcare practitioner is in a position to impact several of these factors. Nonadherence can have a root cause in a lack of understanding of therapy, adverse effects of the therapy, or the number of medications on discharge, among other factors.

CONCLUSION

Treatment of stroke requires a team approach to provide an accurate diagnosis to guide treatment and select therapies proven to improve outcomes. Careful patient selection for pharmacologic and nonpharmacologic therapies is paramount. Monitoring treatment helps assure goals of therapy are met.

ABBREVIATIONS

ACE	angiotensin-converting enzyme
ADP	adenosine diphosphate
AHA	American Heart Association
aPTT	activated partial thromboplastin time
ATP	adenosine triphosphate
AVM	arteriovenous malformation
ASA	American Stroke Association
ASCVD	atherosclerotic cardiovascular disease
BP	blood pressure
cAMP	cyclic adenosine monophosphate
CD	carotid Doppler
cGMP	cyclic guanosine monophosphate
COX	cyclooxygenase
CNS	central nervous system
CT	scan computed tomography
CTA	computed tomography angiography
CYP2C19	cytochrome P450 isoenzyme 2C19
DBP	diastolic blood pressure
DCI	delayed cerebral ischemia
DOAC	direct-acting oral anticoagulants
DWI	diffusion-weighted imaging
ECG	electrocardiogram
EVD	external ventricular drainage
FFP	fresh frozen plasma
GCS	Glasgow Coma Scale
GI	gastrointestinal
GLP1	glucagon-like peptide 1
HgA1c	hemoglobin A1c
ICA	internal carotid artery
ICH	intracerebral hemorrhage
INR	international normalized ratio
IPC	intermittent pneumatic compression
IV	intravenous
LDL	low-density lipoprotein
MCA	middle cerebral artery
MI	myocardial infarction

MRI	magnetic resonance imaging
mRS	modified Rankin score
NIHSS	National Institutes of Health Stroke Scale
NSAID	nonsteroidal anti-inflammatory drug
NVAF	nonvalvular atrial fibrillation
PFO	patent foramen ovale
P2Y12	purinergic receptor P2Y, G-protein coupled 12
PCC	prothrombin complex concentrate
PCSK9	proprotein convertase subtilisin/kexin type 9
PGI2	prostacyclin
PT	prothrombin time
SAH	subarachnoid hemorrhage
SBP	systolic blood pressure
TCD	transcranial Doppler
TEE	transesophageal echocardiography
TIA	transient ischemic attack
TTE	transthoracic echocardiography
TXA2	thromboxane A2

REFERENCES

1. Heron M. Deaths: Leading causes for 2018. *Natl Vital Stat Rep.* 2021;70(4):1–115. 34029179.
2. Virani SS, Alonso A, Aparicio HJ, et al. Heart disease and stroke statistics—2021 update. *Circulation.* 2021;143:e254–e743. 10.1161/cir.0000000000000950.
3. Unnithan AKA, Mehta P. *Hemorrhagic Stroke.* Treasure Island, FL: StatPearls Publishing; 2021. https://www.ncbi.nlm.nih.gov/books/NBK559173/.
4. Meschia JF, Bushnell C, Boden-Albala B, et al. Guidelines for the primary prevention of stroke: A statement for health professionals from the American Heart Association/American Stroke Association. *Stroke.* 2014;45: 3754–3832.
5. Feske SK. Ischemic stroke. *Am J Med.* 2021;134:1457–1464. 10.1016/j.amjmed.2021.07.027.
6. Hemphill JC, Greenberg SM, Anderson CS, et al. Guidelines for the management of spontaneous intracerebral hemorrhage: A guideline for healthcare professionals from the American Heart Association/American Stroke Association. *Stroke.* 2015;46:2032–2060.
7. Powers WJ, Rabinstein AA, Ackerson T, et al. Guidelines for the early management of patients with acute ischemic stroke: 2019 update to the 2018 guidelines for the early management of acute ischemic stroke: A guideline for healthcare professionals from the American Heart Association/American Stroke Association. *Stroke.* 2019;50:e344–e418. 10.1161/str.0000000000000211.
8. Kleindorfer DO, Towfighi A, Chaturvedi S, et al. 2021 Guideline for the prevention of stroke in patients with stroke and transient ischemic attack: A guideline from the American Heart Association/American Stroke Association. *Stroke.* 2021;52:e364–e467. 10.1161/str.0000000000000375.
9. Mojadidi MK, Zaman MO, Elgendy IY, et al. Cryptogenic stroke and patent foramen ovale. *J Am Coll Cardiol.* 2018;71:1035–1043. 10.1016/j.jacc.2017.12.059.
10. Kernan WN, Viera AJ, Billinger SA, et al. Primary care of adult patients after stroke: a scientific statement from the American Heart Association/American Stroke Association. *Stroke.* 2021;52:e558–e571. 10.1161/str.0000000000000382.
11. Serebruany VL, Malinin AI, Sane DC. Rapid platelet inhibition after a single capsule of Aggrenox: Challenging a conventional full-dose aspirin antiplatelet advantage? *Am J Hematol.* 2003;72:280–281.
12. Iqbal AM, Lopez RA, Hai O. *Antiplatelet Medications.* Treasure Island, FL: StatPearls Publishing; 2021. https://www.ncbi.nlm.nih.gov/books/NBK537062/.
13. Alhazzani A, Venkatachalapathy P, Padhilahouse S, et al. Biomarkers for antiplatelet therapies in acute ischemic stroke: A clinical review. *Front Neurol.* 2021;12:667234. 10.3389/fneur.2021.667234.
14. Wiśniewski A. Multifactorial background for a low biological response to antiplatelet agents used in stroke prevention. *Medicina.* 2021;57:59. 10.3390/medicina57010059.
15. Cai G, Zhou W, Lu Y, et al. Aspirin resistance and other aspirin-related concerns. *Neurol Sci.* 2016;37:181–189.
16. Del Giovane C, Boncoraglio GB, Bertù L, et al. Antiplatelet drugs for secondary prevention in patients with ischemic stroke or transient ischemic attack: A systematic review and network meta-analysis. *BMC Neurol.* 2021;21:319. 10.1186/s12883-021-02341-2.
17. Kubisa MJ, Jezewski MP, Gasecka A, et al. Ticagrelor—toward more efficient platelet inhibition and beyond. *Ther Clin Risk Manag.* 2018;14: 129–140.
18. Dean L, et al. Clopidogrel therapy and CYP2C19 genotype. *Medical Genetics Summaries.* Bethesda, MD: National Center for Biotechnology Information; 2018.
19. Bristol-Myers Squibb/Sanofi Pharmaceuticals Partnership. *Plavix Product Information.* Bridgewater, NJ: Author; 2021.
20. CAPRIE Steering Committee. A randomized, blinded trial of clopidogrel versus aspirin in patients at risk of ischaemic events (CAPRIE). *Lancet.* 1995;348:1329–1339.
21. Diener HC, Cunha L, Forbes C, et al. European Stroke Prevention Study 2: Dipyridamole and acetylsalicylic acid in the secondary prevention of stroke. *J Neurol Sci.* 1996;143:1–13.
22. Sacco RL, Diener HC, Yusuf S, et al. Aspirin and extended-release dipyridamole versus clopidogrel for recurrent stroke. *N Engl J Med.* 2008;359:1238–1251.
23. Johnston SC, Amarenco P, Albers GW, et al. Ticagrelor versus aspirin in acute stroke or transient ischemic attack. *New Engl J Med.* 2016;375: 35–43.
24. Amarenco P, Albers GW, Denison H, et al. Efficacy and safety of ticagrelor versus aspirin in acute stroke or transient ischaemic attack of atherosclerotic origin: A subgroup analysis of SOCRATES, a randomised, double-blind, controlled trial. *Lancet Neurol.* 2017;16: 301–310.
25. Brown DL, Levine DA, Albright K, et al. Benefits and risks of dual versus single antiplatelet therapy for secondary stroke prevention: A systematic review for the 2021 guideline for the prevention of stroke in patients with stroke and transient ischemic attack. *Stroke.* 2021;52:e468–e479. 10.1161/str.0000000000000377.
26. Johnston SC, Amarenco P, Denison H, et al. Ticagrelor and aspirin or aspirin alone in acute ischemic stroke or TIA. *N Engl J Med.* 2020;383:207–217. 10.1056/nejmoa1916870.
27. Amarenco P, Denison H, Evans SR, et al. Ticagrelor added to aspirin in acute nonsevere ischemic stroke or transient ischemic attack of atherosclerotic origin. *Stroke.* 2020;51:3504–3513. 10.1161/strokeaha.120.032239.
28. Bath PM, Woodhouse LJ, Appleton JP, et al. Triple versus guideline antiplatelet therapy to prevent recurrence after acute ischaemic stroke or transient ischaemic attack: The TARDIS RCT. *Health Technol Assess.* 2018;22(48):1–76.
29. January CT, Wann LS, Calkins H, et al. 2019 AHA/ACC/HRS focused update of the 2014 AHA/ACC/HRS guideline for the management of patients with atrial fibrillation: A report of the American College of Cardiology/American Heart Association task force on clinical practice guidelines and the Heart Rhythm Society in collaboration with the Society of Thoracic Surgeons. *Circulation.* 2019;140:e125–e151. 10.1161/cir.0000000000000665.
30. Pisters R, Lane DA, Nieuwlaat R, de Vos CB, Crijns HJ, Lip GY. A novel user friendly score (HAS-BLED) to assess 1-year risk of major bleeding in patients with atrial fibrillation: The Euro Heart Survey. *Chest.* 2010;138:1093–1100.
31. Hart RG, Benavente O, McBride R, et al. Antithrombotic therapy to prevent stroke in patients with atrial fibrillation. *Ann Intern Med.* 1999;131:492–501. 10.7326/0003-4819-131-7-199910050-00003.
32. Martin K, Beyer-Westendorf J, Davidson BL, et al. Use of the direct oral anticoagulants in obese patients: Guidance from the SSC of the ISTH. *J Thromb Haemost.* 2016;14:1308–1313.
33. Sebaaly J, Kelley D. Direct oral anticoagulants in obesity: An updated literature review. *Ann Pharmacother.* 2020;54:1144–1158. 10.1177/1060028020923584.
34. Whelton PK, Carey RM, Aronow WS, et al. 2017 ACC/AHA/AAPA/ABC/ACPM/AGS/APhA/ASH/ASPC/NMA/PCNA guideline for the prevention, detection, evaluation, and management of high blood pressure in adults: Executive summary. *Hypertension.* 2018;71: 1269–1324.
35. Bhatt DL, Steg PG, Miller M, et al. Cardiovascular risk reduction with icosapent ethyl for hypertriglyceridemia. *N Engl J Med.* 2019;380:11–22. 10.1056/nejmoa1812792.
36. Pollack CV Jr, Reilly PA, van Ryn J, et al. Idarucizumab for dabigatran reversal: Full cohort analysis. *N Engl J Med.* 2017;377:431–441.
37. Connolly SJ, Gibson CM, Crowther M, et al. Andexanet alfa for factor Xa inhibitor reversal. *N Engl J Med.* 2016;375:2499–500.
38. John S, Katzan I. Recurrent stroke while on antiplatelet therapy. *Neurol Clin.* 2015;33:475–489.

40

Arrhythmias

Jessica J. Tilton, Stephen T. Phillips, and Jerry L. Bauman

KEY CONCEPTS

1. The use of antiarrhythmic drugs (AADs) in the United States has declined because clinical trials have shown increased mortality with their use due to proarrhythmic adverse medication reactions and limited efficacy. AADs have been increasingly replaced by nonpharmacologic approaches such as ablation and the implantable cardioverter defibrillator (ICD). However, AADs remain a key tool in the management of many rhythm disorders.
2. AADs frequently cause adverse medication reactions and are complex in their pharmacokinetic characteristics. Close monitoring is required of all of these medications to assess for adverse reactions as well as potential medication interactions.
3. The most commonly prescribed AAD is amiodarone, which is effective in terminating and preventing a wide variety of symptomatic supraventricular and ventricular arrhythmias. However, amiodarone is plagued by frequent adverse medication reactions and requires close monitoring. The most concerning toxicity is pulmonary fibrosis. The side effect profiles of the intravenous (IV) (acute, short-term) and oral (chronic, long-term) forms of amiodarone differ substantially.
4. In patients with atrial fibrillation (AF), therapy is traditionally aimed at controlling the ventricular rate, preventing thromboembolic (TE) complications, and restoring and maintaining sinus rhythm (SR). Traditionally, many have pointed to the AFFIRM trial that maintenance of SR was often not necessary. However, several recent studies challenge this idea, particularly for patients with heart failure with reduced ejection fraction (HFrEF). AADs are also useful in reducing early AF recurrence in the periprocedural period and may improve long-term post-ablation outcomes.
5. Paroxysmal supraventricular tachycardia (PSVT) is usually a result of either reentry (involving either the atrioventricular [AV] node or incorporating an accessory pathway) or ectopic atrial activity (atrial tachycardia). Common supraventricular tachycardias are often terminated acutely with AV nodal-blocking medications, such as adenosine. For most patients, catheter ablation effectively cures this arrhythmia.
6. Patients with Wolff-Parkinson-White (WPW) syndrome may have several different tachycardias that are acutely treated by different strategies: orthodromic reentry (adenosine), antidromic reentry (adenosine or procainamide), and AF (procainamide or ibutilide). AV nodal-blocking medications are contraindicated in patients with WPW syndrome and AF. The mainstay of long-term therapy for WPW remains catheter ablation.
7. AADs (except for β-blockers) should not be used routinely in patients with prior myocardial infarction (MI) or left ventricular (LV) dysfunction for the treatment of premature ventricular complexes (PVCs). More specifically, the routine suppression of asymptomatic PVCs with AADs is not recommended.
8. Patients with hemodynamically significant ventricular tachycardia (VT) or ventricular fibrillation (VF) not associated with an acute MI who are successfully resuscitated (with electrical cardioversion, epinephrine, amiodarone, and/or lidocaine) are at high risk for sudden cardiac death (SCD). In most cases, implantation of an ICD is recommended for "secondary prevention." AADs can be useful to prevent recurrent ICD shocks, particularly when catheter ablation is not an option or has been unsuccessful.
9. Implantation of an ICD should be considered for the primary prevention of SCD in certain high-risk patient populations. High-risk patients include those with a history of MI and LV dysfunction (regardless of whether they have inducible sustained ventricular arrhythmias) as well as those with New York Heart Association (NYHA) class II or III HFrEF.
10. Life-threatening medication-induced ventricular proarrhythmia generally takes two forms: sinusoidal or incessant monomorphic VT (caused by class Ic AADs) and torsades de pointes (TdP) (caused by class Ia or III AADs and many other noncardiac medications).

BEYOND THE BOOK

Watch the video entitled "Normal Sinus Rhythm on an EKG" in Khan Academy (duration: 8:52) by Bianca Yoo. This video provides a brief overview of the cardiac conduction system and how it translates to an electrocardiogram. The video is useful to enhance student understanding regarding the COLLECT and ASSESS steps in the patient care process.

INTRODUCTION

The heart has two basic properties, namely, an electrical property and a mechanical property. The synchronous interaction between these two properties is complex, precise, and relatively enduring. The study of the electrical properties of the heart has grown at a steady rate, interrupted by periodic salvos of scientific breakthroughs. Einthoven's pioneering work allowed graphic electrical tracings of cardiac rhythm and probably represents the first of these breakthroughs. This discovery of the surface electrocardiogram (ECG) has remained the cornerstone of diagnostic tools for cardiac rhythm disturbances. Since then, intracardiac recordings and programmed cardiac stimulation have advanced our understanding of arrhythmias, and microelectrode, voltage clamping, and patch clamping techniques have allowed considerable insight into the electrophysiologic actions and mechanisms of antiarrhythmic drugs (AADs). The new era of molecular biology and mapping of the human genome promises even greater insights into mechanisms (and potential therapies) of arrhythmias. Noteworthy in this regard is the discovery of genetic abnormalities in the ion channels that control electrical repolarization (heritable long QT syndrome) or depolarization (Brugada syndrome).

1 There was some expectation that advances in AAD discovery would lead to a highly effective and nontoxic agent that would be effective for a majority of patients. Instead, significant problems with medication toxicity and proarrhythmia (provoking a new arrhythmia or exacerbating a preexisting arrhythmia) have resulted in a decline in AAD usage in the United States since 1989. The other phenomenon that has significantly contributed to the decline in AAD use is the development of extremely effective nonpharmacologic therapies. Technical advances have made it possible to permanently interrupt reentry circuits with radiofrequency ablation, which renders long-term AAD use unnecessary in certain arrhythmias. Furthermore, the impressive survival data associated with the use of implantable cardioverter defibrillators (ICDs) for the primary and secondary prevention of SCD have led most clinicians to choose "device" therapy as the first-line treatment for patients who are at high risk for life-threatening ventricular arrhythmias. These nonpharmacologic therapies have become increasingly popular for the management of arrhythmias, avoiding the potential proarrhythmic effects and organ toxicities associated with AADs.

PATHOPHYSIOLOGY

Normal Conduction

Electrical activity is initiated by the sinoatrial (SA) node and moves through cardiac tissue through a specialized conduction system that rapidly propagates the electrical wavefront through the ventricular muscle (Fig. 40-1, panel A). The SA node initiates cardiac rhythm under normal circumstances because this tissue possesses the highest degree of automaticity or rate of spontaneous impulse generation at a rate of 60 to 100 beats/min. The degree of automaticity of the SA node is largely influenced by the autonomic nervous system in that both cholinergic and sympathetic innervations control the sinus rate (Fig. 40-1, panel C). Most tissues within the conduction system also possess varying degrees of inherent automatic properties. However, the rates of spontaneous impulse generation of these tissues are generally less than that of the SA node. Thus, these latent automatic pacemakers are continuously overdriven by impulses arising from the SA node (primary pacemaker) and do not become clinically apparent.

From the SA node, electrical activity moves in a wave front through a specialized atrial conducting system and eventually gains entrance to the ventricle via the AV node and a large bundle of conducting tissue referred to as the bundle of His. The AVN and bundle of His are largely influenced by autonomic input and possess a relatively high degree of inherent automaticity at about 40 beats/min. From the bundle of His, the cardiac conduction system bifurcates into several (usually three) bundle branches: one right bundle and two left bundles. These bundle branches further arborize into a conduction network referred to as the Purkinje system. The conduction system innervates the mechanical myocardium and serves to initiate excitation–contraction coupling and the contractile process in a precise and organized fashion. Following electrical stimulation, cells within the heart enter a brief period during which they cannot again be excited, referred to as the refractory period. As the electrical wave front moves down the conduction system, the impulse eventually encounters tissue refractory to stimulation (recently excited) and subsequently dies out. The SA node subsequently recovers, fires spontaneously, and begins the process again.

Prior to cellular excitation, an electrical gradient, referred to as the resting membrane potential (RMP), results from differences in ion concentrations inside and outside of the cell. At RMP, the cell is polarized primarily by the action of active membrane ion pumps, the most notable of these being the sodium–potassium pump. For example, this specific pump (in addition to other systems) attempts to maintain the intracellular sodium concentration at 5 to 15 mEq/L (mmol/L), the extracellular sodium concentration at 135 to 142 mEq/L (mmol/L), the intracellular potassium concentration at 135 to 140 mEq/L (mmol/L), and the extracellular potassium concentration at 3 to 5 mEq/L (mmol/L).

Electrical stimulation (or depolarization) of the cell will result in changes in membrane potential over time or a characteristic action potential (AP) curve (Fig. 40-2). The AP curve results from the transmembrane movement of specific ions and is divided into different phases. Phase 0 or initial, rapid depolarization of atrial and ventricular tissues is caused by an abrupt increase in the permeability of the membrane to sodium influx. This rapid depolarization more than equilibrates (overshoots) the electrical potential, resulting in a brief initial repolarization or phase 1. Phase 1 (initial repolarization) is caused by a transient and active potassium efflux (ie, the I_{Kto} current). Calcium begins to move into the intracellular space during phase 0, causing a slower depolarization. Calcium influx continues throughout phase 2 of the AP (plateau phase) and is balanced to some degree by potassium efflux. Calcium entrance (only through L channels in myocardial tissue) distinguishes cardiac conducting cells from nerve tissue and provides the critical ionic link to excitation–contraction coupling and the mechanical properties of the heart as a pump. The membrane remains permeable to potassium efflux during phase 3, resulting in cellular repolarization. Phase 4 of the action potential is the gradual depolarization of the cell and is related to a constant sodium leak into the intracellular space balanced by a decreasing (over time) efflux of potassium. As the cell is slowly depolarized during phase 4, an abrupt increase in sodium permeability occurs, allowing the rapid cellular depolarization of phase 0. The juncture of phase 4 and phase 0, where initiation of rapid sodium influx occurs, is referred to as the threshold potential of the cell.

Not all cells in the cardiac conduction system rely on sodium influx for initial depolarization. Some tissues depolarize (phase 0) in response to a slower inward ionic current caused by calcium influx (L channels). These "calcium-dependent" tissues are found primarily in the SA and AV nodes (both L and T channels) and possess distinct conduction properties in comparison to "sodium-dependent" fibers (Fig. 40-2). Calcium-dependent cells generally have a slower conduction velocity and a less negative RMP. The RMP in nodal tissue is referred to as the slow depolarization phase or the pacemaker potential. This phase is initiated by the activation of funny current made up of sodium and potassium ions. It is referred to as the "funny" current because unlike most voltage-sensitive currents, it is activated by hyperpolarization. This phase is highly influenced by the autonomic system as seen in Fig. 40-1, panel C. Furthermore, in calcium-dependent tissues, recovery of excitability outlasts full repolarization, whereas in sodium-dependent tissues, recovery is prompt after repolarization. These two types of electrical tissues also differ dramatically in how medications modify their conduction properties.

Ion conductance across the lipid bilayer of the cell membrane occurs via the formation of membrane pores or "channels" (Fig. 40-3). Selective ion channels probably form in response to specific electrical potential differences between the inside and the outside of

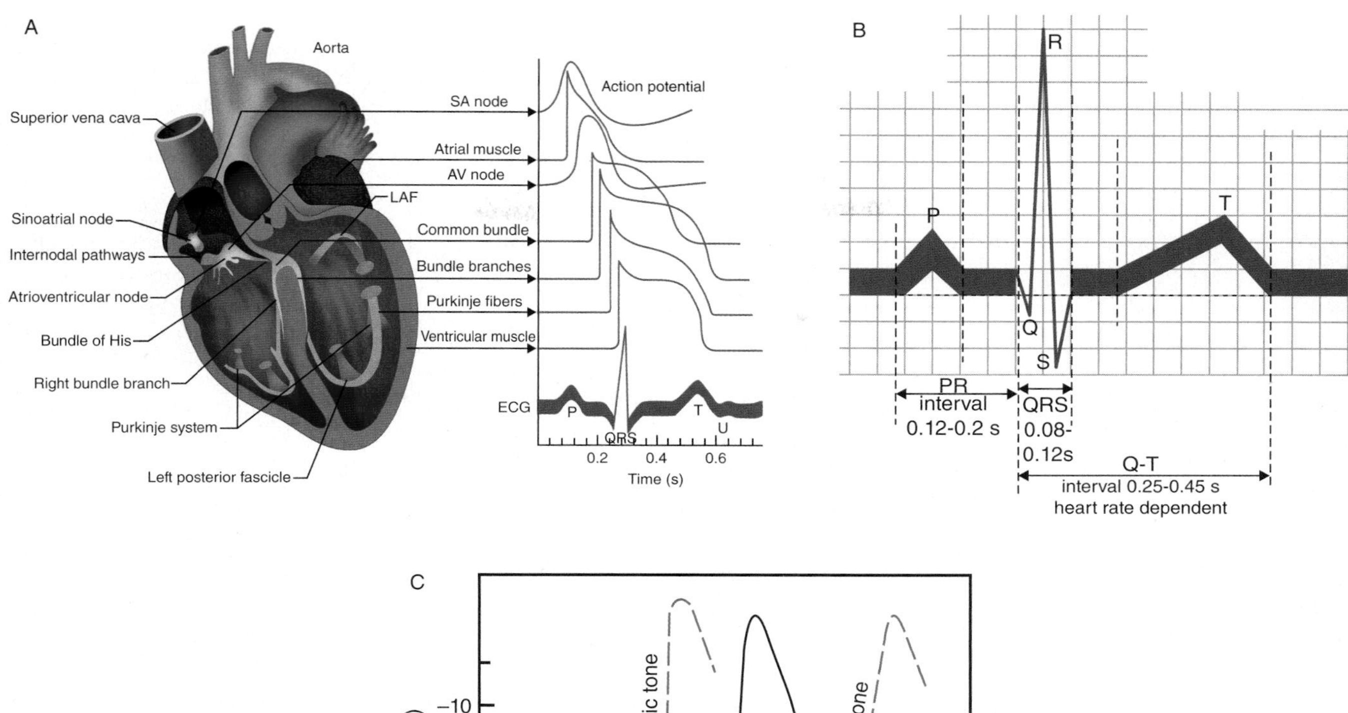

FIGURE 40-1 Cardiac action potentials and electrocardiogram tracing. LAF, left anterior fascicle; SA, sinoatrial; AV, atrioventricular. (*A*) Characterizes the action potentials from different areas of the heart and how those action potentials are illustrated on an ECG. (*B*) Describes the different intervals of an ECG. Normal interval ranges for PR, QRS, and QT are provided. (*C*) Describes the influence the autonomic system has on cardiac pacemaker potentials.

the cell (voltage dependence). Changes in equilibrium occur and permit the formation of activated ion channels. Besides channel formation and membrane composition, intrachannel proteins or phospholipids, referred to as gates, also regulate the transmembrane movement of ions. These gates are thought to be positioned strategically within the channel to modulate ion flow. Each ion channel conceptually has two types of gates: an activation gate and an inactivation gate (see Fig. 40-3). The activation gate opens during depolarization to allow the ion current to enter or exit from the cell, and the inactivation gate later closes to stop ion movement. When the cell is in a rested state, the activation gates are closed and the inactivation gates are open. The activation gates then open to allow ion movement through the channel, and the inactivation gates later close to stop ion conductance. Thus, the cell cycles between three states: resting, activated, and inactivated. Activation of SA and AV nodal tissue is dependent on a slow depolarizing current through calcium channels and gates, whereas the activation of atrial and ventricular tissues is dependent on a rapid depolarizing current through sodium channels and gates.

The impulse that is generated by the SA node disseminates to adjacent cells through gap junctions. The gap junctions provide a pathway for ions to travel to neighboring cells for AP propagation. The compilation of all the cardiac APs is presented on an ECG (Fig. 40-1, panel A). During a normal cardiac conduction cycle the ECG will have a P wave (atrial depolarization), QRS (ventricular depolarization and atrial repolarization), and T wave (ventricular repolarization). It is also important to note the PR interval, or the time from atrial depolarization to ventricular depolarization, and the QT interval, the duration of the ventricular AP (Fig. 40-1, panel B). Augmentation of the ECG is a product of alterations in the cardiac APs.

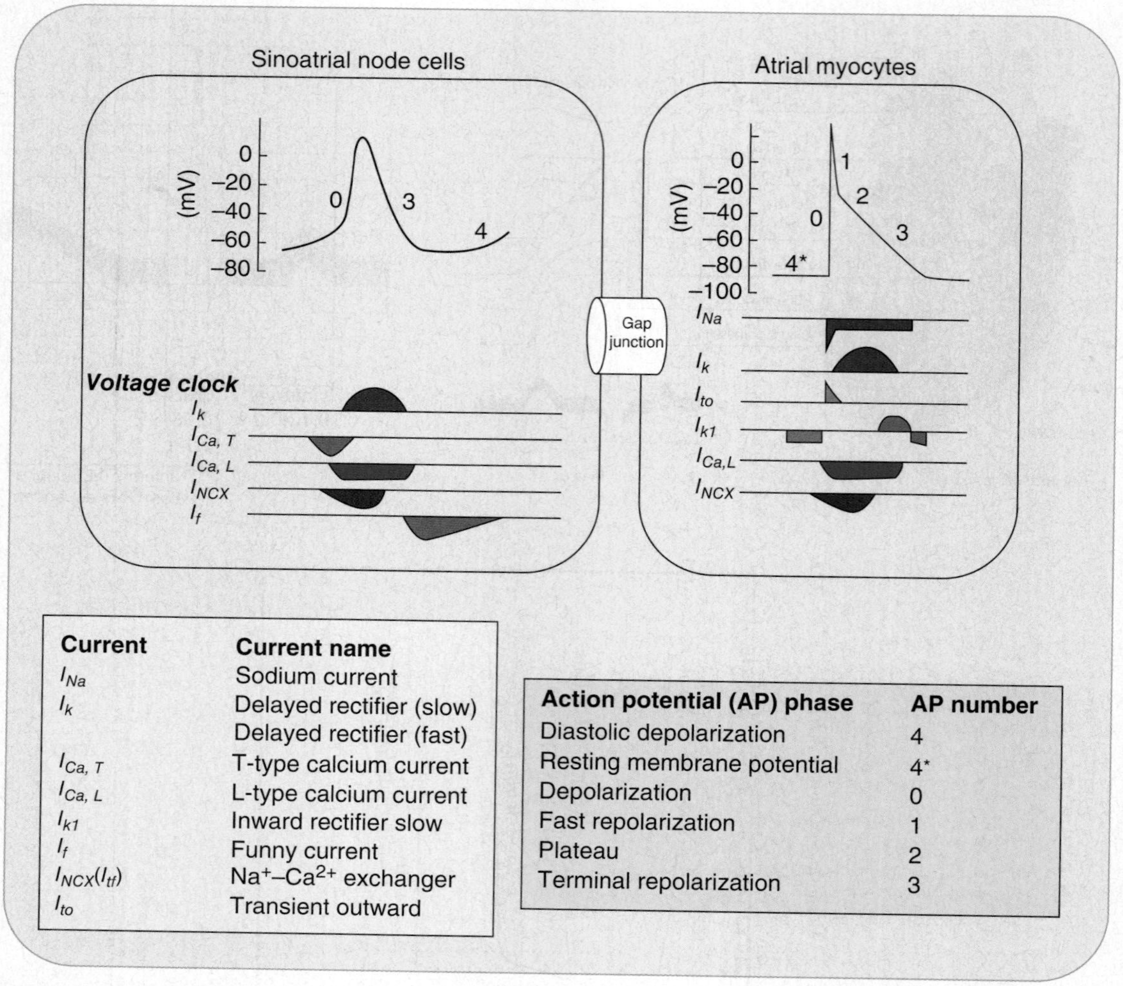

Sinoatrial node cells
Atrial myocytes
(mV)
0
−20
−40
−60
−80
−100
4*
Gap junction
Voltage clock
I_k
$I_{Ca,\,T}$
$I_{Ca,\,L}$
I_{NCX}
I_f
I_{Na}
I_{to}
I_{k1}
Current
Current name
I_{Na} Sodium current
I_k Delayed rectifier (slow)
Delayed rectifier (fast)
$I_{Ca,\,T}$ T-type calcium current
$I_{Ca,\,L}$ L-type calcium current
I_{k1} Inward rectifier slow
I_f Funny current
$I_{NCX}(I_{ti})$ Na^+–Ca^{2+} exchanger
I_{to} Transient outward
Action potential (AP) phase
AP number
Diastolic depolarization 4
Resting membrane potential 4*
Depolarization 0
Fast repolarization 1
Plateau 2
Terminal repolarization 3

FIGURE 40-2 Cardiac action potentials and responsible ion currents. While there are similarities between cardiac nodal and muscle action potentials there are many differences in how the phases are influenced by particular ion currents.

Resting
Activated
Inactivated
Extracellular
Intracellular
Na^+
m
h
Membrane potential (mV)
40
0
−40
−60
Threshold
Recovery

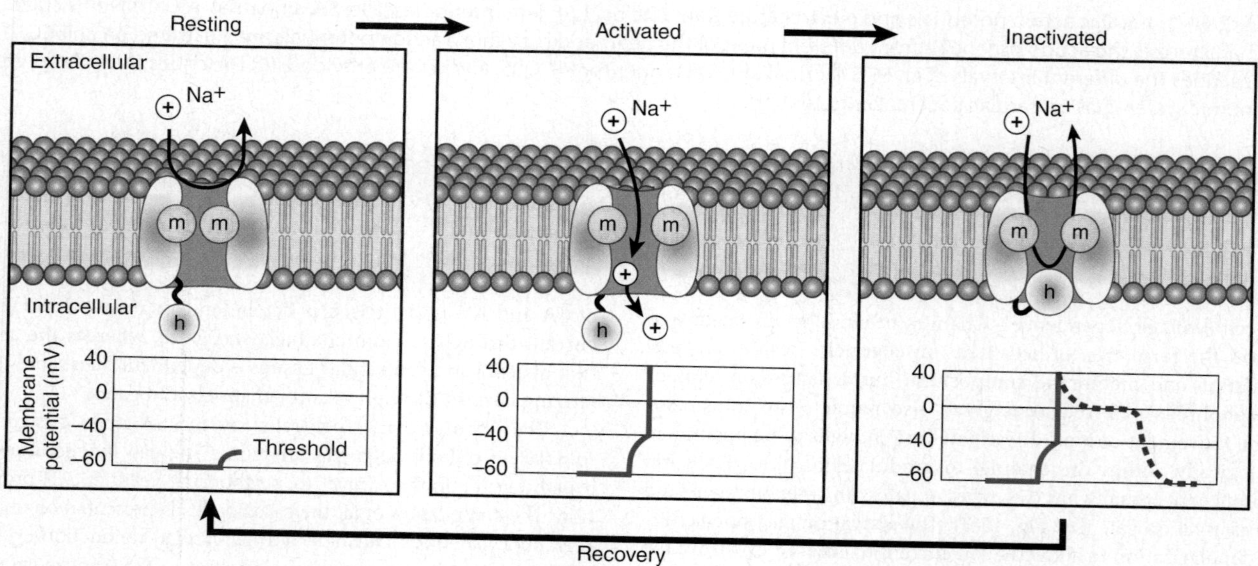

FIGURE 40-3 States of sodium (Na^+) channels cycling through the cardiac action potential. Transitions between resting, activated, and inactivated states are dependent on membrane potential and time. The activation gate is shown as m and the inactivation gate as h. Potentials typical for each state are shown under each channel schematic as a function of time. The dashed line indicates that part of the action potential during which most Na^+ channels are completely or partially inactivated and unavailable for reactivation. *(Reproduced, with permission, from Katzung BG, ed. Basic & Clinical Pharmacology. 15th ed. New York: McGraw Hill; 2021.)*

Abnormal Conduction

The mechanisms of tachyarrhythmias have been classically divided into two general categories: those resulting from an abnormality in impulse generation ("automatic" tachycardia and triggered automaticity) and those resulting from an abnormality in impulse conduction ("reentrant" tachycardias).[1]

Automatic tachycardias depend on spontaneous impulse generation in latent pacemakers and may be a result of several different mechanisms. Medications, such as digoxin or catecholamines, and conditions, such as hypoxia, electrolyte abnormalities (eg, hypokalemia), and fiber stretch (cardiac dilation), may lead to an increased slope of phase 4 depolarization in cardiac tissues other than the SA node.[1] These factors are associated with abnormal automaticity in experimental models and arrhythmogenesis in clinical situations. The increased slope of phase 4 causes heightened automaticity of these tissues and competition with the SA node for dominance of cardiac rhythm. If the rate of spontaneous impulse generation of the abnormally automatic tissue exceeds that of the SA node, then an automatic tachycardia may result. Automatic tachycardias have the following characteristics: (a) the onset of the tachycardia is unrelated to an initiating event such as a premature beat; (b) the initiating beat is usually identical to subsequent beats of the tachycardia; (c) the tachycardia cannot be initiated by programmed cardiac stimulation; and (d) the onset of the tachycardia is usually preceded by a gradual acceleration in rate and termination is usually preceded by a gradual deceleration in rate. Clinical tachycardias resulting from the classic forms of enhanced automaticity are not as common as once thought. Examples are sinus tachycardia and junctional tachycardia.

Triggered automaticity is also a possible mechanism for abnormal impulse generation. Briefly, triggered automaticity refers to transient membrane depolarizations that occur during repolarization (early afterdepolarizations [EADs]) or after repolarization (delayed afterdepolarizations [DADs]) but prior to phase 4 of the AP (Fig. 40-4).[1] Afterdepolarizations may be related to abnormal calcium and sodium influx during or just after full cellular repolarization. Experimentally, EADs may be precipitated by hypokalemia, class Ia AADs, or slow stimulation rates—any factor that blocks the ion channels (eg, potassium) responsible for cellular repolarization. EADs provoked by medications that block potassium conductance and delay repolarization are the underlying cause of TdP. DADs may be precipitated by digoxin or catecholamines and suppressed by non-dihydropyridine (non-DHP) calcium channel blockers (CCBs). DADs have been suggested as the mechanism for multifocal atrial tachycardia, digoxin-induced tachycardias, and exercise-provoked VT. Triggered automatic rhythms possess some of the characteristics of automatic tachycardias and some of the characteristics of reentrant tachycardias (description follows).

Reentry is a concept that involves indefinite propagation of the impulse and continued activation of previously refractory tissue. There are three conduction requirements for the formation of a viable reentrant focus: (1) two pathways for impulse conduction, (2) an area of unidirectional block (prolonged refractoriness) in one of these pathways, and (3) slow conduction in the other pathway (Fig. 40-5, panel A).[1] Usually, a critically timed premature beat initiates reentry. This premature impulse enters both conduction pathways but encounters refractory tissue in one of the pathways at the area of unidirectional block. The impulse dies out because the tissue is still refractory from the previous (sinus) impulse. Although it fails to propagate in one pathway, the impulse may still proceed in a forward direction (antegrade) through the other pathway because of this pathway's relatively shorter refractory period. The impulse may then proceed through a loop of tissue and "reenter" the area of unidirectional block in a backward direction (retrograde). Because the antegrade pathway has slow conduction characteristics, the area of unidirectional block has time to recover its excitability. The impulse can proceed in a retrograde fashion through this previously refractory tissue and continue around the loop of tissue in a circular fashion. Thus, the key to the formation of a reentrant focus is crucial conduction discrepancies in the electrophysiologic characteristics of the two pathways. The reentrant focus may excite surrounding tissue at a rate greater than that of the SA node, leading to the formation of a clinical tachycardia. The above model is anatomically determined in that there is only one pathway for impulse conduction with a fixed circuit length.

Another model of reentry, referred to as a functional reentrant loop, may also occur (Fig. 40-5, panel B).[1] In a functional reentrant focus, the length of the circuit may vary depending on the conduction velocity and recovery characteristics of the impulse. The area in the middle of the loop is continually kept refractory by the inwardly moving impulse. The length of the circuit is not fixed but is the smallest circle possible, such that the leading edge of the wave front is continuously exciting tissue just as it recovers. It differs from the anatomic model in that the leading edge of the impulse is not preceded by an excitable gap of tissue, and it does not have an obstacle in the middle or a fixed anatomic circuit.

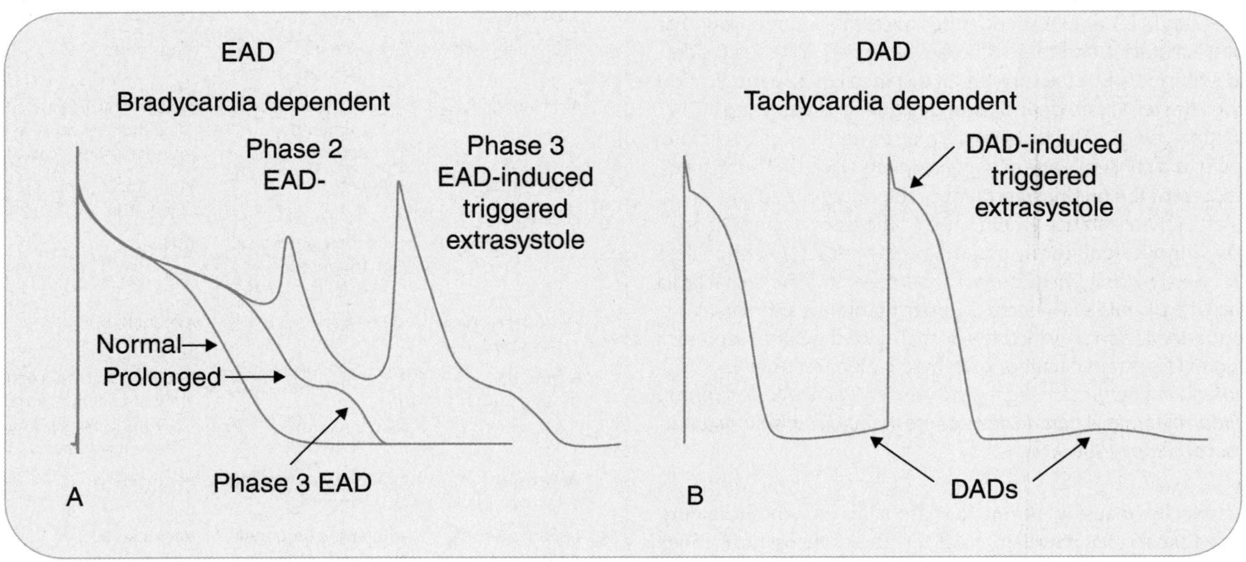

FIGURE 40-4 Afterdepolarizations. (EAD early afterdepolarization; DAD delayed afterdepolarization.)

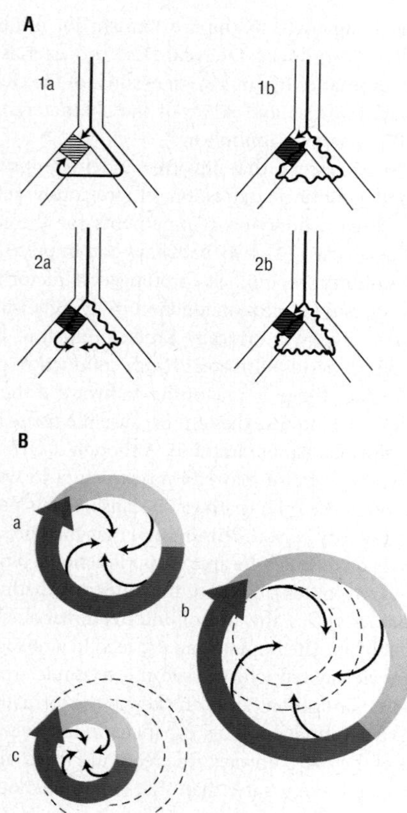

FIGURE 40-5 *(A)* Possible mechanism of proarrhythmia in the anatomic model of reentry. (1a) Nonviable reentrant loop due to bidirectional block (*shaded area*). (1b) Instance where a medication slows conduction velocity without significantly prolonging the refractory period. The impulse is now able to reenter the area of unidirectional block (*shaded area*) because slowed conduction through the antegrade pathway allows recovery of the block. A new reentrant tachycardia may result. (2a) Nonviable reentrant loop due to a lack of a unidirectional block. (2b) Instance where a medication prolongs the refractory period without significantly slowing conduction velocity. The impulse moving antegrade meets refractory tissue (*shaded area*), allowing for unidirectional block. A new reentrant tachycardia may result. *(B)* Mechanism of functional reentry and proarrhythmia. (a) Functionally determined reentrant circuit. This model should be contrasted with anatomic reentry; here, the circuit is not fixed (it does not necessarily move around an anatomic obstacle), and there is no excitable gap. All tissue inside is held continuously refractory. (b) An instance where a medication prolongs the refractory period without significantly slowing conduction velocity. The tachycardia may terminate or slow in rate as shown as a consequence of a greater circuit length. The *dashed lines* represent the original reentrant circuit prior to medication treatment. (c) An instance where a medication slows conduction velocity without significantly prolonging the refractory period (ie, class Ic *antiarrhythmic medications*) and accelerates the tachycardia. The tachycardia rate may increase (proarrhythmia) as shown as a consequence of a shorter circuit length. The dashed lines represent the original reentrant circuit prior to medication treatment. (*Reprinted, with permission, from McCollam PL, Parker RB, Beckman KJ, et al. Proarrhythmia: A paradoxic response to antiarrhythmic agents. Pharmacotherapy 1989;9:146.*)

Clinically, many reentrant foci probably have both anatomic and functional characteristics. All of these theoretical models require a critical balance of refractoriness and conduction velocity within the circuit and, as such, have helped to explain the effects of medications on terminating, modifying, and causing cardiac rhythm disturbances (eg, proarrhythmia).

What causes reentry to become clinically manifest? Reentrant foci may occur at any level of the conduction system: within the branches of the specialized atrial conduction system, within the Purkinje network, and even within portions of the SA and AV nodes. The anatomy of the Purkinje system appears to provide a suitable substrate for the formation of microreentrant loops and is often used as a model to facilitate the understanding of reentry concepts. Of course, because reentry does not usually occur in normal, healthy conduction tissue, various forms of heart disease or conduction abnormalities are typically present before reentry becomes manifest. An often-used example is reentry occurring as a consequence of ischemic or hypoxic damage. With inadequate cellular oxygenation, high-energy phosphate concentrations diminish, the activity of the transmembrane ion pumps declines, and RMP rises. This rise in RMP causes inactivation in the voltage-dependent sodium channel, and the tissue begins to assume slow conduction characteristics. If changes in the tissue's conduction parameters occur in a discordant manner due to varying degrees of ischemia or hypoxia, then a reentry circuit may become manifest. Furthermore, an ischemic, dying cell releases intracellular potassium, which also causes a rise in RMP. In other cases, reentry may occur because of anatomic or functional variants in the normal conduction system. For instance, patients may possess two (instead of one) conduction pathways near or within the AV node or have an anomalous extranodal AV pathway that possesses different electrophysiologic characteristics from the normal AV nodal pathway. Reentry in these cases may occur within the AV node or encompass both atrial and ventricular tissues. Reentrant tachycardias have the following characteristics: (a) the onset of the tachycardia is usually related to an initiating event (ie, premature beat); (b) the initiating beat is usually different in morphology from subsequent beats of the tachycardia; (c) the initiation of the tachycardia can usually be incited with programmed cardiac stimulation; and (d) the initiation and termination of the tachycardia is usually abrupt without an acceleration or deceleration phase. There are many examples of reentrant tachycardias, including AF, atrial flutter (AFl), AV nodal reentrant tachycardia (AVNRT), AV reentrant tachycardia (AVRT), and recurrent VT (Table 40-1).

TABLE 40-1 Characteristics and Presumed Mechanisms of Arrhythmias

Tachycardia	Mechanism	Origin
Sinus tachycardia	Automatic (normal)	Sinus node
Atrial fibrillation	Reentry, automatic, triggered activity	Atria, thoracic veins, pulmonary veins, and superior vena cava
Atrial flutter	Reentry	Right (most common) and left atria
Atrial tachycardia	Reentry, automatic, triggered activity	Atria
AV nodal reentry tachycardia	Reentry	AV junction
AV reentry tachycardia	Reentry	Circuit includes accessory AV connection, atria, AV node, His-Purkinje system, ventricles
Ventricular tachycardia	Reentry, automatic, triggered	Ventricles
Torsades de Pointes	Reentry, triggered activity	Ventricles

AV, atrioventricular.

PHARMACOLOGIC THERAPY

In a theoretical sense, medications have antiarrhythmic activity by directly altering electrical conduction in several ways. First, a medication may depress the automatic properties of abnormal pacemaker cells. If the rate of spontaneous impulse generation of the abnormally automatic foci becomes less than that of the SA node, normal cardiac rhythm can be restored. Second, medications may alter the conduction characteristics of a reentrant loop (Fig. 40-5).[1,2] A medication may facilitate conduction (shorten refractoriness) in the area of unidirectional block, allowing antegrade conduction to proceed. On the other hand, a medication may further depress conduction (prolong refractoriness) either in the area of unidirectional block or in the pathway with slowed conduction and a relatively shorter refractory period. If refractoriness is prolonged in the area of unidirectional block, retrograde propagation of the impulse is not permitted, causing a "bidirectional" block. In the anatomic model, if refractoriness is prolonged in the pathway with slow conduction, antegrade conduction of the impulse is not permitted. In either case, medications that reduce the discordance and cause uniformity in conduction properties of the two pathways may suppress the reentrant substrate. In the functionally determined model, if refractoriness is prolonged without significantly slowing conduction velocity, the tachycardia may terminate or slow in rate because of a greater circuit length (see Fig. 40-5, panel B). There are other theoretical ways to stop reentry: (a) a medication may eliminate the critically timed premature impulse that triggers reentry; (b) a medication may slow conduction velocity to such an extent that conduction is extinguished; or (c) a medication may reverse the underlying form of heart disease that was responsible for the conduction abnormalities that led to the arrhythmia (ie, "reverse remodeling").

AADs have specific electrophysiologic actions that alter cardiac conduction in patients with or without heart disease. These actions form the basis of grouping AADs into specific categories based on their electrophysiologic actions in vitro. Vaughan Williams proposed the most frequently used classification system (Table 40-2).[2] This classification has been criticized for the following reasons: (a) it is incomplete and does not allow for the classification of medications such as digoxin or adenosine; (b) it is not pure, and many agents have properties of more than one class of medications; (c) it does not incorporate medication characteristics such as mechanisms of tachycardia termination/prevention, clinical indications, or side effects; and (d) medications become "labeled" within a class, although they may be distinct in many regards. Despite these criticisms, the Vaughan Williams classification remains the most frequently used for categorizing the electrophysiologic actions of AADs.

Class I AADs are grouped together because of their common action in blocking sodium conductance. The receptor site for these AADs is probably inside the sodium channel so that, in effect, the medication plugs the pore. The AAD may gain access to the receptor either via the intracellular space through the membrane lipid bilayer or directly through the channel (Fig. 40-3). Several principles are inherent in antiarrhythmic sodium channel receptor theories[3,4]:

1. Class I AADs have predominant affinity for a particular state of the channel (eg, during activation or inactivation). For example, lidocaine blocks sodium current primarily when the cell is in the inactivated state, whereas quinidine, flecainide, and propafenone are predominantly open (or activated) channel blockers.
2. Class I AADs have specific binding and unbinding characteristics to the receptor, which has led to the subclassification (Ia, Ib, Ic) of these AADs. For example, lidocaine binds to and dissociates from the channel receptor quickly ("fast on–off") but flecainide has very "slow on–off" properties. This explains why flecainide has such potent effects on slowing ventricular conduction, whereas lidocaine has little effect on normal tissue (at normal heart rates). In general, the class Ic AADs are "slow on–off," the class Ib AADs are "fast on–off,"

TABLE 40-2 Classification of Antiarrhythmic Medications

Class	Medication	Conduction Velocity[a]	Refractory Period	Automaticity	Ion Block
Ia	Quinidine	↓	↑	↓	Sodium (intermediate) Potassium
	Procainamide				
	Disopyramide				
Ib	Lidocaine	0/↓	↓	↓	Sodium (fast on–off)
	Mexiletine				
Ic	Flecainide	↓↓	↑ (atrial)	↓	Sodium (slow on–off)
	Propafenone[b]				
II[c]	β-blockers	↓	↑	↓	Calcium (indirect)
III	Amiodarone[d]	0	↑↑	0	Potassium
	Dofetilide				
	Dronedarone[d]				
	Sotalol[b]				
	Ibutilide				
IV[c]	Verapamil	↓	↑	↓	Calcium
	Diltiazem				

[a]Variables for normal tissue models in ventricular tissue.

[b]Also has β-blocking actions.

[c]Variables for sinoatrial (SA) and atrioventricular (AV) nodal tissue only.

[d]Also has sodium, calcium, and β-blocking actions; see Table 40-3.

and the class Ia AADs are intermediate in their binding kinetics.

3. Class I AADs possess use dependence (ie, sodium channel blockade and slowed conduction are greatest at fast heart rates and least during bradycardia). For "slow on–off" medications, sodium channel blockade is evident at normal rates (60 to 100 beats/min), but for "fast on–off" agents, slowed conduction is only apparent at fast heart rates.
4. Class I AADs are weak bases with a pKa > 7 and block the sodium channel in their ionized form. Consequently, pH will alter these actions: acidosis accentuates, and alkalosis diminishes sodium channel blockade.
5. Class I AADs appear to share a single receptor site in the sodium channel. It should be noted, however, that a number of class I AADs have other electrophysiologic properties. For instance, quinidine has potent potassium channel blocking activity (manifests predominantly at low concentrations) as does N-acetylprocainamide (manifests predominantly at high concentrations), the primary metabolite of procainamide. Additionally, propafenone has β-blocking actions.

The class Ia AADs, quinidine, procainamide, and disopyramide, slow conduction velocity, prolong refractoriness, and decrease the automatic properties of sodium-dependent (normal and diseased) conduction tissue. Although class Ia AADs are primarily considered sodium channel blockers, their electrophysiologic actions can also be attributed to blockade of potassium channels. In reentrant tachycardias, these medications generally depress conduction and prolong refractoriness, theoretically transforming the area of unidirectional block into a bidirectional block. Clinically, class Ia medications are broad-spectrum AADs that are indicated for both supraventricular and ventricular arrhythmias. However, their use tends to be infrequent in clinical practice because of their limited efficacy and significant toxicities.

The class Ib AADs, lidocaine and mexiletine were historically categorized separately from quinidine-like medications. Early work demonstrated that lidocaine had distinctly different electrophysiologic actions. In normal tissue models, lidocaine generally facilitates actions on cardiac conduction by shortening refractoriness and having little effect on conduction velocity. Thus, it was postulated that these agents could improve antegrade conduction, eliminating the area of unidirectional block. Arrhythmias do not usually arise from normal tissue. However, lidocaine possesses class Ia quinidine-like properties in diseased tissues. Therefore, it is probable that lidocaine acts in a similar fashion to the class Ia AADs (ie, prolongs refractoriness) in diseased ischemic tissues leading to bidirectional block in a reentrant circuit. Lidocaine and similar agents have accentuated effects in ischemic tissue caused by the local acidosis and potassium shifts that occur during cellular hypoxia. Changes in pH alter the time that local anesthetics, like lidocaine, occupy the sodium channel receptor, affecting the agent's electrophysiologic actions. In addition, the intracellular acidosis that ensues due to ischemia could cause lidocaine to become "trapped" within the cell, allowing increased access to the receptor. The class Ib AADs are considerably more effective in ventricular arrhythmias than supraventricular arrhythmias. As a group, these medications are relatively weak sodium channel blockers (at normal stimulation rates).

The class Ic AADs, propafenone and flecainide, are extremely potent sodium channel blockers, profoundly slowing conduction velocity while leaving refractoriness relatively unaltered. The class Ic AADs theoretically eliminate reentry by slowing conduction to a point where the impulse is extinguished and cannot propagate further. Although the class Ic AADs are effective for both ventricular and supraventricular arrhythmias, their use for ventricular arrhythmias has been limited by the risk of proarrhythmia.

The β-blockers are classified as class II AADs. For the most part, the clinically relevant acute antiarrhythmic mechanisms of the β-blockers result from their antiadrenergic actions.[4] Because the SA and AV nodes are heavily influenced by adrenergic innervation, β-blockers would be most useful in tachycardias in which these nodal tissues are abnormally automatic or are a portion of a reentrant loop. These medications are also helpful in slowing ventricular response in atrial arrhythmias (eg, AF) by their effects on the AV node. Furthermore, some tachycardias are exercise-related or precipitated by states of high sympathetic tone (perhaps through triggered activity), and β-blockers may be useful in these instances. Beta-adrenergic stimulation results in increased conduction velocity, shortened refractoriness, and increased automaticity of the nodal tissues; β-blockers will antagonize these effects. In the nodal tissues, β-blockers interfere with calcium entry into the cell by altering catecholamine-dependent channel integrity and gating kinetics. In sodium-dependent atrial and ventricular tissues, β-blockers shorten repolarization somewhat but otherwise have little direct effect. The antiarrhythmic properties of β-blockers observed with long-term, chronic therapy in patients with heart disease are less well understood. Although it is clear β-blockers decrease the likelihood of SCD (presumably arrhythmic death) after MI, the mechanism for this benefit remains unclear; this benefit may relate to the complex interplay of changes in sympathetic tone, damaged myocardium, and ventricular conduction. In patients with HF, medications such as β-blockers, angiotensin-converting enzyme inhibitors, and angiotensin II receptor blockers may prevent arrhythmias such as AF by attenuating the structural and/or electrical remodeling process in the myocardium.[5]

The class III AADs include those agents that specifically prolong refractoriness in atrial and ventricular tissues. This class includes amiodarone, dronedarone, sotalol, ibutilide, and dofetilide. These medications share the common effect of delaying repolarization by blocking potassium channels. Amiodarone and sotalol are effective in most supraventricular and ventricular arrhythmias. Amiodarone displays electrophysiologic characteristics of all four Vaughan Williams classes; it is a sodium channel blocker with relatively "fast on–off" kinetics, has nonselective β-blocking actions, blocks potassium channels, and has a small degree of calcium channel blocking activity (Table 40-3). At normal heart rates and with chronic use, its predominant effect is to prolong repolarization. With IV administration, its onset is relatively quick (unlike the oral form) and beta blockade predominates initially. Theoretically, amiodarone, like class I AADs, may interrupt the reentrant substrate by transforming an area of unidirectional block into an area of bidirectional block. However, amiodarone may leave the reentrant loop intact. The impressive effectiveness of amiodarone coupled with its low proarrhythmic potential has challenged the notion that selective ion channel blockade by AADs is preferable. Sotalol is a potent inhibitor of outward potassium movement during repolarization and possesses nonselective β-blocking actions. Unlike amiodarone and sotalol, dronedarone, ibutilide, and dofetilide are only approved for the treatment of supraventricular arrhythmias. Both ibutilide (only available IV) and dofetilide (only available orally) can be used for the acute conversion of AF or AFl to SR. Dofetilide can also be used to maintain SR in patients with AF or AFl of longer than 1 week's duration who have been converted to SR. Dronedarone is approved to reduce the risk of hospitalization in patients with a history of paroxysmal or persistent AF who are currently in SR. Although structurally related to amiodarone, dronedarone's structure has been modified through the addition of a methylsulfonyl group and the removal of iodine. Dronedarone is also similar to amiodarone in exhibiting electrophysiologic characteristics of all four Vaughan Williams classes (sodium channel blocker with relatively "fast on–off" kinetics, nonselective β-blocker, potassium channel blocker, and calcium channel antagonist). However, amiodarone is more effective than dronedarone.

TABLE 40-3 Time Course and Electrophysiologic Effects of Amiodarone

				IV		Oral	
Class	Mechanism	EP	ECG	Minutes–Hours	Hours–Days	Days–Weeks	Weeks–Months
Class I	Na^+ block	↑HV	↑QRS	0	+	+	++
Class II	β-block	↑AH	↑PR ↓HR	++	++	++	++
Class III	K^+ block	↑VERP ↑AERP	↑QT	0	+	++	++++
Class IV	Ca^{2+} block[a]	↑AH	↑PR ↓HR	+	+	+	+

AERP, atrial effective refractory period; AH, atria–His interval; ECG, electrocardiographic effects; EP, electrophysiologic actions; HR, heart rate; HV, His–ventricle interval; IV, intravenous; VERP, ventricular effective refractory period.

[a]Rate-dependent (for amiodarone).

There are several different potassium channels that function during normal conduction; all approved class III AADs inhibit the delayed rectifier current (I_K) responsible for phase 2 and phase 3 repolarization. Subcurrents make up I_K: an ultrarapid component (I_{Kur}), a rapid component (I_{Kr}), and the slow component (I_{Ks}). Sotalol, ibutilide, and dofetilide selectively block I_{Kr}, whereas amiodarone and dronedarone block both I_{Kr} and I_{Ks}. Potassium channel blockers (particularly those with selective I_{Kr} blocking properties) display "reverse use dependence" (ie, their effects on repolarization are greatest at low heart rates). Sotalol and medications like it also appear to be much more effective in preventing VF (in dog models) than the traditional sodium channel blockers. The safety concern of all class III AADs is an extension of their underlying ionic mechanism; that is, by blocking potassium channels and delaying repolarization, these medications may also cause proarrhythmia in the form of TdP by provoking EADs.

The non-DHP CCBs, verapamil and diltiazem, are categorized as class IV AADs. They block L-type calcium channels in SA and AV nodal tissues, slowing conduction, prolonging refractoriness, and decreasing automaticity (eg, due to EADs or DADs). Thus, these agents are effective in automatic or reentrant tachycardias which arise from or use the SA or AV nodes. In supraventricular arrhythmias (eg, AF or AFl), these medications can slow ventricular response by slowing AV nodal conduction. Furthermore, because calcium entry seems to be integral to exercise-related tachycardias and/or tachycardias caused by some forms of triggered automaticity, these agents may be effective in the treatment of these types of arrhythmias. The DHP CCBs (eg, nifedipine) do not have significant antiarrhythmic activity as they do not affect AV nodal conduction.

2 All AADs currently available have an impressive side effect profile (Table 40-4). A considerable percentage of patients cannot tolerate long-term therapy with these medications and will have to discontinue therapy because of adverse drug reactions. Flecainide, propafenone, quinidine, procainamide, disopyramide, sotalol, non-DHP CCBs, and dronedarone may worsen HF symptoms in patients with underlying LV systolic dysfunction. Consequently, these medications should be avoided in patients with HFrEF. The class Ib AAD, mexiletine, causes neurologic and/or gastrointestinal toxicity in a high percentage of patients. One of the most frightening adverse effects related to AADs is the aggravation of underlying ventricular arrhythmias or the precipitation of new, life-threatening ventricular arrhythmias.[4]

3 Amiodarone has assumed a prominent place in the treatment of both acute and chronic supraventricular and ventricular arrhythmias and is the most commonly prescribed AAD.[6] Once considered a medication of last resort, it is often the first AAD considered for the treatment of many arrhythmias. Yet amiodarone is a peculiar and complex medication, displaying unusual pharmacologic effects, pharmacokinetics, dosing regimens, and multiorgan adverse drug reactions. Amiodarone has an extremely long elimination half-life (approximately 60 days) and a large volume of distribution. Consequently, the onset of action with the oral form is delayed (days to weeks) despite the use of a loading regimen, and the duration of effect may persist for months after discontinuation. Amiodarone is a substrate of the cytochrome P450 (CYP) 3A4 isoenzyme, a moderate inhibitor of many CYP isoenzymes (eg, CYP2C9, CYP2D6,

TABLE 40-4 Adverse Drug Reactions of Class I and III Antiarrhythmic Medications

Disopyramide	Anticholinergic symptoms (dry mouth, urinary retention, constipation, blurred vision), nausea, anorexia, HF, conduction disturbances, ventricular arrhythmias (eg, TdP)
Procainamide	Hypotension, worsening HF, conduction disturbances, ventricular arrhythmias (eg, TdP)
Quinidine	Cinchonism, diarrhea, abdominal cramps, nausea, vomiting, hypotension, worsening HF, conduction disturbances, ventricular arrhythmias (eg, TdP), fever
Lidocaine	Dizziness, sedation, slurred speech, blurred vision, paresthesia, muscle twitching, confusion, nausea, vomiting, seizures, psychosis, sinus arrest, conduction disturbances
Mexiletine	Dizziness, sedation, anxiety, confusion, paresthesia, tremor, ataxia, blurred vision, nausea, vomiting, anorexia, conduction disturbances, ventricular arrhythmias
Flecainide	Blurred vision, dizziness, dyspnea, headache, tremor, nausea, worsening HF, conduction disturbances, ventricular arrhythmias
Propafenone	Dizziness, fatigue, blurred vision, bronchospasm, headache, taste disturbances, nausea, vomiting, bradycardia or AV block, worsening HF, ventricular arrhythmias
Amiodarone	Tremor, ataxia, paresthesia, insomnia, corneal microdeposits, optic neuropathy/neuritis, nausea, vomiting, anorexia, constipation, TdP (<1%), bradycardia or AV block (IV and oral use), pulmonary fibrosis, liver function test abnormalities, hypothyroidism, hyperthyroidism, photosensitivity, blue-gray skin discoloration, hypotension (IV use), phlebitis (IV use)
Dofetilide	Headache, dizziness, TdP
Dronedarone	Nausea, vomiting, diarrhea, serum creatinine elevations, bradycardia, worsening HF, hepatotoxicity, pulmonary fibrosis, acute renal failure, TdP (<1%)
Ibutilide	Headache, TdP, bradycardia or AV block, hypotension
Sotalol	Dizziness, weakness, fatigue, nausea, vomiting, diarrhea, bradycardia or AV block, TdP, bronchospasm, worsening HF

AV, atrioventricular; HF, heart failure; IV, intravenous; TdP, torsades de pointes.

CYP3A4), and a P-glycoprotein (P-gp) inhibitor, which can result in numerous medication interactions.[7] By inhibiting P-gp, amiodarone can increase digoxin concentrations by approximately twofold; therefore, the digoxin dose should be empirically reduced by 50% when initiating amiodarone. By inhibiting CYP2C9 and CYP3A4, amiodarone can increase warfarin concentrations and the international normalized ratio (INR). Consequently, when amiodarone and warfarin are initiated concurrently, an empiric warfarin dose reduction is necessary. When amiodarone is initiated in a patient already receiving warfarin, close INR monitoring is needed and the dose of warfarin may need to be reduced by approximately 30%.[8]

Acute administration of amiodarone is usually well tolerated by patients; however, severe organ toxicities may result with chronic use. Severe bradycardia, hyperthyroidism, hypothyroidism, peripheral neuropathy, gastrointestinal discomfort, and photosensitivity are common. Fulminant hepatitis (uncommon) and pulmonary fibrosis (2% of patients) have caused death.[6] While amiodarone can cause benign corneal microdeposits in virtually every patient, it has also been associated with the development of optic neuropathy/neuritis which can lead to blindness. Even though amiodarone may markedly prolong the QT interval, proarrhythmia (ie, TdP) is rare. All of these adverse drug reactions mandate close, continued monitoring (liver enzymes, thyroid function tests, eye examinations, chest radiographs, pulmonary function tests), leading to a proliferation of "amiodarone clinics" designed for patients treated chronically with amiodarone (Table 40-5).[6]

Dronedarone has a considerably shorter half-life (approximately 24 hours) when compared with amiodarone which allows for steady state to be achieved in 5 to 7 days without the need for loading doses. Like amiodarone, dronedarone is a substrate of the CYP3A4 isoenzyme and a moderate inhibitor of the CYP2D6 and CYP3A4 isoenzymes. Its use with potent CYP3A4 inhibitors or inducers should be avoided. Dronedarone may increase plasma concentrations of (*S*)-warfarin; therefore, the INR should be closely monitored with concurrent use of these medications. Dronedarone also inhibits P-gp and can increase digoxin concentrations by about 2.5-fold. Consequently, when concomitantly using dronedarone and digoxin, the digoxin dose should be empirically reduced by 50%. Additionally, dronedarone can increase dabigatran concentrations in patients with renal impairment. To minimize the risk of bleeding when concomitantly using dronedarone and dabigatran in patients with moderate renal impairment (creatinine clearance [CrCl] 30-50 mL/min [0.5-0.83 mL/s]), the dose of dabigatran should be reduced to 75 mg twice daily. The concomitant use of dronedarone and dabigatran should be avoided in patients with severe renal impairment (CrCl less than 30 mL/min [0.5 mL/s]).

Modifications to the chemical structure of dronedarone (addition of a methylsulfonyl group, deletion of the iodine moiety) result in it being less lipophilic than amiodarone. Consequently, dronedarone is supposed to be less likely to accumulate in tissues and cause various organ toxicities. However, like amiodarone, several post-marketing reports have linked dronedarone to significant organ toxicities, including severe hepatic injury, interstitial lung disease (ie, pulmonary fibrosis), and acute kidney injury.[9-11]

Table 40-6 summarizes potential sites/mechanisms for drug interactions with the AADs and Table 40-7 lists recommended dosages of the oral dosage forms of the AADs. Table 40-8 lists the dosing recommendations for the IV forms of various AADs.

Supraventricular Arrhythmias

The common supraventricular tachycardias that often require medication treatment are: (a) AF or AFl; (b) PSVT; and (c) automatic

CLINICAL PRESENTATION Superventricular Tachycardias

Atrial Fibrillation/Flutter

General

- These arrhythmias are usually not directly life-threatening and do not generally cause hemodynamic collapse or syncope; 1:1 AFl (ventricular response approximately 300 beats/min) is an exception. Also, patients with underlying forms of heart disease who are heavily reliant on atrial contraction to maintain adequate cardiac output (eg, mitral stenosis, obstructive cardiomyopathy) display more severe symptoms of AF or AFl.

Symptoms

- Most often, patients complain of rapid heart rate/palpitations, chest pain, dyspnea, dizziness, and fatigue. Medical emergencies are severe HF (ie, pulmonary edema, hypotension) or AF occurring in the setting of acute MI.

ECG Findings

- AF is an irregularly irregular supraventricular rhythm with no discernible, consistent atrial activity (P waves). Ventricular rate is usually 90 to 170 beats/min and the pulse is irregular (Fig. 40-6).
- AFl is (usually) a regular supraventricular rhythm with characteristic flutter waves (or sawtooth pattern) reflecting more organized atrial activity. Commonly, the ventricular rate 150 beats/min (Fig. 40-6).

Paroxysmal Supraventricular Tachycardia Caused by Reentry

General

- This arrhythmia can be transient.

Symptoms

- Patients can complain of intermittent episodes of rapid heart rate/palpitations that abruptly start and stop, usually without provocation (but occasionally as a result of exercise). Severe symptoms include syncope. Often (in particular, those with AV nodal reentry), patients complain of a chest pressure or neck sensation. This is caused by simultaneous AV contraction with the right atrium contracting against a closed tricuspid valve. Life-threatening symptoms (syncope, hemodynamic collapse) are associated with an extremely rapid heart rate (eg, greater than 200 beats/min) and AF associated with an accessory pathway.

ECG Findings

- Most commonly, PSVT is a rapid, narrow QRS tachycardia (regular in rhythm) that starts and stops abruptly (Fig. 40-6). Atrial activity, although present, is difficult to ascertain on surface ECG because P waves are "buried" in the QRS complex or T wave.

TABLE 40-5 Amiodarone Monitoring

Adverse Drug Reaction	Monitoring Recommendations	Management of Adverse Drug Reactions
Pulmonary fibrosis	Chest radiograph (baseline, and then every 12 months)	Discontinue amiodarone immediately; may consider corticosteroid therapy
	Pulmonary function tests (baseline, and then if symptoms develop)	
	High-resolution CT (if symptoms develop)	
Hypothyroidism	TFTs (baseline, and then every 6 months)	Thyroid hormone supplementation (eg, levothyroxine)
Hyperthyroidism	TFTs (baseline, and then every 6 months)	Antithyroid medications (eg, methimazole, propylthiouracil) or corticosteroids; may need to discontinue amiodarone
Optic neuritis/ neuropathy	Ophthalmologic examination (baseline [only if visual impairment present], and then if symptoms develop)	Discontinue amiodarone immediately
Corneal microdeposits	Slit-lamp examination (routine monitoring not necessary)	No treatment necessary
Hepatotoxicity	LFTs (baseline, and then every 6 months)	Lower the dose or discontinue amiodarone if LFTs >2× the upper limit of normal
Bradycardia/heart block	ECG (baseline, and then every 6 months or as clinically indicated)	Lower the dose, if possible, or discontinue amiodarone if severe (or continue amiodarone and implant permanent pacemaker)
Tremor, ataxia, peripheral neuropathy	History/physical examination (each office visit)	Lower the dose, if possible, or discontinue amiodarone if severe
Photosensitivity	History/physical examination (each office visit)	Lower the dose; advise patients to wear sunblock while outdoors

ECG, electrocardiogram; LFTs, liver function tests; TFTs, thyroid function tests.

TABLE 40-6 Potential Mechanisms for Drug-Drug Interactions with Antiarrhythmic Medications

Medication	Substrate	Inhibitor
Disopyramide	CYP3A4 (M)	—
Procainamide	NAT CYP2D6 (M)	—
Quinidine	CYP3A4 (M) CYP2C9	CYP2D6 (S) CYP3A4 (S) CYP2C9 P-gp
Lidocaine	CYP3A4 (M) CYP2D6 (M) CYP1A2 CYP2C9	CYP1A2 (S) CYP2D6
Mexiletine	CYP2D6 (M) CYP1A2 (M)	CYP1A2 (S)
Flecainide	CYP2D6 (M) CYP1A2	CYP2D6
Propafenone[a]	CYP2D6 (M) CYP1A2 CYP2D6	CYP1A2 CYP2D6
Amiodarone	CYP3A4 (M) CYP1A2 CYP2C19 CYP2D6	CYP2C9 CYP2D6 CYP3A4 CYP1A2 CYP2C19 P-gp
Dofetilide	CYP3A4	—
Dronedarone	CYP3A4	CYP2D6 CYP3A4
Ibutilide	—	—
Sotalol	—	—
Diltiazem	CYP3A4 (M) CYP2C9 CYP2D6	CYP3A4 CYP2C9 CYP2D6 P-gp
Verapamil	CYP3A4 (M) CYP1A2 CYP2C9	CYP3A4 CYP1A2 CYP2C9 CYP2D6 P-gp

[a]Variables for parent compound (not 5-OH-propafenone).

CYP, cytochrome P450 isoenzyme; M, major; NAT, N -acetyltransferase; P-gp, P-glycoprotein; S, strong.

atrial tachycardias. Other common supraventricular arrhythmias that usually do not require medication therapy include premature atrial complexes and sinus tachycardia. For example, premature atrial complexes rarely cause symptoms and never cause hemodynamic compromise; therefore, medication therapy is usually not indicated. Likewise, the cause of sinus tachycardia is often an underlying metabolic or hemodynamic disorder (eg, infection,

TABLE 40-7 Typical Maintenance Doses of Class I and Class III Oral Antiarrhythmic Medications

Medication	Dose	Dose Adjustments
Disopyramide	Immediate-release: 100-150 mg every 6 hours Controlled-release: 200-300 mg every 12 hours	**Chronic kidney disease** CrCl 30-40 mL/min (0.5-0.67 mL/s): 100 mg every 8 hours CrCl 15-30 mL/min (0.25-0.5 mL/s): 100 mg every 12 hours CrCl < 15 mL/min (0.25 mL/s): 100 mg daily *Note:* Avoid controlled release formulation if CrCl <40 mL/min (0.67 mL/s) **Hepatic impairment** Immediate-release: 100 mg every 6 hours Controlled-release: 200 mg every 12 hours

(*continued*)

TABLE 40-7 Typical Maintenance Doses of Class I and Class III Oral Antiarrhythmic Medications (*Continued*)

Medication	Dose	Dose Adjustments
Quinidine	200-600 mg sulfate every 6 hours 324-648 gluconate every 8-12 hours	**Chronic kidney disease** No dosage adjustment. Use with caution. The following guidelines have been used by some clinicians[12]: CrCl ≥10 mL/min (0.17 mL/s): No dosage adjustment CrCl <10 mL/min (0.17 mL/s): Administer 75% of normal dose. Hemodialysis: Dose following hemodialysis. **Hepatic impairment** No dosage adjustment. Use with caution due to reduced clearance.
Mexiletine	200-300 mg every 8 hours	**Hepatic impairment** No dose adjustment provided. Use caution as half-life doubles with hepatic impairment.
Flecainide	50-200 mg every 12 hours	**Chronic kidney disease** CrCl >35 mL/min (0.58 mL/s): Initial: 100 mg every 12 hours. Dose increases should be made very cautiously at intervals >4 days. CrCl ≤35 mL/min (0.58 mL/s): Initial: 100 mg once daily or 50 mg every 12 hours. Dose increases should be made very cautiously at intervals >4 days. **Hepatic impairment** No dose adjustment provided. Use caution.
Propafenone	150-300 mg every 8 hours 225-425 mg every 12 hours (SR form)	**Chronic kidney disease** No dose adjustment provided. Use caution. **Hepatic impairment** No dose adjustment provided. Use caution.
Amiodarone	400 mg one to three times daily until 10 g total, then 100-400 mg daily	None
Dofetilide	500 µg every 12 hours	**Chronic kidney disease** CrCl >60 mL/min (1.0 mL/s): No dosage adjustment. CrCl 40 to 60 mL/min (0.67-1.0 mL/s): 250 µg twice daily. CrCl 20 to 39 mL/min (0.33-0.65 mL/s): 125 µg twice daily. CrCl <20 mL/min (0.33 mL/s): Use is contraindicated. **Hepatic impairment** Child-Pugh class A or B: No dosage adjustment. Child-Pugh class C: Use caution.
Dronedarone	400 mg twice daily (with meals)	**Hepatic impairment** Severe impairment: Contraindicated.
Sotalol	80-320 mg every 12 hours	**Chronic kidney disease** *Atrial fibrillation/flutter* CrCl >60mL/min: No dosage adjustment CrCl 30 to 60 mL/min: Administer every 24 hours CrCl <30 mL/min: Avoid use *Ventricular arrhythmia* CrCl >60 mL/min: No dosage adjustment CrCl 30 to 60 mL/min: Administer every 24 hours CrCl 10 to 29 mL/minute: Administer every 36 to 48 hours CrCl <10 mL/min: Individualized **Hepatic impairment** No dosage adjustment.

SR, sustained release.

TABLE 40-8 Typical Doses of IV Antiarrhythmic Medications

Medication	Clinical Situation	Dose
Amiodarone	Pulseless VT/VF	300 mg IV/IO push (can give additional 150 mg IV/IO push if persistent VT/VF or if VT/VF recurs), followed by infusion of 1 mg/min for 6 hours, and then 0.5 mg/min × 18 hours
	Stable VT (with a pulse)	150 mg IV over 10 minutes, followed by infusion of 1 mg/min for 6 hours, and then 0.5 mg/min × 18 hours
	AF (termination)	150 mg IV over 10 minutes, followed by infusion of 1 mg/min for 6 hours, and then 0.5 mg/min × 18 hours
	AF (rate control)	300 mg IV over 1 hour, then 10-50 mg/hour over 24 hours
Diltiazem	PSVT; AF (rate control)	0.25 mg/kg IV over 2 minutes (may repeat with 0.35 mg/kg IV over 2 minutes), followed by infusion of 5-15 mg/hr
Ibutilide	AF (termination)	1 mg IV over 10 minutes (may repeat once, if needed, 10 minutes after initial dose)
Lidocaine	Pulseless VT/VF	1-1.5 mg/kg IV/IO push (can give additional 0.5-0.75 mg/kg IV/IO push every 5-10 minutes if persistent VT/VF [maximum cumulative dose = 3 mg/kg]), followed by infusion of 1-4 mg/min (1-2 mg/min if liver disease or HF)
	Stable VT (with a pulse)	1-1.5 mg/kg IV push (can give additional 0.5-0.75 mg/kg IV push every 5-10 minutes if persistent VT [maximum cumulative dose = 3 mg/kg]), followed by infusion of 1-4 mg/min (1-2 mg/min if liver disease or HF)
Procainamide	AF (termination); stable VT (with a pulse)	15-18 mg/kg IV over 60 minutes, followed by infusion of 1-4 mg/min
Verapamil	PSVT; AF (rate control)	2.5-5 mg IV over 2 minutes (may repeat up to maximum cumulative dose of 20 mg); can follow with infusion of 2.5-10 mg/hr

AF, atrial fibrillation; HF, heart failure; IO, intraosseous; IV, intravenous; PSVT, paroxysmal supraventricular tachycardia; VF, ventricular fibrillation; VT, ventricular tachycardia.

dehydration, hypotension); therapy should focus on treating the underlying cause, not the tachycardia. Of course, there are exceptions to these suggestions. For example, sinus tachycardia may be deleterious in patients after cardiac surgery or MI. Therefore, AADs, such as β-blockers, may be indicated in these situations. Stated in another way, although many arrhythmias generally do not require therapy, clinical judgment and patient-specific variables play an important role in this decision. AF, AFl, and PSVT tend to be the most common supraventricular arrhythmias seen in clinical practice; therefore, this discussion will focus only on these arrhythmias.

Atrial Fibrillation and Atrial Flutter

AF continues to be the most common sustained arrhythmia encountered in clinical practice, affecting approximately 5 million Americans.[13] The overall prevalence of AF is 2% to 4%, and increases with age (eg, approximately an 8% prevalence in patients greater than 65 years old). The prevalence of AF is expected to increase dramatically to an estimated 12 million by the year 2030. The general lifetime risk for AF in White people is 1 in 3 and 1 in 5 among Black people. Hypertension carries the highest risk of developing AF, followed by obesity, smoking, cardiac disease, diabetes, CKD, alcohol consumption, and sleep apnea.[13]

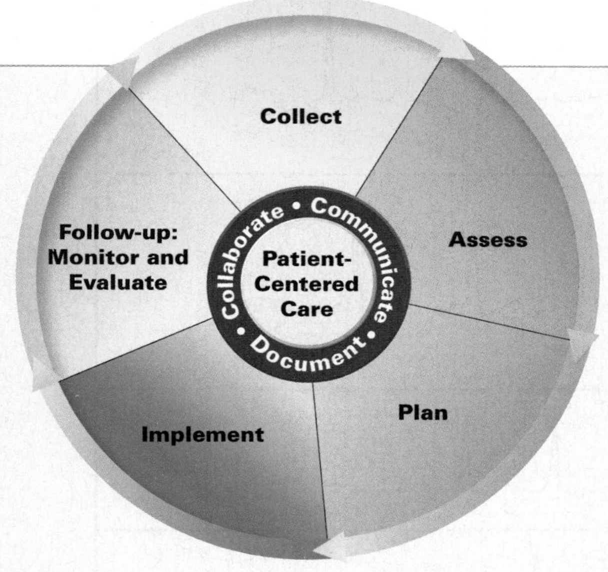

Patient Care Process: Atrial Fibrillation

Collect

- Patient characteristics (eg, age, sex)
- History of present illness (eg, signs/symptoms of AF, duration of AF symptoms) and patient medical history
- Social history (eg, tobacco/ethanol use) and dietary habits including intake of vitamin K–containing foods (for warfarin)
- Current and previous medications including prescription, over-the-counter, aspirin/nonsteroidal anti-inflammatory medications, herbal products, and dietary supplements
- Objective data
    - o Blood pressure (BP), ventricular rate (ie, heart rate), height, weight
    - o Labs: electrolytes (potassium, magnesium), serum creatinine (SCr), hemoglobin, hematocrit, platelets, activated partial thromboplastin time, prothrombin time (PT), international normalized ratio (INR), thyroid function tests
    - o 12-lead electrocardiogram and echocardiogram

Assess

- Hemodynamic instability (eg, systolic BP <90 mm Hg), evidence of decompensated heart failure, or angina
- Duration of AF symptoms (unknown, less than 48 hours, or greater than 48 hours)
- Left ventricular systolic function (ie, left ventricular ejection fraction)
- Risk of stroke (CHA_2DS_2-VASc score) and risk of bleeding (HAS-BLED score)
- Presence of potentially reversible causes of AF (eg, thyrotoxicosis, alcohol withdrawal, infection, electrolyte abnormalities [hypokalemia, hypomagnesemia])
- Ability/willingness to pay for anticoagulation treatment options
- Ability/willingness to obtain laboratory monitoring tests (eg, PT/INR [warfarin], SCr [direct oral anticoagulants (DOACs)])
- Potential medication interactions with anticoagulants and/or antiarrhythmics

Plan*

- Medication therapy regimen including anticoagulant, and/or antiarrhythmic as well as dose, route, frequency, and duration; see Figs. 40-7 and 40-8 and Tables 40-7, 40-8, 40-10, and 40-11.
- Monitoring parameters including efficacy (eg, ventricular rate, rhythm, PT/INR [warfarin], signs/symptoms of stroke) and safety (eg, proarrhythmia [ventricular tachycardia, torsades de pointes], sign/symptoms of bleeding, SCr); frequency and timing of follow-up
- Patient education (eg, purpose of treatment, medication-specific information, monitoring/follow-up)

Implement*

- Provide patient education regarding all elements of treatment plan
- Use motivational interviewing and coaching strategies to maximize adherence
- Schedule follow-up (eg, PT/INR [warfarin], SCr [DOACs], adherence assessment (all medications), bleeding risk assessment [warfarin and DOACs], serum digoxin concentration [digoxin], pertinent laboratory/radiologic tests [amiodarone])

Follow-up: Monitor and Evaluate

- Ventricular rate and rhythm
- Symptoms
- Presence of adverse medication reactions (eg, bradycardia [ventricular rate control medications], bleeding [warfarin and DOACs], organ toxicities [antiarrhythmics]) (see Table 40-4)
- INR [warfarin only] (adjust warfarin dose as needed to maintain target INR in range of 2-3) and determine time in therapeutic range (TTR)
- Patient adherence to treatment plan using multiple sources of information

**Collaborate with patient, caregivers, and other healthcare professionals.*

AF and AFl may present as a chronic, established tachycardia, an acute tachycardia, or a self-terminating, paroxysmal form. The following terms may be used to further define AF: first diagnosed AF (never diagnosed before, irrespective of its duration or symptoms), paroxysmal AF (terminates spontaneously or with intervention within 7 days of onset), persistent AF (duration longer than 7 days), long-standing persistent AF (duration longer than 12 months), and permanent AF (patient and provider jointly decide to stop attempts to restore or maintain SR).[14] AF is characterized by extremely rapid (atrial rate of 400-600 beats/min) and disorganized atrial activation. With this disorganized atrial activity, the contribution of synchronized atrial contraction (atrial kick) is lost, potentially decreasing forward cardiac output. Moreover, the impulses penetrate the AV conduction system in variable degrees resulting in an irregular activation of the ventricles and an irregularly irregular pulse (Fig. 40-6). The AV node will not conduct most of the supraventricular impulses,

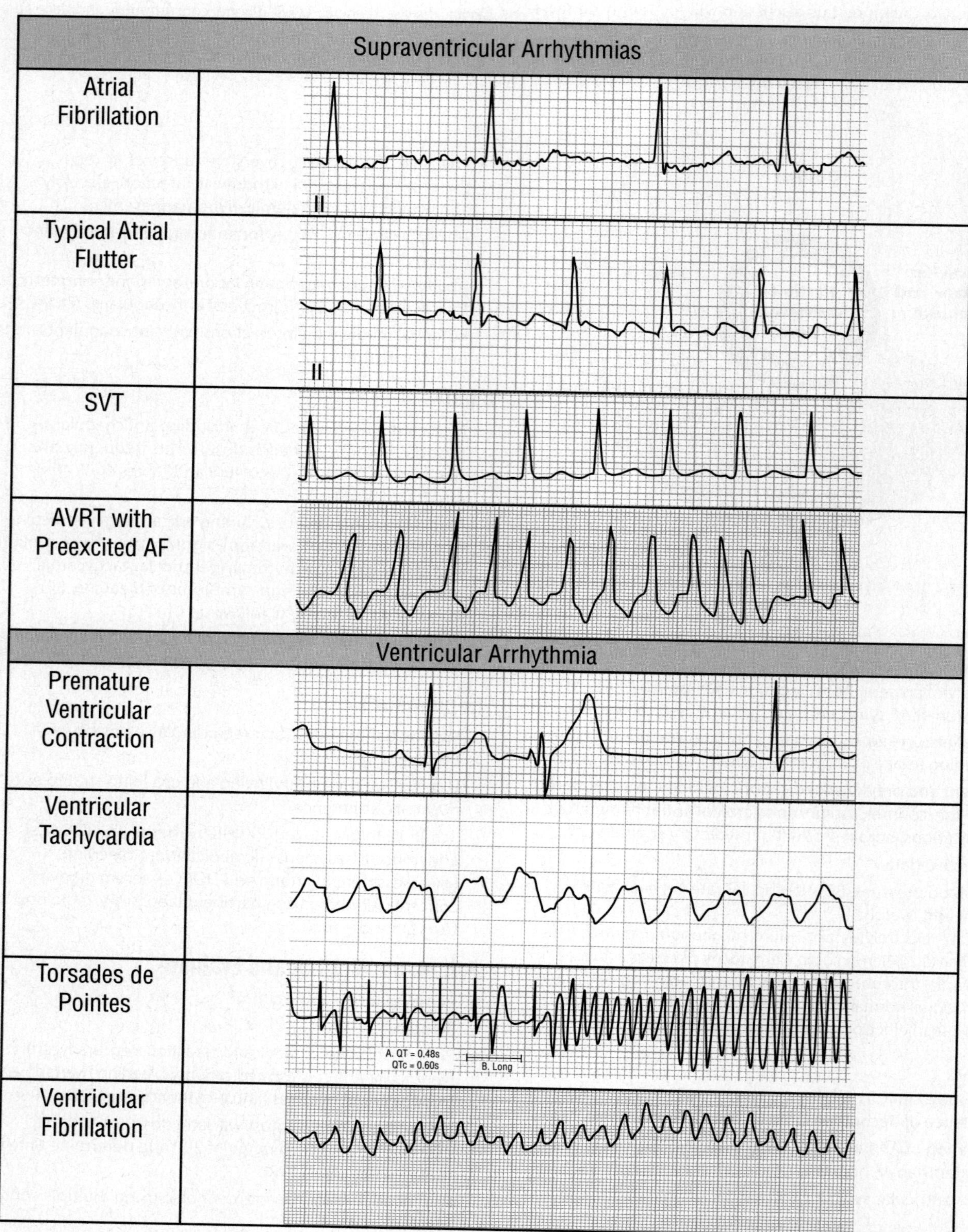

FIGURE 40-6 Electrocardiographic findings of common arrhythmias. (SVT, supraventricular tachycardia; AVRT, atrioventricular reentrant tachycardia; AF, atrial fibrillation.)

causing the ventricular response to be considerably slower than the atrial rate. It is sometimes stated that "AF begets AF," that is, the arrhythmia tends to perpetuate itself. Long episodes are more difficult to terminate perhaps because of tachycardia-induced changes in atrial function (mechanical and/or electrical "remodeling").

AFl occurs less frequently than AF but is similar in its precipitating factors, consequences, and medication therapy approach. This arrhythmia is characterized by rapid (atrial rate of 270 to 330 beats/min) but regular atrial activation. The slower and regular electrical activity results in a regular ventricular response that is in approximate factors of 300 beats/min (ie, 1:1 AV conduction = ventricular rate of 300 beats/min; 2:1 AV conduction = ventricular rate of 150 beats/min; 3:1 AV conduction = ventricular rate of 100 beats/min). AFl may be characterized as "typical" or "atypical." "Typical" flutter is the more common form, which involves the cavotricuspid isthmus. The characteristic "sawtooth" pattern of atrial activation is seen on the surface ECG (Fig. 40-6). The ventricular rate for "atypical" flutter can vary. There are times when a coarse AF can regularize into AFl and then degenerates into AF.

AF may result from multiple atrial reentrant loops (or wavelets), triggered, or abnormal automaticity, whereas AFl is caused by a single, dominant, reentrant substrate ("typical" AFl counterclockwise or clockwise circus movement in the right atrium around the tricuspid annulus). AF or AFl usually occurs in association with various forms of structural heart disease (SHD) that cause left atrial distension, including myocardial ischemia or infarction, hypertensive heart disease, valvular disorders such as mitral stenosis or mitral insufficiency, congenital abnormalities such as septal defects, dilated or hypertrophic cardiomyopathy, and obesity. Disorders that cause right atrial stretch and are associated with AF or AFl include acute pulmonary embolism and chronic lung disease resulting in pulmonary hypertension and right-sided heart failure. AF may also occur in association with states of high adrenergic tone such as thyrotoxicosis, surgery, alcohol withdrawal, sepsis, and excessive physical exertion. Other states in which patients are predisposed to episodes of AF are the presence of an accessory pathway and sinus node dysfunction (SND).

Patients with AF or AFl may experience the entire range of symptoms associated with other supraventricular tachycardias, although syncope as a presenting symptom is uncommon. Because left atrial kick is lost with the onset of AF, patients with HFrEF, HF with preserved ejection fraction (HFpEF) or critical valvular heart disease, particularly mitral stenosis, may develop worsening signs and symptoms of HF as they often depend on the contribution of their atrial kick to maintain an adequate cardiac output. Thromboembolic (TE) events resulting from atrial stasis, predominantly in the left atrial appendage (LAA), and poorly adherent mural thrombi are an additional complication of AF. The risk of stroke is increased fivefold in patients with AF.[14] Stroke can precede the onset of documented AF, probably because of undetected paroxysms prior to the onset of established AF. The risk of stroke significantly increases with age, with the annual attributable risk increasing from 1.5% in individuals 50 to 59 years of age to almost 24% in those 80 to 89 years of age.[15] The risk of stroke in patients with only AFl has been traditionally believed to be lower than AF. Yet, the same risk stratification scheme and antithrombotic recommendations used in patients with AF should also be applied to those with AFl.[14]

General Approach to Treatment 4 The Atrial Fibrillation Better Care (ABC) approach to the treatment of AF can be organized into several sequential goals: "A" Anticoagulation/Avoid stroke; "B" Better symptom management; "C" Cardiovascular and Comorbidity optimization. This approach improves outcomes and reduces cardiovascular events and health-related costs.[5] A review of the management of AF and AFl follows, organized according to the ABCs.

A—Anticoagulation/Avoid Stroke Historically, warfarin has been the standard of care for stroke prevention in patients considered to be at moderate or high risk for stroke due to AF. However, while warfarin is undoubtedly effective in preventing strokes in patients with AF, its use is associated with several potential limitations, including a narrow therapeutic window, requirement for routine INR monitoring, food and drug interactions, and pharmacogenetic influences. Over the past decade, the Food and Drug Administration (FDA) has approved several oral antithrombotic therapies for stroke prevention in patients with AF not due to valvular heart disease (moderate-to-severe mitral stenosis or mechanical heart valve). These oral anticoagulant medications, commonly referred to as direct oral anticoagulants (DOAC), include the direct thrombin inhibitor, dabigatran, and the factor Xa inhibitors, apixaban, edoxaban, and rivaroxaban.

When initiating chronic antithrombotic therapy in patients with AF, the CHEST and American College of Cardiology (ACC)/American Heart Association (AHA) guidelines recommend assessing the patient's risk for stroke and bleeding before selecting the most appropriate regimen.[16,17] The CHA_2DS_2-VASc risk scoring system is used for stroke risk stratification in patients with AF.[16] CHA_2DS_2-VASc is an acronym for each of these risk factors as seen in Fig. 40-7. The points are added up, and the total score is then used to determine the most appropriate antithrombotic therapy for the patient. No antithrombotic therapy is recommended for males with a CHA_2DS_2-VASc score of 0 and females with a CHA_2DS_2-VASc score of 1, as these patients are considered to be at low risk for stroke.[16] For patients with one non-sex CHA_2DS_2-VASc stroke risk factor (ie, CHA_2DS_2-VASc score of 1 in males or 2 in females), oral anticoagulant therapy is suggested by the ACC/AHA and recommended by the CHEST guidelines over no antithrombotic therapy.[16,17] For patients with 2 or more non-sex CHA_2DS_2-VASc stroke risk factors (ie, CHA_2DS_2-VASc score of 2 or higher in males or 3 or higher in females), oral anticoagulant therapy is recommended. If anticoagulation is indicated, the patient's risk for bleeding should also be evaluated. There are several tools to assess bleeding risk, but the most predictive is the HAS-BLED score (Table 40-09).[16] A score of 3 or more is considered high-risk for bleeding. The score should be used to manage modifiable bleeding risk factors and increase surveillance for bleeding in patients with nonmodifiable risk factors.

The efficacy and safety of two dabigatran doses (110 mg and 150 mg twice daily) were compared with those of warfarin in patients with AF.[18] For the primary endpoint of stroke or systemic embolism, both dabigatran groups were shown to be noninferior to warfarin. Furthermore, the dabigatran 150-mg group was shown to be superior to warfarin in reducing this endpoint. The rate of major bleeding was similar between the dabigatran 150-mg and warfarin groups, while the rate of major bleeding was significantly lower in the dabigatran 110-mg group than in the warfarin group. The rate of intracranial hemorrhage (ICH) was significantly lower in both dabigatran groups than in the warfarin group. Even though the 110- and 150-mg dosing regimens of dabigatran were evaluated in this trial, only the 150-mg dose was initially approved by the FDA for AF. A lower 75-mg dose was also approved for patients with a CrCl of 15 to 30 mL/min (0.25 to 0.5 mL/s) even though this dose has not been evaluated in a randomized, prospective clinical trial in patients with AF; this dose has only pharmacokinetic data to support its use.[19] It is important to note that the trial excluded patients with a CrCl less than 30 mL/min (0.5 mL/s). A 110-mg dose of dabigatran has been approved for prophylaxis of venous thromboembolism in patients following hip replacement surgery. Although this dose has not been FDA-approved for stroke prevention in AF, the CHEST guidelines suggest using this dose (or apixaban or edoxaban) in patients with a history of or who are at high risk of bleeding.[16] Dabigatran is contraindicated in patients with mechanical heart valves because its use in this population has been associated with an increased risk of TE complications and bleeding.[20]

The efficacy and safety of rivaroxaban were compared with those of warfarin in patients with AF in the Rivaroxaban Once Daily Oral Direct Factor Xa Inhibition Compared with Vitamin K Antagonism for Prevention of Stroke and Embolism Trial in Atrial Fibrillation (ROCKET AF).[21] In this study, patients were randomized to receive rivaroxaban 20 mg daily or adjusted-dose warfarin.

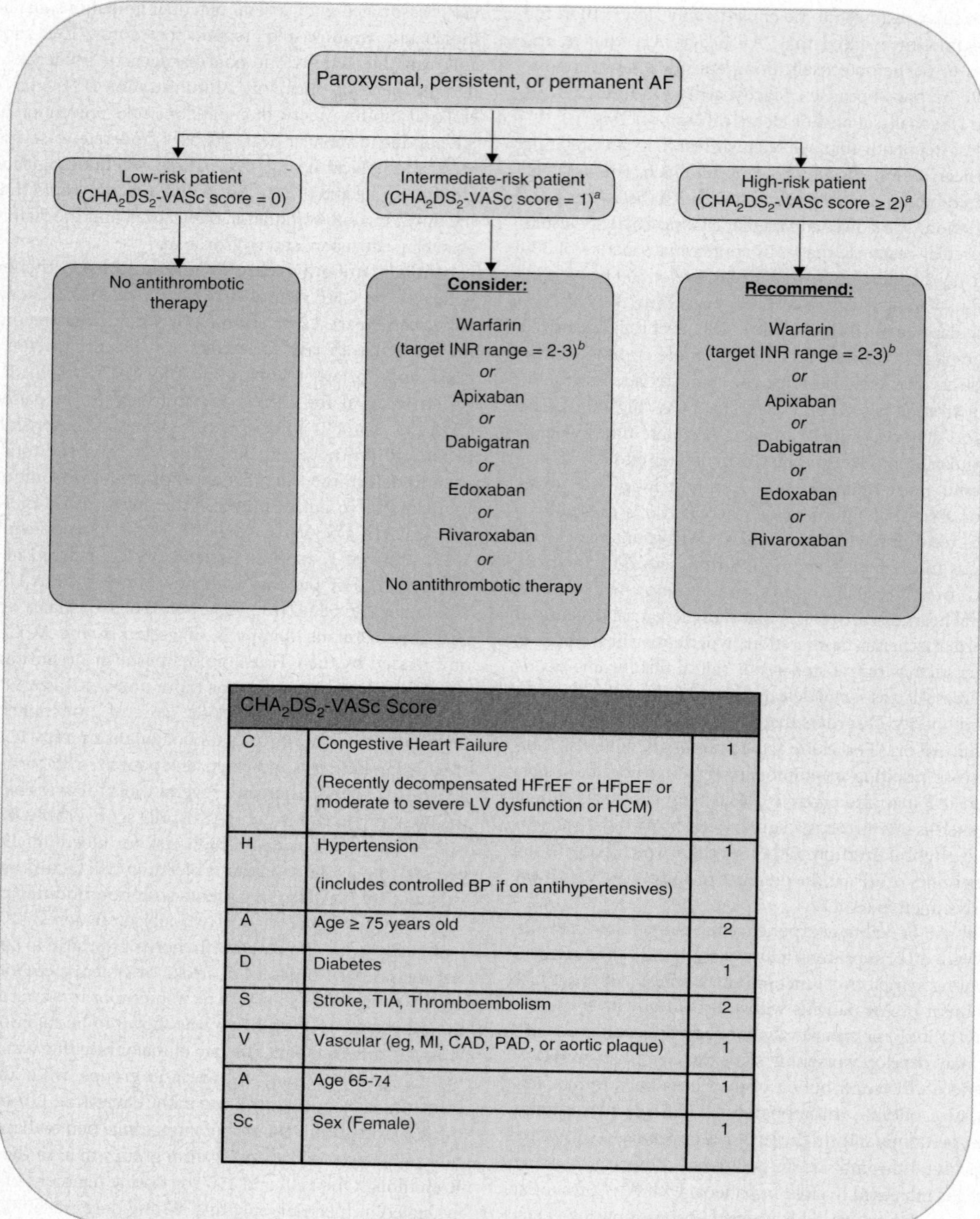

CHA_2DS_2-VASc Score		
C	Congestive Heart Failure (Recently decompensated HFrEF or HFpEF or moderate to severe LV dysfunction or HCM)	1
H	Hypertension (includes controlled BP if on antihypertensives)	1
A	Age ≥ 75 years old	2
D	Diabetes	1
S	Stroke, TIA, Thromboembolism	2
V	Vascular (eg, MI, CAD, PAD, or aortic plaque)	1
A	Age 65-74	1
Sc	Sex (Female)	1

FIGURE 40-7 Algorithm for the prevention of thromboembolism in atrial fibrillation.
[a]Score based on non-sex risk factors.
[b]The target INR for patients with prosthetic heart valves should be based on the type of valve that is present. (AF, atrial fibrillation; INR, international normalized ratio; MI, myocardial infarction; PAD, peripheral arterial disease.)

For the primary endpoint of stroke or systemic embolism, rivaroxaban was shown to be noninferior to warfarin. The rate of major and nonmajor clinically relevant bleeding was similar between the rivaroxaban and warfarin groups. Significantly fewer ICHs occurred in the rivaroxaban group compared with the warfarin group.

The efficacy and safety of apixaban were compared with those of warfarin in patients with AF in the Apixaban for Reduction in Stroke and Other Thromboembolic Events in Atrial Fibrillation (ARISTOTLE) trial.[22] Overall, apixaban was shown to be noninferior and superior to warfarin with regard to the primary endpoint of stroke or systemic embolism. The rate of major bleeding in this trial was significantly lower in the apixaban group than in the warfarin group. Additionally, significantly fewer ICHs occurred in the apixaban group compared with the warfarin group.

The efficacy and safety of edoxaban were compared with those of warfarin in patients with AF in the Effective Anticoagulation with Factor Xa Next Generation in Atrial Fibrillation-Thrombolysis in Myocardial Infarction (ENGAGE AF-TIMI) 48 trial.[23] In this study, patients were randomized to receive edoxaban 60 mg daily, edoxaban 30 mg daily, or adjusted-dose warfarin. Overall, both doses of edoxaban were shown to be noninferior to warfarin with regard to the primary endpoint of stroke or systemic embolism. However, the edoxaban 60-mg dosing regimen was also shown to be superior to warfarin with regard to this endpoint. The rate of major bleeding and

TABLE 40-9 HAS-BLED Score to Predict Bleeding Risk in Patients with Atrial Fibrillation

Letter	Risk Factor	Points
H	Uncontrolled hypertension (systolic blood pressure >160 mm Hg)	1
A	Abnormal renal +/− hepatic function (dialysis, transplant, serum creatinine >2.26 mg/dL (200 μmol/L), cirrhosis, bilirubin >2× normal with AST/ALT/AP >3× normal)	1 point each
S	Stroke (ischemic or hemorrhagic)	1
B	Bleeding (history of major hemorrhage or anemia or severe thrombocytopenia)	1
L	Labile INR on warfarin (TTR <60%)	1
E	Elderly (>65 years old or extremely frail)	1
D	Drugs or alcohol use (concomitant use of antiplatelet or NSAID and/or ≥8 alcoholic drinks/week)	1 point each

HAS-BLED score assesses a patient's 1-year risk of major bleeding when taking anticoagulants for atrial fibrillation. A score of 3 or greater is considered high risk for bleeding. The maximum score is 9. (AST, aspartate aminotransferase; ALT, alanine aminotransferase; AP, alkaline phosphatase; INR, international normalized ratio; NSAID, nonsteroidal anti-inflammatory drug; TTR, time in therapeutic range.)

the risk of ICH were significantly lower in both edoxaban groups than in the warfarin group. However, the risk of major gastrointestinal bleeding was significantly higher in the edoxaban 60-mg group, but significantly lower in the edoxaban 30-mg group when compared to the warfarin group.

Guidelines recommend therapy with a DOAC over warfarin.[16,17] However, it is essential that anticoagulant therapy be individualized for each patient, with consideration given to medication cost, insurance coverage, INR monitoring options, patient preference, drug interaction potential, anticipated medication adherence, and necessary follow-up. Specifically with warfarin, the target INR range should be 2 to 3 and the time in therapeutic range (TTR) should ideally be greater than 70%.[16] The TTR is an important metric when evaluating the efficacy of warfarin therapy as the risk of TE events, major bleeding, and death is lower in patients with a TTR of at least 65% compared to patients with a TTR of less than 65%.[24] The CHEST guidelines have recommended the use of the SAMe-TT_2R_2 score to assist in the identification of patients who are likely or not likely to achieve good anticoagulation control with warfarin (ie, TTR of at least 65%).[16] With this scoring system, patients with AF are given two points each if they use tobacco or are of a non-white race. Patients are given one point each for being female, being younger than 60 years of age, having at least two of the specified medical conditions (hypertension, diabetes, CAD/MI, congestive HF, previous stroke, pulmonary disease, hepatic disease, or renal disease), or receiving treatment with a medication that interacts with warfarin. SAMe-TT_2R_2 is an acronym for each of these risk factors. Once the points for this scoring system are added up, a score of 0 to 2 suggests that patients are likely to achieve a TTR of at least 65%. Patients with a score of more than 2 are less likely to achieve a TTR of at least 65% and should be educated on strategies that could improve their TTR including more frequent INR monitoring and medication reviews, adherence counseling, and dietary guidance. Alternatively, these patients could be considered for DOAC therapy. Additionally, if a patient has previously taken warfarin, the time that his/her INR has been within the therapeutic range should also be considered before making the decision to switch the patient to a DOAC.

If a patient is unable to maintain a therapeutic INR while on warfarin, therapy with a DOAC is recommended. Strict adherence with the DOACs is important because missing a single dose could result in an increased risk of TE events.[25] If treatment with warfarin must be temporarily interrupted for the patient to undergo a medical procedure, coverage with a parenteral anticoagulant (eg, unfractionated heparin, low molecular weight heparin [LMWH]) should be considered in patients with a high risk of stroke and/or have a mechanical heart valve. Moreover, warfarin is the anticoagulant of choice for patients with moderate to severe mitral stenosis or a mechanical heart valve; the INR should be based on the type and location of the valve placed. Dabigatran, edoxaban, and rivaroxaban should be avoided in patients with a CrCl less than 15 mL/min (0.25 mL/s). In this particular population, anticoagulant options are warfarin and apixaban. Edoxaban should also be avoided in patients with a CrCl greater than 95 mL/min (1.58 mL/s) because of the potential for reduced efficacy.

Although it was previously an acceptable practice to discontinue antithrombotic therapy 4 weeks after successful cardioversion (with the belief that a patient's risk for thromboembolism had abated since he/she was in SR), data from the RACE and AFFIRM trials strongly suggest that patients with AF and other risk factors for stroke continue to be at risk for stroke even when maintained in SR.[26,27] It is possible that these patients may be having undetected episodes of paroxysmal AF, placing them at risk for stroke. Consequently, the decision regarding chronic antithrombotic therapy should be based on a patient's risk for stroke using the CHA_2DS_2-VASc scoring system.[14]

Should a patient have an increased risk of stroke, but have a contraindication to long-term anticoagulation, a LAA occluder may be an alternative.[5,14,17] The Watchman, the only FDA-approved device, is deployed into the left atrial appendage and designed to conform to the anatomy of the LAA, permanently sealing it off and reducing the risk of emboli. Although postimplantation antithrombotic practice patterns vary, patients should initiate aspirin the day before the procedure and an oral anticoagulant upon implantation. If an adequate seal has been formed at 45 days postimplant, oral anticoagulation should be discontinued, aspirin should be continued, and a $P2Y_{12}$ inhibitor should be started. At 6 months postimplant, the $P2Y_{12}$ inhibitor is stopped while aspirin is continued life long.

B—Better Symptom Management Should patients receive rate control (regulate only the ventricular rate and remain in AF) or rhythm control (restoring and maintaining normal sinus rhythm)? Six landmark clinical trials have compared the efficacy of rate control and rhythm control treatment strategies in patients with AF.[26-31] The Atrial Fibrillation Follow-Up Investigation of Rhythm Management (AFFIRM) trial is the largest rate control versus rhythm control study conducted to date in patients with AF.[27] In this trial, patients with AF and at least one risk factor for stroke were randomized to either a rate control or a rhythm control group. Rate-control treatment involved AV nodal blocking medications (digoxin, β-blockers, and/or non-DHP CCBs) first, and then nonpharmacologic treatment (AV nodal ablation with pacemaker implantation), if necessary. All patients in this group were anticoagulated. In the rhythm control group, class I or III AADs were used to maintain SR. The choice of AAD therapy was left up to each patient's physician. By the end of the trial, more than 60% of patients had received at least one trial of amiodarone, and approximately 40% of patients had received at least one trial of sotalol. In the rhythm control group, anticoagulation was encouraged but could be discontinued if SR had been maintained for at least 4 weeks. Overall mortality was not statistically different between the two strategies. However, patients in the rhythm-control group were significantly more likely to be hospitalized or experience an adverse drug reaction. The results of the other four trials were consistent with those of the AFFIRM trial.[26,28-30] In addition, a meta-analysis of these data demonstrated no significant difference in overall mortality between rate control and pharmacological rhythm control strategies, which persisted even when the results from the AFFIRM trial were excluded from this analysis.[32]

Collectively, these trials demonstrate that a rate control strategy is a viable alternative to a rhythm control strategy in patients with persistent AF. However, only a small proportion of patients enrolled in these trials had HFrEF. Thus, a trial was conducted to specifically evaluate the safety and efficacy of rate control and rhythm control strategies in patients with HFrEF.[31] Consistent with other rate control versus rhythm control studies, no significant difference in the primary endpoint of death from cardiovascular (CV) causes was observed between treatment groups. Though not statistically significant, patients in the rhythm control group tended to have more hospitalizations, primarily due to repeated cardioversions and adjustment of AAD therapy. It is important to note that the results of this trial should not be applied to patients with HFpEF. Together, these trials suggest that a pharmacological rhythm control strategy does not confer any advantage over a rate control strategy in patients with AF, with or without HFrEF.

4 Clearly, these important findings temper the old approach of aggressively attempting to maintain SR. Because a rhythm control strategy does not offer any significant advantage over a rate control strategy in the management of patients with AF, the decision to utilize one strategy over another is primarily driven by the goal of improving a patient's quality of life (Table 40-10).

Rate Control Once the decision has been made to rate control a patient, the next important question is: What defines "adequate" ventricular rate control? A lenient rate control strategy targeting a resting heart rate less than 110 beats/min is recommended for asymptomatic patients with a preserved LV systolic function (LVEF greater than 40% [0.40]).[14,33] In patients who are symptomatic or have LV systolic dysfunction (LVEF less than or equal to 40% [0.40]), a stricter rate control approach targeting a resting heart rate less than 80 beats/min should be considered.

The selection of an AV nodal-blocking medication to control ventricular rate is primarily based on the patient's LV function.[14] In patients with preserved LV function or in patients with stable HFpEF, a β-blocker or non-DHP CCB (diltiazem or verapamil) is preferred over digoxin because of their relatively quick onset and maintained efficacy during exercise. When adequate ventricular rate control cannot be achieved with one of these medications, the addition of digoxin may result in an additive lowering of the heart rate. However, digoxin tends to be ineffective for controlling ventricular rate under conditions of increased sympathetic tone (ie, surgery, thyrotoxicosis) because it slows AV nodal conduction primarily through vagotonic mechanisms. Verapamil and diltiazem should be avoided in patients with HFrEF (LVEF less than or equal to 40% [0.40]) because of their potent negative inotropic effects.[14] Instead, β-blockers and digoxin are preferred. Specifically, in patients with NYHA class II or III HF, β-blockers should be considered over digoxin because of their survival benefits in patients with HFrEF. If patients are having an episode of decompensated HF (NYHA class IV), digoxin is preferred as first-line therapy to achieve ventricular rate control because of the potential for worsening HF symptoms with the initiation and subsequent titration of β-blocker therapy. Several analyses have associated digoxin with a significant increase in the risk of mortality in patients with AF.[34] The risk is highest when serum digoxin concentrations are 1.2 ng/mL (mcg/L; 1.5 nmol/L) or greater.[35]

If adequate ventricular rate control during rest and exercise cannot be achieved with β-blockers, non-DHP CCBs, and/or digoxin in patients with normal or depressed LV function, amiodarone can be used as an alternative therapy to control the heart rate (Table 40-11). However, clinicians should be aware that the use of amiodarone for controlling ventricular rate may also stimulate the conversion of AF to SR and place the patient at risk for a TE event, especially if the AF has persisted for at least 48 hours or is of unknown duration.

TABLE 40-10 Considerations for Selecting a Rate-Control Versus Rhythm-Control Strategy in Patients with Atrial Fibrillation

Rate-Control	Rhythm-Control
No or minimal symptoms	Paroxysmal or persistent AF
Treatment of choice for permanent AF	Symptomatic despite adequate rate control
	Hemodynamically unstable
	Exacerbating heart failure
	Tachycardia-mediated cardiomyopathy
	Other factors • Younger age • First episode of AF • Patient preference

AF, atrial fibrillation.

Rhythm Control In those whose decision has been made to restore SR, one must consider that this very act (regardless of whether an electrical or pharmacologic method is chosen) places the patient at risk for a TE event. The heightened risk is because the return of SR restores effective contraction in the atria, which may dislodge poorly adherent thrombi. Administering anticoagulant therapy prior to cardioversion not only prevents clot growth and the formation of new thrombi but also allows existing thrombi to become organized and well adherent to the atrial wall. It is a generally accepted principle that the risk of thrombus formation and a subsequent embolic event increases if the duration of the AF exceeds 48 hours. Therefore, it is vital for clinicians to estimate the duration of the patient's AF so that appropriate anticoagulant therapy can be administered prior to cardioversion if needed.

For patients undergoing elective cardioversion (electrical or pharmacologic) for AF lasting at least 48 hours or for an unknown duration, guidelines recommend that therapeutic anticoagulation with warfarin or DOAC should be given for at least 3 weeks before cardioversion is performed; this recommendation applies to patients regardless of their CHA_2DS_2-VASc score.[16,37] If 3 weeks of therapeutic oral anticoagulant therapy is not feasible in these patients, a screening transesophageal echocardiogram (TEE) can be performed prior to cardioversion to evaluate for the presence of thrombus in the heart chambers (particularly the atria or atrial appendage). Overall, there is no difference in the efficacy and safety between DOACs and warfarin in patients undergoing TEE-guided cardioversion.[38]

If cardioversion is successful (ie, patient is now in SR), therapeutic anticoagulation with warfarin (INR target range 2 to 3) or a DOAC should be continued for at least 4 weeks, regardless of the patient's baseline risk of stroke.[16,37] The reason for continuing anticoagulation for this additional 4-week time period is that after restoration of SR, full atrial contraction does not occur immediately. Rather, it returns gradually to a maximum contractile force over a 3- to 4-week period. Decisions regarding long-term antithrombotic therapy after this 4-week period should be based on the patient's risk for stroke and not on whether the patient is in SR. If a thrombus is seen on TEE, cardioversion should not be performed and the patient should be anticoagulated for another 4 to 12 weeks.[16]

In patients with AF that is less than 48 hours in duration, a prolonged period of anticoagulation prior to cardioversion is unnecessary because there has not been sufficient time to form atrial thrombi. However, an oral anticoagulant, LMWH or unfractionated heparin should be started as soon as possible.[5,16,37]

After anticoagulation needs and/or TEE have been addressed, the process of restoring SR can be considered. There are two methods of restoring SR in patients with AF or AFl: pharmacologic cardioversion and DCCV. The decision to use either of these methods is generally based on clinical preference and the

TABLE 40-11 Evidence-Based Pharmacologic Treatment Recommendations for Controlling Ventricular Rate, Restoring Sinus Rhythm, and Maintaining Sinus Rhythm in Patients with Atrial Fibrillation

Treatment Recommendations	ACC/AHA Guideline Recommendation
Ventricular rate control (acute setting)	
In the absence of an accessory pathway, an IV β-blocker or IV non-DHP CCB is recommended for patients without HF.	Class I
In the absence of an accessory pathway, IV digoxin or IV amiodarone is recommended to control the ventricular rate in patients with HF.	Class I
In the absence of an accessory pathway, an IV β-blocker is recommended to control the ventricular rate in patients with stable HFrEF.	Class I
In the absence of an accessory pathway, an IV non-DHP CCB is recommended to control the ventricular rate in patients with stable HFpEF.	Class I
In the absence of an accessory pathway, IV amiodarone is recommended to control the ventricular rate in critically ill patients.	Class IIa
IV amiodarone can be useful to control the ventricular rate when other measures are unsuccessful or contraindicated.	Class IIa
Digoxin, non-DHP CCBs, or IV amiodarone should not be used in patients with an accessory pathway.	Class III
IV β-blockers or IV non-DHP CCBs are not recommended in patients with decompensated HF.	Class III
Ventricular rate control (chronic setting)	
An oral β-blocker or non-DHP CCB is recommended to control the ventricular rate in patients with paroxysmal, persistent, or permanent AF.	Class I
An oral β-blocker or non-DHP CCB is recommended to control the ventricular rate in patients with persistent or permanent AF and compensated HFpEF.	Class I
Digoxin is effective for controlling resting heart rate in patients with HFrEF.	Class I
A combination of digoxin and a β-blocker is reasonable to control resting and exercise heart rate in patients with HFrEF.	Class IIa
A combination of digoxin and a non-DHP CCB is reasonable to control resting and exercise heart rate in patients with HFpEF.	Class IIa
Oral amiodarone can be used when the ventricular rate cannot be adequately controlled at rest and during exercise with an oral β-blocker, non-DHP CCB, and/or digoxin.	Class IIb
Oral non-DHP CCBs and dronedarone are not recommended to control the ventricular rate in patients with decompensated HF.	Class III
Dronedarone should not be used to control the ventricular rate in patients with permanent AF.	Class III
Restoration of sinus rhythm	
In the absence of contraindications, flecainide, dofetilide, propafenone, or ibutilide is recommended for pharmacologic cardioversion of AF.	Class I
Oral amiodarone is a reasonable option for pharmacologic cardioversion of AF.	Class IIa
The "pill-in-the-pocket" approach with flecainide or propafenone can be used to terminate persistent AF on an outpatient basis once the treatment has been used safely in the hospital, in patients without sinus or AV node dysfunction, bundle-branch block, QT interval prolongation, Brugada syndrome, or SHD (*Note*: AV node must be adequately blocked with β-blocker or non-DHP CCB therapy before initiating this therapy).	Class IIa
Dofetilide should not be initiated on an outpatient basis.	Class III
Maintenance of sinus rhythm	
The following AADs are recommended for maintaining SR, depending on underlying SHD and other comorbidities: amiodarone, dofetilide, dronedarone, flecainide, propafenone, and sotalol.	Class I
Because of its potential toxicities, amiodarone should only be used after consideration of its risks and when other agents have failed or are contraindicated.	Class I
The risk of the AAD, including proarrhythmia, should be considered before initiating treatment with that medication.	Class I
Antiarrhythmic therapy can be useful for maintaining SR for the treatment of tachycardia-induced cardiomyopathy.	Class IIa
It may be reasonable to continue current AAD therapy in the setting of infrequent, well-tolerated recurrences of AF when the medication has reduced the frequency or symptoms of AF.	Class IIb
An AAD should not be continued when the AF becomes permanent.	Class III
Dronedarone should not be used in patients with class III or IV HF or patients who have had an episode of decompensated HF in the last 4 weeks.	Class III

AAD, antiarrhythmic medication; ACC, American College of Cardiology; AF, atrial fibrillation; AHA, American Heart Association; AV, atrioventricular; CCB, calcium channel blocker; DHP, dihydropyridine; HF, heart failure; HFpEF, heart failure with preserved ejection fraction; HFrEF, heart failure with reduced ejection fraction; HRS, Heart Rhythm Society; IV, intravenous; SHD, structural heart disease; SR, sinus rhythm.

Data from Reference 36.

hemodynamic stability of the patient. In situations of hemodynamic instability (eg, severe hypotension, angina, or pulmonary edema), direct current cardioversion is indicated as first-line therapy in an attempt to immediately restore SR (without regard to the risk of thromboembolism). The disadvantages of pharmacologic cardioversion are the risk of significant adverse drug reactions (eg, drug-induced TdP), the potential for drug-drug interactions (eg, digoxin–amiodarone), and the lower efficacy of AADs when compared with DCCV. The advantages of DCCV are that it is quick and more often successful (80% to 90% success rate) compared to pharmacologic cardioversion. The disadvantages of DCCV are the need for periprocedural sedation/anesthesia and the risk (albeit small) of serious complications such as sinus arrest or ventricular arrhythmias.

Nonetheless, despite the relatively high success rate associated with DCCV, clinicians and patients may elect to use AADs first, and then resort to DCCV if these medications fail. Pharmacologic cardioversion appears to be most effective when initiated within 7 days after the onset of AF.[14] There is relatively strong evidence for the efficacy of class III pure I_K blockers (ibutilide and dofetilide), the class Ic AADs (flecainide and propafenone), and amiodarone (oral or IV) for cardioversion of AF.[14] Class Ia AADs have limited efficacy or have not been adequately studied in this setting. Sotalol is not effective for cardioversion of paroxysmal or persistent AF. Single, oral loading doses of propafenone (body weight greater than 70 kg: 600 mg; less than 70 kg: 450 mg) and flecainide (body weight greater than 70 kg: 300 mg; less than 70 kg: 200 mg) are effective compared with placebo for conversion of recent-onset AF and have been incorporated into the "pill-in-the-pocket" approach endorsed by treatment guidelines.[14,39] With this method, patient-controlled, self-administration of a single, oral loading dose of flecainide or propafenone in the outpatient setting is relatively safe and effective for the termination of recent-onset AF in the absence of sinus or AV node dysfunction, bundle-branch block, or SHD.[39] This approach should be considered in patients who have previously been successfully cardioverted with these medications on an inpatient basis.

Overall, when considering pharmacologic cardioversion, the selection of an AAD should be based on whether the patient has SHD (eg, LV dysfunction, CAD, valvular heart disease, LV hypertrophy).[14] In the absence of any type of SHD, the use of a single, oral loading dose of flecainide or propafenone is a reasonable approach for cardioversion. Ibutilide can also be used as an alternative in this patient population; however, the use of this agent is restricted to a monitored setting in the hospital because it requires QT interval monitoring. In patients with underlying SHD, flecainide, propafenone, and ibutilide should be avoided because of the increased risk of proarrhythmia; amiodarone or dofetilide should be used instead. Although amiodarone can be administered safely on an outpatient basis because of its low proarrhythmic potential, dofetilide therapy can only be initiated in the hospital (for QT interval monitoring and assessment of renal function). Additionally, a patient's ventricular rate should be adequately controlled with AV nodal blocking medications prior to administering a class Ic AAD for cardioversion. The class Ic AADs may paradoxically increase ventricular response. The most likely mechanism for this effect is that by slowing atrial conduction, the class Ic AADs decrease the number of impulses reaching the AV node. Consequently, the AV node paradoxically allows more impulses to gain entrance to the ventricular conduction system, thereby increasing ventricular rate.

Class Ic or III AADs are reasonable to consider to maintain patients in SR (Table 40-12).[14] The role of the class Ia AADs for maintenance of SR has been deemphasized compared with the class Ic and III AADs. While a systematic review of AADs for the maintenance of SR after cardioversion in patients with AF demonstrated that AF recurrences were significantly reduced with the use of class Ia, Ic, and III AADs, mortality was significantly increased with the class Ia medications.[40] The class Ic AADs, flecainide and propafenone, are effective for maintaining SR. However, because of the increased risk for proarrhythmia, these medications should be avoided in patients with SHD.

Although all oral class III AADs have demonstrated efficacy in preventing AF recurrences, amiodarone is clearly the most effective agent and the most frequently used AAD despite its potential for causing significant organ toxicity.[41] The superiority of amiodarone over other AADs for maintaining patients in SR has been demonstrated in a number of clinical trials. Amiodarone was significantly more effective than sotalol or propafenone in maintaining SR in patients with persistent or paroxysmal AF.[42] Amiodarone was also found to be significantly more effective than sotalol at maintaining SR in all patient subgroups, except for those with CAD where the efficacy of these two medications was comparable.[43] Furthermore, amiodarone appears to be the most effective AAD in maintaining SR.[44]

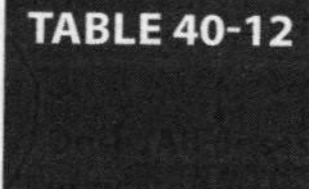

TABLE 40-12 Guidelines for Selecting Antiarrhythmic Medication Therapy to Maintain Sinus Rhythm in Patients with Recurrent Paroxysmal or Recurrent Persistent Atrial Fibrillation

No structural heart disease[a] (absence of heart failure, coronary artery disease, or significant LVH)
First line[b]: dofetilide, dronedarone, flecainide, propafenone, or sotalol
Second line[c]: amiodarone
Heart failure[a]
First line[b]: amiodarone or dofetilide
Second line: catheter ablation
Coronary artery disease[a]
First line[b]: dofetilide, dronedarone,[d] or sotalol[d]
Second line[c]: amiodarone

LVH, left ventricular hypertrophy.

[a]Medications are listed alphabetically and not in order of suggested use.

[b]Catheter ablation may also be considered first-line therapy in select patients with paroxysmal atrial fibrillation.

[c]Catheter ablation may also be considered when patients are refractory or intolerant to at least one antiarrhythmic medication.

[d]Should only be used in this situation if the patient has normal left ventricular systolic function.

Although sotalol is not effective for the conversion of AF, it is an effective medication for maintaining SR. Sotalol appears to be at least as effective as propafenone in preventing recurrences of AF.[42] However, treatment with sotalol is associated with TdP. Because TdP occurs primarily with higher doses of sotalol, it may be easier to predict and avoid. Nonetheless, sotalol may increase mortality in patients with AF.[45]

Dofetilide is effective in preventing AF recurrences but has not been directly compared with either amiodarone or sotalol. In a large, multicenter trial, dofetilide was more effective than placebo in maintaining SR (approximately 35% to 50% at 1 year).[46] The efficacy of dofetilide for maintenance of SR has also specifically been demonstrated in patients with HFrEF.[47] Like sotalol and quinidine, dofetilide also has significant potential to cause TdP (in a dose-related fashion).

In two similarly designed trials, dronedarone was more effective than placebo in maintaining SR in patients with paroxysmal or persistent AF or AFl.[48] In another trial, the use of dronedarone in patients with persistent or paroxysmal AF or AFl was associated with significantly fewer hospitalizations due to CV events or death when compared with placebo.[49] In another study, dronedarone was shown to be significantly less effective than amiodarone in reducing AF recurrences.[50] However, tolerability was significantly better in the dronedarone group than the amiodarone group as evidenced by higher rates of premature medication discontinuation due to adverse events in the amiodarone group.[50] Most recently, a trial that enrolled patients with permanent AF and risk factors for major vascular events was terminated prematurely after significantly more patients in the dronedarone group died (primarily from CV causes), or hospitalized for HF, or suffered a stroke compared with the placebo group.[51] Based on the results of this trial, dronedarone is contraindicated (black box warning) in patients with permanent AF.

One study evaluated the safety and efficacy of dronedarone to prevent death and heart failure hospitalizations in patients with NYHA class III or IV HFrEF (presumably due to decreasing arrhythmia occurrence).[52] This trial was prematurely terminated because all-cause mortality (primarily due to worsening HF) was significantly higher in the dronedarone group compared with the placebo group. Consequently, dronedarone is contraindicated (black box warning) in advanced HF (NYHA class IV or NYHA class II or III with a recent hospitalization for decompensated HF).

Overall, the selection of an AAD to maintain SR should be primarily based on whether the patient has SHD.[14] However, other factors, including renal and hepatic function, concomitant disease states and medications, and the AAD's side effect profile also need to be considered. Dofetilide, dronedarone, flecainide, propafenone, or sotalol should be considered initially for those patients with no underlying SHD because these medications have the most optimal long-term safety profile in this setting.[14] However, amiodarone could be used as an alternative therapy if the patient fails or does not tolerate one of these initial AADs. In the presence of SHD, flecainide and propafenone should be avoided because of the risk of proarrhythmia. For those patients with HFrEF (LVEF less than or equal to 40% [0.40]), amiodarone or dofetilide should be considered the AADs of choice. Only amiodarone and dofetilide have been shown to be mortality-neutral in patients with AF and HFrEF. Both dronedarone and sotalol should be avoided in patients with HFrEF because of the risk for increased mortality (dronedarone) or worsening HF (dronedarone and sotalol). In patients with CAD, dofetilide, dronedarone, or sotalol can be used initially. Amiodarone could be used as an alternative therapy if the patient fails or does not tolerate one of these initial AADs. The presence of LV hypertrophy may predispose the myocardium to proarrhythmic events. Because of their low proarrhythmic potential, amiodarone or dronedarone should be considered first-line AAD therapy in these patients.

Figure 40-8 shows an algorithm for the management of AF and AFl.

Nonpharmacologic forms of therapy, designed to maintain SR, are becoming increasingly popular treatment options for patients with AF or AFl. For patients who have "typical" AFl, not associated with concurrent AF, ablation of the reentrant substrate with radiofrequency current is highly effective (more than 90%) and should be first-line treatment of AFl to prevent recurrences.[53] Catheter ablation for patients with AF is much more technically difficult for a variety of reasons, including the lack of a single, identifiable, and ablatable reentrant focus (as in AFl). Patients with AF have been found to have arrhythmogenic foci that occur in atrial tissue near and within the pulmonary veins. The ablation procedure most commonly used is a pulmonary vein isolation (PVI) ablation, where the foci originating in these areas are abolished by locally delivering heat (radiofrequency energy) or freezing the tissue (cryoablation). Historically, PVI ablation was often considered last-line therapy for patients who had failed all AADs, including amiodarone. However, in some trials, the use of PVI ablation in patients with AF has been associated with a significant reduction in recurrent episodes of AF and an improvement in quality of life when compared with AAD therapy.[54,55] In patients with AF and concomitant HFrEF who did not respond to, were intolerant of, or were unwilling to take AADs, the use of PVI ablation has been associated with a significant reduction in all-cause mortality or hospitalization for worsening HF.[56] There is also evidence to suggest that this procedure may be superior to AADs as first-line therapy of symptomatic AF.[57,58] Moreover, ablation is an appropriate option for patients with tachycardia-induced cardiomyopathy. Controlling comorbidities (ie, OSA, obesity, HTN) highly contributes to the success of maintaining normal sinus rhythm post ablation. This procedure is not without risks, as major complications, such as pulmonary vein stenosis, TE events, cardiac tamponade, and new AFl, have been reported in 4.5% of patients.[59]

C—Cardiovascular and Comorbidity Optimization Cardiovascular burden and comorbidities, such as obesity, hypertension, diabetes, and sleep apnea, play a role in atrial structural and electrical remodeling; thus, the development of AF.[5] Weight loss can reduce AF episodes and reoccurrence after ablation. Furthermore, weight loss can reduce blood pressure, Hgb A1C, and cholesterol, which leads to better cardiovascular health. Other lifestyle interventions a patient should engage in are abstaining from alcohol and incorporating physical activity, except for endurance training, as this can precipitate AF.

Patients with hypertension have a 1.7-fold higher risk of AF than a patient with normal blood pressure and should be treated to a goal blood pressure of ≤130/80 mm Hg.[5] Patients with diabetes have a twofold higher prevalence of AF than those without diabetes. Moreover, diabetes places patients at a higher risk for stroke. Roughly 50% of patients with AF have sleep apnea. When managed with continuous positive airway pressure, the recurrence of AF may be ameliorated. Controlling these disease states reduces a patient's risk of developing AF, the number of occurrences the patient experiences, and the success of rhythm control management.

Paroxysmal Supraventricular Tachycardia

5 PSVT generated by reentrant mechanisms includes AV nodal reentry (ie, AVNRT), AV reentry incorporating an accessory pathway (ie, AVRT), SA nodal reentry, and intra-atrial reentry. AVNRT and AVRT are, by far, the most common of these tachycardias.

AVNRT is usually seen in middle-aged adults without heart disease and more than 60% of cases occur in females.[60] The ventricular rate can range from 110 beats/min to more than 250 beats/min. This arrhythmia can spontaneously occur or be provoked by exertion, coffee, tea, or alcohol. Patients generally tolerate AVNRT hemodynamically; however, many are highly symptomatic.[53]

The underlying substrate of AVNRT is the functional division of the AV node into two (or more) longitudinal conduction pathways or "dual" AV nodal pathways.[61] There are not two distinct anatomic pathways inside the AV node itself; rather, it is likely that a fan-like network of perinodal fibers inserts into the AV node and represents the second pathway. The pathways possess key differences in conduction characteristics: one is a fast-conducting pathway with a relatively long refractory period (fast pathway) and the other is a slower-conducting pathway with a shorter refractory period (slow pathway). The presence of dual pathways does not necessarily imply that the patient will have clinical PSVT. In fact, it is estimated that between 10% and 50% of patients have discernible dual pathways, but the incidence of AVNRT is considerably lower.[61] Sustenance of the tachycardia depends on the critical electrophysiologic discrepancies and the ability of one pathway (usually the slow) to allow repetitive antegrade conduction, and the ability of the other pathway (usually the fast) to allow repetitive retrograde conduction. During SR, a patient with dual pathways conducts the impulses antegrade through both pathways but reaches the distal common pathway first through the fast AV nodal route and continues to depolarize the ventricles in an antegrade direction (Fig. 40-9).

The mechanism behind AVNRT may occur by the following sequence of events. The occurrence of a properly timed premature atrial impulse penetrates the AV node but is blocked in the fast pathway that is still refractory from the previous beat. However, the slow pathway, which has a shorter refractory period, permits antegrade conduction of the premature impulse. By the time the impulse has reached the distal common pathway, the fast pathway has recovered its excitability and now will permit retrograde conduction. The

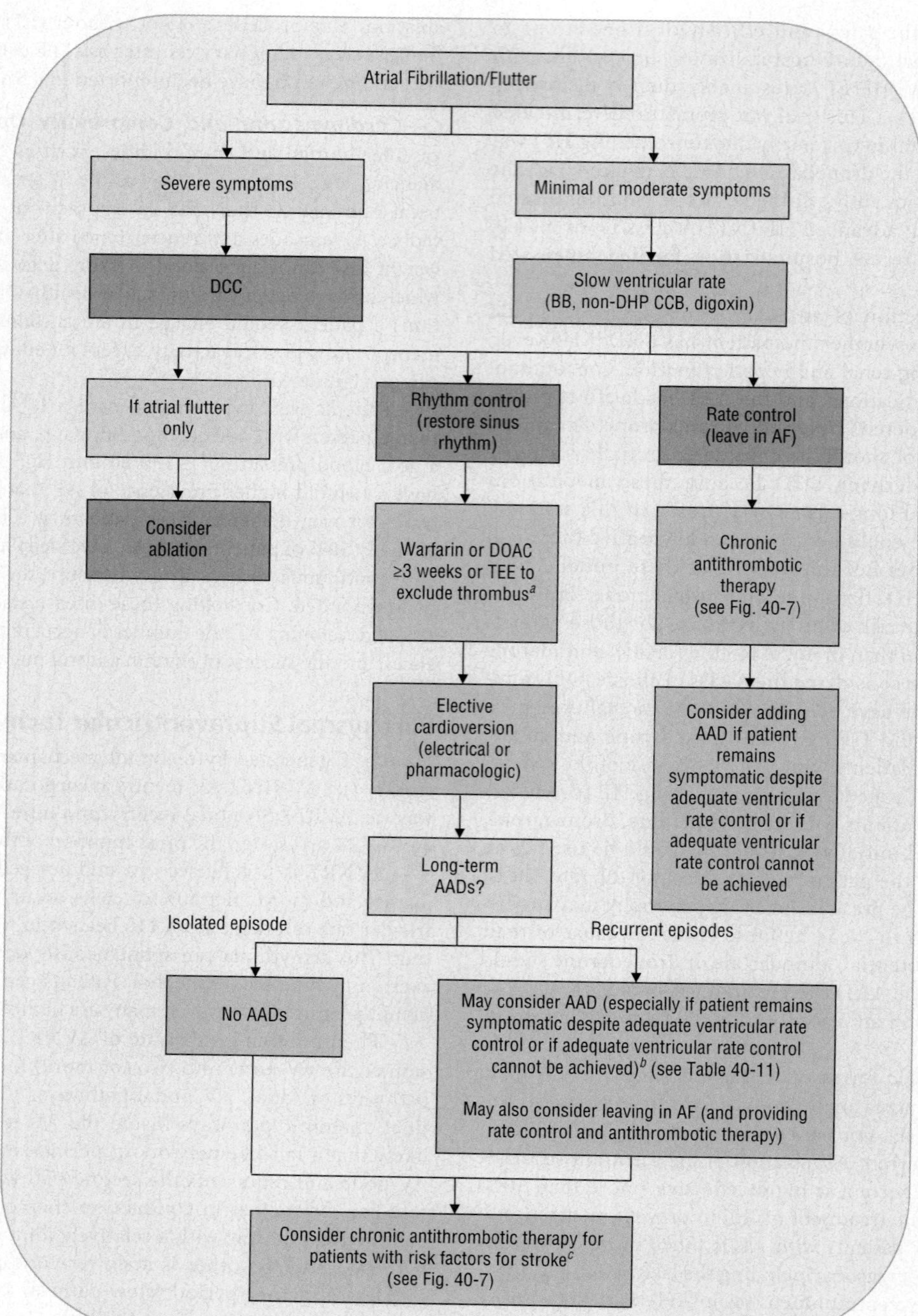

FIGURE 40-8 Algorithm for the treatment of AF and AFl. [a]If AF is less than 48 hours in duration, anticoagulation prior to cardioversion is unnecessary; initiate anticoagulation with unfractionated heparin, a low-molecular-weight heparin, apixaban, dabigatran, edoxaban, or rivaroxaban as soon as possible either before or after cardioversion for stroke prevention (this anticoagulant regimen or no antithrombotic therapy may be considered in low-risk patients). [b]Ablation may be considered for patients who fail or do not tolerate at least one AAD or as first-line therapy (before AAD therapy) for select patients with recurrent symptomatic paroxysmal AF or any classification of AF and heart failure with reduced left ventricular ejection fraction. [c]Chronic antithrombotic therapy should be considered in all patients with AF and risk factors for stroke regardless of whether or not they remain in sinus rhythm. (AAD, antiarrhythmic medication; AF, atrial fibrillation; AFl, atrial flutter; BB, beta-blocker; non-DHP CCB, non-dihydropyridine calcium channel blocker; DCCV, direct current cardioversion; DOAC, direct oral anticoagulant; TEE, transesophageal echocardiogram.)

impulse then reaches the common proximal pathway, reenters the slow pathway, and the tachycardia is initiated. This reentrant circuit that does not require atrial or ventricular tissue; it is completed within the AV node. The common form of this tachycardia uses the slow pathway for antegrade conduction and the fast pathway for retrograde conduction; an uncommon form exists in which the reentrant impulse travels in the opposite direction.

AVRT is generally seen in young adults, and like AVNRT, it is generally well tolerated. However, it can be less benign than AVNRT as it can cause syncope. AVRT depends on the presence of an accessory

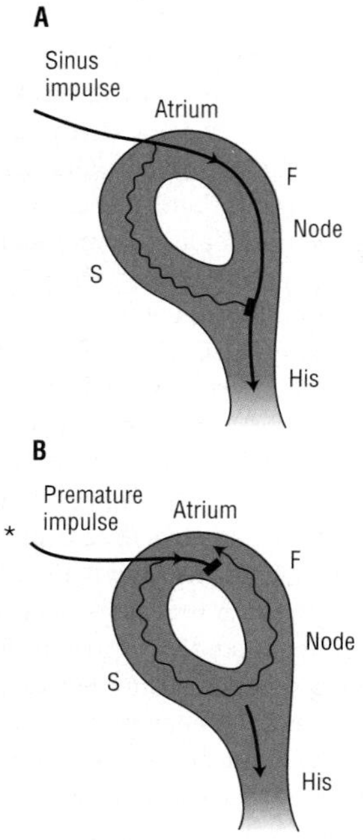

FIGURE 40-9 Reentry mechanism of dual AV nodal pathway PSVT. (*A*) Sinus rhythm: the impulse travels from the atrium through the fast pathway, F, and then to the distal common pathway and the His-Purkinje system (*His*). The impulse also travels through the slow pathway, S, but is stopped when refractory tissue is encountered. (*B*) Dual AV nodal reentry: a critically timed premature impulse, *, is stopped in the fast pathway, F (because of prolonged refractoriness) but is able to travel antegrade down the slow pathway, S, and retrograde through the fast pathway. (AV, atrioventricular; PSVT, paroxysmal supraventricular tachycardia.)

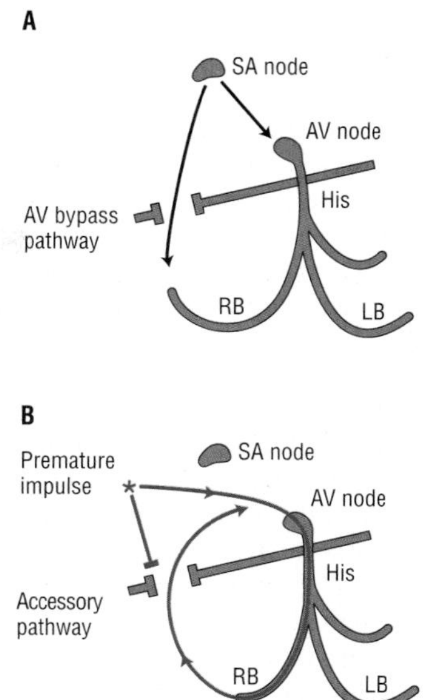

FIGURE 40-10 Reentry mechanism for AV accessory pathway PSVT in Wolff-Parkinson-White syndrome. (*A*) Sinus rhythm: the impulse travels from the atrium to the ventricle by two pathways—the AV node and an accessory bypass pathway. (*B*) AV reentry: a critically timed premature impulse (*) is stopped in accessory pathway (because of prolonged refractoriness) but travels antegrade through the AV node and retrograde through accessory pathway. (AV, atrioventricular; His, His-Purkinje system; LB, left bundle branch; PSVT, paroxysmal supraventricular tachycardia; RB, right bundle branch; SA, sinoatrial.)

pathway that bypasses the normal AV conduction pathway. Several different types of accessory pathways have been described, depending on the specific anatomic areas they connect (eg, AV or nodoventricular tracts). During SR (Fig. 40-10), patients with an accessory pathway that can conduct antegrade depolarize the ventricles simultaneously through both the AV nodal and accessory pathway, causing ventricular preexcitation and creating a fusion pattern on the early portion of the QRS complex (known as a delta wave). Patients may have an accessory pathway that is not evident on ECG, which is referred to as a "concealed" accessory pathway. These concealed accessory pathways are often incapable of antegrade conduction and can only accept electrical stimulation in a retrograde fashion. The electrocardiographic expression of a delta wave depends on the location of the accessory pathway, the distance from the wave front of sinus activation, and the conduction characteristics of the various structures involved. Similar to patients with dual AV nodal pathways, not all patients with an accessory AV pathway are capable of having clinical PSVT, characterized as Wolff-Parkinson-White (WPW) syndrome.

6 WPW syndrome can occur as orthodromic AVRT, antidromic AVRT, and/or AF. AVRT usually occurs by the following sequence of events. Analogous to AVNRT, two pathways (eg, the normal AV nodal pathway and the accessory AV pathway) exist that have different electrophysiologic characteristics. The AV nodal pathway usually has a relatively slower conduction velocity and shorter refractory period, and the accessory pathway has a faster conduction velocity and a longer refractory period. A critically timed premature atrial impulse may be blocked in the accessory pathway because this area is still refractory from the previous sinus beat. However, the AV nodal pathway, with a relatively shorter refractory period, may accept antegrade conduction of the premature atrial impulse. Meanwhile, the accessory pathway may recover its excitability and now allow retrograde conduction. A macroreentrant tachycardia is thereby initiated in which the antegrade pathway is the AV nodal pathway, the distal common pathway is the ventricle, the retrograde pathway is the accessory pathway, and the proximal common pathway is the atrium (see Fig. 40-10). Additionally, this macroreentrant tachycardia could also be initiated by a premature ventricular impulse that first conducts retrograde over the accessory pathway, then antegrade through the AV nodal pathway. This sequence of events (down the AV node, up the accessory pathway), termed *orthodromic AVRT*, is the common variety of reentry in patients with an accessory AV pathway, resulting in a narrow QRS tachycardia (Fig. 40-6). In the uncommon variety, conduction proceeds in the opposite direction (down the accessory pathway, up the AV node), resulting in a wide QRS tachycardia, which is termed *antidromic AVRT*. Patients with WPW syndrome can have a third type of tachycardia, namely, AF. The occurrence of AF in the setting of an accessory AV pathway can be extremely serious. As AF is an extremely rapid atrial tachycardia, conduction can proceed down the accessory AV pathway, resulting in a very fast ventricular response or even VF and SCD. Unlike the AV nodal pathway, the refractory period of the accessory pathway shortens in response to rapid stimulation rates.

General Approach to Treatment Both pharmacologic and nonpharmacologic methods have been used to treat patients with PSVT. Medications used in the treatment of these arrhythmias can be divided into three broad categories: (a) those that directly or indirectly increase vagal tone to the AV node (eg, digoxin);

(b) those that depress conduction through slow, calcium-dependent tissue (eg, adenosine, β-blockers, and non-DHP CCBs); and (c) those that depress conduction through fast, sodium-dependent tissue (eg, quinidine, procainamide, disopyramide, and flecainide). Medications within these categories alter the electrophysiologic characteristics of the reentrant substrate so that PSVT cannot be sustained. In PSVT caused by AVNRT, class I AADs, such as flecainide, act primarily on the retrograde fast pathway. Digoxin and β-blockers may work on either the retrograde fast or the antegrade slow pathway. Verapamil, diltiazem, and adenosine prolong conduction time and increase refractoriness, primarily in the slow antegrade pathway of the reentrant loop. In PSVT caused by AVRT, class I AADs increase refractoriness in the fast accessory pathway or within the His-Purkinje system. β-Blockers, digoxin, adenosine, and verapamil all act by their effects on the AV nodal (antegrade, slow) portion of the reentrant circuit. Regardless of the mechanism, treatment measures are directed first at terminating an acute episode of PSVT and then at preventing symptomatic recurrences of the arrhythmia.

Acute management (Fig. 40-11) for patients with AVNRT or orthodromic AVRT include vagal maneuvers and/or adenosine.[53] Vagal techniques, such as unilateral carotid sinus massage, Valsalva maneuver, ice water facial immersion, or induced retching, are about 20% successful in terminating these PSVTs. Carotid massage and Valsalva maneuver are the simplest, least obtrusive, and most frequently used of these techniques. Should these techniques and/or adenosine be ineffective or unfeasible in a hemodynamically unstable patient (ie, syncope, pre-syncope, angina, or severe HF), synchronized DCCV is the next step. Even at low energy levels (such as 25 J), DCCV is almost always effective in quickly restoring SR and correcting symptomatic hypotension. If vagal techniques and/or adenosine are ineffective or unfeasible in patients who are hemodynamically stable, the next course of action would be administration of IV β-blockers or non-DHP CCBs (oral could be used with AVNRT). Approximately 80% to 98% of patients with a narrow QRS, regular arrhythmia (AVNRT or orthodromic AVRT) given adenosine (6 to 12 mg) will revert to SR within seconds; and, those given IV verapamil (5 to 10 mg), IV diltiazem (15 to 25 mg) will revert to SR within 5 minutes.[62] However, if AVNRT is unable to be corrected with these measures, IV amiodarone can be utilized.[53] For patients with AVRT, the next step would be synchronized cardioversion.

Should a patient have preexcited AF, synchronized cardioversion should be used if hemodynamically unstable.[53] If the patient is hemodynamically stable, IV ibutilide or procainamide can be administered. IV digoxin, IV amiodarone, oral or IV β-blockers, diltiazem, and verapamil should be avoided in patients with preexcited AF as they may increase conduction over the accessory pathway leading to an increase in the ventricular rate and enhance the risk of provoking a life-threatening ventricular arrhythmia.

Once the acute episode of AVNRT or AVRT is terminated, a decision on long-term preventive therapy must follow (Fig. 40-11). Preventive treatment is indicated if: (a) frequent episodes occur that necessitate therapeutic intervention (ie, emergency department visits) or cause symptoms that interfere with the patient's lifestyle; or (b) episodes are infrequent but cause severe symptoms. If preventive treatment is deemed necessary, either medication therapy or catheter ablation can be used.

AADs are no longer the treatment of choice to prevent recurrences of reentrant PSVT for the following reasons: (a) lifelong treatment is necessary in these generally young, but otherwise healthy, individuals; (b) there are few, if any, large controlled or comparative trials to assist the clinician in rationally choosing effective agents; and (c) most importantly, other nonpharmacologic treatments are clearly more effective. Nevertheless, medication therapy may occasionally be necessary in some patients, particularly those with mild symptoms and infrequent recurrences. A trial-and-error approach may be used, complemented by the use of ambulatory electrocardiographic recordings (Holter) or telephonic transmissions of cardiac rhythm (event monitors) to objectively document the efficacy or failure of the chosen medication regimen. Medications known to be effective in preventing recurrences of these arrhythmias are the AV nodal blocking medications (digoxin, β-blockers, non-DHP CCBs, and combinations of these agents) and the class Ic AADs (flecainide, propafenone).[53] Sotalol, dofetilide, and amiodarone can be considered alternatives. Although rarely used, digoxin is only indicated in orthodromic AVRT without preexcitation.

5 Catheter ablation using radiofrequency current on the PSVT substrate has dramatically altered the traditional treatment of these patients (Fig. 40-12). Radiofrequency ablation is highly effective, preventing the recurrences of PSVT in more than 90% of patients.[63,64] The procedure was originally used in patients with WPW syndrome.[63] In these patients, the extranodal pathway is most often located at the left lateral free wall between the left atrium and ventricle at the level of the mitral valve (see Fig. 40-12). During invasive electrophysiologic studies, portions of the reentrant circuit can be located (or mapped) using several catheters. Once this is completed, either radiofrequency or cryo ablation is performed, causing cell death in the tissue necessary for reentry. In this way, the substrate for reentry is destroyed, "curing" the patient of recurrent episodes of PSVT and obviating the need for chronic medication therapy. Thereafter, a similar approach was developed for patients with AVNRT, placing the catheter just anterior to the coronary sinus, below the His bundle and in the region of the slow pathway.[64] The preferred method in these individuals is to apply lesions to the slow pathway of the reentrant circuit in order to modify its properties enough so that AVNRT cannot recur. Complications, although unusual, include cardiac tamponade, pericarditis, valvular insufficiency, and AV block. Ablation of the extranodal connection occurs promptly, and evidence of preexcitation (delta waves) disappears.

Catheter ablation is the preferred treatment strategy (over AADs) for patients with symptomatic PSVT because the procedure is highly effective and curative, rarely results in complications, and obviates the need for chronic AAD therapy.[53]

Ventricular Arrhythmias

The common ventricular arrhythmias include (a) premature ventricular complexes (PVCs), (b) VT, and (c) VF. These arrhythmias may result in a wide variety of symptoms. PVCs often cause no symptoms or only mild palpitations. VT may be a life-threatening situation associated with hemodynamic collapse or may be totally asymptomatic. VF, by definition, is an acute medical emergency necessitating cardiopulmonary resuscitation (CPR).

Premature Ventricular Complexes and Sudden Cardiac Death

PVCs (Fig. 40-6) are very common ventricular rhythm disturbances that occur in patients with or without SHD. Experimental models show that PVCs may be elicited by abnormal automaticity, triggered activity, or reentrant mechanisms. PVCs are commonly observed in healthy individuals; in these patients, the PVCs seem to have little, if any, prognostic significance. PVCs occur more frequently and in more complex forms in patients with SHD than in healthy individuals. The prognostic meaning of PVCs has been well studied in patients with MI (acute or remote) with several consistent themes. Patients with some forms of PVCs (ie, multifocal or couplets) are at higher risk for SCD, defined as unexpected death (without an obvious noncardiac cause) occurring in a patient within 1 hour of experiencing symptoms (witnessed episodes) or within 24 hours of last being observed in normal health (unwitnessed episodes).[65] Studies of patients who experienced SCD (and happened to be wearing an electrocardiographic monitor at the time) often demonstrate the cause to be VF preceded by a short run of VT and frequent PVCs.[66]

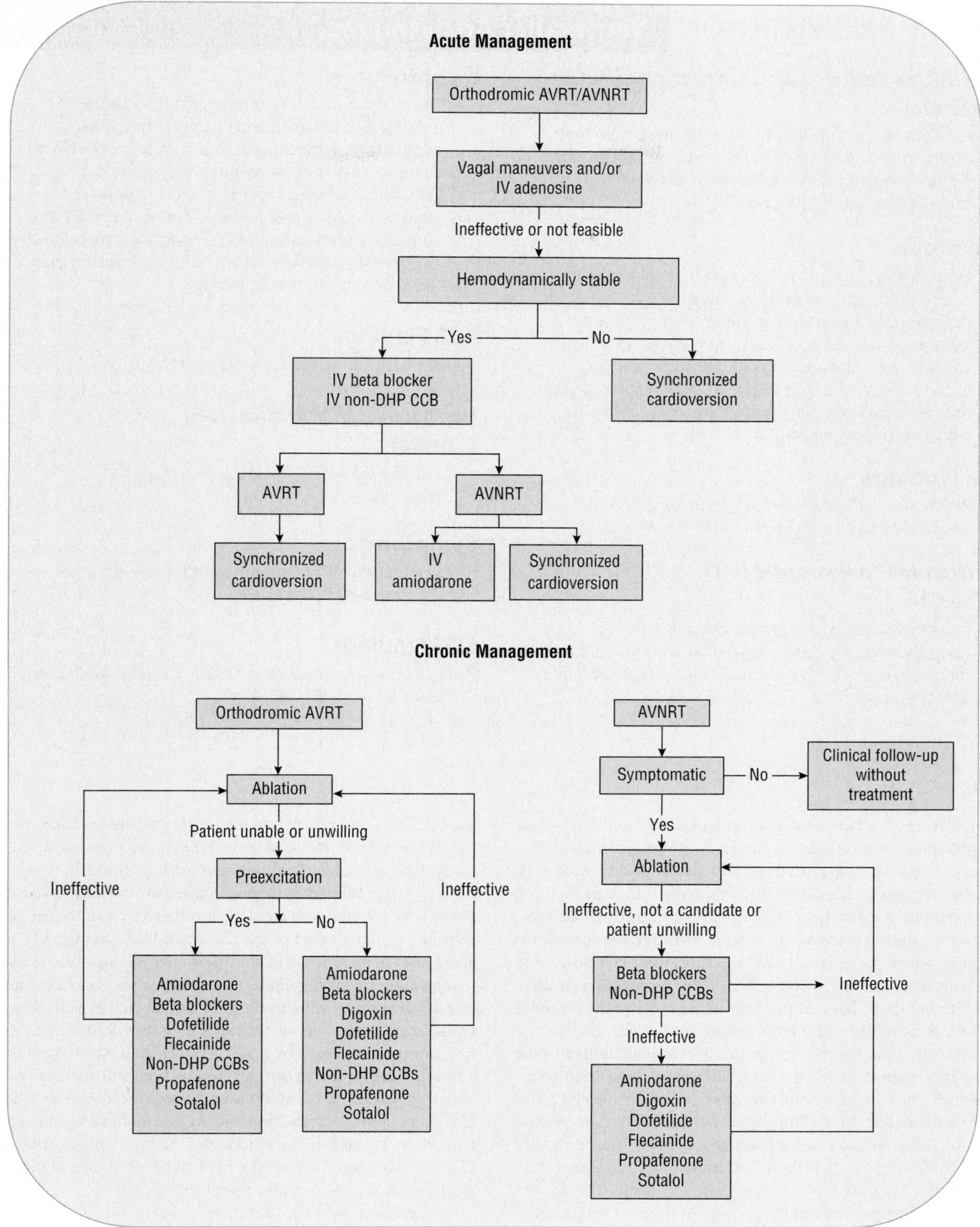

FIGURE 40-11 Algorithm for the treatment of acute (*top panel*) orthodromic AVRT/AVNRT and chronic prevention of recurrences (*bottom panel*). (AVNRT, atrioventricular nodal reentrant tachycardia; AVRT, atrioventricular reentrant tachycardia; IV, intravenous; non-DHP CCBs, non-dihydropyridine calcium channel blockers.) *Note*: Medications are listed in alphabetical order, not in order of preference.

General Approach to Treatment Historically, investigators promoted the concept that patients in the acute phase of MI may have types of PVCs that are predictive of VF and SCD. These types of PVCs were referred to as "warning arrhythmias" and included frequent ventricular ectopy (more than 5 beats/min), multiform configuration (different morphology), couplets (two in a row), and R-on-T phenomenon (PVCs occurring during the repolarization phase of the preceding sinus beat in the vulnerable period of

CLINICAL PRESENTATION Ventricular Arrhythmias

Premature Ventricular Contractions (PVCs)

General

- PVCs are not acutely life-threatening in a patient with a structurally normal heart and usually asymptomatic. A high frequency of PVCs (>20% of all beats) can cause ventricular dysfunction.

Symptoms

- Occasionally, patients will complain of palpitations or uncomfortable heartbeats. Since the PVC, by definition, occurs early and the ventricle contracts when it is incompletely filled, often the aortic valve will not open. The ensuing compensatory pause allows for an increase in left ventricular filling causing the next sinus beat have a more forceful contraction which can result in symptoms.

ECG Findings

- Premature, oddly shaped QRS complex that is unusually wide (Fig. 40-6).

Ventricular Tachycardia (VT)

General

- Patients can be asymptomatic or become hemodynamically compromised depending on their degree of underlying structural heart disease and rate of tachycardia.

Symptoms

- The symptoms of VT (monomorphic VT or TdP), if prolonged (ie, sustained), can vary from nearly completely asymptomatic to pulseless, hemodynamic collapse. Fast heart rates and underlying poor LV function will result in more severe symptoms. Symptoms of nonsustained, self-terminating VT also correlate with duration of episodes (eg, patients with 15-second episodes will be more symptomatic than those with three-beat episodes).

ECG Findings

- Wide QRS complexes at a rate >100 beats/min (Fig. 40-6).

Ventricular Vibrillation (VF)

General

- Cardiac output and blood pressure are not recordable.

Symptoms

- By definition, VF results in hemodynamic collapse, syncope, and cardiac arrest.

ECG Findings

- Lack of organized electrical activity, coarse fibrillation waves are seen. (Fig. 40-6).

ventricular recovery). However, as a result of using continuous electrocardiographic monitoring techniques, it is apparent that almost all patients have warning arrhythmias in the acute MI setting. In those patients who experience VF, warning arrhythmias are no more common than in those without VF. Consequently, warning arrhythmias observed during acute MI are neither sensitive nor specific for determining which patients will have VF. Thus, there is little need to direct medication therapy specifically at PVC suppression in these patients. Studies show that effective prevention of VF in the acute MI setting may be achieved without the abolition of PVCs.

Conversely, data strongly imply that PVCs documented in the convalescence period of MI do carry important long-term prognostic significance.[67] PVCs occurring after an MI seem to be a risk factor for patient death that is independent of the degree of LV dysfunction or the extent of coronary atherosclerosis. Using a classification of PVCs (simple or benign [infrequent and monomorphic] versus complex [at least 5 PVCs/min, couplets, R-on-T beats, and multiform]), investigators found that complex (but not simple) ventricular ectopy in the setting of CAD was associated with a higher incidence of overall mortality and cardiac death.[67]

PVCs carry little or no risk when the frequency is low and individuals are without SHD; thus, medication therapy is unnecessary. However, because of the prognostic significance of complex PVCs in patients with SHD, the use of AAD therapy to suppress them has been controversial. Historically, many supported the aggressive use of AAD therapy to suppress PVCs, based on the underlying premise of eliminating a risk factor for SCD in patients with CAD (namely, the presence of complex PVCs). However, others favored a more conservative approach and disregarded the use of AAD therapy in the absence of significant symptoms. An important study, the Cardiac Arrhythmia Suppression Trial (CAST), abruptly put an end to this debate in noteworthy fashion. This trial was conducted to determine if suppression of ventricular ectopy with encainide, flecainide, or moricizine could decrease the incidence of death from arrhythmia in patients who had suffered an MI.[68] In the trial, patients with an LVEF less than or equal to 55% (0.55) (if recruited within 90 days of the MI) or an LVEF less than or equal to 40% (0.40) (if recruited at least 90 days after the MI) were randomized to receive encainide, flecainide, moricizine, or placebo. Compared with placebo, treatment with encainide or flecainide was associated with a significantly higher rate of total mortality and death due to arrhythmia, presumably caused by proarrhythmia. Analysis of the moricizine arm indicated neither harm nor benefit from this therapy; therefore, only this portion of the study was allowed to continue as CAST II.[69] However, CAST II was also prematurely discontinued because there was a trend toward an increase in mortality in moricizine-treated patients. Moreover, quinidine and sotalol have also been shown to increase the risk of death in patients with a HFrEF and PVCs.[70]

Currently, only two AADs have been shown *not* to increase mortality in post-MI patients with long-term use: amiodarone and dofetilide. A number of trials have shown amiodarone to decrease the incidence of sudden (or arrhythmic) death, but not total mortality, in post-MI patients with complex ventricular ectopy.[71,72] Clearly, because of its impressive side effect profile and its inability to improve survival, amiodarone should not routinely be recommended in patients with heart disease such as remote MI and complex PVCs. Two randomized controlled trials have also shown that chronic therapy with dofetilide has no effect on overall mortality in post-MI patients with LV dysfunction.[73,74]

These results have clearly had a negative influence on the long-term use of all AADs, causing a broad skepticism in the

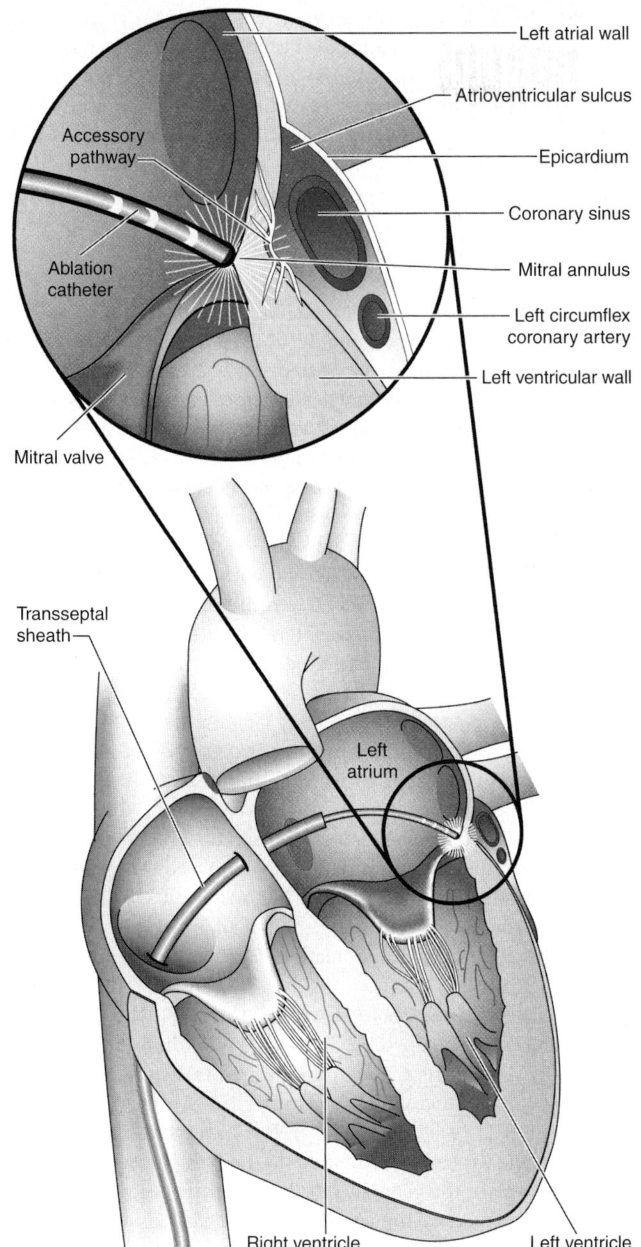

FIGURE 40-12 Drawing showing catheter placement for radiofrequency ablation of a left lateral free wall accessory pathway. Here, a venous (atrial) transseptal puncture to gain access to accessory pathway is shown; a retrograde arterial approach has also been used. (*Reprinted with permission from Lerman BB, Basson CT. High risk patients with ventricular preexcitation: A pendulum in motion. N Engl J Med 2003;349:1787–1789. Copyright © 2003 Massachusetts Medical Society. All rights reserved.*)

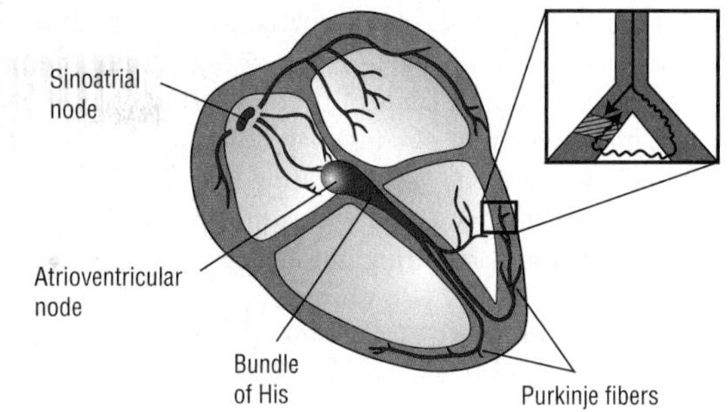

FIGURE 40-13 Conduction system of the heart. The magnified portion shows a bifurcation of a Purkinje fiber traditionally explained as the etiology of reentrant VT. A premature impulse travels to the fiber which is damaged by heart disease or ischemia. It encounters a zone of prolonged refractoriness (area of unidirectional block; *cross-hatched area*) but fails to propagate because the fiber remains refractory to stimulation from the previous impulse. However, the impulse may slowly travel (*squiggly line*) through the other portion of the Purkinje twig and will "reenter" the cross-hatched area if the refractory period is concluded and the fiber is now excitable. Thus, the premature impulse never meets refractory tissue; circus movement ensues. If this site stimulates the surrounding ventricle repetitively, clinical reentrant VT results. (VT, ventricular tachycardia.)

risk-versus-benefit analysis of these medications. Consequently, pharmaceutical companies have shifted their medication discovery and investigative efforts away from potent sodium channel blockers. The findings of the CAST have also provided additional fuel for the pursuit of nonpharmacologic therapies for arrhythmias, such as catheter ablation and implantable devices.

7 How should the clinician approach the patient with documented asymptomatic PVCs? Clearly, attempts to suppress asymptomatic PVCs should *not* be made with any AAD. Indeed, those patients who are at risk for arrhythmic death (recent MI, LV dysfunction, complex PVCs) should also *not* be routinely given *any* class I or III AAD.[70] In post-MI patients, the use of β-blockers is associated with a reduction in mortality and SCD, especially in the presence of LV dysfunction. β-Blockers and non-DHP CCBs can be used in patients without underlying SHD to suppress symptomatic PVCs. If neither is effective in reducing recurrence and symptoms, class Ic AADs, amiodarone, or sotalol can be used. Uncommonly, patients have such frequent PVCs that are either extremely bothersome or result in the development of cardiomyopathy leading to a decline in left ventricular function (usually when the PVCS greater than 20% of all beats).[70] In these patients, ablation of the PVCs can be pursued.

Ventricular Tachycardia

VT is a wide QRS tachycardia (Fig. 40-6) that may acutely occur because of metabolic abnormalities, ischemia, or medication toxicity, or chronically recur as a paroxysmal form. On the ECG, VT may appear as repetitive monomorphic or polymorphic ventricular complexes. The definition of VT is three or more consecutive PVCs occurring at a rate of greater than 100 beats/min. An acute episode of VT may be precipitated by severe electrolyte abnormalities (hypokalemia or hypomagnesemia), hypoxia, or digoxin toxicity, or (most commonly) may occur in patients presenting with acute MI or myocardial ischemia complicated by HF. In these cases, correction of the underlying precipitating factors will usually prevent further recurrences of VT. As an example, if VT occurs during the first 24 hours of an acute MI, it will probably not reappear on a chronic basis after the infarcted area has been reperfused or healed with scar formation. This form of acute VT may be caused by a transient reentrant mechanism within temporarily ischemic or dying ventricular tissue. In contrast, some patients have a chronic, recurrent form of VT that is almost always associated with some type of underlying SHD. Common examples are paroxysmal VT associated with idiopathic dilated cardiomyopathy or remote MI with an LV aneurysm. In chronic, recurrent VT, microreentry within the distal Purkinje network and myocardium is responsible for the underlying substrate in a large majority of patients (see Fig. 40-13). Theoretically, electrophysiologic abnormalities occur as a result of structural damage and heart disease within the ventricular conducting system. The reentrant circuit may possess both anatomically determined and functional properties coursing through normal tissue, damaged (but not dead) tissue, and islands of necrosed tissue. In a minority of patients, macroreentrant circuits may be responsible for recurrent VT, including reentry incorporating the bundle branches. Patients with acute VT associated with a precipitating factor often suffer severe symptoms, requiring immediate treatment measures. Chronic, recurrent VT may also cause severe hemodynamic compromise but may also be associated with only mild symptoms that are generally well tolerated. The severity of symptoms is reliant upon the rate of the tachycardia and the patient's underlying heart disease and ventricular function.

Sustained VT is that which requires therapeutic intervention to restore a stable rhythm or persists for a relatively long time (usually more than 30 seconds). Nonsustained VT is that which self-terminates after a brief duration (usually less than 30 seconds). Patients who experience VT more frequently than SR (ie, VT is the dominant rhythm) are considered to have incessant VT. In monomorphic VT, the QRS complexes are similar in morphologic characteristics from beat to beat. In polymorphic VT, the QRS complexes vary in shape and/or size between beats. A characteristic type of polymorphic VT, in which the QRS complexes appear to undulate around a central axis and that is associated with evidence of delayed ventricular repolarization (long QT interval or prominent U waves), is referred to as TdP.

Most, but not all forms of recurrent VT occur in patients with extensive SHD. VT occurring in a patient without SHD is sometimes referred to as idiopathic VT and may take several forms including fascicular VT and ventricular outflow tract VT.[75-77] Fascicular VT arises from a fascicle of the left bundle branch (usually posterior) and is usually not associated with severe underlying SHD. Non-DHP CCBs are effective in terminating an acute episode of fascicular VT. Ventricular outflow tract VT (usually originating from the right ventricular outflow tract) originates from near the pulmonic valve (or uncommonly the aortic valve or LV outflow tract) and also occurs in patients with normal LV function without discernible SHD.[77] Unlike other forms of VT, right ventricular outflow tract VT often terminates with adenosine and may be prevented with β-blockers and/or non-DHP CCBs.

Some unusual forms of VT are congenital or heritable. TdP can be associated with heritable defects in the flux of ions that govern ventricular repolarization. Although multiple syndromes and genetic mutations have been described, the more common examples are long QT syndrome 1 (depressed I_{Ks}), long QT syndrome 2 (depressed I_{Kr}), and long QT syndrome 3 (enhanced, inward sodium ion flux during repolarization).[78] Polymorphic VT (without a prolonged QT interval) or VF may also occur due to a heritable defect in the sodium channel. This is the case in Brugada syndrome, which is described as a typical ECG pattern (ST-segment elevation in leads V_1 to V_3) in SR that is associated with SCD, and commonly occurs in young males.[70]

General Approach to Treatment Consider the patient with the more common form of sustained monomorphic VT (ie, those with SHD, usually ischemic in nature). Like other rapid tachycardias, the initial management of an acute episode of VT (with a pulse) requires a quick assessment of the patient's signs and symptoms. An investigation should be made into possible precipitating factors which should be corrected if possible. The diagnosis of acute MI should always be entertained. If the episode of VT is thought to be an isolated electrical event associated with a transient initiating factor (such as acute myocardial ischemia or digoxin toxicity), there is no need for long-term AAD therapy once the precipitating factors are corrected (eg, an MI has been reperfused and healed and the patient is stable). Nevertheless, the patient should be monitored closely for possible recurrences of VT.

Patients presenting with an acute episode of sustained monomorphic VT and hemodynamically instability should have advanced cardiovascular life support (ACLS) initiated immediately, including DCCV to restore SR.[79] In patients with stable monomorphic VT treatment is driven by the presence of SHD. If a patient has SHD, cardioversion should be implemented and IV procainamide, amiodarone, or sotalol can be considered. For patients without SHD, verapamil and β-blockers are first-line options. See Fig. 40-14 for an algorithm to acutely manage monomorphic VT.

Once an acute episode of sustained VT has been successfully terminated by electrical or pharmacologic means and an acute MI has been ruled out, the possibility of a patient having recurrent episodes of VT should be considered. Evidence for the possibility of VT recurrence can often be gleaned from invasive electrophysiologic studies using programmed ventricular stimulation. Patients who survive an acute episode of sustained VT are at extremely high risk for death and the yield for finding an effective AAD via electrophysiologic testing is low. Amiodarone is the most effective (approximately 50% effective after 2 years) AAD in patients with recurrent VT. However, nonpharmacologic approaches have demonstrated impressive effectiveness in the treatment of recurrent VT/VF.[70] For instance, some forms of recurrent VT are amenable to catheter ablation therapy using radiofrequency current. This approach is highly effective (approximately 90%) in idiopathic VT (right ventricular outflow tract or fascicular VT), but less so in recurrent VT associated with a cardiomyopathic process or remote MI with LV aneurysm. In the latter patients, ablation is usually regarded as second-line therapy after other methods have failed.[80] Numerous trials have established ICDs as a superior treatment over AADs not only for the prevention of SCD in patients who have been resuscitated from an episode of cardiac arrest or had sustained VT ("secondary prevention") but also for the prevention of an initial episode of SCD in certain high-risk patient populations ("primary prevention").

Implantable Cardioverter-Defibrillator 8 The introduction of and advances in the ICD (Fig. 40-15) have obviated the need for AADs to prevent episodes of life-threatening ventricular arrhythmias.[70,81] Numerous advancements in device technology have allowed the ICD to become smaller, less invasive to implant, and programmable with advanced functions. Early ICDs required a thoracotomy to place the generator in the abdomen, whereas with the newer, smaller models, the leads are implanted transvenously with the generator placed into the pectoral region in a manner similar to cardiac pacemakers. Modern ICDs now employ a "tiered-therapy approach," meaning that overdrive or antitachycardia pacing (stimulates the heart to go faster than the rate induced by the VT) can be attempted first to terminate the tachyarrhythmia (no shock delivered), followed by low-energy cardioversion, and, finally, by high-energy defibrillation shocks. In addition, backup antibradycardia pacing and extended battery lives have made these newer devices much more attractive. All models store recordings during delivery of pacing shocks, which is extremely important in discerning appropriate shocks (ie, delivers shock for serious ventricular arrhythmia) from inappropriate shocks (ie, delivers shock for AF with rapid ventricular rate) and in documenting true recurrences of the patient's tachycardia.

Although ICDs are highly effective for preventing SCD due to recurrent VT or VF, several problems remain. First, the device itself, the implantation procedure, electrophysiologic studies, hospitalization, and physician fees are costly. Second, many patients with ICDs end up receiving concomitant AAD therapy (usually amiodarone or sotalol).[81,83] AADs can be initiated in these patients for a number of reasons, including: (a) decreasing the frequency of VT/VF episodes to subsequently reduce the frequency of appropriate shocks; (b) reducing the rate of VT so that it can be terminated with antitachycardia pacing; and (c) decreasing episodes of concomitant

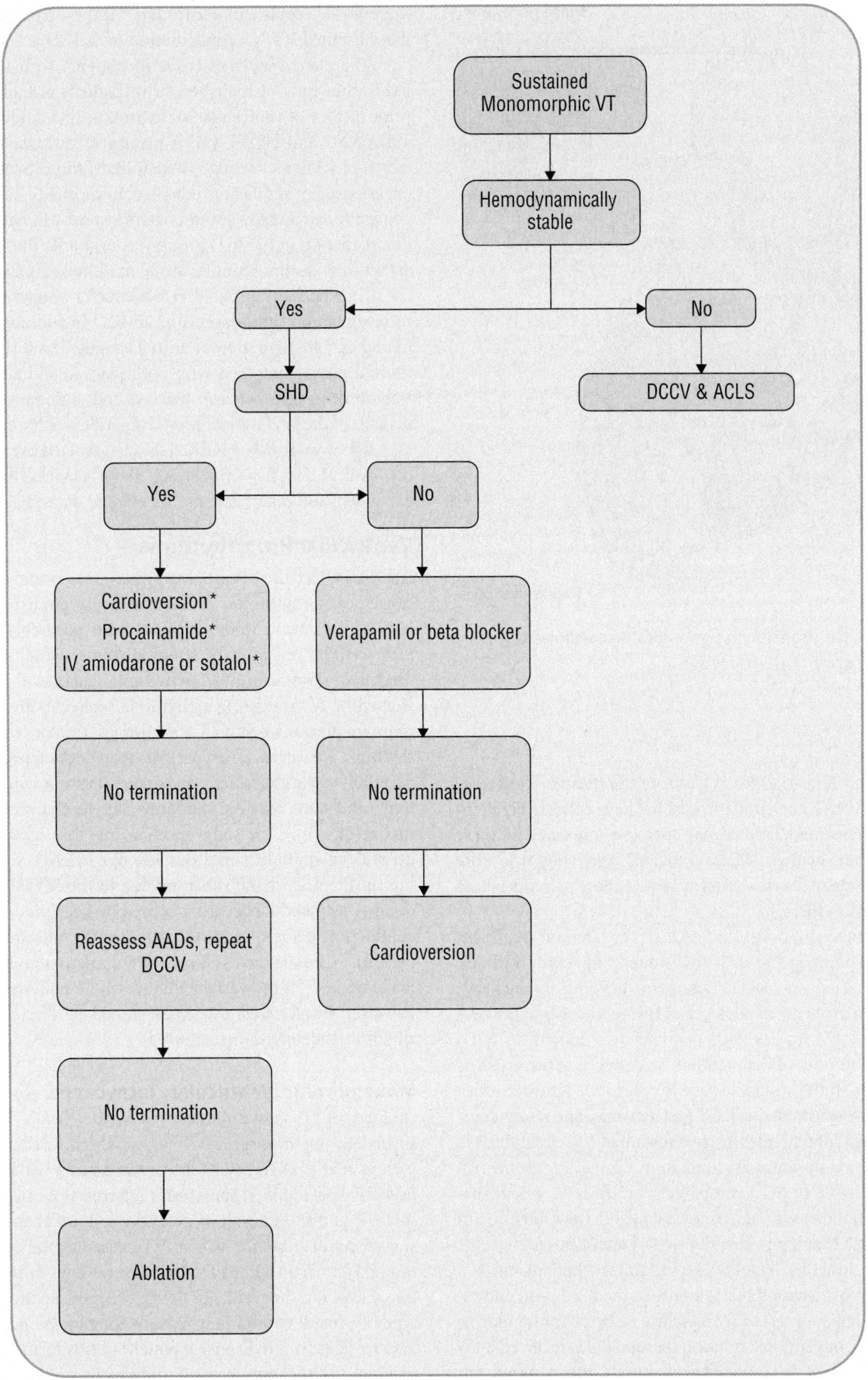

FIGURE 40-14 Acute management of ventricular tachycardia. *Treatment listed in order of level of evidence. (ACLS, acute cardiovascular life support; AAD, antiarrhythmic drug; DCCV, direct current cardioversion; SHD, structural heart disease; VT, ventricular tachycardia.) *(Data from Reference 70.)*

supraventricular arrhythmias (eg, AF, AFl) that may trigger inappropriate shocks. As a result of these potential benefits, the concomitant use of AADs can minimize patient discomfort and prolong the battery life of the ICD. The decision to initiate concomitant AAD therapy should be individualized, with treatment usually being reserved for those patients with frequent shocks because of VT or AF.

Prevention of Sudden Cardiac Death First-line therapy for the secondary prevention of SCD is ICD implantation as the rate of survival is superior to that of AADs in patients who are at high risk for recurrent, life-threatening ventricular arrhythmias.[84-86] Patient populations at high risk for a first episode of SCD include those with a prior MI, HFrEF, and nonsustained VT. The use of AADs to

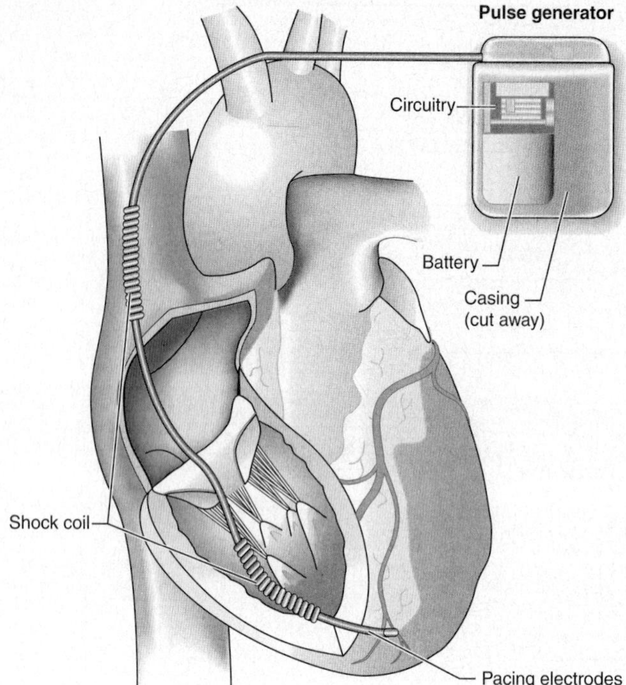

FIGURE 40-15 Drawing showing implantable cardioverter-defibrillator. (*Data from Reference 82.*)

prevent SCD in this high-risk group has been significantly limited by the results of the CAST and similar trials that have collectively demonstrated that these medications may increase mortality in these patients. As a result of these trials, clinicians have sought a more clearly defined strategy for risk stratification in these patients before initiating medication therapy.

9 For patients with nonsustained VT, there are four treatment strategies based upon symptoms and underlying comorbidities: (a) conservative (ie, no AAD treatment beyond β-blockers); (b) empiric amiodarone or sotalol; (c) ablation; and (d) aggressive (ie, electrophysiologic studies with possible insertion of an ICD) (Fig. 40-16).[70] A number of early studies suggested that tests such as electrophysiologic studies could be used to determine long-term risk in patients with nonsustained VT.[87,88] For instance, one study demonstrated that post-MI patients with nonsustained VT and inducible sustained VT after programmed stimulation were at increased risk for subsequent VT/VF or SCD compared with those in whom sustained VT could not be induced.[87] These data led to the evaluation of the efficacy of ICD therapy in this high-risk patient population.[89,90] The first trial to test this hypothesis randomized patients with a previous MI, HFrEF, asymptomatic nonsustained VT, and inducible VT that was not suppressed with the use of IV procainamide to receive an ICD or conventional medical therapy (74% received amiodarone).[89] This trial was terminated prematurely after a significant survival benefit was detected in the ICD group. A subsequent study randomized patients with a history of MI, HFrEF, and either asymptomatic nonsustained VT or inducible sustained VT to treatment using a conservative approach (no AAD therapy beyond β-blockers) or electrophysiologically guided therapy (AADs and/or ICD).[90] The conservative approach had a significantly higher event rate (cardiac arrest or death from arrhythmia). Furthermore, patients in the electrophysiologically guided group receiving only AADs (no ICD) had similar event rates to the conservative therapy group. In other words, only those treated with an ICD had a significantly lower event rate and greater survival. Based on the results of these trials, it is reasonable for patients with CAD, HFrEF, and nonsustained VT to undergo electrophysiologic testing.[70] If these patients do have inducible sustained VT/VF, implantation of an ICD is warranted.

The effectiveness of ICDs in patients with nonsustained VT led to the study of their benefit in patients at high risk for but no prior history of ventricular arrhythmias. In a study of patients with a prior MI and HFrEF (prior history of ventricular arrhythmia or electrophysiologic testing not required), those treated with an ICD experienced a significant reduction in mortality compared with the conventional therapy group (routine post-MI and HF therapy).[91] The reduction in the ICD group was primarily due to a reduction in arrhythmic death. A similar study randomized patients with NYHA class II or III HFrEF (of either ischemic or nonischemic etiology) to receive placebo, amiodarone, or an ICD in addition to standard HF therapies.[92] Implantation of an ICD resulted in a significantly lower mortality rate compared with both placebo and amiodarone (there was no difference between placebo and amiodarone). The survival benefits of the ICD were observed regardless of the etiology of the HF.

9 Overall, as the ICD trials have evolved over the past decade, the indications for implanting these devices have significantly expanded, and many patients are eligible for an ICD.[70,93]

Ventricular Proarrhythmia

All AADs have the potential to aggravate existing arrhythmias or to cause new arrhythmias. AADs may cause proarrhythmia in nearly 30% of patients.[94] Many definitions for proarrhythmia have been proposed; however, in the simplest terms, it indicates the development of a significant new arrhythmia (such as VT, VF, or TdP) or worsening of an existing arrhythmia (episodes are longer, faster, or more frequent). As with all arrhythmias, the consequences of proarrhythmia are varied. Some patients who develop proarrhythmia may be totally asymptomatic, others may notice a worsening of symptoms, and some may die suddenly. The development of proarrhythmia results from the same mechanisms that cause arrhythmias in general (eg, quinidine-induced TdP due to EADs) or from an alteration in the underlying substrate due to the AAD (eg, development of an accelerated tachycardia caused by flecainide, which decreases conduction velocity without significantly altering the refractory period).[67] The diagnosis of proarrhythmia is sometimes difficult to make because of the variable nature of the underlying arrhythmias. However, in all cases, the AAD should be discontinued if proarrhythmia is detected or suspected.

Monomorphic Ventricular Tachycardia 10 The prototypical form of proarrhythmia caused by the class Ic AADs is a rapid, sustained, monomorphic VT with a characteristic sinusoidal QRS pattern that is often resistant to resuscitation with cardioversion or overdrive pacing. It is sometimes referred to as sinusoidal or incessant VT and is the result of excessive sodium channel blockade and slowed conduction. Sinusoidal VT caused by the class Ic AADs was thought to occur within the first several days of medication initiation. However, the results of the CAST indicate that the risk for this type of proarrhythmia may exist as long as the AAD is continued. Factors that can predispose a patient to this form of proarrhythmia include: (a) the presence of underlying ventricular arrhythmias; (b) CAD; and (c) LV dysfunction. Provocation of proarrhythmia by the class Ic AADs is sometimes reported during exercise, which is most likely a result of augmented slowed conduction at rapid heart rates (ie, rate-dependent sodium blockade). The incidence of proarrhythmia caused by class Ic AADs is greatest in patients with all three of the above risk factors (approximately 10%-20%) and extremely uncommon in those without these risk factors, such as patients with supraventricular tachycardias and normal LV function. Other factors that have a less well-defined association with proarrhythmia are elevated AAD serum concentrations and rapid dosage escalation of the AAD. The presence of underlying ventricular conduction delays may also pose a risk for proarrhythmia. As mentioned

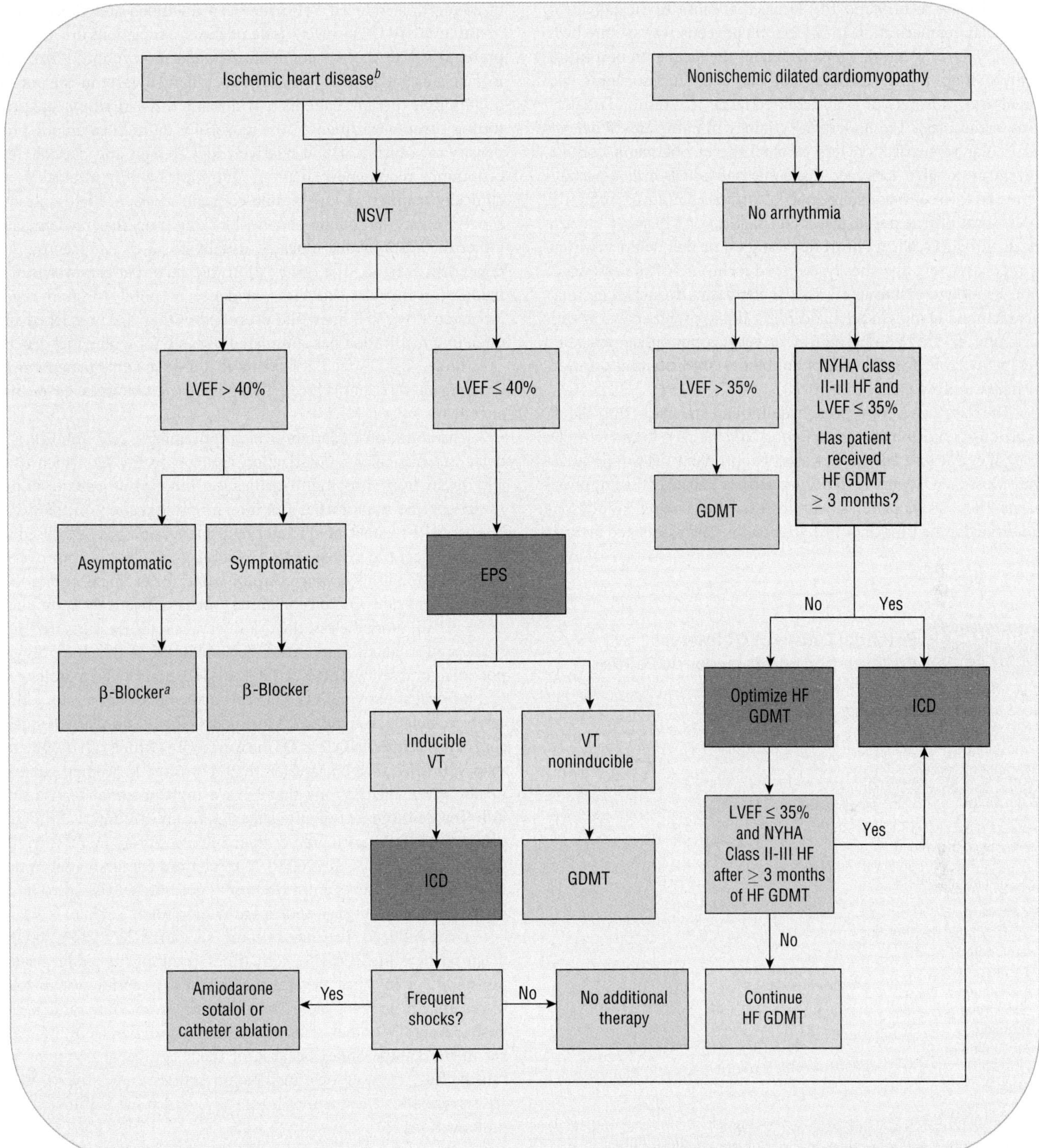

FIGURE 40-16 Algorithm for the primary prevention of SCD in patients with a history of MI or with a nonischemic dilated cardiomyopathy. LVEF of 35% is equivalent to 0.35 expressed as a fraction. (a) In these patients, the β-blocker is being used to reduce post-MI mortality. (b) Patients should be >40 days post-MI and at least 90 days postrevascularization prior to insertion of the ICD. (EPS, electrophysiologic study; GDMT, guideline-directed medical therapy; HF, heart failure; ICD, implantable cardioverter-defibrillator; LVEF, left ventricular ejection fraction; MI, myocardial infarction; NSVT, nonsustained VT; SCD, sudden cardiac death; VT, ventricular tachycardia.)

earlier, incessant monomorphic VT is often resistant to resuscitation. However, some have had success with lidocaine ("fast on–off" AAD, which successfully competes with a "slow on–off" agent such as flecainide for sodium channel receptor) or sodium bicarbonate (reverses the excessive sodium channel blockade).

Torsades de Pointes 10 TdP is a rapid form of polymorphic VT (Fig. 40-6) that is associated with evidence of delayed ventricular repolarization (long QT interval) on ECG. Most forms of polymorphic VT occurring in the setting of a normal QT interval are similar to monomorphic VT in terms of etiology and treatment strategies (thus, a long QT interval is crucial to the diagnosis of TdP). Much has been learned about the underlying etiology of TdP. Basic defects (genetic, medications, or diseases) that delay repolarization by influencing ion movement (usually by blocking potassium efflux) provoke EADs preferentially in cells deep in the heart muscle, which, in turn, trigger reentry and TdP. Drugs that cause TdP usually delay ventricular repolarization in an inhomogeneous way (termed *dispersion of refractoriness*), which facilitates the formation of multiple reentrant loops in the ventricle.[95] TdP may occur in association with hereditary syndromes or as an acquired form (ie, a result of medications or diseases). The underlying etiology in both cases is delayed ventricular repolarization due to blockade of potassium conductance. It is possible, however, that some individuals have a partially expressed form of these congenital syndromes but never suffer TdP unless some other external factor (eg, medications, diseases, electrolyte disturbances, abrupt heart rate changes) further delays ventricular repolarization. Specifically, acquired forms of TdP are associated with electrolyte disturbances (hypokalemia or hypomagnesemia), subarachnoid hemorrhage, myocarditis, liquid protein diets, arsenic poisoning, severe hypothyroidism, or, most commonly, medication therapy (notably phenothiazines, antibiotics, antihistamines, antidepressants, and AADs) (Table 40-13).

The class Ia AADs (especially quinidine) and class III I_{Kr} blockers are most notorious for precipitating TdP; the class Ib and Ic AADs rarely, if ever, cause TdP as they do not appreciably delay repolarization. Most AADs with I_{Kr} blocking activity cause TdP in approximately 2% to 4% of patients, with the exceptions being amiodarone and dronedarone (less than 1%). Risk factors and associated features of medication-induced TdP have been identified and summarized in Table 40-14.[96] However, none of these associations are absolute prerequisites to the development of medication-induced TdP. For instance, although TdP is usually documented early in the course of quinidine therapy, patients may develop this arrhythmia anytime during chronic treatment.[97] The reason for quinidine's unique propensity for causing TdP at relatively low dosages and plasma concentrations requires explanation. Quinidine's ability to block I_{Kr} is clinically manifest at low plasma concentrations; at higher plasma concentrations, its sodium channel blocking properties predominate. Other medications that block I_{Kr} usually do so in a concentration-dependent fashion. The observation that most patients who suffer medication-induced TdP have evidence of mildly delayed repolarization (long QT intervals) even before they are prescribed the offending medication has stimulated a search for a potential genetically linked risk. Indeed, it appears that at least some patients with acquired medication-induced TdP possess mutations of genes that encode for I_{Kr} or I_{Ks}.[96]

The common underlying electrophysiologic cause of TdP is a delay in ventricular repolarization (provoking EADs), which usually results from inhibition (medication-induced or genetic) of the I_K current and manifests as QT interval prolongation on the ECG. Therefore, the extent of QT interval prolongation has been used as a measurement of risk of TdP. However, considerable controversy exists regarding this practice. Amiodarone, for example, commonly causes significant QT prolongation but is a relatively infrequent cause of TdP. Nonetheless, the QT interval should be measured and monitored in all patients prescribed medications that have a high potential for causing TdP (see Table 40-3). Patients with a prolonged QT_c interval at baseline (QT interval corrected for heart rate, which can be calculated using Bazett's formula: QTc = QTmeasured/square root of R − R IntervalQTc = QTmeasured/R − RInterval) (ie, greater than 450 msec in men; greater than 470 msec in women) should not be given medications that have a high potential for causing TdP. The development of clinically significant QTc interval prolongation (ie, QTc interval greater than 500 msec or an increase in the QTc interval of more than 60 to 70 msec from baseline) after initiation of a medication is an indication to discontinue the agent or, at least, to reduce its dosage and carefully monitor.[98]

Drug-induced TdP has become an extremely visible hazard plaguing new medications, sometimes resulting in public health disasters. For instance, several medications (cisapride, astemizole, levomethadyl, grepafloxacin, sparfloxacin, terfenadine, and high-dose [32 mg] IV ondansetron) have been withdrawn from the market in the United States because of their significant potential for causing TdP. Thus, all new medication entities under investigation are screened for their ability to block I_K and cause significant QT prolongation.

TABLE 40-13 Potential Causes of QT Interval Prolongation and Torsades de Pointes

Conditions
Congenital long QT syndromes
Heart failure
Hypokalemia
Hypomagnesemia
Myocardial ischemia/infarction
Myocarditis
Severe bradycardia (<50 beats/min)
Severe hypothermia
Severe starvation/liquid protein diets
Subarachnoid hemorrhage

Medications
Antiarrhythmic medications
- Amiodarone (<1%)
- Disopyramide
- Dofetilide
- Dronedarone
- Ibutilide
- Procainamide
- Quinidine
- Sotalol

Antiinfectives
- Azole antifungals (eg, fluconazole, voriconazole)
- Fluoroquinolones (eg, levofloxacin, moxifloxacin, gemifloxacin)
- Macrolides
- Pentamidine
- Chloroquine

Cancer chemotherapy or biologic agents
- Oxaliplatin
- Vandetanib

Methadone
Ondansetron (IV)
Psychotropics
- Citalopram
- Escitalopram
- Droperidol
- Haloperidol
- Phenothiazines (eg, thioridazine, chlorpromazine)
- Pimozide

Toxins
- Arsenic
- Organophosphate insecticides

IV, intravenous
Note: For a complete list, see www.crediblemeds.org.

TABLE 40-14 Risk Factors Associated with Drug-Induced Torsades de Pointes

High dosages or plasma concentrations of the offending medication
Concurrent SHD (eg, CAD, HF, and/or LV hypertrophy)
Prolonged QT interval at baseline
Prolonged QT interval shortly after initiation of the offending medication
Concomitant electrolyte disturbances (ie, hypokalemia or hypomagnesemia)
Female gender
A characteristic long-short initiating sequence of the TdP episode ()
Bradycardia
Concomitant QT interval prolonging medications

CAD, coronary artery disease; HF, heart failure; LV, left ventricular; SHD, structural heart disease; TdP, torsades de pointes.

Acute treatment of TdP is different than treatment for the more common acute monomorphic VT. For an acute episode of TdP, most patients will require and respond to defibrillation. However, TdP tends to be paroxysmal in nature and often will rapidly recur after defibrillation. Therefore, after the initial restoration of a stable rhythm, therapy designed to prevent recurrences of TdP should be instituted. AADs that further prolong repolarization, such as IV procainamide, are absolutely contraindicated. Lidocaine is usually ineffective. Although there are no true efficacy trials, IV magnesium sulfate, by suppressing EADs, is considered the medication of choice in preventing recurrences of TdP.[70] If IV magnesium sulfate is ineffective, treatment strategies designed to increase heart rate, shorten ventricular repolarization, and prevent the pause dependency should be initiated. Either temporary transvenous pacing (105-120 beats/min) or pharmacologic pacing (isoproterenol) can be initiated for this purpose. All medications that prolong the QT interval should be discontinued, and exacerbating factors (eg, hypokalemia or hypomagnesemia) should be corrected.

Ventricular Fibrillation

VF (Fig. 40-6) is electrical anarchy of the ventricle resulting in no cardiac output and CV collapse. Death will ensue rapidly if effective treatment measures are not taken. Patients who die abruptly (within 1 hour of initial symptoms) and unexpectedly (ie, "sudden death") usually have VF recorded at the time of death.[99] SCD accounts for more than 360,000 deaths per year in the United States.[13] It occurs most commonly in patients with CAD or LV dysfunction, but occasionally in those without associated heart disease (eg, Brugada syndrome). When a patient experiences sudden cessation of cardiac activity with no normal breath or signs of circulation, they are said to have sudden cardiac arrest. CPR, medications, and defibrillation can be corrective measures to prevent SCD. If the event is not associated with acute MI, sustained VT and/or VF during electrophysiologic studies are often inducible. These individuals are at high risk for the recurrence of VT and/or VF. In contrast, patients who have VF associated with acute MI (ie, within 48 hours of hospital presentation) usually have little risk of recurrence.

In the presence of acute coronary syndrome, CAD should be treated. The patient's LVEF should be reevaluated 40 days post-MI and 90 days postrevascularization.[70] If the LVEF is greater than 35% (0.35), the patient should be treated with medical management; however, if the LVEF is less than 35% (0.35), an ICD should be considered. Without acute coronary syndrome, the patient should be evaluated for SHD and inherited arrhythmia syndrome. Regardless, reversible causes should be eliminated (ie, discontinue the offending medication or correct electrolytes) and avoided. If no reversible cause is identified, an ICD can be considered.

Acute Management A patient with pulseless VT or VF should have advanced cardiovascular life support (ACLS) initiated immediately, including defibrillation to restore SR.[100] A detailed discussion regarding the acute management of pulseless VT/VF can be found in Chapter 41, "Cardiopulmonary Arrest."

Bradyarrhythmias

For the most part, the symptoms of bradyarrhythmias result from a decline in cardiac output. Because cardiac output decreases as heart rate decreases (to a point), patients with bradyarrhythmias may experience symptoms in association with hypotension, such as dizziness, syncope, fatigue, and confusion. If LV dysfunction exists, patients may experience worsening HF symptoms. Except in the case of recurrent syncope, symptoms associated with bradyarrhythmias are often subtle and nonspecific.

Sinus Bradycardia

Sinus bradyarrhythmias (heart rate less than 60 beats/min) are a common finding, especially in young, athletically active individuals, and usually are neither symptomatic nor in need of therapeutic intervention. On the other hand, some patients, particularly the elderly, have SND. This may be the result of underlying SHD and the normal aging process that attenuate SA nodal function over time resulting in symptomatic sinus bradycardia and/or periods of sinus arrest.[93] SND is usually reflective of diffuse conduction disease and accompanying AV block is relatively common. Furthermore, symptomatic bradyarrhythmias may be accompanied by alternating periods of paroxysmal tachycardias such as AF. In this instance, AF sometimes presents with a rather slow ventricular response (in the absence of AV nodal blocking medications) because of diffuse conduction disease. The occurrence of alternating bradyarrhythmias and tachyarrhythmias is referred to as the tachy-brady syndrome. The occurrence of paroxysmal AF in a patient with SND may be a result of underlying SHD with atrial dysfunction or atrial escape in response to reduced sinus node automaticity. In fact, because the rate of impulse generation by the sinus node is generally depressed or may fail altogether, other automatic pacemakers within the conduction system may "rescue" the sinus node. These rescue rhythms often present as paroxysmal atrial rhythms (eg, AF) or as a junctional escape rhythm.

The treatment of SND involves eliminating the symptomatic bradycardia and potentially managing alternating tachycardias such as AF. In general, the long-term therapy of choice is permanent pacemaker implantation.[81,93] Pacing clearly improves symptoms and overall quality of life and decreases the incidence of paroxysmal AF and systemic embolism. Drugs commonly employed to treat supraventricular tachycardias should be used with caution, if at all, in the absence of a functioning pacemaker. AADs prescribed to prevent AF recurrences may also suppress the escape or rescue rhythms that appear in severe sinus bradycardia or sinus arrest. Consequently, these medications may transform an asymptomatic patient with bradycardia into a symptomatic one. Other medications that depress SA or AV nodal function, such as β-blockers, non-DHP CCBs, and ivabradine, may also significantly exacerbate bradycardia. Drugs with indirect sympatholytic actions, such as methyldopa and clonidine, may also worsen SND. The use of digoxin in these patients is controversial; however, in most cases, it can be used safely.

Another reason for paroxysmal bradycardia and sinus arrest, not directly due to SND, is carotid sinus syndrome.[101,102] This syndrome occurs commonly in the elderly with underlying SHD and may precipitate falls and hip fractures. Symptoms occur when the carotid sinus is stimulated, resulting in an accentuated baroreceptor reflex. Often, however, symptoms are not well correlated with the obvious physical manipulation of the carotid sinus (in the lateral neck region). Patients may experience intermittent episodes of dizziness or syncope because of sinus arrest caused by increased vagal tone (the cardioinhibitory type), a drop in systemic blood pressure caused by sympathetic withdrawal (the vasodepressor type), or both (mixed cardioinhibitory and vasodepressor types). The diagnosis can be confirmed by performing carotid sinus massage with ECG and blood pressure monitoring in a controlled setting. Symptomatic carotid sinus hypersensitivity should be treated with permanent pacemaker therapy.[93] However, some patients, particularly those with a significant vasodepressor component, still experience syncope or dizziness even after pacemaker implantation.

Vasovagal syndrome, by causing bradycardia, sinus arrest, and/or hypotension, is the cause of syncope in many patients who present with recurrent fainting of unknown origin.[102] Many individuals can recount rare instances of fainting spells at times of duress or fear while others may have extremely frequent, unexpected syncopal episodes that interfere with the patient's quality of life and cause physical danger (sometimes referred to as neurocardiogenic syncope syndrome or malignant vasovagal syndrome). Although the true mechanism is uncertain, vasovagal syncope is presumed to be a neurally mediated, paradoxical reaction involving stimulation of cardiac mechanoreceptors, forceful contraction of the ventricle (eg, as with adrenergic stimulation), and low ventricular volumes (eg, with upright posture or dehydration) leading to transient hypotension (sympathetic withdrawal), bradycardia (vagotonia), and syncope. Patients believed to have frequent episodes of vasovagal syncope may undergo an upright body-tilt test to establish the diagnosis, although the value of this test has been questioned.[102]

Patients with vasovagal syncope should receive education targeting awareness and trigger avoidance (ie, prolonged standing or warm environments).[102] First-line treatment includes counterpressure maneuvers (ie, laying on the ground, squatting, etc.), followed by increasing salt and fluid intake, when not contraindicated. The drug of choice is midodrine, which has been associated with a 43% reduction in syncope recurrence. Midodrine is an alpha-agonist that reduces the peripheral sympathetic neural outflow that causes venous pooling and vasodepression. Although it may seem inappropriate to treat a syndrome resulting from vasodilation and bradycardia with a medication that slows heart rate and reduces blood pressure, β-blockers are used to prevent episodes of vasovagal syncope in patients 42 years of age and older. The rationale for their use is that they inhibit the sympathetic surge that causes forceful ventricular contraction and precedes the onset of hypotension and bradycardia. Other medications that have been used successfully include mineralocorticoids as volume expanders (fludrocortisone) and selective serotonin receptor antagonists (sertraline, paroxetine). Dual-chamber pacemakers can be used but should be reserved for at least 40 years of age with recurrent episodes and prolonged spontaneous pauses.

Atrioventricular Block

Conduction delay or block may occur in any area of the AV conduction system: the AV node, the His bundle, or the bundle branches. AV block is usually categorized into three different types based on ECG findings (Table 40-15). First-degree AV block is 1:1 AV conduction with a prolonged PR interval. Second-degree AV block is divided into two forms: Mobitz I AV block (Wenckebach periodicity) is less than 1:1 AV conduction with progressively lengthening PR intervals until a ventricular complex is dropped; Mobitz II AV block is intermittently dropped ventricular beats in a random fashion without progressive PR lengthening. Third-degree AV block is complete heart block where AV conduction is totally absent (AV dissociation). First-degree AV block usually represents prolonged conduction in the AV node. Mobitz I, second-degree AV block is also usually caused by prolonged conduction in the AV node. In contrast, Mobitz II, second-degree AV block is usually caused by conduction disease below the AV node (ie, His bundle). Third-degree AV block may be caused by disease at any level of the AV conduction system: complete AV nodal block, His bundle block, or trifascicular block. In this situation, the ventricle beats independently of the atria (AV dissociation), and the rate of ventricular activation and QRS configuration are determined by the site of the AV block. The usual degree of automaticity of ventricular pacemakers progressively declines as the site of impulse generation moves down the ventricular conduction system. Therefore, the ventricular escape rate in cases of trifascicular block will be significantly less than complete AV nodal block. Consequently, trifascicular block is a much more dangerous form of AV block. For instance, complete AV block at the level of the AV node usually results in the ventricular rhythm being controlled by the stable AV junctional pacemaker (rate approximately 40 beats/min). In contrast, in complete AV block due to trifascicular or His bundle block, a much less reliable pacemaker with slower rates below the site of block controls ventricular rhythm.

TABLE 40-15 Forms of Atrioventricular Block

Type	Criteria	Site of Block
First-degree block	Prolonged PR interval (>0.2 second) 1:1 AV conduction	Usually AVN
Second-degree block: Mobitz I	Progressive PR prolongation until QRS is dropped; <1:1 AV conduction	AVN
Second-degree block: Mobitz II	Random nonconducted beats (absence of QRS); <1:1 AV conduction	Below AVN
Third-degree block	AV dissociation; absence of AV conduction	AVN or below

AV, atrioventricular; AVN, atrioventricular node.

AV block may be found in patients without underlying SHD, such as trained athletes or during sleep when vagal tone is high. Also, AV block may be transient where the underlying etiology is reversible such as in myocarditis, myocardial ischemia, after CV surgery, or during medication therapy. β-Blockers, digoxin, or non-DHP CCBs may cause AV block, primarily in the AV nodal area. Class I AADs may exacerbate conduction delays below the level of the AV node (sodium-dependent tissue). In other cases, AV block may be irreversible, such as that caused by acute MI, rare degenerative diseases, primary myocardial disease, or congenital heart disease.

If patients with second-degree or third-degree AV block develop signs or symptoms of poor perfusion (eg, altered mental status, chest pain, hypotension, shock), IV atropine (0.5 mg given every 3-5 minutes, up to 3 mg total dose) should be administered.[79] If these patients do not respond to atropine, transcutaneous or transvenous pacing can be initiated. Sympathomimetic infusions such as epinephrine (2-10 μg/min) or dopamine (2-10 μg/kg/min) can also be used in the event of atropine failure and are particularly effective in sinus bradycardia/arrest and AV nodal block. An isoproterenol infusion (2-10 μg/min) may be considered if the patient does not respond to dopamine or epinephrine; however, this medication should be used with caution because of its vasodilating properties and ability to increase myocardial oxygen consumption (particularly during active MI). As would be expected, these medications usually do not help when the site of the AV block is below the AV node (eg, Mobitz II or trifascicular AV block) because their primary mechanism is to accelerate conduction through the AV node. If patients with bradycardia or AV block present with signs and symptoms of adequate perfusion, no acute therapy other than close observation is recommended.

Patients with chronic symptomatic AV block should be treated with the insertion of a permanent pacemaker.[93] Patients without symptoms can sometimes be followed closely without the need for a pacemaker. Patients with acute MI and evidence of new AV block or conduction disturbances will often require the insertion of a temporary transvenous pacemaker. AV block more commonly occurs as a complication of inferior wall MIs because of high vagal innervation at this site, and the coronary blood flow to the nodal areas usually supplies the inferior wall. However, the AV block may only be transient, obviating the need for permanent pacing.

EVALUATION OF THERAPEUTIC OUTCOMES

Generally, patients who suffer from tachyarrhythmias can be monitored for one or several possible therapeutic outcomes. Obviously, the presence or recurrence of any arrhythmia can be documented by electrocardiographic means (eg, surface ECG, Holter monitor, event monitor, or implantable loop recorder). Furthermore, patients may experience a decrease in blood pressure that may result in symptoms ranging from lightheadedness to abrupt syncope, depending

TABLE 40-16 Arrhythmia Outcomes

Mortality
• Total, all-cause mortality
• Arrhythmia-related death (ie, sudden cardiac death)
Signs and symptoms
• Recurrences documented by electrocardiogram
• Time to recurrence
• Frequency of recurrences
• Exercise tolerance
• Lightheadedness
• Blood pressure
• Heart rate
Surrogate markers used to determine efficacy
• Number of premature ventricular complexes per day
• Inducibility of tachycardia with programmed stimulation
• Need for nonpharmacologic interventions (eg, ICD)
• ICD shocks
• Adverse drug reactions/treatment complications
• Quality of life
Economics
Arrhythmia specific (eg, systemic embolism in atrial fibrillation)

ICD, implantable cardioverter-defibrillator.

on the rate of the arrhythmia and the status of the underlying heart disease. For some patients, the potential alteration in hemodynamics may result in death if the arrhythmia is not detected and treated immediately. Besides these clinical outcomes, many patients with tachyarrhythmias experience alterations in quality of life as a result of recurrent symptoms of the arrhythmia or from adverse drug reactions.

There are some therapeutic outcomes that are unique to certain arrhythmias. For instance, patients with AF or AFl need to be monitored for thromboembolism and complications of antithrombotic therapy (bleeding, medication interactions). Ultimately, the most important monitoring parameters for most patients fall into the following categories: (a) mortality (total and sudden cardiac death); (b) arrhythmia recurrence (duration, frequency, symptoms); (c) hemodynamic consequences (heart rate, blood pressure, symptoms); and (d) treatment complications (adverse drug reactions or need for alternative or additional medications, devices, surgery) (Table 40-16).

ABBREVIATIONS

AAD	antiarrhythmic medication
ACC	American College of Cardiology
ACLS	advanced cardiovascular life support
AF	atrial fibrillation
AFl	atrial flutter
AHA	American Heart Association
AV	atrioventricular
AVNRT	atrioventricular nodal reentrant tachycardia
AVRT	atrioventricular reentrant tachycardia
CAD	coronary artery disease
CCB	calcium channel blocker
CPR	cardiopulmonary resuscitation
CrCl	creatinine clearance
CV	cardiovascular
CYP	cytochrome P450
DAD	delayed afterdepolarization
DCCV	direct current cardioversion
DHP	dihydropyridine
DOAC	direct oral anticoagulants
EAD	early afterdepolarization
ECC	emergency cardiovascular care
ECG	electrocardiogram
FDA	Food and Drug Administration
HF	heart failure
HFpEF	heart failure with preserved ejection fraction
HFrEF	heart failure with reduced ejection fraction
HRS	Heart Rhythm Society
ICD	implantable cardioverter-defibrillator
INR	international normalized ratio
ICH	intracranial hemorrhage
IV	intravenous
J	joules
LMWH	low-molecular-weight heparin
LV	left ventricular
LVEF	left ventricular ejection fraction
MI	myocardial infarction
NYHA	New York Heart Association
P-gp	P-glycoprotein
PSVT	paroxysmal supraventricular tachycardia
PVC	premature ventricular complex
PVI	pulmonary vein isolation
RMP	resting membrane potential
SA	sinoatrial
SCD	sudden cardiac death
SHD	structural heart disease
SND	sinus node dysfunction
SR	sinus rhythm
TdP	torsades de pointes
TE	thromboembolic
TEE	transesophageal echocardiography
TTR	time in therapeutic range
VF	ventricular fibrillation
VT	ventricular tachycardia
WPW	Wolff-Parkinson-White

REFERENCES

1. Enriquez A, Frankel DS, Baranchuk A Pathophysiology of ventricular tachyarrhythmias. *Herzschr Elektrophys.* 2017;28:149–156. doi:10.1007/s00399-017-0512-4.
2. Vaughan Williams EM. A classification of antiarrhythmic actions reassessed after a decade of new medications. *J Clin Pharmacol.* 1984;24:129–147.
3. Hondeghem LM, Katzung BG. Antiarrhythmic agents: The modulated receptor mechanism of action of sodium and calcium channel-blocking medications. *Annu Rev Pharmacol Toxicol.* 1984;24:387–423.
4. Lei M, Wu L, Terrar DA, et al. Modernized classification of cardiac antiarrhythmic drugs. *Circulation.* 2018;138:1879–1896. doi:10.1161/circulationaha.118.035455.
5. Hindricks G, Potpara T, Dagres N, et al. 2020 ESC Guidelines for the diagnosis and management of atrial fibrillation developed in collaboration with the European Association for Cardio-Thoracic Surgery (EACTS). *Eur Heart J.* 2020;42:373–498. doi:10.1093/eurheartj/ehaa612.
6. Epstein AE, Olshansky B. Naccarelli GV, et al. Practical management guide for clinicians who treat patients with amiodarone. *Am J Med.* 2016;129:468–475.
7. Oetgen WJ, Sobol SM, Tri TB, et al. Amiodarone-digoxin interaction. *Chest.* 1984;86:75–79. doi:10.1378/chest.86.1.75.
8. Sanoski CA, Bauman JL. Clinical observations with the amiodarone/warfarin interaction: Dosing relationships with long-term therapy. *Chest.* 2002;121:19–23.
9. Jahn S, Zollner G, Lackner C, Stauber B. Severe toxic hepatitis associated with dronedarone. *Curr Drug Saf.* 2013;8:201–202.
10. Siu CW, Wong MP, Ho CM, et al. Fatal lung toxic effects related to dronedarone use. *Arch Intern Med.* 2012;172:516–517.
11. Young C, Maruthappu M, Wayne RP, Leaver L. Reversible acute kidney injury requiring haemodialysis five days after starting dronedarone in a stable 71-year-old man at risk of cardiovascular polypharmacy. *J R Coll Physicians Edinb.* 2013;43:122–125.
12. Aronoff GR, Bennett WM, Berns JS, et al. *Drug Prescribing in Renal Failure: Dosing Guidelines for Adults and Children.* 5th ed. Philadelphia, PA: American College of Physicians; 2007.
13. Virani SS, Alonso A, Aparicio HJ, et al. Heart disease and stroke statistics—2021 update. *Circulation.* 2021;143. doi:10.1161/cir.0000000000000950.

14. January CT, Wann LS, Alpert JS, et al. 2014 AHA/ACC/HRS guideline for the management of patients with atrial fibrillation: A report of the American College of Cardiology/American Heart Association Task Force on Practice Guidelines and the Heart Rhythm Society. *J Am Coll Cardiol.* 2014;(64):e1–e76.
15. Wolf PA, Abbott RD, Kannel WB. Atrial fibrillation as an independent risk factor for stroke: The Framingham Study. *Stroke.* 1991;22:983–988.
16. Lip GYH, Banerjee A, Boriani G, et al. Antithrombotic therapy for atrial fibrillation: CHEST guideline and expert panel report. *Chest.* 2018;154:1121–1201.
17. January CT, Wann LS, Calkins H, et al. 2019 AHA/ACC/HRS focused update of the 2014 AHA/ACC/HRS guideline for the management of patients with atrial fibrillation. *J Am Coll Cardiol.* 2019;74:104–132. doi:10.1016/j.jacc.2019.01.011.
18. Connolly SJ, Ezekowitz MD, Yusuf S, et al. Dabigatran versus warfarin in patients with atrial fibrillation. *N Engl J Med.* 2009;361:1139–1151.
19. Liesenfeld KH, Lehr T, Dansirikul C, et al. Population pharmacokinetic analysis of the oral thrombin inhibitor dabigatran etexilate in patients with non-valvular atrial fibrillation from the RE-LY trial. *J Thromb Haemost.* 2011;9:2168–2175. doi:10.1111/j.1538-7836.2011.04498.x.
20. Eikelboom JW, Connolly SJ, Brueckmann M, et al. Dabigatran versus warfarin in patients with mechanical heart valves. *N Engl J Med.* 2013;369:1206–1214.
21. Patel MR, Mahaffey KW, Garg J, et al. Rivaroxaban versus warfarin in nonvalvular atrial fibrillation. *N Engl J Med.* 2011;365:883–891.
22. Granger CB, Alexander JH, McMurray JJ, et al. Apixaban versus warfarin in patients with atrial fibrillation. *N Engl J Med.* 2011;365:981–992.
23. Giugliano RP, Ruff CT, Braunwald E, et al. Edoxaban versus warfarin in patients with atrial fibrillation. *N Engl J Med.* 2013;369:2093–2104.
24. Haas S, Ten Cate H, Accetta G, et al. Quality of vitamin K antagonist control and 1-year outcomes in patients with atrial fibrillation: A global perspective from the GARFIELD-AF registry. *PloS One.* 2016;11(10):e0164076. doi:10.1371/journal.pone.0164076.
25. Patel MR, Hellkamp AS, Lokhnygina Y, et al. Outcomes of discontinuing rivaroxaban compared with warfarin in patients with nonvalvular atrial fibrillation: Analysis from the ROCKET AF trial (Rivaroxaban Once-Daily, Oral, Direct Factor Xa Inhibition Compared With Vitamin K Antagonism for Prevention of Stroke and Embolism Trial in Atrial Fibrillation). *J Am Coll Cardiol.* 2013;61:651–658.
26. Van Gelder IC, Hagens VE, Bosker HA, et al. The Rate Control Versus Electrical Cardioversion for Persistent Atrial Fibrillation Study Group. A comparison of rate control and rhythm control in patients with recurrent persistent atrial fibrillation. *N Engl J Med.* 2002;347:1834–1840.
27. The Atrial Fibrillation Follow-Up Investigation of Rhythm Management (AFFIRM) Investigators. A comparison of rate control and rhythm control in patients with atrial fibrillation. *N Engl J Med.* 2002;347:1825–1833.
28. Hohnloser SH, Kuck KH, Lilienthal J. Rhythm or rate control in atrial fibrillation—Pharmacological Intervention in Atrial Fibrillation (PIAF): A randomised trial. *Lancet.* 2000;356:1789–1794.
29. Carlsson J, Miketic S, Windeler J, et al. Randomized trial of rate control versus rhythm control in persistent atrial fibrillation: The Strategies of Treatment of Atrial Fibrillation (STAF) study. *J Am Coll Cardiol.* 2003;41:1690–1696.
30. Opolski G, Torbicki A, Kosior DA, et al. Rate control vs rhythm control in patients with nonvalvular persistent atrial fibrillation: The results of the Polish How to Treat Chronic Atrial Fibrillation (HOT CAFE) Study. *Chest.* 2004;126:476–486.
31. Roy D, Talajic M, Nattel S, et al. Rhythm control versus rate control for atrial fibrillation and heart failure. *N Engl J Med.* 2008;358:2667–2677.
32. de Denus S, Sanoski CA, Carlsson J, Opolski G, Spinler SA. Rate vs rhythm control in patients with atrial fibrillation: A meta-analysis. *Arch Intern Med.* 2005;165:258–262.
33. Van Gelder IC, Groenveld HF, Crijns HJ, et al. Lenient versus strict rate control in patients with atrial fibrillation. *N Engl J Med.* 2010;362:1363–1373.
34. Baker WL, Sobieraj DM, DiDomenico RJ. Influence of digoxin on mortality in patients with atrial fibrillation: Overview of systematic reviews. *Pharmacotherapy.* 2021;41(4):394–404. doi:10.1002/phar.251033544894.
35. Lopes RD, Rordorf R, De Ferrari GM, et al. Digoxin and mortality in patients with atrial fibrillation. *J Am Coll Cardiol.* 2018;71:1063–1074. doi:10.1016/j.jacc.2017.12.060.
36. January CT, et al. 2014AHA/ACC/HRS guideline for the management of patients with atrial fibrillation: A report of the American College of Cardiology/American Heart Association TaskForce on Practice Guidelines and the Heart Rhythm Society. *J Am Coll Cardiol.* 2014(64):e1–e76.
37. January CT, Wann LS, Calkins H, et al. 2019 AHA/ACC/HRS focused update of the 2014 AHA/ACC/HRS guidelines for the management of patients with atrial fibrillation: A report of the American College of Cardiology/American Heart Association Task Force on Clinical Practice Guidelines and the Heart Rhythm Society. *Circulation.* 2019. doi:10.1161/CIR.0000000000000665.
38. Caldeira D, Costa J, Ferreira JJ, Lip GYH, Pinto FJ. Non-vitamin K oral anticoagulants in the cardioversion of patients with atrial fibrillation: Systemic review and meta-analysis. *Clin Res Cardiol.* 2015;104:582–590.
39. Alboni P, Botto GL, Baldi N, et al. Outpatient treatment of recent-onset atrial fibrillation with the "pill-in-the-pocket" approach. *N Engl J Med.* 2004;351:2384–2391.
40. Lafuente-LaFuente C, Mouly S, Longás-Tejero MA, et al. Antiarrhythmic medications for maintaining sinus rhythm after cardioversion of atrial fibrillation. *Arch Intern Med.* 2006;166:719–728.
41. Fang MC, Stafford RS, Ruskin JN, et al. National trends in antiarrhythmic and antithrombotic medication use in atrial fibrillation. *Arch Intern Med.* 2004;164:55–60.
42. Zimetbaum P. Antiarrhythmic drug therapy for atrial fibrillation. *Circulation.* 2012;125:381–389. doi:10.1161/circulationaha.111.019927.
43. Singh BN, Singh SN, Reda DJ, et al. Amiodarone versus sotalol for atrial fibrillation. *N Engl J Med.* 2005;352:1861–1872.
44. AFFIRM First Antiarrhythmic Drug Substudy Investigators. Maintenance of sinus rhythm in patients with atrial fibrillation: An AFFIRM substudy of the first antiarrhythmic medication. *J Am Coll Cardiol.* 2003;42:20–29.
45. Valembois L, Audureau E, Takeda A, et al. Antiarrhythmics for maintaining sinus rhythm after cardioversion of atrial fibrillation. *Cochrane Database Syst Rev.* 2019;9:CD005049. doi:10.1002/14651858.cd005049.pub5.
46. Singh S, Zoble RG, Yellen L, et al. Efficacy and safety of oral dofetilide in converting and maintaining sinus rhythm in patients with chronic atrial fibrillation or atrial flutter. The Symptomatic Atrial Fibrillation Investigative Research on Dofetilide (SAFIRE-D) Study. *Circulation.* 2000;102:2385–2390.
47. Pedersen OD, Bagger H, Keller N, et al. Efficacy of dofetilide in the treatment of atrial fibrillation-flutter in patients with reduced left ventricular function, a Danish Investigation of Arrhythmia and Mortality on Dofetilide (DIAMOND) Substudy. *Circulation.* 2001;104:292–296.
48. Singh BN, Connolly SJ, Crijns HJGM, et al. Dronedarone for maintenance of sinus rhythm in atrial fibrillation or flutter. *N Engl J Med.* 2007;357:987–999.
49. Hohnloser SH, Crijns HJGM, van Eickels M, et al. Effect of dronedarone on cardiovascular events in atrial fibrillation. *N Engl J Med.* 2009;360:668–678.
50. Le Heuzey JY, De Ferrari GM, Radzik D, et al. A short-term, randomized, double-blind, parallel-group study to evaluate the efficacy and safety of dronedarone versus amiodarone in patients with persistent atrial fibrillation: The DIONYSOS study. *J Cardiovasc Electrophysiol.* 2010;21:597–605.
51. Connolly SJ, Camm AJ, Halperin JL, et al. Dronedarone in high-risk permanent atrial fibrillation. *N Engl J Med.* 2011;365:2268–2276.
52. Køber L, Torp-Pedersen C, McMurray JJV, et al. Increased mortality after dronedarone therapy for severe heart failure. *N Engl J Med.* 2008;358:2678–2687.
53. Page RL, Joglar JA, Caldwell MA, et al. 2015 ACC/AHA/HRS guideline for the management of adult patients with supraventricular tachycardia: A report of the American College of Cardiology/American Heart Association Task Force on Clinical Practice Guidelines and the Heart Rhythm Society. *Circulation.* 2016;133:e506–e574.
54. Andrade JG, Wells GA, Deyell MW, et al. Cryoablation or drug therapy for initial treatment of atrial fibrillation. *N Engl J Med.* 2021;384:305–315. doi:10.1056/nejmoa2029980.
55. Wazni OM, Dandamudi G, Sood N, et al. Cryoballoon ablation as initial therapy for atrial fibrillation. *N Engl J Med.* 2021;384:316–324. doi:10.1056/nejmoa2029554.
56. Marrouche NF, Brachmann J, Andresen D, et al. Catheter ablation for atrial fibrillation with heart failure. *N Engl J Med.* 2018;378:417–427.
57. Morillo C, Verma A, Kuck A, et al. Radiofrequency ablation vs antiarrhythmic medications as first-line treatment of paroxysmal atrial fibrillation (RAAFT 2): A randomized trial. *JAMA.* 2014;311:692–700.
58. Cosedis NJ, Johannessen A, Raatkainen P, et al. Radiofrequency ablation as initial therapy in paroxysmal atrial fibrillation. *N Engl J Med.* 2012;367:1587–1595.

59. Cappato R, Calkins H, Chen SA, et al. Updated worldwide survey on the methods, efficacy, and safety of catheter ablation for human atrial fibrillation. *Circ Arrhythm Electrophysiol.* 2010;3:32–38.
60. Porter MJ, Morton JB, Denman R, et al. Influence of age and gender on the mechanism of supraventricular tachycardia. *Heart Rhythm.* 2004;1:393–396.
61. Sung RJ, Lauer MR, Chun H. Atrioventricular node reentry: Current concepts and new perspectives. *Pacing Clin Electrophysiol.* 1994;17:1413–1430.
62. DiMarco JP, Miles W, Akhtar M, et al. Adenosine for paroxysmal supraventricular tachycardia: Dose ranging and comparison with verapamil. Assessment in placebo-controlled, multicenter trials. *Ann Intern Med.* 1990;1113:104–110.
63. Jackman WM, Wang Z, Friday KJ, et al. Catheter ablation of accessory atrioventricular pathways (Wolff-Parkinson-White syndrome) by radiofrequency current. *N Engl J Med.* 1991;324:1605–1611.
64. Jackman WM, Beckman KJ, McClelland JH, et al. Treatment of supraventricular tachycardia due to atrioventricular nodal reentry by radiofrequency catheter ablation of slow pathway conduction. *N Engl J Med.* 1992;327:313–318.
65. Meyer L, Stubbs B, Fahrenbruch C, et al. Incidence, causes, and survival trends from cardiovascular related sudden cardiac arrest in children and young adults 0 to 35 years of age: A 30-year review. *Circulation.* 2012;126:1363–1372.
66. Bayes deLuna A, Coumel P, LeClercq IF. Ambulatory sudden cardiac death: Mechanisms of production of fatal arrhythmia on the basis of data from 157 cases. *Am Heart J.* 1989;117:151–159.
67. Ruberman W, Weinblatt E, Goldberg JD, et al. Ventricular premature beats and mortality after myocardial infarction. *N Engl J Med.* 1977;297:750–757.
68. Echt DS, Liebson PR, Mitchell B, et al. Mortality and morbidity in patients receiving encainide, flecainide, or placebo. The Cardiac Arrhythmia Suppression Trial. *N Engl J Med.* 1991;324:781–788.
69. The Cardiac Arrhythmia Suppression Trial II Investigators. Effect of the antiarrhythmic agent moricizine on survival after myocardial infarction. *N Engl J Med.* 1992;327:227–233.
70. Al-Khatib SM, Stevenson WG, Ackerman MJ, et al. 2017 AHA/ACC/HRS guideline for management of patients with ventricular arrhythmias and the prevention of sudden cardiac death: A report of the American College of Cardiology Foundation/American Heart Association Task Force on Clinical Practice Guidelines and the Heart Rhythm Society. *Circulation.* 2018;138:e272–e391.
71. Julian DG, Camm AJ, Frangin G, et al. Randomized trial of effect of amiodarone on mortality in patients with left ventricular dysfunction after recent myocardial infarction: EMIAT. *Lancet.* 1997;349:667–674.
72. Cairns JA, Connolly SJ, Roberts R, et al. Randomized trial of outcome after myocardial infarction in patients with frequent or repetitive ventricular premature depolarizations: CAMIAT. *Lancet.* 1997;349:675–682.
73. Torp-Pederson C, Moller M, Bloch-Thomsen PE, et al. Dofetilide in patients with congestive heart failure and left ventricular dysfunction. *N Engl J Med.* 1999;341:857–865.
74. Kober L, Block-Thomsen PE, Moller M, et al. Effect of dofetilide in patients with recent myocardial infarction and left ventricular dysfunction: A randomized trial. *Lancet.* 2000;356:2052–2058.
75. Edhouse J, Morris F. Broad complex tachycardia—Part I. *BMJ.* 2002;312:719–722.
76. Edhouse J, Morris F. Broad complex tachycardia—Part II. *BMJ.* 2002;324:776–779.
77. Cole CR, Marrouche NF, Natale A. Evaluation and management of ventricular outflow tract tachycardias. *Card Electrophysiol Rev.* 2002;6:442–447.
78. Wallace E, Howard L, Liu M, et al. Long QT syndrome: Genetics and future perspective. *Pediatr Cardiol.* 2019;40:1419–1430. doi:10.1007/s00246-019-02151-x.
79. 2010 American Heart Association guidelines for cardiopulmonary resuscitation and emergency cardiovascular care science. *Circulation.* 2010;122:5640–5933.
80. Sapp JL, Wells GA, Parkash R, et al. Ventricular tachycardia ablation versus escalation of antiarrhythmic medications. *N Engl J Med.* 2016;375:111–121.
81. Wilkoff BL, Fauchier L, Stiles MK, et al. 2015 HRS/EHRA/APHRS/SOLAECE expert consensus statement on optimal implantable cardioverter-defibrillator programming and testing. *J Arrhythm.* 2016;32(1):1–28. doi:10.1016/j.joa.2015.12.00126949427.
82. Data from Pacifico A, et al. Prevention of implantable-defibrillator shocks by treatment with sotalol. *N Engl J Med.* 1999;340:1855–1862. Copyright © 2003 Massachusetts Medical Society. All rights reserved.
83. Abboud J, Ehrlich JR, et al. Antiarrhythmic drug therapy to avoid implantable cardioverter defibrillator shocks. *Arrhyth Electrophys Rev.* 2016;5:117. doi:10.15420/aer.2016.10.2.
84. The AVID Investigators. A comparison of antiarrhythmic-medication therapy with implantable defibrillators in patients resuscitated from near-fatal ventricular arrhythmias. *N Engl J Med.* 1997;337:1576–1583.
85. Connolly SJ, Gene M, Roberts TS, et al. Cardiac Implantable Defibrillator Study (CIDS): A randomized trial of the implantable cardioverter-defibrillator against amiodarone. *Circulation.* 2000;101:1297–1302.
86. Kuck KH, Cappato R, Siebels J, et al. Randomized comparison of antiarrhythmic medication therapy with implantable defibrillators in patients resuscitated from cardiac arrest: The Cardiac Arrest Study Hamburg (CASH). *Circulation.* 2000;102:748–754.
87. Wilber DJ, Olshansky B, Moran JF, et al. Electrophysiological testing and nonsustained VT. Use and limitations in patients with coronary artery disease and impaired ventricular function. *Circulation.* 1990;82:350–358.
88. Buxton AE, Leek KL, DiCarlo L, et al. Electrophysiologic testing to identify patients with coronary artery disease who are at risk for sudden death. Multicenter Unsustained Tachycardia Trial. *N Engl J Med.* 2000;342:1937–1945.
89. Moss AJ, Hall WJ, Cannom DS, et al. Improved survival with an implanted defibrillator in patients with coronary disease at high risk for ventricular arrhythmia. *N Engl J Med.* 1996;335:1933–1940.
90. Buxton AE, Lee KL, Fisher JD, et al. A randomized study of the prevention of sudden death in patients with coronary artery disease. *N Engl J Med.* 1999;341:1882–1890.
91. Moss AJ, Zareba W, Hall WJ, et al. Prophylactic implantation of a defibrillator in patients with myocardial infarction and reduced ejection fraction. *N Engl J Med.* 2002;346:877–883.
92. Bardy GH, Lee KL, Mark DB, et al. Amiodarone or an implantable cardioverter-defibrillator for congestive heart failure. *N Engl J Med.* 2005;352:225–237.
93. Epstein AE, DiMarco JP, Ellenbogen KA, et al. 2012 ACCF/AHA/HRS focused update incorporated into the ACCF/AHA/HRS 2008 guidelines for device-based therapy of cardiac rhythm abnormalities: A report of the American College of Cardiology/American Heart Association Task Force on Practice Guidelines and the Heart Rhythm Society. *J Am Coll Cardiol.* 2013;61:e6–e75.
94. Podrid PJ. Proarrhythmia, a serious complication of antiarrhythmic medications. *Curr Cardiol Rep.* 1999;1:289–296.
95. Antzelevitch C. Heterogeneity of cellular repolarization in LQTS: The role of M cells. *Eur Heart J.* 2001;3:K2–K16.
96. Roden DM, Long QT. Syndrome: Reduced repolarization reserve and the genetic link. *J Intern Med.* 2006;259:59–69.
97. Oberg KC, O'Toole MF, Gallastegui JL, Bauman JL. "Late" proarrhythmia due to quinidine. *Am J Cardiol.* 1994;74:192–194.
98. Schwartz PJ, Woosley RL. Predicting the unpredictable: Drug-induced QT prolongation and torsades de pointes. *J Am Coll Cardiol.* 2016;67:1639–1650.
99. Koplan BA, Stevenson WG. Ventricular tachycardia and sudden cardiac death. *Mayo Clin Proc.* 2009;84:289–297.
100. Panchal AR, Berg KM, Kudenchuk PJ, et al. 2018 American Heart Association focused update on advanced cardiovascular life support use of antiarrhythmic medications during and immediately after cardiac arrest: An update to the American Heart Association guidelines for cardiopulmonary resuscitation and emergency cardiovascular care. *Circulation.* 2018(138):e740–e749.
101. Kusumoto FM, Schoenfeld MH, Barrett C, et al. 2018 ACC/AHA/HRS guideline on the evaluation and management of patients with bradycardia and cardiac conduction delay: A Report of the American College of Cardiology/American Heart Association Task Force on Clinical Practice Guidelines and the Heart Rhythm Society. *Heart Rhythm.* 2019;16(9):e128–e226. doi:10.1016/j.hrthm.2018.10.03730412778.
102. Shen WK, Sheldon RS, Benditt DG, et al. 2017 ACC/AHA/HRS guideline for the evaluation and management of patients with syncope: a report of the American College of Cardiology/American Heart Association task force on clinical practice guidelines and the Heart Rhythm Society. *Circulation.* 2017;136. doi:10.1161/cir.0000000000000499.

41

Cardiopulmonary Arrest

Jeffrey F. Barletta

KEY CONCEPTS

1. High-quality cardiopulmonary resuscitation with minimal interruptions in chest compressions should be delivered to all patients following cardiac arrest.
2. The American Heart Association (AHA) algorithm for basic life support emphasizes circulation, airway, and breathing, forming the mnemonic "CAB."
3. The purpose of using vasopressor therapy following cardiac arrest is to augment coronary and cerebral perfusion pressures.
4. Successful treatment of both pulseless electrical activity (PEA) and asystole largely depends on determining the underlying cause. Epinephrine should be administered as soon as possible.
5. Following the return of spontaneous circulation (ROSC) from a cardiac arrest, patient management should be directed toward the postcardiac arrest syndrome. Post-resuscitation care often requires several interventions including, but not limited to, targeted temperature management, stabilization of respiratory and cardiovascular systems, interventions to achieve hemodynamic stability, control of blood glucose, and treatment of seizures and infectious complications.
6. Intravenous (IV) administration is the preferred route for medication delivery; intraosseous (IO) can be considered when IV access cannot be readily obtained or is not feasible.

BEYOND THE BOOK

Review the American Heart Association (AHA) algorithms for BLS and ACLS. Create a table that lists the medications used during a cardiac arrest and after the ROSC, when those medications might be used, and the intended purpose of each medication. All guidelines for cardiopulmonary resuscitation and emergency cardiac care can be found at https://tinyurl.com/zy2efpq.

INTRODUCTION

Cardiac arrest is defined as the cessation of cardiac mechanical activity as confirmed by the absence of signs of circulation (eg, a detectable pulse, unresponsiveness, and apnea).[1] While there is wide variation in the reported incidence of cardiac arrest, there are more than 350,000 people in the United States who are assessed by EMS for a suspected out-of-hospital cardiac arrest each year.[1] Survival to hospital discharge following out-of-hospital cardiac arrest is only 10.5% and survival with good neurologic function is even lower.[1] While there has been a minimal change over the last 40 years, the survival rate for out-of-hospital cardiac arrest improved slightly during the last reported observation period between 2005 and 2012.[2] This improvement was seen in both prehospital and in-hospital survival.

The incidence of in-hospital cardiac arrests is roughly 10 per 1,000 hospital admissions in the United States annually.[1] Similar to out-of-hospital arrests, some progress has also been made over the past decade with in-hospital cardiac arrests, where survival rates to hospital discharge have increased from 17% in 2000 to 27% in 2019.[1] Survival rates are substantially higher in victims with a shockable rhythm (ie, those who are treated with electrical defibrillation).

EPIDEMIOLOGY

Cardiac arrest can arise from either cardiac or noncardiac origins (eg, submersion, asphyxia, trauma, and overdose). In adult patients, cardiac arrest usually results from the development of an arrhythmia. Historically, ventricular fibrillation (VF) and pulseless ventricular tachycardia (PVT) have been the most common initial rhythms seen in out-of-hospital arrests, but these are now seen in less than one-quarter of cases.[1] In fact, data from the Cardiac Arrest Registry to Enhance Survival (CARES) project reported asystole to be the most common presenting rhythm (53%), which is similar to other registry data whereby nonshockable rhythms (ie, asystole, PEA) were more prevalent.[3] It is unclear why there has been a change in the types of arrhythmias that most commonly lead to cardiac arrest. Possible explanations include the increasing incidence of noncardiac causes of arrest that present with apnea leading to bradycardia and then pulseless electrical activity (PEA) or asystole. A second explanation might be the increasing role of implantable pacemakers and defibrillators.[4] Finally, beta-blockers and ACE inhibitors may shorten the duration of VF, and the expanded use of these drug classes for ischemic heart disease and heart failure may account for the increased occurrence of non-VF/PVT rhythms.[4] This change in the presenting rhythm types is concerning because survival rates to hospital discharge are substantially higher with shockable rhythms like VF and PVT (26%) compared to nonshockable rhythms like PEA (10%) and asystole (2%).[3]

A similar finding has been observed with in-hospital cardiac arrest. One study using the "Get With The Guidelines-Resuscitation" registry reported that 79% of patients had an initial rhythm of asystole or PEA and only 21% had VF or PVT.[5] Survival rates were 12.2% for asystole/PEA and 35% for VF/PVT.

In pediatric patients, cardiac arrest typically results from respiratory failure and asphyxiation. As such, the initial rhythm most often encountered in out-of-hospital arrest is PEA or asystole. Similar to the adult population, survival rates have increased over the past decade from 28% in 2000 to 52% in 2019 according to one registry.[1] Survival rate with out-of-hospital pediatric arrests is roughly 15% and is lower in infants when compared to children and

CLINICAL PRESENTATION Cardiopulmonary Arrest

General:

- Cardiac arrest is characterized by the cessation of cardiac mechanical activity. General signs and symptoms are consistent with a sudden cessation of circulation.

Symptoms (occurring prior to the event)

- Anxiety
- Crushing chest pain
- Nausea
- Vomiting
- Diaphoresis

Signs

- Apnea
- Hypotension
- Lack of a detectable pulse
- Cyanosis
- Cold, clammy extremities
- Loss of consciousness
- Syncope

adolescents.[1] Survival following in-hospital cardiac arrest is much higher (45%), and most survivors have a favorable neurologic outcome (89%).[6]

ETIOLOGY

The most common clinical finding in adult patients who suffer cardiac arrest is coronary artery disease, accounting for roughly 75% of sudden cardiac deaths.[7] Other causes of sudden cardiac death include cardiomyopathies, valvular heart disease, myocarditis, left ventricular hypertrophy, primary electrical heart disease, and noncardiac causes. Unfortunately, in many patients (up to 69%), cardiac arrest is the first clinical sign of coronary artery disease with no preceding signs or symptoms.[7]

In pediatric patients, cardiac arrest is often the terminal event of respiratory failure or progressive shock.[8] Out-of-hospital cardiac arrests frequently are associated with trauma, sudden infant death syndrome, drowning, poisoning, choking, severe asthma, and pneumonia. In-hospital cardiac arrests, on the other hand, are associated with sepsis, respiratory failure, drug toxicity, metabolic disorders, and arrhythmias.

PATHOPHYSIOLOGY

There are two distinct pathophysiologic conditions associated with cardiac arrest. The first is primary cardiac arrest whereby arterial blood is fully oxygenated at the time of arrest. As forward blood flow ceases, arterial blood oxygenation remains normal for about 10 minutes and subsequently declines due to the lack of ventilation.[9] Alternatively, respiratory failure can lead to severe hypoxemia, hypotension, and secondary cardiac arrest. It is important to identify the underlying pathophysiology as different treatment approaches are required.[9]

TREATMENT

Desired Outcome

The global goals of resuscitation are to preserve life, restore health, relieve suffering, limit disability, and respect the individual's decisions, rights, and privacy.[10] Providing high-quality CPR and quickly achieving the ROSC with effective perfusion and ventilation can minimize hypoxic damage to vital organs and achieve these goals. Survival to hospital discharge with good neurologic function should be the primary treatment outcome sought by clinicians. Survival to hospital discharge in a vegetative or comatose state cannot be classified as a success and can impose a tremendous economic burden on the healthcare system.

The presence of a healthcare advanced directive allows patients to communicate their wishes and preferences regarding medical care and may lead to a "do not attempt resuscitation" order. These orders should explicitly state the resuscitation interventions that are to be performed and should have been clearly communicated by the patient, their family, or a surrogate decision-maker.

General Approach to Treatment

Cardiopulmonary Resuscitation

Resuscitation techniques have been studied for many years. In 1960, Kouwenhoven described positive outcomes in 14 of 20 patients with in-hospital cardiac arrest who were given closed chest compressions at a rate of 60 per minute.[11] Following the publication of this landmark article, chest compressions integrated with expired air ventilation (ie, mouth-to-mouth) became the fundamentals of basic life support known as the "ABC's."[11]

Cardiopulmonary resuscitation employs chest compressions to restore threshold blood flows, particularly to the heart and brain. There are two proposed explanations to describe how chest compression improves blood flow during CPR.[11] The original explanation is known as the cardiac pump theory whereby compression of the heart between the sternum and vertebrae creates forward flow. However, echocardiography during chest compressions has revealed that the left ventricular size does not always change and the mitral valve may not close.[11] The second explanation is the thoracic pump theory whereby intrathoracic pressure changes during chest compressions promote blood flow while the heart merely acts as a passive conduit. It is likely that both cardiac compression and intrathoracic pressure changes contribute.

Since 1966, the AHA has published guidelines for the treatment of cardiac arrest in 5-year increments. In 2015, this process transitioned to an online format that is continuously updated in an attempt to expedite the most current evidence-based practices to the bedside. The most recent document, the 2020 guidelines, reflects alignment with the International Liaison Committee on Resuscitation and reviews scientific questions considered of greatest significance and new evidence.[12]

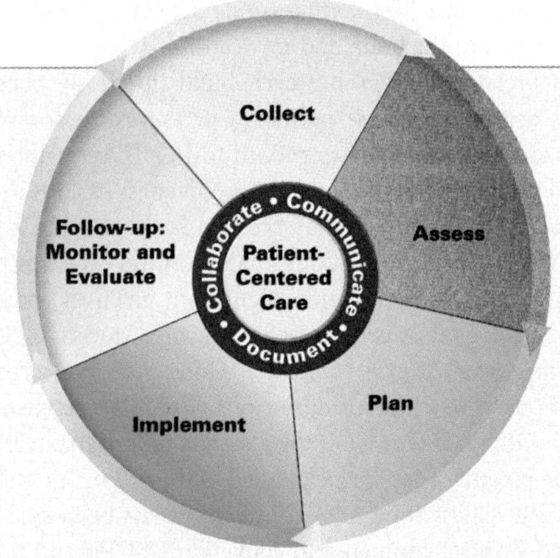

Patient Care Process for Cardiac Arrest

The image shows the five fundamental steps included in The Pharmacist's Care Process endorsed by the Joint Commission for Pharmacy Practitioners (2014). The tagline of this process reads collaborate, communicate, and document. The five fundamental steps listed here are collect, assess, plan, implement, and follow-up: monitor and evaluate. All these steps are listed in a circular block diagram.

Collect*

- Patient characteristics (eg, sex, age)
- Patient medical history (if available)
- Current and past medications that could have contributed to the arrest or serve as a clue to the underlying medical history
- Objective data
  - o Presence of a pulse
  - o Cardiac rhythm

Assess*

- Is the patient responsive?
- Is there a pulse present?
- Are the electrocardiogram (ECG) leads correctly placed on the patient?
- Is the rhythm shockable?

Plan*

- Activate emergency medical services (EMS) and obtain an automated external defibrillator (AED) if one is nearby (for out-of-hospital arrest) (Fig. 41-2)
- Call for "code blue" and obtain crash cart (for in-hospital arrest)
- Immediately begin chest compressions and follow basic life support (BLS) algorithm
- Administer electrical therapy (ie, defibrillation) if indicated
- Drug therapy per advanced cardiac life support (ACLS) algorithm if indicated (Table 41-1)
- Monitor for the return of spontaneous circulation (ROSC), cardiac rhythm, and pulse

Implement*

- Perform high-quality chest compressions with minimal interruptions
- Administer defibrillations and drug therapy as indicated by cardiac rhythm

Follow-up: Monitor and Evaluate*

- Monitor end-tidal CO_2 as an indicator of cardiopulmonary resuscitation (CPR) quality
- Implement postresuscitative care plan
- ECG and percutaneous coronary intervention (PCI) when an acute coronary syndrome is suspected
- Review patient history for identification of other contributors or underlying cause of the arrest
- Diligent monitoring of blood pressure, oxygen saturation, temperature, urine output, and glucose
- Evaluate and monitor for seizure

Collaborate with patient, caregivers, and other healthcare professionals.

1 High-quality CPR continues to be emphasized in the latest guidelines published by the AHA. Clinicians must focus on proper technique, including adequate rate and depth of compressions, allowing full chest recoil after each compression, avoiding excessive ventilation, and minimizing interruptions. There is an association between survival to hospital discharge and chest compression rate (optimally between 100 and 120 beats/minute), chest compression depth (optimally 40-54 mm), and chest compression fraction (optimally the proportion of resuscitation time without spontaneous circulation when chest compressions are administered should be ≥60%).[13] Unfortunately, the provision of CPR is frequently sub-optimal, particularly when rescuers become fatigued.[14] Real-time audiovisual feedback mechanisms during CPR have been encouraged. These can include voice prompts (eg, "push harder"), visual displays (for compression quality), audio prompts (eg, metronome to guide CPR rate) or an analog "clicker" feedback device that emits a noise and sensation when sufficient pressure is applied during CPR. One study reported a 25% absolute increase in survival to hospital discharge with the use of an analog "clicker" device.[15]

The 2020 guidelines continue to emphasize the "chain of survival" to highlight the treatment approach and illustrate the importance of a timely response. The updated guidelines include two separate chains (one for out-of-hospital cardiac arrest and another for in-hospital cardiac arrest), both having six links.[16] The two chains reflect the differences in the steps needed to respond to a cardiac arrest in the in-patient and out-patient settings. The links in each chain of survival are as follows:

Out-of-hospital

1. Activation of emergency response
2. High-quality CPR
3. Defibrillation
4. Advanced resuscitation
5. Postcardiac arrest care
6. Recovery

In-hospital

1. Early recognition and prevention
2. Activation of emergency response
3. High-quality CPR
4. Defibrillation
5. Postcardiac arrest care
6. Recovery

Activation of emergency response systems and early recognition and prevention are the first links in the chain of survival for out-of-hospital and in-hospital cardiac arrests, respectively. For out-of-hospital cardiac arrests, activation of emergency response systems allows for dispatcher-assisted CPR whereby instructions are delivered to a community bystander over the telephone. Further, mobile phone technology is increasingly being used to summon nearby bystanders who might assist with out-of-hospital events. For in-hospital cardiac arrests, clinical deterioration typically precedes a cardiac arrest; therefore, early warning systems based on vital sign abnormalities, advanced scoring systems, or staff concerns are advised.[17] High-quality CPR and rapid defibrillation for shockable rhythms are the foundation for good resuscitation outcomes after cardiac arrest.[18] Advanced resuscitation interventions, which include pharmacotherapy, advanced airways, and extracorporeal CPR, may improve outcomes in special situations. Postcardiac arrest care consists of important therapies such as targeted temperature management, mechanical ventilation, and other crucial critical care support modalities including pharmacotherapy. Recovery is the newest link added to both chains of survival. Recognizing that recovering from cardiac arrest continues long after hospital discharge, measures to support physical, cognitive, emotional well-being, and psychosocial needs are recommended.[16]

Sequence of Resuscitation

Basic Life Support 2 The mnemonic for the CPR sequence is "CAB" which stands for circulation, airway, and breathing. Historically, BLS and ACLS providers have been taught the mnemonic, "ABC." The change to CAB was made to stress the importance of maintaining blood flow to the heart and brain and to avoid delays or interruptions to chest compressions.

When first encountering a cardiac arrest victim, the initial action is to determine if the patient is responsive. If there is no response, the rescuer should immediately activate the EMS team, obtain (or call for) an AED, and then immediately start CPR with chest compressions. A cardiac arrest victim will be unresponsive, and it can be difficult for rescuers to determine if the victim is breathing normally. Thus, "look, listen, and feel" for respirations is no longer recommended as part of the initial assessment.[16] Similarly, lay rescuers may have difficulty in detecting a pulse leading to delays in chest compressions; thus, a pulse check is not recommended. In situations where the rescuer is unsure if the victim has suffered a cardiac arrest (eg, when agonal breathing is present), CPR should be promptly initiated. The risk of chest compressions in a patient who is not in cardiac arrest is low compared to the high potential for harm should CPR be withheld in a pulseless victim.[16] Healthcare providers could assess for a pulse but take no more than 10 seconds to do so. If one is not detected within this short time frame, then chest compressions should be immediately initiated.[16]

The prompt provision of chest compressions is of paramount importance, and rescuers should attempt them regardless of rescuer experience or skill. High-quality chest compressions should be delivered at a rate of 100 to 120 compressions per minute, with adequate depth (at least 2 in. [~50 mm] in an adult), while allowing full chest recoil and minimizing any interruptions.

While the provision of high-quality chest compressions is essential, the role of ventilation (ie, rescue breaths) in the initial management of cardiac arrest is less clear. Chest compressions deliver a small but critical amount of oxygen to the brain and myocardium. Cerebral and coronary perfusion pressure (CPPs), however, build up slowly once chest compressions are begun. These perfusion pressures are lost if chest compressions are stopped to deliver mouth-to-mouth ventilation resulting in reduced blood flow and decreased effectiveness of CPR. In fact, the time it takes to deliver two rescue breaths has been reported to range between 10 seconds and 16 seconds based on the experience of the rescuer.[19] These interruptions can be significant given the proportion of time chest compressions are being performed during CPR is associated with improvements in survival.[20] Along with concerns related to interruptions with chest compressions, some lay rescuers may be reluctant to initiate CPR at all, if they are uncomfortable with administering rescue breaths. These principles led to the origin of chest compression-only CPR. Chest compression-only CPR has been associated with increased survival compared to conventional CPR and no bystander CPR.[21] However, if ventilations are withheld, arterial oxygen content will decrease as CPR duration increases.

Based on a recent systematic review, CPR recommendations have been updated.[16,22] Chest compression-only CPR is appropriate for lay rescuers who are untrained or unwilling to provide respirations. Lay rescuers who are trained, able, and willing to give rescue breaths should do so using a compression to breath ratio of 30:2. For EMS-delivered CPR, providers should perform CPR in cycles of 30 compressions and 2 breaths or alternatively 1 breath every 6 seconds for asynchronous ventilation during continuous chest compressions.

In all cases, CPR should continue until an AED arrives. The AED leads should be immediately placed on the victim so that the device can determine if the rhythm is shockable. If so, then one shock should be delivered, and CPR immediately resumed for 2 minutes or until prompted by the AED for another rhythm check. If the rhythm is not shockable, CPR should resume immediately for 2 minutes or until prompted by the AED. This cycle should be continued until advanced life support providers take over or the victim starts to move (Fig. 41-1). In settings where more than one rescuer is present, rotating the provider performing chest compressions should occur every 2 minutes to minimize rescuer fatigue, which can lead to poor quality chest compressions.

Defibrillation is crucial for survival in cardiac arrests caused by VF or PVT, especially when administered as soon as possible after the onset of the arrest. When the duration of VF/PVT is more prolonged (eg, an unwitnessed or an unmonitored arrest due to the arrival of an AED), the efficacy of defibrillation is compromised due to depletion of myocardial oxygen reserves and the presence of global tissue ischemia. A short period of CPR to replenish blood flow (via chest compressions) and "flush out" deleterious metabolic factors may be beneficial. Intentional, prolonged periods of chest compressions (90-180 seconds) before defibrillation have not been shown to improve outcomes.[22] Therefore, in unmonitored cardiac arrests, a brief period of CPR can be administered while the defibrillator is being obtained and readied for use.

CPR can be physically demanding, and rescuer fatigue can lead to poor quality chest compressions. As a result, mechanical devices have been developed with the aim of providing consistent high-quality chest compressions that can be sustained throughout the entire arrest period. Animal studies have shown that cerebral blood flow is greater with these devices compared to manual compression. Studies in humans, however, have not demonstrated improved survival or survival with good neurological function.[16] Lack of survival benefit may be due to time delays associated with their deployment. While the routine use of mechanical CPR devices is not recommended, their use may be considered in specific settings where the delivery of high-quality manual compressions may be challenging such as ambulance or helicopter transfers.

Advanced Cardiac Life Support Once EMS- or other ACLS-certified providers arrive, additional therapy may be given. Either a

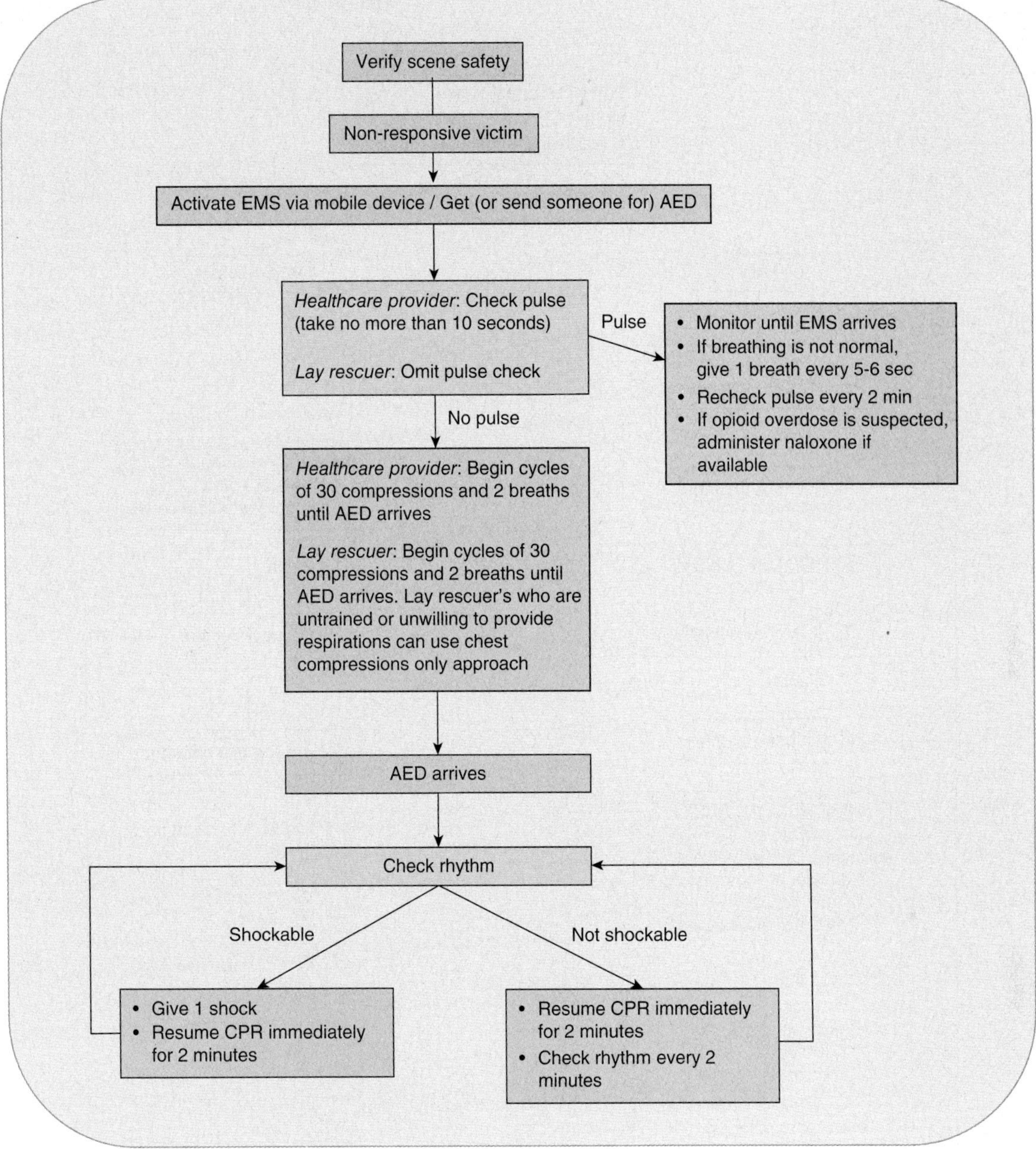

FIGURE 41-1 Treatment algorithm for adult cardiac arrest: Basic life support (BLS).

bag-mask device or an advanced airway such as a supraglottic device or an endotracheal tube may be utilized to provide ventilation. If an advanced airway is used, supraglottic airways are preferred in settings with low tracheal intubation success rates or when minimal training opportunities exist. Once an airway is established, one provider can deliver 1 breath every 6 seconds while continuous chest compressions are being performed by a second provider.

Monitoring of CPR quality may be performed using end-tidal carbon dioxide ($ETCO_2$) monitoring or arterial blood pressure assessment when feasible. $ETCO_2$ is the concentration of carbon dioxide in exhaled air at the end of expiration. During cardiac arrest, the level of $ETCO_2$ decreases because there is no flow through the pulmonary circulation. Thus, a persistently low $ETCO_2$ (ie, <10 mm Hg [1.3 kPa]) during CPR in intubated patients makes ROSC unlikely.[16] One large study using the "Get with the Guidelines-Resuscitation" registry reported a higher rate of ROSC when physiologic monitoring with either $ETCO_2$ or arterial blood pressure was performed.[23] Physiologic monitoring with $ETCO_2$ or arterial blood pressure is, therefore, suggested.

If not already placed, an AED should be attached and access for administration of parenteral medications should be obtained. Cardiac arrest victims who are in VF or PVT should be administered one shock with the immediate resumption of chest compressions.[16] If there is still a shockable rhythm, then an additional shock should be delivered every 2 minutes. After two cycles, epinephrine is indicated. Chest compressions continue while medications are being prepared and administered. This cycle is repeated until either a pulse is obtained with effective circulation, the rhythm changes or the patient expires. If the cardiac rhythm is not deemed to be shockable, then the patient is likely to be in either asystole or PEA. In this circumstance, epinephrine should be administered as soon as possible and the rescuer must consider reversible causes (Fig. 41-2).

Extracorporeal CPR is the use of cardiopulmonary bypass during the resuscitation of a cardiac arrest victim. It entails the rapid deployment of veno-arterial extracorporeal membrane oxygenation (ECMO) to provide circulatory support when conventional CPR is unsuccessful. The goal is to provide end-organ support while reversible conditions are addressed. ECMO is a highly specialized therapy

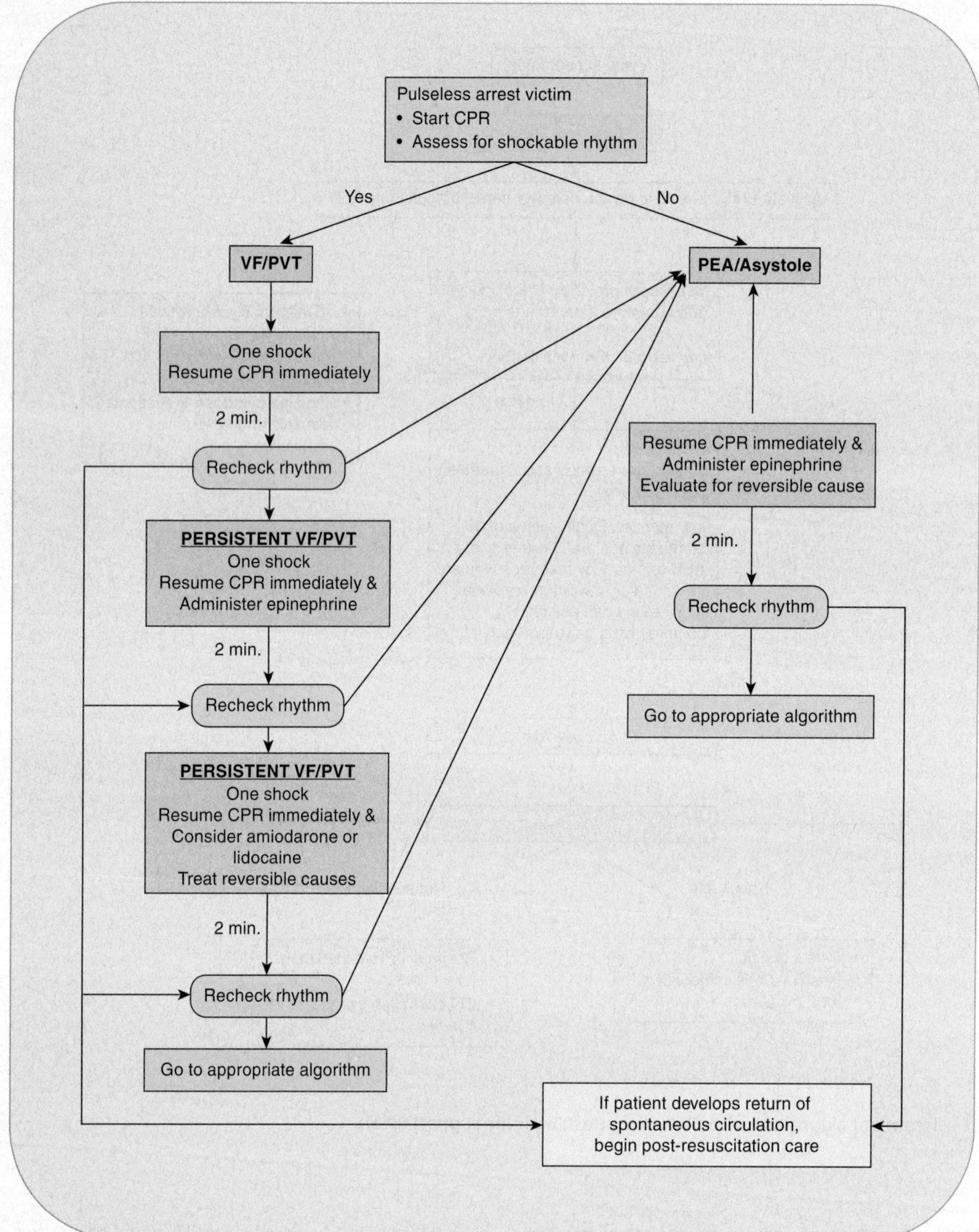

FIGURE 41-2 Treatment algorithm for adult cardiac arrest: Advanced cardiac life support (ACLS).

that requires a dedicated team of specialized experts. While there is insufficient evidence to support the routine use of extracorporeal CPR, it may be considered as rescue therapy if there is a reversible cause of the arrest.

Ventricular Fibrillation/Pulseless Ventricular Tachycardia

Nonpharmacologic Therapy

Ventricular fibrillation and PVT are "shockable rhythms." Thus, defibrillation combined with cardiopulmonary resuscitation are crucial components in the care of cardiac arrest victims. CPR provides critical blood flow to the heart and brain, prolongs the time VF/PVT is present (prior to the deterioration to asystole), and increases the likelihood that a shock will terminate VF/PVT and result in a rhythm compatible with life. The brain can normally survive for only 3 to 5 minutes before damage occurs; thus, delays in the provision of CPR can worsen outcomes. With immediate CPR, the rate of survival decreases by 3% to 4% per minute between the onset of the arrest and defibrillation.[24] Without bystander CPR, survival rates decrease by 7% to 10% per minute.[24] In effect, CPR can increase the likelihood of survival threefold from arrest to survival. Basic CPR alone is not likely to terminate VF/PVT; electrical defibrillation is often necessary to restore a cardiac rhythm.

Pre-hospital systems of care remain an area of emphasis for communities to improve outcomes following a cardiac arrest.[18,25]

In one large study, the rate of bystander CPR was only 34% while only 2.3% of cardiac arrests utilized an AED.[26] Community programs are necessary to provide education and raise awareness of the importance of early CPR. Examples of these programs include dispatcher-assisted CPR, whereby instructions are provided via mobile telephone. Mobile phone technology can also be used to alert a bystander that an arrest has occurred within their geographic vicinity. Education programs on the use of public access defibrillators can promote the early use of AEDs by lay responders. One systematic review reported survival rates of 53% with the early use of defibrillation using an AED administered by lay responders.[27] Finally, specialized cardiac arrest centers with experienced clinicians who are well versed in the evidence-based management of post-resuscitation care could be important. While data reporting improvements in survival to hospital discharge are mixed, these centers often have the capability to perform ECMO and other advanced forms of organ support.

Pharmacologic Therapy

Vasopressors Vasopressors continue to be the first pharmacologic agents administered in the setting of cardiac arrest despite limited evidence demonstrating improvements in neurologic function postarrest. Nevertheless, vasopressors have been associated with an increased rate of ROSC and play a major role in the pharmacotherapy of cardiac arrest.

3 The primary goal of vasopressor therapy is to augment low coronary and cerebral perfusion pressures encountered during CPR. Chest compressions can improve blood flow to the heart and the brain but only to about 25% of normal. Even with optimally performed chest compressions, CPPs are only 10 to 15 mm Hg, and systolic arterial pressure is rarely above 80 mm Hg.[28] Clinical data have indicated that ROSC is unlikely when the CPP is less than 15 mm Hg.[29,30] Vasopressors, therefore, work to increase these pressures through their vasoconstrictive properties.

Epinephrine continues to be the drug of first choice for the treatment of VF, PVT, asystole, and PEA. Epinephrine is an alpha- and beta-receptor agonist causing vasoconstriction as well as increasing the rate and forcefulness of heart contractions.

In a large randomized controlled trial of patients with out-of-hospital cardiac arrest (18% with VF or PVT), epinephrine was compared to saline placebo.[31] Epinephrine use was associated with a significant improvement in survival at 30-days, and the benefit was more pronounced in patients with a nonshockable initial rhythm. Favorable neurologic outcome (at discharge), however, was no different in the epinephrine group. In fact, there were more patients with severe neurologic impairment with epinephrine. A second randomized, controlled trial compared epinephrine with placebo in patients with cardiac arrest (fewer than 50% had VT or PVT as the initial rhythm).[32] ROSC and survival to hospital admission were significantly higher with epinephrine but there was no difference in survival to hospital discharge. Similar to the previous trial, the effect of epinephrine was greater in those with non-shockable rhythms. A subsequent meta-analysis found that epinephrine was associated with significant improvements in ROSC, survival to hospital discharge, and survival at 30 days.[33] There was no difference, however, in neurological outcome at discharge. When stratified by initial rhythm, these differences were greater in the cohort of patients with nonshockable rhythms. Most notably, survival at 30-days was significant with nonshockable rhythms but not with VF/PVT.

Several large observational studies have evaluated the impact of epinephrine on survival. One large registry study failed to demonstrate a survival benefit with prehospital administration of epinephrine.[34] Despite a significant improvement in ROSC with epinephrine, 1-month survival and survival with good neurologic function were both lower in patients who received epinephrine. A second study evaluated outcomes in patients with witnessed out-of-hospital cardiac arrest.[35] Epinephrine was associated with improvements in survival at 1 month or discharge in patients with VF/PVT but there was no difference in neurologically intact survival.

Timing of epinephrine administration could be an important confounder and contribute to the heterogeneity observed with survival data. In a posthoc analysis of data from the largest randomized controlled trial conducted to date, the odds of ROSC decreased in both epinephrine and placebo groups over time, but at a greater rate with placebo.[36] A second study revealed survival and favorable functional status decreased with delayed administration.[37] Specifically, ROSC was highest in the cohort who received epinephrine within 5 minutes after the provision of advanced life support. Similarly, other studies have reported the association with delays in epinephrine administration and a reduction in the odds of survival and the odds of hospital discharge with good neurologic function are reduced.[38-42]

Despite notable improvements in survival, epinephrine does not improve survival with good neurologic function, which may be related to its mechanism of action. Epinephrine causes alpha-mediated vasoconstriction which increases coronary perfusion but may also decrease perfusion to other vital organs. Animal research has linked epinephrine to a decrease in cerebral microvascular blood flow and an increase in brain tissue ischemia during and after CPR.[43] One study in humans measured cerebral oxygenation in patients who experienced an in-hospital cardiac arrest, before-and-after epinephrine administration.[44] A small increase in cerebral oxygenation (1.4%) was noted but the clinical importance of this small change is questionable. Alternatively, the negligible effect on neurologic function could be due to the brain being more sensitive to ischemia compared to other organs and less able to recover once ROSC is achieved.

Epinephrine also stimulates beta-receptors, which can increase myocardial oxygen demand, impair lactate clearance, and contribute to post-resuscitation myocardial dysfunction.[45] Studies have compared epinephrine with other adrenergic agonists with less beta-activity (eg, pure alpha-1 agonists such as phenylephrine and methoxamine or more potent alpha-agonists like norepinephrine).[46] When compared to pure alpha-1 agonists, there is no advantage in terms of long-term survival. One potential reason could be the potent alpha-2 effects of epinephrine and the fact that these receptors lie extrajunctionally in the intima of the blood vessels making them more accessible to circulating catecholamines. Furthermore, during ischemia, the number of postsynaptic alpha-1-receptors decreases which suggests a greater role for alpha-2 agonists during CPR. Epinephrine has also been compared with norepinephrine, a potent alpha-agonist (both alpha-1 and alpha-2) with some beta-1 effects. In the only large-scale randomized, double-blind, prospective trial comparing epinephrine and norepinephrine use in patients with an out-of-hospital cardiac arrest, there were no significant differences in ROSC, hospital admission, or discharge.[47] A second, smaller study demonstrated higher resuscitation rates with norepinephrine compared to epinephrine (64% vs 32%) but no significant difference in survival to hospital discharge.[48]

The recommended dose for epinephrine is 1 mg administered by intravenous (IV) or intraosseous (IO) injection every 3 to 5 minutes[16] (Table 41-1). The recommended dose for epinephrine was derived from animal studies (0.1 mg/kg in a 10 kg dog) and equates to approximately 0.015 mg/kg for a 70 kg human.[49] Animal studies have demonstrated a positive dose-response relationship with epinephrine, suggesting that higher doses might improve hemodynamics and resuscitation success.[46] However, human studies have reported increased morbidity with high-dose epinephrine. The hemodynamic findings are consistent with catecholamine toxicity, including decreased cardiac indices, left ventricular dysfunction, and decreased oxygen delivery. This discrepancy between animal and human studies could be related to most victims of cardiac arrest having coronary artery disease, which is not encountered in an animal model. Additionally, atherosclerotic plaques in humans can aggravate the balance between myocardial oxygen supply and demand,

TABLE 41-1 Evidence-Based Recommendations

Recommendations	Recommendation Grades[a]
Epinephrine	
Epinephrine is recommended for patients in cardiac arrest	Class I, LOE B-R
Standard dose epinephrine (1 mg IV/IO every 3-5 minutes) may be reasonable for patients with cardiac arrest	Class IIa, LOE B-R
In patients with cardiac arrest with a shockable rhythm, it may be reasonable to administer epinephrine after initial defibrillation attempts have failed	Class IIb, LOE C-LD
In patients with cardiac arrest with a nonshockable rhythm, it may be reasonable to administer epinephrine as soon as feasible after the onset of cardiac arrest	Class IIa, LOE C-LD
High-dose epinephrine is not recommended for routine use in cardiac arrest	Class 3, LOE B-R
Vasopressin	
Vasopressin alone or in combination with epinephrine may be considered but offers no advantage as a substitute for standard dose epinephrine	Class IIb, LOE C-LD
Amiodarone	
Amiodarone may be considered in patients with VF/PVT unresponsive to defibrillation	Class IIb, LOE B-R
Lidocaine	
Lidocaine may be considered in patients with VF/PVT unresponsive to defibrillation	Class IIb, LOE B-R
Magnesium	
Magnesium is not routinely recommended for VF/PVT	Class III: No benefit, LOE B-R
Thrombolysis	
Thrombolysis may be considered when cardiac arrest is suspected to be caused by pulmonary embolism	Class IIb, LOE C-LD
Sodium bicarbonate	
Routine use of sodium bicarbonate is not recommended	Class III: No benefit, LOE B-R
Corticosteroids	
For out-of-hospital cardiac arrest, use of corticosteroids during CPR is of uncertain benefit	Class IIb, LOE C-LD

CPR, cardiopulmonary resuscitation; IV, intravenous; IO, intraosseous; VF, ventricular fibrillation; PVT, pulseless ventricular tachycardia; LOE, level of evidence.

[a]Key for evidence-based classifications:
Class of recommendations:
- Class I (Strong). Benefit >>>Risk
- Class IIa (Moderate). Benefit >> Risk
- Class IIb (Weak). Benefit ≥ Risk
- Class III: No Benefit (Moderate). Benefit = Risk
- Class III: Harm (Strong). Risk > Benefit

Levels of Evidence (LOE):
- Level A: High-quality evidence from more than one RCT, meta-analyses of high-quality RCTs, one or more RCT corroborated by high-quality registry studies.
- Level B-R (Randomized): Moderate-quality evidence from one or more RCTs, meta-analyses of moderate-quality RCTs.
- Level B-NR (Nonrandomized): Moderate-quality evidence from one or more well-designed nonrandomized studies, observational studies, or registry studies, meta-analyses of such studies.
- Level C-LD (Limited data): Randomized or nonrandomized observational or registry studies with limitations of design or execution, meta-analyses of such studies, physiological or mechanistic studies in human subjects.
- Level C-EO (Expert opinion): Consensus of expert opinion based on clinical experience.

Data from Reference 16.

and the interval from arrest to treatment is longer in human studies than that encountered in an animal model. Thus, high-dose epinephrine is not recommended for routine use in cardiac arrest.

Vasopressin Vasopressin, also known as antidiuretic hormone, is a potent, nonadrenergic vasoconstrictor that increases blood pressure and systemic vascular resistance. Although it acts on various receptors throughout the body, its vasoconstrictive properties are due primarily to its effects on the V_1 receptor. Measurement of vasopressin levels in patients undergoing CPR has shown a high correlation between the levels of endogenous vasopressin released and the potential for ROSC.[50] In one study, plasma vasopressin concentrations were approximately three times as high in survivors compared with nonsurvivors, suggesting that vasopressin is released as an adjunct to epinephrine in life-threatening events such as cardiac arrest.[51]

Vasopressin is proposed to have several advantages over epinephrine. First, the metabolic acidosis that frequently accompanies cardiac arrest can blunt the vasoconstrictive effect of adrenergic agents such as epinephrine. This effect does not occur with vasopressin. Second, the stimulation of beta-receptors caused by epinephrine can increase myocardial oxygen demand and complicate the post-resuscitation phase of CPR. This is not seen with vasopressin use because it does not act on beta-receptors. Vasopressin also may have a beneficial effect on renal blood flow by stimulating V_2 receptors in the kidney, causing vasodilation and increased water reabsorption. With regard to splanchnic blood flow (ie, blood flow to the gastrointestinal tract), however, vasopressin has a detrimental effect when compared to epinephrine.[50] Despite these theoretical advantages with vasopressin, clinical outcomes are not superior to that achieved with epinephrine alone.[52] Furthermore, vasopressin in combination with epinephrine offers no advantage over epinephrine alone.

A multidrug regimen that included vasopressin plus corticosteroid therapy has been evaluated in the setting of in-hospital cardiac arrest.[53-55] The rationale is based on the hemodynamic effects of steroids alone with their potential to impact the intensity of the post-resuscitation systemic inflammatory response and organ dysfunction. A recent meta-analysis observed a favorable effect on ROSC and survival to hospital discharge with good neurologic function using this multidrug regimen.[56] The largest randomized controlled trial to evaluate this multidrug approach combined vasopressin (20 units administered after each dose of epinephrine, maximum cumulative dose of 80 units) plus a single dose of methylprednisolone 40 mg.[55] A significant difference in ROSC was detected in the study group but no difference in 30-day survival or survival with favorable neurologic function was detected. Possible reasons for these disparate results could include the lack of corticosteroid use in the post-resuscitation phase and the time to trial drug administration, which was longer in this trial.

In summary, vasopressin may be considered in cardiac arrest but offers no benefit when used as a substitute for or in combination with epinephrine compared to the standard dose of epinephrine alone.[16] The combination of methylprednisolone, vasopressin, and epinephrine will require further study before this approach could be routinely recommended.

Antiarrhythmics Amiodarone or lidocaine are suggested in adults with VF/PVT refractory to defibrillation and epinephrine therapy. The purpose of antiarrhythmic drug therapy following unsuccessful defibrillation and vasopressor administration is to prevent the development or recurrence of VF and PVT. However, clinical evidence demonstrating improved survival to hospital discharge is lacking.[57,58]

A large, randomized, double-blind trial in patients with out-of-hospital cardiac arrest secondary to VF or PVT reported a higher incidence of survival to hospital admission but no difference in survival to hospital discharge.[59] This was the first trial to demonstrate the benefit of any antiarrhythmic agent over placebo in patients with out-of-hospital cardiac arrest. A subsequent trial compared amiodarone with lidocaine in patients with out-of-hospital cardiac arrest due to VF.[60] In this trial, amiodarone was associated with improved survival to hospital admission compared with lidocaine but there was no difference in survival to hospital discharge. A most recent trial compared amiodarone and lidocaine to placebo in patients with an out-of-hospital arrest with shock-resistant VF/PVT.[61] Both agents were associated with an increase in survival to hospital admission compared to placebo. However, no significant difference in survival to hospital discharge was observed for amiodarone versus placebo, lidocaine versus placebo, or amiodarone versus lidocaine. A subgroup analysis noted higher rates of survival to hospital discharge with both agents (versus placebo) in patients with bystander-witnessed cardiac arrest.

Magnesium Severe hypomagnesemia has been associated with VF/PVT, but the routine administration of magnesium during a cardiac arrest has not demonstrated any benefit in clinical outcomes. Two observation trials noted an improvement in ROSC in patients with arrests associated with torsades de pointes.[16] Therefore, magnesium should only be administered in the setting of torsades de pointes.

Thrombolytics Since most cardiac arrests are related to either myocardial infarction or pulmonary embolism (PE), several investigators have evaluated the role of thrombolytics during CPR. Initial studies evaluating the use of thrombolytics in cardiac arrest yielded mixed results. The most rigorous study performed to date randomized patients with out-of-hospital cardiac arrest to receive either tenecteplase or placebo.[62] Both ROSC and survival to hospital discharge were similar between groups, criteria for futility were met, and the trial was terminated. The incidence of intracranial hemorrhage was significantly greater with tenecteplase versus placebo (2.7% vs 0.4%). Given these results, fibrinolytic therapy should not be used routinely in cardiac arrest. When PE is suspected, its use may be warranted.[16]

Pulseless Electrical Activity and Asystole

Nonpharmacologic Therapy

4 Pulseless electrical activity is defined as the absence of a detectable pulse and the presence of some type of electrical activity other than VF or PVT. Patients with PEA have mechanical cardiac contractions but they are too weak to produce a palpable pulse or blood pressure. Although PEA is classified as a "rhythm of survival," the likelihood of successful resuscitation is much lower than seen with VF/PVT.[1] PEA is often caused by a treatable underlying cause, and the resuscitation team must quickly identify and correct it if the resuscitation is to be successful (Table 41-2). Asystole occurs when there is a lack of electrical activity in the heart and appears as a flat line on the ECG. Asystole is often not amenable to treatment. Like

TABLE 41-2 Underlying Causes of Pulseless Electrical Activity and Asystole

Condition	Clues	Treatment
Hypovolemia	History, flat neck veins	Intravenous fluids
Hypoxia	Cyanosis, blood gases, airway problems	Ventilation, oxygen
Hydrogen ion (acidosis)	History of bicarbonate-responsive preexisting acidosis	Sodium bicarbonate, hyperventilation
Hyper (Hypo) kalemia	History of renal failure, diabetes, recent dialysis, dialysis fistulas, medications	Calcium chloride, insulin, glucose, sodium bicarbonate, sodium polystyrene sulfonate, dialysis
Hypothermia	History of exposure to cold, central body temperature	Rewarming, oxygen, intravenous fluids
Hypoglycemia	History of diabetes	Glucose infusion
Toxin (Drug overdose)	Bradycardia, history of ingestion, empty bottles at the scene, pupils, neurologic exam	Drug screens, intubation, lavage, activated charcoal
Tamponade (Cardiac)	History (trauma, renal failure, thoracic malignancy), no pulse with CPR, vein distention, impending tamponade-tachycardia, hypotension, low pulse pressure changing to sudden bradycardia as terminal event	Pericardiocentesis
Tension pneumothorax	History (asthma, ventilator, chronic obstructive pulmonary disease, trauma), no pulse with CPR, neck vein distention, tracheal deviation	Needle decompression
Thrombosis, coronary	History, ECG, enzymes	PCI, thrombolytics, oxygen, nitroglycerin, heparin, aspirin, morphine
Thrombosis, pulmonary	History, no pulse with CPR, distended neck veins	Pulmonary arteriogram, surgical embolectomy, thrombolytics
Trauma	History, examination	Volume infusion, intracranial pressure monitoring, bleeding control, surgical intervention

Data from Reference 16.

PEA, successful treatment of asystole depends almost entirely on diagnosing the underlying cause.

The algorithm for treating PEA and asystole is the same. Both conditions require CPR, airway control, and IV access. Asystole should be reconfirmed by checking a second lead on the cardiac monitor. Defibrillation should be avoided because the parasympathetic discharge that occurs with defibrillation may reduce the chance of ROSC and worsen the chance of survival. High-quality CPR without interruption remains an emphasis along with identifying a correctable cause.

Pharmacologic Therapy

The primary pharmacologic agent used in the treatment of asystole or PEA is epinephrine. In a systematic review of randomized controlled trials evaluating epinephrine in out-of-hospital cardiac arrest due to nonshockable rhythms, significant improvements were observed in ROSC, survival to hospital admission, and 3-month survival.[33] Survival with good neurologic function at 3-months improved, albeit not statically significant. Nevertheless, the global benefits of epinephrine were most apparent in patients with nonshockable versus shockable rhythms.

Similar to shockable rhythms, the time to epinephrine administration is an important confounder related to its efficacy. One large study of patients with out-of-hospital cardiac arrest from nonshockable rhythms reported a 4% decrease in the odds of survival to hospital discharge with each minute delay in epinephrine administration.[63] Furthermore, the odds of surviving with good neurologic function decreased by 6% with each minute delay. Other observational studies have yielded similar results. In a large North American registry trial, survival to hospital discharge was highest when epinephrine was administered within 5 minutes after EMS arrival and decreased with each 5-minute period thereafter.[37] A study from a Japanese database revealed worse neurological outcomes when the time to epinephrine administration exceeded 10 minutes.[64] Early epinephrine administration is also important after in-hospital cardiac arrests with nonshockable rhythms. In one large study using the Get with the Guidelines-Resuscitation database, a step-wise decrease in survival was observed with each incremental delay in epinephrine administration.[39] Thus, epinephrine should be administered as soon as possible.

Acid/Base Management

Acidosis seen during cardiac arrest results from decreased blood flow and inadequate ventilation. Chest compressions generate only approximately 25% of normal cardiac output, leading to inadequate organ perfusion, tissue hypoxia, and metabolic acidosis. In addition, the lack of ventilation causes retention of carbon dioxide, leading to respiratory acidosis. Acidosis produces not only reduced myocardial contractility but also lowers the fibrillation threshold. Despite the deleterious effects of acidosis on normal physiology, sodium bicarbonate has not been shown to improve ROSC or survival to hospital discharge.[65] One large observational study reported sodium bicarbonate use was associated with a lower probability of both ROSC and a favorable neurologic outcome.[66] In addition, this negative association persisted in the subgroup of patients having arrests of long duration (defined as >22.6 minutes of resuscitation) conflicting with some beliefs that sodium bicarbonate may be useful in this setting.

Sodium bicarbonate may have detrimental effects because of the following reaction: $[HCO_3^-] + [H^+] \leftrightarrow [H_2O] + [CO_2]$.[67] When sodium bicarbonate is added to an acidic environment, the reaction will shift to the right, thereby increasing tissue and venous hypercarbia. The carbon dioxide generated by this reaction will diffuse into the cell and decrease intracellular pH. The accumulation of intracellular carbon dioxide, specifically within the myocardium, is inversely correlated with CPP produced by CPR. Intracellular acidosis also will decrease myocardial contractility, further complicating the low-flow state associated with CPR. Furthermore, treatment with sodium bicarbonate often overcorrects extracellular pH because sodium bicarbonate has a greater effect when the pH is closer to normal. The induced alkalosis causes an increase in the affinity of oxygen to hemoglobin ("left shift"), thus interfering with oxygen release into the tissues.

Sodium bicarbonate is not recommended for routine use in patients with cardiac arrest.[16] It can be considered in special circumstances such as patients with hyperkalemia, tricyclic antidepressant overdose, or salicylate toxicity.

Postresuscitative Care

5 Following the ROSC from a cardiac arrest, patient management should be directed toward the postcardiac arrest syndrome.[68] There are four main components of the postcardiac arrest syndrome which highlight succinct pathophysiologic processes and potential areas for treatment: hypoxic brain injury, myocardial dysfunction, systemic ischemia-reperfusion response, and the underlying precipitating pathology (Table 41-3).[69] Many of the concepts within these four components surround the principles of basic ICU care (eg, adequate oxygenation, circulatory support, hemodynamic optimization, and prevention of secondary brain injury). Similar to other ICU patients, a systems-based approach should be used to assess the role of drug therapy. Key components of pharmacotherapy related to postcardiac arrest care are described below.

Neurologic Management and Prevention of Secondary Brain Injury

Following the restoration of blood flow after a cardiac arrest, there is a sequence of chemical cascades and destructive enzymatic reactions that result in edema, cerebral hypoxia, and neuronal injury. These reactions include free-radical production, excitatory amino acid release, and calcium shifts, which lead to mitochondrial damage and apoptosis (programmed cell death).[70] In addition, seizures,

TABLE 41-3 Postcardiac Arrest Syndrome

Syndrome	Pathophysiology	Clinical Manifestation
Hypoxic brain injury	• Impaired cerebrovascular autoregulation • Cerebral edema • Postischemic neurodegeneration	• Seizures • Coma • Myoclonus • Cognitive dysfunction • Cortical/Spinal Stroke • Brain death
Myocardial dysfunction	• Global hypokinesis • Acute coronary syndrome	• Reduced cardiac output • Cardiogenic shock • Dysrhythmias
Systemic ischemia-reperfusion response	• Systemic inflammatory response syndrome • Impaired vasoregulation • Hypercoagulability • Microcirculatory dysfunction • Adrenal suppression • Immunosuppression	• Tissue hypoxia • Hypotension • Fever • Hyperglycemia • Infection • Multi-system organ failure
Underlying precipitating pathology	• Cardiovascular disease • Pulmonary disease • Hypovolemia/Hemorrhage • Stroke • Pulmonary embolism • Poisoning/overdose • Infection • Electrolyte disturbances	• Clinical manifestation will be specific to the underlying cause

Data from Reference 69.

hyperglycemia, and hyperthermia can increase metabolic demand and further contribute to secondary hypoxic brain injury. The severity of hypoxic brain injury is a key determinant for survival; thus, appropriate preventative or treatment strategies are crucial.

Targeted Temperature Management Targeted temperature management (TTM) has been a cornerstone of post-resuscitation care for the last 20 years. TTM can protect against cerebral injury by suppressing the chemical reactions associated with cerebral injury. Additionally, TTM can decrease cerebral metabolism and oxygen consumption. For each 1°C drop in temperature, cerebral metabolism decreases by 6% to 10%.[70]

Early success with TTM was described in two pivotal trials.[71,72] In the first trial, patients who had been resuscitated after cardiac arrest due to VF but remained comatose were assigned randomly to undergo TTM through therapeutic hypothermia, targeting a temperature of 32°C to 34°C (89.6°F to 93.2°F), for 24 hours.[71] More patients in the hypothermia group achieved a favorable neurologic outcome compared to the normothermia group. The second study targeted 33°C (91.4°F) maintained for 12 hours.[72] Likewise, more patients in the hypothermia group had good neurologic function at the time of hospital discharge (to either home or a rehabilitation facility) compared to patients in the normothermia group.

Since the publication of these landmark articles, several randomized controlled trials evaluating TTM have produced mixed results. One randomized controlled trial compared TTM delivered at 33°C versus 36°C (91.4°F vs 96.8°F) for 36 hours to assess whether the benefits of TTM were related to hypothermia or prevention of hyperthermia, which occurred periodically in a previous trial.[73] Overall, this study reported no significant differences in all-cause mortality, end-of-trial mortality, or poor neurologic function. A second randomized controlled trial evaluated the impact of prehospital cooling on survival.[74] Although the target temperature (less than 34°C [89.6°F]) was reached approximately 1 hour sooner in the intervention group compared to controls, prehospital cooling was not associated with increased survival to hospital discharge or improvement in neurological status. Another study found that the duration of TTM (24 hours compared to 48 hours) had no impact on neurologic outcomes assessed at 6 months.[75] In one trial, patients with nonshockable rhythms who achieved ROSC and who were randomized to TTM targeting hypothermia (33°C [91.4°F]) had improved survival with a favorable neurologic outcome at day 90 compared to those who received normothermia (37°C [98.6°F]).[76] The most recent trial (TTM-2 trial) compared hypothermia (33°C [91.4°F]) versus normothermia (37°C [98.6°F]) in patients with both shockable and nonshockable rhythms and found no significant differences in 6-month mortality or poor functional outcome.[77] Similarly, there were no differences based on the initial rhythm being shockable or nonshockable. A subsequent systematic review evaluated the impact of TTM at 32-34°C (89.6-93.2°F) versus normothermia and found no differences in hospital survival, survival to 90 or 180 days, and survival with good neurologic outcome.[78]

One potential reason for these discordant results could be the influence of initial illness severity assessed immediately post-ROSC. One study evaluated survival to hospital discharge in patients who received TTM at 33°C or 36°C (91.4°F or 96.8°F), stratified by illness severity using the Pittsburgh Cardiac Arrest Category (PCAC) score.[79] There was a robust interaction between PCAC score and the effect of TTM at 33°C (91.4°F) whereby a greater benefit was observed in patients with higher severity of illness. In contrast, in patients with lower severity of illness, 36°C (96.8°F) was associated with higher survival rates. Further prospective research will have to validate these findings.

Current guidelines (published before the TTM-2 trial data were available) recommend TTM between 32 and 36°C (89.6°F and 96.8°F) for at least 24 hours.[16] Following the TTM period, fever should be prevented. However, a draft of the Consensus on Science with Treatment Recommendations (CoSTR) for TTM suggests preventing fever by targeting a temperature less than 37.5°C (99.5°F), acknowledging that the benefit of targeting hypothermia (32-34°C [89.6-93.2°F]) in subpopulations surviving cardiac arrest is unknown.[80]

Inducing hypothermia is not without risk. Shivering occurs during the induction phase, increasing metabolic rate and myocardial oxygen demand. Several strategies exist to blunt the thermoregulatory response to hypothermia, and these measures should be implemented accordingly.[81] These measures include acetaminophen, buspirone, magnesium, meperidine, sedation with dexmedetomidine or propofol, and analgesia with fentanyl. In some cases, neuromuscular blocking agents (NMBA) may be required. Neuromuscular blockade, however, may mask the appearance of seizures which are common postcardiac arrest. One randomized study showed no difference in serum lactate levels, survival, or neurologic function with continuous NMBA.[82] In contrast, a large observational study found that as-needed NMBA increased the odds of good outcomes compared to escalating sedation doses without NMBA.[83] When an NMBA is required, as-needed, intermittent dosing regimens are preferred over continuous infusions.

Hypothermia can also affect drug metabolism and clearance resulting in supratherapeutic concentrations.[84] These alterations may persist even upon rewarming into the posttreatment period. This is particularly relevant for sedatives and analgesics, which could confound prognostication. In fact, midazolam clearance is estimated to decrease by up to 11% for each degree Celsius.[84] Propofol clearance is 23% lower in hypothermic compared to normothermic patients. A 45% decrease in clearance has been noted with fentanyl. Careful dose titration should occur to minimize drug accumulation induced by TTM.

Other potential complications described with TTM include coagulopathy, dysrhythmias, bradycardia, diuresis, electrolyte disorders, hyperglycemia, and infections.[81] An intracellular shift of electrolytes like potassium can occur with hypothermia therefore frequent assessment and supplementation are required. Aggressive repletion, however, should be avoided because hyperkalemia may occur during rewarming as sequestered potassium is released from the intracellular compartment.

Seizures Seizures postcardiac arrest are an indicator of severe brain injury and are associated with poor prognosis. The incidence of seizures is approximately 10% to 30%.[85,86] Seizures usually occur within 8 to 24 hours postarrest but can occur later, especially after rewarming in patients treated with TTM. Continuous electroencephalogram monitoring for at least 72 hours is suggested. Either valproic acid or levetiracetam should be used as first-line therapy for the treatment of seizures. Medications for prophylaxis of seizures are not indicated.

Respiratory Management

After ROSC, it is imperative to ensure a secure airway is in place (ie, an endotracheal tube) and oxygenation is appropriate. Rearrest is common in the first minutes after resuscitation (occurring in roughly one of five cases). Hypoxia and hypotension are also frequently seen.[81] Both hypoxia and hyperoxia are associated with adverse outcomes after cardiac arrest and should be avoided.[81] Initially, 100% oxygen should be used during the resuscitation effort. If ROSC is obtained, the fraction of inspired oxygen can be titrated down as tolerated to maintain an oxygen saturation of 92-98% (0.92-0.98).[16] Overventilation, which leads to hypocapnia, should be avoided since hypocapnia causes vasoconstriction and may lead to cerebral ischemia.

Cardiovascular and Hemodynamic Management

Given that cardiac ischemia is the most common cause of cardiac arrest, a rapid search for ECG changes consistent with acute myocardial infarction should be undertaken immediately.[81] If an acute myocardial infarction is present, urgent revascularization should be performed.

Shock will be present in 50% to 70% of patients post-ROSC.[87] Cardiac echocardiography should be performed to evaluate myocardial dysfunction and can guide pharmacotherapy decisions. Volume management should be individualized for each patient based on underlying organ dysfunction, the hemodynamic target chosen, and the etiology of the arrest. Inotropes and vasopressors should be used accordingly. Steroids should not be routinely given but can be considered in refractory cases or when adrenal insufficiency is evident.

The choice for a target blood pressure is a balance between overall heart function (eg, presence of left ventricular dysfunction) and the need to maintain adequate cerebral perfusion. This is complicated by the fact that following ROSC, cerebral hypoperfusion is common, lasting several hours to days after resuscitation. During this time, cerebral vascular resistance is increased and autoregulation is impaired. Autoregulation is the ability of the cerebral vasculature to regulate constant blood flow to the brain across a range of systemic blood pressures. In the post-resuscitation phase, increased systemic pressures are needed to maintain adequate blood flow to the brain. While an optimal goal of mean arterial pressure (MAP) target has not been determined, augmenting blood pressure to achieve a goal of MAP of more than 80 mm Hg has been recommended, especially when advanced cerebral monitoring is not in use.[81]

Glucose Management

Both hyperglycemia and hypoglycemia are associated with poor outcomes in critically ill patients. Hyperglycemia is particularly common postcardiac arrest and can be influenced by TTM.[88] During therapeutic hypothermia, insulin sensitivity is significantly lower and highly variable. Upon rewarming, insulin sensitivity increases which could increase the risk for hypoglycemia. One small study compared strict (72-108 mg/dL [4-6 mmol/L]) with moderate (108-144 mg/dL [6-8 mmol/L]) glycemic control in patients with ROSC after out-of-hospital cardiac arrest.[89] There was no survival benefit recognized with strict glucose control but hypoglycemic events were higher. Maintaining glucose between 81 and 180 mg/dL (4.5 and 10 mmol/L) after cardiac arrest is suggested.

Infectious Disease Management

Therapeutic hypothermia is associated with an increased risk for infectious complications, particularly ventilator-associated pneumonia. A large trial evaluated the benefit of a short course (48 hours) of antibiotic therapy (amoxicillin-clavulanate) in patients who received TTM at 32-34°C (89.6-93.2°F).[90] Patients who received antibiotic prophylaxis had a lower incidence of early-onset pneumonia but no differences were observed in the incidence of late-onset pneumonia, number of ventilator-free days, ICU length of stay, or mortality. Routine use of antibiotic prophylaxis, therefore, is not recommended.[18]

Special Populations

Asthma

Asthma is a common disorder, and despite modern therapies, there are still in excess of 3,500 asthma-related deaths annually in the United States.[16] True cardiac arrest in asthma is infrequent, as the primary pathophysiology is respiratory compromise and poor ventilation.[91] Asthma exacerbations are a combination of bronchoconstriction, airway inflammation, and mucous plugging. This leads to severe air trapping, hyperinflation, and hemodynamic compromise. While wheezing is common in an asthma exacerbation, it does not correlate with the degree of airway obstruction. In contrast, with worsening disease (and subsequent decrease in airflow), wheezing may disappear. Further, several disease states cause wheezing, including pulmonary edema, pneumonia, anaphylaxis, foreign bodies, and tumors.

Patients with life-threatening asthma need to be treated aggressively with bronchodilators and corticosteroids. Adjunctive therapies include anticholinergics, magnesium sulfate, ketamine, helium/oxygen mixtures, or inhaled anesthetics.[92-96] Noninvasive ventilation can be attempted if the patient is deteriorating and still awake. This may prevent the need for mechanical ventilation.[97] The decision to intubate is a clinical judgment. However, the endotracheal tube will not solve the airway problem and aggressive asthma management needs to continue after intubation. In addition, intubation and positive airway pressure can trigger further bronchoconstriction or hemodynamic compromise.

The provision of BLS and standard ACLS measures should be followed in patients with acute asthma.[16] However, since the effect of auto-positive end-expiratory pressure, known as breath stacking, can be severe, a strategy of low respiratory rate and volume ventilation may be appropriate.[16] Similarly, for cardiac arrest in patients with acute asthma, especially when ventilation is difficult, tension pneumothorax should be strongly considered.[16]

Anaphylaxis

Anaphylaxis is a severe allergic reaction that can lead to airway obstruction and cardiovascular collapse. In the United States, at least 1.6% of adults have experienced anaphylaxis with about 200 individuals dying each year.[16] The initial signs can be nonspecific, but a "sense of impending doom" is common. Rhinitis often leads to laryngeal edema with stridor in the upper airway. Bronchoconstriction often mimics an acute asthma attack.

Cardiovascular collapse is common in severe anaphylaxis due to vasodilation and increased capillary permeability. This can rapidly lead to myocardial hypoperfusion and ischemia and to full cardiac arrest. There are no randomized trials comparing strategies to manage arrest due to anaphylaxis.[16] Therefore, standard basic and advanced life support measures should be followed.

Clinicians are advised to stop any drug or remove any trigger (eg, stinger after a bee sting) suspected of causing anaphylaxis. Early advanced airway management is recommended due to the potential for rapidly developing laryngeal edema. Epinephrine remains the cornerstone of the treatment.[16] The recommended dose is 0.2 to 0.5 mg and should be administered via intramuscular injection to all patients with signs of systemic allergy.[16] This can be repeated every 5 to 15 minutes if there is no clinical improvement. About 10% of patients will require more than one dose and 98% will respond with two or three doses.[98] Fluid resuscitation is usually required for restoration of circulation and is supported by one study in which the combination of fluid resuscitation and epinephrine was effective in treating hypotension unresponsive to vasoactive drugs.[99] Other agents such as antihistamines, inhaled beta-agonists, and IV corticosteroids have been used successfully in anaphylaxis and may be considered in cardiac arrest due to anaphylaxis but there are no data illustrating their benefit.[16]

Opioid Overdose

Opioid-associated cardiac arrests are responsible for approximately 115 deaths per day in the United States, largely affecting individuals aged 25 to 65 years.[16] Opioid overdose is characterized by central nervous system and respiratory depression that ultimately progresses to respiratory arrest and then cardiac arrest. Maintaining an airway and ventilation are, therefore, the highest priorities. Naloxone is an effective antidote to reverse the effect of opioids, but there are no studies demonstrating improvements in outcomes during cardiac arrest.[16] Naloxone should be administered along with standard basic and advanced life support measures but should not delay components of high-quality CPR. Repeat doses may be necessary with ingestion of long-acting or sustained release opioids. Naloxone is ineffective for arrests caused by nonopioids or other overdose scenarios.

Pregnancy

Pregnancy is a unique situation where the survival of both the fetus and the mother depends on CPR. Despite the fact that pregnant patients are younger than most cardiac arrest victims, the incidence of cardiac arrest during pregnancy appears to be on the rise in the United States.[16] Historically, survival has been poor but survival rates of nearly 60% have been reported.[100] Survival is largely dependent on the underlying etiology. The most common causes of cardiac arrest during pregnancy are anesthetic complications, accidents, bleeding, cardiovascular, drugs, embolism, fever, and hypertension.[101]

The best hope for survival of the fetus is maternal survival. Fetal monitoring is not advised during cardiac arrest because of potential interference with maternal resuscitation. High-quality chest compressions are essential and hand placement is similar to a nonpregnant patient. Because the vena cava and aorta can be obstructed by the uterus in the second and third trimesters during pregnancy, CPR procedures should be modified. Manual lateral uterine displacement (ie, pulling the uterus to the side) is recommended.[16] Alternatively, tilting the patient laterally by approximately 30 degrees can be used but the quality of chest compressions is compromised.

Pregnant patients are more prone to hypoxia; thus, oxygenation and airway management are important. The airway may be smaller because of the hormonal changes and edema.[101] Similarly, because of increased intra-abdominal pressure exerted by the uterus, as well as hormonal changes that change the resting state of the gastroesophageal sphincter, there is an increased risk of aspiration. The rescuer may need to give smaller respiration volumes than normal.

The ACLS provider should follow the standard guidelines for the pregnant patient, including the same use of chest compressions, defibrillation, and medications.[101] Epinephrine remains the vasopressor of first choice despite concerns that it can diminish uterine blood flow. Antiarrhythmics should be considered for refractory, shock-resistant VF/PVT. No medication should be withheld in the setting of cardiac arrest because of concerns about fetal teratogenicity. While there are clear changes in pharmacokinetic parameters (ie, the volume of distribution and clearance) during pregnancy, there are limited data to justify alternative dosing strategies. Standard doses, therefore, are recommended.

Although the etiology of arrest in pregnancy is often the same as in the nonpregnant patient, there are several unique causes that need to be considered.[101] Excess magnesium sulfate administration (ie, iatrogenic from treating eclampsia) can prompt cardiac arrest. In such cases, the therapeutic administration of calcium can be lifesaving. An amniotic embolism can lead to complete cardiovascular collapse during labor and delivery. Pre-eclampsia/eclampsia developing after the 20th week of gestation can produce hypertension and multiple organ dysfunction, including cardiac arrest. Vascular events including acute coronary syndromes and acute PE can also be a cause.

It is paramount to remember that unless circulation is restored to the mother, both the mother and the fetus will succumb. The resuscitation leader should consider the need for emergent cesarean delivery if ROSC is not obtained within 5 minutes.[16] In patients who achieve ROSC but remain comatose, TTM with fetal monitoring is recommended.

Accidental Hypothermia

Accidental (unintentional) hypothermia (not therapeutic hypothermia used postarrest) occurs when the body temperature is less than 30°C (86°F). It is associated with marked derangements in body function. Because it can depress virtually every body system, including pulse and respiration, the patient may appear to be dead. If the patient still has a perfusing rhythm, therapy is directed toward rewarming techniques. For mild hypothermia (ie, >34°C [93.2°F]), passive rewarming is recommended.[102] For moderate hypothermia (ie, 30°C–34°C [86°F–93.2°F]), active external rewarming is recommended, and for severe hypothermia (ie, <30°C [86°F]), active internal rewarming is recommended. Patients need to be manipulated very gently as VF is sometimes precipitated by movement.

If the patient is in cardiac arrest, then the standard BLS algorithm should be followed. Pulse and respiratory rates may be slow or difficult to detect and ECG may show asystole. If the victim displays no signs of life, then chest compressions and rescue breaths should ensue immediately. If the patient is in VF or PVT, electrical therapy should be given in a standard manner and CPR should immediately resume. Source of heat loss should be minimized (ie, removal of wet clothing, protection from the environment). The role for medications is unclear. Some resources recommended withholding epinephrine when the body temperature is less than 30°C (86°F). Current recommendations state it is reasonable to administer epinephrine according to standard ACLS practices.[16]

It is debatable when to stop resuscitative efforts in hypothermic patients. Many authors have proposed that a patient should not be pronounced dead until the core temperature has been restored to near normal.[102]

Trauma

Cardiac resuscitation of the trauma arrest patient should follow standard BLS and ACLS practices. Survival rates following an out-of-hospital cardiac arrest due to trauma are low.[98] Survival is higher in young patients with treatable penetrating injuries. Common reversible causes of traumatic cardiac arrest are hemorrhage, tension pneumothorax, asphyxia, and pericardial tamponade.

Trauma patients often suffer head or cervical injuries; thus, cervical spine precautions should be used. A jaw thrust maneuver is the preferred way to open the airway, with in-line stabilization during attempts at advanced airway placement.[16] Inadequate ventilation of one side is usually due to tube malposition, tension pneumothorax, or hemothorax. These conditions are usually treated by medical personnel at the hospital after transport.

Chest compressions should be performed in a standard manner. Chest compressions are less likely to be effective when cardiac arrest is due to hypovolemia, cardiac tamponade, or tension pneumothorax. Treatment for these "reversible causes" should be prioritized.

Ongoing hemorrhage must be controlled with either temporizing or definitive measures. Restoration of blood volume with blood products is essential as resuscitation is unlikely if the patient has severe hypovolemia. Tranexamic acid can be considered for patients with traumatic hemorrhage who present within 3 hours from injury.[103] Resuscitative endovascular balloon occlusion of the aorta is being evaluated in both traumatic and nontraumatic cardiac arrest to improve the effectiveness of chest compressions. Available data suggest this technique may be beneficial.[104]

Open thoracotomy for trauma-induced arrest may be indicated for select patients.[105] Open thoracotomy can allow relief of tamponade, control of major vessel hemorrhage, or direct repair. Open thoracotomy is a strong recommendation for patients who are pulseless but have signs of life after penetrating thoracic injury.[105] In the setting of penetrating extra-thoracic injury or blunt injury, open thoracotomy is a conditional recommendation.

A unique cause of cardiac arrest caused by a blow to the anterior chest or sternum during the repolarization part of the cardiac cycle is called "Commotio Cordis."[106] These events are commonly seen in young athletes and can be caused by a fall or a baseball or hockey puck striking the sternum. Prompt recognition and rapid defibrillation are often lifesaving. Provision of BLS, the use of an AED, and standard ACLS procedures are appropriate for this type of arrest.

Drowning

Drowning is the result of primary respiratory impairment following immersion/submersion in a liquid. It is a common, preventable cause of morbidity and mortality. Cardiac arrest in this setting is due to hypoxia. The most powerful predictor of outcome, therefore, is the duration of submersion. In one study, the probability of a good outcome was only 2% when the submersion duration exceeded 10 minutes.[107] With submersion durations that exceed 25 minutes, resuscitation efforts may be futile.

Because hypoxia is the underlying etiology of cardiac arrest in drowning victims, the traditional A-B-C approach should be used instead of C-A-B.[102] Early care consists of immediate rescue breathing, even before they are removed from the water. Once the victim is removed from the water, immediate chest compressions should be started if they are pulseless. Drowning victims can present with any of the pulseless rhythms; standard guidelines for these rhythms should be followed. A "Drowning Chain of Survival" has been proposed to improve outcomes.[108] The five links in the chain are as follows: prevent drowning, recognize distress, provide flotation, remove from water, and provide care as needed.

Electrocution/Lightning

There are many etiologies of electrical shock injuries including a lightning strike, high-tension current, or household current. The severity of injury depends on the site, type of current, duration of contact, pathway, and the magnitude of delivered electricity.

Cardiac arrest is common in electrical injury due to the current passing through the heart during the "vulnerable period" of the cardiac cycle. In large-current events, such as lightning strikes, the heart undergoes massive depolarization. In some cases, the intrinsic pacemaker can restore an organized cardiac electrical cycle. Injury to other muscles, however, particularly the thoracic musculature, and suppression of the respiratory center can lead to inadequate ventilation, hypoxia, and subsequent cardiac arrest. Ventilatory support, therefore, must be maintained after ROSC is achieved.

When approaching a victim of electrocution, the rescuer must first be certain of his or her own safety. Prompt CPR and ACLS, when available, is indicated. Electric shock is often associated with multiple trauma, including spinal injury, multiple injuries to the skeletal muscles, as well as fractures. These factors need to be evaluated by the resuscitation team.

Airway control may be difficult due to the edema that often accompanies electrical injuries; thus, an advanced airway early in the treatment process is recommended.[102] With soft tissue swelling, there is often a need for aggressive fluid resuscitation in these patients. The underlying tissue, or visceral organ damage, is often worse than the external appearance. It is usually recommended that these patients can be transferred to centers with expertise in dealing with these types of injuries.

Drug Administration

The routes of administration available for drug delivery during CPR include IV (both central and peripheral access), IO, and endotracheal. Each route represents a compromise between access and efficacy in introducing the drug into the central circulation. When selecting a route for drug administration, it is important to minimize any interruptions in chest compressions during CPR.

The traditional access site for parenteral medication administration during a cardiac arrest is a peripheral IV line. Peripheral drug administration yields a peak concentration in the major systemic arteries in roughly 1.5 to 3 minutes but this time can be shortened by up to 40% if the drug is followed by a 20-mL fluid bolus and elevating the extremity.[109] Central venous access will result in a faster and higher peak drug concentration than peripheral access but central line access is not needed in most resuscitation attempts. If a central line is already present, it should be the access site of choice. An appropriately trained provider may consider placing a central line if one is not present and attempts to establish IV or IO access are unsuccessful, but CPR should not be interrupted. Central lines located above the diaphragm are preferable to those located below the diaphragm because of poor blood flow during CPR.

6 If IV access cannot be obtained, IO is the next preferred route for drug and fluid administration.[16] Several IO access devices are commercially available that allow for rapid insertion and are easy to use. Pharmacokinetic data have demonstrated similar areas under the curve and times to peak concentration for sternal IO and central IV administration.[110] Clinical data, however, have suggested outcomes may be worse with IO administration versus IV.[18] IO administration should only be used if initial attempts at IV access are unsuccessful. Potential anatomic sites for insertion of an IO needle are the sternum, tibia, and humerus.[110] The need for cessation of chest compressions, however, along with the risk of injury to the heart or great vessels makes the sternum a less desirable site for insertion. As such, the proximal tibia is typically preferred because it is easy to locate, provides a flat, wide surface for insertion, has minimal subcutaneous layers overlying the bone, and does not interfere with CPR.

If neither IV nor IO access can be established, a few drugs can be administered through an endotracheal tube. These drugs are atropine, lidocaine, epinephrine, naloxone, and vasopressin.[109] There are no data with amiodarone. Medications administered through the endotracheal route will have both a lower and delayed peak concentration than when drugs are administered by the IV or IO routes. In one clinical trial, lower rates of ROSC, hospital admission, and hospital discharge were observed with endotracheal drug administration compared to IV.[109] If the endotracheal route is to be used, the recommended medication dose is 2 to 2.5 times larger than the IV/IO dose. Providers should dilute the medication in 5 to 10 mL of either sterile water or normal saline. Better drug absorption may be achieved with sterile water.[109]

EVALUATION OF THERAPEUTIC OUTCOMES

The optimal outcome following CPR is an awake, responsive, spontaneously breathing patient. Patients must remain neurologically intact with minimal morbidity following the resuscitation if it is to be considered a success.

Monitoring during cardiac arrest includes both CPR performance and physiologic. CPR performance can be assessed using devices that provide real-time feedback on CPR quality. In many cases, rhythm assessment via ECG and pulse checks are the only physiologic parameters available to guide therapy. Palpating a pulse to determine the efficacy of blood flow during CPR, however, has not been shown to be useful. Invasive hemodynamic monitoring (eg, CPP, central venous oxygenation) can provide useful information during CPR but these are seldom available. Arterial diastolic pressure may be a reasonable surrogate for CPP; values less than 20 mm Hg are generally considered suboptimal, and a goal of more than 25 mm Hg is suggested.[111] An arterial central venous oxygen saturation of less than 30% (0.30) is indicative of poor CPR quality.[109]

$ETCO_2$ monitoring is a useful method to assess cardiac output during CPR and has been associated with ROSC. The main determinant of carbon dioxide excretion is the rate of delivery from the peripheral tissues to the lungs. Increasing cardiac output through effective CPR will yield higher $ETCO_2$ levels. Therefore, $ETCO_2$ levels reflect the cardiac output generated by CPR. Persistently low $ETCO_2$ values (<10 mm Hg [1.3 kPa]) during CPR in intubated patients suggest ROSC is unlikely.[16] $ETCO_2$ levels that exceed 20 mm Hg (2.7 kPa) may be associated with a higher chance for ROSC.[18]

Evaluation of outcomes in the post-resuscitation phase should be directed toward the components of the postcardiac arrest syndrome. Because the postcardiac arrest syndrome can affect practically every organ system, a review-of-systems approach for assessment (ie, "head-to-toe") is strongly suggested. Neuroprognostication should occur at least 5 days after ROSC (or 72 hours after normothermia) for patients who receive TTM because of the prolonged effects of sedatives noted with hypothermia.

The latest link added to the "chain of survival" is recovery. Many patients who survive cardiac arrest suffer from prolonged emotional, cognitive, physical, and neurologic symptoms. In fact, one-third of survivors experience symptoms of anxiety, depression, and posttraumatic stress disorder.[16] Family members and caregivers may also experience stress during the recovery period. A multimodal plan should be provided at hospital discharge that includes instructions for treatment, rehabilitation, and surveillance. In addition, both short-term and long-term expectations should be clearly defined with appropriate action plans for each phase of the recovery.

CONCLUSION

Cardiac arrest is often fatal, but rapid recognition and treatment can result in a favorable outcome. The "Chains of Survival" as described by the AHA provides a framework for treatment. Early recognition and response including high-quality chest compressions with minimal interruptions, early defibrillation, and post-resuscitation care remain major hallmarks of therapy. Nevertheless, there are many areas of uncertainty including the optimal approach for oxygenation and ventilation, the role of drug therapy (eg, epinephrine), the value of TTM, resuscitation targets, and the role of extracorporeal therapies (ie, cardiopulmonary bypass), and the value of neuroprotective agents.[112] A comprehensive research approach, consisting of randomized controlled trials, registry-based studies, pragmatic trials, and animal/laboratory research will be necessary to advance our understanding and improve outcomes.

ABBREVIATIONS

ACLS	advanced cardiac life support
AED	automated external defibrillator
AHA	American Heart Association
BLS	basic life support
CI	confidence interval
CPP	coronary perfusion pressure
CPR	cardiopulmonary resuscitation
ECC	emergency cardiovascular care
ECG	electrocardiogram
EMS	emergency medical services
$ETCO_2$	end-tidal carbon dioxide
IO	intraosseous
IV	intravenous
MAP	mean arterial pressure
OR	odds ratio
PCI	percutaneous coronary intervention
PEA	pulseless electrical activity
PE	pulmonary embolism
ROSC	return of spontaneous circulation
PVT	pulseless ventricular tachycardia
SBP	systolic blood pressure
VF	ventricular fibrillation

REFERENCES

1. Virani SS, Alonso A, Aparicio HJ, et al. Heart disease and stroke statistics—2021 update: A report from the American Heart Association. *Circulation.* 2021;143(8):e254–e743. 10.1161/CIR.0000000000000950 33501848.
2. Chan PS, McNally B, Tang F, et al. Recent trends in survival from out-of-hospital cardiac arrest in the United States. *Circulation.* 2014;130:1876–1882.
3. Cardiac Arrest Registry to Enhance Survival (CARES) 2020 Annual Report. https://mycares.net/sitepages/uploads/2021/2020_flipbook/index.html?page=1. 2020. Accessed 11/26/2021.
4. Patil KD, Halperin HR, Becker LB. Cardiac arrest: Resuscitation and reperfusion. *Circ Res.* 2015;116(12):2041–2049. 10.1161/CIRCRESAHA.116.304495 26044255.
5. Girotra S, Nallamothu BK, Spertus JA, et al. Trends in survival after in-hospital cardiac arrest. *N Engl J Med.* 2012;367(20):1912–20. 10.1056/NEJMoa1109148 23150959.
6. Berg RA, Nadkarni VM, Clark AE, et al. Incidence and outcomes of cardiopulmonary resuscitation in PICUs. *Crit Care Med.* 2016;44:798–808.
7. Hayashi M, Shimizu W, Albert CM. The spectrum of epidemiology underlying sudden cardiac death. *Circ Res.* 2015;116:1887–1906.
8. Topjian AA, Raymond TT, Atkins D, et al. Part 4: Pediatric basic and advanced life support: 2020 American Heart Association guidelines for cardiopulmonary resuscitation and emergency cardiovascular care. *Circulation.* 2020;142(16_suppl_2):S469–S523. 10.1161/CIR.0000000000000901 33081526.
9. Ewy GA. Cardiocerebral and cardiopulmonary resuscitation—2017 update. *Acute Med Surg.* 2017;4:227–234.
10. Mancini ME, Diekema DS, Hoadley TA, et al. Part 3: Ethical issues: 2015 American Heart Association guidelines update for cardiopulmonary resuscitation and emergency cardiovascular care. *Circulation.* 2015;132:S383–S396.
11. Cooper JA, Cooper JD, Cooper JM. Cardiopulmonary resuscitation: History, current practice, and future direction. *Circulation.* 2006;114:2839–2849.
12. Merchant RM, Topjian AA, Panchal AR, et al. Part 1: Executive summary: 2020 American Heart Association guidelines for cardiopulmonary resuscitation and emergency cardiovascular care. *Circulation.* 2020;142(16_suppl_2):S337–S357. 10.1161/CIR.0000000000000918 33081530.
13. Harris AW, Kudenchuk PJ. Cardiopulmonary resuscitation: The science behind the hands. *Heart.* 2018.;104:1056–1061.
14. Soar J, Edelson DP, Perkins GD. Delivering high-quality cardiopulmonary resuscitation in-hospital. *Curr Opin Crit Care.* 2011;17:225–230.
15. Goharani R, Vahedian-Azimi A, Farzanegan B, et al. Real-time compression feedback for patients with in-hospital cardiac arrest: A multi-center randomized controlled clinical trial. *J Intensive Care.* 2019;7:5–5. 10.1186/s40560-019-0357-5 30693086.
16. Panchal AR, Bartos JA, Cabañas JG, et al. Part 3: Adult basic and advanced life support: 2020 American Heart Association guidelines for cardiopulmonary resuscitation and emergency cardiovascular care. *Circulation.* 2020;142(16_suppl_2):S366–S468. 10.1161/CIR.0000000000000916 33081529.
17. Andersen LW, Holmberg MJ, Berg KM, et al. In-hospital cardiac arrest: A review. *JAMA.* 2019;321(12):1200–1210. 10.1001/jama.2019.1696 30912843.
18. Berg KM, Soar J, Andersen LW, et al. Adult advanced life support: 2020 international consensus on cardiopulmonary resuscitation and emergency cardiovascular care science with treatment recommendations. *Circulation.* 2020;142(16_suppl_1):S92–S139. 10.1161/CIR.0000000000000893 33084390.
19. Ewy GA. Cardiocerebral and cardiopulmonary resuscitation—2017 update. *Acute Med Surg.* 2017;4(3):227–234. 10.1002/ams2.281 29123868.
20. Christenson J, Andrusiek D, Everson-Stewart S, et al. Chest compression fraction determines survival in patients with out-of-hospital ventricular fibrillation. *Circulation.* 2009;120(13):1241–1247. 10.1161/CIRCULATIONAHA.109.852202 19752324.
21. Bobrow BJ, Spaite DW, Berg RA, et al. Chest compression-only CPR by lay rescuers and survival from out-of-hospital cardiac arrest. *JAMA.* 2010;304(13):1447–1454. 10.1001/jama.2010.1392 20924010.
22. Olasveengen TM, Mancini ME, Perkins GD, et al. Adult basic life support: 2020 international consensus on cardiopulmonary resuscitation and emergency cardiovascular care science with treatment recommendations. *Circulation.* 2020;142(16_suppl_1):S41–S91. 10.1161/CIR.0000000000000892 33084391.
23. Sutton RM, French B, Meaney PA, et al. Physiologic monitoring of CPR quality during adult cardiac arrest: A propensity-matched cohort study. *Resuscitation.* 2016;106:76–82. 10.1016/j.resuscitation.2016.06.018 27350369.
24. Link MS, Atkins DL, Passman RS, et al. Part 6: electrical therapies: Automated external defibrillators, defibrillation, cardioversion, and pacing: 2010 American Heart Association guidelines for cardiopulmonary resuscitation and emergency cardiovascular care. *Circulation.* 2010;122:S706–S719.

25. Böttiger BW, Becker LB, Kern KB, et al. BIG FIVE strategies for survival following out-of-hospital cardiac arrest. *Eur J Anaesthesiol.* 2020;37(11):955–958. 10.1097/EJA.0000000000001247 32467418.
26. Girotra S, van Diepen S, Nallamothu BK, et al. Regional variation in out-of-hospital cardiac arrest survival in the United States. *Circulation.* 2016;133(22):2159–2168. 10.1161/CIRCULATIONAHA.115.018175 27081119.
27. Bækgaard JS, Viereck S, Møller TP, et al. The effects of public access defibrillation on survival after out-of-hospital cardiac arrest: A systematic review of observational studies. *Circulation.* 2017;136(10):954–965. 10.1161/CIRCULATIONAHA.117.029067 28687709.
28. Robinson LA, Brown CG, Jenkins J, et al. The effect of norepinephrine versus epinephrine on myocardial hemodynamics during CPR. *Ann Emerg Med.* 1989;18:336–340.
29. Paradis NA, Martin GB, Rivers EP, et al. Coronary perfusion pressure and the return of spontaneous circulation in human cardiopulmonary resuscitation. *JAMA.* 1990;263:1106–1113.
30. Reynolds JC, Salcido DD, Menegazzi JJ. Conceptual models of coronary perfusion pressure and their relationship to defibrillation success in a porcine model of prolonged out-of-hospital cardiac arrest. *Resuscitation.* 2012;83:900–906.
31. Perkins GD, Ji C, Deakin CD, et al. A randomized trial of epinephrine in out-of-hospital cardiac arrest. *N Engl J Med.* 2018;379(8):711–721. 10.1056/NEJMoa1806842 30021076.
32. Jacobs IG, Finn JC, Jelinek GA, et al. Effect of adrenaline on survival in out-of-hospital cardiac arrest: A randomised double-blind placebo-controlled trial. *Resuscitation.* 2011;82(9):1138–1143. 10.1016/j.resuscitation.2011.06.029 21745533.
33. Perkins GD, Kenna C, Ji C, et al. The effects of adrenaline in out of hospital cardiac arrest with shockable and non-shockable rhythms: Findings from the PACA and PARAMEDIC-2 randomised controlled trials. *Resuscitation.* 2019;140:55–63. 10.1016/j.resuscitation.2019.05.007 31116964.
34. Hagihara A, Hasegawa M, Abe T, Nagata T, Wakata Y, Miyazaki S. Prehospital epinephrine use and survival among patients with out-of-hospital cardiac arrest. *JAMA.* 2012;307:1161–1168.
35. Nakahara S, Tomio J, Takahashi H, et al. Evaluation of pre-hospital administration of adrenaline (epinephrine) by emergency medical services for patients with out of hospital cardiac arrest in Japan: Controlled propensity matched retrospective cohort study. *BMJ.* 2013;347:f6829.
36. Perkins GD, Kenna C, Ji C, et al. The influence of time to adrenaline administration in the Paramedic 2 randomised controlled trial. *Intensive Care Med.* 2020;46(3):426–436. 10.1007/s00134-019-05836-2 31912202.
37. Okubo M, Komukai S, Callaway CW, et al. Association of timing of epinephrine administration with outcomes in adults with out-of-hospital cardiac arrest. *JAMA Netw Open.* 2021;4(8):e2120176 –e2120176. 10.1001/jamanetworkopen.2021.20176 34374770.
38. Andersen LW, Berg KM, Saindon BZ, et al. Time to epinephrine and survival after pediatric in-hospital cardiac arrest. *JAMA.* 2015;314:802–810.
39. Donnino MW, Salciccioli JD, Howell MD, et al. Time to administration of epinephrine and outcome after in-hospital cardiac arrest with non-shockable rhythms: Retrospective analysis of large in-hospital data registry. *Br Med J.* 2014;348:g3028.
40. Ewy GA, Bobrow BJ, Chikani V, et al. The time dependent association of adrenaline administration and survival from out-of-hospital cardiac arrest. *Resuscitation.* 2015;96:180–185.
41. Koscik C, Pinawin A, McGovern H, et al. Rapid epinephrine administration improves early outcomes in out-of-hospital cardiac arrest. *Resuscitation.* 2013;84:915–920.
42. Dumas F, Bougouin W, Geri G, et al. Is epinephrine during cardiac arrest associated with worse outcomes in resuscitated patients? *J Am Coll Cardiol.* 2014;64:2360–2367.
43. Ristagno G, Tang W, Huang L, et al. Epinephrine reduces cerebral perfusion during cardiopulmonary resuscitation. *Crit Care Med.* 2009;37:1408–1415.
44. Deakin CD, Yang J, Nguyen R, et al. Effects of epinephrine on cerebral oxygenation during cardiopulmonary resuscitation: A prospective cohort study. *Resuscitation.* 2016;109:138–144.
45. Rivers EP, Wortsman J, Rady MY, Blake HC, McGeorge FT, Buderer NM. The effect of the total cumulative epinephrine dose administered during human CPR on hemodynamic, oxygen transport, and utilization variables in the postresuscitation period. *Chest.* 1994;106:1499–1507.
46. Larabee TM, Liu KY, Campbell JA, Little CM. Vasopressors in cardiac arrest: A systematic review. *Resuscitation.* 2012;83:932–939.
47. Callaham M, Madsen CD, Barton CW, Saunders CE, Pointer J. A randomized clinical trial of high-dose epinephrine and norepinephrine vs standard-dose epinephrine in prehospital cardiac arrest. *JAMA.* 1992;268:2667–2672.
48. Lindner KH, Ahnefeld FW, Grunert A. Epinephrine versus norepinephrine in prehospital ventricular fibrillation. *Am J Cardiol.* 1991;67:427–428.
49. Redding JS, Pearson JW. Evaluation of drugs for cardiac resuscitation. *Anesthesiology.* 1963;24:203–207.
50. Wenze IV, Raab H, Dunser MW. Role of arginine vasopressin in the setting of cardiopulmonary resuscitation. *Best Pract Res Clin Anaesthesiol.* 2008;22:287–297.
51. Lindner KH, Haak T, Keller A, Bothner U, Lurie KG. Release of endogenous vasopressors during and after cardiopulmonary resuscitation. *Heart.* 1996;75:145–150.
52. Holmberg MJ, Issa MS, Moskowitz A, et al. Vasopressors during adult cardiac arrest: A systematic review and meta-analysis. *Resuscitation.* 2019;139:106–121. 10.1016/j.resuscitation.2019.04.008 30980877.
53. Mentzelopoulos SD, Malachias S, Chamos C, et al. Vasopressin, steroids, and epinephrine and neurologically favorable survival after in-hospital cardiac arrest: A randomized clinical trial. *JAMA.* 2013;310:270–279.
54. Mentzelopoulos SD, Zakynthinos SG, Tzoufi M, et al. Vasopressin, epinephrine, and corticosteroids for in-hospital cardiac arrest. *Arch Intern Med.* 2009;169:15–24.
55. Andersen Lars W, Isbye Dan, Kjærgaard Jesper, et al. Effect of vasopressin and methylprednisolone vs placebo on return of spontaneous circulation in patients with in-hospital cardiac arrest. *JAMA.* 2021;326:1586. 10.1001/jama.2021.16628.
56. Shah K, Mitra AR. Use of corticosteroids in cardiac arrest: A systematic review and meta-analysis. *Crit Care Med.* 2021;49(6):e642–e650. 10.1097/CCM.0000000000004941 33729721.
57. Huang Y, He Q, Yang M, Zhan L. Antiarrhythmia drugs for cardiac arrest: A systemic review and meta-analysis. *Crit Care.* 2013;17:R173.
58. Ong ME, Pellis T, Link MS. The use of antiarrhythmic drugs for adult cardiac arrest: A systematic review. *Resuscitation.* 2011;82:665–670.
59. Kudenchuk PJ, Cobb LA, Copass MK. Amiodarone for resuscitation after out-of-hospital cardiac arrest due to ventricular fibrillation. *N Engl J Med.* 1999;341:871–878.
60. Dorian P, Cass D, Schwartz B, Cooper R, Gelaznikas R, Barr A. Amiodarone as compared with lidocaine for shock-resistant ventricular fibrillation. *N Engl J Med.* 2002;346:884–890.
61. Kudenchuk PJ, Brown SP, Daya M, et al. Amiodarone, lidocaine, or placebo in out-of-hospital cardiac arrest. *N Engl J Med.* 2016;374:1711–1722.
62. Bottiger BW, Arntz HR, Chamberlain DA, et al. Thrombolysis during resuscitation for out-of-hospital cardiac arrest. *N Engl J Med.* 2008;359:2651–2662.
63. Hansen M, Schmicker RH, Newgard CD, et al. Time to epinephrine administration and survival from nonshockable out-of-hospital cardiac arrest among children and adults. *Circulation.* 2018;137(19):2032–2040. 10.1161/CIRCULATIONAHA.117.033067 29511001.
64. Goto Y, Maeda T, Goto Y. Effects of prehospital epinephrine during out-of-hospital cardiac arrest with initial non-shockable rhythm: An observational cohort study. *Crit Care.* 2013;17(5):R188–R188. 10.1186/cc12872 24004456.
65. Alshahrani MS, Aldandan HW. Use of sodium bicarbonate in out-of-hospital cardiac arrest: A systematic review and meta-analysis. *Int J Emerg Med.* 2021;14(1):21–21. 10.1186/s12245-021-00344-x 33849429.
66. Kawano T, Grunau B, Scheuermeyer FX. Prehospital sodium bicarbonate use could worsen long term survival with favorable neurological recovery among patients with out-of-hospital cardiac arrest. *Resuscitation.* 2017;119:63–69.
67. Velissaris D, Karamouzos V, Pierrakos C, Koniari I, Apostolopoulou C, Karanikolas M. Use of sodium bicarbonate in cardiac arrest: Current guidelines and literature review. *J Clin Med Res.* 2016;8:277–283.
68. Callaway CW, Donnino MW, Fink EL, et al. Part 8: Post-cardiac arrest care: 2015 American Heart Association guidelines update for cardiopulmonary resuscitation and emergency cardiovascular care. *Circulation.* 2015;132:S465–482.
69. Neumar RW, Nolan JP, Adrie C, et al. Post-cardiac arrest syndrome: Epidemiology, pathophysiology, treatment, and prognostication. A consensus statement from the International Liaison Committee on Resuscitation (American Heart Association, Australian and New Zealand Council on Resuscitation, European Resuscitation Council, Heart and Stroke Foundation of Canada, InterAmerican Heart Foundation, Resuscitation Council of Asia, and the

Resuscitation Council of Southern Africa); the American Heart Association Emergency Cardiovascular Care Committee; the Council on Cardiovascular Surgery and Anesthesia; the Council on Cardiopulmonary, Perioperative, and Critical Care; the Council on Clinical Cardiology; and the Stroke Council. *Circulation*. 2008;118:2452–2483.

70. Nolan JP, Soar J, Cariou A, et al. European Resuscitation Council and European Society of Intensive Care Medicine 2015 guidelines for post-resuscitation care. *Intensive Care Med.* 2015;41:2039–2056.
71. The Hypothermia After Cardiac Arrest Study Group. Mild therapeutic hypothermia to improve the neurologic outcome after cardiac arrest. *N Engl J Med.* 2002;346:549–556.
72. Bernard SA, Gray TW, Buist MD, et al. Treatment of comatose survivors of out-of-hospital cardiac arrest with induced hypothermia. *N Engl J Med.* 2002;346:557–563.
73. Nielsen N, Wetterslev J, Cronberg T, et al. Targeted temperature management at 33 degrees C versus 36 degrees C after cardiac arrest. *N Engl J Med.* 2013;369:2197–2206.
74. Kim F, Nichol G, Maynard C, et al. Effect of prehospital induction of mild hypothermia on survival and neurological status among adults with cardiac arrest: A randomized clinical trial. *JAMA*. 2014;311:45–52.
75. Kirkegaard H, Soreide E, deHaas I, et al. Targeted temperature management for 48 vs 24 hours and neurologic outcome after out-of-hospital cardiac arrest: A randomized clinical trial. *JAMA*. 2017;318:341–350.
76. Lascarrou JB, Merdji H, Le Gouge A, et al. Targeted temperature management for cardiac arrest with nonshockable rhythm. *N Engl J Med.* 2019;381(24):2327–2337. 10.1056/NEJMoa1906661 31577396.
77. Dankiewicz J, Cronberg T, Lilja G, et al. Hypothermia versus normothermia after out-of-hospital cardiac arrest. *N Engl J Med.* 2021;384(24):2283–2294. 10.1056/NEJMoa2100591 34133859.
78. Granfeldt A, Holmberg MJ, Nolan JP, et al. Targeted temperature management in adult cardiac arrest: Systematic review and meta-analysis. *Resuscitation.* 2021;167:160–172. 10.1016/j.resuscitation.2021.08.040 34474143.
79. Callaway CW, Coppler PJ, Faro J, et al. Association of initial illness severity and outcomes after cardiac arrest with targeted temperature management at 36 °C or 33 °C. *JAMA Netw Open.* 2020;3(7):e208215 –e208215. 10.1001/jamanetworkopen.2020.8215 32701158.
80. Soar J, Nolan JP, Andersen LW, et al. Temperature Management in Adult Cardiac Arrest Consensus on Science with Treatment Recommendations. Brussels, Belgium: International Liaison Committee on Resuscitation (ILCOR) Advanced Life Support Task Force, 2021 August 30. Available from: http://ilcor.org
81. Elmer J, Polderman KH. Emergency neurological life support: Resuscitation following cardiac arrest. *Neurocrit Care.* 2017;27:134–143.
82. Moskowitz A, Andersen LW, Rittenberger JC, et al. Continuous neuromuscular blockade following successful resuscitation from cardiac arrest: A randomized trial. *J Am Heart Assoc.* 2020;9(17):e017171–e017171. 10.1161/JAHA.120.017171 32851921.
83. May TL, Riker RR, Fraser GL, et al. Variation in sedation and neuromuscular blockade regimens on outcome after cardiac arrest. *Crit Care Med.* 2018;46(10):e975–e980. 10.1097/CCM.0000000000003301 29979225.
84. Anderson KB, Poloyac SM, Kochanek PM, et al. Effect of hypothermia and targeted temperature management on drug disposition and response following cardiac arrest: A comprehensive review of preclinical and clinical investigations. *Ther Hypothermia Temp Manag.* 2016;6(4):169–179. 10.1089/ther.2016.0003 27622966.
85. Perkins GD, Callaway CW, Haywood K, et al. Brain injury after cardiac arrest. *Lancet.* 2021;398(10307):1269–1278. 10.1016/S0140-6736(21)00953-3 34454687.
86. Mayasi Y, Geocadin RG. Updates on the management of neurologic complications of post-cardiac arrest resuscitation. *Semin Neurol.* 2021;41(4):388–397. 10.1055/s-0041-1731310 34412143.
87. Jozwiak M, Bougouin W, Geri G, et al. Post-resuscitation shock: Recent advances in pathophysiology and treatment. *Ann Intensive Care.* 2020;10(1):170–170. 10.1186/s13613-020-00788-z 33315152.
88. Sah Pri A, Chase JG, Pretty CG, et al. Evolution of insulin sensitivity and its variability in out-of-hospital cardiac arrest (OHCA) patients treated with hypothermia. *Crit Care.* 2014;18(5):586–586. 10.1186/s13054-014-0586-x 25349023.
89. Oksanen T, Skrifvars MB, Varpula T, et al. Strict versus moderate glucose control after resuscitation from ventricular fibrillation. *Intensive Care Med.* 2007;33(12):2093–2100. 10.1007/s00134-007-0876-8 17928994.
90. François B, Cariou A, Clere-Jehl R, et al. Prevention of early ventilator-associated pneumonia after cardiac arrest. *N Engl J Med.* 2019;381(19):1831–1842. 10.1056/NEJMoa1812379 31693806.
91. McFadden ER, Jr., Warren EL. Observations on asthma mortality. *Ann Intern Med.* 1997;127:142–147.
92. Petrillo TM, Fortenberry JD, Linzer JF, Simon HK. Emergency department use of ketamine in pediatric status asthmaticus. *J Asthma.* 2001;38:657–664.
93. Rodrigo GJ, Castro-Rodriguez JA. Anticholinergics in the treatment of children and adults with acute asthma: A systematic review with meta-analysis. *Thorax* 2005;60:740–746.
94. Schultz TE. Sevoflurane administration in status asthmaticus: A case report. *AANA J.* 2005;73:35–36.
95. Silverman RA, Osborn H, Runge J, et al. IV magnesium sulfate in the treatment of acute severe asthma: A multicenter randomized controlled trial. *Chest.* 2002;122:489–497.
96. Hess DR, Acosta FL, Ritz RH, Kacmarek RM, Camargo CA. The effect of heliox on nebulizer function using a beta-agonist bronchodilator. *Chest.* 1999;115:184–189.
97. Soroksky A, Stav D, Shpirer I. A pilot prospective, randomized, placebo-controlled trial of bilevel positive airway pressure in acute asthmatic attack. *Chest.* 2003;123:1018–1025.
98. Soar J, Becker LB, Berg KM, et al. Cardiopulmonary resuscitation in special circumstances. *Lancet.* 2021;398(10307):1257–1268. 10.1016/S0140-6736(21)01257-5 34454688.
99. Brown SG, Blackman KE, Stenlake V, Heddle RJ. Insect sting anaphylaxis; prospective evaluation of treatment with intravenous adrenaline and volume resuscitation. *Emerg Med J.* 2004;21:149–154.
100. Mhyre JM, Tsen LC, Einav S, Kuklina EV, Leffert LR, Bateman BT. Cardiac arrest during hospitalization for delivery in the United States, 1998–2011. *Anesthesiology.* 2014;120:810–818.
101. Jeejeebhoy FM, Zelop CM, Lipman S, et al. Cardiac arrest in pregnancy: A scientific statement from the American Heart Association. *Circulation.* 2015;132:1747–1773.
102. Vanden Hoek TL, Morrison LJ, Shuster M, et al. Part 12: Cardiac arrest in special situations: 2010 American Heart Association guidelines for cardiopulmonary resuscitation and emergency cardiovascular care. *Circulation.* 2010;122:S829–S861.
103. Roberts I, Shakur H, Folabi AA, et al. The importance of early treatment with tranexamic acid in bleeding trauma patients: An exploratory analysis of the CRASH-2 randomised controlled trial. *Lancet.* 2011;377(9771):1096-1101, 1101.e1–2. 10.1016/S0140-6736(11)60278-X 21439633.
104. Teeter W, Haase D. Updates in traumatic cardiac arrest. *Emerg Med Clin North Am.* 2020;38(4):891–901. 10.1016/j.emc.2020.06.009 32981624.
105. Seamon MJ, Haut ER, VanArendonk K, et al. An evidence-based approach to patient selection for emergency department thoracotomy: A practice management guideline from the Eastern Association for the Surgery of Trauma. *J Trauma Acute Care Surg.* 2015;79:159–173.
106. Link MS, Maron BJ, VanderBrink BA, Zhu W, Estes NA 3rd. Upper and lower limits of vulnerability to sudden arrhythmic death with chest-wall impact (commotio cordis). *J Am Coll Cardiol.* 2003;41:99–104.
107. Quan L, Mack CD, Schiff MA. Association of water temperature and submersion duration and drowning outcome. *Resuscitation.* 2014;85:790–794.
108. Szpilman D, Webber J, Quan L, et al. Creating a drowning chain of survival. *Resuscitation.* 2014;85:1149–1152.
109. Neumar RW, Otto CW, Link MS, et al. Part 8: Adult advanced cardiovascular life support: 2010 American Heart Association guidelines for cardiopulmonary resuscitation and emergency cardiovascular care. *Circulation.* 2010;122:S729–S767.
110. Hoskins SL, doNascimento P, Jr., Lima RM, Espana-Tenorio JM, Kramer GC. Pharmacokinetics of intraosseous and central venous drug delivery during cardiopulmonary resuscitation. *Resuscitation.* 2012;83:107–112.
111. Meaney PA, Bobrow BJ, Mancini ME, et al. Cardiopulmonary resuscitation quality: Improving cardiac resuscitation outcomes both inside and outside the hospital. A consensus statement from the American Heart Association. *Circulation.* 2013;128:417–435.
112. Nolan JP, Berg RA, Bernard S, et al. Intensive care medicine research agenda on cardiac arrest. *Intensive Care Med.* 2017;43:1282–1293.

e42

Shock Syndromes

Seth R. Bauer, Robert MacLaren, and Brian L. Erstad

KEY CONCEPTS

1. Shock is a clinical syndrome characterized by inadequate global tissue perfusion. Low blood pressures are not required to define shock.
2. Shock is typically classified into one of four etiologic mechanisms: (1) hypovolemic, (2) cardiogenic, (3) obstructive, or (4) vasodilatory/distributive.
3. Shock syndromes can be differentiated based on the evaluation of preload, cardiac output, and afterload or assessment of surrogate markers.
4. Inadequate oxygen delivery leads to organ damage in critical illness.
5. Blood lactate should be measured in all patients in whom shock is suspected.
6. Treatment of the patient with circulatory shock can be divided into four phases: salvage, optimization, stabilization, and de-escalation. Each phase has different but sometimes overlapping goals and therapeutic strategies.
7. Crystalloid solutions are the first-line fluid of choice for forms of circulatory insufficiency that are associated with hemodynamic instability.
8. Vasopressors and inotropes are required in patients with shock when volume resuscitation fails to maintain adequate blood pressure and tissues remain hypoperfused.
9. The choice of a particular vasopressor or inotrope agent depends on the underlying shock pathophysiology, goals of therapy, and clinical pharmacology.
10. Norepinephrine is the preferred initial vasopressor for shock.

BEYOND THE BOOK

Develop a table that has two columns, one titled *crystalloid solutions* and one titled *colloid solutions*. In each column, list at least four potential advantages and four potential disadvantages of the solution. There are several crystalloid and colloid solutions commercially available, so you will need to be specific about the solutions included in the table. The purpose of this exercise is to help students choose a preferred resuscitation fluid for a critically ill patient based on patient-specific data.

INTRODUCTION

Circulatory shock is a medical emergency requiring prompt recognition and treatment because it can quickly lead to serious consequences, including death. Shock is a broad term for a heterogeneous group of syndromes that cause an acute, generalized circulatory failure associated with inadequate oxygen utilization by the cells.[1] Typically, shock is characterized as systolic blood pressure (SBP) <90 mm Hg (or acute reduction of at least 40 mm Hg from baseline) or mean arterial blood pressure (MAP) <70 mm Hg with tachycardia and organ perfusion abnormalities.[2] The key feature of all shock syndromes is inadequate tissue and organ perfusion.

Learners are strongly encouraged to read Chapter e29 "Evaluation of Cardiovascular Function" and Chapter 142 "Sepsis and Septic Shock" to augment their understanding of the content in this chapter.

EPIDEMIOLOGY

Hemodynamic compromise necessitating the use of vasopressors is common in the intensive care unit (ICU), with about one-third of critically ill patients receiving vasopressors during their clinical course.[3] Shock is not a reportable cause of death to state and federal agencies and, thus, the true incidence is unknown. Reported mortality of patients with shock in clinical studies from the 1980s exceeded 70% but now ranges from 20% to 55%.[4–7] However, estimates of deaths due to shock are complicated by differences in definitions and classification systems. Normal compensatory mechanisms may reverse the processes leading to irreversible organ dysfunction. However, progressive circulatory insufficiency may result in the loss of these compensatory responses. Identification of when this occurs can be problematic as this varies from patient to patient and is not always readily apparent during the initial patient presentation. Therefore, forms of shock, such as hemorrhagic shock, are often subsumed by more readily identifiable categories of death, such as accidental injuries and homicides.

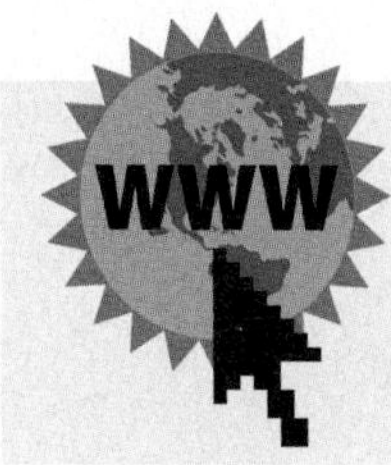

The complete chapter, learning objectives, and other resources can be found at **www.pharmacotherapyonline.com.**

Evaluation of Respiratory Function

e43

Megan L. Carreon, Maria I. Velez, Stephanie M. Levine, and Jay I. Peters

KEY CONCEPTS

1. The function of the lungs is to maintain the arterial partial pressure of oxygen (PaO_2) and arterial partial pressure of carbon dioxide ($PaCO_2$) within normal ranges (ie, normal ventilation-perfusion ratio).
2. The air in the lung is divided into four compartments: tidal volume—air exhaled during non-exertional breathing; inspiratory reserve volume (IRV)—maximal air *inhaled* above tidal volume; expiratory reserve volume (ERV)—maximum air *exhaled* after tidal volume; and residual volume (RV)—air remaining in the lung after maximal exhalation. The sum of all four components is the total lung capacity (TLC). Pulmonary function tests will produce values consistent with normal lungs or an obstructive or restrictive disease: recognition of these values is key.
3. Obstructive lung disease is defined as an inability to get air out of the lung. It is identified on spirometry when forced expiratory volume in the first second of expiration (FEV_1) compared to the forced vital capacity (FVC) (total amount of air that can be exhaled during a forced exhalation) (FEV_1/FVC) is less than 70% to 75% (0.70-0.75) in adults (or below the lower limit of normal [LLN] based on population studies).
4. An increase in FEV_1 of 12% (and greater than 0.2 L in adults) after an inhaled β-agonist suggests an acute bronchodilator response.
5. Restrictive lung disease is defined as an inability to get enough air into the lung and is best defined as a reduction in TLC (usually less than 80% of predicted).
6. Restrictive lung disease can be produced by a number of diseases, such as increased elastic recoil (interstitial lung disease), respiratory muscle weakness (myasthenia gravis), and mechanical restrictions (pleural effusion or kyphoscoliosis). It can also be the result of poor effort during the pulmonary function tests (PFTs).
7. The shape of the flow-volume loop, which includes inspiratory and expiratory flow-volume curves, and the ratio of forced expiratory and inspiratory flow at 50% of VC ($FEF_{50\%}/FIF_{50\%}$ greater than 1) may be useful in the diagnosis of upper airway obstruction.
8. Cardiopulmonary exercise testing allows for the assessment of multiple organs involved in exercise.
9. Spirometry and other pulmonary function tests in children are possible and can successfully be done with proper coaching methods and modified reference values.

BEYOND THE BOOK

Watch this brief video about when and how to perform spirometry: "Taking a Spirometry Test" from the National Heart, Lung & Blood Institute: http://https://youtu.be/Zs8Fs5HaJHs.

INTRODUCTION

The primary function of the respiratory system is to maintain normal arterial blood gases, that is, arterial partial pressure of oxygen (PaO_2) and arterial partial pressure of carbon dioxide ($PaCO_2$). To achieve this goal, several processes must be accomplished, including alveolar ventilation, pulmonary perfusion, ventilation-perfusion matching, and gas transfer across the alveolar-capillary membrane. Alveolar ventilation is achieved by the cyclic process of air movement in and out of the lung. During inspiration, the inspiratory muscles contract and generate a negative pressure in the pleural space. This pressure gradient between the mouth and the alveoli draws fresh air (tidal volume [V_T]) into the lung. Approximately one-third of the inspired gas stays in the conducting airways (dead space), and two-thirds reach the alveoli.

1 The human lung contains a series of branching, progressively tapering airways that originate at the glottis and terminate in a matrix of thin-walled alveoli. Coursing through this matrix of alveoli is a rich network of capillaries that originates from the pulmonary arterioles and terminates in the pulmonary venules. The adequacy of respiration in each gas exchange unit depends on the apposition of a thin film of mixed venous blood with just the right amount of fresh alveolar gas. During "ideal" gas exchange, blood flow and ventilation are uniform; accordingly, there is no alveolar-arterial difference (or gradient) in the partial pressure of oxygen ($P[A\text{–}a]O_2$, sometimes called the A–a gradient). However, gas exchange is not perfect, even in the normal lung. Normally, alveolar ventilation is less than pulmonary blood flow, and the overall ventilation-perfusion ratio is 0.8 (not 1.0).

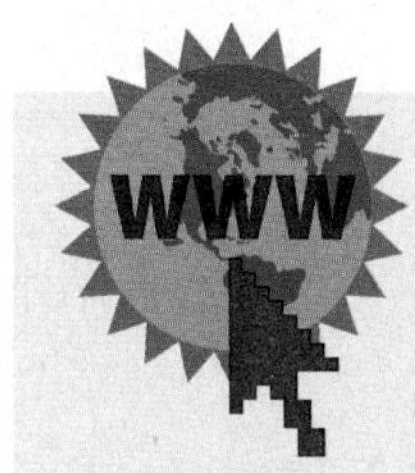

The complete chapter, learning objectives, and other resources can be found at **www.pharmacotherapyonline.com.**

44

Asthma

Kathryn V. Blake and Jean Y. Moon

KEY CONCEPTS

1. Asthma is a highly prevalent disease that is a result of genetic predisposition and environmental interactions; it is one of the most common chronic diseases of childhood.
2. Asthma is primarily a chronic inflammatory disease of the airways of the lung for which there is no known cure or primary prevention; the immunohistopathologic features include cell infiltration by neutrophils, eosinophils, T-helper type 2 lymphocytes, mast cells, and epithelial cells.
3. Chronic asthma is characterized by either the intermittent or persistent presence of highly variable degrees of airflow obstruction from airway wall inflammation and bronchial smooth muscle constriction; in some patients, persistent changes in airway structure occur.
4. Variability in response to medications requires individualization of therapy within existing evidence-based guidelines for management. This is most evident in patients with severe asthma phenotypes.
5. Ongoing patient education, for a partnership in asthma care, is essential for optimal patient outcomes and includes trigger avoidance and self-management techniques.
6. The inflammatory process in asthma is treated most effectively with corticosteroids, with the inhaled corticosteroids (ICS) having the greatest efficacy and safety profile for long-term management.
7. Acute bronchial smooth muscle constriction is prevented or treated most effectively with inhaled short-acting β_2-adrenergic receptor agonists (SABA); long-acting β_2-adrenergic receptor agonists (LABA) and long-acting muscarinic agonists (LAMA) are effective as daily maintenance bronchodilators when used in combination with ICS.
8. Intermittent as-needed SABA and an ICS used concomitantly in mild persistent asthma or the combination of ICS with formoterol (a long-acting β_2-adrenergic receptor agonist) used as daily maintenance and reliever therapy in moderate persistent asthma reduce exacerbation frequency.

BEYOND THE BOOK

Watch the five short videos in the series Asthma Management Academy https://www.youtube.com/watch?v=pC2BrtVTYrU. These videos provide a brief overview of the following topics:

- Module 1 Scope of Asthma
- Module 2 Triggers
- Module 3 Medications
- Module 4 Medication Devices
- Module 5 Monitoring and Assessment

The videos are useful to enhance students understanding of the consequences of asthma, triggers, medications, delivery devices, and monitoring. These videos are also useful for patient education.

INTRODUCTION

Asthma has been known since antiquity, yet it is a disease that still defies precise definition. The word asthma is of Greek origin and means "panting." More than 2,000 years ago, Hippocrates used the word asthma to describe episodic shortness of breath; however, the first detailed clinical description of a person with asthma was made by Aretaeus in the second century.[1]

The Global Initiative for Asthma (GINA) provides a practical definition of asthma[2]: "Asthma is a heterogeneous disease, usually characterized by chronic airway inflammation. It is defined by the history of respiratory symptoms such as wheeze, shortness of breath, chest tightness, and cough that vary over time and in intensity, together with variable expiratory airflow limitation." The National Institutes of Health, National Asthma Education and Prevention Program (NAEPP) Expert Panel Report 3 (EPR3), adds that the variable airflow obstruction is often reversible either spontaneously or with treatment although reversibility may not be complete in some patients with asthma.[3] To guide our current understanding and clinical management of asthma, healthcare providers in the United States often turn to the NAEPP and GINA guidelines.

EPIDEMIOLOGY

1 An estimated 25.1 million persons in the United States have asthma (about 7.8% of the population).[4] Asthma is the most common chronic disease among children in the United States affecting approximately 5 million children in 2019.[4] Self-reported asthma is more common in persons with incomes below $25,000 per year (prevalence rate 17%-20%) and among certain race and ethnic groups such as those who self-identify as multirace non-Hispanic (22.5%) and non-Hispanic Black (16.7%).[4] Adults are nearly five times more likely to die from asthma than children. The rate of death from asthma is highest in those aged 65 years and older, females, and non-Hispanic Black people (who have two to three times the death rate of non-Hispanic Whites or non-Hispanic others).[4] Biological differences in asthma factors between racial and ethnic groups have been observed (albuterol response, airway eosinophilia, low birth weight).[5-7] However, because asthma is a genetic disease strongly

influenced by environmental exposures, it is not fully understood if such differences are related to environmental factors that may be tied to sociodemographic characteristics.[5,7]

Influenza infection can result in serious complications in people with asthma, even those with mild disease and those who are well-controlled on medication. An annual influenza vaccination is an essential preventative measure in people with asthma. However, in 2015, only 47% of adults and 64% of children with asthma received the influenza vaccination. A higher percentage (80%) of children under 5 years received the influenza vaccine perhaps because they are more likely to have regular visits to the pediatrician.[4]

Approximately 65% of adults and 60% of children describe themselves as having persistent (vs intermittent) asthma. However, only 40% of adults and children report using long-term controller medications that are fundamental for the prevention and control of symptoms. Nearly 20% of children and 24% of adults report using a quick-relief medication (such as an inhaled short-acting inhaled β_2-agonist [SABA]) more than twice weekly, which is a marker for poorly controlled asthma.[4]

The estimated economic costs of asthma in the United States from 2008 to 2013 in US dollars was $80 billion in direct medical expenses, missed work or school, and death.[8] The societal burden of asthma (indirect medical expenditures such as loss of productivity and death) in the United States was $33 billion. Prescription drugs were the largest single direct medical expenditure per person.[8]

The natural history of asthma is still not well defined. Although asthma can develop at any age, it is principally a pediatric disease, with most patients with asthma being diagnosed by 5 years of age and up to 50% having symptoms by 2 years of age. Asthma is more common in boys until adolescence and between 30% and 70% of children with asthma will have marked improvement or become symptom-free by early adulthood but is more common in adult women than men. Asthma persists and becomes chronic in about 30% to 40% of patients. Generally, 20% or less develop severe chronic disease.[9] Atopy, a form of hypersensitivity to allergens, is present in 50% to 60% of children and adults with asthma; it is more common in adults who had the onset of disease during childhood and children with more severe asthma.[9]

In adults, most longitudinal studies have suggested a more rapid rate of decline in lung function in people with asthma when measured using forced expiratory volume in 1 second (FEV_1) and is more pronounced in those with severe disease.[9] Individuals with less-frequent asthma exacerbations and normal lung function on initial assessment have higher remission rates. Conversely, smokers have the lowest remission and highest relapse rates.[9] In those with persistent airway obstruction, asthma may become irreversible and worsen over time due to airway remodeling (described below). However, most patients do not die from disease progression and their life span is not different from the general population.

The worldwide prevalence, morbidity, and mortality from acute exacerbations of asthma have been relatively stable over the past 10 years.[10] However, those in the lowest sociodemographic groups are at a fivefold greater risk of death when compared to those in the highest sociodemographic group.[9] Most asthma deaths are preventable with appropriate recognition and treatment.[9]

Most deaths from asthma occur outside the hospital; death is rare after hospitalization. The most common cause of death from asthma is inadequate assessment of the severity of airway obstruction by the patient or healthcare professional and inadequate therapy. Thus, the key to preventing death from asthma is education to both patients and providers.[11,12]

ETIOLOGY

1 Epidemiologic studies strongly support the concept of a genetic predisposition plus environmental interaction to the development of asthma, yet the picture remains complex and incomplete.[13] Asthma represents a complex genetic disorder, in that the asthma phenotype is likely a result of polygenic inheritance of different combinations of genes. The initial genetic research focused on establishing links between atopy (genetically determined state of hypersensitivity to environmental allergens) and asthma. Genome-wide analyses found links with genes on multiple chromosomes that differ by racial groups.[13] Although genetic predisposition to atopy is a significant risk factor for developing asthma, not all atopic individuals develop asthma, nor do all patients with asthma exhibit atopy. Current efforts to identify asthma susceptibility are focused on epigenetics which are heritable characteristics that are modified by environmental influences.[13]

1 Environmental risk factors for the development of asthma include socioeconomic status, family size, exposure to secondhand tobacco smoke in infancy, and in utero, allergen exposure, ambient air pollution, urbanization, viral respiratory infections including respiratory syncytial virus (RSV) and rhinovirus, and decreased exposure to common childhood infectious agents.[9] The timing of and exposure to certain environmental factors during early childhood in genetically susceptible individuals is thought to predispose them to develop allergies and asthma by triggering the allergic immunologic system (T-helper cell type 2 [Th_2] [Th_2 high asthma] lymphocytes) to develop instead of the system to fight infections (T-helper type 1 [Th_1] [Th_2 low asthma] lymphocytes).[9,14] The first 2 to 3 years of life are most important for the exposures to produce an alteration in the immune response system.[14]

Risk factors for early (less than 3 years of age) recurrent wheezing associated with viral infections include preterm birth, low birth weight, male gender, and parental smoking. However, this early pattern is due to smaller airways, and these risk factors are not believed to be risk factors for developing asthma in later life.[14] Atopy is the predominant risk factor for children to subsequently develop asthma.[14] Asthma can begin later in life in adults. Occupational asthma in previously healthy individuals emphasizes the effect of the environment on the development of asthma.[9] The heterogeneity of the asthma phenotype is most obvious when reviewing the diverse list of protective factors and risk factors (Fig. 44-1).[14] These factors have relative degrees of importance. Environmental exposures are the most important precipitants of severe asthma exacerbations. Epidemics of severe asthma in cities have followed exposures to high concentrations of aeroallergens. Viral respiratory tract infections remain the single most common precipitant of severe asthma in children and are an important trigger in adults as well.[15] Other factors precipitating asthma exacerbations include air pollution, emotions, exercise, occupational exposures, and drugs.

PATHOPHYSIOLOGY

Asthma is a chronic airway inflammatory disease stemming from the effects of numerous inflammatory cells and mediators to manifest in clinical characteristics and pathophysiological changes leading to expiratory airflow limitation.[2] Airway narrowing is the ultimate endpoint of the inflammatory processes and is a function of airway smooth muscle contraction, with potential remodeling due to structural changes, and airway plugging by mucus hypersecretion which leads to the common symptoms of asthma, wheeze, shortness of breath, chest tightness, and/or cough. Symptoms may be intermittent (weeks or months between symptoms) or may occur frequently and may resolve spontaneously or following treatment. Over time, asthma can progress to persistent airflow limitations. In addition, bronchial hyperresponsiveness (BHR) is a characteristic functional abnormality of asthma and is the heightened response to a stimulus (eg, cat dander) not observed in healthy individuals that enhances the susceptibility to airway narrowing.[2]

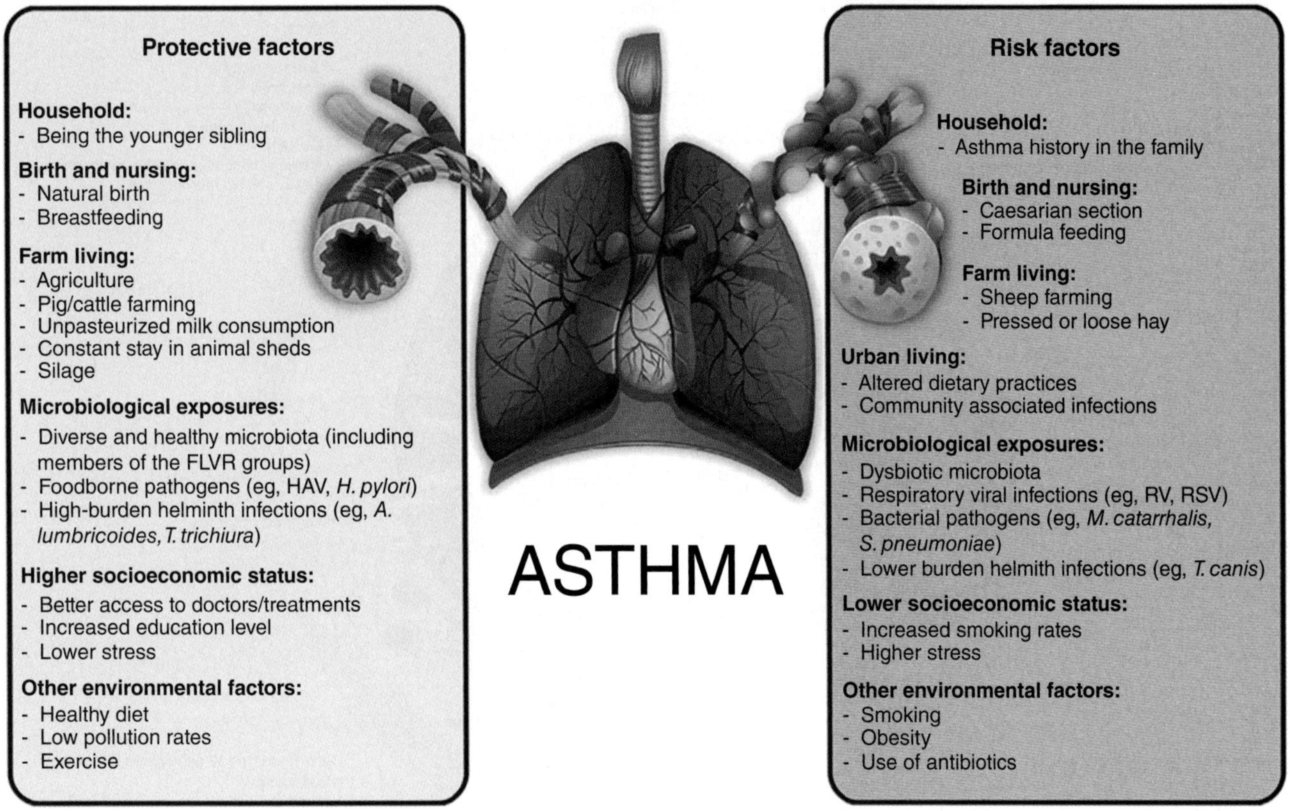

FIGURE 44-1 Factors that are associated with protecting against, or risk for, developing asthma. These various factors have relative degrees of importance from patient to patient. *(Reprinted from van Tilburg Bernardes E, Arrieta MC. Hygiene hypothesis in asthma development: Is hygiene to blame? Arch Med Res. 2017;48(8):717–726.)*

To understand the pathogenetic mechanisms that underlie the many asthma phenotypes, it is critical to identify factors that initiate, intensify, and modulate the inflammatory response of the airways and to determine how these processes produce the characteristic airway abnormalities. Current and evolving treatments target these inflammatory processes (Fig. 44-2).

Inflammatory Processes

Airway inflammation is multifaceted and the primary focus of asthma management and prevention. It has been demonstrated in all forms of asthma, and an association between the extent of inflammation and the clinical severity of asthma has been demonstrated in selected studies. Both central and peripheral airways are inflamed.

The use of inhaled allergen challenge models has contributed significantly to understanding the inflammatory cascade in the airways. Allergen inhalation in allergic patients causes an early-phase reaction (within minutes) that, in some cases, may be followed by a late-phase reaction (hours later). The early phase is initiated by the activation of cells bearing allergen-specific immunoglobulin E (IgE). It is characterized by the rapid activation of airway mast cells and macrophages leading to the rapid release of pro-inflammatory mediators such as histamine, eicosanoids, and reactive oxygen (O_2) species that induce contraction of airway smooth muscle, mucus secretion, and edema. The bronchial microcirculation has an essential role in this inflammatory process. Inflammatory mediators induce microvascular leakage with the exudation of plasma in the airways. Acute plasma protein leakage induces a thickened, engorged, and edematous airway wall and a consequent narrowing of the airway lumen. Plasma exudation may compromise epithelial integrity, and the presence of plasma in the lumen may reduce mucus clearance. Plasma proteins also may promote the formation of exudative plugs mixed with mucus and inflammatory and epithelial cells. Together these effects contribute to airflow obstruction (see Fig. 44-2).

The late-phase inflammatory reaction occurs 6 to 9 hours after allergen provocation and involves the recruitment and activation of eosinophils, $CD4^+$ thymically derived lymphocytes (T-cells), basophils, neutrophils, and macrophages.[16] There is selective retention of airway T-cells, the expression of adhesion molecules, and the release of selected pro-inflammatory mediators and cytokines involved in the recruitment and activation of inflammatory cells.[16] The activation of T-cells after allergen challenge leads to the release of Th_2-related cytokines that may modulate the late-phase response.[16] The release of preformed cytokines by mast cells is the likely initial trigger for the early recruitment of inflammatory cells that then recruit and induce the more persistent involvement by T-cells.[9,16] The enhancement of nonspecific BHR usually can be demonstrated after the late-phase reaction but not after the early-phase reaction following allergen or occupational challenge.

In asthma, all cells of the airways are involved and become activated (Fig. 44-2). Included are eosinophils, neutrophils, T-cells, mast cells, alveolar macrophages, and dendritic cells, epithelial cells, fibroblasts, and bronchial smooth muscle cells. These cells also regulate airway inflammation and initiate the process of remodeling by the release of cytokines and growth factors.[17]

Inflammatory Cells

Epithelial Cells Bronchial epithelial cells participate in mucociliary clearance and removal of noxious agents. Stimuli such as allergens and air pollution stimulate epithelial cells to release various cytokines such as eicosanoids, peptidases, matrix proteins, periostin,

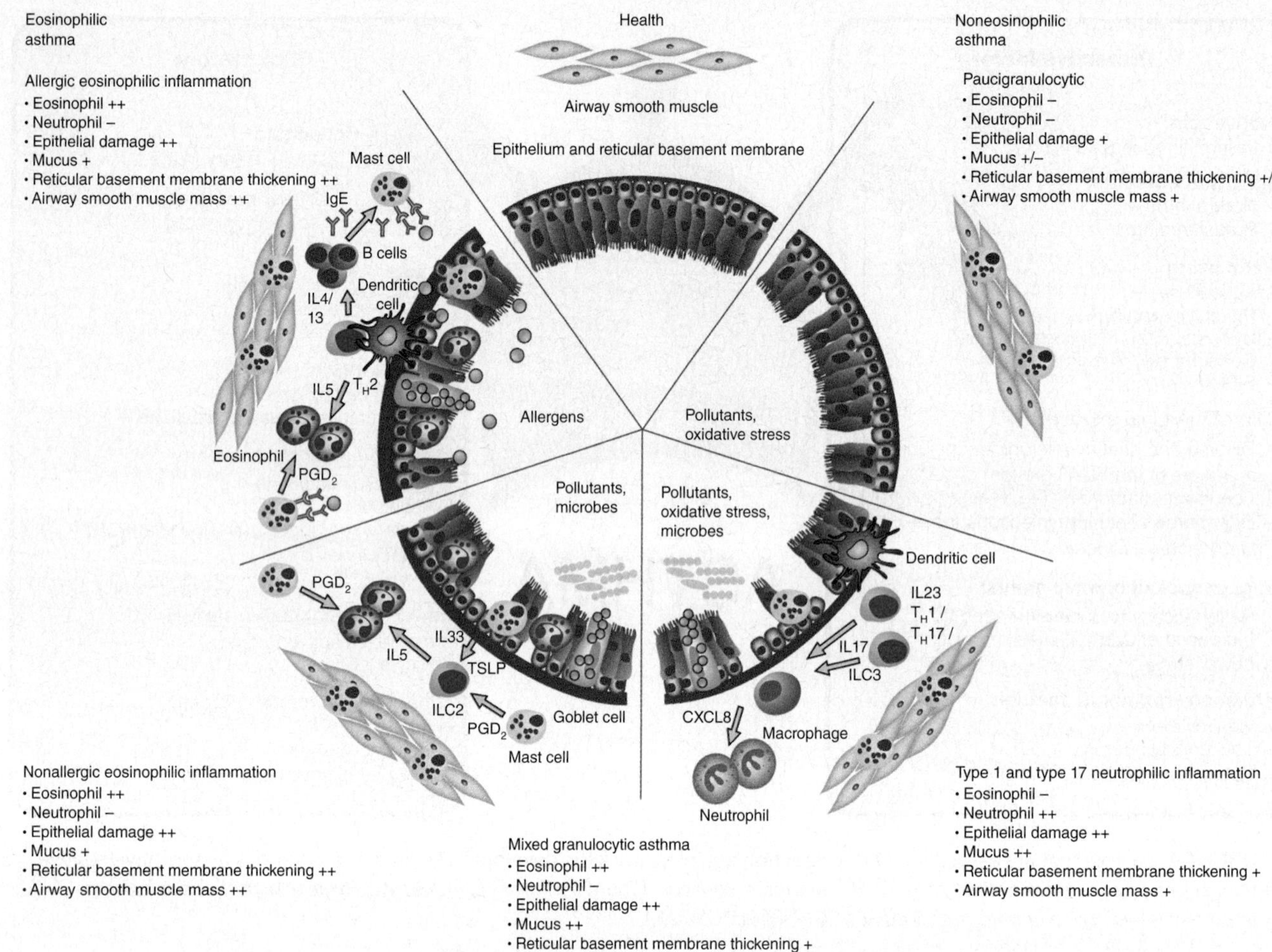

FIGURE 44-2 Diagrammatic presentation of the relationship between inflammatory cells, lipid and preformed mediators, inflammatory cytokines, and proposed pathogenesis and clinical presentation in asthma. (See text for details.) (IL, interleukin; PG, prostaglandin; TSLP, thymic stromal lymphopoietin; CXCL8, C-X-C motif chemokine ligand 8; ILC2, type 2 innate lymphoid cells; Th, T helper.) *(Reprinted from Papi A, Brightling C, Pedersen SE, Reddel HK. Asthma. Lancet. 2018;391(10122):783–800.)*

cytokines, chemokines, and nitric oxide (NO).[16] Periostin is an extracellular matrix protein secreted by epithelial cells that induces the inflammatory cytokines, interleukin 4 (IL-4), and interleukin 13 (IL-13).[18] It has become important more recently as a biomarker of persistent eosinophilic airway inflammation and may have an integral role in airway remodeling, subepithelial fibrosis, and mucus regulation.[18,19] Epithelial cells can be activated by IgE-dependent mechanisms, viruses, pollutants, or histamine. In asthma, especially fatal asthma, extensive epithelial shedding occurs. The functional consequences of epithelial shedding may include heightened BHR, the release of the chemokine eotaxin that attracts eosinophils, altered permeability of the airway mucosa, depletion of epithelial-derived relaxant factors, and loss of enzymes responsible for degrading proinflammatory neuropeptides. The integrity of airway epithelium may influence the sensitivity of the airways to various provocative stimuli. Epithelial cells may also be important in the regulation of airway remodeling and fibrosis.[9,16]

Eosinophils Eosinophils play an effector role in asthma by releasing pro-inflammatory mediators, cytotoxic mediators, and cytokines.[9] Circulating eosinophils migrate to the airways by cell rolling, through interactions with selectins, and eventually adhere to the endothelium through the binding of integrins to adhesion proteins (vascular cell adhesion molecule 1 [VCAM-1] and intercellular adhesion molecule 1 [ICAM-1]). As eosinophils enter the matrix of the membrane, their survival is prolonged by IL-5 and granulocyte-macrophage colony-stimulating factor (GM-CSF). On activation, eosinophils release inflammatory mediators such as leukotrienes (LTs) and granule proteins to injure airway tissue.[9]

Lymphocytes Mucosal biopsy specimens from patients with asthma contain lymphocytes, many of which express surface markers of inflammation. There are two types of T-helper CD4+ cells. Th_1 cells produce IL-2 and interferon-γ (IFN-γ), both essential for cellular defense mechanisms. Th_2 cells produce cytokines (IL-4, IL-5, and IL-13) that mediate allergic inflammation. It is known that Th_1 cytokines inhibit the production of Th_2 cytokines, and vice versa. It is hypothesized that allergic asthmatic inflammation results from a Th_2-mediated mechanism (an imbalance between Th_1 and Th_2 cells).[16] However, it has also been observed that there exists a low Th_2 cytokine phenotype of asthma in adults that appears more resistant to usual therapies for asthma.[16]

Th_1 and Th_2 Endotypes Th_2 high asthma is characterized by activation of mediators such as IL-25 and IL-33 which subsequently activate IL-4, IL-5, and IL-13, as well as non-interleukin-dependent factors such as thymic stromal lymphopoietin (TSLP).[18,19] Inflammation occurs as a result of exposure of the airway epithelium to inhaled allergens, microbes, and inhaled pollutants (thus encompassing allergic and non-allergic inflammation) and occurs in approximately half of all patients with asthma.[19] The effects of these mediators result in inflammatory cell activation and secretion of IgE as well as the airway epithelium and smooth muscle.

Th_2 low asthma is described as neutrophilic asthma or mixed, pauci-granulocytic asthma, and is less well understood.[18,19] Patients are typically less responsive to corticosteroids, have fewer allergic symptoms, and are diagnosed later in life.

The T-cell population in the cord blood of newborn infants is skewed toward a Th_2 phenotype. The extent of the imbalance between Th_1 and Th_2 cells (as indicated by diminished IFN-γ production) during the neonatal phase may predict the subsequent development of allergic disease, asthma, or both. It has been suggested that infants at high risk of asthma and allergies should be exposed to stimuli that upregulate Th_1-mediated responses in order to restore the balance during a critical time in the development of the immune system and the lungs.

The basic premise of the Th_1 and Th_2 imbalance is that the newborn's immune system needs timely and appropriate environmental stimuli to create a balanced immune response. Factors that enhance Th_1-mediated responses include endotoxin exposure, such as increased exposure to infections through contact with older siblings and daycare attendance during the first 6 months of life.[20] Restoration of the balance between Th_1 and Th_2 cells may be impeded by frequent administration of oral antibiotics, with concomitant alterations in GI flora. Other factors favoring the Th_2 phenotype include residence in an industrialized country, urban environment exposure, diet, and sensitization to house dust mites and cockroaches.[18,19]

Mast cells Mast cell degranulation is important in the initiation of immediate responses following exposure to allergens.[3] Mast cells reside throughout the walls of the respiratory tract, and increased numbers of these cells (threefold to fivefold) have been observed in the airways of patients with asthma and atopy.[21] Once binding of allergen to cell-bound IgE occurs, mediators such as histamine; eosinophil and neutrophil chemotactic factors; LTs C_4, D_4, and E_4; prostaglandins; platelet-activating factor (PAF); and others are released from mast cells (see Fig. 44-2). Histologic examination has revealed decreased numbers of granulated mast cells in the airways of patients who have died from acute asthma attacks, suggesting that mast cell degranulation is a contributing factor. Sensitized mast cells are also activated by osmotic stimuli to account for exercise-induced bronchospasm (EIB).[22]

Alveolar Macrophages The primary function of alveolar macrophages in the normal airway is to serve as "scavengers," engulfing and digesting bacteria and other foreign materials. Macrophages are found in large and small airways, ideally located for affecting the asthmatic response. A number of mediators produced and released by macrophages have been identified, including pro-inflammatory and anti-inflammatory cytokines, reactive oxygen species, and eicosanoids.[23] In addition, alveolar macrophages are able to produce neutrophil chemotactic factor and eosinophil chemotactic factor, which in turn amplify the inflammatory process.

Neutrophils The role of neutrophils in the pathogenesis of asthma remains somewhat unclear because they normally reside in low numbers in the airway. Though they usually do not infiltrate tissues showing chronic allergic inflammation, they are instrumental in the inflammation arising from occupational exposures such as particulate matter, ozone, and diesel exhaust. Neutrophils can be involved in late-phase inflammatory reactions. However, high numbers of neutrophils have been observed in the airways of patients who died from sudden-onset fatal asthma and in those with severe disease.[24] This suggests that neutrophils may play a pivotal role in the disease process, at least in some patients with long-standing or corticosteroid-resistant asthma.[24] The neutrophil can also be a source for a variety of mediators, including PAF, prostaglandins, thromboxanes, and LTs, that contribute to BHR and airway inflammation.[24]

Fibroblasts and Myofibroblasts Fibroblasts are found frequently in connective tissue. Human lung fibroblasts may behave as inflammatory cells on activation by IL-4 and IL-13. The myofibroblast may contribute to the regulation of inflammation via the release of cytokines and to tissue remodeling. In asthma, myofibroblasts are increased in numbers beneath the reticular basement membrane, and there is an association between their numbers and the thickness of the reticular basement membrane.[9]

Inflammatory Mediators

Associated with asthma for many years, histamine is capable of inducing smooth muscle constriction and bronchospasm and is thought to play a role in mucosal edema and mucus secretion.[21] Lung mast cells are an important source of histamine. The release of histamine can be stimulated by exposure of the airways to a variety of factors, including physical stimuli (airway drying with exercise) and relevant allergens.[21] Histamine is involved in acute bronchospasm following allergen exposure; however, other mediators such as LTs are also involved.

Besides histamine release, mast cell degranulation releases ILs, proteases, and other enzymes that activate the production of other mediators of inflammation. Several classes of important mediators, including arachidonic acid and its metabolites (ie, prostaglandins, LTs, and PAF), are derived from cell membrane phospholipids.[21]

Once arachidonic acid is released, it can be metabolized by the enzyme cyclooxygenase to form prostaglandins. Prostaglandin D_2 is a potent bronchoconstricting agent; however, it is unlikely to produce sustained effects and its role in asthma remains to be determined. Similarly, prostaglandin $F_2\alpha$ is a potent bronchoconstrictor in patients with asthma and can enhance the effects of histamine.[21] However, its pathophysiologic role in asthma is unclear. Another cyclooxygenase product, prostacyclin (prostaglandin I_2), is known to be produced in the lung and may contribute to inflammation and edema owing to its effects as a vasodilator.

Thromboxane A_2 is produced by alveolar macrophages, fibroblasts, epithelial cells, neutrophils, and platelets within the lung.[25] It may have several effects, including bronchoconstriction, involvement in the late asthmatic response, and involvement in the development of airway inflammation and BHR.

The 5-lipoxygenase pathway of arachidonic acid metabolism is responsible for the production of the cysteinyl LTs.[25] LTC_4, LTD_4, and LTE_4 are released during inflammatory processes in the lung. LTs D_4 and E_4 share a common receptor (LTD_4 receptor) that, when stimulated, produces bronchospasm, mucus secretion, microvascular permeability, and airway edema, whereas LTB_4 is involved with granulocyte chemotaxis.

Thought to be produced by macrophages, eosinophils, and neutrophils within the lung, PAF is involved in the mediation of bronchospasm, sustained induction of BHR, edema formation, and chemotaxis of eosinophils.[26]

Adhesion Molecules

Adhesion molecules are glycoproteins that facilitate infiltration and migration of inflammatory cells to the site of inflammation by enhancing cell-cell communication.[27] Adhesion molecules are divided into families on the basis of their chemical structure. These families are the integrins, cadherins, immunoglobulin supergene family, selectins, vascular adressins, and carbohydrate ligands.[27] Those thought to be important in inflammation include the integrins, immunoglobulin supergene family, selectins, and carbohydrate ligands, including ICAM-1 and VCAM-1.[27] Adhesion molecules are found on a variety of cells, such as neutrophils, monocytes, lymphocytes, basophils, eosinophils, granulocytes, platelets, endothelial cells, and epithelial cells, and can be expressed or activated by the many inflammatory mediators present in asthma.[27]

Nitric Oxide

NO is produced by cells within the respiratory tract. It has been thought to be a neurotransmitter of the nonadrenergic, noncholinergic (NANC) nervous system.[28] Endogenous NO is generated from the amino acid L-arginine (L-Arg) by the enzyme NO synthase.[28] Three isoforms of NO synthase exist. One isoform is induced in response to pro-inflammatory cytokines, inducible NO synthase (iNOS), in airway epithelial cells and inflammatory cells of asthmatic airways.[28] NO produces smooth muscle relaxation in the vasculature and bronchials. However, it amplifies the inflammatory process and is unlikely to be of therapeutic benefit. Investigations measuring the fraction of exhaled NO (FeNO) concentrations have suggested that it may be a useful measure of ongoing allergic lower airway inflammation in patients with asthma and for guiding asthma therapy.[28]

Airway Smooth Muscle

The airway smooth muscle extends from the trachea through the respiratory bronchioles. Total smooth muscle mass decreases rapidly past the terminal bronchioles to the alveoli, so the contribution of smooth muscle tone to airway diameter in this region is relatively small. It is possible that the increased smooth muscle mass of the asthmatic airways is important in magnifying and maintaining BHR in persistent disease. However, the hypertrophy and hyperplasia are secondary processes caused by chronic inflammation and are not the primary cause of BHR.[29]

The airway smooth muscle is innervated by parasympathetic, sympathetic, and nonadrenergic inhibitory nerves.[30] Parasympathetic innervation of the smooth muscle consists of efferent motor fibers in the vagus nerves and sensory afferent fibers in the vagus and other nerves.[30] Normal resting tone of human airway smooth muscle is regulated by vagal nerve activity. Bronchoconstriction caused by vagal stimulation occurs in the small bronchi but is absent in the small bronchioles. The nonmyelinated C fibers are the predominate nerves of the afferent system are present throughout the airways with terminals in airway smooth muscle cells, epithelial cells, and airway ganglia.[30] These nerve endings probably represent the irritant receptors of the airways. Stimulation of these irritant receptors by mechanical stimulation, chemical, and particulate irritants, and pharmacologic agents such as histamine produces reflex bronchoconstriction.[30]

The NANC nervous system has been described in the trachea and bronchi. Substance P, neurokinin A, neurokinin B, and vasoactive intestinal peptide (VIP) are the best-characterized neurotransmitters in the NANC nervous system.[30] VIP is an inhibitory neurotransmitter. Inflammatory cells in asthma can release peptidases that can degrade VIP, producing exaggerated reflex cholinergic bronchoconstriction. NANC excitatory neuropeptides such as substance P and neurokinin A are released by stimulation of C-fiber sensory nerve endings.

Remodeling of the Airways

Acute inflammation is a beneficial response to tissue injury and generally leads to repair and restoration of the normal structure and function. In contrast, asthma is a chronic inflammatory process that leads to abnormal airway healing referred to as *remodeling*.[17] Repair involves replacing parenchymal cells with connective tissue that mature into scar tissue. In asthma, remodeling leads to extracellular matrix fibrosis, an increase in smooth muscle and mucous gland mass, and angiogenesis.[17]

The precise mechanisms of remodeling the airways are under intense study. Airway remodeling is of concern because it may represent an irreversible process that can have serious sequelae including the development of chronic obstructive pulmonary disease (COPD).[17] Observations in children with asthma indicate that some loss of lung function may occur during the first 5 years of life.[17] Importantly, no current therapies have been shown to alter either lung growth or the progressive loss of lung function.

Mucus Production

The mucociliary system is the lung's primary defense mechanism against irritants and infectious agents. Mucus, composed of 95% water and 5% glycoproteins, is produced by bronchial epithelial glands and gobleT-cells.[27] The lining of the airways consists of a continuous aqueous layer controlled by active ion transport across the epithelium in which water moves toward the lumen along the concentration gradient. Catecholamines and vagal stimulation enhance the ion transport and fluid movement. Mucus transport depends on its viscoelastic properties. Mucus that is either too watery or too viscous will not be transported optimally. The exudative inflammatory process and sloughing of epithelial cells into the airway lumen impair mucociliary transport. The bronchial glands are increased in size and the goblet cells are increased in size and number in asthma. Expectorated mucus from patients with asthma tends to have a high viscosity. The mucous plugs in the airways of patients who died in status asthmaticus are tenacious and tend to be connected by mucous strands to the goblet cells.[27] The airways of persons with asthma also may become plugged with casts consisting of epithelial and inflammatory cells. Although it is tempting to speculate that death from asthma attacks is a result of the mucous plugging resulting in irreversible obstruction, there is no direct evidence for this. Autopsies of asthmatics who died from other causes have shown similar pathology. In addition, some patients who have died of sudden severe asthma did not show the characteristic mucous plugging on necropsy.

Bronchial Hyperresponsiveness

Chronic inflammation is associated with nonspecific BHR and increases the risk of asthma exacerbations. Exacerbations are characterized by increased symptoms and worsening airway obstruction over a period of days or even weeks, and rarely, hours. Hyper-responsiveness of the airways to physical, chemical, and pharmacologic stimuli is a hallmark of asthma.[3] BHR also occurs in some patients with chronic bronchitis and allergic rhinitis.[3] Normal healthy subjects may also develop a transient BHR after viral respiratory infections or ozone exposure. However, the degree of BHR in patients with asthma is quantitatively greater than in other populations. Bronchial responsiveness of the general population fits a unimodal distribution that is skewed toward increased reactivity; individuals with clinical asthma represent the extreme end of this distribution. The degree of BHR within asthma correlates with its clinical course and medication requirement necessary to control symptoms.[3] Patients with mild symptoms or in remission demonstrate lower levels of BHR. The current understanding is that the BHR seen in asthma is at least in part due to and correlative with the extent of airway inflammation.[9]

Factors Contributing to Asthma Severity and Persistence

Viral Respiratory Infections

Viral respiratory infections are primarily responsible for exacerbations of asthma, particularly in children younger than 10 years.[15] Children aged 5 years or younger may have wheezing (which may or may not be asthma) associated with upper respiratory tract infections.[2] Infants are particularly susceptible to airway obstruction and wheezing with viral infections because of their small airways. Approximately 30% to 40% of infants who have severe RSV bronchiolitis will have recurrent wheezing but the subsequent prevalence of asthma is 5% to 10% in children.[15] The most common cause of exacerbations in both children and adults is the rhinovirus, which is the most frequent virus associated with the common cold and distributed worldwide.[15] Other viruses isolated include RSV, parainfluenza virus, adenoviruses, coronavirus, and influenza viruses. Certain viruses (RSV and parainfluenza virus) are capable of inducing specific IgE antibodies, and rhinovirus can activate eosinophils directly in asthmatics.[15] The increase in asthma symptoms and BHR that occurs may last for days or weeks following the resolution of the symptoms of the viral infection. Evidence does not support a beneficial effect of the influenza vaccine for preventing asthma exacerbations from subsequent influenza infections.[3] However, patients with moderate-to-severe asthma should be vaccinated against influenza annually.[31]

Coronavirus Disease (COVID-19)

Asthma does not appear to predispose patients with asthma or make them at increased susceptibility to COVID-19 infection. Nor does it increase the risk of severe infection or death.[12] However, the epidemiology of COVID-19 infection and its relationship to preexisting conditions, such as asthma, is continuing to be explored as new data emerge. Nonetheless, the use of oral corticosteroids, which are used for the treatment of an asthma exacerbation and severe chronic asthma, may increase the risk of death from COVID-19.[12] Patients who have severe asthma requiring long-term daily oral corticosteroids should not discontinue treatment abruptly due to the risk of serious withdrawal symptoms and even death resulting from long-term adrenal gland suppression. Other treatments for severe asthma such as biologics or immunosuppressants may need to be considered if oral corticosteroids are tapered and discontinued under the supervision of their provider.

Some data indicate that patients who used inhaled corticosteroids (ICS) chronically to treat asthma and were hospitalized with COVID-19 had a lower risk of death than those without an underlying respiratory disease.[12] Therefore, patients should continue their prescribed inhaled ICS if they become infected with COVID-19. It may be difficult to distinguish symptoms of worsening asthma induced by a viral respiratory infection versus COVID-19 symptoms; therefore, an asthma action plan should be instituted or reinforced.

For patients who become infected with COVID-19 and who use a nebulizer for delivery of asthma medications, every effort should be made to transition the patient to an inhaler with a valved spacer and tight-fitting face mask if appropriate. Nebulizers can transmit respiratory viral particles for at least 1 m from the patient which places others at risk of infection.[12] Importantly, inhalers and spacers should not be shared between patients, and spacers should be regularly cleaned and disinfected.

Patients with asthma should be encouraged to receive a COVID-19 vaccination. There are no data to indicate an increased risk of adverse effects in patients with asthma who are vaccinated.[12] However, vaccinations should be administered in a setting where treatment of anaphylaxis is available. Those who have a history of severe allergic reactions to polyethylene glycol or other vaccine ingredients should not be vaccinated with the Pfizer/BioNTech or Moderna vaccines. Biologic drugs used for the treatment of asthma should not be administered on the same day as the COVID-19 vaccination simply to distinguish any emergent adverse effects between the two medications.[12] Patients with asthma can receive the annual influenza vaccination concurrently with the COVID-19 vaccination.

Environmental and Occupational Factors

The development and heterogeneity of persistent asthma are driven by complex gene-environment interactions. Agents and events that are known to trigger asthma are listed in Table 44-1. The mechanisms for inducing symptoms are as varied as the exposure factor and include both IgE- and cell-mediated reactions.[31] The World Allergy Organization (WAO) predicts an increase in the incidence and prevalence of asthma due to environmental exposures from climate change.[32] Greater temperature variability, industrial pollution, more frequent forest fires, a higher concentration of ground-level ozone, increased transboundary movement of respiratory infectious agents, and changes in aeroallergen distribution are all cited

TABLE 44-1 List of Agents and Events Triggering Asthma Exacerbations

Respiratory infection
Respiratory syncytial virus (RSV), rhinovirus, coronavirus, influenza, parainfluenza, *Mycoplasma pneumonia*, *Chlamydia*, chronic rhinosinusitis
Allergens
Airborne pollens (grass, trees, weeds), house dust mites, animal dander, rodents, cockroaches, fungal spores
Environment
Cold air, fog, ozone, sulfur dioxide, nitrogen dioxide, tobacco smoke (including second and third hand), wood smoke, energy-efficient buildings (increase indoor air pollution), meteorological conditions related to climate change, scented home products, cleaners, and perfumes
Emotions
Anxiety, stress, laughter
Exercise
Particularly in a cold, dry climate
Drugs/preservatives
Acetaminophen, Aspirin, NSAIDs (cyclooxygenase inhibitors), sulfites, benzalkonium chloride, nonselective β-blockers, higher airway reversibility to β_2-agonist
Occupational stimuli
Bakers (flour dust); farmers (hay mold); spice and enzyme workers; occupational cleaners, printers (Arabic gum); chemical workers (azo dyes, anthraquinone, ethylenediamine, toluene diisocyanates, polyvinyl chloride); plastics, rubber, and wood workers (formaldehyde, western cedar, dimethylethanolamine, anhydrides)
Host factors
Obesity, African American race, Hispanic ethnicity, low socioeconomic status

factors. Sulfur dioxide in the ambient atmosphere is highly irritating and presumably induces bronchoconstriction through mast cell or irritant-receptor involvement.[33] Asthma produced by repeated prolonged exposure to industrial inhalants is a significant health problem. It has been estimated that 25% of adult-onset asthma worldwide is occupationally related.[33] Occupational asthma can be difficult to diagnose as the latency between exposure and symptom development can extend from months to years.[33] Persons with occupational asthma have the typical symptoms of asthma with cough, dyspnea, and wheezing. Typically, the symptoms are related to workplace exposure and improve on days off and during vacations.[33] Once occupational asthma has developed, the symptoms persist in most patients even after exposure is no longer present.[33]

Stress, Depression, and Psychosocial Factors

Observational studies demonstrate an association between increased stress and worsening asthma, but the role is not clearly defined.[3] Bronchoconstriction from psychological factors is mediated primarily through excess parasympathetic input. Atropine has been shown to block experimental psychogenic bronchoconstriction. Persons with asthma are more likely to have depression than those without asthma. The episodic nature of both diseases may be related to abnormal expression of Th2 cytokines that have effects in the brain as well as the airway. It is most important to emphasize to both patients and parents of children with asthma that asthma is not an emotional disease. However, coping skills may benefit the patient who becomes emotionally distraught during an asthma exacerbation.

Chronic Rhinosinusitis

Disorders of the upper respiratory tract, particularly rhinitis and sinusitis, have been linked with asthma. The prevalence of allergic sensitization increases with asthma severity; nasal polyposis is often seen in those with allergic rhinitis. It has been postulated that the transport of mucus chemotactic factors and inflammatory mediators from nasal passages during allergic rhinitis into the lungs may accentuate BHR. However, chronic sinusitis may just represent a nonbacterial coexisting condition in patients with asthma and allergies because the histologic changes in the paranasal sinuses are similar to those seen in the lung and nose. Thus, it would seem that treatment of rhinosinusitis could improve asthma control. However, a large study of children and adults found that treatment of chronic sinonasal disease with intranasal corticosteroids for 6 months improved neither asthma control nor BHR, suggesting that the treatment of sinus disease and asthma should be separately managed.[12]

Gastroesophageal Reflux Disease

Symptoms of gastroesophageal reflux disease (GERD), as well as asymptomatic reflux, are common in both children and adults who have asthma.[12] Nocturnal asthma may be associated with nighttime reflux. Reflux of acidic gastric contents into the esophagus is thought to initiate a vagally mediated reflex bronchoconstriction. Also of concern is that most medications that decrease airway smooth muscle tone have a relaxant effect on gastroesophageal sphincter tone. There is no benefit from screening or treating asymptomatic reflux in patients with asthma (Evidence A).[12] However, for patients who have asthma and symptoms of reflux, a trial of anti-reflux medication may improve reflux symptoms; if there is no resolution, further evaluation is warranted.[12] Treatment with proton pump inhibitors does not improve asthma control even in those with documented reflux.[12]

Microbiome

As the role of microbes in human health and disease continues to unfold, there is an increased investigation into the airway and gastrointestinal microbiome's relationship to asthma.[34] Patients with asthma and other obstructive lung diseases have shown differences in the lower airway microbiome compared with healthy individuals.[34] Evidence suggests that treatment-resistant asthma and worse lung function of select patients may be correlated to microbiota differences in the sputum. The upper airway microbiome has different microbiota than the lower airway by which pressure and temperature changes favor certain bacterial populations.[34] In a population-based study following infants to children, those with an altered nasal microbiota (eg, persistent *Moraxella* sparsity) were found to be at higher risk for developing asthma.[35] The gut microbiota is better studied and correlates to the risk of allergic sensitization and infant response to viral respiratory tract infections. As these relationships of the microbiome are further studied, the potential for developing strategies for the prevention and development of asthma may be possible.

Female Hormones

Asthma symptoms may vary significantly during different stages of the menstrual cycle. Premenstrual worsening of asthma symptoms has been reported in 20% of women and worsening of pulmonary function has been observed in women who do not report worsening symptoms.[36] Women with premenstrual symptoms tend to be older, have a higher body mass index, more severe asthma, aspirin sensitivity, and a longer duration of asthma.[36] The pathophysiology is uncertain because estrogen replacement in postmenopausal women has been shown to worsen asthma, whereas estradiol and progesterone administration has been reported to both improve or have no effect on asthma in women with premenstrual asthma.[36] Some studies have reported an increase in ED visits by women who were premenstrual, whereas others have reported no association with the menstrual phase.[36] Pregnancy may cause worsening, improvement, or no change in asthma symptoms, and the changes seem to occur with equal frequency.[36]

Foods, Additives, Supplements, and Vitamins

Food chemicals, specifically sulfites used as preservatives, can trigger life-threatening asthma exacerbations. Beer, wine, dried fruit, and open salad bars, in particular, have high concentrations of metabisulfites.[3] Food avoidance is only recommended when there is clear documentation of allergy or food chemical sensitivity.[12]

Aspirin and other nonsteroidal anti-inflammatory drugs can cause severe asthma exacerbations (aspirin-exacerbated respiratory disease).[12] The mechanism is related to cyclooxygenase-1 (COX-1) inhibition. Inhaled corticosteroids (ICSs) are the primary preventive treatment although oral corticosteroids may be required; leukotriene receptor antagonists (LTRAs) may be useful.[12] Aspirin sensitivity occurs in 7% of adults with asthma and is associated with a more severe disease.[12] While nonselective β-blocking agents do not precipitate bronchospasm, they can prevent reversal.

Vitamin D supplementation may be beneficial to reduce asthma exacerbations in patients who require oral corticosteroids and have low 25-hydroxyvitamin D plasma concentrations (<10 ng/mL [25 nmol/L]).[12] However, high-quality studies confirming improvements in asthma control or reductions in exacerbations are lacking.[12]

The impact of the maternal diet on allergy and asthma development has been a research focus of interest. In a systematic review, fish oil supplementation or dietary intake of fish during pregnancy had no consistent effects on the risk of wheeze, asthma, or atopy in the child.[12] Some evidence indicates that maternal intake of peanut and milk products are associated with decreases in allergy and asthma in the offspring. Due to limited evidence, dietary changes during pregnancy are not recommended now.

Obesity

Epidemiologic data suggest that obesity increases the prevalence of asthma and may reduce asthma control, although it is difficult to distinguish obesity-induced respiratory symptoms from true asthma symptoms because obesity often precedes the onset of asthma. Lung volume and tidal volume are reduced in obesity, promoting airway narrowing. Obesity also produces low-grade systemic inflammation that may act on the lung to worsen asthma. The mechanism may include the release of adipose-derived pro-inflammatory mediators such as IL-6, IL-10, eotaxin, tumor necrosis factor-α, transforming growth factors-β_1, C-reactive protein, leptin, and adiponectin or a result of common predisposing dietary factors. Being overweight or obese is a risk factor for childhood asthma, particularly in females; conversely, there is no evidence that having asthma increases the risk for obesity.[12]

Exposure to Tobacco Smoke and COPD Overlap

A thorough history that considers age, respiratory symptoms, past medical history, previous diagnoses, and treatments, as well as social and occupational risk factors, may identify relevant a smoking history or exposure to environmental tobacco smoke. The clinician is then faced with distinguishing asthma from COPD. First termed Asthma COPD Overlap Syndrome (ACOS) and more recently Asthma COPD Overlap (ACO), some patients have clinical features of both asthma and COPD.[37] Physical examination findings, lung function measures, and radiology data are then combined with the history to confirm this syndromic diagnosis. GINA and the Global Initiative for Chronic Obstructive Lung Disease (GOLD) provide recommendations for initial therapy of ACO if the diagnostic features are equally balanced between asthma and COPD.[37] However, GOLD no longer refers to ACOS due to a misperception that ACOS is a distinct disorder. Rather, GOLD emphasizes that asthma and COPD are different disorders with common traits and features and may coexist in the same patient. Given that patients with features of both asthma and COPD are most often excluded from clinical studies, the pathophysiology and treatment remain less defined for these patients. Compared to patients with either asthma or COPD alone, those with ACO have a greater symptom burden, physical impairment, and hospitalizations with worse quality of life.[38] The origins of ACO may begin in childhood regardless of smoking history, but smoke may have more severe effects on lung function in patients with asthma. Referral for expert advice and further diagnostic evaluation for ACO patients may be necessary. GOLD recommends clinicians prioritize asthma treatment for patients with ACO.[37]

CLINICAL PRESENTATION

Chronic Asthma

3 Classically, asthma is characterized by episodic and variable respiratory symptoms; however, the clinical presentation of asthma is as diverse as the number of triggering events (see "Clinical Presentation: Chronic Asthma"). Although wheezing is the characteristic symptom of asthma, the medical literature is replete with the warning that "not all that wheezes is asthma." A wheeze is a high-pitched, whistling sound created by turbulent airflow through an obstructed airway, so any condition that produces significant obstruction can result in wheezing as a symptom. In addition, "all of asthma does not wheeze" is an equally justifiable warning. Patients may present with a chronic persistent cough (cough variant asthma) as their only symptom.[12]

There is no single diagnostic test for asthma. The diagnosis is based primarily on a thorough history gathered from the patient.[12] The patient may have a family history of allergy or asthma or have symptoms of allergic rhinitis, or atopic dermatitis. Reversibility of airway obstruction following administration of a SABA or excessive variability in twice-daily peak expiratory flow (PEF) over 1 to 2 weeks are diagnostic criteria. Patients with normal spirometry values can be challenged with exercise or substances that produce bronchoconstriction, such as methacholine or mannitol, to determine if they have BHR, but again, a positive challenge test is not diagnostic. Newer tests of inflammation in the airways such as induced sputum eosinophil and neutrophil counts or FeNO measurements are consistent with but not diagnostic of asthma. According to the 2020 Asthma Focused Updates, when the diagnosis is uncertain, a FeNO is recommended as an adjunctive diagnostic test.[11] FeNO results should be interpreted in conjunction with other conditions or factors that influence FeNO levels in patients with asthma (eg, smoking, obesity, and corticosteroid use are associated with lower levels whereas atopy, eosinophilic bronchitis is associated with higher levels).

GINA recommends confirmation of the diagnosis of asthma in patients already taking controller treatment using objective testing. The process depends on the patient's symptoms and lung function and may include a trial of either a lower or a higher dose of controller treatment.[12]

The frequency and severity of asthma symptoms vary widely. The intervals between symptoms can be days, weeks, months, or years. Asthma also can vary in its severity and is related to the intrinsic intensity of the disease process. Asthma severity is determined by lung function, symptoms, nighttime awakenings, rescue SABA use, interference with normal activity prior to therapy, and frequency of exacerbations requiring systemic corticosteroids.[39] Severity is most easily and directly measured in a patient who is not currently receiving asthma treatment. The NAEPP has provided a means of classifying asthma severity that is divided into two domains: impairment and risk.[3] This classification system is individualized for three age groups (0-4, 5-11, and greater than or equal to 12 years) and summarized in Table 44-2. Based on these domains, an individual's severity category is based on the greatest level of either impairment or risk. For example, a patient with several features consistent with mild persistent severity but who has one feature in the moderate persistent category is classified as having moderate persistent asthma. Although classifying severity is helpful for determining the initial treatment, subsequent management is determined by the level of symptom control. GINA has provided a slightly different framework for determining chronic therapy for children and adults based on symptom control and future risk of adverse outcomes.[12]

The frequency or chronicity of the symptoms is not necessarily associated with the severity of symptoms during exacerbations. Patients can present with a range from intermittent symptoms that require no medications or only occasional SABA use to severe

CLINICAL PRESENTATION Chronic Asthma

General

- Asthma is a disease of exacerbation and remission, so the patient may not have any signs or symptoms at the time of examination.

Symptoms

- The patient may complain of episodes of shortness of breath, chest tightness, coughing (particularly at night), wheezing, or a whistling sound from the chest when breathing. These often occur in association with exercise, but also occur spontaneously or in association with known allergens.

Signs

- Wheezing on auscultation (more typically on expiration), prolonged expiratory phase on auscultation dry hacking cough or signs of atopy (allergic rhinitis and/or atopic dermatitis) may occur.

Laboratory

- Spirometry demonstrates obstruction (reduced FEV_1/forced vital capacity [FVC]) with reversibility following inhaled β_2-agonist administration (FEV_1 increases by more than 12% and 200 mL). The FEV_1/FVC ratio is normally more than 75% to 80% (0.75-0.80) in adults and more than 85% (0.85) in children.

Other diagnostic tests

- Excessive variability in twice-daily peak expiratory flow (PEF) over 2 weeks (greater than 10% in adults and greater than 13% in children). A fall in FEV_1 of at least 10% following 6 minutes of near-maximal exercise. Elevated eosinophil count and IgE concentration in blood. FeNO less than 20 ppb in children younger than 12 years and less than 25 ppb in adults suggest a diagnosis other than asthma. Positive methacholine challenge (PC20 FEV_1 less than 12.5 mg/mL) or mannitol challenge (FEV_1 decrease of at least 15% from baseline after 635 mg or less).

CLINICAL PRESENTATION Acute Severe Asthma

General

- Although an episode can progress over several days or hours (usual scenario), it can progress rapidly over 1 to 2 hours.

Symptoms

- The patient is anxious in acute distress and complains of severe dyspnea, shortness of breath, chest tightness, or burning. The patient is only able to say a few words with each breath. Symptoms are unresponsive to usual measures (short-acting inhaled β_2-agonist administration).

Signs

- Signs include expiratory and inspiratory wheezing on auscultation (breath sounds may be diminished with very severe obstruction), dry hacking cough, tachypnea, tachycardia, pale or cyanotic skin, hyper-inflated chest with intercostal and supraclavicular retractions, and hypoxic seizures if very severe.

Laboratory tests

- Peak expiratory flow and/or FEV_1 less than 40% of normal predicted values. Decreased arterial O_2 (PaO_2), and O_2 saturations by pulse oximetry (SaO_2 less than 90% [0.90] on room air is severe). Decreased arterial or capillary CO_2 if mild, but in the normal range or increased in moderate-to-severe obstruction.

Other diagnostic tests

- Blood gases to assess metabolic acidosis (lactic acidosis) in severe obstruction. Complete blood count if there are signs of infection (fever and purulent sputum). Serum electrolytes as therapy with β_2-agonist and corticosteroids can lower serum potassium, magnesium, and phosphate, and increase glucose. Chest radiograph if signs of consolidation on auscultation.

persistent asthma symptoms despite treatment with multiple medications.

Acute Severe Asthma

Uncontrolled asthma, with its inherent variability, can progress to an acute state where inflammation, airway edema, excessive mucus accumulation, and severe bronchospasm result in a profound airway narrowing that is poorly responsive to usual bronchodilator therapy (see "Clinical Presentation: Acute Severe Asthma").[40] Although this progression is a common scenario, some patients experience rapid-onset or hyper-acute exacerbations.[40] Hyper-acute exacerbations are associated with neutrophilic as opposed to eosinophilic infiltration and resolve rapidly with bronchodilator therapy, suggesting that smooth muscle spasm is the major pathogenic mechanism.[40] In most cases, emergency department (ED) visits for acute severe asthma represent the failure of an adequate therapeutic regimen to control persistent asthma. Underutilization of anti-inflammatory drugs and excessive reliance on SABA are the major risk factors for severe exacerbations.[40] However, frequent exacerbations may represent a specific phenotype of asthma. A blunted perception of airway obstruction may predispose certain individuals to fatal asthma attacks.[40]

Exercise-Induced Bronchospasm

During vigorous exercise, pulmonary function measurements (FEV_1 and PEF) in patients with asthma increase during the first few minutes but then begin to decrease after 6 to 8 minutes.[2] Exercise-induced bronchospasm (EIB) is defined as a drop in FEV_1 of 10% or greater from baseline (pre-exercise value).[2] Most studies suggest that many patients with persistent asthma experience EIB.[3] The exact pathogenesis of EIB is unknown, but heat loss and/or water loss from the central airways play an important role.[41] EIB is provoked more easily in cold, dry air, ambient ozone, and airborne particulate matter; alternatively, warm, humid air can blunt or block it.[42] Studies have demonstrated increased plasma histamine, cysteinyl LTs, prostaglandins, and tryptase concentrations during EIB, suggesting a role for mast cell degranulation.[41] These findings led to the development of inhaled mannitol, an osmotic agent, as an indirect pharmacologic bronchoprovocation test to assist in the diagnosis of asthma.

A refractory period following EIB lasts up to 4 hours after exercise in some patients. The refractory period is thought to be caused by an acute depletion of mast cell mediators and the time required for their repletion.

EIB is believed to be a reflection of increased BHR associated with asthma. A correlation, though not perfect, exists between EIB and reactivity to histamine, methacholine, and mannitol. During periods of remission, a decreased sensitivity to the same degree of exercise is often observed. Many children and adults with EIB report no symptoms and have normal pulmonary function except in association with exercise.[2] Interestingly, elite athletes have a higher prevalence of EIB than the general population.[41]

Nocturnal Asthma

3 Worsening of asthma during sleep is referred to as *nocturnal asthma*. Patients with nocturnal asthma have significant declines in pulmonary function between bedtime and awakening.[2] Typically, their lung function reaches a nadir at 3 to 4 am. Although the pathogenesis of this phenomenon is unknown, it has been associated with diurnal patterns of endogenous cortisol secretion and circulating epinephrine and is associated with an increase in airway inflammation.[2]

Numerous other factors may affect nocturnal worsening of asthma, including allergies and improper environmental control, gastroesophageal reflux, obstructive sleep apnea, and sinusitis. Experts consider nocturnal symptoms to be a sign of inadequately treated persistent asthma. Awakening from nocturnal asthma is a sensitive indicator of both severity and inadequate control.

TREATMENT

Desired Outcomes

GINA's long-term goals for asthma management are: (1) to achieve good control of symptoms and maintain normal activity levels and

TABLE 44-2 Classifying Asthma Severity for Patients Who Are Not Currently Taking Long-Term Control Medications

	Children 0-4 and 5-11 Years of Age				
			Persistent		
	Components	**Intermittent**	**Mild**	**Moderate**	**Severe**
Impairment	Symptoms	≤2 days/week	>2 days/week but not daily	Daily	Throughout the day
	Nighttime awakenings (0-4 years)	0	1-2 × month	3-4 × month	>1 × week
	Nighttime awakenings (5-11 years)	≤2 × month	3-4 × month	>1 × week, but not nightly	Often 7 × week
	SABA use for symptom control	≤2 days/week	>2 days/week but not daily	Daily	Several times per day
	Interference with normal activity	None	Minor limitation	Some limitation	Extremely limited
	Lung function	FEV_1 > 80%	FEV_1 > 80%	FEV_1 60%-80%	FEV_1 < 60%
	5-11 years	FEV_1/FVC > 85% (0.85)	FEV_1/FVC > 80% (0.80)	FEV_1/FVC 75%-80% (0.75-0.80)	FEV_1/FVC < 75% (0.75)
	Exacerbations	**Intermittent**	**Persistent**		
Risk	0-4 years	0-1/year	≥2 in 6 months or ≥4 wheezing episodes/1 year lasting >1 day		
	5-11 years	0-2/year	>2 in 1 year		
	Recommended initial treatment	Step 1	Step 2	Step 3 and consider short-course of oral corticosteroids	
	Youths ≥12 Years of Age and Adults				
			Persistent		
	Components	**Intermittent**	**Mild**	**Moderate**	**Severe**
Impairment	Symptoms	≤2 days/week	>2 days/week but not daily	Daily	Throughout the day
	Nighttime awakenings	≤2 × month	3-4 × month	>1 × week, but not nightly	Often 7 × week
	SABA use for symptom control	≤2 days/week	>2 days/week, but not >1 × day	Daily	Several times per day
	Interference with normal activity	None	Minor limitation	Some limitation	Extremely limited
	Lung function	FEV_1 > 80%	FEV_1 > 80%	FEV_1 60%-80%	FEV_1 < 60%
		[a]FEV_1/FVC normal	[a]FEV_1/FVC normal	[a]FEV_1/FVC reduced 5% (0.05)	[a]FEV_1/FVC reduced > 5% (0.05)
	Exacerbations	Intermittent	Persistent		
Risk		0-2/year	>2 in 1 year		
	Recommended initial treatment	Step 1	Step 2	Step 3 and consider short course of oral corticosteroids	Step 4 or 5 and consider course of oral corticosteroid

SABA, short-acting β-agonist.

[a]Normal FEV_1/FVC: 8 to 19 years 85% (0.85); 20 to 39 years 80% (0.80); 40 to 59 years 75% (0.75); 60 to 80 years 70% (0.70).

(2) to minimize future risk of exacerbations, fixed airflow limitation, and medication-related side effects.[12] The importance of eliciting the patient's own goals is critical through an ongoing patient-healthcare provider partnership. Key components are strategies to facilitate effective communication and reduce the impact of impaired health literacy.[12] Self-management education reduces asthma morbidity in both adults and children (Evidence A).[12] GINA and NAEPP recommend control-based asthma management, adjusting pharmacological and nonpharmacological treatment in a continuous cycle of assessment, treatment adjustment, and review. Assessment includes symptom control, risk factors, inhaler technique and adherence, and patient preferences. Response review includes symptoms, exacerbations, medication side effects, patient satisfaction, and lung function.[11,12]

GINA differentiates between the preferred treatment options at a population level (based on efficacy, effectiveness, safety, availability, and cost) versus appropriate treatment options for individual patients. A shared decision-making approach is recommended and should include a discussion of preferred treatment options, patient characteristics or phenotype, patient/parent preferences, and practical issues (inhaler technique, adherence, and cost).[12] Evidence suggests that a shared decision-making approach may be associated with better outcomes.[12]

General Approach to Treatment

The NAEPP[3,11] and GINA[12] outline sound strategies for the management and treatment of asthma. The NAEPP EPR3 guideline was last published in 2007 and updated in 2020. The NAEPP 2020 Asthma Focused Updates specifically reviewed six topics for clinical management of asthma, but did not comprehensively revise the 2007 EPR3.[11] Therefore, healthcare professionals may need to use both the EPR3 and 2020 Focused Updates when managing a patient with asthma.

The GINA guidelines and the 2020 Asthma Focused Updates use different approaches in evaluating the literature and determining recommended treatment approaches. The NAEPP continues to utilize the Grading of Recommendations Assessment, Development

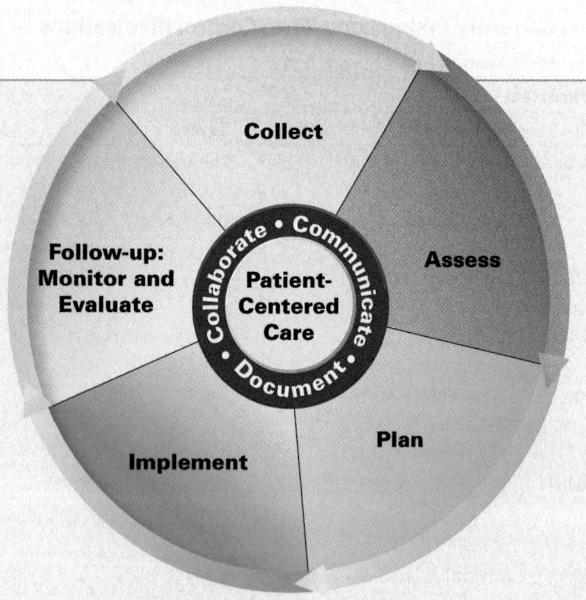

Patient Care Process for the Management of Persistent Asthma

Collect

- Patient characteristics (eg, age, race/ethnicity, sex, pregnancy status)
- Patient history (eg, past medical, known triggers, psychosocial history, gastroesophageal reflux disease)
- Family history (eg, asthma, allergy, atopic dermatitis)
- Home/work environment (eg, environmental, occupational, tobacco smoke, carpet/bedding, pets) (see Table 44-1)
- Current medications and prior response to controller therapies (eg, ICS+/−LABA; montelukast; LAMA; biologic therapies)
- Subjective and objective data (see Table 44-2)
    - Symptoms (description and frequency)
    - Nocturnal awakenings
    - Albuterol use frequency for symptom control
    - Activity limitation
    - Exacerbation frequency
    - Peak expiratory flow readings

Assess

- Comorbid conditions (eg, allergies, rhinosinusitis, obesity, obstructive sleep apnea, gastroesophageal reflux, smoking)
- Symptom frequency including exercise tolerance (see Tables 44-2)
- Exacerbation history (eg, oral corticosteroid use, emergency department visits, hospitalization)
- Current medications that may contribute to or worsen asthma (eg, nonsteroidal anti-inflammatory drug [NSAID], aspirin) (see Table 44-1)
- Appropriateness and effectiveness of current medications in controlling symptoms and preventing exacerbations
- Inhaler technique (see Fig. 44-10) and adherence; potential barriers
- Socioeconomic barriers to obtaining medications
- Adherence to nonpharmacologic recommendations (eg, allergen avoidance, environmental control)

Plan*

- Tailored environmental modifications (eg, pet removal, carpet removal, pillow and mattress covers, exercise pretreatment, occupational exposures) (see Table 44-1)
- Medication therapy regimen: dose, route, frequency, duration, and MDI spacer; specify the continuation and discontinuation of existing therapies (see Tables 44-4, 44-7, 44-8, 44-10, and 44-13)
- Monitoring parameters include efficacy (eg, daily symptoms, nocturnal awakenings, albuterol use, exercise tolerance, peak expiratory flow [in selected patients]), and time frame (see Table 44-2)
- Patient/family education (eg, purpose of treatment, environmental modifications, drug therapies, inhaler technique)
- Self-monitoring of symptoms, albuterol use, peak expiratory flow (in selected patients)—where and how to record results (see Fig. 44-6)
- Referrals to other providers when appropriate (eg, specialist physician)

Implement*

- Provide patient/family education regarding all elements of the treatment plan
- Use motivational interviewing and coaching strategies to maximize adherence
- Schedule follow-up based on symptoms and medication changes

Follow-up: Monitor and Evaluate

- Determine symptom control and exacerbation outcomes
- Presence of adverse effects
- Patient adherence to treatment plan using multiple sources of information

**Collaborate with patient, caregivers, and other healthcare professionals.*

and Evaluation (GRADE) approach, an internationally accepted framework to determine the strength of a recommendation, however, is generally less nimble for incorporating new evidence. The GINA guidelines are updated every year, and thus, GINA is generally more current and can indicate emerging treatment strategies.[12] Thus, clinicians may consult both guidelines for these reasons. With the release of the 2020 Asthma Focused Updates, the GINA and the NAEPP overall guidance have become more similar and will be described in further detail for the management of chronic asthma.

General Approach to the Management of Chronic Asthma

As outlined in the 2020 Asthma Focused Updates, a stepped approach to managing persistent asthma is used for all ages

(Figs. 44-3-44-5)[11]. Step of care depends upon whether the individual is newly diagnosed (treatment naïve) or if therapy is being adjusted to achieve control. If newly diagnosed, the initial step is based upon levels of impairment and risk which determine asthma severity (Table 44-2)[39]. All patients with persistent asthma (mild, moderate, or severe) should also be initiated on inhaled corticosteroid therapy. 5 An ICS is the preferred long-term controller therapy for persistent asthma in all patients due to potency and consistent effectiveness.[11,12] ICSs reduce BHR, improve lung function, and reduce severe exacerbations leading to ED visits and hospitalizations. ICS therapy is more effective than theophylline or the LTRAs. In addition, ICS therapy is the only treatment that has been documented to reduce the risk of dying from asthma.[11,12] Therapy is escalated as needed by increasing the dose of ICS or the addition of a second and then a third inhaled controller medication, typically a long-acting β_2-adrenergic receptor agonist (LABA) (preferred choice) or a long-acting muscarinic agonist (LAMA) (Fig. 44-3-44-5). All patients with asthma should have quick-relief medication (reliever therapy), available for acute symptoms. It is important to ensure that the patient can correctly use both the reliever and controller delivery devices. Once therapy has been initiated, patients are then evaluated 2 to 6 weeks later to rate their level of control (ie, well-controlled, not well-controlled, or very poorly controlled) using the same domains of impairment and risk in severity classification.[39] Based on their level of control, step therapy should be adjusted accordingly and follow-up should continue every 2 to 3 months as indicated by clinical urgency.

The primary therapeutic differences between GINA and the 2020 Asthma Focused Updates are in Steps 1 and 2 therapy for adolescents and adults. For adolescents and adults, Step 1 therapy in the 2020 Asthma Focused Updates begins with as-needed rescue therapy (ie, SABA). Step 2 progresses to adding a controller therapy of low-dose ICS or as needed concomitant ICS and SABA. GINA, on the other hand, recommends the use of ICS-formoterol taken as-needed in Steps 1 and 2. Both guidelines recommend the use of ICS-formoterol therapy for maintenance and as-needed use, known as Single Maintenance And Reliever Therapy (SMART) as the preferred therapy, for Steps 3 and 4 in patients aged 4 years[11] or 6 years[12] and older. Add-on LAMA with ICS-LABA (2020 Asthma Focused Updates) or SMART (GINA) is recommended for Step 5 in patients 12 years and older.

When asthma remains poorly controlled with ICS-LABA with LAMA or SMART with LAMA, the addition of biologics can be considered.[11,12] There are currently no studies that support the selection of one biologic over another other than by criteria included in the labeling (eg, serum IgE or eosinophil levels).

SMART therapy reduces exacerbation rates and corticosteroid use but has inconsistent effects on asthma control and quality of life.[11] SMART therapy has only been used with formoterol as the LABA component due to its rapid onset of action and maximum allowable total daily dose. The maximum formoterol dose in children aged 4 to 11 years for SMART is eight inhalations of 4.5 μg/inhalation (total dose 36 μg formoterol). Budesonide was the inhaled corticosteroid studied in this age group. In patients aged

	Intermittent Asthma	Management of Persistent Asthma in Individuals Ages 0–4 Years				
Treatment	STEP 1	STEP 2	STEP 3	STEP 4	STEP 5	STEP 6
Preferred	PRN SABA and At the start of RTI: Add short course daily ICS[a]	Daily low-dose ICS and PRN SABA	Daily medium-dose ICS and PRN SABA	Daily medium-dose ICS-LABA and PRN SABA	Daily high-dose ICS-LABA and PRN SABA	Daily high-dose ICS-LABA + oral systemic corticosteroid and PRN SABA
Alternative		Daily montelukast[b] or Cromolyn,[b] and PRN SABA		Daily medium-dose ICS + montelukast[b] and PRN SABA	Daily high-dose ICS + montelukast[b] and PRN SABA	Daily high-dose ICS + montelukast[b]+ oral systemic corticosteroid and PRN SABA
			For children age 4 years only, see Step 3 and Step 4 on Management of Persistent Asthma in Individuals Ages 5–11 Years diagram.			

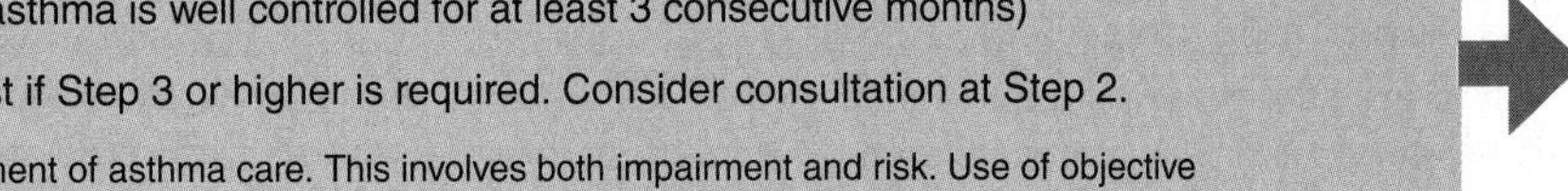

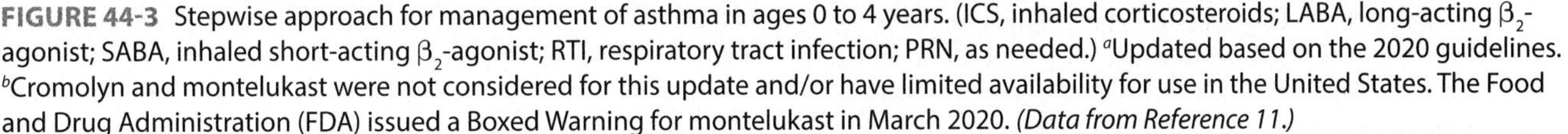

FIGURE 44-3 Stepwise approach for management of asthma in ages 0 to 4 years. (ICS, inhaled corticosteroids; LABA, long-acting β_2-agonist; SABA, inhaled short-acting β_2-agonist; RTI, respiratory tract infection; PRN, as needed.) [a]Updated based on the 2020 guidelines. [b]Cromolyn and montelukast were not considered for this update and/or have limited availability for use in the United States. The Food and Drug Administration (FDA) issued a Boxed Warning for montelukast in March 2020. *(Data from Reference 11.)*

	Intermittent Asthma	Management of Persistent Asthma in Individuals Ages 5–11 Years				
Treatment	**STEP 1**	**STEP 2**	**STEP 3**	**STEP 4**	**STEP 5**	**STEP 6**
Preferred	PRN SABA	Daily low-dose ICS and PRN SABA	Daily and PRN combination low-dose ICS-formoterol[a]	Daily and PRN combination medium-dose ICS-formoterol[a]	Daily high-dose ICS-LABA and PRN SABA	Daily high-dose ICS-LABA + oral systemic corticosteroid and PRN SABA
Alternative		Daily LTRA,[b] or Cromolyn,[b] or Nedocromil,[b] or Theophylline,[b] and PRN SABA	Daily medium-dose ICS and PRN SABA or Daily low-dose ICS-LABA, or daily low-dose ICS + LTRA,[b] or daily low-dose ICS +Theophylline,[b] and PRN SABA	Daily medium-dose ICS-LABA and PRN SABA or Daily medium-dose ICS + LTRA[b] or daily medium-dose ICS + Theophylline,[b] and PRN SABA	Daily high-dose ICS + LTRA[b] or daily high-dose ICS + Theophylline,[b] and PRN SABA	Daily high-dose ICS + LTRA[b] + oral systemic corticosteroid or daily high-dose ICS + Theophylline[b] + oral systemic corticosteroid, and PRN SABA
		Steps 2–4: Conditionally recommend the use of subcutaneous immunotherapy as an adjunct treatment to standard pharmacotherapy in individuals ≥ 5 years of age whose asthma is controlled at the initiation, build up, and maintenance phases of immunotherapy[b]			Consider Omalizumab[c,a]	

Assess Control

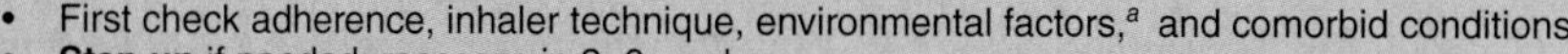

- First check adherence, inhaler technique, environmental factors,[a] and comorbid conditions.
- **Step up** if needed; reassess in 2–6 weeks
- **Step down** if possible (if asthma is well controlled for at least 3 consecutive months)

Consult with asthma specialist if Step 4 or higher is required. Consider consultation at Step 3.

Control assessment is a key element of asthma care. This involves both impairment and risk. Use of objective measures, self-reported control, and health care utilization are complementary and should be employed on an ongoing basis, depending on the individual's clinical situation.

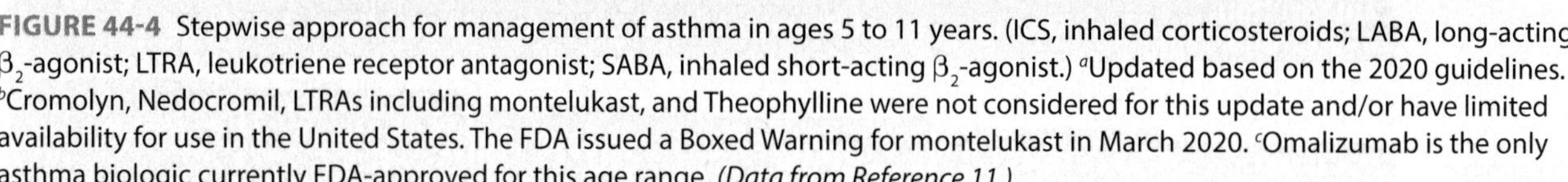

FIGURE 44-4 Stepwise approach for management of asthma in ages 5 to 11 years. (ICS, inhaled corticosteroids; LABA, long-acting β_2-agonist; LTRA, leukotriene receptor antagonist; SABA, inhaled short-acting β_2-agonist.) [a]Updated based on the 2020 guidelines. [b]Cromolyn, Nedocromil, LTRAs including montelukast, and Theophylline were not considered for this update and/or have limited availability for use in the United States. The FDA issued a Boxed Warning for montelukast in March 2020. [c]Omalizumab is the only asthma biologic currently FDA-approved for this age range. *(Data from Reference 11.)*

12 years and older, the SMART maintenance dose is one to two puffs once or twice daily plus a rescue dose of one to two puffs as needed up to a combined maximum of 12 puffs per day (total dose 54 μg formoterol). Importantly, ICS-formoterol reliever therapy is not to be used concomitantly with ICS-salmeterol maintenance therapy.[11,12]

Although the alternative long-term control therapies (eg, LTRAs and theophylline), used as either monotherapy or concomitantly with ICS, improve symptoms, lung function, and reduce as-needed SABA use, they do not reduce BHR, suggesting minimal anti-inflammatory activity.[11,12] There are minimal to no differences in efficacy between these alternatives.

Other therapies reserved for the treatment of uncontrolled severe asthma after an optimal trial of high-dose ICSs in combination with LABA or LAMA or biologic therapy include bronchial thermoplasty and oral corticosteroids. The GINA guidelines also suggest considering treatment with azithromycin for its anti-inflammatory effects in adults whose asthma is uncontrolled despite higher doses of ICS-formoterol.[12] Due to significant adverse effects that occur with their long-term use, oral corticosteroids are prescribed at the lowest dose that maintains asthma control and administered daily or every other day. Bronchial thermoplasty reduces the airway smooth muscle mass by targeting the hypertrophied smooth muscle in the airways and delivers thermal energy in a controlled manner to the airway wall. This results in a reduced response to bronchoconstrictive stimuli. Bronchial thermoplasty is not recommended in the 2020 Asthma Focused Updates due to the relatively small improvements in asthma control and the moderate risk of harm observed in clinical trials. Moreover, there is an insufficient long-term follow-up in large numbers of patients to adequately assess its benefits and harms.[11] Both guidelines recommend a very careful selection of patients before using bronchial thermoplasty.

Patients with documented allergen sensitization with clinical symptoms can be considered for allergen immunotherapy, given either by subcutaneous injections or sublingually. The 2020 Asthma Focused Updates do not recommend sublingual therapy except in those who also have allergic rhinoconjunctivitis. Data regarding immunotherapy will continue to expand and be reviewed.[11,12] Patients suitable for subcutaneous therapy are those children aged 5 years and older who demonstrate allergic sensitization and adults with allergic asthma who have worsening asthma symptoms temporally related to allergen exposure and who have testing that confirms sensitization. Subcutaneous therapy is not recommended in patients with severe asthma due to the risk of systemic reactions. Subcutaneous treatment must be administered in a setting that is prepared to manage anaphylactic reactions. Sublingual treatment must initially be supervised by health professionals but may be continued at home if there are no systemic adverse effects observed.[11] Because treatment may involve weekly appointments for several years, patients need to carefully consider the burden of treatment before initiating allergy immunotherapy.

	Intermittent Asthma	Management of Persistent Asthma in Individuals Ages 12+ Years				
Treatment	**STEP 1**	**STEP 2**	**STEP 3**	**STEP 4**	**STEP 5**	**STEP 6[d]**
Preferred	PRN SABA	Daily low-dose ICS and PRN SABA or PRN concomitant ICS and SABA[a]	Daily and PRN combination low-dose ICS-formoterol[a]	Daily and PRN combination medium-dose ICS-formoterol[a]	Daily medium-high dose ICS-LABA + LAMA and PRN SABA[a]	Daily high-dose ICS-LABA + oral systemic corticosteroids + PRN SABA
Alternative		Daily LTRA[b] and PRN SABA or Cromolyn,[b] or Nedocromil,[b] or Zileuton,[b] or Theophylline,[b] and PRN SABA	Daily medium-dose ICS and PRN SABA or Daily low-dose ICS-LABA, or daily low-dose ICS + LAMA,[a] or daily low-dose ICS + LTRA,[b] and PRN SABA or Daily low-dose ICS + Theophylline[b] or Zileuton,[b] and PRN SABA	Daily medium-dose ICS-LABA or daily medium-dose ICS + LAMA, and PRN SABA[a] or Daily medium-dose ICS + LTRA,[b] or daily medium-dose ICS + Theophylline,[b] or daily medium-dose ICS + Zileuton,[b] and PRN SABA	Daily medium-high dose ICS-LABA or daily high-dose ICS + LTRA,[b] and PRN SABA	
		Steps 2–4: Conditionally recommend the use of subcutaneous immunotherapy as an adjunct treatment to standard pharmacotherapy in individuals ≥ 5 years of age whose asthma is controlled at the initiation, build up, and maintenance phases of immunotherapy[a]			Consider adding Asthma Biologics (e.g., anti-IgE, anti-IL5, anti-IL5R, anti-IL4/IL13)[c]	

Assess Control

- First check adherence, inhaler technique, environmental factors,[a] and comorbid conditions.
- **Step up** if needed; reassess in 2–6 weeks
- **Step down** if possible (if asthma is well controlled for at least 3 consecutive months)

Consult with asthma specialist if Step 4 or higher is required. Consider consultation at Step 3.

Control assessment is a key element of asthma care. This involves both impairment and risk. Use of objective measures, self-reported control, and health care utilization are complementary and should be employed on an ongoing basis, depending on the individual's clinical situation.

FIGURE 44-5 Stepwise approach for management of asthma in ages 12 years and older. (ICS, inhaled corticosteroids; LABA, long-acting β_2-agonist; LAMA, long-acting muscarinic antagonist; LTRA, leukotriene receptor antagonist; SABA, inhaled short-acting β_2-agonist.) [a]Updated based on the 2020 guidelines. [b]Cromolyn, nedocromil, LTRAs including zileuton and montelukast, and theophylline were not considered for this update and/or have limited availability for use in the United States, and/or have an increased risk of adverse consequences and need for monitoring that makes their use less desirable. The FDA issued a Boxed Warning for montelukast in March 2020. [c]The AHRQ systematic reviews that informed this report did not include studies that examined the role of asthma biologics (eg, anti-IgE, anti-IL5, anti-IL5R, anti-IL4/IL13). Thus this report does not contain specific recommendations for the use of biologics in asthma in Steps 5 and 6. [d]Data on the use of LAMA therapy in individuals with severe persistent asthma (Step 6) were not included in the AHRQ systematic review and thus no recommendation is made. *(Data from Reference 11.)*

GINA provides general principles for stepping-down controller treatments.[12] Step-down therapy is warranted if symptoms have been well controlled and lung function has been stable for at least 3 months (Evidence Grade D). Step-down therapy should only be initiated when the patient is expected to remain stable; for example, at a time when the patient has no evidence of a respiratory infection, will not be traveling, and is not pregnant. When engaging in a trial of treatment step-down, the patient should regularly monitor symptoms and PEF, and a follow-up visit with the provider should be scheduled (Evidence Grade D). Stepping down ICS doses by 25% to 50% at 3-month intervals is considered feasible and safe for most patients (Evidence Grade A).

GINA emphasizes three components of personalized asthma management: ASSESS, ADJUST, and REVIEW RESPONSE.[12] It is important to ASSESS and document symptom control and risk factors at every patient encounter. If symptoms are uncontrolled, check inhaler technique and adherence, and consider whether symptoms are due to a comorbid condition such as allergic rhinitis, GERD, or obesity rather than asthma. ADJUST therapy (intensify or de-escalate)—both drug therapy and nonpharmacological strategies; treat modifiable risk factors. REVIEW RESPONSE—assess and optimize asthma control about every 3 months.

Special Populations

Infants and Children Younger Than 5 Years The management of asthma in children younger than 5 years follows the same stepwise approach as in older children and adults but many treatments have not been studied adequately (Fig. 44-3). Thus, many of the recommendations in this age group are extrapolated from older children and adults.[11,12] Because viral respiratory tract infections are a common cause of wheezing in young children, the 2020 Asthma Focused Updates now recommend starting a short (7-10 day) course of ICS with as-needed SABA at the start of a respiratory tract infection.[11] A suggested regimen is budesonide inhalation suspension, 1 mg, twice daily.[11] The primary differences in chronic management in this age group are that no controller treatment is necessarily indicated for Step 1 and the recommended treatment in Step 3 is doubling the dose of ICS rather than adding LABA as is recommended for older children and adults.[11,12] There is insufficient evidence to recommend ICS-LABA in young children at any step of therapy.[12] Most of the available ICS have been studied in young children but not all have marketing approval from the FDA in this age group. Lack of an approved indication in children younger than 5 years could affect insurance coverage for specific products. ICSs are available as MDI, DPI, and nebulized formulations but the preferred method of delivery is by MDI with a valved spacer and facemask in children younger than 3 years and valved spacer for older children, if needed.[12] Smaller spacers (less than 350 mL) are preferred because 5 to 10 breaths after actuation are required to inhale the complete dose. It is also recommended to not change the spacer type once a child is stable on a specific dose of ICS due to large differences in delivery between devices.[12] ICS use, even with low doses, causes reductions in growth velocity in children who are clinically important.[11,12] Thus, the lowest effective should be used and height should be regularly measured during treatment.[11,12]

The 2020 Asthma Focused Updates now recommends that a short course of daily ICS be initiated at the start of a respiratory tract infection in children who have had three or more episodes of wheezing triggered by presumed respiratory tract infections in their lifetime.[11] Treatment of moderate-to-severe asthma exacerbations may require the use of oral corticosteroids but nebulized budesonide at a dose of 1 mg twice daily for 7 days is effective at preventing exacerbations requiring treatment with oral corticosteroids. This dose did not affect linear growth but higher doses of other ICS (eg, fluticasone 750 μg twice daily for 10 days) may reduce the growth rate.[11] Therefore, the growth rate should be monitored regularly.

The FDA approval for montelukast (an LTRA) in children younger than 6 years was based on safety and pharmacokinetic studies establishing doses but not on efficacy, although improvement in symptoms and as-needed bronchodilators was noted. Montelukast is less effective than ICS in preschoolers with asthma or recurrent wheezing.[12] If montelukast is considered for therapy, parents should be counseled that the FDA has required a boxed warning of the risk of serious mental health side effects; a decision to use montelukast should be based on shared decision making between the provider and caregiver.

Older Adults Older adults are at the highest risk of dying from asthma due to multiple contributing factors.[4] As in very young children, there have been few prospective studies evaluating drug therapies. In addition, older adults have a high comorbidity burden which may impact response to therapies differently than younger patients, and adherence to treatment can be more challenging when multiple medications for different diseases are prescribed. Control of comorbid conditions (obesity, smoking, depression, and rhinosinusitis) may be required to improve treatment outcomes.[12] Arthritis, vision impairment, and muscle weakness which may affect the inspiratory flow should be considered when selecting inhaler devices.[12] In addition, older adults may have difficulty distinguishing breathlessness due to aging or cardiovascular disease from symptoms of asthma.[12] Given their increased risk of osteoporosis and cataracts, older adults who require high doses of ICSs should have routine height measurements, bone mineral density determinations, and ophthalmic examinations.[12] Appropriate therapies for the prevention of osteoporosis should be instituted.[12] ICS use may contribute to skin bruising in older adults.

Pregnant Women Asthma control may change during pregnancy; either improving or worsening and control may vary during each trimester.[12] Maternal asthma increases the risk of perinatal mortality, preeclampsia, preterm birth, and low-birth-weight infants.[12] More severe asthma is associated with increased risks, whereas better-controlled asthma is associated with decreased risks. The advantages of actively treating asthma during pregnancy far outweigh any risks of using ICS or albuterol and these medications are not associated with fetal abnormalities.[12] The safety of the newer biological treatments in pregnancy is unknown. Proper monitoring and control of asthma should enable a woman with asthma to maintain a normal pregnancy with little or no risk to the mother or her fetus. Patients should be monitored monthly to assess asthma control. ICS should not be discontinued in women planning a pregnancy or who are pregnant.[12]

Pregnant women are particularly susceptible to viral infections leading to exacerbations and worsening asthma symptoms. These asthma exacerbations should be aggressively treated to avoid fetal hypoxia.[12] Moderate-to-severe exacerbations should be treated with SABA, oxygen, and early administration of systemic corticosteroids.[12] Hyperventilation during labor may induce bronchoconstriction and should be treated with SABA.[31]

General Approach to the Management of Acute Severe Asthma

The primary goal in the treatment of acute severe asthma is to prevent death by recognizing the signs of deterioration and providing rapid treatment. Initial assessment includes history, physical examination, and objective assessments. It is important that therapy not be delayed, so the history and physical examination should be obtained while therapy is being initiated. The brief history will assess for onset and causes of the exacerbation; severity of symptoms and if associated with anaphylaxis; medication use, adherence, and response to current therapy; and risk factors for asthma-related death. Guidance for the self-management of acute asthma exacerbation should be provided to patients and caregivers using a written asthma action plan (Fig. 44-6).[43] This tool provides an individualized plan of action for patients based on symptoms and peak flow measurements. The action to be taken is based on whether the patient is in the green ("doing well"), yellow ("getting worse"), or red ("medical alert") zone.[43] For patients in the yellow or red zones, instructions for rescue treatment, including the dose and frequency, are provided. Most importantly, the asthma action plan should clearly state when to seek emergency care. The asthma-related risk factors for death include a history of near-fatal asthma requiring intubation and mechanical ventilation; hospitalization or emergency care in the past year; current or recent use of oral corticosteroids; no current use of ICSs; poor medication adherence; overuse of SABA therapy (more than one canister per month); history of psychiatric disease or psychosocial problems; lack of a written asthma action plan; food allergy in a patient with asthma; and comorbidities such as pneumonia, diabetes, and arrhythmias.[12]

The physical examination should include the measurement of vital signs and the history to pay careful attention to complicating factors such as anaphylaxis and comorbid conditions that could be causing acute shortness of breath such as an inhaled foreign body, congestive heart failure, pulmonary infection, and pulmonary embolism.[12]

Objective assessments are keys to monitoring response to therapy and should be made before initiation of oxygen or drug treatment. Lung function testing by PEF or FEV_1 should be measured before treatment if possible and thereafter at 1 hour after starting treatment and then periodically until a response is achieved or no

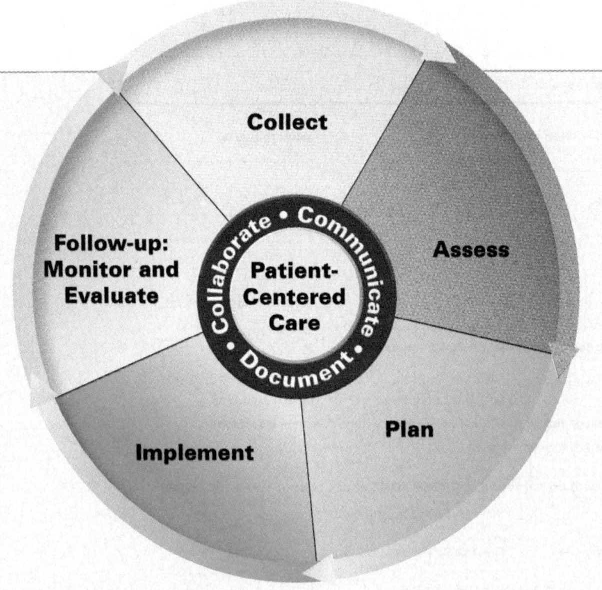

Patient Care Process for the Management of Acute Asthma

Collect

- Initial assessments
  - o **A**irway, **B**reathing, **C**irculation
  - o If signs of extreme distress, drowsiness, confusion, silent chest → start SABA, oxygen, consult ICU, consider intubation
- Patient characteristics (eg, age, race/ethnicity, sex, pregnancy status)
- Patient history (eg, past medical, known triggers, psychosocial history)
- Past exacerbation history (eg, past need for hospitalization, intensive care, or intubation). History of food allergy
- Current medications and prior response to controller therapies (eg, ICS+/−LABA; montelukast; LAMA; biologic therapies)

Assess

- Degree of severity of exacerbation—MILD or MODERATE (see Fig. 44-8). Can talk in phrases or sentences
  - o Can sit up
  - o Not agitated
  - o Respiratory rate elevation mild to moderate
  - o No sign of accessory muscle use
  - o Oxygen saturation 90% to 95% (0.90-0.95)
  - o PEF rate>50% of predicted (or previous best)
- Degree of severity of exacerbation—SEVERE (see Fig. 44-8)
  - o Can only talk in single words
  - o Hunched forward. Agitated
  - o Respiratory rate elevation severe (>30/min for adults)
  - o Accessory muscle use evidence
  - o Oxygen saturation <90% (0.90)
  - o PEF rate ≤50% of predicted (or previous best)

Plan and Implement

- If MILD-MODERATE (see Fig. 44-8)
  - o Start SABA
  - o Consider ipratropium bromide
  - o Titrate oxygen to keep 94% (0.94) or higher
  - o Oral corticosteroids
- If SEVERE, use a team-based approach to immediately and simultaneously start SABA, oxygen, ICU involvement, and preparation for possible intubation (see Fig. 44-8)
  - o Start SABA and ipratropium bromide
  - o Titrate oxygen to keep 94% (0.94) or higher; use continuous oximetry and cardiac monitoring
  - o IV corticosteroids (consider IV magnesium and high-dose ICS)

Follow-up: Monitor and Evaluate (see Fig. 44-8)

- Assess symptoms frequently
- If continuing deterioration, consider intubation and ICU transfer
- Measure lung function in all patients 1 hour after initial treatment if able
- Disposition
  - o If continued signs/symptoms of distress and FEV_1 or PEF minimally improved, <60% predicted or personal best → continue treatment as above and reassess frequently
  - o If significantly improved clinical signs/symptoms and FEV_1 or PEF improved to 60% to 80% predicted or personal best → consider for discharge planning

further improvement is evident.[12] Oxygen saturation is also monitored closely preferably by pulse oximetry and is a key parameter in young children who may not be able to perform lung function. Arterial blood gases are typically reserved for patients who are poorly responsive to initial treatment or deteriorating. A chest x-ray is rarely indicated unless there are physical signs of other or additional complicating features such as foreign body aspiration.

Oxygen therapy is initiated to achieve an arterial oxygen saturation of 93% to 95% in adolescents and adults and 94% to 98% in school-aged children and pregnant women or those with cardiac disease.[12] Oxygen therapy is continued until the patient has stabilized with continued use of pulse oximetry to monitor further oxygen need and response to medications.

The primary therapy of acute exacerbations is pharmacologic, which includes SABA and, depending on the severity, systemic corticosteroids, inhaled ipratropium, intravenous magnesium sulfate, and O_2. Treatments are typically administered concurrently to facilitate rapid improvement.

Serum electrolytes should be monitored in patients who take diuretics regularly and in patients with coexistent cardiovascular disease, as SABA can produce transient decreases in potassium, magnesium, and phosphate. The combination of high-dose β_2-agonists and systemic corticosteroids occasionally may result in excessive elevations of glucose and lactic acid.

The initial response is measured 1 hour after the first three inhaled bronchodilator treatments are administered and provide

ASTHMA ACTION PLAN

For: ______________________ Doctor: ______________________ Date: ____________

Doctor's Phone Number: ______________ Hospital/Emergency Department Phone Number: ______________

GREEN ZONE

DOING WELL

- No cough, wheeze, chest tightness, or shortness of breath during the day or night
- Can do usual activities

And, if a peak flow meter is used,

Peak flow: more than ____________ (80 percent or more of my best peak flow)

My best peak flow is: ____________

Daily Medications

Medicine	**How much to take**	**When to take it**
____________	____________	____________
____________	____________	____________
____________	____________	____________
____________	____________	____________
____________	____________	____________

Before exercise	❑ ____________	❑ 2 or ❑ 4 puffs	5 minutes before exercise

YELLOW ZONE

ASTHMA IS GETTING WORSE

- Cough, wheeze, chest tightness, or shortness of breath, or
- Waking at night due to asthma, or
- Can do some, but not all, usual activities

-Or-

Peak flow: ________ to ________ (50 to 79 percent of my best peak flow)

1st **Add: quick-relief medicine—and keep taking your GREEN ZONE medicine.**

____________ (quick-relief medicine) ________ Number of puffs **or** ❑ Nebulizer, once — Can repeat every _____ minutes up to maximum of _____ doses

2nd **If your symptoms (and peak flow, if used) return to GREEN ZONE after 1 hour of above treatment:**

❑ Continue monitoring to be sure you stay in the green zone.

-Or-

If your symptoms (and peak flow, if used) do not return to GREEN ZONE after 1 hour of above treatment:

❑ Take: ____________ (quick-relief medicine) ________ Number of puffs **or** ❑ Nebulizer

❑ Add: ____________ (oral steroid) mg per day For _____ (3–10) days

❑ Call the doctor ❑ before/ ❑ within _____ hours after taking the oral steroid.

RED ZONE

MEDICAL ALERT!

- Very short of breath, or
- Quick-relief medicines have not helped,
- Cannot do usual activities, or
- Symptoms are same or get worse after 24 hours in Yellow Zone

-Or-

Peak flow: less than ____________ (50 percent of my best peak flow)

Take this medicine:

❑ ____________ (quick-relief medicine) ________ Number of puffs **or** ❑ Nebulizer

❑ ____________ (oral steroid) mg

Then call your doctor NOW. Go to the hospital or call an ambulance if:

- You are still in the red zone after 15 minutes AND
- You have not reached your doctor.

DANGER SIGNS

- **Trouble walking and talking due to shortness of breath**
- **Lips or fingernails are blue**

- **Take ________ puffs of ____________ (quick relief medicine) AND**
- **Go to the hospital or call for an ambulance ____________ (phone) NOW!**

See the reverse side for things you can do to avoid your asthma triggers.

HOW TO CONTROL THINGS THAT MAKE YOUR ASTHMA WORSE

This guide suggests things you can do to avoid your asthma triggers. Put a check next to the triggers that you know make your asthma worse and ask your doctor to help you find out if you have other triggers as well. Keep in mind that controlling any allergen usually requires a combination of approaches, and reducing allergens is just one part of a comprehensive asthma management plan. Here are some tips to get started. These tips tend to work better when you use several of them together. Your health care provider can help you decide which ones may be right for you.

ALLERGENS

❑ Dust Mites

These tiny bugs, too small to see, can be found in every home—in dust, mattresses, pillows, carpets, cloth furniture, sheets and blankets, clothes, stuffed toys, and other cloth-covered items. If you are sensitive:

- Mattress and pillow covers that prevent dust mites from going through them should be used along with high efficiency particulate air (HEPA) filtration vacuum cleaners.
- Consider reducing indoor humidity to below 60 percent. Dehumidifiers or central air conditioning systems can do this.

❑ Cockroaches and Rodents

Pests like these leave droppings that may trigger your asthma. If you are sensitive:

- Consider an integrated pest management plan.
- Keep food and garbage in closed containers to decrease the chances for attracting roaches and rodents.
- Use poison baits, powders, gels, or paste (for example, boric acid) or traps to catch and kill the pests.
- If you use a spray to kill roaches, stay out of the room until the odor goes away.

❑ Animal Dander

Some people are allergic to the flakes of skin or dried saliva from animals with fur or hair. If you are sensitive and have a pet:

- Consider keeping the pet outdoors.
- Try limiting to your pet to commonly used areas indoors.

❑ Indoor Mold

If mold is a trigger for you, you may want to:

- Explore professional mold removal or cleaning to support complete removal.
- Wear gloves to avoid touching mold with your bare hands if you must remove it yourself.
- Always ventilate the area if you use a cleaner with bleach or a strong smell.

❑ Pollen and Outdoor Mold

When pollen or mold spore counts are high you should try to:

- Keep your windows closed.
- If you can, stay indoors with windows closed from late morning to afternoon, when pollen and some mold spore counts are at their highest.
- If you do go outside, change your clothes as soon as you get inside, and put dirty clothes in a covered hamper or container to avoid spreading allergens inside your home.
- Ask your health care provider if you need to take or increase your anti-inflammatory medicine before the allergy season starts.

IRRITANTS

❑ Tobacco Smoke

- If you smoke, visit smokefree.gov or ask your health care provider for ways to help you quit.
- Ask family members to quit smoking.
- Do not allow smoking in your home or car.

❑ Smoke, Strong Odors, and Sprays

- If possible, avoid using a wood-burning stove, kerosene heater, or fireplace. Vent gas stoves to outside the house.
- Try to stay away from strong odors and sprays, such as perfume, talcum powder, hair spray, and paints.

❑ Vacuum Cleaning

- Try to get someone else to vacuum for you once or twice a week, if you can. Stay out of rooms while they are being vacuumed and for a short while afterward.
- If you must vacuum yourself, using HEPA filtration vacuum cleaners may be helpful.

❑ Other Things That Can Make Asthma Worse

- Sulfites in foods and beverages: Do not drink beer or wine or eat dried fruit, processed potatoes, or shrimp if they cause asthma symptoms.
- Cold air: Cover your nose and mouth with a scarf on cold or windy days.
- Other medicines: Tell your doctor about all the medicines you take. Include cold medicines, aspirin, vitamins and other supplements, and nonselective beta-blockers (including those in eye drops).

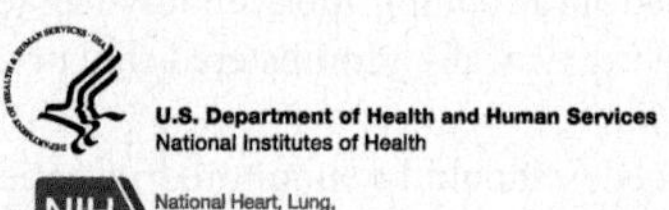

NIH National Heart, Lung, and Blood Institute

NIH Publication No. 20-HL-5251
February 2021

For more information and resources on asthma, visit *nhlbi.nih.gov/BreatheBetter.*

LEARN MORE BREATHE BETTER®

FIGURE 44-6 Asthma Action Plan. *(Reprinted from National Heart, Lung, and Blood Institute. Digital Toolkit: Asthma Action Plan [updated December 2000].)*

the best indicator for the need for hospitalization.[12] Indicators for hospitalization typically rely on the degree of respiratory distress, oxygen requirement, and frequency of need for inhaled β_2-agonists. Adjunctive indicators may include an initial FEV_1 less than 25% predicted or PEF that is less than 40% of their personal best, and post-treatment FEV_1 or PEF that is 40% to 60%.[12] Other indicators of severe asthma include monosyllabic speech, inaudible breath sounds, sitting hunched forward, and use of accessory muscles. Patients with lung function that is 40% to 60% predicted may be considered for discharge after assessment of risk factors for death from asthma and the likelihood for follow-up care. Those with higher lung function can be discharged after risk factor and follow-up care assessment.[12]

Discharge planning after an ED visit or hospitalization includes arranging follow-up care within 1 week as well as reviewing strategies to improve asthma management. Referral to a specialist is suggested for those who have been hospitalized or frequently seek care in the ED despite having regular primary care. Strategies for preventing future urgent care visits include ensuring the patient understands the cause of the exacerbation, how to modify risk factors, how to correctly use medications and for what purpose, and having a written asthma action plan that includes self-assessment of worsening symptoms and home PEF values.[12]

Figures 44-7 and 44-8 illustrate the recommended therapies for the treatment of acute asthma exacerbations in-home and ED/hospital settings.[12] Note that Fig. 44-7 is from the GINA guidelines and includes a recommendation to increase the frequency of ICS-formoterol which is not yet standard practice in the United States and is Evidence Grade A. The dosages of the drugs for acute severe exacerbations are provided in Table 44-3.[3,12]

Special Populations

Infants and Children Under 5 Years Old Infants and children younger than 5 years of age may be at greater risk of respiratory failure than older children and adults. Although treated with the same drugs, these younger children require the use of a pressurized MDI with a spacer or face mask as opposed to a mouthpiece for delivery of aerosolized medication. The face mask should be sized appropriately and should fit snugly over the nose and mouth. The pressurized MDI with spacer is preferred over a nebulizer because of its greater effectiveness and nebulizers can spread infectious particles.[12]

Children with severe exacerbations present with oxygen saturation of 92% (0.92) or less, speak in monosyllabic words, and have increased heart rate (above 180 beats/min if 0-3 years or above 150 beats/min if 4-5 years), central cyanosis, and inaudible breath sounds which indicate minimal ventilation sufficient to cause wheezing.[12] Hypoxemia is treated with oxygen to achieve oxygen saturation of 94% to 98% (0.94-0.98). Avoidance of hypoxemia is critical and treatment should be initiated with nebulized β_2-agonists delivered by an oxygen-driven nebulizer. Treatment should begin immediately even if a full assessment has not been taken. Initial SABA treatment is two puffs of albuterol, or if the exacerbation is severe, six inhalations of albuterol with a spacer/facemask. Treatment with 2 to 6 puffs of albuterol (severity dependent) may be repeated every 20 minutes for three doses with reassessment at the end of this treatment. Subsequent doses by nebulizer or two to three inhalations by spacer/facemask can be given every hour, but if symptoms do not resolve after 10 inhalations administered over 3 to 4 hours then a hospital admission is advised.[12] For nebulizer therapy, a dose of 2.5 mg albuterol every 20 minutes for 1 hour is administered and appropriate infection control measures must be followed.[12] Ipratropium bromide 1 to 2 puffs by pressurized MDI and spacer or nebulizer (250 μg) can be administered concurrently with albuterol during the first hour only.[12] Oral corticosteroids are administered at the time of inhaled β_2-agonists or intravenously in children unable to swallow. Nebulized magnesium sulfate may be administered as three doses in the first hour in children aged 2 years and older with severe exacerbations.[12] As in older children and adults, young children should be discharged with a prescription for oral corticosteroids for a 3- to 5-day treatment course and followed up within 7 days by a primary care provider.

Nonpharmacologic Therapy

Chronic Asthma

Although the mainstay of the management of asthma is pharmacologic therapy, it is likely to fail without concurrent attention to relevant environmental control and management of comorbidities that may contribute to respiratory symptoms and poor quality of life. Nonpharmacologic therapies are incorporated into GINA's recommendations for initiation of regular daily controller treatment, as well as the stepwise approach for adjusting treatment in adults, adolescents, and children.[11,12] The guidelines were designed to give healthcare providers a framework with which to develop the proper approach to the individualized therapy of patients. The heterogeneity of asthma demands an individualized approach to therapy with the basic goals of therapy as primary outcome measures.[11,12] The focus of controller therapy is the reduction of airway inflammation, control of symptoms, and reduction of future risks. Thus, current therapeutic options in asthma consist of acute reliever (rescue) medications for as-needed relief of breakthrough symptoms and exacerbations, and long-term control medications used for the prevention of symptoms and exacerbations and the suppression of inflammation and reduction of BHR.[11,12] Guidelines emphasize the importance of concurrently identifying and treating modifiable risk factors, such as active smoking and exposure to tobacco smoke, obesity, major psychological problems, major socioeconomic problems, confirmed food allergy, and allergen exposure if sensitized.[11,12] Occupational exposures, indoor allergens, and medications that may make asthma worse and should be evaluated when relevant.

In patients with known allergic triggers for their asthma, allergen avoidance has resulted in an improvement in symptoms, a reduction in medication use, and a decrease in BHR.[11] A multicomponent approach to environmental control is recommended in the 2020 Asthma Focused Updates because single-component interventions often are ineffective at improving asthma control.[11] Interventions should be tailored for individuals who have symptoms and/or positive allergy tests and who are exposed to specific allergens.[11] The 2020 Asthma Focused Updates provide a comprehensive evaluation of allergen mitigation strategies.[11] Some long-standing practices such as the use of acaricides to remove dust mites, carpet removal, use of air filtration systems, and purifiers are not effective even when included in a multi-component strategy.[11] However, if a home has pests (eg, cockroaches and mice) or a mold problem, a single component strategy to address the problem is warranted.[11] The use of HEPA vacuum cleaners, particularly for children, and impermeable pillow and mattress covers are recommended as part of a multicomponent strategy.[11]

Allergen-specific immunotherapy as either subcutaneous injections or sublingual administration is discussed in the section "General Approach to the Management of Chronic Asthma." Allergen treatment should be directed to specific allergens to which the patient has documented sensitivity. The 2020 Asthma Focused Updates only recommends subcutaneous therapy for asthma management which may improve symptom scores and reduce medication use in patients with documented allergen sensitivity.[11] In addition, it may have a disease-modifying effect and reduce clinical asthma severity over time.[11] The efficacy of multiple-allergen (vs single-allergen) subcutaneous immunotherapy is an area identified for future study.[11] The burden of frequent healthcare visits for immunotherapy administration must be considered before starting therapy as treatment will need to be continued for several years before there is sustained improvement in symptoms.

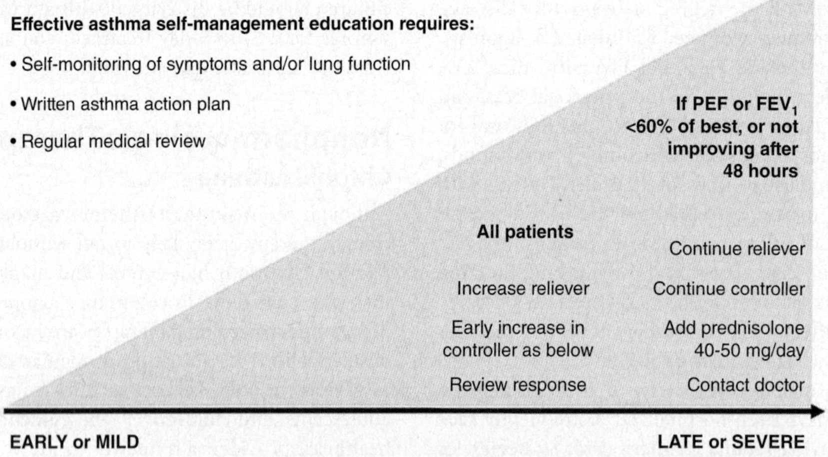

Effective asthma self-management education requires:

- Self-monitoring of symptoms and/or lung function
- Written asthma action plan
- Regular medical review

If PEF or FEV_1 <60% of best, or not improving after 48 hours

All patients

Increase reliever

Early increase in controller as below

Review response

Continue reliever

Continue controller

Add prednisolone 40-50 mg/day

Contact doctor

EARLY or MILD → **LATE or SEVERE**

Medication	Short-term change (1-2 weeks) for worsening asthma	Evidence Level
Increase usual reliever:		
Low dose ICS/formoterol[a]	Increase frequency of reliever use (maximum formoterol total 72 mcg/day	A
Short-acting beta2-agonist (SABA)	Increase frequency of SABA use For pMDI, add spacer	A A
Increase usual controller:		
Maintenance and reliever ICS/formoterol[a]	Continue maintenance ICS/formoterol and increase reliever ICS/formoterol as needed[a] (maximum formoterol total 72 mcg/day)	A
Maintenance ICS with SABA as reliever	At least double ICS; consider increasing ICS to high dose (maximum 2000 mcg/day BDP equivalent)	B
Maintenance ICS/formoterol with SABA as reliever	Quadruple maintenance ICS/formoterol (maximum formoterol 72 mcg/day)	B
Maintenance ICS/other LABA with SABA as reliever	Step up to higher dose formulation of ICS/other LABA, or consider adding a separate ICS inhaler (to maximum total 2000 mcg/day BDP equivalent)	D
Add oral corticosteroids (OCS) and contact doctor		
OCS (prednisone or prednisolone)	Add OCS for severe exacerbations (eg, PEF or FEV_1 <60% personal best or predicted), or patient not responding to treatment over 48 hours. Once started, morning dosing is preferable.	A
	Adults: prednisolone 40-50 mg/day (maximum 50 mg) usually for 5-7 days. *Children 6-11 years:* 1-2 mg/kg/day (maximum 40 mg) usually for 3-5 days	D
	Tapering is not needed if OCS are prescribed for <2 weeks	B

FIGURE 44-7 Self-management of worsening asthma in adults and adolescents with a written asthma action plan. BDP: beclomethasone dipropionate: FEV_1: forced expiratory volume in 1 second: ICS: inhaled corticosteroid: PEF: peak expiratory flow: SABA short-acting $beta_2$-against. Options are listed in order of evidence. [a]ICS-formoterol as-needed for relief of symptoms in mild asthma, or as part of maintenance and reliever regimen with low dose budesonide or beclomethasone with formoterol. Based on product information, the maximum recommended dose of ICS-formoterol in a single day is a total of 48 mcg formoterol, for beclomethasone-formoterol, and 72 mcg for budesonide-formoterol. *(© 2022 Global Initiative for Asthma, used with express permission, www.ginasthma.org.)*

Acute Asthma

Infants and young children may be mildly dehydrated owing to increased insensible loss, vomiting, and decreased intake.[44] Unless dehydration has occurred, increased fluid therapy is not indicated in acute asthma management because the capillary leak from cytokines and increased negative intrathoracic pressures may promote edema in the airways.[44] Correction of significant dehydration is always indicated, and the physical examination and urine specific gravity may help to guide therapy in young children, in whom the state of hydration may be difficult to determine.

Oxygen therapy is the primary nonpharmacologic therapy for the management of acute asthma and is discussed in the section "General Approach to the Management of Acute Severe Asthma." Sedatives should not be given because anxiety may be a sign of hypoxemia, which could be worsened by central nervous system depressants.[44] Antibiotics are also not indicated routinely because viral respiratory tract infections are the primary cause of asthma exacerbations.[44] Antibiotics should be reserved for patients who have signs and symptoms of pneumonia (eg, fever, pulmonary consolidation, and purulent sputum from polymorphonuclear leukocytes).

Respiratory failure or impending respiratory failure as measured by rising $PaCO_2$ (greater than or equal to 45 mm Hg [6 kPa]) or failure to correct hypoxemia with supplemental O_2 therapy is treated first with noninvasive ventilation and eventually with intubation and mechanical ventilation if needed. Oral

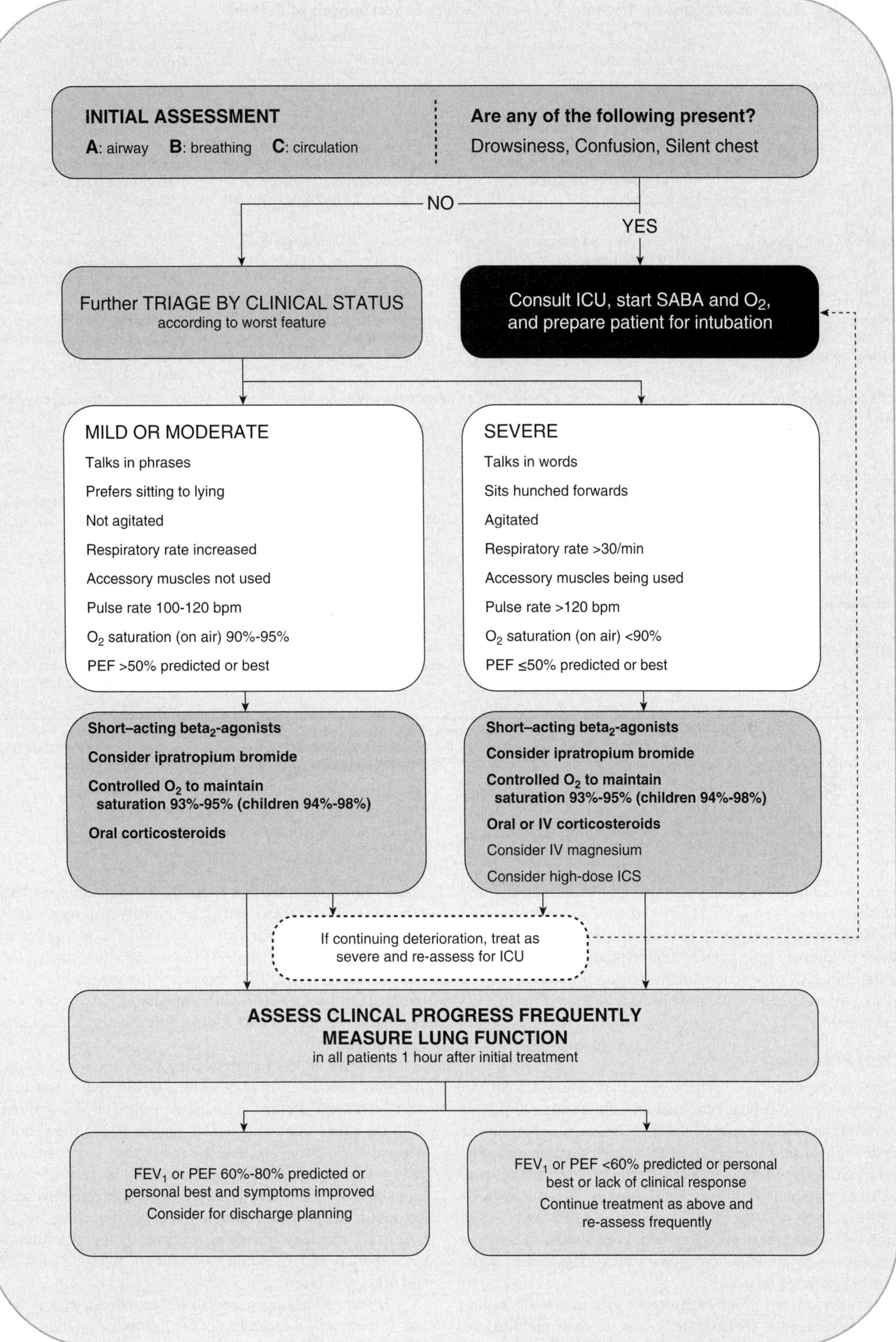

FIGURE 44-8 Management of asthma exacerbations in an acute care facility, for example, the emergency department. To obtain O_2 saturation in SI units (fraction) multiply the results expressed as a percentage by 0.01. *(© 2022 Global Initiative for Asthma, used with express permission, www.ginasthma.org.)*

TABLE 44-3 Dosages of Drugs for Treatment of Acute Severe Exacerbations of Asthma

Medications	Dosages ≥12 Years Old	Dosages <12 Years Old	Comments
Inhaled β-Agonists			
Albuterol nebulizer solution (5 mg/mL, 0.63 mg/3 mL, 1.25 mg/3 mL, 2.5 mg/3 mL)	2.5-5 mg every 20 minutes for three doses, and then 2.5-10 mg every 1-4 hours as needed, or 10-15 mg/hr continuously if in the emergency department or hospitalized	0.15 mg/kg (minimum dose 2.5 mg) every 20 minutes for three doses, and then 0.15-0.3 mg/kg up to 10 mg every 1-4 hours as needed, or 0.5 mg/kg/hr by continuous nebulization if in the emergency department or hospitalized	Only selective β_2-agonists are recommended. For optimal delivery, dilute aerosols to a minimum of 4 mL at gas flow of 6-8 L/min. Use face mask if <4 years
Albuterol MDI (90 µg/puff)	4-8 puffs every 30 minutes up to 4 hours, and then every 1-4 hours as needed	4-8 puffs every 20 minutes for three doses, and then every 1-4 hours as needed	In patients in severe distress, nebulization is preferred; use a VHC-type spacer with face mask if <4 years old
Levalbuterol nebulizer solution (0.31 mg/3 mL, 0.63 mg/3 mL, 2.5 mg/1 mL, 1.25 mg/3 mL)	Give one-half the milligram dose of albuterol above	Give one-half the milligram dose of albuterol above	The single isomer of albuterol is twice as potent on a milligram basis Not recommended
Levalbuterol MDI (45 µg/puff)	See albuterol MDI dose above	See albuterol MDI dose above	See albuterol MDI dose one-half as potent as albuterol on a microgram basis Not recommended
Anticholinergics			
Ipratropium bromide nebulizer solution (0.25 mg/mL)	500 µg every 30 minutes for three doses, and then every 2-4 hours as needed	250 µg every 20 minutes for three doses, and then 250 µg every 2-4 hours	May mix in the same nebulizer with albuterol; only add to β_2-agonist therapy
Ipratropium bromide MDI (18 µg/puff)	8 puffs every 20 minutes as needed for up to 3 hours	4-8 puffs as needed every 2-4 hours	Not to be continued once hospitalized
Corticosteroids[a]			
Prednisone, methylprednisolone, prednisolone	50 mg in one or two divided doses (prednisone equivalent)	1 mg/kg (maximum 40 mg/day) in two divided doses (prednisone equivalent)	For outpatient "burst" use 1-2 mg/kg/day, maximum 60 mg, for 3-5 days in children and 40-60 mg/day in one or two divided doses for 5-7 days in adults

[a]No advantage has been found for very-high-dose corticosteroids in acute severe asthma, nor is there any advantage for IV administration over oral therapy. The usual regimen is to continue the oral corticosteroid for the duration of hospitalization. The final duration of corticosteroid therapy for an acute exacerbation may be from 3 to 10 days. If patients are then started on ICSs, there is no need to taper the systemic corticosteroid dose. ICSs can be started at any time during the exacerbation.

Data from Reference 3.

intubation facilitates secretion removal and bronchoscopy and decreases airway resistance.[45] Heavy sedation and neuromuscular blockade may be needed to reduce ventilatory dyssynchrony in order to improve lung volume and respiratory rate.[45] Oxygen consumption, CO_2 production, and lactate accumulation may be mitigated by using neuromuscular blockade in mechanically ventilated patients.[45]

Patient Education

7 The development of a patient–healthcare provider partnership in care through patient education and the teaching of patient self-management skills should be the cornerstone of any treatment program.[12] There are a number of published self-management programs for children and adults available through the American Lung Association, Asthma and Allergy Foundation of America, asthma treatment centers, and the guidelines from NAEPP and GINA. Asthma self-management programs have been shown to improve patient adherence to medication regimens, self-management skills, and use of healthcare services.[12]

Self-management programs instruct patients in the pathogenesis of asthma and the appropriate use of their medications (including the rationale for treatment and why controllers and relievers are needed), teach patients to recognize triggers for their asthma and early signs of deterioration, how to keep track of symptoms (with or without a diary), and take action.[12] Short-term home PEF monitoring can be used following an exacerbation to assess response to treatment, determine if symptoms seem excessive, assess a baseline for asthma action plans, or evaluate triggers (such as occupational triggers) and is typically recorded for a few weeks.[12] Longer-term PEF monitoring is generally only recommended for those patients with a history of sudden severe asthma exacerbations, difficult-to-control severe asthma, or poor symptom perception.[12]

The NAEPP has recommended a PEF monitoring system or symptom-based action plan using a traffic light scenario (based on a percentage of normal predicted values or personal best values): the green zone is equal to 80% to 100%, the yellow zone is equal to 50% to 79%, and the red zone is less than 50%. The yellow zone is cautionary and requires increasing as-needed bronchodilator use and possibly beginning prednisone if not improved, whereas the red zone warrants contacting the patient's healthcare provider.[43] Samples of clinically tested written action plans that are PEF or symptom-based are available from NAEPP and other sources.[43]

Patient education is essential before monitoring can be effective. It is successful regardless of the healthcare provider who provides it. The NAEPP and GINA advocate significant involvement of all points of patient care in the educational process. The provision of written action plans enhances the success of education and is considered an essential component of care.

Pharmacologic Therapy

β_2-Agonists

5 2 The β_2-agonists are the most effective bronchodilators available. β_2-Agonists do not inhibit the late asthmatic response to allergen challenge or the subsequent BHR. Long-term administration of β_2-agonists does not reduce BHR, confirming a lack of significant anti-inflammatory activity. β_2-Adrenergic stimulation also activates Na^+-K^+-ATPase, produces gluconeogenesis, and enhances insulin secretion, resulting in a mild-to-moderate decrease in serum potassium concentration by driving potassium intracellularly. The chronotropic response to β_2-agonists is mediated in part by baroreceptor reflex mechanisms as a result of the drop in blood pressure from vascular smooth muscle relaxation, as well as by direct stimulation of cardiac β_2-receptors and some β_1 stimulation at high concentrations.

Table 44-4 compares the various short-, long-, and ultra-long-acting β-adrenergic agonists used in asthma in terms of onset and duration of action.[46] The β_2-agonists are functional or physiologic antagonists, in that they relax airway smooth muscle regardless of the mechanism for constriction. When administered in equipotent doses, all the short-acting drugs produce the same intensity of response; the only differences are in duration of action and cardiac toxicity.[46] All the β_2-agonists are more bronchoselective when administered by the aerosol route. Aerosol administration of a SABA provides more rapid response and greater protection against provocations that induce bronchospasm such as exercise and allergen challenges than does systemic administration.[46]

Both the intensity and duration of response to β_2-agonists are dose-dependent, and, more important, the dose-response relationship is dynamic. At increasing levels of baseline bronchoconstriction (irrespective of the stimulus), the dose-response curve is shifted to the right, and the duration of bronchodilation is decreased. This shift is reflected in the need for higher, more frequent doses in acute asthma exacerbations; the duration of protection against significant provocation is much less than the duration of bronchodilation in chronic stable asthma for short-acting inhaled β_2-agonists (see Table 44-4).[46]

Chronic administration of β_2-agonists leads to downregulation (decreased number of β_2-receptors) and a decreased binding affinity (desensitization) for these receptors.[46] Systemic corticosteroid therapy can both prevent and partially reverse this phenomenon.

TABLE 44-4 Onset and Duration of Action of β-Adrenergic Agonists

	Onset and Duration of Action[a]		
Agent	**Bronchodilation (hours)**	**Protection (hours)[a]**	**Onset of bronchodilation**
SABA			
Albuterol/levalbuterol	4-8	2-4	1-2 minutes
Terbutaline	4-6	2-4	1-2 minutes
LABA			
Formoterol	≥12	≥12	1-2 minutes
Salmeterol	≥12	≥12	10 minutes
Ultra-LABA			
Indacaterol	≥24	≥24	1-2 minutes
Olodaterol	≥24	≥24	1-2 minutes
Vilanterol	≥24	≥24	1-2 minutes

[a]Protection refers to the prevention of bronchoconstriction induced by exercise or nonspecific bronchial challenges.

However, the use of ICSs has minimal ability to prevent tolerance to β_2-agonists.[46] Tolerance primarily reduces the duration of bronchodilation as opposed to diminishing the peak response, although the latter can occur as well. A significantly greater tolerance develops in other tissues (eg, lymphocytes and cardiac and skeletal muscle) compared with the lung, primarily as a result of the surplus β_2-receptors found in respiratory smooth muscle. Tolerance to the extra-pulmonary effects (cardiac stimulation and hypokalemia) may account for a lack of significant cardiac effects despite chronic inhaled β_2-agonist therapy. Thus, chronic β_2-agonist administration produces a tolerance that can be easily overcome by increasing the dose or by administering systemic corticosteroids. Most of the tolerance occurs within 1 to 2 weeks of regular administration and does not worsen with continued administration. As would be expected from a receptor phenomenon, cross-tolerance to all β_2-agonists develops.

Short-Acting β_2-Agonists 4 The short-acting inhaled β_2-agonists are the most effective bronchodilators and the treatment of first choice for the management of acute severe asthma.[12] In adults, administration as either continuous nebulization in a large volume nebulizer or intermittent administration (every 20 minutes for three doses) over 1-hour results in equivalent improvement.[12] Systematic reviews of continuous versus intermittent SABA in severe acute asthma have conflicting findings.[12] There is no role for intravenous β_2-agonists in patients with severe asthma (Evidence A).[12] Effective doses of aerosolized β_2-agonists can be delivered successfully through mechanical ventilator circuits to infants, children, and adults in respiratory failure secondary to severe airway obstruction.

The doses of inhaled β_2-agonists for acute severe asthma exacerbations (see Table 44-3) have been derived empirically. The β_2-agonists follow a log-linear dose-response curve. In addition, the dose-response curve is shifted to the right by more severe bronchospasm or by increased concentrations of bronchospastic mediators, which is characteristic of functional antagonists. The ability to increase the dose of SABA by as much as 5- to 10-fold over doses producing adequate bronchodilation in chronic stable asthma is what contributes to their efficacy in reversing the bronchospasm of acute severe exacerbations. The nebulizer dose of inhaled β_2-agonists for children often is listed on a weight basis (milligrams per kilogram). The preferred method from both an efficiency and economic perspective with an MDI and spacer.[12]

The inhaled β_2-agonists produce similar efficacy whether delivered by MDI plus valved holding chamber (VHC) or nebulization in treating acute severe exacerbations in the ED and hospital. The preferred choice is an MDI with a valved spacer, particularly considering the risk of spreading infectious viral particles via nebulization.[12] Most DPIs are not used for acute severe asthma exacerbations due to the higher inspiratory flows required for adequate drug delivery.[12]

Unlike in children, nebulized albuterol is administered in adults in a fixed-dose (vs a weight-based dose) in order to avoid excessive cardiac stimulation.[3] Conversely, children younger than 5 years are dosed based on weight and should have a fixed minimal dose (2.5 mg albuterol or equivalent) due to the resultant underdosing when weight-based dosing is used; higher doses (up to 10 mg based on weight) can be administered every 1 to 4 hours as needed (Table 44-3). Initial doses of inhaled β_2-agonists can produce vasodilation, worsening ventilation-perfusion mismatch, slightly lowering O_2 saturation or PaO_2.[12] High doses of inhaled β_2-agonists can produce a decrease in serum potassium concentration, an increase in heart rate, and an increase in serum glucose and lactic acid concentration. Electrolyte monitoring may be needed in patients with preexisting heart disease who receive frequent doses for an acute exacerbation.[9] Both children and adults receiving continuously nebulized β_2-agonists (not a recommended treatment)[12] have demonstrated decreased heart rate as their lung function improves which indicates elevated heart rate is not an indication to use lower doses or to avoid using inhaled β_2-agonists.

β_2-Agonists can exist as racemic mixtures (eg, albuterol, salmeterol, formoterol) or as single enantiomers (eg, levalbuterol, indacaterol, olodaterol, vilanterol). There is no evidence to support the use of levalbuterol over albuterol for the treatment of acute severe exacerbations in either children or adults with respect to efficacy or adverse effects.[47]

Primatene Mist® MDI is the only inhaled asthma medication available without a prescription and was reintroduced onto the market in late 2018 as an MDI with a hydrofluoroalkane propellant. Primatene Mist® should only be used for the temporary relief of mild symptoms of intermittent asthma in patients 12 years and older. If improvement is not seen within 20 minutes or symptoms become worse, or the patient requires more than eight inhalations in a 24-hour period or has a recurrence of symptoms within a week, the patient should see a physician for additional evaluation and treatment. Primatene Mist® is less effective than prescription SABAs.

A SABA is also indicated for the as-needed treatment of intermittent episodes of bronchospasm. They inhibit EIB in a dose-dependent fashion and provide complete protection for a 2-hour period following inhalation with varying levels of patient-dependent protection over 4 hours.[12] Although the regular administration of β2-agonists slightly decreases the protective effect, two inhalations prior to exercise still essentially block EIB completely (1% vs 5% drop in FEV_1).[12] The GINA guidelines also recommend low-dose ICS-formoterol taken before exercise but this treatment is not recommended by NAEPP.[11,12]

Long-Acting and Ultra Long-Acting Inhaled β_2-Agonists

The two LABAs, formoterol and salmeterol, provide long-lasting bronchodilation (greater than or equal to 12 hours) and are dosed twice daily[48] (see Table 44-4). Formoterol, in combination with an ICS, may be dosed on a daily and as-needed basis (thus, more frequently than twice daily). Unlike the more water-soluble SABA, the long-acting agents are lipid-soluble, readily partitioning into the outer phospholipid layer of the cell membrane.[48] In addition, ultra-LABAs (indacaterol, vilanterol, and olodaterol) have a 24-hour bronchodilator duration of effect permitting once-daily dosing. Only vilanterol in combination with fluticasone furoate (with and without umeclidinium, an anticholinergic) is available for once-daily dosing for asthma in adults aged 18 years and older in the United States. Products containing indacaterol and olodaterol are only indicated for COPD but are being evaluated for asthma.

The LABAs and ultra-LABAs are more β_2-selective than albuterol and more bronchoselective by virtue of their property of remaining in the lung tissue cell membrane, which produces its longer duration.[48] The onset of action (time required to increase FEV_1 by 12% over baseline) is similar to that of albuterol for LABAs and ultra-LABAs with the exception of salmeterol which has an onset of approximately 10 minutes. LABAs are available as a single entity and as fixed-dose combinations with ICSs (see below) though single-entity LABA products are FDA-approved for use only with ICS. Patients need to be counseled to continue to use their SABA for acute exacerbations while receiving the ICS/LABA combination products.

As with SABA, tolerance can occur with chronic administration of LABAs and seems to plateau after about 1 week of regular therapy but response recovers rapidly after only 2 to 3 days of nonuse.[48] Long-term trials have shown no diminution in bronchodilator response but a partial loss of the bronchoprotective effect against methacholine, histamine, and exercise challenge.[48] These effects do not seem to have a significant impact on the quality of asthma control with chronic daily use.

Concern for risks with LABA use began shortly after approval of the first available LABA, salmeterol, with reports of respiratory deaths in salmeterol users, and risks were evaluated in multiple meta-analyses which resulted in Boxed Warnings on the labeling of products containing an ICS-LABA.[12] In response to these findings, the FDA mandated several large clinical trials by the manufacturers to evaluate the risk of ICS-LABA therapy on serious asthma-related adverse effects. The results of these trials which included over 41,000 patients aged 12 years and older, and a single trial in children 4 to 11 years old, indicate that there is no significantly increased risk of asthma-related hospitalizations, intubations, or asthma-related deaths with ICS-LABA compared to ICS; the FDA has removed the Boxed Warning for ICS-LABA products but has retained it for single-ingredient LABA products.[49]

Corticosteroids

4 Corticosteroids are the most effective anti-inflammatories available to treat asthma.[11,12] Actions useful in treating asthma include: (a) increasing the number of β_2-adrenergic receptors and improving the receptor responsiveness to β_2-adrenergic stimulation, (b) reducing mucus production and hypersecretion, (c) reducing BHR, and (d) reducing airway edema and exudation. The glucocorticoid receptor is found in the cytoplasm of most body cells, explaining the multiple effects of systemic corticosteroids. There is no difference between glucocorticoid receptors found throughout the body; however, genetic differences in the glucocorticoid receptor among individuals may explain some of the variations in response.[50] The corticosteroids are lipophilic, readily cross the cell membrane, and combine with the glucocorticoid receptor. The activated glucocorticoid receptor complex then enters the nucleus, where it acts as a transcription factor leading to gene activation or suppression.[50] This leads to specific mRNA production, resulting in increased production of anti-inflammatory mediators and suppression of genes regulating the expression of several pro-inflammatory cytokines such as tumor necrosis factor-α, GM-CSF, interferon-γ, IL-1, IL-4, IL-5, IL-6, IL-8, IL-10, and IL-13.[50] In addition, the activated glucocorticoid receptor complex can act directly with transcription factors, nuclear factor-κB, and activating protein 1 to prevent the action of pro-inflammatory cytokines on the cell.[50]

Given that glucocorticoids work by altering gene expression, the time required to see a particular effect depends on the time required for new protein synthesis, decreased formation of the particular mediator, and resolution of the inflammatory response. While the cellular and biochemical effects are immediate, variable amounts of time are required to produce a clinical response. β_2-Receptor density increases within hours of corticosteroid administration leading to improved responsiveness to β2-agonists. In acute severe asthma, 3 to 8 hours may be required before any clinical response is noted.[51] The chronic use of corticosteroids does not induce a state of corticosteroid dependence and there is no evidence of tolerance produced by chronic administration.

The systemic and inhaled corticosteroids most commonly used in the treatment of asthma are compared in Table 44-5.[51,52] The pharmacokinetic and pharmacodynamic parameters (receptor binding affinity, bioavailability, clearance) influence the therapeutic index of inhaled corticosteroids. Higher receptor binding affinities and longer half-lives contribute to both improved efficacy but also increase the potential for systemic adverse effects. These factors affect the relative efficacy between products and thus may influence treatment decisions.

Systemic Corticosteroids Systemic corticosteroids are indicated in all patients with acute severe asthma exacerbations not responding completely to initial SABA administration (every 20 minutes for three doses) and should be administered within 1 hour of presentation to reduce the risk of hospitalization.[12] Clinical improvement is

TABLE 44-5 Pharmacodynamic/Pharmacokinetic Comparison of the Corticosteroids

Systemic	Anti-inflammatory Potency	Mineralocorticoid Potency	Duration of Biologic Activity (hours)
Hydrocortisone	1	1	8-12
Prednisone	4	0.8	12-36
Methylprednisolone	5	0.5	12-36
Dexamethasone	25	0	36-72
	Receptor Binding Affinity[a]	**Oral Bioavailability (%)**	**Systemic Clearance (L/hr)**
Beclomethasone dipropionate/ monoproprionate[b]	0.4/13.5	20/40	150/120
Budesonide	9.4	11	84
Ciclesonide/des-ciclesonide[b]	0.12/12	<1/<1	152/228
Flunisolide	1.8	20	58
Fluticasone proprionate	18	≤1	66
Mometasone furoate[c]	23	<1	53

[a]Receptor binding affinities are relative to dexamethasone equal to 1.

[b]Beclomethasone diproprionate and ciclesonide are prodrugs that are activated in the lung to their active metabolites beclomethasone monopropionate and des-ciclesonide, respectively.

[c]Mometasone furoate was studied in a different receptor system. Value estimated from relative values of beclomethasone dipropionate and fluticasone proprionate in that system.

noted after approximately 4 hours.[12] IV therapy offers no therapeutic advantage over oral administration except in patients who are too dyspneic to swallow, vomiting, or intubated.[12] This therapy usually is continued until hospital discharge. There is no need to taper the systemic corticosteroid dose following discharge from the hospital in patients who are prescribed an ICS for outpatient therapy (Evidence B).[12] Adults are effectively treated with a 5- to 7-day course of therapy but children typically require only 3-5 days (Evidence A).[12] Very short courses (3-5 days) are effective in reducing hospitalization from acute exacerbations.[12] Use of the shorter-acting corticosteroids such as prednisone will produce less adrenal suppression than the longer-acting dexamethasone.[12] Dexamethasone for 1 or 2 days versus a 5-day course of prednisone/prednisolone may be an option for children and has the benefit of causing less vomiting.[12] If there is an inadequate response to dexamethasone, switching to prednisone should be considered.[12] Multiple daily dosing of systemic corticosteroids for the initial therapy of acute asthma exacerbations is warranted because receptor binding affinities of lung corticosteroid receptors are decreased in the face of airway inflammation. However, patients with less-severe exacerbations may be treated adequately with once-daily administration.[2]

The beneficial and adverse effects of corticosteroids in asthma are dose- and duration-dependent. Adverse effects can occur in adults and children even after a short duration (<14 days) of therapy. In adults, there is an increased risk of 1.8- to 5.3-fold in fracture, gastrointestinal bleeding, sepsis, venous thromboembolism, and heart failure (the only adverse events evaluated) in the 30 days following a short course of systemic corticosteroids.[53,54] A similar pattern is observed in children with a 1.8- to 2.2-fold increased risk in gastrointestinal bleeding, sepsis, and pneumonia.[55] Adverse effects of chronic daily use of oral corticosteroids are well known (Table 44-6). The clinician must continually balance the toxicity of chronic systemic corticosteroid therapy with the control of asthma symptoms. The ideal use is to administer the systemic corticosteroids in a short "burst" (<7 days) and then to maintain the patient on appropriate long-term control therapy with ICSs.[12]

TABLE 44-6 Adverse Effects of Chronic Systemic Glucocorticoid Administration

Hypothalamic-pituitary-adrenal suppression	Hypertension
Growth retardation	Skin striae
Skeletal muscle myopathy	Impaired wound healing
Osteoporosis/fractures	Inhibition of leukocyte and monocyte function
Aseptic necrosis of bone	Subcutaneous tissue atrophy
Pancreatitis	Glaucoma
Pseudotumor cerebri	Posterior subcapsular cataracts
Psychiatric disturbances	Moon facies
Sodium and water retention	Central redistribution of fat
Hypokalemia/hyperglycemia	

Inhaled Corticosteroids The principal advantage of the ICSs is their high topical potency to reduce inflammation in the lung and low systemic activity.[51] The ICSs have high receptor binding affinity which is related to potency, and ICS products differ from each other in binding affinity by as much as 10- to 100-fold.[51] However, potency differences can be overcome simply by giving different microgram dosages of the drug (Table 44-5). Depending upon the microgram per inhalation, the potency differences between products will be reflected by the number of inhalations required to achieve the same therapeutic effect. Products that require more inhalations per dose or that must be administered twice daily may result in poorer adherence.

In the low-to-medium doses recommended (Tables 44-7 and 44-8), ICSs are safe for long-term administration. They do not reduce airway remodeling or prevent the loss of lung function seen in some patients with persistent asthma.[56] ICS therapy does not prevent the development of asthma in high-risk infants or induce asthma remission as BHR and other measures of inflammation return to pretreatment levels soon after the discontinuation of therapy.[12] The sensitivity and consequent clinical response to ICSs can vary among patients.[11,12]

Aerosol delivery of the corticosteroid is variable and is influenced by the nominal dose from the specific device (eg, that dose that leaves the actuator) and any device attached to MDIs to improve inhalation technique. Different devices which contain the same chemical entity may result in twofold differences in delivery. Thus, the delivery method can make a significant difference in the relative dose or therapeutic index.[12]

TABLE 44-7 Inhaled Corticosteroids and Comparative Daily Dosages in Adults and Adolescents (12 Years and Older)

	Comparative Daily Dosages (μg) of Inhaled Corticosteroids		
	Low Dose	Medium Dose	High Dose
Beclomethasone dipropionate DPI[a]	80-240	>240-480	>480
Budesonide DPI	180-540	>540-1,080	>1,080
Budesonide Nebules	unknown	unknown	unknown
Ciclesonide HFA[b] MDI[c]	160-320	320-640	>640
Flunisolide HFA MDI	320	320-640	>640
Fluticasone furoate DPI		100	200
Fluticasone propionate HFA MDI	888-264	264-440	>440
Fluticasone propionate DPI	100-300	300-500	>500
Mometasone furoate DPI	110-220	>220-440	>440

[a]Dry powder inhaler.
[b]Hydrofluoroalkane
[c]Metered-dose inhaler.
Data from Reference 57.

TABLE 44-8 Inhaled Corticosteroids and Comparative Daily Dosages in Children (6 to 11 Years)

	Comparative Daily Dosages (μg) of Inhaled Corticosteroids		
	Low Dose	Medium Dose	High Dose
Beclomethasone DPI[a] dipropionate DPI[a]	80-160	>160-320	>320
Budesonide DPI	180-360	>360-720	>720
Budesonide Nebules	500	1,000	2,000
Ciclesonide HFA[b] MDI[c]	80-160	>160-320	>320
Flunisolide HFA MDI	160	320	>320
Fluticasone furoate DPI		100	200
Fluticasone propionate HFA MDI	88-176	176-352	>352
Fluticasone propionate DPI	100-200	200-400	>400
Mometasone furoate DPI	110	220-440	>440

[a]Dry powder inhaler.
[b]Hydrofluoroalkane.
[c]Metered-dose inhaler.
Data from Reference 57.

All ICSs are approved for once- or twice-daily dosing. The ICSs have pharmacokinetic differences that result in different topical/systemic activity.[51] Most evidence is consistent with log-linear dose-response curves for both indirect (measures to assess efficacy such as lung function, BHR, symptom control) and direct responses (receptor activity). The log-linear nature of the dose-response curve for ICS clinical effects makes dose-response relationships for efficacy difficult to establish. Alternatively, comparative potency effects may be based upon the dose-response adverse effects on hypothalamic-pituitary-adrenal axis suppression.[51] Comparable ICS doses (see Tables 44-3 and 44-4) are based on extensive clinical trial data.[12] Clinically comparable doses take into consideration drug potency differences as well as device delivery differences but not the potential for systemic activity and potential adverse effects.

TABLE 44-9 Effects of Inhaled Corticosteroids

Beneficial Effects	Potential Adverse Effects
• Decrease eosinophil numbers • Decrease mast cell numbers • Decrease T-lymphocyte cytokine production • Inhibit transcription of inflammatory genes in airway epithelium • Reduce endothelial cell leak • Upregulate β_2-receptor production • Reduce airway epithelial subbasement membrane thickening	• Hoarseness, dysphonia, thrush • Growth retardation, skeletal muscle myopathy • Osteoporosis, fractures, and aseptic necrosis of the hip • Posterior subcapsular cataract formation and glaucoma • Adrenal axis suppression, immunosuppression • Impaired wound healing, easy bruising, skin striae • Hyperglycemia/hypokalemia, hypertension • Psychiatric disturbances

Because the glucocorticoid receptors within the various tissues are the same, differences in the pharmacokinetic profile are required to produce differences in the topical/systemic effect ratio (therapeutic index).[51] Pharmacokinetic properties that enhance topical selectivity include higher potency, rapid systemic clearance, poor oral bioavailability, and prolonged residence time in the lung.[51] Due to their high lipophilicity, systemic clearance of the available ICSs is very rapid, approaching the rate of liver blood flow with the exception of beclomethasone diproprionate and ciclesonide, which are prodrugs metabolized in the lung by esterases to the active compounds, beclomethasone monopropionate, and des-ciclesonide.[51] However, the ICSs differ markedly in their oral bioavailability, although they all undergo rather extensive first-pass metabolism to less active substances when absorbed.[51] The ICSs produce dose-dependent systemic effects, contributed by the orally absorbed fraction and the fraction absorbed from the lung. (Table 44-9). Essentially, all the drug that reaches the lung is absorbed systemically; thus, a slow absorption from the lung results in an apparent long elimination half-life and enhances topical selectivity by lowering the systemic concentration. The potential advantage of the drugs with low oral bioavailability is obviated by using an MDI plus spacer device for the drugs with higher oral bioavailability because appropriate spacers substantially reduce the oral amount delivered.[12] The use of VHCs also can increase systemic activity by increasing lung delivery of drugs that are not absorbed significantly orally.[51] Mouth rinsing and spitting will also reduce oral absorption and are particularly useful for DPI devices.[12]

The response to ICSs is somewhat delayed. Most patients' symptoms will improve in the first 1 to 2 weeks of therapy and will reach maximum improvement in 4 to 8 weeks.[3] Improvement in baseline FEV_1 and PEF may require 3 to 6 weeks for maximum improvement, whereas improvement in BHR requires 2 to 3 weeks and approaches maximum in 1 to 3 months but may continue to improve over 1 year.[2] Most of the improvement in these parameters occurs at low-to-medium doses, and there is a large variability in response, with 10% of patients not demonstrating an improvement in either parameter.

Local adverse effects from ICSs include oropharyngeal candidiasis and dysphonia that are dose-dependent. The dysphonia (reported in 5%-20% of patients) is due to a local corticosteroid-induced myopathy of the vocal cords. The use of a spacer device with MDIs can decrease oropharyngeal deposition and thus decrease the incidence and severity of local side effects.[12] In infants who require ICS delivery through a face mask, the parent should clean the nasal-perioral area with a damp cloth following each treatment to prevent oropharyngeal candidiasis.

Systemic adverse effects can occur with any of the ICSs given in a sufficiently high dose.[12] Long-term adverse effects of greatest concern include growth suppression in children, osteoporosis, cataracts, dermal thinning, easy bruising, and adrenal insufficiency and crisis.[2] Growth retardation may occur with low-to-medium ICS doses. However, the growth reduction is transient, in that growth velocity is reduced in the first 6 months to 2 years of therapy and then returns to normal.[12] The effect is small (1-2 cm total) and not cumulative, but does persist into adulthood (difference of 0.7% from adult height).[12] The suppression of the HPA axis and decreased bone mineralization are dose-dependent and are not significant clinically except at high doses. The risks, therefore, depend on the therapeutic index of each ICS and its delivery device.

Many of the ICSs, including fluticasone propionate, budesonide, ciclesonide, and mometasone furoate, are metabolized in the GI tract and liver by cytochrome (CYP) 3A4 isoenzymes. Potent inhibitors of CYP3A4 such as ritonavir, itraconazole, and ketoconazole have the potential for increased systemic concentrations of these ICSs by increasing oral availability and decreasing systemic clearance.[12] Some cases of clinically significant Cushing's syndrome and secondary adrenal insufficiency have been reported.[12]

There is no specific pharmacologic or pharmacokinetic aspect of the current ICSs that allows for once-daily dosing because all the agents studied (both the older low-potency ICSs and newer high-potency ICSs) have been effective, provided that patients had relatively mild-to-moderate asthma. More severe patients may require multiple daily dosing. The inflammatory response of asthma has been shown to inhibit corticosteroid-receptor binding. Once asthma is controlled, many patients are able to reduce the ICS dose and maintain control.

Anticholinergics

Anticholinergic agents have a long history of use for asthma, with an evolving role in the chronic management of asthma.[58] Anticholinergics are competitive inhibitors of muscarinic receptors. Unlike β_2-agonists, they are not functional antagonists, rather they reverse cholinergic-mediated bronchoconstriction. This difference in mechanism supports the combined use of anticholinergics and β_2-agonists in the treatment of severe acute asthma exacerbations. The normal bronchial tone is maintained through parasympathetic innervation of the airways via the vagus nerve.[58] A number of the triggers and mediators of asthma (ie, histamine, prostaglandins, sulfur dioxide, exercise, and allergens) produce bronchoconstriction in part through vagal reflex mechanisms.[58] Studies consistently demonstrate that anticholinergics are effective bronchodilators in asthma. There is some evidence that anticholinergics may reduce allergen-induced and methacholine-induced airway responsiveness.[58]

Five muscarinic receptor subtypes (M_1 through M_5) have been identified; M_1, M_2, and M_3 are the principal receptors in the airway.[58] Available anticholinergics ipratropium, aclidinium (not indicated for asthma), glycopyrrolate (not indicated for asthma), and tiotropium are nonselective antagonists of M1, M2, and M3 receptors; umeclidinium bromide which is indicated for persistent asthma is selective for the M3 receptor. M1 receptors are found in epithelial cells and the ganglia and regulate electrolyte and water secretion; M2 receptors, on airway smooth muscle and parasympathetic neurons, have a limited role on smooth muscle constriction; M3 receptors are the primary subtype responsible for smooth muscle bronchoconstriction and mucus secretion.[58] Ipratropium bromide has a duration of action of 4 to 8 hours and is used for the relief of acute asthma symptoms in combination with SABA. The time to reach maximum bronchodilation for ipratropium is considerably slower than for aerosolized SABA (30-60 minutes vs 5-10 minutes). However, this difference is of little clinical consequence because some bronchodilation is seen within 30 seconds; 50% of maximum response occurs within 3 minutes. Ipratropium bromide is useful as adjunctive therapy in acute severe asthma not completely responsive to SABA alone.[12] Care should be taken when administering ipratropium bromide by nebulizer. If a tight mask or mouthpiece is not used, the ipratropium bromide that deposits in the eyes may produce pupillary dilation and difficulty in accommodation. There is no benefit to continuing combined anticholinergic therapy during hospitalization on the duration of stay or clinical outcomes.[12] In patients with persistent asthma who are intolerant to adverse effects from short-acting β_2-agonists may be prescribed ipratropium for rescue inhaler use.

Tiotropium bromide and umeclidinium bromide are long-acting inhaled anticholinergics with a duration of 24 hours. Tiotropium may be considered an add-on therapy in patients whose asthma is not well controlled with a medium-to-high dose of ICS and LABA combination therapy per the GINA guidelines in those 6 years and older and in those 12 years and older per the 2020 Asthma Focused Updates.[11,12] The addition of tiotropium modestly improves lung function and severe exacerbation requiring oral corticosteroid treatment.[11,12] Umeclidinium bromide is available as a combination inhaler with fluticasone and vilanterol and is indicated in patients aged 18 years and older.

Leukotriene Modifiers

Two cysteinyl LTRAs (zafirlukast and montelukast) and one 5-lipoxygenase inhibitor (zileuton) are available in the United States. These drugs have modest effects on bronchodilation, lung function, exacerbation frequency, and exercise-induced bronchoconstriction; patients with aspirin-induced asthma may benefit.[2] Clinical use of zileuton is limited due to the potential for elevated liver enzymes (especially in the first 3 months of therapy), and the potential inhibition of drugs metabolized by the CYP3A4 isoenzymes. They are not preferred alternatives in mild persistent asthma nor as alternative add-on therapy for moderate persistent asthma (see Tables 44-3 and 44-4).[11,12]

One major advantage of the LT modifiers is that they are effective orally, and can be administered once or twice a day. However, they are less effective in asthma than low doses of ICSs.[11,12] Although montelukast is approved for EIB in adults, it is significantly less effective than SABA. They are not as effective as LABAs when added to ICSs for moderate persistent asthma.[11,12] It is not yet possible to assuredly predict which patients respond best to LT modifiers, although there is some evidence that patients with aspirin-sensitive asthma do well. Other predictors may include preschool age, females, short duration of disease, minimal atopy, high cotinine levels, or high urinary LTE4 levels may respond favorably.[59] It is possible that genetic polymorphisms in the 5-lipoxygenase or LTC_4 synthase pathways or in cys-LT_1 receptors might predict better responders in the future.[59]

The use of montelukast and zafirlukast has fallen out of favor due to the increased observance of unusual adverse effects and modest therapeutic efficacy. Eosinophilic granulomatosis with polyangiitis (formerly known as Churg–Strauss syndrome) is a rare antineutrophil cytoplasmic antibody vasculitis characterized by eosinophil involvement and granulomatous necrotizing effects on small and medium vessels.[60] Other inflammatory skin reactions have been reported that resolve upon discontinuation of montelukast.[60]

Also worrisome are reports of adverse neuropsychiatric events which resulted in the FDA issuing mental health warnings with the use of montelukast beginning in 2008 and updated in 2009 and, most recently, in 2020. In children, the relative risk of neuropsychiatric adverse reactions associated with montelukast is 12 times greater than with ICS.[61] The risks are greatest within a few weeks of starting therapy, resulting in approximately 16% of children discontinuing therapy. Therefore, patients should be closely monitored when initiating treatment with montelukast.[61] The most frequently reported reactions are irritability, aggressiveness, and sleep disturbance; suicidality, though rare, has also been reported.[61]

Reports of fatal hepatic failure associated with zafirlukast have prompted an FDA warning for patients to be made aware of signs and symptoms of hepatic dysfunction.

Zileuton can be administered twice daily as controlled-release tablets. Efficacy data are more limited, liver function monitoring is recommended, and drug interactions are reported with warfarin and theophylline.

Biologic Agents

Table 44-10 outlines the available biologic agents as well as the biomarkers predicting therapeutic responses and the biomarkers modulated by therapy.[62] These agents are targeting the IgE pathway (relevant to allergic asthma) or IL-4, IL-13, and IL-5 pathways (relevant to the Th2 pathway and eosinophilic disorders) and are indicated for patients with moderate or severe asthma (depending upon the drug) along with other biomarker or other clinical indicator associated with treatment response. Tezepelumab blocks TSLP and is potentially a first in class drug.

These products are typically reserved for patients with moderate-to-severe persistent asthma who have poor symptom control despite treatment on high-dose ICS-LABA with relevant allergic (or eosinophilic) biomarkers or need maintenance oral corticosteroids. Defining which patients have severe asthma and are candidates for biologic therapy consideration is important. The European Respiratory Society (ERS) and the American Thoracic Society (ATS) define severe asthma as "asthma which requires treatment with high-dose inhaled corticosteroids plus a second controller (and/or systemic corticosteroids) to prevent it from becoming 'uncontrolled' or which remains uncontrolled despite this therapy."[64] According to the GINA guidelines approximately, 3% to 10% of people with asthma have severe disease.[2]

The 2020 Asthma Focused Updates did not include an evaluation of biologic therapy because at the time the topics were identified, the only biologic available was omalizumab. GINA provides step-wise guidance for treating difficult-to-treat asthma, which after optimizing management delineates patients with severe asthma and when to consider add-on biologic treatment.[12] Having severe asthma incurs significant healthcare costs.[12] Affordability, availability, predictors of response, and patient preferences should be considered prior to the selection of a biologic agent. Eligibility for biologic therapy will also be determined by age and other specific criteria. In general, criteria for most biologic studies have included pre-bronchodilator FEV_1 between 40% and 80% of predicted and one or more exacerbations in the past year despite moderate-to-high dose ICS.[65] Although some biologics are available for use in children younger than 12 years, limited numbers of pediatric patients have been included in trials. After the biologic agent is initiated, a trial of at least 4 months is recommended. If the trial results in an unclear response, the trial should be continued for 6 to 12 months, and for those with little to no response, a different biologic should be considered (if eligible). In those patients demonstrating a positive response, biologic therapy should continue and be reassessed every 3 to 6 months. With each assessment, considerations for decreasing or stopping oral corticosteroid therapy first and then other inhaled treatments are recommended, though patients should be on at least a moderate ICS dose. Testing for parasitic infections should be considered prior to starting biologic therapy as these infections can cause blood eosinophilia and untreated infections with a biologic on board can lead to disseminated disease.[12]

TABLE 44-10 Targeted Biologic Therapies for Asthma and Potential Biomarkers

Pathway	Biologic Agents Approved	Biomarkers Predicting Therapeutic Response	Route of Administration
IgE	Omalizumab	FeNO Blood eosinophils	Subcutaneous
IL-5	Mepolizumab Reslizumab	Blood eosinophils	Mepolizumab: subcutaneous Reslizumab: intravenous
IL-5Rα	Benralizumab	Blood eosinophils	Subcutaneous
IL-4Rα (IL-4/IL-13)	Dupilumab	Blood eosinophils	Subcutaneous
TSLP	Tezepelumab	–	Subcutaneous

CRTh2, chemoattractant receptor-homologous molecule expressed on Th2 cells; FeNO, the fraction of exhaled nitric oxide; Ig, immunoglobulin; IL, interleukin; R, receptor; TSLP, thymic stromal lymphopoietin.

Data from Reference 63.

Anti-IgE Omalizumab is a recombinant anti-IgE antibody approved for the treatment of allergic asthma not well controlled on oral corticosteroids or ICSs.[66] It is a humanized monoclonal antibody directed at IgE. Omalizumab binds to the Fc portion of the IgE antibody preventing the binding of IgE to its high-affinity receptor (FcεRI) on mast cells and basophils.[65] The decreased binding of IgE on the surface of mast cells leads to a decrease in the release of mediators in response to allergen exposure.

Omalizumab is administered subcutaneously every 2 to 4 weeks and the dosage is determined by the patient's baseline total serum IgE level (international units per milliliter [kIU/L]) and body weight (kilograms).[12] Treatment must be administered in a clinical setting for observation for anaphylaxis after each dose, so patient selection must be judicious to ensure commitment to therapy. Omalizumab is currently recommended for the treatment in patients greater than 6 years of age with moderate-to-severe asthma, which is not adequately controlled by ICS, ICS-LABA, and in some cases, oral corticosteroids. Elevated levels of FeNO (24 ppb or greater) and eosinophil levels greater than 260 eosinophils/μg/L while taking high dose ICS are predictive of exacerbation reduction response.[2]

Omalizumab is the biological agent with the greatest safety data in children and long-term safety data has been reassuring.[65] Patients taking omalizumab reported local injection site reactions (similar to all subcutaneous biologics) and rates of anaphylaxis at 0.1% which carries a Boxed Warning. Initial reports indicated increases in malignant neoplasms, however, observational studies have shown rates similar to placebo.

Anti-IL-5 Mepolizumab and reslizumab target IL-5 which regulates the terminal differentiation of eosinophils as well as eosinophil activation and recruitment to the airway.[65] These drugs are monoclonal antibodies directed against IL-5 to block activation of the IL-5 receptor on eosinophils. Benralizumab binds to the alpha subunit of the IL-5 receptor of eosinophils and prevents the binding of IL-5, thus mitigating downstream eosinophilic inflammation.[65]

Mepolizumab is approved for children 6 years and older and has demonstrated long-term safety data in children aged 6 to 11 years.[65] Benralizumab is approved for patients aged 12 years and older; reslizumab is approved for those with severe asthma, 18 years and older, and is the only biologic available that is administered intravenously. Mepolizumab and reslizumab are dosed every 4 weeks; benralizumab is dosed every 4 weeks for 3 months then every 8 weeks. Doses are to be administered in a healthcare setting by professionals who are prepared to manage anaphylaxis. Each of these drugs is indicated for patients with an "eosinophilic phenotype" which has not been formally defined by the FDA or any professional society. However, reductions in exacerbation rate of approximately 50% is observed when patients have a certain minimum peripheral blood eosinophil count which varies by drug.[65] Blood eosinophil counts may be a better predictor of response compared with sputum (airway) eosinophil numbers (airway eosinophils are the ideal biomarker but are difficult to measure clinically).[65] Responsiveness to exacerbation reduction appears to be more likely with blood eosinophil levels above 150 cells/μL (0.15×10^9/L) with mepolizumab, above 400 cells/μL (0.4×10^9/L) with reslizumab, and above 300 cells/μL (0.3×10^9/L) for benralizumab.[65] Benefits in reduced exacerbation rate have been observed in patients who require daily oral corticosteroid therapy while also having an oral corticosteroid-sparing effect.[65]

Patients aged 50 years or older who are to be treated with mepolizumab should receive a recombinant zoster vaccination (preferably not a live virus) 4 weeks prior to starting treatment.[65] Similar to omalizumab, reslizumab had some initial concerns with malignancy that have been mitigated by event rates similar to placebo. Also, as intravenous therapy, the risk of anaphylaxis is higher with reslizumab and includes a Boxed Warning. In addition to injection site reactions, common adverse effects for all three include respiratory tract infections, headache, and asthma worsening.[65]

Anti-IL-4/IL-13 (Dupilumab) Dupilumab targets the IL-4α receptor, thus blocking IL4 and IL-13 signaling which are key cytokines that promote IgE synthesis and inflammatory cell recruitment. Dupilumab is approved for patients with moderate-to-severe asthma aged 12 years and older with an eosinophilic phenotype and is administered subcutaneously every 2 weeks. Unlike mepolizumab, reslizumab, and benralizumab, FeNO levels above 25 ppb in addition to blood eosinophil levels of at least 150 cells/μL (0.15×10^9/L) is predictive of a response in reducing asthma exacerbation rate by approximately 50%; in those on maintenance OCS, it reduces exacerbation rate and maintenance oral corticosteroid doses.[65] Injection site reactions with dupilumab are relatively higher compared to other biologic agents. Patients have also developed eosinophilia (>3,000 cells/μg/L) and patients should be monitored for vasculitic-appearing rashes, worsening pulmonary or cardiac symptoms, or neuropathy with peripheral eosinophilia.[65]

Magnesium Sulfate

Intravenous and nebulized magnesium sulfate have been used in addition to standard therapies (β_2-agonists, systemic corticosteroids, anticholinergics, and oxygen) in children and adults with severe or life-threatening asthma. Magnesium sulfate is a moderately potent bronchodilator, producing relaxation of smooth muscle by blocking calcium ion influx into smooth muscles and it may have anti-inflammatory effects.[44] For patients with severe asthma exacerbations, current guidelines suggest that a single 2 g intravenous infusion can be helpful in reducing hospital admissions in adults who have an FEV_1 less than 25% to 30% predicted upon arrival in the ED, children and adults who have persistent hypoxemia after standard treatment, and children whose FEV_1 remains below 60% predicted after 1 hour of standard treatment (Evidence A).[12] There appears to be little benefit to adding intravenous or nebulized magnesium in patients with less severe asthma.[12] In children 2 years and older with acute severe asthma and symptoms for 6 hours or less, nebulized (or intravenous) magnesium may be considered during the first hour of standard treatment with nebulized albuterol plus ipratropium.[12] The adverse effects of magnesium sulfate include hypotension, facial flushing, sweating, depressed deep tendon reflexes, hypothermia, cardiac, CNS, and respiratory depression.

Methylxanthines

Methylxanthines have been used for asthma therapy for more than 50 years, but are rarely used owing to the high risk of severe life-threatening toxicity and numerous drug interactions, as well as decreased efficacy compared with ICSs, LABAs, and biologics. Theophylline, the primary methylxanthine of interest, is a moderately potent bronchodilator with mild anti-inflammatory properties and is available for oral and intravenous administration but is not recommended in the GINA guidelines for acute exacerbations or persistent asthma.[12]

TABLE 44-11 Factors Affecting Theophylline Clearance

Decreased Clearance	% Decrease	Increased Clearance	% Increase
Cimetidine	−25 to −60	Rifampin	+53
Macrolides: erythromycin, TAO, clarithromycin	−25 to −50	Carbamazepine	+50
		Phenobarbital	+34
		Phenytoin	+70
Allopurinol	−20	Charcoal-broiled meat	+30
Propranolol	−30		
Quinolones ciprofloxacin, enoxacin	−20 to −50	High-protein diet	+25
Perfloxacin		Smoking	+40
Interferon	−50	Sulfinpyrazone	+22
Thiabendazole	−65	Moricizine	+50
Ticlopidine	−25	Aminoglutethimide	+50
Zileuton	−35		
Systemic viral illness	−10 to −50		

Theophylline has a log-linear dose-response curve and dosing requires monitoring of blood concentrations for both efficacy and toxicity (excessive blood concentrations can cause seizures and death). In addition, theophylline is eliminated primarily by metabolism via the hepatic CYP 450 mixed-function oxidase microsomal enzymes (primarily the CYP1A2 and CYP3A4 isozymes), and drug interactions affecting metabolism will significantly affect blood concentrations (see Table 44-11).

Alternative Therapies

Complementary therapies that patients might report using include acupuncture, homeopathy, herbal medicines, ayurvedic medicine, ionizers, osteopathy, and chiropractic manipulations. However, there are no studies of sufficient rigor to assess their efficacy.[2] Breathing and relaxation exercises have shown to provide small improvements in symptoms, quality of life, and psychological outcomes but not in exacerbation frequency.[2] Benefits may be due to relaxation effects, voluntary reduction in SABA use, and engagement in self-care, but the costs of certain intervention measures may be expensive.[2] In patients with low serum levels of Vitamin D, supplementation may be effective in reducing exacerbations requiring systemic corticosteroids (high-quality evidence).[2] Vitamin D is an inexpensive treatment alternative that may be useful only in those who are Vitamin D deficient.[2] There is little evidence to support using immunosuppressants such as methotrexate due to marginal steroid-sparing effects and the risk of significantly severe adverse effects.[2]

General Principles of Aerosol Therapy for Asthma

4 5 Aerosol delivery of drugs for asthma has the advantage of being site-specific and thus enhancing the therapeutic ratio. Inhalation of short-acting β_2-agonists provides more rapid bronchodilation than either parenteral or oral administration, as well as the greatest degree of protection against EIB and other challenges.[46]

TABLE 44-12 Factors Determining Lung Deposition of Aerosols

Device	Device Factors	Patient Factors
Metered-dose inhaler (MDI)	Canister held inverted Formulation (solution or suspension) Actuator cleanliness Addition of a spacer device	Inspiratory flow (slow, deep) Breath-holding Tilting head back Coordinating actuation with inhalation Priming and shaking the device
Dry powder inhaler (DPI)	Device cleanliness Resistance to inhalation; Humidity	Inspiratory flow (deep, forceful); Tilting head back Maintaining parallel to ground once activated
Jet nebulizer (small volume)	Volume fill (3-6 mL) Gas flow (6-12 L/min); Dead space volume; Open vs closed system Thumb-activating valve; Mouthpiece vs face mask	Inspiratory flow (slow, deep) Breath-holding Tapping nebulizer
Ultrasonic nebulizer	Volume fill Not effective for suspensions Mouthpiece vs face mask	Inspiratory flow (slow, deep) Breath-holding Tapping nebulizer
Spacer device	Volume (≥650 mL) One-way valves Holding chamber vs open-ended Antistatic lining Mouthpiece vs face mask	Inspiratory flow (slow, deep) Time between actuation and inhalation (<5 seconds) Cleaning with detergent to reduce static Multiple actuations (all at once) decrease delivery Coordination of actuation and inhalation for the simple open-tube spacers

ICSs have been developed with rapid oral and systemic clearance to enhance lung activity and reduce systemic activity.[52] Specific agents (eg, formoterol, salmeterol, and ipratropium bromide) are only effective by inhalation. Therefore, an understanding of aerosol drug delivery is essential to optimal asthma therapy. Table 44-12 lists the factors determining lung deposition of therapeutic aerosols.

Using the appropriate inhalation technique is essential to achieving optimal drug delivery and therapeutic effect.[12] The components are illustrated in Fig. 44-9. Approximately 50% to 80% of a dose from MDIs and DPIs deposits on the oropharynx and is then swallowed; the rest is either left in the device or exhaled.[67] It is important that MDI actuation occurs during inhalation.[67] Many patients do not use their MDIs optimally, and patient instruction with demonstration is the most effective means of improving inhaler technique.[12] Even with instruction, up to 80% of patients, particularly young children and older adults, cannot master the use of an MDI.[12] For these patients, attachment of a VHC to the MDI can improve efficacy significantly. However, the addition of a VHC offers no advantage in patients who can use an MDI optimally alone.[67] Mouth rinsing following treatment with MDI- and DPI-ICSs is important to minimize local adverse effects and oral absorption.[12]

Medication Delivery: Device Determinants Devices used to generate therapeutic aerosols include jet nebulizers, ultrasonic nebulizers, MDIs, and DPIs. The single most important device factor determining the site of aerosol deposition is particle size.[67] Devices for delivering therapeutic aerosols generate particles with mass median aerodynamic diameters (MMAD) from 0.5 to 35 μm.[67] Particles larger than 10 μm deposit in the oropharynx, particles between 5 and 10 μm deposit in the trachea and large bronchi, particles 1 to 5 μm in size reach the lower airways, and particles smaller than 0.5 μm act as a gas and are exhaled. The available MDIs, particularly for corticosteroid inhalers, are solution aerosols (vs suspensions) with extra-fine particle size distributions (MMAD of 1.1 μm) and high lung deposition.

In asthma, the target for drug delivery is the airways and not the alveoli. Respirable particles are deposited in the airways by three mechanisms: (a) inertial impaction, (b) gravitational sedimentation, and (c) Brownian diffusion.[67] The first two mechanisms are the most important for therapeutic aerosols and probably are the only factors that can be manipulated by patient technique.

Each delivery device within a classification generates specific aerosol characteristics, so the extrapolation of delivery data from one device cannot be applied to the other devices in the class. For instance, MDIs can deliver 15% to 50% of the actuated dose; DPIs, 10% to 30% of the labeled dose; and nebulizers 2% to 15% of the starting dose.[67] MDIs and DPIs are portable and convenient, unlike jet nebulizers. Small portable ultrasonic nebulizers have also been developed.

MDIs consist of a pressurized canister with a metering valve; the canister contains the active drug, low-vapor-pressure propellants such as HFA, co-solvents, and/or surfactants.[67] With any change in the components of an MDI, the FDA considers it to be a new drug that requires stability, safety, and efficacy studies prior to approval. The MDI drug is either in solution or a suspended micronized powder. In order to disperse the suspension for accurate delivery, the canister must be shaken. The metering chamber measures a liquid volume, and, therefore, the device must be held with the valve stem downward so that the chamber is covered with liquid[67] (Fig. 44-10). If not used for a period of time the drug in the chamber evaporates which could lead to an inadequate therapeutic dose. Some inhalers have to be primed before first use to fill the chamber and after an interval of nonuse.[67] When the canister is actuated, the device releases the propellant and drug in a forceful spray whose particles are large (MMAD = 45 μm)[67] (see Fig. 44-10). As evaporation occurs, the particle size is reduced to a final MMAD of 0.5 to 5.5 μm depending on the MDI. The aerosol-cloud extends about 6 inches beyond the MDI at the lowest MMAD.[67] Each MDI has different conditions for storage, priming, and durations to expiration, so the clinician must become familiar with and counsel the patient on these factors.

Spacer devices are used frequently with an MDI to decrease oropharyngeal deposition and enhance lung delivery.[12] However, not all spacer devices produce similar effects. The design of spacers varies from simple open-ended tubes that separate the MDI from the mouth to the VHC with one-way valves that open during inhalation (the preferred system); some VHCs have a face mask to accommodate drug delivery in children 5 years or younger. A VHC allows evaporation of the propellant prior to inhalation permitting a greater number of drug particles to achieve a respirable droplet size. VHC use also allows inhalation after actuation of the MDI, obviating the need for good hand-lung coordination.[67] Additionally, the large particles that normally would deposit in the oropharynx "rain out" in the spacer.[67] Spacer size may affect the amount of drug available for inhalation; a lower volume spacer (less than 350 mL) is advantageous in very young children.[12]

All the available spacers significantly reduce oropharyngeal deposition from MDIs, with the VHCs being superior to the open-ended tubes.[67] Reducing oropharyngeal deposits is an important factor in reducing local adverse effects (eg, hoarseness and oropharyngeal candidiasis) from ICSs.[67] The change in lung delivery depends on both the MDI and the drug, where one spacer device may enhance delivery with one MDI preparation and decrease delivery with others.[67] Therefore, once a patient is stabilized on a drug and chamber combination, the chamber should not be substituted in order to avoid changes in the dose delivered to the lungs. Finally,

EMERGENCY DEPARTMENT—ASTHMA DISCHARGE PLAN: HOW TO USE YOUR METERED-DOSE INHALER

Using an inhaler seems simple, but most patients do not use it the right way. When you use your inhaler the wrong way, less medicine gets to your lungs.

For the next few days, read these steps aloud as you do them or ask someone to read them to you. Ask your doctor, nurse, other health care provider, or pharmacist to check how well you are using your inhaler.

Use your inhaler in one of the three ways pictured below. A or B is the best, but C can be used if you have trouble with A and B. Your doctor may give you other types of inhalers.

Steps for Using Your Inhaler

Getting ready

1. Take off the cap and shake the inhaler.
2. Breathe out all the way.
3. Hold your inhaler the way your doctor said (A, B, or C below).

Breathe in slowly

4. As you start breathing in slowly through your mouth, press down on the inhaler one time. (If you use a holding chamber, first press down on the inhaler. Within 5 seconds, begin to breathe in slowly.)
5. Keep breathing in slowly, as deeply as you can.

Hold your breath

6. Hold your breath as you count to 10 slowly, if you can.
7. For inhaled quick-relief medicine (short-acting beta$_2$-agonists), wait about 15–30 seconds between puffs. There is no need to wait between puffs for other medicines.

L. Hold inhaler 1 to 2 inches in front of your mouth (about the width of two fingers).

M. Use a spacer/holding chamber. These come in many shapes and can be useful to any patient.

N. Put the inhaler in your mouth. Do not use for steroids.

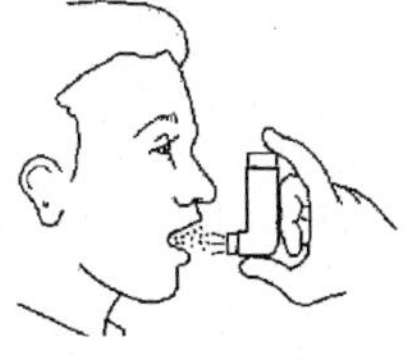

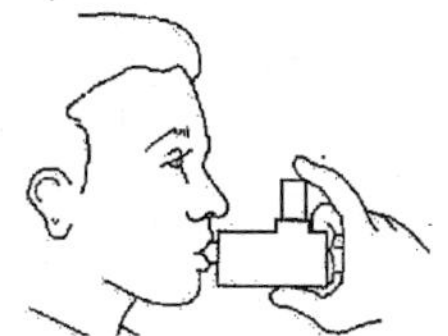

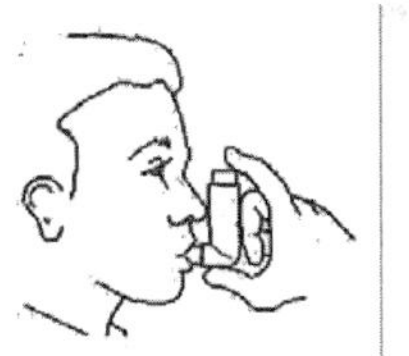

Clean your inhaler as needed, and know when to replace your inhaler. For instructions, read the package insert or talk to your doctor, other healthcare provider, or pharmacist.

FIGURE 44-9 Instructions for inhaler use. *(Reprinted from NIH Publication No. 07-4051. Expert Panel Report 3: Guidelines for the Diagnosis and Management of Asthma Full Report 2007.)*

over time, holding chambers (eg, plastic) can build up static electricity that attracts small particles to the sides of the chamber, significantly reducing aerosol availability. Some spacers should be washed with household detergent with a single rinse and allowed to drip dry.[12] Other VHCs have been developed with antistatic materials.

Dry micronized powders can be inhaled directly into the lungs. A number of DPIs are now available for use in the United States.[67] Each DPI has unique characteristics with advantages and disadvantages (Table 44-13). The primary advantage of DPIs is that they are breath-actuated and require minimal hand-lung coordination, and it is thus easier to teach patients proper technique.[67] Some DPIs are more flow-dependent than others.[67] Thus, similar to MDIs and spacers, delivery data from one DPI cannot be extrapolated to another.

Reported adherence to inhaled asthma medications has been less than 50% for adolescents and adults.[68] Adherence barriers are different in each patient population and should include a personalized approach. Device ease-of-use and ability to perform proper inhaler technique should be considered and assessed. Electronic sensors either attached to or integrated with MDIs and DPIs used in conjunction with smartphone applications have been developed to track and promote adherence. Although these technological advances will likely become commonplace in the future, the current cost (~$300 per device or for a 1-year subscription) for these devices and monitoring services are a significant barrier.

Nebulizer devices come in two basic types: the jet nebulizer and the ultrasonic nebulizer. Jet nebulizers produce an aerosol

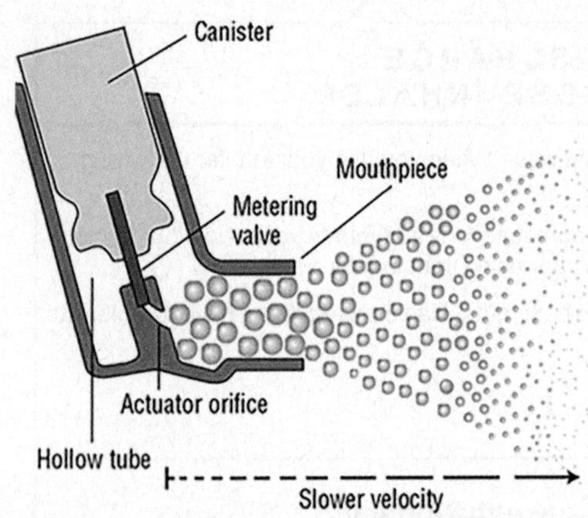

FIGURE 44-10 Illustration of a metered-dose inhaler demonstrating the particle size difference as the aerosol-cloud extends outward.

from a liquid solution or suspension placed in a cup. A tube connected to a stream of compressed air or O_2 flows up through the bottom and draws the liquid up an adjacent open-ended tube.[67] The air and liquid strike a baffle, creating a droplet cloud that is then inhaled.[67] Ultrasonic nebulizers produce an aerosol by vibrating liquid lying above a transducer at speeds of about 1 MHz.[67] Both produce similar degrees of lung deposition, with the exception that ultrasonic nebulizers are ineffective for nebulizing currently available micronized suspensions.[67] The aerosol output and lung delivery vary significantly among the commercially available jet nebulizers even when operated in the same manner.[67] Increasing fill volume will increase the total amount of drug delivered; however, it also will take longer for the patient to nebulize the dose.[67] The MMAD of the droplets is related directly to the gas flow, with flows of 5 to 12 L/min providing an aerosol cloud with an MMAD of 4 to 8 μm for most jet nebulizers.[67] Each jet nebulizer comes with optimal operating and cleaning instructions.

TABLE 44-13 Characteristics of Commonly Used Inhalation Devices

Device	Drugs	Breath Activated	Dose Counter	Other Excipients	Disadvantages
MDI	All classes	No	No/yes	Propellants, surfactants, cosolvents	Requires coordination of actuation and inhalation. Large pharyngeal deposition. Difficult to teach. Priming and cleaning considerations
Pressair (DPI)	Aclidinium	Yes	Yes	Lactose filler	Requires rapid inhalation to activate
Respiclick (DPI)	Albuterol	Yes	Yes	Lactose filler	Requires rapid inhalation to activate
MDI plus valved holding chamber	All classes	No	No		More expensive than MDI alone; less portable; some payers will not pay; inconsistent effect on delivery; nonstatic prefer red
Jet nebulizers	All classes	No	—	Preservatives in some solutions	Significant interbrand variability; expensive and time-consuming; less efficient than MDIs; contamination possible; preparations may be light and temperature-sensitive (short shelf life)
Ultrasonic nebulizer	Cromolyn solution, short-acting β_2-agonist solutions	No	—	Preservatives in some solutions	Same as for jet nebulizers and cannot be used for suspensions; battery-operated are portable
Flexhaler (DPI)	Budesonide	Yes	Yes	Lactose filler	Requires high inspiratory flow (60 L/min) Pharyngeal deposition Not approved for <6 years of age
Diskus (DPI)	Fluticasone; salmeterol; fluticasone/salmeterol	Yes	Yes	Lactose filler	Not approved for <4 years of age Requires inspiratory flow of 30-60 L/min
Ellipta (DPI)	Fluticasone furoate Fluticasone/vilanterol	Yes	Yes	Lactose filler	Not approved for <12 years of age (18 years for fluticasone/vilanterol) Requires inspiratory flow of 60 L/min
Aerolizer (DPI)	Formoterol	Yes	—	Lactose filler	Single-dose capsules. Not approved for <5 years of age Requires flow of 30-60 L/min
Neohaler (DPI)	Indacaterol	Yes	—	Lactose filler	Single-dose capsules. Not approved for children. Requires flow of 60 L/min
Handihaler (DPI)	Tiotropium	Yes	—	Lactose filler	Single-dose capsule. Not approved for children. Requires flow of 20 L/min. Not FDA-approved in asthma
Twisthaler (DPI)	Mometasone	Yes	Yes	Lactose filler	Not approved for <4 years of age
Respimat (SMI)	Tiotropium Albuterol/Ipratropium Olodaterol	No	Yes	Preservative	Requires slow deep breath. Not approved for <12 years of age

Medication Delivery: Patient Determinants 6 7 The most important patient factor determining aerosol deposition is inspiratory flow (see Table 44-12).[67] High inspiratory flows with MDIs increase the degree of deposition owing to impaction of particles of any size, thereby increasing deposition centrally (ie, throat and large airways) and decreasing peripheral deposition. The optimal inspiratory flow for most MDIs is slow and deep (approximately 30 L/min or 5 seconds for a full inhalation).[67] In general, DPIs require higher inspiratory flows (greater than or equal to 60 L/min) and a change in inhalation technique (ie, deep, forceful inspiration) for optimal dispersion of the powder, which, in turn, increases the amount of drug delivered to the larger central airways.[67] Patients should be cautioned not to exhale into DPIs because this causes loss of dose and moistens the dry powder, causing aggregation into larger particles. Patient factors that cannot be controlled include interpatient variability in airway geometry (particularly the differences between children and adults)[67] and the effects of bronchospasm, edema, and mucus hypersecretion. Mild obstruction increases aerosol deposition; however, severe obstruction probably leads to increased central deposition from impaction.[67] The absolute delivery to the lung is not as important as the consistency of delivery, assuming that a sufficient dose to produce the desired therapeutic effect is achieved. No single inhalation device is the best for all patients. Table 44-13 lists the differing characteristics of inhalation devices.

Delivery from high-resistance DPIs is more flow-dependent than from low-resistance DPIs. Thus, younger children and possibly older adults will have more variability in delivery from high-resistance devices.[67] Most children younger than 4 years of age cannot generate a sufficient inspiratory flow to use DPIs. Young children (younger than 4 years) and infants generally require the use of a face mask attached to either an MDI plus VHC or a nebulizer. The use of a face mask results in a reduction in lung delivery due to the portion of the aerosol inhaled nasally, so the doses of drugs used in these patients are often not decreased.

EVALUATION OF THERAPEUTIC OUTCOMES

The two domains of asthma control are "symptom control" and "future risk of adverse outcomes."[12] Symptom control is assessed by asking about the frequency of daytime and night-time asthma symptoms, reliever medication use, and activity limitations. Poor symptom control is also an indicator of future risk for exacerbations.[12] However, even when perceived symptom control is good, an assessment of the future risk of exacerbations is critical. Determining the risk of future adverse patient outcomes includes assessment of the risk of future exacerbations, fixed airflow limitation (and thus diminished response to therapy), and medication adverse effects.[12] To assess the risk for future exacerbations (defined as a worsening of asthma requiring the use of systemic corticosteroids or an increase in the use of systemic corticosteroids), lung function should be measured before the start of treatment and then 2 months later when the maximum response to controller medications is likely attained.[12] This benchmark of "personal best" can then be used for ongoing risk assessment. Other factors that affect future risk of exacerbations include exacerbation history in the previous year (define as one or more exacerbations requiring systemic corticosteroids is a risk factor), history of intubation or intensive care unit stay for asthma, or asthma-related ED visits for urgent care.[12] Fixed airflow limitation can be affected by lack of ICS treatment, smoking exposure, and poor lung function. During ongoing care, spirometry should be measured yearly but long-term PEF monitoring is typically reserved for those with severe asthma.[12] The risk of adverse effects is influenced by oral drug administration, ICS dose, and potential drug interactions with cytochrome P450 inhibitors.[12] In addition, poor inhaler technique (such as not rinsing and spitting after ICS use) can lead to oral candidiasis or an increase in the swallowed fraction of the dose that could influence linear growth in children.

There are several simple screening questionnaires that can be used to assess asthma symptom control quickly in a clinic setting. The Asthma Control Test is a validated simple five-question survey for patients 12 years and older that yields a numerical score; a score of 19 or less indicates poor asthma control and several institutions have incorporated the survey into the electronic health record in order to evaluate changes over time.[12] There is a companion Childhood Asthma Control Test survey for children 4 to 11 years.[12] A number of other validated questionnaires exist such as the Asthma Control Questionnaire (ACQ) and the Test for Respiratory and Asthma Control in Kids (TRACK).[12]

Patients should also be asked about exercise tolerance but perceived good exercise tolerance may be biased by a sedentary lifestyle due to frequent bothersome symptoms. All patients on inhaled drugs should have their inhalation delivery technique evaluated periodically—monthly initially and then every 3 to 6 months. Before stepping up therapy, adherence, environmental factors, and comorbid conditions should be reviewed.[12]

Following initiation of anti-inflammatory therapy or an increase in dosage, most patients should begin experiencing a decrease in symptoms in 1 to 2 weeks and achieve maximum improvement within 4 to 8 weeks. The use of higher ICS doses or more potent agents may accelerate symptom improvement. Increases in FEV_1 and PEF should follow a similar time frame; however, a decrease in BHR, as measured by morning PEF, PEF variability, and exercise tolerance, may take 1 to 3 months.[12] Patients should be informed that following a viral respiratory infection, they may experience decreased exercise tolerance for up to 4 weeks.

Initial visits with the patient should focus on the patient's concerns, expectations, and goals of treatment. Initial patient education should focus on asthma as a chronic lung disease, the types of medications, how they are to be used including inhaler technique, and when to seek medical advice. Written action plans should be provided. Both peak flow-based and symptom-based self-monitoring plans can be effective.[12] The first follow-up visit should include a repetition of the educational messages from the first visit, as well as a review of the patient's current medications, adherence, barriers, and challenges.

CONCLUSION

Asthma is a complex disease with a multitude of clinical presentations. The exact defect in asthma has not been defined, and it may be that asthma is a common presentation of a heterogeneous group of diseases. Asthma is defined and characterized by excessive reactivity of the bronchial tree to a wide variety of noxious stimuli. The reaction is characterized by bronchospasm, excessive mucus production, and inflammation. The central role of inflammation in inducing and maintaining BHR is now becoming widely appreciated. The goal of asthma therapy is to normalize, as much as possible, the patient's life and prevent chronic irreversible lung changes. Drugs are the mainstay of asthma management. The goal of drug therapy is to use the minimum amount of medications possible to control the disease. In persistent asthma, therapy should be aimed at both bronchospasm and inflammation in order to produce the best results. Patients should be followed and monitored diligently for toxicities. Although death from asthma is an uncommon event, the most common cause of death is under-estimating the severity of obstruction either by the patient or by the clinician; the next common cause is under-treatment. A cornerstone of therapy is education and the realization that most asthma deaths are avoidable.

ABBREVIATIONS

ACOS	Asthma COPD Overlap Syndrome
ACQ	Asthma Control Questionnaire
ACTH	adrenocorticotropic hormone
Arg	arginine
BHR	bronchial hyper-responsiveness
CFC	chlorofluorocarbon
COPD	chronic obstructive pulmonary disease
CYP	cytochrome P450
DPI	dry powder inhaler
ED	emergency department
EIB	exercise-induced bronchospasm
EPR3	Expert Panel Report 3
FeNO	fraction of exhaled nitric oxide
FEV_1	forced expiratory volume in 1 second
FVC	forced vital capacity
GERD	gastroesophageal reflux disease
GINA	Global Initiative for Asthma
GM-CSF	granulocyte-macrophage colony-stimulating factor
HFA	hydrofluoroalkane
HPA	hypothalamic-pituitary–adrenal
ICAM-1	intercellular adhesion molecule 1
ICS	inhaled corticosteroid
IFN-γ	interferon-γ
IgE	immunoglobulin E
IL	interleukin
iNOS	inducible nitric oxide synthase
LABA	long-acting inhaled β_2-agonist
LAMA	long-acting muscarinic antagonist
LT	leukotriene
MDI	metered-dose inhaler
MMAD	mass median aerodynamic diameter
NAEPP	National Asthma Education and Prevention Program
NANC	nonadrenergic, noncholinergic
NO	nitric oxide
O_2	oxygen
PAF	platelet-activating factor
PEF	peak expiratory flow
RCT	randomized controlled trial
RSV	respiratory syncytial virus
SABA	short-acting beta-agonist
T-cells	thymically derived lymphocytes
Th_1	type 1 T-helper cell
Th_2	type 2 T-helper cell
TSLP	thymic stromal lymphopoietin
VCAM-1	vascular cell adhesion molecule 1
VHC	valved holding chamber
VIP	vasoactive intestinal peptide

REFERENCES

1. Rosenblatt MB. History of bronchial asthma. In: Weiss EB, Segal MS, eds. *Bronchial Asthma: Mechanisms and Therapeutics*. 2nd ed. Boston: Little, Brown; 1976:5–17.
2. *Global Initiative for Asthma*. Global Strategy for Asthma Management and Prevention: Online Appendix 2020 [updated 2020 May 26, 2021]. Available at: http://www.ginasthma.org/.
3. National Asthma Education and Prevention Program. Expert Panel Report 3: Guidelines for the diagnosis and management of asthma Bethesda, MD: U.S. Department of Health and Human Services, Public Health Service, National Institutes of Health, National Heart, Lung, and Blood Institute, publication no. 08-4051; 2007.
4. Centers for Disease Control and Prevention Most Recent Asthma Data: Centers for Disease Control and Prevention; 2019 [updated March 25, 2019; May 25, 2021]. Available at: https://www.cdc.gov/asthma/most_recent_data.htm.
5. Alexander D, Currie J. Is it who you are or where you live? Residential segregation and racial gaps in childhood asthma. *J Health Econ.* 2017;55:186–200. doi:10.1016/j.jhealeco.2017.07.003.
6. Mak ACY, White MJ, Eckalbar WL, et al. Whole-genome sequencing of pharmacogenetic drug response in racially diverse children with asthma. *Am J Respir Crit Care Med.* 2018;197(12):1552–1564. doi:10.1164/rccm.201712-2529OC.
7. Nyenhuis SM, Krishnan JA, Berry A, et al. Race is associated with differences in airway inflammation in patients with asthma. *J Allergy Clin Immunol.* 2017;140(1):257–265 e11. doi:10.1016/j.jaci.2016.10.024.
8. Nurmagambetov T, Kuwahara R, Garbe P. The economic burden of asthma in the United States, 2008-2013. *Ann Am Thorac Soc.* 2018;15(3):348–356. doi:10.1513/AnnalsATS.201703-259OC.
9. Papi A, Brightling C, Pedersen SE, Reddel HK. Asthma. *Lancet.* 2018;391(10122):783–800. doi:10.1016/S0140-6736(17)33311-1.
10. Collaborators GBDCoD. Global, regional, and national age-sex-specific mortality for 282 causes of death in 195 countries and territories, 1980-2017: A systematic analysis for the Global Burden of Disease Study 2017. *Lancet.* 2018;392(10159):1736–1788. doi:10.1016/S0140-6736(18)32203-7.
11. 2020 Focused Updates to the Asthma Management Guidelines Bethesda, MD: U.S. Department of Health and Human Services, Public Health Service, National Institutes of Health, National Heart, Lung, and Blood Institute; 2020 [updated December 3, 2020; cited December 2020]. Available from: https://www.nhlbi.nih.gov/health-topics/asthma-management-guidelines-2020-updates.
12. Global Initiative for Asthma. *Global Strategy for Asthma Management and Prevention 2021* [October 20, 2021]. Available at: www.ginaasthma.org.
13. Ntontsi P, Photiades A, Zervas E, Xanthou G, Samitas K. Genetics and epigenetics in asthma. *Int J Mol Sci.* 2021;22(5). doi:10.3390/ijms22052412.
14. van Tilburg Bernardes E, Arrieta MC. Hygiene hypothesis in asthma Development: Is hygiene to blame? *Arch Med Res.* 2017;48(8):717–726. doi:10.1016/j.arcmed.2017.11.009.
15. Jartti T, Gern JE. Role of viral infections in the development and exacerbation of asthma in children. *J Allergy Clin Immunol.* 2017;140(4):895–906. doi:10.1016/j.jaci.2017.08.003.
16. Lambrecht BN, Hammad H, Fahy JV. The cytokines of asthma. *Immunity.* 2019;50(4):975–991. doi:10.1016/j.immuni.2019.03.018.
17. Hough KP, Curtiss ML, Blain TJ, Liu RM, Trevor J, Deshane JS, et al. Airway remodeling in asthma. *Front Med (Lausanne).* 2020;7:191. doi:10.3389/fmed.2020.00191.
18. Robinson D, Humbert M, Buhl R, et al. Revisiting Type 2-high and Type 2-low airway inflammation in asthma: Current knowledge and therapeutic implications. *Clin Exp Allergy.* 2017;47(2):161–175. doi:10.1111/cea.12880.
19. Kuruvilla ME, Lee FE, Lee GB. Understanding asthma phenotypes, endotypes, and mechanisms of disease. *Clin Rev Allergy Immunol.* 2019;56(2):219–233. doi:10.1007/s12016-018-8712-1.
20. Tung HY, Li E, Landers C, et al. Advances and evolving concepts in allergic asthma. *Semin Respir Crit Care Med.* 2018;39(1):64–81. doi:10.1055/s-0037-1607981.
21. Mendez-Enriquez E, Hallgren J. Mast cells and their progenitors in allergic asthma. *Front Immunol.* 2019;10:821. doi:10.3389/fimmu.2019.00821.
22. Kim KB, Kwak YS. Dehydration affects exercise-induced asthma and anaphylaxis. *J Exerc Rehabil.* 2019;15(5):647–650. doi:10.12965/jer.1938470.235.
23. van der Veen TA, de Groot LES, Melgert BN. The different faces of the macrophage in asthma. *Curr Opin Pulm Med.* 2020;26(1):62–68. doi:10.1097/MCP.0000000000000647.
24. Crisford H, Sapey E, Rogers GB, et al. Neutrophils in asthma: The good, the bad and the bacteria. *Thorax.* 2021. doi:10.1136/thoraxjnl-2020-215986.
25. Peebles RS Jr. Prostaglandins in asthma and allergic diseases. *Pharmacol Ther.* 2019;193:1–19. doi:10.1016/j.pharmthera.2018.08.001.
26. Munoz-Cano RM, Casas-Saucedo R, Valero Santiago A, Bobolea I, Ribo P, Mullol J. Platelet-activating factor (PAF) in allergic rhinitis: Clinical and therapeutic implications. *J Clin Med.* 2019;8(9). doi:10.3390/jcm8091338.
27. Hammad H, Lambrecht BN. The basic immunology of asthma. *Cell.* 2021;184(9):2521–2522. doi:10.1016/j.cell.2021.04.019.
28. Antosova M, Mokra D, Pepucha L, et al. Physiology of nitric oxide in the respiratory system. *Physiol Res.* 2017;66(Suppl 2):S159–S172. doi:10.33549/physiolres.933673.
29. Ijpma G, Panariti A, Lauzon A-M, Martin JG. Directional preference of airway smooth muscle mass increase in human asthmatic airways.

American Journal of Physiology-Lung Cellular and Molecular Physiology. 2017;312(6):L845–L854. doi:10.1152/ajplung.00353.2016.
30. Kistemaker LEM, Prakash YS. Airway innervation and plasticity in asthma. *Physiology (Bethesda).* 2019;34(4):283–298. doi:10.1152/physiol.00050.2018.
31. *Global Initiative for Asthma.* Global Strategy for Asthma Management and Prevention 2018 [August 3, 2018]. Available at: http://www.ginasthma.org/.
32. D'Amato G, Holgate ST, Pawankar R, et al. Meteorological conditions, climate change, new emerging factors, and asthma and related allergic disorders. A statement of the World Allergy Organization. *World Allergy Organ J.* 2015;8(1):25. doi:10.1186/s40413-015-0073-0.
33. Tiotiu AI, Novakova S, Labor M, et al. Progress in occupational asthma. *Int J Environ Res Public Health.* 2020;17(12). doi:10.3390/ijerph17124553.
34. Hufnagl K, Pali-Scholl I, Roth-Walter F, Jensen-Jarolim E. Dysbiosis of the gut and lung microbiome has a role in asthma. *Semin Immunopathol.* 2020;42(1):75–93. doi:10.1007/s00281-019-00775-y.
35. Toivonen L, Karppinen S, Schuez-Havupalo L, Waris M, He Q, Hoffman KL, et al. Longitudinal changes in early nasal microbiota and the risk of childhood asthma. *Pediatrics.* 2020;146(4). doi:10.1542/peds.2020-0421.
36. Yung JA, Fuseini H, Newcomb DC. Hormones, sex, and asthma. *Ann Allergy Asthma Immunol.* 2018;120(5):488–494. doi:10.1016/j.anai.2018.01.016.
37. *2021 Global Strategy for Prevention, Diagnosis and Management of COPD 2021* [updated 2021; May 26, 2021]. Available at: https://goldcopd.org/2021-gold-reports/.
38. Woodruff PG, van den Berge M, Boucher RC, et al. American Thoracic Society/National Heart, Lung, and Blood Institute Asthma-Chronic Obstructive Pulmonary Disease Overlap Workshop Report. *Am J Respir Crit Care Med.* 2017;196(3):375–381. doi:10.1164/rccm.201705-0973WS.
39. National Asthma Education and Prevention Program. Expert Panel Report 3: Guidelines for the diagnosis and management of asthma. Bethesda, MD: U.S. Department of Health and Human Services, Public Health Service, National Institutes of Health, National Heart, Lung, and Blood Institute, publication no. 08-4051; 2007.
40. Serrano-Pariente J, Plaza V. Near-fatal asthma: A heterogeneous clinical entity. *Curr Opin Allergy Clin Immunol.* 2017;17(1):28–35. doi:10.1097/ACI.0000000000000333.
41. Cote A, Turmel J, Boulet LP. Exercise and asthma. *Semin Respir Crit Care Med.* 2018;39(1):19–28. doi:10.1055/s-0037-1606215.
42. Parsons JP, Hallstrand TS, Mastronarde JG, et al. An official American Thoracic Society clinical practice guideline: Exercise-induced bronchoconstriction. *Am J Respir Crit Care Med.* 2013;187(9):1016–1027. doi:10.1164/rccm.201303-0437ST.
43. National Heart, Lung, and Blood Institute. Digital Toolkit: Asthma Action Plan [updated December 2020]. Available at: https://www.nhlbi.nih.gov/health-topics/all-publications-and-resources/asthma-action-plan-2020.
44. Agnihotri NT, Saltoun C. Acute severe asthma (status asthmaticus). *Allergy Asthma Proc.* 2019;40(6):406–409. doi:10.2500/aap.2019.40.4258.
45. Vatrella A, Maglio A, Pelaia C, Pelaia G, Vitale C. Pharmacotherapeutic strategies for critical asthma syndrome: A look at the state of the art. *Expert Opin Pharmacother.* 2020;21(12):1505–1515. doi:10.1080/14656566.2020.1766023.
46. Billington CK, Penn RB, Hall IP. Beta2 agonists. *Handb Exp Pharmacol.* 2017;237:23–40. doi:10.1007/164_2016_64.
47. Virk MK, Hotz J, Khemani RG, Newth CJ, Ross PA. Change in oxygen consumption following inhalation of albuterol in comparison with levalbuterol in healthy adult volunteers. *Lung.* 2017;195(2):233–239. doi:10.1007/s00408-017-9982-8.
48. Cazzola M, Rogliani P, Matera MG. Ultra-LABAs for the treatment of asthma. *Respir Med.* 2019;156:47–52. doi:10.1016/j.rmed.2019.08.005.
49. FDA Drug Safety Communication: FDA review finds no significant increase in risk of serious asthma outcomes with long-acting beta agonists (LABAs) used in combination with inhaled corticosteroids (ICS) Silver Spring, MD: Food and Drug Administration; 2017 [updated December 20, 2017; cited 2018 November 15, 2018]. Available at: https://www.fda.gov/Drugs/DrugSafety/ucm589587.htm.
50. Cazzola M, Rogliani P, Calzetta L, Matera MG. Pharmacogenomic response of inhaled corticosteroids for the treatment of asthma: Considerations for therapy. *Pharmgenomics Pers Med.* 2020;13:261–271. doi:10.2147/PGPM.S231471.
51. Williams DM. Clinical pharmacology of corticosteroids. *Respir Care.* 2018;63(6):655–670. doi:10.4187/respcare.0631463/6/655.
52. Matera MG, Rinaldi B, Calzetta L, Rogliani P, Cazzola M. Pharmacokinetics and pharmacodynamics of inhaled corticosteroids for asthma treatment. *Pulm Pharmacol Ther.* 2019;58:101828. doi:10.1016/j.pupt.2019.101828.
53. Yao TC, Huang YW, Chang SM, Tsai SY, Wu AC, Tsai HJ. Association between oral corticosteroid bursts and severe adverse events: A Nationwide Population-Based Cohort Study. *Ann Intern Med.* 2020;173(5):325–330. doi:10.7326/M20-0432.
54. Waljee AK, Rogers MA, Lin P, et al. Short term use of oral corticosteroids and related harms among adults in the United States: Population based cohort study. *BMJ.* 2017;357:j1415. doi:10.1136/bmj.j1415.
55. Yao TC, Wang JY, Chang SM, et al. Association of oral corticosteroid bursts with severe adverse events in children. *JAMA Pediatr.* 2021. doi:10.1001/jamapediatrics.2021.0433.
56. Boulet LP. Airway remodeling in asthma: Update on mechanisms and therapeutic approaches. *Curr Opin Pulm Med.* 2018;24(1):56–62. doi:10.1097/MCP.0000000000000441.
57. Raissy HH, Kelly HW, Harkins M, et al. Inhaled corticosteroids in lung diseases. *Am J Respir Crit Care Med.* 2013;187(8):798–803. 10.1164/rccm.201210-1853PP 23370915.
58. Gosens R, Gross N. The mode of action of anticholinergics in asthma. *Eur Respir J.* 2018;52(4). doi:10.1183/13993003.01247-2017.
59. Rodriguez-Martinez CE, Sossa-Briceno MP, Castro-Rodriguez JA. Predictors of response to medications for asthma in pediatric patients: A systematic review of the literature. *Pediatr Pulmonol.* 2020;55(6):1320–1331. doi:10.1002/ppul.24782.
60. Di Salvo E, Patella V, Casciaro M, Gangemi S. The leukotriene receptor antagonist Montelukast can induce adverse skin reactions in asthmatic patients. *Pulm Pharmacol Ther.* 2020;60:101875. doi:10.1016/j.pupt.2019.101875.
61. Benard B, Bastien V, Vinet B, Yang R, Krajinovic M, Ducharme FM. Neuropsychiatric adverse drug reactions in children initiated on montelukast in real-life practice. *Eur Respir J.* 2017;50(2). doi:10.1183/13993003.00148-2017.
62. Struss N, Hohlfeld JM. Biologics in asthma management: Are we out of breath yet? *Allergol Select.* 2021;5:96–102. doi:10.5414/ALX02192E.
63. McGregor MC, Krings JG, Nair P, Castro M. Role of biologics in asthma. *Am J Respir Crit Care Med.* 2018. doi:10.1164/rccm.201810-1944CI.
64. Holguin F, Cardet JC, Chung KF, et al. Management of severe asthma: A European Respiratory Society/American Thoracic Society guideline. *Eur Respir J.* 2020;55(1). doi:10.1183/13993003.00588-2019.
65. Doroudchi A, Pathria M, Modena BD. Asthma biologics: Comparing trial designs, patient cohorts and study results. *Ann Allergy Asthma Immunol.* 2020;124(1):44–56. doi:10.1016/j.anai.2019.10.016.
66. McGregor MC, Krings JG, Nair P, Castro M. Role of biologics in asthma. *American Journal of Respiratory and Critical Care Medicine.* 2019;199(4):433–445. doi:10.1164/rccm.201810-1944CI.
67. Dolovich MB, Dhand R. Aerosol drug delivery: Developments in device design and clinical use. *Lancet.* 2011;377(9770):1032–1045. doi:10.1016/S0140-6736(10)60926-9.
68. Blake KV. Improving adherence to asthma medications: Current knowledge and future perspectives. *Curr Opin Pulm Med.* 2017;23(1):62–70. doi:10.1097/MCP.0000000000000334.

Chronic Obstructive Pulmonary Disease

45

Sharya V. Bourdet and Dennis M. Williams

KEY CONCEPTS

1. Chronic obstructive pulmonary disease (COPD) is a treatable and preventable disease characterized by progressive airflow limitation that is not fully reversible and is associated with an abnormal inflammatory response of the lungs to noxious particles or gases.
2. Mortality from COPD has increased steadily over the past three decades; it is the fourth leading cause of death in the United States.
3. The primary cause of COPD is cigarette smoking, implicated in 75% of diagnosed cases in the United States. Other risks include genetic predisposition, environmental exposures (including occupational dust and chemicals), and air pollution.
4. In patients with COPD, staging of airflow limitation (GOLD 1-4) is classified by spirometry measurements. Disease severity (Category A-D) is classified using a combined assessment of symptom score, as measured by a validated questionnaire, and risk for future exacerbations.
5. Smoking cessation and avoidance of other known toxins are the only management strategies proven to slow COPD progression.
6. Oxygen therapy can reduce mortality in selected patients with COPD. Oxygen therapy is indicated for patients with a resting PaO_2 of less than 55 mm Hg (7.3 kPa) or a PaO_2 of less than 60 mm Hg (8.0 kPa) and evidence of right-sided heart failure, polycythemia, or impaired neurologic function.
7. Inhaled bronchodilators are the mainstay of drug therapy for COPD and are used to relieve patient symptoms and improve exercise tolerance and quality of life. Guidelines recommend short-acting bronchodilators as initial therapy for patients with occasional symptoms and all patients as rescue therapy to relieve symptoms.
8. For patients experiencing persistent symptoms, either a long-acting β_2-agonist (LABA) or long-acting anticholinergic (LAMA) offers significant benefits, and both are of comparable efficacy. If a patient has continued symptoms, combining long-acting bronchodilator agents (LABA plus LAMA) is recommended.
9. For patients at high risk for future exacerbations, either a long-acting β_2-agonist (LABA) or long-acting anticholinergic (LAMA) is effective at reducing exacerbation frequency. Anticholinergic agents are more effective at reducing exacerbation frequency and should be considered first-line. If a patient has continued exacerbations or has more severe disease, combining long-acting bronchodilator agents (LABA plus LAMA) is recommended.
10. The role of inhaled corticosteroid (ICS) therapy in COPD is controversial. Patients with frequent and severe exacerbations may benefit from ICS therapy, although the risk of pneumonia is increased.
11. Acute exacerbations of COPD (AECOPD) have a significant impact on disease progression and mortality. Treatment of acute exacerbations includes intensification of bronchodilator therapy and a short course of systemic corticosteroids.
12. Antimicrobial therapy should generally be used during AECOPD if the patient exhibits at least two of the following: increased dyspnea, increased sputum volume, and increased sputum purulence. A C-reactive protein (CRP) test may be helpful to guide the decision to treat a COPD exacerbation with antibiotics.

BEYOND THE BOOK

Watch the video entitled "Pathophysiology of Large and Small Airway Disease in COPD" in AccessPharmacy by Scott Stern, MD. This 5-minute video provides a visual explanation of pathophysiologic changes occurring in lungs of patients with COPD. This video assists with comprehension of physiologic changes and correlation with clinical presentation in COPD.

Watch the video "Gasping for Air: Life with COPD" (*The New York Times*, July 31, 2008). This 6-minute video provides the perspective of a patient diagnosed with COPD. This video helps remind clinicians of patient experiences with the disease, how physiologic changes are correlated with symptoms, and challenges to optimal diagnosis and treatment.

INTRODUCTION

1 Chronic obstructive pulmonary disease (COPD) is a common lung disease characterized by airflow limitation that is not fully reversible, in contrast to the reversibility of airflow limitation in asthma. COPD is both chronic and progressive and is associated with an abnormal inflammatory response of the lungs to noxious particles or gases.[1] COPD is preventable and treatable and causes significant extrapulmonary effects that contribute to disease severity in a subset of patients.

To standardize the care of patients with COPD and present evidence-based recommendations, the National Heart, Lung, and Blood Institute (NHLBI) and the World Health Organization (WHO) launched the Global Initiative for Chronic Obstructive Lung Disease (GOLD) in 2001. The GOLD expert panel revises their recommendations annually, typically in December.[1] The goals of the

GOLD organization are to increase awareness of COPD and reduce morbidity and mortality associated with the disease. In addition to GOLD, other international organizations have developed consensus guidelines focusing on preventing and managing acute exacerbations associated with COPD. The American College of Chest Physicians (ACCP) and the Canadian Thoracic Society collaborated on guidelines for the prevention of COPD exacerbations which were published in 2015.[2] In 2017, the American Thoracic Society (ATS) and European Respiratory Society (ERS) jointly published guidelines for both the prevention and management of acute exacerbations of COPD (AECOPD).[3,4]

International guidelines emphasize the terms *preventable* and *treatable* to support a positive approach to managing the patient with COPD. Support is also reflected in advocacy and availability of research funding to improve understanding about this disease and its management. Examples include the creation of the Division of Lung Diseases of the NHLBI to promote and fund multidisciplinary research and collaboration as well as the Centers for Disease Control and Prevention's COPD National Action Plan, which outlines strategic goals for empowering patients and caregivers, preventing and managing disease, supporting research initiatives, and developing educational and public health policies related to COPD.[5,6]

COPD has historically described a group of pulmonary diseases with a fixed airflow limitation. The two principal conditions are chronic bronchitis and emphysema, which are phenotypes. Chronic bronchitis is associated with chronic or recurrent episodes of excessive mucus secretion into the bronchial tree with a cough present on most days for at least 3 months of the year for at least 2 consecutive years in a patient in whom other causes of chronic cough have been excluded.[1] While chronic bronchitis is defined in clinical terms, emphysema is defined in terms of anatomic pathology. Historically, emphysema was diagnosed based on histologic findings at autopsy. Given that this histologic definition has limited clinical value, emphysema also has been defined as abnormal permanent enlargement of the airspaces distal to the terminal bronchioles accompanied by destruction of their walls without obvious fibrosis.[1]

Differentiating COPD as either chronic bronchitis or emphysema as distinct subsets of COPD is no longer considered relevant because both are caused by a common risk factor (cigarette smoking), and most patients exhibit features of both. Emphasis is placed on the pathophysiologic features of small airways disease and parenchymal destruction as contributors to chronic airflow limitation. Chronic inflammation affects the integrity of the airways, causes damage, and promotes the destruction of the parenchymal structures. The underlying problem is persistent exposure to noxious particles or gases that sustain the inflammatory response. The airways of both the lung and the parenchyma are susceptible to inflammation, and the result is the chronic airflow limitation that characterizes COPD (Fig. 45-1).

EPIDEMIOLOGY

2 In the United States, approximately 16 million Americans are estimated to have COPD, although the true prevalence of people with chronic airflow obstruction as measured by spirometry may

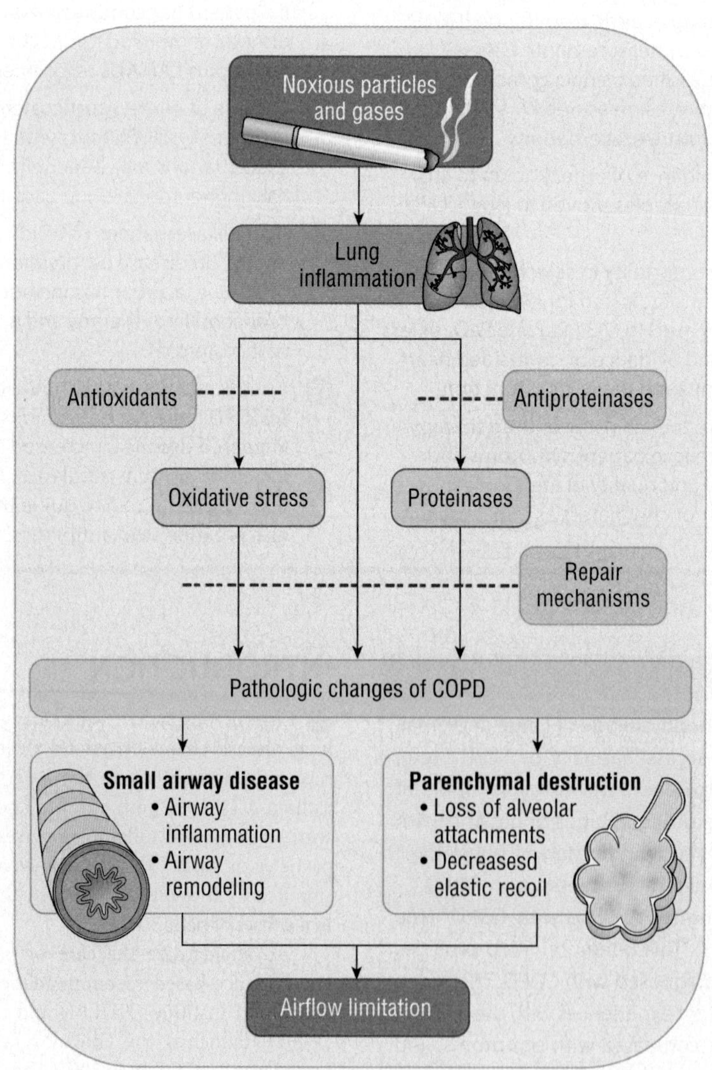

FIGURE 45-1 Pathogenesis of COPD.

exceed 28 million.[7] Despite a decline in the rate of cigarette smoking among adults in the United States, the prevalence of airflow obstruction and COPD is not expected to significantly decrease in the future. Approximately 14% of the population in the United States currently smoke cigarettes. While cessation of cigarette smoking has steadily decreased over the last 10 years, the use of e-cigarettes and smokeless tobacco products has increased.[8] Historically considered a disease primarily affecting White men, women in the United States are now more likely to have a diagnosis of COPD than men. The prevalence of COPD diagnosis also varies among ethnic and racial groups and by state or region of the country. Among ethnic and racial groups, American Indians/Alaskan Natives are more affected than others, and the prevalence is higher in some southeastern states.[9,10]

Chronic obstructive pulmonary disease is the fourth leading cause of death in the United States, exceeded only by cancer, heart disease, and unintentional injuries. Over 150,000 deaths are attributed to COPD annually.[9,10] In contrast to other leading causes of death, which have declining mortality rates, the mortality rate attributable to COPD has increased over the last 40 years. The trend of increasing COPD mortality likely reflects the long latency period between smoking exposure and complications associated with COPD. Between 1969 and 1985, the mortality rate due to COPD increased for men and then plateaued between 1985 and 1999.[11] From 1999 to 2014, the mortality rate due to COPD decreased among men but remained unchanged among women.[11,12] The magnitude difference is likely reflective of changes in smoking status among women in the first decades of the 20th century, although other gender-based differences may also contribute.[13]

While the mortality associated with COPD is significant, morbidity and costs associated with the disease also have a significant impact on patients, their families, and the healthcare system. Annually, patients with COPD account for over 15 million physician office visits and 700,000 hospitalizations. Surveys indicate that individuals with COPD are more likely to report physical activity limitations and be unable to work compared to individuals without COPD.[14] In the United States, an estimated $32 billion was spent on services related to COPD care in 2010 and increasing to $49 billion in the year 2020.[6] Costs associated with the disease are directly related to the severity of COPD and frequency of exacerbations.

ETIOLOGY

3 Cigarette smoking is the most common risk factor and accounts for approximately 75% of cases of COPD in the United States.[1,10] Although the remaining 25% of patients who develop COPD do not have a history of smoking, these patients may have exposure to environmental tobacco smoke or secondhand smoke through their occupation or family. Components of tobacco smoke activate inflammatory cells, which produce and release the inflammatory mediators characteristic of COPD. Smokers are 12 to 13 times more likely to die from COPD than nonsmokers.[15] Although the risk is lower in pipe and cigar smokers, it is still higher than in nonsmokers. Age of starting, total pack-years, and current smoking status are predictive of COPD mortality.

Chronic obstructive pulmonary disease is attributed to a combination of risk factors that results in lung injury and tissue destruction, as evidenced by the fact that less than 50% of all smokers develop COPD, but not all smokers who have equivalent smoking histories develop the same degree of pulmonary impairment.[16] Risk factors can be divided into host factors and environmental factors (Table 45-1), and the interaction between these risks leads to the expression of the disease. Host factors, such as genetic predisposition, may not be modifiable but are important for identifying patients at high risk of developing the disease.

Environmental factors, such as tobacco smoke, occupational dust, and chemicals, are modifiable factors that, if avoided, may reduce the risk of disease development. Environmental exposures associated with COPD are particles that are inhaled by the individual, which result in inflammation and cell injury. Exposure to multiple environmental toxins increases the risk of COPD. Thus, the total burden of inhaled particles (eg, cigarette smoke as well as occupational and environmental particles and pollutants) plays a significant role in the development of COPD. It is helpful to assess an individual's total burden of inhaled particles. For example, an individual who smokes and works in a textile factory has a higher total burden of inhaled particles than an individual who smokes and has no occupational exposure.

TABLE 45-1 Risk Factors for Development of Chronic Obstructive Pulmonary Disease (COPD)

Exposures	Host Factors
Environmental tobacco smoke	Genetic predisposition (AAT deficiency)
Occupational dust and chemicals	Airway hyperresponsiveness
Air pollution	Impaired lung growth

In nonindustrialized countries, occupational exposures may be a more common risk than cigarette smoking. These exposures include dust and chemicals such as vapors, irritants, and fumes. Reduced lung function and deaths from COPD are higher for individuals who work in gold and coal mining, in the glass or ceramic industries with exposure to silica dust, and in jobs that expose them to cotton dust or grain dust, toluene diisocyanate, or asbestos. Other occupational risk factors include chronic exposure to open cooking or heating fires. It is unclear whether air pollution alone is a significant risk factor for the development of COPD in smokers and nonsmokers with normal lung function. However, in individuals with existing pulmonary dysfunction, significant air pollution worsens symptoms.

Individuals exposed to the same environmental risk factors do not have the same chance of developing COPD, suggesting that host factors play an important role in pathogenesis. Specific genes, such as matrix metalloproteinase 12 (MMP12), α_1-antitrypsin, and other genetic markers, have been implicated with the decline of lung function and potential risk of developing COPD.[1] However, only hereditary deficiency of α_1-antitrypsin (AAT) has been definitively shown to correlate with the development of emphysema and pulmonary dysfunction.[17] AAT-associated emphysema is an example of a purely genetic disorder inherited in an autosomal recessive pattern. A primary role of AAT, a plasma protein synthesized in hepatocytes, is to protect cells, especially those in the lung, from destruction by elastase released by neutrophils. Deficiency of AAT results in a protease–antiprotease imbalance and accelerated decline in lung function. Several types of AAT deficiency have been identified and are due to mutations in the AAT gene. True AAT deficiency accounts for less than 1% of COPD cases.[1]

Patients with AAT deficiency develop COPD at an early age (20-50 years) primarily owing to an accelerated decline in lung function. Compared with an average annual decline in forced expiratory volume in 1 second (FEV_1) of 25 mL/year in healthy nonsmokers, patients with homozygous AAT gene deficiency have been reported to have declines of 54 mL/year for nonsmokers and 108 mL/year for current smokers. Effective diagnosis is dependent on clinical suspicion, diagnostic testing of serum concentrations, and genotype confirmation.[17] Patients developing COPD at an early age or those with a strong family history of COPD should be screened for AAT deficiency.

Additional host factors that may influence the risk of developing COPD include airway hyperresponsiveness and lung growth. Individuals with airway hyperresponsiveness, such as asthma, to various inhaled particles may have an accelerated decline in lung function compared with those without airway hyperresponsiveness. Additionally, individuals who do not attain maximal lung growth owing to low-birth weight, prematurity at birth, or childhood illnesses may be at risk for COPD in the future.[1]

PATHOPHYSIOLOGY

Chronic obstructive pulmonary disease is characterized by chronic inflammatory changes that lead to destructive tissue changes and chronic airflow limitation. The inflammatory process is widespread and involves airways, pulmonary vasculature, and lung parenchyma. Exposure to noxious gas and particles activate inflammatory cells to release a variety of chemical mediators. While both asthma and COPD result from inflammatory responses, it is helpful to contrast the types of inflammatory cells and mediators involved because the response to anti-inflammatory therapy differs between the two diseases. The inflammation seen in COPD is often referred to as *neutrophilic* in nature, but macrophages and CD8+ lymphocytes also play major roles.[1,18] In a small subset of patients with COPD, there may be inflammation common to both COPD and asthma, and such patients may be classified as having "asthma-COPD overlap syndrome."[19] Characteristics of inflammation for the two diseases are summarized in Table 45-2.

Other processes proposed to play a major role in the pathogenesis of COPD include increased oxidative stress and imbalance between destructive and protective defense systems in the lungs (proteases and antiproteases).[1,20] Altered interaction between airway oxidants and antioxidants is responsible for the increased oxidative stress present in COPD. Increases in oxidant markers (eg, hydrogen peroxide and nitric oxide) are seen in the epithelial lining fluid and are generated by cigarette smoke or noxious particles.[1]

Oxidants react with and damage various proteins and lipids, leading to cell and tissue damage. Oxidants also promote inflammation directly and exacerbate the protease–antiprotease imbalance by inhibiting antiprotease activity.[20] These processes may be the result of ongoing inflammation or occur because of environmental pressures and exposures (Fig. 45-1).

Pathologic changes of COPD are widespread, affecting large and small airways, lung parenchyma, and the pulmonary vasculature.[1] An inflammatory exudate is often present that leads to an increase in the number and size of goblet cells and mucus glands. Mucous secretion is increased, and ciliary motility is impaired. There is also a thickening of smooth muscle and connective tissue in the airways. Inflammation is present in central and peripheral airways. The chronic inflammation results in a repeated injury and repair process that leads to scarring and fibrosis. Diffuse airway narrowing is present and is more prominent in smaller peripheral airways. Airflow obstruction is attributed to airway inflammation, while the blood gas abnormalities result from impaired gas transfer due to parenchymal damage and loss of alveolar-capillary networks.

TABLE 45-2 Features of Inflammation in COPD Compared with Asthma

	COPD	Asthma
Cells	Neutrophils Large increase in macrophages Increase in CD8+ T lymphocytes	Eosinophils Small increase in macrophages Increase in CD4+ Th2 lymphocytes Activation of mast cells
Mediators	LTB4 IL-8 TNF-α	LTD4 IL-4, IL-5 (Plus many others)
Consequences	Squamous metaplasia of the epithelium Parenchymal destruction Mucus metaplasia Glandular enlargement	Fragile epithelium Thickening of basement membrane Mucus metaplasia Glandular enlargement
Response to treatment	Glucocorticosteroids have a variable effect	Glucocorticosteroids inhibit inflammation

TABLE 45-3 Etiology of Airflow Limitation in COPD

Reversible
Presence of mucus and inflammatory cells and mediators in bronchial secretions
Bronchial smooth muscle contraction in peripheral and central airways
Dynamic hyperinflation during exercise

Irreversible
Fibrosis and narrowing of airways
Reduced elastic recoil with loss of alveolar surface area
Destruction of alveolar support with reduced patency of small airways

Mucus hypersecretion is present early in the course of the disease and is associated with an increased number and size of mucus-producing cells. The presence of chronic inflammation perpetuates the process, although resulting airflow obstruction and chronic airflow limitation may be reversible or irreversible. The various causes of airflow obstruction are summarized in Table 45-3.

Parenchymal changes affect the gas-exchanging units of the lungs, including the alveoli and pulmonary capillaries. As the disease progresses, abnormalities in gas exchange lead to hypoxemia and/or hypercapnia, although there is not a strong correlation between pulmonary function and arterial blood gas (ABG). Significant changes in ABGs usually are not present until airflow limitation is very severe.[1] In such patients, hypoxemia, or low arterial oxygen tension (pressure exerted by oxygen gas in arterial blood [PaO_2] = 45-60 mm Hg [6.0-8.0 kPa]), and hypercapnia, or elevated arterial carbon dioxide tension (pressure exerted by carbon dioxide gas in arterial blood [$PaCO_2$] = 50-60 mm Hg [6.7-8.0 kPa]), can become chronic problems. Initially, when present, hypoxemia is associated with exertion. As the disease progresses, hypoxemia develops at rest. Hypoxemia is attributed to hypoventilation (V) of lung tissue relative to perfusion (Q) of the area. This low (V/Q) ratio will progress over a period of several years, resulting in a consistent decline in the PaO_2. Some COPD patients lose the ability to increase the rate or depth of respiration in response to persistent hypoxemia.

As COPD progresses and gas exchange worsens, patients may exhibit chronic hypercapnia and are referred to as carbon dioxide retainers. In such patients, central respiratory response to chronically increased $PaCO_2$ is blunted. These changes in PaO_2 and $PaCO_2$ are subtle and progress over a period of many years. As a result, serum pH usually is near normal because the kidneys compensate by retaining bicarbonate. If acute respiratory distress develops, such as seen with significant pneumonia or COPD exacerbation with respiratory failure, $PaCO_2$ may rise sharply, and the patient presents with a worsening respiratory acidosis.

The vascular changes of COPD include loss of pulmonary capillary beds, thickening of pulmonary vessels, and vasoconstriction of pulmonary arteries in response to hypoxemia.[1,21] Chronic hypoxemia and permanent changes in pulmonary vasculature lead to increases in pulmonary pressures, especially during exercise. When elevated pulmonary pressures are sustained, right-sided heart failure, or cor pulmonale, develops and is characterized by right ventricle hypertrophy in response to increased pulmonary vascular resistance. Pulmonary hypertension is the most common cardiovascular complication of COPD and can result in significant morbidity.

Thoracic over-inflation is a relevant feature in the pathophysiology of COPD because it is a central factor in causing dyspnea. Chronic airflow obstruction leads to air trapping, resulting in thoracic hyperinflation that can be detected on chest radiograph. Hyperinflation results in several dynamic changes in the chest,

CLINICAL PRESENTATION Chronic Obstructive Pulmonary Disease

Symptoms

- Chronic cough—may be intermittent; may be unproductive
- Chronic sputum production
- Dyspnea—worse with exercise; progressive over time
  - Decreased exercise tolerance or decline in physical activity
  - Chest tightness or wheezing

Risk Factors

- Tobacco smoke exposure
- Indoor air pollution (eg, burning wood and biofuel for cooking or heating)
- Occupational and environmental hazards (eg, organic and inorganic dusts, chemical fumes)
- α_1-Antitrypsin deficiency

Physical Examination

- Shallow breathing
- Increased resting respiratory rate
- Pursed lips during exhalation
- Use of accessory respiratory muscles
- Cyanosis of mucosal membranes (seen in later stages of disease)

Diagnostic Tests

- Spirometry with postbronchodilator testing
- Radiograph of chest (to rule out other diagnoses)
- Arterial blood gas (not routinely obtained in chronic management; has utility in acute decompensation). Lab abnormalities may include pH <7.35, PaO_2 <80 mm Hg (10.6 kPa), $PaCO_2$ >50 mm Hg (6.7 kPa), and bicarbonate >26 mEq/L (mmol/L)

including flattening of diaphragmatic muscles. Under normal circumstances, diaphragms are dome-shaped muscles tethered at the lung bases. When diaphragms contract, the muscles become shorter and flatter, creating the negative inspiratory force through which air flows into lungs during inspiration. With thoracic hyperinflation, diaphragmatic muscles are placed at a disadvantage and are less efficient muscles of ventilation. Increased work required by diaphragmatic contractions predisposes patients to muscle fatigue, especially during periods of exacerbations.

Another consequence of thoracic hyperinflation is the change in lung volumes. For patients with COPD exhibiting thoracic hyperinflation, there is an increase in functional residual capacity (FRC), which is the amount of air left in the lung after exhalation at rest. Therefore, these patients are breathing at higher lung volumes that perturb gas exchange. Increased FRC limits the inspiratory reserve capacity, which is the amount of air that the patient can inhale to fill the lungs. Increased FRC limits the duration of inhalation time and has been associated with increased complaints of dyspnea by patients.[1] Pharmacotherapy for COPD, especially bronchodilators, can reduce thoracic hyperinflation by reducing airflow obstruction and air trapping. This explains symptom improvement reported by patients with COPD despite minimal improvements in expiratory lung function.

Another important systemic consequence of COPD is loss of skeletal muscle mass and a general decline in the overall health status. These changes are partially attributed to systemic inflammation and can have devastating effects on overall health status and comorbidities. Systemic effects include cardiovascular events associated with ischemia, cachexia, weight loss, osteoporosis, anemia, and muscle wasting.[1] There has been interest in measuring C-reactive protein as a marker to assess systemic inflammation and its correlation with disease severity; however, it is premature to recommend its use in practice for chronic management.[22] Instead, C-reactive protein may have a role in identifying patients with acute exacerbation of COPD who should receive treatment with antibiotics.

The diagnosis of COPD is made based on the patient's symptoms, history of exposure to risk factors, and confirmed by pulmonary function testing, such as spirometry. Patients may experience cough for several years before dyspnea develops and often will not seek medical attention until dyspnea is significant. A diagnosis of COPD should be considered for any patient, age 40 years or older, with persistent or progressive dyspnea, with chronic cough productive of sputum, and who exhibits an unusual or abnormal decline in activity, especially in the presence of exposure to environmental tobacco smoke. In addition, the presence of genetic factors, including AAT deficiency, and occupational exposures should be evaluated as approximately 15% of patients with COPD do not have a history of cigarette smoking. Current preventative guidelines do not endorse routine screening tests for asymptomatic patients with risk factors for COPD, although some medical societies advocate proactively identifying patients early in the stages of the disease.[23]

Spirometry combined with physical examination improves the diagnostic accuracy of COPD.[1] Spirometry represents a comprehensive assessment of lung volumes and capacities. Patients with all levels of severity of COPD exhibit the hallmark finding of airflow obstruction; specifically, a reduction in FEV_1/FVC ratio to less than 70% (0.70). FVC is the total volume of air exhaled after maximal inhalation and FEV_1 is the total volume of air exhaled in 1 second. A fixed ratio of less than 70% (0.70) may be problematic because normal aging may affect this result; however, it continues to be the current standard. Previous criteria for the diagnosis of COPD included measuring the degree of airflow limitation before and after inhaled bronchodilator challenge. It is no longer recommended to obtain prebronchodilator values or to calculate the degree of reversibility to diagnose COPD (Table 45-4).[1] Postbronchodilator spirometry results should be used in assessing lung function in patients with COPD.

TABLE 45-4 Procedures for Postbronchodilator Testing

Preparation

Tests should be performed when patients are clinically stable and free from a respiratory infection.

Patient must be able to participate with maximal effort during the test

Spirometry

Bronchodilators can be given by either a metered-dose inhaler or nebulization

Usual doses are 400 mcg of β-agonist, 160 mcg of anticholinergic, or the two combined

FEV_1 should be measured 10-15 minutes after a short-acting β-agonist or 30-45 minutes after a short-acting anticholinergic or combination

Results

Airflow limitation is confirmed by a postbronchodilator FEV_1/FVC <0.70

Data from Reference 1.

TABLE 45-5 Spirometric Grades: Classification of Severity of Airflow Obstruction (Based on Postbronchodilator FEV_1)

GOLD 1: mild $FEV_1/FVC < 70\%$ (0.70) $FEV_1 \geq 80\%$ With or without symptoms
GOLD 2: moderate $FEV_1/FVC < 70\%$ (0.70) $50\% \leq FEV_1 < 80\%$ With or without symptoms
GOLD 3: severe $FEV_1/FVC < 70\%$ (0.70) $30\% \leq FEV_1 < 50\%$ With or without symptoms
GOLD 4: very severe $FEV_1/FVC < 70\%$ (0.70) $FEV_1 < 30\%$

Data from Reference 1.

Spirometry is useful to confirm the presence of airflow limitation and to determine the severity of obstruction.[24] GOLD consensus guidelines suggest a four-grade classification of airflow limitation (Table 45-5). The use of peak expiratory flow measurements as a diagnostic tool or to classify severity is not adequate for COPD due to low specificity and the high degree of effort dependence; however, a low peak expiratory flow is consistent with the clinical presentation of COPD. A comprehensive discussion about spirometry and interpretation can be found in Chapter e43, "Evaluation of Respiratory Function."

Dyspnea is typically the most troublesome complaint for patients with COPD and often is the stimulus for seeking medical attention. It can impair exercise performance and functional capacity and is frequently associated with depression and anxiety. Together, these have a significant effect on health-related quality of life.[1] As a subjective symptom, dyspnea is often difficult for the clinician to assess. Various tools are available to evaluate the severity of dyspnea. The modified Medical Research Council (mMRC) scale is commonly employed and categorizes dyspnea grades from 0 to 4.[1] Patients with COPD may experience a variety of symptoms, not limited only to dyspnea. Therefore, the impact of COPD on other measures of health status has been recognized and newer patient assessment tools, such as COPD assessment Test (CAT) and COPD Control Questionnaire (CCQ), include items related to overall symptoms and activities. Other patient assessment questionnaires, such as the Chronic Respiratory Questionnaire (CRQ) and St. George's Respiratory Questionnaire (SGRQ), are comprehensive measures of disease impact on health status and are used frequently in clinical trials; however, use in clinical practice is limited by their length and complexity. There are three patient assessment questionnaires amenable to use in routine clinical practice and recommended by international guidelines (Table 45-6).[1]

Classification Based on Severity

4 Previously, therapy guidelines have defined disease severity solely by spirometry. Observations that patients with similar spirometric parameters exhibit variations in symptom severity and risk of adverse health events, such as exacerbations, led to a revision in severity classification. The GOLD consensus guidelines recommend using multiple factors to determine disease severity, and that spirometric severity (ie, GOLD spirometric grade 1-4, see Table 45-5) be evaluated separately from symptom and exacerbation risk. A combined "ABCD" classification system is now used and the classification is based on the patient's symptom severity and risk of future exacerbation (Table 45-7). This classification system acknowledges

TABLE 45-6 Comparison of Patient Assessment Questionnaires Used in COPD

Name	Description of Scoring System	Link to Assessment Tool
COPD Assessment Test (CAT)	• Includes 8 items related to health status and impact of COPD on daily activities • Each item scored 0-5 with a maximum total score of 40 • Score of <10 means less symptoms • Score of ≥10 means more symptoms	http://catestonline.org
Modified Medical Research Council Dyspnea Questionnaire (mMRC)	• Includes 5 descriptive statements related to dyspnea only • Patient chooses the most appropriate statement • Each statement corresponds to a score of 0-4 • Score of <2 means less symptoms • Score of ≥2 means more symptoms	http://www.goldcopd.org
COPD Control Questionnaire (CCQ)	• Includes 10 items in 3 domains related to symptoms, functional state, mental state • Assesses clinical control of disease in the past week • Score weighted for each domain • Score <1 means less symptoms[a] • Score ≥1 means more symptoms[a]	http://www.ccq.nl

[a]Exact cut point values have not yet been established for this assessment questionnaire.

TABLE 45-7 Combined Assessment of COPD Severity

Patient Group	Description	Exacerbations in Last Year[a]	CAT	mMRC
A	Less symptoms; low risk	0-1	<10	0-1
B	More symptoms; low risk	0-1	≥10	≥2
C	Less symptoms; high risk	≥2	<10	0-1
D	More symptoms; high risk	≥2	≥10	≥2

[a]greater than 1 exacerbation, or one requiring hospitalization equals high risk (eg, Patient Group C or D)

Data from Reference 1.

that symptom management and prevention of exacerbations should be used to guide therapy. Classification of airflow limitation severity and spirometric grade predicts disease outcomes such as mortality and exacerbations and is useful when considering therapies such as lung reduction surgery or transplantation.

Symptom assessment should be measured at baseline and then during routine visits using CAT or mMRC. Defined cut points for patients exhibiting "more symptoms" and "less symptoms" have been established for CAT and mMRC but are not as well defined for CCQ. The frequency of exacerbations can be assessed by a review of exacerbation history for the past 12 months. Patients with at least two exacerbations in the last 12 months, or one exacerbation requiring hospitalization, are considered high risk for future exacerbations

TABLE 45-8 Selected Prognostic Indices Used in COPD

Name	Description of Tool
BMI, Obstruction, Dyspnea, Exercise (BODE) Index	• Composite score of body mass index, measured FEV_1, mMRC score, and 6MWT distance • Score provides an estimate of 4-year survival • Well-known and validated tool
Age, Dyspnea, Obstruction (ADO) Index	• Composite score of age, mMRC score, and measured FEV_1 • Score provides an estimate for 3-year survival • Maybe more helpful in primary care if 6MWT cannot be measured
COPD Specific Comorbidity Test (COTE) Index	• Includes 12 comorbidities observed to contribute to mortality in COPD patients • Better predictive power if combined with ADO or BODE index

FEV_1, forced expiratory volume in one second; mMRC, modified Medical Research Council scale; 6MWT, six-minute walk test.

(category C or D). Patients are then assigned to an ABCD category based on these two assessments. Classifying patients according to ABCD categories helps inform treatment decisions as guideline-recommended initial and escalation therapy is based on ABCD category classification.

Prognosis

Patients with COPD are a heterogeneous group and multiple factors, such as airflow limitation, age, frequency and severity of exacerbations, and comorbidities, have been implicated in the rate of disease progression and prognosis. The rate of COPD progression is variable and not easily predicted for individual patients. Several prognostic indices have been shown to be useful in predicting survival among populations of patients with COPD (Table 45-8).[25,26] Based on prognostic indices, mortality for patients with COPD increases with worsening airflow limitation (lower FEV_1 percent of predicted), greater age, lower body mass index (BMI), higher dyspnea score (mMRC), shorter 6-minute walk distance, continued smoking, frequent and severe exacerbations, and presence of selected comorbidities. The primary causes of death of patients with COPD include respiratory failure, cardiovascular events or diseases, and lung cancer.[1] Advanced directives, palliative care coordination and end-of-life care are appropriate options to consider for patients with significant progression and comorbidities.

Complications of Progressive COPD

Pulmonary Hypertension

Pulmonary hypertension associated with COPD (PH-COPD) may occur in up to 30% of patients and is associated with increased mortality.[27] Given the management complexity of patients with pulmonary hypertension, referral to expert centers specializing in PH is recommended. Investigations of pharmacologic therapy typically used in the treatment of pulmonary arterial hypertension (ie, endothelin receptor antagonists, phosphodiesterase type 5 [PDE5] inhibitors, prostacyclin analogs) for patients with PH-COPD are limited and provide conflicting results. Due to concerns of worsening gas exchange in patients with COPD, pulmonary vasodilators are not recommended outside of clinical trials or specialized pulmonary hypertension centers.

Cor Pulmonale

Cor pulmonale is right-sided heart failure secondary to pulmonary hypertension. Long-term oxygen therapy and diuretics are mainstays of therapy for cor pulmonale. Increasing PaO_2 above 60 mm Hg (8.0 kPa) with supplemental oxygen therapy decreases pulmonary hypertension and resistance against which the right ventricle must work. While diuretics may help decrease fluid overload, caution should be used because patients with significant right-sided heart failure are highly dependent on preload for cardiac output. Digitalis glycosides have no role in the treatment of cor pulmonale.

Beta-blocker therapy is indicated to treat systolic heart failure including patients who have experienced a myocardial infarction. Beta-blocker therapy can present unique challenges for patients with airway disease but are generally well tolerated by patients with COPD who do not exhibit bronchial hyperreactivity. Patients with COPD should generally be treated with β_1-selective agents, although there is some evidence the non-selective agents can be tolerated. Use of beta-blocker therapy for patients with COPD and cardiac disease has been associated with improved overall survival.[28]

Polycythemia

Polycythemia secondary to chronic hypoxemia in COPD patients can be improved by either continuous oxygen therapy (COT) or periodic phlebotomy if oxygen therapy alone is not sufficient. Acute phlebotomy is indicated if the hematocrit is above 55% to 60% (0.55-0.60) and the patient is experiencing CNS effects suggestive of sludging from high blood viscosity. Long-term oxygen then can be used to maintain a lower hematocrit.

TREATMENT

Chronic Obstructive Pulmonary Disease

Desired Outcome

Given the significant clinical and economic impact of COPD, a major focus in healthcare should be on its prevention in patients at risk of the disease. Limiting or eliminating exposure to tobacco smoke and other environmental irritants should be the goal of prevention efforts. For patients already with a diagnosis of COPD, the primary goal is to prevent or slow disease progression. Specific goals are listed in Table 45-9. Optimally, these goals can be accomplished with minimal risks or adverse effects. Therapy of the patient with COPD is multifaceted and includes pharmacologic and nonpharmacologic strategies.

Unfortunately, most treatments for COPD have not been shown to improve survival or to slow the progressive decline in lung function. However, many therapies do improve pulmonary function and quality of life as well as reduce the risk of COPD exacerbations and duration of hospitalization. While earlier studies of COPD therapies focused primarily on relief of symptoms and improvements in pulmonary function measurements such as FEV_1, more recent studies also measure disease-specific quality-of-life and the frequency and severity of exacerbations. A reduction in exacerbation frequency is an important outcome to consider when evaluating the role and benefit of chronic therapies used in COPD management.

General Approach to Treatment

To be effective, clinicians should address four major components of management: assess and monitor the condition, avoid or reduce

TABLE 45-9 Goals of COPD Management

1. Prevent disease progression
2. Relieve symptoms
3. Improve exercise tolerance
4. Improve overall health status
5. Prevent and treat exacerbations
6. Prevent and treat complications
7. Reduce morbidity and mortality

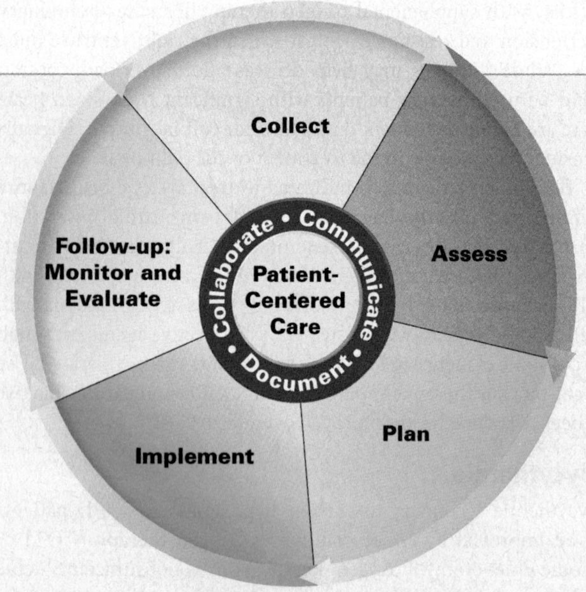

Patient Care Process for the Management of Chronic Obstructive Pulmonary Disease (COPD)

The image shows the five fundamental steps included in patient care process for nausea and vomiting. The tagline of this process reads collaborate, communicate, and document. The five fundamental steps listed here are collect, assess, plan, implement, and follow-up: monitor and evaluate. All these steps are listed in a circular block diagram.

Collect

- Patient characteristics (eg, age, gender)
- History of present illness including a history of COPD exacerbations in last 12 months and management (eg, home, Primary Care Provider visit, Emergency Department visit, or hospitalization)
- Patient history (past medical, family, social-environmental exposures, tobacco use, exercise tolerance, and capacity)
- Current medications including immunizations (eg, influenza, pneumococcus, tetanus/diphtheria/pertussis) and any prior pulmonary medication use
- Objective data (see Tables 45-5 to 45-7)
  - Symptom scores using validated questionnaire (eg, CAT, mMRC)
  - Current and previous spirometry/pulmonary function tests (eg, FEV_1)

Assess

- Severity of symptoms (eg, "more symptoms" or "less symptoms" based on questionnaires, Table 45-6)
- Risk of future exacerbation (eg, high risk or low risk)
- Degree of airflow limitation (eg, GOLD spirometry group, Table 45-5)
- Patient category based on GOLD Combined Assessment (eg, Category ABCD, Table 45-7)
- Readiness to quit, if current tobacco use (see Tables 45-10 to 45-12)
- Appropriateness and effectiveness of current pulmonary medication regimen
- Ability to administer/participate with inhaled therapies (eg, dexterity, vision, coordination)
- Ability to pay for medications (eg, insurance, formulary considerations, self-pay)

Plan

- Patient-specific goals of therapy (see Tables 45-13 and 45-19)
- Preventative health measures (eg, immunizations, smoking cessation)
- Drug therapy regimen including specific medication, dose, route, frequency, and duration; specify the continuation and discontinuation of existing therapies (see Tables 45-13 and 45-14)
- Oxygen therapy if severe airflow limitation
- Monitoring parameters including efficacy (eg, symptoms, exacerbations), safety (medication-specific adverse effects), and time frame
- Patient education (eg, purpose of medications, administration technique, recognition of exacerbations)
- Referrals to other providers when appropriate (eg, physician, pulmonary rehabilitation)

Implement*

- Provide patient education regarding all elements of the treatment plan
- Use motivational interviewing and coaching strategies to maximize adherence
- Schedule follow-up

Follow-up: Monitor and Evaluate

- Determine goal attainment (eg, symptoms, exacerbations, complications)
- Presence of treatment-related adverse effects
- Patient adherence to treatment plan using multiple sources of information

**Collaborate with patient, caregivers, and other healthcare professionals.*

exposure to risk factors, manage stable disease, and treat exacerbations.[1] These components are addressed through a variety of nonpharmacologic and pharmacologic approaches.

Nonpharmacologic Therapy and Health Maintenance Strategies

Patients with COPD should receive education about their disease, treatment plans, and strategies to slow progression and prevent complications. For those patients who smoke and who are exposed to environmental smoke, advising and counseling patients about smoking cessation are essential for patients in all stages of the disease. Because the natural course of the disease leads to respiratory failure, clinicians should address end-of-life decisions and advanced directives prospectively with the patient and family. Increasingly, palliative care services, which include both end-of-life and hospice care for patients with all types of life-threatening acute and chronic illnesses, have been utilized for patients with severe COPD.[29]

Smoking Cessation 5 Smoking cessation represents the single most important intervention in preventing the development, as well as progression, of COPD. A primary component of COPD management is avoidance of or reduced exposure to risk factors. Smoking cessation leads to decreased symptomatology and slows the rate of decline of pulmonary function even after significant abnormalities in pulmonary function tests have been detected. As confirmed by the Lung Health Study, smoking cessation is the only intervention proven to affect long-term decline in FEV_1 and slow the progression of COPD.[30] In this 5-year prospective trial, smokers with early COPD were randomly assigned to one of three groups: smoking-cessation intervention plus inhaled ipratropium three times a day, smoking-cessation intervention alone, or no intervention. During an 11-year follow-up, the rate of decline in FEV_1 among subjects who continued to smoke was more than twice the rate in sustained quitters.[31] Smokers who underwent smoking-cessation intervention had fewer respiratory symptoms and a smaller annual decline in FEV_1 compared with smokers who had no intervention.

Tobacco cessation has mortality benefits beyond those related to COPD. A follow-up analysis of the Lung Health Study data conducted more than 14 years later demonstrated an 18% reduction in all-cause mortality in patients who received the intervention compared with usual care.[32] Intervention patients had lower death rates due to cardiovascular diseases (the leading cause of mortality) and lung cancer.

Every clinician has a responsibility to advise smokers regarding smoking cessation and should take an active role in assisting patients with tobacco dependence to reduce the burden on the individual, their family, and the healthcare system. Counseling that is provided by clinicians is associated with greater success rates than self-initiated efforts. The major findings from recent clinical practice guidelines for treating tobacco dependence are summarized in Table 45-10. Since 2004, reports from the Surgeon General on the health consequences of smoking have emphasized the detrimental effects of cigarette smoking on the general health of smokers and individuals exposed to secondhand smoke. Over 20 million Americans have died prematurely from exposure to cigarette smoking since 1964.

Evidence from long-term trials shows that tobacco cessation, either sustained or intermittent, is of benefit at any point. For patients with COPD, maximum benefit is seen with early and sustained cessation; however, incremental benefit is seen at all time points. Given that approximately 40% of patients with COPD continue to smoke, patients and clinicians should understand it is never too late to quit, and repeated attempts at cessation may be necessary. Approximately 70% of smokers want to quit, and over half have made a cessation attempt in the last year. Yet complete and sustained tobacco cessation is difficult.[33,34] Understanding that tobacco dependence is a chronic disease, the focus should be on congratulating and encouraging patients for any behavior changes that result in reduced exposure to tobacco smoke rather than admonishing patients for unsuccessful attempts, relapses, or incomplete cessation.

The guidelines recommend that clinicians take a comprehensive approach to smoking cessation assessment. All patients should be routinely assessed for tobacco use and advice given to smokers even if they have no symptoms of smoking-related disease or if they are receiving care for reasons unrelated to smoking. Clinicians should be persistent in their motivational efforts to determine the patient's readiness and support cessation attempts. Even brief interventions (3 minutes) of counseling have been shown to be effective. There are several stages that influence patient decision making. Based on this, a five-step intervention program is proposed (Table 45-11).

There is strong evidence to support the use of pharmacotherapy to assist in smoking cessation, and therapy should be offered

TABLE 45-10 Key Guideline Recommendations Regarding Tobacco Use and Dependence

- Tobacco dependence is a chronic disease that often requires repeated intervention and multiple attempts to quit. Effective treatments are available that can significantly improve rates of long-term abstinence
- Clinicians and healthcare delivery systems should systemically identify tobacco use and dependence and treat every patient who uses tobacco
- Tobacco-dependence treatments are effective over a broad range of populations. Clinicians should encourage every patient willing to quit to use counseling and medications recommended in the guideline
- Brief tobacco-dependence treatments are effective. Clinicians should offer every patient who uses tobacco at least these brief treatments
- Individual, group, and telephone counseling are effective, and their effectiveness increases with treatment intensity. Practical counseling (problem-solving and/or skills training) and social support are very effective and should be part of treatment
- There are numerous effective medications for tobacco dependence, and clinicians should encourage their use by patients during a quit attempt, except when medically contraindicated or with populations in which the evidence of effectiveness is insufficient (pregnancy). Seven first-line medications (five nicotine and two non-nicotine) consistently increase long-term abstinence rates. Clinicians should also consider the use of combinations as identified in the guideline
- Counseling and medication are effective when used by themselves for treating tobacco dependence. The combination of the two is more effective than either alone. Patients should be encouraged to use both counseling and medication
- Telephone quitline counseling is effective for diverse populations and offers the advantage of broad reach. Clinicians should ensure patient access to quitlines and promote quitline use
- For a patient with tobacco dependence who is currently unwilling to make a quit attempt, clinicians should use motivational treatments that have been shown to be effective in increasing future quit attempts
- Tobacco-dependence treatments are both clinically effective and highly cost-effective relative to interventions for other clinical disorders. Providing coverage for these treatments increases quit rates. Insurers and purchasers should ensure that all insurance plans include the counseling and medications identified as effective in the guideline as covered benefits

Data from References 33 and 34.

TABLE 45-11 Five-Step Strategy for Smoking-Cessation Program (5 A's)

Ask	Use a systematic approach to identify all patients who use tobacco at every visit
Advise	Strongly urge all patients who use tobacco to quit
Assess	Determine willingness and motivation to make a cessation attempt
Assist	Provide support for the patient to quit smoking
Arrange	Schedule follow-up and monitor for continued abstinence

to most patients as part of a cessation attempt. In general, available pharmacotherapies will double the effectiveness of a cessation effort when combined with behavioral counseling. Agents considered first line are listed in Table 45-12. The usual duration of therapy is 8 to 12 weeks, although some individuals may require longer courses of treatment. Precautions to consider before using bupropion include a history of seizures or an eating disorder. Nicotine replacement therapies are contraindicated for patients with recent (less than 2 weeks) myocardial infarction or stroke. Varenicline, a nicotine acetylcholine receptor partial agonist, relieves physical withdrawal symptoms and reduces the rewarding properties of nicotine. Nausea and headache are the most frequent complaints associated with varenicline. Second-line agents are less effective or associated with greater adverse effects; however, they may be useful in selected clinical situations. These therapies include clonidine and nortriptyline, a tricyclic antidepressant. Given the significant increase in the use of e-cigarettes and other electronic nicotine delivery systems (ENDS), there is

TABLE 45-12 First-Line Pharmacotherapies for Smoking Cessation

Agent	Usual Dose	Duration	Common Complaints
Bupropion SR	150 mg orally daily for 3 days, then twice daily	12 weeks, up to 6 months	Insomnia, dry mouth
Nicotine gum or lozenge	2-4 mg prn, up to 24 pieces daily	12 weeks	Sore mouth, dyspepsia
Nicotine inhaler	6-16 cartridges daily	Up to 6 months	Sore mouth and throat
Nicotine nasal spray	8-40 doses daily	3-6 months	Nasal irritation
Nicotine patches	Various, 7-21 mg every 24 hr	Up to 8 weeks	Skin reaction, insomnia
Varenicline	0.5 mg daily orally for 3 days, then 0.5 mg twice daily for 4 days, then 1 mg twice daily	12 weeks	Nausea, sleep disturbances

interest in the potential role of these nicotine delivery systems as smoking cessation strategies. It is not clear if substituting ENDS for traditional cessation therapy produces similar or greater tobacco cessation rates, and long-term safety outcomes of these systems have not been determined.[1,34] ENDS should not be recommended as part of a smoking cessation strategy until additional evidence is available. A comprehensive discussion of tobacco cessation can be found in Chapter 86, "Substance Use Disorders II: Alcohol Nicotine and Caffeine."

Other Environmental Triggers Although cigarette smoke is by far the most common risk for developing COPD in most patients, exposure to other environmental toxins also confers risks.[1] Exposure to occupational dust and fumes has been implicated as a cause of COPD in 19% of smokers and 31% of nonsmokers with COPD in the United States. In the case of known environmental hazards, primary prevention is appropriate. Policies to limit airborne exposures in the workplace and outdoors, as well as education efforts of workers and policymakers, are recommended.

Pulmonary Rehabilitation Exercise training is beneficial in the treatment of COPD to improve exercise tolerance and to reduce symptoms of dyspnea and fatigue.[1] Pulmonary rehabilitation programs are an integral component in the management of COPD and should include exercise training along with smoking cessation, breathing exercises, optimal medical treatment, psychosocial support, and health education. Pulmonary rehabilitation has no direct effect on lung function or gas exchange. Instead, it optimizes other body systems so that the impact of poor lung function is minimized. Exercise training reduces the CNS response to dyspnea, ameliorates anxiety and depression, reduces thoracic hyperinflation, and improves skeletal muscle function.[35]

High-intensity training (70% maximal workload) is possible even in advanced COPD patients, and level of intensity improves peripheral muscle and ventilatory function. Studies have demonstrated that pulmonary rehabilitation with exercise three to seven times per week can produce long-term improvement in activities of daily living, quality of life, exercise tolerance, and dyspnea for patients with moderate-to-severe COPD.[36] Improvements in dyspnea do not always result in improvements in spirometry. While rehabilitation programs vary in length as well as exercise frequency and intensity, optimal benefits result from programs of 6 to 8 weeks in duration and including at least twice a week supervised sessions with targeted feedback.[1]

Surgical Intervention

Various surgical options have been employed in the management of COPD.[1] These include bullectomy, lung volume reduction surgery (LVRS), and lung transplantation. Presence of bullae may contribute to complaints of dyspnea, and their removal can improve lung function and reduce symptoms, although there is no evidence of a mortality benefit. Lung volume reduction surgery removes sections of lung to reduce hyperinflation and may improve survival in selected patients. Lung transplantation, either single or double, may improve exercise capacity and health status but median survival is only 5.5 years after transplant.[1]

Long-Term Oxygen Therapy 6 The use of supplemental oxygen therapy increases survival in COPD patients with chronic hypoxemia at rest. Patients receiving oxygen therapy for at least part of the day have lower rates of mortality than those not receiving oxygen. Long-term oxygen therapy provides more benefit in terms of survival after at least 5 years of use and improves the quality of life for patients by increasing walking distance, improving neuropsychological condition, and reducing time spent in the hospital.[1] Before patients are considered for long-term oxygen therapy, they should be stabilized in the outpatient setting, and pharmacotherapy should be optimized. Once optimized, long-term oxygen therapy should be instituted if either of the following conditions is observed and documented twice in a 3-week period:

1. A resting PaO_2 of less than 55 mm Hg (7.3 kPa) or SaO_2 less than 88% (0.88) with or without hypercapnia.
2. A resting PaO_2 between 55 and 60 mm Hg (7.3 and 8.0 kPa) or SaO_2 less than 88% (0.88) with evidence of right-sided heart failure, polycythemia, or pulmonary hypertension.

The most practical means of administering long-term oxygen is with a nasal cannula, at 1 to 2 L/min, providing 24% to 28% (0.24 to 0.28) fraction of inspired oxygen (FiO_2) with a goal to raise PaO_2 above 60 mm Hg (8.0 kPa). There are three different ways to deliver oxygen, including (a) in liquid reservoirs, (b) compressed into a cylinder, and (c) via an oxygen concentrator. Although conventional liquid oxygen and compressed oxygen are quite bulky, smaller, portable tanks are available to permit greater patient mobility. Oxygen concentrator devices separate nitrogen from room air and concentrate oxygen. These are the most convenient and the least expensive method of oxygen delivery. Oxygen-conservation devices are available that allow oxygen to flow only during inspiration, making the supply last longer. These may be particularly useful to prolong the oxygen supply for mobile patients using portable cylinders. However, devices are bulky and subject to failure. Patient education about flow rates and avoidance of flames (ie, smoking) is of the utmost importance.

Adjunctive Therapies In addition to supplemental oxygen, adjunctive therapies to consider as part of a pulmonary rehabilitation program are psychoeducational care and nutritional support. Psychoeducational care (such as relaxation) has been associated with improvement in the functioning and well-being of adults with COPD.[1] The role of nutritional support for patients with COPD is controversial. Several studies have shown associations of malnutrition, low BMI, and impaired pulmonary status among patients with COPD. However, results from multiple studies suggest that the effect of nutritional support on physical and functional outcomes in COPD is small and may be most beneficial for malnourished patients.[37]

Vaccinations The GOLD guidelines include specific recommendations about vaccines.[1] The CDC also provides advice about vaccines for COPD patients in the United States and these are updated periodically based on new evidence and as new vaccines become available. Recommended vaccines can reduce the likelihood of respiratory infections that lead to COPD exacerbations. Influenza is a common complication in COPD that can lead to exacerbations and respiratory failure. Therefore, annual vaccination with the inactivated intramuscular influenza vaccine is recommended.[1,38] Immunization against influenza can reduce exacerbations, hospitalization, all-cause death, and respiratory death in COPD patients.[39] Influenza vaccine should be administered annually during each influenza season. Vaccination against influenza can begin as early as August, with most patients being vaccinated during regular medical visits or at vaccination clinics in October and November. The oral antiviral agent, oseltamivir, can be considered for non-immunized patients with COPD during an outbreak; however, this therapy is less effective and causes more adverse effects.

Vaccination against pneumococcal infection is recommended for all adults with COPD. For individuals who have not previously received a pneumococcal conjugate vaccine (PCV), either PCV20 or PCV15 followed by a pneumococcal polysaccharide vaccine (PPSV23) at least 1 year later is recommended.[38] If the patient has previously received PPSV23, either PCV15 or PCV20 should be administered at least 1 year later. Individuals with COPD who have not received the tetanus toxoid, reduced diphtheria toxoid, and acellular pertussis (Tdap) vaccine, the CDC and GOLD guidelines recommend Tdap and then subsequent tetanus and diphtheria boosters, with or without acellular pertussis, every 10 years.[1,40] Herpes zoster vaccine is recommended for adults with COPD at age 50 or older.[1]

After the global outbreak of novel coronavirus SARS-Co-V-2, the CDC recommend all individuals over the age of 5 years receive a viral vector or mRNA vaccine to prevent severe illness and death associated with coronavirus infection and disease (COVID-19).

Pharmacologic Therapy

In contrast to survival benefit conferred by supplemental oxygen therapy and tobacco cessation, there is no medication available for the treatment of COPD that has been conclusively shown to modify lung function decline or prolong survival.[1] There is some evidence that chronic treatment with pharmacotherapy may reduce the rate of lung function decline in a subset of patients, although more definitive studies are needed to confirm these observations. The primary goal of pharmacotherapy is to improve patient symptoms, reduce the frequency and severity of exacerbations, and improve the patient's exercise tolerance.

Currently available therapies for COPD are summarized in Tables 45-13 to 45-15. International guidelines recommend a stepwise approach to the use of pharmacotherapy based on disease severity determined by an assessment of symptom burden and exacerbation risk.[1] The impact of recurrent exacerbations on accelerating disease progression is increasingly recognized as an important factor to be considered. There is inadequate evidence to support the routine use of more aggressive pharmacotherapy early in the course of the disease because of the lack of a disease-modifying benefit. Due to the progressive nature of COPD, pharmacotherapy tends to be chronic and cumulative. Step-down approaches in stable patients may be considered if adverse effects outweigh therapeutic benefits or if patients do not demonstrate a sufficient response. Patients exhibit varied responses to available therapies and the treatment approach must be individualized.

Pharmacotherapy for COPD involves the use of inhaled medications that require patient knowledge and skill using various inhalation devices. Several delivery devices are available (ie, metered-dose inhalers [MDIs], dry powder inhalers [DPIs], soft-mist inhalers [SMIs], nebulizers, and ancillary devices such as holding chambers), and instructions about proper use vary (see Chapter 44, "Asthma" for information about inhalation devices). There is no clear advantage

TABLE 45-13 Recommended Initial Pharmacologic Therapy for Stable COPD and Evaluation of Therapeutic Outcomes

Patient Group	Initial Therapy	Assessment
A (less symptoms, less risk)	Offer bronchodilator, either short- or long-acting depending on symptoms	Assess symptomatic benefit of therapy after initiation (ie, mMRC or CAT score) Assess exacerbation history Assess inhaler technique regularly Assess technique and adherence before modifying therapy Assess tobacco cessation readiness, if continued smoking Assess immunization status (influenza, pneumococcal)
B (more symptoms, less risk)	Start either LAMA or LABA for symptom control	Assess symptomatic benefit of therapy after initiation (ie, mMRC or CAT score) Assess exacerbation history Assess inhaler technique regularly Assess technique and adherence before modifying therapy Assess tobacco cessation readiness, if continued smoking Assess immunization status (influenza, pneumococcal)
C (less symptoms, more risk)	• Start long-acting bronchodilator for exacerbation prevention • LAMA is preferred over LABA for initial monotherapy	Assess symptomatic benefit of therapy after initiation (ie, mMRC or CAT score) Assess exacerbation history Assess inhaler technique regularly Assess technique and adherence before modifying therapy Assess tobacco cessation readiness, if continued smoking Assess immunization status (influenza, pneumococcal)
D (more symptoms, more risk)	• LAMA is preferred over LABA for initial monotherapy • For severe breathlessness, may start with dual LAMA/LABA. If less symptoms, may start only LAMA monotherapy and add LABA at a later time • If blood eosinophils ≥ 300 cells/microliter (0.3 x 10^9/L), start ICS/LABA as initial dual therapy	Assess symptomatic benefit of therapy after initiation (ie, mMRC or CAT score) Assess exacerbation history Assess inhaler technique regularly Assess technique and adherence before modifying therapy Assess tobacco cessation readiness, if continued smoking Assess immunization status (influenza, pneumococcal)

CAT, COPD assessment test; ICS, inhaled corticosteroids; LABA, long-acting beta-agonist; LAMA, long-acting muscarinic antagonists; mMRC, modified Medical Respiratory Council questionnaire; SABA, short-acting beta-agonist; SAMA, short-acting muscarinic antagonists.

TABLE 45-14 Recommended Escalation Pharmacologic Therapy for Stable COPD and Evaluation of Therapeutic Outcomes

Target Symptom	Current Therapy	Assessment	Escalation Therapy
Dyspnea	LABA or LAMA monotherapy	Assess symptomatic benefit of therapy after initiation (ie, mMRC or CAT score) Assess exacerbation history Assess inhaler technique regularly Assess technique and adherence before modifying therapy Assess tobacco cessation readiness, if continued smoking Assess immunization status (influenza, pneumococcal) Assess other causes of dyspnea	Add additional long-acting bronchodilator if persistent symptoms on monotherapy. New regimen = LAMA + LABA If dual bronchodilators do not improve symptoms, consider changing device or active ingredient and/or stepping back to monotherapy If a patient becomes high risk for future exacerbations, choose escalation therapy based on the target symptom of "Exacerbations"
Dyspnea	LABA + ICS	Assess symptomatic benefit of therapy after initiation (ie, mMRC or CAT score) Assess exacerbation history Assess inhaler technique regularly Assess technique and adherence before modifying therapy Assess tobacco cessation readiness, if continued smoking Assess immunization status (influenza, pneumococcal)	Add additional long-acting bronchodilator if persistent symptoms on dual therapy. New regimen = LAMA + LABA + ICS If pneumonia, inappropriate indication or lack of response to ICS, consider de-escalation back to LABA + LAMA only
Exacerbations	LABA or LAMA monotherapy	Assess symptomatic benefit of therapy after initiation (ie, mMRC or CAT score) Assess exacerbation history Assess inhaler technique regularly Assess technique and adherence before modifying therapy Assess tobacco cessation readiness, if continued smoking Assess immunization status (influenza, pneumococcal)	Add long-acting bronchodilator if persistent exacerbations on monotherapy. New regimen = LABA + LAMA If current therapy is LABA and blood eosinophils ≥300, consider adding ICS to LABA. New regimen = LABA + ICS If current therapy is LABA and blood eosinophils ≥100 AND ≥2 moderate exacerbations/1 hospitalization, consider adding ICS to LABA. New regimen = LABA + ICS
Exacerbations	LABA + ICS	Assess symptomatic benefit of therapy after initiation (ie, mMRC or CAT score) Assess exacerbation history Assess inhaler technique regularly Assess technique and adherence before modifying therapy Assess tobacco cessation readiness, if continued smoking Assess immunization status (influenza, pneumococcal)	Add long-acting bronchodilator if persistent exacerbations on dual therapy. New regimen = LAMA + LABA + ICS If pneumonia, inappropriate indication or lack of response to ICS, consider de-escalation back to LABA + LAMA only
Exacerbations	LABA + LAMA + ICS	Assess symptomatic benefit of therapy after initiation (ie, mMRC or CAT score) Assess exacerbation history Assess inhaler technique regularly Assess technique and adherence before modifying therapy Assess tobacco cessation readiness, if continued smoking Assess immunization status (influenza, pneumococcal)	If FEV_1 <50% and presence of chronic bronchitis, consider adding roflumilast If a former or never smoker, consider adding azithromycin daily or three times a week for 12 months If pneumonia, inappropriate indication or lack of response to ICS, consider de-escalation and withdrawal of ICS

CAT, COPD assessment test; ICS, inhaled corticosteroids; LABA, long-acting beta-agonist; LAMA, long-acting muscarinic antagonists; mMRC, modified Medical Respiratory Council questionnaire; SABA, short-acting beta-agonist; SAMA, short-acting muscarinic antagonists.

of one delivery system over another, and all devices are associated with administration errors.[41] Comorbidities common for patients with COPD, including physical and cognitive impairments, can have a significant effect on the patient's ability to use devices, and it is recommended that patient-specific factors and preferences be considered.[1] Periodic and frequent reinforcement and observation by clinicians are required to assess optimal use and determine if alternative devices or therapy are needed.

Treatment regimens with multiple inhalation devices add complexity and may adversely impact adherence and disease management. In one cohort study, patients prescribed multiple types of inhalation devices had worse outcomes (increased exacerbations and rescue therapy use) compared to patients using devices of a similar type or administration technique.[42] For patients requiring therapy with multiple inhaled medications, clinicians should prescribe devices with a similar administration technique or containing combinations of medications. Formulary restrictions and healthcare payer reimbursement issues often make this recommendation difficult to apply in practice.

Bronchodilators

7 Bronchodilators represent the mainstay of drug therapy for COPD and are used to relieve patient symptoms, improve exercise tolerance, and quality of life. For patients with COPD, clinical benefits of bronchodilators include increased exercise capacity, decreased air trapping in lungs, and relief of symptoms such as dyspnea. However, the use of bronchodilators does not produce significant improvements in pulmonary function measurements of expiratory

TABLE 45-15 COPD Medication Chart

	Active Ingredient	Dosage Form; Route	Usual Frequency	Proprietary Name	Device Type
Short-Acting Bronchodilators					
Short-acting beta-agonist (SABA)	Albuterol sulfate	Aerosol, metered; inhalation	Four to six times a day as needed	Proventil-HFA; Ventolin-HFA; Proair HFA	MDI
	Albuterol sulfate	Solution; inhalation	Four to six times a day as needed	Accuneb; generic	Nebulization
	Levalbuterol hydrochloride	Solution; inhalation	Three to four times a day as needed	Xopenex; generic	Nebulization
	Levalbuterol tartrate	Aerosol, metered; inhalation	Three to four times a day as needed	Xopenex HFA	MDI
Short-acting anticholinergics (SAMA)	Ipratropium bromide	Aerosol, metered; inhalation	Four times a day as needed	Atrovent HFA	MDI
	Ipratropium bromide	Solution; inhalation	Four times a day as needed	generic	Nebulization
Long-Acting Bronchodilators					
Long-acting beta-agonist (LABA)	Arformoterol tartrate	Solution; inhalation	Twice daily	Brovana	Nebulization
	Formoterol fumarate	Solution; inhalation	Twice daily	Perforomist	Nebulization
	Olodaterol hydrochloride	Spray metered; inhalation	Once daily	Striverdi Respimat	SMI
	Salmeterol xinafoate	Powder; inhalation	Twice daily	Serevent Diskus	DPI
Long-acting anticholinergics (LAMA)	Aclidinium bromide	Powder; inhalation	Twice daily	Tudorza Pressair	DPI
	Tiotropium bromide	Spray metered; inhalation	Once daily	Spiriva Respimat	SMI
	Tiotropium bromide	Powder; inhalation	Once daily	Spiriva Handihaler	DPI
	Glycopyrrolate	Solution; inhalation	Twice daily	Lonhala Magnair	Nebulization
	Glycopyrrolate	Powder; inhalation	Twice daily	Seebri Neohaler	DPI
	Umeclidinium bromide	Powder; inhalation	Once daily	Incruse Ellipta	DPI
	Revefenacin	Solution; inhalation	Once daily	Yupelri	Nebulization
Inhaled Corticosteroids					
Inhaled Corticosteroids (ICS)	Beclomethasone dipropionate	Aerosol, metered; inhalation	Twice daily	Qvar Redihaler	MDI
	Budesonide	Powder; inhalation	Twice daily	Pulmicort Flexhaler	DPI
	Budesonide	Suspension; inhalation	Once or twice daily	Pulmicort Respules; generic	Nebulization
	Fluticasone propionate	Aerosol, metered; inhalation	Twice daily	Flovent HFA	MDI
	Fluticasone furoate	Powder; inhalation	Twice daily	Arnuity Ellipta	DPI
	Mometasone furoate	Powder; inhalation	Twice daily	Asmanex Twisthaler	DPI
	Mometasone furoate	Aerosol; metered; inhalation	Twice daily	Asmanex HFA	MDI
Combination Inhalers					
Dual combination (SABA/SAMA)	Albuterol sulfate; ipratropium bromide	Solution; inhalation	Four to six times a day as needed	Duoneb; generic	Nebulization
	Albuterol sulfate; ipratropium bromide	Spray metered; inhalation	Four to six times a day as needed	Combivent Respimat	SMI
Dual combination (LAMA/LABA)	Umeclidium bromide; vilanterol trifenatate	Powder; inhalation	Once daily	Anoro Ellipta	DPI
	Tiotropium bromide; olodaterol hydrochloride	Spray metered; inhalation	Once daily	Stiolto Respimat	SMI
	Glycopyrrolate; formoterol fumarate	Aerosol, metered; inhalation	Twice daily	Bevespi Aerosphere	MDI
	Aclidinium; formoterol fumarate	Powder; metered; inhalation	Twice daily	Duaklir Pressair	DPI
Dual combination (ICS/LABA)	Budesonide; formoterol fumarate dihydrate	Aerosol, metered; inhalation	Twice daily	Symbicort	MDI
	Fluticasone furoate; vilanterol trifenatate	Powder; inhalation	Once daily	Breo Ellipta	DPI
	Fluticasone propionate; salmeterol xinafoate	Powder; inhalation	Twice daily	Advair Diskus; Airduo Respiclick; Airduo Digihaler	DPI
	Fluticasone propionate; salmeterol xinafoate	Aerosol, metered; inhalation	Twice daily	Advair HFA	MDI
	Mometasone furoate; formoterol fumarate	Aerosol, metered; inhalation	Twice daily	Dulera	MDI

(continued)

TABLE 45-15 COPD Medication Chart (*Continued*)

	Active Ingredient	Dosage Form; Route	Usual Frequency	Proprietary Name	Device Type
Triple combination (ICS/LAMA/LABA)	Fluticasone furoate; umeclidinium bromide; vilanterol trifenatate	Powder; inhalation	Once daily	Trelegy Ellipta	DPI
	Budesonide; formoterol fumarate; glycopyrrolate	Aerosol; metered; inhalation	Twice daily	Breztri Aerosphere	DPI
Oral Medications					
	Roflumilast	Tablet; oral	Once daily	Daliresp	Oral
	Theophylline	Tablet; capsule; oral	Once or twice daily (extended-release)	Theo-24; generic	Oral

airflow such as FEV_1. Bronchodilator classes available for the treatment of COPD include short- and long-acting β_2-agonists, short- and long-acting anticholinergics, and methylxanthines. Short-acting bronchodilators relieve symptoms and increase exercise tolerance. Long-acting bronchodilators relieve symptoms, reduce exacerbation frequency, and improve quality of life and health status. In general, adverse effects of bronchodilator medications are related to their pharmacologic effects and are dose dependent. Because COPD patients are older and more likely to have comorbid conditions, the risk for adverse effects and drug interactions is higher compared with patients with asthma.

Short-Acting Bronchodilators The initial recommended therapy for COPD patients who experience occasional symptoms (category A) is a bronchodilator, either long- or short-acting (Tables 45-13 and 45-14). Short-acting bronchodilators are also recommended for all patients for use as rescue or as-needed therapy to manage symptoms (category A, B, C, D). Among short-acting bronchodilators, choices include short-acting β_2-agonist or short-acting anticholinergic agents. Both classes of agents have a relatively rapid onset of action, relieve symptoms, and improve exercise tolerance and lung function. Of note, short-acting bronchodilators do not reduce the frequency or severity of exacerbations in COPD. Both classes are equally effective for symptom management. When a patient does not achieve adequate management of symptoms with one agent, a combination of a short-acting β_2-agonist and short-acting anticholinergic is reasonable.

Short-Acting Sympathomimetics (β_2-Agonists) β_2-agonists cause bronchodilation by stimulating adenyl cyclase to increase the formation of cyclic adenosine monophosphate (cAMP), which is responsible for mediating the relaxation of bronchial smooth muscle. In addition, β_2-agonists may improve mucociliary clearance within the airways. In COPD patients, short-acting β_2-agonists exert a rapid onset of effect, although response generally is less than that seen in asthma. Short-acting inhaled β_2-agonists cause only a small improvement in FEV_1 acutely but may improve respiratory symptoms and exercise tolerance despite the small improvement in spirometric measurements.

Choices for short-acting, selective β_2-agonists are albuterol and levalbuterol. Racemic epinephrine is available as an over-the-counter product but is not appropriate for chronic treatment. Albuterol is the most frequently used short-acting β_2-agonist and is a racemic mixture of (*R*)-albuterol, which is responsible for the bronchodilator effect, and (*S*)-albuterol, which has no therapeutic effect. (*S*)-Albuterol is considered by some clinicians to be inert, whereas others believe that it may be implicated in worsening airway inflammation and antagonizing the response to (*R*)-albuterol. Levalbuterol is a single-isomer formulation of (*R*)-albuterol. Despite years of clinical use, there is no compelling evidence to suggest that levalbuterol offers a clear advantage in terms of clinical effectiveness or safety over albuterol, and it is more expensive.[1]

The preferred route of administration for short-acting, selective β_2-agonists is inhalation. The use of oral and parenteral β-agonists in COPD is discouraged because they are no more effective than properly used inhalation devices, and the incidence of systemic adverse effects such as tachycardia and hand tremor is greater. Administration of β_2-agonists in outpatient and emergency room settings via inhalers (MDIs or DPIs) is at least as effective as nebulization therapy and is usually favored for reasons of cost and convenience.[1,4] Chapter 44 includes information about the devices used for delivering aerosolized medication and a comparison of β_2-agonist therapies.

Inhaled β_2-agonists are generally well tolerated. They can cause sinus tachycardia and rhythm disturbances in predisposed patients, but these are rarely reported. Skeletal muscle tremors can occur initially but generally subside as tolerance develops. Older patients may be more sensitive and may experience palpitations, skeletal muscle tremors, and "jittery" feelings after β_2-agonist use.

Short-Acting Anticholinergics When given by inhalation, anticholinergics, also referred to as antimuscarinics, produce bronchodilation by competitively inhibiting muscarinic receptors, subtypes M_1, M_2, and M_3, in bronchial smooth muscle and mucus glands. This activity blocks acetylcholine, with the net effect being a reduction in cyclic guanosine monophosphate (cGMP), which normally acts to constrict bronchial smooth muscle and decreased mucus secretion.

Ipratropium is the most prescribed short-acting anticholinergic agent for COPD in the United States. Studies comparing ipratropium with inhaled β_2-agonists have generally reported similar improvements in pulmonary function, although ipratropium has a slower onset of action and a more prolonged bronchodilator effect. Because of the slower onset of effect (15-20 minutes compared with 5 minutes for albuterol), ipratropium may be less suitable for as-needed use; however, it is often prescribed in that manner. In contrast to albuterol, ipratropium exhibits a dose-response effect with increasing dose rather than increasing frequency. Patients may experience additional symptom improvement with a higher number of inhalations (ie, 6 puffs Q6 hours, maximum 24 puffs/day), whereas no additional improvement is seen with increasing the frequency (ie, more frequent than Q6 hours).[1]

Lack of systemic absorption of ipratropium greatly diminishes anticholinergic adverse effects such as blurred vision, constipation, urinary retention, nausea, and tachycardia associated with the prototype anticholinergic, atropine. The most frequent patient complaints with ipratropium are dry mouth, nausea, and an occasional metallic taste. In rare instances, inhaled anticholinergics may precipitate narrow-angle glaucoma symptoms. Compared to albuterol, ipratropium has a lower incidence of skeletal muscle tremor and tachycardia.

Long-Acting Bronchodilators 8 9 For patients with COPD who experience persistent symptoms, or in whom short-acting therapies do not provide adequate relief, long-acting bronchodilator therapies are recommended (Tables 45-13 and 45-14). Long-acting agents are also recommended as initial therapy for patients at high risk for exacerbation (category C and D). Long-acting inhaled bronchodilator therapy can be administered as an inhaled β_2-agonist (LABA) or an anticholinergic (LAMA). Compared with short-acting agents, long-acting inhaled bronchodilator therapy is more convenient for patients with persistent symptoms and has shown superior outcomes in improving lung function, relieving symptoms, reducing exacerbation frequency, and improving quality of life. For symptom management, both LABAs and LAMAs are equally effective. However, LAMAs appear to be slightly more effective at preventing exacerbations. Treatment selection should consider the individual patient's response, tolerability, adherence, and economic factors.

Long-Acting Inhaled β_2-Agonists Multiple LABAs are currently available in the United States (Table 45-15) and differ primarily by dosing frequency (twice daily vs once daily) and device type (SMI, DPI, nebulizer). One LABA, vilanterol, is currently available in the United States only in combination with an inhaled corticosteroid (fluticasone) or long-acting anticholinergic (umeclidinium). Arformoterol, formoterol, indacaterol, and olodaterol have an onset of action similar to albuterol (less than 5 minutes), whereas salmeterol has a slower onset (15-20 minutes). However, none of these agents are recommended for acute relief of symptoms in COPD. There is no dose titration for any of these agents; the starting dose is the effective and recommended dose for all patients.

Clinical benefits of LABAs compared with short-acting bronchodilators include similar or superior improvements in lung function and symptoms, as well as reduced exacerbation rates and need for hospitalization.[1] The use of the long-acting agents should be considered for patients with frequent and persistent symptoms and those at higher risk for exacerbation (see Tables 45-13 and 45-14). When patients require short-acting β_2-agonists on a scheduled basis, LABAs are more convenient based on dosing frequency but may be more expensive. In contrast to their use in asthma, LABA monotherapy for COPD is not associated with increased mortality and is recommended as part of international guidelines.

Long-acting β_2-agonists are similar with regard to the impact on disease outcomes. Salmeterol and formoterol improve lung function, symptoms, exacerbation frequency, and associated hospitalizations.[1] Indacaterol improves symptoms, health status, and frequency of exacerbations.[1] Olodaterol also decreases symptoms and improves lung function, but evidence for exacerbation outcomes is limited. Effect of olodaterol on exacerbation frequency has not been evaluated when used as monotherapy; however, when used with tiotropium, it moderately reduces exacerbations requiring systemic corticosteroids compared to tiotropium monotherapy alone.[43]

Long-Acting Anticholinergics Several LAMAs are currently available in the United States (Table 45-15) and differ in terms of dosing frequency (twice daily vs once daily) and device type (SMI, DPI, nebulizer). Long-acting anticholinergic agents are more selective than ipratropium at blocking important muscarinic receptors. They dissociate slowly from M_3 receptors, resulting in prolonged bronchodilation with once or twice a day dosing.[44] Aclidinium, glycopyrrolate, and umeclidinium have a faster onset of action (5-15 minutes) compared to tiotropium (80 minutes); however, none of these agents are recommended for acute relief of symptoms. There is no dose titration for any of these agents; the starting dose is the effective and recommended dose for all patients.

Clinical benefits of LAMAs compared with placebo or short-acting bronchodilators include superior improvements in lung function and symptoms, as well as reduced exacerbation rates and hospitalization.[44,45] Available in the United States since 2004, tiotropium is the most extensively studied LAMA with regard to comparative outcomes. In clinical trials, aclidinium and glycopyrrolate have been shown to have similar improvements in lung function and symptoms compared to tiotropium and also reduce the frequency of exacerbations.[46-48] Clinical benefits of umeclidinium have primarily been evaluated as part of combination bronchodilator regimens.

8 9 Long-acting anticholinergics provide similar improvements ins symptoms and health status when compared to long-acting β_2-agonists. Either class is an appropriate choice for patients with persistent symptoms or those needing a step-up from short-acting agents. When evaluating exacerbation outcomes, LAMAs (primarily tiotropium) provide a greater reduction in exacerbation frequency compared to LABAs and should be considered as first-line monotherapy for patients at high risk for exacerbation (Tables 45-13 and 45-14).

Long-acting anticholinergics have been evaluated in clinical trials to determine the potential impact of bronchodilator therapy on the progression of lung function decline. In the landmark clinical trial understanding potential long-term impacts on function with tiotropium (UPLIFT), patients were randomized to therapy with either placebo or inhaled tiotropium, and lung function decline was followed for 4 years.[49] Tiotropium was not shown to have significant effect on lung function decline over time but was effective for reducing symptoms and frequency of exacerbations. Patients in this trial were in more advanced stages of COPD as reflected by the mean postbronchodilator FEV_1 of 1.32 L, corresponding to 48% of predicted FEV_1 or GOLD spirometric stage 3. More recently, tiotropium has again been evaluated for its effect on lung function, but this time in patients in earlier stages of the disease. In the Tie-COPD trial, patients with an FEV_1 > 50% of predicted (GOLD spirometric grade 1 or 2) were randomized to placebo or tiotropium, and lung function decline followed for 2 years.[50] At the end of the trial, patients in the tiotropium group had a higher measured FEV_1 and slower annual decline compared to patients in the placebo group. Application of these results to clinical practice may be difficult given that current goals for inhaled therapy are targeted at patients with symptoms or those at high risk of future exacerbation. Slowing lung function has not yet been a therapeutic target with inhaled therapy. If used in early-stage disease, it would require patients who do not yet have symptoms or experienced an exacerbation to commit to long-term maintenance therapy. Future studies are needed to determine optimal timing and length of bronchodilator therapy.

Previously, retrospective analyses have reported an increased risk of cardiovascular events associated with ipratropium and tiotropium use.[51] However, the UPLIFT study, which was a prospective trial over 4 years, did not report an increased cardiovascular risk associated with tiotropium use.[49] Additionally, a prospective, non-inferiority trial (TIOSPIR) has been published which compared the effects of tiotropium delivered via Handihaler or Respimat devices among 17,000 patients with COPD over a median 2.3-year period.[52] Primary outcomes in this trial were risk of death and risk of first COPD exacerbation. Secondary outcomes included cardiovascular safety. No significant differences were seen in any of the primary or secondary outcomes when comparing tiotropium delivery devices. Further studies are needed to evaluate the cardiovascular safety of ipratropium.

Combination Anticholinergics and β-Agonists (Dual Bronchodilators) Combination regimens of bronchodilators are often used in the treatment of COPD as symptoms worsen over time. Combining bronchodilators with different mechanisms of action allows the lowest possible effective doses to be used and reduces potential adverse effects from individual agents.[1] Short-acting bronchodilators may be combined for patients experiencing persistent symptoms, although step-up to long-acting bronchodilator monotherapy is usually preferred (Tables 45-13 and 45-14).

Current clinical practice guidelines recommend combining long-acting bronchodilators for patients who have persistent symptoms or recurrent exacerbations on bronchodilator monotherapy (Tables 45-13 and 45-14). Combination of long-acting bronchodilators (LAMA/LABA) provides significant improvement in lung function, symptoms, and quality-of-life measures compared with LABA or LAMA monotherapy.[1,53] In addition, dual long-acting bronchodilator therapy has been shown to decrease the frequency of moderate-to-severe exacerbations compared to either LAMA or LABA monotherapy.

Methylxanthines Methylxanthines, including theophylline and aminophylline, may produce bronchodilation through numerous mechanisms, including (a) inhibition of phosphodiesterase, thereby increasing cAMP levels, (b) inhibition of calcium ion influx into smooth muscle, (c) prostaglandin antagonism, (d) stimulation of endogenous catecholamines, (e) adenosine receptor antagonism, and (f) inhibition of release of mediators from mast cells and leukocytes.[1] Chronic theophylline use for patients with COPD may offer improvements in lung function and gas exchange. Subjectively, theophylline has been shown to reduce dyspnea, increase exercise tolerance, and improve respiratory drive in COPD patients.[1]

Methylxanthines have been available for the treatment of COPD for at least five decades and at one time were considered first-line therapy. However, with the availability of LABAs and LAMAs, the role of methylxanthine therapy has become more limited. Because of the risk for drug interactions and significant intrapatient and interpatient variability in dosage requirements, theophylline therapy generally is considered for patients who are intolerant or unable to use an inhaled bronchodilator. Theophylline is considered an alternative to commonly used inhaled therapies for bronchodilation and improving symptoms.[1] However, the evidence does not support the use of theophylline to prevent exacerbations.[54]

Although theophylline is available in a variety of oral dosage forms, sustained-release preparations are most appropriate for the long-term management of COPD. These products have the advantage of improving medication adherence and achieving more consistent serum concentrations over rapid-release theophylline and aminophylline preparations. However, caution must be used in switching from one sustained-release preparation to another because there is considerable variability in their sustained-release characteristics.

Therapy can be initiated at 200 mg twice daily and titrated upward every 3 to 5 days to the target dose. Most patients require daily doses of 400 to 900 mg. Dosage adjustments generally should be made based on serum concentration results. Traditionally, the therapeutic range of theophylline has been 10 to 20 mcg/mL (mg/L; 55-111 μmol/L); however, because of the frequency of dose-related adverse effects and a lack of a clear benefit when used in higher concentrations, a more conservative therapeutic range of 8 to 15 mcg/mL (mg/L; 44-83 μmol/L) is now targeted, especially in the elderly. When concentrations are measured, trough measurements should be obtained.

Once a dose is established, serum concentrations should be monitored once or twice a year unless the patient's disease worsens, medications that interfere with theophylline metabolism are added to therapy, or toxicity is suspected. Adverse effects are dose-related; however, there is an overlap between therapeutic and toxic ranges. Minor adverse effects include dyspepsia, nausea, vomiting, diarrhea, headache, dizziness, and tachycardia. More serious toxicities, which typically do not occur until concentrations exceed 20 mcg/mL (mg/L; 111 μmol/L), include arrhythmias and seizures.

Factors that decrease theophylline clearance and lead to reduced maintenance dose requirements include advanced age, bacterial or viral pneumonia, left or right ventricular failure, liver dysfunction, hypoxemia from acute decompensation, and use of drugs such as cimetidine, macrolides, and fluoroquinolone antibiotics. Factors that may enhance theophylline clearance and result in the need for higher maintenance doses include tobacco and marijuana smoking, hyperthyroidism, and the use of such drugs as phenytoin, phenobarbital, and rifampin.

Theophylline is a challenging medication to dose, monitor, and manage due to the significant intrapatient and interpatient variability in pharmacokinetics and the potential for drug interactions and toxicities. Consequently, inhaled bronchodilator therapy is currently preferred based on superior efficacy and safety, as well as ease of use. Current guidelines recommend theophylline only when inhaled bronchodilators are unavailable or unaffordable.[1]

Corticosteroids Anti-inflammatory mechanisms whereby corticosteroids exert their beneficial effect in COPD include: (a) reduction in capillary permeability to decrease mucus, (b) inhibition of release of proteolytic enzymes from leukocytes, and (c) inhibition of prostaglandins. The benefits of chronic systemic corticosteroid therapy in the chronic management of COPD are not clear, and the risk of toxicity is significant. Long-term adverse effects associated with systemic corticosteroid therapy include osteoporosis, muscular atrophy, thinning of the skin, development of cataracts, and adrenal suppression and insufficiency. Therefore, chronic therapy with oral steroids should be avoided in COPD patients.[1] While a small number of COPD patients are responders to oral steroids, many of these patients may have an asthmatic, or reversible, component to their disease. Asthma-COPD overlap syndrome (ACOS) is now a recognized condition affecting both asthma and COPD patients, and patients exhibiting this syndrome may benefit from therapies traditionally considered for asthma alone.[19] Inhaled corticosteroids may be considered in patients with chronic stable COPD who are at high risk of exacerbation (category C or D) and used short-term as systemic therapy for acute exacerbations (Tables 45-13, 45-14, and 45-22).

10 It has been postulated that inhaled corticosteroid therapy might be beneficial in COPD to slow disease progression. Unfortunately, the results of major clinical trials have failed to demonstrate any clear benefit from chronic treatment with ICS in modifying long-term decline in lung function.[1] ICS have been associated with improvements in clinical endpoints related to exacerbations, including a decrease in exacerbation frequency and time to first exacerbation.[1,55] Clinical benefits of ICS therapy in COPD have been observed with combination therapy, primarily as an addition to LABA monotherapy. Given the lack of supporting evidence and in contrast to evidence in patients with asthma, ICS monotherapy for patients with COPD is not recommended.

Although a dose-response relationship for ICS has not been demonstrated in COPD, initial clinical trials employed moderate-to-high doses for chronic treatment. At these doses, adverse effects must be considered with long-term therapy. Recent trials have reported an increased risk of pneumonia and mycobacterial pulmonary infections in patients with COPD who receive inhaled corticosteroids, and there is increasing recognition for utilizing lower doses of ICS and withdrawing therapy in selected patients.[55-57] Risk factors for developing pneumonia include age >55 years, body mass index (BMI) less than 25 kg/m^2, current smoker, history of exacerbation or pneumonia (last 12 months), or severe airflow limitation.[1] Other adverse effects associated with inhaled corticosteroids include hoarseness, sore throat, oral candidiasis, and skin bruising. Severe adverse effects, such as adrenal suppression, osteoporosis, and cataract formation, have been reported less frequently than with systemic corticosteroids, but clinicians should monitor patients who are receiving high-dose chronic inhaled therapy.

There has been conflicting evidence supporting a dose relationship between ICS use and risk of fractures among patients with COPD. A recent nested, case-control analysis of over 200,000 patients observed an increased risk of fracture with higher daily doses of ICS and long-term use (>4 years).[58] Given this evidence, it appears prudent to treat patients with the lowest effective dose of ICS to minimize the risk of fracture. Clinicians should also recommend adequate intake of calcium and vitamin D and consider periodic bone mineral density testing for patients at risk of osteopenia.

ICS therapy is recommended for initial treatment in patients at high risk of exacerbation and with a blood eosinophil count greater than 300 cells per microliter (category D).[1] For escalation therapy, inhaled corticosteroids may be considered for patients who have recurrent exacerbations despite optimal therapy with inhaled bronchodilators (Table 45-14). Given the risks associated with long-term ICS therapy, clinicians should appropriately identify patients who will receive the best benefit, and patient-specific factors should be considered when making the decision to initiate ICS therapy (Table 45-16). Evaluations of current practice have shown that many patients with COPD may be inappropriately prescribed an ICS (ie, not high risk for exacerbations nor elevated blood eosinophil count), exposing them to unnecessary adverse effects.[59,60]

Given concern for increased pulmonary infections among patients treated with ICS and growing evidence for benefit of dual bronchodilator therapy, clinicians have advocated for withdrawing ICS therapy in selected patients (Table 45-17). Recent trials have reported that ICS can be safely withdrawn from combination ICS/LABA therapy in patients with no initial indication for ICS (ie, FEV_1 > 50% and low risk of exacerbation), without an increase in exacerbation frequency.[60] For patients with more severe disease or at high risk of exacerbation, ICS may also be safely withdrawn from combination ICS/LABA/LAMA therapy in selected situations. These situations may include patients experiencing adverse effects, such as recurrent pneumonia, or those who do not appear to benefit from ICS therapy. For patients with blood eosinophil counts greater than 300 cells/μL (0.3 × 10^9/L), the benefit of continuing ICS therapy may outweigh the risk of adverse effects.

TABLE 45-16 Considerations for Initiating Inhaled Corticosteroid Therapy in COPD

Recommend ICS Initiation	Consider ICS Initiation	Recommend Against ICS Initiation
History of hospitalization(s) for acute exacerbation of COPD despite appropriate long-acting bronchodilator therapy Two or more moderate exacerbations of COPD per year despite appropriate long-acting bronchodilator therapy Blood eosinophils greater than 300 cells/μL (0.3 × 10^9/L) History of or concomitant asthma	One moderate exacerbation of COPD per year despite appropriate long-acting bronchodilator therapy Blood eosinophils between 100 and 300 cells/μL(0.1 × 10^9/L – 0.3 × 10^9/L)	Repeated pneumonia events Blood eosinophils less than 100 cells/μL (0.1 × 10^9/L) History of mycobacterial infection

ICS, inhaled corticosteroid.

TABLE 45-17 Considerations for Withdrawing Inhaled Corticosteroid Therapy in COPD

Recommend ICS Withdrawal	Consider ICS Withdrawal	Recommend Against ICS Withdrawal
Patients initiated on ICS therapy with no clear guideline-based indication Patients experiencing adverse effects with ICS therapy and limited therapeutic benefit Patients experiencing no perceived therapeutic benefit with ICS Blood eosinophils less than 100 cells/μL (0.1 × 10^9/L)	Patients experiencing adverse effects with ICS therapy and some therapeutic benefit Blood eosinophils between 100 and 300 cells/μL (0.1 × 10^9/L – 0.3 × 10^9/L)	Blood eosinophils greater than 300 cells/μL (0.3 × 10^9/L) History of concomitant asthma

ICS, inhaled corticosteroid

Combination Therapy: Dual Therapy (LAMA/LABA or ICS/LABA) For most patients with recurrent exacerbations despite optimal long-acting bronchodilator monotherapy, combination therapy with dual long-acting bronchodilators (LAMA/LABA) is preferred over combination therapy with ICS/LABA (Table 45-14).[1,61] This recommendation is based on results of the FLAME trial which reported superior efficacy with regard to exacerbation prevention with LAMA/LABA (glycopyrrolate/indacaterol) therapy compared to ICS/LABA (fluticasone/salmeterol) and a lower rate of pneumonia (3.2% for LAMA/LABA vs 4.8% for ICS/LABA).[6,62] Subgroup analyses of several trials have indicated that patients with elevated sputum and blood eosinophil counts and those with concomitant asthma have greater therapeutic benefit with ICS therapy compared to other patients.[63] Consequently, guidelines recommend combination therapy with ICS/LABA instead of LAMA/LABA for patients with blood eosinophil ≥300 cells/μL (0.3 × 10^9/L) or ≥100 cells/μL (0.1 × 10^9/L) and ≥ two moderate exacerbations or one exacerbation requiring hospitalization in the last year (high risk).[1]

A more recent study appears to contradict the superiority of LAMA/LABA over ICS/LABA for exacerbation prevention. In the IMPACT trial, which was a three-arm study designed to evaluate the benefit of escalation to triple therapy (LAMA/LABA/ICS) versus dual therapy with ICS/LABA or LAMA/LABA, exacerbation prevention was greater in the ICS/LABA group compared to the LAMA/LABA group.[64] While these results are in contrast to the outcomes of the FLAME trial, 70% of patients enrolled in the IMPACT trial were already receiving ICS prior to randomization and the run-in period after randomization was only 2 weeks. Thus, patients on ICS and randomized to the LAMA/LABA group effectively discontinued ICS therapy without tapering and may account for the higher number of exacerbations seen initially after randomization. Additionally, patients with asthma were not excluded from this study, which may account for the lower exacerbation rate observed in the ICS/LABA group compared to the LAMA/LABA group.

Combination Therapy: Triple Therapy (LAMA/LABA/ICS) For patients with persistent symptoms and recurrent exacerbations on dual inhaled therapy, triple therapy with LAMA/LABA/ICS is recommended as initial escalation therapy for patients with blood eosinophil counts greater than 100 cells/μL (0.1 × 10^9/L) (Table 45-14). Evidence for the benefit of triple therapy has emerged from recent studies evaluating combination therapy within a single device, and there is also limited evidence supporting triple therapy given by multiple devices.[64-67] Compared to dual therapy with either LAMA/LABA or ICS/LABA, triple therapy with LAMA/LABA/ICS provides additional benefit in reducing the frequency of moderate-to-severe exacerbations in patients with COPD. Given the risk of adverse effects with ICS, clinicians may consider bypassing triple inhalation therapy (LAMA/LABA/ICS) for those patients with persistent exacerbations and lower blood eosinophil count (<100 cells/μL [0.1 × 10^9/L]) in favor of oral alternatives such as roflumilast or azithromycin.[1]

Post-hoc analyses from two recent trials have reported a potential association between triple therapy with LAMA/LABA/ICS and reduction in mortality.[68,69] Early information suggests that the addition of ICS may provide a survival benefit when compared to combination therapy with LAMA/LABA alone in some patients. Definitive causation and conclusions cannot yet be determined until more prospective studies are conducted. As has been seen with therapeutic outcomes from ICS treatment in COPD patients, it is likely that any potential survival benefit may vary based on patient-specific factors and considerations.

Phosphodiesterase Inhibitors

Phosphodiesterase 4 (PDE4) is the major phosphodiesterase found in airway smooth muscle cells and inflammatory cells and is responsible for degrading intracellular cAMP. Inhibition of PDE4 results in relaxation of airway smooth muscle cells and diminished inflammatory mediators such as TNF-α and IL-8. Roflumilast, an oral PDE4 inhibitor available in the United States, is recommended for patients with recurrent exacerbations despite treatment with triple inhalation therapy (LAMA/LABA/ICS) (Table 45-14).[1] It may also be considered as escalation therapy for patients with recurrent exacerbations on dual long-acting bronchodilators (LAMA/LABA) who are not candidates for ICS, such as those with low blood eosinophil count (<100 cells/μL [0.1×10^9/L]) or who are at higher risk of adverse effects associated with ICS. Given both theophylline and roflumilast have similar mechanisms of action through inhibition of phosphodiesterases, both should not be used together for the management of COPD.

Roflumilast has bothersome adverse effects that may limit therapy in some patients.[70] Major effects include diarrhea, nausea, decreased appetite, weight loss, headache, and neuropsychiatric effects such as suicidal thoughts, insomnia, anxiety, and new or worsened depression. Most symptoms such as diarrhea, nausea, and headache occur early after initiation and usually resolve over time. The starting dose should be 250 mcg orally for 4 weeks and then increase to a maintenance dose of 500 mcg orally once a day to avoid adverse effects that may lead to early discontinuation of therapy. Weight loss (average of 2 kg) may be of concern in patients with low BMI, and discontinuation may be necessary if significant weight loss is observed. The use of roflumilast is cautioned in patients with a history of depression or suicidality. Both patients and family members should be counseled regarding the potential for mood and behavior changes and to alert healthcare providers if they occur.

Roflumilast is metabolized by CYP3A4 and 1A2, and coadministration with strong inducers of cytochrome P450 is not recommended due to the potential for subtherapeutic plasma concentrations. Although there are no recommended dose adjustments, caution should also be used when administering roflumilast with strong inhibitors of cytochrome P450 due to the potential for adverse effects.

Azithromycin

In certain pulmonary conditions such as cystic fibrosis and bronchiectasis, chronic therapy with macrolide antibiotics, specifically azithromycin, has proven clinical benefit due to their anti-inflammatory and antimicrobial properties. Studies evaluating chronic azithromycin therapy (either 250 mg orally daily or 500 mg orally three times a week for 12 months) in patients with COPD have reported lower rates of exacerbations among treated patients.[71,72] In a subgroup analysis, patients who continued to smoke did not have a reduction in exacerbation frequency with azithromycin. Therapy with azithromycin was associated with a higher rate of colonization with macrolide-resistant bacteria and hearing deficits. In 2012, a retrospective, observational study reported an increase in cardiac events with short courses of azithromycin.[73] The Food and Drug Administration (FDA) has since updated product labeling to include a precaution about QT prolongation.

Given limited evidence supporting the use of long-term treatment with azithromycin, it would be prudent to wait for more safety data before routinely recommending this therapy for more than 12 months in patients with COPD who are at high risk for exacerbations. Current guidelines recommend considering the addition of chronic azithromycin for patients with recurrent exacerbations despite optimal therapy and who are not active smokers (Table 45-14). Clinicians may choose to consider azithromycin for individual patients at high risk for exacerbations but must carefully weigh the risks and benefits of therapy.

α_1-Antitrypsin Replacement Therapy

For patients with inherited AAT deficiency (AATD)–associated emphysema, treatment focuses on the reduction of risk factors such as smoking, symptomatic treatment with bronchodilators, and augmentation therapy with replacement AAT. Based on knowledge about the relationship between serum concentrations of AAT and the risk of developing emphysema, augmentation therapy is intended to maintain serum concentrations above the protective threshold throughout the dosing interval.[1,17] Augmentation therapy consists of weekly infusions of pooled human AAT to maintain AAT plasma levels over 10 μmol/L (0.54 g/L). Much of the data supporting the use of AAT replacement are based on evidence of biochemical efficacy (eg, administering the product and demonstrating protective serum concentrations of AAT).

Clinical evidence for slowing lung function decline or improving outcomes with augmentation therapy is sparse. Stated challenges to performing randomized clinical trials include the large sample size and long duration of follow-up required, and the expense of conducting such a trial. A systematic review of available trials found an association between intravenous augmentation therapy and reduction in disease progression, as measured by computed tomography (CT) density, and decrease in exacerbation frequency.[74] Augmentation therapy with AAT remains the mainstay of treatment for patients with AATD-associated lung disease.

The recommended dosing regimen for replacement AAT is 60 mg/kg administered IV once a week at a rate of 0.08 mL/kg/min, adjusted to patient tolerance. Augmentation therapy can cost over $50,000 annually. In the absence of alternative treatments, it is difficult to assess the cost-effectiveness using conventional criteria. Based on the high cost and limited availability of therapy in some countries, consensus guidelines have suggested that therapy be considered for patients with an FEV_1 35% to 60% predicted. AAT replacement therapy is derived from pooled blood donors. There have been repeated problems with the supply of this product due to production and contamination issues. There are several products available, which should minimize interruption in product supply in the future. Development of recombinant products and AAT replacement via inhalation continues.

Other Pharmacologic Considerations

Several other treatments have been explored over the years. Among these therapies, either there is insufficient evidence to warrant recommending their use, or they have been proven to not be beneficial in the management of COPD. A summary is provided because the clinician likely will encounter patients who are receiving or inquire about these treatments.

Expectorants, Mucolytics, and Antioxidants

Adequate water intake generally is sufficient to maintain hydration and assist in the removal of airway sections. Mucolytics and expectorants such as N-acetylcysteine and guaifenesin have been evaluated as adjunctive therapy for patients with COPD. In one trial, patients with moderate-to-severe COPD were randomized to either placebo or oral N-acetylcysteine 600 mg twice daily for 1 year. Patients were not required to be on ICS prior to randomization. N-acetylcysteine was associated with a significant decrease in exacerbation rate among patients with moderate disease only.[75] Strong evidence of clinical benefit is lacking for the routine use of mucolytics in the treatment of COPD.[76]

In 2011, FDA removed unapproved cough and cold preparations, including several containing guaifenesin, from the market due to safety and efficacy concerns. Several extended-release tablet formulations are currently approved by the FDA. Other approved formulations of guaifenesin contain dextromethorphan or pseudoephedrine and should not be used for COPD maintenance therapy.

Opioids

Systemic (oral and parenteral) opioids, especially morphine, can relieve dyspnea for patients with end-stage COPD. Nebulized therapy is sometimes used in clinical practice, although data about clinical benefit are lacking. Opioids should be used carefully, if at all, to avoid reducing ventilatory drive.

Emerging Therapies

Based on knowledge about the importance of neutrophilic inflammation in COPD and potential therapeutic benefit of inhibition of neutrophil activity, several anti-inflammatory compounds have been explored. Many studies of these strategies have been disappointing or report inconsistent results. Therapy with mepolizumab, an anti-interleukin 5 antibody, and benralizumab, an anti-interleukin 5 receptor-alpha antibody, has been shown to decrease exacerbations among COPD patients and may be associated with a greater effect among patients with elevated blood eosinophils.[1] Other current areas of investigation immunoglobulin E, inhibitors of interleukin 5, interleukin 4, interleukin 13, and tyrosine kinases.[77]

The role of HMG-CoA reductase inhibitors for patients with COPD has garnered interest due to known pleiotropic effects statins and the role of systemic inflammation in COPD. Retrospective and observational trials have reported previous associations with simvastatin therapy and reduction in exacerbation frequency, although this effect was not confirmed in a prospective, randomized trial.[78]

In a meta-analysis of trials, vitamin D supplementation for patients with COPD and low baseline levels of 25-hydroxyvitamin D (less than 25 nmol/L [10 ng/mL]) significantly reduced the rate of moderate and severe exacerbations but was not associated with a reduction in exacerbations in patients with levels of 25-hydroxyvitamin D greater than 25 nmol/L (10 ng/mL).[79] Given the low cost and multiple benefits of vitamin D supplementation, it is recommended to check 25-hydroxyvitamin D concentrations for patients hospitalized with AECOPD and supplement if below 25 nmol/L (10 ng/mL).[1]

Acute Exacerbation of COPD

Pathophysiology

The natural history of COPD is characterized by recurrent acute exacerbations associated with increased symptoms and a decline in overall health status. An exacerbation is defined as a change in the patient's baseline symptoms (dyspnea, cough, or sputum production) beyond day-to-day variability sufficient to warrant a change in management.[1] Exacerbations have a significant impact on the natural course of COPD and occur more frequently in patients with advanced age, significant airflow limitation, and comorbid conditions. Because many patients experience chronic symptoms, diagnosis of an exacerbation is based, in part, on subjective measures and clinical judgment; thus, it can be considered a syndrome. Exacerbations are significant events associated with significant morbidity, including worsening health status, increased risk for acute cardiovascular events, impairment of daily activities, and acceleration of lung function decline. Additionally, exacerbations, especially those requiring hospitalization, are associated with increased mortality risk. Acute exacerbations have a significant impact on the economics of treating COPD, estimated at 35% to 45% of the total costs of the disease in some settings.[2-4]

There is limited data about the pathophysiology of COPD exacerbation due to the chronic nature of the disease and the poor health of patients. Inflammatory mediators, including neutrophils and eosinophils, may be increased in sputum during an exacerbation. Airflow limitation may not change remarkably during an exacerbation compared to chronic baseline limitation.[1] Lung hyperinflation, if present, is worsened during an exacerbation, which contributes to increasing dyspnea and poor gas exchange.

The primary physiologic change is often a worsening of ABG values due to poor gas exchange and increased muscle fatigue. For a patient experiencing a severe exacerbation, profound hypoxemia and hypercapnia can be accompanied by respiratory acidosis and respiratory failure.

Criteria used to define acute exacerbation of COPD (AECOPD) among clinicians vary widely; however, most rely on a change in one or more of the following clinical findings: worsening symptoms of dyspnea, increase in sputum volume, or purulence (Table 45-18). With an exacerbation, patients using rapid-acting bronchodilators may report an increase in the frequency of use and may seek additional medical care. Acute exacerbations can range from mild to severe and are classified based on the level of treatment and intervention required (Table 45-19).

An important complication of a severe exacerbation is acute respiratory failure. In the emergency department or hospital, an ABG usually is obtained to assess the severity of an exacerbation. The diagnosis of acute respiratory failure in COPD is made based on an acute change in the ABGs. Defining acute respiratory failure as a PaO_2 of less than 50 mm Hg (6.7 kPa) or a $PaCO_2$ of greater than 50 mm Hg (6.7 kPa) often may be incorrect and inadequate because these values may not represent a significant change from a patient's baseline values. A more precise definition is an acute drop in PaO_2 of 10 to 15 mm Hg (1.3-2.0 kPa) or any acute increase in $PaCO_2$ that decreases the serum pH to 7.3 or less. Additional acute clinical manifestations of respiratory failure include restlessness, confusion, tachycardia, diaphoresis, cyanosis, hypotension, irregular breathing, miosis, and unconsciousness.

Prognosis

AECOPD are associated with significant morbidity and mortality. While mild exacerbations may be managed at home, mortality rates are higher for patients admitted to the hospital with the highest rates among those admitted to the intensive care unit. COPD

TABLE 45-18 Staging Acute Exacerbations of COPD[a]

Mild (type 1)	One cardinal symptom[a] plus at least one of the following: URTI[b] within 5 days, fever without other explanation, increased wheezing, increased cough, increase in respiratory or heart rate >20% above baseline
Moderate (type 2)	Two cardinal symptoms[a]
Severe (type 3)	Three cardinal symptoms[a]

[a]Cardinal symptoms include worsening of dyspnea, increase in sputum volume, and increase in sputum purulence.

[b]URTI, upper respiratory tract infection.

TABLE 45-19 Classification of Acute Exacerbation of COPD

Severity	Definition
Mild	Treated with short-acting bronchodilators only No treatment with antibiotics or systemic corticosteroids required
Moderate	Treated with short-acting bronchodilators Treatment with antibiotics and/or systemic corticosteroids required
Severe	Treated with short-acting bronchodilators Treatment with antibiotics and/or systemic corticosteroids required Treatment requires hospitalization or a visit to an emergency department May be associated with acute respiratory failure

CLINICAL PRESENTATION COPD Exacerbations

Symptoms

- Increased sputum volume
- Acutely worsening dyspnea
- Chest tightness
- Presence of purulent sputum
- Increased need for bronchodilators
- Malaise, fatigue
- Decreased exercise tolerance

Physical Examination

- Fever
- Wheezing, decreased breath sounds

Diagnostic Tests

- Sputum sample for Gram stain and culture
- Chest radiograph to evaluate for new infiltrates

exacerbations contribute to in-hospital mortality, deaths after discharge, and the decline of lung function. Many patients experiencing an exacerbation do not return to their baseline clinical status for several weeks, significantly affecting their quality of life.

As many as 50% of patients hospitalized for an exacerbation are readmitted within 6 months.[2-4] Risk factors for relapse and potential readmission include FEV_1 less than 50% of predicted, the severity of exacerbation, previous exacerbation frequency, presence of comorbidities, and inadequate antibiotic therapy.[80] As part of the 2010 Affordable Care Act, the Hospital Readmission Reduction Program was established by the Centers for Medicare & Medicaid Services (CMS) that incentivize healthcare organizations to reduce readmission rates for selected conditions, including COPD. The most important predictor for a future exacerbation is past exacerbation history; thus, prevention of AECOPD is a major therapeutic goal for patients with a history of frequent exacerbations (ie, high risk).

TABLE 45-21 Assessment of Patients Hospitalized for Acute Exacerbations of COPD

Assessment	Presentation
No respiratory failure	Respiratory rate 20-30 bpm No use of accessory muscles No changes in mental status Hypoxemia improved with supplemental oxygen No increase in $PaCO_2$
Acute respiratory failure—not life-threatening	Respiratory rate >30 bpm Using accessory muscles No changes in mental status Hypoxemia improved with supplemental oxygen Increase in $PaCO_2$ compared to baseline or 50-60 mm Hg (6.7-8.0 kPa)
Acute respiratory failure—life-threatening	Respiratory rate >30 bpm Using accessory muscles Acute changes in mental status Hypoxemia not improved with supplemental oxygen or need for FIO_2 > 40% (0.40) Increase in $PaCO_2$ compared to baseline or >60 mm Hg (8.0 kPa) or acidosis (pH < 7.25)

bpm, beats per minute.

TREATMENT

Copd Exacerbations

Desired Outcomes (11) The goals of therapy for patients experiencing AECOPD are to minimize the negative consequences of the acute exacerbation (ie, reduce symptoms, prevent hospitalization, shorten hospital stay, prevent acute respiratory failure or death), and prevent future exacerbations.[1] Factors that influence severity, and subsequently the level of care required, include the severity of airflow limitation, presence of comorbidities, and history of previous exacerbations. Table 45-20 includes factors that warrant treatment in the hospital, and Table 45-21 describes the assessment of hospitalized patients for the presence of acute respiratory failure.

Various therapeutic options for exacerbation management are summarized in Table 45-22. Pharmacotherapy consists of intensification of bronchodilator therapy and a short course of systemic corticosteroids. Antimicrobial therapy is indicated in the presence of selected symptoms. Since the frequency and severity of exacerbations are closely related to each patient's overall health status, all patients should receive optimal chronic treatment, including smoking cessation, appropriate pharmacologic therapy, and preventative therapy such as vaccinations.

TABLE 45-20 Factors Favoring Hospitalization for Treatment of COPD Exacerbation

Presence of high-risk comorbidity (eg, pneumonia, arrhythmia, CHF, diabetes, renal or hepatic failure)
Suboptimal response to outpatient management
Marked worsening of dyspnea
Inability to eat or sleep due to symptoms
Worsening hypoxemia or hypercapnia
Mental status changes
Lack of home support for care
Uncertain diagnosis

Nonpharmacologic Therapy Noninvasive positive-pressure ventilation (NPPV) provides ventilatory support with oxygen and pressurized airflow using a face or nasal mask with a tight seal but without endotracheal intubation. There have been numerous trials reporting the benefits of NPPV for patients with acute respiratory failure due to COPD exacerbations. NPPV has been associated with lower mortality, lower intubation rates, and shorter hospital stays for COPD exacerbations. A recent analysis regarding NPPV in patients with respiratory failure, in general, included a subset of patients with COPD and reported that the risk of hospital-based mortality and long-term mortality was reduced by 56%.[81] Benefits seen with NPPV generally can be attributed to a reduction in the complications that often arise with invasive mechanical ventilation. Not all patients with COPD exacerbations are appropriate candidates for NPPV. Patients with altered mental status may not be able to protect their airway and thus may be at increased risk for aspiration. Patients with severe acidosis (pH < 7.25), respiratory arrest, or cardiovascular instability should not be considered for NPPV. Patients who fail a trial of NPPV or those considered poor candidates should be considered for intubation and mechanical ventilation if appropriate based on the patient's goals of care.

Pharmacologic Therapy

Bronchodilators During exacerbations, intensification of bronchodilator regimens is used commonly. Short-acting β_2-agonists are preferred due to their rapid onset of action. The doses and frequency of bronchodilator administration can be increased to provide symptomatic relief. Anticholinergic agents may be added if symptoms persist despite increased doses of β_2-agonists. Combinations of

TABLE 45-22 Therapeutic Options for Acute Exacerbations of COPD

Therapy	Comments
Antibiotics	Recommended if all three of the following cardinal symptoms are present: • Increased dyspnea • Increased sputum production • Increased sputum purulence Recommended if at least two of the following cardinal symptoms are present as long as one of the symptoms is increased sputum purulence: • Increased dyspnea • Increased sputum production • Increased sputum purulence Recommended for patients requiring mechanical ventilation (either noninvasive or invasive) regardless of symptoms present Recommended treatment duration is 5-7 days
Corticosteroids	Oral or IV therapy may be used for a total duration of 5-7 days. If IV is used, it should be changed to oral after improvement in pulmonary status. Longer courses of therapy are associated with increased risk of pneumonia and adverse effects
Bronchodilators	MDIs and DPIs equal in efficacy to nebulization β-Agonists also may increase mucociliary clearance Long-acting β-agonists or long-acting antimuscarinics should not be used for quick relief of symptoms or on an as-needed basis
Controlled oxygen therapy	Titrate oxygen to desired oxygen saturation (>90% [0.90]) Monitor arterial blood gas for the development of hypercapnia
Noninvasive mechanical ventilation	Consider for patients with acute respiratory failure Not appropriate for patients with altered mental status, severe acidosis, respiratory arrest, or cardiovascular instability

these agents are often employed, although data are lacking about their benefit versus using higher doses of a single agent. Bronchodilators may be administered via MDIs or nebulization with equal efficacy.[1] Nebulization may be considered for patients with severe dyspnea who cannot hold their breath after the actuation of an MDI. Evidence supporting the use of theophylline during exacerbations is lacking, and thus theophylline generally should be avoided due to concern for adverse effects.

Corticosteroids Treatment with systemic corticosteroids in AECOPD has been shown to improve oxygenation, recovery time, shorten hospitalization, and reduce the risk of relapse.[4,82] Studies have varied with regards to the severity of exacerbation (ie, moderate or severe), clinical setting (ie, outpatient management or hospitalization), and dosing regimen (ie, dose, route, frequency, and duration). Several trials enrolling hospitalized patients have used high initial doses (often intravenous) before tapering to a lower oral dose to complete the duration of therapy. Adverse effects such as hyperglycemia, insomnia, and hallucinations may occur at higher doses. Depending on the patient's clinical status, treatment may be initiated at a lower dose or tapered more quickly if these effects occur.

The optimal corticosteroid dosing regimen for each presentation of AECOPD is unknown. However, a regimen of prednisone 40 mg orally daily (or equivalent) for 5 days can be effective for most patients. The REDUCE trial evaluated a 5-day course of prednisone 40 mg versus 14 days in a noninferiority study.[83] Shorter treatment duration was noninferior to longer treatment duration for the primary outcome of time to next exacerbation and resulted in less systemic corticosteroid exposure. Longer courses of systemic steroids have been associated with increased risk of pneumonia, hospitalization, and all-cause mortality, and shorter courses (5-7 days) are preferred to avoid adverse effects.[84] Areas of emerging evidence in the treatment of AECOPD include using nebulized corticosteroid (budesonide) rather than systemic administration and correlation of blood eosinophil counts and benefits of therapy.[1]

Antimicrobial Therapy 12 Viral or bacterial infections cause most AECOPD. However, as many as 30% of exacerbations are caused by unknown factors.[1] Data supporting the use of antibiotics for COPD exacerbations are remarkably sparse. To limit unnecessary use, antibiotics should be initiated in any of these clinical situations: (1) patients presenting with three cardinal symptoms of AECOPD, (2) patients presenting with two cardinal symptoms as long as one is increased sputum purulence, and (3) patients requiring mechanical ventilation (noninvasive or invasive) regardless of symptoms (Table 45-22).[1] Utility of sputum Gram stain and culture is questionable, as some patients have chronic bacterial colonization of the bronchial tree between exacerbations.

C-reactive protein (CRP) has been evaluated as a potential biomarker to assist with decisions regarding the use of antimicrobial therapy for COPD exacerbations. An open-label randomized controlled trial evaluated the use of CRP measurement versus no CRP measurement when deciding whether to use antibiotics for AECOPD. The primary outcome was the percentage of antibiotic prescriptions issued within 4 weeks of initial exacerbation. Antibiotic prescriptions were issued less frequently when CRP levels were used to guide decisions compared to usual care. Moreover, patients in the CRP-guided group had improved COPD health status scores. The risk of hospitalization was similar in both groups. These results support the use of CRP measurements to guide antimicrobial decisions for AECOPD, and it supports antimicrobial stewardship efforts.[85]

The emergence of drug-resistant organisms has mandated that antibiotic regimens be chosen judiciously. The selection of empirical antimicrobial therapy should be based on the most likely organism(s) thought to be responsible for the infection based on the patient's presentation and site-specific sensitivities. The most common organisms for acute exacerbation of COPD are *Haemophilus influenzae, Moraxella catarrhalis, Streptococcus pneumoniae,* and *Haemophilus parainfluenzae.* More virulent bacteria may be present for patients with more complicated AECOPD, including drug-resistant pneumococci, β-lactamase–producing *H. influenzae* and *M. catarrhalis*, and enteric gram-negative organisms, including *Pseudomonas aeruginosa.* Table 45-23 summarizes recommended antimicrobial therapy for exacerbations of COPD and the most common organisms based on patient presentation. Therapy with antibiotics generally should be continued for at least 5 to 7 days. If the patient deteriorates or does not improve as anticipated, hospitalization may be necessary, and more aggressive attempts should be made to identify potential pathogens.

Controlled Oxygen Therapy Oxygen therapy should be provided for patients with significant hypoxemia during an exacerbation (eg, oxygen saturation less than 90% [0.90]). Caution must be used, however, because many patients with COPD rely on mild hypoxemia to trigger their drive to breathe. In healthy individuals, drive to breathe is triggered by carbon dioxide accumulation. For patients with COPD who retain carbon dioxide due to disease progression, hypoxemia rather than hypercapnia becomes the main trigger for the respiratory drive. Overly aggressive administration of oxygen to patients with chronic hypercapnia may result in respiratory depression and respiratory failure. Oxygen therapy should be used to achieve a PaO_2 of greater than 60 mm Hg (8.0 kPa) or oxygen saturation of greater than 90% (0.90). An ABG should be obtained after oxygen initiation to monitor carbon dioxide retention resulting from hypoventilation.

Discharge Planning and Follow-up

Patients hospitalized for AECOPD are at high risk for relapse and readmission to the hospital; therefore, appropriate planning should take place prior to discharge to ensure therapy issues, and post-discharge care coordination are clearly addressed. Patients should be initiated or restarted on appropriate maintenance therapy (such as long-acting bronchodilators) before discharge. Patient assessment

TABLE 45-23 Recommended Antimicrobial Therapy in Acute Exacerbations of COPD

Patient Characteristics	Likely Pathogens	Recommended Therapy
Uncomplicated exacerbations <4 exacerbations per year No comorbid illness	*S. pneumoniae* *H. influenzae* *M. catarrhalis* *H. parainfluenzae* Resistance uncommon	Macrolide (azithromycin, clarithromycin) Second- or third-generation cephalosporin Doxycycline Therapies not recommended[a]: TMP/SMX, amoxicillin, first-generation cephalosporins, and erythromycin
Complicated exacerbations Age ≥65 and >4 exacerbations per year Presence of comorbid illness	As above plus drug-resistant pneumococci, β-lactamase–producing *H. influenzae,* and *M. catarrhalis*	Amoxicillin/clavulanate Fluoroquinolone with enhanced pneumococcal activity (levofloxacin, gemifloxacin, and moxifloxacin)
Presence of risk factors for colonization and infection with multidrug-resistant pathogens Need for chronic corticosteroid therapy Recent hospitalization (90 days) Recent antibiotic treatment (90 days) Resident of long-term care facility	Some enteric gram-negatives As above plus *P. aeruginosa*	Fluoroquinolone with enhanced pneumococcal and *P. aeruginosa* activity (levofloxacin) IV therapy if required: β-lactamase–resistant penicillin with antipseudomonal activity third- or fourth-generation cephalosporin with antipseudomonal activity

[a]TMP/SMX should not be used due to increasing pneumococcal resistance; amoxicillin and first-generation cephalosporins are not recommended due to β-lactamase susceptibility; erythromycin is not recommended due to insufficient activity against *H. influenzae.*

and education regarding new or continuing therapy should also occur before discharge and be reinforced during post-discharge follow-up. Some patients may require supplemental oxygen during their exacerbation and for a period of time after discharge. The continued need for long-term oxygen therapy should be assessed as part of post-discharge follow-up (Table 45-24). Other critical elements of discharge planning and follow-up include medication reconciliation, self-management plans, when to seek medical attention, assessment of symptoms and activities of daily living, and status of other comorbid conditions. Early follow-up after discharge (within

TABLE 45-24 Discharge Planning and Post-Discharge Follow-up in Acute Exacerbations of COPD

Timeline	Assessment	Plans
Prior to discharge	Assess maintenance therapy and optimize per therapeutic goals and patient factors Assess inhaler technique Assess technique and adherence before modifying therapy Assess understanding of AECOPD medications (steroids and/or antibiotics) and when to stop taking after discharge Assess the need for vitamin D supplementation to prevent future exacerbations Assess tobacco cessation readiness, if continued smoking Assess immunization status (influenza, pneumococcal) Assess need for oxygen therapy after discharge Assess needed follow-up for comorbid conditions	Ensure patient will be able to obtain and afford prescriptions for therapy Utilize motivational interviewing and teach-back for education and counseling Ensure understanding of medications to continue and/or stop (ie, antibiotics, systemic corticosteroids) Coordinate referral to outpatient tobacco cessation services, if indicated Provide immunizations while hospitalized Coordinate outpatient services for supplemental oxygen, if indicated Ensure follow-up care plans are communicated and appointments scheduled (ie, within 1-4 weeks post-discharge)
1-4 weeks post-discharge	Assess symptoms (ie, mMRC or CAT score) Assess patient ability to cope in their usual environment Assess physical activity and ability to do activities of daily living (ADLs) Assess inhaler technique Assess technique and adherence before modifying therapy Assess tobacco cessation readiness, if continued smoking Assess immunization status (influenza, pneumococcal) Assess continued need for oxygen therapy, if continued after discharge Assess the status of comorbidities	Ensure patient completes mMRC or CAT before or during a visit Coordinate home care services for assistance with ADLs, if indicated Ensure patient will be able to obtain and afford prescriptions for therapy Utilize motivational interviewing and teach-back for education and counseling Ensure understanding of medications Coordinate referral to outpatient tobacco cessation services, if indicated Provide immunizations, if appropriate Coordinate outpatient services for supplemental oxygen, if indicated Ensure follow-up care plans are communicated and appointments scheduled
12-16 weeks post-discharge	Assess symptoms (ie, mMRC or CAT score) Assess patient ability to cope in their usual environment Assess physical activity and ability to do activities of daily living Assess airflow limitation via spirometry Assess inhaler technique Assess technique and adherence before modifying therapy Assess tobacco cessation readiness, if continued smoking Assess immunization status (influenza, pneumococcal) Assess continued need for oxygen therapy, if continued after discharge Assess the status of comorbidities	Ensure patient completes mMRC or CAT before or during a visit Coordinate home care services for assistance with ADLs, if indicated Refer the patient for spirometry testing Ensure patient will be able to obtain and afford prescriptions for therapy Utilize motivational interviewing and teach-back for education and counseling Ensure understanding of medications Coordinate referral to outpatient tobacco cessation services, if indicated Provide immunizations, if appropriate Coordinate outpatient services for supplemental oxygen, if indicated Ensure follow-up care plans are communicated and appointments scheduled

1-4 weeks) is associated with a reduction in readmission due to exacerbations of COPD, and lack of post-discharge follow-up is associated with an increase in 90-mortality.[1]

It is important to assess medication understanding and potential barriers to adherence, inhaler technique, optimal pharmacotherapy, tobacco cessation readiness, and immunization status before discharge. In acute care or ambulatory care settings, clinical pharmacists are often called on to educate patients, recommend appropriate therapy changes, assist patients with formulary and insurance barriers, and complete prior authorization requests. The focus of COPD exacerbation management and prevention has shifted from only clinician-delivered education to patient-clinician collaboration that integrates motivation, engagement, and support to develop self-management interventions and target behaviors.[1,86] Key elements that should be addressed in self-management programs include risk factor management, inhaler technique, management of breathlessness, and a written action plan for acute exacerbations.[1] Incorporating an action plan for AECOPD within a self-management program has been shown to decrease respiratory-related hospital admissions and increase health-related quality of life indicators.[87] Dedicated programs targeting recently discharged patients have shown improvements in health outcomes, such as readmissions, when combined with clinical pharmacy services.[88-90]

PALLIATIVE CARE, END-OF-LIFE CARE, AND HOSPICE

Based on the natural course of COPD, characterized by a progressive decline in lung function and the development of complications, it is important to periodically reconsider the goals of care, end-of-life decisions, and advanced directives.[1] Involvement of palliative care services is recommended once symptoms become significantly limiting or disabling or if repeated hospitalizations occur. An effective strategy to discuss end-of-life care involves the patient's participation in identifying advanced directives and goals of care. Clinicians reassure patients that their symptoms, including pain, will be managed, and their dignity will be preserved. Specific issues that are addressed include the location and provider for terminal care, desire to use or withhold mechanical ventilation, and involvement of other family members in decisions on behalf of the patient.

EVALUATION OF THERAPEUTIC OUTCOMES

To evaluate therapeutic outcomes of COPD, the practitioner must first delineate between chronic stable COPD and acute exacerbations. In chronic stable COPD, pulmonary function tests should be annually assessed as recommended by guidelines and following any treatment additions or discontinuations. The average rate of decline of FEV_1 is a useful objective measure to assess the course of COPD over time. However, patients with similar FEV_1 values may differ in the frequency and severity of symptoms and exacerbation history, thus emphasizing the need for a combined assessment for all patients. The average rate of decline in FEV_1 for healthy, nonsmoking patients attributable to age alone is 25 to 30 mL/year. The rate of decline in smokers is steeper, especially for heavy smokers compared with light smokers. The decline in pulmonary function is a curvilinear path. The more severely diminished the FEV_1 at diagnosis, the steeper the rate of decline. Greater numbers of years of smoking and the number of cigarettes smoked correlate with a steeper decline in pulmonary function.[1]

Objective improvements in PFTs often are minimal—therefore, subjective assessments are important. These include symptom scores and quality-of-life assessments. In addition, exacerbation rates, visits to the emergency department, and hospitalizations should be quantified and evaluated. During AECOPD, the patient's white blood cell count, vital signs, chest x-ray, and changes in dyspnea, sputum volume, and sputum purulence should be assessed at presentation and periodically throughout the treatment of an exacerbation. In severe exacerbations, ABGs and oxygen saturation also should be monitored. As with any drug therapy, adherence, adverse effects, and potential drug interactions should also be evaluated.

To date, there is limited evidence that any available pharmacotherapies for COPD impact disease progression. Removal of the primary causative factor for COPD (eg, cessation of cigarette smoking) does improve survival, as does supplemental oxygen therapy in a subset of patients. The most pertinent clinical outcomes that have emerged from clinical trials over the past decade are symptom improvement and reductions in exacerbation frequency. While it is important to continue to explore strategies to improve survival, consideration should be given to these two relevant and important outcome measures when initiating, continuing, and monitoring therapy.

ABBREVIATIONS

AAT	α_1-antitrypsin
AATD	α_1-antitrypsin deficiency
ABG	arterial blood gas
ACCP	American College of Chest Physicians
ACIP	Advisory Committee on Immunization Practices
ACOS	asthma and COPD overlap syndrome
AECOPD	acute exacerbations of COPD
ATS	American Thoracic Society
BMI	body mass index
cAMP	cyclic adenosine monophosphate
CAT	COPD Assessment Test
CCQ	Clinical COPD Questionnaire
CDC	Centers for Disease Control and Prevention
cGMP	cyclic guanosine monophosphate
COPD	chronic obstructive pulmonary disease
COT	continuous oxygen therapy
COVID-19	coronavirus disease 2019
CRQ	Chronic Respiratory Questionnaire
CT	computed tomography
DPI	dry powder inhaler
ENDS	electronic nicotine delivery systems
ERS	European Respiratory Society
FEV_1	forced expiratory volume in 1 second
FRC	functional residual capacity
FVC	forced vital capacity
GOLD	Global Initiative for Chronic Obstructive Lung Disease
HPA	hypothalamic–pituitary–adrenal
ICS	inhaled corticosteroid
IL	interleukin
LABA	long-acting inhaled β_2-agonist
LTB_4	leukotriene B_4
LVRS	lung volume reduction surgery
MDI	metered-dose inhaler
MMP12	matrix metalloproteinase 12
mMRC	modified Medical Research Council
NETT	National Emphysema Treatment Trial
NHLBI	National Heart, Lung, and Blood Institute
NOT	nocturnal oxygen therapy
NPPV	noninvasive positive-pressure ventilation
$PaCO_2$	pressure exerted by carbon dioxide gas in arterial blood
PaO_2	pressure exerted by oxygen gas in arterial blood
PDE4	phosphodiesterase 4

PDE5	phosphodiesterase type 5
PHS	Public Health Service
PH-COPD	pulmonary hypertension associated with COPD
SARS-CoV-2	severe acute respiratory syndrome coronavirus
SCCOPE	Systemic Corticosteroids in Chronic Obstructive Pulmonary Disease Exacerbations
SGRQ	St. George's Respiratory Questionnaire
Tdap	tetanus toxoid, reduced diphtheria toxoid, and acellular pertussis vaccine
TNF-α	tumor necrosis factor-α
TORCH	Towards a Revolution in COPD Health
UPLIFT	understanding potential long-term impacts on function with tiotropium
VC	vital capacity
WHO	World Health Organization

REFERENCES

1. Global Initiative for Chronic Obstructive Lung Disease. Global Strategy for the Diagnosis, Management, and Prevention of Chronic Obstructive Pulmonary Disease (GOLD). 2021. Available at: http://www.goldcopd.
2. Criner GJ, Bourbeau J, Diekemper RL, et al. Prevention of acute exacerbations of COPD: American College of Chest Physicians and Canadian Thoracic Society Guideline. *Chest.* 2015;147(4):894–942. doi:10.1378/chest.14-1676.
3. Wedzicha JA, Calverley PMA, Albert RK, et al. Prevention of COPD exacerbations: A European Respiratory Society/American Thoracic Society guideline. *Eur Respir J.* 2017;50:1602265. http://www.thoracic.org/statements/copd.php.
4. Papi A, Rabe KF, Rigau D, et al. Management of COPD exacerbations: A European Respiratory Society/American Thoracic Society guideline. *Eur Respir J.* 2017;49:1600791. http://www.thoracic.org/statements/copd.php.
5. Mannino DM. Fifty years of progress in the epidemiology of chronic obstructive pulmonary disease: A review of National Heart, Lung, and Blood Institute-sponsored studies. *Chronic Obstr Pulm Dis.* 2019;6(4):350–358. 10.15326/jcopdf.6.4.2019.0145. PMID: 31647857; PMCID: PMC7006703.
6. U.S. Department of Health and Human Services. COPD National Action Plan. National Heart, Lung, and Blood Institute. Bethesda, MD. Publication NO. 17-HL-8031. Available at: http://copd.nih.gov.
7. Ford ES, Mannino DM, Wheaton AG, Giles WH, Presley-Cantrell LR, Croft JB. Trends in the prevalence of obstructive and restrictive lung function among adults in the United States: Findings from the National Health and Nutrition Examination Survey from 1988-1994 to 2007-2010. *Chest.* 2013;143(5):1395–1406.
8. Creamer MR, Wang TW, Babb S, et al. Tobacco product use and cessation indicators among adults—United States, 2018. *MMWR Morb Mortal Wkly Rep.* 2019;68:1013–1019. doi:http://dx.doi.org/10.15585/mmwr.mm6845a2.
9. Sullivan J, Pravosud V, Mannino DM, Siegel K, Choate R, Sullivan T. National and state estimates of COPD morbidity and mortality—United States, 2014–2015. *Chronic Obstr Pulm Dis.* 2018;5(4):324–333. 10.15326/jcopdf.5.4.2018.0157. PMID: 30723788; PMCID: PMC6361472.
10. Wheaton AG, Liu Y, Croft JB, VanFrank B, et al. Chronic obstructive pulmonary disease and smoking status—United States, 2017. *MMWR.* 2019;68(24):553–538.
11. Ma J, Ward EM, Siegel RL, Jemal A. Temporal trends in mortality in the United States, 1969–2013. *JAMA.* 2015;314:1731–1739.
12. COPD Death Rates in the United States, 1999–2014. National Vital Statistics System. Available at: https://www.cdc.gov/copd. Accessed May 2, 2021.
13. Jenkins CR, Chapman KR, Donohue JF, Roche N, Tsiligianni I, Han MK. Improving the management of COPD in women. *Chest* 2017;151(3):686–696. 10.1016/j.chest.2016.10.031. Epub 2016 Nov 2. PMID: 27816445.
14. Wheaton AG, Cunningham TJ, Ford ES, Croft JB. Employment and activity limitations among adults with chronic obstructive pulmonary disease—United States, 2013. *MMWR.* 2015:64(11):290–295.
15. U.S. Department of Health and Human Services. The Health Consequences of Smoking—50 Years of Progress: A Report of the Surgeon General. Atlanta, GA: U.S. Department of Health and Human Services, Centers for Disease Control and Prevention, National Center for Chronic Disease Prevention and Health Promotion, Office on Smoking and Health, 2014.
16. Rennard SI, Vestbo J. COPD: The dangerous underestimate of 15%. *Lancet.* 2006;367(9518):1216–1219. doi:10.1016/S0140-6736(06)68516-4.
17. Sandhaus RA, Turino G, Brantly ML, et al. The diagnosis and management of alpha-1 antitrypsin deficiency in the adult. *Chronic Obstr Pulm Dis.* 2016;3(3):668–682. 10.15326/jcopdf.3.3.2015.0182. PMID: 28848891; PMCID: PMC5556762.
18. Barnes PJ. Inflammatory mechanisms in patients with chronic obstructive pulmonary disease. *J Allergy Clin Immunol.* 2016;138:16–27.
19. Global Initiative for Asthma. Asthma, COPD and Asthma-COPD Overlap. 2017. Available at: http://www.ginasthma.org.
20. Domej W, Oettl K, Renner W. Oxidative stress and free radicals in COPD—Implications and relevance for treatment. *Int J Chron Obstruct Pulmon Dis.* 2014;9:1207–1224.
21. Sakao S, Voelkel NF, Tatsumi K. The vascular bed in COPD: Pulmonary hypertension and pulmonary vascular alterations. *Eur Respir Rev.* 2014;23:350–355.
22. Patel N, Belcher J, Thorpe G, Forsyth NR, Spiteri MA. Measurement of C-reactive protein, procalcitonin and neutrophil elastase in saliva of COPD patients and healthy controls: Correlation to self-reported well-being parameters. *Respir Res.* 2015;16:62–69.
23. Guirguis-Blake JM, Senger CA, Webber EM, Mularski RA, Whitlock EP. Screening for chronic obstructive pulmonary disease: Evidence report and systematic review for the US Preventive Services Task Force. *JAMA.* 2016;315:1378–1393.
24. Dempsey TM, Scanlon PD. Pulmonary function tests for the generalist: A brief review. *Mayo Clin Proc.* 2018;93:763–771.
25. de Torres JP, Casanova C, Marín JM, et al. Prognostic evaluation of COPD patients: GOLD 2011 versus BODE and the COPD comorbidity index COTE. *Thorax.* 2014;69:799–804.
26. Morales DR, Flynn R, Zhang J, Trucco E, Quint JK, Zutis K. External validation of ADO, DOSE, COTE and CODEX at predicting death in primary care patients with COPD using standard and machine learning approaches. *Respir Med.* 2018;138:150–155.
27. Grimminger J, Ghofrani HA, Weissmann N, Klose H, Grimminger F. COPD-associated pulmonary hypertension: Clinical implications and current methods for treatment. *Expert Rev Respir Med.* 2016;10:755–766.
28. Rezaei SS, Rinner C, Ratajczak P, Grossmann W, Gall W, Wolzt M. Use of beta-blocker is associated with lower mortality in patients with coronary artery disease with or without COPD. *Clin Respir J.* 2018;12(12):2627–2634. 10.1111/crj.12968. Epub 2018 November 4. PMID: 30276967.
29. Vermylen JH, Szmuilowicz E, Kalhan R. Palliative care in COPD: An unmet area for quality improvement. *Int J Chron Obstruct Pulmon Dis.* 2015;10:1543–1551.
30. Anthonisen NR, Connett JE, Kiley JP, et al. Effects of smoking intervention and the use of an inhaled anticholinergic bronchodilator on the rate of decline in FEV1: The Lung Health Study. *JAMA.* 1994;272:1497–1505.
31. Anthonisen NR, Connett JE, Murray RP. Smoking and lung function of Lung Health Study participants after 11 years. *Am J Respir Crit Care Med.* 2002;166:675–679.
32. Anthonisen NR, Skeans MA, Wise RA, et al. The effects of a smoking cessation intervention on 14.5-year mortality: A randomized clinical trial. *Ann Intern Med.* 2005;142:233.
33. Leone FT, Zhang Y, Evers-Casey S, et al. Initiating pharmacologic treatment in tobacco-dependent adults. An official American Thoracic Society Clinical Practice Guideline. *Am J Respir Crit Care Med.* 2020;202(2):e5–e31. 10.1164/rccm.202005-1982ST. PMID: 32663106; PMCID: PMC7365361.
34. Krist AH, Davidson KW, Mangione CM, et al., US Preventive Services Task Force. Interventions for tobacco smoking cessation in adults, including pregnant persons: US Preventive Services Task Force Recommendation Statement. *JAMA.* 2021;325(3):265–279. 10.1001/jama.2020.25019. PMID: 33464343.
35. McCarthy B, Casey D, Devane D, Murphy K, Murphy E, Lacasse Y. Pulmonary rehabilitation for chronic obstructive pulmonary disease. *Cochrane Database Syst Rev.* 2015;2:CD003793.
36. Spruit MA, Singh SJ, Garvey C, et al. An official American Thoracic Society/European Respiratory Society statement: Key concepts and advances in pulmonary rehabilitation. *Am J Respir Crit Care Med.* 2013;188(8):e13–e64.
37. van Beers M, Rutten-van Mölken MPMH, van de Bool C, et al. Clinical outcome and cost-effectiveness of a 1-year nutritional intervention

programme in COPD patients with low muscle mass: The randomized controlled NUTRAIN trial. *Clin Nutr.* 2020;39(2):405–413. 10.1016/j.clnu.2019.03.001. Epub 2019 March 18. PMID: 30954363.
38. Centers for Disease Control and Prevention (CDC). Adult Immunization Schedule by Vaccine and Age Group. Available at: https://www.cdc.gov/vaccines/schedules/hcp/imz/adult.html. Accessed May 9, 2021.
39. Bekkat-Berkani R, Wilkinson T, Buchy P, et al. Seasonal influenza vaccination in patients with COPD: A systematic literature review. *BMC Pulmonary Medicine.* 2017;17(1):79.
40. Centers for Disease Control and Prevention Mortality and Morbidity Weekly Report. Use of Tetanus Toxoid, Reduced Diptheria Toxoid, and Acellular Pertussis Vaccines: Updated Recommendations of the Advisotry Committee on Immunization Practices – United States, 2019. Available at: https://www.cdc.gov/mmwr/volumes/69/wr/mm690a5.html. Accessed May 9, 2021.
41. Chrystyn H, van der Palen J, Sharma R, et al. Device errors in asthma and COPD: Systematic literature review and meta-analysis. *NPJ Primary Care Respiratory Medicine.* 2017;27:1–10.
42. Bosnic-Anticevich S, Chrystyn H, Costello R, et al. The use of multiple respiratory inhalers requiring different inhalation techniques has an adverse effect on COPD outcomes. *Int J Chron Obstruct Pulmon Dis.* 2016;12:59–71.
43. Calverley PMA, Anzueto AR, Carter K, et al. Tiotropium and olodaterol in the prevention of chronic obstructive pulmonary disease exacerbations (DYNAGITO): A double-blind, randomised, parallel-group, active-controlled trial. *Lancet Respir Med.* 2018;6:337–344. doi:10.1001/jama.2018.14432.
44. Melani AS. Long-acting muscarinic antagonists. *Expert Rev Clin Pharmacol.* 2015;8(4):479–501. doi:10.1001/jama.2018.14432.
45. Cheyne L, Irvin-Sellers MJ, White J. Tiotropium versus ipratropium bromide for chronic obstructive pulmonary disease. *Cochrane Database Syst Rev.* 2015;9:CD009552.
46. Wedzicha JA, Agusti A, Donaldson G, Chuecos F, Lamarca R, Garcia Gil E. Effect of aclidinium bromide on exacerbations in patients with moderate-to-severe COPD: A pooled analysis of five phase III, randomized, placebo-controlled studies. *COPD: J Chron Obstruct Pulmon Dis.* 2016;13:669–676.
47. Tashkin DP, Gross NJ. Inhaled glycopyrrolate for the treatment of chronic obstructive pulmonary disease. *Int J Chron Obstruct Pulmon Dis.* 2018;13:1873–1888.
48. Chen W, Huang C, Sheu C, et al. Long-acting beta2-agonists versus long-acting muscarinic antagonists in patients with stable COPD: A systematic review and meta-analysis of randomized controlled trials. *Respirology.* 2017;22:1313–1319.
49. Tashkin DP, Celli B, Senn S, et al. A 4-year trial of tiotropium in chronic obstructive pulmonary disease (UPLIFT). *N Engl J Med.* 2008;359:1543–1554.
50. Zhou Y, Zhong N, Li X, et al. Tiotropium in early-stage chronic obstructive pulmonary disease. *N Eng J Med.* 2017;377:923–935.
51. Celli B, Decramer M, Leimer I, Vogel U, Kesten S, Tashkin DP. Cardiovascular safety of tiotropium in patients with COPD. *Chest.* 2010;137:2–30.
52. Wise RA, Anzueto A, Cotton D, et al.; TIOSPIR Investigators. Tiotripium Respimat inhaler and the risk of death in COPD. *N Engl J Med.* 2013;369(16):1491–1501.
53. Oba Y, Sarva ST, Dias S. Efficacy and safety of long-acting β-agonist/long-acting muscarinic antagonist combinations in COPD: A network meta-analysis. *Thorax.* 2016;71:15.
54. Devereux G, Cotton S, Fielding S, et al. Effect of theophylline as adjunct to inhaled corticosteroids on exacerbations in patients with COPD: A randomized clinical trial. *JAMA.* 2018;320(15):1548–1559. 10.1001/jama.2018.14432.
55. Tashkin DP, Strange C. Inhaled corticosteroids for chronic obstructive pulmonary disease: What is their role in therapy? *Int J Chron Obstruct Pulmon Dis.* 2018;13:2587–2601. doi:10.2147/COPD.S172240. PMID: 30214177; PMCID: PMC6118265.
56. Izquierdo JL, Cosio BG. The dose of inhaled corticosteroids in patients with COPD: When less is better. *Int J Chron Obstruct Pulmon Dis.* 2018;13:3539–3547. doi:10.2147/COPD.S175047. PMID: 30498343; PMCID: PMC6207269.
57. Castellana G, Castellana M, Castellana C, et al. Inhaled corticosteroids and risk of tuberculosis in patients with obstructive lung diseases: A systematic review and meta-analysis of non-randomized studies. *Int J Chron Obstruct Pulmon Dis.* 2019;14:2219–2227. 10.2147/COPD.S209273. PMID: 31576118; PMCID: PMC6769028.
58. Gonzalez AV, Coulombe J, Ernst P, Suissa S. Long-term use of inhaled corticosteroids in COPD and the risk of fracture. *Chest.* 2018;153:321–328.
59. Chalmers JD, Tebboth A, Galyle A, et al. Determinants of initial inhaled corticosteroid use in patients with GOLD A/B COPD: A retrospective study of UK general practice. *NPJ Prim Care Respir Med.* 2017;27(1):43.
60. Avdeev S, Aisanov Z, Arkhipov V, et al. Withdrawal of inhaled corticosteroids in COPD patients: Rationale and algorithms. *Int J Chron Obstruct Pulmon Dis.* 2019;14:1267–1280. 10.2147/COPD.S207775. PMID: 31354256; PMCID: PMC6572750.
61. Beeh KM, Burgel P, Franssen FME, et al. How do dual long-acting bronchodilators prevent exacerbations of chronic obstructive pulmonary disease? *Am J Respir Crit Care Med.* 2017;196:139–149.
62. Wedzicha JA, Banerji D, Chapman KR, et al. Indacaterol-glycopyrronium versus salmeterol-fluticasone for COPD (FLAME). *N Eng J Med.* 2016;374:2222–2234.
63. Cheng SL. Blood eosinophils and inhaled corticosteroids in patients with COPD: Systematic review and meta-analysis. *Int J Chron Obstruct Pulmon Dis.* 2018;13:2775–2784. doi:10.2147/COPD.S175017. PMID: 30233168; PMCID: PMC6132232.
64. Lipson DA, Barnhart F, Brealey N, et al. Once-daily single-inhaler triple versus dual therapy in patients with COPD (IMPACT). *N Eng J Med.* 2018;378:1671–1680.
65. Papi A, Vestbo J, Fabbri L, et al. Extrafine inhaled triple therapy versus dual bronchodilator therapy in chronic obstructive pulmonary disease (TRIBUTE): A double-blind, parallel group, randomised controlled trial. *Lancet.* 2018;391:1076–1084.
66. Vestbo J, Papi A, Corradi M, et al. Single inhaler extrafine triple therapy versus long-acting muscarinic antagonist therapy for chronic obstructive pulmonary disease (TRINITY): A double-blind, parallel group, randomised controlled trial. *Lancet.* 2017;389:1919–1929.
67. Siler TM, Kerwin E, Sousa AR, Donald A, Ali R, Church A. Efficacy and safety of umeclidinium added to fluticasone furoate/vilanterol in chronic obstructive pulmonary disease: Results of two randomized studies. *Respir Med.* 2015;109(9):1155–1163.
68. Vestbo J, Fabbri L, Papi A, et al. Inhaled corticosteroid containing combinations and mortality in COPD. *Eur Respir J.* 2018;52(6):1801230. 10.1183/13993003.01230-2018. PMID: 30209195.
69. Lipson DA, Crim C, Criner GJ, et al. Reduction in all-cause mortality with fluticasone furoate/umeclidinium/vilanterol in patients with chronic obstructive pulmonary disease. *Am J Respir Crit Care Med.* 2020;201(12):1508–1516. 10.1164/rccm.201911-2207OC. PMID: 32162970; PMCID: PMC7301738.
70. Wedzicha JA, Calverley PM, Rabe KF. Roflumilast: A review of its use in the treatment of COPD. *Int J Chron Obstruct Pulmon Dis.* 2016;11:81–90.
71. Albert RK, Connett J, Bailey WD, et al. Azithromycin for prevention of exacerbation in COPD. *N Engl J Med.* 2011;365:689–698.
72. Uzun S, Djamin RS, Kluytmans JA, et al. Azithromycin maintenance treatment in patients with frequent exacerbations of chronic obstructive pulmonary disease (COLUMBUS): A randomised, double-blind, placebo-controlled trial. *Lancet Respir Med.* 2014;2(5):361–368. 10.1016/S2213-2600(14)70019-0. Epub 2014 April 15. PMID: 24746000.
73. Ray WA, Murray KT, Hall K, et al. Azithromycin and the risk of cardiovascular death. *N Engl J Med.* 2012;366:1881–1890.
74. Edgar RG, Patel M, Bayliss S, Crossley D, Sapey E, Turner AM. Treatment of lung disease in alpha-1 antitrypsin deficiency: A systematic review. *Int J Chron Obstruct Pulmon Dis.* 2017;12:1295–1308. doi:10.2147/COPD.S130440. PMID: 28496314; PMCID: PMC5422329.
75. Zheng JP, Wen FQ, Bai CX, et al.; PANTHEON study group. Twice daily N-acetylcysteine 600 mg for exacerbations of chronic obstructive pulmonary disease (PANTHEON): A randomised, double-blind placebo-controlled trial. *Lancet Respir Med.* 2014;2(3):187–194.
76. Poole P, Sathananthan K, Fortescue R. Mucolytic agents versus placebo for chronic bronchitis or chronic obstructive pulmonary disease. *Cochrane Database Syst Rev.* 2019;5(5):CD001287. doi:10.1002/14651858.CD001287.pub6. PMID: 31107966; PMCID: PMC6527426.
77. Wechsler ME. Current and emerging biologic therapies for asthma and COPD. *Respir Care.* 2018;63(6):699–707. 10.4187/respcare.06322. PMID: 29794205.
78. Criner GJ, Connett JE, Voelker H. Simvastatin in moderate-to-severe COPD. *N Eng J Med.* 2014;371:970.
79. Jolliffe DA, Greenberg L, Hooper RL, et al. Vitamin D to prevent exacerbations of COPD: Systematic review and meta-analysis of individual participant data from randomised controlled trials. *Thorax.* 2019;74(4):337–345. 10.1136/thoraxjnl-2018-212092. Epub 2019 January 10. PMID: 30630893.
80. Mantero M, Rogliani P, DiPasquale M, et al. Acute exacerbations of COPD: Risk factors for failure and relapse. *Int J COPD.* 2017;12:2687–2693.
81. Cabrini L, Landoni G, Oriani A, et al. Noninvasive ventilation and survival in acute care settings: A comprehensive systematic review

and meta-analysis of randomized controlled trials. *Crit Care Med.* 2014;43(4):880–888.

82. Hernandez JM, Edmonds M. Do systemic corticosteroids improve outcomes in chronic obstructive pulmonary disease exacerbations? *Ann Emerg Med.* 2016;67(2):258–259. doi:10.1016/j.annemergmed.2015.07.009.
83. Leuppi JD, Schuetz P, Bingisser R, et al. Short-term vs conventional glucocorticoid therapy in acute exacerbations of chronic obstructive pulmonary disease: The REDUCE clinical trial. *JAMA.* 2013;309(21):2223–2231.
84. Sivapalan P, Ingebrigtsen TS, Rasmussen DB, et al. COPD exacerbations: The impact of long versus short courses of oral corticosteroids on mortality and pneumonia: Nationwide data on 67 000 patients with COPD followed for 12 months. *BMJ Open Respir Res.* 2019;6(1):e000407. 10.1136/bmjresp-2019-000407. PMID: 31179005; PMCID: PMC6530506.
85. Butler CC, Gillespie D, White P, et al. C-reactive protein testing to guide antibiotic prescribing for COPD exacerbations. *N Engl J Med.* 2019;381(2):111–120. doi:10.1056/NEJMoa1803185.
86. Effing TW, Vercoulen JH, Bourbeau J, et al. Definition of a COPD self-management intervention: International Expert Group consensus. *Eur Respir J.* 2016;48(1):46–54. 10.1183/13993003.00025-2016. Epub 2016 April 13. PMID: 27076595.
87. Lenferink A, Brusse-Keizer M, van der Valk PD, et al. Self-management interventions including action plans for exacerbations versus usual care in patients with chronic obstructive pulmonary disease. *Cochrane Database Syst Rev.* 2017;8(8):CD011682. 10.1002/14651858.CD011682.pub2. PMID: 28777450; PMCID: PMC6483374.
88. Fathima M, Bawa Z, Mitchell B, Foster J, Armour C, Saini B. COPD management in community pharmacy results in improved inhaler use, immunization rate, COPD action plan ownership, COPD knowledge, and reductions in exacerbation rates. *Int J Chron Obstruct Pulmon Dis.* 2021;16:519–533. 10.2147/COPD.S288792. PMID: 33688177; PMCID: PMC7936701.
89. Cavanaugh JJ, Lindsey KN, Shilliday BB, Ratner SP. Pharmacist-coordinated multidisciplinary hospital follow-up visits improve patient outcomes. *J Manag Care Spec Pharm.* 2015;21:256–260.
90. Sanchez GM, Douglass MA, Mancuso MA. Revisiting project re-engineered discharge (RED): The impact of a pharmacist telephone intervention on hospital readmission rates. *Pharmacotherapy.* 2015;35:805–812.

Pulmonary Arterial Hypertension

46

Rebecca L. Attridge, Rebecca Moote, and Deborah J. Levine

KEY CONCEPTS

1. Pulmonary arterial hypertension (PAH) is defined as a mean pulmonary artery pressure (mPAP) ≥20 mm Hg at rest with a pulmonary capillary wedge pressure (PCWP) or left ventricular end-diastolic pressure ≤15 mm Hg and a pulmonary vascular resistance (PVR) >3 Wood units (24 MPa·s/m^3) measured by right heart catheterization.
2. Patients with PAH most commonly present with exertional dyspnea, fatigue, weakness, and exercise intolerance. As the disease progresses, symptoms of right heart dysfunction and failure, such as dyspnea at rest, lower extremity edema, chest pain, and syncope, may be present.
3. The definitive diagnosis of PAH is done with a right heart catheterization. The right heart catheterization provides important prognostic information and can be used to assess pulmonary vasoreactivity prior to initiating therapy.
4. Treatment goals are to achieve low-risk status; alleviate symptoms; improve quality of life, functional class, and exercise capacity; slow disease progression; and improve survival.
5. Nonpharmacologic therapy, including counseling on pregnancy avoidance, structured pulmonary or cardiac rehabilitation, immunizations, and low-sodium diets, should be provided to all patients with PAH.
6. Conventional therapy options for PAH include oral anticoagulants, diuretics, oxygen, and digoxin.
7. Prostacyclin analogs such as epoprostenol, treprostinil, and iloprost induce potent vasodilation of pulmonary vascular beds. These therapies can be administered through different routes, including oral, inhaled, subcutaneous, and intravenous. Intravenous therapies are typically reserved for high-risk patients and are used in combination with endothelin receptor antagonists, phosphodiesterase-5 inhibitors, and riociguat. Only epoprostenol has demonstrated improved survival.
8. Oral combination therapy is recommended initially for patients with PAH at low-to-intermediate risk for mortality at 1 year. Options include endothelin-receptor antagonists, phosphodiesterase-5 inhibitors, riociguat, and selexipag. These agents improve exercise capacity, functional class, and hemodynamics in PAH.
9. Calcium channel blockers (CCBs) are only considered in a small number of patients who have a positive response to acute vasoreactivity testing. A small number of patients have a long-term response to CCBs.

BEYOND THE BOOK

The mechanism of action of medications used in pulmonary arterial hypertension (PAH) is directly tied to the pathophysiology of the disease. Create a concept map of the site of action of the major medication classes utilized in PAH—prostacyclin analogs, endothelin-receptor antagonists (ERAs), phosphodiesterase-5 inhibitors, and guanylate cyclase stimulators. This activity is intended to prepare you to understand the role of the medications in the treatment of PAH as well as to increase critical thinking skills related to evaluating side effects and monitoring parameters of these medications.

INTRODUCTION

1 Pulmonary arterial hypertension (PAH) is a group of conditions relating to elevated blood pressure measured within the pulmonary arteries. Pulmonary hypertension (PH) is not a specific diagnosis; rather it is a complex group of disorders relating to the pulmonary circulation. PH is classified into five groups according to the World Health Organization (WHO); see Table 46-1.[1] PAH, or Group 1 PH, is a progressive disease characterized by an elevation in pulmonary arterial pressure and pulmonary vascular resistance. PAH may be defined as a mean pulmonary artery pressure (mPAP) ≥20 mm Hg at rest, with a pulmonary capillary wedge pressure (PCWP) or left ventricular end-diastolic pressure ≤15 mm Hg and a pulmonary vascular resistance (PVR) >3 Wood units (24 MPa·s/m^3) measured by cardiac catheterization.[1-3]

PAH may occur in the setting of underlying medical conditions or as an idiopathic disease (idiopathic PAH [IPAH]). Historically, medical treatment of PAH has been limited due to lack of effective, targeted therapy. Without medical therapy, IPAH portends a poor prognosis (median survival 2.8 years) after diagnosis.[4] Prior to the availability of disease-specific therapy for IPAH, survival rates at 1, 3, and 5 years were 68%, 48%, and 34%, respectively.[5] Since the approval of epoprostenol in 1995, a number of new therapeutic options have been developed. A recent study shows survival rates at 1 and 3 years were 85% and 68%, respectively, in patients with PAH, and 91% and 74%, respectively, in patients with IPAH.[6] Overall 5-year survival rates in that registry were 65% in previously diagnosed patients versus 61% in newly diagnosed patients with PAH.[7]

EPIDEMIOLOGY

The prevalence of PAH is 15 to 26 patients per million individuals.[8] One registry study found that the most common cause of PAH was

TABLE 46-1 World Health Organization Classification of Pulmonary Hypertension

Group 1—Pulmonary Arterial Hypertension (PAH)

- Idiopathic (IPAH)
- Heritable
  - BMPR-2
  - Other mutations: ALK-1, ENG, SMAD9, CAV1, KCNK3
- Medications and toxin-induced PAH
- PAH associated with
  - Connective tissue diseases
  - HIV infection
  - Portal hypertension
  - Congenital heart diseases
  - Schistosomiasis
- PAH long-term responders to calcium channel blockers
- PAH with overt features of venous/capillaries (PVOD/PCH) involvement
- Persistent pulmonary hypertension (PH) of the newborn

Group 2—PH due to Left Heart Disease

- PH due to heart failure with preserved ejection fraction or heart failure with reduced ejection fraction
- Valvular disease
- Congenital/acquired cardiovascular conditions leading to post-capillary PH

Group 3—PH due to Lung Diseases and/or Hypoxia

- Obstructive pulmonary disease
- Restrictive lung disease
- Other lung diseases with a mixed restrictive and obstructive pattern
- Hypoxia without lung disease
- Developmental lung disorders

Group 4—PH due to pulmonary artery obstructions

- Chronic thromboembolic pulmonary hypertension (CTEPH)
- Other pulmonary artery obstructions
  - Sarcoma or angiosarcoma
  - Other intravascular tumors
  - Arteritis without connective tissue disease
  - Congenital pulmonary arteries stenosis
  - Parasites (hydatidosis)

Group 5—Pulmonary Hypertension with Unclear and/or Multifactorial Mechanisms

- Hematological disorders: chronic hemolytic anemia, myeloproliferative disorders
- Systemic disorders: sarcoidosis, pulmonary Langerhans cell histiocytosis, Gaucher disease, glycogen storage disease, neurofibromatosis
- Others: fibrosing mediastinitis, chronic renal failure (with/without dialysis)
- Complex congenital heart disease

ALK-1, activin receptor-like kinase type-1; BMPR-2, bone morphogenetic protein receptor 2; CAV1, caveolin-1; ENG, endoglin; EIF2AK4, eukaryotic translation initiation factor 2 alpha kinase 4; HIV, human immunodeficiency virus; PVOD, pulmonary veno-occlusive disease; PCH, pulmonary capillary hemangiomatosis.

Data from Reference 1.

IPAH (approximately 40%), followed by PAH associated with connective tissue diseases (15.3%), congenital heart disease (11.3%), portal hypertension (10.4%), and familial PAH (FPAH) (3.9%).[9] The US-based REVEAL (Registry to Evaluate Early and Long-Term Pulmonary Arterial Hypertension Disease Management) registry found that 46% of PAH was idiopathic, 25% was associated with connective tissue diseases, and 10% was associated with congenital heart diseases.[10] The incidence of IPAH is 2.0 to 7.6 per 1 million in North America and Europe, with a marked female predominance (male-to-female ratio, 1:1.7), and mean age at the time of recognition is approximately 37 years, although there is considerable variation.[11]

The diagnosis of PAH is growing due to increased awareness and knowledge of the disease state, leading to earlier and improved evaluation and identification. Based on recent registry data, PAH is now being diagnosed more commonly in older patients, with a mean age at diagnosis ranging from 50 to 65 years.[11]

ETIOLOGY

PAH most often originates with a predisposing state and one or more inciting factors that could be genetic or environmental exposures.[12] Once a permissive environment exists, multiple mechanisms can be activated leading to vascular constriction, cellular proliferation, and a prothrombotic state resulting in PAH and its sequelae.[13] PAH can be associated with numerous conditions as well as being an idiopathic condition (IPAH). Although uncommon in the United States, the most common form of PAH worldwide is schistosomiasis followed by congenital heart disease and pulmonary hypertension of early childhood.[2] Rheumatologic diseases such as scleroderma, systemic lupus erythematosus, rheumatoid arthritis, and myositis are also associated with the development of PAH. Patients with scleroderma who develop PAH, between 7% and 12% of patients, have markedly worse outcomes in comparison to other PAH subgroups. Patients with human immunodeficiency virus (HIV) infection can develop PAH with a prevalence of 0.5%. In patients with liver disease, portal hypertension may cause concurrent pulmonary hypertension in 2% to 6% of patients.[2] Multiple medications and toxins have been associated with PAH but those that definitively precipitate PAH include anorexigens such as aminorex, fenfluramine, benfluorex, and dexfenfluramine.[1,3,11] Other precipitants include toxic rapeseed oil and selective serotonin reuptake inhibitors (SSRIs), specifically in newborns of pregnant patients exposed to SSRIs after 20 weeks of gestation.[2,3] Other medications considered to be likely or possible causative agents for PAH include amphetamines, L-tryptophan, cocaine, interferon α and β, leflunomide, and certain chemotherapeutic agents (dasatanib, mitomycin C, carmustine, etoposide, cyclophosphamide, bleomycin).[1-3] Heritable PAH (HPAH) includes both IPAH with germline mutations and familial cases without an identified mutation. Germline mutations seen in PAH include bone morphogenetic protein receptor 2 (BMPR-2) and activin receptor-like kinase 1 (ALK-1). About 75% of patients with HPAH have BMPR-2 mutations.[14] Genetic testing for these mutations may be offered, and professional genetic counseling should be provided at expert centers.[2,14]

PATHOPHYSIOLOGY

PAH is characterized by progressive vasoconstriction of the small pulmonary arteries that eventually leads to right ventricular hypertrophy and failure. The right ventricle is thin-walled and accustomed to the much lower pressures of the pulmonary system and, therefore, does not have the reserve that the left ventricle does.[15] Regardless of etiology, all subgroups of PAH are based on similar clinical and pathologic physiology. The pathobiology of PAH involves several key biologic events, including endothelial cell dysfunction, thrombotic lesions, platelet activation, the gain of constricting factors, loss of relaxing factors, intimal proliferation, medial hypertrophy, fibrosis, and inflammation—all combining to produce progressive and deleterious vascular remodeling (Fig. 46-1).[16,17] Multiple genetic mutations are known to contribute to the pathophysiology of PAH, including BMPR-2, ALK-1, Caveolin-1, KCNK3, nitric oxide synthase (ec-NOS), and 5-hydroxytryptamine (serotonin [5-HT]) transporter (5-HTT).[2,16,18]

Molecular, cellular, and genetic mechanisms are mediated by a variety of biologically active compounds, including prostacyclin (PGI_2), endothelin-1 (ET-1), nitric oxide (NO), and 5-HT. PGI_2 is a vasodilatory and antiproliferative substance that is produced by the endothelial cells. The synthesis of PGI_2 and its circulating levels is reduced in PAH. Furthermore, thromboxane, a vasoconstrictor, is increased in PAH. ET-1 is produced in the endothelium and possesses potent vasoconstrictor and mitogenic effects. ET-1 levels are increased in PAH, and clearance is reduced. ET-1 acts via the endothelin receptors (ET_A and ET_B) to promote vascular smooth muscle proliferation and vasoconstriction.[17,19] Plasma levels of ET-1 are correlated with the severity of PAH and prognosis.[20] NO is produced in the endothelium via NO synthase, leading to vasodilation. NO also leads to the opening of potassium channels in the cell membrane,

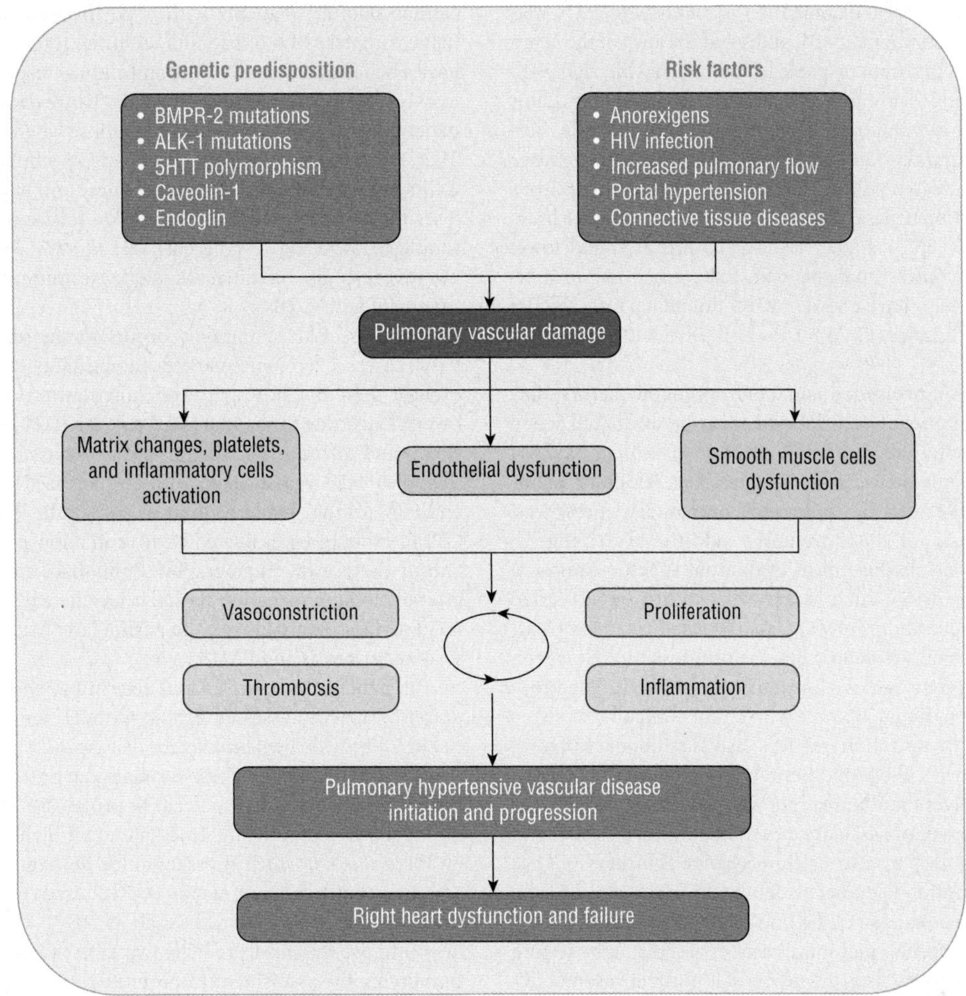

FIGURE 46-1 Pathophysiology of pulmonary arterial hypertension. Pulmonary arterial hypertension; potential pathogenetic and pathobiologic mechanisms. (5-HTT, serotonin transporter gene; ALK-1, activin receptor-like kinase 1 gene; BMPR-2, bone morphogenetic receptor 2 gene; HIV, human immunodeficiency virus.) *(Reproduced from Galiè N, Torbicki A, Barst R, et al. Guidelines on diagnosis and treatment of pulmonary arterial hypertension. The Task Force on Diagnosis and Treatment of Pulmonary Arterial Hypertension of the European Society of Cardiology. Eur Heart J. 2004;25(24):2243–2278.)*

allowing potassium efflux, membrane depolarization, and calcium channel inhibition. In PAH, there is evidence of decreased NO synthase expression, leading to vasoconstriction and cell proliferation.[21] Elevated 5-HT has been observed and vasoconstriction mediated via the increased expression of the 5-HT_{1B} receptor is seen in PAH.[2]

Autoantibodies, proinflammatory cytokines, and inflammatory infiltrates may also participate in the pathogenesis of PAH. Coagulation is disordered in PAH as evidenced by increased levels of von Willebrand factor, plasma fibrinopeptide A, plasminogen activator inhibitor-1, 5-HT, and thromboxane. Furthermore, tissue plasminogen activator, thrombomodulin, NO, and PGI_2 are decreased, leading to an imbalance favoring thrombosis. Endothelial dysfunction is the common denominator of mechanisms for PAH, and a variety of injuries, such as shear stress, inflammation, toxins, and hypoxia, are thought to be involved.[2,16]

CLINICAL PRESENTATION

2 The signs and symptoms of PAH are highly variable depending on the stage of the disease and comorbidities. The impact of these signs and symptoms on functional capacity can be generally described using the WHO functional classification (Table 46-2). Symptoms are often related to right ventricular dysfunction and may include exertional dyspnea, fatigue, and weakness.[3] As the disease progresses, patients may experience dyspnea at rest, chest pain, presyncope, syncope, lower extremity edema, and abdominal bloating

TABLE 46-2 World Health Organization Functional Classification of Pulmonary Arterial Hypertension

Class	Description
I	Patients with PAH in whom there is no limitation of usual physical activity; ordinary physical activity does not cause increased dyspnea, fatigue, chest pain, or presyncope
II	Patients with PAH who have mild limitation of physical activity. There is no discomfort at rest, but normal physical activity causes increased dyspnea, fatigue, chest pain, or presyncope
III	Patients with PAH who have marked limitation of physical activity. There is no discomfort at rest, but less than normal physical activity causes increased dyspnea, fatigue, chest pain, or presyncope
IV	Patients with PAH who are unable to perform any physical activity at rest and who may have signs of right ventricular failure. Dyspnea and/or fatigue may be present at rest, and symptoms are increased by almost any physical activity

Data from Reference 4.

and distension. On physical examination, patients with PAH may have an accentuated component of S_2 audible at the apex of the heart, midsystolic ejection murmur, palpable left parasternal lift, right ventricular S_4 gallop, and a prominent "a" wave.[2] Hepatojugular reflux, a diastolic murmur of pulmonary regurgitation, and a systolic murmur of tricuspid regurgitation may be present in advanced disease.[2] Patients with an increased risk of mortality are more likely to have a higher WHO functional class, older age, male gender, higher brain natriuretic peptide (BNP), higher right atrial pressure, and lower cardiac output. In contrast, patients with a decreased risk of mortality are more likely to have a lower WHO functional class, higher 6-minute walking distance (6MWD), lower BNP, and higher cardiac output.[13]

3 Several comorbidities and environmental factors play a role in the development of PAH and must be evaluated when establishing an initial diagnosis of PAH (Fig. 46-2). If PAH is suspected, a noninvasive screening test (eg, Doppler echocardiography) may detect increased pulmonary pressures. However, diagnosis of PAH requires additional testing.[22,23] Echocardiography is also useful in evaluating specific causes of pulmonary hypertension, such as a cardiac shunt or left-sided heart disease. Echocardiography can also be used to assess treatment interventions and to follow disease progression.[2] However, right heart catheterization is the definitive study to diagnose PAH and evaluate patients who are worsening clinically.[18]

Right heart catheterization is used to assess pulmonary vasoreactivity in patients with idiopathic, heritable, or medication-induced PAH. This test involves the administration of fast-acting vasodilators to determine the extent of vascular smooth muscle constriction and predict vasodilator response to calcium channel blockers (CCBs; class of recommendation I, level of evidence C).[4] Table 46-3 lists the classes of recommendations [COR] and levels of evidence [LOE], and Table 46-4 lists agents commonly used for vasoreactivity testing and their doses. The consensus definition of a positive vasoreactivity response is defined as a reduction of mPAP by at least 10 mm Hg to a value of 40 mm Hg or less with an unchanged or increased cardiac output.[24] Patients with a positive vasoreactivity response (approximately 13% of patients on initial testing) are most likely to have a beneficial hemodynamic and clinical response. These patients may be able to be treated with CCBs. However, about half of these patients lose an acute vasodilator response when tested 1 year later.[25] Therefore, even this small group of patients who may be treated with CCBs must be followed closely for safety and efficacy. If the patient loses the acute vasodilator response on follow-up assessment, they should be switched to different PAH therapy. Patients who have a negative response on initial vasodilator testing are not candidates for treatment with CCBs.[2,26]

Because PAH commonly occurs in the setting of connective tissue disease, serologic markers should be obtained to confirm or exclude these diagnoses.[2,28] Liver function tests (LFTs) should also be evaluated due to the increased risk for PAH in patients with cirrhosis and portal hypertension and as a baseline for certain PAH therapies. HIV is associated with an increased prevalence of PAH, and HIV testing should be done as part of the initial PAH workup.[2] CTEPH should be evaluated with ventilation-perfusion lung scans and/or pulmonary angiography. Pulmonary function testing and arterial blood oxygenation should be evaluated. The diffusing capacity of carbon monoxide may be particularly helpful in patients with systemic sclerosis and PAH.[2]

In patients with PAH, serial determinations of functional class, exercise capacity (assessed by the 6MWD), and serial biomarkers (ie, BNP) provide benchmarks for disease severity, response to therapy, and progression.[2,28] These variables can be used to determine the risk level in patients and may aid in prognosis. Table 46-5 outlines the calculation of low-, intermediate-, and high-risk patients based on these factors, which is essential for determining initial therapy and assessing treatment response. Risk assessment tools continue to be developed and refined (such as REVEAL 2.0 and REVEAL Lite 2) to use the most predictive variables to assess risk while also simplifying the assessment to promote routine use in daily clinical practice.[29,30] Table 46-6 provides guidelines for initial and follow-up assessments and their timing.

CLINICAL PRESENTATION Pulmonary Arterial Hypertension

Symptoms

- Exertional dyspnea
- Fatigue
- Weakness
- Exertional chest pain
- Complaints of general exertion intolerance
- Dyspnea at rest as the disease progresses
- Syncope
- Lower extremity edema

Symptoms of Related Conditions

- Paroxysmal nocturnal dyspnea as a result of left-sided heart disease
- Raynaud's phenomenon, arthralgia, or swollen hands and other symptoms of connective tissue disease
- Orthopnea

Symptoms of Disease Progression

- Leg swelling
  - Abdominal bloating and distension
  - Anorexia
  - Profound fatigue
  - May develop as right ventricular dysfunction and tricuspid valve regurgitation evolve

Signs of Advanced Disease

- Diastolic murmur of pulmonary regurgitation
- A pansystolic murmur of tricuspid regurgitation
- Hepatojugular reflux
- Right ventricular S_3 gallop
- Marked distension of jugular veins
- Peripheral edema
- Hypotension
- Cool extremities suggesting markedly reduced cardiac output and peripheral vasoconstriction

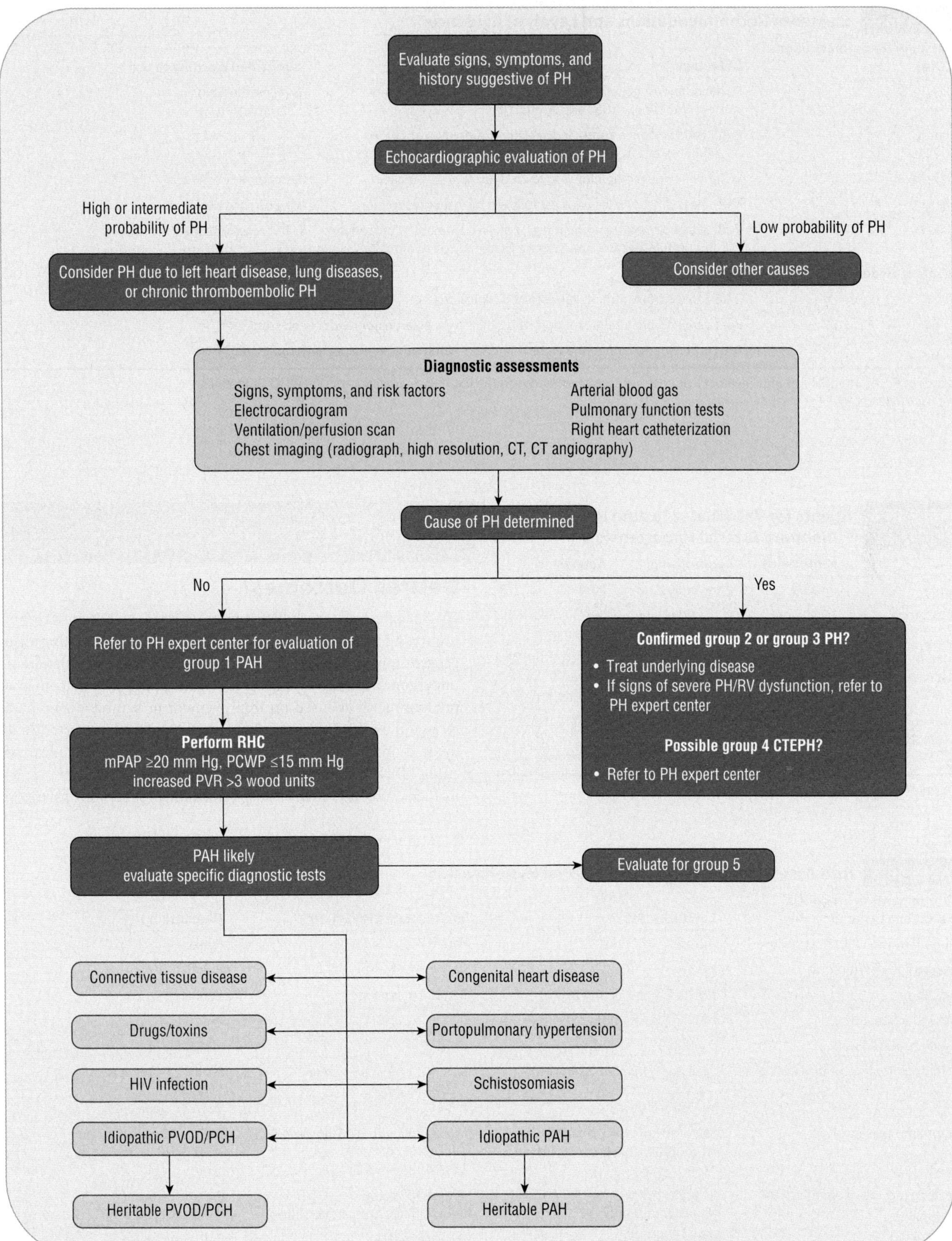

FIGURE 46-2 Diagnostic algorithm of pulmonary arterial hypertension. (PH, pulmonary hypertension; PAH, pulmonary arterial hypertension; CT, computed tomography; RV, right ventricular; mPAP, mean pulmonary artery pressure; CTEPH, chronic thromboembolic pulmonary hypertension; HIV, human immunodeficiency virus; PVOD/PCH, pulmonary veno-occlusive disease or pulmonary capillary hemangiomatosis; RHC, right heart catheterization.) *(Adapted from Galiè N, Humbert M, Vachiery JL, et al. 2015 ESC/ERS Guidelines forthe diagnosis and treatment of pulmonary hypertension. Eur Respir J. 2015;46:903–975.)*

TABLE 46-3 Classes of Recommendations and Levels of Evidence[a]

Classes of Recommendations (CORs)	Definition	Suggested Wording to Use
Class I	Evidence and/or general agreement that a given treatment or procedure is beneficial, useful, effective.	Is recommended/ Is indicated
Class II	Conflicting evidence and/or a divergence of opinion about the usefulness/efficacy of the given treatment or procedure.	
Class IIa	Weight of evidence/opinion is in favor of usefulness/efficacy.	Should be considered
Class IIb	Usefulness/efficacy is less well established by evidence/opinion.	May be considered
Class III	Evidence or general agreement that a given treatment or procedures is not useful/effective, and in some cases may be harmful.	Is not recommended
Levels of Evidence (LOE)	**Definition**	
A	Data derived from multiple randomized clinical trials or meta-analyses.	
B	Data derived from a single randomized clinical trial or large nonrandomized studies.	
C	The consensus opinion of the experts and/or small studies, retrospective studies, registries.	

[a]Classes of Recommendations and Levels of Evidence are consistent between the ESC/ERS Guidelines and the WHO Guidelines.

Data from Reference 4.

TABLE 46-4 Agents for Vasodilator Testing in Pulmonary Arterial Hypertension

	Nitric Oxide	Epoprostenol	Adenosine
Route	Inhaled	Intravenous	Intravenous
Dose range	10-80 ppm	2-10 ng/kg/min	50-250 mcg/kg/min
Dosing increments	10-80 ppm for 5 minutes	2 ng/kg/min every 15 minutes	50 mcg/kg/min every 2 minutes
Common side effects	None	Headache, flushing, nausea	Chest tightness, dyspnea

Data from Reference 27.

TREATMENT

Desired Outcomes

4 Specific goals in the treatment of PAH include lowering risk, improving quality of life and symptoms, and preventing disease progression and mortality.[13] Trials in the PAH population have undergone a change over the last decade. In the past, outcomes were predominantly focused on improvement in hemodynamic parameters and exercise tolerance.[31,32] However, more recent studies have focused on clinical outcomes, particularly combined clinical worsening. This outcome may differ among clinical trials but typically includes outcomes such as hospitalization, progression of symptoms,

TABLE 46-5 Risk Assessment in Pulmonary Arterial Hypertension

Determinants of Prognosis[a] (estimated 1-year mortality)	Low Risk <5%	Intermediate Risk 5%-10%	High Risk >10%
Clinical signs of right heart failure	Absent	Absent	Present
Progression of symptoms	No	Slow	Rapid
Syncope	No	Occasional syncope[b]	Repeated syncope[c]
WHO functional class	I, II	III	IV
6-minute walk distance	>440 m	165-440 m	<165 m
Cardiopulmonary exercise testing	Peak VO_2 >15 mL/min/kg (>65% pred.) Ve/VCO_2 slope <36	Peak VO_2 11-15 mL/min/kg (35%-65% pred.) Ve/VCO_2 slope 36-44.9	Peak VO_2 <11 mL/min/kg (<35% pred.) Ve/VCO_2 slope ≥45
NT-proBNP plasma levels	BNP <50 ng/L (14.5 pmol/L) NT-proBNP <300 ng/L (35.4 pmol/L)	BNP 50-300 ng/L (14.5-86.7 pmol/L) NT-proBNP 300-1,400 ng/L (35.4-165 pmol/L)	BNP >300 ng/L (86.7 pmol/L) NT-proBNP >1,400 ng/L (165 pmol/L)
Imaging (echocardiography, CMR imaging)	RA area <18 cm^2 No pericardial effusion	RA area 18-26 cm^2 No or minimal, pericardial effusion	RA area >26 cm^2 Pericardial effusion
Hemodynamics	RAP <8 mm Hg CI ≥2.5 L/min/m^2 (0.042 L/s/m^2) SvO_2 >65% (0.65)	RAP 8-14 mm Hg CI 2.0-2.4 L/min/m^2 (0.033-0.040 L/s/m^2) SvO_2 60%-65% (0.60-0.65)	RAP >14 mm Hg CI ≤2.0 L/min/m^2 (0.033 L/s/m^2) SvO_2 <60% (0.60)

WHO, World Health Organization; VO_2, oxygen consumption; Ve, ventilation; VCO_2, volume of exhaled carbon dioxide; NT, n-terminal; BNP, b-type natriuretic peptide; CMR, cardiac magnetic resonance; RA, right atrial, RAP, right atrial pressure; CI, cardiac index; SvO_2, venous oxygen saturation.

[a]Most of the proposed variables and cut-off values are based on expert opinion. They may provide prognostic information and are used to guide therapeutic decisions, but applications to individual patients must be done carefully. One must also note that most of these variables have been validated for IPAH and the cut-off values used above may not apply to other forms of PAH. Furthermore, the use of approved therapies and their influence on the variables should be considered in the evaluation of the risk.

[b]Occasional syncope during brisk or heavy exercise, or occasional orthostatic syncope in the otherwise stable patient.

[c]Repeated episodes of syncope, even with little or regular physical activity.

Data from Reference 4.

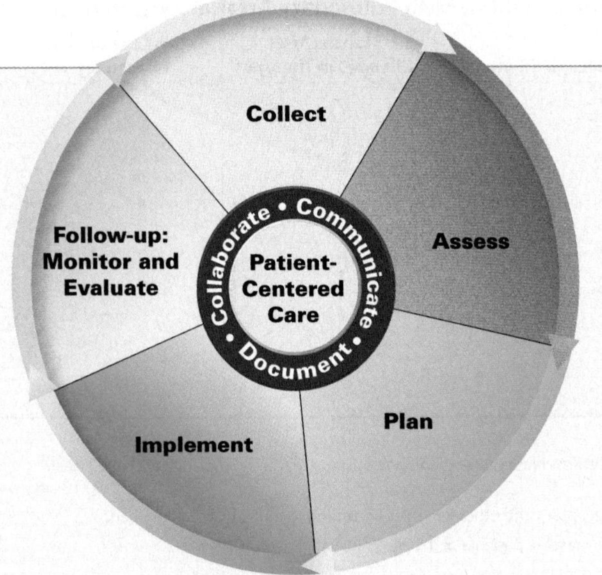

Patient Care Process for Pulmonary Arterial Hypertension

The illustration shows that patient-centered care includes collaboration, communication, and documentation. The actions associated with the care are collect, assess, plan, implement, and follow-up by monitoring and evaluating.

Collect

- Patient characteristics (eg, age, race, gender, pregnancy status)
- Patient history: past medical (eg, connective tissue diseases), family (eg, family history of pulmonary arterial hypertension), social (eg, use of cocaine or amphetamines)
- Current medications (eg, particularly anorexigen use such as fenfluramine)
- Immunization history (eg, influenza, pneumococcal vaccination)
- Socioeconomic factors that may affect access to treatment
- Lifestyle assessment: smoking status, exercise, diet, alcohol intake, sexual activity
- Symptoms (eg, exertional dyspnea or chest pain, syncope, volume overload) and WHO functional class (Table 46-2)
- Objective data (Table 46-6)
    - Height, weight, BMI, blood pressure, and heart rate
    - Echocardiography and electrocardiogram
    - Right heart catheterization (with acute vasoreactivity testing if idiopathic, heritable, or anorexigen-associated PAH)
    - Labs (eg, AST/ALT, BNP)

Assess

- Rule out secondary causes (eg, left heart disease [Group 2], lung diseases and/or hypoxia [Group 3], CTEPH hypertension [Group 4], PH with unclear multifactorial mechanisms [Group 5])
- Assess groups with special considerations such as pregnant women
- Presence of comorbid conditions: atrial tachyarrhythmias, depression, anxiety, anemia
- Current medications that may affect PAH-targeted therapy (eg, drug-drug interactions)
- Recommended treatment options based on risk assessment (see Fig 46-3 and Table 46-5)
- Appropriateness and effectiveness of current PAH therapy (eg, current risk status [Table 46-5], WHO functional class [Table 46-2], exercise capacity, change in pulmonary pressures, if any)

Plan*

- Therapeutic lifestyle changes (eg, diet and nutrition)
- Medication therapy regimen including specific PAH medication, dose, route, frequency, and duration; specify the continuation and discontinuation of existing therapies (see Table 46-7)
- Evaluate current therapy for drug-drug interactions at each visit (see Table 46-9)
- Monitoring parameters including efficacy (eg, risk status [Table 46-5], WHO functional class [Table 46-2], exercise capacity, change in pulmonary pressures), safety (medication-specific adverse effects [Table 46-8]), and time frame (3-month initial follow-up intervals, followed by 6-12 month intervals once at goal) (see Table 46-6)
- Patient education (eg, the purpose of treatment, dietary and lifestyle modification, medication therapy, immunizations, counseling on pregnancy and air travel)
- Self-monitoring of weight, exercise, diet, medication adherence/adverse effects
- Referral to PAH specialty center for coordination of care

Implement*

- Provide patient education regarding all elements of the treatment plan
- For parenteral prostacyclin analogs, coordinate with specialty company to ensure appropriate education on agents, including reconstitution, safety, back-up supplies
- Use motivational interviewing and coaching strategies to maximize adherence
- Schedule follow-up and time frame to achieve goals of therapy (eg, low-risk status [Table 46-5], improvement in WHO functional class [Table 46-2] and exercise capacity, symptom improvement, euvolemia [see Table 46-6])
- Educate patient on when to seek medical care (eg, worsening edema or dyspnea)

Follow-up: Monitor and Evaluate

- Determine response to PAH therapy and volume management
- Presence of medication-induced adverse effects (eg, elevated transaminases on ERAs, headache, flushing, edema, pump issues with parenteral prostacyclin analogs [see Table 46-8])
- Routine pregnancy screening for females (especially if receiving ERAs or riociguat)
- The occurrence of PAH worsening (eg, worsening symptoms or hospitalizations for PAH)
- Patient adherence to the treatment plan

**Collaborate with patient, caregivers, and other healthcare professionals.*

TABLE 46-6 Suggested Assessment and Timing for the Follow-up of Patients with Pulmonary Arterial Hypertension

	At Baseline	Every 3-6 Months	Every 6-12 Months[a]	3-6 Months After Changes in Therapy[a]	In Case of Clinical Worsening
Medical assessment and determination of functional class	+	+	+	+	+
ECG	+	+	+	+	+
6MWT/Borg dyspnea score	+	+	+	+	+
CPET	+		+		+[a]
Echocardiogram	+		+	+	+
Basic labs[b]	+	+	+	+	+
Extended labs[c]	+		+		+
Blood gas analysis[d]	+		+	+	+
Right heart catheterization	+		+[e]	+[f]	+[f]

[a]Intervals to be adjusted according to patient needs.

[b]Basic labs includes complete blood count, INR (in patients receiving vitamin K antagonists), serum creatinine, sodium, potassium, AST/ALT (in patients receiving ERAs), bilirubin, and BNP/NT-proBNP

[c]Extended labs includes TSH, troponin, uric acid, iron status (iron, ferritin, soluble transferrin receptor), and other variables according to individual patient need.

[d]From arterial or arterialized capillary blood; may be replaced by peripheral oxygen saturation in stable patients or if BGA is not available.

[e]Some centers perform RHCs at regular intervals during follow-up.

[f]Should be considered.

ALT, alanine aminotransferase; AST, aspartate aminotransferase; BGA, blood gas analysis; BNP, brain natriuretic peptide; CPET, cardiopulmonary exercise testing; Echo, echocardiography; ECG, electrocardiogram; ERAs, endothelin-receptor antagonists; FC, functional class; INR, international normalized ratio; lab, laboratory assessment; NT-proBNP, N-terminal pro-brain natriuretic peptide; RHC, right heart catheterization; TSH, thyroid stimulating hormone; 6MWT, 6-minute walking test.

Data from Galiè N, Humbert M, Vachiery JL, et al. 2015 ESC/ERS Guidelines for the diagnosis and treatment of pulmonary hypertension. Eur Respir J. 2015;43:903–975.

treatment escalation to prostacyclin therapy, transplantation, atrial septostomy, and death.[31]

General Approach to Treatment

Treatment of PAH may be categorized into nonpharmacologic, pharmacologic, and surgical interventions. The principal pathophysiologic abnormalities that are current pharmacologic therapeutic targets include the following: (1) supplementing endogenous vasodilators, (2) inhibiting endogenous vasoconstrictors, and (3) reducing endothelial platelet interaction and limiting thrombosis. Nonpharmacologic therapy can be quite broad and should be used when clinically appropriate. Surgical therapy is indicated in certain situations and includes atrial septostomy, pulmonary thromboendarterectomy for CTEPH, and lung or heart-lung transplantation (for disease that is not responsive to medical therapy). Bilateral lung and lung-heart transplantation improves survival rates in patients with PAH.[4]

Selection of targeted pharmacologic therapy should consider many factors, such as disease severity, safety profile, cost, and patient preference.[3] In 2019, the Sixth World Symposium on Pulmonary Hypertension published an updated series on PAH recommendations.[3] These guidelines recommend combination therapy as initial management for many patients with PAH, particularly WHO functional class II and higher. For patients on monotherapy with an inadequate response, an additional agent should be added to current therapy. Many patients with PAH will require combination therapy with two or three medications. Specific combination therapies will be discussed later on in this chapter.

Not all patients with PAH should be started on combination therapy. Those who are considered low risk may have improvement in symptoms with monotherapy. Other patient groups who may be candidates for monotherapy initially include those with multiple comorbidities, those at higher risk of adverse events, and populations of patients who were not included in the randomized controlled trials of initial combination therapy, such as patients with HIV or portal hypertension.[33]

Nonpharmacologic Therapy

5 Nonpharmacologic therapy is frequently used to address comorbid conditions that often accompany PAH. Patients with PAH should be counseled on several important points. Pregnancy should be avoided due to high morbidity and mortality rates in females with PAH during pregnancy and in the postpartum course (COR I, LOE C).[3,4] Immunization against influenza and pneumococcal disease should be provided (COR I, LOE C).[3,4] Hypoxemia may aggravate pulmonary vasoconstriction in patients with PAH; therefore, patients with PAH may require supplemental oxygen (COR IIa, LOE C), particularly when using air travel.[4] Patients should adhere to a low-sodium diet to avoid fluid retention predisposing to right heart failure.[34] Counseling on smoking cessation should be provided to all patients who are active smokers. Cardiopulmonary rehabilitation improves functional status, exercise capacity, and quality of life in patients with PAH.[3]

Pharmacologic Therapy

The number of potential therapies for PAH has expanded dramatically in the last decade. In addition to adjunctive background therapy, multiple medications have been developed specifically for the treatment of PAH. Figure 46-3 illustrates the recommended treatment algorithm based on the most recent guidelines.[3,33]

Conventional Pharmacologic Treatment

6 Conventional therapy includes oral anticoagulants, diuretics, oxygen, and digoxin.[33] Anticoagulation with warfarin may be considered on a case-by-case basis in patients with idiopathic, heritable, or drug-induced PAH (COR IIb, LOE C).[4] The rationale for oral anticoagulants is based on the presence of traditional risk factors for venous thromboembolism, such as heart failure and immobility, as well as thrombotic changes in the pulmonary microcirculation. Meta-analyses of small cohort studies demonstrate a 31% mortality risk reduction with anticoagulation.[35] However, recent observational studies report conflicting results regarding the benefit of

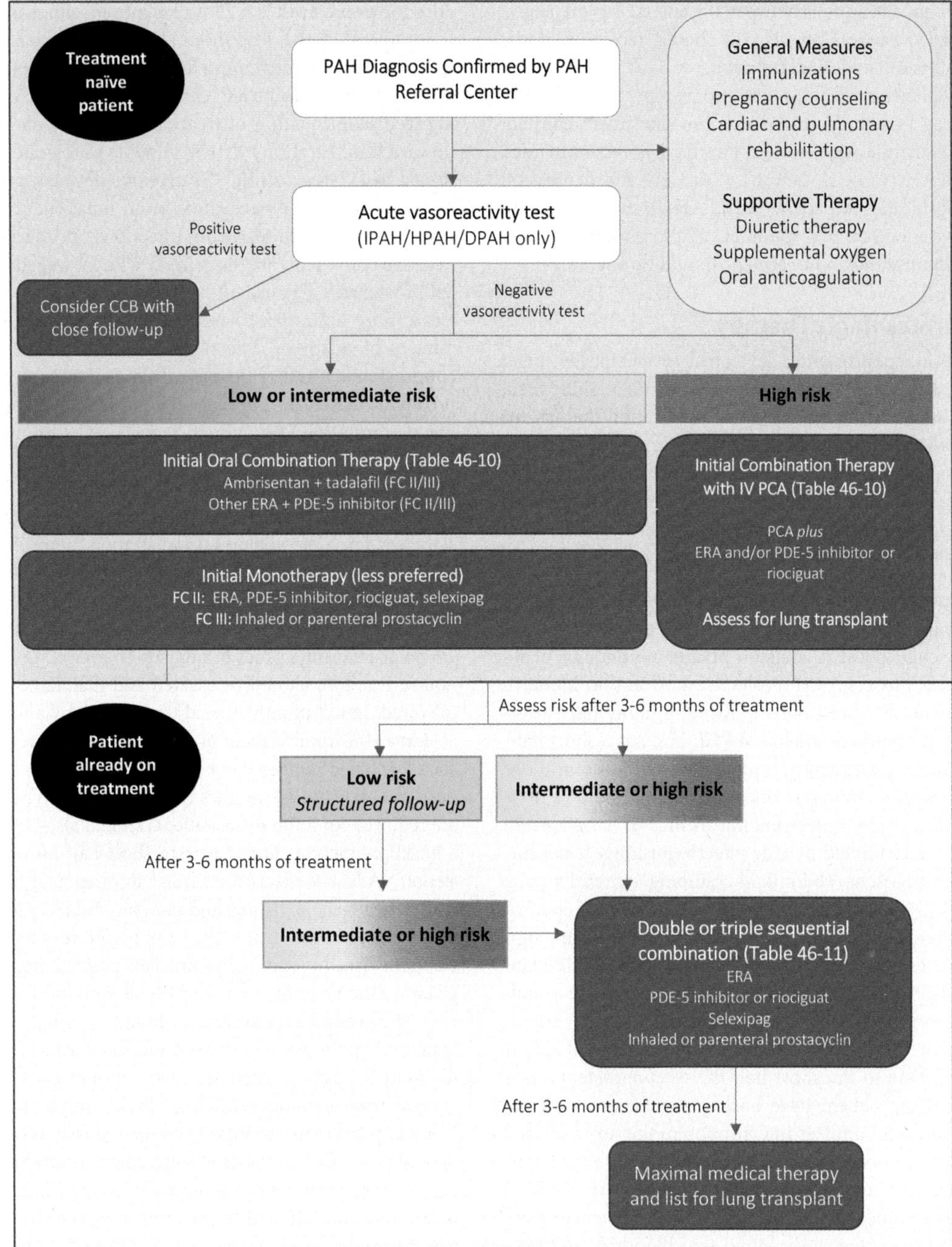

FIGURE 46-3 Treatment algorithm. (CCB, calcium channel blocker; DPAH, drug-induced pulmonary arterial hypertension; ERA, endothelin receptor antagonist; FC, functional class; HPAH, heritable pulmonary arterial hypertension; IPAH, idiopathic pulmonary arterial hypertension; PCA, prostacyclin analog; PDE, phosphodiesterase.) *(Reprinted from Risk stratification and medical therapy of pulmonary arterial hypertension. Galiè N, Channick RN, Frantz RP et al. European Respiratory Journal Jan 2019, 53 (1) 1801889; DOI: 10.1183/13993003.01889-2018. Published 24 January 2019.)*

anticoagulation in IPAH and associated PAH (APAH).[36,37] When warfarin is used, the target international normalized ratio (INR) in most centers is 1.5 to 2.5.[2,24] Anticoagulation is not recommended for patients with APAH due to HIV or portal hypertension.[33]

Loop diuretics such as furosemide are helpful adjunctive therapy in patients with decompensated right heart failure and associated findings of increased central venous pressure, abdominal organ congestion, peripheral edema, and ascites.[2] Appropriate diuretic therapy in right heart failure and volume overload provides symptomatic and clinical benefits in patients with PAH (COR I, LOE C).[4] Patients should be maintained at as close to a euvolemic state as possible.

Oxygen therapy with a goal oxygen saturation greater than 90% (0.90) may be beneficial in some patients with a PaO_2 <60 mm Hg (8.0 kPa), although no data exist regarding long-term benefit of oxygen treatment in PAH (COR I, LOE C).[4] Oxygen treatment is controversial in patients with PAH associated with shunts (ie, Eisenmenger's syndrome).

Digoxin may be used for patients with PAH with right heart failure as adjunctive therapy along with diuretics to control symptoms as well as in patients with atrial arrhythmias (COR I, LOE C).[4] There are no long-term trials, and clinical benefit is uncertain. Optimal plasma concentrations are unknown; however, based on data for digoxin use in heart failure with reduced ejection fraction, the typical target concentration is between 0.5 and 0.8 ng/mL (μg/L; 0.64 and 1 nmol/L). Patients on digoxin should receive periodic monitoring of potassium and renal function.

Lastly, iron-deficiency anemia is commonly reported in patients with PAH and may lead to decreased exercise capacity. Treatment of iron-deficiency anemia with iron replacement is recommended in patients with PAH (COR II, LOE b).[3,4] Anxiety and depression are frequent comorbidities in patients with PAH, occurring in up to 50%, with negative effects on perception of symptoms and quality of life. Appropriate counseling and treatment should be offered.[38]

Targeted Pharmacologic Therapy

The first medication, epoprostenol, developed to specifically target the disease process causing PAH was approved in 1995. Since then, there has been a surge in the availability of medication therapy for the treatment of PAH with five classes of medications now available. Specific pharmacologic therapy targets the disease process while conventional therapy is used for the management of symptoms and/or comorbid conditions. Specific information concerning individual medications used for PAH is shown in Tables 46-7–46-9.

Synthetic Prostacyclin and Prostacyclin Analogs 7 PGI_2 is produced predominantly by endothelial cells, inducing potent vasodilation of all vascular beds. It is also a potent inhibitor of platelet aggregation and possesses cytoprotective and antiproliferative activities. PGI_2 synthase expression is reduced in pulmonary arteries. Epoprostenol is a synthetic analog of PGI_2 and has a short half-life of 3 to 5 minutes; consequently, it must be given by continuous intravenous (IV) infusion. Initiation of epoprostenol should be done in a hospital setting at low doses ranging from 2 to 4 ng/kg/min and increased at a rate limited by side effects (flushing, headache, diarrhea, jaw pain, backache, abdominal cramping, extremity pain, and hypotension). During initiation and initial titration of epoprostenol, patients may require inotropic and/or blood pressure support for hemodynamic stability.[39] The two available products, Flolan® (generic formulation available) and Veletri®, have unique stability and reconstitution parameters; both pharmacists and patients should be aware of the differences and follow the manufacturer recommendations. Due to the short half-life of epoprostenol, it is recommended that the patient have backup supplies of both the medication and infusion pump, as interruption of therapy may lead to life-threatening pulmonary vasoconstriction.[40] Because the medication must be administered by continuous infusion with a central venous catheter and pump, bacteremia and catheter obstruction are potential complications. One study found that bloodstream infections occurred with epoprostenol and treprostinil in the range of 0.3 to 2.1 per 1,000 medicine days (approximately one infection every 3 years) when these medications are given IV.[41] The target dose for the first 2 to 4 weeks is around 10 to 15 ng/kg/min, and periodic dose increases are then required to maximize efficacy. Maintenance doses are variable but are often in the range of 25 to 80 ng/kg/min.[4] Multiple observational studies have documented an improvement in survival in patients with IPAH treated with epoprostenol.[4,42,43] Based on current guidelines, epoprostenol is indicated for WHO functional class III and IV (COR I, LOE A).[3,4]

Treprostinil is a stable analog of PGI_2 administered by subcutaneous (SC) or IV infusion and approved for WHO functional class II, III, and IV.[44] The major advantages of treprostinil over epoprostenol include ease of use and increased safety due to a longer half-life. Because of the longer half-life, the risk of rebound vasoconstriction that may occur if therapy is interrupted is lower, resulting in an improved safety profile.[19] Treprostinil improves 6MWD and hemodynamics with outcomes that are similar to epoprostenol.[45,46] In clinical trials, the greatest exercise improvement was observed in patients who were more compromised at baseline and who could tolerate doses in the upper quartile (>13.8 ng/kg/min). The initial dose for treprostinil is 1.25 ng/kg/min by either the SC or IV route. If not tolerated, the dose should be reduced to 0.625 ng/kg/min and dose titration again attempted at 4 weeks. Infusion site pain is common with the SC route and can occur in up to 85% of patients, leading to discontinuation of treatment in 8% of patients and limiting upward dose titration.[4] Patients unable to tolerate SC can be transitioned to IV treprostinil.[24] Transitions between prostacyclin agents or routes should be performed in an inpatient setting at an expert referral center. Bloodstream infections, primarily due to gram-negative pathogens, are more likely with IV treprostinil than with IV epoprostenol.[47] The use of the diluent used for epoprostenol, which has a more basic pH, to reconstitute IV treprostinil may decrease rates of bloodstream infections to a rate similar to that seen with epoprostenol.[48] Other adverse drug reactions are similar to epoprostenol. Based on international guidelines, treprostinil is recommended for WHO functional class III (SC administration—COR I, LOE B; IV administration—COR IIa, LOE C) and functional class IV (SC and IV administration—COR IIb, LOE C).[3,4]

To prevent complications and use of pumps and central venous catheters for PGI_2 analog administration, aerosolized formulations were developed. The first approved formulation, iloprost (Ventavis), is a PGI_2 analog that is given by inhalation using a dosing system provided by the manufacturer (ADD system). The initial inhaled dose is 2.5 mcg six to nine times per day up to every 2 hours during waking hours. The dose should be titrated and maintained at 5 mcg/dose if tolerated. In a 3-month clinical trial, iloprost via inhalation provided at least a 10% improvement in 6MWD and improvement in functional class.[49] Inhaled iloprost can be cumbersome to use as each inhalation dose can take 4 to 10 minutes to administer, and multiple inhalations are required for a full dose. Patients should also be instructed to have a backup supply as iloprost has a short half-life, similar to epoprostenol.[24] Adverse effects are similar to other PGI_2 analogs, including cough, headache, flushing, and jaw pain. Inhaled iloprost is indicated for functional class III (COR I, LOE B) and functional class IV (COR IIb, LOE C), although many clinicians prefer using PAH medications given via the IV or SC route in patients with more severe disease.[3]

The second aerosolized formulation, inhaled treprostinil, was approved by the Food and Drug Administration (FDA) in July 2009 to improve exercise capacity in functional class III patients. In a clinical trial, patients receiving inhaled treprostinil experienced a 20-m improvement in 6MWD compared with those on placebo. All patients included in the trial were concurrently receiving bosentan or sildenafil for at least 3 months.[50] An open-label extension of the trial found that inhaled treprostinil provided sustained benefit and was safe and efficacious over a 2-year period.[51] The approved dosing of inhaled treprostinil is three breaths (18 mcg each) four times daily during waking hours. The dose may be titrated based on patient tolerance at 1- to 2-week intervals to a maximum dose of nine breaths four times daily. Inhaled treprostinil requires less time to administer, but the formulation is more complicated to prepare than inhaled iloprost.[24] While inhaled treprostinil avoids the infusion-related complications of the other PGI_2 analogs, use is cautioned in patients with acute pulmonary infections or underlying lung disease. The most common adverse effects seen in clinical trials include throat irritation, cough, headache, nausea, dizziness, and flushing. Inhaled treprostinil may also cause systemic hypotension, and patients should be monitored carefully if they are concurrently on diuretics, antihypertensives, or other vasodilators. Inhaled treprostinil is indicated for patients with WHO functional class III (COR I, LOE B) and IV (COR IIb, LOE C).[3,4]

Finally, the first oral prostacyclin analog, sustained-release treprostinil (Orenitram), was approved by the FDA in December 2013 for patients with WHO functional class II and III PAH. Oral treprostinil monotherapy for 12 weeks was associated with a significant increase of 23 m in 6MWD.[52] No differences were observed between treprostinil and placebo in time to clinical worsening or

WHO functional class. Two randomized controlled trials followed evaluating the use of oral treprostinil in addition to ERAs and/or phosphodiesterase-5 inhibitors (PDE-5i). Neither study demonstrated a significant improvement in 6MWD with oral treprostinil therapy.[53,54] The average increase in 6MWD did correspond to treprostinil dose, with patients receiving higher doses demonstrating more improvement. Adverse events in studies included headache, nausea, diarrhea, and jaw pain; it is not well-tolerated overall, resulting in a high discontinuation rate of over 30%. Like other prostacyclin analogs, oral treprostinil inhibits platelet aggregation and may increase the risk of bleeding, especially in patients treated with anticoagulants. Oral treprostinil must be taken with food to improve absorption and cannot be crushed due to the osmotic release formulation. Oral treprostinil is indicated for patients with WHO functional class III (COR IIb, LOE B).[4]

Prostacyclin IP Receptor Agonist Selexipag is a novel prostacyclin IP receptor agonist that was approved for use in patients with WHO functional class II and III PAH in 2015. Selexipag works by agonizing the prostacyclin IP receptor coupled with G_s protein, leading to increased cyclic adenosine monophosphate and relaxation of vascular smooth muscle. This leads to pulmonary vasodilation, as well as antiproliferative effects on smooth muscle cells and inhibition of platelet aggregation. The initial clinical trial evaluating the use of selexipag showed efficacy in decreasing pulmonary vascular resistance and improving cardiac index and 6MWD.[55] In a large clinical trial, patients with IPAH and APAH treated with selexipag experienced less disease progression, fewer hospitalizations for PAH, and reduced complications from PAH compared to placebo.[56] These outcomes were similar in patients on no background therapy and when added to background eERAs, PDE-5i, or both. This finding supports the use of triple oral combination therapy.[57] Similar benefits were seen with selexipag in a subgroup of patients with PAH associated with connective tissue diseases.[58] An additional substudy of this trial demonstrated that patients initiating therapy within 6 months of their PAH diagnosis demonstrated more pronounced reduction of morbidity and mortality with the addition of oral selexipag, further supporting oral combination therapy early in the disease.[59] Dose titration is similar to the prostacyclin analogs where the patient is initiated on a starting dose and titrated to the maximum tolerated dose. The initial starting dose is 200 mcg orally twice daily; this dose can be increased by 200 mcg twice daily increments to a maximum dose of 1,600 mcg twice daily. The median dose tolerated was 1,000 mcg twice daily in the clinical trial.[56] Patients with treatment interruptions greater than 3 days require re-titration of selexipag. Adverse drug reactions are common, especially during dose titration, and similar to those caused by prostacyclin analogs, including flushing, headache, diarrhea, nausea, jaw pain, and myalgias. Selexipag may also cause anemia; periodic monitoring of the complete blood cell count is warranted. Selexipag has also been associated with an increased incidence of hyperthyroidism. Current guidelines do not provide a recommendation on the role of selexipag in therapy.

Endothelin-Receptor Antagonists 8 ET-1, a peptide produced primarily by the vascular endothelial cells, is characterized as a powerful vasoconstrictor and mitogen for smooth muscle. Activation of the ET-1 system has been shown in both plasma and lung tissue of patients with PAH. There are three FDA-approved oral ERAs available for the treatment of PAH—bosentan, ambrisentan, and macitentan. All ERAs are orally administered and teratogenic. Patients must be enrolled in a Risk Evaluation and Mitigation Strategy (REMS) program for all ERAs. All ERAs can cause liver toxicity, although the incidence is highly variable across the class. ERAs are metabolized through cytochrome p450 (CYP) enzyme system and are, therefore, targets for drug-drug interactions, requiring providers to evaluate for potential drug-drug interactions.[44]

Ambrisentan is a once-daily selective ET_A receptor antagonist that improves exercise capacity and hemodynamics and delays clinical worsening in PAH.[60,61] Two large trials demonstrated a significant improvement in functional capacity with ambrisentan (at doses of 2.5, 5, and 10 mg daily) compared to placebo.[44,61] However, a greater response was seen with higher doses. All doses were well tolerated, and no patients on therapy experienced an increase in LFTs more than three times the upper limit of normal. Unlike bosentan, liver toxicity occurs rarely with ambrisentan (0.8% in 12-week trials and 2.8% for up to 1 year).[4] Common side effects include peripheral edema, nasal congestion, flushing, anemia, and palpitations. Treatment should be initiated with 5 mg once daily and increased to 10 mg once daily, if required. Ambrisentan is recommended for WHO functional class II and III (COR I, LOE A/B) as well as functional class IV (COR IIb, LOE C).[4]

Macitentan (Opsumit) is a once-daily dual ERA. In a phase III clinical trial, patients with PAH (primarily functional class II and III), including those on stable therapy with oral or inhaled prostanoids, CCBs, or oral PDE-5i, were randomized to macitentan 3 mg daily, 10 mg daily, or placebo.[62] Both macitentan doses demonstrated statistically significant decreases in composite events related to PAH or death compared to placebo, primarily due to less frequent worsening of PAH (defined as a decrease in 6MWD, worsening symptoms, and need for additional treatment). Increased LFTs occurred with similar frequency in all groups, about 3.5%-4.5%. More patients in the macitentan groups experienced nasopharyngitis, headache, and anemia than with placebo. The FDA-approved dose is 10 mg by mouth daily. Macitentan is recommended for WHO functional class II and III (COR I, LOE B) as well as functional class IV (COR IIb, LOE C).[4]

Bosentan is an orally active dual ET_A and ET_B receptor antagonist that improves exercise capacity, functional class, hemodynamics, echocardiographic and Doppler variables, and time to clinical worsening.[63-65] In one of the larger studies with bosentan, patients were started on 62.5 mg twice daily for 4 weeks followed by 125 or 250 mg twice daily for a minimum of 12 weeks. Both doses improved 6MWD, WHO functional class, and increased time to clinical worsening compared to placebo. Increases in hepatic aminotransferases occurred in 9% of patients and were dose-dependent.[64] The mechanism of increased liver enzymes is thought to be competition by bosentan and its metabolites with the biliary excretion of bile salts, resulting in the retention of bile salts that can be cytotoxic to hepatocytes. Because of this toxicity, bosentan is only available through a distribution program.[24] Bosentan should be started at 62.5 mg twice daily for 4 weeks. After 4 weeks of therapy, the dose should be increased to 125 mg twice daily. If LFTs are confirmed to be in the range of three to five times the upper limit of normal, reduce the daily dose or interrupt treatment. If LFTs return to pretreatment levels, bosentan may be continued or reintroduced if indicated. LFTs should be monitored at baseline and monthly thereafter. A complete blood count should be monitored every 3 months as bosentan has been associated with anemia. Bosentan is indicated for WHO functional class II and III (I-A/B) as well as functional class IV (COR IIb, LOE C).[1,4]

Phosphodiesterase Inhibitors There are two PDE-5i available for the treatment of PAH—sildenafil and tadalafil. PDE-5i increase the intracellular concentration of cyclic guanosine monophosphate, leading to vasorelaxation and antiproliferative effects on vascular smooth muscle cells. PDE-5i commonly cause headaches and flushing as well as systemic hypotension. Both are contraindicated in combination with nitrates and riociguat due to increased risk of hypotension. Sildenafil and tadalafil both interact with bosentan, which is a potent CYP3A4 inducer.[66] Bosentan can decrease sildenafil and tadalafil concentrations by up to 50%, necessitating higher doses of PDE-5i when used in combination. PDE-5i are unique compared to other PAH therapies, as they are the only class that does not require enrollment in a REMS program nor acquisition through a specialty pharmacy.[62]

Sildenafil is a potent and highly specific PDE-5i that is approved for erectile dysfunction but also reduces mPAP and improves functional class. In one clinical trial, sildenafil added to conventional therapy significantly improved 6MWD and hemodynamic parameters at 12 weeks compared with placebo.[67] The FDA-approved dose is 20 mg orally three times per day; however, much higher doses are routinely used clinically. Common adverse drug reactions include headaches, flushing, epistaxis, dyspepsia, and diarrhea. Changes in vision have been reported, including blue-tinted vision and sudden loss of vision. In the event of sudden loss of vision, sildenafil should be stopped. Current guidelines recommend sildenafil for WHO functional class II and III patients with PAH (COR I, LOE A) in addition to functional class IV patients (COR IIb, LOE C).[4]

Another PDE-5i, tadalafil, was approved by the FDA in 2009 for the treatment of PAH. In a trial of patients with symptomatic PAH, more than 50% of whom were treated with bosentan at baseline, tadalafil 40 mg daily significantly improved exercise capacity, quality of life, and time to clinical worsening.[68] Treatment-naïve patients demonstrated not only greater improvement in exercise capacity than those on bosentan therapy but also greater improvement in all secondary outcomes. One possible explanation is decreased tadalafil levels as bosentan is a potent CYP3A4 inducer.[66] The most common adverse drug reactions were headache, myalgia, and flushing. Similar to sildenafil, tadalafil can also cause vision changes and dyspepsia. The recommended dose is 40 mg by mouth once a day.[68] Current guidelines recommend tadalafil for functional class II and III (COR I, LOE B) and functional class IV (COR IIb, LOE C).[4]

Guanylate Cyclase Stimulator Riociguat is a soluble guanylate cyclase stimulator approved by the FDA in 2013. Riociguat works synergistically with nitric oxide and directly stimulates soluble guanylate cyclase. In a phase 3 study of patients with PAH, many of whom were on an ERA or non-IV prostacyclin analog at baseline, riociguat 2.5 mg by mouth three times daily improved 6MWD, hemodynamic parameters, and WHO functional class compared to placebo.[69] Syncope, the most frequent serious adverse event, occurred in 1% of riociguat patients compared to 4% in the placebo group. The recommended starting dose is 1 mg orally, three times daily (TID), titrated by 0.5 mg TID every 2 weeks to a maximum dose of 2.5 mg by mouth TID. An initial starting dose of 0.5 mg TID may be used in patients with baseline hypotension. The use of riociguat is contraindicated in patients treated with PDE-5i due to the additive risk of hypotension. Riociguat is teratogenic and female patients must go through a REMS program to receive the medication. Smoking status should also be evaluated prior to initiation of riociguat because smoking reduces riociguat concentrations by 50% to 60%, potentially requiring dose adjustment to achieve the same effect. Riociguat is recommended for WHO functional class II and III (COR I, LOE B), functional class IV (COR IIb, LOE C), and is also approved for patients with Group 4 CTEPH.[4]

Calcium Channel Blockers 9 Since such a small number of patients with PAH have a positive response to acute vasodilator testing, CCBs are infrequently used. Approximately 13% of patients with IPAH will demonstrate an acute vasodilator response and may be initiated on CCB therapy. However, the number responding to long-term therapy is low (7%).[25] For the small group of patients that are long-term responders (at least 1 year on CCB monotherapy), a new clinical classification was added to the guidelines in group 1 PAH (Table 46-1).[1] Many long-term responders will lose the response to CCBs; therefore, patient response should be monitored closely with follow-up hemodynamic assessment with vasoreactivity testing. CCBs should not be used in the absence of demonstrated acute vasoreactivity.[3] If used in patients without acute vasoreactivity, CCBs are associated with systemic hypotension leading to reflex tachycardia, sympathetic stimulation, and right ventricular ischemia, ultimately increasing patient morbidity.[4] When used, dihydropyridine CCBs are preferred as they lack the negative inotropic effects seen with verapamil. Diltiazem may be used in patients who also have tachycardia to slow heart rate through atrioventricular node blockade. If left ventricular systolic dysfunction is present, diltiazem and verapamil should not be used. Assessment of CCB therapy should occur soon after initiation, and if improvement in functional class to class I or II is not seen, additional or alternative PAH therapy must be initiated. In acute responders, CCBs may be used in WHO functional class I to IV (COR I, LOE C).[4] Compared to CCB doses used to treat other conditions (eg, hypertension), doses for PAH are relatively high—that is, up to 20 to 30 mg/day for amlodipine, 120 to 240 mg/day for nifedipine, and 240 to 720 mg/day for diltiazem. However, initial doses should be much lower and titrated upward to response.[4] The most common adverse drug reaction is peripheral edema.

Combination Therapy

Combination therapy is an attractive treatment option that targets multiple pathophysiologic mechanisms in PAH. This approach improves hemodynamics, symptoms, and exercise capacity. A significant portion of patients require combination therapy with either two- or three-drug regimens. Two meta-analyses found that combination therapy decreased time to clinical worsening by 35% to 40%.[32,70] Several trials have evaluated different combination therapies. The first-line recommended combination therapy in treatment-naïve patients is an ERA with a PDE-5i. In a clinical trial of patients with newly diagnosed PAH, initial combination therapy with ambrisentan and tadalafil was associated with a significant reduction in time to clinical failure and PAH hospitalizations compared to either therapy alone.[71] Peripheral edema, headache, nasal congestion, and anemia were more common in the combination group than either monotherapy group. However, there was no difference in medication discontinuation due to adverse events.[71] This initial combination is considered a class I recommendation (LOE B) for WHO functional class II and III patients and a class IIb recommendation (LOE C) for WHO functional class IV patients.[4]

While not specifically evaluated as initial combination therapy, the addition of macitentan to a PDE-5i or nonparenteral prostanoid therapy delayed clinical worsening in one trial.[72] Another study found a 40% decrease in clinical worsening when selexipag was added to background therapy; clinical improvements were similar regardless of the type of background therapy (ERA, PDE-5i, or a combination).[73] In a post hoc analysis, investigators found a more profound effect in patients who were started on selexipag within 6 months of diagnosis.[74] Sildenafil added to epoprostenol provided significant improvements in clinical outcomes and delay in clinical worsening.[75] Riociguat combined with ERAs showed benefit at 12 weeks.[69]

Current guidelines state the combination therapies with the strongest evidence and guideline support include the following: macitentan and sildenafil, riociguat and bosentan, and selexipag and ERA and/or PDE-5i.[33] A recent study compared an initial triple therapy (macitentan, tadalafil, and selexipag) to initial dual therapy (macitentan and tadalafil) in patients with PAH and found no difference in pulmonary vascular resistance but reduced the risk of disease progression with initial triple therapy.[76] Adverse drug reactions occurring more frequently in the triple therapy group included headache, diarrhea, nausea, pain in extremity, jaw pain, and vomiting.[76]

Tables 46-10 and 46-11 show current treatment recommendations for initial combination and sequential combination therapy, respectively.

TABLE 46-7 Dosing Recommendations for Common Treatments for Pulmonary Arterial Hypertension

Medication	Initial Dose	Usual Range	Other
Epoprostenol	2-4 ng/kg/min by IV infusion	Titrate up to 20-40 ng/kg/min	
Treprostinil (IV or SC)	1.25 ng/kg/min by continuous subcutaneous or IV infusion	Decrease to 0.625 ng/kg/min if not tolerated Increase by no more than 1.25 ng/kg/min weekly for the first 4 weeks of therapy and no more than 2.5 ng/kg/min weekly for the duration of therapy	
Treprostinil (inhaled)	Three inhalations (18 mcg) four times daily during waking hours (approximately 4 hours apart)	Reduce to one to two breaths if three breaths not tolerated; increase to three breaths when tolerance improves The goal maintenance dose is nine breaths (54 mcg) per treatment four times daily; titrate by increasing three breaths at 1- to 2-week intervals as tolerated	
Treprostinil (oral)	0.25 mg every 12 hours or 0.125 mg every 8 hours	Titrate dose in increments of 0.25-0.5 mg every 12 hours or 0.125 mg every 8 hours every 3-4 days The maximum dose is determined by tolerability Avoid abrupt discontinuation; if not tolerated, decrease dose stepwise in 0.25-0.5 mg increments	If unable to continue oral therapy temporarily while inpatient, consider initiation of IV or SC treprostinil; 1/5 of the total daily oral dose is an estimate of total daily parenteral dose
Iloprost	2.5 mcg inhaled six to nine times daily (dosing at ≥2-hour intervals while awake)	Titrate to 5 mcg per dose with a maximum daily dose of 45 mcg	
Bosentan	62.5 mg orally twice daily	Increase to 125 mg orally twice daily	Available through Tracleer Access Program
Ambrisentan	5 mg orally daily	Titrate to maximum dose of 10 mg daily	Available through Letairis Education and Access Program
Macitentan	10 mg orally daily	Maximum dose of 10 mg orally daily	Available through Opsumit Risk Evaluation and Mitigation Strategy Program
Sildenafil	20 mg orally three times daily, taken at least 4-6 hours apart	Maximum FDA-approved dose is 20 mg orally three times a day; higher doses frequently used clinically	
Tadalafil	40 mg orally once daily, with or without food	40 mg orally once daily	Not recommended to divide the dose
Riociguat	0.5-1 mg orally three times daily	Maximum dose is 2.5 mg orally three times daily Titrate by 0.5 mg every 2 weeks to maximum tolerated dose; dose limited by hypotension	Use is contraindicated with PDE-5 inhibitors due to the risk of hypotension Available through Adempas Risk Evaluation and Mitigation Program
Selexipag	200 mcg orally twice daily	Titrate to maximally tolerated dose in 200 mcg increments; maximum dose 1,600 mcg orally twice daily	

IV, intravenous; SC, subcutaneous; FDA, Food and Drug Administration; PDE-5, phosphodiesterase-5.

TABLE 46-8 Monitoring Recommendations for Adverse Drug Reactions

Medication	Adverse Drug Reaction	Monitoring Parameter	Comments
Synthetic Prostacyclin and Prostacyclin Analogs			
Epoprostenol, Treprostinil (IV/SC/oral)	Pain (chest and jaw), flushing, headache	Patient reported symptoms	Occurs with dose titration; titrate to balance efficacy and adverse effect
	GI (nausea, vomiting, diarrhea, anorexia)	Patient reported symptoms	
	Hypotension	Blood pressure	Occurs with dose titration; additive hypotensive effects with other antihypertensives, vasodilators, and diuretics
	Thrombocytopenia	Platelets; signs and symptoms of bleeding	Monitor with concurrent anticoagulant and antiplatelet agents
Treprostinil (SC-specific)	SC site pain	Local pain at SC administration site	Frequent site rotation may improve; may also use cool compresses, lidocaine-based creams or patches, or pluronic lecithin organogel (PLO) to relieve pain
Treprostinil (inhaled)	Cough and throat irritation	Patient reported symptoms	
Iloprost	Cough and throat irritation	Patient reported symptoms	
Prostacyclin IP Receptor Agonist			
Selexipag	Pain (chest and jaw), flushing, headache	Titrate to balance efficacy and adverse effect	Occurs with dose titration
	GI (nausea, diarrhea)	Patient reported symptoms	
	Anemia	Hemoglobin	Monitor at baseline and then periodically throughout treatment
	Hyperthyroidism	Thyroid stimulating hormone	May monitor if associated symptoms

(continued)

TABLE 46-8 Monitoring Recommendations for Adverse Drug Reactions (*Continued*)

Medication	Adverse Drug Reaction	Monitoring Parameter	Comments
Endothelin-Receptor Antagonists			
Bosentan, Ambrisentan, Macitentan	Anemia	Hemoglobin	Usually resolves after the first 3 months of therapy
	Edema	Edema on physical exam	May require a dose increase of diuretic therapy
Bosentan (specific)	Hepatotoxicity	Baseline and monthly liver function tests required	Black box warning for liver injury
Phosphodiesterase-5 Inhibitors			
Sildenafil, Tadalafil	Headache	Patient reported symptoms; occurs due to vasodilation	
	Nasal congestion	Patient reported symptoms	
	Hypotension	Blood pressure	Concurrent use with nitrates potentiates effects
	Visual changes	Consider baseline exam; repeat exam if visual changes occur	
Soluble Guanylate Cyclase Stimulator			
Riociguat	Headache	Patient reported symptoms	
	Hypotension	Blood pressure	
	Peripheral edema	Edema on physical exam	
	Major bleeding	Hemoglobin and hematocrit Signs and symptoms of bleeding	
	Gastroesophageal reflux disease (GERD)	Patient reported symptoms; heart burn/reflux symptoms	

IV, intravenous; SC, subcutaneous; GI, gastrointestinal.

TABLE 46-9 Potentially Significant Drug Interactions with Pulmonary Arterial Hypertension Medications

PAH Medication	Mechanism of Interaction	Interacting Medication	Interaction
Ambrisentan	Unknown	Cyclosporine Ketoconazole	Caution is required in the coadministration of ambrisentan with ketoconazole and cyclosporine.
Bosentan	CYP3A4 inducer	Sildenafil	Sildenafil levels fall 50%; bosentan levels increase 50%. May not require dose adjustments of either medication.
	CYP3A4 substrate	Cyclosporine	Cyclosporine levels fall 50%; bosentan levels increase fourfold. Combination contraindicated.
	CYP3A4 substrate	Erythromycin	Bosentan levels increase. May not require dose adjustment of bosentan during a short course.
	CYP3A4 substrate	Ketoconazole	Bosentan levels increase twofold.
	CYP3A4 substrate + bile salt pump inhibitor	Glibenclamide	Increase incidence of elevated aminotransferases. Potential decrease of hypoglycemic effect of glibenclamide. Combination contraindicated.
	CYP2C9 & CYP3A4 substrate	Fluconazole, amiodarone	Bosentan levels increase considerably. Combination contraindicated.
	CYP2C9 & CYP3A4 inducers	Rifampin, phenytoin	Bosentan levels decrease by 50%. Need for dose adjustment uncertain.
	CYP2C9 inducer	HMG CoA reductase inhibitors	Simvastatin levels reduce 50%; similar effects likely with atorvastatin. Cholesterol level should be monitored.
	CYP2C9 inducer	Warfarin	Increases warfarin metabolism, may need to adjust warfarin dose. Intensified monitoring of warfarin recommended following initiation but dose adjustment usually unnecessary.
	CYP2C9 & CYP3A4 inducers	Hormonal contraceptives	Hormone levels decrease. Contraception unreliable.
Macitentan			Not yet determined.
Selexipag			Not yet determined.
Sildenafil[47]	CYP3A4 substrate	Bosentan	Sildenafil levels fall 50%; bosentan levels increase 50%. May not require dose adjustments of either medication.
	CYP3A4 substrate	HMG CoA reductase inhibitors (statins)	May increase simvastatin/atorvastatin levels through competition for metabolism, Sildenafil levels may increase. Possible increased risk of rhabdomyolysis.
	CYP3A4 substrate	HIV protease inhibitors	Ritonavir and saquinavir increase sildenafil levels markedly.
	CYP3A4 inducer	Phenytoin	Sildenafil levels may fall.
	CYP3A4 substrate	Erythromycin	Sildenafil levels increase. May not require dose adjustment for a short course.

(*continued*)

TABLE 46-9 Potentially Significant Drug Interactions with Pulmonary Arterial Hypertension Medications (*Continued*)

PAH Medication	Mechanism of Interaction	Interacting Medication	Interaction
	CYP3A4 substrate	Ketoconazole	Sildenafil levels increase. May not require dose adjustment.
	CYP3A4 substrate	Cimetidine	Sildenafil levels increase. May not require dose adjustment.
	cGMP	Nitrates, Nicorandil Molsidomine	Profound systemic hypotension, combination contraindicated.
Tadalafil[48]	CYP3A4 substrate	Bosentan	Tadalafil exposure decreases by 42%, no significant changes in bosentan levels.[48] May not require dose adjustment.
	cGMP	Nitrates, Nicorandil	Profound systemic hypotension, combination contraindicated.
Riociguat[18]	cGMP	Sildenafil, other PDE-5 inhibitors	Hypotension, severe side effects, combination contraindicated.
	cGMP	Nitrates, Nicorandil	Profound systemic hypotension, combination contraindicated.

HMG CoA, 3-hydroxy-3-methylglutaryl coenzyme A; HIV, human immunodeficiency virus; GMP, guanosine monophosphate.

Data from Reference 4.

TABLE 46-10 Recommendations for Efficacy of Initial Medication Combination Therapy for Pulmonary Arterial Hypertension (Group 1) According to World Health Organization Functional Class

	Class of Recommendations/Level of Evidence					
Treatment	COR	LOE	COR	LOE	COR	LOE
Ambrisentan + tadalafil[a]	I	B	I	B	IIb	C
Other ERA + PDE-5i	IIa	C	IIa	C	IIb	C
Bosentan + sildenafil + iv epoprostenol	-	-	IIa	C	IIa	C
Bosentan + iv epoprostenol	-	-	IIa	C	IIa	C
Other ERA or PDE-5i + sc treprostinil			IIb	C	IIb	C
Other ERA or PDE-5i + other iv prostacyclin analogs			IIb	C	IIb	C

ERA, endothelin-receptor antagonist; iv, intravenous; PDE-5i, phosphodiesterase type 5 inhibitor; RCT, randomized controlled trial; sc, subcutaneous; WHO-FC, World Health Organization functional class; COR, class of recommendation; LOE, level of evidence.

[a]Time to clinical failure as primary endpoint in RCTs or medications with demonstrated reduction in all-cause mortality (prospectively defined).

TABLE 46-11 Recommendations for Efficacy of Sequential Medication Combination Therapy for Pulmonary Arterial Hypertension (Group 1) According to World Health Organization Functional Class

	Class of Recommendation/Level of Evidence					
Treatment	COR	LOE	COR	LOE	COR	LOE
Macitentan added to sildenafil[a]	I	B	I	B	IIa	C
Riociguat added to bosentan	I	B	I	B	IIa	C
Selexipag added to ERA[b] and/or PDE-5i[a]	I	B	I	B	IIa	C
Sildenafil added to epoprostenol	-	-	I	B	IIa	B
Treprostinil inhaled added to sildenafil or bosentan	IIa	B	IIa	B	IIa	C
Iloprost inhaled added to bosentan	IIb	B	IIb	B	IIb	C
Tadalafil added to bosentan	IIa	C	IIa	C	IIa	C
Ambrisentan added to sildenafil	IIb	C	IIb	C	IIb	C
Bosentan added to epoprostenol	-	-	IIb	C	IIb	C
Bosentan added to sildenafil	IIb	C	IIb	C	IIb	C
Sildenafil added to bosentan	IIb	C	IIb	C	IIb	C
Other double combinations	IIb	C	IIb	C	IIb	C
Other triple combinations	IIb	C	IIb	C	IIb	C
Riociguat added to sildenafil or other PDE-5i	III	B	III	B	III	B

EMA, European Medicines Agendy; ERA, endothelin-receptor antagonist; PAH, pulmonary arterial hypertension; PDE-5i, phosphodiesterase type 5 inhibitor; RCT, randomized controlled trial; WHO-FC, World Health Organization functional class; COR, class of recommendation; LOE, level of evidence.

[a]Time to clinical failure as primary endpoint in RCTs or medications with demonstrated reduction in all-cause mortality (prospectively defined).

[b]This medication was not approved by the EMA at the time of publication of these guidelines.

Fusion Protein

An emerging treatment option in development is sotatercept. Sotatercept is a fusion protein composed of the extracellular domain of the human activin receptor type IIA linked to the Fc domain of human IgG1.[77] Sotatercept impairs activation in the transforming growth factor ß (TGF-ß) pathway, thereby restoring the balance between proproliferative and antiproliferative pathways. Mutations in the TGF-ß pathway, specifically BMPR2, are present in 70% to 80% of heritable PAH and in 10% to 20% of IPAH.[14] In a phase 2 trial, sotatercept dosed at 0.3 mg/kg or 0.7 mg/kg SC every 3 weeks reduced pulmonary vascular resistance at 24 weeks in patients with PAH on background therapy, the majority of whom were on double or triple therapy while many others were on intravenous prostacyclin therapy.[77] Thrombocytopenia occurred in 6% of the lower dose group and 12% in the higher dose. An increase in hemoglobin was also seen in 3% of patients on the lower dose and 17% of patients on higher dose, perhaps because the TGF-ß pathway is involved in hematopoiesis. In 2020, the FDA granted Breakthrough Therapy status for sotatercept for the treatment of PAH, and phase 3 trials are ongoing.

Special Populations

Pregnancy

Pregnancy confers an increased risk of mortality in patients with PAH. Guidelines recommend encouraging patients with PAH to actively avoid pregnancy.[4] There is no consensus on the best birth control method for patients with PAH, but the use of two methods should be considered. Estrogen-containing products should be avoided. Patients who do become pregnant need to be referred as soon as possible to a PH center where there are expert high-risk obstetricians and PAH specialists who have experience in this area.[4] All ERAs (bosentan, ambrisentan, and macitentan) are teratogenic, as is riociguat. These medications should be discontinued immediately if a patient becomes pregnant and therapy needs to be adjusted. Monthly pregnancy tests are required for use of ERAs and riociguat. It is also important to note that bosentan may decrease the efficacy of oral birth control medications (Table 46-9).

Evaluation of Therapeutic Outcomes

All patients with PAH, regardless of risk status, should be reevaluated within 3 to 6 months of starting therapy.[33] Current guidelines recommend the use of a comprehensive risk assessment tool to assess prognosis and inform therapy (Table 46-5). Additionally, recent studies have reported successful use of refined risk assessment tools that use the most predictive variables and simplify assessment for clinicians.[29,30] If a patient has achieved a low-risk status, therapy should be continued. If a patient is considered intermediate risk, additional therapy should be considered. This may result in initial combination therapy escalating to triple therapy in some patients. Patients who are high risk on follow-up should be initiated on IV prostacyclin therapy and referred for lung transplant evaluation. Table 46-6 provides recommendations regarding specific baseline and follow-up assessments and when they should be performed.

CONCLUSION

PAH is an uncommon disease state with complex therapies. Significant advances have been made in elucidating the pathogenesis of PAH as well as in the evaluation and treatment of these patients over the past three decades. With targeted therapies such as ERAs, PDE-5i, and PGI_2 analogs, clinical improvement is possible in most patients, leading to a higher quality of life and delayed disease progression. Patient education is important to improve acceptance of this disease and referral to specialty care centers may provide the best outcomes.

ABBREVIATIONS

6MWD	6-minute walking distance
5-HT	serotonin
5-HTT	5-hydroxytryptamine transporter
ALK-1	activin receptor-like kinase 1
APAH	associated pulmonary arterial hypertension
BMPR-2	bone morphogenetic protein receptor 2
BNP	brain natriuretic peptide
CCB	calcium channel blocker
COR	class of recommendation
CTEPH	chronic thromboembolic pulmonary hypertension
CYP	cytochrome p450
ERA	endothelin-receptor antagonist
ET-1	endothelin-1
FDA	Food and Drug Administration
HIV	human immunodeficiency virus
HPAH	heritable pulmonary arterial hypertension
INR	international normalized ratio
IPAH	idiopathic pulmonary arterial hypertension
IV	intravenous
LOE	level of evidence
LFT	liver function test
NO	nitric oxide
NOS	nitric oxide synthase
PAH	pulmonary arterial hypertension
PAP	pulmonary artery pressure
PCWP	pulmonary capillary wedge pressure
PDE-5i	phosphodiesterase-5 inhibitors
PGI2	prostacyclin
REMS	Risk Evaluation and Mitigation Strategy
SC	subcutaneous
SSRIs	selective serotonin reuptake inhibitors
TGF-β	transforming growth factor-β
WHO	World Health Organization

REFERENCES

1. Simonneau G, Montani D, Celermajer DS, et al. Haemodynamic definitions and updated clinical classification of pulmonary hypertension. *Eur Respir J.* 2019;53:1801913. 10.1183/13993003.01913-2018.
2. McLaughlin VV, Shah SJ, Souza RHM. Management of pulmonary arterial hypertension. *J Am Coll Cardiol.* 2015;65(18):1976–1997.
3. Klinger JR, Elliott CG, Levine DJ, et al. Therapy for pulmonary arterial hypertension in adults: Update of the CHEST guideline and expert panel report. *Chest.* 2019;155:565–586. 10.1016/j.chest.2018.11.030.
4. Galiè N, Humbert M, Vachiery J-L, et al. 2015 ESC/ERS guidelines for the diagnosis and treatment of pulmonary hypertension. *Eur Respir J.* 2015;46:903–975. doi: 10.1183/13993003.01032-2015.
5. D'Alonzo GE. Survival in patients with primary pulmonary hypertension. *Ann Intern Med.* 1991;115(5):343. doi: 10.7326/0003-4819-115-5-343.
6. Benza RL, Miller DP, Gomberg-Maitland M, et al. Predicting survival in pulmonary arterial hypertension: Insights from the Registry to Evaluate Early and Long-Term Pulmonary Arterial Hypertension Disease Management (REVEAL). *Circulation.* 2010;122(2):164–172. doi: 10.1161/CIRCULATIONAHA.109.898122.
7. Farber HW, Miller DP, Poms AD, et al. Five-year outcomes of patients enrolled in the REVEAL registry. *Chest.* 2015;148(4):1043–1054. doi: 10.1378/chest.15-0300.
8. McGoon MD, Benza RL, Escribano-Subias P, et al. Pulmonary arterial hypertension. *J Am Coll Cardiol.* 2013;62(25):D51–D59. doi: 10.1016/j.jacc.2013.10.023.
9. Humbert M, Sitbon O, Chaouat A, et al. Pulmonary arterial hypertension in France: Results from a national registry. *Am J Respir Crit Care Med.* 2006;173(9):1023–1030. doi: 10.1164/rccm.200510-1668OC.

10. Badesch DB, Raskob GE, Elliott CG, et al. Pulmonary arterial hypertension: Baseline characteristics from the REVEAL Registry. *Chest.* 2010;137(2):376–387. doi: 10.1378/chest.09-1140.
11. McLaughlin VV, Shah SJ, Souza R, Humbert M. Management of pulmonary arterial hypertension. *J Am Coll Cardiol.* 2015;65(18):1976–1997. doi: 10.1016/J.JACC.2015.03.540.
12. Yuan JX-J. Pathogenesis of pulmonary arterial hypertension: The need for multiple hits. *Circulation.* 2005;111(5):534–538. doi: 10.1161/01.CIR.0000156326.48823.55.
13. McGoon MD, Benza RL, Escribano-Subias P, et al. Pulmonary arterial hypertension: Epidemiology and registries. *J Am Coll Cardiol.* 2013;62(25 Suppl):D51–D59. doi: 10.1016/j.jacc.2013.10.023.
14. Morrell NW, Aldred MA, Chung WK, et al. Genetics and genomics of pulmonary arterial hypertension. *Eur Respir J.* 2019;53:1801899. 10.1183/13993003.01899-2018.
15. Shah SJ. Pulmonary hypertension. *JAMA.* 2012;308(13):1366. doi: 10.1001/jama.2012.12347.
16. Schermuly RT, Ghofrani HA, Wilkins MR, Grimminger F. Mechanisms of disease: Pulmonary arterial hypertension. *Nat Rev Cardiol.* 2011;8(8):443–455. doi: 10.1038/nrcardio.2011.87.
17. Olsson KM, Hoeper MM. Novel approaches to the pharmacotherapy of pulmonary arterial hypertension. *Drug Discov Today.* 2009;14(5-6):284–290. doi: 10.1016/j.drudis.2008.12.003.
18. Humbert M. Update in pulmonary hypertension 2008. *Am J Respir Crit Care Med.* 2009;179(8):650–656. doi: 10.1164/rccm.200901-0136UP.
19. Park MH. Advances in diagnosis and treatment in patients with pulmonary arterial hypertension. *Catheter Cardiovasc Interv.* 2008;71(2):205–213. doi: 10.1002/ccd.21389.
20. Rubens C, Ewert R, Halank M, et al. Big endothelin-1 and endothelin-1 plasma levels are correlated with the severity of primary pulmonary hypertension. *Chest.* 2001;120(5):1562–1569. Available at http://www.ncbi.nlm.nih.gov/pubmed/11713135. Accessed October 20, 2015.
21. Giaid A, Saleh D. Reduced expression of endothelial nitric oxide synthase in the lungs of patients with pulmonary hypertension. *N Engl J Med.* 1995;333(4):214–221. doi: 10.1056/NEJM199507273330403.
22. Janda S, Shahidi N, Gin K, Swiston J. Diagnostic accuracy of echocardiography for pulmonary hypertension: A systematic review and meta-analysis. *Heart.* 2011;97(8):612 LP–622. Available at http://heart.bmj.com/content/97/8/612.abstract.
23. Frost A, Badesch D, Gibbs JSR, et al. Diagnosis of pulmonary hypertension. *Eur Respir J.* 2019;53:1801904. 10.1183/13993003.01904-2018.
24. Bishop BM, Mauro VF, Khouri SJ. Practical considerations for the pharmacotherapy of pulmonary arterial hypertension. *Pharmacother J Hum Pharmacol Drug Ther.* 2012;32(9):838–855. doi: 10.1002/j.1875-9114.2012.01114.x.
25. Olivier S, Marc H, Xavier J, et al. Long-term response to calcium channel blockers in idiopathic pulmonary arterial hypertension. *Circulation.* 2005;111(23):3105–3111. doi: 10.1161/CIRCULATIONAHA.104.488486.
26. O'Callaghan DS, Savale L, Montani D, et al. Treatment of pulmonary arterial hypertension with targeted therapies. *Nat Rev Cardiol.* 2011;8:526. Available athttps://doi.org/10.1038/nrcardio.2011.104.
27. Calderone A, Stevens W, Prior D, et al. Multicentre randomised placebo-controlled trial of oral anticoagulation with apixaban in systemic sclerosis-related pulmonary arterial hypertension: The SPHInX study protocol. *BMJ Open.* 2016;6(12):e011028. http://bmjopen.bmj.com/content/6/12/e011028.abstract.
28. Agarwal R, Gomberg-Maitland M. Current therapeutics and practical management strategies for pulmonary arterial hypertension. *Am Heart J.* 2011;162(2):201–213. doi: 10.1016/J.AHJ.2011.05.012.
29. Benza RL, Kanwar MK, Raina A, et al. Development and Validation of an Abridged Version of the REVEAL 2.0 Risk Score Calculator, REVEAL Lite 2, for Use in Patients with Pulmonary Arterial Hypertension. *Chest.* 2021;159:337–346. 10.1016/j.chest.2020.08.2069.
30. Benza RL, Gomberg-Maitland M, Elliott CG, et al. Predicting survival in patients with pulmonary arterial hypertension. *Chest.* 2019;156:323–337. 10.1016/j.chest.2019.02.004.
31. Lajoie AC, Bonnet S, Provencher S. Combination therapy in pulmonary arterial hypertension: Recent accomplishments and future challenges. *Pulm Circ.* 2017;7(2):312–325. doi: 10.1177/2045893217710639.
32. Fox BD, Shtraichman O, Langleben D, Shimony A, Kramer MR. Combination therapy for pulmonary arterial hypertension: A systematic review and meta-analysis. *Can J Cardiol.* 2016;32(12):1520–1530. doi: 10.1016/j.cjca.2016.03.004.
33. Galiè N, Channick RN, Frantz RP, et al. Risk stratification and medical therapy of pulmonary arterial hypertension. *Eur Respir J.* 2019;53:1801889. 10.1183/13993003.01889-2018.
34. McGoon M, Gutterman D, Steen V, et al. Screening, early detection, and diagnosis of pulmonary arterial hypertension: ACCP evidence-based clinical practice guidelines. *Chest.* 2004;126(1 Suppl):14S–34S. doi: 10.1378/chest.126.1_suppl.14S.
35. Caldeira D, Loureiro MJ, Costa J, Pinto FJ, Ferreira JJ. Oral anticoagulation for pulmonary arterial hypertension: Systematic review and meta-analysis. *Can J Cardiol.* 2014;30(8):879–887.
36. Preston IR, Roberts K, Miller DP. Effect of warfarin treatment on survival of patients with pulmonary arterial hypertension (PAH) in the registry to evaluate early and long-term PAH disease management (REVEAL). *Circulation.* 2015;132:2403–2411.
37. Olsson KM, Delcroix M, Ghofrani H-A. Anticoagulation and survival in pulmonary arterial hypertension: Results from the comparative, prospective registry of newly initiated therapies for pulmonary hypertension (COMPERA). *Circulation.* 2014;129(1):57–65.
38. Bussotti M, Sommaruga M. Anxiety and depression in patients with pulmonary hypertension: Impact and management challenges. *Vasc Health Risk Manag.* 2018;14:349–360. 10.2147/vhrm.s147173.
39. Akagi S, Ogawa A, Miyaji K, Kusano K, Ito H, Matsubara H. Catecholamine support at the initiation of epoprostenol therapy in pulmonary arterial hypertension. *Ann Am Thorac Soc.* 2014;11(5):719–727. doi: 10.1513/AnnalsATS.201308-268OC.
40. Coons JC, Clarke M, Wanek MR, Bauer A, Bream-Rouwenhorst HR. Safe and effective use of prostacyclins to treat pulmonary arterial hypertension. *Am J Heal Pharm.* 2013;70(19):1716 LP–1723. http://www.ajhp.org/content/70/19/1716.abstract.
41. Kallen AJ, Lederman E, Trevino I, et al. Bloodstream infections in patients given treatment with intravenous prostanoids. *Infect Control Hosp Epidemiol.* 2008;29(4):342–349.
42. Badesch DB, Tapson VF, McGoon MD, et al. Continuous intravenous epoprostenol for pulmonary hypertension due to the scleroderma spectrum of disease. A randomized, controlled trial. *Ann Intern Med.* 2000;132(6):425–434. http://www.ncbi.nlm.nih.gov/pubmed/10733441.
43. Sitbon O, Humbert M, Nunes H, et al. Long-term intravenous epoprostenol infusion in primary pulmonary hypertension: Prognostic factors and survival. *J Am Coll Cardiol.* 2002;40(4):780–788. http://www.ncbi.nlm.nih.gov/pubmed/12204511.
44. Coons JC, Pogue K, Kolodziej AR, et al. Pulmonary arterial hypertension: A pharmacotherapeutic update. *Curr Cardiol Rep.* 2019;21:141. 10.1007/s11886-019-1235-4.
45. Simonneau G, Barst RJ, Galiè N, et al. Continuous subcutaneous infusion of treprostinil, a prostacyclin analogue, in patients with pulmonary arterial hypertension: A double-blind, randomized, placebo-controlled trial. *Am J Respir Crit Care Med.* 2002;165(6):800–804. doi: 10.1164/ajrccm.165.6.2106079.
46. Gomberg-Maitland M, Tapson VF, Benza RL, et al. Transition from intravenous epoprostenol to intravenous treprostinil in pulmonary hypertension. *Am J Respir Crit Care Med.* 2005;172(12):1586–1589. doi: 10.1164/rccm.200505-766OC.
47. Kitterman N, Poms A, Miller DP, Lombardi S, Farber HW, Barst RJ. Bloodstream infections in patients with pulmonary arterial hypertension treated with intravenous prostanoids: Insights from the REVEAL REGISTRY®. *Mayo Clin Proc.* 2012;87(9):825–834. doi: 10.1016/j.mayocp.2012.05.014.
48. Rich JD, Glassner C, Wade M, et al. The effect of diluent pH on bloodstream infection rates in patients receiving IV treprostinil for pulmonary arterial hypertension. *Chest.* 2012;141(1):36–42. doi: 10.1378/chest.11-0245.
49. Olschewski H, Simonneau G, Galiè N, et al. Inhaled iloprost for severe pulmonary hypertension. *N Engl J Med.* 2002;347(5):322–329. doi: 10.1056/NEJMoa020204.
50. McLaughlin VV, Benza RL, Rubin LJ, et al. Addition of inhaled treprostinil to oral therapy for pulmonary arterial hypertension: A randomized controlled clinical trial. *J Am Coll Cardiol.* 2010;55(18):1915–1922. doi: 10.1016/J.JACC.2010.01.027.
51. Benza RL, Seeger W, McLaughlin VV, et al. Long-term effects of inhaled treprostinil in patients with pulmonary arterial hypertension: The TReprostinil sodium Inhalation Used in the Management of Pulmonary arterial Hypertension (TRIUMPH) study open-label extension. *J Hear Lung Transplant.* 2011;30(12):1327–1333. doi: 10.1016/J.HEALUN.2011.08.019.
52. Jing Z-C, Parikh K, Pulido T, et al. Efficacy and safety of oral treprostinil monotherapy for the treatment of pulmonary arterial hypertension. *Circulation.* 2013;127(5):624–633. doi: 10.1161/CIRCULATIONAHA.112.124388.
53. Tapson VF, Torres F, Kermeen F, et al. Oral treprostinil for the treatment of pulmonary arterial hypertension in patients on background endothelin receptor antagonist and/or phosphodiesterase

type 5 inhibitor therapy (The FREEDOM-C Study): A randomized controlled trial. *Chest.* 2012;142(6):1383–1390. doi: 10.1378/CHEST.11-2212.

54. Tapson VF, Jing Z-C, Xu K-F, et al. Oral treprostinil for the treatment of pulmonary arterial hypertension in patients receiving background endothelin receptor antagonist and phosphodiesterase type 5 inhibitor therapy (The FREEDOM-C2 Study): A randomized controlled trial. *Chest.* 2013;144(3):952–958. doi: 10.1378/CHEST.12-2875.
55. Simonneau G, Torbicki A, Hoeper MM, et al. Selexipag: An oral, selective prostacyclin receptor agonist for the treatment of pulmonary arterial hypertension. *Eur Respir J.* 2012;40(4):874 LP–880. http://erj.ersjournals.com/content/40/4/874.abstract.
56. Sitbon O, Channick RC, Chin KM, et al. Selexipag for the treatment of pulmonary arterial hypertension. *N Engl J Med.* 2015;373(26):2522–2533. doi: 10.1056/NEJMoa1503184.
57. Coghlan JG, Channick R, Chin K, et al. Targeting the prostacyclin pathway with selexipag in patients with pulmonary arterial hypertension receiving double combination therapy: Insights from the randomized controlled GRIPHON study. *Am J Cardiovasc Drugs.* 2018;18(1):37–47. doi: 10.1007/s40256-017-0262-z.
58. Gaine S, Chin K, Coghlan G, et al. Selexipag for the treatment of connective tissue disease-associated pulmonary arterial hypertension. *Eur Respir J.* 2017;50(2):1602493. doi: 10.1183/13993003.02493-2016.
59. Gaine S, Sitbon O, Channick RN, et al. Relationship between time from diagnosis and morbidity/mortality in pulmonary arterial hypertension. *Chest.* 2021;160:277–286. 10.1016/j.chest.2021.01.066.
60. Galié N, Badesch D, Oudiz R, et al. Ambrisentan therapy for pulmonary arterial hypertension. *J Am Coll Cardiol.* 2005;46(3):529–535. doi: 10.1016/j.jacc.2005.04.050.
61. Barst RJ. A review of pulmonary arterial hypertension: Role of ambrisentan. *Vasc Health Risk Manag.* 2007;3(1):11–22. http://www.pubmedcentral.nih.gov/articlerender.fcgi?artid=1994051&tool=pmcentrez&rendertype=abstract.
62. Pulido T, Adzerikho I, Channick RN, et al. Macitentan and morbidity and mortality in pulmonary arterial hypertension. *N Engl J Med.* 2013;369(9):809–818. doi: 10.1056/NEJMoa1213917.
63. Hoeper MM, Leuchte H, Halank M, et al. Combining inhaled iloprost with bosentan in patients with idiopathic pulmonary arterial hypertension. *Eur Respir J.* 2006;28(4):691 LP–694. http://erj.ersjournals.com/content/28/4/691.abstract.
64. Humbert M, Barst RJ, Robbins IM, et al. Combination of bosentan with epoprostenol in pulmonary arterial hypertension: BREATHE-2. *Eur Respir J.* 2004;24(3):353 LP–359. http://erj.ersjournals.com/content/24/3/353.abstract.
65. Bishop BM, Mauro VF, Khouri SJ. Practical considerations for the pharmacotherapy of pulmonary arterial hypertension. *Pharmacother.* 2012;32:838–855. 10.1002/j.1875-9114.2012.01114.x.
66. Abraham T, Wu G, Vastey F, Rapp J, Saad N, Balmir E. Role of combination therapy in the treatment of pulmonary arterial hypertension. *Pharmacotherapy.* 2010;30(4):390–404. doi: 10.1592/phco.30.4.390.
67. Galiè N, Ghofrani HA, Torbicki A, et al. Sildenafil citrate therapy for pulmonary arterial hypertension. *N Engl J Med.* 2005;353(20):2148–2157. doi: 10.1056/NEJMoa050010.
68. Galiè N, Brundage BH, Ghofrani HA, et al. Tadalafil therapy for pulmonary arterial hypertension. *Circulation.* 2009;119:2894–2903. 10.1161/circulationaha.108.839274.
69. Ghofrani H-A, D'Armini AM, Grimminger F, et al. Riociguat for the treatment of chronic thromboembolic pulmonary hypertension. *N Engl J Med.* 2013;369(4):319–329. doi: 10.1056/NEJMoa1209657.
70. Lajoie AC, Lauziere G, Lega J-C, et al. Combination therapy versus monotherapy for pulmonary arterial hypertension: A meta-analysis. *Lancet Respir Med.* 2016;4(4):291–305.
71. Galiè N, Barberà JA, Frost AE, et al. Initial use of ambrisentan plus tadalafil in pulmonary arterial hypertension. *N Engl J Med.* 2015;373:834–844. 10.1056/nejmoa1413687.
72. Pulido T, Adzerikho I, Channick RN, et al. Macitentan and morbidity and mortality in pulmonary arterial hypertension. *N Engl J Med.* 2013;369:809–818. 10.1056/nejmoa1213917.
73. Sitbon O, Channick R, Chin KM, et al. Selexipag for the treatment of pulmonary arterial hypertension. *N Engl J Med.* 2015;373:2522–2533. 10.1056/nejmoa1503184.
74. Gaine S, Sitbon O, Channick RN, et al. Relationship between time from diagnosis and morbidity/mortality in pulmonary arterial hypertension. *Chest.* 2021;160:277–286. 10.1016/j.chest.2021.01.066.
75. Simonneau G, Rubin LJ, Galiè N, et al. Addition of sildenafil to long-term intravenous epoprostenol therapy in patients with pulmonary arterial hypertension: A randomized trial. *Ann Intern Med.* 2008;149(8):521–530. http://www.ncbi.nlm.nih.gov/pubmed/18936500.
76. Chin KM, Sitbon O, Doelberg M, et al. Three- versus two-drug therapy for patients with newly diagnosed pulmonary arterial hypertension. *J Am Coll Cardiol.* 2021;78:1393–1403. 10.1016/j.jacc.2021.07.057.
77. Humbert M, McLaughlin V, Gibbs JSR, et al. Sotatercept for the treatment of pulmonary arterial hypertension. *N Engl J Med.* 2021;384:1204–1215. 10.1056/nejmoa2024277.

47

Cystic Fibrosis

Kim G. Adcock, Ha K. Phan, and David Josey Jr.

KEY CONCEPTS

1. Cystic fibrosis (CF) is caused by a functional loss of the cystic fibrosis transmembrane conductance regulator (CFTR) gene. This leads to reduced chloride and bicarbonate secretion and a buildup of thick mucus throughout the body affecting the lungs, pancreas, liver, intestine, and reproductive tract. Thus, CF is a multisystem disease with most patients experiencing a wide range of symptoms and diverse organ complications.
2. Three classes of CFTR modulators play an important role in the treatment of CF. Although there is no cure for CF, the CFTR modulator class of medications alleviates and corrects the underlying pathophysiology.
3. Infection is one of the main causes of morbidity and mortality in patients with CF and contributes to CF lung disease. Treating infections in CF involves not only antibiotics but chest physiotherapy and inhaled mucolytics play an important adjunction role. Strategies should be employed to prevent *Pseudomonas aeruginosa* acquisition including measures to prevent transmission between CF patients and early eradication of both *P. aeruginosa* and *Staphylococcus aureus* with appropriate treatment regimens. Chronic colonization with *P. aeruginosa* necessitates chronic treatment with inhaled antibiotics.
4. Pancreatic exocrine insufficiency occurs in CF patients as a result of pancreatic duct obstruction. If left untreated, pancreatic insufficiency leads to growth failure, weight loss, abdominal bloating, foul-smelling stools, or diarrhea. Pancreatic enzyme replacement therapy is the treatment of choice.
5. Dosing of antibiotics in CF patients can be a challenge to ensure adequate lung penetration and maximum bactericidal activity. In addition, the pharmacokinetics of antibiotics in CF patients differ compared to most other individuals. The volume of distribution and total body clearance is increased in CF patients for hydrophilic drugs such as aminoglycosides, penicillins, and cephalosporins. Specifically, the initial dose of aminoglycosides is higher in CF patients when compared to the general population and adjusted based on patient-specific pharmacokinetic parameters.
6. CF is a multi-system disease requiring a multimodal treatment approach administered through a multidisciplinary team to provide optimal care and the best patient outcomes. With the advancements in science and treatment options, not only is the quality of life for cystic fibrosis patients increasing but their lifespan is extending.

BEYOND THE BOOK

1. Create a concept map that interlinks cystic fibrosis pathophysiology and its complications with appropriate medication regimens. This activity will help develop the learner's application of treatment strategies with the underlying pathophysiology and complications of the disease.
2. Review the case study "Cystic Fibrosis: Blood, Sweat, Lungs, and Gut Level III," by Novak, Kimberly J. in *Pharmacotherapy Casebook: A Patient-Focused Approach*, 11e Eds. Terry L. Schwinghammer, et al. McGraw Hill, 2020. Write a pharmacokinetic SOAP note based on the serum tobramycin concentrations obtained in the case. This activity will help develop the learner's application of pharmacokinetic principles and practice communication of recommendations based on patient-specific pharmacokinetic parameters.

INTRODUCTION

Cystic fibrosis (CF) is the most common autosomal recessive disease in the Caucasian population with a prevalence of approximately 1/3,500 live births.[1] First described in 1938, CF was initially thought to be a disease of malnutrition since malnutrition was the cause of death in these children in early childhood but is now known to be a genetic disorder.[2] Mutations of a gene that encodes the cystic fibrosis transmembrane conductance regulator (CFTR), a chloride-conducting transmembrane channel, impairs the regulation of chloride and other anion transport and results in thickened, viscous secretions in many organ systems, including the pulmonary, biliary, pancreatic, intestinal, and reproductive systems.[3] The resultant organ dysfunction not only encapsulated the initial findings of malnutrition due to maldigestion and malabsorption but also signifies the progressive lung disease that now highlights the major cause of morbidity and mortality in most patients.

CF currently affects more than 30,000 people in the United States and approximately 80,000 people worldwide. However, CF is no longer exclusively a childhood disease. Advancements in therapy have enabled most CF patients to live into adulthood.[2] More than half of the CF patients in the United States are adults.[4] The median predicted survival age has steadily increased over the past decade and was approximately 48 years in 2019. It is likely the median survival age will continue to increase as the impact of newer therapies such as the CFTR modulators are realized.

EPIDEMIOLOGY

Cystic fibrosis occurs in a classic single-gene (Mendelian) autosomal recessive pattern.[5,6] Autosomal recessive patterns of inheritance require both parents to be carriers of the gene. CF occurs most commonly in the populations of people of northern European ancestry where the predominant mutation is delta F508 (which is a deletion of phenylalanine at position 508 on the long arm of chromosome 7 also known as F508del).[5,6] This mutation accounts for approximately 70% of all mutations. The disease incidence in other populations is less defined but has been reported to be 1 in 17,033 live births for Black American patients, 1 in 12,000 in mixed-race South Africans, and 1 in 90,000 in Asian populations (Chinese, Japanese, and Filipino) living in Hawaii.[7] To date more than 2,000 gene variants have been identified many of which have been associated with disease causation.[8]

ETIOLOGY

The gene for CF, localized to the long arm of chromosome 7, encodes a protein of 1,480 amino acids residues.[9] This CFTR protein is found in the apical membrane of epithelial cells and regulates the transepithelial transport of chloride, other ions, and water.

The CFTR mutations can be grouped into six classes (Fig. 47-1).[6,10] Classes 1 to 3 are known as minimal function mutations as they confer no, or hardly any, CFTR function. Class 1 mutations, referred to as protein production mutations, affect the transcription of CFTR by the formation of premature stop codons into the messenger RNA. This results in a total absence of the CFTR protein. Class 2 mutations, protein processing mutations, or trafficking defects, involve intracellular processing of the CFTR protein. CFTR protein is produced but is misfolded, making it unstable and leading to degradation. The most notable Class 2 mutation is delta F 508. Class 3 mutations (defective channel regulation or gating mutations) alter the regulation of CFTR. While the CFTR is intact and incorporated into the cell membrane surface, this mutation affects channel activation, reducing its opening probability. Class 4 mutations, referred to as conduction mutations, affect the chloride conductance of CFTR. The CFTR protein channel can be activated to open and secrete chloride but the conductance is reduced. Class 5 mutations result in the production of CFTR protein with normal chloride secretion but a decreased number of CFTR channels. Finally, Class 6 mutations result in an accelerated CFTR turnover from the cell surface resulting in decreased CFTR stability.

Patients with at least one mutation of class 4, 5, or 6 typically have a later onset of disease, lower sweat chloride values, slower decline in lung function, less chronic *Pseudomonas aeruginosa* infections, less CF-related diabetes, and lower treatment burden.[11] Together, these mutations are called residual function mutations.

PATHOPHYSIOLOGY

CF is caused by a mutation in the CF transmembrane conductance regulator gene.[12] The CFTR protein produced by this gene regulates

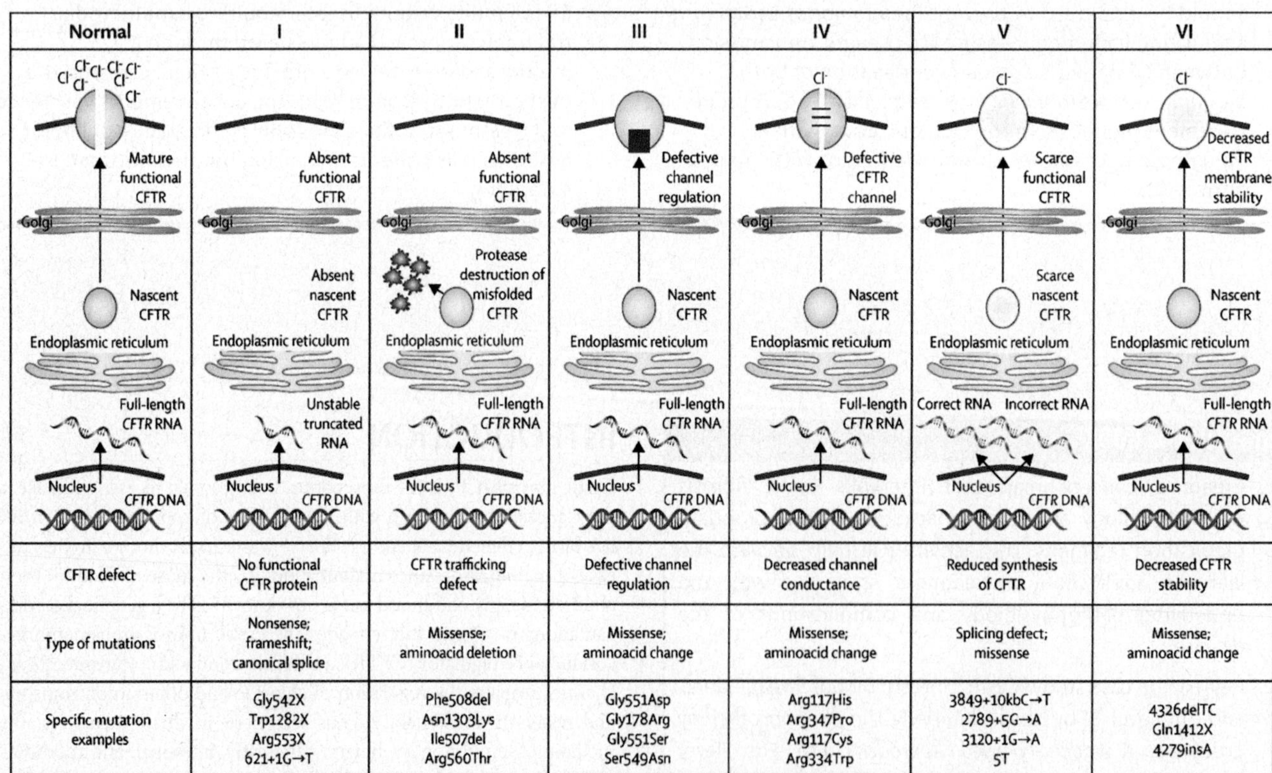

FIGURE 47-1 Mutations in the cystic fibrosis transmembrane conducatance regulator (CFTR) gene can be divided into six classes. Class I mutations result in no protein production. Class II mutations (including the most prevalent, Phe508del) cause retention of a misfolded protein at the endoplasmic reticulum, and subsequent degradation in the proteasome. Class III mutations affect channel regulation, impairing channel opening (eg, Gly551Asp). Class IV mutants show reduced conduction—ie, decreased flow of ions (eg, Arg117His). Class V mutations cause substantial reduction in mRNA or protein, or both, Class VI mutations cause substantial plasma membrane instability and and include Phe508del when rescued by most correctors (fPhe508del). *(Reproduced with permission from Boyle MP, De Boeck K. A new era in the treatment of cystic fibrosis: correction of the underlying CFTR defect. Lancet Respir Med 2013;1:158-163.)*

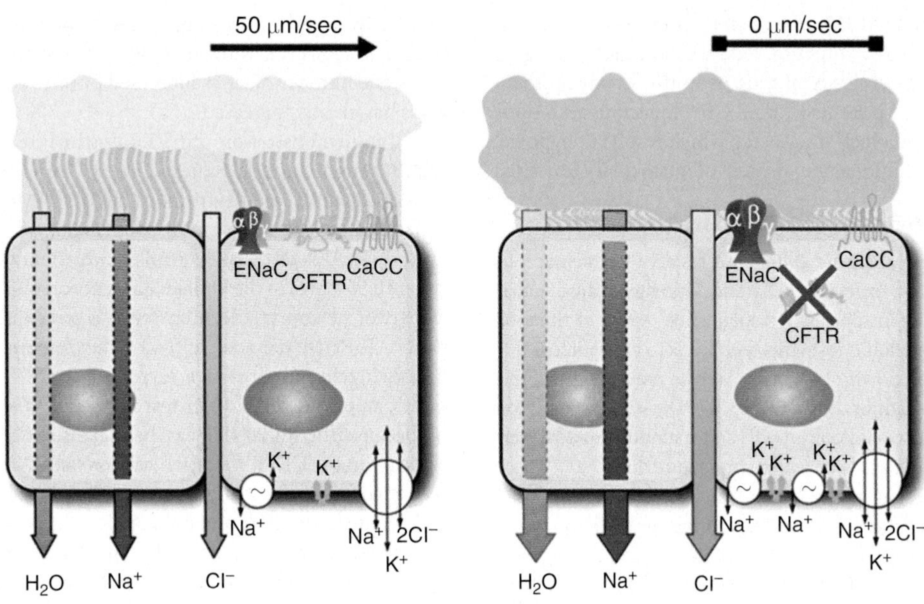

FIGURE 47-2 Illustration of the normal and abnormal movement of chloride and sodium ions across epithelial cell membranes. ENaC, amiloride sensitive epithelial Na+ channel; CFTR, cystic fibrosis transmembrane conductance regulator; CaCC, calcium-activated Cl− channels.

the movement of chloride and sodium ions across epithelial cell membranes (Fig. 47-2). CFTR functions primarily as an apical anion channel of chloride and bicarbonate, rather than an active pump. Loss of apical CFTR leads to reduced chloride and bicarbonate secretion, resulting in a buildup of thick mucus throughout the body including in the lungs, pancreas, liver, intestine, and reproductive tract. This defect also leads to increased salt content in sweat gland secretions. Thus, cystic fibrosis is a multisystem disease with most patients experiencing a wide range of symptoms and diverse organ complications.

Pulmonary Manifestations

Although CFTR mainly functions as an anion transporter, it also regulates numerous processes, including fundamental aspects of airway defense and inflammatory cell function.[13] The release of water and electrolytes onto the airway surface is driven in large measure by CFTR-dependent fluid secretion through both the sweat glands and the surface epithelia. A CFTR deficiency leads to diminished airway surface hydration, thickened mucus secretions, and accumulation that compromises the airway lumen, submucosal gland hyperplasia, and impaired mucociliary transport.[14,15] Airway disease likely begins in the small airways with the development of bronchiectasis whereby the walls of the bronchioles are thickened from infection and inflammation. This leads to irreversible changes that encourage continued infection, accelerate disease pathogenesis, and ultimately, obstructive pulmonary disease.[15]

The inflammatory response contributes to a pro-inflammatory state that sets up chronic infections and further tissue damage.[16] The massive influx of neutrophils to the airways further exacerbates inflammatory cell recruitment, perpetuating a cycle of inflammation and damage. In addition, in the CF airways, neutrophils undergo necrosis instead of apoptosis and clearance by alveolar macrophages that occurs in healthy lung tissue. This necrosis leads to the release of intracellular contents further eliciting a persistent inflammatory response. This exaggerated inflammatory process plays an essential role in the progression of airway wall remodeling, lung damage, and lung function decline in CF patients. With the colonization by bacterial pathogens, overly exaggerated protective mechanisms result in the release of proteases, reactive oxygen/nitrogen species, and proinflammatory chemokines. CFTR also regulates anion secretions through other chloride channels such as transmembrane member 16a (TMEM16a; also known as anoctamin-1) and contributes to airway pH regulation through chloride exchangers, such as anion exchanger type 2. Dysfunction of these mechanisms results in diminished or absent bicarbonate secretion leading to an acidic pH airway surface liquid in cystic fibrosis. This may lead to changes in the highly pH-sensitive innate defensins and defective bacterial killing.[17,18] CFTR also has a direct effect on neutrophil killing, as it affects degranulation by interfering with granule trafficking as peripheral neutrophils release fewer secondary and tertiary granule components compared with control cells. Activation of the low-molecular-mass GTP-binding protein Rab27a, involved in the regulation of granule trafficking, is also defective.

Chronic pulmonary infections adversely impact the quality of life and can lead to respiratory failure which is the leading cause of death in patients with CF.[19] The decreased airway surface liquid volume leads to a collapse of respiratory cilia, impaired mucociliary clearance, and mucus retention on the lower airways. Under these conditions, inhaled microorganisms cannot be efficiently cleared and this predisposes CF patients to chronic bacterial infection and recurrent pulmonary exacerbations. The most common microorganisms that cause chronic pulmonary infections are *P. aeruginosa*, *Staphylococcus aureus*, *Stenotrophomonas maltophilia*, and *Burkholderia cepacia*. CF patients are not infected at birth but acquire these organisms over time. Viral infections such as Rhinovirus and Influenza A and B and fungal infections such as Aspergillus fumigatus are also prevalent in the population.

Finally, mucus accumulation in the lower airways is the main feature of CF lung disease. The major component of mucus in CF is not mucin from mucus-producing cells but rather a pus that includes viscous materials such as polymerized DNA from degraded neutrophils.

Upper Airway Manifestations

Due to the increased viscous mucus that accumulates in the sinuses, chronic rhinosinusitis is common and nasal polyposis is a complication noted in up to 45% of patients.[15] Imbalance of electrolyte transport from CFTR dysfunction reduces airway surface liquid depth and increases the viscosity of mucins in the airway 30 to 60 times higher than seen in patients without CF.[20] Tenacious secretions and tissue inflammation block sinus ostia, which results in hypoxia, mucosal edema, and additional impairment of mucociliary function.

Gastrointestinal Manifestations

Defective CFTR in the pancreatic epithelium results in proteinaceous secretions that block the exocrine ducts and ultimately cause acinar destruction.[14] Pancreatic insufficiency results when >95% of the total pancreatic exocrine function is lost. This then leads to nutrient loss due to the inability to break down nutrients as well as reduced fat-soluble vitamin absorption (Vitamins A, D, E, and K). The early recognition of nutritional deficits is vital. Poor growth and malnutrition adversely affect pulmonary function and can lead to premature death.

CFTR is also present in the GI epithelium and, like the lung, reduced chloride and fluid secretion lead to mucus buildup in the intestines resulting in obstruction of the intestines. Impaired bowel transit can lead to frequent gastro-esophageal reflux, distal intestinal obstruction syndrome, and constipation, depending on the site of obstruction.

Hepatic involvement is also common. Up to one in three patients have evidence of hepatic steatosis, cholelithiasis, ductal stenosis, or focal biliary cirrhosis due to the accumulation of viscous secretions that clog the biliary tract.[21] Biliary cirrhosis typically becomes evident in late childhood or early adolescence and leads to portal hypertension. Patients with liver disease may be classified into the following categories: (1) liver involvement with cirrhosis/portal hypertension or (2) liver involvement without cirrhosis or portal hypertension. Advanced liver disease may be found in patients with PI. Risk factors for advanced liver disease include male gender and the presence of alpha-1 antitrypsin Z allele. Typically, patients with a CFTR mutation that belongs to class I to III are more likely to have abnormalities of the hepatobiliary system.

Endocrine Manifestations

Cystic fibrosis-related diabetes (CFRD) is increasingly common as more patients with CF live longer. CFRD is clinically distinct from type 1 and type 2 diabetes mellitus. CFRD is thought to be related to loss of insulin-producing islet cells due to autolysis and fatty infiltration of the pancreas, pancreatic duct obstruction from the accumulation of viscous secretions, and decreased islet cell mass, all of which lead to both insulin and glucagon deficiency, altered intestinal motility, and delayed gastric emptying.[22] Unlike type 1 diabetes, the loss of islet cells in CFRD is not due to an autoimmune process.[23] The course is progressive in nature, and patients may move back and forth between an impaired state and CFRD. Uncontrolled CFRD may correlate with pulmonary function decline, weight loss, and *P. aeruginosa*.

Other endocrinological complications of cystic fibrosis include delayed menarche in malnourished adolescent females and reduced bone mineral density, increasing the risk of bone fractures. A bilateral absence of the vas deferens occurs in 98% of males with cystic fibrosis and results in azoospermia. Most males with CF are infertile.

Renal Manifestations

Nephrocalcinosis due to salt and water depletion can result in acute kidney injury and proteinuria.[14] Chronic kidney disease is more common in adult patients and risk factors for its development include diabetes, prior episodes of acute kidney injury, and immunosuppressive regimens associated with prior organ transplantation.

CLINICAL PRESENTATION

Historically, cystic fibrosis was diagnosed based on presenting symptoms such as meconium ileus, respiratory symptoms (persistent productive cough, wheezing, or any breathing difficulty), or failure to thrive. However, with the newborn screening programs now in place, the number of cases identified prior to presenting with symptoms has greatly increased.

The demonstration of CFTR dysfunction using a "sweat test" requires high chloride values in sweat (≥60 mmol/L) in two independent measurements on the same day.[24] Molecular genetic tests constitute the second stage of confirmatory diagnostic testing (see Fig. 47-3). This test also determines which mutations are present.

All 50 states in the United States now require cystic fibrosis tests as part of newborn screening.[26] It is a screening test and not diagnostic. The first-tier screen in all state screening programs involves measuring immunoreactive trypsinogen (IRT), a marker of pancreatic injury. A second-tier test is needed to improve test specificity because the initial IRT can be increased due to perinatal stress, critical illness, CFTR mutation carrier status, and other causes. The second-tier test differs between state newborn screening programs and can include CFTR mutation analysis, measurement of pancreas-associated protein, or repeat IRT. The diagnosis must be confirmed by a positive sweat test or, alternatively, by genetic tests demonstrating two disease-causing mutations.

With the increase in newborn screening, new categories of infants who do not meet the classic definition of CF have arisen. Infants identified at risk for CF through newborn screening who have an in-determinate sweat chloride (30-59 mmol/L) and less than two known disease-causing CFTR mutations are classified as having Cystic Fibrosis–Related Metabolic Syndrome (CRMS).[27] An additional diagnostic category, CFTR-Related Disorder, is used for patients who do not meet diagnostic criteria for CF, but have clinical disease limited to an isolated CF-related condition or organ system, such as congenital bilateral absence of the vas deferens (CBAVD).[28] Many of these patients have mutations in the CFTR gene that are not considered the classic disease-causing mutations. For example, some patients with CFTR-Related Disorder have the 5T variant which is a common mild variant and causes abnormal splicing of the CFTR gene transcript. Most individuals with two copies of this variant are asymptomatic but some may have an absence of the vas deferens or bronchiectasis. Patients without a definitive diagnosis of CF are continued to be followed for symptom progression and potentially reclassification later in life.

Diagnosis of liver disease can include a physical exam which may reveal ascites, palmar erythema, digital clubbing, scleral icterus, spider hemangiomas, and hepatosplenomegaly.[21] Additionally, evaluation of liver function panel and obtaining lab work for alpha-1 antitrypsin deficiency, Wilson disease, and hemochromatosis should be included. Imaging and a liver biopsy may also be performed to determine the extent of the liver disease and exclude other causes. There are annual labs that can identify CFLD early; these include complete blood count (CBC), prothrombin time, liver function panel, gamma-glutamyl-transferase (GGTP), albumin, cholesterol, and glucose.

In CFRD, patients often do not present with the classic symptoms of diabetes such as polyuria and polydipsia.[23] There may be no symptoms, or there may be poor growth velocity, delayed progression of puberty, and unexplained chronic decline in pulmonary function. Screening for CFRD should occur annually in patients aged 10 and older as recommended by the American Diabetes Association (ADA). Additionally, women with CF who are not previously known to have CFRD and who are contemplating pregnancy should be evaluated for CFRD utilizing a 2-hour, 75-g oral glucose tolerance test (OGTT). If screening has not occurred within the last 6 months, screening should occur in women prior to conception because women with CF are at higher risk for developing hyperglycemia. Screening is typically done as an OGTT for all patients with CF. An A1c reading of ≥6.5% (48 mmol/mol) may indicate CFRD; however, an A1c should be used in combination with an OGTT as

CLINICAL PRESENTATION Cystic Fibrosis

General

- Typical respiratory manifestations include persistent productive cough, hyperinflation of the lung fields, and obstructive findings on pulmonary function tests. Other manifestations may include GI, endocrine, and renal abnormalities.

Diagnosis

- Two diagnostic components and a combination of criteria.[24]
- At least one clinical feature of the disease (such as failure to thrive, malabsorption, chronic sinopulmonary disease), a history of a sibling with the disease, or a positive neonatal screening test.
- The second diagnostic component is the demonstration of CFTR dysfunction which can be established either by sweat testing or by molecular genetic testing (Fig. 47-3).[25]
  - The demonstration of CFTR dysfunction using a "sweat test" requires high chloride values in sweat (≥60 mmol/L) in two independent measurements on the same day.[24] Values below 29 mmol/L make cystic fibrosis unlikely; values between 30 and 59 mmol/L require further diagnostic testing.
  - Infants identified at risk for CF through newborn screening who have an in-determinate sweat chloride (30-59 mmol/L) and less than two known disease-causing CFTR mutations are classified as having Cystic Fibrosis–Related Metabolic Syndrome (CRMS).[27]
  - CFTR-Related Disorder is used for patients who do not meet diagnostic criteria for CF but have clinical disease limited to an isolated CF-related condition or organ system, such as the congenital bilateral absence of the vas deferens (CBAVD).[28]

Signs and Symptoms

- Disease progression results in acute exacerbations with cough, tachypnea, dyspnea, increased sputum production, malaise, anorexia, and weight loss.
- Digital clubbing is often seen in advanced disease as well. Sinus involvement can present with chronic nasal congestion, headaches, cough, and sleep disturbance.
- Common signs and symptoms of pancreatic insufficiency include steatorrhea, poor weight gain, and failure to thrive.
- In CFRD, patients often do not present with the classic symptoms of diabetes such as polyuria and polydipsia.[23] There may be no symptoms, or there may be poor growth velocity, delayed progression of puberty, and unexplained chronic decline in pulmonary function.

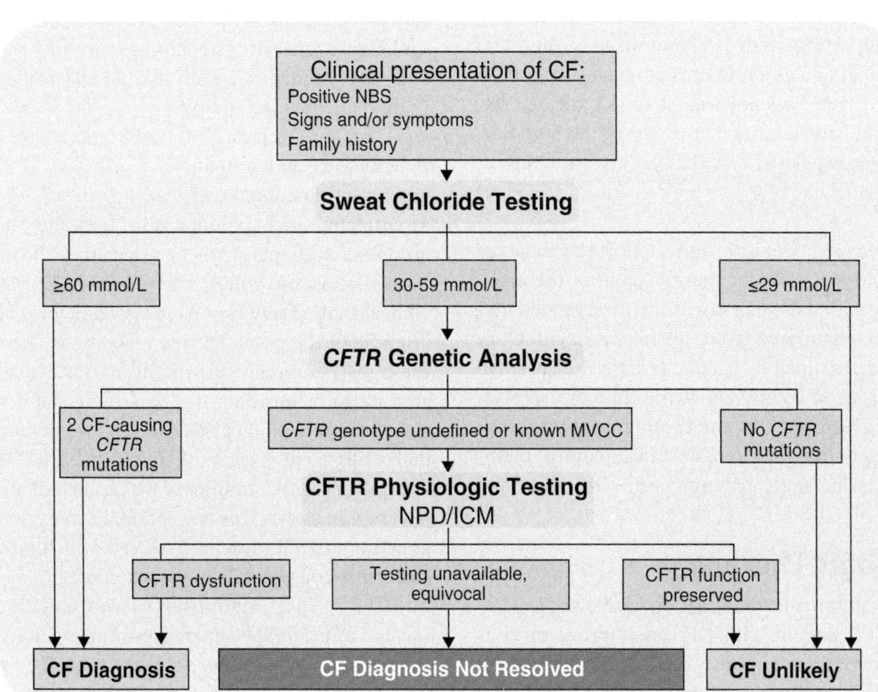

FIGURE 47-3 CFF diagnostic algorithm. (CFTR, cystic fibrosis transmembrane conductance regulator; ICM, intestinal current measurements; MVCC, mutation of varying clinical consequence; NBS, newborn screen; NPD, nasal potential difference.)

a confirmation of CFRD. Fructosamine, urine glucose, and random glucose levels have low sensitivity in patients with CF. The OGTT should be administered following stable baseline health for at least 6 weeks and patients should consume at least 150 carbohydrates for 3 days prior and fast for 8 hours prior to the OGTT.

TREATMENT

Desired Outcome(s)

The overall goal of treatment is to enable each person with cystic fibrosis to live a full and productive life. Optimizing treatment to reduce pulmonary exacerbations, delaying colonization by pathogens, and maintaining lung health is key to improving survival. In addition, maximizing adequate nutrition with appropriate dosing of pancreatic enzymes and vitamin supplementation contributes to accomplishing the desired outcomes. Furthermore, with the development of the CFTR modulators and as other disease-modifying therapies become available, every patient should receive treatments that address the underlying pathophysiology of the disease.

General Approach to Treatment

Pulmonary and Sinus

The goal of treatment is to prevent and treat sinusitis and acute pulmonary exacerbations. Routine care goals are to maintain the FEV1 and promote optimal pulmonary function tests. Effective airway clearance is promoted with counseling on the use of appropriate medications and airway clearance techniques (ACT) at least twice a day. Prevention and treatment of bacterial colonization with oral and inhaled therapies are also keys to maintaining lung function.

Gastrointestinal

Optimizing growth and nutrition is done primarily with the use of pancreatic enzyme supplementation. This in turn will promote healthy bowel habits and maintenance of appropriate fat-soluble vitamin levels (Vitamins A, D, E, and K). Vitamin levels are checked at least yearly and some such as Vitamin D can have seasonal variations. Evaluating and supporting needed caloric intake is important to promote good lung function and symptoms of malabsorption are evaluated at every clinic visit. Patients' weight for length or body mass index (BMI) should be maintained at or above the 50th percentile because it has been associated with the best lung functions.

Psychosocial

Each patient will need ongoing education and support to encourage adherence to pharmacological and nonpharmacological therapies. Counseling to help cope with a lifelong disease, as well as guidance to live a fulfilling life, are paramount to successful treatment. Once patients' mutations are determined by genetic testing, it is essential to provide appropriate genetic counseling at the time of diagnosis and periodically thereafter. As patients and significant others reach reproductive age it is key to offer both possible birth control methods and support couples in family planning with education and resources.

Nonpharmacologic Therapy

Exercise, infection prevention control, nutrition, and airway clearance are ways in which a patient with CF can improve mucous obstruction and avoid chronic infections. There is not a specified length of time in which exercise is recommended by the Cystic Fibrosis Foundation; however, the purpose is to loosen mucous and clear the airways.[29] Shorter exercises that are enjoyable and tolerated by patients are the best exercises. Sodium loss may occur during intense exercise, and repletion is necessary to avoid dehydration.

The Cystic Fibrosis Foundation sets forth several recommendations for infection prevention. Patients with CF should engage in regular hand hygiene throughout the day using an antimicrobial soap or alcohol-based hand rub. All patients with CF should adhere to the six-foot rule to reduce droplet transmission. Patients with CF should wear a surgical mask when in a healthcare setting to reduce transmission or acquisition of CF pathogens.[30]

Patients with CF often need 1.5 to 2 times the number of calories as patients without CF. Nutrition plays an essential role in pulmonary function and bone health. Weight for length is a measure that is used to track patients who are under the age of two and body mass index (BMI) is typically used after the age of two. The CF Foundation recommends that children younger than 2 should reach a weight-for-length >50th percentile by 2 years of age and children and adolescents 2- to 20 years old should be at or above the 50th percentile for BMI.[31] In adults, women should be encouraged to maintain a BMI of at least 22 and for men, a BMI of 23 is recommended.

Airway clearance techniques (ACT) include percussion and postural drainage, positive expiratory pressure (PEP), active-cycle-of-breathing technique, autogenic drainage, oscillatory PEP, high-frequency chest compression, and exercise. One way to facilitate airway clearance is through the use of a vest. A vest uses high-frequency chest wall oscillation that is performed by a machine. Use of the vest loosens and thins mucus. These sessions typically last about 20 to 30 minutes. Airway clearance may also be done manually by a parent or caregiver. The caregiver uses a variety of hand-to-chest techniques, typically lasting 3-5 minutes, to help loosen and drain the mucus. These techniques can include clapping with a cupped hand and creating vibration with a flattened hand. The best times to complete chest physical therapy (CPT) is before meals or one and a half hours to two hours after eating. CPT may be performed more frequently if the patient is congested or getting sick.

Pharmacologic Therapy

Genetic Therapies

CFTR Modulators Understanding the defect with each class of mutations helps identify the role the three classes of CFTR modulators play in the treatment of CF.[32] Even though no cure to treat the underlying cause of cystic fibrosis currently exists, the CFTR modulator class of medications is used to alleviate and correct part of the underlying pathophysiology.

The three classes of CFTR modulators include correctors, potentiators, and amplifiers. Correctors work by increasing the amount of functional CFTR at the cell surface. Medications labeled as correctors include lumacaftor, tezacaftor, and elexacaftor. There are a few additional correctors that are in the pipeline which include posenacaftor, dirocaftor, and ABBV-2222, which are currently in clinical trials. There is only one potentiator on the market, ivacaftor. The role of the potentiator is to keep the channel open to increase the transport of chloride in and out of the cell. VX-561 is deuterated ivacaftor meaning that it is more stable in the body than the current formulation of ivacaftor and would be able to be taken once daily. This agent is currently in phase 2 trial. The last class of CFTR modulators is the amplifiers which include one agent in the pipeline, nesolicafator. This class of medications works by increasing the amount of CFTR protein in the cell, which provides more CFTR for correctors and potentiators to act upon.

The CFTR modulators have mutation-specific and age-specific indications. General recommendations for the selection of a CF modulator are therefore based on the age of the patient and the mutation. For delta F508 homozygotes older than 6 years of age, elexacaftor/tezacaftor/ivacaftor combination is recommended. For delta F508 homozygous children between 2 and 5 years of age should be started on lumacaftor/ivacaftor combination. Patients can be transitioned from dual therapy to triple therapy as they increase

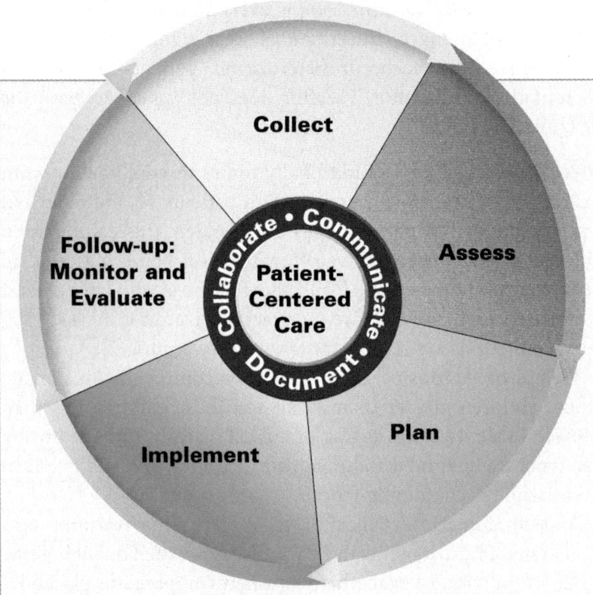

PATIENT CARE PROCESS

Collect

- Patient characteristics
  - o Age
  - o Race/ethnicity
  - o Sex assignment
  - o Gender preferred pronouns
- Symptoms
  - o Sputum production color and production
  - o Cough
  - o Shortness of breath
  - o Stool frequency and description
- Diagnostic Screening
  - o Newborn screening
  - o Genetic mutations
  - o Sweat test
- Patient history (past medical history, family history, birth history)
  - o History of hospitalizations
  - o History of infections (particularly resistant organisms)
  - o Complications of CF (eg, CF renal disease, CF lung disease)
  - o Past surgical history (eg, G-tube placement)
  - o Reproductive history
- Social history
  - o Home and work environment (infection control, dedicated space, and time for treatments)
  - o Insurance status and income history may be used to qualify for grants
  - o Eating habits
- Current medication and history of past medication use, herbals, dietary supplements, and over the counter products
- Objective data
  - o Respiratory function (FEV1, oxygen saturation)
  - o Nutritional status (height, weight, BMI)
  - o Mental status (PHQ-9 and GAD-7)
  - o Labwork: CBC, CMP, Lipids, Liver function, Vitamin D
- Immunization status and history

Assess

- Medication effectiveness and safety (reduction in symptoms, ADEs)
- Medication adherence to prescribed medications (schedule, costs, dietary supplements)
- Barriers to medication use
- Adherence to respiratory therapy (vest and technique)
- Nutritional status (BMI, calorie intake)
- Lung function (exacerbations)
- Emotional well-being of patient, family, and caregivers
- Exercise tolerance
- Comorbidities

Plan*

- Infection control and environmental modifications
- Medication plan (timing, order of medications, doses, route, formulation, frequency, duration)
- Labs
  - o CBC and CMP yearly
  - o Sputum culture quarterly
  - o Liver panel quarterly for the first year of modulator therapy
  - o 25-hydroxyvitamin D, retinol, alpha-tocopherol, prothrombin time, PIVKA II, and OGTT annually
- Referrals (endocrinology, urology, gastroenterology, ob-gyn, transplant, infectious disease, audiology, ophthalmology)

Implement*

- Patient/family education on the purpose of each medication
- Use motivational interviewing and coaching strategies to maximize adherence
- Schedule follow-up

Follow-up: Monitor and Evaluate

- Results of lab work and sputum cultures
- Medication access and adherence
- Medication changes based on results of lab work
- Sick visits to decrease the need for hospitalization
- Home infusions of antibiotics when necessary and available

**In collaboration with the patient, caregiver, and other healthcare professionals on the team (social worker, dietitian, respiratory therapist, pulmonologist, nurses).*

in age. For delta F508 heterozygous patients who are 6 years of age or older, triple therapy is recommended. Tezacaftor/ivacaftor may be used for children 6 and older, whereas ivacaftor alone may be used in infants greater than 4 months old. As the FDA approves additional modulators and adjusts the age-specific labeling of current modulators, recommendations for a CF modulator will need to follow suit.

Even though adverse effects with the CFTR modulators are often mild, monitoring for the elevation of transaminases and cataracts is currently recommended. Assessments of transaminases (ALT, AST, and/or bilirubin) are recommended for all patients prior to initiating the currently approved CF modulators, every 3 months during the first year of treatment, and annually thereafter.

In addition, baseline and follow-up ophthalmological examinations are recommended in pediatric patients initiating treatment with these agents. Of particular note, a subgroup of patients develops chest discomfort and dyspnea after initiating the combination of lumacaftor/ivacaftor.[33] These patients tend to have worse baseline lung function. Initiating treatment with a one-half dose for the first 1-2 weeks may help prevent treatment discontinuations in patients with severe lung disease.[34] However, there was no increase in chest discomfort, bronchospasm, dyspnea, or wheezing with tezacaftor as seen with lumacaftor/ivacaftor.[35,36]

Caution should also be used when CFTR modulator medications are used concomitantly with CYP3A4 inducers or inhibitors. Even though tezacaftor/ivacaftor are substrates of CYP3A and co-administration with strong CYP3A inducers is not recommended, texacaftor/ivacaftor combination appears to have fewer drug interactions than the lumacaftor/ivacaftor combination.

Current CFTR modulators are administered with a high-fat meal to improve absorption. Some examples of high-fat foods include eggs, peanut butter, avocado, butter, cheese pizza, and whole-milk dairy products.

CFTR Correctors

Lumacaftor Lumacaftor is manufactured in combination with ivacaftor which works to potentiate and enhance chloride transport.[37] This combination product is currently approved for use in patients homozygous for delta F 508 for ages two and up. The formulation usually is dosed as two tablets of lumacaftor 200 mg/ivacaftor 125 mg every 12 hours with fat-containing food to help with medication absorption. See Table 47-1 for dosing and dosing formulations.

The outcomes that were studied when looking at the efficacy of lumacaftor/ivacaftor included FEV1, BMI, and exacerbations.[38] In homozygous delta F508 participants, clinical studies demonstrated statistically significant improvements in percent predicted FEV1 along with improvements in body mass index and quality-of-life measures at both low and high doses (400 or 600 mg of lumacaftor in combination with ivacaftor 250 mg every 12 hours for 24 weeks). In addition, pulmonary exacerbations were significantly reduced when compared to placebo. In heterozygous patients for the delta F508 mutation, lumacaftor/ivacaftor does not appear to have the same clinical benefits.[39]

Tezacaftor Tezacaftor is additionally found in combination with ivacaftor.[36] It was previously approved in patients 12 and older but has now expanded to patients ages 6 and older. This combination is different from lumacaftor/ivacaftor due to it being indicated in patients that are homozygous for F508del or those who have at least one mutation that is responsive to tezacaftor/ivacaftor. At least 150 different mutations are eligible for tezacaftor/ivacaftor.

Weight-based dosing is used with recommendations made for those children greater than 30 kg and those children less than 30 kg. See Table 47-2 for dosing of tezacaftor/ivacaftor. The dosing is also twice daily, similar to lumacaftor/ivacaftor, and still needs to be taken with fat-containing food.

As with lumacaftor/ivacaftor trials, tezacaftor/ivacaftor also demonstrated improvements in FEV1, disease-related quality of life, and rate of pulmonary exacerbations when compared to placebo.[36] Additionally, it was found that BMI had improved slightly. These effects were seen in both delta F508 homozygous and heterozygous patients.

Elexacaftor The newest approved CFTR modulator is the first triple combination that includes elexacaftor/tezacaftor/ivacaftor.[40] Elexacaftor and tezacaftor have slightly different mechanisms although both are still known as correctors. Elexacaftor corrects a flaw during the formation of the delta F508 CFTR protein that helps get more functioning CFTR proteins to the surface. This is known as a next-generation CFTR when compared to tezacaftor. Additionally, the triple combination only requires a single delta F508 mutation. Elexacaftor/tezacaftor/ivacaftor is currently only approved in those ages 6 and older. See Table 47-3.

Clinical trials, in both homozygous and heterozygous delta F 508 patients, evaluating the efficacy of the triple combination demonstrated an increase in percent predicted FEV1, a decrease in pulmonary exacerbations, and sweat chloride concentrations, and an

TABLE 47-1 Lumacaftor Dosing and Dosing Formulations

Dosage Form	Age	Recommended Dose	Counseling Points
Granules	2-5 years old	• <14 kg one packet lumacaftor 100 mg/ivacaftor 125 mg every 12 hours • >14 kg one packet lumacaftor 150 mg/ivacaftor 188 mg every 12 hours	• Take with fat-containing food • Shake the packet gently to settle the granules, after opening the packet, pour the granules into 1 teaspoon of soft food or liquid in a small container, food or liquid should be at or below room temperature, and once mixed should be given within 1 hour, the entire dose should be consumed
Tablets	6 years and older	• 6-11 years old • 2 tablets lumacaftor 100 mg/ivacaftor 125 mg every 12 hours • 12 years and older • 2 tablets lumacaftor 200 mg/ivacaftor 125 mg every 12 hours	

TABLE 47-2 Tezacaftor/Ivacaftor Dosing

Weight Based, Ages 6-11	Morning	Evening
<66 lbs or less than 30 kg	One tezacaftor 50 mg/ ivacaftor 75 mg tablet	One ivacaftor 75 mg tablet
≥66 lbs or greater than 30 kg	One tezacaftor 100 mg/ 150 ivacaftor tablet	One ivacaftor 150 mg tablet
Patients who are greater than 12 years of age		
Ages greater than 12	One tezacaftor 100/ ivacaftor 150 mg tablet	One ivacaftor 150 mg tablet

TABLE 47-3 Elexacaftor Dosing

Age	Morning	Evening
6-12 years weighing less than 30 kg	Two tablets, each containing elexacaftor 50 mg/ tezacaftor 25 mg/ivacaftor 37.5 mg	One tablet of ivacaftor 75 mg
6-12 years weighing more than 30 kg	Two tablets, each containing elexacaftor 100 mg/ tezacaftor 50 mg/ivacaftor 75 mg	One tablet of ivacaftor 75 mg
12 years and older	Two tablets, each containing elexacaftor 100 mg/ tezacaftor 50 mg/ivacaftor 75 mg	One tablet of ivacaftor 150 mg

improvement in respiratory symptoms as measured by a standardized questionnaire.[41,42] When compared to dual therapy, tezacaftor/ivacaftor, improvements were still noted in FEV1, sweat chloride concentrations, and respiratory symptoms.

Similar outcomes were noted in patients with advanced lung disease (<40% percent predicted FEV1).[41,43,44] These patients experienced an increase in FEV1, a decrease in chronic oxygen therapy and noninvasive ventilation, an increase in mean body weight, and a decrease in enteral feeding requirements.

CFTR Potentiator

Ivacaftor Ivacaftor was the first medication approved for patients with CF that targeted the CFTR protein.[45] It is a CFTR potentiator that keeps the channels open at the cell surface to increase the transport of chloride in and out of the cell. Ivacaftor needs the CFTR protein to be present at the cell surface in order to be efficacious. The mutation first studied with ivacaftor was the missense mutation, G551D. Approximately 4% to 5% of patients with cystic fibrosis have the G551D mutation on one allele of the CFTR protein. Ivacaftor is indicated in patients who have one mutation in the CFTR gene that is responsive to ivacaftor potentiation based on clinical and/or in vitro assay data. The FDA approved 97 additional mutations for use with ivacaftor based on in vitro demonstration of modulator-induced increase chloride transport and clinical benefit. The in vitro-responsive mutations did show clinical benefits in a small randomized trial. Ivacaftor is approved for patients as young as four months old and is available as granule packets for children 4 months to 5 years and tablets for patients 6 years of age or older. As with the other agents, dose reductions are needed in patients with hepatic impairment. See dosing Table 47-4.

In patients with a G551D mutation, ivacaftor increased the FEV1, decreased sweat chloride, reduced pulmonary exacerbations, improved pulmonary symptoms, and increased body weight.[46] The long-term effects demonstrated lower risks of death, hospitalizations, and transplantations.[47] Lower prevalence of *P. aeruginosa* along with lower acquisition rates and higher clearance rates have also been noted in patients on ivacaftor monotherapy.[48-50]

As with the correctors, elevations in hepatic enzyme concentrations and noncongenital lens opacities have also been reported with ivacaftor. Therefore, ivacaftor monitoring includes cataracts at baseline and then annually, as well as liver function tests at baseline and every 3 months during the first year of treatment and then annually thereafter.

TABLE 47-4 Ivacaftor Dosing

Dosage Form	Age	Recommended Dose	Counseling Points
Granules	4 months to 6 months	One 25 mg packet every 12 hours	Shake the packet, and pour into 1 teaspoon (5 mL) with soft food or liquid that is at or below room temperature. (Ex: breast milk, formula, applesauce, milk, yogurt, juice)
	6 months to 6 years old	• 11 pounds (5 kg) to less than 15 pounds (6.8 kg): one 25 mg packet every 12 hours • 15 pounds (6.8 kg) to less than 31 pounds (14 kg): one 50 mg packet every 12 hours • 31 pounds (14 kg) or more: one 75 mg packet every 12 hours	
Tablet	6 years and older	One tablet 150 mg twice daily	With fat-containing food

CFTR Amplifiers Amplifiers work by increasing the amount of CFTR protein in the cell and stabilizing CFTR mRNA through translational elongation.[51] In phase II trials, nesolicaftor appears well-tolerated and did increase the production of CFTR; however, it did not impact lung function in patients taking tezacaftor/ivacaftor with two copies of the F508del mutation.

Airway Clearance Therapy

Airway clearance therapies are recommended for all patients with CF for clearance of sputum, maintenance of lung function, and improved quality of life.[52] Cystic fibrosis is characterized by dehydration of the airway surface liquid and impaired mucociliary clearance. Dehydration occurs as a direct result of the inherited abnormality in the cystic fibrosis transmembrane regulator protein which leads to a reduced chloride section and increased absorption of sodium and water from the airway surface liquid.[53] The dehydrated mucus layer eventually becomes adherent to the airway surface.[54] This tenacious adhesive mucus, leading to airway obstruction, creates an environment conducive to the growth of bacteria followed by a neutrophilic host response in the airway lumen. Subsequently, the DNA from dead neutrophils left in the airways further increases the viscosity of already abnormal secretions. Dehydration of the airway surface liquid layer is the primary initiating event in CF-related lung disease; therefore, therapeutic interventions to improve mucus clearance and reduce the obstruction, infection, and inflammation remains a cornerstone of treatment in CF.[29]

In addition to non-pharmacological measures to facilitate mucus clearance, pharmacologic therapies including mucolytics such as dornase-alfa and hyperosmolar agents such as aerosolized hypertonic saline are also used to improve mucus clearance. In addition, bronchodilators are utilized to support ACT by opening the airway to facilitate the removal of secretions along with deeper deposition of other inhaled medications into the smaller airways. Bronchodilators should be administered prior to CPT or other ACT techniques.

Mucoactive Agents

Dornase alfa (Recombinant human DNase) Dornase alfa (recombinant human DNase, rhDNase), an enzyme that selectively hydrolyzes the extracellular DNA in the sputum of CF patients and reduces sputum viscoelasticity, is FDA-indicated in conjunction with standard therapies for the management of CF patients to improve pulmonary function.[55] The recommended dosage is one 2.5 mg single-use ampule inhaled once daily using a recommended nebulizer; however, some patients may benefit from twice-daily administration. The most common adverse reactions (occurring in ≥3% of patients treated with dornase alfa over placebo) seen in clinical trials in CF patients were: voice alteration, pharyngitis, rash, laryngitis, chest pain, conjunctivitis, rhinitis, decrease in FVC of ≥10%, fever, and dyspnea.

Both short-term and long-term clinical trials have demonstrated improvement in lung function as measured by FEV_1 as well as reductions in exacerbations requiring the use of parenteral antibiotics compared to placebo.[56-60] Increases in FEV1 have been noted in both short-term studies lasting from 1 to 2 weeks in duration and in long-term studies lasting from 24 weeks to 3 years.

The CF guidelines recommend the chronic use of dornase alfa to improve lung function and reduce exacerbations in all cystic fibrosis patients >6 years of age and older with asymptomatic/mild disease as well as moderate to severe disease.[61]

Hypertonic Saline (Nebusal™ 4 mL 7%) Hypertonic saline acts as an osmotic agent which draws water into luminal secretions resulting in the restoration of airway hydration.[54] It is a solution possessing an osmotic pressure greater than that of a physiologic isotonic salt solution (0.9%NaCl).[62] By drawing water from CFTR defective airway epithelial cells, the periciliary layer becomes rehydrated and mucociliary clearance reestablished.[63,64]

In CF patients, 7% hypertonic saline has been shown to be safe, well-tolerated, and effective in restoring mucus clearance, reducing disease exacerbations, and slowing progressive airway obstruction. Short-term administration is associated with improved lung function, increased mucociliary clearance for at least 8 hours in a dose-dependent manner, and increased sputum expectoration.[65] Among infants and children with cystic fibrosis less than 6 years old, the use of inhaled hypertonic saline compared with isotonic saline did not reduce the rate of pulmonary exacerbations over 48 weeks of treatment.[66] In the majority of trials hypertonic saline was used after pre-treatment with bronchodilators and as an adjunct to chest physiotherapy; in both cases, this may be important to ensure its efficacy.[67]

As intolerability due to oropharyngeal irritation and bronchospasm generally relates to the concentration of hypertonic saline and its rate of delivery, the selection of a dose for an individual patient is typically made by determining the maximally tolerated concentration.[54] For individuals with CF, 6 years of age and older, the Cystic Fibrosis Foundation recommends twice-daily use of inhaled hypertonic saline to improve lung function and quality of life and reduce exacerbations.[61]

Mannitol Inhaled mannitol, an osmotic agent with a high molecular weight, has been proposed as an additional strategy to improve the airway surface hydration by the slow influx of water through a pericellular pathway and mucociliary clearance in patients with CF.[62]

A two-week course of inhaled mannitol in patients with CF resulted in an increase in mean FEV1 from baseline as well as mean FEF_{25-75} compared with placebo.[68] While an international trial assessing the effect of inhaled dry powder mannitol on lung function in CF showed a sustained clinical benefit, there have been no large randomized trials comparing the effect of hypertonic saline versus mannitol.[69]

Inhaled mannitol is considered a second line as a replacement for hypertonic saline in adult patients who fail the combination of hypertonic saline and dornase alpha. Inhaled mannitol was only recently approved by the FDA for use in cystic fibrosis adult patients.

Antibiotics Infection is one of the main influences on the morbidity and mortality of CF and CF lung disease. Treating infections in CF involves not only antibiotics but chest physiotherapy and inhaled mucolytics play an important adjunction role. Most patients with CF develop chronic bacterial infections; however, the goal of antibiotic treatment is to delay the colonization by pathogens as long as possible. The prevalence of bacterial type varies with age; the most common pathogens include *P. aeruginosa, Staphylococcus aureus,* methicillin-resistant *Staphylococcus* (MRSA), *Burkholderia cepacia complex,* and *nontuberculous mycobacteria.*

CF patients have an increased susceptibility to *P. aeruginosa* which is an independent risk factor for a decline in pulmonary function and decreased survival.[70,71] With chronic infection, *P. aeruginosa* converts from "dry" to a "mucoid" phenotype with the production of an alginate biofilm and becomes much more difficult to treat leading to a worse prognosis. *S. aureus* is another pathogen commonly found in the respiratory secretions of CF patients. Co-infection with *S. aureus* and *P. aeruginosa* has an independent and additive effect on airway inflammation.[72] As with *P. aeruginosa*, chronic infection with *B. cepacia* complex is associated with an accelerated decline in pulmonary function and shortened survival.

Strategies should be employed to prevent *P. aeruginosa* acquisition including measures to prevent transmission between CF patients and early eradication of both *P. aeruginosa* and *S. aureus* with appropriate treatment regimens. The CF Foundation recommends a 28-day cycle of inhaled tobramycin for the treatment of patients with newly acquired *P. aeruginosa.* Other regimens have been evaluated but were not as effective as inhaled tobramycin or had similar outcomes as inhaled tobramycin. Eradication protocols for MRSA are more difficult but can be offered to highly selected patients who are capable of following the protocol. The regimen typically includes oral rifampin, oral trimethoprim-sulfamethoxazole, nasal mupirocin, chlorhexidine oral rinses, body wipes, and environmental decontamination.[73]

Inhaled Antibiotics Chronic colonization with *P. aeruginosa* necessitates chronic treatment with inhaled antibiotics. Currently available regimens include tobramycin, aztreonam lysine, and colistin with all of these agents administered initially in a cyclic phase (28 days on followed by 28 days off) or alternatively as continuous treatment by alternating in 28-day cycles between two different inhaled antibiotics.

Inhaled tobramycin is recommended as a first-line treatment. Inhaled aztreonam may be used in patients who do not tolerate tobramycin, whose pulmonary status is declining while on inhaled tobramycin, or who is or attempting to become pregnant. Adherence may be better with inhaled tobramycin because it is administered twice daily versus three times a day with aztreonam. Conversely, the aztreonam dose is delivered in less than 3 minutes, whereas tobramycin requires a 15 to 20-minute nebulization. If patients do not tolerate either tobramycin or aztreonam or pulmonary function continues to decline on either agent or both agents, inhaled colistin is an alternative. Inhaled colistin does not have the renal toxicity or neurotoxicity typically seen when administered intravenously and is administered twice daily for 28 days, alternating with 28 days off treatment.

Oral Azithromycin Azithromycin has demonstrated clinical benefits in CF patients with chronic infection with *P. aeruginosa.* These benefits do not appear to be exclusively related to its antimicrobial effects but also an anti-inflammatory effect.[74-77] The antimicrobial effects center around the ability of macrolides to reduce the ability of *Pseudomonas* to produce biofilms, whereas the anti-inflammatory effect relates to azithromycin's ability to suppress the excessive inflammatory response noted in CF patients. In CF patients 6 years of age and older who are chronically infected with *P. aeruginosa,* azithromycin is typically prescribed as a 10 mg/kg dose administered three times a week. Smaller daily dosing rather than three times a week dosing could also be used with similar efficacy. Azithromycin may also be initiated at the time of a first positive culture for *P. aeruginosa* in children as young as 6 months and continued for 18 months rather than waiting until becoming chronically infected in order to initiate therapy.[78] Azithromycin therapy can be discontinued after multiple negative cultures over the previous year. Macrolide therapy should not be initiated in patients with a positive sputum sample for nontuberculous mycobacteria. The use of oral azithromycin may reduce the efficacy of inhaled and intravenous tobramycin. In retrospective studies, the concurrent use of tobramycin (either acute or chronic therapy) and azithromycin were associated with less improvement in lung function based on FEV1 when compared to tobramycin use alone.[79-82]

Anti-inflammatory Agents Oral ibuprofen has also been used in cystic fibrosis for its anti-inflammatory properties and limited data has demonstrated a slower decline in lung function when used at a high dose in children who have good lung function (FEV1 > 60% [0.6] predicted).[61,83,84] However, the need for pharmacokinetic monitoring and the risk of side effects have restricted its use. A serum concentration between 50 and 100 mcg/mL (mg/L: 242-485 μmol/L) is needed.[85]

Inhaled glucocorticoids are only recommended in cystic fibrosis patients with a co-diagnosis of asthma.[61,86] These agents should not be routinely used in patients with cystic fibrosis without definite signs of asthma. Other agents that are not recommended in cystic fibrosis include chronic use of systemic glucocorticoids and cromolyn due to a lack of efficacy, potential for adverse effects, and increased expense.

Pancreatic Disease

Pancreatic exocrine insufficiency (PI) occurs in cystic fibrosis patients as a result of pancreatic duct obstruction due to a viscous exocrine fluid that congeals in the proximal pancreatic ducts.[87] Pancreatic function correlates strongly with genotype with 60% of infants being affected at birth. Patients with two "severe" CFTR mutations usually are associated with PI.[88-90] If left untreated, PI can lead to growth failure, weight loss, abdominal bloating, foul-smelling stools, or diarrhea.

The most common way to screen and diagnose pancreatic insufficiency in patients with cystic fibrosis is the use of the fecal pancreatic elastase-1 test. When values of the fecal pancreatic elastic-1 test result in a value of less than 100 micrograms/gram, it is likely, given the specificity and sensitivity of the elastase test, that the patient is pancreatic insufficient. Patients are often tested for PI at diagnosis and annually if deemed to be pancreatic sufficient.

Pancreatic Enzymes Pancreatic enzyme replacement therapy (PERT) is the treatment of choice. PERTs are a combination of lipase, protease, and amylase. The PERT dose is generally expressed in lipase units. Typically, PERTs are known to increase fat absorption and provide more consistency in stool frequency and consistency when compared to placebo. There are multiple formulations of PERTs; however, the formulations are not interchangeable as recommended by the Cystic Fibrosis Foundation Guidelines.[91] High doses of PERT could lead to colonic stricture; therefore doses of PERT should not exceed 25,000 lipase units per kilogram per meal. Recommended doses are provided with three meals a day and with two to three snacks a day. The snack doses are traditionally half the dose at meal times. It is important to ensure the doses are taken prior to eating and not during or after eating. Enzymes can always be opened, and the contents may be mixed with small amounts of applesauce or alkaline food but should not be crushed or allowed to sit in food. Doses may be titrated based on symptoms of malabsorption such as foul-smelling stools, weight loss, abdominal bloating, or diarrhea. Prior to increasing the dose always take into consideration adherence, dietary factors, liver disease, intestinal hyperacidity, and abnormal intestinal motility. Dosing is also provided similarly when patients are on continuous overnight gastrostomy tube feedings.

There are six different FDA-approved pancreatic enzymes each consisting of various amounts of the combination of lipase, protease, and amylase. Most products are proprietary and there is only one generic pancreatic enzyme formulation available. Each formulation of pancreatic enzymes has different characteristics. Some are delayed-release capsules. One product contains bicarbonate-buffered enteric-coated microspheres; this raises the pH of the duodenal environment to help delay the enzymes' inactivation by the stomach acid. Another product has a non-enteric coat and thus must be taken with a proton pump inhibitor to reduce the enzymes from being broken down in the stomach too quickly.

Common adverse events from pancreatic enzymes include headache, abdominal pain, flatulence, and cough. Some of these events may be related to malabsorption and may require dose increases. A dose-limiting side effect is fibrosing colonopathy as previously described.

Vitamins

Patients with CF, especially those that are pancreatic insufficient are at increased risk for fat-soluble vitamin deficiency. The fat-soluble vitamins include A, D, E, and K. Supplementation of these vitamins should begin as soon as CF is diagnosed and at typically higher doses than recommended for the general population. Monitoring of serum retinol, 25-hydroxyvitamin D, alpha-tocopherol, prothrombin time, and PIVKA II for assessment of vitamin K deficiency should occur at least annually.

Vitamin D deficiency is probably the most commonly studied vitamin deficiency in CF patients and appears to have an impact on inflammation and maintenance of bone health. The cystic fibrosis foundation has guidelines specifically for vitamin D to ensure that the serum 25-hydroxyvitamin D levels remain at least at 30 ng/mL (75 nmol/L) or higher in all patients with cystic fibrosis.[92] Vitamin D3 or cholecalciferol is the currently recommended oral supplement by the CF Foundation as opposed to vitamin D2, ergocalciferol.

Specific CF-formulated vitamins come in all formulations from drops, chewables, soft gels, and tablets. In addition, individual supplements may also be needed for continued vitamin-specific deficiency.

Pulmonary Exacerbations

Pulmonary infection is a major contributor to CF lung disease. A typical clinical course in most CF patients includes acute episodes of worsening pulmonary status with a decrease in FEV1 along with worsening symptoms such as increased cough and sputum production. Although viruses such as coxsackie/echovirus, rhinovirus, respiratory syncytial virus, parainfluenza, adenovirus, and influenza are often detected during acute exacerbations in children, most patients with CF also have a bacterial infection of the airways that are the same pathogens associated with chronic infections. These bacterial pathogens include *P. aeruginosa, S. aureus, B. cepacia* complex, non-typeable *Haemophilus influenzae, Stenotrophomonas maltophilia, Achromobacter* species, and nontuberculous mycobacteria. Treatment of pulmonary exacerbations requires a multimodal approach including antibiotics, chest physiotherapy, inhaled medications, anti-inflammatory agents, optimization of nutrition, and exercise as tolerated.

Systemic antibiotics are the mainstay of therapy for an acute exacerbation. The severity of the infection dictates the route of administration. Mild exacerbations can be treated with oral antibiotics, whereas severe exacerbations require the use of intravenous antibiotics. In general, the CF guidelines recommend using one antibiotic to cover each pathogenic bacteria and two antibiotics to cover *P. aeruginosa*.[93] Treatment with antipseudomonal antibiotics has demonstrated an improvement in pulmonary function tests, reduction in sputum bacterial density, and inflammatory markers.

The specific antibiotic selection should be patient-specific based on historic sputum culture and sensitivities and then narrowed or altered based on sputum cultures and sensitivities obtained at the onset of the exacerbation. Oral therapy with antipseudomonal coverage includes ciprofloxacin or levofloxacin. For moderate to severe exacerbations, an antibiotic combination of a beta-lactam along with either a fluoroquinolone or tobramycin should be used. If clinical response is inadequate after approximately 5 days of treatment, consideration should be given to switching the beta-lactam. Other alternatives may include switching the fluoroquinolone to tobramycin or exchanging tobramycin with amikacin. Colistimethate may also be an option when there is treatment failure.

The selection of antibiotic coverage for *S. aureus* will be dependent on if it is methicillin-sensitive or methicillin-resistant. Mild exacerbations with methicillin-sensitive *S. aureus* may be treated with trimethoprim-sulfamethoxazole, doxycycline, or amoxicillin-clavulanate. Trimethoprim-sulfamethoxazole and doxycycline may still be used for methicillin-resistant *S. aureus* in mild infections; however, severe exacerbations require the use of oral linezolid, intravenous vancomycin, or intravenous ceftaroline. When culture results reveal both *Pseudomonas* and *Staphylococcus*, a combination of the above agents is required. Due to the lack of sensitivity of ceftaroline against *P. aeruginosa* and the use of another beta-lactam for *Pseudomonas* coverage, ceftaroline is generally not encouraged in these situations in order to avoid using two beta-lactams simultaneously. In addition, the combination of piperacillin-tazobactam with vancomycin and tobramycin should be avoided due to the increased risk of renal toxicity.

Dosing of antibiotics in CF patients can be a challenge to ensure adequate lung penetration and maximum bactericidal activity. For instance, beta-lactam's effect is based upon time above the minimum inhibitory concentration, whereas aminoglycosides and fluoroquinolones killing effect is dependent upon the peak antimicrobial tissue concentration along with the post-antibiotic effect. In addition, the pharmacokinetics of antibiotics in CF patients differ compared to most other individuals. The volume of distribution and total body clearance is increased in CF patients for hydrophilic drugs such as aminoglycosides, penicillins, and cephalosporins. Specifically, the aminoglycoside's initial dose is higher than the general population and adjusted based on patient-specific pharmacokinetic parameters. The CF guidelines also support the use of extended-interval dosing or once-daily dosing of aminoglycosides in patients with normal renal function. The recommended target peak concentration differs between once-daily dosing and conventional dosing. The target peak concentration for once-daily dosing is 20 to 30 mcg/mL (mg/L) versus the 8 to 12 mcg/mL (mg/L) for conventional dosing. The calculated concentration at 18 hours should be <0.5 mcg/mL (mg/L) to minimize toxicity and to ensure at least a 6-hour period with low serum concentrations prior to the next dose.

Vancomycin, on the other hand, can be dosed and monitored in CF patients similar to the general population. The pharmacokinetics of vancomycin appears to be unaltered in CF patients. Patient-specific pharmacokinetic calculations should be used to maintain a trough concentration of 15 to 20 mcg/mL (mg/L; 10.4-13.8 μmol/L) in adults and 7 to 10 mcg/mL (mg/L; 4.8-6.9 μmol/L) in children. AUC-guided dosing may also be used instead of trough-driven dosing.[94] A target AUC between 400 and 600 × h/L is suggested for adults and pediatric patients.

The duration of treatment for an acute exacerbation is not standardized. Some centers continue antibiotic regimens until the resolution of symptoms and others continue therapy until there are improvements in the FEV1. Typically, antibiotics are continued for 10 days to 3 weeks depending upon the clinical course.

Bone Disease

Bone disease is a common complication of CF and is characterized by low bone mineral density (BMD). Factors that may contribute to bone disease over time may include malabsorption of vitamin D, poor nutritional status, physical inactivity, glucocorticoid therapy, and delayed pubertal maturation. It is thought that loss of bone mass occurs in childhood and worsens around puberty. Puberty plays a role in bone development and peak bone accruals usually occur during the growth velocity. Delay can be seen in patients with poor nutrition and poor control of CF. Dual-energy x-ray absorptiometry (DXA) scans should be performed routinely on adults and children older than 8 years if they are less than 90% of their ideal body weight, their FEV1 is less than 50% (0.5) of predicted, they received systemic glucocorticoids for more than 90 days in the previous year, have delayed puberty, or a history of fracture.[95] Osteoporosis is defined as having a BMD T score > −2.5, and osteopenia with a score between −1 and −2.5. Low BMD is common among adults with CF. A T-score less than −1 has been observed in 85% of adult patients with CF. As much as 34% of adult CF patients have a Z score less than −2 and 10% have T-scores less than −2.5. In pediatric patients, osteopenia is found in up to 47% of patients and osteoporosis in up to 34% of patients. Z scores are typically used for children less than 18. T scores are not meaningful in children. Both T and Z scores are useful in patients 18 to 30 years of age and T scores should be used in those 30 years and older.

Strategies for preventing the loss of bone minerals in patients with CF include maintaining good lung function, treatment of pulmonary exacerbations in a timely manner, optimizing nutritional care, and promoting the maintenance of lean body mass. Oral and inhaled steroids should be avoided as much as possible. Weight-bearing activities and exercise are recommended. Vitamin D and calcium supplementation should be continued as directed by the Cystic Fibrosis Foundation guidelines. Specifically, vitamin D3 (cholecalciferol) should be supplemented to achieve and maintain serum 25-hydroxyvitamin D concentration of 30 to 60 ng/mL (75-150 nmol/L) along with 1,300 to 1,500 mg of calcium per day.

An area of active research includes the use of growth hormone (GH) in patients with CF. With the use of GH, improvement in height and bone mineral content has been demonstrated. Long-term studies are still in progress to determine the optimal management of GH in patients with CF.

If DXA T score is greater than −1 or Z score is greater than −2.0, fragility fractures have occurred, or a patient is awaiting transplant, or BMD loss is greater than 3% to 5% a year, bisphosphonates are indicated in these patients. If the T/Z score is less than or equal to 2.0 then bisphosphonates are indicated. Bisphosphonates have been studied in trials in adults with CF and trials have yet to be heavily studied in children with CF. Pamidronate resulted in gains in the lumbar spine and total hip after 6 months; however, there were significant adverse effects from bone pain, fever, and phlebitis in 75% of the patients, some of which required hospitalization. The IV bisphosphonate, zoledronic acid, showed benefit; however, the patient dropout rate was 20% due to bone pain.[96]

In patients aged 5 to 30 years old with CF and low BMD, oral alendronate, 5 mg/day and 10 mg/day based on weight, increased BMD by 16.5% and was well-tolerated.[97] Additionally, alendronate is the only bisphosphonate available in liquid formulation. Risedronate 35 mg once weekly in patients older than 18 with CF was found to improve lumbar spine BMD.[98] There were reports of bone pain in the first 56 days of risedronate use, with some leading to discontinuation of risedronate.

Denosumab is a monoclonal antibody that works to inhibit osteoclasts differentiation and activation and functions as an anti-resorptive therapy to reduce bone breakdown. It is approved for the treatment of osteoporosis in men and post-menopausal women and glucocorticoid-induced osteoporosis. There are no studies published evaluating the use of denosumab in patients with CF. Until more studies can be conducted denosumab is considered second-line for patients who cannot tolerate, have a contraindication, or fail bisphosphonate therapy.

There are other adverse effects to monitor when initiating an oral bisphosphonate such as esophageal ulcers, osteonecrosis, and hypocalcemia. IV bisphosphonates appear to have that acute-phase reaction after the initial infusion leading to flu-like symptoms but have been seen to be more severe in patients with CF for an unknown reason. A short course of NSAIDs or acetaminophen was found to mitigate the effect.

Long-term data is lacking for the safety of bisphosphonates in children and young adults, the general approach is to minimize bisphosphonate treatment to typically less than 5 years with periods of off treatment or bisphosphonate holidays.[99] Following this off-treatment period, patients may be monitored via DXA scans every 1 to 2 years to assess for interval bone loss. If no treatment is needed following a DXA scan, DXA scores may be repeated every 5 years unless there is a change in risk factors if T or Z scores are

−1 or better. Individuals between −1 and −2 should have a repeat DXA every 2 to 4 years and annually for scores greater than −2.

Cystic Fibrosis–Related Diabetes

CFRD is the most common comorbidity in patients with CF, occurring in 20% of adolescents and 50% of adults. The course is progressive in nature, and patients may move back and forth between an impaired state and CFRD. Uncontrolled CFRD may correlate with pulmonary function decline, weight loss, and *P. aeruginosa*. This comorbidity is difficult to manage as patients are directed to have high caloric intake due to having CF. Diabetes ketoacidosis (DKA) is rare.[22] CFRD may present like in the honeymoon period when compared to type 1 diabetes patients because they may still have endogenous insulin secretion.

Following the diagnosis of CFRD, patients should be treated with insulin therapy instead of oral anti-hyperglycemic medications. Data suggests that therapies such as sulfonylureas, metformin, meglitinides, and thiazolidinediones are not as effective as insulin. After an acute illness or systemic glucocorticoid treatment, insulin requirements may increase and take about 4 to 6 weeks to return to baseline. Close monitoring is required to ensure that hypoglycemia does not occur in these patients following acute illness. Dosing for insulin is usually between 0.5 and 0.8 units/kg/day in both adolescents and adults. If a patient has fasting hyperglycemia a basal/bolus regimen is recommended. The starting dose for basal insulin is 0.125/units/kg and may be titrated up to 0.25/units/kg. For meal coverage doses start at 0.5 to 1 unit for every 15 grams of carbohydrates consumed. The doses may be titrated by 0.5 units per 15 grams of carbohydrates to achieve 2 hours postprandial blood glucose. Carbohydrate counting is recommended to best determine a pre-meal insulin dose. Correction doses are typically 0.5 to 1 unit of rapid-acting insulin based on a insulin sensitivity factor of 1 unit for every 50 mg/dL (2.8 mmol/L) above 150 mg/dL (8.3 mmol/L). Some lifestyle recommendations differ in patients with CFRD when compared to patients with diabetes mellitus. Carbohydrate intake is individualized, there is no restriction on fat intake, protein intake is doubled, sodium intake is liberalized, and regular supplementation with ADEK vitamins is needed. Weight loss is not recommended.

Blood glucose (BG) should be self-monitored at least three times daily and goals should be individualized. Monitoring can also occur using a continuous glucose monitoring (CGM). Plasma glucose goals for CFRD are similar to patients with diabetes as recommended by ADA but some patients may benefit from higher or lower goals. Glucose monitoring may be useful to detect early glucose abnormalities that the OGTT and A1c cannot detect. While CGM's are not approved to diagnosis diabetes, they can be useful in detecting glucose excursions when titrating insulin therapy. The patient's A1c may falsely indicate good glycemic control despite the fact that the patient may have frequent hyperglycemia or hypoglycemia.[23] Like other patients with diabetes mellitus, the A1c treatment goal should be ≤7% (53 mmol/mol) to reduce the risk of microvascular complications; however, goals must be individualized. An A1c should be ordered quarterly. Monitoring of microvascular complications such as nephropathy, retinopathy, and neuropathy is important. Screening for these complications should be initiated 5 years after diagnosis of CFRD.[22] The use of ACEI or ARBs are appropriate, and cough associated with ACEI use is seen in ~10% of patients. Nephropathy should be monitored using urine protein testing, with an albumin to creatinine ratio of 300 µg/mg (33.9 mg/mmol) or greater indicating macroalbuminuria and progression toward renal failure. Retinopathy is seen in 10% to 20% of patients with CFRD and should be monitored through regular dilated retinal exams. Neuropathy may be less severe in patients with CFRD but annual foot evaluations are still recommended. An annual lipid profile is recommended for patients with CFRD.

Cystic Fibrosis Liver Disease

Cystic fibrosis liver disease (CFLD) is the third leading cause of death among patients with CF.[21] There is a wide variety of presentations of liver disease from steatosis, cholelithiasis, and multilobular cirrhosis.

The aim of the treatment of CFLD is to prevent further liver damage and complications related to portal hypertension and cirrhosis. There is currently no long-term treatment that has proven efficacy; however, there are treatments for the complications of CFLD. Ursodiol displaces toxic bile from enterohepatic circulation, has a cytoprotective effect on cells that are exposed to toxic bile acids, stimulates Ca-activated chloride channels, and has immunoregulatory properties. It may delay the progression of cirrhotic changes in patients with CFLD. It is dosed 20 to 30 mg/kg/day. Table 47-5 for medical management of complications of CFLD. In patients with advanced CFLD with decompensated liver failure, transplantation is the treatment of choice.

TABLE 47-5 Medical Management of Complications Related to Cystic Fibrosis Liver Disease

Indication	Treatment of choice
Hepatic steatosis	Optimize nutritional status and evaluate for deficiencies of essential fatty acids, carnitine, and choline
Hepatic congestion	Optimize cardiopulmonary function
Cholestasis	Treatment of fat-soluble vitamin deficiency
Portal hypertension	Beta-blocker use with caution, variceal band ligation
Ascites	Salt restriction, or transjugular intrahepatic portosystemic shunt

Cystic Fibrosis GI Disease

Gastrointestinal complications have become a common cause of morbidity in the cystic fibrosis population and include conditions such as gastroesophageal reflux (GERD), constipation, distal intestinal obstruction syndrome, and fibrosing colonopathy along with others.

GERD in the CF patient is similar to that of the general population. Even though there has been some association between GERD and pulmonary disease, there is not overwhelming evidence to support a causal association, nor that treatment has a beneficial effect on pulmonary function. There are pros and cons to the management of GERD with proton pump inhibitors (PPIs) including improving fat absorption in patients with pancreatic insufficiency, whereas potential harm would be the negative effects on bone health in a population already at increased risk for osteoporosis. A clear goal should be determined when initiating PPIs in cystic fibrosis patients with GERD and therapy discontinued if no improvement in symptoms is noted. Patients should be monitored for increased pulmonary exacerbations, vitamin B12 deficiency, hypomagnesemia, and bone health while receiving PPI treatment.

Constipation affects 25% to 50% of cystic fibrosis patients and is a common cause of flatulence and abdominal pain. Constipation in the CF patient results from abnormal intestinal fluid composition, dysmotility, and pancreatic insufficiency even though pancreatic sufficient patients have a relatively dehydrated bowel. Treatment generally consists of osmotic laxatives with or without electrolytes along with an assessment of the PERT dosing to ensure an adequate dose. Lubiprostone may be considered a second-line option in adult cystic fibrosis patients with severe refractory constipation.

Distal intestinal obstruction syndrome (DIOS) results from either a complete or incomplete obstruction of the ileocecum by thickened intestinal contents and is manifested by cramping abdominal pain, abdominal distention, flatulence, weight loss, and poor appetite. Unlike constipation which is a gradual onset of fecal impaction, DIOS occurs acutely to intermittently with symptoms becoming progressively more severe over time. DIOS is more common in those with pancreatic insufficiency and having the F 508 del genotype. Others at risk of DIOS include patients with poorly controlled malabsorption, dehydration, and opioid use. Treatment should target fluid and electrolyte abnormalities along with a regimen of either oral/nasogastric rehydration and osmotic laxatives or hyperosmolar enemas with or without laxatives. Prevention should be the goal once the impaction is removed by optimizing the pancreatic enzymes and sufficient hydration.

Fibrosing colonopathy, a dose-limiting side effect of pancreatic enzymes, is a severe intestinal process involving fibrosis and strictures. First detected in patients receiving large doses of pancreatic enzymes, pancreatic enzyme dosing recommendations now limit the maximum dose to 2,500 lipase units/kg/meal or 10,000 lipase units/kg/day. Adjunctive therapy with H2 blockers or proton pump inhibitors helps maintain the recommended dosing range while boosting the stability of the pancreatic enzymes in the acidic environment of the GI tract and increasing the efficiency of the prescribed pancreatic dose in managing the fat malabsorption.

Mental Health

Managing CF is complex and takes about 2 to 4 hours of the day, especially, if other complications arise which may increase this time. The burden of this disease may lead to patient and parent depression and anxiety. Depression prevalence ranges from 8% to 29% in children and adolescents and 13% to 33% in adults.[100,101] Similarly, 22% of the adolescent population and 32% of the adult population reported anxiety.[102] Reports of depression and anxiety have been associated with decreased lung function, lower body mass index, worse adherence, and worse health-related quality of life.[103] It is recommended by the Cystic Fibrosis Foundation that all children with CF who are 7 to 11 years old be assessed for depression and anxiety or when there is a concern for the child exhibiting symptoms of depression or anxiety by his/her team or caregivers. Annual screening for depression and anxiety is recommended for all individuals with CF beginning at 12 years of age utilizing the PHQ-9 and GAD-7. Screening is also recommended for caregivers.

When caring for patients with CF it is important to provide behavioral interventions to help alleviate distress when it relates to medical procedures. Additionally, to provide supportive intervention when PHQ/GAD scores are elevated. Patients who are aged 7 to 11 who present with clinically significant or elevated PHQ and GAD scores may undergo evidence-based psychological interventions such as cognitive-behavioral therapy (CBT) with continued monitoring. For those that are 12 years of age and older with mild symptoms of depression or anxiety, education can be provided, as well as preventative and supportive interventions and to continue to follow up at the next scheduled visit. For those 12 years of age and older with moderate symptoms it is appropriate to engage in CBT, if this treatment is not alleviating symptoms, psychotropic medication may be considered next. For those 12 and older, selective serotonin reuptake inhibitors (SSRIs) are recommended for the treatment of depression and anxiety. Doses of SSRIs may need to be increased when used in combination with lumacaftor. Additionally, linezolid is not recommended for use with SSRIs when alternatives are available. QTc prolongation may be more significant with the use of citalopram and may require EKG monitoring when used with other medications that may cause QT prolongation.

EVALUATION OF THERAPEUTIC OUTCOMES

CF patients are typically monitored every month for the first year after diagnosis and then every 1 to 3 months, depending on the stability of their illness. Clinicians should evaluate the patient's pulmonary function and lung volumes using pulmonary function tests (PFTs) quarterly and assess for unusual or increased respiratory symptoms at each clinic visit to determine if the current pharmacotherapy regimen is effective. Quarterly sputum cultures are typically collected to determine which organisms are growing in the patient's lungs. Airway clearance, inflammation, and bacterial colonization must be under control for optimal pulmonary function. Weight and height should be measured at every visit to assure adequate growth (pediatrics) and nutrition (pediatrics and adults). A BMI greater than the 50th percentile in children and greater than 22 in female adults and 23 in male adults is associated with optimal lung function. The pharmacist is integral to the multidisciplinary CF team to ensure optimization of pharmacotherapy and to evaluate and encourage patient/family adherence to recommended treatments, both nonpharmacologic and pharmacologic.

CONCLUSION

Cystic fibrosis is a multi-system disease requiring a multi-modal treatment approach administered through a multidisciplinary team to provide optimal care and the best patient outcomes. This multidisciplinary team consists of nurses, physicians, respiratory therapists, dietitians, social workers, and an overall program coordinator as required team members. The CF Foundation recommends that pharmacists, physical therapists, psychologists, and a research coordinator also be a part of these teams.

With the advancements in science and treatment options, not only is the quality of life for cystic fibrosis patients increasing but their overall lifespan is also expanding. Thus, it is crucial that the healthcare team optimizes treatment to reduce pulmonary exacerbations, delay colonization by pathogens and maintain lung health; maximizes adequate nutrition with appropriate dosing of pancreatic enzymes and vitamin supplementation; and initiates CFTR modulators to target the underlying pathology and advance the management of cystic fibrosis.

ABBREVIATIONS

ACT	Airway Clearance Technique
ADA	American Diabetes Association
ADEs	adverse drug events
ALT	alanine transaminase
AST	aspartate aminotransferase
BMD	bone mineral density
BMI	body mass index
CBAVD	congenital bilateral absence of the vas deferens
CBT	cognitive behavioral therapy
CF	cystic fibrosis
CGM	continuous glucose monitoring
CFLD	cystic fibrosis liver disease
CFMS	cystic fibrosis metabolic syndrome
CFRD	cystic fibrosis–related diabetes
CFTR	cystic fibrosis transmembrane conductance regulator
CMP	comprehensive metabolic panel
CPT	chest physical therapy
DIOS	distal Intestinal obstruction syndrome
DXA	dual-energy x-ray absorptiometry
EKG	electrocardiogram
FDA	Food and Drug Administration
FEF_{25-75}	forced expiratory flow at 25% and 75%
FVC	forced vital capacity
FEV1	forced expiratory volume in 1 second
GAD-7	generalized anxiety disorder assessment
GERD	gastroesophageal reflux disease

GGTP	gamma-glutamyl transpeptidase
GGT	gamma-glutamyl transferase
GH	growth hormone
G-tube	gastrostomy tube
H2 Blockers	histamine 2 receptor antagonist
HTS	hypertonic saline
IRT	immunoreactive trypsinogen
MRSA	methicillin-resistant *Staphylococcus aureus*
OGTT	oral glucose tolerance test
PEP	positive expiratory pressure
PERT	pancreatic enzyme replacement therapy
PHQ-9	Patient Health Questionnaire
PI	pancreatic insufficiency
PIVKA II	protein induced by vitamin K absence-II
PPI	proton pump inhibitor
QTc	corrected QT interval
SMBG	self-monitoring blood glucose
SOCAP	subjective, objective, calculations, assessment plan note

REFERENCES

1. Mehta G, Macek M Jr, Mehta A; European Registry Working Group. Cystic fibrosis across Europe: EuroCareCF analysis of demographic data from 35 countries. *J Cyst Fibros.* 2010 Dec;9(suppl 2):S5–S21. doi:10.1016/j.jcf.2010.08.002. Epub 2010 Nov 1. PMID: 21041121.
2. Spoonhower KA, Davis PB. Epidemiology of cystic fibrosis. *Clin Chest Med.* 2016 Mar;37(1):1–8. doi:10.1016/j.ccm.2015.10.002. PMID: 26857763.
3. Elborn JS. Cystic fibrosis. *Lancet.* 2016 Nov 19;388(10059):2519–2531. doi:10.1016/S0140-6736(16)00576-6. Epub 2016 Apr 29. PMID: 27140670.
4. Cystic Fibrosis Foundation. 2019 Patient Registry: Annual Data Report. Avilable at: https://www.cff.org/Research/Researcher-Resources/Patient-Registry/2019-Patient-Registry-Annual-Data-Report.pdf Accessed July 26, 2021.
5. De Boeck K, Zolin A, Cuppens H, Olesen HV, Viviani L. The relative frequency of CFTR mutation classes in European patients with cystic fibrosis. *J Cyst Fibros.* 2014 Jul;13(4):403–409. doi:10.1016/j.jcf.2013.12.003. Epub 2014 Jan 16. PMID: 24440181.
6. Boyle MP, De Boeck K. A new era in the treatment of cystic fibrosis: Correction of the underlying CFTR defect. *Lancet Respir Med.* 2013 Apr;1(2):158–163. doi:10.1016/S2213-2600(12)70057-7. Epub 2013 Jan 30. Erratum in: *Lancet Respir Med.* 2013 Apr;1(2):101. PMID: 24429096.
7. Hamosh A, FitzSimmons SC, Macek M Jr, Knowles MR, Rosenstein BJ, Cutting GR. Comparison of the clinical manifestations of cystic fibrosis in black and white patients. *J Pediatr.* 1998 Feb;132(2):255–259. doi:10.1016/s0022-3476(98)70441-x. PMID: 9506637.
8. Castellani C, Cuppens H, Macek M Jr, et al. Consensus on the use and interpretation of cystic fibrosis mutation analysis in clinical practice. *J Cyst Fibros.* 2008 May;7(3):179–196. doi:10.1016/j.jcf.2008.03.009. PMID: 18456578; PMCID: PMC2810954.
9. Orenstein DM, Rosenstein BJ, Stern RC. *Cystic Fibrosis Medical Care.* USA: Lippincott Williams & Wilkins, 2000.
10. Amin R, Ratjen F. Cystic fibrosis: A review of pulmonary and nutritional therapies. *Adv Pediatr.* 2008;55:99–121. doi:10.1016/j.yapd.2008.07.015. PMID: 19048729.
11. De Boeck K. Cystic fibrosis in the year 2020: A disease with a new face. *Acta Paediatr.* 2020 May;109(5):893–899. doi:10.1111/apa.15155. Epub 2020 Jan 22. PMID: 31899933.
12. Brown SD, White R, Tobin P. Keep them breathing: Cystic fibrosis pathophysiology, diagnosis, and treatment. *JAAPA.* 2017 May;30(5):23–27. doi:10.1097/01.JAA.0000515540.36581.92. PMID: 28441669.
13. Garnett JP, Hickman E, Burrows R, et al. Novel role for pendrin in orchestrating bicarbonate secretion in cystic fibrosis transmembrane conductance regulator (CFTR)-expressing airway serous cells. *J Biol Chem.* 2011 Nov 25;286(47):41069–41082. doi:10.1074/jbc.M111.266734. Epub 2011 Sep 13. PMID: 21914796; PMCID: PMC3220502.
14. Ratjen F, Bell SC, Rowe SM, Goss CH, Quittner AL, Bush A. Cystic fibrosis. *Nat Rev Dis Primers.* 2015 May 14;1:15010. doi:10.1038/nrdp.2015.10. PMID: 27189798; PMCID: PMC7041544.
15. Ratjen F, Grasemann H. New therapies in cystic fibrosis. *Curr Pharm Des.* 2012;18(5):614–627. doi:10.2174/138161212799315984. PMID: 22229570.
16. Ghigo A, Prono G, Riccardi E, De Rose V. Dysfunctional inflammation in cystic fibrosis airways: From mechanisms to novel therapeutic approaches. *Int J Mol Sci.* 2021 Feb 16;22(4):1952. doi:10.3390/ijms22041952. PMID: 33669352; PMCID: PMC7920244.
17. Pezzulo AA, Tang XX, Hoegger MJ, et al. Reduced airway surface pH impairs bacterial killing in the porcine cystic fibrosis lung. *Nature.* 2012 Jul 4;487(7405):109–113. doi:10.1038/nature11130. PMID: 22763554; PMCID: PMC3390761.
18. Pohl K, Hayes E, Keenan J, et al. A neutrophil intrinsic impairment affecting Rab27a and degranulation in cystic fibrosis is corrected by CFTR potentiator therapy. *Blood.* 2014 Aug 14;124(7):999–1009. doi:10.1182/blood-2014-02-555268. Epub 2014 Jun 16. PMID: 24934256; PMCID: PMC4133506.
19. Castellani C, Assael BM. Cystic fibrosis: A clinical view. *Cell Mol Life Sci.* 2017 Jan;74(1):129–140. doi:10.1007/s00018-016-2393-9. Epub 2016 Oct 5. PMID: 27709245.
20. Illing EA, Woodworth BA. Management of the upper airway in cystic fibrosis. *Curr Opin Pulm Med.* 2014 Nov;20(6):623–31. doi:10.1097/MCP.0000000000000107. PMID: 25250804; PMCID: PMC4301682.
21. Debray D, Narkewicz MR, Bodewes FAJA, et al. Cystic fibrosis-related liver disease: Research challenges and future perspectives. *J Pediatr Gastroenterol Nutr.* 2017 Oct;65(4):443–448. doi:10.1097/MPG.0000000000001676. PMID: 28753176.
22. Moran A, Pillay K, Becker D, Granados A, Hameed S, Acerini CL. ISPAD Clinical Practice Consensus Guidelines 2018: Management of cystic fibrosis-related diabetes in children and adolescents. *Pediatr Diabetes.* 2018 Oct;19(suppl 27):64–74. doi:10.1111/pedi.12732. PMID: 30094886.
23. Chan CL, Ode KL, Granados A, Moheet A, Moran A, Hameed S. Continuous glucose monitoring in cystic fibrosis: A practical guide. *J Cyst Fibros.* 2019 Oct;18(suppl 2):S25–S31. doi:10.1016/j.jcf.2019.08.025. PMID: 31679725.
24. Naehrig S, Chao CM, Naehrlich L. Cystic fibrosis. *Dtsch Arztebl Int.* 2017 Aug 21;114(33-34):564–574. doi:10.3238/arztebl.2017.0564. PMID: 28855057; PMCID: PMC5596161.
25. Farrell PM, White TB, Ren CL, et al. Diagnosis of cystic fibrosis: Consensus Guidelines from the Cystic Fibrosis Foundation. *J Pediatr.* 2017 Feb;181S:S4–S15.e1. doi:10.1016/j.jpeds.2016.09.064. Erratum in: *J Pediatr.* 2017 May;184:243. PMID: 28129811.
26. De Boeck K, Vermeulen F, Dupont L. The diagnosis of cystic fibrosis. *Presse Med.* 2017 Jun;46(6 Pt 2):e97–e108. doi:10.1016/j.lpm.2017.04.010. Epub 2017 May 31. PMID: 28576637.
27. Davis PB. Cystic fibrosis since 1938. *Am J Respir Crit Care Med.* 2006 Mar 1;173(5):475–482. doi:10.1164/rccm.200505-840OE. Epub 2005 Aug 26. PMID: 16126935.
28. Cystic Fibrosis Foundation, Borowitz D, Parad RB, Sharp JK, Sabadosa KA, Robinson KA, Rock MJ, Farrell PM, Sontag MK, Rosenfeld M, Davis SD, Marshall BC, Accurso FJ. Cystic Fibrosis Foundation practice guidelines for the management of infants with cystic fibrosis transmembrane conductance regulator-related metabolic syndrome during the first two years of life and beyond. *J Pediatr.* 2009 Dec;155(6 suppl):S106–S116. doi:10.1016/j.jpeds.2009.09.003. PMID: 19914443; PMCID: PMC6326077.
29. Radtke T, Nevitt SJ, Hebestreit H, Kriemler S. Physical exercise training for cystic fibrosis. *Cochrane Database Syst Rev.* 2017 Nov 1;11(11):CD002768. doi:10.1002/14651858.CD002768.pub4. PMID: 29090734; PMCID: PMC6485991.
30. Saiman L, Siegel JD, LiPuma JJ, et al.; Cystic Fibrous Foundation; Society for Healthcare Epidemiology of America. Infection prevention and control guideline for cystic fibrosis: 2013 Update. *Infect Control Hosp Epidemiol.* 2014 Aug;35(suppl 1):S1–S67. doi:10.1086/676882. Epub 2014 Jul 1. PMID: 25025126.
31. Stallings VA, Stark LJ, Robinson KA, Feranchak AP, Quinton H; Clinical Practice Guidelines on Growth and Nutrition Subcommittee; Ad Hoc Working Group. Evidence-based practice recommendations for nutrition-related management of children and adults with cystic fibrosis and pancreatic insufficiency: Results of a systematic review. *J Am Diet Assoc.* 2008 May;108(5):832–839. doi:10.1016/j.jada.2008.02.020. PMID: 18442507.
32. Cystic Fibrosis Foundation. Types of CFTR Mutations [Internet]. Bethesda, MD: Cystic Fibrosis Foundation [cited 2021 December 11]. Available from: https://www.cff.org/What-is-CF/Genetics/Types-of-CFTR-Mutations/
33. Clancy JP, Rowe SM, Accurso FJ, et al. Results of a phase IIa study of VX-809, an investigational CFTR corrector compound, in subjects with

cystic fibrosis homozygous for the F508del-CFTR mutation. *Thorax.* 2012 Jan;67(1):12–8. doi:10.1136/thoraxjnl-2011-200393. Epub 2011 Aug 8. PMID: 21825083; PMCID: PMC3746507.

34. Konstan MW, McKone EF, Moss RB, et al. Assessment of safety and efficacy of long-term treatment with combination lumacaftor and ivacaftor therapy in patients with cystic fibrosis homozygous for the F508del-CFTR mutation (PROGRESS): A phase 3, extension study. *Lancet Respir Med.* 2017 Feb;5(2):107–118. doi:10.1016/S2213-2600(16)30427-1. Epub 2016 Dec 21. PMID: 28011037.
35. Rosenfeld M, Cunningham S, Harris WT, et al.; KLIMB study group. An open-label extension study of ivacaftor in children with CF and a CFTR gating mutation initiating treatment at age 2-5 years (KLIMB). *J Cyst Fibros.* 2019 Nov;18(6):838–843. doi:10.1016/j.jcf.2019.03.009. Epub 2019 Apr 30. PMID: 31053538; PMCID: PMC6821553.
36. Vertex Pharmaceuticals Incorporated. Symdeko (tezacaftor and ivacaftor) tablet. 2018 [rev. 2021 Aug; cited 2021 Dec]. In: DailyMed [Internet]. [2005]. [about 44 p.]. Bethesda (MD): National Library of Medicine (US). Available from: https://dailymed.nlm.nih.gov/dailymed/drugInfo.cfm?setid=302ae804-37db-44fd-ac2f-3dbdeda9aa4b
37. Vertex Pharmaceuticals Incorporated. Orkambi (lumacaftor and ivacaftor) tablet, film coated. 2015 [rev. 2020 May; cited 2021 Dec]. In: DailyMed [Internet]. [2005]. [about 41 p.]. Bethesda (MD): National Library of Medicine (US). Available from: https://dailymed.nlm.nih.gov/dailymed/drugInfo.cfm?setid=3fc1c40e-cfac-47a1-9e1a-61ead3570600
38. Wainwright CE, Elborn JS, Ramsey BW, et al.; TRAFFIC Study Group; TRANSPORT Study Group. Lumacaftor-ivacaftor in patients with cystic fibrosis homozygous for Phe508del CFTR. *N Engl J Med.* 2015 Jul 16;373(3):220–231. doi:10.1056/NEJMoa1409547. Epub 2015 May 17. PMID: 25981758; PMCID: PMC4764353.
39. Ren CL, Morgan RL, Oermann C, et al. Cystic Fibrosis Pulmonary Guidelines: Use of CFTR modulator therapy in patients with cystic fibrosis. *Ann Am Thorac Soc.* 2018 Mar. doi:10.1513/AnnalsATS.201707-539OT. PMID: 29342367.
40. Vertex Pharmaceuticals Incorporated. Trikafta (elexacaftor, tezacaftor, and ivacaftor) tablet. 2019 [rev. 2021 Oct; cited 2021 Dec]. In: DailyMed [Internet]. [2005]. Bethesda (MD): National Library of Medicine (US). Available from: https://dailymed.nlm.nih.gov/dailymed/drugInfo.cfm?setid=f354423a-85c2-41c3-a9db-0f3aee135d8d
41. Middleton PG, Mall MA, Dřevínek P, et al.; VX17-445-102 Study Group. Elexacaftor-tezacaftor-ivacaftor for cystic fibrosis with a single Phe508del allele. *N Engl J Med.* 2019 Nov 7;381(19):1809–1819. doi:10.1056/NEJMoa1908639. Epub 2019 Oct 31. PMID: 31697873; PMCID: PMC7282384.
42. Heijerman HGM, McKone EF, Downey DG, et al.; VX17-445-103 Trial Group. Efficacy and safety of the elexacaftor plus tezacaftor plus ivacaftor combination regimen in people with cystic fibrosis homozygous for the F508del mutation: A double-blind, randomised, phase 3 trial. *Lancet.* 2019 Nov 23;394(10212):1940–1948. doi:10.1016/S0140-6736(19)32597-8. Epub 2019 Oct 31. Erratum in: *Lancet.* 2020 May 30;395(10238):1694. PMID: 31679946; PMCID: PMC7571408.
43. Jennings MT, Dezube R, Paranjape S, et al. An observational study of outcomes and tolerances in patients with cystic fibrosis initiated on lumacaftor/ivacaftor. *Ann Am Thorac Soc.* 2017 Nov;14(11):1662–1666. doi:10.1513/AnnalsATS.201701-058OC. PMID: 28406713.
44. Iacobucci G. Cystic fibrosis: NHS England strikes deal to offer triple combination treatment. *BMJ.* 2020 Jul 1;370:m2643. doi:10.1136/bmj.m2643. PMID: 32611555.
45. Vertex Pharmaceuticals Incorporated. Kalydeco (ivacaftor) tablet. 2012 [rev. 2020 Dec; cited 2021 Dec]. In: DailyMed [Internet]. [2005]. [about 42 p.]. Bethesda (MD): National Library of Medicine (US). Available from: https://dailymed.nlm.nih.gov/dailymed/drugInfo.cfm?setid=0ab0c9f8-3eee-4e0f-9f3f-c1e16aaffe25
46. Skilton M, Krishan A, Patel S, Sinha IP, Southern KW. Potentiators (specific therapies for class III and IV mutations) for cystic fibrosis. *Cochrane Database Syst Rev.* 2019 Jan 7;1(1):CD009841. doi:10.1002/14651858.CD009841.pub3. PMID: 30616300; PMCID: PMC6353056.
47. Heltshe SL, Mayer-Hamblett N, Burns JL, et al.; GOAL (the G551D Observation-AL) Investigators of the Cystic Fibrosis Foundation Therapeutics Development Network. Pseudomonas aeruginosa in cystic fibrosis patients with G551D-CFTR treated with ivacaftor. *Clin Infect Dis.* 2015 Mar 1;60(5):703–712. doi:10.1093/cid/ciu944. Epub 2014 Nov 25. PMID: 25425629; PMCID: PMC4342673.
48. Sawicki GS, McKone EF, Pasta DJ, et al. Sustained Benefit from ivacaftor demonstrated by combining clinical trial and cystic fibrosis patient registry data. *Am J Respir Crit Care Med.* 2015 Oct 1;192(7):836–842. doi:10.1164/rccm.201503-0578OC. Erratum in: *Am J Respir Crit Care Med.* 2016 Jun 1;193(11):1317–1320. PMID: 26132840.
49. Rowe SM, Heltshe SL, Gonska T, et al.; GOAL Investigators of the Cystic Fibrosis Foundation Therapeutics Development Network. Clinical mechanism of the cystic fibrosis transmembrane conductance regulator potentiator ivacaftor in G551D-mediated cystic fibrosis. *Am J Respir Crit Care Med.* 2014 Jul 15;190(2):175–84. doi:10.1164/rccm.201404-0703OC. PMID: 24927234; PMCID: PMC4226057.
50. Bessonova L, Volkova N, Higgins M, et al. Data from the US and UK cystic fibrosis registries support disease modification by CFTR modulation with ivacaftor. *Thorax.* 2018 Aug;73(8):731–740. doi:10.1136/thoraxjnl-2017-210394. Epub 2018 May 10. PMID: 29748252; PMCID: PMC6204955.
51. Dukovski D, Villella A, Bastos C, et al. Amplifiers co-translationally enhance CFTR biosynthesis via PCBP1-mediated regulation of CFTR mRNA. *J Cyst Fibros.* 2020 Sep;19(5):733–741. doi:10.1016/j.jcf.2020.02.006. Epub 2020 Feb 15. PMID: 32067958.
52. Flume PA, Robinson KA, O'Sullivan BP, et al.; Clinical Practice Guidelines for Pulmonary Therapies Committee. Cystic fibrosis pulmonary guidelines: Airway clearance therapies. *Respir Care.* 2009 Apr;54(4):522–537. PMID: 19327189.
53. Yang C, Montgomery M. Dornase alfa for cystic fibrosis. *Cochrane Database Syst Rev.* 2018 Sep 6;9(9):CD001127. doi:10.1002/14651858.CD001127.pub4. Update in: *Cochrane Database Syst Rev.* 2021 Mar 18;3:CD001127. PMID: 30187450; PMCID: PMC6513278.
54. Goralski JL, Donaldson SH. Hypertonic saline for cystic fibrosis: Worth its salt? *Expert Rev Respir Med.* 2014 Jun;8(3):267–269. doi:10.1586/17476348.2014.896203. Epub 2014 Mar 26. PMID: 24666113.
55. Genetech Inc. Pulmozyme (dornase alfa) solution. 2010 [rev. 2021 Aug; cited 2021 Dec]. In: DailyMed [Internet]. [2005]. [about 26 p.]. Bethesda (MD): National Library of Medicine (US). Available from: https://dailymed.nlm.nih.gov/dailymed/drugInfo.cfm?setid=d8c78a7e-ff99-48f3-8952-643ec2ea0f86
56. Ramsey BW, Astley SJ, Aitken ML, et al. Efficacy and safety of short-term administration of aerosolized recombinant human deoxyribonuclease in patients with cystic fibrosis. *Am Rev Respir Dis.* 1993 Jul;148(1):145–151. doi:10.1164/ajrccm/148.1.145. PMID: 8317790.
57. Shah PL, Scott SF, Knight RA, Marriott C, Ranasinha C, Hodson ME. In vivo effects of recombinant human DNase I on sputum in patients with cystic fibrosis. *Thorax.* 1996 Feb;51(2):119–125. doi:10.1136/thx.51.2.119. PMID: 8711640; PMCID: PMC473012.
58. Shah PI, Bush A, Canny GJ, et al. Recombinant human DNase I in cystic fibrosis patients with severe pulmonary disease: a short-term, double-blind study followed by six months open-label treatment. *Eur Respir J.* 1995 Jun;8(6):954–958. PMID: 7589382.
59. Robinson TE, Goris ML, Zhu HJ, et al. Dornase alfa reduces air trapping in children with mild cystic fibrosis lung disease: A quantitative analysis. *Chest.* 2005 Oct;128(4):2327–2335. doi:10.1378/chest.128.4.2327. PMID: 16236891.
60. Paul K, Rietschel E, Ballmann M, et al.; Bronchoalveolar Lavage for the Evaluation of Antiinflammatory Treatment Study Group. Effect of treatment with dornase alpha on airway inflammation in patients with cystic fibrosis. *Am J Respir Crit Care Med.* 2004 Mar 15;169(6):719–725. doi:10.1164/rccm.200307-959OC. Epub 2003 Dec 18. PMID: 14684561.
61. Mogayzel PJ Jr, Naureckas ET, Robinson KA, et al.; Pulmonary Clinical Practice Guidelines Committee. Cystic fibrosis pulmonary guidelines. Chronic medications for maintenance of lung health. *Am J Respir Crit Care Med.* 2013 Apr 1;187(7):680–689. doi:10.1164/rccm.201207-1160oe. PMID: 23540878.
62. Reeves EP, Molloy K, Pohl K, McElvaney NG. Hypertonic saline in treatment of pulmonary disease in cystic fibrosis. *ScientificWorldJournal.* 2012;2012:465230. doi:10.1100/2012/465230. Epub 2012 May 3. PMID: 22645424; PMCID: PMC3356721.
63. Donaldson SH, Bennett WD, Zeman KL, Knowles MR, Tarran R, Boucher RC. Mucus clearance and lung function in cystic fibrosis with hypertonic saline. *N Engl J Med.* 2006 Jan 19;354(3):241–250. doi:10.1056/NEJMoa043891. PMID: 16421365.
64. Robinson M, Hemming AL, Regnis JA, et al. Effect of increasing doses of hypertonic saline on mucociliary clearance in patients with cystic fibrosis. *Thorax.* 1997 Oct;52(10):900–903. doi:10.1136/thx.52.10.900. PMID: 9404379; PMCID: PMC1758438.
65. Enderby B, Doull I. Hypertonic saline inhalation in cystic fibrosis—salt in the wound, or sweet success? *Arch Dis Child.* 2007 Mar;92(3):195–196. doi:10.1136/adc.2006.094979. PMID: 17337677; PMCID: PMC2083400.
66. Rosenfeld M, Ratjen F, Brumback L, et al.; ISIS Study Group. Inhaled hypertonic saline in infants and children younger than 6 years with cystic fibrosis: the ISIS randomized controlled trial. *JAMA.* 2012 Jun

6;307(21):2269–2277. doi:10.1001/jama.2012.5214. PMID: 22610452; PMCID: PMC3586815.
67. Wark P, McDonald VM. Nebulised hypertonic saline for cystic fibrosis. *Cochrane Database Syst Rev.* 2018 Sep 27;9(9):CD001506. doi:10.1002/14651858.CD001506.pub4. PMID: 30260472; PMCID: PMC6513595.
68. Jaques A, Daviskas E, Turton JA, et al. Inhaled mannitol improves lung function in cystic fibrosis. *Chest.* 2008 Jun;133(6):1388–1396. doi:10.1378/chest.07-2294. Epub 2008 Mar 13. PMID: 18339790.
69. Bilton D, Robinson P, Cooper P, et al.; CF301 Study Investigators. Inhaled dry powder mannitol in cystic fibrosis: An efficacy and safety study. *Eur Respir J.* 2011 Nov;38(5):1071–1080. doi:10.1183/09031936.00187510. Epub 2011 Apr 8. PMID: 21478216.
70. Rosenfeld M, Gibson RL, McNamara S, et al. Early pulmonary infection, inflammation, and clinical outcomes in infants with cystic fibrosis. *Pediatr Pulmonol.* 2001 Nov;32(5):356–366. doi:10.1002/ppul.1144. PMID: 11596160.
71. Emerson J, Rosenfeld M, McNamara S, Ramsey B, Gibson RL. Pseudomonas aeruginosa and other predictors of mortality and morbidity in young children with cystic fibrosis. *Pediatr Pulmonol.* 2002 Aug;34(2):91–100. doi:10.1002/ppul.10127. PMID: 12112774.
72. Sagel SD, Gibson RL, Emerson J, et al.; Inhaled Tobramycin in Young Children Study Group; Cystic Fibrosis Foundation Therapeutics Development Network. Impact of Pseudomonas and Staphylococcus infection on inflammation and clinical status in young children with cystic fibrosis. *J Pediatr.* 2009 Feb;154(2):183–188. doi:10.1016/j.jpeds.2008.08.001. Epub 2008 Sep 25. PMID: 18822427; PMCID: PMC2654617.
73. Dolce D, Neri S, Grisotto L, et al. Methicillin-resistant Staphylococcus aureus eradication in cystic fibrosis patients: A randomized multicenter study. *PLoS One.* 2019 Mar 22;14(3):e0213497. doi:10.1371/journal.pone.0213497. PMID: 30901344; PMCID: PMC6430412.
74. Southern KW, Barker PM, Solis-Moya A, Patel L. Macrolide antibiotics for cystic fibrosis. *Cochrane Database Syst Rev.* 2012 Nov 14;11(11):CD002203. doi:10.1002/14651858.CD002203.pub4. PMID: 23152214; PMCID: PMC7098459.
75. Saiman L, Anstead M, Mayer-Hamblett N, et al.; AZ0004 Azithromycin Study Group. Effect of azithromycin on pulmonary function in patients with cystic fibrosis uninfected with Pseudomonas aeruginosa: A randomized controlled trial. *JAMA.* 2010 May 5;303(17):1707–1715. doi:10.1001/jama.2010.563. PMID: 20442386.
76. Moskowitz SM, Foster JM, Emerson J, Burns JL. Clinically feasible biofilm susceptibility assay for isolates of Pseudomonas aeruginosa from patients with cystic fibrosis. *J Clin Microbiol.* 2004 May;42(5):1915–1922. doi:10.1128/JCM.42.5.1915-1922.2004. PMID: 15131149; PMCID: PMC404629.
77. Hoffmann N, Lee B, Hentzer M, et al. Azithromycin blocks quorum sensing and alginate polymer formation and increases the sensitivity to serum and stationary-growth-phase killing of Pseudomonas aeruginosa and attenuates chronic P. aeruginosa lung infection in Cftr(-/-) mice. *Antimicrob Agents Chemother.* 2007 Oct;51(10):3677–3687. doi:10.1128/AAC.01011-06. Epub 2007 Jul 9. PMID: 17620382; PMCID: PMC2043275.
78. Mayer-Hamblett N, Retsch-Bogart G, Kloster M, et al.; OPTIMIZE Study Group. Azithromycin for Early Pseudomonas Infection in Cystic Fibrosis. The OPTIMIZE Randomized Trial. *Am J Respir Crit Care Med.* 2018 Nov 1;198(9):1177–1187. doi:10.1164/rccm.201802-0215OC. Erratum in: *Am J Respir Crit Care Med.* 2019 Mar 15;199(6):809. PMID: 29890086; PMCID: PMC6221579.
79. Nick JA, Moskowitz SM, Chmiel JF, et al. Azithromycin may antagonize inhaled tobramycin when targeting Pseudomonas aeruginosa in cystic fibrosis. *Ann Am Thorac Soc.* 2014 Mar;11(3):342–350. doi:10.1513/AnnalsATS.201310-352OC. PMID: 24476418; PMCID: PMC4028742.
80. Nichols DP, Happoldt CL, Bratcher PE, et al. Impact of azithromycin on the clinical and antimicrobial effectiveness of tobramycin in the treatment of cystic fibrosis. *J Cyst Fibros.* 2017 May;16(3):358–366. doi:10.1016/j.jcf.2016.12.003. Epub 2016 Dec 24. PMID: 28025037; PMCID: PMC5492972.
81. Somayaji R, Russell R, Cogen JD, et al. Oral Azithromycin use and the recovery of lung function from pulmonary exacerbations treated with intravenous tobramycin or colistimethate in adults with cystic fibrosis. *Ann Am Thorac Soc.* 2019 Jul;16(7):853–860. doi:10.1513/AnnalsATS.201811-773OC. PMID: 30840835; PMCID: PMC6600836.
82. Nichols DP, Odem-Davis K, Cogen JD, et al. Pulmonary outcomes associated with long-term azithromycin therapy in cystic fibrosis. *Am J Respir Crit Care Med.* 2020 Feb 15;201(4):430–437. doi:10.1164/rccm.201906-1206OC. PMID: 31661302; PMCID: PMC7049934.
83. Flume PA, O'Sullivan BP, Robinson KA, et al.; Cystic Fibrosis Foundation, Pulmonary Therapies Committee. Cystic fibrosis pulmonary guidelines: Chronic medications for maintenance of lung health. *Am J Respir Crit Care Med.* 2007 Nov 15;176(10):957–969. doi:10.1164/rccm.200705-664OC. Epub 2007 Aug 29. PMID: 17761616.
84. Lands LC, Stanojevic S. Oral non-steroidal anti-inflammatory drug therapy for lung disease in cystic fibrosis. *Cochrane Database Syst Rev.* 2019 Sep 9;9(9):CD001505. doi:10.1002/14651858.CD001505.pub5. PMID: 31499593; PMCID: PMC6733592.
85. Arranz I, Martín-Suárez A, Lanao JM, et al. Population pharmacokinetics of high dose ibuprofen in cystic fibrosis. *Arch Dis Child.* 2003 Dec;88(12):1128–1130. doi:10.1136/adc.88.12.1128. PMID: 14670788; PMCID: PMC1719401.
86. Lahiri T, Hempstead SE, Brady C, et al. Clinical Practice Guidelines From the Cystic Fibrosis Foundation for Preschoolers With Cystic Fibrosis. *Pediatrics.* 2016 Apr;137(4):e20151784. doi:10.1542/peds.2015-1784. Epub 2016 Mar 23. PMID: 27009033.
87. Nakajima K, Oshida H, Muneyuki T, Kakei M. Pancrelipase: An evidence-based review of its use for treating pancreatic exocrine insufficiency. *Core Evid.* 2012;7:77–91. doi:10.2147/CE.S26705. Epub 2012 Jul 19. PMID: 22936895; PMCID: PMC3426252.
88. Walkowiak J, Sands D, Nowakowska A, et al. Early decline of pancreatic function in cystic fibrosis patients with class 1 or 2 CFTR mutations. *J Pediatr Gastroenterol Nutr.* 2005 Feb;40(2):199–201. doi:10.1097/00005176-200502000-00022. PMID: 15699697.
89. Ahmed N, Corey M, Forstner G, et al. Molecular consequences of cystic fibrosis transmembrane regulator (CFTR) gene mutations in the exocrine pancreas. *Gut.* 2003 Aug;52(8):1159–1164. doi:10.1136/gut.52.8.1159. PMID: 12865275; PMCID: PMC1773762.
90. The Clinical and Functional TRanslation of CFTR (CFTR2) [Internet]. Bethesda, MD: US CF Foundation, Johns Hopkins University, The Hospital for Sick Children; 2021 September [cited 2021 December 11]. Available from: http://cftr2.org
91. Borowitz DS, Grand RJ, Durie PR. Use of pancreatic enzyme supplements for patients with cystic fibrosis in the context of fibrosing colonopathy. Consensus Committee. *J Pediatr.* 1995 Nov;127(5):681–684. doi:10.1016/s0022-3476(95)70153-2. PMID: 7472816.
92. Tangpricha V, Kelly A, Stephenson A, et al.; Cystic Fibrosis Foundation Vitamin D Evidence-Based Review Committee. An update on the screening, diagnosis, management, and treatment of vitamin D deficiency in individuals with cystic fibrosis: Evidence-based recommendations from the Cystic Fibrosis Foundation. *J Clin Endocrinol Metab.* 2012 Apr;97(4):1082–1093. doi:10.1210/jc.2011-3050. Epub 2012 Mar 7. PMID: 22399505.
93. Flume PA, Mogayzel PJ Jr, Robinson KA, et al.; Clinical Practice Guidelines for Pulmonary Therapies Committee. Cystic fibrosis pulmonary guidelines: Treatment of pulmonary exacerbations. *Am J Respir Crit Care Med.* 2009 Nov 1;180(9):802–808. doi:10.1164/rccm.200812-1845PP. Epub 2009 Sep 3. PMID: 19729669.
94. Rybak MJ, Le J, Lodise TP, et al. Therapeutic monitoring of vancomycin for serious methicillin-resistant Staphylococcus aureus infections: A revised consensus guideline and review by the American Society of Health-System Pharmacists, the Infectious Diseases Society of America, the Pediatric Infectious Diseases Society, and the Society of Infectious Diseases Pharmacists. *Am J Health Syst Pharm.* 2020;77(11):835–864. 10.1093/ajhp/zxaa036 32191793.
95. Aris RM, Merkel PA, Bachrach LK, et al. Guide to bone health and disease in cystic fibrosis. *J Clin Endocrinol Metab.* 2005 Mar;90(3):1888–1896. doi:10.1210/jc.2004-1629. Epub 2004 Dec 21. PMID: 15613415.
96. Sermet-Gaudelus I, Castanet M, Retsch-Bogart G, Aris RM. Update on cystic fibrosis-related bone disease: A special focus on children. *Paediatr Respir Rev.* 2009 Sep;10(3):134–142. doi:10.1016/j.prrv.2009.05.001. Epub 2009 Jul 17. PMID: 19651384.
97. Bianchi ML, Colombo C, Assael BM, et al. Treatment of low bone density in young people with cystic fibrosis: A multicentre, prospective, open-label observational study of calcium and calcifediol followed by a randomised placebo-controlled trial of alendronate. *Lancet Respir Med.* 2013 Jul;1(5):377–385. doi:10.1016/S2213-2600(13)70064-X. Epub 2013 Jun 2. PMID: 24429202.
98. Haworth CS, Sharples L, Hughes V, et al. Multicentre trial of weekly risedronate on bone density in adults with cystic fibrosis. *J Cyst Fibros.* 2011 Dec;10(6):470–476. doi:10.1016/j.jcf.2011.07.007. Epub 2011 Aug 16. PMID: 21849264.
99. Putman MS, Anabtawi A, Le T, Tangpricha V, Sermet-Gaudelus I. Cystic fibrosis bone disease treatment: Current knowledge and future directions. *J Cyst Fibros.* 2019 Oct;18(suppl 2):S56–S65. doi:10.1016/j.jcf.2019.08.017. PMID: 31679730.

100. Smith BA, Modi AC, Quittner AL, Wood BL. Depressive symptoms in children with cystic fibrosis and parents and its effects on adherence to airway clearance. *Pediatr Pulmonol.* 2010 Aug;45(8):756–763. doi:10.1002/ppul.21238. PMID: 20597082.
101. Latchford G, Duff AJ. Screening for depression in a single CF centre. *J Cyst Fibros.* 2013 Dec;12(6):794–796. doi:10.1016/j.jcf.2013.04.002. Epub 2013 Apr 26. PMID: 23628513.
102. Quittner AL, Goldbeck L, Abbott J, et al. Prevalence of depression and anxiety in patients with cystic fibrosis and parent caregivers: Results of The International Depression Epidemiological Study across nine countries. *Thorax.* 2014 Dec;69(12):1090–1097. doi:10.1136/thoraxjnl-2014-205983. Epub 2014 Sep 21. PMID: 25246663.
103. Quittner AL, Abbott J, Georgiopoulos AM, et al.; International Committee on Mental Health; EPOS Trial Study Group. International Committee on Mental Health in Cystic Fibrosis: Cystic Fibrosis Foundation and European Cystic Fibrosis Society consensus statements for screening and treating depression and anxiety. *Thorax.* 2016 Jan;71(1):26–34. doi:10.1136/thoraxjnl-2015-207488. Epub 2015 Oct 9. PMID: 26452630; PMCID: PMC4717439.

Drug-Induced Pulmonary Diseases

e48

Margaret A. Miklich and Mojdeh S. Heavner

KEY CONCEPTS

1. The most common drug-induced pulmonary diseases (DIPDs) are interstitial pneumonitis and pulmonary fibrosis.
2. DIPD is a diagnosis of exclusion.
3. The occurrence of DIPD is unpredictable, but there are agent- and population-specific risk factors including extremes of age, the dose of the offending agent, and preexisting lung conditions.
4. Prevention includes avoiding causative agents in high-risk patients.
5. Early recognition of DIPD is essential to improving long-term outcomes.
6. Management of DIPD commonly involves discontinuation of the causative agent and treatment with corticosteroids.

BEYOND THE BOOK

Watch the video entitled "Lung Disease and Double Lung Transplantation" at Stanford: "Jen Julian's Story" (https://stanfordhealthcare.org/stanford-health-care-now/2012/julian-interstitial-lung-disease.html) from Stanford Health Care. This 5-minute video shares the patient perspective of living with a severe interstitial lung disease ultimately necessitating transplantation. While the etiology of this patient's chronic hypersensitivity pneumonitis is believed to have been from an inhaled environmental exposure, certain medications can cause a similar condition. The video adds a personal connection to the impact healthcare providers can have on patients with DIILD.

INTRODUCTION

Clinicians should be familiar with drug-induced pulmonary diseases (DIPD) to promptly identify cases and manage complications to minimize potential morbidity and mortality. In the United States, over 2 million adverse drug reactions (ADRs) and 100,000 drug-associated deaths are reported annually. Pulmonary complications may represent the largest proportion of fatalities from ADRs.[1,2] Certain medications and patient-specific situations carry a greater risk for pulmonary ADRs. As an example, up to 10% of patients receiving chemotherapy and up to 40% of patients receiving chemotherapy with bleomycin may develop pulmonary toxicity.[1] The Website pneumotox.com and associated Android and iPhone applications list over 1,500 medications reported to cause DIPD, 650 patterns of DIPD, and 10,000 references. This resource functions as a free searchable database for clinicians. The true rate of drug-induced reactions is likely underestimated because there is a challenge in reaching a definitive diagnosis of DIPD, and estimates largely rely on case reports and observational studies.

DIPD may result from direct or indirect drug effects. Direct effects may present as an idiosyncratic reaction or through direct pulmonary toxicity from a drug or its metabolites. DIPD can affect a variety of pulmonary tissues and structures. The clinical presentation and patient symptoms associated with DIPD are often nonspecific. Patients may complain of pleuritic chest pain, dyspnea, cough, wheezing, and fever. Symptoms may be present at rest or during activity. When DIPD affects the vasculature, it often presents with pulmonary hemorrhage or vasculitis, hemoptysis, hematoma, or alveolar hemorrhage. DIPD is a diagnosis of exclusion. It should be considered when a patient has had a known drug exposure and subsequently develops new signs and symptoms consistent with DIPD clinical presentation. The resolution of symptoms after drug withdrawal is particularly informative. Radiographic imaging, including X-rays and CT scans, can help rule out other potential causes of pulmonary disease and establish the diagnosis of DIPD.[3] Table e48-1 summarizes DIPD diagnostic considerations and general management strategies.

The clinical spectrum of DIPD is heterogeneous; narrowing down the affected region of the lung can assist with identifying a distinct diagnosis and subsequent management approach. DIPD most frequently impacts the pulmonary parenchyma, but can affect the pleura, airways, pulmonary vasculature, mediastinum, and neuromuscular respiratory system (see Fig. e48-1). Notable manifestations can include interstitial pneumonitis, fibrosis, pleural effusions, or drug-induced lupus.[3]

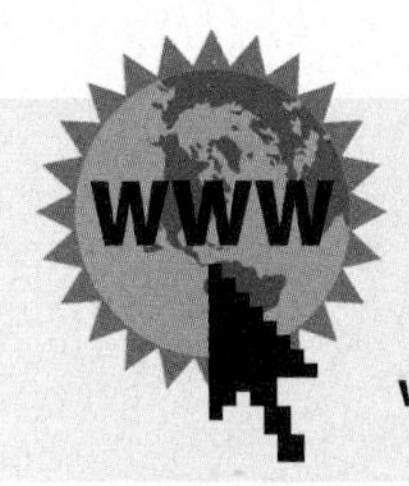

The complete chapter, learning objectives, and other resources can be found at **www.pharmacotherapyonline.com.**

Evaluation of the Gastrointestinal Tract

e49

Keith M. Olsen

KEY CONCEPTS

1. The patient history is key to evaluating gastrointestinal (GI) tract disorders and should include the problem onset, the setting in which it developed, and its presentation. Patient warning signs and alarm symptoms should be identified quickly and referral for further evaluation should be obtained in a prompt manner.
2. A complete physical examination should be performed, the severity and location of symptoms directing the focus of the examination.
3. Contrast agents, barium sulfate and Gastrografin® (diatrizoate meglumine and diatrizoate sodium solution), have gradually been replaced by endoscopy, but allow evaluation of the hollow organs of the digestive tract for mucosally based lesions as well as narrowing or strictures involving the GI tract.
4. The upper GI series involves radiographic visualization of the esophagus, stomach, and duodenum; whereas the lower GI series involves visualization of the colon and rectum.
5. Enteroclysis is used to evaluate the small bowel by introducing contrast agents by tube through the nose or mouth directly into the small intestine.
6. Transabdominal ultrasound, computed tomography, and magnetic resonance imaging provide images of the gallbladder, liver, pancreas, and abdominal wall and are increasingly utilized for assessing small bowel and colonic diseases.
7. Radionuclide imaging is sometimes useful to visualize and evaluate the liver, spleen, bile ducts, and gallbladder.
8. The endoscope, an illuminated optical instrument, remains the cornerstone of GI diagnosis and most importantly therapy. Common examples of endoscopic procedures include esophagogastroduodenoscopy, colonoscopy, enteroscopy, endoscopic retrograde cholangiopancreatography, and endoscopic ultrasound.
9. Capsule endoscopy, a newer less invasive endoscopic technique, takes pictures of the GI tract in the assessment of the small bowel in particular.
10. Ambulatory esophageal pH measurement is an important diagnostic test for gastroesophageal reflux disease and is often performed in conjunction with upper endoscopy. Most systems today are completely wireless and patient friendly.
11. Multichannel intraluminal impedance and pH monitoring combines acid exposure with impedance changes in resistant flow to aid the diagnosis of reflux in patients receiving a proton pump inhibitor and other antisecretory medications.

BEYOND THE BOOK

This activity will encourage students to review the chapter to determine the most useful approach for diagnostic or therapeutic interventions for each gastrointestinal disease. With each of the following gastrointestinal diseases, determine which laboratory, radiologic, mechanical test, or patient history is required to confirm the diagnosis: unexplained diarrhea, bowel obstruction, Barrett esophagus, reflux disease treated with a proton pump inhibitor.

INTRODUCTION

The GI tract is an organ system responsible for nutrient absorption, waste excretion, and immunity. It is composed of the upper GI tract (oral cavity, esophagus, and duodenum), lower GI tract (small intestine, cecum, colon, rectum, and anus), and associated glandular organs (gallbladder, pancreas, and liver). A variety of symptoms can arise from GI tract dysfunction, including heartburn, dyspepsia, abdominal pain, nausea, vomiting, diarrhea, constipation, and GI bleeding. Signs and symptoms of malabsorption, hepatitis, and GI infection are also commonly seen. All clinicians must recognize warning or alarm symptoms including weight loss, intractable vomiting, anemia, dysphagia, odynophagia, and bleeding; and a patient presenting with any of these symptoms should be immediately referred for further diagnostic interventions.

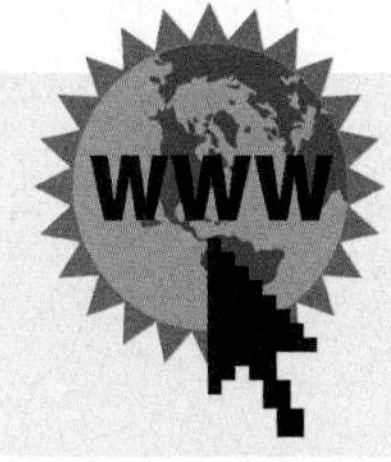

The complete chapter, learning objectives, and other resources can be found at **www.pharmacotherapyonline.com.**

Gastroesophageal Reflux Disease

50

Dianne W. May, Devin L. Lavender, and Satish C. Rao

KEY CONCEPTS

1. Gastroesophageal reflux disease (GERD) can be described on the basis of either esophageal symptoms or esophageal tissue injury. The common symptoms include heartburn, regurgitation, chest pain, and dysphagia.
2. Endoscopy is commonly used to evaluate mucosal injury from GERD and to assess for the presence of Barrett's esophagus or other complications, such as strictures or adenocarcinoma.
3. Whereas ambulatory reflux monitoring only measures acid reflux, combined impedance–pH monitoring measures both acid and nonacid reflux.
4. The goals of GERD treatment are to alleviate symptoms and improve health-related quality of life, decrease the frequency of recurrent disease, promote healing of mucosal injury, and prevent complications.
5. GERD treatment is determined by disease severity and includes: (a) lifestyle changes and patient-directed therapy with antacids, nonprescription H2-receptor antagonists (H2RAs), and/or nonprescription proton pump inhibitors; (b) pharmacologic treatment with prescription-strength acid suppression therapy; (c) surgery; and (d) endoscopic therapies.
6. Patients with typical GERD symptoms should be treated with lifestyle modifications as appropriate and a trial of empiric acid suppression therapy. Those who do not respond to empiric therapy or who present with alarm symptoms such as dysphagia, weight loss, or gastrointestinal (GI) bleeding should undergo endoscopy.
7. Surgical intervention is a viable alternative treatment for select patients when long-term pharmacologic management is undesirable or when patients have complications.
8. Acid suppression is the mainstay of GERD treatment. Proton pump inhibitors provide the greatest symptom relief and the highest healing rates, especially for patients with erosive disease or moderate-to-severe symptoms or with complications.
9. Many patients with GERD will relapse if medication is withdrawn; so, long-term maintenance treatment may be required. A proton pump inhibitor is the drug of choice for maintenance of patients with moderate-to-severe GERD, erosive disease, or other complications such as Barrett's esophagus.
10. Patient medication profiles should be reviewed for drugs that may aggravate GERD. Patients should be monitored for adverse drug reactions and potential drug–drug interactions. Deprescribing PPIs or tapering to the lowest effective dose is a key strategy in preventing adverse effects.

BEYOND THE BOOK

Watch video entitled, "GERD" in AccessPharmacy. This ~6-minute video summarizes the normal function of the esophagus and stomach compared to that seen with acid reflux, complications of GERD, process of acid production, and pharmacologic therapy for GERD. Students' understanding regarding the Collect, Assess, and Plan steps of the Patient Care Process are addressed with this video.

INTRODUCTION

Gastroesophageal reflux disease (GERD) is a common medical disorder.[1] GERD has been described based on its physiological, functional, and symptomatic attributes.[2,3] The Lyon consensus highlighted the physiological attributes of GERD, such as esophageal motor dysfunction and esophageal permeability issues. However, these abnormalities are nonspecific for GERD. The Rome IV conference described the functional syndromes with GERD characteristics. However, reflux causality cannot be made based on clinical presentation mimicking GERD.[2] The Montreal consensus defines GERD as "symptoms or complications resulting from refluxed stomach contents into the esophagus or beyond, into the oral cavity (including the larynx) or lung."[1] The key is that these troublesome symptoms, defined as symptoms occurring twice weekly or more, is that they adversely affect the well-being of the patient.[4] Episodic heartburn that is not frequent enough or painful enough to be considered bothersome by the patient is not included in this definition of GERD.

GERD can be further classified as either symptom-based or tissue injury–based depending on how the patient presents.[1] Symptom-based GERD may exist with or without esophageal injury, and most commonly presents as heartburn, regurgitation, or dysphagia (difficulty swallowing). Less commonly, odynophagia (painful swallowing), water brash, belching, bloating, or hypersalivation may also occur. The absence of tissue injury or erosions is commonly termed nonerosive reflux disease (NERD). The presence of abnormal acid exposure on ambulatory reflux monitoring differentiates NERD from functional heartburn where no abnormalities are seen.[5] NERD should also be differentiated from reflux hypersensitivity where patients have physiologic (normal) acid production but are symptomatic. Functional heartburn or reflux hypersensitivity may not respond well to acid suppression therapy since the underlying cause is not acid related.

Tissue injury-based GERD may exist with or without symptoms. The spectrum of injury includes esophagitis (inflammation of the lining of the esophagus), Barrett's esophagus (when tissue lining the esophagus is replaced by tissue similar to the lining of the intestine), esophageal strictures, and esophageal adenocarcinoma.[1] Esophagitis occurs when the esophagus is repeatedly exposed to refluxed gastric contents for prolonged periods of time.[1] This can progress to erosion of the squamous epithelium of the esophagus (erosive esophagitis). Esophagitis is classified as low grade (grade A or B) or high grade (grade C or D) based on the Los Angeles classification system. Complications of long-term reflux may include the development of esophageal strictures, Barrett's esophagus, or possibly adenocarcinoma of the esophagus.

Gastroesophageal reflux symptoms associated with disease processes in organs other than the esophagus are referred to as extraesophageal reflux syndromes. Patients with extraesophageal reflux syndromes may present with chest pain, hoarseness, chronic cough, or asthma. An association between these syndromes and GERD should only be considered when they occur along with esophageal GERD syndrome because these extraesophageal symptoms are nonspecific and have many other causes.[1]

Many patients suffering from mild GERD do not go on to develop erosive esophagitis and are often managed with lifestyle changes, antacids, and nonprescription histamine-2 receptor antagonists (H2RAs) or nonprescription proton pump inhibitors (PPIs). Those with more severe symptoms (with or without tissue injury) predictably follow a course of relapsing disease, requiring more intensive treatment with acid suppression therapy followed by long-term maintenance therapy. Periodic assessment is important to assure the lowest effective medication dose is being used. Antireflux surgery offers an alternative for select patients in whom prolonged medical management is undesirable, those with refractory GERD, or those with complications. Bariatric surgery may be an option in obese patients. Endoscopic therapies continue to be evaluated in an effort to find a less invasive alternative therapy that bridges the gap between pharmacologic management and more invasive surgery.

EPIDEMIOLOGY

GERD occurs most commonly in those older than 50 years of age.[6] Although mortality is rare, GERD may have a significant economic impact and decrease the quality of life. The true prevalence of GERD is difficult to assess because many patients do not seek medical treatment, symptoms do not always correlate well with the severity of the disease, and there is no standardized definition or universal gold standard method for diagnosing the disease. However, the prevalence has risen significantly over the last 20 years with approximately 20% of adults in the United States suffering from GERD symptoms on a weekly basis.[7-9] The prevalence of GERD varies depending on the geographic region.[7,8] Over 50% of those taking a PPI still had persistent symptoms.[9]

Two contributing factors for the increased prevalence of GERD in females include pregnancy and the presence of NERD.[10] The prevalence of erosive esophagitis is higher in men.[10] Gender is an important factor in the development of Barrett's esophagus and esophageal adenocarcinoma, which are both more common in men. As such, screening for Barrett's esophagus is only considered in men, except in unique circumstances, such as women with scleroderma and esophageal involvement.[11] Adenocarcinoma of the esophagus is more common in those with chronic GERD symptoms than those who do not have GERD. The relationship of adenocarcinoma with Barrett's esophagus, or long-standing GERD symptoms (as an independent risk factor for esophageal adenocarcinoma), remains to be clearly defined.

Established risk factors that may contribute to the development or worsening of GERD symptoms include obesity, tobacco smoking, and genetic predisposition.[12] Obesity is associated with a 2.5 times increased risk for developing GERD.[13] Tobacco smoking may increase the prevalence of GERD 1.26 times compared to nonsmokers.[6] Other risk factors or comorbidities for GERD include alcohol consumption, certain medications and foods, respiratory diseases, and reflux chest pain syndrome. More recently, nonalcoholic fatty liver disease and major depressive disorder have been reported as worsening GERD symptoms.[14]

PATHOPHYSIOLOGY

The key factor in the development of GERD is the abnormal reflux of gastric contents from the stomach into the esophagus, oral cavity, and/or the lung.[1] An incompetent antireflux barrier at the esophagogastric junction (EGJ) plays a major role in GERD pathophysiology.[3] In some cases, gastroesophageal reflux is associated with defective lower esophageal sphincter (LES) pressure or function (Fig. 50-1). Patients may have decreased gastroesophageal sphincter pressures related to (a) spontaneous transient LES relaxations (TLESRs), (b) transient increases in intra-abdominal pressure, or (c) an atonic LES, all of which may lead to the development of gastroesophageal reflux. Problems with other normal mucosal defense mechanisms,

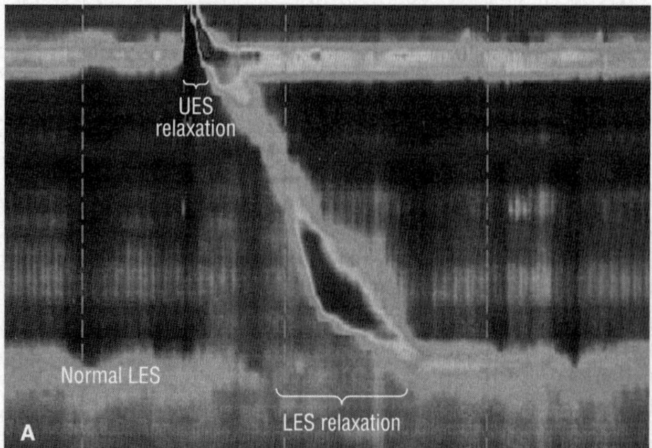

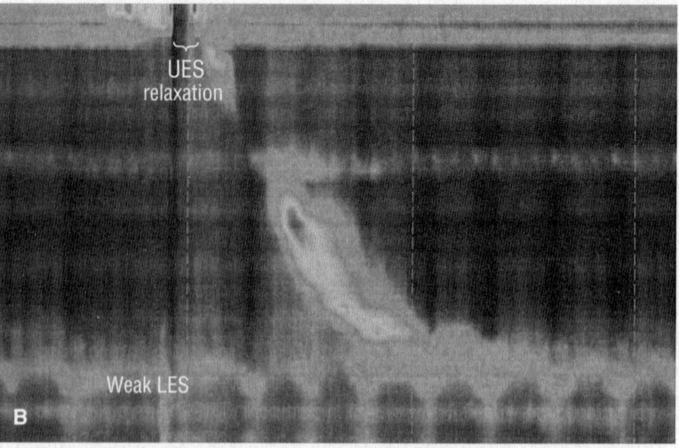

FIGURE 50-1 Normal versus weak lower esophageal sphincter pressure and relaxations via high resolution manometry.

such as abnormal esophageal anatomy, improper esophageal clearance of gastric fluids, reduced mucosal resistance to acid, delayed or ineffective gastric emptying, inadequate production of epidermal growth factor, and reduced salivary buffering of acid, may also contribute to the development of GERD. Substances that may promote esophageal damage on reflux into the esophagus include gastric acid, pepsin, bile acids, and pancreatic enzymes. Thus, the composition and the volume of the refluxate, as well as duration of exposure, are important aggressive factors in determining the consequences of gastroesophageal reflux.

The presence of an "acid pocket" is a potential explanation for postprandial reflux symptoms and may represent a target for treatment of reflux disease. While gastric acidity is buffered by food, ambulatory pH reflux monitoring has shown that this buffering effect may vary in different parts of the stomach and esophagus. The acid pocket is thought to be an area of unbuffered acid in the proximal stomach that accumulates after a meal and may contribute to GERD symptoms postprandially.[15] It occurs due to meal-stimulated acid not mixing well with the chyme in the proximal stomach. Gastric secretions form a distinct layer above the chyme. GERD patients are predisposed to upward migration of acid from the acid pocket. In addition, the acid pocket may also be positioned above the diaphragm in patients, especially in those with hiatal hernia, which increases the risk for acid reflux.

Lower Esophageal Sphincter Pressure

The LES is a specialized thickening of the smooth muscle lining of the distal esophagus with an elevated basal resting pressure.[13] The sphincter is normally in a tonic, contracted state, preventing the reflux of gastric material from the stomach, but relaxes on swallowing to permit the passage of food into the stomach. There are three mechanisms by which defective LES pressure may cause gastroesophageal reflux. First, and probably most importantly, reflux may occur following spontaneous TLESRs that are not associated with swallowing. Although the exact mechanism is unknown, esophageal distension, vomiting, belching, and retching cause relaxation of the LES. While not thought to contribute significantly to erosive esophagitis, these transient relaxations, which are normal postprandially, may play an important role in symptom-based esophageal reflux syndromes. Transient decreases in sphincter pressure are responsible for more than half of the reflux episodes in patients with GERD. The propensity to develop gastroesophageal reflux secondary to transient decreases in LES pressure is probably dependent on numerous factors, including the degree of sphincter relaxation, efficacy of esophageal clearance, patient position (more common in recumbent position), gastric volume, and intragastric pressure. Second, reflux may occur following transient increases in intra-abdominal pressure (stress reflux). An increase in intra-abdominal pressure such as that occurring during straining, bending over, coughing, eating, or a Valsalva maneuver may overcome a weak LES, and thus may lead to reflux. Third, the LES may be atonic, thus permitting free reflux as seen in patients with scleroderma.

Various foods and medications may aggravate esophageal reflux by decreasing LES pressure or by precipitating symptomatic reflux by direct mucosal irritation (Table 50-1). Pregnancy is a condition in which reflux is common. There are many postulated reasons for the increased incidence of heartburn during pregnancy, including hormonal effects on esophageal muscle, LES tone, and physical factors (increased intra-abdominal pressure) resulting from an enlarging uterus. A decrease in LES pressure resulting from any of the previously mentioned causes is not always associated with gastroesophageal reflux. Likewise, individuals who experience decreases in sphincter pressures and subsequently reflux do not always develop GERD. The other natural defense mechanisms (anatomic factors, esophageal clearance, mucosal resistance, and other gastric factors) must be evoked to explain this phenomenon.

TABLE 50-1 Foods and Medications That May Worsen GERD Symptoms

Foods/Beverages	Medications
Decreased Lower Esophageal Sphincter Pressure	
Fatty meal	Anticholinergics
Carminatives (peppermint, spearmint)	Barbiturates Caffeine
Chocolate	Dihydropyridine calcium channel blockers
Coffee, cola, tea	Dopamine
Garlic	Estrogen
Onions	Nicotine
Chili peppers	Nitrates
Alcohol	Progesterone
	Tetracycline
	Theophylline
Direct Irritants to the Esophageal Mucosa	
Spicy foods	Aspirin
Orange juice	Bisphosphonates
Tomato juice	Nonsteroidal anti-inflammatory drugs
Coffee	Iron
Tobacco	Quinidine
	Potassium chloride

Anatomic Factors

Disruption of the normal anatomic barriers by a hiatal hernia (when a portion of the stomach protrudes through the diaphragm into the chest) was once thought to be a primary etiology of gastroesophageal reflux and esophagitis. Now it appears that a more important factor related to the presence or absence of symptoms in patients with hiatal hernia is the LES pressure. Patients with hypotensive LES pressures and large hiatal hernias are more likely to experience gastroesophageal reflux following abrupt increases in intra-abdominal pressure compared with patients with a hypotensive LES and no hiatal hernia.

Esophageal Clearance

In many patients with GERD, the problem is not that they produce too much acid but that the acid spends too much time in contact with the esophageal mucosa. Contact time is dependent on the rate at which the esophagus clears the noxious material, as well as the frequency of reflux. Swallowing contributes to esophageal clearance by increasing salivary flow. Saliva contains bicarbonate that buffers the residual gastric material on the surface of the esophagus. The production of saliva decreases with increasing age, making it more difficult to maintain a neutral intraesophageal pH. In addition, swallowing is decreased during sleep, making nocturnal GERD a problem in many patients.

Mucosal Resistance

Within the esophageal mucosa and submucosa, there are mucus-secreting glands that may contribute to the protection of the esophagus. Bicarbonate moving from the blood to the lumen can neutralize acidic refluxate in the esophagus. When the mucosa is repeatedly exposed to the refluxate in GERD, or if there is a defect in the normal mucosal defenses, hydrogen ions diffuse into the mucosa, leading to the cellular acidification and necrosis that ultimately cause esophagitis. In theory, mucosal resistance may be related not only to esophageal mucus but also to tight epithelial junctions, epithelial cell turnover, nitrogen balance, mucosal blood flow, tissue prostaglandins, and the acid–base status of the tissue. Saliva is also rich in epidermal growth factor, stimulating cell renewal.

Gastric Emptying/Increased Intra-abdominal Pressure

Delayed gastric emptying can contribute to gastroesophageal reflux. An increase in gastric volume may increase both the frequency of reflux and the amount of gastric fluid available to be refluxed. Gastric volume is related to the volume of material ingested, rate of gastric secretion, rate of gastric emptying, and amount and frequency of duodenal reflux into the stomach. Factors that increase gastric volume and/or decrease gastric emptying, such as smoking and high-fat meals, are often associated with gastroesophageal reflux. This partially explains the prevalence of postprandial gastroesophageal reflux. Fatty foods may increase postprandial gastroesophageal reflux by increasing gastric volume, delaying the gastric emptying rate, and decreasing the LES pressure. Patients with gastroesophageal reflux, particularly infants, may have a defect in gastric antral motility. The delay in emptying may promote regurgitation of feedings, which might, in turn, contribute to two common complications of GERD in infants (eg, failure to thrive and pulmonary aspiration).[16]

Increased GERD symptoms and complications occur in obese patients. Obesity is considered an independent risk factor for GERD due to increased intra-abdominal pressure and reduced LES pressure.[17] An increased risk for developing both erosive esophagitis and Barrett's esophagus can be attributed to obesity. A gain in body mass index (BMI) of greater than 3.5 kg/m^2 is associated with increased new-onset GERD symptoms, regardless of baseline BMI.[18] TLESRs, incompetent LES, and impaired esophageal motility have been attributed to obesity.[19,20]

Composition of Refluxate

The composition, pH, and volume of the refluxate are important aggressive factors in determining the consequences of gastroesophageal reflux. If the pH of the refluxate is less than 2, esophagitis may develop secondary to protein denaturation. In addition, pepsinogen is activated to pepsin at this pH and may also cause esophagitis. Duodenogastric reflux esophagitis, or "alkaline esophagitis," refers to esophagitis induced by the reflux of bilious and pancreatic fluid. The term "alkaline esophagitis" may be a misnomer in that the refluxate may be either weakly alkaline or acidic in nature. Although bile acids have both a direct irritant effect on the esophageal mucosa and an indirect effect of increasing hydrogen ion permeability of the mucosa, symptoms are more often related to acid reflux than to bile reflux. Specifically, the percentage of time that the esophageal pH is less than 4 is greater for patients with severe disease as compared with that for patients with mild disease. Nevertheless, the combination of acid, pepsin, and/or bile is a potent refluxate in producing esophageal damage.

The pathophysiology of gastroesophageal reflux is a complex cyclic process. It is difficult, if not impossible, to determine which occurs first: gastroesophageal reflux leading to defective peristalsis with delayed clearing or an incompetent LES pressure leading to gastroesophageal reflux. Understanding the factors associated with the development of GERD provides insight into the treatment modalities currently used to manage patients suffering from this disease.

Complications

Several complications may occur with gastroesophageal reflux, including esophagitis, esophageal strictures, Barrett's esophagus, and esophageal adenocarcinoma. Strictures are common in the distal esophagus and are 1 to 2 cm in length. The use of nonsteroidal anti-inflammatory drugs (NSAIDs) or aspirin is an additional risk factor that may contribute to the development or worsening of GERD complications. In some patients, the reparative process leads to the replacement of the squamous epithelial lining of the esophagus by specialized columnar-type epithelium (Barrett's esophagus), which increases the incidence of esophageal strictures by as much as 30%. Screening for Barrett's esophagus is indicated in men with chronic GERD symptoms (more than 5 years) and/or heartburn or acid regurgitation occurring at least weekly; and two or more of the following risk factors for Barrett's esophagus or esophageal adenocarcinoma: (1) over 50 years old; (2) White race; (3) central obesity (waist circumference greater than 102 cm or waist-hip ratio greater than 0.9); (4) tobacco use (current or previous use); and (5) family history of Barrett's esophagus or esophageal adenocarcinoma.[21] Women with scleroderma and esophageal involvement may also benefit from screening for Barrett's esophagus.[11] The risk of esophageal adenocarcinoma may be higher for patients with Barrett's esophagus as compared with that for the general population. The annual risk of esophageal adenocarcinoma was 0.2% to 05% in those with nondysplastic Barrett's esophagus.[21] The annual risk of cancer progression increases to 0.7% in those with low-grade dysplasia and as high as 7% in those with high-grade dysplasia.[14,21]

Helicobacter pylori

The role of *H. pylori* status for patients with GERD is uncertain. As a consequence of the controversy surrounding *H. pylori* and GERD, specific guidelines on how to handle patients who are *H. pylori* positive are lacking. Most clinicians would probably opt to eradicate *H. pylori* infections once detected. However, routine screening for *H. pylori* is not recommended as part of the diagnosis and management of GERD. Further studies are needed to determine the role of *H. pylori* for patients with GERD.

CLINICAL PRESENTATION: GERD

1 GERD can be described on the basis of either esophageal symptoms or esophageal tissue injury. The common symptoms include heartburn, regurgitation, chest pain, and dysphagia. Dysphagia and odynophagia are considered alarm symptoms that require further evaluation. The severity or frequency of the symptoms of gastroesophageal reflux does not always correlate with the degree of esophageal tissue injury, but it does correlate with the duration of reflux. The clinical presentation of GERD overlaps with other conditions such as eosinophilic esophagitis, functional heartburn, and gastroparesis leading to challenges in managing GERD patients.[7] Reflux hypersensitivity may contribute to the patient's perception of symptom severity despite normal esophageal reflux exposure.[15] It is important to distinguish GERD symptoms from those of other diseases.

Diagnostic Tests

The most useful tool in the diagnosis of gastroesophageal reflux is the clinical history, including presenting symptoms and associated risk factors.[1] Patients presenting with typical symptoms of reflux, such as heartburn or regurgitation, do not usually require invasive esophageal evaluation. These patients benefit from an initial empiric trial of acid suppression therapy. A clinical diagnosis of GERD can be assumed in patients who respond to appropriate therapy.[1] However, response to an empiric course of PPI was only 71% sensitive and 44% specific as compared to the combination of endoscopy and ambulatory pH monitoring.[22] This is due to the diverse symptom profile seen in GERD with variable responses to PPIs. PPIs are the most effective in patients with erosive esophagitis and are less effective with regurgitation, extraesophageal symptoms, gastroparesis, achalasia, eosinophilic esophagitis, reflux hypersensitivity,

CLINICAL PRESENTATION GERD Syndromes[1,22,26-28]

Symptom-Based GERD Syndromes (With or Without Esophageal Tissue Injury)

Typical symptoms (may be aggravated by activities that worsen gastroesophageal reflux such as recumbent position, bending over, or eating a meal high in fat):

- Heartburn (hallmark symptom described as a substernal sensation of warmth or burning rising up from the abdomen that may radiate to the neck; may be waxing and waning in character)
- Regurgitation/belching
- Reflux chest pain

Alarm symptoms (these symptoms may be indicative of complications of GERD such as Barrett's esophagus, esophageal strictures, or esophageal adenocarcinoma and require further diagnostic evaluation):

- Dysphagia (common)
- Odynophagia
- Bleeding
- Weight loss

Tissue Injury-Based GERD Syndromes (With or Without Esophageal Symptoms)

Symptoms (may present with alarm symptoms such as dysphagia, odynophagia, or unexplained weight loss):

- Esophagitis
- Esophageal strictures
- Barrett's esophagus
- Esophageal adenocarcinoma

Extraesophageal GERD Syndromes

These symptoms have an association with GERD, but causality should only be considered if a concomitant esophageal GERD syndrome is also present:

- Chronic cough
- Laryngitis
- Wheezing
- Asthma (~50% with asthma have GERD)

Diagnostic Tests for GERD

Clinical History

- Used to make a clinical diagnosis of GERD in patients with typical symptoms.

Endoscopy

- Preferred for assessing mucosal injury and complications. Biopsies are needed to identify Barrett's esophagus, adenocarcinoma, and eosinophilic esophagitis (a nonacid-related esophageal disorder that does not respond well to acid suppression therapy).
- Indications for endoscopy: (1) persistent or progressive GERD symptoms despite appropriate therapy; (2) presence of dysphagia or odynophagia; (3) unexplained weight loss of more than 5%; (4) presence of GI bleeding and strictures; (5) screening for Barrett's esophagus in high-risk patients; (6) placement of wireless pH monitoring; (7) prior to endoscopic or surgical antireflux procedures or after procedures in those with recurrent symptoms.[26]
- Note: Noninflammatory GERD and major motor disorders may be missed by endoscopy.

Ambulatory Reflux Monitoring With or Without Impedance

- Useful for (a) patients not responding to acid suppression therapy when endoscopy is normal; (b) those with atypical/extraesophageal symptoms; or (c) those contemplating surgery.
- Assesses the acid exposure time (AET) and frequency of reflux episodes and helps determine if symptoms are acid-related.
  - An AET of less than 4% is considered normal, while greater than 6% is considered abnormal.[22]
  - Less than 40 reflux episodes in a 24-hour period is considered normal, while more than 80 reflux episodes per 24-hour period is considered abnormal.
- Reflux hypersensitivity is defined as positive symptom association in the absence of breakthrough acid.[27]
- Monitoring without impedance measures only acid reflux; adding impedance measures both acid and nonacid reflux
  - Testing patients off PPI therapy is recommended (1) to evaluate the AET in patients with normal endoscopy or low-grade esophagitis and no previously positive pH testing and (2) in those considering antireflux surgery.[22]
  - Testing patients on double-dose PPI therapy is recommended in patients with (1) prior Los Angeles grade C or D esophagitis; (2) long segment Barrett's esophagus; or (3) prior abnormal ambulatory pH monitoring. In these cases, pH–impedance monitoring is recommended to correlate refractory symptoms with reflux episodes or to identify inadequate acid suppression.

Manometry/High-Resolution Esophageal Pressure Topography

- Useful in those who have failed twice-daily PPI therapy with normal endoscopic findings to identify motor disorders, to evaluate peristaltic function in those who are candidates for antireflux surgery, and to assure proper placement of pH probes. Tubeless pH monitoring using endoscopic landmarks for placement may negate the need for manometry for ensuring proper placement of esophageal pH probes.

Impedance Manometry

- Evaluates bolus transit esophageal clearance/retention.
- Evaluates LES and UES pressures and peristalsis.

Empiric Proton Pump Inhibitor as a Diagnostic Test for GERD

- Less expensive and more convenient than ambulatory reflux monitoring but lacks standardized dosing regimen and duration of the diagnostic trial. This is not recommended as a diagnostic tool.

Barium Radiography

- Not routinely used to diagnose GERD because it lacks sensitivity and specificity; cannot identify Barrett's esophagus. Can detect hiatal hernia.

or functional gastrointestinal (GI) disorders. A strategy based on symptom domain and assessment of esophageal function testing may better define therapy.[23] The presence of erosive esophagitis (grade B, C, or D) or Barrett's esophagus per endoscopy, or abnormal pH testing defines "proven" GERD.[24] In addition having a "proven" diagnosis of GERD helps limit PPI use to those who are most likely to respond and avoid unnecessary adverse effects such as renal failure, enteric infections, vitamin/mineral deficiencies, bone fractures, and hypomagnesemia.[22,23] Proven GERD should be established before long-term acid suppression therapy is considered. In the case of functional heartburn, eosinophilic esophagitis, reflux hypersensitivity, or other nonreflux GI disorders, acid suppression therapy may not be the most appropriate choice for treatment as these are not acid-related disorders.

Diagnostic evaluation is useful to prevent misdiagnosis, identify complications, and assess treatment failures.[20] Diagnostic tests should be performed in those patients who do not respond to therapy and in those who present with alarm symptoms (eg, dysphagia, odynophagia, and weight loss), which may be more indicative of complicated disease. Additional diagnostic testing can help stratify patients with GERD into management categories that help guide clinicians to the most appropriate therapy.[24]

2 Useful diagnostic tests for GERD include upper endoscopy, ambulatory reflux (pH) monitoring, combined impedance–pH monitoring, manometry/high-resolution esophageal pressure topography, and impedance manometry. Endoscopy is commonly used to evaluate mucosal injury and to assess for the presence of Barrett's esophagus or other complications, such as strictures or adenocarcinoma. Biopsies are necessary to diagnose Barrett's esophagus. A camera-containing capsule swallowed by the patient offers visualizing the esophageal mucosa via endoscopy. This is less invasive than traditional endoscopy and takes less than 15 minutes to perform in the clinician's office, but biopsies cannot be obtained. Unfortunately, the presence or absence of mucosal damage does not prove whether the patient's symptoms are reflux related; for that, ambulatory reflux monitoring is useful.

3 Whereas ambulatory reflux monitoring (24-hour pH monitoring) only measures acid reflux, combined impedance–pH monitoring measures both acid and nonacid reflux. Ambulatory reflux monitoring is performed by passing a small pH probe transnasally and placing it approximately 5 cm above the LES. Patients are asked to keep a diary of symptoms that later are correlated with the pH measurement corresponding to the time the symptom was reported (Fig. 50-2). Approximately 24 hours of data can be obtained using this method. The wireless pH monitoring involves attaching a radiotelemetry capsule to the esophageal mucosa. The advantages of this method are that a longer period of monitoring is possible (48-96 hours), it may demonstrate superior recording accuracy compared with some catheter designs, and it is more comfortable for the patient because a nasogastric tube is unnecessary.[1,22] Ambulatory reflux monitoring is especially useful in patients with symptoms that are refractory to PPIs.[25]

TREATMENT

Therapeutic modalities used in the treatment of gastroesophageal reflux are targeted at reversing the various pathophysiologic abnormalities.

Desired Outcomes

4 The goals of treatment are to (a) alleviate or eliminate the patient's symptoms and improve health-related quality of life, (b) decrease the frequency or recurrence and duration of gastroesophageal reflux, (c) promote healing of the injured mucosa, and (d) prevent complications. Therapy is directed at augmenting defense mechanisms that prevent reflux and/or decrease the aggressive factors that worsen reflux or mucosal damage. Therapy is directed at (a) decreasing the acidity of the refluxate, (b) decreasing the gastric volume available to be refluxed, (c) improving gastric emptying, (d) increasing LES pressure, (e) enhancing esophageal acid clearance, and (f) protecting the esophageal mucosa.

General Approach to Treatment

5 GERD treatment is determined by disease severity and includes: (a) lifestyle changes and patient-directed therapy with antacids, nonprescription H2RAs, and/or nonprescription PPIs; (b) pharmacologic treatment with prescription-strength acid suppression therapy; (c) surgery; and (d) endoscopic therapies (Table 50-2).[1,29] The initial therapeutic modality used is in part dependent on the patient's condition (frequency of symptoms, degree of esophagitis, and presence of complications) (Table 50-3). A step-down approach, starting with a PPI, instead of an H2RA, is most often advocated. Once esophageal healing has occurred or symptoms improved, patients should be stepped down to the lowest effective dose of PPI or switched to an H2RA. The clinician should determine the most appropriate approach for the individual patient. Every attempt should be made to aggressively control symptoms and to prevent relapses early in the course of the patient's disease in order to prevent the complications. For patients with moderate-to-severe GERD, especially those with erosive disease, starting with a PPI as initial therapy is advocated because of its superior efficacy over H2RAs.

While weight loss in obese patients and elevation of the head end of the bed are beneficial for most GERD patients, recommending all lifestyle modifications to all patients is not recommended.[1] Instead, education on lifestyle modifications should be tailored to the individual needs of the patient. Table 50-4 lists some of the lifestyle modifications that can be recommended on an individualized basis.

6 Patients with typical GERD symptoms should be treated with lifestyle modifications as appropriate and a trial of empiric acid suppression therapy. Those who do not respond to empiric therapy or who present with alarm symptoms such as dysphagia, weight loss, or GI bleeding should undergo endoscopy. Acid suppression therapy with PPIs or H2RAs is the mainstay of GERD treatment. Patients presenting with moderate-to-severe symptoms (with or without esophageal erosions) should be started on a PPI as initial therapy because it provides the most rapid symptomatic relief and healing in the highest percentage of patients.[1] H2RAs in divided doses are effective for patients with milder GERD symptoms. However, when standard doses of H2RA therapy are not effective at relieving symptoms, it is more cost effective and efficacious to switch to a PPI.

Promotility agents (such as metoclopramide) are not as effective as acid suppression agents. Combining a promotility agent with acid suppression medications offer only modest improvements in symptoms over standard doses of H2RAs and should not be routinely recommended. In addition, the availability of a promotility agent that has an acceptable adverse effect profile is lacking. Mucosal protectants, such as sucralfate, have a limited role in the treatment of GERD.

Maintenance therapy may be necessary to control symptoms and to prevent complications. For patients with more severe symptoms (with or without esophageal erosions) or for patients with other complications, maintenance therapy with a PPI is most effective. Routine use of combination therapy is not recommended in GERD maintenance therapy. In cases of refractory GERD, the diagnosis should be confirmed through further diagnostic tests before long-term, high-dose acid suppression therapy is considered.[1]

Nonpharmacologic Therapy

Nonpharmacologic treatment of GERD includes lifestyle modifications, antireflux surgery, bariatric surgery (in obese patients), and endoscopic therapies.

A

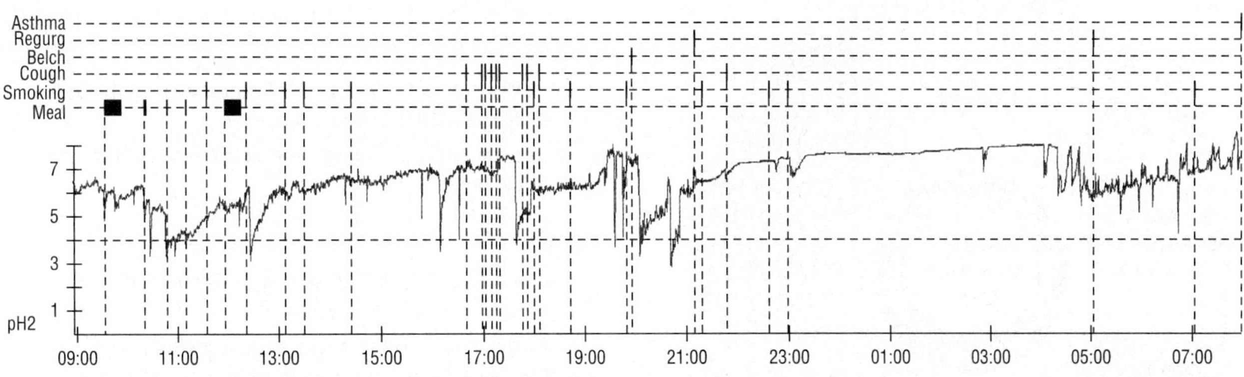

Normal 24 hour ambulatory esophageal pH test						
	Total	Normal	Upright	Normal	Supine	Normal
• Fraction time pH <4 (%)	1.9	<4.2	1.9	<6.3	0%	<1.2
• Number of refluxes	81		81		0	
• Number of long refluxes (>5 min)	0		0		0	
• Duration of longest reflux (min)	2.3		2.3		0	
• Time pH <4 (min)	25.9		25.9		0	

B

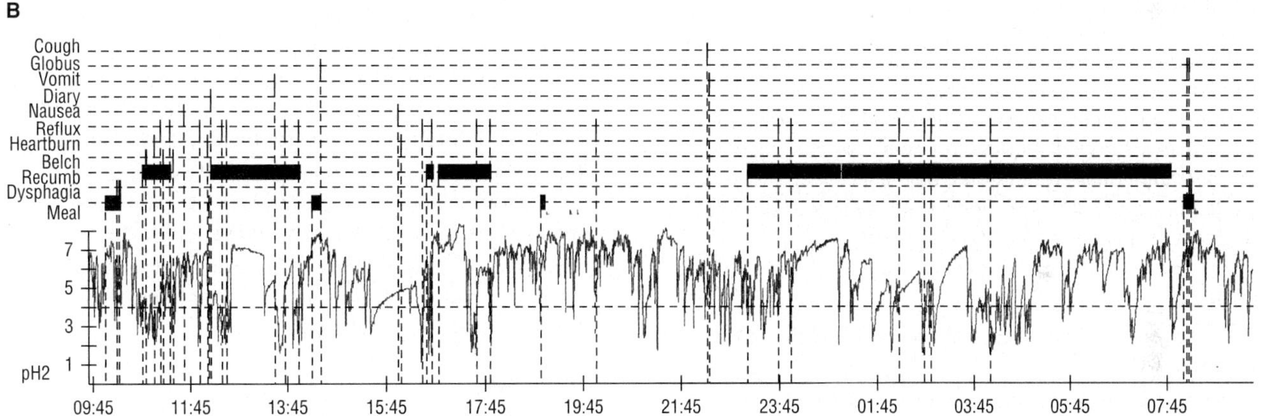

Abnormal 24-hour ambulatory esophageal pH test						
	Total	Normal	Upright	Normal	Supine	Normal
• Fraction time pH <4 (%)	16	<4.2	10.6	<6.3	20.6	<1.2
• Number of refluxes	332		143		189	
• Number of long refluxes (>5 min)	10		6		4	
• Duration of longest reflux (min)	7.9		7.1		7.9	
• Time pH <4 (min)	220.5		66.8		153.7	

FIGURE 50-2 Graphical representation of a normal 24-hour esophageal pH test profile compared to an abnormal 24-hour ambulatory esophageal pH test profile.

Lifestyle Modifications

The most common lifestyle modifications for GERD include weight loss in obese patients and elevation of the head end of the bed, especially for those patients who have symptoms while in a recumbent position.[1] Other lifestyle modifications should be individualized based on the patient's specific situation. These include consumption of smaller meals and not sleeping for at least 3 hours after eating, avoidance of foods or medications that exacerbate GERD, smoking cessation, avoidance of tight-fitting clothes, and avoidance of alcohol (see Table 50-4).[30]

Obesity increases the risk of GERD symptoms and complications including Barrett's esophagus. There is a clear association between BMI, waist circumference, and weight gain.[1] Surprisingly, weight gain in those considered to have a normal BMI is also associated with new onset GERD symptoms.[1] Even more alarming is the potential association between BMI and cancer in the esophagus and gastric cardia.[1] A high-fat meal will decrease LES pressure for 2 hours or more postprandially. In contrast, a high-protein, low-fat meal will elevate LES pressure. A weight loss goal of at least 10% is recommended to help to improve GERD symptoms.[30]

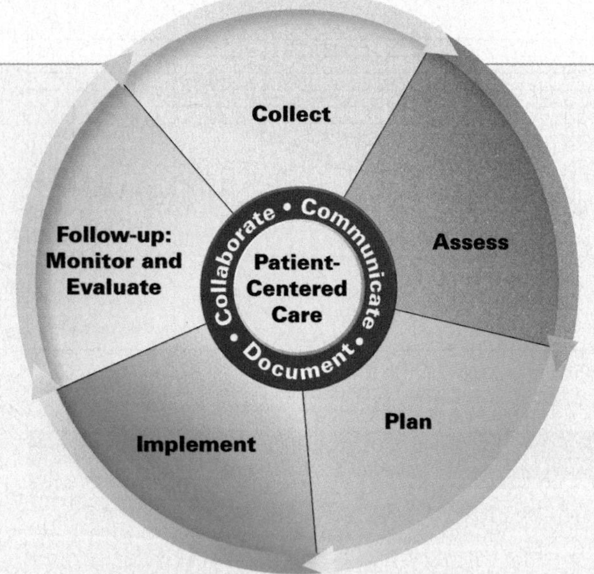

Patient Care Process for the Management of Gastroesophageal Reflux Disease

The image shows the five fundamental steps included in The Pharmacist's Care Process endorsed by the Joint Commission for Pharmacy Practitioners (2014).[32] The tagline of this process reads collaborate, communicate, and document. The five fundamental steps listed here are collect, assess, plan, implement, and follow-up: monitor and evaluate. All these steps are listed in a circular block diagram.

Collect

- Patient characteristics (eg, age, race, sex, weight, BMI, pregnant)
- Patient history (past medical, family, social, dietary habits, tobacco use)
- Health literacy and barriers to medication access
- Thorough history of prescription, nonprescription, and natural medication use
- Medication allergies and intolerances (including actual reaction to medication)
- Laboratory results for major organ function (eg, SCr to calculate CrCL, liver enzymes to assess hepatic function)

Assess

- Assess major organ function (eg, creatinine clearance, hepatic impairment)
- Determine the type, frequency, duration of symptoms, and identify exacerbating factors
- Identify alarm symptoms or extraesophageal symptoms that require further diagnostic evaluation by clinician (see section "Clinical Presentation")
- Review lifestyle factors, including foods that may be contributing to symptoms (see Table 50-1)
- Review medication profile for medications that may be contributing to symptoms (see Table 50-1) and potential drug–drug interactions
- Assess what has been done so far (including medications and lifestyle modifications)
- Establish goals of therapy and if they are currently being met (see section "Desired Outcomes")
- Assess the appropriateness and effectiveness of current GERD regimen

Plan*

- Identify individualized lifestyle modifications that may improve symptoms (see Table 50-4)
- Determine appropriate therapy (may include both nonpharmacologic and pharmacologic) based on patient's presentation (see Table 50-2)
- For pharmacologic therapy, include medication name, dose, route, frequency, and duration of therapy recommendation (see Table 50-3)
- Establish monitoring parameters for safety (eg, drug–drug, drug–food, drug–disease, and drug–lab interaction checking; short- and long-term adverse effects, and prevention of complications)
- Establish monitoring parameters for efficacy (eg, resolution of symptoms, improvement of symptoms, and healing of injured mucosa) (see Table 50-5)
- Identify patient education that may be needed (eg, purpose of medication, individualized lifestyle modifications, adverse effects, administration clinical pearls, adherence, potential need for long-term maintenance therapy, and so on)
- For refractory symptoms, seek potential causes such as medication adherence, timing of medication, drug interactions, nonacid related disorders, and so on
- Screen for symptoms that would require further diagnostic evaluation from clinician (eg, alarm symptoms, atypical symptoms, or complications)

Implement*

- Counsel patient on individualized lifestyle modifications that may improve symptoms (eg, elevating head of the bed with a wedge, weight management, and so on) (see Table 50-4)
- Initiate appropriate nonpharmacologic and pharmacologic therapy based on patient presentation (see Tables 50-2 and 50-3)
- Recommend additions, modifications, or discontinuations to therapy based on patient response
- Provide patient education with regard to disease state, lifestyle modifications, and treatment plan. Counsel patient on (a) what causes GERD and things to avoid; (b) when to take their medication (eg, 30 minutes before meal); (c) what potential adverse effects (including long-term adverse effects) or drug interactions may occur
- Use motivational interviewing techniques to maximize medication adherence
- Schedule follow-up as appropriate

Follow-up: Monitor and Evaluate

- Follow-up after 8 to 16 weeks to assess effectiveness of acid-suppression therapy. Recommend alternative therapy when necessary; attempt to deprescribe PPIs if possible
- Monitor patient for safety goals established above
- Evaluate the need for maintenance therapy based on patient presentation and response to therapy

(continued)

- Assess improvement in quality-of-life measures such as physical, psychological, and social functioning and well-being
- Evaluate patient for the presence of adverse drug reactions, complications or new drug–drug interactions
- Stress the importance of medication adherence to treatment plan to patient as indicated

*Collaborate with patient, caregivers, and other healthcare professionals.

TABLE 50-2 Evidence-Based Treatment Recommendations for GERD in Adults

Recommendation	Level of Evidence and Strength of Evidence[a]
Lifestyle Modifications	
• Weight loss in overweight GERD patients or those who have recently gained weight.	Moderate, Conditional
• Elevation of the head end of the bed and avoidance of food 2-3 hours before bedtime if nocturnal GERD symptoms present.	Low, Conditional
• Routine elimination of foods that can trigger reflux is not recommended in the treatment of GERD.	Low, Conditional
Acid Suppression Therapy	
• Therapy of choice for symptom relief and healing of erosive esophagitis is an 8-week PPI course. There is similar efficacy among all PPIs.	High, Strong
• For maximal pH control, delayed-release PPIs should be administered 30-60 minutes before meals.	Moderate, Strong
• PPIs should be started at once-daily dosing prior to the first meal each day.	Moderate, Strong
• Patients with Barrett's esophagus can be treated similarly to those with GERD who do not have Barrett's esophagus.	Moderate, Strong
• Flexibility with meal-time administration may be seen with newer PPIs (eg, dexlansoprazole).	Moderate, Conditional
• When clinically indicated, PPIs are considered safe in pregnancy.	Moderate, Conditional
• Adjustments of dose timing and/or twice-daily dosing may be beneficial in patients with night-time symptoms, variable schedules, and/or sleep disturbances who are partial responders to PPI therapy.	Low, Strong
• In patients with typical GERD symptoms who also have extraesophageal symptoms, a PPI trial is recommended.	Low, Strong
• Optimization of PPI therapy should be assessed in anyone with refractory GERD symptoms.	Low, Strong
• Increasing to twice-daily dosing or switching PPI may be beneficial in partial responders to PPI therapy.	Low, Conditional
• Further evaluation is recommended for nonresponders to PPI therapy.	Low, Conditional
• If adverse effects occur with PPI, may consider switching to an alternative PPI.	Low, Conditional
• Patients with osteoporosis can use a PPI.	Moderate, Conditional
• Concern for hip fracture with PPI should be considered in those with osteoporosis AND other risk factors for hip fracture.	Moderate, Conditional
• PPIs are a risk factor for development of *Clostridium difficile*.	Moderate, Moderate
• PPIs are a risk factor for development of community-acquired pneumonia with short-term use (but not long-term use).	Moderate, Conditional
• PPIs can be used in patients on clopidogrel, and there is not an increased risk for adverse cardiovascular events.	High, Strong
Promotility Therapy and Other Nonacid Suppression Therapies	
• Prokinetic medications and/or baclofen should not be used to manage GERD without diagnostic evaluation.	Moderate, Conditional
• Sulcralfate is not recommended in nonpregnant GERD patients.	Moderate, Conditional
Maintenance Therapy	
• Maintenance therapy is recommended for (1) patients with continued symptoms after PPI discontinuation and (2) patients with complications including erosive esophagitis and Barrett's esophagus.	Moderate, Strong
• The lowest effective dose should be used when long-term PPI therapy is indicated for maintenance. Strategies such as on-demand and intermittent therapy may be beneficial.	Low, Conditional
• H2RAs may be used as maintenance therapy in patients without erosive disease when the goal is heartburn relief.	Moderate, Conditional
Surgery	
• Antireflux surgery is a long-term treatment option in GERD patients.	High, Strong
• Antireflux surgery is not recommended in PPI nonresponders.	High, Strong
• Antireflux surgery is not recommended in patients with extraesophageal symptoms not responding to PPI therapy.	Moderate, Strong
• Endoscopic therapy or transoral incisionless fundoplication not recommended as alternative to medical or traditional surgical procedures.	Moderate, Strong
• Bariatric surgery (gastric bypass) should be considered in obese patients contemplating surgical therapy.	Moderate, Conditional

GERD, gastroesophageal reflux disease; PPI, proton pump inhibitor.

[a]Level of evidence per Grades of Recommendation, Assessment, Development, and Evaluation (GRADE) system: High = further research not likely to change authors' confidence in the estimate of effect; Moderate = further research would likely have an impact on the confidence in the estimate of effect; Low = further research would be expected to have an important impact on the confidence in the estimate of the effect and would be likely to change the evidence. Strength of evidence per GRADE system: Strong = desired effects of an intervention clearly outweigh the undesirable effects; Conditional = there is uncertainty about the trade-offs between desirable effects and undesirable effects.

Data from References 1 and 29.

TABLE 50-3 Therapeutic Approach to GERD in Adults

Recommended Treatment Regimen	Oral Dose	Comments
Intermittent, mild heartburn (individualized lifestyle modifications + patient-directed therapy with antacids and/or nonprescription H2RAs *or* nonprescription PPIs)		
Individualized lifestyle modifications		Lifestyle modifications should be individualized for each patient.
Patient-directed therapy with antacids (12 years of age or older)		
Magnesium hydroxide/aluminum hydroxide with simethicone	10-20 mL as needed or after meals and at bedtime	If symptoms are unrelieved with lifestyle modifications and nonprescription medications after 2 weeks, patient should seek medical attention; do not exceed 16 teaspoonfuls per 24 hours.
Antacid/alginic acid	2-4 tablets or 10-20 mL after meals and at bedtime	Note: Content of alginic acid varies greatly among products; the higher the alginic acid the better (at least 500 mg).
Calcium carbonate	500 mg, 2-4 tablets as needed	
Patient-directed therapy with nonprescription H2RAs (up to twice daily) (12 years of age or older)		
Cimetidine Famotidine Nizatidine	200 mg 10-20 mg 75 mg	If symptoms are unrelieved with lifestyle modifications and nonprescription medications after 2 weeks, patient should seek medical attention.
Patient-directed therapy (over 18 years old) with nonprescription PPIs (taken once daily)		
Esomeprazole Lansoprazole Omeprazole Omeprazole/sodium bicarbonate	20 mg 15 mg 20 mg 20 mg/1,100 mg	If symptoms are unrelieved with lifestyle modifications and nonprescription medications after 2 weeks, patient should seek medical attention.
Symptomatic relief of GERD (individualized lifestyle modifications + prescription-strength H2RAs *or* prescription-strength PPIs)		
Individualized lifestyle modifications		Lifestyle modifications should be individualized for each patient.
Prescription-strength H2RAs		
Cimetidine (off-label use) Famotidine Nizatidine	400 mg four times daily or 800 mg twice daily 20 mg twice daily 150 mg twice daily	• For typical symptoms, treat empirically with prescription-strength acid suppression therapy. • If symptoms recur, consider maintenance therapy. Note: Most patients will require standard doses for maintenance therapy.
Prescription-strength PPIs		
Dexlansoprazole Esomeprazole Lansoprazole Omeprazole Omeprazole/sodium bicarbonate Pantoprazole (Off-label use) Rabeprazole	30 mg once daily for 4 weeks 20-40 mg once daily 15 mg once daily 20 mg once daily 20 mg once daily 40 mg once daily 20 mg once daily	• For typical symptoms, treat empirically with prescription-strength acid suppression therapy. • Patients with moderate-to-severe symptoms should receive a PPI as initial therapy. • If symptoms recur, consider maintenance therapy.
Healing of erosive esophagitis or treatment of patients with moderate-to-severe symptoms or complications (individualized lifestyle modifications + high-dose H2RAs *or* PPIs *or* antireflux surgery)		
Individualized lifestyle modifications		Lifestyle modifications should be individualized for each patient.
PPIs (up to twice daily for up to 8 weeks)		
Dexlansoprazole Esomeprazole Lansoprazole Omeprazole Rabeprazole Pantoprazole	60 mg daily 20-40 mg daily 30 mg once or twice daily 20 mg once or twice daily 20 mg once or twice daily 40 mg once or twice daily	• For extraesophageal or alarm symptoms, obtain endoscopy with biopsy to evaluate mucosa. • If symptoms are relieved, consider maintenance therapy. PPIs are the most effective maintenance therapy for patients with extraesophageal symptoms, complications, and erosive disease. Start with twice-daily PPI therapy if reflux chest syndrome is present. • Patients not responding to pharmacologic therapy, including those with persistent extraesophageal symptoms, should be evaluated via manometry and/or ambulatory reflux monitoring.
High-dose H2RAs (for 8-12 weeks)		
Cimetidine Famotidine Nizatidine	400 mg four times daily or 800 mg twice daily 20-40 mg twice daily 150 mg two to four times daily	Note: If high-dose H2RA is needed, may consider using PPI to lower cost, increase convenience, and increase tolerability. Note: Four times daily H2RA is considered off-label use for nizatidine.
Interventional therapy		
Antireflux surgery Bariatric surgery Endoscopic therapies		

TABLE 50-4 Nonpharmacologic Treatment of GERD with Lifestyle Modifications

- Elevate the head end of the bed (increases esophageal clearance). Use 6- to 8-inch (15-20 cm) blocks under the head side of the bed.
- Weight reduction (reduces symptoms) in obese patients.
- Avoid foods that may decrease lower esophageal sphincter pressure or increase transient lower esophageal sphincter relaxation (fats, chocolate, alcohol, peppermint, and spearmint).
- Include protein-rich meals in diet (augments lower esophageal sphincter pressure).
- Avoid foods that have a direct irritant effect on the esophageal mucosa (spicy foods, orange juice, tomato juice, and coffee).
- Behaviors that may reduce esophageal acid exposure.
- Eat small meals and avoid sleeping immediately after meals (sleep after 3 hours if possible; decreases gastric volume).
- Stop smoking (decreases spontaneous esophageal sphincter relaxation).
- Avoid alcohol (increases amplitude of the lower esophageal sphincter, peristaltic waves, and frequency of contraction).
- Avoid tight-fitting clothes.
- Always take drugs in the sitting upright or standing position and with plenty of liquid, especially for those that have a direct irritant effect on the esophageal mucosa (eg, bisphosphonates, tetracyclines, quinidine, potassium chloride, iron salts, aspirin, nonsteroidal anti-inflammatory drugs).

Data from Reference 20.

Elevating the head end of the bed by approximately 6 to 8 inches (15-20 cm) with a foam wedge under the mattress (not just elevating the head with pillows) decreases nocturnal esophageal acid contact time and should be recommended. In general, anything that improves sleep hygiene may reduce GERD symptoms because TLESRs are reduced during sleep.[31] Many foods have been linked to worsening GERD symptoms; however, the evidence is weak for this association. Some foods decrease LES pressure (eg, fats and chocolates), while other foods can act as direct contact irritants to the esophageal mucosa (citrus juice, tomato juice, coffee, and pepper) (see Table 50-1).

Evaluate patient profiles to identify potential medications that may exacerbate GERD symptoms (see Table 50-1). Some medications decrease LES pressure, while other medications can act as direct contact irritants to the esophageal mucosa. Proper patient education can help prevent dysphagia or esophageal ulceration. Closely monitor patients for worsening symptoms when any of these medications are started. If symptoms worsen, alternative therapies may be warranted. Clinicians must weigh the risks and benefits of continuing a medication known to worsen GERD and esophagitis.

Smoking can cause aerophagia (eg, air swallowing), which leads to increased belching and regurgitation. Patients with GERD should be encouraged to quit smoking because it may be a risk factor for Barrett's esophagus and esophageal adenocarcinoma.[21] Alcohol decreases LES pressure and may exacerbate symptoms such as heartburn.

Many patients are noncompliant with lifestyle modifications, and even those who do comply continue to have symptoms that require acid suppression therapy. Nonetheless, it is important to stress the potential benefits of lifestyle modifications that would benefit each individual patient.

Interventional Approaches

Interventional approaches include antireflux surgery, bariatric surgery, magnetic sphincter augmentation, and endoscopic therapies. These are discussed in more detail below.

Antireflux Surgery

7 The goal of antireflux surgery is to reestablish the antireflux barrier, to position the LES within the abdomen where it is under positive (intra-abdominal) pressure, and to close any associated defect in the diaphragmatic hiatus by reinforcing the crural muscles. Surgical intervention is a viable alternative treatment for select patients. It is indicated when (1) long-term pharmacologic management is undesirable, (2) persistent proven GERD symptoms or esophageal mucosal damage despite appropriate pharmacologic therapy, and (3) significant EGJ disruption (eg, hiatal hernia).[22] Antireflux surgery does not impact the progression of Barrett's esophagus to esophageal adenocarcinoma.[13] The most common antireflux surgery performed is laparoscopic Nissen fundoplication. Patients should undergo ambulatory reflux pH monitoring and manometry prior to antireflux surgery.[31] Patients with typical symptoms who are responsive to PPIs and those with abnormal ambulatory pH monitoring showing positive correlation with GERD symptoms show the most benefit from antireflux surgery, while those with extraesophageal symptoms show a lower response to antireflux surgery. The major complications with antireflux surgery include gas bloat syndrome (inability to belch or vomit), dysphagia, vagal denervation, and splenic trauma. Long-term effectiveness of antireflux surgery is uncertain.[33]

Success of antireflux surgery in patients with PPI-refractory heartburn depends on careful screening and ruling out nonacid related causes of heartburn, such as eosinophilic esophagitis, achalasia, and biliary disease. Seventy-eight percent of the patients with "refractory GERD" evaluated did not have reflux-related disease. Instead, they had non-GERD esophageal disorders or functional heartburn. In those who were PPI-refractory and had reflux-related heartburn, surgery was superior to medical treatment (67% versus 12%-28%, respectively).[34]

Bariatric surgery, specifically laproscopic Roux-en-Y gastric bypass, should be considered in obese patients (BMI greater than 35 kg/m^2) contemplating surgery.[1] The consideration of bariatric surgery in obese patients for improvement of GERD symptoms is a result of the proposed difference in pathophysiology in this patient population. Abdominal pressure may play a greater role in the development of GERD in obese patients. Reflux symptoms were decreased from 31% to 5%, esophagitis was decreased from 24% to 10%, and incidence of GERD was decreased from 34% to 12% with laparoscopic Roux-en-Y gastric bypass surgery in morbidly obese patients.[13]

Magnetic Sphincter Augmentation

This minimally invasive alternative to antireflux surgery involves surgically implanting a ring of titanium-encased magnets at the EGJ to improve lower esophageal resistance and reduce symptoms of GERD.[24,35] Long-term effectiveness of magnetic sphincter augmentation is uncertain.

Endoscopic Therapies

Endoscopic therapies are less invasive than surgical fundoplication and aim for a similar efficacy. Two endoscopic therapies are radiofrequency ablation of the LES and endoscopic suturing of the LES (transoral incisionless fundoplication). Radiofrequency ablation is recommended in patients with Barrett's esophagus with esophageal high-grade dysplasia. Guidelines also acknowledge radiofrequency ablation as a treatment option in low-grade dysplasia.[21] Transoral incisionless fundoplication creates a valve at the EGJ and is beneficial in patients with chronic GERD with abnormal ambulatory pH monitoring or low-grade erosive esophagitis with either no hiatal hernia or a hiatal hernia less than or equal to 2 cm.[31] However, it was less effective than laparoscopic Nissen fundoplication.[36]

Pharmacologic Therapy

Pharmacologic treatment consists of (a) patient-directed therapy with nonprescription antacids, H2RAs, or PPIs and (b) prescription-strength acid suppression therapy, or (c) promotility medications. Because of clinical similarities to other GI disorders, such as functional heartburn, eosinophilic esophagitis, and reflux hypersensitivity, which are not acid-related disorders, "proven" GERD should be diagnosed prior to committing a patient to long-term acid suppression therapy. Considering alternative therapies may be more appropriate for these non-GERD indications that may be more affiliated with modulating effects of anxiety or visceral and central hypersensitivity.[3]

Patient-Directed Therapy

Patient-directed therapy, where patients self-treat themselves with nonprescription medications, is appropriate for mild, intermittent symptoms. Patients with continuous symptoms lasting longer than 2 weeks should seek medical attention.[4] Self-treatment without further evaluation should also be avoided when the duration of severe or nocturnal heartburn exceeds 3 months, patient is symptomatic while taking prescription strength acid suppression therapy, or in the presence of alarm symptoms.[4]

Antacids and Antacid–Alginic Acid Products Patients should be educated that antacids are an appropriate component of treating milder GERD symptoms, even though documentation of their efficacy in placebo-controlled clinical trials is lacking. Antacids may offer immediate symptomatic relief and help maintain the intragastric pH greater than 4, which decreases the activation of pepsinogen to pepsin, a proteolytic enzyme. The neutralization of gastric fluid may also lead to increased LES pressure. Patients who require frequent use of antacids for chronic symptoms should be treated with prescription strength acid suppression therapy.

Some antacid products are combined with alginic acid, which is not a potent-neutralizing agent and does not enhance LES pressure; however, it does form a highly viscous solution or "raft" that floats on the surface of the gastric contents. This viscous solution serves as a protective barrier for the esophagus against reflux of gastric contents and reduces the frequency of the reflux episodes. The alginic acid "raft" can adapt to the acid pocket, continuously floating above newly secreted acid near the EGJ. The combination product may be superior to antacids alone in relieving the symptoms of GERD.[37] There was a significant benefit favoring alginate therapy when compared to antacids in GERD; however, with moderate heterogeneity.[37] Alginate may also improve symptoms in patients on once-daily PPI still having residual reflux symptoms.[38] Liquid containing sodium alginate 1,000 mg/20 mL was more effective than an antacid without sodium alginate in controlling esophageal acid exposure after meals.[39] Efficacy data indicating endoscopic healing are lacking. There are many products with varying amounts of alginic acid. Some of the products contain lower amounts of alginic acid or list alginic acid under inactive ingredients with no amounts specified. Products with a higher alginic acid component are preferred (eg, 500 mg or higher amount of alginc acid). Patients should be encouraged to check medication labels for ingredients.

Antacid or antacid combination products interact with a variety of medications by altering gastric pH, increasing urinary pH, adsorbing medications to their surfaces, providing a physical barrier to absorption, or forming insoluble complexes with other medications. Antacids have clinically significant drug interactions with tetracycline, ferrous sulfate, isoniazid, sulfonylureas, and quinolone antibiotics. Antacid–drug interactions are influenced by composition, dose, dosage schedule, and formulation of the antacid. They may also cause constipation or diarrhea depending on the magnesium or aluminum content.

Dosage recommendations for antacids in the management of GERD are somewhat difficult to derive from the literature. Doses range from hourly to an as-needed basis (see Table 50-3). In general, antacids have a short duration of action, which necessitates frequent administration throughout the day to provide continuous neutralization of acid. Taking antacids after meals can increase the duration of action from about 1 to 3 hours; however, nighttime acid suppression cannot be maintained with bedtime doses.

Nonprescription H2RAs and Proton Pump Inhibitors Nonprescription H2RAs (cimetidine, famotidine, and nizatidine) are effective in diminishing gastric acid secretion when taken prior to meals and decrease GERD symptoms associated with exercise. Antacids may have a slightly faster onset of action, while the H2RAs have a much longer duration of action compared with antacids.

The PPIs esomeprazole, omeprazole (alone or combined with sodium bicarbonate), and lansoprazole are available without a prescription for the short-term treatment of heartburn.

Acid Suppression Therapy

8 Acid suppression is the mainstay of GERD treatment. PPIs provide the greatest symptom relief and the highest healing rates, especially for patients with erosive disease, moderate-to-severe symptoms, or complications.

Proton Pump Inhibitors PPIs (dexlansoprazole, esomeprazole, lansoprazole, omeprazole [with or without sodium bicarbonate], pantoprazole, and rabeprazole) block gastric acid secretion by inhibiting gastric H^+/K^+-adenosine triphosphatase in gastric parietal cells. This produces a profound, long-lasting antisecretory effect capable of maintaining the gastric pH greater than 4, even during postprandial acid surges. A correlation exists between the percentage of time the gastric pH remains greater than 4 during the 24-hour period and healing erosive esophagitis.

The efficacy in treating GERD is similar among all of the PPIs.[31] Symptomatic relief is seen in approximately 83% of patients with endoscopic evidence of injury after 8 weeks treated with a PPI, whereas the endoscopic healing rate at 8 weeks is 78%.[1] Symptom response to NERD is less robust with approximately 60% of patients experiencing complete relief with PPI therapy.[1] PPIs are superior to H2RAs in treating moderate-to-severe GERD and should be given empirically to those with troublesome symptoms. This includes not only patients with esophageal tissue injury (eg, Barrett's esophagus, strictures, or esophagitis) but also patients with symptom-based GERD syndromes. Patients with uncomplicated GERD who respond well to a short-term course of PPI therapy should attempt to discontinue or to lower to the lowest effective dose.[40,41] Rebound acid hypersecretion may occur when PPIs are withdrawn making deprescribing of PPIs difficult. While no specific deprescribing or tapering regimen is recognized, strategies could include tapering dose down over 4 to 6 weeks, on-demand dosing, or abrupt discontinuation. One approach is to lower the dose by going from twice daily to once daily or halving the dose; or stopping the PPI and using an on-demand-regimen.[42] Up to 30% of patients on long-term PPI therapy could discontinue use and up to 80% were able to lower the dose.[43] PPI on-demand dosing was just as effective as low dose maintenance therapy for GERD symptoms.[44,45] Abrupt discontinuation of PPI therapy, while not ideal due to increased risk of rebound GERD symptoms, could be a reasonable option in select patients.

Twice-daily PPI use is indicated in those not responding to a standard once-daily course of therapy. Before increasing the frequency to twice daily, optimization of PPI therapy should be assessed (eg, taken 30-60 minutes prior to largest meal each day). In patients who are partial responders to initial PPI therapy, a trial of an alternative PPI may also be considered. Either strategy (twice-daily PPI or switching to an alternative PPI) has resulted in about a 20% improvement in symptoms with neither strategy demonstrating a clear advantage.[1] Partial response may also be due to abnormal patient perception, altered motility, or impaired LES dynamics where adjunctive therapy addressing the underlying cause may be helpful.[46] Patients with Barrett's esophagus should be treated similar to patients without Barrett's esophagus.[1] Further diagnostic evaluation is indicated for patients not responding to twice-daily PPI therapy.

The most common adverse effects associated with PPIs include headache, diarrhea, nausea, and abdominal pain. Increasing concerns regarding PPI safety continue to be reported. Community-acquired pneumonia may occur with short-term use in GERD patients.[1] Enteric infections, vitamin B12 deficiency, hypomagnesemia, and bone fractures are potential long-term adverse effects associated with PPIs (Table 50-5).[28,40,47,48] Gastric acidity plays an important role in the absorption of minerals such as calcium and magnesium, as well as with vitamin B12. While PPIs do not have a direct effect on the pH in the colon, they do have a downstream effect on colonic bacteria increasing the risk for *Clostridioides difficile* infections.[40,48] There is no evidence to support the use of probiotics in patients on long-term PPIs to prevent infection.[40] Despite potential concerns, data are lacking to recommend calcium, vitamin B12, or magnesium intake above the recommended daily allowance, unless there are other risk factors that warrant additional supplementation. Likewise, routine screening or monitoring of bone mineral density, serum creatinine, magnesium, or vitamin B12 levels are not recommended just because the patient is on long-term PPI therapy.[40] Another concern is chronic kidney disease. Proposed mechanisms for kidney injury include repeated bouts of acute interstitial nephritis, concurrent NSAID use, diabetes, and hypomagnesemia. Chronic kidney disease occurred in 3.68% of patients started on a PPI over a 5-year period compared to 2.56% in patients on an H2RA (Hazard ratio [HR] = 1.28). No association between PPI use and myocardial infarction has been clearly demonstrated.[48]

An increased risk of PPI-induced hepatic encephalopathy has been suggested.[48] The mechanism of this toxicity is related to alterations in the gut microbiota. Hypochlorhydria may lead to small bowel bacterial overgrowth which may contribute to hepatic adverse events. The risk of dementia or cognitive decline in patients receiving PPIs has raised concerns in the lay press; however, the evidence for this association is weak.[40] Vitamin B12 deficiency and enhanced beta-amyloid levels are potential contributing factors related to the potential cognitive decline associated with PPI use.[48]

Most of this data on these long-term adverse events are from observational studies and results have been variable. The first and largest prospective, randomized trial that examined PPI safety for up to 3 years found no difference in most adverse outcomes previously associated with long-term PPI use.[49] The one outcome that occurred more often in the PPI group was non-*Clostridioides difficile* enteric infections. Based on the results of this trial, limiting use of PPIs due to concerns regarding long-term effects is not warrented.[49] Overuse of PPI should still be minimized until the clinical implications of chronic therapy are better elucidated as more patients remain on PPI therapy for more than 3 years. Best practice advice from the American Gastroenterology Association states there is no convincing evidence to rank PPI formulations on potential risks.[40] More importantly, changing the paradigm to a more individualized approach to diagnosing GERD has been advocated based on careful assessment of anatomy, motor function, reflux burden, and symptomatic phenotype as a strategy to reduce the overuse of PPIs.[22] Clinicians should strive to identify a clear indication for PPI use before long-term therapy is considered. Deprescribing PPIs to reduce the potential for long-term adverse effects is important. Proper patient education should be done to ensure that appropriate patients are selected for PPI dose reductions or discontinuations to avoid adverse outcomes.[50,51]

Drug interactions with the PPIs vary slightly with each agent. All PPIs can decrease the absorption of medications such as ketoconazole or itraconazole, which require an acidic environment to be absorbed. Concerns have been raised regarding the concomitant use of PPIs, particularly omeprazole, with clopidogrel since it is the strongest inhibitor of CYP2C19.[52] Clopidogrel, a prodrug, is converted to its active metabolite via the CYP2C19 and CYP3A4

TABLE 50-5 Drug Monitoring

Drug	Adverse Drug Reaction	Monitoring Parameter	Comments
Antacids			
Magnesium hydroxide/aluminum hydroxide Antacid/alginic acid Calcium carbonate	• Diarrhea or constipation (depending on product) • Alterations in mineral metabolism • Acid–base disturbances	• Periodic calcium and phosphate levels in patients on chronic therapy	• Use caution with aluminum- and calcium-containing antacids in patients with renal impairment • Aluminum-containing antacids may bind to phosphate in the gut and lead to bone demineralization
H2RAs			
Cimetidine Famotidine Nizatidine	• Headache, somnolence, fatigue, dizziness, and either constipation or diarrhea	• Monitor for CNS effects, especially in older patients	• May see increased CNS effects (rare) in those over 50 years of age or in those with renal or hepatic dysfunction • May be associated with vitamin B12 deficiency with longer duration therapy and in higher doses
Proton Pump Inhibitors			
Dexlansoprazole Esomeprazole Lansoprazole Omeprazole Omeprazole/sodium bicarbonate Pantoprazole Rabeprazole	*Most common adverse effects:* • Headache, dizziness, diarrhea, flatulence, abdominal pain, and nausea *Other important adverse effects:* • Enteric infections • Community-acquired pneumonia *Long-term adverse effects:* • Hypomagnesemia • Bone fractures • Vitamin B12 deficiency • Chronic kidney disease	• Number and type of diarrhea episodes • Periodic magnesium levels warranted in those on higher doses or who are on therapy for greater than 1 year • Routine bone density studies or calcium supplementation should only be considered if other risk factors for osteoporosis or bone fractures are present • Respiratory symptoms within first 30 days of therapy • Periodic (not routinely) vitamin B12 serum concentration with long-term use	• Acid suppression may result in loss of host defense against ingested spores and bacteria permitting a higher burden of exposure • Hypomagnesemia is uncommon but can be serious; more likely in those on PPIs greater than 1 year • May increase risk for osteoporosis-related fractures of the hip, wrist, or spine; most common with high-dose (eg, multiple daily doses) and long-term use (eg, more than 1 year) and patients with osteoporosis can remain on PPI • PPIs may inhibit secretion of intrinsic factor, which potentially can lead to vitamin B12 deficiency; this is not common and usually associated with use for greater than 3 years • May increase risk of community-acquired pneumonia, particularly within the first 30 days of therapy

Data from References 28, 40, 47, and 48.

enzymes. Inhibition of CYP2C19 by PPIs, specifically omeprazole, may possibly decrease the effectiveness of clopidogrel.

Another consideration, particularly with omeprazole, is the potential polymorphic gene variations seen in the hepatic activity of CYP2C19. This is especially true for patients who are considered "slow metabolizers" of omeprazole, which is not only more common in Asian patients but also found in approximately 3% of White patients. Unfortunately, it is unclear which patients have the polymorphic gene variation that makes them slow metabolizers. Like omeprazole, the metabolism of esomeprazole may also be altered for patients with this polymorphic gene variation. Despite these concerns, there are certain patients with upper GI bleeding or those with multiple risk factors for GI bleeding who require antiplatelet therapy would benefit from PPI therapy. Risk factors for GI bleeding include advanced age, use of anticoagulants, steroids or NSAIDs, presence of *H. pylori*, or previous history of bleeding or peptic ulcer disease complications.[53] For patients on clopidogrel, using an alternative acid suppression agent, such as an H2RA, or a PPI other than omeprazole and esomeprazole or using an alternative antiplatelet agent may be an acceptable alternative if there are concerns.

The PPIs degrade in acidic environments and therefore are formulated in a delayed-release capsule or tablet formulation. Dexlansoprazole, esomeprazole, lansoprazole, and omeprazole contain enteric-coated (pH-sensitive) granules in a capsule form. Dexlansoprazole is unique in that the capsule is a dual delayed-release formulation, with the first release occurring 1 to 2 hours after the dose and the second release occurring 4 to 5 hours after the dose. The clinical significance of this dual release is to allow the medication to have a longer lasting benefit, at least 16 to 18 hours. Patients taking pantoprazole or rabeprazole should be instructed not to crush, chew, or split the delayed-release tablets.

For patients who are unable to swallow the capsule or tablet, or for pediatric patients, there are several alternative administration methods available. The contents of the delayed-release capsules can be mixed in applesauce or placed in orange juice. If a patient has a nasogastric tube, the contents of an omeprazole capsule can be mixed in 8.4% sodium bicarbonate solution. Esomeprazole granules can be dispersed in water. Esomeprazole, omeprazole, and pantoprazole are also available in a delayed-release oral suspension powder packet, while lansoprazole is available as a delayed-release, orally disintegrating tablet. Esomeprazole and pantoprazole are available in an IV formulation, which offers an alternative route of administration for patients who are unable to take an oral PPI. Importantly, the IV product is not more efficacious than oral PPIs and is significantly more expensive. The IV product should not be routinely used in GERD.

Omeprazole is also available as a delayed-release tablet and in a combination product with sodium bicarbonate as an immediate-release capsule and oral suspension. This is the only immediate-release PPI, and it should be taken on an empty stomach at least 1 hour before a meal. Omeprazole powder for oral suspension offers an alternative to the delayed-release capsules, or IV formulation in adult patients with a nasogastric tube. The immediate-release capsule should be swallowed whole and not opened, sprinkled on food, or administered via nasogastric tube. The 20- and 40-mg immediate-release capsules have the same amount of sodium bicarbonate; therefore, two 20-mg capsules cannot be substituted for a 40-mg capsule.

Patients should be instructed to take their PPI in the morning, 30 to 60 minutes before breakfast or before their biggest meal of the day, to maximize efficacy. Dexlansoprazole can be taken without regard to meals. Patients with nocturnal symptoms may benefit from taking their PPI prior to the evening meal. If dosed twice daily, the second dose should be administered approximately 10 to 12 hours after the morning dose and prior to a meal or snack.

H2RAs H2RAs (cimetidine, famotidine, and nizatidine) in divided doses are effective in treating patients with mild-to-moderate GERD.[1]

The efficacy of H2RAs in the management of GERD is extremely variable and is frequently lower than desired. Response to the H2RAs is dependent on the (a) severity of disease, (b) dosage regimen used, and (c) duration of therapy. These factors are important when comparing clinical trials and/or assessing a patient's response to therapy. The severity of esophagitis at baseline has a profound impact on the patient's response to H2RAs. For symptomatic relief of mild GERD, low-dose, nonprescription H2RAs or standard doses given twice daily may be beneficial. Patients who do not respond to standard doses may be hypersecreters of gastric acid and will require higher doses. Although higher doses of H2RAs may provide higher symptomatic and endoscopic healing rates, limited information exists regarding the safety of these regimens, and they can be less effective and more costly than once-daily PPIs. Unlike duodenal ulcer disease, in which the duration of therapy is relatively short (eg, 4-6 weeks), prolonged courses of H2RAs are frequently required in the treatment of GERD.

Because all of the H2RAs have similar efficacy, selection of the specific agent to use in the management of GERD should be based on factors such as differences in pharmacokinetics, safety profile, and cost. Patients should be monitored for the presence of adverse effects, as well as potential drug interactions, especially when taking cimetidine. Cimetidine may inhibit the metabolism of theophylline, warfarin, phenytoin, nifedipine, and propranolol, among others. An alternate H2RA should be selected if the patient is on any of these medications. Headache, fatigue, dizziness, and constipation/diarrhea are the most common adverse effects associated with the use of H2RAs. Tachyphylaxis commonly occurs with H2RAs rendering them ineffective after a period of time in some patients. Ranitidine was taken off the US market in 2020 due to contamination with N-nitrosodimethylamine. The age of the product and storage temperatures were noted to accelerate production of this contaminant linked to cancer.

Promotility Agents

Promotility agents may be useful as an adjunct to acid suppression therapy for patients with a known motility defect (eg, LES incompetence, decreased esophageal clearance, and delayed gastric emptying). Unfortunately, all available promotility agents are fraught with undesirable adverse effects and are not as effective as acid suppression therapy.

Metoclopramide Metoclopramide, a dopamine antagonist, increases LES pressure in a dose-related manner and accelerates gastric emptying in gastroesophageal reflux patients. However, it does not improve esophageal clearance. Metoclopramide provides symptomatic improvement for some patients with GERD; however, substantial data supporting endoscopic healing are lacking. In addition, metoclopramide's adverse effect profile, including extrapyramidal effects, tardive dyskinesia, and other central nervous system (CNS) effects, limits its usefulness in treating many patients with GERD. The risk of adverse effects is much greater for older patients and for patients with renal dysfunction because the drug is primarily eliminated by the kidneys. Contraindications include Parkinson's disease, mechanical obstruction, concomitant use of other dopamine antagonists or anticholinergic agents, and pheochromocytoma.

Bethanechol Bethanechol, a promotility drug, has limited value in the treatment of GERD because of unwanted adverse effects, such as urinary retention, abdominal discomfort, nausea, and flushing. It is not routinely recommended for the treatment of GERD.

Mucosal Protectants

Sucralfate, a nonabsorbable aluminum salt of sucrose octasulfate, has limited value in the treatment of GERD. It may not be useful in the routine treatment of acid reflux but may be useful in the management of radiation esophagitis and bile or nonacid reflux GERD.

Combination Therapy

Combination therapy with an acid suppression agent and a promotility agent or a mucosal protectant agent would seem logical given the multifactorial nature of the disease, particularly in light of the disappointing results seen with many monotherapy regimens. However, data to support combination therapy are limited, and this approach should not routinely be recommended unless a patient has GERD plus motor dysfunction occurring. The effectiveness of the addition of an H2RA at bedtime to PPI therapy for the treatment of nocturnal symptoms may decrease over time due to tachyphylaxis with H2RAs. Therefore, "as needed" use of bedtime H2RA may be a more appropriate approach if combination with a PPI is deemed necessary. Using the omeprazole–sodium bicarbonate immediate-release product in addition to once-daily PPIs may offer an alternative for nocturnal GERD symptoms.

Maintenance Therapy

9 Many patients with GERD will relapse if medication is withdrawn; therefore, long-term maintenance treatment may be required. A PPI is the drug of choice for maintenance of patients with moderate-to-severe GERD, erosive disease, or other complications such as Barrett's esophagus. Patients who have symptomatic relapse following discontinuation of therapy or lowering of medication doses should be considered for long-term maintenance therapy to prevent complications or worsening of esophageal function.[1]

In patients with uncomplicated GERD who respond to short-term PPI therapy, lowering the PPI dose or discontinuing the PPI should be considered. If this is not possible, ambulatory reflux pH with or without impedance monitoring should be performed to assure symptoms are GERD-related prior to committing to lifelong PPI use.[40] Patients receiving chronic PPI therapy should be periodically evaluated to assure the lowest possible effective dose is used.[40,60] The goal of maintenance therapy is to improve quality of life by controlling the patient's symptoms and preventing complications. Patients should be counseled on the importance of complying with lifestyle changes and long-term maintenance therapy in order to prevent recurrence or worsening of disease. H2RAs may be an effective maintenance therapy for patients with mild disease.[1] Low doses of a PPI or alternate-day dosing may be effective in some patients with mild symptoms, thereby allowing dose reduction in some cases. "On-demand" or intermittent maintenance therapy, by which patients take their PPI only when they have symptoms, may be effective for patients with endoscopy-negative GERD.[1,31] Many patients with only mild-to-moderate symptoms may decide on their own to use "on-demand" for the financial benefit and patient satisfaction.[31] However, patients with persistent symptoms and/or complications require standard doses of PPIs.

Studies evaluating the efficacy of the H2RAs in maintaining patients with GERD in remission have been disappointing. No currently available H2RA regimen is FDA-approved for maintenance of healing of erosive esophagitis. Antireflux surgery may also be considered a viable alternative to long-term drug therapy for maintenance of healing for patients who are candidates.

Special Populations

There are several special populations that should be considered when discussing GERD, such as patients with extraesophageal symptoms, pediatric patients, older patients, and patients with refractory symptoms.

Patients with Extraesophageal GERD

Extraesophageal symptoms (such as asthma, laryngitis, or chest pain) should prompt investigation for other possible causes outside of GERD. Because there are many causes of asthma and laryngeal symptoms, a concomitant esophageal GERD syndrome must also be present to associate these symptoms with GERD. A trial of PPI therapy is recommended for those with extraesophageal symptoms with concurrent typical GERD symptoms. Patients with extraesophageal symptoms without typical GERD symptoms should undergo ambulatory reflux monitoring prior to initiation of PPI therapy. If symptoms continue, patients should be evaluated with manometry or ambulatory reflux monitoring with or without impedance to rule out dysmotility or refractory symptoms, respectively.[1] Ambulatory reflux monitoring while on PPI is useful for those with "proven" GERD while testing while off PPI is useful when the goal is to identify moderate-to-severe reflux at baseline.[54]

In patients with chronic cough suspected to be reflux related, lifestyle modifications are recommended.[55] Acid suppression therapy is unlikely to be beneficial if heartburn or regurgitation is not also present. If the patient does have concomitant heartburn or regurgitation with a chronic cough, PPI therapy may be beneficial but may take up to 3 months before resolution of cough.[55] After 3 months, more diagnostic evaluation is needed.

Pediatric Patients with GERD

Many infants have physiologic reflux with little or no clinical consequence. Uncomplicated gastroesophageal reflux usually manifests as regurgitation or "spitting up" and resolves without incident by about 12 months of life.[16] When evaluating a child for GERD, conduct a history and physical examination. If alarm signs are present, clinicians should tailor testing to address the alarm signs and refer appropriately. If no alarm signs are present, lifestyle and dietary education should be initiated. Symptoms usually respond to supportive therapy, including dietary adjustments, postural management, and reassurance for the parents. Thickened feedings may be useful in milder cases. While this does not decrease reflux episodes, it may decrease the incidence of regurgitation.[16] This strategy of thickening feedings may be appropriate for full-term infants; however, may be associated with necrotizing enterocolitis in preterm infants. Chronic vomiting associated with gastroesophageal reflux must be distinguished from other causes, such as neurologic, metabolic, eating, and rumination disorders. Smaller, more frequent feedings may be beneficial. In formula-fed infants, an extensively hydrolyzed protein may help identify milk protein sensitivity as the cause of unexplained GERD-like symptoms, likewise, exclusion of milk and eggs in the maternal diet for breastfeeding infants may be appropriate.[16] Additionally, a trial of an amino acid-based formula should occur prior to a trial of acid suppression therapy. If lifestyle and dietary education do not resolve the GERD symptoms, a 4- to 8-week trial of acid suppression therapy is recommended.[16] Once a 4- to 8-week course is complete, referral to a pediatric GI specialist is recommended if symptoms are not improved or recur upon weaning therapy.[16]

Developmental immaturity of the LES is one suspected cause of gastroesophageal reflux in infants. Like adults, TLESRs seem to be the most common cause of gastroesophageal reflux in children. Other causes include impaired luminal clearance of gastric acid, neurologic impairment, and type of infant formula. Complications, although rare, include distal esophagitis, failure to thrive, esophageal peptic strictures, Barrett's esophagus, and pulmonary disease. Further diagnostic evaluation is indicated in all who experience apnea or an apparent life-threatening event.

The benefits of using promotility medications, such as metoclopramide, erythromycin, bethanechol, and baclofen, are outweighed by the potential adverse effects that may occur and, therefore, cannot be routinely recommended.[16] Careful consideration should be made before medication is recommended, especially in children younger than 1 year of age.

PPI use in children is increasing, especially in those with esophagitis. Most patients will respond to once-daily PPI dosing. In

TABLE 50-6 Oral Proton Pump Inhibitor Therapy in Pediatric Patients

Drug	Indication	Age	Recommended Oral Dose (daily)	
Dexlansoprazole	Symptomatic GERD, erosive esophagitis	≥12 years		30 mg
		≥12 years		60 mg
Esomeprazole	Erosive esophagitis	1 month-1 year	3-5 kg	2.5 mg
			>5-7.5 kg	5 mg
			>7.5	10 mg
		1-11 years	<20 kg	10 mg
			≥20 kg	10-20 mg
		≥12 year		20-40 mg
	Symptomatic GERD		<20 kg	10 mg
			>20 kg	20 mg
Lansoprazole	Symptomatic GERD	Infants >3 months		7.5 mg twice daily or 15 mg daily
		1-11 years	≤30 kg	15 mg
			>30 kg	30 mg
		≥12 year		15 mg
	Erosive esophagitis	Infants >3 months		7.5 mg twice daily or 15 mg daily
		1-11 years	≤30 kg >30 kg	15-30 mg
		≥12 year		30 mg
Omeprazole	GERD, erosive esophagitis, maintenance of healing of erosive esophagitis	≥1 year	5 to <10 kg	5 mg
			10 to <20 kg	10 mg
			≥20 kg	20 mg
Pantoprazole	Symptomatic GERD			1-2 mg/kg/day
	Erosive esophagitis	≥5 years	≥15 to <40 kg	20 mg
			≥40 kg	40 mg
Rabeprazole	Symptomatic GERD	1-11 years	<15 kg	5-10 mg
			≥15 kg	10 mg
		≥12 years		20 mg

*Note: Omeprazole also has dosing for treatment of erosive esophagitis in infants 3 kg to <5 kg of 2.5 mg daily. Otherwise, dosing is the same for children and adolescents for all GERD indications.

Duration of therapy depends on age and indication.

Data from Reference 56.

infants with reflux-related esophagitis, the use of PPIs is the first-line treatment option.[16] Table 50-6 details indications and dosing of PPIs in pediatric patients. Dexlansoprazole and pantoprazole have not been adequately studied in younger pediatric patients. When examining adverse effect data from currently available trial data the authors noted that overall PPI therapy was well tolerated with mostly mild-to-moderate adverse effects in the short term. Adverse effects with individual agents included diarrhea, abdominal pain, and vomiting with headache noted in older age groups and upper and lower respiratory tract infections noted in infants. Long-term use of a PPI without a clear diagnosis of GERD is not recommended.[16]

Older Patients with GERD

Many older patients have decreased host defense mechanisms, such as saliva production. In addition, they have more comorbidities, medications, and physiologic changes that put them at higher risk. Often these patients do not seek medical attention because they feel their symptoms are part of the normal aging process. They may also present with atypical symptoms such as chest pain, asthma, poor dentition, or jaw pain. Decreased GI motility is a common problem in older patients. Unfortunately, there are no good promotility agents available to these patients. Older patients are especially sensitive to the CNS effects of metoclopramide. They may also be sensitive to the CNS effects of H2RAs. PPIs appear to be the most useful treatment modality, because they have superior efficacy and are dosed once daily, which is beneficial in all patients, but is especially beneficial in the older population. Long-term risk of bone fractures may be of concern in this population. Patients at risk for bone fractures should be monitored appropriately.

Patients with Refractory GERD

What constitutes refractory GERD is not well defined. Prior to increasing the dose to twice daily, adherence and proper administration timing of PPI therapy should be optimized. Refractory GERD should be considered in patients who have not responded to a standard course of twice-daily PPI therapy over a 12-week period. The most likely causes associated with PPI-refractory GERD include: (1) abnormal acid reflux despite PPI therapy; (2) reflux hypersensitivity where physiologic (normal) reflux causes symptoms; (3) esophageal disorders other than GERD (eg, achalasia); (4) extraesophageal disorders (eg, lung disease or heart disease); and (5) functional heartburn.[57,58] In some situations, variations in drug metabolism in certain patients may contribute to refractory GERD. Switching to another PPI or increasing the dose to twice daily may be beneficial; however, the latter may reduce compliance.[31] Rabeprazole is least affected by CYP enzymes and improves acid suppression in patients considered to be slow metabolizers of CYP 2C19.[57] Reeducating patients regarding lifestyle modifications is recommended.[31] Manometry or ambulatory esophageal reflux monitoring is useful for patients who are not responding to therapy who have normal endoscopic findings.

Patients with Los Angeles Grade C or D esophagitis, peptic stricture, Barrett's esophagus or pathologic acid exposure seen on ambulatory reflux pH monitoring (while off PPI) indicate "proven" GERD. These patients should undergo ambulatory reflux pH-impedance monitoring while on PPI therapy to determine if they are truly PPI-refractory or if contents are nonacidic in nature.[57] PPI-refractory GERD is associated with esophageal exposure time greater than 6% on PPI.[57] AET represents the percentage of time the esophageal pH is less than 4 over the monitoring period. If AET is normal then consider other non-GERD causes such as functional heartburn or reflux hypersensitivity. Patients with hypersensitive esophagus or functional heartburn do not respond as well to acid suppression therapy.[2]

The majority of patients with refractory symptoms experience nocturnal acid breakthrough. Dexlansoprazole offers greater dosing flexibility since it does not need to be administered with food so may provide effective control of nocturnal symptoms.[59] Likewise, omeprazole-sodium bicarbonate immediate-release products can be given without regard to meals and may be useful in controlling nocturnal symptoms.[59]

Antireflux surgery, magnetic sphincter augmentation, and endoscopic therapies may have a role in refractory GERD, depending on the scenario. If ambulatory reflux monitoring tests are negative, the patient is unlikely to have GERD and PPI therapy should be discontinued and alternative diagnosis should be investigated.[1] Baclofen may be beneficial for patients with residual acid or weakly acidic reflux by decreasing TLESRs, although with potential adverse effects seen in some patients.[31] Functional heartburn or reflux hypersensitivity may be treated with tricyclic antidepressants, selective serotonin reuptake inhibitors, serotonin-norepinephrine reuptake inhibitors, or trazodone.[5,31] Eosinophilic esophagitis or dysmotility syndromes are causes of nonacid-related esophageal symptoms and require therapies other than a PPI.[31,60]

EVALUATION OF THERAPEUTIC OUTCOMES

The long-term benefits of treatment are difficult to assess because of the limited information known about the epidemiology and natural history of GERD. Consequently, successful outcomes are measured in terms of three separate end points: (a) relieving symptoms, (b) healing the injured mucosa, and (c) preventing complications.

10 The short-term goal of therapy is to relieve symptoms such as heartburn and regurgitation to the point at which they do not impair the patient's quality of life. Patients should be educated regarding specific lifestyle modifications that are applicable to their individual situation including weight loss and raising the head end of the bed. Patient medication profiles should be reviewed for medications that may aggravate GERD. Patients should be monitored for adverse drug reactions and potential drug interactions. Deprescribing PPIs or tapering to the lowest effective dose is a key strategy in preventing adverse effects. Table 50-5 reviews common adverse drug reactions and monitoring of medications used in GERD. The frequency and severity of symptoms should be monitored, and patients should be counseled on symptoms that suggest the presence of complications requiring immediate medical attention, such as dysphagia. Patients should also be monitored for the presence of extraesophageal symptoms, such as laryngitis asthma or chest pain. These symptoms require further diagnostic evaluation. Long-term maintenance treatment is indicated for patients who have strictures as they commonly recur if reflux esophagitis is not treated.

The second goal is to heal the injured mucosa. Again, individualized lifestyle modifications and the importance of complying with the therapeutic regimen chosen to heal the mucosa should be stressed. Patients should be educated about the risk of relapse and the need for long-term maintenance therapy to prevent recurrence or complications.

The final, long-term goal of therapy is to decrease the risk of complications (esophagitis, strictures, Barrett's esophagus, and esophageal adenocarcinoma). A small subset of patients may continue to fail treatment despite therapy with high doses of H2RAs or a PPI. Patients should be monitored for the presence of continual pain, dysphagia, or odynophagia.

ABBREVIATIONS

AET	acid exposure time
BMI	body mass index
EGJ	esophagogastric junction
GERD	gastroesophageal reflux disease
GI	gastrointestinal
HR	hazard ratio
H2RA	histamine-2 receptor antagonist
LES	lower esophageal sphincter
NERD	nonerosive reflux disease
NSAID	nonsteroidal anti-inflammatory drug
PPI	proton pump inhibitor
TLESR	transient lower esophageal sphincter relaxation
UES	upper esophageal sphincter

REFERENCES

1. Katz PO, Gerson LB, Vela MF. Guidelines for the diagnosis and management of gastroesophageal reflux disease. *Am J Gastroenterol.* 2013;108:308–328. 10.1038/ajg.2012.444.
2. Katzka DA, Kahrilas PJ. Advances in the diagnosis and management of gastroesophageal reflux disease. *BMJ.* 2020;374:m3786. doi: 10.1136/bmj.m3786.
3. Katzka DA, Pandolfino JE, Kahrilas PJ. Phenotypes of gastroesophageal reflux disease: Where Rome, Lyon, and Montreal meet. *Clin Gastroenterol Hepatol.* 2020;18:767–776. doi: 10.1016/j.cgh.2019.07.015.
4. Hunt R, Armstrong D, Katelaris P, et al. World Gastroenterology Organisation Global Guidelines. GERD global perspective on gastroesophageal reflux disease. *J Clin Gastroenterol.* 2017;51(6):467–478. doi: 10.1097/MCG.0000000000000854.
5. Fass R, Zerbib F, Gyawali CP. AGA clinical practice update on functional heartburn: Expert review. *Gastroenterology.* 2020;158:2286–2293. doi: 10.1053/j.gastro.2020.01.034.
6. Eusebi LH, Ratnakumaran R, Yuan Y, et al. Global prevalence of and risk factors for gastro-oesophageal reflux symptoms: A meta-analysis. *Gut.* 2018;67(3):430–440. doi: 10.1136/gutjnl-2016-313589.
7. Richter JE, Rubenstein JH. Presentation and epidemiology of gastroesophageal reflux disease. *Gastroenterology.* 2018;154(2):267–276. doi: 10.1053/j.gastro.2017.07.045.
8. El-Serag HB, Sweet S, Winchester CC, Dent J. Update on the epidemiology of gastro-oesophageal reflux disease: A systematic review. *Gut.* 2014;63(6):871–880. doi: 10.1136/gutjnl-2012-304269.
9. Delshad SD, Almario CV, Chey WD, Spiegel BMR. Prevalence of gastroesophageal reflux disease and proton pump inhibitor-refractory symptoms. *Gastroenterology.* 2020;158:1250–1261. doi: 10.1053/j.gastro.2019.12.014.
10. Kim YS, Kim N, Kim GH. Sex and gender differences in gastroesophageal reflux disease. *J Neurogastroenterol Motil.* 2016;22(4):575–588. doi: 10.5056/jnm16138.
11. Shaukat A, Oxentenko AS. The time is now to understand and address sex-related disparities in gastroenterology and hepatology. Official journal of the American College of Gastroenterology | ACG. *Am J Gastroenterol.* 2021;116(3):441–443. doi: 10.14309/ajg.0000000000001185.

12. Maret-Ouda J, Markar SR, Lagergren J. Gastroesphageal reflux disease: A review. *JAMA*. 2020;324(24):2536–2547. doi: 10.1001/jama.2020.21360.
13. Park S, Weg R, Enslin S, Kaul V. Ten things every gastroenterologist should know about antireflux surgery. *Clin Gastroenterol Hepatol.* 2020;18:1923–1929. doi: 10.1016/j.cgh.2020.02.041.
14. Yang HJ, Chang Y, Park SK, et al. Nonalcoholic fatty liver disease is associated with increased risk of reflux esophagitis. *Dig Dis Sci.* 2017;62:3605–3613. doi: 10.1007/s10620-017-4805-6.
15. Tack J, Pandolfino JE. Pathophysiology of gastroesophageal reflux disease. *Gastroenterology.* 2018;154:277–288. doi: 10.1053/j.gastro.2017.09.047.
16. Rosen R, Vandenplas Y, Singendonk M et al. Pediatric Gastroesophageal Reflux Clinical Practice Guidelines: Joint recommendations of the North American Society for Pediatric Gastroenterology, Hepatology, and Nutrition and the European Society for Pediatric Gastroenterology, Hepatology, and Nutrition. *J Pediatr Gastroenterol Nutr.* 2018;66(3):516–554. doi: 10.1097.0000000000001889.
17. Camilleri M, Malhi H, Acosta A. Gastrointestinal complications of obesity. *Gastroenterology.* 2017;152:1656–1670. doi: 10.1053/j.gastro.2016.12.052.
18. Hallan A, Bomme M, Hveem K, et al. Risk factors on the development of new-onset gastroesophageal reflux symptoms. A population-based prospective cohort study: The HUNT study. *Am J Gastroenterol.* 2015;110:393–400. doi: 10.1038/ajg.2015.18.
19. Khan A, Kim A, Sanossian C, et al. Impact of obesity treatment on gastroesophageal reflux disease. *World J Gastroenterol.* 2016;22:1627–1638. doi: 10.3748/wjg.v22.i4.1627.
20. Pandit S, Boktor M, Alexander JS, et al. Gastroesophageal reflux disease: A clinical overview for primary care physicians. *Pathophysiology.* 2018;25:1–11. doi: 10.1016/j.pathophys.2017.09.001.
21. Shaheen NJ, Falk GW, Iyer PS, Gerson L. ACG Clinical Guideline: Diagnosis and management of Barrett's esophagus. *Am J Gastroenterol.* 2016;111:30–50. doi: 10.1038/ajg.2015.322.
22. Gyawali CP, Kahrilas PJ, Savarino E, et al. Modern diagnosis of GERD: The Lyon Consensus. *Gut.* 2018;67:1351–1362. doi: 10.1136/gutjnl-2017-314722.
23. Vaezi MF, Pandolfino JE, Vela MF, Shaheen NJ. White Paper AGA: Optimal strategies to define and diagnose gastroesophageal reflux disease. *Clin Gastroenterol Hepatol.* 2017;15(8):1162–1172. doi: 10.1016/j.cgh.2017.03.021.
24. Gyawali CP, Fass R. Management of gastroesophageal reflux disease. *Gastroenterology.* 2018;154(2):302–318. doi: 10.1053/j.gastro.2017.07.049.
25. Vaezi MF, Sifrim D. Assessing old and new diagnostic tests for gastroesophageal reflux disease. *Gastroenterology.* 2018;154:289–301. doi: 10.1053/j.gastro.2017.07-040.
26. American Society for Gastrointestinal Endoscopy. The role of endoscopy in the management of GERD. *Gastrointest Endosc.* 2015;81(6):1305–1310. doi: 10.1016/j.gie.2015.02.021.
27. Yadlapati R, Vaezi MF, Vela MF, et al. Management options for patients with GERD and persistent symptoms on proton pump inhibitors: Recommendations from an expert panel. *Am J Gastroenterol.* 2018;1–7. 10.1038/s41395-018-0045-4.
28. Young A, Kumar MA, Thota PN. GERD: A practical approach. *Cleve Clin J Med.* 2020;87(4):223–230. doi: 10.3949/ccjm.87a.19114.
29. GRADE Working Group. Grading quality of evidence and strength of recommendations. *BMJ.* 2004;328:1490–1494. doi: 10.1136/bmj.328.7454.1490.
30. Garvey WT, Mechanick JI, Brett EM. American Association of Clinical Endocrinologists and American College of Endocrinology comprehensive clinical practice guidelines for medical care of patients with obesity. *Endocr Pract.* 2016;22(7): 842–884. doi: 10.4158/EP161356.ESGL.
31. Sandhu DS, Fass R. Current trends in the management of gastroesophageal reflux disease. *Gut Liver.* 2018;12(1):7–16. doi: 10.5009/gnl16615.
32. Joint Commission of Pharmacy Practitioners. Pharmacists' Patient Care Process. May 29, 2014. Available at: https://jcpp.net/wp-content/uploads/2016/03/PatientCareProcess-with-supporting-organizations.pdf. Accessed May 11, 2021.
33. Katz PO, Katzka DA. Getting into a TIF(F) over fundoplication. *Gastroenterology.* 2018;154:1227–1228. doi: 10.1053/j.gastro.2018.03.005.
34. Spechler SJ, Hunter JG, Jones KM, et al. Randomized trial of medical versus surgical treatment for refractory heartburn. *N Engl J Med.* 2019;381(16):1513–1523. doi: 10.1056/NEJMoa1811424.
35. Bell R, Lipham J, Louie B, et al. Laparoscopic magnetic sphincter augmentation versus double-dose proton pump inhibitors for management of moderate-to-severe regurgitation in GERD: A randomized controlled trial. *Gastrointest Endosc.* 2019;89(1):14–22. e1. doi: 10.1016/j.gie.2018.07.007.
36. Richter JE, Kumar A, Lipka S, et al. Efficacy of laparoscopic Nissen fundoplication vs transoral incisionless fundoplication or proton pump inhibitors in patients with gastroesophageal reflux disease: A systematic review and meta-analysis. *Gastroenterology.* 2018;154:1298–1308. doi: 10.1053/j.gastro.2017.12.021.
37. Leiman DA, Riff BP, Morgan S, et al. Alginate therapy is effective treatment for gastroesophageal reflux disease symptoms: A systematic review and meta-analysis. *Dis Esophagus.* 2017;30:1–8. doi: 10.1093/dote/dow020.
38. Reimer C, Lodrup AB, Smith G, et al. Randomised clinical trial: Alginate (Gaviscon Advance) vs placebo as add-on therapy in reflux patients with inadequate response to a once daily proton pump inhibitor. *Aliment Pharmacol Ther.* 2016;43:899–909. doi: 10.1111/apt.13567.
39. De Ruigh A, Roman S, Chen J, et al. Gaviscon double action liquid (antacid & alginate) is more effective than antacid in controlling post-prandial oesophageal acid exposure in GERD patients: A double-blind cross-over study. *Aliment Pharmacol Ther.* 2014;40:531–537. doi: 10.1111/apt.12857.
40. Freedberg DE, Kim LS, Yang YX. The risks and benefits of long-term use of proton pump inhibitors: Expert review and best practice advice from the American Gastroenterological Association. *Gastrenterology.* 2017;152:706–715. doi: 10.1053/j.gastro.2017.01.031.
41. Kim J, Blackett JW, Jodorkovsky D. Strategies for effective discontinuation of proton pump inhibitors. *Curr Gastroenterol Rep.* 2018;20(6):27. doi: 10.1007/s11894-018-0632-y.
42. Farrell B, Pottie K, Thompson W, et al. Deprescribing proton pump inhibitors: Evidence-based clinical practice guideline. *Can Fam Physician.* 2017;63:354–364.
43. Helgadottir H, Bjornsson ES. Problems associated with deprescribing of proton pump inhibitors. *Int J Mol Sci.* 2019;20(21):5469. doi: 10.3390/ijms20215469.
44. Cho JH, Koo JY, Kim KO, Lee SH, Jang BI, Kim TN. On-demand versus half-dose continuous therapy with esomeprazole for maintenance treatment of gastroesophageal reflux disease: A randomized comparative study. *Medicine.* 2018;97(43):e12732. doi: 10.1097/MD.0000000000012732.
45. Chiang H, et al. Clinical efficacy of 60-mg dexlansoprazole and 40-mg esomeprazole after 24 weeks for the on-demand treatment of gastroesophageal reflux disease grades A and B: A prospective randomized trial. *Drug Des Devel Ther.* 2019;26(13):1347–1356. doi: 10.2147/DDDT.S193559.
46. Triadafilopoulos G, Clarke JO, Hawn M. Precision GERD management for the 21st century. *Dis Esophagus.* 2017;30:1–6. doi: 10.1093/dote/dox079.
47. Gyawali CP. Proton pump inhibitors in gastroesophageal reflux disease: Friend or foe. *Curr Gastroenterol Rep.* 2017;19:46. doi: 10.1007/s11894-017-0586-5.
48. Vaezi MF, Yang YX, Howden CW. Complications of proton pump inhibitor therapy. *Gastroenterology.* 2017;153:35–48. doi: 10.1053/j.gastro.2017.04.047.
49. Moayyedi P, Eikelboom JW, Bosch J, et al. Safety of proton pump inhibitors based on a large, multi-year, randomized trial of patients receiving rivaroxaban or aspirin. *Gastroenterology.* 2019;157(3):682–691.e682. doi: 10.1053/j.gastro.2019.05.056.
50. Kurlander JE, Rubenstein JH, Richardson CR, et al. Physicians' perceptions of proton pump inhibitor risks and recommendations to discontinue: A national survey. *Am J Gastroenterol.* 2020;115(5):689–696. doi: 10.14309/ajg.0000000000000061.
51. Longstreth GF. Internists' misconceptions about PPIs: Increasing knowledge and implementing guidelines. *Am J Gastroenterol.* 2020;115(5):681–682. doi: 10.14309/ajg.0000000000000561.
52. Bouziana SD, Tziomalos K. Clinical relevance of clopidogrel-proton pump inhibitors interaction. *World J Gastrointest Pharmacol Ther.* 2015;6:17–21.
53. Abraham NS, Hlatky MA, Antman EM, et al. ACCF/ACG/AHA 2010 expert consensus document on the concomitant use of proton pump inhibitors and thienopyridines: A focused update of the ACCF/ACG/AHA 2008 expert consensus document on reducing the gastrointestinal risks of antiplatelet therapy and NSAID use: A report of the American College of Cardiology Foundation Task Force on Expert Consensus Documents. *Circulation.* 2010;122:2619–2633. doi: 10.1161/CIR.0b013e318202f701.

54. Vaezi MF, Katzka D, Zerbib F. Extraesophageal symptoms and diseases attributed to GERD: Where is the pendulum swinging now? *Clin Gastroenterol Hepatol.* 2018;16:1018–1029. doi: 10.1016/j.cgh.2018.02.001.
55. Kahrilas PJ, Altman KW, Chang AB, et al. Chronic cough due to gastroesophageal reflux in adults: CHEST Guideline and Expert Panel Report. *Chest.* 2016;150(6):1341–1360. doi: 10.1016/j.chest.2016.08.1458.
56. Lexicomp Online, Pediatric and Neonatal Lexi-Drugs Online, Hudson, Ohio. Accessed May 12, 2021.
57. Yadlapati R, DeLay K. PPI refractory gastroesophageal reflux disease. *Med Clin North Am.* 2019;103(1):15–27. doi: 10.1016/j.mena.2018.08.002.
58. Spechler SJ, Hunter JG, Jones KM, et al. Randomized trial of medical versus surgical treatment for refractory heartburn. *N Engl J Med.* 2019;381:1513–1523. doi: 10.1056/NEJMoa1811424.
59. Kung YM, Hsu WH, Wu MC, et al. Recent advances in the pharmacological management of gastroesophageal reflux disease. *Dig Dis Sci.* 2017;62:3298–3316. doi: 10.1016/j.cgh.2018.02.001.
60. Subramanian CR, Triadafilopoulos G. Refractory gastroesophageal reflux disease. *Gastroenterol Rep.* 2015;3:41–53. doi: 10.1093/gastro/gou061.

Peptic Ulcer Disease and Related Disorders

51

Bryan L. Love

KEY CONCEPTS

1. Psychological stress, cigarette smoking, nonsteroidal anti-inflammatory drug (NSAID) use, and certain foods/beverages can exacerbate ulcer symptoms and should be avoided.
2. Eradication of *Helicobacter pylori* (*H. pylori*) is recommended for all patients who test positive, especially in those patients with an active ulcer, a documented history of a prior ulcer, or a history of ulcer-related complications.
3. The selection of an *H. pylori* eradication regimen should be based on several factors, including efficacy, safety, antibiotic resistance, cost, and the likelihood of medication adherence. The recommended initial treatment options with the strongest level of evidence include bismuth quadruple and concomitant therapy, both administered for 10 to 14 days. Empiric clarithromycin-based triple therapy is no longer recommended due to increasing resistance and reduced eradication rates.
4. When first-line therapy fails, salvage treatment for *H. pylori* should contain different antibiotics due to potential resistance. Patients with reported penicillin allergy should be considered for penicillin skin testing after failing first-line therapy since many can safely be treated with amoxicillin containing salvage regimens.
5. PPI co-therapy reduces the risk of NSAID-related gastric and duodenal ulcers and is at least as effective as misoprostol and superior to histamine-2 receptor antagonists (H2RAs).
6. Standard PPI dosages and a nonselective NSAID are as effective as a selective cyclooxygenase-2 (COX-2) inhibitor in reducing the risk of NSAID-induced ulcers and upper gastrointestinal (GI) complications.
7. Patients with peptic ulcer disease (PUD), especially those receiving *H. pylori* eradication or misoprostol co-therapy, require patient education regarding their disease and drug treatment to successfully achieve a positive therapeutic outcome.
8. Treatment for severe peptic ulcer bleeding after appropriate endoscopic treatment includes administration of a PPI either orally or parenterally via intermittent or continuous infusion targeting cumulative daily doses of 80 to 160 mg.
9. Coagulopathy and respiratory failure requiring mechanical ventilation are the most notable risk factors for developing stress-related mucosal bleeding (SRMB). Prophylactic drug therapy should be administered to critically ill patients with either of these risk factors.
10. Selection of a PPI over an IV H2RA for SRMB prophylaxis should be based on individual patient characteristics (eg, nothing by mouth, presence of nasogastric tube, thrombocytopenia, renal failure).

BEYOND THE BOOK

Create a table with two columns, one titled PPI and one titled H2RA. Create rows for Prevention of NSAID-induced ulcer disease and Stress Ulcer Prophylaxis. In each new cell, list advantages and disadvantages of using each medication class for these conditions. The purpose of this exercise is to familiarize students with the relative safety and efficacy for medications commonly used to treat PUD.

PEPTIC ULCER DISEASE

Gastric acid is a critical component of upper gastrointestinal (GI) tract complications including gastritis, erosions, and peptic ulcer.[2-4] Peptic ulcer disease (PUD) differs from gastritis and erosions in that ulcers are larger (greater than or equal to 5 mm) and extend deeper into the muscularis mucosa. The three common forms of peptic ulcers can be grouped according to their etiology: *Helicobacter pylori*–positive, NSAID-induced, and stress-related mucosal damage (SRMD) (Table 51-1).

H. pylori–positive and NSAID-induced ulcers are chronic peptic ulcers that differ in etiology, clinical presentation, and tendency to recur (see Table 51-1). These ulcers develop most often in the stomach and duodenum of ambulatory patients (Fig. 51-1). Occasionally, ulcers develop in the esophagus, jejunum, ileum, or colon. The natural course of chronic PUD is characterized by frequent ulcer recurrence. The cause of ulcer recurrence is often multifactorial, although *H. pylori* infection and NSAID use are commonly associated. In addition, cigarette smoking, alcohol use, gastric acid hypersecretion, and medication nonadherence are frequently related.

Conditions such as Zollinger-Ellison syndrome (ZES), radiation, chemotherapy, vascular insufficiency, and other chronic diseases (Table 51-2) are associated with development and recurrence of peptic ulcers.[2,3] Ulcer development at the gastro-jejunal anastomosis, termed marginal ulcers, occurs in patients with history of Roux-en-Y gastric bypass surgery and shares risk factors with PUD; however, the pathogenesis is not fully understood.[5] Although a strong association exists between chronic pulmonary diseases, chronic kidney disease, and cirrhosis, the pathophysiologic mechanisms of these associations remain unclear.[3] In contrast, SRMD occurs primarily in the stomach of critically ill patients (see Table 51-1).[2]

TABLE 51-1 Comparison of Common Forms of Peptic Ulcer

Characteristic	*H. pylori*–Induced	NSAID-Induced	SRMD
Condition	Chronic	Chronic	Acute
Site of damage	Duodenum > stomach	Stomach > duodenum	Stomach > duodenum
Intragastric pH	More dependent	Less dependent	Less dependent
Symptoms	Usually epigastric pain	Often asymptomatic	Asymptomatic
Ulcer depth	Superficial	Deep	Most superficial
GI bleeding	Less severe, single vessel	More severe, single vessel	More severe, superficial mucosal capillaries

GI, gastrointestinal; NSAID, nonsteroidal anti-inflammatory drug; SRMD, stress-related mucosal damage.

TABLE 51-2 Potential Causes of Peptic Ulcer

Common causes
Helicobacter pylori infection
NSAIDs
Critical illness (stress-related mucosal damage)

Uncommon causes of chronic peptic ulcer
Idiopathic (non–*H. pylori*, non-NSAID peptic ulcer)
Hypersecretion of gastric acid (eg, Zollinger-Ellison syndrome)
Viral infections (eg, cytomegalovirus)
Vascular insufficiency (eg, crack cocaine associated)
Radiation therapy
Chemotherapy (eg, hepatic artery infusions)
Infiltrating disease (eg, Crohn's disease)
Roux-en-Y gastric bypass surgery

Diseases and medical conditions associated with chronic peptic ulcer
Cirrhosis
Chronic kidney disease
Chronic obstructive pulmonary disease
Cardiovascular disease
Organ transplantation

NSAIDs, nonsteroidal anti-inflammatory drugs.

EPIDEMIOLOGY

4 The epidemiology of PUD is complicated, and the prevalence is difficult to estimate given the variability in *H. pylori* infection, NSAID use, and cigarette smoking. In addition, endoscopy, radiology, symptoms, or other methods have different sensitivity and specificity to detect ulcers.[2] Gastroduodenal ulcers occur in 0.1% to 0.3% of the general population annually, and the lifetime prevalence of PUD is between 5% and 10%.[3] The prevalence and incidence of PUD in the United States has decreased, reflecting improvements in drug therapy, the dramatic shift to ambulatory management, and changes in the criteria and coding system for mortality and hospitalization data. Mortality, hospitalization, and emergency department and ambulatory care visits have declined, but 30-day readmissions for upper GI hemorrhage have increased.[6] Mortality rates are higher among those 65 years and older and in males compared to females.[6] PUD remains a common GI disease, resulting in impaired quality of life, work loss, and high-cost medical care.

7 The prevalence of *H. pylori* varies by geographic location, resource limitations, ethnicity, and age. In the United States and other industrialized countries, *H. pylori* prevalence has declined with successive birth cohorts and is thought to correlate with improved hygiene and living conditions compared with developing countries.[7,8] In the United States, *H. pylori* prevalence is approximately 30% to 40%, but it is much higher in adults older than 60 years (50%-60%) than in children younger than 12 years (10%-15%). The rate of *H. pylori* acquisition in children is declining due to improved environmental conditions in Western populations, but maternal colonization remains an important transmission factor. Disparities in *H. pylori* prevalence continue to exist among Black and Hispanic persons with infection rates approximately two to three times that of non-Hispanic White persons.[8,9] Adults with some college education have reduced prevalence of *H. pylori*, probably related to improved access to resources and living conditions.[9] Infection rates do not differ with gender or smoking status. Among Hispanic persons overall *H. pylori* seroprevalence was 38% in US born and 62% among non-US born individuals.[10]

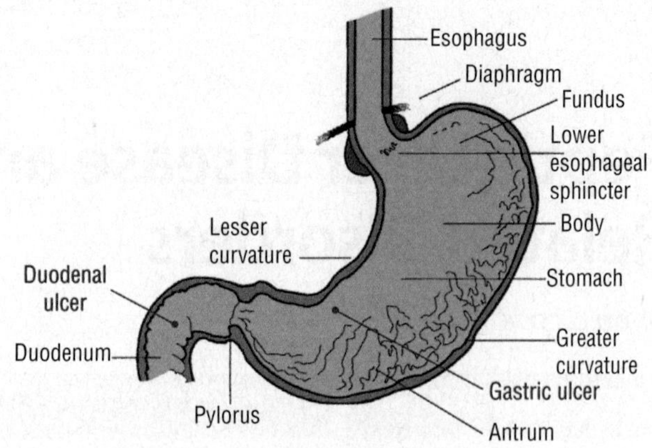

FIGURE 51-1 Anatomic structure of the stomach and duodenum and most common locations of gastric and duodenal ulcers.

Nonsteroidal Anti-Inflammatory Drugs

Gastroduodenal lesions including erosions, petechiae, and ulcers are visible upon endoscopy in an estimated 30% to 50% of chronic NSAID users. In most cases, the gastric mucosa adapts, and no clinical manifestations are observed. NSAIDs and low-dose aspirin increase the relative risk of PUD by an estimated 2.7 and 1.7 times, respectively. Despite the introduction of gastroprotective medications, NSAIDs represent an important cause of morbidity and mortality. NSAIDs and low-dose aspirin contribute to significant GI events, including ulceration and bleeding, in 122 per 100,000 persons/year, and 5% of deaths result from upper GI complications. Low-dose aspirin represents approximately 10% of all complications and deaths.[12]

ETIOLOGY

H. pylori infection and NSAID use are the most common risk factors for PUD. Less common factors, including ZES with hypersecretion of acid (see Table 51-2), can also be involved.[2] Disruptions in normal mucosal defense and healing mechanisms allow acid and pepsin to reach the gastric epithelium.[2] Benign gastric ulcers, erosions, and gastritis can occur anywhere in the stomach, although the antrum and lesser curvature represent the most common locations (see Fig. 51-1). Most duodenal ulcers occur in the first part of the duodenum (duodenal bulb).

Helicobacter pylori

H. pylori are spiral, microaerophilic, gram-negative bacteria with flagella that have urease, catalase, and oxidase activity. These factors allow the bacterium to survive in the acidic environment of the stomach. Bacterial urease converts urea to ammonia that neutralizes gastric acid, thereby alkalinizing the microenvironment. Catalase activity enables the bacterium to survive reactive oxidation by

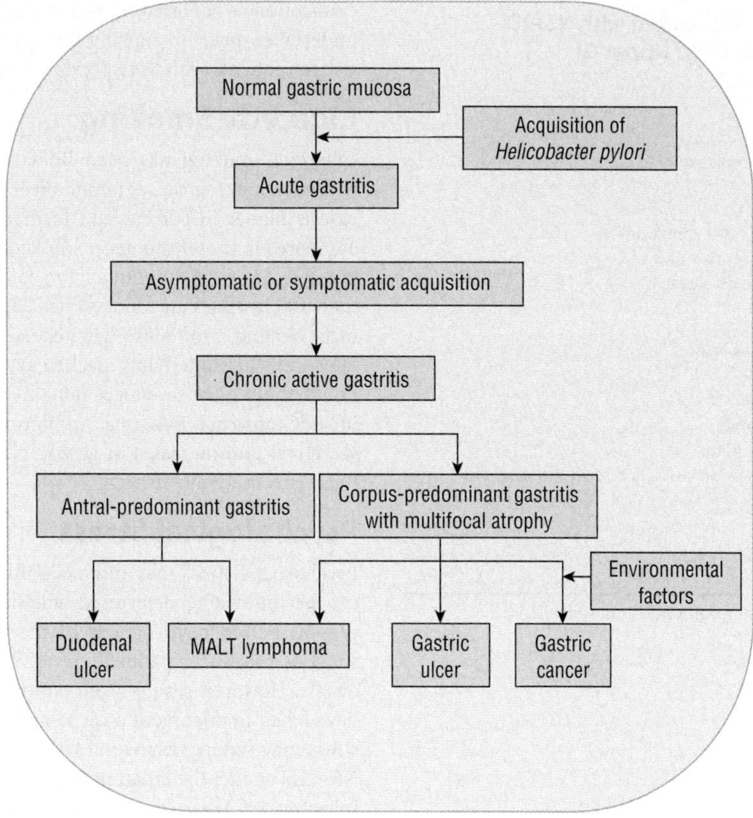

FIGURE 51-2 The natural history of *Helicobacter pylori* infection in the pathogenesis of gastric ulcer and duodenal ulcer, mucosa-associated lymphoid tissue (MALT) lymphoma, and gastric cancer.

phagocytes attempting to kill the organism, but the resulting inflammation damages the gastric epithelial lining allowing *H. pylori* to thrive. Bacterial flagella facilitate the initial infection and allows for colonization of the gastric mucosa.[13] *H. pylori* is primarily transmitted via person-to-person routes by either gastro–oral (vomitus) or fecal–oral (diarrhea) contact. Risk factors for acquiring *H. pylori* include close contact within households, low income status, and country of origin.[2,8]

H. pylori infection can cause both acute and chronic gastritis in infected individuals and is associated with multiple GI complications. PUD, mucosa-associated lymphoid tissue (MALT) lymphoma, and gastric cancer (Fig. 51-2) have all been linked to *H. pylori* infection.[2,7,8] Most infected individuals remain asymptomatic, but 10% to 20% will develop PUD during their lifetime and about 1% will develop gastric cancer. Environmental factors, host genetics, and *H. pylori* strain virulence factors play an important role in the pathogenesis of PUD and gastric cancer.[3] *H. pylori* infection increases the risk of GI bleeding and peptic ulcers by threefold to sevenfold.[8] No specific link has been established between *H. pylori* and dyspepsia, nonulcer dyspepsia (NUD), or gastroesophageal reflux disease (GERD).[8] However, some patients with dyspepsia and NUD have symptom improvement from *H. pylori* eradication. Conversely, eradication of *H. pylori* may worsen GERD symptoms in some patients, but eradication should be attempted due to the known gastric cancer risk. *H. pylori* is also associated with iron deficiency anemia, although the benefit of eradication remains unknown.[8]

Nonsteroidal Anti-Inflammatory Drugs

Prescription and nonprescription NSAIDs (Table 51-3) are widely used in the United States, and have been linked to PUD. There is overwhelming evidence linking chronic NSAID (including low-dose aspirin) use to upper GI tract injury, PUD, gastritis, and superficial erosion.[2,14,15] In susceptible individuals, NSAIDs cause superficial mucosal damage consisting of petechiae (intramucosal hemorrhages) within minutes of ingestion, and progress to erosions with continued use.[11] These lesions typically heal within a few days and rarely cause ulcers or acute upper GI bleeding. NSAID-induced ulcers occur less frequently in the esophagus, small bowel, and colon.[11,12] The mechanisms by which NSAIDs damage the lower GI tract is not clear, but the enteropathy is associated with lower GI bleeding.

Table 51-4 lists the risk factors associated with NSAID-induced ulcers and upper GI complications. Combinations of factors confer an additive risk.[2,12,16-19] Advanced age is an independent risk factor, and the incidence of NSAID-induced ulcers increases linearly with the age of the patient.[2] The high incidence of ulcer complications in older individuals may be explained by age-related changes in gastric mucosal defense. The relative risk of NSAID complications is increased for patients with a previous peptic ulcer and may be as high as 14-fold in those with a history of an ulcer-related complication.[2,18] Although the risk of ulcer complications is greatest during

TABLE 51-3 Selected NSAIDs and COX-2 Inhibitors

Nonsalicylates[a]
Nonselective (traditional) NSAIDs: indomethacin, piroxicam, ibuprofen, naproxen, sulindac, ketoprofen, ketorolac, flurbiprofen, diclofenac
Selective COX-2 inhibitors: etodolac, nabumetone, meloxicam, celecoxib, rofecoxib,[b] valdecoxib[b]

Salicylates
Acetylated: aspirin
Nonacetylated: salsalate, trisalicylate

COX-2, cyclooxygenase-2; NSAIDs, nonsteroidal anti-inflammatory drugs.
[a]Based on COX-1-to-COX-2 selectivity ratio.
[b]Withdrawn from US market.

TABLE 51-4 Risk Factors Associated with NSAID-Induced Ulcers and Upper GI Complications[a]

Age >65
Previous peptic ulcer
Previous ulcer-related upper GI complication
High-dose NSAIDs
Multiple NSAID use
Selection of NSAID (eg, COX-1 vs COX-2 inhibition)
NSAID-related dyspepsia
Aspirin (including cardioprotective dosages)
Concomitant use of
Low-dose aspirin
Oral bisphosphonates (eg, alendronate)
Systemic corticosteroids
Anticoagulant or coagulopathy
Antiplatelet drugs (eg, clopidogrel)
Selective serotonin reuptake inhibitor
Chronic debilitating disorders (eg, cardiovascular disease, rheumatoid arthritis)
Helicobacter pylori infection
Cigarette smoking
Alcohol consumption

COX-2, cyclooxygenase-2; GI, gastrointestinal; NSAIDs, nonsteroidal anti-inflammatory drugs.

[a]Combinations of risk factors are additive.

Data from References 2 and 18–20.

the first few months after initiating continuous NSAID therapy, it does not vanish with long-term treatment.[20]

NSAID ulcers and related complications are dependent upon the dose, duration of use, and type of NSAID. Although dose is important, low doses of nonprescription NSAIDs and low cardioprotective dosages of aspirin (81-325 mg/day) increase risk of ulcer formation.[2,3,12,17,20] Factors such as NSAID potency, longer duration of effect, and a greater propensity to inhibit cyclooxygenase-1 (COX-1) versus cyclooxygenase-2 (COX-2) isoenzymes are associated with increased risk (see Table 51-3).[2,12,20] NSAID-related dyspepsia, in itself, does not correlate directly with mucosal injury or clinical events. However, new-onset dyspepsia, changes in severity, or dyspepsia not relieved by antiulcer medications may suggest an ulcer or ulcer complication.[2] Nonacetylated salicylates (eg, salsalate) may be associated with decreased GI toxicity.[1,11,21] Buffered or enteric-coated aspirin confers no added protection from upper GI events.[12] NSAID ulcer and GI complication risk are increased with the use of multiple NSAIDs or the concomitant use of low-dose aspirin, oral bisphosphonates, systemic corticosteroids, anticoagulants, antiplatelet drugs, and selective serotonin reuptake inhibitors.[17,19,21] The risk of an ulcer-related GI complication is 10-fold greater when an NSAID or COX-2 inhibitor (see Table 51-3) is coadministered with low-dose aspirin than when either drug is taken alone.[3] The NSAID may also reduce the antiplatelet effects of aspirin, although NSAIDs vary in their effects on platelet function. Corticosteroids, when used alone, do not potentiate the risk of ulcer or complications, but the relative risk is increased twofold in corticosteroid users who are also taking concurrent NSAIDs.[2] The relative risk of GI bleeding increases up to 20-fold when NSAIDs are taken concomitantly with anticoagulants (eg, warfarin) and up to sixfold with the concurrent use of serotonin reuptake inhibitors.[21,22] Coadministration of aspirin with clopidogrel or an anticoagulant increases the risk of GI bleeding compared with either agent taken alone.[15,23]

H. pylori and NSAIDs act independently to increase ulcer risk and ulcer-related bleeding and appear to have additive effects.[8] Thus, the incidence of peptic ulcer is higher in *H. pylori*–positive individuals who use NSAIDs. Whether *H. pylori* infection is actually a risk factor for NSAID ulcers remains controversial.[8] However, eradication is reported to reduce the incidence of peptic ulcer if undertaken prior to starting the NSAID, but does not reduce the risk for patients who were previously taking an NSAID.[8]

Cigarette Smoking

Cigarette smoking has been linked to PUD, but it is uncertain whether smoking causes peptic ulcers. The prevalence of ulcer disease is higher in current and former smokers (11.4% and 11.5%) compared to those who never smoked (6%). The risk of peptic ulcers is greatest in smokers with a large daily use, but modest when fewer than 10 cigarettes are smoked per day.[27] Cigarette smoking impairs ulcer healing, promotes ulcer recurrence, and increases ulcer risk. However, the underlying mechanisms by which cigarette smoking exerts these adverse effects remain unclear. Possible mechanisms include mucosal ischemia, inhibition of pancreatic bicarbonate secretion, and increases in gastric acid and mucous secretion, but these effects are inconsistent.[28]

Psychological Stress

Psychosocial stress may influence the pathogenesis of PUD, but it can be difficult to determine whether the stressful exposure was present before development of ulceration.[29] Clinical observation suggests that ulcer patients are adversely affected by stressful life events. However, results from controlled trials are conflicting and have failed to document a cause-and-effect relationship. Emotional stress may induce behavioral risks such as smoking and the use of NSAIDs or alter the inflammatory response or resistance to *H. pylori* infection.[29,30] The role of stress and how it affects PUD is complex and probably multifactorial.

Dietary Factors

The effects of diet and nutrition on the pathophysiology PUD is uncertain. Carbonated beverages, coffee, tea, beer, milk, and spices often cause dyspepsia, but they do not appear to increase the risk of PUD.[2] Dietary interventions such as bland or restricted diets do not alter the frequency of ulcer recurrence. Although caffeine is a gastric acid stimulant, constituents in decaffeinated coffee or tea, caffeine-free carbonated beverages, beer, and wine may also increase gastric acid secretion. In high concentrations, alcohol ingestion is associated with acute gastric mucosal damage and upper GI bleeding; however, there is insufficient evidence to confirm that alcohol causes ulcers.[2]

PATHOPHYSIOLOGY

The pathophysiology of gastric and duodenal ulcers is determined by the imbalance between aggressive (gastric acid and pepsin) and protective (mucosal defense and repair) factors.[2] Gastric acid is secreted by the parietal cells, which contain receptors for histamine, gastrin, and acetylcholine.[2] Acid (as well as *H. pylori* infection and NSAID use) is an independent factor that contributes to the disruption of mucosal integrity.[2] Acid secretion is increased in patients with duodenal ulcers and may be a consequence of *H. pylori* infection.[31] In contrast, patients with gastric ulcers usually have normal or reduced rates of acid secretion (hypochlorhydria).

The amount of acid secreted under basal or fasting conditions is referred to as basal acid output (BAO); after maximal stimulation, maximal acid output (MAO). Basal and maximal acid secretion varies with time of day and the individual's psychological state, age, gender, and health status. The BAO follows a circadian rhythm, with the highest acid secretion occurring at night and the lowest in the morning.[2] An increase in the BAO:MAO ratio suggests a basal hypersecretory state such as ZES.

Pepsin is an important enzyme cofactor in the proteolytic activity involved in ulcer formation. Pepsinogen, the inactive precursor of pepsin, is secreted by the chief cells in the gastric fundus (see Fig. 51-1).

Pepsin activity is determined by pH as it is activated by acid pH (optimal pH of 1.8-3.5), reversibly inactivated at pH 4, and irreversibly destroyed at pH 7.[2]

Mucus and bicarbonate secretion, intrinsic epithelial cell defense, and mucosal blood flow protect the gastroduodenal mucosa from noxious endogenous and exogenous substances.[2] The viscous nature and near-neutral pH of the mucus–bicarbonate barrier protect the stomach from the acidic contents in the gastric lumen. Mucosal repair after injury is related to epithelial cell restitution, growth, and regeneration. Endogenous prostaglandins' (PGs) production facilitate mucosal integrity and repair. The term *cytoprotection* is often used to describe this process, but *mucosal defense* and *mucosal protection* are more accurate terms, as PGs prevent deep mucosal injury and not superficial damage to individual cells.[11] Gastric hyperemia and increased PG synthesis characterize adaptive cytoprotection, the short-term adaptation of mucosal cells to mild topical irritants that enables the stomach to initially withstand the damaging effects of irritants. Alterations in mucosal defense that are induced by *H. pylori* or NSAIDs are the most important cofactors in the formation of peptic ulcers.[11,32]

Helicobacter pylori

In infected people, *H. pylori* resides between the gastric mucus layer and surface epithelial cells, or any location where gastric-type epithelium is found. The bacterium binds to gastric-type epithelium by adherence pedestals, which prevent the organism from being shed during cell turnover and mucus secretion. Colonization of the antrum and corpus (body) of the stomach is associated with gastric ulcer and cancer. Antral organisms colonize gastric tissue that develops in the duodenum secondary to changes in gastric acid or bicarbonate secretion leading to duodenal ulcer (see Fig. 51-2). Although *H. pylori* causes chronic gastric mucosal inflammation in all infected individuals, only a minority actually develop an ulcer or gastric cancer. The difference in the diverse clinical outcomes is related to variations in bacterial pathogenicity and host susceptibility.

Bacterial enzymes (urease, lipases, and proteases), bacterial adherence, and *H. pylori* virulence factors produce gastric mucosal injury. Lipases and proteases degrade gastric mucus, ammonia produced by urease may be toxic to gastric epithelial cells, and bacterial adherence enhances the uptake of toxins into gastric epithelial cells. *H. pylori* induces gastric inflammation by altering the host inflammatory response and damaging epithelial cells directly by cell-mediated immune mechanisms or indirectly by activated neutrophils or macrophages attempting to phagocytize bacteria or bacterial products. However, *H. pylori* strains are genetically diverse and account for differences in adaptation within the human host. Two of the most important are cytotoxin-associated gene protein (CagA) and vacuolating cytotoxin (VacA). About 60% of *H. pylori* strains in the United States possess CagA, but CagA-positive strains increase the risk for severe PUD, gastritis, and gastric cancer compared with CagA-negative strains. The VacA gene codes for the VacA cytotoxin, a vacuolating toxin. Although VacA is present in most *H. pylori* strains, strains vary in cytotoxicity and increased risk for peptic ulcer and gastric cancer. Host polymorphisms are important markers of disease susceptibility and may identify high-risk patients.[32,33]

Nonsteroidal Anti-Inflammatory Drugs

NSAIDs, including aspirin (see Table 51-3), cause gastric mucosal damage by local and systemic mechanisms, but systemic inhibition of endogenous mucosal PG synthesis is believed to be the primary mechanism.[20] The onset of injury is initiated by the acidic properties of many of the NSAIDs, while systemic inhibition of the protective PGs limits the ability of the mucosa to defend against injury and thus plays the predominant role in the development of gastric ulcer.[20] Acidic NSAIDs (eg, aspirin) have topical irritant properties and they decrease the hydrophobicity of the mucous gel layer in the gastric mucosa. Most non-aspirin NSAIDs have topical irritant effects, but aspirin is the most damaging. Although NSAID prodrugs, enteric-coated aspirin tablets, salicylate derivatives, and parenteral or rectal preparations are associated with less acute gastric mucosal injury, they can cause ulcers and related GI complications because of systemic inhibition of endogenous PGs.

COX is the rate-limiting enzyme in the conversion of arachidonic acid to PGs and is inhibited by NSAIDs (Fig. 51-3). Two similar COX isoforms have been identified: COX-1 is found in most body tissue, including the stomach, kidney, intestine, and platelets; COX-2 is undetectable in most tissues under normal physiologic conditions, but its expression can be induced during acute inflammation and arthritis (Fig. 51-4). COX-1 produces protective PGs that regulate physiologic processes such as GI mucosal integrity,

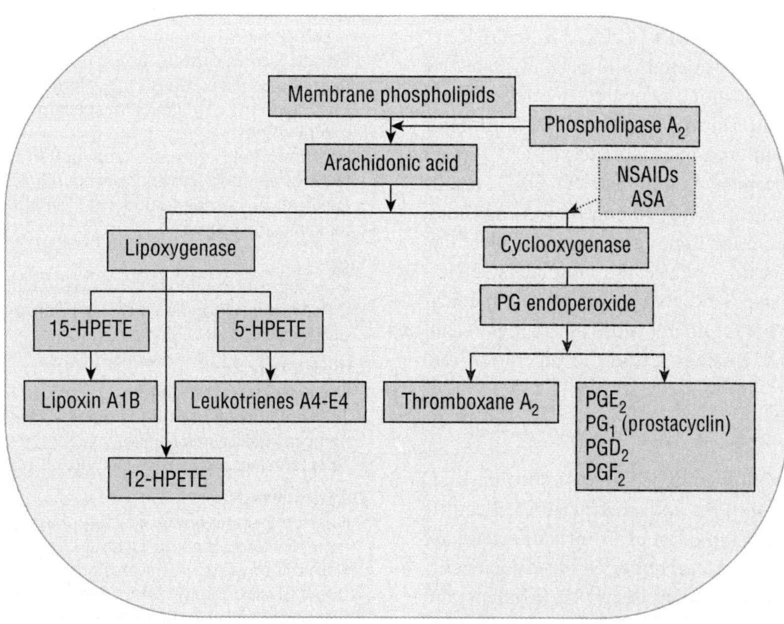

FIGURE 51-3 Metabolism of arachidonic acid after its release from membrane phospholipids. Broken arrow indicates inhibitory effects. (ASA, aspirin; HPETE, hydroperoxyeicosatetraenoic acid; NSAIDs, nonsteroidal anti-inflammatory drugs; PG, prostaglandin.)

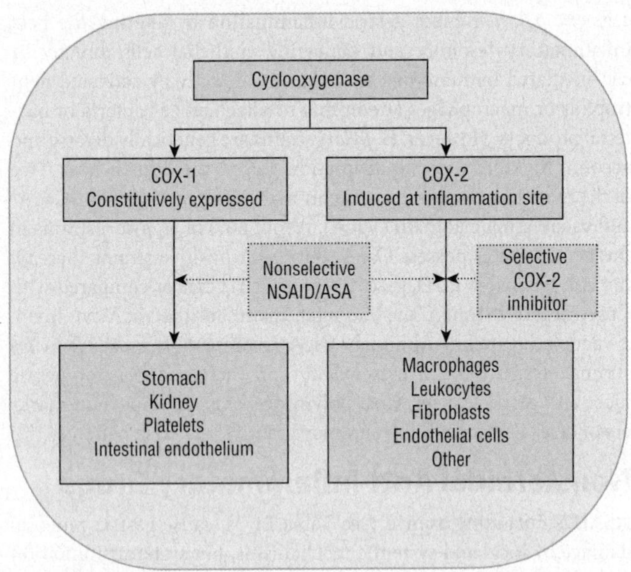

FIGURE 51-4 Tissue distribution and actions of cyclooxygenase (COX) isoenzymes. Nonselective nonsteroidal anti-inflammatory drugs (NSAIDs) including aspirin (ASA) inhibit COX-1 and COX-2 to varying degrees; COX-2 inhibitors inhibit only COX-2. Broken arrow indicates inhibitory effects.

platelet homeostasis, and renal function. COX-2 is induced (unregulated) by inflammatory stimuli such as cytokines and produces PGs involved with inflammation, fever, and pain. It is also constitutionally expressed in organs such as the brain, kidney, and reproductive tract. Adverse effects (eg, GI or renal toxicity) of NSAIDs are primarily associated with the inhibition of COX-1, whereas anti-inflammatory actions result primarily from NSAID inhibition of COX-2.[11]

The COX-1-to-COX-2 inhibitory ratio determines the relative GI toxicity of a specific NSAID. Nonselective NSAIDs, including aspirin (see Table 51-3), inhibit both COX-1 and COX-2 to varying degrees and are associated with an increased propensity to cause gastric ulcers. In contrast, the selective COX-2 inhibitors preferentially inhibit COX-2 in vitro resulting in a reduced risk of ulcers and related GI complications (see Table 51-3). The selectivity for the COX-2 isoenzyme varies among NSAIDs. Celecoxib, meloxicam, etodolac, and nabumetone are considered only partially selective and have more risk of GI complications compared to rofecoxib and valdecoxib.[34] The addition of aspirin to a selective COX-2 inhibitor reduces its ulcer-sparing benefit and increases ulcer risk.[12] Aspirin and non-aspirin NSAIDs irreversibly inhibit platelet COX-1, resulting in decreased platelet aggregation and prolonged bleeding times, thereby increasing the potential for upper and lower GI bleeding. Coadministration of NSAIDs may reduce the antiplatelet effects of aspirin. Clopidogrel, prasugrel, ticagrelor, and related medications that affect platelet aggregation do not cause ulcers, per se, but may impair healing of gastric erosions leading to ulceration and bleeding.[15,25,26]

Complications

The most serious, life-threatening complications of chronic PUD are upper GI bleeding, perforation, and obstruction.[2] Bleeding peptic ulcers, caused by the erosion of an ulcer into an artery, are the most common cause of non-variceal upper GI bleeding, occurring in 26% to 59% of patients.[35] It may be occult (hidden) and insidious or may present as melena (black-colored that combine clarithromycin with amoxicillin stools) or hematemesis (vomiting of blood). NSAID use (especially in older adults) is the most important risk factor for upper GI bleeding. Mortality is highest in patients with uncontrolled bleeding or who have a rebleeding event after the initial bleeding has stopped (see section "Upper Gastrointestinal Bleeding" below).[35]

Gastric perforation into the peritoneal cavity is the second most common ulcer-related complication, occurring in 4 to 14 cases per 100,000 patients.[36] Depending on location, the ulcer may penetrate into an adjacent structure (pancreas, biliary tract, or liver) rather than opening freely into a cavity. Although the incidence of perforated peptic ulcers has decreased with the availability of PPIs, the mortality and morbidity remain high. Mortality from perforated ulcers is five times higher compared with bleeding peptic ulcer and 30-day mortality is approximately 24%. Older patients and those with comorbidities have a worse prognosis.[36] The pain of perforation is usually sudden, sharp, and severe, beginning first in the epigastrium, but quickly spreading over the entire abdomen. Most patients experience ulcer symptoms prior to perforation; however, older patients who experience perforation in association with NSAID use may be asymptomatic. The duodenum can be narrowed due to chronic inflammation and scaring from ulcers, resulting in gastric outlet obstruction. Although gastric outlet obstruction is rare, patients often present with severe vomiting and hematemesis.[37] Perforation, penetration, and gastric outlet obstruction occur most often with long-standing PUD.

CLINICAL PRESENTATION

There is significant variability in the clinical presentation of PUD depending on the severity of epigastric pain and the presence of complications (Table 51-5). Pain related to duodenal ulcer often

TABLE 51-5 Clinical Presentation of PUD

General
- Mild epigastric pain or acute life-threatening upper GI complications

Symptoms
- Abdominal pain that is often epigastric and described as burning but may present as vague discomfort, abdominal fullness, or cramping
- A typical nocturnal pain that awakens the patient from sleep (especially between 12 and 3 AM)
- The severity of ulcer pain varies between patients and may be seasonal, occurring more frequently in the spring or fall; episodes of discomfort usually occur in clusters, lasting up to a few weeks and followed by a pain-free period or remission lasting from weeks to years
- Changes in the character of the pain may suggest the presence of complications
- Heartburn, belching, and bloating often accompany the pain
- Nausea, vomiting, and anorexia are more common for patients with gastric ulcer than with duodenal ulcer but may also be signs of an ulcer-related complication

Signs
- Weight loss associated with nausea, vomiting, and anorexia
- Complications including ulcer bleeding, perforation, penetration, or obstruction

Laboratory tests
- Gastric acid secretory studies
- The hematocrit and hemoglobin are low with bleeding, and stool hemoccult tests are positive
- Tests for *Helicobacter pylori* (see Table 51-6)

Diagnostic tests
- Fiber-optic upper endoscopy (esophagogastroduodenoscopy) detects more than 90% of peptic ulcers and permits direct inspection, biopsy, visualization of superficial erosions, and sites of active bleeding
- Upper GI radiography with barium has been replaced with upper endoscopy as the diagnostic procedure of choice for suspected peptic ulcer

GI, gastrointestinal; PUD, peptic ulcer disease.

occurs 1 to 3 hours after meals and is usually relieved by food, but this is variable. Food may precipitate or accentuate gastric ulcer pain. Antacids usually provide immediate pain relief in most ulcer patients. Pain usually diminishes or disappears during treatment; however, recurrence of epigastric pain after healing often suggests an unhealed or recurrent ulcer.

The presence or absence of epigastric pain does not define an ulcer and ulcer healing does not necessarily render the patient asymptomatic. Symptoms may remain because of sensitization of afferent nerves in response to mucosal injury. Conversely, the absence of pain does not preclude an ulcer diagnosis, especially in older patients who may present with a "silent" ulcer complication possibly related to differences in the way they perceive pain or the analgesic effect of NSAIDs.

Dyspepsia alone is of little clinical value when assessing subsets of patients who are most likely to have an ulcer. Patients taking NSAIDs often report dyspepsia, but these symptoms do not always correlate with an ulcer. Functional dyspepsia (FD), or nonulcer dyspepsia (NUD), refers to the lack of an ulcer upon endoscopy in a patient with ulcer-like symptoms.[40] *H. pylori* gastritis or duodenitis may cause ulcer-like symptoms in the absence of peptic ulceration. There is no one sign or symptom that differentiates between *H. pylori*–positive and NSAID-induced ulcer.

Diagnosis

Symptoms of PUD are nonspecific and are of limited predictive value for diagnosis. The diagnosis of PUD depends on visualizing the ulcer crater (see Table 51-5).[2,19] Upper endoscopy has replaced radiography as the diagnostic procedure of choice because it provides a more accurate diagnosis and permits direct visualization of the ulcer and implementation of therapeutic maneuvers to control bleeding such as injection of epinephrine or deployment of hemostatic clips.

Tests for *Helicobacter pylori*

The diagnosis of *H. pylori* infection can be made using endoscopic or nonendoscopic tests (Table 51-6). All patients with active PUD, past history of PUD without documentation of prior cure, low-grade gastric MALT lymphoma, or history of endoscopic resection for early gastric cancer should be tested for *H. pylori*.[8] Testing that requires upper endoscopy is invasive, more expensive, and usually requires a mucosal biopsy for histology, culture, or detection of urease activity. The updated Sydney system recommends taking five tissue samples from different sites within the stomach, as patchy distribution of *H. pylori* infection can lead to false-negative results.[41] Because antibiotics, including bismuth salts, and proton pump inhibitors (PPIs) may decrease the sensitivity of rapid urease test, they should be withheld prior to endoscopic testing for 4 weeks and 2 weeks, respectively.[13,42,43] If the patient has been taking these medications, then a gastric biopsy for histology is preferred.[43]

Nonendoscopic tests (urea breath test [UBT], serologic antibody detection tests, and the fecal antigen test) may identify active infection or detect antibodies (see Table 51-6) and are less invasive, more convenient, and less expensive than the endoscopic tests.[43] However, antibody tests do not differentiate between active infection and previously eradicated *H. pylori*.

The UBT is the most accurate noninvasive test and is based on *H. pylori* urease activity.[41] The ^{13}Carbon (nonradioactive isotope) and ^{14}Carbon (radioactive isotope) tests require that the patient ingest radiolabeled urea, which is then hydrolyzed by *H. pylori* (if present in the stomach) to ammonia and radiolabeled bicarbonate.

TABLE 51-6 Tests for Detection of *Helicobacter pylori*

Test	Description	Comments
Endoscopic tests		
Histology	Microbiologic examination using various stains	Gold standard; greater than 95% sensitive and specific; permits classification of gastritis; results are not immediate; not recommended for initial diagnosis; tests for active *H. pylori* infection
Culture	Culture of biopsy	Enables sensitivity testing to determine appropriate treatment or antibiotic resistance; 100% specific; results are not immediate; not recommended for initial diagnosis; used after failure of second-line treatment; tests for active *H. pylori* infection
Biopsy (rapid) urease	*H. pylori* urease generates ammonia, which causes a color change	Test of choice at endoscopy; greater than 90% sensitive and specific; easily performed; rapid results (usually within 24 hours); tests for active *H. pylori* infection
Polymerase chain reaction	*H. pylori* DNA detected in gastric tissue	Test is highly specific and sensitive; high rate of false-positives and false-negatives; positive DNA does not directly equate to presence of the organism; considered a research technique
Nonendoscopic tests		
Antibody detection (laboratory-based)	Detects antibodies to *H. pylori* in serum using laboratory-based ELISA tests and latex agglutination techniques	Quantitative; less sensitive and specific than endoscopic tests; more accurate than in office; unable to determine if antibody is related to active or cured infection; antibody titers vary markedly among individuals and take 6 months to 1 year to return to the uninfected range; not affected by PPIs or bismuth; antibiotics given for unrelated indications may cure the infection, but antibody test will remain positive
Antibody detection (can be performed in office or near patient)	Detects IgG antibodies to *H. pylori* in whole blood or finger stick	Qualitative; quick (within 15 minutes); unable to determine if antibody is related to active or cured infection; most patients remain seropositive for at least 6 months to 1 year after *H. pylori* eradication; not affected by PPIs, bismuth, or antibiotics
Urea breath test	*H. pylori* urease breaks down ingested labeled C-urea, patient exhales labeled CO_2	Tests for active *H. pylori* infection; 95% sensitive and specific; results take about 2 days; antibiotics, bismuth, PPIs, and H2RAs may cause false-negative results; withhold PPIs or H2RAs (1-2 weeks) and bismuth or antibiotics (4 weeks) prior to testing; recommended test to confirm posttreatment eradication of *H. pylori*
Fecal antigen	Identifies *H. pylori* antigen in stool by enzyme immunoassay using polyclonal anti–*H. pylori* antibody	Tests for active *H. pylori* infection; sensitivity and specificity comparable to urea breath test when used for initial diagnosis; antibiotics, bismuth, and PPIs may cause false-negative results, but to a lesser extent than with the urea breath test; may be used posttreatment to confirm eradication, but patients may have a reluctance to obtain stool samples

ELISA, enzyme-linked immunosorbent assay; H2RA, H_2-receptor antagonist; PPIs, proton pump inhibitors.

Data from References 13, 38, and 39.

The radiolabeled bicarbonate is absorbed in the blood and excreted in the breath. In addition to being noninvasive, another advantage of UBT over biopsy is that it overcomes the possible sampling error associated with endoscopic biopsy secondary to irregular distribution of *H. pylori*.[41] The fecal antigen test is less expensive and easier to perform than the UBT, and may be useful in children.

Serologic tests are a cost-effective alternative for the initial diagnosis of *H. pylori* infection in the untreated patient. Antibodies to *H. pylori* usually develop about 3 weeks after infection and remain present after successful eradication. Therefore, serology should not be used to confirm *H. pylori* eradication. Office-based tests are less expensive, widely available, and provide rapid results, but the results are less accurate and more variable than the laboratory-based tests.

Testing for *H. pylori* is only recommended if eradication therapy is planned. Serologic antibody testing is a reasonable choice if endoscopy is not planned. The diagnostic accuracy of *H. pylori* tests for patients with an active bleeding ulcer has been questioned because of the potential for false-negative results. However, endoscopic biopsy-based tests such as the rapid urease test have a high degree of specificity in these patients (see section "Peptic Ulcer–Related Bleeding").[8]

Confirmation of eradication is indicated posttreatment whenever *H. pylori* is identified and treated.[8] Endoscopic biopsy-based tests, UBT and fecal antigen are the recommended tests to confirm *H. pylori* eradication. Testing for eradication should be delayed at least 4 weeks after the completion of antibiotics and after PPI has been discontinued for 2 weeks to avoid confusing bacterial suppression with eradication.[8]

Clinical Course and Prognosis

Untreated PUD is characterized by periods of exacerbations and remissions.[2] Ulcer pain is usually recognizable and episodic, but symptoms are varied, especially in older adults and for patients taking NSAIDs. Antiulcer medications, including the histamine-2 receptor antagonists (H2RAs), PPIs, and sucralfate, relieve symptoms, accelerate ulcer healing, and reduce the risk of ulcer recurrence, but they do not cure the disease. Both duodenal and gastric ulcers recur unless the underlying cause (*H. pylori* or NSAID) is addressed. Successful *H. pylori* eradication markedly decreases ulcer recurrence and complications. Prophylactic co-therapy or a COX-2 inhibitor decreases the risk of upper GI events for patients who are taking NSAIDs. GI bleeding, perforation, and obstruction remain troublesome complications of chronic PUD. Mortality for patients with gastric ulcer is slightly higher than in duodenal ulcer and the general population. The development of gastric cancer in *H. pylori*–infected individuals is a slow process that occurs over 20 to 40 years and is associated with a lifetime risk of less than 1%.[1]

TREATMENT

General Approach to Treatment

The treatment of PUD varies depending on the etiology of the ulcer (*H. pylori* or NSAID), whether the ulcer is initial or recurrent, and whether complications have occurred (Fig. 51-5). Treatment is aimed at relieving ulcer pain, healing the ulcer, preventing ulcer recurrence, and reducing ulcer-related complications. Antimicrobials in combination with antisecretory drugs (PPIs or H2RAs) eradicate *H. pylori* infection allowing for ulcer healing and relief of ulcer symptoms. PPIs accelerate ulcer healing and provide more effective relief of symptoms compared to H2RAs or sucralfate, and are preferred for healing *H. pylori*–negative NSAID-induced ulcers. In patients taking NSAIDs for pain, alternative agents such as acetaminophen or nonacetylated salicylate (eg, salsalate) should be used for relief of pain when possible. Patients requiring continuation of NSAID therapy at high risk of developing peptic ulcers should be switched to a selective COX-2 inhibitor NSAID or receive prophylactic co-therapy to reduce ulcer risk and related complications.

Dietary modifications can be considered for patients unable to tolerate certain foods and beverages. Lifestyle modifications such as reducing stress and smoking cessation are encouraged. Surgery is rarely necessary and is used only for patients with ulcer-related complications.[2,19]

Desired Outcome

The goal for patients with PUD, regardless of the cause, is to relieve ulcer symptoms, heal the ulcer, and prevent recurrence. In patients with NSAID-induced ulcer, withdrawal of the offending agent and careful consideration of the need for continued NSAID therapy can reduce the risk of ulcer recurrence. In *H. pylori*–positive patients with an active ulcer, a previously documented ulcer, or a history of an ulcer-related complication, the goal is to eradicate *H. pylori*, heal the ulcer, and cure the disease. Successful eradication heals ulcers and reduces the risk of recurrence for most patients.

Nonpharmacologic Therapy

1 Lifestyle modifications, including stress reduction and smoking cessation, should be implemented in patients with PUD. There is no specific recommended diet for patients with current or history of PUD; however, patients should avoid foods and beverages (eg, spicy foods, caffeine, and alcohol) that cause dyspepsia or that exacerbate ulcer symptoms. Emergent surgery for patients with ulcer-related complications, including bleeding, perforation, or obstruction, is necessary in 5% to 10% of hospitalized patients.[2]

Pharmacologic Therapy

Recommendations

2 Table 51-7 presents guidelines for the eradication of infection in *H. pylori*–positive individuals. Table 51-8 lists regimens used to eradicate *H. pylori* infection.

3 The most cost-effective drug regimen should be used whenever feasible. Several first-line therapies are recommended, but bismuth quadruple therapy for 10 to 14 days has the strongest level of recommendation and should be used preferentially. Another recommended first-line therapy is concomitant therapy (PPI, clarithromycin, amoxicillin, and metronidazole) for 10 to 14 days. Clarithromycin triple therapy is no longer recommended in areas where *H. pylori* resistance exceeds 15%, which includes all of North America.[45] If a second course of treatment is required, the salvage regimen should contain different antibiotics and patients with reported penicillin allergy should be considered for allergy testing.

H. pylori testing should be performed in patients with NSAID-induced ulcers to determine their status. If *H. pylori*–positive, treatment should be initiated with a recommended first-line regimen (see Table 51-8). If *H. pylori*–negative, the NSAID should be discontinued, and the patient treated with a PPI, H2RA, or sucralfate (see Table 51-9). If the NSAID is continued, co-therapy with a PPI or misoprostol should be implemented. Patients at highest risk of recurrent ulcers or ulcer-related complications should be switched to a selective COX-2 inhibitor.

Maintenance therapy with a PPI or H2RA should be limited to high-risk patients with ulcer complications, patients who fail eradication, and those with *H. pylori*–negative ulcers. Treatment failure is associated with poor medication adherence, antimicrobial resistance, NSAID use, cigarette smoking, acid hypersecretion, or tolerance to the antisecretory effects of an H2RA.

Treatment of *Helicobacter pylori*–Positive Ulcers

This chapter focuses on the eradication of *H. pylori* in adults. A discussion of the treatment of *H. pylori* infection in children is found elsewhere.[46]

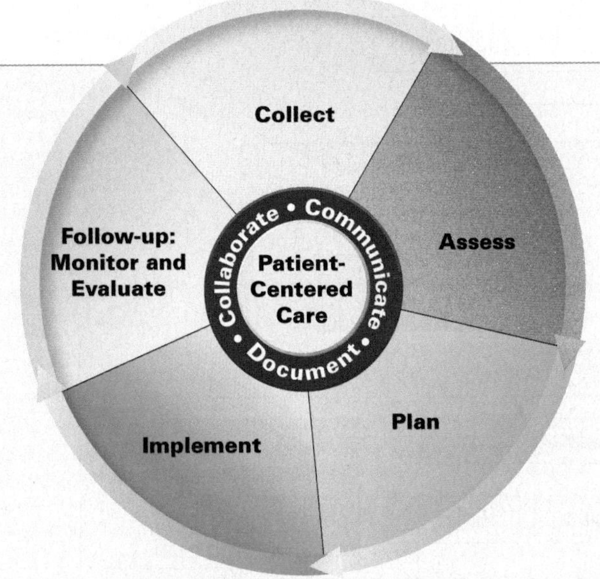

Patient Care Process for Peptic Ulcer Disease (PUD)

The image shows the five fundamental steps included in The Pharmacist's Care Process endorsed by the Joint Commission for Pharmacy Practitioners (2014). The tagline of this process reads collaborate, communicate, and document. The five fundamental steps listed here are collect, assess, plan, implement, and follow-up: monitor and evaluate. All these steps are listed in a circular block diagram.

Collect

- Patient characteristics (eg, age, sex, pregnant)
- Patient medical history (personal and family) especially prior history of *H. pylori* infection, previous peptic ulcers, or previous upper GI disorders (see Table 51-4)
- Social history (eg, tobacco and ethanol use) as well as recent medical procedures and stress levels (see Table 51-2)
- Current medications, especially NSAIDs (nonprescription and prescription) use of nonprescription proton pump inhibitors (PPIs), other acid reflux treatments, anticoagulants, and antiplatelet medications. If prior NSAID use, note medication, dosage, and duration of use
- Pain: presence or absence, rating (1-10), quality, and location (see Table 51-5)
- Objective Data
  - Blood pressure (BP), heart rate (HR), respiratory rate (RR), height, weight, O_2-saturation
  - Labs including hemoglobin (Hgb), hematocrit, assessment of kidney and liver function, gastric acid secretory studies, and stool hemoccult
  - Urea breath test (UBT) for detection of *H. pylori*. Follow-up culture with endoscopy recommended (see Table 51-6)
  - Imaging studies: Upper endoscopy

Assess

- Hemodynamic stability (eg, systolic BP >90 mm Hg, Hr >110 bpm, O_2 sat <90% [0.90])
- Presence of active gastric bleeding based on imaging studies
- Presence of GI-bleed provoking factors (low platelets, anticoagulant/antiplatelet use, NSAID use, age >65, recent surgery, severe co-morbidities, eg, cardiovascular disease) (see Table 51-4)
- Presence/absence of *H. pylori*
- Emotional status (eg, anxiety, depression, stress levels)
- Ability/willingness to pay for ulcer treatment options
- Ability/willingness to discontinue NSAIDs and switch to another pain reliever, if applicable
- Ability/willingness to obtain laboratory monitoring tests (eg, *H. pylori* status to confirm eradication) (see Table 51-7)
- Ability/willingness to follow a multiple drug regimen for 10 to 14 days, with some doses to be taken at specific times

Plan

- Drug therapy regimen based on ulcer classification and patient's antibiotic tolerance (eg, penicillin allergy) see Tables 51-7 and 51-8
- Patient education (eg, purpose of treatment, dietary and lifestyle modification, drug-specific information, medication administration)
- Self-monitoring for resolution of symptoms such as epigastric pain, dyspepsia, when to seek emergency medical attention

Implement*

- Provide patient education regarding all elements of treatment plan
- Use motivational interviewing and coaching strategies to maximize adherence
- Schedule follow-up (endoscopic *H. pylori* culture, lab tests: CBC, serum electrolytes, renal/liver function; see Table 51-12)

Follow-up: Monitor and Evaluate

- Resolution of PUD symptoms such as epigastric pain and dyspepsia
- Presence of adverse effects (eg, N/V/D [PPIs, H2RAs, metronidazole, other antibiotics]), headaches (PPIs and H2RAs)
- Patient adherence to treatment plan using multiple sources of information
- Monitor patient for symptoms of PUD recurrence, especially if their risk factors change

**Collaborate with patient, caregivers, and other healthcare professionals.*

Ideally, treatment of *H. pylori*–positive PUD should be highly effective, free of significant side effects, easy to adhere to, and cost-effective. Unfortunately, available treatments are lacking in one or more of these areas, making it difficult to identify an ideal treatment regimen.[2] The most important predictor of *H. pylori* eradication is antimicrobial resistance.[8] Additional factors that may also be important include duration of therapy, medication adherence, and genetic polymorphism.[47] The initial eradication regimen offers the highest

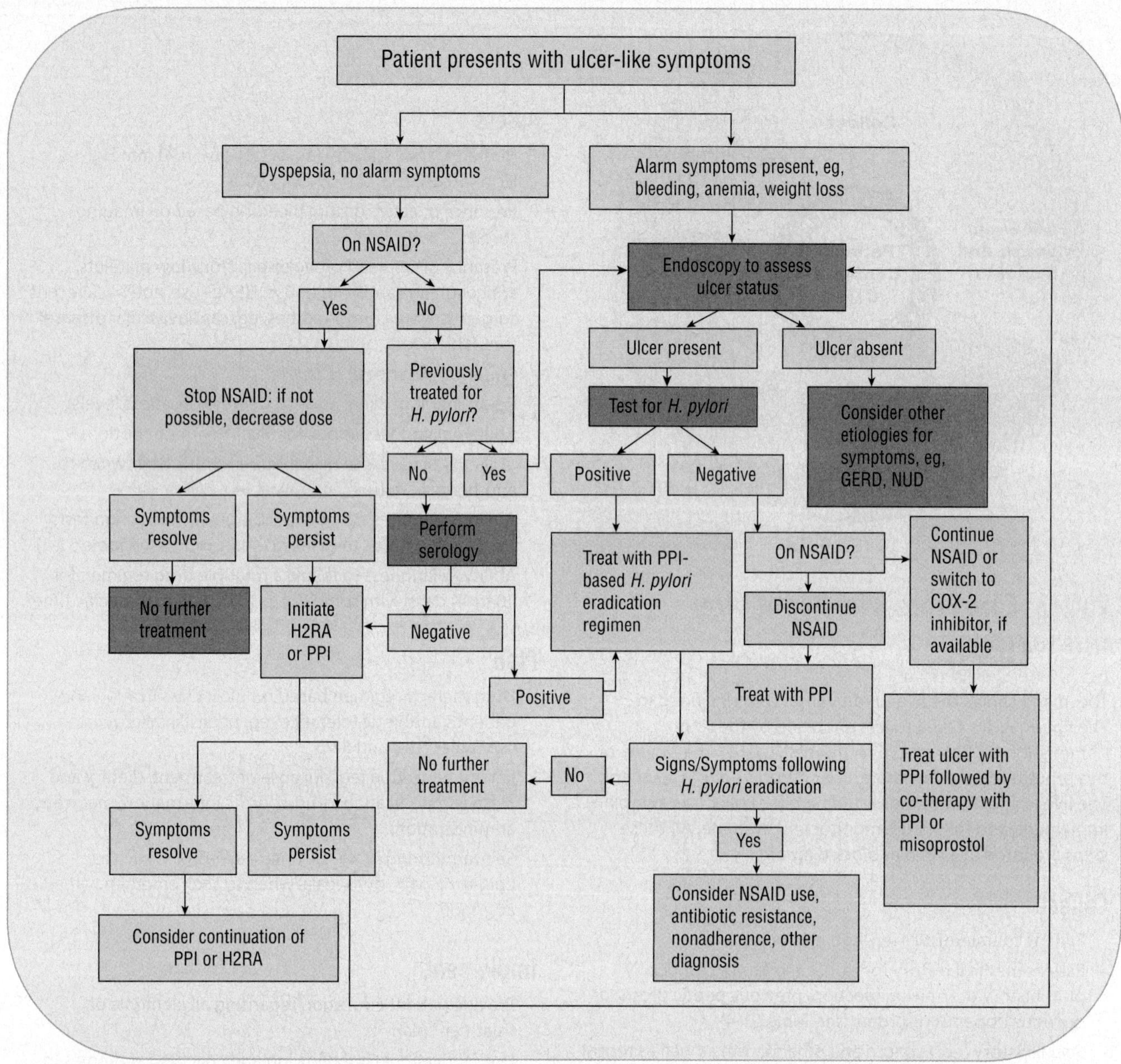

FIGURE 51-5 Guidelines for the evaluation and management of a patient who presents with dyspeptic or ulcer-like symptoms. (COX-2, cyclooxygenase-2; GERD, gastroesophageal reflux disease; H2RA, H_2-receptor antagonist; NSAID, nonsteroidal anti-inflammatory drug; NUD, nonulcer dyspepsia; PPI, proton pump inhibitor.)

likelihood of eradication; therefore, selection of an appropriate first-line regimen is important. No available regimen offers assurance of 100% eradication, and few recommended regimens consistently exceed 90% eradication in studies.[8,48]

Table 51-8 summarizes available first-line drug regimens with antisecretory drug, usually a PPI, in combination with multiple antibiotics and/or bismuth. The use of only one antibiotic is associated with a higher rate of antimicrobial resistance and is therefore not recommended. Clarithromycin, amoxicillin, metronidazole, and tetracycline have in vitro activity against *H. pylori* and have been extensively studied in various combinations and dosing strategies. Bismuth salts have a topical antimicrobial effect. Lesser studied antibiotics with activity include rifabutin, doxycycline, and minocycline.[49,50]

Antisecretory drugs hasten ulcer healing, relieve pain in patients with an active ulcer, and enhance antibiotic activity by increasing intragastric pH and by decreasing intragastric volume, thereby enhancing the topical antibiotic concentration. *PPIs generally produce higher H. pylori eradication rates and are preferred over H2RA.* The PPI is an integral part of the regimen and should be taken 30 to 60 minutes before a meal (see Table 51-8). Prolonged PPI treatment beyond 2 weeks after eradication is usually not necessary for ulcer healing. A single daily dose of a PPI may be less effective than a twice-daily dose. Substitution of one PPI for another is acceptable and does not enhance or diminish *H. pylori* eradication.[51] An H2RA should not be substituted for a PPI unless there are significant tolerability issues. Pretreatment with a PPI does not influence *H. pylori* eradication regardless of the pretreatment duration.[52]

Proton Pump Inhibitor–Based Three-Drug Regimens

PPI-based triple therapy remains an option in regions where clarithromycin resistance is <15% and no prior macrolide exposure is documented, but these regimens are no longer recommended in

TABLE 51-7 Guidelines for the Eradication of *Helicobacter pylori* Infection

Indications for treatment of *H. pylori* infection

- Established indications for the treatment of *H. pylori* include active PUD, past history of PUD (unless eradication previously documented), MALT lymphoma, or after endoscopic resection of gastric cancer
- Controversial indications for the treatment of *H. pylori* infection include individuals with functional dyspepsia, gastroesophageal reflux disease, unexplained iron deficiency anemia, or idiopathic thrombocytopenic purpura; individuals taking long-term low-dose aspirin or initiating chronic treatment with NSAIDs; and individuals at high risk for gastric cancer

Initial treatment of *H. pylori* infection

- Bismuth quadruple therapy and concomitant (non-bismuth quadruple therapy), both administered for 10-14 days, are recommended first-line treatments
- In penicillin-allergic patients, bismuth quadruple therapy is the preferred initial treatment. Consider referral for allergy testing in patients who fail initial therapy, since many patients who report penicillin allergy are not truly allergic
- Alternate initial therapies (conditionally recommended) include: Sequential, hybrid, levofloxacin-triple, levofloxacin sequential, and LOAD therapies (see Table 51-8 for a full description)

Eradication of *H. pylori* after initial treatment failure

- Bismuth quadruple therapy or levofloxacin regimens are preferred if the patient received initial treatment with clarithromycin
- Clarithromycin- or levofloxacin-containing regimens are preferred if patients received initial treatment with bismuth quadruple therapy
- Selection of the optimal salvage regimen should be based on local antibiotic resistance profile, if available, and the patient's prior antibiotic history

MALT, mucosa-associated lymphoid tissue; NSAIDs, nonsteroidal anti-inflammatory drugs; PPI, proton pump inhibitor.

Data from References 8, 13, and 39.

North America due to high clarithromycin resistance rates.[8,39,48,53] If use is indicated, regimens that combine clarithromycin with amoxicillin or metronidazole are more effective than the amoxicillin–metronidazole regimen. The clarithromycin–amoxicillin regimen is preferred initially (see Table 51-7), but metronidazole can be substituted for amoxicillin for penicillin-allergic patients unless alcohol is consumed.[8,39] In most cases, increasing the antibiotic dosage does not improve eradication rates. Since the first treatment regimen offers the highest probability of *H. pylori* eradication, the recommended duration of triple therapy is 14 days.[8] Shorter treatment durations, including 7- to 10-day courses, should no longer be used because of increased resistance and lower overall eradication rates.[8]

Bismuth-Based Quadruple Therapy

Bismuth-based quadruple therapy (bismuth salicylate, metronidazole, tetracycline, and either a PPI or H2RA) (see Table 51-8) is a recommended first-line option (see Table 51-7), particularly for those patients who are allergic to penicillin.[8] The mean eradication rate for bismuth-based quadruple therapy given for 10 days was 91%, which is considerably higher compared with PPI-based triple therapy.[8] Bismuth quadruple therapy for 10 to 14 days was superior to 7 days of clarithromycin triple therapy (85% vs 73%, RR = 1.17).[54] Eradication rates are comparable for different bismuth preparations used (see Table 51-8).[50] All medications except the PPI should be taken with meals and at bedtime. Limitations of this regimen include four times per day dosing, potential for poor medication adherence, and frequent minor side effects.[50]

Sequential Therapy Sequential therapy is a form of eradication therapy in which the antibiotics are administered in a sequence

TABLE 51-8 Drug Regimens Used to Eradicate *Helicobacter pylori*

Regimen	Duration	Drug #1	Drug #2	Drug #3	Drug #4
Proton pump inhibitor–based triple therapy[a]	14 days	PPI once or twice daily[b]	Clarithromycin 500 mg twice daily	Amoxicillin 1 g twice daily *or* metronidazole 500 mg twice daily	
Bismuth quadruple therapy[a]	10-14 days	PPI or H2RA once or twice daily[b,c]	Bismuth subsalicylate[d] 525 mg four times daily	Metronidazole 250-500 mg four times daily	Tetracycline 500 mg four times daily
Non-bismuth quadruple or "concomitant" therapy[e]	10-14 days	PPI once or twice daily on days 1-10[b]	Clarithromycin 250-500 mg twice daily on days 1-10	Amoxicillin 1 g twice daily on days 1-10	Metronidazole 250-500 mg twice daily on days 1-10
Sequential therapy[e]	10 days	PPI once or twice daily on days 1-10[b]	Amoxicillin 1 g twice daily on days 1-5	Metronidazole 250-500 mg twice daily on days 6-10	Clarithromycin 250-500 mg twice daily on days 6-10
Hybrid therapy[e]	14 days	PPI once or twice daily on days 1-14[b]	Amoxicillin 1 g twice daily on days 1-14	Metronidazole 250–500 mg twice daily on days 7-14	Clarithromycin 250-500 mg twice daily on days 7-14
Levofloxacin triple	10-14 days	PPI twice daily	Levofloxacin 500 mg daily	Amoxicillin 1 g twice daily	
Levofloxacin sequential	10 days	PPI twice daily on days 1-10	Amoxicillin 1 g twice daily on days 1-5	Levofloxacin 500 mg once daily on days 6-10	Metronidazole 500 mg twice daily on days 6-10
Levofloxacin, omeprazole, nitazoxanide, doxycycline (LOAD)	7-10 days	Levofloxacin 250 mg once daily	Omeprazole (or other PPI) at high dose once daily	Nitazoxanide (Alinia) 500 mg twice daily	Doxycycline 100 mg once daily
Rifabutin-based triple therapy	14 days	Omeprazole 40 mg every 8 hours	Amoxicillin 1 g every 8 hours	Ribabutin 50 mg every 8 hours	

H2RA, H_2-receptor antagonist; PPI, proton pump inhibitor.

[a]Although treatment is minimally effective if used for 7 days, 10 to 14 days is recommended. The antisecretory drug may be continued beyond antimicrobial treatment for patients with a history of a complicated ulcer, for example, bleeding, or in heavy smokers.

[b]Standard PPI peptic ulcer healing dosages given once or twice daily.

[c]Standard H2RA peptic ulcer healing dosages may be used in place of a PPI.

[d]Bismuth subcitrate potassium (biskalcitrate) 140 mg, as the bismuth salt, is contained in a prepackaged capsule (Pylera), along with metronidazole 125 mg and tetracycline 125 mg; three capsules are taken with each meal and at bedtime; a standard PPI dosage is added to the regimen and taken twice daily. All medications are taken for 10 days.

[e]Requires validation as first-line therapy in the United States.

Data from References 4, 8, 13, 39, and 44.

TABLE 51-9 Drug Dosing Table

Drug	Brand Name	Initial Dose	Usual Range	Special Population Dose	Other
Proton Pump Inhibitors					
Omeprazole, sodium bicarbonate	Prilosec, Zegerid	40 mg daily	20-40 mg/day	Consider adjustment for hepatic disease	Pregnancy Category C
Lansoprazole	Prevacid, various	30 mg daily	15-30 mg/day	Consider adjustment for hepatic disease	Pregnancy Category B
Rabeprazole	Aciphex	20 mg daily	20-40 mg/day	Use with caution in severe hepatic disease	Pregnancy Category B
Pantoprazole	Protonix, various	40 mg daily	40-80 mg/day	Consider adjustment for severe hepatic disease	Pregnancy Category B
Esomeprazole	Nexium	40 mg daily	20-40 mg/day	Limit dose to 20 mg/day in severe hepatic disease	Pregnancy Category B
Dexlansoprazole	Dexilant	30-60 mg daily	30-60 mg/day	Consider dose limit of 30 mg/day in moderate hepatic impairment, dose not established in severe hepatic disease	Pregnancy Category B
H2-Receptor Antagonists					
Cimetidine	Tagamet, various	300 mg four times daily, 400 mg twice daily, or 800 mg at bedtime	800-1,600 mg/ day in divided doses	Adjust dose for renal and severe hepatic impairment	Pregnancy Category B
Famotidine	Pepcid, various	20 mg twice daily, or 40 mg at bedtime	20-40 mg/day	Adjust dose for renal impairment	Pregnancy Category B
Nizatidine	Axid, various	150 mg twice daily, or 300 mg at bedtime	150-300 mg/day	Adjust dose for renal impairment	Pregnancy Category B
Ranitidine[a]	Zantac, various	150 mg twice daily, or 300 mg at bedtime	150-300 mg/day	Adjust dose for renal impairment	Pregnancy Category B
Mucosal Protectants					
Sucralfate	Carafate, various	1 g four times daily, or 2 g twice daily	2-4 g/day		Aluminum may accumulate in renal failure, Pregnancy Category B
Misoprostol	Cytotec	100-200 mcg four times daily	400-800 mcg/day		Pregnancy Category X

[a]Ranitidine products are no longer available in the United States.

Data from References 2 and 4.

rather than together.[8,55] The basis for sequential therapy is to initially treat with antibiotics that rarely promote resistance (eg, amoxicillin) to reduce the bacterial load and any preexisting resistant organisms that are susceptible. The second sequence follows with different antibiotics (eg, clarithromycin and metronidazole) to kill any remaining organisms.[8,55,56] See Table 51-8 for a typical treatment regimen. Although this regimen has achieved eradication rates that are superior to the PPI-based three-drug regimens containing clarithromycin,[56] the regimen requires a change in medication mid-treatment, which may contribute to nonadherence. Though promising, the advantages of sequential therapy have yet to be fully validated in the United States, and is only conditionally recommended within guidelines as a first-line *H. pylori* eradication therapy (see Table 51-7).[8]

Non-Bismuth Quadruple "Concomitant" Therapy and Hybrid Therapy

Non-bismuth quadruple therapy, also called "concomitant" therapy, is a regimen with a PPI, amoxicillin, clarithromycin, and metronidazole taken together at standard doses for 10 to 14 days. Hybrid therapy combines the strategies of concomitant and sequential therapy. Patients take dual therapy (PPI and amoxicillin) followed by 7 days of quadruple therapy (PPI, amoxicillin, clarithromycin, and metronidazole). Although clarithromycin resistance may impact efficacy rates, both concomitant and hybrid therapy may be impacted less than clarithromycin triple therapy. Both regimens are first-line alternatives to clarithromycin triple therapy, but there is a lack of evidence in North America with these regimens.[8]

Levofloxacin-Based Therapy

Levofloxacin has been studied as first-line and salvage therapy for *H. pylori* eradication, but data are scarce for levofloxacin-based first-line treatment regimens. Three regimens using levofloxacin have been studied (see Table 51-8). Eradication is similar with 7 days of clarithromycin-based or levofloxacin triple therapy; however, levofloxacin-based triple therapy for 10 to 14 days is superior to clarithromycin triple therapy for 7 days.[54] Levofloxacin sequential therapy has eradication rates higher than pooled clarithromycin-based triple and sequential regimens (87.8% vs 71.1%).[8] A first-line quadruple regimen, termed "LOAD," is not recommended within the guidelines due to cost and lack of data.[8] Concerns about using fluoroquinolones to treat *H. pylori* include development of resistance and adverse effects (eg, tendonitis and hepatotoxicity).

Probiotics

Probiotics (eg, strains of *Lactobacillus* and *Bifidobacterium*) limit *H. pylori* colonization and when taken as a supplement to antibiotic therapy, increase eradication rates compared to placebo and may reduce the adverse effects of antibiotic eradication therapy.[57,58] However, the administration of probiotics alone does not eradicate

H. pylori infection. The optimal probiotic strains, dose, timing, and duration has yet to be determined.

Eradication of *Helicobacter pylori* After Initial Treatment Failure

H. pylori eradication is often more difficult after initial treatment fails and successful eradication after retreatment is extremely variable.[8] Treatment failures should be referred to a gastroenterologist for further diagnostic evaluation. Second-line (salvage) treatment should (a) use antibiotics that were not used during initial therapy or recently for another infection; (b) be guided by region-specific or individual antibiotic resistance testing, if available; and (c) use an extended duration of treatment up to 10 to 14 days.[8] Ideally, culture and sensitivity or molecular resistance data would be available to guide salvage regimen selection; however, these modalities may be unavailable (eg, the United States) and empiric treatment decisions are necessary. European guidelines recommend obtaining antimicrobial sensitivity information following the second failed attempt to eradicate *H. pylori*. Preferred regimens are provided in Table 51-7. A 10-day therapy containing PPI, bismuth, tetracycline, and levofloxacin achieved a high eradication rate after failure of first-line treatment with standard clarithromycin triple or non-bismuth quadruple therapy.[59] High-dose dual therapy using amoxicillin plus a PPI with both administered three-to-four times daily for 14 days is an acceptable therapy.[8] Other salvage regimens that include rifabutin are also effective, but these are discussed in more detail elsewhere.[60,61] Penicillin skin testing is now recommended for patients after failing one or two eradication attempts since amoxicillin is an important component of therapy with low prevalence of resistance and many patients reporting penicillin allergy are not truly allergic.[8]

Factors That Predict *Helicobacter pylori* Eradication Outcomes

Factors that predict successful *H. pylori* eradication can be divided into host-related and *H. pylori*–related factors. Medication adherence and pharmacogenomic factors are important host-related considerations, and antibiotic resistance is the most important and consistent predictor of *H. pylori* eradication.[39]

Medication adherence decreases with multiple medications, increased frequency of administration, intolerable adverse effects, and costly drug regimens—all of which can be issues with recommended treatment options. Tolerability varies with different regimens, but common adverse effects include nausea, vomiting, abdominal pain, diarrhea, and taste disturbances (metronidazole and clarithromycin). Adverse effects with metronidazole are dose-related (especially when more than 1 g/day) and include a disulfiram-like reaction with alcohol. Tetracycline may cause photosensitivity and should not be used in children because of possible tooth discoloration. Bismuth salts may cause darkening of the stool and tongue. Antibiotic-associated diarrhea and *Clostridioides difficile*–associated disease can occur. Oral thrush and vaginal candidiasis may also occur.

An increasingly important predictor of eradication is the presence or absence of resistant *H. pylori* strains.[8] The following are worldwide antibiotic resistance rates among *H. pylori* strains (n = 818 isolates): clarithromycin (30.8%), metronidazole (30.5%), amoxicillin (2%), tetracycline (0%), and levofloxacin (14.2%).[45] Although amoxicillin and tetracycline resistance remains low in available surveillance, prevalence of clarithromycin resistance exceeding 20% negatively impacts successful empiric *H. pylori* eradication therapy.[53] Increasing clarithromycin resistance may explain the decrease in efficacy of triple therapy clarithromycin-containing regimens. Prior exposure to macrolide antibiotics adversely affected the success of eradication using clarithromycin-based triple therapy.[62] Bismuth-containing, concomitant, or sequential therapies may be preferred in patients with prior macrolide exposure.[8,62] Therefore, prior antibiotic use should prompt consideration for possible *H. pylori* resistance. The clinical importance of metronidazole resistance remains uncertain, as resistance can be overcome by using higher dosages and by combining metronidazole with other antibiotics. Resistance to tetracycline and amoxicillin is uncommon. Resistance to bismuth has not been reported.[8] Although the role of antibiotic sensitivity testing prior to initiating *H. pylori* treatment has not been formally established, molecular-based tests may offer quick and easy determination of *H. pylori* resistance to macrolides and fluoroquinolones allowing optimal regimen selection.[63]

Treatment of Nonsteroidal Anti-Inflammatory Drug–Induced Ulcers

NSAID therapy should be interrupted upon confirmation of an active ulcer. Once stopped, most uncomplicated NSAID ulcers heal with standard 8-week regimens of an H2RA, PPI, or sucralfate (see Table 51-9).[20] Generally, PPIs are preferred due to more rapid symptom relief and ulcer healing. In patients where the NSAID is continued despite ulceration, treatment with a PPI or misoprostol should be initiated.[64] PPIs are the drugs of choice when the NSAID is continued, as potent acid suppression is required to accelerate ulcer healing. PPI treatment duration should be extended 12 weeks if the NSAID must be continued. In addition, consideration should be given to reducing the NSAID dose, switching to acetaminophen or a nonacetylated salicylate, or using a selective COX-2 inhibitor (see Table 51-3). If the ulcer is *H. pylori*–positive, eradication should be initiated with a regimen that contains a PPI.[20]

Prevention of NSAID-Related Peptic Ulcers

Among patients who use NSAIDs, several therapeutic strategies are available to prevent gastroduodenal ulcers and related upper GI complications. These strategies include co-therapy of an NSAID with a PPI, H2RA, or misoprostol; preferential use of a COX-2 selective NSAID; or combination of a gastroprotective agent with a COX-2 selective NSAID (see Table 51-10). COX-2 selective NSAID in combination with a PPI offers the greatest protection against upper GI complications. This regimen is followed in effectiveness by COX-2 selective NSAIDs alone, nonselective NSAIDs with a PPI, and medical co-therapy with misoprostol.[12,65] Unfortunately, these strategies may not eliminate ulcers and complications for patients at the "highest risk." Nonselective NSAID and co-therapy with an H2RA is effective at preventing duodenal but not gastric ulcers.[12] Selection of a gastroprotective strategy should consider both the

TABLE 51-10 Potential Risks and Safety Issues Associated with the PPIs

Gastric cancers or malignancy
Carcinoid tumors
Atrophic gastritis
Adenocarcinoma
Bacterial overgrowth
Increase in *N*-nitroso compounds from ingested nitrates (carcinogenic)
Enteric infections (*Clostridioides difficile, Salmonella typhimurium*, and *Campylobacter jejuni*)
Community-acquired pneumonia
Decreased nutrient absorption:
Iron
Calcium
Cyanocobalamin (vitamin B_{12})
Magnesium
Osteoporosis and related fractures
Chronic kidney disease and acute kidney injury

PPI, proton pump inhibitor.

Data from References 51, 79, and 97.

GI benefits and the cardiovascular risks associated with NSAIDs.[20] Strategies aimed at reducing the topical irritant effects of nonselective NSAIDs, for example, prodrugs, slow-release formulations, and enteric-coated products, are not effective at preventing ulcers or GI complications.

Misoprostol Co-therapy

Misoprostol, a synthetic analog of prostaglandin E1, has dual gastroprotective effects by improving mucosal blood flow and by stimulating gastric mucous and bicarbonate secretion. It has a short half-life requiring doses to be administered three-to-four times daily. Misoprostol's efficacy increases with higher doses, with prevention trials demonstrating significantly fewer endoscopically confirmed gastric and duodenal ulcers compared with placebo. Misoprostol also decreases the risk of PUD complications including perforation, gastric outlet obstruction, and bleeding.[66] Misoprostol is associated with high-rates of nausea, diarrhea, and abdominal cramping that increase with the dose, limiting its clinical utility.[3,12]

H2-Receptor Antagonist Co-therapy

Standard doses of H2RA are effective at reducing endoscopically confirmed duodenal ulcers compared to placebo, but higher doses (eg, famotidine 80 mg/day) are needed to prevent gastric ulcers.[19] In both cases, H2RAs are less effective when compared with PPI or misoprostol.[66] For this reason, H2RAs are relegated to second-line therapy for prevention of NSAID-induced gastric ulcer and related complications. Patients at higher risk (eg, prior ulcer or older patients) should receive PPIs preferentially over H2RA.[64] Candidates for H2RA as co-therapy include patients who have significant nonmodifiable drug interactions or are intolerant of PPIs or misoprostol.

Proton Pump Inhibitor Co-therapy

4 PPI co-therapy reduces NSAID-related gastric and duodenal ulcer risk and is better tolerated than misoprostol.[12,18,20] PPI co-therapy is more effective than misoprostol and H2RA at preventing NSAID-induced gastric ulcer and related complications.[66] All PPIs are considered equally effective when used in standard dosages (see Table 51-9) for ulcer prevention. There is not an incremental benefit with higher doses for ulcer prevention, even among higher risk patients (ie, age >60 years, prior gastric/duodenal ulcer).[67] PPIs reduce the risk of NSAID-related upper GI bleeding, but do not protect against lower GI bleeding.[18]

Cyclooxygenase-2 Inhibitors

COX-2 inhibitors preferentially act on the cyclooxygenase-2 enzyme, exhibiting equivalent anti-inflammatory activity of traditional NSAIDs with a lower risk of gastric or duodenal ulcers. Avoidance of COX-1 isoenzyme inhibition preserves prostaglandin production and its beneficial gastroprotective effects. Celecoxib preferentially inhibits COX-2, but carries the same GI and cardiovascular thrombotic black-box warnings as nonselective NSAIDs. The pooled relative risk for GI bleeding is lower with celecoxib (RR 1.45) compared to nonselective NSAIDs, but it is not without some risk. Gastroprotective benefits of celecoxib are lessened in aspirin users, thus if low-dose aspirin is needed, co-therapy with PPI is necessary and a longer duration of treatment. Thus, the lowest effective celecoxib dose should be used for the shortest duration of time. Dyspepsia and abdominal pain, fluid retention, hypertension, and renal toxicity are associated with the COX-2 inhibitors and nonselective NSAIDs. Patients taking NSAIDs or COX-2 inhibitors should be counseled about signs and symptoms of adverse events, including upper GI bleeding and cardiovascular risks, and what to do should they occur.

COX-2 Inhibitor Versus NSAID Plus PPI

5 For high GI risk, low CV risk, *H. pylori*–negative patients, a COX-2 selective NSAID alone is at least as beneficial as a nonselective NSAID plus PPI co-therapy in reducing NSAID-related ulcer complications.[20] However, neither the COX-2 selective NSAID nor the NSAID plus a PPI guarantees elimination of upper GI events for high GI risk patients. Combining a COX-2 selective NSAID with a PPI can be considered for very high GI risk patients as it offers the best protection against PUD complications. Patients with complicated peptic ulcer history or presence of multiple risk factors are candidates for COX-2 selective NSAID combined with a PPI.[20]

Treatment of Non–*Helicobacter pylori*, Non-Nonsteroidal Anti-Inflammatory Drug Ulcers

Peptic ulcers unrelated to *H. pylori* or use of NSAIDs, including low-dose aspirin, are considered a distinct diagnosis and referred to as idiopathic ulcers. In North America, between 11% and 44% of peptic ulcers were determined to be idiopathic.[68] With more effective acid suppressive therapy, the incidence of idiopathic ulcers is believed to be increasing worldwide. Patients with idiopathic ulcer have a worse prognosis due to high relapse rate, recurrent ulcer bleeding, and increased risk of death. Possible explanations for *non–H. pylori*, non-NSAID ulcers include gastric hypersecretion, gastric outlet obstruction, genetic predisposition, concomitant diseases (see Table 51-2), and heavy tobacco use. Treatment includes conventional ulcer healing therapies (see Table 51-9). Maintenance therapy may be required to prevent PUD complications since there is a high rate of recurrent bleeding within 1 year. No significant difference was seen in recurrent bleeding between famotide 40 mg daily and lansoprazole 30 mg daily for up to 24 monhts.[68]

Long-Term Maintenance of Ulcer Healing

Long-term maintenance of ulcer healing and the prevention of ulcer-related complications may be necessary in some patients. Because *H. pylori* eradication dramatically decreases ulcer recurrence, continuous maintenance therapy is primarily used to treat high-risk patients who failed *H. pylori* eradication, have a history of ulcer-related complications, have frequent recurrences of *H. pylori*–negative ulcers, and are heavy smokers or NSAID users. For most patients, standard maintenance dosages (see Table 51-9) are effective.

Treatment of Refractory Ulcers

Refractory peptic ulcers are ulcers that persist after 8 to 12 weeks of standard antisecretory drug treatment. Persistent *H. pylori* infection and use of NSAIDs are the most common causes of refractory ulcers. Additional contributing factors may include poor patient compliance, cigarette smoking, gastric acid hypersecretion, or tolerance to the antisecretory effects of an H2RA (see section "Antiulcer Agents" below). Patients with refractory ulcers should undergo upper endoscopy to confirm a nonhealing ulcer, exclude malignancy, and reassess *H. pylori* status with two or more diagnostic methods to increase sensitivity.[69] *H. pylori*–positive patients should receive eradication therapy (see "Treatment of *Helicobacter pylori*–Positive Ulcers" above). Fasting plasma gastrin levels can be checked if Zollinger-Ellison syndrome is suspected. Refractory ulcers, despite a complete standard PPI course, should be retreated with double-dose of PPI. Consideration can be given to using a different PPI.[69]

Antiulcer Agents

Proton Pump Inhibitors

PPIs (see Tables 51-9 and 51-11) dose-dependently inhibit basal and stimulated gastric acid secretion. The duration of acid suppression is a function of binding to the H^+/K^+-adenosine triphosphatase (ATPase) enzyme.[3] When PPI therapy is initiated, the degree of acid suppression increases over the first 3 to 4 days of therapy, as more proton pumps are inhibited. PPIs inhibit only those proton pumps that are actively secreting acid, thus they are most effective when taken 30 to 60 minutes before meals.[4] Symptomatic acid rebound on

TABLE 51-11 PPI Formulations and Options for Administration

	Omeprazole	Esomeprazole	Lansoprazole	Pantoprazole	Rabeprazole	Dexlansoprazole
Commercially available oral formulations						
Capsule	X[a]	X	X			X[b]
Tablet	X[c]			X	X	
Oral disintegrating tablet			X			
Packet for oral suspension	X[d]	X[e]				
Extemporaneous oral preparations						
Pellets from capsule in water		X				
Pellets from capsule in applesauce	X		X			X
Pellets from capsule in juice	X	X[e]	X			
Extemporaneous preparation of delayed-release PPI in bicarbonate (omeprazole-sodium bicarbonate)	X		X	X		
Parenteral formulations						
IV	X (not available in the United States)	X		X		

PPI, proton pump inhibitor; X, product is available.

[a]Omeprazole is available as delayed-release enteric-coated pellets in a capsule or as immediate-release capsule that contains 20 or 40 mg of omeprazole with 1,100 mg sodium bicarbonate (equivalent to 304 mg of sodium). Because 20 and 40 mg dosages contain the same amount of bicarbonate, two 20 mg capsules should not be substituted for the 40 mg immediate-release omeprazole-sodium bicarbonate capsule.

[b]Dexlansoprazole is available as a dual delayed-release formulation in capsules for oral administration. The capsule contains dexlansoprazole in a mixture of two types of enteric-coated granules with different pH-dependent dissolution profiles.

[c]Omeprazole oral tablets are available as 20 mg delayed-release nonprescription tablets.

[d]Omeprazole oral suspension is available as 20 or 40 mg omeprazole with 1,680 mg sodium bicarbonate (equivalent to 460 mg of sodium). Because 20 and 40 mg dosages contain the same amount of bicarbonate, two 20 mg packets should not be substituted for the 40 mg immediate-release omeprazole-bicarbonate packet.

[e]No published information; based on omeprazole data.

withdrawal of a PPI has been reported in healthy volunteers after 8 weeks of treatment.[70]

PPIs are formulated as delayed-release enteric-coated dosage forms that have pH-sensitive granules contained in gelatin capsules (omeprazole, esomeprazole, prescription and nonprescription lansoprazole, and dexlansoprazole), rapidly disintegrating tablets (lansoprazole), and delayed-release enteric-coated tablets (rabeprazole, pantoprazole, and nonprescription omeprazole) (see Table 51-11). The pH-sensitive enteric coating prevents degradation and premature protonation of the drug in stomach allowing the drug to be dissolved then absorbed in the duodenum at a higher pH. Dexlansoprazole is formulated with a dual-release mechanism that provides inhibition of proton pumps that become activated after initial release of the medication while omeprazole is also available as an immediate-release formulation (oral suspension, oral capsule) containing sodium bicarbonate, which can control intragastric pH in the absence of food.[71] Parenteral formulations include omeprazole (not available in the United States), esomeprazole, and pantoprazole.

PPIs provide similar rates of ulcer healing, symptom relief, and maintenance of ulcer healing when used in recommended dosages (see Table 51-9).[3] Higher than indicated daily doses should be divided to obtain better 24-hour control of intragastric pH. Older adults and patients with renal impairment do not require dosage reductions, but dosage reductions should be considered in patients with severe hepatic disease.[72] Short-term adverse effects of PPIs are like those observed with the H2RAs (headache, nausea, and abdominal pain). Immediate-release formulations contain sodium bicarbonate, and thus are contraindicated for patients with metabolic alkalosis and hypokalemia.

Drug Interactions Since PPIs increase intragastric pH, they may alter the bioavailability of orally administered drugs that are weak bases (eg, ketoconazole), digoxin, or pH-dependent dosage forms. This interaction is especially important with antiretroviral therapies for treatment of HIV and direct acting antivirals for hepatitis C, as reduced absorption can lead to therapeutic failure due to development of viral resistance.[73,74] Omeprazole and esomeprazole selectively inhibit the hepatic CYP2C19 pathway and may decrease the elimination of several drugs (eg, phenytoin, warfarin, diazepam, and carbamazepine).[51] PPIs may increase the metabolic clearance and decrease the GI absorption of levothyroxine resulting in increased thyroid-stimulating hormone levels and a corresponding increase in the levothyroxine dose.[75] Few drug-drug interactions (eg, phenytoin, warfarin, methotrexate) involving PPIs are clinically significant and constitute a major clinical risk.[51]

A controversial PPI drug interaction involves the antiplatelet drug clopidogrel. Clopidogrel is converted to its active form through CYP2C19. PPIs may attenuate the antiplatelet effect of clopidogrel by inhibiting or competing for this metabolic pathway. FDA safety guidelines recommend that the coadministration of omeprazole, omeprazole/sodium bicarbonate, or esomeprazole with clopidogrel be avoided because they reduce the effectiveness of clopidogrel. Warnings regarding omeprazole, esomeprazole, and other interacting drugs (eg, cimetidine) are contained in the clopidogrel package insert as well. This interaction is further complicated since genetic polymorphisms of the CYP2C19 gene leading to decreased biotransformation of clopidogrel to its active form may also explain reduced effectiveness of clopidogrel. Whether the use of other PPIs such as pantoprazole, lansoprazole, dexlansoprazole, and rabeprazole interacts with clopidogrel remains uncertain as the capacity to inhibit CYP2C19 varies among these PPIs.[76] Although pharmacodynamic studies suggest attenuated anti-platelet effects of clopidogrel with omeprazole, it does not appear to translate to increased cardiovascular risk in most studies. In randomized, double-blind, placebo-controlled studies of clopidogrel and omeprazole, there was no increased cardiovascular risk noted; however, the combination reduced the risk of upper GI bleeding.[77] Given the limitations of existing studies, administration of clopidogrel with PPIs should be balanced based upon cardiovascular and gastrointestinal risk.[76,78]

Potential Long-Term Safety Issues Prolonged hypergastrinemia and chronic hypochlorhydria from long-term PPI use has been associated with numerous potential risks and safety issues (see Table 51-10).[79] Issues with study design, confounding, and subject selection make it difficult to attribute direct causality of PPIs for these potential safety issues. Patients receiving long-term PPIs can develop increases in serum gastrin levels, which exerts tropic effects on enterochromaffin-like cells. These cells have potential for inducing carcinoid tumors within the stomach during or after chronic acid suppression; however, there is very limited evidence (ie, case reports) of this effect, and a causal relationship between PPI use and gastric cancers has not yet been established.[2] There is also no evidence to support an association between PPIs and colonic polyps or colorectal cancer. Chronic PPI use is also associated with alterations of the intestinal microbiome, including small intestinal overgrowth and *C. difficile* infection because of inhibition of gastric acid and bacterial proton pumps. The full impact of changes in gastric and intestinal bacterial diversity and composition is unclear.[79,80]

Gastric acid is an important factor in nutrient absorption and protects against bacterial colonization of the stomach. Chronic acid suppression has been associated with increased risk of nutrient malabsorption and enteric infections. Acid suppression has been implicated as a risk factor for community-acquired pneumonia (CAP) and enteric infections (*C. difficile*, *Salmonella*, *Campylobacter*). There is a higher adjusted relative risk of CAP for patients using PPIs compared with controls, particularly in patients receiving higher doses or within the first 30 days of therapy.[79] The results of these retrospectively designed studies need to be interpreted cautiously because of the variability in the length of therapy for current PPI users and the inclusion of older (older than 60 years) patients with concomitant comorbidities. PPIs are linked with various enteric infections, but the most convincing data were with *C. difficile*. Sustained elevations in intragastric pH may facilitate the survival of *C. difficile* spores. However, the magnitude of risk varies and causality is difficult to establish. The risk of various infections associated with PPI therapy cannot be firmly established until the results of large prospective studies are made available.

The absorption of vitamin B_{12}, dietary iron, and calcium requires an acidic environment and may be adversely affected by long-term use of PPIs (see Table 51-12). The clinical importance of PPIs on absorption has not been established, and routine monitoring of B_{12} and iron levels cannot be routinely recommended. Adequate supplementation and monitoring should be considered in high-risk populations (eg, older patients, vegetarians, alcohol misuse) who may be already depleted. Hypomagnesemia, both symptomatic and asymptomatic, has been reported with PPI use with serious adverse events including tetany, arrhythmias, and seizures (see Table 51-12). In most cases it occurs in patients taking PPIs more than 1 year but can occur with as little as 3 months of therapy. High PPI dosage and long-term therapy have been associated with an increased risk of hip, wrist, and spine fractures related to reduction in calcium absorption. The FDA has revised the warnings and precautions of prescription and nonprescription PPIs to reflect these potential risks. Routine bone density tests for osteoporosis screening, calcium supplementation, or other precautions cannot be recommended solely based on chronic PPI therapy.[51]

H2-Receptor Antagonists

Ulcer healing is comparable among H2RAs with equipotent multiple daily doses or a single full dose given after dinner or at bedtime (see Table 51-9), but tolerance to their antisecretory effect may occur. Twice-daily administration may be beneficial in patients with daytime ulcer pain while patients who smoke cigarettes may require higher doses or a longer duration of treatment. H2RAs are renally eliminated, thus a dosage reduction is recommended for patients with moderate-to-severe renal impairment. The short- and long-term safety of all H2RAs is similar. Thrombocytopenia is a common yet likely overestimated hematologic adverse effect that occurs with all H2RAs and is reversible (see Table 51-12). The H2RAs decrease acid secretion and may alter the bioavailability of orally administered drugs. Cimetidine inhibits several CYP450 isoenzymes, resulting in numerous drug interactions (eg, theophylline, lidocaine, phenytoin, warfarin, and clopidogrel). Famotidine and nizatidine do not interact with drugs metabolized by the hepatic CYP450 pathway. In April 2020, the Food and Drug Administration (FDA) recommended withdrawal of all ranitidine products from the US market following a report that, when stored at higher than recommended temperatures, products could contain unsafe quantities of N-nitrosodimethylamine (NDMA), a probable human carcinogen.[81]

Sucralfate

Sucralfate heals peptic ulcers but is not widely used today for this indication. Deterrents to its use include the requirement for multiple doses per day, large tablet size, and the need to separate the

TABLE 51-12 Drug Monitoring Table

Drug	Adverse Drug Reaction	Monitoring Parameter	Comments
PPIs	Headache, N/V/D, flatulence Less common: thrombocytopenia, neutropenia, hypomagnesemia, hypocalcemia, liver function abnormalities, renal impairment	Baseline and periodic CBC, serum electrolytes, renal/liver function	Well tolerated; may be associated with increased risk of fractures, pneumonia, *Clostridioides difficile* infection
H2RA	Headache, dizziness, diarrhea, somnolence, gynecomastia (cimetidine) Less common: thrombocytopenia, neutropenia, liver function abnormalities, renal impairment, pancreatitis	Baseline and periodic CBC, serum electrolytes, renal/liver function	
Sucralfate	Constipation, aluminum toxicity, gastric bezor		
Misoprostol	Diarrhea, abdominal pain, headache, nausea/vomiting, flatulence, dysmenorrhea, hypophosphatemia	Pregnancy test Serum phosphate	Avoid in pregnancy

CBC, complete blood count; H2RA, H_2-receptor antagonists; PPIs, proton pump inhibitors.

Data from References 4 and 11.

drug from meals and potentially interacting medications (eg, fluoroquinolones). Drug interactions can be minimized by giving the interacting drug at least 2 hours before sucralfate, or avoidance as with fluoroquinolones. Constipation may be troublesome especially in older individuals, and seizures have been observed in dialysis patients taking aluminum-containing antacids. Hypophosphatemia may develop with long-term treatment. Rarely, gastric bezoar formation has been reported (see Table 51-12).

Prostaglandins

The synthetic PGE_1 analogue, misoprostol, moderately inhibits acid secretion and enhances mucosal defense. Antisecretory effects are dose dependent over the range of 50 to 200 mcg, and cytoprotective effects occur in humans at doses of greater than 200 mcg. The most troublesome adverse effect is diarrhea which is dose dependent; develops in 10% to 30% of patients; and is accompanied by abdominal cramping, nausea, flatulence, and headache.[3] Taking the drug with or after meals and at bedtime may minimize the diarrhea (see Table 51-12). Misoprostol is contraindicated in pregnant women because it produces uterine contractions that may endanger pregnancy. If misoprostol is prescribed to women in their childbearing years, contraceptive measures must be confirmed, and a negative serum pregnancy test should be documented within 2 weeks of initiating treatment (see Table 51-12).

Bismuth Preparations

Bismuth subsalicylate and bismuth subcitrate potassium are the only available bismuth salts in the United States. Possible ulcer healing mechanisms include an antibacterial effect, a local gastroprotective effect, and stimulation of endogenous PGs. Bismuth salts do not inhibit or neutralize acid. Bismuth subsalicylate is regarded as safe and has few adverse effects when taken in recommended dosages. Bismuth salts should be used with caution in older patients and in patients with renal failure as renal insufficiency may decrease bismuth elimination. Bismuth subsalicylate may cause salicylate sensitivity or bleeding disorders and should be used with caution for patients receiving concurrent salicylate therapy. Bismuth salts impart a black color to stool and possibly the tongue with liquid preparations. Long-term use of bismuth salts is not recommended due to the potential for bismuth toxicity.

Antacids

Antacids neutralize gastric acid, inactivate pepsin, and bind bile salts. Aluminum-containing antacids also suppress *H. pylori* and enhance mucosal defense. The GI adverse effects are most common and are dose dependent: Aluminum-containing antacids cause constipation, and magnesium salts can cause an osmotic diarrhea. Aluminum-containing antacids (except aluminum phosphate) form insoluble salts with dietary phosphorus and interfere with phosphorus absorption. Hypophosphatemia occurs most often for patients with low dietary phosphate intake (eg, malnutrition or alcoholism). Combined treatment with sucralfate may amplify the hypophosphatemia and aluminum toxicity.

Magnesium excretion is impaired in patients with a creatinine clearance of less than 30 mL/min (0.5 mL/s) that may lead to toxicity; thus, magnesium-containing antacids should be avoided in these patients. Hypercalcemia may occur for patients with normal renal function taking more than 20 g/day of calcium carbonate and for patients with renal failure who are taking more than 4 g/day. The milk-alkali syndrome (ie, hypercalcemia, alkalosis, renal stones, increased blood urea nitrogen, and increased serum creatinine concentration) occurs with high calcium intake for patients with systemic alkalosis produced by either ingestion of absorbable antacids (sodium bicarbonate) or prolonged vomiting. Antacids may alter the absorption and excretion of drugs when administered concomitantly (eg, iron, warfarin, tetracycline, digoxin, quinidine, isoniazid, ketoconazole, or the fluoroquinolones). Most interactions can be avoided by separating the antacid from the oral drug by at least 2 hours.

EVALUATION OF THERAPEUTIC OUTCOMES

6 Table 51-13 lists the recommendations for treating and monitoring patients with PUD. Relief of epigastric pain should be monitored throughout the course of treatment for patients with either *H. pylori*– or NSAID-related ulcers. Ulcer pain typically resolves in a few days when NSAIDs are discontinued and within 7 days upon initiation of antiulcer therapy. Patients with uncomplicated PUD are usually symptom free after treatment with any of the recommended antiulcer regimens. Persistent or recurrent symptoms within 14 days following treatment completion suggests failure of ulcer healing

TABLE 51-13 Recommendations for Treating and Monitoring Patients with *Helicobacter Pylori*–Associated and NSAID-Induced Ulcers

***H. pylori*–associated ulcer**

1. Recommend drug treatment as presented in the chapter text. See Table 51–7 and Table 51–8
2. Assess patient allergies to determine if allergic to penicillin (or other antibiotics) so that drug regimens that contain penicillin (or other antibiotics) can be avoided. Avoid regimens that contain tetracycline in children
3. Assess patient use of alcohol or alcohol-containing products with metronidazole and oral birth control medications with antibiotics and counsel appropriately
4. Assess likelihood of nonadherence to the drug regimen as a cause of treatment failure
5. Recommend a different antibiotic combination if *H. pylori* eradication fails and a second treatment is planned
6. Inform the patient of change in stool color when bismuth salicylate is included in an *H. pylori* eradication regimen
7. Assess and monitor patients for potential adverse effects, especially those associated with metronidazole, clarithromycin, and amoxicillin
8. Assess and monitor patients for potential drug interactions, especially those receiving metronidazole, clarithromycin, or cimetidine
9. Monitor patients for salicylate toxicity, especially patients receiving co-therapy with other salicylates and anticoagulants and patients with renal insufficiency
10. Monitor patients for persistent or recurrent symptoms within 14 days after completion of a course of *H. pylori* eradication therapy
11. Provide education to patients who are receiving *H. pylori* eradication therapy and include why antibiotic and antiulcer combinations are used; when and how to take medications; adverse effects; alarm symptoms; the importance of adherence to the entire course of drug treatment; and contact their healthcare provider if alarm symptoms develop (eg, blood in the stools, black tarry stools, vomiting, severe abdominal pain), or if symptoms persist or return after *H. pylori* eradication

NSAID-induced ulcer

1. Recommend drug treatment as presented in the chapter text
2. Assess risk factors for NSAID-induced ulcers and ulcer-related complications and recommend appropriate strategies for reducing ulcer risk (see Table 51-14)
3. Weigh patient risk factors for NSAID-related GI bleeding and cardiovascular events when selecting a strategy to reduce ulcer risk
4. Recommend eradication treatment for *H. pylori*–positive patients taking NSAIDs
5. Monitor patients for signs and symptoms of NSAID-related upper GI complications
6. Assess and monitor patients for potential drug interactions and adverse effects (especially misoprostol)
7. Provide patient education to patients who are at risk of NSAID-induced ulcers or GI-related complications and include why co-therapy is used with nonselective NSAIDs, when and how to take medications, adverse effects, alarm symptoms, when to contact their healthcare provider, and the importance of adherence to drug treatment

TABLE 51-14 Prevention of Peptic Ulcer Disease in Patients Receiving Chronic NSAID Therapy

	Low Gastrointestinal Risk[a]	High Gastrointestinal Risk[b,c]
Low Cardiovascular Risk	Nonselective NSAIDs	Nonselective NSAIDs plus PPI; celecoxib plus PPI[d]
High Cardiovascular Risk[e]	Naproxen; add PPI if patient is taking aspirin	No NSAIDs; naproxen plus PPI; low-dose celecoxib plus aspirin plus PPI may be an alternative option[f]

[a]No risk factors.

[b]Presence of risk factors (patients 60 years or older, history of peptic ulcers, receiving concomitant antiplatelet agents, anticoagulants, corticosteroids, or selective serotonin reuptake inhibitors).

[c]In patients with prior history of ulcers, adopt test-and-treat strategy to exclude *H. pylori* infection.

[d]Consider when patients have complicated ulcer history or presence of multiple risk factors.

[e]Use risk calculator (eg, Framingham or atherosclerotic cardiovascular disease [ASCVD] risk calculators) to estimate cardiovascular risk on the basis of several variables. Patients with a history of cardiovascular events or diabetes are considered high cardiovascular risk.

[f]NSAIDs with increasing selectivity for Cyclooxygenase-2 (COX-2) (ie, celecoxib) have been associated with increased cardiovascular risk, and this risk appears to be increased in patients with established cardiovascular disease. Patients with cardiovascular disease or risk factors, recommendations for pain management (in the order listed) include: acetaminophen, aspirin, tramadol, opioids (short-term), nonacetylated salicylates (eg, diflunisal), NSAIDs with low COX-2 selectivity (eg, naproxen), NSAIDs with some COX-2 selectivity (eg, nabumetone), and COX-2 selective agents (ie, celecoxib).

NSAID, nonsteroidal anti-inflammatory drug; PPI, proton pump inhibitor.

Data from Reference 4.

or *H. pylori* eradication or presence of an alternate diagnosis such as GERD. Eradication should be confirmed after treatment in all patients, particularly among individuals who are at risk for complications (eg, prior bleeding ulcer). The UBT and fecal antigen are the preferred methods to confirm *H. pylori* eradication when endoscopy is not indicated. Medication adherence should be assessed for patients who fail therapy. Many at-risk patients treated with NSAIDs do not receive adequate prophylaxis for GI complications; however, therapeutic outcomes can be improved by advocating preventive strategies. Any signs or symptoms of bleeding, obstruction, penetration, or perforation require prompt investigation to avoid complications. A follow-up endoscopy is justified for patients with frequent symptomatic recurrence, refractory disease, complications, or suspected hypersecretory states.

RELATED DISORDERS

Upper Gastrointestinal Bleeding

Upper GI bleeding is one of the most common GI emergencies with more than 200,000 hospital admissions annually.[6] There are about 48 to 160 cases of upper GI bleeding per 100,000 adults annually in the United States, and the in-hospital mortality rate associated with acute hemorrhage remains relatively high at 2% despite a decreased incidence of PUD and improvements in the management of upper GI bleeding.[6] Upper GI bleeding is categorized as variceal or nonvariceal bleeding. A complete discussion of variceal bleeding is found elsewhere (Chapter 55). Two common types of nonvariceal bleeding are bleeding from chronic peptic ulcers, often related to antithrombotic therapy, and bleeding from SRMD.[82] Upper GI bleeding associated with chronic PUD usually precedes hospital admission. Bleeding associated with SRMD develops in critically ill patients during hospitalization.[83,84] The underlying pathophysiology of bleeding from a peptic ulcer or from SRMD is similar in that impaired mucosal defense in the presence of gastric acid and pepsin leads to mucosal damage. In chronic PUD, *H. pylori* infection and NSAID use are the most important etiologic factors. The primary pathogenic factor of SRMD in critically ill patients is thought to be mucosal ischemia, which is a result of reduced gastric blood flow resulting from splanchnic hypoperfusion.[83,84] Stress-related mucosal lesions are characteristically asymptomatic, numerous, located in the proximal stomach, and unlikely to perforate. Bleeding from SRMD occurs from superficial mucosal capillaries, whereas bleeding associated with chronic PUD usually results from a single vessel.[83,84] The mortality rate associated with clinically important stress-related mucosal bleeding (SRMB) is approximately 50% and is related to disease severity and comorbidities in this patient population. The mortality associated with chronic PUD-related bleeding is approximately 5% but can increase dramatically in select patient populations.[83,84] Initial management of acute upper GI bleeding focuses on aggressive resuscitation and hemodynamic stability.

Peptic Ulcer–Related Bleeding

Clinical Presentation and Diagnosis

Hematemesis (vomiting up blood), melena (dark, tarry stools), or both are the most common presenting signs and symptoms of PUD-related bleeding. Risk for adverse outcomes must be rapidly assessed to determine if the patient's condition constitutes a medical emergency.[84] Two risk stratification tools exist for early assessment and triage. The Blatchford score is used to evaluate the need for urgent endoscopic intervention for patients presenting with PUD-related bleeding. The scale values range from 0 to 23, with higher scores indicating higher risk. The Rockall score is composed of two assessments: the clinical score, which is performed prior to endoscopy, and the endoscopic score. The use of these risk stratification tools can reduce the requirement of endoscopic procedures and lead to early discharge for low-risk patients while ensuring rapid intervention for patients at higher risk.[84] When considering the risk of death due to PUD bleeding, the following patients generally have poorer prognoses and usually require more aggressive intervention including admission to an intensive care unit (ICU): older age (>60 years), hypotension (SBP <100 mm Hg), tachycardia (HR <100 BPM), shock, poor overall health, comorbid conditions, low initial hemoglobin/hematocrit, active bleeding (red blood per rectum or hematemesis), sepsis, and elevated serum creatinine or serum transaminases.[85] Diagnostic endoscopy is usually performed within 24 hours of presentation to identify the source of the bleeding, assess the potential risk for rebleeding using the Forrest classification of lesions, and, if appropriate, employ therapeutic interventions to promote hemostasis.[85,86]

The appearance of the ulcer at the time of endoscopy is a prognostic indicator for the risk of rebleeding. Clean-based (Forrest type III) and flat spot (pigmented; Forrest type IIc) ulcers are most commonly seen and are associated with a low risk of rebleeding (5% and 10%, respectively). In most cases, patients with clean-based ulcers can be treated as an outpatient on antiulcer therapy, while patients with flat spot ulcers may be admitted to the general hospital ward for brief observation.[84] Patients with an adherent clot overlying the ulcer base (Forrest type IIb) are at intermediate risk of rebleeding (22%-33%), and controversy exists as to the appropriate management of these patients. Patients with a visible vessel (Forrest type IIa) or active bleeding (Forrest type Ia or Ib) are at the highest risk of rebleeding (43%-50% and 55%-90%, respectively) and should receive ICU care for at least 24 hours followed by monitoring on a general medical/surgical service for an additional 48 hours as rebleeding significantly increases mortality.[84]

Treatment

Initial therapy for patients with defined hemostatic instability should focus on correcting fluid volume loss through appropriate volume resuscitative measures. This is usually accomplished with a continuous 0.9% sodium chloride infusion or blood products if clinically indicated.[82] The use of nasogastric (NG) tubes as an aid in early assessment remains controversial, but nasogastric lavage has no impact on transfusion requirements, surgery, or mortality.[82,84] Several endoscopic treatment approaches (eg, thermocoagulation, argon plasma coagulation therapy, injection sclerotherapy, hemostatic clips, and ligation) can be used.[35]

Antisecretory agents are often used as adjuvant therapy to endoscopic procedures to prevent PUD rebleeding in high-risk patients because acid impairs clot stability. PPIs reduce the incidence of rebleeding and need for surgery but have no significant impact on overall mortality.[84] There is no difference in recurrent bleeding, need for surgery, or mortality when comparing equivalent dosing of oral and intravenous PPI therapy.[88] Oral or intermittent IV dosing of PPIs (at cumulative daily omeprazole doses of 80-160 mg) may be preferred over continuous fusion (eg, omeprazole 8 mg/hr) in order to provide a greater ease of administration. PPI therapy is not a replacement for interventional endoscopy in patients with a high risk of rebleeding, as data demonstrate that the combination of a PPI with therapeutic endoscopy is superior to either strategy alone. The risk of rebleeding is greatest within the first 72 hours, and thus antisecretory therapy to prevent rebleeding in high-risk patients should be employed in this time frame. Patients with high-risk endoscopic lesions should be transitioned to twice-daily PPI for 14 days. Patients with low-risk endoscopic lesions can be treated with once-daily PPI. Once-daily PPI treatment should be continued for 4 to 8 weeks in all patients with peptic ulcer bleeding.[84]

Patients with upper GI bleeding should be tested for *H. pylori* at the time of endoscopy (see section "Tests for *Helicobacter pylori*" above). However, the tests are associated with an increased rate of false-negatives when obtained during acute bleeding episodes. If the initial results of the rapid urease test and/or histology are negative, a confirmatory test should be performed following the acute bleeding episode. Ulcer treatment, including *H. pylori* eradication, should be initiated after the acute bleeding episode has resolved (see "Treatment of *H. Pylori*–Positive Ulcers" and "Treatment of NSAID-Induced Ulcers" above).

Stress-Related Mucosal Bleeding

Epidemiology and Risk Factors

Clinically important bleeding increases ICU length of stay, results in excessive healthcare costs, and is associated with increased mortality. Thus, attempts to prevent SRMB are warranted in high-risk patients. Prophylactic therapy to prevent bleeding is most effective if initiated early in the patient's course.[83] The majority (75%-100%) of critically ill patients develop SRMD within the first 1 to 3 days of admission to an ICU, but the incidence of clinically important SRMB (defined as overt bleeding with concomitant hemodynamic instability and likely requirement for blood products) has decreased to 2% to 5%.[83]

Patients who are at risk for SRMB include those with respiratory failure (ie, need for mechanical ventilation for longer than 48 hours), coagulopathy (ie, INR greater than 1.5, platelet count less than 50,000/mm^3 [50 × 10^9/L]), hypotension, sepsis, hepatic failure, acute renal failure, high-dose corticosteroid therapy (ie, more than 250 mg/day hydrocortisone or equivalent), multiple trauma, severe burns (ie, more than 35% of body surface area), head injury, traumatic spinal cord injury, major surgery, prolonged ICU admission (ie, more than 7 days), or history of GI bleeding. The relative importance of the various risk factors remains controversial, but most clinicians concur that patients with respiratory failure or coagulopathy should receive prophylaxis, as these two factors are independent risk factors for SRMB.[89]

Prevention and Treatment

Prevention of SRMB includes resuscitative measures that restore mucosal blood flow, and pharmacotherapy that either maintains an intragastric pH of greater than 4 or provides gastric mucosal protection.[83,90] Although the benefits of enteral nutrition to patient outcome (eg, improved nutritional status enhances mucosal integrity) are of overall critical importance, its precise role as a sole modality to prevent SRMB remains controversial. Patients receiving enteral nutrition may not require medications for SRMB prophylaxis, and such therapies may increase the risk of adverse complications, particularly nosocomial pneumonia, over enteral nutrition alone.[91,92] Therapeutic options for the prevention of SRMB include antisecretory drugs (H2RAs and PPIs), and sucralfate.[83,89]

Sucralfate is an option for SRMB but requires multiple daily dosage administration (up to four times daily). Also, it may occlude nasogastric (NG) tubes, and possibly cause adverse effects previously discussed. Although sucralfate may have a lower risk of pneumonia compared to antisecretory therapy, these factors limit its use for SRMB prophylaxis. PPIs have become the most widely used therapy since they are more potent in inhibiting acid secretion and, unlike H2RAs, tolerance does not develop. Improved efficacy for SRMB when the PPIs are used as prophylaxis must be balanced against adverse events including increased risk of enteric infections, namely *C. difficile*–associated diarrhea and evidence-based nosocomial pneumonia, which are associated with increased healthcare costs.[89,93] A decision analytic model determined H2RA stress ulcer prophylaxis reduced costs, increased survival, and avoided complications compared with PPI therapy.[94] There are several evidence-based dosing regimens for SRMB prophylaxis (see Table 51-15).[83]

Even though PPIs have become the most widely used prevention therapy, numerous studies and years of experience support the use of H2RAs, and they remain a recommended option for the prevention of SRMB.[83] Parenteral H2RAs may be administered as either continuous infusions or intermittent bolus doses (see Table 51-15). Cimetidine, given as a continuous IV infusion, is the only

TABLE 51-15 Pharmacotherapy Options for Prophylaxis of Stress-Related Mucosal Bleeding

Drug and Route	Dosage
Parenteral H2RAs	
Cimetidine	300 mg IV loading dose followed by 50 mg/hr as a continuous infusion[a] or 300 mg IV every 6-8 hours
Ranitidine[b]	6.25 mg/hr as a continuous infusion or 50 mg IV every 6-8 hours
Famotidine	1.7 mg/hr as a continuous infusion or 20 mg IV every 12 hours
Oral/NG Tube PPIs	
Omeprazole	20-40 mg orally/NG tube[c] every 12-24 hours
Omeprazole/ bicarbonate powder for oral suspension	40 mg orally/NG tube to start, then followed by an additional 40 mg in 6-8 hours as a loading dose, and then 40 mg every 24 hours
Lansoprazole	30 mg orally/NG tube[c,d] every 12-24 hours
Pantoprazole	40 mg orally/NG tube[c] every 12-24 hours
Parenteral PPIs	
Pantoprazole	40-80 mg IV every 12-24 hours
Esomeprazole	40 mg IV every 12-24 hours

[a]Product is FDA-approved for the prevention of stress-related mucosal bleeding.

[b]All ranitidine products were removed from the US market effective April 2020.

[c]Administered as an extemporaneously compounded suspension made with sodium bicarbonate.

[d]Administered as a rapidly disintegrating tablet given orally or by NG tube dissolved in 10 mL of water.

H2RA, histamine-2 receptor antagonist; NG, nasogastric; PPI, proton pump inhibitor.

FDA-labeled H2RA for the prevention of SRMB. Drug interactions are more common with cimetidine, thus the other H2RAs (famotidine, ranitidine) have been used more frequently.[83] Adverse events associated with the use of H2RAs for the critically ill patient include thrombocytopenia, mental status changes (more common in older patients or individuals with renal or hepatic compromise), and tachyphylaxis (especially with parenteral or high-dose therapy). Given that the H2RAs are renally eliminated, dosage reductions are recommended for patients with renal dysfunction.

When deciding on the most appropriate pharmacotherapy plan for the prevention of SRMB for a specific patient, the clinical presentation, risk factors, and medication costs should be used as a guide. Oral H2RA or PPI suspension is safe and cost-effective for patients who can take oral medication or have a working NG tube in place. For patients who are not able to utilize one of these routes, parenteral antisecretory therapies are appropriate. However, if the patient has any relative or absolute contraindications to an H2RA, then an IV PPI may be the most appropriate prophylaxis option.

Improvement in the patient's overall medical condition (resolution of risk factors, discharge from the ICU, extubation, and oral intake) suggests that prophylactic therapy can be discontinued. Often patients are continued on SRMB prophylaxis on transition to the general medical/surgical unit and frequently discharged on oral PPI therapy without an appropriate indication. This results in unnecessary costs for the patient and the healthcare system.[89] Patients in whom SRMB prophylaxis is no longer indicated should be identified. If a patient develops clinically important bleeding, endoscopic evaluation of the GI tract is indicated along with aggressive antisecretory therapy (see section "Peptic Ulcer–Related Bleeding" above).

Zollinger-Ellison Syndrome

ZES, characterized by hypersecretion of gastric acid and severe gastroesophageal PUD, is caused by a neuroendocrine tumor (gastrinoma) that is present in the duodenum or pancreas. Gastrinoma has a yearly incidence of approximately 0.1 to three cases per million in the United States with ZES being the underlying cause of PUD in 0.1% to 1% of patients. ZES occurs spontaneously in 75% to 80% of patients, but 25% to 30% of patients have the familial form associated with multiple endocrine neoplasia type 1 (MEN1), an autosomal-dominant syndrome due to a variant in the *MEN1* gene. Patients with MEN1 commonly develop hyperparathyroidism, pituitary adenomas, and neuroendocrine tumors. Half (50%) of patients with MEN1 have ZES making gastrinoma and ZES the most common functional neuroendocrine tumor and syndrome in MEN1. Gastrinomas are usually slow growing, but approximately 60% to 90% are malignant with metastases to regional lymph nodes, liver, and other distant sites at time of diagnosis.[95]

Pathophysiology

Gastrinomas are derived from the enteroendocrine cells, form tumors mainly in the pancreas and proximal small intestine, and are generally classified under the larger term of neuroendocrine tumors. Most gastrinomas arise in the duodenum. Gastrinomas located in the pancreas carry a greater malignant potential. ZES pathophysiology is related to the trophic action of gastrin on parietal cells of the gastric antrum and the resulting hypersecretion of gastric acid. Most patients consequently develop large peptic ulcers frequently in the distal duodenum and even proximal jejunum, which is an uncommon location for ulcers resulting from *H. pylori* or the use of NSAIDs.[95]

Clinical Presentation and Diagnosis

Historically, patients with ZES presented with refractory PUD or complications of acid hypersecretion (perforation, penetration, bleeding, and esophageal stricture). Due to the widespread use of PPIs and H2RAs, this form of presentation has decreased drastically.[95] Patients commonly present with severe refractory heartburn, epigastric pain, and profound diarrhea. Diarrhea may be the only symptom in 10% to 20% of patients and is due to the osmotic load of high gastric acid, inhibition of sodium and water reabsorption by the intestinal brush border of high gastric acid secretion, and a malabsorptive component from inactivation of pancreatic digestive enzymes by gastric acid.[95]

ZES diagnosis is established when the serum gastrin is greater than 1,000 pg/mL (ng/L; 481 pmol/L) and the basal acid output (BAO) is more than or equal to 15 mEq/hr (mmol/hr) for patients with an intact stomach (BAO more than or equal to 5 mEq/hr [mmol/hr] for patients with previous gastric surgery) or when hypergastrinemia is associated with a gastric pH value of more than or equal to 2.[95] In situations in which the serum gastrin is between 100 and 1,000 pg/mL (ng/L; 48 and 481 pmol/L) and gastric pH is less than or equal to 2, a secretin or calcium proactive test is used to aid the diagnosis.[95] Identification of the location of the tumor with imaging techniques is essential, as early surgical resection prior to liver metastases is often curative.[96] The widespread use of PPIs, although effective in reducing symptoms, may mask the clinical presentation and PPI-related hypergastrinemia may further complicate the diagnosis.

TREATMENT

With the development of H2RAs and PPIs, medical management of ZES is feasible in almost all patients. Because of their long duration of action and potency, PPIs are now the drugs of choice for treating gastric acid hypersecretion in patients with ZES.[95] Many of the PPIs (omeprazole, esomeprazole, lansoprazole, esomeprazole, rabeprazole, and pantoprazole) are effective in ZES. Initial doses of 80 mg/day of pantoprazole (or an equivalent dose of other available PPIs) given every 8 to 12 hours is most effective at controlling gastric acid hypersecretion and reliving symptoms. IV PPIs can be used for those patients who do not tolerate oral therapy. PPIs must be dose-adjusted in patients with ZES to normalize BAO levels to less than 15 mEq/hr (mmol/hr) or less than 5 mEq/hr (mmol/hr) in patients with reflux esophagitis or prior operations to reduce acid secretion, such as subtotal gastrectomy. PPI therapy can be gradually decreased after adequate control of hypersecretion is achieved.[95] Since 60% to 90% of gastrinomas are malignant, management of advanced disease may include surgical resection of primary and metastatic gastrinomas. Nonsurgical therapy may include treatment with chemotherapy, somatostatin analogues such as octreotide, interferon, and targeted-molecular therapies such as an mTor inhibitor (everolimus) or a tyrosine-kinase inhibitor (sunitinib).[95]

ABBREVIATIONS

ATPase	adenosine triphosphatase
BAO	basal acid output
CAP	community-acquired pneumonia
CLASS	Celecoxib Long-Term Arthritis Safety Study
COX	cyclooxygenase
COX-1	cyclooxygenase-1
COX-2	cyclooxygenase-2
CYP450	cytochrome P450
ECL	enterochromaffin-like
GERD	gastroesophageal reflux disease
H2RA	histamine-2 receptor antagonist
ICU	intensive care unit
IL	interleukin
INR	international normalized ratio
MALT	mucosa-associated lymphoid tissue
MAO	maximal acid output
MEN 1	multiple endocrine neoplasia type 1

NG	nasogastric
NSAID	nonsteroidal anti-inflammatory drug
NUD	nonulcer dyspepsia
PG	prostaglandin
PPI	proton pump inhibitor
PUD	peptic ulcer disease
SRMB	stress-related mucosal bleeding
SRMD	stress-related mucosal damage
TNF-α	tumor necrosis factor-α
UBT	urea breath test
ZES	Zollinger-Ellison syndrome

REFERENCES

1. Leja M, Grinberga-Derica I, Bilgilier C, Steininger C. Review: Epidemiology of *Helicobacter pylori* infection. *Helicobacter.* 2019;24 (Suppl 1):e12635.
2. Valle JD. Peptic ulcer disease and related disorders. In: Jameson JL, Fauci AS, Kasper DL, Hauser SL, Longo DL, Loscalzo J, eds. *Harrison's Principles of Internal Medicine, 20e.* New York, NY: McGraw Hill Education; 2018.
3. McQuaid KR. Peptic ulcer disease. In: Papadakis MA, McPhee SJ, Rabow MW, eds. *Current Medical Diagnosis & Treatment 2021.* New York, NY: McGraw Hill Education; 2021.
4. Love BL. Upper gastrointestinal disorders. In: Sutton SS, ed. *McGraw Hill's NAPLEX® Review Guide, 4e.* New York, NY: McGraw Hill Education; 2020.
5. Susstrunk J, Wartmann L, Mattiello D, Kostler T, Zingg U. Incidence and prognostic factors for the development of symptomatic and asymptomatic marginal ulcers after Roux-en-Y gastric bypass procedures. *Obes Surg.* 2021.
6. Peery AF, Crockett SD, Murphy CC, et al. Burden and cost of gastrointestinal, liver, and pancreatic diseases in the United States: Update 2018. *Gastroenterology.* 2019;156(1):254–272 e211.
7. Mentis A, Lehours P, Megraud F. Epidemiology and diagnosis of *Helicobacter pylori* infection. *Helicobacter.* 2015;20(Suppl 1):1–7.
8. Chey WD, Leontiadis GI, Howden CW, Moss SF. ACG Clinical Guideline: Treatment of *Helicobacter pylori* infection. *Am J Gastroenterol.* 2017;112(2):212–239.
9. Nguyen T, Ramsey D, Graham D, et al. The prevalence of *Helicobacter pylori* remains high in African American and Hispanic veterans. *Helicobacter.* 2015;20(4):305–315.
10. Tsang SH, Aviles-Santa ML, Abnet CC, et al. Seroprevalence and determinants of *Helicobacter pylori* infection in the Hispanic Community Health Study/Study of Latinos. *Clin Gastroenterol Hepatol.* 2021.
11. Bjarnason I, Scarpignato C, Holmgren E, Olszewski M, Rainsford KD, Lanas A. Mechanisms of damage to the gastrointestinal tract from nonsteroidal anti-inflammatory drugs. *Gastroenterology.* 2018;154(3):500–514.
12. Melcarne L, Garcia-Iglesias P, Calvet X. Management of NSAID-associated peptic ulcer disease. *Expert Rev Gastroenterol Hepatol.* 2016;10(6):723–733.
13. Kamboj AK, Cotter TG, Oxentenko AS. *Helicobacter pylori*: The past, present, and future in management. *Mayo Clin Proc.* 2017;92(4):599–604.
14. Mo C, Sun G, Lu ML, et al. Proton pump inhibitors in prevention of low-dose aspirin-associated upper gastrointestinal injuries. *World J Gastroenterol.* 2015;21(17):5382–5392.
15. Lanas A, Gargallo CJ. Management of low-dose aspirin and clopidogrel in clinical practice: A gastrointestinal perspective. *Journal of Gastroenterology.* 2015;50(6):626–637.
16. Lin XH, Young SH, Luo JC, et al. Risk factors for upper gastrointestinal bleeding in patients taking selective COX-2 inhibitors: A nationwide population-based cohort study. *Pain Medicine (Malden, Mass).* 2018;19(2):225–231.
17. Chen WC, Lin KH, Huang YT, et al. The risk of lower gastrointestinal bleeding in low-dose aspirin users. *Aliment Pharmacol Ther.* 2017;45(12):1542–1550.
18. Gwee KA, Goh V, Lima G, Setia S. Coprescribing proton-pump inhibitors with nonsteroidal anti-inflammatory drugs: Risks versus benefits. *J Pain Res.* 2018;11:361–374.
19. Sverden E, Agreus L, Dunn JM, Lagergren J. Peptic ulcer disease. *BMJ.* 2019;367:l5495.
20. Lanas A, Chan FKL. Peptic ulcer disease. *Lancet.* 2017;390(10094):613–624.
21. Masclee GM, Valkhoff VE, Coloma PM, et al. Risk of upper gastrointestinal bleeding from different drug combinations. *Gastroenterology.* 2014;147(4):784–792 e789; quiz e713-e784.
22. Jiang HY, Chen HZ, Hu XJ, et al. Use of selective serotonin reuptake inhibitors and risk of upper gastrointestinal bleeding: A systematic review and meta-analysis. *Clin Gastroenterol Hepatol.* 2015;13(1):42–50 e43.
23. Abrignani MG, Gatta L, Gabrielli D, et al. Gastroprotection in patients on antiplatelet and/or anticoagulant therapy: A position paper of National Association of Hospital Cardiologists (ANMCO) and the Italian Association of Hospital Gastroenterologists and Endoscopists (AIGO). *Eur J Intern Med.* 2021;85:1–13.
24. Cardoso RN, Benjo AM, DiNicolantonio JJ, et al. Incidence of cardiovascular events and gastrointestinal bleeding in patients receiving clopidogrel with and without proton pump inhibitors: An updated meta-analysis. *Open Heart.* 2015;2(1):e000248.
25. Alfredsson J, Neely B, Neely ML, et al. Predicting the risk of bleeding during dual antiplatelet therapy after acute coronary syndromes. *Heart (British Cardiac Society).* 2017;103(15):1168–1176.
26. Li JJ, Wu XY, Chen JL, et al. Antiplatelet drug ticagrelor delays gastric ulcer healing in rats. *Exp Ther Med.* 2017;14(4):3774–3779.
27. Li LF, Chan RL, Lu L, et al. Cigarette smoking and gastrointestinal diseases: The causal relationship and underlying molecular mechanisms (review). *Int J Mol Med.* 2014;34(2):372–380.
28. Zhang L, Ren JW, Wong CC, et al. Effects of cigarette smoke and its active components on ulcer formation and healing in the gastrointestinal mucosa. *Curr Med Chem.* 2012;19(1):63–69.
29. Melinder C, Udumyan R, Hiyoshi A, Brummer RJ, Montgomery S. Decreased stress resilience in young men significantly increases the risk of subsequent peptic ulcer disease—A prospective study of 233093 men in Sweden. *Aliment Pharmacol Ther.* 2015;41(10):1005–1015.
30. Lee YB, Yu J, Choi HH, et al. The association between peptic ulcer diseases and mental health problems: A population-based study: A STROBE compliant article. *Medicine (Baltimore).* 2017;96(34):e7828.
31. Waldum HL, Kleveland PM, Sordal OF. *Helicobacter pylori* and gastric acid: An intimate and reciprocal relationship. *Therap Adv Gastroenterol.* 2016;9(6):836–844.
32. Nejati S, Karkhah A, Darvish H, Validi M, Ebrahimpour S, Nouri HR. Influence of *Helicobacter pylori* virulence factors CagA and VacA on pathogenesis of gastrointestinal disorders. *Microb Pathog.* 2018;117:43–48.
33. Baj J, Forma A, Sitarz M, et al. *Helicobacter pylori* virulence factors—Mechanisms of bacterial pathogenicity in the gastric microenvironment. *Cells.* 2020;10(1).
34. Yang M, Wang HT, Zhao M, et al. Network meta-analysis comparing selective COX-2 inhibitors versus Coxibs for the prevention of NSAID-induced gastrointestinal injury. *Medicine (Baltimore).* 2015;94(40):e1592.
35. Samuel R, Bilal M, Tayyem O, Guturu P. Evaluation and management of gastrointestinal bleeding. *Dis Mon.* 2018.
36. Stern E, Sugumar K, Journey JD. Peptic ulcer perforated. In: *StatPearls.* Treasure Island (FL) 2021.
37. Kumar A, Annamaraju P. Gastric outlet obstruction. In: *StatPearls.* Treasure Island (FL) 2021.
38. Fashner J, Gitu AC. Diagnosis and treatment of peptic ulcer disease and *H. pylori* infection. *Am Fam Physician.* 2015;91(4):236–242.
39. Siddique O, Ovalle A, Siddique AS, Moss SF. *Helicobacter pylori* infection: An update for the internist in the age of increasing global antibiotic resistance. *Am J Med.* 2018;131(5):473–479.
40. Moayyedi PM, Lacy BE, Andrews CN, Enns RA, Howden CW, Vakil N. ACG and CAG Clinical Guideline: Management of dyspepsia. *Official Journal of the American College of Gastroenterology / ACG* 2017;112(7):988–1013.
41. Ferwana M, Abdulmajeed I, Alhajiahmed A, et al. Accuracy of urea breath test in *Helicobacter pylori* infection: Meta-analysis. *World J Gastroenterol.* 2015;21(4):1305–1314.
42. Kilincalp S, Ustun Y, Akinci H, Coban S, Yuksel I. Letter: Effect of proton pump inhibitor use on invasive detection of *Helicobacter pylori* gastritis. *Aliment Pharmacol Ther.* 2015;41(6):599.
43. Calvet X. Diagnosis of *Helicobacter pylori* infection in the proton pump inhibitor era. *Gastroenterol Clin North Am.* 2015;44(3):507–518.
44. Graham DY, Canaan Y, Maher J, Wiener G, Hulten KG, Kalfus IN. Rifabutin-Based Triple Therapy (RHB-105) for *Helicobacter pylori* eradication: A double-blind, randomized, controlled trial. *Ann Intern Med.* 2020;172(12):795–802.

45. Ghotaslou R, Leylabadlo HE, Asl YM. Prevalence of antibiotic resistance in *Helicobacter pylori*: A recent literature review. *World J Methodol.* 2015;5(3):164–174.
46. Aguilera Matos I, Diaz Oliva SE, Escobedo AA, Villa Jimenez OM, Velazco Villaurrutia YDC. *Helicobacter pylori* infection in children. *BMJ Paediatr Open.* 2020;4(1):e000679.
47. Dos Santos AA, Carvalho AA. Pharmacological therapy used in the elimination of *Helicobacter pylori* infection: A review. *World J Gastroenterol.* 2015;21(1):139–154.
48. Malfertheiner P, Megraud F, O'Morain CA, et al. Management of *Helicobacter pylori* infection—The Maastricht V/Florence Consensus Report. *Gut.* 2017;66(1):6–30.
49. Zhang L, Lan Y, Wang Q, Zhang Y, Si X. Application of minocycline-containing bismuth quadruple therapies as first-line regimens in the treatment of *Helicobacter pylori*. *Gastroenterol Res Pract.* 2019;2019:9251879.
50. Graham DY, Lee SY. How to effectively use bismuth quadruple therapy: The good, the bad, and the ugly. *Gastroenterol Clin North Am.* 2015;44(3):537–563.
51. Scarpignato C, Gatta L, Zullo A, et al. Effective and safe proton pump inhibitor therapy in acid-related diseases—A position paper addressing benefits and potential harms of acid suppression. *BMC Med.* 2016;14(1):179.
52. Yoon SB, Park JM, Lee JY, et al. Long-term pretreatment with proton pump inhibitor and *Helicobacter pylori* eradication rates. *World J Gastroenterol.* 2014;20(4):1061–1066.
53. Park JY, Dunbar KB, Mitui M, et al. Helicobacter pylori clarithromycin resistance and treatment failure are common in the USA. *Dig Dis Sci.* 2016;61(8):2373–2380.
54. Li BZ, Threapleton DE, Wang JY, et al. Comparative effectiveness and tolerance of treatments for *Helicobacter pylori*: Systematic review and network meta-analysis. *BMJ.* 2015;351:h4052.
55. Nyssen OP, McNicholl AG, Megraud F, et al. Sequential versus standard triple first-line therapy for *Helicobacter pylori* eradication. *Cochrane Database Syst Rev.* 2016(6):CD009034.
56. He L, Deng T, Luo H. Meta-analysis of sequential, concomitant and hybrid therapy for Helicobacter pylori eradication. *Intern Med.* 2015;54(7):703–710.
57. Song HY, Zhou L, Liu DY, Yao XJ, Li Y. What roles do probiotics play in the eradication of *Helicobacter pylori*? Current knowledge and ongoing research. *Gastroenterol Res Pract.* 2018;2018:9379480.
58. Ji J, Yang H. Using probiotics as supplementation for *Helicobacter pylori* antibiotic therapy. *Int J Mol Sci.* 2020;21(3):1136. doi: 10.3390/ijms21031136.
59. Hsu PI, Tsai FW, Kao SS, et al. Ten-day quadruple therapy comprising proton pump inhibitor, bismuth, tetracycline, and levofloxacin is more effective than standard levofloxacin triple therapy in the second-line treatment of *Helicobacter pylori* infection: A randomized controlled trial. *Am J Gastroenterol.* 2017;112(9):1374–1381.
60. Molina-Infante J, Shiotani A. Practical aspects in choosing a *Helicobacter pylori* therapy. *Gastroenterol Clin North Am.* 2015;44(3):519–535.
61. Fiorini G, Zullo A, Vakil N, et al. Rifabutin triple therapy is effective in patients with multidrug-resistant strains of *Helicobacter pylori*. *J Clin Gastroenterol.* 2018;52(2):137–140.
62. Boltin D, Levi Z, Gingold-Belfer R, et al. Impact of previous exposure to macrolide antibiotics on *Helicobacter pylori* infection treatment outcomes. *Am J Gastroenterol.* 2019;114(6):900–906.
63. Megraud F, Benejat L, Ontsira Ngoyi EN, Lehours P. Molecular approaches to identify *Helicobacter pylori* antimicrobial resistance. *Gastroenterol Clin North Am.* 2015;44(3):577–596.
64. Satoh K, Yoshino J, Akamatsu T, et al. Evidence-based clinical practice guidelines for peptic ulcer disease 2015. *J Gastroenterol.* 2016;51(3):177–194.
65. Bakhriansyah M, Souverein PC, de Boer A, Klungel OH. Gastrointestinal toxicity among patients taking selective COX-2 inhibitors or conventional NSAIDs, alone or combined with proton pump inhibitors: A case-control study. *Pharmacoepidemiol Drug Saf.* 2017;26(10):1141–1148.
66. Scally B, Emberson JR, Spata E, et al. Effects of gastroprotectant drugs for the prevention and treatment of peptic ulcer disease and its complications: A meta-analysis of randomised trials. *Lancet Gastroenterol Hepatol.* 2018;3(4):231–241.
67. Ali Khan M, Howden CW. The role of proton pump inhibitors in the management of upper gastrointestinal disorders. *Gastroenterol Hepatol (NY).* 2018;14(3):169–175.
68. Wong GLH, Lau LHS, Ching JYL, et al. Prevention of recurrent idiopathic gastroduodenal ulcer bleeding: A double-blind, randomised trial. *Gut.* 2020;69(4):652–657.
69. Kim HU. Diagnostic and treatment approaches for refractory peptic ulcers. *Clin Endosc.* 2015;48(4):285–290.
70. Kim J, Blackett JW, Jodorkovsky D. Strategies for effective discontinuation of proton pump inhibitors. *Curr Gastroenterol Rep.* 2018;20(6):27.
71. Orbelo DM, Enders FT, Romero Y, et al. Once-daily omeprazole/sodium bicarbonate heals severe refractory reflux esophagitis with morning or nighttime dosing. *Dig Dis Sci.* 2015;60(1):146–162.
72. Weersink RA, Bouma M, Burger DM, et al. Safe use of proton pump inhibitors in patients with cirrhosis. *British J Clin Pharmacol.* 2018;84(8):1806–1820.
73. Lewis JM, Stott KE, Monnery D, et al. Managing potential drug-drug interactions between gastric acid-reducing agents and antiretroviral therapy: Experience from a large HIV-positive cohort. *Int J STD AIDS.* 2016;27(2):105–109.
74. Lee TH, Chan A, Bryan W, et al. Proton pump inhibitor usage reduces sustained viral response rates for veterans with HIV/HCV coinfection on ledipasvir/sofosbuvir: A real-world study from a multicentre VA cohort. *J Viral Hepat.* 2021;28(4):630–636.
75. Skelin M, Lucijanic T, Amidzic Klaric D, et al. Factors affecting gastrointestinal absorption of levothyroxine: A review. *Clin Ther.* 2017;39(2):378–403.
76. Bouziana SD, Tziomalos K. Clinical relevance of clopidogrel-proton pump inhibitors interaction. *World J Gastrointest Pharmacol Ther.* 2015;6(2):17–21.
77. Vaduganathan M, Cannon CP, Cryer BL, et al. Efficacy and safety of proton-pump inhibitors in high-risk cardiovascular subsets of the COGENT trial. *Am J Med.* 2016;129(9):1002–1005.
78. Han YY, Li ZX, Duan R. Efficacy and safety of proton pump inhibitors combined with clopidogrel in patients undergoing percutaneous coronary intervention: A meta-analysis. *Rev Cardiovasc Med.* 2021;22(1):167–174.
79. Savarino V, Marabotto E, Furnari M, Zingone F, Zentilin P, Savarino E. Latest insights into the hot question of proton pump inhibitor safety—A narrative review. *Dig Liver Dis.* 2020;52(8):842–852.
80. Tsuda A, Suda W, Morita H, et al. Influence of proton-pump inhibitors on the luminal microbiota in the gastrointestinal tract. *Clin Transl Gastroenterol.* 2015;6:e89.
81. FDA Requests Removal of All Ranitidine Products (Zantac) from the Market. 2020; https://www.fda.gov/news-events/press-announcements/fda-requests-removal-all-ranitidine-products-zantac-market.
82. Wilkins T, Wheeler B, Carpenter M. Upper gastrointestinal bleeding in adults: Evaluation and management. *Am Fam Physician.* 2020;101(5):294–300.
83. Bardou M, Quenot JP, Barkun A. Stress-related mucosal disease in the critically ill patient. *Nat Rev Gastroenterol Hepatol.* 2015;12(2):98–107.
84. Klein A, Gralnek IM. Acute, nonvariceal upper gastrointestinal bleeding. *Curr Opin Crit Care.* 2015;21(2):154–162.
85. Laine L. CLINICAL PRACTICE. Upper gastrointestinal bleeding due to a peptic ulcer. *New Eng J Med.* 2016;374(24):2367–2376.
86. Alhazzani W, Alshamsi F, Belley-Cote E, et al. Efficacy and safety of stress ulcer prophylaxis in critically ill patients: A network meta-analysis of randomized trials. *Intensive Care Med.* 2018;44(1):1–11.
87. Laine L. Upper gastrointestinal bleeding due to a peptic ulcer. *New Eng J Med.* 2016;375(12):1198.
88. Tringali A, Manta R, Sica M, Bassotti G, Marmo R, Mutignani M. Comparing intravenous and oral proton pump inhibitor therapy for bleeding peptic ulcers following endoscopic management: A systematic review and meta-analysis. *British Journal of Clinical Pharmacology.* 2017;83(8):1619–1635.
89. Cook D, Guyatt G. Prophylaxis against upper gastrointestinal bleeding in hospitalized patients. *New Eng J Med.* 2018;378(26):2506–2516.
90. Barletta JF, Bruno JJ, Buckley MS, Cook DJ. Stress ulcer prophylaxis. *Crit Care Med.* 2016;44(7):1395–1405.
91. El-Kersh K, Jalil B, McClave SA, et al. Enteral nutrition as stress ulcer prophylaxis in critically ill patients: A randomized controlled exploratory study. *J Crit Care.* 2018;43:108–113.
92. Huang HB, Jiang W, Wang CY, Qin HY, Du B. Stress ulcer prophylaxis in intensive care unit patients receiving enteral nutrition: A systematic review and meta-analysis. *Crit Care.* 2018;22(1):20.
93. Lewis PO, Litchfield JM, Tharp JL, Garcia RM, Pourmorteza M, Reddy CM. Risk and severity of hospital-acquired *Clostridium difficile* infection in patients taking proton pump inhibitors. *Pharmacotherapy.* 2016;36(9):986–993.
94. Hammond DA, Kathe N, Shah A, Martin BC. Cost-effectiveness of histamine-2 receptor antagonists versus proton pump inhibitors for stress ulcer prophylaxis in critically ill patients. *Pharmacotherapy.* 2017;37(1):43–53.

95. Cho MS, Kasi A. Zollinger Ellison syndrome. In: *StatPearls*. Treasure Island (FL) 2021.
96. Shao QQ, Zhao BB, Dong LB, Cao HT, Wang WB. Surgical management of Zollinger-Ellison syndrome: Classical considerations and current controversies. *World J Gastroenterol.* 2019;25(32):4673–4681.
97. Ziyad Al-Aly, Maddukuri Geetha, Xie Yan. Proton pump inhibitors and the kidney: Implications of current evidence for clinical practice and when and how to deprescribe. *Am J Kidney Dis.* 2020;75(4):497–507.

52

Inflammatory Bowel Disease

Brian A. Hemstreet

KEY CONCEPTS

1 The exact cause of inflammatory bowel disease (IBD) is unknown. Proposed causes include infectious, genetic, and environmental factors, as well as alterations in intestinal epithelium function and systemic immune dysregulation.

2 Ulcerative colitis (UC) is confined to the rectum and colon, causes continuous lesions, and affects primarily the mucosa and the submucosa. Crohn's disease (CD) can involve any part of the GI tract, often causes discontinuous (skip) lesions, and is a transmural process that can result in fistulas, perforations, abscesses, or strictures.

3 Common GI complications of IBD include rectal fissures, fistulas (CD), perirectal abscess (UC), toxic megacolon (UC), and colon cancer. Extraintestinal manifestations include hepatobiliary complications, arthritis, uveitis, skin lesions (including erythema nodosum and pyoderma gangrenosum), osteoporosis, anemia, and aphthous ulcerations of the mouth.

4 The severity of UC may be assessed by stool frequency, presence of blood in stool, fever, pulse, hemoglobin, erythrocyte sedimentation rate (ESR), C-reactive protein (CRP), abdominal tenderness, and radiologic or endoscopic findings. The severity of CD can be assessed using similar parameters, in addition to the CD Activity Index, which includes stool frequency, presence of blood in stool, endoscopic appearance, and physician's global assessment.

5 The goals of IBD treatment are resolution of acute inflammation and complications, alleviation of systemic manifestations, maintenance of remission, and improvement in quality of life (QOL).

6 The first line of treatment for mild-to-moderate extensive UC consists of oral aminosalicylates (ASAs) or oral controlled-release budesonide with prednisone as an alternative. Mesalamine enemas or suppositories are preferred for distal disease. Mesalamine is less effective for CD. Controlled-release budesonide or a tapering course of prednisone with or without azathioprine is preferred as a first-line agent for mild-to-moderate CD confined to the terminal ileum and/or ascending colon. Patients with more diffuse disease can be managed by a tapering course of prednisone with or with azathioprine.

7 Systemic corticosteroids are often required for acute moderate to severe UC or CD. The duration of steroid use should be minimized and the dose tapered gradually over 3 to 4 weeks if possible.

8 Infliximab, adalimumab, golimumab, ozanimod, and vedolizumab are treatment options for high-risk or moderate-to-severe active UC in outpatients and for those patients with UC who are corticosteroid dependent. Azathioprine or mercaptopurine may be used for maintenance of remission in UC as an alternative to or in combination with tumor necrosis factor-alpha (TNF-α) inhibitors, and in patients failing ASAs or with corticosteroid dependency. Vedolizumab with or without an immunomodulator may also be used as initial therapy or for patients failing TNF-α inhibitors. Tofacitinib is used for patients with moderate-to-severe UC who have failed TNF-α inhibitors.

9 IV continuous infusion of cyclosporine or infliximab may be effective in treating severe colitis that is refractory to corticosteroids as an option to delay or prevent the need for surgery.

10 Aminosalicylates may prevent recurrence of acute UC in many patients, while corticosteroids are ineffective for this purpose.

11 Treatments for high-risk or moderate-to-severe CD include infliximab, adalimumab, certolizumab, and vedolizumab. Methotrexate, azathioprine, or mercaptopurine may be used for inadequate response or to reduce steroid dosage and in combination with TNF-α inhibitors; ustekimumab (patients failing other therapies); metronidazole (for perineal or colonic disease); and cyclosporine (for refractory disease) may be used.

BEYOND THE BOOK

Several online resources about IBD are available for both patients and providers. Visit the Crohn's and Colitis Foundation webcast (http://www.crohnscolitisfoundation.org/resources/webcasts.html) and watch one the following videos.

a. IBD: Diet and nutrition
b. "Ulcerative Colitis 101"
c. "Crohn's Disease 101"
d. Comprehensive Care for IBD Wellness: Integrating Diet and Complementary Therapies

Identify three things you would use to educate a patient with IBD based on the information provided in the video.

INTRODUCTION

There are two forms of idiopathic inflammatory bowel disease (IBD): (a) ulcerative colitis (UC), a mucosal inflammatory condition confined to the rectum and colon, and (b) Crohn's disease (CD), a transmural inflammation of the GI tract that can affect any part, from the mouth to the anus.

EPIDEMIOLOGY

IBD is most prevalent in Western countries and in areas of northern latitude.[1] Rates of IBD are highest in North America, Northern Europe, and Great Britain.[1,2] The incidence of IBD is increasing worldwide, especially in Westernized and newly industrialized countries.[2-4] CD has an incidence of 6 to 15.5 cases per 100,000 persons per year and a prevalence of 3.6 to 214 per 100,000 persons per year.[1,2] The incidence of UC ranges from 1.2 to 20 cases per 100,000 persons per year with a prevalence of 7.6 to 246 per 100,000 persons per year.[1] Although most epidemiologic studies combine ulcerative proctitis with UC, 17% to 49% of cases are classified as proctitis.

Both sexes are affected somewhat equally with IBD, although 20% to 30% more women are affected with CD and slightly more males (60%) are affected with UC.[2] Both UC and CD tend to have bimodal distributions in age of initial presentation. The peak incidence generally occurs in the second (CD) or third (UC) decade of life, with a second peak occurring between 60 and 70 years of age.[1-3] A higher incidence of IBD occurs in the Jewish population, while Black and Asian patients have a relatively similar, and possibly lower, incidence of IBD compared to White pateints.[2-4]

ETIOLOGY

1 The exact etiology of UC and CD is unknown; however, there are similar factors believed responsible for both conditions. The major theories behind the cause of IBD involve a combination of infectious, genetic, environmental, and immunologic factors. This may involve abnormal regulation of the innate immune response or a reaction to various antigens.[4-7] The microflora of the GI tract may provide an environmental trigger to activate inflammation in genetically susceptible individuals and is highly implicated in the development of IBD.[4,7]

Infectious Factors

Microorganisms are proposed to be a major factor in the initiation of inflammation in IBD. In general, there is thought to be shift toward the presence of more proinflammatory bacteria in the GI tract, often referred to as dysbiosis.[5-7] Patients with IBD have a decreased number, richness, and diversity of intestinal microbiotica compared with those without IBD as well as increases in aggressive bacterial groups and presence of mucosal and intraepithelial bacteria.[1,5-7] The development and composition of the intestinal microbiotica may also be influenced by dietary factors.[8] The pathogenesis of IBD may involve a loss of tolerance toward normal GI bacterial flora.[1,5-7]

Microorganisms may play a key role in the development of IBD. Suspect infectious agents include viruses, protozoans, mycobacteria such as *Mycobacterium paratuberculosis* or *avium*, and other bacteria such as *Ruminococcus gnavus*, *Ruminococcus torques*, *Listeria monocytogenes*, *Fusobacterium varium*, *Chlamydia trachomatis*, and adherent invasive *Escherichia coli*.[4-10] Patients with CD typically have circulating antibodies to *Saccharomyces cerevisiae*, which demonstrates some immunologic response to intestinal organisms.[5] Bacterial gene products may promote alteration of the intestinal barrier while bacterial antigens or ligands may include and propagate the inflammatory response.[5-7,10] Appendectomy has been associated with an increase in the risk of CD in White and Middle Eastern patients, while being protective against UC in White patients.[2]

Genetic Factors

Genetic factors play a significant role in the predisposition to IBD. Studies of monozygotic twins demonstrate a high concordance rate of IBD in both individuals (particularly CD).[1,12] First-degree relatives of patients with IBD may have up to a 20-fold increase in the risk of disease and risk is extended to second- and third-degree relatives.[5,13] The nucleotide-binding oligomerization domain protein 2 (NOD2), a key component involved in pathogen recognition in the innate immune system, is a major contributor of genetic predisposition to CD.[4,10,11] Other genes involved in the innate immune system autophagy, such as ATG16L1 and IRGM, as well as genes involved in the interleukin (IL) biologic pathway such as polymorphisms of the IL-23 receptor IL-23R, and IL-12B, STAT3, and CCR6, are strongly associated with CD and possibly UC (IL-23R).[1,5,10,11] The major genetic region for UC is on chromosome 6p21, in the major histocompatibility region, near human leukocyte antigen (HLA) class II genes.[10] Alterations in the genes encoding for IL-10 and the IL-10 receptor have been implicated in UC.[10,11] Emerging areas of interest in IBD pathogenesis are the role of microRNAs and the interface between environmental factors and peroxisome proliferator-activated receptors (PPARs).[12,13]

Immunologic Mechanisms

Potential immunologic mechanisms contributing to IBD include both autoimmune and nonautoimmune phenomena. NOD proteins involved in recognition of organisms and toll-like membrane receptors (TLRs) are involved in intestinal surveillance and can lead to release of antibacterial peptides such as defensins, among other functions.[1,5] Reduction in defensin secretion by Paneth cells is thought to be one contributing factor in the loss of effective intestinal barrier function.[5,14] Consequently, the bowel wall in CD is infiltrated with lymphocytes, plasma cells, mast cells, macrophages, and neutrophils, often leading to formation of granulomas. Similar infiltration has been observed in the colonic mucosal layer in patients with UC. Given that inflammation is limited to the colon in UC, dysfunction of colonocytes is highly implicated.[1] The colonic mucosal layer in UC may be thinner and less effective in protecting the epithelial cells. This may be due to reduced mucin secretion secondary to defective goblet cell differentiation.[1,5] Autoimmune features may be directed against mucosal epithelial cells or against neutrophil cytoplasmic elements. Innate lymphoid cells are also thought to possibly play a role in IBD pathogenesis.[1,5]

Antineutrophil cytoplasmic antibodies are found in a high percentage of patients with UC (70%) and less frequently in CD.[1,3,6,10] Overproduction of circulating IgG1 antibodies in UC may react with epithelium in the eyes, skin, joints, and biliary tract.[1] Dysfunction or reduced expression of the PPAR γ in colonocytes may play a role in this process.[1,13]

Th1 cytokine activity is excessive in CD and increased expression of interferon-γ in the intestinal mucosa and excess production of IL-12, IL-17A, and IL-22 are features of the immune response in CD.[3,5,10] In contrast, Th2 cytokine activity is excessive with UC.[1,5] This is mediated by excess production of IL-13, which contributes to epithelial cell dysfunction by enhancing natural killer T-cell cytotoxicity, and IL-5, which is involved with eosinophil recruitment and activation.[1] Activated epithelial cells secrete a variety of substances involved in the recruitment of inflammatory cells, including IL-1β, epithelial neutrophil-activating peptide 78, IL-8, and monocyte chemoattractant protein 1.[1]

Tumor necrosis factor-alpha (TNF-α) is a pivotal proinflammatory cytokine that is increased in the mucosa and intestinal lumen of patients with CD and UC. TNF-α can recruit inflammatory cells to inflamed tissues, activate coagulation, promote the formation of granulomas in patients with CD, and possibly modify epithelial cell apoptosis.[1,3,5,10]

Psychological Factors

Complex interactions between the enteric and central nervous systems, as well as contributions from the endocrine and immune systems can lead to alterations in secretion, mobility, and alterations in the intestinal barrier in patients with IBD.[15,16] Mental health changes, particularly stress, possibly correlate with disease flares in IBD, but whether psychological factors are true etiologic factors in the pathophysiologic process is unclear.[15-17] Pain, anxiety, and depression are more common in patients with IBD compared to the general population, and are reported in up to 19% to 21% of patients.[15] In some instances symptoms of mood disorders, such as anxiety, may precede the onset of IBD symptoms.[16] Perceived stress has a great bearing on frequency of symptomatic flares.[17] While perceived stress and psychological factors may not be a direct cause of IBD, they significantly affect QOL.[16] This is compounded by the need for surgical intervention and temporary or permanent ostomy placement in young patients. Patients should be screened for the presence of anxiety and depression as part of their ongoing assessment, and have ongoing assessment of their QOL. Stress reduction should be an integral part of the treatment approach for IBD symptoms.[16]

Lifestyle, Dietary, and Drug-Related Causes

Several theories regarding dietary influence on the development of IBD have been proposed. Intake of refined sugars and animal fats has been associated with development of CD, while increased protein intake has been associated with a higher risk of developing IBD.[8,9] Diet composition and food derivatives may directly influence the makeup of the gut microbiotica, alter intestinal permeability, and affect immune function possibly triggering IBD.[8,9] Diets low in fruits and vegetables and high in ω-6 polyunsaturated fats may increase the risk of CD.[8] Changes in expression of the aryl hydrocarbon receptor, a transcription factor activated by dietary ligands and involved in the maintenance of the innate immune response, may increase development of IBD.[8] Interest has arisen in vitamin D deficiency as a possible cause of IBD given that vitamin D is involved with NOD2 gene induction.[9] Diets low in fermentable oligo-, di-, and monosaccharides and polyols, referred to as FODMAPs, improve IBD symptoms in some patients by reducing the osmotic load and fermentation of these sugars.[8] Tea or coffee consumption are protective against development of IBD in Asian patients.[2,8]

Smoking plays an important but contrasting role in UC and CD. It appears to be protective for UC and is associated with fewer disease flare-ups and reduced disease severity.[1,2,10] The risk of developing UC is increased for 2 to 3 years after smoking cessation in patients without IBD. In contrast, smoking is associated with increased frequency and severity of CD, and appears to worsen ileal disease more than colonic.[4,10] Patients with CD who stop smoking have a disease severity that is similar to nonsmokers. Smoking cessation should be offered to all patients. There are data to support transdermal nicotine replacement as an adjunctive therapy in UC.[18]

Use of nonsteroidal anti-inflammatory drugs (NSAIDs) may trigger disease occurrence or lead to disease flares by impairing mucosal barrier protective mechanisms.[25,30] Alteration in platelet function, release of inflammatory mediators, and alteration in the microvascular response to stress are other potential mechanisms of worsening of IBD. Cyclooxygenase-2 inhibitors and cyclooxygenase-1 inhibitors increase risk; however, it is unclear whether cyclooxygenase-2 inhibitors may be safer in select patients with IBD.[2] Despite the association between NSAID use and IBD flares, there is conflicting evidence regarding the consistency of this association.[19] There was no major impact on clinical outcomes with daily use of aspirin in patients with IBD.[20] Use of NSAIDs may be warranted in some patients with IBD, particularly those with arthritic symptoms, if the benefit outweighs the potential risk of disease flare. Oral contraceptives may also confer increased risk of IBD in susceptible patients.[22,23]

Development of IBD in White patients is associated with antibiotic use in childhood, while risk may be reduced in Asian and Middle Eastern patients.[2] There is a higher association of antibiotic use with development of CD.[21] Since antibiotics alter the intestinal flora, this appears to be a viable mechanism; however, delineating antibiotics as a causative factor is difficult given that symptoms may not manifest for several weeks to years following a treatment course. Furthermore, antibiotics may induce *Clostridioides difficile* infection, which is a cause of colitis. Patients presenting with severe diarrhea for whom a diagnosis of IBD is being entertained should be asked about recent antibiotics, and should be tested for *C. difficile* infection.

PATHOPHYSIOLOGY

UC and CD differ in two general respects: the extent and distribution of inflammation within the GI tract and depth of involvement within the bowel wall. Confusion in the diagnosis can occur, particularly when the inflammation is limited to the colon. For patients in whom it cannot be determined whether they have UC or CD, they are often classified as indeterminate colitis.[1] Table 52-1 compares pathologic and clinical findings of the two diseases.

Ulcerative Colitis

2 Ulcerative colitis is confined to the rectum and colon and affects the mucosal and the submucosal layers. The disease distribution upon initial diagnosis is 30% to 60% proctitis, 16% to 45% left-sided colitis, and 14% to 35% have extensive colitis, also referred to as pancolitis.[1] In some instances, a short segment of terminal ileum may be inflamed; this is referred to as *backwash ileitis*. Unlike CD, the deeper longitudinal muscular layers, serosa, and regional lymph nodes are not usually involved.[1] Fistula, perforation, or obstruction is uncommon because of the more superficial pattern of inflammation.

In UC, abscesses form in the crypts of the mucosa occurs (crypts of Lieberkuhn) secondary to infiltration of lymphocytes, plasma cells, and granulocytes.[1] Crypt abscesses are usually visible only with microscopy but may be visible when coalescence results in ulceration. Extension and coalescence of ulcers may surround

TABLE 52-1 Comparison of the Clinical and Pathologic Features of Crohn's Disease and Ulcerative Colitis

Feature	Crohn's Disease	Ulcerative Colitis
Clinical		
Malaise, fever	Common	Uncommon
Rectal bleeding	Common	Common
Abdominal tenderness	Common	May be present
Abdominal mass	Common	Absent
Abdominal pain	Common	Unusual
Abdominal wall and internal fistulas	Common	Absent
Distribution	Discontinuous	Continuous
Aphthous or linear ulcers	Common	Rare
Pathologic		
Rectal involvement	Rare	Common
Ileal involvement	Very common	Rare
Strictures	Common	Rare
Fistulas	Common	Rare
Transmural involvement	Common	Rare
Crypt abscesses	Rare	Very common
Granulomas	Common	Rare
Linear clefts	Common	Rare
Cobblestone appearance	Common	Absent

areas of uninvolved mucosa, causing *pseudopolyp* formation. Mucosal damage and friability in UC can result in significant diarrhea and bleeding, although a small percentage of patients experience constipation.

3 Complications of UC may be local, including hemorrhoids, anal fissures, or perirectal abscesses, and are more likely to be present during active colitis.

A major complication is toxic megacolon, which is a segmental or total colonic distension of greater than 6 cm with acute colitis and signs of systemic toxicity.[1,24] It occurs in up to 7.9% of UC patients admitted to hospitals and results in death rates of up to 8% if not medically or surgically treated.[24] Patients typically have a high fever, tachycardia, distended abdomen, elevated white blood cell count, and a dilated colon observed on x-ray.[24] Colonic perforation may occur with or without toxic megacolon and is a greater risk with the first episode. Another infrequent major complication is massive colonic hemorrhage. Colonic stricture, sometimes with clinical obstruction, may also complicate long-standing UC.

The risk of colonic dysplasia with transition to colorectal carcinoma (CRC) is two to six times greater for patients with chronic UC with colonic involvement compared with the general population.[25] CRC is responsible for 10% to 15% of deaths in patients with UC.[26] Patients with ulcerative proctitis or proctosigmoiditis are generally not considered to be at increased risk.[25,26] The cumulative risk of developing CRC in patients with chronic UC may be as high as 8% at 20 years.[26] Risk factors for CRC include young age at onset, longer duration of disease, greater extent of colonic involvement, presence of primary sclerosing colangitis (PSC), active histological inflammation, family history of a first-degree relative diagnosed with CRC prior to age 50, history of dysplasia, colonic strictures, pseudopolyps, a shortened tubular colon, and male gender.[26] Screening colonoscopy with multiple biopsies should be performed at 8 years after onset of pancolitis or 15 years following onset of left-sided UC or CD-related colitis.[32,33] Patients with PSC, extensive colitis with active endoscopic or histologic inflammation, a history of dysplasia, or a family history of a first-degree relative diagnosed with CRC prior to age 5 should undergo yearly colonoscopy.[26]

Crohn's Disease

Crohn's disease is characterized as a transmural inflammatory process. The terminal ileum is the most common site of the disorder, but it may occur in any part of the GI tract from mouth to anus.[3,10,27,28] Patients often have areas of normal bowel separating segments of diseased bowel resulting in discontinuous disease. The "cobblestone" appearance of the bowel wall results from deep mucosal ulceration intermingled with nodular submucosal thickening.

Small bowel stricture and subsequent obstruction is a complication that may require surgery. Fistula formation is also common, occurring much more frequently than with UC.[10,27] Fistulas often occur in highly inflamed areas, where loops of bowel become matted together by fibrous adhesions. Perianal fistulas may occur in up to 26% of patients within 20 years of diagnosis.[27] Fistulas may connect a segment of the GI tract to skin (enterocutaneous), two segments of the GI tract (enteroenteric), or the intestinal tract with the bladder (enterovesicular) or vagina.

Bleeding with CD is usually not as severe as with UC, although patients with CD may develop hypochromic anemia. The risk of carcinoma is increased but not as greatly as with UC; however, patients with CD and a personal history of dysplasia or PSC are at higher risk, and chromoendoscopy should be used during colonscopy.[26]

Nutritional deficiencies are common with CD.[28-30] Reported deficiencies include folate, vitamin B_{12}, vitamins A and D, calcium, magnesium, iron, and zinc.[37] Major contributing factors include decreased food intake, intestinal loss, malabsorption, hypermetabolic state, drug-nutrient interactions, and those receiving long-term total parenteral nutrition.[28-30]

Extraintestinal Manifestations of IBD

Both forms of IBD are associated with development of symptoms and organ involvement outside of the GI tract referred to as extraintestinal manifestations.

Hepatobiliary Complications

Hepatobiliary complications are commonly found in patients with IBD.[1,27,31-33] Hepatic complications include non-alcoholic fatty liver disease, pericholangitis, autoimmune hepatitis, liver abscess, and cirrhosis. Biliary complications include PSC, cholangiocarcinoma, and cholelithiasis.[1,31,32] Fatty infiltration of the liver may result from malabsorption, protein-losing enteropathy, or corticosteroid use, and may be found in up to 50% of patients with IBD.[31] PSC is associated with progressive fibrosis of intrahepatic and extrahepatic bile ducts in 4% of patients with UC.[31] Cirrhosis may result from cholangitis or chronic active hepatitis. Often the severity of hepatic disease does not correlate with GI disease activity. Gallstones occur in up to 34% of patients with CD (particularly with terminal ileal disease) and are related to bile salt malabsorption.[31,32]

Joint Complications

Both peripheral and axial arthropathies may be present in patients with IBD. Peripheral arthritis is typically asymmetric, oligoarticular, non-erosive, and occurs in 5% to 20% of patients.[32,33] Symptoms may present prior to GI symptoms of IBD. Axial arthropathies include sacroiliitis, ankylosing spondylitis, and IBD-associated spondyloarthropathy. The prognosis is not as favorable as peripheral arthritis, as progression is common. Patients with axial involvement should be referred to a rheumatologist in order to assist in the disease management.[32]

Ocular Complications

Ocular complications including dry eye, blepharitis, iritis, uveitis, episcleritis, and conjunctivitis occur in up to 29% of patients with IBD.[1,32,33] Commonly reported symptoms with iritis and uveitis include blurred vision, eye pain, and photophobia. Episcleritis is associated with scleral injection, burning, and increased secretions. These complications may parallel the severity of intestinal disease, and recurrence after colectomy with UC is uncommon.

Dermatologic and Mucocutaneous Complications

Skin and mucosal lesions associated with IBD include erythema nodosum, pyoderma gangrenosum, aphthous ulceration, and Sweet's syndrome.[32,33] Raised, red, tender nodules on the tibial surfaces of the legs and arms that vary in size from 1 to 5 cm are manifestations of erythema nodosum, and may occur in 4.2% to 7.5% of patients with IBD.[39]

Pyoderma gangrenosum occurs in 0.6% to 2% of patients with IBD and is characterized by skin pustules that progress to a burrowing ulcer with violaceous edges, ranging between 2 and 20 cm.[1,32,33] They can be seen on any part of the body but commonly occur on the lower extremities.

Oral lesions are found in 4% to 20% of patients with IBD.[32,33] The most common lesion seen with CD is aphthous stomatitis. The severity of these lesions tends to parallel the disease course. Sweet's syndrome, also known as acute febrile neutrophilic dermatosis, is characterized by tender erythematous skin lesions secondary to dermal neutrophil infiltration, and is often associated with fever and a distribution on the upper trunk, face, neck, and arms.[32,33]

Hematologic, Coagulation, Pulmonary, and Metabolic Abnormalities

Patients with IBD may develop anemia, with a prevalence reported up to 74%.[1,29,32,33] The anemia may present as iron deficiency related to chronic blood loss, ongoing inflammation, malnutrition, hemolysis, or bone marrow suppression from drug treatment.[32,33] Alternatively, it may be more characteristic of anemia of chronic disease. Patients with IBD are at a 1.5 to 3.6 times higher risk of venous thromboembolism (VTE) compared with the general population.[32] This is secondary to activation of the clotting cascade and platelet activation secondary to inflammation. Occurrence of VTE is higher during disease flares and occurs more often in peripheral veins.[1,32,33] Patients should be considered for pharmacologic VTE prophylaxis when admitted to the hospital for a disease flare. Patients with IBD may be at increased risk for metabolic bone disease. Osteopenia may be present in 32% to 36% of patients, while osteoporosis is reported in 2% to 15%.[33,34] Bone disease may be related to a combination of nutritional deficiencies, especially calcium and vitamin D, chronic cytokine-related inflammatory effects on bone, disease-associated hypogonadism, and use of corticosteroids.[33,34] Pulmonary manifestations occur from the glottis all the way to the small airways, but most commonly involve the large airways and may include cryptogenic organizing pneumonia, bronchiectasis, and bronchiolitis obliterans.[32]

CLINICAL PRESENTATION

Inflammatory Bowel Disease

The patterns of clinical presentation of IBD can vary widely. Patients may have a single acute episode that resolves and does not recur, but most patients experience acute flares with alternating periods of remission.

Ulcerative Colitis

There is a wide range of presenting symptoms in UC, ranging from mild abdominal cramping with frequent small-volume bowel movements to profuse diarrhea (Table 52-2). Most patients with UC experience intermittent bouts of illness after varying intervals of remission.

4 While various disease classifications for UC exist, a standard disease severity scoring system is not universally accepted.[1,18,35] The American College of Gastroenterology (ACG) UC Activity Index uses designations of mild, moderate-severe, and fulminant disease activity using clinical signs and symptoms and laboratory data[18]:

1. Mild: Fewer than four stools daily, with intermittent blood, mild or occasional urgency, normal erythrocyte sedimentation rate (ESR <30 mm/hr [8.3 μm/s]), normal hemoglobin, and elevated C-reactive protein (CRP) and fecal calprotectin (FC).
2. Moderate-Severe: More than six stools per day with frequent blood and urgency, fever, tachycardia, anemia, elevated CRP and FC, ESR greater than 30 mm/hr (8.3 μm/s).
3. Fulminant: More than 10 bowel movements per day with continuous bleeding and urgency, toxicity, abdominal tenderness, requirement for transfusion, elevated CRP and FC, and possible colonic dilation.

Guidelines from the American Gastroenterological Association (AGA) focusing specifically on moderate-to-severe UC utilize similar definitions; however, they define a subset of severe patients with acute severe UC (ASUC) as requiring hospitalization and having greater than six bloody stools per day and at least one marker of systemic toxicity, including heart rate greater than 90 beats per minutes, temperature greater than 37.8°C, hemoglobin less than 10.5 g/dL (105 g/L; 6.52 mmol/L), and/or ESR greater than 30 mm/hr (8.3 μm/s).[35]

A clinical care pathway for UC assesses the severity of UC based on risk for colectomy.[36] Patients are stratified according to low risk for colectomy (limited anatomic extent and mild endoscopic disease) or high risk for colectomy (extensive colitis, age less than 40 years, deep ulcers, high ESR/CRP, steroid dependence, history of hospitalization, and *C. difficile* or cytomegalovirus infection).

Determining disease extent, that is, which sections of the colon are involved, is important. This is accomplished via endoscopy. Patients with "distal" disease have inflammation limited to areas distal to the splenic flexure (also referred to as *left-sided* disease), while those with "extensive disease" have inflammation extending proximal to the splenic flexure.[1,18] Inflammation confined to the rectal area is referred to as *proctitis*, while disease involving the rectum and sigmoid colon is referred to as *proctosigmoiditis*. Inflammation of the majority of the colon is called *extensive disease*, sometimes referred to as *pancolitis*. Disease activity may be assessed upon endoscopy using common scoring systems, such as the UCEIS or Mayo Score.[18]

The diagnosis of UC is made on clinical suspicion and confirmed by biopsy, stool examinations, sigmoidoscopy or colonoscopy, or barium radiographic contrast studies.[35,37] Evaluation of CRP, and FC, a protein released during leukocyte trafficking, may also assist in identifying the presence of intestinal inflammation, and are also helpful in monitoring response to therapy.[37] The presence of extraintestinal manifestations may also aid in establishing the diagnosis.[1,18,32,33]

Crohn's Disease

The time between the onset of CD complaints and the initial diagnosis may be as long as 3 years. The patient typically presents with diarrhea and abdominal pain. Hematochezia occurs in about one-half of patients with colonic involvement and much less frequently when there is no colonic involvement. A patient may first present with a perirectal or perianal lesions, or extraintestinal manifestations in up to 50% of cases[10] (Table 52-3). The diagnosis should also be suspected in children with growth retardation, especially with abdominal complaints.

TABLE 52-2 Clinical Presentation of Ulcerative Colitis

Signs and symptoms
- Abdominal cramping
- Frequent bowel movements, often with blood in the stool
- Weight loss
- Fever and tachycardia in severe disease
- Blurred vision, eye pain, and photophobia with ocular involvement
- Arthritis
- Raised, red, tender nodules that vary in size from 1 cm to several centimeters

Physical examination
- Hemorrhoids, anal fissures, or perirectal abscesses may be present
- Iritis, uveitis, episcleritis, and conjunctivitis with ocular involvement
- Dermatologic findings with erythema nodosum, pyoderma gangrenosum, or aphthous ulceration

Laboratory tests
- Decreased hematocrit/hemoglobin
- Increased ESR, CRP, and fecal calprotectin
- Leukocytosis and hypoalbuminemia with severe disease
- (+) perinuclear antineutrophil cytoplasmic antibodies

TABLE 52-3 Clinical Presentation of Crohn's Disease

Signs and symptoms
- Malaise and fever
- Abdominal pain
- Frequent bowel movements
- Hematochezia
- Fistula
- Weight loss and malnutrition
- Arthritis

Physical examination
- Abdominal mass and tenderness
- Perianal fissure or fistula

Laboratory tests
- Increased white blood cell count, ESR, CRP, and fecal calprotectin
- (+) anti-*Saccharomyces cerevisiae* antibodies

Much like UC, global classification guidelines for scoring severity of active CD are not available. For patients with luminal nonfistulizing CD, the Crohn's Disease Activity Index (CDAI) is used most often to gauge response to therapy and determine remission and is employed mostly in the research setting. This score system ranges from 0 to 600, with score greater than 150 defined as active disease. The Harvey-Bradshaw Index (HBI) is another scoring system that is also used for CD, and tends to correlate well with the CDAI. A decrease of 3 points in the HBI is defined as a clinical response with complete remission defined as a score of less than 4. Treatment guidelines use the presence of signs and symptoms as their marker for disease activity and severity.[27]

The classification of CD severity is similar to UC.[3,10,27] Patients with mild-to-moderate CD are typically ambulatory and have no evidence of dehydration, systemic toxicity, less than 10% loss of body weight, or abdominal tenderness, mass, or obstruction. This correlates to a CDAI of 150 to 220. Moderate-to-severe disease is considered in patients who fail to respond to treatment for mild-to-moderate disease or those with fever, weight loss, abdominal pain or tenderness, vomiting, intestinal obstruction, or significant anemia. Severe-to-fulminant CD is classified as the presence of persistent symptoms or evidence of systemic toxicity despite corticosteroid or biologic treatment or presence of cachexia, rebound tenderness, intestinal obstruction, or abscess with a CDAI more than 450. Disease activity may be assessed and correlated by evaluation of CRP concentrations.

Similar to UC, the AGA has developed a clinical decision support tool for assessing CD severity.[38] Patients are stratified as low risk (age at initial diagnosis over 30 years, limited anatomic involvement, no perianal and/or severe rectal disease, superficial ulcers, no prior surgical resection, and no stricturing and/or penetrating disease) or moderate to high risk (age at initial diagnosis less than 30 years, extensive anatomic involvement, perianal and/or severe rectal disease, deep ulcers, prior surgical resection, stricturing and/or penetrating disease).

The course of CD is characterized by periods of remission and exacerbation. Patients may be symptom-free for years, while others experience chronic symptoms in spite of medical therapy. As with UC, the diagnosis of CD involves a thorough evaluation using laboratory, endoscopic, and radiologic testing to detect the extent and characteristic features of the disease.[10,27,37,38] Small bowel involvement, strictures detected on radiographs, and presence of fistulae are characteristic of CD.

TREATMENT

Desired Outcomes

5 The clinician must have a clear concept of realistic therapeutic goals for each patient with IBD. Goals may relate to resolution of acute inflammatory processes, resolution and prevention of complications (eg, fistulae, abscesses, and CRC), alleviation of extraintestinal manifestations, maintenance of remission, or surgical palliation or cure.

When determining goals of therapy and selecting therapeutic regimens, it is important to understand the natural history of IBD.[1,18,27,39] Some cases of acute UC are self-limited. Following remission, up to 43% of patients may experience relapse in the first year, and almost half may require hospitalization at some point during their disease course.[39] Being young at the time diagnosis, female sex, presence of extraintestinal manifestations, nonsmoking status, and higher levels of education have been associated with higher risk of relapse.[39] With severe colitis, improvement without treatment cannot be expected. The response to medical management of toxic megacolon is variable and emergent colectomy may be required. CD tends to be progressive and destructive, with only 20% to 30% having an indolent course.[3,9,27] Patients at risk for progression of CD include young age at diagnosis, extensive bowel involvement, perianal or severe rectal disease, or stenosis.[27] Up to 80% of patients will require hospitalization at some point during their disease course, and there are high rates of steroid dependence and the need for surgical intervention.

There has been a movement toward use of the "Treat-to-Target" approach.[10,40] This involves use of specific targets, such as mucosal healing and endoscopic remission, or resolution of symptoms such as abdominal pain and diarrhea, as the main indicators of treatment efficacy. Mucosal healing, defined as the absence of ulceration, has become an important target and is accessed via endoscopy with specific scoring systems used to determine if this outcome has been assessed. Mucosal healing can be used as a monitoring parameter for treatment efficacy, particularly in CD, and if achieved may be predictive of steroid-free sustained remission.[27,40] Biomarkers, such as CRP and FC, have also become important adjunctive monitoring parameters to endoscopic approaches.[27,37,40]

General Approach to Treatment

6 Treatment of IBD centers on agents used to suppress the inflammatory process, induce, and then maintain disease remission. The severity and extent of the disease should be taken into account, as this will often dictate the dose, route, frequency, and formulation of drug therapies that will be most effective. Patient preference for different drug formulations and cost of therapies should also be taken into account.

Surgical procedures are sometimes performed when active disease is inadequately controlled with drugs, or when the required drug dosages pose an unacceptable risk of adverse effects. Nutritional considerations are also important because many patients may develop malnutrition. A variety of adjunctive therapies may be used to address complications or symptoms of IBD.

Nonpharmacologic Therapy

Nutritional Support

Malabsorption or maldigestion may occur secondary to the catabolic effects of the disease process. Patients with IBD have a five-fold higher risk of malnutrition compared to those without IBD.[28] Patients with CD have continued risk, even when their disease is quiescent, while patients with UC are more at risk during times of active disease.[30] Unnecessary food restriction during hospitalization also places patients at higher risk for malnutrition.[28] Patients who have undergone multiple small bowel resections may have reduction in the absorptive surface of the intestine (ie, "short gut"). Maldigestion with accompanying diarrhea can also occur if there is a bile salt deficiency in the gut. Patients should be screened for malnutrition upon diagnosis and assessed intermittently for the presence of micronutrient deficiencies.[30]

Elimination of specific foods that appear to exacerbate symptoms can be tried; however, exclusion diets are generally not endorsed, even in the setting of severe disease.[30] Increased intake of red meat, protein, sulfur and sulfates, and alcoholic beverages have been associated with disease flares.[8] If attempted, the elimination process must be conducted cautiously, as patients may exclude a wide range of nutritious products without adequate justification. Some patients with IBD may have lactase deficiency as well; therefore, diarrhea may be associated with intake of dairy products. For these patients, avoidance of dairy products or supplementation with lactase generally improves the patient's symptoms. Patients with small bowel strictures due to CD should avoid excessive high-residue foods, such as citrus fruits and nuts, in order to prevent obstruction. Increases in soluble fiber may induce the production of intestinal short chain fatty acids, which may have intrinsic anti-inflammatory effects.[8]

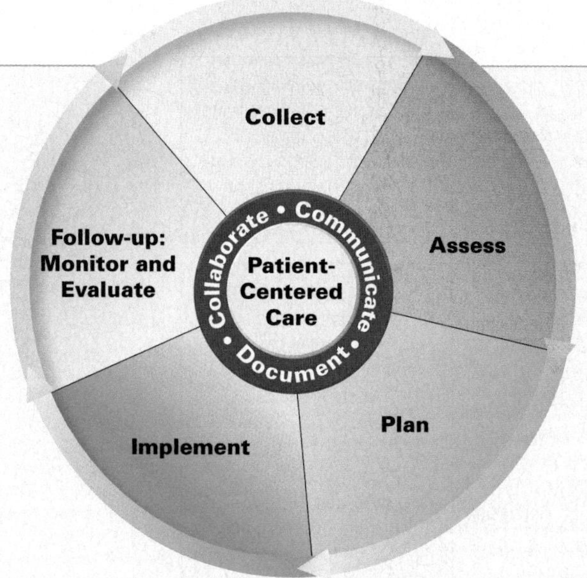

Patient Care Process for Inflammatory Bowel Disease

The image shows the five fundamental steps included in The Pharmacist's Care Process endorsed by the Joint Commission for Pharmacy Practitioners (2014). The tagline of this process reads collaborate, communicate, and document. The five fundamental steps listed here are collect, assess, plan, implement, and follow-up: monitor and evaluate. All these steps are listed in a circular block diagram.

Collect

- Patient characteristics (eg, age, sex, weight, vital signs)
- Patient symptoms, including evidence of abdominal pain, stool frequency, presence of hematochezia, weight loss, or extraintestinal manifestations
- Patient medical, family, and social history (in particular tobacco use)
- Surgical operations (site, date, procedure) and abdominal imaging findings (CT, MRI, ultrasound)
- Thorough medication history at hospital admission (include prescription, non-prescription medications, and other substances), and drug allergies and intolerances
- Laboratory results for evidence of inflammation (CRP, ESR, WBC), major organ function (particularly kidney and liver), hemoglobin and hematocrit, nutritional status (serum albumin and transferrin), vaccination status, pregnancy status, and pANCA or anti-*Saccharomyces cerevisiae* antibodies if initial diagnostic workup, and pharmacogenomics status for TPMT, if applicable

Assess

- Determine severity of illness based on symptoms, vital signs, stool frequency, and inflammatory markers. Consider use of Crohn's Disease Activity Index to assess disease progress. Include assessment of fluid and electrolyte status
- Determine extent and location of inflammation in the gastrointestinal tract based on endoscopic and imaging procedures
- Assess if extraintestinal disease manifestations and comorbidities are present that may affect section and outcomes of medication regimens
- Evaluate current medication regimen for potential drug-induced exacerbating factors and for efficacy and toxicity of current IBD treatment regimen
- Assess if disease complications are present that may require surgical intervention (abscess or fistulae)
- Estimate creatinine clearance for drug dosing

Plan*

- Determine goals of therapy with monitoring parameters for each goal
- Based on severity and location of Illness, determine the appropriate medications to induce and maintain remission considering severity and site of disease (Figs. 52-1 and 52-2)
- Initiate adjunctive medications for pain and diarrhea, if needed
- Check for adverse drug reactions and interactions and dose adjustments based on end-organ function (Table 52-4)

Implement

- Initiate medications for short-term induction of remission and subsequent maintenance
- Discontinue medications that may be exacerbating symptoms
- Provide patient education on appropriate use of oral, parenteral, or rectally administered medications
- Assure that corticosteroids doses are tapered during discontinuation

Follow-up: Monitor and Evaluate

- Determine if patient shows improvement in the signs and symptoms within 24 to 48 hours for hospitalized patients, and 7 to 14 days for outpatients
- Evaluate laboratory parameters for evidence of drug efficacy and potential toxicity
- Monitor for adverse effects of medications
- Assess adherence to current medication regimen and address barriers to medication use
- Determine the need for dose reduction or tapering of medications intended for short-term use, such as corticosteroids

Collaborate with patient, caregivers, and other healthcare professionals.

Many specific diets have been tried to improve nutritional status and symptoms in IBD. Use of diets low in FODMAPs may help improve IBD symptoms. The specific carbohydrate diet (SCD) is another option that involves restriction of all carbohydrates except monosaccharides (glucose, fructose, and galactose), as well as restriction of milk, canned fruits and vegetables, and processed meats.[9,28,30] Some studies have demonstrated improvement in symptoms and inflammation; however, these diets are difficult to follow

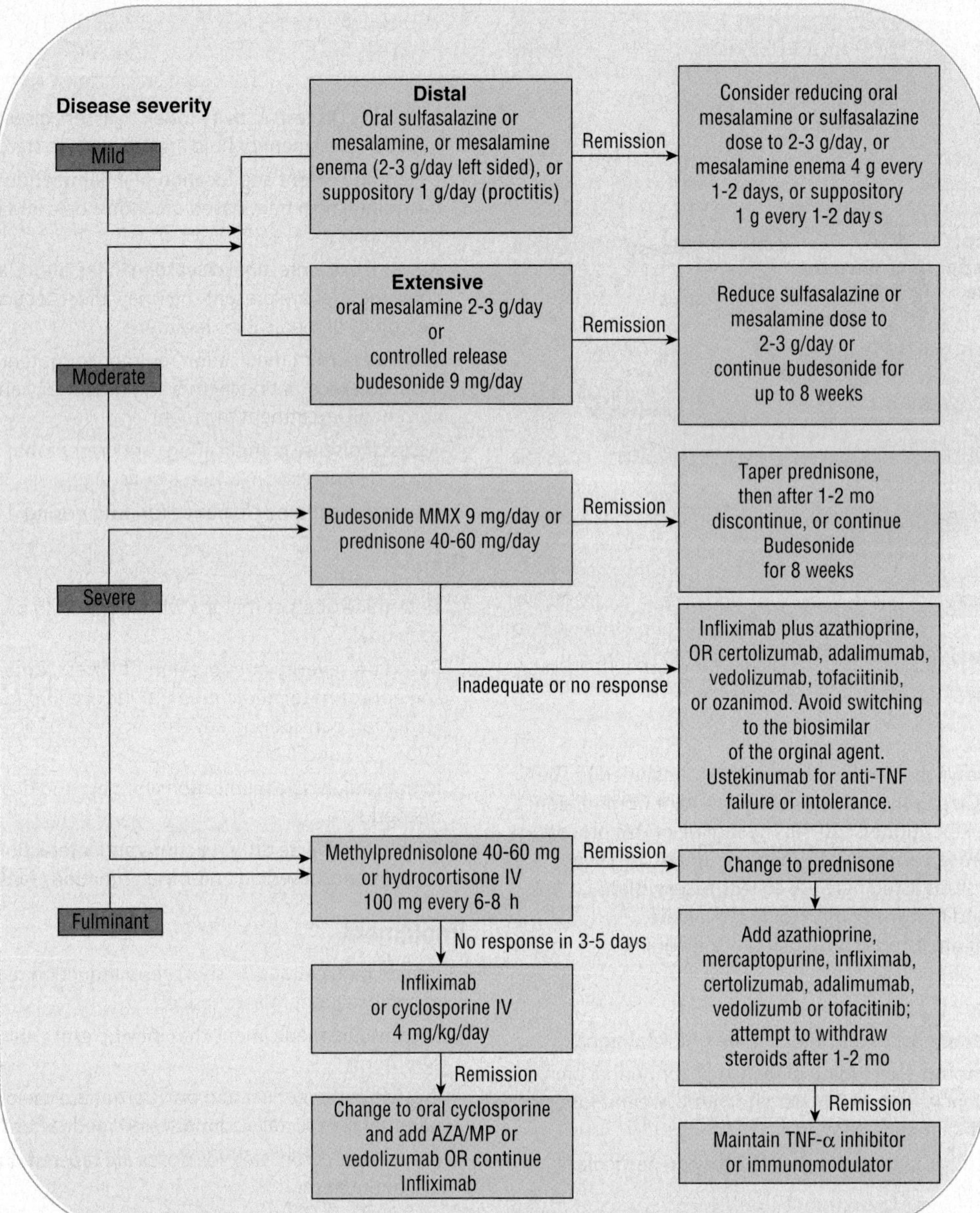

FIGURE 52-1 Treatment approaches for ulcerative colitis.

and patient adherence may by problematic.[28,30] Exclusive enteral nutrition, which involves use of elemental, semi-elemental, and defined formulas, has shown some benefit in increasing nutritional status and reducing intestinal inflammation and cytokine production.[8,28,30] While this approach may lead to a greater chance of induction of remission, particularly in patients with CD, most data are in pediatric patients and are lacking regarding its use as a maintenance diet.[28,30]

Parenteral nutrition is generally reserved for patients with severe malnutrition or those who fail enteral therapy or have a contraindication to receiving enteral therapy, such as perforation, protracted vomiting, short-bowel syndrome, or severe intestinal stenosis.[30] Parenteral therapy is not preferred as primary therapy for IBD even in the setting of acute disease flares in hospitalized patients, and should be reserved for those patients with the most complicated disease.[30] Home parenteral nutrition may be necessary for patients requiring long-term therapy, particularly those with short-bowel syndrome. Parenteral nutrition is more costly and is associated with more complications, such as serious infections, compared with enteral nutrition.

Probiotic administration as an adjunctive treatment of IBD has been explored. Postulated mechanisms for using probiotics in IBD include reestablishment of normal bacterial flora within the gut, reduction in bacterial adhesion and competition for nutrients with pathogenic bacteria, production of antibacterial substances, and promotion of favorable effects on the host immune response.[7] Probiotic preparations often contain various organisms such as nonpathogenic *E. coli Nissle*, bifidobacteria, lactobacilli, *Streptococcus thermophilus*, or *Saccharomyces boulardii*. While probiotics were effective in inducing and maintaining remission in some trials for patients with UC, differences in methodology, probiotics used, and underlying treatments for IBD make comparison of trials difficult.[40,41] A formulation of *Bifidobacterium*, lactobacilli, and streptococci (VSL #3) is marketed specifically for use in UC as an adjunctive therapy and for patients who have a surgically constructed ileal pouch anal anastomosis (IPAA) to prevent or treat pouchitis.[18,41,42] Evidence of probiotic use for the induction and maintenance of CD is

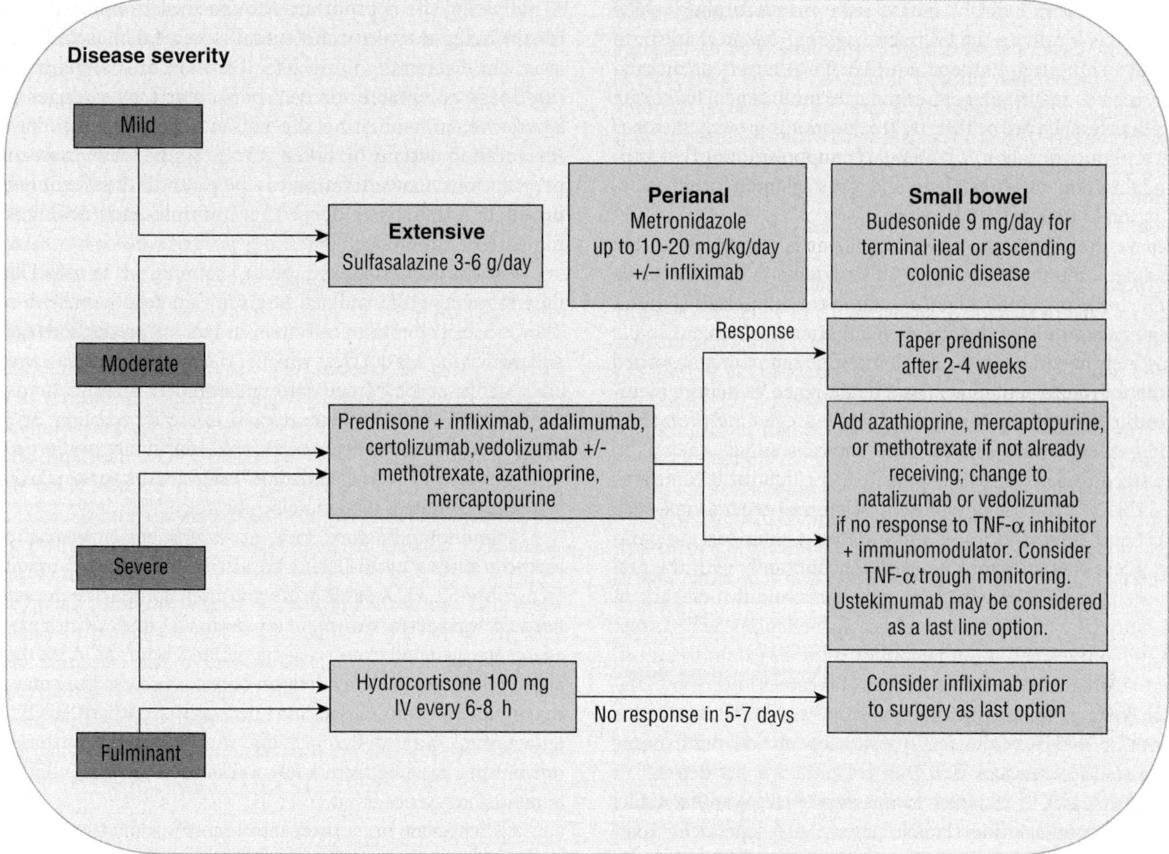

FIGURE 52-2 Treatment approaches for Crohn's disease.

less compelling and has led to recommendations not supporting widespread use, but rather further investigation.[27,42] While probiotics are considered to be generally safe in patients with IBD, the added cost, requirement to take multiple doses per day, coupled with the lack of quality data to support their use, should also weigh into the decision to use them in IBD.

Surgery

Patients with IBD often require surgery. Surgical procedures may involve resection of segments of intestine that are affected, as well as correction of complications (eg, fistulas) or drainage of abscesses.

Rates of colectomy over 20 years UC are reported as 0.55% to 20%.[1,18,39,43] Colectomy may be necessary when the patient has disease uncontrolled by maximum medical therapy or when there are complications of the disease such as colonic perforation, toxic megacolon, uncontrolled colonic hemorrhage, or colonic strictures.[1,24,43] Colectomy may be indicated for patients with long-standing disease (greater than 8-10 years), as a prophylactic measure against the development of CRC, and for patients with premalignant changes (severe dysplasia) on surveillance mucosal biopsies.[42] Proctocolectomy, after which the patient is left with a permanent ileostomy, is generally considered curative for UC; however, the decision to perform this should take into account the effects on the patient's QOL. Restorative proctocolectomy with construction of an IPAA is the most common surgical procedure performed in UC. This procedure is typically well tolerated with approximately 29% of patients developing long-term complications such as pouchitis, pelvic floor abscess, or bowel obstruction.[43]

Surgery in patients with CD is usually reserved for patients with intractable hemorrhage, perforation, persistent or recurrent obstruction, abscess, dysplasia, cancer, or medically refractory disease.[27,44,45] The 10-year cumulative risk of surgical intervention is 40% to 55%, with the 5-year postoperative recurrent rate reported as approximately 50%.[27] The surgical procedures performed most often include resections of the major intestinal areas of involvement. Patients who undergo multiple resections of the small intestine may develop malabsorption related to short-bowel syndrome. For some patients with severe rectal or perianal disease, particularly abscesses, diversion of the fecal stream is performed with a colostomy.

Pharmacologic Therapy

The approach to treatment of IBD should consider all aspects of each individual patient in order to maximize therapy, improve patient symptoms and QOL, and prevent complications. To ensure optimal drug therapy, an assessment of each patient's health literacy and potential barriers to understanding and adherence should be performed. Involving the patient in the care process will help to keep him or her engaged. Since patients with IBD are often seen by GI specialists or surgeons, ensuring that each provider has a current, accurate, and complete medication list will help to prevent potential medication errors. Female patients of childbearing age should discuss with their providers their goals for becoming pregnant, as this may dictate the choice of drugs used.

None of the drugs used for IBD are curative; therefore, reasonable goals of drug therapy are resolution of acute disease symptoms and induction and maintenance of remission.

Sulfasalazine is the prototypical ASA, and is composed of a sulfonamide moiety (sulfapyridine) and mesalamine (5-aminosalicylate acid [5-ASA]) joined by a diazo bond in the same molecule.[46] Sulfasalazine has been used for years to treat IBD but was originally intended to treat arthritis. It is cleaved by gut bacteria in the colon to sulfapyridine (which is mostly absorbed and excreted in the urine) and mesalamine (which mostly remains in the colon and is excreted in stool).[46,47]

The active component of sulfasalazine is mesalamine, which exerts its effects locally in the GI tract; however, the mechanism of action is not completely understood. Beneficial effects of mesalamine may include scavenging of free radicals, inhibition of leukocyte motility, interference with TNF-α, transforming growth factor-β (TGF-β) and nuclear factor κ B (NF-κ β), suppression of IL-1 production, inhibition of leukotriene and prostaglandin production, and induction of PPARγ.[13,18,46,47]

Because the effectiveness of sulfasalazine is not related to the sulfapyridine component and since sulfapyridine is believed to be responsible for many of the adverse reactions to sulfasalazine, mesalamine can be administered alone. Given that mesalamine is rapidly and completely absorbed in the small intestine but poorly absorbed in the colon, drug formulations must be designed to deliver mesalamine to the affected areas in the GI while preventing premature absorption. Mesalamine can be used topically as an enema, to treat left-sided disease, or as a suppository for treatment of proctitis (Fig. 52-3).[48-50] The use of topical mesalamine preparations, such as enemas and suppositories, is more effective than oral preparations.[48-50] These therapies may be used concomitantly with the oral mesalamine preparations, which may result in additive efficacy in patients with UC.[49,50] Oral slow-release formulations will deliver mesalamine to the small intestine and/or colon based on the product design (Table 52-5). Slow-release oral formulations of mesalamine (eg, Pentasa) release mesalamine from the duodenum to the ileum, with up to 59% of the drug passing into the colon.[46,47] Some dose forms (Asacol, Asacol HD, Delzicol) utilize a pH-dependent coating that releases in response to intestinal pH.[46] Another tablet formulation of mesalamine (Lialda) uses a pH-dependent coating that releases at a pH of 7, in combination with a polymeric matrix core, referred to as the Multi-MatriX (MMX) system, and releases drug evenly throughout the colon also allowing for once-daily dosing.[51] A capsule formulation of mesalamine (Apriso) utilizes enteric-coated mesalamine granules in a polymer matrix for delayed and extended delivery of mesalamine to the colon and also allows for once-daily dosing.[46] Use of once-daily oral mesalamine preparations may enhance adherence, which may help to prevent relapse.[46-48] Olsalazine is a dimer of two mesalamine molecules linked by an azo bond. Mesalamine is released in the colon after colonic bacteria cleave the azo bond.[46] Balsalazide is a mesalamine prodrug that couples mesalamine with the inert carrier molecule 4-aminobenzoyl-β-alanine and is also enzymatically cleaved in the colon to release mesalamine.[46] Because the oral mesalamine formulations are delayed-release coated tablets or granules, they should not be crushed or chewed. Unlike sulfasalazine, all of these agents are safe to use for patients with sulfonamide allergies.

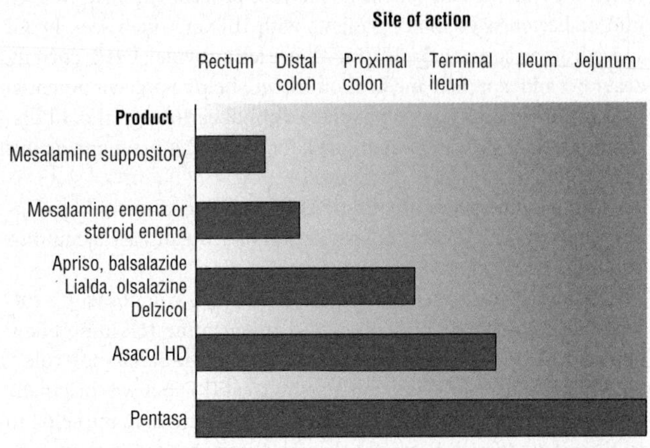

FIGURE 52-3 Site of activity of various agents used to treat inflammatory bowel disease.

Picking the appropriate ASA formulation and dose of drug for the disease severity and extent is key. Enemas and suppositories, while generally more effective than oral preparations, may not be as acceptable for use, particularly by younger patients. Therefore, individuating the patient's preference for a specific formulation should be taken into account when choosing ASA preparations. Consideration can be given to the use of once-daily products if there is evidence that multiple-daily dosing is affecting patient adherence.[18,46-51]

7 Corticosteroids are used to suppress acute inflammation in the treatment of IBD, and may be given parenterally, orally, or rectally.[52] They modulate the immune system and inhibit production of cytokines and mediators. It is not clear whether the most important steroid effects are systemic or local (mucosal). Budesonide is a corticosteroid that is administered orally in a controlled-release formulation designed to release in the terminal ileum or the colon depending on the product, or as a rectal foam. The drug undergoes extensive first-pass metabolism; so systemic exposure is thought to be minimized.[50,52]

Immunomodulators such as azathioprine, mercaptopurine, methotrexate, or cyclosporine are also used for the treatment of IBD (see Table 52-4). Azathioprine and mercaptopurine are effectively used in long-term treatment of both CD and UC.[1,18,27,53,54] These agents are generally reserved for patients who fail ASA therapy or are refractory to or dependent on corticosteroids. They may be used in conjunction with mesalamine derivatives, corticosteroids, TNF-α antagonists, and vedolizumab, and must be used for extended periods of time, ranging from a few weeks up to several months, before benefits may be observed.[53,54]

Cyclosporine has a short-term benefit in the treatment of acute, severe UC to avoid colectomy in patients failing corticosteroids, but has little efficacy in CD.[1,18,35] It is used initially as a continuous IV infusion of 2 to 4 mg/kg daily.[35] Cyclosporine poses a risk of nephrotoxicity and neurotoxicity. Studies evaluating tacrolimus for the treatment of IBD suggest a potential role for short-term use in patients with perianal or fistulizing CD; however, results have been variable with few data to support its routine use.[27] There are limited data to suggest routine use of tacrolimus in UC as well.[18] Methotrexate 15 to 25 mg given intramuscularly or subcutaneously once weekly may useful for maintenance therapy of CD and may result in steroid-sparing effects, while data supporting use in UC are lacking.[27,55]

Antimicrobial agents have limited roles as adjunctive therapies in IBD. Metronidazole can be used as adjunctive therapy for simple perianal fistulaes and may be combined with infliximab.[27] Risks of long-term antibiotic use include the development of antibiotic resistance, predisposition to *C. difficile* infection, and adverse effects such as neurotoxicity secondary to metronidazole use.

Biologic agents that target TNF-α have become a key class of agents in the treatment and maintenance of IBD.[56-58] Infliximab is an IgG1 chimeric monoclonal antibody that utilizes 25% murine variable regions and is administered IV. Infliximab binds TNF-α and inhibits its inflammatory effects, resulting in reductions in pro-inflammatory cytokines, such as IL-1 and IL-6. Adalimumab is also an IgG1 antibody to TNF-α; however, this agent, unlike infliximab, is fully humanized and contains no murine sequences. It is administered subcutaneously. Theoretically, the lack of a murine component in adalimumab reduces antibody development seen with use of infliximab. Certolizumab pegol is a humanized pegylated Fab fragment directed against TNF-α that is also administered subcutaneously. Golimumab is similar in structure to adalimumab and offers similar efficacy to the currently approved agents.

Biosimilars are highly similar to the FDA-approved biologic agents. There are no clinically meaningful differences in efficacy or adverse effects from the reference products. Biosimilars have a nonproprietary name plus an FDA-designated suffix consisting of four lowercase letters that have no intended meaning. Some are considered to be interchangeable with the reference product.[56] Several infliximab biosimilar agents are approved for use in UC and CD,

TABLE 52-4 Drug Monitoring Guidelines

Drug(s)	Adverse Drug Reaction	Monitoring Parameters	Comments
Sulfasalazine	Nausea, vomiting, headache Rash, anemia, pneumonitis Hepatotoxicity, nephritis Thrombocytopenia, lymphoma	Folate, complete blood count Liver function tests, Scr, BUN	Increase the dose slowly, over 1-2 weeks
Mesalamine	Nausea, vomiting, headache	GI disturbances	
Corticosteroids	Hyperglycemia, dyslipidemia	Blood pressure, fasting lipid panel	Avoid long-term use if possible or consider budesonide
	Osteoporosis, hypertension, acne	Glucose, vitamin D, bone density	
	Edema, infection, myopathy, psychosis		
Azathioprine/ mercaptopurine	Bone marrow suppression, pancreatitis, lymphoma	Complete blood count	Check TPMT activity or NUDT15 phenotype
	Liver dysfunction, rash, arthralgia	Scr, BUN, liver function tests, genotype/phenotype	May monitor TGN
Methotrexate	Bone marrow suppression, pancreatitis	Complete blood count, Scr, BUN	Check baseline pregnancy test
	Pneumonitis, pulmonary fibrosis, hepatitis	Liver function tests	Chest x-ray
Infliximab Adalimumab Certolizumab Golimumab	Infusion-related reactions (infliximab), infection Heart failure, optic neuritis, demyelination, injection site reaction, signs of infection	Blood pressure/heart rate (infliximab) Neurologic exam, mental status Trough concentrations (infliximab) Antidrug antibodies (all agents)	Need negative PPD and viral serologies
Natalizumab Vedolizumab	Infusion-related reactions	Brain MRI, mental status, progressive multifocal leukoencephalopathy	Vedolizumab not associated with PML
Ustekinumab	Infections, skin cancers	Signs/symptoms of infection, annual skin exam	Rare instances of reversible posterior leukoencephalopathy syndrome (RPLS) Avoid live vaccines
Tofacitinib	Infection, thrombosis, lymphoma, elevated cholesterol, CPK, LFTs, lymphopenia, neutropenia, anemia	Symptoms of Infection or thrombosis	Avoid live vaccines. Screen for baseline TB. Do not initiate in patients with lymphocytes < 500/mm^3(0.5 x 10^9/L), ANC <1000/mm^3(1 x 10^9/L), or hemoglobin <9 g/dL (90 g/L; 5.59 mmol/L). Monitor lipids and LFTs every 4-8 weeks. Gastrointestinal perforation has been reported with use of the XR formulation. Drug interactions with CYP3A4 and 2C19 inhibitor
Ozanimod	Infection, heart rate, blood pressure, LFTs, respiratory rate, fetal abnormalities, macular edema, headache	Symptoms of infection or respiratory dysfunction, changes in vision	Need baseline ECG, WBC, LFTs, ophthalmic assessment, and testing for varicella zoster antibodies. Contraindicated if patient has experienced MI, unstable angina, stroke, TIA, decompensated heart failure, or Mobitz type II second- or third-degree AV block, sick sinus syndrome in the last 6 months, presence of sleep apnea, and concomitant use of MAOI. Women of childbearing age should use effective contraception during and for 3 months after use

including infliximab-dyyb, infliximab-abda, infliximab-qbtx, and infliximab-axxq. There are several adalimumab biolsimilars, including adalimumab-adbm, adalimumab-atto, adalimumab-adaz, adalimumab-afzb, and adalimumab-bwwd. Legal disputes involving the manufacturers of the adalimumab reference products have led to delays in the commercial availability of the biosimilar products.

Natalizumab and vedolizumab are biologic agents that inhibit leukocyte adhesion and migration by targeting the α_4 subunit of integrin.[59,60,70] Vedolizumab works similar to natalizumab but is more specific for the $\alpha_{4\beta7}$ subunit of integrin, which targets leukocyte trafficking in the gut.[59] Ustekinumab is a biologic agent that blocks IL-21 and IL-23 action by binding to the p40 protein subunit used by these cytokines.[61,62] It is approved for use in moderate-to-severe CD in patients who failed immunomodulators or corticosteroids but have not received anti-TNF therapy. It can also be used for patients who have failed anti-TNF therapy and in combination with immunomodulators. Tofacitinib inhibits intracellular Janus kinases (JK) proteins, which are responsible for the signal transduction of multiple cytokines involved in the inflammatory cascade.[63] It is approved for patients with moderate-to-severe UC who are unresponsive to TNF-α inhibitors. Ozanimod is a small molecule that inhibits sphingosine-1 phosphate (S1P) which inhibits lymphocyte egress from lymph nodes and subsequent migration to the intestinal tract.[57] It is approved for the treatment of moderate to severely active UC in adult patients.

Ulcerative Colitis

Induction Therapy for Mild-to-Moderate Active Disease

Most patients with mild-to-moderate active UC can typically be managed on an outpatient basis with oral and/or topical ASAs or oral or rectal budesonide (Fig. 52-1; Table 52-6). Mesalamine preparations are typically better tolerated than sulfasalazine and thus are

TABLE 52-5 Agents for the Treatment of Inflammatory Bowel Disease

Drug	Brand Name	Initial Dose	Usual Range
Sulfasalazine	Azulfidine Azulfidine EN	500 mg to 1 g 500 mg to 1 g	4-6 g/day 4-6 g/day
Mesalamine suppository	Canasa	1 g	1 g daily to three times weekly
Mesalamine enema	Rowasa	4 g	4 g daily to three times weekly
Mesalamine (oral)	Asacol HD Apriso Lialda Pentasa Delzicol	1.6 g/day 1.5 g/day 1.2-2.4 g/day 2 g/day 1.2 g/day	2.8-4.8 g/day 1.5 g/day once daily 1.2-4.8 g/day once daily 2-4 g/day 2.4-4.8 g/day
Olsalazine	Dipentum	1.5 g/day	1.5-3 g/day
Balsalazide	Colazal	2.25 g/day	2.25-6.75 g/day
Azathioprine	Imuran, Azasan	50-100 mg	1-2.5 mg/kg/day
Cyclosporine	Gengraf Neoral, Sandimmune	2-4 mg/kg/day IV 2-8 mg/kg/day oral	2-4 mg/kg/day IV
Mercaptopurine	Purinethol, Purixan	50-100 mg	1-2.5 mg/kg/day
Methotrexate	No branded IM injection	15-25 mg IM weekly	15-25 mg IM weekly
Adalimumab	Humira	160 mg SC day 1	80 mg SC 2 (day 15), and then 40 mg every 2 weeks
Adalimumab-atto	Amjevita[a]		
Adalimumab-abdm	Cyltezo[a]		
Adalimumab-adaz	Hyrimoz[a]		
Adalimumab-afzb	Abrilada[a]		
Adalimumab-bwwd	Hadlima[a]		
Certolizumab	Cimzia[a]	400 mg SC	400 mg SC weeks 2 and 4, and then 400 mg SC monthly
Infliximab	Remicade	5 mg/kg IV	5 mg/kg weeks 2 and 6, 5-10 mg/kg every 8 weeks
Infliximab-dyyb	Inflectra		
Infliximab-abda	Renflexis		
Infliximab-qbtx	IXIFI		
Infliximav-axxq	AVSOLA		
Natalizumab	Tysabri	300 mg IV	300 mg IV every 4 weeks
Budesonide	Entocort EC capsule, Uceris tablet	9 mg orally once daily	6-9 mg daily
	Uceris rectal foam	2 mg twice daily	2 mg daily
Vedolizumab	Entyvio	300 mg IV	300 mg IV weeks 2 and 6 and then every 8 weeks
Golimumab	Simponi	200 mg SC	100 mg SC weeks 2 and 4
Ustekinumab	Stelara	Weight based initial IV dose <55 kg (260 mg), 55-85 kg (390 mg), >85 kg (520 mg)	90 mg SC every 8 weeks
Tofacitinib	Xeljanz, Xeljanz XR	10 mg twice daily or 22 mg XR for 8 weeks; may continue for max of 16 weeks	5 mg twice daily or 11 mg once daily
Ozanimod	Zeposia	0.23 mg orally once daily days 1-4, then 0.46 mg once daily days 5-7	0.92 mg orally once daily starting day 8 of therapy

[a]Not available until 2023

SC, subcutaneous; IM, intramuscular.

often chosen preferentially as first-line therapies. For patients with extensive disease, oral once daily mesalamine is generally preferred at a dose of 2 to 3 g/day (see Table 52-2).[18,64] Doses of greater than 3 g/day are reserved for lack of response to standard doses. Topical mesalamine in an enema or suppository formulation is more effective than oral mesalamine or topical steroids for distal disease. Mesalamine suppositories will only reach to approximately 10 to 20 cm within the lower GI tract and thus are reserved for patients with proctitis. Enemas will reach to the splenic flexure and are preferred for left-sided disease. Combining suppositories or enemas with oral mesalamine preparations has additive effects and is preferred in patients with extensive or left-sided disease if patients are willing to use both preparations.[18,64] Sulfasalazine, at doses of 2 to 4 g/day, may be considered in patients already receiving it in remission, or in those with prominent arthritic symptoms.[44]

Controlled-release budesonide (Uceris) is an alternative for mildly active extensive UC, and is typically recommended in patients unresponsive to mesalamine. While budesonide foam may be used for distal disease, it has a limited role and is reserved for patients who are intolerant or unresponsive to topical mesalamine.[1,18,52,64] Oral budesonide MMX at a dose of 9 mg/day is preferred for patients who are unresponsive to optimized doses of mesalamine.[18,64] Oral corticosteroids in doses of 40 to 60 mg/day prednisone equivalent can be used as an alternative to budesonide for patients with moderately active extensive disease who are refractory to oral ASAs or require more rapid control of symptoms.[18,64] Topical corticosteroids, given as

TABLE 52-6 Levels of Evidence for Therapeutic Interventions in Inflammatory Bowel Disease

Interventions	Evidence Grades[a]
Ulcerative Colitis	
Rectal mesalamine is recommended at a dose of 1 g/day for induction of remission in mildly active UC	Strong
Mesalamine enemas at a dose of 1 g/day is preferred over rectal steroids for induction of remission in mildly active left-sided colitis	Strong
Rectal mesalamine at a dose of 1 g/day in combination with oral mesalamine at a dose of 2 g/day is preferred for induction of remission of mildly active left-sided UC	Conditional
Oral budesonide 9 mg/day is preferred in patients who fail or are intolerant of oral or rectal mesalamine for induction of remission in mildly active UC	Strong
High-dose mesalamine (>3 g/day) is suggested in patients who have suboptimal response to standard dose mesalamine	Conditional
Oral mesalamine at a dose of at least 2 g/day is recommended for induction of remission in patients with mildly active extensive colitis	Strong
Oral systemic corticosteroids are recommended for induction of remission in patients with UC of any extent who fail to respond to mesalamine	Strong
Sulfasalazine, mesalamine, or balsalazide is effective in maintenance of remission of distal disease; combining oral and topical mesalamine is more effective than is either alone	Strong
Sulfasalazine, olsalazine, mesalamine, and balsalazide are effective in preventing relapses in patients with mild-to-moderate extensive disease	Strong
Corticosteroids are not effective as maintenance treatment	Strong
Oral budesonide is recommended for induction of remission in patients with moderately active UC	Strong
Monotherapy with thiopurines or methotrexate is not recommended for induction therapy in patients with moderate-to-severe active UC	Strong
Infliximab, adalimumab, and golimumab are effective for induction of remission in moderate-to-severe active UC	Strong
Infliximab combined with a thiopurine is effective for induction therapy in moderately severe active UC	Strong
Tofacitinib is effective for induction and maintenance of remission for patients with moderate to severely active UC	Strong
Vedolizumab is effective for induction of remission in moderate-to-severe active UC	Strong
Tofacitinib is effective for induction of remission in patients with moderate-to-severe UC	Strong
Crohn's Disease	
Sulfasalazine is effective for treating mild-to-moderate active colonic CD	Conditional
Mesalamine has not consistently been demonstrated to be effective in active CD	Strong
Ileal release budesonide is effective for mild-to-moderate ileal or right-sided colonic disease	Strong
Metronidazole is not effective for treatment of luminal CD	Conditional
Ciprofloxacin should not be used for treatment of luminal CD	Conditional
Systemic corticosteroids are effective for short-term treatment of moderate to severely active CD	Strong
Conventional corticosteroids do not consistently achieve mucosal healing	Weak
Thiopurines should be considered for steroid sparing in CD	Strong
Azathioprine and mercaptopurine are not effective to induce short-term remission	Strong
Azathioprine and mercaptopurine are effective for maintenance of remission	Strong
TPMT testing should be considered prior to use of azathioprine or mercaptopurine	Strong
Anti-TNF agents should be given in patients refractory to azathioprine or methrotrexate	Strong
Vedolizumab with or without an immunomodulator should be considered for induction of remission in symptomatic patients	Strong
Natalizumab can be considered for induction of remission	Strong
Infliximab, adalimumab, and certolizumab are effective in lowering or eliminating corticosteroid use in corticosteroid-dependent patients	Strong
Ustekinumab should be given in moderate to severe CD in patients who fail treatment with corticosteroids, thiopurines, methotrexate, or anti-TNF agents or who have no prior exposure to anti-TNF agents	Strong
Cyclosporine, mycophenolate mofetil, and tacrolimus should not be used for CD	Strong
Methotrexate maintenance therapy (15-25 mg IM weekly) is effective for steroid sparing and for maintenance of remission	Conditional
Intravenous corticosteroids should be used for severe to fulminant CD	Conditional
Infliximab, adalimumab, and certolizumab are effective in severely active CD	Strong
Infliximab can be administered for treatment of fulminant CD	Conditional
Infliximab is effective for perianal fistulas	Strong

[a]Strong (desirable effects outweigh undesirable), conditional (uncertainty about trade-offs).

Data from References 6, 8, 18, 27, and 35.

foams, enemas, and suppositories, while effective for patients with distal disease, are generally less effective than mesalamine but can be used for patients with tenesmus or intolerance to meslamine.[18,52,64]

Induction therapy for Moderate-to-Severe Active Disease Patients with moderate-to-severe active disease require prompt initiation of therapies to quickly suppress inflammation. While oral mesalamine products may be effective for moderately severe UC, oral budesonide MMX is the preferred alternative prior to use of more systemic corticosteroids and for moderate disease.[18,35,64] Systemic corticosteroids are an alternative for the treatment of moderate-to-severe active UC regardless of disease location or in those patients who are unresponsive to maximal doses of oral and/or topical mesalamine derivatives.[18,35] Oral doses of 40 to 60 mg prednisone equivalent daily are recommended.[18,52,64]

Use of TNF-α inhibitors or vedolizumab are the main options for patients with moderate-to-severe disease who are unresponsive to aminosalicylates or corticosteroids, or are corticosteroid dependent, and are more effective than immunomodulator monotherapy for induction of remission.[18,35] The choice of agent depends on previous exposure to biologic agents. For treatment-naive patients, infliximab or vedolizumab in combination with an immunomodulator (eg, azathioprine) is recommended preferentially.[18,35] Vedolizumab is superior to adalimumab in this setting.[65] Certolizumab is not approved for use in UC in the United States. Combining infliximab or vedolizumab with a thiopurine is more effective in inducing corticosteroid-free remission in patients with moderate-to-severe UC and is the preferred approach.[35,60] Vedolizumab should not be used in combination with TNF-α inhibitors. For patients previously exposed to infliximab, ustekinumab or tofacitinib is preferentially recommended over vedolizumab or adalimumab.[35] Ozanimod is an alternative for induction and subsequent maintenance therapy in moderate to severely active UC.[66]

Therapy for Acute Severe or Fulminant Disease Patients with ASUC or those with incapacitating symptoms require hospitalization for effective management. Under these conditions, patients generally receive nothing by mouth to promote bowel rest. Medications are given by the parenteral route, and oral sulfasalazine or mesalamine derivatives are not typically beneficial in this setting because of rapid elimination of these agents from the colon with diarrhea. Patients should be tested for *C. difficile* infection and receive VTE prophylaxis.

Systemic corticosteroids are used in the treatment of severe disease and may allow some patients to avoid colectomy. Methylprednisolone IV at a dose of 40-60 mg daily is considered a first-line agent.[35] A trial of corticosteroids is warranted in most patients before proceeding to colectomy, unless the condition is grave or rapidly deteriorating. The length of corticosteroid therapy before consideration of surgery is open to debate, with recommendations ranging from 3 to 5 days.[1,18,52] Steroids do increase surgical risk, particularly infectious, if an operation is required later.

8 Patients, who are unresponsive to parenteral corticosteroids, have the option of receiving higher-potency agents such as cyclosporine or infliximab.[18,35] Among those unresponsive to corticosteroids, 76% to 85% will typically respond to IV cyclosporine.[64] Infliximab as a single 5 mg/kg IV dose or a continuous IV infusion of cyclosporine 2 to 4 mg/kg/day, with goal serum levels of 200-400 ng/mL (mcg/L), is the typical dose range utilized and may delay the need for colectomy.[1,18,35] Patients with ASUC who respond to infliximab should be continued on this agent, while those who are controlled on IV cyclosporine can be transitioned to maintenance therapy with azathioprine.

Maintenance of Remission

9 After remission from active disease is achieved, the goal of therapy is to maintain remission for as long as possible. Various agents can be used and the choice may depend on the initial response to treatment, patient specific factors, and safety.

For patients with previously mildly active extensive or left side disease the oral aminosalicylate agents are preferred for maintenance therapy at a dose of at least 2 g/day.[18] The newer mesalamine derivatives are generally better tolerated than sulfasalazine and are associated with fewer adverse effects, making them a preferred choice.[1,18] For patients with proctitis, mesalamine suppositories are preferred at a dose of 1 g/day.[1,18,48,49] The frequency of administration of topical agents may be lessened to every third night over time.[1,18,48,49] For patients with previously moderate-to-severe active disease, the aminosalicylate products can be continued if remission is achieved initially with an aminosalicylate agent; however, the likelihood of sustaining remission is significantly lower, especially if more severe disease is present. Thiopurine monotherapy is recommended for maintenance in the setting of corticosteroid induced remission for moderate-to-severe disease.[18,35]

Corticosteroids have no role in the maintenance of remission, as they are ineffective and are associated with serious adverse effects with long-term use.[1,18,35,52] Budesonide oral MMX may be continued for up to 8 weeks for patients with moderate disease; however, systemic corticosteroids should be tapered over 4-12 weeks in moderately active UC patients achieving remission.[18,35,52] For patients who are steroid dependent, there is a strong justification for use of alternative therapies to allow for steroid withdrawal. Azathioprine may be effective in preventing relapse of UC for patients who fail ASAs or who are steroid dependent.[52-54] Approximately one-third of patients will maintain remission on azathioprine; however, the onset of action is slow and 3 to 6 months may be required before beneficial effects are noted.[52-54]

The TNF-α inhibitors, vedolizumab, ustekinumab, or tofacitinib are all options for maintenance in patients with moderate-to-severe UC following successful induction of remission, and in those who are steroid dependent or have failed azathioprine. Once patients with moderate-to-severe disease achieve remission with a biologic therapy or azathioprine there is no further role for aminosalicylate agents, so these should be discontinued.[35] For patients with ASUC, if remission with infliximab is achieved, this agent can be continued as maintenance therapy, while azathioprine or vedolizumab are recommended as maintenance therapies in patients achieving remission with cyclosporine.[35]

Crohn's Disease

Management of CD often proves more difficult than management of UC because of the greater complexity of presentation and the aggressive nature of the disease (Fig. 52-2; see Table 52-3). There is a greater potential for reliance on drug therapy with CD because resection of involved areas of the GI tract may not be possible. Surgical intervention is often required with rates of recurrence of CD following surgery reported in up to 80% of patients.[10]

Drug treatment of CD involves many of the same agents used for UC. While the treatment strategy for CD has often followed a similar "step-up" pattern as seen with UC, there has been more interest in the Treat-to-Target approach in patients with severe disease, which often involves more of a "step-down" approach of using more effective agents earlier in the disease course.[10,27,40]

Mild-to-Moderate Active Crohn's Disease

While effective in UC, ASAs have not demonstrated significant efficacy in CD. Sulfasalazine is reported to have marginal efficacy when compared with placebo for patients with mild-to-moderate CD, while the newer mesalamine derivatives are generally considered to have minimal efficacy.[27] Despite limited and variable effectiveness, the mesalamine derivatives are often tried as an initial therapy for mild-to-moderate CD in low-risk patients given their more favorable adverse effect profile.[67] Since CD often involves the small intestine, formulations such as Pentasa, which release in the small intestine, may be used to target areas of inflammation.

Systemic corticosteroids are frequently used for the treatment of moderate-to-severe active CD; however, controlled-release budesonide (Entocort) at a dose of 9 mg daily is a preferred first-line option for patients with mild-to-moderate ileal or right-sided (ascending colonic) disease.[27,52] This agent is superior to placebo and has demonstrated superiority to mesalamine and is preferred for patients with ileal disease.[27,52,67]

Antibiotics have little to no efficacy in treating luminal CD and are not recommended.[6,7,27] Broad-spectrum agents may be used for treatment of abscess formation in CD.[34] Metronidazole may have some role in prevention of postoperative recurrence of CD, and is also recommended for use in patients with perianal fistulas, particularly in combination with infliximab.[27]

Moderate-to-Severe Active Crohn's Disease

Patients with moderate-to-severe active CD require rapid suppression of inflammation for symptom improvement and prevention of complications. Oral corticosteroids, such as prednisone 40 to 60 mg/day, are generally considered first-line therapies for moderate-to-severe active CD who are unresponsive to ASAs.[10,27,52,60] Traditional oral systemic steroids have greater efficacy in inducing remission compared with budesonide in patients with moderate disease; however, the potential for adverse effects is greater, even with short-term use.[10,27,52] Hospitalized patients with moderate-to-severe disease who are unable to tolerate oral therapy are candidates for administration of parenteral steroids, with methylprednisolone or hydrocortisone being first-line options.[10,27] Systemic steroids do not appear to be effective for treatment of perianal fistulas, nor do they induce mucosal healing.[27,58]

10 Azathioprine, mercaptopurine, and methotrexate are generally not recommended for induction of remission as monotherapy in moderate-to-severe CD.[6,7,10,27] These agents are largely used for maintenance of remission, and are effective in maintaining steroid-induced remission and reducing steroid dependency, either as monotherapy or in combination with TNF-α inhibitors or vedolizumab.[10,27,53,54] Clinical response to azathioprine and mercaptopurine may be related to whole-blood concentrations of the metabolite 6-thioguanine (TGN). Concentrations of TGN between 230 and 450 pmol/8 × 10^8 erythrocytes have beneficial effects when used as monotherapy, but monitoring is not routinely performed or may not be available at some sites.[54,68]

11 Methotrexate given weekly intramuscularly or subcutaneously in doses of 15 to 25 mg is effective in reducing steroid dependency and maintaining remission, and may be considered as an alternative to azathioprine or mercaptopurine.[27]

The TNF-α inhibitors, including the biosimilar agents, are the preferred agents in the management of moderate-to-severe CD, especially those with high-risk features.[27,55,60,67] All agents in this class, with the exception of golimumab, which is not approved for use in CD in the United States, have similar rates of efficacy. The choice of agent depends on patient preference, route of administration, and cost. Adalimumab and certolizumab have the advantage of subcutaneous administration and may be considered alternates to infliximab as initial therapy or in those patients losing response to infliximab. Collectively these agents have demonstrated higher likelihood of induction of remission, reductions in hospitalization and the need for surgery, and lower rates of endoscopic recurrence.[10,27,57,58,60,67]

The use of TNF-α inhibitors in combination with thiopurines has quickly become the preferred approach to treatment of moderate-to-severe CD. Combination therapy results in added efficacy and reduction in antibody formation to the TNF-α inhibitor, which extends the duration of efficacy. Studies comparing infliximab to azathioprine combined with infliximab demonstrate greater rates of remission, steroid-free remission, and mucosal healing.[10,27,58] For this reason combination therapy is preferred unless patients have contraindications.

The integrin antagonists are options for patients who do not respond to steroids or have lost efficacy to or are intolerant of TNF-α inhibitors. Vedolizumab is also considered a first-line alternative to TNF-α inhibitors for moderate-to-severe disease.[27,59,60] These agents should not be used in combination with TNF-α inhibitors, but may be used with immunomodulators, which will also result in lower rates of antibody development.[27] Vedolizumab is preferred over natalizumab due to the reduced risk of adverse effects, particularly progressive multifocal leukoencephalopathy (PML) and has similar efficacy and safety outcomes compared to anti–TNF-α therapies.[59,60,69] If natalizumab is used, a baseline John Cunningham (JC) virus antibody must be negative prior to initiating therapy, and then should be monitored every 6 months. Therapy should be discontinued if a positive JC virus antibody is detected.[27]

Ustekinumab can be considered for moderate-to-severe CD in patients who have failed previous treatment with corticosteroids, immunomodulators, or TNF-α inhibitors, in patients with no prior exposure to TNF-α inhibitors.[27] This agent may be a preferred option for patients at higher risk of infections, those with advance age or multiple comorbidities, or in patients with prior malignancies.[27,56,60,62,67]

Severe/Fulminant Active Disease

Patients with severe or fulminant disease require prompt management in the inpatient setting and are often considered for surgical intervention. Parenteral corticosteroids at a dose equivalent of 40 to 60 mg prednisone should be instituted once the presence of abscess has been excluded.[27] TNF-α inhibitors may be used in severe disease, and infliximab may be considered in fulminant disease.[27] There are no data to support the use of cyclosporine, tacrolimus, or mycophenolate in patients with severe or fulminant disease.[27] TNF-α inhibitors are also considered first-line agents for fistulizing disease, with azathioprine and mercaptopurines as alternatives.[27] Patients may require surgical intervention in the setting of medically refractory disease.

Maintenance of Remission

Maintaining remission is typically more difficult with CD than with UC. Sulfasalazine may be considered in low-risk patients with disease confined to the colon who initially respond.[66] There is minimal evidence that oral mesalamine derivatives are effective therapies for maintenance of CD following medically induced remission, and therefore these agents are not preferred.[27,70] Mesalamine appears to have limited efficacy in preventing postsurgical relapse following resection, but can be considered in patients with isolated ileal resection with no risk factors for recurrence.[27] Metronidazole, 1 to 2 g/day, may also be used to prevent postoperative recurrence, but is not recommended for use in medically induced remission.[27]

Systemic corticosteroids have no role in maintenance of remission or prevention of recurrence of CD. These agents do not alter the long-term course of the disease and predispose patients to serious adverse effects with long-term use.[27] Despite a lower potential for systemic adverse effects, use of budesonide as maintenance therapy is only recommended for a duration of up to 4 months.[27]

All of the TNF-α inhibitors currently approved for use in CD are viable options for maintenance of remission.[27] Combination therapy with a thiopurine should be highly considered to further improve efficacy and to extend the duration of TNF-α inhibitor efficacy by reducing the immunogencity.[27] If surgical resection is being considered, TNF-α inhibitors should be started within 4 weeks of surgery in high-risk patients (age 2 prior resections for penetrating disease) in order to prevent postoperative recurrence.[71] Methotrexate may be considered as an alternative to thiopurines to maintain corticosteroid-induced remission.[27] Vedolizumab, natalizumab, and ustekinumab can be used for maintenance in patients who initially achieve induction of remission with these agents.[34]

Selected Complications

Toxic Megacolon

The treatment required for toxic megacolon includes general supportive therapy, consideration for early surgical intervention, and drug therapy.[24] Perforation can significantly worsen outcomes, with up to 44% of patients requiring surgery.[24] Aggressive fluid and electrolyte management is required for dehydration. Transfusion may be necessary if significant blood loss has occurred. Opiates and medications with anticholinergic properties should be discontinued because these agents enhance colonic dilation, thereby increasing the risk of bowel perforation. Broad-spectrum antimicrobials that include coverage for gram-negative bacilli and intestinal anaerobes should be used as preemptive therapy in the event that perforation occurs. If the patient is not receiving corticosteroids, then high-dose IV therapy with hydrocortisone 100 mg every 6 to 8 hours should be administered to reduce acute inflammation.[24] Emergent surgical intervention, mainly an abdominal colectomy with formation of an ileostomy, is an important consideration for patients with toxic megacolon and prevents death in some patients.[43-45]

Extraintestinal Manifestations

For some extraintestinal manifestations of IBD, specific therapies can be instituted, whereas for others the treatment that is used for the GI inflammatory process also addresses the systemic manifestations.

Anemia secondary to blood loss from the GI tract can be treated with oral ferrous sulfate. If the patient is unable to take oral medication and the patient's hematocrit is sufficiently low, blood transfusions or IV iron infusions may be required.[32] Anemia may also be related to malabsorption of vitamin B_{12} or folic acid, particularly for patients who have had ileal resection, so supplementation may be required.[28,29] Screening for osteoporosis does not differ significantly from the general population. Patients with conventional risk factors for abnormal bone density should be screened for osteoporosis with dual x-ray absorptiometry and then periodically thereafter.[72] Screening should also occur in patients starting oral corticosteroids, particularly in patients who have received greater than 7.5 mg/day equivalent of prednisone for longer than three consecutive months.[72] If the patient is deemed high risk for osteoporosis, such as those receiving corticosteroids, or exhibits a reduced serum vitamin D concentration, vitamin D supplementation should be instituted.[29] If osteoporosis is present, then calcium, vitamin D, and a bisphosphonate or possibly teriparatide are recommended.[32] Corticosteroid use should be avoided or limited, and weight-bearing exercise initiated if possible.

There are no consistently recommended therapies for aphthous ulcers; however, topical viscous lidocaine may provide symptom relief while topical corticosteroids may promote healing.[32] Episcleritis or uveitis is often worse during exacerbations of the intestinal disease, and measures improving intestinal disease will improve these systemic manifestations. Cool compresses and topical corticosteroids or NSAIDs may provide symptomatic relief, while immunomodulators and TNF-α inhibitors when in use may also provide benefit.[32] For arthritis associated with IBD, short-term NSAID or corticosteroids may be considered. However, NSAID use may exacerbate the underlying IBD and predispose patients to GI bleeding, so COX-2 inhibitors may be considered.[33,73] Intra-articular corticosteroids may be tried to limit the adverse effects of systemically administered agents.[32] Skin manifestations often require local wound care and use of topical or systemic corticosteroids.[32,33] Anti–TNF-α therapies may also improve severe dermatologic manifestations.

Adverse Drug Effects

Compared with mesalamine, sulfasalazine is more often associated with adverse drug effects, and these effects may be classified as either dose related or idiosyncratic (Table 52-4).[18,27,46,47,74] The sulfapyridine portion of the sulfasalazine molecule is believed to be responsible for much of the sulfasalazine toxicity.[18] Dose-related side effects usually include GI disturbances such as nausea, vomiting, diarrhea, or anorexia but may also include headache and arthralgia. These adverse reactions tend to occur more commonly on initiation of therapy and decrease in frequency as therapy is continued. Approaches to the management of these adverse effects include discontinuing the agent for a short period and then reinstituting therapy at a reduced dosage with subsequent slower dose escalation, administration with food, or substituting another enteric-coated 5-ASA product. Folic acid absorption is impaired by sulfasalazine, which may lead to anemia, so oral folic acid supplementation should be administered.

Idiosyncratic effects commonly include rash, fever, or hepatotoxicity, as well as relatively uncommon but serious reactions such as bone marrow suppression, thrombocytopenia, pancreatitis, pneumonitis, interstitial nephritis, and hepatitis. For most patients with idiosyncratic reactions, sulfasalazine must be discontinued. Mesalamine has been associated with development of interstitial nephritis as well; therefore, intermittent monitoring of serum creatinine is warranted.[74]

Up to 80% of patients who are intolerant to sulfasalazine will tolerate oral mesalamine derivatives.[18] The most commonly encountered adverse effects are nausea, vomiting, and headache. However, olsalazine may cause watery diarrhea in up to 25% of patients, often requiring drug discontinuation.

Adverse effects of corticosteroids include hyperglycemia, hypertension, osteoporosis, acne, fluid retention, electrolyte disturbances, myopathies, muscle wasting, increased appetite, psychosis, infection, and adrenocortical suppression.[18,52,74] To minimize corticosteroid effects, clinicians may use alternate-day steroid therapy; however, some patients do not do well clinically on the days when no steroid is given. For most patients a single daily corticosteroid dose suffices, and divided daily doses are unnecessary. Adrenal insufficiency after abrupt steroid withdrawal often necessitates gradual tapering of steroid therapy for patients using these agents daily for more than 2 to 3 weeks. Budesonide is preferred in CD involving the ileum or right colon, or in UC, and may also be substituted for prednisone in CD patients who are steroid dependent or require long-term therapy.[27,60]

Azathioprine and mercaptopurine may be associated with serious adverse effects such as lymphomas, pancreatitis, or nephrotoxicity.[18,27,53,54,74] Adverse events to thiopurines are typically divided into two groups: type A and type B.[27,35,54] Type A reactions are dose related and include malaise, nausea, infectious complications, hepatitis, and myelosuppression. Complete blood counts with differential should be monitored every 2 weeks while doses are being titrated. Type B reactions are considered idiosyncratic and include fever, rash, arthralgia, and pancreatitis (3%-15% of patients).[35,53,54] Predisposition to development of these adverse effects may be related to polymorphisms in the enzyme thiopurine methyltransferase (TPMT), which is partially responsible for activation and metabolism of these drugs. Determination of TPMT activity is recommended prior to initiation of therapy to determine which patients require lower doses of these agents.[54,74,75] Alternatively, evaluating TPMT genotype or phenotype can also assist in assessing a patient's risk for toxicity.[61,62,74,75] Doses may need to be reduced by 30% to 80% if low TPMT activity is present.[75] Adjusting azathioprine and mercaptopurine doses by measuring concentrations of metabolites, particularly TGN, may be useful, with target concentrations of 230 to 450 pmol/8 $\times$ 10^8 erythrocytes considered optimal.[61,62,68,75-77]

Variations in the NUDT15 allele also predisposes patients using mercaptopurine to excess myelosuppresion.[75,76] Assessment of the NUDT15 phenotype can be performed as well if Mercaptopurine is used, with similar recommendations for dose reductions if poor or intermediate metabolizer status is present.[75] Since the initial dosing of these agents is weight based, obtaining a current accurate weight for the patient is necessary as well. Obtaining a family history regarding lymphoproliferative disorders or lymphoma is important for determining if the potential risks outweigh the benefits of long-term use. Women receiving immunosuppressive therapy should undergo annual cervical cancer screening and all patients should be screened annually for melanoma.[72]

With the advent of coadministration of azathioprine with infliximab, development of hepatosplenic T-cell lymphoma (HSTCL) has become a concern. The overall impact of using both drugs together, the contribution of drug classes to the development of lymphoma, and the risk and effects of both drugs are unclear. Those most at risk appear to be younger male patients (<35 years) and most of the risk is thought to be conferred by the thiopurine component.[53,74] Thiopurines are also associated with the development of non-melanoma squamous cell carcinoma, with the risk being higher during combination therapy with TNF-α inhibitors.[72,74] Methotrexate is associated with the development of nausea, vomiting, pulmonary fibrosis, pneumonitis, hepatotoxicity, anemia, and renal dysfunction, and is a known abortifacient. Patients should have baseline liver function tests, serum creatinine, BUN, complete blood count, and chest x-ray prior to use. Female patients should have a negative pregnancy test prior to use. Some patients may require supplementation with folic acid. Female patients of childbearing age opting to use methotrexate should have a safe and effective method of birth control available that is based on their preference.

Most patients receiving metronidazole for CD tolerate the agent fairly well; however, mild adverse effects occur frequently. They commonly include nausea, metallic taste, urticaria, and glossitis.[27,74] More serious effects that occur with long-term use include development of paresthesias and reversible peripheral neuropathy. Other effects include a disulfiram-like reaction if alcohol is ingested in conjunction.

The TNF-α inhibitors may be associated with development of serious adverse effects and carry similar adverse effect profiles for the available agents. Patients who receive infliximab often develop antibodies to infliximab (ATIs), also referred to as antidrug antibodies (ADAs). These ADAs can develop in response to administration of the other TNF-α inhibitors as well. Overall up to 50% of patients may lose efficacy after 1 year of treatment due to ADA development.[68] The development of ADAs also results in increases in the occurrence of serious infusion-related reactions in up to 2.8% of patients.[75] Up to 10% of patients per year require discontinuation of infliximab due to adverse effects and loss of efficacy related to development of ATIs.[55,58,74,76]

Strategies to reduce ATI formation include administration of a second dose within 8 weeks of the first dose, concurrent administration of steroids (hydrocortisone 200 mg IV on the day of the infusion or oral prednisone the day prior), and use of concomitant immunomodulators agents such as thiopurines.[18,27,58,74] Loss of efficacy may be managed by a dose escalation to 10 mg/kg, reducing the dosing interval, or switching to another TNF-α inhibitor.[27,55,74,77] Delayed hypersensitivity reactions may also occur up to 14 days after administration, with 5 to 7 days being the most common time frame. Autoimmune phenomena, such as lupus and hemolytic anemia, may also occur during infliximab therapy but are uncommon, as are adverse neurologic events such as optic neuritis and demyelinating syndrome.[74,76] Anti-TNF agents may also cause worsening of heart failure and should be avoided in patients with New York Heart Association Class III or IV heart failure.

All TNF-α inhibitors predispose patients to development of serious infections, including fungal, bacterial, and viral. Patients with clinically significant active infections should not receive TNF-α inhibitors. While the overall risk of hospitalization for serious infections may be less than previously suspected, development of infection remains a serious concern and increases with age.[67,74,76] Reactivation of latent mycobacterial infections may occur because of the inhibition of TNF-protective mechanisms; therefore, patients should receive a tuberculin skin test (purified protein derivative [PPD] test) and a chest x-ray prior to initiating therapy to rule out undiagnosed tuberculosis.[67,74,76] Reactivation of hepatitis B may occur; thus, patients should also be screened for hepatitis B virus infection prior to initiating therapy. Patients should also be screened for hepatitis C infection, although it does not appear that use of TNF-α inhibitors is unsafe or significantly alters the disease course. Natalizumab is associated with development of PML and is only available via the manufacturer's TOUCH prescribing program. Patients receiving natalizumab should be monitored for development of adverse neurologic events and undergo MRI of the brain should development of PML be suspected. Vedolizumab has not been associated with development of PML and may be associated with a lower risk of infection compared to TNF-α inhibitors.[69,74,76] Ustekinumab and tofacitinib carry many of the same adverse effect profile as the TNF-α inhibitors, and baseline screening for TB and hepatitis should be performed; however, overall risk of serious infection appears to be lower compared to TNF-α inhibitors.[67,69,74,76] Tofacitinib is also associated with development of thrombosis and lymphoma, as well as neutropenia, lymphopenia, and anemia.[60,63,74,76] The risk of thrombosis was observed at the higher doses of 10 mg twice daily, and in trials of patients with rheumatoid those greater than 50 years of age with at least one cardiovascular risk factor were at higher risk.[78] Tofacitinib should be avoided in patients with risks for thrombosis or history of pulmonary, deep vein, or arterial thrombosis.[78] Ozanimod is associated with the development of several potentially serious adverse effects. These include increased rate of infection, macular edema, fetal abnormalities, bradycardia or atrioventricular block, liver injury, and respiratory dysfunction. This necessitates a thorough patient history be obtained for presence of cardiovascular or cerebrovascular events within the last 6 months, as well as a history of sleep apnea.

For patients receiving ustekinumab and tofacitinib, baseline screening for latent infections should be performed. If patients appear to be losing response to TNF-α inhibitors, evaluating for ADAs, if assays are available, in addition to evaluating serum trough concentrations may assist the clinician in determining if dose and frequency need to be altered. Recommendation trough concentrations for TNF-α inhibitors include >5 μg/mL (mg/L) for infliximab, >7.5 μg/mL (mg/L) for adalimumab, >20 μg/mL (mg/L) for certolizumab, while optimal concentrations for golimumab are unknown.[68]

Patients should be evaluated for use of recommended vaccines; however, if patients are receiving immunosuppressants or biologic agents, the use of live or attenuated vaccines may be contraindicated.[72] Patients who currently use tobacco should be encouraged to undergo tobacco cessation, as tobacco use will worsen CD.[27,72] Since nicotine often improves symptoms in UC, it may be more difficult to cease tobacco use in this patient population. Choice of tobacco cessation products should also be based on current nicotine consumption and patient preference.

Special Populations

Pregnancy and Breastfeeding

The occurrence or consideration of pregnancy may cause significant concerns for the patient with IBD. Patients with IBD have similar infertility rates as the general female population, and the rate of involuntary childlessness in IBD patients who have not undergone surgery is similar.[79-81] There is a greater risk of adverse pregnancy outcomes such as spontaneous abortion, low birth weight, cesarean section, congenital abnormalities, low Apgar scores, preterm rupture of membranes, and preeclampsia.[79-81] However, most patients can conceive normally and have a normal pregnancy. The impact of IBD disease activity on pregnancy still remains unclear. In patients in remission at the time of conception the rates of reported flares are 20% in CD and 33% in UC, and postpartum rates of relapse are reported as 14%.[78-81] Preconception counseling in patients with IBD is recommended, in addition to objective assessment of disease activity in order to optimize therapy.[1,8] Overall patients should optimally achieve at least 3 to 6 months of corticosteroid-free remission prior to conceiving.[7,9] Patients should be managed by a gastroenterologist throughout their pregnancy, and also be referred to an obstetrician who manages high-risk patients if they have active or complicated disease.[80,81]

Diligence should be given to reviewing current medications in patients with IBD who are both contemplating pregnancy or have already conceived. Sulfasalazine is generally well tolerated; however, it does interfere with folate absorption, so supplementation with folic acid 1 mg twice daily should be used during the pregnancy.[74,79,80] Sulfasalazine causes decreased sperm counts and reduced fertility in males and corticosteroids may adversely affect fertility as well.[82] This effect is reversible on discontinuation of the drug, and it is not reported with mesalamine. Other ASAs can be used as well; however, there are concerns regarding the presence of dibutyl phthalate in the coating of Asacol.[7,9] Mesalamine preparations not containing dibutyl phthalate should be preferentially used.[7,80] Steroids given systemically do not appear to be detrimental to the fetus, and in general can be used in the same manner as in non-pregnant patients.[4,7,8,80] Due to its lower systemic bioavailability budesonide may be considered safer than other systemic corticosteroids for pregnant patients.[4,7] Azathioprine and mercaptopurine appear to carry an overall minimal risk in pregnant patients, and should be continued in patients receiving these agents as maintenance therapy.[74,80] Given pharmacokinetic changes in azathioprine metabolism occur during pregnancy, monitoring of 6-TGN during and after pregnancy is indicated.[80] Use of TNF-α inhibitors in pregnant patients appear to carry an overall low risk, and continuation of therapy is warranted in most patients. Infliximab, adalimumab, and golimumab do cross the placenta and there are some concerns with increased exposure to the fetus in the third trimester. While the risk is low, consideration can be given to administering the last dose at 22 to 24 weeks of gestation to minimize drug transfer to the fetus in patients considered low risk for relapse.[75,80,81] For newborns of women who were receiving TNF-α inhibitors during pregnancy it is recommended that use of live vaccines be avoided.[80] In patients receiving combination therapy with azathioprine and a TNF-α inhibitor, consideration of switching to monotherapy can be given, with use of a TNF-α inhibitor as preferred therapy.[80] Natalizumab, vedolizumab, and ustekinumab appear to carry low risk when used as monotherapies; however, consideration can also be given to administering the last dose at 8 to 10 weeks prior to delivery to minimize fetal exposure.[7,9] Tofacitinib does not appear to cause birth defects, miscarriage, or adverse fetal outcomes. There is a pregnancy registry that women who become pregnant while receiving tofacitinib are encouraged to enroll in. Metronidazole and ciprofloxacin may be used for short courses for treatment of perianal disease, and should be avoided during the first trimester if possible.[74,79,81] Methotrexate should not be used during pregnancy, and should be stopped 3 months prior to conception. It should be stopped immediately in patients who become pregnant while taking it, with referral for obstetric counseling.[1,8]

Use of agents in breastfeeding women is also a consideration. Sulfasalazine does pose a small risk of kernicterus, as levels of sulfapyridine in breast milk are low or undetectable, and thus monitoring for this symptom should be implemented.[79-81] Other mesalamine derivatives are considered safe in breastfeeding.[78,79] Corticosteroids can be detected in breast milk, with fetal levels approximately 10% to 12% of maternal levels.[79] However, breastfeeding is believed to be safe, but mothers should optimally wait at least 4 hours after an oral dose of systemic corticosteroids before breastfeeding to limit exposure to the child.[7,9] The anti-TNF-α agents and thiopurines are generally considered safe for use in breastfeeding and carry minimal risk of adverse effects.[74,81] Methotrexate should be avoided in breastfeeding mothers.[1,8] Metronidazole and cyclosporine should not be given to nursing mothers because these agents are excreted into breast milk and may cause adverse effects.[74,78-81]

Children and Adolescents

IBD can present early in life, with 6% to 15% of patients being diagnosed prior to 6 years of age, and CD being more prevalent than UC.[83,84] This distinction in pediatric patients is referred to as very-early-onset IBD (VEO-IBD).[83] Due to the aggressive nature of CD, patients may be at risk for poor nutritional status, growth failure, micronutrient deficiencies, anemia, and pubertal delay.[84,85] Patients should be assessed for nutrient deficiencies, particularly iron and vitamin D, and replacement implemented if needed.[83-87]

Drug treatment in pediatric patients is similar to adults, with mesalamine, azathioprine, and the TNF-α inhibitors all being viable options. Due to the association with development of lymphoma and pharmacokinetic changes in metabolism as patients get older, thiopurines are used less often in pediatric patients.[83] Due to the potential for adverse effects, corticosteroid use should be limited to short-term use as induction therapy. The TNF-α inhibitors have become a major drug class used in the management of pediatric patients with IBD for both induction and maintenance of remission. Infliximab is approved for use in the United States for patients 6-17 years of age with moderate-to-severe active CD. Adalimumab is also approved for use in patients 6 years of age or older with CD. Studies indicate that early use significantly improves clinical outcomes, such as remission and mucosal healing.[88] However, initial response rates in patients to infliximab with VEO-IBD may actually be lower due to differences in pharmacokinetics and immune pathways of the disease.[83] This may necessitate higher and more frequent dosing to optimize therapy. Data are lacking to support routine use of vedolizumab, ustekinumab, and tofacitinib in pediatric patients.

Older Adults

Up to 30% of patients with IBD develop symptoms after age 60, and prevalence in older patients appears to be increasing.[89,90] In North America the incidence of IBD is reported as 4-8 per 100,000 persons greater than age 60 and 15% of cases are diagnosed after age 60.[90] One of the difficulties in diagnosis of IBD is that patients greater than 60 years of age may have other conditions present that may mimic IBD symptoms. This includes ischemic colitis, diverticular disease, microscopic colitis, CRC, NSAID-induced intestinal changes, or radiation induced enteritis or colitis.[89,90] Older patients with CD may present more often with isolated colonic disease, while left-sided disease is more common in elderly patients with UC.[90]

The approach to drug therapy in older adults is similar to younger individuals; however, a multidisciplinary approach is favored given the greater number of comorbidities and medications that may be present.[90] Overall patient fitness and frailty should be assessed, as this may impact the potential for serious adverse effects from medications, such as infection.[89,90] The aminosalicylates can be used for both induction and maintenance therapy; however, routine monitoring of renal function should be implemented, as interstitial nephritis is a potential adverse effect.[90] Corticosteroids should still be reserved for short courses as induction therapy, as older patients may have conditions that corticosteroids may worsen, such as diabetes, hypertension, heart failure, glaucoma, or osteoporosis.[89,90] Budesonide may be preferred, if possible, due to the lower systemic bioavailability.

Thiopurines are an attractive option due to their oral route of administration; however, there are concerns about increases in hepatotoxicity and nonmelanoma skin cancers in older patients.[90,91] They should be used cautiously in this population, and methotrexate may be an alternative in some instances.[90,91] The TNF-α inhibitors can be used for induction and maintenance; however, more frail patients may be at higher risk for infection and malignancy, especially if used in combination with a thiopurine. Combination therapy should be reserved for patients with severe disease.[90] Use of ustekinumab or vedolizumab may be preferred for more frail patients due to the lower overall risk for infection.[74,76,90] Tofacinib is largely reserved as a second-line agent in elderly patients, due to both lack of data and increases in risk of thromboembolic disease. Lastly, older patients with IBD should have routine health screening and maintenance performed. This is important in this patient population due to the need for maintaining appropriate vaccinations and implementing screenings for osteoporosis and CRC.[72,92]

PATENTS WITH COVID-19 INFECTION

Given that patients with IBD are often receiving one or more immunosuppressive agents, concerns with the COVID-19 pandemic were that patients would be at higher risk for infection and potentially worse outcomes. In order to communicate information rapidly, an international reporting website, https://covidibd.org/, was formed to allow clinicians and investigators to report outcomes related to COVID infection in both adult and pediatric patients with IBD. This resulted in an initial report of outcomes in over 500 patients in 33 countries.[93] Based on the analysis, patients with IBD who were older, had multiple comorbidities, or were receiving corticosteroids had more severe COVID-19 disease. Interestingly, TNF-α use was not associated with severe COVID-19 disease. A subsequent meta-analysis demonstrated that the risk of acquiring COVID-19 in patients with IBD is not significantly different than the general population and does also not differ based on subtype of IBD.[93] Worse outcomes, such as hospitalization and increased mortality was seen more in patients with UC and in patients receiving 5-ASA products or corticosteroids. TNF-α use was actually found to be a protective factor in this trial, indicating that the anti-inflammatory effects of these drugs may actually attenuate some aspects of COVID-induced inflammation. With regard to the COVID-19 vaccines, the Crohns and Colitis Foundation have released recommendations that patients with IBD should receive the vaccine, regardless of current medication use (https://www.crohnscolitisfoundation.org/coronavirus/vaccines). Both international and British guidelines also advocate for the same approach, indicating that the benefit of vaccination as soon as possible in patients with IBD outweighs the risk of potential reduced response in those receiving immunosuppressive therapies.[94-96]

EVALUATION OF THERAPEUTIC OUTCOMES

The success of therapeutic regimens to treat IBD can be measured by patient-reported complaints, signs, and symptoms; by direct clinician examination (including endoscopy); by history and physical examination; by selected laboratory tests; and by QOL measures. Evaluation of IBD severity is difficult because much of the assessment is subjective. Disease rating scales, such as the CDAI or other indices, have been created to make disease assessment more objective. The CDAI is a commonly used scale for patients with nonfistulizing disease and for evaluation of patients during clinical trials.[10,27] The scale incorporates eight elements: (a) number of stools in the past 7 days, (b) sum of abdominal pain ratings from the past 7 days, (c) rating of general well-being in the past 7 days, (d) use of antidiarrheals, (e) body weight, (f) hematocrit, (g) finding of abdominal mass, and (h) a sum of extraintestinal symptoms present in the past week. Elements of this index provide a guide for those measures that may be useful in assessing the effectiveness of treatment regimens. A decrease in CDAI of 100 points is considered a clinically significant response, with a score of less than 150 considered to be disease remission.[10,27] A subsequent scale was developed specifically for perianal CD, known as the *Perianal Crohn's Disease Activity Index* (PDAI). The PDAI includes five items: presence of discharge, pain, restriction of sexual activity, type of perianal disease, and degree of induration. The HBI may also be used in place of the CDAI.

Standardized assessment tools have also been constructed for UC.[1,18] Elements in these scales vary and include (a) stool frequency, (b) presence of blood in the stool, (c) mucosal appearance (from endoscopy), and (d) physician's global assessment based on physical examination, endoscopy, and laboratory data. While these tools are often used for assessment of patients in clinical trials, they are sometimes used in the clinical setting as well.

Additional studies that are often useful include direct endoscopic examination of affected areas and/or radiocontrast studies. Mucosal healing is considered a major end point for patients with luminal disease. For patients with acute disease, assessment of fluid and electrolyte status is important, because these may be lost during diarrheal episodes. Other laboratory tests, such as serum albumin, transferrin, or other markers of visceral protein status as well as markers of inflammation such as ESR or CRP, and fecal calprotectin, are used to monitor disease and drug therapy. Lastly assessing for both trough concentrations and presence of ADAs can help guide therapy in patients who are not responding to normal doses of TNF-α inhibitors.

Finally, a patient QOL assessment should be performed regularly.[1,18,27] Inquiry should be made regarding the patient's general well-being, emotional function, and social function. Social function may include assessment of the ability to perform routine daily functions and to maintain occupational activities, sexual function, and recreation. The most common tool used to assess QOL is the Inflammatory Bowel Disease Questionnaire (IBDQ), a 32-item questionnaire that covers four disease dimensions: bowel function, emotional status, systemic symptoms, and social function. The IBDQ has shown good correlation with the CDAI.[27] The standard short form 36 (SF-36) is often used as a measure of QOL in IBD intervention trials.

ABBREVIATIONS

ADA	antidrug antibody
ASA	aminosalicylate
ATI	antibody to infliximab
CD	Crohn's disease
CDAI	Crohn's Disease Activity Index
CRC	colorectal carcinoma
CRP	C-reactive protein
ESR	erythrocyte sedimentation rate
FC	fecal calprotectin
FODMAPS	fermentable oligo-, di-, and monosaccharides and polyols
HBI	Harvey-Bradshaw Index
HLA	human leukocyte antigen
HSTCL	hepatosplenic T-cell lymphoma
IBD	inflammatory bowel disease
IBDQ	Inflammatory Bowel Disease Questionnaire
IL	interleukin
IPAA	ileal pouch anal anastomosis
JAK	Janus Kinase
MMX	Multi-MatriX
NF-κ B	nuclear factor κ B
NOD2	nucleotide-binding oligomerization domain protein 2
NSAID	nonsteroidal anti-inflammatory drug
PDAI	perianal Crohn's Disease Activity Index
PML	progressive multifocal leukoencephalopathy
PPD	purified protein derivative
PSC	primary sclerosing cholangitis
QOL	quality of life
SCD	specific carbohydrate diet
S1P	sphingosine-1 phosphate

TGF-β	transforming growth factor-β
TGN	thioguanine
TLR	toll-like membrane receptor
TNF-α	tumor necrosis factor-α
TPMT	thiopurine methyltransferase
UC	ulcerative colitis
VTE	venous thromboembolism

REFERENCES

1. Ungaro R, Mehandru S, Allen PB, et al. Ulcerative colitis. *Lancet.* 2017;389(18):1756–1770.
2. Ng SC. Understanding and preventing the global increase of inflammatory bowel diseases. *Gastroenterology.* 2017;152(152):313–321.
3. Gajendra M, Priyadarshini L, Catinella, AP, et al. A comprehensive review and update on Crohn's disease. *Dis Mon.* 2018 Feb;64(2):20–57. doi:10.1016/j.disamonth.2017.07.001.
4. Kaplan GG, Ng SC. Inflammatory bowel disease: Innovations and changing paradigms. *Gastroenterology.* 2017;152:309–312.
5. Chang JT. Pathophysiology of inflammatory bowel diseases. *N Engl J Med.* 2020;383:2652–64. 10.1056/NEJMra2002697.
6. Sartor RB, Wu GD. Role for intestinal bacteria, viruses, and fungi in pathogenesis of inflammatory bowel diseases and therapeutic approaches. *Gastroenterlgy.* 2017;152:327–329.
7. Yoshimatsuet Y, Mikami Y, Kanai T. Bacteriotherapy for inflammatory bowel disease. *Inflammation and Regeneration.* 2021;41:3. https://doi.org/10.1186/s41232-020-00153-4.
8. Lewis JD, Abreu MT. Diet as a trigger or therapy for inflammatory bowel disease. *Gastroenterology.* 2017;152:398–414.
9. Guo AY, Stevens BW, Wilson RG, et al. Early life environment and natural history of inflammatory bowel disease. *BMC Gastroenterol.* 2014;14:216.
10. Torres J, Mehandru S, Colombel JF, et al. Crohn's disease. *Lancet.* 2017;389:1741–1755.
11. Moller FT, Andersen V, Wohlfahrt J, et al. Familial risk if inflammatory bowel disease: A population-based cohort study 1977–2011. *Am J Gastroenterol.* 2015;110:564–571.
12. Chapman CG, Pekow J. The emerging role of miRNAs in inflammatory bowel disease: A review. *Ther Adv Gastroenterol.* 2015;8(1):4–22.
13. Caioni G, Viscido A, d'Angelo M, et al. Inflammatory bowel disease: New insights into the interplay between environmental factors and PPARy. *Int J Mol Sci.* 2021;22:985. https://doi.org/10.3390/ijms22030985.
14. Stappenbeck TS, McGovern DP. Paneth cell alterations in the development and phenotype of Crohn's disease. *Gastroenterology* 2017;152:322–326.
15. Regueiro M, Greer JB, Szigethy E. Etiology and treatment of pain and pyschosocial issues in patients with inflammatory bowel disease. *Gastroenterology.* 2017;152(152):430–439.
16. Yue S, Lu Li, Runxiang X, et al. Stress triggers flare of inflammatory bowel disease in children and adults. *Front Pediatr.* 24 October 2019. https://doi.org/10.3389/fped.2019.00432.
17. Sweeney L, Moss-Morris R, Czuber-Dochan W, et al. Systematic review: Psychosocial factors associated with pain in inflammatory bowel disease. *Aliment Pharmcol Ther.* 2018;47:715–729. doi:10.1111/apt.14493.
18. Rubin DT, Ananthakrishnan AN, Siegel CA, et al. ACG Clinical Guideline: Ulcerative colitis in adults. *Am J Gastroenterol.* 2019;114:384–413.
19. Moninuloa OO, Milligan W, Lochhead P, et al. Systemic review with meta-analysis: Association between acetaminophen and nonsteroidal anti-inflammatory drugs (NSAIDs) and risk of Crohn's disease and ulcerative colitis. *Aliment Pharmacol Ther.* 2018;47:1428–1439. doi:10.1111/apt.14606.
20. Patel P, Gao G, Gulotta G, et al. Daily aspirin use does not impact clinical outcomes in patients with inflammatory bowel disease. *Inflamm Bowel Dis.* 2021;27(2). doi:10.1093/ibd/izaa060.
21. Theochari NA, Stefanopoulos A, Mylonas KS, Economopoulos KP. Antibiotics exposure and risk of inflammatory bowel disease: A systematic review. *Scand J Gastroenterol.* 2018;53(1):1–7. doi:10.1080/00365521.2017.1386711. Epub 2017 Oct 12. PMID: 29022402.
22. Ortizo R, Lee SY, Nguyen ET, Jamal MM, Bechtold MM, Nguyen DL. Exposure to oral contraceptives increases the risk for development of inflammatory bowel disease: A meta-analysis of case-controlled and cohort studies. *Eur J Gastroenterol Hepatol* 2017;29(9):1064–1070. 10.1097/MEG.0000000000000915. PMID: 28542115.
23. Wang X, Fan X, Deng H, Zhang X, Zhang K, Xu J, Li N, Han Q, Liu Z. Use of oral contraceptives and risk of ulcerative colitis—A systematic review and meta-analysis. *Pharmacol Res.* 2019;139: 367–374. doi:10.1016/j.phrs.2018.11.036. Epub 2018 Nov 28. PMID: 30502529.
24. Desai J, Elnaggar M, Hanfy AA, Doshi R. Toxic megacolon: Background, pathophysiology, management, challenges and solutions. *Clin Exp Gastroenterol.* 2020;13:203–210. Published 2020 May 19. doi:10.2147/CEG.S200760.
25. Keller DS, Windsor A, Cohen R, Chand M. Colorectal cancer in inflammatory bowel disease: Review of the evidence. *Tech. Coloproctol.* 2019;23(1):3–13. https://doi.org/10.1007/s10151-019-1926-2.
26. Limdi JK, Farraye FA. An update on surveillance in ulcerative colitis. *Curr Gastroenterol Rep.* 2018;20:112.
27. Lichtenstein GR, Loftus EV, Isaacs KI, et al. ACG Clinical Guideline: Management of Crohn's disease in adults. *Am J Gastroenterol.* 2018;113:481–517.
28. Schreiner P, Martinho-Grueber M, Studerus D, et al., on behalf of Swiss IBDnet, an official working group of the Swiss Society of Gastroenterology. Nutrition in inflammatory bowel disease digestion. *Digestion.* 2020;101(Suppl 1):120–135. 10.1159/000505368. Epub 2020 Jan 10. PMID: 31927540.
29. Ghishan FK, Kiela PR. Vitamins and minerals in inflammatory bowel disease. *Gastroenterol Clin North Am.* 2017;46(4):797–808. 10.1016/j.gtc.2017.08.011. Epub 2017 Oct 3. PMID: 29173522; PMCID: PMC6342481.
30. Forbes A, Escher J, Hébuterne X, Kłęk S, Krznaric Z, Schneider S, Shamir R, Stardelova K, Wierdsma N, Wiskin AE, Bischoff SC. ESPEN guideline: Clinical nutrition in inflammatory bowel disease. *Clin Nutr.* 2017;36(2):321–347. doi:10.1016/j.clnu.2016.12.027. Epub 2016 Dec 31. Erratum in: Clin Nutr. 2019 Jun;38(3):1486. Erratum in: Clin Nutr. 2019 Jun;38(3):1485. PMID: 28131521.
31. Fousekis FS, Thropistos VI, Katsanos KH. Hepatobiliary manifestations and complications in inflammatory bowel disease: A review. *Gastroenterol Res.* 2018;11(2):83–94.
32. Rogler G, Singh A, Kavanaugh A, Rubin DT. Extraintestinal manifestations of inflammatory bowel disease: Current concepts, treatment, and implications for disease management. *Gastroenterology.* 2021;161(4):1118–1132. 10.1053/j.gastro.2021.07.042.
33. Marotto D, Atzeni F, Ardizzone S, et al. Extra-intestinal manifestations of inflammatory bowel diseases. *Pharmacol Res.* 2020;161:105–206. doi:10.1016/j.phrs.2020.105206. Epub 2020 Sep 28. PMID: 32998068.
34. Kärnsund S, Lo B, Bendtsen F, Holm J, Burisch J. Systematic review of the prevalence and development of osteoporosis or low bone mineral density and its risk factors in patients with inflammatory bowel disease. *World J Gastroenterol.* 2020;26(35):5362–5374. doi:10.3748/wjg.v26.i35.5362.
35. Feuerstein Joseph D, Isaacs Kim L, Schneider Y, et al. AGA Clinical Practice Guidelines on the management of moderate to severe ulcerative colitis. *Gastroenterology.* 2020;158:1450–1461. 10.1053/j.gastro.2020.01.006.
36. American Gastroenterological Association. Ulcerative colitis clinical care pathway. Available at: https://s3.amazonaws.com/agaassets/pdf/guidelines/UlcerativeColitis/index.html. Accessed May 7, 2021.
37. Panes J, Jairath V, Levesque BG. Advances in use of endoscopy, radiology, and biomarkers to monitor inflammatory bowel diseases. *Gastroenterology.* 2017;152:362–373.
38. AGA Institute Guidelines for the identification, assessment and initial medical treatment in Crohn's disease clinical care pathway. Available at: https://s3.amazonaws.com/agaassets/pdf/guidelines/IBDCarePathway.pdf. Accessed May 7, 2021.
39. Fumery M, Singh S, Dulai PS, et al. Natural history of adult ulcerative colitis in population based cohorts: A systematic review. *Clin Gastroenterol Hepatol.* 2018;16:343–356.
40. Colombel JF, Narula N, Peyrin-Biroulet L. Management strategies to improve outcomes of patients with inflammatory bowel diseases. *Gastroenterology.* 2017;152:351–361.
41. Derwa Y, Gracie DJ, Hamlin PJ, et al. Systematic review with meta analysis: The efficacy of probiotics in inflammatory bowel disease. *Aliment Pharmacol Ther.* 2017;46:389–400.
42. Su Grace L, Ko Cynthia W, Bercik P, et al. AGA Clinical Practice Guidelines on the role of probiotics in the management of gastrointestinal disorders. *Gastroenterology.* 2020;159:697–705. 10.1053/j.gastro.2020.05.059.
43. Sarigoz T. Surgical treatment of ulcerative colitis: A review. *Int J Surg Res Pract.* 2020;3:14–19. 10.23937/2378-3397/1410116.

44. Adamina M, Bonovas S, Raine T, et al. ECCO Guidelines on therapeutics in Crohn's disease: Surgical treatment. *J Crohns Colitis.* 2020;14(2):155–168. 10.1093/ecco-jcc/jjz187. PMID: 31742338.
45. Lightner AL, Vogel JD, Carmichael JC, et al. The American Society of Colon and Rectal Surgeons Clinical Practice Guidelines for the surgical management of Crohn's disease. *Dis Colon Rectum.* 2020;63(8): 1028–1052. 10.1097/DCR.0000000000001716.
46. Naganuma M. Solving the questions regarding 5-aminosalitylate formulation in the treatment of ulcerative colitis. *J Gastroenterol.* 2020;55:1013–1022. 10.1007/s00535-020-01713-8.
47. Bayan MF, Bayan RF. Recent advances in mesalamine colonic delivery systems. *Futur J Pharm Sci* 2020;34(6):1–7. https://doi.org/10.1186/s43094-020-00057-.
48. Kato S, Ishibashi A, Kani K, et al. Optimized management of ulcerative proctitis: When and how to use mesalazine suppository. *Digestion.* 2018;97:59–63.
49. Cohen RD, Dalal SR. Systematic review: Rectal therapies for the treatment of distal forms of ulcerative colitis. *Inflamm Bowel Dis.* 2015;21:1719–1736.
50. Christophi G, Rengarajan A. Ciorba Matthew Rectal budesonide and mesalamine formulations in active ulcerative proctosigmoiditis: Efficacy, tolerance, and treatment approach. *Clinical and Experimental Gastroenterology.* 2016;9:125. doi:10.2147/ceg.s80237.
51. Nardelli S, Pisani LF, Tontini GE. MMX technology and its applications in gastrointestinal diseases. *Ther Adv Gastroenterol.* 2017;7:545–552.
52. Dorrington Alexander M, Selinger Christian P, Parkes Gareth C, et al. The historical role and contemporary use of corticosteroids in inflammatory bowel disease. *J Crohn's Colitis.* 2020;14:1316–1329. 10.1093/ecco-jcc/jjaa053.
53. van Gennep S, de Boer NK, d'Haens GR, et al. Thiopurine treatment in ulcerative colitis: A critical review of the evidence for current clinical practice. *Inflamm Bowel Dis.* 2018;24:67–77.
54. Louis E, Irving P, Beaugerie L. Use of azathioprine in IBD: Modern aspects of an old drug. *Gut.* 2014;63(11):1695–1699.
55. Terdiman JP, Gruss CB, Heidelbaugh JJ, et al. American Gastroenterological Association Institute guideline on the use of thiopurines, methotrexate, and anti-TNF-α biologic drugs for the induction and maintenance of remission in Crohn's disease. *Gastroenterology.* 2013;145:1459–1463.
56. Rawlal P, Sunkara T, Raj JP. Role of biologics and biosimilars in inflammatory bowel disease: Current trends and future perspectives. *J Inflamm Res.* 2018;11:215–226. doi:10.2147/JIR.S165330.
57. Baumgart DC, Le Berre C. Newer biologic and small-molecule therapies for inflammatory bowel disease. *N Engl J Med.* 2021;385(14):1302–1315. 10.1056/NEJMra1907607.PMID: 34587387.
58. Mao EJ, Hazlewood GS, Kaplan GG. Systematic review with meta-analysis: Comparative efficacy of immunosuppressants and biologics for reducing hospitalization and surgery in Crohn's disease and ulcerative colitis. *Aliment Pharmacol Ther.* 2017;45:3–13.
59. Dotan Iris AM, Danese S, et al. The role of integrins in the pathogenesis of inflammatory bowel disease: Approved and investigational anti-integrin therapies. *Med Res Rev.* 2019;40:245–262. 10.1002/med.21601.
60. Honap S, Cunningham G, Tamilarasan AG, Irving PM. Positioning biologics and new therapies in the management of inflammatory bowel disease. *Curr Opin Gastroenterol.* 2019;35(4):296–301. doi:10.1097/MOG.0000000000000546. PMID: 31021925.
61. Gionata F, Mariangela A, Carmen C, et al. Positioning ustekinumab in moderate-to-severe ulcerative colitis: New kid on the block. *Expert Opin Biol Ther.* 2020;20:421–427. 10.1080/14712598.2020.1727437.
62. Honap S, Meade S, Ibraheim H, et al. Effectiveness and safety of ustekinumab in inflammatory bowel disease: A systematic review and meta-analysis. *Dig Dis Sci.* 2021 Mar 16. 10.1007/s10620-021-06932-4. Epub ahead of print. PMID: 33723700.
63. Siegmund B. Janus Kinase inhibitors in the new treatment paradigms of inflammatory bowel disease. *J Crohn's Colitis.* 2020;14:S761–S766. 10.1093/ecco-jcc/jjaa003.
64. Ko CW, Singh S, Feurerstein JD, et al. AGA Clinical Practice Guidelines on the management of mild-moderate ulcerative colitis. *Gastroenterology.* 2019;156:748–764.
65. Sands Bruce E, Peyrin-Biroulet L, Loftus EV, et al. Vedolizumab versus adalimumab for moderate-to-severe ulcerative colitis. *New Eng J Med.* 2019;381:1215–1226. 10.1056/nejmoa1905725.
66. Sandborn WJ, Feagan BG, D'Haens G, et al., True North Study Group. Ozanimod as induction and maintenance therapy for ulcerative colitis. *N Engl J Med.* 2021;385(14):1280–1291. 10.1056/NEJMoa2033617. PMID: 34587385.
67. Nguyen Nghia H, Singh S, Sandborn WJ. Positioning therapies in the management of Crohn's disease. *Clin Gastroenterol Hepatol.* 2020;18:1268–1279. 10.1016/j.cgh.2019.10.035.
68. Feuerstein JD, Nguyen GC, Kupfer SS, et al. American Gastroenterological Association Institute guideline on therapeutic drug monitoring in inflammatory bowel disease. *Gastroenterology.* 2017;153:827–834.
69. Bohm M, Xu R, Zhang Y, et al. Comparative safety and effectiveness of vedolizumab to tumour necrosis factor antagonist therapy for Crohn's disease. *Aliment Pharmacol Ther.* 2020;52(4):669–681. doi:10.1111/apt.15921. Epub 2020 Jul 13. Erratum in: Aliment Pharmacol Ther. 2020 Nov;52(9):1534. Erratum in: Aliment Pharmacol Ther. 2021 Apr;53(8):963. PMID: 32656800; PMCID: PMC7496810.
70. Gordon M. 5-Aminosalicylates to maintain remission in Crohn's Disease: Interpreting conflicting systematic review evidence. *World J Gastrointest Pharmacol Ther.* 2017;8(2):99–102.
71. Nguyen GD, Loftus EV, Hirano I, et al. American Gastroenterological Association Institute Guideline on the management of Crohn's disease after surgical resection. *Gastroenterology.* 2017;152:271–275.
72. Farraye FA, Melmed GY, Lichtenstein GR, et al. ACG Clinical Guideline: Preventative care in inflammatory bowel disease. *Am J Gastroenterol.* 2017;112:241–258.
73. Miao XP, Li JS, Ouyang Q, Hu RW, Zhang Y, Li HY. Tolerability of selective cyclooxygenase 2 inhibitors used for the treatment of rheumatological manifestations of inflammatory bowel disease. *Cochrane Database of Syst Rev.* 2014;(10):CD007744. doi:10.1002/14651858.CD007744.pub2.
74. Biancone L, Annese V, Ardizzone S, et al. Safety of treatments for inflammatory bowel disease: Clinical practice guidelines of the Italian Group for the study of Inflammatory Bowel Disease (IG-IBD). *Dig and Liver Dis.* 2017;49:338–358.
75. Relling MV, Schwab M, Whirl-Carrillo M, et al. Clinical Pharmacogenetics Implementation Consortium Guideline for thiopurine dosing based on TPMT and NUDT15 genotypes: 2018 update. *Clin Pharmacol Ther.* 2019;105(5):1095–1105. 10.1002/cpt.1304. Epub 2019 Jan 20. PMID: 30447069; PMCID: PMC6576267.
76. Queiroz NSF, Regueiro M. Safety considerations with biologics and new inflammatory bowel disease therapies. *Curr Opin Gastroenterol.* 2020;36(4):257–264. doi:10.1097/MOG.0000000000000607. PMID: 31895234.
77. Papamichael K, Cheifetz AS. Therapeutic drug monitoring in inflammatory bowel disease: For every patient and every drug? *Curr Opin Gastroenterol.* 2019;35(4):302–310. doi:10.1097/MOG.0000000000000536. PMID: 30973355; PMCID: PMC6785387.
78. Chimenti MS, Conigliaro P, Biancone L, et al. Update on the therapeutic management of patients with either psoriatic arthritis or ulcerative colitis: Focus on the JAK inhibitor tofacitinib. *Ther Adv Musculoskelet Dis.* 2021;13:1759720X20977777. doi:10.1177/1759720X20977777. PMID: 33680096; PMCID: PMC7897839.
79. Mahadevan U, McConnell RA, Chambers CD. Drug safety and risk of adverse outcomes for pregnant patients with inflammatory bowel disease. *Gastroenterology.* 2017;152:451–462.
80. Nguyen G, Seow CH, Maxwell C, et al. The Toronto Consensus Statements for the management of inflammatory bowel disease in pregnancy. *Gastroenterology.* 2016;150:734–757.
81. Mahadevan Uma RC, Bernasko N, et al. Inflammatory bowel disease in pregnancy clinical care pathway: A report from the American Gastroenterological Association IBD Parenthood Project Working Group. *Gastroenterology.* 2019;156:1508–1524. 10.1053/j.gastro.2018.12.022.
82. Sands K, Jansen RZ, et al. Review article: The safety of therapeutic drugs in male inflammatory bowel disease patients wishing to conceive. *Aliment Pharmacol Ther.* 2015;41:821–834.
83. Kelsen JR, Sullivan KE, Rabizadeh S, Singh N, et al. North American Society for Pediatric Gastroenterology, Hepatology, and Nutrition Position Paper on the evaluation and management for patients with very early-onset inflammatory bowel disease. *J Pediatr Gastroenterol Nutr.* 2020;70(3):389–403. 10.1097/MPG.0000000000002567.
84. Yu YR, Rodriguez JR. Clinical presentation of Crohn's, ulcerative colitis, and indeterminate colitis: Symptoms, extraintestinal manifestations, and disease phenotypes. *Semin Pediatr Surg.* 2017;26(6):349–355. 10.1053/j.sempedsurg.2017.10.003. Epub 2017 Oct 5.
85. Rempel J, Grover K, El-Matary W. Micronutrient deficiencies and anemia in children with inflammatory bowel disease. *Nutrients.* 2021;13(1):236. 10.3390/nu13010236. PMID: 33467587; PMCID: PMC7830649.
86. Cabrera JM, Sato TT. Medical and surgical management of pediatric ulcerative colitis. *Clin Colon Rectal Surg.* 2018;31(2):71–79. doi:10.1055/s-0037-1609021. Epub 2018 Feb 25.
87. Turner D, Ruemmele FM, Orlanski-Meyer E, Griffiths AM, et al. Management of paediatric ulcerative colitis, part1: ambulatory

care—An evidence-based guideline from European Crohn's and Colitis Organization and European Society of Paediatric Gastroenterology Hepatology and Nutrition. *J Pediatr Gastroenterol Nutr.* 2018;67(2): 257–291. 10.1097/MPG.0000000000002035.

88. Ungaro RC, Aggarwal S, Topaloglu O, et al. Systematic review and meta-analysis: efficacy and safety of early biologic treatment in adult and paediatric patients with Crohn's disease. *Aliment Pharmacol Ther.* 2020;51(9):831–842. 10.1111/apt.15685. Epub 2020 Mar 23. PMID: 32202328; PMCID: PMC7160034.
89. Robertson DJ, Grimm IS. Management of inflammatory bowel disease in the elderly patient: Challenges and opportunities. *Inflamm Bowel Dis.* 2017;23:882–893.
90. Ananthakrishnan AN, Nguyen GC, Bernstein CN. AGA clinical practice update on management of inflammatory bowel disease in elderly patients: Expert review. *Gastroenterology.* 2021;160(1):445–451. 10.1053/j.gastro.2020.08.060. Epub 2020 Oct 1. PMID: 33011177.
91. Calafat M, Mañosa M, Cañete F, Domènech E. Clinical considerations regarding the use of thiopurines in older patients with inflammatory bowel disease. *Drugs Aging.* 2021;38(3):193–203. 10.1007/s40266-020-00832-4. Epub 2021 Jan 13. PMID: 33438138.
92. Manser CN, Maillard MH, Rogler G, et al. Vaccination in patients with inflammatory bowel diseases. *Digestion.* 2020;1–11.
93. Brenner EJ, Ungaro RC, Gearry RB, et al. Corticosteroids, but not TNF antagonists, are associated with adverse COVID-19 outcomes in patients with inflammatory bowel diseases: Results from an international registry. *Gastroenterology.* 2020;159:481–491.e3.
94. Singh AK, Jena A, Kumar-M P, Sharma V, Sebastian S. Risk and outcomes of coronavirus disease in patients with inflammatory bowel disease: A systematic review and meta-analysis. *United European Gastroenterol J.* 2021;9(2):159–176. 10.1177/2050640620972602. Epub 2021 Mar 23. PMID: 33210980.
95. Alexander JL, Moran GW, Gaya DR, et al., Inflammatory Bowel Disease section of the British Society of Gastroenterology and the Inflammatory Bowel Disease Clinical Research Group. SARS-CoV-2 vaccination for patients with inflammatory bowel disease: A British Society of Gastroenterology Inflammatory Bowel Disease section and IBD Clinical Research Group position statement. *Lancet Gastroenterol Hepatol.* 2021;6(3):218–224. 10.1016/S2468-1253(21)00024-8. Epub 2021 Jan 26. PMID: 33508241; PMCID: PMC7834976.
96. Siegel CA, Melmed GY, McGovern DP, et al., International Organization for the Study of Inflammatory Bowel Disease (IOIBD). SARS-CoV-2 vaccination for patients with inflammatory bowel diseases: Recommendations from an international consensus meeting. *Gut.* 2021;70(4):635–640. 10.1136/gutjnl-2020-324000. Epub 2021 Jan 20. PMID: 33472895; PMCID: PMC7818789.

53

Nausea and Vomiting

Leigh Anne H. Gravatt, Krista L. Donohoe, and Mandy L. Gatesman

KEY CONCEPTS

1. Nausea and/or vomiting is often a part of the symptom complex for a variety of gastrointestinal (GI), cardiovascular, infectious, neurologic, metabolic, or psychogenic processes.
2. Nausea or vomiting is caused by a variety of medications or other noxious agents.
3. The overall goal of treatment should be to prevent or eliminate nausea and vomiting regardless of etiology.
4. Treatment options for nausea and vomiting include drug and nondrug modalities such as relaxation, biofeedback, and hypnosis.
5. The primary goal with chemotherapy-induced nausea and vomiting (CINV) is to prevent nausea and vomiting throughout the entire risk period; the emetic risk of the chemotherapeutic regimen is a major factor to consider when selecting a prophylactic regimen.
6. Patients at high risk of vomiting should receive prophylactic antiemetics for postoperative nausea and vomiting (PONV).
7. Antihistaminic–anticholinergic agents are the most effective therapy for balance disorders.

BEYOND THE BOOK

Drug Information Question: Can you use medical marijuana for nausea and vomiting in your state? Research your state laws and the evidence-based literature for using medical marijuana for nausea and vomiting.

INTRODUCTION

Nausea and vomiting are common complaints from individuals of all ages. Management can be simple or detailed and complex, depending on the etiology. This chapter provides an overview of nausea and vomiting, two multifaceted problems. Nausea is defined as the inclination to vomit or as a feeling in the throat or epigastric region alerting an individual that vomiting is imminent. Vomiting is the ejection or expulsion of gastric contents through the mouth and is often a forceful event. Either condition may occur transiently with no other associated signs or symptoms; however, these conditions may be part of a more complex clinical presentation.

ETIOLOGY

1 Nausea and vomiting may be associated with a variety of conditions, including gastrointestinal (GI), cardiovascular, infectious, neurologic, or metabolic disease processes. Nausea and vomiting may be a feature of conditions such as pregnancy, or may follow operative procedures or administration of certain medications such as those used in treating cancer. Psychogenic etiologies of these symptoms may be present. Anticipatory etiologies may be involved, such as in patients who have experienced poor nausea and/or vomiting control with previous antineoplastic agents. Table 53-1 lists specific etiologies associated with nausea and vomiting.[1]

The etiology of nausea and vomiting may vary with the age of the patient. For example, vomiting in the newborn during the first day of life suggests upper digestive tract obstruction or an increase in intracranial pressure.

2 Nausea or vomiting is caused by a variety of medications or other noxious agents. Drug-induced nausea and vomiting is of particular concern, especially with the increasing number of patients receiving antineoplastic agents. A four-level classification system defines the risk for emesis with agents used in oncology (Table 53-2).[2] Although some agents may have greater emetic risk than others, combinations of agents, higher doses, clinical settings, psychological conditions, prior treatment experiences, and unusual stimulus of sight, smell, or taste may alter a patient's response to antiemetic treatment. In this setting, nausea and vomiting may be unavoidable and some patients experience these problems so intensely that chemotherapy is postponed or discontinued.

PATHOPHYSIOLOGY

The three consecutive phases of emesis include nausea, retching, and vomiting. Nausea, the subjective feeling of the need to vomit, may be considered a separate and singular symptom. Retching is the labored movement of abdominal and thoracic muscles before vomiting. The final phase of emesis is vomiting, the forceful expulsion of gastric contents caused by GI retroperistalsis. The act of vomiting is coordinated by the brainstem, but requires the contractions of the abdominal muscles, pylorus, and antrum, a raised gastric cardia, diminished lower esophageal sphincter pressure, and esophageal dilation.[1] Vomiting should not be confused with regurgitation, an act in which the gastric or esophageal contents rise to the pharynx but is not usually associated with forceful ejection seen with vomiting. Accompanying autonomic symptoms of pallor, tachycardia, and diaphoresis account for many of the distressing feelings associated with emesis.

Vomiting is triggered by afferent impulses to the vomiting center (VC), a nucleus of cells in the medulla. Impulses are received from sensory centers, which include the chemoreceptor trigger zone (CTZ), cerebral cortex, and visceral afferents from the pharynx and

TABLE 53-1 Etiologies of Nausea and Vomiting

Intraperitoneal
- Mechanical obstruction
  - Gastric outlet obstruction
  - Bowel obstruction
- Altered sensorimotor function
  - Gastroparesis
  - Gastroesophageal reflux
  - Intestinal pseudo-obstruction
- Irritable bowel syndrome
- Chronic idiopathic nausea
- Functional vomiting
- Cyclic vomiting syndrome
- Cannabinoid hyperemesis syndrome
- Rumination syndrome
- Inflammatory diseases
- Pancreatitis
- Pyelonephritis
- Cholecystitis
- Appendicitis
- Hepatitis
- Acute gastroenteritis
  - Viral
  - Bacterial
  - Biliary colic
  - Liver failure

Cardiovascular diseases
- Acute myocardial infarction
- Cardiomyopathy

Neurologic processes
- Increased intracranial pressure
- Migraine headache
- Vestibular disorders
- Intracerebral hemorrhage
- Intracerebral malignancy

Metabolic disorders
- Diabetes mellitus (diabetic ketoacidosis)
- Addison's disease
- Renal disease (uremia)

Psychiatric causes
- Depression
- Anxiety disorders
- Anorexia and bulimia nervosa

Therapy-induced causes
- Antineoplastic agents
- Radiation therapy
- Anticonvulsant preparations
- Digoxin, Cardiac antiarrhythmics
- Opiates
- Oral hypoglycemics
- Oral contraceptives
- Antibiotics
- Volatile general anesthetics
- Lubiprostone

Drug withdrawal
- Opiates
- Benzodiazepines

Miscellaneous causes
- Pregnancy
- Noxious odors
- Postoperative vomiting

Data from Reference 1.

GI tract. The VC integrates the afferent impulses, resulting in efferent impulses to the salivation center, respiratory center, and the pharyngeal, GI, and abdominal muscles, leading to vomiting.

The CTZ, located in the area postrema of the fourth ventricle of the brain, is a major chemosensory organ for emesis and is usually associated with chemically induced vomiting. Because of its location, blood-borne and cerebrospinal fluid toxins have easy access to the CTZ. Antineoplastic agents primarily stimulate this area rather

TABLE 53-2 Emetic Risk of Agents Used in Oncology and Treatment Options

Antiemetic Agent	Antiemetic Dose on Day 1 of Chemotherapy	Antiemetic Dose on Subsequent Days
High Risk (>90%): Anthracycline/Cyclophosphamide combination, Carmustine, Cisplatin, Cyclophosphamide >1,500 mg/m², Dacarbazine, Mechlorethamine, Streptozocin		
NK-1 Antagonist		
Aprepitant	125 mg oral or 130 mg IV	80 mg oral on days 2-3
Fosaprepitant	150 mg IV	
Netupitant-palonosetron	300 mg/0.5 mg oral	
Fosnetupitant-palonosetron	235 mg fosnetupitant/0.25 mg palonosetron IV	
Rolapitant	180 mg oral	
5-HT$_3$ Antagonist[a]		
Granisetron	2 mg oral or 1 mg IV or 10 mcg/kg IV or 1 patch or 10 mg SQ	
Ondansetron	24 mg oral or 8 mg IV or 0.15 mg/kg IV	
Palonosetron	0.5 mg oral	
Ramosetron	0.3 mg IV	
Tropisetron	5 mg oral OR 5 mg IV	
Dexamethasone[b]	12 mg or 20 mg oral/IV	8 mg oral/IV daily or twice daily on days 2-4
Olanzapine	5 mg or 10 mg oral	5 mg or 10 mg oral on days 2-4
Moderate Risk (30%-90%): Aldesleukin, Alemtuzumab, Arsenic trioxide, Azacitidine, Bendamustine, Busulfan, Carboplatin, Clofarabine, Cyclophosphamide <1,500 mg/m², Cytarabine >1,000 mg/m², Daunorubicin, Daunorubicin and cytarabine liposomal, Doxorubicin, Epirubicin, Fam-trastuzumab deruxtecan-nxki, Idarubicin, Ifosfamide, Irinotecan, Irinetecan liposomal injection, Oxaliplatin, Romidepsin, Temozolomide, Thiotepa, Trabectidin		
5-HT$_3$ Antagonist		
Granisetron	2 mg oral or 1 mg IV or 10 mcg/kg IV or 1 patch or 10 mg SQ	
Ondansetron	8 mg oral twice daily or 8 mg IV or 0.15 mg/kg IV	
Palonosetron	0.5 mg oral or 0.25 mg IV	
Ramosetron	0.3 mg IV	
Tropisetron	5 mg oral or 5 mg IV	
Dexamethasone	8 mg oral/IV	8 mg oral/IV on days 2-3[c]
Low Risk (10%-30%): Aflibercept, Axicabtogene ciloleucel, Belinostat, Blinatumomab, Bortezomib, Brentuximab, Cabazitaxel, Carfilzomib, Cetuximab, Copanlisib, Cytarabine <1,000 mg/m², Decitabine, Docetaxel, Elotuzumab, Enfortumab vedotin-ejfv, Eribulin, Etoposide, Fluorouracil, Gemcitabine, Gemcitabine ozogamicin, Inotuzumab ozogamicin, Ixabepilone, Methotrexate, Mitomycin, Mitoxantrone, Moxetumomab pasudotox, Nab-paclitaxel, Necitumumab, Nelarabine, Paclitaxel (conventional and albumin-bound), Panitumumab, Pegylated liposomal doxorubicin, Prmetrexed, Pertuzumab, Tagraxofusp-erzs, Topotecan, Trastuzumab emtansine, Vinflunine		
Choose One:		
5-HT$_3$ Antagonist		
Granisetron	2 mg oral or 1 mg IV or 10 mcg/kg IV or 1 patch or 10 mg SQ	
Ondansetron	8 mg oral or IV	
Palonosetron	0.5 mg oral or 0.25 mg IV	

(continued)

TABLE 53-2 Emetic Risk of Agents Used in Oncology and Treatment Options (*Continued*)

Antiemetic Agent	Antiemetic Dose on Day 1 of Chemotherapy	Antiemetic Dose on Subsequent Days
Ramosetron	0.3 mg IV	
Tropisetron	5 mg oral or IV	
OR		
Dexamethasone	8 mg oral or IV	
Minimal Risk (<10%): Avelumab, Atezolizumab, Bevacizumab, Bleomycin, Cemiplimab, 2-Chlorodeoxyadenosine, Cladribine, Daratumumab, Durvalumab, Emapalumab, Fludarabine, Ipilimumab, Nivolumab, Obinutuzumab, Ofatumumab, Pembrolizumab, Pralatrexate, Ramucirumab, Rituximab (IV and SQ), Trastuzumab, Vinblastine, Vincristine (conventional and liposomal), Vinorelbine		
No routine prophylactic antiemetics are needed		

[a]No additional 5-HT_3-RA is needed if netupitant/palonosetron is used.

[b]Dexamethasone dose on day 1 should be reduced to 12 mg when given with aprepitant, fosaprepitant, and netupitant/palonosetron due to drug interactions. Dexamethasone dose on days 2-4 should be omitted when used as antiemetic with anthracycline/cyclophosphamide combination regimen or carboplatin AUC ≥4.

[c]Only if regimen is known to cause delayed nausea/vomiting (eg, cyclophosphamide, doxorubicin, oxaliplatin).

Data from Reference 2.

than the cerebral cortex and visceral afferents. Pregnancy-associated vomiting probably occurs through stimulation of the CTZ.

Numerous neurotransmitter receptors are located in the VC, CTZ, and GI tract, including cholinergic, histaminic, dopaminergic, opiate, serotonergic, neurokinin (NK), and benzodiazepine receptors. Antineoplastic agents, their metabolites, or other emetic compounds theoretically trigger the process of emesis through stimulation of one or more of these receptors. Antiemetics have been developed to antagonize or block these emetogenic receptors.[3] See Fig. 53-1.

CLINICAL PRESENTATION

Nausea and vomiting is commonly seen in many clinical situations. Patients may present in varying degrees of distress summarized in the Patient Care Process (PCP). See box below for clinical presentation of nausea and vomiting.

TREATMENT

Desired Outcomes

3 The overall goal of antiemetic therapy is to prevent or eliminate nausea and vomiting. This should be accomplished without adverse effects or with clinically acceptable adverse effects. In addition to these clinical goals, appropriate cost issues should be considered, particularly in the management of chemotherapy-induced nausea and vomiting (CINV) and postoperative nausea and vomiting (PONV).

General Approach to Treatment

3 Treatment options include drug and nondrug modalities such as relaxation, biofeedback, and hypnosis. Initially patients may choose to not treat or to self-medicate with nonprescription drugs. As symptoms become worse or are associated with more serious medical problems, patients are more likely to utilize prescription antiemetic drugs. When prescribed and used appropriately, these agents can provide relief; however, some patients will never be totally free of symptoms. This lack of relief is most disabling when it is associated with an unresolved medical problem or when the necessary therapy for this condition is the cause of the nausea or vomiting, as in the case of patients who are receiving antineoplastic agents of moderate or high emetic risk.

Nonpharmacologic Management

4 Nonpharmacologic management of nausea and vomiting involves dietary, physical, or psychological strategies that are

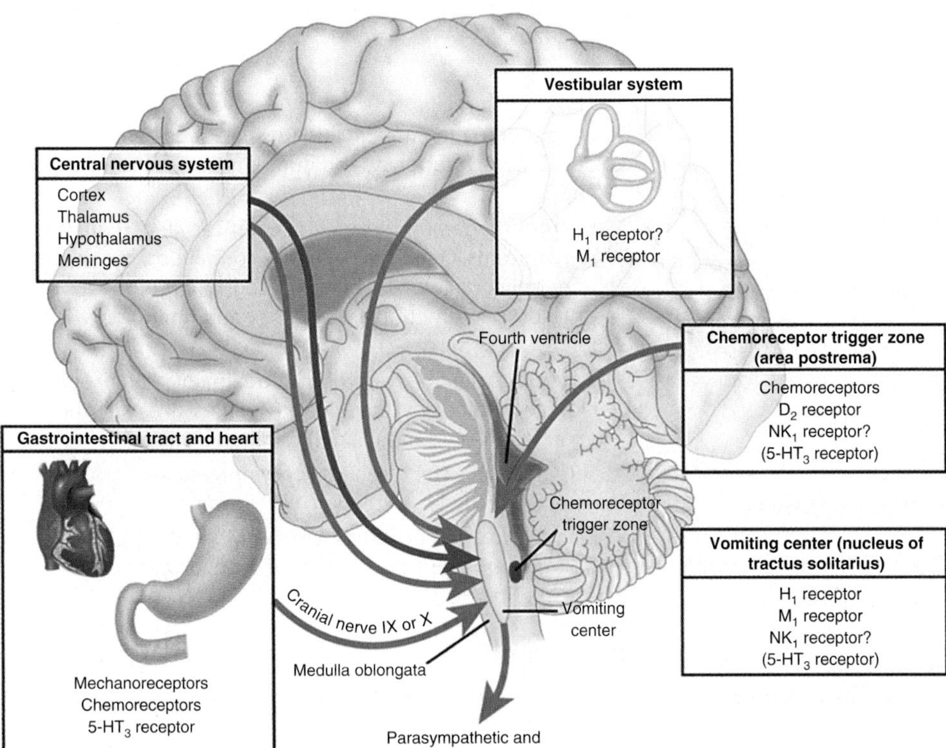

FIGURE 53-1 Pathogenesis of nausea and vomiting: neurologic pathways involved in pathogenesis of nausea and vomiting (see text). (*Reprinted, with permission, from Krakauer EL, et al. Case records of the Massachusetts General Hospital.* Weekly clinicopathological exercises. Case 6-2005. A 58-year-old man with esophageal cancer and nausea, vomiting, and intractable hiccups. *N Engl J Med. 2005;352:817. © Massachusetts Medical Society.*)

CLINICAL PRESENTATION Nausea and Vomiting

General

- Depending on severity of symptoms, patients may present in mild to severe distress.

Symptoms

- *Simple:* Self-limiting, resolves spontaneously, and requires only symptomatic therapy.
- *Complex:* Not relieved after administration of antiemetics; progressive deterioration of patient secondary to fluid-electrolyte imbalances; usually associated with noxious agents or psychogenic events.

Signs

- *Simple:* Patient complaint of queasiness or discomfort.
- *Complex:* Weight loss; fever; abdominal pain.

Laboratory Tests

- *Simple:* None.
- *Complex:* Serum electrolyte concentrations; upper/lower GI evaluation .

Other Information

- Fluid input and output.
- Medication history.
- Recent history of behavioral or visual changes, headache, pain, or stress.
- Family history positive for psychogenic vomiting.

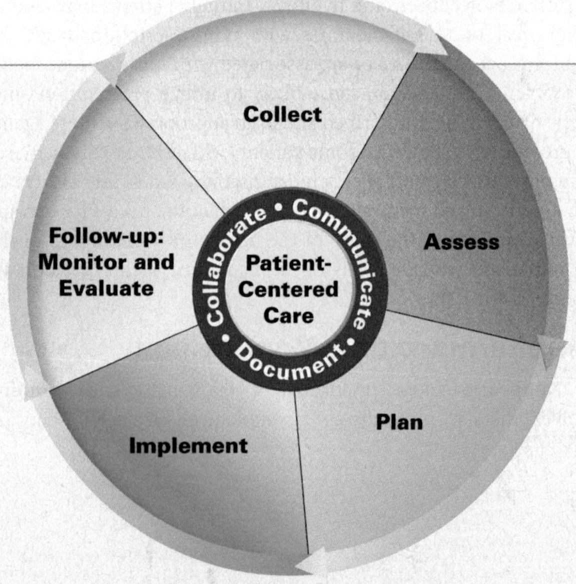

Patient Care Process for Nausea and Vomiting

The image shows the five fundamental steps included in patient care process for nausea and vomiting. The tagline of this process reads collaborate, communicate, and document. The five fundamental steps listed here are collect, assess, plan, implement, and follow-up: monitor and evaluate. All these steps are listed in a circular block diagram.

Collect

- Patient characteristics (eg, age, sex, pregnancy status, triggers)
- Patient medical history (personal and family), history of NV
- Social history (eg, tobacco/ethanol/cannabis use) and dietary habits
- Current medications including prescription and nonprescription medications, herbal products, dietary supplements
- Objective data (eg, QTc prolongation, BP/pulse, complete metabolic panel, CBC, liver function, weight, skin turgor, urine output)

Assess

- Duration, frequency, severity of nausea and vomiting
- Ability/willingness to pay for treatment options
- Emotional status (eg, presence of anxiety, depression)
- Assess ability of the patient to use oral, rectal, injectable, or transdermal medications
- Success of previous antiemetic regimens
- For CINV: Assess emetic risk of chemotherapy (see Table 53-6)
- For PONV: Assess risk factors for developing PONV (see Table 53-5)

Plan*

- Drug therapy regimen including specific antiemetic(s), dose, route, frequency, and duration (see Tables 53-3 and 53-6)
- Monitoring parameters including efficacy (eg, reduction in symptoms, resolution of lab abnormalities, resumption of normal oral intake) and safety (eg, QTc prolongation, drug-drug interactions); frequency and timing of follow-up
- Patient education (eg, purpose of treatment, dietary and lifestyle modification, invasive procedures, drug-specific information, medication administration technique)
- Self-monitoring for resolution of symptoms, when to seek emergency medical attention
- Referrals to other providers when appropriate (eg, gastroenterologist, dietitian, OBGYN, oncologist, anesthesiologist)

Implement*

- Provide patient education regarding all elements of treatment plan

(continued)

- Use motivational interviewing and coaching strategies to maximize adherence
- Schedule follow-up, adherence assessment

Follow-up: Monitor and Evaluate

- Resolution of nausea and vomiting symptoms
- Need for rescue antiemetics
- Presence of adverse effects
- Patient adherence to treatment plan

Collaborate with patient, caregivers, and other healthcare professionals.

consistent with the etiology of nausea and vomiting. For patients who are suffering due to excessive or disagreeable food or beverage consumption, avoidance or moderation in dietary intake may lead to symptom resolution. Patients suffering from symptoms of systemic illness may quickly improve as their underlying condition resolves. Patients in whom these symptoms result from labyrinthine changes produced by motion may benefit quickly by assuming a stable physical position.

Nonpharmacologic interventions include relaxation, biofeedback, hypnosis, cognitive distraction, optimism, guided imagery, acupuncture, yoga, transcutaneous electrical stimulation, chewing gum, and systematic desensitization.[4-8] Chewing gum after certain surgical procedures improves bowel function and decreases time to first flatus as well as decreases the incidence of postoperative ileus.[6,7] Some of these modalities, such as acupuncture, are effective at preventing nausea and vomiting in the surgical population.[8] Other therapies, such as ginger and pyridoxine, may be beneficial in specific situations as with pregnancy associated nausea and vomiting.

Changes in diet such as restricting oral intake, eating smaller meals, avoiding spicy or fried foods, and instead eating bland foods such as with the BRAT diet (**B**ananas, **R**ice, **A**pplesauce, and **T**oast) can help alleviate symptoms.

Pharmacologic Therapy

Although many approaches to the treatment of nausea and vomiting have been suggested, antiemetic drugs (nonprescription and prescription) are most often recommended. These agents work in various ways and may be used singularly or in conjunction with each other, and have a number of delivery methods.

Factors that enable the clinician to choose the appropriate regimen include: (a) the suspected etiology of the symptoms; (b) the frequency, duration, and severity of the episodes; (c) the ability of the patient to use oral, rectal, injectable, or transdermal medications; and (d) the success of previous antiemetic medications. See Table 53-3 for dosing information of commonly available antiemetic preparations.

TABLE 53-3 Common Antiemetic Preparations and Adult Dosage Regimens[a]

Drug	Adult Dosage Regimen	Dosage Form/Route	Availability
Antacids: Useful with simple nausea/vomiting *Adverse drug reactions: Magnesium products—diarrhea; Aluminum or calcium products—constipation*			
Antacids (various)	15-30 mL every 2-4 hr prn	Liquid/oral	Nonprescription
Antihistaminic–Anticholinergic Agents: Especially problematic in the elderly; increased risk of complications in patients with benign prostatic hyperplasia (BPH), narrow angle glaucoma, or asthma *Adverse drug reactions: Drowsiness, confusion, blurred vision, dry mouth, urinary retention*			
Dimenhydrinate (Dramamine)	50-100 mg every 4-6 hr prn	Tab, chew tab, cap	Nonprescription
Diphenhydramine (Benadryl)	25-50 mg every 4-6 hr prn 10-50 mg every 2-4 hr prn	Tab, cap, liquid IM, IV	Prescription/Nonprescription
Hydroxyzine (Vistaril, Atarax)	25-100 mg every 4-6 hr prn	Tab (unlabeled use)	Prescription
Meclizine (Bonine, Antivert)	12.5-25 mg 1 hr before travel; repeat every 12-24 hr prn	Tab, chew tab	Prescription/Nonprescription
Scopolamine (Transderm Scop)	1.5 mg every 72 hr	Transdermal patch	Prescription
Trimethobenzamide (Tigan)	300 mg three to four times daily 200 mg three to four times daily	Cap IM	Prescription
Benzodiazepine: Used for ANV but is contraindicated with olanzapine *Adverse drug reactions: Dizziness, sedation, appetite changes, memory impairment; observe for additive sedation especially if used with narcotic analgesics*			
Lorazepam (Ativan)	0.5-2 mg on night before and morning of chemotherapy	Tab, IV	Prescription (C-IV)
Butyrophenones: Used for breakthrough CINV; Droperidol has limited use *Adverse drug reactions: Haloperidol—sedation, constipation, hypotension, extrapyramidal symptoms (EPS); Droperidol—QTc prolongation and/or torsade de pointes, 12-lead electrocardiogram prior to administration, followed by cardiac monitoring for 2-3 hr after administration*			
Haloperidol (Haldol)	0.5-2 mg every 4-6 hr prn	Tab, liquid, IM, IV	Prescription
Droperidol (Inapsine)[b]	2.5 mg; additional 1.25 mg may be given	IM, IV	Prescription
Cannabinoids: Used for breakthrough CINV *Adverse drug reactions: Eurphoria, somnolence, xerostomia*			
Dronabinol (Marinol, Syndros)	5-15 mg/m^2 every 2-4 hr prn 4.2-12.6 mg/m^2 every 2-4 hr prn	Cap Oral solution	Prescription (C-III)
Nabilone (Cesamet)	1-2 mg twice daily	Cap	Prescription (C-II)
Corticosteroids: Useful as a single agent or combination therapy for prophylaxis of CINV or PONV *Adverse drug reactions: Insomnia, GI symptoms, agitation, appetite stimulation, hypertension, and hyperglycemia*			

(Continued)

TABLE 53-3 Common Antiemetic Preparations and Adult Dosage Regimens[a] (*Continued*)

Drug	Adult Dosage Regimen	Dosage Form/Route	Availability
Dexamethasone	See Table 53-6 for CINV dosing and Table 53-5 for PONV dosing	Tab, IV	Prescription
Histamine (H2) Antagonists: Useful with nausea secondary to heartburn or GERD *Adverse drug reactions: Headache, constipation, or diarrhea*			
Cimetidine (Tagamet HB)	200 mg twice daily prn	Tab	Nonprescription
Famotidine (Pepcid AC)	10 mg twice daily prn	Tab	Nonprescription
Nizatidine (Axid AR)	75 mg twice daily prn	Tab	Nonprescription
5-Hydroxytryptamine-3 Receptor Antagonists: Useful as a single-agent or combination therapy for prophylaxis of CINV or PONV *Adverse drug reactions: Asthenia, constipation, headache*			
	See Table 53-6 for CINV dosing and Table 53-5 for PONV dosing	Tab, IV	Prescription
Miscellaneous Agents • **Metoclopramide:** Prokinetic activity useful in diabetic gastroparesis. *Adverse drug reactions: Asthenia, headache, somnolence, EPS* • *Amisulpride: Mainly used in PONV; avoid use in severe renal impairment. Adverse drug reactions: Increased serum prolactin, prolonged QTc interval* • **Olanzapine:** Use with caution in elderly; contraindicated with benzodiazepines. *Adverse drug reactions: Sedation, prolonged QTc interval, EPS* • **Pyridoxine:** Used in NVP. May be used alone or in combination with doxylamine 12.5 mg. Combination product available as prescription. *Adverse drug reactions: Drowsiness, headache*			
Metoclopramide (Reglan)	10-20 mg (0.5-2 mg/kg) four times daily	Tab, IV	Prescription
Olanzapine (Zyprexa)	5-10 mg daily	Tab	Prescription
Pyridoxine (Vitamin B_6)	10-25 mg orally three to four times daily	Tab, cap	Nonprescription
Amisulpride	5-10 mg once either before or after surgery	5-10 mg once either before or after surgery	Prescription
Phenothiazines: Useful in simple nausea/vomiting or breakthrough CINV *Adverse drug reactions: Prolonged QTc interval, constipation, dizziness, tachycardia, tardive dyskinesia, drowsiness*			
Chlorpromazine (Thorazine)	10-25 mg every 4-6 hr prn	Tab, liquid	Prescription
	25-50 mg every 4-6 hr prn	IM, IV	
Prochlorperazine (Compazine)	5-10 mg every 4-6 hr prn	Tab, liquid	Prescription
	5-10 mg every 3-4 hr prn	IM	
	2.5-10 mg every 3-4 hr prn	IV	Prescription
	25 mg twice daily prn	Supp	Prescription
Promethazine (Phenergan)	12.5-25 mg every 4-6 hr prn	Tab, liquid, IM, IV, supp	Prescription
Substance P/Neurokinin-1 Receptor Antagonist: Useful in combination therapy for prophylaxis of CINV and PONV *Adverse drug reactions: Constipation, diarrhea, headache, hiccups, dyspepsia, and fatigue*			
Aprepitant	See Table 53-6 for CINV dosing and Table 53-5 for PONV dosing	Cap, IV	Prescription
Fosaprepitant		IV	Prescription
Fosnetupitant-palonosetron		IV	Prescription
Netupitant/palonosetron		Cap	Prescription
Rolapitant		Cap	Prescription

[a]All regimens should be monitored for resolution or occurrence of nausea and vomiting as well as maintaining an adequate hydration status.

[b]See text for warnings.

ANV, anticipatory nausea and vomiting; C-II, C-III, and C-IV, controlled substance schedule 2, 3, and 4, respectively; cap, capsule; chew tab, chewable tablet; CINV, chemotherapy-induced nausea and vomiting; GI, gastrointestinal; GERD, gastroesophageal reflux disease; liquid, oral syrup, concentrate, or suspension; NVP, nausea and vomiting of pregnancy; PONV, postoperative nausea and vomiting; supp, rectal suppository; tab, tablet.

The treatment of simple nausea and vomiting often involves self-care from a list of nonprescription products. Both nonprescription and prescription drugs are useful in the treatment of simple nausea and vomiting in small, infrequently administered doses and are associated with minimal side effects. As the symptoms persist or become worse, prescription medications may be chosen, either as single-agent therapy or in combination.

The management of complex nausea and vomiting, such as in patients who are receiving antineoplastic agents, may require initial combination therapy. In combination regimens, the goal is to achieve symptomatic control through administration of agents with different pharmacologic mechanisms of action.

Antacids

Patients who are experiencing simple nausea and vomiting may initially use antacids, as many of these products are readily available without a prescription. Single or combination products, especially those containing magnesium hydroxide, aluminum hydroxide, and/or calcium carbonate, may provide rapid relief, primarily through gastric acid neutralization. These agents are most effective for those with symptoms related to acid reflux or heartburn and must be used with caution in those who experience acute or chronic kidney disease due to the risk of accumulation. These agents may exacerbate other GI complaints that accompany nausea and vomiting, such as diarrhea or constipation, so attention must be paid to which of these agents may worsen these other conditions.

Antihistamine–Anticholinergic Drugs

Antiemetic drugs from the antihistaminic–anticholinergic category work on muscarinic and histamine receptors in the VC and the vestibular system that stimulate nausea and vomiting. These agents are frequently initiated as self-care to prevent nausea and vomiting associated with motion disturbances such as vertigo and motion sickness.

Benzodiazepines

Benzodiazepines are relatively weak antiemetics and are primarily used for their anxiolytic activity to prevent anxiety or anticipatory nausea and vomiting (ANV) that may occur in patients experiencing suboptimal CINV control. Lorazepam may be used as an adjunct to other antiemetics in patients experiencing ANV.

Butyrophenones

Haloperidol and droperidol work by blocking dopaminergic stimulation of the CTZ, which in turn decreases the incidence of nausea and vomiting. The use of these agents may be complicated by their propensity to cause extrapyramidal symptoms and QTc prolongation. For these reasons, haloperidol is not considered first-line therapy for uncomplicated nausea and vomiting but has been used in breakthrough CINV and palliative care situations.[9] Droperidol use is limited to rescue antiemetic for PONV. The current labeling of droperidol recommends that all patients should undergo a 12-lead electrocardiogram prior to administration, followed by cardiac monitoring for 2 to 3 hours after administration because of the possibility of the development of potentially fatal QT prolongation and/or torsade de pointes.[10]

Cannabinoids

Cannabinoids have complex effects on the CNS and their effects at cannabinoid receptor 1 (CB1) in neural tissues may explain efficacy in CINV. Medicinal cannabis can be in the use of cannabis or cannabinoids in order to treat various conditions, including nausea and vomiting. Cannabinoids can be administered in a variety of methods including orally, topically, or sublingually. Oral dronabinol and nabilone, FDA-approved synthetic analogs of delta-9-tetrahydrocannabinol (THC), may be therapeutic options when CINV is refractory to other antiemetics. Medicinal marijuana has been approved for use in over half of states in the United States; however, its use remains debatable.[11] There is limited data to support the use of smoked or ingested cannabis for CINV. FDA-approved cannabinoids and medicinal cannabis improved symptoms in comparison to placebo or active comparators in some trials.[12] The combination of dronabinol and prochlorperazine was significantly more effective when used in combination for the treatment of CINV versus either agent alone.[11] Cannabinoids have the advantage of being effective for other cancer-related side effects such as pain or use as an appetite stimulant.[11-13] Despite these advantages, cannabinoids are not indicated as first-line agents. There is also concern that chronic cannabis use can lead to cyclic nausea and vomiting, which is called cannabinoid hyperemesis syndrome. This syndrome is primarily treated by supportive care, frequent hot showers, and cannabis cessation.[14]

Corticosteroids

Corticosteroids have demonstrated antiemetic efficacy since the initial recognition that patients who received prednisone as part of their Hodgkin's disease protocol appeared to develop less nausea and vomiting than did those patients who were treated with protocols that excluded this agent. The site and mechanism of action of corticosteroids for CINV and PONV are unknown.

Dexamethasone is the most commonly studied and used corticosteroid in the management of CINV and PONV, either as a single agent or in combination with 5-hydroxytryptamine-3 receptor antagonists (5-HT_3-RAs). Dexamethasone is effective in the prevention of both CINV acute emesis and delayed nausea and vomiting when used alone or in combination.[15,16] Given the risk of corticosteroids such as hyperglycemia, fluid retention, and even psychosis, steroids are not indicated for the treatment of simple nausea and vomiting.

H2-Receptor Antagonists

Histamine-2 receptor antagonists (H2RA) work by decreasing gastric acid production and are used to manage simple nausea and vomiting associated with heartburn or gastroesophageal reflux. Except for potential drug interactions with a variety of oral chemotherapy agents, these agents cause few side effects when used for episodic relief.

5-Hydroxytryptamine-3 Receptor Antagonists

5-Hydroxytryptamine-3 receptor antagonists (5-HT_3-RAs) block serotonin receptors on sensory vagal fibers in the gut wall; thus, blocking the acute phase of CINV. These agents do not completely block the acute phase of CINV and are less efficacious in preventing the delayed phase, but they are considered the standard of care in the management of CINV, PONV, and radiation-induced nausea and vomiting (RINV).[2,16]

The 5-HT_3-RAs are considered equivalent when used in equipotent doses/schedules so any agent may be used for CINV. Intravenous doses of ondansetron should not exceed 16 mg due to QTc prolongation.[17] Palonosetron has less effect on QTc and a significantly longer half-life compared to other 5-HT_3-RAs. Granisetron is available in two nonoral formulations: a transdermal patch and an extended-release subcutaneous injection. The granisetron patch should be applied 24 to 48 hours prior to chemotherapy and may be worn for up to 7 days. The choice of 5-HT_3-RAs for CINV should be based on route of administration, potential side effects, and cost concerns.

Metoclopramide

Metoclopramide works by blocking dopaminergic receptors centrally in the CTZ. It also increases lower esophageal sphincter tone, aids gastric emptying, and accelerates transit through the small bowel, possibly through the release of acetylcholine. The prokinetic activity of metoclopramide makes it useful in patients with nausea and vomiting associated with diabetic gastroparesis. Due to the risk of extrapyramidal symptoms, metoclopramide should be used with caution if used in combination with other dopamine antagonists such as olanzapine or haloperidol.

Neurokinin-1 Receptor Antagonists

Substance P is a peptide neurotransmitter in the NK family whose preferred receptor is the NK_1 receptor. The acute phase of CINV is thought to be mediated by both serotonin and substance P, where substance P is believed to be the primary mediator of the delayed phase. An NK_1 receptor antagonist in combination with other antiemetics is now standard of care for prevention of CINV in both adults and children receiving highly emetogenic chemotherapy.[2] Aprepitant, fosaprepitant, and rolapitant are NK_1 receptor antagonists currently in clinical use, along with two combination NK_1 receptor antagonist/5-HT_3-RA co-formulated products, netupitant/palonosetron (NEPA) and fosnetupitant-palonosetron.[18]

Aprepitant has the potential for numerous drug interactions because it is a substrate and moderate inhibitor of cytochrome isoenzyme CYP3A4 as well as a weak inducer of CYP2C9. It can increase serum concentrations of many drugs, including chemotherapeutic agents metabolized by CYP3A4 such as anthracyclines, bosutinib, cabazitaxel, cyclophosphamide, and ifosfamide.[19] Other significant drug interactions include decreased effectiveness of estrogen-containing contraceptives (oral, patches, vaginal rings), and a decrease in the international normalized ratio when used with warfarin.[20] The dose of oral dexamethasone within the antiemetic regimen should be reduced 50% when coadministered with aprepitant, because of the 2.2-fold increase in observed area under the plasma-concentration-versus-time curve.[21] Conversely, if dexamethasone is used as part of the chemotherapy regimen, the dexamethasone dose should remain the same.

Fosaprepitant is an injectable form of aprepitant approved by the FDA as an IV substitute for oral aprepitant, given on day 1 only of the CINV prevention regimen.[22] Drug interactions are likely reduced with fosaprepitant compared to oral aprepitant.[19]

Rolapitant has a significantly longer half-life in comparison with aprepitant (7 days vs 9 hours) and therefore should only be administered once in a 2-week period.[23] Although rolapitant has no effects on CYP3A4, it does inhibit p-glycoprotein/ABCB1 and CYP2D6, which may lead to drug interactions with certain antineoplastic agents, including doxorubicin, liposomal vincristine, pazopanib, topotecan, and venetoclax. Postmarketing reports of anaphylaxis, anaphylactic shock, and severe hypersensitivity reactions during or shortly after initiation of IV rolapitant resulted in an FDA warning for this product. Patients with known hypersensitivity to components of IV rolapitant, including soybean oil, may be at an increased risk of reactions. All patients should be screened for cross-reactive allergens including soybeans and other legumes prior to administration.[23]

NEPA, when given in one dose combined with dexamethasone, was noninferior to a combination regimen of aprepitant, granisetron, and dexamethasone regimen in individuals receiving moderate or highly emetogenic chemotherapy.[24] Netupitant is also a moderate inhibitor of CYP3A4, and requires a significant decrease in the dexamethasone dose when used together. Drug interactions with other CYP3A4 substrates would also be expected with NEPA.[18]

Olanzapine

Olanzapine is an antipsychotic that blocks several neurotransmitters including dopamine, serotonin, adrenergic, histamine (H_1), and 5-HT_3-RA. Olanzapine in combination with aprepitant/fosaprepitant, 5-HT_3-RA, and dexamethasone significantly improved nausea control after highly emetogenic chemotherapy.[25] The American Society of Clinical Oncology (ASCO) antiemesis practice guidelines include olanzapine as part of the standard four drug combination antiemetic regimen for highly emetogenic chemotherapy.[2] Sedation is the most common side effects with olanzapine; it should be used with caution in older adults and dose reductions may be necessary in this population.[26-28]

Phenothiazines

Phenothiazines have been the most widely prescribed antiemetic agents and appear to block dopamine receptors, most likely in the CTZ. They are marketed in an array of dosage forms, none of which appears to be more efficacious than the other. These agents may be most practical for long-term treatment and are inexpensive in comparison with newer drugs. Rectal administration is a reasonable alternative for patients in whom oral or parenteral administration is not feasible.

Phenothiazines are most useful in adult patients with simple nausea and vomiting. Intravenously administered prochlorperazine provided faster and more complete relief with less drowsiness than IV promethazine in adult patients treated in an emergency department for nausea and vomiting associated with uncomplicated gastritis or gastroenteritis.[28]

CHEMOTHERAPY-INDUCED NAUSEA AND VOMITING

There are five categories of CINV: acute, delayed, anticipatory, breakthrough, and refractory. Nausea and vomiting that occurs within 24 hours of chemotherapy administration is defined as acute CINV, whereas when it starts more than 24 hours after chemotherapy administration, it is defined as delayed CINV.[29]

Nausea or vomiting that occurs prior to receiving chemotherapy is termed anticipatory nausea and vomiting (ANV). ANV is believed to be a learned, conditioned, or psychological response that occurs in about 14% of patients by the third cycle of chemotherapy.[4,31,32] ANV triggers include tastes, odors, sights, or thoughts associated with chemotherapy. Risk factors associated with ANV include experiencing CINV with prior chemotherapy cycles and anxiety before receiving chemotherapy.[4] In the setting of optimal antiemetic prophylaxis and no prior history of emesis, reported chemotherapy-induced ANV is rare. Use of newer antiemetic regimens appears to have resulted in a decreased rate of ANV.[30]

TABLE 53-4 Nonchemotherapy Etiologies of Nausea and Vomiting in Cancer Patients

Fluid and electrolyte abnormalities
Hypercalcemia
Volume depletion
Water intoxication
Adrenocortical insufficiency
Drug induced
Opiates
Anti-infectives
GI obstruction
Increased intracranial pressure
Peritonitis
Malignancy (primary tumor or metastases)
Brain
Meninges
Hepatic
Gastrointestinal
Uremia
Infections (septicemia, local)
Radiation therapy

Data from Reference 25.

Breakthrough nausea and vomiting is defined as emesis occurring despite prophylactic administration of antiemetics and requiring the use of rescue antiemetics. Breakthrough emesis occurs in 10% to 40% of patients treated with antiemetics.[29]

Refractory nausea and vomiting is evident when there is a poor response to antiemetic regimens in prior cycles of chemotherapy. It is also important to rule out other potential causes of nausea and vomiting in the cancer population that are listed in Table 53-4.[2]

5 The primary goal with CINV is to prevent nausea and/or vomiting, and the emetic risk of the chemotherapeutic regimen is a major factor to consider when selecting a prophylactic regimen.[2]

Clinical practice guidelines for the use of antiemetics in CINV have been published by the National Comprehensive Cancer Network (NCCN), the Multinational Association of Supportive Care in Cancer/European Society of Medical Oncology (MASCC/ESMO), and ASCO.[2,28,32] The NCCN guidelines are updated annually, while the ASCO and ESMO guidelines are updated less frequently. Despite the demonstrated improvement in outcomes with the use of these practice guidelines, they are underutilized by a high percentage of practitioners.[32] Product availability and recommended doses are often institution-specific and may vary considerably from the doses listed in Table 53-2.

Principles of Antiemetic Use for CINV

The ASCO, MASCC, and NCCN consensus groups share several of the principles listed below that are important for the effective prevention of CINV in adults.[2,27,31,28,32]

1. The primary goal of emesis prevention is no nausea and/or vomiting throughout the period of emetic risk.
2. The duration of emetic risk is 2 days for patients receiving moderately emetogenic chemotherapy and 3 days for highly emetogenic chemotherapy. Emetic prophylaxis should be provided through the entire period of risk.
3. The selection of the antiemetic regimen should be based on the chemotherapy drug with highest emetogenicity (see

Table 53-2). Prior emetic experience and patient-specific factors should also be considered.

4. When given in equipotent doses, oral and IV 5-HT_3-RAs are equivalent in efficacy.
5. The toxicities of antiemetics should be considered and managed appropriately.

Prophylaxis of CINV

Each of the practice guidelines states that the most effective classes of drugs for the prevention of acute emesis, anticipatory, breakthrough, and refractory CINV are the 5-HT_3-RAs, NK_1 receptor antagonists, olanzapine, and glucocorticoids (especially dexamethasone). Treatment recommendations for the different categories of emesis are outlined in Table 53-2. For a full treatment algorithm, see Chapter 150, "Supportive Care."

RADIATION-INDUCED NAUSEA AND VOMITING

Nausea and vomiting associated with radiation therapy (RT) is not well understood and often underestimated by radiation oncologists.[34] RINV is neither as predictable nor as severe as CINV, and many patients receiving RT will not experience nausea or vomiting. RINV occurs in approximately one-third of patients, is site dependent, and can have a substantial impact on a patient's quality of life. Risk factors associated with the development of RINV include combination chemoradiotherapy, prior CINV, upper abdomen RT, and field size.[27] For more information on treatment options for the prevention of RINV, see Chapter 150, "Supportive Care."

POSTOPERATIVE NAUSEA AND VOMITING

PONV in adults occurs in 30% of patients and usually within 24 hours of undergoing anesthesia.[35] Patients with multiple risk factors are at highest risk for PONV (Table 53-5). In adults with 0, 1, 2, 3, and 4 of the risk factors in Table 53-5, the incidence of PONV is 10%, 20%, 40%, 60%, and 80%, respectively. Those who are found to have 0 to one risk factors are considered low risk, those with two risk factors are considered medium risk, and those with three or more risk factors are considered high risk. In children, those with no risk factors are considered low risk, those with one to two risk factors are considered as medium risk, and those with three or more risk factors are considered high risk. The use of a risk assessment tool can help identify patients most likely to benefit from prophylaxis.[16,36,37]

TABLE 53-5 Risk Factors for Postoperative Nausea and Vomiting (PONV)

Patient-related factors
Age less than 50 years old
Female sex (two to three times greater incidence of PONV vs male sex)
Nonsmoker
History of PONV or motion sickness (threefold increase in incidence of PONV)
Hydration status
Factors related to anesthesia
Use of general anesthesia
Use of volatile anesthetics
Nitrous oxide use for >1 hr
Use of opioids (intraoperative or postoperative)
Factors related to surgery
Type of surgical procedure (laparoscopic, gynecological, cholecystectomy)
Duration of surgery

Data from References 36 and 37.

In addition to using prophylactic antiemetics in moderate- and high-risk patients, other strategies to prevent PONV include using regional rather than systemic anesthesia, propofol, and hydration, as well as avoiding the use of extended duration nitrous oxide, volatile anesthetics, or opioids.[16]

Prophylaxis of PONV

6 Patients at highest risk of vomiting (>2 risk factors) should receive three or four prophylactic antiemetics from different pharmacologic classes, while those at moderate risk (1-2 risk factors) should receive a two-drug regimen. Adherence to consensus guidelines for prophylaxis and treatment of PONV decrease emetic episodes.[16] Timing the administration of the antiemetic is vital to the efficacy with PONV and may vary dependent upon the agent. Scopolamine patches must be initiated the evening before the surgery or at least 2 hours prior, whereas NK_1 antagonists should be given during the induction of anesthesia; all other agents are recommended to be administered at the end of the surgery. Pharmacological options for the prevention of PONV include 5-HT_3-RAs, an NK_1 antagonist, corticosteroids, droperidol, haloperidol, amisulpride, antihistamines, and anticholinergics.

Ondansetron is considered the "gold standard" 5-HT3-RA and has the most data supporting its use at the end of surgical procedures. It has greater antivomiting activity versus antinausea activity and is as effective as dexamethasone and IV haloperidol. However, it is less effective than longer acting agents such as aprepitant, ramosetron, granisetron, and fosaprepitant in decreasing emesis beyond 24 hours, and less effective than palonosetron for decreasing the incidence of PONV.[16,38-41,42-45]Ondansetron has greater efficacy compared to metoclopramide.[16]

Steroids, such as dexamethasone and methylprednisolone, are useful low-cost agents for preventing PONV. The recommended dose of dexamethasone ranges from 4 to 10 mg; however, there is limited evidence to support the use of doses greater than 8 mg. Dexamethasone should be administered after the induction of anesthesia, and when given in a single dose, has low risk of postoperative infections and only a mild increase in blood glucose values.[16,34,46] Palonosetron is more efficacious than dexamethasone in reducing PONV over a 24-hour interval.[47] One unique advantage dexamethasone has over other agents is that it decreases the need for other analgesic agents.[48] In patients undergoing hip and knee arthroplasty, methylprednisolone in doses from 40 mg to 125 mg decreased both PONV and pain.[16,49-51]

When evaluating antiemetics for PONV, there are several options including agents with antidopaminergic, antihistaminic, or anticholinergic activity. Intravenous amisulpride at 5 mg was more effective when compared to placebo in decreasing nausea severity. While it may lead to small increases in prolactin levels at lower doses, it was not found to be associated with QTc prolongation or a high risk of extrapyramidal symptoms, but may lead to small increases in prolactin levels.[53] Droperidol can be effective for PONV when administered at the end of surgery; however, its use has been limited due to the risk of sudden cardiac death.[16] Haloperidol, while not an FDA-approved agent for PONV, was efficacious and safe at low doses (0.5-2 mg) for prevention of PONV when compared to 5-HT3 antagonist.[42] Diphenhydramine at a dose of 50 mg decreased the incidence of PONV following outpatient laparoscopic gynecologic surgery.[43]

Several other agents have been studied to decrease the incidence of PONV including gabapentin and midazolam. When used 1 to 2 hours before laparoscopic cholecystectomy gabapentin decreased both pain and the incidence of PONV.[54] When administered at induction of anesthesia midazolam reduced the incidence of PONV, and when combined with other antiemetics has increased efficacy.[55]

Guidelines advocate the use of a combination of antiemetics; however, the optimal regimen when using more than two agents is

TABLE 53-6 Recommended Prophylactic Doses of Selected Antiemetics for Postoperative Nausea and Vomiting in Adults and Postoperative Vomiting in Children

Drug	Adult Dose	Pediatric Dose (IV)	Timing of Dose[a]
Amisulpride	5 mg	Not included in consensus guidelines	At induction
Aprepitant	40 mg orally	3 mg/kg up to 125 mg	At induction
Dexamethasone	4-8 mg IV	150 mcg/kg up to 5 mg	At induction
Dimenhydrinate	1 mg/kg IV	0.5 mg/kg up to 25 mg	Not specified
Droperidol[b]	0.625 mg IV	10-15 mcg/kg up to 1.25 mg	At end of surgery
Granisetron	0.35-3 mg IV	40 mcg/kg up to 0.6 mg	At end of surgery
Haloperidol	0.5-2 mg (IM or IV)	Not included in consensus guidelines	Not specified
Methylprednisolone	40 mg IV	Not included in consensus guidelines	Not specified
Metoclopramide	10 mg	Not included in consensus guidelines	Not specified
Ondansetron	4 mg IV, 8 mg orally or orally disintegrating tablet	50-100 mcg/kg up to 4 mg	At end of surgery
Palonosetron	0.075 mg IV	0.5-1.5 mcg/kg	At induction
Promethazine[b]	6.25 mg IV	Not included in consensus guidelines	At induction
Ramosetron	0.3 mg IV	Not included in consensus guidelines	At end of surgery
Rolapitant	70-200 mg orally	Not included in consensus guidelines	At induction
Scopolamine	Transdermal patch	Not included in consensus guidelines	Prior evening or 24 hr before surgery
Tropisetron	2 mg IV	0.1 mg/kg up to 2 mg	At end of surgery

[a]Based on recommendations from consensus guidelines.

[b]See FDA "black box" warning.

Data from Reference 16.

more ambiguous.[16] The choice should be based on the use of different mechanisms of action, adverse effect profiles, and cost. When evaluating two-drug regimens, the combination of a 5-HT3-RA plus dexamethasone 4 to 8 mg is considered the cornerstone of therapy.[44] There is also strong evidence to support the use of aprepitant plus dexamethasone. The addition of low-dose midazolam has increased efficacy, and amisulpride plus either ondansetron or dexamethasone was beneficial when compared to either ondansetron or dexamethasone alone.[16,45] Table 53-6 summarizes the doses for prophylactic antiemetics from the consensus guidelines.[16]

In children, those with no risk factors who are considered low risk can either use no antiemetic or either a 5-HT3- RA or dexamethasone. In those with one to two risk factors and are at a medium risk for PONV, it is recommended to use a combination of a 5-HT_3-RA plus dexamethasone. For those with three or more risk factors and at a high risk for developing PONV, the recommendation is to use a 5-HT_3-RA plus dexamethasone, or consider total intravenous anesthesia.[16]

Treatment of PONV

Patients who experience PONV after receiving prophylactic treatment with a combination of a 5-HT_3-RA plus dexamethasone should be given rescue therapy from a different drug class such as a phenothiazine, metoclopramide, or droperidol. Repeating the agent given for PONV prophylaxis within 6 hours of surgery offers no additional benefit. A repeated dose of a 5-HT_3-RA is not effective in treatment of PONV.[58,59] If an emetic episode occurs more than 6 hours postoperatively, a second dose of a 5-HT_3-RA can be used; however, it is not recommended to repeat doses of either dexamethasone or transdermal scopolamine.[16]

If no prophylaxis was given initially, the recommended treatment is low-dose 5-HT_3-RA such as ondansetron 4 mg orally or IV or ramosetron 0.3 mg IV. Alternative treatments for established PONV include haloperidol 1 mg, vestipitant 4 to 36 mg, amisulpride 5 to 10 mg, droperidol 0.625 mg IV, and promethazine 6.25 mg IV.[50-52]

DISORDERS OF BALANCE

Disorders of balance include vertigo, dizziness, and motion sickness. The etiology of these complaints may include diseases that are infectious, postinfectious, demyelinative, vascular, neoplastic, degenerative, traumatic, toxic, psychogenic, or idiopathic. Symptoms of imbalance perceived by the patient present a particular clinical challenge.

7 Beneficial therapy for patients with balance disorders can most reliably be found among the antihistaminic–anticholinergic agents. However, the precise mechanisms of action of these agents are unknown. Oral regimens of antihistaminic–anticholinergic agents given one to several times each day may be effective, especially when the first dose is administered prior to motion.

Motion sickness may be associated with nausea and vomiting; however, medication is more effective when given prophylactically. Scopolamine is effective for the prevention of motion sickness and is considered first line for this indication.[56] The usefulness of scopolamine in preventing motion sickness was enhanced with the development of the transdermal system (patch) that increased patient satisfaction and decreased untoward side effects. The patch should be placed several hours before the anticipated motion exposure. First-generation sedating antihistamines are also effective. However, second-generation nonsedating antihistamines, ondansetron, and ginger root are not effective in the prevention and treatment of motion sickness.[56]

ANTIEMETIC USE DURING PREGNANCY

As many as 80% of pregnant females experience nausea and 50% will have vomiting or retching.[56] The severity of the symptoms varies considerably, from mild nausea to incapacitating nausea and vomiting. The etiology of nausea and vomiting of pregnancy (NVP) is not well understood, but theories proposed include hormonal stimulus, evolutionary adaptation, and psychological predisposition.[56,57] Symptoms are self-limited for a majority of females, although up to 3% develop hyperemesis gravidarum, a serious condition marked by severe physical symptoms and/or medical complications requiring hospitalization.[58] Hyperemesis gravidarum may result in volume contraction, starvation, and electrolyte abnormalities.

Treatment recommendations for the management of NVP are available from the American College of Obstetricians and Gynecologists (ACOG).[59,60] Prevention of NVP should be the initial treatment approach. A prenatal vitamin should be started 1 month prior to becoming pregnant, which may help reduce the incidence and severity of NVP.[60] Dietary changes and/or lifestyle modifications such as eating smaller, more frequent meals every 1 to 2 hours, and avoiding foods or odors that trigger symptoms are recommended. Ginger is beneficial in reducing nausea but not vomiting.[59] Persistent nausea and/or vomiting leads to the consideration of drug therapy at a time when teratogenic potential of each agent must be considered. Pyridoxine (vitamin B_6), with or without doxylamine, is recommended as first-line therapy.[59] A delayed-release formulation of doxylamine and pyridoxine hydrochloride (Diclegis®) is available as a prescription product.[59] Dimenhydrinate, diphenhydramine, prochlorperazine, or promethazine may also be considered in the treatment of NVP.

Patients with persistent NVP or who show signs of dehydration should receive intravenous hydration with thiamine administered before dextrose to prevent Wernicke encephalopathy. Enteral tube feedings should be considered in females with hyperemesis gravidarum not responsive to medical therapy and who cannot maintain weight.[59] Ondansetron, promethazine, and metoclopramide have similar effectiveness for hyperemesis gravidarum, although ondansetron may be better tolerated due to less adverse effects.[61-64] Glucocorticoids, like methylprednisolone, may be used in patients with severe NVP or hyperemesis gravidarum, but should only be used after 10 weeks of gestation due to the increased risk of cleft lip.[56]

ANTIEMETIC USE IN SPECIAL POPULATIONS

Gastroenteritis in Children

Nausea and vomiting associated with pediatric gastroenteritis is usually self-limited and improves with correction of dehydration. The majority of patients can be successfully treated with oral rehydration therapy. Pediatric practitioners may prescribe antiemetics for intractable vomiting due to gastroenteritis. The use of promethazine is contraindicated in patients less than 2 years old and should be used with caution in older children due to the potential risk of fatal respiratory depression.[65] Administration of ondansetron is associated with decreased vomiting, a reduced need for intravenous rehydration therapy, and preventing hospital admissions.[66,67,69,70]

Antiemetic Use in Older Patients

Many of the commonly used antiemetics are on the Beers Criteria list, which are medications that may be inappropriate in older adults due to the risks outweighing the benefits.[68] These include first-generation antihistamines and scopolamine due to their highly anticholinergic side effects. Metoclopramide is also on the Beers list because it may cause extrapyramidal effects including tardive dyskinesia especially in frail older adults.[69] Ondansetron may be considered a preferred antiemetic in older adults; however, consider drug-drug interactions and potential adverse effects before prescribing.[70]

EVALUATION OF EMETIC OUTCOMES

In assessing emetic outcomes, standardized monitoring criteria should include a subjective assessment and objective parameters. For patients on chemotherapy, evaluation of emetic outcomes should occur after the administration of each chemotherapy cycle. In regards to PONV, the patient should be monitored both immediately post procedure as well as for delayed symptoms.

ABBREVIATIONS

ACOG	American College of Obstetricians and Gynecologists
ANV	anticipatory nausea and vomiting
ASCO	American Society of Clinical Oncology
BRAT	bananas, rice, applesauce, or toast
CINV	chemotherapy-induced nausea and vomiting
CTZ	chemoreceptor trigger zone
GI	gastrointestinal
ESMO	European Society of Medical Oncology
HEC	high emetogenic chemotherapy
5-HT_3-RA	5-hydroxytryptamine-3 receptor antagonist
MASCC	Multinational Association of Supportive Care in Cancer
NCCN	National Comprehensive Cancer Network
NEPA	netupitant/palonosetron
NK_1	neurokinin-1
NVP	nausea and vomiting of pregnancy
PONV	postoperative nausea and vomiting
RINV	radiation-induced nausea and vomiting
RT	radiation therapy
TBI	total-body irradiation
VC	vomiting center

REFERENCES

1. Hasler WL. Nausea, vomiting, and indigestion. In: Kasper D, Fauci A, Hauser S, Longo D, Jameson J, Loscalzo J, eds. *Harrison's Principles of Internal Medicine*. 19th ed. New York, NY: McGraw-Hill; 2014. http://accessmedicine.mhmedical.com/content.aspx?bookid=1130§ionid=79726154.
2. Hesketh PJ, Kris MG, et al. Antiemetics: ASCO guideline update. *J Clin Oncol*. 2020 Aug 20;38(24):2782–2797.
3. Krakauer EL, Zhu AX, Bounds BC, Sahani D, McDonald KR, Brachtel EF. Case records of the Massachusetts General Hospital. *N Engl J Med*. 2005;352:817. Massachusetts Medical Society.
4. Kamen C, Tejani MA, Chandwani K, et al. Anticipatory nausea and vomiting due to chemotherapy. *Eur J Pharmacol*. 2014;722:172–179.
5. Morehead A, Salmon G. Acupressure in the prevention and treatment of nausea and vomiting across multiple patient populations: Implications for practice. *Nurs Clin N Am*. 2020;55:571–580.
6. Craciunas L, Sajid MS, Ahmed AS. Chewing gum in preventing postoperative ileus in women undergoing caesarean section: A systematic review and meta-analysis of randomised controlled trials. *BJOG*. 2014;121:793–799.
7. Short V, Herbert G, Perry R, et al. Chewing gum for postoperative recovery of gastrointestinal function. *Cochrane Database of Syst Rev*. 2015;(2):CD006506.
8. Acar HV. Acupuncture and related techniques during perioperative period: A literature review. *Complement Ther Med*. 2016 Dec;29:48–55.
9. Murray-Brown F, Dorman S. Haloperidol for the treatment of nausea and vomiting in palliative care patients. *Cochrane Database Syst Rev*. 2015;11:CD006271.
10. Droperidol [package insert]. Lake Forest, IL: Hospira, Inc.; 2004.
11. Wilkie G, Sakr B, Rizack T. Medical marijuana use in oncology: A review. *JAMA Oncol*. 2016;2(5):670–675.
12. Whiting PF, Wolff RF, Deshpande S, et al. Cannabinoids for medicinal use: A systematic review and meta-analysis. *JAMA*. 2015;313:2456–2473.
13. Inglet S, Winter B, Yost SE, et al. Clinical data for the use of cannabis-based treatments: A comprehensive review of the literature. *Ann Pharmacother*. 2020;54(11):1109–1143.
14. Sorensen CJ, DeSanto K, Borgelt L, Phillips KT, Monte AA. Cannabinoid hyperemesis syndrome—diagnosis, pathophysiology, and treatment: A systematic review. *J Med Toxicol*. 2017;13:71–87.
15. Italian Group for Antiemetic Research. Double-blind, dose-finding study of four intravenous doses of dexamethasone in the prevention of cisplatin-induced acute emesis. *J Clin Oncol*. 1998;16:2937–2942.
16. Gan T, Kumar G, Bergese S, et al. Fourth Consensus Guidelines for the management of postoperative nausea and vomiting. *Anesth Analg*. 2020;131(2):411–448.

17. Ondansetron [package insert]. Research Triangle Park, NC: GlaxoSmithKline; 2017.
18. Akynzeo (netupitant and palonosetron) [package insert]. Iselin, NJ: Helsinn Therapeutics, Inc.; 2018.
19. Patel P, Leeder JS, Piquette-Miller M, et al. Aprepitant and fosaprepitant drug interactions: A systematic review. *Br J Clin Pharmacol.* 2017;83(10):2148–2162.
20. Emend (aprepitant) [package insert]. Whitehouse Station, NJ: Merck & Co, Inc.; 2017.
21. McCrea JB, Majumdar AK, Goldberg MR, et al. Effects of the neurokinin-1 receptor antagonist aprepitant on the pharmacokinetics of dexamethasone and methylprednisolone. *Clin Pharmacol Ther.* 2003;74:17–24.
22. Emend (fosaprepitant) [package insert]. Whitehouse Station, NJ: Merck & Co, Inc.; 2018.
23. Varubi (rolapitant) [package insert]. Waltham, MA: Tesaro, Inc.; 2018.
24. Zhang L, Lu S, Feng J, et al. A randomized phase III study evaluating the efficacy of single-dose NEPA, a fixed antiemetic combination of netupitant and palonosetron, versus an aprepitant regimen for prevention of chemotherapy-induced nausea and vomiting (CINV) in patients receiving highly emetogenic chemotherapy (HEC). *Ann Oncol.* 2018;29:452–458.
25. Navari RM, Qin R, Ruddy KJ, et al. Olanzapine for the prevention of chemotherapy-induced nausea and vomiting. *N Engl J Med.* 2016;375:134–142.
26. Yanai T, Iwasa S, Hashimoto H, et al. A double-blind randomized phase II dose-finding study of olanzapine 10 mg or 5 mg for the prophylaxis of emesis induced by highly emetogenic cisplatin-based chemotherapy. *Int J Clin Oncol.* 2018;23:382–388.
27. National Comprehensive Cancer Network (NCCN) Clinical Practice Guidelines in Oncology. Management of immunotherapy related toxicites. v3.2021. Available at: https://www.nccn.org/professionals/physician_gls/pdf/immunotherapy.pdf. Last accessed September 1, 2021.
28. Ernst A, Weiss SJ, Park S, et al. Prochlorperazine versus promethazine for uncomplicated nausea and vomiting in the emergency department: A randomized, double-blind clinical trial. *Ann Emerg Med.* 2000;36:89–94.
29. Navari RM, Aapro M. Antiemetic prophylaxis for chemotherapy-induced nausea and vomiting. *N Engl J Med.* 2016;374:1356–1367.
30. Molassiotis A, Lee PH, Burke TA. Anticipatory nausea, risk factors, and its impact on chemotherapy-induced nausea and vomiting: Results from the Pan European Emesis Registry Study. *J Pain Symptom Manage.* 2016;51:987–993.
31. Roila F, Molassiotis A, Herrstedt J, et al. 2016 MASCC and ESMO guideline update for the prevention of chemotherapy- and radiotherapy-induced nausea and vomiting and of nausea and vomiting in advanced cancer patients. *Ann Oncol.* 2016;27(Suppl 5):v119–v133.
32. Jordan K, Gralla R, Jahn F, Molassiotts A. International antiemetic guidelines on chemotherapy induced nausea and vomiting (CINV): Content and implementation in daily practice. *Eur J Pharmacol.* 2014;722:197–222.
33. Enblom A, Bergius Axelsson B, Steineck G, et al. One third of patients with radiotherapy-induced nausea consider their antiemetic treatment insufficient. *Support Care Cancer.* 2009;17:23–32.
34. Polderman JA, Farhang-Razi V, Van Dieren S, et al. Adverse side effects of dexamethasone in surgical patients. *Cochrane Database Syst Rev.* 2018;8(8):CD011940.
35. Wiesmann T, Kranke P, Eberhart L. Postoperative nausea and vomiting—A narrative review of pathophysiology, pharmacotherapy and clinical management strategies. *Expert Opin Pharmacother.* 2015;16:1069–1077.
36. Shaikh SI, Nagarekha D, Hegade G, Marutheesh M. Postoperative nausea and vomiting: A simple yet complex problem. *Anesth Essays Res.* 2016;10:388–396.
37. Apfel CA, Karttila K, Abdalla M, et al. A factorial trial of six intervention for the prevention of postoperative nausea and vomiting. *N Engl J Med.* 2004;350:2441–2451.
38. Diemunsch P, Gan TJ, Philip BK, et al. Single-dose aprepitant vs. ondansetron for the prevention of postoperative nausea and vomiting: A randomized, double-blind phase III trial in patient undergoing open abdominal surgery. *Br J Anaesth.* 2007;99:202–211.
39. Park SK, Cho EJ. A randomized, double-blind trial of palonosetron compared with ondansetron in preventing postoperative nausea and vomiting after gynaecological laparoscopic surgery. *J Int Med Res.* 2011;39:399–407.
40. Okafor D, Kaye AD, Kaye RJ, Urman RD. The role of neurokinin-1 (substance P) antagonists in the prevention of postoperative nausea and vomiting. *J Anaesthesiol Clin Pharmacol.* 2017;33:441–445.
41. Janicki PK, Schuler HG, Jarzembowski TM, Ross M II. Prevention of postoperative nausea and vomiting with granisetron and dolasetron in relation to CYP2D6 genotype. *Anest Analg.* 2006;102:1127–1133.
42. Singh PM, Borle A, Makkar JK, et al. Haloperidol versus 5-HT_3 receptor antagonists for postoperative vomiting and QTc prolongation: A noninferiority meta-analysis and trial sequential analysis of randomized controlled trials. *J Clin Pharmacol.* 2018;58(2):131–143.
43. De Oliveira GS Jr, Bialek J, Marcus RJ, McCarthy R. Dose-ranging effect of systemic diphenhydramine on postoperative quality of recovery after ambulatory laparoscopic surgery: A randomized, placebo-controlled, double-blinded, clinical trial. *J Clin Anesth.* 2016 Nov;34:46–52.
44. Som A, Bhattacharjee S, Maitra S, et al. Combination of 5-HT3 antagonist and dexamethasone is superior to 5-HT3 antagonist alone for PONV prophylaxis after laparoscopic surgeries: A meta-analysis. *Anesth Analg.* 2016;123(6):1418–1426.
45. Kranke P, Bergese SD, Minkowitz HS, et al. Amisulpride prevents postoperative nausea and vomiting in patients at high risk: A randomized, double-blind, placebo-controlled trial. *Anesthesiology.* 2018;128(6):1099–1106.
46. Fan Z, Ma J, Ma X, et al. The efficacy of dexamethasone on pain and recovery after total hip arthroplasty: A systematic review and meta-analysis of randomized controlled trials. *Medicine (Baltimore).* 2018;97(13):e0100.
47. Paul AA, George SK, Ranjan RV, et al. Randomised control study of palonosetron versus dexamethasone in preventing postoperative nausea and vomiting flowing ear and nose surgeries under general anesthesia. *J Clin Diagn Res.* 2018;12(11):UC10–UC13.
48. Singh PM, Borle A, Panwar R, et al. Perioperative antiemetic efficacy of dexamethasone versus 5-HT3 receptor antagonists: A meta-analysis and trial sequential analysis of randomized controlled trials. *Eur J Clin Pharmacol.* 2018;74:1201–1214.
49. Liu G, Gong M, Wang Y, Xiang Z. Effect of methylprednisolone on pain management in total knee or hip arthroplasty: A systematic review and meta-analysis of randomized controlled trials. *Clin J Pain.* 2018;34(10):967–974.
50. Candiotti KA, Kranke P, Bergese SD, et al. Randomized, double-blind, placebo-controlled study of intravenous amisulpride as treatment of established postoperative nausea and vomiting in patients who have had no prior prophylaxis. *Anesth Analg.* 2019;128(6):1098–1105.
51. Kranke P, Thompson JP, Dalby PL, et al. Comparison of vestipitant with ondansetron for the treatment of breakthrough postoperative nausea and vomiting after failed prophylaxis with ondansetron. *Br J Anaesth.* 2015 Mar;114(3):423–429.
52. Yazbeck-Karam VG, Siddik-Sayyid SM, Barakat HB, Korjian S, Aouad MT. Haloperidol versus ondansetron for treatment of established nausea and vomiting following general anesthesia: A randomized clinical trial. *Anesth Analg.* 2017;124(2):438–444.
53. Gan TJ, Kranke P, Minkowitz HS, et al. Intravenous amisulpride for the prevention of postoperative nausea and vomiting: Two concurrent, randomized, double-blind, placebo-controlled trials. *Anesthesiology.* 2017;126(2):268–275.
54. Wang L, Dong Y, Zhang J, Tan H. The efficacy of gabapentin in reducing pain intensity and postoperative nausea and vomiting following laparoscopic cholecystectomy: A meta-analysis. *Medicine (Baltimore).* 2017;96(37):e8007.
55. Ahn EJ, Kang H, Choi GJ, Baek CW, Jung YH, Woo YC. The effectiveness of midazolam for preventing postoperative nausea and vomiting: A systematic review and meta-analysis. *Anesth Analg.* 2016;122(3):664–676.
56. Brainard A, Gresham C. Prevention and treatment of motion sickness. *Am Fam Physician.* 2014;90:41–46.
57. Flaxman SM, Sherman PW. Morning sickness: A mechanism for protecting mother and embryo. *Q Rev Biol.* 2000;75:113–148.
58. Simpson SW, Goodwin TM, Robins SB, et al. Psychological factors and hyperemesis gravidarum. *J Womens Health Gend Based Med.* 2001;10:471–477.
59. Matthews A, Haas DM, O'Mathúna DP, Dowswell T. Interventions for nausea and vomiting in early pregnancy. *Cochrane Database Syst Rev.* 2015;(9):CD007575.
60. Committee on Practice Bulletins-Obstetrics. ACOG Practice Bulletin No. 189: Nausea and vomiting of pregnancy. *Obstet Gynecol.* 2018;131:e15–e30.
61. Herrell HE. Nausea and vomiting of pregnancy. *Am Fam Physician.* 2014;89(12):965–970.
62. Committee on Practice Bulletins-Obstetrics. Practice Bulletin No. 187: Neural tube defects. *Obstet Gynecol.* 2017;130:e279–e290.
63. Koren G, Clark S, Hankins GD, et al. Maternal safety of the delayed-release doxylamine and pyridoxine combination for nausea and vomiting of pregnancy: A randomized placebo controlled trial. *BMC Pregnancy Childbirth.* 2015;15:59.

64. Abas MN, Tan PC, Azmi N, Omar SZ. Ondansetron compared with metoclopramide for hyperemesis gravidarum: A randomized controlled trial. *Obstet Gynecol.* 2014;123(6):1272–1279.
65. Phenergan [package insert]. Philadelphia, PA. Wyeth Pharmaceuticals Inc. 2004.
66. Danewa AS, Shah D, Batra P, et al. Oral ondansetron in management of dehydrating diarrhea and vomiting in children aged 3 months to 5 years: A randomized controlled trial. *J Pediatr.* 2016;169:105–109.
67. Nino-Serna LF, Acosta-Reyes J, Veroniki AA, Florez ID. Antiemetics in children with acute gastroenteritis: A meta-analysis. *Pediatrics.* 2020;145(4):e20193260.
68. Danewa AS, Shah D, Batra P, et al. Oral ondansetron in management of dehydrating diarrhea and vomiting in children aged 3 months to 5 years: A randomized controlled trial. *J Pediatr.* 2016;169:105–109.
69. The 2019 American Geriatrics Society Beers Criteria Update Expert Panel. American Geriatrics Society 2019 updated Beers Criteria for potentially inappropriate medication use in older adults. *J Am Geriatr Soc.* 2019;67(4):674–694.
70. Reuben DB, Herr KA, Pacala JT, et al. *Geriatrics at Your Fingertips 2021.* 23rd ed. New York, NY: The American Geriatrics Society; 2021.

Diarrhea, Constipation, and Irritable Bowel Syndrome

54

Patricia H. Fabel and Kayce M. Shealy

KEY CONCEPTS

1. Diarrhea is caused by many viral and bacterial organisms. It is most often a minor discomfort, not life-threatening, and usually self-limited.
2. The four pathophysiologic mechanisms of diarrhea have been linked to the four broad diarrheal groups, which are secretory, osmotic, exudative, and altered intestinal transit. The three mechanisms by which absorption occurs from the intestines are active transport, diffusion, and solvent drag.
3. Management of diarrhea focuses on preventing excessive water and electrolyte losses, dietary care, relieving symptoms, treating curable causes, and treating secondary disorders.
4. Bismuth subsalicylate is marketed for indigestion, relieving abdominal cramps, and controlling diarrhea, including traveler's diarrhea, but may cause interactions with several components if given excessively.
5. Constipation is defined as difficult or infrequent passage of stool, at times associated with straining or a feeling of incomplete defecation.
6. Underlying causes of constipation should be identified when possible and corrective measures taken (eg, alteration of diet or treatment of diseases such as hypothyroidism).
7. The foundation of treatment of constipation is dietary fiber or bulk-forming laxatives that provide 20 to 25 g/day of raw fiber.
8. Irritable bowel syndrome (IBS) is one of the most common GI disorders characterized by lower abdominal pain, disturbed defecation, and bloating. Many non-GI manifestations also exist with IBS. Visceral hypersensitivity is a major culprit in the pathophysiology of the disease.
9. Diarrhea-predominant IBS should be managed by dietary modification and drugs such as rifaximin or eluxadoline when diet changes alone are insufficient to promote control of symptoms.
10. Several drug classes are involved in the treatment of the pain associated with IBS including tricyclic compounds and the gut-selective calcium channel blockers.

BEYOND THE BOOK

Go to www.loperamidesafety.org/resources and review the fact sheets for healthcare providers aimed at helping identify potential loperamide misuse. Reflecting on your role on the healthcare team, what can you do to ensure safe and appropriate loperamide use?

DIARRHEA

Diarrhea is a troublesome discomfort that affects most individuals in the United States at some point in their lives and can be thought of as both a symptom and a sign. Usually diarrheal episodes begin abruptly and subside within 1 or 2 days without treatment. This chapter focuses primarily on noninfectious diarrhea, with only minor reference to infectious diarrhea (see Chapter 136 for a discussion of gastrointestinal infections). Diarrhea is often a symptom of a systemic disease, and not all possible causes of diarrhea are discussed in this chapter. Acute diarrhea is commonly defined as less than 14-day duration, persistent diarrhea as more than 14-day duration, and chronic diarrhea as more than 30-day duration.

To understand diarrhea, one must have a reasonable definition of the condition; unfortunately, the literature is extremely variable on this. Simply put, diarrhea is an increased frequency and decreased consistency of fecal discharge as compared with an individual's normal bowel pattern. Frequency and consistency are variable within and between individuals. For example, some individuals defecate as often as three times per day, whereas others defecate only two or three times per week. A Western diet usually produces a daily stool weighing between 100 and 300 g, depending on the amount of nonabsorbable materials (mainly carbohydrates) consumed. Patients with serious diarrhea may have a daily stool weight in excess of 300 g; however, a subset of patients experience frequent small, watery passages. Additionally, vegetable fiber-rich diets, such as those consumed in some Eastern cultures (eg, those in Africa), produce stools weighing more than 300 g/day.

Diarrhea may be associated with a specific disease of the intestines or secondary to a disease outside the intestines. For instance, bacillary dysentery directly affects the gut, whereas diabetes mellitus causes neuropathic diarrheal episodes. Furthermore, diarrhea can be considered as acute or chronic disease. Infectious diarrhea is often acute; diarrhea secondary to diabetes is chronic. Congenital disorders in GI ion transport mechanisms are another cause of chronic diarrhea.[1] Whether acute or chronic, diarrhea has the same pathophysiologic causes that help in identification of specific treatments.

Epidemiology

The epidemiology of diarrhea varies in developed versus developing countries.[2] In the United States, diarrheal illnesses are usually not reported to the Centers for Disease Control and Prevention (CDC) unless associated with an outbreak or an unusual organism or condition. For example, the acquired immune deficiency syndrome (AIDS) has been identified with protracted diarrheal illness. Diarrhea is a major problem in daycare centers and nursing homes, probably because early childhood and senescence plus environmental conditions are risk factors. Although an exact epidemiologic profile in the United States is not available through the CDC or published literature, 25% of individuals in the United States experience an episode of acute diarrhea annually with increased incidence in children and older adults.[3] In developing countries, diarrhea is a leading cause of illness and death in children, creating a tremendous economic strain on healthcare costs.

1 Most cases of acute diarrhea are self-limiting infections caused by food or waterborne organisms, such as viruses, bacteria, or protozoa.[4] Although viruses are more commonly associated with acute gastroenteritis, bacteria are responsible for more cases of acute diarrhea. Evaluation of a noninfectious cause is considered if diarrhea persists and no infectious organism can be identified, or if the patient falls into a high-risk category for metabolic complications with persistent diarrhea. Common causative bacterial organisms include *Shigella*, *Salmonella*, *Campylobacter*, *Staphylococcus*, and *Escherichia coli*. Foodborne bacterial infection is a major concern, as several major food poisoning episodes have occurred that were traced to poor sanitary conditions in meat processing plants. Acute viral infections are attributed mostly to the Norwalk and rotavirus groups.

Physiology

In the fasting state, 9 L of fluid enters the proximal small intestine each day. Of this fluid, 2 L is ingested through diet, while the remainder consists of internal secretions. Because of meal content, duodenal chyme is usually hypertonic. When chyme reaches the ileum, the osmolality adjusts to that of plasma, with most dietary fat, carbohydrate, and protein being absorbed. The volume of ileal chyme decreases to about 1 L/day on entering the colon, which is further reduced by colonic absorption to 100 mL daily. If the small intestine water absorption capacity is exceeded, chyme overloads the colon, resulting in diarrhea. In humans, the colon absorptive capacity is about 5 L daily. Colonic fluid transport is critical to water and electrolyte balance.

Absorption of fluid from the intestines back into the blood occurs by three mechanisms: active transport, diffusion, and solvent drag. Active transport and diffusion are the mechanisms of sodium transport. Because of the high luminal sodium concentration (142 mEq/L [mmol/L]), sodium diffuses from the sodium-rich gut into epithelial cells, where it is actively pumped into the blood and exchanged with chloride to maintain an isoelectric condition across the epithelial membrane. Hydrogen ions are transported by an indirect mechanism in the upper small intestine. As sodium is absorbed, hydrogen ions are secreted into the gut. Hydrogen ions then combine with bicarbonate ions to form carbonic acid, which then dissociates into carbon dioxide and water. Carbon dioxide readily diffuses into the blood for expiration through the lung. The water remains in the chyme.

Paracellular pathways are major routes of ion movement. As ions, monosaccharides, and amino acids are actively transported, an osmotic pressure is created, drawing water and electrolytes across the intestinal wall. This pathway accounts for significant amounts of ion transport, especially sodium. Sodium plays an important role in stimulating glucose absorption. Glucose and amino acids are actively transported into the blood via a sodium-dependent cotransport mechanism. Cotransport absorption mechanisms of glucose–sodium and amino acid–sodium are extremely important for treating diarrhea.

Gut motility influences absorption and secretion. The amount of time in which luminal content is in contact with the epithelium is under neural and hormonal control. Neurohormonal substances, such as angiotensin, vasopressin, glucocorticoid, aldosterone, and neurotransmitters, also regulate ion transport.

Pathophysiology

2 Four general pathophysiologic mechanisms disrupt water and electrolyte balance, leading to diarrhea, and are the basis of diagnosis and therapy. These are (a) a change in active ion transport by either decreased sodium absorption or increased chloride secretion; (b) change in intestinal motility; (c) increase in luminal osmolarity; and (d) increase in tissue hydrostatic pressure. These mechanisms have been related to four broad clinical diarrheal groups: secretory, osmotic, exudative, and altered intestinal transit.

Secretory diarrhea occurs when a stimulating substance either increases secretion or decreases absorption of large amounts of water and electrolytes. Substances that cause excess secretion include vasoactive intestinal peptide (VIP) from a pancreatic tumor, unabsorbed dietary fat in steatorrhea, laxatives, hormones (such as secretion), bacterial toxins, and excessive bile salts. Many of these agents stimulate intracellular cyclic adenosine monophosphate and inhibit Na^+/K^+-adenosine triphosphatase (ATPase), leading to increased secretion. Also, many of these mediators inhibit ion absorption simultaneously. Secretory diarrhea is recognized by large stool volumes (more than 1 L/day) with normal ionic contents and osmolality approximately equal to plasma. Fasting does not alter the stool volume in these patients.

Poorly absorbed substances retain intestinal fluids, resulting in osmotic diarrhea. This process occurs with malabsorption syndromes, lactose intolerance, administration of divalent ions (eg, magnesium-containing antacids), or consumption of poorly soluble carbohydrate (eg, lactulose). As a poorly soluble solute is transported, the gut adjusts the osmolality to that of plasma; in so doing, water and electrolytes flux into the lumen. Clinically, osmotic diarrhea is distinguishable from other types, as it ceases if the patient resorts to a fasting state.

Inflammatory diseases of the GI tract discharge mucus, serum proteins, and blood into the gut. Sometimes bowel movements consist only of mucus, exudate, and blood. Exudative diarrhea affects other absorptive, secretory, or motility functions to account for the large stool volume associated with this disorder.

Altered intestinal motility produces diarrhea by three mechanisms: (1) reduction of contact time in the small intestine, (2) premature emptying of the colon, and (3) bacterial overgrowth. Chyme must be exposed to intestinal epithelium for a sufficient time period to enable normal absorption and secretion processes to occur. If this contact time decreases, diarrhea results. Intestinal resection or bypass surgery and drugs (such as metoclopramide) cause this type of diarrhea. On the other hand, an increased time of exposure allows fecal bacteria overgrowth. A characteristic small intestine diarrheal pattern is rapid, small, coupling bursts of waves. These waves are inefficient, do not allow absorption, and rapidly dump chyme into the colon. Once in the colon, chyme exceeds the colonic capability to absorb water.

Examination of the Stool

Stool characteristics are important in assessing the etiology of diarrhea. A description of the frequency, volume, consistency, and color provides diagnostic clues. For instance, diarrhea starting in the small intestine produces a copious, watery or fatty (greasy), and foul-smelling stool; contains undigested food particles; and is usually free from gross blood. Colonic diarrhea appears as small, pasty, and sometimes bloody or mucoid movements. Rectal tenesmus with flatus accompanies large intestinal diarrhea.

Clinical Presentation

Table 54-1 outlines the clinical presentation of diarrhea, and Table 54-2 shows common drug-induced causes of diarrhea. A medication history is extremely important in identifying drug-induced diarrhea. Many agents, including antibiotics and other drugs, cause diarrhea or, less commonly, pseudomembranous colitis. Self-inflicted laxative abuse for weight loss is common.

Most acute diarrhea is self-limiting, subsiding within 72 hours. However, infants, young children, older patients, and debilitated persons are at risk for morbid and mortal events in prolonged or

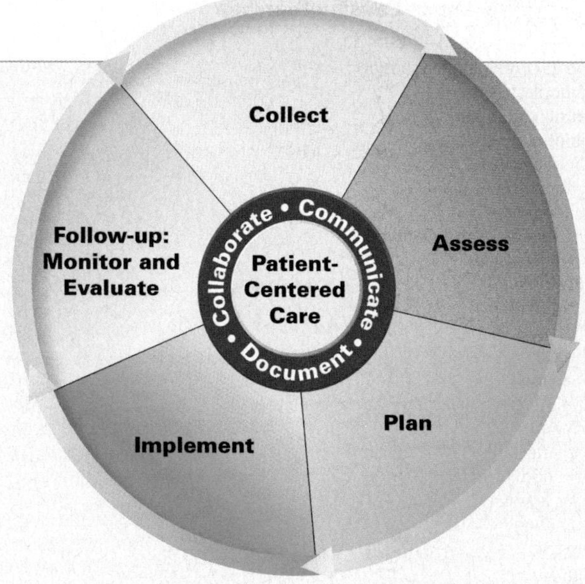

Patient Care Process for Diarrhea

The image shows the five fundamental steps included in The Pharmacist's Care Process endorsed by the Joint Commission for Pharmacy Practitioners (2014). The tagline of this process reads collaborate, communicate, and document. The five fundamental steps listed here are collect, assess, plan, implement, and follow-up: monitor and evaluate. All these steps are listed in a circular block diagram.

Collect

- Patient characteristics
- Patient medical, family, social history, and dietary habits
- Current medications, including nonprescription
- Vital signs and weight
- Laboratory tests depending upon medical history and other presenting symptoms
  - o Thyroid function tests, complete blood count, glucose, serum electrolytes

Assess

- Underlying causes of diarrhea (see Tables 54-1 and 54-2)
- Severity and duration of symptoms
- Patient preference for symptom resolution
- Ability/willingness to pay for treatment options

Plan*

- Treat specific cause of diarrhea (ie, diabetes, infectious)
- Increase fluid intake using oral rehydration solutions (ORS) (Table 54-3)
- Antidiarrheal medication (Table 54-4)
- Monitor symptom resolution for efficacy, and pronounced constipation for safety
- Patient education regarding importance of prevention dehydration
- Referral to other providers when appropriate

Implement

- Educate the patient on all aspects of the treatment plan
- Schedule follow-up to monitor safety and efficacy of treatment plan

Follow-up: Monitor and Evaluate

- Determine resolution of diarrhea and related symptoms
- Evaluate for signs and symptoms of dehydration
- Assess for presence of adverse effects (eg, abdominal pain, constipation)
- Assess patient adherence to treatment plan
- Reevaluate periodically until resolution

**Collaborate with patient, caregivers, and other healthcare professionals.*

voluminous diarrhea. These groups are at risk for water, electrolyte, and acid-base disturbances, and potentially cardiovascular collapse and death. The prognosis for chronic diarrhea depends on the cause; for example, diarrhea secondary to diabetes mellitus waxes and wanes throughout life.

TREATMENT AND PREVENTION

Acute viral diarrheal illness often occurs in daycare centers and nursing homes. Because person-to-person contact is the mechanism by which viral disease spreads, isolation techniques must be initiated. For bacterial, parasitic, and protozoal infections, strict food handling, sanitation, water, and other environmental hygiene practices can prevent transmission. If diarrhea is secondary to another illness, controlling the primary condition is necessary. Antibiotics and bismuth subsalicylate are advocated to prevent traveler's diarrhea, in conjunction with treatment of drinking water and caution with consumption of fresh vegetables.[5,6]

Desired Outcome

3 If prevention is unsuccessful and diarrhea occurs, therapeutic goals are to (a) manage the diet; (b) prevent excessive water, electrolyte, and acid-base disturbances; (c) provide symptomatic relief; (d) treat curable causes; and (e) manage secondary disorders causing diarrhea (Figs. 54-1 and 54-2).

Clinicians must clearly understand that diarrhea, like a cough, may be a body defense mechanism for ridding itself of harmful substances or pathogens. The correct therapeutic response is not necessarily to stop diarrhea at all costs.

Nonpharmacologic Management

Dietary management is a first priority in the treatment of diarrhea. Feeding should continue in children with acute bacterial diarrhea. Fed children have less morbidity and mortality, whether or not they receive oral rehydration fluids. Studies are not available in older patients or in other high-risk groups to determine the value of continued feeding in bacterial diarrhea.

Water and Electrolytes

Rehydration and maintenance of water and electrolytes are primary treatment goals until the diarrheal episode ends. If the patient is volume depleted, rehydration should be directed at replacing water and electrolytes to normal body composition. Then water and electrolyte composition are maintained by replacing losses. Many patients will

TABLE 54-1 Clinical Presentation of Diarrhea

General
- Usually, acute diarrheal episodes subside within 72 hours of onset, whereas chronic diarrhea involves frequent attacks over extended time periods.

Signs and symptoms
- Abrupt onset of nausea, vomiting, abdominal pain, headache, fever, chills, and malaise.
- Bowel movements are frequent and never bloody, and diarrhea lasts 12-60 hours.
- Intermittent periumbilical or lower right quadrant pain with cramps and audible bowel sounds is characteristic of small intestinal disease.
- When pain is present in large intestinal diarrhea, it is a gripping, aching sensation with tenesmus (straining, ineffective, and painful stooling). Pain localizes to the hypogastric region, right or left lower quadrant, or sacral region.
- In chronic diarrhea, a history of previous bouts, weight loss, anorexia, and chronic weakness are important findings.

Physical examination
- Typically demonstrates hyperperistalsis with borborygmi and generalized or local tenderness.

Laboratory tests
- Stool analysis studies include examination for microorganisms, blood, mucus, fat, osmolality, pH, electrolyte and mineral concentration, and cultures.
- Stool test kits are useful for detecting GI viruses, particularly rotavirus.
- Antibody serologic testing shows rising titers over a 3- to 6-day period, but this test is not practical and is nonspecific.
- Occasionally, total daily stool volume is also determined.
- Direct endoscopic visualization and biopsy of the colon may be undertaken to assess for the presence of conditions such as colitis or cancer.
- Radiographic studies are helpful in neoplastic and inflammatory conditions.

TABLE 54-2 Drugs Causing Diarrhea

Laxatives
Antacids containing magnesium
Antineoplastics
Auranofin (gold salt)
Antibiotics
- Clindamycin
- Tetracyclines
- Sulfonamides
- Any broad-spectrum antibiotic

Antihypertensives
- Reserpine
- Guanethidine
- Methyldopa
- Guanabenz
- Guanadrel
- Angiotensin-converting enzyme inhibitors

Cholinergics
- Bethanechol
- Neostigmine

Cardiac agents
- Quinidine
- Digitalis
- Digoxin

Nonsteroidal anti-inflammatory drugs
Misoprostol
Colchicine
Proton pump inhibitors
H_2-receptor blockers

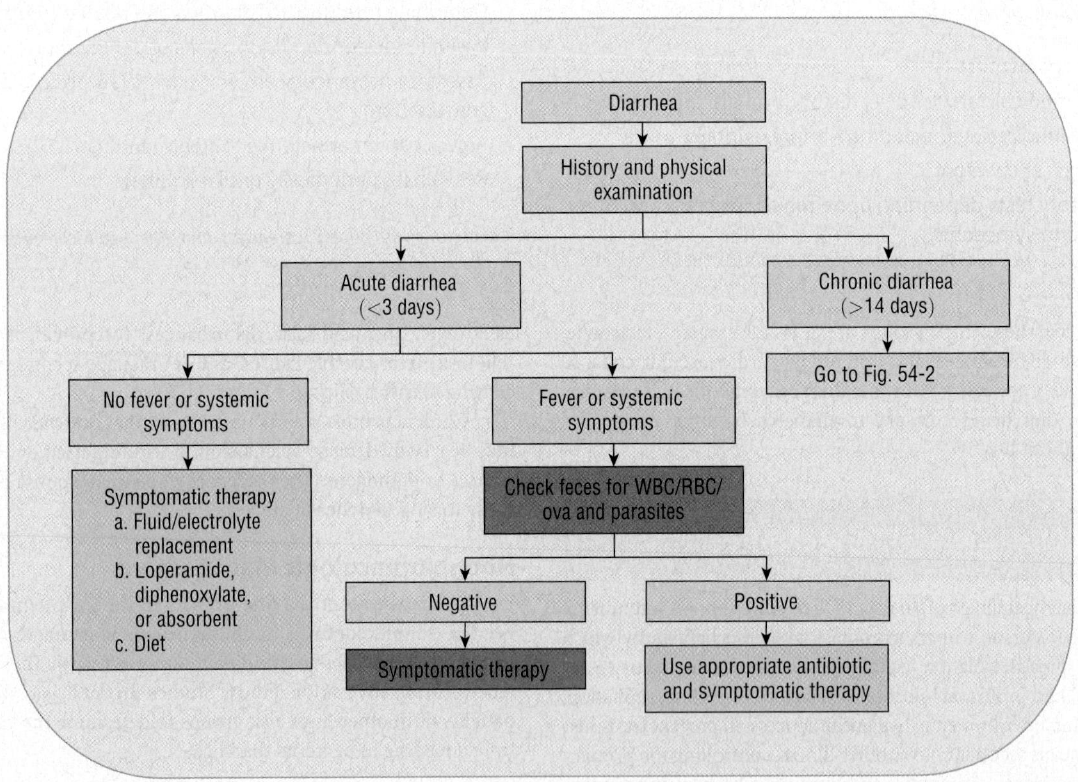

FIGURE 54-1 Recommendations for treating acute diarrhea. Follow the following steps: (a) Perform a complete history and physical examination. (b) Is the diarrhea acute or chronic? If chronic diarrhea, go to Fig. 54-2. (c) If acute diarrhea, check for fever and/or systemic signs and symptoms (ie, toxic patient). If systemic illness (fever, anorexia, or volume depletion), check for an infectious source. If positive for infectious diarrhea, use appropriate antibiotic/anthelmintic drug and symptomatic therapy. If negative for infectious cause, use only symptomatic treatment. (d) If no systemic findings, then use symptomatic therapy based on severity of volume depletion, oral or parenteral fluid/electrolytes, antidiarrheal agents (see Table 54-4), and diet. (RBC, red blood cells; WBC, white blood cells.)

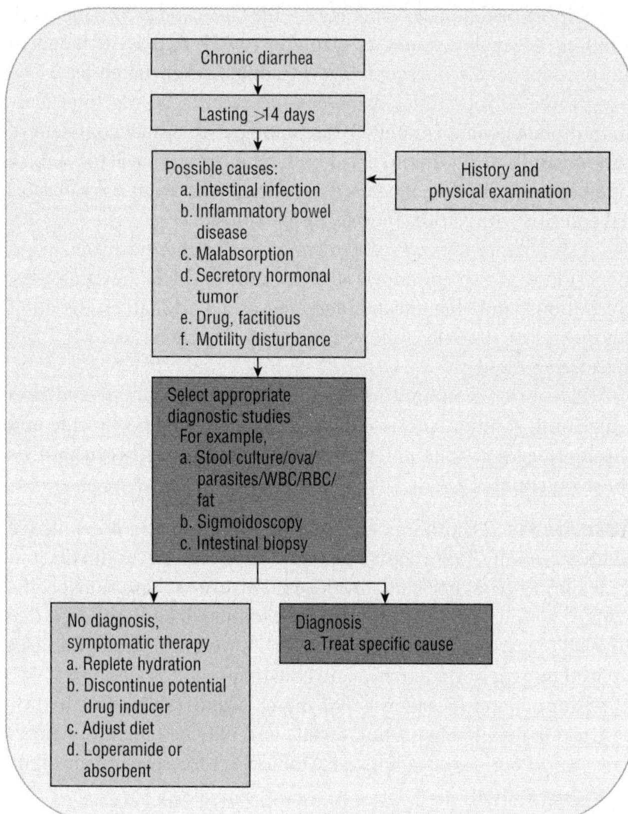

FIGURE 54-2 Recommendations for treating chronic diarrhea. Follow the following steps: (a) Perform a careful history and physical examination. (b) The possible causes of chronic diarrhea are many. These can be classified into intestinal infections (bacterial or protozoal), inflammatory disease (Crohn's disease or ulcerative colitis), malabsorption (lactose intolerance), secretory hormonal tumor (intestinal carcinoid tumor or vasoactive intestinal peptide-secreting tumor [VIPoma]), drug (antacid), factitious (laxative abuse), or motility disturbance (diabetes mellitus, irritable bowel syndrome, or hyperthyroidism). (c) If the diagnosis is uncertain, selected appropriate diagnostic studies should be ordered. (d) Once diagnosed, treatment is planned for the underlying cause with symptomatic antidiarrheal therapy. (e) If no specific cause can be identified, symptomatic therapy is prescribed. (RBC, red blood cells; WBC, white blood cells.)

not develop volume depletion and therefore will only require maintenance fluid and electrolyte therapy. Parenteral and enteral routes may be used for supplying water and electrolytes. If vomiting and dehydration are not severe, the enteral route is the less costly and preferred. In the United States, many commercial oral rehydration preparations are available (Table 54-3).

Because of concerns about hypernatremia, physicians continue to hospitalize patients and use IV fluids to correct fluid and electrolyte deficits in severe dehydration. Oral solutions are strongly recommended when tolerated to limit side effects, reduce costs, and improve recovery.[7] In developing countries, the WHO oral rehydration solution (WHO-ORS) saves the lives of millions of children annually.

During diarrhea, the small intestine retains its ability to actively transport monosaccharides such as glucose. Glucose actively carries sodium with water and other electrolytes. The WHO recommends an ORS with a lower osmolarity, sodium content, and glucose load (see Table 54-3).[8] A separate oral supplement of zinc 20 mg daily for 10 days in addition to ORS significantly reduces the severity and duration of acute diarrhea in developing countries.[2] ORS is a lifesaving treatment for millions afflicted in developing countries. Acceptance in developed countries is less enthusiastic; however, the advantage of this product in reducing hospitalizations may prove its use as a cost-effective alternative, saving millions of dollars in healthcare expenditures.

Pharmacologic Therapy

Various drugs have been used to treat diarrheal attacks (Table 54-4), including antimotility agents, adsorbents, antisecretory compounds, antibiotics, enzymes, and intestinal microflora. Usually these drugs are not curative but palliative.

Opiates and Their Derivatives

Opiates and opioid derivatives (a) delay the transit of intraluminal contents or (b) increase gut capacity, prolonging contact and absorption. Enkephalins, which are endogenous opioid substances, regulate fluid movement across the mucosa by stimulating absorptive processes. Limitations to the use of opiates include an addiction potential (a real concern with long-term use) and potential for worsening of diarrhea in selected infectious diarrhea.

Most opiates act through peripheral and central mechanisms with the exception of loperamide, which acts only peripherally. Loperamide is antisecretory; it inhibits the calcium-binding protein calmodulin, controlling chloride secretion. Loperamide, available

TABLE 54-3 Oral Rehydration Solutions

	WHO-ORS[a]	Pedialyte[b] (Ross)	CeraLyte (Cera Products)	Enfalyte (Mead Johnson)
Osmolality (mOsm/kg or mmol/kg)	245	250	220	167
Carbohydrates[b] (g/L)	13.5	25	40[c]	30[c]
Calories (cal/L [J/L])	65 (272)	100 (418)	160 (670)	126 (527)
Electrolytes (mEq/L; mmol/L)				
Sodium	75	45	50-90	50
Potassium	20	20	20	25
Chloride	65	35	40-80	45
Citrate	—	30	30	34
Bicarbonate	30	—	—	—
Calcium	—	—	—	—
Magnesium	—	—	—	—
Sulfate	—	—	—	—
Phosphate	—	—	—	—

[a]The World Health Organization (WHO) reduced osmolarity oral rehydration solution.

[b]Carbohydrate is glucose.

[c]Rice syrup solids are carbohydrate source.

TABLE 54-4 Selected Antidiarrheal Preparations

	Dose Form	Adult Dose
Antimotility		
Diphenoxylate	2.5 mg/tablet 2.5 mg/5 mL	5 mg four times daily; do not exceed 20 mg/day
Loperamide	2 mg/capsule	Initially 4 mg, and then 2 mg after each loose stool; do not exceed 16 mg/day
Paregoric	2 mg/5 mL (morphine)	5-10 mL one to four times daily
Opium tincture	10 mg/mL (morphine)	0.6 mL four times daily
Difenoxin	1 mg/tablet	Two tablets, and then one tablet after each loose stool; up to eight tablets per day
Adsorbents		
Kaolin-pectin mixture	5.7 g kaolin + 130.2 mg pectin/30 mL	30-120 mL after each loose stool
Polycarbophil	500 mg/tablet	Chew 2 tablets four times daily or after each loose stool; do not exceed 12 tablets per day
Attapulgite	750 mg/15 mL 300 mg/7.5 mL 750 mg/tablet 600 mg/tablet 300 mg/tablet	1,200-1,500 mg after each loose bowel movement or every 2 hours; up to 9,000 mg/day
Antisecretory		
Bismuth subsalicylate	1,050 mg/30 mL 262 mg/15 mL 524 mg/15 mL 262 mg/tablet	Two tablets or 30 mL every 30 minutes to 1 hour as needed up to eight doses per day
Enzymes		
Lactase	1,250 neutral lactase units/4 drops 3,300 FCC lactase units per tablet	Three to four drops taken with milk or dairy product
Bacterial replacement (*Lactobacillus acidophilus, Lactobacillus bulgaricus*)		Two tablets or one granule packet three to four times daily; give with milk, juice, or water
Octreotide	0.05 mg/mL 0.1 mg/mL 0.5 mg/mL	Initial: 50 mcg subcutaneously One to two times per day and titrate dose based on indication up to 600 mcg/day in two to four divided doses

as 2 mg capsules or 1 mg/5 mL solution (both are nonprescription products), is suggested for managing acute and chronic diarrhea. The usual adult dose for acute diarrhea is initially 4 mg orally, followed by 2 mg after each loose stool, up to 16 mg/day. Used correctly, this agent has rare side effects, such as dizziness and constipation. If the diarrhea is concurrent with a high fever or bloody stool, the patient should be referred to a physician. Also, diarrhea lasting 48 hours beyond initiating loperamide warrants medical attention. Loperamide can also be used in traveler's diarrhea. It is comparable to bismuth subsalicylate for treatment of this disorder.[5] The Food and Drug Administration (FDA) has released a warning about using high doses of loperamide for euphoria as it can lead to serious side effects including cardiovascular problems.[9] The packaging of loperamide has been reduced to minimize abuse.[10]

Diphenoxylate is available as a 2.5-mg tablet and as a 2.5 mg/5 mL solution. A small amount of atropine (0.025 mg) is included in the product to discourage abuse. In adults, when taken as 2.5 to 5 mg three or four times daily, not to exceed a 20 mg total daily dose, diphenoxylate is rarely toxic. Some patients may complain of atropinism (blurred vision, dry mouth, and urinary hesitancy). Like loperamide, it should not be used in patients who are at risk of bacterial enteritis with *E. coli*, *Shigella*, or *Salmonella*.

Difenoxin, a diphenoxylate derivative also chemically related to meperidine, is also combined with atropine and has the same uses, precautions, and side effects. Marketed as a 1-mg tablet, the adult dosage is 2 mg initially, followed by 1 mg after each loose stool, not to exceed 8 mg/day.

Paregoric, camphorated tincture of opium, is marketed as a 2 mg/5 mL solution and is indicated for managing both acute and chronic diarrhea. It is not widely prescribed today because of its abuse potential.

Adsorbents Adsorbents are used for symptomatic relief. These products, many not requiring a prescription, are nontoxic, but their effectiveness remains unproven. Adsorbents are nonspecific in their action; they adsorb nutrients, toxins, drugs, and digestive juices. Polycarbophil absorbs 60 times its weight in water and can be used to treat both diarrhea and constipation. It is a nonprescription product and is sold as a 500-mg chewable tablet. This hydrophilic, nonabsorbable product is safe and may be taken four times daily, up to 6 g/day in adults. See Table 54-4 for selected antidiarrheal preparations.

Antisecretory Agents Bismuth subsalicylate have antisecretory, anti-inflammatory, and antibacterial effects. As a nonprescription product, it is marketed for indigestion, relieving abdominal cramps, and controlling diarrhea, including traveler's diarrhea. Bismuth subsalicylate dosage strengths are a 262-mg chewable tablet, 262-mg/5 mL liquid, and 524-mg/15 mL liquid. The usual adult dose is two tablets or 30 mL every 30 minutes to 1 hour up to eight doses per day.

(4) Bismuth subsalicylate contains multiple components that might be toxic if given in excess to prevent or treat diarrhea. For instance, an active ingredient is salicylate, which may interact with anticoagulants or may produce salicylism (tinnitus, nausea, and vomiting). Bismuth reduces tetracycline absorption and may interfere with select GI radiographic studies. Patients may complain of a darkening of the tongue and stools with repeat administration. Salicylate can induce gout attacks in susceptible individuals.

Bismuth subsalicylate suspension is useful in the treatment of secretory diarrhea of infectious etiology as well. With a dose of 30 mL every 30 minutes for eight doses, unformed stools decrease in the first 24 hours. Bismuth subsalicylate may also be effective in preventing traveler's diarrhea.

Octreotide, a synthetic octapeptide analog of endogenous somatostatin, is effective for the symptomatic treatment of carcinoid tumors and other peptide-secreting tumors, dumping syndrome, and chemotherapy-induced diarrhea.[11] It has had limited success in patients with AIDS-associated diarrhea and short-bowel syndrome, does not appear to have an advantage over various opiate derivatives in the treatment of chronic idiopathic diarrhea, and has the disadvantage of being administered by injection.[4] Metastatic intestinal carcinoid tumors secrete excessive amounts of vasoactive substances, including histamine, bradykinin, serotonin (5-hydroxytryptamine, 5-HT), and prostaglandins. Primary carcinoid tumors occur throughout the GI tract, with most in the ileum. Predominant signs and symptoms experienced by patients with these tumors are attributable to excessive concentrations of 5-hydroxytryptophan and 5-HT. The totality of their clinical effects is termed the carcinoid syndrome. Some patients have a violent, watery diarrhea with abdominal cramping. Initially, diarrhea might be managed with various agents such as codeine, diphenoxylate, cyproheptadine, methysergide, phenoxybenzamine, or methyldopa, but octreotide is now considered first-line therapy for carcinoid syndrome.

Octreotide blocks the release of 5-HT and many other active peptides and has been effective in controlling diarrhea and flushing. It is reported to have direct inhibitory effects on intestinal secretion and stimulatory effects on intestinal absorption. Non-gastrin-secreting adenomas of the pancreas are tumors associated with profuse watery diarrhea. This condition has been referred to as Verner–Morrison syndrome, watery diarrhea, hypokalemia, and achlorhydria (WDHA) syndrome, pancreatic cholera, watery diarrhea syndrome, and vasoactive intestinal peptide-secreting tumor (VIPoma). Excessive secretion of VIP from a retroperitoneal or pancreatic tumor produces most of the clinical features. Surgical tumor dissection is the treatment of choice. In nonsurgical candidates, the profuse watery diarrhea and other symptoms commonly encountered are managed with octreotide.

The dose of octreotide varies with the indication, disease severity, and patient response.[11] For managing diarrhea and flushing associated with carcinoid tumors in adults, the initial dosage range is 100 to 600 mcg/day in two to four divided doses subcutaneously for 2 weeks. For controlling secretory diarrhea of VIPomas, the dosage range is 200 to 300 mcg/day in two to four divided doses for 2 weeks. Some patients may require higher doses for symptomatic control. Patients responding to these initial doses may be switched to Sandostatin LAR Depot, a long-acting octreotide formulation. Initial doses consist of 20 mg given intramuscularly intragluteally at 4-week intervals for 2 months. During the first 2 weeks of therapy the short-acting formulation should be administered subcutaneously. At the end of 2 months, patients with good symptom control may have the dose reduced to 10 mg every 4 weeks, while those without sufficient symptom control may have the dose increased to 30 mg every 4 weeks. For patients experiencing recurrence of symptoms on the 10 mg dose, dosage adjustment to 20 mg should be made. Patients with carcinoid tumors or VIPomas may experience periodic exacerbation of symptoms. Subcutaneous octreotide for several days should be reinstituted in these individuals. In so-called carcinoid crisis, octreotide is given as an IV infusion at 50 mcg/hr for 8 to 24 hours.

Because octreotide inhibits many other GI hormones, it has a variety of intestinal side effects. With prolonged use, gallbladder and biliary tract complications such as cholelithiasis may occur. Approximately 5% to 10% of patients complain of nausea, diarrhea, and abdominal pain. Local injection pain occurs with about an 8% incidence. With high doses, octreotide may reduce dietary fat absorption, leading to steatorrhea.

Two other somatostatin analogs, lanreotide and vapreotide, have been studied.[4] Lanreotide is approved for use in the United States for acromegaly. The starting dose is 90 mg subcutaneously every 4 weeks for 3 months, and then the dose is adjusted based on growth hormone and insulin-like growth factor levels.[12] Vapreotide is an orphan drug that is indicated for pancreatic and GI fistulas as well as esophageal variceal bleeding.

Miscellaneous Products Probiotics are microorganisms given to reestablish normal colonic microflora. This supposedly restores normal intestinal function and suppresses the growth of pathogenic microorganisms. There is conflicting evidence on whether *Saccharomyces boulardii*, *Lactobacillus* GG, and *Lactobacillus acidophilus* decrease the duration of infectious and antibiotic-induced diarrhea in adults and children.[13] Probiotics may prevent antibiotic-associated diarrhea (AAD).[14] However, a randomized control trial in hospitalized patients over the age of 65 years found no difference in cases of AAD between a probiotic preparation (two strains of lactobacillus acidophilus and Bifidobacterium) and placebo.[15] The dosage of probiotic preparations varies depending on the brand used. Intestinal flatus is the primary patient complaint experienced with this modality.

Anticholinergic drugs such as atropine block vagal tone and prolong gut transit time. Drugs with anticholinergic properties are present in many nonprescription products. Their value in controlling diarrhea is questionable and limited because of side effects. Angle-closure glaucoma, selected heart diseases, and obstructive uropathies are relative contraindications to the use of anticholinergic agents.

Lactase enzyme products are helpful for patients who are experiencing diarrhea secondary to lactose intolerance. Lactase is required for carbohydrate digestion. When a patient lacks this enzyme, eating dairy products causes an osmotic diarrhea. Several products are available for use each time a dairy product, especially milk or ice cream, is consumed.

Vaccines Vaccines are a new therapeutic frontier in controlling infectious diarrheas, especially in developing countries.[16] An oral vaccine for cholera (Vaxchora®) is licensed for use in the United States. The Advisory Committee for Immunization Practices (ACIP) recommends the vaccine for adults aged 18 to 64 years old who are traveling to an endemic area.[17] Studies in the United States suggest the vaccine can reduce the risk of severe diarrhea by about 90%, but data in endemic areas is lacking.[18]

Oral *Shigella* vaccine, although effective under field conditions, requires five weekly oral doses and repeat booster doses, thereby limiting its practicality for use in developing nations. With about 1,500 serotypes for *Salmonella*, a vaccine is not available for humans. There are two newer typhoid vaccine formulations, one a parenteral inactivated whole-cell vaccine and the other an oral live-attenuated (Ty21a) vaccine that is administered in four doses on days 1, 3, 5, and 7, to be completed at least 1 week before exposure. Two rotavirus vaccines prevent gastroenteritis due to rotavirus infection in infants and children in the United States.[19] The pentavalent human-bovine reassortant vaccine (RotaTeq from Merck) is administered as a three-oral-dose sequence, and the monovalent human vaccine (Rotarix from GlaxoSmithKline) is administered as a two-oral-dose sequence. Two additional vaccines were prequalified by the WHO in 2018 and are being utilized in India (Rotavac from Bharat Biotech and ROTASIL from Serum Institute of India Pvt. Ltd.).[20]

Evaluation of Therapeutic Outcomes

Therapeutic outcomes are directed toward key symptoms, signs, and laboratory studies. Constitutional symptoms usually improve within 24 to 72 hours. Monitoring for changes in the frequency and character of bowel movements on a daily basis in conjunction with vital signs and improvement in appetite are of utmost importance. Also, the clinician needs to monitor body weight, serum osmolality, serum electrolytes, complete blood cell counts, urinalysis, and culture results (if appropriate).

Acute Diarrhea

Most patients with acute diarrhea experience mild-to-moderate distress. In the absence of moderate-to-severe dehydration, high fever, and blood or mucus in the stool, this illness is usually self-limiting within 3 to 7 days. Mild-to-moderate acute diarrhea is usually managed on an outpatient basis with oral rehydration, symptomatic treatment, and diet. Older patients with chronic illness as well as infants may require hospitalization for parenteral rehydration and close monitoring.

Severe Diarrhea

In the urgent/emergent situation, restoration of the patient's volume status is the most important outcome. Toxic patients (fever dehydration, hematochezia, or hypotension) require hospitalization, IV fluids and electrolyte administration, and empiric antibiotic therapy while awaiting culture and sensitivity results. With timely management, these patients usually recover within a few days.

CONSTIPATION

5 Constipation is a common complaint among the general population and accounts for many medical visits each year in the United States.[21] It is generally defined by the American Gastroenterology Association (AGA) as difficult or infrequent passage of stool, at times associated with straining or a feeling of incomplete defecation.[22]

Constipation may be further defined by quantitative or qualitative measures. For instance, physicians often use stool frequency to define constipation (most commonly fewer than three bowel movements per week); however, the "normal" frequency of bowel movement is not well established and can vary from person to person. Patients more often describe constipation in terms of symptoms or a combination of quantitative and qualitative descriptors that are difficult to quantify: bowel movement frequency, stool size or consistency (hard or lumpy stools), straining on defecation, inability to defecate at will, and symptoms such as sensation of incomplete evacuation. The condition is considered chronic if symptoms last for at least 3 months. Many people believe that daily bowel movements are required for normal health or that accumulation of toxic substances will occur with infrequent defecation. Inappropriate laxative use by the general public may result from these misconceptions.

Though often considered more of a minor uncomfortable or unpleasant problem, constipation can have serious consequences and be costly to the healthcare system. Patients with constipation spend approximately $8,700 more in overall medical costs compared to patients without constipation.[21]

Epidemiology

The prevalence of constipation depends on the definition used and whether the condition is self-reported or provider-diagnosed. The prevalence of chronic constipation in adults (older than or equal to 15 years old) worldwide is estimated to be 15%.[23]

Constipation is more common in women (2.4-fold more likely) and older patients.[23] Other factors associated with constipation in some reports include inactivity, resource limited populations, lower income, non-White race, symptoms of depression, and history of physical or sexual abuse.

Pathophysiology

Constipation may be primary or secondary. Primary, or idiopathic, constipation occurs without an identifiable underlying cause, whereas secondary constipation may be the result of constipating drugs, lifestyle factors, or medical disorders (Table 54-5).[23] Primary constipation can be further divided into three categories—normal transit, slow transit, and pelvic floor dysfunction, or disordered defecation.[23,24] Normal transit constipation, often referred to as functional, is the most common type. These patients have normal GI motility and stool frequency but may experience difficulty evacuating, passage of hard stools, or bloating and abdominal discomfort. Slow transit constipation represents an abnormality of GI transit time that leads to infrequent defecation. Dysfunction of the pelvic floor muscles and/or anal sphincter is the most frequently encountered reason for disordered defecation. In patients with defecatory disorders, these muscles or sphincter contract during defecation instead of relax and impede evacuation of stool. It is common for patients to have and present with more than one type of constipation.

Factors associated with the increased prevalence of constipation in older patients include a higher number of daily medications, particularly anticholinergic agents, increased incidence of chronic comorbidities, and changes in mobility status.[25] Changes in diet such as decreased fluid and/or fiber intake, diminished physical activity, and institutionalization can lead to constipation. Physiologic changes such as mesenteric dysfunction and changes in anorectal function, including loss of rectal wall elasticity, are also thought to predispose older patients to constipation.

TABLE 54-5 Possible Causes of Constipation

Conditions	Possible Causes
GI disorders	Irritable bowel syndrome
	Diverticulitis
	Upper GI tract diseases
	Anal and rectal diseases
	Hemorrhoids
	Anal fissures
	Ulcerative proctitis
	Tumors
	Hernia
	Volvulus of the bowel
	Syphilis
	Tuberculosis
	Helminthic infections
	Lymphogranuloma venereum
	Hirschsprung's disease
Metabolic and endocrine disorders	Diabetes mellitus with neuropathy
	Hypothyroidism
	Panhypopituitarism
	Pheochromocytoma
	Hypercalcemia
	Enteric glucagon excess
Cardiac disorders	Heart failure
Pregnancy	Depressed gut motility
	Increased fluid absorption from colon
	Use of iron salts
Lifestyle factors	Dietary changes
	Inadequate fluid intake
	Low dietary fiber
	Decreased physical activity
Neurogenic causes	CNS diseases
	Trauma to the brain (particularly the medulla)
	Spinal cord injury
	CNS tumors
	Cerebrovascular accidents
	Parkinson's disease
Psychogenic causes	Ignoring or postponing urge to defecate
	Psychiatric diseases
Drug induced	See Table 54-6

Drug-Induced Constipation

Use of drugs that inhibit the neurologic or muscular function of the GI tract, particularly the colon, may result in secondary constipation.[23] Medications that are commonly associated with causing constipation include opiates, anticholinergic agents, and certain antacids.[23] With most of the agents listed in Table 54-6, the inhibitory effects on bowel function may be dose dependent, with larger doses causing constipation more frequently.

Opiates have effects on all segments of the bowel, but effects are most pronounced on the colon. The major mechanism by which opiates produce constipation has been proposed to be prolongation of intestinal transit time by causing spastic, nonpropulsive contractions. Additionally, anal sphincter tone may be increased with an accompanying decrease in reflex relaxation leading to difficult rectal evacuation.[26]

TABLE 54-6 Drugs Causing Constipation

Analgesics
Inhibitors of prostaglandin synthesis
Opiates
Nonsteroidal anti-inflammatory agents
Anticholinergics
Antihistamines
Antiparkinsonian agents (eg, benztropine or trihexyphenidyl)
Phenothiazines
Tricyclic antidepressants
Antacids containing calcium carbonate or aluminum hydroxide
Barium sulfate
Calcium channel antagonists
Clonidine
Diuretics (non–potassium-sparing)
Ganglionic blockers
Iron preparations
Muscle blockers (d-tubocurarine, succinylcholine)
Polystyrene sodium sulfonate

While all opiate derivatives are associated with constipation, the degree of intestinal inhibitory effects seems to differ between agents. Orally administered opiates appear to have greater inhibitory effects than parenterally administered products.

Other medications may increase the risk of constipation by a variety of mechanisms. Anticholinergic agents decrease contractility of intestinal muscle while calcium channel blockers are thought to cause rectosigmoid dysfunction, leading to constipation. Nonsteroidal anti-inflammatory drugs (NSAIDs) may lead to constipation due to their inhibition of prostaglandin synthesis.[29]

Clinical Presentation

A symptom-based system for classifying functional constipation (and other functional GI disorders) is often used to define constipation in clinical trials. The Rome criteria encompass both quantitative (frequency) and qualitative (stool consistency, etc.) symptoms associated with constipation.[27] Table 54-7 outlines general clinical presentation of patients with constipation. According to the Rome IV criteria, patients should have at least two of the signs and symptoms listed in Table 54-7 apply to a minimum of 25% of bowel movements.

Evaluation of constipation should attempt to clarify the patient's specific symptoms (ie, exactly what the patient means by constipation).[23] A complete and thorough history should be obtained from the patient, including frequency of bowel movements and duration of symptoms. Constipation occurring abruptly in an adult may indicate significant colon pathology such as malignancy. Constipation present since early infancy may be indicative of neurologic disorders. The patient should also be carefully questioned about usual diet and laxative regimens. Does the patient have a diet consistently deficient in high-fiber items and containing mainly high refined foods? What laxatives or cathartics has the patient used to attempt relief of constipation? The patient should be questioned about other concurrent medications, with interest focused on agents that might cause constipation.

Evaluation should also include perianal and anal examinations to identify fecal impaction or other anatomical obstructions that may be contributing to or causing constipation. General health status, signs of underlying medical illness (ie, hypothyroidism), and psychological status (eg, depression or other psychological illness) should also be assessed. Laboratory tests may be performed, particularly if the patient is presumed to suffer from secondary causes and is still experiencing symptoms after a trial of fiber supplementation or other nonprescription therapies.[23]

TABLE 54-7 Clinical Presentation of Constipation

Signs and symptoms
- Infrequent bowel movements (<3 per week)
- Stools that are hard, small, or dry
- Straining
- Feeling of incomplete evacuation
  - Feeling of anorectal obstruction or blockage
  - Physical tactics needed for defecation
  - Loose stools rarely occur without laxative use

Alarm signs and symptoms
- Hematochezia
- Melena
- Family history of colon cancer
- Family history of inflammatory bowel disease
- Anemia
- Unintentional weight loss >10% body weight
- Anorexia
- Nausea and vomiting
- Severe, persistent constipation that is refractory to treatment
- New-onset or worsening constipation in elderly without evidence of primary cause

Physical examination
- Perform rectal exam for presence of anatomical abnormalities (such as fistulas, fissures, hemorrhoids, rectal prolapse) or abnormalities of perianal descent
- Digital examination of rectum to check for fecal impaction, anal stricture, or rectal mass

Laboratory and other diagnostic tests
- No routine recommendations for lab testing—as indicated by clinical discretion
- In patients with signs and symptoms suggestive of organic disorder, specific testing may be performed (ie, thyroid function tests, electrolytes, glucose, complete blood count) based on clinical presentation
- In patients with alarm signs and symptoms or when structural disease is a possibility, select appropriate diagnostic studies:
  1. Rectal Balloon Expulsion Test (BET)
  2. Anorectal manometry
  3. Colonoscopy
  4. Barium defecography

Specific attention should be given to identify any "alarm symptoms" that would warrant further diagnostic workup (see Table 54-7).[23] Patients with alarm symptoms, a family history of colon cancer, or those more than 50 years old with new symptoms may need further diagnostic evaluation.

TREATMENT

Desired Outcome

The major goals of treatment are to (a) relieve symptoms, (b) reestablish normal bowel habits, and (c) improve quality of life by minimizing adverse effects of treatment.

General Approach to Treatment

Figure 54-3 presents a general treatment algorithm for the management of constipation.

6 Approaches to the treatment of constipation should begin with attempts to determine its cause. If an underlying disease is recognized as the cause of constipation, attempts should be made to correct it. Malignancies may be removed via surgical resection. Endocrine and metabolic derangements should be corrected by the appropriate methods. For example, when hypothyroidism is the cause of constipation, cautious institution of thyroid replacement therapy is the most important treatment measure. If a patient is consuming medications known to cause constipation, consideration should be given to alternative agents. If a patient must remain

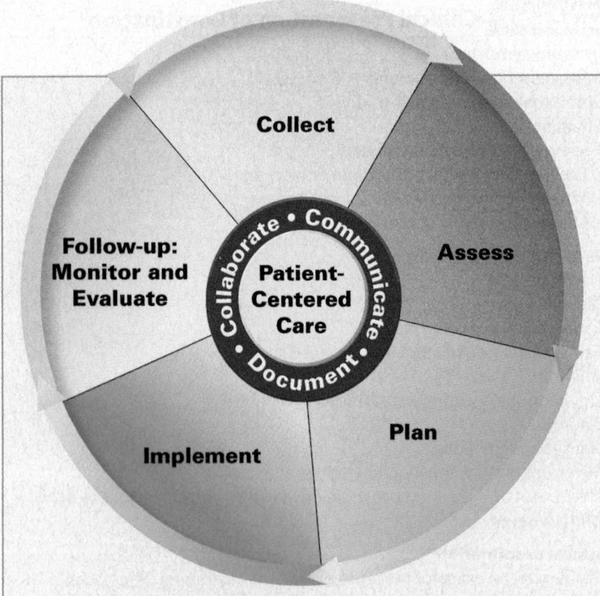

Patient Care Process for Constipation

The image shows the five fundamental steps included in The Pharmacist's Care Process endorsed by the Joint Commission for Pharmacy Practitioners (2014). The tagline of this process reads collaborate, communicate, and document. The five fundamental steps listed here are collect, assess, plan, implement, and follow-up: monitor and evaluate. All these steps are listed in a circular block diagram.

Collect

- Patient characteristics
- Patient medical, social, and family history including dietary habits
- Current medications, including nonprescription
- Vital signs and weight
- Laboratory tests depending upon medical history and other presenting symptoms
    - Thyroid function tests, complete blood count, glucose, serum electrolytes

Assess

- Underlying causes of constipation (see Tables 54-5 and 54-6)
- Presence of alarm symptoms (Table 54-7)
- Severity of symptoms
- Patient preference for symptom resolution
- Ability/willingness to pay for treatment options

Plan*

- Treat specific cause of constipation (ie, thyroid dysfunction)
- Dietary modification to increase fiber (Fig. 54-3)
- Laxative or cathartic option if quick resolution desired and no contraindications (Fig. 54-3; Table 54-8)
- Other pharmacologic therapy (Fig. 54-3; Table 54-8)
- Monitor symptom resolution for efficacy, and pronounced diarrhea for safety
- Patient education regarding lifestyle and dietary modifications, drug-specific information, etc.
- Referral to other providers when appropriate (unresolved symptoms or alarm symptoms present)

Implement

- Educate the patient on all aspects of the treatment plan
- Schedule follow-up to monitor safety and efficacy of treatment plan

Follow-up: Monitor and Evaluate

- Determine resolution of constipation and related symptoms
- Assess for presence of adverse effects (eg, abdominal pain, diarrhea)
- Assess patient adherence to treatment plan
- Reevaluate periodically until resolution

Collaborate with patient, caregivers, and other healthcare professionals.

on constipating medications, then more attention must be given to general measures for prevention of constipation, as discussed in the next section. Also, patients with opioid-induced constipation (OIC) may require the routine use of pharmacologic agents, also discussed below.

The proper management of constipation will require a combination of nonpharmacologic and pharmacologic therapies. Osmotic laxative therapy is considered the preferred first line for the treatment of constipation, in addition to increasing dietary fiber or using fiber supplementation.[27,28] Patients are often encouraged to increase daily fluid intake and physical activity as well dedicate time to respond to the urge to defecate, although efficacy data are conflicting for these measures.[23]

Nonpharmacologic Therapy

Dietary Modification The most important aspect of therapy for constipation for the majority of patients is dietary modification to increase the amount of fiber consumed. Fiber, the portion of vegetable matter not digested in the human GI tract, increases stool bulk, retention of stool water, and rate of transit of stool through the intestine. The result of fiber therapy is an increased frequency of defecation. Also, fiber decreases intraluminal pressures in the colon and rectum, which is thought to be beneficial for diverticular disease and for irritable bowel syndrome (IBS).

7 The specific physiologic effects of fiber are not well understood. Patients should be advised to gradually increase daily fiber intake to 20 to 30 g, through either dietary changes or fiber supplement products (see section "Bulk-Forming Agents" below), a strong recommendation from the American College of Gastroenterology.[30] Fruits, vegetables, and cereals typically have the highest fiber content. Bran, a by-product of milling of wheat, is often added to foods to increase fiber content and contains a high amount of soluble fiber, which may be extremely constipating in larger doses. Raw bran is generally 40% fiber.

A trial of dietary modification with high-fiber content should be continued for at least 1 month before effects on bowel function

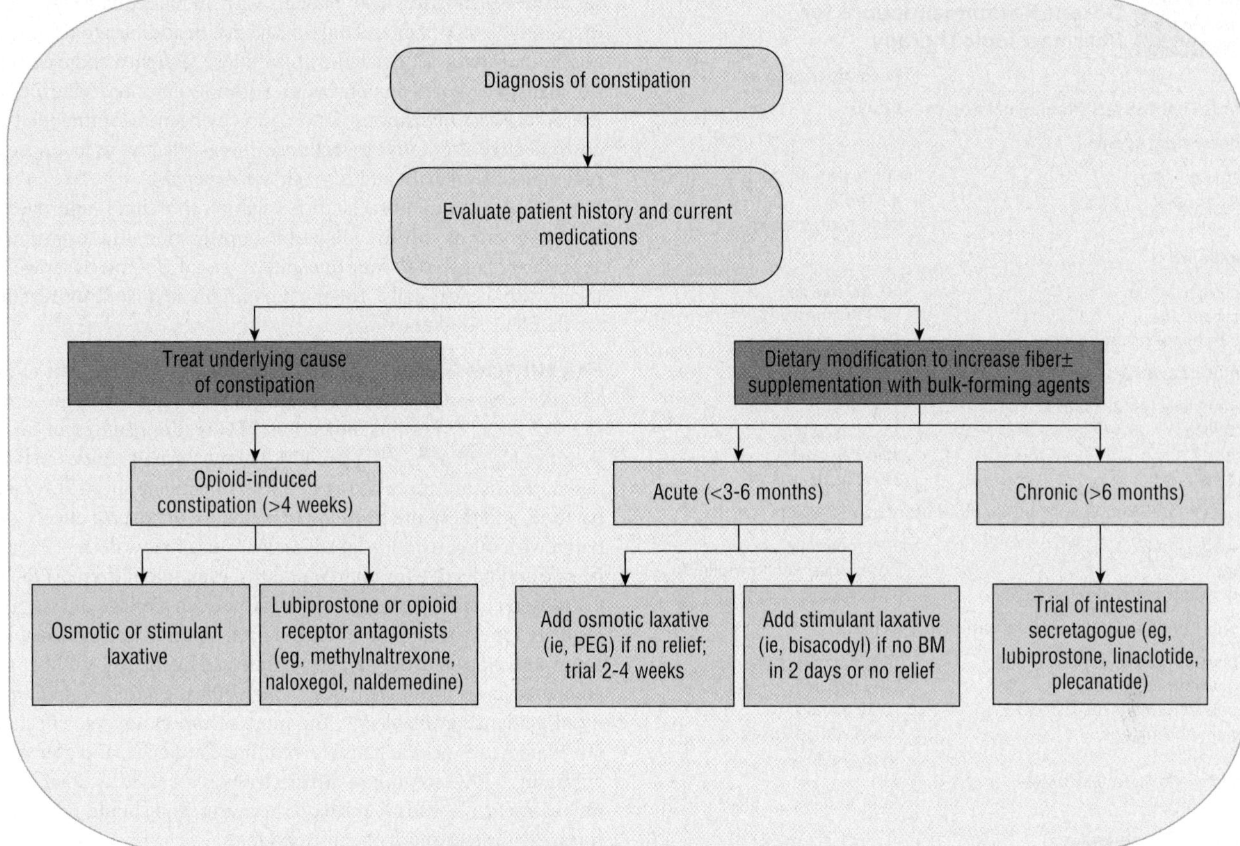

FIGURE 54-3 A general treatment algorithm for constipation.

are determined. Most patients begin to notice effects on bowel function 3 to 5 days after beginning a high-fiber diet, but some patients may require a considerably longer period of time. Patients should be cautioned that abdominal distension and flatulence may be particularly troublesome in the first few weeks of fiber therapy, especially with high bran consumption. Gradually increasing dietary fiber over a few weeks to the goal of 20 to 30 g may help reduce some of the adverse abdominal effects, as well as ensuring adequate fluid intake. In most cases these problems resolve with continued use.

Surgery In a small percentage of patients who present with complaints of constipation, surgical procedures are necessary because of the presence of colonic malignancies or GI obstruction from a number of other causes. Patients who have slow-transit-type primary constipation that is refractory to treatment are also surgical candidates.[23,28] Surgery may be required in some endocrine disorders that cause constipation, such as pheochromocytoma, which requires removal of a tumor. In each case, the involved segment of intestine may be resected or revised.

Biofeedback Patients with constipation due to pelvic floor dysfunction/disordered defecation may have a less favorable response to fiber therapy than other constipation subtypes.[30] Many adult patients with functional defecatory disorders appear to benefit from pelvic floor retraining with biofeedback therapy. The goals of biofeedback are to improve pelvic floor relaxation to facilitate the passage of stool and the procedure is typically performed over 4- to 6-hour-long sessions. Success rates of 65% to 80% have been reported in controlled and uncontrolled studies, and improvement has been sustained for up to 1 year. The value of biofeedback in children with chronic constipation has not been well demonstrated.

Electrical Stimulation Sacral nerve stimulation is a minimally invasive technique that has been used for treatment of fecal incontinence and there are some reports of its use in severe refractory chronic constipation.[31] However, clinical data supporting the use of electrical stimulation for this purpose are limited and there are no recommendations for general practice.

Pharmacologic Therapy

Three general classes of laxatives are discussed in this section: (a) those causing softening of feces in 1 to 3 days; (b) those that result in soft or semifluid stool in 6 to 12 hours; and (c) those causing watery evacuation in 1 to 6 hours (Table 54-8). Other pharmacologic agents available for the treatment of constipation include a calcium channel activator, guanylate cyclase C agonist, and serotonergic agents.

Bulk-Forming Agents Medicinal products, often called "bulk-forming agents," such as psyllium hydrophilic colloids, methylcellulose, or polycarbophil, have properties similar to those of dietary fiber and may be taken as tablets, powders, or granules.[25] These agents increase the water content of stool to increase stool bulk and weight and relieve the symptoms of constipation within 3 days of initiating therapy.

Bulk-forming laxatives have few adverse effects. The most common effects include flatulence, abdominal bloating, and distention. Rarely, these agents may lead to bowel obstruction. Patients should also be cautioned to consume sufficient fluid while supplementing with bulk-forming agents to avoid obstruction of the esophagus, stomach, small intestine, and colon.

Emollient Laxatives Emollient laxatives, including docusate in its various salts, are surfactant agents that work by facilitating mixing

TABLE 54-8 Dosage Recommendations for Pharmacologic Therapy

Agent	Recommended Dose
Agents That Cause Softening of Feces in 1-3 Days	
Bulk-forming agents	
Methylcellulose	Varies with product
Polycarbophil	4-6 g/day
Psyllium	Varies with product
Emollients	
Docusate sodium	50-360 mg/day
Docusate calcium	50-360 mg/day
Docusate potassium	100-300 mg/day
Osmotic Laxatives	
Polyethylene glycol 3350	17 g/dose
Lactulose	15-30 mL orally
Lacitol	20 g/day orally
Sorbitol	30-50 g/day orally
Agents That Result in Soft or Semifluid Stool in 6-12 Hours	
Bisacodyl (oral)	5-15 mg orally
Senna	Dose varies with formulation
Magnesium sulfate (low dose)	<10 g orally
Agents That Cause Watery Evacuation in 1-6 Hours	
Magnesium citrate	18 g 300 mL water
Magnesium hydroxide	2.4-4.8 g orally
Magnesium sulfate (high dose)	10-30 g orally
Sodium phosphates	Varies with salt used
Bisacodyl	10 mg rectally
Polyethylene glycol-electrolyte preparations	4 L
Intestinal Secretagogues	
Lubiprostone	24 mcg orally twice daily
Linaclotide	145 mcg orally daily
Plecanatide	3 mg orally daily
Opioid Antagonists	
Methylnaltrexone	450 mg orally daily or 12 mg subcutaneously daily
Naloxegol	25 mg daily
Naldemedine	0.2 mg daily
Prokinetics	
Prucalopride	2 mg daily

of aqueous and fatty materials within the intestinal tract; these are commonly referred to as stool softeners.[23,25,32] Increased stool moisture content should lead to a softer, easier-to-pass stool. These products are generally given orally, although docusate potassium has also been used rectally. With these products, softening of stools occurs within 1 to 3 days of therapy. Docusate has little evidence to support efficacy in treating constipation.[23] Although docusates are generally safe, a few adverse drug reactions have been noted.

Hyperosmolar Agents

Nonabsorbable Carbohydrates Lactulose is a nonabsorbable disaccharide that is metabolized by colonic bacteria to low-molecular-weight acids, resulting in an osmotic effect whereby fluid is retained in the colon.[33] The fluid retained in the colon lowers the pH and increases colonic peristalsis within 2 to 3 days of use. Lactulose increases stool frequency and consistency in patients with chronic constipation (vs placebo) and may be more effective than fiber alone. In comparison to polyethylene glycol (PEG), lactulose is slightly less effective in increasing stool frequency per week and patients are more likely to need additional products for constipation relief. The most common adverse effects include flatulence, nausea, and abdominal discomfort or bloating—although lactulose can be useful in some patients. It may be justified as an alternative for acute constipation or in patients with an inadequate response to increased dietary fiber and bulking agents. In addition to the adverse abdominal effects associated with lactulose, diarrhea and electrolyte imbalances can occasionally occur. Sorbitol, a monosaccharide, also exerts its effect by osmotic action and has been recommended as a cost-effective alternative to lactulose. It is as effective as lactulose but may cause less nausea and is much less expensive.

Lactitol is a monosaccharide sugar alcohol that is approved for the treatment of chronic idiopathic constipation. The oral powder should be dissolved in four to eight ounces of a liquid beverage and taken with a meal daily. The most common adverse drug reactions are flatulence and diarrhea.[34]

Polyethylene Glycol PEG is FDA-approved for treatment of constipation at low doses and is expected to produce a bowel movement in 1 to 3 days.[23,33] For this indication, PEG is administered in smaller volumes (10-30 or 17-34 g per 120-240 mL) usually once (or twice) daily. PEG is not absorbed systemically or metabolized by colonic bacteria, and therefore has a lower incidence of adverse effects compared with other osmotic laxatives. Daily use in low dose (17 g) may be safe and effective for up to 6 months, even in children.[35] PEG has a strong recommendation from the American College of Gastroenterology for the treatment of chronic constipation and is available as a nonprescription drug.[27] It is also preferred by the AGA if fiber supplementation is insufficient due to high efficacy based on high quality of evidence available.[28,30] The most common adverse effects are GI-related and include nausea, vomiting, flatulence, and abdominal cramping.[23] PEG solutions with electrolytes are used as bowl cleansing regimens prior to GI-related procedures, and should not be used routinely for treatment of constipation.

Magnesium Salts Magnesium salts, including hydroxide, phosphate, and citrate, and sodium phosphate, are frequently used as bowel preparations prior to diagnostic procedures such as colonoscopy.[23,32] Milk of magnesia (an 8% suspension of magnesium hydroxide), though, may be used occasionally to treat constipation in otherwise healthy adults, but efficacy data are limited. These agents should not be used on a routine basis as they may cause fluid and electrolyte depletion. Also, magnesium or sodium accumulation may occur in patients with renal dysfunction or congestive heart failure. These risks increase with long-term use.

Glycerin Glycerin is usually administered as a suppository and exerts its effect by osmotic action in the rectum. As with most agents given as suppositories, the onset of action is usually less than 30 minutes. Glycerin is considered a safe laxative, although it may occasionally cause rectal irritation. Its use is acceptable on an intermittent basis for constipation or fecal impaction, particularly in children.[35]

Stimulant Laxatives Stimulant laxatives such as diphenylmethane (bisacodyl) and anthraquinone (senna and others) derivates primarily affect the colon.[23] These agents stimulate the mucosal nerve plexus of the colon and may also affect intestinal fluid secretion by altering fluid and electrolyte transport, and are expected to cause a bowel movement within 8 to 12 hours of administration. Stimulant laxatives may cause severe abdominal cramping and electrolyte imbalances, particularly with chronic use. Compared with placebo, bisacodyl is effective in treatment of constipation.[30] These agents are typically reserved for intermittent use or in patients who fail to respond adequately to bulking and osmotic laxatives. Some patients, though, with severe chronic constipation and nonmodifiable risk factors may use these agents on a more regular basis.[24]

Intestinal Secretagogues

Lubiprostone Lubiprostone is a chloride channel activator that acts locally in the gut to open chloride channels on the GI luminal epithelium, which, in turn, stimulates chloride-rich fluid secretion into the intestinal lumen. Increased intraluminal fluid secretion helps to soften stool and accelerate GI transit time.[24] Lubiprostone is FDA-approved for adults with chronic idiopathic constipation as well as treatment of patients with OIC at a recommended dose of one 24-mcg capsule twice daily with food.[24] Patients treated with lubiprostone have a significant increase in spontaneous bowel movements versus placebo as well as improvement in straining, stool consistency, and overall constipation severity.[30] For most patients, bowel movements occur within 24 to 48 hours of lubiprostone administration. Common adverse effects include nausea, headache, and diarrhea and may be dose dependent.[32] Because of its high cost (especially relative to other available laxative agents) and lack of comparative data with other laxative therapies, lubiprostone is reserved for patients with chronic constipation who fail conventional first-line agents such as osmotic laxatives and fiber supplementation, or for those with OIC.

Linaclotide Linaclotide is approved for the treatment of constipation and constipation-predominant irritable bowel syndrome (IBS-C).[23] It is a synthetic 14-amino-acid peptide that binds to and activates the guanylate cyclase C receptor found on the intestinal epithelium. This increases intestinal fluid secretion and quickens intestinal motility. Doses of 72 mcg and 145 mcg are approved for treatment of constipation, and patients should be instructed to take linaclotide on an empty stomach at least 30 minutes before the first meal of the day. Diarrhea was the most commonly reported adverse event in clinical trials, followed by flatulence and abdominal pain. Linaclotide should not be used in patients under the age of 18.[36]

Plecanatide Plecanatide is approved for the treatment of adults with chronic idiopathic constipation.[37] It activates the guanylate cyclase C receptor that increases intestinal fluid secretion and motility similarly to linaclotide. Plecanatide is given once daily without regard to food at a dose of 3 mg. The most common side effect is diarrhea. Plecanatide is contraindicated in patients less than 6 years of age or those with mechanical gastrointestinal obstruction, and should not be used in patients under the age of 18.

Opioid Receptor Antagonists Alvimopan is an oral GI-specific μ-opioid antagonist approved for short-term use in hospitalized patients to accelerate recovery of bowel function after large or small bowel resection.[38] It antagonizes the GI (peripheral) effects of opioids without affecting analgesia because it does not cross the blood–brain barrier. Alvimopan is only available through a special use program (ENTEREG access support and education [EASE]), which requires hospitals to register and meet all requirements before the drug can be administered. Additionally, alvimopan is contraindicated in patients receiving therapeutic doses of opioids for more than seven consecutive days prior to surgery as they may be more sensitive to the drug's effects. Dosing for alvimopan is as follows: 12-mg capsule administered 30 minutes to 5 hours before surgery and then 12 mg twice daily for up to 7 days or until discharge (maximum of 15 doses).

Methylnaltrexone is μ-receptor antagonist approved for OIC in patients with advanced disease receiving palliative care or when response to laxative therapy has been insufficient for patients with OIC with chronic noncancer pain.[26,38] This agent does not cross the blood–brain barrier or antagonize analgesia; it acts on peripheral μ-receptors to block unwanted opioid side effects such as constipation. It is administered at a weight-based dose as a subcutaneous injection in patients with advanced illness, usually every other day (no more than once daily). For patients with noncancer pain, methlynaltrexone can be given as a 12-mg subcutaneous injection or 450-mg oral dose daily. Laxative use should be discontinued upon initiation of methlnaltrexone, and its use is contraindicated in patients with known or suspected GI obstruction. Patients with reduced creatinine clearance (<60 mL/min [1 mL/s]) or moderate-to-severe hepatic impairment should receive reduced dosing of methlnaltrexone (ie, 150 mg orally or 6 mg subcutaneously).

Naloxegol is approved by the FDA for the treatment of OIC in adult patients with noncancer pain.[39] It is an oral pegylated naloxone molecule and antagonizes the μ-receptor. Pegylation reduces naloxegol's passive permeability of the blood–brain barrier. The recommended dose is 25 mg by mouth once daily, 1 hour before or 2 hours after a meal. The dose should be reduced by half in patients with diminished renal function (CrCl <60 mL/min [1 mL/s]) or in those unable to tolerate 25 mg. The most common side effects are abdominal pain, diarrhea, and nausea. In clinical trials, naloxegol significantly increased the number and frequency of bowel movements compared to placebo at 12 weeks.[38]

Naldemedine is a peripherally acting opioid antagonist approved for treatment of OIC in patients with chronic noncancer pain.[26] The recommended dose is 0.2 mg by mouth once daily, and there are no dose adjustments for renal or hepatic impairment. However, patients with severe hepatic impairment (ie, Child-Pugh class C) should not use naldemedine. The most common adverse effects are abdominal pain and diarrhea. Naldemedine increased the frequency of bowel movements compared to placebo in clinical trials.[26]

Other Agents Prucalopride is a selective 5-hydroxytryptamine-4 (5-HT_4) receptor agonist approved for treatment of chronic constipation in the United States and Europe.[40] It demonstrates proenterokinetic effects (increased colonic motility and transit), specifically in the GI tract. Prucalopride is more selective than the previously available serotonergic agonists cisapride and tegaserod with higher affinity for the 5-HT_4 receptor. Receptor selectivity is thought to improve the safety profile of prucalopride over cisapride and tegaserod, which were removed from the market due to concerns for adverse cardiovascular events. In clinical trials, prucalopride significantly increased the number of complete, spontaneous bowel movements in adults with chronic constipation. Constipation symptoms and quality of life were also improved with prucalopride. This agent has been safely tolerated in clinical trials with no adverse cardiovascular effects versus placebo (although data are limited).

Probiotics may be useful in the treatment of constipation. Several randomized controlled trials conducted in children and adults revealed that certain strains of probiotics increased weekly stool frequency.[30] However, these trials were small (370 patients total) and only slight improvement was realized (one additional stool per week). More studies are needed to strengthen evidence involving probiotics, but these may be an option for patients seeking alternative treatment.[23]

Prevention

For patients recovering from myocardial infarction (MI) or rectal surgery, straining at defecation should be avoided. The basis of preventive therapy in these patients should be bulk-forming laxatives or PEG. Additionally, the use of docusate is popular, although its effectiveness is debated. In pregnant patients, constipation may result because of alterations in hormones or iron supplementation.

Evaluation of Therapeutic Outcomes

The ultimate goal of treatment for constipation is to prevent further episodes of constipation. Short-term goals include alleviation of acute constipation with relief from symptoms. For patients with chronic constipation, the goals include use of proper diet and decreased reliance on laxatives in addition to relief of symptoms for the patient so that quality of life is not diminished. Effective treatment of constipation requires the patient to become more knowledgeable about the causes of constipation, proper diet, and appropriate use of laxatives.

IRRITABLE BOWEL SYNDROME

Irritable bowel syndrome is a GI syndrome that is the most commonly diagnosed GI condition, and is characterized by chronic abdominal pain and altered bowel habits in the absence of any organic cause.

Epidemiology

The prevalence of IBS is approximately 10% to 12% based on North American population-based studies; however, there is a wide variation in prevalence by individual country.[41] IBS affects men and women, young and older patients, with an overall 2:1 female predominance in North America.[42] However, younger patients and women are more likely to be diagnosed with IBS, and IBS has been linked with reduced quality of life.[41,43]

Pathophysiology

Although the exact pathophysiologic abnormalities with IBS are still being actively investigated, IBS likely results from altered somatovisceral and motor dysfunction of the intestine from a variety of causes. Abnormal CNS processing of afferent signals may lead to visceral hypersensitivity, with the specific nerve pathway affected determining the exact symptomatology expressed. This visceral hypersensitivity is a neuroenteric phenomenon that is independent of motility and psychological disturbances.[44] Factors known to contribute to these alterations include genetics, motility factors, inflammation, colonic infections, mechanical irritation to local nerves, stress, and other psychological factors.

The enteric nervous system contains a significant percentage of the body's 5-HT receptors.[45] Two types of 5-HT receptors exist within the gut: serotonin type 3 (HT_3) and serotonin type 4 (HT_4), which are responsible for secretion, sensitization, and motility. There is an increase in the postprandial levels of 5-HT in the GI tract in those diagnosed with diarrhea-predominant IBS compared to those who are not.[45] Therefore, stimulation and antagonism of these 5-HT receptors have become a focused area for research on new drug therapies for both diarrhea- and constipation-predominant diseases.

Clinical Presentation

8 Irritable bowel syndrome presents as either diarrhea- or constipation-predominant disease and can be defined as lower abdominal pain, disturbed defecation (constipation, diarrhea, or an alternating pattern of both), and bloating in the absence of structural or biochemical factors that might explain these symptoms (Table 54-9). Table 54-10 provides the diagnostic criteria for the Rome IV symptom-based criteria.[43]

Additional diagnostic steps that can be taken include testing for fecal lactoferrin and C-reactive protein to rule out inflammatory bowel disease and serologic testing to rule out celiac disease.[43] Routine colonoscopy, examination of the stool for occult blood and ova and parasites, or testing for food allergies are not recommended.

TABLE 54-9 Clinical Presentation of Irritable Bowel Syndrome

Signs and symptoms
- Lower abdominal pain
- Abdominal bloating and distension
- Diarrhea symptoms, >3 stools/day
- Extreme urgency
- Passage of mucus
- Constipation symptoms, <3 stools/week, straining, incomplete evacuation
- Psychological symptoms such as depression and anxiety

Non-GI symptoms
- Urinary symptoms
- Fatigue
- Dyspareunia

Other concurrent conditions
- Fibromyalgia
- Functional dyspepsia
- Chronic fatigue syndrome
- Reduced health-related quality of life

TABLE 54-10 Rome IV Diagnostic Criteria for Irritable Bowel Syndrome

Recurrent abdominal pain or discomfort at least 3 days per month in the last 3 months associated with two or more of the following:
1. Relieved with defecation
2. Onset associated with a change in frequency of stool
3. Onset associated with a change in form (appearance) of stool

Data from Reference 43.

TREATMENT

General Approach to Treatment

The treatment approach to IBS is based on the predominant symptoms and their severity (Fig. 54-4). Exercise and a limited trial of a diet with reduced fermentable oligosaccharides, disaccharides, and monosaccharides, and polyols (FODMAPs) are recommended for overall symptom improvement.[41] More persistent disease may require pharmacologic agents, such as secretagogues, rifaximin, or eluxadoline.

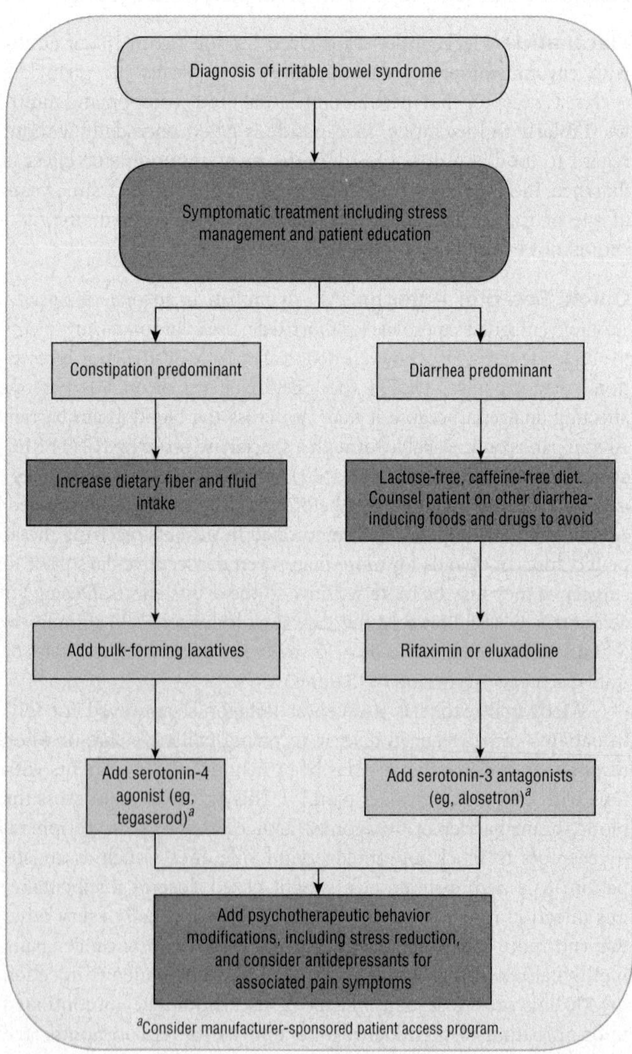

FIGURE 54-4 A general stepwise approach to the management of both constipation- and diarrhea-predominant irritable bowel syndrome.

Constipation-Predominant Disease

In the constipation-predominant patient, dietary fiber may be beneficial. Patients should be instructed to begin with one tablespoonful of fiber with one meal daily and gradually increase the dose to include fiber with two and three meals a day until the desired outcome is achieved. End points that the patient should aim for include bulkier and more easily passed stools. For patients unable to tolerate dietary bran, bulking agents such as psyllium may be substituted.[46] PEG laxatives may be used; however, the AGA does not recommend its use for global symptom relief.[43] When lifestyle modifications alone do not control symptoms, intestinal secretagogues such as linaclotide (290 mcg daily), plecanatide (6 mg daily), and lubiprostone (8 mcg twice daily) should be recommended.[41]

The 5-HT_4 partial agonist tegaserod is approved specifically for short-term, intermittent treatment of IBS-C in women.[43] Tegaserod is available in the United States through a restricted-access program due to a small, yet significant, increase in ischemia events (MI, cerebrovascular accident [CVA], and unstable angina) in patients with preexisting cardiovascular disease and/or cardiovascular risk factors. It is given as 2- or 6-mg doses given twice daily 30 minutes prior to a meal with water for up to 12 weeks. Stimulation of the 5-HT_4 receptors by tegaserod increases gastric secretions and promotes motility, with improvement in symptoms generally occurring within the first week of therapy. Diarrhea was the most common adverse effect, resulting in drug discontinuation in 1.6% of study subjects.

Diarrhea-Predominant Disease

9 For patients in whom diarrhea is the primary complaint, avoidance of certain food products may be necessary. Caffeine, alcohol, and artificial sweeteners (sorbitol, fructose, and mannitol) are known to irritate the gut and produce a laxative effect. Lactose intolerance should be considered in certain patients; however, the prevalence of this condition may be exaggerated.

Herbal medicines or teas often contain senna, which may produce diarrhea. In patients with disease persistence following dietary modification, loperamide may be used for episodic management of urgent diarrhea, or in situations in which the patient wishes to avoid the possibility of an acute onset of symptoms.[42] Loperamide decreases intestinal transit, enhances water and electrolyte absorption, and strengthens rectal sphincter tone. However, loperamide is not likely to address other symptoms of IBS such as abdominal pain.[43]

Diarrhea-predominant IBS caused by excessive stimulation of the 5-HT_3 receptor can be relieved by the drug alosetron, a 5-HT3-receptor antagonist. Its use is limited to an FDA-approved restricted-use program, and requires extensive postmarketing surveillance due to association with serious adverse effects, including severe constipation and ischemic colitis.[42] Additional information can be found at http://www.lotronex.com. It is indicated for women with diarrhea-predominant symptoms of longer than 6 months' duration that are not relieved by conventional therapy at a dose of 0.5 mg twice daily.

Other agents, eluxadoline and rifaximin, are approved and recommended for use in IBS-D.[43] Rifaximin is a rifamycin antibacterial indicated for the treatment of travelers' diarrhea that is indicated for the treatment of IBS-D in adults based on several randomized control trials demonstrating improvement in abdominal pain, stool consistency, and bloating.[42,47] The recommended dose is 550 mg orally three times a day for 2 weeks. Recurrences may be retreated up to two times; however, there is no evidence to support repeating the regimen. Eluxadoline is a μ-opioid receptor agonist indicated for adults with IBS-D. The recommended dose is 100 mg orally twice a day with food. A lower dose of 75 mg twice daily is recommended for patients who cannot tolerate the 100 mg dose and if they have hepatic impairment; eluxadoline should be avoided in patients without a gallbladder.[48] Its main benefits are improvement in abdominal pain and stool consistency. The main side effect seen is constipation.

Use of Antidepressants in Irritable Bowel Syndrome

Tricyclic antidepressants have some benefit in treatment of diarrhea-predominant IBS associated with moderate-to-severe abdominal pain, by modulating perception of visceral pain, altering GI transit time, and treating underlying comorbidities.[49,50] Selective 5-HT reuptake inhibitors (SSRI), fluoxetine, citalopram, and paroxetine have been studied, but the results are conflicting. Large randomized control trials lasting longer than 3 months are needed to determine the place of SSRIs in therapy.[51]

Duloxetine, a serotonin-norepinephrine reuptake inhibitor, has been used in the management of IBS with comorbid generalized anxiety disorder and major depressive disorder. Although the effect was gradual over 12 weeks, both symptom severity and quality of life significantly improved.[52,53]

Pain in Irritable Bowel Syndrome

10 Some patients with IBS suffer significant pain associated with their disease. Data supporting the use of antispasmodic agents in these patients are conflicting, and these are not recommended for global IBS symptoms.[43] A trial of low-dose antidepressant therapy is indicated, especially if pain is associated with eating. Both tricyclic antidepressants and 5-HT reuptake inhibitors produce analgesia and may relieve depressive symptoms if present. Preprandial doses of drugs containing anticholinergic properties may suppress pain (and/or diarrhea) associated with an overactive postprandial gastrocolonic response. Tricyclic antidepressants should be avoided in patients with pain and constipation. In addition, psychotherapy, including cognitive behavioral therapy, relaxation therapy, and hypnotherapy, decreases IBS symptoms.[41]

Evaluation of Therapeutic Outcomes

Irritable bowel syndrome is usually classified as constipation-predominant, diarrhea-predominant, or IBS with mixed symptoms, or unclassified. Therapeutic goals in IBS should focus on the patient's primary complaint. Additionally, global symptoms may be treated with antidepressants, relaxation/stress management, cognitive behavior treatment, and/or hypnosis aimed at specific affective disorders.[41] Lastly, the 5-HT receptor agonists and antagonists can be used in carefully selected patients whose symptoms are not adequately controlled with other agents.

ABBREVIATIONS

AAD	antibiotic-associated diarrhea
AGA	American Gastroenterology Association
AIDS	acquired immune deficiency syndrome
ATPase	adenosine triphosphatase
CDC	Centers for Disease Control and Prevention
CVA	cerebrovascular accident
EASE	ENTEREG access support and education
5-HT	serotonin
HT_3	serotonin type 3
HT_4	serotonin type 4
5-HT_4	5-hydroxytryptamine-4
IBS	irritable bowel syndrome
IBS-C	constipation-predominant irritable bowel syndrome
MI	myocardial infarction
NSAID	nonsteroidal anti-inflammatory drug
OIC	opioid-induced constipation
ORS	oral rehydration solution
PEG	polyethylene glycol
VIP	vasoactive intestinal peptide
VIPoma	vasoactive intestinal peptide-secreting tumor
WDHA	watery diarrhea, hypokalemia, and achlorhydria
WHO	World Health Organization
WHO-ORS	World Health Organization oral rehydration solution

REFERENCES

1. DuPont HL. Persistent diarrhea: A clinical review. *JAMA.* 2016;315(24):2712–2723.
2. Farthing M, Salam M, Lindberg G, et al. Acute diarrhea in adults and children: A global perspective. World Gastroenterology Organization Guidelines. 2012. Available at http://www.worldgastroenterology.org/acute-diarrhea-in-adults.html. Accessed May 31, 2021.
3. Troeger C, Blacker BF, Khalil IA, et al. Estimates of the global, regional, and national morbidity, mortality, and aetiologies of diarrhoea in 195 countries: A systematic analysis for the Global Burden of Disease Study 2016. *Lancet Infect Dis.* 2018;18(11):1211–1228. 10.1016/S1473-3099(18)30362-1.
4. Schiller LR. Antidiarrheal drug therapy. *Curr Gastroenterol Rep.* 2017;19(5):18. 10.1007/s11894-017-0557-x.
5. Lalani T, Maguire JD, Grant EM, et al. Epidemiology and self-treatment of traveler's diarrhea in a larger, prospective cohort of department of defense beneficiaries. *J Travel Med.* 2015;22(3):152–160.
6. Steffen R, Hill DR, Dupont HL. Traveler's diarrhea: A clinical review. *JAMA.* 2015;313(1):71–80.
7. Guarino A, Vecchio AL, Dias JA, et al. Universal recommendations for the management of acute diarrhea in nonmalnourished children. *J Pediatr Gastroenterol Nutr.* 2018;67(5):586–593. 10.1097/MPG.0000000000002053.
8. World Health Organization. *WHO/UNICEF Joint Statement: Clinical Management of Acute Diarrhea (WHO/FCH/CAH/04.7).* Geneva, Switzerland: World Health Organization; 2004.
9. US Food and Drug Administration. Drug Safety Communication: FDA warns about serious heart problems with high doses of the antidiarrheal medicine loperamide (Imodium), including from abuse and misuse. Available at https://www.fda.gov/Drugs/DrugSafety/ucm504617.htm. Accessed May 31, 2021.
10. US Food and Drug Administration. Drug Safety Communication: FDA limits packaging for anti-diarrhea medicine loperamide(Imodium) to encourage safe use. Available at https://www.fda.gov/Drugs/DrugSafety/ucm594232.htm. Accessed May 31, 2021.
11. Harris AG, Odorisio TM, Woltering EA, et al. Consensus statement—Octreotide dose titration in secretory diarrhea—Diarrhea Management Consensus Development Panel. *Dig Dis Sci.* 1995;40(7):1464–1473.
12. Giustina A, Mazziotti G, Cannavo S, et al. High-dose and high-frequency lanreotide autogel in acromegaly: A randomized, multicenter study. *J Clin Endocrinol Metab.* 2017;102(7):2454–2464.
13. Collinson S, Deans A, Padua-Zamora A, et al. Probiotics for treating acute infectious diarrhoea. *Cochrane Database of Systematic Reviews.* 2020;(Issue 12). Art. No.: CD003048. doi:10.1002/14651858.CD003048.pub4. Accessed July 1, 2021.
14. Blaabjeg S, Artzi DM, Aabenhus R. Probiotics for the prevention of antibiotic-associated diarrhea in outpatients: A systematic review and meta-analysis. *Antibiotics (Basel).* 2017;6(4):21. 10.3390/antibiotics6040021.
15. Allen SJ, Wareham K, Wang D, et al. A high-dose preparation of lactobacilli and bifidobacteria in the prevention of antibiotic-associated and Clostridium difficile diarrhoea in older people admitted to hospital: A multicentre, randomised, double-blind, placebo-controlled, parallel arm trial (PLACIDE). *Health Technol Assess.* 2013;17(57):1–140.
16. Thompson RF, Bass DM, Hoffman SL. Travel vaccines. *Infect Dis Clin North Am.* 1999;13(1):149–167.
17. CDC. Vaxchora® (lypholized CVD 103-HgR). Available at https://www.cdc.gov/cholera/vaccines.html. Accessed 1 July 2021.
18. Cabrera A, Lepage JE, Sullivan KM, et al. Vaxchora: A single-dose oral cholera vaccine. *Ann Pharmacother.* 2017;51(7):584–589. 10.1177/1060028017698162.
19. CDC. Prevention of rotavirus gastroenteritis among infants and children: Recommendations of the Advisory Committee on Immunization Practices (ACIP). *MMWR.* 2009;58(RR-2):1–26.
20. Burke RM, Tate JE, Kirkwood CD, et al. Current and new rotavirus vaccines. *Curr Opin Infect Dis.* 2019;32(5):435–444. doi:10.1097/QCO.0000000000000572.
21. Bharucha AE, Wald A. Chronic constipation. *Mayo Clin Proc.* 2019 Nov;94(11):2340–2357. 10.1016/j.mayocp.2019.01.031.
22. Ford AC, Moayyedi P, Lacy BE, et al. Task Force on the Management of Functional Bowel Disorders. American College of Gastroenterology monograph on the management of irritable bowel syndrome and chronic idiopathic constipation. *Am J Gastroenterol.* 2014 Aug;109(Suppl 1):S2–S26. doi:10.1038/ajg.2014.187.
23. Bharucha AE, Lacy BE. Mechanisms, evaluation, and management of chronic constipation. *Gastroentero.* 2020;158:1232–1249. doi:10.1053/j.gastro.2019.12.034.
24. Wald A. Constipation: Advances in diagnosis and treatment. *JAMA.* 2016;315(2):185191. 10.1001/jama.2015.16994.
25. Mounsey A, Raleigh M, Wilson A. Management of constipation in older adults. *Am Fam Physician.* 2015;92(6):500–504.
26. Murphy JA, Sheriden EA. Evidence based review of pharmacotherapy for opioid-induced constipation in noncancer pain. *Ann Pharmacother.* 2018;52(4):370–379.
27. Lacy BE, Mearin F, Chang L, et al. Bowel disorders. *Gastroenterology.* 2016;150:1393–1407.
28. Barucha AE, Dorn SD, Lembo A, Pressman A. American Gastroenterological Association medical position statement on constipation. *Gastroenterology.* 2013;144:211–217.
29. Gallegos-Orozco JF, Foxx-Orenstein AE, Sterler SM, Stoa JM. Chronic constipation in the elderly. *Am J Gastroenterol.* 2012;107:18–25.
30. Ford AC, Moayyedi P, Lacy BE, et al. American College of Gastroenterology monograph on the management of irritable bowel syndrome and chronic idiopathic constipation. *Am J Gastroenterol.* 2014;109(Suppl 1):S2–S26.
31. Thaha MA, Abukar AA, Thin NN, Ramsanahie A, Knowles CH. Sacral nerve stimulation for faecal incontinence and constipation in adults. *Cochrane Database Syst Rev.* 2015;8:CD004464. doi:10.1002/14651858.CD004464.pub3.
32. Costilla VC, Foxx-Orenstein AE. Constipation in adults: Diagnosis and management. *Curr Treat Options Gastroenterol.* 2014;12:310–321. doi:10.1007/s11938-014-0025-8.
33. Lee-Robichaud H, Thomas K, Morgan J, Nelson RL. Lactulose versus polyethylene glycol for chronic constipation. *Cochrane Database Syst Rev.* 2010;(7):CD007570. doi:10.1002/14651858.CD007570.pub2.
34. Product information for Pizensy. Braintree Labs. Braintree, MA 02185. February 2020.
35. Tabbers MM, DiLorenzo C, Berger MY, et al. Evaluation and treatment of functional constipation in infants and children: Evidence-based recommendations from ESPGHAN and NASPGHAN. *J Pediatr Gastroenterol Nutr.* 2014;58(2):258–274.
36. Linzess (linaclotide) [prescribing information]. Madison, NJ: Allergan USA, Inc; April 2021.
37. Trulance (plecanatide) [prescribing information]. Bridgewater, NJ: SalixPharmaceuticals; April 2021.
38. Nee J, Zakari M, Sugarman MA, et al. Efficacy of treatments for opioid-induced constipation: Systematic review and meta-analysis. *Clin Gastroenterol Hepatol.* 2018;16(10):1569–1584. doi:10.1016/j.cgh.2018.01.021.
39. Leonard J, Baker DE. Naloxegol: Treatment for opioid-induced constipation in chronic non-cancer pain. *Ann Pharmocother.* 2015;49(3):360–365.
40. Shin A, Camilleri M, Kolar G, Erwin P, West CP, Murad MH. Systematic review with meta analysis: Highly selective 5-HT4 agonists (prucalopride, velusetrag, or naronapride) in chronic constipation. *Aliment Pharmacol Ther.* 2014;39:239–253.
41. Ford AC, Moayyedi P, Chey WD, et al. for the ACG Task Force on Management of Irritable Bowel Syndrome. American College of Gastroenterology monograph on the management of irritable bowel syndrome. *Am J Gastroenterol.* 2018; 113 (Suppl 2):1–18. doi:10.1038/s41395-018-0084-x.
42. Weinberg DS, Smalley W, Heidelbaugh JJ, Sultan S. American Gastroenterological Association Institute Guideline on the pharmacological management of irritable bowel syndrome. *Gastroenterology.* 2014;147(5):1146–1148.
43. Lacy BE, Pimentel M, Brenner DM, et al. ACG clinical guideline: Management of irritable bowel syndrome. *Am J Gastroenterol.* 2021; 116(1): 1744. doi:10.14309/ajg.0000000000001036.
44. Canavan C, West J, Card T. The epidemiology of irritable bowel syndrome. *Clin Epidemiol.* 2014;6:71–80.
45. Dothel G, Barbaro MR, Raschi E, et al. Advancements in drug development for diarrhea-predominant irritable bowel syndrome. *Expert Opin Investig Drugs.* 2018;27(3):251–263.
46. National Institute for Health and Care Excellence. Addendum to Guideline CG61. Irritable bowel syndrome in adults: Diagnosis and management of irritable bowel syndrome in primary care. 2015. Available at http://www.nice.org.uk/guidance/cg61/chapter/1-recommendations#clinical-management-of-ibs. Accessed July 1, 2021.
47. Xifaxan® [package insert]. Bridgewater, NJ: Salix Pharmaceuticals Inc; October 2020.
48. Viberzi® [package insert]. Madison, NJ: Allergan USA; June 2020.
49. Iskandar HN, Cassell B, Kanuri N, et al. Tricyclic antidepressants for management of residual symptoms in inflammatory bowel disease. *J Clin Gastroenterol.* 2014;48(5):423–429.

50. Xie C, Tang Y, Wang Y. Efficacy and safety of antidepressants for the treatment of irritable bowel syndrome: A meta-analysis. *PLoS ONE.* 2015;10(8):e0127815.
51. Bundeff AW, Woodis CB. Selective serotonin reuptake inhibitors for the treatment of irritable bowel syndrome. *Ann Pharmacother.* 2014;46(6):777–784.
52. Lewis-Fernandex R Lam R, Lam P, Lucak S, et al. An open-label pilot study of duloxetine in patients with irritable bowel syndrome and comorbid major depressive disorder. *J Clin Psychopharmacol.* 2016;36(6):710–715.
53. Kaplan A, Franzen MD, Nickell PV, et al. An open-label trial of duloxetine in patients with irritable bowel syndrome and comorbid generalized anxiety disorder. *Int J Psychiatry Clin Pract.* 2014;18(1):11–15.

55

Portal Hypertension and Cirrhosis

Julie M. Sease

KEY CONCEPTS

1. Cirrhosis is a severe, chronic, potentially irreversible disease associated with significant morbidity and mortality. The progression of cirrhosis secondary to alcohol intake, both in those with alcoholic cirrhosis and cirrhosis due to other causes, can be interrupted by abstinence from alcohol. It is therefore imperative for the clinician to educate and support abstinence from alcohol as part of the overall treatment strategy of the underlying liver disease.
2. Patients with cirrhosis, except those screened and considered to be at low risk, should receive endoscopic evaluation looking for the presence of varices. Patients with medium to large varices, or small varices with risk factors, should receive primary prophylaxis with nonselective β-adrenergic blockade therapy to prevent variceal hemorrhage.
3. When nonselective β-adrenergic blocker therapy with propranolol or nadolol is used to prevent rebleeding, therapy should be titrated to achieve a goal heart rate of 55 to 60 beats/min, but systolic blood pressure must also be maintained above 90 mm Hg.
4. Octreotide is the preferred vasoactive agent for the medical management of variceal bleeding in the United States. Endoscopic band ligation is the primary therapeutic tool for the management of acute variceal bleeding.
5. The combination of spironolactone and furosemide is recommended by clinical guidelines in the United States as the initial diuretic therapy for patients with ascites.
6. All patients who have survived an episode of spontaneous bacterial peritonitis (SBP) should receive long-term antibiotic prophylaxis.
7. The mainstay of treatment of hepatic encephalopathy (HE) involves therapy to lower blood ammonia concentrations and includes diet modifications, lactulose, and rifaximin alone or in combination with lactulose.

BEYOND THE BOOK

Watch the short Medscape video "Cirrhosis Overview Clinical Presentation" (https://www.youtube.com/watch?v=XJQn8MXnTWg). This video reviews the basic pathophysiology of cirrhosis and connects it to the most common complications of decompensated cirrhosis. Create a summary table of treatment options for each complication associated with decompensated cirrhosis: portal hypertension (primary prophylaxis against bleeding, acute bleeding, and secondary prophylaxis against bleeding), ascites, spontaneous bacterial peritonitis (SBP) (acute treatment and secondary prophylaxis), and hepatic encephalopathy. Use the below table as a guide.

Complication	Treatment/drug of choice (to include dose, route, and frequency)	Common adverse effects	Monitoring parameters	Patient counseling points/ pharmacy pearls
Portal hypertension				
Primary prophylaxis against bleeding				
Acute bleeding				
Secondary prophylaxis of bleeding				
Ascites				
SBP				
Acute treatment				
Secondary prophylaxis				
Hepatic encephalopathy				

INTRODUCTION

Chronic liver injury causes damage to normal liver tissue resulting in the development of regenerative nodules surrounded by dense fibrotic material, which are diagnostic hallmarks of cirrhosis.[1] The distorted architecture of the cirrhotic liver impedes portal blood flow, interferes with hepatocyte perfusion, and disrupts hepatic synthetic functions such as the production of albumin. Clinical consequences of cirrhosis include increased intrahepatic resistance leading to portal hypertension, varices, and variceal bleeding; ascites; infection; encephalopathy; and hepatocellular carcinoma. When advanced, cirrhosis can also lead to the development of both renal and pulmonary dysfunction.

TABLE 55-1 Etiology of Cirrhosis

Alcoholism
Chronic hepatitis C
Metabolic liver disease
Hemochromatosis
Wilson disease
Nonalcoholic fatty liver disease
Immunologic disease
Autoimmune hepatitis
Primary biliary cirrhosis
Primary biliary cholangitis
Vascular disease
Budd–Chiari
Drug-induced liver injury (below list not all-inclusive)
Isoniazid, macrolides, amoxicillin-clavulanate, nitrofurantoin, fluoroquinolones, amiodarone, nonsteroidal anti-inflammatory drugs, allopurinol, sulfasalazine, methotrexate, interferon-β, interferon-α, anti-tumor necrosis factor inhibitors, valproate, lamotrigine, phenytoin, carbamazepine, green tea extract

Data from References 1-3.

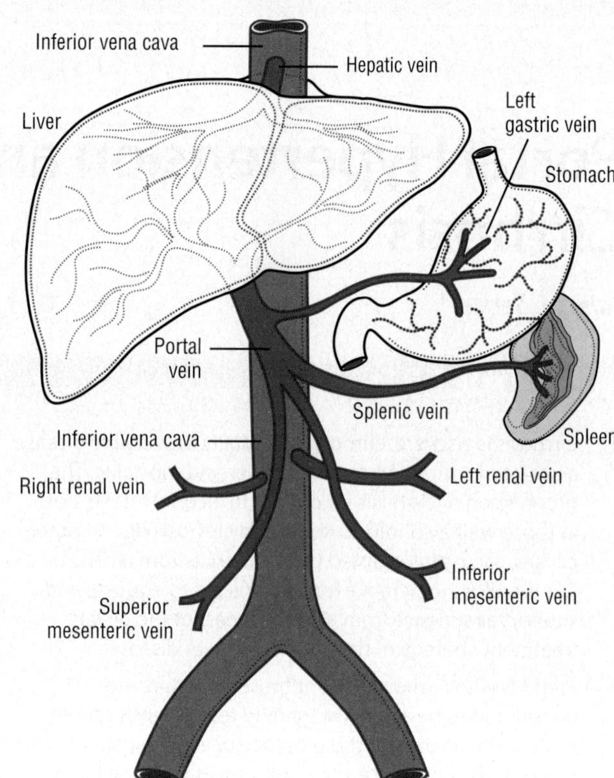

FIGURE 55-1 The portal venous system.

1 While cirrhosis has many causes (Table 55-1),[1-3] in industrialized countries, primary etiologies include hepatitis C, excessive alcohol intake, and nonalcoholic fatty liver disease.[1,2] Treatment strategies for managing the most commonly encountered clinical complications of cirrhosis are discussed. Fibrosis, even significant enough to have caused cirrhosis, is known to regress when anti-viral therapy for hepatitis B and C is instituted.[1] The reader is referred to Chapter 58, "Viral Hepatitis" for a detailed discussion of the treatment of cirrhosis secondary to hepatitis.

EPIDEMIOLOGY

Chronic liver disease and cirrhosis were responsible for nearly 42,838 deaths in America in 2018 making it the 11th leading cause of death.[4] Acute variceal bleeding and spontaneous bacterial peritonitis (SBP) are among the immediately life-threatening complications of cirrhosis. Associated conditions causing significant morbidity include ascites and hepatic encephalopathy (HE).

PATHOPHYSIOLOGY OF CIRRHOSIS

Any discussion of cirrhosis must be based on a firm understanding of hepatic anatomy and vascular supply. Conceptually, the liver can be thought of as an elaborate blood filtration system receiving blood from the hepatic artery and the portal vein (Fig. 55-1), with portal blood originating from the small intestines.[5] Blood enters the liver via the portal triad, which contains branches of the portal vein, hepatic artery, and bile ducts. It then drains through the sinusoidal space (also known as the space of Disse) of the hepatic lobule (Fig. 55-2), which is lined by the workhorses of the liver, the hepatocytes. Individual hepatocytes are arranged in plates that are one cell thick and organized around individual central veins. The six or more surfaces of each individual hepatocyte make contact with adjacent hepatocytes, border the bile canaliculi, or are exposed to the sinusoidal space. Filtered blood travels into the terminal hepatic venules, also called central veins, and then empties into larger hepatic veins and eventually into the inferior vena cava. There are functional gradients of hepatocytes based on oxygen saturation. Hepatocytes closest to the portal triad, which contains the hepatic artery, have greater oxygen saturation than those hepatocytes nearer to the terminal hepatic venule. Blood flows past hepatocytes in zone one, then zone two, and finally zone three before entering the central vein. Hepatocytes in zone one are involved in gluconeogenesis, urea synthesis, and oxidative energy metabolism while those in zone three carry out the functions of glycolysis and lipogenesis.

Hepatic stellate cells (HSCs), located in the space of Disse and surrounded by hepatocytes and endothelial cells, are the cell type primarily responsible for the formation of liver fibrosis.[6] Normally, HSCs function to store vitamin A and maintain the normal matrix of the sinusoidal space. Quiescent HSCs become proliferative and transform into myofibroblasts when they are stimulated to do so by hepatocytes, Kupffer cells, platelets, leukocytes, and sinusoidal endothelial cells in reaction to exposure to toxic agents, viruses, or other insults. As myofibroblasts, HSCs lose the ability to store retinoids and upregulate synthesis of extracellular matrix components. When pro-fibrogenic triggers are persistently present, excessive extracellular matrix components accumulate which alter the liver's architecture, reduce its elasticity, and impact the flow of blood through the liver which leads to elevated sinusoidal pressure and portal hypertension, hallmarks of cirrhosis.

Portal hypertension leads to changes in the splanchnic vasculature and circulation.[7] Splanchnic vasodilation and the formation of new blood vessels contribute to an increased splanchnic blood flow, formation of gastroesophageal varices, and variceal bleeding. Additionally, splanchnic and systemic vasodilation leads to hypoperfusion of the renal system that causes activation of the renin-angiotensin-aldosterone system and the sympathetic nervous system which subsequently result in functional renal impairment as well as sodium and water retention presenting as ascites.[8] Therein lies the pathophysiology of ascites and renal dysfunction that often accompany chronic liver disease. Portosystemic shunting may also occur and is involved in HE and other complications.[7]

ANATOMIC AND PHYSIOLOGIC EFFECTS OF CIRRHOSIS

Cirrhosis and the pathophysiologic abnormalities that cause it result in the commonly encountered problems of ascites, portal hypertension, esophageal varices, HE, and coagulation disorders. Other less common problems in patients with cirrhosis include hepatorenal

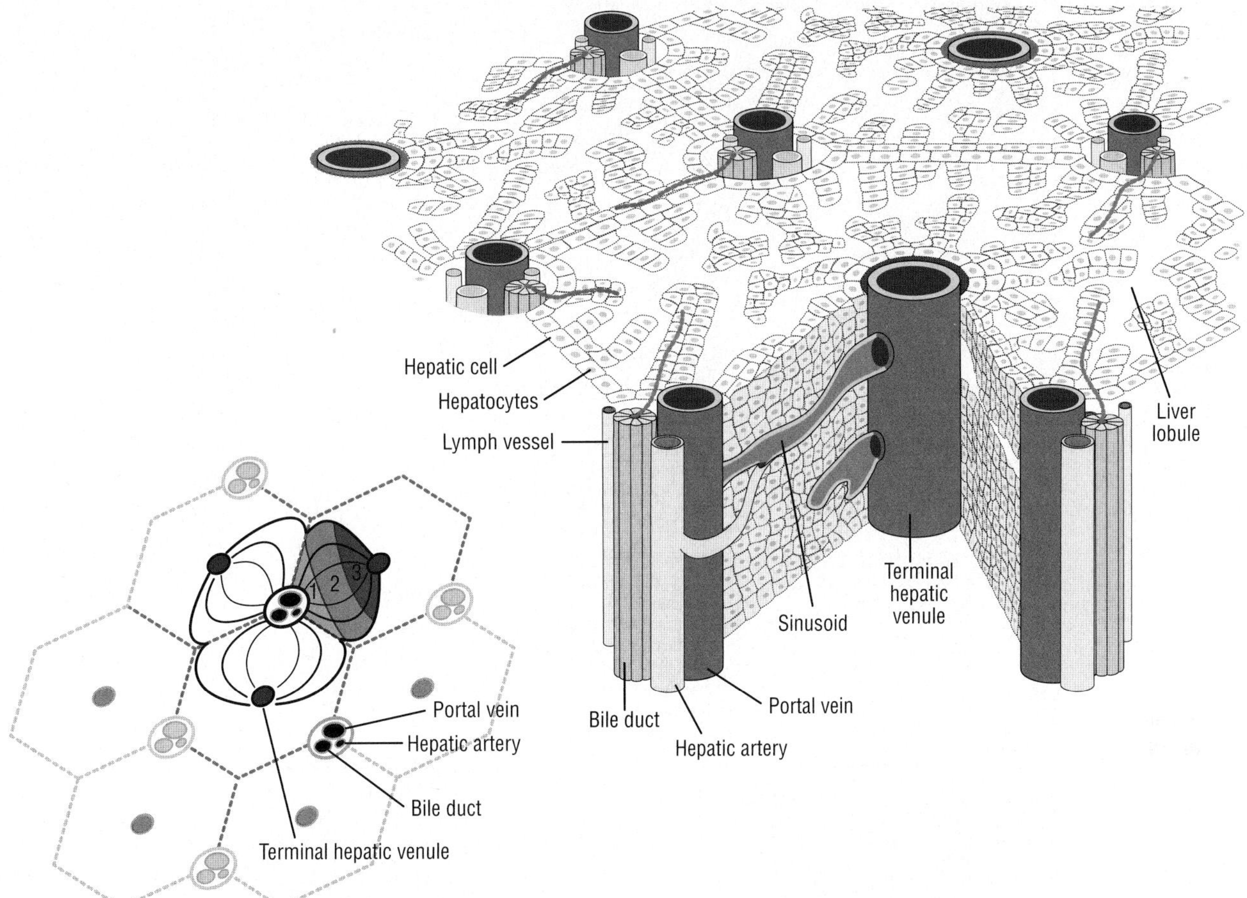

FIGURE 55-2 The hepatic lobule.

syndrome, hepatopulmonary syndrome, and endocrine dysfunction. These are discussed under section "Management of Portal Hypertension and Variceal Bleeding."

Ascites

Ascites is the accumulation of an excessive amount of fluid within the abdomen. It is the most common major complication of cirrhosis with approximately 20% of patients presenting with ascites at the time of their cirrhosis diagnosis.[9] As noted above, portal hypertension activates vasodilatory mechanisms leading to splanchnic and systemic vasodilation and a resultant drop in mean arterial pressure.[8] Portal hypertension is also thought to lead to bacterial translocation of gut bacteria causing local and systemic inflammation and the generation of vasodilatory nitric oxide and prostacyclins in the splanchnic vasculature which further reduces mean arterial pressure. This drop in mean arterial pressure is recognized by arterial baroreceptors activating endogenous vasoconstrictor systems including the sympathetic nervous system, the renin-angiotensin-aldosterone system, as well as a nonosmotic vasopressin release.[10] Renal vasoconstriction and sodium and water retention ensue resulting in the formation of edema and ascites. The excess fluid shifts from the intravascular compartment into the abdominal cavity. Hypoalbuminemia, which results from the decreased synthetic function of the diseased liver, contributes further to fluid leakage into the abdomen. The end result of this complex process is the sustained peritoneal ascites of end-stage liver disease (Fig. 55-3).

Portal Hypertension and Varices

Sinusoidal portal hypertension is most often caused by cirrhosis.[11] It is associated with acute variceal bleeding, a medical emergency that is among the most severe complications of cirrhosis.[12] Portal hypertension is defined by the presence of a gradient of greater than 5 mm Hg (0.7 kPa) between the portal and central venous pressures (see Fig. 55-1).[11] This gradient is called the hepatic venous pressure gradient (HVPG). Esophageal and gastric varices and variceal bleeding may arise after an HVPG pressure gradient of 10 mm Hg (1.3 kPa) is reached.

Progression to bleeding can be predicted by Child-Pugh score, size of varices, and the presence of red wale markings on the varices. First variceal hemorrhage occurs at an annual rate of about 15% and carries a mortality of 7% to 15%. Rebleeding is common following initial hemorrhage with a median rate of 60% and carries a mortality rate as high as 33%. Prevention of bleeding is a major goal in the therapy of portal hypertension, and strategies include both pharmacologic and surgical approaches.

Hepatic Encephalopathy

Hepatic encephalopathy is a functional disturbance of the brain caused by liver insufficiency or portal systemic shunting that presents on a wide spectrum of symptom severity ranging from subclinical alterations to coma.[13] Symptoms of HE result from an accumulation of gut-derived nitrogenous substances in the systemic circulation as a consequence of decreased hepatic functioning.[14] Once these substances enter the CNS, they cause alterations of neurotransmission that affect consciousness and behavior. Ammonia is the most commonly cited culprit in the pathogenesis of HE, but glutamine, benzodiazepine receptor agonists, and aromatic amino acids are also potential causes.[13,14] Arterial ammonia levels are commonly increased in both acute and chronic liver diseases, but an established correlation between blood ammonia levels and mental status does

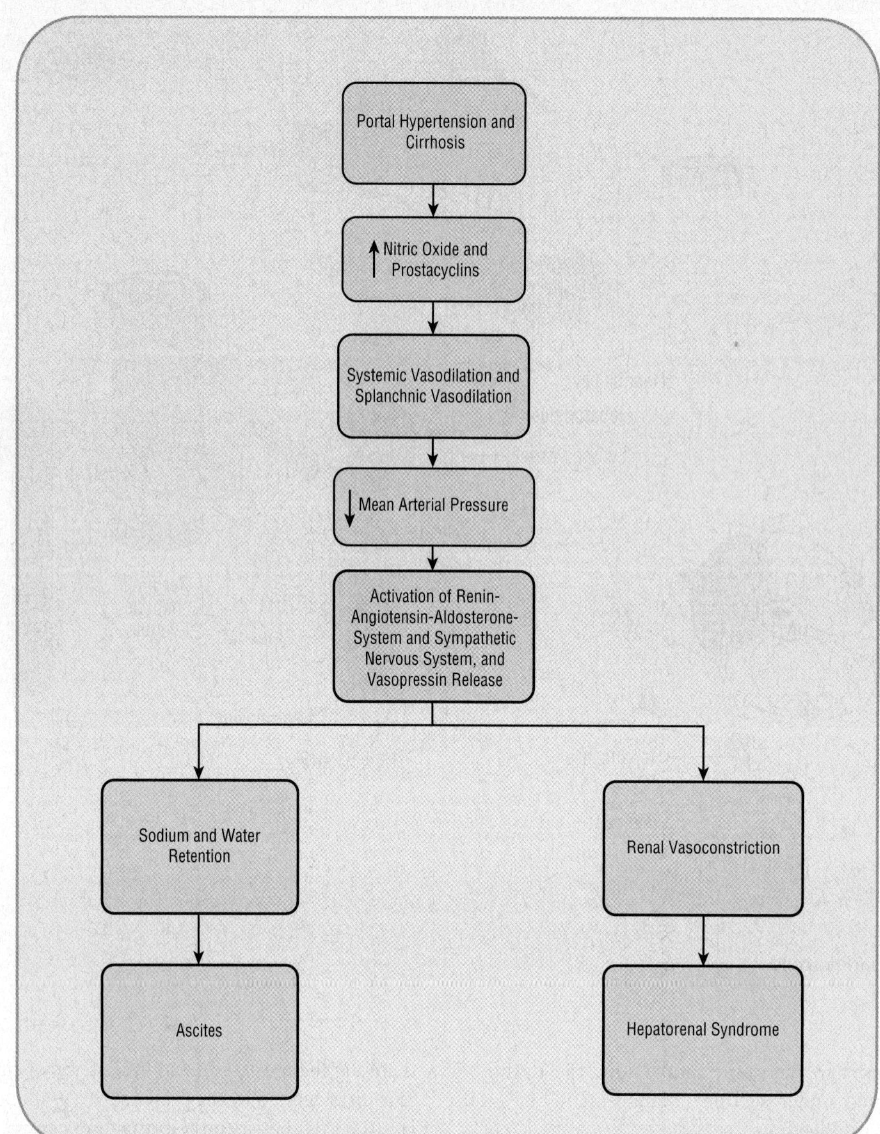

FIGURE 55-3 Pathogenesis of ascites.

not exist.[14] A normal ammonia level finding brings the diagnosis of HE into question.[13] Interventions to lower blood ammonia levels remain the mainstay of treatment for HE.[13,14]

Hepatic encephalopathy is categorized as type A, B, or C.[13] Type A is HE induced by acute liver failure, type B is due to portal-systemic bypass without associated intrinsic liver disease, and type C is HE that occurs in patients with cirrhosis. The severity of HE symptoms, time course (whether episodic, recurrent, or persistent), and whether incited by precipitating factors (such as infection, GI bleeding, an electrolyte disorder, or constipation) are additional ways in which HE is classified. The majority of episodic cases of HE secondary to cirrhosis are associated with a precipitant. It is important that precipitating factors be sought and treated when present.

Coagulation Defects

End-stage chronic liver disease is associated with decreased synthetic capability of the liver leading to decreased levels of most procoagulant factors as well as the naturally occurring anticoagulants, antithrombin, protein C, and protein S.[15] However, two procoagulant factors, factor VIII and von Willebrand factor, are actually elevated in chronic liver disease. It was thought that chronic liver disease induced an acquired bleeding disorder owing to the decrease in most procoagulant factors, but it is now believed that these patients actually live in a tenuous state of rebalanced hemostasis. This is due to increased levels of factor VIII and von Willebrand factor and the decreased levels of natural anticoagulants (antithrombin, protein C, and protein S). The rebalanced homeostasis seen in chronic liver disease can be tipped toward either thrombosis or clinically significant bleeding at any time depending on the circumstances experienced by the patient at the time. The prothrombin time (PT) is a standard component of the Child-Pugh scoring system and the international normalized ratio (INR) is utilized in the model for end-stage liver disease, a prognostic evaluation tool. The ability of the PT and INR to accurately measure bleeding risk and assist with estimation of the severity of a patient's liver disease has been called into question.[15]

Both platelet number and function may be affected in cirrhosis. Thrombocytopenia, a common finding in cirrhosis, could promote bleeding. However, von Willebrand factor, the binding site for platelets, is not decreased by cirrhosis and thrombin generation assays show that platelet procoagulant activity is actually preserved in patients with cirrhosis. Fibrinolysis is another process that is likely rebalanced in cirrhosis. While α-2-antiplasmin and

CLINICAL PRESENTATION Cirrhosis

Signs and Symptoms
- Asymptomatic
- Splenomegaly
- Jaundice, palmar erythema, and spider nevi
- Gynecomastia
- Ascites and edema
- Malaise, anorexia, and weight loss
- Encephalopathy

Laboratory Tests
- Hypoalbuminemia
- Elevated prothrombin time (PT)
- Thrombocytopenia
- Elevated alkaline phosphatase
- Elevated aspartate transaminase (AST), alanine transaminase (ALT), and γ-glutamyl transpeptidase (GGT)

thrombin-activatable fibrinolysis inhibitor levels are reduced, tissue plasminogen activator levels are increased. These changes would be expected to increase the risk for bleeding. However, procoagulant changes, including reduced plasminogen levels and normal to increased platelet activator inhibitor levels, occur concurrently, which provide a homeostasis in the fibrinolysis process.

CLINICAL PRESENTATION

Portal Hypertension

Patients with compensated cirrhosis are usually asymptomatic.[17] Initial symptoms may be nonspecific including fatigue, loss of appetite, and weight loss. Patients may also present with much more significant symptomatology secondary to decompensation related to cirrhosis complications such as ascites (abdominal distention) and HE (confusion, lethargy).

The approach to a patient with suspected liver disease begins with a thorough history and physical examination. In addition to fatigue, loss of appetite, and weight loss, patients may also experience other nonspecific signs. Muscle wasting, palmar erythema, spider nevi, parotid gland enlargement, white nails, Dupuytren contracture, asterixis and metabolic complications including gynecomastia, testicular atrophy, and axillary hair loss are all possibly related to cirrhosis.

Diagnostics for cirrhosis include liver function tests, coagulation tests, complete blood count, and serologic tests for viral causes including hepatitis B and C. A thorough history is key in determining if alcoholism is the likely cause of a patient's cirrhosis. A basic history and physical may also uncover the presence of obesity and history of diabetes that are suggestive of nonalcoholic fatty liver disease. Additional testing may include an antinuclear antibody titer to evaluate for the presence of autoimmune hepatitis; serum iron and transferrin saturation, possibly in conjunction with genetic testing, to look for hemochromatosis; and alpha-1 antitrypsin level and genotyping to test for alpha-1 antitripysin deficiency, a rare disease, but one that can lead to liver disease as well as lung damage. When the underlying cause is still unable to be elucidated, additional testing for antimitochondrial antibodies or a magnetic resonance cholangiopancreatography to look for strictures and dilations of the bile ducts indicating primary biliary cholangitis may be completed. Wilson disease can be screened for using serum ceruloplasmin and copper levels.

Liver Chemistries

Liver chemistries or liver tests are actually markers of liver injury rather than function, though they are commonly referred to as liver function tests.[19] A comprehensive metabolic profile includes AST, ALT, alkaline phosphatase, bilirubin, and albumin. Additionally, the PT and GGT are needed. Liver chemistries are part of the initial evaluation of a patient with symptoms or signs suggestive of cirrhosis.[18] The use of liver function tests in the diagnosis and management of cirrhosis is discussed in the following sections. It may be useful to group the tests into two broad categories: (1) markers of liver injury such as AST, ALT and alkaline phosphatase and (2) markers of hepatocellular function such as PT, bilirubin, and albumin.[19]

Aminotransferases

The aminotransferases, AST and ALT, are enzymes involved in the transfer of amino groups of aspartate and alanine to ketoglutaric acid. Also referred to as transaminases, their presence in serum is a marker of hepatocellular injury. While AST is present in the liver, cardiac tissue, skeletal muscle, kidney, and brain, ALT is primarily in the liver. Liver injury, whether acute or chronic, results in increases in the serum concentrations of the aminotransferase enzymes. The degree of elevation, rate of rise, and whether AST > ALT or ALT > AST are helpful in suggesting possible etiologies.

Transaminases will typically be severely elevated as a result of acute insults including conditions like acute viral hepatitis, autoimmune hepatitis, ischemic hepatitis/shock liver, acute Budd-Chiari syndrome, hepatic artery occlusion, diffuse infiltration of cancer into the liver, acute biliary obstruction, liver trauma, eclampsia, and Wilson disease. The highest elevations (>10,000 units per liter [167 μkat/L]) are most apt to occur in shock liver and drug- or toxin-induced hepatitis. Borderline and mild transaminase elevations are seen in a variety of liver and nonliver disease states.

The ratio of AST to ALT with AST>ALT is more likely when cirrhosis of any etiology exists but also occurs in alcoholic and ischemic liver disease. Seventy percent of patients with alcoholic liver disease had ratios greater than two and 92% of patients had ratios greater than one.[20]

Alkaline Phosphatase and γ-Glutamyl Transpeptidase

Elevated serum levels of alkaline phosphatase and GGT occur in cases of liver injury with a cholestatic pattern and therefore often accompany conditions such as primary biliary cirrhosis, primary sclerosing cholangitis, drug-induced cholestasis, and bile duct obstruction.[19] Alkaline phosphatase is not found solely in the liver. When elevations of alkaline phosphatase occur with subsequent elevations of transaminases, confirmation of hepatic origin is not needed. When alkaline phosphatase is elevated without other concurrent liver test abnormalities, the GGT is evaluated since combined elevations of both alkaline phosphatase and GGT levels increase clinical suspicion of hepatic etiology.

A mixed pattern liver injury is evidenced by elevations of both AST/ALT levels and alkaline phosphatase. An R ratio can be calculated in these cases which is achieved by utilization of the following formula: R = (ALT value/ALT upper limit of normal)/(alkaline phosphatase value/alkaline phosphatase upper limit of normal). An R ratio above 5 indicates hepatocellular injury. An R ratio below 2 indicates cholestatic disease. Ratios between 2 and 5 represent a mixed pattern.

Bilirubin

Bilirubin is the product of the breakdown of hemoglobin molecules.[19] Elevations in serum conjugated (or direct) bilirubin indicate hepatocellular dysfunction or cholestasis. When total bilirubin elevation exists, it should be fractionated into direct (conjugated) and indirect (unconjugated) levels. Indirect bilirubin elevations occur due to over-production (as seen with hemolysis), decreased uptake, or decreased hepatic conjugation of bilirubin and can be found in conditions like Gilbert's syndrome. Direct hyperbilirubinemia is the result of liver injury or biliary obstruction and is associated with a number of hepatic diseases including cirrhosis. When cirrhosis has been established, the degree of bilirubin elevation has prognostic significance and is used as a component of the Child-Pugh and MELD scoring systems for quantifying the severity of cirrhosis.[16,21]

Albumin and Coagulation Factors

Albumin and coagulation proteins are markers of hepatic synthetic activity and are therefore used to estimate the level of hepatic functioning in cirrhosis. Albumin and PT are used in the Child-Pugh system for quantifying liver disease, and the INR is used in the MELD scoring system as a marker of coagulation.[16,21] Reduction in albumin usually indicates a disease duration of more than 3 weeks whereas severe liver disease can cause PT elevation in less than 24 hours. These tests are not specific to liver disease as any significant illness can reduce albumin levels and the PT can be elevated for a variety of reasons including anticoagulation with warfarin, vitamin K deficiency, and steatorrhea.

Thrombocytopenia

Thrombocytopenia is a common feature of chronic liver disease.[15] The platelet count is rarely below 30,000/mm^3 to 40,000/mm^3 (30×10^9/L to 40×10^9/L) though. When liver abnormality is suspected, a complete blood cell count that includes platelets should be evaluated.

Child-Pugh Classification and Model for End-Stage Liver Disease Score

The Child-Pugh classification system has gained widespread acceptance as a means of quantifying the myriad of effects of the cirrhotic process on the laboratory and clinical manifestations of this disease.[16] Recommended drug dosing adjustments for patients in liver failure are normally based on the Child-Pugh score. The newer MELD-Na scoring system is now the accepted classification scheme used by the Organ Procurement and Transplantation United Network for Organ Sharing (OPTN/UNOS) in the allocation livers for transplantation.[17] The Child-Pugh classification system employs a combination of physical and laboratory findings (Table 55-2), whereas the MELD score calculation takes into account a patient's serum creatinine, bilirubin, INR, and etiology of liver disease, omitting the more subjective reports of ascites and encephalopathy used in the Child-Pugh system.

The MELD scoring calculation is as follows[21]:

$$\text{MELD score}^* = 9.57 \times \log_e(\text{creatinine [mg/dL]}) + 3.78 \times \log_e(\text{bilirubin [mg/dL]}) + 11.20 \times \log_e(\text{INR}) + 6.43$$

or using SI units:

$$\text{MELD score}^* = 9.57 \times \log_e(\text{creatinine [}\mu\text{mol/L]} \times 0.01131) + 3.78 \times \log_e(\text{bilirubin [}\mu\text{mol/L]} \times 0.05848) + 11.20 \times \log_e(\text{INR}) + 6.43$$

$$\text{MELD-Na score} = \text{MELD} - (\text{sodium [mEq/L]}) - (0.025 \times \text{MELD} \times (140 - \text{sodium [mEq/L]})) + 140$$

or using SI units:

$$\text{MELD-Na score} = \text{MELD} - (\text{sodium [mmol/L]}) - (0.025 \times \text{MELD} \times (140 - \text{sodium [mmol/L]})) + 140$$

These classification systems are important because they are used to assess and define the severity of cirrhosis, and predict patient survival, surgical outcome, and risk of variceal bleeding.

Imaging and Biopsy

Ultrasound technology can be used to detect more advanced cirrhosis as well as to evaluate the presence of portal hypertension and ascites. A liver in the stage of advanced cirrhosis will appear nodular on ultrasound.[18] Ultrasound may also be used to evaluate the presence of portal hypertension and ascites. Elastography via ultrasound or magnetic resonance may be useful in early cirrhosis or when other imaging is not definitive. Sometimes a liver biopsy is required when less invasive testing is inconclusive or when the results of biopsy may dictate the most appropriate management for the patient.

TREATMENT

General Approaches to Treatment

General approaches to therapy in cirrhosis should include the following:

1. Identify and eliminate, where possible, the causes of cirrhosis (eg, alcohol misuse).
2. Assess the risk for variceal bleeding and begin pharmacologic prophylaxis when indicated. Prophylactic endoscopic therapy can be used for patients with high-risk medium and large varices as well as in patients with contraindications or intolerance to nonselective β-adrenergic blockers. Endoscopic therapy is also appropriate for patients suffering acute bleeding episodes. Variceal obliteration with endoscopic techniques in conjunction with pharmacologic intervention is the recommended treatment of choice in patients with acute bleeding.
3. Evaluate the patient for clinical signs of ascites and manage with pharmacologic therapy (eg, diuretics) and paracentesis. Careful monitoring for SBP should be used in patients with ascites who experience acute deterioration of their clinical status.

TABLE 55-2 Criteria and Scoring for the Child-Pugh Grading of Chronic Liver Disease

Score	1	2	3
Total bilirubin (mg/dL)	<2 (34.2 μmol/L)	2-3 (34.2-51.3 μmol/L)	>3 (51.3 μmol/L)
Albumin (g/dL)	>3.5 (35 g/L)	2.8-3.5 (28-35 g/L)	<2.8 (28 g/L)
Ascites	None	Mild	Moderate
Encephalopathy (grade)	None	1 and 2	3 and 4
Prothrombin time (seconds prolonged)	<4	4-6	>6

Grade A, <7 points; grade B, 7-9 points; grade C, 10-15 points.

Data from Reference 16.

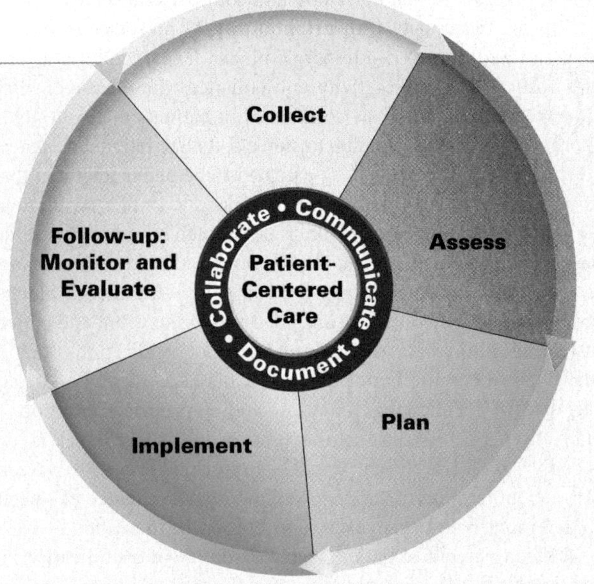

Patient Care Process for Cirrhosis

The image shows the five fundamental steps included in The Pharmacist's Care Process endorsed by the Joint Commission for Pharmacy Practitioners (2014). The tagline of this process reads collaborate, communicate, and document. The five fundamental steps listed here are collect, assess, plan, implement, and follow-up: monitor and evaluate. All these steps are listed in a circular block diagram.

Collect

- Patient medical history
  - Recent history of anorexia or weight loss
  - Risk factors for hepatitis B and C
  - Personal and family history of autoimmune or hepatic diseases
- Social history (specifically ethanol use—quantity and duration)
- Current medications including nonprescription medications
- Objective data
  - Blood pressure (BP), heart rate (HR), respiratory rate (RR), height, weight, O_2-saturation
  - Laboratory findings including albumin, bilirubin, complete blood count (CBC) with platelets, prothrombin time (PT), international normalized ratio (INR), alkaline phosphatase, aspartate transaminase (AST), alanine transaminase (ALT), gamma-glutamyl transpeptidase (GGT)

Assess

- Presence of jaundice, palmar erythema, and spider nevi
- Presence of medications that can cause cirrhosis (see Table 55-1)
- Presence of complications of cirrhosis (ascites, portal hypertension, esophageal varices, hepatic encephalopathy, coagulation disorders)
- Child-Pugh score (see Table 55-2) for need for medication dosage adjustments
- Patient's willingness to stop drinking alcohol

Plan*

- Identify and treat possible causes of cirrhosis (ie, hepatitis C)
- Remove offending medications that may cause or exacerbate cirrhosis or complications of cirrhosis
- Create a plan to treat acute complications of cirrhosis, if present
  - Ascites: sodium restriction and furosemide + spironolactone (see Table 55-3)
  - Portal hypertension
    Primary prevention of esophageal varices: beta-blocker (nadolol, propranolol, or carvedilol) and/or EVL for prevention
    Treatment of acute variceal bleeding: octreotide + EVL, SBP prophylaxis (eg, ceftriaxone) × 7 days (see Fig. 55-4 and Table 55-4)
    Secondary prevention: nadolol or propranolol + EVL
  - Spontaneous bacterial peritonitis
    Treatment: empiric antibiotic therapy with appropriate antibiotic (eg, cefotaxime) based on ascitic fluid PMN count and/or symptoms (see Table 55-3)
    Secondary prevention: ciprofloxacin daily (see Table 55-3)
  - Hepatic encephalopathy: dietary protein restriction and lactulose +/− rifaximin

Implement

- Provide patient education and assistance for achieving abstinence from alcohol, if applicable
- Discuss all elements of treatment plan (medications and dietary modifications) with patient
- Provide vaccines as indicated
- Adjust medication doses as needed based on major organ function and patient characteristics
- Plan to assess progress of treatment including efficacy and adverse effects of treatments (see Table 55-5)

Follow-up: Monitor and Evaluate

- Monitor for long-term efficacy and adverse effects
- Patient's adherence to alcohol abstinence, prescribed medications, and dietary modifications
- Resolution of complications of cirrhosis
- Evaluate for possibility of liver transplant and need for dietitian (ie, sodium and protein restriction)

Collaborate with patient, caregivers, and other healthcare professionals.

4. Recognize that HE is a common complication of cirrhosis that requires clinical vigilance and treatment with dietary restriction, elimination of precipitating factors, and therapy to lower ammonia levels.
5. Monitor patients for signs of hepatorenal syndrome, pulmonary insufficiency, and endocrine dysfunction.

Desired Outcomes

Portal hypertension and cirrhosis can be classified as compensated versus decompensated.[23] In compensated portal hypertension, though HVPG may be elevated and varices may be present, the patient does not experience complications of cirrhosis such as variceal bleeding, ascites, SBP, or encephalopathy. The desired therapeutic outcomes during the compensated stage include *prevention of complications* through therapeutic modalities such as lowering of portal pressure with medical therapy using nonselective β-adrenergic blocker therapy and supporting abstinence from alcohol. In patients with decompensated cirrhosis, *resolution of acute complications* becomes the desired therapeutic outcome. Treatment modalities and therapeutic goals are presented below for each of the primary complications of decompensated portal hypertension. Recommended therapies and therapeutic goals are discussed.

Management of Portal Hypertension and Variceal Bleeding

The management of varices involves three strategies: (a) primary prophylaxis (prevention of the first bleeding episode), (b) treatment of acute variceal hemorrhage, and (c) secondary prophylaxis (prevention of rebleeding in patients who have previously bled).[11] It is also possible for a patient to have been diagnosed with cirrhosis and portal hypertension but have no varices. These patients would be considered to be in a preprimary prophylaxis stage. No specific treatment is recommended for preprimary prophylaxis and, for that reason, the focus of this chapter will be primary prophylaxis, treatment of acute variceal bleeding, and secondary prophylaxis.

Primary Prophylaxis

β-Adrenergic Blockade The mainstay of primary prophylaxis is the use of nonselective β-adrenergic blocking agents such as propranolol, nadolol, or carvedilol.[11,12,23] These agents reduce portal pressure by reducing portal venous inflow via two mechanisms: a decrease in cardiac output through β_1-adrenergic blockade and a decrease in splanchnic blood flow through β_2-adrenergic blockade that results in unopposed α-1 activity.[11]

Endoscopic Variceal Ligation (EVL) Endoscopic variceal ligation is an endoscopic therapy that consists of placing rubber bands around varices until the varices are obliterated.

Treatment Recommendations: Variceal Bleeding—Primary Prophylaxis

2 All patients with cirrhosis should be screened for varices at the time of diagnosis.[11,12] Transient elastography that shows liver stiffness below 20 kPa in patients with platelets over 150,000/mm^3 (150 × 10^9/L) do not require screening endoscopy.[12,23] Others should undergo screening endoscopy to identify and evaluate varices. β-Adrenergic blocker therapy is not indicated in patients without varices to prevent the formation of varices.[11,12,23] Patients with small varices plus risk factors for variceal hemorrhage including red wale marks or Child-Pugh grade C should receive prophylactic therapy with a nonselective β-adrenergic blocker. β-Adrenergic blocker therapy is recommended preferentially to EVL in this situation due to the technical difficulty of EVL in the treatment of small varices. β-Adrenergic blocker therapy is optional for patients with small varices in the absence of risk factors, but additional studies to confirm benefit in this population are needed. All patients found to have medium to large varices that have not bled should receive primary prophylaxis therapy with a nonselective β-adrenergic blocker or EVL. The choice of treatment should be based on a consideration of resources and expertise as well as patient preferences and characteristics with a particular emphasis on side effects and contraindications.[12] If β-adrenergic blocker therapy is chosen, initiate therapy with oral propranolol 20 to 40 mg twice daily or nadolol 20 to 40 mg once daily and titrate every 2 to 3 days to a resting heart rate of 55 to 60 beats/min.[23] The daily dose of propranolol should not exceed 320 mg for patients without ascites or 160 mg for patients with ascites. The maximum daily dose of nadolol should not exceed 160 mg for patients without ascites or 80 mg for those with ascites. Systolic blood pressure should be maintained above 90 mm Hg. Rather than propranolol or nadolol, carvedilol could be chosen and started at 3.125 mg twice daily with titration to 6.25 mg twice daily after 3 days. In addition to β-adrenergic blockade, carvedilol also provides anti-α-adrenergic activity and enhances the release of nitric oxide.[24,25] Carvedilol may be considered in patients unable to tolerate propranolol or nadolol due to side effects like fatigue, weakness, and shortness of breath as it is perceived to be better tolerated than the pure nonselective β-adrenergic blockers.[23] Unlike propranolol and nadolol, titration of carvedilol is not guided by resting heart rate measurement, though systolic blood pressure should be maintained above 90 mm Hg while on carvedilol as well. β-Adrenergic blocker therapy should generally be continued indefinitely, but the patient must be monitored for development of contraindications such as renal impairment and hypotension that may accompany end-stage liver disease.[12] Following initiation and appropriate titration of the β-adrenergic blocker, further endoscopic surveillance is not needed.[11,23] If EVL is chosen, it will be performed every 2 to 8 weeks until the obliteration of varices.[23] Follow-up surveillance will occur at 3 to 6 months and again every 6 to 12 months thereafter.

Fifteen percent of patients have absolute contraindications to nonselective β-adrenergic blockers (ie, those with asthma or those with hypoglycemia unawareness while receiving antihyperglycemic therapy) and another 15% have common side effects such as fatigue, weakness, and shortness of breath that contribute to medication nonadherence.[11] Patients who qualify for β-adrenergic blocker therapy as primary prophylaxis, but who are unable to take or continue it, should be considered for alternative therapy with EVL.[12,23] Also, EVL may be considered as a possible first option for primary prophylaxis in patients with high-risk medium to large varices.

Acute Variceal Hemorrhage

Variceal hemorrhage is a medical emergency that carries a mortality rate of 7% to 15%, requires admission to an intensive care unit, and is one of the most feared complications of cirrhosis.[11] Treatment of acute variceal bleeding includes general stabilizing and assessment measures as well as specific measures to control the acute hemorrhage and prevent complications.

Initial treatment goals include (a) adequate blood volume resuscitation, (b) protection of airway from aspiration of blood, (c) prophylaxis against SBP and other infections, (d) control of bleeding, (e) prevention of re-bleeding, (f) preservation of liver function/prevention of HE, and (g) prevention of acute kidney injury.[25] Prompt stabilization of blood volume, with administration of packed red blood cells at a hemoglobin threshold of 7 g/dL (70 g/L; 4.34 mmol/L) and a goal hemoglobin of 7 g/dL (70 g/L; 4.34 mmol/L) to 9 g/dL (90 g/L; 5.59 mmol/L), should be undertaken.[22] Use of recombinant factor VIIa therapy is not recommended in patients with cirrhosis with GI hemorrhage.[11,23] Combination pharmacologic therapy plus endoscopic therapy with EVL (preferred), or sclerotherapy if EVL is not technically feasible, is considered the most rational approach to the treatment of acute variceal bleeding.[11,23,25] Endoscopy should be performed as soon as possible, but at least within 12 hours of admission.

Vasoactive drug therapy is used to stop or slow bleeding as soon as a diagnosis of variceal bleeding is suspected and is started before endoscopy.[11,23] The vasoactive drug used to manage acute variceal bleeding in the United States is the somatostatin analogue octreotide. Antibiotic therapy to prevent SBP and other infections should be implemented upon admission.[12] Intravenous ceftriaxone 1 g/24 hours is recommended.[12,23] A 250 mg dose of intravenous erythromycin prior to endoscopy may be used to accelerate gastric emptying of clots and improve visibility during the endoscopic procedure.[12,25] Should episodic HE occur secondary to acute GI bleeding, lactulose may be utilized. Figure 55-4 presents an algorithm for the management of variceal hemorrhage.

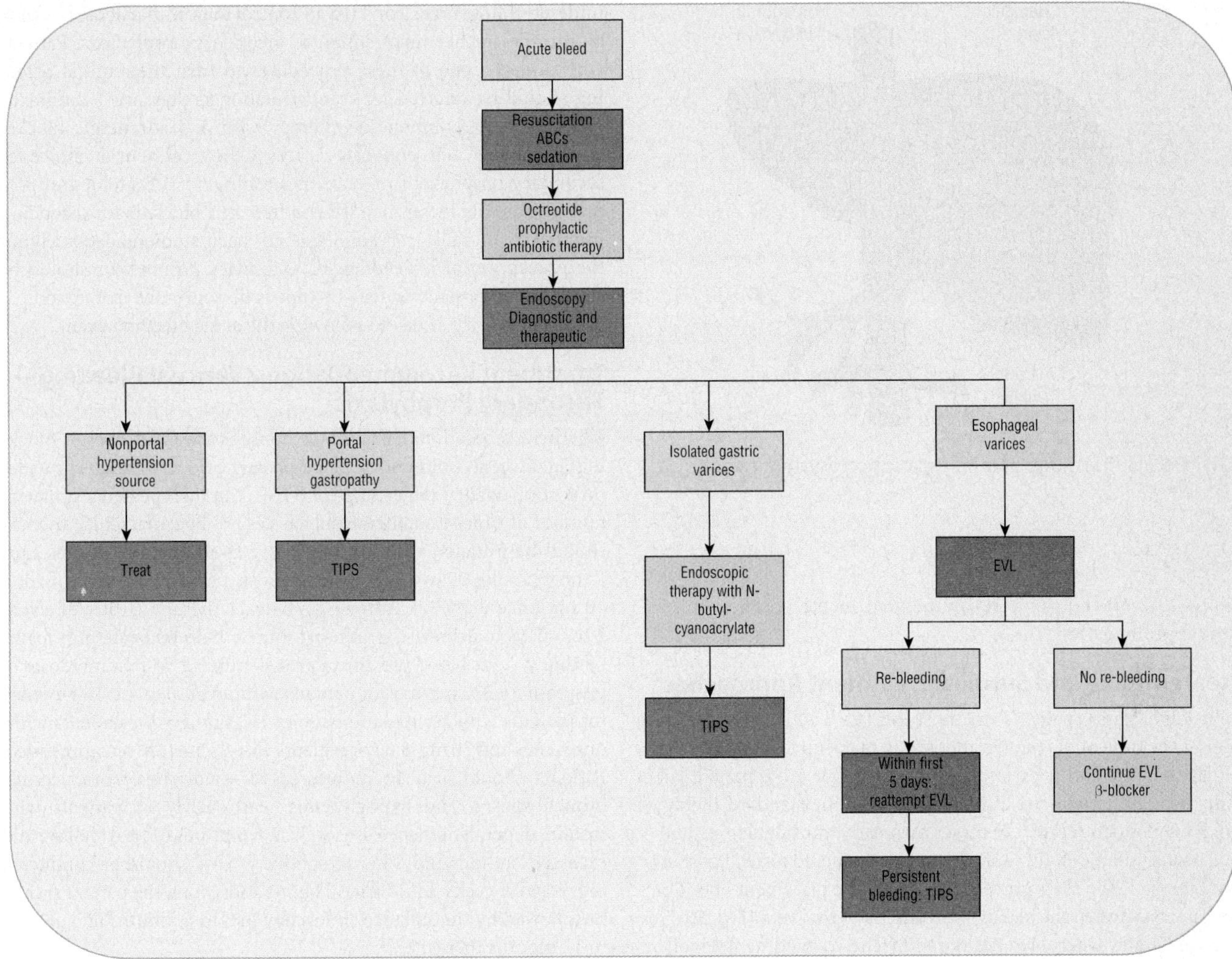

FIGURE 55-4 Management of acute variceal hemorrhage. (ABCs, Airway Breathing Circulation; EVL, endoscopic variceal ligation; TIPS, transjugular intrahepatic portosystemic shunt.)

Octreotide

The splanchnic vasoconstriction from octreotide therapy is due to inhibition of the release of vasodilatory peptides such as glucagon; however, a local vasoconstrictive effect also exists.[26] Somatostatin analogues, including octreotide, are associated with fewer side effects as compared with the most potent splanchnic vasoconstrictor, vasopressin. The primary side effects of octreotide therapy are hyperglycemia, vomiting, bradycardia, hypertension, arrhythmia, and abdominal pain.[11,25] The recommended dosing of octreotide for variceal bleeding consists of an initial IV bolus of 50 μg followed by a continuous IV infusion of 50 μg/h.[11,23] Octreotide can be continued for 2 to 5 days after acute variceal bleeding in an effort to prevent re-bleeding. Vasoactive therapy discontinuation can be considered once the patient is free of bleeding for at least 24 hours.

Prevention of Spontaneous Bacterial Peritonitis

Patients with cirrhosis with active bleeding are at high risk of severe bacterial infections.[23] Short-term prophylactic antibiotic therapy to reduce the risk of infection during episodes of bleeding not only reduces the likelihood of infections but also reduces the incidence of rebleeding and increases survival.[27] For these reasons, a short course (7 days maximum) of IV ceftriaxone 1 g daily is recommended.[12,27,28] Oral norfloxacin was once recommended as an alternative to IV ceftriaxone in cases where the patient had not been previously receiving quinolone therapy and when the prevalence of quinolone-resistant bacteria was low, but norfloxacin is no longer available.[23] Oral ciprofloxacin could be considereded instead, but ceftriaxone is typically used today and is preferred in patients with advanced cirrhosis, in areas of high quinolone resistance, and in patients who have received quinolone therapy for ongoing SBP prophylaxis.

Endoscopic Interventions: Sclerotherapy and Band Ligation

Guidelines recommend that endoscopy be performed within 12 hours of admission in cases of upper GI bleeding.[12,23] Endoscopy is used to diagnose variceal bleeding, and endoscopic techniques, particularly EVL, are used to stop variceal bleeding. EVL can be repeated if hemorrhage is not controlled or in the event of early recurrence of bleeding (within the first 5 days).[12] EVL is more effective than sclerotherapy with greater control of hemorrhage, less risk for rebleeding, lower likelihood of adverse events, and lower mortality.[11] Consensus recommendation calls for EVL (in conjunction with pharmacologic therapy) as the recommended form of endoscopic therapy for acute variceal bleeding.[12] Endoscopic injection of the tissue adhesive *N*-butyl cyanoacrylate is recommended to control acute *gastric* variceal bleeding from isolated gastric varices and gastroesophageal varices type 2 that extend beyond the cardia. EVL or tissue adhesive can be used for bleeding from gastroesophageal varices type 1. A pre-endoscopy infusion of erythromycin 250 mg IV, 30 to 120 minutes

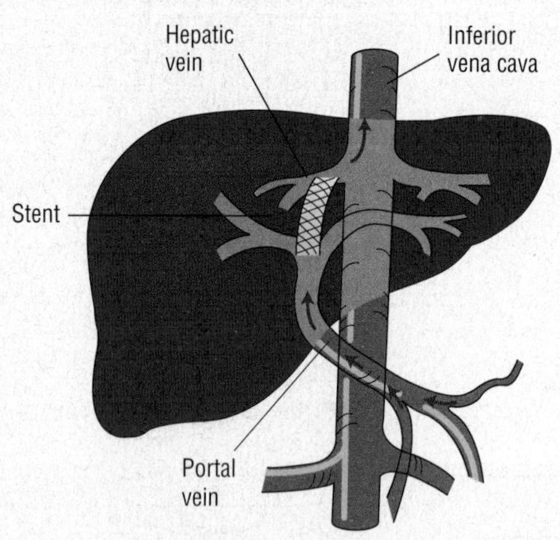

FIGURE 55-5 Transjugular intrahepatic portosystemic shunt.

prior to the procedure, is recommended in the absence of QT interval prolongation.

Interventional and Surgical Treatment Approaches

Child-Pugh Class C patients and those in Class B with active hemorrhage at the time of diagnostic endoscopy make up less than 20% of patients admitted with variceal hemorrhage, but these patients do comprise a group who are at high risk for failing standard therapy with EVL plus octreotide.[11] In these cases, early transjugular intrahepatic portosystemic shunt (TIPS) may be considered instead of standard therapy.[23] The TIPS procedure involves the placement of one or more stents between the hepatic vein and the portal vein (Fig. 55-5). TIPS (preferably with polytetrafluoroethylene-covered stents) is also recommended for patients who fail to achieve or maintain hemostasis despite combined endoscopic and pharmacologic therapy.[23]

Balloon tamponade may be used as a bridge therapy to control variceal bleeding temporarily (maximum of 24 hours).[12,23] It should be reserved as a temporizing measure until a more definitive treatment, such as TIPS, can be performed.

Treatment Recommendations: Variceal Hemorrhage

4 Patients require cautious resuscitation with blood products to correct intravascular losses.[23] Drug therapy with octreotide should be initiated early to control bleeding and facilitate diagnostic and therapeutic endoscopy. Therapy is initiated with an IV bolus of 50 μg and is followed by a continuous infusion of 50 μg/hr for 2 to 5 days.[11,23] Patients should be monitored for bradycardia, hypertension, arrhythmia, and abdominal pain.[11,25] Endoscopy is recommended in any patient with suspected upper GI bleeding due to ruptured varices.[12,23] EVL is the recommended form of endoscopic therapy. An additional endoscopic therapy option is injection of the tissue adhesive *N*-butyl cyanoacrylate for gastric varices.[12] Short-term antibiotic prophylaxis (maximum 7 days) is recommended.[12,23] Ceftriaxone 1 g IV daily is the preferred antibiotic selection for this indication.[23] Surgical procedures like TIPS are employed as salvage therapy in patients who have failed repeated endoscopy and vasoactive drug therapy.[12,23] In patients at highest risk for standard treatment failure, a preemptive decision to utilize early TIPS may occur.

Secondary Prophylaxis

Because rebleeding after initial control of variceal hemorrhage occurs in a median of 60% of patients, and because rebleedingg carries a mortality rate of 33%, it is inappropriate to simply observe patients for evidence of further bleeding.[11,23] Only patients who undergo shunt surgery or TIPS to control their initial acute bleeding require no further intervention as secondary prophylaxis. Patients who undergo one of these procedures to treat their initial bleeding should be referred for transplantation if they are a candidate. For all others, combination therapy with a β-adrenergic blocker and chronic EVL to eradicate varices is the treatment of choice for secondary prophylaxis of variceal bleeding.[11,12,23] Nadolol and propranolol are the recommended β-adrenergic blockers for secondary prophylaxis because carvedilol has not been studied adequately for the prevention of rebleeding.[12,23] Secondary prophylaxis should be started once vasoactive drug therapy is discontinued and as soon as possible (as early as day 6) following the acute bleeding event.[11]

Treatment Recommendations: Variceal Bleeding—Secondary Prophylaxis

3 The combination of EVL and a nonselective β-adrenergic blocking agent is recommended since pharmacologic therapy provides protection against rebleeding until EVL can be repeated a sufficient number of times to obliterate all varices.[11,23] Pharmacologic therapy should be initiated with a nonselective β-adrenergic blocker such as propranolol 20 to 40 mg twice daily or nadolol at a dose of 20 to 40 mg once daily.[23] β-Adrenergic blocker therapy is titrated every 2 to 3 days to achieve a goal heart rate of 55 to 60 beats/min maintaining systolic blood pressure above 90 mm Hg. Maximum doses of propranolol 320 mg/day for patients without ascites and 160 mg/day for patients with ascites, and nadolol 160 mg/day for patients without ascites and 80 mg/day for patients with ascites are recommended. Patients should also be monitored for evidence of bradycardia, bronchospasm, and hypoglycemia, particularly in patients with insulin-dependent diabetes, as well as symptoms of heart failure and excessive sodium and water retention.[11,24] EVL should be conducted every 1 to 4 weeks until variceal obliteration, then the patient should be followed by surveillance endoscopy in 3 to 6 months and every 6 to 12 months thereafter.[23]

The addition of isosorbide mononitrate to nonselective β-adrenergic blocker therapy reduces portal pressure more than a β-adrenergic blocker alone, but there is no difference in the overall rate of rebleeding with this combination and side effects are more likely than with β-adrenergic blocker monotherapy (namely, headache and light-headedness).[23] Pharmacologic therapy (either isosorbide mononitrate plus nonselective β-adrenergic blocker therapy or β-adrenergic blocker therapy alone) plus EVL is associated with lower rebleeding rates than EVL therapy alone, but is only moderately more effective than isosorbide mononitrate plus nonselective β-adrenergic blocker therapy.[29] Thus, drug therapy is considered the cornerstone for secondary prophylaxis against variceal bleeding and patients who cannot tolerate nonselective β-adrenergic blocker therapy should be considered for TIPS.[23]

The lowest rate of variceal rebleeding occurs in patients when pharmacologic therapy leads to a reduction in HVPG of greater than 20% of baseline or to a measurement less than 12 mm Hg (1.6 kPa).[23] Ideally, portal pressure monitoring would be used to assess the response to nonselective β-adrenergic blocker therapy and identify responders from nonresponders earlier in the treatment course.

There is ongoing debate regarding the use of β-adrenergic blockers for prophylaxis against variceal bleeding in patients with refractory ascites.[24] The Baveno VI Consensus statement recommends reduction or temporary discontinuation of β-adrenergic blockers in patients receiving secondary prophylaxis with systolic blood pressure <90 mm Hg, serum sodium <130 mEq/L (mmol/L), or acute kidney injury.[12] This recommendation assumes that other precipitating drug therapies have already been removed. Reinitiation of β-adrenergic blocker therapy can be considered if the patient's circulatory dysfunction improves. A summary of evidence-based treatment recommendations regarding portal hypertension and variceal bleeding is presented in Table 55-4.

TABLE 55-3 Evidence-Based Table of Selected Treatment Recommendations: Ascites and Spontaneous Bacterial Peritonitis

Recommendation	Grade
Ascites	
Paracentesis should be performed in patients with apparent new-onset ascites	IC
Sodium restriction of 2,000 mg/day should be instituted as well as oral diuretic therapy with spironolactone and furosemide	IIaA
Diuretic-sensitive patients should be treated with sodium restriction and diuretics rather than serial paracentesis	IIaC
Refractory ascites	
Serial therapeutic paracenteses may be performed	IC
Postparacentesis albumin infusion of 6-8 g/L of fluid removed can be considered if more than 5 L is removed during paracentesis	IIaA
Treatment of SBP	
If ascitic fluid PMN counts are >250 cells/mm^3 (0.25 × 10^9/L), empiric antibiotic therapy should be instituted (cefotaxime 2 g every 8 hours)	IA
If ascitic fluid PMN counts are <250 cells/mm^3 (0.25 × 10^9/L), but signs or symptoms of infection exist, empiric antibiotic therapy should be initiated while awaiting culture results	IB
If ascitic fluid polymorphonuclear leukocyte counts are >250 cells/mm^3 (0.25 × 10^9/L), clinical suspicion of SBP is present, and the patient has a serum creatinine >1 mg/dL (88 μmol/L), blood urea nitrogen >30 mg/dL (10.7 mmol/L), or total bilirubin over 4 mg/dL (68.4 μmol/L), 1.5 g/kg albumin should be infused within 6 hours of detection and 1 g/kg albumin infusion should also be given on day 3	IIaB
Prophylaxis against SBP	
Short-term antibiotic prophylaxis should be used for 7 days to prevent SBP in cirrhosis patients with GI hemorrhage	IA
Patients who survive an episode of SBP should receive long-term prophylaxis with ciprofloxacin	IA
Patients with low-protein ascites (<1.5 g/dL [15 g/L]) plus at least one of the following: serum creatinine ≥1.2 mg/dL (106 μmol/L), blood urea nitrogen ≥25 mg/dL (8.9 mmol/L), serum sodium ≤ 130 mEq/L (mmol/L), or Child-Pugh score of ≥9 with bilirubin ≥3 mg/dL (51.3 μmol/L) may also justifiably receive long-term ciprofloxacin as prophylaxis	IA

Recommendation grading: Class I—Conditions for which there is evidence and/or general agreement; Class II—Conditions for which there is conflicting evidence and/or a divergence of opinion; Class IIa—Weight of evidence/opinion is in favor of efficacy; Class IIb—Efficacy less well established; Class III—Conditions for which there is evidence and/or general agreement that treatment is not effective and/or potentially harmful; Level A—Data from multiple randomized trials or meta-analyses; Level B—Data derived from single randomized trial or nonrandomized studies; Level C—Only consensus opinion, case studies, or standard of care.

Data from Reference 22.

TABLE 55-4 Evidence-Based Table of Selected Treatment Recommendations: Variceal Bleeding in Portal Hypertension

Recommendation	Grade
Prevention of variceal bleeding	
Nonselective β-blocker therapy should be initiated in:	
Patients with small varices and criteria for increased risk of hemorrhage	1b
Patients with medium/large varices	1a
EVL may be recommended for prevention in patients with medium/large varices at high risk of hemorrhage instead of nonselective β-blocker therapy	1a
Treatment of variceal bleeding	
Short-term antibiotic prophylaxis should be instituted on admission	1a
Vasoactive drugs should be started as soon as possible, prior to endoscopy, and maintained for up to 5 days	1a
Endoscopy should be performed to diagnose variceal bleeding and treat bleeding with EVL	1b
Endoscopy should be performed within 12 hours of presentation	5
Unless contraindicated, erythromycin 250 mg IV should be administered 30-120 minutes prior to endoscopy	1b
Secondary prophylaxis of variceal bleeding	
Nonselective β-blocker therapy plus EVL is the best therapeutic option for prevention of recurrent variceal bleeding	1a

Recommendation grading:

1a Systematic review (with homogeneity) of randomized controlled trials

1b Individual randomized controlled trial with narrow confidence interval

1c All or none

2a Systematic review (with homogeneity) of cohort studies

2b Individual cohort study (including low-quality randomized controlled trial)

2c Outcomes research; ecological studies

3a Systematic review (with homogeneity) of case-controlled studies

3b Individual case-control study

4 Case-series (and poor quality cohort and case-control studies)

5 Expert opinion

Data from Reference 12.

Management of Ascites and Spontaneous Bacterial Peritonitis

Ascites is the most common first sign of decompensation in patients with cirrhosis and represents a clinically important milestone in the natural progression of the disease.[10] The classic physical examination findings of ascites are a bulging abdomen with shifting flank dullness.[9,22] The development of ascites in patients with cirrhosis is an indication of advanced liver disease and is a poor prognostic sign.[10] Workup includes a history and physical examination, abdominal paracentesis and/or ultrasound, and ascitic fluid analysis.[9,22]

Spontaneous bacterial peritonitis is an infection of ascitic fluid that occurs in the absence of any evidence of an intraabdominal, surgically treatable source of infection. It is a common complication that develops in 1.5% to 3.5% of outpatients with cirrhosis and 10% of inpatients with cirrhosis.[9] The altered intestinal permeability and resultant bacterial translocation, in addition to changes in intestinal microbiota and immune system dysfunction place these patients at risk for developing SBP.[30] Most episodes of SBP have traditionally been caused by *Escherichia coli, Klebsiella pneumonia*, and pneumococci.[22] Concerns over quinolone-resistant bacteria and multidrug-resistant organisms have been recognized in clinical guidelines.[31] Symptoms and signs of SBP include abdominal pain, diarrhea, vomiting, and nonspecific symptoms, and patients may be asymptomatic.[32] Diagnostic paracentesis with analysis of ascitic fluid should be performed in all patients newly diagnosed with ascites.[9,22] SBP is diagnosed when there is positive ascitic fluid bacterial culture and ascitic fluid cell counts show an absolute polymorphonuclear (PMN) leukocyte count of greater than or equal to 250 cells/mm^3 (0.25 × 10^9/L).

Treatment guidelines for the management of adult patients with ascites and SBP were updated and approved by the Practice Guidelines Committee of the American Association for the Study of Liver Diseases (AASLD) in 2012.[22] The European Association for the Study of the Liver (EASL) published ascites guidelines in 2018. A synopsis of these guidelines follows.[31]

Ascites

In adult patients with new-onset ascites as determined by physical examination or radiographic studies, abdominal paracentesis should

TABLE 55-5 Drug Monitoring Guidelines

Drug	Adverse Drug Reaction	Monitoring Parameter	Comments
Nonselective β-adrenergic blocker	Heart failure, bronchospasm, glucose intolerance	BP, HR Goal BP: Sytolic >90 mm Hg Goal HR: 55-60 beats/min or maximal tolerated dose	Nadolol, propranolol
Nonselective β-adrenergic blocker; alpha-blocker	Similar to nonselective β-adrenergic blocker, but potentially better tolerated	Goal BP: Sytolic > 90 mm Hg	Carvedilol
Octreotide	Bradycardia, hypertension, arrhythmia, abdominal pain	BP, HR, EKG, abdominal pain	
Spironolactone/furosemide	Electrolyte disturbances, dehydration, renal insufficiency, hypotension	Serum electrolytes (especially potassium), SCr, blood urea nitrogen, BP Goal sodium excretion: >78 mmol/day	Spot urine sodium concentration greater than potassium concentration correlates well with daily sodium excretion >78 mmol/day
Lactulose	Electrolyte disturbances	Serum electrolytes Goal number of soft stools per day: 2-3	
Neomycin	Ototoxicity, nephrotoxicity	SCr, annual auditory monitoring	
Metronidazole	Neurotoxicity	Sensory and motor neuropathy	
Rifaximin	Nausea, diarrhea		

BP, blood pressure; HR, heart rate; beats/min, beats per minute; EKG, electrocardiogram; SCr, serum creatinine; mmol, millimole.

be performed, and ascitic fluid analysis should include a cell count with differential, ascitic fluid total protein, and a serum-ascites albumin gradient (SAAG).[22] If infection is suspected, ascitic fluid cultures should be obtained at the time of the paracentesis. The SAAG can accurately determine whether ascites is a result of portal hypertension or another process. If the SAAG is greater than or equal to 1.1 g/dL (11 g/L), the patient almost certainly has portal hypertension. The treatment of ascites secondary to portal hypertension is relatively straightforward and includes abstinence from alcohol, sodium restriction, and diuretics.

1 Abstinence from alcohol is an essential element of the overall treatment strategy. Abstinence from alcohol can result in improvement of the reversible component of alcoholic liver disease, resolution of ascites, or improved responsiveness of ascites to medical therapy. Patients with cirrhosis not caused by alcohol have less reversible liver disease, and, by the time ascites is present, these patients may be best managed with liver transplantation rather than protracted medical therapy.

Beyond avoidance of alcohol, the primary treatment of ascites due to portal hypertension and cirrhosis is sodium restriction to 2,000 mg/day and oral diuretic therapy. Fluid loss and weight change depend directly on sodium balance in these patients. A goal of therapy is to increase urinary excretion of sodium to greater than 78 mmol/day. Evaluation of urinary sodium excretion, preferably utilizing a 24-hour urine collection, may be helpful, although this collection can be difficult. A random spot urine sodium concentration that is greater than the potassium concentration correlates well with a 24-hour urinary sodium excretion over 78 mmol/day and is an easier test to complete. Severe hyponatremia, defined as serum sodium less than a threshold of 120 mEq/L (mmol/L), does warrant fluid restriction. However, hyponatremia of this severity is rare among patients with cirrhosis and ascites and, for this reason, rarely requires specific treatment.

Diuretic Therapy 5 The AASLD practice guidelines recommend that diuretic therapy be initiated with the combination of spironolactone 100 mg and furosemide 40 mg by mouth daily in the morning, titrated every 3 to 5 days utilizing a ratio of 100:40 to attain adequate natriuresis and weight loss (reasonable daily weight loss goal is 0.5 kg). Maximum daily doses are 400 mg spironolactone and 160 mg furosemide. The EASL guidelines recommend initiation of diuretic therapy with spironolactone alone for the first occurrence of ascites with titration every 3 days to a maximum of 400 mg daily.[31] Subsequent addition of furosemide is recommended by the EASL in those with insufficient weight loss, hyperkalemia, or longstanding or recurring ascites. Due to the likelihood for development of drug-induced hyperkalemia with spironolactone when used as monotherapy at doses sufficient to illicit a sufficient diuresis, combination therapy is most typically employed in this country, except in patients with minimal fluid overload.[29] Furosemide as lone diuretic therapy is inferior to spironolactone in the treatment of ascites and is not recommended. Serum potassium and renal function should be monitored frequently and rapid correction of asymptomatic hyponatremia in patients with cirrhosis should be avoided. Diuretic therapy should be discontinued in patients who experience uncontrolled or recurrent encephalopathy, severe hyponatremia (serum sodium <120 mEq/L [mmol/L]) despite fluid restriction, or renal insufficiency (serum creatinine >2 mg/dL [177 μmol/L]).

If tense ascites is present, paracentesis should be performed prior to institution of diuretic therapy and salt restriction. For patients who respond to diuretic therapy, this approach is preferred over the use of serial paracenteses. In patients with refractory ascites, serial paracenteses may be employed. Albumin infusion of 6 to 8 g for each liter of ascitic fluid removed can be considered post-paracentesis when more than 5 L of ascitic fluid is removed from the patient. Referral for liver transplantation should be made in patients with refractory ascites. TIPS is a therapeutic modality for the treatment of refractory ascites that may be considered in appropriately selected patients. Peritoneovenous shunting may be considered in treatment-refractory patients who are not candidates for paracenteses, transplant, or TIPS.

Patients with cirrhosis and ascites should avoid nonsteroidal anti-inflammatory drugs, angiotensin converting enzyme inhibitors, and angiotensin receptor blockers except under special circumstances. Angiotensin converting enzyme inhibitors and angiotensin receptor blockers should not be used in patients with refractory ascites. While these therapies are not part of the standard therapies of the complications of cirrhosis, nonselective β-adrenergic blocker therapy is indicated for primary and secondary prophylaxis against variceal bleeding in portal hypertension. Unfortunately, nonselective β-adrenergic blocker therapy can cause hypotension in patients with refractory ascites making the condition worse. For this reason, the risks versus benefits of nonselective β-adrenergic blocker therapy in refractory ascites must be carefully weighed, and nonselective β-adrenergic blockers avoided or not started in this population unless the benefit of bleeding prophylaxis outweighs the risk of worsening ascites. The daily dose of propranolol should not exceed 160 mg for patients with ascites.[22] The maximum daily dose of nadolol should not exceed 80 mg for those with ascites. Systolic blood pressure should be maintained above 90 mm Hg.

Spontaneous Bacterial Peritonitis

Relatively broad-spectrum antibiotic therapy that adequately covers the most commonly encountered pathogens (*E. coli, K. pneumoniae*, and pneumococci) has been recommended in patients with documented or suspected SBP.[22] Patients with ascitic fluid PMN counts greater than or equal to 250 cells/mm^3 (0.25×10^9/L) should receive empiric antibiotic therapy.[22,31] The AASLD guidelines specify IV cefotaxime 2 g every 8 hours or a similar third-generation cephalosporin.[22] The EASL guidelines recommend a third-generation cephalosporin (eg, cefotaxime or ceftriaxone) or piperacillin/tazobactam when SBP is community-acquired (ie, when diagnosed at time of admission or within 48 hours of admission).[30,31] Piperacillin/tazobactam is recommended in areas of low MDRO rates for patients without sepsis who are diagnosed within 90 days of previous contact with a hospital system or who live in a residential healthcare facility. In areas of high MDRO rates, or in cases of nosocomial-associated SBP (ie, SBP diagnosed after 48 hours of hospitalization or earlier in a patient who spent at least 48 hours admitted within the past 90 days), carbapenems alone or in combination with daptomycin, vancomycin, or linezolid are recommended. Patients with SBP who previously received quinolone therapy as prophylaxis should be treated with an alternative agent because patients who have received quinolone therapy may become infected with quinolone-resistant flora.[22]

Empiric therapy should not be delayed while awaiting culture results. In some patients, signs and symptoms of infection are present such as fever, abdominal pain, and unexplained encephalopathy at the bacterascites stage (ie, signs and symptoms are present before the PMN count in the ascitic fluid is elevated). In these patients, signs and symptoms of infection justify empiric antibiotic therapy until culture results are known, regardless of the PMN count in the ascitic fluid. An antibiotic course of 5 to 7 days is currently recommended for the treatment of SBP.[30,31]

AASLD and EASL also recommend albumin infusion in patients with SBP who, in addition to PMN counts of 250 cells/mm^3 (0.25×10^9/L) or greater, also have at least one of the following: SCr over 1 mg/dL (88 μmol/L), BUN over 30 mg/dL (10.7 mmol/L), or total bilirubin over 4 mg/dL (68.4 μmol/L).[22,31] Albumin IV 1.5 g/kg body weight within 6 hours of SBP detection followed by 1 g/kg on day 3 (maximum dose 100 g) is recommended. This is then followed by an additional albumin IV infusion of 1 g/kg on day 3 (maximum dose 100 g). (6) All patients who have survived an episode of SBP should receive long-term antibiotic prophylaxis with daily ciprofloxacin 500 mg daily (since norfloxacin is no longer available).[22,28,31] Long-term prophylaxis should also be considered for the prevention of SBP in patients with low-protein ascites (<1.5 g/dL [15 g/L]) who also have one of the following: serum creatinine greater than or equal to 1.2 mg/dL (106 μmol/L), blood urea nitrogen greater than or equal to 25 mg/dL (8.9 mmol/L), serum sodium less than or equal to 130 mEq/L (mmol/L), or Child-Pugh score of greater than or equal to 9 with bilirubin greater than or equal to 3 mg/dL (51.3 μmol/L).[22,31] Short-term prophylaxis (7 days) is indicated in patients with cirrhosis and GI hemorrhage.[12,23] Rifaximin, a synthetic antibiotic which is not systemically absorbed and acts locally within the gastrointestinal tract, is superior to no antibiotic therapy for primary and secondary prophylaxis against SBP.[33] However, it remains undetermined if rifaximin is superior to systemically absorbed antibiotics for SBP prophylaxis. A summary of evidence-based treatment recommendations regarding ascites and SBP is given in Table 55-3.

Management of Hepatic Encephalopathy

Hepatic encephalopathy will occur in 30% to 40% of patients with cirrhosis at some point during the course of their disease.[13] The clinical manifestations of HE vary widely from subclinical alterations to coma. In addition to classification based on underlying disease, HE is also classified based on severity, time course, and the presence of precipitating factors. To determine the severity of HE, a grading system that relates neurologic and neuromuscular signs can be used (Table 55-6). The time course of HE is classified as episodic, persistent, or recurrent. Recurrent HE refers to HE episodes that occur in time intervals less than 6 months apart. Persistent HE refers to behavioral symptoms that are always present and periodically interspersed with episodes of overt HE relapses. A precipitating factor or factors such as constipation, infection, diuretic overuse, GI bleeding, or electrolyte abnormalities can be identified in most episodic cases of HE related to cirrhosis, but spontaneous episodic HE can occur as well. The general approach to the management of HE is four pronged and includes the following: care for patients with altered consciousness, identify and treat any other causes besides HE for altered mental status, identify and treat any precipitating factors, and begin empiric HE treatment. Treatment for HE is primarily focused on reducing ammonia blood concentrations through drug therapy aimed at inhibiting ammonia production or enhancing its removal. Treatment for HE should include avoidance and prevention of precipitating factors in an effort to avoid acute decompensation. In cases where a precipitant of episodic HE has been identified and adequately treated or removed, long-term prophylaxis against another acute HE episode may not be required. Otherwise, chronic therapy to prevent acute decompensation is often required.

TABLE 55-6 Grading System for Hepatic Encephalopathy

Grade	Level of Consciousness	Personality/Intellect	Neurologic Abnormalities
Unimpaired	Normal	Normal	Normal
Minimal	No clinical evidence of change	No clinical evidence of change/alterations identified on psychometric or neuropsychological testing	No clinical evidence of change
I	Trivial lack of awareness; shortened attention span	Euphoria or anxiety; impairment of addition or subtraction	Altered sleep rhythm
II	Lethargic	Obvious personality changes; inappropriate behavior; apathy	Asterixis; dyspraxia; disoriented for time
III	Somnolent but arousable	Bizarre behavior	Responsive to stimuli; confused; gross disorientation to time and space
IV	Coma/unarousable	None	Does not respond to stimuli

Data from Reference 13.

Hyperammonemia

7 Treatment interventions to reduce ammonia blood concentrations are recommended in patients with HE. Decreasing ammonia blood concentrations by reducing the nitrogenous load from the gut remains a mainstay of therapy for patients with HE. Treatment options most commonly used to decrease ammonia load from the gut include nutritional management, nonabsorbable disaccharides, and antibiotics.

Guidelines for nutritional support of patients with liver disease have been published by the International Society for Hepatic Encephalopathy and Nitrogen Metabolism.[34] Protein withdrawal is a cornerstone of treatment for patients during acute episodes of HE.[13] However, prolonged restriction can lead to malnutrition and poorer prognosis among HE patients. Once successful reversal of HE symptoms is achieved, protein is added back to the diet in combination with other therapies until a target of 1.2 to 1.5 g/kg/day of protein is reached. Vegetable-source and dairy-source protein may be preferable to meat-source protein because the latter contains a higher calorie-to-nitrogen ratio. Also, the higher fiber content of vegetable protein lowers colonic pH, increasing catharsis. Oral branched-chain amino acid formulations improve symptoms in episodic HE and may be considered as alternative or add-on therapy in patients who do not respond to conventional measures.

The use of lactulose, a nonabsorbable disaccharide, is the standard therapy for both acute and chronic HE. Lactulose removes nitrogenous waste from the gastrointestinal tract through its laxative effect.[35] In addition, when it reaches the colon, it is metabolized by the microbiota in the lower gastrointestinal tract producing short-chain organic acids. These acids inhibit the growth of ammonia-producing bacteria further reducing the overall ammonia load in the gut. Another laxative, polyethylene glycol 3350, has been compared with lactulose for the treatment of acute HE.[36] Patients receiving polyethylene glycol 3350 had higher rates of HE symptom improvement after 24 hours and their acute HE resolved 1 day sooner than those who received lactulose. Polyethylene glycol may be considered for patients suffering an acute HE episode.

Neomycin has activity against most gram-negative bacteria and inhibits intestinal glutaminase thereby reducing bacterial production of glutamate and ammonia.[37] For this reason, oral neomycin can be used for the treatment of HE. However, this agent is rarely used due to the severity of its potential adverse effects including ototoxicity and nephrotoxicity. Anaerobic bacteria produce urease that hydrolyzes urea to ammonia in the gut. Metronidazole targets these gram-negative anaerobic gut bacteria and, as a result, can be utilized in the management of HE as well. However, neurotoxicity may be problematic so metronidazole is only considered as an alternative agent for HE.

Rifaximin 550 mg twice daily is effective in the treatment of HE.[13] It maintains remission better than lactulose alone and reduces the number of hospitalizations for HE as well; however, 90% of patients in this study received concomitant lactulose.[38] Rifaximin has also been shown in one study to decrease the incidence of overt HE in patients who underwent TIPS for intractable ascites or variceal bleeding prevention.[39]

Zinc is a cofactor for the urea cycle enzymes and is important for ammonia detoxification.[34] Zinc supplementation may be considered in patients with HE.[13] Zinc levels are frequently deficient in patients with cirrhosis. However, supplementation cannot be recommended in the absence of deficiency. Since zinc can inhibit copper absorption leading to anemia, care should be taken in recommending zinc unless truly indicated.

Drugs Affecting Neurotransmission

Flumazenil, a benzodiazepine receptor antagonist, may be considered for short-term therapy in refractory encephalopathy with suspected or confirmed benzodiazepine intake.

Treatment Recommendations: Hepatic Encephalopathy

7 The mainstay of therapy of HE involves measures to lower blood ammonia concentrations and includes diet therapy, lactulose, and antibiotics alone or in combination with lactulose. Other adjunctive therapies include zinc replacement in patients with zinc deficiency and flumazenil in cases of refractory HE with the possibility of benzodiazepine use.

The target daily protein intake for patients with HE is recommended to be within 1.2 to 1.5 g/kg/day. Consideration may be made to substitute meat-source protein with vegetable or dairy protein. Supplementation with elemental zinc may be considered in patients with cirrhosis who are zinc deficient. A typical dose of elemental zinc is 50 mg/day.

In episodic HE, lactulose is initiated at a dose of 30 mL (20 g) orally every 1 to 2 hours until catharsis begins and the patient experiences one to two bowel movements. The dose is then adjusted to produce two to three soft stools per day for chronic therapy. Patients are monitored for changes to their electrolytes periodically as well as for changes in mental status.

Rifaximin 550 mg twice daily plus lactulose is superior to lactulose alone in patients with a history of recurrent HE.[38] Rifaximin is usually well tolerated. Because of its more favorable adverse effect profile, rifaximin is now considered the next line of therapy for recurrent HE over either metronidazole or neomycin.[13]

Systemic Complications

In addition to the more common complications of chronic liver disease discussed earlier, other complications can occur, including hepatorenal syndrome, hepatopulmonary syndrome, coagulation disorders, and endocrine dysfunction.

Hepatorenal syndrome, a functional renal failure in the setting of cirrhosis, occurs in the absence of structural kidney damage.[40] Portal hypertension leads to the release of vasodilators that results in blood pooling in the splanchnic vasculature reducing renal blood flow causing renal hypoperfusion. This causes activation of the renin-angiotensin-aldosterone system that results in severe renal vasoconstriction and fluid retention leading to ascites. As liver disease progresses, systemic vasodilation worsens and, subsequently, increased renal vasoconstriction occurs and renal blood flow is further decreased. The result is hepatorenal syndrome that can be separated into two main types. Type 1 occurs rapidly and has a precipitating cause such as SBP. Type 2 occurs more slowly and does not have a precipitating event.

Management of hepatorenal syndrome begins with discontinuing diuretics and any other medication that could potentially decrease effective blood volume and to expanding the intravascular volume with IV albumin at a dose of 1 g/kg up to a maximum of 100 g.[22,31,40] Precipitating factors, such as infection, fluid loss, and blood loss, should be investigated and treated if found.[40] Liver transplantation is the only definitive treatment for hepatorenal syndrome and the only therapy that will prolong survival. Medications used to bridge patients until transplantation includes arteriolar vasoconstrictor-based treatment with midodrine plus octreotide and IV albumin infusion as already discussed.

Hepatopulmonary syndrome affects up to 50% of patients with cirrhosis.[41] This abnormality is characterized by a defect in arterial oxygenation, which is caused by the pulmonary vascular dilatation that occurs in the presence of liver disease. These patients present with insidious onset of dyspnea, dyspnea upon standing, clubbing, and cyanosis. Patients with cirrhosis with these findings should be evaluated for hepatopulmonary syndrome, which is diagnosed based on the presence of arterial hypoxemia. Arterial hypoxemia is defined by measurements of the partial pressure of oxygen, testing for an increased alveolar–arterial oxygen gradient, and contrast-enhanced echocardiography. There is no effective medical management for hepatopulmonary syndrome. Liver transplantation offers the best chance for long-term recovery.

Patients with cirrhosis who are actively bleeding receive resuscitation with packed red blood cells targeting a hemoglobin of 7 to 9 g/dL (70-90 g/L; 4.34 to 5.59 mmol/L).[15,23] Platelet transfusion is used to maintain platelets over 50,000/mm^3 (50 × 10^9/L) during the period of active bleeding.[15] Cryoprecipitate to maintain fibrinogen levels over 100 mg/dL (1 g/L) is also usually recommended.

The presence of cirrhosis can produce abnormal circulating levels of various hormones.[42] Hypogonadism, diabetes mellitus, osteoporosis, and thyroid disorders are among the endocrine disorders that may develop related to advanced liver disease.

Liver Transplantation

The complications seen in patients with chronic liver disease are essentially secondary effects of the circulatory and metabolic changes that accompany liver failure. Unless the underlying etiology of a patient's fibrosis can be cured, cirrhosis generally progresses. Consequently, liver transplantation is often the only treatment that can offer a cure for the most severe complications of end-stage cirrhosis.

ALTERED DRUG PHARMACOKINETICS AND PHARMACODYNAMICS

Cirrhosis modulates the behavior of drugs in the body by inducing kinetic alterations in drug absorption, distribution, and clearance.[43] Patients with cirrhosis may exhibit pharmacodynamic changes with increased sensitivity to the effects of certain drugs including opiates, benzodiazepines, and nonsteroidal anti-inflammatory drugs (NSAIDs). These pharmacodynamic changes are separate and distinct from the enhancement of drug effects seen in patients with cirrhosis as a result of pharmacokinetic changes. The pathophysiologic changes that have particular impact on drug handling within the body include reduced liver blood flow, decreased first-pass extraction, systemic shunting, hypoalbuminemia, ascites, portal gastropathy, loss of cytochrome P450 enzymatic metabolic activity, reduced glutathione stores, impaired biliary excretion, and impaired renal excretion. Reduced hepatic blood flow, lower first-pass extraction, and portosystemic shunting result in higher bioavailability and serum levels of drugs. Hypoalbuminemia results in higher concentrations of free drug due to less protein binding. Ascites increases the volume of distribution of hydrophilic drugs. Serum levels of various drugs can be higher after normal dosing secondary to impaired biliary and renal excretion that is possible in cirrhosis. Reduced enzymatic clearance by hepatocytes can also lead to reduced first-pass metabolism and reduced hepatic clearance.

Drugs with a high extraction ratio (high-extraction drugs) are dependent on blood flow for metabolism, and the rate of metabolism will be sensitive to changes in blood flow. Drugs with a low extraction ratio (low-extraction drugs) are dependent on intrinsic metabolic activity for metabolism, and the rate of metabolism will reflect changes in intrinsic clearance and protein binding. Furthermore, hepatic biotransformation involves two types of metabolic processes: phase I and phase II reactions. Phase I reactions involve the cytochrome P450 system and include hydrolysis, oxidation, dealkylation, and reduction reactions. Phase II reactions involve conjugation of the drug with an endogenous molecule, such as sulfate or amino acid, rendering it more water soluble and enhancing its elimination. Drug metabolism by phase I reactions, especially oxidation, tend to be significantly impaired in patients with cirrhosis, whereas drugs eliminated by conjugation are relatively unaffected.

The variability and complexity of the interaction between the extent and severity of liver disease and individual characteristics of the drug make it difficult to predict the degree of pharmacokinetic perturbation in an individual patient. There are no sensitive and specific clinical or biochemical markers that allow us to quantify the extent of liver insufficiency or degree of metabolic activity. In addition, renal insufficiency and alterations that commonly accompany cirrhosis further complicate empiric dosing recommendations in these patients. Dosing recommendations are most commonly nonspecific, with recommendations labeled for patients with mild-to-moderate liver impairment. Dosing information for patients with more severe liver impairment is not available. As a result, when patients with cirrhosis require therapy with drugs that undergo hepatic metabolism (eg, benzodiazepines), monitoring response to therapy and anticipating drug accumulation and enhanced effects is essential. In the case of benzodiazepines, selection of an agent such as lorazepam, an intermediate-acting agent that is metabolized via conjugation and has no active metabolites, is easier to monitor than a drug such as diazepam, a long-acting benzodiazepine that is oxidized in the liver and has an active metabolite with a long half-life of its own.

EVALUATION OF THERAPEUTIC OUTCOMES

Table 55-5 summarizes the management approach for patients with cirrhosis and includes possible adverse drug effects. Cirrhosis is generally a chronic progressive disease that requires aggressive medical management to prevent or delay common complications. Table 55-5 also lists monitoring criteria that need to be carefully followed in order to achieve the maximum benefit from the medical therapies employed and prevent adverse effects. A therapeutic plan including therapeutic end points for each medical and diet therapy needs to be developed and discussed with patients who have cirrhosis.

ABBREVIATIONS

AASLD	American Association for the Study of Liver Diseases
ALT	alanine transaminase
AST	aspartate transaminase
EASL	European Association for the Study of the Liver
EVL	endoscopic variceal ligation
GABA	γ-aminobutyric acid
GGT	γ-glutamyl transpeptidase
HE	hepatic encephalopathy
HSC	hepatic stellate cell
HVPG	hepatic venous pressure gradient
INR	international normalized ratio
MDRO	multi-drug resistant organism
MELD	model for end-stage liver disease
PMN	polymorphonuclear
PT	prothrombin time
SAAG	serum-ascites albumin gradient
SBP	spontaneous bacterial peritonitis
TIPS	transjugular intrahepatic portosystemic shunt

REFERENCES

1. Tsochatzis EA, Bosch J, Burroughs AK. Liver cirrhosis. *Lancet.* 2014;383(9930):1749–1761.
2. Zhou WC, Zhang QB, Qiao L. Pathogenesis of liver cirrhosis. *World J Gastroenterol.* 2014;20(23):7312–7324.
3. Chalasani NP, Hayashi PH, Bonkovsky HL, Navarro VJ, Lee WM, Fontana RJ; Practice Parameters Committee of the American College of Gastroenterology. ACG clinical guideline: The diagnosis and management of idiosyncratic drug-induced liver injury. *Am J Gastroenterol.* 2014;109(7):950–966.
4. Murphy SL, Xu J, Kochanek KD, Arias E, Tejada-Vera B. Deaths: Final data for 2018. *Natl Vital Stat Rep.* 2021;69(13).

5. Khalili M, Burman B. Liver disease. In: Hammer GD, McPhee SJ, eds. *Pathophysiology of Disease: An Introduction to Clinical Medicine.* 7th ed. New York: McGraw-Hill; 2014:385–426.
6. Khomich O, Ivanov AC, Bartosch B. Metabolic hallmarks of hepatic stellate cells in liver fibrosis. *Cells.* 2020;9:24.
7. McConnell M, Iwakiri Y. Biology of portal hypertension. *Hepatol Int.* 2018;12(suppl 1):S11–S23.
8. Amin AA, Alabsawy EI, Jalan R, Davenport A. Epidemiology, pathophysiology, and management of hepatorenal syndrome. *Semin Nephrol.* 2019;39(1):17–30.
9. Aithal GP, Palaniyappan N, China L, et al. Guidelines on the management of ascites in cirrhosis. *Gut.* 2021;70:9–29.
10. Adebayo D, Neong SF, Wong F. Ascites and hepatorenal syndrome. *Clin Liver Dis.* 2019;23:559–682.
11. Bari K, Garcia-Tsao G. Treatment of portal hypertension. *World J Gastroenterol.* 2012;18(11):1166–1175.
12. de Franchis R; Baveno VI Faculty. Expanding consensus in portal hypertension report of the Baveno VI consensus workshop: Stratifying risk and individualizing care for portal hypertension. *J Hepatol.* 2015;63:743–752.
13. Vilstrup H, Amodio P, Bajaj J, et al. Hepatic encephalopathy in chronic liver disease: 2014 Practice guideline by AASLD and EASL. *Hepatology.* 2014;60(2):715–735.
14. Wijdicks EFM. Hepatic encephalopathy. *N Engl J Med.* 2016;375:1660–1670.
15. Kujovich JL. Coagulopathy in liver disease: A balancing act. *Hematology.* 2015;2015(1):243–249.
16. Pugh RNH, Murray-Lyon IM, Dawson JL, et al. Transection of the oesophagus for bleeding oesophagus varices. *Br J Surg.* 1973;60:646–649.
17. Smith A, Baumgartner K, Bositis C. Cirrhosis: Diagnosis and management. *Am Fam Physician.* 2019;100(12):759–770.
18. About the MELD/PELD Calculator. Available at http://optn.transplant.hrsa.gov/resources/allocation-calculators/meld-calculator/. Accessed September 28, 2021.
19. Kwo PY, Cohen SM, Kim JK. ACG practice guideline: Evaluation of abnormal liver chemistries. *Am J Gastroenterol.* 2017;112(1):18–35.
20. Cohen JA, Kaplan MM. The SGOT/SGPT ratio—An indicator of alcoholic disease. *Dig Dis Sci.* 1979;24:835–838.
21. MELD/PELD Calculator Documentation. Available at https://www.ssa.gov/disability/professionals/documents/MELD_PELD_Calculator_Documentation.pdf. Accessed October 5, 2021.
22. Runyon BA. Management of adult patients with ascites due to cirrhosis: Update 2012. Available at https://www.aasld.org/sites/default/files/2019-06/141020_Guideline_Ascites_4UFb_2015.pdf. Accessed October 7, 2021.
23. Garcia-Tsao G, Abraldes JG, Berzigotti A, et al. Portal hypertensive bleeding in cirrhosis: Risk stratification, diagnosis, and management: 2016 Practice guidance by the American Association for the Study of Liver Diseases. *Hepatology.* 2017;65:310–335.
24. Giannelli V, Lattanzi B, Thalheimer U, Merli M. Beta-blockers in liver cirrhosis. *Ann Gastroenterol.* 2014;27(1):1–7.
25. Brunner F, Berzigotti A, Bosch J. Prevention and treatment of variceal haemorrhage in 2017. *Liver International.* 2017;37(suppl 1):104–115.
26. Well M, Chande N, Adams P, et al. Meta-analysis: Vasoactive medications for the management of acute variceal bleeds. *Aliment Pharmacol Ther.* 2012;35(11):1267–1278.
27. Chavez-Tapia NC, Barrientos-Gutierrez T, Tellez-Avila F, et al. Meta-analysis: Antibiotic prophylaxis for cirrhotic patients with upper gastrointestinal bleeding—An updated Cochrane review. *Aliment Pharmacol Ther.* 2011;34:509–518.
28. Garcia-Tsao G. Current management of the complications of cirrhosis and portal hypertension: Variceal hemorrhage, ascites, and spontaneous bacterial peritonitis. *Dig Dis.* 2016;34:382–386.
29. Puente A, Hernandez-Gea V, Graupera I, et al. Drugs plus ligation to prevent rebleeding in cirrhosis: An updated systematic review. *Liver Int.* 2014;34:823–833.
30. Marciano S, Diaz JM, Dirchwolf M, Gadano A. Spontaneous bacterial peritonitis in patients with cirrhosis: Incidence, outcomes, and treatment strategies. *Hepat Med Evidence Res.* 2019;11.
31. European Association for the Study of the Liver. EASL clinical practice guidelines for the management of patients with decompensated cirrhosis. *J Hepatol.* 2018;69:406–450.
32. Ginès P, Krag A, Abraldes JG, Solá E, Fabrellas N, Kamath PS. Liver cirrhosis. *Lancet.* 2021;398:1359–1376.
33. Goel A, Rahim U, Nguyen LH, Stave C, Nguyen MH. Systematic review with meta-analysis: Rifaximin for the prophylaxis of spontaneous bacterial peritonitis. *Aliment Pharmacol Ther.* 2017;46:1029–1036.
34. Amodio P, Bemeur C, Butterworth R, et al. The nutritional management of hepatic encephalopathy in patients with cirrhosis: ISHEN practice guidelines. *Hepatology.* 2013;58:325–336.
35. Hudson M, Schuchmann M. Long-term management of hepatic encephalopathy with lactulose and/or rifaximin: A review of the evidence. *Eur J Gastroenterol Hepatol.* 2018;31:434–450.
36. Rahimi RS, Singal AG, Cuthbert JA, Rockey DC. Lactulose vs polyethylene glycol 3350-electrolyte solution for treatment of overt hepatic encephalopathy: The HELP randomized clinical trial. *JAMA Intern Med.* 2014;174:1727–1733.
37. Patidar KR, Bajaj JS. Antibiotics for the treatment of hepatic encephalopathy. *Metab Brain Dis.* 2013;28(2):307–312.
38. Bass NM, Mullen KD, Sanyal A, et al. Rifaximin treatment in hepatic encephalopathy. *N Engl J Med.* 2010;362:1071–1081.
39. Bureau C, Thabut D, Jezequel C, et al. The use of rifaximin in the prevention of overt hepatic encephalopathy after transjugular intrahepatic portosystemic shunt. *Ann Intern Med.* 2021;Epub10.7326/m20-0202.
40. Erly B, Carey WD, Kapoor B, McKinney JM, Tam M, Wang W. Hepatorenal syndrome: A review of pathophysiology and current treatment options. *Semin Intervent Radiol.* 2015;32(4):445–454.
41. Moller S, Henriksen JH, Bendtsen F. Extrahepatic complications to cirrhosis and portal hypertension: Haemodynamic and homeostatic aspects. *World J Gastroenterol.* 2014;20(42):15499–15517.
42. Eshraghian A, Taghavi SA. Systematic review: Endocrine abnormalities in patients with liver cirrhosis. *Arch Iran Med.* 2014;17(10):713–721.
43. Lewis JH, Stine JG. Review article: Prescribing medications in patients with cirrhosis—A practical guide. *Aliment Pharmacol Ther.* 2013;37:1132–1156.

e56

Drug-Induced Liver Injury

William R. Kirchain and Rondall E. Allen

KEY CONCEPTS

1. Through its normally functioning enzymes and processes the liver often causes a drug to become toxic through a process known as bioactivation.
2. Drug-induced liver injury (DILI) can have many different clinical presentations: idiosyncratic reactions, allergic hepatitis, toxic hepatitis, chronic active toxic hepatitis, toxic cirrhosis, and liver vascular disorders.
3. The mechanisms of DILI are diverse, representing many phases of biotransformation, and are susceptible to genetic polymorphism.
4. The assessment of a possible liver injury caused by drugs should include what is known in the literature, the timing involved, the clinical course, and, always, an exploration for preexisting conditions that may have encouraged the lesion's development.
5. Liver enzyme assays in serum can help to determine if a particular type of liver damage is present.
6. Monitoring for DILI must be tailored to the drug and the patient's potential risk factors.

BEYOND THE BOOK

Because it is important to compare cases of liver injury across the world and across time, we use common designations for each type of liver injury. You can see a concise and commonly accepted approach in LiverTox which is part of the NCBI Bookshelf at https://www.ncbi.nlm.nih.gov/books/NBK547852/. Look under "Phenotypes."

It is important to stratify the likelihood that a particular drug has caused this liver injury and decide what are likely candidates. The text provides the RUCAM scoring system and references some supporting literature for its use. The authors of LiverTox at https://www.ncbi.nlm.nih.gov/books/NBK547852/ have a less favorable view of RUCAM and provide several other choices for you to consider, you can score the above case and see how each approach differs. Look under "Causality."

INTRODUCTION

The range of drugs associated with adverse reactions involving the liver is extensive, but in clinical practice is dominated by alcohol, antibiotics, antiseizure medications, and acetaminophen.[1] Complementary and herbal medicines also contribute disproportionately to this disease burden. Drug-induced liver injury (DILI) is a potentially fatal, often debilitating outcome of drug treatment. DILI is responsible for 11% to 13% of all cases of acute liver failure in the United States.[1,2]

Drug-induced liver injury accounts for as much as 20% of acute liver failure in pediatric populations and a similar percentage of adults with acute liver failure.[3] In approximately 75% of these cases, liver transplantation is ultimately required for patient survival.[4] Of patients who required liver transplantation according to the United Network for Organ Sharing, acetaminophen, isoniazid, antiepileptics, and antibiotics collectively account for just over 60% of cases.[5]

The liver's function affects every other organ system in the body; it in turn is exposed to every substance absorbed from the gut and every injected substance that enters the bloodstream.

MECHANISMS OF DRUG-INDUCED LIVER INJURY

Stimulation of Autoimmunity

Autoimmune injuries involve antibody-mediated cytotoxicity or direct cellular toxicity.[6,7] This type of injury occurs when enzyme-drug complexes migrate to the cell surface and form neoantigens. The liver plays host to all of the cells that make up the innate immune response in the body along with Kupffer cells, which act as a type of macrophage, derived from the reticuloendothelial cells. These Kupffer cells sit in anticipation along the lumen of the liver sinusoids waiting for glycoproteins, substances coated with immunoglobulins or complement factors to present themselves.[8] The reticuloendothelial cells that create the porous frame around the hepatocytes are constantly monitoring and communicating via cytokines to stimulate or regulate an immune response.[8] Neoantigens also serve as targets for cytolytic attack by killer T cells, and others.[9] Halothane, sulfamethoxazole, carbamazepine, nevirapine, fluoroquinolones, and anti-tumor necrosis factor (TNF) alpha inhibitors are associated with autoimmune injuries.[2,10]

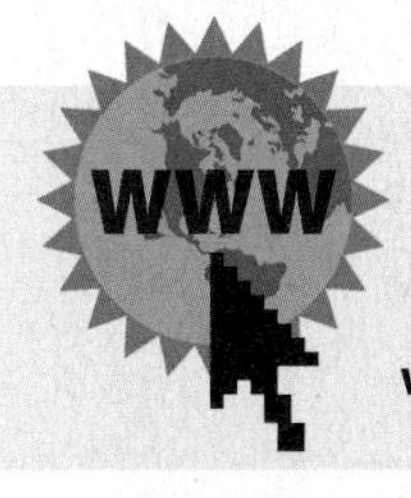

The complete chapter, learning objectives, and other resources can be found at **www.pharmacotherapyonline.com.**

57

Pancreatitis

Scott Bolesta

KEY CONCEPTS

ACUTE PANCREATITIS

1. Factors that can contribute to acute pancreatitis should be identified and corrected, including discontinuation of medications that could be potential causes.
2. Patients with acute pancreatitis should receive goal-directed fluid management to reduce the risks of persistent systemic inflammatory response syndrome (SIRS) and organ failure.
3. Parenteral opioid analgesics are used to control abdominal pain associated with acute pancreatitis despite a lack of high-quality evidence to support the practice.
4. Use of prophylactic antibiotics is not recommended in patients with acute pancreatitis without signs or symptoms of infection, including those with predicted severe acute pancreatitis or necrotizing pancreatitis.

CHRONIC PANCREATITIS

5. Chronic pain, malabsorption with resultant steatorrhea, and diabetes mellitus are the hallmark symptoms and complications of chronic pancreatitis.
6. Pain from chronic pancreatitis may initially be treated with nonopioid analgesics, but adjuvant agents may be necessary as the disease progresses.
7. Pancreatic enzyme and fat-soluble vitamin supplementation are the primary treatments for malabsorption due to chronic pancreatitis.
8. Enteric-coated pancreatic enzyme supplements are the preferred dosage form in the treatment of malabsorption and steatorrhea due to chronic pancreatitis.
9. The addition of a histamine-2 receptor antagonist or proton pump inhibitor to pancreatic enzyme supplementation may increase the effectiveness of enzyme therapy for malabsorption and steatorrhea due to chronic pancreatitis.

BEYOND THE BOOK

1. Robert Whipple is a 48-year-old man admitted to the intensive care unit (ICU) for acute pancreatitis. He weighs 89 kg. He has no signs or symptoms of infection. Which resuscitation fluid would you recommend for Mr. Whipple and why? What volume and rate of infusion would you recommend for his resuscitation fluid? What are the endpoints you recommend monitoring to determine adequate fluid resuscitation? These are the key decisions regarding the assess, plan, implement, and monitor aspects of the Pharmacist Patient Care Process concerning fluid resuscitation in patients with acute pancreatitis.
2. Using available resources, determine the monthly cash prescription payment for a patient with exocrine pancreatic insufficiency from chronic pancreatitis who requires 60,000 USP units of lipase with each meal; the patient eats five meals a day, along with three snacks. Do this for all Food and Drug Administration (FDA)-approved pancrelipase products available in the United States. How would this information affect your recommendation of a pancrelipase product for this patient? Now locate the online formulary of a third-party prescription plan in your area. Determine if the plan's coverage of the same pancrelipase products alters your decision in any way. This activity is to make you aware of not only the pill burden of patients with exocrine pancreatic insufficiency but also the cost related to these medications.

INTRODUCTION

Pancreatitis is inflammation of the pancreas with variable involvement of regional tissues or remote organ systems.[1,2] Acute pancreatitis is characterized by severe pain in the upper abdomen and elevations of pancreatic enzymes in the blood.[3,4] In the majority of patients, acute pancreatitis is a self-limiting disease that resolves spontaneously without complications. Approximately 20% of adults with acute pancreatitis have a severe course.[3] While the overall mortality of acute pancreatitis is low, severe pancreatitis is associated with a mortality as high as 40%.[3,5,6] The risk for progression to chronic pancreatitis after an initial episode of acute pancreatitis is related to the etiology. Patients with acute pancreatitis due to gallstone disease have little risk for progression to chronic disease, whereas patients with alcohol-related acute pancreatitis have a risk of 13% to 38% based on whether or not they continue to consume alcohol.[7]

Chronic pancreatitis is characterized by long-standing inflammation that eventually leads to a loss of pancreatic exocrine and endocrine functions.[8-11] It is a progressive disease that often goes unnoticed for many years. The usual initial presentation is complaints of chronic abdominal pain. Later in the disease process malabsorption with resultant steatorrhea occurs. This leads to malnutrition and weight loss. Finally, patients develop diabetes mellitus due to a loss of pancreatic endocrine function.[8,9,11]

EPIDEMIOLOGY

Acute pancreatitis is one of the most common gastrointestinal disorders causing hospitalization in the United States with admission rates of approximately 13 to 45 per 100,000 per year.[3,5,7] The incidence of hospitalization has increased with a 13.3% rise occurring within the first decade of the century.[12] The risk for acute pancreatitis varies widely with geographic, etiologic (eg, alcohol consumption and smoking), environmental, and genetic factors. In adults and children, the increase in acute pancreatitis is often attributed to rising rates of obesity.[4,13] The annual incidence of chronic pancreatitis in the United States is 5 to 14 per 100,000, and the prevalence is 42 to75 per 100,000.[8,10,11] The prevalence increases with age, with an average onset in the fifth to sixth decade of life, and it is 4.5 times more common in males than females.[8,10,11] Also, the prevalence of chronic pancreatitis varies widely based on geographic location.[9] There is also racial disparity with the disease, with Black patients having two to three times the risk than White patients, and being more than twice as likely to be hospitalized.[8,10,11]

PANCREATIC EXOCRINE PHYSIOLOGY

The pancreas possesses both endocrine and exocrine functions. The islets of Langerhans, which contain the cells of the endocrine pancreas, secrete insulin, glucagon, somatostatin, and other polypeptide hormones. The exocrine pancreas is composed of acini and ductules that secrete about 2.5 L/day of isotonic fluid that contains water, electrolytes, and pancreatic enzymes necessary for digestion. Bicarbonate and other electrolytes are secreted primarily by the centroacinar (ductular) cells in order to neutralize gastric acid. Pancreatic juice is delivered to the duodenum via the pancreatic ducts (Fig. 57-1) where the alkaline secretion neutralizes gastric acid and provides an appropriate pH for maintaining the activity of pancreatic enzymes.[14]

The major pancreatic exocrine enzyme groups are as follows:

1. Amylolytic: α-amylase
2. Lipolytic: lipase, procolipase, prophospholipase A2, and carboxylesterase
3. Proteolytic: trypsinogens, chymotrypsinogen, procarboxypeptidase A and B, proelastase and mesotrypsin
4. Nucleolytic: ribonuclease and deoxyribonuclease
5. Other: trypsin inhibitor

Amylase is responsible for digestion of starches and glycogen through hydrolysis. The lipolytic enzymes break down triglycerides, cholesterol, and other fats in the digestive tract. Specifically, lipase hydrolyzes triglycerides into fatty acids and monoglycerides. Colipase and bile acids facilitate this process by allowing lipase to act on the hydrophobic surface of fat droplets in the mainly hydrophilic environment. Phospholipase A2 and carboxylesterase continue to break down fatty acids, cholesterol, monoglycerides, and other products of fat digestion. Proteolytic enzymes digest proteins into oligopeptides and free amino acids, while nucleases break down nucleic acids.[14]

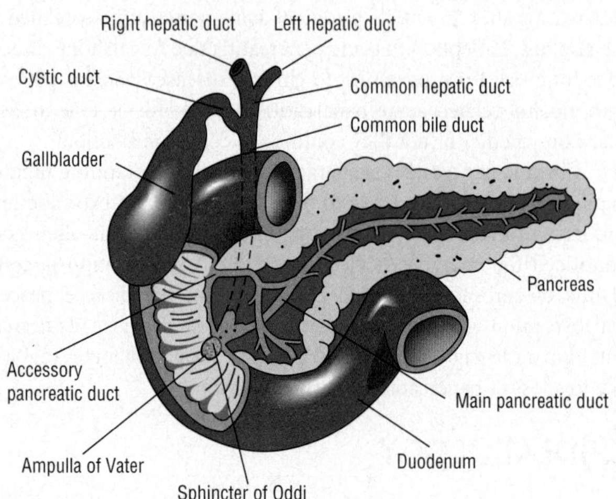

FIGURE 57-1 Anatomic structure of the pancreas and biliary tract.

The production of proteolytic enzymes in the pancreas occurs in a manner that prevents self-digestion of the pancreas. These enzymes are synthesized within the acinar cells, stored in vacuoles, and secreted into the duodenum as zymogens (inactive enzymes). Enterokinase secreted by the duodenal mucosa converts trypsinogen to trypsin, which then activates all other proteolytic zymogens along with procolipase and prophospholipase A2. Thus, two important mechanisms protect the pancreas from the potential degradative action of its own digestive enzymes. First, the synthesis of proteolytic enzymes as zymogens requires extrapancreatic activation by trypsin. Second, pancreatic juice contains a low concentration of trypsin inhibitor, which inactivates any autocatalytically formed trypsin within the pancreas. Proteolytic activity of trypsin in the intestinal lumen is not inhibited because the concentration of trypsin inhibitor is minimal. Lipase, amylase, ribonuclease, and deoxyribonuclease are secreted by the acinar cells in their active form.[14]

The regulation of exocrine pancreatic secretion is a complex interplay of neurohormonal feedback with three distinct phases. The first phase is the cephalic phase where the sight, smell, and taste of food cause pancreatic enzyme secretion through stimulus of the vagus nerve. Vasoactive intestinal peptide (VIP) and gastrin-releasing peptide released from efferent vagus nerve terminals bind to receptors on the acinar cells stimulating enzyme release.[14] Water and bicarbonate are also released from ductal cells due to VIP stimulation. The gastric phase occurs due to gastric distension from food entering the stomach. This results primarily in secretion of digestive enzymes from the pancreas. Once chyme enters the duodenum, the intestinal phase begins. The chyme causes secretin to be released from the duodenal mucosa when its pH is less than 4.5. Secretin results in water and bicarbonate secretion from the pancreas to increase intestinal pH for stable lipolytic enzyme activity. Digestive enzymes are released from the pancreas due to the presence of fatty acids, peptides, amino acids, and glucose in the duodenum.[14]

The feedback mechanism for continued release of pancreatic enzymes involves the hormone cholecystokinin (CCK). When products of fat, protein, and starch digestion enter the upper small intestine, they stimulate the release of CCK from I cells into the blood. Elevated levels of CCK in the serum activate a vasovagal reflex causing further release of VIP and gastrin-releasing peptide, leading to enhanced pancreatic enzyme secretion. Inhibition of this feedback loop is thought to be due to trypsin. After digestion is complete, unoccupied trypsin is thought to inhibit the release of CCK.[14] A more in-depth discussion of pancreatic physiology can be found elsewhere.[14]

ACUTE PANCREATITIS

Acute pancreatitis may be mild or may be associated with complications including organ failure and pancreatic necrosis. Prognosis and management vary according to the severity of the disease. There are several causes of acute pancreatitis, but the most common are obstruction due to gallstones and alcohol-induced pancreatitis. Patients generally present with abdominal pain and other gastrointestinal symptoms with diagnosis being made based on presenting signs and symptoms, lab abnormalities, and imaging studies as necessary. Treatment focuses on providing fluid resuscitation and treating the pain and complications associated with acute pancreatitis.

Etiology

Table 57-1 lists the etiologic risk factors associated with acute pancreatitis. Obstruction caused by gallstones is the most common

TABLE 57-1 Etiologic Risk Factors Associated with Acute Pancreatitis

Structural	Gallstone disease, sphincter of Oddi dysfunction, pancreas divisum, pancreatic tumors
Toxins	Alcohol (ethanol) consumption, scorpion bite, organophosphate insecticides
Infectious	Bacterial, viral (including HIV and H1N1 influenza), parasitic
Metabolic	Hypertriglyceridemia, chronic hypercalcemia
Genetic	Cystic fibrosis, α1-antitrypsin deficiency, hereditary (trypsinogen gene mutations)
Medications	See Table 57-2 for specific drugs
Iatrogenic	Abdominal surgery, ERCP
Kidney disease	Chronic kidney disease, dialysis-related
Trauma	Blunt abdominal trauma
Vascular	Vasculitis, atherosclerosis, cholesterol emboli, coronary artery bypass surgery
Other etiologies	Congenital, Crohn's disease, autoimmune, tropical, solid organ transplantation (eg, liver, kidney, heart), refeeding syndrome
Idiopathic	Undetermined cause

HIV, human immunodeficiency virus; ERCP, endoscopic retrograde cholangiopancreatography.

Data from References 3, 4, 7, and 13.

cause of acute pancreatitis in the United States, with alcohol misuse being the second most common. Abdominal obesity increases the risk for both gallstone- and nongallstone-related acute pancreatitis. Moderate elevations in lipid levels are associated with nonalcohol-related pancreatitis, and smoking has emerged as a strong risk.[4,7,12,13,15] There is also an autoimmune form of pancreatitis.[3,7] Diabetes mellitus is also associated with an increase in acute pancreatitis as are autoimmune disorders such as inflammatory bowel disease.[3,7,13,16,17] Most remaining cases are classified as idiopathic.[4,13] Acute pancreatitis can occur as a result of undergoing an endoscopic retrograde cholangiopancreatography (ERCP) with overall rates up to 5%.[4,7] Pregnancy is not considered a cause of acute pancreatitis; however, pregnant women develop pancreatitis as a result of a coincident process, most commonly cholelithiasis.[18] The reported incidence of acute pancreatitis in children has increased in recent years, and the common etiologies are biliary disease, systemic illness, medications, trauma, and idiopathic.[19,20]

Medications

1 Factors that can contribute to acute pancreatitis should be identified and corrected, including discontinuation of medications that could be potential causes. Drug-induced acute pancreatitis should be considered when other causes have been excluded and there is a temporal relationship with the initiation of a medication that has been implicated as a cause. Most experts consider drug-induced pancreatitis to be rare, although some reports include higher estimates.[4,7,13] The difficulty in diagnosing drug-induced pancreatitis has led to an underestimation of the rate.[13] Most information on drug-induced acute pancreatitis is obtained from case reports, which do not provide reliable information on incidence. The most convincing case reports involve recurrence on rechallenge; however, rechallenge is rare, occurring only when alternative therapy is not available. Further complicating the evaluation of some reports is the use of medications associated with pancreatitis in patient populations with an increased risk of pancreatitis.[13] Adverse events attributed to newly introduced medications may be reported more frequently.[21] Many medications have been frequently reported to cause acute pancreatitis. Patients with human immunodeficiency virus (HIV) have an increased risk of pancreatitis and there are many reports of pancreatitis attributed to antiretroviral agents.[4,7,13,21] Pancreatitis due to azathioprine is reported more frequently in patients with Crohn's disease than in patients taking the medication for other indications, suggesting an interaction between the disease and medication. Patients with Crohn's disease often take other medications that can cause pancreatitis, including 5-aminosalycilates, corticosteroids, and sulfasalazine.[24] Patients with type 2 diabetes mellitus have an increased risk of acute pancreatitis. Case reports and some observational studies have linked antihyperglycemic agents, including metformin, sulfonylureas, and incretin mimetics, with pancreatitis. There is no increase in pancreatitis with incretin mimetics compared to sulfonylureas, metformin, or insulin.[25,26] Mixed results have been reported in meta-analyses evaluating the risk of pancreatitis from dipeptidyl peptidase-4 inhibitors.[26,27] Complicating comparisons between agents used to treat diabetes mellitus is that the medications are often used in obese patients and patients with different durations of disease, both of which may also influence disease-associated pancreatitis.[28] Polypharmacy is associated with an increased risk of acute pancreatitis.[29]

The onset of drug-induced pancreatitis after initiation of medications ranges from a few months to several years, with a median of 5 weeks; onset after rechallenge can occur within hours. The onset may differ according to the mechanism. Clinicians should be especially suspicious of a drug as a cause of acute pancreatitis in high-risk patients, such as those receiving immunomodulating drugs or who have HIV infection, the elderly, or those with diabetes mellitus.[23]

Mechanisms of drug-induced pancreatitis have been proposed for some medications but remain poorly defined. Possible mechanisms include direct toxic effects of the drug or its metabolites, hypersensitivity, drug-induced hypertriglyceridemia, and alterations of cellular function in the pancreas and pancreatic duct.[22] Ultimately, drug-induced pancreatitis causes damage to the pancreas, which produces a response similar to other causes of pancreatitis. It is prudent to withdraw a medication when an association is suspected.

Numerous drugs are believed to cause acute pancreatitis, but ethical and practical considerations often prevent rechallenge with suspected agents. Table 57-2 lists specific agents associated with acute pancreatitis. Classification schemes consider rechallenge, the number of case reports, consistency with respect to the onset of symptoms following initiation of the suspect medication, and exclusion of other causes.

Pathophysiology

The pathophysiology of acute pancreatitis is based on events that initiate injury and secondary events that establish and perpetuate the injury (Fig. 57-2). Gallstones, alcohol misuse, and other causes of pancreatitis produce different initial insults to the pancreas. However, the resulting pathophysiologic process may be similar and include autodigestion, abnormal acinar calcium signaling, and inflammatory response. In acinar cells, the separation of zymogens and lysosomes can be disrupted, resulting in exposure of trypsinogen to lysosomal enzymes such as cathepsin B. The premature activation of trypsinogen to trypsin within the pancreas leads to activation of other digestive enzymes and autodigestion of the gland.[4,7]

In addition to activation of digestive enzymes within the pancreas, enzymes are also released into surrounding fat, vascular endothelium, and other surrounding tissues and structures causing further damage and necrosis. Lipase damages fat cells, producing noxious substances that cause further pancreatic and peripancreatic injury. There may be an independent response from intra-acinar activation of inflammatory factors. The release of cytokines by acinar cells directly causes their injury and enhances the inflammatory response.[30] Injured acinar cells liberate chemoattractants that recruit neutrophils, macrophages, and other cells to the area of inflammation. These immune responses cause a systemic inflammatory

TABLE 57-2 Medications Associated with Acute Pancreatitis

Well-Supported Association	Probable Association	Possible Association	
5-Aminosalicylic acid	Acetaminophen	Aldesleukin	Indinavir
Asparaginase	Hydrochlorothiazide	Amiodarone	Indomethacin
Azathioprine	Itraaconazole	Atorvastatin	Infliximab
Bortezomib	Ifosfamide	Calcium	Ketoprofen
Carbamazepine	Interferon α2b	Ceftriaxone	Ketorolac
Cimetidine	Maprotiline	Capecitabine	Lipid emulsion
Corticosteroids	Methyldopa	Carboplatin	Liraglutide
Cisplatin	Oxaliplatin	Celecoxib	Lisinopril
Cytarabine		Clozapine	Mefenamic acid
Didanosine		Cholestyramine	Metformin
Enalapril		Ciprofloxacin	Metolazone
Erythromycin		Clarithromycin	Metronidazole
Estrogens		Clonidine	Nitrofurantoin
Furosemide		Cyclosporine	Omeprazole
Lamivudine		Danazol	Ondansetron
Mercaptopurine		Diazoxide	Paclitaxel
Mesalamine		Etanercept	Pravastatin
Octreotide		Ethacrynic acid	Propofol
Olsalazine		Exenatide	Propoxyphene
Opiates		Famciclovir	Rifampin
Pentamidine		Glyburide	Sertraline
Pentavalent antimonials		Gold therapy	Simvastatin
Sulfasalazine		Granisetron	Sitagliptin
Sulfamethoxazole and trimethoprim		Ibuprofen	Sorafenib
Tamoxifen		Imatinib	Sulindac
Tetracyclines			Zalcitabine
Valproic acid/salts			

Data from References 4, 7, 13, 21, 22, and 23.

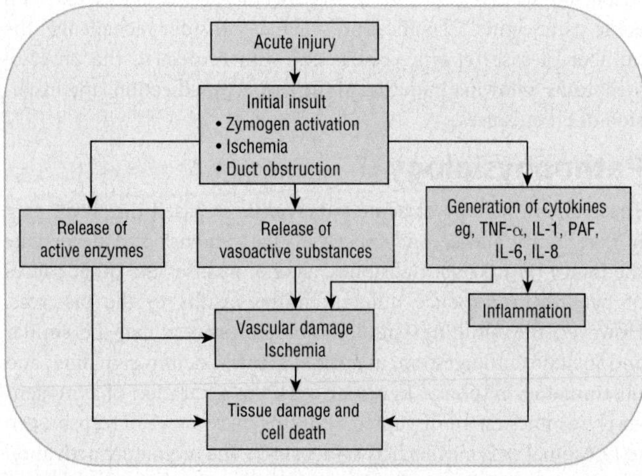

FIGURE 57-2 Pathophysiology of acute pancreatitis: initiating and secondary events. (IL-1β, interleukin-1β; IL-6, interleukin-6; IL-8, interleukin-8; PAF, platelet-activating factor; TNF-α, tumor necrosis factor-α.)

response syndrome (SIRS). Vascular damage and ischemia causes the release of kinins, which makes capillary walls permeable and promotes tissue edema. Finally, pancreatic infection may result from increased intestinal permeability and translocation of colonic bacteria.[30]

Clinical Presentation

Signs and Symptoms

The clinical presentation of acute pancreatitis varies depending on the severity of the inflammatory process and whether damage is confined to the pancreas or involves local and systemic complications (Table 57-3).[7]

Diagnosis

The diagnosis of acute pancreatitis requires two of the following three: upper abdominal pain, a serum lipase or amylase concentration at least three times greater than the upper limit of normal, or characteristic findings on imaging studies.[3,4,13] Lipase is more sensitive and specific than amylase and is the preferred laboratory test. Although used in the diagnosis of acute pancreatitis, the degree of amylase and lipase elevations is not predictive of patient outcome. Imaging studies are not necessary for diagnosis if the other two findings are positive. Contrast-enhanced computed tomography (CECT) of the abdomen may be used to confirm the diagnosis in patients with amylase or lipase that is not three times the upper limit of normal, or in sedated patients. Patients should be monitored for SIRS organ failure for the first 48 hours.[3,13] For further information on laboratory tests and abdominal imaging, refer to Table 57-3. Pertinent history includes previous history of pancreatitis, gallstone disease, alcohol use, medication use, recent surgery or ERCP, hyperlipidemia, recent infections, trauma, and family history. Magnetic resonance cholangiopancreatography (MRCP) is useful for detecting retained common bile duct stones. Laboratory tests should

TABLE 57-3 Presentation and Diagnosis of Acute Pancreatitis

General

- The patient may have acute mild symptoms or present with a severe acute attack with life-threatening complications.

Symptoms

- The patient may present initially with moderate abdominal discomfort to excruciating pain, nausea, shock, and respiratory distress.
- Abdominal pain occurs in 95% of patients. The pain is usually epigastric and radiates to either of the upper quadrants or the back in two-thirds of patients. In gallstone pancreatitis, the pain is typically sudden and quite severe and the intensity is often described as "knife-like" or "boring." The pain usually reaches its maximum intensity within 30 minutes and may persist for hours or days. Repositioning the patient relieves very little of the pain. In alcohol misuse and other cases, the onset of pain may be less abrupt and poorly localized. Pain may not be the dominant symptom if it is masked by multiorgan failure.
- Nausea and vomiting occur in 85% of patients and usually follow the onset of abdominal pain. Vomiting does not provide relief of the abdominal pain.

Signs

- Marked epigastric or diffuse tenderness on palpation with rebound tenderness and guarding in severe cases. The abdomen is often distended and tympanic, with bowel sounds decreased or absent in severe disease.
- Vital signs may be normal, but hypotension, tachycardia, and low-grade fever are often observed, especially with widespread pancreatic inflammation and necrosis.
- Dyspnea and tachypnea are often signs of acute respiratory complications. Jaundice and altered mental status may be present and have multiple causes. Other signs of alcohol-induced liver disease may be present in patients with alcohol-induced pancreatitis.

Laboratory tests

- Leukocytosis is frequently present; hyperglycemia or hypoalbuminemia may be present. Liver transaminases, alkaline phosphatase, and bilirubin are usually elevated in gallstone pancreatitis and in patients with intrinsic liver disease. Elevated serum triglycerides may also be a possible etiology.
- The hematocrit may be normal, but hemoconcentration results from multiple factors (eg, vomiting). In patients with third-space fluid loss, hemoconcentration is present and a reasonably accurate marker of severe disease. A hematocrit of greater than 44% predicts severe acute pancreatitis. Further, failure to reverse hemoconcentration has been associated with pancreatic necrosis.
- Blood urea nitrogen (BUN) that is elevated (greater than 20 mg/dL [7.1 mmol/L]) or rising over the first 24 hours has been associated with increased mortality.
- The total serum calcium is usually normal initially, but hypocalcemia disproportionate to the hypoalbuminemia may develop. Marked hypocalcemia is an indication of severe necrosis and a poor prognostic sign.
- The serum amylase concentration usually rises within 4-8 hours of the initial attack, peaks at 24 hours, and returns to normal over the next 8-14 days. Serum amylase concentrations greater than three times the upper limit of normal are highly suggestive of acute pancreatitis. Persistent elevations suggest extensive pancreatic necrosis and related complications. Normal concentrations may be observed if testing is delayed (ie, amylase may have returned to normal) or in patients with hyperlipidemic pancreatitis (ie, marked triglyceride elevations may interfere with amylase assay). In addition, many nonpancreatic diseases may be associated with hyperamylasemia, including salivary, kidney, hepatobiliary, metabolic, female reproductive tract, and neoplastic diseases.
- Serum lipase is specific to the pancreas and concentrations are elevated and parallel the elevations in serum amylase. Levels remain elevated with pancreatic inflammation and return to normal when the inflammatory process resolves. Because of its longer half-life, elevations of serum lipase can be detected after the serum amylase has returned to normal.
- Additional biomarkers: C-reactive protein is a widely available test and levels greater than 190 mg/L at 48 hours predict severe acute pancreatitis.

Abdominal imaging

- Transabdominal ultrasound should be performed in all patients to detect dilated biliary ducts and stones in the gallbladder.
- CECT is used if the diagnosis cannot be made from clinical and laboratory findings. It is less accurate for evaluating the gallbladder and biliary ducts. The test distinguishes interstitial from necrotizing pancreatitis, but does not distinguish between fat necrosis and acute fluid collection. Tests that are performed in the first few days may miss necrosis. Tests should be performed at least 72-96 hours after symptom onset; tests performed too early may result in unnecessary exposure to risk and increased cost.
- Magnetic resonance imaging is used to grade the severity of acute pancreatitis, identify biliary duct problems that are not seen on CT, or if there are contraindications to CECT. Patients over the age of 40 with pancreatitis of an unknown etiology should be evaluated for pancreatic malignancy with CT or endoscopic ultrasonography.

APACHE, Acute Physiology and Chronic Health Evaluation; CECT, contrast-enhanced computed tomography; CT, computed tomography.

Data from References 4, 7, 13, and 30.

include liver enzymes, triglycerides, and calcium. Transabdominal ultrasound of the right upper quadrant is recommended to assess for gallstones.[3,4,7,13]

Acute pancreatitis is categorized according to the revised Atlanta classification. The revised Atlanta Classification defines acute pancreatitis as mild disease (not associated with organ failure, local complications, or systemic complications), moderately severe (transient organ failure, local complications or systemic complications), and severe (persistent organ failure).[3,7,13,31] An alternative classification system was proposed by an international multidisciplinary group using factors that have a causal association with severity (ie, distant organ failure or pancreatic necrosis) rather than events that may be associated with severity.[3,7,13,32] This determinant-based classification includes mild (no organ dysfunction or necrosis), moderate (sterile necrosis or transient organ dysfunction or both), severe (either infected necrosis or persistent organ dysfunction), and critical (infected necrosis and persistent organ dysfunction).

Prediction of severity of acute pancreatitis is useful for decisions involving the need for aggressive treatment, including admission to an ICU.[2,4,13] Multiple scoring systems have been developed to predict which patients with acute pancreatitis are at greatest risk for persistent organ failure.[2,4,13] Validated systems include the Acute Physiologic and Chronic Health Evaluation II (APACHEII) system, Bedside Index of Severity in Acute Pancreatitis, Harmless Acute Pancreatitis Score, the Ranson criteria, Japanese Severity Score, Pancreatitis Outcome Prediction, and Modified Glasgow Acute Pancreatitis Severity Score. They are used in determining aggressiveness of initial therapy as well as in developing clinical trials of interventions. However, development and validation of such systems remain an ongoing area of research. BISAP and APACHE II were similar in predicting severity of pancreatitis, organ failure and mortality.[33,34] Despite this, many are too complicated for bedside use or rely on measurements that are not widely available.[4] Also, some scoring systems have not been validated in prospective trials or have poor predictive ability.[3,13] The American Gastroenterological Association guidelines note a lack of demonstrated clinical benefit from the scoring systems and supports the use of a combination of clinical judgment and a variety of scoring tools.[2]

Clinical Course and Prognosis

The clinical course of acute pancreatitis varies from a mild transitory disorder to severe necrotizing disease. Mild acute pancreatitis is self-limiting and subsides spontaneously within 3 to 5 days. Mortality is influenced by etiology, as idiopathic and postoperative acute pancreatitis have higher rates than gallstone- or alcohol-related disease. First and second occurrences also carry a higher mortality than subsequent episodes. Mortality increases with unfavorable early prognostic signs, local complications, and organ failure. Persistent organ failure is a greater risk than transient organ failure.[6] Severe pancreatitis with either organ failure or infected necrosis is associated with a mortality of approximately 30%, and increases when both are present.[3,4,6,7,13]

Complications

Early complications are a result of SIRS and organ failure. The most common systemic complication of acute pancreatitis is respiratory failure.[4,13,21] In addition, patients may experience systemic complications due to exacerbation of preexisting renal, lung, or heart disease.[13,31] A second phase occurs in patients with moderately severe or severe disease. These patients have persistent organ failure and may have local complications including interstitial pancreatitis (acute peripancreatic fluid collection and pancreatic pseudocysts) and collection of necrosis. These develop approximately 3 to 4 weeks after the initial attack.[3,4,13] Long-term complications include recurrence of acute pancreatitis, development of pancreatic exocrine and endocrine insufficiency, and progression to chronic pancreatitis.[3,4,13,35] Exocrine and endocrine insufficiency develops in approximately 20% to 30% of patients following acute pancreatitis, with about one-third of those patients progressing to chronic pancreatitis.[3,4,13,36] Some patients with peripancreatic necrosis will develop secondary infections that usually require invasive intervention.[3,13]

TREATMENT

Desired Outcome

Treatment of acute pancreatitis is aimed at relieving abdominal pain and nausea, replacing fluids, correcting electrolyte, glucose, and lipid abnormalities, minimizing systemic complications, and managing pancreatic necrosis and infection. Management varies depending on the severity of the attack (Fig. 57-3). Patients with mild acute pancreatitis respond very well to the initiation of supportive care. Patients with severe acute pancreatitis should be treated aggressively and monitored closely.

General Approach to Treatment

All patients with acute pancreatitis should receive supportive care, including IV fluid resuscitation, adequate nutrition, and effective relief of pain and nausea. Patients should be evaluated for admission to the ICU. Patients predicted to follow a severe course may require treatment of systemic complications.[3,4] Fluid therapy is recommended and may help prevent organ failure.[1,2] Patients with pancreatitis and SIRS should be treated according to SIRS guidelines. IV potassium, calcium, and magnesium are used to correct electrolyte deficiency states. Insulin is used to treat hyperglycemia.

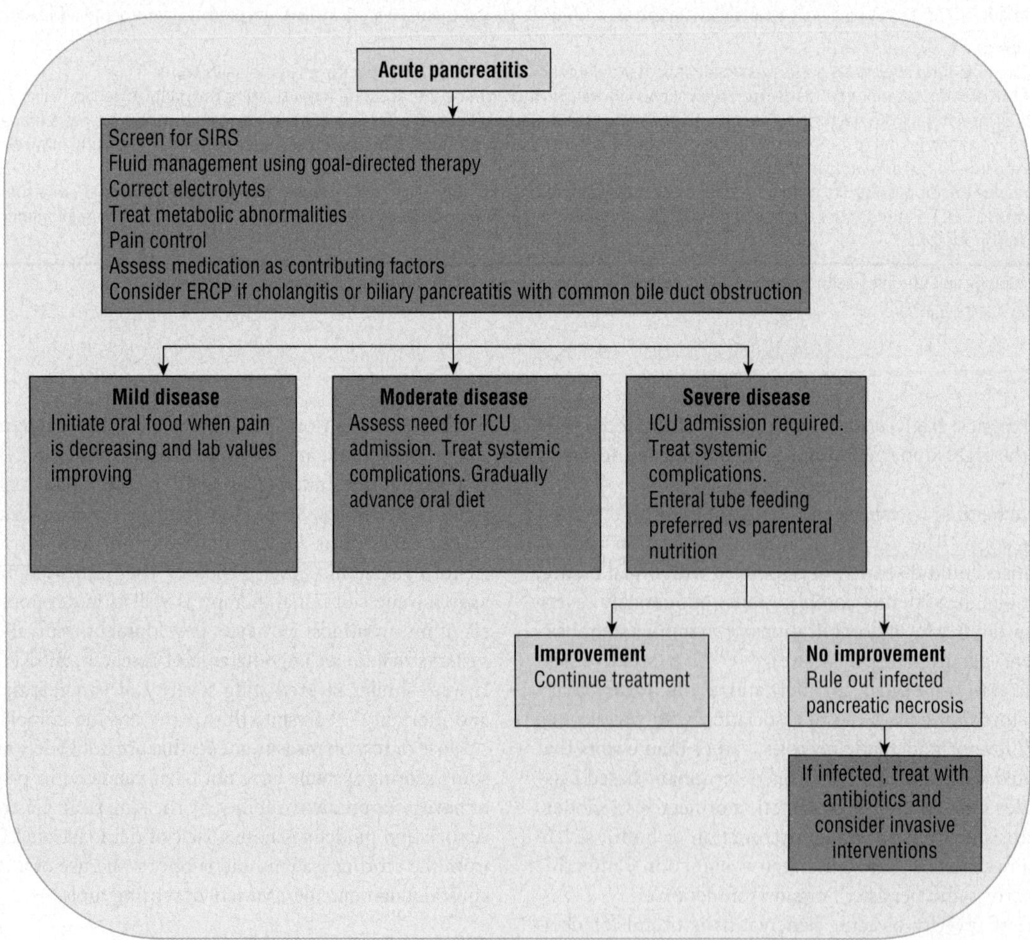

FIGURE 57-3 Algorithm of guidelines for evaluation and treatment of acute pancreatitis. (SIRS, systemic inflammatory response syndrome; ERCP, endoscopic retrograde cholangiopancreatography; ICU, intensive care unit.)

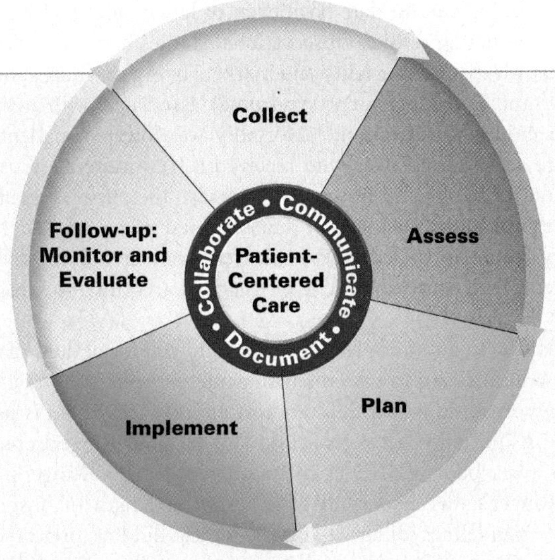

Patient Care Process for Pancreatitis

Collect

- Patient characteristics (eg, age, sex, pregnant)
- Patient history (past medical—hyperlipidemia, recent surgery, gallstone disease or ERCP; social—dietary habits, alcohol use, tobacco use)
- Current and recent (for acute pancreatitis; see Table 57-2) medications
- Medication allergies
- Review of systems for the abdomen and gastrointestinal system (eg, abdominal pain, nausea and vomiting, stool frequency and consistency for chronic pancreatitis; see Tables 57-3 and 57-5)
- Objective data
  - Acute pancreatitis (see Table 57-3)
    Vital signs (eg, BP, heart rate, temperature, respiratory rate)
    Labs (eg, CBC, Chem-7, calcium, albumin, amylase, lipase, transaminases, bilirubin, triglycerides)
    Microbiology results
    Intake/output
  - Chronic pancreatitis (see Table 57-5)
    Physical exam (eg, weight; assessment for neuropathy, nephropathy, and retinopathy with diabetes)
    Labs (eg, fasting serum glucose, bilirubin, transaminases, pancreatic function tests, fat-soluble vitamins, zinc, magnesium, calcium, albumin)

Assess

- Acute pancreatitis
  - Causative medications (see Table 57-2)
  - Nutrition and fluid status
  - Abdominal pain: location, radiation, severity, onset
  - Infectious etiologies
  - Continuous hemodynamic monitoring
- Chronic pancreatitis
  - Alcohol and tobacco use
  - Abdominal pain
  - Trends in weight, nutrition status, serum glucose, and stool consistency and frequency (assess for constipation if patient is taking opioids)

Plan*

- Acute pancreatitis
  - Fluid support including choice and dose
  - Discontinue suspected causal medications
  - Nutrition support including route and caloric requirements
  - Pain management with specific medication choice, route, and dose
  - Antimicrobial therapy regimen for suspected or identified infection(s)
- Chronic pancreatitis
  - Tailored lifestyle modifications (eg, abstinence from alcohol, smoking cessation; see Fig. 57-4)
  - Nutrition support and dietetic counseling
  - Therapy for abdominal pain (see Fig. 57-4) with analgesics (see Table 57-6) and pancreatic enzymes (see Table 57-7), including the need for treatment of constipation if opioids are utilized
  - Therapy for malabsorption (see Fig. 57-5, and Tables 57-6 and 57-7)
  - Treatment of concomitant diabetes mellitus if present

Implement

- Consultation with additional providers as necessary (eg, dietician, pain management specialist, infectious diseases, gastroenterology, endocrinology) and consider transfer to a specialty center if severe disease
- Pain therapy with clearly identified goals for both the provider and patient
- Fluid and nutrition support as appropriate
- Necessary lifestyle modifications (eg, alcohol and smoking cessation)
- For patients with acute pancreatitis consider antimicrobial therapy if suspected or known infection and narrow coverage based on cultures and sensitivities
- For patients with malabsorption due to chronic pancreatitis initiate appropriate pancreatic enzyme therapy

Follow-up: Monitor and Evaluate

- Pain control and constipation if opioids utilized
- Acute pancreatitis
  - Fluid and electrolytes along with kidney and liver function (eg, serum creatinine, BUN, bilirubin, transaminases)
  - Signs and symptoms of infection along with microbiology culture and sensitivity results
  - Hemodynamic parameters for signs of decreased intravascular volume and shock
  - Nutrition status and support (eg, prealbumin, albumin, changes in caloric requirements and delivery route)
  - Discontinuation of causative medication(s) on discharge and identification of necessary therapeutic alternative(s)
  - Brief alcohol cessation intervention prior to discharge for alcohol-related acute pancreatitis
- Chronic pancreatitis
  - Alcohol intake and smoking status utilizing motivational interviewing
  - Weight and effects of diet on abdominal pain and malabsorption symptoms
  - Efficacy of pancreatic enzymes on symptoms of malabsorption (see Fig. 57-5)
  - Serum blood glucose along with signs and symptoms of diabetes mellitus

**Collaborate with patients, caregivers, and other healthcare professionals.*

Local complications resolve as the inflammatory process subsides. However, patients with necrotizing pancreatitis may require procedural intervention.[37] Medications listed in Table 57-2 should be reviewed and discontinued if other etiologies are unlikely.

Nonpharmacologic Therapy

Nonpharmacologic therapy includes ERCP for removal of any underlying biliary tract stones, procedural interventions, and nutritional support. The need for admission to an ICU should be addressed. Advances in minimally invasive surgical techniques are changing practice with respect to timing and approach to managing infected necrotizing pancreatitis, and may help lower the risk of mortality in the most critical patients.[2,37] Patients with alcohol-related pancreatitis should receive abstinence interventions during the inpatient stay.[1]

Nutrition and Probiotics Nutritional support plays an important role in the management of patients with mild or severe disease as acute pancreatitis creates a catabolic state that promotes nutritional depletion. This can impair recovery, increase the risk of complications, and prolong hospitalization.[38] Enteral nutrition results in decreased multiple organ failure, complications, duration of hospitalization, mortality, and need for surgical intervention compared with parenteral nutrition.[38,39] Possible mechanisms for this include protection of the gut barrier and prevention of colonization with pathogenic bacteria, both of which may prevent translocation of bacteria and subsequent infection.[3,4] Patients with mild to moderate acute pancreatitis should begin oral feeding as soon as clinically tolerated regardless of serum lipase concentrations, usually within 24 hours of admission.[1,38] In severe or complicated disease, nutritional deficits develop rapidly and are complicated by tissue necrosis, organ failure, and surgery. Despite this guideline, recommendations support beginning oral or enteral nutrition within 24 to 72 hours of admission.[38,40] If the enteral route is used due to intolerance of an oral diet, based on guidelines make preference for nasogastric feeding tube placement over nasojejunal.[1,38,41] If enteral feeding is not possible or if the patient is unable to obtain sufficient nutrients, total parenteral nutrition should be implemented before protein and calorie depletion become advanced.[1,2,38]

Probiotics have mixed results in several randomized controlled trials for the treatment of severe acute pancreatitis. A meta-analysis, however, did not support the use of probiotics in the treatment of acute pancreatitis, as they have no benefit.[42] Therefore, use of probiotic agents for acute pancreatitis is not recommended by guidelines.[38]

Pharmacologic Therapy

Patients with acute pancreatitis often require IV antiemetics for nausea. Those requiring ICU admission should be treated with antisecretory agents (such as famotidine or pantoprazole) if they are at risk of stress-related mucosal bleeding. Patients also require appropriate fluid resuscitation and pain management, but there is controversy surrounding both of these therapies (see Fig. 57-3). Clinical trials have also failed to identify a group of patients that benefit from prophylactic antibiotics.

Fluid Resuscitation 2 Vasodilation from the inflammatory response, vomiting, and nasogastric suction contributes to hypovolemia and fluid and electrolyte abnormalities, thus necessitating replacement. Patients with acute pancreatitis should receive goal-directed fluid management to reduce the risks of persistent SIRS and organ failure.[1] Recommendations regarding the volume of fluid differ, with anywhere from 250 to 500 mL/hr to 5 to 10 mL/kg/hr in the first 12 to 24 hours.[3,4,13] Goals for fluid therapy in the management of acute pancreatitis are not well-defined but include one or more of the following: heart rate less than 120/min, mean arterial pressure 65 to 85 mm Hg, urinary output greater than 0.5 to 1 mL/kg/hr, or hematocrit 35% to 44% (0.35-0.44) with transfusion of blood.[3,4]

Studies completed to date have been of low quality and have somewhat conflicting results. Observational studies have identified both benefit (decreased mortality and markers of organ failure) and harm (abdominal compartment syndrome) associated with early aggressive fluid administration.[1,2] Mortality was lower in patients with severe acute pancreatitis who received 6 L or more of resuscitation fluid in the first 24 hours.[43] In contrast, there is no benefit to mortality and a greater risk of acute kidney injury and acute respiratory failure in patients who received aggressive fluid therapy.[44] Patients with sepsis should be resuscitated according to sepsis guidelines.[45]

In addition to questions about the rate and volume of fluid that should be administered to patients with acute pancreatitis, there is also debate regarding which fluid is most appropriate. There is no difference in mortality between saline and lactated Ringer's, but did find a lower odds of SIRS at 24 hours with lactated Ringer's.[46] Lactated Ringer's was associated with a shorter length of hospitalization.[47] Guidelines differ regarding which fluid is preferred with most recommending lactated Ringer's in adult patients.[4] The American Gastroenterological Association Institute Guideline on Initial Management of Acute Pancreatitis also recommends against the use of hydroxyethyl starch solutions because there are no benefits beyond saline and lactated Ringer's, and an association with an increase in multiple organ failure.[1]

Relief of Abdominal Pain 3 Parenteral opioid analgesics are used to control abdominal pain associated with acute pancreatitis despite a lack of high-quality evidence to support the practice. Pentazocine led to lower rescue analgesic use and a longer pain-free period compared to parenteral diclofenac.[48]

NSAIDs, however, may be sufficient in patients with mild or moderate pain due to acute pancreatitis and can be used if not otherwise contraindicated.[49] Parenteral morphine is often recommended for pain control because it provides a longer duration of pain relief than other opioids. Although morphine increases biliary pressure, it is contraindicated for use in acute pancreatitis. Patient-controlled analgesia should be considered in patients who require frequent opioid dosing (eg, every 2-3 hours). There was a reduction in 30-day mortality in patients with acute pancreatitis who received thoracic epidural analgesia compared to those who received a standard approach to pain management.[50]

Antimicrobial Use in Acute Pancreatitis

4 Use of prophylactic antibiotics is not recommended in patients with acute pancreatitis without signs or symptoms of infection, including those predicted to develop acute pancreatitis or necrotizing pancreatitis.[1,2] Several small, randomized clinical trials have compared antibiotic prophylaxis with no prophylaxis in patients with severe acute and necrotizing pancreatitis with varying results. Prophylactic antibiotics do not reduce infected necrosis or mortality.[2,51] In addition, overuse of antibiotics increases microbial resistance.

Because the source of bacterial contamination is most likely translocation of organisms from the colon, the antibiotic regimen for patients with known or suspected infected pancreatitis should be broad-spectrum, covering the range of enteric aerobic gram-negative bacilli and anaerobic microorganisms. Imipenem–cilastatin (500 mg IV every 8 hours) has been widely used because of its good penetration into the pancreas and one positive prophylaxis study.[52] However, it has been replaced on many hospital formularies by one of the newer carbapenems (eg, meropenem). Fluoroquinolones, such as ciprofloxacin or levofloxacin, combined with metronidazole should be considered for penicillin-allergic patients.[53] Patients with infected necrotic pancreatitis are generally treated with a combination of invasive interventions and antibiotics. Antibiotics alone may be sufficient in some cases or at least delay the need for an invasive procedure long enough for the necrotic areas to be walled off.[3]

Post-ERCP Pancreatitis

The clinical characteristics of post-ERCP pancreatitis are similar to those of acute pancreatitis from other causes. In most cases, the disease course is mild and resolves in several days. The incidence of post-ERCP pancreatitis has decreased in recent decades, most likely due to better patient selection. Several classes of medications have been studied for prevention of post-ERCP pancreatitis. The best data are with nonsteroidal anti-inflammatory drugs (NSAIDs) administered rectally prior to or immediately following the procedure.[54] The most common beneficial NSAIDs are indomethacin and diclofenac. The combination of rectal diclofenac and sublingual isosorbide dinitrate was superior to diclofenac alone in prevention of post-ERCP pancreatitis, but this finding needs to be validated in additional studies.[55] Another agent that reduced post-ERCP pancreatitis is gabexate mesilate; however, this agent is not approved in the United States.[56] In addition to NSAIDs more aggressive peri-procedural hydration with intravenous crystalloids reduces the occurrence of post-ERCP pancreatitis.[57,58]

CHRONIC PANCREATITIS

Chronic pancreatitis results from long-standing pancreatic inflammation resulting in irreversible destruction of pancreatic tissue with fibrin deposition, leading to a loss of exocrine and endocrine functions.[5-11] It has four different stages beginning with a preclinical inflammatory stage where patients remain asymptomatic or have indistinguishable symptoms.[9] In the second-stage patients present with acute attacks that often resemble those of acute pancreatitis. The third stage consists of episodes of intermittent or constant abdominal pain. Finally, in the burnout stage patients present with diminished or absent pain, but develop malabsorption syndrome due to loss of pancreatic exocrine function and may develop diabetes mellitus from loss of endocrine function.

Etiology

Chronic alcohol consumption remains the leading cause of chronic pancreatitis in Western society, accounting for up to two-thirds of cases.[10,11,59,60] The consumption of 40 g/day or more of alcohol poses a significant risk of chronic pancreatitis.[60] Most of the remaining cases can be classified as idiopathic, while a small percentage of cases are due to rare causes, such as autoimmune, hereditary, and tropical pancreatitis.[10,11,61] Various genetic alterations have also been associated with the occurrence of chronic pancreatitis, including mutations of the following genes: protease serine 1 (trypsin 1) (*PRSS1*), serine peptidase inhibitor Kazal type 1 (*SPINK1*), cystic fibrosis transmembrane conductance regulator (*CFTR*), chymotrypsin C, chymotrypsin B1/B2, carboxypeptidase A1, and carboxyl ester lipase (CEL).[8,10,11,59,62,63] There is also a risk of chronic pancreatitis with cigarette smoking that appears to be dose-dependent and may contribute to mortality from chronic pancreatitis.[8,11,15,59,61,64] There are two classification systems for chronic pancreatitis that take into account the various risk factors associated with the disease (Table 57-4).[59]

TABLE 57-4 Classification of Etiology and Risk Factors for Chronic Pancreatitis

M-ANNHEIM	
***M**ultiple*	Risk factors
***A**lcohol*	Excessive consumption (>80 g/day), increased consumption (20-80 g/day), moderate consumption (<20 g/day)
***N**icotine*	Quantitated in pack-years for current smokers
***N**utritional factors*	High-fat and protein diet, hyperlipidemia (especially hypertriglyceridemia)
***H**ereditary factors*	Hereditary pancreatitis, familial pancreatitis, early and late-onset idiopathic pancreatitis, tropical pancreatitis, possible gene mutations (eg, *PRSS1*, *SPINK1*, and *CFTR*)
***E**fferent duct factors*	Pancreas divisum, annular pancreas/congenital abnormalities, pancreatic duct obstruction (eg, tumors), posttraumatic pancreatic duct scars, sphincter of Oddi dysfunction
***I**mmunologic factors*	Autoimmune pancreatitis
***M**iscellaneous and rare factors*	Hypercalcemia and hyperparathyroidism, chronic kidney disease, medications, toxins
TIGAR-O	
***T**oxic-metabolic*	Alcohol, tobacco smoking, hypercalcemia, hyperlipidemia, chronic kidney disease, medications, toxins
***I**diopathic*	Early onset, late-onset, tropical pancreatitis
***G**enetic mutations*	*PRSS1, CFTR, SPINK1*, others
***A**utoimmune*	Isolated, syndromic
***R**ecurrent and severe associated acute pancreatitis*	Postnecrotic (severe acute pancreatitis), vascular disease/ischemic, postirradiation
***O**bstructive*	Pancreas divisum, sphincter of Oddi dysfunction, pancreatic duct obstruction (eg, tumor), posttraumatic pancreatic duct scars

Reprinted, with permission, from Conwell DL, Lee LS, Yadav D, et al. American Pancreatic Association Practice Guidelines in Chronic Pancreatitis: Evidence-Based Report on Diagnostic Guidelines. Pancreas. 2014;43(8):1162.

Pathophysiology

Although the exact mechanism for the pathogenesis of chronic pancreatitis is unknown, several theories have been proposed. One of the main theories is that repeated episodes of acute pancreatitis lead to the occurrence of chronic pancreatitis.[10,11,59,65] Repeated episodes of acute pancreatitis initiate inflammation and necrosis that leads to ductal scarring and fibrosis. This leads to ductal obstruction and eventually results in acinar atrophy and fibrin deposition.

Regardless of the pathophysiologic mechanism, activation of pancreatic stellate cells is the cause of fibrin deposition in chronic pancreatitis. Various toxins, oxidative stress, and inflammatory mediators activate pancreatic stellate cells.[10,11,61,65] Activated pancreatic stellate cells then initiate fibrinogenesis. Other mediators generated by the stellate cells themselves perpetuate continued stellate cell activation.

The pathogenesis of pain in chronic pancreatitis has long been thought to be the result of increased pancreatic parenchymal pressure from obstruction, inflammation, and necrosis.[10] However, there is a neurogenic origin of pain. There is abnormal pain processing in the central nervous system of patients with chronic pancreatitis, with functional reorganization of the insular cortex.[10,61] Also, visceral nerves in these patients are sensitized. This may explain the hyperalgesia often experienced by these patients, and the need for various methods of pain management.[11] Patients with chronic pancreatitis may also experience pain in areas distant to the pancreas due to impaired inhibition of somatic and visceral pain pathways.

5 Chronic pain, malabsorption with resultant steatorrhea, and diabetes mellitus are the hallmark symptoms and complications of chronic pancreatitis. Although abdominal pain is the most common symptom at any stage, patients may present with various signs and symptoms depending on the stage of the disease. A more comprehensive list of the common signs and symptoms is presented in Table 57-5.

Diagnosis

The diagnosis of chronic pancreatitis is based primarily on presenting signs and symptoms in combination with either imaging, pancreatic function studies, or histological examination (see Table 57-5).

TABLE 57-5 Signs, Symptoms, and Diagnosis of Chronic Pancreatitis

Signs
- Malnutrition (especially in chronic alcohol misuse)
- Abdominal mass (may indicate a pancreatic pseudocyst)
- Jaundice may be seen
- Splenomegaly (rare)

Symptoms
- Abdominal pain
  - Commonly in epigastric area
  - May radiate to the back
  - Described as deep and penetrating
  - May be relieved by bending/leaning forward or bringing knees to the chest
  - Often occurs with meals and at night
  - May be associated with nausea and vomiting
- Steatorrhea
  - Patients describe bulky or foul-smelling stools often with obvious oil droplets
  - Usually have an average of three to four stools per day
  - May be associated with deficiencies in fat-soluble vitamins
  - Watery diarrhea, excess gas, and abdominal cramps are uncommon
- Pancreatic diabetes mellitus
- Diarrhea (associated with steatorrhea)
- Weight loss
  - May be due to severe malabsorption or acute/chronic pain
  - Substantial loss may be due to associated or unrelated malignancy
- Osteopenia/Osteoporosis (from vitamin D malabsorption and increased bone resorption)
- Bone fractures
- Dyspepsia

Laboratory studies
- CBC to rule out infection (ie, infected pseudocyst)
- Serum amylase and lipase
  - Low specificity for chronic pancreatitis
  - May be elevated in acute exacerbations
  - Usually are normal or only slightly elevated
- Total bilirubin, alkaline phosphatase, and hepatic transaminases may be elevated with ductal obstruction
- Fasting serum glucose or hemoglobin A_{1c}
- Screening for fat-soluble vitamin (ie, A, D, E, and K) and mineral (ie, magnesium, iron, selenium, and zinc) deficiency
- Pancreatic function tests
  - Indirect
    Serum trypsinogen (<20 ng/mL [mcg/L] is abnormal)
    Fecal elastase (<200 mcg/g of stool is abnormal)
    Fecal chymotrypsin (<3 units/g of stool is abnormal)
    Fecal fat estimation (>7 g/day is abnormal; need to collect 72 hours of stool)
    ^{13}C-mixed triglyceride breath test (conducted over 6 hours; not available in the United States)
  - Direct
    Secretin stimulation (evaluates duodenal bicarbonate secretion)
    Cholecystokinin stimulation (evaluates pancreatic lipase secretion)
  - Serum albumin (may be low with malnutrition)
  - Serum calcium (may be low with malnutrition)

Imaging studies
- Noninvasive
  - Abdominal ultrasound
  - Computed tomography (CT)
  - Magnetic resonance imaging (MRI)
  - Secretin-enhanced magnetic resonance cholangiopancreatography
- Invasive
  - Endoscopic ultrasonography (EUS)
  - Endoscopic retrograde cholangiopancreatography (ERCP)
- Dual-energy X-ray absorptiometry to assess for osteopenia and osteoporosis

CBC, complete blood count.

Data from References 8–11, 23, 38, 63, 66, 67, and 79.

Although histology would be the best diagnostic test, it is recommended only in high-risk patients with strong clinical and functional evidence, but inconclusive imaging studies.[61,63] Therefore, testing usually begins with noninvasive or invasive imaging studies. Abdominal ultrasonography, computed tomography (CT), and magnetic resonance imaging may be used first, but are limited in their ability to produce detailed imaging of pancreatic ductal abnormalities.[8,11,63,68] Invasive studies, such as endoscopic ultrasonography (EUS), are recommended when noninvasive studies are inconclusive.[8,11,63] Secretin-enhanced magnetic resonance cholangiopancreatography produces more detailed images of the pancreatic ducts, and is recommended if all other imaging studies cannot confirm a diagnosis and clinical suspicion remains high.[8,11,59,63,68,69] While ERCP is the gold standard invasive study, it is rarely used due to inter- and intra-observer variability, the risk of post-ERCP pancreatitis, and lack of high-quality evidence comparing it to other imaging studies such as CT, MRI, and EUS.[59,63,68,69] In addition to imagining studies, pancreatic function tests are used when imagining is inconclusive, as adjunctive diagnostic studies or to quantify the degree of exocrine insufficiency.[63,68] The most sensitive studies are the secretin and CCK stimulation tests.[59,68,69] However, these are not widely available and are uncomfortable for patients. Indirect studies of pancreatic function are most sensitive during late chronic pancreatitis.[59]

Clinical Course and Prognosis

The clinical course of chronic pancreatitis depends on the etiology. Exocrine insufficiency occurs when lipase secretion is less than 10% of normal.[9,63,69] Patients with hereditary chronic pancreatitis typically have exocrine insufficiency occur at an early age, while those with alcohol-induced disease have exocrine insufficiency occur about 5 years after disease onset, with "burnout" of the pancreas in about 10 to 20 years.[69,70] Patients with early-onset idiopathic chronic pancreatitis have delayed progression to exocrine insufficiency compared to those with alcohol-induced or late-onset idiopathic disease.[66] Diabetes mellitus occurs later than exocrine insufficiency and has a reported prevalence of 25% to 80%.[8,71]

The median survival of patients with chronic pancreatitis is estimated to be 15 to 20 years after diagnosis.[11] One of the most significant complications of long-standing disease is pancreatic cancer. Patients with chronic pancreatitis have a 16-fold increased risk of pancreatic cancer.[72] This risk increases depending on the etiology, with patients who smoke having twice the risk.[69]

TREATMENT

Desired Outcome

The major goals in the treatment of uncomplicated chronic pancreatitis are relief of abdominal pain, treatment of any associated complications such as malabsorption and diabetes mellitus, and improvement in quality of life. Secondary goals include delaying development of complications and treating associated disorders such as depression and malnutrition.

General Approach to Treatment

Treatment of chronic pancreatitis and its complications involves various nonpharmacologic and pharmacologic interventions. Lifestyle modifications should include abstinence from alcohol and smoking cessation.[8,11,63,68,69] In addition, patients with steatorrhea may need to eat smaller, more frequent meals and reduce dietary fat intake.[9,38,63,69] The majority of patients require analgesics and pancreatic enzyme replacement therapy (PERT).[8,11,38,63,68,69] Pain can initially be controlled with medications, but may require more aggressive medical and surgical therapies as the disease progresses. Patients with malabsorption require pancreatic enzymes to reduce steatorrhea and maintain adequate nutrient absorption.[8,11,38,63,68,69] An antisecretory agent may be added to the regimen when enzymes alone provide an inadequate reduction in steatorrhea.[8-10,38,63,69]

Nonpharmacologic Therapy

In addition to medical management, the treatment of chronic pancreatitis includes both lifestyle and dietary modifications. Patients should be counseled to abstain from alcohol use, and smoking cessation should be advocated. Cessation of alcohol use may reduce pain in patients with alcohol-induced chronic pancreatitis, and hastens disease progression and reduces the risk of developing pancreatic cancer.[8,9,11,63,68,69] Smoking has been associated with pain relapses and progression of disease, so cessation should be advocated.[8,11,63] Patients with steatorrhea should be counseled to eat small and frequent meals.[38,63,69] A reduction in dietary fat is not needed routinely, but may be needed in those whose symptoms are uncontrolled with enzyme PERT.[38,68,73] Enteral nutrition via a feeding tube is recommended for patients with malnutrition who do not have an adequate response to oral nutrition support.[38] For patients with chronic pancreatitis requiring tube feeding, use of a jejunal feeding tube is recommended.[38,66]

Invasive procedures and surgery are primarily used to treat uncontrolled pain and the associated complications of chronic pancreatitis. Stents placed via ERCP may be used to treat pancreatic duct strictures in order to relieve parenchymal pressure and reduce pain.[8,63,68,74] Extracorporeal shock wave lithotripsy can be used to break up pancreatic stones with ultrasonic vibration prior to removal by ERCP.[8,11,74,75] Blockade of pain signals through the celiac plexus may be achieved utilizing EUS.[11,63,68,74] The various complications of chronic pancreatitis that can be treated endoscopically include common bile duct strictures, duodenal obstructions, and pancreatic pseudocysts.[8,11,63,68,74] Various surgical techniques including total pancreatectomy may also be used to relieve pain associated with chronic pancreatitis.[23,67,76] Surgery is more effective at relieving pain than endoscopic procedures, but is usually reserved when endoscopic therapy fails.[8,11,63,68,76,77] Finally, total pancreatectomy with transplantation of pancreatic islet cells to reduce the need for exogenous insulin is recommended as a last-line option for the treatment of pain due to chronic pancreatitis.[8,11,63,68]

Pharmacologic Therapy

General Recommendations Pharmacologic therapy of chronic pancreatitis is aimed at controlling pain, treating malabsorption and associated steatorrhea, and controlling diabetes mellitus. Once other causes have been excluded, acetaminophen with or without NSAIDs should be tried initially for pain management (Fig. 57-4).[8,11,61,65,66] Patients with inadequate relief from these agents should have adjuvant agents added to their regimen, with opioid analgesics reserved for patients with refractory pain.[8,11,65,66,68,69] The addition of pancreatic enzyme supplements for pain control has been studied, but is not recommended based on available evidence.[8,9,11,61,63,65,68,69] Antioxidants are recommended for relief of pain due to chronic pancreatitis based on some trials.[8,11,63]

Most patients with malabsorption will require pancreatic enzyme supplementation in order to achieve adequate nutritional status and reduction in steatorrhea (Fig. 57-5). An antisecretory agent (ie, histamine-2 receptor antagonist or proton pump inhibitor) should be added to the regimen when there is an inadequate response to enzyme therapy alone.[8,38,63,68,69,73] If these measures are ineffective, documentation of the diagnosis and exclusion of other diseases should be undertaken. Exogenous insulin is the primary pharmacologic agent used in the treatment of diabetes mellitus associated with chronic pancreatitis.[8,9,61,65] Metformin may be initiated in early chronic pancreatitis, and has the added benefit of significantly reducing the risk of pancreatic cancer.[8,61,65]

Relief of Chronic Abdominal Pain

6 ***Analgesics*** Pain from chronic pancreatitis may initially be treated with nonopioid analgesics, but adjuvant agents may be necessary as the disease progresses. Regimens should be individualized

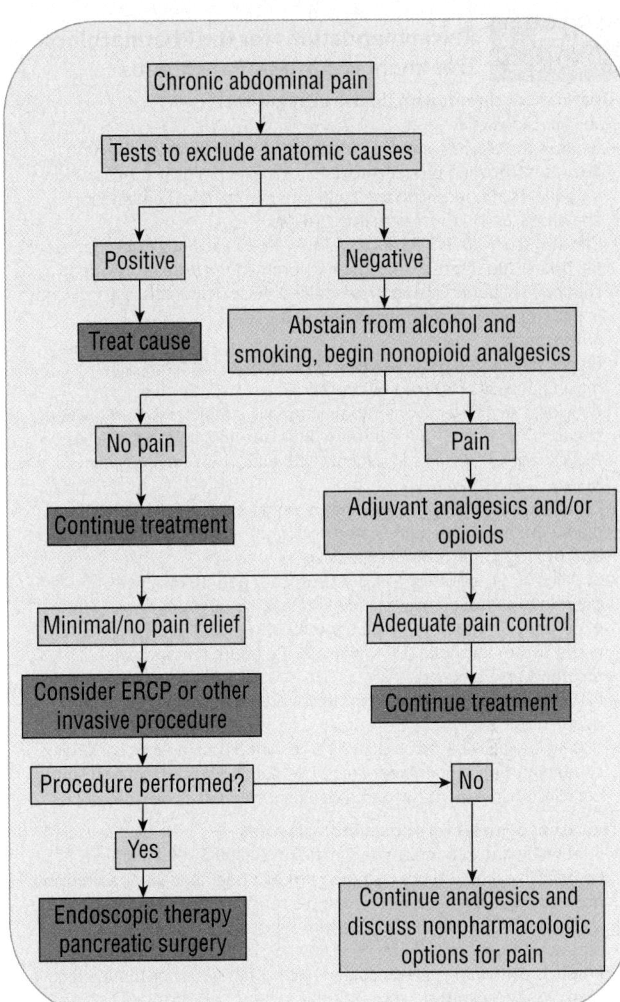

FIGURE 57-4 Algorithm for the treatment of abdominal pain in chronic pancreatitis. (ERCP, endoscopic retrograde cholangiopancreatography.)

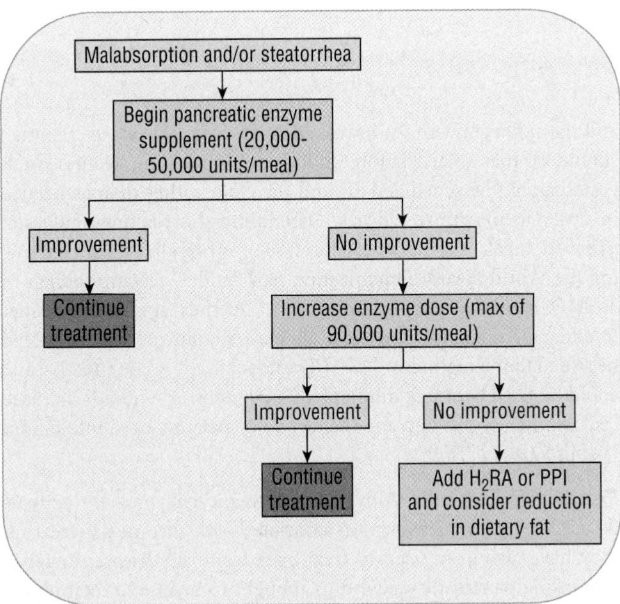

FIGURE 57-5 Algorithm for the treatment of malabsorption and steatorrhea in chronic pancreatitis. (H_2RA, histamine-2 receptor antagonist; PPI, proton pump inhibitor.)

TABLE 57-6 Recommendations for the Pharmacologic Treatment of Chronic Pancreatitis

Treatment of chronic pain (oral drug regimens)

Nonopioid analgesics

- Begin with acetaminophen at doses of 500-650 mg per dose every 4-6 hours following product labeling for maximum daily dose; caution for patients also receiving acetaminophen from other combination analgesics, and in those with liver disease
- Can also start with NSAIDs at low doses (ie, 200-400 mg ibuprofen every 6-8 hours) and titrate to maximum recommended doses as needed; caution in patients with cardiovascular disease or high disease risk, and in patients with kidney impairment or disease

Adjuvant agents

- Pregabalin has the best evidence; begin with 75 mg twice daily; maximum dose of 300 mg twice daily
- Consider use of selective serotonin reuptake inhibitors (eg, paroxetine), serotonin/norepinephrine reuptake inhibitors (eg, duloxetine) and tricyclic antidepressants in patients with difficult-to-manage pain

Opioids

- Tramadol: 50-100 mg every 4-6 hours, not to exceed 400 mg/day; has opioid-like effect; contraindicated in alcohol or hypnotic intoxication; be aware of drug interactions; expensive
- Codeine 30-60 mg every 6 hours; hydrocodone 5-10 mg every 4-6 hours; morphine sulfate (extended-release) 30-60 mg every 8-12 hours; oxycodone 5-10 mg every 6 hours; methadone 2.5-10 mg every 8-12 hours; hydromorphone 0.5-1 mg every 4-6 hours; fentanyl patch 25-100 mcg/hr every 72 hours
- Risk of potentiation with alcohol; impaired respiration; constipation; hypotension; allergy
- Dosing is usually based on providing continuous pain relief; consider combining with acetaminophen; opioid dependence is common; abuse is a concern in patients who misuse alcohol; tolerance may develop

Treatment of malabsorption and steatorrhea

- Start with pancreatic enzymes containing 20,000-50,000 USP units of lipase with each meal of a preferred product (see Table 57-7); administer dose during meals; administer multiple capsules/tablets throughout the meal; use half the mealtime dose with snacks
- Increase dose to a maximum of 90,000 USP units of lipase per meal
- Products containing enteric-coated microspheres may be more effective than other dose forms

Acid-suppression agents

- May improve efficacy of enzyme therapy for malabsorption and steatorrhea
- Preferred for use with nonenteric-coated dose forms

USP, United States Pharmacopeia.

Data from References 8, 9, 11, 61, 63, 66, 68, 69, 73, and 79.

and should begin with the lowest effective dose. The dosage regimen should be maximized before adding or substituting agents. Analgesics should be scheduled around the clock rather than as needed in order to maximize efficacy. Scheduling short-acting analgesics prior to meals should help decrease postprandial pain. Following the World Health Organization pain ladder, acetaminophen or NSAIDs should be used initially.[8,11,61,65-67] As the response diminishes to adequate doses of nonopioid analgesics, adjuvant agents should be added to the regimen.[8,11,61,65,67] Tramadol may also be effective and could be tried before adding opioid analgesics.[11,67] Opioids are used last as other agents become ineffective or patients have intolerance (Table 57-6).[8,11,61,63,65,66,73]

Pancreatic Enzymes Although pancreatic enzymes are primarily used to treat malabsorption associated with chronic pancreatitis, they have also been used to treat pain from the disease. Relief of pain using pancreatic enzymes is thought to be due to their ability to break down CCK.[9,66,68] Release of CCK is normally inhibited by trypsin, but patients with chronic pancreatitis have decreased trypsin production. The proteases in pancreatic enzyme supplements are thought to act as substitutes for endogenous trypsin, leading to a decrease in CCK release. However, there are mixed results from trials investigating pancreatic enzyme supplements for the treatment of pain from chronic pancreatitis. This may be due to the differences between the various enzyme formulations used in the trials as well as the small number of subjects enrolled.[9,11,63,68,69] However, trials that used nonenteric-coated enzyme formulations have a benefit in the treatment of pain.[65,66,79] Enteric-coated formulations may not release enough proteases in the duodenum to inhibit CCK release. Despite their intuitive mechanism current guidelines do not recommend the use of pancreatic enzyme therapy for the treatment of pain from chronic pancreatitis due to lack of beneficial outcomes.[63,73]

Other Agents Various adjuvant agents are also used in patients experiencing pain from chronic pancreatitis. Selective serotonin reuptake inhibitors and tricyclic antidepressants are used both for treating the concomitant depression that often occurs in patients with chronic pancreatitis and for their potential effects on pain (see Table 57-6).[8,9,11,61,65] Gabapentin and pregabalin are effective adjunct analgesics.[8,9,11,61,80] Patients with chronic pancreatitis have increased oxidative stress, and the use of antioxidants, such as selenium, vitamins C and E, and β-carotene, has some benefit in relieving pain and improving quality of life in these patients.[11,63,81-83] The details of their benefit remains variable, but due to their low cost and relative safety, the American College of Gastroenterology guidelines for chronic pancreatitis considers their use for treatment of pain.[63]

7 **Treatment of Malabsorption** Pancreatic enzyme and fat-soluble vitamin supplementation are the primary treatments for malabsorption due to chronic pancreatitis. Treatment should begin when steatorrhea is documented and persistent weight loss occurs despite any dietary modifications. The utilization of pancreatic enzymes enhances the patient's nutritional status and reduces steatorrhea and resultant abdominal symptoms. Malabsorption is minimized if the concentration of lipase delivered to the duodenum with supplementation is about 10% of normal pancreatic output.[9] This requires that 20,000 to 50,000 units of lipase be administered with each meal to start (see Table 57-6).[38,61,68,73,78,84] Half of the necessary mealtime dose is recommended with snacks.[38,73,78] In many cases the lipase dose will need to be increased due to insufficient lipolytic activity, but doses greater than 90,000 units per meal are not recommended. In addition to enzyme replacement therapy, patients with chronic pancreatitis have deficiencies in fat-soluble vitamins.[38,63,85] Thus, they should be assessed for vitamin deficiencies and provided necessary supplementation as required.[9,38,63,69,73,78]

8 There is little evidence regarding the optimal dosage form and administration of pancreatic enzyme supplements. Most studies have compared them with placebo rather than other enzyme products, and used quantitation of fat absorption or elimination as a primary measure of efficacy rather than weight gain.[63,86] While they may not completely eliminate steatorrhea, they improve nutritional parameters and quality of life of patients with chronic pancreatitis.[8,11,63,69] Since most exogenous lipase is rapidly and irreversibly destroyed at low intragastric pH, enteric-coated products are preferred for the treatment of malabsorption and steatorrhea. The enteric coating only dissolves at a pH greater than 5.5, which allows a sufficient quantity of enzymes to remain intact until dissolution of the coating in the duodenum.[38,69] However, enzymes must also be emptied from the stomach into the duodenum at the same rate and time as ingested food. The size of the enteric-coated enzyme preparation influences the rate of enzyme delivery to the duodenum.[9] Likewise, the administration time relevant to a meal influences the timing of enzyme delivery. Products containing enzymes in small enteric-coated microspheres are preferred, and they should be administered with meals.[38,61,69,73,84] Ideally, patients should eat five to six small meals per day, and if patients need to take more than one capsule/tablet per meal, the doses should be distributed throughout the meal.[38,61,73]

Despite enzyme therapy, patients may continue to have steatorrhea and fail to have improvement in nutritional parameters. Adherence should be assessed in these patients as the number of capsules required with each meal can lead to reduced adherence. Alternative products with higher lipase content can be tried in order to reduce the number of capsules needed. If this fails, the dose of lipase should be increased. Finally, addition of an antisecretory agent (ie, histamine-2 receptor antagonist or proton pump inhibitor) may be tried to increase the availability of active enzymes in the duodenum.[8,38,69,73,78,84]

Pancreatic Enzyme Supplements Five pancreatic enzyme products are approved by the FDA, but only two of these products are specifically approved for exocrine pancreatic insufficiency associated with chronic pancreatitis.[87,88] Dosage forms of approved products include regular-release tablets, enteric-coated beads, bicarbonate-buffered enteric-coated microspheres, enteric-coated microspheres, and enteric-coated minitablets or microtablets encased in a cellulose or gelatin capsule (Table 57-7). Enzymes are easily administered to patients who are able to swallow the capsules or their contents. However, administration to patients with enteral feeding tubes presents a challenge. Products containing microspheres may be administered through feeding tubes in food or solutions with a pH of 4.5 or less.[38,84] Clinicians must be aware, however, that available products are not equivalent and should consider this before substituting products in patients who require administration through a nonoral route.

TABLE 57-7 Commercially Available Pancreatic Enzyme (Pancrelipase) Preparations

	Enzyme Content Per Unit Dose (USP Units)		
Product	**Lipase**	**Amylase**	**Protease**
Tablets			
Viokace™ 10,440 lipase units	10,440	39,150	39,150
Viokace™ 20,880 lipase units	20,880	78,300	78,300
Enteric-coated beads			
Zenpep® 3,000 lipase units	3,000	14,000	10,000
Zenpep® 5,000 lipase units	5,000	24,000	17,000
Zenpep® 10,000 lipase units	10,000	42,000	32,000
Zenpep® 15,000 lipase units	15,000	63,000	47,000
Zenpep® 20,000 lipase units	20,000	84,000	38,000
Zenpep® 25,000 lipase units	25,000	105,000	79,000
Zenpep® 40,000 lipase units	40,000	168,000	126,000
Enteric-coated microspheres with bicarbonate buffer			
Pertzye 4,000 lipase units	4,000	15,125	14,375
Pertzye 8,000 lipase units	8,000	30,250	28,750
Pertzye 16,000 lipase units	16,000	60,500	57,500
Enteric-coated microspheres			
Creon® 3,000 lipase units	3,000	15,000	9,500
Creon® 6,000 lipase units	6,000	30,000	19,000
Creon® 12,000 lipase units	12,000	60,000	38,000
Creon® 24,000 lipase units	24,000	120,000	76,000
Creon® 36,000 lipase units	36,000	180,000	114,000
Enteric-coated minitablets/microtablets			
Pancreaze® 2,600 lipase units	2,600	10,850	6,200
Pancreaze® 4,200 lipase units	4,200	24,600	14,200
Pancreaze® 10,500 lipase units	10,500	61,500	35,500
Pancreaze® 16,800 lipase units	16,800	98,400	56,800
Pancreaze® 21,000 lipase units	21,000	83,900	54,700

USP, United States Pharmacopeia.

Careful consideration should also be given to this issue in patient care facilities with limited formularies.

Adverse reactions from pancreatic enzyme supplements are generally benign. High doses can lead to nausea, diarrhea, and intestinal upset.[69] One of the more serious adverse effects of these products is fibrosing colonopathy. It occurs when the enzymes cause deposition of fibrin in the colon leading to colonic stricture. This reaction is uncommon and has been reported mostly in children with cystic fibrosis who received high doses of enzymes for prolonged periods.[38,69] Another concern with pancreatic enzymes is the risk of possible viral infection due to contamination of these porcine-derived products.[69]

9 ***Adjuncts to Enzyme Therapy*** The addition of a histamine-2 receptor antagonist or proton pump inhibitor to pancreatic enzyme supplementation may increase the effectiveness of enzyme therapy for malabsorption and steatorrhea. The beneficial effects of these agents result from an increase in gastric and duodenal pH.[38,69,84] This results in an increase in the amount of active enzymes available in the duodenum. Their use has been mainly recommended with nonenteric-coated enzyme products.[9,68,73,78] In fact, the only nonenteric-coated formulation approved by the FDA is indicated for administration with a proton pump inhibitor.[88]

EVALUATION OF THERAPEUTIC OUTCOMES

Acute Pancreatitis

Hydration status, serum electrolytes, pain control, and nutritional status should be assessed periodically in patients with mild acute pancreatitis, depending on the degree of abdominal pain and fluid loss. Patients with severe acute pancreatitis should receive intensive care and close monitoring of vital signs, fluid and electrolyte status, white blood cell count, blood glucose, lactate dehydrogenase, aspartate aminotransferase, serum albumin, hematocrit, BUN, serum creatinine, and international normalized ratio. Continuous hemodynamic and arterial blood gas monitoring is essential. Serum lipase, amylase, and bilirubin require less frequent monitoring. The patient should also be monitored for signs of infection, relief of abdominal pain, and adequate nutritional status. Severity of disease and patient response should be assessed using an evidence-based method.

Chronic Pancreatitis

The severity and frequency of abdominal pain should be assessed periodically in patients with chronic pancreatitis using a standardized scale in order to determine the efficacy of pain therapy. Patients receiving opioids should be prescribed laxatives on an as-needed or scheduled basis and be monitored for constipation. Patients receiving pancreatic enzymes for malabsorption should have their weight and stool frequency and consistency monitored periodically. More objective assessments of fecal fat content, such as the ^{13}C-mixed triglyceride breath test, can be utilized, but are usually unnecessary and impractical in general clinical practice.[9,38,69] Blood glucose must be closely monitored in patients with diabetes mellitus, and those with long-standing disease should receive appropriate monitoring for nephropathy, retinopathy, and neuropathy.[9]

ABBREVIATIONS

APACHE	Acute Physiology and Chronic Health Evaluation
BISAP	besdside index of severity in acute pancreatitis
BUN	blood urea nitrogen
CCK	cholecystokinin
CECT	contrast-enhanced computed tomography
CEL	carboxyl ester lipase

CFTR	cystic fibrosis transmembrane conductance regulator gene
CT	computed tomography
ERCP	endoscopic retrograde cholangiopancreatography
EUS	endoscopic ultrasonography
HIV	human immunodeficiency virus
ICU	intensive care unit
MRCP	magnetic resonance cholangiopancreatography
MRI	magnetic resonance imaging
NSAID	nonsteroidal anti-inflammatory drug
PERT	pancreatic enzyme replacement therapy
PRSS1	protease serine 1 (trypsin 1) gene
SIRS	systemic inflammatory response syndrome
SPINK1	serine peptidase inhibitor Kazal type 1 gene
VIP	vasoactive intestinal peptide

REFERENCES

1. Crockett SD, Wani S, Gardner TB, et al. American Gastroenterological Association Institute Guideline on initial management of acute pancreatitis. *Gastroenterology*. 2018;154(4):1096–1101. doi:10.1053/j.gastro.2018.01.032
2. Vege SS, DiMagno MJ, Forsmark CE, Martel M, Barkun AN. Initial medical treatment of acute pancreatitis: American Gastroenterological Association Institute Technical Review. *Gastroenterology*. 2018;154(4):1103–1139. doi:10.1053/j.gastro.2018.01.031
3. Boxhoorn L, Voermans RP, Bouwense SA, et al. Acute pancreatitis. *Lancet*. 2020;396(10252):726–734. doi:10.1016/S0140-6736(20)31310-6
4. Mederos MA, Reber HA, Girgis MD. Acute pancreatitis: A review. *JAMA - J Am Med Assoc*. 2021;325(4):382–390. doi:10.1001/jama.2020.20317
5. Peery AF, Crockett SD, Barritt AS, et al. Burden of gastrointestinal, liver, and pancreatic diseases in the United States. *Gastroenterology*. 2015;149(7):1731–1741e3. doi:10.1053/j.gastro.2015.08.045
6. Koutroumpakis E, Slivka A, Furlan A, et al. Management and outcomes of acute pancreatitis patients over the last decade: A US tertiary-center experience. *Pancreatology*. 2017;17(1):32–40. doi:10.1016/j.pan.2016.10.011
7. Lankisch PG, Apte M, Banks PA. Acute pancreatitis. *Lancet*. 2015;386(9988):85–96. doi:10.1016/S0140-6736(14)60649-8
8. Beyer G, Habtezion A, Werner J, Lerch MM, Mayerle J. Chronic pancreatitis. *Lancet*. 2020;396(10249):499–512. doi:10.1016/S0140-6736(20)31318-0
9. Forsmark CE. Chronic pancreatitis. In: Feldman M, LS F, LJ B, eds. *Sleisenger and Fordtran's Gastrointestinal and Liver Disease: Pathophysiology, Diagnosis, Management*. Vol 10th. Philadelphia: Elsevier Saunders; 2016:994–1026.
10. Muniraj T, Aslanian HR, Farrell J, Jamidar PA. Chronic pancreatitis, a comprehensive review and update. Part I: epidemiology, etiology, risk factors, genetics, pathophysiology, and clinical features. *Dis Mon*. 2014;60(12):530–550.
11. Singh VK, Yadav D, Garg PK. Diagnosis and management of chronic pancreatitis: A review. *JAMA - J Am Med Assoc*. 2019;322(24):2422–2434. doi:10.1001/jama.2019.19411
12. Krishna SG, Kamboj AK, Hart PA, Hinton A, Conwell DL. The changing epidemiology of acute pancreatitis hospitalizations: A decade of trends and the impact of chronic pancreatitis. *Pancreas*. 2017;46(4):482–488. doi:10.1097/MPA.0000000000000783
13. Forsmark CE, Vege SS, Wilcox CM. Acute pancreatitis. *N Engl J Med*. 2016;375(20):1972–1981. doi:10.1056/NEJMra1505202
14. Pandol SJ. Pancreatic secretion. In: Feldman M, LS F, LJ B, eds. *Sleisenger and Fordtran's Gastrointestinal and Liver Disease: Pathophysiology, Diagnosis, Management*. Vol 10th. Philadelphia: Elsevier Saunders; 2016:934–943.
15. Aune D, Mahamat-Saleh Y, Norat T, Riboli E. Tobacco smoking and the risk of pancreatitis: A systematic review and meta-analysis of prospective studies. *Pancreatology*. 2019;19(8):1009–1022. doi:10.1016/j.pan.2019.09.004
16. Pedersen JE, Ängquist LH, Jensen CB, Kjærgaard JS, Jess T, Allin KH. Risk of pancreatitis in patients with inflammatory bowel disease: A meta-analysis. *Dan Med J*. 2020;67(3).
17. Garcia Garcia de Paredes A, Rodriguez de Santiago E, Rodriguez-Escaja C, et al. Idiopathic acute pancreatitis in patients with inflammatory bowel disease: A multicenter cohort study: Idiopathic acute pancreatitis in IBD. *Pancreatology*. 2020;20(3):331–337. doi:10.1016/j.pan.2020.02.007
18. Ducarme G, Maire F, Chatel P, Luton D, Hammel P. Acute pancreatitis during pregnancy: A review. *J Perinatol*. 2014;34(2):87–94.
19. Liu QY, Abu-El-Haija M, Husain SZ, et al. Risk factors for rapid progression from acute recurrent to chronic pancreatitis in children: Report from INSPPIRE. *J Pediatr Gastroenterol Nutr*. 2019;69(2):206–211. doi:10.1097/MPG.0000000000002405
20. Gariepy CE, Heyman MB, Lowe ME, et al. Causal evaluation of acute recurrent and chronic pancreatitis in children: Consensus from the INSPPIRE group. *J Pediatr Gastroenterol Nutr*. 2017;64(1):95–103. doi:10.1097/MPG.0000000000001446
21. Hung WY. Contemporary review of drug-induced pancreatitis: A different perspective. *World J Gastrointest Pathophysiol*. 2014;5(4):405–415. doi:10.4291/wjgp.v5.i4.405
22. Jones MR, Hall OM, Kaye AM, Kaye AD. Drug-induced acute pancreatitis: A review. *OchsnerJ*. 2015;15(1):45–51.
23. Wolfe D, Kanji S, Yazdi F, et al. *Drug Induced Pancreatitis: A Systematic Review of Case Reports to Determine Potential Drug Associations*. Vol 15. 2020. doi:10.1371/journal.pone.0231883
24. Jasdanwala S, Babyatsky M. Crohn's disease and acute pancreatitis. A review of literature. *JOP*. 2015;16(2):136–142.
25. Li L, Shen J, Bala MM, et al. Incretin treatment and risk of pancreatitis in patients with type 2 diabetes mellitus: Systematic review and meta-analysis of randomised and non-randomised studies. *BMJ*. 2014;348:g2366.
26. Singh AK, Gangopadhyay KK, Singh R. Risk of acute pancreatitis with incretin-based therapy: A systematic review and updated meta-analysis of cardiovascular outcomes trials. *Expert Rev Clin Pharmacol*. 2020;13(4):461–468. doi:10.1080/17512433.2020.1736041
27. Dicembrini I, Montereggi C, Nreu B, Mannucci E, Monami M. Pancreatitis and pancreatic cancer in patients treated with dipeptidyl peptidase-4 inhibitors: An extensive and updated meta-analysis of randomized controlled trials. *Diabetes Res Clin Pract*. 2020;159:107981. doi:10.1016/j.diabres.2019.107981
28. Faillie JL, Azoulay L, Patenaude V, Hillaire-Buys D, Suissa S. Incretin based drugs and risk of acute pancreatitis in patients with type 2 diabetes: Cohort study. *BMJ*. 2014;348:g2780.
29. Razavi D, Lindblad M, Bexelius T, Oskarsson V, Sadr-Azodi O, Ljung R. Polypharmacy and risk of acute pancreatitis. *Pharmacoepidemiol Drug Saf*. 2016;25(11):1337–1341. doi:10.1002/pds.4109
30. Tenner S, Steinberg WM. Acute Pancreatitis. In: Feldman M, Friedman L, Brandt L, eds. *Sleisenger and Fordtran's Gastrointestinal and Liver Disease: Pathophysiology, Diagnosis, Management*. 10th ed. Philadelphia: Elsevier Saunders; 2016:969–993.
31. Banks PA, Bollen TL, Dervenis C, et al. Classification of acute pancreatitis—2012: Revision of the Atlanta classification and definitions by international consensus. *Gut*. 2013;62(1):102–111.
32. Dellinger EP, Forsmark CE, Layer P, et al. Determinant-based classification of acute pancreatitis severity: An international multidisciplinary consultation. *Ann Surg*. 2012;256(6):875–880.
33. Vasudevan S, Goswami P, Sonika U, Thakur B, Sreenivas V, Saraya A. comparison of various scoring systems and biochemical markers in predicting the outcome in acute pancreatitis. *Pancreas*. 2018;47(1):65–71. doi:10.1097/MPA.0000000000000957
34. Hagjer S, Kumar N. Evaluation of the BISAP scoring system in prognostication of acute pancreatitis: A prospective observational study. *Int J Surg*. 2018;54(Pt A):76–81. doi:10.1016/j.ijsu.2018.04.026
35. Das SL, Singh PP, Phillips AR, Murphy R, Windsor JA, Petrov MS. Newly diagnosed diabetes mellitus after acute pancreatitis: A systematic review and meta-analysis. *Gut*. 2014;63(5):818–831.
36. Hollemans RA, Hallensleben NDL, Mager DJ, et al. Pancreatic exocrine insufficiency following acute pancreatitis: Systematic review and study level meta-analysis. *Pancreatology*. 2018;18(3):253–262. doi:10.1016/j.pan.2018.02.009
37. Rohan JD, Osman HG, Patel S. Advances in management of pancreatic necrosis. *Curr Probl Surg*. 2014;51(9):374–408.
38. Arvanitakis M, Ockenga J, Bezmarevic M, et al. ESPEN guideline on clinical nutrition in acute and chronic pancreatitis. *Clin Nutr*. 2020;39(3):612–631. doi:10.1016/j.clnu.2020.01.004
39. Li W, Liu J, Zhao S, Li J. Safety and efficacy of total parenteral nutrition versus total enteral nutrition for patients with severe acute pancreatitis: A meta-analysis. *J Int Med Res*. 2018;46(9):3948–3958. doi:10.1177/0300060518782070

40. Qi D, Yu B, Huang J, Peng M. Meta-analysis of early enteral nutrition provided within 24 hours of admission on clinical outcomes in acute pancreatitis. *J Parenter Enter Nutr*. 2018;42(7):1139–1147. doi:10.1002/jpen.1139
41. Dutta AK, Goel A, Kirubakaran R, Chacko A, Tharyan P. Nasogastric versus nasojejunal tube feeding for severe acute pancreatitis. *Cochrane Database Syst Rev*. 2020;2020(3):CD010582. doi:10.1002/14651858.CD010582.pub2
42. Gou S, Yang Z, Liu T, Wu H, Wang C. Use of probiotics in the treatment of severe acute pancreatitis: A systematic review and meta-analysis of randomized controlled trials. *Crit Care*. 2014;18(2):1–10. doi:10.1186/cc13809
43. Yamashita T, Horibe M, Sanui M, et al. Large volume fluid resuscitation for severe acute pancreatitis is associated with reduced mortality: A multicenter retrospective study. *J Clin Gastroenterol*. 2019;53(5):385–391. doi:10.1097/MCG.0000000000001046
44. Gad MM, Simons-Linares CR. Is aggressive intravenous fluid resuscitation beneficial in acute pancreatitis? A meta-analysis of randomized control trials and cohort studies. *World J Gastroenterol*. 2020;26(10):1098–1106. doi:10.3748/wjg.v26.i10.1098
45. Rhodes A, Evans LE, Alhazzani W, et al. *Surviving Sepsis Campaign: International Guidelines for Management of Sepsis and Septic Shock: 2016*. Vol 45. 2017. doi:10.1097/CCM.0000000000002255
46. Iqbal U, Anwar H, Scribani M. Ringer's lactate versus normal saline in acute pancreatitis: A systematic review and meta-analysis. *J Dig Dis*. 2018;19(6):335–341. doi:10.1111/1751-2980.12606
47. Farrell PR, Farrell LM, Hornung L, Abu-El-Haija M. Use of lactated ringers solution compared with normal saline is associated with shorter length of stay in pediatric acute pancreatitis. *Pancreas*. 2020;49(3):375–380. doi:10.1097/MPA.0000000000001498
48. Mahapatra SJ, Jain S, Bopanna S, et al. Pentazocine, a kappa-opioid agonist, is better than diclofenac for analgesia in acute pancreatitis: A randomized controlled trial. *Am J Gastroenterol*. 2019;114(5):813–821. doi:10.14309/ajg.0000000000000224
49. Stephan Schorn, Güralp O. Ceyhan, Elke Tieftrunk HF and IED. Pain management in acute pancreatitis. *Pancreapedia*. 2015.Available at http://www.pancreapedia.org/reviews/pain-management-in-acute-pancreatitis. Accessed April 22, 2016. doi:10.3998/panc.2015.15
50. Jabaudon M, Belhadj-Tahar N, Rimmel T, et al. Thoracic epidural analgesia and mortality in acute pancreatitis: A multicenter propensity analysis. *Crit Care Med*. 2018;46(3):e198-e205. doi:10.1097/CCM.0000000000002874
51. Poropat G, Radovan A, Peric M, et al. Prevention of infectious complications in acute pancreatitis: Results of a single-center, randomized, controlled trial. *Pancreas*. 2019;48(8):1056–1060. doi:10.1097/MPA.0000000000001368
52. Rokke O, Harbitz TB, Liljedal J, et al. Early treatment of severe pancreatitis with imipenem: a prospective randomized clinical trial. *Scand J Gastroenterol*. 2007;42(6):771–776.
53. Schubert S, Dalhoff A. Activity of moxifloxacin, imipenem, and ertapenem against *Escherichia coli*, *Enterobacter cloacae*, *Enterococcus faecalis*, and *Bacteroides fragilis* in monocultures and mixed cultures in an in vitro pharmacokinetic/pharmacodynamic model simulating concentrations in the human pancreas. *Antimicrob Agents Chemother*. 2012;56(12):6434–6436.
54. Pekgöz M. Post-endoscopic retrograde cholangiopancreatography pancreatitis: A systematic review for prevention and treatment. *World J Gastroenterol*. 2019;25(29):4019–4042. doi:10.3748/wjg.v25.i29.4019
55. Tomoda T, Kato H, Ueki T, et al. Combination of diclofenac and sublingual nitrates is superior to diclofenac alone in preventing pancreatitis after endoscopic retrograde cholangiopancreatography. *Gastroenterology*. 2019;156(6):1753–1760.e1. doi:10.1053/j.gastro.2019.01.267
56. Chiu YJ, Chen SC, Kang YN, Hou SK, Chao CC, Chang CC. Efficacy of gabexate mesilate in preventing post endoscopic retrograde cholangiopancreatography pancreatitis: A meta-analysis of randomized clinical trials. *J Formos Med Assoc*. 2021;120(4):1090–1099. doi:10.1016/j.jfma.2020.10.034
57. Radadiya D, Devani K, Arora S, et al. Peri-procedural aggressive hydration for post endoscopic retrograde cholangiopancreatography (ERCP) pancreatitis prophylaxsis: Meta-analysis of randomized controlled trials. *Pancreatology*. 2019;19(6):819–827. doi:10.1016/j.pan.2019.07.046
58. Park CH, Paik WH, Park ET, et al. Aggressive intravenous hydration with lactated Ringer's solution for prevention of post-ERCP pancreatitis: A prospective randomized multicenter clinical trial. *Endoscopy*. 2018;50(4):378–385. doi:10.1055/s-0043-122386
59. Conwell DL, Lee LS, Yadav D, et al. American Pancreatic Association Practice Guidelines in Chronic Pancreatitis: Evidence-based report on diagnostic guidelines. *Pancreas*. 2014;43(8):1162.
60. Samokhvalov AV, Rehm J, Roerecke M. Alcohol consumption as a risk factor for acute and chronic pancreatitis: A systematic review and a series of meta-analyses. *EBioMedicine*. 2015;2(12):1996–2002. doi:10.1016/j.ebiom.2015.11.023
61. Majumder S, Chari ST. Chronic pancreatitis. *Lancet*. 2016;387(10031):1957–1966. doi:10.1016/S0140-6736(16)00097-0
62. Hegyi E, Sahin-Tóth M. Genetic risk in chronic pancreatitis: The trypsin-dependent pathway. *Dig Dis Sci*. 2017;62(7):1692–1701. doi:10.1007/s10620-017-4601-3
63. Gardner TB, Adler DG, Forsmark CE, Sauer BG, Taylor JR, Whitcomb DC. ACG Clinical Guideline: Chronic pancreatitis. *Am J Gastroenterol*. 2020;115(3):322–339. doi:10.14309/ajg.0000000000000535
64. Sankaran SJ, Xiao AY, Wu LM, Windsor JA, Forsmark CE, Petrov MS. Frequency of progression from acute to chronic pancreatitis and risk factors: A meta-analysis. *Gastroenterology*. 2015;149(6):1490–1500.e1. doi:10.1053/j.gastro.2015.07.066
65. Lew D, Afghani E, Pandol S. Chronic pancreatitis: Current status and challenges for prevention and treatment. *Dig Dis Sci*. 2017;62(7):1702–1712. doi:10.1007/s10620-017-4602-2
66. Singh VK, Drewes AM. Medical management of pain in chronic pancreatitis. *Dig Dis Sci*. 2017;62(7):1721–1728. doi:10.1007/s10620-017-4605-z
67. Anderson MA, Akshintala V, Albers KM, et al. Mechanism, assessment and management of pain in chronic pancreatitis: Recommendations of a multidisciplinary study group. *Pancreatology*. 2016;16(1):83–94. doi:10.1016/j.pan.2015.10.015
68. Muniraj T, Aslanian HR, Farrell J, Jamidar PA. Chronic pancreatitis, a comprehensive review and update. Part II: Diagnosis, complications, and management. *Disease-a-Month*. 2015;61(1):5–37. http://www.sciencedirect.com/science/article/pii/S0011502914001692.
69. Afghani E, Sinha A, Singh VK. An overview of the diagnosis and management of nutrition in chronic pancreatitis. *Nutr Clin Pract*. 2014;29(3):295–311.
70. Hirth M, Weiss C, Hardt P, et al. Analysis of the course of chronic pancreatitis: Pancreatic burnout rates are only increased in a subgroup of patients with alcoholic chronic pancreatitis. *Pancreas*. 2019;48(5):726–733. doi:10.1097/MPA.0000000000001302
71. Zhu X, Liu D, Wei Q, et al. New-onset diabetes mellitus after chronic pancreatitis diagnosis: A systematic review and meta-analysis. *Pancreas*. 2019;48(7):868–875. doi:10.1097/MPA.0000000000001359
72. Kirkegård J, Mortensen FV, Cronin-Fenton D. Chronic pancreatitis and pancreatic cancer risk: A systematic review and meta-analysis. *Am J Gastroenterol*. 2017;112(9):1366–1372. doi:10.1038/ajg.2017.218
73. Hoffmeister A, Mayerle J, Beglinger C, et al. English language version of the S3-consensus guidelines on chronic pancreatitis: Definition, aetiology, diagnostic examinations, medical, endoscopic and surgical management of chronic pancreatitis. *Z Gastroenterol*. 2015;53(12):1447–1495. doi:10.1055/s-0041-107379
74. Adler JM, Gardner TB. Endoscopic therapies for chronic pancreatitis. *Dig Dis Sci*. 2017;62(7):1729–1737. doi:10.1007/s10620-017-4502-5
75. Moole H, Jaeger A, Bechtold ML, Forcione D, Taneja D, Puli SR. Success of extracorporeal shock wave lithotripsy in chronic calcific pancreatitis management: A meta-analysis and systematic review. *Pancreas*. 2016;45(5):651–658. doi:10.1097/MPA.0000000000000512
76. Kempeneers MA, Issa Y, Ali UA, et al. International consensus guidelines for surgery and the timing of intervention in chronic pancreatitis. *Pancreatology*. 2020;20(2):149–157. doi:10.1016/j.pan.2019.12.005
77. Tillou JD, Tatum JA, Jolissaint JS, et al. Operative management of chronic pancreatitis: A review. *Am J Surg*. 2017;214(2):347–357. doi:10.1016/j.amjsurg.2017.03.004
78. Ramsey ML, Conwell DL, Hart PA. Complications of chronic pancreatitis. *Dig Dis Sci*. 2017;62(7):1745–1750. doi:10.1007/s10620-017-4518-x
79. Yaghoobi M, McNabb-Baltar J, Bijarchi R, Cotton PB. Pancreatic enzyme supplements are not effective for relieving abdominal pain in patients with chronic pancreatitis: Meta-analysis and systematic review of randomized controlled trials. *Can J Gastroenterol Hepatol*. 2016;2016:8541839. doi:10.1155/2016/8541839
80. Gurusamy KS, Lusuku C, Davidson BR. Pregabalin for decreasing pancreatic pain in chronic pancreatitis. *Cochrane database Syst Rev*. 2016;2:CD011522. doi:10.1002/14651858.CD011522.pub2
81. Rustagi T, Njei B. Antioxidant therapy for pain reduction in patients with chronic pancreatitis: A systematic review and meta-analysis. *Pancreas*. 2015;44(5):812–818. doi:10.1097/MPA.0000000000000327

82. Zhou D, Wang W, Cheng X, Wei J, Zheng S. Antioxidant therapy for patients with chronic pancreatitis: A systematic review and meta-analysis. *Clin Nutr*. 2015;34(4):627–634. doi:10.1016/j.clnu.2014.07.003
83. Ahmed AU, Jens S, Busch OR, et al. Antioxidants for pain in chronic pancreatitis. *Cochrane Database Syst Rev*. 2014;8:CD008945:CD008945.
84. Trang T, Chan J, Graham DY. Pancreatic enzyme replacement therapy for pancreatic exocrine insufficiency in the 21(st) century. *World J Gastroenterol*. 2014;20(33):11467–11485.
85. Martínez-Moneo E, Stigliano S, Hedström A, et al. Deficiency of fat-soluble vitamins in chronic pancreatitis: A systematic review and meta-analysis. *Pancreatology*. 2016;16(6):988–994. doi:10.1016/j.pan.2016.09.008
86. De La Iglesia-García D, Huang W, Szatmary P, et al. Efficacy of pancreatic enzyme replacement therapy in chronic pancreatitis: Systematic review and meta-analysis. *Gut*. 2017;66(8):1474–1486. doi:10.1136/gutjnl-2016-312529
87. Laboratories A. Creon (pancrelipase) package insert. March 2020.
88. Aptalis Pharma US I. Viokace (pancrelipase) package insert. March 2012.

58

Viral Hepatitis

Paulina Deming

KEY CONCEPTS

1. Hepatitis A virus (HAV) is transmitted via the fecal–oral route, most often from ingestion of contaminated food or water, or through contact with an infected person.
2. HAV causes an acute, self-limiting illness and does not lead to chronic infection. There are three stages of infection: incubation, acute hepatitis, and convalescence. Rarely, the infection progresses to liver failure.
3. HAV vaccination is highly effective. There is no pharmacological treatment specifically for HAV; treatment consists of supportive care.
4. Hepatitis B virus (HBV) causes both acute and chronic infection. Chronic infections are responsible for high rates of liver disease, liver cancer, and death.
5. Vaccination can prevent HBV and is the most effective strategy in preventing complications of HBV infections. Prevention of HBV infections focuses on immunization of all children and at-risk adults.
6. The purpose of anti-HBV drug therapy is for viral suppression and immune control and to prevent progression of liver disease and the complications associated with HBV infections.
7. Initial therapy of chronic HBV is with tenofovir or entecavir because these agents have a high barrier to resistance. Therapy is often long term.
8. Patients undergoing immunosuppressive therapy or chemotherapy should be screened for HBV infections and may require HBV therapy to reduce the risks of reactivating their HBV and developing fulminant liver failure.
9. The hepatitis C virus (HCV) is an insidious, blood-borne infection. Universal, one-time screening is recommended for all persons aged 18 and over.
10. Hepatitis C infections can cause significant morbidity (including extrahepatic manifestations) and mortality. Patients with chronic hepatitis C are at risk for end-stage liver disease, cirrhosis, liver transplant, and death as a result of their infection.
11. The goal of anti-hepatitis C virus (HCV) drug treatment is cure. Drug therapy with direct-acting antivirals (DAAs) is highly effective and well tolerated.

BEYOND THE BOOK

Watch "Hepatitis C: Test, Treat, Cure" available at: Npaihb.org/hcv/

This short video includes a review of epidemiology of HCV infections, risks for HCV infection, tests for HCV diagnosis, and patient experiences with HCV as well as with HCV treatment.

INTRODUCTION

The major hepatotrophic viruses responsible for viral hepatitis are hepatitis A, hepatitis B, hepatitis C, delta hepatitis (hepatitis D), and hepatitis E. All share clinical, biochemical, immunoserologic, and histologic findings. Hepatitis A and E are spread through fecal–oral contamination, whereas hepatitis B, C, and delta are transmitted parenterally. Infection with delta hepatitis requires coinfection with hepatitis B. This chapter focuses on hepatitis A, B, and C.

Viral hepatitis remains a major cause of morbidity and mortality with a significant impact on healthcare costs in the United States. Compared with human immunodeficiency virus (HIV), there are three to five times as many people infected with chronic viral hepatitis. In the United States, a national strategy for the elimination of hepatitis B and C was established by the National Academies of Science, Engineering, and Medicine.[1] Despite the national strategy, many challenges persist in achieving elimination goals. Although unprecedented therapeutic advances occurred for the treatment for hepatitis C; the rates of acute infection are on the rise and challenges in screening and access to treatment persist. Both hepatitis A and B are vaccine preventable, yet many vulnerable patients remain unvaccinated and susceptible to infection.

HEPATITIS A

Hepatitis A virus (HAV) is often a self-limiting and acute viral infection of the liver posing a health risk worldwide. The infection is rarely fatal. According to the Centers for Disease Control and Prevention (CDC), rates of reported cases of acute clinical HAV infection in the United States were declining until multi-state outbreaks were reported in 2013 and 2016. Since 2016, 38 multi-state outbreaks were reported with an increase of over 1,300% in the number of acute cases. As of May 2021, nearly 40,000 cases were reported with a 61% hospitalization rate and 374 deaths.[2]

Epidemiology

1 Infection primarily occurs through the fecal–oral route, by person-to-person, or by ingestion of contaminated food or water. HAV's prevalence is linked to resource-limited regions and specifically to those with poor sanitary conditions and overcrowding. Travel to areas with poor sanitation poses a risk for travelers. In areas with good sanitation and hygiene, HAV outbreaks are observed among specific patient

groups, such as persons who inject drugs (PWID) and in men who have sex with men (MSM). Household or close personal contacts of an infected person are at high risk for infection. Children can contribute to the spread of the disease because they often remain asymptomatic and are infectious for longer periods of time than adults.

In the United States, recent HAV outbreaks were identified in persons who use drugs, persons experiencing homelessness, and in MSM.[3] Foodborne outbreaks occur with local and widespread outbreaks reported annually. Although HAV infections were previously mostly identified in children, since 2018 adults aged 30 to 39 accounted for the highest number of cases, followed by adults aged 40 to 49.[2] In 2019, HAV rates were highest among White, non-Hispanic males aged 30 to 39. Of patients with a known history of risk factors, 46% were linked with injection drug use. Mortality rates are low and were previously recognized to be most likely in elderly patients with underlying comorbid conditions. However, in 2019 death was most likely to occur in males aged 45 and above.[2] Patients with preexisting chronic liver disease, such as HCV, are at an increased risk of developing fulminant HAV.[4]

Despite low endemic rates and successful vaccination programs in the United States, travel to HAV endemic areas is a recognized risk for acquiring acute HAV infections and includes "standard" tourist itineraries. Rural and backcountry travel or consumption of food or drink in areas of poor sanitation pose the highest travel-related risk.[5]

Etiology

1 Hepatitis A is a nonenveloped ribonucleic acid (RNA) virus in the *Picornaviridae* family. The virus is stable in low pH environments and in freezing to moderate temperatures.[5] Inactivation requires disinfecting with a 1:100 dilution of sodium hypochlorite (bleach) in tap water or heating foods to a minimum of 85°C (185°F) for 1 minute.[5] Chlorination of water also effectively kills HAV in water systems. Transmission occurs primarily through the fecal–oral route because HAV is shed in the feces of infected people.[5] Contaminated water or ice are common modes of transmission, as are any foods which may be prepared using contaminated water including shellfish harvested from contaminated water. Access to clean water and proper handwashing are critical in preventing the transmission of HAV.

Pathophysiology

HAV infection is usually acute, self-limiting, and confers lifelong immunity. HAV's life cycle in the human host classically begins with ingestion of the virus. Absorption in the stomach or small intestine allows entry into the circulation and uptake by the liver. Replication of the virus occurs within hepatocytes and gastrointestinal epithelial cells. New virus particles are released into the blood and secreted into bile by the liver. The virus is then either reabsorbed to continue its cycle or excreted in the stool. The enterohepatic cycle will continue until interrupted by antibody neutralization.[5]

Clinical Presentation

2 The incubation period of HAV is approximately 28 days, with a range of 15 to 50 days.[5] Table 58-1 summarizes the clinical features of acute hepatitis. There are no specific distinguishing features of HAV compared to other types of hepatitis; thus, serological testing for immunoglobulin (Ig) M antibody to HAV (anti-HAV) is needed to confirm a diagnosis of acute HAV. In the majority of patients, IgM anti-HAV will be detectable within 5 to 10 days of symptom onset. Symptom severity varies according to age. Children younger than 6 years typically are asymptomatic and can shed the virus for long periods of time, serving as a reservoir for the spread of HAV. Peak fecal shedding of the virus precedes the onset of clinical symptoms and elevated liver enzymes. Acute hepatitis follows, beginning with the preicteric or prodromal period. The phase is marked by an abrupt onset of nonspecific symptoms, some mild.[6] More unusual symptoms include chills, myalgia, arthralgia, cough, constipation, diarrhea, pruritus, and urticaria. The phase generally lasts 2 months.

Liver enzyme levels rise in serum within the first weeks of infection, peaking approximately in the fourth week and normalizing by the eighth week. Conjugated bilirubinemia, clinically evident as dark urine, precedes the onset of the icteric period. Gastrointestinal symptoms may persist or subside during this time and some patients may have hepatomegaly. Duration of the icteric period varies and corresponds to disease duration, averaging between 7 and 30 days.[6]

The diagnosis of acute HAV is made through the IgM anti-HAV which is detectable 5 to 10 days prior to symptomatic HAV infections in the majority of patients. The IgG anti-HAV replaces IgM and indicates host immunity following the acute phase of the infection.[6] Serological testing is available for IgM anti-HAV, IgG anti-HAV, and total (anti-IgM and IgG) anti-HAV. Patients who have detectable total anti-HAV with a negative IgM have resolved their infection. Concentrations of antibody often fall to 10 to 100 times lower than what would be expected after a natural course of infection. Detectable antibodies may persist for over 40 years. Although a positive anti-HAV result confirms protection, undetectable concentration of anti-HAV may not necessarily imply that protective levels were not achieved.[6] Booster, or challenge doses, may be given after

TABLE 58-1 Clinical Presentation of Acute Hepatitis

	Hepatitis A (HAV)	Hepatitis B (HBV)	Hepatitis C (HCV)
Signs and symptoms	>70% of patients are symptomatic with fever, jaundice, and scleral icterus. Hepatomegaly is evident on physical exam. Less common signs include splenomegaly, skin rash, arthralgia.	Approximately 70% of patients are anicteric or subclinical. Younger patients most likely to be asymptomatic. If symptoms occur, jaundice, dark urine, white stool, abdominal pain, fatigue, fever, chills, loss of appetite, and pruritus are possible.	Approximately 70% of patients are asymptomatic. If symptoms occur, jaundice, dark urine, white stool, abdominal pain, fatigue, fever, chills, loss of appetite, and pruritus are possible.
Laboratory Findings in Acute Phase of Infection			
Aminotransferase (ALT, AST) Elevations	• >1,000 IU/L (16.7 μkat/L) • ALT>AST	• 1,000-2,000 IU/L (16.7-33.3 μkat/L) • ALT>AST	• Highly variable, can be approximately 1,000 IU/L (16.7 μkat/L) • ALT>AST
Bilirubin	Elevated and preceded by aminotransferase elevations	Can be normal or elevated	Elevated and preceded by aminotransferase elevations
Virus Specific Tests	IgM anti-HAV for acute HAV; IgG anti-HAV for prior infection or vaccination	IgM anti-HBc (+), HBsA g (+) for active, acute infection	HCV RNA (+) or quantifiable; HCV antibody reactive within 12 weeks of exposure

ALT, alanine aminotransferase; anti-, antibody; AST, aspartate aminotransferase; HBc, hepatitis B core; HBsAg, hepatitis B surface antigen; IU, international units; L, liter.

an HAV vaccine series is completed to provide rapid immunity when there is concern for serious infection.[6]

HAV does not lead to chronic infections; however, some patients may experience symptoms for up to 9 months. Rarely, patients experience complications from HAV including relapsing hepatitis, cholestatic hepatitis, and fulminant hepatitis. These severe effects are more likely in patients who are immunocompromised, have underlying liver disease, or are greater than 40 years of age.[6] Fatalities from HAV are generally rare, although more likely in patients older than 50 years and in persons with preexisting liver disease.[6]

A diagnosis of HAV is based on clinical criteria of an acute onset of fatigue, abdominal pain, loss of appetite, intermittent nausea and vomiting, jaundice or elevated serum aminotransferase levels, and serologic testing for IgM anti-HAV. Testing for IgM anti-HAV in the absence of symptoms is not recommended.[6] Serologic testing is necessary to differentiate the diagnosis from other types of hepatitis.

TABLE 58-2 Recommendations for Hepatitis A Virus Vaccination

- All children at 1 year of age
- Any unvaccinated children ages 2-18 years
- Persons traveling to or working in countries that have high or intermediate endemicity of infection[a]
- Men who have sex with men
- Users of injection and noninjection drugs
- Persons with occupational risk for infection (eg, persons who work with HAV-infected primates or with HAV in a research laboratory)
- Persons with chronic liver disease including persons with hepatitis B virus infection, hepatitis C virus infection
- All previously unvaccinated persons anticipating close personal contact (eg, household contact or regular babysitter) with an international adoptee from a country of high or intermediate endemicity within the first 60 days following the arrival of the adoptee
- Anyone who would like HAV vaccine

[a]Travelers to Canada, Western Europe, Japan, Australia, or New Zealand are at no greater risk for infection than they are in the United States. All other travelers should be assessed for HAV risk.

Data from Reference 6.

TREATMENT

Desired Outcomes

The majority of people infected with HAV can be expected to fully recover without clinical sequelae.[7] Nearly all individuals will have clinical resolution within 6 months of the infection and a majority will have done so by 2 months. Rarely, symptoms persist for longer or patients relapse. The ultimate goal of therapy is complete clinical resolution. Other goals include reducing complications from the infection, normalization of liver function, and reducing infectivity and transmission. Prevention of HAV infection is important because significant costs are accrued during acute HAV infections, including costs of administration and use of immunoglobulin and vaccine, hospitalizations, and indirect costs from loss of workdays.

General Approach to Treatment

3 Prevention and prophylaxis are keys to managing this vaccine-preventable virus. No specific treatment options exist for HAV infections. Instead, patients should receive general supportive care. The importance of good hand hygiene should be emphasized in preventing disease transmission. Passive immunity with Ig is used for preexposure and postexposure prophylaxis. Active immunity is achieved through vaccination. Vaccines were approved for use since 1995 and implemented in the routine vaccination of children, as well as at-risk adults, to reduce the overall incidence of HAV.[6] Despite HAV vaccine availability, vaccine coverage in adults is low.

Prevaccination serologic testing to determine susceptibility is generally not recommended. In some cases, testing may be cost-effective if the cost of the test is less than that of the vaccine and if the person is from a moderate-to-high endemic area and likely to have prior immunity. Similarly, because of high vaccine response, postvaccine serologic testing is not recommended.[6]

Prevention of Hepatitis A

HAV is easily preventable with vaccination. Because children often serve as reservoirs of the disease, vaccine programs have targeted children as the most effective means to control HAV. Two vaccines for HAV are available and are incorporated into the routine childhood vaccination schedule. The Advisory Committee on Immunization Practices (ACIP) recommends expanding vaccine coverage to all children, including catch-up programs for children not previously vaccinated. Vaccination is also recommended for adults. The recommendations were enacted in the attempt to further reduce HAV incidence rates and possibly to eradicate the virus.[6] Complete HAV vaccination recommendations are available from the CDC (Table 58-2).

Persons at risk for worse outcomes with HAV infection are also recommended to receive vaccination and include persons over the age of 40, persons with immunocompromising conditions, persons with chronic liver disease planning on traveling, and persons with HIV. In response to the HAV outbreaks beginning in 2016, ACIP revised its vaccination recommendations to persons ≥1 year of age who are at risk for HAV infection including PWIDs, persons experiencing homelessness, MSM, or persons at risk for severe outcomes with HAV infection such as persons with chronic liver disease or persons with HIV. Vaccination is recommended in settings providing services to adults in which a high proportion have risk factors for HAV infection such as healthcare settings with a focus on injection or noninjection drug use, group homes, and non-residential day care facilities for developmentally disabled persons.

TABLE 58-3 Recommended Dosing of Hepatitis A Vaccines

Vaccine	Age (Years)	Dose of Hepatitis A Antigen (Volume)	No. of Doses	Schedule[a]
HAVRIX	1-18	720 ELISA units (0.5 mL)	2	0, 6-12 months
	≥19	1,440 ELISA units (1 mL)	2	0, 6-12 months
VAQTA	1-18	25 units (0.5 mL)	2	0, 6-18 months
	≥19	50 units (1 mL)	2	0, 6-18 months
TWINRIX[b]	≥18	720 ELISA units (1 mL)	3	0, 1, 6 months
	≥18 (accelerated schedule)	720 ELISA units (1 mL)	4	0, 7 days, 21-30 days, +12 months

[a]Zero (0) denotes initial dose, subsequent numbers denote time after initial dose for timing of additional doses.

[b]Combination hepatitis A and B vaccine, also contains 20 mcg of hepatitis B surface antigen and requires a three-dose schedule for adequate HBV response.

Data from Reference 6.

Vaccines to Prevent Hepatitis A

The inactivated virus vaccines licensed in the United States are the single-antigen HAVRIX® and VAQTA® and the combination of HAV and HBV antigen vaccine TWINRIX®. Both single-antigen vaccines are available for pediatric (12 months and older) and adult (18 years and older) use, while the TWINRIX® is indicated for adults only (Table 58-3). The differences in the vaccines are in the

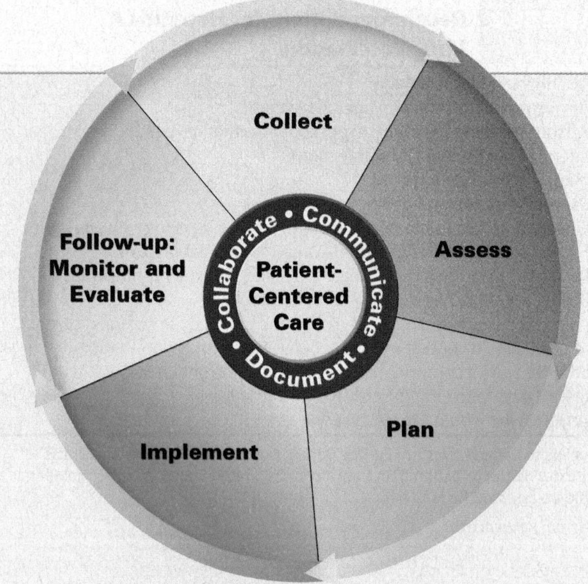

Patient Care Process for Hepatitis C

The image shows the five fundamental steps included in The Pharmacist's Care Process endorsed by the Joint Commission for Pharmacy Practitioners (2014). The tagline of this process reads collaborate, communicate, and document. The five fundamental steps listed here are collect, assess, plan, implement, and follow-up: monitor and evaluate. All these steps are listed in a circular block diagram.

Collect

- Patient history (past medical, family, social) and medical record summary
- Thorough medication history (include prescription, nonprescription medications, and other substances) and drug allergies and intolerances. Previous HCV therapy, if applicable
- Laboratory results (see Table 58-1)
- Laboratory results to assess if patient has cirrhosis (see Table 58-2)
- Abdominal imagining or transient elastography results (if available)

Assess

- Determine if the patient is a candidate for the simplified treatment algorithm (see Table 58-3)
- If the patient has cirrhosis, assess the level of liver dysfunction using the Child-Pugh Score to determine options for HCV therapy
- Review insurance company formulary preferences for HCV therapy
- Review national guidelines for updated treatment recommendations
- Assess if patient assistance programs may be utilized

Plan

- Determine goals of therapy with monitoring parameters for each goal
- Based on severity of underlying liver disease, determine the appropriate therapy, treatment duration, and monitoring plan
- Counsel patients on avoiding pregnancy and need for contraception during treatment
- Identify potential obstacles to treatment success such as insurance requirements regarding refills
- Check for drug interactions with prescribed medications, any over-the-counter medications, herbals, or supplements

Implement

- Initiate HCV direct-acting antiviral (DAA) therapy
- Discontinue or modify adjunct medications if drug interactions anticipated with HCV DAAs
- Discuss with the patient and patient's family what to expect for monitoring while on therapy, strategies to address any potential adverse effects and strategies to minimize likelihood for therapy interruptions

Follow-up: Monitor and Evaluate

- Continually reassess patient's use of HCV antivirals, any changes in other medications or herbals and supplements which could compromise HCV therapy, and any adverse effects
- Patients not on the simplified algorithm require monitoring of laboratory tests
- Monitor for any interruptions in therapy which could risk treatment failure
- Evaluate patient for cure at least 12 weeks after completion of therapy
- Reassess patient's risk for reinfection and counsel on harm-reduction strategies

**Collaborate with patients, caregivers, and other healthcare professionals.*

use of a preservative and in expression of antigen content. VAQTA® is formulated without a preservative and uses units of HAV antigen to express potency. HAVRIX® and TWINRIX® use 2-phenoxyphenol as a preservative and antigen content is expressed as enzyme-linked immunosorbent assay (ELISA) units.[6] High seroconversion rates of more than or equal to 94% are achieved with the first dose; however, VAQTA® and HAVRIX® recommend a booster shot to achieve the highest possible antibody titers. Although seroconversion exceeds 90% for HAV after the first dose of TWINRIX®, the full three-dose series is required for maximal HBV seroconversion. An accelerated dosing schedule of TWINRIX® is available but requires four doses for optimal response. The combined vaccine offers the advantage of immunization against both types of hepatitis in a single vaccine.

In situations of postexposure prophylaxis, either the vaccine or Ig can be used, although vaccine is preferred because it confers the benefit of long-term immunity against HAV. In patients older than 40 years or with underlying medical conditions, vaccine experience is limited, thus vaccine and immunoglobulin may be preferred for optimal protection.[5] Both vaccines may be given concomitantly with Ig and the two brands are interchangeable.[6]

Vaccination is recommended for international travel to areas of high or intermediate endemicity and can be given regardless of scheduled dates of departure. For older patients, immunocompromised, or any patients with chronic liver disease or any other chronic medical conditions traveling within 2 weeks, both Ig and vaccine are recommended.[5] Vaccination is preferred because it confers long-term protection.

The most common side effects of the vaccines include soreness and warmth at the injection site, headache, malaise, and pain. More than 65 million doses of the HAV vaccine have been administered and despite routine monitoring for adverse events, there are no data to suggest a greater incidence of serious adverse events among vaccinated people compared with nonvaccinated. The vaccine is considered safe.[4-6]

Post serological testing after vaccination is not recommended due to the high efficacy of vaccination. However, anti-HAV levels can be measured against a World Health Organization (WHO) standard. Although the lowest level of protective anti-HAV has not been established, a general standard is ≥10 mIU/mL (IU/L).[6]

Immunoglobulin

Immunoglobulin (Ig) is a sterile preparation of concentrated antibodies against HAV that provides protection by passive transfer of antibody. In 2017, recommendations for increased dose of Ig were established due to concerns for declining HAV antibody from donors. Active immunity is achieved through vaccination, although preexposure prophylaxis is used in situations where protective effects of vaccine may either be inadequate or take too long to develop. Specifically, Ig is recommended with vaccination if travel to an HAV high or intermediate risk country will begin in <2 weeks and the individual is an older adult, immunocompromised, or has chronic liver disease or other chronic medical condition. Ig is used when preexposure or postexposure prophylaxis against HAV infection is needed in persons for whom vaccination is not an option. Vaccination is preferred for multiple reasons, including that it induces active immunity and, therefore, a longer time of protection against HAV than Ig.

Immunoglobulin is most effective if given in the incubation period of the infection. Receipt of Ig within the first 2 weeks of infection will reduce infectivity and moderate the infection in 85% of patients. Patients who receive at least one dose of the HAV vaccine at least 1 month prior to exposure do not need preexposure or postexposure prophylaxis with Ig.[6] Although Ig is available as both an intravenous (IV) and intramuscular (IM) injection, for HAV exposure only the IM formulation is used.

Serious adverse events from Ig are rare. Anaphylaxis has been reported in patients with IgA deficiency. Patients who had an anaphylaxis reaction to Ig should not receive it. There is no contraindication for use in pregnancy or lactation.

Dosing of Ig is the same for adults and children. For postexposure prophylaxis and for short-term preexposure coverage of less than 3 months, a single dose of 0.02 mL/kg IM is given. For long-term preexposure prophylaxis of less than or equal to 5 months, a single dose of 0.06 mL/kg is used. Either the deltoid or gluteal muscle may be used. In children younger than 24 months, Ig can be given in the anterolateral thigh muscle.[6]

Vaccination is also preferred in most patients who were recently exposed to HAV and who had not been previously vaccinated. In contrast, prophylaxis with Ig may be preferred in patients younger than 12 months or who have an allergy to a vaccine component.[5]

Ig can be given concomitantly with the HAV vaccine. Although the antibody titer will be significantly lower than with the vaccine administered alone, the response is still protective and coadministration should be considered for the advantages of long-term HAV protection. However, Ig can interfere with the response of other live-attenuated vaccines and should be delayed.

Vaccine efficacy may be reduced in certain patient populations. In HIV-infected patients, greater immunogenic response may correlate with higher baseline CD4-cell counts. Patients with lower CD4 counts or HIV viremia at vaccination have a reduced response rate.[7]

HEPATITIS B

4 Viral hepatitis B infections pose a substantial global disease burden. Hepatitis B is highly infectious, approximately 50 to 100 times more so than HIV.[8] In 2015, 3.5% of the population, or 257 million people, had chronic HBV. In comparison, 0.8% of the adult population, or 38 million people, were living with HIV. Screening and diagnosis also vary between the two viral infections; only 10% of patients with chronic HBV are aware of their infection in comparison to 79% of people living with HIV.

Globally, the majority of adults with chronic HBV were infected prior to the availability and use of the HBV vaccine in infancy.[9,10] Chronic infection with HBV is a major public health issue as it serves as a reservoir for continued HBV transmission and poses a significant risk of death resulting from liver disease including liver cirrhosis and hepatocellular carcinoma (HCC). According to the WHO, 650,000 people per year die as a result of complications from HBV.[10] In the United States, there is no national chronic hepatitis surveillance program; however, estimates suggest between 850,000 and 2.2 million people have chronic HBV.[1] Although HBV infection is uncommon among the general population in the United States, prevalence is high among certain groups.

Low public awareness, low perceived risk, and misinformation about HBV can result in discrimination and stigma.[1] In 2013, the Department of Justice recognized patients with chronic HBV infection to be protected under the Americans with Disabilities Act after students with HBV were denied enrollment in health professional schools. Although not curable, HBV infections can be successfully managed with viral suppression. Importantly, vaccination prevents HBV infection. In 2021, the CDC's ACIP recommended universal HBV vaccination for all adults aged 19 to 59.

Epidemiology

According to the WHO, chronic HBV infections disproportionately affect low- and middle-income countries.[9,10] Prevalence can vary regionally; however, areas commonly associated with high infectivity rates include sub-Saharan Africa, East Asia, followed by the Amazon and southern parts of Eastern and Central Europe.[10] Most new HBV infections are in children in areas of high HBV prevalence, approximately 45% of the global population. Infections of infants and children are of special concern because more than 90% of cases lead to chronic infections and serve as ongoing source of infectivity. Major public health initiatives focused on pediatric vaccination have successfully reduced HBV infection. In the United States, acute HBV cases declined by approximately 90% since vaccination recommendations were first issued in the 1980s.[11] Annual rates of acute cases vary but in 2019, the number of new HBV cases was 20,700. Substantial increases in the number of cases of acute HBV were first reported in 2016 and were attributed to injection drug use and the opioid epidemic. The highest rates of acute HBV continue to be among White non-Hispanic or Black non-Hispanic men between the ages of 30 to 49 years.[2] Injection drug use continues to be the most commonly identified risk factor for new HBV infections, followed by sexual contact.

HBV is transmitted sexually, parenterally, and perinatally because concentration of HBV is high in blood, serum, and wound exudates of infected persons. The virus can be stable in the environment for at least 7 days and can cause infection during this time. Even in the absence of visible blood, HBV can cause infection and transmission may occur through the reuse of contaminated needles, syringes, or sharp objects. In areas of high HBV prevalence, perinatal transmission from mother to child at birth is most common. Horizontal transmission, such as from an infected child to an uninfected child, is also common. In the United States, perinatal transmission and sexual contact continue to be key routes of transmission. Lack of infection control practices specifically related to

TABLE 58-4 Persons at High Risk for HBV: Recommended Screening

Individuals from the Following Areas	Other Groups
• Africa (all countries) • Asia (all countries in North, Southeast, East Asia) • South Pacific Islands (all countries except Australia and New Zealand) • Middle East (all countries except Cyprus and Israel) • Malta • Spain • Arctic (indigenous populations of Alaska, Canada, Greenland) • South America (Ecuador, Guyana, Suriname, Venezuela, and Amazonian areas) • Central America (Mexico, Guatemala, and Honduras) • Eastern Europe (all countries except Hungary) • Caribbean (Antigua-Barbuda, Dominica, Granada, Haiti, Jamaica, St. Kitts and Nevis, St. Lucia, Turks and Caicos)	• US-born persons not vaccinated as infants whose parents were born in high HBV endemic regions • Household, needle-sharing, and sexual contacts of HBsAg-positive patients • Infants born to HBsAg-positive mother • Persons who have ever injected drugs • Persons not in a long-term mutually monogamous relationship (>1 partner in previous 6 months) • Persons seeking evaluation or treatment for an STD • Men who have sex with men • Inmates of correctional facilities • Individuals with chronic liver disease • Individuals with elevated AST or ALT of unknown etiology • Individuals with HIV or HCV • Patients with end-stage kidney disease including those receiving dialysis • All pregnant women • Persons requiring immunosuppressive therapy (chemotherapy, organ transplantation, rheumatological, or gastroenterologic) • Donors of blood, plasma, organs, tissues, or semen • Unvaccinated persons with diabetes aged 19-59 years (clinical discretion for persons >60 years) • Residents/staff of facilities for developmentally disabled persons • Travelers to countries of high or intermediate HBV prevalence • Healthcare, public safety workers at risk for occupational exposure to blood or blood-contaminated body fluids • Persons who may require postexposure prophylaxis following blood or fluid exposures

ALT, alanine aminotransferase; AST, aspartate aminotransferase; HBsAg, hepatitis B surface antigen; STD, sexually transmitted disease.

Data from Reference 11.

TABLE 58-5 Interpretation of Serologic Tests in Hepatitis B Virus

Tests	Result	Interpretation
HBsAg	(–)	Susceptible
Anti-HBc	(–)	
Anti-HBs	(–)	
HBsAg	(–)	Past HBV infection, resolved
Anti-HBc	(+)	No further management needed unless undergoing immunosuppressive therapy or chemotherapy
Anti-HBs	(+)	
HBsAg	(–)	Immune because of vaccination (valid only if test performed 1-2 months after third vaccine dose)
Anti-HBc	(–)	
Anti-HBs	(+)	
HBsAg	(+)	Acute infection
Anti-HBc	(+)	
IgM anti-HBc	(+)	
Anti-HBs	(–)	
HBsAg	(+)	Chronic infection
Anti-HBc	(+)	Further evaluation needed
IgM anti-HBc	(–)	
Anti-HBs	(–)	
HBsAg	(–)	Possible interpretations: (1) Resolved infection or (2) false positive. If patient immunocompromised, check
Anti-HBc	(+)	HBV DNA[a]
Anti-HBs	(–)	

[a]Some patients may experience occult HBV infection, defined by the presence of low-level HBV DNA levels in the setting of negative HBsAg.

Note: Unless otherwise specified, anti-HBc includes total (both IgM anti-HBc and IgG anti-HBc) or IgG anti-HBc. IgM anti-HBc is present during acute phase of infection.

Anti-, antibody; HBc, hepatitis B core; HBs, hepatitis B surface; HBsAg, hepatitis B surface antigen.

Data from References 12 and 58.

blood glucose monitoring also contributed to HBV outbreaks in the 2000s and 2010s.[10] Screening recommendations focus on individuals at high risk for HBV including household contacts of an HBV-positive person (Table 58-4).[11]

Up to half of all children infected before the age of 6 will develop chronic HBV.[9] Children infected in the first year of life have a 90% likelihood of developing chronic HBV infection; thus, prevention of perinatal transmission and pediatric vaccination is critical.

Etiology

The HBV is a deoxyribonucleic acid (DNA) virus that infects hepatocytes.[12] There are at least 10 HBV genotypes (GTs) (A-J) with distinct geographic and ethnic distribution. Although particular HBV GTs can affect the course of HBV infections, testing for HBV GT is not recommended for clinical practice.[13]

Pathophysiology

On infection, replication of the virus begins by attachment of the virion to the hepatocyte cell surface receptors. The virion contains an internal capsid shielding a partially double stranded DNA which is released within the hepatocyte nucleus and integrates into the host chromosomal DNA.[12] In the nucleus the DNA is converted into closed, circular DNA that serves as a template for pregenomic RNA to transcribe various viral proteins and begins the viral life cycle. The viral genome has four reading frames coding for various proteins and enzymes required for viral replication. Several of these proteins are used diagnostically (Table 58-5).

The hepatitis B surface antigen (HBsAg) is the most abundant of the three surface antigens and is detectable at the onset of clinical symptoms. Its persistence past 6 months after initial detection corresponds to chronic infection and indicates an increased risk for cirrhosis, hepatic decompensation, and HCC. Patients with detectable HBsAg are considered to have active HBV infection. The loss of HBsAg (defined as negative or non-reactive HBsAg) is a goal of therapy and considered an optimal endpoint because it indicates that viral replication and protein expression is suppressed. The loss of HBsAg may occur with or without the development of antibody to HBsAg (anti-HBs).[13]

The precore polypeptide encodes for the secretory protein hepatitis B e-antigen (HBeAg) and the hepatitis B core antigen (HBcAg) proteins. HBeAg is present in an acute infection. In children, HBeAg is responsible for chronic HBV infection because it promotes immune tolerance to HBV.[12] In patients where HBeAg is replaced by antibodies (anti-HBe), the HBV DNA is undetectable, and alanine aminotransferase (ALT) levels normalize, the HBV infection is considered to be resolving. If after a year the patient continues to have HBeAg seroconversion (HBeAg is replaced by anti-HBe), the HBV DNA remains undetectable and the ALT levels remain in the normal range, antiviral therapy may be discontinued with close follow to monitor for HBV reactivation.[14]

The HBcAg is a nucleocapsid protein that, when expressed on hepatocytes, promotes immune-mediated cell death. It is not readily detectable by current laboratory techniques, instead antibodies to HBcAg (anti-HBc) are used for diagnostic purposes. High levels of antibodies (IgM anti-HBc) are detectable during acute infections. Patients who were infected with HBV at any point will be anti-HBc positive (either as total or IgG anti-HBc). Patients who respond to vaccine will have anti-HBs only.[10]

Some patients can have HBeAg negative chronic HBV infections. Due to substantial genetic variability of HBV and propensity for viral mutation, there are viral mutants that have down-regulated expression of HBeAg without affecting viral replication.[12] HBeAg-negative mutants pose a particular clinical challenge because they are refractory to treatment and have been implicated in acute liver failure.[12] Patients with HBeAg-negative mutants will continue to have detectable HBV DNA.

Immune response to HBV affects patient outcomes. In patients who have acute resolving infections, a robust immune response is necessary to quickly neutralize and destroy infected cells before the virus can infect other hepatocytes.[13] Chronic infections are associated with a progressive impairment in immune response. Liver injury is likely caused by secondary, nonspecific inflammation activated by the initial cytotoxic lymphocyte response and as an attempt by the immune system to clear the virus by destroying HBV antigen–presenting hepatocytes. HBV itself is not pathogenic to hepatocytes.[12] Destruction of hepatocytes results in release of circulating, and hence increased ALT levels.

Chronic Hepatitis B Virus

4 Chronic HBV is defined as detectable HBsAg for more than 6 months.[11] Chronic infections can be controlled in many cases, but cure is not possible because the HBV template is integrated into the host genome. The most predictive factor for developing a chronic infection is age. Perinatal infections almost always result in chronic infections because of immune tolerance to the virus. The risk of chronicity declines to less than 5% in adult-onset infections. Importantly, chronic HBV infections are often dynamic and disease progression may not necessarily be sequential.[13]

Clinical Presentation and Phases of Infection

The clinical symptoms and course of an HBV infection are indistinguishable from other types of viral hepatitis (Table 58-4).

During the initial phase of the infection, profuse HBV DNA replication results in high levels of HBV DNA and HBeAg secretion (positive or detectable levels of HBeAg). Patients with HBV >1 million IU/ml (kIU/L) are highly contagious.[13] This phase has been described as "immune tolerant" because hepatic injury is limited.[11] ALT levels remain within normal limits (historically defined as <40 IU/L [0.67 μkat/L]) and no or minimal evidence of fibrosis is seen on liver biopsy.[13] In perinatal or early childhood infections, the phase can persist for years and the likelihood for spontaneous HBeAg seroconversion (loss of HBeAg) is low.[13]

As the immune system responds to HBV-infected hepatocytes, ALT elevants may be intermittent or persist. This immune activity against HBV-infected hepatocytes can lead to liver injury with progression of fibrosis.[11,13] During this time high levels HBeAg and HBV DNA may be present. This phase is more likely in adults and progresses more rapidly.[13] With the increase in immune activity against HBV-infected hepatocytes, the outcome can include HBV DNA suppression. Another scenario where immune response is minimized to the infection is characterized by undetectable or low (<2,000 IU/mL [kIU/L]) HBV DNA, reactive antibody to HBeAg (anti-HBe positive), and normal ALT. Progression of liver disease is unlikely in this phase if ALT remains persistently normal. However, some patients will not see immune control of HBV.

A less common state, described as HBeAg negative chronic HBV, is characterized by viral mutation. Mutations within the virus result in loss of HBeAg production but viral replication is not affected and HBV DNA levels range from moderate to high. ALT levels can also fluctuate or be elevated and patients have more advanced liver disease. Guidelines recognize this mutation in HBV with a lower threshold for initiating HBV treatment.

An uncommon but important clinical state is the "occult HBV infection," where HBcAg (anti-HBC) antibody is positive with negative HBsAG, yet HBV DNA is present, frequently in low levels. Patients may or may not have detectable anti-HBs and the ALT levels are often within normal limits. The risk of ongoing liver damage is minimal unless HBV reactivation occurs, such as if a patient is started on immunosuppressive therapies which may allow rapid increases in HBV replication.[14-16]

Reactivation of hepatitis B, defined as the recurrence or abrupt rise in HBV replication by an increase in serum HBV DNA of at least 1 $\log_{10}$ and a marked increase in transaminase levels, is well described in the literature in patients receiving cancer chemotherapy, steroids, and other immunosuppressive agents.[15,16] Reactivation is the loss of HBV immune control and can occur in anyone with a prior or current HBV infection, but patients who are HBsAg positive are at particular risk. Patients who are HBsAg positive and undergoing treatment with B-cell depleting agents (eg, rituximab), anthracycline derivatives (eg, doxorubicin), or moderate-to-high dose steroid therapy (10-20 mg per day of prednisone or equivalent for 4 weeks or longer) are considered high risk for reactivation.[15] Risk of reactivation is especially high among patients undergoing B-cell depleting therapy (eg, rituximab), where reactivation can occur even in the setting of HBsAg negativity but anti-HBc positivity.[15] Antiviral prophylactic therapy is often indicated to prevent reactivation and continued for at least 6 months, or at least 12 months for B cell–depleting agents, after discontinuation of immunosuppressive therapy.[15]

Cirrhosis

Cirrhosis results as the liver attempts to regenerate while in an environment of persistent inflammation, such as HBV or HCV infections. The development of cirrhosis is mostly insidious and patients can remain stable for years before disease progression. Most patients with compensated cirrhosis either are asymptomatic or have mild symptoms of epigastric pain. The diagnosis is made by laboratory or imaging findings. A decline in albumin, increase in bilirubin, and/or increase in prothrombin time (PT)/international normalized ratio (INR), and/or evidence of portal hypertension (thrombocytopenia) typically demonstrate a gradual decline in synthetic function as blood perfusion through the liver is affected. On imaging, the classical appearance of a small and knobby liver reflects nodules of regenerating cells integrated with infiltrates of inflammation-induced fibrous tissue. Progression of liver disease is variable and affected by both viral and host factors; in particular, the immune response to HBV plays a key role in clinical outcomes (Table 58-6). Patients without cirrhosis have a 5% to 20% risk of progression to cirrhosis over a 5-year period. Subsequently, 20% of all patients with chronic hepatitis B infection and cirrhosis progress to decompensated cirrhosis within a 5-year period.[13] Progression to decompensated cirrhosis is marked by the development of clinical complications of hepatic insufficiency and portal hypertension such as ascites or hepatic encephalopathy. Risks for death and decompensation increase with underlying liver disease. All patients with cirrhosis, irrespective of severity or receipt of HBV treatment, are at an

TABLE 58-6 Factors Associated with Hepatitis B Virus Cirrhosis and Risk of HCC

Host Factors	Viral Factors
Older age at diagnosis African ancestry (greater likelihood for early onset HCC)	Persistence of high HBV serum DNA and or HBsAg levels Infection with genotype C > B
Asian ethnicity	Specific HBV mutations
Alcohol misuse	
Chronic coinfection with HCV, delta hepatitis, or HIV	
Diabetes or metabolic syndrome	
Active smoking	
Family history of cirrhosis/HCC Presence of cirrhosis (as a risk for HCC)	

Data from References 13 and 17.

annual risk of developing HCC and require routine surveillance for HCC as per guidelines.[11]

Hepatocellular Carcinoma

HBV is a known risk factor for the development of HCC and in areas of high HBV endemicity, a major complication of the infection.[9] There is a known annual risk of developing HCC in patients with cirrhosis because of the years of inflammatory processes provoked by ongoing HBV infection. Several factors influence the development of HCC (Table 58-6), in particular, the presence of cirrhosis. In the United States, the majority of cases of HCC are in patients >60 years of age, male, with cirrhosis, and of Asian race. Patients of African ancestry are more likely to develop HCC at a younger age (median 44 years).[17] HBV itself is an oncogenic virus and HCC can occur in patients with HBV who do not have cirrhosis.[9]

Vaccine Prevention of Hepatitis B

5 Vaccination is the most effective strategy to prevent HBV infection. Despite substantial declines in HBV, gaps in HBV vaccination persist that contribute to ongoing HBV transmission. Birth dose vaccination of infants born to HBsAg-positive women remains below the 85% target for Healthy People 2020.[18] Similarly, the three-dose vaccine coverage for adults, including patients with chronic liver disease, travelers, persons with diabetes, and healthcare personnel, are lower and far below target levels.[19] Vaccination for HBV is less effective than for HAV and requires multiple doses for improved response. Many patients start a vaccine series but do not complete it. All infants and all previously unvaccinated children less than 19 years of age should receive HBV vaccine. Additionally, in 2021 ACIP voted to recommend universal HBV vaccination for all adults aged 19 to 59. Adults 60 and older are recommended for vaccination based on risk factors (Table 58-7).

The development of the HBV vaccine represented the first vaccine against a major human cancer.[9] Vaccines use HBsAg to prompt active immunity. The HBsAg is produced using recombinant DNA technology using yeast. The HBsAg itself is not infectious; only the complete HBV is infectious. Available vaccines include HBV antigen only products and combination products. The two single-antigen products are Recombivax® HB and Engerix-B®. The PreHevbrio™ vaccine, approved in 2021, contains three hepatitis B surface antigens to elicit a more robust vaccine response. TWINRIX® is a combination vaccine for HAV and HBV in adults. Comvax® and Pediarix® are used for children along with other scheduled vaccines. Unlike the HAV vaccine, the HBV vaccine response is generally lower and often requires at least three doses for optimal protection. Most

TABLE 58-7 Risk Factors for Hepatitis B Virus Infections: Adult 60 and Older Vaccination Recommendations

- All unvaccinated adults aged 19-59 with diabetes; those aged >60 should be vaccinated at the discretion of treating clinician
- Sex partners of persons who are HBsAg positive
- Sexually active persons not in a long-term monogamous relationship (>1 partner/6 months)
- Men who have sex with men
- STD clinic patients
- Persons with HIV
- Current or recent injection drug use
- Household contacts of persons with chronic hepatitis B infection; clients and staff of institutions for the developmentally disabled
- Healthcare and public safety workers with anticipated risk for exposure to blood or blood-contaminated fluid in the workplace
- Chronic dialysis/ESRD patients including predialysis, peritoneal dialysis, and home dialysis patients
- Correctional facilities inmates
- International travelers to regions with high or intermediate levels (HBsAg prevalence >2%) of endemic HBV infection
- Persons with chronic HCV infection
- Persons with chronic liver disease (eg, patients with alcoholic liver disease, cirrhosis, fatty liver disease, autoimmune hepatitis)
- All unvaccinated adults seeking vaccination (specific risk factor not required)

ESRD, end-stage renal disease.

Data from Reference 19.

TABLE 58-8 Recommended Dosing of Hepatitis B Vaccines (HBV Antigen Vaccines)

Vaccine	Age (Years)	Dose (Volume)	No. of Doses	Schedule[a]
Engerix-B	0-19	10 mcg IM (0.5 mL)	3	0, 1, 6 months
	>20	20 mcg IM (1 mL)	3	0, 1, 6 months
Recombivax	1-19	10 mcg IM (0.5 mL)	3	0, 1, 6 months
	>20	10 mcg IM (1 mL)	3	0, 1, 6 months
Heplisav-B[b,c]	≥18	0.5 mL	2	0, 1 months
PreHevbrio[c]	≥18	1 mL	3	0, 1, 6 months

[a]Zero (0) denotes initial dose, subsequent numbers denote time after initial dose for timing of additional doses.

[b]Utilizes different adjuvant; cannot be interchanged with other HBV vaccines.

[c]Cannot be interchanged with other HBV vaccines.

Data from Reference 6.

vaccines use aluminum as an adjunct; however in 2017 the Food and Drug Administration approved the Heplisav-B® vaccine which uses a novel adjuvant for immunogenicity, a toll-like receptor ligand to enhance immunity that allows for a two-dose vaccine schedule in adults (Table 58-8).

The most commonly reported adverse events for single-antigen vaccine are nausea/dizziness, and fever/headache; for combination vaccines, fever, injection site erythema, and vomiting. For Heplisav-B, the most common adverse reactions reported within 7 days of vaccination included injection site pain, fatigue, and headache.

Vaccination is the standard for HBV prevention. Passive immunity with hepatitis B Ig offers temporary protection against HBV and is used in conjunction with the hepatitis B vaccine for postexposure prophylaxis in infants born to HBsAg-positive mothers and for select other prophylaxis.[19]

TREATMENT

Desired Outcomes

6 Prevention of HBV, in particular preventing mother-to-child transmission, is a primary goal with substantial public health benefits. HBV infections are not curable; thus, the goals of therapy are to suppress HBV replication and prevent disease progression to cirrhosis and HCC. Another important goal is preventing HBV reactivation in patients with inactive HBV infections.

General Approach to Treatment

6 HBV viral suppression is a goal of all therapies.[13] In patients who are HBeAg positive, HBeAg loss, with or without seroconversion to anti-HBeAg, indicates immune control. Normalization of ALT is another goal associated with viral suppression. An ultimate goal of therapy is the loss of HBsAg with or without anti-HBs seroconversion. This is a goal not often realized but one associated with suppression of HBV replication and viral protein expression and indicates antiviral therapy that can be safely discontinued.

Indications for treatment consider HBV DNA levels, ALT levels, and whether or not the patient has cirrhosis (Table 58-10). All patients with cirrhosis require HBV treatment, irrespective of DNA or ALT levels. In patients without cirrhosis, HBV DNA and ALT levels can determine the need for treatment because active viral replication predicts disease progression.[13] In persons without cirrhosis, elevated ALT levels are used to recognize inflammation within the liver and thus the need for HBV treatment to minimize disease progression. Not all persons with chronic HBV are candidates for treatment. Persons without cirrhosis who have low levels of HBV DNA (<2,000 IU/mL [kIU/L]) may be managed by periodic monitoring. The rationale for deferring HBV treatment includes the concern that therapeutic response is unlikely and does not outweigh the risks and costs associated with treatment. The major organizations providing comprehensive guidelines on the management of HBV infections are the WHO, American Association for the Study of Liver Diseases (AASLD), the European Association for the Study of the Liver, and the Asian Pacific Association for the Study of the Liver. A more simplified approach to treatment for primary care providers is also available through the online resource from the HBV Primary Care Workgroup (https://www.hepatitisb.uw.edu/page/primarycareworkgroup/guidance).

Patient Counseling and Nonpharmacologic Therapy

All persons with chronic HBV should be counseled on preventing disease transmission. Sexual and household contacts should be vaccinated against HBV. Barrier protection methods are recommended for sex partners who have not completed vaccination series.[11] Concomitant metabolic syndrome and insulin resistance increase hepatic liver disease progression and the development of HCC.[20,21] Other lifestyle factors known to potentiate liver disease include alcohol use and smoking.[11,20] Herbal medicines are an intriguing option to many patients, although no data support their use and some may have harmful effects on liver function.

TABLE 58-10 Generally Accepted Criteria for Treatment of HBV

Characteristics:
Anyone with HBeAg (+) or HBeAg (−) active HBV defined as:
• HBV DNA >2,000 IU/mL (kIU/L)
• ALT 2 × upper limit of normal[a] and/or with evidence of histological disease[b]
Anyone with compensated or decompensated cirrhosis with HBV DNA >2,000 IU/mL (kIU/L)[c]
Anyone not fulfilling above criteria with ALT < 2 × ULN and any detectable HBV DNA (<2,000 IU/mL [kIU/L]), consider:
Patient's age
Family history of HCC
Prior history of HBV treatment
• Extrahepatic manifestations of HBV

[a]Per European guidelines, any elevations in ALT.

[b]Moderate or greater fibrosis as determined by biopsy or noninvasive measures.

[c]Per European guidelines, any detectable HBV DNA.

Pharmacologic Therapy

HBV virological cure, or HBV virus eradication, is not an achievable goal of therapy because of persistence of the closed, circular DNA in hepatocytes and lifelong risk for HBV reactivation. Instead, the loss of HBsAg and the development of anti-HBs is considered a "functional cure" because it indicates a loss of HBV replication. This is a rare event even in patients on HBV therapy and rarely occurs spontaneously in the absence of HBV therapy.[10]

Because hepatic damage is sustained by ongoing viral replication, drug therapy aims to suppress viral replication by either antivirals—the nucleos(t)ide agents (NAs)—or immunomodulating agents. A major difference in therapy between the NAs and the immune-mediating agents is duration of use: interferon (IFN)-based therapies are typically administered for a predefined duration, whereas NAs are used until a specific end point is achieved. Antiviral agents are the preferred therapy for several reasons, including that they are all oral agents, are well tolerated, and can be safely used even in patients with decompensated cirrhosis.[22]

The preferred NAs are those considered to have a high barrier to resistance and include entecavir, tenofovir diprovoxil, and tenofovir alafenamide. All of these agents also have some level of activity against HIV; thus, it is important to understand a patient's HIV status before starting HBV therapy.

In the United States, the immune-mediating agents approved for use are pegylated interferon (peg-IFN)-alfa and IFN-alfa. These agents are injectable. Due to the substantial side effects, need for monitoring, and toxicities of IFN-based therapies, their role in HBV treatment is limited. IFN is not recommended as a first-line therapy by the WHO.[9]

Entecavir 7 Entecavir is an oral guanosine analogue that inhibits the HBV polymerase, thus preventing HBV replication. It has weak activity against HIV.[9] Entecavir is considered to be a first-line agent for HBV therapy because of its efficacy and low rates of resistance.[8,10,12,13] It is more potent than lamivudine and adefovir in suppressing serum HBV DNA levels, improving liver histology, and normalizing ALT levels.[9] Rates of HBeAg seroconversion increase with subsequent years of treatment.[13] The dose is 0.5 mg orally daily for adults with treatment-naïve or non–lamivudine-resistant infections and 1 mg daily in lamivudine-experienced patients or patients with decompensated cirrhosis. Entecavir resistance remains low in treatment-naïve persons, demonstrating the high barrier to resistance of the drug.[13] However, resistance to lamivudine is a risk factor for entecavir resistance; thus, guidelines do not recommend use of entecavir in patients with prior lamivudine experience.[11] Entecavir is safe and well tolerated.

Tenofovir 7 Due to its high barrier to resistance, tenofovir is considered a first-line therapy in the treatment of HBV.[11,13] For HBV, it is available as a single-agent oral tablet. Tenofovir is a nucleotide analog which competitively inhibits HBV polymerase, thus interrupting viral replication. There are two forms of tenofovir available: tenofovir disoproxil fumarate (tenofovir DF) and tenofovir alafenamide. Tenofovir DF is available as a 300-mg dose for HBV. Tenofovir alafenamide is a prodrug converted to the active tenofovir in the hepatocyte, allowing for a lower dose at 25 mg. Tenofovir DF was used for HBV where it was highly effective in HBV DNA viral suppression demonstrating regression of fibrosis.[10,23] It is effective even in patients previously treated with other HBV therapies. Tenofovir DF is associated with acute renal injury and hypophosphatemia, thus renal function should be monitored before and during treatment.[11] It is also associated with decreased bone mineral density. In persons with suspected tenofovir DF renal or bone disease, HBV treatment should be switched to entecavir or tenofovir alafenamide.

Tenofovir alafenamide offers several advantages over tenofovir DF as it allows more efficient delivery of tenofovir directly to the hepatocytes and thus a more direct action against HBV replication. In both HBeAg-positive and HBeAg-negative patients, tenofovir alafenamide was as effective as tenofovir DF and was more likely to result in normalization of ALT.[24] The ability to reduce the systemic exposure to tenofovir allows for an improved safety profile. Compared to tenofovir DF, tenofovir alafenamide demonstrated improved bone safety and smaller changes in estimated glomerular filtration rates.[24]

Resistance to tenofovir has not been seen in clinical studies. No resistance was identified to tenofovir DF through a 7-year study period and viral suppression was seen in nearly all patients, regardless of HBeAg status.[23] Similarly, there was no resistance to tenofovir alafenamide with 96 weeks of follow-up.[25]

Alternative Drug Treatments

Other available NAs which have a low barrier to resistance and are thus not preferred for treatment of HBV include lamivudine, telbivudine, and adefovir.[11] Lamivudine has antiviral activity against both HIV and HBV but is not recommended as first-line therapy for chronic HBV infections. The main limitation to lamivudine use is its likelihood for resistance, which is considered inevitable and can undermine the value of treatment. Adefovir's role in HBV therapy is unclear. It is no longer recommended as monotherapy because it also has a relatively low barrier to resistance. Telbivudine is similar to lamivudine and also has a high rate of mutations that limits its efficacy. It has been discontinued in the US market. Combination therapy has been proposed for chronic HBV treatment; however, it is not recommended for initial HBV treatment.[13] Patients who are treatment adherent but have incomplete HBV DNA viral control on entecavir or tenofovir DF/tenofovir alafenamide should be switched to the other drug. In rare instances combination therapy can be considered, such as if adherent patients continue to have suboptimal HBV DNA viral suppression or in patients with multiple underlying HBV resistance mutations.[11,13,26] If combination therapy is considered, guidance should be sought from a clinician with expertise in HBV treatment.

Special Populations

Cirrhosis All patients with cirrhosis should receive HBV treatment irrespective of HBV DNA, HBeAg status, or ALT elevations. The presence of cirrhosis is a risk for worsening complications of end-stage liver disease thus an independent reason to initiate HBV treatment. Patients with decompensated cirrhosis should be on HBV therapy and evaluated for liver transplant.[11] Recommended therapies in patients with decompensated cirrhosis include entecavir and tenofovir DF. There are no data using tenofovir alafenamide in patients with decompensated cirrhosis; however, if renal function or bone disease is a concern, it is reasonable to use tenofovir alafenamide. Treatment in these patients is continued indefinitely.[11]

Coinfection with Hepatitis C Virus Coinfection with HCV increases the progression of liver disease including the risk of HCC; thus, all patients with HBV should be screened for HCV. Moreover, reactivation of HBV can occur in patients undergoing treatment with direct-acting antivirals (DAAs) for HCV and may require HBV prophylaxis.[11,13] The exact mechanism of this is unknown but is primarily a concern in patients undergoing HCV DAA therapy who also have detectable HBsAg. Patients with both HBV and HCV should be evaluated for HBV treatment according to HBV treatment criteria.

Coinfection with Hepatitis D Infection with hepatitis D requires infection with hepatitis B. No NAs have demonstrated efficacy against HDV; however, IFN does have some efficacy against HDV and treatment may include either IFN monotherapy or a combination of IFN with an NA.[9,13]

Coinfection with Human Immunodeficiency Virus In HIV-coinfected patients, initiation of highly active antiretroviral therapy (HAART) is strongly recommended as it may improve overall survival. Therapy should include either tenofovir alafenamide or tenofovir DF since both have efficacy against HIV and HBV.[13]

Pediatric Patients Most children with chronic HBV are asymptomatic and do not meet the established criteria for HBV treatment.[13] Treatment is recommended in HBeAg-positive children aged 2 to 18 who have elevated ALT and measurable HBV DNA.[11] A limitation to the recommendations is a lack of clarity regarding the upper limit of normal for ALT in pediatric patients with guidelines using an upper limit of normal of 35 IU/L (0.58 μkat/L) for males and 25 IU/L (0.42 μkat/L) for females.[11] Entecavir and tenofovir DF are approved for children 2 years and older and are preferred due to their high barrier to resistance. Adefovir and lamivudine are not preferred due to the low barrier to resistance. Although IFN is approved for use in children 1 year and older, its side effect profile and need for injection limit its use.

Chronic HBV in Pregnancy Perinatal transmission of HBV is a major cause of chronic HBV. In pregnant females who are HBeAg positive and have an HBV DNA >200,000 IU/mL (kIU/L), tenofovir DF is recommended in the third trimester. Tenofovir alafenamide has been shown to prevent transmission with no safety concerns in one small retrospective study, and may be a potential option once additional evidence is available.[27] To prevent mother-to-child transmission, all infants born to HBsAg-positive women should receive HBV vaccination and immunoglobulin within 12 hours of birth.[19] Assessment of HBsAg status, a complete HBV vaccine series, and post-vaccination serological testing to document vaccine response (anti-HBs) is recommended. Revaccination is recommended in infants who are HBsAg negative and do not have a post-vaccination anti-HBs titer ≥10 mIU/mL (IU/L). Infants born to females with an unknown HBsAg status should also receive the first dose of vaccine within 12 hours of birth while maternal serological tests are pending. The rationale for this birth dose vaccination approach is that timely prophylaxis against HBV can disrupt the vertical transmission associated with perinatal HBV infections. Completion of the vaccine series is critical to long-term HBV prevention.

Immunosuppressive or Cytotoxic Therapy 8 Patients who will undergo chemotherapy or immunosuppressive therapy should be assessed for risk of HBV. The American Gastroenterological Association recommends antiviral prophylaxis for persons who are at high risk of HBV including persons who are (1) HBsAg-positive or negative and anti-HBc-positive and undergoing B-cell depleting agents such as rituximab; (2) HBsAg-positive and anti-HBc-positive treated with anthracycline derivatives such as doxorubicin; (3) HBsAg-positive and anti-HBc-positive undergoing 10 to 20 mg prednisone daily or equivalent therapy or on high-dose (>20 mg prednisone daily or equivalent) corticosteroids for 4 weeks or more.[15,16] Due to moderate risks of reactivation, other immunosuppressive therapies such as tumor necrosis factor alpha inhibitors, cytokine or integrin inhibitors, tyrosine kinase inhibitors, and corticosteroids are also identified as requiring antiviral prophylaxis in patients with specific HBV serological results.[15,16] The CDC recommends testing for hepatitis B for all patients who are to receive chemotherapy or other immunosuppressive agents.

8 Patients who are at high risk of HBV reactivation and are expected to be on chemotherapy or immunosuppressive treatment for 1 year or less should receive prophylactic HBV antiviral therapy and be treated for at least 6 months after completion of chemotherapy or immunosuppressive therapy.[15]

Hepatitis B Virus Mutations and Resistance Concerns

Although a DNA virus, HBV uses reverse transcriptase, similar to a retrovirus such as HIV. The similarities between HIV reverse transcriptase and HBV polymerase prompted the development of NAs for the treatment of HBV. The preferred therapies have a high barrier to resistance. Resistance potential in HBV is evaluated by an antiviral agent's genetic barrier to resistance, or the number of primary mutations needed for antiviral drug resistance to occur. Other factors include cross-resistance and drug potency. Treatment adherence is important.

Viral resistance in HBV is a concern given HBV's high replication rate and an estimated 10 mutations generated daily.[9-11] Viral suppression is important because the HBV virus mutates and risks the development of resistance when ongoing viral replication occurs in the setting of antiviral drug pressure.

Patients who experience treatment interruptions risk treatment failure because HBV can archive drug-resistant mutations that allow the virus to quickly select the mutation if the antiviral agent is reintroduced. Cross-resistance among antiviral agents also occurs, further limiting therapeutic options. Lamivudine is most commonly associated with resistance due to (1) its low barrier for developing resistance with a single mutation able to overcome efficacy and (2) widespread use of lamivudine in some regions.[9]

Resistance to the NA agents occurs by alteration of the active site of the HBV DNA polymerase. Long-term use of lamivudine is associated with resistance mutations of this active site and cross-resistance occurs which also affects telbivudine.[28] Prior treatment with lamivudine and the expected resistance with ongoing lamivudine therapy is an established risk for entecavir resistance. In these patients with prior lamivudine experience, a tenofovir-based therapy is preferred due to concerns for entecavir resistance. Resistance to tenofovir alafenamide was not identified in clinical trials and is rare is clinical practice.[25]

Guidelines favor the use of entecavir, tenofovir DF, and tenofovir alafenamide because these are potent agents able to suppress viral replication and maintain a high barrier to resistance. However, another major factor in resistance is patient adherence to therapy. Barriers to adherence include forgetting doses, limited understanding of the importance of adherence, and changes to routine.[29]

HEPATITIS C

Approximately 2.4 million people in the United States are chronically infected with HCV.[2] Considering that HCV infection is prevalent in high-risk populations such as prisoners, PWIDs, and homeless individuals, and that this population is generally excluded from most surveys, the actual number of chronically infected people is not known. Routine screening for HCV remains a barrier to diagnosis given the substantial stigma associated with HCV. Most acute HCV infections are asymptomatic. Chronic infections are often insidious, leading to delays in HCV diagnosis and significant disease progression. The current HCV epidemic is linked to the opioid crisis. HCV therapies are curative in the overwhelming majority of patients. These treatments are all-oral and well tolerated with few adverse effects or laboratory abnormalities. However, HCV treatment access is variable and may include a number of stipulations which act as barriers to care and ultimately, the ability to cure HCV.

Epidemiology

9 10 HCV is the most common blood-borne pathogen. Since 2010, the number of acute HCV cases increased, due to both improved surveillance and increase in incidence. There were 50,300 new HCV infections in 2018 compared to 16,500 in 2011.[2] Since 2014, acute HCV cases increased by 71% and most were among people aged 20 to 39. Universal HCV screening is recommended for all persons aged 18 and older by the CDC and the United States Prevention Services Task Force, in an attempt to address this rising epidemic.[30]

Transmission of HCV occurs through percutaneous exposure.[31] Injection-drug use is a major factor in the cycle of HCV transmission and the most common reason for the current increase in new infections. In Indiana in 2015, an outbreak of 135 new cases of HIV among PWIDs identified coinfection with HCV in over 84% of patients.[32] Some experts also consider other illicit drug use, for example, intranasal cocaine, as a risk factor because of the possible contamination of drug paraphernalia not limited to syringes and needles. Unsafe injection practices are associated with HCV transmission and include tattoos received in a nonregulated setting and needle stick injuries. Less common routes of transmission include sexual transmission and infants born to HCV-infected women.[33] Although sexual contact is considered an inefficient means of HCV transmission, anal sex, multiple sexual partners, and coinfection with sexually transmitted diseases, including HIV, increase the risk for HCV sexual transmission. Outbreaks of HCV were demonstrated in MSM with guidelines recommending annual HCV screening for adolescent and adult MSM including HIV-uninfected men seeking HIV preexposure prophylaxis.[31] Blood transfusion posed a major risk for infection, but improved screening of blood in 1992 decreased the risk of transfusion-related HCV.[31] Healthcare-associated transmission is rare; however, unsafe injection practices are often identified as the cause of HCV transmission.

9 The CDC recommends hepatitis C screening at least once in all adults aged 18 and above.[30] More frequent screening is recommended if there are risk factors for infection (Table 58-11). Because of the increase in HCV infections among women of reproductive age, HCV screening should also be done with each pregnancy.[30] The AASLD, in conjunction with the Infectious Diseases Society of America (IDSA), publish online guidelines for testing, managing, and treating HCV (see www.hcvguidelines.org).[31] The AASLD recommends children born to mothers with HCV be screened at or after 18 months of age. More frequent screening is also warranted in persons who are at high risk for infection, especially among PWIDs or who have a history of injection drug use (Table 58-11).[31] Any needle-borne exposure in an unregulated setting poses a risk for infection.

The initial test for HCV infection is the anti-HCV or antibody test (Fig. 58-1). Patients who are antibody positive for HCV require confirmatory testing for HCV RNA to verify current HCV infection. Some laboratories offer reflex testing where confirmatory testing is done on all samples where the anti-HCV is reactive. Patients who are anti-HCV positive but who do not have a detectable HCV RNA do not have a current HCV infection and no further workup is required

TABLE 58-11 Recommendations for Hepatitis C Virus Screening

All adults ≥18 years
All pregnant females during each pregnancy
Routine periodic testing for persons with ongoing risk factors:
• Persons who inject drugs, share needles, syringes, or other drug preparation equipment
• Persons undergoing maintenance hemodialysis
• Sexually active MSM with HIV
• MSM at initiation of HIV pre-exposure prophylaxis

Data from References 30 and 31.

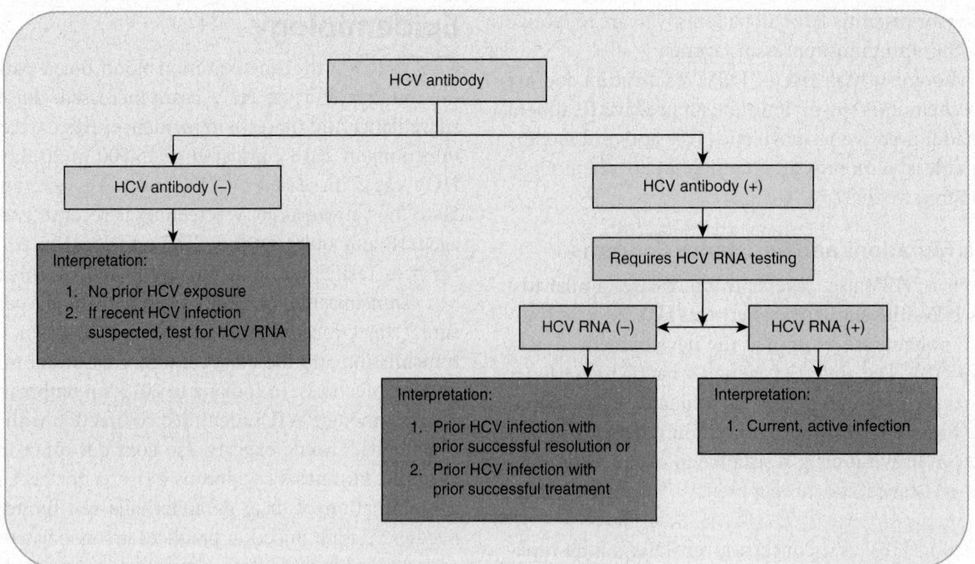

FIGURE 58-1 HCV testing.

in the majority of cases.[34] The presence of antibody does not infer immunity and patients are at risk for HCV infection should they be reexposed.[35]

Etiology

HCV is a single-stranded RNA virus notable for lacking a proofreading polymerase which enables frequent viral mutations and poses a challenge for vaccine development.[35] The virus replicates within hepatocytes and, like hepatitis B, is not directly cytopathic. HCV replicates copiously posing an immense challenge for host immune control.[35] Viral mutations can affect DAA therapy.

HCV is differentiated into seven major GTs, numbered 1 to 7. GTs are further classified into subtypes (a, b, c, etc.). The most widely distributed GTs are 1 and 2, with GT1 being the most common. In the United States, GT1a and GT1b, followed by GT2 and GT3, cause most infections. Chronic HCV infection with any of the GTs can lead to cirrhosis, end-stage liver disease (ESLD), or HCC. Preferred therapies on most formularies are those that are pan-genotypic (active against all GTs).

Pathophysiology

In most cases, an acute HCV infection leads to chronic infection. The immune response in an acute HCV infection is mostly insufficient to eradicate the virus. HCV poses a daunting challenge for immune control because of its rapid viral diversification. Resolved cases of HCV are defined by a vigorous T-cell response with highly active CD8 and persistent CD4-cell response. CD8 activity mediates protective immunity but requires the aid of CD4 cells to maintain the response during viral mutations.[35]

Clinical Presentation

In an acute HCV infection, most patients are asymptomatic and thus undiagnosed. HCV RNA is detectable within 1 to 2 weeks of exposure and levels rise quickly during the initial weeks. Approximately one-third of adults will experience some mild and nonspecific symptoms of hepatitis, including fatigue, anorexia, weakness, jaundice, abdominal pain, or dark urine.[36] Acute infections rarely progress to fulminant hepatitis, although the course can be severe and prolonged. Patients who have self-limiting infections may experience symptoms as the immune response attempts to clear the infection. This can result in clinical symptoms and elevated ALT levels. If symptomatic, patients generally see symptom improvement as ALT and HCV RNA levels subside. In patients who are immunosuppressed or have been infected with HCV for less than 6 months, antibody testing could be negative because the immune system is unable or has not yet developed an antibody response. In these cases, confirmation of HCV infection requires HCV RNA testing.[31]

Up to 85% of acutely infected patients will go on to develop a chronic HCV infection, defined as persistently detectable HCV RNA for 6 months or more. HCV RNA levels and ALT levels can fluctuate. Most patients will have few, if any, specific symptoms of chronic HCV infection. Chronic inflammation of the liver from chronic HCV infection may result in fibrosis. Fibrosis is defined by altered hepatic perfusion creating a distorted structure and affecting normal function. Fibrosis leads to cirrhosis, although the speed of fibrosis progression is variable. Patients with cirrhosis require follow-up care specifically for management of the complications associated with cirrhosis. Once a patient is diagnosed with cirrhosis, staging is necessary to differentiate patients who have compensated cirrhosis (Child's class A cirrhosis) versus decompensated (Child's class B or C cirrhosis). Patients with decompensated cirrhosis generally require management by specialists due to severe liver damage and potential complications.

10 The development of HCV cirrhosis poses a 30% risk over 10 years for the development of ESLD, as well as a 1% to 2% risk per year of developing HCC.[30] Progression to cirrhosis is the primary concern in patients infected with HCV for two decades or longer. Disease progression is not uniform or linear, making it difficult to identify which patients will have progressive liver damage and when. Other concomitant viral infections, comorbidities, and lifestyle factors can contribute to disease progression. Ongoing alcohol use, obesity, and metabolic syndrome can potentiate fibrosis.[31] Viral load is not a factor for disease progression and not associated with degree of fibrosis. Coinfection with HIV or HBV is associated with disease progression as is infection with HCV GT3.[31,37]

10 Although HCV is thought of as a liver disease, chronic HCV is associated with extrahepatic manifestations, or HCV-associated systemic disease. The most common is cryoglobulinemia, a local deposition of immune complexes that cause vasculitis.[31] Typical manifestations involve the skin and internal organ damage, predominantly affecting the kidneys and associated with worsening renal function. Other systemic diseases associated with HCV include

cardiovascular disease, diabetes, B-cell non-Hodgkin lymphoma, Sjögren syndrome, glomerulonephritis, arthritis, corneal ulcers, thyroid disease, neuropathies, and skin diseases such as vasculitis, porphyria cutanea tarda, and lichen planus.[38]

TREATMENT

Desired Outcomes

11 The primary goal of therapy is to eradicate HCV infection. Virologic cure, or sustained virologic response (SVR), is defined as a nondetectable HCV RNA at least 12 weeks after completing HCV therapy. Patients who achieve SVR will continue to have detectable HCV antibody indefinitely. The persistence of HCV antibody should not be confused with the potential to reactivate HCV and it does not confer protection against subsequent exposure to HCV. Patients can be reinfected with the same or different HCV GT. Resolving the infection prevents the development of chronic HCV infection sequelae including ESLD, HCC, and death. Patients with extrahepatic manifestations of HCV are expected to benefit with reductions in symptoms and disease severity of their extrahepatic disease while experiencing improvements in quality of life measures.[31] As more patients are cured, the risk of transmission is expected to decline and reduce HCV disease prevalence.[31]

General Approach to Treatment

Treatment for HCV is recommended for all persons with HCV. Initiating HCV therapy early in the disease state can provide substantial benefit by preventing complications of liver disease as well as preventing extrahepatic manifestations of HCV. In persons at high risk of transmitting HCV such as PWIDs, HCV treatment may help reduce rates of HCV transmission.[31] There are no clearly identified contraindications for HCV therapy. Patients with a short-life expectancy who are unlikely to benefit from HCV therapy, liver transplantation, or other directed therapy are the only populations for whom treatment is not recommended.[31]

The initial evaluation for HCV treatment is intended to stage the patient's level of liver disease, specifically to differentiate patients with cirrhosis from those without (Table 58-12). Patients without cirrhosis may be candidates for a much more simplified treatment approach if the patient does not have cirrhosis, is HCV treatment naïve, has no history or suspicion of HCC, has not received a liver transplant, and has no evidence of HIV or active HBV infection (Table 58-13). In contrast, patients with cirrhosis must be further evaluated to determine if the cirrhosis is compensated (Child–Turcotte–Pugh [CTP] A) or decompensated (CTP B or C). Patients with cirrhosis will likely require on-treatment monitoring as well as additional post-treatment follow-up to manage the complications associated with cirrhosis (eg, need for endoscopy or screening and surveillance for HCC). Patients with decompensated cirrhosis should be treated by clinicians with expertise in managing advanced liver disease.[31]

The suggested laboratory tests prior to treatment are listed in Table 58-14. Quantitative HCV RNA testing is performed to confirm HCV infection. Genotyping is often performed although not required per national guidelines. Patients should be evaluated for HAV and HBV and offered vaccinations if not previously vaccinated. On-treatment laboratory monitoring is not necessary for patients without cirrhosis who meet the criteria for the simplified algorithm. Patients with cirrhosis may need on-treatment monitoring, with the most monitoring required for patients undergoing HCV therapy with the addition of ribavirin.

TABLE 58-12 Tools Used for Assessment of Cirrhosis

Any of the Following	
FIB-4 score[a]	Scores >3.25 suggestive of cirrhosis
Transient elastography	Scores >12.5 kPa indicate cirrhosis
Clinical evidence of cirrhosis	Liver nodularity and/or splenomegaly on imaging; thrombocytopenia (platelets <150,000/mm^3 [150 × 10^9/L]); etc.
Serological tests (eg. FibroSure)	Scores above specific test thresholds
Prior biopsy findings[b]	

[a]FIB-4 includes age, AST, ALT, and platelet level.

[b]Biopsy not required for diagnosis of cirrhosis.

TABLE 58-13 Simplified Treatment Candidates

Candidates for Simplified Treatment Approach		
HCV treatment naïve	AND	• No cirrhosis • No coinfection with HIV or active HBV infection • Not pregnant • No history or suspicion of HCC • No history of liver transplant

TABLE 58-14 Suggested Laboratories Prior to Initiating HCV Treatment

Test	Timeframe	Comments
HCV RNA	Any point before starting HCV therapy	Confirm HCV infection
Complete blood count	Within 6 months of starting HCV therapy	Thrombocytopenia (platelets <150,000/mm^3 [150 × 10^9/L] suggest cirrhosis)
Liver function tests	Within 6 months of starting HCV therapy	Albumin, bilirubin used to assess synthetic function of liver and for calculating Child Pugh in patients with cirrhosis; AST/ALT used to assess level of liver inflammation
International normalized ratio	Within 6 months of starting HCV therapy	In patients with cirrhosis used to assess synthetic function of the liver and for calculating Child–Pugh score
Estimated glomerular filtration rate	Within 6 months of starting HCV therapy	Renal insufficiency may indicated extrahepatic manifestations of HCV
HIV antigen/antibody	Any point before starting HCV therapy	Patients with HIV are not candidates for simplified algorithm; HIV and HCV share common routes of transmission (injection drug use)
Hepatitis B serologies (anti-HBs, anti-HBc, HBsAg)	Any point before starting HCV therapy	Patients with detectable HBsAg are at risk for HBV reactivation; patients who are HBV susceptible should be offered HBV vaccine
Anti-HAV	Any point before starting HCV therapy	Patients susceptible to HAV should be offered HAV vaccine

Data from Reference 31.

Counseling and Nonpharmacologic Therapy

Lifestyle changes are an important factor in reducing health consequences in hepatitis C. Continued alcohol use is a known risk factor for disease progression and severity. There is no established lower limit of alcohol consumption at which disease progression is not seen. Obesity is also a factor and patients should be encouraged to eat a balanced diet and exercise regularly to maintain a normal weight. Progression of fibrotic changes is associated with obesity. The use of herbal therapy is ineffective and potentially a source of drug interaction with HCV therapies. Patients should be counseled on minimizing HCV transmission risks and harm reduction strategies are recommended by national guidelines.[31]

Pharmacologic Therapy

11 The treatment of chronic HCV was revolutionized with the approval of DAAs. The DAAs act on one of three targets on the HCV virion. The DAAs must be used in combination with at least two drugs acting on different targets. The drug nomenclature identifies where the drug is inhibiting viral replication: the N3/4A protease inhibitors end with –previr; NS5A inhibitors end with –asvir; and the NS5B polymerase inhibitors end with –buvir. Early DAAs acted on specific HCV GTs. Sofosbuvir/velpatasvir, glecaprevir/pibrentasvir, and sofosbuvir/velpatasvir/voxilaprevir are pangenotypic, meaning they are effective in all HCV GTs. The ability to treat without pretreatment GT testing favors the use of these agents and is an increasingly appealing strategy because it can streamline HCV treatment and reduce costs. As a group, the DAAs are well tolerated and cause few laboratory abnormalities.

The guidelines offer a simplified treatment algorithm which takes advantage of the safety and efficacy of pangenotypic therapies and shortened duration of therapy with either an 8- or 12-week treatment course (Table 58-15).[31] Patients who do not have cirrhosis or any other major medical comorbidity are candidates for the simplified treatment (see Table 58-16 for exclusion criteria). Laboratory monitoring is not necessary; patients are re-assessed 12 weeks after the end of therapy with an HCV RNA and LFTs. A negative HCV RNA 12 weeks after completing treatment is consistent with cure, or sustained virologic response (SVR or SVR12 to denote that the HCV RNA was done 12 weeks after completing treatment). The LFTs are determined to confirm resolution of inflammation and identify patients which may need further workup of their liver disease if inflammation persists.[31]

Patients without cirrhosis or those with compensated cirrhosis are treated similarly with no difference in treatment duration. A main difference in the treatment approach is the necessary monitoring. Patients with cirrhosis may have laboratories (eg, AST/ALT) checked every 4 weeks while on treatment to monitor their underlying liver disease. In contrast, patients with decompensated cirrhosis (CTP class B or C) often require concomitant ribavirin and have fewer treatment options due to the underlying level of liver disease and concerns for safety. In general, patients with decompensated cirrhosis should be managed by clinicians with experience with end-stage liver disease due to the potential for complications related to cirrhosis (eg, ascites, encephalopathy) developing while on HCV treatment.[31]

Prior treatment experience does not substantially alter retreatment except that there are more limited options for retreatment if patients were previously treated with more recent DAA therapies. Patients previously treated with IFN or IFN and a first generation protease inhibitor (boceprevir, teleaprevir, or simeprevir) who did not achieve cure can be retreated with a DAA therapy and expect cure rates comparable to those in patients who are treatment naïve. As a result the national guidelines no longer recognize separate recommendations for IFN-experienced patients. For patients previously treated with a DAA therapy (sofosbuvir- or NS5A-based regimen) who experience treatment failure, the only recommended retreatment is with the combination of sofosbuvir/velpatasvir/voxilaprevir.[31]

Clinically significant drug-drug interactions are expected with carbamazepine, phenobarbital, phenytoin, oxcarbazepine, rifampin, and St. John's wort and concurrent use of these agents with any of the HCV therapies is expected to result in HCV treatment failure. The use of statins is variable and clinical management can vary from holding statins during HCV therapy to changing or dose reducing the statin. An important resource for timely and updated guidance on HCV-drug interactions is available for free through the University of Liverpool: https://www.hep-druginteractions.org/checker.

Previously, HCV treatment included the injection of peg-IFN and was associated with a substantial side-effect profile as well as a prolonged duration of therapy. The current standard of care for all chronic HCV infections, regardless of GT, is an all-oral drug regimen. Despite the change in pharmacological therapy, many patients are aware of the substantial side effects associated with IFN-based therapy and are wary of all HCV therapy. For patients familiar with IFN treatment, it

TABLE 58-15 AASLD/IDSA Recommended Treatment Regimens for Treatment-Naïve Patients with Hepatitis C (All Genotypes)

Simplified Treatment Algorithm		
Glecaprevir/pibrentasvir 3 tabs orally daily with food × 8 weeks	Or	Sofosbuvir/velpatasvir 1 tab orally daily with or without food × 12 weeks
Repeat HCV RNA and LFTs 12 weeks after completing HCV therapy to assess for cure (SVR) and resolution of hepatic inflammation		

Data from Reference 31.

TABLE 58-16 AASLD/IDSA Recommended Treatment Regimens for Treatment-Naïve Patients with No Cirrhosis (NC) or Compensated Cirrhosis (CC) and Hepatitis C Genotypes 1-6

	GT1a NC	GT1a CC	GT1b NC or CC	GT2 NC or CC	G3 NC	GT3 CC	GT4 NC or CC	GT5, 6 NC or CC
DAA Therapy								
Glecaprevir/Pibrentasvir	Yes	Yes	Yes	Yes	Yes	Yes	Yes	Yes
Ledipasvir/Sofosbuvir	Yes	Yes	Yes	No	No	No	Yes	Yes
Sofosbuvir/Velpatasvir	Yes	Yes	Yes	Yes	Yes	Yes[b]—but with RAS testing	Yes	Yes
Elbasvir/Grazoprevir	No[a]	No	Yes	No	No	No	Yes	No

[a]Considered an alternative regimen because NS5A resistance testing is required prior to treatment start.

[b]Pre-treatment resistance testing for NS5A resistance-associated substitutions (RAS) should be done; if the Y93 RAS is identified, an alternative therapy is recommended.

Data from Reference 31.

is important to clearly distinguish current therapies from IFN-based ones as the concern for side effects of IFN-based HCV therapy can prevent patients from seeking HCV treatment with DAAs.

Sofosbuvir Sofosbuvir was approved in 2013 for HCV GT1 to 4 at a dose of 400 mg. Although available as a single product, its use is mostly as the backbone of combination therapies including ledipasvir/sofosbuvir, sofosbuvir/velpatasvir, and sofosbuvir/velpatasvir/voxilaprevir. Sofosbuvir is metabolized to its primary circulating active metabolite GS-331007. Sofosbuvir is well tolerated and has few drug-drug interactions; the majority of drug interactions are related to the agents used in combination with sofosbuvir. Serious symptomatic bradycardia was identified in patients treated with sofosbuvir and taking amiodarone in combination with other DAAs; thus, this combination is not recommended.

Ledipasvir/Sofosbuvir The fixed dose combination tablet of ledipasvir/sofosbuvir (90 mg/400 mg) is a recommended therapy in patients with HCV GT1 or 4. A 12-week treatment course is highly effective in treatment-naïve patients with or without cirrhosis with an estimated SVR of 95%.[39] Initial studies also demonstrated a high SVR of 94% in patients without cirrhosis, treatment-naïve, and with a baseline viral load of less than 6 million IU/mL (kIU/L) treated for 8 weeks. However, due to limited data the level of evidence to support this shorter course of therapy is lower than the 12-week course of treatment and the shorter course is not recommended in patients who have cirrhosis, have a viral load greater than 6 million IU/mL (kIU/L), are Black, or have HIV–HCV coinfection.[31,40] There are no differences in treatment whether patients have GT1a, 1b, or 4; however, there are differences in treatment duration depending on underlying cirrhosis.[41,42] The use of ribavirin did not affect SVR rates and is not routinely recommended. Patients with decompensated cirrhosis are more difficult to treat with lower SVR rates. In these patients, ledipasvir/sofosbuvir plus ribavirin is recommended for 12 weeks of treatment. If patients are unable to tolerate ribavirin due to its hematological effects, ledipasvir/sofosbuvir for 24 weeks is an alternative.[31,43] National guidelines also recommend ledipasvir/sofosbuvir for treatment of HCV GT4 for a 12-week course of therapy.[31]

The combination of ledipasvir/sofosbuvir is well tolerated and can be used in patients with cirrhosis, including CTP Class A, B, and C cirrhosis. It may also be used in patients with renal insufficiency including patients with end-stage renal disease on dialysis. Headache and fatigue are the most common side effects. Laboratory abnormalities do not frequently occur. The drug-drug interaction potential is also limited, although amiodarone use is not recommended because of the symptomatic bradycardia observed with the concomitant use of sofosbuvir. Acid suppressive therapy poses a challenge to treatment because ledipasvir requires an acidic environment for absorption. Antacids must be spaced apart by 4 hours whereas histamine blockers should be taken either at the same time or 12 hours apart from ledipasvir/sofosbuvir. The use of proton pump inhibitors is controversial with omeprazole 20 mg once daily recommended by the manufacturer; however, more frequent dosing or higher dosages are expected to compromise the efficacy of ledipasvir.[44] The effect of other proton pump inhibitors is not established and concomitant histamine blockers or antacids must be timed appropriately to avoid a clinically significant drug-drug interaction.

Sofosbuvir/Velpatasvir Sofosbuvir/velpatasvir is a pan-genotypic agent with activity against GT1 to 6. It is available as a fixed-dose tablet (400 mg/100 mg for adult dosing or 200 mg/50 mg for pediatric dosing) and as oral pellets for pediatric use (200 mg/50 mg or 150 mg/37.5 mg). In patients with HCV GT1, 2, 4, 5, and 6, 99% SVR was achieved with sofosbuvir/velpatasvir, irrespective of prior treatment experience or whether patients had cirrhosis or not.[40] In GT3 patients, pretreatment resistance testing is recommended for any patients with cirrhosis or prior treatment experience with peg-INF and ribavirin. If the Y93 substitution is detected, ribavirin should be added or an alternative therapy chosen.[31] Studies showed a numerically higher SVR in patients with HCV GT3 and cirrhosis who had received concomitant ribavirin, although this did not reach statistical significance.[45]

Sofosbuvir/velpatasvir is well tolerated with few side effects or laboratory abnormalities. It is recommended for use in patients with all levels of liver disease including decompensated cirrhosis where it is used in combination with ribavirin in order to maximize SVR. Patients with HCV GT1, 2, 3, 4, or 6 and decompensated liver disease treated with sofosbuvir/velpatasvir and ribavirin for 12 weeks achieved an SVR of 94%.[46] Patients with decompensated cirrhosis who cannot tolerate ribavirin may be treated with an extended duration of sofosbuvir/velpatasvir alone for 24 weeks. Most patients with decompensated cirrhosis also demonstrated an improvement in their liver disease (eg, reductions in their Child–Pugh score) as a result of treatment. Sofosbuvir/velpatasvir may also be used in patients with renal impairment, including patients on dialysis. Velpatasvir, like ledipasvir, requires an acidic environment for absorption; thus, patients must be appropriately counseled to avoid the use of proton pump inhibitors and on timing of other acid suppressive therapy to minimize the drug-drug interaction.

Elbasvir/Grazoprevir Elbasvir/grazoprevir as a fixed-dose tablet (50 mg/100 mg) is approved for use in patients with HCV GT1 and 4. In treatment-naïve patients with HCV GTs 1, 4, and 6, the overall SVR rate was 95%.[47] Among patients with HCV GT1a, SVR rates were lower than for GT1b and this difference was attributed to the presence of baseline resistance–associated substitutions (RASs). When comparing patients with GT1a versus 1b who did not have any RASs, there was no difference in SVR (99 vs 100% SVR, respectively). For patients with baseline RASs and GT1a, the SVR rate dropped to 58%. Therefore, in patients with HCV GT1a, pretreatment resistance testing is required. If specific mutations are identified, treatment must be modified to include ribavirin and extended to 16 weeks, thus making it an alternative treatment as per guidelines in favor of shorter, ribavirin-free treatments.[31] Elbasvir/grazoprevir is approved for use in patients with HCV GT1 or 4, including those with renal insufficiency receiving hemodialysis. Because it contains a protease inhibitor, it should not be used in patients with decompensated cirrhosis.

Glecaprevir/Pibrentasvir Glecaprevir/pibrentasvir is a pangenotypic agent with activity against the major HCV GTs. It is available as a combination tablet (100 mg/40 mg) and as oral pellets (50 mg/20 mg) for pediatric use. It is recommended for use in both treatment-naïve and treatment-experienced patients with HCV GTs1 to 6. It is also recommended for use in patients with renal insufficiency including patients on hemodialysis. For patients who are treatment naïve, without cirrhosis or with compensated cirrhosis (CTP class A), the combination is recommended for an 8-week treatment regimen.[31] The approved combination tablet demonstrated the highest SVR rates ranging from 94% to 100% in patients with HCV GTs1 to 6. The lowest SVR at 94% was seen in patients with HCV GT3.[48] An 8-week treatment course is recommended for patients with cirrhosis and HCV GT1 to 6 due to SVR results comparable to those seen in patients without cirrhosis.[49] A smaller number of patients with cirrhosis and HCV GT3 in the clinical trial led to a lower level of recommendation for the use of the 8-week treatment course in these patients.[31] Baseline mutations for NS3 or NS5A did not affect SVR in clinical trials.[50] Because it contains a protease inhibitor, glecaprevir/pibrentasvir should not be used in patients with decompensated cirrhosis due to concerns for worsening liver injury, including liver failure.

Although approved for use in patients with prior DAA failure, guidelines limit the use of glecaprevir/pibrentasvir in this patient population pending further data.[31] Glecaprevir/pibrentasvir is recommended in patients with prior NS3/4A treatment experience (eg, boceprevir or simeprevir). However, it is an alternative treatment for patients with prior NS5A (eg, ledipasvir) treatment in part due to limited data and the need for an extended 16-week treatment duration in this patient population.[31]

Similar to other DAAs, glecaprevir/pibrentasvir is not associated with laboratory abnormalities and is well tolerated. The most common adverse events include headache and nausea. It is contraindicated with ethinyl estradiol products including hormone replacement and oral contraceptives due to a potential for ALT increases.

Sofosbuvir/Velpatasvir/Voxilaprevir The addition of the pangenotypic protease inhibitor voxilaprevir to sofosbuvir/velpatasvir represents the first triplet regimen against all three targets on the HCV virion. It is available as a combination tablet (100 mg voxilaprevir/400 mg sofosbuvir/100 mg velpatasvir). Although effective in both treatment-naïve and treatment-experienced patients, the triplet regimen is reserved for patients who have failed prior DAA therapies and represents the last available combination for HCV therapy.[31] Although sofosbuvir/velpatasvir can be safely used in patients with decompensated cirrhosis, due to the presence of the protease inhibitor voxilaprevir, the triplet regimen cannot be used in patients with decompensated cirrhosis.

In patients with HCV GT1 to 6 who were previously treated with a DAA course including an NS5A agent, a retreatment course of sofosbuvir/velpatasvir/voxilaprevir achieved an SVR of 99%.[51] A lower SVR was seen in patients with cirrhosis at 93%; however, baseline resistance mutations were not associated with reduced SVR. The combination is also recommended in patients with HCV GT3 who are more difficult to treat including patients with cirrhosis or a known Y93 mutation (ie, patients with prior treatment experience with peg-INF and ribavirin tested for GT3 mutations).[31]

Ribavirin Ribavirin continues to be used in combination with DAAs, although its use has been minimized when alternative treatments are available that are highly effective and ribavirin-free. There are some situations that continue to require ribavirin in order to improve SVR rates, such as in patients with decompensated cirrhosis or those with HCV GT3. The mechanism of action of ribavirin is not well understood. Ribavirin is a synthetic guanosine analog and is ineffective as a monotherapy for HCV. The most common adverse effect of ribavirin is hemolytic anemia, necessitating close monitoring during HCV therapy and contributing to complaints of fatigue during treatment. In addition, ribavirin is a teratogenic agent, Pregnancy Category X, and women of childbearing age as well as female partners of male patients who undergo HCV treatment with ribavirin need to practice two forms of contraception during HCV treatment and for 6 months after to avoid pregnancy.[31]

Special Populations

Clinical trials are conducted with a patient population that generally does not reflect the patient spectrum encountered in clinical practice. HCV infections are associated with patients who may be less likely to be engaged in routine healthcare and underrepresented in clinical trials. Treatment guidelines address some of these higher-risk populations and include recommendations for enhanced screening as well as treatment.[31] Published recommendations for treatment in various populations are as follows.

Patients with Decompensated Cirrhosis Patients with decompensated cirrhosis, defined as CTP class B or C cirrhosis, are at high risk for developing complications of their end-stage liver disease and thus are recommended to be treated by clinicians with expertise in managing decompensated cirrhosis.[31] As a class, the protease inhibitors are not recommended in patients with decompensated cirrhosis due to the risk of further decompensation including liver failure. The only therapies recommended for use in decompensation include ledipasvir/sofosbuvir and sofosbuvir/velpatasvir.

Persons Who Inject Drugs Injection drug use is not a contraindication to therapy and treatment of PWIDs will be necessary to reduce HCV transmission.[52] Treatment of PWIDs is recommended as part of a comprehensive harm-reduction effort, ideally in a multidisciplinary setting.[31,52] Treatment outcomes are comparable to rates in those in clinical trials among persons without injection drug use and reinfection rates among PWID are low.[53] However, access to HCV therapies is limited as many insurers refuse coverage of HCV therapies in the setting of active drug use.

Persons with Ongoing Alcohol Use Alcohol cessation is recommended for all patients with liver disease. However, due to the short-treatment course, safety profile of the DAAs, and the ability to cure HCV, ongoing alcohol use is not a reason to withhold or defer HCV treatment.[31]

End-Stage Renal Disease There are no dose adjustments needed for the DAAs in patients with chronic kidney disease including for patients on hemodialysis. In contrast, ribavirin elimination is dependent on renal function and significant dose adjustments may be necessary.

Patients with HCV GT3 In patients with HCV GT3 and cirrhosis, a more aggressive treatment strategy may be recommended due to the concerns for lower SVR rates in some patients. For patients who are to be treated using sofosbuvir/velpatasvir and who have cirrhosis or prior TE, pretreatment resistance testing is recommended.[31] If the Y93 mutation is identified, ribavirin should be added to the treatment course. Alternatively, a different regimen should be used, such as sofosbuvir/velpatasvir/voxilaprevir. In contrast, glecaprevir/pibrentasvir is recommended for an 8-week treatment course for patients with HCV GT3 and cirrhosis although the level of evidence to support the 8-week treatment duration in patients with cirrhosis is lower than the 12-week course.[31] As a result, some clinicians will prefer to use a 12-week course of glecaprevir/pibrentasvir in patients with cirrhosis and HCV GT3. Guidelines do recommend a 12-week treatment course for HIV-HCV coinfection in persons with cirrhosis and HCV GT3 infection.[31]

DAA-Experienced Patients Patients without cirrhosis or those with compensated cirrhosis who failed any course of DAA therapy (eg, elbasvir/grazoprevir, glecaprevir/pibrentasvir) or any prior HCV regimen which included sofosbuvir can be retreated with sofosbuvir/velpatasvir/voxilaprevir. For patients with cirrhosis who were previously treated with glecaprevir/pibrentasvir and experienced treatment failure, the addition of ribavirin may be considered to sofosbuvir/velpatasvir/voxilaprevir. Glecaprevir/pibrentasvir is an alternative retreatment strategy; however, its use is limited to specific patient populations and to specific prior treatment experience and requires an extended treatment duration of 16 weeks. For patients who failed multiple prior DAA therapies, including sofosbuvir/velpatasvir/voxilaprevir or the combination of sofosbuvir plus glecaprevir/pibrentasvir, there are limited options for retreatment. Using available therapies, the recommended retreatment in these unique circumstances includes the addition of ribavirin and retreatment for a longer duration of therapy.[31,51] There are no recommendations for pretreatment resistance testing in this population, and given the small number of patients who failed DAA therapy, it is difficult to predict who will fail DAA treatments.

HIV Coinfection Patients with HIV HCV coinfection should be treated as having HCV monoinfection. Despite this, patients with HIV HCV coinfection are not candidates for the simplified algorithm. Similarly, the 8-week treatment duration is not recommended for patients with compensated cirrhosis and HCV and HIV coinfection. Potential drug-drug interaction concerns between HCV DAAs and HIV antivirals do merit careful scrutiny and may necessitate antiretroviral drug changes.[31] The University of Liverpool HCV drug interaction checker is a useful resource for up to date information on drug interactions.

Preferred HCV therapies for treatment-naïve patients with HIV coinfection are the pan-genotypic agents—sofosbuvir/velpatasvir or glecaprevir/pibrentasvir. Elbasvir/grazoprevir and ledipasvir/sofosbuvir may also be used. Sofosbuvir/velpatasvir has few clinically significant drug-drug interactions but should be avoided with efavirenz, etravirine, or nevirapine. Ledipasvir and velpatasvir increase tenofovir disoproxil levels and may increase the risk of tenofovir-associated renal toxicity especially if combined with cobicistat or ritonavir; however, this risk is minimized with tenofovir alafenamide and thus is the preferred formulation of tenofovir. Glecaprevir/pibrenasvir can be used in patients concurrently on abacavir, bictegravir, cabotegravir, dolutegravir, doravirine, emtricitabine, fostemsavir, ibalizumab-uiyk, lamivudine, maraviroc, raltegravir, rilpivirine, and tenfovir. Glecaprevir/pibrenasvir exposure can increase when combined with elvitegravir/cobicistat with a concern for potential resultant hepatic toxicity. Pending more data, concomitant use necessitates more frequent monitoring for worsening liver function. For patients who are DAA treatment experienced, sofosbuvir/velpatasvir/voxilaprevir is recommended.

HIV treatment poses additional problems because of hepatotoxicity issues associated with HAART, hepatic complications from HIV-associated diseases, as well as flares in hepatitis as CD4 counts recover. In general, treatment is recommended with coadministration of HIV and HCV therapies and is considered a priority due to more liver-related morbidity and mortality than in HCV monoinfected patients.

Children Although the number of pediatric HCV cases is low, there are no good epidemiological studies to determine the actual prevalence of HCV in the pediatric population. Mother-to-child transmission is possible and of concern given the rise in HCV prevalence among younger females of childbearing age. Because maternal HCV antibody can persist and thus interfere with an infant's HCV antibody test, testing in newborns is not recommended until 18 months of age.[31] This delay in testing raises concerns for loss to follow up and potential missed opportunities for HCV diagnosis. Although fibrosis progression is generally considered slow in children, there is a general lack of data on the impact of persistent viremia on child development. Children with HCV as well as their families may face stigma and discrimination due to a general lack of knowledge about HCV and HCV transmission.

HCV DAA treatment is available; however, it is deferred until age 3 due to limited data in children. Both pan-genotypic agents are approved (sofosbuvir/velpatasvir and glecaprevir/pibrentasvir) as is ledipasvir/sofosbuvir. Pediatric dosing may be done with reduced dose tablets and pellets/granules which may be sprinkled over food.

Similar to adult clinical trial data, glecaprevir/pibrentasvir is highly effective in pediatric patients and is approved for children 3 years of age and older. The overall SVR was 96% in 80 children ranging in age from 3 to 12 years and with HCV GT1, 2, 3, or 4 infection.[54] The most common side effect was headache with patients also reporting vomiting and diarrhea. Glecaprevir/pibrentasvir is available as oral pellets for pediatric use.

Sofosbuvir/velpatasvir is also highly effective in pediatric patients and approved for children 3 years of age and older. SVR rates were 92% overall in 216 patients ranging in age from 3 to 17 years.[55] Virological failure was 1%, of the 17 patients who did not have a document SVR. The adverse effect profile was similar to what was observed in adult trials. Younger patients were more likely to report vomiting.

Ledipasvir/sofosbuvir is also an option and is available in a smaller dose tablet (45 mg/200 mg) as well as oral pellets (45 mg/200 mg or 33.75 mg/150 mg). The expected SVR is high at 98%.[56] The main limitation of this combination therapy is that it is not pan-genotypic; it is indicated for patients with HCV GT1, 4, 5, or 6.

Pregnancy Transmission of HCV can occur during pregnancy and children born to mothers with HCV should be tested for HCV. HCV screening is recommended for each pregnancy; however, HCV therapy is not recommended during pregnancy.[31]

Post-Organ Transplant Given the high efficacy of the DAAs and the number of HCV-positive organ donors, some organ transplant centers are offering HCV-positive organs to HCV-negative patients. Pan-genotypic agents are preferred in the transplant setting. Both glecaprevir/pibrentasvir and sofosbuvir/velpatasvir are recommended as soon as the patient is clinically stable but preferably within the first week after transplant. Experience in the transplant setting is increasing and includes liver, heart, lung, and kidney transplant.[31,57]

Prevention

No vaccine is available for HCV. It is unlikely that a vaccine will be developed in the near future because of the mutagenesis of the virus. Although the likelihood of household transmission is small, patients should minimize risks by avoiding possible blood or mucus exposure, such as not sharing razors or toothbrushes and covering open wounds. Sharing of any drug paraphernalia poses a risk of transmission. Where legally allowed, patients should be provided with resources for needle and syringe exchange programs.

Targeted HCV treatment in specific patient groups can reduce transmission and offer substantial public health benefits. Patients who achieve cure (SVR) cannot transmit virus, thus interrupting HCV transmission. Improved access to HCV DAA therapy and scale-up of treatment efforts is critical to prevention of new infections.

Treatment Interruptions

In real-world settings, treatment interruptions occur for a number of reasons. It is important to minimize treatment interruptions and identify solutions to help patients be successful in obtaining refills in a timely manner. Disruptions in the treatment course can cause treatment failure. It is important to review the most current guidance available.[31] Patients who miss a week or less of therapy should restart treatment immediately and complete the originally scheduled treatment course. Patients who miss 8 or more days during the first month of treatment should continue DAA therapy and ideally also obtain an HCV RNA. If the HCV RNA is negative, the original treatment duration should be completed. In contrast, if the HCV RNA is positive or unable to be obtained, or if the patient has HCV GT3 infection or cirrhosis, DAA therapy should be extended by an additional 4 weeks.

If a patient misses 8 to 20 days of therapy after receiving at least the first month of treatment, DAA therapy should be restarted immediately and an HCV RNA checked. If the RNA is negative, the originally scheduled therapy should be continued or extended by 4 weeks if the patient has GT3 or cirrhosis. If the RNA is positive or not obtained, treatment should be stopped.

If patients experience a treatment interruption of more than 20 days, DAA therapy should be stopped. Although not common, it is possible that some patients may experience cure. The recommendation is to wait and recheck HCV RNA 12 weeks after the last known dose of medication was taken to assess for possible cure (SVR12).[31]

ABBREVIATIONS

AASLD	American Association for the Study of Liver Diseases
ACIP	Advisory Committee on Immunization Practices
ALT	alanine aminotransferase
Anti-HAV	antibody to hepatitis A virus
Anti-HBsAg	antibody to HBsAg
CDC	Centers for Disease Control and Prevention
CTP	Child–Turcotte–Pugh
DAA	direct-acting antiviral
DF	disoproxil fumarate
DNA	deoxyribonucleic acid
ELISA	enzyme-linked immunosorbent assay
ESLD	end-stage liver disease
GT	genotype
HAART	highly active antiretroviral therapy
HAV	hepatitis A virus
HBcAg	hepatitis B core antigen
HBeAg	hepatitis B e-antigen
HBsAg	hepatitis B surface antigen
HBV	hepatitis B virus
HCC	hepatocellular carcinoma
HCV	hepatitis C virus
HIV	human immunodeficiency virus
IDSA	Infectious Diseases Society of America
IFN	interferon
Ig	immunoglobulin
IM	intramuscular
IV	intravenous
MSM	men who have sex with men
NAs	nucleos(t)ide analogs
peg-IFN	pegylated interferon
PWID	persons who inject drugs
RAS	resistance–associated substitution
RNA	ribonucleic acid
SVR	sustained virologic response
WHO	World Health Organization

REFERENCES

1. Department of Health and Human Services. *National Viral Hepatitis Action Plan 2021-2025*. Available at: https://www.hhs.gov/sites/default/files/Viral-Hepatitis-National-Strategic-Plan-2021-2025.pdf. Accessed November 10, 2021.
2. Centers for Disease Control and Prevention. Surveillance for Viral Hepatitis—United States. Available at: https://www.cdc.gov/hepatitis/statistics/2019surveillance/index.htm. Accessed July 28, 2021.
3. Centers for Disease Control and Prevention. Hepatitis A outbreaks in the United States. Available at: https://www.cdc.gov/hepatitis/outbreaks/hepatitisaoutbreaks.htm. Accessed June 1, 2021.
4. Centers for Disease Control and Prevention. Hepatitis A. In: Hall E, Wodi AP, Hamborsky J, et al., eds. *Epidemiology and Prevention of Vaccine-Preventable Diseases*. 14th ed. Washington, DC: Public Health Foundation; 2021.
5. Centers for Disease Control and Prevention. Hepatitis A. In: *CDC Yellow Book 2020: Health Information for International Travel*. 13th ed. New York: Oxford University Press; 2017.
6. Centers for Disease Control and Prevention. Prevention of hepatitis A through active or passive immunizations: Recommendations of the Advisory Committee on Immunization Practices (ACIP). *MMWR Morb Mortal Wkly Rep*. 2020;69(5):1–38.
7. Huang SH, Huang CH, Wang NC. Taiwan HIV Study Group. Early seroconversion after 2 doses of hepatitis A vaccination in human inmmunodeficiency virus positive patients: Incidence and associated factors. *Hepatology*. 2019;70:465–475.
8. World Health Organization. Hepatitis B. July 21, 2021. Available at: http://www.who.int/news-room/fact-sheets/detail/hepatitis-b. Accessed September 14, 2021.
9. World Health Organization. Guidelines for the prevention, care, and treatment of persons with chronic hepatitis B infection. 2015. Available at: http://apps.who.int/iris/bitstream/10665/154590/1/9789241549059_eng.pdf?ua=1ua=1. Accessed September 25, 2021.
10. Centers for Disease Control and Prevention. Hepatitis B. In: Hall E, Wodi AP, Hamborsky J, et al., eds. *Epidemiology and Prevention of Vaccine-Preventable Diseases*. 14th ed. Washington, DC: Public Health Foundation; 2021.
11. Terrault NA, Lok ASF, McMahon BJ, et al. Update on prevention, diagnosis, and treatment of chronic hepatitis B; AASLD 2018 Hepatitis B Guidance. *Hepatology*. 2018;67:1560–1599.
12. Tong S, Revill P. Overview of hepatitis B viral replication and genetic variability. *J Hepatol*. 2016;64:S41–S48.
13. European Association for the Study of the Liver. EASL 2017 clinical practice guidelines on the management of hepatitis B virus infection. *J Hepatol*. 2017;67:370–398.
14. Tang AS, Thornton K, HBV Primary Care Workgroup. Hepatitis B management: Guidance for the primary care provider. February 25, 2020. Available at: https://www.hepatitisb.uw.edu/page/primary-care-workgroup/guidance. Accessed October 25, 2021.
15. Reddy RK, Beavers KL, Hammond SP, et al. American Gastroenterological Association Institute guideline on prevention and treatment of hepatitis B reactivation during immunosuppressive drug therapy. *Gastroenterology*. 2015;148:215–219.
16. Perrillo RP, Gish R, Falck-Ytter YT. American Gastroenterological Association Institute technical review on prevention and treatment of hepatitis B virus reactivation during immunosuppressive drug therapy. *Gastroenterology*. 2015;148:221–244.
17. Kennedy K, Graham SM, Arora N, et al. Hepatocellular carcinoma among US and non–US-born patients with chronic hepatitis B: Risk factors and age at diagnosis. *PLoS One*. 2018;13:e0204031.
18. U.S. Department of Health and Human Services, Office of Disease Prevention and Health Promotion. Healthy People 2020. Washington, DC. Available at: https://www.healthypeople.gov/2020/topics-objectives/topic/immunization-and-infectious-diseases/objectives. Accessed September 15, 2018.
19. Schillie S, Vellozzi C, Reingold A, et al. Centers for Disease Control and Prevention (CDC). Prevention of hepatitis B virus infection in the United States: Recommendations of the Advisory Committee on Immunization Practices. *MMWR Morb Mortal Wkly Rep*. 2018;67:1–31.
20. Yu MW, Lin CL, Yang SH, et al. Influence of metabolic risk factors on risk of hepatocellular carcinoma and liver-related death in men with chronic hepatitis B: A large cohort study. *Gastroenterology*. 2017;153:1006–1017.
21. Kim JH, Sinn DH, Gwak GY, et al. Insulin resistance and the risk of hepatocellular carcinoma in chronic hepatitis B patients. *J Gastroenterol Hepatol*. 2017;32:1100–1106.
22. Terrault N, Bzowej NH, Chang KM, et al. AASLD guidelines for treatment of chronic hepatitis B. *Hepatology*. 2016;63:261–283.
23. Buti M, Tsai N, Petersen J, et al. Seven-year efficacy and safety of treatment with tenofovir disoproxil fumarate for chronic hepatitis B virus infection. *Dig Dis Sci*. 2015;60(5):1457–1464.
24. Agarwal K, Brunetto M, Seto WK, et al. 96 weeks treatment of tenofovir alafenamide vs tenofovir disoproxil fumarate for hepatitis B virus infection. *J Hepatol*. 2018;68:672–681.
25. Cathcart AL, Chan HL, Bhardwaj N, et al. No resistance to tenofovir alafenamide detected through 96 weeks of treatment for chronic hepatitis B infection. *Antimicrob Agents Chemother*. 2018;62(10):e01064–18. doi:10.1128/AAC.01064-18.
26. Lim YS, Yoo BC, Byun KS, et al. Tenofovir monotherapy versus tenofovir and entecavir combination therapy in adefovir-resistant chronic hepatitis B patients with multiple drug failure: Results of a randomized trial. *Gut*. 2016;65:1042–1051.
27. Ding Y, Cao L, Zhu L, et al. Efficacy and safety of tenofovir alafenamide fumarate for preventing mother-to-child transmission of hepatitis B virus: A national cohort study. *Alimentary Pharmacol Ther*. 2020 Aug 27;52(8):1–10. doi:10.1111/apt.16043.
28. Gupta N, Goyal M, Wu CH, Wu GY. The molecular and structural basis of HBV-resistance to nucleos(t)ide analogs. *J Clin Transl Hepatol*. 2014;2:201–211.
29. Ford N, Scourse R, Lemoine M, Hutin Y, Bulterys M. Adherence to nucleos(t)ide analogue therapies for chronic hepatitis B infection: A systematic review and meta-analysis. *Hepatol Commun*. 2018;25:1160–1167.

30. Schillie S, Wester C, Osborne M, Wesolowski L, Ryerson AB. CDC recommendations for hepatitis C screening among adults—United States, 2020. *MMWR Recomm Rep.* 2020;69(RR-2):1–17.
31. AASLD/IDSA. Recommendations for testing, managing, and treating hepatitis C. Available at: http://www.hcvguidelines.org. Accessed August 20, 2021.
32. U.S. Preventive Services Task Force. Final Recommendation Statement: Hepatitis C Virus Infection in Adolescents and Adults: Screening. March 2020. Available at: http://www.uspreventiveservicestaskforce.org/uspstf/recommendation/hepatitis-c-screening. Accessed August 27, 2021.
33. Terrault NA, Dodge JL, Murphy EL, et al. Sexual transmission of HCV among monogamous heterosexual couples: The HCV partners study. *Hepatology.* 2013;57:881–889.
34. Centers for Disease Control. Testing for HCV infection: An update of guidance for clinicians and laboratorians. *MMWR.* 2013;62(18):362–365.
35. Kanto T, Hayashi N. Immunopathogenesis of hepatitis C virus infection: Multifaceted strategies subverting innate and adaptive immunity. *Intern Med.* 2006;45:183–191.
36. Centers for Disease Control and Prevention. Hepatitis C FAQs for health professionals. Available at: http://www.cdc.gov/hepatitis/hcv/hcvfaq.htm. Accessed September 17, 2021.
37. Kanwal F, Kramer JR, Ilyas J, Duan Z, El-Serag HB. HCV genotype 3 is associated with an increased risk of cirrhosis and hepatocellular cancer in a national sample of U.S. veterans with HCV. *Hepatology.* 2014;60(1):98–105.
38. Sherman AC, Sherman KE. Extrahepatic manifestations of hepatitis C: Navigating CHASM. *Curr HIV/AIDS Rep.* 2015;12(3):353–361.
39. Kowdley KV, Gordon SC, Reddy KR, et al. Ledipasvir and sofosbuvir for 8 or 12 weeks for chronic HCV without cirrhosis. *N Engl J Med.* 2014;370:1879–1888.
40. Feld JJ, Jacobson IM, Hézode C, et al. Sofosbuvir and velpatasvir for HCV genotype 1, 2, 4, 5, and 6 infection. *N Engl J Med.* 2015;373(27):2599–2607.
41. Afdhal N, Zeuzem S, Kwo P, et al. Ledipasvir and sofosbuvir for untreated HCV genotype 1 infection. *N Engl J Med.* 2014;370(20):1889–1898.
42. Afdhal N, Reddy KR, Nelson DR, et al. Ledipasvir and sofosbuvir for previously treated HCV genotype 1 infection. *N Engl J Med.* 2014;370(16):1483–1493.
43. Charlton M, Everson GT, Flamm SL, et al. Ledipasvir and sofosbuvir plus ribavirin for treatment of HCV infection in patients with advanced liver disease. *Gastroenterology.* 2015;149:649–659.
44. Tapper EB, Bacon BR, Curry MP, et al. Real-world effectiveness for 12 weeks of ledipasvir-sofosbuvir for genotype 1 hepatitis C: The Trio Health Study. *J Viral Hepat.* 2017;24:22–27.
45. Esteban R, Pineda JA, Calleja L, et al. Efficacy of sofosbuvir and velpatasvir, with or without ribavirin, in patients with HCV genotype 3 infection and cirrhosis. *Gastroenterology.* Oct 2018;155(4):1120–1127. doi:10.1053/j.gastro.2018.06.042.
46. Curry MP, O'Leary JG, Bzowej N, et al. Sofosbuvir and velpatasvir for HCV in patients with decompensated cirrhosis. *N Engl J Med.* 2015b;373(27):2618–2628.
47. Zeuzem S, Ghalib R, Reddy KR, et al. Grazoprevir-elbasvir combination therapy for treatment-naive cirrhotic and noncirrhotic patients with chronic hepatitis C virus genotype 1, 4, or 6 infection: A randomized trial. *Ann Intern Med.* 2015;163(1):1–13.
48. Kwo PY, Poordad F, Asatryan A, et al. Glecaprevir and pibrentasvir yield high response rates in patients with HCV genotype 1-6 without cirrhosis. *J Hepatol.* 2017;67:263–271.
49. Brown RS, Buti M, Rodrigues L, et al. Glecaprevir/pibrentasvir for 8 weeks in treatment naïve patients with chronic HCV genotype 1-6 and compensated cirrhosis. *J Hepatol.* 2020;72:441–449.
50. Gane E, Poordad F, Wang S, et al. High efficacy of ABT-493 and ABT-530 treatment in patients with HCV genotype 1 or 3 infection and compensated cirrhosis. *Gastroenterology.* 2016b;151:651–659.
51. Bourliere M, Gordon SC, Flamm SL, et al. Sofosbuvir, velpatasvir, and voxilaprevir for previously treated HCV infection. *N Engl J Med.* 2017;376:2134–2146.
52. Doyle JS, Aspinall EJ, Hutchinson SJ, et al. Global policy and access to new hepatitis C therapies for people who inject drugs. *Int J Drug Policy.* 2015;26(11):1064–1071.
53. Aspinall EJ, Corson S, Doyle JS, et al. Treatment of hepatitis C virus infection among people who are actively injecting drugs: A systematic review and meta-analysis. *Clin Infect Dis.* 2013;57(suppl 2):S80–S89.
54. Jonas MM, Rhee S, Kelly DA, et al. Pharmacokinetics, safety, and efficacy of glecaprevir/pibrentasvir in children with chronic HCV: Part 2 of the DORA study. *Hepatology.* 2021;74:19–27.
55. Sokal E, Schwarz K, Rosenthal P, et al. Safety and efficacy of sofosbuvir/velpatasvir for the treatment of chronic hepatitis C infection in adolescents and children aged 3 to 17 years old through 24 weeks posttreatment. Poster session presented at: The American Association for the Study of Liver Diseases (AASLD) Liver Meeting Digital Experience 2020; 2020 November 13-16.
56. Balistreri WF, Murray KF, Rosenthal P, et al. The safety and effectiveness of ledipasvir-sofosbuvir in adolescents 12-17 years old with hepatitis C virus genotype 1 infection. *Hepatology.* 2017;66:371–378.
57. American College of Obstetricians and Gynecologists. Practice Advisory: Routinehepatitis C virus screening in pregnant individuals. May 2021. Available at: acog.org/clinical-guidance/practice-advisory/articles/2021/05/routine-hepatitis-c-virus-screening-inpregnant individuals. Accessed November 11, 2021.
58. Hepatitis B Serology, Centers for Disease Control and Prevention. https://www.cdc.gov/hepatitis/hbv/pdfs/serologicchartv8.pdf.

59

Celiac Disease

Priti N. Patel and Robert A. Mangione

KEY CONCEPTS

1. Celiac disease is a chronic, small intestinal immune-mediated enteropathy caused by intolerance to gluten found in wheat, barley, rye, and other foods when a genetically predisposed person is exposed to the environmental trigger, gluten.
2. The prevalence of celiac disease is 0.7% in America and is increasing in prevalence worldwide.
3. The integrity of the tissue junctions of the intestinal epithelium is compromised in patients with celiac disease; this enables gluten to reach the lamina propria. The presence of gluten in the lamina propria and an inherited combination of genes contribute to the heightened immune sensitivity to gluten that is found in patients with celiac disease.
4. The classic presenting symptom is diarrhea, which may be accompanied by abdominal pain or discomfort; however, during the past decade diarrhea has been reported as the main presenting symptom of celiac disease in less than 50% of cases.
5. Dermatitis herpetiformis is a skin manifestation of small intestinal immune-mediated enteropathy caused by exposure to dietary gluten.
6. The frequency of diagnosis of patients with celiac disease has increased; however, the majority of patients with this condition remain undiagnosed.
7. The confirmation of a diagnosis of celiac disease should be based on a combination of findings from the medical history, physical examination, serology, and duodenal biopsy. The recommended serologic marker that is used for screening patients is serum antitissue transglutaminase antibody.
8. Strict, lifelong adherence to a gluten-free diet is the only treatment for celiac disease that is available.
9. Clinicians must evaluate the patient with celiac disease for nutritional deficiencies (including folic acid, vitamin B_{12}, fat-soluble vitamins, iron, and calcium) due to malabsorption.

BEYOND THE BOOK

Read "Gluten in Medicine, Vitamins & Supplements" from the Celiac Disease Foundation at https://celiac.org/gluten-free-living/gluten-in-medicine-vitamins-and-supplements/. This provides a patient-centered guide for understanding the risks of gluten in medications and how patients with celiac disease may identify drugs that could pose problems for them. This is important information for pharmacists as well.

Read "Questions and Answers on the Gluten-Free Food Labeling Final Rule" from the Food and Drug Administration (FDA) at https://www.fda.gov/food/food-labeling-nutrition/questions-and-answers-gluten-free-food-labeling-final-rule. This question-and-answer format guide provides information on the FDA's gluten-free food-labeling regulation.

INTRODUCTION

1 Celiac disease is a small intestinal immune-mediated enteropathy caused by intolerance to ingested gluten, a storage protein found in wheat, barley, and rye. Genetic, environmental, and immune factors all play a role in the development of celiac disease. The mainstay of treatment of the disease is strict, lifelong adherence to a gluten-free diet.[1]

A disease resembling celiac disease was first described by a Greek physician in the second century AD. In the mid-1900s, the connection between the ingestion of cereals and celiac disease was made. For many years, celiac disease was considered a disease of childhood with primarily gastrointestinal (GI) symptoms. It is now recognized as a disease of all ages with varied presentations.

Celiac disease has been known as celiac sprue, nontropical sprue, and gluten-sensitive enteropathy; however, these terms are not recommended. The nonspecific use of celiac disease-related terminology may lead to misunderstandings. Accepted terms associated with celiac disease should be used and understood when engaging in patient consultations or discussions with other healthcare providers. The publication of the Oslo Definitions of celiac disease helped to address this concern and further refining of appropriate terminology continues as new information is learned.[1] The Oslo classification used terminology such as "classic" and "non-classic" symptoms while more recent literature cites intestinal and extra-intestinal symptoms.[1]

The disease is characterized by both GI and extra-intestinal symptoms. Chronic inflammation caused by exposure to gluten leads to GI discomfort, nutrient malabsorption, and systemic complications. GI symptoms, including diarrhea, cramping, bloating, and flatulence, are the "classic" symptoms; however, a patient with celiac disease may initially present with a variety of extra-intestinal symptoms. Patients with subclinical celiac disease have no or minimal symptoms but manifest mucosal damage on biopsy and have positive serologic testing. Patients with celiac disease classified as potential are asymptomatic patients who may show positive serology and have the human leukocyte antigen (HLA)-DQ2 and/or DQ8 haplotype, but have normal mucosa on biopsy.[1,3]

Adherence to a gluten-free diet is essential because it improves symptoms and prevents long-term complications of celiac disease, which include T-cell lymphomas, small bowel adenocarcinoma, and esophageal and oropharyngeal carcinomas.[4]

EPIDEMIOLOGY

2 Originally thought to be a pediatric disease, celiac disease is now being diagnosed in increasing numbers of both adult and pediatric patients due to increased awareness and improved diagnostic techniques.[5] Celiac disease is common in Europe and North America. The prevalence of the disease is 0.71% to 0.79% in the United States, affecting up to 1% of White patients.[6] The prevalence of celiac disease is higher in females than in males at a rate of 1.5:1.[7] In Finland and the United States, the prevalence of celiac disease has increased fivefold during the past 50 years.[8]

Celiac disease has been less well studied in other parts of the world. Previously believed to rarely occur in racial groups other than White patients, improved screening and diagnostic techniques prove that the prevalence of celiac disease in many non-Western nations is similar to that in Europe and North America.[9] The common and increasing use of wheat in diets, coupled with the prevalence of HLA-DQ2, may lead to an increase in the prevalence of celiac disease in the global population in coming years in areas where celiac disease is rarely diagnosed.[10,11]

ETIOLOGY

Celiac disease is known to occur when a genetically predisposed person ingests gluten. Wheat gluten proteins exist in two fractions: gliadins and glutenins. Wheat, barley, and rye are all derived from the Triticeae tribe of the grass (Gramineae) family. Proteins similar to glutenins, called hordeins and secalins, are found in barley and rye, respectively. Table 59-1 refers to grains and other foods that do and do not contain gluten and related proteins. Ingestion of any of these proteins will lead to an autoimmune response in patients with celiac disease. Oats, from the Aveneae tribe, are distantly related and therefore contain fewer disease-activating proteins.[13] One concern with oats is that they may be contaminated with gluten during the manufacturing process.[13]

Genetic factors, in combination with exposure to gluten, are necessary for the development of celiac disease. There is a concordance rate of 85% in monozygotic twins indicating that genetics play a large role in the disease, but other factors also are likely to involved.[13,15]

Most patients with celiac disease have variants of HLA-DQ2 or HLA-DQ8 molecules that are expressed on the surface of antigen-presenting cells.[3,4] Other non-HLA genes may also play a role in enhancing genetic susceptibility to celiac disease.[16]

Various infections and compounds may contribute to the development of celiac disease. There is an association between change in the gut microbiome and celiac disease; however, experts caution against suggesting that the gut microbiome causes celiac disease since many environmental factors that play a role in celiac disease also affect the gut microbiome.[1,17] GI, upper respiratory, and lower respiratory infections are risk factors for the development of celiac disease. Various drugs, such as olmesartan, azathioprine, methotrexate, as well as others, may play a role in the development of sprue-like bowel disease.[2]

In Sweden, increased rates of diagnosis of celiac disease in the mid-1980s was thought to correspond to a change in infant feeding practices. However, the timing of gluten introduction or duration of breastfeeding did not avoid the eventual diagnosis of celiac disease, even at children at higher risk due to the presence of one of the high-risk HLA haplotypes.[16]

PATHOPHYSIOLOGY

3 During normal digestion, peptides that remain from gastric or pancreatic digestion are broken down into amino acids, dipeptides, or tripeptides by the small intestinal brush-border membrane enzymes.[16] These GI proteases that are found in the intestinal lumen are one of the body's first defenses against potentially toxic dietary proteins.[18] The intestinal epithelium, with its intact intercellular tight junctions, functions as the primary barrier to the passage of macromolecules into the lamina propria. Gluten is unusually rich in the amino acids glutamine and proline, which enable part of the molecule to withstand the digestive processes. These peptides are kept within the GI tract and are primarily excreted before they can illicit an immune reaction. Small fractions of gluten do cross this important defense barrier in patients without celiac disease; however, the quantity of gluten that passes across the GI lining is generally insufficient to illicit a significant response from a normally functioning immune system.[18]

Pathophysiology of celiac disease is associated with an interaction between gluten and immune, genetic, and environmental factors.[18] In celiac disease, the integrity of the tissue junctions of the intestinal epithelium is compromised, enabling gluten to reach the lamina propria through different routes. The presence of gluten in the lamina propria and an inherited combination of genes contribute to the heightened immune sensitivity to gluten found in patients with celiac disease (Table 59-2).[18] The notable immune

TABLE 59-1 Grains and Other Foods That Do and Do Not Contain Gluten

Contain Gluten	Do Not Contain Gluten
Wheat	Amaranth
Barley	Buckwheat
Rye	Corn
Bran	Flax
Graham flour	Millet
Spelt	Potato flour
Wheat germ	Quinoa
Triticale	Rice
Oats[a]	Sorghum
	Soybeans
	Tapioca
	Teff

[a]Oats are in a different plant family, but they have also been regarded as problematic, although the ingestion of certified pure gluten-free oats is safe in most patients with celiac disease.[12] Due to the continued difference of opinion regarding the safety of oats, patients are generally advised to discuss the risks and benefits associated with consuming oats with their healthcare provider before they include oats in their diet.

TABLE 59-2 Proposed Pathophysiology of Celiac Disease

- Enterocytes release the protein zonulin in response to the presence of indigestible fragments of gluten in the intestine.
- Zonulin loosens the intercellular tight junctions.
- Abundant quantities of gluten fragments cross the intestinal lining and accumulate under the enterocytes (epithelial cells).
- Gluten induces the enterocytes to secrete interleukin-15 (IL-15).
- IL-15 induces an immune response of intraepithelial lymphocytes against the enterocytes.
- The damaged cells release the enzyme tissue transglutaminase (tTG), which modifies the gluten.
- Antigen-presenting cells of the immune system join the modified gluten to HLA molecules and display the resulting complexes to other immune cells (ie, helper T cells).
- Helper T cells that recognize the complexes secrete molecules that attract other immune cells, which may result in damage to the enterocytes.
- Helper T cells spur killer T cells that directly attack the enterocytes.
- B cells release antibody molecules that are targeted to gluten and tTG (the role that these antibodies play remains to be further clarified; however, they may cause further damage when they contact their targets on or near the enterocytes).
- Enterocytes are disabled or killed.

Data from Reference 18.

response to gluten consists of both adaptive and innate immune responses that occur only in individuals who carry the HLA type DQ2 or DQ8.[18] The precise mechanism by which the immune system leads to damage of the intestinal lining of patients with celiac disease continues to be studied.

Nonceliac gluten sensitivity is a condition in which the ingestion of gluten results in morphological or symptomatic manifestations in the absence of celiac disease.[19] This disorder must therefore be considered in the differential diagnosis of celiac disease. Symptoms alone cannot reliably differentiate celiac disease from nonceliac gluten sensitivity. Therefore, a diagnostic evaluation including celiac serology and small-intestinal biopsy (while the patient is including gluten in their diet) is needed. If these tests are negative, HLA-DQ typing is required to differentiate between the two disorders. Differentiating between these disorders is important as it will impact the implications of the level of adherence to the gluten-free diet, approach to continued disease-state monitoring and evaluation, and the counseling of family members (as nonceliac disease sensitivity does not have a strong hereditary basis).[4]

The primary toxic components of wheat gluten are a family of closely related proteins called gliadins.[18] The gliadin peptides induce changes in the epithelium through innate immunity and in the lamina propria through adaptive immunity.[18]

Tissue transglutaminase (tTG), a ubiquitous enzyme that catalyzes posttranslational modification of proteins and is released during inflammation, may play at least two crucial roles in celiac disease by serving as the main target autoantigen for antiendomysial enzymes and as a deaminating enzyme that raises the immunostimulatory effect of gluten. This enzyme, by deaminating glutamine to glutamic acid, makes the gliadin peptides become negatively charged and therefore more capable of fitting into pockets of the HLA-DQ2 (or HLA-DQ8) antigen-binding groove on the antigen-presenting cells.[21] Gliadin is presented to gliadin-reactive CD4 T cells through a T-cell receptor, which then results in the production of cytokines that cause tissue damage. This then leads to villous atrophy, crypt hyperplasia, and the expansion of antibody-producing B cells found in celiac disease.[21]

TABLE 59-3 Selected Signs and Symptoms of Celiac Disease

Children	Adults
Symptoms	**Symptoms**
• Fatigue	• Abdominal pain
• Bloating	• Chronic diarrhea
• Constipation	• Abdominal distension
• Abdominal pain	• Recurrent spontaneous abortion
• Chronic diarrhea	• Peripheral neuropathy
• Irritability	• Depression
• Vomiting	• Fatigue/malaise
Signs	• Ataxia
• Muscle wasting	**Signs**
• Failure to thrive/weight loss	• Weight loss
• Short stature	• Infertility
• Delayed puberty	• Dermatitis herpetiformis
• Osteopenia/osteoporosis	• Hepatitis
• Hepatitis	• Anemia
• Dental anomalies	• Aphthous ulcers
• Anemia	• Alopecia
	• Malignancy
	• Seizures
	• Osteopenia/osteoporosis
	• Arthritis

Data from Reference 22.

TABLE 59-4 Selected Common Misdiagnoses

- Irritable bowel syndrome
- Viral gastroenteritis
- Lactose intolerance
- Amoebic/parasitic infection
- Inflammatory bowel disease
- Psychological dysfunction
- Gallbladder disease
- Chronic fatigue syndrome
- Gastroesophageal reflux disease
- Allergies
- Ulcers
- Cystic fibrosis
- Colitis

Data from Reference 4.

CLINICAL PRESENTATION

4 The recognition of celiac disease may be quite challenging due to the wide range of presenting symptoms, which includes patients who are asymptomatic.[1] Clinical manifestations of celiac disease significantly vary with age group (Table 59-3) in that pediatric patients are more likely to experience classic GI symptoms while adults are more likely to have extra-intestinal symptoms.[2] Infants and young children generally experience diarrhea, abdominal distention, and failure to thrive. Vomiting, irritability, anorexia, and even constipation are also common in these young patients. Extra-intestinal manifestations such as short stature, neurologic findings (eg, peripheral neuropathy, ataxia, seizure, migraine, and dementia), or anemia are often found in older children and adolescents.[23] The classic presenting symptom in adults is diarrhea, which may be accompanied by abdominal pain or discomfort; however, during the past decade diarrhea has been reported as the main presenting symptom of celiac disease in less than 50% of cases.[19,20] Adults may exhibit iron-deficiency anemia or osteoporosis. Less common presentations of celiac disease in adults include abdominal pain, constipation, weight loss, neurologic symptoms, dermatitis herpetiformis, hypoproteinemia, hypocalcemia, and elevated liver enzymes. Patients with celiac disease without GI symptoms often experience symptoms for a long period of time before celiac disease is diagnosed.[24]

5 Dermatitis herpetiformis is a skin manifestation of small intestinal immune-mediated enteropathy caused by the ingestion of gluten.[25] This extremely pruritic, bullous skin rash should prompt testing for celiac disease.[25]

6 The diagnosis of celiac disease is based on clinical suspicion and confirmation with laboratory tests and duodenal biopsy.[4] Although the prevalence of celiac disease has increased, many patients with this condition remain undiagnosed.[4] This is particularly concerning as undiagnosed celiac disease has been associated with a nearly fourfold increased risk of death compared with subjects without serologic evidence of disease.[12]

Healthcare providers should recognize the many and diverse possible symptoms of celiac disease.[19] A delay in diagnosis is often reported, with longer times to diagnosis in patients who primarily exhibit extra-intestinal symptoms.[24] Clinicians can help reduce the time from the onset of symptoms to the diagnosis of celiac disease by being aware of the common diseases that may also coexist with celiac disease (Table 59-4).[24]

Individuals with certain disorders are more likely to have celiac disease than the general population. Examples include other autoimmune diseases, such as thyroid disease, diabetes mellitus (type 1), multiple sclerosis, myasthenia gravis, Raynaud's disease, rheumatoid arthritis, Addison's disease, chronic active hepatitis, cystic fibrosis, scleroderma, and Sjögren's syndrome; Down's syndrome; neurologic conditions such as ataxia, epilepsy, and cerebral calcifications; and primary biliary cirrhosis. Although patients with these disorders are more frequently found to have celiac disease than the general population, these associated conditions are not believed to cause celiac disease.[26]

7 Diagnostic testing for celiac disease must be performed while the patient continues to consume gluten; patients who have already started on a gluten-free diet prior to diagnosis should consume three slices of wheat bread daily for 1 to 3 months before testing commences.[5,27] A confirmed diagnosis of celiac disease requires both a positive finding on duodenal biopsy and a positive response to a gluten-free diet.[4] The identification of villous atrophy with small bowel endoscopy and biopsy is generally regarded as the diagnostic gold standard (although according to the guidelines from the European Society of Paediatric Gastroenterology, Hepatology, and Nutrition a small intestinal biopsy may not be required in children with typical symptoms, titers of anti-tTG greater than 10 times the upper normal limit and predisposing HLA genotype).[28] Although villous atrophy is associated with celiac disease, clinicians must consider that this may also be found in other diseases, including giardiasis, autoimmune enteropathy, tuberculosis, Crohn's disease, intolerance to food other than gluten, intestinal lymphoma, and Zollinger–Ellison syndrome.[4]

Histologic changes seen on biopsy are categorized according to one of several classification systems including the Marsh, Marsh modified, or the Corazza, all of which examine intraepithelial lymphocytes, crypt hyperplasia and villous atrophy.[4] Histologic findings lead to a diagnosis that is followed by placing the patient on a gluten-free diet. Dermatitis herpetiformis is diagnosed by skin biopsy.[29]

Serologic test results provide clinicians with a useful non-invasive tool that helps to determine if symptomatic patients, or patients who are at risk for celiac disease, require a biopsy.[4] Available tests include those for deamidated gliadin peptide (DGP) IgA or IgG antibodies, anti-endomysial antibodies, and antibodies against tTG. The American College of Gastroenterology recommends tTG IgA testing for patients 2 years and older and DGP IgA and IgG combined with IgA tTG for patients younger than 2 years.[4] Although serology is a good method to identify patients who will benefit from endoscopy and biopsy, negative serology should not preclude a biopsy examination in individuals for whom disease is suspected on clinical grounds.[4] Positive serology should be followed with confirmatory testing via biopsy, with the exception of some children who may be diagnosed based on serology alone.[4,28]

Genetic testing can be performed as a means of determining which family members of a diagnosed patient may develop the disease (the prevalence of celiac disease is 10% to 12% in first-degree relatives and is also higher than that found in the general population in second-degree relatives).[4] Patients and their family members can be tested for HLA-DQ2 and HLA-DQ8 as HLA-DQ2 is found in up to 95% of patients with celiac disease, with most other patients being HLA-DQ8 positive.[4] Although nearly all patients with celiac disease carry one of these alleles, they are also found in 30% to 40% of the general population. When these alleles are absent, it is extremely unlikely that the individual has celiac disease (ie, the test has a high negative predictive value).[4] A patient-administered saliva-based test for HLA-DQ2/DQ8 was released for direct sale to consumers but is not recommended for use in the diagnosis of celiac disease.[4]

In 2017, the US Preventive Services Taskforce stated that the evidence on hand is "insufficient to assess the balance and harms of screening for celiac disease in asymptomatic persons."[30]

Forms of celiac disease that have been identified in practice since the publication of the Oslo classification include seronegative celiac disease, in which a patient experiences symptoms and positive findings in biopsy but is negative for serum markers, and gluten-free diet-nonresponsive celiac disease, in which a patient does not respond to 12 months of strict gluten-free diet.[2] Potential celiac disease is an additional new term indicating the presence of serum antibodies and HLA-DQ2/8 but normal intestinal mucosa.[31]

TREATMENT

Desired Outcomes

The main goals of treatment include relieving symptoms, healing the intestine, and prevent complications. In children, increases in height and weight are additional goals.[27]

General Approach to Treatment

The mainstay of treatment of celiac disease is the strict, lifelong adherence to the gluten-free diet. Supportive care of nutrient deficiencies should be addressed through drug therapy and preventive care, such as vaccines, should be recommended.

Nonpharmacologic

8 Table 59-5 presents a mnemonic that summarizes the major principles of the treatment of celiac disease. Strict lifelong adherence to a gluten-free diet is the only proven treatment for celiac disease.[1] Patients must recognize that adhering to a gluten-free diet includes not ingesting anything that contains gluten or has been contaminated with gluten. Wheat, barley, and rye must be avoided.[3] Although oats are in a different plant family, they may be problematic; however, the ingestion of certified pure gluten-free oats is safe.[25] Due to the continued difference of opinion regarding the safety of oats, they should be added to the diet cautiously and with monitoring.[4] Patients must also commit to avoiding the ingestion of gluten found in nonfood items such as toothpaste, lip balm, lipstick, etc.[12] A list of gluten-free grains can be found in Table 59-1.

Oral prescription drugs, nonprescription drugs, vitamin and mineral supplements, and health and beauty aids and cosmetics that have oral ingestion potential must not be overlooked as sources of gluten due to its presence in their formulation or due to contamination or contact.[12] Lack of reliable information can be confusing and although there are published lists of gluten-free drugs, it is often difficult to obtain information about the gluten content of medications.[33] Patients with celiac disease are concerned about the possibility of gluten in medications causing disease-related symptoms.[34] Also, the FDA issued draft guidance on "Gluten in Drug Products and Associated Label Recommendations" encouraging drug manufacturers to have accurate information about their products' gluten content available so they can respond to questions from consumers. Healthcare professionals and some researchers have advocated that all medications should be gluten-free.[35] Clinicians should realize that conflicting data regarding drug absorption requires careful selection and use of drugs in patients with celiac disease.[36]

The FDA determined the tolerable daily intake level for gluten in individuals with celiac disease to be 0.4 mg gluten/day for adverse morphologic effects and 0.015 mg gluten/day for adverse clinical effects and ruled that foods labeled on or after August 5, 2014 as gluten-free must contain less than 20 ppm gluten.[37,38] Although the

TABLE 59-5 Mnemonic for Celiac Disease

C	**C**onsultation with a skilled dietician
E	**E**ducation about the disease
L	**L**ifelong adherence to a gluten-free diet
I	**I**dentifying and treating nutritional deficiencies
A	**A**ccess to an advocacy group
C	**C**ontinuous long-term follow-up by a multidisciplinary team

Data from Reference 32.

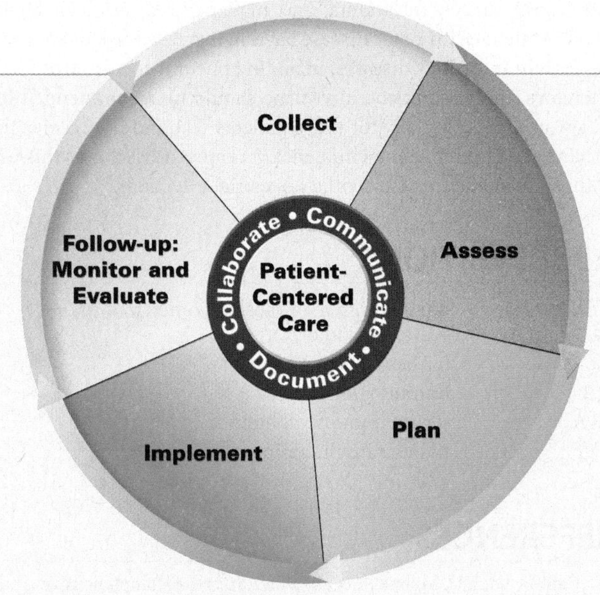

Patient Care Process for Celiac Disease

The image shows the five fundamental steps included in The Pharmacist's Care Process endorsed by the Joint Commission for Pharmacy Prac, communicate, and document. The five fundamental steps listed here are collect, assess, plan, implement, and follow-up: monitor and evaluate. All these steps are listed in a circular block diagram.

Collect

- Patient characteristics (eg, age, sex, height, weight)
- Patient medical history (personal and family)
- Social history (eg, tobacco/ethanol use) and dietary habits including intake of gluten-containing grains (see Table 59-1)
- Current medications including nonprescription, herbal products, dietary supplements
- Objective data
  - Results of diagnostic testing (HLA typing, serology, and/or biopsy)
  - Results of testing for nutritional deficiencies (eg, iron, folic acid, vitamin D, vitamin B_{12})
  - Results of other testing (eg, DEXA)

Assess

- Presence of signs and symptoms of malnutrition or nutrient deficiency
- Ability/willingness to follow gluten-free diet
- Ability/willingness to pay for treatment options (gluten-free food, dietary supplements)
- Emotional status (eg, presence of anxiety, depression)
- Family/caregiver support

Plan*

- Patient education (purpose of treatment, dietary and lifestyle modification)
- Self-monitoring for symptoms of celiac disease (intestinal and extra-intestinal)
- Referral to dietician
- Dietary supplement regimen including specific product(s), dose, route, frequency, and duration
- Medication regimen including identification of gluten-free oral medications

Implement

- Provide patient education regarding all elements of treatment plan
- Use motivational interviewing and coaching strategies to maximize adherence
- Schedule follow-up (eg, adherence assessment)

Follow-up: Monitor and Evaluate

- Resolution of celiac disease symptoms (eg, intestinal and extra-intestinal)
- Patient's adherence to treatment plan
- Resolution of nutritional deficiencies
- Repeat testing as needed (serology, biopsy, labs for nutritional deficiencies, DEXA)

**Collaborate with patients, caregivers, and other healthcare professionals.*

ruling pertains to food only, the concerns regarding low-level exposure emphasize why healthcare providers must check to determine whether prescription drugs contain gluten in their formulation or have been contaminated with gluten before these drugs are provided to the patient with celiac disease.

9 Newly diagnosed patients should be evaluated for nutritional deficiencies associated with vitamin and mineral malabsorption, including folic acid, vitamin B_{12}, fat-soluble vitamins, iron, and calcium.[4] Monitoring for potential nutritional deficiencies should also continue during subsequent follow-up visits.

Most adults with celiac disease have some degree of bone loss. Therefore, all patients must be screened for osteoporosis or osteopenia.[39,40] Supplementing a gluten-free diet with calcium, magnesium, and vitamin D may arrest or reverse celiac-related bone loss. Although their use has not been extensively studied in patients with celiac disease, bisphosphonates and other drugs have been prescribed for patients with bone disease.[36]

Implementing a gluten-free diet presents some challenges. Consultation with a registered dietician is recommended for dietary evaluation and education.[4] Patients are advised to initiate a complete gluten-free lifestyle immediately after diagnosis. Partial adherence to this diet is not adequate. In order to accomplish this objective, patients must be aware of what foods are gluten-free and when in doubt must know how to confirm whether a food contains gluten. Reading labels is extremely important; however, it may be difficult to identify hidden sources of gluten listed among the ingredients. Patients with celiac disease must also determine whether products were processed on equipment shared with wheat, barley, or rye. It may be necessary to call the manufacturers or check their website to obtain the needed information.[41] Patients should seek guidance from a dietitian in order to avoid incurring nutritional deficiencies such as with fiber, vitamins and minerals, or overconsumption of fats, both of which can occur with gluten-free diets.[1]

Individuals with celiac disease must also be advised to maintain a gluten-free kitchen. A dedicated toaster, bread maker, waffle iron, and other appliances should be obtained for use in preparing gluten-free meals. Utensils and dishes must be carefully cleaned to avoid gluten contamination. Care must also be taken when dining in restaurants and homes of family and friends. The individuals who prepare and serve the food must be knowledgeable about gluten-free foods and food preparation.[12] The economic burden associated with maintaining a gluten-free diet may present some challenges.[42] The relatively low availability and high cost of these foods contribute to the challenges associated with adhering to the required strict diet and may lead to varying degrees of noncompliance.[43,44] Patients also find that the extra cost associated with the special diet is not reimbursed by healthcare plans, and most policies do not pay for consultations with a dietician.[44] These challenges with compliance are particularly concerning as noncompliance with the gluten-free diet is associated with an increased mortality rate and compromised quality of life.[43] Hypervigilance to a strict gluten-free diet may negatively impact upon the patient's quality of life and clinicians should therefore also promote the social and emotional well-being of the patient while counseling about the importance of adhering to the gluten-free diet.[45] Patients are also encouraged to investigate their personal circumstances as to whether some of the costs of maintaining a gluten-free diet are eligible for approval as a tax deduction.[44]

Pharmacologic

Dietary avoidance of gluten remains the mainstay of treatment of celiac disease. Novel pharmacologic treatment modalities are under investigation. Most reports related to pharmacotherapy for celiac disease focus on the treatment of refractory disease.

In case reports, corticosteroids, azathioprine, cyclosporine, tacrolimus, infliximab, and alemtuzumab have been reported as effective treatments for refractory celiac disease. Patients characterized to have refractory celiac disease have persistent or recurrent malabsorptive symptoms and signs with villous atrophy despite maintaining a gluten-free diet for more than 12 months.[1] Less than 5% of adult patients have refractory celiac disease.

Based on the pathophysiology of celiac disease, novel targets for the treatment of the disease have been identified: decreasing the antigenic load and modulation of the immune response. Methods of decreasing the antigenic load include blocking the activity of tTG, GI destruction of proline peptides via enzyme therapy, blocking the binding of deaminated proteins to HLA-DQ2 and HLA-DQ8, detoxification of gluten peptides, and decreasing intestinal permeability in patients with celiac disease, in particular through inhibition of zonulin.[2] A zonulin inhibitor, larazotide, was well tolerated and had efficacy in three phase-2 studies, allowing patients to tolerate small amounts of gluten through symptom control in patients who did not respond fully to a gluten-free diet.[1,47] Latiglutenase is a combination of recombinant proteases which aims to digest small amounts of gluten.[1]

EVALUATION OF THERAPEUTIC OUTCOMES

Clinical improvement will often be observed within days or weeks of instituting a strict gluten-free diet.[47] Repeat biopsy may be a helpful tool to monitor mucosal healing, particularly in patients with ongoing symptoms.[1,27]

Healthcare providers must also be mindful of conditions that are related to celiac disease and that are potential complications of the disease, including certain forms of cancer, neurologic manifestations, osteoporosis, depression, diabetes, infertility, as well as other autoimmune and related illnesses. Cancers that are of particular concern include thyroid cancer, adenocarcinoma of the small intestine, lymphoma (predominantly non-Hodgkin's lymphoma of any type), esophageal cancer, melanoma, and malignancies found in childhood.[3] Patients with celiac disease have an increased risk of developing certain infectious diseases, including pneumococcal infection.[48] Therefore, the pneumococcal vaccine should be recommended for all age groups, especially for those patients who did not receive the vaccine as a child.[48] Annual influenza vaccine is advisable as this will reduce the incidence of secondary bacterial infections.[49]

ABBREVIATIONS

DEXA	dual-energy X-ray absorptiometry
GI	gastrointestinal
HLA	human leukocyte antigen
IgA	immunoglobulin A
SIgA	serum immunoglobulin A
tTG	tissue transglutaminase

REFERENCES

1. Caio G, Volta U, Sapone A, et al. Celiac disease: A comprehensive current review. *BMC Medicine.* 2019;17(1):142.
2. Freeman HJ. Celiac disease: A disorder emerging from antiquity, its evolving classification and risk, and potential new treatment paradigms. *Gut Liver.* 2015;9(1):28–37.
3. Kelly CP, Bai JC, Liu E, et al. Advances in diagnosis and management of celiac disease. *Gastroenterology.* 2015;148(6):1175–1186.
4. Rubio-Tapia A, Hill I, Kelly CP. ACG clinical guidelines: Diagnosis and management of celiac disease. *Am J Gastroenterol.* 2013;108(5):656–676.
5. Catassi C, Gatti S, Fasano A. The new epidemiology of celiac disease. *J Pediatr Gastroenterol Nutr.* 2014;59(Suppl 1):S7–S9.
6. Mardini H, Westgate P. Racial differences in the prevalence of celiac disease in the US population: National Health and Nutrition Examination Survey (NHANES) 2009-2012. *Dig Dis Sci.* 2015;60:1738–1742.
7. Choung RS, Ditah I, Nadeau A, et al. Trends and racial/ethnic disparities in gluten-sensitive problems in the United States: Findings from the National Health and Nutrition Examination Surveys from 1988 to 2012. *Am J Gastroenterol.* 2015;110:455–461.
8. Catassi C, Kryszak D, Bhatti B, et al. Natural history of celiac disease autoimmunity in a USA cohort followed since 1974. *Ann Med.* 2010;42:530–538.
9. Lionetti E, Gatti S, Pulivirenti A, et al. Celiac disease from a global perspective. *Best Pract Res Clin Gastroenterol.* 2015;29:365–379.
10. Kang JY, Kang AHY, Green A, et al. Systematic review: Worldwide variation in the frequency of coeliac disease and changes over time. *Aliment Pharmacol Ther.* 2013;38:226–245.
11. Singh P, Arora S, Singh A, et al. Prevalence of celiac disease in Asia: A systematic review and meta- analysis. *J Gastroenterol Hepatol.* 2016;31(6):1095–1101.
12. See JA, Kaukinen K, Makharia GK, et al. Practical insights into gluten-free diets. *Nat Rev Gastroenterol Hepatol.* 2015;12(10):580–591.
13. Comino I, Moreno Mde L, Sousa C. Role of oats in celiac disease. *World J Gastroenterol.* 2015;21(41):11825–11831.
14. Nistico L, Fagnani C, Coto I, et al. Concordance, disease progression, and heritability of coeliac disease in Italian twins. *Gut.* 2006;55:803–808.
15. Kuja-Halkola R, Lebwohl B, Halfvarson J. Heritability of non-HLA genetics in coeliac disease: A population-based study in 107 000 twins. *Gut.* 2016;65(11):1793–1798.
16. Lebwohl B, Sanders DS, Green PHR. Coeliac disease. *The Lancet.* 2018;391(10115):70–81.
17. Valitutti F, Cucchiara S, Fasano A. Celiac disease and the microbiome. *Nutrients* 2019;11(10):2403.
18. Green PHR, Lebwohl B, Greywoode R. Celiac disease. *J Allergy Clin Immunol.* 2015;135(5):1099–1106.
19. DiSabatino A, Vanoli A, Giuffrida P, et al. The function of tissue transglutaminase in celiac disease. *Autoimmunity Rev.* 2012;11:746–753.
20. Leonard MM, Sapone A, Catassi C, et al. Celiac disease and nonceliac gluten sensitivity: A review. *JAMA.* 2017;318(7):647–656.
21. Green PHR, Cellier C. Celiac disease. *N Engl J Med.* 2007;357:1731–1743.
22. Aronsson CA, Lee H, Liu E, et al. Age at gluten introduction and risk of celiac disease. *Pediatrics.* 2015;135(2):239–245.

23. Vivas S, Vaquero L, Rodríguez-Martín L, et al. Age-related differences in celiac disease: Specific characteristics of adult presentation. *World J Gastrointest Pharmacol Ther.* 2015;6(4):207–212.
24. Paez MA, Gramelspacher AM, Sinacore J. Delay in diagnosis of celiac disease in patients without gastrointestinal complaints. *Am J Med.* 2017;130(11):1318–1323.
25. Al-Toma A, Volta U, Auricchio R, et al. European Society for the Study of Coeliac Disease (ESsCD) guideline for coeliac disease and other gluten-related disorders. *United Eur Gastroenterol J.* 2019;7(5):583–613.
26. Lauret E, Rodrigo L. Celiac disease and autoimmune-associated conditions. *Biomed Res Int.* 2013;2013:127589.
27. Husby S, Murray JA, Katzka DA. AGA Clinical practice update on diagnosis and monitoring of celiac disease – Changing utility of serology and histologic measures: Expert review. *Gastroenterol.* 2019;156:885–889.
28. Husby S, Koletzko S, Korponay-Szabo IR, et al. European Society for Pediatric Gastroenterology, Hepatology, and Nutrition guidelines for the diagnosis of coeliac disease. *J Pediatr Gastroenterol Nutr.* 2012;54(1):136–160.
29. Collin P, Salmi TT, Hervonen K. Dermatitis herpetiformis: A cutaneous manifestation of coeliac disease. *Ann Med.* 2017;49(1):23–31.
30. US Preventive Services Task Force. Screening for celiac disease: US preventive services task force recommendation statement. *JAMA.* 2017;317(12):1252–1257.
31. Trovato CM, Montuori M, Valitutti F, et al. The challenge of treatment in potential celiac disease. *Gastroenterol Res Pract,* 2019;2019: 8974751.
32. NIH consensus development conference on celiac disease. *NIH Consens State Sci Statements.* 2004;21:1–23.
33. King AR, Gluten content of the top 200 medications: Follow-up to the influence of gluten on a patient's medication choices. *Hosp Pharm.* 2013;48(9):736–743.
34. Choung RS, Jay L, Al-Lami HS, et al. Concerns regarding gluten presence in medicines is common among individuals with celiac disease, dermatitis herpetiformis, and non-celiac gluten sensitivity. *Gastroenterology.* 2017;152(2):S484–S485.
35. Shah AV, Serajuddin ATM, Mangione RA. Making all medications gluten free. *J Pharmaceut Sci.* 2018;107:1263–1268.
36. Tran T, Smith C, Mangione RA. Drug absorption in celiac disease. *Am J Health-Syst Pharm.* 2013;70:2199–2206.
37. Office of Food Safety Center of Food Safety and Applied Nutrition, Food and Drug Administration Health Hazard Assessment for Gluten Exposure in Individuals with Celiac Disease: Determination of Tolerable Daily Intake Levels and Levels of Concern for Gluten. Health Hazard Assessment for Gluten Exposure in Individuals with Celiac Disease: Determination of Tolerable Daily Intake Levels and Levels of Concern for Gluten. 2011. Available at: https://www.fda.gov/media/81500/download. Accessed May 1, 2018.
38. FDA. Questions and Answers: Gluten-Free Food Labeling Final Rule. Available at: https://www.fda.gov/Food/GuidanceRegulation/GuidanceDocumentsRegulatoryInformation/Allergens/ucm362880.htm. Accessed May 1, 2018.
39. Micic D, Rao VL, Semrad CD. Celiac disease and its role in the development of metabolic bone disease. *J Clin Densitometry.* 2020;23(2):190–199.
40. Krupa-Kozak U. Pathologic bone alterations in celiac disease: Etiology, epidemiology, and treatment. *Nutrition.* 2014;30(1):16–24.
41. Mangione RA, Patel PN. Caring for patients with celiac disease: The role of the pharmacist. *J Am Pharm Assoc.* 2008;48(4):e125–e135.
42. Mogul D, Nakamura Y, Seo J, et al. The unknown burden and cost of celiac disease in the U.S. *Expert Rev Pharmacoecon Outcomes Res.* 2017;17(2):181–188.
43. Lee A, Ng D, Zivin J, Green H. Economic burden of a gluten-free diet. *J Hum Nutr Diet.* 2007;20:423–430.
44. Stevens L, Rashid M. Gluten-free and regular foods: A cost comparison. *Can J Diet Pract Res.* 2008;69:147–150.
45. Wolf RL, Lebwohl B, Zybert P, et al. Hypervigilance to a gluten-free diet and decreased quality of life in teenagers and adults with celiac disease. *Dig Dis Sci.* 2018;63(6):1438–1448.
46. Khaleghi S, Ju JM, Lamba A. The potential utility of tight junction regulation in celiac disease: Focus on larazotide acetate. *Therap Adv Gastroenterol.* 2016;9(1):37–49.
47. Thom S, Longo BM, Running A, Ashley J. Celiac disease: A guide to successful diagnosis and treatment. *J Nurse Pract.* 2009;5:244–253.
48. Simons M, Scott-Sheldon LAJ, Risech-Neyman Y, et al. Celiac disease and increased risk of pneumococcal infection: A systematic review and meta-analysis. *Am J Med.* 2018;131(1):83–89.
49. Ludvigsson JF, Montgomery SM, Ekbom A, et al. Small-intestinal histopathology and mortality risk in celiac disease. *JAMA.* 2009;302:1171–1178.

Evaluation of Kidney Function

e60

Linda Awdishu and Thomas C. Dowling

KEY CONCEPTS

1. The stage of chronic kidney disease (CKD) should be determined for all individuals based on the level of kidney function, independent of etiology, in accordance with the Kidney Disease: Improving Global Outcomes (KDIGO) classification system.
2. Persistent proteinuria indicates the presence of CKD and is associated with mortality and risk of end-stage kidney disease (ESKD).
3. Assessment of urine protein excretion, including measurement of a spot urine albumin-to-creatinine ratio, is critical for determining the severity of CKD and monitoring the rate of disease progression.
4. The glomerular filtration rate (GFR) is the single best indicator of kidney function.
5. Measurement of the GFR is most accurate when performed following administration of iohexol, iothalamate, or radioisotopes such as technetium-99m diethylenetriamine pentaacetic acid (^{99m}Tc-DTPA).
6. Equations to estimate creatinine clearance (CL_{cr}) or GFR (eGFR) are commonly used in ambulatory and inpatient settings, and incorporate patient laboratory and demographic variables such as serum creatinine concentration (S_{cr}), cystatin C, age, sex, and weight.
7. Assessments of kidney structure and function, such as radiography, computed tomography, magnetic resonance imaging, sonography, and biopsy, are predominantly used for determining the diagnosis of a given condition.

BEYOND THE BOOK

Using the Drugs@FDA Website <https://www.accessdata.fda.gov/scripts/cder/daf/> or tertiary databases like Micromedex identify two commonly used drugs that require drug dose adjustments in patients with impaired kidney function. Compile a summary table of the dosing information including drug name, kidney estimation method and categories, and dose adjustment recommendation. Now consider the following patient scenarios: (1) 49-year-old Caucasian man with Scr 1.7 mg/dL (150 μmol/L), height 72 in. (183 cm), weight 100 kg; (2) 67-year-old female of African ancestry with Scr 1.5 mg/dL (133 μmol/L), height 65 in. (165 cm), weight 90 kg.

Calculate kidney function for each patient utilizing the Cockcroft–Gault equation, and the CKD EPI race free equation using Scr with and without indexing to body surface area. Compare and contrast the corresponding doses for the drugs identified using each kidney function equation. This activity is intended to build upon your understanding of kidney function and to familiarize you with how the various estimating equations may impact your dosing recommendations.

INTRODUCTION

Chronic kidney disease (CKD) continues to be a worldwide health concern, with over 2 million people in the United States estimated to require hemodialysis or kidney transplantation by 2030.[1,2] In response to this widespread problem, standardized approaches are now used for the identification of individuals with CKD and their subsequent stratification into risk categories for the development of end-stage kidney disease (ESKD) (see Chapter 62, Chronic Kidney Disease).[1,2] These efforts have heightened the awareness of the need for early identification of patients with CKD and the importance of monitoring the progression of kidney disease.

Comprehensive evaluation of kidney function requires use of qualitative, quantitative, and semi-quantitative methods. Estimation of creatinine clearance (CL_{cr}) was the clinical standard for assessment of kidney function for over 50 years. Although it continues to be used to assess kidney function for renal drug dosing purposes in pharmacokinetic studies, recent FDA guidance recommended use of estimated glomerular filtration rate (GFR) in addition to or in lieu of CL_{cr} for renal dosing recommendations.[3] Estimated GFR is routinely used across clinical settings to identify patients with CKD, and in large epidemiology studies to evaluate risks of mortality and progression to stage 5 CKD or ESKD.[4,5]

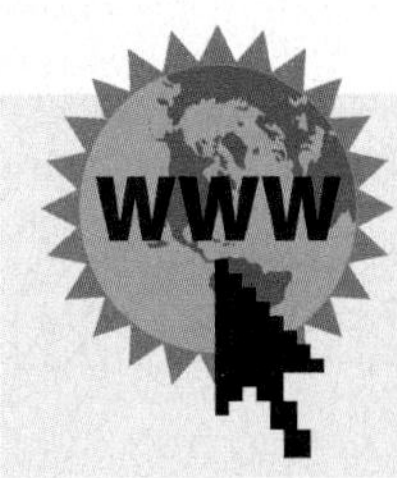

The complete chapter, learning objectives, and other resources can be found at **www.pharmacotherapyonline.com.**

Acute Kidney Injury

Jenana H. Maker, Lauren K. Roller, and William Dager

61

KEY CONCEPTS

1. Kidney Disease: Improving Global Outcomes (KD!GO) clinical practice guidelines provide a classification system for diagnosing and staging acute kidney injury (AKI). This classification system is based on separate criteria for serum creatinine (S_{cr}) and urine output.
2. AKI is a common complication in critically ill patients that is different than chronic kidney disease and is associated with high morbidity and mortality.
3. AKI is typically categorized based on three types of injury: (a) prerenal—decreased renal blood flow, (b) intrinsic—structural damage within the kidney, and (c) postrenal—an obstruction within the urine collection system.
4. Serum creatinine, urea, and urine output are commonly used markers of kidney function in clinical practice. However, advances in AKI research have led to the development of multiple novel biomarkers that can be used for risk assessment, early detection, classification, and prognosis in AKI.
5. Conventional formulas used to estimate glomerular filtration rate (eGFR) are not recommended in AKI patients. In addition, medication dose adjustment recommendations are typically based on limited pharmacokinetic studies conducted in chronic kidney disease (CKD) patients and may not be reflective of pharmacokinetic changes and dosing requirements in AKI patients.
6. The most effective prevention strategies for AKI include limiting exposure to nephrotoxic medications and optimizing the patient's hemodynamic and fluid status. Incorporation of electronic health alerts may increase early detection and decrease risk of AKI progression.
7. Supportive management remains the primary approach to prevent or reduce complications associated with AKI or comorbid conditions. Supportive therapies include renal replacement therapy (RRT), nutritional support, identifying potential causes and avoidance of nephrotoxins, blood pressure management, and fluid management.
8. For patients with prolonged or severe AKI, RRT is the cornerstone of support along with aggressive fluid and electrolyte management.
9. Medication dosing for AKI patients receiving continuous renal replacement therapy (CRRT) or prolonged RRT is poorly characterized. Dosing requirements of agents primarily eliminated by the kidney may require individualization and may be higher than observed in CKD. Dosing requirements may need to be adjustment downward as kidney function declines, and then subsequently increase as AKI resolves. Therapeutic drug monitoring should be utilized whenever possible for any agent with a narrow therapeutic index.

BEYOND THE BOOK

Watch the video entitled "Changing Glomerular Filtration Rate" in Khan Academy (https://youtu.be/x0pFo1RxTzM). This 4 min video provides a brief overview of how changes in afferent and efferent arteriolar tone control the glomerular filtration rate. This video is useful to enhance student understanding of the pathophysiology and medication-induced causes of AKI, as well as the COLLECT and ASSESS steps in the patient care process.

INTRODUCTION

Acute kidney injury (AKI) is a clinical syndrome generally defined by an abrupt reduction in kidney function as evidenced by changes in serum creatinine (S_{cr}), blood urea nitrogen (BUN), and urine output. The consequences of AKI can be serious, especially in hospitalized patients. Early recognition along with supportive therapy is the focus of management for those with established AKI, as there is no pharmacologic therapy that directly reverses the injury. Individuals at risk, such as those with history of chronic kidney disease (CKD), need to have their hemodynamic status carefully monitored and their exposure to nephrotoxins minimized. A thorough patient assessment including medical and surgical history, medication use, physical examination, and multiple laboratory tests is essential. Management goals include maintenance of blood pressure, fluid and electrolyte homeostasis, all of which may be dramatically altered in the presence of AKI, as well as the use of diuretics and renal support therapies. Additional therapies designed to eliminate or minimize the insult that precipitated AKI include discontinuation of any offending agents (ie, nephrotoxins), hydration, maintenance of renal perfusion, and renal replacement therapy (RRT).

In this chapter, the definition, classification, epidemiology, and common etiologies of AKI are presented. Methods to recognize and assess the extent of kidney function loss are also discussed. Unique considerations for medication dosing adjustments and finally, preventive strategies for patients at risk and management approaches for those with established AKI are reviewed.

DEFINITION AND CLASSIFICATION OF ACUTE KIDNEY INJURY

1 Several different definitions and classifications of AKI have been published, including the *Risk, Injury, Failure, Loss* of Kidney

Function, and End-Stage Kidney Disease (RIFLE), Acute Kidney Injury Network (AKIN), and Kidney Disease: Improving Global Outcomes (KDIGO) classifications. Among these, the KDIGO criteria are the most commonly used for diagnosing and staging AKI (Table 61-1).[1-3] The KDIGO criteria have been validated across different patient populations and their staging correlates closely with hospital mortality, cost, and length of stay.[4-6]

Since the KDIGO staging system depends on S_{cr} and urine output as the main diagnostic criteria, it is associated with some inherent weaknesses. An increase in S_{cr} is usually evident roughly 1 or 2 days after development of AKI. This lag time in S_{cr} rise may delay diagnosis of AKI and adversely affect patient outcomes. Urine output decreases earlier and often is the first indicator of AKI but it is a fairly nonspecific marker. Documentation can be challenging, especially with patients able to independently void without ability to document urine output. In fact, patients with AKI can be nonoliguric (urine output greater than 500 mL/day), oliguric (urine output less than 500 mL/day), or anuric (urine output less than 50 mL/day). Urine output will also vary with volume status, diuretic administration or omission, and the presence of an obstruction.[7]

AKI becomes acute kidney disease (AKD) if kidney function is impaired beyond 7 days, and can ultimately transition into CKD if the duration exceeds 90 days (Fig. 61-1).[8] As such, there has been a growing recognition of the need to standardize AKI recovery. The Acute Disease Quality Initiative (ADQI) proposed to further subclassify AKI into those who recover within 48 hours of injury (rapid

TABLE 61-1 RIFLE, AKIN, and KDIGO Classification Schemes for AKI[a]

RIFLE Category	S_{cr} and GFR[b] Criteria	Urine Output Criteria
Risk	S_{cr} increase to 1.5-fold or GFR decrease >25% from baseline	<0.5 mL/kg/hr for ≥6 hours
Injury	S_{cr} increase to twofold or GFR decrease >50% from baseline	<0.5 mL/kg/hr for ≥12 hours
Failure	S_{cr} increase to threefold or GFR decrease >75% from baseline, or S_{cr} ≥4 mg/dL (354 μmol/L) with an acute increase of at least 0.5 mg/dL (44 μmol/L)	Anuria for ≥12 hours
Loss	Complete loss of function (RRT) for >4 weeks	
ESKD	RRT >3 months	
AKIN Criteria	**S_{cr} Criteria**	**Urine Output Criteria**
Stage 1	S_{cr} increase ≥0.3 mg/dL (27 μmol/L) or 1.5- to 2-fold from baseline	<0.5 mL/kg/hr for ≥6 hours
Stage 2	S_{cr} increase >2- to 3-fold from baseline	<0.5 mL/kg/hr for ≥12 hours
Stage 3	S_{cr} increase >3-fold from baseline, or S_{cr} ≥4 mg/dL (354 μmol/L) with an acute increase of at least 0.5 mg/dL (44 μmol/L), or need for RRT	<0.3 mL/kg/hr for ≥24 hours or anuria for ≥12 hours
KDIGO Criteria	**S_{cr} Criteria**	**Urine Output Criteria**
Stage 1	S_{cr} increase ≥0.3 mg/dL (27 μmol/L) or 1.5-1.9 times from baseline	<0.5 mL/kg/hr for 6-12 hours
Stage 2	S_{cr} increase 2-2.9 times from baseline	<0.5 mL/kg/hr for ≥12 hours
Stage 3	S_{cr} increase three times from baseline, or S_{cr} ≥4 mg/dL (354 μmol/L), or need for RRT, or eGFR[c] <35 mL/min/1.73 m² in patients <18 years	Anuria for ≥12 hours

[a]For all staging systems, the criterion that leads to worst possible diagnosis should be used.

[b]GFR calculated using the Modification of Diet in Renal Disease (MDRD) equation.

[c]GFR calculated using the Schwartz formula.

AKI, acute kidney injury; AKIN, Acute Kidney Injury Network; ESKD, end-stage kidney disease; eGFR, estimated glomerular filtration rate; hr, hours; KDIGO, Kidney Disease: Improving Global Outcomes; RIFLE, Risk, Injury, Failure, Loss of Kidney Function, and End-Stage Kidney Disease; RRT, renal replacement therapy; S_{cr}, serum creatinine.

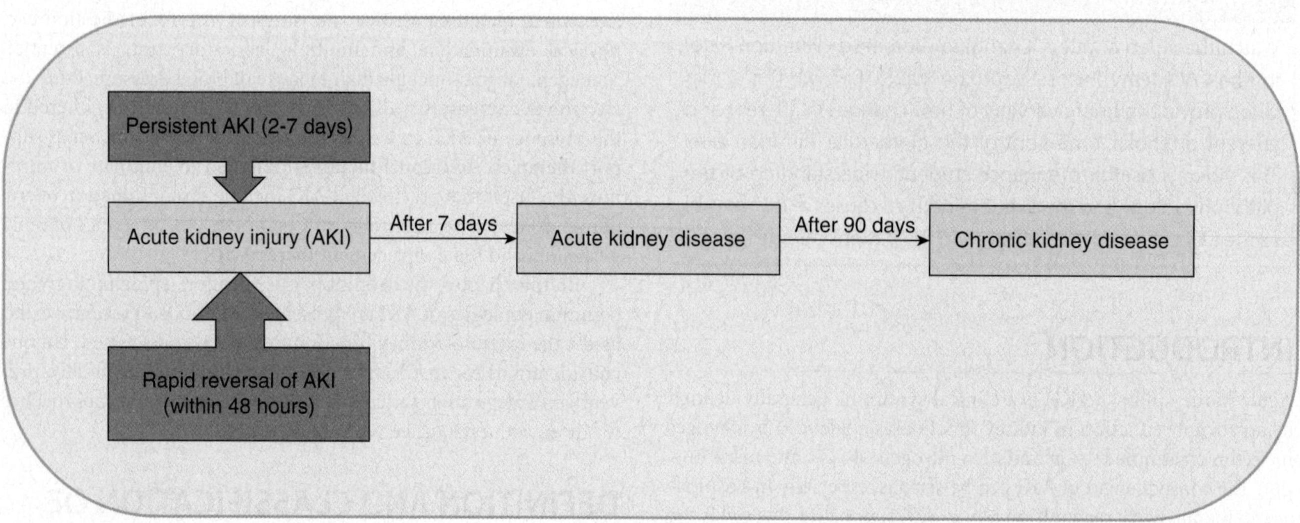

FIGURE 61-1 Continuum of impaired kidney function. Acute kidney injury is an abrupt decrease in kidney function that can either rapidly reverse within the first 48 hours or persist over a period of up to 7 days. Kidney impairment that persists beyond 7 days is termed acute kidney disease and can lead to chronic kidney disease if its duration exceeds 90 days.

reversal of AKI) and those whose injury persists beyond 48 hours (persistent AKI).[8]

EPIDEMIOLOGY

The epidemiology of AKI varies widely depending on the patient population studied and the criteria used to evaluate the patient. A recent CDC analysis from the National Inpatient Sample and the National Health Interview Surveys noted that the total number of AKI-related hospitalizations increased fourfold over the last two decades (from 953,926 in 2000 to 3,959,560 in 2014). Age-standardized rates of AKI hospitalizations increased 139% (23-55 per 1,000 persons) among diabetic adults and rose by 230% (3.5-11.7 per 1,000 persons) among non-diabetic adults.[9]

AKI occurs in 3.0% to 18.3% of hospitalized non-critically ill patients and 30% to 60% of critically ill adults.[10] Risk factors associated with AKI include the presence of CKD, diabetes, heart or liver disease, albuminuria, major surgery (especially cardiac surgery), acute decompensated heart failure, sepsis, hypotension, volume depletion (diarrhea, vomiting, or dehydration), medications (exposure to angiotensin-converting enzyme [ACE] inhibitors, angiotensin receptor blockers [ARBs], aminoglycosides, etc.), advanced age, male gender, and African American race.[3,10-12]

2 Severity, duration, and frequency of AKI are important predictors of poor patient outcomes. Any degree of AKI is associated with an increased risk of death, and the odds increase with the severity of the insult.[10,12] For survivors of AKI, the development of some degree of CKD and need for RRT are other important considerations. In addition, AKI is associated with increased length of hospital stay, mortality, cost, readmission, ventilator days, and need for post-hospitalization care.[10,12,13]

ETIOLOGY

3 The etiology of AKI can be divided into three broad categories based on the anatomic location of the injury associated with the precipitating factor(s). The management of patients presenting with this disorder is largely predicated on identification of the specific etiology responsible for the patient's AKI (Fig. 61-2). Traditionally, the causes of AKI have been categorized as (a) prerenal, which results

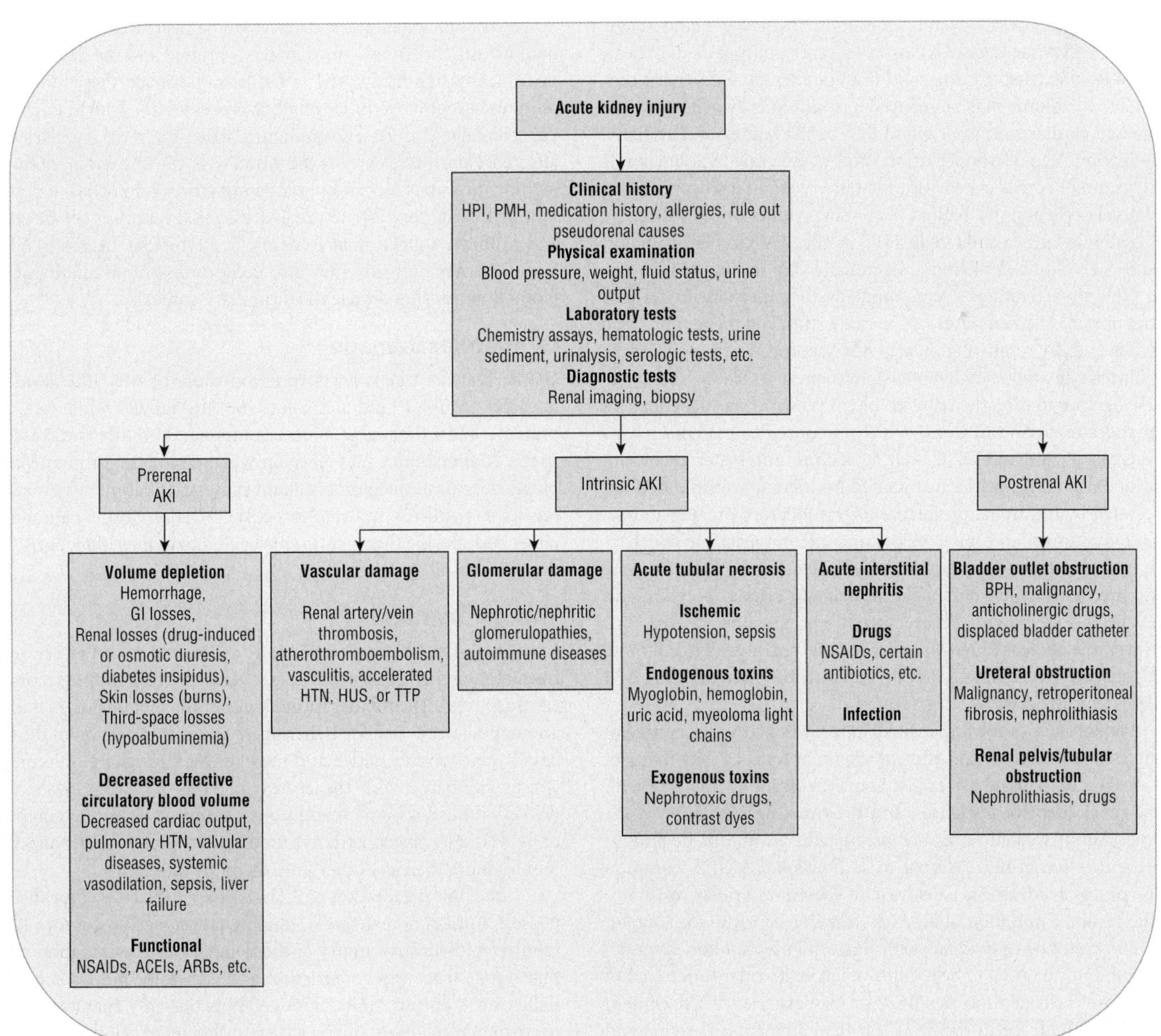

FIGURE 61-2 Classification of acute kidney injury (AKI) based on etiology. (ACEIs, angiotensin-converting enzyme inhibitors; ARBs, angiotensin receptor blockers; BPH, benign prostatic hyperplasia; HPI, history of present illness; HTN, hypertension; HUS, hemolytic uremic syndrome; NSAIDs, nonsteroidal anti-inflammatory drugs; PMH, past medical history; TTP, thrombotic thrombocytopenic purpura.)

from decreased renal perfusion in the setting of undamaged parenchymal tissue, (b) intrinsic, the result of structural damage to the kidney, most commonly the tubule from an ischemic or toxic insult, and (c) postrenal, caused by obstruction of urine flow downstream from the kidney.

The risk of AKI increases substantially with decreasing glomerular filtration rate (GFR) and presence of albuminuria and underlying CKD. A history of AKI has also been associated with high risk for developing additional episodes of AKI and subsequent complications such as CKD.[10,14]

PATHOPHYSIOLOGY

The pathophysiologic processes involved in the development of the three traditional categories of AKI: prerenal AKI, intrinsic AKI, and postrenal AKI are described below.

Prerenal Acute Kidney Injury

Prerenal AKI or prerenal azotemia results from hypoperfusion of the renal parenchyma, with or without systemic arterial hypotension. Renal hypoperfusion associated with systemic arterial hypotension may be caused by a decline in either the intravascular volume or the effective circulating blood volume. Intravascular volume depletion may result from several conditions, including hemorrhage, excessive gastrointestinal (GI) losses (severe vomiting or diarrhea), dehydration, extensive burns, and diuretic therapy. Effective circulating blood volume may be reduced in conditions associated with a decreased cardiac output or blood flow to the kidney and systemic vasodilation. Renal hypoperfusion without systemic hypotension is most commonly associated with bilateral renal artery occlusion or unilateral occlusion in a patient with a single functioning kidney.

Patients with a mild reduction in effective circulating blood volume or volume depletion are generally able to maintain a normal GFR by activating several compensatory mechanisms. Those initial physiologic responses by the body stimulate the sympathetic nervous and the renin–angiotensin–aldosterone system and release antidiuretic hormone if hypotension is present. These responses work together to directly maintain blood pressure via vasoconstriction and stimulation of thirst, which in conscious patients results in increased fluid intake, as well as sodium and water retention. Additionally, GFR may be maintained by afferent arteriole dilation (mediated by intrarenal production of vasodilatory prostaglandins, kallikrein, kinins, and nitric oxide) and efferent arteriole constriction (mainly mediated by angiotensin II). In concert, these homeostatic mechanisms are often able to maintain arterial pressure and renal perfusion, potentially averting the progression to AKI.[15] If, however, the decreased renal perfusion is severe or prolonged, these compensatory mechanisms may be overwhelmed, and prerenal AKI will be clinically evident.

Patients at risk for prerenal AKI are particularly susceptible to changes in the afferent and efferent arteriolar tone, as they may not be able to compensate as readily. Some medications interfere with these renal adaptive responses, and the resulting reduction in the glomerular hydrostatic pressure precipitates an abrupt decline in GFR and is sometimes referred to as *functional AKI*. A common cause of this syndrome is a decrease in efferent arteriolar resistance as the result of initiation of an ACE inhibitor or ARB (see Chapter 65). For example, individuals with heart failure are often given an ACE inhibitor or ARB to help improve left ventricular function, but if the dose is titrated too rapidly, they may experience a decline in GFR. If the increase in the S_{cr} is less than 30% from baseline and potassium serum levels are within normal range, the medication can generally be continued. Nonsteroidal anti-inflammatory drugs (NSAIDs) may also precipitate AKI in susceptible individuals due to their impact on renal prostaglandin production and afferent arteriolar vasodilation, which some patients rely on to maintain GFR.[16]

Sepsis is one of the leading clinical conditions associated with AKI. The exact mechanism by which sepsis causes AKI is poorly understood. A complex interplay of different mechanisms may be involved in its pathogenesis, including disturbances in renal microcirculation, inflammation, and metabolic reprogramming.[17,18]

Intrinsic Acute Kidney Injury

Intrinsic AKI results from direct damage to the kidney and is categorized on the basis of the injured structures within the kidney: vasculature, glomeruli, tubules, and interstitium.

Renal Vasculature Damage

Occlusion of the larger renal vessels resulting in AKI is not common but can occur if large atheroemboli or thromboemboli occlude the bilateral renal arteries or one vessel of the patient with a single kidney. Atheroemboli most commonly develop during vascular procedures that cause atheroma dislodgement, such as angioplasty and aortic manipulations. Thromboemboli may arise from dislodgement of a mural thrombus in the left ventricle of a patient with severe heart failure or from the atria of a patient with atrial fibrillation. Renal artery thrombosis may occur in a similar fashion to coronary thrombosis, in which a thrombus forms in conjunction with an atherosclerotic plaque.

Although smaller vessels can also be obstructed by atheroemboli or thromboemboli, the damage is limited and the development of clinically significant AKI is unlikely. However, these small vessels are susceptible to inflammatory processes that lead to microvascular damage and vessel dysfunction when the renal capillaries are affected. Neutrophils invade the vessel wall, causing damage that can include thrombus formation, tissue infarction, and collagen deposition within the vessel structure. Diffuse renal vasculitis can be severe and promote concomitant ischemic acute tubular necrosis (ATN). Untreated hypertension may also compromise renal microvascular blood flow, causing diffuse renal capillary damage.

Glomerular Damage

Glomerular damage is an uncommon cause of AKI. The glomerulus serves to filter fluid and solute into the tubules while retaining proteins and other large blood components in the intravascular space. Kidney injury may develop when circulating immune complexes deposit in the glomeruli and cause an inflammatory reaction (eg, lupus nephritis, IgA nephropathy).[19] Details on the pathophysiology and specific therapeutic approaches to glomerulonephritis are described in Chapter e66.

Tubular Damage

Most intrinsic AKI cases are due to ATN, which can either result from renal ischemia or nephrotoxin exposure (eg, aminoglycosides, contrast dyes). The tubules located within the medulla of the kidney are particularly at risk for ischemic injury, as this portion of the kidney is metabolically active and thus has high oxygen requirements, yet, as compared with the cortex, receives relatively low oxygen delivery. Thus, ischemic conditions caused by severe hypotension or exposure to vasoconstrictive medications preferentially affect the tubules more than any other portion of the kidney.

The clinical evolution of ATN is characterized by four distinct phases: initiation, extension, maintenance, and recovery. Renal tubular epithelial cell injury is the hallmark of the initiation phase that results from vasoconstriction and ischemia, and leads to GFR reduction. Contrary to its name, ATN is not only characterized by necrosis and cell death but by a large spectrum of cellular injury that usually involves sublethal damage to the cells. The extent of injury depends not only on the severity and duration of ischemia but also on the sensitivity of renal cells to the insult which may vary based on the cells' metabolic demands, physical location within the kidney, degree of regional blood perfusion, oxygenation status, and membrane permeability. Further, alterations in cytoskeletal structure lead to a loss of epithelial polarity and barrier function. As a result, the glomerular filtrate starts leaking back into the interstitium and is reabsorbed into the systemic circulation. Additionally, urine flow is obstructed by accumulation of sloughed epithelial cells, cellular debris, and formation of casts.[19,20]

The extension phase is characterized by continued hypoxia following the initial ischemic event and an inflammatory response. Both events are more pronounced in the outer medullary region and the GFR continues to decrease. During the maintenance phase, GFR reaches a nadir during which cellular repair processes are initiated in an attempt to reestablish and maintain cellular and tubular integrity. The surviving cells undergo repair, migration, dedifferentiation, and proliferation. The maintenance phase is eventually followed by a recovery phase, during which new tubule cells are regenerated through redifferentiation and epithelial polarity is reestablished.[19,20]

Interstitial Damage

Acute interstitial nephritis (AIN) is an idiosyncratic delayed hypersensitivity immune reaction that is most commonly caused by medications (see Chapter 65) and less commonly by infections, autoimmune diseases, or idiopathic causes. AIN is characterized by tubular and interstitial inflammation, and edema with lesions composed of mononuclear cells, with a predominance of lymphocytes (primarily CD4+ T lymphocytes) and monocytes or macrophages. The specific pathogenic process depends on the cause of AIN. Medication-induced disease is characterized by renal interstitial dendritic and renal tubular epithelial cells recognition of the offending agent as immunogenic and their activation of T lymphocytes which induce proinflammatory molecules. Once acute interstitial inflammation sets in, it can progress rapidly to a more destructive fibrogenic process marked by increased interstitial matrix, ischemia, tubular atrophy, and interstitial fibrosis.[21,22] The prognosis of AIN varies depending on the specific cause, baseline kidney function, and timely detection of the offending agent; however, it is estimated that almost a quarter of patients may not recover their baseline kidney function.[22]

Postrenal Acute Kidney Injury

Postrenal AKI accounts for less than 5% of all cases of AKI and may develop as the result of obstruction at any level within the urinary collection system (see Fig. 61-2). However, if the obstructing process is above the bladder, it must involve both kidneys (one kidney in a patient with a single functioning kidney) to cause clinically significant AKI, as one functioning kidney can generally maintain a near-normal GFR. Bladder outlet obstruction, the most common cause of obstructive nephropathy, is often the result of a prostatic process in males (hypertrophy, cancer, or infection), producing a physical impingement on the urethra and thereby preventing the passage of urine. It may also be the result of an improperly placed urinary catheter. Blockage may also occur at the ureter level secondary to nephrolithiasis, blood clots, sloughed renal papillae, or physical compression by an abdominal process. Crystal deposition within the tubules from oxalate and some medications severe enough to cause AKI is uncommon, but it is possible in patients with severe volume contraction and in those receiving large doses of a medication with relatively low urine solubility (see Chapter 65).[19] Typically, these patients have insufficient urine volume to prevent crystal precipitation in the urine. Extremely elevated uric acid concentrations from chemotherapy-induced tumor lysis syndrome can cause obstruction and direct tubular injury as well.[23] Wherever the location of the obstruction, urine will accumulate in the renal structures above the obstruction and cause increased pressure upstream. The ureters, renal pelvis, and calyces all expand, and the net result is a decline in GFR. If renal vasoconstriction ensues, a further decrement in GFR will be observed.

CLINICAL PRESENTATION

The initiating signs or symptoms of AKI are highly variable and largely dependent on the underlying etiology. It may be a change in urinary character (eg, decreased urine output or urine discoloration), edema, electrolyte disturbances, sudden weight gain, or severe abdominal or flank pain. Early recognition and cause identification are critical, as they directly affect the outcome of AKI. One of the first steps in the diagnostic process is to determine if the change in kidney function is acute, chronic, or the result of an acute change in a patient with known CKD (also called acute-on-chronic kidney failure). Patients should also be promptly evaluated for any changes in their fluid and electrolyte status. Patients presenting with AKI in the outpatient environment may have nonspecific or seemingly unrelated symptoms so that the time of onset of the injury can be difficult to determine. On the other hand, AKI in hospitalized patients is often detected much earlier in its course due to frequent laboratory studies and daily (or hourly) patient assessments.

Patient Assessment

The assessment of a patient with AKI starts with a thorough review of his or her medical records, with a particular focus on chronic conditions, laboratory studies, procedures, and surgeries. An exhaustive review of prescription and nonprescription medicines, herbal products, and drugs of abuse may help determine if AKI was potentially precipitated by drug ingestion.

During the initial patient evaluation, presumptive signs and symptoms of AKI need to be differentiated from a potential new diagnosis of CKD. A medical history for kidney disease–related chronic conditions (eg, poorly controlled hypertension or diabetes mellitus), previous laboratory data documenting the presence of proteinuria or an elevated S_{cr}, and the finding of bilateral small kidneys on renal ultrasonography suggest the presence of new onset CKD rather than AKI. However, it is important to note that patients with CKD may develop episodes of AKI as well. In these patients, an abrupt rise in the baseline S_{cr} is one of the most useful indicators of the presence of an acute insult to the kidneys. The staging of AKI should also be assessed including the initial insult and decline in kidney function, stabilization of the decline in function, and recovery period.

An acute change in urinary habitus is another common and noticeable symptom associated with AKI. The presence of cola-colored urine is indicative of blood in the urine, a finding commonly associated with acute glomerulonephritis. In hospitalized patients, changes in urine output may be helpful in characterizing the cause of the patient's AKI. Acute anuria is typically caused by either complete urinary obstruction or a catastrophic event (eg, shock or acute cortical necrosis). Oliguria, which often develops over several days, suggests prerenal azotemia, whereas nonoliguric kidney failure usually results from acute intrinsic kidney failure or incomplete urinary obstruction.

Depending on the underlying cause of AKI, patients may present with a variety of symptoms affecting virtually any organ system of the body. Constitutional symptoms such as nausea, vomiting, fatigue, malaise, and weight gain are common but nonspecific. The onset of flank pain is suggestive of a urinary stone; however, if bilateral, it may suggest swelling of the kidneys secondary to acute glomerulonephritis or AIN. Complaints of severe headaches may suggest the presence of severe hypertension and vascular damage. The presence of fever, rash, and arthralgia may be indicative of medication-induced AIN or lupus nephritis.

A thorough physical examination is an important step in evaluating individuals with AKI, as clues regarding the etiology can be evident from the patient's head (eye examination) to toe (evidence of dependent edema) assessment. Evaluation of the patient's volume and hemodynamic status is critical as well, as it will guide management. For example, patients with prerenal AKI can present with either volume depletion or fluid overload. Volume depletion may be evidenced by the presence of postural hypotension, decreased jugular venous pressure (JVP), and dry mucous membranes. Fluid overload, on the other hand, is often reflected by elevated JVP, pitting edema, ascites, and pulmonary crackles.

Conventional Markers of Kidney Function

4 Common laboratory tests used to evaluate the patient with impaired kidney function are described in Chapter e60. Over the past four decades, S_{cr} has been the most widely used laboratory test for estimating creatinine clearance (CL_{cr}) and eGFR. However, there are several limitations associated with its use since it is affected by age, gender, muscle mass or evidence of acute breakdown, diet, hydration status, and stability of the values (eg, S_{cr}) utilized. For example, patients with reduced creatinine production, such as those with low muscle mass, may have low values (less than 0.6 mg/dL [53 μmol/L]); thus, the presence of a gradual rise to normal values (0.8-1.2 mg/dL [71-106 μmol/L]) may actually suggest the presence of AKI. However, in the presence of improved nutrition and a large muscle mass, a S_{cr} of 1.2 mg/dL (106 μmol/L) may be a true representation of a person's current renal status. Instead of using only the most current value to determine kidney function, changes in the value from a patient's baseline over the past few days need to be considered. S_{cr} is normally inversely proportional to GFR. However, rapid changes in GFR disrupt this equilibrium and make S_{cr} an insensitive marker. In fact, changes in S_{cr} will lag behind the GFR's decline by 1 to 2 days due to slow accumulation, increased tubular secretion, and increased extrarenal clearance.[24,25] This can lead to an overestimation of the patient's GFR in the early stages of AKI and consequently a potential delay in the diagnosis of the syndrome.

5 Because S_{cr} steady-state values are assumed when one uses several GFR calculation methods, such as the Cockcroft-Gault and Chronic Kidney Disease Epidemiology Collaboration (CKD-EPI) equations, they should not be used to estimate GFR in AKI patients with unstable kidney function. These equations will typically overestimate GFR when the AKI is worsening and underestimate it when the AKI is resolving. Instead, it may be useful to evaluate changes in S_{cr} values from the patient's baseline and also consider the S_{cr} sequence values to determine if kidney function is potentially improving or worsening. The most recent S_{cr} reflects the time-averaged kidney function over the preceding time period. Several mathematical approaches to estimate GFR in patients with unstable S_{cr} that incorporate the principles of creatinine accumulation and elimination have been proposed and are discussed in detail in Chapter e60. However, these methods have not been extensively validated in the setting of AKI, and their value for adjusting medication dosing is questionable. Additionally, these equations are complex and are not commonly used in the clinical setting.

Two other widely available markers of kidney function are BUN and urine output. The value of the BUN in AKI is limited because urea production and renal clearance are heavily influenced by extrarenal factors such as critical illness, volume status, protein intake, and medications. Urine output measured over a specified period of time (eg, 4-24 hours) allows for short-term assessment of kidney function, but its utility is limited to cases in which it is significantly decreased. The presence of anuria suggests complete kidney failure, whereas oliguria indicates some degree of kidney damage. Urine output needs to be interpreted with caution, as it is dependent on several factors, such as hydration status and medications. As mentioned earlier in the chapter, a patient may have AKI and still maintain a normal urine output; this condition is referred to as *nonoliguric AKI*. Another approach to estimating kidney function is to directly measure CL_{cr} over a short period of time, for example, 4 to 12 hours.[26] Although, potentially precise and simple to do, its accuracy is questionable if the urine output is low or the urine collection is incomplete.

TABLE 61-2 Diagnostic Parameters for Differentiating Causes of AKI[a]

Laboratory Test	Prerenal AKI	Intrinsic AKI	Postrenal AKI
Urine sediment	Hyaline casts, may be normal	Granular casts, cellular debris	Cellular debris
Urinary RBC	None	2-4+	Variable
Urinary WBC	None	2-4+	1+
Urine Na (mEq/L or mmol/L)	<20	>40	>40
FE_{Na} (%)	<1	>2	Variable
Urine specific gravity	>1.018	<1.012	Variable

[a]Common laboratory tests are used to classify the cause of AKI. Functional AKI, which is not included in this table, would have laboratory values similar to those seen in prerenal AKI. The laboratory results listed under intrinsic AKI are those seen in acute tubular necrosis, the most common cause of intrinsic AKI.

AKI, acute kidney injury; FE_{Na}, fractional excretion of sodium; S_{cr}, serum creatinine; RBC, red blood cell; WBC, white blood cell.

In addition to BUN and S_{cr}, selected blood and urine tests, and urinary sediment are routinely evaluated to differentiate the cause of AKI and guide patient management. For example, a complete blood cell count with differential can help rule out infectious causes of AKI. Serum electrolyte values may be abnormal because of the acute decline of the kidney's ability to regulate electrolyte excretion. Particular attention should be paid to serum potassium, calcium, magnesium, and phosphorus values, which can be markedly elevated and cause life-threatening complications.

Given the limited usefulness of solely using S_{cr} or BUN concentrations to differentiate the etiology of AKI, urinary electrolytes and osmolality should be determined, and both a microscopic and chemical analysis of the urine should be performed (Table 61-2). The finding of a high urinary specific gravity, in the absence of glucosuria or mannitol administration, suggests an intact urinary concentrating mechanism and that the cause of the patient's AKI is likely prerenal azotemia. The presence of urinary protein is often difficult to interpret, especially in the setting of acute or chronic kidney failure. A patient with CKD may have a baseline proteinuria, thus clouding the clinical presentation, unless this is known at the time of AKI assessment. Classically, proteinuria is a hallmark of glomerular damage. However, tubular damage can also result in proteinuria, as the tubules are responsible for reabsorbing small proteins that are normally filtered by all glomeruli. The presence of blood also results in a positive urine protein test, so this confounder must always be assessed when a positive urine protein is obtained. Hematuria suggests acute intrinsic AKI secondary to glomerular injury, catheter-related trauma, infection, or a kidney stone. On microscopic examination, the key findings are cells, casts, and crystals, and the presence of one or more of these may suggest specific etiologies of the AKI (Table 61-3). The finding of urinary crystals may indicate nephrolithiasis and a postrenal obstruction. If red blood cells or red blood cell casts are present, one should consider the presence of a physical injury to the glomerulus, renal parenchyma, or vascular beds. The finding of white blood cells or white blood cell casts suggests interstitial inflammation (ie, interstitial nephritis), which can be secondary to an allergic, granulomatous, or infectious process.

Simultaneous measurement of urine and serum electrolytes is also helpful in the setting of AKI (see Table 61-3). From these values, a fractional excretion of sodium (FE_{Na}) can be calculated. The equation for the calculation of the FE_{Na} is as follows:

$$FE_{NA} = \frac{\text{Excreted Na}}{\text{Filtered Na}} \times 100 = \frac{U_{vol} \times U_{Na}}{GFR \times S_{Na}} \times 100$$

TABLE 61-3 Urinary Findings as a Guide to the Etiology of AKI

Type of Urinary Evaluation	Presence of	Suggestive of
Urinalysis	Leukocyte esterases	Pyelonephritis
	Nitrites	Pyelonephritis
	Protein	
	Mild (<0.5 g/day)	Tubular damage
	Moderate (0.5-3 g/day)	Glomerulonephritis, pyelonephritis, tubular damage
	Large (>3 g/day)	Glomerulonephritis, nephrotic syndrome
	Hemoglobin	Glomerulonephritis, pyelonephritis, renal infarction, renal tumors, kidney stones
	Myoglobin	Rhabdomyolysis-associated tubular necrosis
	Urobilinogen	Hemolysis-associated tubular necrosis
Urine sediment	Microorganisms	Pyelonephritis
Cells	Red blood cells	Glomerulonephritis, pyelonephritis, renal infarction, papillary necrosis, renal tumors, kidney stones
	White blood cells	Pyelonephritis, interstitial nephritis
	Eosinophils	Drug-induced interstitial nephritis, renal transplant rejection
	Epithelial cells	Tubular necrosis
Casts	Granular casts	Tubular necrosis
	Hyaline casts	Prerenal azotemia
	White blood cell casts	Pyelonephritis, interstitial nephritis
	Red blood cell casts	Glomerulonephritis, renal infarct, lupus nephritis, vasculitis
Crystals	Urate	Postrenal obstruction
	Calcium phosphate	Postrenal obstruction

AKI, acute kidney injury.

where

$$GFR = \frac{U_{vol} \times U_{cr}}{S_{cr} \times t}$$

Thus:

$$FE_{Na} = \frac{U_{Na} \times S_{cr} \times 100}{U_{cr} \times S_{Na}}$$

where U_{vol} is the urine volume, U_{cr} is the urine creatinine concentration, U_{Na} is the urine sodium concentration, S_{cr} is the serum creatinine concentration, S_{Na} is the serum sodium concentration, which usually does not vary much, GFR is the glomerular filtration rate, and t is the time period over which the urine is collected.

The FE_{Na} is one of the better diagnostic parameters to differentiate the cause of AKI. A low urinary sodium concentration (less than 20 mEq/L [mmol/L]) and low FE_{Na} (less than 1%) in a patient with oliguria suggest that there is stimulation of the sodium-retentive mechanisms in the kidney and that tubular function is intact. These findings are most characteristic of prerenal azotemia. Unfortunately, diuretic use in the preceding days limits the usefulness of the FE_{Na} calculation by increasing natriuresis, even in hypovolemic patients. The fractional excretion of urea (FE_{Urea}), which can be calculated like FE_{Na}, is sometimes used as an alternative means to assess tubular function in patients receiving diuretics. The inability to concentrate urine results in a high FE_{Na} (greater than 2%), suggesting tubular damage as the primary cause of the intrinsic AKI. However, this is also not an absolute finding, as there are some intrinsic causes that can be associated with a low FE_{Na} (eg, contrast nephropathy, myoglobinuria, and interstitial nephritis). Highly concentrated urine (greater than 500 mOsm/kg [mmol/kg]) suggests stimulation of antidiuretic hormone and intact tubular function. These findings are consistent with prerenal azotemia.

Novel Biomarkers of Kidney Damage

A variety of biomarkers have been investigated to detect and predict the clinical outcomes of AKI. While they vary in their origin, function, distribution, and time of release following kidney injury, the large majority are molecules that are released as a result of direct kidney cell damage. The performance of most biomarkers is variable and depends on the patient population, cause of AKI, presence of comorbidities, and timing of biomarker measurements. In general, their ability to detect AKI is better within homogenous patient populations where the time of AKI is known than in heterogeneous populations with multiple comorbidities and unknown AKI time or cause such as critically ill patients. Even though some biomarker tests are now commercially available, these tests are not routinely available at most clinical practice sites.[27,28]

Two of the most promising biomarkers for use in AKI are tissue inhibitor of metalloproteinases 2 (TIMP-2) and insulin-like growth factor binding protein 7 (IGFBP7). Both molecules inhibit specific proteins that result in G1 cell cycle arrest noted to occur during the early phases of cellular stress or injury.[29] The combination of TIMP-2 and IGFBP7 was approved by the Food and Drug Administration (FDA) as the first point-of-care device (Nephrocheck®) to detect early AKI. The Nephrocheck® test uses a fluorescent immunoassay and reveals test results expressed as an AKI risk score within 20 minutes. A score over 0.3 $(ng/mL)^2/1{,}000$ indicates high risk for developing moderate to severe AKI within 12 hours of testing. The cutoff value of 0.3 has a sensitivity of 95% and a specificity of only 46%. TIMP-2 and IGFBP7 have greatest predictability in patients at high risk for AKI, particularly patients who are critically ill, septic, or undergoing major surgery.[30] Nephrocheck® is not to be used as a standalone test for the diagnosis of AKI and should be used in conjunction with other diagnostic and clinical findings. Further, Nephrocheck® should be avoided in patients experiencing severe albuminuria and hyperbilirubinuria, as they interfere with the test results.[31]

Other biomarkers of kidney damage include neutrophil gelatinase–associated lipocalin (NGAL), kidney injury molecule 1 (KIM-1), interleukin 18 (IL-18), liver-type fatty acid binding protein (L-FABP), and N-acetyl-beta-D-glucosaminidase (NAG). They have been used for risk assessment, early detection, classification, and prognosis of AKI.[28,32] Since novel AKI biomarkers are still not widely utilized in clinical practice, the ADQI published a consensus statement on how AKI biomarkers can be integrated into a patient-centered approach to improve AKI care.[33] The panel recommends using AKI biomarkers to identify patients at risk who would benefit from preventative treatment. Further, they suggest using biomarkers to guide AKI management and predict AKI recovery and duration. It is important to note that these biomarkers would be used in addition to and not as a replacement for clinical assessment and standardized tests for kidney function such as S_{cr} and urine output.[32,33]

The advances in our knowledge of AKI pathophysiology as well as the advent of biomarkers has prompted ADQI to propose the use of two new terms "functional change" and "kidney damage."

TABLE 61-4 Classification of AKI Based on Functional and Kidney Damage Biomarkers

Loss of function	Kidney Damage	
	No	Yes
No	No loss of function or damage Biomarker negative KDIGO negative	Kidney damage without loss of function Biomarker positive KDIGO negative
Yes	Loss of function but no kidney damage KDIGO positive Biomarker negative	Loss of function and presence of kidney damage KDIGO positive Biomarker positive

AKI, acute kidney injury; KDIGO, Kidney Disease Improving Renal Outcomes.

Functional change refers to changes in glomerular and tubular function and includes markers such as S_{cr}, eGFR, and cystatin C. Kidney damage describes the presence of tubular and/or glomerular injury and includes markers such as TIMP-2 and IGFBP7. The rationale behind the proposed changes in terminology stems from the recognition of subclinical kidney injury. According to this, kidney injury may be detected by changes in the plasma or urinary levels of specific biomarkers before overt changes in kidney function (decreased eGFR or increased S_{cr}) have occurred. As a result, a patient may have kidney damage without a change in kidney function. Since this patient group is at a greater risk of complications, a longer stay in intensive care unit, and has a higher risk of dying when compared with the group without kidney damage, they may benefit from preventative interventions geared toward minimizing progression and toxicity (ie, avoidance or cessation of nephrotoxic drugs). The ADQI group has proposed the use of functional and damage markers, along with clinical information, to improve diagnostic accuracy, etiology, and staging of AKI.[33] Table 61-4 summarizes the relationship between functional change and kidney damage.[34,35]

Diagnostic Considerations

When the source of kidney injury is unclear after reviewing the patient's history, physical examination, and assessment of laboratory values, imaging techniques such as abdominal radiography, including the kidneys, ureters, and bladder (KUB), computed tomography (CT), and ultrasonography may be helpful. These may reveal small, shrunken kidneys indicative of CKD. Postrenal obstruction can often be identified with a renal ultrasonography and/or CT scan. Renal ultrasonography is also useful in detecting obstruction or hydronephrosis. Nephrolithiasis as small as 5 nm or a narrowing of the ureteral tract can be detected by ultrasonography or more sensitive tests, such as KUB and CT. When the cause of AKI is not evident, renal biopsies are useful in determining the cause in most patients. Because of the associated risk of bleeding, a renal biopsy is rarely undertaken and should only be performed in those circumstances when a definitive diagnosis is needed to guide therapy, such as the precise etiology of glomerulonephritis (see Chapter e66).

PREVENTION OF ACUTE KIDNEY INJURY

Prevention of AKI is critical since there is no treatment to reverse the insult once it has developed. Several nonpharmacologic and pharmacologic options to reduce the risk of AKI are described below.

Desired Outcomes

The goals of AKI prevention are to (a) screen and identify patients at risk, (b) monitor high-risk patients until the risk has subsided, and (c) implement prevention strategies when appropriate.

General Approach to Prevention

6 The choice of preventive strategy depends on the patient's risk factors for AKI such as comorbidities, planned procedures, and medications, to name a few.

Sometimes, the risk of kidney injury is predictable, such as in the setting of decreased perfusion secondary to compromised cardiac function (eg, post coronary bypass surgery) or secondary to the administration of a nephrotoxic agent like radiocontrast dye. In these situations, the potential insult to the kidneys cannot be avoided but may be preventable or minimized with intravenous fluids and/or avoidance or removal of any additional insults. In the inpatient setting, volume status optimization, hemodynamic support, and careful assessment of the risk versus benefit of potentially nephrotoxic medications are commonly recommended strategies for the prevention of AKI.

Nonpharmacologic and Pharmacologic Strategies for Prevention of AKI

Electronic Alert Systems

Advances in electronic health record (EHR) systems have led to the development of clinical decision support systems and electronic alerts designed to improve and standardize care in certain high-risk patient populations. Electronic alerts have been used for early detection of AKI and increased surveillance of patients on nephrotoxic medications. In general, alerts lead to greater implementation of the intervention, lower loss of kidney function, and decreased exposure to nephrotoxins.[36-38] For example, use of an EHR generated screening tool to identify pediatric patients receiving nephrotoxic medications and to recommend daily S_{cr} monitoring, switching a nephrotoxic drug to a non-nephrotoxic alternative or therapeutic drug monitoring, as appropriate has resulted in a 23% decrease in AKI rates and 42% decrease in AKI intensity.[39] Electronic alerts have the potential to reduce AKI by focusing on more appropriate medication prescribing and monitoring.

In addition to EHR systems, advances in machine learning technology have led to development of AKI risk prediction models. So far, there is an increasing amount of evidence that these machine learning models are effective in predicting AKI, typically within the following 24 to 72 hours.[40-42] While the application of machine learning in nephrology is still relatively new and not widely available in clinical practice, it has potential to improve patient outcomes in the future.

Intravenous Fluids

Intravenous fluids are one of the primary interventions that have consistently shown benefit and are routinely used in the prevention of AKI, particularly in patients with hemodynamic instability secondary to intravascular volume depletion as well as in patients receiving radiocontrast agents before a radiologic procedure.

Hemodynamic instability and systemic hypotension increase the risk of AKI as they can lead to decreased renal perfusion and subsequent kidney injury. Both isotonic crystalloids and colloid-containing solutions have been used for intravascular volume replacement. Among colloids, synthetic products such as hyperoncotic hydroxyethyl starch (HES) have been associated with impaired kidney function and should generally be avoided.[43] Albumin does not increase the risk of AKI and specific patient populations such as those with cirrhosis and spontaneous bacterial peritonitis may benefit from its therapy.[44] It has been hypothesized that albumin may offer additional advantages to septic patients as it is the main protein responsible for maintaining plasma colloid osmotic pressure, it has antioxidant and anti-inflammatory properties, and acts as a scavenger for reactive oxygen and nitrogen species. However, major patient outcomes such as risk of AKI, need for RRT, and mortality are comparable between albumin replacement therapy and isotonic saline.[45]

Now, the 2012 KDIGO guidelines recommend isotonic crystalloids over colloids for intravascular volume expansion in patients at risk for AKI.[3]

When using crystalloid solutions, options include either balanced solutions or isotonic saline. Use of balanced fluids over normal saline in acutely ill individuals likely decreases risk of AKI, need for RRT, and death.[46–48] The main concerns associated with the use of large amounts of saline are hyperchloremic acidosis since the chloride content in isotonic saline is 1.5 times that of plasma (154 mEq/L [mmol/L]). Hyperchloremia in turn can decrease renal artery blood flow and renal tissue perfusion. Further, saline infusions cause a greater increase in interstitial fluid volume than balanced solutions, which may result in increased renal volume and intracapsular pressure, decreased microvascular blood flow, and impaired kidney function.[49] On the other hand, balanced solutions such as Ringer's lactate, Hartmann's solution, and PlasmaLyte have an electrolyte composition similar to human plasma, and do not increase risk of hyperchloremic acidosis.

In addition to correcting hemodynamic instability and hypovolemia, fluids are the mainstay of therapy for the prevention of contrast-induced acute kidney injury (CI-AKI). CI-AKI is a common cause of ATN in the inpatient setting (see Chapter 65 for a detailed discussion of CI-AKI).[50]

While administration of intravenous fluids clearly has a critical role in AKI prevention, fluids need to be used judiciously as volume overload can have deleterious effects on the kidneys. The majority of crystalloid solutions redistribute into the interstitial space and can lead to interstitial edema, increased intraabdominal pressure, decreased renal oxygen delivery, and decreased GFR. In fact, poorer outcomes may be observed in patients with fluid overload including increased risk of AKI and decreased recovery of kidney function.[51] Hence, fluid administration beyond reestablishing euvolemia is generally not recommended.

Glycemic Control

In critical illness, both hyper- and hypoglycemia are associated with adverse patient outcomes.[52] Hyperglycemia can occur secondary to stress, inflammation, or medications (eg, steroids) while hypoglycemia can develop secondary to decreased clearance of insulin, interruptions in nutrition support prior to procedures, or tight insulin protocols. Tight glycemic control with target glucose levels of 80 to 110 mg/dL (4.4-6.1 mmol/L) may significantly decrease the risk of AKI and this has been adopted in the ICU setting.[53,54] However, tight glycemic control protocols may also increase risk of hypoglycemia and mortality.[52,55,56] As a result, a more moderate approach to glycemic control is favored in the critically ill. Guidelines from the American Diabetes Association and Surviving Sepsis Campaign recommend a glycemic target range of 140 to 180 mg/dL (7.8-10 mmol/L) and less than 180 mg/dL (10 mmol/L), respectively, in critically ill patients.[57,58]

TREATMENT OF ACUTE KIDNEY INJURY

7 Since there is no specific treatment that can reverse AKI or hasten its recovery, supportive measures that focus on hemodynamics, fluid balance, acid-base balance, and electrolyte homeostasis are the mainstays of therapy.

Desired Outcomes

Short-term goals of AKI management include minimizing the degree of insult to the kidney, reducing extrarenal complications, and expediting the patient's recovery of kidney function. Therapy should focus on maintaining organ functions while sustaining mean arterial pressure goals. The ultimate goal is to have the patient's kidney function restored to pre-AKI baseline.

General Approach to Treatment

Identification and management of AKI should be prompt. At times, the most effective method for managing AKI may be treatment of the precipitating event. A review of a patient's medications should be conducted to determine if a nephrotoxic agent could be the potential cause of AKI. Additionally, if possible, exposure to nephrotoxic agents should be limited either by discontinuation or switching to a less nephrotoxic option. Prerenal AKI should be managed with hemodynamic support and volume replacement, intrinsic AKI management relies on managing the cause and providing supportive care, and postrenal AKI therapy should focus on removing the cause of the obstruction. At the same time, patient's comorbidities need to be reviewed, as disease states such as cardiac and liver failure may require introduce additional management challenges.

Pharmacologic and Nonpharmacologic Strategies for Treatment of AKI

There is no cure for AKI. Thus, management of AKI focuses on supportive care and managing resultant complications, which includes hemodynamic instability, fluid overload, electrolyte imbalances, and acid-base abnormalities. In initial stages of AKI or mild disease, pharmacologic therapy may be sufficient, but patients with more severe AKI, RRT may be necessary to maintain fluid, electrolyte, and acid-base balance while removing accumulating waste products or toxins.

Fluid Management

Maintaining an adequate fluid status is imperative but also challenging, working to balance the need for volume resuscitation and fluid overload. First-line therapies for volume resuscitation consist of intravenous fluids, while fluid overload may need to be treated with loop diuretics or RRT.[3] Additionally, administration of all intravenous fluids should also be evaluated to determine if any notable reduction in daily intake can be achieved. This can be accomplished by concentrating intravenous medications to deliver less fluid overall or switching intravenous medication to the enteral route.

Intravenous Fluids

The principle of fluid therapy is to maintain or restore effective intravascular volume to assure adequate renal perfusion. In selected settings such as sepsis, low oncotic pressures and leaky vasculature can pose a challenge by leading to excessive extracellular fluid and anasarca with intravenous fluid administration. Similar to preventative hydration strategies, intravenous fluids need to be used judiciously as both volume depletion and fluid overload can adversely affect kidney function and increase morbidity and mortality.

Intravenous fluids should be administered to patients who have a prerenal AKI caused by hypovolemia or patients experiencing hemodynamic instability resulting from hypovolemia. The goal of fluid administration should be to restore and maintain euvolemia. In order to reduce the risk for fluid overload, slower correction strategies with either small intravenous boluses or short-term infusions of crystalloid fluids should be administered. Frequent reassessment of volume and hemodynamic status should be completed to determine further need for or changes to fluid therapy. As previously noted, balanced crystalloid solutions may be preferred for patients requiring IV fluids (eg, resuscitation) since isotonic saline has been associated with hyperchloremic metabolic acidosis and death in critically ill adults.[47,59,60] The patient should be monitored for fluid intake (both enteral and intravenous), urine output, insensible losses (ie, vomiting, diarrhea, excessive perspiration) which may not be captured in overall documented daily totals of fluid loss, pulmonary and peripheral edema, blood pressure (target mean arterial pressure ≥65 mm Hg), and serum electrolytes. Urine output ≥0.5 mL/kg/hr is generally targeted during the initial fluid resuscitation phase.[57] Assessing

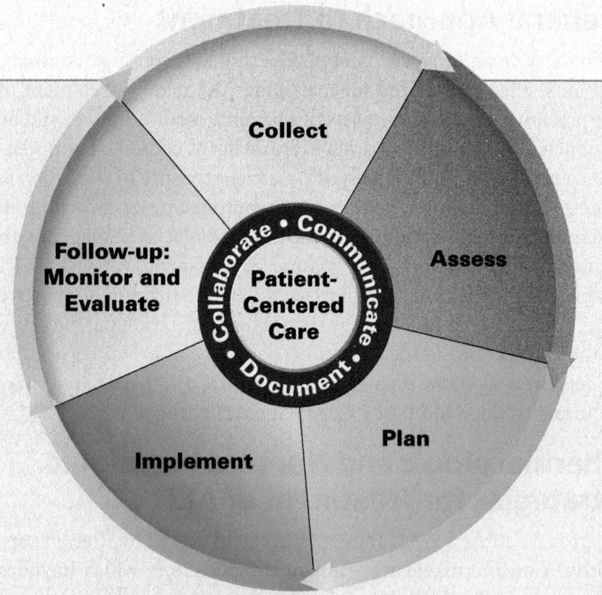

Patient Care Process for Acute Kidney Injury

Collect

- Patient characteristics (eg, age, sex)
- Chief complaint/reason for admission
- Patient medical history including other relate comorbid conditions (eg, CKD, diabetes, HTN, cirrhosis)
- Current medication list
- Baseline serum creatinine (if available)
- Volume status (low fluid volume eg, dehydration), urine output
- Hemodynamic (eg, blood pressure, mean arterial pressure)
- Urinalysis results (eg, WBCs, RBCs, protein, granular casts, FE_{Na}) (see Table 61-2)
- Kidney imaging results (eg, obstruction, hydronephrosis)

Assess

- Stage and severity of AKI using KDIGO criteria (Table 61-1)
- Most likely type of AKI (Fig. 61-2)
- Presence of baseline CKD
- Presence of sepsis, severe sepsis, or septic shock
- Presence of electrolyte disturbances
- RRT modality and parameters if applicable (Fig. 61-3)

Plan*

- Assess direction and degree of changing kidney function
- Review all medications for appropriateness and ensure doses and frequencies are adjusted for patient's current kidney function and RRT
- Evaluate presence and eliminate any potential nephrotoxins
- Need for electrolyte corrections
- Identify any renally eliminated medications with narrow therapeutic indexes. Recommend therapeutic drug monitoring when necessary

Implement*

- Formulate a management plan for any necessary medication additions, deletions or dose alterations
- Communicate treatment plant to the patient's primary team and nephrology team (if consulted)
- Document therapy recommendations including dose adjustments and follow-up assessment plans in the patient's electronic health record or chart
- Provide patient education regarding all elements of treatment plan (when possible)

Follow-up: Monitor and Evaluate (Table 61-7)

- Changes in kidney function (eg, changes in S_{cr}, urine output, continued need for RRT or changes in the RRT approach)
- Hemodynamic and volume status
- Electrolytes, acid-base status
- Response to the medication regimen including any potential adverse events
- Patient adherence to treatment plan using multiple sources of information
- Overall clinical status and management progression

Collaborate with patient, caregivers, and other healthcare professionals.

documentation of fluid balance in the EHR should consider that a patient's independent drinking or urinary voiding or excessive perspiration may not be captured. When this occurs, changes in a patient's weight can assist in validating fluid status.

If AKI is a result of blood loss or is complicated by symptomatic anemia, red blood cell transfusion to a hemoglobin >7 g/dL (70 g/L; 4.34 mmol/L) is the treatment of choice.[57] Once a hemoglobin of >7 g/dL (70 g/L; 4.34 mmol/L) is reached, balanced solutions or normal saline can be used to restore intravascular volume. In patients with cardiac failure, fluids should only be administered if intravascular volume is depleted. Albumin is typically preferred in individuals with severe hypoalbuminemia secondary to cirrhosis or nephrotic syndrome.[44] In critically ill patients with vasodilatory shock, vasopressors such as norepinephrine and vasopressin may be used in conjunction with fluids in order to maintain adequate hemodynamics and renal perfusion.[3]

Diuretics

Loop diuretics are frequently prescribed for the management of fluid overload in patients with established kidney injury and often as a precursor to RRT. Loop diuretics have several theoretical advantages: increased urine output, decreased risk of ischemic injury by inhibiting the Na-K-Cl cotransporter and thus decreasing oxygen demand, and enhanced renal blood flow due to increased availability of renal prostaglandins. Enhancing urine output from oliguric to nonoliguric may be beneficial in itself, as nonoliguric AKI is associated with better outcomes than oliguric AKI.[61] However, even though loop diuretics increase urine output, they may not improve patient outcomes (ie, mortality, need for RRT) for patients with established AKI.[61,62] Therefore, the KDIGO guidelines recommend limiting the use of loop diuretics to the management of fluid overload and avoiding their use for the purpose of treatment of AKI.[3]

Diuretic resistance is a relatively common problem in patients with AKI for several reasons. Excessive sodium administration (eg, normal saline) may override the ability of the diuretics to eliminate sodium. Also, patients with ATN have a reduced number of functioning nephrons on which the diuretic may exert its action upon. In other clinical states such as glomerulonephritis, heavy proteinuria can occur. In these patients, intraluminal loop diuretics cannot exert their effect in the loop of Henle if they are extensively bound to proteins present in the urine. Still other patients may have greatly reduced bioavailability of oral furosemide because of intestinal edema, often associated with high preload states, which further reduces oral furosemide absorption. Lastly, the braking phenomenon, which is a progressively decreasing response to natriuresis associated with repeated administration of a loop diuretic, may also lead to diuretic resistance.[61,63] Table 61-5 includes possible therapeutic options to counteract each form of diuretic resistance.

The most common therapeutic option to overcome diuretic resistance is to use higher doses of intravenous loop diuretics. Often, patients with impaired kidney function have lower rates of diuretic secretion into the tubular fluid; consequently, higher doses of loop diuretics are prescribed. Caution must be taken when increasing intermittent bolus doses as the risk of adverse reactions such as ototoxicity also increases due to higher corresponding peak concentrations achieved too quickly. To avoid rapid high peak concentrations when using furosemide, doses of less than 160 mg can be administered undiluted no faster than a rate of 20 to 40 mg/minute, whereas doses exceeding 160 mg can be diluted and administered via a short infusion at a rate no faster than 4 mg/min. Another option to avoid high peak concentrations and post-diuretic sodium retention is to administer loop diuretics as a continuous infusion. Administration via a continuous infusion can achieve the same degree of diuresis with lower doses and results in no difference in mortality or hospital length of stay. An initial loading dose is recommended prior to the initiation of a continuous infusion of furosemide or its equivalent to decrease the time to the medication's onset of action.[63] One disadvantage of using a continuous infusion is it requires more extensive and frequent monitoring, as infusion rates are usually based on an hourly urine output goal. Typically, increasing intermittent bolus doses or increasing dosing frequency are trialed before implementing the more labor-intensive continuous infusion strategy.

Another approach to overcome diuretic resistance in AKI is to use a loop diuretic in combination with a diuretic from a different pharmacologic class. Diuretics that work at the distal convoluted tubule (chlorothiazide and metolazone) or the collecting duct (amiloride, triamterene, and spironolactone) may have a synergistic effect when administered with loop diuretics by blocking the compensatory increase in sodium and chloride reabsorption (see Chapter 68, Disorders of Sodium and Water Homeostasis). Thiazide diuretics are most commonly used in combination with loop diuretics. Oral metolazone is used most often because, unlike other thiazides, it produces effective diuresis at a CL_{cr} less than 20 mL/min (0.33 mL/s). Oral metolazone is frequently given 30 minutes prior to intravenous loop diuretics to achieve peak effects at the same time to potentially enhance diuresis. The combination of thiazide and thiazide-type diuretics and a loop diuretic has been used successfully in the management of fluid overload. When such combinations are used, the regimen should be assessed for any improved or enhanced diuresis and determine if the regimen should be continued.[63]

While diuretic strategies are being used, symptoms of ototoxicity, fluid status, and serum creatinine and electrolytes (ie, potassium, sodium, magnesium, calcium, BUN) should be closely monitored, especially with aggressive strategies such as larger doses of diuretics and continuous infusions. The goal of diuretic therapy in the setting of fluid overload is to achieve adequate urine output to accomplish a net negative diuresis. Net negative diuresis, or achieving a fluid output that is higher than fluid intake, is desired. Strict intake and output measures are best accomplished when a patient has a urinary catheter to monitor urine volume or is located in the intensive care unit where any changes are frequently assessed and documented. In patients who do not have a urinary catheter, accurate assessment of urine output can be challenging and a patient's weight should be closely followed. Daily goals for diuretic therapy should be a net negative diuresis of 500 to 1,000 mL of urine per day or a weight loss of 0.5 to 1 kg per day as tolerated. Once a patient has reached euvolemic status, diuretics should either be discontinued or dose adjusted to maintain the patient's fluid balance.

TABLE 61-5 Common Causes of Diuretic Resistance in Patients with AKI

Causes of Diuretic Resistance	Potential Therapeutic Solutions
Excessive sodium intake (sources may be dietary, IV fluids, and drugs)	Remove sodium from nutritional sources and medications
Inadequate diuretic dose or inappropriate regimen	Increase dose, increase frequency, use continuous infusion or add thiazide
Reduced oral bioavailability (usually furosemide)	Use parenteral therapy, switch to oral torsemide or bumetanide
Nephrotic syndrome (loop diuretic protein binding in tubule lumen)	Increase dose, add thiazide
Reduced renal blood flow	
Drugs (NSAIDs, ACEIs, vasodilators)	Discontinue these drugs if possible
Intravascular depletion	Intravascular volume expansion
Increased sodium resorption	
Distal nephron hyperthrophy	Add thiazide, sodium restriction
Postdiuretic sodium retention	Dietary sodium restriction, use continuous infusion
Heart failure	Assess effective circulatory volume, increase dose, increase frequency, use continuous infusion
Cirrhosis	Assess effective circulatory volume, consider paracentesis
Acute tubular necrosis	Increase diuretic dose, diuretic combination therapy

ACEIs, angiotensin-converting enzyme inhibitors; NSAIDs, nonsteroidal anti-inflammatory drugs.

Electrolyte and Acid-Base Management

The most common electrolyte disorder encountered in AKI patients is hyperkalemia, as >90% of potassium is renally eliminated. Life-threatening cardiac arrhythmias may occur with serum potassium concentrations greater than 6 mEq/L (mmol/L), so frequent monitoring of potassium is essential. Medications and foods with high amounts of potassium (antibiotics, oral phosphorous replacement powders, alkalinizers, potassium salt substitutes) should be avoided (see Chapter 70, Disorders of Potassium and Magnesium Homeostasis). Some medications may promote potassium retention by the kidneys (spironolactone, eplerenone, finerenone) and should also be avoided or closely monitored if used (see Chapter 70). In general, exogenous potassium supplementation should be avoided in patients with AKI unless warranted by the presence of hypokalemia. Medications that can cause an increase of potassium such as ACE inhibitors, ARBs, and sulfamethoxazole-trimethoprim should be avoided.

Other electrolytes abnormalities include hyperphosphatemia and hypocalcemia. These electrolytes are eliminated by the kidneys and, unlike potassium, are not efficiently removed by dialysis. Hyperphosphatemia can be particularly high in patients with tissue destruction (eg, trauma, rhabdomyolysis, and tumor lysis syndrome) due to substantial amounts of phosphorus released from the destroyed tissue. Typically, the dietary intake of phosphorus needs to be restricted in advanced stages of AKI. When phosphorus is particularly high, phosphate binding agents (eg, calcium acetate, sevelamer hydrochloride) may be considered. Caution should be taken when using calcium-containing phosphate binding agents or calcium-containing antacids in situations where hypercalcemia is present to prevent precipitation of calcium phosphate which can lead to soft tissue calcification. In contrast to the patient with CKD, AKI patients do not usually develop calcium imbalance secondary to the limited duration of the illness. Hypocalcemia can develop as a result of hyperphosphatemia; thus, the treatment of hyperphosphatemia should correct the imbalance. Additionally, hypocalcemia can be seen in patients who are receiving continuous renal replacement therapy (CRRT) along with a concomitant infusion of regional citrate being used for anticoagulation. Typically, citrate is infused before the renal replacement machine's dialyzer/hemofilter to bind serum calcium in order to prevent the extracorporeal circuit from clotting which leaves less calcium to return to circulation. Since severe hypocalcemia can result in arrhythmias or even death, frequent monitoring of unbound serum calcium concentrations and supplementation with parenteral calcium is necessary to maintain normocalcemia.

Metabolic acidosis can also occur in patients with severe AKI due to the kidney's inability to adequately excrete acid. This can be a result of AKI itself or from other conditions that are common in critically ill patients, such as shock due to severe hypoperfusion. Determining and correcting the underlying cause of the acid-base imbalance is imperative. Supplementation with bicarbonate therapy can be utilized in patients with mild acidosis to temporarily correct the derangement. RRT may need to be initiated if the underlying cause cannot be reversed promptly or in patients with severe life-threatening acidosis.

Nutritional Considerations in AKI

Nutritional management of critically ill patients with AKI can be extremely complex, as it needs to account for metabolic derangements resulting from both impaired kidney function and underlying disease processes, as well as the effects of RRT on nutrient balance. Loss of the normal physiologic and metabolic functions of the kidney and the hypercatabolic response to stress and injury will have an impact on the metabolism of nutrients. Derangements in glucose, lipid, and protein metabolism result in hyperglycemia and insulin resistance, hypertriglyceridemia, protein catabolism, and negative nitrogen balance. The latter, in particular, is problematic to manage, as increased amino acid turnover and skeletal muscle breakdown lead to muscle wasting and malnutrition that does not respond well to increasing exogenous protein supplementation. The KDIGO guidelines recommend a caloric intake goal of 20 to 30 kcal/kg/day (84-126 kJ/kg/day) irrespective of the stage of kidney impairment and preferentially through the enteral route. In the setting of noncatabolic AKI without need for dialysis, 0.8 to 1 g/kg/day of protein is suggested and 1 to 1.5 g/kg/day if patient is receiving RRT.[3] CRRT is associated with an increased removal of small water-soluble molecules such as amino acids and certain nutrients. As a result, hypercatabolic patients receiving CRRT will typically have higher protein requirements up to a maximum of 1.7 g/kg/day.[3] The Society of Critical Care Medicine (SCCM) and American Society for Parenteral and Enteral Nutrition (ASPEN) guidelines for nutrition in patients with AKI recommend a caloric intake goal of 25 to 30 kcal/kg/day (105-126 kJ/kg/day). In the ICU setting, up to 2.5 g/kg/day of protein is suggested if patient is receiving RRT.[64]

Renal Replacement Therapy

8 Renal replacement therapy is often utilized to treat life threatening indications resulting from severe AKI. These indications include fluid overload, electrolyte disturbances (eg, hyperkalemia), acid-base imbalances, uremic complications, oliguria or anuria, and pulmonary edema from fluid overload. Multiple factors influence decisions to initiate dialysis including specific timing and type of modality.[3,65-69] The most common indications for initiation of RRT are summarized in Table 61-6. In the setting of AKI, the mode of delivery of RRT can be either intermittent hemodialysis or continuous RRT and the chosen modality usually depends on physician preference and the resources (ie, healthcare professionals, machines) available. No difference in mortality or dialysis dependence has been shown between patients who received continuous or intermittent forms of RRT; however, continuous RRT is generally preferred in hemodynamically unstable patients.[3,67,70]

TABLE 61-6 Common Indications for RRT

Indication for RRT	Clinical Setting
A: *acid-base abnormalities*	Metabolic acidosis (especially if pH <7.2)
E: *electrolyte imbalance*	Severe hyperkalemia and/or hypermagnesemia
I: *intoxications*	Salicylates, lithium, methanol, ethylene glycol, theophylline, phenobarbital
O: fluid overload	Fluid overload (especially pulmonary edema unresponsive to diuretics)
U: uremia	Uremia or associated complications (neuropathy, encephalopathy, pericarditis)

RRT, renal replacement therapy.

Intermittent Hemodialysis Intermittent hemodialysis (IHD) is the most frequently used RRT (see Chapter 64). Hemodialysis treatments usually last 3 to 4 hours and thus can achieve the rapid removal of volume and solutes and thereby contribute to correction of most of the electrolyte abnormalities associated with AKI. The primary challenge with this modality is hypotension, which is typically caused by the rapid removal of intravascular volume over a short period of time. Achieving prompt venous access for dialysis can be difficult in hypotensive patients and can limit the effectiveness of IHD. This can result in a lack of solute clearance, an inability to correct metabolic derangements, continued volume overload, and can lead to delayed recovery because of further ischemic insults to the kidneys. Patients with dialysis-dependent CKD generally achieve adequate solute and volume control with three times weekly dialysis, but hypercatabolic, fluid-overloaded patients with AKI may require more frequent hemodialysis treatments. Chapter 64 provides a detailed explanation of the principles and processes of IHD.

Continuous Renal Replacement Therapy CRRT is a viable option to manage hemodynamically unstable patients with AKI, especially those who cannot tolerate rapid volume removal. Unlike IHD treatments that last a few hours, CRRT runs continuously 24 hours a day, providing a slower and more consistent removal of solutes and fluid over time. In general, CRRT can achieve a greater amount of solute removal with higher mean arterial pressures compared with IHD in critically ill patients with AKI.[70] CRRT use is most commonly considered for those patients with higher acuity because of their intolerance of IHD-associated hypotension. The KDIGO guidelines suggest using CRRT over IHD in hemodynamically unstable patients.[3]

Several CRRT variants have been developed, including continuous venovenous hemofiltration (CVVH), continuous venovenous hemodialysis (CVVHD), and continuous venovenous hemodiafiltration (CVVHDF). These modalities differ in the degree of both their solute removal as well as fluid clearance and the modality chosen is based on an individual patient's needs. The removal of solutes and fluid can be achieved via three different mechanisms: diffusion, convection, and membrane adsorption. In CVVH, solute and fluid clearance is primarily a result of convection, the active transport of drug molecules at the concentration at which they exist in plasma water into the ultrafiltrate using a pump-driven pressure gradient, known as "solvent drag," then fluid absent of solutes is replaced (Fig. 61-3). CVVHD provides a more extensive solute removal that works primarily by diffusion, where solute molecules passively move down a concentration gradient from an area of higher concentration (plasma) pass through the dialysis membrane to an area of lower concentration (dialysate). CVVHDF combines both convection and hemodialysis, achieving even higher solute and fluid removal rates (Fig. 61-3).

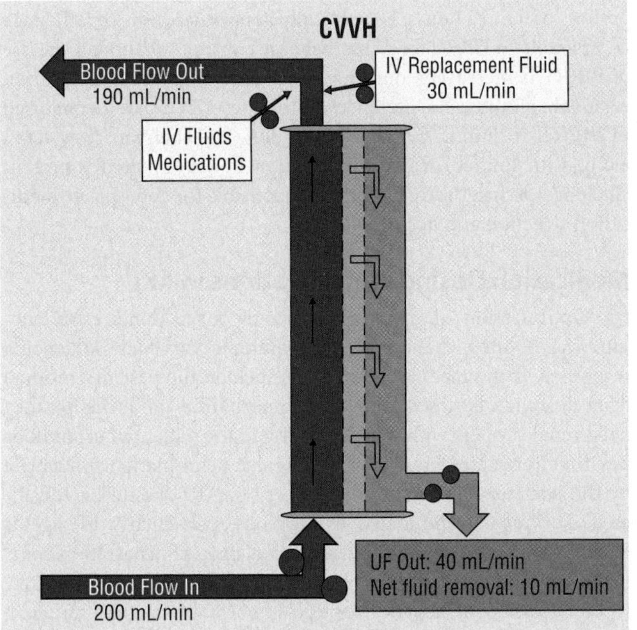

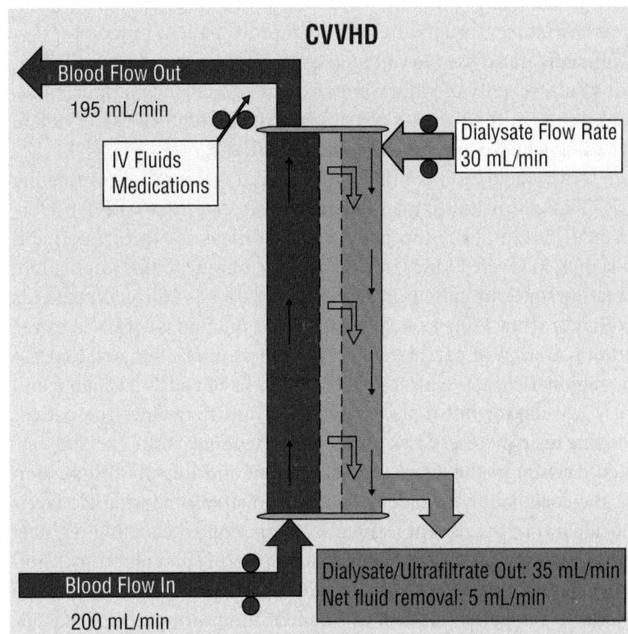

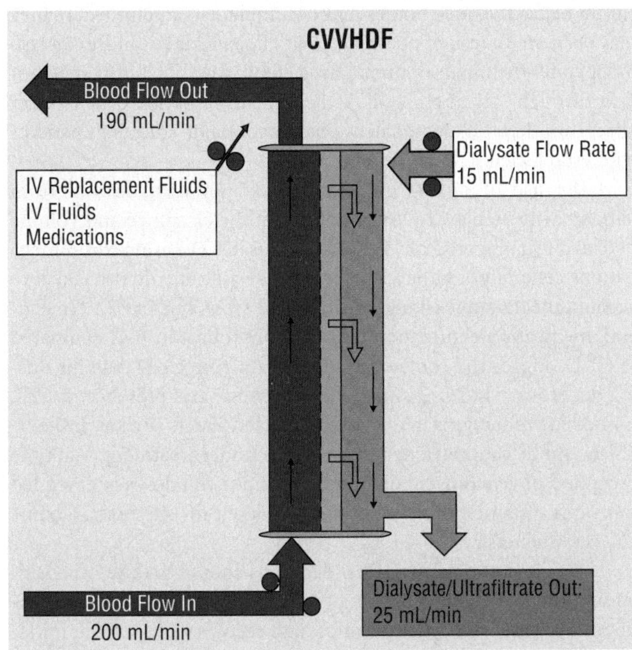

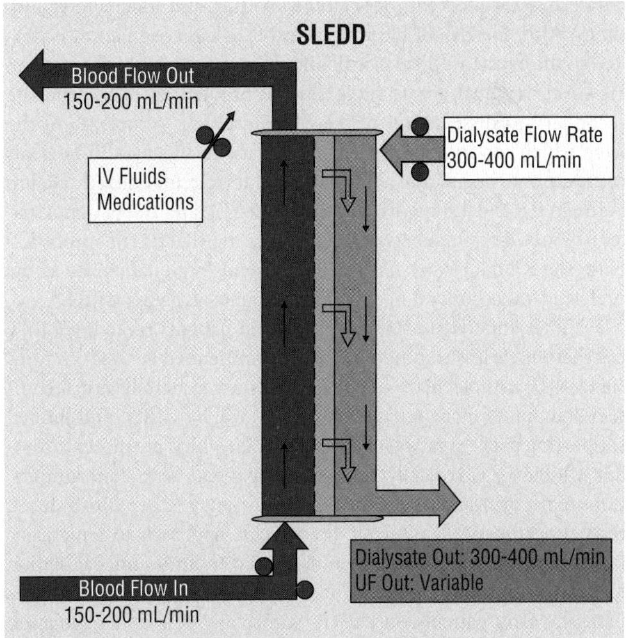

FIGURE 61-3 Several renal replacement therapies are commonly used in patients with acute kidney injury (AKI), including one of the three primary continuous renal replacement therapy (CRRT) variants: (a) continuous venovenous hemofiltration (CVVH), (b) continuous venovenous hemodialysis (CVVHD), (c) continuous venovenous hemodiafiltration (CVVHDF), and the hybrid intermittent hemodialysis therapy, and (d) sustained low-efficiency daily dialysis (SLEDD). The blood circuit in each diagram is represented in red, the hemofilter/dialyzer membrane is yellow, and the ultrafiltration/dialysate compartment is brown. Excess body water and accumulated endogenous waste products are removed solely by convection when CVVH is employed. With CVVHD, waste products are predominantly removed as the result of passive diffusion from the blood, where they are in high concentration to the dialysate. The degree of fluid removal that is accomplished by convection is usually minimal. CVVHDF uses convection to a degree similar to that employed during CVVH as well as diffusion, and thus is often associated with the highest clearance of medications and waste products. Finally, SLEDD employs lower blood and dialysate flow rates than intermittent hemodialysis (IHD), but because of its extended duration, it is a gentler means of achieving adequate waste product and fluid removal.

Optimal timing of CRRT initiation has not been clearly established. Whether early initiation of RRT has improved morbidity and mortality benefit versus delaying RRT to allow for the possibility for a patient to recover function without needing RRT has been the subject of considerable debate. In situations when severe or life-threatening complications of AKI are present such as oliguria, pulmonary edema, or metabolic disorders (eg, acidosis, hyperkalemia, uremia), the indication for CRRT is clear. However, in the absence of such complications, the exact timing of CRRT initiation is uncertain. In fact, early initiation of CRRT at the onset of AKI may not demonstrate a mortality benefit or improve patient outcomes.[66,71,72] Clinicians are advised to carefully consider the patient's overall clinical status, severity of kidney impairment and related complications, and trends in the patient's physiologic and laboratory values before deciding whether and when to initiate CRRT.[68]

Anticoagulation is a major consideration for patients receiving CRRT as circuit clotting and filter patency can limit CRRT performance. It is important to note that the drivers for thrombosis and bleeding in severe kidney impairment are unique to this population, creating some limitations in applying approaches utilized in patients with more intact function. Typical anticoagulation is achieved by the administration of parenteral agents such as unfractionated heparin or regional citrate. Unfractionated heparin is widely available and easy to monitor but it also systemically anticoagulates the patient leading to an increased risk of bleeding. Regional citrate chelates ionized calcium in the extracorporeal circuit and impairs progression of the coagulation cascade. In order to maintain physiologic levels of calcium in the patient's systemic circulation when using regional citrate, most protocols require infusion of parenteral calcium (ie, calcium chloride or calcium gluconate) prior to returning the blood to the patient as well as frequent monitoring of ionized calcium levels. When compared to unfractionated heparin, regional citrate is associated with less circuit clotting and longer filter lifetimes. Also, the risk of bleeding is lower as anticoagulation is limited to the extracorporeal circuit and does not extend to the patient. However, regional citrate increases the production of bicarbonate secondary to dissociation of the calcium-citrate complexes in the liver, which can increase the risk of metabolic alkalosis.[73] The goals of citrate anticoagulation are to maintain the circuit ionized calcium between 0.8 and 1.6 mg/dL (0.2-0.4 mmol/L), and the patient's systemic ionized calcium between 4.4 and 5.2 mg/dL (1.1-1.3 mmol/L).[3] Now, the KDIGO Work Group recommends regional citrate as the preferred anticoagulant of choice for patients receiving CRRT.[3]

Other anticoagulants may be used in patients receiving CRRT but their use is less common or only recommended in select circumstances. Low-molecular weight heparins are generally not recommended due to increased cost, poor removal by CRRT, and limited supporting data. Argatroban or bivalirudin, which are direct thrombin inhibitors, is typically reserved for patients with contraindications to heparin such as antithrombin deficiency or heparin-induced thrombocytopenia.[3,73] Overall, the specific approach to anticoagulation depends on whether there is a need to limit anticoagulation to the circuit alone or extend it to systemically anticoagulate the patient. Many patients on CRRT require systemic anticoagulation for an underlying comorbidity (eg, atrial fibrillation and artificial heart valve) and will not need additional anticoagulation for RRT. As a result, the need for anticoagulation and the specific anticoagulant of choice should be tailored to individual patient requirements and corresponding indications.

Challenges with CRRT may include limited availability of the specialized equipment and other resources necessary to provide the treatments and to individualize the IV replacement, dialysate fluids, and medication therapy adjustments. Also, medication dosing requirements for patients who are receiving CRRT are complex and not clearly defined.[74] CRRT use is most commonly considered for those patients with higher acuity because of their intolerance of IHD-associated hypotension. The KDIGO guidelines suggest using CRRT over IHD in hemodynamically unstable patients.[3]

Prolonged Intermittent Renal Replacement Therapies An alternative to CRRT is prolonged intermittent RRT (PIRRT), which has had a variety of names including extended-duration IHD, hybrid IHD, sustained low-efficiency dialysis (SLED), or sustained low efficiency daily dialysis (SLEDD) (see Fig. 61-3). These therapies use conventional dialysis machines but lower blood (150-200 mL/min) and dialysate (300-400 mL/min) flow rates with extended treatment periods of 6 to 12 hours. For critically ill patients with AKI, they are comparable to CRRT for hemodynamic control.[69] Although the use of PIRRT is increasing, our knowledge of its impact on medication removal is limited.[75] Differences in the prescribed parameters used in PIRRT, including frequency, duration, and dialysate flow rates, along with limited data on medication dosing in PIRRT present challenges to healthcare providers responsible for appropriate medication selection and dosing.[76-78]

Medication Dosing Considerations in AKI

9 Optimization of medication therapy for patients experiencing AKI is often challenging. The multiple variables influencing responses to the medication regimen include the patient's residual drug clearance, fluid accumulation, comorbidities, and whether they need renal support with RRT. In addition, the patient's current kidney function state and corresponding drug elimination influenced by the decline, stabilization or recovery of AKI should be considered. For renally eliminated medications, particularly for agents with a narrow therapeutic range, serum drug concentration measurements and assessment of pharmacodynamic responses are likely to be necessary. If hepatic function is normal, choosing an agent eliminated primarily by the liver may be preferred. However, renally eliminated active metabolites may accumulate to a point where they may elicit an undesired pharmacologic effect. Kidney failure can also independently impair nonrenal drug elimination including metabolism through "organ crosstalk," where the dysfunction of one organ affects another.[79] Unfortunately, pharmacokinetic studies in patients with established AKI are limited.

The use of dosing guidelines based on data derived from patients with stable CKD may not reflect the clearance and volume of distribution in critically ill AKI patients. CKD dosing recommendations generally assume a stable rate of decline and do not take into account the dynamic changes seen in AKI (see Chapter 67).[74] In general, medication elimination may be more robust in AKI compared to CKD, suggesting some caution with utilizing CKD data for dosing decisions.[80] In some situations with sepsis and presence of AKI, immediate reductions in dosing for selected agents such as antibiotics should be cautioned as it may lead to under treatment. With the exception of vancomycin or aminoglycosides, full doses or extended infusions of antibiotics should be considered for the first 24 hours and reevaluated.[81]

Pharmacotherapy regimen decisions should take into consideration the four distinct phases of AKI described earlier, specifically initiation, extension, maintenance, and recovery phase. The initiation and extension phases occur right after the kidney insult. First, a clinical determination should be made about the severity of AKI and degree of residual renal clearance. Then, in order to determine if medication therapy modifications are needed, the clinician should consider the goals of therapy, the specific pharmacokinetics of the medication, the potential for increased risk for an adverse drug event, and therapeutic drug monitoring (if available) (see Fig. 61-4). In AKI, the severity and timing of the decline in kidney function is relatively unpredictable, so frequent monitoring and reevaluation of medication dosing is necessary. Urine output is a good surrogate marker to monitor kidney function and prospectively assess where kidney function is trending. S_{cr} measurements lag behind

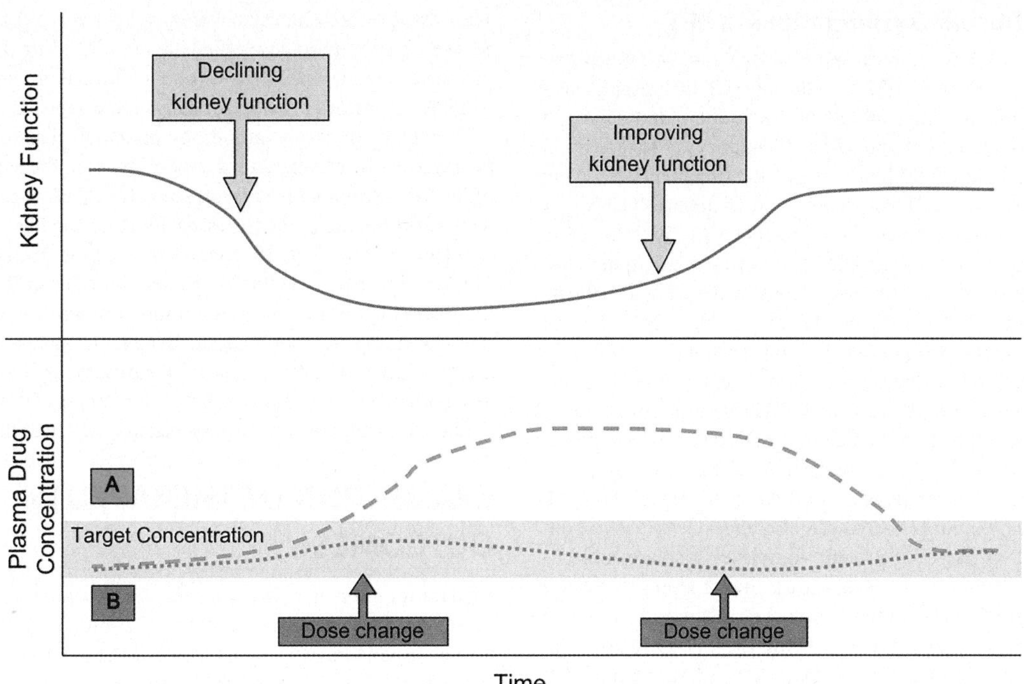

FIGURE 61-4 Relationship between kidney function changes in AKI and dosing of renally eliminated drugs. As kidney function fluctuates in AKI, plasma drug concentrations will be affected. (A) If no dosing adjustments are made, then this will lead to supratherapeutic concentrations [depicted by green line] which can lead to adverse effects. In order to maintain target drug concentrations, dosing adjustments should be made as fluctuations occur. (B) When kidney function declines, a dosing regimen should be adjusted by decreasing the dose or frequency to maintain plasma drug concentrations in the therapeutic range [depicted by red line]. When kidney function improves, the dosing regimen should be changed by increasing the dose or frequency.

kidney function; that is, today's S_{cr} measurements typically reflect yesterday's kidney function, and thus, S_{cr} is not a good marker for monitoring kidney function. In the next phase, maintenance, kidney function stabilizes and medication therapy regimens may require fewer alterations. The fourth and final phase is recovery, where AKI begins to resolve and there may be a need to increase the medication dose due to enhanced renal clearance. It is critically important to follow the patient closely and recognize trends for decreasing or improving kidney function in an effort to achieve and maintain medication therapy management goals.

Edema, which is common in AKI, can increase the volume of distribution of many medications, particularly water-soluble compounds with relatively small volumes of distribution. Increased fluid distribution into the tissues (ie, sepsis and anasarca in heart failure) can also contribute to a larger volume of distribution for many medications and thereby reduce the proportion of medication in the plasma that is available to be removed by the kidneys. Because AKI frequently occurs in critically ill patients, multisystem organ failure is often an accompanying problem. In addition to volume overload, reductions in cardiac output or liver function can alter the pharmacokinetic profile of most medications. For selected renally eliminated medications or related metabolites with narrow therapeutic windows, close follow-up and dosing adjustments may be necessary.[74,75]

If rapid onset of activity is desired, a loading dose may be necessary to promptly achieve desired serum concentrations because the expanded volume of distribution and the prolonged elimination half-life extend the time (3.5 times the half-life) needed to reach steady-state concentrations. Maintenance dosing regimens should be reviewed frequently and be based on the assessment of the patient's most current kidney function. A dose that provides the desired serum concentration on 1 day may be inappropriate a few days later if there is a change in the patient's fluid status or kidney function has dramatically changed, or if RRT is initiated, changed, or discontinued (see Fig. 61-4).[74]

Medication therapy individualization in patients with AKI is complicated by the fact that patients with AKI may have a higher residual nonrenal clearance than patients with CKD who have a similar CL_{cr}.[74] Alterations in the activity of some, but not all, cytochrome P450 enzymes have been demonstrated in patients with CKD.[79,80] This may be the result of less accumulation of uremic waste products that may alter hepatic function. If a patient with AKI has higher than anticipated nonrenal clearance, this would result in more robust elimination leading to lower than expected, possibly subtherapeutic, serum concentrations. For example, to maintain comparable serum concentrations, the imipenem dose requirement in patients with AKI would be 2,000 mg divided daily as compared with the recommended dosage for patients with ESRD of 1,000 mg daily. As AKI persists, the nonrenal clearance values approach those observed in patients with CKD.[82] Another challenge associated with medication dosing in patients with AKI is that much of the dosing-related data were acquired in patients with CKD, with initial pharmacokinetic assessments done after single-dose administration. The determination of pharmacokinetic parameters using a single-dose model may result in overestimated initial medication removal secondary to simultaneous distribution from the plasma to the tissue.[83] In conclusion, the application of dosing regimens derived from patients with CKD and ESRD in addition to the use of more aggressive RRT approaches may result in underdosing of certain medications and thereby contribute to less than optimal clinical outcomes.

Medication Dosing Considerations in RRT

There are several physicochemical and pharmacokinetic characteristics that can alter medication clearance during RRT, including molecular weight, protein binding, volume of distribution, and degree of renal clearance or fraction eliminated by the kidneys.[83,84] Medication dosage regimen design considerations specific to patients receiving peritoneal dialysis and IHD are presented in Chapter 67. However, medication-dosing requirements for patients with AKI or CKD who are receiving CRRT are complex and not as clearly defined as in IHD.[74,81] Inadequately dosed medications in critically ill patients with AKI requiring RRT may be one factor contributing to the lack of improving outcomes with newer RRT approaches.

In general, RRT-mediated medication clearance is inversely related to molecular weight, such that RRT medication clearance decreases as the weight of a medication increases. IHD efficiently clears medications with a small molecular weight (ie, <500 Da), whereas CRRTs can efficiently clear much larger solutes (ie, <15,000 Da). High protein binding (>80%) can also affect clearance in both IHD and CRRT as the drug-protein complexes increase molecular weight significantly (eg, >50,000 Da), thus making it difficult for the complexes to pass through the pores in the hemofilter.[83,84] Conversely, patients who are experiencing hypoalbuminemia will have a higher fraction of unbound drug, thus a larger amount of the agent may be removed during RRT depending on the weight of the drug and its primary mode of elimination (eg, liver, kidney). Compounds with a large volume of distribution (V_D) of >1 L/kg are extensively distributed to extravascular tissues, leaving only a small fraction of the drug in the vascular compartment and thereby limiting drug removal.[74,81,83] Renal clearance of a drug also plays a role in determining RRT removal. In general, medications that are predominantly cleared by the kidney are more likely to be cleared via CRRT than medications that are eliminated primarily by nonrenal mechanisms.

There are marked differences in medication removal between the different CRRT modalities. Since CVVH relies on convection, medication removal is independent of molecular size of the medication or presence of a concentration gradient. Thus, it is the most efficient means of removing larger molecules (<15,000 Da) and those that are primarily not protein bound in the plasma. Another parameter that can assist in determining the likelihood of medication removal during use of convective RRT modalities is the sieving coefficient (SC), which is the ratio of a solute or medication in the ultrafiltrate to that in plasma. An SC of 1 indicates free transport across the membrane where an SC of 0 indicates no transport across the membrane. The SC is often approximated by the fraction unbound (f_u), or the fraction of drug unbound to protein in the plasma, because the ratios are often similar, and this information may be more readily available than SC. In CVVHD, medication removal relies on diffusion, which is an efficient means of removal of smaller molecules (<500 Da). Since CVVHDF is a combination of both convection and diffusion, medication removal is enhanced.

Limitations of using IHD-based dosing recommendations in patients receiving RRT for AKI include variability in the patient's individual pharmacokinetic parameters, differences in the dialysis prescription, such as dialyzer blood flow or duration, unpredictability of dialysis timing based on availability, use of new hemodialyzers, and advances in the technology without knowing how medications are impacted. Pharmacokinetic and medication dosing assessments in patients with impaired kidney function often are performed after single dose administration to stable CKD subjects. Distribution and clearance estimates in this setting may not reflect those observed at steady and may be over-estimated.[84,85] The RRT approach used may also change on an hourly or daily basis, especially in hemodynamically unstable individuals. The approach can also be affected by a failure of the circuit, the need for a procedure, or the availability of a machine. Individualization of a dosing regimen may require daily assessment of the clinical status of the patient and any planned or administered hemodialysis. Renally eliminated drugs with narrow therapeutic ranges may benefit from additional orders to contact the patient's healthcare providers if dialysis is stopped.[86]

Overall, there are numerous potential pharmacokinetic and pharmacodynamic alterations to be aware of in the patient with AKI. Individualization of pharmacotherapy for a patient receiving RRT is dependent on the patient's residual kidney function, the clearance of the medication by CRRT, as well as the properties of the medication (ie, molecular weight, V_D, protein binding, and SC). In CRRT, the frequency of therapy interruptions will also impact medication removal and corresponding dosing requirements. Unfortunately, there is still a scarcity of data to quantify these changes, and even less evidence demonstrating that if one incorporates these considerations into patient care, the associated outcomes will be improved.

EVALUATION OF THERAPEUTIC OUTCOMES

Vigilant monitoring of patients with AKI is essential, particularly in those who are critically ill. Table 61-7 summarizes the main monitoring parameters for patients with established AKI.

Once the laboratory-based tests (eg, urinalysis and FE_{Na} calculations) have been conducted to diagnose the cause of AKI, they usually do not have to be repeated. In established AKI, daily measurements of fluid intake and output are usually adequate. Urine output should be measured more frequently in critically ill, hemodynamic instability, or more severe AKI. Monitoring diuretic response is also important. Vital signs should be monitored at least daily, and more often if the acuity of illness warrants. Electrolytes, BUN, and S_{cr} should be considered routine and measured at least daily for hospitalized patients. Electrolytes may need to be monitored more frequently in patients who are receiving enhanced diuretic strategies

TABLE 61-7 Key Monitoring Parameters for Patients with Established AKI[a]

Parameter	Frequency
Fluid ins & outs	Hourly/Every shift
Patient weight	Daily
Hemodynamics (blood pressure, heart rate, mean arterial pressure, etc.)	Hourly/Every shift
Blood chemistries	
Sodium, potassium, chloride, bicarbonate, calcium, phosphate, magnesium	Daily
Blood urea nitrogen/serum creatinine	Daily
Drugs and their dosing regimens	Daily
Nutritional regimen	Daily
Blood glucose	Daily (minimum)
Therapeutic drug monitoring of renally cleared drugs (eg, vancomycin aminoglycosides)	Highly variable, about three times weekly
Times of administered doses	Daily
Doses relative to administration of renal replacement therapy	Daily (unless unanticipated changes occur)
Urinalysis	
Calculate measured creatinine clearance	Every time measured urine collection performed
Calculate fractional excretion of sodium	Every time measured urine collection performed
Plans for renal replacement therapy	Daily

[a]Phlebotomy should be coordinated to minimize excessive blood draws.

or on RRT. For medications influenced by RRT, the need for dose adjustments should be assessed daily or anytime RRT is interrupted, discontinued, or a change in modality or rate has been made.

The presence of renally eliminated medications should be assessed frequently. Therapeutic drug monitoring should be performed for medications that have a narrow therapeutic index if results can be obtained in a timely fashion. For patients receiving IHD, measuring a pre-dialysis serum drug concentration has the advantage of allowing time for the result to be reported and the next dose calculated so that it can be administered soon after dialysis. This is especially important if the desired pharmacologic effects are lost during or after hemodialysis because the serum concentration has become subtherapeutic. Serum concentrations drawn right after hemodialysis may reflect plasma concentrations that are transiently depressed until the medication can reequilibrate from the tissues (ie, a redistribution or rebound effect). The advantage of collecting a post-dialysis sample is the greater accuracy in determining how much medication was removed during hemodialysis. The down side of this strategy is that it delays dosing calculations and the administration of the next dose and ultimately delays the reestablishment of the target concentrations.

CONCLUSION

The unique characteristics of AKI can lead to notable differences in how kidney function is measured and how treatment regimens are developed. Most management approaches involve both prevention and supportive strategies, so as to minimize the potential for additional harm to the kidney. Understanding the constantly changing status inherent to AKI and how to adjust medication regimens is a key component to optimizing therapy.

ABBREVIATIONS

ACE	angiotensin-converting enzyme
ADQI	acute dialysis quality initiative
AIN	acute interstitial nephritis
AKD	acute kidney disease
AKI	acute kidney injury
AKIN	Acute Kidney Injury Network
ARB	angiotensin receptor blocker
ATN	acute tubular necrosis
BUN	blood urea nitrogen
CI-AKI	contrast-induced acute kidney injury
CKD	chronic kidney disease
CKD-EPI	Chronic Kidney Disease Epidemiology Collaboration
CL_{cr}	creatinine clearance
CRRT	continuous renal replacement therapy
CT	computed tomography
CVVH	continuous venovenous hemofiltration
CVVHD	continuous venovenous hemodialysis
CVVHDF	continuous venovenous hemodiafiltration
eGFR	estimated glomerular filtration rate
EHR	electronic health record
ESKD	end-stage kidney disease
FDA	Food and Drug Administration
FE_{Na}	fractional excretion of sodium
FE_{Urea}	fractional excretion of urea
GI	gastrointestinal
GFR	glomerular filtration rate
IGFBP7	insulin growth-like factor binding protein 7
IHD	intermittent hemodialysis
JVP	jugular venous pressure
KDIGO	Kidney Disease: Improving Global Outcomes
KUB	kidneys, ureters, and bladder
NAC	*N*-acetylcysteine
NGAL	neutrophil gelatinase-associated lipocalin
NSAID	nonsteroidal anti-inflammatory drug
PIRRT	prolonged intermittent renal replacement therapy
RIFLE	Risk, Injury, Failure, Loss of kidney Function, and End-stage kidney disease
RRT	renal replacement therapy
SC	sieving coefficient
S_{cr}	serum creatinine
SLED	sustained low-efficiency dialysis
TIMP-2	tissue inhibitor of metalloproteinases 2
UFR	ultrafiltration rate

REFERENCES

1. Bellomo R, Ronco C, Kellum JA, et al. Acute renal failure—Definition, outcome measures, animal models, fluid therapy and information technology needs: The Second International Consensus Conference of the Acute Dialysis Quality Initiative (ADQI) Group. *Crit Care.* 2004;8:R204–R212.
2. Mehta RL, Kellum JA, Shah SV, et al. Acute Kidney Injury Network: Report of an initiative to improve outcomes in acute kidney injury. *Crit Care.* 2007;11:R31.
3. Kidney Disease: Improving Global Outcomes (KDIGO) Acute Kidney Injury Workgroup. KDIGO clinical practice guideline for acute kidney injury. *Kidney Int Suppl.* 2012;2:1–138.
4. Zeng X, McMahon GM, Brunelli SM, et al. Incidence, outcomes, and comparisons across definitions of AKI in hospitalized individuals. *Clin J Am Soc Nephrol.* 2014;9(1):12–20.
5. Pereira M, Rodrigues N, Godinho I, et al. Acute kidney injury in patients with severe sepsis or septic shock: a comparison between the 'Risk, Injury, Failure, Loss of kidney function, End-stage kidney disease' (RIFLE), Acute Kidney Injury Network (AKIN) and Kidney Disease: Improving Global Outcomes (KDIGO) classifications. *Clin Kidney J.* 2017; 10(3):332–340.
6. Luo X, Jiang L, Du B, et al. A comparison of different diagnostic criteria of acute kidney injury in critically ill patients. *Crit Care.* 2014 Jul;18(4):R144.
7. Lin J, Fernandez H, Shashaty MG et al. False positive rate of AKI using consensus creatinine-based criteria. *Clin J Am Soc Nephrol.* 2015 Oct;10(10):1723–1731.
8. Chawla LS, Bellomo R, Bihorac A, et al. Acute kidney disease and renal recovery: Consensus report of the Acute Disease Quality Initiative (ADQI) 16 Workgroup. *Nat Rev Nephrol.* 2017 Apr;13(4):241–250.
9. Pavkov ME, Harding JL, Burrows NR. Trends in hospitalizations for acute kidney injury—United States, 2000–2014. *MMWR.* 2018;67:289–293.
10. Hoste EA, Kellum JA, Selby NM, et al. Global epidemiology and outcomes of acute kidney injury. *Nat Rev Nephrol.* 2018 Aug; doi:10.1038/s41581-018-0052-0.
11. Grams ME, Sang Y, Ballew SH, et al. A meta-analysis of the association of estimated GFR, albuminuria, age, race, and sex with acute kidney injury. *Am J Kidney Dis.* 2015 Oct;66(4):591–601.
12. Hoste EA, Bagshaw SM, Bellomo R, et al. Epidemiology of acute kidney injury in critically ill patients: The multinational AKI-EPI study. *Intensive Care Med.* 2015 Aug;41(8):1411–1423.
13. Horkan CM, Purtle SW, Mendu ML, et al. The association of acute kidney injury in the critically ill and postdischarge outcomes: A cohort study. *Crit Care Med.* 2015 Feb;43(2):354–364.
14. Horne KL, Packington R, Monaghan J, et al. Three-year outcomes after acute kidney injury: Results of a prospective parallel group cohort study. *BMJ Open.* 2017 Mar 29;7(3):e015316.
15. Badr KF, Ichikawa I. Prerenal failure: A deleterious shift from renal compensation to decompensation. *N Engl J Med.* 1988;319:623–629.
16. Ungprasert P, Cheungpasitporn W, Crowson CS, Matteson EL. Individual non-steroidal anti-inflammatory drugs and risk of acute kidney injury: A systematic review and meta-analysis of observational studies. *Eur J Intern Med.* 2015 May;26(4):285–291.
17. Gomez H, Kellum JA. Sepsis-induced acute kidney injury. *Curr Opin Crit Care.* 2016 Dec;22(6):546–553.
18. Bellomo R, Kellum JA, Ronco C, et al. Acute kidney injury in sepsis. *Intensive Care Med.* 2017 Jun;43(6):816–828.

19. Ostermann M, Liu K. Pathophysiology of AKI. *Best Pract Res Clin Anaesthesiol.* 2017 Sep;31(3):305–314.
20. Bevc S, Ekart R, Hojs R. The assessment of acute kidney injury in critically ill patients. *Eur J Intern Med.* 2017;45:54–58.
21. Krishnan N, Perazella MA. Drug-induced acute interstitial nephritis: Pathology, pathogenesis, and treatment. *Iran J Kidney Dis.* 2015 Jan;9(1):3–13.
22. Joyce E, Glasner P, Ranganathan S, et al. Tubulointerstitial nephritis: Diagnosis, treatment and monitoring. *Pediatr Nephrol.* 2017 Apr;32(4):577–587.
23. Lameire N, Vanholder R, Van Biesen W, et al. Acute kidney injury in critically ill cancer patients: An update. *Crit Care.* 2016 Aug;20(1):209.
24. Ostermann M. Diagnosis of acute kidney injury: Kidney disease improving global outcomes and beyond. *Curr Opin Crit Care.* 2014 Dec;20(6):581–587.
25. Macedo E, Mehta RL. Measuring renal function in critically ill patients: Tools and strategies for assessing glomerular filtration rate. *Curr Opin Crit Care.* 2013 Dec;19(6):560–566.
26. Baumann TJ, Staddon JE, Horst HM, Bivins BA. Minimum urine collection periods for accurate determination of creatinine clearance in critically ill patients. *Clin Pharm.* 1987;6:393–398.
27. Wasung ME, Chawla LS, Madero M. Biomarkers of renal function, which and when? *Clin Chim Acta.* 2015 Jan;438:350–357.
28. Teo SU, Endre ZH. Biomarkers in acute kidney injury. *Best Prac Res Clin Anesthesiol.* 2017;31:331–344.
29. Kellum JA, Chawla LS. Cell-cycle arrest and acute kidney injury: The light and the dark sides. *Nephrol Dial Transplant.* 2015;0:1–7.
30. Nalesso F, Cattarin L, Gobbi L, et al. Evaluating Nephrocheck as a predictive tool for acute kidney injury. *Int J Nephrol Renovasc Dis.* 2020;13:85–96.
31. Nephrocheck Test Kit package insert. http://www.astutemedical.com/documents/US-English/NephroCheck-Test-Kit-Package-Insert-US-PN-300152.pdf. Last accessed, July 15, 2021.
32. Mehta R. Moderator's view: Patient-centered approaches for optimizing AKI management: The role of kidney biomarkers. *Nephrol Dial Transplant.* 2017;32:419–422.
33. Ostermann M, Zarbock A, Goldstein S, et al. Recommendations on acute kidney injury biomarkers from the acute disease quality initiative consensus conference: A consensus statement. *JAMA Netw Open.* 2020;3(10):e2019209. doi:10.1001/jamanetworkopen.2020.19209.
34. McCullough PA, Shaw AD, Haase M, et al. Diagnosis of acute kidney injury using functional and injury biomarkers: Workgroup statements from the tenth Acute Dialysis Quality Initiative Consensus Conference. *Contrib Nephrol.* 2013;182:13–29.
35. Kane-Gill SL, Smithburger PL, Kashani K, et al. Clinical relevance and predictive value of damage biomarkers of drug-induced kidney injury. *Drug Saf.* 2017;40:1049–1074.
36. Haase M, Kribben A, Zidek W, et al. Electronic alerts for acute kidney injury. *Dtsch Arztebl Int.* 2017;114:1–8
37. Martin M, Wilson FP. Utility of electronic medical record alerts to prevent drug nephrotoxicity. *Clin J Am Soc Nephrol.* 2018 Apr; doi:10.2215/CJN.13841217.
38. Hodgson LE, Roderick PJ, Venn RM, et al. The ICE-AKI study: Impact analysis of a Clinical prediction rule and Electronic AKI alert in general medical patients. *PLoS One.* 2018 Aug;13(8):e0200584.
39. Goldstein SL, Kirkendall E, Nguyen H, et al. Electronic health record identification of nephrotoxin exposure and associated acute kidney injury. *Pediatrics.* 2013 Sep;132:756–767.
40. Gameiro J, Branco T, Lopes JA. Artificial intelligence in acute kidney injury risk prediction. *J Clin Med.* 2020;9(3):678. doi:10.3390/jcm9030678.
41. Li Q, Fan Q, Han Q, et al. Machine learning in nephrology: Scratching the surface. *Chin Med J (Engl).* 2020;133(6):687–698. doi:10.1097/CM9.0000000000000694.
42. Tomasev N, Glorot X, Rae J, et al. A clinically applicable approach to continuous prediction of future acute kidney injury. *Nature.* 2019;572(7767):116–119. doi:10.1038/s41586-019-1390-1.
43. Joannidis M, Druml W, Forni LG, et al. Prevention of acute kidney injury and protection of renal function in the intensive care unit: Update 2017: Expert opinion of the Working Group on Prevention, AKI section, European Society of Intensive Care Medicine. *Intensive Care Med.* 2017 Jun;43(6):730–749.
44. Caraceni P, Domenicali M, Tovoli A, et al. Clinical indications for the albumin use: Still a controversial issue. *Eur J Intern Med.* 2013 Dec;24:721–728.
45. Caironi P, Tognoni G, Masson S, et al. Albumin replacement in patients with severe sepsis or septic shock. *N Engl J Med.* 2014;370:1412–1421.
46. Self WH, Semler MW, Wanderer JP, et al. Balanced crystalloids versus saline in noncritically ill adults. *N Engl J Med.* 2018 Mar;378:819–828.
47. Semler MW, Self WH, Wanderer JP, et al.; SMART Investigators and the Pragmatic Critical Care Research Group. Balanced crystalloids versus saline in critically ill adults. *N Engl J Med.* 2018;378:829–839.
48. Semler MW, Wanderer JP, Ehrenfeld JM, et al.; SALT Investigators; Pragmatic Critical Care Research Group. Balanced crystalloids versus saline in the intensive care unit: The SALT randomized trial. *Am J Respir Crit Care Med.* 2017;195:1362–1372.
49. Semler MW, Kellum JA. Balanced crystalloid solutions. *Am J Respir Crit Care Med.* 2019;199(8):952–960.
50. Mehran R, Dangas GD, Weisbord SD. Contrast-induced acute kidney injury. *N Engl J Med.* 2019;380:2146–2155.
51. Heung M, Wolfgram DF, Kommareddi M, et al. Fluid overload at initiation of renal replacement therapy is associated with lack of renal recovery in patients with acute kidney injury. *Nephrol Dial Transplant.* 2012 Mar;27:956–961.
52. Fiaccadori E, Sabatino A, Morabito S, et al. Hyper/hypoglycemia and acute kidney injury in critically ill patients. *Clin Nutr.* 2016;35:317–321.
53. Van den Berghe G, Wouters P, Weekers F, et al. Intensive insulin therapy in critically ill patients. *N Engl J Med.* 2001 Nov;345:1359–1367.
54. Van den Berghe G, Wilmer A, Hermans G. Intensive insulin therapy in the medical ICU. *New Engl J Med.* 2006 Feb;354:449–461.
55. Finfer S, Chittock DR, Su SY, et al. Intensive versus conventional glucose control in critically ill patients. *N Engl J Med.* 2009 Mar;360:1283–1297.
56. Ling Y, Li X, Gao X. Intensive versus conventional glucose control in critically ill patients: A meta-analysis of randomized controlled trials. *Eur J Intern Med.* 2012 Sep;23:564–574.
57. Rhodes A, Evans LE, Alhazzani W, et al. Surviving Sepsis Campaign: International Guidelines for Management of Sepsis and Septic Shock: 2016. *Crit Care Med.* 2017 Mar;45:486–552.
58. American Diabetes Association. Diabetes care in the hospital: Standards of Medical Care in Diabetes—2021. *Diabetes Care.* 44(Suppl. 1):S211–S222.
59. Hammond DA, Lam SW, Rech MA, et al. Balanced crystalloids versus saline in critically ill adults: A systematic review and meta-analysis. *Ann Pharmacother.* 2020 Jan;54:5–13.
60. Ostermann M, Liu K, Kashani K. Fluid management in acute kidney injury. *Chest.* 2019 Sep;156:594–603.
61. Nadeau-Fredette AC, Bouchard J. Fluid management and use of diuretics in acute kidney injury. *Adv Chr Kidney Dis.* 2013 Jan;20:45–55.
62. Krzych ŁJ, Czempik PF. Impact of furosemide on mortality and the requirement for renal replacement therapy in acute kidney injury: A systematic review and meta-analysis of randomised trials. *Ann Intensive Care.* 2019;9(1):85. doi:10.1186/s13613-019-0557-0.
63. Asare K. Management of loop diuretic resistance in the intensive care unit. *Am J Health-Syst Pharm.* 2009 Sep;66:1635–1640.
64. McClave SA, Taylor BE, Martindale RG, et al. Guidelines for the Provision and Assessment of Nutrition Support Therapy in the Adult Critically Ill Patient: Society of Critical Care Medicine (SCCM) and American Society for Parenteral and Enteral Nutrition (A.S.P.E.N.). *J Parenter Enteral Nutr.* 2016;40(2):159–211.
65. Zarbock A, Kellum JA, Schmidt C, et al. Effect of early vs delayed initiation of renal replacement therapy on mortality in critically ill patients with acute kidney injury: The ELAIN randomized clinical trial. *JAMA.* 2016 May;315:2190–2199.
66. Gaudry S, Hajage D, Schortgen F, et al. Initiation strategies for renal-replacement therapy in the intensive care unit. *N Engl J Med.* 2016 Jul;375:122–133.
67. Negi S, Koreeda D, Kobayashi S, et al. Acute kidney injury: Epidemiology, outcomes, complications, and therapeutic strategies. *Semin Dial.* 2018;31(5):519–527. doi:10.1111/sdi.12705.
68. Bagshaw SM, Wald R. Strategies for the optimal timing to start renal replacement therapy in critically ill patients with acute kidney injury. *Kidney Int.* 2017;91:1022–1032.
69. Heung M, Yessayan L. Renal replacement therapy in acute kidney injury: Controversies and consensus. *Crit Care Clin.* 2017;33:365–378.
70. Villa G, Ricci Z, Ronco C. Renal replacement therapy. *Crit Care.* 2015 Oct;31:839–848.
71. Barbar SD, Clere-Jehl R, Bourredjem A, et al. Timing of renalreplacement therapy in patients with acute kidney injury and sepsis. *N Engl J Med.* 2018;379:1431–1442.
72. The STARRT-AKI Investigators. Timing of initiation of renal-replacement therapy in acute kidney injury. *N Engl J Med.* 2020;383(3):240–251.
73. Brandenburger T, Dimski T, Slowinski T, et al. Renal replacement therapy and anticoagulation. *Best Pract Res Clin Anesthesiol.* 2017 Sep;31:387–401.
74. Heintz BH, Matzke GR, Dager WE. Antimicrobial dosing concepts and recommendations for critically ill adult patients receiving

continuous renal replacement therapy or intermittent hemodialysis. *Pharmacotherapy*. 2009;29:562–577.

75. Dager WE. Filtering out important considerations for developing drug-dosing regimens in extended daily dialysis. *Crit Care Med.* 2006;34:240–241.
76. Keough LA, Krauss A, Hudson JQ. Inadequate antibiotic dosing in patients receiving sustained low efficiency dialysis. *Int J Clin Pharm.* 2018;45(5):1250–1256. doi:10.1007/s11096-018-0697-6.
77. Sethi SK, Krishnappa V, Nagethu N, et al. Antibiotic dosing in sustained low-efficiency dialysis in critically ill patients. *Can J Kidney Health Dis.* 2018;5:2054358118792229. doi:10.1177/2054358118792229.
78. Brown P, Battistella M. Principles of drug dosing in sustained low efficiency dialysis (SLED) and review of antimicrobial dosing literature. *Pharmacy (Basel)*. 2020;8:33. doi:10.3390/pharmacy8010033.
79. Philips BJ, Lane K, Dixon J, et al. The effects of acute renal failure on drug metabolism. *Expert Opin Drug Metabol Toxicol.* 2014 Jan;10:11–23.
80. Dager WE, King JH. Aminoglycosides in intermittent hemodialysis: Pharmacokinetics with individual dosing. *Ann Pharmacother.* 2006;40:9–14.
81. Hoff BM, Maker JH, Dager WE, et al. Antibiotic dosing for critically ill adult patients receiving intermittent hemodialysis, prolonged intermittent renal replacement therapy, and continuous renal replacement therapy: An update. *Ann Pharmacother.* 2020;54(1):43–55.
82. Vilay AM, Churchwell MD, Mueller BA. Clinical review: Drug metabolism and nonrenal clearance in acute kidney injury. *Crit Care.* 2008;12:235.
83. Bugge JF. Pharmacokinetics and drug dosing adjustments during continuous venovenous hemofiltration or hemodiafiltration in critically ill patients. *Acta Anaesthesiol Scand.* 2001;45:929–934.
84. Dager WE. What are the important drug use errors in dialysis patients? Pharmacokinetic and pharmacodynamic principles. *Semin Dial.* 2010 Sep-Oct;23:466–469.
85. Mavrakanas TA, Samer CF, Nessim SJ, et al. Apixaban pharmacokinetics at steady state in hemodialysis patients. *J Am Soc Nephrol.* 2017 Jul;28:2241–2248.
86. Thompson A, Li F, Gross AK. Considerations for medication management and anticoagulation during continuous renal replacement therapy. *AACN Adv Crit Care*. 2017;28:51–63.

Chronic Kidney Disease

62

Lori D. Wazny

KEY CONCEPTS

1. Chronic kidney disease (CKD) is classified based on the cause of kidney disease, assessment of glomerular filtration rate, and extent of albuminuria over at least a 3-month period.
2. Guidelines from the Kidney Disease: Improving Global Outcomes (KDIGO) provide information to assist healthcare providers in clinical decision making and the design of appropriate therapy to manage CKD progression and the associated complications.
3. Patient education and shared decision making play a critical role in the appropriate management of patients with CKD. Studies of multidisciplinary teams in CKD clinics have demonstrated significant benefits in slowing progression of CKD and reduced mortality.
4. Angiotensin-converting enzyme inhibitors (ACEIs) and angiotensin receptor blockers (ARBs) are primary pharmacologic treatments to delay progression of CKD in patients with category A2-A3 albuminuria because of their effects on renal hemodynamics to reduce intraglomerular pressure and albuminuria.
5. Sodium Glucose Transport-2 inhibitors (SGLT2i) have emerged as the latest treatment to prevent progression to later stages of CKD and ESRD in patients with Type 2 diabetes and other kidney diseases associated with albuminuria.

BEYOND THE BOOK

Visit The Kidney Failure Risk Equation Website (available at https://kidneyfailurerisk.com/). Watch the video then practice using the Kidney Failure Risk Equation to calculate the 2-year and 5-year probability of treated kidney failure (dialysis or transplantation) for a potential patient with CKD Stage G3 to G5. The video is useful to enhance student understanding regarding the COLLECT and ASSESS steps in the patient care process.

INTRODUCTION

1 Chronic kidney disease (CKD) is defined as abnormalities in kidney structure or function, present for 3 months or longer. Lower glomerular filtration rate (GFR) and a higher urinary albumin to creatinine ratio (ACR) are both independently associated with adverse events.[1] The Kidney Disease: Improving Global Outcomes (KDIGO) guidelines for evaluation and management of CKD classification system stages kidney disease by cause, GFR, and albuminuria. Figure 62-1 shows the KDIGO GFR and albuminuria categories along with the prognosis based on these factors.

The prognosis of CKD is dependent on the following factors: (a) cause of kidney disease; (b) GFR at time of diagnosis; (c) degree of albuminuria measured by ACR; and (d) presence of other comorbid conditions. Patients with any of the following should be referred to a nephrologist for evaluation and collaborative management: persistent and significant albuminuria (ACR >100 mg/g [>11.3 mg/mmol]), progression of CKD (eg, a marked but nonacute decline in GFR), presence of a non-surgical cause of hematuria, hypertension refractory to treatment (eg, ≥4 antihypertensive agents), persistent abnormalities of serum potassium, recurrent or extensive nephrolithiasis, GFR less than 30 mL/min/1.73 m^2 (0.29 mL/s/m^2), or hereditary kidney disease such as polycystic kidney disease even in the presence of normal GFR and ACR.[1]

CKD is often unrecognized and this contributes to significant morbidity, premature mortality, and a poorer prognosis when it is finally diagnosed. This chapter primarily covers the epidemiology, etiology, pathophysiology, clinical presentation, and treatment of progressive CKD. The reader is referred to Chapter 63 for a detailed discussion of management and monitoring strategies for secondary complications of CKD.

EPIDEMIOLOGY

CKD is recognized as a significant global public health problem.[2] People with CKD experience high morbidity and mortality rates with a resulting economic burden to healthcare systems due to frequent hospitalizations and the high cost of chronic dialysis and kidney transplantation. CKD affects more than 697 million individuals worldwide. In 2017, 1.2 million deaths and 35.8 million disability-adjusted life years were attributed to CKD. As a result, many countries have implemented public health initiatives to reduce the proportion of the population with CKD; increase CKD patient awareness through targeted screening programs; reduce the rate of new cases of CKD G5; and reduce mortality in persons with CKD.[2]

Diabetic kidney disease is the most frequent cause of end-stage (G5) kidney failure worldwide. Approximately 25% to 50% of all patients receiving dialysis have diabetic kidney disease.[3] In first-world countries, the leading cause of CKD is diabetes mellitus followed by hypertension.[4] It is projected that the aging population and other changes in the demographics will result in an increased incidence and subsequent increase in prevalence of Stage 5 CKD by 2030.[5] The prevalence of CKD increases with age, with the highest prevalence in individuals over 60 years mainly attributed to a decrease in estimated GFR (eGFR, less than 60 mL/min/1.73 m^2).[6]

Prognosis of CKD by GFR and Albuminuria Categories

GFR categories (mL/min/1.73 m^2) Description and range			Persistent albuminuria categories Description and range: A1 Normal to mildly increased <30 mg/g <3 mg/mmol	A2 Moderately increased 30-300 mg/g 3-30 mg/mmol	A3 Severely increased >300 mg/g >30 mg/mmol
G1	Normal or high	≥90			
G2	Mildly decreased	60-89			
G3a	Mildly to moderately decreased	45-59			
G3b	Moderately to severely decreased	30-44			
G4	Severely decreased	15-29			
G5	Kidney failure	<15			

FIGURE 62-1 KDIGO GFR and albuminuria categories and prognosis of CKD by category. To meet criteria for CKD there must be a significant reduction in GFR (categories 3a-5) or there must also be evidence of kidney damage (categories 1 and 2) for 3 months or greater. Prognosis Scale—Green: low risk (if no other markers of kidney disease, no CKD); Yellow: moderately increased risk; Orange: high risk; Red: very high risk. (CKD, chronic kidney disease; GFR, glomerular filtration rate; KDIGO, Kidney Disease Improving Global Outcomes.)

While there is some debate as to whether the eGFR decline in older individuals as a consequence of the normal physiological aging process should be considered a *disease* necessitating the label of CKD, the fact remains that patients with reduced eGFR and albuminuria suffer from worse health outcomes regardless of age.[1]

Specific racial, social, and environmental factors are important to consider when evaluating risk of progressive CKD in individual patients. Racial health disparities in CKD also exist and contribute to differing CKD rates. There is evidence for higher risk of CKD progression in patients of African, Hispanic, and Asian (South, East, and Pacific Islanders) descent and Indigenous people compared to Caucasians. This is partly explained by biological factors (eg, blood pressure) and comorbidities such as diabetes, and cardiovascular disease. However, despite a higher risk of CKD progression, there is a lower risk of mortality for patients of Asian and Hispanic descent compared to Caucasians, and a key gap in the literature is understanding why they live longer despite having a higher prevalence of comorbidities such as diabetes, cardiovascular disease, and heart failure.[7] Increased risk of CKD in high-risk ethnic groups may be tackled through closer monitoring and management of renal comorbidities such as diabetes and cardiovascular disease, for example, through albuminuria and blood pressure measurement.[7]

With regards to socioeconomic factors, the likelihood of CKD is higher in individuals with lower income and education.[8] Multiple studies conducted in the United States, Canada, and Europe have shown a strong association between low-socioeconomic status and higher incidence, prevalence and more complications related to CKD. Poverty is known to affect some of the most important social determinants of health, such as developing healthy habits, getting healthcare in a timely manner and environmental exposure to nephrotoxic agents such as lead, cadmium, and arsenic. A higher prevalence of births with low-birth weight promotes not only less development in terms of renal mass but also an increased risk of hypertension and CKD. Depression, anxiety, and increased exposure to addictions also promote the activation of the sympathetic nervous system and an increased release of cytokines that can influence the pathogenesis of kidney damage. An increased intake of sodium, sweetened beverages, and foods with phosphorus has also been reported, and the chances of receiving proper treatment to slow the progression of kidney damage are lower. A clearer understanding of the situations of vulnerable populations could allow for better public health measures to reduce the burden of kidney disease.[9]

ETIOLOGY

Susceptibility and Initiation Risk Factors

Clinical and sociodemographic risk factors for susceptibility to and initiation of CKD are listed in Table 62-1 and are useful for identifying individuals at high risk of developing CKD.[10]

Predicting Risk of Progression

KIDGO recommends that all patients with CKD be staged according to eGFR and ACR and that their prognosis be considered to help

TABLE 62-1 Risk Factors for Susceptibility to and Initiation of Chronic Kidney Disease

Clinical Factors
Diabetes
Hypertension
Obesity
Smoking
Autoimmune diseases, such as lupus, rheumatoid arthritis, connective tissue disease, vasculitis
Systemic infections, such as group A *streptococcus* causing post-infectious glomerulonephritis (PIGN)
Artherosclerotic vascular disease
Urinary tract infections, such as recurrent pyelonephritis
Lower urinary tract obstruction from prostatic hypertrophy, neurogenic bladder, kidney stones
Neoplasia, such as multiple myeloma, renal cell carcinoma
First degree relative with CKD
History of acute kidney injury (AKI) including recurrent episodes of dehydration
Reduction in kidney mass, such as congenital single kidney, post nephrectomy, scarring from reflux nephropathy
Exposure to nephrotoxic drugs, such as chronic use acetaminophen, NSAIDs, COX-2 inhibitors, lithium, cyclosporine, tacrolimus, contrast dyes, certain chemotherapy drugs, etc.
Pregnancy complications including edema, hypertension, proteinuria
Low-birth weight
Chronic viral infections, such as Hepatitis B and C, HIV
Hereditary polycystic kidney disease
Sociodemographic Factors
Older age
Ethnic minority status
Exposure to certain chemical and environmental conditions
Low income/education

Data from References 1 and 10.

guide further testing and treatment decisions (Fig. 62-1). Estimating equations such as the kidney failure risk equation (KFRE), which incorporates urine data, sex, age, and GFR, have also been used and provide an accurate 2- and 5-year risk of progression to kidney failure for individuals with stage 3 to 5 CKD.[11] The KFRE has been widely validated in multiple international cohorts and pediatric populations and provides the best current evidence-based approach to point-of-care risk of progression to be used in combination with expert clinical judgment.[12] Risk equations may also be beneficial to help align resources with risk in assigning priority for referral to nephrologists.

Progression Risk Factors

Progression risk factors are those associated with further decline in kidney function. Persistence of the underlying initiation factors (eg, diabetes mellitus, hypertension) is the most important predictor of progressive CKD.

Diabetes mellitus

Type 2 diabetes accounts for about 90% of the 460 million people with diabetes in the world. About half of these patients will develop kidney disease.[3] The KDIGO Clinical Practice Guideline for Diabetes Management in CKD recommends an individualized hemoglobin A_{1C} (HbA1c) target ranging from <6.5% (0.065; 48 mmol/mol) to <8.0% (0.08; 64 mmol/mol) in patients with diabetes and CKD[13] (Evidence level 1C). Achieving HbA1c targets prevents the surrogate endpoints of microalbuminuria and macroalbuminuria associated with diabetic chronic kidney disease (DIABETIC CKD).

Hypertension

The 2021 KDIGO guideline for the management of blood pressure in CKD recommends control blood pressure at all categories of CKD regardless of the underlying cause since early treatment of hypertension and achievement of target blood pressure have been demonstrated to slow the rate of progression of CKD.[14]

Albuminuria

Albuminuria is a strong independent predictor of accelerated progression of CKD and also a risk factor for CV mortality and morbidity.[1] Albuminuria remains the primary modifiable risk factor associated with CKD progression in most patients.

Smoking

Smoking is associated with kidney damage in the general population as well as in patients with diabetes and hypertension.[15] Acute reductions in GFR and an increase in urinary albumin excretion, heart rate, and blood pressure, likely secondary to nicotine exposure, have been reported.[16] Smoking is also associated with an increase in CV events in people with CKD.[1]

Obesity

Population data have demonstrated an increased risk of CKD G5 in overweight and obese subjects.[17] The risk of CKD 5 was directly related to the magnitude of obesity and remained even after adjustment for diabetes and hypertension. A body mass index (BMI) greater than or equal to 25 kg/m^2 at the age of 20 years has been associated with a threefold increase in risk of CKD compared with a BMI lower than 25 kg/m^2.[18] This association has also been shown in healthy young and middle-aged individuals without CKD or albuminuria.[19] Intentional weight loss in individuals with CKD was associated with decreases in albuminuria, systolic blood pressure, and stabilization in GFR.[20] These data suggest that weight reduction be included as part of the treatment of CKD (Table 62-2).

TABLE 62-2 Recommendations for Individuals with Chronic Kidney Disease

Nonpharmacologic
Exercise 30 minutes five times per week [1D]
Weight loss if BMI >25 kg/m^2 [1D]
Smoking cessation [1D]
Alcohol: Two standard drinks per day for men and one standard drink per day for women[a] [2D]
If hypertension: Low-sodium diet (<2 g/day, <90 mmol/day) [1C]
Pharmacologic
Adjust medication doses for kidney function [1A]
Seek pharmacist or medical advice before using over-the-counter medicines or nutritional protein supplements [1B]
Herbal medicines are not recommended [1B]
Temporarily discontinue potentially nephrotoxic/renally excreted drugs if eGFR <60 mL/min/1.73 m^2 in patients who are acutely unwell or hypovolemic (eg, metformin, RAAS blockers, diuretics, NSAIDs/COX II inhibitors, lithium, digoxin) [1C]
Vaccines
Influenza yearly [1B]
Pneumococcal vaccine if eGFR <30 mL/min/1.73 m^2, nephrotic syndrome, diabetes, or receiving immunosuppression. Single booster dose at year 5 [1B]
Hepatitis B vaccine if eGFR <30 mL/min/1.73 m^2 and risk of progression of CKD [1B]
ASA suggested for patients at risk for atherosclerotic events unless there is an increased bleeding risk [2B]
Avoid oral phosphate-containing bowel preparations in people with a GFR <60 mL/min/1.73 m^2 (0.58 mL/s/m^2) or in those known to be at risk of phosphate nephropathy [1A]

BMI, body mass index; CKD, chronic kidney disease; COX, cyclooxygenase; eGFR, estimated glomerular filtration rate; NSAIDs, nonsteroidal anti-inflammatory drugs; RAAS, renin–angiotensin–aldosterone system.

See Table 62-3 for definitions of evidence grading in brackets.

[a]Standard drink: 30 mL spirits, 100 mL wine, 285 mL full-strength beer, and 425 mL light beer.

Data from References 1 and 13.

PATHOPHYSIOLOGY

Chronic Kidney Disease

Progression of CKD to more advanced stages (G4-G5) typically occurs over decades in the majority of people, with the precise mechanism of kidney damage dependent on the etiology of the disease and strongly associated with age, sex, and urine ACR. As evidenced by the variety of initiation and progression factors, kidney damage can result from an array of heterogeneous causes. Diabetic CKD is characterized by glomerular mesangial expansion while with hypertensive nephrosclerosis, the kidney's arterioles have arteriolar hyalinosis. Polycystic kidney disease is characterized by the development and expansion of renal cysts. While the initial structural damage depends on the primary disease affecting the kidney, the key elements of the pathway to ESRD are (a) loss of nephron mass, (b) glomerular capillary hypertension, and (c) albuminuria (Fig. 62-2).

Exposure to any of the initiation risk factors can result in loss of nephron mass. In response to the decrease in nephron function, the remaining nephrons compensate through the process of autoregulation. With nephron loss and the resulting reduction in perfusion pressure and GFR, renin release from the juxtaglomerular apparatus increases and converts angiotensinogen to angiotensin I, which is then converted to angiotensin II (ATII). ATII is a potent vasoconstrictor of both afferent and efferent arterioles, but it preferentially affects the efferent arterioles, leading to increased pressure within the glomerular capillaries and consequent increased filtration fraction. Initially, this compensatory action may be adaptive and beneficial; however, over time it can lead to the development of intraglomerular hypertension and hypertrophy and a further decline in the number of functioning nephrons. High intraglomerular capillary pressure impairs the size-selective function of the glomerular permeability barrier, resulting in increased urinary excretion of albumin and albuminuria. The development of intraglomerular hypertension usually parallels the development of systemic hypertension. ATII as well as aldosterone may also mediate CKD progression through nonhemodynamic effects by increasing growth factors (eg, transforming growth factor beta [TGF-β]) and causing cellular proliferation and hypertrophy of the glomerular endothelial cells, epithelial cells, and fibroblasts ultimately resulting in further inflammation and fibrosis.[21]

Proteinuria alone may promote progressive loss of nephrons as a result of direct cellular damage. Filtered proteins such as albumin, transferrin, complement factors, immunoglobulins, cytokines, and ATII are toxic to kidney tubular cells. Studies have demonstrated that the presence of these proteins in the renal tubule leads to increased production of inflammatory and vasoactive cytokines such as endothelin and monocyte chemoattractant protein-1 (MCP-1).[22] Proteinuria is also associated with the activation of complement components on the apical membrane of proximal tubules. Intratubular complement activation may be the key mechanism of damage in the progressive proteinuric nephropathies.[22] Furthermore, these events ultimately lead to scarring of the interstitium, progressive loss of structural nephron units, and a reduction in GFR.

CLINICAL PRESENTATION

CKD is often asymptomatic, which is a reason many patients are not diagnosed with the disease until they reach CKD G4-G5 and may be near the point of requiring renal replacement therapy such as dialysis or kidney transplantation. This problem has prompted automated reporting by clinical laboratories of the eGFR as determined by the estimating equations [Chronic Kidney Disease Epidemiology Collaboration equation (CKD-EPI equation)] for the purpose of identifying individuals with CKD earlier (see Chapter e60). Comprehensive screening for CKD includes analysis of eGFR and ACR (Fig. 62-1) and risk stratification for progression using the Kidney Failure Risk Equation. Clinicians must understand how to interpret the eGFR and values for urine albumin excretion to appropriately stage individuals with CKD. Chapter e60 provides a detailed discussion of the methods available for detection of urinary albumin and protein.

CLINICAL PRESENTATION CKD Stages G1-G5

Symptoms (usually not observed until Stage G4-G5)

- Fatigue, weakness, shortness of breath, mental confusion, nausea and vomiting, and loss of appetite, itching, cold intolerance, and peripheral neuropathies are common

Signs

- Edema, weight gain (from accumulation of fluid), changes in urine output (volume and consistency), "foaming" of urine (indicative of albuminuria), elevated blood pressure (hypertension is a common cause and result of CKD)

Laboratory Tests

- *Decreased*: eGFR, bicarbonate (metabolic acidosis), Hb/hematocrit (Hct) (anemia), transferrin saturation (TSat) and/or ferritin (iron deficiency; note: ferritin may be increased due to inflammatory conditions), vitamin D levels, albumin (malnutrition)
- *Increased*: Serum creatinine, blood urea nitrogen, potassium, phosphorus, PTH, ACR, glucose/HbA1c (diabetes is a cause of CKD), low-density lipoprotein (LDL), and triglycerides

Other Diagnostic Tests

- Urine sediment abnormalities (hematuria, red blood cell and white blood cell casts, renal tubular epithelial cells)
- Pathologic abnormalities indicating glomerular, vascular, tubulointerstitial disease, or cystic and congenital diseases
- Structural abnormalities such as polycystic kidneys, renal masses, renal artery stenosis, cortical scarring due to infarcts and pyelonephritis, or small kidneys (common in more severe CKD) detected by imaging studies (eg, ultrasound, computed tomography, magnetic resonance imaging, angiography)

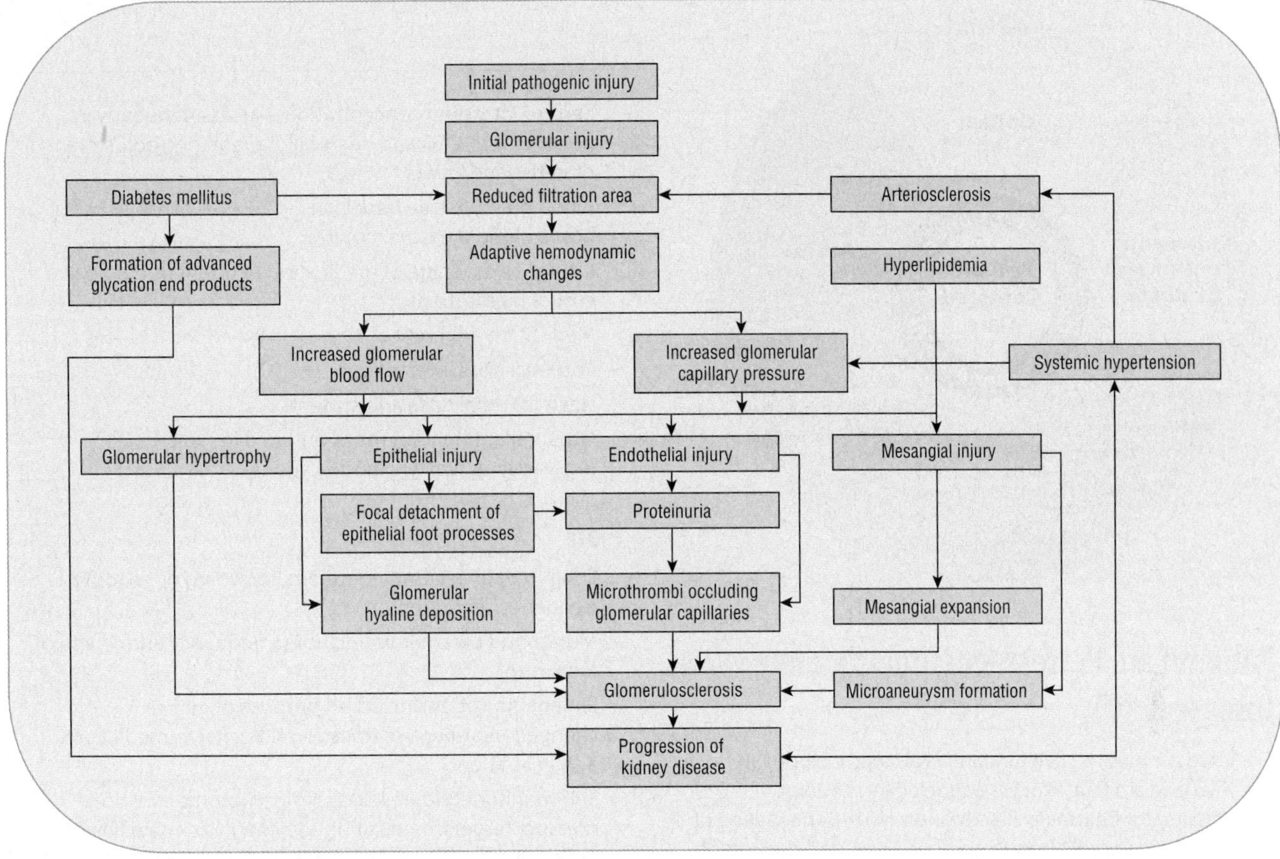

FIGURE 62-2 Proposed mechanisms of progression of kidney disease.

TREATMENT

Desired Outcome

The overall goal of treatment is to delay or prevent progression of CKD.

General Approach to Treatment

Individuals with CKD should be evaluated frequently to assess the risk of progression of CKD, to identify the presence and causes of secondary complications and comorbid conditions, and to receive treatment for these complications prior to development of Stage G5 CKD. Many nonpharmacologic and pharmacologic recommendations can be broadly applied as part of the general approach to care for all CKD patients (Table 62-2).

2 Management of CKD should be based on the KDIGO consensus guidelines (available at www.kdigo.org) which are based on evidence and expert recommendations. The available KDIGO clinical practice guidelines relevant to CKD address evaluation and management of CKD, blood pressure, diabetes, glomerulonephritis, lipid management, and hepatitis C in CKD. Table 62-3 provides a guide to the grading and strength of recommendations used in these guidelines.

3 Appropriate management of CKD ideally involves a multidisciplinary approach to address the nonpharmacologic and pharmacologic interventions, dietary education, and social/financial concerns. Multidisciplinary CKD team models that have included members such as a nephrologist, nurse, dietitian, pharmacist, and social worker have demonstrated significant slowing of CKD progression, longer time to start of renal replacement therapy (dialysis or kidney transplant), and reduction in all-cause mortality.[23] Estimates in the pediatric CKD population indicate that the additional salary costs of the multidisciplinary team (pharmacist, nurse,

TABLE 62-3 KDIGO Guidelines: Grading and Strength of Recommendations

Grade	Description	Implications for Clinicians
Level 1	"We recommend"	Most patients should receive the recommended course of action.
Level 2	"We suggest"	Different choices will be appropriate for different patients. Each patient needs help arrive at a management decision consistent with her or his values and preferences.
Grade	**Quality of Evidence**	**Meaning**
A	High	We are confident that the true effect lies close to that of the estimate of the effect.
B	Moderate	The true effect is likely to be close to the estimate of the effect, but there is a possibility that it is substantially different.
C	Low	The true effect may be substantially different from the estimate of the effect.
D	Very low	The estimate of effect is very uncertain, and often will be far from the truth.

The strength of recommendation is indicated as Level 1, Level 2, or Not Graded. The quality of the supporting evidence is shown as A, B, C, or D.

Data from Reference 1.

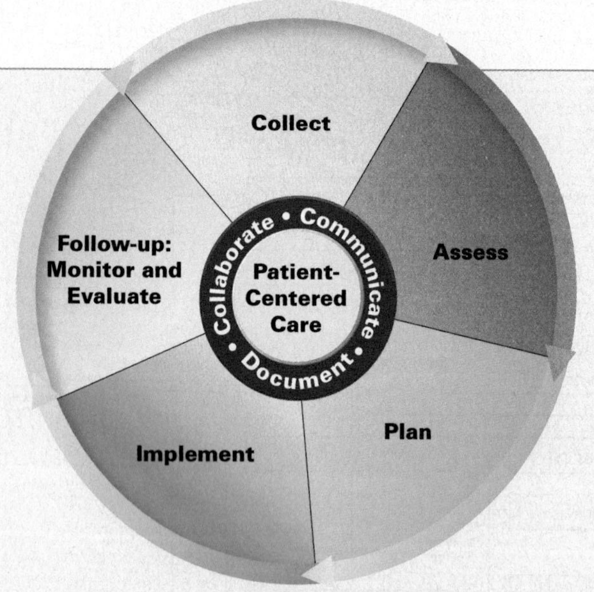

Patient Care Process for Chronic Kidney Disease (CKD)

The image shows the five fundamental steps included in The Pharmacist's Care Process endorsed by the Joint Commission for Pharmacy Practitioners (2014). The tagline of this process reads collaborate, communicate, and document. The five fundamental steps listed here are collect, assess, plan, implement, and follow-up: monitor and evaluate. All these steps are listed in a circular block diagram.

Collect

- Patient characteristics (eg, age, CKD stage [see Fig. 62-1] and cause of CKD, medication allergies)
- Past medical history
- Social history (eg, smoking), family/friend supports
- Current medications including OTC (eg, NSAID use), herbals, dietary supplements
- Objective data:
  - Blood pressure, heart rate, weight
  - Labs as outlined in Table 62-4

Assess

- Serum creatinine, glomerular filtration rate (GFR), or creatinine clearance
- Presence of albuminuria (see Fig. 62-1)
- Serum potassium concentration—assess frequently in patients with CKD and heart failure requiring adjustment of diuretics and/or ACEI
- Blood pressure (see targets in Fig. 62-3)—consider use of home blood pressure monitor
- Insurance coverage of medications, current out of pocket cost of medications
- Medication adherence
- Potential drug interactions
- Need for renal dose adjustments
- Other recommendations as outlined in Table 62-2 (eg, vaccines, lifestyle modifications)

Plan

- Drug therapy recommendations, including dose, route, frequency, and duration
- Monitoring parameters, including frequency and timing of follow-up
- Patient education, including purpose of new or changed treatment, medication side effects, medication administration
- Self-monitoring for resolution of symptoms and blood pressure targets, medication to hold on sick days if vomiting or diarrhea occur (eg, ACEI/ARB; SGLT2 inhibitors)
- Referrals to other providers when appropriate (eg, dietitian, occupational therapist, social worker, endocrinologist, CKD clinic)

Implement*

- Provide patient education on all elements of the treatment plan
- Use motivational interviewing strategies to maximize adherence
- Schedule follow-up labs, adherence assessment

Follow-up: Monitor and Evaluate

- Resolution of CKD symptoms
- Presence of adverse effects (eg, dizziness, hypoglycemia)
- Patient adherence to treatment plan using multiple sources of information

Communicate with patient, caregivers, and CKD multidisciplinary team.

social worker, dietician, data manager) could be recovered in 1 year if dialysis was delayed by 1 year in only 2% of patients.[24]

Drug-dosing guidelines based on the degree of kidney function should be followed, and a complete medication history of prescription and nonprescription medications, as well as herbals and nutritional supplements, should be obtained and routinely updated. Appropriate measures should also be taken for patients with CKD to decrease the risk of nephrotoxicity from radiocontrast agents, antibiotics such as aminoglycosides, as well as from nonsteroidal anti-inflammatory drugs and ACEIs (Chapter 65).[25]

Nonpharmacologic Therapy

Nonpharmacologic therapies for CKD include diet and lifestyle interventions targeted at reducing the risk for CKD progression and are outlined in Table 62-2.

Pharmacologic Therapy

Pharmacologic therapies used to slow CKD progression include drugs with demonstrated benefits to reduce albuminuria and to manage the causal factors for CKD primarily hypertension and

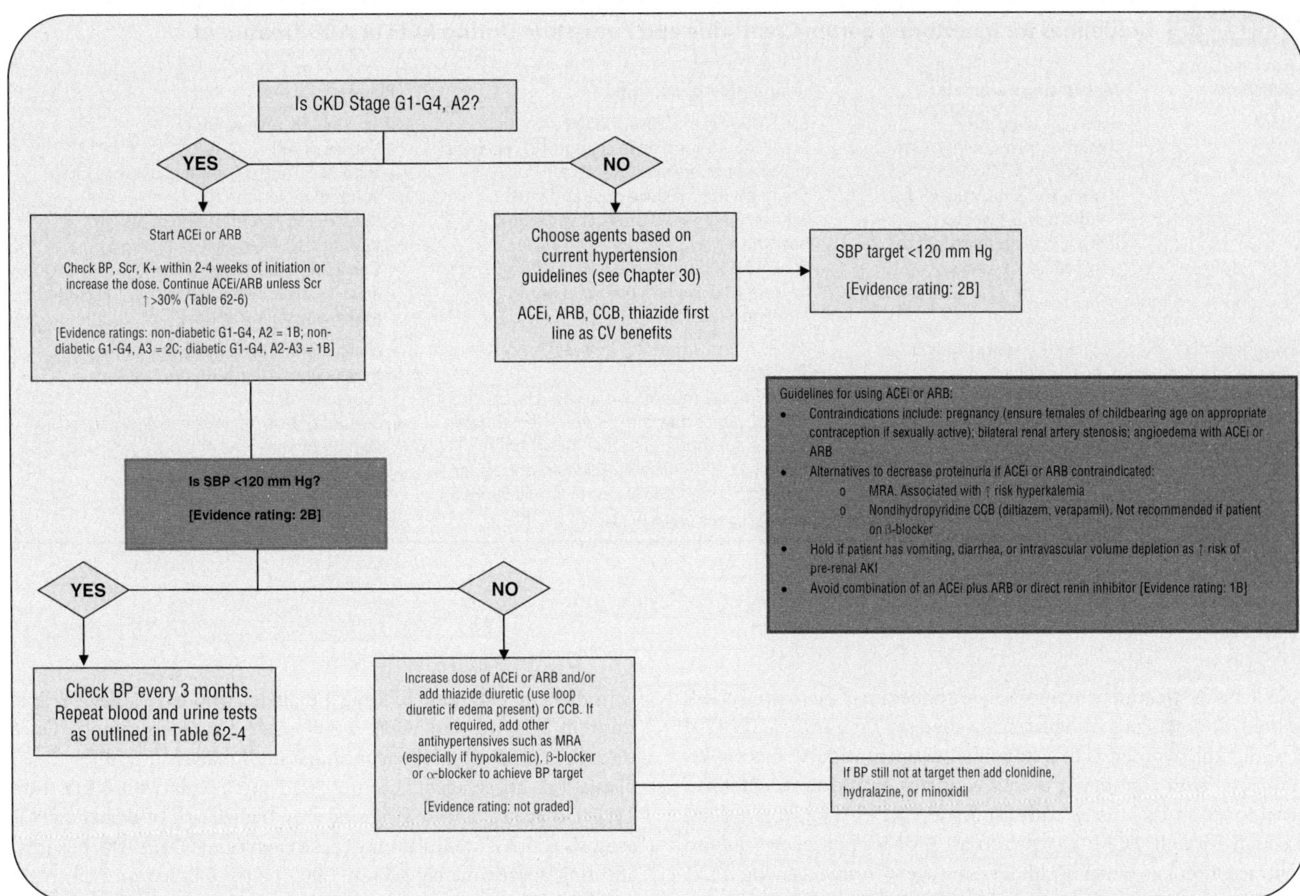

FIGURE 62-3 Treatment of hypertension in chronic kidney disease. (ACEI, angiotensin-converting enzyme inhibitor; ACR, albumin-to-creatinine ratio; AKI, acute kidney injury; ARB, angiotensin receptor blocker; BP, blood pressure; CCB, calcium channel blocker; eGFR, estimated glomerular filtration rate; SBP, systolic blood pressure; CV, cardiovascular.)

diabetes. The next sections focus on pharmacologic therapy targeting these factors. Glomerular disease is the third leading cause of CKD and a review of the treatment strategies for glomerulonephritis is provided in Chapter e66.

Albuminuria

ACEIs and ARBs

4 Evidence from clinical trials has confirmed the beneficial effects of ACEIs and ARBs on kidney function for patients with albuminuria. A meta-analysis has shown that the effects of ACEIs or ARBs on key CKD outcomes such as doubling of serum creatinine and prevention of progression of micro- to macroalbuminuria are equivalent and, thus, they can be used interchangeably.[26] An ACEI or an ARB should be used as first-line therapy if the patient urine albumin excretion is in category A2 or greater (ACR >30 mg/g (>3.4 mg/mmol)) (see Fig. 62-3 and Table 62-4). The antiproteinuric effect of ACEIs and ARBs is a class effect and not specific to any one agent.[26] For patients with hypertension, the primary goal is to achieve the target blood pressure while a secondary goal is to control albuminuria. Specific dosing recommendations for ACEIs and ARBs for the treatment of albuminuria have not been established; consequently, the lowest recommended dose should be initiated and titrated up to the maximally tolerated dose. The dose is usually increased until albuminuria is reduced by 30% to 50% or side effects such as a greater than 30% increase in serum creatinine (Scr) concentration or elevation in serum potassium occur or the maximum dose for hypertension is achieved (see Table 62-5). When these drugs are used in patients with eGFR <30 mL/min per 1.73 m², close monitoring of serum potassium level is required. However, in patients with CKD G5 who are experiencing uremic symptoms or very high serum potassium levels (eg, K ≥ 6 mEq/L [mmol/L]), it is reasonable to discontinue

TABLE 62-4 Recommended Monitoring Intervals for Outcome Measure in Patients with Chronic Kidney Disease (Evidence Rating: Not Graded)

		Albuminuria Stage (based on ACR in mg/g)		
KDIGO GFR Category	eGFR (mL/min/1.73 m²)	A1: <30 mg/g (3 mg/mmol)	A2: 30-300 mg/g (3-30 mg/mmol)	A3: >300 mg/g (30 mg/mmol)
1	≥90	12 months	12 months	6 months
2	60-89	12 months	12 months	6 months
3a	45-59	12 months	6 months	4 months
3b	30-44	6 months	4 months	4 months
4	15-29	4 months	4 months	2-3 months
5	<15	1-3 months	1-3 months	1-3 months

Blood tests to monitor: CBC, Na, K, Cl, bicarbonate, urea, creatinine, and eGFR. If DKD, add HbA1c. Fasting lipid profile at least yearly. At CKD category 3b or later: also add albumin, calcium, phosphorus, parathyroid hormone, serum iron, TIBC, and ferritin.

Urine tests to monitor: uACR (or uPCR if indicated), standard urinalysis, and urine culture and sensitivity only if symptoms suggestive of urinary tract infection.

Data from Reference 1.

TABLE 62-5 Guidelines for Monitoring Serum Creatinine and Potassium During ACEI or ARB Treatment

Adverse Drug Reaction	Monitoring Parameter	Therapeutic Adjustments	Review
↑ Scr	Scr to calculate eGFR If eGFR ≥ 60 mL/min/1.73 m², repeat in 4-12 weeks If eGFR 30-59 mL/min/1.73 m², repeat in 2-4 weeks If eGFR <30 mL/min/1.73 m², repeat in ≤2weeks	• Scr ↑0%-15%, no dose change • Scr ↑15%-30%, no dose change but repeat Scr in 2 weeks to ensure it is stable • Scr ↑31%-50%, reduce dose and repeat Scr every 1-2 weeks until Scr within 30% of baseline • Scr ↑>50%, discontinue ACE or ARB and repeat Scr every 1-2 weeks until Scr is within 15% of baseline value	If Scr ↑>30%, review for: • Causes of AKI • Hold ACEI/ARB if vomiting, diarrhea, or volume depletion • Reassess any contributing meds (eg, diuretics, NSAIDs, COX 2 inhibitors) • Consider renal artery stenosis • If Scr ↑<30%, increase dose of ACEI/ARB to maximally tolerated dose
Hyperkalemia	Serum K+ at same intervals as eGFR above	If K+>5 mEq/L (mmol/L), advise dietary K+ restriction If K+>6 mEq/L (mmol/L), consider treatment with diuretics that can lower K+ (eg, thiazide, loop) if appropriate; sodium bicarbonate tablets for patients with acidosis; potassium binders. If unable to lower K+ to <5.5 mEq/L (mmol/L), decrease or stop ACEI/ARB	• Concurrent drugs which may cause hyperkalemia (eg, MRAs, potassium supplements) • Dietary potassium intake review preferable by a dietitian

Data from Reference 13.

ACEI or ARB treatment temporarily with the aim of increasing eGFR to hold off starting renal replacement therapy. The STOP-ACEi Trial is testing the hypothesis that stopping treatment with ACEi, or ARB compared with continuing these treatments, improves or stabilizes renal function in patients with G4 or G5 CKD.[27] If patients exhibit a cough with an ACEI, a switch to an ARB is appropriate. Advise contraception in women of childbearing age who are receiving ACEI or ARB therapy and discontinue these agents in women who are considering pregnancy or who become pregnant as these drugs can impair fetal kidney function especially with exposure during the second and third trimester.[13] Patients should be counseled to hold ACEI or ARB on sick days (ie, vomiting or diarrhea). A thorough discussion of dose, dose titration, monitoring, and adverse effects of ACEIs and ARBs is presented in Chapter 30.

The lack of response of some patients to ACEI or ARB therapy may be due to aldosterone escape from renin–angiotensin–aldosterone system (RAAS) blockade. Combination therapy with an ACEI plus an ARB or direct renin inhibitor (eg, aliskiren) produces a more complete blockade of the RAAS and results in a greater reduction in macroalbuminuria.[28] However, several trials have failed to show that dual blockade of the RAAS either slowed progression of CKD or decreased CV events.[29-32] Combination therapy in these trials was also associated with increased risks of hyperkalemia and AKI. Thus, the combination of an ACEI plus an ARB or aliskiren for the treatment of albuminuria is to be avoided (Evidence level 1B).[14]

Sodium Glucose Transport-2 Inhibitors

4 Sodium glucose transport-2 inhibitors (SGLT2i) slow progression of both Type 2 diabetic and nondiabetic proteinuric CKD with benefits that are independent of the glucose lowering effect.[33] By reducing glucose and sodium reabsorption in the proximal tubule of the kidney, these agents decrease glomerular hyperfiltration and reduce glomerular hypertension. Recent trials have demonstrated the benefits of these agents (Table 62-6). These trials have shown that SGLT2i significantly slow progression of kidney disease, reduce the need for dialysis or transplantation, and decrease mortality.[33,34] The slowing of progression of CKD equates to a gain of 15.1 years before the average CREDENCE trial patient (age 63 years; eGFR = 56 mL/min/1.83 m²; receiving an ACEI/ARB) would reach an eGFR = 10 mL/min/1.73 m².[34] Hence, SGLT2i could significantly reduce the need for dialysis or kidney transplant in many patients with diabetic CKD and are an exciting advance in treatment for clinicians. SGLT2i should be considered after ACEI/ARB in all patients with diabetic CKD due to Type 2 diabetes who have an eGFR ≥20 mL/min/1.73 m² and ACR >200 mg/g (22.6 mg/mmol). Once started, SGLT2i should be continued until dialysis or kidney transplantation. These agents are not used in patients with CKD from Type 1 diabetes due to a significantly higher risk of diabetic ketoacidosis (DKA).[35] SGLT2i may cause euglycemic DKA which is rare, affecting approximately one in 1,000 patients based on real world data with 40% of cases occurring during a hospital stay. Blood glucose is typically less than 252 mg/dL (14 mmol/L) (range 216-324 mg/dL [12-18 mmol/L]). There is a higher risk for euglycemic DKA in Type 2 diabetics who are receiving insulin. Most patients will present with DKA within 2 months of starting a SGLT2i with some cases occurring shortly after SGLT2i discontinuation. Most patients with SGLT2i induced DKA will have a precipitating event such as dehydration, infection, surgery, and changes in insulin dose being commonly reported.[36] Symptoms of DKA associated with SGLT2i use are similar to DKA in general, with nausea, vomiting, and abdominal pain most commonly reported. However, these patients may not present with symptoms of dehydration to the same degree as other DKA patients due to the lack of hyperglycemia.[37]

Patients at increased risk of volume depletion, mycotic genital infections (eg, vaginal yeast infections, Fournier's gangrene), women with a history of urinary tract infections, those with indwelling foley catheters may not be good candidates for this class of medications. Genital mycotic infections occur in approximately one in three patients and may be treated with topical or oral antifungals with no need to discontinue the SGLT2i.[39] The exception to this is Fournier's gangrene which requires incision and drainage and IV antibiotics. Patients should seek urgent medical care if pain, tenderness, erythema, swelling in genital or perineal area with fever and/or malaise. Patients should be counseled to hold SGLT2i on sick days (ie, vomiting or diarrhea). However, the SGLT2i groups in the clinical trials were less likely to discontinue drug versus placebo. Lower eGFR also did not result in increased adverse drug reactions and the SGLT2i group had a reduced the risk of AKI.[37] For surgery and procedures requiring one or more days in hospital, or requiring bowel preparation including colonoscopy, stop the SGLT2i at least 3 days pre-procedure (2 days prior to surgery and the day of surgery/procedure) to decrease the risk of DKA. This may require increasing other glucose-lowering drugs during that time. For day procedures, SGLT2i can be stopped on the day of procedure.[40] More details on the use of SGLT2i for the treatment of Type 2 diabetes may be found in Chapter 94.

TABLE 62-6 SGLT2 Inhibitor and MRA CKD Trials

Study	CREDENCE	Dapa-CKD	FIDELIO-DKD
Populations			
Age (mean±SD)	63±9.2	61.9±12.1	65.6±9.1
CKD inclusion criteria	ACR >300-5,000 mg/g + eGFR 30-<90 mL/min/1.73 m²; Type 2 DM	eGFR 25-75 mL/min/1.73 m²; ACR 200-5,000 mg/g (22.6-566 mg/mmol); Type 2 DM & nondiabetics included	ACR 30-<300 mg/g (3.4-34 mg/mmol) + eGFR 25-<60 mL/min/1.73 m² OR ACR 300-5,000 mg/g (34-566 mg/mmol) + eGFR 25-<75 mL/min/1.73 m²; Type 2 DM
Race distribution	White 66.6%; Asian 19.9%; Black 5.15%	White 53.2%; Asian 34.1%; Black 4.4%	White 63.3%; Asian 25.4%; Black 4.7%
Mean eGFR	56.2±18.2	43.1±12.4	44.3±12.6
Median UACR (IQR)	927 (463-1833 mg/g) or 105 (52-207 mg/mmol)	965 (472-1,903 mg/g) or 109 (53-215 mg/mmol)	852 (446-1,634 mg/g) or 96 (50-185 mg/mmol)
Baseline medications	ACEi or ARB; no MRAs or DRIs	ACEI or ARB	ACEI or ARB
Study medication	Canagliflozin 100 mg daily	Dapagliflozin 10 mg daily	Finerenone 10 mg daily if eGFR <60 mL/min/1.73 m², increased to 20 mg daily if tolerated OR 20 mg daily if eGFR >60 mL/min/1.73 m²
Results			
Number of participants	4,401	4,304	5,674
Primary outcome	Occurrence of: ESKD (established dialysis, transplant or eGFR persistently <15 mL/min/1.73 m²) + doubling of baseline creatinine + death from renal or CV cause (HR 0.7 [0.59-0.82])	Time to event of: ESKD (established dialysis, transplant or eGFR persistently <15 mL/min/1.73 m²) + decline in eGFR by at least 50% + death from renal or CV cause (HR 0.61 [0.51-0.72])	Time to event of: ESKD (established dialysis, transplant or eGFR persistently <15 mL/min/1.73 m²) + decline in eGFR by 40% from baseline + death from renal (HR 0.82 [0.73-0.93])
NNT to prevent primary outcome	22 (15-38) patients over 2.5 years	19 (14-29) patients over 3 years	29 (16-166) patients over 3 years
Key secondary outcome	CV death + hospitalization for HF (HR 0.69 [0.57-0.83])	Composite kidney outcome (50% decline, ESKD or renal death); composite CV outcome; death from any cause (HR 0.56, 0.71, 0.69, respectively)	CV death + hospitalization for HR + nonfatal MI + nonfatal stroke (HR 0.86 [0.75-0.99])
Adverse effects	Genital mycotic infections, euglycemic DKA (rare)	Genital mycotic infections, euglycemic DKA (rare)	Hyperkalemia

CREDENCE, Canagliflozin and Renal Outcomes in Type 2 Diabetes and Nephropathy; Dapa-CKD, Dapagliflozin in Patients with Chronic Kidney Disease; FIDELIO-DKD, Effect of Finerenone on Chronic Kidney Disease Outcomes in Type 2 Diabetes.

Data from References 33, 34, and 38.

Mineralcorticoid Receptor Antagonists (MRA)

The concept of aldosterone escape has led to the search for other drug combinations to further suppress the RAAS to improve kidney outcomes. A Cochrane systematic review examined the addition of the MRA spironolactone to an ACEI or ARB in patients with CKD Stage G1-G4.[41] Spironolactone significantly reduced albuminuria and blood pressure but doubled the risk of hyperkalemia and significantly increased the risk of gynecomastia. However, it is unknown whether adding spironolactone or eplerenone to ACEI or ARB will reduce the risk of major CV events or ESKD as a large efficacy trial in diabetic CKD has never been performed.[42]

Finerenone is a novel, more selective, nonsteroidal MRA. The FIDELIO-DKD trial examined kidney and cardiovascular outcomes in patients with CKD due to Type 2 diabetes (Table 62-6).[38] The risk of hyperkalemia was higher in patients receiving finerenone with an absolute risk increase (ARI) of 12% for serum potassium greater than 5.5 mEq/L (mmol/L) and 3% for serum potassium greater than 6 mEq/L (mmol/L). More patients in the finerenone group needed potassium binding agents for hyperkalemia (307 vs 184 in placebo).[3] Finerenone, unlike spironolactone, is not a blood pressure–lowering drug as mean systolic blood pressure decreased by 2 mm Hg. The patient centric quality of life results of this trial have not been reported yet.[38] Only 4.4% of patients were also on an SGLT2i; therefore, a study examining finerenone in combination with SGLT2i plus ACEI/ARB is ongoing (CONFIDENCE trial). However, finerenone can be considered in patients who cannot tolerate SGLT2i.

Nondinydropyridine Calcium Channel Blockers

Nondihydropyridine calcium channel blockers (diltiazem and verapamil) have yielded beneficial effects on albuminuria, although not as profoundly as ACEIs.[43] The postulated mechanisms for this decrease in kidney injury include suppression of glomerular hypertrophy, inhibition of platelet aggregation, and a decrease in salt accumulation. These agents have been used to reduce albuminuria in combination with an ACEI or ARB even though there are limited data to support this strategy. In general, nondihydropyridine CCBs should be considered fourth-line antiproteinuric drugs when an ACEI/ARB, finerenone SGLT2 inhibitor is contraindicated or not tolerated (Fig. 62-3).[57]

Hypertension

Figure 62-3 provides an algorithm for recommended blood pressure goals based on the degree of albuminuria present and the choice of antihypertensive agent.

The Systolic Blood Pressure Intervention Trial (SPRINT) is the largest trial testing BP targets in CKD. SPRINT assessed whether a lower systolic blood pressure goal of less than 120 mm Hg versus a target of less than 140 mm Hg was desirable.[44] In the 2,646 participants with

CKD, the composite renal outcome of a decrease in eGFR of 50% or more or the need for chronic dialysis or kidney transplantation was not significant over the 3.3 years duration of this trial but CV events and all-cause mortality were reduced.[14] Within the CKD subgroup, SPRINT reported no significant difference in serious adverse events. There were increased risks for hypokalemia and hyperkalemia, presumably because of the greater use of antihypertensive medications. Intensive BP lowering increased the risk of AKI in people with moderate CKD (eGFR <45 mL/min/1.73 m^2) and advanced age (>75 years), but the episodes were infrequent and tended to be mild and reversible.[14] There were potential harms to all participants (with and without CKD) in the intensive systolic blood pressure group that included significantly increased risks of syncope, hypotension, electrolyte abnormalities, AKI, and CKD progression.[44] However, the CV and mortality benefits outweigh the risks of harm even in frail and elderly patients.[14]

A SBP target <120 mm Hg may be appropriate in patients who achieve SBP in the 120s without requiring a high number of antihypertensives and who are not experiencing adverse effects of therapy. It is reasonable to consider a change in medications or less-intensive therapy if the patient is symptomatic or BP is excessively low (eg, SBP <100 mm Hg).[14] In practice, adoption of this recommendation in a population of patients with CKD will result in a median SBP around 120 mm Hg, meaning that 50% of patients will have SBP greater than 120 mm Hg.[14] The mean achieved SBP in SPRINT was 121.4 mm Hg.[44] Patients prescribed ACEI/ARBs or diuretics who are targeting an SBP below 120 mm Hg need to be reliable and able to follow instructions to hold these medications when they are unable to maintain adequate fluid intake (eg, vomiting/diarrhea) due to the risk of AKI. The adoption of an SBP target less than 120 mm Hg is an ideal topic for shared decision making between individual patients and clinicians. There is likely to be marked variability in how individual patients weigh and value the potential benefits and harms of intensive BP control. This may vary with age, culture, number of drugs (both BP-lowering and other drugs), and other factors.[14]

Diabetes

Patients with diabetes should be screened annually for CKD starting at the time of diagnosis of Type 2 diabetes and 5 years after the diagnosis of Type 1 diabetes by ordering a serum creatinine, eGFR, and a urine albumin-to-creatinine ratio (ACR).[13]

The management of diabetes in patients with CKD includes reduction of albuminuria and achievement of desired blood pressure and HbA1c (Chapter 94). An individualized HbA1c target ranging from <6.5% (0.065; 48 mmol/mol) to <8.0% (0.08; 64 mmol/mol) is recommended[13] (Evidence Level 1C). Clinicians may consider a target greater than 7% (0.07; 53 mmol/mol) if there is a risk of hypoglycemia, multiple comorbidities, lack of hypoglycemia symptoms or awareness, or limited life expectancy.[13,45] A lower HbA1c target (eg, <6.5% [0.065; 48 mmol/mol] or <7% [0.07; 53 mmol/mol]) is preferred in patients where prevention of complications is the main goal. It should be noted that HbA1c measurements are based on an assumed red blood cell life span of 90 days. In later stage, CKD G4-G5, the red blood cell life span is decreased, so HbA1c values may be falsely low.[45] Hence, in patients with CKD, the HbA1c should be interpreted along with the patient's home blood glucose readings when assessing diabetic control. It is also important to note that patients with CKD G4-G5 are at higher risk of developing hypoglycemia because of the reduction in metabolism of insulin by the kidney as GFR declines. As a result, these patients may require reduced doses of oral or injectable hypoglycemic agents and using agents associated with a lower risk of hypoglycemia (metformin, SGLT2i, GLP-1 receptor agonists, DPP-4 inhibitors). Metformin is still considered a first-line agent in individuals with Type 2 diabetes and CKD[14] (Evidence level 1B). As previously discussed, most patients with CKD due to Type 2 diabetes should also be treated with an SGLT-2 inhibitor if eGFR is greater than or equal to 20 to 25 mL/min/1.73 m^2 and the patient is already receiving an ACEI or ARB. Metformin can be initiated and/or continued in individuals with an eGFR greater than or equal to 30 mL/min/1.73 m^2. The metformin dose should be reduced to 500 mg once or twice daily in patients with an eGFR between 30 and 44 mL/min/1.73 m^2.[46] Metformin is contraindicated in individuals with an eGFR less than 30 mL/min/1.73 m^2 due to the rare but serious risk of lactic acidosis and should be temporarily discontinued before administering contrast agents for imaging studies. Monitor patients for vitamin B12 deficiency when they are treated with metformin for more than 4 years, as metformin interferes with intestinal vitamin B12 absorption.[13] Dose adjustments or avoidance of other renally eliminated hypoglycemic agents may also be necessary; the dosing, monitoring, and goals of therapies to treat diabetes mellitus are detailed in Chapter 94.

Evaluation of Therapeutic Outcomes

Frequency of laboratory and urine testing based on CKD category and degree of albuminuria as defined by KDIGO are shown in Table 62-4. The monitoring necessary for patients with hypertension and diabetes is the same in the CKD population as it is in the non-CKD population.

CONCLUSION

The prevalence of CKD continues to increase especially in high-risk populations. Although efforts to delay progression of CKD, including prudent use of ACEI/ARB and SGLT2i in diabetic patients are paramount, measures to diagnose and manage the associated secondary complications and comorbid conditions early in the course of the disease are also essential.

A multidisciplinary team structure is a rational approach to effectively design and implement individual patient care plans often required in the CKD population given the extensive nonpharmacologic and pharmacologic interventions. Pharmacists are well positioned to actively participate in the chronic disease and medication management of ambulatory CKD patients as well as those who are hospitalized.

ABBREVIATIONS

ACEI	angiotensin-converting enzyme inhibitor
ACR	urinary albumin-to-creatinine ratio
AKI	acute kidney injury
ARB	angiotensin receptor blocker
ATII	angiotensin II
CCB	calcium channel blocker
CKD	chronic kidney disease
CKD-EPI equation	Chronic Kidney Disease Epidemiology Collaboration equation
CREDENCE	Canagliflozin and Renal Outcomes in Type 2 Diabetes and Nephropathy
CV	cardiovascular
CVD	cardiovascular disease
Dapa-CKD	Dapagliflozin in Patients with Chronic Kidney Disease
DKA	diabetic ketoacidosis
eGFR	estimated glomerular filtration rate
ESRD	end-stage renal disease
FIDELIO-DKD	Effect of Finerenone on Chronic Kidney Disease Outcomes in Type 2 Diabetes
GFR	glomerular filtration rate
HbA1c	glycated hemoglobin or hemoglobin A_{1c}
KDIGO	Kidney Disease: Improving Global Outcomes
MDRD	Modification of Diet in Renal Disease
MRA	mineralcorticoid receptor antagonist

NNT	number needed to treat
PIGN	post-infectious glomerulonephritis
PTH	parathyroid hormone
RAAS	renin–angiotensin–aldosterone system
Scr	serum creatinine
SGLT2i	sodium glucose transport-2 inhibitors
SPRINT	Systolic Blood Pressure Intervention Trial

REFERENCES

1. Kidney Disease: Improving Global Outcomes (KDIGO) CKD Work Group. KDIGO 2012 clinical practice guideline for the evaluation and management of chronic kidney disease. *Kidney Int.* Suppl. 2013;3:1–150.
2. US Department of Health and Human Services. Healthy People 2020 Objectives for Chronic Kidney Disease. Available at: http://www.healthypeople.gov/2020/topicsobjectives2020/overview.aspx?topicid=6. Accessed February 28, 2022.
3. Raj R. Can Finerenone Fiddle the Forgotten A of the RAAS String? Available at: http://www.nephjc.com/news/fidelio. Accessed June 25, 2021.
4. United States Renal Data System. 2019 USRDS Annual Data Report: Epidemiology of kidney disease in the United States. National Institutes of Health, National Institute of Diabetes and Digestive and Kidney Diseases. 2019. Available at: https://www.usrds.org/annual-data-report/. Accessed June 25, 2021.
5. McCullough KP, Morgenstern H, Saran R, Herman WH, Robinson BM. Projecting ESRD Incidence and prevalence in the United States through 2030. *J Am Soc Nephrol.* 2019;30(1):127–135. 10.1681/asn.2018050531
6. United States Renal Data System, 2018 USRDS Annual Data Report: Epidemiology of Kidney Disease in the United States. National Institutes of Health, National Institute of Diabetes and Digestive and Kidney Diseases, Bethesda, MD, 2018.
7. Hounkpatin HO, Fraser SDS, Honney R, Dreyer G, Brettle A, Roderick PJ. Ethnic minority disparities in progression and mortality of pre-dialysis chronic kidney disease: A systematic scoping review. *BMC Nephrol.* 2020;21(1):217. 10.1186/s12882-020-01852-3
8. Norton JM, Moxey-Mims MM, Eggers PW, et al. Social determinants of racial disparities in CKD. *J Am Soc Nephrol.* 2016;27(9):2576–2595. 10.1681/asn.2016010027
9. Robles-Osorio ML, Sabath E. Social disparities, risk factors and chronic kidney disease. *Nefrol (English Ed).* 2016;36(5):577–579. 10.1016/j.nefroe.2016.05.004
10. Inker LA, Astor BC, Fox CH, et al. KDOQI US commentary on the 2012 KDIGO clinical practice guideline for the evaluation and management of CKD. *Am J Kidney Dis.* 2014;63(5):713–735. 10.1053/j.ajkd.2014.01.416
11. Tangri N, Stevens LA, Griffith J, et al. A predictive model for progression of chronic kidney disease to kidney failure. *JAMA.* 2011;305(15):1553–1559. 10.1001/jama.2011.451
12. Tangri N, Grams ME, Levey AS, et al. Multinational assessment of accuracy of equations for predicting risk of kidney failure: A meta-analysis. *JAMA.* 2016;315(2):164–174. 10.1001/jama.2015.18202
13. Caramori ML, Chan JCN, Heerspink HJL, et al. KDIGO 2020 clinical practice guideline for diabetes management in chronic kidney disease. *Kidney Int.* 2020;98(4S):S1–S115. 10.1016/j.kint.2020.06.019
14. Cheung AK, Chang TI, Cushman WC, et al. KDIGO 2021 clinical practice guideline for the management of blood pressure in chronic kidney disease. *Kidney Int.* 2021;99(3S):S1–S87. 10.1016/j.kint.2020.11.003
15. Orth SR, Hallan SI. Smoking: A risk factor for progression of chronic kidney disease and for cardiovascular morbidity and mortality in renal patients: Absence of evidence or evidence of absence? *Clin J Am Soc Nephrol.* 2008;3(1):226–236. CJN.03740907
16. Hogan SL, Vupputuri S, Guo X, et al. Association of cigarette smoking with albuminuria in the United States: The third National Health and Nutrition Examination Survey. *Ren Fail.* 2007;29(2):133–142. 10.1080/08860220601098888
17. Hsu CY, McCulloch CE, Iribarren C, Darbinian J, Go AS. Body mass index and risk for end-stage renal disease. *Ann Intern Med.* 2006;144(1):21–28. http://www.ncbi.nlm.nih.gov/entrez/query.fcgi?cmd=Retrieve&db=PubMed&dopt=Citation&list_uids=16389251
18. Ejerblad E, Fored CM, Lindblad P, Fryzek J, McLaughlin JK, Nyren O. Obesity and risk for chronic renal failure. *J Am Soc Nephrol.* 2006;17(6):1695–1702. 10.1681/asn.2005060638
19. Chang Y, Ryu S, Choi Y, et al. Metabolically healthy obesity and development of chronic kidney disease: A cohort study. *Ann Intern Med.* 2016;164(5):305–312. 10.7326/M15-1323
20. Navaneethan SD, Yehnert H, Moustarah F, Schreiber MJ, Schauer PR, Beddhu S. Weight loss interventions in chronic kidney disease: A systematic review and meta-analysis. *Clin J Am Soc Nephrol.* 2009;4(10):1565–1574. doi:10.2215/CJN.02250409 [doi]
21. Gajjala PR, Sanati M, Jankowski J. Cellular and molecular mechanisms of chronic kidney disease with diabetes mellitus and cardiovascular diseases as its comorbidities. *Front Immunol.* 2015;6:340. 10.3389/fimmu.2015.00340
22. Abbate M, Zoja C, Remuzzi G. How does proteinuria cause progressive renal damage? *J Am Soc Nephrol.* 2006;17(11):2974–2984. 10.1681/asn.2006040377
23. Wang SM, Hsiao LC, Ting IW, et al. Multidisciplinary care in patients with chronic kidney disease: A systematic review and meta-analysis. *Eur J Intern Med.* 2015;26(8):640–645. 10.1016/j.ejim.2015.07.002
24. Filler G, Lipshultz SE. Why multidisciplinary clinics should be the standard for treating chronic kidney disease. *Pediatr Nephrol.* 2012;27(10):1831–1834. 10.1007/s00467-012-2236-3
25. St. Peter WL, Wazny LDD, Patel UDD, St Peter WL, Wazny LDD, Patel UDD. New models of chronic kidney disease care including pharmacists: Improving medication reconciliation and medication management. *Curr Opin Nephrol Hypertens.* 2013;22(6):656–662. 10.1097/MNH.0b013e328365b364
26. Strippoli GF, Bonifati C, Craig M, Navaneethan SD, Craig JC. Angiotensin converting enzyme inhibitors and angiotensin II receptor antagonists for preventing the progression of diabetic kidney disease. *Cochrane Database Syst Rev.* 2006;(4)(4):CD006257. doi:10.1002/14651858.CD006257
27. Multi-centre Randomised Controlled Trial of Angiotensin Converting Enzyme inhibitor (ACEi)/Angiotensin Receptor Blocker (ARB) withdrawal in advanced renal disease (STOP ACEi). Available at: https://www.birmingham.ac.uk/research/bctu/trials/renal/stopacei/index.aspx. Accessed June 25, 2021.
28. Tylicki L, Lizakowski S, Rutkowski B. Renin-angiotensin-aldosterone system blockade for nephroprotection: Current evidence and future directions. *J Nephrol.* 2012;25(6):900–910. 10.5301/jn.5000134
29. Mann JF, Schmieder RE, McQueen M, et al. Renal outcomes with telmisartan, ramipril, or both, in people at high vascular risk (the ONTARGET study): A multicentre, randomised, double-blind, controlled trial. *Lancet.* 2008;372(9638):547–553. 10.1016/s0140-6736(08)61236-2
30. Fried LF, Emanuele N, Zhang JH, et al. Combined angiotensin inhibition for the treatment of diabetic nephropathy. *N Engl J Med.* 2013;369(20):1892–1903. 10.1056/NEJMoa1303154
31. Parving HH, Brenner BM, McMurray JJ, et al. Cardiorenal end points in a trial of aliskiren for type 2 diabetes. *N Engl J Med.* 2012;367(23):2204–2213. 10.1056/NEJMoa1208799
32. Imai E, Haneda M, Yamasaki T, et al. Effects of dual blockade of the renin-angiotensin system on renal and cardiovascular outcomes in type 2 diabetes with overt nephropathy and hypertension in the ORIENT: A post-hoc analysis (ORIENT-Hypertension). *Hypertens Res.* 2013;36(12):1051–1059. 10.1038/hr.2013.86;10.1038/hr.2013.86
33. Heerspink HJL, Stefánsson BV, Correa-Rotter R, et al. Dapagliflozin in patients with chronic kidney disease. *N Engl J Med.* 2020;383(15):1436–1446. 10.1056/NEJMoa2024816
34. Perkovic V, Jardine MJ, Neal B, et al. Canagliflozin and renal outcomes in type 2 diabetes and nephropathy. *N Engl J Med.* 2019;380(24):2295–2306. 10.1056/NEJMoa1811744
35. Musso G, Sircana A, Saba F, Cassader M, Gambino R. Assessing the risk of ketoacidosis due to sodium-glucose cotransporter (SGLT)-2 inhibitors in patients with type 1 diabetes: A meta-analysis and meta-regression. *PLOS Med.* 2020;17(12):e1003461. doi:10.1371/journal.pmed.1003461
36. Goldenberg RM, Berard LD, Cheng AYY, et al. SGLT2 inhibitor–associated diabetic ketoacidosis: Clinical review and recommendations for prevention and diagnosis. *Clin Ther.* 2016;38(12):2654–2664.e1. doi:10.1016/j.clinthera.2016.11.002
37. Neuen BL, Young T, Heerspink HJL, et al. SGLT2 inhibitors for the prevention of kidney failure in patients with type 2 diabetes: A systematic review and meta-analysis. *Lancet Diabetes Endocrinol.* 2019;7(11):845–854. 10.1016/S2213-8587(19)30256-6
38. Bakris GL, Agarwal R, Anker SD, et al. Effect of finerenone on chronic kidney disease outcomes in type 2 diabetes. *N Engl J Med.* 2020;383(23):2219–2229. 10.1056/NEJMoa2025845
39. Unnikrishnan A, Kalra S, Purandare V, Vasnawala H. Genital infections with sodium glucose cotransporter-2 inhibitors: Occurrence

and management in patients with type 2 diabetes mellitus. *Indian J Endocrinol Metab.* 2018;22(6):837. 10.4103/ijem.IJEM_159_17

40. Society AD. ALERT UPDATE January 2020 Periprocedural Diabetic Ketoacidosis (DKA) with SGLT2 Inhibitor Use. 2020. Available at: https://diabetessociety.com.au/documents/ADS_DKA_SGLT2i_Alert_update_2020.pdf. Accessed June 25, 2021.
41. Bolignano D, Palmer SC, Navaneethan SD, Strippoli GF. Aldosterone antagonists for preventing the progression of chronic kidney disease. *Cochrane Database Syst Rev.* 2014;4:Cd007004. 10.1002/14651858.CD007004.pub3
42. Hou J, Xiong W, Cao L, Wen X, Li A. Spironolactone add-on for preventing or slowing the progression of diabetic nephropathy: A meta-analysis. *Clin Ther.* 2015;37(9):2086–2103 e10. doi:10.1016/j.clinthera.2015.05.508
43. Hart P, Bakris GL. Calcium antagonists: Do they equally protect against kidney injury? *Kidney Int.* 2008;73(7):795–796. 10.1038/sj.ki.5002773
44. Wright JT Jr., Williamson JD, Whelton PK, et al. A randomized trial of intensive versus standard blood-pressure control. *N Engl J Med.* 2015;373(22):2103–2116. 10.1056/NEJMoa1511939
45. Tuttle KR, Bakris GL, Bilous RW, et al. Diabetic kidney disease: A report from an ADA Consensus Conference. *Am J Kidney Dis.* 2014;64(4):510–533. 10.1053/j.ajkd.2014.08.001
46. Lalau J-D, Kajbaf F, Bennis Y, Hurtel-Lemaire A-S, Belpaire F, De Broe ME. Metformin treatment in patients with type 2 diabetes and chronic kidney disease stages 3A, 3B, or 4. *Diabetes Care.* 2018;41(3):547–553. 10.2337/dc17-2231

Chronic Kidney Disease: Management of Secondary Complications

63

Joanna Q. Hudson

KEY CONCEPTS

1 Chronic kidney disease (CKD) affects many other organ systems leading to secondary complications. The most common complications include fluid and electrolyte disorders, anemia, mineral and bone disorder, metabolic acidosis, and increased incidence of cardiovascular disease.

2 Anemia of CKD is multifactorial with loss of erythropoietin synthesis by the kidney, iron deficiency, and chronic inflammation all implicated.

3 CKD-mineral and bone disorder (CKD-MBD) includes abnormalities in parathyroid hormone (PTH), fibroblast growth factor-23 (FGF-23), phosphorus, calcium, vitamin D, and bone turnover, and contributes to soft-tissue and extravascular calcifications.

4 Guidelines from the Kidney Disease: Improving Global Outcomes (KDIGO) provide information to assist healthcare providers in clinical decision making and the design of appropriate therapy to manage complications of CKD.

5 Patient education, an interdisciplinary team, and shared decision making play critical roles in the appropriate management of complications of CKD.

6 Management of anemia includes administration of erythropoiesis-stimulating agents (ESAs) and regular iron supplementation to maintain the target hemoglobin concentration and prevent the need for blood transfusions. There is a higher risk of cardiovascular events when ESAs are used to target hemoglobin values greater than 11 g/dL (110 g/L; 6.83 mmol/L).

7 Management of CKD-MBD includes dietary phosphorus restriction, phosphate-binding agents, activated vitamin D supplementation, and calcimimetic therapy.

8 Initiation of statins for primary prevention of hyperlipidemia in patients receiving dialysis is not recommended due to a lack of benefit from randomized controlled trials and meta-analyses, while benefit still may exist in those with non-dialysis dependent CKD.

9 CKD-associated pruritus is a secondary complication that significantly affects patients' quality of life and has limited treatment options. Difelikefalin is a selective kappa opioid receptor agonist with antipruritic effects approved for pruritus in hemodialysis patients and is the only approved treatment option.

BEYOND THE BOOK

Read and evaluate the case presented in Chapter 56—End-Stage Kidney Disease: Urine Trouble Level II. In: Schwinghammer TL, Koehler JM, Borchert JS, Slain D, Park SK. eds. *Pharmacotherapy Casebook: A Patient-Focused Approach*, 11e. Mcgraw Hill; 2020. Available at https://accesspharmacy.mhmedical.com/content.aspx?bookid=2868§ionid=242182546.

This activity is useful to enhance student understanding regarding the COLLECT, ASSESS, PLAN, and IMPLEMENT steps in the patient care process.

INTRODUCTION

1 Chronic kidney disease (CKD) affects many organ systems and processes leading to secondary complications. While the primary goal is to prevent CKD progression and the resultant complications (see Chapter 62 for a more in-depth discussion of CKD progression and management), ultimately many individuals progress to the more advanced stages of CKD (CKD G4—end-stage kidney disease, ESKD). The most common complications of CKD include fluid and electrolyte disorders (hypervolemia, hyperkalemia), anemia, mineral and bone disorder, metabolic acidosis, and increased incidence of cardiovascular disease (CVD). Complications of CKD are frequently unrecognized or are inappropriately managed, and for many patients, this contributes to significant morbidity, premature mortality, or a poorer prognosis if and when they require renal replacement therapy. This chapter primarily covers the pathophysiology and treatment of anemia, CKD-mineral and bone disorder (CKD-MBD), select cardiovascular complications, and CKD-associated pruritus in adult patients with CKD. The reader is referred to Chapters 68, 70, and 71 for a more detailed discussion of management and monitoring strategies for CKD patients with hypervolemia, hyperkalemia, and metabolic acidosis, respectively. A list of complications of advanced CKD is provided in Table 63-1.

EPIDEMIOLOGY

Anemia of Chronic Kidney Disease

As a common complication of CKD, anemia prevalence increases with age in individuals with non-dialysis (ND) CKD with reports of 50% prevalence in older Medicare patients (aged 66-85 years) and 28% in younger individuals (aged 18-63 years).[1] This prevalence increases as CKD progresses with estimates of 44% in CKD G3 increasing to 73% in CKD G5 for the older individuals and 22% increasing to 54% in the younger individuals. Despite the fact that

TABLE 63-1 Complications of Chronic Kidney Disease[a]

Organ System or Complication	Clinical Manifestations[a]
Amyloidosis	Accumulation of β_2-microglobulin Carpal tunnel syndrome
Cardiovascular disease	Atherosclerosis-related complications (arrhythmias, heart failure, myocardial infarction, stroke)
Endocrine	Hypoglycemic episodes (result of decreased degradation of insulin by the kidney)
Gastrointestinal	Nausea, vomiting, anorexia (from uremia) Delayed gastric emptying Gastroesophageal reflux GI bleeding
Hematologic	Anemia Bleeding diathesis Platelet dysfunction
Hyperkalemia	Arrhythmias/ECG changes Metabolic acidosis Muscle weakness or paralysis
Hypervolemia	Edema Heart failure Hypertension
Immune disorders	Impaired cell-mediated immunity Lymphopenia
Metabolic acidosis	Bone disease Hyperkalemia Reduced respiratory reserve Skeletal muscle catabolism
Mineral and bone disorder	Bone fractures Calciphylaxis
Neurologic	Peripheral neuropathies Restless leg syndrome Uremic encephalopathy
Protein–energy wasting	Malnutrition
Uremic pruritus	Generalized itching predominantly of back, face, and extremity used for vascular access, but may affect any area (May be more severe during or immediately after hemodialysis)

ECG, electrocardiogram.

[a]Not all inclusive.

anemia is a well-recognized complication of CKD, management is suboptimal, particularly in the ND-CKD population where patients who meet criteria for treatments including erythropoiesis stimulating agents (ESAs) and iron often do not receive an intervention.[2] This is supported by the fact that the average hemoglobin (Hb) among incident (new) ESKD patients in the United States in 2018 was 9.3 g/dL (93 g/L; 5.77 mmol/L) with levels less than 9 g/dL (90 g/L; 5.59 mmol/L) in many areas throughout the United States. Only 14.6% of incident patients had received an ESA prior to ESKD.[3] Furthermore, iron deficiency is present in more than half of ND-CKD patients and up to 25% of dialysis patients, in part, due to the fact that iron supplementation is not a standard treatment approach for ND-CKD patients.[4] For prevalent dialysis patients (on dialysis for at least 90 days), the majority of patients maintain Hb levels between 10 and 11.9 g/dL (100 and 119 g/L; 6.21 and 7.39 mmol/L), due in large part to protocol-driven approaches that lead to ESA and iron use.[5] This does not negate the fact that suboptimal anemia management at initiation of dialysis is associated with increased mortality, even if corrected in the subsequent months after dialysis initiation.[6] Anemia of CKD is also associated with increased morbidity with greater likelihood of hospitalization, cardiovascular (CV) disease, cognitive impairment, and decreased quality of life.[7]

Chronic Kidney Disease–Related Mineral and Bone Disorder

CKD-MBD collectively includes abnormalities in parathyroid hormone (PTH), calcium, phosphorus, active vitamin D, and fibroblast growth factor 23 (FGF23) and is considered one of the most common CKD-related secondary complications with significant implications on patient morbidity and mortality. Abnormalities in these parameters, particularly elevations in PTH and FGF23, may be observed in earlier stages of CKD (stage G3) with hyperphosphatemia and calcium abnormalities more prevalent as kidney function declines to stage G4.[8,9] Data regarding prevalence are limited in the ND-CKD population. Based on data from dialysis patients from the Dialysis Outcomes and Practice Patterns Study (DOPPS) approximately 24% of ESKD patients on HD have hyperparathyroidism (defined as a PTH >600 pg/mL [ng/L; 64.2 pmol/L]) and 43% have phosphorus above goal (phosphorus >5.6 mg/dL [1.81 mmol/L]).[5] CKD-MBD worsens as kidney function declines with more resistant disease associated with worsening kidney function.[9] Severity of this secondary complication is also indicated by control of associated parameters (PTH, albumin corrected calcium and phosphorus) and use of pharmacologic therapy. Based on data from US hemodialysis patients, approximately 70% of patients had at least one parameter out of control PTH (>600 pg/mL [ng/L; 64.2 pmol/L], corrected calcium >10.2 mg/dL [2.55 mmol/L], serum phosphorus >5.5 mg/dL [1.78 mmol/L]).

ETIOLOGY AND PATHOPHYSIOLOGY

Anemia of Chronic Kidney Disease

2 The primary cause of anemia of CKD is a relative deficiency in production of erythropoietin by interstitial fibroblasts in the outer renal cortex and medulla of the kidney where approximately 90% of production occurs (the remainder occurs in the liver). Erythropoietin is a glycoprotein hormone that stimulates erythropoiesis (red blood cell production) by binding to receptors on early erythroid progenitor cells, burst-forming units, and colony-forming units in the bone marrow, thus preventing apoptosis and allowing cell division and maturation into mature red blood cells. In individuals with normal kidney function, plasma concentrations of erythropoietin increase exponentially in response to hypoxia to promote erythropoiesis; however, this response is lost as kidney disease progresses.[10]

Impaired oxygen sensing in the kidneys leads to disrupted signaling of specific hypoxia inducible factors (HIFs). HIF is a transcription factor composed of oxygen regulated α subunits (HIF-1α and HIF-2α) and a β subunit. The β subunit is present consistently in the HIF complex and binds with one of the three isoforms of the α subunit to induce expression of target genes depending on the complex formed. Erythropoietin gene transcription for all hypoxia-induced genes is initiated by HIF-α with the HIF-2α subunit being the main subunit involved in erythropoietin production and iron transport. In the presence of normal oxygen levels, an enzyme known as HIF-prolyl hydroxylase (HIF-PH) is activated and causes HIF-α to be hydroxylated which leads to its degradation and no stimulation of erythropoietin production by erythropoietin producing cells. In hypoxic conditions, the HIF-PH enzyme is inactive allowing HIF-α to translocate to the cell nucleus where it forms a heterodimer with the β subunit causing activation of gene transcription to increase erythropoietin production, promote iron absorption and transport, and decrease hepcidin levels. This is a nicely regulated system that is altered in CKD. With CKD, oxygen consumption in the kidneys is decreased due to disease-related changes (Fig. 63-1). Despite the fact that hypoxia is present systemically, the erythropoietin producing cells do not detect the

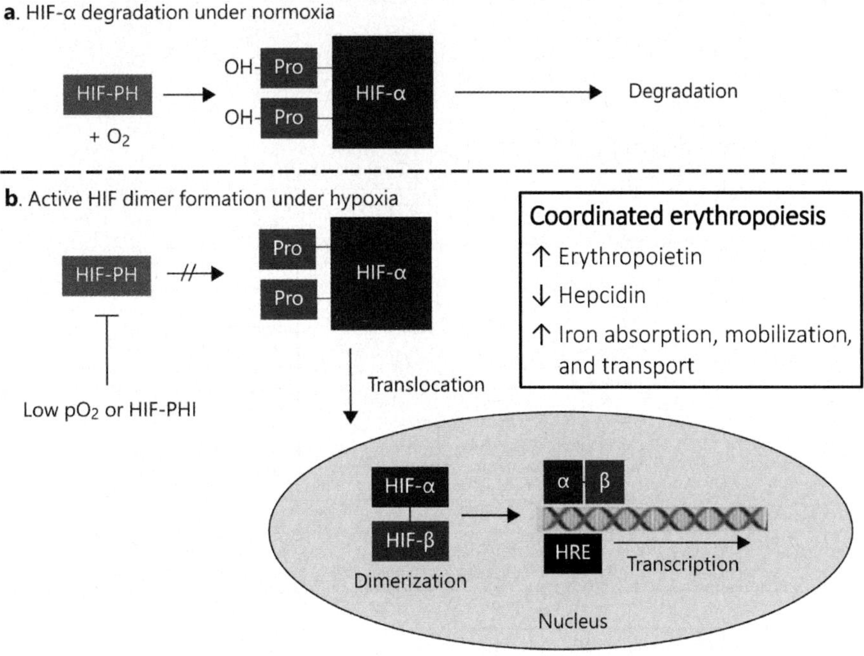

FIGURE 63-1 HIF activity under normoxia and hypoxia. Under normoxia (normal oxygen conditions) oxygen binds with the HIF-PH enzyme to form a complex with HIF-α which is then degraded. With hypoxia (reduced oxygen conditions) the HIF-PH enzyme is inactive and the HIF-α subunit can translocate to the cell nucleus where it forms a heterodimer with the β subunit. This leads to gene transcription and expression of multiple genes resulting in increased endogenous erythropoietin production, decreased hepcidin, and improved iron absorption, mobilization, and transport. (HIF-PH, hypoxia inducible factor prolyl hydroxylase enzyme; HRE, HIF responsive element, Pro, proline.) *(Reprinted, with permission, from Locatelli F, Fishbane S, Block GA, MacDougall IC. Targeting hypoxia-inducible factors for thetreatment of anemia in chronic kidney disease patients. Am J Nephrol. 2017;45:187–199.)*

extent of hypoxia since there is sufficient oxygen in the immediate environment (in the kidney relative to oxygen needs). This results in a disruption in HIF signaling and a relative deficiency in erythropoietin production.[11-13]

In addition to impaired erythropoietin production, iron deficiency is common in individuals with advanced kidney disease (ie, CKD stages G4, G5, and ESKD) due to decreased gastrointestinal (GI) absorption of iron, inflammation, frequent blood testing, blood loss from hemodialysis (HD) for patients with ESKD, and increased iron demands from ESA therapy when treatment is initiated. Iron deficiency is the leading cause of resistance to ESAs and the reason frequent iron supplementation is necessary.[10,14] Hepcidin, a hormone produced by the liver, is a primary regulator of iron homeostasis. This hormone directly binds to and inhibits the protein ferroportin that transports iron out of storage cells and into circulation. When iron stores are high, hepcidin production is increased and results in a decrease in intestinal iron absorption, impairment of iron recycling from macrophages, and decreased mobilization of stored iron from hepatocytes. Hepcidin production is also induced by inflammation or infection. As a result, the increase in hepcidin in inflammatory conditions leads to sequestering of iron, decreased iron absorption, and ineffective red blood cell production. Conversely, hepcidin production is decreased when iron stores are low. The fact that hepcidin plays such a role in iron regulation has prompted the development of agents to target hepcidin and potentially alter iron transport.[15]

Additional factors contributing to the development of anemia of CKD are the decreased red cell life span (from the normal 120 days to approximately 60 days in individuals with CKD 5D), the effects of accumulation of uremic toxins and inflammatory cytokines, and vitamin B_{12} and folate deficiencies.

Chronic Kidney Disease–Related Mineral and Bone Disorder

3 Disorders of mineral and bone metabolism are common in the CKD population and include abnormalities in PTH, calcium, phosphorus, vitamin D, fibroblast growth factor-23 (FGF-23), bone turnover, as well as soft-tissue calcifications. These abnormalities have been described as characteristics of secondary hyperparathyroidism (sHPT) and renal osteodystrophy (ROD). The term CKD-MBD encompasses these abnormalities in mineral and bone metabolism as well as associated calcifications.

The pathophysiology of CKD-MBD is complex (Fig. 63-2). Calcium and phosphorus homeostasis is mediated through the effects of PTH, 1,25-dihydroxyvitamin D_3 (calcitriol), and FGF-23 on bone, the GI tract, kidney, and the parathyroid gland. As kidney function declines, there is a decrease in phosphate elimination, which results in hyperphosphatemia and a decrease in serum calcium concentration. Hypocalcemia is the primary stimulus for secretion of PTH by the parathyroid glands. Hyperphosphatemia also increases PTH synthesis and release through its direct effects on the parathyroid gland and production of prepro-PTH messenger RNA.[16] In an attempt to normalize ionized calcium, PTH increases calcium reabsorption by the distal tubules and decreases phosphate reabsorption in the proximal tubules of the kidney (at least until the GFR falls to less than 30 mL/min/1.73 m^2 [0.29 mL/s/m^2]) and also increases calcium mobilization from bone. FGF-23 production in bone also increases in response to high phosphate levels and increased PTH and promotes phosphate excretion by the kidney. The result is a relative normalization of calcium and phosphorus, at least in the early stages of CKD; however, this occurs at the expense of an elevated PTH and FGF-23 ("the trade-off hypothesis").

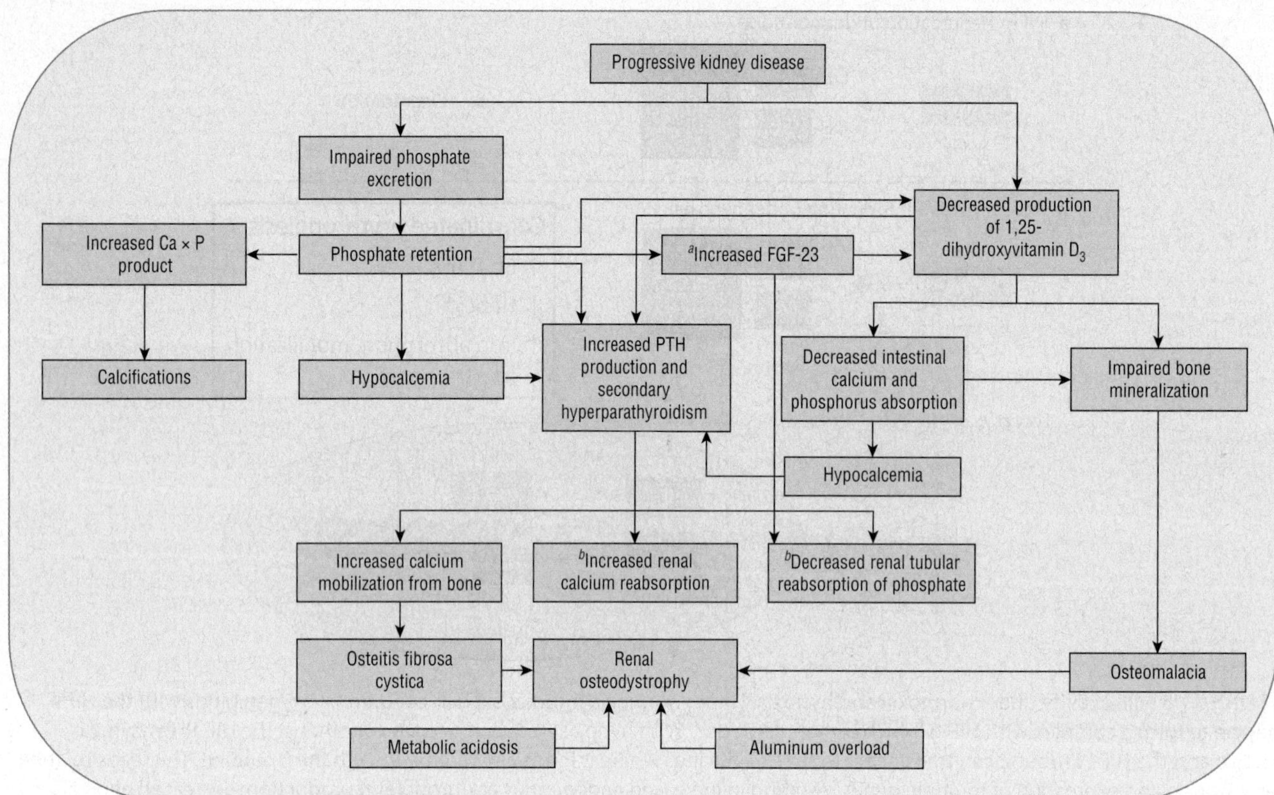

FIGURE 63-2 Pathophysiology of CKD-MBD. (Ca, calcium; FGF-23, fibroblast growth factor-23; PTH, parathyroid hormone.) [a]FGF-23 also increases in response to 1,25-dihydroxyvitamin D_3. [b]These adaptations are lost as kidney disease progresses.

The increase in PTH is most notable when GFR is less than 60 mL/min/1.73 m^2 (0.58 mL/s/m^2) (CKD G3a and higher) and worsens as kidney function further declines.[16] With advanced kidney disease, the kidney fails to respond to PTH or to FGF-23 and abnormalities in calcium and phosphorus worsen. Over time the negative effects of sustained hyperparathyroidism on bone are realized as calcium resorption from bone persists.

1,25-Dihydroxyvitamin D_3 or calcitriol promotes increased intestinal absorption of calcium and phosphorus, which helps normalize ionized calcium. Calcitriol also works directly on the parathyroid gland to suppress PTH production. The enzyme 1-α-hydroxylase is responsible for the final hydroxylation and conversion of the vitamin D precursor, 25-hydroxyvitamin D or 25(OH)D, to calcitriol in the kidney (Fig. 63-3). As kidney disease progresses, the concentrations of calcitriol decline due to loss of 1-α-hydroxylase activity. The resultant vitamin D deficiency leads to reduced intestinal calcium and phosphorus absorption and worsening hyperparathyroidism. Increases in FGF-23 also promote calcitriol deficiency.[16] Calcitriol deficiency is more prevalent in individuals with CKD G4-G5. Deficiency in 25(OH)D (levels of <30 ng/mL [75 nmol/L]) is also common in individuals with CKD due to decreased dermal synthesis of vitamin D, decreased exposure to sunlight, and reduced dietary intake of vitamin D.

The abnormalities of CKD-MBD lead to alterations in structural integrity of bone and other associated consequences. The continuous high rate of production of PTH by the parathyroid glands promotes parathyroid hyperplasia. Nodular tissue demonstrates more rapid growth potential and is associated with fewer vitamin D and calcium-sensing receptors, resulting in resistance to exogenous calcitriol therapy. Bone abnormalities are almost universal in dialysis patients and observed in the majority of those with CKD G3-G5.[17] The bone abnormalities include osteitis fibrosa cystica (high bone turnover disease), osteomalacia (low bone turnover disease), and adynamic bone disease. Osteitis fibrosa cystica is most common and is characterized by areas of peritrabecular fibrosis. Bone marrow fibrosis and decreased erythropoiesis are also consequences of severe osteitis fibrosa cystica. Osteomalacia was historically noted in HD patients with aluminum toxicity, a finding less common today due to the decreased use of aluminum-containing phosphate binders and changes in the processing of dialysate solutions to decrease aluminum content. Adynamic lesions are characterized by low amounts of fibrosis or osteoid tissue and low bone formation rates. Multiple risk factors for the development of this bone disease include high concentrations of dialysate calcium along with high doses of calcium-containing phosphate binders, aggressive management with vitamin D therapy, diabetes, and aluminum toxicity.[16]

The morbidity and mortality of CKD patients are increased in individuals with both severe hypo- and hyperparathyroidism.[17] Elevations of serum phosphorus, even within the upper limits of the normal range, have been associated with increased risk of CV events and/or mortality (all-cause or CV mortality) in patients with CKD G3-G5.[18] FGF-23 has also been associated with increased mortality and CV events in individuals with CKD. The incidence of calciphylaxis, or rapid calcification of subcutaneous tissue, in patients with advanced kidney disease has increased over the past decade and has been associated with CKD-MBD, an elevated calcium times phosphorus product, and warfarin use.[17,19] Warfarin inhibits the matrix Gla protein, which is a vitamin-K-dependent protein that prevents calcium deposition in arteries, and may therefore promote vascular calcification in individuals at risk.[20] The decision to initiate warfarin therapy in patients with advanced kidney disease with a clinical indication (eg, atrial fibrillation) should take into account this additional

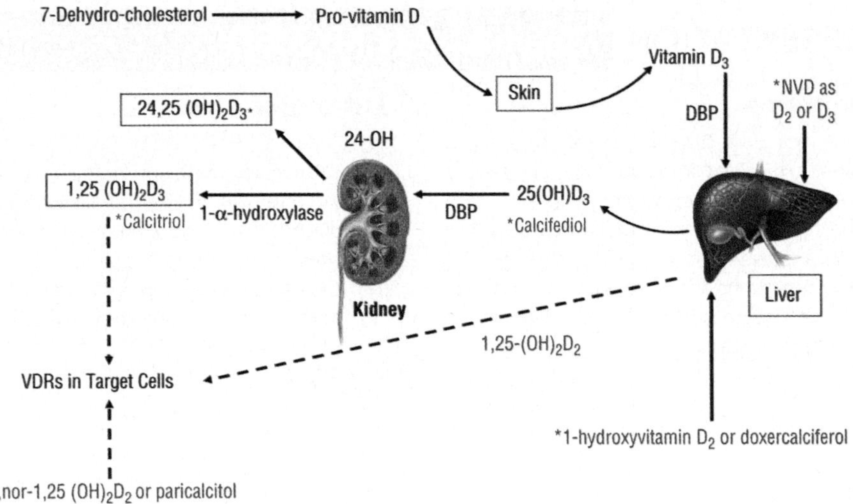

FIGURE 63-3 Vitamin D metabolism. Production of active vitamin D requires conversion of 7-dehydrocholesterol to cholecalciferol (vitamin D_3) by sunlight, followed by the first hydroxylation step in the liver to form 25-hydroxyvitamin D_3 or 25(OH)D_3, and the final conversion step in the kidney to form 1,25-dihydroxyvitamin D_3 or calcitriol. Within the kidney vitamin D may also be converted to an inactive form 24,25$(OH)_2D_3$. *Vitamin D therapies include calcitriol which is the active compound 1,25$(OH)_2D_3$ made endogenously, nutritional vitamin D (NVD) as ergocalciferol (a D_2 compound) or cholecalciferol (a D_3 compound), calcifediol which is 25(OH)D_3, and the vitamin analogs paricalcitol and doxercalciferol. If NVD is administered, the compound requires conversion to the active form as either a 1,25(OH)D_2 (as with ergocalciferol) or a 1,25(OH)D_3 (as with cholecalciferol). Calcitriol and paricalcitol are active as given. Doxercalciferol requires conversion to the active form [1,25$(OH)_2D_2$] by the liver. Agents in red are vitamin D agents. (DBP, vitamin D binding protein; NVD, nutritional vitamin D; VDRs, vitamin D receptors.)

risk of calcifications. Intake of calcium from calcium-based binders may also contribute to coronary artery calcification. These data underscore the need to consider all the consequences of elevated PTH, calcium, and phosphorus, not just their effects on bone.

CLINICAL PRESENTATION

Diagnostic Considerations for Anemia of Chronic Kidney Disease

Since individuals with anemia of CKD may be asymptomatic, laboratory evaluation is commonly the initial approach to diagnosing anemia of CKD. According to the KDIGO guidelines, Hb concentrations should be measured annually in CKD 3, biannually in CKD 4-5, and at least every 3 months in CKD 5D patients.[14] The diagnosis of anemia is made and further workup of anemia is required when the Hb is less than 13 g/dL (130 g/L; 8.07 mmol/L) for adult males and less than 12 g/dL (120 g/L; 7.45 mmol/L) for adult females. As iron deficiency is the primary cause of resistance to treatment of anemia with ESAs, assessment of the iron status is necessary. The TSat provides information on iron immediately available for use in the bone marrow for red blood cell production and the serum ferritin is in indirect measure of storage iron. The TSat is calculated as follows: (serum iron/total iron-binding capacity [TIBC]) × 100. Transferrin is the carrier protein for iron and may be affected by nutritional status. Serum ferritin is an indirect measure of storage iron and an acute-phase reactant, meaning it may be elevated under certain inflammatory conditions and give a false indication of storage iron. Patients may be diagnosed with *absolute iron deficiency* when both circulating iron and stored iron are low (low TSat and ferritin). In CKD patients absolute iron deficiency has been defined as a TSat <20% (0.20) and a ferritin of <100 ng/mL (μg/L; 225 pmol/L) in ND-CKD patients and <200 ng/mL (μg/L; 449 pmol/L) in HD patients.[7] The term *functional iron deficiency* describes a situation when the TSat is low, but the serum ferritin is not considered low (TSat <20% [0.20], ferritin >100 and 200 ng/mL [μg/L; 225 and 449 pmol/L] for ND-CKD and HD patients, respectively). In this situation, iron is not released rapidly enough to satisfy the demands for erythropoiesis and further evaluation is warranted. While there is some controversy regarding the reliability of these definitions, particularly for functional iron deficiency, they do provide a working definition used in clinical practice. The KDIGO guideline for anemia does suggest TSat and serum ferritin thresholds that warrant iron supplementation (Table 63-2).[14]

Additional workup should be done to evaluate other causes of anemia such as blood loss, deficiencies in vitamin B_{12} or folate, or other disease states that contribute to anemia, including human immunodeficiency virus infection and malignancies (see Chapter 122). Red blood cell indices (mean corpuscular volume, mean corpuscular Hb concentration), white blood cell count, differential and platelet count, and absolute reticulocyte count should also be assessed. A stool guaiac test should be performed to rule out GI bleeding. Measurement of serum erythropoietin concentrations is not generally useful since levels may fall into what is considered a "normal" range but are insufficient relative to the degree of decline in Hb.

Diagnostic Considerations for Chronic Kidney Disease–Related Mineral and Bone Disorder

Symptoms of CKD-MBD are often not evident until significant skeletal damage has developed; consequently, prevention is the key to minimize the risk of long-term complications. When signs and symptoms such as bone pain and skeletal fractures are evident, the disease is not easily amenable to treatment. Thus, the identification of

CLINICAL PRESENTATION Anemia and CKD-MBD

Signs and Symptoms

- Anemia: Fatigue, weakness, dizziness, headache, shortness of breath, mental confusion, cold intolerance, cold hands and feet, tingling in the extremities, chest pain, pale skin, irregular heartbeat.
- CKD-MBD: *Clinical presentation varies depending on the prevailing metabolic abnormality and characteristic bone disease (see Chapter 69, Calcium and Phosphorus Homeostasis).

Laboratory Tests

- Anemia: Decreased Hb/hematocrit (Hct), transferrin saturation (TSat), and/or ferritin (iron deficiency; note: ferritin may be increased due to inflammatory conditions), may be hemoccult-positive if GI bleeding present. Increased hepcidin.
- CKD-MBD: Decreased vitamin D levels, albumin, and calcium (in early stages of CKD). Increased: phosphorus, PTH, FGF-23, and calcium (more likely in CKD G5 and ESKD).

TABLE 63-2 KDIGO Recommendations for Initiation of Erythropoiesis Stimulating Agents and Iron in Adults with Anemia of Chronic Kidney Disease

	ND-CKD	ESKD
ESA initiation	If Hb <10 g/dL (100 g/L; 6.21 mmol/L). Consider rate of fall of Hb, prior response to iron, risk of needing a transfusion, risk of ESA therapy, and presence of anemia symptoms before initiating an ESA. [2C] Do not initiate if Hb ≥10 g/dL (100 g/L; 6.21 mmol/L). [2D]	Use ESAs to avoid drop in Hb to <9 g/dL (90 g/L; 5.59 mmol/L) by starting an ESA when Hb is between 9 and 10 g/dL (90 and 100 g/L; 5.59 and 6.21 mmol/L). [2B]
Hb level	Do not use ESAs to *intentionally* increase Hb above 13 g/dL (130 g/L, 8.07 mmol/L). [1A] Do not use ESAs to maintain Hb above 11.5 g/dL (115 g/L; 7.14 mmol/L). [2C]	Do not use ESAs to *intentionally* increase Hb above 13 g/dL (130 g/L, 8.07 mmol/L). [1A] Do not use ESAs to maintain Hb above 11.5 g/dL (115 g/L; 7.14 mmol/L). [2C]
Iron initiation[a]	If TSat is ≤30% (0.30) and ferritin is ≤500 ng/mL (µg/L; 1,120 pmol/L). [2C]	If TSat is ≤30% (0.30) and ferritin is ≤500 ng/mL (µg/L; 1,120 pmol/L). [2C]

CKD, chronic kidney disease; ESA, erythropoiesis stimulating agent; ESKD, end-stage kidney disease; Hb, hemoglobin; ND-CKD, non-dialysis CKD patients; QOL, quality of life; TSat, transferrin saturation.

See Chapter 62 for definitions of evidence grading in brackets.

[a]If TSat and serum ferritin are below suggested levels, consider iron supplementation if goal is to increase Hb and/or decrease ESA dose. *Note*: Serum ferritin is an acute-phase reactant-use clinical judgment when above 500 ng/mL (µg/L; 1120 pmol/L).

Data from Reference 14.

biochemical or imaging abnormalities which typically precede clinical manifestations is an essential component of patient evaluation. The biochemical abnormalities of CKD-MBD that are commonly present in patients with CKD include alterations in serum phosphorus, calcium, PTH, 25(OH)D (D represents either D2 or D3), and 1,25$(OH)_2D_3$ or calcitriol. Because of deficiency in the vitamin D precursor, 25(OH)D, is common and has been associated with negative outcomes in the CKD population, measurement of 25(OH) D levels in patients with CKD 3-5D is suggested.[17] The assay methods for 25(OH)D are not standardized, which creates a challenge regarding the clinical implications of abnormal values and limits its value as an indicator of therapeutic response.[21] Current monitoring recommendations and goals of therapy are covered in the "Treatment of CKD-MBD" section.

In addition to evaluating biochemical indices that define CKD-MBD, evaluation of bone architecture may be desirable. The gold standard test for diagnosing bone manifestations of CKD-MBD is a bone biopsy for histologic analysis; however, this is an invasive test that is not easily performed. KDIGO guidelines recommend bone biopsy only in patients in whom the etiology of clinical symptoms and biochemical abnormalities is not clear and the results may lead to changes in therapy.[17] This includes patients experiencing unexplained fractures, persistent hypercalcemia, osteomalacia, an atypical response to standard therapies for elevated PTH, or progressive decreases in bone mineral density despite therapy. Bone biopsy findings are described on the basis of turnover rate, mineralization, and volume. Bone mineral density testing is recommended in patients with CKD G3-G5 and ESKD with evidence of CKD-MBD and/or risk factors for osteoporosis.[17] CKD-MBD is also highly associated with vascular and soft-tissue calcifications, known risk factors for mortality; therefore, diagnostic testing for calcifications should be considered in the evaluation for CKD-MBD.

TREATMENT OF SECONDARY COMPLICATIONS

General Approach to Treatment of CKD Complications

4 Management of complications of CKD should be based on the KDIGO consensus guidelines which are based on evidence, when available, and expert recommendations. There are guidelines provided by the Kidney Disease Outcome Quality Initiative (KDOQI) for many of the associated complications; however, this chapter emphasizes KDIGO guidelines, which are international guidelines and, in most cases, based on data or expert opinion. Chapter 62 includes a guide to the grading and strength of recommendations used in these guidelines.

5 An interdisciplinary approach to care should emphasize patient-centered care and at minimum include a team of nephrologists, nurses, dietitians, pharmacists, and social workers. This team approach puts the patient at the center and includes individuals trained to address many of the complex secondary complications of CKD and provide patient education about CKD, the associated complications, and their management. Treatment of secondary complications of CKD requires a number of pharmacologic intervention, thus adding to the number of medications required for patients with advanced CKD. Pharmacists are readily accessible medication experts equip to address medication-related problems and provide comprehensive medication management.

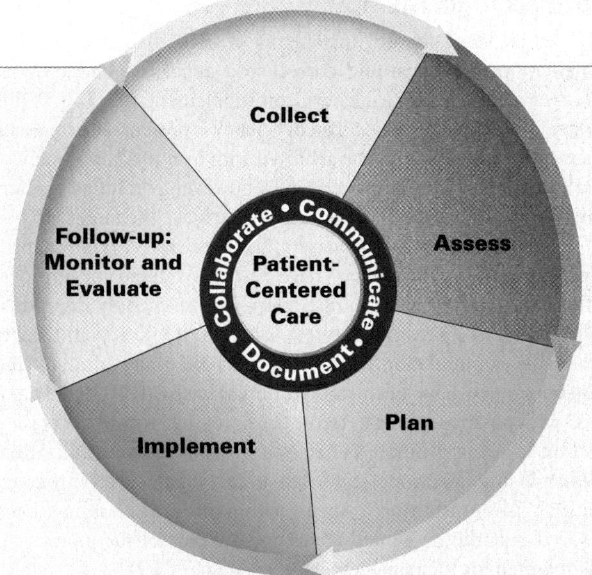

Patient Care Process for Secondary Complications of Chronic Kidney Disease (CKD)

Collect

- Patient characteristics (eg, age, sex, CKD stage [see Chapter 62], medication allergies)
- Past medical history
- Social history (eg, smoking), family/friend supports
- Dietary intake (eg, phosphate-containing foods/sources, iron sources, sodium intake)
- Current medications including OTC medications, herbals, dietary supplements
- Objective data:
  - Blood pressure, heart rate, weight
  - Labs as defined under "Assess"

Assess

- CKD stage (see Chapter 62 for staging criteria)
- Reported symptoms: see Clinical Presentation for signs and symptoms of secondary complications
- Serum potassium concentration—assess frequently in CKD stage 4, 5, and end-stage kidney disease (ESKD)
- Volume status—peripheral and pulmonary edema versus hypovolemia (may need to alter diuretic regimen)
- Hemoglobin concentration (see Table 63-2 for ESA initiation)
- Iron indices (transferrin saturation and ferritin) for patients on an ESA, assess transferrin saturation (TSAT) and ferritin at least every 3 months and assess when clinically indicated (eg, following blood loss)
- Concentrations of calcium, albumin (to calculate corrected calcium), phosphorus, and parathyroid hormone (PTH) (see Table 63-6)
- Insurance coverage of medications, current out of pocket cost of medications
- Medication adherence
- Other recommendations as outlined in Chapter 62

Plan

- Drug therapy recommendations, including dose, route, frequency, and duration
- Dietary recommendations (consider sodium, potassium, phosphorus, and fluid intake)
- Monitoring parameters, including frequency and timing of follow-up
- Patient education, including purpose of new or changed treatment, lifestyle modifications, medication administration (eg, timing of phosphate binders with meals), injection technique
- Self-monitoring for resolution of symptoms
- Referrals to other providers when appropriate (eg, clinical pharmacist, dietitian, nephrologist, nephrology nurse, social worker, endocrinologist)

Implement*

- Provide patient education on all elements of the treatment plan
- Use motivational interviewing strategies to maximize adherence
- Schedule follow-up labs and appointment, adherence assessment

Follow-up: Monitor and Evaluate

- Resolution of symptoms
- Presence of adverse effects
- Patient adherence to treatment plan using multiple sources of information

**Communicate with patient, caregivers, and CKD multidisciplinary team.*

Anemia

Desired Outcome

The desired outcomes of anemia management are to safely achieve target Hb levels that increase oxygen-carrying capacity to decrease signs and symptoms of anemia and reduce the need for blood transfusions. Hb is the preferred monitoring parameter for red blood cell production because, unlike Hct, its concentration is not affected by blood storage conditions and instrumentation used for analysis. Initiation of iron or ESA therapy is guided by the patient's Hb, TSat, and ferritin (Table 63-2).[14] The risk of mortality and CV events is higher in CKD patients treated to higher Hb target values with an ESA. There are discrepancies, however, in the FDA-approved labeling for ESAs and the KDIGO anemia guidelines in terms of target Hb, with more conservative Hb of 10 to 11 g/dL (100-110 g/L; 621-683 mmol/L) recommended by the FDA for individuals with ESKD.[14]

Despite associations of development of left ventricular hypertrophy (LVH) with worsening anemia, there are no prospective studies demonstrating that early and aggressive treatment improves CV end points or reduces LVH in CKD patients. Improvements in the quality of life are not universally observed with increases in Hb and such perceived improvements must be weighed against reported risks associated with using ESAs in the CKD population.[22]

Target Hemoglobin and Use of Erythropoiesis Stimulating Agents

The target range for Hb in the CKD population has been a topic of much debate. Although the benefits of achieving a normal or near normal Hb seemed rational when ESAs became available in the late 1980s, the Normal Hematocrit Cardiac Trial (NHCT),[23,24] the Correction of Hb and Outcomes in Renal Insufficiency (CHOIR),[25] and the Cardiovascular Risk Reduction by Early Anemia Treatment with Epoetin-Beta (CREATE)[26] trials later proved otherwise, and the suggested target Hb at the time of those trials of 11 to 12 g/dL (110-120 g/L; 6.83-7.45 mmol/L) was subsequently lowered. Several FDA advisories have been released and changes were made to the precautions, black box warning, and dosing sections of ESA product labeling promoting more conservative use of ESAs.[27] The current labeling for all ESAs warns that dosing ESAs to target Hb levels greater than 11 g/dL (110 g/L; 6.83 mmol/L) for CKD patients increases the risk for death, serious CV reactions, and stroke. Practitioners are advised to consider ESAs in patients with CKD only when the Hb is below 10 g/dL (100 g/L; 6.21 mmol/L) and to individualize therapy to use the lowest ESA dose necessary to decrease the need for red blood cell transfusions.

Of concern is the fact that CHOIR demonstrated that targeting Hb levels above 11 g/dL (110 g/L; 6.83 mmol/L) with ESA therapy in individuals with CKD not requiring dialysis resulted in increased risk of mortality and CV events compared with patients maintained in a lower Hb range (trial was terminated early).[25] CREATE demonstrated no benefit of targeting a higher Hb target (13-15 g/dL [130-150 g/L; 8.07-9.31 mmol/L]) to reduce CV events in the ND-CKD patients.[26] An increased risk of all-cause mortality with ESA treatment was also reported in a meta-analysis of nine randomized controlled trials that included over 5,100 CKD patients treated to Hb targets in the range of 12 to 16 g/dL (120-160 g/L; 7.45-9.93 mmol/L).[28] There was also a higher risk of dialysis access thrombosis and uncontrolled blood pressure in the higher Hb groups. Results from the Trial to Reduce Cardiovascular Events with Aranesp Therapy (TREAT) also failed to support a higher Hb.[29] In addition, there was also an almost twofold increase in the risk of stroke (5% in the treatment group vs 2.6% in the placebo group), a finding that was not associated with baseline characteristics of the patients or other potential risk factors. Those patients with a history of cancer in the higher Hb group also had a higher risk of death.

The overall negative CV outcomes observed with higher Hb targets in the randomized trials have prompted much discussion about the potential causes, including not only ESA dose and Hb target, but also the rate of rise in Hb and the variability in Hb over time (eg, degree of fluctuation in Hb). Individuals in the CHOIR study who were able to achieve the target Hb did not have worse outcomes. Further analysis of the NHCT data also showed a reduction in mortality by 60% for those individuals who responded to epoetin therapy compared with nonresponders.[24] Resistance to ESAs was associated with higher 1-year mortality and hospitalization for CV events.[30] Such findings have led to discussion of whether hyporesponsiveness to ESAs due to other conditions such as inflammation may explain the higher event rates in this group of individuals.

Nonpharmacologic Therapy

Nonpharmacologic therapy for anemia of CKD includes maintaining adequate dietary intake of iron as well as folate and B_{12}. A relatively small amount of dietary iron, approximately 1 to 2 mg, is absorbed each day, primarily in the duodenum. While oral intake or iron should be encouraged, iron from dietary sources alone is insufficient to meet the increased iron requirements from initiation of ESA therapy.

Pharmacologic Therapy

6 Pharmacologic therapy for anemia of CKD includes iron supplementation to prevent and correct iron deficiency and ESAs to correct erythropoietin deficiency. Iron supplementation is first-line therapy for anemia of CKD if iron deficiency is present, and for some patients, the target Hb may be achieved with iron therapy alone. For most individuals with advanced CKD, however, combined therapy with iron and an ESA will be necessary to achieve the target Hb.

The HIF prolyl hydroxylase inhibitors (HIF-PHIs) (daprodustat, roxadustat, vadadustat) have been considered for approval by the Food and Drug Administration. Currently, only daprodustat has received a favorable review in terms of efficacy and safety in the dialysis population. These HIF-PHIs are orally administered medications that have been studied in patients with ND-CKD and ESKD with positive results in terms of improving Hb and decreasing hepcidin levels to promote better iron distribution and utilization, without raising erythropoietin levels to levels achieved with exogenous ESA administration.[31] Agents within this drug class have been approved outside the United States and are part of the pharmacologic regimen for the management of anemia of CKD.

Iron Supplementation Iron formulations are available for administration orally, intravenously, or through the dialysate used for hemodialysis. Iron supplements provide the elemental iron required for production of Hb and its subsequent incorporation in red blood cells, the net result of which is an increase in the transportation of oxygen to tissues. Iron supplementation is necessary to treat *absolute iron deficiency*, but may also be warranted in individuals with a TSat less than 30% (0.30) and a ferritin less than 500 ng/mL (μg/L; 1,120 pmol/L) in whom an increase in Hb or a decrease in ESA dose is desired (KDIGO suggestion).[14] Patients with *functional iron deficiency* may also benefit from iron supplementation. The optimal upper limit for these iron indices is not clearly defined and clinicians must balance achieving adequate iron for erythropoiesis with safety in terms of preventing adverse consequences such as iron overload and concerns with nontransferrin (unbound) iron.

The preferred route of administration depends on CKD stage, severity of iron deficiency, tolerability of and prior response to oral iron, history of adverse reactions to IV iron, availability of IV access, and cost (see the "Therapeutic Options" section). KDIGO recommends either oral or IV iron administration in non-HD patients (eg, CKD stage G3 or higher) and IV supplementation for patients with ESKD.[14] The National Institute for Health Care Excellence (NICE) guidelines suggest a trial of oral iron (for up to 3 months) in ND-CKD patients not receiving an ESA and IV iron for patients treated with and ESA and/or on HD.[32] Oral iron supplementation is more convenient for ND-CKD patients since they do not have regular IV access; however, at some point they are likely to require IV iron supplementation to correct absolute iron deficiency, especially if they are receiving an ESA. If oral therapy is initiated, a 1- to 3-month trial is recommended to assess response. In patients with CKD on hemodialysis, GI absorption of iron is often inadequate to meet the increase in iron demand from ESA therapy and chronic blood loss, due largely to the effects of hepcidin on GI absorption. Thus, the IV route is preferred for almost all HD patients.[14] IV administration is also recommended in the peritoneal dialysis (PD) population, although the desire to preserve potential future venous access sites for HD (if needed) must be considered. Parenteral iron improves the responsiveness to ESA therapy and, thus, lower ESA doses can be used to maintain the target Hb in HD patients.[14] In the FIND-CKD trial, 624 ND-CKD patients were randomized to IV ferric carboxymaltose administered at high dose (1,000 mg every 4 weeks) to target a ferritin of 400 to 600 ng/mL (μg/L; 899-1348 pmol/L), low dose (200 mg every 4 weeks) to target a ferritin of 100 to 200 ng/mL (μg/L; 225-449 pmol/L), or oral iron administered as 200 mg/day. After 56 weeks, the high ferritin IV iron group had better outcomes in terms of the increase in mean Hb at 12 months and time to achieve that level, but no differences in adverse events. Iron administration in patients with functional iron deficiency (ie, low TSat, high serum ferritin) should be decided on an individual basis. A trial of IV iron therapy may be warranted if the Hb is less than desired despite high-dose ESA therapy as long as potential risks of IV therapy are considered (see the "Adverse Effects" section).

Therapeutic Options Multiple oral and IV products are marketed in the United States. Oral iron preparations include ferrous and ferric salts (ferrous sulfate, ferrous fumarate, ferrous gluconate, ferric citrate, and ferric maltol), polysaccharide iron complex, and carbonyl iron. These forms of iron differ in terms of the amount of elemental iron (Table 63-3). A heme iron polypeptide formulation is also available and contains 12 mg of elemental iron. Numerous nonprescription products that contain ferrous salts and iron polysaccharide are available. Ferric maltol is a newer agent available by prescription containing 100% elemental iron that is approved for iron deficiency anemia in adults. Ferric citrate was originally developed as a phosphate binding agent but was subsequently shown to improve iron status and Hb levels also, leading to its approval for treatment of iron-deficiency anemia in ND-CKD patients.[33]

Iron is absorbed from the GI tract via the divalent metal transporter 1 in the duodenum and upper jejunum where approximately 10% of orally administered iron is absorbed. Ferroportin transports iron across the mucosal cell to the blood where it is bound to transferrin. Immediate release oral iron agents are preferred over enteric coated and slow or sustained release products, which are absorbed more distally in the GI tract and not as readily absorbed. Absorption of iron is decreased by food and achlorhydria. Some oral iron formulations also include ascorbic acid to enhance iron absorption, although data to support this practice are lacking. The role of hepcidin to decrease GI absorption is also a significant factor that influences iron regulation and a reason that oral therapy may be inadequate to meet iron needs, particularly in HD patients.

Soluble ferric pyrophosphate citrate (Triferic) is an iron compound approved for iron replacement in patients with ESKD on HD and may be administered via the dialysate during HD or intravenously using the IV formulation (Triferic AVNU). When administered in the dialysate, this agent crosses to the blood side of the dialyzer by diffusion to allow for continuous iron administration during the procedure. Ferric pyrophosphate citrate is a mixed-ligand iron complex with iron bound to pyrophosphate and citrate. Once in the systemic circulation ferric pyrophosphate binds directly to transferrin, bypassing the reticuloendothelial system, and is delivered to the bone marrow for use in red blood cell production. Studies to date have shown an increase in Hb concentration and a reduction in ESA dose and IV iron requirements, but no significant increase in ferritin or in nontransferrin bound iron.[34,35] These findings are important when considering the potential adverse effects associated with iron accumulation and free (unbound) iron.

Most IV iron preparations are colloids that consist of an iron-containing core that is surrounded by a carbohydrate shell to stabilize the iron complex. Available agents differ in the size of the core and the composition of the surrounding carbohydrate. Such differences affect the rate of dissociation of iron from the complex, the rate of distribution, and the maximum tolerated dose and rate of infusion. The IV iron products that are currently available in the United States are shown in Table 63-4.

Adverse Effects Adverse effects of oral iron are primarily GI in nature and include constipation, nausea, and abdominal cramping (see Chapter 122). These adverse effects are more likely as the dose is escalated. These unfavorable effects often discourage patients from taking these medications on a chronic basis. Some of these GI side effects can be minimized if oral iron products are taken with food; however, food may decrease absorption of oral iron.

Adverse effects of IV iron include allergic reactions, hypotension, dizziness, dyspnea, headaches, lower back pain, arthralgia, syncope, and arthritis. Some of these reactions, in particular hypotension, can be minimized by decreasing the dose or rate of infusion of iron. The most concerning potential consequence of IV iron administration is anaphylaxis. Serious reactions to iron dextran including respiratory complications and CV collapse have been reported in approximately 0.6% to 0.7% of patients.[14] Such reactions are believed to be partly a response to antibody formation to the dextran component. Adverse reactions were reported more frequently with the brand product Dexferrum (no longer available) compared with INFeD.[14] Iron dextran carries a black box warning of the risk of anaphylactic-type reactions, including fatalities, and a 25-mg test dose is required. An analysis of anaphylaxis risk in patients newly exposed to IV iron products (including dextran, gluconate, sucrose, or ferumoxytol) reported the highest risk for iron dextran and the lowest risk with iron sucrose.[36]

The non-dextran IV iron formulations have a better safety record than either of the iron dextran products. The labeling for these formulations also includes a warning of the risk of hypersensitivity reactions. Following the approval of ferumoxytol in 2009, there were 79 cases of anaphylactic reactions, of which 18 were fatal.[37] Almost half of the cases occurred with the first dose and approximately 75% occurred during the infusion or within 5 minutes of completion. In 2015, the FDA required a black box warning for ferumoxytol noting that fatal and serious hypersensitivity reactions including anaphylaxis have occurred and that the risks and benefits should be considered in patients with a history of multiple drug allergies. Ferumoxytol should not be administered IV push, but should be diluted and administered as an IV infusion (see Table 63-4). As a superparamagnetic oxide, ferumoxytol may alter the diagnostic

TABLE 63-3 Oral Iron Agents

Preparation	Brand Names[a]	[c]% Elemental Iron	Commonly Rx'd Unit Size in mg (Amount elemental iron)
Carbonyl iron	Feosol, Ferralet (combo with ferrous gluconate, docusate)	100	45 (45)
Ferric citrate[b]	Auryxia	21	1,000 (210)
Ferric maltol[b]	Accufer	100	30 (30)
Ferrous fumarate	Femiron, Feostat	33	200 (66)
Ferrous gluconate	Simron, Fergon	12	325 (38)
Ferrous sulfate	Feosol, Fer-In-Sol	20	325 (65)
Iron Polysaccharide	Niferex, Nu-Iron	100	150 (150)

[a]Not all inclusive for over-the-counter medications (ie, ferrous salts).

[b]Available by prescription only.

[c]Generally target a dose of 200 mg elemental iron per day. Ferric citrate and ferric maltol approved at different doses [ferric citrate - 210 mg (one tablet) three times daily; ferric maltol - 30 mg (one capsule) twice daily].

TABLE 63-4 Intravenous Iron Agents

Iron Compounds	Brand Names	Molecular Weight (Daltons)	FDA-Approved Indications	FDA-Approved Dosing[a,b]
Ferric carboxymaltose	Injectafer	150,000	Adult patients with intolerance to oral iron or who have had an unsatisfactory response to oral iron and in adult patients with CKD not on dialysis	Give 2 doses separated by at least 7 days of 750 mg per dose (if body weight is ≥50 kg) or 15 mg/kg per dose (if body weight is <50 kg) not to exceed 1,500 mg per course. Give either IV push (100 mg/min) or diluted in not more than 250 mL of 0.9 NaCl as an infusion over at least 15 minutes
Ferric derisomaltose	Monoferric	155,000	Treatment of iron deficiency anemia in adults with ND-CKD or who have intolerance to oral iron or unsatisfactory response to oral iron	If weight ≥50 kg: 1,000 mg as a single dose If weight <50 kg administer 20 mg/kg actual body weight as a single dose
Ferric pyrophosphate citrate	Triferic AVNU	1,313	Iron replacement to maintain Hb in adult patients with ESKD on hemodialysis	6.75 mg iron over 3 to 4 hours at each HD session via pre-dialyzer infusion line, post-dialyzer infusion line, or a separate connection to the venous blood line
	Triferic			Add the appropriate ampule or powder packet* to the bicarbonate concentrate solution to achieve a final concentration of ferric pyrophosphate citrate of 110 μg/L *add one 5 mL ampule to 2.5 gallons (9.5 L) of bicarbonate concentrate or one 50 mL ampule to 25 gallons (95 L) of bicarbonate or one packet of powder to each 25 gallons ampule (95 L)
Ferumoxytol	Feraheme	750,000	Adult patients with iron-deficiency anemia associated with chronic kidney disease	510 mg (17 mL) as a single dose, followed by a second 510 mg dose 3-8 days after the initial dose. Dilute in 50-200 mL of 0.9% NaCl or 5% dextrose and administer as an IV infusion over 15 minutes
Iron dextran	INFeD	96,000	Patients with iron deficiency in whom oral iron is unsatisfactory or impossible	100 mg over 2 minutes (25-mg test dose required) Note: Equation provided by manufacturer to calculate dose based on desired Hb
Iron sucrose	Venofer	43,000	Adult and pediatric ESKD patients on HD age 2 years and older	Adult: 100 mg over 2-5 minutes or 100 mg in maximum of 100 mL of 0.9% NaCl over 15 minutes per consecutive HD session Pediatric: 0.5 mg/kg not to exceed 100 mg per dose over 5 minutes or diluted in 25 mL of 0.9% NaCl administered over 5-60 minutes (give dose every 2 weeks for 12 weeks)
			Adult and pediatric ND-CKD patients age 2 years and older	Adult: 200 mg over 2-5 minutes on five different occasions within 14-day period. There is limited experience with administration of 500 mg diluted in a maximum of 250 mL of 0.9% NaCl over 3.5-4 hours on days 1 and 14 Pediatric: see pediatric dosing for CKD 5HD (give dose every 4 weeks for 12 weeks)
			Adult and pediatric ESKD patients on PD, age 2 years and older	Adult: give 3 divided doses within 28 days as 2 infusions of 300 mg over 1.5 hours 14 days apart followed by one 400 mg infusion over 2.5 hours 14 days later. Dilute in a maximum of 250 mL of 0.9% NaCl Pediatric: see pediatric dosing for CKD 5HD (give dose every 4 weeks for 12 weeks)
Sodium ferric gluconate	Ferrlecit	350,000	Adult and pediatric ESKD patients on HD age 6 years and older receiving ESA therapy	Adult: 125 mg over 10 minutes or 125 mg in 100 mL of 0.9% NaCl over 60 minutes Pediatric: 1.5 mg/kg in 25 mL of 0.9% NaCl over 60 minutes; maximum dose 125 mg per dose

CKD, chronic kidney disease; ESA, erythropoiesis stimulating agent; ESKD, end-stage kidney disease; HD, hemodialysis; ND-CKD, non-dialysis CKD patients.

[a]Monitor for 30 minutes following an infusion; KDIGO guidelines recommend monitoring for 60 minutes (1B recommendation for iron dextran, 2C recommendation for non-dextran products).

[b]With the exception of ferric carboxymaltose, ferric derisomaltose, and ferumoxytol, small doses (eg, 25-150 mg/wk) are generally used for maintenance regimens. Larger doses (eg, 1 g) should be administered in divided doses. The IV form of ferric pyrophosphate citrate (Triferic AVNU) is administered in smaller increments (6.75 mg)

ability of magnetic resonance imaging studies for up to 3 months after administration; therefore, they should be done prior to administration of ferumoxytol whenever possible.

Long-term administration of IV iron also introduces a risk of iron overload. Deposition of excess iron may affect several organ systems, leading to hepatic, pancreatic, and cardiac dysfunction. Bone marrow biopsy provides the most definitive diagnosis of iron overload, but because it is an extremely invasive procedure, it is not widely employed in most clinical settings. Maintaining target serum ferritin and TSat values is the most reasonable approach to minimize the risk of iron toxicity. The challenge is in defining what should be the upper limit, particularly for serum ferritin, which may be elevated in inflammatory conditions and not reflective of true iron stores in such situations. If symptomatic overload does occur, iron chelating agents such as deferoxamine (Desferal), deferiprone (Ferriprox), deferasirox (Exjade), or phlebotomy may be necessary.

More conservative use of ESAs has led to an increase in iron supplementation. This has raised some concerns regarding the potential detrimental effects of increased iron exposure and higher TSat and ferritin targets on patient outcomes (eg, infection, mortality, hospitalizations). Specific concerns relate to the ability of iron to promote infection since iron is essential for infectious microorganisms, increased risk of oxidative stress, and subsequent cardiovascular complications, as well as the concerns of other effects of non-transferrin bound iron (unbound/free iron). Data from clinical trials do not confirm unequivocally that exposure to IV iron in CKD patients treated with ESA therapy increases patient morbidity or mortality.[7,38-42]

A large randomized controlled trial in the United Kingdom (PIVOTAL trial) evaluated the safety of high-dose IV iron (400 mg/month) administered proactively (with the upper TSat limit 40% [0.40] and ferritin of 700 ng/mL [μg/L; 1,573 pmol/L]) and low-dose IV iron (0-400 mg monthly) administered reactively (with a TSat <20% [0.20] or a ferritin <200 ng/mL [μg/L; 449 pmol/L] prompting the need for IV iron administration) in 2,141 dialysis patients over a median of 2 years.[38] There were significantly fewer deaths and nonfatal CV events (nonfatal MI, stroke, hospitalization for heart failure) in the high-dose group compared to the low-dose group and a lower requirement for ESAs and transfusions. The high-dose and low-dose IV iron groups exhibited identical infection rates.[42] This is the most robust evidence to date that IV iron at this dose level and prespecified iron targets is safe in HD patients. Caution is recommended with the use of IV iron doses higher than those used in the PIVOTAL trial as observational data have suggested associations with increased risk of mortality and infection. Although more data are needed to draw conclusions, the general consensus is that administration of IV iron in the setting of an active infection is not recommended.[7] The benefits of correcting iron deficiency in patients with CKD should also be considered in the clinical decision process.

Drug Interactions Drug interactions with oral iron are common. Iron absorption is decreased by other elements (eg, calcium in calcium-containing phosphate binders), medications that increase the pH of the GI tract such as proton pump inhibitors and H_2-antagonists, and antibiotics including doxycycline and tetracycline. Iron also decreases absorption of other drugs such as antibiotics (fluoroquinolones, doxycycline).

If oral therapy is initiated, the suggested dose is 200 mg of elemental iron per day for most available agents. The approved dose of ferric maltol is 30 mg twice daily. The recommended dose of ferric citrate in ND-CKD patients is 210 mg three times daily. With numerous oral agents to choose from, the best option is one that provides adequate elemental iron with the fewest number of dosage units required per day and the lowest incidence of adverse effects. Strategies to improve absorption and potentially minimize adverse GI events have been evaluated in non-CKD patients and include single-dose administration of ferrous sulfate on alternate days, which resulted in a decrease in hepcidin and improved iron absorption, although such data in CKD patients are not available.[43] KDIGO guidelines suggest a 1- to 3-month trial of oral therapy in the non-HD CKD population prior to initiating IV therapy.[14]

For the HD population, IV therapy is preferred with administration of a 1-g course of IV iron (in divided doses) historically used to replete patients with an absolute iron deficiency. The amount per dose and rate at which to administer IV iron depends on the product (see Table 63-4). Typical repletion dosing regimens for IV iron are 100 mg as iron sucrose over 10 dialysis sessions or 125 mg of sodium ferric gluconate over eight dialysis sessions to provide a total of 1 g. As a general practice, if IV iron doses higher than those currently approved are needed, they should be infused over a longer period of time (eg, at least 2-4 hours) due to the risk of hypersensitivity reactions, hypotension, dizziness, and nausea. The newer agents, ferumoxytol, ferric carboxymaltose, and ferric derisomaltose differ in terms of how rapidly iron is released from the compound, which allows for higher single doses to be administered compared to the other IV iron agents (Table 63-4). Ferric pyrophosphate citrate when given IV is approved at smaller doses of 6.75 mg given over 2 to 4 hours during each HD session. When administered via the dialysate used for HD, the ampule or powder is added to the bicarbonate concentrate solution used for dialysis to achieve a final concentration of 110 μg/L.

Without ongoing iron supplementation, many patients quickly become iron deficient. To prevent iron deficiency and the need for intermittent repletion doses, maintenance doses of IV iron should be administered in HD patients (eg, iron sucrose 25-100 mg/wk; sodium ferric gluconate 62.5-125 mg/wk).[14] There are many different maintenance dosing protocols in clinical practice for CKD patients and some controversy as to the maximum monthly doses given safety concerns (see the "Adverse Events" section). The main consideration is to provide enough iron to help achieve goal hemoglobin levels and to reduce the need for ESAs and transfusions, while minimizing risks of IV iron.

Administration of a 25-mg test dose is required for all iron dextran products. This test dose should be administered over at least 30 seconds. It is recommended that patients be observed for at least 1 hour before administering the remainder of the dose. For this reason, the non-dextran agents are predominantly used in the CKD population. Regardless of which IV iron agent is used, all patients should be monitored for signs and symptoms of hypersensitivity for at least 30 minutes following completion of a dose. KDIGO clinical practice guidelines suggest monitoring patients for at least 60 minutes following administration of IV iron; a 1B recommendation for iron dextran products and a 2C recommendation for non-dextran formulations.[14] These agents should only be administered when personnel and therapies are immediately available for the treatment of anaphylaxis and other hypersensitivity reactions.

Erythropoiesis-Stimulating Agent Therapy Since FDA approval of epoetin-alfa in 1989, ESA therapy has become an integral part of the care for patients with CKD. ESAs available in the United States are listed in Table 63-5. The biosimilar epoetin-alfa epbx is approved in the United States. As a biosimilar, this agent has the same indications as the biological drug, epoetin-alfa.

Pharmacology and Mechanism of Action Epoetin-alfa is a glycoprotein manufactured by recombinant DNA technology that has the same amino acid sequence as endogenous erythropoietin. Darbepoetin alfa has two additional *N*-linked carbohydrate chains that decrease the affinity for the erythropoietin receptor, but yield a longer duration of activity compared with erythropoietin. Methoxy PEG-epoetin-beta was created by the addition of an amide bond between the N-terminal or ε-amino group of epoetin-beta and methoxy polyethylene glycol butanoic acid. The compound, which is referred to as a continuous erythropoietin receptor activator (CERA), has a much longer half-life than the other ESAs. All ESAs have the same biologic activity as endogenous erythropoietin in that they bind to and activate the erythropoietin receptor to stimulate erythropoiesis.

Pharmacokinetics and Pharmacodynamics All available ESAs may be administered via either the IV or the subcutaneous (SUBQ) route. Although bioavailability is less with SUBQ than with IV administration, the prolonged absorption phase leads to an extended half-life (see Table 63-5). Thus, the same target Hb can be achieved and maintained at SUBQ epoetin doses 15% to 30% lower than IV doses.[14] The prolonged half-lives of darbepoetin-alfa and methoxy PEG-epoetin-beta offer the advantage of less-frequent dosing. This is of particular benefit for individuals with CKD who are not yet receiving dialysis and those receiving PD since these patients are not in a

TABLE 63-5 Erythropoiesis-Stimulating Agents in Chronic Kidney Disease

Drug Name	Brand Name(s)	Starting Dose	Route of Administration	Half-Life (Hours)
Epoetin-alfa	Epogen, Procrit	Adults: 50-100 units/kg three times per week Pediatrics: 50 units/kg three times per week	IV or SUBQ	8.5 (IV) 24 (SUBQ)
Epoetin-alfa-epbx	Retacrit	See epoetin-alfa information		
Darbepoetin alfa	Aranesp	Adults: ND-CKD: 0.45 μg/kg once every 4 weeks ESKD: 0.45 μg/kg once per week or 0.75 μg/kg every 2 weeks Pediatrics: 0.45 μg/kg once weekly; may give 0.75 μg/kg once every 2 weeks in ND-CKD patients	IV or SUBQ	25 (IV) 48 (SUBQ)
Methoxy PEG-epoetin-beta	Mircera	All adult CKD patients: 0.6 μg/kg every 2 weeks; Once Hb stabilizes, double the dose and administer monthly (eg, if administering 0.6 μg/kg every 2 weeks, give 1.2 μg/kg every month)	IV or SUBQ	134 (IV) 139 (SUBQ)

CKD, chronic kidney disease; ESKD, end-stage kidney disease; ND-CKD, non-dialysis CKD patients; PEG, polyethylene glycol; SUBQ, subcutaneous.

clinical setting as frequently as HD patients and do not have regular IV access.

The pharmacodynamic effect of ESAs is important to consider when evaluating response to therapy. With initiation of ESA therapy or a change in dose, the Hb may begin to rise as the result of demargination of reticulocytes; however, it takes approximately 10 days before erythrocyte progenitor cells mature and are released into the circulation. The Hb continues to increase until the life span of the cells stimulated by ESA therapy is reached (mean 2 months; range 1-4 months in patients with ESKD). At this point, a new steady state is achieved (ie, the rate at which red blood cells are being produced equals the rate at which they are leaving the circulation). For this reason, evaluate the Hb response over several weeks and not make dosing changes too soon.

Efficacy Patients will generally respond to ESA therapy in a dose-related fashion. The most common causes of resistance are iron deficiency, acute illness, inflammation, infection, chronic bleeding, aluminum toxicity, malnutrition, hyperparathyroidism, cancer, and chemotherapy.[14] Deficiencies in folate and vitamin B_{12} should also be considered as potential causes of resistance to ESA therapy, as both are essential for optimal erythropoiesis. Use of ACEIs and ARBs has also been associated with hyporesponsiveness to ESA therapy.[14]

Hypertension is the most common adverse event reported with ESAs and may be associated with the rate of rise in Hb.[10] Hypertensive encephalopathy has also been observed. According to FDA-approved product labeling, ESAs should not be used in those with uncontrolled blood pressure. Protocols established in some clinical settings recommend withholding ESA therapy if blood pressure is above a defined threshold; however, others advocate more judicious use of antihypertensive agents and dialysis to control blood pressure. Seizures have occurred in patients treated with ESAs, particularly within the first 90 days of starting therapy. Thrombosis of the HD vascular access site and other thromboembolic events were reported when ESAs were used to target Hb greater than 13 g/dL (130 g/L; 8.07 mmol/L).[44] The potential for these adverse effects calls for close monitoring of the rate of rise in Hb, changes in blood pressure, and neurologic symptoms following initiation of therapy or a change in ESA dose.

Antibody-associated pure red cell aplasia (PRCA), caused by induction of antibodies directed against the ESA molecule, was reported in the late 1990s and early 2000 and was primarily associated with subcutaneous administration of Eprex, an epoetin-alfa formulation manufactured outside the United States.[45] This reaction was potentially a result of organic compounds being formed when the stabilizing agent polysorbate was used in combination with uncoated rubber stoppers in the prefilled syringes. There have been few cases since changes in the packaging of this product were made; however, the cause of PRCA with this formulation has been disputed.[46] Of note, there have been reports of PRCA with methoxy PEG-epoetin-beta.[47] An evaluation for PRCA should be considered for patients receiving ESA therapy for more than 8 weeks who develop either a rapid decrease in Hb level (rate of 0.5-1 g/dL/wk [5-10 g/L/wk; 0.31-0.62 mmol/L/wk]) or require one to two blood transfusions per week, and have an absolute reticulocyte count of less than 10,000/μL (10×10^9/L) with a normal platelet and white blood cell count.[14] Discontinuation of ESA therapy is recommended if antibody-mediated PRCA develops because antibodies are cross-reactive and continued exposure may lead to anaphylactic reactions (a grade 1A recommendation).

ESAs have also been associated with a reduction in overall survival and increased risk of progression of certain tumor types among CKD patients (eg, head and neck). ESAs are not indicated in patients receiving myelosuppressive chemotherapy when the anticipated outcome is cure. These are important effects to consider when managing a CKD patient with an oncologic disorder.[48]

Drug-Drug Interactions No significant drug interactions have been reported with the available ESAs.

Dosing and Administration Recommended starting doses of ESA are listed in Table 63-5. Less-frequent dosing of epoetin-alfa (eg, every 1-2 weeks) is effective and may be preferred for ND-CKD patients since these individuals are seen in the outpatient clinical setting on a relatively infrequent basis. Subcutaneous dosing is also more convenient in this population and in PD patients who do not have regular IV access. Conversion tables for patients who are to be switched from epoetin-alfa (units/wk) to darbepoetin-alfa (μg/wk) are available in the labeling information for darbepoetin.[49] There is also a conversion chart for patients being converted from epoetin-alfa or darbepoetin-alfa to methoxy PEG-epoetin-beta.[47]

When starting an ESA, Hb levels should be monitored at least monthly (weekly may be preferred) until stable and then monthly thereafter. Dose adjustments should be made based on Hb response with a goal of avoiding an excessively quick rise or the achievement of values above the recommended target values. An acceptable rate of increase in Hb is 1 to 2 g/dL (10-20 g/L; 0.62-1.24 mmol/L) per month. As a general rule, ESA doses should not be increased more frequently than every 4 weeks, although decreases in dose may occur more frequently in response to a rapid rate of rise in Hb. The dose should be reduced by at least 25% if the Hb increases by more than 1 g/dL (10 g/L; 0.62 mmol/L) in a 2-week period.[10] The dose should be reduced or temporarily discontinued if the Hb level approaches or exceeds 11 g/dL (110 g/L; 6.83 mmol/L) in dialysis patients or 10 g/dL

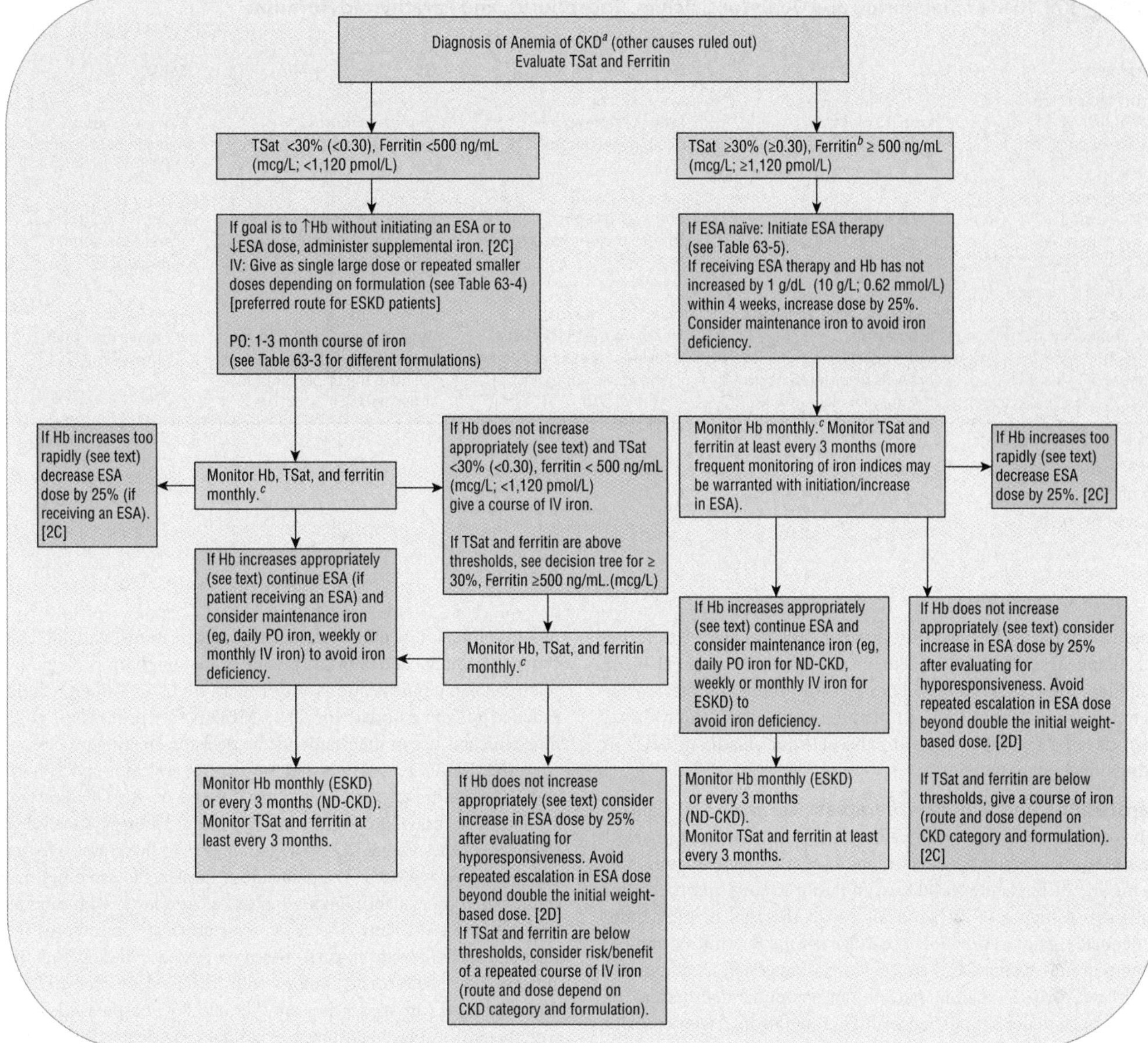

FIGURE 63-4 Algorithm for management of anemia of CKD in adults.[14,44] (CKD, chronic kidney disease; ESKD, end-stage kidney disease; ESA, erythropoiesis-stimulating agent; Hb, hemoglobin; ND-CKD, non-dialysis CKD patients; TSat, transferrin saturation.) Evidence grading in brackets. [a]See Table 63-2 and text for discussion of Hb levels. [b]Clinical judgment should be used to determine if iron supplementation should be continued when ferritin >500 ng/mL (μg/L; 1,120 pmol/L). [c]Weekly monitoring of Hb may be warranted. Wait at least 1 week after an IV dose of iron to measure TSat and ferritin.

(100 g/L; 6.21 mmol/L) in patients with CKD not requiring dialysis. KDIGO recommendations advocate a decrease in dose as opposed to withholding the ESA when a decrease in Hb concentration is desired (2C grade recommendation).[14] A 25% increase in dose may be considered if the Hb has not increased by 1 g/dL (10 g/L; 0.62 mmol/L) after 4 weeks of ESA treatment and if no causes of hyporesponsiveness to the ESA have been identified. For patients who do not respond adequately over a 12-week escalation period, an increase in ESA dose is unlikely to improve response and may increase risks. Initial hyporesponsiveness to ESAs should be considered when there is no increase in Hb from baseline after the first month of appropriate weight-based dosing. In this situation escalations in ESA dose beyond double the initial weight-based dose should be avoided (a grade 2D recommendation). Acquired ESA hyporesponsiveness may be suspected when patients previously on a stable ESA dose require two increases in ESA doses up to 50% beyond the previously utilized stable dose.[14] In this situation, repeat escalations in ESA dose beyond double the dose at which they had been stable should be avoided (a grade 2D recommendation). The lowest dose of ESA should be used to maintain an Hb level sufficient to reduce the need for red blood cell transfusions. Figure 63-4 provides an approach to management of anemia using ESAs and iron therapy in patients with CKD.

Hypoxia-Inducible Factor Prolyl-Hydroxylase Inhibitors A key target for anemia management in CKD is the development of HIF-prolyl-hydroxylase (HIF-PH) inhibitors or HIF stabilizers that mimic the conditions of hypoxia to prevent the hydroxylation process. The HIF-PH inhibitors in development in the United States include roxadustat, daprodustat, and vadadustat.[11,50] Demonstrated benefits include improvement in hemoglobin levels and induction of physiologic blood levels of erythropoietin. These agents also decrease hepcidin, increase iron absorption, and improve functional iron deficiency. There is some concern that long-term use of these agents and sustained HIF activation may promote tumor

TABLE 63-6 KDIGO Monitoring and Goals for Calcium, Phosphorus, and Parathyroid Hormone

	Chronic Kidney Disease Stage			
Parameter	**G3**	**G4**	**G5**	**ESKD**
Corrected calcium[a]				
Monitoring frequency[b] / Goal	Every 6-12 months Avoid hypercalcemia [2C]	Every 3-6 months Avoid hypercalcemia [2C]	Every 1-3 months Avoid hypercalcemia [2C]	Every 1-3 months Avoid hypercalcemia [2C]
Phosphorus				
Monitoring frequency[b] / Goal	Every 6-12 months Toward the normal range [2C]	Every 3-6 months Toward the normal range [2C]	Every 1-3 months Toward the normal range [2C]	Every 1-3 months Toward the normal range [2C]
Intact PTH				
Monitoring frequency[b] / Goal	Based on baseline level and CKD progression Avoid progressively rising levels or levels persistently above the upper limit of normal [2C]	Every 6-12 months Avoid progressively rising levels or levels persistently above the upper limit of normal [2C]	Every 3-6 months Avoid progressively rising levels or levels persistently above the upper limit of normal [2C]	Every 3-6 months 2-9 times the upper normal limit [2C]

Evidence grading in brackets.
[a]Corrected for albumin.
[b]Not graded.
Data from Reference 17.

progression due to the effects on vascular endothelial growth factor and angiogenesis. While there remains much to learn about HIF-PH inhibitors, these agents are likely to become an integral therapy for anemia management in CKD. At the present time, only daprodustat has received a favorable review by the FDA for anemia of CKD in dialysis-dependent patients.

Transfusions and Adjunct Therapies Red blood cell transfusions carry many risks and therefore should only be used in select situations, such as acute management of symptomatic anemia, following significant acute blood loss, and prior to surgical procedures that carry a high risk of blood loss, with the goal of preventing inadequate tissue oxygenation or cardiac failure. L-carnitine supplementation and vitamin C were previously suggested as adjunctive treatments of CKD anemia, but are not recommended because of the lack of evidence supporting improved anemia management with these therapies.[14]

Evaluation of Therapeutic Outcomes

Important therapeutic outcomes to monitor in patients with anemia of CKD include Hb, iron status, as well as the need for blood transfusions. Iron status should be assessed at least every 3 months in patients receiving a stable ESA regimen.[14] Iron status should be monitored more frequently (eg, every month) when initiating or increasing the ESA dose, following a course of IV iron, or when other factors put the patient at risk for iron loss (eg, bleeding). Hb levels should be monitored at least every 3 months in patients with ND-CKD or PD patients and at least monthly in HD patients. Hb should be monitored at least monthly in patients started on ESA therapy until the Hb is stable. Of note, FDA labelling for ESAs recommends weekly monitoring of Hb with initiation of therapy or a change in dose until the Hb is stable.[44,47,49]

Mineral and Bone disorder

Management of PTH, phosphorus, and calcium is important in preventing CKD-MBD and CV and extravascular calcifications. Patients with CKD-MBD usually require a combination of dietary intervention, phosphate-binding medications, vitamin D, and calcimimetic therapy (for ESKD patients) to achieve these goals.

Desired Outcome

7 The desired outcomes for management of CKD-MBD are to "normalize" the biochemical parameters and prevent bone manifestations, CV and extravascular calcifications, and the associated morbidity and mortality with both nonpharmacologic and pharmacologic interventions. At present, the 2017 KDIGO clinical practice guideline update for CKD-MBD is the most recent guideline clinicians use in their patient care decision-making process.[17]

The KDIGO-recommended targets for calcium, phosphorus, and PTH and frequency of monitoring based on the CKD category are shown in Table 63-6.[17] The most appropriate strategy is to evaluate trends in all these key CKD-MBD parameters to determine a reasonable treatment approach. The guideline emphasizes to avoid hypercalcemia based on evidence linking higher calcium levels with mortality and nonfatal CV events. The recommendation for phosphorus is to maintain levels "toward normal" based on evidence linking both high and low phosphate concentrations with increased mortality. Despite this association with higher mortality, the effect of phosphorus lowering with therapy (ie, phosphate binders) has not consistently demonstrated improved hard outcomes such as reduced mortality.[51,52]

Clinicians involved in the care of patients with CKD should know which PTH assays are available in their facilities. PTH is secreted from the parathyroid gland as intact PTH, an 84-amino-acid peptide chain (1-84 PTH) that is biologically active, and as smaller carboxy-terminal PTH fragments.[53] Circulating levels of these fragments (eg, 7-84 PTH) may increase substantially in patients with CKD and actively antagonize the effects of 1 to 84 PTH. The available immunoradiometric assays measure not only the intact PTH molecule but also fragments, which may lead to overestimation of biologically active PTH. While correction factors have been proposed, they cannot be uniformly applied to all commercially available assays and thus inconsistent results are common. The variability in PTH measurements and lack of evidence to support a specific target are part of the rationale for the KDIGO recommendation to monitor trends in serum PTH to guide treatment decisions. The optimal PTH in patients with CKD stages G3a-G5 is unclear. An increase in PTH is expected in response to declining kidney function and the desired phosphaturic effects; therefore, the guideline specifies that PTH levels *persistently* above the upper limit of normal and *progressively rising* should warrant a treatment decision. KDIGO recommends that PTH values for ESKD patients be within two to nine times the upper limit of the normal range, which corresponds to a PTH of approximately 130 to 600 pg/mL (ng/L; 14-64 pmol/L).[17] PTH values above 600 pg/mL (ng/L; 64 pmol/L) have been associated with higher CV mortality and hospitalizations.[54]

Monitoring of alkaline phosphatase activity is also recommended as this test may serve as a gauge of a patient's response to therapy and/or bone turnover status. Avoiding the development of vascular calcification and calciphylaxis is also important as treatment options for this complication once it develops are extremely limited and the associated mortality is high.

Nonpharmacologic Therapy

Dietary Phosphorus Restriction Dietary phosphorus restriction is a first-line intervention for management of hyperphosphatemia and should be initiated for most patients with CKD G3-G5.[17] The challenge with dietary restriction of phosphorus is providing enough protein to prevent malnutrition, a common problem in the ESKD population because dialysis patients require a higher protein intake (1.2-1.3 g/kg/day) and foods high in phosphorus are generally high in protein. An additional consideration is the source of phosphorus, organic versus inorganic. Inorganic sources such as from frozen meals and processed foods include preservatives or additives used during food processing, whereas organic sources such as from meat and plant sources typically do not and may be a better option. Dietary supplements and certain brands of medications also contain phosphate (eg, amlodipine, codeine) and may contribute to phosphate intake.[55] One of the most common obstacles to dietary phosphorus restriction is patient nonadherence because of the poor palatability of the allowed foods. Regular counseling by a dietitian is ideal to design a realistic diet that works with the patient's lifestyle and considers nutritional goals.

Dialysis HD and PD lower serum phosphorus and calcium, the extent of which is dependent on the concentration of each in the dialysate and the duration of dialysis. It is suggested that the dialysate calcium concentration be between 2.5 and 3 mEq/L (1.25 and 1.5 mmol/L).[17] Removal of phosphorus does occur with dialysis (~2.5-3.5 g/wk, dependent on the dialysis prescription); however, conventional dialysis alone does not usually control hyperphosphatemia.[56] Patients on daily HD or nocturnal HD who typically have longer and/or more frequent dialysis sessions have better phosphorus control and require fewer phosphate-binding agents and in some cases may even require phosphate supplementation.

Parathyroidectomy Parathyroidectomy is a therapeutic option for those patients with persistently elevated PTH associated with hypercalcemia and/or hyperphosphatemia who are refractory to medical therapy (a grade 2B recommendation).[17] Surgical approaches include either subtotal parathyroidectomy or total parathyroidectomy with autotransplantation of parathyroid tissue to an accessible site, such as the forearm. Postoperative hypocalcemia, hypophosphatemia, and hypomagnesemia may occur because of a marked increase in bone production in relation to bone absorption ("hungry bone syndrome"). Following surgery, frequent monitoring of calcium and phosphorus is necessary. Treatment with supplemental calcium and vitamin D may be required for weeks or months.

While a parathyroidectomy is indicated for refractory patients, these patients may experience significant morbidity following the procedure. In a study of over 4,400 ESKD patients who underwent a parathyroidectomy, there was an increase in hospitalizations (particularly for acute myocardial infarction and dysrhythmia) and emergency room visits for treatment of hypocalcemia in the year following the procedure.[57] For some patients, a parathyroidectomy may be ineffective and there is also the risk of over suppression of PTH and prolonged hypocalcemia.[58]

Pharmacologic Therapy Patients with CKD-MBD usually require a combination of dietary intervention, phosphate-binding medications, vitamin D, and calcimimetic therapy (for ESKD patients).

Phosphate-Binding Agents Phosphate-binding agents are used in addition to dietary phosphorus restriction to limit GI absorption. These agents are indicated for CKD patients with progressive or persistent hyperphosphatemia. For many patients, the pill burden with phosphate-binding agents contributes to nonadherence and efforts should be made to simplify the regimen when possible. The cost of phosphate binders is also significant, contributing to over 1.5 billion in Medicare costs for US dialysis patients and CKD patients with Medicare Part D.[52]

Pharmacology and Mechanism of Action Drugs that bind dietary phosphorous in the GI tract form insoluble phosphate compounds that are excreted in feces, thus reducing dietary phosphorus absorption. Patients must be instructed to take these agents with meals to maximize the binding of phosphorus from dietary sources. A variety of phosphate-binding agents with varying binding affinity are available including elemental calcium, iron, and lanthanum-containing compounds, and the nonelemental agent sevelamer (Table 63-7). Estimates of phosphate-binding equivalent doses relative to 1 g of calcium carbonate have been reported based on the commonly available tablet or capsule strengths of each binder (calcium acetate 667 mg = 0.67; lanthanum 500 mg = 1.0, sevelamer carbonate 800 mg = 0.60, sucroferric oxyhydroxide 500 mg = 1.6, ferric citrate 210 mg = 0.64, aluminum hydroxide 500 mg = 0.75, and aluminum carbonate 500 mg = 0.95).[52,59]

Efficacy Oral calcium compounds are commonly used agents for control of serum phosphorus. Calcium carbonate and calcium acetate are the primary preparations used. Calcium citrate is also available but not used as a binder since the citrate component increases aluminum absorption and may cause more GI side effects. Calcium carbonate is marketed in a variety of dosage forms and is relatively inexpensive. Unfortunately, many calcium carbonate products are considered food supplements and thus do not meet US Pharmacopeia (USP) disintegration and dissolution requirements. In general, nationally advertised brands do meet these requirements, but it is difficult to determine whether private labels or house brands conform to these standards. Variability in gastric pH may also affect disintegration or dissolution, and thus phosphate-binding efficacy. Calcium carbonate is more soluble in an acidic medium and should be administered prior to meals when stomach acidity is highest. In addition, acid-suppressing agents such as ranitidine and proton pump inhibitors may reduce the phosphate-binding activity of calcium carbonate by increasing gastric pH. For patients with hypocalcemia, calcium carbonate or calcium acetate may also be given as a calcium supplement taken between meals to promote calcium absorption. This is a common scenario for patients following a parathyroidectomy.

Sevelamer is a nonabsorbable, nonelemental hydrogel phosphate-binding agent approved for ESKD patients, which effectively lowers phosphorus and has also been shown to lower LDL and increase HDL cholesterol. Sevelamer hydrochloride carries the risk of metabolic acidosis, a problem that has been overcome with development of the carbonate formulation. Sevelamer carbonate also comes in a powder formulation, which is a good option for many patients unable to swallow tablets.

Most of the comparative studies to date have focused on calcium-based binders versus sevelamer, which was the first non-calcium binder made available in the United States. The chronic use of calcium-containing phosphate binders promotes progression of vascular calcification; however, not all studies support this finding and this effect may occur with non-calcium–containing binders as well.[52] Available studies have more consistently shown a significant increase in coronary artery calcification with calcium-containing binders compared to sevelamer.[60] The effect of binder choice on mortality, particularly on CV mortality, is also controversial as studies evaluating this outcome are limited. Results of a meta-analysis showed that all cause death and risk of

TABLE 63-7 Phosphate-Binding Agents for Treatment of Hyperphosphatemia in Chronic Kidney Disease Patients

Category	Drug	Brand Name	Compound Content	Starting Doses	Dose Titration[a]	Comments[b]
Calcium-based binders	Calcium acetate (25% elemental calcium)	PhosLo	25% Elemental calcium (169 mg elemental calcium per 667 mg capsule)	1,334 mg three times a day with meals	Increase or decrease by 667 mg meal (169 mg elemental calcium)	Comparable efficacy to calcium carbonate with lower dose of elemental calcium Approximately 45 mg phosphorus bound per 1 g calcium acetate Evaluate for drug interactions with calcium
		Phoslyra	667 mg calcium acetate per 5 mL			
	Calcium carbonate[c]	Tums, Os-Cal, Caltrate	40% Elemental calcium	0.5-1 g (elemental calcium) three times a day with meals	Increase or decrease by 500 mg/ meal (200 mg elemental calcium)	Dissolution characteristics and phosphate binding may vary from product to product Approximately 39 mg phosphorus bound per 1 g calcium carbonate Evaluate for drug interactions with calcium
Iron-based binders	Ferric citrate	Auryxia	210 mg elemental iron per tablet (= 1 g ferric citrate)	420 mg ferric iron three times daily with meals	Increase or decrease dose by 1 or 2 tablets per meal	May increase serum iron, ferritin, and TSat May cause discolored (dark) stools Evaluate for drug interactions with iron
	Sucroferric oxyhydroxide	Velphoro	500 mg elemental iron per chewable tablet (= 2.5 g succroferric oxyhydroxide)	500 mg three times daily with meals	Increase or decrease by 500 mg/day	May cause discolored (dark) stools Evaluate for drug interactions with iron
Resin binders	Sevelamer carbonate	Renvela	800 mg tablet 0.8 and 2.4 g powder for oral suspension	800-1,600 mg three times a day with meals (once-daily dosing also effective)	Increase or decrease by 800 mg/meal	Also lowers low-density lipoprotein cholesterol Consider in patients at risk for extraskeletal calcification Risk of metabolic acidosis with sevelamer hydrochloride (less risk with carbonate formulation) May interact with cipro and mycophenolate mofetil
	Sevelamer hydrochloride	Renagel	400 and 800 mg caplets	800-1,600 mg three times a day with meals	Increase or decrease by 800 mg/meal	
Other elemental binders	Lanthanum carbonate	Fosrenol	500, 750, and 1,000 mg chewable tablets 750 and 1,000 mg oral powder	1,500 mg daily in divided doses with meals	Increase or decrease by 750 mg/day	Potential for accumulation of lanthanum due to GI absorption (long-term consequences unknown) Evaluate for drug interactions (eg, cationic antacids, quinolone antibiotics)
	Aluminum hydroxide (NOT PREFERRED)	AlternaGel	Content varies (range 100-600 mg/unit)	300-600 mg three times a day with meals	Not for long-term use requiring titration	Not a first-line agent; risk of aluminum toxicity; do not use concurrently with citrate-containing products Reserve for short-term use (4 weeks) in patients with hyperphosphatemia not responding to other binders Evaluate for drug interactions

TSat, transferrin saturation.

[a]Based on phosphorus levels, titrate every 2 to 3 weeks until phosphorus goal is reached.

[b]GI side effects are possible with all agents (eg, nausea, vomiting, abdominal pain, diarrhea, or constipation).

[c]Multiple preparations available that are not listed.

hypercalcemia were lower in dialysis patients receiving sevelamer when compared with calcium-based binders.[51] Fatal and nonfatal cardiovascular events, however, did not differ for ESKD patients receiving sevelamer compared to calcium acetate in an observational cohort study.[61] KDIGO suggests restricting the dose of calcium-based binders (a grade 2B recommendation); however, a maximum dose was not defined and this is left to clinical judgement.[17]

Lanthanum carbonate is a phosphate binder approved for patients with ESKD and has demonstrated efficacy in controlling phosphorus and maintaining PTH in the target range with less risk of hypercalcemia than calcium-containing binders.[17] The initial daily dose of 1,500 mg (administered in divided doses with meals) is often titrated to a range of 1,500 to 3,000 mg to maintain target phosphorus. The poor GI absorption, which limits systemic effects, and high binding capacity with phosphorus make this an attractive phosphate-binding agent, particularly when calcium-containing binders are not recommended due to hypercalcemia. Lanthanum is available as a chewable tablet, which may be appealing for some patients.

Ferric citrate and sucroferric oxyhydroxide are the newest iron-based phosphate-binding agents approved for ESKD patients. Sucroferric oxyhydroxide effectively lowers phosphorus over a long-term (1-year) period and may have a lower pill burden compared to other agents.[62] It is also available as a chewable tablet. Ferric citrate effectively lowers phosphorus and also offers the advantage of increasing iron indices (TSat and ferritin) while lowering IV iron and ESA use when compared to other binders and ferrous sulfate.[63-65] This agent is approved for treatment of both hyperphosphatemia in ESKD patients and for iron deficiency anemia in patients with CKD not on dialysis. Another potential advantage of ferric citrate (and of iron supplementation in general) being explored is reduction in FGF23 that has been observed.[64] This finding is of interest given the associated between FGF23 and adverse outcomes.

Aluminum salts were widely used in the 1980s as phosphate-binding agents because of their high binding potency. Due to the potential for accumulation and toxicities in patients with CKD, they should not be used as first-line agents. KDIGO recommends avoiding the long-term use of aluminum-containing binders in all patients with CKD stage G3a-G5D (a 1C recommendation).[17]

Magnesium-containing antacids are also effective phosphate binders and may decrease the amount of calcium-containing binders necessary for control of phosphorus; however, they are not preferred due to the frequent occurrence of GI side effects (ie, diarrhea) and the potential for magnesium accumulation.

Other agents that have been evaluated for their phosphate binding effects and potential use for prevention and treatment of hyperphosphatemia in CKD patients include nicotinamide and tenapanor. Nicotinamide is a metabolite of nicotinic acid that inhibits the gastrointestinal sodium-dependent phosphate transporter, NaPi2b. This agent has been studied in hemodialysis patients with some promising results in terms of phosphorus-lowering effects; however, lack of robust clinical data to support consistent phosphate lowering and adverse effects may limit effectiveness and tolerability.[66-68] Tenapanor is an inhibitor of intestinal sodium/hydrogen exchanger 3 (NHE3) that blocks paracellular transport of phosphate across the intestinal lumen. This agent is approved for treatment of irritable bowel syndrome with constipation, but has also been studied in hemodialysis patients as a single agent and as an add-on therapy to current phosphate binder treatments.[69-71] Phosphate-lowering effects have been consistently demonstrated with diarrhea as the most frequent adverse effect. In 2021, the FDA did not grant approval of this agent for control of phosphorus in dialysis patients due to what was considered a small treatment effect with unclear clinical significance.

Adverse Effects Adverse effects of all available phosphate binders are generally limited to constipation, diarrhea, nausea, vomiting, and abdominal pain. The risk of hypercalcemia may necessitate restriction of calcium-containing binder use and/or a reduction in dietary intake. Aluminum binders have been associated with CNS toxicity and the worsening of anemia, whereas magnesium binder use may lead to hypermagnesemia and hyperkalemia; therefore, aluminum and magnesium are not recommended for regular use in patients with kidney disease. The potential for iron overload should also be considered with ferric citrate given the effects on increasing iron indices. Accumulation of lanthanum tablets in the GI tract of a patient who swallowed these tablets resulted in severe complications; therefore, counsel patients to chew these tablets.[72] The same counseling point applies for sucroferric oxyhydroxide.

Drug-Drug and Drug-Food Interactions Calcium-containing phosphate-binding agents interfere with the absorption of several oral medications that are commonly prescribed for CKD patients, including iron, zinc, and quinolone antibiotics. Coadministration of sevelamer with ciprofloxacin and mycophenolate did result in a reduction in bioavailability of these agents and they should be taken at least 2 hours before sevelamer. Coadministration of lanthanum with tetracyclines, fluoroquinolones, levothyroxine, or drugs known to bind with cationic antacids may result in decreased bioavailability of these agents. The iron-containing products ferric citrate and sucroferric oxyhydroxide also have the potential for drug interactions due to the iron component. In general, it is rational to separate the administration time of oral medications for which a reduction in bioavailability has a clinically significant effect (eg, quinolones) from phosphate binders by at least 1 hour before or 3 hours after administration of the phosphate binder. Many phosphate binders are marketed as antacids or calcium supplements, and often CKD patients do not know why they have been prescribed these agents. Regular patient counseling is essential to improve adherence and minimize the potential for drug interactions.

Dosing and Administration Initial dosing regimens for phosphate-binding agents and suggested dose titration schemes are shown in Table 63-7. Doses should be titrated to achieve the recommended serum phosphorus concentrations in conjunction with dietary intervention and dialysis (for ESKD patients).

Vitamin D Therapy Vitamin D compounds available in the United States include nutritional vitamin D (ergocalciferol [D_2] and cholecalciferol [D_3]), the prohormone calcifediol [25(OH)D_3], active vitamin D (calcitriol [D_3]), and vitamin D analogs (paricalcitol and doxercalciferol [both D_2]) (Table 63-8). Nutritional vitamin D (NVD) is derived from dietary plant (D_2) and animal (D_3) sources, or from supplements. While this chapter focuses on the role of NVD and FDA-approved vitamin D formulations for the management of mineral homeostasis, there are several other therapeutic uses for vitamin D (eg, for CV and immune-related effects) and other analogs available outside the United States which are not discussed (eg, alfacalcidol).

Pharmacology and Mechanism of Action Vitamin D is a cholesterol derivative and is transported in the circulation by vitamin D–binding protein. The process of vitamin D metabolism is shown in Fig. 63-3. Both endogenously synthesized D_3 and NVD compounds (as D_2 or D_3) are converted in the liver to 25(OH)D, by the 25-hydroxylase enzyme. The 25(OH)D form is subsequently converted to the biologically active form 1,25-dihydroxyvitamin D (either D_2 or D_3 depending on the parent compound) by the 1-α-hydroxylase enzyme. This conversion occurs primarily in the kidney, but this enzyme is also present in extrarenal tissues. It is not clear whether active vitamin D produced in extrarenal tissue exerts its effects only locally or contributes to the systemic endocrine functions. It is the concentration of 25(OH)D that is most commonly measured clinically to diagnose vitamin D deficiency. The 25(OH)D form is available as calcifediol, an extended release oral formulation of the prohormone, indicated for patients with CKD G3 or G4 with low 25(OH)D levels (<30 ng/mL [75 nmol/L]).

Calcitriol and the vitamin D analogs bind to the vitamin D receptors (VDRs), which are located in many organ systems including the parathyroid glands, intestine, bone, kidney, heart, nervous, and immune systems. When vitamin D binds to the VDR, there is a conformational change in the VDR that allows for interaction of the receptor with the retinoid X receptor (RXR), a transcriptional factor.[73] The VDR-RXR complex binds to DNA sequences in target genes to either promote or inhibit transcription depending on the

TABLE 63-8 Vitamin D Agents

Generic Name	Brand Name	Form of Vitamin D	Dosage Forms	Initial Dose	Dosage Range	Frequency of Dosing or Dose Titration[a]
Nutritional Vitamin D						
Ergocalciferol	Drisdol	D_2	po	Varies based on 25(OH)D levels	400-50,000 international units	Daily (doses of 400-2,000 international units)
Cholecalciferol[b]	Generic	D_3	po			Weekly or monthly for higher doses (50,000 international units)
Calcifediol	Rayaldee	D_3	po	30 μg daily	30-60 μg	Increase after 3 months if PTH above desired range
Vitamin D and Analogs						
Generic Name	**Brand Name**	**Form of Vitamin D**	**Dosage Forms**	**Initial Dose[c,d]**	**Dosage Range**	**Dose Titration[a]**
Calcitriol	Rocaltrol	D_3	po	0.25 μg daily	0.25-5 μg	Increase by 0.25 μg/day at 4- to 8-week intervals
	Calcijex		IV	1-2 μg three times per week	0.5-5 μg	Increase by 0.5-1 μg at 2 to 4-week intervals
Doxercalciferol[e]	Hectorol	D_2	po	ND-CKD: 1 μg daily ESKD: 10 μg three times per week	5-20 μg	Increase by 0.5 μg at 2-week intervals for daily dosing or by 2.5 μg at 8-week intervals for three times per week dosing
			IV	ESKD: 4 μg three times per week	2-8 μg	Increase by 1-2 μg at 8-week intervals
Paricalcitol	Zemplar	D_2	po	ND-CKD: 1 μg daily or 2 μg three times per week if PTH ≤500 pg/mL (ng/L; 54 pmol/L); 2 μg daily or 4 μg three times per week if PTH >500 pg/mL (ng/L; 54 pmol/L)	1-4 μg	Increase by 1 μg (for daily dosing) or 2 μg (for three times per week dosing) at 2- to 4-week intervals
			IV	ESKD: 0.04-1 μg three times per week	2.5-15 μg	Increase by 2-4 μg at 2- to 4-week intervals

ESKD, end-stage kidney disease; ND-CKD, non-dialysis chronic kidney disease; PTH, parathyroid hormone.

[a]Based on PTH, calcium and phosphorus levels. Decreases in dose are necessary if PTH is oversuppressed and/or if calcium and phosphorus are elevated.

[b]Multiple preparations are available that are not listed.

[c]Dose ratios are as follows: 1:1 for IV paricalcitol to oral doxercalciferol, 1.5:1 for IV paricalcitol to IV doxercalciferol, and 1:1 for IV to oral calcitriol.

[d]Daily orally dosing most common for ND- CKD patients, IV dosing three times per week more often used in the hemodialysis population.

[e]Prodrug that requires activation by the liver.

organ system. Vitamin D inhibits or suppresses PTH synthesis and also stimulates absorption of serum calcium by intestinal cells. As a result, the serum calcium concentration is raised, which decreases PTH secretion by the parathyroid glands. The set point for calcium (ie, the calcium concentration at which PTH secretion is decreased by 50%), which is generally raised in those with CKD-MBD, is lowered when active vitamin D therapy is initiated. This results in a lower ionized calcium concentration becoming effective at suppressing secretion of PTH. Unfortunately, the enhanced GI absorption of calcium and phosphorus associated with calcitriol therapy may lead to hypercalcemia and hyperphosphatemia, which are associated with soft-tissue and vascular calcifications.

The unique interactions of vitamin D with the VDRs have led to the development of vitamin D analogs that vary in their affinity for the VDRs. Paricalcitol and doxercalciferol retain activity with vitamin D receptors on the parathyroid gland to effectively lower PTH, but have less risk of hypercalcemia and hyperphosphatemia due to their lower intestinal activity. Paricalcitol differs from calcitriol by the absence of the exocyclic carbon 19 and the fact that it is a vitamin D_2 derivative (19-nor-1,25-dihydroxyvitamin D_2). This compound is active as given. Doxercalciferol, however, is a prohormone that does require activation by CYP27 in the liver to form the major active D_2 metabolite 1,25-dihydroxyvitamin D_2 (see Fig. 63-3).

Pharmacokinetics Oral absorption of calcitriol occurs rapidly; therefore, both oral and IV therapies are reasonable options for treatment of CKD-MBD. The half-life of active calcitriol ranges from 15 to 38 hours in patients with ESKD.[74] The half-lives of paricalcitol and doxercalciferol are approximately 15 hours and 32 to 37 hours, respectively.[75,76] These agents are extensively bound to plasma proteins and not removed by dialysis.

Efficacy Calcitriol, paricalcitol, and doxercalciferol are all effective in lowering PTH in patients with CKD; however, the trade-off is the undesired effect of raising calcium and phosphorus concentrations due to increased intestinal absorption. Although these effects are less likely with paricalcitol and doxercalciferol, elevated calcium concentrations have been observed. An all-cause and CV survival benefit has also been reported with these agents in both CKD and ESKD patients in observational studies.[77] These survival benefits, however, have not been substantiated in randomized clinical trials based on meta-analysis of available data.[78] KDIGO does not advocate for routine use of calcitriol and vitamin D analogs in the ND-CKD population (a 2C recommendation) and suggests that they be reserved for patients with CKD stages G4-G5 (a recommendation that was not graded). These agents may be used in conjunction with calcimimetics when warranted in the dialysis population (a 2B recommendation).

A review and meta-analysis in CKD patients (including ESKD patients) reported that NVD supplementation was associated with an improvement in 25(OH)D levels and decreased PTH without significant hypercalcemia or hyperphosphatemia in ND-CKD patients[79]; however, this has not been a consistent finding. In ESKD patients, NVD has resulted in increased levels of 25(OH)D and a decrease in PTH, which suggests a potential role of extrarenal pathways of vitamin D activation; however, these patients typically also require active vitamin D or analog therapy. Calcifediol has been shown to lower PTH with relatively minimal effects on serum calcium and phosphorus in stage G3-G4 CKD, which is the reason it has gained approval in ND-CKD patients to treat 25(OH)D deficiency.[80] The survival benefit of correcting vitamin D deficiency with NVD in the CKD population is unknown. The recommendation by KDIGO is that confirmed 25(OH)D deficiency in patients with CKD G3a-G5D be corrected using treatment strategies in the general population (a 2C recommendation), which includes NVD therapies.[17,81]

Adverse Effects Although all agents are effective in suppressing PTH, they may cause hypercalcemia and hyperphosphatemia, an effect that is most likely with calcitriol. Oversuppression of PTH and inducement of adynamic bone disease are also distinct possibilities.

Drug-Drug and Drug-Food Interactions Cholestyramine may reduce the absorption of orally administered calcitriol and doxercalciferol. In vitro data suggest that paricalcitol is metabolized by the hepatic enzyme CYP3A4 and thus it has the potential to interact with other agents that are metabolized by this enzyme. Caution is also advised when CYP3A4 inhibitors are given to those receiving doxercalciferol since hydroxylation of this precursor agent may be inhibited.

Dosing and Administration Despite limited evidence, KDIGO guidelines support administering NVD to patients with CKD G3a-G5 and ESKD with vitamin D deficiency or insufficiency (a grade 2C recommendation).[17] Calcitriol, doxercalciferol, or paricalcitol should be administered when PTH remains elevated despite the achievement of adequate 25(OH)D levels. ESKD patients require calcitriol, doxercalciferol, or paricalcitol.

Calcitriol by either the oral or the IV route may be administered daily (usually 0.25-1 μg/day) or using a pulse dosing (0.5-2 μg 2 to 3 times/wk) approach. Recommended doses of available NVD and analogs and suggested dose titration schemes are shown in Table 63-8. Prior to starting therapy, the serum calcium and phosphorus should be within the normal range. This does not mean that vitamin D therapy should be withheld or discontinued in all patients with elevated calcium and phosphorus values, but rather that use of agents with a lower risk of hypercalcemia and hyperphosphatemia and more prudent use of phosphate binders to lower calcium and phosphorus may be necessary in such patients. Dose adjustments of vitamin D should be made every 2 to 4 weeks based on PTH concentrations and trends in calcium and phosphorus.

Calcimimetics Cinacalcet hydrochloride (Sensipar) and etelcalcetide (Parsabiv) are calcimimetic agents approved for treatment of secondary hyperparathyroidism in CKD patients on dialysis. Cinacalcet is available as an oral agent, whereas etelcalcetide is an IV formulation. Both agents are approved for use only in dialysis patients.

Pharmacology and Mechanism of Action Cinacalcet and etelcalcetide work through their interactions on the calcium-sensing receptor (CSR) located on the surface of the chief cells of the parathyroid gland. Cinacalcet works as an allosteric modulator of the CSR though binding to the transmembrane domain of the receptor while etelcalcetide binds directly to the extracellular domain resulting in increased sensitivity of the receptor to extracellular calcium (ie, lowering the threshold for receptor activation by calcium) and subsequently reducing PTH secretion.[82]

Pharmacokinetics Cinacalcet peak concentrations are observed 2 to 6 hours following oral administration. Its elimination half-life is approximately 30 to 40 hours and steady-state plasma concentrations are achieved in approximately 7 days. It has a large volume of distribution (~1,000 L) and is 93% to 97% bound to plasma proteins, thus removal by dialysis is negligible. Cinacalcet is metabolized by the liver, specifically by the cytochrome P450 isoenzymes CYP3A4, CYP2D6, and CYP1A2.[83] Etelcalcetide has a half-life of 3 to 4 days and plasma levels reach steady state in several weeks.[84] This agent is not metabolized by CYP isoenzymes, but is cleared by renal excretion. Unlike cinacalcet this agent is cleared by hemodialysis.

Efficacy In clinical trials conducted predominantly in dialysis patients, cinacalcet significantly decreased PTH, calcium, and phosphorus, regardless of the severity of secondary hyperparathyroidism. In ND-CKD patients cinacalcet reduced PTH, but was associated with a high incidence of hypocalcemia and hyperphosphatemia; thus, this agent is not approved for use in non-dialysis CKD patients. Cinacalcet may be used as a single agent to control hyperparathyroidism in ESKD patients; however, combined therapy with vitamin D is often necessary to achieve target PTH, calcium, and phosphorus values. In the ADVANCE trial, cinacalcet plus low-dose active vitamin D increased coronary artery calcification scores but to a lesser degree than its comparator calcitriol alone.[85] A decrease in all-cause and CV mortality was also suggested by results of an observational study in HD patients prescribed cinacalcet in addition to vitamin D compared with those on vitamin D alone.[86] While these findings were promising, they were not supported by the EVOLVE trial (the Evaluation of Cinacalcet Therapy to Lower CV Events), a prospective study which revealed that cinacalcet did not significantly reduce the risk of all-cause mortality or major CV events in patients with CKD 5HD.[87] There has been much debate with regard to the design and analysis of the EVOVLE trial and the interpretation of the findings with subsequent sub-analyses of the data to evaluate other outcomes such as reduction in FGF23 and risk of hypocalcemia.[88-90]

Etelcalcetide is effective in lowering PTH in hemodialysis patients with more long-term data (up to 12 months) showing sustained efficacy and safety.[91-93] Like cinacalcet, this agent also lowers calcium and phosphorus but has also been shown to lower FGF23 to a greater extent.[91,94,95] There have not been clinical studies to evaluate the effect of etelcalcetide on mortality or cardiovascular events; however, a small study in HD patients did show improvement in left ventricular hypertrophy that was associated with FGF23-lowering effects.[96]

Adverse Effects The most frequent adverse events associated with cinacalcet are nausea and vomiting, which may account for nonadherence. Nausea and vomiting were reported with etelcalcetide in both the placebo-controlled trials and in the comparison trial with cinacalcet at a rate that was not significantly different compared with cinacalcet.[91,97] Since these agents lower serum calcium they should not be started if the corrected serum calcium is less than the lower limit of normal, approximately 8.4 mg/dL (2.10 mmol/L). Serum calcium should be measured within 1 week after initiation or following a dose adjustment. Once the maintenance dose is established, serum calcium should be measured monthly. Potential manifestations of hypocalcemia include paresthesia, myalgia, cramping, tetany, and convulsions. Hypocalcemia may also lead to Q-T interval prolongation and ventricular arrhythmias, which further emphasizes the importance of regular calcium monitoring.

Drug-Drug and Drug-Food Interactions Because cinacalcet is partially metabolized by CYP3A4, there is potential for drug interactions with agents that inhibit this pathway. Coadministration of cinacalcet and ketoconazole, a strong inhibitor of CYP3A4, results in a twofold increase in the area under the curve and maximum concentration. Cinacalcet is also a potent inhibitor of CYP2D6. As a result, dose adjustments of concomitant medications that are predominantly metabolized by this enzyme and have a narrow therapeutic index, such as flecainide, thioridazine, vinblastine, and most tricyclic antidepressants (eg, amitriptyline, desipramine), may be necessary. Concurrent administration of cinacalcet with desipramine increased desipramine exposure by approximately 260% in CYP2D6-extensive metabolizers.[83] Food has been shown to increase absorption of cinacalcet by up to 82% compared with fasting; therefore, this medication should be taken with meals to achieve the maximal effect.

There are no drug interactions reported with etelcalcetide. Of note, this agent is not a substrate or inhibitor of CYP isoenzymes or transporter proteins (eg, *P*-glycoprotein, organic anionic/cationic transporters).

Dosing and Administration The recommended starting dose of cinacalcet is 30 mg orally once daily. Calcium and phosphorus should be measured at 1 week and PTH should be measured within 1 to 4 weeks after starting cinacalcet or adjusting the dose. The dose should be titrated every 2 to 4 weeks to a maximum dose of 180 mg once daily until the desired PTH values are achieved and to maintain goal serum calcium concentrations. Patients with hepatic disease may require lower doses, since the cinacalcet half-life is approximately doubled in those with severe liver disease.[83] Cinacalcet is available as film-coated tablets containing 30, 60, or 90 mg.

Etelcalcetide should be initiated at a dose of 5 mg administered intravenously three times per week at the end of the hemodialysis treatment. Calcium and phosphorus should be measured 1 week after initiation and then every 4 weeks for maintenance therapy. PTH levels should be measured 4 weeks after initiation and then per protocol based on the practices of the dialysis center. If PTH levels are above the recommended target range and the corrected serum calcium is within the normal range, the dose of etelcalcetide should be increased in 2.5 or 5 mg increments up to a maximum dose of 15 mg. The dose should be decreased or temporarily discontinued in patients with PTH levels below the target range or in patients with a corrected calcium at or above 7.5 mg/dL (1.88 mmol/L) but less the lower limit of normal (8.4 mg/dL), without symptoms of hypocalcemia. Other interventions to increase calcium may be initiated if necessary (eg, altering vitamin D therapy and calcium supplementation). Etelcalcetide may be resumed once the PTH is within the target range and hypocalcemia has resolved, but at a lower dose. If the corrected calcium is below 7.5 mg/dL (1.88 mmol/L), then etalcalcitide should be discontinued and reinitiated at a dose 5 mg lower than the last administered dose once hypocalcemia has resolved. Patients who were receiving 2.5 or 5 mg should reinitiate therapy at a dose of 2.5 mg.[84]

Since etelcalcetide is removed by hemodialysis it should be administered at the end of the hemodialysis treatment and injected into the venous line of the dialysis circuit during or after rinse back. If a dose is missed (eg, due to a missed hemodialysis treatment), then that missed dose should not be administered, but the patient should resume the regular treatment schedule at the next hemodialysis session. If doses are missed for more than 2 weeks, then etelcalcetide should be restarted at the 5 mg dose.[84] If switching a patient from cinacalcet to etelcalcetide, then cinacalcet should be discontinued for at least 7 days prior to starting etelcalcetide. If switching patients from etelcalcetide to cinacalcet, etalcalcetide should be discontinued for at least 4 weeks prior to starting cinacalcet due to the long half-life of etalcalcetide.

Cardiovascular Complications of Chronic Kidney Disease

Cardiovascular Disease Patients with CKD are at increased risk of CVD, independent of the etiology of their kidney disease. This greater burden of CVD in patients with CKD is illustrated in Fig. 63-5.[3] The prevalence of any form of CVD is greater as kidney disease progresses from CKD stages G1-G5 (Fig. 63-5a) and is highest in patients with ESKD (Fig. 63-5b). This burden of CVD is associated with much higher mortality rates. In general, CKD patients have a lower probability of survival for all of the CVD conditions reported, with late stages of CKD being associated with the worst outcomes.[98] For example, the adjusted 2-year survival probability for patients with an AMI without a diagnosis of CKD is 71% versus 60% for CKD Stage 1 to 2 patients and 54% for CKD Stage 4 to 5 patients.[3] In addition to traditional risk factors for CVD such as diabetes mellitus/insulin resistance, dyslipidemia, hypertension, LVH, smoking, and obesity patients with CKD have other nontraditional risk factors including proteinuria, inflammation, anemia, and abnormal calcium and phosphate metabolism resulting in vascular calcification and oxidative stress.[98,99]

Unfortunately, the lack of randomized trials treating CVD in patients with CKD often leads to treatment decisions that are based on extrapolation from trials in non-CKD populations and from observational data in CKD patients and not robust evidence. Treatment approaches for CVD include strategies to mitigate the traditional and non-traditional risk factors for CVD. The lack of data specific to CKD is a reason for the absence of guidelines on management of CVD in patients with CKD. The 2013 KDIGO CKD guideline did include statement regarding select CVDs including ischemic heart disease and recommended that the level of care for ischemic heart disease offered to people with CKD should not differ from people without CKD (grade 1A recommendation) as the treatment of traditional risk factors in CKD patients is of benefit.[100] These patients should also receive the standard assessments and treatments such as statins for CKD 1-5 (non-dialysis), beta-blockers, ACEIs/ARBs, and antiplatelet agents (see Chapters 33 and 34). Clinicians should note that in the diagnosis of acute coronary syndrome, elevated serum troponins should be interpreted with caution in individuals with a GFR less than 60 mL/min/1.73 m^2 (<0.58 mL/s/m^2) because these markers are often elevated as a result of reduced kidney excretion (a grade 1B recommendation).

With regard to heart failure, KDIGO suggested that patients with CKD should receive standard heart failure therapies (Chapter 36); however, clinicians should be aware that RAAS blockade (eg, ACEI, ARB, neprilysin inhibitor/ARB, spironolactone, eplerenone) and diuretic therapy (eg, furosemide, metolazone) may lead to significant changes in GFR and serum potassium concentrations. Such therapy should not be avoided, but closely monitored and put into the context of individual risks and benefits. With regard to the cardiac biomarkers of B-type natriuretic peptide (BNP) and N-terminal pro-BNP (NT-pro-BNP) in individuals with a GFR less than 60 mL/min/1.73 m^2 (<0.58 mL/s/m^2) (CKD G3a-G5), it is recommended that serum concentrations be interpreted with caution with respect to diagnosis of heart failure and assessment of volume status (a grade 1B recommendation).

Aspirin (ASA) is recommended for secondary prevention in all patients with CKD based on decreased mortality in observational studies.[100,101] ASA is generally not recommended for primary prevention as compared to placebo or no treatment as it reduces the risk of myocardial infarction but not all-cause mortality, CV mortality, or stroke and increases the risk of major and minor bleeding.[102,103]

Also of importance with regard to cardiovascular disease in patients with CKD is the fact that non-dialysis CKD patients now have more therapies available to delay CKD progression including sodium-glucose co-transporter type 2 (SGLT2) inhibitors (eg, canagloflozin, dapagloflozin), glucagon-like-peptide-1 (GLP-1) receptor agonists, and mineralocorticoid receptor antagonists (eg, finerenone) (see Chapter 62 for further discussion). While the primary reason these agents are prescribed relates to slowing CKD

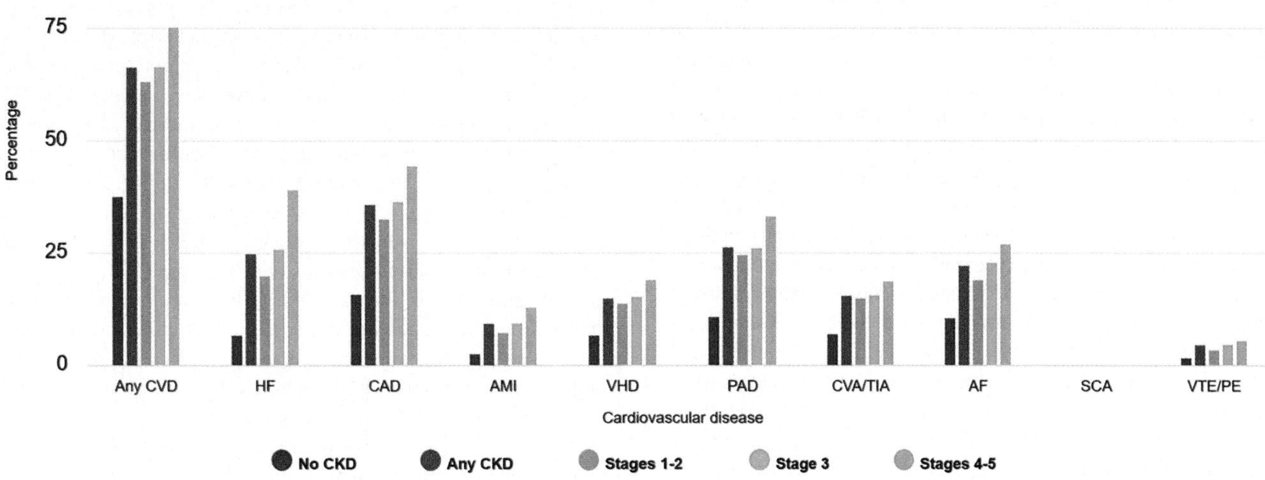

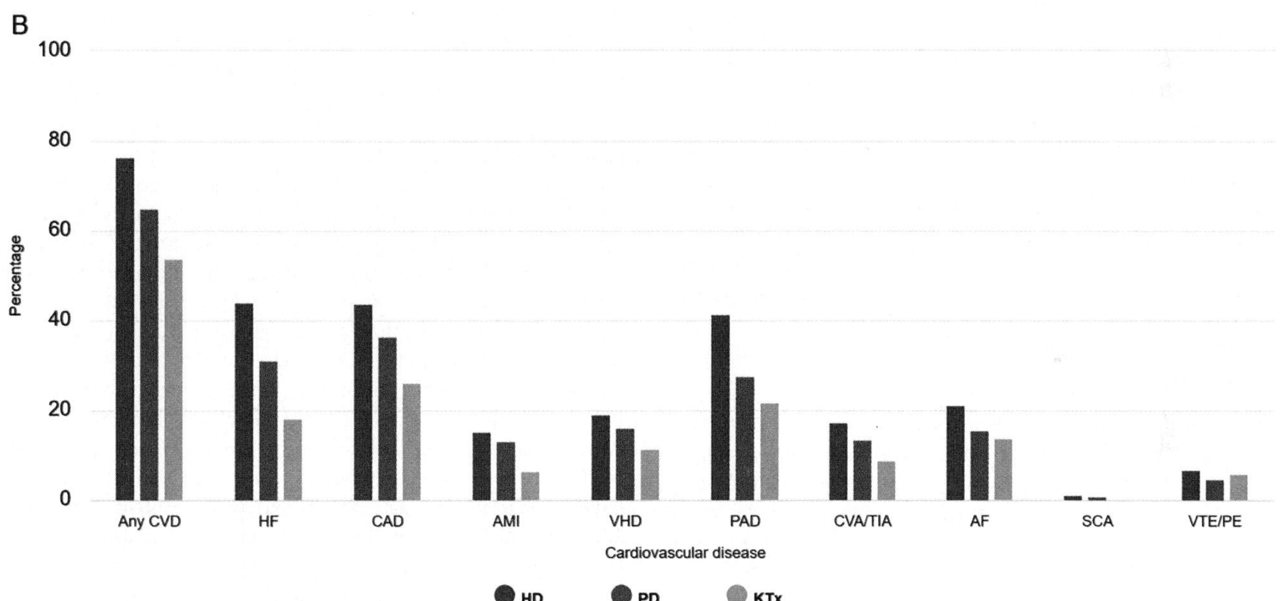

FIGURE 63-5 Prevalence of cardiovascular diseases in (A) Medicare patients ≥66 years by CKD status and stage, 2018 and (B) patients with ESKD by treatment modality.[3] (AF, atrial fibrillation; AMI, acute myocardial infarction; CAD, coronary artery disease; CKD, chronic kidney disease; CVA/TIA, cerebrovascular accident/transient ischemic attack; CVD, cardiovascular disease; HD, hemodialysis; HF, heart failure; KTx, kidney transplant; PAD, peripheral arterial disease; PD, peritoneal dialysis; SCA/VA, sudden cardiac arrest and ventricular arrhythmias; VHD, valvular heart disease; VTE/PE, venous thromboembolism and pulmonary embolism. *(Medicare 5% sample of patients aged 66 years and older, alive, without ESKD, and residing in the United States on 12/31/2018. Note: The data reported here have been supplied by the United States Renal Data System [USRDS].)*

progression, the positive cardiovascular outcomes associated with use of these agents are important when considering the potential benefits of selecting a given agent.

Hyperlipidemia CKD with or without nephrotic syndrome is frequently accompanied by abnormalities in lipoprotein metabolism. Although the concentrations of LDL are not uniformly increased in patients with kidney disease, these patients produce small, dense LDL particles that are more susceptible to oxidation and more atherogenic than larger LDL subfractions. Other lipid abnormalities include low HDL, increased VLDL, and increased triglycerides.[104,105] In patients with nephrotic syndrome, the major lipid abnormalities are elevation of plasma total and LDL cholesterol, with or without low HDL cholesterol, and elevated triglycerides. See Chapter e66 for a detailed discussion of the management of proteinuria in patients with glomerular disease.

The KDIGO Lipid Guideline recommends that a complete fasting lipid profile be performed in all adults with newly identified CKD (a grade 1C recommendation).[106] Follow-up lipid levels are not recommended unless the information may alter management (eg, assessing adherence to therapy or assessing CV risk in a patient <50 years and not currently on a statin). Reduction in the risk of CV events in patients with CKD has only been demonstrated with statins or a statin plus ezetimibe combination.[107]

Statins in Chronic Kidney Disease

8 Statins have been shown to decrease mortality and CV events in ND-CKD patients; however, data are not as compelling in the ESKD population. Two trials (4D and AURORA) conducted in ESKD patients on hemodialysis did not show a benefit of statin therapy for primary prevention of cardiovascular events including nonfatal myocardial infarction, nonfatal stroke, and death from cardiac causes.[105,106] The Study of Heart and Renal Protection (SHARP) trial was conducted after these trials and was a primary prevention trial that evaluated the effects of combined simvastatin (20 mg) and ezetimibe (10 mg) compared with placebo on time to first major vascular event (nonfatal MI or cardiac death, any stroke, or revascularization) in patients with no history of MI or coronary revascularization and included patients with CKD (6,247) and ESKD (3,023).[107] In all patients receiving combined therapy during the 4.9-year follow-up period, there was a significant 17% reduction in the relative risk (RR) of major vascular events and a 32% reduction in LDL in the patients who were assessed as compliant with therapy (two-thirds were compliant). While overall these results are positive, the reduction in major atherosclerotic events was not significant for the dialysis subgroup, although the study was not powered to evaluate ESKD patients as a separate group. A subgroup analysis comparing dialysis versus non-dialysis patients showed no differences in the RR of CV events even after adjustment for the reduction in LDL. A subsequent meta-analysis of statins in dialysis patients indicated that they had no significant beneficial effect on major CV events, all-cause mortality, CV death, or myocardial infarction, and a trend toward increased strokes despite clinically relevant reductions in LDL cholesterol.[108] In contrast, a meta-analysis of statins in ND-CKD showed significant reductions in major CV events, CV death, all-cause mortality; myocardial infarction but uncertain effects on stroke.[109] Now there are also more data to support statins in non-dialysis CKD patients than in ESKD patients for secondary prevention of atherosclerotic cardiovascular events.[105,110]

The KDIGO Lipid guidelines[106] make the following recommendations:

1. In adults aged 18 to 49 years with CKD but not treated with chronic dialysis or kidney transplantation, we suggest statin treatment in people with one or more of the following (Level 2A): known coronary disease (myocardial infarction or coronary revascularization); diabetes mellitus; prior ischemic stroke; estimated 10-year incidence of coronary death or nonfatal myocardial infarction greater than 10%.
2. In adults older than 50 years with eGFR less than 60 mL/min/1.73 m^2 but not treated with chronic dialysis or kidney transplantation, we recommend treatment with a statin or statin/ezetimibe combination (Level 1A).
3. In adults with dialysis-dependent CKD, we suggest that statins or statin/ezetimibe combination not be initiated (Level 2A). However, in patients already receiving statins or statin/ezetimibe combination at the time of dialysis initiation, we suggest that these agents be continued (Level 2C).

The 2018 American Heart Association and the American College of Cardiology (AHA/ACC) guidelines on cholesterol recognize CKD as a risk factor for CV events and recommend that treatment with a moderate-intensity statin (or moderate-intensity statin therapy plus ezetimibe) can be considered in patients with non-dialysis CKD between the ages of 40 and 75 years and 10-year CV risk of 7.5% or higher.[111]

In addition to some of the controversies with statin therapy in CKD, the newer cholesterol lowering agents for the management of hyperlipidemia to reduce atherosclerotic CVD such as the PCSK9 inhibitors have not been evaluated across the spectrum of CKD except in secondary analyses and further data are needed to evaluate potential benefits beyond lipid lowering in CKD patients.[105,110]

Pruritus

Chronic pruritus (or uremic pruritus/itching) is among the many complications that patients with advanced CKD endure and has long been a problem without a directly linked etiology, which has made determination of treatment options a challenge. The diagnosis is made in patients with CKD when all other potential comorbid conditions associated with pruritus have been ruled out. CKD-associated pruritus is estimated to occur in approximately 40% of ESKD patients, but this is thought to be an underestimate.[112] There is much variability in time of onset relative to dialysis, frequency of symptoms, and body distribution with up to 50% of patients experiencing generalized pruritis that is often symmetrical. Some patients experience more localized pruritus with the face, back, and access arm, but common sites include the legs, back, and scalp. Over time other complications may occur such as impetigo, ulcerations, and increased risk of infections.[113,114] Regardless of location pruritus has a negative effect on patient quality of life with sleep disturbances and depression associated with this condition.[112-114]

The mechanisms of pruritus are not fully understood, which is part of the reason multiple interventions have been attempted. The release of compounds by keratinocytes, immune cells, or neurons in the skin that promote inching (pruritogens) including histamine, prostaglandins, cytokines, neuropeptides, and protases has been proposed.[114] Imbalances in the endogenous opioid system, particularly peripherally distributed kappa opioid receptors, have been explored as playing a key role.[113] Pruritus has also been associated with inadequate dialysis, elevated PTH, calcium, and phosphorus; however, these associations are inconsistent and their correction does not necessarily correlate with resolution of pruritus.[113] Pharmacologic interventions that have been implemented to address CKD-associated pruritus include gabapentinoids, capsaicin, sertraline, mirtazapine, antihistamines, among other strategies, with variable success.[113]

9 Until recently, there was no approved therapy for uremic pruritus in the United States. Difelikefalin, a peripheral kappa opioid receptor agonist, exerts antipruritic effects by means of activation of kappa opioid receptors on peripheral neurons and immune cells. Reductions in itch intensity and improvements in sleep and quality of life were demonstrated in phase 3 clinical trials which lead to the larger scale trial to evaluate efficacy and safety of difelikefalin in 378 adult HD patients with moderate to severe pruritus. Patients received either difelikefalin 0.5 μg/kg or placebo three times per week and improvements in itching intensity scores compared to baseline over a 12-week period were evaluated. Significantly more patients receiving difelikeflain (52%) had what was deemed a clinically significant (3 point) decrease in itching intensity score compared to 31% in the placebo group (primary outcome). There was also improvement in quality of life.[115] Adverse effects included diarrhea, dizziness, and vomiting. Based on these data difelikefalin was approved in 2021 for treatment of moderate to severe CKD associated pruritus in HD patients. This agent is approved at a dose of 0.5 μg/kg administered intravenously into the venous line of the dialysis circuit at the end of each HD treatment since this agent is extensively removed by HD.[116] Post approval data and patient-reported outcomes with use of this agent will be of interest as difelikefalin begins to be used in clinical practice in the ESKD population.

CONCLUSION

Although efforts to delay progression of CKD are paramount, measures to diagnose and manage the associated secondary complications and comorbid conditions early in the course of the disease are also essential. There are many secondary complications of advanced CKD that worsen as kidney disease progresses. This chapter focused on common complications of advanced CKD for which pharmacologic therapies are available including anemia, CKD-MBD, and uremic pruritus. CV complications are also prevalent in the population with CKD and although data are sparse compared to the general population, mitigation strategies should be considered as CVD is the leading cause of mortality in patients with ESKD.

Involving a multidisciplinary team to address not only CKD but to effectively design and implement individual patient care plans often required in the CKD population that include extensive nonpharmacologic and pharmacologic interventions is logical. Pharmacists are well positioned to actively participate in the chronic disease and medication management of CKD and ESKD patients and should be part of the current and developing kidney care models within the nephrology environment.

ABBREVIATIONS

CERA	continuous erythropoietin receptor activator
CHOIR	Correction of Hb and Outcomes in Renal Insufficiency
CKD	chronic kidney disease
CREATE	Cardiovascular Risk Reduction by Early Anemia Treatment with Epoetin Beta
CV	cardiovascular
CVD	cardiovascular disease
eGFR	estimated glomerular filtration rate
ESA	erythropoiesis stimulating agent
ESKD	end-stage kidney disease
FGF-23	fibroblast growth factor-23
GFR	glomerular filtration rate
GI	gastrointestinal
Hb	hemoglobin
Hct	hematocrit
HD	hemodialysis
HIF	hypoxia inducible factor
HIF-PHI	HIF-prolyl hydroxylase inhibitors
KDIGO	Kidney Disease: Improving Global Outcomes
LDL	low-density lipoprotein
LVH	left ventricular hypertrophy
MBD	mineral and bone disorder
ND-CKD	non-dialysis CKD patients
NHCT	Normal Hematocrit Cardiac Trial
NVD	nutritional vitamin D
25(OH)D	25-hydroxyvitamin D
PRCA	pure red cell aplasia
PD	peritoneal dialysis
PTH	parathyroid hormone
ROD	renal osteodystrophy
RXR	retinoid X receptor
SUBQ	subcutaneous
sHPT	secondary hyperparathyroidism
TIBC	total iron-binding capacity
TREAT	Trial to Reduce Cardiovascular Events with Aranesp Therapy
TSat	transferrin saturation
USRDS	United States Renal Data System
VDRs	vitamin D receptors
VLDL	very low-density lipoprotein

REFERENCES

1. St Peter WL, Guo H, Kabadi S, Gilbertson DT, Peng Y, Pendergraft T, et al. Prevalence, treatment patterns, and healthcare resource utilization in Medicare and commercially insured non-dialysis-dependent chronic kidney disease patients with and without anemia in the United States. *BMC Nephrol.* 2018;19. https://doi.org/10.1186/s12882-018-0861-1.
2. Lopes MB, Tu C, Zee J, Guedes M, Pisoni RL, Robinson BM, et al. A real-world longitudinal study of anemia management in non-dialysis-dependent chronic kidney disease patients: A multinational analysis of CKDopps. *Sci Rep.* 2021;11. https://doi.org/10.1038/s41598-020-79254-6.
3. United States Renal Data System, 2020 USRDS annual data report: Epidemiology of kidney disease in the United States. National Institutes of Health, National Institute of Diabetes and Digestive and Kidney Diseases, Bethesda, MD, 2020.
4. Del Vecchio L, Minutolo R. ESA, iron therapy and new drugs: Are there new perspectives in the treatment of anaemia? *J Clin Med.* 2021;10:839. https://doi.org/10.3390/jcm10040839.
5. The DOPPS Practice Monitor. www.dopps.org. Accessed August 1, 2021. n.d.
6. Karaboyas A, Morgenstern H, Waechter S, Fleischer NL, Vanholder R, Jacobson SH, et al. Low hemoglobin at hemodialysis initiation: An international study of anemia management and mortality in the early dialysis period. *Clin Kidney J.* 2020;13:425–433. https://doi.org/10.1093/ckj/sfz065.
7. Babitt JL, Eisenga MF, Haase VH, Kshirsagar AV, Levin A, Locatelli F, et al. Controversies in optimal anemia management: Conclusions from a kidney disease: Improving Global Outcomes (KDIGO) Conference. *Kidney Int.* 2021;99:1280–1295. https://doi.org/10.1016/j.kint.2021.03.020.
8. Gutiérrez OM. Fibroblast growth factor 23 and disordered vitamin D metabolism in chronic kidney disease: Updating the "trade-off" hypothesis. *Clin J Am Soc Nephrol.* 2010;5:1710–1716. https://doi.org/10.2215/CJN.02640310.
9. KDIGO clinical practice guideline for the diagnosis, evaluation, prevention, and treatment of Chronic Kidney Disease-Mineral and Bone Disorder (CKD-MBD). *Kidney Int Suppl.* 2009:S1–130.
10. Fishbane S, Spinowitz B. Update on anemia in ESRD and earlier stages of CKD: Core Curriculum 2018. *Am J Kidney Dis.* 2018;71:423–435. https://doi.org/10.1053/j.ajkd.2017.09.026.
11. Gupta N, Wish JB. Hypoxia-inducible factor prolyl hydroxylase inhibitors: A potential new treatment for anemia in patients with CKD. *Am J Kidney Dis.* 2017;69:815–826. https://doi.org/10.1053/j.ajkd.2016.12.011.
12. Locatelli F, Del Vecchio L. Are prolyl-hydroxylase inhibitors potential alternative treatments for anaemia in patients with chronic kidney disease? *Nephrol Dial Transplant.* 2020;35. https://doi.org/10.1093/ndt/gfz031.
13. Locatelli F, Fishbane S, Block GA, MacDougall IC. Targeting hypoxia-inducible factors for the treatment of anemia in chronic kidney disease patients. *Am J Nephrol.* 2017;45:187–199. https://doi.org/10.1159/000455166.
14. Kidney Disease: Improving Global Outcomes (KDIGO) Anemia Work Group. KDIGO Clinical Practice Guideline for Anemia in Chronic Kidney Disease. *Kidney Inter Suppl.* 2012;2:279–335.
15. Sheetz M, Barrington P, Callies S, Berg PH, McColm J, Marbury T, et al. Targeting the hepcidin-ferroportin pathway in anemia of chronic kidney disease. *Br J Clin Pharmacol.* 2019. https://doi.org/10.1111/bcp.13877.
16. Moorthi RN, Moe SM. CKD-mineral and bone disorder: Core curriculum 2011. *Am J Kidney Dis.* 2011;58:1022–1036. https://doi.org/10.1053/j.ajkd.2011.08.009.
17. KDIGO 2017 Clinical Practice Guideline Update for the Diagnosis, Evaluation, Prevention, and Treatment of Chronic Kidney Disease-Mineral and Bone Disorder (CKD-MBD). *Kidney Int Suppl.* 2017;7:1–59. https://doi.org/10.1016/j.kisu.2017.04.001.
18. Isakova T, Ix JH, Sprague SM, Raphael KL, Fried L, Gassman JJ, et al. Rationale and approaches to phosphate and fibroblast growth factor 23 reduction in CKD. *J Am Soc Nephrol.* 2015;26:2328–2339. https://doi.org/10.1681/asn.2015020117.
19. Nigwekar SU, Thadhani R, Brandenburg VM. Calciphylaxis. *N Engl J Med.* 2018;379:399–400. https://doi.org/10.1056/NEJMc1807324.
20. Portales-Castillo I, Kroshinksy D, Malhotra CK, Culbert-Costley R, Cozzolino MG, Karparis S, et al. Calciphylaxis—as a drug induced adverse event. *Expert Opin Drug Saf.* 2018. https://doi.org/10.1080/14740338.2019.1559813.
21. Jones G. Interpreting vitamin D assay results: Proceed with caution. *Clin J Am Soc Nephrol.* 2015;10:331–334. https://doi.org/10.2215/CJN.05490614.
22. Collister D, Komenda P, Hiebert B, Gunasekara R, Xu Y, Eng F, et al. The effect of erythropoietin-stimulating agents on health-related quality of life in anemia of chronic kidney disease: A systematic review and meta-analysis. *Ann Intern Med.* 2016;164:472–478. https://doi.org/10.7326/m15-1839.
23. Besarab A, Bolton WK, Browne JK, Egrie JC, Nissenson AR, Okamoto DM, et al. The effects of normal as compared with low hematocrit

values in patients with cardiac disease who are receiving hemodialysis and epoetin. *N Engl J Med.* 1998;339:584–590.

24. Besarab A, Goodkin DA, Nissenson AR. The normal hematocrit study—follow-up. *N Engl J Med.* 2008;358:433–434.
25. Singh AK, Szczech L, Tang KL, Barnhart H, Sapp S, Wolfson M, et al. Correction of anemia with epoetin-alfa in chronic kidney disease. *N Engl J Med.* 2006;355:2085–2098.
26. Drueke TB, Locatelli F, Clyne N, Eckardt KU, Macdougall IC, Tsakiris D, et al. Normalization of hemoglobin level in patients with chronic kidney disease and anemia. *N Engl J Med.* 2006;355:2071–2084.
27. FDA Drug Safety Communication: modified dosing recommendations to improve the safe use of erythropoiesis-stimulating agents (ESAs) in chronic kidney disease. Last updated 8/4/2017. http://www.fda.gov/Drugs/DrugSafety/ucm259639.htm.
28. Phrommintikul A, Haas SJ, Elsik M, Krum H. Mortality and target haemoglobin concentrations in anaemic patients with chronic kidney disease treated with erythropoietin: A meta-analysis. *Lancet.* 2007;369:381–388.
29. Pfeffer MA, Burdmann EA, Chen CY, Cooper ME, de Zeeuw D, Eckardt KU, et al. A trial of darbepoetin alfa in type 2 diabetes and chronic kidney disease. *N Engl J Med.* 2009;361:2019–2032.
30. Cizman B, Smith HT, Camejo RR, Casillas L, Dhillon H, Mu F, et al. Clinical and economic outcomes of erythropoiesis-stimulating agent hyporesponsiveness in the post-bundling era. *Kidney Med.* 2020;2. https://doi.org/10.1016/j.xkme.2020.06.008.
31. Souza E, Cho KH, Harris ST, Flindt NR, Watt RK, Pai AB. Hypoxia-inducible factor prolyl hydroxylase inhibitors: A paradigm shift for treatment of anemia in chronic kidney disease? *Expert Opin Investig Drugs.* 2020;29. https://doi.org/10.1080/13543784.2020.1777276.
32. Ratcliffe LEK, Thomas W, Glen J, Padhi S, Pordes BAJ, Wonderling D, et al. Diagnosis and management of iron deficiency in CKD: A summary of the NICE guideline recommendations and their rationale. *Am J Kidney Dis.* 2016;67:548–558. https://doi.org/10.1053/j.ajkd.2015.11.012.
33. Fishbane S, Block GA, Loram L, Neylan J, Pergola PE, Uhlig K, et al. Effects of ferric citrate in patients with nondialysis-dependent CKD and iron deficiency anemia. *J Am Soc Nephrol.* 2017;28:1851–1858. https://doi.org/10.1681/ASN.2016101053.
34. Fishbane SN, Singh AK, Cournoyer SH, Jindal KK, Fanti P, Guss CD, et al. Ferric pyrophosphate citrate (Triferic) administration via the dialysate maintains hemoglobin and iron balance in chronic hemodialysis patients. *Nephrol Dial Transpl.* 2015;30:2019–2026. https://doi.org/10.1093/ndt/gfv277.
35. Gupta A, Lin V, Guss C, Pratt R, Ikizler TA, Besarab A. Ferric pyrophosphate citrate administered via dialysate reduces erythropoiesis-stimulating agent use and maintains hemoglobin in hemodialysis patients. *Kidney Int.* 2015;88:1187–1194. https://doi.org/10.1038/ki.2015.203.
36. Wang C, Graham DJ, Kane RC, Xie D, Wernecke M, Levenson M, et al. Comparative risk of anaphylactic reactions associated with intravenous iron products. *JAMA.* 2015;314:2062–2068. https://doi.org/10.1001/jama.2015.15572.
37. FDA drug safety communication: FDA strengthens warnings and changes prescribing instructions to decrease the risk of serious allergic reactions with anemia drug Feraheme (ferumoxytol). http://www.fda.gov/Drugs/DrugSafety/ucm440138.htm. Last accessed August 17, 2021.
38. Macdougall IC, White C, Anker SD, Bhandari S, Farrington K, Kalra PA, et al. Intravenous iron in patients undergoing maintenance hemodialysis. *N Engl J Med.* 2019;380:447–458. https://doi.org/10.1056/NEJMoa1810742.
39. Avni T, Bieber A, Grossman A, Green H, Leibovici L, Gafter-Gvili A. The safety of intravenous iron preparations: Systematic review and meta-analysis. *Mayo Clin Proc.* 2015;90:12–23. https://doi.org/10.1016/j.mayocp.2014.10.007.
40. Hougen I, Collister D, Bourrier M, Ferguson T, Hochheim L, Komenda P, et al. Safety of intravenous iron in dialysis: A systematic review and meta-analysis. *Clin J Am Soc Nephrol.* 2018;13:457–467. https://doi.org/10.2215/cjn.05390517.
41. Ganz T, Aronoff GR, Gaillard CAJM, Goodnough LT, Macdougall IC, Mayer G, et al. Iron administration, infection, and anemia management in CKD: Untangling the effects of intravenous iron therapy on immunity and infection risk. *Kidney Med.* 2020;2:341–353. https://doi.org/10.1016/j.xkme.2020.01.006.
42. Macdougall IC, Bhandari S, White C, Anker SD, Farrington K, Kalra PA, et al. Intravenous iron dosing and infection risk in patients on hemodialysis: A prespecified secondary analysis of the PIVOTAL trial. *J Am Soc Nephrol.* 2020;31:1118–1127. https://doi.org/10.1681/ASN.2019090972.
43. Stoffel NU, Cercamondi CI, Brittenham G, Zeder C, Geurts-Moespot AJ, Swinkels DW, et al. Iron absorption from oral iron supplements given on consecutive versus alternate days and as single morning doses versus twice-daily split dosing in iron-depleted women: Two open-label, randomised controlled trials. *Lancet Haematol.* 2017;4:e524–e533. https://doi.org/10.1016/S2352-3026(17)30182-5.
44. Epogen. Package Insert. Amgen. Thousand Oaks, CA. 2018.
45. Macdougall IC, Roger SD, de Francisco A, Goldsmith DJ, Schellekens H, Ebbers H, et al. Antibody-mediated pure red cell aplasia in chronic kidney disease patients receiving erythropoiesis-stimulating agents: New insights. *Kidney Int.* 2012;81:727–732. https://doi.org/10.1038/ki.2011.500.
46. Macdougall IC, Casadevall N, Locatelli F, Combe C, London GM, Di Paolo S, et al. Incidence of erythropoietin antibody-mediated pure red cell aplasia: The Prospective Immunogenicity Surveillance Registry (PRIMS). *Nephrol Dial Transpl.* 2015;30:451–460. https://doi.org/10.1093/ndt/gfu297.
47. Mircera. Package Insert. Hoffmann-La Roche, Inc, South San Francisco, CA. 2018.
48. Hazzan AD, Shah HH, Hong S, Sakhiya V, Wanchoo R, Fishbane S. Treatment with erythropoiesis-stimulating agents in chronic kidney disease patients with cancer. *Kidney Int.* 2014;86:34–39. https://doi.org/10.1038/ki.2013.528.
49. Aranesp. Package Insert. Amgen, Thousand Oaks, CA, 2018.
50. Wish JB. Hypoxia-inducible factor–prolyl hydroxylase inhibitors for the treatment of anemia in CKD: Additional pieces of the jigsaw puzzle. *Kidney Int Rep.* 2021;6:1751–1754. https://doi.org/10.1016/j.ekir.2021.05.017.
51. Ruospo M, Palmer SC, Natale P, Craig JC, Vecchio M, Elder GJ, et al. Phosphate binders for preventing and treating chronic kidney disease-mineral and bone disorder (CKD-MBD). *Cochrane Database Syst Rev.* 2018;8:Cd006023. https://doi.org/10.1002/14651858.CD006023.pub3.
52. St Peter WL, Wazny LD, Weinhandl ED. Phosphate-binder use in US dialysis patients: Prevalence, costs, evidence, and policies. *Am J Kidney Dis.* 2018;71:246–253. https://doi.org/10.1053/j.ajkd.2017.09.007.
53. Soliman M, Hassan W, Yaseen M, Rao M, Sawaya BP, El-Husseini A. PTH assays in dialysis patients: Practical considerations. *Semin Dial.* 2019;32:9–14. https://doi.org/10.1111/sdi.12743.
54. Tentori F, Wang M, Bieber BA, Karaboyas A, Li Y, Jacobson SH, et al. Recent changes in therapeutic approaches and association with outcomes among patients with secondary hyperparathyroidism on chronic hemodialysis: The DOPPS study. *Clin J Am Soc Nephrol.* 2015;10:98–109. https://doi.org/10.2215/cjn.12941213.
55. Nelson SM, Sarabia SR, Christilaw E, Ward EC, Lynch SK, Adams MA, et al. Phosphate-containing prescription medications contribute to the daily phosphate intake in a third of hemodialysis patients. *J Ren Nutr.* 2017;27:91–96. https://doi.org/10.1053/j.jrn.2016.09.007.
56. Daugirdas JT. Removal of phosphorus by hemodialysis. *Semin Dial.* 2015;28:620–623. https://doi.org/10.1111/sdi.12439.
57. Ishani A, Liu J, Wetmore JB, Lowe KA, Do T, Bradbury BD, et al. Clinical outcomes after parathyroidectomy in a nationwide cohort of patients on hemodialysis. *Clin J Am Soc Nephrol.* 2015;10:90–97. https://doi.org/10.2215/cjn.03520414.
58. Wetmore JB, Liu J, Do TP, Lowe KA, Ishani A, Bradbury BD, et al. Changes in secondary hyperparathyroidism-related biochemical parameters and medication use following parathyroidectomy. *Nephrol Dial Transpl.* 2016;31:103–111. https://doi.org/10.1093/ndt/gfv291.
59. Daugirdas JT, Finn WF, Emmett M, Chertow GM. The phosphate binder equivalent dose. *Semin Dial.* 2011;24:41–49. https://doi.org/10.1111/j.1525-139X.2011.00849.x.
60. St. Peter WL, Wazny LD, Weinhandl E, Cardone KE, Hudson JQ. A review of phosphate binders in chronic kidney disease: Incremental progress or just higher costs? *Drugs.* 2017;77:1155–1186. https://doi.org/10.1007/s40265-017-0758-5.
61. Spoendlin J, Paik JM, Tsacogianis T, Kim SC, Schneeweiss S, Desai RJ. Cardiovascular outcomes of calcium-free vs calcium-based phosphate binders in patients 65 years or older with end-stage renal disease requiring hemodialysis. *JAMA Intern Med.* 2019;179:741–749. https://doi.org/10.1001/jamainternmed.2019.0045.
62. St. Peter WL, Wazny LD, Weinhandl E, Cardone KE, Hudson JQ. A review of phosphate binders in chronic kidney disease: Incremental progress or just higher costs? *Drugs.* 2017;77:1155–1186. https://doi.org/10.1007/s40265-017-0758-5.
63. Choi YJ, Noh Y, Shin S. Ferric citrate in the management of hyperphosphataemia and iron deficiency anaemia: A meta-analysis in patients with chronic kidney disease. *Br J Clin Pharmacol.* 2021;87:414–426. https://doi.org/10.1111/bcp.14396.

64. Yokoyama K, Fukagawa M, Akiba T, Nakayama M, Ito K, Hanaki K, et al. Randomised clinical trial of ferric citrate hydrate on anaemia management in haemodialysis patients with hyperphosphataemia: ASTRIO study. *Sci Rep.* 2019;9:8877. https://doi.org/10.1038/s41598-019-45335-4.
65. Womack R, Berru F, Panwar B, Gutiérrez OM. Effect of ferric citrate versus ferrous sulfate on iron and phosphate parameters in patients with iron deficiency and CKD: A randomized trial. *Clin J Am Soc Nephrol.* 2020;15:1251–1258. https://doi.org/10.2215/CJN.15291219.
66. Cozzolino M, Ketteler M, Wagner CA. An expert update on novel therapeutic targets for hyperphosphatemia in chronic kidney disease: Preclinical and clinical innovations. *Expert Opin Ther Targets.* 2020;24:477–488. https://doi.org/10.1080/14728222.2020.1743680.
67. Ketteler M, Wiecek A, Rosenkranz AR, Pasch A, Rekowski J, Hellmann B, et al. Efficacy and safety of a novel nicotinamide modified-release formulation in the treatment of refractory hyperphosphatemia in patients receiving hemodialysis—A randomized clinical trial. *Kidney Int Rep.* 2021;6:594–604. https://doi.org/10.1016/j.ekir.2020.12.012.
68. Lenglet A, Liabeuf S, El Esper N, Brisset S, Mansour J, Lemaire-Hurtel AS, et al. Efficacy and safety of nicotinamide in haemodialysis patients: The NICOREN study. *Nephrol Dial Transplant.* 2017;32:870–879. https://doi.org/10.1093/ndt/gfw042.
69. Pergola PE, Rosenbaum DP, Yang Y, Chertow GM. A randomized trial of tenapanor and phosphate binders as a dual-mechanism treatment for hyperphosphatemia in patients on maintenance dialysis (AMPLIFY). *J Am Soc Nephrol.* 2021;32:1465–1473. https://doi.org/10.1681/ASN.2020101398.
70. Akizawa T, Sato Y, Ikejiri K, Kanda H, Fukagawa M. Effect of tenapanor on phosphate binder pill burden in hemodialysis patients. *Kidney Int Rep.* 2021;6:2371–2380. https://doi.org/10.1016/j.ekir.2021.06.030.
71. Sprague SM, Martin KJ, Coyne DW. Phosphate balance and CKD–mineral bone disease. *Kidney Int Rep.* 2021;6:2049–2058. https://doi.org/10.1016/j.ekir.2021.05.012.
72. Moazzam AA, Boongird S. Ingestion of lanthanum carbonate tablets. *Am J Kidney Dis.* 2013;62:844. https://doi.org/10.1053/j.ajkd.2013.06.019.
73. Wan LY, Zhang YQ, Chen MD, Liu CB, Wu JF. Relationship of structure and function of DNA-binding domain in vitamin D receptor. *Molecules.* 2015;20:12389–12399. https://doi.org/10.3390/molecules200712389.
74. Bailie GR, Johnson CA. Comparative review of the pharmacokinetics of vitamin D analogues. *Semin Dial.* 2002;15:352–357.
75. Zemplar Capsules Package Insert. AbbVie, Inc. North Chicago, IL. 2018.
76. Hectorol Injection. Package Insert. Genzyme Corporation, Cambridge, MA 2018.
77. Zheng Z, Shi H Fau - Jia J, Jia J Fau - Li D, Li D Fau - Lin S, Lin S, Nephrol BMC. Vitamin D supplementation and mortality risk in chronic kidney disease: A meta-analysis of 20 observational studies. *BMC Nephrol.* 2013;14:199.
78. Lu RJ, Zhu SM, Tang FL, Zhu XS, Fan ZD, Wang GL, et al. Effects of vitamin D or its analogues on the mortality of patients with chronic kidney disease: An updated systematic review and meta-analysis. *Eur J Clin Nutr.* 2017;71:683–693. https://doi.org/10.1038/ejcn.2017.59.
79. Kandula P, Dobre M, Schold JD, Schreiber MJ Jr., Mehrotra R, Navaneethan SD. Vitamin D supplementation in chronic kidney disease: A systematic review and meta-analysis of observational studies and randomized controlled trials. *Clin J Am Soc Nephrol.* 2011;6:50–62. https://doi.org/10.2215/cjn.03940510.
80. Sprague SM, Strugnell SA, Bishop CW. Extended-release calcifediol for secondary hyperparathyroidism in stage 3-4 chronic kidney disease. *Expert Rev Endocrinol Metab.* 2017;12:289–301. https://doi.org/10.1080/17446651.2017.1347501.
81. Melamed ML, Chonchol M, Gutierrez OM, Kalantar-Zadeh K, Kendrick J, Norris K, et al. The role of vitamin D in CKD stages 3 to 4: Report of a Scientific Workshop Sponsored by the National Kidney Foundation. *Am J Kidney Dis.* 2018;72:834–845. https://doi.org/10.1053/j.ajkd.2018.06.031.
82. Harada K, Fujioka A, Konno M, Inoue A, Yamada H, Hirota Y. Pharmacology of Parsabiv((R)) (etelcalcetide, ONO-5163/AMG 416), a novel allosteric modulator of the calcium-sensing receptor, for secondary hyperparathyroidism in hemodialysis patients. *Eur J Pharmacol.* 2019;842:139–145. https://doi.org/10.1016/j.ejphar.2018.10.021.
83. Sensipar (cinacalcet HCl) Tablets Package Insert. Amgen Inc., Thousand Oaks, CA 2019.
84. Parsabiv (etelcalcetide) Injection Package Insert. Amgen Inc., Thousand Oaks, CA 2021.
85. Raggi P, Chertow GM, Torres PU, Csiky B, Naso A, Nossuli K, et al. The ADVANCE study: A randomized study to evaluate the effects of cinacalcet plus low-dose vitamin D on vascular calcification in patients on hemodialysis. *Nephrol Dial Transpl.* 2011;26:1327–1339. https://doi.org/10.1093/ndt/gfq725.
86. Block GA, Zaun D, Smits G, Persky M, Brillhart S, Nieman K, et al. Cinacalcet hydrochloride treatment significantly improves all-cause and cardiovascular survival in a large cohort of hemodialysis patients. *Kidney Int.* 2010;78:578–589. https://doi.org/10.1038/ki.2010.167.
87. Chertow GM, Block GA, Correa-Rotter R, Drueke TB, Floege J, Goodman WG, et al. Effect of cinacalcet on cardiovascular disease in patients undergoing dialysis. *N Engl J Med.* 2012;367:2482–2494. https://doi.org/10.1056/NEJMoa1205624.
88. Bover J, Urena P, Ruiz-Garcia C, daSilva I, Lescano P, del Carpio J, et al. Clinical and practical use of calcimimetics in dialysis patients with secondary hyperparathyroidism. *Clin J Am Soc Nephrol.* 2016;11:161–174. https://doi.org/10.2215/cjn.01760215.
89. Block GA, Chertow GM, Cooper K, Xing S, Fouqueray B, Halperin M, et al. Fibroblast growth factor 23 as a risk factor for cardiovascular events and mortality in patients in the EVOLVE trial. *Hemodial Int.* 2021;25:78–85. https://doi.org/10.1111/hdi.12887.
90. Floege J, Tsirtsonis K, Iles J, Drueke TB, Chertow GM, Parfrey P. Incidence, predictors and therapeutic consequences of hypocalcemia in patients treated with cinacalcet in the EVOLVE trial. *Kidney Int.* 2018;93:1475–1482. https://doi.org/10.1016/j.kint.2017.12.014.
91. Block GA, Bushinsky DA, Cunningham J, Drueke TB, Ketteler M, Kewalramani R, et al. Effect of etelcalcetide vs placebo on serum parathyroid hormone in patients receiving hemodialysis with secondary hyperparathyroidism: Two randomized clinical trials. *JAMA.* 2017;317:146–155. https://doi.org/10.1001/jama.2016.19456.
92. Karaboyas A, Muenz D, Fuller DS, Desai P, Lin T-C, Robinson BM, et al. Etelcalcetide utilization, dosing titration, and chronic kidney disease–mineral and bone disease (CKD-MBD): Marker responses in US hemodialysis patients. *Am J Kidney Dis.* 2021. https://doi.org/10.1053/j.ajkd.2021.05.020.
93. Bushinsky DA, Chertow GM, Cheng S, Deng H, Kopyt N, Martin KJ, et al. One-year safety and efficacy of intravenous etelcalcetide in patients on hemodialysis with secondary hyperparathyroidism. *Nephrol Dial Transplant.* 2020;35:1769–1778. https://doi.org/10.1093/ndt/gfz039.
94. Friedl C, Zitt E. Role of etelcalcetide in the management of secondary hyperparathyroidism in hemodialysis patients: A review on current data and place in therapy. *Drug Des Devel Ther.* 2018;12:1589–1598. https://doi.org/10.2147/dddt.s134103.
95. Wolf M, Block GA, Chertow GM, Cooper K, Fouqueray B, Moe SM, et al. Effects of etelcalcetide on fibroblast growth factor 23 in patients with secondary hyperparathyroidism receiving hemodialysis. *Clin Kidney J.* 2019;13:75–84. https://doi.org/10.1093/ckj/sfz034.
96. Dörr K, Kammer M, Reindl-Schwaighofer R, Lorenz M, Prikoszovich T, Marculescu R, et al. Randomized trial of etelcalcetide for cardiac hypertrophy in hemodialysis. *Circ Res.* 2021;128:1616–1625. https://doi.org/10.1161/CIRCRESAHA.120.318556.
97. Block GA, Bushinsky DA, Cheng S, Cunningham J, Dehmel B, Drueke TB, et al. Effect of etelcalcetide vs cinacalcet on serum parathyroid hormone in patients receiving hemodialysis with secondary hyperparathyroidism: A randomized clinical trial. *JAMA.* 2017;317:156–164. https://doi.org/10.1001/jama.2016.19468.
98. Jankowski J, Floege J, Fliser D, Böhm M, Marx N. Cardiovascular disease in chronic kidney disease: Pathophysiological insights and therapeutic options. *Circulation.* 2021;1157–1172. https://doi.org/10.1161/CIRCULATIONAHA.120.050686.
99. Ardhanari S, Alpert MA, Aggarwal K. Cardiovascular disease in chronic kidney disease: Risk factors, pathogenesis, and prevention. *Adv Perit Dial.* 2014;30:40–53.
100. Kidney Disease: Improving Global Outcomes (KDIGO) CKD Work Group. KDIGO 2012 clinical practice guideline for the evaluation and management of chronic kidney disease. *Kidney Int Suppl.* 2013;3:1–150.
101. Goicoechea M, de Vinuesa SG, Quiroga B, Verde E, Bernis C, Morales E, et al. Aspirin for primary prevention of cardiovascular disease and renal disease progression in chronic kidney disease patients: A Multicenter Randomized Clinical Trial (AASER Study). *Cardiovasc Drugs Ther.* 2018;32:255–263. https://doi.org/10.1007/s10557-018-6802-1.
102. Pallikadavath S, Ashton L, Brunskill NJ, Burton JO, Gray LJ, Major RW. Aspirin for the primary prevention of cardiovascular disease in individuals with chronic kidney disease: A systematic review and

meta-analysis. *Eur J Prev Cardiol.* 2021. https://doi.org/10.1093/eurjpc/zwab132.
103. Palmer SC, Di Micco L, Razavian M, Craig JC, Perkovic V, Pellegrini F, et al. Antiplatelet agents for chronic kidney disease. *Cochrane Database Syst Rev.* 2013:Cd008834. https://doi.org/10.1002/14651858.CD008834.pub2.
104. Noels H, Lehrke M, Vanholder R, Jankowski J. Lipoproteins and fatty acids in chronic kidney disease: Molecular and metabolic alterations. *Nat Rev Nephrol.* 2021;17:528–542. https://doi.org/10.1038/s41581-021-00423-5.
105. Mathew RO, Rosenson RS, Lyubarova R, Chaudhry R, Costa SP, Bangalore S, et al. Concepts and controversies: Lipid management in patients with chronic kidney disease. *Cardiovasc Drugs Ther.* 2021;35:479–489. https://doi.org/10.1007/s10557-020-07020-x.
106. KDIGO clinical practice guideline for lipid management in chronic kidney disease. *Kidney Int Suppl.* 2013;3:259–305.
107. Baigent C, Landray MJ, Reith C, Emberson J, Wheeler DC, Tomson C, et al. The effects of lowering LDL cholesterol with simvastatin plus ezetimibe in patients with chronic kidney disease (Study of Heart and Renal Protection): A randomised placebo-controlled trial. *Lancet.* 2011;377:2181–2192. https://doi.org/10.1016/S0140-6736(11)60739-3.
108. Palmer SC, Navaneethan SD, Craig JC, Johnson DW, Perkovic V, Nigwekar SU, et al. HMG CoA reductase inhibitors (statins) for dialysis patients. *Cochrane Database Syst Rev.* 2013;9:CD004289. https://doi.org/10.1002/14651858.CD004289.pub5.
109. Palmer SC, Navaneethan SD, Craig JC, Johnson DW, Perkovic V, Hegbrant J, et al. HMG CoA reductase inhibitors (statins) for people with chronic kidney disease not requiring dialysis. *Cochrane Database Syst Rev.* 2014;5:CD007784. https://doi.org/10.1002/14651858.CD007784.pub2.
110. Ali S, Dave N, Virani SS, Navaneethan SD. Primary and secondary prevention of cardiovascular disease in patients with chronic kidney disease. *Curr Atheroscler Rep.* 2019;21:32. https://doi.org/10.1007/s11883-019-0794-6.
111. Grundy SM, Stone NJ, Bailey AL, Beam C, Birtcher KK, Blumenthal RS, et al. 2018 AHA/ACC/AACVPR/AAPA/ABC/ACPM/ADA/AGS/APhA/ASPC/NLA/PCNA Guideline on the Management of Blood Cholesterol: A Report of the American College of Cardiology/American Heart Association Task Force on Clinical Practice Guidelines. *J Am Coll Cardiol.* 2019;73:e285–e350. https://doi.org/10.1016/j.jacc.2018.11.003.
112. Rayner HC, Larkina M, Wang M, Graham-Brown M, van der Veer SN, Ecder T, et al. International comparisons of prevalence, awareness, and treatment of pruritus in people on hemodialysis. *Clin J Am Soc Nephrol.* 2017;12:2000–2007. https://doi.org/10.2215/CJN.03280317.
113. Makar M, Smyth B, Brennan F. Chronic kidney disease-associated pruritus: A review. *Kidney Blood Press Res.* 2021:1–11. https://doi.org/10.1159/000518391.
114. Verduzco HA, Shirazian S. CKD-associated pruritus: New insights into diagnosis, pathogenesis, and management. *Kidney Int Rep.* 2020;5:1387–1402. https://doi.org/10.1016/j.ekir.2020.04.027.
115. Fishbane S, Jamal A, Munera C, Wen W, Menzaghi F. A phase 3 trial of difelikefalin in hemodialysis patients with pruritus. *N Engl J Med.* 2020;382:222–232. https://doi.org/10.1056/nejmoa1912770.
116. Lipman ZM, Yosipovitch G. An evaluation of difelikefalin as a treatment option for moderate-to-severe pruritus in end stage renal disease. *Expert Opin Pharmacother.* 2021;22:549–555. https://doi.org/10.1080/14656566.2020.1849142.

Hemodialysis and Peritoneal Dialysis

64

Kevin M. Sowinski and Mariann D. Churchwell

KEY CONCEPTS

1. Hemodialysis (HD) involves the perfusion of blood and dialysate on opposite sides of a semipermeable membrane. Solutes are removed from the blood by diffusion and convection. Excess plasma water is removed by ultrafiltration.
2. Native arteriovenous (AV) fistulas are the preferred access for HD because of fewer complications and a longer survival rate. Venous catheters are plagued by complications such as infection and thrombosis and often deliver low blood flow rates.
3. Adequacy of HD can be assessed by the *Kt/V* and urea reduction ratio (URR). The National Kidney Foundation's Kidney Disease Outcomes Quality Initiative minimum goal *Kt/V* is greater than 1.2 per treatment and the URR is greater than 65%.
4. During HD, patients commonly experience hypotension and cramps. Other more serious complications include infection and thrombosis of the vascular access.
5. Peritoneal dialysis (PD) involves the instillation of dialysate into the peritoneal cavity via a permanent peritoneal catheter. The peritoneal membrane lines the highly vascularized abdominal viscera and acts as the semipermeable membrane. Solutes are removed from the blood across the peritoneum via diffusion and ultrafiltration. Excess plasma water is removed via ultrafiltration created by osmotic pressure generated by various dextrose or icodextrin concentrations.
6. Patients on PD are required to instill and drain, manually or via automated systems, several liters of fresh dialysate each day. The more exchanges completed each day results in greater solute removal.
7. Peritonitis is a common complication of PD. Initial empiric therapy for peritonitis should include intraperitoneal antibiotics that are effective against both gram-positive and gram-negative organisms.
8. Nasal carriage of *Staphylococcus aureus* is associated with an increased risk of catheter-related infections and peritonitis. Prophylaxis with a topical antimicrobial agent (mupirocin 2% or polysporin triple ointment) applied to the catheter exit site after each dialysis session can reduce catheter-related infections.

BEYOND THE BOOK

Visit the National Institute of Diabetes and Digestive and Kidney Diseases Website <https://www.niddk.nih.gov/health-information/kidney-disease/kidney-failure>. Review the information provided in the "Hemodialysis" and "Peritoneal Dialysis" links. Watch the video titled "What Is Dialysis?" <https://www.youtube.com/watch?v=mi34xCfmLhw>. The video provides a brief description of hemodialysis and peritoneal dialysis. This Website and video are useful to enhance student understanding of and potential treatments for end-stage kidney disease.

INTRODUCTION

The three primary treatment options for patients with end-stage renal disease (ESRD) are hemodialysis (HD), peritoneal dialysis (PD), and kidney transplantation. The United States Renal Data System (USRDS) is the national system that "collects, analyzes, and distributes" data relating to patients with ESRD or Stage 5 chronic kidney disease (CKD) in the United States and releases these data yearly.[1] According to the 2020 USRDS, at the end of 2018, there were 785,883 patients in the United States with ESRD. Of whom, 62.7% were being treated with in-center HD, 1.6% home HD, 7.6% PD, and nearly 29.7% had a functioning kidney transplant. Each of these represents an increase in the actual number of patients in each treatment modality. In 2018, 131,636 new patients started therapy for ESRD. In 2018, the prevalence of ESRD was 3.4 times greater in Black patients than White patients. In addition, the percentage of Black patients treated with in-center HD is higher in Black people than White people.[1]

Since 1972, the cost of treating ESRD has been covered by Medicare. In 2015, Medicare fee-for-service spending for patients with ESRD was $49.2 billion, which make up approximately 7% of all Medicare claim costs. ESRD consumes a vastly disproportionate amount of resources as only 1% of Medicare patients have the disease. Although total spending for ESRD treatment continues to climb by 2.1% each year, per-patient spending (after adjusting for inflation) increased by only 1.1% in 2018.[1] The prevalence of ESRD continues to climb, reflective of reduced mortality and enhanced patient care. The two primary diagnoses and underlying etiologies of kidney disease for new patients with ESRD are diabetes and hypertension.[1] Chapter 62 provides a thorough discussion on the epidemiology of chronic kidney disease.

This chapter serves as a primer on the principles and practice of dialysis and the complications associated with the delivery of dialysis treatments. HD and PD as the modalities most commonly employed for the management of ESRD (see Chapter 61 for a discussion of the role of renal replacement therapies in the management of acute kidney injury). The pertinent factors that should be considered before the initiation of dialysis are described. The morbidity and mortality associated with HD and PD are compared, as these considerations may influence the dialysis method chosen by patients and clinicians. The variants of HD and PD are detailed, and the multiple types of vascular and peritoneal access used with each (ie, catheters and surgical techniques) are illustrated. The concept of dialysis adequacy for each modality is briefly reviewed. Finally, the clinical presentation of common complications of both dialytic therapies is presented, along with pertinent nonpharmacologic and pharmacologic therapeutic approaches. Information resources that describe the influence of CKD on patient's quality of life, as well as the patient perspective on dialysis and dialysis-related therapies, are presented to highlight the human consequences of chronic disease.

Morbidity and Mortality in Dialysis

Morbidity in patients receiving dialysis can be assessed in a number of different ways including the number of hospitalizations per patient-year, the number of days hospitalized per patient-year, or the incidence of certain complications. The number of all-cause hospital admissions, 1.58 hospitalizations per patient-year, has fallen in recent years from greater than 1.82 hospitalizations per patient-year in 2009. Trends in hospitalization demonstrate an increase in hospitalization as a consequence of infection and cardiovascular disease and a decrease in hospitalizations as a consequence of vascular access problems. Patients with a functioning kidney transplant have a lower rate of hospitalization and shorter length of stay. Hospitalizations are more frequent in women than men, and in White people than Black people, and the frequency and duration increase with age in both dialysis modality groups.[1]

The life expectancy of US dialysis patients is markedly lower than that of healthy subjects of the same age and sex. In dialysis patients older than 75 years, the risk of dying is greater than four-fold higher when compared to all Medicare patients not receiving dialysis.[1] Adjusted all-cause mortality is greater for dialysis patients compared with age-matched individuals. Greater than 50% of deaths in dialysis patients are cardiovascular related. In fact, those with CKD are more likely to die from cardiovascular disease before they reach ESRD. Infections, usually related to the dialysis access, are the second-most common cause of death in dialysis patients. Although mortality remains high in this patient population, the overall patient mortality rate has fallen among dialysis patients since 2009. The reductions are dependent on treatment type and are smallest for HD and greatest for transplantation. In the United States, only 58% of HD patients and 68% of PD patients are alive 3 years after ESRD diagnosis and initiation of dialysis treatment.[1]

In addition to high morbidity and mortality, a dialysis patient's quality of life is generally poor. For example, restrictions caused by thrice weekly HD and/or associated treatments have been shown to impact many areas of a patient's life. These include, but are not limited to, physical endurance, sex, employment, social life, and diet. Patients often complain of fatigue and fear of the unknown related to their disease and its progression. The PD patient or the home HD patient may have some freedom from these restrictions, but this freedom comes with its own constraints.

Indications for Dialysis

Since first published in 2002, The National Kidney Foundation's Kidney Disease Outcome Quality Initiative (KDOQI) has been the primary treatment guideline for CKD. Although the Kidney Diseases: Improving Global Outcomes (KDIGO) guidelines[2] published in 2013, the updated 2015 version of the KDOQI guidelines serves as the most up-to-date recommendations.[3] Planning for dialysis initiation should occur when a patient's kidney function declines to CKD stage 4 (estimated glomerular filtration rate [eGFR] below 30 mL/min/1.73 m^2).[3] Beginning the preparation process at this point allows adequate time for proper education of the patient and family and for the creation of a suitable vascular or peritoneal access.

TABLE 64-1 Advantages and Disadvantages of Hemodialysis

Advantages

1. Higher solute clearance allows intermittent treatment.
2. Parameters of adequacy of dialysis are better defined and therefore underdialysis can be detected early.
3. Technique failure rate is low.
4. Even though intermittent heparinization is required, hemostasis parameters are better corrected with hemodialysis than peritoneal dialysis.
5. In-center hemodialysis enables closer monitoring of the patient.

Disadvantages

1. In-center hemodialysis requires multiple visits each week to the hemodialysis center, which translates into loss of patient independence.
2. Disequilibrium, dialysis-induced hypotension, and muscle cramps are common. May require months before the patient adjusts to hemodialysis.
3. Infections in hemodialysis patients may be related to the choice of membranes, the complement-activating membranes being more deleterious.
4. Vascular access is frequently associated with infection and thrombosis.
5. Decline of residual kidney function is more rapid compared to peritoneal dialysis.

For patients choosing HD, a permanent arteriovenous (AV) access (preferably a fistula) should be surgically created when eGFR falls below 25 mL/min/1.73 m^2, serum creatinine is greater than 4 mg/dL (354 μmol/L), or 1 year prior to the anticipated need for dialysis.[4] The KDIGO and KDOQI guidelines provide recommendations for referral to a specialist in kidney care services and for planning for RRT. The recommendation for timely referral is for patients with progressive CKD in whom the risk of kidney failure within 1 year is greater than 10% based on validated risk prediction tools.[2]

The KDIGO guidelines and commentaries addressing them agree that the primary criterion for initiation of dialysis is the patient's clinical status, rather than a specific level of kidney function.[2,5] Namely, dialysis should be initiated when one or more of the following are present: signs or symptoms of kidney failure (eg, serositis, acid-base or electrolyte abnormalities, pruritis); inability to control volume status or blood pressure; a progressive deterioration in nutritional status or cognitive impairment. The guidelines suggest that these signs and symptoms are patient specific but tend to be evident once the patient's eGFR is in the range of 5 to 10 mL/min/1.73 m^2. The guidelines specifically indicate that RRT should be initiated to manage signs and symptoms and not to treat an arbitrary kidney function measurement.[2] The advantages and disadvantages of HD and PD are depicted in Tables 64-1 and 64-2, respectively. These factors, along with the patients' concomitant diseases, personal preferences, and support environments, are the principal determinants of the dialysis mode they will receive. The timing of dialysis initiation is a compromise between maximizing patient quality of life by extending the dialysis-free period while avoiding complications that will decrease the length and quality of dialysis-assisted life.[3]

There is considerable debate in the literature regarding the mortality differences between HD and PD.[6-8] Most observational trials suggest that PD is associated with a survival advantage early in therapy, which wanes with increased treatment time. Prospective trials have reported conflicting results relative to efficacy of one modality over another. If there is a survival advantage for PD, the consensus is that the advantage is early in therapy and may not with continued therapy. Well-designed studies are extremely difficult to conduct in this population, and thus the question of superiority of one modality over the other is controversial and continues to be debated. Differences in outcomes may be related to a wide array of confounding factors, such as the dose of dialysis, baseline patient health status, physician bias in modality selection, patient

TABLE 64-2 Advantages and Disadvantages of Peritoneal Dialysis

Advantages

1. Hemodynamic stability due to slow ultrafiltration rate.
2. Higher clearance of larger solutes, which may explain good clinical status in spite of lower urea clearance.
3. Better preservation of residual kidney function.
4. Convenient intraperitoneal route for administration of drugs such as antibiotics and insulin.
5. Suitable for elderly and young patients who may not tolerate hemodialysis well.
6. Freedom from the "machine" gives the patient a sense of independence (for continuous ambulatory peritoneal dialysis).
7. Less blood loss and iron deficiency, resulting in easier management of anemia or reduced requirements for erythropoietin and parenteral iron.
8. No systemic heparinization required.
9. Subcutaneous versus intravenous erythropoietin or darbepoetin may reduce overall doses and be more physiologic.

Disadvantages

1. Protein and amino acid losses through peritoneum and reduced appetite from continuous glucose load and sense of abdominal fullness predispose patients to malnutrition.
2. Risk of peritonitis.
3. Catheter malfunction, and exit-site and tunnel infection.
4. Inadequate ultrafiltration and solute clearance in patients with a large body size, unless large volumes and frequent exchanges are employed.
5. Patient burnout and high rate of technique failure.
6. Risk of obesity with excessive glucose absorption.
7. Mechanical problems such as hernias, dialysate leaks, hemorrhoids, or back pain are more common than HD.
8. Extensive abdominal surgery may preclude peritoneal dialysis.
9. No convenient access for intravenous iron administration.

compliance with dialysis and medication therapy, or other unknown factors. For example, healthier patients tend to be directed toward PD, and factors such as age, duration of dialysis, and comorbidities play an important role in the complex relationship between patient outcomes and mortality. Without clear distinction between modalities in terms of many important outcomes, the selection of the optimal therapy for a given patient is challenging. The selection of one modality over the other should be based upon patient motivation, desire, geographic distance from an HD unit, healthcare team preference, and patient education rather than survival advantages alone.

HEMODIALYSIS

Although HD was first successfully used in 1940, the procedure was not used widely until the Korean War in 1952. Permanent dialysis access was developed in the 1960s, which allowed routine use of HD in patients with ESRD. Subsequent decades brought advances in dialysis technology, including the introduction of more efficient and biocompatible dialyzer membranes and safer techniques. HD is the most common type of renal replacement therapy for patients with ESRD.

Principles of Hemodialysis

1 Hemodialysis consists of the perfusion of blood and a physiologic solution on opposite sides of a semipermeable membrane. Multiple substances, such as water, urea, creatinine, potassium, uremic toxins, and drugs, move from the blood into the dialysate, by either passive diffusion or convection as the result of ultrafiltration. Diffusion is the movement of substances down a concentration gradient. The rate of diffusion depends on the difference between the concentration of the solute in blood and dialysate, solute characteristics, that is, size, water solubility, and charge, the dialyzer membrane composition, and blood and dialysate flow rates. Diffusive transport is rapid for small solutes but decreases with increasing molecular size. Other important diffusive solute transport factors include the membrane thickness, porosity, and the steric hindrance between the membrane pores and solute. Ultrafiltration is the movement of water across the dialyzer membrane because of hydrostatic or osmotic pressure and is the primary means for removal of excess fluid. Convection occurs when dissolved solutes move across a membrane with water transport. This occurs only if the pores in the dialyzer are large enough to allow them to pass along with water. Convection can be maximized by increasing the hydrostatic pressure gradient across the dialysis membrane or by using a dialyzer that is more permeable to water transport. Diffusion and convection can be controlled independently, and thus, a patient's HD prescription can be individualized to attain the desired degree of solute and fluid removal.[9]

Hemodialysis Access

2 Obtaining and maintaining access to the circulation has been a challenge for long-term use and success of HD. Permanent access to the circulation may be accomplished by several techniques, including the creation of an AV fistula, an AV graft, or by venous catheters (Fig. 64-1).[10] As shown in Fig. 64-1, the native AV fistula is created by the anastomosis of a vein and artery (ie, the radial artery to the cephalic vein or the brachial artery to the cephalic vein). The native AV fistula has many advantages including providing the longest survival time of all blood-access devices and the lowest rate of complications such as infection and thrombosis. Patients with fistulas have increased survival and lower hospitalization rates compared to other HD patients. Finally, AV fistulas are the most cost-effective in terms of placement and long-term maintenance. Ideally, the most distal site (the wrist) is used to construct the first fistula; it is the easiest to create, and in the case of access failure, more proximal sites on the arm are preserved for later use. Unfortunately, fistulas require at least 1 to 2 months to mature before they can be routinely utilized for dialysis. Creation of an AV fistula, however, may be difficult in elderly patients and in patients with peripheral vascular disease, which is a particularly common comorbidity in patients with diabetes.

Synthetic AV grafts, usually made of polytetrafluoroethylene, are another permanent AV access option. These grafts require 2 to 3 weeks before they can be routinely used. Their primary disadvantages are shorter survival of the graft, and higher rates of infection and thrombosis. The least-desirable and least permanent HD access option involves the placement of a central venous catheter. Venous catheters can be placed in the femoral, subclavian, or internal jugular veins. Their main advantage is that they can be used immediately, and they are often used in small children, diabetic patients with severe vascular disease, the morbidly obese, and patients who have no viable sites for permanent AV access. Late referrals to a nephrology specialist for HD initiation and delayed placement of a more appropriate long-term access contribute to the use of venous catheters in chronic HD patients. The major problem with all venous catheters is that they have shorter survival and are more prone to infection and thrombosis than either AV grafts or fistulas. Furthermore, some catheters are not able to provide adequate blood flow rates, which may limit the deliverable dose of dialysis.[10,11] Regardless, tunneled dialysis catheters are used frequently because of the ease of insertion, pain-free dialysis needle placement and availability for immediate use. They are, however, associated with increased morbidity, mortality, and cost.

Hemodialysis Procedures

The HD system consists of an external vascular circuit through which the patient's blood is transferred in sterile tubing to the dialyzer via a mechanical pump (Fig. 64-2).[10] The patient's blood then passes through the dialyzer on one side of the semipermeable membrane and is returned to the patient. The dialysate solution, which consists of purified water and electrolytes, is pumped through the dialyzer countercurrent to the flow of blood on the opposite side of

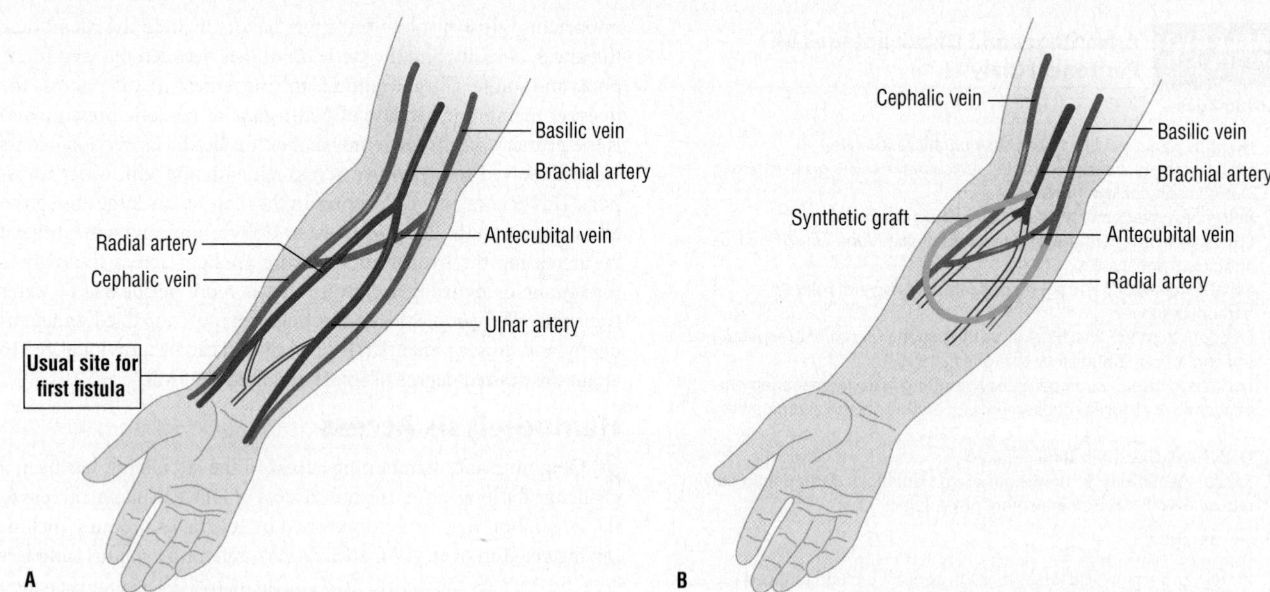

FIGURE 64-1 The predominant types of vascular access for chronic dialysis patients are (*A*) the arteriovenous fistula and (*B*) the synthetic arteriovenous forearm graft. The first primary arteriovenous fistula is usually created by the surgical anastomosis of the cephalic vein with the radial artery. The flow of blood from the higher-pressure arterial system results in hypertrophy of the vein. The most common AV graft (depicted in green) is between the brachial artery and the basilic or cephalic vein. The flow of blood may be diminished in the radial and ulnar arteries since it preferentially flows into the low-pressure graft.

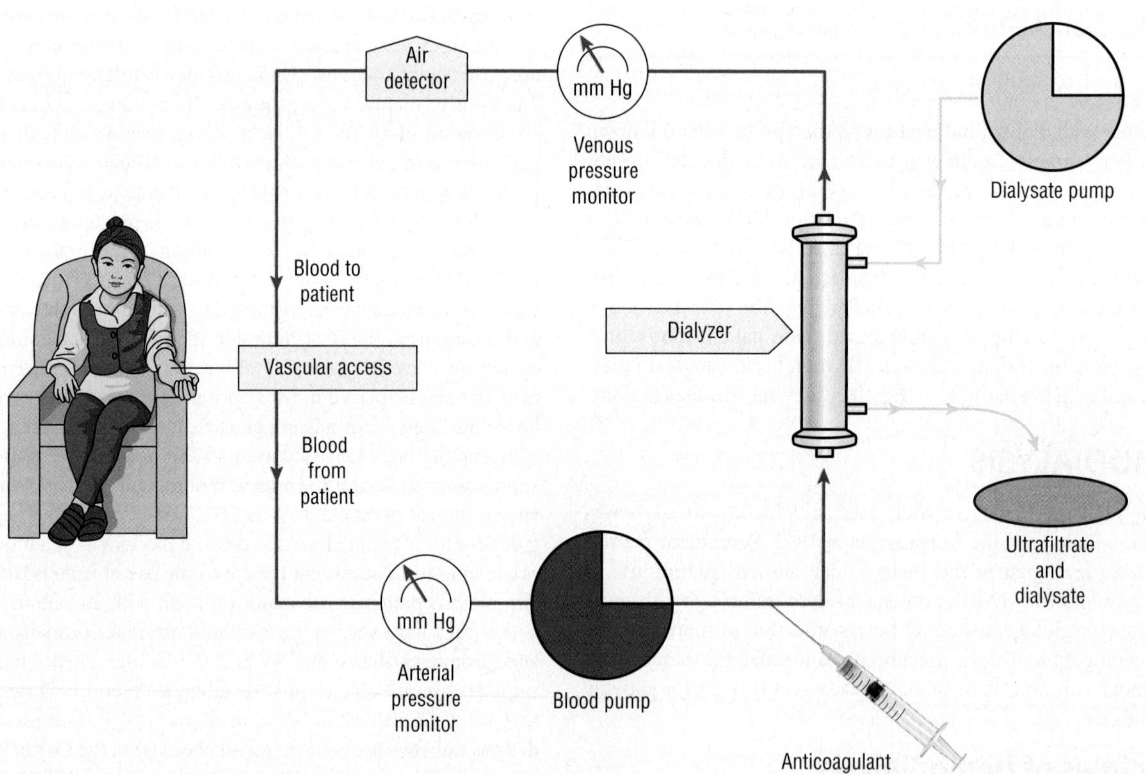

FIGURE 64-2 In hemodialysis, the patient's blood is pumped to the dialyzer at a rate of 300 to 600 mL/min. An anticoagulant is administered to prevent clotting in the dialyzer. The dialysate is pumped at a rate of 500 to 800 mL/min through the dialyzer countercurrent to the flow of blood. The rate of fluid removal from the patient is controlled by adjusting the pressure in the dialysate compartment.

the semipermeable membrane. In most cases, systemic anticoagulation (usually unfractionated heparin in the United States) is used to prevent blood clotting in the HD circuit tubing. The process of dialysis results in the removal of metabolic waste products, medications, and water and replenishment of body buffers, such as acetate and bicarbonate.

Hemodiafiltration (HDF), another variant of traditional HD, enhances convective solute and water transport in addition to diffusive clearance to a much greater extent than high-flux HD.[10,12,13] When fluid losses exceed those desired for the patient, an IV infusion referred to as replacement fluid may be administered. HDF may improve outcomes due to its ability to remove middle molecular weight uremic solutes more efficiently than the other HD variants. HDF improves survival compared to conventional HD.[13,14] Preliminary information suggests that HDF enhances clearance of phosphate, beta-2 microglobulin, and pro-inflammatory solutes. This procedure is not used extensively in the United States. Barriers to its use are the high cost and logistic issues associated with providing the fluid replacement needs.

Dialyzers are made up of a polyurethane container containing hollow fibers which are suspended in dialysate. These hollow fibers, or dialysis membranes, are made up of three substances, unmodified cellulose (cuprophan), substituted cellulose (cellulose acetate), and cellulosynthetic materials. The permeability of these membranes varies and the membranes are divided into three general types: low flux, high efficiency, and high flux. Low-flux and high-efficiency membranes have small pores that limit clearance to relatively small molecules (size less than or equal to 500 daltons) such as urea and creatinine and are utilized for less than 20% of chronic HD procedures.[10] High-flux membranes are now used in the vast majority of patients because they are capable of removing high-molecular-weight endogenous substances, such as β2-microglobulin, and medications such as vancomycin.[10] The primary reason for using high-flux membranes is that clearance of water as well as low- and high-molecular-weight substances is much greater, allowing for shorter treatment times. To maximize the clearance capacity of high-flux dialyzers, the blood flow rates should be 400 to 600 mL/min, and dialysate flow rates greater than 500 mL/min, which necessitates strict controls and active monitoring of the rate of fluid removal. Typically, these dialyzers are composed of polysulfone, polymethylmethacrylate, polyamide, cellulose triacetate, and polyacrylonitrile.[10]

HD is usually prescribed as three sessions per week for 3 to 5 hours/session. These sessions are usually performed in "in-center" dialysis units. This is a large time commitment for any patient undergoing HD and results in substantial loss of control over their life. Several alternatives to this type of HD have been explored in an effort to balance dialysis adequacy with patient outcomes and quality of life. These alternatives include procedures that increase dialysis frequency, enhance dialysis duration, or both.[15-18] Examples are as follows: (1) frequent HD (5-7 sessions/week), which can be frequent short (less than 3 hours/session), frequent standard (3-5 hours/session), or frequent long sessions (longer than 5 hours/session); (2) long HD (more than 5 hours/session given 3-7 times/week, which can be long thrice weekly (administered either at night or during the day), long every other night (administered at night), and long frequent (administered at night 5-7 nights/week). Many of these alternatives are suggested to be associated with improved survival.[16-18] For example, in-center, thrice weekly HD was associated with a higher risk of the composite outcome of death, left-ventricular mass, and change in health composite score than in-center six times per week HD.[19] Intensive dialysis has been associated with reductions in left-ventricular mass and improved blood pressure control, both surrogates for improved cardiovascular outcomes, and improved phosphate removal. Lastly, and perhaps most importantly, these procedures are associated with a reduction in dialysis-related symptoms and improved quality of life.[16-18] Despite the perceived advantages and more frequent use in other countries such as New Zealand and Canada, the use of home HD is uncommon, albeit increasing in use in the United States, still less than 2% of dialysis patients receiving HD care at home at the end of 2018.[1] Potential obstacles to home HD include patient factors (eg, lack of self-efficacy, fear of self-cannulation, fear of catastrophic event, and fear of lack of quality care) and a lack of awareness of the availability of this type of dialysis. Finally, there are suggestions that patients receiving intensive dialysis may be at higher risk of access infections and need for vascular access procedures. Further clinical trials are needed to elucidate the role of these types of dialysis therapy. The 2015 KDOQI guidelines provide suggestions and/or recommendations that all patients be offered short frequent HD as an alternative to standard HD in addition to providing patients with information about the potential risk associated with them.[3]

Adequacy of Hemodialysis

The optimal dose of HD, the patient's dialysis prescription, is that amount of therapy above which there is no cost-effective increment in the patient's quality-adjusted life expectancy. The two primary goals of the dialysis prescription are to achieve the patient's dry weight and the adequate removal of endogenous waste products such as urea. Dry weight is the target post-dialysis weight at which the patient is normotensive and free of edema. Measurement of urea removal, while imperfect, is the typical method used to quantify dialysis adequacy. Urea removal reflects the "delivered dose" of dialysis and is utilized as the surrogate for removal of other toxins.

The delivered or desired dose of dialysis in terms of solute removal can be expressed as the urea reduction ratio (URR) or the *Kt/V* (pronounced "K-T-over-V"). The URR is a simple concept and is easily calculated as follows:

$$\text{URR} = \frac{\text{Predialysis BUN} - \text{Postdialysis BUN}}{\text{Predialysis BUN}} \times 100$$

The URR is frequently used to measure the delivered dialysis dose; however, it does not account for the contribution of convective removal of urea. The *Kt/V* is a unitless index based on the dialyzer clearance of urea (*K*) in L/h multiplied by the duration of dialysis (*t*) in hours, divided by the urea distribution volume of the patient (*V*) in liters.[10] The *Kt/V* is thus the fraction of the patient's total body water that is cleared of urea during a dialysis session. Urea kinetic modeling, using computer software, is the optimal means to calculate the *Kt/V*.[10] An in-depth discussion of the pros and cons of various methods of calculating and interpreting *Kt/V* is beyond the scope of this chapter. The reader is referred to other sources for more in-depth information.[10]

3 For patients who receive thrice weekly HD, KDOQI recommends that the minimally adequate delivered dose of dialysis is a *Kt/V* of 1.2 (equivalent to an average URR of 65%).[3] To achieve this goal, the recommended target prescribed *Kt/V* is 1.4 (equivalent to an average URR of 70%).[3] For patients who receive HD on a schedule other than thrice weekly, the KDOQI suggests a target standard *Kt/V* of 2.3 volumes/week with a minimum delivered dose of 2.1. Lower doses of dialysis treatment are thought to be associated with increased morbidity and mortality. Many nephrologists believe that even greater doses of dialysis would have positive outcomes in dialysis patients, and so the average dose of dialysis has been increasing in the United States although the evidence for this is not strong. The results of HEMO study, a prospective, randomized trial that assigned patients to either standard ($Kt/V = 1.25$) or high-dose ($Kt/V = 1.65$) dialysis with high-flux or low-flux membranes, revealed that the risk of death was similar in both the standard and high-dose therapy and the low- and high-flux groups. Thus, there is no benefit in increasing the dose of dialysis above the current recommendations. The HEMO study only enrolled patients who were on traditional thrice-weekly dialysis, so the applicability of these findings to patients on more intensive regimens such as daily or nocturnal HD regimens remains to be determined. However, intensive HD regimens may result in better control of blood pressure, anemia, phosphate, and sleep apnea.[15] In those relatively few patients who are below the adequacy goal, the deficiency may be related to patient compliance with the dialysis prescription (ie, ending dialysis early)

TABLE 64-3 Common Complications During Hemodialysis

	Incidence (%)	Etiology/Predisposing Factors
Hypotension	20-30	Hypovolemia and excessive ultrafiltration
		Antihypertensive medications prior to dialysis
		Target dry weight too low
		Diastolic dysfunction
		Autonomic dysfunction
		Low calcium and sodium in dialysate
		High dialysate temperature
		Meal ingestion prior to or during dialysis
Hypertension	5-15	Plasma sodium concentration
		Intravascular volume
		Dialytic removal of antihypertensive medications
		Activation of the Renin Angiotensin Aldosterone system
Cramps	5-20	Muscle hypoperfusion due to ultrafiltration and hypovolemia
		Hypotension
		Electrolyte imbalance
		Acid–base imbalance
Nausea and vomiting	5-15	Hypotension
		Dialyzer reaction
Headache	5	Disequilibrium syndrome
		Caffeine withdrawal due to dialysis removal
Chest and back pain	2-5	Unknown
Pruritus	5	Inadequate dialysis
		Skin dryness
		Secondary hyperparathyroidism
		Abnormal skin concentrations of electrolytes
		Histamine release
		Mast cell proliferation
Fever and chills	<1	Endotoxin release; infection of dialysis catheter

Data from Reference 10.

or low blood flow rates caused by access stenosis or thrombosis, or due to the use of catheters. Adequate dialysis may not be achieved in some patients despite compliance and sufficient blood flow. For these patients, there are two options to increase urea clearance: use a larger membrane or increase the treatment time.

Complications of Hemodialysis

4 HD is a life-extending therapy for patients with kidney failure but HD is associated with short- and long-term complications. Complications associated with HD can decrease the efffectiveness of therapy, quality of life and life expectancy. This chapter discusses complications that occur during an HD session (intradialytic) and complications associated with vascular access.

Hemodialysis Procedure Complications

The most common complications that occur during HD include hypotension, hypertension, cramps, nausea and vomiting, headache, chest pain, back pain, and fever or chills.[20] Table 64-3 lists these complications and their etiology and predisposing factors.

TABLE 64-4 Management of Hypotension

Acute treatment	Place patient in Trendelenburg position
	Decrease ultrafiltration rate
	Give 100-200 mL bolus of normal saline intravenous
	Give 10-20 mL of hypertonic saline (23.4%) intravenous over 3-5 minutes
	Give 12.5 g mannitol
Prevention	
Nonpharmacologic	Accurately set "dry weight"
	Use steady constant ultrafiltration rate
	Keep dialysate sodium >serum sodium
	Lower dialysate temperatures
	Bicarbonate dialysate
	Avoid food before or during hemodialysis
Pharmacologic	Midodrine 2.5-10 mg orally 30 minutes before hemodialysis (start at 2.5 mg and titrate)
	Droxidopa 100-600 mg orally 1 hour before hemodialysis (start at 100 mg and titrate up to 600 mg)
	Other options (limited evidence):
	Levocarnitine 20 mg/kg IV after hemodialysis
	Sertraline 50-100 mg daily
	Fludrocortisone 0.1 mg before hemodialysis
	DDAVP 1-2 intranasal sprays (150 μg/spray)
Counsel patients	Administer antihypertensive medications in the evening or after hemodialysis
	Minimize intradialytic weight gain by decreasing salt content in their diet

Intradialytic hypotension (IDH) as defined by the National Kidney Foundation Kidney Disease Outcomes Quality Initiative (NKF KDOQI) is a decrease in systolic blood pressure by ≥20 mm Hg or a decrease in mean arterial pressure (MAP) by 10 mm Hg. A patient with IDH may experience abdominal discomfort, yawning, sighing, nausea, vomiting, muscle cramps, restlessness, dizziness or fainting, and anxiety. A decrease in BP can increase the risk of vascular access thrombosis, induce a cardiac arrhythmia, or predispose a patient to a coronary or cerebral ischemic event. Hypotension during HD can decrease the effectiveness of a dialysis session resulting in a lower Kt/V_{urea}.[21] A systolic blood pressure <90 mm Hg has been associated with increased mortality.[22]

A primary cause of IDH is related to the rate and amount of fluid removed during[10,23] typical HD treatments, although other causes, as listed in Table 64-4, may also play a role.[10,23] Symptoms such as nausea and cramping are often present during acute hypotensive episodes. The replacement of acetate with bicarbonate as the dialysate buffer, the use of volumetric ultrafiltration controllers, and individualized or modeled dialysate sodium concentrations have helped reduce the incidence of IDH. Sodium modeling uses a higher initial dialysate sodium concentration (145-155 mmol/L [mEq/L]) and tapers sodium concentration down (135-140 mmol/L [mEq/L]) over the dialytic session. Dialytic treatment modifications such as sodium individualization or modeling may decrease post-HD thirst and subsequent intradialytic weight gain. This modification may decrease the need for aggressive dialytic fluid removal and the incidence of IDH.[24-26]

Intradialytic or post-HD hypertension can occur in 5% to 15% of patients receiving HD and may increase post-HD fatigue and the risk of cardiovascular and all-cause mortality.[27] Underlying causes include, not achieving post-HD dry weight goal, over-estimation of dry weight, dialytic removal of antihypertensive medications, or the activation of the renin-angiotensin system secondary to abrupt hypovolemia.[28]

Skeletal muscle cramps complicate 5% to 20% of HD treatments. Although the pathogenesis of cramps is multifactorial, plasma volume contraction and decreased muscle perfusion caused by excessive ultrafiltration are frequently the initiating events.[10] Pruritus may increase in severity during the HD treatment and is a complication of CKD. The management of pruritus is discussed in Chapter 63.

Vascular Access Complications

The most common vascular access complications in patients receiving HD are thrombosis and infection. The highest occurrence of complications is found in patients with a central venous catheter (CVC) compared with those with an AV graft or AV fistula.[10,29] A majority of patients initiate HD with a CVC (80.8%), and of those patients 65.2% did so without a maturing AV fistula or graft. In prevalent patients receiving HD, 82.4% had either an AV fistula or graft.[1] The maintenance of vascular access patency is critical for patients receiving HD. Predisposing factors are often described using Virchow's triad of blood flow stasis, hypercoagulability, and endothelial injury. An aneurysm or stenosis of an AV fistula, graft or surrounding vasculature generally require a surgical intervention. Several pharmacologic therapies have been evaluated to maintain vascular access patency but results are conflicting.[30] Vascular access stenosis can contribute to decreases in blood flow (blood flow <300 mL/min) and increase the risk of thrombus formation within the access. A decrease in blood flow through the access can occur abruptly, or over days to weeks or intermittently and may require ultrasound, venography, or computed tomography scans for a definitive diagnosis.[29,30] Catheter-related thrombosis can form either inside (intrinsic) or outside (extrinsic) the catheter. An occlusion can form within the lumen, at the tip or develop a fibrin sleeve around the catheter where this fibrin sleeve can serve as a nidus for infection and ultimately require catheter removal.[31,32]

Infection is a leading cause of mortality in HD patients.[1] The risk of sepsis-related death is 100 times greater in patients receiving HD than the general population, and those with an indwelling catheter have the highest risk.[32] A comparison of patients receiving HD with a catheter compared to those without a catheter found a higher rate of bloodstream infections in patients with a catheter.[33] An examination of the United States Renal Data System identified patients initiating HD with a central venous catheter (CVC), AV fistula or graft from 2006 through 2014 who developed sepsis. The highest rate of sepsis was found in patients with a CVC (31.2%) followed by an AV graft (30.6%) and an AV fistula (22.9%, $P < 0.001$).[34]

The National Healthcare Safety Network (NHSN) dialysis event surveillance report found that 69.8% of access-related blood stream infections (ARBSIs) were in patients with an indwelling CVC.[35] The most prevalent pathogens for blood stream infections (BSIs) were gram-positive (64%) followed by gram-negative (35%) and Candida species (0.2%). The most frequently isolated micro-organisms in ARBSIs were as follows: *S. aureus* (31.8%), *S. epidermidis* (15.6%), coagulase-negative staphylococcus (9.7%), *E. faecalis* (4.9%), and *E. coli* (2.9%). The incidence with methicillin-resistant *S. aureus* (39.5%) and cephalosporin-resistant *E. coli* (17.8%) organisms were highest in patients with a CVC.[35]

Catheter-related infections can develop at the insertion site, hub, or both. The infection source for long-term catheters such as a tunneled cuffed catheter is usually the hub where bacteria can enter the blood leading to a BSI.[29,32] Overall, HD access with a catheter is associated with higher rates of bacteremia, osteomyelitis, septic arthritis, endocarditis, thrombus, and death, as well as increased treatment costs compared with an AV fistula or AV graft.[36]

Complications of CKD

Patients receiving HD are likely to have at least one additional comorbid disease such as diabetes, hypertension, cardiovascular disease, or obesity (BMI greater than or equal to 30 kg/m^2) and older age (greater than or equal to 60). The pharmacotherapy management of most CKD complications and comorbid diseases that persist in patients receiving HD are discussed in Chapter 63. The daily medication burden for HD patients is one of the highest for any chronic disease state. The pill burden in HD patients was reported as an average of 15.1 ± 7.6 pills/day of which phosphate binder medications accounted for 6.44 ± 4.78 pills/day.[37] Adherence to phosphate binder regimens is reported to be 43% in US patients receiving dialysis. Patients taking more than the average pills/day of phosphorus binders were more likely to miss a dose than patients taking less than the average pills/day. The increased pill burden is associated with a lower quality of life in patients receiving dialysis.[38]

Management of Hemodialysis Complications

The management of HD complications is discussed in this section. The most common causes of HD complications and appropriate management are reviewed.

Hypotension

Acute management of intradialytic hypotension (IDH) includes decreasing the ultrafiltration rate or stopping ultrafiltration, placing the patient in the Trendelenburg position, lowering the dialysate temperature, modifying dialysate electrolyte concentrations, and/or administering normal or hypertonic saline.[23,39,40] IDH may not occur during each HD session and a patient's response to therapeutic modifications can be variable, which could necessitate modification of their HD prescription. Patients with IDH will need a careful review of all medications including antihypertensive medications. Evaluation should consider the timing of antihypertensive medication administration and may require adjustments to medications administered the day prior to and the day of HD therapy.[23] Patients with IDH should be counseled to take their blood pressure medications after HD and avoid the consumption of food during HD.

IDH is often due to an insufficient cardiac response to reduced circulating blood volume, which may occur when aggressive ultrafiltration is required to restore dry weight. Most treatments for IDH are directed toward restoring or maintaining adequate blood vessel perfusion in these patients. One approach is to limit interdialytic weight gain (IDWG) that may decrease the rate and volume of fluid removal during HD. Patients are counseled to limit dietary salt intake especially hidden sodium in processed foods. A reduction in dietary sodium could decrease a patient's thirst and subsequent fluid intake.[10] Another approach, decreasing the dialysate temperature to 36.5°C (97.7°F), may help reduce core body temperature, which can decrease vasodilation.[30,41] If nonpharmacologic interventions are not adequate to prevent or reduce the incidence of symptomatic IDH, then pharmacologic interventions should be considered (see Table 64-4).

Oral midodrine (5-10 mg) given two to three times daily can increase blood pressure in patients receiving HD with chronic hypotension. Midodrine, an alpha-1 adrenergic agonist, can also be administered 30 minutes prior to initiating HD to increase intradialytic blood pressure. It is rapidly absorbed in the gastrointestinal tract and will begin to increase blood pressure within 60 minutes. Midodrine's half-life during HD can be less than 2 hours but on nondialysis days it is approximately 10 hours. HD will remove the prodrug and metabolite of midodrine which contributes to the drug's decreased half-life during HD. It is important to note that the effects of midodrine are probably best in patients with hypotension related to autonomic dysfunction. Patients with peripheral vascular disease should be monitored for digital or lower limb ischemia.[42]

Droxidopa is an oral synthetic amino acid analog metabolized by the catecholamine pathway to norepinephrine, resulting in vasoconstriction of peripheral veins and arteries. Droxidopa is FDA-approved for neurogenic orthostatic hypotension. Droxidopa was studied in patients with a history of IDH that were randomized to receive droxidopa 400 mg, 600 mg, or placebo 1 hour prior to HD. The patients receiving droxidopa when compared to placebo had a lower rate of early HD termination due to IDH. Gastrointestinal disorders were the most frequent adverse effect reported in the treatment groups.[43]

Fludrocortisone is a potential agent for symptomatic IDH, including patients with an inadequate response to midodrine. It increases blood pressure through several mechanisms including enhancing blood vessel sensitivity to circulating catecholamines. Fludrocortisone dosing for orthostatic hypotension generally ranges from 0.1 mg to 1.0 mg/day but IDH dosing has not been determined. A case report described a patient receiving HD with IDH and a decreased response to midodrine that resulted in early termination of HD sessions. Fludrocortisone 0.2 mg was administered with 10 mg of midodrine 30 minutes prior to the start of HD. Prior to initiating fludrocortisone, 6 out of 45 HD sessions were terminated early but after fludrocortisone initiation, no HD sessions were terminated early in the subsequent 45 HD sessions.[44] The use of fludrocortisone may be beneficial in select patients with IDH but adverse effects such as sodium and water retention could increase edema in patients with congestive heart failure.

The treatment of IDH with levocarnitine, sertraline, and intranasal desmopressin acetate (DDAVP) have been reported to improve IDH. Administration of levocarnitine (20 mg/kg IV at the end of each HD session) may reduce hypotensive episodes, particularly in patients with carnitine deficiency.[45] High cost and limited efficacy precludes a strong recommendation for routine levocarnitine use. The administration of sertraline 50 mg daily titrated to 100 mg daily after 1 week improved systolic and diastolic blood pressure in a small trial.[46] Sertraline 50 mg was administered daily to patients receiving HD, but sertraline did not increase in post-HD blood pressure.[47] The mixed results do not support routine sertraline administration for hypotension. Overall, the use of DDAVP increased post-HD blood pressure and decreased the incidence of IDH.[48] These medications have limited clinical evidence and should be used with caution in patients receiving HD with IDH. Overall, the best evidence for an oral pharmacological treatment of IDH is with midodrine. Alternative agents have been studied but the evidence is limited for each of these agents as many of the studies had a small sample size and did not have a placebo control.

Hypertension

An elevated blood pressure in a patient prior to receiving HD is often attributed to volume expansion. A decline in blood pressure is expected during and after HD and improves survival, but a dramatic increase or decrease in blood pressure during or after HD decreases overall survival.[49] An increase in blood pressure of >10 mm Hg either during or post-HD may require a change in the delivery of an HD session, antihypertensive medications or adjustments to the timing of medication administration.[28] Although the underlying mechanism may be multifactorial, antihypertensive medication dialyzability could play a role in HD-related increases in blood pressure.[50] HD enhances the clearance of metoprolol, atenolol, and angiotensin-converting enzyme inhibitors (ACE-Is). An angiotensin receptor blocker (ARB), carvedilol or amlodipine is minimally removed during HD and may be an option in patients experiencing a rise in blood pressure during or post-HD. Antihypertensive medication regimes need to be individualized based on a patient's comorbid conditions and risk of HD-related blood pressure changes. A retrospective cohort examined patients with heart failure receiving HD and either taking a daily beta-blocker (carvedilol, bisoprolol, or metoprolol CR/XL) or those patients not taking a daily beta-blocker. Patients receiving either carvedilol, bisoprolol, or metoprolol had lower all-cause mortality at 5 years.[51] However, in patients at risk of IDH, a large retrospective study found an increased rate of IDH and risk of all-cause mortality in patients taking carvedilol compared to metoprolol.[52] Initiation of any antihypertensive medication in patients at high-risk should be followed with close monitoring pre- and post-HD in addition to during HD. One small study found an improvement in patients with intradialytic hypertension when low-dose carvedilol (6.25 mg twice daily) was initiated and titrated as tolerated.

Muscle Cramps

The cause of muscle cramps in patient receiving HD may be multifactorial and include aggressive removal of fluid and electrolyte imbalances. Nonpharmacologic interventions related to dialytic therapy may help alleviate muscle cramps. These measures include adjusting the ultrafiltration rate to avoid hypotension, volume contraction, or hypoosmolality. Other methods to reduce muscle cramps, including compression devices, moist heat, massage, exercise, stretching, or muscle flexing, should be considered first to minimize adverse consequences (Table 64-5).[10,23]

Pharmacologic interventions include increasing the magnesium concentration in dialysate, supplementation with oral magnesium, vitamin E, or vitamin C or a trial of gabapentin or quinine. Vitamin E and quinine can reduce the incidence of muscle cramps.[53,54] Quinine is associated with temporary sight and hearing disturbances, thrombocytopenia, or gastrointestinal distress. Quinine is FDA-approved for malaria only and the FDA has warned against the off-label use of quinine for muscle cramps.[55]

In a small prospective study of patients receiving HD with at least six episodes of intradialytic muscle cramps in the 30 days prior to enrollment, patients received either placebo or gabapentin 300 mg three times a week administered 5 minutes prior to HD. After 1 month, patients experienced less episodes of muscle cramps in the treatment arm.[56] Both vitamin E (400 mg) and vitamin C (250 mg) reduced the frequency of cramps in patients receiving dialysis.[57] The combination of these two drugs had an additive effect. Although these data further strengthen the case for vitamin E and vitamin C, long-term therapy must be used with caution. Doses of vitamin E greater than 400 U/day have been reported to increase mortality and high doses of vitamin C increase the risk of oxalate accumulation and developing oxalosis. Pharmacologic interventions to diminish muscle cramps are limited and vitamin E has the strongest evidence-based efficacy and safety profile.

Vascular Access Thrombosis

Vascular access patency is key to maintaining effective dialytic therapy for patients receiving HD. Multiple pharmacologic agents have been studied including oral and intravenous anticoagulant and

TABLE 64-5 Management of Cramps

Acute treatment	Give 100-200 mL bolus of intravenous normal saline
	Give 10-20 mL of intravenous hypertonic saline (23.4%) over 3-5 minutes
	Give 50 mL of 50% intravenous glucose (nondiabetic patients)
Prevention	
Nonpharmacologic	Accurately set "dry weight"
	Keep dialysate sodium >serum sodium
	Stretching exercises, massage, flexing, or compression devices
Pharmacologic	Vitamin E 400 international units at bedtime
	Quinine sulfate 324 mg daily (second-line therapy)

antiplatelet agents and intravenous thrombolytic agents to assess their clinical value.

The efficacy of oral antiplatelet therapy for the prevention of vascular access thrombosis has not been well established. Studies in patient receiving HD have shown an increased risk of bleeding with minimal benefit in maintaining vascular access patency. Therapy with antiplatelet agents should be individualized based on the patient's risk factors and comorbidities.[30] A meta-analysis of randomized controlled trials for the prevention of vascular access failure identified nine trials assessing antiplatelet therapy and dialysis access patency in AV fistula ($n = 6$) and graft ($n = 3$).[58] This analysis found a lower rate of thrombosis or patency failure in patients with an AV fistula taking either aspirin, ticlopidine, or clopidogrel for up to 6 months (RR, 0.49; 95% CI, 0.30-0.81). In patients with an AV graft, there was no benefit with any of these antiplatelet therapies (RR, 0.94; 95% CI, 0.80-1.10). A post-hoc analysis identified that patients receiving aspirin prior to AV graft placement had improved graft patency but not graft survival.[59] An observational study in patients undergoing surgery for the creation of an HD-related vascular access examined primary patency at 12 months and compared antiplatelet therapy (aspirin or a platelet adenosine diphosphate receptor [$P2Y_{12}$] inhibitor) versus no antiplatelet therapy. There was no difference in primary patency between antiplatelet versus no antiplatelet therapy in patients receiving an AV fistula. There was a significant increase in primary patency in patients receiving an AV graft and antiplatelet therapy ($P = 0.04$). In hospital bleeding was assessed but long-term bleeding and bleeding risk were not reported and these results need to be interpreted with caution as previous studies have found an increased risk of bleeding with $P2Y_{12}$ inhibitors.[60] Overall, the studies have reported conflicting results, and patients with an AV graft taking antiplatelet therapy prior to a procedure may have some benefit but initiating aspirin post-surgery may increase the risk of thrombosis.

The use of anticoagulation to maintain vascular access patency remains controversial with some trials suggesting an increase in morbidity and mortality.[61,62] Patients receiving HD generally require a lower dose of anticoagulation and are at a much higher risk of a major hemorrhagic event.[61,62] An examination of patients receiving a new AV fistula or graft from 2011 to 2019 were identified in the Vascular Quality Initiative database. Patients received either no anticoagulation or anticoagulation (warfarin, dabigatran, or rivaroxaban) post-procedure. At 6 months post procedure patients who received anticoagulation had a higher rate of wound infections (3.8% vs 2.3%) and a lower rate of access patency (84.3% vs 85.7%) compared to patients receiving no anticoagulation.[63] The decision to initiate anticoagulation in patients receiving HD should be individualized for a patient's comorbid diseases and bleeding risk.

The effect of fish oil supplementation, a combination of eicosapentaenoic acid (EPA) 400 mg and docosahexaenoic acid (DHA) 200 mg, on AV graft patency for 12 months after graft placement revealed that the loss of patency was lower in the fish oil (48%) than the placebo (62%). Fish oil thus may benefit some patients with an AV graft since time to thrombus was longer and thrombus rates were about half that of placebo.[64] Based on this evidence, the KDOQI guidelines are suggesting the use of fish oil supplements in patients with a newly created AV graft to reduce morbidity and the frequency of thrombosis. The guidelines state there is inadequate evidence to recommend fish oil supplementation in patients with an AV graft to prolong graft patency.

Fish oil supplements were also studied in patients scheduled to receive surgery for an AV fistula. Patients were randomized to receive either placebo (olive oil) or fish oil 4 g/day (EPA 46% and DHA 38%) starting the day prior to surgery for 12 weeks. The patients receiving aspirin 100 mg/day were similar in each study arm. The AV fistula failure rate during the first 12 months post-surgery was 47% in both groups with similar rates of thrombus formation in patients receiving fish oil versus placebo (22% vs 23%) including those receiving aspirin or placebo (20% vs 18%).[65] The KDOQI guidelines do not recommend the use of fish oil supplementation to prevent flow dysfunction in an AV fistula.[30]

Catheter-locking solutions have been associated with a reduction in catheter thrombosis. The instillation of unfractionated heparin (UFH), recombinant tissue plasminogen activator (rt-PA), or sodium citrate in each HD catheter lumen between HD sessions have demonstrated efficacy in reducing catheter thrombosis. Sodium citrate 4% is as effective as UFH but may offer a better safety profile at a reduced cost.[66] A systematic review and meta-analysis of randomized controlled trials of HD locking solutions containing UFH and citrate found significantly fewer bleeding episodes in the patients receiving citrate. The analysis found no difference between citrate and UFH for catheter patency.[67] Unfractionated heparin 5,000 units/mL twice weekly and recombinant tissue plasminogen activator (rt-PA) 1 mg/catheter lumen once weekly were instilled in patients receiving HD with a CVC. Alternating the catheter-locking solution regimen with rt-PA significantly decreased catheter malfunction compared to the patients receiving UFH only for catheter patency. The cost of catheter replacement and hospitalization may offset the cost of once weekly administration of rt-PA.

Based on their medical history, patients at high risk for catheter malfunction or bacteremia ($n = 373$) received post-HD catheter-locking solutions of rt-PA (1 mg/lumen) once weekly plus routine care with either sodium citrate 4% or UFH on the remaining post-HD sessions. Catheter malfunction significantly declined with weekly rt-PA treatment from 18.4 to 10.1 days/1,000 catheter days and the episodes of bacteremia declined from 0.28 to 0.25/1,000 catheter days. Most patients (96%) received routine care with sodium citrate 4%, which may account for the small decline in bacteremia episodes. Overall, the increased cost of weekly rt-PA was not offset by the decline in catheter malfunction or bacteremia.[68] Taurolidine-based catheter solutions were examined in patients with a tunneled catheter ($n = 177$). Patients were randomized to receive either taurolidine citrate with urokinase (Tauro/U) once weekly plus taurolidine citrate with heparin (Tauro/Hep) twice a week ($n = 84$) or Tauro/Hep ($n = 93$) three times a week. During the 6-month study, no patients in the Tauro/U group required catheter replacement compared with three patients in the Tauro/Hep group. The use of rt-PA to restore catheter patency occurred at a lower rate with Tauro/U ($n = 5$) compared to Taurolock/Hep ($n = 12$). This was a short-term study; therefore, it is difficult to extrapolate long-term benefits until further studies are completed.[69] A catheter locking solution of taurolidine (1.35%), citrate (3.5%), and heparin (1,000 units) is seeking FDA approval for the prevention of CRBSI in patients receiving HD.

A prospective cohort study in patients ($n = 451$) receiving HD with a tunneled or non-tunneled catheter and either sodium bicarbonate 7.5% or 8.4%, or 0.9% normal saline as a catheter locking solution. Patients receiving the sodium bicarbonate locking solution had a significantly lower rate of thrombosis and blood stream infections compared the 0.9% NaCl group ($P < 0.0001$).[70] UFH and citrate (concentrations less than 5%) are listed by KDOQI as catheter locking solution options. The KDOQI guidelines consider citrate and UFH to have similar efficacy for survival and maintaining patency. Catheter locking solutions to prevent infections with taurolidine, tinzaparin, or gentamicin are not recommended by KDOQI based on the current evidence. In patients with an indwelling catheter at high risk for a catheter-related blood stream infection (CRBSI) defined as patients with multiple prior CRBSIs and/or an *S. aureus* nasal carriers may benefit from prophylactic instillation of rt-PA once weekly.[30]

The therapeutic alternatives for the management of venous catheter thrombosis are listed in Table 64-6. If a catheter-related thrombus is suspected, a forced saline flush should be used to clear the catheter, followed by installation of a thrombolytic. A number of studies have been published using alteplase and reteplase and initial

TABLE 64-6 Management of Hemodialysis Catheter Thrombosis

Nonpharmacologic therapy
Forced saline flush
Referral to vascular surgeon
Pharmacologic therapy
Alteplase: instill 2 mg/2 mL/catheter lumen port; attempt to aspirate after 30 minutes; may repeat dose if catheter function is not restored in 120 minutes; longer durations of instillation have been used.
Reteplase: instill 0.4 U/0.4 mL in each lumen, attempt to aspirate after 20-30 minutes, may repeat if necessary.

reperfusion rates for both were approximately 90%, respectively.[71] The efficacy, safety, and cost of alteplase, reteplase, and tenecteplase were compared, and venous catheter clearance rates were similar with reteplase (88% ± 4%) and alteplase (81% ± 37%), but markedly lower with tenecteplase (41% ± 5%).[71] The cost analysis favored the use of reteplase, however, to attain these savings, reteplase must be batch-prepared. Reteplase is not FDA-approved for this indication which may limit it use.[71] The instillation of a tissue plasminogen activator once weekly in a catheter may reduce catheter dysfunction and could be considered in select patients at a high risk of thrombosis.[30]

Alteplase is available commercially and is the only agent that is FDA-approved, for venous catheter clearance, and is administered as a short dwell for 30 to 60 minutes, as a long dwell, or left in the catheter between treatments. No difference in patency rates between the short or long dwells has been demonstrated. Alteplase has also been given as a short infusion of 2 mg/h over 4 hours for a blocked catheter and 1 mg/h over 4 hours for sluggish blood flow. Infusions may theoretically be more efficacious than the dwell technique because the thrombus is only exposed to the thrombolytic at the tip of the catheter. Another consideration is dwell versus push techniques for thrombolytic therapy, with recent data indicating that a push protocol with alteplase is as effective and safe for managing HD catheter dysfunction and might be more practical than a dwell technique.[72]

A retrospective single-center study evaluated the dose of alteplase in patients receiving HD with a catheter requiring a thrombolytic for catheter dysfunction. Patients during the first 3 years of the study received alteplase 2 mg/lumen and during the last 3 years received alteplase 1 mg/lumen. Dwell time was 30 minutes and independent of dose. Patients receiving alteplase 2 mg dose had a lower rate of catheter removal due to dysfunction (10.2% vs 19.4%). Overall, the instillation of alteplase 2 mg compared to 1 mg resulted in a 89.2% success rate at resolving catheter occlusions versus 80.6% ($P = 0.036$).[73]

Infection

Patients who develop a fever during dialysis should immediately be evaluated for infection; blood cultures should be collected prior to the administration of any antibiotics. When an AV fistula infection is suspected, empiric broad-spectrum antimicrobial therapy must be initiated usually with vancomycin plus an aminoglycoside or extended spectrum beta-lactamase inhibitor. Antimicrobial therapy, if the infection is confirmed, should continue for a total of 6 weeks and should be tailored to culture sensitivities. Unfortunately, a suspected infection in an AV graft may require a surgical procedure to remove the infected graft material in addition to antimicrobial therapy. A suspected infection in a temporary catheter may warrant catheter removal and a culture of the catheter tip should be obtained.[31,74] Catheter-related infections are more common than infections of an AV fistula or graft; therefore, preventative care approaches are paramount. Preventative care includes minimizing the use and duration of catheters, proper disinfection and sterile technique, and the use of an antimicrobial ointment at the exit site (mupirocin 2%, povidone-iodine).[75] Dialysis unit protocols that employ universal precautions, limit the manipulation of the catheter, and utilize an antiseptic wash (tincture of iodine, chlorhexidine, etc.) for skin preparation, and the use of facemasks by the patient and caregiver can significantly reduce the incidence of catheter-related bacteremia.[31,74,76] Topical application of 2% mupirocin ointment to a tunneled HD catheter exit site after each HD session can increase infection-free days. Current recommendations are to apply either povidone-iodine antiseptic ointment or polysporin triple ointment (bacitracin/gramicidin/polymyxin B) to the exit site after each HD session. Long-term monitoring of infection rates of patients receiving HD with a catheter did not reveal an increase in antibiotic resistance with a once-a-week application of a topical polysporin triple ointment to catheter exit sites.[77]

The Infectious Disease Society of America (IDSA) and KDOQI guidelines address catheter care and the diagnosis and management of catheter-related infections.[30,76] Peripheral blood draws, although recommended by IDSA, are often avoided in patients receiving HD to protect potential or future HD vascular access sites. Blood cultures are generally obtained from the blood tubing connecting the catheter to the HD machine. A prospective study examined blood cultures (n = 178) obtained from patients receiving HD suspected of a CRBSI. The blood cultures obtained from the HD circuit and venous catheter hub were the most sensitive, specific, and accurate for diagnosing CRBSI compared to blood cultures taken from a peripheral vein and either catheter hub or HD circuit.[78] A full-course of antimicrobial treatment is warranted if blood cultures are positive.[31,76] Empiric therapy with coverage for both gram-positive and gram-negative bacteria should be initiated after the blood cultures are obtained. The incidence of MRSA bacteremia warrants initial treatment for gram-positive coverage with vancomycin or daptomycin. If gram-negative antimicrobial coverage is warranted, an aminoglycoside or third-generation cephalosporin should be initiated depending on a center's protocols and antimicrobial susceptibilities.[31,76] Antimicrobial therapy de-escalation should occur once blood cultures identify an organism and antimicrobial susceptibility. For example, if the isolated organism is methicillin-sensitive *S. aureus*, administer IV cefazolin (20 mg/kg, rounded to the nearest 500 mg) after each dialysis session. Antibiotic selection should be based on bacterial coverage and the ability to optimize pharmacokinetics by administering a dose either during the last 30 to 60 minutes of HD treatment or during the rinse bath. This method minimizes additional dosages between HD sessions. Examples of antimicrobial agents that meet these objectives are vancomycin, cefazolin, ceftazidime, daptomycin, and aminoglycosides.[76,79]

The IDSA guidelines recommend removal of an infected catheter if *S. aureus*, *Pseudomonas* species, or *Candida* species are the infectious cause. Although removal of the catheter is warranted, this is not always possible in patients receiving HD because of limited vascular access options. Retaining an infected catheter significantly increases a patient's risk of bacteremia recurrence after completing a course of antibiotics; therefore, other options need to be considered. Options such as replacing the catheter over a guidewire or using a catheter-lock solution in conjunction with IV antibiotics are alternatives.[31,76]

The catheter salvage success rate when a catheter-lock solution is used in addition to systemic antibiotics is highly variable and pathogen dependent.[31,76] The IDSA guidelines recommend the use of catheter-lock solutions as adjunctive therapy after each dialysis session for 10 to 14 days in a patient whose catheter was not removed and bacteremia symptoms resolved in 2 to 3 days. The IDSA recommendations for antibiotic therapy are listed in Table 64-7.[76]

Microbial colonization of a catheter could affect patency and a patient's access to dialytic treatment. An examination of the

TABLE 64-7 Management of Hemodialysis Access Infection

1. Primary arteriovenous fistula
   Treat as subacute bacterial endocarditis for 6 weeks.
   Initial antibiotic choice should always cover gram-positive organisms (eg, vancomycin 20 mg/kg IV with serum concentration monitoring or cefazolin 20 mg/kg IV three times/week or after each dialysis session).
   Gram-negative coverage is indicated for patients with diabetes, human immunodeficiency virus infection, prosthetic valves, or those receiving immunosuppressive agents, gentamicin 2 mg/kg IV with serum concentration monitoring.
2. Synthetic arteriovenous grafts
   Local infection—empiric antibiotic coverage for gram-positive, gram-negative, and Enterococcus (eg, gentamicin plus vancomycin then individualized after culture results available). Continue for 2-4 weeks.
   Extensive infection—antibiotics as above plus total resection.
   If access is less than 1-month-old, antibiotics as above plus remove the graft.
3. Tunneled cuffed catheters (internal jugular, subclavian)
   Infection localized to catheter exit site.
   - No drainage—topical antibiotics (eg, mupirocin ointment).
   - Drainage present—gram-positive antibiotic coverage, vancomycin 20 mg/kg IV with serum concentration monitoring or cefazolin 20 mg/kg IV three times/week.

   Bacteremia with or without systemic signs or symptoms.
   - Gram-positive antibiotic coverage as above.
   - If symptomatic at 36 hours, remove the catheter.
   - If stable and asymptomatic, change catheter and provide culture-specific antibiotic coverage for a minimum of 3 weeks.

Data from References 76 and 80.

catheter-lock solutions, UFH 5,000 U/mL and tetra-sodium EDTA, found an increased rate of microbial colonization with UFH but the tetra-sodium EDTA solution had an increased rate of thrombosis.[81] Alternative solutions to UFH and tetra-sodium EDTA including catheter-lock solutions containing ethanol 30% combined with sodium citrate 4% or ethanol 70% with UFH 2,000 U/mL have been effective at decreasing CRBSI and improving catheter survival.[82]

Catheter-locking solutions have been utilized to prevent infection and thrombosis in HD catheters. A meta-analysis of randomized control trials of catheter-related bacteremia and antimicrobial lock solutions identified eight studies with 829 patients and more than 90,100 catheter days. Overall analysis found that the use of an antimicrobial locking solution significantly reduced the risk of a catheter-related infection (relative risk [RR] 0.32; 95% confidence interval [CI] 0.10-0.42).[83] A comparison of UFH 1,000 U/mL to the combination solution of 4% sodium citrate with gentamicin 320 μg/mL as a catheter-lock solution significantly reduced the incidence of catheter-related bloodstream infections.[84] The value of catheter-locking solutions for treatment and prevention of catheter-related infections is increasingly becoming evident, but the possibility of antibiotic resistance with the wide use of antibiotics in catheter locks remains a concern. Gentamicin resistance to coagulase-negative *Staphylococcus* was reported in a retrospective study using routine post-HD administration of gentamicin (4 mg/mL) combined with UFH (5,000 U/mL) as a catheter-lock solution. Over the 4-year study, there were 80 CRBSIs with 21 episodes (26%) of gentamicin resistance identified. The increase in gentamicin resistance led to a discontinuation of the gentamicin-heparin catheter-lock solutions.[85]

PERITONEAL DIALYSIS

Although the concept of peritoneal lavage has been described as far back as the 1700s, it wasn't until the 1920s that PD was first employed as an acute treatment for uremia. It was used infrequently during subsequent years until the concept of PD as a chronic therapy for ESRD was proposed in the 1960s. Over the ensuing years, the number of patients receiving PD increased slowly until the early 1980s. At that time, several innovations in PD delivery systems were introduced, such as improved catheters and dialysate bags. These innovations led to improved outcomes, decreased morbidity, mortality, and a corresponding increase in the use of PD as a viable alternative to HD for the treatment of ESRD. However, the worldwide use of PD has declined over the past decade. Some patients, such as those with more hemodynamic instability (eg, hypotension) or significant residual renal function (RRF), and perhaps patients who desire to maintain a significant degree of self-care may be better suited to PD than to HD. Table 64-2 shows the advantages and disadvantages of PD.

Principles of Peritoneal Dialysis

5 The three basic components of HD—namely, a blood-filled compartment separated from a dialysate-filled compartment by a semipermeable membrane—are also present in PD.[4] In PD, the dialysate-filled compartment is the peritoneal cavity, into which dialysate is instilled via a peritoneal catheter that traverses the abdominal wall. The contiguous peritoneal membrane surrounds the peritoneal cavity. The cavity, which normally contains about 100 mL of lipid-rich lubricating fluid, can expand to a capacity of several liters. The peritoneal membrane that lines the cavity functions as the semipermeable membrane, across which diffusion and ultrafiltration occur. The peritoneal dialyzing membrane is comprised of a monocellular layer of peritoneal mesothelial cells, the basement membrane, and underlying connective and interstitial tissue. The peritoneal membrane has a total area that approximates body surface area (approximately 1-2 m^2). Blood vessels supplying and draining the abdominal viscera, musculature, and mesentery constitute the blood-filled compartment.

Unlike HD, the crucial components of PD cannot be manipulated to maximize solute and fluid removal. Because the blood is not in intimate contact with the dialysis membrane as it is in HD, metabolic waste products must travel a considerable distance to the dialysate-filled compartment. In addition, unlike HD, there is no easy method to regulate blood flow to the surface of the peritoneal membrane, nor is there a countercurrent flow of blood and dialysate to increase diffusion and ultrafiltration via changes in hydrostatic pressure. Similarly, there is no easy means available to manipulate the peritoneal membrane. Thus, to enhance PD clearance involve alterations in dialysate volume, dwell time, and the number of exchanges per day. For these reasons, PD is a less efficient process per unit time compared with HD, and must, therefore, be a virtually continuous procedure to achieve acceptable goals for clearance of metabolic waste products.

Peritoneal Dialysis Access

Access to the peritoneal cavity is via the placement of an indwelling catheter. Many types are available, and Fig. 64-3 shows an example.[4] Most catheters are manufactured from silicone rubber, which is soft, flexible, and biocompatible. A typical adult catheter is 40 to 45 cm long, 20 to 22 cm of which is inside the peritoneal cavity. Placement of the catheter is such that the distal end lies low in a pelvic gutter. The center section of the catheter has one or two cuffs made of a porous material that is tunneled inside the anterior abdominal wall so that the cuffs provide mechanical support and stability to the catheter, serve as a mechanical barrier to skin organisms, and prevent their migration along the catheter into the peritoneal cavity. The cuffs are placed at different sites surrounding the abdominal rectus muscle. The remainder of the central section of the catheter is tunneled subcutaneously before exiting the abdominal surface, usually a few centimeters below and to one side of the umbilicus.

The placement of the catheter exit site is one of the factors related to the development or prevention of exit-site infections and peritonitis. The external section of most peritoneal catheters ends

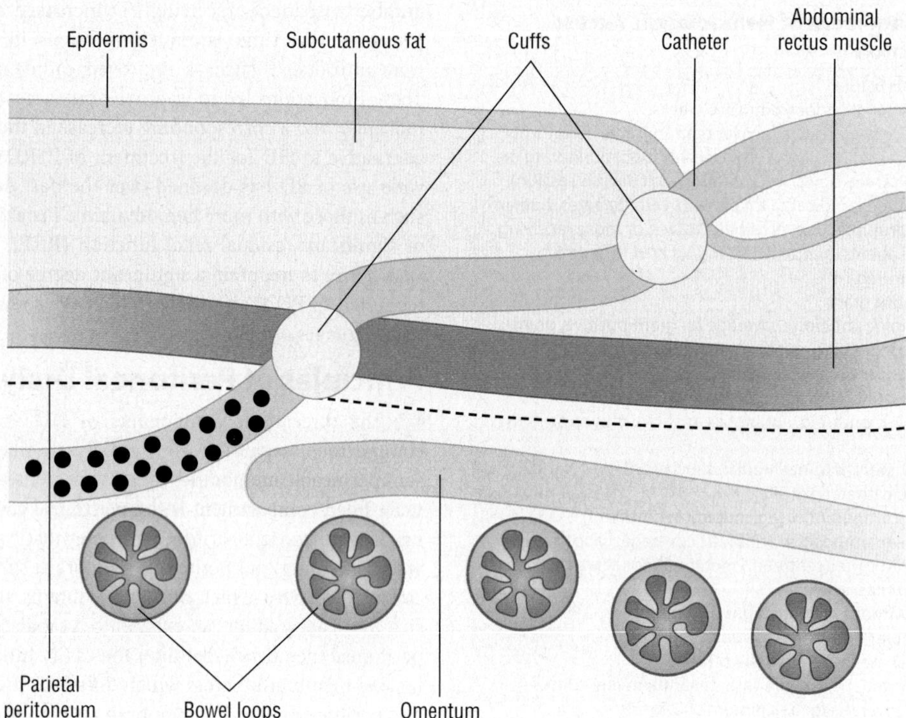

FIGURE 64-3 Diagram of the peritoneal dialysis catheter placement through the abdominal wall into the peritoneal cavity. *(Reprinted, with permission, from Sherman R, Daugirdas J, Ing T. Complications during hemodialysis. In: Daugirdas J, Blake P, Ing T, eds. Handbook of Dialysis. 5th ed. Philadelphia: Wolters Kluwer; 2014.)*

with a Luer-Lok connector, which can be connected to a variety of administration sets. These catheters can be used immediately, if necessary, provided small initial volumes are instilled; however, a maturation period of 2 to 6 weeks is preferred.

Peritoneal Dialysis Procedures

6 Several variants of PD are clinically utilized in the United States. All variants of PD require the placement of a dialysis solution to dwell in the peritoneal cavity for some period, removing the spent dialysate, and then repeating the process. PD prescriptions can be delivered as continuous or intermittent and use manual or automated exchanges. Continuous PD involves intraperitoneal dialysate 24 hours/day, 7 days/week. A continuous ambulatory PD procedure uses manual exchanges, versus a continuous cycling PD procedure uses a cycler to perform the exchanges. Whereas an intermittent procedure involves the use of cycler to deliver PD for a portion of the day.[4] The prescribed dose of PD may be altered by changing the number of exchanges per day, by altering the volume of each exchange, or by altering the strength of dextrose or other osmotic agent in the dialysate for some or all exchanges. Increasing any one of these variables increases the effective osmotic gradient across the peritoneum, leading to increased ultrafiltration and diffusion (solute removal). If the dwell time is extended, equilibrium may be reached, after which time there will be no further water or solute removal. In fact, after a critical period, reverse water movement may occur.[4] In a basic CAPD system, the patient or caregiver is manually responsible for performing the prescribed number of dialysate exchanges. The patient is connected to a bag of prewarmed peritoneal dialysate via the PD catheter, by a length of tubing called a transfer set. The most common transfer set used is the Y transfer set which consists of a Y-shaped piece of tubing that is attached at its stem to the patient's catheter, leaving the remaining two limbs of the Y attached to dialysate bags, one filled with fresh dialysate and the other empty. The spent dialysate from the previous dwell is drained into the empty bag, and the peritoneum is subsequently refilled from the bag containing fresh dialysate. The Y set is then disconnected and the bag containing the spent fluid and the empty bag that had contained fresh dialysate are detached and discarded. Typically, a patient instills 2 to 3 L of dialysate three times during the day with each exchange lasting 4 to 6 hours, and then a single dialysate exchange overnight lasting 8 to 12 hours. At the end of the prescribed dwell period, a new Y set is attached and the process is repeated. The process of outflow, aseptic manipulation of the administration set and catheter, and inflow requires a total time of approximately 30 minutes.

As described earlier, CAPD involves performing the dialysate exchanges manually, whereas automated systems collectively termed automated peritoneal dialysis (APD) performs the exchanges with a cycler. APD systems are designed for patients who are unable or unwilling to perform the necessary aseptic manipulations and for those who require more dialysis. The device is set up in the evening, and the patient attaches the peritoneal catheter to it at bedtime. The machine performs several short-dwell exchanges (usually 1-2 hours) during the night. This permits a long cycle-free daytime dwell of up to 12 to 14 hours. Typical APD regimens involve total 24-hour exchanges of approximately 12 L, which include one or more daytime instillations and dwell periods.[86] This type of regimen is referred to as APD with a "wet" day. The APD variant, nightly intermittent PD, has a similar theme, except that the peritoneal cavity tends to be dialysate-free during the day. This type of regimen is frequently referred to as APD with a "dry" day. A number of variants exist and depend largely on equipment availability, patient and prescriber preference, and whether the patient retains any RRF, which influences the quantity of dialysis prescribed.

The APD systems include continuous cycling PD (CCPD), tidal PD, and nocturnal intermittent PD. The prototypic form of APD is usually a hybrid between CAPD and continuous cycling PD, in which some of the daily exchanges (usually the overnight exchanges) are completed using an automated device. Other advances in PD procedures involve using continuous flow PD. This technique maintains a fixed intraperitoneal volume and rapid, continuous movement of dialysate into and out of the peritoneal cavity. To accomplish this, two PD catheters (an inlet and outlet catheter) and a means of generating a large volume of sterile dialysate are required. Dialysate is generated via conventional HD equipment or sorbent technology. In continuous flow PD, clearance of small solutes is three to eight times greater than with APD and approximates daily HD. Potential applications of continuous flow PD include daily home dialysis, treatment of acute kidney injury in the intensive care unit, and ultrafiltration of ascites.

Peritoneal Dialysis Solutions

All forms of PD use dialysate solutions, which are commercially available in volumes of 1 to 3 L in flexible polyvinyl chloride plastic bags. The most commonly used solutions that are commercially available contain an osmotic agent, electrolytes, and buffer. The solutions contain electrolytes, such as sodium (132-134 mEq/L [mmol/L]), chloride (96 mEq/L [mmol/L]), calcium (2.5-3.5 mEq/L [1.25-1.75 mmol/L]), and magnesium (0.5 mEq/L [0.25 mmol/L]). These solutions may contain dextrose (1.5%, 2.5%, 3.86%, or 4.25%) or icodextrin (a glucose polymer) at a concentration of 7.5%. The dextrose solutions are hyperosmolar (osmolarity range, 345-484 mOsm/L) and induce ultrafiltration (removal of free water) by crystalline osmosis. Dextrose is not the ideal osmotic agent for peritoneal dialysate because these solutions are not biocompatible with peritoneal mesothelial cells or with peritoneal leukocytes. The cytotoxic effects on these cells are mediated by the osmolar load and the low pH of the solutions, as well as the presence of glucose degradation products formed during heat sterilization of these products. Icodextrin PD solution contains icodextrin, a starch-derived glucose polymer. It has an osmolality of 282 to 286 mOsm/kg (mmol/kg), which is isoosmolar with serum. Icodextrin produces prolonged ultrafiltration by a mechanism resembling colloid osmosis resulting in ultrafiltration volumes similar to those with 4.25% dextrose. Icodextrin may have fewer of the metabolic effects associated with dextrose, such as hyperglycemia and weight gain. It is indicated for use during the long (8-16 hours) dwell of a single daily exchange in CAPD and APD patients. Lower glucose degradation product dialysate solutions are also available with similar solute concentrations, but with pH of 7.3.[4] These newer, biocompatible dialysate solutions are described as less harmful to the peritoneal membrane and preserve RRF to a greater extent than the available standard solutions.[4] Preservation of RRF in PD and HD patients is important as it decreases mortality and increases the time to the first episode of peritonitis. However, the putative benefits of the biocompatible dialysate solutions have not been completely borne out: their use has not consistently slowed the rate of decline in glomerular filtration rate as compared to standard solutions, although the incidence of peritonitis has been lower. Finally, the solutions contain buffers, lactate (0-40 mmol/L), and/or bicarbonate (0-34 mmol/L).

Adequacy of Peritoneal Dialysis

The most recent International Society of Peritoneal Dialysis practice guidelines argue that the assessment and prescription of PD should be a shared decision-making process between the patient and the care giving team. Ideally assessments should focus on (1) patient reported outcome measures (well-being, quality of life, symptomatology, etc.), (2) fluid status, (3) nutrition status, and (4) toxin removal (ie, solute clearance determination).[87] As in HD, toxin removal can be quantified by the clearance of urea, by calculating *Kt/V*. The calculations determine a daily *Kt/V*, which is then converted into a weekly value that is relevant to PD patients.

PD adequacy is a major issue that has received considerable attention. The most recent KDOQI guidelines recommend that patients on PD have a total *Kt/V* of at least 1.7/week, including both PD *Kt/V* and residual kidney *Kt/V*.[86] It is important to note that RRF may provide a significant component of the total *Kt/V*. Patients may commence PD with a residual CLcr of approximately 9 to 12 mL/min (0.15-0.20 mL/s), which contributes a renal *Kt/V* of 0.2 to 0.4. Over a period of 1 to 2 years, if RRF progressively deteriorates, the total *Kt/V* will progressively diminish unless PD *Kt/V* is increased (by increasing the prescribed dose of PD) to compensate for the reduced renal *Kt/V*.

For patients producing less than 100 mL urine/day, the weekly *Kt/V* dose of 1.7 must be provided entirely by peritoneal clearance. For patients producing greater than 100 mL urine/day, combined renal and peritoneal urea clearances must exceed the weekly *Kt/V* dose of 1.7.[86] The weekly *Kt/V* dose should be measured within the first month of PD initiation and at least once every 4 months thereafter. It is imperative to detect subtle decreases in RRF along with poor adherence to make necessary alterations to the prescribed PD dose to attain adequate clearance of waste products.

The KDOQI guidelines also stress the importance of preserving RRF in PD patients because it is associated with decreased mortality. Typical measures to preserve RRF include preferential use of ACE-Is or ARBs, regardless of blood pressure, and avoidance of medications or procedures that are associated with insults to the kidney (eg, nonsteroidal anti-inflammatory drugs, cyclooxygenase-2 inhibitors, aminoglycosides, intravenous iodinated radiocontrast dyes, withdrawal of immunosuppressant therapies from a transplanted kidney, hypovolemia, urinary tract obstruction, and hypercalcemia).[86]

Complications of Peritoneal Dialysis

Mechanical, medical, and infectious problems complicate PD therapy. Mechanical complications include kinking of the catheter and inflow and outflow obstruction; excessive catheter motion at the exit site, leading to induration and possible infection and aggravation of tissues; pain from impingement of the catheter tip on the viscera; or inflow pain resulting from a jet effect of too rapid dialysate inflow.

Table 64-8 lists the numerous medical complications of PD. An average PD patient absorbs up to 60% of the dextrose in each exchange. This continuous supply of calories leads to increased adipose tissue deposition, decreased appetite, malnutrition, and altered requirements for insulin in diabetic patients. Fibrin formation in dialysate is common and can lead to obstruction of catheter outflow.

TABLE 64-8 Medical Complications of Peritoneal Dialysis

Cause	Complication	Treatment
Glucose load	Exacerbation of diabetes mellitus	IP insulin
Fluid overload	Exacerbation of heart failure Edema Pulmonary congestion	Increase ultrafiltration Diuretics, if the patient has residual renal function
Electrolyte abnormalities	Hypercalcemia/Hypocalcemia	Alter dialysate calcium content
PD additives	Chemical peritonitis	Discontinue PD additives
Malnutrition	Albumin loss Loss of amino acids Muscle wasting Increased adipose tissue	Dietary changes Parenteral nutrition Discontinue PD
Unknown	Fibrin formation in dialysate	IP heparin

IP, intraperitoneal; PD, peritoneal dialysis.

Infectious complications of PD are a major cause of morbidity and mortality and the transfer of patients from PD to HD therapies. A leading cause of infections is related to technique failure during PD exchanges. The two predominant infectious complications are peritonitis and catheter-related infections, which include both exit-site and tunnel infections.

Peritonitis

7 The incidence of peritonitis is influenced by connector technology, by the composition of patient populations, and by the use of APD versus CAPD. The Peritoneal Dialysis Outcomes and Practice Patterns Study (PDOPPS) is an international cohort study reporting on PD-related peritonitis and potential contributing factors such as exit-site prophylaxis. The rate of peritonitis was 0.26 (95% CI, 0.24-0.27) per patient-year in the United States with the causative organisms as gram-positive (37%), gram-negative (13%), culture-negative (16%), polymicrobial (5%), and yeast (1%). The most common exit-site prophylaxis was topical aminoglycoside (72%) and topical mupirocin (13%).[88]

Peritonitis is a major cause of catheter loss in PD patients. The clinical presentation and diagnosis are listed in Table 64-9. A retrospective cohort study found a mortality rate of 0.07 per patient-year (95% CI, 0.06-0.08). The cause of mortality was identified as cardiovascular (56.3%) and infectious disease (17.6%). Patients who died from an infectious cause, 41.3% were related to peritonitis.[89] A statistically significant correlation between infectious complications and death rates has been reported: patients who had more than 1 peritonitis episode/year, 0.5 to 1 episode/year, or less than 0.5 episode/year, 50% died after 3, 4, and 5 years of therapy, respectively. It is important to note that these relationships are not necessarily cause and effect, as many of these patients succumb to cardiovascular events.[90]

Peritonitis has several imprecise definitions, but guidelines suggest that an elevated dialysate white blood cell count of greater than 100/μL (0.1×10^9/L) with at least 50% polymorphonuclear neutrophils indicates the presence of inflammation, of which peritonitis is the most likely cause.[91] A patient who presents with abdominal pain and a cloudy effluent is usually given a provisional diagnosis of peritonitis. Inherent in this definition is a number of false-positive and false-negative diagnoses, because a small percentage of patients with culture-proven peritonitis will have clear dialysate, and some patients, such as menstruating females, may have cloudy PD effluent without clinical infection. Sterile culture peritonitis remains problematic; it is defined as an episode in which there is clinical suspicion of peritonitis, but for which the culture of the dialysate reveals no organism. There are several postulates for the high incidence (up to 20% of episodes) of culture-negative peritonitis. Many peritonitis-producing organisms are slime producers and may adhere to the peritoneal membrane or to the catheter surface and may be protected from exogenous antibiotics. Sufficient numbers of these bacteria may proliferate to cause peritoneal membrane inflammation and clinical peritonitis, but an inadequate number may seed into the peritoneal cavity to be recovered by conventional microbiologic techniques. In addition, free-floating planktonic bacteria may be rapidly phagocytosed by peritoneal white blood cells, thereby rendering them unavailable for culture.[92]

TABLE 64-9 Clinical Presentation and Diagnosis of Peritoneal Dialysis-Related Peritonitis

General

- Patients generally present with abdominal pain and cloudy effluent

Symptoms

- The patient may complain of abdominal tenderness, abdominal pain, fever, nausea and vomiting, and chills

Signs

- Cloudy dialysate effluent may be observed
- Temperature may or may not be elevated

Laboratory Tests

- Dialysate white blood cell count >100/mm^3 (0.1×10^9/L), of which at least 50% are polymorphonuclear neutrophils
- Gram stain of a centrifuged dialysate specimen

Other Diagnostic Tests

- Culture and sensitivity of dialysate should be obtained

Contemporary methods have increased the recovery rate of organisms and decreased the culture-negative rate. Centrifugation is recommended as the optimum culture method. Centrifugation of a large volume of dialysate (50 mL), resuspension of the sediment in 3 to 5 mL of sterile saline, and subsequent inoculation in culture media produce a culture-negative rate less than 5%. If centrifuge equipment is not available, blood culture bottles can be directly injected with 5 to 10 mL of dialysate effluent. However, this method results in a culture-negative rate of up to 20%.[91]

The majority of infections are caused by gram-positive bacteria, of which *Staphylococcus epidermidis* is the predominant organism. There is no single predominant gram-negative organism. Together, gram-positive and gram-negative organisms account for 80% to 90% of all episodes of peritonitis and constitute the spectrum against which initial empiric therapy is directed.[93]

Catheter-Related Infections

A catheter-related infection in patients receiving PD includes both exit-site infection (ESI) and tunneled infection. Patients with previous infections tend to have a higher subsequent incidence. A case-controlled study found that 69.8% of patients receiving PD had at least one ESI over a 3-year period and are more likely to develop peritonitis (64%) compared to patients without an ESI.[94] The majority of ESIs are caused by *S. aureus*. In contrast to peritonitis, *S. epidermidis* accounts for less than 20% of ESIs. Although gram-negative organisms, such as *Pseudomonas*, are less common, they can result in significant morbidity. The diagnostic characteristics of these infections are somewhat vague but generally include the presence of purulent drainage, with or without erythema at the catheter exit-site. The risk of ESIs is increased several-fold in patients who are nasal carriers of *S. aureus*.[94]

Management

Peritonitis

The International Society of Peritoneal Dialysis (ISPD) updated the Peritoneal Dialysis-Related Infections recommendations in 2016, which provide guidelines for treatments for peritonitis and tunneled and exit-site infections.[91] These PD-related infections are associated with dialysis modality treatment failures and substantial morbidity and mortality; therefore, appropriate pharmacotherapy treatment is essential. The ISPD guidelines specifically address the importance of peritonitis prevention, dialysis center antibiotic selection, and intraperitoneal (IP) antibiotic dosing and treatment duration for peritonitis.[91] In 2017, ISPD published catheter-related infection recommendations to prevent ESIs and described routine catheter care for PD patients.[93] Both guidelines provide a summary of best practices based on available evidence or consensus in areas where evidence exists. Figure 64-4 shows the pharmacotherapy recommendations for the treatment of bacterial peritonitis.

The preferred delivery route for antibiotics is IP over IV therapy for the treatment of peritonitis. Antimicrobial dosing recommendations provided in the ISPD guidelines for CAPD dosing distinguish between intermittent (one exchange per day) and continuous therapy (all exchanges). The 2016 guidelines no longer provide APD IP drug dosing recommendations due to a "substantial knowledge gap" within this treatment area. The ISPD guidelines include oral and IV dosing recommendations that can be dosed either independent of or in conjunction with IP dosing.[91,93]

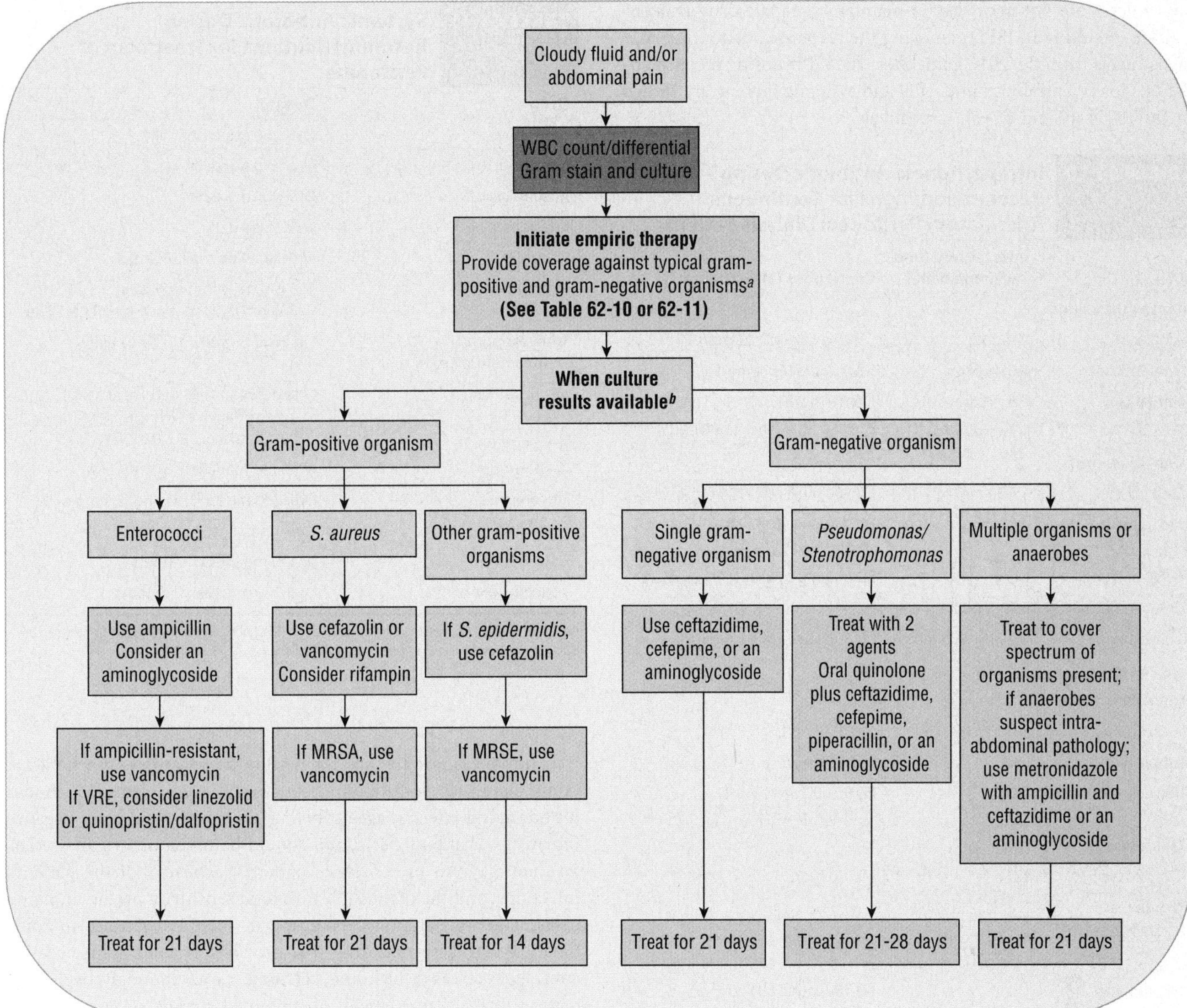

FIGURE 64-4 Pharmacotherapy recommendations for the treatment of bacterial peritonitis in peritoneal dialysis patients. [a]Choice of empiric treatment should be made based on the dialysis center's and the patient's history of infecting organisms and their sensitivities. [b]Final choice of therapy is guided by culture and sensitivity results. (MRSA, methicillin-resistant *Staphylococcus aureus;* MRSE, methicillin-resistant *Staphylococcus epidermidis; S. aureus, Staphylococcus aureus; S. epidermidis, Staphylococcus epidermidis;* VRE, vancomycin-resistant enterococci; WBC, white blood cell.)

Following a single IP antibiotic dose, the drug concentrations achieved in dialysate and serum differ between intermittent and continuous methods. Intermittent IP therapy necessitates that a sufficient amount of drug transfers from the peritoneal cavity to the systemic circulation, thus allowing drug to diffuse back into the peritoneum during drug-free dialysate dwell time(s). Therefore, once daily dosing requires drug(s) be added to the exchange with the longest dwell time (at least 6 hours) to ensure maximum systemic exposure.

Continuous dosing recommendations may require a loading dose with the first IP dose and a maintenance dose for each subsequent exchange. Vancomycin, aminoglycosides, and cephalosporins generally are administered by either dosing method. It is recommended that a continuous dosing method be used for penicillins and fluoroquinolones. No matter which CAPD drug dosing method is used, the goal is to deliver and maintain adequate peritoneum drug concentrations. Intermittent or continuous dosing is effective for CAPD patients but IP dosing for APD patients may require a different dosing schedule. The rapid overnight dialysate exchanges with APD will increase solute clearance over a short time period. This is particularly important for first-generation cephalosporin agents. The ISPD guidelines recommend continuous dosing of a first-generation cephalosporin because of concerns over inadequate IP drug concentration during the shorter APD dialysate dwells. To maintain adequate peritoneum drug concentrations, patients may be advised to temporarily switch to CAPD delivery or manually instill dialysate with an antimicrobial agent during the day or the longest dwell. If a patient is not a good candidate for CAPD, the cycler can be reset to provide a longer dwell period or slower exchange rate to allow for drug transfer during APD.[91] Intermittent dosing of first-generation cephalosporin for APD does not sustain adequate drug concentrations for most organisms; therefore, continuous dosing may be more effective in providing better drug coverage. Oral ciprofloxacin attains adequate IP drug concentrations in patients receiving APD and is a therapeutic option if the pathogen is susceptible. Regarding RRF, in patients with substantial residual renal function, previous ISPD guidelines recommended dose adjustments for antibiotics with renal elimination. Recent studies suggest these dosing adjustments are not necessary to maintain adequate drug concentrations, resulting in ISPD removing the recommendation for dose adjustments from the 2016 guidelines. The ISPD dosing recommendations for IP antibiotics in CAPD and systemic therapy are shown in Tables 64-10 and 64-11, respectively.[91]

TABLE 64-10 Intraperitoneal Antibiotic Dosing Recommendations for Continuous Ambulatory Peritoneal Dialysis Patients

Drug	Intermittent (one exchange daily)	Continuous (all exchanges)
Aminoglycosides		
Amikacin	2 mg/kg	LD 25 mg/L; MD 12 mg/L
Gentamicin	0.6 mg/kg	LD 8 mg/L; MD 4 mg/L
Netilmicin	0.6 mg/kg	MD 10 mg/L
Tobramycin	0.6 mg/kg	LD 3 mg/kg; MD 0.3 mg/kg
Cephalosporins		
Cefazolin	15-20 mg/kg	LD 500 mg/L; MD 125 mg/L
Cefepime	1,000 mg	LD 250-500 mg/L; MD 100-125 mg/L
Cefoperazone	ND	LD 500 mg/L; MD 62.5-125 mg/L
Cefotaxime	500–1,000 mg	ND
Ceftazidime	1,000–1,500 mg	LD 500 mg/L; MD 125 mg/L
Ceftriaxone	1,000 mg	ND
Penicillins		
Amoxicillin	ND	MD 150 mg/L
Ampicillin	ND	MD 125 mg/L
Penicillin G	ND	LD 50,000 units/L; MD 25,000 units/L
Quinolones		
Ciprofloxacin	ND	MD 50 mg/L
Others		
Vancomycin	15-30 mg/kg Q5-7d[a]	LD 30 mg/kg; MD 1.5 mg/kg/bag
Daptomycin	ND	LD 100 mg/L; MD 20 mg/L
Aztreonam	2 g	LD 1,000 mg/L; MD 250 mg/L
Teicoplanin	15 mg/kg q 5 days	LD 400 mg/bag; MD 20 mg/bag
Linezolid	ND	Oral 200-300 mg daily
Clindamycin	ND	600 mg/bag
Polymixin B	ND	MD 300,000 Unit (30 mg)/bag
Meropenem	1 g	ND
Antifungals		
Fluconazole	200 mg IP every 24-48 hours	ND
Voriconzaole	2.5 mg/kg IP	ND
Combinations		
Ampicillin/sulbactam	2 g/1 g q 12 h	LD 750 mg/L/100 mg/L; MD 100 mg/L
Pipercillin/tazobactam	ND	LD 4 g/0.5 g; MD 1 g/0.125 g
Imipenem/cilastatin	500 mg in alternate exchanges	LD 250 mg/L; MD 50 mg/L
Quinupristin/dalfopristin[b]	25 mg/L in alternate exchanges[a]	ND

[a]Supplemental doses may be required for APD patients.

[b]Given in conjunction with 500 mg intravenous twice daily.

LD, loading dose in milligram; MD, maintenance dose in milligram; NA, not applicable; ND, no data.

Adapted from Li PK, Szeto CC, Piraino B, et al. ISPD peritonitis recommendations: 2016 update on prevention and treatment. Perit Dial Int. 2016;36:481–508.

TABLE 64-11 Systemic Antibiotic Dosing Recommendations for Treatment of Peritonitis

Drug	Dosing
Ciprofloxacin	Oral 250 mg twice daily
Levofloxacin	Oral 250 mg daily
Moxifloxacin	Oral 400 mg daily
Ertapenem	IV 500 mg daily
Linezolid	IV or oral 600 mg twice daily
Rifampicin	450 mg daily for body weight ≤50 kg, 600 mg daily for body weight ≥50 kg
Trimethoprim/Sulfamethoxazole	Oral 160 mg/800 mg twice daily
Amphotericin	IV test dose 1 mg; starting dose 0.1 mg/kg/day over 6 hours increase to target dose 0.75-1.0 mg/kg/day
Caspofungin	IV 70 mg load, then 50 mg daily
Fluconazole	Oral 200 mg loading, then 50 mg daily
Flucytosine	Oral 1 g daily
Posaconazole	IV 400 mg every 12 hours
Voriconazole	Oral 200 mg every 12 hours

Adapted from Li PK, Szeto CC, Piraino B, et al. ISPD peritonitis recommendations: 2016 update on prevention and treatment. Perit Dial Int. 2016;36:481–508.

Initial empiric therapy for peritonitis, regardless of whether a Gram stain was performed, or organisms were identified, should include agents effective against both gram-positive and gram-negative organisms. Antibiotic selection should be based on a dialysis center's antibiogram or resistance patterns, a history of the patient's infections, and the organism's antibiotic sensitivity profile. In many cases, a first-generation cephalosporin such as cefazolin in combination with a second drug that provides broader gram-negative coverage, such as ceftazidime, cefepime, or an aminoglycoside, will prove suitable. Patients with documented allergy to cephalosporin antibiotics can be treated with vancomycin and an aminoglycoside. High rates of methicillin resistance have been reported by many dialysis centers, and vancomycin should be used as first-line therapy against gram-positive organisms for patients treated at these centers. Monotherapy with agents providing both gram-positive and gram-negative coverage is an alternative option. Both imipenem-cilastin and cefepime are effective in treating CAPD-related peritonitis.[95]

After culture and sensitivity results are obtained, antibiotic therapy should be adjusted appropriately (see Fig. 64-4). Tables 64-10 and 64-11 list doses for antibiotics. Treatment should be continued for 14 to 21 days. If the patient does not show signs of clinical improvement within 72 hours after antibiotic treatment is initiated, the culture should be repeated, and the patient reevaluated. If the peritoneal dialysate white blood cell count remains high after 4 days of appropriate antibiotic therapy, clinicians should consider removing the peritoneal catheter, starting IV antibiotics, and initiating HD for dialytic maintenance therapy.

Fungal peritonitis is associated with a poor prognosis and high morbidity and mortality. One problem with prospective assessment of antifungal regimens is the infrequency with which these infections occur. This makes it difficult to design and implement comparative studies. Most literature about antifungal treatment is therefore retrospective or limited to reports of local experience. As a result, the ISPD recommendations for treatment of fungal peritonitis are somewhat vague and treatment should be based on culture and sensitivity results. However, one area that has been clarified is the question as to whether the PD catheter should be removed. The ISPD recommendations are to remove the catheter immediately after identifying fungi. If the Gram stain indicates the presence of yeast, treatment may be initiated with IV amphotericin B and oral flucytosine. Once culture and sensitivity results are available, fluconazole, caspofungin, or voriconazole may replace amphotericin B. Guidelines recommend amphotericin B be administered IV and not IP as this agent can cause chemical peritonitis and pain and has poor peritoneal bioavailability. Treatment with an oral agent continues for an additional 10 days after catheter removal. It remains unclear whether there is any benefit from fungal prophylaxis. Recommendations are also provided for the treatment of mycobacterial, or tuberculous peritonitis. Although these infections are rare complications, they can be difficult to diagnose and treatment requires multiple drugs.[91]

Catheter-Site Infections

Topical antibiotics and disinfectants are effective agents for the prevention of ESIs. Gram-positive organisms should be treated with oral penicillinase-resistant penicillin or a first-generation cephalosporin such as cephalexin (Fig. 64-5). Rifampin may be added, if necessary, in slowly resolving or particularly severe *S. aureus* infections. Vancomycin should be avoided in routine or empiric treatment of gram-positive catheter-related infections but will be necessary for methicillin-resistant *S. aureus*. Treatment for gram-negative organisms consists of oral quinolones if the organism is susceptible. The effectiveness of oral quinolones may be diminished owing to chelation interactions with drugs containing divalent and trivalent ions, which are commonly taken by patients receiving dialysis. Administration of quinolones should occur at least 2 hours prior to these drugs. In cases where *Pseudomonas aeruginosa* is the pathogen, a quinolone should not be used as monotherapy. Options for a second antipseudomonal drug include the IP administration of an aminoglycoside, ceftazidime, cefepime, piperacillin, imipenem-cilastatin, or meropenem. In all cases, antibiotics should be continued until the exit site is normal; 2 to 3 weeks of therapy may be necessary. A patient with a catheter-related infection that progresses to peritonitis will usually require catheter removal.[91,93]

Prevention of Peritonitis and Catheter Exit-Site Infections

8 Attempts to prevent peritonitis and catheter-related infections have included refinement of connector system technology (Luer-Lok connectors), enhanced patient training techniques, and the use of prophylactic antibiotic regimens and vaccines. Several antimicrobial agents have been examined as prophylaxis against peritonitis and tunnel-related infections. Rifampin 300 mg orally taken twice a day for 5 days, then repeated every 3 months, decreased the number of catheter-related infections, but not the incidence of peritonitis. The efficacy of other antibiotic prophylaxis for peritonitis and catheter-related infections is limited but long-term, extended-duration prophylaxis with penicillins or cephalosporins is not effective.[91,93]

Nasal carriage of *S. aureus* is associated with an increased risk of catheter-related infections and peritonitis.[91,93] In addition, diabetic patients and those on immunosuppressive therapy are at increased

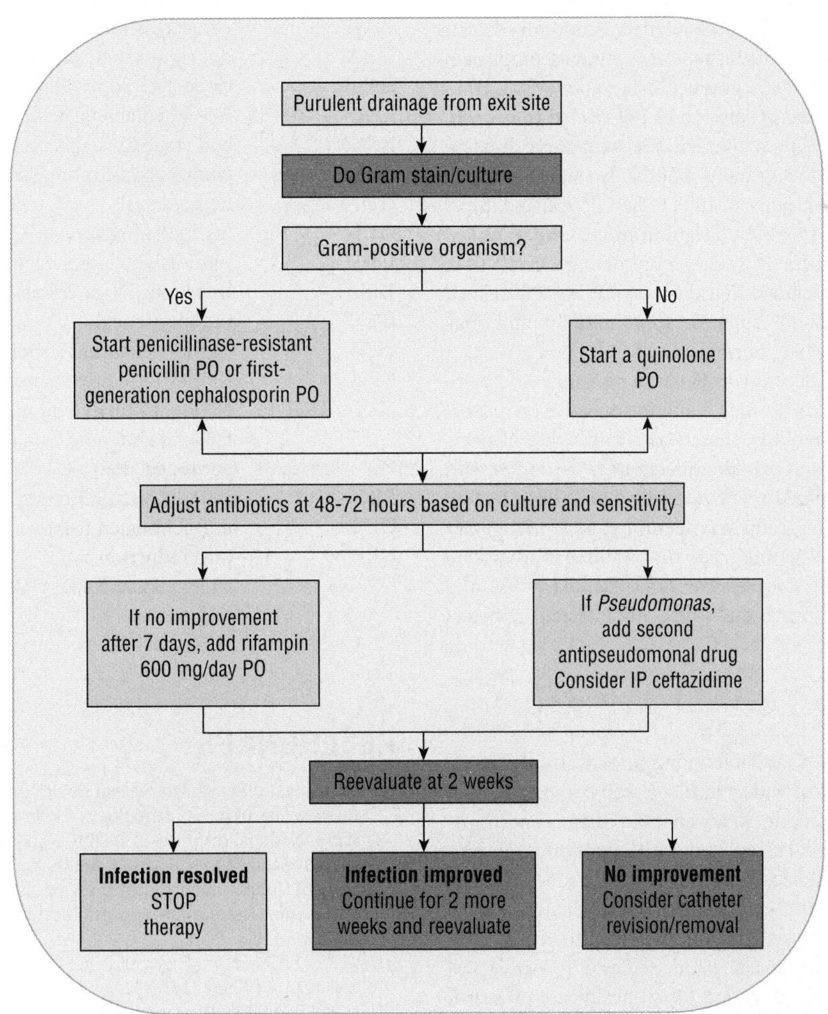

FIGURE 64-5 Management strategy of exit-site infections for peritoneal dialysis patients. (IP, intraperitoneal; PO, orally) (*Data from Reference 93.*)

risk for *S. aureus* catheter infections. Prophylaxis with intranasal mupirocin (twice daily for 5-7 days every month), mupirocin (daily) at the exit site, or oral rifampin can effectively reduce *S. aureus* ESIs. Because of the minimal toxicity of mupirocin and the risk of rifampin resistance, mupirocin regimens are preferred.[91,93] However, it is important to note that *S. aureus* isolates with a high degree of resistance to mupirocin have been isolated from PD patients using prophylactic mupirocin at the peritoneal catheter exit site. A recent study did not observe resistance patterns with the use of mupirocin. Patients in this study applied mupirocin to the exit site either once or thrice weekly. After 3 years, patients in the once-weekly group had an ESI (0.26 episodes/patient/year) and peritonitis (0.36 episodes/patient/year) but patients in the thrice-weekly group had an ESI (0.11 episodes/patient/year) and peritonitis (0.24 episodes/patient/year). The thrice weekly group had a significant reduction in ESIs ($P = 0.030$) and peritonitis ($P = 0.04$).[96] In addition, gentamicin cream applied daily to the exit site has been found to effectively reduce both *S. aureus* and *P. aeruginosa* ESI.[91,93] However, a comparison of mupirocin 2% and gentamicin 0.1% creams for exit-site prophylaxis noted a decrease in gentamicin susceptibility patterns for *Enterobacteriaceae* (12%) and *Pseudomonas* (14%).[97]

A retrospective study of topical chlorhexidine and mupirocin for the prevention of exit-site infections (ESIs) in patients receiving PD. Patients received routine exit-site cleaning with 10% povidone-iodine followed by topical application to the exit site with mupirocin ($n = 162$) or chlorhexidine ($n = 175$). Patients receiving chlorhexidine had a higher rate of ESIs compared to mupirocin (0.22 vs 0.12 episodes/year) ($P = 0.048$). This study found no significant difference in time to first ESI ($P = 0.10$), rate of peritonitis ($P = 0.95$), or hospitalizations ($P = 0.21$).[98] A double-blinded, randomized controlled trial compared the use of the topical ointments mupirocin to polysporin triple (P^3; bacitracin, gramicidin, and polymixin B) in PD patients ($n = 201$) for the prevention of PD-related infections. Patients applied the ointment to the exit site with each dressing change and were followed for up to 18 months. No significant difference was found between groups for time to first PD-related infections ($P = 0.41$) for either agent but a significant increase in fungal infections was observed in the P^3 versus mupirocin group (7 vs 0; $P = 0.01$). The authors concluded that the use of P^3 for PD-related infection prophylaxis was not superior to mupirocin and may increase the risk of fungal infections.[99]

The use of polyhexanide was compared to povidone–iodine to prevent ESIs in PD patients in a single-center prospective open label study ($n = 46$). After 12 months, there was a lower rate of overall infections ($P = 0.037$) and exit-site infections ($P = 0.032$) with use of polyhexanide compared to povidone-iodine. The infection source in the polyhexanide group was identified as *P. aeruginosa* ($n = 3$), but in the povidone–iodine group ($n = 9$) three sources were identified: *S. aureus* ($n = 6$), *Corynebacterium jeikeium* ($n = 2$), and *P. aeruginosa* ($n = 1$). During the study, no infected catheters required removal.[100]

CONCLUSION

Because of the limitation of available kidneys for transplantation, HD and PD remain the most widely available and commonly used ESRD treatments. Despite continual advances in dialysis and transplantation, kidney disease is associated with significant morbidity and mortality. Given the lack of a true cure for kidney disease, emphasis has been placed on the prevention and early detection of kidney disease. Goals set by the KDOQI, the Healthy People 2020 initiative, and the Centers for Medicare and Medicaid Services' CPM Project provide guidance and direction for all healthcare practitioners. In fact, there have been significant reductions in the incidence rate of ESRD, enhanced timing and selection of the preferred access placement, and mortality and morbidity.[101,102] For patients with ESRD, a focus on quality of life and rehabilitation is now a valuable and viable goal toward which the nephrology community should direct its research resources. Several links to patient-related videos that discuss CKD patient experiences are presented in Table 64-12. Although prevention of ESRD is the primary goal for clinicians and adequate access to renal transplantation is secondary, dialysis will likely be a part of the treatment paradigm for ESRD for many years to come.

TABLE 64-12 Patient-Related Videos Relative to Renal Disease, Dialysis Procedures and Therapies

Source	Website
Davita Inc.	www.davita.com/education/videos
NxStage Medical, Inc.	www.nxstage.com/
Fresenius Medical Care	www.freseniuskidneycare.com/tools-and-resources
National Kidney Foundation	www.youtube.com/watch?v=NHS0oyHR4vI

ABBREVIATIONS

APD	automated peritoneal dialysis
AV	arteriovenous
CAPD	continuous ambulatory peritoneal dialysis
CLcr	creatinine clearance
CPM	clinical performance measures
DHA	docosahexaenoic acid
eGFR	estimated glomerular filtration rate
EPA	eicosapentaenoic acid
ESRD	end-stage renal disease
GFR	glomerular filtration rate
HD	hemodialysis
HDF	hemodiafiltration
IDH	intradialytic hypotension
IDSA	Infectious Disease Society of America
IP	intraperitoneal
ISPD	The International Society of Peritoneal Dialysis
KDIGO	Kidney Diseases: Improving Global Outcomes
NKF-KDOQI	National Kidney Foundation's Kidney Disease/Dialysis Outcome Quality Initiative
PD	peritoneal dialysis
RRF	residual renal function
UFH	unfractionated heparin
URR	urea reduction ratio
USRDS	United States Renal Data System

REFERENCES

1. United States Renal Data System (USRDS), 2020 Annual Data Report: An overview of the epidemiology of kidney disease in the United States. National Institutes of Health, National Institute of Diabetes and Digestive and Kidney Diseases, Bethesda, MD; 2020.
2. KDIGO clinical practice guidelines for chronic kidney disease: Evaluation, classification, and stratification. *Kidney Int Suppl.* 2013;3:1–150.
3. KDOQI Clinical Practice Guideline for Hemodialysis Adequacy: 2015 update. *Am J Kidney Dis.* 2015;66:884–930.
4. Yeun JY, Young B, Depner TA, Chin AA. Hemodialysis. In: Yu ASL, Chertow GM, Luyckx VA, Marsden PA, Skorecki K, Taal MW, eds. *Brenner & Rector's The Kidney.* 11th ed. Philadelphia, PA: Elsevier; 2020:2038–2093.

5. Andrassy KM. Comments on 'KDIGO 2012 Clinical Practice Guideline for the Evaluation and Management of Chronic Kidney Disease'. *Kidney Int.* 2013;84:622–623.
6. Sinnakirouchenan R, Holley JL. Peritoneal dialysis versus hemodialysis: Risks, benefits, and access issues. *Adv Chronic Kidney Dis.* 2011;18:428–432.
7. Lee MB, Bargman JM. Survival by dialysis modality—who cares? *Clin J Am Soc Nephrol.* 2016;11:1083–1087.
8. Marshall MR. The benefit of early survival on PD versus HD—why this is (still) very important. *Perit Dial Int.* 2020;40:405–418.
9. Himmelfarb J, Ikizler TA. Hemodialysis. *N Engl J Med.* 2010;363:1833–1845.
10. Daugirdas JT, Blake PG, Ing TS. *Handbook of Dialysis.* 5th ed. Philadelphia, PA: Wolters Kluwer Health; 2015.
11. Hayashi R, Huang E, Nissenson AR. Vascular access for hemodialysis. *Nat Clin Pract Nephrol.* 2006;2:504–513.
12. Tattersall JE, Ward RA, group E. Online haemodiafiltration: Definition, dose quantification and safety revisited. *Nephrol Dial Transplant.* 2013;28:542–550.
13. den Hoedt CH, Mazairac AH, van den Dorpel MA, Grooteman MP, Blankestijn PJ. Effect of hemodiafiltration on mortality, inflammation and quality of life. *Contrib Nephrol.* 2011;168:39–52.
14. Mostovaya IM, Blankestijn PJ, Bots ML, et al. Clinical evidence on hemodiafiltration: A systematic review and a meta-analysis. *Semin Dial.* 2014;27:119–127.
15. Nissenson AR, Fine RN. *Handbook of Dialysis Therapy.* 5th ed. Philadelphia, PA: Elsevier; 2017.
16. Hakim RM, Saha S. Dialysis frequency versus dialysis time, that is the question. *Kidney Int.* 2014;85:1024–1029.
17. Nesrallah GE, Lindsay RM, Cuerden MS, et al. Intensive hemodialysis associates with improved survival compared with conventional hemodialysis. *J Am Soc Nephrol.* 2012;23:696–705.
18. Schachter ME, Chan CT. Current state of intensive hemodialysis: A comparative review of benefits and barriers. *Nephrol Dial Transplant.* 2012;27:4307–4313.
19. Group FHNT, Chertow GM, Levin NW, et al. In-center hemodialysis six times per week versus three times per week. *N Engl J Med.* 2010;363:2287–3000.
20. Saha M, Allon M. Diagnosis, treatment, and prevention of hemodialysis emergencies. *Clinical Journal of the American Society of Nephrology.* 2017;12:357–369.
21. K/DOQI clinical practice guidelines for cardiovascular disease in dialysis patients. *Am J Kidney Dis.* 2005;45:S1–S153.
22. Flythe JE, Inrig JK, Shafi T, et al. Association of intradialytic blood pressure variability with increased all-cause and cardiovascular mortality in patients treated with long-term hemodialysis. *Am J Kidney Dis.* 2013;61:966–974.
23. Morfin JA, Fluck RJ, Weinhandl ED, Kansal S, McCullough PA, Komenda P. Intensive hemodialysis and treatment complications and tolerability. *Am J Kidney Dis.* 2016;68:S43–S50.
24. Thijssen S, Raimann JG, Usvyat LA, Levin NW, Kotanko P. The evils of intradialytic sodium loading. *Contrib Nephrol.* 2011;171:84–91.
25. Mcgill RL, Weiner DE. Dialysate composition for hemodialysis: Changes and changing risk. *Semin Dial.* 2017;30:112–120.
26. Zhou YL, Liu HL, Duan XF, Yao Y, Sun Y, Liu Q. Impact of sodium and ultrafiltration profiling on haemodialysis-related hypotension. *Nephrol Dial Transplant.* 2006;21:3231–3237.
27. Park J, Rhee CM, Sim JJ, et al. A comparative effectiveness research study of the change in blood pressure during hemodialysis treatment and survival. *Kidney Int.* 2013;84:795–802.
28. Denker MG, Cohen DL. Antihypertensive medications in end-stage renal disease. *Semin Dial.* 2015;28:330–336.
29. Hicks CW, Canner JK, Arhuidese I, et al. Mortality benefits of different hemodialysis access types are age dependent. *J Vasc Surg.* 2015;61:449–456.
30. Lok CE, Huber TS, Lee T, et al. KDOQI Clinical practice guideline for vascular access: 2019 Update. *Am J Kidney Dis.* 2020;75:S1–S164.
31. Rupp ME, Karnatak R. Intravascular catheter-related bloodstream infections. *Infect Dis Clin North Am.* 2018;32:765–787.
32. Böhlke M, Uliano G, Barcellos FC. Hemodialysis catheter-related infection: Prophylaxis, diagnosis and treatment. *J Vasc Access.* 2015;16:347–355.
33. Brown RS, Brickel K, Davis RB. Two-year observational study of bloodstream infection rates in hemodialysis facility patients with and without catheters. *Clin J Am Soc Nephrol.* 2018;13:1381–1388.
34. Locham S, Naazie I, Canner J, Siracuse J, Al-Nouri O, Malas M. Incidence and risk factors of sepsis in hemodialysis patients in the United States. *J Vasc Surg.* 2021;73:1016–1021.e3.
35. Nguyen DB, Shugart A, Lines C, et al. National Healthcare Safety Network (NHSN) Dialysis Event Surveillance Report for 2014. *Clin J Am Soc Nephrol.* 2017;12:1139–1146.
36. Xue H, Ix JH, Wang W, et al. Hemodialysis access usage patterns in the incident dialysis year and associated catheter-related complications. *Am J Kidney Dis.* 2013;61:123–130.
37. Nagano N, Ito K, Ono T, et al. Prescription characteristics of phosphate binders in a high pill burden for hemodialysis patients. *Renal Replacement Therapy.* 2021;7:5.
38. Fissell RB, Karaboyas A, Bieber BA, et al. Phosphate binder pill burden, patient-reported non-adherence, and mineral bone disorder markers: Findings from the DOPPS. *Hemodial Int.* 2016;20:38–49.
39. Reeves PB, Mc Causland FR. Mechanisms, clinical implications, and treatment of intradialytic hypotension. *Clin J Am Soc Nephrol.* 2018;13:1297–1303.
40. Gabutti L, Bianchi G, Soldini D, Marone C, Burnier M. Haemodynamic consequences of changing bicarbonate and calcium concentrations in haemodialysis fluids. *Nephrol Dial Transplant.* 2009;24:973–981.
41. Chesterton LJ, Selby NM, Burton JO, McIntyre CW. Cool dialysate reduces asymptomatic intradialytic hypotension and increases baroreflex variability. *Hemodial Int.* 2009;13:189–196.
42. Rubinstein S, Haimov M, Ross MJ. Midodrine-induced vascular ischemia in a hemodialysis patient: A case report and literature review. *Ren Fail.* 2008;30:808–812.
43. Vannorsdall MD, Hariachar S, Hewitt LA. A randomized, placebo-controlled, phase 2 study of the efficacy and safety of droxidopa in patients with intradialytic hypotension. *Postgrad Med.* 2015;127:133–143.
44. Seo Y, Jeung S, Kang SM, Yang WS, Kim H, Kim SB. Use of fludrocortisone for intradialytic hypotension. *Kidney Res Clin Pract.* 2018;37:85–8.
45. Higuchi T, Abe M, Yamazaki T, et al. Levocarnitine improves cardiac function in hemodialysis patients with left ventricular hypertrophy: A randomized controlled trial. *Am J Kidney Dis.* 2016;67:260–270.
46. Razeghi E, Dashti-Khavidaki S, Nassiri S, et al. A randomized crossover clinical trial of sertraline for intradialytic hypotension. *Iran J Kidney Dis.* 2015;9:323–330.
47. Brewster UC, Ciampi MA, Abu-Alfa AK, Perazella MA. Addition of sertraline to other therapies to reduce dialysis-associated hypotension. *Nephrology (Carlton).* 2003;8:296–301.
48. Beladi-Mousavi SS, Beladi-Mousavi M, Hayati F, Talebzadeh M. Effect of intranasal DDAVP in prevention of hypotension during hemodialysis. *Nefrologia.* 2012;32:89–93.
49. Assimon MM, Wang L, Flythe JE. Intradialytic hypertension frequency and short-term clinical outcomes among individuals receiving maintenance hemodialysis. *Am J Hypertens.* 2018;31:329–339.
50. Weir MA, Dixon SN, Fleet JL, et al. β-Blocker dialyzability and mortality in older patients receiving hemodialysis. *J Am Soc Nephrol.* 2015;26:987–996.
51. Tang CH, Wang CC, Chen TH, Hong CY, Sue YM. Prognostic benefits of carvedilol, bisoprolol, and metoprolol controlled release/extended release in hemodialysis patients with heart failure: A 10-year cohort. *J Am Heart Assoc.* 2016;5.
52. Assimon MM, Brookhart MA, Fine JP, Heiss G, Layton JB, Flythe JE. A comparative study of carvedilol versus metoprolol initiation and 1-year mortality among individuals receiving maintenance hemodialysis. *Am J Kidney Dis.* 2018;72:337–348.
53. El-Hennawy AS, Zaib S. A selected controlled trial of supplementary vitamin E for treatment of muscle cramps in hemodialysis patients. *Am J Ther.* 2010;17:455–459.
54. El-Tawil S, Al Musa T, Valli H, et al. Quinine for muscle cramps. *Cochrane Database Syst Rev.* 2015:Cd005044.
55. Houstoun M, Reichman ME, Graham DJ, et al. Use of an active surveillance system by the FDA to observe patterns of quinine sulfate use and adverse hematologic outcomes in CMS Medicare data. *Pharmacoepidemiol Drug Saf.* 2014;23:911–917.
56. Beladi Mousavi SS, Zeraati A, Moradi S, Mousavi MB. The effect of gabapentin on muscle cramps during hemodialysis: A double-blind clinical trial. *Saudi J Kidney Dis Transpl.* 2015;26:1142–1148.
57. Khajehdehi P, Mojerlou M, Behzadi S, Rais-Jalali GA. A randomized, double-blind, placebo-controlled trial of supplementary vitamins E, C and their combination for treatment of haemodialysis cramps. *Nephrol Dial Transplant.* 2001;16:1448–1451.
58. Palmer SC, Di Micco L, Razavian M, et al. Antiplatelet therapy to prevent hemodialysis vascular access failure: Systematic review and meta-analysis. *Am J Kidney Dis.* 2013;61:112–122.
59. Dixon BS, Beck GJ, Dember LM, et al. Use of aspirin associates with longer primary patency of hemodialysis grafts. *J Am Soc Nephrol.* 2011;22:773–781.

60. Locham S, Beaulieu RJ, Dakour-Aridi H, Nejim B, Malas MB. Role of antiplatelet therapy in the durability of hemodialysis access. *J Nephrol.* 2018;31:603–611.
61. Chan KE, Lazarus JM, Thadhani R, Hakim RM. Warfarin use associates with increased risk for stroke in hemodialysis patients with atrial fibrillation. *J Am Soc Nephrol.* 2009;20:2223–2233.
62. Limdi NA, Beasley TM, Baird MF, et al. Kidney function influences warfarin responsiveness and hemorrhagic complications. *J Am Soc Nephrol.* 2009;20:912–921.
63. Kumpfbeck A, Rockman CB, Jacobowitz GR, et al. Anticoagulation therapy is associated with increased access-related wound infections after hemodialysis access creation. *Ann Vasc Surg.* 2021.
64. Lok CE, Moist L, Hemmelgarn BR, et al. Effect of fish oil supplementation on graft patency and cardiovascular events among patients with new synthetic arteriovenous hemodialysis grafts: A randomized controlled trial. *JAMA.* 2012;307:1809–1816.
65. Irish AB, Viecelli AK, Hawley CM, et al. Effect of fish oil supplementation and aspirin use on arteriovenous fistula failure in patients requiring hemodialysis: A randomized clinical trial. *JAMA Intern Med.* 2017;177:184–193.
66. Macrae JM, Dojcinovic I, Djurdjev O, et al. Citrate 4% versus heparin and the reduction of thrombosis study (CHARTS). *Clin J Am Soc Nephrol.* 2008;3:369–374.
67. Zhao Y, Li Z, Zhang L, et al. Citrate versus heparin lock for hemodialysis catheters: A systematic review and meta-analysis of randomized controlled trials. *Am J Kidney Dis.* 2014;63:479–490.
68. Hemmelgarn BR, Manns BJ, Soroka SD, et al. Effectiveness and cost of weekly recombinant tissue plasminogen activator hemodialysis catheter locking solution. *Clin J Am Soc Nephrol.* 2018;13:429–435.
69. Al-Ali F, Hamdy AF, Hamad A, et al. Safety and efficacy of taurolidine/urokinase versus taurolidine/heparin as a tunneled catheter lock solution in hemodialysis patients: a prospective, randomized, controlled study. *Nephrol Dial Transplant.* 2018;33:619–626.
70. El-Hennawy AS, Frolova E, Romney WA. Sodium bicarbonate catheter lock solution reduces hemodialysis catheter loss due to catheter-related thrombosis and blood stream infection: An open-label clinical trial. *Nephrol Dial Transplant.* 2019;34:1739–1745.
71. Hilleman D, Campbell J. Efficacy, safety, and cost of thrombolytic agents for the management of dysfunctional hemodialysis catheters: A systematic review. *Pharmacotherapy.* 2011;31:1031–1040.
72. Vercaigne LM, Zacharias J, Bernstein KN. Alteplase for blood flow restoration in hemodialysis catheters: A multicenter, randomized, prospective study comparing "dwell" versus "push" administration. *Clin Nephrol.* 2012;78:287–296.
73. Yaseen O, El-Masri MM, El Nekidy WS, et al. Comparison of alteplase (tissue plasminogen activator) high-dose vs. low-dose protocol in restoring hemodialysis catheter function: The ALTE-DOSE study. *Hemodial Int.* 2013;17:434–440.
74. Allon M. A patient with recurrent arteriovenous graft thrombosis. *Clin J Am Soc Nephrol.* 2015;10:2255–2262.
75. Golestaneh L, Mokrzycki MH. Prevention of hemodialysis catheter infections: Ointments, dressings, locks, and catheter hub devices. *Hemodial Int.* 2018;22:S75–S82.
76. Mermel LA, Allon M, Bouza E, et al. Clinical practice guidelines for the diagnosis and management of intravascular catheter-related infection: 2009 Update by the Infectious Diseases Society of America. *Clin Infect Dis.* 2009;49:1–45.
77. Battistella M, Bhola C, Lok CE. Long-term follow-up of the hemodialysis infection prevention with polysporin ointment (HIPPO) study: A quality improvement report. *Am J Kidney Dis.* 2011;57:432–441.
78. Quittnat Pelletier F, Joarder M, Poutanen SM, Lok CE. Evaluating approaches for the diagnosis of hemodialysis catheter-related bloodstream infections. *Clin J Am Soc Nephrol.* 2016;11:847–854.
79. Fitzgibbons LN, Puls DL, Mackay K, Forrest GN. Management of gram-positive coccal bacteremia and hemodialysis. *Am J Kidney Dis.* 2011;57:624–640.
80. O'Grady NP, Alexander M, Burns LA, et al. Guidelines for the prevention of intravascular catheter-related infections. *Am J Infect Control.* 2011;39:S1–S34.
81. Kanaa M, Wright MJ, Akbani H, Laboi P, Bhandari S, Sandoe JA. Cathasept line lock and microbial colonization of tunneled hemodialysis catheters: A multicenter randomized controlled trial. *Am J Kidney Dis.* 2015;66:1015–1023.
82. Sofroniadou S, Revela I, Kouloubinis A, et al. Ethanol combined with heparin as a locking solution for the prevention of catheter related blood stream infections in hemodialysis patients: A prospective randomized study. *Hemodial Int.* 2017;21:498–506.
83. Labriola L, Crott R, Jadoul M. Preventing haemodialysis catheter-related bacteraemia with an antimicrobial lock solution: A meta-analysis of prospective randomized trials. *Nephrol Dial Transplant.* 2008;23:1666–1672.
84. Moore CL, Besarab A, Ajluni M, et al. Comparative effectiveness of two catheter locking solutions to reduce catheter-related bloodstream infection in hemodialysis patients. *Clin J Am Soc Nephrol.* 2014;9:1232–1239.
85. Landry DL, Braden GL, Gobeille SL, Haessler SD, Vaidya CK, Sweet SJ. Emergence of gentamicin-resistant bacteremia in hemodialysis patients receiving gentamicin lock catheter prophylaxis. *Clin J Am Soc Nephrol.* 2010;5:1799–1804.
86. Clinical Practice Guidelines for Peritoneal Dialysis Adequacy. *Am J Kidney Dis.* 2006;48:S98–S129.
87. Brown EA, Blake PG, Boudville N, et al. International Society for Peritoneal Dialysis practice recommendations: Prescribing high-quality goal-directed peritoneal dialysis. *Perit Dial Int.* 2020;40:244–253.
88. Perl J, Fuller DS, Bieber BA, et al. Peritoneal dialysis-related infection rates and outcomes: Results From the Peritoneal Dialysis Outcomes and Practice Patterns Study (PDOPPS). *Am J Kidney Dis.* 2020;76:42–53.
89. Ye H, Zhou Q, Fan L, et al. The impact of peritoneal dialysis-related peritonitis on mortality in peritoneal dialysis patients. *BMC Nephrol.* 2017;18:186.
90. Troidle L, Gorban-Brennan N, Finkelstein FO. Outcome of patients on chronic peritoneal dialysis undergoing peritoneal catheter removal because of peritonitis. *Adv Perit Dial.* 2005;21:98–101.
91. Li PK, Szeto CC, Piraino B, et al. ISPD peritonitis recommendations: 2016 Update on prevention and treatment. *Perit Dial Int.* 2016;36:481–508.
92. Piraino B, Bernardini J, Bender FH. An analysis of methods to prevent peritoneal dialysis catheter infections. *Perit Dial Int.* 2008;28:437–443.
93. Szeto CC, Li PK, Johnson DW, et al. ISPD catheter-related infection recommendations: 2017 Update. *Perit Dial Int.* 2017;37:141–154.
94. Lloyd A, Tangri N, Shafer LA, et al. The risk of peritonitis after an exit site infection: A time-matched, case-control study. *Nephrol Dial Transplant.* 2013;28:1915–1921.
95. Ballinger AE, Palmer SC, Wiggins KJ, et al. Treatment for peritoneal dialysis-associated peritonitis. *Cochrane Database Syst Rev.* 2014:Cd005284.
96. Aykut S, Caner C, Ozkan G, et al. Mupirocin application at the exit site in peritoneal dialysis patients: Five years of experience. *Ren Fail.* 2010;32:356–361.
97. Pierce DA, Williamson JC, Mauck VS, Russell GB, Palavecino E, Burkart JM. The effect on peritoneal dialysis pathogens of changing topical antibiotic prophylaxis. *Perit Dial Int.* 2012;32:525–530.
98. Htay H, Johnson DW, Wu SY, Oei EL, Foo MWY, Choo JCJ. Comparison of topical chlorhexidine and mupirocin for the prevention of exit-site infection in incident peritoneal dialysis patients. *Perit Dial Int.* 2017;37:266–272.
99. McQuillan RF, Chiu E, Nessim S, et al. A randomized controlled trial comparing mupirocin and polysporin triple ointments in peritoneal dialysis patients: The MP3 Study. *Clin J Am Soc Nephrol.* 2012;7:297–303.
100. Núñez-Moral M, Sánchez-Álvarez E, González-Díaz I, et al. Exit-site infection of peritoneal catheter is reduced by the use of polyhexanide. Results of a prospective randomized trial. *Perit Dial Int.* 2014;34:271–277.
101. Clinical practice guidelines for vascular access. *Am J Kid Dis.* 2006;2:S176–S247.
102. Mujais S, Story K. Peritoneal dialysis in the US: Evaluation of outcomes in contemporary cohorts. *Kidney Int Suppl.* 2006:S21–S26.

65

Drug-Induced Kidney Disease

Thomas D. Nolin and Mark A. Perazella

KEY CONCEPTS

1. The initial diagnosis of drug-induced kidney disease (DIKD) typically involves detection of elevated serum creatinine (S_{cr}) and blood urea nitrogen, for which there is a temporal relationship between the toxicity and use of a potentially nephrotoxic drug.
2. DIKD is best prevented by avoiding the use of potentially nephrotoxic agents for patients at increased risk for toxicity. However, when exposure to these drugs cannot be avoided, recognition of risk factors and specific techniques, such as hydration, may be used to reduce potential nephrotoxicity.
3. Acute tubular injury/necrosis (ATN) is the most common presentation of DIKD in hospitalized patients. The primary agents implicated are aminoglycosides, radiocontrast media, cisplatin, amphotericin B, and osmotically active agents.
4. Angiotensin-converting enzyme inhibitors (ACEIs), angiotensin-receptor blockers (ARBs), and nonsteroidal anti-inflammatory drugs (NSAIDs) are associated with hemodynamically mediated kidney injury, the pathogenesis of which is a decrease in glomerular capillary hydrostatic pressure.
5. Acute allergic interstitial nephritis (AIN) is observed in up to 27% of kidney biopsies performed for hospitalized patients with unexplained acute kidney injury (AKI). Clinical manifestations of AIN typically (but not always) present approximately 14 days after initiation of therapy and may include fever, maculopapular rash, eosinophilia, arthralgia, as well as pyuria, hematuria, proteinuria, and oliguria.

BEYOND THE BOOK

Visit the National Institute of Diabetes and Digestive and Kidney Diseases Website: https://tinyurl.com/y2pnoj26. This Website is useful to enhance student understanding of risk factors for and commonly used drugs that are associated with nephrotoxicity. Watch the video titled, "Keeping Kidneys Safe: Know How Medicines Affect the Kidneys," https://tinyurl.com/ybjao5qg. The video provides a brief overview of glomerular physiology and hemodynamically mediated nephrotoxic effects of nonsteroidal anti-inflammatory drugs and renin-angiotensin system blockers.

INTRODUCTION

Numerous diagnostic and therapeutic agents have been associated with the development of drug-induced kidney disease (DIKD) or nephrotoxicity. It is a relatively common complication with variable presentations depending on the drug and clinical setting, inpatient or outpatient. Manifestations of DIKD may include acid–base abnormalities, electrolyte imbalances, urine sediment abnormalities, proteinuria, pyuria, and/or hematuria.[1] However, the most common manifestation of nephrotoxicity is a decline in the glomerular filtration rate (GFR) and a corresponding rise in serum creatinine (S_{cr}) concentrations. Initial diagnosis of nephrotoxicity is often delayed because it typically is based on the detection of elevated S_{cr}, for which there is a temporal relationship between the kidney injury (evidenced by the rise in S_{cr}) and exposure to the potentially nephrotoxic drug. This is consistent with contemporary definitions of acute kidney injury (AKI), which rely on either an abrupt increase in S_{cr} or an abrupt decline in urine output (see Chapter e60, "Evaluation of Kidney Function" and Chapter 61, "Acute Kidney Injury").[2]

Nephrotoxicity is often reversible if one discontinues the use of the offending agent, but in some cases it may evolve into AKI and may even progress to stage 5 chronic kidney disease (CKD) and end-stage kidney disease (ESKD). Many different mechanisms are responsible for the pathogenesis of DIKD, and the introduction of new drugs with novel mechanisms of action provides the potential for the identification of new presentations of AKI and CKD. This chapter reviews the epidemiology, pathophysiology, risk factors, and basic principles of prevention of DIKD. Detailed discussions of these issues plus management strategies are presented for the most commonly used agents that have been associated with a moderate-to-high likelihood of DIKD.

EPIDEMIOLOGY

The incidence and characteristics of outpatient or community-acquired DIKD are not well understood since mild toxicity is often unrecognized in this setting. The incidence of community-based AKI requiring dialysis is as high as 29.5 per 100,000 person years and 522.4 per 100,000 person years for patients not requiring dialysis.[3] Although the incidence of drug-induced AKI was not specifically reported, up to 20% of hospital admissions due to AKI have been attributed to nephrotoxicity acquired in the community setting.[4] The incidence of AKI is even higher in hospitalized patients and increases over time.[3,5] As many as 22% of adults and 34% of children worldwide experience AKI during a hospital admission.[6] While up to 30% of critically ill patients experience AKI during their hospitalization, one in four cases is associated with nephrotoxic medication exposure.[7] Indeed, drugs have been implicated in 26% of all cases of in-hospital AKI and as such are a recognized source of significant morbidity and mortality.[1]

(1) Because the most common manifestation of DIKD is a decline in GFR leading to a rise in S_{cr} and blood urea nitrogen (BUN), the onset of toxicity in hospitalized, acutely ill patients is most often recognized by routine laboratory monitoring. Decreased urine output may also be an early sign of toxicity, particularly with radiographic contrast media, nonsteroidal anti-inflammatory drugs

CLINICAL PRESENTATION Drug-Induced Kidney Disease

General

- The most common manifestation is a decline in GFR leading to a rise in S_{cr} and BUN.
- Alterations in renal tubular function without loss of glomerular filtration may be evident.

Symptoms

- Patients may complain of malaise, anorexia, nausea, vomiting, shortness of breath, or edema, particularly in the outpatient setting.

Signs

- Decreased urine output may be an early sign of toxicity, particularly with radiographic contrast media, NSAIDs, and ACEIs, with progression to volume overload and hypertension.
- Proximal tubular injury: Metabolic acidosis with bicarbonaturia; glycosuria in the absence of hyperglycemia; and reductions in serum phosphate, uric acid, potassium, and magnesium due to increased urinary losses.
- Distal tubular injury: Polyuria from failure to maximally concentrate urine, metabolic acidosis from impaired urinary acidification, and hyperkalemia from impaired potassium excretion.

Laboratory Tests

- An abrupt (within 48 hours) reduction in kidney function defined as an absolute increase in S_{cr} of greater than or equal to 0.3 mg/dL (27 μmol/L), a percentage increase in S_{cr} of greater than or equal to 50% (1.5-fold from baseline) within 7 days, or a reduction in urine output (documented oliguria of less than 0.5 mL/kg/hr for more than 6 hours), when correlated temporally with the initiation of drug therapy may indicate drug-induced AKI.[1]
- Electrolyte (hyponatremia, hyperkalemia, hypo/hyperphosphatemia) and acid-base disturbances (metabolic acidosis) may also develop.

Other Diagnostic Tests

- Urinary excretion of *N*-acetyl-β-glucosaminidase, γ-glutamyl transpeptidase, glutathione *S*-transferase, and interleukin-18 are markers of proximal tubular injury and have been used for the early detection of AKI in critically ill patients.
- Kidney injury molecule-1 (KIM-1) is expressed in the proximal tubule and is upregulated for patients with ischemic acute tubular necrosis (ATN), appearing in the urine within 12 hours after the ischemic insult.
- Neutrophil gelatinase–associated lipocalin (NGAL) protein may be detected in the urine within 3 hours of ischemic injury.
- The urinary cell-cycle arrest biomarkers insulin-like growth factor–binding protein 7 (IGFBP7) and tissue inhibitor of metalloproteinase 2 (TIMP-2) can predict AKI in high-risk surgical patients, and clinical outcomes (death and the need for dialysis) in critically ill adults. These biomarkers may have an emerging role in detecting and/or minimizing DIKD.

(NSAIDs), and angiotensin-converting enzyme inhibitors (ACEIs). Other laboratory abnormalities such as electrolyte and acid-base disturbances often follow an increase in S_{cr}. In the outpatient setting, nephrotoxicity is often recognized by the development of symptoms such as malaise, anorexia, vomiting, volume overload (shortness of breath or edema), and hypertension. S_{cr} or BUN concentrations and urine collection for creatinine clearance may subsequently be measured to quantify the degree of decline in GFR. Marked intrasubject between-day variability of S_{cr} values has been noted (±20% for values within the normal range; see Chapter e60). Furthermore, they may be altered as the result of dietary changes and initiation of drug therapy, which may interfere with the assay procedure. Nevertheless, changes in S_{cr} or urine output consistent with the diagnostic criteria for AKI (see Chapter e60), when correlated temporally with the initiation of drug therapy, are a common threshold for the identification of DIKD.[1]

CLINICAL PRESENTATION

Nephrotoxicity may also be evidenced by primary alterations in renal tubular function without a corresponding loss of glomerular filtration. In this setting, urinary enzymes and low-molecular-weight proteins may be used as earlier and more specific biomarkers of nephrotoxicity compared with S_{cr} and BUN, which are relatively insensitive markers of kidney injury.[8,9] S_{cr} and BUN are used as surrogates of kidney function, not injury per se, and typically significant kidney injury must have occurred days before a rise in either is evident. The emergence of novel biomarkers of kidney injury represents an important opportunity for earlier detection of DIKD. Urinary excretion of KIM-1, *N*-acetyl-β-glucosaminidase, γ-glutamyl transpeptidase, glutathione *S*-transferase, NGAL, and interleukin-18 (markers of proximal tubular injury) have been used for the early detection of acute kidney damage in several patient populations.[8-10] For example, the transmembrane protein KIM-1 is upregulated for patients with ischemic ATN, appearing in the urine within 12 hours after the ischemic insult. Urinary *N*-acetylglucosamine concentrations are a highly sensitive indicator of AKI and can detect AKI in critically ill patients up to 4 days prior to a rise in S_{cr}. Similarly, urinary NGAL is an early marker of AKI, preceding a rise observed in S_{cr} by up to 3 days.[11]

The urinary cell-cycle arrest biomarkers IGFBP7 and TIMP-2 predict AKI in high-risk surgical patients,[12] and clinical outcomes (death and the need for dialysis) in critically ill adults.[13] The clinical utility of IGFBP7 and TIMP-2 in detecting and/or minimizing DIKD remain unclear, but several preclinical studies suggest a potential clinical role and utility of monitoring TIMP or IGFBP for this purpose. For example, TIMP-1 is an effective biomarker of cisplatin-induced nephrotoxicity in human kidney cells,[14] and is useful in predicting aristolochic acid–induced kidney injury in rats.[15] The urinary biomarkers may facilitate the earlier detection of kidney injury and diagnosis of nephrotoxicity and minimize the long-term consequences of this common drug-induced disorder.

PRINCIPLES FOR PREVENTION OF DRUG-INDUCED NEPHROPATHY

2 The primary principle for prevention of DIKD is to avoid the use of nephrotoxic agents for patients at increased risk for toxicity. Therefore, an awareness of potentially nephrotoxic drugs and knowledge of risk factors that increase kidney vulnerability are essential.[16] Exposure to these drugs often cannot be avoided; so, several interventions have been proposed to reduce the potential for the development of nephrotoxicity, for example, adjustment of medication dosage regimens based on accurate estimates of kidney function, and careful and adequate hydration to establish high urine flow rates.[17] Other preventative strategies are still theoretical and/or investigational and relate directly to the specific nephrotoxic mechanisms of a given drug.

The several specific drug-induced kidney structural-functional alterations that are responsible for the vast majority of cases of DIKD are listed in Table 65-1. This chapter discusses the pathophysiologic mechanisms responsible for the development of DIKD with these agents in detail, along with clinical presentation, prevention strategies, therapeutic management approaches, and relevant monitoring plans.

TABLE 65-1 Drug-Induced Kidney Structural-Functional Alterations

Tubular epithelial cell damage	
Acute tubular injury/necrosis	Osmotic nephropathy
• Aminoglycoside antibiotics	• Mannitol
• Radiographic contrast media	• Dextran
• Cisplatin, carboplatin	• IV immunoglobulin (sucrose)
• Ifosfamide	• Hydroxyethyl starch
• Amphotericin B	• SGLT-2 inhibitors
• Cyclosporine, tacrolimus	
• Adefovir, cidofovir, tenofovir	
• Pentamidine	
• Foscarnet	
• Zoledronate	
• Chimeric antigen receptor T-cells	
Hemodynamically mediated kidney injury	
• Angiotensin-converting enzyme inhibitors	• NSAIDs
• Angiotensin II receptor blockers	• Cyclosporine, tacrolimus
• SGLT-2 inhibitors	• OKT3
• Chimeric antigen receptor T-cells	• High dose interleukin-2
Obstructive nephropathy	
Crystal nephropathy	Nephrolithiasis
• Acyclovir	• Sulfonamides
• Sulfonamides	• Triamterene
• Indinavir, atazanavir	• Indinavir, atazanavir
• Foscarnet	Nephrocalcinosis
• Methotrexate	• Oral sodium phosphate solution
• Ascorbic acid, ethylene glycol, orlistat	
• Ciprofloxacin	
Glomerular disease	
Minimal change disease	Focal segmental glomerulosclerosis
• NSAIDs, COX-2 inhibitors	• Pamidronate
• Lithium	• Interferon-α and β
• Pamidronate	• Lithium
• Interferon-α and β	• Sirolimus
Membranous disease	• Anabolic steroids
• NSAIDs	• Tyrosine kinase inhibitors
• Penicillamine	
• Captopril	
Tubulointerstitial disease	
Acute allergic interstitial nephritis	Chronic interstitial nephritis
• β-Lactams	• Cyclosporine
• Ciprofloxacin	• Lithium
• NSAIDs, cyclooxygenase-2 inhibitors	• Aristolochic acid
• Proton pump inhibitors	• Combination analgesics
• Loop diuretics	Papillary necrosis
• Immune checkpoint inhibitors	• NSAIDs, combined phenacetin, aspirin, and caffeine analgesics
Renal vasculitis, thrombotic microangiopathy, and cholesterol emboli	
Vasculitis	Thrombotic microangiopathy
• Hydralazine	• Cyclosporine, tacrolimus
• Propylthiouracil	• Gemcitabine
• Allopurinol	• Bevacizumab
• Penicillamine	• Mitomycin C
• Adalimumab	• Quinine
• Minocycline	Cholesterol emboli
• Sulfasalazine	• Warfarin
	• Thrombolytic agents

COX-2, cyclooxygenase-2; SGLT-2, sodium-glucose co-transporter 2

TUBULAR EPITHELIAL CELL DAMAGE

3 Drugs that lead to renal tubular epithelial cell (RTEC) damage typically do so via direct cellular toxicity or ischemia. Damage is most often localized in the proximal and distal tubular epithelia and is termed "ATN" when cellular degeneration and sloughing from proximal and distal tubular basement membranes are observed. This classically manifests as cellular debris-filled, RTECs and RTEC casts and/or muddy brown granular casts in the urinary sediment.[18] Specific indicators of proximal tubular injury include metabolic acidosis with bicarbonaturia; glycosuria in the absence of hyperglycemia; and reductions in serum phosphate, uric acid, potassium, and magnesium as a result of increased urinary losses.[19] Indicators of distal tubular injury include polyuria from failure to maximally concentrate urine (ie, nephrogenic diabetes insipidus), metabolic acidosis from impaired urinary acidification, and hyperkalemia from impaired potassium excretion.[20]

Acute Tubular Injury/Necrosis

Acute tubular injury/necrosis (ATN) is the most common presentation of DIKD in the inpatient setting. The primary agents associated with this type of injury are aminoglycosides, radiocontrast media, cisplatin, amphotericin B, foscarnet, and osmotically active agents such as immunoglobulins, dextrans, hydroxyethyl starch, and mannitol.[21]

Aminoglycoside Nephrotoxicity

Incidence Aminoglycoside antibiotic–associated nephrotoxicity may occur in between 10% and 25% of patients receiving a therapeutic course.[22,23] Critically ill patients appear to have a higher risk for nephrotoxicity with rates as high as 58%.[24] The large variance is in part a result of the use of different definitions of toxicity, variability between agents in the class, and the risk factors present in the study population.

Clinical Presentation Clinical evidence of aminoglycoside-associated nephrotoxicity is typically seen within 5 to 7 days after initiation of therapy and manifests as a gradual progressive rise in S_{cr} and BUN and decrease in creatinine clearance.[23] Patients usually present with non-oliguria, that is, they maintain urine volumes greater than 500 mL/day and sometimes have microscopic hematuria and proteinuria.[21] Although renal magnesium wasting can occur (ie, daily excretion of more than 10-30 mg), the risk of symptomatic hypomagnesemia is generally low. Full recovery of kidney function is common if aminoglycoside therapy is discontinued immediately upon discovering signs of toxicity. However, severe AKI may develop occasionally, and for these individuals renal replacement therapy may be required (see Chapter 61). The diagnosis of aminoglycoside-associated nephrotoxicity is often difficult, particularly in critically ill patients with multiple comorbidities and is confounded by other factors that are independently associated with the development of AKI.[24] For instance, concurrent dehydration, sepsis, hypotension, ischemia, and use of other nephrotoxic drugs frequently contribute to AKI in patients who are receiving aminoglycosides.

Pathogenesis Aminoglycoside-associated ATN is primarily due to accumulation of high drug concentrations within proximal tubular epithelial cells, and subsequent generation of reactive oxygen species that produce mitochondrial injury, which leads to cellular apoptosis and necrosis.[22] This results in cell sloughing from proximal tubular basement membranes into the tubular lumen, which can result in tubular obstruction and back leakage of the glomerular filtrate across the damaged tubular epithelium. Toxicity is related to cationic charge of the drugs in this class, which facilitates their binding to negatively charged renal tubular epithelial membrane phospholipids in the proximal tubules, followed by intracellular transport and concentration in lysosomes. The number of cationic groups on the drug molecule correlates with the degree of nephrotoxicity, which is consistent with the observation of higher rates of toxicity with neomycin versus gentamicin, followed by tobramycin, then amikacin.[23]

Risk Factors Multiple risk factors for aminoglycoside-associated nephrotoxicity have been identified: the aggressiveness of aminoglycoside dosing, synergistic toxicity as the result of combination drug therapy, and preexisting clinical conditions of the patient (Table 65-2).[22,24]

Prevention Aminoglycoside-associated ATN may be prevented by careful and cautious selection of patients and the use of alternative antibiotics whenever possible and as soon as microbial sensitivities are known. Commonly used alternatives include fluoroquinolones (eg, ciprofloxacin or levofloxacin) and third- or fourth-generation cephalosporins (eg, ceftazidime or cefepime). When aminoglycosides are necessary, gentamicin, tobramycin, and amikacin are most commonly used, but therapy should be selected to optimize antimicrobial efficacy. Furthermore, it is imperative to avoid volume depletion, limit the total aminoglycoside dose administered, and avoid concomitant therapy with other nephrotoxic drugs.[22] Future therapeutic alternatives may include new aminoglycoside congeners that retain the desired bactericidal activity and yet are devoid of nephrotoxicity, and may also include concurrent use of antioxidant compounds such as alpha-lipoic acid, vitamin E, and *N*-acetylcysteine.[25,26]

Prospective, individualized pharmacokinetic monitoring has been associated with a decrease in the incidence of aminoglycoside-associated nephrotoxicity.[27] High-dose intermittent administration of aminoglycosides, termed once daily dosing, used in combination with other antibiotics, has been intensively investigated as a practical cost-effective method to maintain antimicrobial efficacy while reducing the risk of AKI.[27,28] The reduction in incidence may be the result of limited proximal tubular aminoglycoside uptake during the transient, high-peak serum concentrations, and because of the presence of low aminoglycoside concentrations for a greater proportion of the dosing interval, which facilitates excretion of the aminoglycoside.[22] Although greater clinical efficacy and reduced nephrotoxicity may be realized with once daily compared with standard dosing, seriously ill, immunocompromised, and elderly patients, as well as those with preexisting kidney disease, are not ideal candidates for this approach.

Management Aminoglycoside use should be discontinued or the dosage regimen revised if AKI is evident (ie, there is an S_{cr} increase of 0.5 mg/dL [44 μmol/L] or more that is not attributable to another cause). Other nephrotoxic drugs should be discontinued if possible, and the patient should be maintained adequately hydrated and hemodynamically stable.[28] Short-term renal replacement therapy may be necessary, but ESKD is rarely the result of aminoglycoside toxicity alone.

TABLE 65-2 Potential Risk Factors for Aminoglycoside-Associated Nephrotoxicity

(A) Related to aminoglycoside dosing:
Large total cumulative dose
Prolonged therapy
Trough concentration exceeding 2 mg/L[a]
Recent previous aminoglycoside therapy
(B) Related to synergistic nephrotoxicity—Aminoglycosides in combination with:
Cyclosporine
Amphotericin B
Vancomycin
Diuretics
Iodinated radiographic contrast agents
Cisplatin
NSAIDs
(C) Related to predisposing conditions in the patient:
Preexisting kidney disease
Diabetes mellitus
Increased age
Poor nutrition
Shock
Gram-negative bacteremia
Liver disease
Hypoalbuminemia
Obstructive jaundice
Dehydration
Hypotension
Potassium or magnesium deficiencies

[a]The equivalent concentration in SI molar units is 4.3 μmol/L for tobramycin and 4.2 μmol/L for gentamicin.

Radiographic Contrast Media Nephrotoxicity

Incidence Radiographic contrast media–induced AKI (CI-AKI) is the third leading cause of hospital-acquired AKI, accounting for 10% to 13% of cases.[29] Estimates of the incidence varies widely depending on the population studied and presence of risk factors; rising from less than 2% for patients with normal kidney function, to 17% in patients with impaired kidney function, and 23% to 50% of critically ill patients.[21,30,31] However, the incidence of AKI in patients receiving radiocontrast is commonly overestimated, with the true incidence approximately 5.5%.[32] CI-AKI is extremely rare with intravenous contrast administration in patients with an eGFR >30 mL/min/1.73 m^2.[33] As the number of risk factors associated with CI-AKI increases, there is a corresponding increase in the incidence of nephrotoxicity and mortality rates. Approximately fivefold increased risk of death is seen in patients who develop CI-AKI compared with those who do not, with the highest mortality rates observed for patients who developed AKI and required renal replacement therapy. Specifically, in-hospital mortality for patients who developed CI-AKI was 34% versus only 7% of patients who received contrast but did not develop AKI.[29] Moreover, a two-year mortality rate of 81% has been observed for patients who developed CI-AKI and required dialysis.[29]

Clinical Presentation CI-AKI is usually transient in nature, presenting most commonly as nonoliguria with kidney injury apparent within the first 24 to 48 hours after the administration of contrast. The S_{cr} concentration usually peaks between 3 and 4 days after exposure, with recovery after 7 to 10 days.[23] However, irreversible oliguric (urine volume less than 500 mL/day) AKI requiring dialysis is seenin high-risk patients.[34] Urinalysis typically reveals tubular enzymuria with hyaline and granular casts but may also be completely void of casts. The urine sodium concentration and fractional excretion of sodium are frequently low, with the latter typically less than 1% (0.01).

Pathogenesis The primary mechanisms by which contrast media induces nephrotoxicity are renal ischemia and direct cellular toxicity.[35] Renal ischemia likely results from systemic hypotension and simultaneous acute vasoconstriction caused by disruption of normal prostaglandin synthesis and the release of adenosine, endothelin, and other renal vasoconstrictors. Subsequently, a sustained reduction in renal blood flow of up to 25% that lasts for several hours immediately following contrast administration may be evident.[35] This reduced renal blood flow leads to a 50% reduction in oxygen partial pressure and renal ischemia, along with increased concentrations of contrast in the renal tubules, which exacerbates the direct cytotoxicity.[35,36] The extent of cellular toxicity is directly related to the duration of tubular cell exposure to contrast. Thus, preservation of high urinary flow rates with adequate hydration before, during, and after contrast administration is vital to keep renal blood flow as high as reasonably possible to minimize tubular cell exposure to the contrast agent.[36] In humans, plasma osmolality is normally between 275 and 290 mOsm/kg (mmol/kg). Since low- and high-osmolar contrast agents are hyperosmolar to plasma (ie, 600-800 mOsm/kg [mmol/kg] and ~2,000 mOsm/kg [mmol/kg], respectively), their use may result in osmotic diuresis, dehydration, renal ischemia, and increased blood viscosity caused by red blood cell aggregation.[37] Oxidative stress has also been implicated in the development of ATN after contrast administration, which may explain the possible benefit of the antioxidants *N*-acetylcysteine and ascorbic acid.[38]

Risk Factors Decreased renal blood flow exacerbates the ischemic and direct cytotoxic effects of contrast media on the renal tubules. Therefore, preexisting kidney disease, particularly in those with estimated GFR less than 60 mL/min/1.73 m^2, is the most important risk factor, since lower GFR is associated with increasing levels of risk.[31] Other patient-specific risk factors include conditions associated with decreased renal blood flow (ie, congestive heart failure, dehydration/volume depletion, and hypotension), and patients with atherosclerosis and reduced effective circulating arterial blood volume appear to also have an elevated risk.[39,40] Diabetes is also a significant risk factor, likely due to coexisting kidney disease (diabetic nephropathy). The presence of multiple myeloma has traditionally been considered a relative contraindication for contrast use, but the risk is associated with concomitant dehydration, kidney disease, or hypercalcemia rather than the diagnosis itself. Larger volumes or doses of contrast and the use of low- as well as high-osmolar contrast agents are also independent predictors of CI-AKI.[39,40] Intra-arterial administration of contrast confers greater risk than IV administration.[31] Lastly, concurrent use of nephrotoxins and drugs that alter renal hemodynamics such as NSAIDs and ACEIs also increases risk. Risk factors are additive, and there is a proportional increase in the incidence of CI-AKI and associated mortality as the number of risk factors increases.[40]

Prevention CI-AKI can be anticipated in the majority of patients who are at risk; so the use of preventative procedures is justified for virtually all patients. Table 65-3 lists the recommended interventions for prevention of contrast nephrotoxicity. All patients scheduled to receive contrast media should be assessed for risk factors, and the risk-to-benefit ratio should be considered.[29,39,40] High-risk patients can be identified by evaluating medical history and indication for the contrast procedure, along with their most recent S_{cr} concentrations. Nephrotoxicity is best prevented in high-risk patients by using alternative imaging procedures (eg, ultrasound, noncontrast magnetic resonance imaging, and nuclear medicine scans). However, if contrast media must be used, the smallest adequate volume should be administered.[29] If the ratio of the volume of contrast to be infused relative to the patient's creatinine clearance is greater than or equal to 3.7 (222 if creatinine clearance is expressed in units of mL/s), the likelihood of nephrotoxicity is markedly increased.[40]

TABLE 65-3 Recommended Interventions for Prevention of Contrast Media-Induced AKI[38-41]

Intervention	Recommendation	Recommendation Grade[a]
Contrast	• Minimize contrast volume/dose	A-1
	• Use noniodinated contrast	A-2
	• Use low- or iso-osmolar contrast agents	A-2
Medications	• Avoid concurrent use of potentially nephrotoxic drugs (eg, NSAIDs, aminoglycosides)	A-2
Isotonic sodium chloride (0.9%)	• Initiate infusion 3-12 hours prior to contrast exposure and continue 6-24 hours postexposure • Infuse at 1-1.5 mL/kg/hr adjusting postexposure as needed to maintain a urine flow rate of 150 mL/hr • Alternatively, in urgent cases, initiate infusion at 3 mL/kg/hr, beginning 1 hour prior to contrast exposure, then continue at 1 mL/kg/hr for 6 hours postexposure	A-1

[a]*Strength of recommendations*: A, B, and C are good, moderate, and poor evidence to support recommendation, respectively. *Quality of evidence*: (1) evidence from more than one properly randomized, controlled trial; (2) evidence from more than one well-designed clinical trial with randomization, from cohort or case-controlled analytic studies or multiple time series, or dramatic results from uncontrolled experiments; and (3) evidence from opinions of respected authorities, based on clinical experience, descriptive studies, or reports of expert communities.

Therefore, in general, the volume of contrast administered should not be greater than twice the baseline estimated creatinine clearance.

Low-osmolar (600-800 mOsm/kg [mmol/kg]) nonionic (iohexol and iopamidol) and ionic (ioxaglate) contrast agents may be used to minimize the incidence of nephrotoxicity. Standard hyperosmolar contrast media (eg, low- and high-osmolar agent) are not reabsorbed in the kidney and cause osmotic diuresis, which contributes to the renal toxicity observed with these agents. Low-osmolar contrast agents have less than half the osmolality of high-osmolar (~2,000 mOsm/kg [mmol/kg]) agents and are associated with less toxicity, especially when used for patients with preexisting kidney disease.[37] However, use of low-osmolar agents does not preclude the development of nephrotoxicity. Even low-osmolar agents are hyperosmolar relative to plasma, which is likely the reason they have been associated with greater nephrotoxicity than the iso-osmolar nonionic contrast agent iodixanol. The relative differences in nephrotoxicity between the class of low-osmolar agents and iodixanol are unclear.[40,41]

Volume expansion and correction of dehydration prior to contrast administration is a mainstay of preventive therapy.[36] Parenteral hydration with isotonic saline before and after contrast administration reduces the incidence of toxicity, particularly in high-risk patients, and is the most widely accepted preventative intervention.[40] Volume expansion may exert its beneficial effects through dilution of contrast media, prevention of renal vasoconstriction, preservation of high urine flow rates, decreased tubular cell exposure to contrast, and avoidance of tubular obstruction. There is no benefit in using sodium bicarbonate or the thiol-containing antioxidant *N*-acetylcysteine over saline.[42] The guidelines recommend hydration with isotonic saline for CI-AKI prevention.[40,41] The use of oral hydration is also not recommended in lieu of parenteral hydration.[40,41]

Renal replacement therapy, including intermittent hemodialysis and continuous modalities, for example, continuous venovenous hemofiltration, effectively removes iodinated contrast, and was considered by some to be a therapeutic option for the prevention of CI-AKI. However, because of the logistical issues (eg, technical difficulty), potential infectious and noninfectious risks, high cost of renal replacement therapy, and lack of consistent clinical efficacy, renal replacement therapy is not recommended.[31,41]

Management There is no specific therapy available for managing established CI-AKI. Other nephrotoxic drugs should be discontinued if possible, and subsequent contrast studies must be appropriately timed to minimize cumulative toxicity. Care is supportive as described in Chapter 61. Kidney function (eg, S_{cr} and urine output), electrolytes (eg, sodium and potassium), and volume status should be closely monitored.

Cisplatin Nephrotoxicity

Incidence Cisplatin is one of the most important and widely used antineoplastic drugs for the treatment of solid tumors, often demonstrating exceptional efficacy (ie, cure rates over 90% in testicular cancers).[43] The primary dose-limiting toxicity of platin-containing compounds is nephrotoxicity. Cisplatin nephrotoxicity occurs in up to one-third of patients receiving the drug and is a significant cause of morbidity.[43,44] Carboplatin, a second-generation platinum analog, is associated with a lower incidence of nephrotoxicity than cisplatin and thus is the preferred agent in high-risk patients.[45]

Clinical Presentation Cisplatin administration results in impaired tubular reabsorption and decreased urinary concentration ability, leading to increased excretion of salt and water (ie, polyuria) within 24 hours of treatment. Polyuria persists and a decrease in GFR evidenced by a rise in S_{cr} concentration may be seen within 72 to 96 hours after cisplatin administration.[46] S_{cr} peaks approximately 10 to 14 days after initiation of therapy, with recovery by 21 days.[47] As many as 25% of patients may have reversible elevations in S_{cr} and BUN for 2 weeks after cisplatin treatment. However, kidney damage is dose related and cumulative with subsequent cycles of therapy, so the S_{cr} concentration may continue to rise, and irreversible kidney injury may result.[45] Hypomagnesemia is a hallmark finding of cisplatin nephrotoxicity, due to impaired magnesium reabsorption and thus increased urinary losses.[48] Hypomagnesemia is often accompanied by hypocalcemia and hypokalemia and may be severe, leading to seizures, neuromuscular irritability, or personality changes. Urinalysis typically reveals leukocytes, RTECs, and granular casts.

Pathogenesis The pathogenesis of cisplatin nephrotoxicity is multifactorial in nature and likely begins with cellular uptake and accumulation of the drug in proximal tubular epithelial cells to concentrations that may reach five times the serum concentration.[49] Tubular cell exposure to cisplatin then activates a series of cell signaling pathways, including the mitogen-activated protein kinase pathway, p53, caspase, and the generation of reactive oxygen species, that collectively promote tubular cell injury and death via necrosis and/or apoptosis.[43,44] Simultaneous production of proinflammatory cytokines such as tumor necrosis factor-α (TNF-α) within tubular cells activates an inflammatory response, which may worsen the renal insult. Although tubular damage is evident in both the proximal and distal segments, the majority occurs in the proximal tubules and is followed by a progressive loss of glomerular filtration capacity and impaired distal tubular function. Kidney biopsies generally reveal necrosis-apoptosis of proximal and distal tubules and collecting ducts, with no obvious morphological changes to the glomeruli.[47]

Risk Factors Risk factors include age more than 65 years, dehydration, preexisting kidney disease, renal irradiation, concurrent use of nephrotoxic drugs, large cumulative doses, and alcohol abuse.[50]

Prevention The best renoprotective strategy is a combination of interventions, including prospective dose reduction and decreased frequency of administration, which usually requires using the platin compounds in combination with other chemotherapeutic agents, avoiding concurrent use of other nephrotoxic drugs, and ensuring patients are euvolemic or somewhat hypervolemic prior to initiating treatment.[50,51] Vigorous hydration with isotonic saline should be used for all patients with a goal of maintaining at least 100 to 150 mL/hr of urine output during and after cisplatin treatment. Hydration should be initiated 12 to 24 hours prior to and continued for 2 to 3 days after cisplatin administration at rates of 100 to 250 mL/hr, as tolerated, to maintain a urine flow of 3 to 4 L/day.[46]

Amifostine, an organic thiophosphate that is converted to an active metabolite, chelates cisplatin in normal cells and reduces the nephrotoxicity, neurotoxicity, ototoxicity, and myelosuppression associated with cisplatin and carboplatin therapy. It is also thought to serve as a thiol donor, thereby reducing intracellular reactive oxygen species and corresponding oxidative stress that plays a critical role in the development of cellular injury.[44] Amifostine is Food and Drug Administration (FDA)-approved to reduce nephrotoxicity associated with repeated cisplatin treatment in patients with advanced ovarian cancer. Pretreatment with amifostine should be considered for patients who are at high risk for kidney injury, particularly patients who are elderly, volume depleted, have CKD, or are receiving other nephrotoxic drugs concurrently. The recommended dose of amifostine is 910 mg/m^2 administered IV over 15 minutes, beginning 30 minutes prior to cisplatin administration. Common toxicities include acute hypotension, nausea, and fatigue.

Other renoprotective strategies include the use of hypertonic saline (eg, administration of each dose in 250 mL of 3% saline) to reduce tubular cisplatin uptake. Classic antioxidants such as ascorbic acid, thiol-based antioxidants such as α-lipoic acid and *N*-acetylcysteine, which reduce oxidative damage by acting as a sulfhydryl donor, and the disulfiram metabolite diethyldithiocarbamate to reduce cytochrome P450 2E1–mediated generation of hydroxyl radicals have also been evaluated.[49,52] Intravenous magnesium infusion has also been administered to prevent cisplatin-related AKI with mixed effects. Finally, reduced renal exposure can be achieved with the use of localized intraperitoneal administration in conjunction with systemic administration of sodium thiosulfate for those with peritoneal tumors.[46]

Management AKI caused by cisplatin therapy is usually partially reversible with time and supportive care, including dialysis. Kidney function indices should be closely followed, with S_{cr} and BUN concentrations checked daily. Serum magnesium, potassium, and calcium concentrations should be monitored daily and corrected as needed.[45] Hypocalcemia and hypokalemia may be difficult to reverse until hypomagnesemia is corrected. There is no role for dialysis to remove cisplatin. Progressive kidney disease caused by cumulative nephrotoxicity may be irreversible and in some cases may lead to ESKD and require chronic dialysis support.[45]

Amphotericin B Nephrotoxicity

Incidence Variable rates of amphotericin B nephrotoxicity are seen that correspond in large part to the cumulative dose administered. Nephrotoxicity may be seen in nearly 30% of patients receiving median cumulative doses as low as 240 mg and reaches an incidence of greater than 80% when cumulative doses approach 5 g.[53-55] Although numerous studies demonstrate lower rates of nephrotoxicity with liposomal formulations compared with conventional amphotericin B, it is difficult to compare rates of toxicity between products and studies because of the variability in the study populations, doses administered, and inconsistent definitions of nephrotoxicity and methods of assessment.[53,54,56]

Clinical Presentation Dose-dependent nephrotoxicity is often evident after administration of cumulative doses of 2 to 3 g as nonoliguria, renal tubular potassium, sodium, and magnesium wasting, impaired urinary concentrating ability, and distal renal tubular acidosis.[23,56] Although the cumulative dose is a significant risk factor, the time to onset of kidney injury varies considerably, ranging from a few days to weeks. Tubular dysfunction usually manifests 1 to 2 weeks after treatment is begun, and potassium and magnesium replacement may be necessary.[53] This is typically followed by a decrease in GFR and a rise in S_{cr} and BUN concentrations. Consequently, kidney function indices should be closely followed, with S_{cr} and BUN concentrations checked daily, and serum magnesium, potassium, and calcium concentrations monitored every other day and corrected as needed.

Pathogenesis Amphotericin B nephrotoxicity occurs predominantly via two mechanisms. The first is direct tubular epithelial cell toxicity resulting from interaction of amphotericin B with ergosterol in the cell membrane, leading to increased tubular cell membrane permeability, lipid peroxidation, and eventual necrosis of proximal tubular cells.[56] The second mechanism is afferent arteriolar vasoconstriction leading to a reduction in renal blood flow and GFR, and ischemic tubular injury.[23,56]

Risk Factors Risk factors that impact the likelihood of developing amphotericin B nephrotoxicity include preexisting kidney disease, large individual and cumulative doses, short infusion times, volume depletion, hypokalemia, increased age, and concomitant administration of diuretics and other nephrotoxins, including vancomycin and cyclosporine.[53,56]

Prevention Permanent decrements in GFR are best prevented by incorporating a low threshold (ie, if S_{cr} reaches 2 mg/dL [177 μmol/L] on 2 consecutive days) for stopping amphotericin B or switching to a liposomal formulation. Several lipid formulations of amphotericin B (eg, amphotericin B lipid complex, liposomal amphotericin B) are available and should be used in most high-risk patients as they reduce nephrotoxicity by enhancing drug delivery to sites of infection and reducing interaction with tubular epithelial cell membranes.[54,56] Nephrotoxicity can also be minimized by limiting the cumulative dose, increasing the infusion time, ensuring the patient is well hydrated, and avoiding concomitant administration of other nephrotoxins.[56] Administration of 1 L IV 0.9% sodium chloride daily during the course of therapy reduces toxicity and a single infusion of saline 10 to 15 mL/kg prior to administration of each dose of amphotericin B is generally recommended.[56] A number of other antifungal agents such as itraconazole, voriconazole, and caspofungin are viable alternatives and are now routinely used in lieu of amphotericin B for patients at high risk of developing nephrotoxicity. Administration of the antioxidant *N*-acetylcysteine (600 mg orally twice daily in adults) during amphotericin treatment may be nephroprotective.[57]

Management Amphotericin B nephrotoxicity is best treated by discontinuation of therapy and substitution of alternative antifungal therapy, if possible. Renal tubular dysfunction and glomerular filtration will improve gradually to some degree in most patients, but damage may be irreversible. Kidney function indices should be closely followed, with S_{cr} and BUN concentrations checked daily, and serum magnesium, potassium, and calcium concentrations should be monitored daily and corrected as needed.

Osmotic Nephropathy

Several drugs, including mannitol, low-molecular-weight dextran, hydroxyethyl starch, and radiographic contrast media, or drug vehicles, such as sucrose, maltose, and propylene glycol, are associated with osmotic nephropathy, which may rarely lead to ATN and AKI.[58] Since osmotic nephropathy does not necessarily negatively affect proximal tubular function, its presence may often go undetected in patients without overt signs of ATN. This likely contributes to the extremely low incidence of osmotic nephropathy reported for causative agents. IV immunoglobulin solutions containing hyperosmolar sucrose may cause osmotic nephropathy and AKI in 1% to 10% of cases, which is usually reversible shortly after discontinuing therapy.[59,60] Maltose-based IV immunoglobulin solutions have also been implicated in the development of osmotic nephropathy. Although IV immunoglobulin-induced AKI is the modern prototype for osmotic nephropathy, the vehicle (ie, sucrose or maltose) is the culprit and not the immunoglobulins themselves.[60] The SGLT-2 inhibitors have been associated with a kidney lesion reminiscent of osmotic nephropathy. Presumably, the proximal tubule encounters massive glucose loads that are reabsorbed (SGLT-1 transporter) and overwhelm cellular metabolism, though this is rare.[61]

Clinical Presentation

The clinical presentation of osmotic nephropathy is often subtle. While tubular proteinuria or vacuolated tubular cells may be observed on urinalysis for patients with AKI, the definitive diagnosis of osmotic nephropathy is only made via a kidney biopsy.[59] IV immunoglobulin-induced AKI typically presents as oliguria after 2 to 4 days of treatment and may persist for up to 2 weeks. Kidney injury occurs via uptake of the offending agent through pinocytosis into proximal tubular epithelial cells, subsequent formation of vacuoles, and accumulation of lysosomes, which collectively results in an oncotic gradient and thus cellular swelling, tubular luminal occlusion, and compromised cellular integrity.[62] Renal replacement therapy may be necessary for up to 40% of patients developing osmotic nephropathy-associated AKI.[59] However, it is usually reversible, with nearly all patients recovering normal kidney function following withdrawal of the offending drug.

Risk Factors

Risk factors for osmotic nephropathy include excessive doses of offending agents, preexisting kidney disease, ischemia, older age (greater than 65 years), and concomitant use of other nephrotoxins. Nephrotoxicity may be prevented by limiting the dose, reducing the rate of infusion, and avoiding dehydration and concomitant nephrotoxins.[60,62]

HEMODYNAMICALLY MEDIATED KIDNEY INJURY

4 Hemodynamically mediated kidney injury generally refers to any cause of AKI resulting from an acute decrease in intraglomerular pressure, including "prerenal" states leading to reduced effective renal blood flow (eg, hypovolemia and congestive heart failure) and medications that affect the renin–angiotensin system (RAS).[23,63] The kidneys receive approximately 25% of resting cardiac output, which renders them particularly susceptible to alterations in renal blood flow and enhances their exposure to circulating drugs.[16,64] Within each nephron, blood flow and pressure are regulated by glomerular afferent and efferent arterioles to maintain intraglomerular capillary hydrostatic pressure, glomerular filtration, and urine output. Afferent and efferent arteriolar vasoconstrictions are primarily mediated by angiotensin II, whereas afferent vasodilation is primarily mediated by prostaglandins (Fig. 65-1). This specialized blood flow is precisely regulated by interrelations between arachidonic acid metabolites, natriuretic factors, nitric oxide, the sympathetic nervous system, the RAS, and the macula densa response to distal tubular solute delivery.[64] Drug-induced causes of hemodynamic kidney injury typically stem from constriction of glomerular afferent arterioles and/or dilation of glomerular efferent arterioles. ACEIs, angiotensin II receptor blockers (ARBs), and NSAIDs are the agents that have been most commonly implicated.[23,65] Capillary leak syndrome due to a severe cytokine release syndrome (CRS) is associated with hemodynamically mediated AKI with high-dose interleukin-2 and the chimeric antigen receptor (CAR) T-cells.[66]

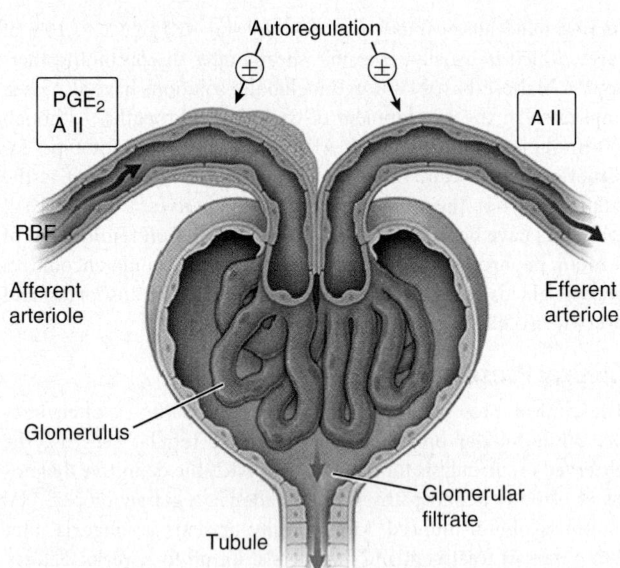

FIGURE 65-1 Normal glomerular autoregulation serves to maintain intraglomerular capillary hydrostatic pressure, glomerular filtration rate, and, ultimately, urine output. (A II, angiotensin II; PGE_2, prostaglandin E_2; RBF, renal blood flow.)

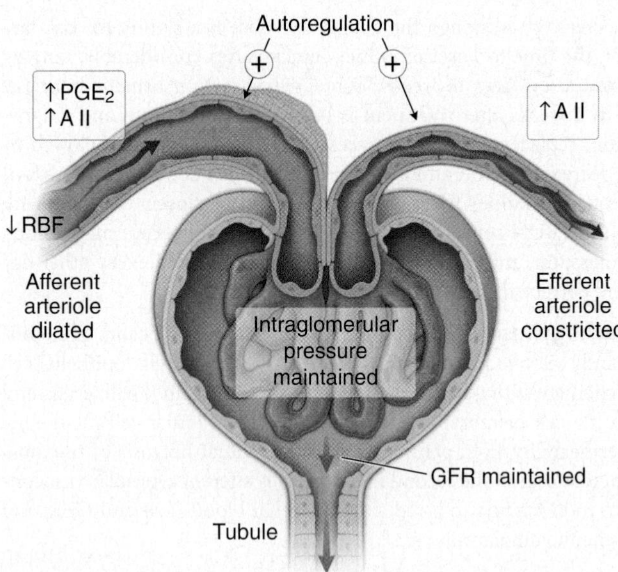

FIGURE 65-2 Glomerular autoregulation during "prerenal" states (ie, reduced blood flow).

Angiotensin-Converting Enzyme Inhibitors and Angiotensin II Receptor Blockers

ACEIs and ARBs are extensively utilized for the management of hypertension and prevention of the progression of CKD even though they have been associated with the development of AKI.

Incidence

Patients with renal artery stenosis, volume depletion, and congestive heart failure and those with preexisting kidney disease, including diabetic nephropathy, are most likely to experience a significant decline in kidney function when therapy with one of these agents is initiated.[23] For example, up to 25% of hospitalized patients with congestive heart failure develop AKI within weeks after beginning treatment with ACEIs.[67] Moreover, ACEIs and ARBs are among the most commonly implicated medications in emergency hospitalizations, contributing to nearly 3% of emergency room visits for adverse drug events.[68]

Clinical Presentation

Therapy with ACEIs and ARBs will acutely reduce GFR; so a moderate rise in S_{cr} after initiation of therapy should be anticipated.[69] Importantly, a distinction must be made between a potentially detrimental reduction in GFR and a normal, predictable rise in S_{cr}. An increase in S_{cr} of up to 30% is commonly observed within 3 to 5 days of initiating therapy and is an indication that the drug has begun to exert its desired pharmacologic effect.[69] The increase in S_{cr} typically stabilizes within 1 to 2 weeks and is usually reversible upon stopping the drug. Furthermore, an association exists between acute increases in S_{cr} of less than or equal to 30% from baseline that stabilize within the first 2 months of initiating therapy and preservation of kidney function. The S_{cr} threshold for discontinuation of ACEI or ARB therapy is unclear. However, an increase in S_{cr} of more than 30% above baseline in the course of 1 to 2 weeks may necessitate discontinuation of the offending drug.[69]

Pathogenesis

ACEIs—or ARB-mediated kidney injury—is primarily the result of disruption of normal autoregulation of intraglomerular capillary hydrostatic pressure.[23] Normally, the kidney attempts to maintain GFR by dilating the afferent arteriole and constricting the efferent arteriole in response to a decrease in renal blood flow. During states of reduced blood flow, the juxtaglomerular apparatus increases renin secretion. Plasma renin converts angiotensinogen to angiotensin I, and ultimately angiotensin II by angiotensin-converting enzyme. Angiotensin II constricts the afferent and efferent arterioles, but has a greater effect on the efferent arterioles, resulting in a net increase in intraglomerular pressure.[64] Additionally, renal prostaglandins, prostaglandin E_2 in particular, are released and induce a net dilation of the afferent arteriole, thereby improving blood flow into the glomerulus. Together these processes maintain GFR and urine output (Fig. 65-2).

When ACEI therapy (eg, enalapril or ramipril) is initiated, the synthesis of angiotensin II is decreased, thereby preferentially dilating the efferent arteriole. This reduces outflow resistance from the glomerulus and decreases hydrostatic pressure in the glomerular capillaries, which alters Starling forces across the glomerular capillaries to decrease intraglomerular pressure and GFR. This in turn often leads to nephrotoxicity, particularly in the setting of reduced renal blood flow or effective arterial blood volume (Fig. 65-3), that is, prerenal settings (eg, congestive heart failure) in which glomerular afferent arteriolar blood flow is reduced and the efferent arteriole is vasoconstricted to maintain sufficient glomerular capillary hydrostatic pressure for ultrafiltration.[23]

Risk Factors

Patients at greatest risk are those dependent on angiotensin II and renal efferent arteriolar constriction to maintain blood pressure and GFR. These include patients with bilateral renal artery stenosis or stenosis in a single kidney (ie, renal transplant); patients with decreased effective arterial blood volume (ie, prerenal states), especially those with decompensated congestive heart failure, volume depletion from excess diuresis or GI fluid loss, hepatic cirrhosis with ascites, and nephrotic syndrome; patients with preexisting kidney disease; and patients receiving concurrent nephrotoxic drugs, particularly other drugs that affect intraglomerular autoregulation such as NSAIDs.[23,65,70]

Prevention

Hemodynamically mediated AKI caused by ACEIs or ARBs is frequently preventable by recognizing the presence of preexisting

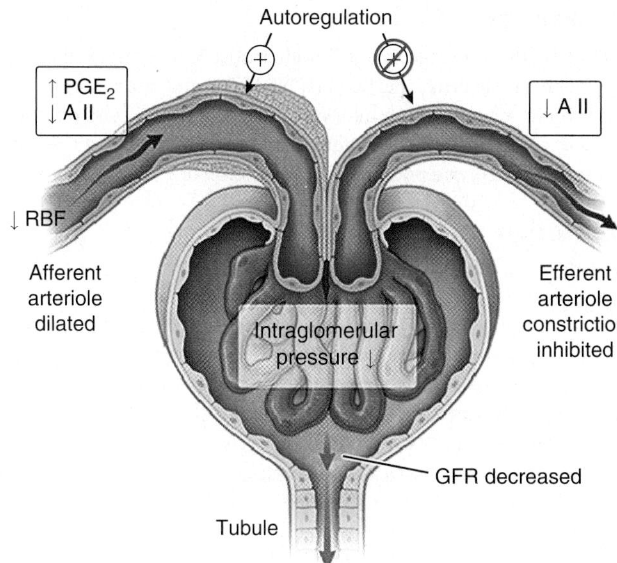

FIGURE 65-3 Pathogenesis of angiotensin-converting enzyme inhibitor (ACEI) nephropathy.

kidney disease or decreased effective renal blood flow as a result of volume depletion, heart failure, or liver disease. A common strategy for at-risk patients is to initiate therapy with low doses of a short-acting ACEI (eg, captopril 6.25-12.5 mg), then gradually titrate the dose upward, and convert to a longer-acting agent after patient tolerance has been demonstrated. Outpatients may be started on low doses of long-acting ACEIs (eg, enalapril 2.5 mg) with gradual dose titration every 2 to 4 weeks until the maximum dose or desired response is achieved.[69] Kidney function indices and serum potassium concentrations must be monitored carefully, daily for hospitalized patients and every 2 to 3 days for outpatients. Monitoring may need to be more frequent during outpatient initiation of ACEI or ARB therapy for patients with preexisting kidney disease, congestive heart failure, or suspected renovascular disease. Use of concurrent hypotensive agents and other drugs that affect renal hemodynamics (eg, NSAIDs, diuretics) should be discouraged and dehydration avoided.[69]

Management

Acute decreases in kidney function and the development of hyperkalemia usually resolve over several days after ACEI or ARB therapy is discontinued. Occasionally patients will require management of severe hyperkalemia, as described in detail in Chapter 70, "Potassium and Magnesium Homeostasis."

ACEIs or ARB therapy may frequently be reinitiated, particularly for patients with congestive heart failure, after intravascular volume depletion has been corrected or diuretic doses reduced. Slight reductions in kidney function (maintenance of a S_{cr} concentration of 2-3 mg/dL [177-265 μmol/L]) may be an acceptable trade-off for hemodynamic improvement in certain patients with severe congestive heart failure or renovascular disease not amenable to revascularization.

Nonsteroidal Anti-Inflammatory Drugs and Selective Cyclooxygenase-2 Inhibitors

The overall safety of NSAIDs is evidenced by the nonprescription availability in the United States of several drugs in the class (eg, ibuprofen, naproxen, ketoprofen). Although potential adverse renal effects from nonprescription NSAIDs had been a concern, conventional nonselective NSAIDs and selective cyclooxygenase-2 (COX-2) inhibitors are unlikely to acutely affect kidney function in the absence of renal ischemia or excess renal vasoconstrictor activity. Nevertheless, given their general safety and widespread availability, NSAIDs are among the most commonly used drugs, with approximately 111 million prescriptions worldwide and 30 billion over-the-counter doses of NSAIDs administered annually in the United States.[71]

Incidence

The incidence of NSAID-induced kidney injury is unclear. As many as 500,000 to 2.5 million people may develop some degree of NSAID nephrotoxicity in the United States annually.[72]

Clinical Presentation

NSAID- and COX-2-induced AKI usually occurs within 2 to 7 days of initiating therapy,[63,71] particularly with a short-acting agent such as ibuprofen, or within days of some other precipitating event (eg, intravascular volume depletion). Patients typically present with complaints of diminished urine output, weight gain, and/or edema. Urine sodium concentrations (less than 20 mEq/L [mmol/L]) and fractional excretion of sodium (less than 1% [0.01]) are usually low, and BUN, S_{cr}, potassium, and blood pressure are typically elevated. The urine sediment is usually bland and unchanged from baseline but may show occasional RTECs and granular casts.[63,71]

Pathogenesis

The pathogenesis of NSAID- and COX-2-induced AKI lies in the disruption of normal intraglomerular autoregulation.[63] Specifically, NSAIDs inhibit COX-catalyzed synthesis of vasodilatory prostaglandins, including prostaglandins I_2 (prostacyclin) and E_2, from arachidonic acid.[71] These prostaglandins are synthesized in the renal cortex and medulla by vascular endothelial and glomerular mesangial cells, and their effects are primarily local and result in net afferent arteriolar vasodilation. Vasodilatory prostaglandins have limited activity in states of normal renal blood flow, but in states of decreased renal blood flow, their synthesis is increased and they serve a vital autoregulatory role in the protection against renal ischemia and hypoxia by antagonizing renal arteriolar vasoconstriction due to angiotensin II, norepinephrine, endothelin, and vasopressin. Thus, administration of NSAIDs in the setting of reduced renal blood flow will blunt the usual compensatory increase in prostaglandin activity, altering the normal autoregulatory balance in favor of renal vasoconstrictors, thereby promoting renal ischemia and a reduction in glomerular filtration.[71]

Risk Factors

Risk factors for NSAID- and COX-2-induced AKI include age more than 60 years, preexisting kidney disease, hepatic disease with ascites, congestive heart failure, intravascular volume depletion/dehydration, systemic lupus erythematosus, or concurrent treatment with diuretics, ACEIs, or ARBs.[65,70,71] Use of ACEIs, diuretics, and NSAIDs concurrently is associated with a greater than 30% increased risk for AKI, which increases to greater than 60% in patients over age 75 or with preexisting kidney disease.[65,70] The elderly people are at higher risk because of multiple comorbidities, multiple-drug therapies, and reduced renal hemodynamics. Combined use of NSAIDs or COX-2 inhibitors and concurrent nephrotoxic drugs, particularly other drugs that affect intraglomerular autoregulation, should be avoided in high-risk patients.

Prevention

NSAID- and COX-2 inhibitor–induced AKI can be prevented by recognizing high-risk patients, avoiding potent compounds such as indomethacin and using analgesics with less prostaglandin inhibition, such as acetaminophen, nonacetylated salicylates, aspirin, and possibly nabumetone. Nonnarcotic analgesics (eg, tramadol) may also be useful but do not provide anti-inflammatory activity. When NSAID therapy is essential for high-risk patients, the minimal effective dose should be used for the shortest duration possible, and NSAIDs with short half-lives should be considered (eg, sulindac) along with optimal management of predisposing medical problems and frequent kidney function monitoring. Moreover, use of concurrent hypotensive agents and other drugs that affect renal hemodynamics (eg, ACEIs, ARBs, diuretics) should be discouraged in high-risk patients and dehydration avoided.[71]

Management

NSAID-induced AKI is treated by discontinuation of therapy and supportive care. Use of other nephrotoxic drugs should be avoided. Kidney injury is rarely severe, and kidney function generally recovers within 3 to 5 days.[63] Occasionally, the hemodynamic insult is sufficiently severe to cause ATN, which can prolong injury.

Cyclosporine and Tacrolimus

The calcineurin inhibitors cyclosporine and tacrolimus have dramatically enhanced the success of solid-organ transplantation. As many as 94% of kidney transplant patients are prescribed a calcineurin inhibitor–based immunosuppressive regimen.[73] Nephrotoxicity, however, remains a major dose-limiting adverse effect of both drugs. Although delayed chronic interstitial nephritis also is possible,[74] acute hemodynamically mediated kidney injury is an important mechanism of calcineurin inhibitor–induced nephrotoxicity.

Incidence

The reversible AKI occurred frequently in transplant recipients during the first 6 months of cyclosporine therapy. The five-year risk of CKD after transplantation of a nonrenal organ ranges from 7% to 21%, depending on the type of organ transplanted, and the occurrence of CKD in these patients is associated with more than a fourfold increase in the risk of death.[75]

Clinical Presentation

The clinical presentation of acute nephrotoxicity associated with calcineurin inhibitors (ie, hemodynamically mediated AKI) is quite different from the presentation of chronic nephrotoxicity (see "Chronic Interstitial Nephritis" section).[76] AKI may occur within days of initiating therapy, manifesting as a rise in S_{cr} concentration and a corresponding decline in creatinine clearance. Hypertension, hyperkalemia, sodium retention, oliguria, renal tubular acidosis, and hypomagnesemia are frequently observed in the absence of urine sediment abnormalities or morphologic lesions.[73] On the other hand, renal biopsy may reveal thickening of arterioles, mild focal glomerular sclerosis, proximal tubular epithelial cell vacuolization and atrophy, and interstitial fibrosis. Biopsy is most useful to distinguish acute calcineurin inhibitor nephrotoxicity from acute cellular rejection of the transplanted kidney, the latter being evidenced by interstitial infiltrates composed of activated lymphocytes (see Chapter 110, "Osteoarthritis").[77]

Pathogenesis

The acute hemodynamic changes associated with calcineurin inhibitor nephrotoxicity result from an increase in potent vasoconstrictors including thromboxane A_2 and endothelin, activation of the RAS and sympathetic nervous systems, as well as a reduction in the vasodilators nitric oxide, prostacyclin, and prostaglandin E_2.[73,75,76] The net effect is an imbalance in afferent and efferent tone, resulting in predominantly afferent vasoconstriction with reduced renal plasma flow and GFR. The mechanism of acute nephrotoxicity is generally thought to be dose related, since kidney function improves rapidly following dose reduction.[76]

Risk Factors

Risk factors include age over 65, higher dose, concomitant therapy with nephrotoxic drugs (particularly NSAIDs), and interacting drugs that inhibit calcineurin inhibitor metabolism and transport and thus increase systemic exposure, older kidney allograft age, salt depletion, diuretic use, and polymorphic expression of P-glycoprotein.[73,77]

Prevention

Because acute hemodynamically mediated kidney injury secondary to cyclosporine and tacrolimus is concentration related, pharmacokinetic and pharmacodynamic monitoring is an important means of preventing toxicity.[73] However, the persistent presence of therapeutic or low cyclosporine concentrations does not totally preclude the development of nephrotoxicity. Calcium channel blockers may antagonize the vasoconstrictor effect of cyclosporine by dilating glomerular afferent arterioles and preventing acute decreases in renal blood flow and glomerular filtration.[73] Lastly, decreased doses of cyclosporine or tacrolimus, primarily when used in combination with other nonnephrotoxic immunosuppressants, may minimize the risk of toxicity, but this may increase the risk of chronic rejection.

Management

AKI usually improves with dose reduction and treatment of contributing illness or the discontinuation of interacting drugs. CKD is usually irreversible, but progressive toxicity may be limited by discontinuation of cyclosporine (or tacrolimus) therapy or dose reduction, with the continuation of other immunosuppressants.[73,76] S_{cr} and BUN should be closely monitored (daily if possible), as should cyclosporine or tacrolimus concentrations, to ensure that serum concentrations are within the narrow therapeutic range.

SGLT-2 Inhibitors

The sodium-glucose co-transporter-2 (SGLT-2) inhibitors (eg, empagliflozin, canagliflozin, dapagliflozin) are now being employed frequently to enhance serum glucose control in patients with type 2 diabetes mellitus.[78] SGLT-2 inhibitor drugs are nephroprotective.[79,80] As such, they are FDA-approved and now used in addition to metformin to help with glucose control in patients with type 2 diabetes mellitus. The estimated GFR cutoffs for use of these drugs is <60 mL/min/1.73 m^2 for dapagliflozin and <45 mL/min/1.73 m^2 for empagliflozin and canagliflozin. However, AKI is one complication of canagliflozin and dapagliflozin that has been reported to the FDA Adverse Event Reporting System (FAERS). This led the FDA to issue an FDA Drug Safety Communication, http://www.fda.gov/downloads/Drugs/DrugSafety/UCM506772.pdf, for these two SGLT-2 inhibitors.

Incidence

There is no estimated incidence of AKI available for these drugs. However, over 100 cases of AKI associated with the SGLT-2 inhibitors have been reported to FAERS. This contrasts with the randomized controlled trials that do not note AKI as a complication of these drugs.[79,80] In addition, a propensity-matched analysis also showed no signal for AKI with these drugs.[81]

Pathogenesis

The increase in S_{cr} and development of AKI are likely related to a number of processes. As these drugs induce glucosuria due to inhibition of proximal tubular glucose reabsorption, they induce an osmotic diuresis (natriuresis) that can lead to volume depletion, especially when used along with diuretics. SGLT-2 inhibitor related volume depletion in the setting of RAS blocker therapy (ie, ACEI or ARB therapy) can lead to prominent hemodynamic (prerenal) AKI. When severe, acute tubular injury may develop leading to a classic form of ATN. In addition, the delivery of sodium chloride to the macula densa also induces a phenomenon known as tubuloglomerular feedback, which vasoconstricts glomerular afferent arterioles and reduces GFR, ultimately causing an increase in S_{cr}. The increase in S_{cr} may be interpreted by clinicians as indicative of AKI. However, over the long term, this effect is thought to be one of the major nephroprotective mechanisms of the SGLT-2 inhibitors by reducing hyperfiltration-related injury. The SGLT-2 inhibitors may cause direct tubular injury. Uricosuria induced by these drugs may cause both crystal-related tubular injury (crystal nephropathy) and crystal-independent mechanisms of injury.[82] Also, increased urinary glucose may promote intratubular oxidative stress by activating aldose reductase and sorbitol and fructose generation.[82]

Risk Factors

According to the FAERS reports, many patients developing AKI with these drugs were older, were also treated with RAS blockers and diuretics, and sometimes were also taking other nephrotoxins such as NSAIDs. Clearly, combining these drugs with the SGLT-2 inhibitors may lead to AKI when volume depletion occurs. Also, concurrent illness that leads to volume depletion (nausea, vomiting, diarrhea) may also increase risk for AKI.

Prevention

Prevention of AKI in patients with type 2 diabetes mellitus taking these drugs requires careful follow-up in patients who are also taking RAS blockers and diuretics. Patients should be counseled to avoid other nephrotoxins, in particular NSAIDs and COX-2 inhibitors, and contact their care provider when a concurrent illness develops. This will allow timely adjustment of the medications.

Management

When AKI develops, stopping the SGLT-2 inhibitor often is enough to allow kidney recovery. However, in patients with volume depletion on exam, holding the SGLT-2 inhibitor (and RAS blocker and diuretic if also prescribed) and giving intravenous fluids typically resolve AKI. In cases where ATN develops, the SGLT-2 inhibitor should be held and usual supportive care, including RRT when required, should be undertaken. The SGLT-2 inhibitor can likely be restarted in patients where kidney function recovers to baseline and eGFR is above the FDA-recommended threshold.

Chimeric Antigen Receptor T-Cells

Incidence

CAR T-cell therapy is a highly efficacious immunotherapy that employs the principle of adoptive cell transfer. T-cells are collected from patients and re-engineered to express selective tumor-targeted receptors (CARs) on cell surfaces. CARs function irrespective of any major histocompatibility complex restriction, making them immune to any T-cell evading mechanisms of tumor cells. The CAR T-cell therapy tisagenlecleucel is a CD-19 targeted therapy for B-cell acute lymphoblastic leukemia while axicabtagene ciloleucel is used to treat large B-cell lymphoma and brexucabtagene autoleucel is employed for relapsed/refractory mantle cell lymphoma.[83,84] CAR T-cell therapy is complicated by severe systemic inflammatory disorders that lead to AKI in 18.6% of patients, with up to 4.4% of patients developing AKI requiring dialysis.[85]

Pathogenesis

One of the most common toxicities observed with CAR-T therapy is CRS, which is characterized by high fever, hypotension, hypoxia, and multi-organ toxicity including AKI. CRS is triggered by a surge of cytokines and chemokines released by activated T-cells and by bystander immune cells. CRS typically manifests in the first week (median 2-3 days) after the CAR T-cell infusion and peaks within 1 to 2 weeks.[86] Patients at highest risk have bulky disease and multiple comorbidities. AKI is due to primarily to either hemodynamic (prerenal) kidney dysfunction or ischemic acute tubular injury (with severe hypotension and high grade CRS). Cytokine-mediated kidney injury, hemophagocytic lymphohistiocytosis (hyperactivation of lymphocytes and macrophages), and tumor lysis syndrome may also play a role, but have not been verified with kidney biopsy evidence. Infectious complications with sepsis and nephrotoxic medications (antibiotics, NSAIDs, etc.) may also contribute to AKI in these patients.[66,86]

Management

Management of AKI from CAR T-cell treatment is primarily focused on the severity (grade) of CRS with the overall goal to balance treatment of CRS complications and end-organ injury with beneficial effects of the anti-cancer therapy. Supportive care includes vasopressors and intravenous fluids for hypotension, while anti–interleukin-6 therapy with tocilizumab or siltuximab with/without corticosteroids is used for severe CRS.[66,86]

OBSTRUCTIVE NEPHROPATHY

Numerous medications may cause obstructive nephropathy, or kidney injury from deposition or precipitation within the renal tubules and/or collecting system. For example, the precipitation of drug crystals in distal tubular lumens can lead to intratubular obstruction, interstitial nephritis, and occasionally superimposed ATN, collectively termed "crystal nephropathy." Nephrolithiasis, the formation of stones within the kidney, results from abnormal crystal precipitation in the renal collecting system, potentially causing urinary tract obstruction with kidney injury. Several medications that have been associated with development of obstructive nephropathy are listed in Table 65-1.

Crystal Nephropathy

Incidence

The incidence of crystal nephropathy is unclear for most of the implicated agents because histologically confirmed cases are rare, and many drugs cause kidney injury via multiple mechanisms.[87] For example, AKI develops in approximately 2% of patients who receive high-dose methotrexate, likely due to a combination of direct toxic effects and crystal nephropathy.[88,89] Similarly, crystalluria is observed in 20% of patients receiving indinavir, but the number of patients developing crystal nephropathy is unknown.[90]

Pathogenesis

Drugs may induce intratubular obstruction and AKI by direct (precipitation of the drug itself) and indirect means (ie, promoting release and precipitation of tissue-degradation products or cellular casts). For example, antineoplastic drugs may cause acute renal tubular obstruction indirectly by inducing tumor lysis syndrome, hyperuricemia, and intratubular precipitation of uric acid crystals.[50] The diagnosis is supported by a urine uric acid-to-creatinine ratio greater than 1. Uric acid precipitation can be prevented by vigorous hydration with normal saline, beginning at least 48 hours prior to chemotherapy, to maintain urine output 100 mL/hr in adults. Administration of allopurinol 100 mg/m^2 thrice daily (maximum of 800 mg/day) started 2 to 3 days prior to chemotherapy, and urinary alkalinization to pH 7 may also be of value. In patients at high risk of developing tumor lysis syndrome (ie, large tumor burden, preexisting kidney disease, and older age), a single fixed dose of 3 mg rasburicase may be beneficial.[91]

Drug-induced rhabdomyolysis is another form of indirect toxicity, which can lead to intratubular precipitation of myoglobin and, if severe, AKI.[92] The most common cause of drug-induced rhabdomyolysis is direct myotoxicity from 3-hydroxy-3-methylglutaryl-coenzyme A (HMG-CoA) reductase inhibitors or statins, including lovastatin and simvastatin.[93] The risk of rhabdomyolysis is increased when these drugs are administered concurrently with gemfibrozil, niacin, or inhibitors of the CYP3A4 metabolic pathway (eg, erythromycin and itraconazole).

Anticoagulant nephropathy, including warfarin-related nephropathy, is characterized by glomerular hemorrhage with subsequent intratubular obstruction by red blood cell casts. Patients with underlying CKD appear to be at greatest risk. The incidence of warfarin-related nephropathy may be as high as 33% in CKD versus 16.5% in non-CKD patients. Other risk factors included age, diabetes mellitus, hypertension, and cardiovascular disease.[94]

Intratubular precipitation of drugs or their metabolites can also directly cause AKI. Precipitation of drug crystals is due primarily to supersaturation of a low urine volume with the offending drug or relative insolubility of the drug in either alkaline or acidic urine.[90] Volume depletion is an important risk factor for the development of AKI. Urine pH decreases to approximately 4.5 during maximal stimulation of renal tubular hydrogen ion secretion. Certain solutes can precipitate and obstruct the tubular lumen at this acid pH, particularly when urine is concentrated, such as for patients with volume depletion. For example, several antiviral drugs have been associated with intratubular precipitation and AKI.[95,96] Acyclovir is relatively insoluble at physiologic urine pH and is associated with intratubular precipitation in dehydrated oliguric patients.[90] Foscarnet complexation with ionized calcium may result in precipitation of calcium-foscarnet salt crystals in renal glomeruli, causing primarily a crystalline glomerulonephritis. The salt crystals may then secondarily precipitate in the renal tubules causing tubular necrosis.[23] The protease inhibitors indinavir and atazanavir have been associated with symptomatic crystalluria or nephrolithiasis in 20% to 33% of patients receiving chronic treatment.[90,96] Intratubular indinavir or atazanavir crystal precipitation can be prevented in most patients if the patient consumes adequate hydration to obtain a urinary output of at least 1,500 mL/day.[95] Sulfadiazine, when used at high doses, and methotrexate may also precipitate in acidic urine and can cause oligoanuric kidney injury.[90] Massive administration of ascorbic acid can also result in obstruction of renal tubules with calcium oxalate crystals, leading to "oxalate nephropathy."[90] Triamterene and the quinolone antibiotic ciprofloxacin may also precipitate in renal tubules and cause kidney injury.[23,87]

Kidney injury caused by intratubular precipitation of most tissue-degradation products or drugs and their metabolites can be largely prevented and possibly treated by administering the drug after vigorously prehydrating the patient, maintaining a high urine volume, and urinary alkalinization.[95,96]

Vancomycin Cast Nephropathy

Vancomycin-associated AKI may also be due to the formation of obstructive tubular casts composed of noncrystal nanospheric vancomycin aggregates admixed with uromodulin.[97] These distinctive casts are observed in some patients with AKI associated with high vancomycin trough concentrations. On kidney biopsy, acute tubulointerstitial inflammation is associated with these tubular casts. Co-precipitation of vancomycin and uromodulin occurs.[98]

Acute Phosphate Nephropathy

Nephrocalcinosis is a clinical pathologic condition characterized by extensive tubulointerstitial precipitation and deposition of calcium phosphate crystals leading to marked tubular calcification.[99] It is most commonly seen in clinical conditions associated with hypercalcemia and hypercalciuria, such as hyperparathyroidism, malignancy, and less frequently increased intake of calcium or vitamin D. However, nephrocalcinosis can also result from hyperphosphatemia and hyperphosphaturia in the absence of hypercalcemia, as is known to occur for patients who have received oral sodium phosphate solution (OSPS) as a bowel preparation.[100]

The term "acute phosphate nephropathy" was coined specifically to describe OSPS-induced nephrocalcinosis, as its pathogenesis is the result of increased phosphate intake rather than hypercalcemia.[100] Nephrocalcinosis is associated with use of OSPS for bowel preparation prior to GI procedures, and strong associations are present between exposure to OSPS and a decline in kidney function, particularly in the elderly and those with preexisting kidney disease.[100,101]

Incidence

The incidence of acute phosphate nephropathy is between 1 in 1,000 and 1 in 5,000 exposures, translating to roughly 1,400 to 7,000 new cases annually.[102]

Clinical Presentation

Patients usually present with AKI several days to months after exposure to OSPS. Low-grade proteinuria (less than 1 g/day), normocalcemia, and bland urinary sediment are usually observed. Extensive deposition of calcium phosphate in the distal tubules and collecting ducts without glomerular or vascular injury is the hallmark of acute phosphate nephropathy.[90]

Risk Factors

Risk factors include advanced age, preexisting kidney disease, female sex, hypertension, diabetes, bowel conditions associated with prolonged intestinal transit, high sodium phosphate dosage, volume depletion, and medications that affect renal perfusion or function (eg, diuretics, lithium, NSAIDs, ACEIs, or ARBs).[100]

Nephrolithiasis

Nephrolithiasis (formation of renal calculi or kidney stones) does not present as classic nephrotoxicity since GFR is usually not decreased. Drug-induced nephrolithiasis can be the result of abnormal crystal precipitation in the renal collecting system, potentially causing pain, hematuria, infection, or, occasionally, urinary tract obstruction with kidney injury. The overall prevalence of drug-induced nephrolithiasis is about 1% to 2% of all cases of nephrolithiasis.[96]

Kidney stone formation, possibly also accompanied by intratubular precipitation of crystalline material, has been a rare complication of drug therapy. Until the development of antiretroviral drugs, triamterene had been the drug most frequently associated with kidney stone formation, with a prevalence of 0.4%.[87] Sulfadiazine is a poorly soluble sulfonamide that may cause symptomatic acetylsulfadiazine crystalluria with stone formation and flank or back pain, hematuria, or kidney injury.[90] A high urine volume and urinary alkalinization to pH greater than 7.15 may be protective. Numerous other drugs have been implicated in the development of nephrolithiasis, including the antibacterial agents ciprofloxacin, amoxicillin, and nitrofurantoin, and various products containing ephedrine, norephedrine, pseudoephedrine, and melamine. Moreover, nephrolithiasis has become a well-known complication of antiretroviral agents, including the protease inhibitors indinavir, atazanavir, nelfinavir, amprenavir, saquinavir, ritonavir, and darunavir.[96]

GLOMERULAR DISEASE

Proteinuria, particularly nephrotic range proteinuria (defined as urine protein excretion greater than 3.5 g/day) with or without a decline in the GFR is a hallmark sign of glomerular injury (see Chapter e66, "Glomerulonephritis"). Glomerular injury associated with drug exposure is broadly classified into either direct cellular toxicity or immune-mediated injury. Glomerular lesions associated with direct cellular toxicity include thrombotic microangiopathy (see "Renal Vasculitis" section), minimal change glomerular disease, and focal segmental glomerulosclerosis (FSGS). Lesions from immune-mediated injury include vasculitis (see "Renal Vasculitis" section) and membranous nephropathy.[103,104] Although drug-induced glomerular disease is uncommon, a variety of agents have been implicated.

Minimal Change Glomerular Disease

Drug-induced minimal change glomerular disease is frequently accompanied by interstitial nephritis and is most common during NSAID therapy. Lithium, pamidronate, interferon-α, and interferon-β have also been implicated.[103] Patients present abruptly with nephrotic range proteinuria, hypoalbuminemia, and hyperlipidemia and rarely with hematuria and hypertension. The pathogenesis is unknown, but nephrotic range proteinuria as a consequence of NSAID therapy is frequently associated with a T-lymphocytic interstitial infiltrate, suggesting disordered cell-mediated immunity.[71] Proteinuria usually resolves rapidly after discontinuation of the offending drug, and a course of corticosteroids (eg, prednisone) may help resolve the lesion. That said, the majority of adults with NSAID-induced minimal change glomerular disease achieve complete remission over the course of several months, even in the absence of corticosteroid treatment.[103]

Focal Segmental Glomerulosclerosis

FSGS is characterized by patchy areas (ie, only some glomeruli are partially affected by the disease) of glomerular sclerosis with interstitial inflammation and fibrosis (see Chapter e66). It represents a pattern of glomerular injury, not a disease per se, and is the final common pathway by which normal glomerular components are replaced by fibrous scar tissue. FSGS has been described in the setting of chronic heroin abuse (known as *heroin nephropathy*).[105] The pathogenesis is unknown but may include direct toxicity by heroin or adulterants and injury from bacterial or viral infections accompanying IV drug use. The bisphosphonates pamidronate and zoledronate, commonly used to treat osteoporosis, malignancy-associated hypercalcemia, and Paget's disease, are associated with the development of a particularly aggressive variant of FSGS called *collapsing glomerulopathy*.[103] It presents with massive proteinuria (greater than 8 g/day), and it is typically characterized by rising S_{cr} at diagnosis and rapid progression to ESKD. Patients receiving IV formulations, high doses, or prolonged therapy are at highest risk. Interferon-α, interferon-β, lithium, sirolimus, and anabolic steroids have also been associated with FSGS.

Membranous Nephropathy

Membranous nephropathy is the most common etiology of nephrotic syndrome in Caucasian adults.[104] It is characterized by subepithelial immune complex formation along glomerular capillary loops and, although rarely seen, has classically been associated with gold therapy, penicillamine, captopril, and NSAID use.[104] Patients present with nephrotic range proteinuria and microscopic hematuria, with hypertension and elevated S_{cr} apparent for patients with more advanced disease. The pathogenesis may involve damage to proximal tubule epithelium with antigen release, antibody formation, and glomerular immune complex deposition.[104] Proteinuria usually resolves slowly after discontinuing the offending drug. Patients who remain nephrotic after 6 months should be treated with a 6- to 12-month course of immunosuppressive therapy, which typically consists of prednisone with or without cyclophosphamide.

TUBULOINTERSTITIAL NEPHRITIS

Tubulointerstitial nephritis refers to diseases in which the predominant changes occur in the renal interstitium rather than the tubules. The presentation may be acute and reversible with interstitial edema, rapid loss of kidney function, and systemic symptoms or chronic and irreversible, associated with interstitial fibrosis and minimal to no systemic symptoms.[106]

Acute Allergic Interstitial Nephritis

Incidence

5 The incidence of drug-induced acute allergic interstitial nephritis (AIN) is unclear and likely varies with clinical setting. For example, pathology registries indicate AIN as the histologic lesion in only 2% to 5% of kidney biopsies, but from 10% to 27% of kidney biopsies performed in hospitalized patients with unexplained AKI demonstrate AIN.[63] Multiple drugs have been implicated in the development of AIN (Table 65-4). It usually manifests 2 weeks after exposure to a drug but may occur sooner if the patient was previously sensitized.[107]

Clinical Presentation

Although methicillin-induced AIN is the prototype for AIN, AIN is associated with all β-lactam antibiotics (including cephalosporins) and numerous other antimicrobials. Clinical signs present approximately 14 days after initiation of therapy and include (with their approximate incidence) fever (27%-80%), maculopapular rash (15%-25%), eosinophilia (23%-80%), arthralgia (45%), and oliguria (50%).[107] The systemic hypersensitivity findings of the classic

TABLE 65-4 Drugs Associated with Allergic Interstitial Nephritis

Antimicrobials	
Acyclovir	Indinavir
Aminoglycosides	Rifampin
Amphotericin B	Sulfonamides
β-Lactams	Tetracyclines
Ciprofloxacin	Trimethoprim–sulfamethoxazole
Ethambutol	Vancomycin
Diuretics	
Acetazolamide	Loop diuretics
Amiloride	Triamterene
Chlorthalidone	Thiazide diuretics
Neuropsychiatric	
Carbamazepine	Phenytoin
Lithium	Valproic acid
Phenobarbital	
Nonsteroidal anti-inflammatory drugs	
Aspirin	Ketoprofen
Indomethacin	Phenylbutazone
Naproxen	Diclofenac
Ibuprofen	Zomepirac
Diflunisal	Cyclooxygenase-2 inhibitors
Piroxicam	
Miscellaneous	
Acetaminophen	Immune checkpoint inhibitors
Allopurinol	Lansoprazole
Interferon-α	Methyldopa
Aspirin	Omeprazole
Azathioprine	P-aminosalicylic acid
Captopril	Phenylpropanolamine
Cimetidine	Propylthiouracil
Clofibrate	Radiographic contrast media
Cyclosporine	Ranitidine
Glyburide	Sulfinpyrazone
Gold	Warfarin sodium

triad of fever, rash, and arthralgia, often along with eosinophilia and eosinophiluria, supported the diagnosis of AIN. However, this constellation of findings is not consistently reliable as one or more are frequently absent. In fact, the triad is seen in only 5% to 10% of patients with AIN, so caution is warranted in basing diagnosis on hypersensitivity findings alone.[108] Eosinophilia alone is insensitive, and eosinophiluria is insensitive and nonspecific, so urinary eosinophils are not considered a useful sign of AIN and are no longer recommended as a diagnostic test.[108] Anemia, leukocytosis, and elevated immunoglobulin E levels may occur. Tubular dysfunction may be manifested by acidosis, hyperkalemia, salt wasting, and concentrating defects.[107]

Nonsteroidal Anti-Inflammatory Drugs NSAID-induced AIN has a different clinical presentation than that seen with most other drugs. Patients are typically over 50 years of age (reflecting NSAID use for degenerative joint disease), the onset is delayed a mean of 6 months from initiation of therapy compared with 2 weeks with β-lactams, and fever, rash, and eosinophilia are typically not observed in patients with NSAID-induced AIN.[100] Concomitant nephrotic syndrome (proteinuria greater than 3.5 g/day) occurs in more than 70% of patients. Prompt diagnosis of AIN is important as discontinuation of the offending drug may prevent irreversible renal damage. Renal biopsy is the most definitive method for diagnosis.

Proton Pump Inhibitors The proton pump inhibitors (PPIs) are widely prescribed to treat acid-related gastrointestinal disease. While they are generally well tolerated and safe, AIN is a complication and it may lead to AKI, and rarely to CKD.[109] In contrast to the classic allergic presentation of AKI seen with the β-lactams, fever, rash, and eosinophilia are rarely seen with PPIs. In addition, the latent period from PPI exposure to AIN is much longer (weeks to months). Kidney biopsy is often required to definitively diagnose PPI-related AIN due to the lack of diagnostic clinical and laboratory findings.[110]

Immune Checkpoint Inhibitors Immune checkpoint inhibitors are a novel class of cancer immunotherapy noted to be associated with AKI, which is due primarily to AIN.[66,111,112] The incidence of AKI associated with these drugs ranges between 1% and 5%, with kidney biopsy showing AIN in more than 80% of patients.[111] These drugs (monoclonal antibodies) target immune pathways, including the receptors cytotoxic T-lymphocyte antigen-4 (CTLA-4), programmed cell death protein-1 (PD-1), and the T-cell receptor ligand (PD-ligand-1), that dampen T-cell activation and effector responses to prevent autoimmunity. Cancer cells, however, use these pathways to escape targeting by the immune system. In inhibiting such pathways, immune checkpoint inhibitors stimulate T-cell responses against cancer cells. Off-target organ injury, termed "immune-related adverse events," including AIN has been described. AIN has been observed in patients receiving anti-PD-1 agents either as monotherapy or in combination with anti-CTLA-4 drugs.[66,111,112] The mechanism underlying immune checkpoint inhibitor–associated AIN is unknown, but may be similar to the previously described mechanisms behind AIN from other drugs. Immune checkpoint inhibitors may also favor development of autoantibodies or encourage a pro-inflammatory cytokine milieu.[66] Patients may present with either other immune-related adverse events or no symptoms. Clinical findings such as rash and eosinophilia may not be encountered, while laboratory tests such as pyuria and white blood cell casts are present only occasionally. Diagnosis of immune checkpoint inhibitor–associated AIN generally requires kidney biopsy.

Pathogenesis

The pathogenesis of the majority of cases of AIN is considered to be an allergic hypersensitivity response. This is supported by the fact that AIN is characterized as a diffuse or focal interstitial infiltrate of lymphocytes, eosinophils, and occasional polymorphonuclear neutrophils.[106] Granulomas and tubular epithelial cell necrosis are relatively common with drug-induced AIN. Occasionally a humoral antibody-mediated mechanism is implicated by the presence of circulating antibody to a drug hapten–tubular basement membrane complex, low serum complement levels, and deposition of immunoglobulin G and complement in the tubular basement membrane. More commonly, a cell-mediated immune mechanism is suggested by the absence of these findings and the presence of a predominantly T-lymphocyte.[106]

Risk Factors

Despite this being an idiosyncratic hypersensitivity reaction, recent studies suggest that underlying CKD, receipt of drugs such as PPIs and NSAIDs, and combination immune checkpoint inhibitor therapy increase risk for AKI.[111] Individuals with other drug allergies may have increased risk and warrant close monitoring.

Prevention

No specific preventive measures are known because of the idiosyncratic nature of these reactions. Patients must be monitored carefully to recognize the signs and symptoms because promptly discontinuing the offending drug often leads to full recovery.[107]

Management

Corticosteroid therapy may be beneficial and should be initiated immediately or soon after diagnosis of AIN along with discontinuance of the offending drug to avoid the risk of incomplete recovery of kidney function. While various regimens have been used, high-dose oral prednisone 1 mg/kg/day for 4 to 6 weeks with a stepwise taper over the next 4 weeks may be considered. However, if there is no significant improvement in kidney function after 3 to 4 weeks of treatment, then steroids should be discontinued.[106] Typical kidney function indices (eg, S_{cr}, BUN) and signs and symptoms of AIN should be monitored closely for improvement. In PPI-induced AIN, drug discontinuation and corticosteroids are effective in most but not all cases, with CKD occurring in a significant number.[109] Management of immune checkpoint inhibitor–associated AIN generally includes drug discontinuation and corticosteroids, although recommendations on dose and duration are lacking.[66] Rechallenge with an immune checkpoint inhibitor is associated with recurrent AKI in approximately 23% of patients.[111]

Chronic Interstitial Nephritis

Lithium, analgesics, calcineurin inhibitors, aristolochic acid, and only a few other drugs cause chronic interstitial nephritis, which is usually a progressive and irreversible lesion.

Lithium

Incidence The prevalence of non-dialysis-dependent CKD stemming from chronic lithium nephrotoxicity in the general population of patients treated with lithium is approximately 1%.[113,114] The prevalence of lithium-induced ESKD among all ESKD patients is between 0.2% and 0.8%.[113] Although several renal tubular lesions are associated with lithium therapy, an impaired ability to concentrate urine (nephrogenic diabetes insipidus) is seen in 20% of all patients receiving lithium therapy.[115]

Clinical Presentation Lithium-induced nephrotoxicity is typically asymptomatic and develops insidiously during years of therapy. Blood pressure is normal and urinary sediment is bland, making detection difficult until the disease progresses significantly.[116] It is usually recognized by rising BUN or S_{cr} concentrations or the onset of hypertension. Polydipsia (excessive thirst) and polyuria (excessive urination) are observed in 40% and 20%, respectively, of patients with nephrogenic diabetes insipidus (see Chapter 68, "Disorders of Sodium and Water Homeostasis"). Although interstitial fibrosis may be observed as early as five years after beginning therapy, lithium-induced CKD usually occurs after 10 to 20 years of lithium treatment.[116]

Pathogenesis The precise mechanism of chronic lithium-induced nephrotoxicity is not well characterized. Impaired ability to concentrate urine is a result of a decrease in collecting duct response to antidiuretic hormone, which may be related to downregulation of aquaporin 2 water channel expression during lithium therapy.[116] Chronic tubulointerstitial nephritis attributed to lithium is evidenced most commonly by kidney biopsy findings of interstitial fibrosis, tubular atrophy, tubular microcysts, and glomerular sclerosis. The tubular microcysts can sometimes be visualized on imaging studies such as MRI. The pathogenesis may involve cumulative direct lithium toxicity, since duration of therapy correlates with the decline in the GFR.[116]

Risk Factors The duration of lithium therapy and cumulative dose was considered the major determinants of chronic nephrotoxicity. However, this is now questionable, as long-term lithium therapy in the absence of episodes of acute intoxication may not be nephrotoxic.[117] Increased age may also be a risk factor, but daily dose is not.[114,116]

Prevention Prevention of acute and chronic toxicity includes maintaining lithium concentrations as low as therapeutically possible, avoiding dehydration, and monitoring kidney function. It is unknown whether progression to CKD can be prevented by stopping lithium use when mild kidney injury is first recognized. This poses a dilemma as lithium is highly effective for affective disorders and the risks and potential benefits of discontinuing such a beneficial drug need to be carefully considered.[116] However, if lithium therapy is continued, kidney function must be monitored and therapy discontinued if it continues to decline. Amiloride has been used for prevention and treatment of lithium-induced nephrogenic diabetes insipidus, since it blocks epithelial sodium transport of lithium into the cortical collecting duct in the distal nephron.[116]

Management Symptomatic polyuria and polydipsia can be reversed by discontinuation of lithium therapy or ameliorated with amiloride 5 to 10 mg daily during continued lithium therapy (see Chapter 68). If polyuria does not resolve within 7 to 10 days of therapy, then the amiloride dose should be increased to 20 mg daily. Progressive chronic interstitial nephritis is treated by discontinuation of lithium therapy, adequate hydration, and avoidance of other nephrotoxic agents. Lithium serum concentrations, as well as kidney function indices, including urine output, BUN, and S_{cr}, should be monitored closely for resolution of signs and symptoms of toxicity.[116]

Cyclosporine and Tacrolimus

Delayed chronic tubulointerstitial nephritis, considered the Achilles' heel of calcineurin inhibitor–based immunosuppressive regimens, may occur after several months of therapy and can result in irreversible kidney disease.[73,74] Toxicity is progressive and usually manifests as a slowly rising S_{cr} concentration and decreased creatinine clearance that may not reflect the severity of histopathologic changes. All three compartments of the kidney can be affected, evidenced by typical biopsy findings that include arteriolar hyalinosis, glomerular sclerosis, and a striped pattern of tubulointerstitial fibrosis.[74] The pathogenesis involves sustained renal arteriolar endothelial cell injury and increased extracellular matrix synthesis, which ultimately result in chronic ischemia of the tubulointerstitial compartment because of increased release of endothelin-1, decreased production of nitric acid, and upregulation of transforming growth factor-β. Unlike acute nephrotoxicity, chronic toxicity is not dose dependent.[73,74]

Aristolochic Acid

Incidence Although the true incidence of aristolochic acid nephropathy is unknown, approximately 3% to 5% of patients who consume the natural product develop interstitial fibrosis with tubular atrophy.[118]

Clinical Presentation Patients with aristolochic acid nephropathy typically present with mild-to-moderate hypertension, mild proteinuria, glucosuria, and moderately elevated S_{cr} concentrations. Anemia and shrunken kidneys are also common on initial presentation.[119] The overwhelming majority of cases to date have been in women. The main pathologic lesions observed in the kidneys are interstitial fibrosis with atrophy and destruction of proximal tubules throughout the renal cortex; in general, the glomeruli are not affected. Perhaps the most remarkable feature of aristolochic acid nephropathy is the rate at which it progresses. In most individuals, ESKD requiring dialysis or transplantation develops within 6 to 24 months of exposure. An alarming high prevalence (approximately 40%-45%) of urothelial transitional cell carcinoma has been observed in Belgian patients who underwent renal transplantation.[118,119]

Pathogenesis The precise mechanism of aristolochic acid nephropathy and urothelial carcinoma has yet to be characterized. The major components of aristolochic acid are metabolized to mutagenic compounds called *aristolactam I* and *aristolactam II*, respectively, which form aristolochic acid–DNA adducts in humans. These adducts cause direct DNA damage and may lead to proximal tubular atrophy and apoptosis.[119]

Prevention The primary means of preventing aristolochic acid nephropathy is the limitation of exposure to compounds containing aristolochic acids. Several countries, including the United States, the United Kingdom, Canada, Australia, and Germany, have banned the use of herbs containing *Aristolochia*.[119] In patients that develop aristolochic acid nephropathy, treatment with corticosteroids along with toxin elimination have beneficial results.

Papillary Necrosis

Papillary necrosis is a form of chronic tubulointerstitial nephritis characterized by necrosis of the renal papillae, the regions of the kidney where the collecting ducts enter the renal pelvis, which leads to progressive kidney disease. Papillary necrosis is associated with diabetes, sickle cell disease, obstruction and infection of the urinary tract, and most commonly analgesic use.[120]

Analgesic Nephropathy

Incidence Prototypical analgesic nephropathy is characterized by chronic tubulointerstitial nephritis with papillary necrosis.[120] Chronic excessive consumption of combination analgesics, particularly those containing phenacetin, was believed to be the major cause and led to the removal of phenacetin and phenacetin mixtures from most world markets. However, contemporary analgesics, particularly aspirin, acetaminophen, and NSAIDs, alone or in combination, are also associated with the development of analgesic nephropathy. The incidence of analgesic nephropathy has declined significantly since removal of phenacetin from many countries, with the prevalence now less than 5% in the US-adult ESKD population.[120]

Clinical Presentation Analgesic nephropathy is a progressive disease that evolves slowly over several years.[120] It is difficult to recognize in the early stages of the disease because patients are often asymptomatic, and it may be underdiagnosed as a cause of ESKD. It is seen more commonly in women than men. Early manifestations are generally nonspecific and may include headache and upper GI symptoms; later manifestations include impaired urinary concentrating ability, dysuria, sterile pyuria, microscopic hematuria, mild proteinuria (less than 1.5 g/day), and lower back pain. As disease progresses, hypertension, atherosclerotic cardiovascular disease, renal calculi, and bladder stones are common, and pyelonephritis is a classic finding in advanced analgesic nephropathy. The most sensitive and specific diagnostic criteria include: (a) a history of chronic daily habitual analgesic ingestion (daily use for at least 3 to 5 years); (b) IV pyelography, renal ultrasound, or renal computed tomography imaging, which reveals decreased renal mass and bumpy renal contours; (c) elevated S_{cr}, that is, up to 4 mg/dL (354 μmol/L); and (d) papillary calcifications.[120]

Pathogenesis Analgesic nephropathy originates in the papillary tip as a result of accumulated toxins, drugs and metabolites, decreased blood flow, and impaired cellular energy production. The metabolism of phenacetin to acetaminophen, which is then oxidized to toxic-free radicals that are concentrated in the papilla, is the initiating factor that causes toxicity by mechanisms analogous to acetaminophen hepatotoxicity via glutathione depletion.[121] Cortical interstitial nephritis develops secondary to papillary necrosis. Salicylates potentiate these effects by also depleting renal glutathione, and inhibiting prostaglandin-mediated vasodilation, thus further predisposing the renal medulla to ischemic injury.[121]

Risk Factors The epidemiology of analgesic use and analgesic nephropathy continues to evolve. The classic concept persists that risk for ESKD increases with cumulative consumption of combination analgesics, phenacetin, or acetaminophen and aspirin or NSAIDs. Caffeine contained in combination analgesics may increase risk, but the role is not clear.[120] Chronic use of therapeutic doses of NSAIDs or high-dose acetaminophen, but not aspirin or salicylates alone, can cause analgesic nephropathy.

Prevention Prevention has depended primarily on public health efforts to restrict the sale of phenacetin and combination analgesics. However, risk continues with ongoing availability of nonprescription combination analgesics containing aspirin, acetaminophen, and caffeine in the United States and throughout the world.

Individuals requiring chronic analgesic therapy may reduce risk by limiting the total dose, avoiding combined use of two or more analgesics, and maintaining good hydration to prevent renal ischemia and decrease the papillary concentration of toxic substances. Acetaminophen remains the preferred nonopiate analgesic for patients with preexisting kidney disease.

Management Treatment of established nephrotoxicity requires cessation of analgesic consumption.[121] This can prevent progression and may improve kidney function. Kidney function indices, including urine output, BUN, and S_{cr}, should be monitored every several months. Patients should also be monitored for the development of transitional cell carcinoma of the renal pelvis, calyces, ureters, and bladder, which may present years after analgesic nephropathy is diagnosed.

RENAL VASCULITIS, THROMBOSIS, AND CHOLESTEROL EMBOLI

Renal Vasculitis

Drug-induced renal vascular disease commonly presents as vasculitis, thrombotic microangiopathy, or cholesterol emboli.[104,122] Vasculitis implies inflammation of the vessel wall, capillaries, or glomeruli and is typically classified according to vessel size (ie, small, medium, or large vessel vasculitis). Small vessel vasculitides usually affect multiple organ systems, including the kidneys and lungs, and are associated with nonspecific inflammatory symptoms such as fever, malaise, myalgias, arthralgias, and weight loss. Numerous drugs are associated with the development of renal vasculitis, including hydralazine, propylthiouracil, allopurinol, phenytoin, sulfasalazine, penicillamine, and minocycline (see Table 65-1).[104,122] Most drug-induced cases of vasculitis, including hydralazine, propylthiouracil, allopurinol, penicillamine, and the anti-TNF-α drug adalimumab, have been implicated in the development of antineutrophil cytoplasmic antibody–positive vasculitis.[104,122,123] Patients present with hematuria, proteinuria, oliguria, and red cell casts, frequently along with fever, malaise, myalgias, and arthralgias.[122] Treatment typically consists of withdrawing the offending drug and administration of corticosteroids or other immunosuppressive therapy, and usually leads to resolution of symptoms within weeks to months.

Thrombotic Microangiopathy

Thrombotic microangiopathy is characterized clinically by microangiopathic hemolytic anemia, fragmented red cells, and thrombocytopenia and pathologically by vascular endothelial proliferation, endothelial cell swelling, and intraluminal platelet thrombi in the small vessels, particularly affecting the renal and cerebral capillaries and arterioles.[103,124] The absence of inflammation in vessel walls distinguishes thrombotic microangiopathy from vasculitis. Numerous medications, including oral contraceptive agents, cyclosporine, tacrolimus, muromonab-CD3, many cancer chemotherapeutic agents including antiangiogenesis drugs (eg, bevacizumab, sunitinib, and sorafenib), mitomycin C, cisplatin, and gemcitabine, interferon-α, ticlopidine, clopidogrel, quinine, and several antimicrobial agents (eg, valacyclovir, penicillins, rifampin, and metronidazole) are associated with the development of thrombotic microangiopathy.[103,124] Patients may present with fever, neurological dysfunction, elevated S_{cr} and BUN, and hypertension, along with microangiopathic hemolytic anemia and thrombocytopenia. Kidney injury can be severe and irreversible, although corticosteroids, antiplatelet agents, plasma exchange, plasmapheresis, and high-dose IV immunoglobulin G have each induced clinical improvement.[124]

Cholesterol Emboli

Anticoagulants (particularly warfarin) and thrombolytics (eg, urokinase, streptokinase, and tissue-plasminogen activator) are associated with cholesterol embolization of the kidney.[125] These drugs act to remove or prevent thrombus formation over ulcerative plaques or may induce hemorrhage within clots, thereby causing showers of cholesterol crystals that lodge in small-diameter arteries of the kidney (renal arterioles and glomerular capillaries). Cholesterol crystal emboli induce an endothelial inflammatory response, which leads to complete obstruction, ischemia, and necrosis of affected vessels within weeks to months after initiation of therapy.[125] Purple discoloration of the toes and mottled skin over the legs are important clinical clues. Treatment is supportive in nature, since kidney injury is generally irreversible.

PHARMACOECONOMICS

The pharmacoeconomic implications of DIKD are enormous. In general, an episode of AKI leads to higher hospital resource use, with increases in the median direct hospital cost of $2,600 and the hospital length of stay by 5 days.[126] An increase in S_{cr} of greater than or equal to 0.5 mg/dL (44 μmol/L) is independently associated with a 6.5-fold increase in the odds of death, a 3.5-day increase in length of hospital stay, and nearly $7,500 in excess hospital costs even after adjusting for age, sex, and measures of comorbidity.[127] Amphotericin B–induced AKI leads to a mean increased length of hospital stay of 8.2 days and adjusted additional costs of $29,823 per patient.[128] The major driver of the increased costs associated with contrast-induced AKI was the cost of the longer initial hospital stay. The increased availability of automated clinical decision support systems and computer-guided medication dosing for hospital inpatients may improve the safety of potentially harmful drugs and minimize the occurrence of nephrotoxicity in this setting, thereby potentially lowering the corresponding economic consequences.[128]

ABBREVIATIONS

ACEI	angiotensin-converting enzyme inhibitor
AIN	allergic interstitial nephritis
AKI	acute kidney injury
ARB	angiotensin II receptor blocker
ATN	acute tubular necrosis
BUN	blood urea nitrogen
CI-AKI	contrast media–induced AKI
CKD	chronic kidney disease
COX	cyclooxygenase
CRS	cytokine release syndrome
CTLA-4	cytotoxic T-lymphocyte antigen-4
DIKD	drug-induced kidney disease
ESKD	end-stage kidney disease
FAERS	FDA Adverse Event Reporting System
FDA	Food and Drug Administration
FSGS	focal segmental glomerulosclerosis
GFR	glomerular filtration rate
IGFBP7	insulin-like growth factor–binding protein 7
KIM-1	kidney injury molecule-1
NGAL	neutrophil gelatinase–associated lipocalin
NSAIDs	nonsteroidal anti-inflammatory drugs
OSPS	oral sodium phosphate solution
PD-1	programmed cell death protein-1
PPI	proton pump inhibitor
RAS	renin–angiotensin system
RTEC	renal tubular epithelial cell
S_{cr}	serum creatinine
SGLT-2	sodium-glucose co-transporter 2
TIMP-2	tissue inhibitor of metalloproteinase 2

REFERENCES

1. Mehta RL, Awdishu L, Davenport A, et al. Phenotype standardization for drug-induced kidney disease. *Kidney Int.* 2015;88:226–234.
2. Thomas ME, Blaine C, Dawnay A, et al. The definition of acute kidney injury and its use in practice. *Kidney Int.* 2015;87:62–73.
3. Siew ED, Davenport A. The growth of acute kidney injury: A rising tide or just closer attention to detail? *Kidney Int.* 2015;87:46–61.
4. Elasy TA, Anderson RJ. Changing demography of acute renal failure. *Semin Dial.* 1996;9:438–443.
5. Hsu RK, McCulloch CE, Dudley RA, Lo LJ, Hsu CY. Temporal changes in incidence of dialysis-requiring AKI. *J Am Soc Nephrol.* 2013;24:37–42.
6. Susantitaphong P, Cruz DN, Cerda J, et al. World incidence of AKI: A meta-analysis. *Clin J Am Soc Nephrol.* 2013;8:1482–1493.
7. Bentley ML, Corwin HL, Dasta J. Drug-induced acute kidney injury in the critically ill adult: Recognition and prevention strategies. *Crit Care Med.* 2010;38:S169–S174.
8. van Meer L, Moerland M, Cohen AF, Burggraaf J. Urinary kidney biomarkers for early detection of nephrotoxicity in clinical drug development. *Br J Clin Pharmacol.* 2014;77:947–957.
9. Gobe GC, Coombes JS, Fassett RG, Endre ZH. Biomarkers of drug-induced acute kidney injury in the adult. *Expert Opin Drug Metab Toxicol.* 2015;11:1683–1694.
10. Chen LX, Koyner JL. Biomarkers in acute kidney injury. *Crit Care Clin.* 2015;31:633–648.
11. Vaidya VS, Ferguson MA, Bonventre JV. Biomarkers of acute kidney injury. *Annu Rev Pharmacol Toxicol.* 2008;48:463–493.
12. Gocze I, Koch M, Renner P, et al. Urinary biomarkers TIMP-2 and IGFBP7 early predict acute kidney injury after major surgery. *PLoS One.* 2015;10:e0120863.
13. Koyner JL, Shaw AD, Chawla LS, et al. Tissue inhibitor metalloproteinase-2 (TIMP-2)IGF-binding protein-7 (IGFBP7) levels are associated with adverse long-term outcomes in patients with AKI. *J Am Soc Nephrol.* 2015;26:1747–1754.
14. Sohn SJ, Kim SY, Kim HS, et al. In vitro evaluation of biomarkers for cisplatin-induced nephrotoxicity using HK-2 human kidney epithelial cells. *Toxicol Lett.* 2013;217:235–242.
15. Fuchs TC, Mally A, Wool A, Beiman M, Hewitt P. An exploratory evaluation of the utility of transcriptional and urinary kidney injury biomarkers for the prediction of aristolochic acid-induced renal injury in male rats. *Vet Pathol.* 2014;51:680–694.
16. Perazella MA. Renal vulnerability to drug toxicity. *Clin J Am Soc Nephrol.* 2009;4:1275–1283.
17. Ghane Shahrbaf F, Assadi F. Drug-induced renal disorders. *J Renal Inj Prev.* 2015;4:57–60.
18. Perazella MA. The urine sediment as a biomarker of kidney disease. *Am J Kidney Dis.* 2015;66:748–755.
19. Curthoys NP, Moe OW. Proximal tubule function and response to acidosis. *Clin J Am Soc Nephrol.* 2014;9:1627–1638.
20. Subramanya AR, Ellison DH. Distal convoluted tubule. *Clin J Am Soc Nephrol.* 2014;9:2147–2163.
21. Ettore B. Adverse effects of drugs on the kidney. *Eur J Intern Med.* 2015;28:1–8.
22. Wargo KA, Edwards JD. Aminoglycoside-induced nephrotoxicity. *J Pharm Pract.* 2014;27:573–577.
23. Pazhayattil GS, Shirali AC. Drug-induced impairment of renal function. *Int J Nephrol Renovasc Dis.* 2014;7:457–468.
24. Oliveira JF, Silva CA, Barbieri CD, et al. Prevalence and risk factors for aminoglycoside nephrotoxicity in intensive care units. *Antimicrob Agents Chemother.* 2009;53:2887–2891.
25. Balakumar P, Rohilla A, Thangathirupathi A. Gentamicin-induced nephrotoxicity: Do we have a promising therapeutic approach to blunt it? *Pharmacol Res.* 2010;62:179–186.
26. Asci H, Saygin M, Cankara FN, et al. The impact of alpha-lipoic acid on amikacin-induced nephrotoxicity. *Ren Fail.* 2015;37:117–121.
27. Destache CJ. Aminoglycoside-induced nephrotoxicity—a focus on monitoring: A review of literature. *J Pharm Pract.* 2014;27:562–566.
28. Pagkalis S, Mantadakis E, Mavros MN, Ammari C, Falagas ME. Pharmacological considerations for the proper clinical use of aminoglycosides. *Drugs.* 2011;71:2277–2294.
29. Keaney JJ, Hannon CM, Murray PT. Contrast-induced acute kidney injury: How much contrast is safe? *Nephrol Dial Transplant.* 2013;28:1376–1383.
30. Lefel N, Janssen L, le Noble J, Foudraine N. Sodium bicarbonate prophylactic therapy in the prevention of contrast-induced nephropathy in patients admitted to the intensive care unit of a teaching hospital: A retrospective cohort study. *J Intensive Care.* 2016;4:5.
31. Weisbord SD, Palevsky PM. Contrast-associated acute kidney injury. *Crit Care Clin.* 2015;31:725–735.
32. Wilhelm-Leen E, Montez-Rath ME, Chertow G. Estimating the risk of radiocontrast-associated nephropathy. *J Am Soc Nephrol.* 2017;28(2):653–659.
33. Davenport MS, Perazella MA, Yee J, et al. Use of intravenous iodinated contrast media in patients with kidney disease: Consensus statements from the American College of Radiology and the National Kidney Foundation. *Radiology.* 2020;294(3):660–668. doi: 10.1148/radiol.2019192094.
34. McCullough PA. Contrast-induced nephropathy: Definitions, epidemiology, and implications. *Intervent Cardiol Clin.* 2014;3:357–362.
35. Geenen RWF, Kingma HJ, van der Molen AJ. Pathophysiology of contrast-induced acute kidney injury. *Intervent Cardiol Clin.* 2014;3:363–367.
36. Rojkovskiy I, Solomon R. Intravenous and oral hydration: Approaches, principles, and differing regimens. *Intervent Cardiol Clin.* 2014;3:393–404.
37. Aqeel I, Garcha AS, Rudnick MR. Relative nephrotoxicity of different contrast media. *Intervent Cardiol Clin.* 2014;3:349–356.
38. Toso A, Leoncini M, Maioli M, Tropeano F, Bellandi F. Pharmacologic prophylaxis for contrast-induced acute kidney injury. *Intervent Cardiol Clin.* 2014;3:405–419.
39. Tao SM, Wichmann JL, Schoepf UJ, et al. Contrast-induced nephropathy in CT: Incidence, risk factors and strategies for prevention. *Eur Radiol.* 2016;26(9):3310–3318.
40. Azzalini L, Spagnoli V, Ly HQ. Contrast-induced nephropathy: From pathophysiology to preventive strategies. *Can J Cardiol.* 2016;32(2):247–255.
41. Ohno I, Hayashi H, Aonuma K, et al. JSN, JRS, and JCS Joint Working Group. Guidelines on the use of iodinated contrast media in patients with kidney disease 2012: Digest version. *Circ J.* 2013;77:1883–1914.
42. Weisbord SD, Gallagher M, Jneid H, et al. Outcomes after angiography with sodium bicarbonate and acetylcysteine. *N Engl J Med.* 2018;378(7):603–614.
43. Yang Y, Liu H, Liu F, Dong Z. Mitochondrial dysregulation and protection in cisplatin nephrotoxicity. *Arch Toxicol.* 2014;88:1249–1256.
44. Peres LA, da Cunha AD Jr. Acute nephrotoxicity of cisplatin: Molecular mechanisms. *J Bras Nefrol.* 2013;35:332–340.

45. Perazella MA. Onco-nephrology: Renal toxicities of chemotherapeutic agents. *Clin J Am Soc Nephrol.* 2012;7:1713–1721.
46. Launay-Vacher V, Rey JB, Isnard-Bagnis C, Deray G, Daouphars M. Prevention of cisplatin nephrotoxicity: State of the art and recommendations from the European Society of Clinical Pharmacy Special Interest Group on Cancer Care. *Cancer Chemother Pharmacol.* 2008;61:903–909.
47. Sanchez-Gonzalez PD, Lopez-Hernandez FJ, Lopez-Novoa JM, Morales AI. An integrative view of the pathophysiological events leading to cisplatin nephrotoxicity. *Crit Rev Toxicol.* 2011;41:803–821.
48. Finkel M, Goldstein A, Steinberg Y, Granowetter L, Trachtman H. Cisplatinum nephrotoxicity in oncology therapeutics: Retrospective review of patients treated between 2005 and 2012. *Pediatr Nephrol.* 2014;29:2421–2424.
49. dos Santos NA, Carvalho Rodrigues MA, Martins NM, dos Santos AC. Cisplatin-induced nephrotoxicity and targets of nephroprotection: An update. *Arch Toxicol.* 2012;86:1233–1250.
50. Shirali AC, Perazella MA. Tubulointerstitial injury associated with chemotherapeutic agents. *Adv Chronic Kidney Dis.* 2014;21:56–63.
51. Oh GS, Kim HJ, Shen A, et al. Cisplatin-induced kidney dysfunction and perspectives on improving treatment strategies. *Electrolyte Blood Press.* 2014;12:55–65.
52. Santabarbara G, Maione P, Rossi A, Gridelli C. Pharmacotherapeutic options for treating adverse effects of cisplatin chemotherapy. *Expert Opin Pharmacother.* 2016;17(4):561–570.
53. Rocha PN, Kobayashi CD, de Carvalho Almeida L, et al. Incidence, predictors, and impact on hospital mortality of amphotericin B nephrotoxicity defined using newer acute kidney injury diagnostic criteria. *Antimicrob Agents Chemother.* 2015;59:4759–4769.
54. Hamill RJ. Amphotericin B formulations: A comparative review of efficacy and toxicity. *Drugs.* 2013;73:919–934.
55. Mistro S, Maciel Ide M, de Menezes RG, Maia ZP, et al. Does lipid emulsion reduce amphotericin B nephrotoxicity? A systematic review and meta-analysis. *Clin Infect Dis.* 2012;54:1774–1777.
56. Bes DF, Rosanova MT, Sberna N, Arrizurieta E. Deoxycholate amphotericin B and nephrotoxicity in the pediatric setting. *Pediatr Infect Dis J.* 2014;33:e198–e206.
57. Karimzadeh I, Khalili H, Sagheb MM, Farsaei S. A double-blinded, placebo-controlled, multicenter clinical trial of *N*-acetylcysteine for preventing amphotericin B-induced nephrotoxicity. *Expert Opin Drug Metab Toxicol.* 2015;11:1345–1355.
58. Martensson J, Bellomo R. Are all fluids bad for the kidney? *Curr Opin Crit Care.* 2015;21:292–301.
59. Dickenmann M, Oettl T, Mihatsch MJ. Osmotic nephrosis: Acute kidney injury with accumulation of proximal tubular lysosomes due to administration of exogenous solutes. *Am J Kidney Dis.* 2008;51:491–503.
60. Dantal J. Intravenous immunoglobulins: In-depth review of excipients and acute kidney injury risk. *Am J Nephrol.* 2013;38:275–284.
61. Phadke Gautam, Kaushal Amit, Tolan Dean R, et al. Osmotic nephrosis and acute kidney injury associated with SGLT2 inhibitor use: A case report. *Am J Kidney Dis.* 2020;76:144–147. doi: 10.1053/j.ajkd.2020.01.015.
62. Nomani AZ, Nabi Z, Rashid H, et al. Osmotic nephrosis with mannitol: Review article. *Ren Fail.* 2014;36:1169–1176.
63. Perazella MA, Luciano RL. Review of select causes of drug-induced AKI. *Expert Rev Clin Pharmacol.* 2015;8:367–371.
64. Carlstrom M, Wilcox CS, Arendshorst WJ. Renal autoregulation in health and disease. *Physiol Rev.* 2015;95:405–511.
65. Dreischulte T, Morales DR, Bell S, Guthrie B. Combined use of nonsteroidal anti-inflammatory drugs with diuretics and/or renin-angiotensin system inhibitors in the community increases the risk of acute kidney injury. *Kidney Int.* 2015;88:396–403.
66. Perazella MA, Shirali AC. Nephrotoxicity of cancer immunotherapies: Past, present and future. *J Am Soc Nephrol.* 2018;29(8):2039–2052.
67. Cruz CS, Cruz LS, Silva GR, Marcilio de Souza CA. Incidence and predictors of development of acute renal failure related to treatment of congestive heart failure with ACE inhibitors. *Nephron Clin Pract.* 2007;105:c77–c83.
68. Budnitz DS, Lovegrove MC, Shehab N, Richards CL. Emergency hospitalizations for adverse drug events in older Americans. *N Engl J Med.* 2011;365:2002–2012.
69. St Peter WL, Odum LE, Whaley-Connell AT. To RAS or not to RAS? The evidence for and cautions with renin-angiotensin system inhibition in patients with diabetic kidney disease. *Pharmacotherapy.* 2013;33:496–514.
70. Lapi F, Azoulay L, Yin H, Nessim SJ, Suissa S. Concurrent use of diuretics, angiotensin converting enzyme inhibitors, and angiotensin receptor blockers with nonsteroidal anti-inflammatory drugs and risk of acute kidney injury: Nested case-control study. *BMJ.* 2013;346:e8525.
71. Rahman S, Malcoun A. Nonsteroidal anti-inflammatory drugs, cyclooxygenase-2, and the kidneys. *Prim Care.* 2014;41:803–821.
72. Whelton A. Nephrotoxicity of nonsteroidal anti-inflammatory drugs: Physiologic foundations and clinical implications. *Am J Med.* 1999;106:13S–24S.
73. Naesens M, Kuypers DR, Sarwal M. Calcineurin inhibitor nephrotoxicity. *Clin J Am Soc Nephrol.* 2009;4:481–508.
74. Chapman JR. Chronic calcineurin inhibitor nephrotoxicity lest we forget. *Am J Transplant.* 2011;11:693–697.
75. Ojo AO, Held PJ, Port FK, et al. Chronic renal failure after transplantation of a nonrenal organ. *N Engl J Med.* 2003;349:931–940.
76. Issa N, Kukla A, Ibrahim HN. Calcineurin inhibitor nephrotoxicity: A review and perspective of the evidence. *Am J Nephrol.* 2013;37:602–612.
77. Pallet N, Djamali A, Legendre C. Challenges in diagnosing acute calcineurin-inhibitor induced nephrotoxicity: From toxicogenomics to emerging biomarkers. *Pharmacol Res.* 2011;64:25–30.
78. Shyangdan DS, Uthman OA, Waugh N. SGLT-2 receptor inhibitors for treating patients with type 2 diabetes mellitus: A systematic review and network meta-analysis. *BMJ Open.* 2016;6(2):e009417.
79. Wanner C, Inzucchi SE, Lachin JM, et al. Empagliflozin and progression of kidney disease in type 2 diabetes. *N Engl J Med.* 2016;375(4):323–334.
80. Neal B, Perkovic V, Mahaffey KW, et al. Canagliflozin and cardiovascular and renal events in type 2 diabetes. *N Engl J Med.* 2017;377(7):644–657.
81. Nadkarni GN, Ferrandino R, Chang A, et al. Acute kidney injury in patients on SGLT2 inhibitors: A propensity-matched analysis. *Diabetes Care.* Nov 2017;40(11):1479–1485.
82. Hahn K, Ejaz AA, Kanbay M, Lanaspa MA, Johnson RJ. Acute kidney injury from SGLT2 inhibitors: Potential mechanisms. *Nat Rev Nephrol.* 2016;12(12):711–712.
83. Park JH, Rivière I, Gonen M, et al. Long-term follow-up of CD19 CAR therapy in acute lymphoblastic leukemia. *N Engl J Med.* 2018;378(5):449–459. doi: 10.1056/NEJMoa1709919.
84. Wang M, Munoz J, Goy A, et al. KTE-X19 CAR T-cell therapy in relapsed or refractory mantle-cell lymphoma. *N Engl J Med.* 2020;382(14):1331–1342. doi: 10.1056/NEJMoa1914347.
85. Kanduri SR, Cheungpasitporn W, Thongprayoon C, et al. Systematic review of risk factors and incidence of acute kidney injury among patients treated with CAR-T cell therapies. *Kidney Int Rep.* 2021;6(5):1416–1422. doi: 10.1016/j.ekir.2021.02.013.
86. Neelapu SS, Tummala S, Kebriaei P, et al. Chimeric antigen receptor T-cell therapy—Assessment and management of toxicities. *Nat Rev Clin Oncol.* 2018;15(1):47–62. doi: 10.1038/nrclinonc.2017.148.
87. Nasr SH, Milliner DS, Wooldridge TD, Sethi S. Triamterene crystalline nephropathy. *Am J Kidney Dis.* 2014;63:148–152.
88. Garneau AP, Riopel J, Isenring P. Acute methotrexate-induced crystal nephropathy. *N Engl J Med.* 2015;373:2691–2693.
89. Faught LN, Greff MJ, Rieder MJ, Koren G. Drug-induced acute kidney injury in children. *Br J Clin Pharmacol.* 2015;80:901–909.
90. Herlitz LC, D'Agati VD, Markowitz GS. Crystalline nephropathies. *Arch Pathol Lab Med.* 2012;136:713–720.
91. Jones GL, Will A, Jackson GH, Webb NJ, Rule S; British Committee for Standards in Haematology. Guidelines for the management of tumour lysis syndrome in adults and children with haematological malignancies on behalf of the British Committee for Standards in Haematology. *Br J Haematol.* 2015;169:661–671.
92. Petejova N, Martinek A. Acute kidney injury due to rhabdomyolysis and renal replacement therapy: A critical review. *Crit Care.* 2014;18:224.
93. Zimmerman JL, Shen MC. Rhabdomyolysis. *Chest.* 2013;144:1058–1065.
94. Brodsky SV, Nadasdy T, Rovin BH, et al. Warfarin-related nephropathy occurs in patients with and without chronic kidney disease and is associated with an increased mortality rate. *Kidney Int.* 2011;80:181–189.
95. Kumar N, Perazella MA. Differentiating HIV-associated nephropathy from antiretroviral drug-induced nephropathy: A clinical challenge. *Curr HIV/AIDS Rep.* 2014;11:202–211.
96. Izzedine H, Lescure FX, Bonnet F. HIV medication-based urolithiasis. *Clin Kidney J.* 2014;7:121–126.
97. Luque Y, Louis K, Jouanneau C, et al. Vancomycin-associated cast nephropathy. *J Am Soc Nephrol.* 2017;28(6):1723–1728. doi: 10.1681/ASN.2016080867.
98. Tantranont N, Luque Y, Hsiao M, et al. Vancomycin-associated tubular casts and vancomycin nephrotoxicity. *Kidney Int Rep.* 2021;6(7):1912–1922. doi: 10.1016/j.ekir.2021.04.035.

99. Shavit L, Jaeger P, Unwin RJ. What is nephrocalcinosis? *Kidney Int.* 2015;88:35–43.
100. Markowitz GS, Perazella MA. Acute phosphate nephropathy. *Kidney Int.* 2009;76:1027–1034.
101. Choi NK, Lee J, Chang Y, et al. Acute renal failure following oral sodium phosphate bowel preparation: A nationwide case-crossover study. *Endoscopy.* 2014;46:465–470.
102. Markowitz GS, Radhakrishnan J, D'Agati VD. Towards the incidence of acute phosphate nephropathy. *J Am Soc Nephrol.* 2007;18:3020–3022.
103. Markowitz GS, Bomback AS, Perazella MA. Drug-induced glomerular disease: Direct cellular injury. *Clin J Am Soc Nephrol.* 2015;10:1291–1299.
104. Hogan JJ, Markowitz GS, Radhakrishnan J. Drug-induced glomerular disease: Immune-mediated injury. *Clin J Am Soc Nephrol.* 2015;10:1300–1310.
105. Lan X, Rao TK, Chander PN, Skorecki K, Singhal PC. Apolipoprotein L1 (APOL1) Variants (Vs) a possible link between Heroin-associated Nephropathy (HAN) and HIV-associated Nephropathy (HIVAN). *Front Microbiol.* 2015;6:571.
106. Krishnan N, Perazella MA. Drug-induced acute interstitial nephritis: Pathology, pathogenesis, and treatment. *Iran J Kidney Dis.* 2015;9:3–13.
107. Perazella MA, Markowitz GS. Drug-induced acute interstitial nephritis. *Nat Rev Nephrol.* 2010;6:461–470.
108. Perazella MA. Diagnosing drug-induced AIN in the hospitalized patient: A challenge for the clinician. *Clin Nephrol.* 2014;81:381–388.
109. Moledina DG, Perazella MA. PPIs and kidney disease: From AIN to CKD. *J Nephrol.* 2016;29(5):611–616.
110. Perazella MA. Clinical approach to diagnosing acute and chronic tubulointerstitial disease. *Adv Chronic Kidney Dis.* 2017;24(2):57–63.
111. Cortazar FB, Kibbelaar ZA, Glezerman IG, et al. Clinical features and outcomes of immune checkpoint inhibitor-associated AKI: A multicenter study. *J Am Soc Nephrol.* 2020;31(2):435–446. doi: 10.1681/ASN.2019070676.
112. Shirali AC, Perazella MA, Gettinger S. Association of acute interstitial nephritis with programmed cell death 1 inhibitor therapy in lung cancer patients. *Am J Kidney Dis.* 2016;68(2):287–291.
113. Bendz H, Schon S, Attman PO, Aurell M. Renal failure occurs in chronic lithium treatment but is uncommon. *Kidney Int.* 2010;77:219–224.
114. Rej S, Herrmann N, Shulman K. The effects of lithium on renal function in older adults—A systematic review. *J Geriatr Psychiatry Neurol.* 2012;25:51–61.
115. Alsady M, Baumgarten R, Deen PM, de Groot T. Lithium in the Kidney: Friend and Foe? *J Am Soc Nephrol.* 2016;27(6):1587–1595.
116. Grunfeld JP, Rossier BC. Lithium nephrotoxicity revisited. *Nat Rev Nephrol.* 2009;5:270–276.
117. Clos S, Rauchhaus P, Severn A, Cochrane L, Donnan PT. Long-term effect of lithium maintenance therapy on estimated glomerular filtration rate in patients with affective disorders: A population-based cohort study. *Lancet Psychiatry.* 2015;2:1075–1083.
118. Debelle FD, Vanherweghem JL, Nortier JL. Aristolochic acid nephropathy: A worldwide problem. *Kidney Int.* 2008;74:158–169.
119. Luciano RL, Perazella MA. Aristolochic acid nephropathy: Epidemiology, clinical presentation, and treatment. *Drug Saf.* 2015;38:55–64.
120. De Broe ME, Elseviers MM. Over-the-counter analgesic use. *J Am Soc Nephrol.* 2009;20:2098–2103.
121. Braden GL, O'Shea MH, Mulhern JG. Tubulointerstitial diseases. *Am J Kidney Dis.* 2005;46:560–572.
122. Radic M, Martinovic Kaliterna D, Radic J. Drug-induced vasculitis: A clinical and pathological review. *Neth J Med.* 2012;70:12–17.
123. Perez-Alvarez R, Perez-de-Lis M, Ramos-Casals M. Biologics-induced autoimmune diseases. *Curr Opin Rheumatol.* 2013;25:56–64.
124. Izzedine H, Perazella MA. Thrombotic microangiopathy, cancer, and cancer drugs. *Am J Kidney Dis.* 2015;66:857–868.
125. Scolari F, Ravani P. Atheroembolic renal disease. *Lancet.* 2010;375:1650–1660.
126. Lameire NH, Bagga A, Cruz D, et al. Acute kidney injury: An increasing global concern. *Lancet.* 2013;382:170–179.
127. Chertow GM, Burdick E, Honour M, Bonventre JV, Bates DW. Acute kidney injury, mortality, length of stay, and costs in hospitalized patients. *J Am Soc Nephrol.* 2005;16:3365–3370.
128. Hug BL, Witkowski DJ, Sox CM, et al. Occurrence of adverse, often preventable, events in community hospitals involving nephrotoxic drugs or those excreted by the kidney. *Kidney Int.* 2009;76:1192–1198.

e66

Glomerular Diseases

Duncan B. Johnstone

KEY CONCEPTS

1. Glomerular diseases vary in causes, clinical symptoms, treatments, and outcomes, but are united because they all affect the glomerulus, which is the filter of the kidney.
2. The five principal clinical features of glomerular disease are hematuria, proteinuria, edema, hypertension, and progressive kidney failure. These features occur to varying degrees among different glomerular diseases and between individual patients.
3. Glomerular diseases can be classified with many different systems, each of which has advantages and disadvantages. A basic classification is whether a glomerular disease is nephritic (reflecting inflammatory injury) or nephrotic (reflecting noninflammatory injury).
4. For some glomerular diseases there are treatments that can induce a remission, which is often based on suppression of the immune system. If disease remission cannot be achieved, we use conservative measures to reduce proteinuria, edema, hypertension, hyperlipidemia, and hypercoagulability, with the aim of stabilizing the loss of kidney function.
5. Patients undergoing treatment for glomerular disease must be monitored closely to assess their therapeutic response and any treatment-induced toxicity.
6. Among all glomerular diseases, minimal-change nephropathy is the most responsive to treatment with steroids.
7. Focal segmental glomerulosclerosis (FSGS) is difficult to treat for two reasons: first, it is difficult to distinguish primary FSGS, which may respond to steroids or other immunosuppressants, from the many causes of secondary FSGS, which will not respond to these treatments; second, the response of primary FSGS to steroids, unlike minimal change disease, is not robust.
8. Systemic lupus erythematosus can cause many different types of kidney disease. The optimal treatment of lupus nephritis depends on the underlying lesion, the disease activity on biopsy, and the patient's symptoms in organs other than the kidney.
9. Post-streptococcal glomerulonephritis arises when the immune response to bacteria damages the glomerular filter. By definition, post-streptococcal glomerulonephritis occurs after the infection, so there is no role for antibiotic therapy. Symptoms are treated aggressively with conservative measures.
10. Membranous nephropathy can be either primary disease, or secondary to a long list of other causes. Within the last 10 years, the cause of primary membranous nephropathy has been identified as auto-antibodies to the phospholipase A2 receptor, resulting in significant improvements in diagnosis, treatment, and outcomes.

BEYOND THE BOOK

Visit the National Kidney Foundation Website <https://www.kidney.org>. This Website is useful to learn about kidney disease from the perspective of both patients and healthcare providers. Watch the video titled "New Insights Regarding Treatment of Membranous Nephropathy" at <https://www.kidney.org/content/new-insights-regarding-treatment>. This video provides an overview of the approach to treating membranous nephropathy, particularly with regards to immunosuppressive therapy, and is useful to enhance student understanding regarding the ASSESS and PLAN steps in the patient care process.

INTRODUCTION

Glomerular disease is one of the most common causes of end-stage kidney disease (ESKD). From the 2018 yearly report of all patients nationwide by US Renal Data Systems, the number of patients who started dialysis that year (incident patients) was 213,588, of whom 7% carried a diagnosis of primary glomerular disease.[1] This under-represents the total burden of glomerular disease because this figure of 7% does not include secondary glomerular diseases such as classic diabetic nephropathy, does not include patients starting dialysis due to undiagnosed glomerular disease that was erroneously labeled "hypertensive nephropathy,"[2] and does not include patients with "ESKD of unknown cause," who never had a biopsy, some of whom likely had glomerular disease. Altogether, if we combine primary, secondary, and undiagnosed glomerular diseases, we account for about 40% to 60% of new ESKD patients starting dialysis each year, which is roughly 100,000 people. A larger number of patients with glomerular disease are receiving treatment and trying to avoid progression of their disease to ESKD.

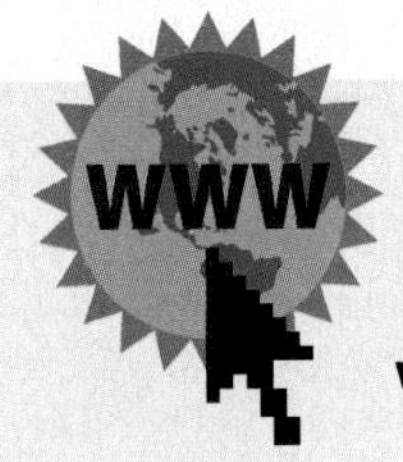

The complete chapter, learning objectives, and other resources can be found at **www.pharmacotherapyonline.com.**

Personalized Pharmacotherapy for Patients with Chronic Kidney Disease

67

Morgan A. Butrovich and Thomas D. Nolin

KEY CONCEPTS

1. Chronic kidney disease (CKD) and related comorbidities can impact processes contributing to medication absorption and bioavailability, but the significance of these changes is ill-defined for most medications.
2. The volume of distribution (V_D) of many medications is increased in the presence of acute kidney injury (AKI) and CKD secondary to volume expansion and/or decreased protein binding.
3. Renal clearance (CL_R) is a composite of renal excretory functions (filtration, secretion, and reabsorption). These functions decline in the setting of CKD, causing accumulation of medications that are predominantly renally excreted.
4. Nonrenal clearance (CL_{NR}) may be altered in CKD, causing accumulation of medications that are predominantly cleared by metabolism and/or transport.
5. Although information on pharmacokinetics and medication dosing in patients with CKD has improved in recent years, dosing guidelines remain highly variable and many are not optimal for clinical use.
6. Individualization of a medication dosage regimen for a patient with CKD is based on the pharmacodynamic/pharmacokinetic characteristics of the medication, the patient's degree of residual kidney function, and the patient's overall clinical condition.
7. The effect of dialysis on medication elimination is dependent on the characteristics of the medication and the dialysis prescription. Hemodialysis (HD) clearance data can be used to guide the initial medication dosage regimen recommendation; however, prospective monitoring of serum concentrations is often warranted, especially for narrow therapeutic index drugs.

BEYOND THE BOOK

Visit the US National Library of Medicine website DailyMed (https://dailymed.nlm.nih.gov/dailymed/index.cfm), which is the official provider of US Food and Drug Administration (FDA)-approved medication label information (i.e., package inserts). Identify two medications that require renal dose adjustment in CKD, including, one that is predominantly renally excreted ($f_e > 0.3$) and one that is not ($f_e < 0.3$). Review the renal dosing adjustment recommendations and develop a table that compares and contrasts the kidney function cutoffs for dose adjustment, the kidney function estimate (i.e., creatinine clearance, glomerular filtration rate) upon which the recommendations are based, and the dosage regimen adjustment strategy used (i.e., decrease dose or increase dosing interval). This activity is useful to enhance student understanding of the ASSESS and PLAN steps in the patient care process.

INTRODUCTION

Chronic kidney disease (CKD) is defined by the presence of abnormalities of kidney function or structure for more than 3 months (see Chapter e60, "Evaluation of Kidney Function" and Chapter 62, "Chronic Kidney Disease").[1] The Kidney Disease: Improving Global Outcomes (KDIGO) CKD categories by GFR cutoff are depicted in Fig. 62-1. About 10% to 15% of the global population and 1 in 7 US adults have CKD.[2-5] CKD patients are characterized by a high prevalence of polypharmacy, with a median of eight prescribed medications per patient and up to 90% of CKD patients taking over five medications daily.[6,7] Therefore, understanding the changes in pharmacokinetics, pharmacodynamics, and medication dosing in this patient population is crucial for personalizing pharmacotherapy and optimizing pharmacotherapeutic outcomes.

CKD patients exhibit altered pharmacokinetics and/or pharmacodynamics due to disease-related physiologic and biochemical changes, including altered renal excretory function, protein binding, and cytochrome P450 enzyme and/or transporter activity.[8-15] Changes to medication absorption and bioavailability are not well quantified, while changes to distribution and elimination are better described. Medications with a high fraction excreted unchanged in the urine ($f_e > 0.3$) may accumulate in CKD patients due to a decline in the renal excretory functions (filtration, secretion, and reabsorption) that compose renal clearance (CL_R). Medications that are not predominantly renally eliminated (i.e., are predominantly eliminated by metabolism and/or transport) may also accumulate in patients with CKD secondary to changes in nonrenal clearance (CL_{NR}).

In CKD patients, the dosage regimens of numerous medications must be altered to prevent toxicity without compromising the desired therapeutic benefit.[11,16] An accurate assessment of patient kidney function is a crucial first step in renal dose adjustment. Despite conduction of more renal impairment studies by industry and improvements in product labeling language, challenges remain for determining medication dose adjustments in CKD patients.[17] If there is no official dosage regimen recommendation in the product labeling, an adjustment may be calculated on the basis of the medication's f_e and the patient's residual kidney function.[18] For medications that are extensively metabolized or for which dramatic changes in protein binding and/or volume of distribution (V_D) have been noted, a complex adjustment strategy may need to be employed.[19,20] For patients receiving chronic renal replacement therapy (i.e., dialysis), medication dosage adjustments will be based on characteristics of the drug, the dialysis prescription, and the clinical setting for which dialysis is being performed, and prospective monitoring of serum drug concentrations may be warranted.[19]

Clinicians will often need to design individualized therapeutic regimens to optimize clinical outcomes in patients with CKD.[11] In this chapter, the influence of CKD on pharmacokinetics and pharmacodynamics is examined. A general approach to personalizing pharmacotherapy, with emphasis on medication selection and dosing strategies for CKD patients, is presented. Finally, the impact of chronic renal replacement therapy on drug disposition is discussed. Medication dosage adjustment strategies for patients with acute kidney injury (AKI), including those who are receiving continuous renal replacement therapy, are presented in Chapter 61, "Acute Kidney Injury."

PHARMACOKINETIC AND PHARMACODYNAMIC CHANGES IN CHRONIC KIDNEY DISEASE

The pharmacokinetics and pharmacodynamics of numerous medications are altered by CKD.[8-14] An understanding of why and how pharmacokinetic processes are impacted by CKD provides a framework to project the influence of CKD on emerging therapies. In addition, these effects can be factored into the clinician's dosage recommendations for individual CKD patients.

Absorption and Bioavailability

1 Bioavailability describes the fraction of medication reaching systemic circulation following extravascular administration. Oral bioavailability is dependent on absorption from the gastrointestinal (GI) tract and pre-systemic (i.e., intestinal and hepatic) metabolism and transport. There is relatively little quantitative information regarding the influence of CKD on medication absorption and bioavailability. Most evaluations of medication absorption in CKD assess changes to peak medication serum concentration (C_{max}) and the time at which the peak serum concentration is achieved (t_{max}) rather than oral bioavailability (ie, a comparison of the area under the concentration-time curve [*AUC*] after oral and intravenous [IV] administration). Changes to absorption processes are likely the result of complex interplay between disease-related physiologic changes and drug-drug interactions.[8-15,21]

Altered absorption and/or bioavailability of medications in CKD patients may be a consequence of changes to GI physiologic and biochemical processes secondary to CKD and related comorbidities. These changes include decreased gastric mobility, decreased gastric acidity, GI edema, and altered pre-systemic metabolism and/or transport.[8-15,21] Decreased GI motility can occur in CKD patients secondary to diabetic gastroparesis and may delay t_{max} and decrease C_{max}, thereby altering a medication's absorption profile without impacting its bioavailability. Gastric acidity may decrease (i.e., an increase in gastric pH) in CKD patients due to urea retention and subsequent conversion to ammonia by gastric urease. This alkalization may alter the dissolution or ionization properties of weakly basic drugs and lead to changes in absorption. Edema of the GI tract secondary to concomitant cirrhosis or congestive heart failure can also decrease the absorption of some medications, such as furosemide. Finally, the bioavailability of some medications (e.g., dihydrocodeine, felodipine, sertraline, and cyclosporine) may be increased in CKD patients due to alterations in pre-systemic (i.e., intestinal and hepatic) metabolism and/or transport that increases the amount of parent drug reaching systemic circulation (i.e., decreased metabolism, increased uptake, and/or decreased efflux, see Nonrenal Clearance below).

Drug interactions can also alter the absorption and/or bioavailability of other medications through a variety of mechanisms.[8] Although not disease-specific effects, these drug-drug interactions are worth noting due to the high medication burden of CKD patients.[6,7] Administration of antacids, H_2-receptor antagonists, proton pump inhibitors, and phosphate binders can decrease gastric acidity and lower the bioavailability of several medications, such as some antibiotics and digoxin. Antacids and vitamin supplements can form insoluble salts or metal ion chelates with some medications and decrease their bioavailability. Finally, drug interactions that modulate pre-systemic intestinal and hepatic metabolism and/or transport may alter bioavailability.

Distribution

A medication's volume of distribution (V_D) reflects the extent of distribution throughout the body.[8,10] Lower V_D values reflect distribution primarily in the vascular space, whereas higher V_D values reflect extensive distribution outside the vascular space (i.e., in the tissues). 2 The V_D of numerous medications is increased in CKD and AKI patients as a result of fluid overload, altered protein binding, and/or altered tissue binding, leading to a decrease in serum drug concentrations. The V_D of a few medications may be decreased in the setting of CKD, likely due to decreased tissue binding (Table 67-1).[8,10,12-14]

TABLE 67-1 Volume of Distribution of Selected Medications in Patients with ESKD

Medication	Normal (L/kg)	ESKD (L/kg)	Change from Normal
Increased			
Amikacin	0.20	0.29	45%
Cefazolin	0.13	0.17	31%
Cefoxitin	0.16	0.26	63%
Ceftriaxone	0.28	0.48	71%
Cefuroxime	0.20	0.26	30%
Doripenem	0.25	0.47	88%
Dicloxacillin	0.08	0.18	125%
Erythromycin	0.57	1.09	91%
Furosemide	0.11	0.18	64%
Gentamicin	0.20	0.32	60%
Isoniazid	0.60	0.80	33%
Minoxidil	2.60	4.90	88%
Naproxen	0.12	0.17	42%
Phenytoin	0.64	1.40	119%
Trimethoprim	1.36	1.83	35%
Vancomycin	0.64	0.85	33%
Decreased			
Atenolol	1.20	0.90	-25%
Chloramphenicol	0.87	0.60	-31%
Ciprofloxacin	2.50	1.95	-22%
Digoxin	7.30	4.00	-45%
Ethambutol	3.70	1.60	-57%
Methicillin	0.45	0.30	-33%
Metoprolol	5.60	1.00	-82%
Pindolol	2.10	1.10	-48%
Propranolol	4.40	3.60	-18%

ESKD, end-stage kidney disease.

Data from References 12 to 14.

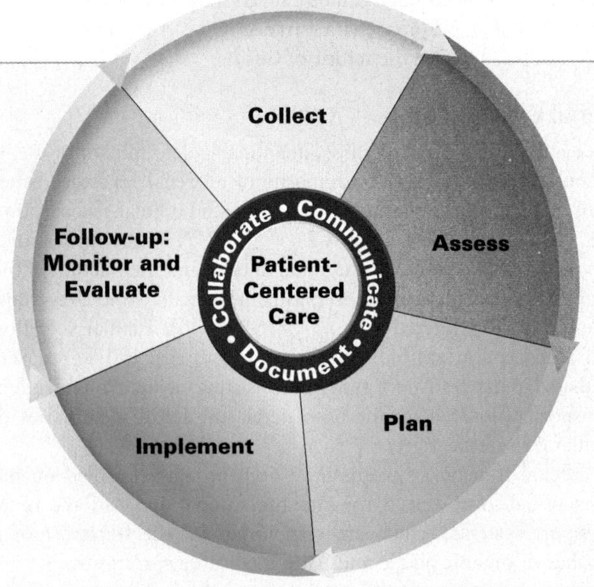

Patient Care Process for Personalizing Pharmacotherapy in Patients with Chronic Kidney Disease

Collect

- Patient characteristics (e.g., age, sex, height, weight)
- Patient medical history (personal and family)
- Social history (e.g., use of tobacco, alcohol, other substances of misuse)
- Current medications including over-the-counter products, and herbal/dietary supplements
- Objective data
    - o Labs, including serum creatinine and/or cystatin C

Assess

- Kidney function
    - o Estimated GFR or CL_{Cr} for medication dosing, based on best available methodology (see Chapter e60)
    - o Measured CL_{Cr} or GFR as confirmatory test if needed
- Medication regimen
    - o Indication and treatment goals for all medications
    - o Potential drug-drug interactions
    - o Identify medications requiring adjustment to the dosage regimen (see Table 67-3)

Plan*

- Adjusted dosage regimen as needed for each medication
    - o Calculate adjusted regimen (dose and frequency) based on pharmacokinetic characteristics and patient's kidney function (see Tables 67-4 and 67-5)
- Treatment goals and corresponding monitoring parameters

Implement*

- Provide patient education regarding all elements of treatment plan
- Discontinue or avoid prescription of nephrotoxic medication if possible

Follow-up: Monitor and Evaluate

- Medication serum concentrations if therapeutic drug monitoring is available/applicable
- Parameters of medication response and toxicity
- Kidney function (every 3 to 5 days for acute therapies, monthly or quarterly for chronic therapies)
- Revise regimen based on medication response or change in patient status (including change in kidney function)
- Patient adherence to treatment plan

** Collaborate with patient, caregivers, and other health professionals.*

Fluid Status

Variability in fluid status is a common issue in patients with AKI and severe CKD (category G4 and G5), especially those who are critically ill. Many critically ill patients receive large volumes of IV fluids for resuscitation from shock, and can subsequently develop edema, pleural effusions, or ascites. Furthermore, AKI and CKD can precipitate decreased water excretion. These factors can lead to fluid overload and, subsequently, an increase in V_D and a decrease in serum concentrations. This is especially problematic with hydrophilic medications, such as aminoglycosides and cephalosporins.[8,10,11]

Altered Plasma Protein Binding

Protein binding limits medication distribution, as only unbound or "free" medication can cross cellular membranes and distribute outside the vascular space. Albumin is a major drug-binding plasma protein that primarily binds acidic medications and exhibits decreased plasma concentrations in CKD.[8] Protein binding of many acidic medications such as penicillins, cephalosporins, aminoglycosides, furosemide, and phenytoin, is therefore decreased in the setting of CKD secondary to hypoalbuminemia, qualitative changes in the conformation of the albumin binding site, and/or competition for binding sites by other medications, metabolites, and endogenous substances.[8,12,13,15] This increases the apparent V_D. Ultimately, a new equilibrium is established as a result of increased medication elimination/distribution, such that the unbound concentrations remain comparable to those observed in patients with normal kidney function despite the fact that total concentrations are decreased. Thus, the net effect is an alteration in the relationship between total medication concentration and pharmacodynamic effect.

For example, protein binding of phenytoin (90% protein-bound, primarily to albumin) is dramatically decreased in CKD secondary to hypoalbuminemia and decreased plasma phenytoin binding affinity for albumin. These changes alter the relationship between total phenytoin concentration and therapeutic and toxic effects.[22] The increase in unbound fraction, from values of 10% in those with normal kidney function to 20% or more in those with G5 CKD, results in increased hepatic clearance and decreased total concentrations. Thus, in patients with CKD, the therapeutic range based on total phenytoin concentration is shifted downward from normal values of 10 to 20 mg/L (μg/mL; 40-79 μmol/L) to values as low as 4 to 8 mg/L (μg/mL; 16-32 μmol/L). Since the unbound concentration therapeutic range is the same for all patients, 1 to

2 mg/L (μg/mL; 4-8 μmol/L), this measurement provides the best target for individualizing phenytoin therapy in patients with CKD.

One can approximate the total phenytoin concentration that would be observed in category G5 CKD patients assuming they had normal plasma protein binding ($C_{\text{normal binding}}$). The estimated total phenytoin concentration can then be interpreted in light of the usual total therapeutic range to assess the patient's response to therapy.[22] For normal or low albumin (concentration expressed in g/dL; albumin expressed in g/L must be multiplied by 0.1 prior to using the following equation) and category G5 CKD:

$$C_{\text{normal binding}} = C_{\text{reported}}/[(0.9)(0.48)(\text{albumin}/4.40)] + 0.1$$

where $C_{\text{normal binding}}$ = total phenytoin concentration that would be observed assuming patient had normal protein binding, and C_{reported} = patient's total phenytoin concentration reported by the laboratory (represents decreased plasma protein binding).

α1-acid glycoprotein is another major drug-binding plasma protein which primarily binds basic medications and exhibits increased plasma concentrations in CKD. For most medications that bind to α1-acid glycoprotein, protein binding is unaffected by CKD. However, for some medications (e.g., bepridil, disopyramide), the unbound fraction may be dramatically decreased and the V_D decreased in CKD patients, especially kidney transplant and HD patients.[8,13,19]

Altered Tissue Binding

Distribution may also be affected by altered tissue binding of medications in CKD patients; this is relatively rare and limited to few medications, such as pindolol, ethambutol, and, most notably, digoxin.[13] The V_D of digoxin is decreased by up to 50% in patients with category G5 CKD, leading to elevated serum concentrations.[23] In this case, the absolute amount of digoxin bound to the receptor is decreased and the resultant serum digoxin concentration is higher than anticipated. Thus, in CKD patients, particularly in those with category G5, a "normal" total medication concentration may be associated with either an adverse reaction secondary to elevated unbound medication concentrations, or a subtherapeutic response because of an altered plasma-to-tissue medication concentration ratio. The monitoring of unbound medication concentrations in CKD patients is thus warranted for those medications that have a narrow therapeutic range, are highly protein bound (unbound fraction of less than 20%), and for which marked variability in the unbound fraction is possible (e.g., phenytoin and disopyramide).

V_D Calculation Method

Finally, determination of the influence of CKD on V_D may depend on the method used to calculate V_D. The three most commonly used volume of distribution terms are: volume of the central compartment (V_c, which relates drug concentration and amount immediately following IV bolus administration), volume of the terminal phase (V_β and V_{area}, which relates drug concentration and amount during the terminal elimination phase), and volume of distribution at steady state (V_{ss}, which relates drug concentration and amount at IV infusion steady state). For many medications, V_c approximates extracellular fluid volume and thus may be increased or decreased by acute changes in fluid status; oliguric AKI is often accompanied by fluid overload and a resultant increased V_c for many medications. V_{area} and V_β are affected by both distribution and the terminal elimination rate constant, whereas V_{ss} has the advantage of being independent of medication elimination. Therefore, V_{ss} is the most appropriate volume term to use when one desires to compare drug distribution volumes between patients with CKD and those with normal kidney function.[24]

Elimination

Elimination of medication from the body is characterized in pharmacokinetic terms as total systemic clearance (CL_T). CL_T is the sum of all organ clearances and can be defined simply as the sum of renal clearance (CL_R) and nonrenal clearance (CL_{NR}).[8,10,13] Both CL_R and CL_{NR} can be altered in the setting of CKD.

Renal Clearance

3 Kidney function is the most quantifiable determinant of medication clearance. CL_R is a composite of all renal excretory functions, namely, filtration, tubular secretion, and tubular reabsorption ($CL_R = CL_{\text{filtration}} + CL_{\text{secretion}} - CL_{\text{reabsorption}}$).[10,12,13] Filtration clearance occurs by diffusion and is a function of GFR and the fraction of the medication that is unbound to plasma proteins (f_u) and thus available to be freely filtered ($CL_{\text{filtration}} = \text{GFR} \times f_u$). Tubular secretion and reabsorption are bidirectional processes that involve carrier-mediated renal transport systems consisting of uptake and efflux transporters located on the basolateral and apical membranes of tubular cells, respectively.[13,25,26]

Renal transport systems have been broadly classified on the basis of substrate selectivity into the anionic and cationic renal transport systems, which are responsible for the transport of a number of organic acidic and basic medications, respectively.[13,25,26] Basolateral uptake of medications into renal tubular cells from the plasma is mediated primarily by organic anion transporters (OATs), organic anion transporting polypeptides (OATPs), and organic cation transporters (OCTs). Apical efflux of medications from renal tubular cells to the tubular lumen is mediated primarily by multidrug resistance proteins (MRPs), breast cancer resistance protein (BCRP), P-glycoprotein (P-gp), multidrug and toxin extrusion proteins (MATEs), and organic cation/carnitine transporters (OCTNs). Many drugs are actively secreted by one or more of these transporter families.[25]

Medications that are majority excreted via the renal route (i.e., $f_e > 0.3$) are likely to have their pharmacokinetics altered by decreases in CL_R secondary to CKD.[17] Reduction in kidney mass, the number of functioning nephrons, renal blood flow, GFR, and/or the rate of tubular secretion and reabsorption all contribute to the decreased renal excretory capacity observed in CKD.[8] The intact nephron hypothesis describes the anatomic and physiologic changes to the nephron population in CKD and states that as CKD progresses, all facets of renal excretory function (filtration, secretion, and reabsorption) will decline in parallel.[27,28] However, CL_R of medications may violate the intact nephron hypothesis in that renal secretory function may decline more quickly or more slowly than renal filtration function.[29-31] For example, OAT1 and OAT3 substrates exhibit a greater decline in $CL_{\text{secretion}}$ than $CL_{\text{filtration}}$ in patients with severe CKD, suggesting that tubular secretion declines more quickly than glomerular filtration.[29,31] The impact of CKD on renal secretory function is dependent on the transporter systems involved in clearance and/or the medication being secreted.[30]

For medications that are primarily filtered, a decrease in GFR will result in a proportional decrease in CL_R. However, for medications that are highly secreted, a decrease in GFR may result in a variable decrease in CL_R depending on the relative decline in secretory function compared to GFR. Therefore, the impact of CKD on CL_R of a medication may depend on the renal excretory profile of the drug (i.e., the relative contributions of filtration, secretion, and reabsorption to overall CL_R, and the relevant transporter pathways involved in secretion and reabsorption).[30]

Nonrenal Clearance

4 CL_{NR} encompasses all routes of medication elimination other than renal excretion of unchanged drug, and broadly includes hepatic and extrahepatic metabolism and transcellular transport pathways. Major CL_{NR} pathways include oxidative metabolism by cytochrome P450s (CYPs), conjugative metabolism by uridine diphosphate-glucuronosyltransferases (UGTs), and transport by OATPs, MRPs, BCRP, and other transporters.[9,10,15,32] CKD, and

TABLE 67-2 Impact of ESKD on CL_{NR} of Selected Medications

Medication	Decrease in CL_{NR}
Acyclovir	50%
Aztreonam	33%
Bupropion	↓
Captopril	50%
Carvedilol	↓
Cefotaxime	40%
Ceftriaxone	↓
Cimetidine	46%
Ciprofloxacin	33%
Doripenem	↓
Erythromycin	↓
Imipenem	58%
Isoniazid	↓
Ketorolac	↓
Losartan	↓
Lovastatin	↓
Metoclopramide	66%
Minoxidil	46%
Morphine	40%
Nicardipine	37%
Nimodipine	87%
Nortriptyline	↓
Procainamide	60%
Quinapril	↓
Raloxifene	↓
Repaglinide	↓
Rosuvastatin	↓
Simvastatin	↓
Valsartan	↓
Vancomycin	43%
Verapamil	54%
Warfarin	50%

CL_{NR}, nonrenal clearance; ESKD, end-stage kidney disease.

↓ a decrease is documented but not quantified.

Data from References 13, 14, and 33.

particularly end-stage kidney disease (ESKD), impacts CL_{NR} of many drugs (Table 67-2), and over 30% of medications with $f_e < 0.3$ require a renal dose adjustment.[13,14,17,33] The impact of CKD on CL_{NR} is due largely to altered activity of drug-metabolizing enzymes and transporters in the liver and other organs. It is believed that these effects are due to accumulation of solutes that would otherwise be renally cleared in CKD patients (i.e., uremic solutes), which may inhibit drug-metabolizing enzymes and/or transporters by down-regulation of mRNA and/or protein expression and/or by direct inhibition.[8,10,13-15]

Importantly, the impact of CKD on CL_{NR} is pathway-specific; not all metabolizing enzymes and transporters are impacted by CKD or altered to the same magnitude by CKD. Generally, Drug metabolizing enzymes are only modestly affected by CKD. For example, the activities of CYP1A2, CYP2C8, CYP2C9, and CYP2C19 do not appear to be altered to a clinically significant extent in CKD. Conversely, the activity of CYP2D6 may be decreased in CKD.[34-36] The activity of CYP3A4 in CKD is of great interest, considering CYP3A4 is responsible for the metabolism of many medications on the market. Although there are conflicting clinical reports, it has been shown that CYP3A4 activity is generally preserved in patients with CKD.[8,10,13-15,36-38] Conversely, the activity of extrarenal transporters may often be affected by CKD. For example, there is a 40% to 60% decrease in hepatic OATP activity in patients with severe CKD.[34,35] Furthermore, the effect of CKD on CL_{NR} may depend partly on whether the decrease in kidney function is acute or chronic. For example, higher residual CL_{NR} has been documented in AKI versus CKD for patients with comparable creatinine clearance (CL_{cr}) receiving vancomycin and imipenem[11,15,39,40]

CKD-associated changes to CL_{NR} are complex and the result of pathway-specific changes to CL_{NR} and overlapping substrate specificity of medication for multiple drug-metabolizing enzymes and/or transporters. Therefore, prediction of the effect of kidney disease on the metabolism of a particular medication is difficult and there is no quantitative strategy to predict changes for one medication based on data from another, even if they are in the same pharmacologic class. However, some qualitative insight can be gained if one knows what enzyme or transporter is involved in the elimination of the drug of interest and how the enzyme or transporter is affected by CKD.

Accumulation of Metabolites

CKD patients who are receiving chronic pharmacotherapy may experience considerable accumulation of metabolite(s) as well as the parent compound, particularly if the ultimate route of metabolite elimination is renal. Metabolites of several medications have significant pharmacologic and/or toxicologic activity. However, the pharmacokinetics and pharmacodynamics of metabolites are not often fully elucidated during the drug development process. Because of the multiplicity of potential interactions of compounds that are primarily metabolized, the practical consequences of metabolite accumulation are difficult to predict and are most often identified in patients at risk serendipitously.

The metabolite may have similar pharmacologic activity to the parent drug and thus contribute significantly to clinical and toxicologic response.[16] For example, the liver rapidly metabolizes morphine into active metabolites, morphine-3-glucuronide (M3G), and morphine-6-glucuronide (M6G), which readily cross the blood-brain barrier, bind to opiate receptors, and exert strong analgesic effects. In CKD patients, morphine is metabolized more slowly, and clearance of M3G and M6G decreases, resulting in prolonged narcosis and respiratory depression.[41] Alternatively, the metabolite may have qualitatively dissimilar pharmacologic action compared to the parent drug. For example, meperidine undergoes *N*-demethylation metabolism by various CYP450 isoforms to form normeperidine. Whereas meperidine has central nervous system depressant effects, normeperidine has stimulatory activity that may produce seizures.[42]

Pharmacodynamics

CKD affects multiple organ systems, and therefore the response to a medication may change beyond what would be predicted based on pharmacokinetic changes alone. For example, enoxaparin dosage reduction is required in category G4 and G5 CKD patients.[43,44] This is due to the accumulation of uremic solutes which results in complex disturbances of the coagulation system leading to an increase in bleeding. Therefore, it seems that dosage adjustment solely based on kidney function may not always lead to optimal anticoagulation outcomes in CKD patients.

Successful antibiotic or antiviral treatment of CKD patients requires not only consideration of pharmacokinetic profiles, but also the medications' pharmacodynamics, which links measures of systemic exposure (such as peak and trough serum concentrations, and *AUC*) to bacteriologic activity.[10] Most antibiotics demonstrate concentration-dependent or time-dependent bacterial killing. For concentration-dependent antibiotics, such as fluoroquinolones or aminoglycosides, a high ratio of the peak serum concentration to the minimum inhibitory concentration (MIC, the minimum concentration required to inhibit bacterial growth) has been associated with increased likelihood of clinical success. Conversely, for time-dependent antibiotics, such as cephalosporins, the percentage of the dosing interval spent above the MIC is the most important pharmacodynamic parameter to maximize clinical success. This has led to the utilization of prolonged infusions or to continuous infusions. Thus, it is necessary to administer anti-infective medications with a time-dependent action more frequently, whereas anti-infective medications with a concentration-dependent action should be administered with a higher maintenance dose and potentially a prolonged dosage interval to increase efficacy while minimizing toxicity. Therefore, both the pharmacodynamics and pharmacokinetics of medications may need to be considered when initiating antimicrobial therapy in CKD patients.

MEDICATION DOSAGE REGIMEN INDIVIDUALIZATION IN CHRONIC KIDNEY DISEASE

Determining the appropriate dose of medication for a patient with CKD is dependent on both patient- and medication-specific factors.[11,16] Obtaining a full clinical picture of the patient, including an accurate assessment of kidney function, is imperative. Furthermore, a thorough understanding of how CKD impacts the pharmacokinetics of the medication being prescribed, and, if available, corresponding dose adjustment recommendations, is necessary to individualize pharmacotherapy. The patient care process for personalizing pharmacotherapy in patients with CKD involves a stepwise approach for adjusting medication dosage.

Estimation of Kidney Function for Personalizing Pharmacotherapy

Accurate assessment of kidney function is a critical step in determining appropriate medication dosing regimens, and the KDIGO guidelines recommend utilizing the most accurate method to assess kidney function for an individual patient.[16] A detailed discussion of the methodologies for assessing kidney function is presented in Chapter e60, "Evaluation of Kidney Function." The most common equations for estimating GFR include the Cockcroft-Gault (CG) equation (which calculates estimated creatinine clearance [eCL_{cr}]) and the several iterations of the Chronic Kidney Disease-Epidemiology Collaboration (CKD-EPI) equations (which calculate estimated GFR [eGFR]).[45-48] CG has been the most commonly used method to estimate kidney function for medication dosing for over 40 years; however, contemporary eGFR equations offer improved accuracy and precision over CG and are automatically reported in the clinical setting.[46,49]

There is considerable debate regarding which equation to estimate kidney function is the most appropriate to use for medication dosing. The CKD-EPI equations offer increased accuracy over CG.[46,47] However, for most medications, any renal pharmacokinetic studies were performed and dosing guidelines were developed using CG, and some argue that renal dose adjustment based on eGFR may be inappropriate.[50,51] Furthermore, the CKD-EPI equations provide eGFR indexed to body surface area (BSA) (i.e., in mL/min/1.73 m^2), whereas CG calculates eCL_{cr} as an absolute value (i.e., in mL/min). Therefore, reported eGFR values can differ significantly from eCL_{cr} if congruent units are not achieved by de-indexing for BSA (i.e., converted to an absolute value by multiplying by patient BSA/1.73 m^2), especially for patients of extreme body size.[51,52] Potential discordance between medication dosing recommendations based on these equations is well established.[51,53-55] Average discordance rates between eGFR equations and CG vary between 10% and 40%. This illustrates that the kidney function-estimating equation used for medication selection and dosing can have important clinical consequences on pharmacotherapy.[56]

Although quantitative assessment of kidney function is a crucial consideration, the output of kidney function-estimating equations should not be the sole determinant for pharmacotherapeutic decision making. Renal dose adjustment should be guided by clinical judgment, including an assessment of the risk-benefit ratio of the medication being prescribed, a complete clinical picture of the patient, and a thorough understanding of the limitations and implications of the various kidney function-estimating equations.[51] The ultimate goal of kidney function assessment and renal dose adjustment of medications is optimized and personalized pharmacotherapy.

Medication Dosing Information Resources

5 The 1998 FDA guidance on Pharmacokinetics in Patients with Impaired Renal Function were the first official guidelines addressing when and how to conduct pharmacokinetic and pharmacodynamic studies of a new medication in patients with impaired kidney function.[57] The 1998 guidance recommended that renal pharmacokinetic studies be conducted for medications with a narrow therapeutic index, medications that are primarily renally excreted, and medications for which the parent drug or active metabolite has high hepatic clearance and significant plasma protein binding. Furthermore, the guidance recommended assessing kidney function using CL_{cr} or serum creatinine (SCr) values.[57] The most recent 2020 draft guidance expands the recommendations of when to conduct renal pharmacokinetic studies to include medications that are predominantly cleared by nonrenal routes. Additionally, the use of eGFR, as calculated by a contemporary GFR-estimating equation, is preferred to assess kidney function.[58] The adoption of the FDA guidance has resulted in increased frequency of renal pharmacokinetic studies and improved availability of renal dosing recommendations, especially for medications with predominantly renal elimination. However, a lack of renal pharmacokinetic and dosing data persists for many medications, including oncology and antiviral agents and medications with $f_e < 0.3$, for which only 56% to 66% of medications approved from 1999 to 2010 have renal pharmacokinetic studies.[17]

The KDIGO guideline group recommends adjusting the dosage of medications in patients with CKD according to FDA- or EMA-approved labeling when such information is available. When this information is not available, the use of peer-reviewed literature is recommended to guide medication dosage adjustment.[16] These resources, along with other commonly used drug information sources such as Drug Prescribing in Renal Failure,[59] The Renal Drug Handbook,[60] Lexicomp,[61] Micromedex,[62] and the American Hospital Formulary Service Drug Information.[63] are excellent sources of information about a medication's pharmacokinetic characteristics. However, they are not without limitation and can yield marked variation in recommendations and the paucity of details of the methods used to generate the dosing advice (Table 67-3).[64,65] In addition, none of these sources consistently provide the explicit relationships of the pharmacokinetic parameters of interest (CL_T, elimination rate constant [k], and V_D) with a continuous index of kidney function (eCL_{cr} or eGFR). To find this information, one may need to identify the primary research study that assessed the medication's disposition, which can be a time-consuming process and difficult to carry out for each medication and patient combination in real time.

MEDICATION DOSAGE REGIMENS FOR NONDIALYSIS CKD PATIENTS

6 Dosage regimen design in CKD patients is dependent on the pharmacodynamic/pharmacokinetic characteristics of the

TABLE 67-3 Comparison of Secondary References Used for Medication Dosing in Patients with CKD

Resource	Pros	Cons
Aronoff's Drug Prescribing in Renal Failure[63]	• Exclusive focus on medication dosing in patients with CKD • Information provided for IHD, PD, CRRT • Tables include medication PK and dosage adjustment based on CL_{cr} (>50, 10-50, <10 mL/min [>0.83, 0.17-0.83, <0.17 mL/s]) • Tables for both adult and pediatric dosing provided • Concise, easy to use • References to primary literature provided	• Updated infrequently; information may not be current, newer medications may not be included • Some dosage recommendations are not feasible for dialysis patients (i.e., q 36 hours dosing interval)
The Renal Drug Handbook[64]	• Easy to access with a subscription • Contains information on clinical use of medications, PK, dose in normal kidney function, dose adjustment in CKD, drug interactions and administration • Specific to CKD patients	• Updated every few years; information may not be current, newer medications may not be included • References not provided
Lexicomp[65]	• Easy to access with a subscription • Easy to navigate • Concise information • Dose adjustment in CKD provided (including HD and PD)	• May be difficult to navigate • No specific focus on CKD patients • References to primary literature for dosing not provided
Micromedex[66]	• Easy to access with a subscription • Comprehensive, detailed information (both "in-depth" and "quick") • Dose adjustment in CKD provided (including HD and PD)	• May be difficult to navigate • No specific focus on CKD patients • References to primary literature for dosing not consistently provided
American Hospital Formulary Service (AHFS)[67]	• Easy to access with a subscription • Detailed medication monographs • "Dosage in Renal and Hepatic Impairment/ Special Populations" section for each medication listed • Online version updated regularly, print version updated yearly	• Hard copy version can be difficult to navigate, cumbersome • Information on dose adjustment in CKD is minimal • No specific focus on CKD patients • References to primary literature for dosing not provided

CKD, chronic kidney disease; CL_{cr}, creatinine clearance; CRRT, continuous renal replacement therapy; HD, hemodialysis; IHD, intermittent hemodialysis; PD, peritoneal dialysis; PK, pharmacokinetics.

Data from References 59-63.

medication, the patient's degree of residual kidney function, and their overall clinical condition. The initial or "loading" dose for CKD patients should be the same as the dose recommended for those with normal kidney function unless the medication's V_D is known to be altered in CKD or a concomitant disease.[11] If V_D is increased, then the dose should be increased proportionally (see Table 67-1). Rapid achievement of therapeutic drug concentrations is important in many patient care situations and thus it is often better to start therapy aggressively rather than conservatively.

If available, maintenance dosage regimen guidelines for CKD patients in FDA- or EMA-approved product labeling should be the foundation for ongoing therapy.[16] Approved product labeling typically includes dose adjustment recommendations for ranges of kidney function. These ranges represent mild (eCL_{Cr} 60-90 mL/min or eGFR 60-90 mL/min/1.73 m^2), moderate (eCL_{Cr} 30-59 mL/min or eGFR 30-59 mL/min/1.73 m^2), and severe (eCL_{Cr} <30 mL/min or eGFR <30 mL/min/1.73 m^2) CKD (see Chapter 62, "Chronic Kidney Disease").[66] Each of these categories encompasses a broad range in kidney function, and thus the recommended dosage regimen may not be optimal for all patients whose kidney function lies within a given kidney function category.

Quantifying the Relationship Between Kidney Function and Medication Clearance

If FDA- or EMA-approved product labeling information is not available or if there is marked variance between these two agencies' recommendations, a stepwise approach for designing a dosage regimen for a patient with CKD can be used. In either case, the design of the optimal dosage regimen is dependent on the availability of an accurate characterization of the relationship between the pharmacokinetic parameters of the medication and kidney function and an accurate assessment of the patient's kidney function.

The "Dettli Method" is a graphical means to generate medication dosing recommendations based on the linear relationship between the elimination rate constant of a renally cleared medication and a patient's creatinine clearance:

$$k = k_{NR} + (\alpha \times CL_{cr})$$

where k is the elimination rate constant of the medication based on a first-order one-compartment model, k_{NR} is the nonrenal elimination rate constant, and α is a constant relating the renal drug elimination rate constant to the patient's creatinine clearance (CL_{cr}).[67] This approach assumes that the overall elimination rate constant (k), relating to CL_T, declines linearly with CL_{cr}, and that the nonrenal elimination rate constant (k_{NR}), relating to CL_{NR}, remains constant as kidney function declines. While the first assumption generally holds true for medications that are mainly renally cleared, the second assumption is flawed, as CL_{NR} can be altered in CKD.[8-15] The relationship between CL_T and CL_{cr} for selected medications is depicted in Table 67-4. This information, along with the patient's eCL_{cr} or eGFR, is the foundation upon which a therapeutic regimen to attain the desired medication concentration-time profile and ultimately the therapeutic outcome can be formulated when renal dosing information is not provided in the approved product labeling information.

However, the linear relationship of kinetic parameters to eGFR or eCL_{cr} is often not explicitly reported. In this case, then the CL_T or k for CKD patients can be estimated using the method of Rowland and Tozer, provided that f_e for subjects with normal kidney function is known.[18] This approach assumes that the changes in CL_T and k are proportional to eCL_{cr}, that CKD does not alter the medication's metabolism, that any metabolites that are formed are inactive and nontoxic, and that the medication obeys first-order (linear) one-compartment kinetic principles. If these assumptions are true, which is rarely the case, then the dosage-adjustment factor (Q) can be calculated as:

$$Q = 1 - [f_e(1 - KF)]$$

where KF is the ratio of the patient's kidney function (ie, eCL_{cr} or eGFR) to the assumed normal value of 120 mL/min. Thus, for a

TABLE 67-4 Relationship Between CL_{cr} and CL_T of Selected Medications

Medication	Total Systemic Clearance[a]
Acyclovir	$CL_T = 3.37\ (CL_{cr}) + 0.41$
Amikacin	$CL_T = 0.6\ (CL_{cr}) + 9.6$
Aztreonam	$CL_T = 0.8\ (CL_{cr}) + 26.6$
Cefazolin	$CL_T = 0.34\ (CL_{cr}) + 6.6$
Ceftazidime	$CL_T = 1.15\ (CL_{cr}) + 10.6$
Ciprofloxacin	$CL_T = 2.83\ (CL_{cr}) + 363$
Digoxin	$CL_T = 0.88\ (CL_{cr}) + 23$
Ganciclovir	$CL_T = 1.24\ (CL_{cr}) + 8.57$
Gentamicin	$CL_T = 0.983\ (CL_{cr})$
Imipenem	$CL_T = 1.42\ (CL_{cr}) + 54$
Lithium	$CL_T = 0.20\ (CL_{cr})$
Ofloxacin	$CL_T = 1.04\ (CL_{cr}) + 38.7$
Piperacillin	$CL_T = 1.36\ (CL_{cr}) + 1.50$
Tobramycin	$CL_T = 0.801\ (CL_{cr})$
Vancomycin	$CL_T = 0.69\ (CL_{cr}) + 3.7$

CL_T, total systemic clearance; CL_{cr}, creatinine clearance.

[a]Clearance in mL/min can be converted to mL/s through multiplication by 0.0167.

medication that is 85% eliminated renally unchanged in a patient who has an eCL_{cr} of 10 mL/min, Q would be:

$$\begin{aligned} Q &= 1 - (0.85[1 - (10/120)]) \\ &= 1 - (0.85[1 - 0.083]) \\ &= 1 - 0.78 \\ &= 0.22 \end{aligned}$$

Designing Adjusted Renal Dosage Regimens

In order to determine the best method for dosage regimen adjustment, a regimen goal must be defined.[10,11] The goal may be pharmacokinetic (maintenance of a similar peak, trough, or average steady-state drug concentration) or pharmacodynamic (time above the MIC [e.g., cephalosporins] or the ratio of the *AUC* relative to the MIC [e.g., fluoroquinolones]). If there is a strong relationship between peak concentration and clinical response (e.g., aminoglycosides) or toxicity (e.g., phenobarbital and phenytoin), then the attainment of specific target values is critical for optimal therapeutic outcomes. If, however, no specific target values for peak or trough concentrations have been reported, then a regimen goal of attaining the same average steady-state concentration is likely to be appropriate.

The options to attain the desired average steady-state concentration profile in CKD patients are to either decrease the dose or increase the dosing interval (τ). If the dose is decreased and the dosing interval remains unchanged, then the average steady-state concentration will be unchanged but the peaks will be lower and the troughs will be higher. Conversely, if the dosing interval is increased and the dose remains unchanged, then the average steady-state, peak, and trough concentrations in the patient with CKD will be similar to those in the patient with normal kidney function (Fig. 67-1).[68] Increasing the dosing interval is the approach used most commonly to adjust dosage regimens in patients with CKD because it translates into a lower daily medication burden in these patients. Moreover, it is likely to yield cost savings as a result of a reduction in pharmacy and nursing time for preparation and administration of fewer (less frequent) doses, as well as a reduction in the corresponding supplies. Lastly, it is important to note that occasionally both the dose and dosing interval may need to be changed for pragmatic reasons (i.e., to allow the administration of a clinically practical dose [500 mg vs a calculated value of 487 mg] or dosing interval [administer every 12 hours vs every 17 hours]).

If the relationships between the pharmacokinetic parameters of the medication and kidney function are known (i.e., equations are available such as those depicted in Table 67-4), then the change in dose and/or dosing interval for a patient with a given kidney function can be calculated and a dosage regimen adjustment can be designed using a stepwise approach. CL_T is calculated for a patient

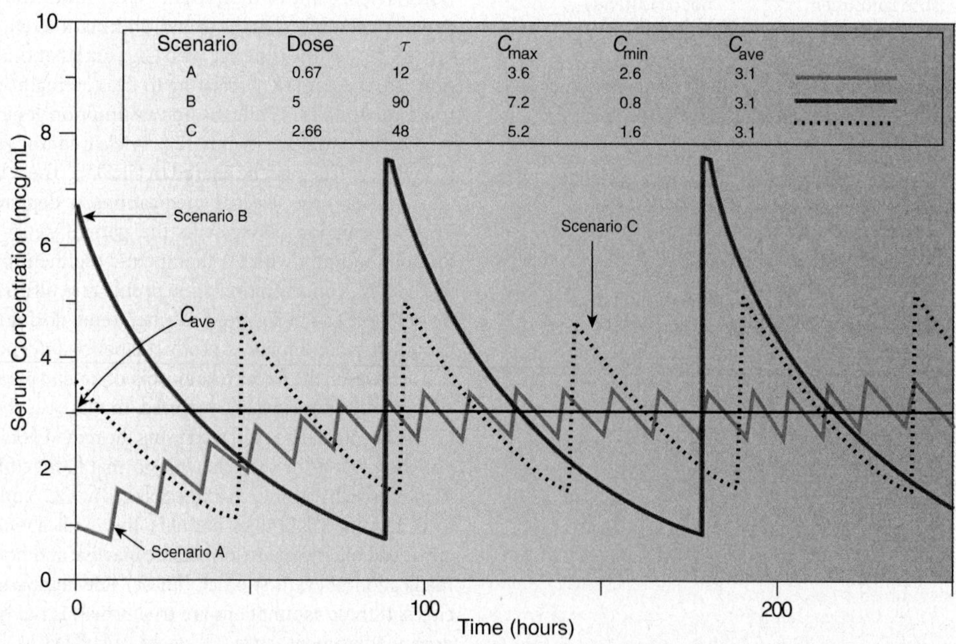

FIGURE 67-1 Although the average steady-state concentrations (C_{ave}) are identical regardless of which dosage-adjustment strategy one decides to implement, the concentration-time profile will be markedly different if one changes the dose and maintains the dosing interval (τ) constant (*Scenario A*), versus changing the dosing interval and maintaining the dose constant (*Scenario B*) or changing both (*Scenario C*).

with normal kidney function (CL_{cr} or eGFR = 120 mL/min) and a patient with CKD based on available equations describing the quantitative relationship between CL_T and CL_{cr} or eGFR (as presented in Table 67-4). In this situation, the dosage-adjustment factor (Q) is calculated as the ratio of the estimated k or CL of the patient with CKD relative to a subject with normal kidney function. The Q is then used to determine the adjusted dose or dosing interval for a patient with CKD, as follows:

$$D_{CKD} = D_{norm} \times Q$$

$$\tau_{CKD} = \tau_{norm}/Q$$

where D_{CKD} is the adjusted dose for a patient with CKD, D_{norm} is the standard dose for a patient with normal kidney function, τ_{CKD} is the adjusted dosing interval for a patient with CKD, τ_{norm} is the standard dosing interval for a patient with normal kidney function, and Q is the dosage-adjustment factor. The strategy for dosing adjustment (i.e., decrease the dose or increase dosing interval) is chosen and the corresponding dosing interval or dose is calculated.

An example of this process is illustrated in Table 67-5 for ciprofloxacin, a commonly used antibiotic for the treatment of infections in CKD and dialysis patients. Ciprofloxacin is a concentration-dependent antibiotic, and thus the peak concentration and *AUC* determine its efficacy. Therefore, extending the interval but keeping the same dose allows for peak concentrations in CKD patients similar to those seen in normal kidney function, allowing for this pharmacodynamic action to be achieved without accumulation of medication that could cause dose-dependent toxicities.

If the V_D of a medication is significantly altered in CKD patients or if one desires to attain a specific maximum or minimum concentration, the estimation of a dosage regimen becomes more complex. If the relationship between V_D and CL_{cr} has been characterized, then V_D may be estimated. If one assumes that a one-compartment linear model can describe the medication, the predicted V_D may then be used with the predicted k of the medication to yield an adjusted-dosing interval and IV dose:

$$\tau_{CKD} = (-1/k)[\ln(C_{min}/C_{max})]$$

$$D_{CKD} = V_D \times (C_{max} - C_{min})$$

where τ_{CKD} is the adjusted dosing interval for a patient with CKD, and D_{CKD} is the adjusted dose for a patient with CKD. These principles have been used to derive dosage recommendations for many commonly used medications for CKD patients. It should be noted, however, that in most dosing guidelines, the "usual" dose or dose for "normal kidney function" represents eGFR greater than 50 mL/min/1.73 m². This assumption, however, could lead to dosing errors for patients with eGFRs of 60 mL/min/1.73 m² versus 90 mL/min/1.73 m² versus 130 mL/min/1.73 m². Augmented renal clearance, defined as CL_{cr} greater than 130 mL/min/1.73 m², has been associated with subtherapeutic antibiotic concentrations and outcomes in critically ill patients when standard doses of antibiotics were administered.[69] Clinicians should be aware of the potential to underdose critically ill patients with documented augmented kidney function and thus should consider the use of higher doses, especially for antibiotics and antivirals.

TABLE 67-5 Stepwise Approach to Calculating a Dosage Regimen Based on a Medication's Pharmacokinetic Properties and a Patient's Kidney Function

	Steps	Calculation Examples with Ciprofloxacin
Step 1	Calculate total systemic clearance of medication in an individual with normal kidney function (CL_{norm}); CL_{cr} = 120 mL/min	CL_{norm} = [2.83 (CL_{cr})] + 363 CL_{norm} = [2.83(120)] + 363 CL_{norm} = 702.6 mL/min
Step 2	Calculate total systemic clearance of medication in a patient with CKD (CL_{CKD})	In patient with CL_{cr} = 15 mL/min CL_{CKD} = [2.83(CL_{cr})] + 363 CL_{CKD} = [2.83(15)] + 363 CL_{CKD} = 405.5 mL/min
Step 3	Calculate the dosage-adjustment factor (Q) for a patient with CKD as the ratio of the *CL* of the patient with CKD relative to an individual with normal kidney function	$Q = CL_{CKD}/CL_{norm}$ Q = 702.6/405.5 Q = 0.58
Step 4	Calculate the maintenance dose (D_{CKD}) or adjusted dosing interval (τ_{CKD}) in a patient with CKD; D_{norm} = normal dose; τ_{norm} = normal dosing interval	D_{norm} = 500 mg; τ_n = 12 h $D_{CKD} = D_{norm} \times Q$ D_{CKD} = 500 mg × 0.58 D_{CKD} = 290 mg $\tau_{CKD} = \tau_{norm}/Q$ τ_{CKD} = 12/0.58 τ_{CKD} = 20.7 h
Step 5	Choose dosing adjustment: Option A. Maintain D_{norm} and use τ_{CKD} Option B. Maintain τ_{norm} and use D_{CKD}	Dosing adjustments: Option A. 500 mg every 21 hr Option B. 290 mg every 12 hr
Step 6	Determine adjusted dosing regimen based on Option A using a practical dosing interval	D_{norm} = 500 mg; τ_{CKD} = 21 h *Practical* τ = 24 h (selected to limit missed doses)
Step 7	Recommend dosing regimen (dependent on product availability and limited risk of missed doses)	500 mg every 24 h

CL_{cr}, creatinine clearance.

Creatinine clearance in mL/min can be converted to mL/s through multiplication by 0.0167. Clearance in mL/min/1.73 m² can be converted to mL/s/m² through multiplication by 0.00963.

MEDICATION DOSAGE REGIMENS FOR DIALYSIS PATIENTS

The rationale and approaches for delivery of renal replacement therapy to patients with ESKD are described in Chapter 64, "Hemodialysis and Peritoneal Dialysis." This section will describe medication dosing regimens for patients on traditional HD, peritoneal dialysis, and alternative HD modalities, including short-daily hemodialysis (SDHD) and nocturnal hemodialysis (NHD). Several forms of continuous renal replacement therapy in clinical use today and corresponding approaches to individualize dosage regimens are described in Chapter 61, "Acute Kidney Injury."

Hemodialysis

Principles of Hemodialytic Clearance of Medications

7 The impact of HD on a patient's pharmacotherapy is dependent on several factors, including the physicochemical characteristics of the medication and the dialysis prescription. Medication-related factors that affect dialyzability include molecular weight, degree of protein binding, and V_D.[19] The permeability of a dialysis filter for medication depends on the composition of the filter and the molecular weight of the medication. The majority of dialysis filters in use in North America up until the mid-1990s were composed of cellulose, cellulose acetate, or regenerated cellulose (cuprophane) and

were generally impermeable to medications with a molecular weight >1,000 Da.[16] Dialysis membranes in the 21st century ("high-flux" dialysis membranes) are predominantly composed of semisynthetic or synthetic materials (e.g., polysulfone, polymethylmethacrylate, or polyacrylonitrile), have larger pore sizes, and more closely mimic the filtration characteristics of the human kidney. This allows for the passage of most solutes, including medications that have a molecular weight up to 20,000 Da, causing larger medications to be more easily removed with high flux dialyzers.[16] Some medications that are cleared in high-flux dialysis, but not through conventional dialysis, include vancomycin, carbamazepine, cisplatin, enoxaparin, ranitidine, valproic acid, sorafenib, and tramadol. The effect of HD on drug disposition is rarely reevaluated after it is initially reported; therefore, information for medications that were developed prior to the advent of high-flux dialysis membranes probably represents an underestimation of the impact of HD on a medication's disposition. Therapeutic drug monitoring for medications such as aminoglycosides and vancomycin should also be performed to ensure adequate dosing for patients on HD. Medications that are highly protein bound (i.e., $f_u < 0.10$) are not well dialyzed because both of the principal drug-binding plasma proteins, α1-acid glycoprotein and albumin, have a high molecular weight. Finally, medications that are widely distributed, with V_D greater than 2 L/kg, are poorly removed by HD.

The dialysis prescription can dramatically affect the total clearance of a medication.[95] HD can occur in a number of clinical settings, including acute management of AKI, intermittent three times a week, daily for an extended period, or some combination thereof for the management of category G5 CKD patients. The primary factors that vary between patients are the composition of the dialysis filter, the filter surface area, the blood, dialysate and ultrafiltration flow rates, and whether or not the dialysis unit reuses the dialysis filter.[16]

Overall, the impact of HD on pharmacotherapy is highly variable. One cannot assume that a certain percentage of a medication is removed with each dialysis session and an "all" or "none" approach regarding the dialyzability of a medication is insufficient information to make therapeutic decisions. Characteristics of the dialysis procedure that were utilized in the drug study, such as membrane composition and surface area and blood and dialysis flow rates, are critical parameters that should be known before one uses the published HD clearance data to prospectively design a medication dosing regimen for an HD patient.

Prospective Monitoring of Medication Concentrations

If medication concentrations can be measured in the clinical setting, the quantitative impact of HD on drug disposition can be calculated in one of the several ways.[19] The most commonly utilized means for assessing the effect of HD is to calculate the dialyzer clearance (CL_D) of the medication. The CL_D^p from blood can be calculated as:

$$CL_D^p = Q_p[(A_p - V_p)/A_p]$$

where Q_b is the blood flow through the dialyzer and Q_p is the plasma flow, which equals Q_b (1 − hematocrit); A_p is the plasma concentration of medication entering the dialyzer, and V_p is the plasma concentration of the medication leaving the dialyzer. This clearance calculation most accurately reflects dialysis drug clearance as most medications do not extensively penetrate red blood cells or bind to formed blood elements. However, for medications that readily partition into and out of erythrocytes, this equation would likely underestimate HD clearance. Furthermore, one must keep in mind that venous plasma concentrations may be artificially high and CL_D^p will be low if plasma water is removed from the blood at a faster rate than the medication. This tends to occur when extensive ultrafiltration is performed simultaneously with diffusion during dialysis.[16,19]

The following principles may be used to generate a medication dosage regimen recommendation for HD patients, if none is available in product labeling or other sources, by using a value of CL_D.[16,19] Because clearance terms are additive, the total clearance during dialysis can be calculated as the sum of the patient's underlying residual systemic clearance stemming from the patient's remaining renal clearance and nonrenal clearance during the interdialytic period (CL_{RES}) and dialyzer clearance (CL_D):

$$CL_T = CL_{RES} + CL_D$$

The half-life during the period between dialysis treatments and during dialysis can then be calculated from the following relationships using an estimate of the medication's V_D (see Table 67-2)[19]:

$$t_{1/2,\ \text{off HD}} = 0.693(V_D/CL_{RES})$$

$$t_{1/2,\ \text{on HD}} = 0.693(V_D/CL_{RES} + CL_D)$$

Once the key pharmacokinetic parameters have been estimated/calculated, they may be used to simulate the plasma concentration-time profile of the medication for the individual patient and then one can ascertain how much medication to administer and when. This approach to personalizing pharmacotherapy can be accomplished in a stepwise fashion assuming first-order elimination of the medication and a one-compartment model.

For medications with a narrow therapeutic index (e.g., vancomycin, phenytoin, and gentamicin), therapeutic drug monitoring (e.g., plasma concentration measurements and dialyzer clearance estimation) should be utilized to guide medication dosing.[19] The ultimate reason for measuring the plasma concentrations of antibacterial agents is to individualize the patient's dosage regimen to achieve a bacteriologic cure while preventing adverse effects and preserving residual kidney function. Vancomycin dosing is primarily based on attaining desired trough concentrations, usually between 15 and 20 mg/L (10-14 μmol/L) as this is likely to attain the target *AUC* of 400 to 600 mg·hr/L in the previous 24 hours.[70,71] It is common practice to administer medications post-dialysis on the premise that it is desirable to minimize the loss of medication that would result from dialyzer clearance. For example, the administration of traditional doses of tobramycin (1.5 mg/kg) or vancomycin (1,000 mg) during dialysis has been associated with markedly lower *AUC*s than those observed when the same dose was administered post-dialysis; consequently, higher dosage regimens are usually necessary to compensate for the additional loss of medication during the dialysis procedure. However, there are clinical scenarios when pre-dialysis or intradialytic medication administration may be optimal. Medications for pain may be given on a precise schedule and thus would be administered irrespective of the time on dialysis. Furthermore, it may be optimal to administer some medications, such as aminoglycosides[72,73] and vancomycin,[74,75] during or immediately prior to the start of a dialysis treatment. For example, pre-dialysis or intradialytic aminoglycoside dosing may obtain similar peak concentrations, a prime indicator of efficacy, but lower *AUC*, a correlate to ototoxicity and nephrotoxicity, compared to post-dialysis dosing.[72] Performing HD immediately after dosing might also be a good option for several anticancer medications. The pre-dialysis administration of a normal dose makes sense when the patient undergoes HD 2 to 12 hours later. This strategy delivers the desired maximum plasma concentration effect while minimizing patient exposure to the toxic drug or metabolite effects.[76,77]

Peritoneal Dialysis

Peritoneal dialysis, like other dialysis modalities, has the potential to affect drug disposition; however, personalizing pharmacotherapy is often less complicated in these patients as a result of the limited clearances of medications achieved with this procedure (see Chapter 64, "Hemodialysis and Peritoneal Dialysis"). In general, HD is more

CLINICAL CASE EXAMPLE Personalizing Pharmacotherapy for a Hemodialysis Patient

A 54-year-old critically ill woman with ESKD was transferred to a medical intensive care unit from the general medical unit, where she was febrile with a temperature of 39°C (102.2°F). Her weight was 64 kg (141 lb) and her height was 65 in (165 cm). She had a residual CL_{cr} of 5 mL/min (0.083 mL/s), and was receiving high-flux hemodialysis (F80 polysulfone dialyzer) for 4 hours on Mondays, Wednesdays, and Fridays. She was started on vancomycin for a methicillin-resistant *Staphylococcus aureus* (MRSA) catheter-associated bacteremia and her first dose of 1,000 mg was administered at the end of her HD treatment. The first step is to estimate this patient's pharmacokinetic parameters of vancomycin using known population data (Table 67-1) and equations (Table 67-4). The V_D in this patient can be estimated to be 54.4 L (0.85 L/kg × 64 kg). Her underlying residual systemic clearance (CL_{RES}) of vancomycin is estimated from the relationship between CL_T and kidney function (where $CL_T = [0.69 \times CL_{cr}] + 3.7$) and is 7.15 mL/min (0.12 mL/s) or 0.43 L/h. The k can be approximated as:

$$k = CL_{RES}/V_D$$
$$= 0.43\ \text{L/h} / 54.4\ \text{L}$$
$$= 0.0079\ \text{h}^{-1}$$

The HD clearance of vancomycin (CL_D) is dependent on the dialyzer and a value of 120 mL/min (2 mL/s; 7.2 L/hr) is a reasonable estimate for this dialyzer.[20]

One can now predict what the plasma concentrations of vancomycin will be over the next 24 to 48 hours, assuming the infusion time for the medication (t') was 1 hour. The concentration at the end of the 1-hour infusion (C_{max}) would be:

$$C_{max} = \frac{(\text{Dose}/t')}{CL_{RES}}(1 - e^{-kt'})$$
$$= \frac{(1.000\ \text{mg/h})}{0.43\ \text{L/h}}(1 - e^{-(0.0079)^{(1)}})$$
$$= (2{,}325.58\ \text{mg/L})(0.0078)$$
$$= 18.1\ \text{mg/L}$$

The plasma concentration prior to the next dialysis session (C_{bD}), which is 44 hours away can be calculated as:

$$C_{bD} = C_{max} \times e^{-(CL_{RES}/V_D) \times t}$$
$$= 18.1 \times e^{-0.0079 \times 44}$$
$$= 12.8\ \text{mg/L}$$

and the concentration 4 hours later after dialysis (C_{aD}) can be calculated as:

$$C_{aD} = C_{bD} \times e^{-[(CL_{RES} + CL_D + CL_D/V_D)] \times t}$$
$$= 12.8 \times e^{-[(0.43 + 7.2)/54.4] \times 4}$$
$$= 12.8 \times e^{-0.14 \times 4}$$
$$= 7.3\ \text{mg/L}$$

On the basis of these data, the second dose, which should be administered after the second dialysis session, was increased in order to maintain vancomycin trough concentrations between 15 and 20 mg/L (10-14 μmol/L) for an MRSA catheter-associated bacteremia, as this is likely to attain the *AUC* target of 400 to 600 mg·h/L in the previous 24 hours.[70,71] The patient received a vancomycin dose of 1,500 mg 4 hours after the end of the second dialysis session. The increase or change in serum concentration (ΔC) at the end of this 1-hour infusion can thus be estimated:

$$\Delta C = \frac{(\text{Dose}/t')}{CL_{RES}}(1 - e^{-kt'})$$
$$= \frac{(1{,}500\ \text{mg/h})}{0.43\ \text{L/h}}(1 - e^{-(0.0079)1})$$
$$= (3{,}488.4\ \text{mg/L})(0.0078)$$
$$= 27.2\ \text{mg/L}$$

Thus, the C_{max} would be approximately 34.5 mg/L (24 μmol/L), the sum of the residual concentration from the first dose of 7.3 mg/L (5 μmol/L) and the ΔC of 27.2 mg/L (18.8 μmol/L). The plasma concentration prior to the third dialysis session (C_{bD}), which is 40 hours away can be estimated as:

$$C_{bD} = C_{max} \times e^{(CL_{RES}/V_D) \times t}$$
$$= 34.5\ \text{mg/L} \times e^{-0.0079 \times 40}$$
$$= 25.2\ \text{mg/L}$$

and the concentration 4 hours later after the third dialysis (C_{aD}) can be estimated as:

$$C_{aD} = C_{bD} \times e^{-[(CL_{RES} + CL_D)/V_D] \times t}$$
$$= 25.2 \times e^{-[(0.43 + 7.2)/54.4] \times 4}$$
$$= 25.2 \times e^{-0.14 \times 4}$$
$$= 14.4\ \text{mg/L}$$

This higher dose would be considered to have achieved concentrations that are too high since the lowest value during the majority of the dosing interval exceeded 25.2 mg/L (17.1 μmol/L). The dose required to maintain vancomycin trough concentrations between 15 and 20 mg/L (10-14 μmol/L) should be determined.

effective in removing medications than peritoneal dialysis, such that if a medication is not removed by HD, it is unlikely to be significantly removed by peritoneal dialysis.

Many of the factors that are important in determining medication dialyzability for other treatment modalities pertain to peritoneal dialysis as well.[78,79] Factors that influence medication dialyzability by peritoneal dialysis include drug-specific characteristics such as molecular weight, solubility, degree of ionization, protein binding, and V_D. The intrinsic properties of the peritoneal membrane that affect medication removal include blood flow and peritoneal membrane surface area, which is approximately equal to the body surface area. There is an inverse relationship between peritoneal clearance of medications and molecular weight, protein binding, and V_D. In addition, medications that are ionized at physiologic pH will diffuse across the membrane more slowly than unionized compounds.[78,79]

Peritoneal dialysis, in current practice, is often prescribed to attain a urea clearance of approximately 10 mL/min (0.17 mL/s), so it is unlikely to significantly impact the *CL* of any medication. In addition, since most medications have a larger molecular size than urea, their resultant *CL* will likely be even lower: probably between 5 and 7.5 mL/min (0.08-0.13 mL/s). Therefore, medication dosing recommendations for the management of conditions other than peritonitis, reported for patients with estimated CL_{cr} or GFR of 10 to 15 mL/min (0.17-0.25 mL/s), are likely suitable for patients receiving peritoneal dialysis.[16]

Alternative Hemodialysis Modalities

Short-daily and nocturnal HD are two alternative HD techniques. Both modalities are administered 5 to 6 days a week but differ primarily in the duration of the treatment and blood-flow rate.[80] Overall small solute removal is more efficient if the frequency of HD is increased. Therefore, SDHD and NHD therapies yield different clearance values compared to intermittent three times per week HD. Furthermore, prolonged HD, such as in the case of NHD, results in less rebound of medication concentrations after the termination of dialysis. This likely occurs because the rate of transfer from the peripheral to central compartment relative to the rate of diffusive removal is lower. Therefore, careful monitoring of pharmacotherapy is necessary when these newer modalities are used to avoid potential errors in designing medication dosing regimens.

Nocturnal Hemodialysis

NHD is performed over 6 to 8 hours on 5 to 6 nights per week.[80] There is a paucity of information related to medication dosing with this modality; however, the principles of medication dosing discussed above with intermittent HD can also be applied here. Although there is an increase in dialysis hours, which would suggest an increase in medication removal, the blood and dialysate flow rates are slower and thus clearance per unit of time will be less. This has been demonstrated with cefazolin where the cefazolin clearance during NHD was slightly lower ($CL = 1.65$ L/hr) than during high-flux intermittent HD ($CL = 1.85$ L/hr); however, a greater percentage of cefazolin was removed in 8 hours of NHD (80%) than conventional 4-hour high-flux HD (60%).[81]

Short-Daily Hemodialysis

SDHD involves 2 to 3 hours of dialysis performed 5 to 6 days per week.[80] As in the case with NHD, there is also limited information on medication dosing with this modality; however, the general principles of medication dosing for HD also apply here. In SDHD, the number of dialysis sessions per week and blood and dialysate flow rates are similar to intermittent HD, which may suggest similar medication removal. However, for certain medications (smaller size and decreased V_D, and protein binding) removal may be increased. For example, the cefazolin clearance rate in SDHD is slightly higher than the value observed during high-flux intermittent HD; the amount of cefazolin removed in 2 hours of SDHD is similar to that after 4 hours of high-flux HD.[82] Therefore, the same amount of medication given over the entire week for patients on intermittent HD could also be given to patients on SDHD but in smaller amounts administered more frequently. For instance, in intermittent HD, the cefazolin dose is typically 2 g IV after each HD for a total of 6 g/week; whereas in SDHD, the dose would be 1 g IV daily (i.e., for 6 days) after each HD.

CONCLUSION

Patients with CKD often exhibit changes to pharmacokinetics and pharmacodynamics, and medication dosage regimen adjustment is often warranted in these patients. When available, the utilization of FDA or EMA medication dosage recommendations in official prescribing information should be used for the initiation of therapy in most clinical situations. However, when these guidelines are unavailable for the relevant clinical setting, the use of pharmacokinetic principles in conjunction with reliable population pharmacokinetic estimates may be used to determine the optimal medication dosage regimen. Prospective monitoring of serum concentrations for medications with a narrow therapeutic index should be undertaken whenever clinical therapeutic monitoring tools are available. The ultimate goal of medication dosage regimen adjustment in CKD is to individualize and optimize pharmacotherapeutic outcomes in this population to maximize therapeutic efficacy while minimizing unnecessary toxicity.

ABBREVIATIONS

α	constant relating the renal drug elimination rate constant to creatinine clearance
A_b	concentration of medication in blood going into the dialyzer (arterial side)
AKI	acute kidney injury
A_p	concentration of medication in plasma going into the dialyzer (arterial side)
AUC	area under the plasma concentration-time curve
$AUC_{0\text{-}t}$	the area under the predialyzer plasma concentration-time curve during hemodialysis
BCRP	breast cancer resistance protein
BSA	body surface area
ΔC	change in plasma concentration
C_{aD}	plasma concentration after dialysis
C_{bD}	plasma concentration prior to the next dialysis session
CG	Cockcroft–Gault
CKD	chronic kidney disease
CKD-EPI	Chronic Kidney Disease Epidemiology Collaboration Equation
CL	clearance
CL_D^b	dialyzer clearance from blood
CL_{CKD}	clearance of a medication in patients with CKD
CL_{cr}	creatinine clearance
CL_D	dialyzer clearance
CL_{filt}	renal filtration clearance
CL_{norm}	clearance of a medication in patients with normal kidney function
CL_{NR}	nonrenal clearance
CL_D^p	dialyzer clearance from plasma
CL_R	renal clearance
$CL_{reabsorption}$	renal tubular reabsorption
CL_{RES}	residual clearance in a dialysis patient
$CL_{secretion}$	renal tubular secretion clearance
CL_T	total clearance
$C_{reported}$	patient's total phenytoin concentration reported by the laboratory
C_{max}	peak or maximum concentration
C_{min}	trough or minimum concentration
$C_{normal\ binding}$	total phenytoin concentration that would be observed if a patient had normal protein binding
C_{ss}	average steady-state plasma concentration
CYP	cytochrome P450
D_{CKD}	maintenance dose for a patient with CKD
D_{norm}	dose for a patient with normal kidney function
eCL_{cr}	estimated creatinine clearance
eGFR	estimated glomerular filtration rate
EMA	European Medicine Agency
ESKD	end-stage kidney disease
FDA	Food and Drug Administration
f_e	fraction of medication eliminated unchanged in the urine

f_u	fraction of medication unbound to plasma proteins
GFR	glomerular filtration rate
GI	gastrointestinal
HD	hemodialysis
IV	intravenous
k	elimination rate constant
k_a	absorption rate constant
k_{NR}	nonrenal elimination rate constant
KDIGO	Kidney Disease: Improving Global Outcomes
KF	ratio of the patient's CL_{cr} to the assumed normal value of 120 mL/min (2 mL/s)
MATE	multidrug and toxin extrusion protein
MIC	minimum inhibitory concentration
mRNA	m ribonucleic acid
MRP	multidrug resistance protein
MRSA	methicillin-resistant *Staphylococcus aureus*
NHD	nocturnal hemodialysis
OAT	organic anion transporter
OATP	organic anion transporting polypeptide
OCT	organic cation transporter
OCTN	organic cation and carnitine transporters
P-gp	P-glycoprotein
Q	kinetic parameter/dosage-adjustment factor
Q_b	blood flow through the dialyzer
Q_p	plasma flow through the dialyzer = Q_b (1 – hematocrit)
R	the total amount of medication recovered unchanged in the dialysate
SCr	serum creatinine
SDHD	short daily hemodialysis
t'	infusion time of medication
Δt	time in hours between two measured concentrations
$t_{1/2}$	half-life
$t_{1/2,\ on\ HD}$	half-life during dialysis
$t_{1/2,\ off\ HD}$	half-life off dialysis
τ_{CKD}	dosing interval in a patient with kidney failure
τ_{norm}	dosing interval in a patient with normal kidney function
t_{max}	time to peak concentration
UGT	uridine diphosphate-glucuronosyltransferase
V_{area}	volume of distribution area
V_b	blood concentration of medication leaving the dialyzer
V_β	volume of terminal phase (serum protein)
V_c	volume of the central compartment
V_D	volume of distribution
V_{ss}	volume of distribution at steady state

REFERENCES

1. Kidney Disease: Improving Global Outcomes (KDIGO) CKD Work Group. 2012 Clinical practice guideline for the evaluation and management of chronic kidney disease. *Kidney Int Suppl.* 2013;2:1–150. DOI:10.1038/kisup.2012.73
2. National Institute of Diabetes and Digestive and Kidney Diseases (NIDDK). Kidney Disease Statistics for the United States. Available at: https://www.niddk.nih.gov/health-information/health-statistics/kidney-disease. Accessed December 1, 2021.
3. GBD Chronic Kidney Disease Collaboration. Global, regional, and national burden of chronic kidney disease, 1990–2017: A systematic analysis for the Global Burden of Disease Study 2017. *Lancet.* 2020;395:709–733. DOI:10.1016/S0140-6736(20)30045-3
4. Mills KT, Xu Y, Zhang W, et al. A systematic analysis of worldwide population-based data on the global burden of chronic kidney disease in 2010. *Kidney Int.* 2015;88:950–957. DOI:10.1038/ki.2015.230
5. Hill NR, Fatoba ST, Oke JL, et al. Global prevalence of chronic kidney disease: A systematic review and meta-analysis. *PLoS One.* 2016;11:e0158765. DOI:10.1371/journal.pone.0158765
6. Schmidt IM, Hubner S, Nadal J, et al. Patterns of medication use and the burden of polypharmacy in patients with chronic kidney disease: The German Chronic Kidney Disease study. *Clin Kidney J.* 2019;12:663–672. DOI:10.1093/ckj/sfz046
7. Laville SM, Metzger M, Stengel B, et al. Evaluation of the adequacy of drug prescriptions in patients with chronic kidney disease: Results from the CKD-REIN cohort. *Br J Clin Pharmacol.* 2018;84:2811–2823. DOI:10.1111/bcp.13738
8. Nolin TD. A synopsis of clinical pharmacokinetic alterations in advanced CKD. *Semin Dial.* 2015;28:325–329. DOI:10.1111/sdi.12374
9. Yeung CK, Shen DD, Thummel KE, et al. Effects of chronic kidney disease and uremia on hepatic drug metabolism and transport. *Kidney Int.* 2014;85:522–528. DOI:10.1038/ki.2013.399
10. Lea-Henry TN, Carland JE, Stocker SL, et al. Clinical pharmacokinetics in kidney disease: Fundamental principles. *Clin J Am Soc Nephrol.* 2018;13:1085–1095. DOI:10.2215/CJN.00340118
11. Roberts DM, Sevastos J, Carland JE, et al. Clinical pharmacokinetics in kidney disease: Application to rational design of dosing regimens. *Clin J Am Soc Nephrol.* 2018;13:1254–1263. DOI:10.2215/CJN.05150418
12. Matzke GR, Frye RF. Drug administration in patients with renal insufficiency. Minimising renal and extrarenal toxicity. *Drug Saf.* 1997;16:205–231. DOI:10.2165/00002018-199716030-00005
13. Verbeeck RK, Musuamba FT. Pharmacokinetics and dosage adjustment in patients with renal dysfunction. *Eur J Clin Pharmacol.* 2009;65:757–773. DOI:10.1007/s00228-009-0678-8
14. Naud J, Nolin TD, Leblond FA, et al. Current understanding of drug disposition in kidney disease. *J Clin Pharmacol.* 2012;52:10S–22S. DOI:10.1177/0091270011413588
15. Lalande L, Charpiat B, Leboucher G, et al. Consequences of renal failure on non-renal clearance of drugs. *Clin Pharmacokinet.* 2014;53:521–532. DOI:10.1007/s40262-014-0146-1
16. Matzke GR, Aronoff GR, Atkinson AJ Jr., et al. Drug dosing consideration in patients with acute and chronic kidney disease: A clinical update from Kidney Disease: Improving Global Outcomes (KDIGO). *Kidney Int.* 2011;80:1122–1137. DOI:10.1038/ki.2011.322
17. Matzke GR, Dowling TC, Marks SA, et al. Influence of kidney disease on drug disposition: An assessment of industry studies submitted to the FDA for new chemical entities 1999–2010. *J Clin Pharmacol.* 2016;56:390–398. DOI:10.1002/jcph.604
18. Rowland M, Tozer TN. *Clinical Pharmacokinetics and Pharmacodynamics: Concepts and Applications.* 4th ed. Baltimore, MD: Lippincott Williams & Wilkins; 2011:403–444.
19. Matzke GR, Comstock TJ. Influence of renal disease and dialysis on pharmacokinetics. In: Evans WE, Schentag JJ, Burton ME, eds. *Applied Pharmacokinetics: Principles of Therapeutic Drug Monitoring.* 4th ed. Baltimore, MD: Lippincott Williams & Wilkins; 2005:187–212.
20. Matzke GR, Dowling TC. Renal drug dosing concepts. In: Murphy JE, ed. *Clinical Pharmacokinetics.* 5th ed. Bethesda, MD: American Society of Health-System Pharmacists; 2012:73–85.
21. Etemad B. Gastrointestinal complications of renal failure. *Gastroenterol Clin North Am.* 1998;27:875–892. DOI:10.1016/s0889-8553(05)70036-4
22. Winter ME. Phenytoin and fosphenytoin. In: Murphy JE, ed. *Clinical Pharmacokinetics.* 5th ed. Bethesda MD: American Society of Health System Pharmacists; 2012:273–283.
23. Page RL. Digoxin. In: Murphy JE, ed. *Clinical Pharmacokinetics.* 5th ed. Bethesda, MD: American Society of Health-System Pharmacists; 2012:185–192.
24. Koup JR. Disease states and drug pharmacokinetics. *J Clin Pharmacol.* 1989;29:674–679. DOI:10.1002/j.1552-4604.1989.tb03401.x
25. Ivanyuk A, Livio F, Biollaz J, et al. Renal drug transporters and drug interactions. *Clin Pharmacokinet.* 2017;56:825–892. DOI:10.1007/s40262-017-0506-8
26. Nigam SK, Wu W, Bush KT, et al. Handling of drugs, metabolites, and uremic toxins by kidney proximal tubule drug transporters. *Clin J Am Soc Nephrol.* 2015;10:2039–2049. DOI:10.2215/CJN.02440314
27. Bricker NS, Morrin PA, Kime SW Jr. The pathologic physiology of chronic Bright's disease. An exposition of the "intact nephron hypothesis." *Am J Med.* 1960;28:77–98. DOI:10.1016/0002-9343(60)90225-4
28. Bricker NS. On the meaning of the intact nephron hypothesis. *Am J Med.* 1969;46:1–11. DOI:10.1016/0002-9343(69)90053-9

29. Hsueh CH, Yoshida K, Zhao P, et al. Identification and quantitative assessment of uremic solutes as inhibitors of renal organic anion transporters, OAT1 and OAT3. *Mol Pharm.* 2016;13:3130–3140. DOI:10.1021/acs.molpharmaceut.6b00332
30. Chapron A, Shen DD, Kestenbaum BR, et al. Does secretory clearance follow glomerular filtration rate in chronic kidney diseases? Reconsidering the intact nephron hypothesis. *Clin Transl Sci.* 2017;10:395–403. DOI:10.1111/cts.12481
31. Hsueh CH, Hsu V, Zhao P, et al. PBPK modeling of the effect of reduced kidney function on the pharmacokinetics of drugs excreted renally by organic anion transporters. *Clin Pharmacol Ther.* 2018;103:485–492. DOI:10.1002/cpt.750
32. Jetter A, Kullak-Ublick GA. Drugs and hepatic transporters: A review. *Pharmacol Res.* 2020;154:104234. DOI:10.1016/j.phrs.2019.04.018
33. Nolin TD, Unruh ML. Clinical relevance of impaired nonrenal drug clearance in ESRD. *Semin Dial.* 2010;23:482–485. DOI:10.1111/j.1525-139x.2010.00775.x
34. Tan ML, Yoshida K, Zhao P, et al. Effect of chronic kidney disease on nonrenal elimination pathways: A systematic assessment of CYP1A2, CYP2C8, CYP2C9, CYP2C19, and OATP. *Clin Pharmacol Ther.* 2018;103:854–867. DOI:10.1002/cpt.807
35. Tan ML, Zhao P, Zhang L, et al. Use of physiologically based pharmacokinetic modeling to evaluate the effect of chronic kidney disease on the disposition of hepatic CYP2C8 and OATP1B drug substrates. *Clin Pharmacol Ther.* 2019;105:719–729. DOI:10.1002/cpt.1205
36. Yoshida K, Sun B, Zhang L, et al. Systematic and quantitative assessment of the effect of chronic kidney disease on CYP2D6 and CYP3A4/5. *Clin Pharmacol Ther.* 2016;100:75–87. DOI:10.1002/cpt.337
37. Nolin TD, Frye RF, Le P, et al. ESRD impairs nonrenal clearance of fexofenadine but not midazolam. *J Am Soc Nephrol.* 2009;20:2269–2276. DOI:10.1681/ASN.2009010082
38. Thomson BK, Nolin TD, Velenosi TJ, et al. Effect of CKD and dialysis modality on exposure to drugs cleared by nonrenal mechanisms. *Am J Kidney Dis.* 2015;65:574–582. DOI:10.1053/j.ajkd.2014.09.015
39. Macias WL, Mueller BA, Scarim SK. Vancomycin pharmacokinetics in acute renal failure: Preservation of nonrenal clearance. *Clin Pharmacol Ther.* 1991;50:688–694. DOI:10.1038/clpt.1991.208
40. Mueller BA, Scarim SK, Macias WL. Comparison of imipenem pharmacokinetics in patients with acute or chronic renal failure treated with continuous hemofiltration. *Am J Kidney Dis.* 1993;21:172–179. DOI:10.1016/s0272-6386(12)81089-4
41. Osborne R, Joel S, Grebenik K, et al. The pharmacokinetics of morphine and morphine glucuronides in kidney failure. *Clin Pharmacol Ther.* 1993;54:158–167. DOI:10.1038/clpt.1993.127
42. Szeto HH, Inturrisi CE, Houde R, et al. Accumulation of normeperidine, an active metabolite of meperidine, in patients with renal failure of cancer. *Ann Intern Med.* 1977;86:738–741. DOI:10.7326/0003-4819-86-6-738
43. Bazinet A, Almanric K, Brunet C, et al. Dosage of enoxaparin among obese and renal impairment patients. *Thromb Res.* 2005;116:41–50. DOI:10.1016/j.thromres.2004.10.004
44. Hulot JS, Vantelon C, Urien S, et al. Effect of renal function on the pharmacokinetics of enoxaparin and consequences on dose adjustment. *Ther Drug Monit.* 2004;26:305–310. DOI:10.1097/00007691-200406000-00015
45. Cockcroft DW, Gault MH. Prediction of creatinine clearance from serum creatinine. *Nephron.* 1976;16:31–41. DOI:10.1159/000180580
46. Levey AS, Stevens LA, Schmid CH, et al. A new equation to estimate glomerular filtration rate. *Ann Intern Med.* 2009;150:604–612. DOI:10.7326/0003-4819-150-9-200905050-00006
47. Inker LA, Schmid CH, Tighiouart H, et al. Estimating glomerular filtration rate from serum creatinine and cystatin C. *N Engl J Med.* 2012;367:20–29. DOI:10.1056/NEJMoa1114248
48. Inker LA, Eneanya ND, Coresh J, et al. New creatinine- and cystatin C-based equations to estimate GFR without race. *N Engl J Med.* 2021;385:1737–1749. DOI:10.1056/NEJMoa2102953
49. Miller WG, Jones GRD. Estimated glomerular filtration rate; laboratory implementation and current global status. *Adv Chronic Kidney Dis.* 2018;25:7–13. DOI:10.1053/j.ackd.2017.09.013
50. Fernandez-Prado R, Castillo-Rodriguez E, Velez-Arribas FJ, et al. Creatinine clearance is not equal to glomerular filtration rate and cockcroft-gault equation is not equal to CKD-EPI collaboration equation. *Am J Med.* 2016;129:1259–1263. DOI:10.1016/j.amjmed.2016.08.019
51. Hudson JQ, Nolin TD. Pragmatic use of kidney function estimates for drug dosing: The tide is turning. *Adv Chronic Kidney Dis.* 2018;25:14–20. DOI:10.1053/j.ackd.2017.10.003
52. Casal MA, Nolin TD, Beumer JH. Estimation of kidney function in oncology: Implications for anticancer drug selection and dosing. *Clin J Am Soc Nephrol.* 2019;14:587–595. DOI:10.2215/CJN.11721018
53. Stevens LA, Nolin TD, Richardson MM, et al. Comparison of drug dosing recommendations based on measured GFR and kidney function estimating equations. *Am J Kidney Dis.* 2009;54:33–42. DOI:10.1053/j.ajkd.2009.03.008
54. Nabiee M, Dashti-Khavidaki S, Khajeh B. Dose discordance of direct acting oral anticoagulants using different equations for estimating GFR: A literature review. *Expert Rev Clin Pharmacol.* 2020;13:857–863. DOI:10.1080/17512433.2020.1798759
55. Shepherd ST, Gillen G, Morrison P, et al. Performance of formulae based estimates of glomerular filtration rate for carboplatin dosing in stage 1 seminoma. *Eur J Cancer.* 2014;50:944–952. DOI:10.1016/j.ejca.2013.12.021
56. Steffl JL, Bennett W, Olyaei AJ. The old and new methods of assessing kidney function. *J Clin Pharmacol.* 2012;52:63S–71S. DOI:10.1177/0091270011420260
57. US Food Drug Administration. Guidance for industry: Pharmacokinetics in patients with impaired renal function—study design, data analysis and impact on dosing and labelling, 1998. Available at: http://www.fda.gov/downloads/Drugs/GuidanceComplianceRegulatoryInformation/Guidances/ucm072127.pdf. Accessed December 1, 2021.
58. US Food Drug Administration. Guidance for industry: Pharmacokinetics in patients with impaired renal function—study design, data analysis and impact on dosing and labelling, 2020. Draft Guidance. Available at: https://www.fda.gov/media/78573/download. Accessed December 1, 2021.
59. Aronoff GR, Bennett WM, Berns JS, et al. *Drug Prescribing in Renal Failure: Dosing Guidelines for Adults and Children.* 5th ed. Philadelphia, PA: American College of Physicians-American Society of Internal Medicine; 2007.
60. *The Renal Drug Handbook.* 4th ed. CRC Press [Internet]. Available at: http://renaldrugdatabase.com. Accessed December 1, 2021.
61. Lexicomp. Wolters Kluwer Clinical Drug Information, Inc [Internet]. Available at: https://www.wolterskluwer.com/en/solutions/lexicomp. Accessed December 1, 2021.
62. IBM Micromedex. Truven Health Analytics, Inc [Internet]. Available at: https://www.micromedexsolutions.com/. Accessed December 1, 2021.
63. AHFS Clinical Drug Information. Bethesda, MD: American Society of Health-System Pharmacists, Inc. Available at: http://www.ahfsdruginformation.com. Accessed December 1, 2021.
64. Vidal L, Shavit M, Fraser A, et al. Systematic comparison of four sources of drug information regarding adjustment of dose for renal function. *BMJ.* 2005;331:263. DOI:10.1136/bmj.38476.471088.3A
65. Mountford CM, Lee T, de Lemos J, et al. Quality and usability of common drug information databases. *Can J Hosp Pharm.* 2010;63:130–137. DOI:10.4212/cjhp.v63i2.898
66. Dowling TC, Matzke GR, Murphy JE, et al. Evaluation of renal drug dosing: Prescribing information and clinical pharmacist approaches. *Pharmacotherapy.* 2010;30:776–786. DOI:10.1592/phco.30.8.776
67. Dettli LC. Drug dosage in patients with renal disease. *Clin Pharmacol Ther.* 1974;16:274–280. DOI:10.1002/cpt1974161part2274
68. Vondracek SF, Teitelbaum I. Principles of kidney pharmacotherapy for the nephrologist: Core Curriculum 2021. *Am J Kidney Dis.* 2021;78:442–458. DOI:10.1053/j.ajkd.2021.02.342, kiserth.
69. Hobbs AL, Shea KM, Roberts KM, et al. Implications of augmented renal clearance on drug dosing in critically ill patients: A focus on antibiotics. *Pharmacotherapy.* 2015;35:1063–1075. DOI:10.1002/phar.1653
70. Rybak MJ, Le J, Lodise TP, et al. Therapeutic Monitoring of Vancomycin for Serious Methicillin-resistant Staphylococcus aureus Infections: A Revised Consensus Guideline and Review by the American Society of Health-system Pharmacists, the Infectious Diseases Society of America, the Pediatric Infectious Diseases Society, and the Society of Infectious Diseases Pharmacists. *Clin Infect Dis.* 2020;71:1361–1364. DOI:10.1093/cid/ciaa303
71. Lewis SJ, Nolin TD. New vancomycin dosing guidelines for hemodialysis patients: Rationale, caveats, and limitations. *Kidney 360.* 2021;2:1313–1315. DOI:10.34067/KID.0000192021
72. Teigen MM, Duffull S, Dang L, et al. Dosing of gentamicin in patients with end-stage renal disease receiving hemodialysis. *J Clin Pharmacol.* 2006;46:1259–1267. DOI:10.1177/0091270006292987
73. Kamel Mohamed OH, Wahba IM, Watnick S, et al. Administration of tobramycin in the beginning of the hemodialysis session: A novel intradialytic dosing regimen. *Clin J Am Soc Nephrol.* 2007;2:694–699. DOI:10.2215/CJN.01600407

74. Zelenitsky SA, Ariano RE, McCrae ML, et al. Initial vancomycin dosing protocol to achieve therapeutic serum concentrations in patients undergoing hemodialysis. *Clin Infect Dis.* 2012;55:527–533. DOI:10.1093/cid/cis458
75. Ariano RE, Fine A, Sitar DS, et al. Adequacy of a vancomycin dosing regimen in patients receiving high-flux hemodialysis. *Am J Kidney Dis.* 2005;46:681–687. DOI:10.1053/j.ajkd.2005.07.018
76. Oguri T, Shimokata T, Inada M, et al. Pharmacokinetic analysis of carboplatin in patients with cancer who are undergoing hemodialysis. *Cancer Chemother Pharmacol.* 2010;66:813–817. DOI:10.1007/s00280-010-1366-1
77. Haubitz M, Bohnenstengel F, Brunkhorst R, et al. Cyclophosphamide pharmacokinetics and dose requirements in patients with renal insufficiency. *Kidney Int.* 2002;61:1495–1501. DOI:10.1046/j.1523-1755.2002.00279.x
78. Taylor CA 3rd, Abdel-Rahman E, Zimmerman SW, et al. Clinical pharmacokinetics during continuous ambulatory peritoneal dialysis. *Clin Pharmacokinet.* 1996;31:293–308. DOI:10.2165/00003088-199631040-00005
79. Manley HJ, Bailie GR. Treatment of peritonitis in APD: Pharmacokinetic principles. *Semin Dial.* 2002;15:418–421. DOI:10.1046/j.1525-139x.2002.00103.x
80. Bieber SD, Young BA. Home hemodialysis: Core Curriculum 2021. *Am J Kidney Dis.* 2021;78:876–885. DOI:10.1053/j.ajkd.2021.01.025
81. Law V, Walker S, Dresser L, et al. Optimized dosing of cefazolin in patients treated with nocturnal home hemodialysis. *Am J Kidney Dis.* 2014;64:479–480. DOI:10.1053/j.ajkd.2014.05.007
82. Palmer K, Walker S, Richardson R, et al. Pharmacokinetic study of cefazolin in short daily hemodialysis. *Ann Pharmacother.* 2019;53:348–356. DOI:10.1177/1060028018809695

Disorders of Sodium and Water Homeostasis

68

Katherine H. Chessman and Jason S. Haney

KEY CONCEPTS

1. Maintenance of normal blood volume and serum osmolality is essential for cellular function and is tightly regulated in the human body. Simply put, water balance determines serum sodium concentration, and sodium balance determines volume status.
2. Total body water (TBW) ranges from 45% to 80% of body weight depending on sex, age, gestational age, and disease states and is distributed primarily into two compartments: the intracellular compartment or intracellular fluid (ICF; two-thirds [67%] of TBW) and the extracellular compartment or extracellular fluid (ECF; one-third [33%] of TBW).
3. Arginine vasopressin (AVP), also known as antidiuretic hormone (ADH), is synthesized in the hypothalamus and secreted by the posterior pituitary in response to both osmotic (serum sodium greater than 135 mEq/L [mmol/L]) and non-osmotic regulators to maintain water balance.
4. Hyponatremia, defined as a serum sodium concentration less than 135 mEq/L (mmol/L), is the most common electrolyte abnormality encountered in clinical practice in both adults and children and is associated with significant morbidity and mortality.
5. Hyponatremia is predominantly the result of an excess of extracellular water relative to sodium because of impaired water excretion.
6. Hypovolemic hypotonic hyponatremia is common in patients taking thiazide diuretics.
7. Euvolemic (isovolemic) hypotonic hyponatremia is associated with a normal or slightly decreased ECF sodium content and increased TBW and ECF volume and is most often caused by the syndrome of inappropriate ADH secretion (SIADH).
8. Hyponatremia with ECF volume expansion (hypervolemia) occurs in conditions in which sodium and water excretion is impaired such as heart failure, cirrhosis, or nephrotic syndrome.
9. The brain's adaptation to chronic serum hypoosmolality or hyperosmolality leads to neurologic symptoms when either hyponatremia (hypoosmolality) or hypernatremia (hyperosmolality) is corrected too rapidly.
10. Hypernatremia, defined as a serum sodium concentration greater than 145 mEq/L (mmol/L), is always associated with hypertonicity and intracellular dehydration, resulting from a water deficit relative to ECF sodium content.
11. Edema, defined as a clinically detectable increase in interstitial fluid volume, is usually due to heart, kidney, or liver failure or a combination of these conditions; although, it can develop with a rapid decrease in serum albumin concentration along with excess fluid intake such as seen in the setting of burns or trauma.

BEYOND THE BOOK

Read and evaluate the case presented in Chapter 57 "Syndrome of Inappropriate Antidiuretic Hormone Release: A Sudden Change of Mind Level I. In: Schwinghammer TL, Koehler JM, Borchert JS, Slain D, Park SK. eds. *Pharmacotherapy Casebook: A Patient-Focused Approach, 11e*. McGraw Hill; 2020." Available at https://accesspharmacy.mhmedical.com/content.aspx?bookid=2868§ionid=242182677.

This activity is useful to enhance student understanding regarding the COLLECT, ASSESS, PLAN, and IMPLEMENT steps in the patient care process.

INTRODUCTION

1 Maintenance of normal blood volume and serum osmolality is essential for cellular function and is tightly regulated in the human body. Simply put, water balance determines serum sodium concentration, and sodium balance determines volume status. Adequate blood volume is required for effective tissue perfusion which is required to deliver oxygen and nutrients to and remove metabolic waste products from tissues. Serum osmolality, determined primarily by the serum sodium concentration, is an important determinant of ICF volume. Maintaining normal ICF volume is particularly critical in the brain, which is 80% water, and where alterations, especially rapid changes, can result in significant dysfunction, and even death.

Homeostatic mechanisms for controlling blood volume focus on controlling sodium balance, and, in contrast, homeostatic mechanisms for controlling serum osmolality (serum sodium concentration) focus on controlling water balance. Disorders of sodium and water balance are common, caused by a variety of diseases, conditions, and medications, and potentially serious. This chapter reviews the etiology, pathophysiology, clinical presentation, and treatment options for disorders of sodium and water homeostasis.

SODIUM AND WATER HOMEOSTASIS

The average daily sodium intake of Americans consuming a typical western diet usually exceeds the recommendations for Chronic Disease Risk Reduction (CDRR) levels established by the

US Department of Agriculture: adults and children older than 13 years, 2.3 g; 9 to 13 years, 1.8 g; 4 to 8 years, 1.5 g; 1 to 3 years, 1.2 g; and, infants and young children 6 to 11 months, 0.37 g (Adequate Intake, AI).[1] Excessive sodium intake is a major risk factor for hypertension as BP rises with increased sodium intake. Appropriately functioning kidneys excrete excess sodium to maintain the serum sodium concentration and osmolality within a tight range. The kidney can also conserve sodium (urine sodium less than 30 mEq/L [mmol/L]) during periods of low sodium intake or in the presence of excessive losses. Both hypo- and hypernatremia are conditions of altered serum tonicity and cell volume that reflect a change in the ratio of total exchangeable body sodium to TBW.

2 TBW ranges from 45% to 80% of body weight depending on sex, age, gestational age, and disease states and is distributed primarily into two compartments: the intracellular compartment or intracellular fluid (ICF; two-thirds [67%] of TBW) and the extracellular compartment or extracellular fluid (ECF; one-third [33%] of TBW). The serum (plasma) volume is approximately 17% of the ECF volume. Sodium contributes more than 90% of the ECF osmolality, whereas ICF osmolality is primarily determined by the ICF potassium concentration. The extra- and intracellular sodium and potassium concentrations are maintained by the sodium–potassium–adenosine triphosphatase (Na^+-K^+-ATPase) pump. Because most cell membranes are freely permeable to water, the free flow of water between compartments ensures that the ICF and ECF osmolalities remain equal.

Effective osmoles are solutes that cannot freely cross cell membranes, such as sodium and potassium, which are kept in their respective compartments by the Na^+-K^+-ATPase pump. The ECF concentration of effective osmoles determines its tonicity, which directly affects water distribution between the ECF and ICF. Addition of an isotonic solution (eg, 0.9% NaCl) to the ECF will result in no change in ICF volume because there will be no change in the effective ECF osmolality. However, addition of a hypertonic solution (eg, 3% NaCl) to the ECF will result in a decrease in ICF (cell) volume. Conversely, addition of a hypotonic solution (eg, 0.45% NaCl) to the ECF will result in an increase in ICF (cell) volume. Thus, administration of both hypertonic and hypotonic solutions can result in cell crenation or hemolysis, respectively. Table 68-1 summarizes the composition and osmolality of commonly used IV solutions and their expected distribution into the ICF and ECF compartments following administration.

Edelman's equation (simplified) defines serum sodium (Na_s) as a function of the total exchangeable sodium and potassium in the body and the TBW:

$$Na_s = Na_{\text{total body}} + K_{\text{total body}} / TBW$$

where $Na_{\text{total body}}$ is the total body sodium content; $K_{\text{total body}}$ is the total body potassium content; and TBW is the total body water (TBW) in liters.[2,3] The usual serum sodium concentration (135-145 mEq/L [mmol/L]) is tightly regulated and thus usually varies by no more than 3%. Serum sodium regulation occurs via mechanisms that control serum osmolality and blood volume. The kidney regulates water excretion through a hypothalamic feedback mechanism, such that the serum osmolality remains relatively constant (275-290 mOsm/kg [mmol/kg]) despite day-to-day variations in water intake. While serum osmolality is primarily determined by the sodium concentration, abnormally high glucose and blood urea nitrogen (BUN) concentrations may contribute significantly. Glucose is an effective osmole, but BUN is not; thus, elevated osmolality due to these two substances will have differing effects. Serum osmolality can be estimated as follows:

$$Osm_s = (2 \times Na_s) + (glucose_s/18) + (BUN/2.8)$$

where Osm_s is the serum osmolality in mOsm/kg [mmol/kg]; Na_s is the serum sodium concentration in mEq/L; $glucose_s$ is the serum

TABLE 68-1 Composition of Common IV Solutions

								Distribution		
Solution	Dextrose g/dL (kcal/L)	[Na^+] (mEq/L or mmol/L)	[K^+] (mEq/L or mmol/L)	[Cl^-] (mEq/L or mmol/L)	Other (mEq/L)	Osmolality (mOsm/kg or mmol/kg)	Tonicity	% ECF	% ICF	Free water (mL/L)
Dextrose 5% in water	5 (170)	0	0	0	---	253	Hypotonic	33	67	1,000 mL
0.2% NaCl[a]	0	34	0	34	---	68	Hypotonic	50	50	750 mL
0.45% NaCl[b]	0	77	0	77	---	154	Hypotonic	67	33	500 mL
0.9% NaCl[c]	0	154	0	154	---	308	Isotonic	100	0	0 mL
Lactated Ringer's[d]	0	130	4	105	Lactate 28 Ca 4.8	273	Isotonic	97	3	0 mL
Plasma-Lyte A[e] Plasma-Lyte 148[e]	0.44 (21)	140	5	98	Acetate 27 Mg 3 Gluc 23	294	Isotonic	100	0	0 mL
Normosol-R[f] Normosol-R pH 7.4	0	140	5	98	Acetate 27 Mg 3 Gluc 23	294	Isotonic	100	0	0 mL
3% NaCl[g]	0	513	0	513	---	1,026	Hypertonic	100	0	−2,331 mL

Ca, calcium; Cl^-, chloride; ECF, extracellular fluid; ICF, intracellular fluid; IV, intravenous; K^+, potassium; Mg, magnesium; NA, not applicable; Na^+, sodium; NaCl, sodium chloride; For conversion of kcal/L to kJ/L multiply by 4.184.

[a]Also referred to as *quarter normal saline*.

[b]Also referred to as *half normal saline*.

[c]Also referred to as *normal saline*.

[d]Also referred to as LR; also available commercially as Dextrose 5% LR.

[e]Plasma-Lyte A pH 7.4; Plasma-Lyte 148 pH 5.5.

[f]Normosol-R available with pH 6.6 and Normosol-R pH 7.4.

[g]Hypertonic solution; results in osmotic removal of water from the ICF.

glucose concentration in mg/dL; BUN is the BUN concentration in mg/dL; and 18 and 2.8 are the factors needed to convert from a weight measurement (mg/dL) to a concentration (mmol/L) for glucose and BUN, respectively. Thus, when using SI units, the equation becomes

$$Osm_s = (2 \times Na_s) + glucose_s + BUN$$

where Osm_s is the serum osmolality in mmol/kg; and Na_s, $glucose_s$, and BUN are the respective concentrations in mmol/L.

3 Arginine vasopressin (AVP), also known as antidiuretic hormone (ADH), is synthesized in the hypothalamus, and secreted by the posterior pituitary in response to both osmotic (serum sodium greater than 135 mEq/L [mmol/L]) and non-osmotic regulators to maintain water balance. When the serum osmolality increases by as little as 1% to 2%, AVP is released and binds to the arginine vasopressin 2 (V_2) receptor, a G protein-coupled receptor, on the basolateral membrane of principal cells lining the renal collecting duct, resulting in the insertion of water channels (aquaporin 2, AQP2) into both the apical cell membrane of the collecting duct principal cells and intracellular vesicles below the apical membrane increasing permeability.[2,4] Water can then pass through the cell into the peritubular capillary space where it is reabsorbed into the systemic circulation. A maximally concentrated urine (1,200 mOsm/L) will be formed when the serum sodium concentration is 145 mEq/L (mmol/L) or above.[2] AVP release also stimulates thirst as an additional means to return serum osmolality toward normal. The combined effect of increased water intake (response to thirst) and decreased water excretion (kidney's response to AVP) results in a decrease in the serum osmolality. Once the serum osmolality is restored to normal, AVP secretion is inhibited, AQP2 water channels are retrieved, water permeability returns to the usual low state, and renal excretion of solute-free water (aquaresis) occurs.

While AVP secretion is regulated primarily by osmolality, non-osmotic AVP release occurs when the brain's osmoreceptors detect as little as a 6% to 10% reduction in the effective circulating volume or arterial BP. The effective circulating volume is the portion of the ECF responsible for organ perfusion. A decrease in the effective circulating volume (more accurately, the arterial BP associated with that volume) activates arterial baroreceptors in the carotid sinus and glomerular afferent arterioles, resulting in stimulation of the renin–angiotensin system and increased angiotensin II synthesis. Angiotensin II stimulates both non-osmotic AVP release and thirst. This non-osmotic volume stimulus can override osmotic AVP inhibition. Water conservation then restores the effective circulating volume and BP at the expense of producing a decreased serum osmolality and hyponatremia.[2] Both hypo- and hypernatremia can be associated with either high, low, or normal ECF sodium or volume. To understand treatment options, differentiating between *dehydration* and *hypovolemia* is important. Dehydration refers to a loss of TBW producing hypertonicity while hypovolemia (volume depletion) is a symptomatic ECF volume deficit. It is important to note that volume depletion and dehydration can exist independently or concurrently. Often these terms are used interchangeably, but they are different processes requiring different types and rates of fluid replacement.[5]

HYPONATREMIA

Epidemiology and Etiology

4 Hyponatremia, defined as a serum sodium concentration less than 135 mEq/L (mmol/L), is the most common electrolyte abnormality encountered in clinical practice in both adults and children and is associated with significant morbidity and mortality.[4] It affects 3 to 6 million persons and 1 million hospitalized patients yearly.[6,7] Although the prevalence is not well established and varies with the patient population studied, it has been estimated to be 15% to 30% of hospitalized patients.[6,7] In one study, the prevalence of mild hyponatremia (serum sodium concentration less than 136 mEq/L [mmol/L]) in hospitalized patients was 42% (28% on admission, 14% during admission); 6.2% of patients evaluated (2.5% on admission, 3.7% during admission) had values less than 126 mEq/L (mmol/L); and 1.2% (0.5% on admission, 0.7% during admission) had a serum sodium concentration less than 116 mEq/L (mmol/L).[8] The prevalence of hyponatremia in the intensive care unit (ICU) is 30% to 40% with an admission serum sodium less than 130 mEq/L (mmol/L) in approximately 14%.[9] In hospital-based ambulatory care clinics and community clinics, the prevalence of hyponatremia (serum sodium concentration less than 136 mEq/L [mmol/L]) is 21% and 1.7% to 9.2%, respectively.[8,10] Medication-induced hyponatremia, especially that associated with thiazide diuretics[11] and psychotropic medications,[12–14] is common.

Advancing age is a risk factor for hyponatremia, independent of sex.[10,15,16] Residents in nursing homes have a twofold higher incidence of hyponatremia than age-matched, community-dwelling individuals. More than 75% of these hyponatremic episodes in long-term care facilities were precipitated by increased intake of hypotonic fluids either orally or through enteral feedings or IV fluids.[17] Similarly, ingestion of excessive volumes of hypotonic fluids (water, sports drinks) has been identified as a key risk factor in the development of exercise-associated hyponatremia occurring during or up to 24 hours after prolonged physical activity. Men and women are at an equal risk for developing exercise-induced hyponatremia when rates are adjusted based on body mass index (smaller body size) and racing time (longer times).[18] Hyponatremia is also the most common electrolyte abnormality seen in pregnancy, frequently seen in patients with hyperemesis gravidarum and preeclampsia.[19]

Recognition of the high prevalence of hyponatremia is essential because this condition is associated with significant morbidity and mortality.[7,9,19-22] Even in asymptomatic patients, chronic hyponatremia has been associated with decreased cognitive function and increased risk of frailty, falls, fractures, and bone loss, particularly in older adults.[23-26] In patients with hyponatremia, transient or permanent brain dysfunction can result from either acute effects of hypoosmolality or too rapid correction.

5 Hyponatremia is predominantly the result of an excess of extracellular water relative to sodium because of impaired water excretion. The kidney normally has the capacity to excrete large volumes of dilute urine after ingestion of a water load. Non-osmotic AVP release, however, can lead to water retention and a decrease in the serum sodium concentration, despite a decrease in ECF and ICF osmolality. Causes of non-osmotic AVP release include hypovolemia and a decreased effective circulating volume (eg, chronic heart failure [HF], nephrotic syndrome, cirrhosis). The syndrome of inappropriate antidiuretic hormone secretion (SIADH), a common cause of hyponatremia, is associated with some cancers, CNS damage, certain lung conditions, medications, and primary or psychogenic polydipsia.

Pathophysiology

Hyponatremia can be associated with normal, increased, or decreased serum osmolality, depending on its cause. Figure 68-1 provides an algorithm for the assessment and treatment of patients with non-emergent hyponatremia.[2,4]

Isotonic Hyponatremia

Hyponatremia (expected low osmolality) with a normal measured serum osmolality (*osmol gap*) can be seen in the setting of markedly elevated serum lipids (hyperlipidemia) or proteins (eg, hyperproteinemia, multiple myeloma) when flame photometry or indirect potentiometry is used to measure the sodium concentration (see Fig. 68-2)

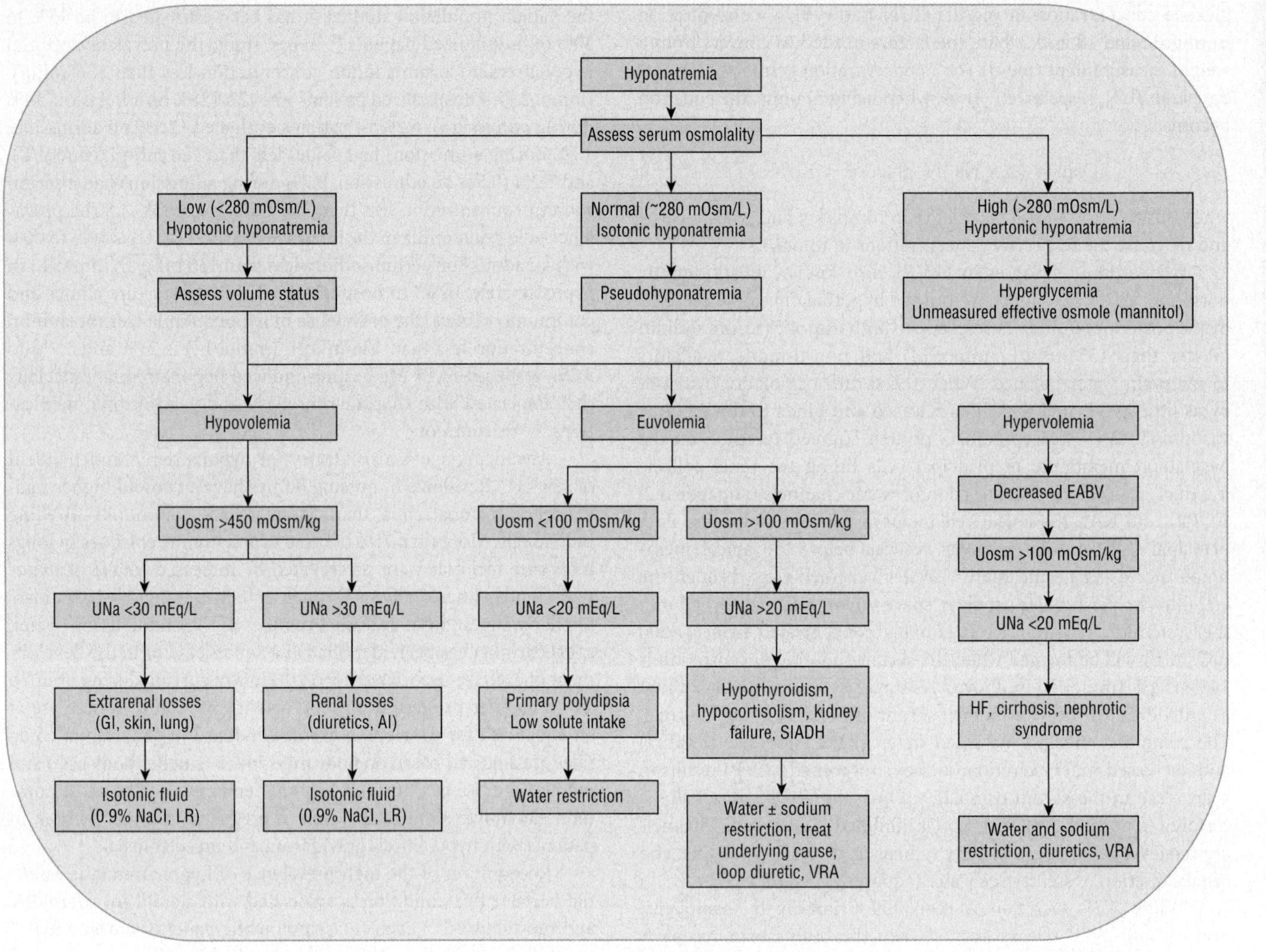

Hyponatremia
Assess serum osmolality
Low (<280 mOsm/L) Hypotonic hyponatremia
Normal (~280 mOsm/L) Isotonic hyponatremia
High (>280 mOsm/L) Hypertonic hyponatremia
Assess volume status
Pseudohyponatremia
Hyperglycemia Unmeasured effective osmole (mannitol)
Hypovolemia
Euvolemia
Hypervolemia
Decreased EABV
Uosm >450 mOsm/kg
Uosm <100 mOsm/kg
Uosm >100 mOsm/kg
Uosm >100 mOsm/kg
UNa <30 mEq/L
UNa >30 mEq/L
UNa <20 mEq/L
UNa >20 mEq/L
UNa <20 mEq/L
Extrarenal losses (GI, skin, lung)
Renal losses (diuretics, AI)
Primary polydipsia Low solute intake
Hypothyroidism, hypocortisolism, kidney failure, SIADH
HF, cirrhosis, nephrotic syndrome
Isotonic fluid (0.9% NaCl, LR)
Isotonic fluid (0.9% NaCl, LR)
Water restriction
Water ± sodium restriction, treat underlying cause, loop diuretic, VRA
Water and sodium restriction, diuretics, VRA

FIGURE 68-1 Algorithm for the assessment and treatment of non-emergent hyponatremia. (AI, adrenal insufficiency; EABV, effective arterial blood volume; GI, gastrointestinal; HF, heart failure; LR, lactated Ringers; NaCl, sodium chloride; SIADH, syndrome of inappropriate secretion of antidiuretic hormone; UNa, urine sodium concentration [values in mEq/L are numerically equivalent to mmol/L]; UOsm, urine osmolality [values in mOsm/kg are numerically equivalent to mmol/kg]; VRA, vasopressin receptor antagonist.)

This *pseudohyponatremia* is an artifact because elevated lipids or proteins account for a larger than usual proportion of the total sample volume, reducing the percentage of water in the serum (Fig. 68-2). Because sodium is distributed in the water component only, the measured serum sodium concentration is falsely decreased, and the calculated osmolality will be low. The measurement of serum osmolality is not affected, leading to a discrepancy between the calculated and measured serum osmolality (*osmolal gap*). Pseudohyponatremia is not seen when the sodium concentration is measured via direct potentiometry using ion-selective electrodes as is most often done in current laboratory practice, including blood gas analyzers, because it does not involve sample dilution. Treatment of *hyponatremia* in a case of pseudohyponatremia can lead to serious consequences.[27]

Hypertonic Hyponatremia

Hypertonic (increased serum osmolality) hyponatremia is due to the presence of excess effective osmoles (other than sodium) in the ECF (Fig. 68-1). Significant hyperglycemia is the most frequent cause. An elevated serum glucose concentration initially causes water diffusion from cells (ICF) into the ECF, thereby decreasing

Pseudohyponatremia
Normal
Hyperlipidemia
Serum water
Serum volume
93%
Proteins/lipids
7%
Serum water
72%
Serum volume
Proteins/lipids
28%
S_{Na} = 154 mEq/L serum water × 0.93 = 143 mEq/L
S_{Na} = 154 mEq/L serum water × 0.72 = 111 mEq/L

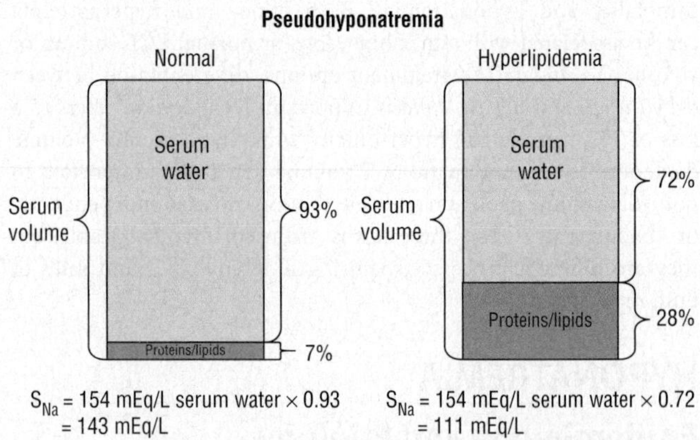

FIGURE 68-2 Elevated serum lipids or proteins result in a larger discrepancy between the volume of the sample and serum water, which leads to a falsely low measurement of the serum sodium concentration when using flame photometry. (S_{Na}, serum sodium concentration [values in mEq/L are numerically equivalent to mmol/L].)

the ICF volume, expanding the ECF volume, and diluting the existing sodium resulting in hyponatremia. The increased ECF volume results in increased urine output (polyuria) which triggers the thirst mechanism (polydipsia). If the hyperglycemia is not corrected and/or extra fluid is not ingested, hypovolemia develops due to excessive urinary losses.

The volume of distribution (V_d) of glucose is a complex function of insulin activity, glucose distribution time, ECF volume, and glucose concentration. Using a clinically relevant glucose V_d of 0.3 to 0.5 L/kg, one would predict a 1.5 to 1.9 mEq/L (mmol/L) decrease in the serum sodium concentration for every 100 mg/dL (5.6 mmol/L) increase in the serum glucose concentration above 100 mg/dL (5.6 mmol/L), and the serum osmolality will increase by 2 mOsm/kg (mmol/kg).[5,28] This correction is only an estimate because of the variability in the V_d of glucose, and clinical practice guidelines recommend simplifying to 1.6 mg/dL as the correction factor using the equation:

$$SNa_{corrected} = SNa_{measured} + (1.6 \times glucose_{measured}/100)$$

where $SNa_{corrected}$ is the serum sodium (mg/dL) corrected for hyperglycemia; $SNa_{measured}$ is the measure serum sodium (mg/dL); and $glucose_{measured}$ is the measured serum glucose in mg/dL.[20]

Alternatively, one would predict a 0.29 mmol/L decrease in the serum sodium concentration for every 1 mmol/L increase in the serum glucose concentration above 5.6 mmol/L using for glucose and sodium expressed in units of mmol/L the following equation:

$$SNa_{corrected} = SNa_{measured} + 0.29 \times glucose_{measured} - 5.6$$

where $SNa_{corrected}$ is the serum sodium (mmol/L) corrected for hyperglycemia; $SNa_{measured}$ is the measure serum sodium (mmol/L); and $glucose_{measured}$ is the measured serum glucose in mmol/L.

The presence of other effective osmoles (eg, mannitol) can also cause hypertonic hyponatremia. The presence of an unmeasured osmole should be suspected in patients with a normal glucose concentration and hypertonic hyponatremia when there is a significant osmolal gap.

Hypotonic Hyponatremia

Hypotonic (decreased osmolality) hyponatremia is the most common form of hyponatremia and has many potential causes (see Fig. 68-1 and Table 68-2). Assessment of ECF volume status is important in the evaluation of a patient with hypotonic hyponatremia. Categorization into one of three groups (decreased, increased, or clinically normal ECF volume) is the essential first step in identifying the pathophysiologic mechanism(s) responsible for the hyponatremia and developing an appropriate treatment plan.

Hypovolemic Hypotonic Hyponatremia

Most patients with ECF volume contraction have lost fluids that are hypotonic relative to the serum and thus may become transiently hypernatremic. This situation includes patients with fluid losses caused by diarrhea, excessive sweating, and diuretics. This transient hypernatremic hyperosmolality results in osmotic AVP release and thirst. If sodium and water losses continue, the resultant hypovolemia results in more AVP release. Patients who then drink water (a hypotonic fluid) or who are given hypotonic IV fluids retain water, and hyponatremia develops. These patients will typically have a concentrated urine (urine osmolality greater than 450 mOsm/kg [mmol/kg]), reflecting AVP action. The urine sodium concentration will be less than 30 mEq/L (mmol/L) when sodium losses are extrarenal (eg, diarrhea, vomiting), and greater than 30 mEq/L (mmol/L) with renal sodium losses (eg, thiazide diuretics, adrenal insufficiency); although, urine sodium concentration is also affected by solute intake.[4,20]

6 Hypovolemic hypotonic hyponatremia is common in patients taking thiazide diuretics.[6,11] Thiazide diuretic-induced hyponatremia is usually mild and relatively asymptomatic but can be severe. Hyponatremia typically develops within 2 weeks of diuretic initiation but can occur at any time during therapy, particularly after dosage increases or if other causes of hyponatremia are present. Older women are at the greatest risk for thiazide diuretic-induced hyponatremia.[6,11]

Thiazide diuretic-induced hyponatremia is related to a balance of direct and indirect effects. These agents block sodium reabsorption in the distal tubules of the renal cortex, thereby increasing sodium and water removal from the body. The resultant decrease in effective circulating volume stimulates AVP release, resulting in increased free water reabsorption in the collecting duct, as well as increased water intake because of thirst stimulation. Hyponatremia develops when the net result of these effects is the loss of more sodium than water.

Conversely, hyponatremia occurs infrequently with loop diuretics due to their different site of action. Loop diuretics block sodium reabsorption in the ascending limb of the loop of Henle. This action decreases medullary osmolality; thus, when loop diuretic use decreases the effective circulating volume and stimulates AVP release, less water reabsorption occurs in the collecting ducts than would occur with normal medullary osmolality. Thiazide diuretics do not alter medullary osmolality because they act in the renal cortex. Additionally, most loop diuretics have a shorter half-life than thiazides, and patients usually replete the urinary sodium and water losses prior to taking the next dose, thereby minimizing AVP stimulation.[29]

Cerebral (renal) salt wasting syndrome is a condition observed most often in patients with intracranial disorders such as subarachnoid hemorrhage and traumatic brain injury or after neurosurgical procedures, but it can occur in patients without CNS pathology. It results in decreased ECF volume due to a profound natriuresis (urinary sodium loss). A high urine sodium, osmolality, and volume; high serum BUN; orthostatic hypotension; and low central venous pressure suggests cerebral salt wasting.[30] In more severe cases, treatment consists of IV volume repletion with 0.9% NaCl. If serum sodium concentration is less than 120 mEq/L (mmol/L), 3% NaCl may be needed to correct the serum sodium concentration. In some cases, careful titration with 3% NaCl and 0.9% NaCl is required to maintain the serum sodium within an acceptable range.[30] In stable patients, oral administration of a salt supplement and a mineralocorticoid such as fludrocortisone may be used to augment serum sodium and intravascular volume until resolution of this typically transient condition.

Euvolemic Hypotonic Hyponatremia

7 Euvolemic (isovolemic) hypotonic hyponatremia is associated with a normal or slightly decreased ECF sodium content and increased TBW and ECF volume and is most often caused by SIADH. The increase in ECF volume is not sufficient to cause peripheral or pulmonary edema or other signs of volume overload, and thus patients will appear euvolemic upon physical examination.

In SIADH, water intake exceeds the kidney's capacity to excrete a water load, either because of increased AVP release via nonosmotic and/or nonphysiologic processes or enhanced sensitivity of the kidney to AVP. In most patients with SIADH, the urine osmolality and sodium concentrations will be greater than 100 mOsm/kg (mmol/kg) and 20 to 30 mEq/L (mmol/L), respectively, and serum osmolality will be less than 275 mOsm/kg (mmol/kg) due to ECF volume expansion (see Fig. 68-1 and Table 68-2).[4,14]

The most common causes of SIADH are certain cancers (eg, small cell lung, pancreatic, brain), CNS disorders (eg, traumatic brain injury, stroke, meningitis, pituitary surgery), and lung disease (eg, tuberculosis, pneumonia, abscess, acute respiratory distress syndrome). A number of medications can cause SIADH by enhancing AVP release or its action on the kidney or by other mechanisms[13-15,31] (see Table 68-3). Patients with kidney and adrenal insufficiency or

TABLE 68-2 Characteristics of Hypotonic Hyponatremic States

Characteristics	Hypovolemic Hyponatremia	Euvolemic (Isovolemic) Hyponatremia	Hypervolemic Hyponatremia
Water and sodium	Sodium loss >> water loss	Water gain only	Water gain > sodium gain
Causes	Renal: thiazide diuretics Nonrenal: diarrhea, cerebral salt wasting	SIADH	Heart failure Liver cirrhosis Kidney failure
Effect on TBW	↓↓	↑	↑↑
Effect on TBNa	↓	↔	↑↑
Additional laboratory findings	Renal: UOsm high, UNa high Nonrenal: UOsm high, UNa low	Renal: UOsm low, UNa variable Nonrenal: UOsm high, UNa variable	UOsm high, UNa high
Clinical presentation	Orthostasis, hypotension, tachycardia, dry mucous membranes, CNS changes	Depends on severity of hyponatremia: seizures, lethargy	Peripheral and pulmonary edema, variable BP
Treatment	0.9% NaCl until vital signs stable; *maintenance* fluids to continue fluid deficit replacement; sodium replacement if cerebral salt wasting; VRA contraindicated	Water restriction, demeclocycline, loop diuretics, VRA, urea	Sodium and water restriction, loop diuretic, VRA, urea

CNS, central nervous system; NaCl, sodium chloride; SIADH, syndrome of inappropriate antidiuretic hormone secretion; TBW, total body weight; UNa, urine sodium; UOsm, urine osmolality; VRA, vasopressin receptor antagonist.

TABLE 68-3 Potential Causes of SIADH

Drug-Induced		Nondrug-Induced
Acetaminophen ACE inhibitors Anti-epileptic agents (barbiturates, carbamazepine, lamotrigine, valproic acid) Anti-infectives (linezolid, moxifloxacin) AVP analogs (desmopressin terlipressin, oxytocin, vasopressin) Bromocriptine Cytotoxic agents (carboplatin, cisplatin, ifosfamide, melphalan, methotrexate, vinca alkaloids)	Chlorpropamide Duloxetine Haloperidol MDMA (ectasy) Monoamine oxidase inhibitors Nicotine NSAIDs Opioids Phenothiazines Proton pump inhibitors Risperidone SSRIs Thioridazine Thiothixene Tolbutamide Tricyclic antidepressants Venlafaxine	Malignancy (lung, pancreatic, duodenal) CNS (trauma, tumor, meningitis, hemorrhage, stroke) Pulmonary (pneumonia, ARDS, TB) Postoperative state Nausea Anxiety

ACE, angiotensin-converting enzyme; ARDS, acute respiratory distress syndrome; AVP, arginine vasopressin; CNS, central nervous system; MDMA, 3,4-methylenedioxymethamphetamin; NSAIDs, nonsteroidal anti-inflammatory drugs; SIADH, syndrome of inappropriate antidiuretic hormone secretion; SSRIs, selective serotonin receptor inhibitors; TB, tuberculosis.

hypothyroidism can also present with euvolemic hyponatremia. The evaluation of a patient with suspected SIADH should include consideration of these disorders or medications.

Euvolemic hypotonic hyponatremia may also be caused by primary or psychogenic polydipsia (water intoxication or compulsive water drinking) where more water (usually more than 20 L/day) is ingested than the kidneys can excrete as solute-free water. Unlike in SIADH, AVP secretion is suppressed, resulting in a urine osmolality less than 100 mOsm/kg (mmol/kg). The urine sodium is typically low (less than 15 mEq/L [mmol/L]) due to dilution.[14] Hyponatremia may develop even with more modest water intakes in individuals who ingest low-solute diets.

Hypervolemic Hypotonic Hyponatremia

8 Hyponatremia with ECF volume expansion (hypervolemia) occurs in conditions in which both sodium and water excretion are impaired such as HF, cirrhosis, or nephrotic syndrome. These patients have an expanded ECF volume and edema but a decreased effective arterial blood volume. The decrease in the effective circulating blood volume results in renal sodium retention and eventual ECF volume expansion and edema. There is concomitant nonosmotic AVP stimulation and water retention in excess of sodium retention, which perpetuates hyponatremia.

Clinical Presentation

Patients with chronic (longer than 48 hours) mild hyponatremia (serum sodium concentration 125-134 mEq/L [mmol/L]) are usually relatively asymptomatic, with hyponatremia often being discovered incidentally when serum electrolytes are measured for other reasons. Mild symptoms of hyponatremia frequently go unnoticed by both clinicians and patients.[32] Chronic, mild hyponatremia, especially in older adults, has been associated with impairment of attention, posture, and gait; all of which contribute to a substantially increased fall risk.[23-26,33] Even *asymptomatic* patients, when formally tested, have impaired attention and gait to a degree that is comparable to symptoms seen with a blood alcohol level of 0.06% (13 mmol/L).[32]

Patients with moderate (serum sodium concentration 115-124 mEq/L [mmol/L]), severe (serum sodium concentration 110-114 mEq/L [mmol/L]), or rapidly developing hypotonic hyponatremia may present with a range of CNS symptoms resulting from hypoosmolality-induced brain cell swelling. Classic neurologic symptoms include nausea, malaise, headache, lethargy, restlessness, and disorientation. In severe cases, seizures, coma, respiratory arrest, brainstem herniation, and death can occur.

The presence and severity of symptoms depend on both the degree of the hyponatremia and the rate at which it develops. The degree of hyponatremia is important because serum osmolality decreases in direct proportion to the serum sodium concentration, and water movement into cells, including brain cells, increases as serum osmolality decreases. The rate of change of the serum osmolality is important because brain cells are not able to rapidly adjust intracellular osmolality to minimize cellular volume changes.[2,34] When decreased serum osmolality causes water movement into brain cells, inorganic Cl^- and K^+ and organic osmolytes (eg, taurine, glutamate, myoinositol, GABA), move out of the cells to decrease intracellular osmolality and minimize the intracellular water shift. The components of this adaptive mechanism occur and dissipate over different time frames, with Cl^- and K^+ efflux occurring and

CLINICAL PRESENTATION Hyponatremia

General

- Severity of symptoms depends on the magnitude and rapidity of onset
- Too rapid correction can lead to severe neurologic symptoms

Symptoms

- Symptoms are primarily neurologic in nature
- Mild: may be asymptomatic; nausea, malaise, gait or cognitive disturbances
- Moderate: headache, lethargy, restlessness, disorientation
- Severe: seizures, coma, respiratory arrest, brainstem herniation, death
- Other symptoms depend on etiology: dry mucous membranes, tachycardia, hypotension, reduced or increased urine output

Laboratory tests

- Serum sodium concentration less than 135 mEq/L (mmol/L)
- Serum osmolality and urine sodium concentration vary depending on etiology
- Altered serum glucose, lipids, proteins, or thyroid function in certain patients

dissipating within minutes to hours and organic osmolyte efflux occurring and dissipating within hours to days.[3,34] Thus, maximal compensation for decreased serum osmolality typically requires up to 48 hours, and acute changes in serum osmolality are more likely to cause symptoms. Gender and age play a role in the response to severe hyponatremia. Young women (pre-menopausal) have been found to have a higher likelihood of death or permanent brain damage compared to men or older women. Female sex hormones may inhibit the Na^+/K^+-ATPase system. Additionally, interleukin-6 which is found in higher concentrations in women than in men influences vasopressin secretion and reduces the expression of aquaporin-2, impairing free water excretion.[3] Hyponatremia is an important risk factor for morbidity and mortality in patients with HF and cirrhosis.[20,35]

In addition to CNS symptoms, patients with hypovolemic hyponatremia present with signs and symptoms of hypovolemia, including dry mucous membranes, decreased skin turgor, tachycardia, decreased jugular venous pressure, hypotension, and orthostatic hypotension. Lactic acidosis and low mixed venous oxygen saturation, indicating decreased tissue perfusion, may be present with severe hypovolemia.

The brain's adaptation to chronic serum hypoosmolality or hyperosmolality leads to neurologic symptoms when either hyponatremia (hypoosmolality) or hypernatremia (hypertonicity) is corrected too rapidly. The combination of the adaptive decrease in ICF osmolality and a rapid increase in ECF osmolality results in rapid and excessive water movement out of cells, including brain cells, and ICF volume depletion. Thus, too rapid correction of the serum sodium concentration can lead to an acute decrease in brain cell volume, which contributes to the pathogenesis of *osmotic demyelination syndrome* (ODS) or central pontine myelinolysis.[3] While demyelinated lesions identified on magnetic resonance imaging most often occur in the central pons, ODS can extend to other areas of the brain. Patients with ODS may be asymptomatic or develop mild to severe symptoms including confusion, disorientation, dysarthria, dysphagia, hyperreflexia, obtundation, para- or quadriparesis, parkinsonism, pseudobulbar palsy, *locked-in syndrome* (a condition in which a patient is aware and awake but cannot move or communicate verbally due to complete paralysis of nearly all voluntary muscles except for the eyes), seizures, coma, and/or death in 1 to 7 days after correction of the serum sodium concentration.[3,36] If recovery from ODS occurs, it can take several months for symptoms to improve. Patients with significant cerebral adaptation (eg, chronic serum sodium concentration less than 110 mEq/L [mmol/L]) are at highest risk of developing ODS because these patients have a lower intracellular osmolality at the initiation of therapy, and there is a greater decrease in brain cell volume when the serum osmolality is raised too rapidly.[3] Other conditions that increase the risk of ODS include alcoholism, liver disease including orthotopic liver transplantation, potassium depletion, and malnutrition. Thus, if the duration of hyponatremia is unknown, it is generally safer to treat as if it is chronic when developing an initial therapy plan.

Treatment: Hyponatremia

General guidelines for the treatment of patients with hyponatremia are shown in Table 68-4. Application of these principles to the treatment of various forms of hyponatremia is discussed in the following sections.

Desired Outcomes

Regardless of the type or cause of hyponatremia, treatment goals for all patients are to resolve the underlying cause of the sodium and ECF volume imbalance, if possible, and to safely correct the sodium and water derangements. The treatment plan depends on the underlying cause and symptom severity. Patients with acute onset hyponatremia with severe symptoms require more aggressive therapy to correct the hypotonicity. The initial treatment goal is to increase serum tonicity just enough to control severe symptoms which typically requires only a small increase (5%) in the serum sodium concentration. Once severe symptoms have abated, then continued serum sodium correction should be achieved at a slower, more controlled rate. Patients who are asymptomatic or who have only mild to moderate symptoms do not require rapid correction of the serum sodium concentration. While treatment is dictated by the underlying cause, in all cases the goal is to avoid an increase in the serum sodium concentration of more than 6 to 12 mEq/L (mmol/L) in 24 hours (0.5 mEq/L [mmol/L] per hour) or 18 mEq/L (mmol/L) in any 48-hour period.[6,20] When the duration of hyponatremia is unknown, a sodium correction rate of no more than 6 to 8 mEq/L (mmol/L) in 24 hours is prudent to avoid ODS.[3]

ACUTE OR SEVERELY SYMPTOMATIC HYPOTONIC HYPONATREMIA

A patient who has or is at high risk of experiencing severe symptoms caused by hyponatremia (serum sodium less than 110-115 mEq/L [mmol/L]) should receive a small amount of 3% NaCl (513 mEq/L [mmol/L]) until severe symptoms resolve.[2,3] While resolution of severe symptoms generally requires approximately a 5% increase in

TABLE 68-4 General Guidelines for Treatment of Hyponatremia

- For both short- and long-term management, treat the underlying cause of hyponatremia, if possible.
- Appropriate treatment of moderate-to-severe hypotonic hyponatremia requires balancing the risks of hyponatremia vs the risk of ODS.
- Patients who acutely develop moderate-to-severe hyponatremia and/or patients who have severe symptoms are at greatest risk and potentially benefit most from more rapid correction of hyponatremia.
- Correction of hypovolemic hypotonic hyponatremia is usually best accomplished with 0.9% NaCl, as these patients have both sodium and water deficits.
- Active correction of euvolemic and hypervolemic hypotonic hyponatremia in patients who do not require rapid correction is usually best accomplished by water restriction. Demeclocycline, VRA, urea, or a loop diuretic can be used if the initial response to water restriction is not adequate.
- In patients with severe symptoms, 3% NaCl should initially be used to correct the hyponatremia more rapidly. A loop diuretic can be administered concurrently with 3% NaCl to enhance the serum sodium correction by increasing free water excretion.
- Long-term management will be required for patients in whom the underlying cause of hyponatremia cannot be corrected. Depending on the cause, water restriction, increasing sodium intake, and/or a VRA may be used.

NaCl, sodium chloride; ODS, osmotic demyelination syndrome; VRA, vasopressin receptor antagonist.

the serum sodium concentration, some clinicians suggest that the initial safe target should be a serum sodium concentration of approximately 120 mEq/L (mmol/L).

The relative concentrations of urine sodium and potassium (osmotically effective urine cations) should be compared with those of the infusate in planning a treatment regimen for patients with hypotonic hyponatremia. For the serum sodium concentration to increase after a NaCl infusion, the sodium concentration of the infusate must exceed the sum of the urinary sodium and potassium concentrations so that an effective net free-water excretion is produced.[6] In SIADH, the urinary concentration of osmotically effective cations often exceeds 154 mEq/L (mmol/L) (sodium concentration of 0.9% NaCl); thus 0.9% NaCl administration could worsen hyponatremia. These patients should be preferentially treated with 3% NaCl.[32,37] The relatively high urinary sodium concentration in patient with SIADH is due to ECF expansion, which minimizes sodium reabsorption along the nephron. When the urine osmolality exceeds 300 mOsm/kg (mmol/kg), it is advisable to administer an IV loop diuretic to increase solute-free water excretion and to prevent volume overload which can result from NaCl administration. Intravenous furosemide 20 to 40 mg given every 6 hours or bumetanide 0.5 to 1 mg given every 2 to 3 hours for several doses is generally sufficient to prevent volume overload and to decrease the urinary concentration of osmotically active cations to less than 150 mEq/L (mmol/L). If intermittent loop diuretic doses are not sufficient to manage volume overload, then either IV furosemide 20 to 40 mg followed by a 10 to 40 mg/hr infusion or IV bumetanide 1 mg followed by a 0.5 to 2 mg/hr infusion can be used.

Patients with hypovolemic hypotonic hyponatremia should be treated initially with 0.9% NaCl. In contrast to SIADH, avid reabsorption of sodium throughout the nephron occurs because the effective circulating blood volume is decreased. Thus, the urine sodium concentration usually will be less than 30 mEq/L (mmol/L), substantially less than the sodium content of 0.9% NaCl. While administration of 3% NaCl will correct hyponatremia, it will not correct the hypovolemia and should be reserved for patients with severe symptoms requiring rapid serum sodium correction.

Acute hypervolemic hypotonic hyponatremia is particularly problematic to manage because the sodium and volume needed to minimize the risk of cerebral edema or seizures can worsen already compromised liver, heart, or kidney function. These patients generally should be treated initially with 3% NaCl and fluid (water) restriction. Loop diuretic or arginine vasopressin receptor antagonist (VRA) therapy is often required to facilitate urinary-free water excretion.

Determination of a NaCl Infusion Regimen

Multiple approaches can be used for determining an empiric NaCl infusion regimen for a patient with hyponatremia.[3,7,20] While several complex equations have been published, improved outcomes have not been demonstrated using these equations. Pragmatically, 150 mL[6] or 1 to 2 mL/kg[2] of 3% NaCl can be infused over 20 minutes. If symptoms do not resolve, then 100 mL or 1 mL/kg of 3% NaCl can be administered over 10 to 20 minutes every 30 minutes until symptoms resolve and/or the target serum sodium concentration is reached (usually 5-8 mEq/L [mmol/L] from baseline). Within the first hour, the serum sodium should not increase by more than 5 mEq/L (mmol/L). After relief of symptoms, 0.9% NaCl can be used to continue the sodium correction.

Another method is to calculate the sodium deficit, then replace one-third of the deficit in the first 6 hours and the remaining two-thirds over the following 24 to 48 hours or longer depending on the acuity of the serum sodium decrease. Sodium deficit can be calculated using the following equation:

$$Na_{deficit}(\text{mEq or mmol}) = [(Na_d - Na_s) \times TBW]$$

where Na_d is the goal or desired serum sodium (usually no higher than 120-125 mEq/L [mmol/L] to avoid too rapid or overcorrection); Na_s is the patient's current serum sodium concentration; and TBW is the patient's current TBW calculated as shown in Table 68-5. The change in serum sodium concentration resulting from the infusion of 1 L of 3% NaCl or 0.9% NaCl can be estimated. An example of this approach is shown in Table 68-5.

Clinicians may disagree whether or not to administer 3% NaCl to patients with symptomatic hypotonicity. An advantage of 3% NaCl is more rapid correction of serum sodium concentration with a smaller infusion volume. A disadvantage of 3% NaCl is a higher risk of too rapid correction of serum sodium concentration and ODS. Another disadvantage of 3% NaCl is its high osmolality (1,026 mOsm/L) which can result in phlebitis and significant tissue damage with extravasation when given via a peripheral IV catheter (~7% complication rate with peripheral administration). Central line administration is preferred but short-term peripheral administration is acceptable if the infusion rate is low and a relatively large peripheral IV catheter is used.[38] The historical use of 5% NaCl has been replaced by 3% NaCl due to these infusion issues. Some clinicians have suggested the use of 2% NaCl to avoid infusion-related issues, but this practice has not been evaluated in clinical trials. Fluid choice depends on the cause and the rapidity of development of the patient's hyponatremia as well as the relative risk of slower correction of the hyponatremia versus the development of ODS.

The appropriate infusion volume for a given patient can be estimated using the amount of fluid needed to provide the calculated sodium deficit or the desired proportion of the estimated change that would result from a 1-L infusion. The final step is to calculate an appropriate infusion rate for the calculated volume that will increase the serum sodium concentration by no more than 6 to 8 mEq/L (mmol/L) in 24 hours in high-risk patients and by 10 to 12 mEq/L (mmol/L) in 24 hours or 18 mEq/L (mmol/L) in 48 hours in others (see Table 68-5).[5] To minimize the risk of too rapid correction of hyponatremia, desmopressin (1-4 mcg) and free water replacement given along with 3% NaCl may be considered in patients with severe hyponatremia until the serum sodium concentration reaches 128 mEq/L (mmol/L).[3,20]

TABLE 68-5 Assessment and Treatment of Euvolemic Hyponatremia

Change in serum sodium concentration after an IV fluid bolus

$\Delta Na_s = (Na_{IV} + K_{IV} - Na_s) / (TBW + volume_{IV})$

ΔNa_s, change in serum sodium concentration; K_{IV}, potassium concentration of infusate; Na_{IV}, sodium concentration of infusate (eg, 154 mEq/L [mmol/L] for 0.9% NaCl; 513 mEq/L [mmol/L] for 3% NaCl); Na_s, initial serum sodium concentration; TBW, total body water (L); and $volume_{IV}$, volume of infused fluid (L)

TBW can be estimated as:

Term newborn infants: 0.7 L/kg × wt (kg); higher in premature infants depending on degree of prematurity
Children and men younger than 70 years: 0.6 L/kg × wt (kg)
Men older than 70 years and women younger than 70 years: 0.5 L/kg × wt (kg)
Women older than 70 years: 0.45 L/kg × wt (kg)
Dehydrated, older patients: 0.4 L/kg × wt (kg)
(Note: wt is the current body weight)

Clinical example

A 76-year-old man (weight, 70 kg [154 lb]; height, 178 cm [5 ft 10 in]) presents with nausea, headache, and confusion which developed over the past 3 days. Ten days ago, he began taking carbamazepine for trigeminal neuralgia. His serum sodium concentration on admission to the emergency department was 109 mEq/L (mmol/L). He is diagnosed with drug-induced SIADH.

Plan of care

1. Discontinue carbamazepine (the likely etiology of his SIADH).
2. Admit to the hospital for correction of hyponatremia.
3. Increase the serum sodium concentration by no more than 6 to 12 mEq/L (mmol/L) during first 24 hours and no higher than 120 mEq/L (mmol/L); thus, the goal is to increase the sodium concentration by 11 mEq/L (mmol/L).
4. Due to degree of hyponatremia (less than 110 mEq/L [mmol/L]) and the presence of moderate-to-severe symptoms, give 3% NaCl.

Calculate the change in serum sodium after 1 L infusion of 3% NaCl:

$$\Delta Na_s = (513\ \text{mEq/L} - 109\ \text{mEq/L})/[(0.5\ \text{L/kg} \times 70\ \text{kg}) + 1\ \text{L}] = 11.2\ \text{mEq/L or } 1.12\ \text{mEq/100 mL}$$

(Note: In SI units, the calculation is the same using mmol/L rather than mEq/L.)

Infusion of 1 L of 3% NaCl will result in a 11.2 mEq/L (mmol/L) rise in the serum sodium concentration. An 11 mEq/L (mmol/L) increase is desired; thus, the appropriate infusion volume is 982 mL [(11 mEq/L/11.2 mEq/L) × 1,000 mL] or [(11 mmol/L/11.2 mmol/L) × 1,000 mL].

(Note: The approach to this calculation would be similar if 0.9% NaCl was used, except that for each 1 L infusion, the expected increase in serum sodium concentration would be only 1.25 mEq/L (mmol/L), and an infusion volume of approximately 8.8 L would be required to achieve the targeted serum sodium concentration.)

5. Moderate-to-severe symptoms: serum sodium concentration should be increased by approximately 1.5 mEq/L/hr (mmol/L/hr) over the first 2 to 4 hours of treatment for a total of 3 to 6 mEq/L [mmol/L] or until the symptoms have resolved. An initial infusion rate of 114 mL/hr for the first 2 to 4 hours is needed.
6. Check serum sodium concentration every 1 to 4 hours depending on rate of rise of serum sodium.
7. Once symptoms subside, continue infusion rate at approximately 23 to 31 mL/hr for the next 20 to 22 hours, to slowly correct hyponatremia. Monitor serum sodium concentration every 4 hours or more often if serum sodium is rapidly changing.

IV, intravenous; SIADH, syndrome of inappropriate antidiuretic hormone secretion; NaCl, sodium chloride.

Evaluation of Therapeutic Outcomes

Patients with severely symptomatic hypotonic hyponatremia should be admitted to the ICU or other setting that will allow frequent monitoring of CNS symptoms and volume status. Examination of the heart, lungs, and neurologic status should be performed frequently during the first 12 hours of therapy. The serum sodium concentration should be measured at least every 2 to 4 hours, and the urine sodium, potassium, and osmolality should be measured every 4 to 6 hours during the first 24 to 48 hours of therapy to allow timely infusion rate adjustment to avoid too rapid correction.

NONEMERGENT HYPOVOLEMIC HYPOTONIC HYPONATREMIA

Most patients with hypovolemic hypotonic hyponatremia are either asymptomatic or have only mild-to-moderate symptoms and do not require rapid sodium correction. Many of these patients are at high risk of developing ODS if serum sodium correction occurs too rapidly because they have chronic hyponatremia and maximum compensation by the brain's osmotic adaptive mechanisms. Treatment should include correction of the underlying condition, if possible, and administration of 0.9% NaCl or other isotonic solution (eg, lactated Ringer's, Plasma-Lyte®, Normosol-R®) to correct the hypovolemia. These solutions will replace the existing sodium and water deficits while conveying a lower risk of too rapid sodium correction than 3% NaCl.

The ECF deficit can be estimated based on the patient's sex, age, and change in body weight. One method and an example of its use is shown in Table 68-6. If the patient's previous weight is unknown, the ECF deficit can be roughly estimated based on clinical signs and symptoms. The presence of hyponatremia suggests an ECF deficit of 5% or more, whereas the presence of orthostatic hypotension suggests an ECF deficit of at least 10% to 15%. Administration of an isotonic solution would be optimal to correct the patient's ECF volume deficit because essentially 100% of it will remain in the ECF space (see Table 68-1). The overriding initial treatment goal is to restore effective circulating volume; thus, it may be necessary to administer an IV bolus (500-1,000 mL in adults; 10-20 mL/kg in children) over a period of 1 hour or less or begin an IV infusion of the isotonic solution at 200 to 400 mL/hr (10-20 mL/kg/hr in children) until symptoms of hypovolemia improve. The infusion rate can then be decreased to 100 to 150 mL/hr (4-6 mL/kg/hr in children) so that the serum sodium concentration does not increase too rapidly. Fluids should be given rapidly enough and in sufficient quantity to restore and maintain adequate tissue perfusion without overloading the cardiovascular or pulmonary system.

It is important to recognize that once hypovolemia is corrected, the serum sodium will increase rapidly if the infusion rate is not adjusted appropriately. When the ECF volume is restored, AVP secretion stops, and a rapid water diuresis can ensue, potentially resulting in a rapid increase in serum sodium. Estimating the patient's ECF deficit at the start of therapy may be helpful. If the serum sodium concentration is increasing at a rate greater than 0.5 mEq/L/hr (mmol/L/hr), the infusate can be changed to 0.45% NaCl, and the infusion rate set to slow the rate of serum sodium increase. In general, 0.45% NaCl should not be infused alone as this hypoosmolar solution (154 mOsm/L) may result in red blood cell hemolysis. Most often, Dextrose 5%/0.45% NaCl is infused

TABLE 68-6 Assessment and Treatment of Hypotonic Hypovolemic Hyponatremia

Calculating ECF deficit

$$\text{ECF deficit (mL)} = \text{ECF}_{\text{normal}} - \text{ECF}_{\text{current}}$$

where ECF volume = 0.33 × TBW

Clinical example

A 75-year-old woman (height, 168 cm [5 ft 6 in]; usual weight, 50 kg [110 lb]) was started on hydrochlorothiazide 25 mg once daily 10 days ago for hypertension. She presents with complaints of mild nausea and dizziness when she stands up. Her current weight is 45 kg (99 lb). Upon physical examination she has dry mucous membranes and orthostatic hypotension. Her serum sodium concentration is 126 mEq/L (mmol/L).

Calculate the ECF deficit

ECF deficit = (50 kg × 0.4 L/kg × 0.33) – (45 kg × 0.4 L/kg × 0.33) = 660 mL

(Note: TBW = 0.4 L/kg used because she is a dehydrated older patient; see Table 68-5.)

Calculate the expected increase in the serum sodium after infusion of 1 L of 0.9% NaCl (see Table 68-1):

ΔNa_s with 1 L of infusate = [154 mEq/L – 126 mEq/L]/[(0.4 L/kg × 45 kg) + 1 L] = 1.47 mEq/L (mmol/L)

The patient's serum sodium concentration will be 127.5 mEq/L (mmol/L) following the infusion of 1 L 0.9% NaCl.

Treatment goals: Restore effective circulating volume and correct serum sodium concentration

Treatment plan:

1. Infuse 0.9% NaCl at 200-250 mL/hr until symptoms of hypovolemia improve; then decrease infusion to 150-200 mL/hr so that the serum sodium concentration increases by no more than 6-12 mEq/L (mmol/L) or 0.5-1 mEq/L/hr (mmol/L/hr) over the initial 24 hours. Rate depends on patient status.
2. Hold thiazide diuretic until volume status is restored.
3. Consider restarting diuretic at lower dose, for example, 12.5 mg once daily, if needed.

ECF, extracellular fluid; NaCl, sodium chloride; TBW, total body water.

to provide a relatively isotonic solution (Dextrose 5% provides 250 mOsm/L to the solution). Potassium depletion or repletion can also affect hyponatremia and its correction. One mEq (mmol) of retained potassium equals 1 mEq (mmol) retained sodium; thus, if hypokalemia is corrected at the same time as hyponatremia, the serum sodium may increase more rapidly.

Evaluation of Therapeutic Outcomes

Patients presenting with hypovolemia should be reexamined frequently during the initial few hours of therapy. Of note, the urine output will often lag behind during fluid resuscitation, so careful monitoring for pulmonary congestion is critical, especially in patients with underlying heart, lung, or kidney dysfunction. The serum sodium concentration should be measured every 2 to 4 hours to allow timely adjustment of the rate and composition of IV fluids to avoid too rapidly increasing the serum sodium concentration. In patients with a history of HF or kidney insufficiency, 0.9% NaCl should be administered judiciously with frequent cardiopulmonary assessments so that the infusion rate can be adjusted at the earliest sign of pulmonary congestion.

NONEMERGENT EUVOLEMIC HYPOTONIC HYPONATREMIA

The fact that neurological performance is restored to normal with correction of even mild hyponatremia provides a rationale for maintaining the serum sodium concentration at 130 mEq/L (mmol/L) or higher, if possible. Long-term management will be required for patients in whom the underlying cause is not readily correctable.

Treatment of SIADH always involves restricting water and correcting the underlying cause (see Table 68-3). Medications that could be contributing should be identified and discontinued, if possible. The primary treatment goal is to induce a negative water balance by initially restricting water intake to 1,000 to 1,200 mL/day so that insensible water loss (skin and lung, 900 mL/day) plus obligate urine (500 mL/day) and stool (200 mL/day) loss exceed water intake. Because approximately 850 mL of water per day is ingested in food, and an additional 350 mL are generated from oxidative processes, this degree of water restriction should result in a negative water balance of several hundred milliliters per day. Further water restriction may be needed but adherence is difficult. An additional goal is to maintain the serum sodium concentration close to 130 mEq/L (mmol/L) to reduce CNS symptoms and avoid iatrogenic hypovolemia.

Patients with chronic SIADH who are unable to restrict water intake sufficiently to maintain an acceptable serum sodium concentration can be treated by increasing solute intake with NaCl supplementation and/or loop diuretic administration. NaCl supplements increase the obligatory daily solute excretion, which augments the kidney's capacity for water excretion. The goal is to increase the daily solute intake and excretion to approximately 900 mOsm (mmol) per day. Because an average diet contains approximately 600 mOsm (mmol), 9 g of NaCl would be required to increase the osmolar excretion to 900 mOsm/day (mmol/day). Each 1 g NaCl tablet contains 17 mmol of sodium and 17 mmol of chloride. Because ECF volume expansion is an expected adverse effect, a loop diuretic should be administered concurrently to avoid volume overload and edema. Loop diuretics will also enhance water excretion by limiting the formation of the medullary concentration gradient.

Vasopressin Receptor Antagonists

VRAs are high-affinity non-peptide antagonists of arginine vasopressin V_2 and V_{1a} receptors, often referred to as *vaptans*.[39] VRAs have dramatic effects on water excretion and were the first significant breakthrough in hyponatremia treatment since loop diuretics. These agents are additional therapeutic options for both euvolemic and hypervolemic hypotonic hyponatremia but are contraindicated in hypovolemic hyponatremia.

Blockade of AVP binding can occur at any of its three distinct receptors: V_{1a}, predominantly in the liver, CNS, and cardiomyocytes; V_2, in the distal nephron; and V_{1b} (formerly V_3), in the anterior pituitary and pancreas.[39] Selective V_2 receptor antagonism prevents AQP2 water channel transport to the apical surface, thereby decreasing AVP-dependent water reabsorption in the collecting duct. AVP inhibition leads to excretion of large water volumes, decreased urine osmolality, and an increase in the serum sodium concentration. These outcomes are achieved without significantly increasing electrolyte excretion; thus, these agents have been called *aquaretics*.

Only two VRAs are currently marketed in the United States, conivaptan and tolvaptan. Conivaptan (Vaprisol®, Astellas Pharma US, Inc., Northbrook, IL), a mixed vasopressin V_1- and V_2-receptor antagonist, is FDA-labeled for use in the treatment of acute euvolemic and hypervolemic hyponatremia in hospitalized patients. Its utility in chronic hyponatremia is limited because it is only available as an IV formulation, FDA-labeled for up to 4 days of use, a moderate CYP3A4 inhibitor, and not FDA-labeled for use in patients with HF.

Tolvaptan (Samsca®, Otsuka Pharmaceutical Co, Ltd, Tokyo, Japan) is an oral selective VRA with a greater affinity for the V_2 receptor than endogenous AVP. It is FDA-labeled for the treatment of clinically significant (serum sodium concentration less than 125 mEq/L [mmol/L]) euvolemic or hypervolemic hyponatremia or less marked symptomatic hyponatremia that is unresponsive to other therapeutic interventions in patients with HF, cirrhosis, and SIADH. When given alone, tolvaptan promotes aquaresis and modestly raises serum sodium concentrations by 3.6 mEq/L (mmol/L) at 4 days and 4.4 mEq/L (mmol/L) at 30 days, respectively (SALT-1 and SALT-2 studies).[40,41] However, the effect of tolvaptan on serum sodium concentrations may have been limited by the high average fluid intake (~2 L/day) in these studies. In fact, mean increases in serum sodium may be double those found in the SALT studies.[42-44] In SALT-1 and SALT-2, the percentage of patients with a normal serum sodium concentration (greater than 135 mEq/L [mmol/L]) after one month of tolvaptan use was 53% and 58%, respectively, versus 25% (both studies) with placebo.[40,41] When used as monotherapy, tolvaptan is superior to either furosemide or water restriction, and when given in combination with furosemide, there are synergistic effects.[45]

The usual starting tolvaptan dosage is 15 mg given orally once daily based on the SALT studies. A greater risk of overcorrection of serum sodium exists in patients with euvolemic compared to hypervolemic hypotonic hyponatremia.[43,46,47] Thus, a lower starting dosage of 7.5 mg once daily may be considered in patients with euvolemic hypotonic hyponatremia due to its equivalent efficacy and lower risk of overcorrection of serum sodium.[48] This lower dosage should also be used for patients older than 90 years of age.[49]

In critically ill neurological patients, who often require more aggressive care to prevent long-term morbidity, a single tolvaptan dose (7.5 or 15 mg) can effectively increase serum sodium concentration by 5 to 7.8 mEq/L (mmol/L) with the effect sustained for up to 96 hours. Multiple doses may be required. Overcorrection (increasing serum sodium concentration by more than 6 to 12 mEq/L [mmol/L] in 24 hours) may occur, particularly when a 15-mg dose is given, thus careful monitoring in these high-risk patients is warranted.[50,51] Reducing the starting dosage to less than 15 mg/day may not eliminate the risk of too rapid sodium correction.[52]

The oral bioavailability of tolvaptan is about 56%, and its activity peaks at 2 to 4 hours after a dose. For patients who cannot swallow tablets, the tablets can be crushed, suspended in water, and the slurry administered orally or via a nasogastric tube, but a 25% average decrease in the tolvaptan area under the concentration-time curve may be seen with this administration method.[53] Fluid restriction should be avoided within the first 24 to 48 hours of starting VRA therapy when active sodium correction is occurring.[20] After 24 hours, if a greater increase in serum sodium concentration is needed, the dosage may be increased to 30 mg once daily, and after another 24 hours, to a maximum of 60 mg once daily.

Approximately 10% to 50% of patients do not significantly respond to VRA therapy.[54,55] Therapeutic resistance or failure to respond to VRA therapy could be due to high circulating AVP concentrations, AVP-independent impaired urinary dilution, excessive water intake, or an activating V_2-receptor mutation causing nephrogenic SIADH.[39] There is currently no pharmacogenomic information available for the G protein-coupled receptor family of AVP receptors or the VRAs that can be used to individualize therapy.[56]

Tolvaptan is primarily metabolized to inactive metabolites by CYP3A4 and less than 1% is eliminated unchanged in the urine; thus, its use should be avoided in patients receiving potent CYP3A4 inhibitors (eg, ketoconazole, clarithromycin, itraconazole, ritonavir). Concomitant therapy with P-glycoprotein inhibitors and grapefruit juice results in increased serum tolvaptan concentrations. Tolvaptan inhibits P-glycoprotein and coadministration with P-glycoprotein substrates should be avoided, if possible.[57] Conversely, optimal tolvaptan benefits may not be achieved on usual dosages in patients who are receiving potent CYP3A4 inducers (eg, phenytoin, phenobarbital, St. John's Wort).

Tolvaptan therapy is contraindicated in patients needing rapid serum sodium correction (due to the 2- to 4-hour delayed onset), those unable to sense or respond appropriately to thirst, patients with hypovolemic hyponatremia, patients taking strong CYP3A4 inhibitors, and patients who are anuric. Tolvaptan has not been studied in patients with severe hyponatremia (severe symptoms or serum sodium less than 120 mEq/L [mmol/L]). Patients with more profound hyponatremia are more likely to experience larger increases in serum sodium concentrations. Tolvaptan should be used cautiously in these patients with serum sodium concentration monitoring every 2 to 4 hours. Tolvaptan effectively produces aquaresis and increases serum sodium concentrations in patients with chronic kidney disease (CKD stages 3, 4, 5) who are not receiving renal replacement therapy.[58,59] VRA use should be avoided with hypertonic saline (eg, 3% NaCl) due to the risk of too rapid and/or overcorrection of the serum sodium concentration. Thirst, dry mouth, weakness, constipation, hyperglycemia, and urinary frequency are the most common adverse medication reactions, and they rarely necessitate therapy discontinuation.[40,41]

Reversible increases in hepatic transaminases have been reported with tolvaptan use; however, concerns for irreversible liver damage arose in the TEMPO 3:4 trial which evaluated tolvaptan in patients with autosomal dominant polycystic kidney disease. Tolvaptan dosages (45-120 mg/day) were much higher than those typically used for hyponatremia, and the duration of therapy was longer than 30 days (up to 3 years in some patients). Increases in hepatic transaminases did not meet Hi's criteria for medication-induced liver injury because the total bilirubin was not elevated to more than twice the upper limit of normal.[60] The FDA issued a warning to avoid tolvaptan use for more than 30 days in anyone with chronic liver disease. Additionally, tolvaptan should be discontinued if any sign of liver injury occurs during therapy. To reduce the ODS risk, tolvaptan therapy should begin or resume only in a hospital where the serum sodium concentration can be closely monitored (boxed warning).

VRAs are more expensive than other treatment options. Multiple economic analyses have determined tolvaptan therapy to be cost-effective for SIADH and HF when compared to fluid restriction or no additional therapy as evidenced by reduced hospital stay, avoidance of ICU admission, and avoidance of hospital readmission.[61-63] However, the cost-effectiveness of VRAs in the management of patients with SIADH is still unclear when considering all therapeutic modalities. Therapy continuation after acute treatment depends on the etiology of SIADH. While many cases are transient, other etiologies require indefinite treatment. The inability to discontinue the offending agent in medication-induced SIADH may also necessitate long-term treatment. When considering long-term VRA treatment, cost and potential liver toxicity must be weighed against potential benefits.

It is unclear whether normalizing the serum sodium concentration improves the morbidity and/or mortality associated with hyponatremia. Additional research is needed to compare VRA use with traditional therapies after fluid restriction in the acute phase of nonemergent euvolemic hyponatremia. Further investigation is also warranted for long-term VRA use in asymptomatic or minimally symptomatic hyponatremia, particularly in older adults, to reduce morbidity (eg, cognitive deficits, gait disturbance, falls, bone fractures).

Sodium-Glucose Co-Transporter-2 Inhibitors

Sodium-glucose co-transporter-2 (SGLT2) inhibitors are oral hypoglycemic medications with cardiovascular and kidney benefits. Through blockade of SGLT2, a glucose transporter in the proximal renal tubule responsible for 90% of glucose reabsorption, SGLT2 inhibitors lead to excretion of 50% to 60% of filtered glucose, approximately 60 to 100 g/day. The resulting glucosuric effect causes an osmotic diuresis and increases free water excretion.[64] The use of SGLT2 inhibitors in addition to standard fluid restriction of less than 1,000 mL/day in patients with euvolemic hypotonic hyponatremia results in an increased median plasma sodium concentration compared to placebo (10 vs 7 mEq/L [mmol/L]), but this difference may not be clinically significant.[65] Further studies are needed before

SGLT2 inhibitors can be routinely recommended for treatment of euvolemic hypotonic hyponatremia.

Demeclocycline

Demeclocycline, a semisynthetic tetracycline antibiotic, is a treatment option for some patients with SIADH whose serum sodium concentration is not adequately controlled by water restriction alone. Demeclocycline use in SIADH is largely based on clinical experience rather than data from clinical trials and it is ineffective in a significant proportion of patients.[4,66] Demeclocycline essentially causes nephrogenic diabetes insipidus (DI) by unpredictably inhibiting tubular AVP activity, which increases free water excretion. Some patients may even develop polyuria and hypernatremia due to this mechanism. The demeclocycline dosage is 300 mg given orally two to four times daily. Because of the delayed onset of action (2-6 days), this agent has no role in the acute management of severe hyponatremia, and dosage adjustments should be made no more frequently than every 3 to 4 days. Demeclocycline should not be used in patients with cirrhosis or compromised fluid intake, who are at high risk for demeclocycline-induced renal tubular toxicity and acute kidney failure,[4] who are pregnant, or who are younger than 8 years unless no other options are available because long-term use may interfere with tooth and bone development. Photosensitivity with skin rash may occur; thus, patients receiving demeclocycline should be counselled to use appropriate UV protection during sun exposure.

Urea

Urea is an osmotic agent that increases urinary-free water excretion and decreases urinary sodium excretion. Urea has been used as an alternative oral treatment for SIADH and other hyponatremic disorders. The administration of urea at a dose ranging from 7.5 to 90 g/day for a median of 4.5 days in the inpatient setting[67] and 15 to 30 g/day for up to 1 year in the outpatient setting[68] is safe and effective for treatment of hyponatremia. Adherence to therapy is a concern due to the bitter taste of urea. The FDA considers urea to be a medical food, thus a prescription is not required. An over-the-counter product, ure-Na™ (Nephcentric LLC, Phoenix, AZ) is available in a pouch that provides 15 g powder that can be dissolved in water or juice (juice usually preferred due to taste). While there is little quality evidence for the efficacy of urea in the treatment of SIADH or other hyponatremic disorders, it is recommended as a second-line agent in the European guidelines.[6]

Evaluation of Therapeutic Outcomes

The serum sodium concentration should be monitored at least every 4 to 6 hours during the active sodium correction phase with treatment other than fluid restriction until reaching a stable value greater than 125 mEq/L (mmol/L). The serum sodium concentration should be measured every 24 to 48 hours when water restriction is initiated until it stabilizes at a concentration at or above 125 mEq/L (mmol/L).[20] Continued decline in the serum sodium concentration would indicate either nonadherence to the prescribed water restriction or the need for more aggressive restriction. If tolvaptan is initiated, the serum sodium concentration should be monitored every 4 to 8 hours for the first 24 to 48 hours.[20]

When the serum sodium has increased by 6 to 8 mEq/L (mmol/L), oral water or IV Dextrose 5% in water (D_5W) should be given to replace urine output to minimize the risk of overcorrecting the serum sodium concentration and ODS. Variable reported rates of sodium overcorrection may be due to differences in baseline serum sodium and definitions of excessive correction. In the SALT trials, only 1.8% of patients exceeded the daily limit for changes in serum sodium; however, most had serum sodium concentrations greater than 130 mEq/L (mmol/L) at the start of treatment and were protected from overcorrection by thirst, so the risk of sodium overcorrection in clinical practice may be greater.[40,41] In a Cochrane review, VRA therapy increased the risk of a rapid increase in serum sodium (greater than 8 mEq/L [mmol/L] in 24 hours) by 67%, with an additional three patients per 100 treated with a VRA experiencing a rapid sodium increase versus placebo.[69] Other studies have shown a ~25% incidence among patients with euvolemic hypotonic hyponatremia. In these studies, patients with profound hyponatremia (baseline serum sodium 121 mEq/L [mmol/L] or less) experienced significantly greater rates of increase; although none developed neurological symptoms or ODS.[42,47] Since 2010, 38 cases of ODS including five deaths have been reported through the FDA Adverse Events Reporting System (FAERS; fis.fda.gov). Once the serum sodium concentration is stable at 125 mEq/L (mmol/L) or higher, the patient should be evaluated every 2 to 4 weeks to assess neurologic status and to obtain serum and urine sodium, potassium, and osmolality values. Volume status (eg, BP, mucous membranes, skin turgor, heart, and lung examination) should also be assessed, particularly in patients who are being treated with NaCl supplements and/or loop diuretics.

NONEMERGENT HYPERVOLEMIC HYPOTONIC HYPONATREMIA

The initial treatment goals for patients with asymptomatic or minimally symptomatic hypervolemic (expanded ECF volume) hypotonic hyponatremia include achieving a negative water balance and minimizing rapid changes in brain cell volume until the serum sodium concentration is 125 mEq/L (mmol/L) or higher. Management involves correction of the underlying cause, when possible, as well as water restriction of 1,000 to 1,500 mL/day.[35] To be effective, the combined daily losses (insensible water, urine, and stool) must exceed fluid intake. Additionally, dietary sodium intake should be restricted to 1,000 to 2,000 mg/day, depending on the degree of ECF volume expansion. On average, only modest changes in serum sodium concentration are seen over the first 5 days of treatment with fluid restriction (2 mEq/L [mmol/L; IQR 0-4] at 24 hours[70,71]; 0.7 ± 2.1 mEq/L [mmol/L] on day 5.[72] This small change may be due to poor adherence to fluid restriction and the frequent patient practice of sucking on ice chips to quench thirst. In moderately severe cases, other options should be considered if serum sodium does not improve in the first 24 to 48 hours.

In patients with HF, the severity of hypervolemic hypotonic hyponatremia is directly related to HF severity and is associated with a poorer short- and long-term prognosis once the serum sodium concentration falls below 137 mEq/L (mmol/L).[73,74] Patients with hypervolemic hypotonic hyponatremia caused by HF should be treated with measures that can potentially improve cardiac contractility and effective circulating volume, thereby limiting non-osmotic AVP release. Therapeutic options include digitalis or afterload reduction with angiotensin-converting enzyme inhibitors (ACEI), angiotensin II receptor blockers (ARB), angiotensin receptor-neprilysin inhibitors (ARNI) SGLT2 inhibitors, or other vasodilators. Of these, only ACEI have proven benefit in partially correcting hyponatremia in patients with HF[75]; however, sodium correction with ACEI does not improve outcomes.[76] No specific ACEI offers any particular advantage for this indication, and the dosage should be titrated in accordance with HF guidelines. Dose-limiting adverse medication reactions of ACEI include hyperkalemia (serum potassium concentration greater than 5.5 mEq/L [mmol/L]) and impaired kidney function. The benefits and risks of continuing ACEI use must be weighed carefully in each case, but a decrease in glomerular filtration rate (GFR) of less than 30% that stabilizes within 2 months of beginning ACEI therapy generally does not require dosage reduction or discontinuation.[73]

Other potentially treatable causes of asymptomatic hypervolemic hyponatremia include nephrotic syndrome and cirrhosis. An ACEI can be used to decrease proteinuria in patients with nephrotic syndrome, leading to partial correction of hypoalbuminemia and to a decrease in non-osmotic AVP release. Management of asymptomatic cases of hyponatremia in patients with cirrhosis includes temporary discontinuation of diuretics and cautious correction of hypokalemia in addition to fluid restriction.[35] Exogenously administered potassium will enter the cells as intracellular sodium is exchanged in the opposite direction. This increase in extracellular sodium must be accounted for to avoid rapid overcorrection of hyponatremia. If hyponatremia persists in patients with cirrhosis, short-term hyper-oncotic albumin solutions (20%-25%) may be administered at dosages of at least 40 g/day.[77,78] Efficacy is likely due to increased urinary-free water clearance following intravascular volume expansion.[35]

VRAs have also been used for the treatment of hypervolemic hypotonic hyponatremia in patients with HF or cirrhosis.[79-84] Conivaptan is not an ideal choice for patients with cirrhosis due to its mixed antagonism of the V_1 and V_2 receptors. V_1 receptor blockade in these patients may worsen hypotension, increase bleeding risk, and compromise kidney function.[80] As previously mentioned, the FDA issued a warning regarding tolvaptan use in patients with impaired liver function due to the potential for further liver injury. However, 25% and 31% of patients in the tolvaptan groups of the SALT-1 and SALT-2 trials, respectively, had underlying liver cirrhosis, and there were no cases of further liver injury.[40,41] Subsequent studies have supported these findings.[81,82] The optimal tolvaptan starting dosage in patients with cirrhosis is unknown. Given the concern for hepatotoxicity, a dose of 3.75 or 7.5 mg may be appropriate; however, usual starting dosages may be recommended based on the SALTWATER study.[35,83,85]

Patients with cirrhosis who receive tolvaptan generally have a more modest increase in serum sodium concentrations compared to patients with euvolemic hyponatremia, and the increase may be more dependent on baseline GFR.[82-85] Patients with advanced cirrhosis may benefit from placement of a transjugular intrahepatic portosystemic shunt, which can increase the effective circulating volume and thus reduce non-osmotic AVP release.[86] This procedure can potentially exacerbate or precipitate hepatic encephalopathy and is not recommended in patients with a history of encephalopathy. Additionally, tolvaptan may be considered in patients with end-stage liver disease awaiting liver transplantation to normalize serum sodium concentrations.[35,87] The benefit of avoiding the need for rapid perioperative sodium correction outweighs the likely negligible effect of tolvaptan-related liver damage in these patients. It is also reasonable to continue treatment until liver transplantation even if the duration is longer than 30 days.

In general, VRA treatment in hyponatremic patients with HF is reserved for refractory patients whose hyponatremia does not adequately respond to other medical management strategies. Tolvaptan dosing for HF-associated hypervolemic hyponatremia is the same as for euvolemic hypotonic hyponatremia. In the short-term management of patients with HF with hypervolemic hyponatremia, tolvaptan use decreases body weight, increases urine output, decreases left ventricular filling pressures, and decreases urine osmolality; however, evidence for clinical benefits such as improved dyspnea is lacking.[88-94] Long-term beneficial effects, reduction in hospitalization or death, or slowed HF progression have not been observed in several pivotal trials. A post-hoc analysis of the EVEREST trial, however, showed patients with severe hyponatremia (less than 130 mEq/L [mmol/L]), who presumably had greater activation of the arginine-vasopressin axis, had reduced cardiovascular morbidity and mortality after discharge.[94] Prolonged tolvaptan use leads to an increased endogenous AVP concentration, and this overstimulation of V_{1a} receptors can lead to increased afterload and HF progression.[95] However, no worsening of left ventricular dilatation was observed after 52 weeks of tolvaptan therapy (30 mg/day).[96] In contrast to European guidelines, an American expert panel on hyponatremia recommended a VRA in non-severe hyponatremia when fluid restriction is unsuccessful.[20] The 2013 American College of Cardiology Foundation/American Heart Association (ACCF/AHA) guidelines recommend short-term use of a VRA in hospitalized patients who have volume overload and persistent severe hyponatremia and who are at risk for or having cognitive symptoms despite fluid restriction and optimization of guideline-directed medical therapy.[97] It is still unknown whether VRAs decrease length of hospitalization, rehospitalization rates, or morbidity or increase quality of life when compared to other treatments.

Various biological markers, such as copeptin, the c-terminal segment of the precursor of provasopressin; apelin; and midregional proatrial natriuretic peptide (MR-proANP), may have diagnostic utility for hyponatremia in HF and improve the overall management.[98] The association between copeptin concentrations and tolvaptan response was investigated in patients with HF and may help determine the most appropriate patients for VRA use.[99] Given the potential vascular and cardiac effects of V_{1a} receptor stimulation and V_{1a} receptor dose-dependent activity (as opposed to maximal V_2 signaling at low AVP activity levels), an oral V_{1a} or nonselective VRA likely would provide greater benefits in patients with HF.[100]

Evaluation of Therapeutic Outcomes

Patients being treated for hypervolemic hyponatremia should initially be evaluated on a daily basis for lung congestion, ascites, peripheral edema, and signs or symptoms of hyponatremia. If water restriction is started, the serum sodium concentration should be measured daily until it stabilizes at 125 mEq/L (mmol/L) or higher. If VRA therapy is initiated, serum sodium concentrations should be monitored every 4 hours to minimize the risk of overcorrection and ODS. Patients should be assessed 1 week following discharge, and then every 2 to 4 weeks to assess adherence to water restriction and other therapies, volume status, and symptoms.

HYPERNATREMIA

Epidemiology and Etiology

10 Hypernatremia, defined as a serum sodium concentration greater than 145 mEq/L (mmol/L), is always associated with hypertonicity and intracellular dehydration, resulting from a water deficit relative to ECF sodium content. This hypertonic state is a potent stimulus for AVP secretion and thirst. Therefore, hypernatremia is most commonly observed in patients with an impaired thirst response or in those who cannot access water. Young infants and children, mechanically ventilated or comatose patients, older adults, and patients with an impaired sensorium or functional status are at highest risk for this disorder.[101] Hypernatremia generally occurs in sicker patients and has a higher mortality.[102] The incidence of hypernatremia in general medical–surgical hospitalized patients and patients in ICUs has been estimated to be at least 1% and as high as 26% to 59%, respectively.[103-107] A marked increase in the incidence of hypernatremia compared to hyponatremia has occurred in ICUs in the past two decades. In critically ill patients, the majority of cases of hypernatremia are iatrogenic, the result of too little free water and too much hypertonic solution along with increased renal water loss.[108] Focusing only on overall fluid balance and not considering the sodium intake from all sources, including excessive isotonic fluids, and evaluating urine sodium excretion leads to hypernatremia, and more free water is needed in most cases.[106,109]

Clinical outcomes in patients with hypernatremia, as in hyponatremia, depend on the severity of the increase and the rapidity with which it develops. In children, mortality from acute hypernatremia developing in less than 72 hours ranges from 10% to 70%; while chronic hypernatremia which develops over 3 or more days

TABLE 68-7 Characteristics of Hypernatremic States

Characteristics	Hypovolemic Hypernatremia	Euvolemic (Isovolemic) Hypernatremia	Hypervolemic Hypernatremia
Water and sodium	Water loss >> sodium loss	Water loss only	Sodium gain > water gain
Causes	Renal: osmotic diuresis, diuretic use, postoperative diuresis, high-output acute tubular necrosis	Congenital or acquired DI Nephrogenic DI Primary polydipsia	Sodium overload (eg, 3% NaCl, sodium bicarbonate, NaCl tablets, concentrated tube feedings, hypertonic dialysate, sodium-containing medications)
Effect on TBW	↓↓	↓	↑
Effect on TBNa	↓	↔	↑↑
Additional laboratory findings	Renal: UOsm high, UNa high Non-renal: UOsm high, UNa low	Renal: UOsm low, UNa variable Non-renal: UOsm high, UNa variable	UOsm high, UNa high
Clinical presentation	Orthostasis, hypotension, tachycardia, dry mucous membranes	Depends on severity of hypernatremia; seizures, lethargy	Peripheral and pulmonary edema, variable BP
Treatment	0.9% NaCl until vital signs stable, then free water replacement	Free water replacement, AVP, or AVP analogue	Free water replacement with loop diuretic, may require hemodialysis to remove volume

AVP, arginine vasopressin; DI, diabetes insipidus; NaCl, sodium chloride; TBNa, total body sodium; TBW, total body weight; UNa, urine sodium concentration; UOsm, urine osmolality.

has a mortality rate of only 10%.[110] In adults, an acute increase in serum sodium concentration to greater than 160 mEq/L (mmol/L) is associated with a 75% mortality rate, and hypernatremia that develops at a slower rate also has a high mortality rate of approximately 60%.[111] Hypernatremia is often associated with a serious underlying illness, which likely contributes to the higher mortality rate.

Pathophysiology

Hypernatremia most often results from water loss by either renal or extrarenal mechanisms. Hypernatremia also results from hypertonic or isotonic fluid administration or excess sodium ingestion. Patients can develop hypovolemic, hypervolemic, or euvolemic (isovolemic) hypernatremia depending on the relative magnitude of sodium and water loss or gain caused by the underlying condition (Table 68-7).

Water loss commonly occurs as a result of insensible losses (evaporative water loss through the skin and lungs) in patients deprived of water. Hospitalized patients who are febrile or being mechanically ventilated are often treated with isotonic IV fluids which contain insufficient free water to replace insensible losses. Hypernatremia can develop in patients with hypotonic GI losses (eg, diarrhea, vomiting, gastric suctioning) or in patients who have been exposed to high temperatures who suffer large water losses from both sweat and insensible losses.

A water diuresis can be caused by DI, which can be classified as either central DI (decreased AVP secretion) or nephrogenic DI (decreased kidney response to AVP). Patients with untreated DI excrete large volumes (3-20 L/day) of dilute urine, resulting in hypernatremia. Various causes of DI are listed in Table 68-8. Lithium, which impairs AVP-mediated water transport, is the most common cause of acquired nephrogenic DI.[112]

Hypertonic NaCl administration can result in hypervolemic (expanded ECF volume) hypernatremia. This type of hypernatremia is typically iatrogenic following excess sodium bicarbonate administration, hypertonic NaCl enemas, or intrauterine injection of hypertonic NaCl. Excessive isotonic infusions (0.9% NaCl, lactated Ringers; see Table 68-1) may lead to sodium accumulation, particularly when dilute urine is excreted. A common cause of hypernatremia in the ICU is sodium intake from IV and enteral fluids and medications.[102,105-113] Sodium balance should be monitored carefully in critically ill patients to avoid iatrogenic hypernatremia. Patients

TABLE 68-8 Causes of DI

Central	Nephrogenic	Other

Familial[a]
Unreplaced insensible losses
  Skin
  Lung
Hypodipsia
Neurogenic
  Neurosurgery
  Tuberculosis
  Head trauma
  CNS malignancy/cyst
  Ethanol ingestion (transient)
  Hypoxic encephalopathy
  Lung tumor
  Sarcoidosis
  Sheehan syndrome[b]
	Familial
	  Inherited aquaporin-2 defect
	  Inherited vasopressin V2 receptor defect
	Hypercalcemia (chronic)
	Hypokalemia
	Kidney disease
	Medication-induced
	  Most common
	  Lithium—most common
	  Foscarnet
	  Clozapine
	  Less common
	  Amphotericin B
	  Cidofovir
	  Didanosine
	  Ifosfamide
	  Orlistat
	  Vasopressin receptor antagonists
		Gestational
		Primary polydipsia (dipsogenic DI)

AVP, arginine vasopressin; CNS, central nervous system; DI, diabetes insipidus.

[a]At least 60 mutations in the AVP gene cause neurohypophyseal DI.

[b]Postpartum hypopituitarism caused by severe bleeding during childbirth.

with hyperaldosteronism also may present with an expanded ECF and mild hypernatremia.

Clinical Presentation

Hypernatremia results in water movement from the ICF to the ECF. Patients with central DI often present with sudden onset of polyuria, whereas patients with nephrogenic DI develop polyuria more gradually. Symptoms are like those seen with hyponatremia and are primarily neurological due to decreased brain cell volume. Symptoms of mild-to-moderate hypernatremia (hypertonicity) include weakness, lethargy, restlessness, irritability, twitching, and confusion. More severe or rapidly developing hypernatremia can lead to seizures, coma, and death. As discussed in the hyponatremia section,

CLINICAL PRESENTATION Hypernatremia

General

- Increased serum sodium concentration and osmolality causes acute water movement from the ICF to the ECF.
- Decreased brain cell volume can cause cerebral vein rupture, leading to focal intracerebral and subarachnoid hemorrhages and irreversible CNS damage.

Symptoms

- Mild: lethargy, weakness, confusion, restlessness, irritability
- Moderate: twitching
- Severe: seizures, coma, death; usually requires acute increase in serum sodium to ≥160 mEq/L (mmol/L)
- Serum sodium ≥180 mEq/L (mmol/L) is associated with high mortality
- Other symptoms (depend on etiology of hypernatremia): postural hypotension, tachycardia, dry mucous membranes, diminished skin turgor, reduced or increased urine output
- Signs and symptoms are difficult to detect in patients with underlying neurologic dysfunction.

Laboratory tests

- Serum sodium concentration greater than 145 mEq/L (mmol/L)
- Serum osmolality is always high.
- Urine osmolality may be helpful in diagnosing the cause.

brain cells adapt to ECF tonicity changes by decreasing or increasing the concentration of inorganic (K^+, Cl^-) and organic (glutamate, taurine, and myoinositol) osmolytes.[2,34] ECF hypertonicity results in intracellular organic osmolyte generation within 24 hours of onset leading to an increase in ICF tonicity that then draws water into brain cells, limiting the decrease in cell volume. Thus, patients with chronic hypernatremia are less likely to be symptomatic than patients with acute hypernatremia.

Hypernatremia is often associated with serious underlying illness, and signs and symptoms related to the illness are often present. Patients with a history of severe diarrhea or vomiting can present with ECF volume depletion. Older patients deprived of water after sustaining a stroke or hip fracture often present with mental status changes and other signs of ECF volume depletion. Clinically detectable ECF volume depletion, however, may not be evident until the serum sodium concentration exceeds 160 mEq/L (mmol/L) because these patients primarily have water loss, two-thirds of which is derived from the ICF. The urine will be concentrated, often exceeding 450 mOsm/kg (mmol/kg), because of osmotic and non-osmotic AVP release. The first step in the evaluation and treatment of hypernatremia is assessment of the ECF and urine volume and the serum and urine osmolality (Fig. 68-3).

Patients with a contracted ECF volume and low urine output include those who have sustained insensible water losses that exceed intake, as well as those with extrarenal losses of hypotonic fluids. On physical examination, the patient will have postural hypotension, diminished skin turgor, and delayed capillary refill. Lactic acidosis and low mixed venous oxygen saturation, indicating decreased tissue perfusion, may be present. The daily urine output is typically less than 1 L.

In older adults, hypotension, tachycardia, dry oral mucosa, decreased skin turgor, and recent changes in consciousness are all more common in patients with hypernatremia. The presence of signs of dehydration are variable, with orthostatic hypotension and decreased subclavicular and forearm skin turgor present in at least 60% of patients.[114]

Osmotic Diuresis

In the presence of an ongoing osmotic diuresis, patients will have a urine volume greater than 3 L/day. Excessive urinary excretion of glucose, sodium, urea, or an exogenously administered solute (eg, mannitol) can be identified either by history or by direct measurement of serum and urinary concentrations of the suspected solute, if possible. Patients with post-obstructive diuresis, such as those with bladder outlet obstruction caused by prostatic hypertrophy, are usually ECF volume expanded because of retained solute because of a reduction in GFR. The osmotic diuresis that follows resolution of the obstruction is appropriate in that it promotes excretion of the excess solute.

Patients with severe hyperglycemia may have a low measured serum sodium concentration (hyponatremia) but a high *corrected* sodium concentration (hypernatremia). Patients with severe hyperglycemia present with signs of hypovolemia, and the diuresis is inappropriate as it further exacerbates the ECF volume contraction associated with hyperglycemia. As previously discussed, the estimated (or corrected) serum sodium concentration can be calculated by adding 1.6 mEq/L (mmol/L) for every 100 mg/dL (5.6 mmol/L) increase in the serum glucose concentration before estimating the water deficit.[5,28]

Diabetes Insipidus

Patients with DI tend to maintain a normal ECF volume if they are conscious, can drink, and have access to water. While hypernatremia can occur with DI, patients typically have serum sodium concentrations of 141-145 mEq/L [mmol/L] and daily urine volumes greater than 3 L.

A water deprivation test has been recommended to aid in the differential diagnosis. This diagnostic test consists of depriving a patient with marked polyuria of water for 8 to 12 hours in a supervised setting to avoid severe hypernatremia and volume depletion. Body weight and urine osmolality and volume are measured before and after administration of desmopressin acetate (4 mcg subcutaneously or intravenously or 10 mcg intranasally). After desmopressin administration, patients with central DI will have a prompt increase in urine osmolality to approximately 600 mOsm/kg (mmol/kg) and decreased urine volume. In patients with nephrogenic DI, the urine osmolality will not increase above 300 mOsm/kg (mmol/kg).[115]

The value of a water deprivation test in patients with polyuria and hypernatremia has been questioned. Because hypernatremia provides a maximal stimulus for AVP secretion, discriminating between nephrogenic and central DI can be based on the serum AVP concentration and urinary response to desmopressin without the need for a water deprivation test. The water deprivation test is likely to be of diagnostic value only in patients with polyuria and a normal serum sodium concentration.[116]

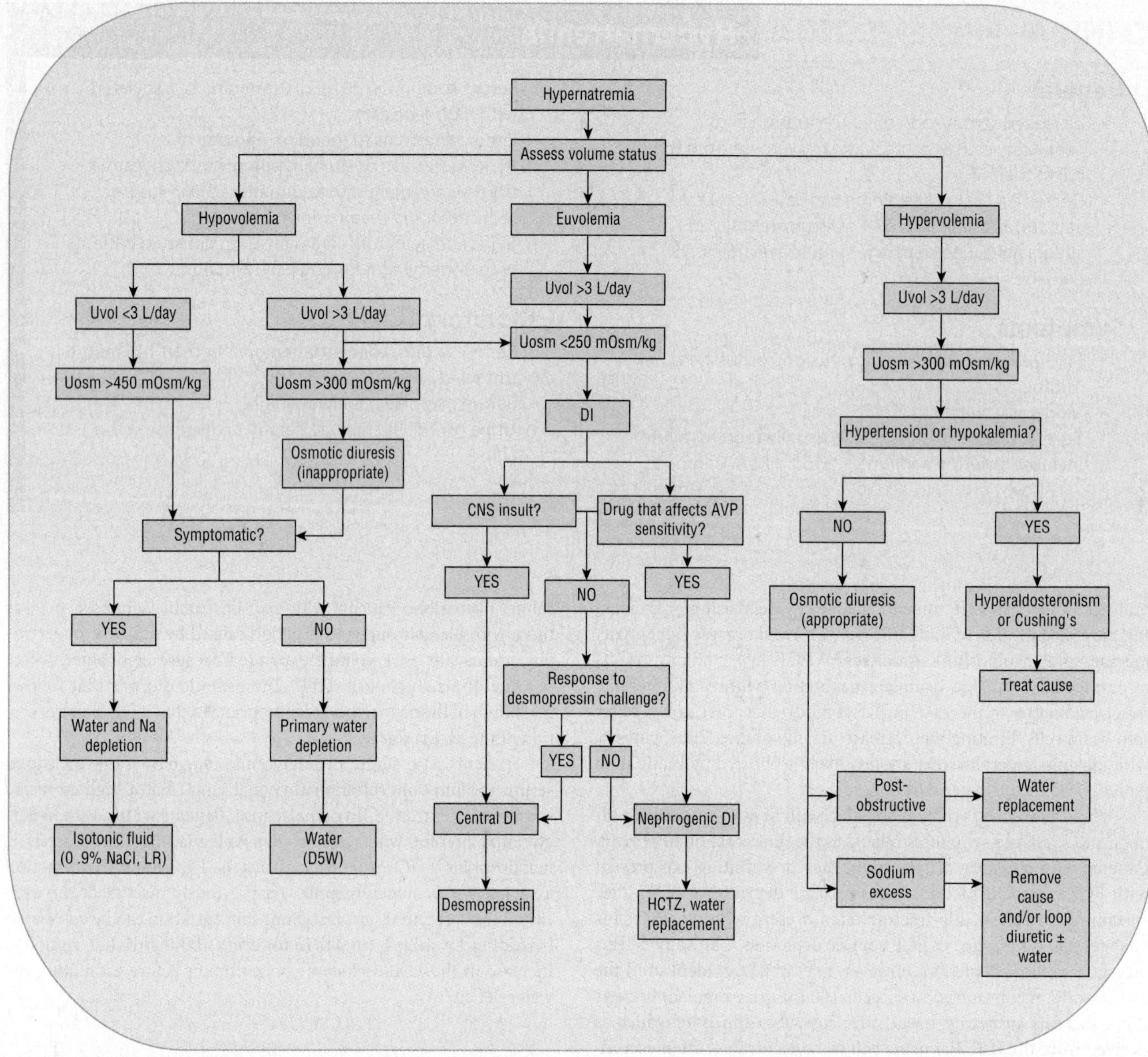

FIGURE 68-3 Algorithm for the assessment and treatment of hypernatremia. (AVP, arginine vasopressin; CNS, central nervous system; D_5W, Dextrose 5% in water; DI, diabetes insipidus; ECF, extracellular fluid; HCTZ, hydrochlorothiazide; LR, lactated Ringers; Na, sodium; NaCl, sodium chloride; Uosm, urine osmolality [values in mOsm/kg are numerically equivalent to mmol/kg]; Uvol, daily urine volume.)

Sodium Overload

Patients who have ingested a large amount of sodium (more than four tablespoons table salt [1,400 mEq or mmol sodium]) or who have received more than 5 L of hypertonic fluids are volume expanded; although, this volume may not always be clinically evident as edema. Volume expansion results in an osmotic diuresis, polyuria, and a urine osmolality greater than 300 mOsm/kg (mmol/kg). In patients with normal perfusion and kidney function, the excess sodium will be excreted in the urine; with organ dysfunction, sodium excretion is compromised, and volume expansion occurs.

TREATMENT

Desired Outcomes

Treatment goals for patients with hypernatremia include correcting the serum sodium concentration to between 145 and 150 mEq/L (mmol/L) at a rate that restores and maintains brain cell volume as close to normal as possible while normalizing ECF volume, if indicated. Hypernatremia is often undertreated; adequate treatment should result in symptom resolution. Although inadvertent overcorrection is more common with hyponatremia, careful titration of fluids and medications should minimize the adverse effects associated with too rapid correction of hypernatremia, including cerebral edema, seizures, neurologic damage, and death. These complications occur almost exclusively in young children with chronic hypernatremia (at least 48 hours duration) and serum sodium concentrations greater than 150 mEq/L (mmol/L).[2] Water replacement and dietary sodium restriction can be necessary to prevent recurrence of hypernatremia.

Physical examination with attention to volume status and laboratory measurement of serum and urine sodium and osmolality should be completed every 2 to 3 months during chronic therapy. A 24-hour urine collection to measure urine volume and sodium excretion may help guide diuretic therapy and determine adherence to sodium restriction.

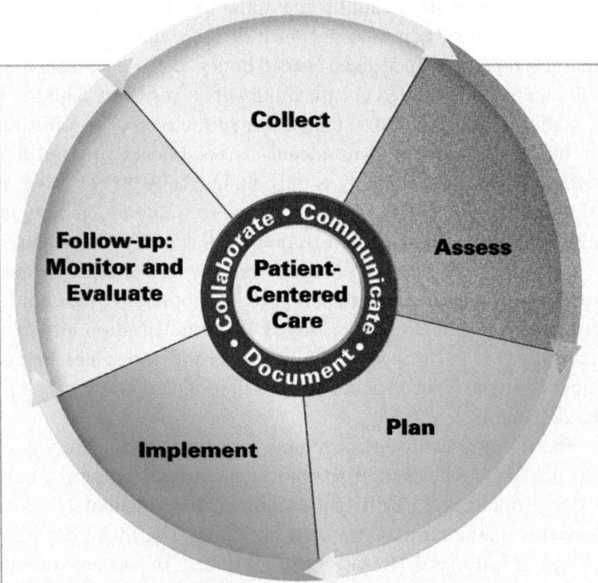

Patient Care Process for the Management of Disorders of Sodium and Water Homeostasis

Collect

- Patient characteristics (eg, age, sex, pregnant)
- Patient history (eg, medical, surgical, diet, recent gastrointestinal [GI] losses; see Tables 68-2 and 68-7)
- Current medications (eg, diuretics, intravenous [IV] fluids, sodium-containing therapies; see Tables 68-3 and 68-8)
- Objective data
  - Body weight (current and historical)
  - Recent intake/output
  - ECF volume status (eg, blood pressure [BP], mucous membranes, skin turgor, cardiopulmonary examination, level of consciousness; see Figs. 68-1 and 68-3)
  - Labs (eg, serum osmolality, electrolytes, glucose, protein, lipids; urine osmolality, sodium, and potassium; thyroid function tests)

Assess

- Chronicity and severity of the disorder
- Potential causative underlying disorders (eg, diarrhea, central nervous system [CNS] disorders, pulmonary disease, cirrhosis, nephrotic syndrome, polydipsia, diabetes insipidus; see Tables 68-2 and 68-7)
- Dysregulated sodium- or fluid-related complications (eg, BP variations, CNS changes, edema; see Clinical Presentation boxes and Tables 68-2 and 68-7)
- Current medications that may affect or worsen the disorder (see Tables 68-2, 68-3, 68-7, and 68-8)
- Goals for sodium and/or volume status and achievement of the goals

Plan*

- Treat the underlying cause of the disorder, if possible
- Develop therapy regimen, including specific medication(s), dose, route, frequency, and duration (see Tables 68-4 to 68-6 and 68-9 to 68-12; Figs. 68-4 to 68-6)
- Balance risks of underlying disorder versus risk of too rapid or overcorrection (see Table 68-4)
- Specify continuation and discontinuation of existing therapies
- Tailor dietary modifications (eg, water and solute intake) and weight management
- Establish monitoring parameters, including efficacy (serum sodium, volume status, urine output), safety (rate of serum sodium correction, medication-specific adverse reactions), and time frame
- Provide patient education (purpose of treatment, dietary and lifestyle modification, medications, self-monitoring of weight and volume status)
- Refer to other providers, when appropriate (eg, physician, dietitian)

Implement*

- Provide patient education regarding all elements of treatment plan
- Schedule follow-up

Follow-up: Monitor and Evaluate

- Attainment of sodium and/or volume status goals
- Presence of adverse medication reactions
- Need for long-term management if disorder cannot be corrected
- Patient adherence to treatment plan using multiple sources of information

**Collaborate with patient, caregivers, and other healthcare professionals.*

Hypovolemic Hypernatremia

Patients with symptomatic hypovolemic hypernatremia should be treated similarly to those with hypovolemic hyponatremia with 0.9% NaCl or another isotonic fluid until hemodynamic stability is restored (Fig. 68-3). An initial infusion rate of 200 to 300 mL/hr or higher will likely be appropriate for most adults; children generally receive 10 to 20 mL/kg/hr. Once intravascular volume is restored, 0.45% NaCl, D_5W, or another hypotonic fluid, may be infused to correct the water deficit. In patients with hypernatremia from water loss, the ECF volume deficit can be estimated as follows:

$$\text{ECF(water)deficit} = \text{TBW}_{\text{current}} \times [1 - (140/\text{Na}_s)]$$

where Na_s is the initial serum sodium concentration (in mEq/L [mmol/L]), and 140 is the normal or goal serum sodium concentration in mEq/L (mmol/L). Although this formula provides an estimate of the water deficit caused by pure free water loss, it underestimates the deficit in patients with hypotonic fluid loss.[2]

The appropriate rate for correcting the water deficit depends on the rapidity with which the hypernatremia developed. Hypernatremia developing in less than 48 hours can be initially corrected at a rate of approximately 1 mEq/L (mmol/L) per hour, whereas a rate of 0.5 mEq/L (mmol/L) per hour or less should be used when hypernatremia has developed more slowly.[2,112] The sodium should be lowered no more than 10 to 12 mEq/L (mmol/L) per day.[2] Renal replacement therapy may be needed for patients with kidney failure; NaCl will be added to the replacement fluid/dialysate to achieve the same sodium content as the goal serum sodium concentration to avoid too rapid overcorrection and cerebral edema.[102]

The serum sodium concentration and volume status should be monitored every 2 to 3 hours during the first 24 hours of treatment in patients with symptomatic hypernatremia to permit appropriate adjustment of the rate of the hypotonic fluid administration. Once symptoms resolve and the serum sodium concentration is less than 148 mEq/L (mmol/L), measuring serum sodium concentrations every 6 to 12 hours and assessing fluid status every 8 to 24 hours is generally adequate.

Recurrent iatrogenic hypernatremia can be prevented by avoiding infusing excessive hypertonic solution, providing adequate *maintenance* fluids, and replacing ongoing abnormal losses. Traditional maintenance fluid for adults and children weighing 40 kg or more is Dextrose 5%/0.45% NaCl with 20 mEq (mmol) KCl/L. Children weighing less than 40 kg typically receive Dextrose 5%/0.2% NaCl with 20 mEq (mmol) KCl/L, except infants younger than 3 months who may receive Dextrose 10%/0.2% NaCl with 20 mEq (mmol) KCl/L. These fluids were chosen to provide a small amount of glucose for CNS function and to replace usual urinary sodium and potassium losses. Estimating daily fluid requirements and calculation of an appropriate maintenance fluid rate is discussed in Chapter 164.

Concerns related to the development of hyponatremia in hospitalized patients have led to the recommendation that an isotonic fluid be used for *maintenance* fluids to reduce the incidence of hyponatremia.[117,118] However, excess administration of 0.9% NaCl can result in ICF dehydration and chloride overload leading to metabolic acidosis. A *balanced* electrolyte solution (eg, lactated Ringer's, Plasma-Lyte®) may be preferred for this reason.[118] Excess sodium administration also carries the risk of hypernatremia and volume overload, especially in vulnerable patients. While isotonic fluids may be appropriate for some hospitalized patients, it is important to remember that *maintenance* fluids are appropriate when used as intended (ie, in patients who are euvolemic with no excess ongoing fluid losses and normal kidney function). Careful attention to the sodium content of IV fluids administered to all hospitalized patients is warranted.

Treatment of hyperglycemia-induced osmotic diuresis consists of correcting the hyperglycemia with insulin, as well as administering 0.9% NaCl until signs of hypovolemia resolve. Once hemodynamic stability is restored, the free water deficit can be corrected as described above.

Hypernatremia in patients undergoing a post-obstructive diuresis should be treated with a hypotonic fluid (eg, 0.45% NaCl [IV], Pedialyte® [oral]) administered at a rate of approximately one-half to two-thirds of the urine output over a similar time point. Oral fluid replacement is preferred, if possible. The common practice of administering IV or oral fluids to replace urine output on a 1:1 volume basis tends to perpetuate the diuresis and generally should be avoided.[119]

Euvolemic (Isovolemic) Hypernatremia

Central Diabetes Insipidus

Patients with central DI should generally receive AVP replacement therapy with desmopressin, an AVP analog (Fig. 68-3). The intranasal formulation, 1-desamino-8-D-arginine vasopressin (DDAVP), is preferred; however, oral tablets are available and may be useful in some patients. Each insufflation of intranasal DDAVP (100 mcg/mL) delivers 10 mcg of desmopressin acetate. A rhinal tube delivery system is preferred in patients requiring doses that are lower than 10 mcg or not in 10-mcg increments. In infants with congenital DI, preparation of a DDAVP dilution may be required to provide the small dosages needed. In adults, the initial intranasal DDAVP dosage is 5 to 10 mcg administered once or twice daily, titrated to a maximum dose of 40 mcg given every 8 hours. The oral starting dosage is 0.05 mg BID titrated to a maximum of 0.4 mg every 8 hours.[115]

Patients may prefer oral tablets due to the ease of administration, but not all patients will adequately respond to the oral formulation as the bioavailability is only about 5%. A 0.1 mg tablet is equivalent to 2.5 to 5 mcg of the intranasal formulation. Sublingual tablets are also available. Re-titration of the dosage is required when transitioning between dosage forms due to the unpredictable absorption. A parenteral formulation of desmopressin (4 mcg/mL) is available for either subcutaneous or IV administration and may be administered in cases when the intranasal and oral routes are not feasible or effective, or in acute settings to initiate therapy in symptomatic patients.

The desmopressin dosage should be adjusted to achieve adequate urinary concentration to control nighttime symptoms during sleep (nocturia), a daily urine volume of approximately 1.5 to 2 L, and a safe serum sodium concentration. The mean duration of action of intranasal DDAVP is 7 to 9 hours. The serum sodium concentration should be measured at 24 hours and every 3 to 4 days during the initial dosage titration period, and then every 2 to 4 months. Desmopressin administration results in non-suppressible AVP activity and presents a risk of water intoxication with excess water intake and retention. Patients must be knowledgeable of the signs and symptoms of both hyponatremia and hypervolemia. Patients who experience water intoxication may minimize the risk of a second episode by delaying one desmopressin dose each week until polyuria and thirst develop, thus demonstrating the continued need for desmopressin therapy.[120]

When there is an inadequate response to desmopressin, additional therapies may be needed. Carbamazepine increases renal sensitivity to AVP, chlorpropamide potentiates the action of circulating AVP and decreases urine output by 50%, and indapamide increases urinary osmolality and decreases serum osmolality. These medications are associated with significant adverse medication reactions and close monitoring is required if added to the patient's therapy.[115]

Nephrogenic Diabetes Insipidus

In patients with nephrogenic DI, concomitant electrolyte disturbances, if present, should be corrected, and any medications that potentially contribute to the pathogenesis should be discontinued, if possible. The free water deficit must be replaced initially. Mild cases may be managed with sufficient water intake only. Because the ongoing urinary losses are essentially free water, patients should receive hypotonic fluids to avoid excess sodium intake which could worsen hypernatremia (Fig. 68-3). Water or milk can be given enterally or D_5W can be given intravenously at a rate that slightly exceeds the urine output with a goal to normalize the serum sodium concentration at a rate no faster than 0.5 mEq/L per hour (mmol/L per hour).[121] A key goal in treating nephrogenic DI is to induce a mild ECF deficit (1-1.5 L) with a thiazide diuretic and dietary sodium restriction (85 mEq [mmol] Na^+ or 2,000 mg NaCl per day), which can decrease urine volume by as much as 50% (Table 68-9). This ECF deficit will increase proximal tubule water reabsorption, decrease the filtrate volume delivered to the distal nephron, and decrease urine volume. In a patient with a maximally dilute urine osmolality (100 mOsm/kg [mmol/kg]), each gram of salt that is avoided will reduce the obligatory urine output by 360 mL because 1 g of table salt provides an osmolar load of approximately 36 mOsm.[121] Indomethacin, 50 mg given orally three times daily, potentiates AVP activity and can be used as adjunctive therapy in patients able to tolerate the gastrointestinal (GI) adverse medication reactions. The relative benefits of other medications for nephrogenic DI, including thiazide diuretics and nonsteroidal anti-inflammatory drugs (NSAIDs), are not well studied; therefore, the choice of agent is primarily based on clinician

TABLE 68-9 Medications Used in Central and Nephrogenic DI

Medication	Indication	Dose
Desmopressin acetate	Central and nephrogenic	IN: 5-20 mcg q12-24hr IV/SQ: Initial, 0.25-1 mcg q12-24hr PO: Initial: 0.05-0.2 mg qhs; usual: 0.1-0.8 mg in 2-3 doses, max 1.2 mg daily SL: 60 mcg TID; usual, 120-720 mcg daily in 2-3 doses
Chlorpropamide	Central	125-250 mg orally daily
Carbamazepine	Central	100-300 mg orally twice daily
Hydrochlorothiazide	Central and nephrogenic	25 mg orally q12-24hr
Amiloride	Nephrogenic	5-10 mg orally daily Pediatrics: 0.2 mg/kg/day in 3 doses or 20 mg/1.73 m²/day
Indomethacin	Central and nephrogenic	50 mg orally q8-12hr

DI, diabetes insipidus; IN, intranasal; IV, intravenous; PO, oral; SL, sublingual; SQ, subcutaneous.

preference. It is unclear if there is a significant difference in the risk of a clinically important GFR decrease when these medications are used to produce a mild ECF volume deficit. Lithium-induced nephrogenic DI can usually be treated with increased water intake because thirst is intact. If water intake is inadequate, amiloride 2.5 mg to 10 mg daily can be used as amiloride decreases lithium entry into the principal cells by inhibiting the amiloride-sensitive epithelial sodium channel (ENaC).[115] Several other medications with antidiuretic properties have been used successfully in the management of central and nephrogenic DI (Table 68-9). They may be used as adjunctive therapy or rarely as an alternative to DDAVP.

Hypervolemic Hypernatremia (Sodium and Water Overload)

Treatment of hypervolemic hypernatremia consists of administration of D_5W and a loop diuretic to facilitate excretion of the excess sodium while replacing free water to prevent worsening of hypernatremia (Fig. 68-3). The volume needed to correct the water deficit and hypernatremia at an appropriate rate can be estimated as described previously. Furosemide, 20 to 40 mg given orally or intravenously every 6 hours, should also be administered.

The serum sodium concentration should initially be measured at least every 2 to 4 hours, and diuresis continued until signs of ECF volume overload (eg, pulmonary congestion, edema) resolve. The serum sodium concentration can be measured every 6 to 12 hours once the serum sodium concentration is less than 148 mEq/L (mmol/L) and symptoms have resolved.[2]

EDEMA

11 Edema, defined as a clinically detectable increase in interstitial fluid volume, is usually due to heart, kidney, or liver failure or a combination of these conditions; although, it can develop with a rapid decrease in serum albumin concentration along with excess fluid intake such as seen in the setting of burns or trauma. In an adult, edema formation is indicative of an interstitial volume increase of at least 2.5 to 3 L.

Pathophysiology

Edema develops when excess sodium is retained either as a primary defect in renal sodium excretion or as a response to a decrease in the effective circulating volume (actually the BP resulting from that volume) despite a normal or expanded ECF volume. Under these conditions, the kidneys retain all the water and sodium ingested until the effective circulating volume is restored to near normal. An increase in dietary sodium is accompanied by an increase in water intake caused by the initial increase in serum osmolality and thirst. The resultant ECF volume increase augments kidney perfusion, resulting in a transient GFR increase, which leads to enhanced sodium filtration and excretion. These homeostatic mechanisms are crucial for maintaining sodium balance, as retention of just a few milliequivalents (millimoles) of sodium per day can eventually lead to an expanded ECF volume and edema formation. An increase in the capillary hydrostatic pressure because of ECF volume expansion or an increase in central venous pressure also can lead to edema formation. Edema may also occur when there is an alteration in Starling forces within the capillary. The Starling equation denotes the relationship between factors affecting fluid movement between the capillary and interstitium. Edema may develop rapidly in patients with an acute decompensation in myocardial contractility, which leads to an elevated pulmonary venous pressure that is transmitted back to the pulmonary capillaries, and ultimately results in acute pulmonary edema.

Patients with nephrotic syndrome may initially present with edema, primarily periorbital, labial/scrotal, and lower extremity which may progress to pulmonary edema, ascites, and anasarca. There are two theories posited to explain edema in nephrotic syndrome: the *underfill* and the *overfill* hypotheses.[122,123] The underfill hypothesis states that high-grade proteinuria leads to decreased oncotic pressure due to hypoalbuminemia (most pronounced with a serum albumin concentration less than 2 g/dL [20 g/L]). Decreased oncotic pressure then leads to excess fluid movement from the intravascular space to the interstitial space (*third spacing*) causing hypovolemia, kidney hypoperfusion, activation of the renin–angiotensin–aldosterone system, and secondary renal sodium retention. The overfill hypothesis is simply that protein loss in the urine leads to primary renal sodium retention causing intravascular volume expansion, leading to fluid overflow into the interstitial space (edema). Edema mechanisms can vary between patients and also vary at different times in an individual patient. Distinguishing the predominant mechanism in individual patients with nephrotic syndrome is often challenging but clinically important, as patients who are primarily underfilled will likely have worsening hypovolemia and an elevated serum creatinine requiring volume repletion after initially tolerating diuresis.

Patients with cirrhosis initially develop ascites because of splanchnic vasodilation resulting in an increase in the pressure in the portal circulation (portal hypertension). This combination of portal hypertension and splanchnic vasodilation increases capillary pressure and permeability and facilitates the accumulation of ascites (fluid in the abdominal cavity). Ascites can cause a decrease in effective circulating volume and activation of the sympathetic nervous system and the renin–angiotensin–aldosterone system, leading to secondary hyperaldosteronism. Subsequent renal sodium retention leads to worsened ascites, edema, and hypervolemic hyponatremia.[124]

Clinical Presentation

Edema is usually first detected in the feet or periorbital or pretibial area in ambulatory patients and in the presacral area of bed-bound individuals. Edema is described as "pitting" when a depression created by exerting pressure for several seconds over a bony prominence, such as the tibia, does not rapidly refill. Edema severity is rated on a semi-quantitative scale of 1+ to 4+ depending on the depth of the pit: 1+ = 2 mm; 2+ = 4 mm; 3+ = 6 mm; and 4+ = 8 mm.

The extent of edema should be quantified according to the areas involved. Pretibial edema, for example, should be quantified according to how far it extends up the lower leg (eg, one-third up the lower leg). Pulmonary edema, an increase in lung interstitial and alveolar water, is often evidenced by crackles (rales) upon auscultation. Rales should be quantified according to how far the crackles extend from the dependent portion of the lung(s). For example, edema limited to the ankles and feet would indicate less severe edema than edema that extends halfway up the lower legs, and crackles limited to the base of both lungs in an upright person would indicate less severe pulmonary edema than crackles throughout both lung fields. *Anasarca* is a term used to refer to a massive amount of edema generalized throughout the body.

Treatment

General Approach

Treatment goals for hypervolemic hypernatremia are to minimize edema and to improve organ function, as well as to relieve symptoms (eg, dyspnea, abdominal distention, extremity pain). The presence of edema does not always dictate the need for diuretic therapy; however, severe pulmonary edema is life-threatening and requires immediate pharmacologic treatment. Other forms of edema may be treated less acutely, with a comprehensive approach that includes not only diuretics but also sodium and water restriction and optimal treatment of the underlying disease. Sodium intake should generally be restricted to 1,000 to 2,000 mg/day. A slow judicious approach in non-life-threatening situations will help minimize complications of diuretic therapy, including excessive diuresis, impaired perfusion, azotemia, impaired cardiac output due to decreased left ventricular end-diastolic filling pressure, and electrolyte abnormalities. Fluid should be removed cautiously in patients with cirrhosis and ascites but no peripheral edema. A goal of 500 mL/day can be safely mobilized in patients with isolated ascites; higher volumes may result in decreased ECF volume and lead to elevated BUN and possibly hepatorenal syndrome.[124]

Diuretic Therapy

Diuretics are the primary pharmacologic therapy for edema when severe or when treatment of the underlying disease and sodium and water restriction are insufficient. Diuretics are categorized according to the site in the nephron where sodium reabsorption is inhibited. Loop diuretics (furosemide, bumetanide, torsemide, ethacrynic acid) inhibit the sodium–potassium–chloride (Na^+–K^+–$2Cl^-$) carrier in the loop of Henle, while thiazide and thiazide-like diuretics (hydrochlorothiazide, chlorothiazide, chlorthalidone, indapamide, metolazone) inhibit the Na^+–Cl^- carrier in the distal tubule. Potassium-sparing diuretics inhibit the sodium channel in the cortical collecting duct either directly (triamterene, amiloride) or by interfering with aldosterone activity (spironolactone, eplerenone). Acetazolamide, a carbonic anhydrase inhibitor, acts in the proximal convoluted tubule and has been used in patients with diuretic resistance. Diuretic efficacy in patients with edema depends on the amount of filtered sodium normally reabsorbed at its site of action, the amount of sodium reabsorbed distal to its site of action, adequate medication delivery to the site of action, and the amount of sodium reaching the site of action.[29]

All diuretics act by inhibiting sodium reabsorption in the renal tubules, increasing the fractional excretion of sodium (FeNa). Loop diuretics are the most potent diuretics, as evidenced by the fact that they increase peak FeNa from normal (1% [0.01] or less) to 20% to 25% (0.20-0.25). Thiazide- and potassium-sparing diuretics are less potent and increase peak FeNa only to 3% to 5% (0.03-0.05) and 1% to 2% (0.01-0.02), respectively.[29] Although a large portion of the filtered sodium is reabsorbed in the proximal nephron, the efficacy of proximal-acting diuretics (acetazolamide) is limited by excess fluid and sodium reabsorption in the loop of Henle. Furthermore, sodium reabsorption by the distal tubule can compensate for reduced reabsorption in the loop of Henle when sodium intake is high.

The pharmacogenomics of diuretic therapy, particularly the thiazides, have been studied extensively in the setting of hypertension therapy.[125] Multiple genetic polymorphisms possibly affecting diuretic activity at the site of action have been identified, but the clinical significance of these genetic variations related to patient outcomes is still being elucidated. It is likely that a complex predictive model utilizing pharmacodynamic, pharmacokinetic, and pharmacogenomic parameters will be necessary to predict significantly different diuretic responses and outcomes due to the potential for compensatory mechanisms in other parts of the nephron. While genetic testing for gene variants is now available, it is not yet a practical option to guide diuretic treatment.

The effectiveness of thiazide and loop diuretics is dependent on the medication concentration in the tubular lumen. These diuretics are delivered to the tubular lumen via active transport by the proximal tubular cells. Osmotic diuretics are freely filtered into the tubular lumen in the proximal tubule, whereas spironolactone reaches mineralocorticoid receptors in the cortical collecting duct via diffusion from the systemic circulation.[29] A threshold concentration of loop or thiazide diuretic must be delivered to the respective site of action to achieve a natriuresis. Once the threshold concentration is achieved, a further diuretic dose increase will not elicit an increased diuretic response. Thus, a *ceiling dose* for these diuretics is recognized. In healthy subjects, administration of IV furosemide 40 mg results in excretion of 200 to 250 mEq (mmol) of sodium in 3 to 4 L of urine over a 3- to 4-hour period.[29]

Loop diuretics, except torsemide, have a rapid onset but short half-life requiring administration every 2 to 3 hours while thiazide diuretics have a longer half-life allowing for less frequent (once daily) dosing (Table 68-10). Table 68-11 lists the maximal effective doses and dosing intervals for loop diuretics in patients with cirrhosis, HF, nephrotic syndrome, and kidney insufficiency.

Patients with kidney insufficiency often require larger diuretic doses to achieve adequate medication concentrations at the site of action. The natriuretic response is decreased in patients with kidney

TABLE 68-10 Characteristics of Thiazide Diuretics

Diuretic	Duration of Action	Initial Daily Dosage	Sequential Nephron Blockade	Maximum Total Daily Dose
Chlorothiazide	6-12 hr	250-500 mg once or twice	500-1,000 mg once plus loop diuretic	1,000 mg
Chlorthalidone	24-72 hr	12.5-25 mg once		100 mg
Hydrochlorothiazide	6-12 hr	25 mg once or twice	25-100 mg once or twice plus loop diuretic	200 mg
Indapamide	36 hr	2.5 mg once		5 mg
Metolazone	12-24 hr	2.5 mg once	2.5-10 mg plus loop diuretic	20 mg

TABLE 68-11 Characteristics of Loop Diuretics

Diuretic	Dosing Interval	Recommended Doses: Normal	Cirrhosis	HF	Nephrotic Syndrome	GFR 10-50 mL/min (0.17-0.83 mL/s)	GFR <10 mL/min (0.17 mL/s)	Maximum Total Daily Dose[a]
Furosemide								
IV	6-8 hr	10-40 mg	40 mg	40-80 mg	120 mg	80 mg	200 mg	200 mg or 160 mg/hr
Oral	6-8 hr	20-80 mg	80 mg	80-160 mg	240 mg	160 mg	320-400 mg	600 mg
Bumetanide								
IV/oral	6-8 hr	1 mg	1 mg	2-3 mg	3 mg	2-3 mg	8-10 mg	10 mg
Torsemide								
IV/oral	24 hr	15-20 mg	10-20 mg	20-50 mg	50 mg	20-50 mg	50-100 mg	200 mg
Ethacrynic acid[b]								
IV	8-12 hr[c]	0.5-1 mg/kg (max 100 mg)						
Oral	12-24 hr	25-100 mg	50-100 mg	50-100 mg				400 mg

HF, heart failure; GFR, glomerular filtration rate.

[a]Although these doses are generally accepted maximal doses, higher doses may be required due to insufficient quantities in the renal tubular fluid.

[b]Rarely used because of higher rates of ototoxicity and relative insolubility; may be used in a patient with a sulfa allergy.

[c]Repeat doses not routinely recommended.

TABLE 68-12 Continuous Infusion Rates for Loop Diuretics

Medication	Initial Infusion Rate Based on Creatinine Clearance (CrCl)			Maximum Infusion Rate	
	CrCl <25 mL/min (0.42 mL/s)	CrCl 25-75 mL/min (0.42-1.25 mL/s)	CrCL >75 mL/min (1.25 mL/s)	Undiluted bolus	Continuous infusion
Bumetanide	1-2 mg/hr	0.5-1 mg/hr	0.5 mg/hr	5 mg/min	0.17 mg/min
Furosemide	20-40 mg/hr	10-20 mg/hr	10 mg/hr	40 mg/min	4 mg/min
Torsemide	10-20 mg/hr	5-10 mg/hr	5 mg/hr	100 mg/min	0.05 mg/min[a]

[a]Studies used a 100-mg total daily dose as a 25-mg injection over 2 minutes (25% of total daily dose) followed by an infusion of 3.1 mg/hr over 24 hours (75% of total daily dose).

insufficiency because the filtered sodium load falls proportionately as GFR declines. This effect can be partially overcome by administering diuretics more frequently or by using a continuous infusion, a method commonly employed in critically ill patients. Continuous delivery will limit the effect of the post-diuresis sodium retention in the distal nephron. Table 68-12 lists initial continuous infusion rates based on creatinine clearance and maximum recommended infusion rates.

Loop diuretic resistance can be caused by pronounced sodium reabsorption in the distal nephron when sodium absorption in the loop of Henle is blocked. If sodium intake is not restricted, this distal sodium reabsorption can compensate entirely for loop diuretic-induced sodium loss. Patients with diuretic-resistant edema can be treated with a loop diuretic and metolazone. Metolazone should be given first and allowed sufficient time to start blocking distal sodium reabsorption to maximize loop diuretic efficacy.

Impaired diuretic delivery to the site of action is another mechanism of diuretic resistance. Patients with HF and a normal GFR may have impaired oral furosemide absorption. An adequate diuresis is most readily sustained by increasing the frequency of diuretic administration, but a higher dose may also be effective (Fig. 68-4). Absorption of orally administered loop diuretics can be compromised by GI edema and delayed gastric emptying, conditions often seen in critically ill patients.

Inadequate medication concentration at the site of action also can be caused by decreased perfusion as might be seen in patients with decompensated HF or those with decreased kidney perfusion. Due to extensive albumin binding (more than 95%), little of these

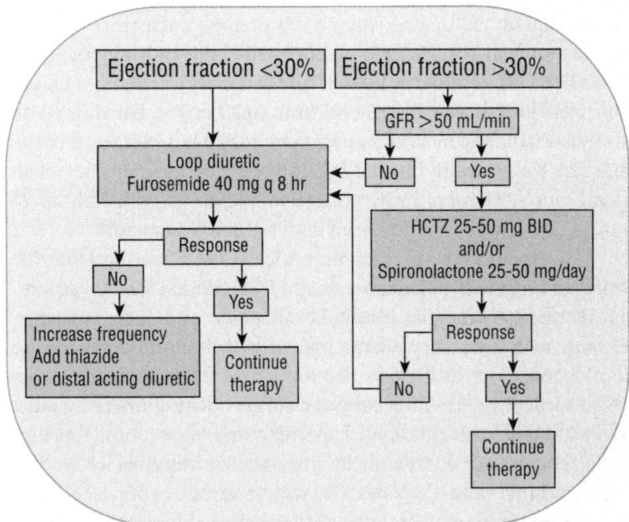

FIGURE 68-4 Algorithm for diuretic use in patients with heart failure. (GFR, glomerular filtration rate [50 mL/min is equivalent to 0.83 mL/s]; HCTZ, hydrochlorothiazide.)

agents reach the tubule lumen by filtration, and they are almost exclusively transported into the proximal tubule lumen by active secretion via the organic acid secretory pathway.[29] When albumin binding is inhibited by concurrent sulfasoxazole administration,

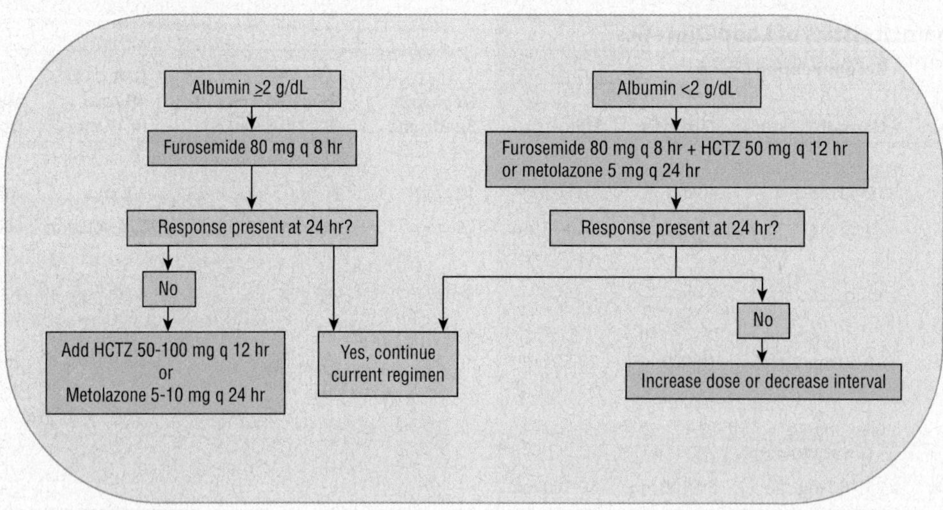

FIGURE 68-5 Algorithm for diuretic therapy in patients with nephrotic syndrome. Albumin concentration of 2 g/dL is equivalent to 20 g/L. (HCTZ, hydrochlorothiazide.)

diuretic resistance persists, suggesting a decrease in intrinsic tubular sensitivity to loop diuretics.[126] This impaired natriuretic response can be overcome by using higher diuretic doses to increase unbound medication delivery to the secretory site in the nephron. Decreased intrinsic diuretic activity with repeated dosing may also play a role in diuretic resistance, the mechanism of which is not well understood. A combination of a loop diuretic with a distally acting diuretic is generally necessary to promote a natriuresis that exceeds distal tubular sodium reabsorption in patients with nephrotic syndrome (Fig. 68-5).[127]

In patients with cirrhosis, secondary hyperaldosteronism from activation of the renin–angiotensin–aldosterone system plays a major role in the pathogenesis of edema. Therefore, these patients should initially be treated with an aldosterone antagonist (eg, spironolactone) in the absence of impaired GFR and hyperkalemia (Fig. 68-6). Thiazides can then be added for patients with a creatinine clearance greater than 50 mL/min (0.83 mL/s). For those with diuretic-resistant edema, a loop diuretic may be used instead of the thiazide. Patients with impaired GFR (creatinine clearance less than 40 mL/min [0.67 mL/s]) will require a loop diuretic, with addition of a thiazide in those who do not achieve adequate diuresis.[128]

Adverse medication reactions associated with loop and thiazide diuretics include hypokalemia, excess ECF volume loss (hypovolemia), hypomagnesemia, metabolic alkalosis, and hyperuricemia. Patients with refractory edema treated with high-dose synergistic combinations are at highest risk for developing hypokalemia. As noted earlier, sodium imbalance is a concern with diuretic therapy: hyponatremia with thiazides, hypernatremia with loops. Calcium imbalance also can occur with diuretic use: hypocalcemia with loops, hypercalcemia with thiazides. Thiazide-induced hypercalcemia is more common in patients with mild subclinical hyperparathyroidism. Loop diuretics cause hypercalciuria and can lead to bone disorders (osteopenia, osteoporosis), kidney stones, or nephrocalcinosis when used chronically. Chronic use of potassium-sparing diuretics can cause a mild metabolic acidosis and hyperkalemia. Patients with moderate-to-severe kidney dysfunction or those receiving NSAIDs, ACEIs, or ARBs are at highest risk for hyperkalemia. In addition, spironolactone can cause reversible gynecomastia in about 10% of men receiving it, and in about 50% of men receiving 150 mg/day or more. This adverse medication reaction has not been associated with eplerenone.[129]

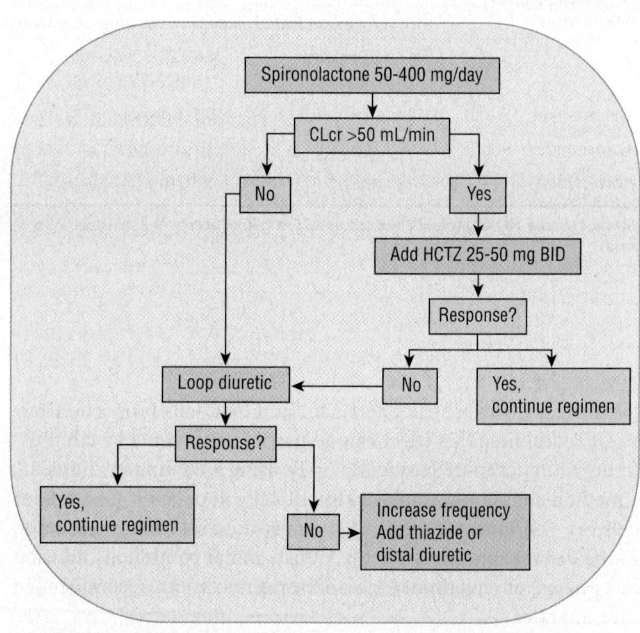

FIGURE 68-6 Algorithm for diuretic use in patients with cirrhosis. (CLcr, creatinine clearance [50 mL/min is equivalent to 0.83 mL/s]; HCTZ, hydrochlorothiazide.)

Evaluation of Therapeutic Outcomes

In patients with significant edema, volume status must be monitored carefully to ensure adequate tissue perfusion. Patients should be monitored by careful history and intermittent physical examination to detect signs and symptoms of edema as well as adverse effects. Physical examination should include measurement of BP and pulse in either supine or seated positions and after standing for 2 to 3 minutes to assess for orthostasis. ECF volume can be estimated based on the height of the jugular venous pressure, extent of edema, heart and lung auscultation, and skin turgor. Follow-up monitoring 10 to 14 days after therapy initiation should include determinations of serum sodium, potassium, chloride, bicarbonate, magnesium, calcium,

BUN, serum creatinine, and uric acid. A new steady-state balance will have developed over that time period and further fluctuations in ECF volume and electrolyte balance generally do not occur in the absence of a change in clinical status, diuretic dosage, or dietary intake. Repeated blood tests generally are not necessary at every visit unless there is a change in the patient's clinical status.

ABBREVIATIONS

ACEI	angiotensin-converting enzyme inhibitor
AQP2	aquaporin 2
ARB	angiotensin receptor blocker
AVP	arginine vasopressin, also known as vasopressin and antidiuretic hormone (ADH)
ATPase	adenosine triphosphatase
BP	blood pressure
BUN	blood urea nitrogen
CNS	central nervous system
D_5W	dextrose 5% in water
DDAVP	1-desamino-8-D-arginine vasopressin
DI	diabetes insipidus
ECF	extracellular fluid
FeNa	fractional excretion of sodium
GFR	glomerular filtration rate
GI	gastrointestinal
HF	heart failure
ICF	intracellular fluid
ICU	intensive care unit
IV	intravenous
NSAID	nonsteroidal anti-inflammatory drug
ODS	osmotic demyelination syndrome
SIADH	syndrome of inappropriate antidiuretic hormone secretion
SGLT2	sodium-glucose co-transporter-2
TBW	total body water
VRA	vasopressin receptor antagonist
V_d	volume of distribution

REFERENCES

1. U.S. Department of Health and Human Services and U.S. Department of Agriculture. *Dietary Guidelines for Americans*. 9th Edition. December 2020. https://www.dietaryguidelines.gov. Accessed January 17, 2022.
2. Sterns RH. Disorders of plasma sodium—causes, consequences, and correction. *N Engl J Med.* 2015;372:55–65. doi:10/1056/NEJMc1501342
3. Kheetan M, Ogu I, Shapiro JI, et al. Acute and chronic hyponatremia. *Front Med.* 2021;8:693738. doi:10.3389/fmed.2021.693738
4. Dineen R, Thompson CJ, Sherlock M. Hyponatremia—presentations and management. *Clin Med (Lond).* 2017;17:263–269. doi:10.7861/clinmedicine.17-3-263
5. Bhave G, Neilson EG. Volume depletion versus dehydration: how understanding the difference can guide therapy. *Am J Kidney Dis.* 2011;58:302–309. doi:10.1053/j.ajkd.2011.02.395
6. Spasovski G, Vanholder R, Allolio B, et al. Clinical practice guideline on diagnosis and treatment of hyponatraemia. *Nephrol Dial Transplant.* 2014;29(Suppl.2):ii1–ii39. doi:10.1093/ndt/gfu040
7. Patterson JH. The impact of hyponatremia. *Pharmacotherapy.* 2011;31 (5 Pt 2):5S–8S. doi:10.1592/phco.31.5.55
8. Hawkins RC. Age and gender as risk factors for hyponatremia and hypernatremia. *Clin Chim Acta.* 2003;337:169–172. doi:10.1016/j.cccn.2004.08.001
9. Friedman B, Cirulli J. Hyponatremia in critical care patients: frequency, outcome, characteristics, and treatment with the vasopressin V2-receptor antagonist tolvaptan. *J Crit Care.* 2013;28:219.e1-e12. doi:10.1016/j.jcrc.2012.06.001
10. Rondon-Berrios H, Berl T. Mild chronic hyponatremia in the ambulatory setting: significance and management. *Clin J Am Soc Nephrol.* 2015;10:2268–2278. doi:10.2215/CJN.00170115
11. Filippone EJ, Ruzieh M, Foy A. Thiazide-associated hyponatremia: clinical manifestations and pathophysiology. *Am J Kidney Dis.* 2020;75:256–264. doi:10.1053/j.ajkd.2019.07.011
12. Gandhi S, Shariff SZ, Al-Jaishi A, et al. Second-generation antidepressants and hyponatremia risk: a population-based cohort study of older adults. *Am J Kidney Dis.* 2017;69:87–96. doi:10.1053/j.ajkd.2016.08.020
13. Sahoo S, Grover S. Hyponatremia and psychotropics. *J Geriatr Ment Health.* 2016;3:108–22. doi:10.4103/2348-9995.195604
14. Pinkhasov A, Xiong G, Bourgeois JA, et al. Management of SIADH-related hyponatremia due to psychotropic medications—an expert consensus from the Association of Medicine and Psychiatry. *J Psychosom Res.* 2021;151:110654. doi:10.1016/j.jpsychores.2021.110654
15. Cumming K, Hoyle GE, Hutchison JD, et al. Prevalence, incidence and etiology of hyponatremia in elderly patients with fragility fractures. *PLoS ONE.* 2014;9(2):e88272. doi:10.1371/journal.pone.0088272
16. Correia L, Ferreira R, Correia I, et al. Severe hyponatremia in older patients at admission in an internal medicine department. *Arch Gerontol Geriatr.* 2014;54:642–647. doi:10.1016/j.archger.2014.08.002
17. Upadhyay A, Jaber BL, Madias NE. Incidence and prevalence of hyponatremia. *Am J Med.* 2006;119(7A):S30–S35. doi:10.1016/j.amjmed.2006.05.005
18. Bennett BL, Hew-Butler T, Rosner MH, et al. Wilderness Medical Society Clinical Practice Guidelines for the Management of Exercise-Associated Hyponatremia: 2019 Update. *Wilderness Environ Med.* 2020;31:50–62. doi:10.1016/j.wern.2019.11.003
19. Morton A, Lumchee M, Kumar S, et al. Pregnancy outcomes in women with hyponatraemia and preeclampsia: case series and literature review. *Pregnancy Hypertens.* 2021;26:38–41. doi:10.1016/j.preghy.2021.08.116
20. Verbalis JG, Goldsmith SR, Greenberg A, et al. Diagnosis, evaluation, and treatment of hyponatremia: expert panel recommendations. *Am J Med.* 2013;126:S1–S42. doi:10.1016/j.amjmed.2013.07.006
21. Koczmara C, Wade AW, Skippen P, et al. Hospital-acquired acute hyponatremia and reports of pediatric deaths. *Dynamics.* 2010;21: 21–26. PMID: 20333891
22. Krummel T, Prinz E, Metten M-A, et al. Prognosis of patients with severe hyponatremia is related not only to hyponatraemia but also to comorbidities and to medical management: results of an observational retrospective study. *BMC Nephrol.* 2016;17:159. doi:10.1186/s12882-016-0370-z
23. Tachi T, Yokoi T, Goto C, et al. Hyponatremia and hypokalemia as risk factors for falls. *Eur J Clin Nutr.* 2015;69:205–210. doi:10.1038/ejcn.2014.195
24. Fehlberg EA, Lucero RJ, Weaver MT, et al. Associations between hyponatraemia, volume depletion and the risk of falls in US hospitalised patients: a case–control study. *BMJ Open.* 2017;7:e017045. doi:10.1136/bmjopen-2017-017045
25. Kuo SCH, Kuo P-J, Rau C-S, et al. Hyponatremia is associated with worse outcomes from fall injuries in the elderly. *Int J Environ Res Public Health.* 2017;14:E460. doi:10.3390/ijerph14050460
26. Karakousis ND, Kostakoupoulos NA. Hyponatremia in the frail. *J Frailty Sarcopenia Falls.* 2021;6:241–245. doi:10.22540/JFSF-06-241
27. Igbinedion SO, Pandit S, Mavuram MS, et al. Pseudohyponatraemia secondary to hyperlipidaemia in obstructive jaundice. *BMJ Case Rep.* 2017 Dec 1;2017:bcr2017221984. doi:10.1136/bcr-2017-221984
28. Palmer BF, Clegg DJ. Electrolyte and acid-base disturbances in patients with diabetes mellitus. *N Engl J Med.* 2015;373:548–559. doi:10.1056/NEJMra1503102
29. Sarafidis PA, Georgianos PI, Lasaridis AN. Diuretics in clinical practice. Part I: mechanisms of action, pharmacological effects and clinical indications of diuretic compounds. *Expert Opin Drug Saf.* 2010;9: 243–257. doi:10.1517/14740330903499240
30. Oh JY, Shin JI. Syndrome of inappropriate antidiuretic hormone secretion and cerebral/renal salt wasting syndrome: similarities and differences. *Front Pediatr.* 2015;2:146. doi:10.3389/fped.2014.00146
31. Liamis G, Milionis H, Elisaf M. A review of drug-induced hyponatremia. *Am J Kidney Dis.* 2008;52:144–153. doi:10.1053/j.ajkd.2008.03.004
32. Decaux G. Is asymptomatic hyponatremia really asymptomatic? *Am J Med.* 2006;119(7A):S79–S82. doi:10.1016/j.amjmed.2006.05.013
33. Kinsella S, Moran S, Sullivan MO, et al. Hyponatremia independent of osteoporosis is associated with fracture occurrence. *Clin J Am Soc Nephrol.* 2010;5:275–280. doi:10.2215/CJN.06120809
34. Fisher SK, Heacock AM, Keep RF, et al. Receptor regulation of osmolyte homeostasis in neural cells. *J Physiol.* 2010;18:3355–3364. doi:10.1113/jphysiol.2010.190777
35. Alukal JJ, John S, Thuluvath PJ. Hyponatremia in cirrhosis: an update. *Am J Gastroenterol.* 2020;115:1775–1785. doi:10.14309/ajg/0000000000000786

36. Yuridullah R, Kumar V, Nanavati S, et al. Clinical resolution of osmotic demyelination syndrome following overcorrection of severe hyponatremia. *Case Rep Nephrol.* 2019;1757656. doi:10.1155/2019/1757656
37. Cuesta M, Thompson CJ. The syndrome of inappropriate antidiuresis (SIAD). *Best Pract Res Clin Endocrinol Metab.* 2016;30:175–187. doi:10.1016/j.beem.2016.02.009
38. Jones GM, Bode L, Riha H, et al. Safety of continuous peripheral infusion of 3% sodium chloride solution in neurocritical care patients. *Am J Crit Care.* 2016;26:37–42. doi:10.4037/ajcc2017439
39. Berl T. Vasopressin antagonists. *N Engl J Med.* 2015;372:2207–2216. doi:10.1056/NEJMra1403672
40. Schrier RW, Gross P, Gheorghiade M, et al. Tolvaptan, a selective oral vasopressin V2-receptor antagonist, for hyponatremia. *N Engl J Med.* 2006;355:2099–2112. doi:10.1056/NEJMoa065181
41. Rozen-Zvi B, Yahav D, Gheorghiade M, et al. Vasopressin receptor antagonists for the treatment of hyponatremia: systematic review and meta-analysis. *Am J Kidney Dis.* 2010;56:325–337. doi:10.1053/j.ajkd.2010.01.013
42. Tzoulis P, Waung JA, Bagkeris E, et al. Real-life experience of tolvaptan use in the treatment of severe hyponatraemia due to syndrome of inappropriate antidiuretic hormone secretion. *Clin Endocrinol (Oxf).* 2016;84:620–6. doi:10.1111/cen.12943
43. Li B, Fang D, Qian C, et al. The efficacy and safety of tolvaptan in patients with hyponatremia: a meta-analysis of randomized controlled trials. *Clin Drug Investig.* 2017;37:327–342. doi:10.1007/s40261-016-0470-3
44. Pose-Reino A, de la Vega IR, de Jong-Laird A, et al. Real-world, non-interventional, retrospective study (SAMPLE) of tolvaptan in patients with hyponatraemia secondary to the syndrome of inappropriate antidiuretic hormone secretion. *Adv Ther.* 2021;38:1055–1067. doi:10.1007/s12325-020-01560-2
45. Shoaf SE, Bramer SL, Bricmont P, et al. Pharmacokinetic and pharmacodynamic interaction between tolvaptan, a non-peptide AVP antagonist, and furosemide or hydrochlorthiazide. *J Cardiovasc Pharmacol.* 2007;50:213–222. doi:10.1097/FJC.0b013e318074f934
46. Kamgar M, Hanna RM, Hasnain H, et al. Risk of serum sodium overcorrection with V2 antagonists in SIADH and other high risk patients. *J Onco-Nephrol.* 2017;1(3):143–146. doi:10.5301/jo-n.5000025
47. Morris JH, Bohm NM, Nemecek BD, et al. Rapidity of correction of hyponatremia due to syndrome of inappropriate secretion of antidiuretic hormone following tolvaptan. *Am J Kidney Dis.* 2018;71:772–782. doi:10.10.1053/j.ajkd.2017.12.002
48. Hanna RM, Velez JC, Rastogi A, et al. Equivalent efficacy and decreased rate of overcorrection in patients with syndrome of inappropriate secretion of antidiuretic hormone given very low-dose tolvaptan. *Kidney Med.* 2019;2:20–28. doi:10.1016/j.xkme.2019.009.004
49. Liu Y-H, Han X-B, Fei Y-H, et al. Long-term low-dose tolvaptan treatment in hospitalized male patients aged >90 years with hyponatremia: report on safety and effectiveness. *Medicine (Baltimore).* 2017;96:e9539. doi:10.1097/MD.0000000000009539
50. Der-Nigoghossian C, Lesch C, Berger K. Effectiveness and tolerability of conivaptan and tolvaptan for the treatment of hyponatremia in neurocritically ill patients. *Pharmacotherapy.* 2017;37:528–534. doi:10.1002/phar.1926
51. Llompart-Pou JA, Pérez-Bárcena J, Novo M, et al. Effect of single-dose of tolvaptan in neurocritical patients with hyponatremia due to syndrome of inappropriate antidiuretic hormone secretion. *Med Intensiva.* 2017;41:501–503. doi:10.1016/j.medin.2016.11.007
52. Shoaf SE, Bricmont P, Dandurand A. Low-dose tolvaptan PK/PD: comparison of patients with hyponatremia due to syndrome of inappropriate antidiuretic hormone secretion to healthy adults. *Eur J Clin Pharmacol.* 2017;73:1399–1408. doi:10.1007/s00228-017-2302
53. McNeely EB, Talameh JA, Adams KF Jr, et al. Relative bioavailability of tolvaptan administered via nasogastric tube and tolvaptan tablets swallowed intact. *Am J Health-Syst Pharm.* 2013;70:1230–1237. doi:10.2146/ajhp120543
54. Decaux G. V2-antagonists for the treatment of hyponatraemia. *Nephrol Dial Transplant.* 2007;22:1853–1855. doi:10.1093/ndt/gfm136
55. Pose A, Almenar L, Gavira JJ, et al. Benefit of tolvaptan in the management of hyponatraemia in patients with diuretic-refractory congestive heart failure: the SEMI-SEC project. *ESC Heart Fail.* 2017;4:130–137. doi:10.1002/ehf2.12124
56. Rosskopf D, Michel MC. Pharmacogenomics of G protein-coupled receptor ligands in cardiovascular medicine. *Pharmacol Rev.* 2008;60:513–535. doi:10.1124/pr.108.000612
57. Shoaf SE, Ohzone Y, Ninomiya S, et al. In vitro P-glycoprotein interactions and steady-state pharmacokinetic interactions between tolvaptan and digoxin in healthy subjects. *J Clin Pharmacol.* 2011:51:761–769. doi:10.1177/0091270010376193
58. Shoaf SE, Bricmont P, Mallikaarjun S. Pharmacokinetics and pharmacodynamics of oral tolvaptan in patients with varying degrees of renal function. *Kidney Int.* 2014;85:953–961. doi:10.1038/ki.2013.350
59. Katsumata M, Hirawa N, Sumida K, et al. Effects of tolvaptan in patients with chronic kidney disease and chronic heart failure. *Clin Exp Nephrol.* 2017;21:858–865. doi:10.1007/s10157-016-1379-0
60. Torres VE, Chapman AB, Devuyst O, et al. Tolvaptan in patients with autosomal dominant polycystic kidney disease. *N Engl J Med.* 2012;367:2407–2418. doi:10.1056/NEJMoa1205511
61. Rondon-Berrios H, Berl T. Vasopressin receptor antagonists in hyponatremia: uses and misuses. *Front Med (Lausanne).* 2017:4:141. doi:10.3389/fmed.2017.00141
62. Ramamohan V, Mladsi D, Ronquest N, et al. An economic analysis of tolvaptan compared with fluid restriction among hospitalized patients with hyponatremia. *Hosp Pract (1995).* 2017;45:111–117. doi:10.1080/21548331.2017.1324227
63. Dasta JF, Sundar S, Chase S, et al. Economic impact of tolvaptan treatment vs. fluid restriction based on real-world data among hospitalized patients with heart failure and hyponatremia. *Hosp Pract (1995).* 2018:46:197–202. doi:10.1080/21548331.2018.1505180
64. Sarafidis P, Loutradis C, Ferro CJ, et al. SGLT-2 inhibitors to treat hyponatremia associated with SIADH: a novel indication? *Am J Nephrol.* 2020;51:553–555. doi:10.1159/000509082
65. Refardt J, Imber C, Sailer CO, et al. A randomized trial of empagliflozin to increase plasma sodium levels in patients with the syndrome of inappropriate antidiuresis. *J Am Soc Nephrol.* 2020;31:615–624. doi:10.1681/ASN/2019090944
66. Miell J, Dhanjal P, Jamookeeah C. Evidence for the use of demeclocycline in the treatment of hyponatraemia secondary to SIADH: a systematic review. *Int J Clin Pract.* 2015;69:1396–1417. doi:10.1111/ijcp.12713
67. Rondon-Berrios H, Tandukar S, Mor MK, et al. Urea for the treatment of hyponatremia. *Clin J Am Soc Nephrol.* 2018;13:1627–1632. doi:10.2215/CJN.04020318
68. Soupart A, Coffernils M, Couturier B, et al. Efficacy and tolerance of urea compared with vaptans for long-term treatment of patients with SIADH. *Clin J Am Soc Nephrol.* 2012;7:742–747. doi:10.2215/CJN.06990711
69. Nagler EV, Haller MC, van Biesen W, et al. Interventions for chronic non-hypovolaemic hypotonic hyponatraemia. *Cochrane Database Syst Rev.* 2018;6:CD010965. doi:10.1002/14651858.CD010965.pub2
70. Sonawane KB, Hansen RA. PHP92—Serious adverse drug events reported to the Food and Drug Administration (FDA): analysis of the FDA adverse event reporting system (FAERS) 2006-2011 database. *Value in Health.* 2015;18:A86. doi:10.1016/j.jval.2015.03.502
71. Gheorghiade M, Gottlieb SS, Udelson JE, et al. Vasopressin v(2) receptor blockade with tolvaptan versus fluid restriction in the treatment of hyponatremia. *Am J Cardiol.* 2006;97:1064–1067. doi:10.1016/j.amjcard.2005.10.050
72. Dunlap ME, Hauptman PJ, Amin AN, et al. Current management of hyponatremia in acute heart failure: a report from the Hyponatremia Registry for Patients with Euvolemic and Hypervolemic Hyponatremia (HN Registry). *J Am Heart Assoc.* 2017;6:e005261. doi:10.1161/JAHA.116.005261
73. Lee WH, Packer M. Prognostic importance of serum sodium concentration and its modification by converting-enzyme inhibition in patients with severe chronic heart failure. *Circulation.* 1986;73:257–267. doi:10.1161/01.cir.73.2.257
74. Klein L, O'Connor CM, Leimberger JD, et al; OPTIME-CHF Investigators. Lower serum sodium is associated with increased short-term mortality in hospitalized patients with worsening heart failure: results from the Outcomes of a Prospective Trial of Intravenous Milrinone for Exacerbations of Chronic Heart Failure (OPTIME-CHF) study. *Circulation.* 2005;111:2454–2460. doi:10.1161/01.CIR.0000165065.82609.3D
75. Bakris GL, Weir MR. Angiotensin-converting enzyme inhibitor-associated elevation of creatinine: Is this a cause for concern? *Arch Intern Med.* 2000;160:685–693. doi:10.1001/archinte.160.5.685
76. Baldasseroni S, Urso R, Orso F, et al. Relation between serum sodium levels and prognosis in outpatients with chronic heart failure: neutral effect of treatment with beta-blockers and angiotensin-converting enzyme inhibitors: data from the Italian network on congestive heart failure (IN-CHF database). *J Cardiovasc Med.* 2011;12:723–731. doi:10.2459/JCM.0b013e32834ae87e
77. Bajaj JS, Tandon P, O'Leary JG, et al. The impact of albumin use on resolution of hyponatremia in hospitalized patients with cirrhosis. *Am J Gastroenterol.* 2018;113:1339–1344. doi:10.1038/s41395-018-0119-3

78. Caraceni P, Riggio O, Angeli P, et al for the ANSWER Study Investigators. Long-term albumin administration in decompensated cirrhosis (ANSWER): an open-label randomised trial. *Lancet.* 2018;391:2417–2429. doi:10.1016/S0140-6736(18)30840-7
79. Gerbes AL, Gülberg V, Ginès P, et al. Therapy of hyponatremia in cirrhosis with a vasopressin receptor antagonist: a randomized double-blind multicenter trial. *Gastroenterology.* 2003;124:933–939. doi:10.1053/gast.2003.50143
80. Urso C, Brucculeri S, Caimi G. Employment of vasopressin receptor antagonists in management of hyponatraemia and volume overload in some clinical conditions. *J Clin Pharm Ther.* 2015;40:376–385. doi:10.1111/jcpt.12279
81. Jia J-D, Xie W, Ding H-G, et al. Utility and safety of tolvaptan in cirrhotic patients with hyponatremia: a prospective cohort study. *Ann Hepatol.* 2017;16:123–132. doi:10.5604/16652681.1226823
82. Tahara T, Mori K, Mochizuki M, et al. Tolvaptan is effective in treating patients with refractory ascites due to cirrhosis. *Biomed Rep.* 2017;7:558–562. doi:10.3892/br.2017.1005
83. Sakaida I, Terai S, Kurosaki M, et al. Effectiveness and safety of tolvaptan in liver cirrhosis patients with edema: interim results of post-marketing surveillance of tolvaptan in liver cirrhosis (START study). *Hepatol Res.* 2017;47:1137–1146. doi:10.1111/hepr.12852
84. Pose E, Solà E, Piano S, et al. Limited efficacy of tolvaptan in patients with cirrhosis and severe hyponatremia: real-life experience. *Am J Med.* 2017;130:372–375. doi:10.1016/j.amjmed.2016.09.011
85. Berl T, Quittnat-Pelletier F, Verbalis JG, et al for the SALTWATER Investigators. Oral tolvaptan is safe and effective in chronic hyponatremia. *J Am Soc Nephrol.* 2010;21:705–712. doi:10.1681/ASN.200908857
86. Jaber BL, Almarzouqi L, Borgi L, et al. Short-term efficacy and safety of vasopressin receptor antagonists for treatment of hyponatremia. *Am J Med.* 2011;124:977.e1-9. doi:10.1016/j.amjmed.2011.04.028
87. Parekh A, Rajaram P, Patel G, et al. Utility of tolvaptan in the perioperative management of severe hyponatremia during liver transplantation: a case report. *Transplant Proc.* 2017;49:2399–2401. doi:10.1016/j.transproceed.2017.09.011
88. Felker GM, Mentz RJ, Cole RT, et al. Efficacy and safety of tolvaptan in patients hospitalized with acute heart failure. *J Am Coll Cardiol.* 2017;69:1399–1406. doi:10.1016/j.jacc.2016.09.004
89. Konstam MA, Kiernan M, Chandler A, et al. Short-term effects of tolvaptan in patients with acute heart failure and volume overload. *J Am Coll Cardiol.* 2017;69:1409–1419. doi:10.1016/j.jacc.2016.12.035
90. Ikeda S, Ohshima K, Miyazaki S, et al. Impact of chronic kidney disease on the diuretic response of tolvaptan in acute decompensated heart failure. *ESC Heart Fail.* 2017;4:614–622. doi:10.1002/ehf2.12190
91. Gheorghaide M, Niazi I, Quyang J, et al. Vasopressin V2-receptor blockage with tolvaptan in patients with chronic heart failure: results from a double-blind randomized trial. *Circulation.* 2003;107: 2690–2696. doi:10.1161/01.CIR.0000070422.41439.04
92. Gheorghaide M, Gattis WA, O'Connor CM, et al. Effects of tolvaptan, a vasopressin antagonist, in patients hospitalized with worsening heart failure: a randomized controlled trial. *JAMA.* 2004;291:1963–1971. doi:10.1001/jama/291.16.1963
93. Gheorghiade M, Konstam MA, Burnett JC Jr, et al. Short-term clinical effects of tolvaptan, an oral vasopressin antagonist, in patients hospitalized for heart failure: the EVEREST Clinical Status Trials. *JAMA.* 2007;297:1332–1343. doi:10.1001/jama.297.12.1332
94. Konstam MA, Gheorghiade M, Burnett JC Jr, et al. Effects of oral tolvaptan in patients hospitalized for worsening heart failure: the EVEREST Outcome Trial. *JAMA.* 2007;297:1319–1331. doi:10.1001/jama.297.12.1319
95. Hauptman PJ, Burnett J, Gheorghiade M, et al. Clinical course of patients with hyponatremia and decompensated systolic heart failure and the effect of vasopressin receptor antagonism with tolvaptan. *J Card Fail.* 2013;19:390–397. doi:10.1016/j.cardfail.2013.04.001
96. Udelson JE, McGrew FA, Flores E, et al. Multicenter, randomized, double-blind, placebo-controlled study on the effect of oral tolvaptan on left ventricular dilation and function in patients with heart failure and systolic dysfunction. *J Am Coll Cardiol.* 2005;49:2151–2159. doi:10.1016/j.jacc.2007.01.091
97. Heidenreich PA, Bozkurt B, Aguilar D, et al. 2022 AHA/ACC/HFSA Guidelines for the Management of Heart Failure: A Report of the American College of Cardiology/American Heart Association Joint Committee on Clinical Practice Guidelines. *Circulation.* 2022;145:e895–e1032. doi:10.1161?CIR.0000000000001063
98. Hoorn EJ, Zietse R. Diagnosis and treatment of hyponatremia: compilation of the guidelines. *J Am Soc Nephrol.* 2017;28:1340–1349. doi:10.1681/ASN.2016101139
99. Adams KF. Tolvaptan treatment to reverse worsening outpatient heart failure: possible role of copeptin in identifying responders (TROUPER). In: ClinicalTrials.gov [Internet]. Bethesda (MD): National Library of Medicine (US). 2000. https://clinicaltrials.gov/ct2/show/NCT02476409, NLM Identifier: NCT02476409. Accessed January 17, 2022.
100. Goldsmith SR. Is there a cardiovascular rationale for the use of combined vasopressin V1a/V2 receptor antagonists? *Am J Med.* 2006;119(7 Suppl 1):S93–S96. doi:10.1016/j.amjmed.2006.05.015
101. Al-Absi A, Gosmanova EO, Wall BM. A clinical approach to the treatment of chronic hypernatremia. *Am J Kidney Dis.* 2012;60: 1032–1038. doi:10.1053/j.ajkd.2012.06.025
102. Overgaard-Steensen C, Ring T. Clinical review: practical approach to hyponatraemia and hypernatraemia in critically ill patients. *Crit Care.* 2013;17:206. doi:10.1186/cc11805
103. Waite MD, Fuhrman SA, Badawi O, et al. Intensive care unit-acquired hypernatremia is an independent predictor of increased mortality and length of stay. *J Crit Care.* 2013;28:405–412. doi:10.1016/j.jcrc.2012.11.013
104. Stelfox HT, Ahmed SB, Khandwala F, et al. The epidemiology of intensive care unit-acquired hyponatraemia and hypernatraemia in medical-surgical intensive care units. *Crit Care.* 2008;12:R162. doi:10.1186/cc7162
105. Mestrom EHJ, van der Stam JA, te Pas ME, et al. Increased sodium intake and decreased sodium excretion in ICU-acquired hypernatremia: a prospective cohort study. *J Crit Care.* 2021;63:68–75. doi:10.1016/j.jcrc.2021.02.002
106. Rugg C, Schmid S, Kreutiziger J, et al. The lack of free water on ICU: mere fluid-balances are not enough with regard to hypernatremia. *J Crit Care.* 2021;65:232–234. doi:10.1016/j.jcrc.2021.07.001
107. Lansink-Hartgring AO, Hessels L, Weigel J, et al. Long-term changes in dysnatremia incidence in the ICU: a shift from hyponatremia to hypernatremia. *Ann Intensive Care.* 2016:6:22. doi:10.1186/s13613-016-0124-x
108. Hoorn EJ, Betjes MG, Weigel J, et al. Hypernatremia in critically ill patients: Too little water and too much salt. *Nephrol Dial Transplant.* 2008;23:1562–1568. doi:10.1093/ndt/gfm831
109. van Regenmortel N, Moers L, Langer T, et al. Fluid-induced harm in the hospital: look beyond volume and start considering sodium. From physiology towards recommendations for daily practice in hospitalized adults. *Ann Intensive Care.* 2021;11:79. doi:10.1186/s13613-021-00851-3
110. Moritz ML, Ayus JC. The changing pattern of hypernatremia in hospitalized children. *Pediatrics.* 1999;104:435–439. doi:10.1542/peds.104.3.435
111. Lindner G, Funk GC. Hypernatremia in critically ill patients. *J Crit Care.* 2013;28:216.e11-20. doi:10.1016/j.jcrc.2012.05.001
112. Qian Q. Hypernatremia. *Clin J Am Soc Nephrol.* 2019;14:432–444. doi:10.2215/CJN.12141018
113. Buckley MS, Leblanc JM, Cawley MJ. Electrolyte disturbances associated with commonly prescribed medications in the intensive care unit. *Crit Care Med.* 2010;38(6 Suppl):S253–S264. doi:10.1097/CCM.0b013e3181dda0be
114. Chassagne P, Druesne L, Capet C, et al. Clinical presentation of hypernatremia in elderly patients: a case control study. *J Am Geriatr Soc.* 2006;54:1225–1230. doi:10.1111/j.1532-5415.2006.00807.x
115. Saifan C, Nasr R, Mehta S, et al. Diabetes insipidus: a challenging diagnosis with new drug therapies. *ISRN Nephrol.* 2013:797620. doi:10.5402/2013/797620
116. Moritz ML. A water deprivation test is not indicated in the evaluation of hypernatremia [letter]. *Am J Kidney Dis.* 2005;46:1150–1151. doi:10.1053/j.ajkd.2005.09.018
117. Feld LG, Neuspiel DR, Foster BA, et al. Clinical practice guideline: maintenance intravenous fluids in children. *Pediatrics.* 2018;142:e20183083. doi:10.1542/peds.2018-3083
118. Semler MW, Self WH, Wanderer JP, et al. Balanced crystalloids versus saline in critically ill adults. *N Engl J Med.* 2018;378:829–839. doi:10.1056/NEJMoa1711584
119. Shah A, Ellis G, Kucheria R. A guide for the assessment and management of post-obstructive diuresis. *Urology News.* 2015; March 1. https://www.urologynews.uk.com/features/features/post/a-guide-for-the-assessment-and-management-of-post-obstructive-diuresis. Accessed January 17, 2022.
120. Reynolds RM, Padfield PL, Seckl JR. Disorders of sodium balance. *BMJ.* 2006;332:702–705. doi:10.1136/bmj.332.6543.702
121. Bockenhauer D, Bichet DG. Pathophysiology, diagnosis and management of nephrogenic diabetes insipidus. *Nat Rev Nephrol.* 2015;11:576–588. doi:10.1038/nrneph.2015.89

122. Downie ML, Gallibois C, Parekh RS, et al. Nephrotic syndrome in infants and children: pathophysiology and management. *Paediatr Int Child Heal.* 2017;37:248–258. doi:10.1080/20469047.2017.1374003
123. Kallash M, Mahan JD. Mechanisms and management of edema in pediatric nephrotic syndrome. *Pediatr Nephrol.* 2021;36:1719–1730. doi:10.1007/s00467-020-04779-x
124. Fortune B, Cardenas A. Ascites, refractory ascites and hyponatremia in cirrhosis. *Gastroenterol Report.* 2017;5:104–112. doi:10.1093/gastro/gox010
125. Rysz J, Franczyk B, Rysz-Górzyńska, et al. Pharmacogenomics of hypertension treatment. *Int J Mol Sci.* 2020;21:4709. doi:10.3390/ijms21134709
126. Agarwal R, Gorski JC, Sundblad K, et al. Urinary protein binding does not affect response to furosemide in patients with nephrotic syndrome. *J Am Soc Nephrol.* 2000;11:1100–1105. doi:10.1681/ASN.V1161100
127. Siddall EC, Radhakrishnan J. The pathophysiology of edema formation in the nephrotic syndrome. *Kidney International.* 2012;82:635–642. doi:10.1038/ki.2012.180
128. Somberg JC, Molnar J. Therapeutic approaches to the treatment of edema and ascites: the use of diuretics. *Am J Ther.* 2009:16:98–101. doi:10.1097/MJT.0b013e318196082e
129. Nappi JM, Sieg A. Aldosterone receptor antagonists in patients with chronic heart failure. *Vasc Heal Risk Manag.* 2011;7:353–363. doi:10.2147/VHRM.S13779

Disorders of Calcium and Phosphorus Homeostasis

69

Angela L. Bingham

KEY CONCEPTS

1. Severe acute hypercalcemia can result in cardiac arrhythmias, whereas chronic hypercalcemia can lead to calcium deposition in soft tissues including blood vessels and the kidney.
2. The correction of hypercalcemia can include multiple pharmacotherapeutic modalities such as hydration, diuretics, bisphosphonates, and corticosteroids, depending on the etiology and acuity of the hypercalcemia.
3. Hypocalcemia is typically associated with an insidious onset; however, some medications such as cinacalcet are associated with rapid decreases in serum calcium.
4. Acute treatment of hypocalcemia requires calcium supplementation, whereas chronic management may require other therapies such as vitamin D to maintain serum calcium concentrations.
5. Hyperphosphatemia occurs most frequently in patients with chronic kidney disease (CKD).
6. Treatment of nonemergent hyperphosphatemia includes the use of phosphate binders to decrease absorption of phosphorus from the gastrointestinal (GI) tract.
7. Hypophosphatemia is a relatively common complication among critically ill patients.
8. Treatment of acute hypophosphatemia usually requires intravenous (IV) phosphorus supplementation.

BEYOND THE BOOK

Watch the video entitled "Skeletal Endocrine Control" in Khan Academy by Tracy Kim Kovach. This ~8-minute video provides a brief overview of calcium and phosphorus homeostasis. The video is useful to enhance students' understanding regarding the COLLECT and ASSESS steps in the patient care process: <https://www.khanacademy.org/test-prep/mcat/organ-systems/the-skeletal-system/v/skeletal-endocrine-control>.

INTRODUCTION

Disorders of calcium and phosphorus are common complications of multiple acute and chronic diseases. These disorders are frequently seen in the acute care setting; however, they are also often present in ambulatory patients, usually in a less severe state. The consequences of electrolyte disorders can range from asymptomatic to life-threatening, requiring hospitalization and emergent treatment. The maintenance of fluid and electrolyte homeostasis requires adequate functioning and modulation by multiple hormones on tissues of multiple organ systems.

Many common medication therapies can disturb the normal homeostatic mechanisms that maintain calcium and phosphorus balance. In addition, with some medication therapies, toxicity is enhanced when underlying electrolyte disorders are present. Medication-induced disorders typically respond well to discontinuation of the offending agent(s); however, additional therapies are sometimes required to correct the disorder. This chapter reviews the etiology, classification, clinical presentation, and therapy for the most common disorders of calcium and phosphorus homeostasis.

DISORDERS OF CALCIUM HOMEOSTASIS

The maintenance of physiologic calcium concentrations in the intracellular and extracellular spaces is vital for the preservation and function of cell membranes, propagation of neuromuscular activity, regulation of endocrine and exocrine secretory functions, blood coagulation cascade, platelet adhesion process, bone metabolism, muscle cell excitation/contraction coupling, and mediation of the electrophysiologic slow-channel response in cardiac and smooth-muscle tissues.

The disorders of calcium homeostasis are related to the calcium content of the extracellular fluid (ECF), which is tightly regulated and comprises less than 0.5% of the total body stores of calcium. Skeletal bone contains more than 99% of total body stores of calcium.[1] ECF calcium is moderately bound to plasma proteins (40%-50%), primarily albumin.[1] Ionized or free calcium is the biologically active form and is the fraction that is homeostatically regulated.[1] Extracellular calcium, however, is most commonly measured as the total serum calcium concentration, which includes both bound and unbound calcium. The normal total calcium serum concentration range is 8.6 to 10.2 mg/dL (2.15-2.55 mmol/L).[1]

Proper assessment of total serum calcium concentration includes measurement of the patient's serum albumin concentration. Hypoalbuminemia, which can be associated with many chronic disease states, is probably the most common cause of "laboratory hypocalcemia." Patients remain asymptomatic because the unbound or ionized fraction of serum calcium remains normal (normal range, 4.48-5.2 mg/dL [1.12-1.30 mmol/L]).[1] A corrected total serum calcium concentration can be calculated based on the measured total serum calcium and the difference between a patient's measured albumin concentration and the normative value of 4 g/dL (40 g/L) by the following equations:

$$\text{Corrected serum calcium (mg/dL)} = \text{Measured serum calcium (mg/dL)} + (0.8 \times [4\text{ g/dL} - \text{measured albumin (g/dL)}])$$

or

$$\text{Corrected serum calcium (mmol/L)} = \text{Measured serum calcium (mmol/L)} + (0.02 \times [40\text{ g/L} - \text{measured albumin (g/L)}])$$

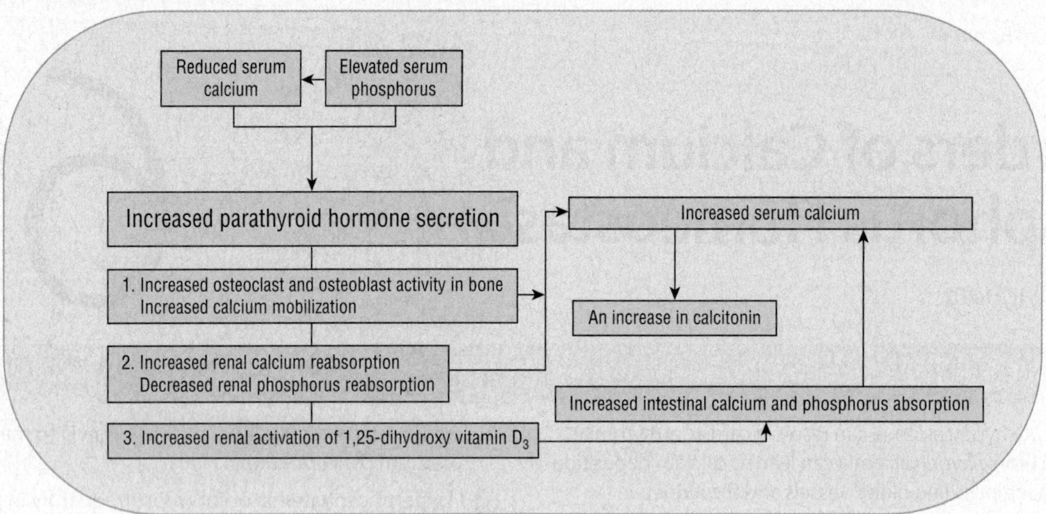

FIGURE 69-1 Homeostatic mechanisms to maintain serum calcium concentrations.

The concentration of ionized calcium is closely regulated by the interactions of parathyroid hormone (PTH), phosphorus, vitamin D, and calcitonin (Fig. 69-1). PTH increases serum calcium concentrations by stimulating calcium release from bone, increasing renal tubular reabsorption, and enhancing absorption in the GI tract secondary to increased kidney production of 1,25-dihydroxyvitamin D_3. Vitamin D directly increases serum calcium, as well as phosphorus concentrations, by increasing GI absorption. Indirectly, it can also lead to calcium release from bone and reduced renal excretion. Calcitonin inhibits osteoclastic bone resorption. Calcitonin plasma concentrations are increased when ionized calcium concentrations are high as the body attempts to return the serum calcium concentration to the normal range. Disruption of these homeostatic mechanisms results in the clinical manifestations of hypercalcemia or hypocalcemia.

Total serum calcium and ionized calcium are poorly correlated in patients with hypoalbuminemia, critical illness, and acid-base disorders.[1] Alteration of the concentration of albumin or its binding of calcium can be expected to change the unbound fraction of total serum calcium. Each 1 g/dL (10 g/L) drop in the serum albumin concentration below 4 g/dL (40 g/L) will result in a decrease of total serum calcium concentration by 0.8 mg/dL (0.20 mmol/L).[1] This approach to calculating an albumin-adjusted calcium concentration has been found to overestimate the degree of hypercalcemia and usually fails to identify hypocalcemia in critically ill patients, because the ionized calcium concentration may be normal despite a low total serum calcium concentration in the setting of hypoalbuminemia. Therefore, ionized calcium values should be used to assess calcium status in critically ill patients.[1] Change in ECF pH is the most significant cause of changes in calcium binding to albumin. In the presence of acute metabolic alkalosis the fraction of calcium bound to albumin is increased, thus reducing the plasma concentration of ionized calcium. This can result in symptomatic hypocalcemia with manifestations such as tetany, paresthesia, muscle cramping, heart block, and seizures.[1] Conversely, metabolic acidosis decreases calcium binding to albumin and results in increased ionized calcium.

HYPERCALCEMIA

There are numerous causes of hypercalcemia (total serum calcium more than 10.2 mg/dL [2.55 mmol/L]) (Table 69-1). The most common causes of hypercalcemia are primary hyperparathyroidism and cancer.

TABLE 69-1 Etiologies of Hypercalcemia

Neoplasms	**Medications**
• Bone metastasis	• Thiazides
• Breast	• Lithium
• Multiple myeloma	• Vitamin D
• Lymphoma	• Vitamin A
• Leukemia	• Calcium
• Humoral induced	• Aluminum/magnesium antacids
• Ovary	• Theophylline
• Kidney	• Tamoxifen
• Pheochromocytoma	• Ganciclovir
• Multiple endocrine neoplasia	**Granulomatous disease**
• Lung	• Sarcoidosis
• Head and neck	• Tuberculosis
• Esophagus	• Cryptococcus
• Cervix	• Berylliosis
• Lymphoproliferative disease	• Histoplasmosis
Hyperparathyroidism	• Coccidioidomycosis
• Primary	• Leprosy
• Tertiary	**Endocrine disease**
Miscellaneous	• Adrenal insufficiency
• Immobilization	• Hyperthyroidism
• Paget's disease	• Acromegaly
• Familial hypocalciuric hypercalcemia	
• Adolescence	
• Rhabdomyolysis	

Epidemiology and Etiology

Primary hyperparathyroidism occurs predominantly after the age of 50 years and affects women 3 to 4 times more than men.[2] Hypercalcemia associated with malignancy occurs in approximately 10% to 30% of patients with cancer at some time during the course of their disease and is dependent on tumor type.[3] Cancer-associated hypercalcemia is predominantly encountered in hospitalized patients, whereas primary hyperparathyroidism accounts for the vast majority of cases in the outpatient setting.[3,4]

Pathophysiology

Hypercalcemia is the result of one or a combination of three primary mechanisms: increased bone resorption, increased GI absorption, or increased tubular reabsorption by the kidneys (see Fig. 69-1).

Many tumors secrete PTH-related protein (PTHrP), which binds to the PTH receptors in bone and kidney tissue, leading to increased bone resorption and tubular reabsorption.[5] Tumors can also secrete substances such as vitamin D, transforming growth factor, interleukins, prostaglandins, interferon, tumor necrosis factor, and granulocyte-macrophage colony-stimulating factor, which are associated with the development of hypercalcemia.[3] Hypercalcemia of malignancy is generally associated with bone metastases and is a common complication of squamous cell carcinomas of the lung, head, and neck, hematologic malignancies such as multiple myeloma and T-cell lymphomas, and carcinomas of ovary, kidney, bladder, and breast. The most frequent types of malignancy associated with hypercalcemia are multiple myeloma, breast, renal, and squamous carcinomas.[3] Breast and squamous cell lung carcinomas secrete PTHrP which binds to the type I PTH receptor (PTHR1) and enhances bone resorption.[5] In contrast, patients with multiple myeloma often develop hypercalcemia principally as the result of osteoclast-mediated bone destruction.[3]

Primary hyperparathyroidism is the most common cause of chronic hypercalcemia in the general population. Benign parathyroid adenomas account for 80% to 85% of these cases of hyperparathyroidism, parathyroid hyperplasia accounts for 15%, and parathyroid carcinoma is the cause in less than 1% of cases.[4]

Other causes of chronic hypercalcemia include medications, endocrine and granulomatous disorders, physical immobilization, high bone-turnover states (eg, adolescence and Paget's disease), and rhabdomyolysis. Increased GI absorption can be the result of excessive ingestion of vitamin D analogs, calcium supplements, and lithium. Lithium and vitamin A therapy can increase bone resorption, whereas increased renal tubular reabsorption of calcium can occur with thiazide and lithium therapy. The exact mechanism of lithium-induced hypercalcemia is unknown but may include competitive inhibition of calcium influx into cells, increasing the threshold sensitivity of the calcium-sensing receptor (CaSr) and subsequent inhibition of PTH gene transcription.[6] Addison's disease, acromegaly, and thyrotoxicosis are endocrine disorders that can lead to hypercalcemia because of increased renal tubular reabsorption and increased bone resorption. Milk-alkali syndrome is the term applied to those situations where an individual develops hypercalcemia following the ingestion of calcium and absorbable alkali (eg, calcium carbonate) and is a frequent cause of hypercalcemia in patients who are not undergoing hemodialysis.[7,8] Finally, the granulomatous disorders (eg, sarcoidosis, tuberculosis, histoplasmosis, leprosy) are associated with hypercalcemia secondary to an increase in GI and renal tubular absorption as the result of granuloma production of 1,25-dihydroxyvitamin D_2.[9]

Clinical Presentation: Hypercalcemia

Patients with mild-to-moderate hypercalcemia, that is, total serum calcium concentrations above the upper threshold of normal but less than 13 mg/dL (3.25 mmol/L) or ionized calcium concentrations less than 6 mg/dL (1.50 mmol/L) can often be asymptomatic. This is typically the case for the vast majority of patients who have medication-induced hypercalcemia or primary hyperparathyroidism.[9,10]

1 The presenting signs and symptoms of severe hypercalcemia that occur if the total serum calcium concentration is more than 13 mg/dL (3.25 mmol/L) may differ depending on the acuity of onset.[1] Hypercalcemia of malignancy usually develops quickly and is accompanied by a classic symptom complex of anorexia, nausea and vomiting, constipation, polyuria, polydipsia, and nocturia.[3] Polyuria and nocturia secondary to a urinary-concentrating defect constitute some of the most frequent renal effects of hypercalcemia.[9] Hypercalcemic crisis is characterized by an acute elevation of total serum calcium to a value more than 15 mg/dL (3.75 mmol/L), acute kidney injury (AKI), and obtundation (inability to arouse).[11] If untreated, hypercalcemic crisis can progress to oliguric AKI, coma, and life-threatening ventricular arrhythmias.[9] The primary complications associated with chronic hypercalcemia (hyperparathyroidism) include metastatic calcification, hypercalciuria, and CKD secondary to interstitial nephrocalcinosis.[9]

Calcium and/or calcium–phosphorus complex deposition in blood vessels and multiple organs is a complication of chronic hypercalcemia and/or concomitant hyperphosphatemia and hyperparathyroidism. Calcium deposits in atherosclerotic lesions contribute to cardiac disease.[12] Intracardiac and arterial calcifications have been found in patients with Paget's disease who have normal kidney function. It is hypothesized that similar calcification processes occur in both bone and vascular tissue, leading to cardiovascular diseases including heart failure, systolic hypertension, and ischemic heart disease.[13]

The electrocardiographic changes associated with hypercalcemia include shortening of the QT interval and coving of the ST-T wave.[9] Very high serum calcium concentrations can cause T-wave widening, indicating a repolarization defect that may be associated with spontaneous ventricular tachyarrhythmias.[9] Hypertension and arrhythmias have occurred in the setting of hypercalcemia. The effects of digoxin on cardiac conduction including lowering of the excitation threshold, shortening of the effective refractory period,

CLINICAL PRESENTATION Hypercalcemia

General

- The signs and symptoms of hypercalcemia depend on the severity and rapidity of onset.

Symptoms

- Symptoms include fatigue, weakness, anorexia, depression, anxiety, cognitive dysfunction, vague abdominal pain, and constipation. Renal symptoms can include polyuria, polydipsia, and nocturia. Rarely, severe hypercalcemia leads to acute pancreatitis.

Signs

- Kidney: Nephrolithiasis; renal tubular dysfunction, particularly decreased concentrating ability; and acute and chronic kidney disease
- Cardiovascular: Hypercalcemia also directly shortens the myocardial action potential, which is reflected in a shortened QT interval and coving of the ST-T wave. Spontaneous ventricular tachyarrhythmias and elevations in blood pressure have also been reported. Chronic hypercalcemia can lead to cardiac calcification
- Musculoskeletal: Rheumatologic complaints related to hyperparathyroidism include gout, pseudogout, and chondrocalcinosis

Laboratory Tests

- Serum calcium concentrations of more than 10.2 mg/dL (2.55 mmol/L) are considered to represent hypercalcemia. Patients with values up to 13 mg/dL (3.25 mmol/L) are generally considered to have mild or moderate hypercalcemia, whereas those with values greater than this indicate the presence of severe hypercalcemia and increased atrioventricular refractoriness can be potentiated by hypercalcemia.[14]

Nephrolithiasis

Nephrolithiasis (ie, kidney stones) and nephrocalcinosis (ie, calcium deposits in the kidney) are the primary renal complications arising from long-standing hypercalcemia, as the result of primary hyperparathyroidism. Stone formation is dependent on a favorable milieu within the kidney or urinary tract, such as oversaturation of the urine and/or reduced concentrations of endogenous inhibitors of crystal formation (eg, citrate or pyrophosphate). About 20% to 30% of patients with primary hyperparathyroidism exhibit nephrolithiasis.[15,16] Of note, in those patients with low glomerular filtration rates (GFRs), the 24-hour urinary calcium will actually diminish secondary to decreased production of 1,25-dihydroxyvitamin D_2. However, the fractional excretion of calcium might increase.[16] Sarcoidosis is the other hypercalcemic condition frequently associated with calcium stones.[9] Other causes of nephrolithiasis with calcium-containing stones include hypocitraturia, renal tubular acidosis, hyperoxaluria, and hyperuricosuria, which are conditions that are prevalent among bariatric surgery patients.[17,18] Stone formers who have primary hyperparathyroidism are more likely to be women, older than 50 years, and have a family history of multiple endocrine disorders.[15] High dietary sodium intake can also raise urinary calcium concentrations, perhaps due to a reduction in calcium reabsorption in the kidney, thus predisposing patients to calcium stones. Although CKD can be the ultimate result of persistent stones, it is the primary cause of kidney disease in less than 2% of the end-stage kidney disease population.

TREATMENT

Desired Outcome

The indications for the treatment of acute hypercalcemia are dependent on the severity of hypercalcemia, acuity of its development, and the presence or absence of symptoms requiring emergent treatment (eg, necrotizing pancreatitis). The therapeutic intervention plan should be crafted to reverse signs and symptoms, restore normocalcemia within hours to days depending on acuity, and correct or manage the underlying cause of hypercalcemia.

General Approach

Chronic hypercalcemia is usually caused by an underlying medical condition or prescribed pharmacotherapies that can be resolved by successful treatment of the condition or withdrawal of the offending agent resulting in a decrease in serum calcium within days or weeks. Acute hypercalcemic episodes induced by malignancies may be mitigated by chemotherapy and/or radiation treatment. Effective surgical or medication treatment of primary hyperparathyroidism should reduce serum calcium concentrations as well as reduce the development of long-term complications such as vascular complications, CKD, and kidney stones. For treatment of nephrolithiasis, the goal in management of serum calcium is prevention of stone formation and diameter. The reduction of serum calcium should be targeted at the underlying disease state causing hypercalcemia (eg, using cinacalcet for primary hyperparathyroidism). Hypercalcemic crisis and acute symptomatic severe hypercalcemia are medical emergencies and require immediate treatment (Fig. 69-2).

These patients may require immediate-acting interventions to promptly reduce the serum calcium concentration if electrocardiogram (ECG) changes, neurologic manifestations, or pancreatitis are present. Pharmacologic therapy consisting of volume expansion and enhancement of urinary calcium excretion with loop diuretics is usually the initial management strategy. Hemodialysis against a zero- or low-calcium dialysate solution should be considered for patients with severely impaired kidney function (CKD stage 4 or 5) who cannot tolerate large fluid loads and in whom diuretics have limited efficacy.[9]

Effective treatment of moderate-to-severe hypercalcemia in the absence of life-threatening symptoms begins with attention to the underlying disorder and correction of associated fluid and electrolyte abnormalities. Patients with primary hyperparathyroidism may require surgery, particularly if they have systemic manifestations.

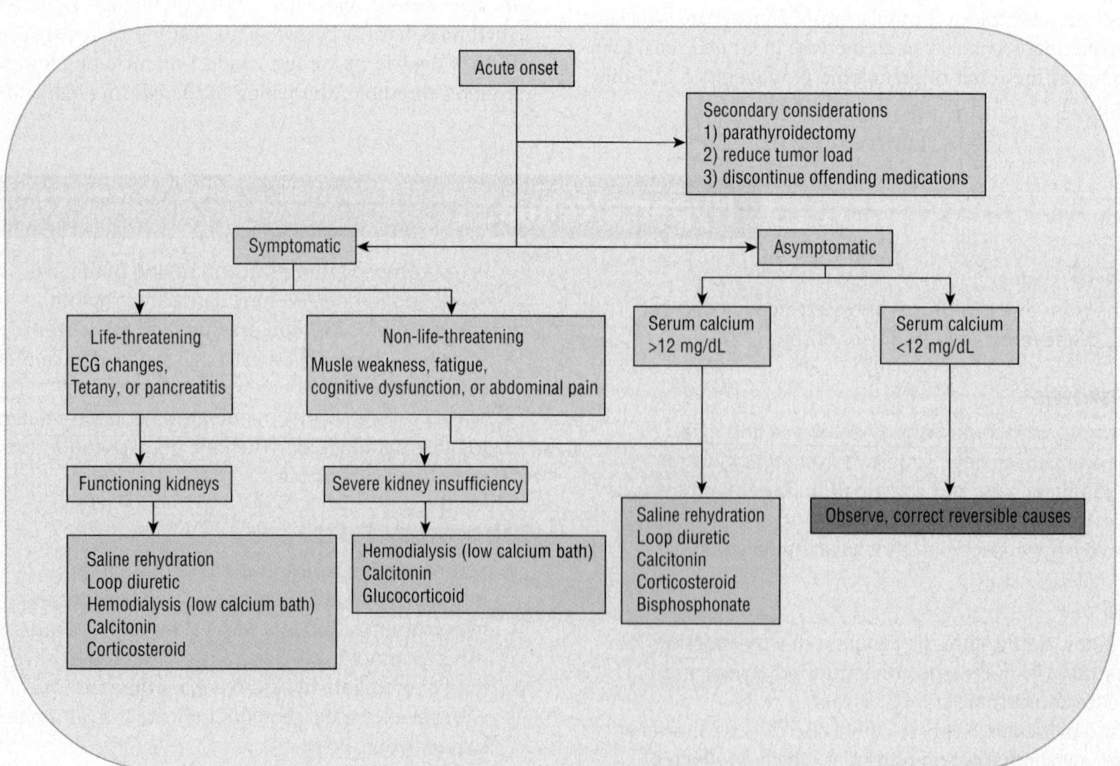

FIGURE 69-2 Pharmacotherapeutic options for the acutely hypercalcemic patient. Serum calcium of 12 mg/dL is equivalent to 3 mmol/L.

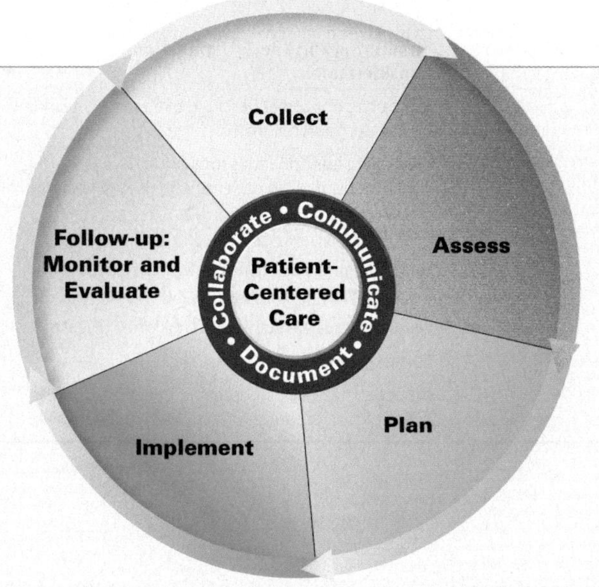

Patient Care Process for the Management of Hypercalcemia

Collect

- Patient characteristics (eg, age, race, sex)
- Patient history (past medical, family, social—dietary habits)
- Evaluate symptoms (see the "Clinical Presentation: Hypercalcemia" section)
- Current medications, including over-the-counter medications, herbal products, nutritional supplements
- Objective data (see the "Clinical Presentation: Hypercalcemia" section)
    - Blood pressure, heart rate, height, weight
    - Labs (serum calcium and albumin, ionized calcium when available)
    - Other diagnostic tests when indicated (eg, ECG)

Assess

- Plausible etiology for hypercalcemia (see Table 69-1)
- Acuity of symptoms and urgency for treatment (see Fig. 69-2)
- Current medications and dietary intake that may contribute to or worsen hypercalcemia
- Kidney function (eg, serum creatinine, creatinine clearance)
- Serum calcium goal

Plan*

- Pharmacotherapy based on etiology of hypercalcemia including specific dose, route of administration, frequency of administration, and anticipated duration of treatment (see Table 69-2)
- Monitoring parameters include efficacy (eg, reduction in serum calcium, resolution of symptoms), safety (adverse medication reactions), and timeframe (see Table 69-2)
- Patient education (eg, purpose of treatment, medication therapy, expected time to reduce calcium, need for future medications)

Implement*

- Provide patient education regarding all elements of treatment plan
- Schedule follow-up based on acuity and symptoms

Follow-up: Monitor and Evaluate

- Measure serum calcium to determine response
- Presence of adverse medication reactions
- Consider alternative medication management if desired reduction in calcium is not achieved

**Collaborate with patient, caregivers, and other healthcare professionals.*

Patients with malignancy often require surgical or chemotherapeutic reduction of tumor load to control the exogenous supply of cytokines and hormones (eg, PTHrP) that cause hypercalcemia. In contrast, patients with medication-induced hypercalcemia generally respond to discontinuation of the offending agent.

Pharmacologic Therapy

Symptomatic Patient Management

2 For those patients with normal to moderately impaired kidney function (CKD stages 3a, 3b, and 4), the cornerstone of initial first-line treatment of severe, acute hypercalcemia or hypercalcemic crisis is volume expansion with normal saline to increase natriuresis and ultimately urinary calcium excretion (Table 69-2). Patients with symptomatic hypercalcemia are often extracellular volume depleted secondary to vomiting and polyuria; thus, rehydration with saline-containing fluids is necessary to interrupt the stimulus for sodium and calcium reabsorption in the renal tubule.[19] Rehydration can be accomplished by the rapid infusion of 1 to 2 L of normal saline followed by a maintenance infusion at 250 to 300 mL/hr, until the patient is fluid resuscitated and serum calcium approaches the upper limit of the normal range.[19] The precise rate depends on concomitant conditions (primarily cardiovascular and kidney) and magnitude of hypercalcemia. The saline infusion rate can be decreased to a rate that approximates the patient's intake of oral or IV fluids. See Chapter 68 for a thorough discussion of how to calculate water deficit and monitor patient's response to saline infusion. Loop diuretics such as furosemide (40-80 mg IV every 1-4 hours) have been used to increase urinary calcium excretion.[19] Loop diuretics block calcium (and sodium) reabsorption in the thick ascending limb of the loop of Henle and augment the calciuric effect of saline alone. Rehydration prior to loop diuretic use is critical because if dehydration persists or becomes worse, the serum calcium can actually increase because of enhanced proximal tubule calcium reabsorption.[20] The primary role for loop diuretics in the setting of hypercalcemia is to minimize the development of volume overload from the administration of saline (Fig. 69-2 and Table 69-2). Furosemide should not be used first-line as there is little evidence that supports the efficacy of furosemide in treatment of hypercalcemia.[20] Potassium chloride, 10 to 20 mEq/L (10-20 mmol/L), should be considered for addition to the saline infusion after rehydration is accomplished to prevent the development of hypokalemia that is a common adverse medication reaction of aggressive diuretic therapy. Serum magnesium concentrations should also

TABLE 69-2 Medication Dosing Table for Hypercalcemia

Medication/Brand Name	Starting Dosage	Time Frame to Initial Response	Monitoring and Special Population Considerations
0.9% Saline ± electrolytes	200-300 mL/hr	24-48 hr	Electrolyte abnormalities, fluid overload CI in kidney disease, heart failure
Loop diuretics • Furosemide/Lasix® • Bumetanide/Bumex® • Torsemide	40-80 mg IV q 1-4 hr of furosemide or equivalent	N/A	Electrolyte abnormalities (potassium and magnesium), CI in patients with allergy to sulfas (use ethacrynic acid)
Calcitonin/Miacalcin®	4 units/kg q 12 hr SC/IM	1-2 hr	Facial flushing, nausea/vomiting, allergic reaction, CI in patients with allergy to calcitonin
Pamidronate/Aredia®	30-90 mg IV over 2-24 hr	2 days	Fever, fatigue, skeletal pain, CI in kidney disease
Zoledronic acid/Reclast®	4 mg IV over 15 minutes	1-2 days	Fever, fatigue, skeletal pain, CI in kidney disease
Corticosteroids	40-60 mg oral prednisone equivalents daily	3-5 days	Diabetes mellitus, osteoporosis, infection, CI in patients with serious infections, hypersensitivity

CI, contraindicated; SC, subcutaneous.

be monitored, and magnesium replacement initiated if magnesium concentrations fall below 1.8 mg/dL (0.74 mmol/L). Rehydration with saline and administration of furosemide may result in normalization total serum calcium within 24 to 48 hours; however, patients should be monitored closely for fluid overload.[19,20] Hemodialysis with low or zero calcium dialysate is a treatment option in the case of failure or when calcium concentrations are life-threatening.[20] It should be noted that preparing a patient for hemodialysis takes time to achieve vascular access; thus, this approach is best suited for patients already receiving hemodialysis chronically.

Asymptomatic Patient Management

Calcitonin In those patients in whom saline hydration therapy is contraindicated (eg, severe heart failure, moderately-to-severely impaired kidney function), short-term therapy with calcitonin is a viable alternative agent to initiate reduction of serum calcium concentrations within 24 to 48 hours. In fact, calcitonin begins to reduce serum calcium concentrations within a few hours; however, the degree and extent of serum calcium concentration reduction are often unpredictable.[1]

Subcutaneous or IM administration of salmon calcitonin, 4 to 8 international units/kg every 12 hours, has been used to manage hypercalcemia in patients with malignancy.[3] The intranasal formulation of calcitonin has been used in doses of 200 to 400 international units daily; unfortunately, this has resulted in only mild decreases in serum calcium. The lack of significant efficacy of the synthetic intranasal formulation is the result of the lower potency and shorter duration of action as compared to salmon calcitonin.

Pharmacology Calcitonin decreases serum calcium concentrations, primarily by inhibiting bone resorption. It can also reduce renal tubular reabsorption of calcium, thus promoting calciuresis.[3] Calcitonin from salmon sources is most commonly administered subcutaneously or intramuscularly (for larger volumes), which may rapidly lower calcium concentrations initially, but the effect can be transient.[3]

Adverse Medication Reactions The adverse medication reactions from calcitonin (facial flushing, nausea, and vomiting) may limit patient acceptability. Allergic reactions, although rare, do occur; therefore, a test dose can be given prior to starting therapy. If marked erythema and/or wheal formation does not occur within 15 minutes after administration, then therapy can be initiated. Salmon calcitonin therapy is associated with tachyphylaxis caused by antibody formation to foreign proteins or molecules resembling the calcitonin polypeptide.[21] The addition of corticosteroid therapy increases effectiveness.[3]

Bisphosphonates Bisphosphonates block bone resorption efficiently, render the hydroxyapatite crystal of bone mineral resistant to hydrolysis by phosphatases, and also inhibit osteoclast precursors from attaching to the mineralized matrix, thus blocking their transformation into mature functioning osteoclasts.[3,9] The antiresorptive properties of this class of agents can provide long-term control of serum calcium and are the first-line therapy for cancer-associated hypercalcemia.

Pharmacology The first-line bisphosphonates to treat hypercalcemia are pamidronate and zoledronic acid.[22] The usual dose of pamidronate is 30 to 90 mg as an IV infusion given over no less than 2 hours and up to 24 hours.[22] Pamidronate also has the advantage of single-day therapy.[22] Zoledronic acid is a high-potency bisphosphonate with demonstrated effectiveness in the treatment of hypercalcemia of malignancy. Complete response has been reported in 88.4% to 86.7% of zoledronic acid-treated versus 69.7% of pamidronate-treated patients.[23] Zoledronic acid IV doses of 4 to 8 mg given over 15 minutes have resulted in normalization of serum calcium concentrations.[3] IV infusions of 0.02 or 0.04 mg/kg diluted in 5% dextrose (given over 20-50 minutes) have also been effective.[24] The onset of serum calcium concentration decline is slower with bisphosphonate therapy (concentrations begin to decline in 2 days and reach a nadir in 7 days); thus calcitonin therapy or other interventions may be necessary if more rapid serum calcium reduction is required.[22] Duration of normocalcemia after treatment is variable and dependent on the severity and treatment response of the underlying malignancy, but usually does not exceed 2 to 3 weeks.

Adverse Medication Reactions Fever is a common adverse medication reaction of IV bisphosphonate therapy. The safety of continuous bisphosphonate therapy in treating hypercalcemia of malignancy is unclear; however, zoledronic acid has been associated with atrial fibrillation.[25] Kidney function monitoring (eg, serum creatinine) is advised with the use of bisphosphonates, as kidney function declines and acute tubular necrosis occurs rarely.[26,27] It is advisable to evaluate serum creatinine within a week after the infusion and just prior to the next scheduled dose.[22] Osteonecrosis of the jaw is a rare, but serious adverse medication reaction. With osteonecrosis of the jaw, there is an area of exposed bone in the maxillofacial or mandibular region that does not heal within 8 weeks after diagnosis.[22] Higher potency bisphosphonates and longer durations of therapy are associated with increased risk.[28]

Denosumab

Pharmacology Denosumab is a monoclonal antibody that inhibits the receptor activator of nuclear factor kappa-light-chain-enhancer of activated B cells (NF-κB) ligand (RANKL), a principal mediator of osteoclast survival. Denosumab is FDA-approved for the treatment of patients with hypercalcemia of malignancy.[3] The medication is effective in treatment of patients with hypercalcemia of malignancy (with or without bone metastases) who are refractory to IV bisphosphonate therapy, that is, their corrected serum calcium remains above 12.5 mg/dL (3.13 mmol/L) after more than 7 days of therapy.[3] Denosumab has also been reported to successfully treat hypercalcemia after successful stem cell transplantation and restitution of osteoclast function in patients with osteopetrosis, a heritable disorder associated with defective osteoclast function.[2,29]

Adverse Medication Reactions Denosumab has been associated with osteonecrosis of the jaw.[30] Although advanced kidney disease has not been shown to affect the pharmacodynamics and pharmacokinetics of denosumab, severe, symptomatic hypocalcemia has been reported in CKD patients receiving the medication.[31] Close monitoring of serum calcium is recommended for patients with creatinine clearance (CrCl) <30 mL/min (0.5 mL/s).[22] This may be due to induction of a hungry bone-like syndrome and warrants careful monitoring.[32]

Corticosteroids Prednisone or an equivalent agent is usually effective in the treatment of hypercalcemia resulting from multiple myeloma, leukemia, lymphoma, sarcoidosis, and hypervitaminoses A and D.[9,33,34] Corticosteroids are effective because they reduce GI calcium absorption.[34] Corticosteroids may also prevent tachyphylaxis to salmon calcitonin.[35] Daily doses of 40 to 60 mg of prednisone or the equivalent have effectively normalized serum calcium values within 3 to 5 days followed by a reduction in urinary calcium excretion within 7 to 10 days. The disadvantages of corticosteroid therapy are its relatively slow onset of action and the potential for diabetes mellitus, osteoporosis, and increased susceptibility to infection.[36]

Cinacalcet The calcimimetic agent cinacalcet is approved for management of parathyroid carcinoma, primary hyperparathyroidism where parathyroidectomy is indicated but cannot be undertaken, and secondary hyperparathyroidism in patients with CKD on dialysis.[3,37] Cinacalcet is an allosteric modulator of the CaSr, and increases the sensitivity for receptor activation by extracellular calcium. This results in reduced PTH and serum calcium concentrations.[3,37] Cinacalcet administered at a starting dose of 30 mg orally twice daily has been used for the treatment of hypercalcemia secondary to parathyroid carcinoma. The dosage is titrated every 2 to 4 weeks in 30 mg increments until the desired serum calcium concentration is achieved. The maximum approved dosage is 90 mg four times daily.[3] Hypocalcemia is a common adverse medication reaction and patients with specific CaSR polymorphisms may be particularly susceptible.[37] Patients should have serum calcium measured within 1 week after starting or increasing the dose of this agent. The role of cinacalcet in the management of nephrolithiasis is still controversial, but it has shown benefits in patients with primary hyperparathyroidism.[38] Etelcalcetide is the first IV calcimimetic that is structurally different from cinacalcet but also acts as an allosteric modulator of the CaSR. Etelcalcetide is only approved to treat secondary hyperparathyroidism in hemodialysis patients (see Chapter 64).[39]

Pharmacoeconomic Considerations

Corticosteroids are inexpensive for treatment of asymptomatic hypercalcemia from a pharmacoeconomic standpoint; however, the low cost of the medication may be offset by the multitude of long-term adverse medication reactions and potential need for additional treatment. Calcitonin is only suitable for short-term therapy and thus the long-term pharmacoeconomic benefits are unknown. Use of bisphosphonates for the management of bone metastases of malignancy is associated with lower morbidity and health gains (quality of life) well below the typical cost-effectiveness threshold.[40] Due to calcitonin's faster onset of action, it may be added to bisphosphonate treatment for rapid serum calcium reduction. However, combination treatment with a bisphosphonate plus calcitonin likely results in similar outcomes and higher costs for moderate-to-severe hypercalcemia of malignancy.[41] The introduction of denosumab and its demonstrated efficacy in preventing and delaying skeletal-related adverse medication reactions while reducing hypocalcemia have prompted questions regarding its cost-effectiveness.[40] Although denosumab is associated with additional health gains compared to zoledronic acid, it may not offer economic advantages.[40] Additional considerations for choice of therapy include co-pay costs and patient assistance program availability for these agents.[42]

Nephrolithiasis from Chronic Hypercalcemia and Hypercalciuria

Patients who develop nephrolithiasis from hypercalciuria are most often treated with sodium citrate to prevent stone formation, thiazide diuretics to decrease urinary calcium excretion, or shock wave lithotripsy (Table 69-3). There are multiple approaches to treating and preventing future nephrolithiasis issues which include stone removal or disintegration, using medications to dissolve or prevent stone formation as well as dietary interventions to prevent stone formation.[18] Procedures such as shockwave lithotripsy are effective in disintegrating stones and subsequently allowing for their urinary removal; however, the procedure is painful and expensive. Urinary alkalinizing agents such as potassium or sodium citrate prevent growth of stone diameter, increasing the likelihood of spontaneous passage. These agents are available in liquid form, but must be taken consistently multiple times per day to maintain an alkaline urine.[15] Thiazide diuretics decrease urinary calcium excretion and reduce the potential for crystal formation and are commonly used for prevention.[18] Other agents such as calcium binding resins, natural plant extracts (*Phyllanthus niruri*), and reduction of dietary calcium offer little benefit.

HYPOCALCEMIA

3 Hypocalcemia (total serum calcium less than 8.6 mg/dL [2.15 mmol/L] or ionized calcium less than 4.4 mg/dL [1.10 mmol/L]) occurs infrequently in the outpatient setting and is most common in older adults, malnourished patients, and those who have received sodium phosphate as a bowel preparation agent.

Epidemiology

Hypocalcemia occurs in 15% to 88% of adult hospitalized patients.[1] Emergent treatment of hypocalcemia is rarely warranted unless life-threatening symptoms are present (eg, frank tetany or seizures).

Pathophysiology

Hypocalcemia is the result of alterations in the effect of PTH and vitamin D on the bone, gut, and kidney (see Fig. 69-1). The primary causes of hypocalcemia are vitamin D deficiency and postoperative hypoparathyroidism. Other causes include magnesium deficiency, critical illness, medications, hypoalbuminemia, blood transfusions, peripheral blood progenitor cell harvesting, tumor lysis syndrome, and mutations in the CaSr.[37,43-47] PTH concentrations are elevated in conditions of hypocalcemia, except hypoparathyroidism and hypomagnesemia.[48]

Vitamin D Deficiency

Vitamin D and its metabolites play an important role in the maintenance of extracellular calcium concentrations and in normal skeletal structure and mineralization. Vitamin D is necessary for the optimal absorption of calcium and phosphorus. On a worldwide basis, the most common cause of chronic hypocalcemia is nutritional vitamin D

TABLE 69-3 Treatment of Nephrolithiasis Associated with Chronic Hypercalcemia and Hypercalciuria

Intervention	Indications	Comments
Extracorporeal Shock Wave Lithotripsy		
Uses sound waves to break up stones, which then can pass spontaneously	Obstruction of the urinary tract, especially with stones >5 mm	Consider adjunctive use of potassium citrate to inhibit aggregation of residual fragments
Prevention of Stone Formation		
Alkalinizing agents	Prevention; Treatment for nonemergent active stones	Potassium citrate is preferred over sodium citrate as it decreases urinary calcium, inhibits calcium oxalate precipitation, and increases urinary citrate more
Potassium citrate PO 20 mEq three times daily or 30 mEq twice daily		
Sodium citrate PO 20-30 mEq twice daily		
Decrease Urinary Calcium Excretion		
Thiazide diuretics	Prevention	Medication of choice in patients with low bone density
Hydrochlorothiazide PO 50 mg daily		
Indapamide PO 2.5 mg daily		
Chlorthalidone PO 25 mg daily		
Binding Intestinal Calcium		
Cellulose sodium phosphate PO 10 g daily in three divided doses with meals	Prevention for those with absorptive hypercalciuria	Restrict dietary intake of oxalate-containing foods, concomitant magnesium therapy recommended, alternative to thiazides if intolerant or ineffective, initial dose dependent on urinary calcium excretion, monitor bone density
Inhibition of Crystal Formation		
Phyllanthus niruri plant extract PO 2 g daily	Prevention, after shock wave lithotripsy	Commercial preparations with *P. niruri* as the sole ingredient can be difficult to obtain, variable dosages reported
Low-Calcium Diet		
Less than 400 mg/day	Prevention	Monitor bone density prior to and periodically during treatment, limit oxalate restriction, can increase hyperoxaluria, high calcium intake may actually be more beneficial

deficiency. In malnourished populations, manifestations include rickets and osteomalacia. Nutritional vitamin D deficiency is uncommon in Western societies because of the fortification of milk with ergocalciferol. The most common cause of vitamin D deficiency in Western societies is GI disease.[9] Gastric surgery, chronic pancreatitis, small-bowel disease, intestinal resection, and bypass surgery are associated with decreased concentrations of vitamin D and its metabolites.[9] Vitamin D replacement therapy might need to be administered by the IV route if poor oral bioavailability is noted. Decreased production of 1,25-dihydroxyvitamin D_3 can occur as a result of a hereditary defect leading to vitamin D-dependent rickets.[48] Polymorphisms of the vitamin D receptor have been identified, and these genetic variations can contribute to increased risk of rickets associated with vitamin D and calcium-deficient diets.[49] It also can occur secondary to CKD if there is insufficient production of the 1-α-hydroxylase enzyme for the production of the 1,25-dihydroxyvitamin D_3. Treatment of hypocalcemia associated with CKD is reviewed in Chapter 62.

Hypoparathyroidism

Hypoparathyroidism can be caused by autoimmune disease, congenital defects, or iatrogenically by inadvertent removal of some or all of the parathyroid glands during thyroidectomy or from damage with radiation therapy. Surgery is the most common cause of chronic hypoparathyroidism, but only occurs in about 3% of patients who have undergone total thyroidectomy.[48] Chronic hypoparathyroidism that persists for more than 6 months may insidiously lead to hypocalcemia and thus most patients remain asymptomatic.[48] The chronic hypocalcemia may ultimately present as visual impairment secondary to cataracts.[50]

Hungry Bone Syndrome

An acute, symptomatic rapid fall in total serum calcium concentration (to values less than 7 mg/dL [1.75 mmol/L]) is common in patients who have recently had a parathyroidectomy or thyroidectomy. Hypocalcemia in these postsurgical patients is generally transient in nature.[48] The "hungry bone syndrome" is a condition of profound hypocalcemia whereby the bone avidly incorporates calcium and phosphorus from the blood in an attempt to recalcify bone.[51] Serum calcium concentrations should be monitored every 6 hours during the 24 to 48 hours following such surgeries, and pharmacologic doses of calcium can be necessary to prevent or minimize the decrease in serum calcium.

Hypomagnesemia

Hypomagnesemia of any cause can be associated with severe symptomatic hypocalcemia that is unresponsive to calcium replacement therapy (see Chapter 70). Reduced serum magnesium concentrations can impair PTH secretion and induce resistance of target organs to the actions of PTH.[48] Normalization of serum calcium concentrations in these patients is thus dependent on appropriate replacement of magnesium.

Critical Illness

During critical illness or postoperatively, hypocalcemia is common but usually mild. It is hypothesized that cytokines impair PTH secretion, decrease production of 1,25-dihydroxyvitamin D_3, and cause PTH end-organ resistance.[48]

Medication-Induced Hypocalcemia

Medication-induced hypocalcemia has been reported due to chelation of calcium (eg, oral sodium phosphate solutions, ethylenediaminetetraacetate, foscarnet), increased enzymatic processing of vitamin D (eg, phenobarbital, phenytoin, ketoconazole), decreased PTH sensitivity (eg, calcitonin), increased sensitivity of the CaSr (eg, cinacalcet), increased excretion of calcium (eg, furosemide), blocked bone resorption (eg, denosumab, bisphosphonates, fluoride), and induction of hypomagnesemia (eg, aminoglycosides).[31,48,52,53]

Chelating agents in blood (citrate) and in radiographic contrast media (ethylenediaminetetraacetate) can cause transient hypocalcemia.[43,44,48] Concentrated citrate is often used in hemodialysis catheter locks and to anticoagulate the dialysis circuit during continuous kidney replacement therapy.[54] Symptomatic hypocalcemia has been reported in patients exposed to citrate solutions, which is related to both the concentration of the citrate solution and capacity to metabolize citrate (ie, impaired metabolism with severe liver failure and tissue hypoperfusion).[55] Injection of citrate solutions greater than the volume of the dead space of the catheter lumen or accidental injection of citrate catheter lock solutions that are not intended for systemic administration has been associated with serious cardiovascular problems such as hypotension or cardiac arrest.[56] Oral phosphorus therapy, commonly used to treat patients with malabsorption syndromes caused by GI diseases, can also result in hypocalcemia by chelation.

The anticonvulsants phenobarbital and phenytoin cause hypocalcemia by increasing catabolism of vitamin D and thereby impairing calcium release from bone and reducing intestinal calcium absorption.[43] By decreasing PTH sensitivity, calcitonin can lead to hypocalcemia.[48] Cinacalcet increases the sensitivity of the CaSr potentially inducing hypocalcemia.[48] Loop diuretics such as furosemide can induce hypocalcemia by increasing calcium excretion.[48] Denosumab and bisphosphonates block bone resorption and can lead to hypocalcemia, especially in the presence of vitamin D deficiency, insufficient calcium intake, or PTH imbalance.[48] Medications that cause hypomagnesemia (eg, aminoglycosides, amphotericin B, cyclosporine, diuretics, foscarnet, and cisplatin) are also associated with an increased risk of hypocalcemia.[57]

Clinical Presentation: Hypocalcemia

The clinical manifestations of hypocalcemia are quite variable. The more acute the decrease in ionized calcium concentration, the more likely the patient will develop symptoms.[48] Increases in plasma pH enhance the binding of calcium to albumin and thus alkalosis can result in rapid decreases in ionized calcium. Concomitant hypomagnesemia, hypokalemia, hyponatremia, and additive adverse medications reactions also increase the likelihood of symptomatic presentation.

Hypocalcemia can manifest as neuromuscular, central nervous system (CNS), dermatologic, and cardiac sequelae.[1] Acute hypocalcemia is more likely to manifest as neuromuscular (paresthesia, muscle cramps, tetany, and laryngeal spasm), and cardiovascular symptoms, whereas chronic hypocalcemia often presents as CNS (eg, depression, anxiety, memory loss, confusion, hallucinations, tonic–clonic seizures) and dermatologic (eg, hair loss, grooved and brittle nails, eczema) symptoms.[43] The hallmark sign of acute hypocalcemia is tetany caused by enhanced peripheral neuromuscular irritability.[1] Tetany manifests as paresthesia around the mouth and in the extremities, muscle spasms and cramps, carpopedal (hands and feet) spasms, and rarely as laryngospasm and bronchospasm.[9] Chvostek and/or Trousseau signs can be elicited during physical examination.[48] Chvostek sign is elicited by tapping the facial nerve anterior to the ear and eliciting twitching of facial muscles. The sensitivity and specificity of Chvostek sign for hypocalcemia are limited; a positive Chvostek sign is observed in 25% of healthy individuals and 29% of patients with hypocalcemia are negative.[48] Trousseau sign is elicited by inflating a blood pressure cuff above systolic blood pressure for 3 minutes and observing whether a carpal spasm is induced. With only 1% of healthy individuals with a positive Trousseau, this sign has greater specificity for hypocalcemia.[48]

CLINICAL PRESENTATION Hypocalcemia

General

- Acute hypocalcemia may result in rapid decreases in serum ionized calcium. Parathyroidectomy and thyroidectomy are also associated with a rapid reduction in serum calcium. In chronic hypocalcemia, vitamin D deficiency should be considered.

Symptoms

- The symptoms of hypocalcemia include tetany, paresthesia, muscle cramps, and laryngeal spasms. Chronic hypocalcemia is usually associated with depression, anxiety, memory loss, and confusion.

Signs

- Neurologic: The hallmark of acute hypocalcemia is tetany, which is characterized by neuromuscular irritability including seizure potential. Extrapyramidal disorders, mainly parkinsonism but also dystonia, hemiballismus, choreoathetosis, and oculogyric crises occur in 5% to 10% of patients with idiopathic hypoparathyroidism. Chvostek and/or Trousseau signs can be elicited during physical examination.
- Dermatologic: The skin can be dry, puffy, and coarse. Other dermatologic manifestations can include hyperpigmentation, dermatitis, eczema, and psoriasis. Hair and skin signs including coarse, brittle, and sparse hair with patchy alopecia and brittle nails can also appear.
- Ophthalmologic: Cataract development has been reported to occur with hypocalcemia.
- Dental manifestations: These are usually associated with the presence of chronic hypocalcemia in early development. Signs include dental hypoplasia, failure of tooth eruption, defective enamel and root formation, and abraded carious teeth.
- Cardiovascular: Hypotension, decreased myocardial performance, and heart failure have been reported. A prolonged QT interval, arrhythmias, and bradycardia can also occur but are more common with acute or severe hypocalcemia.
- GI: Steatorrhea can be associated with chronic hypocalcemia.
- Musculoskeletal: Myopathy has been reported.
- Endocrine: Hypocalcemia alone can impair insulin release. In addition, idiopathic hypoparathyroidism can be associated with polyglandular autoimmune syndromes.

Laboratory Tests

- Serum calcium concentrations of less than 8.6 mg/dL (2.15 mmol/L) are considered to represent hypocalcemia if ionized calcium values are also less than 4.4 mg/dL (1.1 mmol/L).

The cardiovascular manifestations of hypocalcemia result in ECG changes characterized by a prolonged QT interval and symptoms of decreased myocardial contractility often associated with heart failure.[43] Both acute and chronic hypocalcemia can result in a reversible syndrome characterized by acute myocardial failure or refractory heart failure. Other cardiovascular manifestations include arrhythmias, bradycardia, and hypotension that are unresponsive to fluid and vasopressor administration.[43]

TREATMENT

Desired Outcome

4 The goals of therapy for patients with normal kidney function are the resolution of signs and symptoms of hypocalcemia, restoration of normocalcemia, management of associated electrolyte abnormalities, and treatment of the underlying cause of hypocalcemia. The goals for patients with CKD are different and are discussed in Chapter 62. Asymptomatic hypocalcemia associated with hypoalbuminemia requires no treatment because ionized (biologically active) plasma calcium concentrations are normal. Treatment of hypocalcemia is dependent on identification of the pathogenesis of the underlying disorder, acuteness of onset, and presence and severity of symptoms.

Pharmacologic Therapy

Treatment of hypocalcemia is driven by acuity of onset and how significant the ionized calcium is below the normal range. The first approach to treatment is to evaluate causes that will dictate corrective action. Acute symptomatic hypocalcemia will nearly always require parenteral administration of soluble calcium salts (Fig. 69-3).

Acute Treatment

The initial therapeutic intervention for patients with severe, symptomatic hypocalcemia (ionized calcium <4 mg/dL [1 mmol/L]) is to administer 0.5 to 1 g of calcium chloride (1 g calcium chloride = 13.6 mEq calcium) or up to 3 g of calcium gluconate (1 g calcium gluconate = 4.56 mEq calcium) IV slowly over 10 minutes.[1] The treatment of asymptomatic hypocalcemia is controversial, but many practitioners will supplement calcium to avoid negative consequences of hypocalcemia and progression to clinical manifestations.[1] For mild-moderate asymptomatic hypocalcemia (ionized calcium 1-4.48 mg/dL or 1-1.12 mmol/L), 1 to 2 g IV calcium gluconate is recommended, and in the case of severe, asymptomatic hypocalcemia, up to 3 g IV calcium gluconate is indicated as in symptomatic patients.[1] For critically ill patients who are asymptomatic with a serum total calcium less than 7 mg/dL (1.75 mmol/L), 1 to 2 g IV calcium gluconate may be empirically administered with follow-up measurement of ionized calcium.[1] In non-emergent, asymptomatic cases, calcium retention and safety are optimized by infusing calcium gluconate at

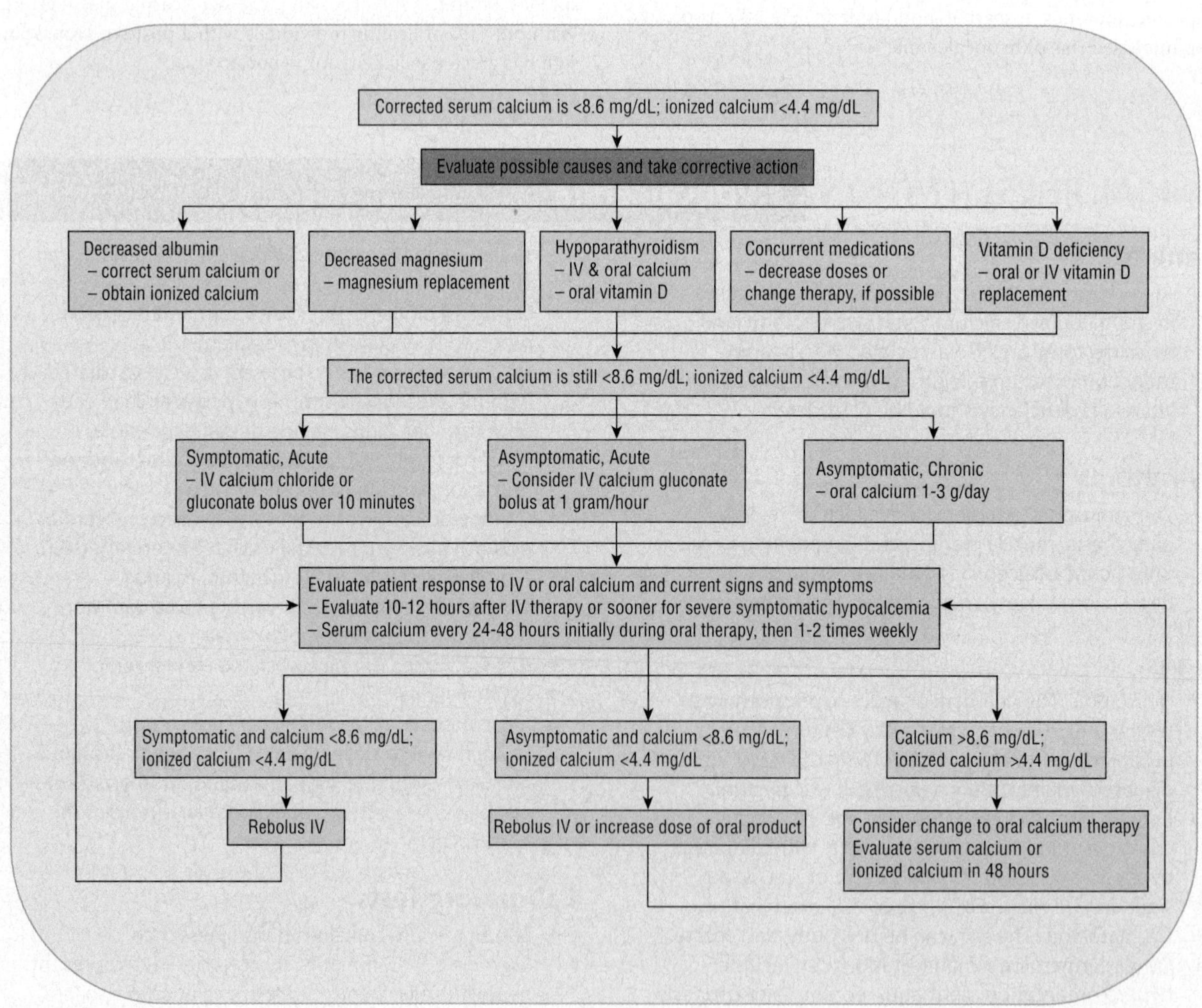

FIGURE 69-3 Hypocalcemia diagnostic and treatment algorithm. Serum calcium of 8.6 mg/dL is equivalent to 2.15 mmol/L and 4.4 mg/dL is equivalent to 1.10 mmol/L.

a rate of 1 g/hr.[1] Since calcium chloride delivers three times more elemental calcium than an equivalent amount of calcium gluconate, clinicians must carefully review dosing to ensure medication errors do not occur. Calcium gluconate is generally preferred over calcium chloride for peripheral venous administration because calcium gluconate is less irritating to veins. To prevent tissue necrosis, calcium chloride should be administered via central venous access. Calcium should not be infused at a rate greater than 60 mg elemental calcium per minute because severe cardiac dysfunction, including ventricular fibrillation, can result, thus ECG monitoring is recommended.[57] IV calcium administration should be used with caution in patients receiving digitalis glycosides because of the possibility of bradycardia or atrioventricular (AV) block.[50] In severe hypokalemia, an acute rise in serum calcium from IV calcium administration can result in cardiac arrhythmias. Bolus doses of calcium are only effective for 1 to 2 hours; therefore, repeat doses should be given hourly as needed until severe, symptomatic patients are stabilized.[1,57] Ionized calcium should be reevaluated approximately 10 to 12 hours after supplementation or sooner for severe, symptomatic hypocalcemia.[1] Calcium should not be added to bicarbonate- or phosphate-containing solutions or infused in the same IV line because of the possibility of precipitation.[57]

Chronic Treatment

Once acute hypocalcemia is corrected by parenteral administration, further treatment modalities should be individualized according to the cause of hypocalcemia. If hypomagnesemia is present, then magnesium supplementation is indicated until concentrations normalize, which will promote successful calcium supplementation regardless of route (see Chapter 70). Hypocalcemia secondary to hungry bone syndrome following parathyroidectomy has been attenuated by pretreatment with bisphosphonates, especially with longer duration use and normalization of alkaline phosphatase prior to surgery.[58] Asymptomatic and chronic hypocalcemia associated with hypoparathyroidism and vitamin D-deficient states can be managed by oral calcium and vitamin D supplementation. Therapy is initiated with 1 to 3 g/day of elemental calcium.[57] Average maintenance doses range from 2 to 8 g of elemental calcium per day in divided doses. If serum calcium does not normalize, a vitamin D supplement may need to be added. In patients with achlorhydria a solution of 10% (1-30 mL) calcium chloride orally every 8 hours can raise serum calcium.[57] Treatment of chronic hypoparathyroidism with PTH formulations such as teriparatide has been shown to better maintain serum calcium concentrations and normalize urinary calcium.[59]

Treatment of chronic asymptomatic hypocalcemia associated with vitamin D-deficient states should be individualized. The optimal 25-hydroxyvitamin D concentration is controversial, but the Endocrine Society defines vitamin D sufficiency as a concentration of at least 30 ng/mL (75 nmol/L).[60] In patients with malabsorption, vitamin D requirements vary markedly, and large doses can be required. In contrast, vitamin D deficiency associated with anticonvulsant medication can be corrected with smaller doses of vitamin D. The usual oral dose of ergocalciferol is 50,000 international units once weekly for 8 weeks followed by decreased maintenance dosing as needed to achieve the goal 25-hydroxyvitamin D concentration.[60] The treatment of vitamin D deficiency associated with CKD generally requires the administration of 1,25-dihydroxyvitamin D_3 or another synthetic vitamin D_2 analog such as paricalcitol or doxercalciferol (see Chapter 61). Patients who have reduced 25-hydroxylase activity (eg, hepatic disease) can also require treatment with calcitriol (1,25-dihydroxyvitamin D_3). Oral doses of 1,25-dihydroxyvitamin D_3 usually range from 0.5 to 2 μg daily. Vitamin D_3 (cholecalciferol) may be more efficacious at raising serum 25-hydroxyvitamin D concentrations compared with plant source vitamin D_2 (ergocalciferol). However, higher loading and maintenance doses of cholecalciferol may be required to maintain serum 25-hydroxyvitamin D concentrations. In selected cases, increasing calcium ingestion can be required if vitamin D replacement alone is ineffective in returning serum calcium concentrations to normal.

Adverse Medication Reactions

Adverse medication reactions of oral calcium and vitamin D supplementation include hypercalcemia and hypercalciuria, especially in patients with hypoparathyroidism, in whom the renal calcium-sparing effect of PTH is absent. Hypercalciuria can increase the risk of calcium stone formation and nephrolithiasis in susceptible patients. One maneuver to help prevent calcium stones is to maintain the urine calcium excretion below 300 mg/day. Intermittently monitoring of 24-hour urine collections for total calcium excretion can help minimize the occurrence of hypercalciuria. The addition of thiazide diuretics for patients at risk for stone formation can increase tubular calcium reabsorption and reduction of vitamin D requirements (see Table 69-3).[57]

DISORDERS OF PHOSPHORUS HOMEOSTASIS

Inorganic phosphorus in the form of phosphate is an essential element in phospholipid cell membranes, nucleic acids, and phosphoproteins, which are required for mitochondrial function.[61] Phosphorus regulates the intermediary metabolism of carbohydrates, fats, and proteins. Phosphorus also regulates enzymatic reactions including glycolysis, ammoniagenesis, and the 1-hydroxylation of 25-hydroxyvitamin D_3.[61] In addition, phosphorus is required for the generation of 2,3-diphosphoglycerate (2,3-DPG) in red blood cells, which is required for normal oxygen–hemoglobin dissociation and delivery of oxygen to the tissues.[61] Phosphorus is the source of the high-energy bonds of adenosine triphosphate (ATP), thus fueling a wide variety of physiologic processes, including muscle contractility, electrolyte transport, neurologic function, and other important biochemical reactions.[61] Considering its diverse biologic importance, it is not difficult to appreciate the clinical implications of disorders of phosphorus homeostasis.

Phosphate, the major intracellular anion, is present in living organisms mainly as organic phosphate esters such as 2,3-DPG, adenosine, guanosine triphosphate, and fructose 1,6-diphosphate.[61] Only a small fraction of intracellular phosphorus exists as inorganic phosphate; however, this fraction is critical because it is the source from which ATP is resynthesized.[61] The majority of inorganic phosphate is located in the extracellular space where it is the prime determinant of intracellular phosphate; thus, small increments in the organic phosphate concentrations can profoundly alter both the extracellular and intracellular phosphate concentrations. Metabolic disturbances (acidosis, alkalosis, and ketoacidosis), hydrogen ion shifts, and hormones (PTH, calcitonin, cortisol, and vitamin D) all can cause transcellular shifts in phosphorus concentrations. Because of these phenomena, the serum phosphorus concentration does not accurately reflect total body stores.[62]

The typical Western diet provides a daily intake of 800 to 1,600 mg of phosphorus. Approximately 60% to 80% of this is absorbed in the GI tract by passive and active transport (vitamin D-mediated). PTH, 1,25-dihydroxyvitamin D_3, and low-phosphate diets mediate increased absorption. Decreased absorption occurs under conditions of increased dietary intake of phosphorus and magnesium, glucocorticoid therapy, and hypothyroidism. The normal serum phosphorus concentration in adults is 2.7 to 4.5 mg/dL (0.87-1.45 mmol/L) and for children younger than 12 years it is 4 to 5.6 mg/dL (1.29-1.81 mmol/L). Influx via the GI tract and bone and tubular reabsorption by the kidney are the most important regulators of steady-state serum phosphorus concentrations. Renal excretion of phosphorus is a two-step process: glomerular filtration and proximal tubular reabsorption by passive transport coupled to sodium. Under normal conditions, 85% to 90% of filtered phosphate is reabsorbed, the majority in the early proximal tubule. Renal tubular reabsorption of phosphate is inhibited by PTH and 1,25-dihydroxyvitamin D_3.[62] Fibroblast growth factor 23 (FGF23) is a key regulator of phosphate homeostasis.[63] FGF23 acts principally to decrease tubular reabsorption of phosphate and inhibit 1-α-hydroxylase, thereby reducing the concentration of active vitamin D. FGF23-mediated receptor activation requires klotho, a transmembrane protein. The tissue specificity for FGF23 effects is defined by klotho–FGF23 coexpression. Conversely, phosphate reabsorption in the renal tubule is increased by growth hormone, insulin, and insulin-like growth factor 1.[61] Internal phosphorus balance (ie, transcellular phosphate distribution) is also of importance in the maintenance of normal serum phosphate. The serum phosphate concentration can vary by as much as 2 mg/dL (0.65 mmol/L) throughout the day, primarily as the result of changes in carbohydrate intake, insulin secretion, and diurnal variation.[61]

HYPERPHOSPHATEMIA

Hyperphosphatemia typically results from either CKD, AKI, or endogenous intracellular phosphate release. Hyperphosphatemia occurs frequently in patients with AKI and is a nearly universal finding in those with advanced CKD (eg, stages 4 and 5). Tumor lysis syndrome, a complication of chemotherapy associated with massive lysis of cells and release of intracellular contents, is also associated with hyperphosphatemia. The incidence of tumor lysis syndrome is highest among patients treated for acute lymphoblastic leukemia, acute myeloid leukemia, and Burkitt's lymphoma (see Chapter 155).[46] Other causes of hyperphosphatemia include hemolysis and rhabdomyolysis.

Pathophysiology

5 The most common cause of hyperphosphatemia is a reduction in renal tubular excretion of phosphate despite elevations in PTH and FGF23 when GFR is markedly impaired (eg, GFR less than 25 mL/min/1.73 m^2 [0.24 mL/s/m^2]).[62,64] Retention of phosphate decreases vitamin D synthesis and induces hypocalcemia, which leads to an increase in PTH, a finding that can be seen in those with stage 2 to 5 CKD. This physiologic response inhibits further tubular reabsorption of phosphorus as the kidney attempts to correct hyperphosphatemia and normalize serum calcium concentrations. Patients with excessive exogenous phosphate administration or who experience massive tissue breakdown or cell lysis in the setting of AKI can rapidly develop moderate-to-severe hyperphosphatemia (serum phosphate more than 6.5 mg/dL [2.10 mmol/L]).[62] Severe hyperphosphatemia (serum phosphate more than 7 mg/dL [2.26 mmol/L]) is commonly encountered in patients with CKD, especially those with GFRs less than 15 mL/min/1.73 m^2 (0.14 mL/s/m^2) (see Chapter 61).

Hyperphosphatemia caused by an increase in renal tubular reabsorption associated with hypoparathyroidism and associated decreases in PTH, is usually less severe than that observed in patients with advanced kidney disease or excessive exogenous or endogenous introduction of phosphate into the ECF. Acromegaly (mediated by growth hormone) and thyrotoxicosis (mediated by catecholamines) can also cause hyperphosphatemia by increasing tubular phosphate reabsorption.

Exogenous Phosphate Loads

Iatrogenic causes of hyperphosphatemia have been widely reported, and clinicians should be aware of the phosphorus content of IV, oral, and rectally administered products.[65] Although less-well recognized, oral and rectal administration of phosphate-containing solutions such as sodium phosphate (Fleet® Phospho-Soda) can also result in severe and life-threatening hyperphosphatemia, especially in patients with moderate-to-severe CKD.[53,65] The risk of mortality is dependent on the amount of phosphorus absorbed from the administered product; however, fatalities have occurred at low phosphate concentrations.[65] Acute phosphate nephropathy and kidney failure have also been reported with the use of oral sodium phosphate bowel preparations. The FDA issued a safety warning regarding the use of these products in patients at risk (ie, older adults, patients with CKD) or on medications known to affect kidney hemodynamics (eg, diuretics, nonsteroidal anti-inflammatory drugs [NSAIDs], or renin–angiotensin–aldosterone system inhibitors).[66] Acute phosphorus poisoning as a result of ingestion of laundry detergents is a rare and often unrecognized cause of elevated phosphate concentrations.

Rapid Tissue Catabolism

Any disorder that results in necrosis of skeletal muscle (ie, rhabdomyolysis) can generate the release of large amounts of intracellular phosphate into the systemic circulation. This condition is frequently associated with AKI (see Chapter 61) and thus severe hyperphosphatemia can develop because of increased endogenous phosphate release coupled with the impaired renal excretion because phosphaturic hormones (eg, PTH, FGF23) become ineffective. Bowel infarction, malignant hyperthermia, and severe hemolysis are also conditions that can increase endogenous release of phosphate.

Moderate hyperphosphatemia is also commonly observed in patients undergoing treatment for acute leukemia and lymphomas.[46] Chemotherapeutic treatment of acute lymphoblastic leukemia can result in the release of large amounts of phosphate into the systemic circulation secondary to lysis of lymphoblasts. Initiation of chemotherapy for Burkitt lymphoma results in tumor lysis syndrome, a rapid lysis of malignant cells that results in hyperphosphatemia, hyperuricemia, hyperkalemia, and hypocalcemia.[46]

Acid–Base Disorders

Lactic acidosis and diabetic ketoacidosis (DKA) can trigger the transcellular shift of endogenous intracellular phosphate into the extracellular space and thereby dramatically increases serum phosphorus concentrations.[67] After the institution of treatment, serum phosphate concentrations should be checked hourly as they can decrease rapidly, and patients can ultimately develop hypophosphatemia.

Clinical Presentation: Hyperphosphatemia

The severe acute onset of hyperphosphatemia can result in calcium and phosphate complexation and lead to the precipitation of calcium phosphate crystals in soft tissues, and within the kidney that can result in nephrolithiasis or obstructive uropathy. Extravascular calcification can result in band keratopathy, "red eye," pruritus, and periarticular calcification, especially in patients with CKD. In addition, soft-tissue calcifications in the conjunctiva, skin, heart, cornea, lung, gastric mucosa, and kidney have been observed, primarily in patients with CKD and chronic disordered mineral metabolism.[62] Extracellular phosphate can form insoluble nanoparticles with both calcium and fetuin-A which are referred to as calciprotein particles.[61] Calcium-phosphate crystals are likely to form in vivo when the product of the serum calcium and phosphate concentrations exceeds 50 to 60 mg^2/dL^2 (4-4.8 mmol^2/L^2). Serum phosphate concentrations greater than 6.5 mg/dL (2.10 mmol/L) have been independently associated with increased morbidity and mortality in patients on maintenance hemodialysis.[68] Other symptoms associated with moderate-to-severe hyperphosphatemia include nausea, vomiting, diarrhea, lethargy, and seizures. The major effects of long-term hyperphosphatemia are related to the development of hypocalcemia

CLINICAL PRESENTATION Hyperphosphatemia

General

- Serum phosphate concentration is primarily determined by the ability of the kidneys to reabsorb phosphate; therefore, hyperphosphatemia is uncommon in patients with normal kidney function.

Symptoms

- Acute symptoms include GI disturbances, lethargy, obstruction of the urinary tract, and rarely seizures. Symptoms associated with chronic hyperphosphatemia include "red eye" and pruritus.

Signs

- The elevated calcium-phosphate product results in precipitation in arteries, joints, soft tissues, and the viscera. This can result in tissue necrosis, termed calciphylaxis or calcemic uremic arteriopathy.

Laboratory Tests

- Serum phosphate concentrations more than 4.5 mg/dL (1.45 mmol/L) represent hyperphosphatemia.

(caused by phosphate inhibition of renal 1-α-hydroxylase) and its related consequences, as well as vascular and organ damage resulting from the deposition of calcium-phosphate crystals. Hyperphosphatemia associated with CKD can result in renal osteodystrophy because of overproduction of PTH. This condition is discussed in detail in Chapter 62.

TREATMENT

Desired Outcome

Management of patients with acutely elevated serum phosphorus concentrations should be directed at avoiding GI and neurologic symptoms and preventing deposition in the urinary tract to avoid the development of AKI. The treatment of hyperphosphatemia is focused on returning serum phosphorus concentrations to the normal or near normal (for patients with CKD) range, with the goal to minimize the long-term cardiovascular consequences of calcium-phosphate deposition in the vasculature. The Kidney Disease Improving Global Outcomes (KDIGO) clinical practice guidelines suggest that for patients with CKD stages 3 to 5, serum phosphorus should be maintained in the normal range. In hemodialysis-dependent patients with stage 5 CKD, KDIGO suggests lowering elevated phosphorus concentrations toward the normal range (see Chapter 62).[69]

Pharmacologic Therapy

Severe symptomatic hyperphosphatemia manifesting as hypocalcemia and tetany may be treated by the IV administration of calcium. Although this can seem counterintuitive and many consider it controversial, for a patient with phosphate of 16 mg/dL (5.17 mmol/L) and calcium of 7 mg/dL (1.75 mmol/L), for example (the calcium–phosphorus product is 112 mg^2/dL^2 [9 $mmol^2/L^2$]), correction of severe hypocalcemia is of primary importance because of the critical nature of this disorder. If serum calcium concentrations are not critically low, the initial management strategy should include limitation of all exogenous sources of phosphate and efforts to block further absorption should be initiated. Hemodialysis can be initiated if the patient remains symptomatic despite these interventions.[57]

6 In general, the most effective way to treat nonemergent hyperphosphatemia is to decrease phosphate absorption from the GI tract by implementing phosphate-binding therapy and altering the dietary content of phosphate.[62] Phosphate binding agents containing divalent and trivalent cations (calcium, lanthanum, magnesium, iron, and aluminum), or sevelamer are the agents most frequently used in the prevention and treatment of hyperphosphatemia (see Chapter 62).[70] Long-term treatment with aluminum hydroxide and aluminum carbonate should be avoided because the use of these agents has been associated with anemia, CNS disorders, and bone disease.[70] Calcium and magnesium agents are available in oral suspension formulations, which can aid administration in acutely ill patients who are receiving enteral nutrition. The most frequent adverse medication reaction from phosphate-binding agents (especially calcium) is constipation. Typically, calcium salts are the preferred initial phosphate-binding agents except when there is concomitant hypercalcemia or evidence of vascular calcification. For long-term therapy with phosphate binders, it is recommended to avoid hypercalcemia and to limit use of calcium-based phosphate binders, and this may require additional non-calcium agents such as sevelamer.[69] Calcium-based phosphate binders may increase vascular calcification, but there is no difference in cardiovascular events for hyperphosphatemia treated with lanthanum carbonate versus calcium carbonate in patients undergoing hemodialysis.[71] The iron-based binders offer the potential advantage of enhancing iron absorption (ferric citrate coordination complex) or reduced pill burden (sucroferric oxyhydroxide).[72] Other mechanistic approaches are being evaluated to manage hyperphosphatemia. Tenapanor is an investigational drug that blocks paracellular absorption of phosphate in the GI tract and may eventually be FDA-approved for hyperphosphatemia treatment in adult patients with CKD undergoing hemodialysis.[73]

HYPOPHOSPHATEMIA

Mild-to-moderate hypophosphatemia is usually asymptomatic and associated with serum phosphate concentrations of 1.5 to 2.7 mg/dL (0.48-0.87 mmol/L), whereas severe hypophosphatemia that is frequently symptomatic is correlated with serum phosphorus concentrations of less than 1.5 mg/dL (0.48 mmol/L).[1]

Incidence

Hypophosphatemia has been observed in approximately 1% to 3% of the laboratory screening panels of patients who have been admitted to a hospital.[74] The incidence in hospitalized critically ill patients is 18% to 28%.[74] Unlike its severe form, mild or moderate hypophosphatemia seldom causes recognizable signs and symptoms.[1]

Pathophysiology

7 Hypophosphatemia can be the result of decreased GI absorption, reduced tubular reabsorption, or extracellular to intracellular redistribution.[61] Although mild-to-moderate hypophosphatemia is common and can occur in inpatients and outpatients, severe

hypophosphatemia is predominantly encountered in the acute care setting and can be associated with life-threatening symptoms, including seizures, coma, and rhabdomyolysis (Table 69-4).

Decreased GI Absorption

Phosphate-binding substances such as sucralfate, calcium carbonate, sevelamer, lanthanum carbonate, sucroferric oxyhydroxide, ferric citrate coordination complex, and aluminum- or magnesium-containing antacids have the potential to bind large amounts of phosphorus in the gut, thereby preventing absorption. If phosphate-binding agents are ingested on a chronic basis in conjunction with a dietary phosphorus deficiency, hypophosphatemia can result.[1] Patients who are receiving long-term phosphate-binding agents, those with peptic ulcer disease or CKD, and those who may be predisposed to moderate hypophosphatemia (eg, alcohol use disorder) are at highest risk for the development of severe hypophosphatemia. Hyperparathyroidism can cause hypophosphatemia as a result of decreased GI absorption of dietary phosphorus.

TABLE 69-4 Conditions Associated with the Development of Hypophosphatemia

Decreased GI absorption
Phosphate-binding drugs
• Sucralfate
• Calcium carbonate
• Aluminum/magnesium antacids
• Sevelamer
• Lanthanum carbonate
• Ferric citrate
• Sucroferric oxyhydroxide
Decreased dietary phosphorus intake
Glucocorticoids
Vitamin D deficiency/resistance
Hyperparathyroidism
Chronic diarrhea
Steatorrhea
Reduced tubular reabsorption
Hyperparathyroidism (primary and secondary)
Elevated FGF23
Recovery from burns
Rickets
Malignant neoplasms
Fanconi syndrome
Acute volume expansion
Metabolic acidosis
Renal transplantation
Vitamin D deficiency and/or resistance
Diuretics
• Loop diuretics
• Thiazide diuretics
• Osmotic agents
• Carbonic anhydrase inhibitors (acetazolamide)
Glucocorticoids
Sodium bicarbonate
Internal redistribution
Refeeding syndrome
Nutrition support
Parathyroidectomy (hungry bone syndrome)
Alcohol use disorder
Respiratory alkalosis
Diabetic ketoacidosis (correction)
Dextrose solutions
Insulin
Catecholamines
Anabolic steroids
Glucagon
Calcitonin
Erythropoietin

Decreased Tubular Reabsorption

Reduced tubular reabsorption of phosphate can occur in patients with hyperparathyroidism (primary and secondary) with normal kidney function and those with vitamin D deficiency or elevated FGF23 concentrations. Elevated PTH concentrations lead to an increase in serum calcium concentrations and decreased serum phosphate concentrations. Serum phosphorus is decreased as the result of a reduction in renal tubular reabsorption.[67] Recovery from extensive third-degree burns is associated with development of an anabolic state as stress levels decrease and nutritional therapies take effect as well as a marked diuretic phase associated with an impressive renal loss of phosphate.[75] Because phosphate is rapidly incorporated into the new cells, this can contribute to the severity of the hypophosphatemia. Medications that cause increased renal elimination of phosphate include diuretics (eg, loop diuretics, thiazide diuretics, osmotic diuretics), carbonic anhydrase inhibitors (eg, acetazolamide), glucocorticoids, and sodium bicarbonate.[1] The IV iron formulation ferric carboxymaltose has been associated with the development of hypophosphatemia in 51% of patients treated, and 13% of cases were severe (serum phosphorus less than 1 mg/dL [0.32 mmol/L]) and prolonged.[76] The mechanism is unclear, however, iron deficiency itself is associated with elevated FGF23.[77]

Internal Redistribution

Rapid refeeding of malnourished patients with high-carbohydrate, high-calorie diets with inadequate amounts of supplemental phosphate can result in severe symptomatic hypophosphatemia. This phenomenon is especially prevalent in patients with other underlying risk factors for the development of hypophosphatemia, such as alcohol use disorder.[75] The etiology of severe hypophosphatemia associated with nutrition support can be separated into two phases: acute, rapid hypophosphatemia secondary to intracellular shifts of phosphate resulting from glucose-induced insulin secretion; and the gradual decrease in serum phosphate concentration over 5 to 10 days secondary to tissue repair in the presence of phosphate deprivation.[78] The development of severe hypophosphatemia secondary to nutrition support can be prevented by appropriate phosphate supplementation. Adult patients with normal kidney function receiving parenteral nutrition require approximately 10-15 mmol of phosphorus per 1,000 kcal (2.4-3.6 mmol per 1,000 kJ) (see Chapter 165).[1] The Recommended Dietary Allowance of phosphorus for healthy adults is provided in one liter of most enteral nutrition formulations (see Chapter 166).[1] In severely malnourished patients, the phosphorus requirements are higher with the initiation of nutrition support.[1] Phosphorus requirements are also typically increased in patients with critical illness, thermal injury, traumatic brain injury, and liver resection.[1] Transcellular shifts in phosphate also occur after parathyroidectomy, causing severe hypocalcemia and hypophosphatemia because of hungry bone syndrome (deposition of phosphate and calcium in the bone).

Severe and prolonged respiratory alkalosis (a result of hyperventilation, pain, anxiety, and sepsis) can cause hypophosphatemia.[74] Respiratory alkalosis is thought to contribute significantly to the hypophosphatemia observed during alcohol withdrawal syndrome.[62] Although patients with DKA may present with hyperphosphatemia, the initiation of therapy to correct it can cause serum phosphate concentrations to decrease rapidly as phosphate shifts back into the intracellular compartment. In addition, the acidosis associated with the DKA state can cause a decomposition of organic compounds inside the cell and a release of inorganic phosphate into the plasma and subsequently into the urine.[79] The combination of intracellular phosphate breakdown and the shift of phosphate into cells on initiation of treatment can lead to severe hypophosphatemia. Medications associated with transcellular shifts in phosphate include dextrose solutions, glucagon, insulin, catecholamines, calcitonin, erythropoietic agents, and anabolic steroids.

Patients with alcohol use disorder are prone to a variety of serum electrolyte disorders including hypocalcemia, hypomagnesemia, hypokalemia, and hypophosphatemia. The etiology of hypophosphatemia in patients with alcohol use disorder is multifactorial. Malnutrition, poor dietary intake, diarrhea, vomiting, and the use of phosphate-binding antacids can all contribute to hypophosphatemia related to alcohol use disorder.[80] In addition, serum phosphate concentrations may decrease after hospitalization in patients with alcohol use disorder with the institution of dextrose-containing IV fluids as a result of an intracellular shift of phosphate.[78,80] Hyperventilation associated with the alcohol withdrawal syndrome can also contribute to the development of hypophosphatemia.[78] Patients with alcohol use disorder are particularly susceptible to the complications of hypophosphatemia such as rhabdomyolysis, which is often seen during withdrawal or refeeding.[78] Thus, serum phosphate concentrations should be routinely monitored in this patient population.

Clinical Presentation: Hypophosphatemia

The clinical manifestations of severe hypophosphatemia are diverse and many organ systems can be affected. It is likely that two primary biochemical abnormalities are responsible for most of the clinical manifestations of severe hypophosphatemia.[74] First, intracellular energy stores may be decreased secondary to depletion of intracellular ATP. This can result in disruptions in cellular function. Second, reduced red blood cell 2,3-DPG concentrations are associated with a shift to the left of the oxyhemoglobin saturation curve. This shift is associated with a decrease in the release of oxygen to peripheral tissues (secondary to increased oxygen affinity for hemoglobin) and may result in tissue hypoxia.[74] These metabolic disorders can be seen in a wide variety of organ systems.

Neurologic manifestations of severe hypophosphatemia can result in a metabolic encephalopathy syndrome characterized by irritability, apprehension, weakness, numbness, paresthesia, dysarthria, confusion, obtundation, seizures, and coma has been described in patients with severe hypophosphatemia.[75,78] Neuropsychiatric disturbances include apathy, delirium, hallucinations, and paranoia. Peripheral neuropathy and symptoms resembling Guillain–Barré syndrome have also been reported.[78]

Severe hypophosphatemia can result in significant dysfunction of skeletal muscle ranging from myalgia, bone pain, and weakness, with chronic hypophosphatemia, to potentially fatal rhabdomyolysis with severe acute hypophosphatemia.[75] Laboratory evaluations can help distinguish between chronic and acute on chronic hypophosphatemia. Elevated alkaline phosphatase, normal creatine phosphokinase, and normal to low phosphate and calcium are present in cases of chronic hypophosphatemia. In contrast, hyperkalemia, hyperuricemia, elevated blood urea nitrogen and creatinine, hypercalcemia, and myoglobinuria are often present in cases in which rhabdomyolysis complicates the acute or chronic hypophosphatemia.[68] Hypophosphatemia can result in acute respiratory failure secondary to respiratory muscle weakness and diaphragmatic contractile dysfunction. Thus, frequent assessment of serum phosphate concentration is indicated in patients at risk for respiratory failure.[74] Likewise, adequate treatment of hypophosphatemia in respiratory

CLINICAL PRESENTATION Hypophosphatemia

General

- Major conditions associated with symptomatic hypophosphatemia are chronic alcohol use disorder, nutrition support without adequate phosphate supplementation, and the chronic ingestion of antacids. Severe hypophosphatemia can also be seen during treatment of DKA and with prolonged hyperventilation.

Symptoms

- Except for the effects on mineral metabolism, the symptoms of hypophosphatemia are caused by two consequences (reduction of red cell 2,3-DPG and reduction of intracellular ATP concentrations), and can impact virtually all organ systems. The symptoms are predominantly neurological and can include irritability, apprehension, weakness, numbness, paresthesia, and confusion. Severe acute development of hypophosphatemia can result in seizures or coma.

Signs

- The initial response of bone to hypophosphatemia contributes to hypercalcemia and hypercalciuria. Prolonged hypophosphatemia can also result in rickets and osteomalacia.
- Neurologic: Severe hypophosphatemia can lead to a metabolic encephalopathy.
- Cardiopulmonary: Impaired myocardial contractility, respiratory failure secondary to ATP depletion, heart failure, new onset or worsening of an existing condition.
- Musculoskeletal: Proximal myopathy, dysphagia, and ileus have been reported. Acute hypophosphatemia superimposed on preexisting severe phosphate depletion can lead to rhabdomyolysis.
- Hematologic: Alterations in the hematopoietic system can also occur, resulting in hemolysis, reduction in phagocytotic and granulocyte chemotactic ability, as well as defective clot retraction and thrombocytopenia.

Laboratory Tests

- Serum phosphate concentrations less than 2.7 mg/dL (0.87 mmol/L) are indicative of hypophosphatemia; however, symptomatic hypophosphatemia typically is not evident until serum phosphate less than 1.5 mg/dL (0.48 mmol/L).

failure can aid in successful weaning from the ventilator.[74] Dysphagia and ileus have also been attributed to hypophosphatemia.[74]

Myocardial dysfunction may be impaired in the setting of hypophosphatemia and can result in congestive cardiomyopathy. This has been observed in patients with alcohol use disorder, and postoperative and critically ill patients. Depletion of cardiac ATP stores may be the cause of this syndrome.[81] Arrhythmias have also been reported in patients with hypophosphatemia. Because hypophosphatemia is a potentially reversible cause of heart failure, it should be considered in patients who experience an acute deterioration in ventricular function.

Hematologic manifestations of hypophosphatemia include decreased concentrations of 2,3-DPG, decreased red blood cell ATP, and membrane rigidity.[81] When red blood cell ATP decreases, cells become spherocytic and rigid, and are trapped and destroyed in the spleen.[81] Therefore, hemolysis can be a manifestation of severe hypophosphatemia. Reduction in ATP content of white blood cells can result in mobility, chemotaxis, phagocytosis, and bactericidal dysfunction.[78,81] These changes can contribute to an increased risk of infection in patients with hypophosphatemia.

Finally, prolonged hypophosphatemia may result in osteopenia and osteomalacia because of enhanced osteoclastic resorption of bone and limited crystallization constituents (phosphate), respectively.[80]

TREATMENT

Desired Outcomes

The goals of therapy are the reversal of signs and symptoms of hypophosphatemia, normalization of serum phosphate concentrations, and management of underlying conditions. Awareness of the clinical situations in which hypophosphatemia is anticipated (eg, alcohol use disorder, DKA, initiation of nutrition support in severely malnourished) is of vital importance in preventing and managing hypophosphatemia.

Pharmacologic Therapy

Pharmacologic treatment for hypophosphatemia will typically involve phosphorus salt supplementation. The acuity and other electrolyte conditions dictate the salt, formulation, and route of administration (Table 69-5).

Mild-to-Moderate Hypophosphatemia

Mild-to-moderate (1.5-2.7 mg/dL [0.48-0.87 mmol/L]) or asymptomatic hypophosphatemia can generally be treated by the administration of oral phosphate salts. Fixed-dose and weight-based phosphate supplementation may be used.[1] Oral phosphate salts in divided doses of 1 to 2 g (32-64 mmol) daily can be provided for mild-to-moderate hypophosphatemia (see Table 69-5). Phosphate concentrations should be monitored daily, with the goal of correcting the reduced phosphate concentration in approximately 7 to 10 days. The primary dose-limiting adverse medication reaction associated with oral phosphate replacement is the development of osmotic diarrhea. For patients who are unable to receive oral supplements, IV phosphorus supplementation may be required. A graduated dosing scheme for IV treatment of hypophosphatemia may be used in patients with normal kidney function.[1] For mild hypophosphatemia (2.3-2.7 mg/dL [0.74-0.87 mmol/L]), an IV phosphate dose of 0.08-0.16 mmol/kg is recommended.[1] In moderate hypophosphatemia (1.5-2.2 mg/dL [0.48-0.71 mmol/L]), an IV phosphate dose of 0.16-0.32 mmol/kg is recommended.[1] Patients with mild-to-moderate hypophosphatemia and impaired kidney function should receive reduced doses, typically ≤50% of the initial empiric dose, with careful monitoring of serum phosphate concentration because they are predisposed to phosphate retention.[1] In the setting of obesity (weight >130% IBW or BMI ≥30 kg/m^2), an adjusted body weight may be used to calculate phosphorus requirements to avoid overdosing. The maximum rate of IV phosphorus infusion is 7.5 mmol/hr.[1] Potassium and sodium are the available salts for IV phosphorus administration. For patients with concomitant hypokalemia, potassium phosphate can be used (1 mmol potassium phosphate = 1.47 mEq K).[1] Patients with hypophosphatemia and normal or elevated serum potassium concentrations should be treated with sodium phosphate (1 mmol sodium phosphate = 1.33 mEq Na).[1] In addition to phosphate supplementation for hypophosphatemia, dipyridamole can decrease renal phosphate leaking and increase serum phosphate. Doses of 75 mg four times daily have resulted in increases in serum 1,25-dihydroxyvitamin D_3 and decreases in serum calcium and urolithiasis events.[82]

Severe Hypophosphatemia

8 Patients with severe (less than 1.5 mg/dL [0.5 mmol/L]) or symptomatic hypophosphatemia should be treated with parenteral phosphate replacement. Thus, dosage and infusion recommendations, as well as response to parenteral phosphate replacement, are highly variable.[83] For severe symptomatic hypophosphatemia (<1.5 mg/dL [0.48 mmol/L]), an IV phosphate dose of 0.32 to 0.64 mmol/kg is recommended for patients with normal kidney function.[1] In critically ill trauma patients, doses up to 1 mmol/kg have been used.[84] IV phosphate therapy produces the desired increase in serum phosphate at 24 hours in 20% to 80% of patients. Response is dependent on the degree of phosphate depletion and replacement dose

TABLE 69-5 Oral Phosphorus Replacement Therapy with Phosphate, Potassium, and Sodium Content Per Packet or Tablet

Product	Phosphate Content	Potassium Content	Sodium Content
Packet			
Phos-NaK®	250 mg (8 mmol)	280 mg (7.1 mEq)	160 mg (6.9 mEq)
Tablet			
Av-Phos 250 Neutral®	250 mg (8 mmol)	45 mg (1.1 mEq)	298 mg (13 mEq)
K-Phos Neutral®	250 mg (8 mmol)	45 mg (1.1 mEq)	298 mg (13 mEq)
K-Phos No. 2®	250 mg (8 mmol)	88 mg (2.3 mEq)	134 mg (5.8 mEq)
Phospha 250 Neutral®	250 mg (8 mmol)	45 mg (1.1 mEq)	298 mg (13 mEq)
Phospho-Trin 250 Neutral®	250 mg (8 mmol)	45 mg (1.1 mEq)	298 mg (13 mEq)
Virt-Phos 250 Neutral®	250 mg (8 mmol)	45 mg (1.1 mEq)	298 mg (13 mEq)

Phosphorus 31 mg = 1 mmol; potassium 39 mg = 1 mEq = 1 mmol; sodium 23 mg = 1 mEq = 1 mmol.

administered.[80] The initial success is often followed in 48 to 72 hours by recurrent hypophosphatemia, necessitating close monitoring of serum phosphate and repeat administration of phosphate products as warranted.

Adverse Medication Reactions of Parenteral Phosphate

Parenteral phosphate supplementation is associated with risks of hyperphosphatemia, metastatic soft tissue deposition of calcium-phosphate product, hypomagnesemia, hypocalcemia, hyperkalemia or hypernatremia (dependent on which IV phosphate formulation is administered), and thrombophlebitis from potassium phosphate. Inappropriate administration of large doses of parenteral phosphate over relatively short time periods has resulted in symptomatic hypocalcemia and soft-tissue calcification.[61] The rate of infusion and choice of initial dosage should therefore be based on severity of hypophosphatemia, presence of symptoms, and coexistent medical conditions. Patients should be closely monitored with frequent serum phosphate determinations for 48 to 72 hours after starting IV therapy. Opinions are mixed regarding the optimal time to reevaluate serum phosphorus after supplementation. Monitoring serum phosphorus 12 to 24 hours after supplementation or daily may be sufficient.[1] However, for patients with severe hypophosphatemia, more frequent monitoring may be warranted.[1] It can be necessary to continue administration of IV phosphate for several days in some patients, although other patients may be able to tolerate an oral maintenance regimen. Monitoring should also include assessment of serum potassium, calcium, and magnesium concentrations. Hypomagnesemia secondary to intracellular shifts occurs frequently (27%-80%) in patients with severe hypophosphatemia.[70] Therapy with parenteral phosphate should be undertaken with great caution and at reduced dosage for patients with hypercalcemia or impaired kidney function.[78]

CONCLUSION

Initial treatment strategy should be based on acuity of onset and severity of symptoms. Because the etiologies of calcium and phosphate disorders are diverse, it is important to integrate the known or anticipated consequences of concomitant diseases into the treatment strategy. The patient's medication history should be comprehensively assessed to determine whether the electrolyte abnormality may be medication induced. After resolution or treatment of the acute calcium or phosphate disorder, the medication regimen should be evaluated periodically. This proactive interventional approach will facilitate the management of mild disorders in the community and can reduce the need for hospitalization.

ABBREVIATIONS

2,3-DPG	2,3-diphosphoglycerate
AKI	acute kidney injury
ATP	adenosine triphosphate
AV	atrioventricular
CaSr	calcium-sensing receptor
CNS	central nervous system
CKD	chronic kidney disease
CrCl	creatinine clearance
DKA	diabetic ketoacidosis
ECF	extracellular fluid
ECG	electrocardiogram
FDA	Food and Drug Administration
FGF23	fibroblast growth factor 23
GFR	glomerular filtration rate
GI	gastrointestinal
IV	intravenous
KDIGO	Kidney Disease Improving Global Outcomes
NSAID	nonsteroidal anti-inflammatory drug
PTH	parathyroid hormone
PTHrP	PTH-related protein
PTHR1	PTH receptor (type I)

REFERENCES

1. Kraft MD. Phosphorus and calcium: A review for the adult nutrition support clinician. *Nutr Clin Pract.* 2015;30(1):21–33. doi:10.1177/0884533614565251.
2. Khan AA, Hanley DA, Rizzoli R, et al. Primary hyperparathyroidism: Review and recommendations on evaluation, diagnosis, and management. A Canadian and international consensus. *Osteoporos Int.* 2017;28(1):1–19. doi:10.1007/s00198-016-3716-2.
3. Asonitis N, Angelousi A, Zafeiris C, et al. Diagnosis, pathophysiology and management of hypercalcemia in malignancy: Review of the Literature. *Horm Metab Res.* 2019;51(12):770–778. doi:10.1055/a-1049-0647.
4. Silva BC, Cusano NE, Bilezikian JP. Primary hyperparathyroidism. *Best Pract Res Clin Endocrinol Metab.* 2018;32(5):593–607. doi:10.1016/j.beem.2018.09.004.
5. McCauley LK, Martin TJ. Twenty-five years of PTHrP progress: From cancer hormone to multifunctional cytokine. *J Bone Miner Res.* 2012;27(6):1231–1239. doi:10.1002/jbmr.1617.
6. Shapiro HI, Davis KA. Hypercalcemia and "primary" hyperparathyroidism during lithium therapy. *Am J Psychiatry.* 2015;172(1):12–15. doi:10.1176/appi.ajp.2013.13081057.
7. Machado MC, Bruce-Mensah A, Whitmire M, et al. Hypercalcemia associated with calcium supplement use: Prevalence and characteristics in hospitalized patients. *J Clin Med.* 2015;4(3):414–424. doi:10.3390/jcm4030414.
8. Bernstein E, Saly DL, Rastegar A. Patient with lethargy and hypercalcemia. *Am J Kidney Dis.* 2019;73(5):A14–A16. doi:10.1053/j.ajkd.2018.06.035.
9. Moe SM. Disorders involving calcium, phosphorus, and magnesium. *Prim Care.* 2008;35(2):215–237, v-vi. doi:10.1016/j.pop.2008.01.007.
10. Shlapack MA, Rizvi AA, Lopez FA. Normocalcemic primary hyperparathyroidism-characteristics and clinical significance of an emerging entity. *Am J Med Sci.* 2012;343(2):163–166. doi:10.1097/MAJ.0b013e31823bbb9b.
11. Ahmad S, Kuraganti G, Steenkamp D. Hypercalcemic crisis: A clinical review. *Am J Med.* 2015;128(3):239–245. doi:10.1016/j.amjmed.2014.09.030.
12. Karwowski W, Naumnik B, Szczepanski M, et al. The mechanism of vascular calcification: A systematic review. *Med Sci Monit.* 2012;18(1):RA1–11.
13. McCarty MF, DiNicolantonio JJ. The molecular biology and pathophysiology of vascular calcification. *Postgrad Med.* 2014;126(2):54–64. doi:10.3810/pgm.2014.03.2740.
14. Vella A, Gerber TC, Hayes DL, et al. Digoxin, hypercalcaemia, and cardiac conduction. *Postgrad Med J.* 1999;75(887):554–556.
15. Cong X, Shen L, Gu X. Current opinions on nephrolithiasis associated with primary hyperparathyroidism. *Urolithiasis.* 2018;46(5):453–457. doi:10.1007/s00240-018-1038-x.
16. Silverberg SJ, Clarke BL, Peacock M, et al. Current issues in the presentation of asymptomatic primary hyperparathyroidism: Proceedings of the Fourth International Workshop. *J Clin Endocrinol Metab.* 2014;99(10):3580–3594. doi:10.1210/jc.2014-1415.
17. Ramaswamy K, Killilea DW, Kapahi P, et al. The elementome of calcium-based urinary stones and its role in urolithiasis. *Nat Rev Urol.* 2015;12(10):543–557. doi:10.1038/nrurol.2015.208.
18. Tarplin S, Ganesan V, Monga M. Stone formation and management after bariatric surgery. *Nat Rev Urol.* 2015;12(5):263–270. doi:10.1038/nrurol.2015.67.
19. Minisola S, Pepe J, Piemonte S, et al. The diagnosis and management of hypercalcaemia. *BMJ.* 2015;350:h2723. doi:10.1136/bmj.h2723.
20. Carrick AI, Costner HB. Rapid fire: Hypercalcemia. *Emerg Med Clin North Am.* 2018;36(3):549–555. doi:10.1016/j.emc.2018.04.008.
21. Grauer A, Ziegler R, Raue F. Clinical significance of antibodies against calcitonin. *Exp Clin Endocrinol Diabetes.* 1995;103(6):345–351. doi:10.1055/s-0029-1211376.
22. Van Poznak C, Somerfield MR, Moy B. Role of bone-modifying agents in metastatic breast cancer: An American Society of Clinical Oncology-Cancer Care Ontario Focused Guideline Update Summary. *J Oncol Pract.* 2017;13(12):822–824. doi:10.1200/JOP.2017.027672.
23. Major P, Lortholary A, Hon J, et al. Zoledronic acid is superior to pamidronate in the treatment of hypercalcemia of malignancy: A pooled

analysis of two randomized, controlled clinical trials. *J Clin Oncol.* 2001;19(2):558–567. doi:10.1200/JCO.2001.19.2.558.
24. Body JJ, Lortholary A, Romieu G, et al. A dose-finding study of zoledronate in hypercalcemic cancer patients. *J Bone Miner Res.* 1999;14(9):1557–1561. doi:10.1359/jbmr.1999.14.9.1557.
25. Kim DH, Rogers JR, Fulchino LA, et al. Bisphosphonates and risk of cardiovascular events: A meta-analysis. *PLoS One.* 2015;10(4):e0122646. doi:10.1371/journal.pone.0122646.
26. Edwards BJ, Usmani S, Raisch DW, et al. Acute kidney injury and bisphosphonate use in cancer: A report from the research on adverse drug events and reports (RADAR) project. *J Oncol Pract.* 2013;9(2):101–106. doi:10.1200/JOP.2011.000486.
27. Yachoui R. Early onset acute tubular necrosis following single infusion of zoledronate. *Clin Cases Miner Bone Metab.* 2016;13(2):154–156. doi:10.11138/ccmbm/2016.13.2.154.
28. Allen MR. Medication-related osteonecrosis of the jaw: Basic and translational science updates. *Oral Maxillofac Surg Clin North Am.* 2015;27(4):497–508. doi:10.1016/j.coms.2015.06.002.
29. Shroff R, Beringer O, Rao K, et al. Denosumab for post-transplantation hypercalcemia in osteopetrosis. *N Engl J Med.* 2012;367(18):1766–1767. doi:10.1056/NEJMc1206193.
30. You T, Lee KH, Lee SH, et al. Denosumab-related osteonecrosis of the jaw: A case report and management based on pharmacokinetics. *Oral Surg Oral Med Oral Pathol Oral Radiol.* 2015;120(5):548–553. doi:10.1016/j.oooo.2015.07.017.
31. Lambe G, Malvathu R, Thomas HM, et al. Hypocalcaemic tetany occurring post a single denosumab dose in a patient with stage 4 chronic kidney disease, followed by calcium- and calcitriol-induced hypercalcaemia. *Nephrology (Carlton).* 2015;20(8):583–584. doi:10.1111/nep.12432.
32. Martin-Baez IM, Blanco-Garcia R, Alonso-Suarez M, et al. Severe hypocalcaemia post-denosumab. *Nefrologia.* 2013;33(4):614–615. doi:10.3265/Nefrologia.pre2013.Apr.11922.
33. Stewart AF. Clinical practice. Hypercalcemia associated with cancer. *N Engl J Med.* 2005;352(4):373–379. doi:10.1056/NEJMcp042806.
34. Malangone S, Campen CJ. Hypercalcemia of Malignancy. *J Adv Pract Oncol.* 2015;6(6):586–592.
35. Lewis MA, Hendrickson AW, Moynihan TJ. Oncologic emergencies: Pathophysiology, presentation, diagnosis, and treatment. *CA Cancer J Clin.* 2011;61(5):287–314. doi:10.3322/caac.20124.
36. Wright JD, Tergas AI, Ananth CV, et al. Quality and outcomes of treatment of hypercalcemia of malignancy. *Cancer Invest.* 2015;33(8):331–339. doi:10.3109/07357907.2015.1047506.
37. Filopanti M, Corbetta S, Barbieri AM, et al. Pharmacology of the calcium sensing receptor. *Clin Cases Miner Bone Metab.* 2013;10(3):162–165.
38. Brardi S, Cevenini G, Verdacchi T, et al. Use of cinacalcet in nephrolithiasis associated with normocalcemic or hypercalcemic primary hyperparathyroidism: Results of a prospective randomized pilot study. *Arch Ital Urol Androl.* 2015;87(1):66–71. doi:10.4081/aiua.2015.1.66.
39. Harada K, Fujioka A, Konno M, et al. Pharmacology of Parsabiv® (etelcalcetide, ONO-5163/AMG 416), a novel allosteric modulator of the calcium-sensing receptor, for secondary hyperparathyroidism in hemodialysis patients. *Eur J Pharmacol.* 2019;842:139–145. doi:10.1016/j.ejphar.2018.10.021.
40. Andronis L, Goranitis I, Bayliss S, et al. Cost-effectiveness of treatments for the management of bone metastases: A systematic literature review. *Pharmacoeconomics.* 2018;36(3):301–322. doi:10.1007/s40273-017-0595-0.
41. Khan AA, Gurnani PK, Peksa GD, et al. Bisphosphonate versus bisphosphonate and calcitonin for the treatment of moderate to severe hypercalcemia of malignancy. *Ann Pharmacother.* 2021;55(3):277–285. doi:10.1177/1060028020957048.
42. Arellano J, Hauber AB, Mohamed AF, et al. Physicians' preferences for bone metastases drug therapy in the United States. *Value Health.* 2015;18(1):78–83. doi:10.1016/j.jval.2014.10.004.
43. Fong J, Khan A. Hypocalcemia: Updates in diagnosis and management for primary care. *Can Fam Physician.* 2012;58(2):158–162.
44. Chung HS, Cho SJ, Park CS. Effects of liver function on ionized hypocalcaemia following rapid blood transfusion. *J Int Med Res.* 2012;40(2):572–582. doi:10.1177/147323001204000219.
45. Kishimoto M, Ohto H, Shikama Y, et al. Treatment for the decline of ionized calcium levels during peripheral blood progenitor cell harvesting. *Transfusion.* 2002;42(10):1340–1347.
46. Wilson FP, Berns JS. Tumor lysis syndrome: New challenges and recent advances. *Adv Chronic Kidney Dis.* 2014;21(1):18–26. doi:10.1053/j.ackd.2013.07.001.
47. Choi KH, Shin CH, Yang SW, et al. Autosomal dominant hypocalcemia with Bartter syndrome due to a novel activating mutation of calcium sensing receptor, Y829C. *Korean J Pediatr.* 2015;58(4):148–153. doi:10.3345/kjp.2015.58.4.148.
48. Bove-Fenderson E, Mannstadt M. Hypocalcemic disorders. *Best Pract Res Clin Endocrinol Metab.* 2018;32(5):639–656. doi:10.1016/j.beem.2018.05.006.
49. Kitanaka S, Isojima T, Takaki M, et al. Association of vitamin D-related gene polymorphisms with manifestation of vitamin D deficiency in children. *Endocr J.* 2012;59(11):1007–1014.
50. De Sanctis V, Soliman A, Fiscina B. Hypoparathyroidism: From diagnosis to treatment. *Curr Opin Endocrinol Diabetes Obes.* 2012;19(6):435–442. doi:10.1097/MED.0b013e3283591502.
51. Tachibana S, Sato S, Yokoi T, et al. Severe hypocalcemia complicated by postsurgical hypoparathyroidism and hungry bone syndrome in a patient with primary hyperparathyroidism, Graves' disease, and acromegaly. *Intern Med.* 2012;51(14):1869–1873.
52. Sensipar (cinacalcet HCL) [package insert]. In: Incorporated A, editor. Thousand Oaks, CA; 2014.
53. Kan WC, Wang HY, Chien CC, et al. Intermediate bioelectrolyte changes after phospho-soda or polyethylene glycol precolonoscopic laxatives in a population undergoing health examinations. *Nephrol Dial Transplant.* 2012;27(2):752–757. doi:10.1093/ndt/gfr189.
54. Yon CK, Low CL. Sodium citrate 4% versus heparin as a lock solution in hemodialysis patients with central venous catheters. *Am J Health Syst Pharm.* 2013;70(2):131–136. doi:10.2146/ajhp120300.
55. Morabito S, Pistolesi V, Tritapepe L, et al. Regional citrate anticoagulation for RRTs in critically ill patients with AKI. *Clin J Am Soc Nephrol.* 2014;9(12):2173–2188. doi:10.2215/cjn.01280214.
56. Polaschegg HD, Sodemann K. Risks related to catheter locking solutions containing concentrated citrate. *Nephrol Dial Transplant.* 2003;18(12):2688–2690.
57. Kelly A, Levine MA. Hypocalcemia in the critically ill patient. *J Intensive Care Med.* 2013;28(3):166–77. doi:10.1177/0885066611411543.
58. Witteveen JE, van Thiel S, Romijn JA, et al. Hungry bone syndrome: still a challenge in the post-operative management of primary hyperparathyroidism: A systematic review of the literature. *Eur J Endocrinol.* 2013;168(3):R45–R53. doi:10.1530/eje-12-0528.
59. Cusano NE, Rubin MR, Irani D, et al. Use of parathyroid hormone in hypoparathyroidism. *J Endocrinol Invest.* 2013;36(11):1121–1127. doi:10.1007/BF03346763.
60. Holick MF. The vitamin D deficiency pandemic: Approaches for diagnosis, treatment and prevention. *Rev Endocr Metab Disord.* 2017;18(2):153–165. doi:10.1007/s11154-017-9424-1.
61. Brown RB, Razzaque MS. Dysregulation of phosphate metabolism and conditions associated with phosphate toxicity. *Bonekey Rep.* 2015;4:705. doi:10.1038/bonekey.2015.74.
62. Felsenfeld AJ, Levine BS, Rodriguez M. Pathophysiology of calcium, phosphorus, and magnesium dysregulation in chronic kidney disease. *Semin Dial.* 2015;28(6):564–577. doi:10.1111/sdi.12411.
63. Kocelak P, Olszanecka-Glinianowicz M, Chudek J. Fibroblast growth factor 23: Structure, function and role in kidney diseases. *Adv Clin Exp Med.* 2012;21(3):391–401.
64. Blaine J, Chonchol M, Levi M. Renal control of calcium, phosphate, and magnesium homeostasis. *Clin J Am Soc Nephrol.* 2015;10(7):1257–1272. doi:10.2215/CJN.09750913.
65. Adamcewicz M, Bearelly D, Porat G, et al. Mechanism of action and toxicities of purgatives used for colonoscopy preparation. *Expert Opin Drug Metab Toxicol.* 2011;7(1):89–101. doi:10.1517/17425255.2011.542411.
66. FDA requires new safety measures for oral sodium phosphate products to reduce risk of acute kidney injury risk associated with both prescription and over-the-counter (OTC) products: Food and Drug Administration; Accessed October 11, 2021. Available at https://www.fda.gov/Drugs/DrugSafety/ucm380757.htm.
67. Kamel KS, Halperin ML. Acid-base problems in diabetic ketoacidosis. *N Engl J Med.* 2015;372(20):1969–1970. doi:10.1056/NEJMc1502745.
68. Block GA, Klassen PS, Lazarus JM, et al. Mineral metabolism, mortality, and morbidity in maintenance hemodialysis. *J Am Soc Nephrol.* 2004;15(8):2208–2218. doi:10.1097/01.ASN.0000133041.27682.A2.
69. Kidney Disease: Improving Global Outcomes CKDMBDUWG. KDIGO 2017 Clinical Practice Guideline Update for the Diagnosis, Evaluation, Prevention, and Treatment of Chronic Kidney Disease-Mineral and Bone Disorder (CKD-MBD). *Kidney Int Suppl. (2011).* 2017;7(1):1–59. doi:10.1016/j.kisu.2017.04.001.

70. Hutchison AJ, Smith CP, Brenchley PE. Pharmacology, efficacy and safety of oral phosphate binders. *Nat Rev Nephrol.* 2011;7(10):578–589. doi:10.1038/nrneph.2011.112.
71. Ogata H, Fukagawa M, Hirakata H, et al. Effect of treating hyperphosphatemia with lanthanum carbonate vs calcium carbonate on cardiovascular events in patients with chronic kidney disease undergoing hemodialysis: The LANDMARK Randomized Clinical Trial. *JAMA.* 2021;325(19):1946–1954. doi:10.1001/jama.2021.4807.
72. Pai AB, Jang SM, Wegrzyn N. Iron-based phosphate binders: A new element in management of hyperphosphatemia. *Expert Opin Drug Metab Toxicol.* 2016;12(1):115–127. doi:10.1517/17425255.2016.1110573.
73. Fishbane SN, Nigwekar S. Phosphate absorption and hyperphosphatemia management in kidney disease: A physiology-based review. *Kidney Medicine.* 2021 Aug 27 Epub. doi:10.1016/j.xkme.2021.07.003.
74. Chang WT, Radin B, McCurdy MT. Calcium, magnesium, and phosphate abnormalities in the emergency department. *Emerg Med Clin North Am.* 2014;32(2):349–366. doi:10.1016/j.emc.2013.12.006.
75. Subramanian R, Khardori R. Severe hypophosphatemia. Pathophysiologic implications, clinical presentations, and treatment. *Medicine (Baltimore).* 2000;79(1):1–8.
76. Hardy S, Vandemergel X. Intravenous iron administration and hypophosphatemia in clinical practice. *Int J Rheumatol.* 2015;2015:468675. doi:10.1155/2015/468675.
77. Wolf M, White KE. Coupling fibroblast growth factor 23 production and cleavage: Iron deficiency, rickets, and kidney disease. *Curr Opin Nephrol Hypertens.* 2014;23(4):411–419. doi:10.1097/01.mnh.0000447020.74593.6f.
78. Amanzadeh J, Reilly RF Jr. Hypophosphatemia: An evidence-based approach to its clinical consequences and management. *Nat Clin Pract Nephrol.* 2006;2(3):136–148. doi:10.1038/ncpneph0124.
79. Konstantinov NK, Rohrscheib M, Agaba EI, et al. Respiratory failure in diabetic ketoacidosis. *World J Diabetes.* 2015;6(8):1009–1023. doi:10.4239/wjd.v6.i8.1009.
80. Felsenfeld AJ, Levine BS. Approach to treatment of hypophosphatemia. *Am J Kidney Dis.* 2012;60(4):655–661. doi:10.1053/j.ajkd.2012.03.024.
81. Gaasbeek A, Meinders AE. Hypophosphatemia: An update on its etiology and treatment. *Am J Med.* 2005;118(10):1094–1101. doi:10.1016/j.amjmed.2005.02.014.
82. Liamis G, Milionis HJ, Elisaf M. Medication-induced hypophosphatemia: A review. *QJM.* 2010;103(7):449–459. doi:10.1093/qjmed/hcq039.
83. Agarwal B, Walecka A, Shaw S, et al. Is parenteral phosphate replacement in the intensive care unit safe? *Ther Apher Dial.* 2014;18(1):31–36. doi:10.1111/1744-9987.12053.
84. Brown KA, Dickerson RN, Morgan LM, et al. A new graduated dosing regimen for phosphorus replacement in patients receiving nutrition support. *JPEN J Parenter Enteral Nutr.* 2006;30(3):209–214. doi:10.1177/0148607106030003209.

Disorders of Potassium and Magnesium Homeostasis

70

Rachel W. Flurie

KEY CONCEPTS

1. Potassium regulates many biochemical processes in the body and is a key cation for electrical action potentials across cellular membranes.
2. The kidney is the primary route of potassium elimination.
3. In patients with concomitant hypokalemia and hypomagnesemia, it is imperative to correct the hypomagnesemia before the hypokalemia.
4. Potassium chloride is the preferred potassium supplement for the most common causes of hypokalemia.
5. Hyperkalemia is a common occurrence in patients with acute kidney injury or chronic kidney disease.
6. Hypomagnesemia is commonly caused by excessive gastrointestinal or renal magnesium wasting.
7. Hypermagnesemia is predominantly observed in patients with acute or chronic kidney disease.
8. Severe hypermagnesemia may affect the neuromuscular and cardiovascular systems.

BEYOND THE BOOK

Watch the video entitled "Hyperkalemia in Primary Care Practice" by the National Kidney Foundation. (https://www.kidney.org/content/hyperkalemia-primary-care-practice) This ~11-minute video provides a brief overview of the risks associated with hyperkalemia, the various causes of hyperkalemia, and prevention and treatment strategies. The video is useful to enhance student understanding of the COLLECT, ASSESS, and PLAN steps in the patient care process.

INTRODUCTION

Potassium and magnesium are electrolytes that are responsible for numerous metabolic activities. Disorders of these electrolytes are frequently seen in both the acute care and community ambulatory care settings. Therefore, clinicians need a firm understanding of the etiology, pathophysiology, symptoms, pharmacotherapy, and monitoring of these disorders. This chapter describes the homeostatic mechanisms that are responsible for the maintenance of normal potassium and magnesium serum concentrations. The clinical disorders responsible for the development of hyperkalemia, hypermagnesemia, hypokalemia, and hypomagnesemia are also reviewed.

POTASSIUM

Potassium is the most abundant cation in the body, with estimated total-body stores of 3,000 to 4,000 mEq (mmol).[1] Ninety-eight percent of this amount is contained within the intracellular compartment, and the remaining 2% is distributed within the extracellular compartment. The sodium-potassium adenosine triphosphatase (Na^+-K^+-ATPase) pump located in the cell membrane is responsible for the compartmentalization of potassium. This pump is an active transport system that maintains increased intracellular stores of potassium by transporting sodium out of the cell and potassium into the cell at a ratio of 3:2. Consequently, the pump maintains a higher concentration of potassium inside the cell.

The normal serum concentration range for potassium is 3.5 to 5 mEq/L (mmol/L), whereas the intracellular potassium concentration is approximately 150 mEq/L (mmol/L).[2] Approximately 75% of the intracellular potassium is located in skeletal muscle; the remaining 25% is located in the liver and red blood cells. Extracellular potassium is distributed throughout the serum and interstitial space. Potassium is dynamic in that it is constantly moving between the intracellular and extracellular compartments according to the body's needs. Thus, the serum potassium concentration alone does not accurately reflect the total-body potassium content.

(1) Potassium has many physiologic functions within cells, including protein and glycogen synthesis and cellular metabolism and growth. It is also a determinant of the electrical action potential across the cell membrane.[1] The ratio of the intracellular-to-extracellular potassium concentration is the major determinant of the resting potential across the cell membrane. Serum potassium concentrations outside the normal range can have disastrous effects on neuromuscular activity, in particular cardiac conduction. Hypo- and hyperkalemia are both associated with potentially fatal cardiac arrhythmias, along with other neuromuscular disturbances. Finally, potassium is integral to maintaining blood pressure, prevention of stroke, and potentially other cardiovascular diseases.[3] Both the National High Blood Pressure Education Program and the Institute of Medicine recommend potassium supplementation as a strategy for preventing and treating hypertension.[4,5]

Control of Potassium Homeostasis

Potassium homeostasis, the maintenance of serum potassium within the normal range, is affected by dietary intake, gastrointestinal (GI) and urinary excretion, hepatic and muscular sequestration, hormones, acid-base balance, body fluid tonicity, central and peripheral circadian clocks, and a highly integrated feedback mechanism.[6,7] Together, these mechanisms usually maintain total-body potassium content within a narrow window without appreciable changes in the serum potassium concentration.[6] Deviations in serum potassium concentrations outside the normal range are a result of nonhomeostatic processes that are not sensitive to changes in potassium balance.[6] The recommended adequate intake of dietary potassium in the United States is 2,600 mg/day for adult females and 3,400 mg/day for adult males.[8] Potassium is considered to be a nutrient of concern, because of its beneficial effects on blood pressure, reduction in the risk of kidney stones, and decrease of bone loss.[9] Potassium is abundant in fruits, vegetables, meats, whole grains, and milk products. Most dietary potassium is absorbed, with only 10 to 20 mEq/day (mmol/day) eliminated in feces. The amount eliminated in the feces increases, however, in patients with diarrhea and in those with chronic kidney disease (CKD).[7]

2 The kidney is the primary route of potassium elimination. Potassium is freely filtered, but almost all of it is reabsorbed passively in the proximal tubule and the thick ascending limb of the loop of Henle.[9] Although the amount of potassium filtered by the glomerulus approaches 700 mEq (mmol) per day, only approximately 10% to 20% is actually excreted in the urine.[9] Potassium excretion is regulated by its secretion into the distal tubule and collecting duct. Variations in potassium excretion are based on dietary intake, serum potassium concentration, and aldosterone activity. For example, more potassium is renally excreted in conditions that result in high aldosterone activity (eg, dehydration) when the body is attempting to conserve sodium or when there is an increase in dietary potassium intake. In addition, enteric solute sensors increase kaliuresis in response to high dietary potassium intake.[1]

Hormones such as insulin, catecholamines, and aldosterone dramatically affect potassium homeostasis. Aldosterone controls renal potassium excretion, which can take several hours to adjust serum potassium concentrations. Rapid buffering of serum potassium concentrations occurs through potassium cellular redistribution, of which insulin and catecholamines play a large role. Insulin is the most important hormonal mediator of potassium balance because it stimulates the cellular Na^+-K^+-ATPase pump to increase transport of potassium into liver, muscle, and adipose tissue.[6] There is a complex negative feedback loop in which insulin secretion tightly regulates serum potassium concentrations: an increase of only a few tenths of a milliequivalent of potassium stimulates pancreatic insulin secretion in an attempt to prevent hyperkalemia from developing.[1] If hyperkalemia does occur, glucagon is released from the liver to protect against insulin-induced hypoglycemia. Conversely, hypokalemia inhibits insulin secretion, a finding that explains why some patients receiving diuretics develop hyperglycemia.

An elevation in circulating catecholamines such as epinephrine usually results in the intracellular movement of potassium by two mechanisms.[9] Stimulation of the β-receptor, which directly activates the Na^+-K^+-ATPase pump and glycogenolysis, which raises blood glucose concentrations, thereby increasing insulin secretion. This dual mechanism is often used therapeutically in patients with hyperkalemia to normalize serum potassium concentrations.

Aldosterone, a mineralocorticoid that is secreted from the adrenal glands in response to high serum potassium concentrations, promotes urinary potassium excretion. Aldosterone acts on the distal tubule and collecting duct to promote the reabsorption of sodium and water in exchange for potassium. It also increases potassium permeability and transport across the luminal membrane of the nephron by stimulating the cellular Na^+-K^+-ATPase pump activity.[7] In patients with impaired kidney function, aldosterone increases potassium excretion in the distal colon.[10]

Changes in acid–base status can dramatically affect the serum potassium concentration. For example, the infusion of metabolic inorganic acids, such as hydrochloric acid, results in an increase in serum potassium. The body compensates for excessive hydrogen ions by moving them from the serum into the cell in exchange for intracellular potassium, to maintain electroneutrality. The processes by which this occurs are highly complex and involve cellular H^+-K^+-ATPase pumps and both Na^+-HCO_3^- and K^+-HCO_3^- cotransporters.[11] The efflux of potassium into the serum can result in hyperkalemia. A commonly quoted approximation of the pH effect is that for every 0.1 unit decrease in pH, serum potassium concentration increases by 0.6 to 0.8 mEq/L (mmol/L) (with a wide range of 0.2-1.7).[12] This is often referred to as *false hyperkalemia* because there is not a true excess of total-body potassium. Metabolic acidosis associated with lactic acidosis and ketoacidosis typically does not lead to clinically significant hyperkalemia, because both cations and anions enter the cell, thus maintaining electroneutrality.[1] Respiratory acidosis also does not significantly affect the serum potassium concentration.

Conversely, metabolic alkalosis has been associated with hypokalemia. As a result of a net loss of hydrogen ion from the serum, intracellular hydrogen ions enter the serum to increase the acidity of the blood. To maintain electroneutrality, extracellular potassium ions are shifted intracellularly. This creates a relative deficiency of potassium in the serum. Serum potassium decreases approximately 0.6 mEq/L (mmol/L) for each 0.1 unit increase in blood pH. This is frequently termed *false hypokalemia* because there is not a true deficiency in total-body potassium.

Finally, hyperosmolality can result in enhanced movement of potassium from the cell into the extracellular fluid. Water movement favors potassium efflux through solvent drag. As cells shrink, intracellular potassium concentrations increase, further promoting potassium efflux.[7] This is seen in conditions such as diabetic ketoacidosis. Conversely, hypoosmolality does not seem to affect potassium distribution.

HYPOKALEMIA

Epidemiology

Hypokalemia (defined as a serum potassium concentration less than 3.5 mEq/L [mmol/L]) is a commonly encountered electrolyte abnormality in clinical practice. Hypokalemia is often categorized as mild (serum potassium 3.1-3.4 mEq/L [mmol/L]), moderate (serum potassium 2.5-3 mEq/L [mmol/L]), or severe (less than 2.5 mEq/L [mmol/L]).[13] When hypokalemia is detected, the diagnostic workup should evaluate the patient's comorbid disease states and concomitant medications. Hypokalemia is virtually nonexistent in healthy adults. This is due in part to the potassium content in the typical Western diet as well as the body's effective potassium-sparing mechanisms, which tightly regulate the serum potassium concentration. However, as many as 20% of hospitalized patients and up to 40% of patients taking thiazide diuretics will develop hypokalemia.[14]

While transient hypokalemia may be thought of as merely a laboratory abnormality, there are serious potential consequences associated with persistent hypokalemia. Hypokalemia increases mortality in patients with heart failure, CKD, or diabetes mellitus, populations typically thought to be more sensitive to the effects of hyperkalemia.[15] Low dietary potassium intake is associated with worsening hypertension and higher risk of stroke.[3]

Etiology and Pathophysiology

Hypokalemia results when there is a total-body potassium deficit, or when serum potassium is shifted into the intracellular compartment. Total-body deficits occur in the setting of poor dietary intake of potassium, or when there are excessive renal and GI losses of potassium. Maintaining a consistent dietary intake of potassium is important because the body has no effective method for storing potassium. At steady state, potassium excretion matches potassium intake; approximately 90% of ingested potassium is renally excreted, whereas 10% is excreted in feces.[9] This underscores the importance of eating a well-balanced diet. Older adults with chronic diseases and those undergoing surgery are at increased risk for developing hypokalemia because of insufficient intake or losses resulting from surgery.

Many medications can cause hypokalemia by a variety of mechanisms including intracellular potassium shifting and increased renal or stool losses (Table 70-1). The most common cause of medication-induced hypokalemia is loop and thiazide diuretic administration as

TABLE 70-1 Mechanism of Medication-Induced Hypokalemia

Transcellular Shift	Enhanced Renal Excretion	Enhanced Fecal Elimination
β_2-Receptor agonists	Diuretics	Laxatives
Epinephrine	Acetazolamide	Sodium polystyrene sulfonate
Albuterol	Thiazides	Sorbitol
Terbutaline	Indapamide	Patiromer
Fomoterol	Metolazone	Sodium zirconium cyclosilicate
Salmeterol	Furosemide	
Isoproterenol	Torsemide	
Ephedrine	Bumetanide	
Pseudoephedrine	Ethacrynic acid	
Theophylline	High-dose penicillins	
Levothyroxine	Nafcillin	
Decongestants	Ampicillin	
Caffeine	Penicillin	
Insulin overdose	Mineralocorticoids	
Verapamil overdose	Miscellaneous	
Barium overdose	Aminoglycosides	
	Amphotericin B	
	Cisplatin	

these agents inhibit sodium reabsorption in the kidney, which results in increased sodium delivery to the distal tubule. Consequently, hypokalemia develops because the distal tubule selectively reabsorbs sodium and excretes potassium. Second, because diuretics result in vascular volume contraction, aldosterone is secreted that further promotes the renal excretion of potassium. If concomitant potassium supplements are not provided to patients receiving loop and thiazide diuretics, mild-to-moderate hypokalemia is inevitable.

The second most common etiology of hypokalemia is excessive loss of potassium-rich GI fluid as a result of diarrhea and/or vomiting. The typical potassium loss in feces is approximately 10 mEq (mmol) per day.[7] In diarrheal states, this amount increases proportionally with the volume of stool output. Fecal potassium losses may be as high as 130 to 170 mEq/L (mmol/L).[16] Vomiting also accounts for substantial potassium losses, which have been estimated to be as high as 30 to 50 mEq (mmol) per liter of vomitus.[17] Metabolic alkalosis which often develops in those with severe diarrhea and vomiting as a result of loss of these bicarbonate-rich fluids causes an intracellular shift of potassium, thereby lowering the serum concentration of potassium even further. Prolonged diarrhea and vomiting tend to affect children and older adults profoundly because their kidneys are unable to effectively maintain adequate fluid status.

3 Hypomagnesemia, which is present in more than 50% of patients with clinically significant hypokalemia, contributes to the development of hypokalemia because it reduces the intracellular potassium concentration and promotes renal potassium wasting.[18] While the precise mechanism of the accelerated renal loss is unknown, many believe that the intracellular potassium concentration may decrease because hypomagnesemia impairs the function of the Na^+-K^+-ATPase pump thereby promoting potassium wasting. Alternatively, the combination of increased sodium delivery to the distal tubule, elevated aldosterone concentrations, and hypomagnesemia may cause the kidney outer medullary potassium channels to excrete more potassium.[18] What is clear is that hypokalemia and hypomagnesemia often coexist as a result of medications (diuretic administration) or disease states (diarrhea). When concomitant hypokalemia and hypomagnesemia occur, the magnesium deficiency should be corrected first; otherwise, full repletion of the potassium deficit is difficult.

TREATMENT

Desired Outcomes

The goals of hypokalemia management are to prevent and/or treat serious life-threatening complications, normalize the serum potassium concentration, identify and correct the underlying cause of hypokalemia, and finally prevent overcorrection of the serum potassium concentration.

General Approach to Therapy

The general approach to therapy depends on the degree and rapidity with which hypokalemia developed and the presence of signs and symptoms. Serum potassium concentrations between 3.5 and 4 mEq/L (mmol/L) are a sign of early potassium depletion. No pharmacologic therapy is recommended; however, patients should be encouraged to increase their dietary intake of potassium-rich foods. When the serum potassium concentration is between 3 and 3.4 mEq/L (mmol/L), the patient's concomitant conditions and medications will largely determine whether pharmacologic therapy should be initiated. Most patients will not have signs or symptoms if serum potassium concentrations remain greater than 3 mEq/L (mmol/L).

CLINICAL PRESENTATION Hypokalemia

General

- The signs and symptoms of hypokalemia are usually nonspecific and highly variable between patients.

Symptoms

- Symptoms are dependent on the degree of hypokalemia and its rapidity of onset.
- Mild hypokalemia is often asymptomatic.
- Moderate hypokalemia is associated with cramping, weakness, malaise, and myalgias.

Signs

- Cardiovascular: In severe hypokalemia, ECG changes often include ST-segment depression or flattening, T-wave inversion, and U-wave elevation. Clinical arrhythmias include heart block, atrial flutter, paroxysmal atrial tachycardia, ventricular fibrillation, and digitalis-induced arrhythmias.
- Musculoskeletal: Cramping and impaired muscle contraction.

Laboratory Tests

- Serum potassium concentration below 3.5 mEq/L (mmol/L) is diagnostic. Hypomagnesemia (serum magnesium concentration below 1.7 mg/dL [1.4 mEq/L; 0.70 mmol/L]) can also be present.

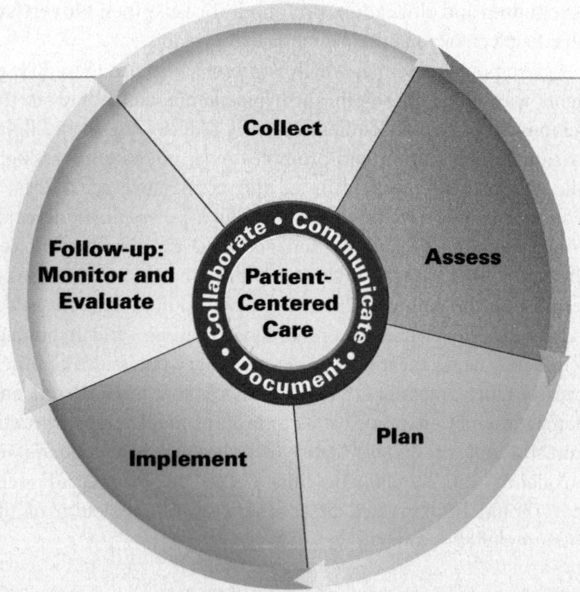

Patient Care Process for the Management of Potassium and Magnesium Disorders

Collect

- Patient characteristics (eg, age, race, sex)
- Patient history (past medical, family, social–dietary habits)
- Current medications including over-the-counter medications, herbals, dietary supplements
- Subjective data
  - Musculoskeletal and neuromuscular review of systems
  - Intake (food and fluid) and output (urine and stool)
- Objective data
  - Blood pressure, heart rate, height, weight
  - Labs (eg, basic metabolic panel, calcium, magnesium, phosphorus)
  - Other diagnostic tests when indicated (eg, electrocardiogram [ECG], urinalysis, urine electrolytes)

Assess

- Presence of symptoms of an electrolyte disorder
- Presence of ECG changes (see Fig. 70-1)
- Severity of electrolyte disorder (eg, change from baseline value, timing of development of electrolyte disorder)
- Kidney function (eg, estimated glomerular filtration rate [GFR], creatinine clearance [CrCl], presence of chronic kidney disease [CKD])
- Current medications that may contribute to electrolyte disorder (see Tables 70-1, 70-6, and 70-8)
- Current diet that may contribute to electrolyte disorder (see Tables 70-2 and 70-9)

Plan*

- Identification of the most likely cause of the electrolyte disorder and discontinuation of offending medication or substance (if applicable)
- Dietary modifications (see Tables 70-2 and 70-9)
- Medication therapy regimen including specific medication, dose, route, frequency, and duration; specify the continuation and discontinuation of existing therapies (see Tables 70-4, 70-5, and 70-7)
- Monitoring parameters including efficacy (eg, potassium, magnesium, serum creatinine [SCr]), safety (medication-specific adverse medication reactions), and need for repeat or additional medication therapy
- Patient education (eg, purpose of treatment, dietary and lifestyle modification, medication therapy)
- Referrals to other providers when appropriate (eg, physician, dietitian)

Implement*

- Provide patient education regarding all elements of treatment plan
- Use motivational interviewing and coaching strategies to maximize adherence
- Schedule follow-up

Follow-up: Monitor and Evaluate

- Resolution of electrolyte disorder and prevention of further episodes
- Presence of adverse medication reactions
- Development/progression of kidney impairment
- Patient adherence to treatment plan using multiple sources of information

**Collaborate with patient, caregivers, and other health professionals*

The presence of signs or symptoms with mild hypokalemia warrants the initiation of potassium supplementation. Oral potassium supplementation should be initiated in patients with underlying cardiac conditions that predispose them to cardiac arrhythmias. Patients with serum potassium concentrations less than 3 mEq/L (mmol/L) should always be treated to achieve values between 4 and 4.5 mEq/L (mmol/L). In asymptomatic patients, oral therapy is the preferred route of administration. Intravenous (IV) potassium may be necessary in symptomatic patients with severe depletion, or in patients who are intolerant to oral supplementation. In patients with concomitant moderate to severe hypomagnesemia, the magnesium deficit should be corrected before potassium supplementation is started.[9,14]

Nonpharmacologic Therapy

The best and most abundant sources of dietary potassium supplementation are fresh fruits and vegetables, fruit juices, and meats (Table 70-2). Increased dietary intake of foods with high potassium content, however, is not recommended long-term because it can add unwanted calories to the patient's diet. Moreover, dietary potassium is almost entirely coupled with phosphate, rather than chloride, so it is not as effective in correcting potassium loss associated with hypochloremic conditions such as vomiting, nasogastric suctioning, and diuretic therapy. Salt substitutes that contain potassium chloride are another effective, inexpensive source of potassium and because they provide chloride as well and are frequently recommended.

TABLE 70-2 Foods That Are High in Potassium

High content (>250 mg)	Very high content (>500 mg)
Kidney beans, cooked	Potato, baked, flesh and skin
Lentils, cooked	Sweet potato, baked in skin
Soybeans, green, cooked	Juice, canned
Lima beans, cooked	Prunes
Soybeans, mature, cooked	Carrot
Pinto beans, cooked	Tomato
Lentils, cooked	Tomato paste
Halibut, cooked	Tomato puree
Rockfish, Pacific, cooked	Beet greens, cooked
Cod, Pacific, cooked	White beans, canned
Tuna, yellowfin, cooked	Plain yogurt, nonfat or low-fat
Rainbow trout, cooked	Clams, canned
Evaporated milk, nonfat	
Low-fat (1%) or reduced fat (2%) chocolate milk	
Skim milk (nonfat)	
Low-fat milk or buttermilk (1%)	
Orange juice, fresh	
Bananas	
Peaches, dried, uncooked	
Prunes, stewed	
Apricots, dried, uncooked	
Plantains, cooked	
Tomato sauce	
Pork loin, center rib, lean, roasted	
Spinach, cooked	

TABLE 70-3 General Consensus Guidelines for Potassium Replacement

Guideline	Comment
Potassium replacement therapy should accompany dietary consumption of potassium-rich foods.	Potassium-rich foods often cannot completely replace potassium associated with chloride losses (vomiting, diuretics, or nasogastric suction) because it is almost entirely coupled to phosphate. Furthermore, increasing dietary intake of these foods can lead to unwanted weight gain.
Potassium replacement is recommended for sodium-sensitive and hypertensive patients.	A high-sodium diet often results in excessive urinary potassium excretion.
Potassium replacement is recommended in patients who are subject to vomiting, diarrhea, or diuretic/laxative misuse.	These conditions promote excessive renal and GI potassium loss.
Potassium supplementation is best administered orally in divided doses over several days to achieve full repletion.	
Laboratory measurement of serum potassium is convenient, but not always accurate.	Clinicians should be aware of the factors that result in transcellular potassium shifts. Monitoring 24-hour urinary potassium excretion can be necessary in high-risk patients.
Patient adherence to potassium replacement can be increased with compliance-enhancing regimens.	Microencapsulated products have no bitter smell or aftertaste and have much better GI tolerance. Regimens should be made as simple as possible to follow.
A potassium dosage of 20 mEq/day (mmol/day) is usually sufficient to prevent hypokalemia from occurring. Doses of 40-100 mEq (mmol) are usually sufficient to treat hypokalemia.	

Pharmacologic Therapy

Formal guidelines for potassium supplementation were last published by the National Council on Potassium in Clinical Practice in 2000 (Table 70-3).[19] While these guidelines are not from a major medical society, they do provide a comprehensive framework for potassium administration as a prophylactic and therapeutic replacement for many patient populations. When deciding how to design the optimal regimen, one must consider: (a) the patient's normal, that is, baseline potassium concentration; (b) underlying medical conditions that can affect potassium balance; (c) concomitant medications that can affect potassium balance; (d) the patient's dietary salt intake; and (e) the patient's ability to comply with the therapeutic regimen.[19]

A general rule for potassium replacement is that for every 1 mEq/L (mmol/L) decrease of serum potassium below 3.5 mEq/L (mmol/L), there is a corresponding total-body potassium deficit of 100 to 400 mEq (mmol). Because of the wide variance in projected deficits, each patient's therapy must be individualized and adjustments made on the basis of the patient's signs, symptoms, and frequent measurements of serum potassium. In the acute care setting, the administration of 10 mEq (mmol) of IV or oral potassium should increase the serum potassium concentration by 0.1 mEq/L (mmol/L). This approximation is used as a basis for dose calculations, with frequent measurements of serum potassium to avoid overestimation. In patients receiving chronic loop or thiazide diuretic therapy, 40 to 100 mEq (mmol) of oral potassium supplementation can correct mild-to-moderate potassium deficits. Doses up to 120 mEq (mmol) can be required in more severe deficiencies. When providing oral potassium supplementation, the total daily dose should be divided into three to four doses to minimize the development of adverse medication reactions in the GI tract. Patients receiving diuretics can become chronically hypokalemic and can benefit from combination potassium-sparing diuretic therapy.

4 Whenever possible, potassium supplementation should be administered by mouth. Four salts are available for oral potassium supplementation: chloride, gluconate, phosphate, and bicarbonate. Potassium phosphate should be used when the patient is both hypokalemic and hypophosphatemic; potassium bicarbonate is most commonly used when potassium depletion occurs in the setting of metabolic acidosis. Potassium chloride, however, is the primary salt form used because it is the most effective treatment for the most common causes of potassium depletion (ie, diuretic and diarrhea-induced) as these conditions are associated with potassium and chloride losses.

Potassium chloride can be administered in either tablet or liquid formulations (Table 70-4). The liquid forms are generally less expensive; however, patient compliance can be low because of their strong, unpleasant taste. Liquid forms should be used when a rapid response to supplementation is desired. Two sustained-release solid dosage forms are currently available in the United States: a wax-matrix formulation, and a microencapsulated formulation. The microencapsulated tablet is generally preferred because it is associated with less GI irritation. IV potassium use should be limited to: (a) severe hypokalemia (serum concentration less than 2.5 mEq/L [mmol/L]);

TABLE 70-4 Differences Among Oral Potassium Supplements

Supplement	Comment
Controlled-release microencapsulated tablet	Disintegrates better in GI tract; fewer GI erosions as compared to wax-matrix tablets
Encapsulated controlled-release microencapsulated particles	Fewer erosions as compared to wax-matrix tablets
Potassium chloride elixir	Inexpensive, poor taste, poor compliance, immediate effect
Potassium chloride effervescent tablets for solution	More expensive than elixir, convenient
Wax-matrix extended-release tablets	Easier to swallow; more GI erosions as compared to other therapies

(b) patients exhibiting signs and symptoms such as ECG changes or muscle spasms; or (c) patients unable to tolerate oral therapy. IV supplementation requires more monitoring than oral therapy because it is more likely to result in hyperkalemia, phlebitis, and pain at the site of infusion.

The vehicle in which IV potassium is administered is important. Whenever possible, potassium should be prepared in saline-containing solutions (eg, 0.9%-0.45% sodium chloride [NaCl]). Dextrose-containing solutions stimulate insulin secretion, which can cause intracellular shifting of potassium, worsening the patient's hypokalemia, and should be avoided whenever possible. Generally, 10 to 20 mEq (mmol) of potassium is diluted in 100 mL 0.9% NaCl for IV administration. These concentrations are safe when administered through a peripheral vein over an hour. When infusion rates exceed 10 mEq/h (mmol/h), ECG monitoring should be performed to detect cardiac changes. The serum potassium concentration should be evaluated following the infusion of each 30 to 40 mEq (mmol) to guide further potassium replacement administration. Multiple doses of potassium can be repeated as needed until the serum potassium concentration normalizes. To allow adequate time for the potassium to equilibrate between the intra- and extracellular spaces, one should wait at least 30 minutes from the end of each infusion and care should be taken to avoid sampling from the same line in which the potassium was infused, as this can result in a spuriously high potassium concentration.

In patients with severe potassium depletion, replacement with as much as 300 to 400 mEq/day (mmol/day) may be needed. In this instance, it is a common practice to dilute 40 to 60 mEq (mmol) in 1,000 mL 0.45% NaCl and infuse at a rate not exceeding 40 mEq/h (mmol/h). The total 24-hour dose should not exceed 400 mEq (mmol). This should be performed in an intensive care unit (ICU) under continuous ECG monitoring. Because of the high potassium concentration and the risk for burning pain and peripheral venous sclerosis, the infusion should be through a central venous catheter into a large vein (eg, superior vena cava) but care must be taken not to place the tip of the catheter into the right atrium.[20] Directly delivering high potassium concentrations into the heart can result in cardiac arrhythmias. Given the volume required to infuse this dose of potassium, this infusion strategy might be impractical in certain clinical situations (eg, patients requiring fluid restriction). A reasonable approach is to split the potassium dose between the oral and IV routes. For example, if a symptomatic patient requires 120 mEq (mmol) of potassium, the clinician can give 60 mEq (mmol) as the immediate-release potassium liquid, and the other 60 mEq (mmol) can be given through the IV route (20 mEq/100 mL/h [mmol/100 mL/h] in three doses). When giving large potassium doses, serum monitoring should be performed following the administration of half the dose to guide the need for additional potassium. This can also help avoid the development of hyperkalemia.

In the rare circumstances when cardiac arrest from hypokalemia is imminent, IV bolus dosing of potassium 10 mEq (mmol) over 5 minutes can be initiated and repeated once, if necessary.[20]

Alternative Therapies

Potassium-sparing diuretics are a viable alternative to chronic exogenous potassium supplementation, especially when patients are concomitantly receiving medications that are known to deplete potassium (eg, diuretics). Spironolactone inhibits the effect of aldosterone in the distal convoluted tubule of the kidney, thereby decreasing potassium elimination in the urine. Spironolactone is especially effective as a potassium-sparing agent in patients with primary or secondary hyperaldosteronism. Amiloride and triamterene are reasonable second-line agents that act by blocking tubular epithelial sodium channels, leading to decreased renal potassium excretion.

Spironolactone is available as 25-, 50-, and 100-mg tablets. The usual starting dose is 25 to 50 mg daily and can be titrated to a maximum dose of 400 mg/day. The potassium-retaining effects generally take 48 hours to be evident. Principal adverse medication reactions include hyperkalemia, gynecomastia, breast tenderness, and impotence in men. Triamterene is available as 50- and 100-mg capsules. The usual starting dose is 50 mg twice daily, which can be titrated to 100 mg twice daily. Triamterene is also available as a combination product with hydrochlorothiazide (37.5/25 mg, 50/25 mg, or 75/50 mg) and is commonly used for the treatment of hypertension. Common adverse medication reactions include hyperkalemia, sodium depletion, and metabolic acidosis. The usual starting dose of amiloride is 5 mg daily; however, 10 mg can be given in those with severe hypokalemia. This is also available as a combination product with hydrochlorothiazide 50 mg. The most common adverse medication reactions are hyperkalemia and metabolic acidosis.

Concomitant use of potassium supplementation with potassium-sparing diuretics is generally not necessary, but when used there is a risk of hyperkalemia, especially in patients with CKD or diabetes mellitus.

Evaluation of Therapeutic Outcomes

Serum potassium concentrations should be monitored regularly while the patient is receiving potassium supplementation. For ambulatory patients receiving prophylactic potassium supplementation during diuretic therapy, the serum potassium and magnesium concentrations, as well as kidney function should be monitored every 1 to 2 months. In hospitalized patients receiving oral therapy for mild hypokalemia, the potassium concentration should be monitored every 2 to 3 days. If it does not increase by at least 1 mEq/L (mmol/L) within 96 hours, the clinician should suspect concomitant magnesium depletion. Patients receiving IV potassium supplementation require close ECG monitoring if the infusion rate is greater than 20 mEq/h (mmol/h): doses greater than this should be administered only in the presence of continuous ECG monitoring. Additionally, the patient should have serum potassium concentrations obtained halfway through, and 30 minutes following completion of the total potassium dose to guide further potassium administration. Finally, the patient should be assessed for adverse medication reactions such as pain at the infusion site or phlebitis.

Clinical Bottom Line

Hypokalemia is a frequent medical condition caused by both biological processes as well as medication therapy. While mild hypokalemia is frequently asymptomatic, severe hypokalemia can cause fatal cardiac dysrhythmias, particularly in patients with underlying cardiac disease. Patients receiving medications that cause potassium wasting (eg, thiazide or loop diuretics) should be closely followed for the development of hypokalemia and appropriate potassium supplementation should be started when necessary. Generally oral potassium is sufficient for the management of mild hypokalemia; IV potassium should be reserved for severe deficiency, and its use should be monitored closely.

HYPERKALEMIA

Hyperkalemia, defined as a serum potassium concentration greater than 5 mEq/L (mmol/L), can be further classified according to its severity: mild hyperkalemia (5.1-5.9 mEq/L [mmol/L]), moderate hyperkalemia (6-7 mEq/L [mmol/L]), and severe hyperkalemia (above 7 mEq/L [mmol/L]).[19]

Epidemiology

5 Hyperkalemia is much less common than hypokalemia. In fact, if all patients with AKI and CKD were excluded, the prevalence of hyperkalemia would be less than 1% in the rest of the population. The incidence of hyperkalemia in hospitalized patients is highly variable, ranging from 1% to 10%.[21] The incidence of hyperkalemia has increased over time likely from the aging of the population, increased prevalence of CKD and diabetes mellitus, and increased use of medications that inhibit the renin-angiotensin-aldosterone system.[22] Severe hyperkalemia occurs more commonly in older adults with impaired kidney function who have been receiving chronic oral potassium supplementation.

Etiology and Pathophysiology

Hyperkalemia develops when potassium intake exceeds excretion (true hyperkalemia) (ie, elevated total-body stores) or when the transcellular distribution of potassium is disturbed (ie, normal total-body stores). The four primary causes of hyperkalemia—(a) increased potassium intake, (b) decreased potassium excretion, (c) tubular unresponsiveness to aldosterone, and (d) redistribution of potassium into the extracellular space—are discussed further.

Hyperkalemia Associated with Increased Potassium Intake

Hyperkalemia in this setting is almost always associated with impaired kidney function. Patients with stage 4 or 5 CKD and dialysis patients who are noncompliant with dietary potassium restrictions often present with life-threatening hyperkalemia. Dietary potassium restrictions are difficult to adhere to since many foods that are considered part of a healthy diet contain potassium. Another common dietary source associated with the development of hyperkalemia is potassium chloride salt substitutes. Many dialysis patients are instructed to use salt substitutes to avoid excessive sodium intake in an attempt to control volume overload. These patients unwittingly become hyperkalemic because these products contain approximately 10 to 15 mEq (mmol) potassium per gram or 200 mEq (mmol) per tablespoon. Finally, some over-the-counter herbal and alternative medicine products may contain large amounts of potassium. It is thus essential for patients with CKD to receive education regarding dietary sources of potassium as well as information on the potassium content of herbal products when available.

Hyperkalemia Associated with Decreased Renal Potassium Excretion

Normally functioning kidneys excrete 90% of the daily potassium intake. Therefore, when the kidney is unable to excrete potassium appropriately, as in AKI and stage 4 to 5 CKD, potassium is retained and often results in hyperkalemia. Finally, because aldosterone is responsible for potassium excretion via the kidney cortical collecting duct, medications and diseases that inhibit this process contribute to hyperkalemia.[23]

Severe hyperkalemia is more common in AKI than in CKD because patients are often hypercatabolic and have underlying disorders, such as rhabdomyolysis or tumor lysis syndrome, which result in release of potassium from injured or lysed cells.[24] Severe hyperkalemia is rare in stable stage 1 to 4 CKD, perhaps because of enhanced GI and renal potassium excretion.[25] Additionally, hyperkalemia directly stimulates renal potassium excretion through an effect that is independent of, and additive to, that of aldosterone.[26] Renal excretion of potassium is also inhibited by various endocrine disorders, including adrenal insufficiency, Addison disease, and selective hypoaldosteronism. All of these disorders involve a decreased production of aldosterone, which results in the retention of potassium.

Several medications have profound effects on the kidney's ability to regulate potassium. These include five medication classes in particular: angiotensin-converting enzyme inhibitors (ACEIs), angiotensin-II receptor blockers (ARBs), direct renin inhibitors, mineralocorticoid receptor antagonists (MRAs) and other potassium-sparing diuretics, and prostaglandin inhibitors such as nonsteroidal anti-inflammatory drugs (NSAIDs). Although hyperkalemia is typically dose-dependent, the rates of hyperkalemia may range from 2% to 10%.[27,28] Finerenone (Kerendia®), a non-steroidal MRA FDA-approved for use in patients with diabetic nephropathy, should not be initiated in patients with a serum potassium greater than 5 mEq/L (mmol/L) and should be withheld if the serum potassium rises above 5.5 mEq/L (mmol/L).[29] It has a novel mechanism of action compared to other medications in the class such as spironolactone and eplerenone but similar rates of hyperkalemia.[30] Other commonly used medications that can cause hyperkalemia are β-blockers, digoxin, cyclosporine, tacrolimus, trimethoprim–sulfamethoxazole, and heparin.

Tubular Unresponsiveness to Aldosterone

Sickle cell anemia, systemic lupus erythematosus, and amyloidosis can produce a defect in renal tubular potassium secretion, possibly as the result of an alteration in the aldosterone-binding site.

Redistribution of Potassium into the Extracellular Space

The efflux of potassium from within the cell into the extracellular space, which is associated with no change in total-body potassium stores, is often observed in the presence of metabolic acidosis, diabetes mellitus, CKD, or lactic acidosis. β-Blockers can also result in a transcellular potassium shift.

The serum potassium concentration can also be falsely elevated in some conditions and not reflect the actual in vivo potassium concentration, that is, pseudohyperkalemia. Pseudohyperkalemia occurs most commonly in the setting of extravascular hemolysis of red blood cells. When a blood specimen is not processed promptly and cellular destruction occurs, intracellular potassium is released into the serum. It can also occur in conditions of thrombocytosis or leukocytosis. If severe hyperkalemia is found in a patient who is asymptomatic with an otherwise normal laboratory report, the hyperkalemia is most likely pseudohyperkalemia, and a repeat blood sample should be collected. Truly elevated potassium concentrations are normally associated with other laboratory abnormalities such as low carbon dioxide (acidosis) or elevated blood urea nitrogen and creatinine concentrations (indicating impaired kidney function).

TREATMENT

Desired Outcomes

The goals of therapy for the treatment of hyperkalemia are to antagonize adverse cardiac effects, reverse signs and symptoms that are present, and return the serum and total-body stores of potassium to

CLINICAL PRESENTATION Hyperkalemia

General

- Related to the effects of excessive potassium on neuromuscular, cardiac, and smooth muscle cell function.

Symptoms

- Frequently asymptomatic.
- The patient might complain of heart palpitations or skipped heartbeats.

Signs

- ECG changes (Fig. 70-1)

Laboratory Tests

- Serum potassium concentration above 5.0 mEq/L (mmol/L) is diagnostic.

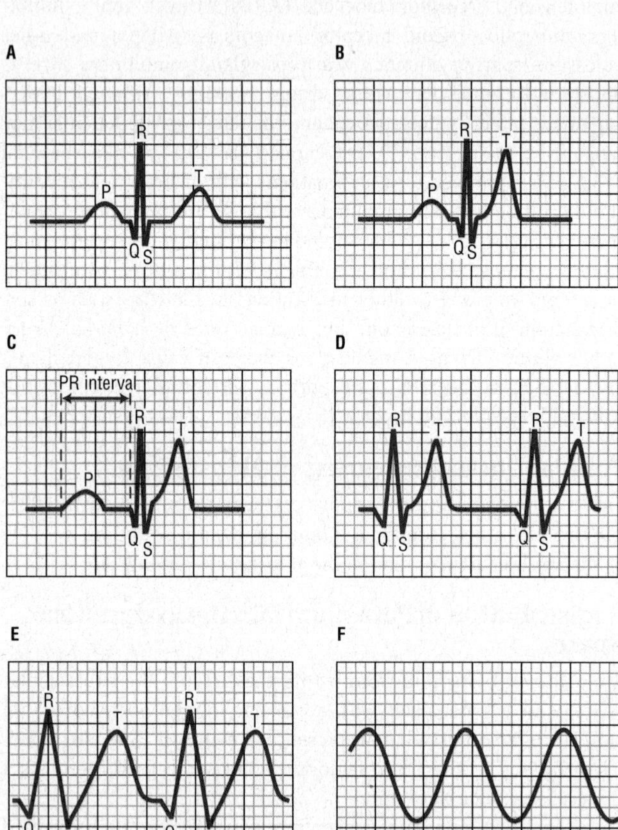

FIGURE 70-1 The earliest electrocardiographic manifestation of hyperkalemia is an increase in the rate of ventricular repolarization, which results in a peaking of the T wave at serum potassium concentrations of ~5.5 to 6 mEq/L (mmol/L) (*B*), relative to the normal ECG presentation (*A*). Further increases in the serum potassium concentration above 6 mEq/L (mmol/L) result in conduction delays through the His-Purkinje system, the atrial myocardium, and the ventricular myocardium. The ECG manifestations of these conduction delays and the sequence in which they occur are a widening of the PR interval (*C*), delay through the His-Purkinje system, a loss of the P wave (*D*), delay through the atrial myocardium, a widening of the QRS complex (*E*), and delay through the ventricular myocardium. Finally, there is a merging of the QRS complex with the T wave (*F*), which results in a sine-wave appearance.

normal. The optimal treatment approach is dependent on the severity of hyperkalemia, the rapidity of its development, and the patient's clinical condition. Cardiac instability and arrhythmias, which can be life-threatening, may be present especially when serum potassium is above 6 mEq/L (mmol/L). Although ECG changes are directly proportional to the serum potassium concentration and its rate of increase, they may not be present in all patients. Asymptomatic patients with mild hyperkalemia usually require no specific therapy other than dietary education to control intake, and monitoring of serum potassium daily if an inpatient or weekly if an outpatient to assure resolution.

Severe hyperkalemia (above 7 mEq/L [mmol/L]) or moderate hyperkalemia (6-6.9 mEq/L [mmol/L]), when associated with clinical symptoms or ECG changes, requires immediate treatment. Initial treatment should be focused on antagonism of the cardiac membrane actions of hyperkalemia (eg, administration of calcium). Secondarily, one should attempt to decrease extracellular potassium concentration by promoting its intracellular movement (eg, with insulin, β_2-receptor agonists, or sodium bicarbonate) or enhance its removal from the body by hemodialysis: the oral administration of cation-exchange resins, and/or the use of loop diuretics may also be considered in some patients. In any case, the underlying cause of hyperkalemia should be identified and reversed, and exogenous potassium must be withheld.

General Approach to Treatment

A treatment approach for patients with hyperkalemia is outlined in Fig. 70-2. In patients who have acute ECG changes, IV calcium should be administered to raise the threshold potential and stabilize the myocardium.[31] At the same time, the serum potassium concentration should be rapidly decreased to below 5 mEq/L (mmol/L) within minutes by administering medications that cause an intracellular shift of potassium, followed by the initiation of those that increase the elimination of potassium from the body.[31] If the patient is asymptomatic, rapid correction may not be necessary and will likely depend on the clinical context associated with the rise in serum potassium concentration. If one anticipates the need to reduce total-body potassium stores, an ion exchange resin that results in removal of potassium from the body over several hours to days may be initiated shortly after the emergent care has been instituted. An IV loop diuretic can be used to facilitate potassium removal through diuresis in patients who are hypervolemic and have preserved kidney function.[31]

Nonpharmacologic Therapy

Hemodialysis patients who ingest foods supplemented with glycyrrhetinic acid, the active ingredient in licorice, may be better able to maintain serum potassium concentrations within the normal range.[32,33] Glycyrrhetinic acid inhibits the enzyme 11β-hydroxysteroid dehydrogenase II, thereby increasing cortisol availability in the colon. The net result is enhanced potassium elimination in the feces. Other nonpharmacologic therapies, specifically available for dialysis-dependent patients are the tailoring of their intermittent

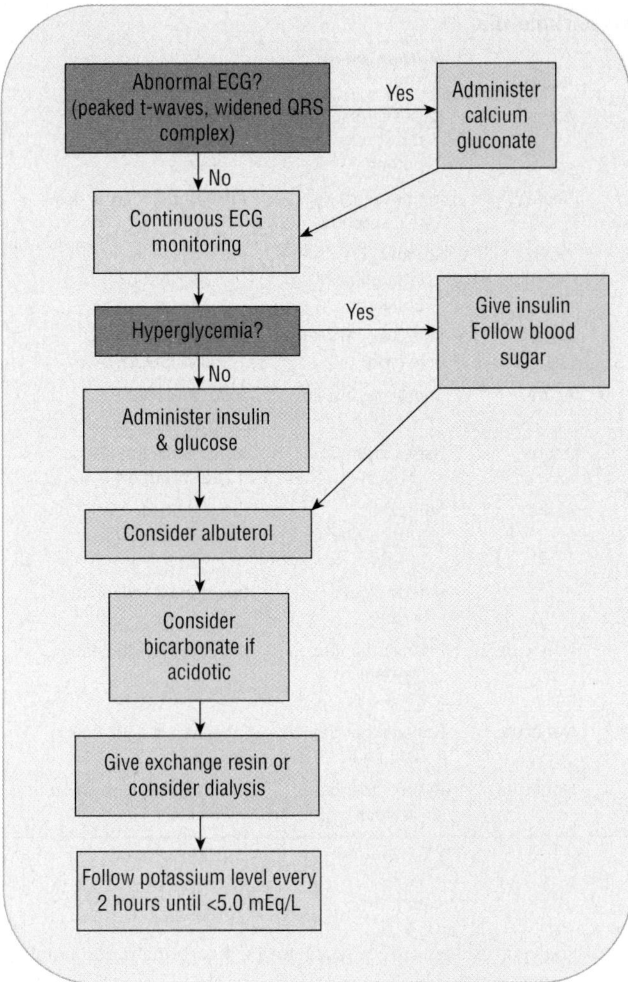

FIGURE 70-2 Treatment approach for hyperkalemia. (Serum potassium of 5.0 mEq/L is equivalent to 5.0 mmol/L.)

dialysis or hemofiltration therapy to include a low potassium dialysate to enhance the removal of potassium (see Chapter 64). Emergency dialysis can be considered in patients with acute kidney injury who have persistent ECG changes or insufficient response to therapies that cause intracellular potassium shifts, although the optimal time to initiate dialysis is not known.[34]

Pharmacologic Therapy

There are several medication therapy options to lower the serum potassium concentration. The optimal regimen for a given patient is dependent on the rapidity and degree of lowering that is necessary. Table 70-5 provides an overview of the available therapies and their respective onset and duration of action.

While specific treatment recommendations vary, it is generally accepted that asymptomatic patients with potassium concentrations below 6 mEq/L (mmol/L) can be treated conservatively. In patients with normal kidney function or those with stage 3 or 4 CKD, this typically involves the administration of furosemide to promote urinary potassium excretion. When given IV at a dosage of 40 to 80 mg, urine flow usually increases within minutes and persists for approximately 4 to 6 hours. Oral furosemide can also be used, keeping in mind the IV:PO dose ratio (1:2) and delayed onset of action compared to IV. Close monitoring of the patient's volume status and other electrolyte concentrations is required while the patient is receiving furosemide. Of note, the effectiveness of diuretics in treating hyperkalemia has not been studied in a randomized, controlled fashion.

In symptomatic patients, or in those with severe hyperkalemia, emergency care is indicated. Initial therapy in this setting is the administration of IV calcium chloride or gluconate 1 g to treat or prevent life-threatening arrhythmias.[31] Calcium antagonizes the cardiac membrane effect of hyperkalemia by reducing the electrical threshold potential for cardiac myocytes and reverses ECG changes within minutes. IV calcium should not be given to patients receiving digoxin as it can lead to digoxin toxicity. Its duration of action is 30 to 60 minutes, and it can be repeated as needed based on ECG findings. IV calcium can be given as either the chloride or gluconate salt; each is available as a 10% solution by weight. Calcium chloride provides approximately three times more calcium than equal volumes of the gluconate salt; however, it can cause tissue necrosis if extravasation occurs. For this reason, calcium gluconate is more commonly administered, with the standard dose being 1 g IV bolus over 5 to 10 minutes.

Rapid correction of hyperkalemia may necessitate the administration of medications that result in an intracellular shift of potassium, such as insulin and dextrose, sodium bicarbonate, and a β_2-adrenergic receptor agonist (eg, albuterol). The treatment of choice depends on the underlying medical disorders accompanying hyperkalemia. For example, in patients with concomitant metabolic acidosis, a sodium bicarbonate bolus or infusion of 50 to 100 mEq (mmol) is the preferred therapy. Sodium bicarbonate helps correct the metabolic acidosis by raising the extracellular pH, in addition to causing a rapid intracellular potassium shift. It should be noted that sodium bicarbonate is much less effective when hyperkalemia is not related to metabolic acidosis.[1] Sodium bicarbonate is also less effective in patients with end-stage renal disease (ESRD), in whom a decrease in serum potassium may not be seen for as long as 4 hours. Use caution in patients sensitive to volume changes as sodium bicarbonate can also lead to hypernatremia and volume overload. Administration of a rapid-acting (eg, Insulin lispro 10 units IV) or regular insulin (10 units IV) and dextrose (10% or 50%) is an effective method of reducing potassium. Insulin increases the activity of the Na^+-K^+-ATPase pump, thereby intracellularly shifting potassium. Insulin therapy results in a reduction in potassium concentration of 0.6 to 1 mEq/L (mmol/L) that is sustained for up to 2 hours.[35] Glucose should be given with insulin because hypoglycemia can develop as a result of the effects of the insulin therapy.[36] Alternative dosing strategies, such as low dose (eg, regular insulin 5 units) or weight-based regimens have been studied to combat hypoglycemia with varying results and cannot be routinely recommended.[37-39] A lower dose insulin strategy may be appropriate for patients with severe kidney impairment.[40] β_2-Adrenergic agonists have a dual mechanism for lowering serum potassium. First, they stimulate the Na^+-K^+-ATPase pump to promote intracellular potassium uptake. Second, they stimulate pancreatic β-receptors to increase insulin secretion. Albuterol can be administered via IV (0.5 mg given over 15 minutes) or via nebulizer (10-20 mg nebulized over 10 minutes). It should be noted that injectable albuterol is not available in the United States.

In patients with ESRD, decreases in the serum potassium concentration of 0.6 mEq/L (mmol/L) and 1 mEq/L (mmol/L) can be anticipated after inhalation of 10 and 20 mg of albuterol, respectively. Notice that the doses of inhaled albuterol used for hyperkalemia are at least four times higher than those typically used for bronchospasm, so adverse medication reactions are of greater concern. Adverse medication reactions include tachycardia, tremors, palpitations, mild anxiety, and increase blood glucose.[35] Furthermore, as many as 40% of patients may be resistant to the hypokalemic effects of albuterol and patients already receiving a nonselective β_2-receptor antagonist may not respond. Inconsistent bioavailability via the inhaled route must also be considered, as it could lead to potential over- or underdosing and an unpredictable response.

While not a fast-acting treatment based on pharmacokinetics, one ion exchange resin, sodium polystyrene sulfonate (SPS),

TABLE 70-5 Therapeutic Alternatives for the Management of Hyperkalemia

Medication	Dose	Route of Administration	Onset/Duration of Action	Acuity	Mechanism of Action	Expected Result
Calcium gluconate or chloride	1 g	IV over 5-10 minutes	1-2 min/ 10-30 min	Acute	Raises cardiac threshold potential	Reverses electrocardiographic effects
Furosemide	20-40 mg	IV	5-15 min/4-6 h	Acute	Inhibits renal Na^+ reabsorption	Increased urinary K^+ loss
Regular insulin	5-10 units	IV or subcut	30 min/2-6 h	Acute	Stimulates intracellular K^+ uptake	Intracellular K^+ redistribution
Dextrose 10%	1,000 mL (100 g)	IV over 1-2 hours	30 min/2-6 h	Acute	Stimulates insulin release	Intracellular K^+ redistribution
Dextrose 50%	50 mL (25 g)	IV over 5 minutes	30 min/2-6 h	Acute	Stimulates insulin release	Intracellular K^+ redistribution
Sodium bicarbonate	50-100 mEq (50-100 mmol)	IV over 2-5 minutes	30 min/2-6 h	Acute	Raises serum pH	Intracellular K^+ redistribution
Albuterol	10-20 mg	Nebulized over 10 minutes	30 min/1-2 h	Acute	Stimulates intracellular K^+ uptake	Intracellular K^+ redistribution
Hemodialysis	4 hours	N/A	Immediate/ variable	Acute	Removal from serum	Increased K^+ elimination
Sodium polystyrene sulfonate	15-60 g	Oral or rectal	1 h/variable	Nonacute	Resin exchanges Na^+ for K^+	Increased K^+ elimination
Patiromer	8.4-25.2 g	Oral	Hours/variable	Nonacute	Resin exchanges Ca^{++} for K^+	Increased K^+ elimination
Sodium zirconium cyclosilicate	5-15 g	Oral	1 h/variable	Nonacute	Resin exchanges Na^+ for K^+	Increased K^+ elimination

is regularly used in hospitalized patients with acute hyperkalemia. It has been used in hospitalized patients for over 60 years. SPS (Kayexalate®) is a cation-exchange resin that can be administered orally or rectally by enema. SPS is available in powder form or prepackaged as a 33% sorbitol suspension. The usual oral SPS dose is 15 to 60 g in the 33% sorbitol suspension. The oral route is more effective than the enema and is better tolerated by patients. As the resin passes through the intestines, each gram of SPS exchanges 1 mEq (mmol) of sodium for 1 mEq (mmol) of potassium, which is in a relatively higher concentration in the large intestine. The onset of action of SPS is within 1 hour, and it can be repeated every 4 hours as needed. The medication should be separated from other oral medications by at least 3 hours as it may bind to and decrease the effectiveness of many oral medications.[41] The sorbitol component of the suspension promotes the excretion of the cationically modified potassium exchange resin by inducing diarrhea. SPS contains a large amount of sodium (100 mg [4.1 mEq or mmol] per gram of SPS) and package labeling advises against its use in patients who cannot tolerate even small increases in sodium loads.[42]

Colonic necrosis is associated with the use of SPS.[43,44] In 2009, the FDA mandated a boxed warning for SPS due to reports of colonic necrosis and other serious GI toxicities.[42] The GI toxicities were believed to be associated with the 70% sorbitol; however, GI toxicity has also occurred with administration of 33% sorbitol solution. Toxicity appears to occur most commonly in patients who have undergone GI surgery or with current or history of bowel dysfunction. Therefore, the 33% sorbitol product is preferred over the 70% sorbitol product, rectal administration should be avoided, and use is contraindicated in patients with bowel dysfunction.

Several years ago, a Cochrane Review evaluated the emergency treatment of hyperkalemia and provided evidence for the efficacy of inhaled and nebulized β-agonists and IV insulin and glucose.[45] The combination of nebulized β-agonists with IV insulin and glucose appeared to be more effective than either agent alone. The meta-analysis results were equivocal for IV bicarbonate, and notably, SPS was not effective by 4 hours. Clinicians should exercise caution when extrapolating these findings to clinical practice. Nonetheless, the Cochrane database review corroborates the approach detailed in Fig. 70-2. Frequently, the management of hyperkalemia will be based on the clinician's personal judgment or institutional protocols. For example, the large majority (95%) of patients being treated for hyperkalemia in academic teaching hospitals receive SPS, with far fewer receiving insulin and IV calcium, and less than 10% of patient receive bicarbonate, albuterol, or hemodialysis.[46] In many emergency departments, insulin/glucose is the most commonly used agent and multimodal therapy is employed for treating initial serum potassium concentrations above 6 mEq/L (mmol/L).[47]

In nonhospitalized patients who have experienced chronic increases in serum potassium concentration, long-term management of hyperkalemia is focused on dietary restriction of potassium-rich foods and supplements, reducing and avoiding medications that impair potassium excretion in the kidney, and using diuretics or other medications to counteract the effects of medications that increase serum potassium concentrations. Medications used for chronic conditions that are known to cause hyperkalemia include NSAIDs, ACEIs, ARBs, direct renin inhibitors, and MRAs. These typically result in asymptomatic hyperkalemia without the need for emergent therapies. To prevent hyperkalemia, clinicians may attempt to lower the dose or switch to another medication without hyperkalemia as an adverse medication reaction (eg, calcium channel blocker). However, medications that inhibit the renin–angiotensin–aldosterone system (RAAS) have significant beneficial effects on morbidity and mortality in patients with chronic diseases such as diabetes mellitus, heart failure, and CKD. Therefore, reducing or avoiding the use of these medications to prevent hyperkalemia is not often appropriate. The use of a combination of ACEI and ARB is generally avoided due to the increased risk of hyperkalemia.[48] Mineralocorticoid receptor antagonists have a different mechanism of action and their use in combination with an ACEI or ARB is considered acceptable. In particular, finerenone has been shown to lower the rates of CKD progression and cardiovascular events in diabetic nephropathy when added to other RAAS inhibitors.[49,50] This provides the strongest evidence to date for the combination of MRA with an ACEI or ARB in patients with diabetic nephropathy and will likely expand the number of patients on dual RAAS inhibitors. As a third-generation non-steroidal MRA, it has equal distribution into cardiac and renal tissues, compared to spironolactone and eplerenone which favor distribution into renal tissue.[30] The starting dose of finerenone is 10 or 20 mg once daily based on eGFR and serum potassium with a target dose of 20 mg once daily. It should not be used with strong CYP3A4 inhibitors and inducers. The most common adverse medication reactions of finerenone are hyperkalemia, hypotension, and hyponatremia.[29] The extent of hyperkalemia is greater with a combination ACEI and MRA than a combination ACEI and ARB in patients with diabetic nephropathy, suggesting an extrarenal mechanism of this adverse medication reaction from MRAs.[51]

To allow for continued use of RAAS inhibitors, especially in patients prone to hyperkalemia, ion exchange resins may be used. A daily dose of SPS in patients with CKD receiving RAAS inhibitors effectively lowers and maintains serum potassium in the normal range.[52,53] Two other cation exchange agents, patiromer and sodium zirconium cyclosilicate, are available as alternatives to SPS in outpatients with hyperkalemia. Patiromer (Veltassa®) is a nonabsorbable polymer that exchanges calcium for potassium in the distal colon to increase the fecal elimination of potassium. The medication effectively achieves and maintains normokalemia in adults with stage 3 or 4 CKD on stable doses of RAAS inhibitors.[54,55] The most common adverse medication reactions of patiromer include constipation, hypomagnesemia, and diarrhea. The usual dose of patiromer is 8.4 to 25.2 g once daily. Patiromer contains sorbitol to increase medication stability, but at amounts 5- to 10-fold lower than SPS in sorbitol.[25] It should not be used to treat life-threatening hyperkalemia due to its delayed onset of action.[56] Additionally, patiromer can bind to many oral medications, which could lead to decreased absorption of other mediations and loss of efficacy. Therefore, it is recommended to administer other oral medications at least 3 hours before or after patiromer.[56]

Sodium zirconium cyclosilicate (ZS-9, Lokelma®) is a nonabsorbable inorganic compound that selectively exchanges sodium for potassium throughout the entire intestinal tract. The medication effectively decreases serum potassium concentrations as soon as 1 hour after administration of the first dose and for up to 48 hours after administration, with an average decrease of approximately 1 mEq/L (mmol/L) for the 10 g dose.[57,58] ZS-9 exhibits an acute onset of action, but is not FDA-approved for emergency treatment of life-threatening hyperkalemia. It is the only ion exchange resin that is approved for treatment of hyperkalemia in patients with ESRD on hemodialysis. The most common adverse medication reaction ZS-9 is edema, likely from the exchange of sodium for potassium. The starting dose is 10 g three times daily for 48 hours followed by 5 to 15 g once daily. The dosing in patients on hemodialysis is 5 to 15 g on nondialysis days. Like SPS and patiromer, ZS-9 must be separated from other oral medications but the separation time is shorter at 2 hours.[59]

Evaluation of Therapeutic Outcomes

The frequency and rigor with which one evaluates patients to ascertain if they have achieved the desired therapeutic outcomes depends on the severity and acuity of hyperkalemia. For example, cautious waiting is more common for those with mild or moderate asymptomatic hyperkalemia compared to those with acute symptomatic, severe hyperkalemia. Many medications such as ACEIs, ARBs, direct renin inhibitors, spironolactone, and finerenone result in asymptomatic hyperkalemia and changes in dosage or to a different agent may be all that is warranted. In patients with normal kidney function, once these medications are initiated and the dose titrated, clinicians should check the potassium concentration at least monthly. More frequent monitoring of serum potassium is warranted with combination MRA and either ACEI or ARB. For those patients with impaired kidney function, monitoring should be biweekly until the dose is stabilized.

In patients who have acute symptomatic hyperkalemia (eg, ECG changes), frequent potassium concentration and ECG monitoring is warranted. The patient should receive continuous ECG telemetry monitoring until the serum potassium concentration decreases below 5 mEq/L (mmol/L), and the ECG abnormalities resolve. Similarly, while the patient is receiving emergent therapy, serial serum potassium concentrations should be obtained hourly until the potassium concentration decreases below 5 mEq/L (mmol/L). For patients who receive insulin and dextrose therapy for hyperkalemia, blood glucose monitoring should be performed hourly or more frequently if patients demonstrate signs and symptoms of hypoglycemia. For patients who receive large doses of sodium bicarbonate therapy for hyperkalemia, an arterial blood gas or serum chemistry profile should be obtained to assess their acid-base status. Furthermore, the patient should be evaluated for signs of fluid overload secondary to the high sodium load. Patients receiving albuterol therapy should be questioned regularly regarding the development of palpitations and tachycardia. The patient's medication records should be reviewed to assure the patient is not receiving medication therapy that increases the serum potassium concentration. Furthermore, the patient should be questioned regarding the occurrence of diarrheal stool output.

Clinical Bottom Line

Hyperkalemia commonly occurs in patients with reduced kidney function or other metabolic disturbances. It can rapidly evolve into a medical emergency; therefore, prompt identification and appropriate pharmacotherapy are needed. In patients with mild hyperkalemia, potassium binding resins or loop diuretics may be useful and should be used as first-line therapy. In severe hyperkalemia with ECG changes, IV calcium should be given to protect against cardiac dysrhythmias. Additionally, rapid-acting therapies such as IV insulin and β_2-adrenergic agonists are indicated to move potassium intracellularly.

DISORDERS OF MAGNESIUM HOMEOSTASIS

Magnesium plays a central role in cellular function and is an important cofactor in more than 300 biochemical reactions in the body, especially those systems that are dependent on adenosine triphosphate. Mitochondrial function, protein synthesis, cell membrane function, parathyroid hormone secretion, and glucose metabolism are just a few important functions affected by magnesium.[60] It is the fourth most abundant extracellular cation and the second most abundant intracellular cation, after potassium. Disorders of magnesium homeostasis are commonly encountered in clinical situations and most frequently are manifested as alterations in cardiovascular and neuromuscular functions. Life-threatening conditions such as paralysis and cardiac arrhythmias can occur, making the proper recognition and treatment of these problems of paramount importance. Altered magnesium balance also plays a key role in chronic disease states such as diabetes mellitus, CKD, osteoporosis, development of kidney stones, as well as heart and vascular disease.[61]

Magnesium is principally distributed in bone (67%) and muscle (20%). Because of its predominantly intracellular distribution, measurement of magnesium in the extracellular compartment may not accurately reflect the total-body magnesium content. The majority of magnesium in the extracellular fluid is in the ionized form as only 30% is bound to serum proteins. The normal range for serum magnesium is 1.4 to 1.8 mEq/L (1.7-2.3 mg/dL or 0.70-0.95 mmol/L).

The recommended daily dietary magnesium intake for adults is approximately 420 mg/day and 320 mg/day for men and women, respectively. The maintenance of magnesium homeostasis depends on the balance between intake and output. Ingested magnesium (30%-40%) is absorbed in the small bowel. The absorption of magnesium decreases as the dietary intake increases. Reductions in absorption have also been noted in older adults and those with CKD. A small amount is present in intestinal secretions and reabsorbed in the sigmoid colon. The kidneys play a major role in maintaining magnesium balance. Approximately 95% of the filtered magnesium is reabsorbed, thus in most patients less than 5% is excreted in the urine.[51] Renal magnesium handling is unique in that approximately 20% of the filtered magnesium is reabsorbed in the proximal tubule; the majority (up to 70%) of reabsorption occurs in the thick ascending limb of the loop of Henle. This explains why loop diuretics often cause profound urinary magnesium wasting. The remaining 10% is reabsorbed in the distal convoluted tubule.[62] Unlike most other important electrolytes, there is no hormonal regulation of the distribution of magnesium between bone and circulating or intracellular magnesium pools. Because of this, both hypomagnesemia and hypermagnesemia commonly occur.

HYPOMAGNESEMIA

Epidemiology

Hypomagnesemia is a common problem in both ambulatory and hospitalized patients. Although the exact prevalence is difficult to estimate, up to 65% of ICU patients may be magnesium-deficient. Although serum magnesium concentrations are not a reliable index of total-body magnesium content, they remain the primary diagnostic tool to evaluate body stores.

Hypomagnesemia is associated with an increase in mortality in critically ill patients. The incidence and associated risks of hypomagnesemia in hospitalized general medicine patients, even though they are at an increased risk of hypomagnesemia given the presence of comorbidities such as heart failure, CKD, and diabetes mellitus. Hypomagnesemia may be observed in as many as 20% of hospitalized general medicine patients and is associated with increased mortality.[63]

Etiology and Pathophysiology

6 Hypomagnesemia is usually associated with disorders of the intestinal tract or kidney.[64] Medications or conditions that interfere with intestinal absorption or increase renal excretion of magnesium can result in hypomagnesemia (Table 70-6). Decreased intestinal absorption as a result of small bowel disease is the most common cause of hypomagnesemia worldwide. These disorders include regional enteritis, radiation enteritis, ulcerative colitis, acute and chronic diarrhea, pancreatic insufficiency and other malabsorptive syndromes, small-bowel bypass surgery, and chronic laxative misuse. Proton pump inhibitors, especially when used chronically, can cause hypomagnesemia through impaired intestinal absorption. Hypomagnesemia is commonly associated with alcohol use disorder, where the etiology is multifactorial, including reduced intake, pancreatic insufficiency, chronic vomiting and diarrhea, and urinary magnesium wasting.

Primary renal magnesium wasting can be caused by a defect in renal tubular magnesium reabsorption, or inhibition of sodium reabsorption in those segments in which magnesium transport follows passively. The former condition is associated with hypercalciuria, nephrolithiasis, and progressive kidney disease, while the latter is associated with Gitelman and Bartter syndromes.[64] Much more common than these is renal magnesium wasting secondary to thiazide and loop diuretics. Other commonly used medications that can cause renal magnesium wasting include aminoglycosides, amphotericin B, cyclosporine, digoxin, tacrolimus, cisplatin, pentamidine, and foscarnet.[65]

TREATMENT

Desired Outcomes

The treatment goals in the management of hypomagnesemia are (a) resolution of the signs and symptoms, (b) restoration of normal magnesium concentrations, (c) correction of concomitant electrolyte abnormalities, and (d) identification and correction of the underlying cause of magnesium depletion.

General Approach to Treatment

Magnesium supplementation can be administered by the oral, intramuscular (IM), or IV route. The severity of the magnesium depletion and the presence of severe signs and symptoms should dictate

CLINICAL PRESENTATION Hypomagnesemia

General

- The dominant organ systems affected by hypomagnesemia are the neuromuscular and cardiovascular systems.

Symptoms

- Neuromuscular symptoms such as tetany, twitching, and generalized convulsions are common.
- Cardiac symptoms include heart palpitations.

Signs

- Neuromuscular: Presence of Chvostek sign, Trousseau sign, tremor, and tetany.
- Cardiovascular: Cardiac arrhythmias (ventricular fibrillation, torsade de pointes, or digoxin-induced arrhythmias), sudden cardiac death, and hypertension can be present. ECG abnormalities include widened QRS complex and peaked T waves with mild hypomagnesemia; and prolonged PR interval, progressive widening of QRS complex, and flattened T waves with moderate to severe hypomagnesemia.

Laboratory Tests

- Serum magnesium concentration less than 1.4 mEq/L (1.7 mg/dL [0.70 mmol/L]). Serum potassium and calcium concentrations can also be low.

TABLE 70-6 Causes of Hypomagnesemia

GI

Reduced intake
- Protein-calorie malnutrition
- Prolonged parenteral fluid administration without magnesium
- Alcohol use disorder

Reduced absorption
- Primary hypomagnesemia
- Malabsorption syndromes (eg, tropical sprue, celiac disease, radiation enteritis, or intestinal lymphectasia)
- Short-bowel syndrome (eg, small-bowel resection or ileal bypass)
- Pancreatic insufficiency
- Proton pump inhibitors (long-term use)

Increased loss
- Excessive vomiting
- Prolonged nasogastric suction
- Excessive laxative use
- Intestinal and biliary fistulas
- Prolonged diarrhea (ulcerative colitis, Crohn disease, or cancer of the colon)

Kidney

Primary tubular disorders
- Primary renal magnesium wasting
- Bartter syndrome
- Renal tubular acidosis
- Diuretic phase of acute tubular necrosis
- Postobstructive diuresis
- Postrenal transplant diuresis

Glomerulonephritis

Pyelonephritis

Drug-induced renal losses
- Aminoglycosides
- Amphotericin B
- Cyclosporine
- Tacrolimus
- Diuretics
- Digitalis
- Cisplatin
- Pentamidine
- Foscarnet

Hormone-induced renal losses
- Primary hyperparathyroidism
- Hyperthyroidism
- Aldosteronism
- "Hungry bone syndrome" after parathyroidectomy

Internal redistribution

Diabetic ketoacidosis
Glucose, amino acid, or insulin administration
Massive blood transfusion (citrate)
Pancreatitis with lipedema (magnesium soap)

Other

Excessive sweating and lactation
Hypercalcemia and hypercalciuria
Phosphate depletion
Chronic alcohol use disorder
Extracellular fluid volume expansion

the route of administration. Because IM administration is painful, it should be reserved for those patients with severe hypomagnesemia and limited venous access. IV bolus administration is associated with flushing, sweating, and a sensation of warmth; thus, bolus administration should be avoided if possible. Additionally, because calcium forms a complex with the sulfate moiety, which is then excreted, large amounts of IV magnesium sulfate should be administered with caution to patients with hypocalcemia, as it can further exacerbate calcium deficiency.[61] It is widely accepted that 8 to 12 g of magnesium sulfate be administered, in divided doses, in the first 24 hours followed by 4 to 6 g/day for 3 to 5 days to adequately replete body stores in those with severe hypomagnesemia.[66] Even if severe magnesium depletion is present, approximately 50% of the administered dose is excreted in the urine. Consequently, magnesium replacement

TABLE 70-7 Common Magnesium Products and Their Elemental Magnesium Content

Product	Elemental Magnesium Content
Magnesium aspartate hydrochloride	122 mg in 1,230 mg dietary supplement granules
Magnesium carbonate	121 mg in 500 mg capsule
Magnesium chloride	64 mg in each 535 mg tablet
Magnesium citrate	48 mg in each 5 mL of the oral solution
Magnesium gluconate	27 mg in a 500 mg tablet
Magnesium glycerophosphate	97 mg in 1 g tablet
Magnesium hydroxide	167 mg in a 400 mg tablet or 5 mL oral suspension
Magnesium lactate	84 mg in an 84 mg tablet
Magnesium oxide	242 mg in a 400 mg tablet

should be performed over 3 to 5 days, and continued supplementation should be provided for patients unable to eat. Table 70-7 lists the commonly used magnesium oral supplements and their respective elemental magnesium content.

Nonpharmacologic Therapy

There are no nonpharmacologic options for the management of hypomagnesaemia.

Pharmacologic Therapy

It is controversial whether all asymptomatic patients require magnesium supplementation when serum magnesium concentration falls below the normal range. In particular, for patients with type 2 diabetes mellitus, hypomagnesemia contributes to diabetic complications by affecting glucose transport and insulin secretion and utilization. Indeed, oral magnesium supplementation in patients with type 2 diabetes mellitus and hypomagnesemia improves insulin sensitivity and metabolic control.[67] On the other hand, hypomagnesemia may be a consequence of diabetes mellitus. Possible mechanisms of hypomagnesemia in these patients include reduced GI absorption, enhanced renal excretion secondary to an increased filtered magnesium load and tubular flow, and reduced tubular reabsorption. Metabolic abnormalities such as hypokalemia, hypophosphatemia, and metabolic acidosis may also contribute to its development.[68] While it seems reasonable to provide a supplement for diabetic patients with low serum magnesium concentrations, improved clinical outcomes have not been demonstrated.

Should treatment be warranted, those patients with serum magnesium concentrations greater than 1 mEq/L (1.2 mg/dL [0.5 mmol/L]) can be treated with oral supplements. Oral supplementation is preferred because magnesium uptake is a slow process that may require prolonged administration. Several magnesium products are available, including magnesium-containing antacids or laxatives, comprising a variety of magnesium salts in tablet or capsule formulations. Many of the oral products contain little magnesium, which necessitates three or four doses per day. As expected, diarrhea is the most common dose-limiting adverse medication reactions of oral therapy, which can greatly reduce patient compliance. Therefore, sustained-release magnesium products are preferred as they not only improve patient compliance but also reduce the occurrence of GI adverse medication reactions.

In patients with severe magnesium depletion (serum concentrations less than 1 mEq/L [1.2 mg/dL; 0.5 mmol/L]) or if signs and symptoms are present regardless of the serum concentration, IV magnesium should be administered. A dose of 4 to 6 g in 50 to 100 mL (maximum concentration 1 g/10 mL) should be administered in divided doses over 12 to 24 hours and repeated as necessary in order to maintain magnesium concentrations above 1 mEq/L (1.2 mg/dL [0.5 mmol/L]). Doses of 2 to 4 g in 50 mL infused over 1 hour are frequently used clinically; however, these result in transient benefit because of the extensive renal excretion and usually have to be repeated daily over 3 to 5 days for adequate repletion. Therapy should be continued until the signs and symptoms have completely resolved. In patients with impaired kidney function, some have reduced the does by 25% to 50%.

Evaluation of Therapeutic Outcomes

In patients with acute, asymptomatic mild-to-moderate hypomagnesemia, serum magnesium concentrations should be obtained at least daily during their hospitalization. Patients receiving oral magnesium therapy should be questioned regarding GI tolerance and the occurrence of diarrhea. Patients being treated for symptomatic severe hypomagnesemia should have their serum magnesium concentration monitored hourly until the serum concentration reaches 1.5 mEq/L (1.8 mg/dL [0.75 mmol/L]) and the symptoms resolve. At that point, the serum magnesium concentration can be monitored every 6 to 12 hours for the next 24 hours while receiving magnesium supplementation. Once the magnesium concentration is stable in the normal range, a concentration can be obtained daily. It should be reiterated that it typically takes 3 to 5 days to fully replete total-body magnesium stores. Patients receiving oral magnesium-containing antacids or supplements should be asked regularly about the occurrence of diarrhea.

Clinical Bottom Line

Hypomagnesemia is generally associated with kidney or GI tract disorders. Patients with mild, chronic magnesium loss, oral magnesium preparations can be used; however, the dose-limiting adverse medication reaction is diarrhea. For more severe hypomagnesemia, IV magnesium sulfate can be safely administered. Repeated doses may be needed as IV magnesium is rapidly eliminated in urine. In such cases, close monitoring of serum magnesium concentrations is needed.

HYPERMAGNESEMIA

Epidemiology

7 Hypermagnesemia (serum magnesium greater than 2 mEq/L [2.4 mg/dL; 1 mmol/L]) is a rare occurrence that is generally seen in patients with stage 4 or 5 CKD when magnesium intake exceeds the excretory capacity of the kidneys. Older adults are prone to hypermagnesemia because of their reduced GFR and because of their tendency to consume magnesium-containing antacids and vitamins.

Etiology and Pathophysiology

Because magnesium excretion decreases as GFR declines, serum magnesium concentrations tend to increase in patients with moderate-to-severe CKD. Indeed, magnesium concentrations steadily increase as the GFR decreases below 30 mL/min/1.73 m^2. As long as the patient maintains a normal diet, the serum magnesium concentration typically stabilizes at approximately 2.5 mEq/L (3 mg/dL [1.25 mmol/L]). If patients with stage 4 or 5 CKD are taking concomitant magnesium-containing antacids, the serum concentration can approach 6 mEq/L (7.3 mg/dL [3 mmol/L]), a value associated with signs and symptoms of toxicity. Critically ill patients with multiorgan system failure receiving enteral or parenteral nutrition are also prone to develop hypermagnesemia. Finally, the parenteral treatment of eclampsia with magnesium sulfate can lead to hypermagnesemia. Table 70-8 lists other causes of hypermagnesemia.

Clinical Presentation

8 The signs and symptoms of hypermagnesemia reflect magnesium's action on the neuromuscular and cardiovascular systems.[66,69] The main symptoms include lethargy, confusion, dysrhythmias, and muscle weakness. Symptoms are rare when the serum concentration is below 4 mEq/L (4.9 mg/dL [2 mmol/L]) (Fig. 70-3).

TABLE 70-8 Causes of Hypermagnesemia

Decreased renal excretion
Acute kidney injury
CKD with exogenous intake
Excessive intake
Treatment of toxemia of pregnancy
Ureteral irrigants (hemiacidrin)
Cathartics
Other
Lithium therapy
Hypothyroidism
Milk-alkali syndrome
Addison disease
Viral hepatitis
Acute diabetic ketoacidosis

CKD, chronic kidney disease.

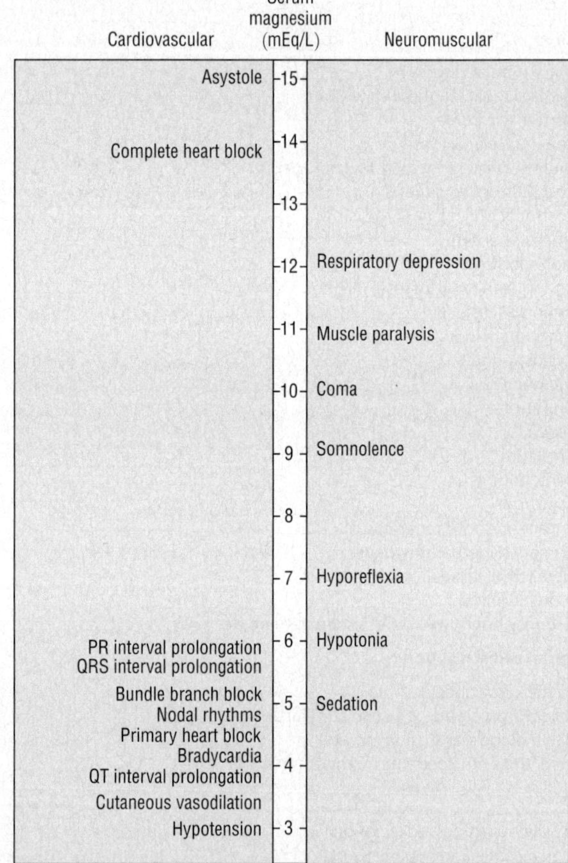

FIGURE 70-3 Clinical findings associated with hypermagnesemia. (Serum magnesium concentrations in mmol/L can be determined by multiplying the serum magnesium value expressed in mEq/L by 0.5.)

TREATMENT

Desired Outcome

The goals of therapy are to (a) reverse the neuromuscular and cardiovascular manifestations of hypermagnesemia, (b) decrease the magnesium concentration toward normal values, and (c) identify and treat the underlying cause of hypermagnesemia.

Nonpharmacologic Therapy

There are no nonpharmacologic options for the management of hypermagnesemia.

Pharmacologic Therapy

There are three primary means of treating hypermagnesemia: (a) reduce magnesium intake, (b) enhance elimination of magnesium, and (c) antagonize the physiologic effects of magnesium. The optimal treatment regimen for the management of hypermagnesemia depends on the severity of the patient's signs and symptoms and the degree of serum concentration elevation. IV elemental calcium doses of 100 to 200 mg directly antagonize the neuromuscular and cardiovascular effects of hypermagnesemia. Oral calcium is not effective because of its relatively poor bioavailability and slow onset of action. The clinical effect of calcium is immediate, but the effect is transient; hence, repeated IV doses of 100 to 200 mg of elemental calcium (eg, 2 g of calcium gluconate) might need to be administered hourly until the signs or symptoms abate and the magnesium concentration is normalized. Supportive care with cardiac pacing, vasopressors, and mechanical ventilation can be necessary in life-threatening situations. In patients with normal kidney function or those with stage 1, 2, or 3 CKD, forced diuresis with 0.45% NaCl and loop diuretics can promote magnesium elimination. An initial IV bolus of furosemide 40 mg or a similar equivalent can be used. Subsequent dosing can be determined based on the patient's clinical response. Patients with CKD can require long-term loop diuretic therapy to maintain adequate fluid and electrolyte balance. In patients with ESRD receiving dialysis, their hemodialysis prescription should be changed to employ magnesium-free dialysate.

Evaluation of Therapeutic Outcomes

Patients who are receiving IV calcium salts for the treatment of severe, symptomatic hypermagnesemia should have their serum magnesium concentration evaluated hourly until symptoms abate and the magnesium concentration decreases below 4 mg/dL (3.3 mEq/L [1.64 mmol/L]). Furthermore, the patient should be continuously monitored to detect ECG changes. In patients with CKD who can produce urine, forced diuresis with saline and furosemide should reduce the serum magnesium concentration within 6 to 12 hours. Close monitoring of the urine output and physical examination for signs of volume overload are important. Emergency hemodialysis will usually correct the hypermagnesemia within 4 hours and is a reasonable option for those who are receiving hemodialysis. To prevent further episodes of hypermagnesemia, the patient should receive dietary education regarding foods and beverages that contain large quantities of magnesium (Table 70-9).

TABLE 70-9 Magnesium Content of Selected Foods

Food	Elemental Magnesium Content per Serving (mg)
Halibut, cooked, 3 oz (85 g)	90
Almonds, dry roasted, 1 oz (28 g)	80
Spinach, boiled, one-half cup (~125 mL)	78
Cashews, dry roasted, 1 oz (28 g)	74
Peanuts, oil roasted, one-fourth cup (~60 mL)	63
Shredded wheat cereal, two large biscuits	61
Soymilk, plain, or vanilla, 1 cup (~250 mL)	61
Black beans, cooked, one-half cup (~125 mL)	60
Edamame, shelled, cooked, one-half cup (~125 mL)	50
Peanuts, dry roasted, 1 oz (28 g)	50
Peanut butter, smooth, 2 tablespoons (~30 mL)	49
Bread, whole wheat, 2 slices	46
Avocado, cubed, 1 cup (~250 mL)	44
Potato, baked with skin, 3.5 oz (~100 g)	43
Yogurt, plain, low fat, 8 oz (~225 g)	42
Rice, brown, cooked, one-half cup (~125 mL)	42
Breakfast cereals, fortified with 10% of the daily value for magnesium	40
Instant oatmeal, 1 cup (~250 mL)	36
Kidney beans, canned, one-half cup (~125 mL)	35
Banana, 1 medium	32

Clinical Bottom Line

Hypermagnesemia is generally associated with advanced CKD. Severe hypermagnesemia can result in neurologic symptoms or cardiac dysrhythmias. Should these symptoms occur, IV calcium can counteract these effects. Forced diuresis with saline and loop diuretics is useful in lowering magnesium in patients with mild to moderate kidney disease; hemodialysis should be reserved for patients with ESRD.

ABBREVIATIONS

ACEI	angiotensin-converting enzyme inhibitor
AKI	acute kidney injury
ARB	angiotensin-II receptor blocker
CKD	chronic kidney disease
ECG	electrocardiogram
ESRD	end-stage renal disease
FDA	Food and Drug Administration
GFR	glomerular filtration rate
GI	gastrointestinal
IM	intramuscular
IV	intravenous
MRA	mineralocorticoid receptor antagonist
NSAID	nonsteroidal anti-inflammatory drug
RAAS	renin–angiotensin–aldosterone system
SPS	sodium polystyrene sulfonate

REFERENCES

1. Palmer BF, Dubose T. Disorders of potassium metabolism. In: Schrier R, ed. *Renal and Electrolyte Disorders.* 8th ed. Wolters Kluwer; 2018:137–161.
2. Palmer BF, Clegg DJ. Physiology and pathophysiology of potassium homeostasis: Core curriculum 2019. *Am J Kidney Dis.* 2019;74(5):682–695. doi:10.1053/j.ajkd.2019.03.427.
3. Kovesdy CP, Appel LJ, Grams ME, et al. Potassium homeostasis in health and disease: A scientific workshop cosponsored by the National Kidney Foundation and the American Society of Hypertension. *Am J Kidney Dis.* 2017;70(6):844–858. 10.1053/j.ajkd.2017.09.003.
4. Whelton PK. Primary prevention of hypertension clinical and public health advisory from the National High Blood Pressure Education Program. *JAMA.* 2002;288(15):1882. 10.1001/jama.288.15.1882.
5. Food and Nutrition Board, Institute of Medicine. *Dietary Reference Intakes for Water, Potassium, Sodium, Chloride, and Sulfate.* National Academies Press; 2005:10925. doi:10.17226/10925.
6. Gumz ML, Rabinowitz L, Wingo CS. An integrated view of potassium homeostasis. *N Engl J Med.* 2015;373(1):60–72. 10.1056/NEJMra1313341.
7. Palmer BF. Regulation of potassium homeostasis. *Clin J Am Soc Nephrol.* 2015;10(6):1050–1060. doi:10.2215/CJN.08580813.
8. U.S. Department of Agriculture and U.S. Department of Health and Human Services. *Dietary Guidelines for Americans, 2020–2025.* 9th ed. Skyhorse Publishing, Inc; 2020.
9. Malnic G, Giebisch G, Muto S, et al. Regulation of K^+ excretion. In: Alpern RJ, Caplan M, Moe OW, eds. *Seldin and Giebisch's the Kidney: Physiology and Pathophysiology.* 5th ed. Elsevier Science & Technology; 2013. Accessed September 30, 2021. http://ebookcentral.proquest.com/lib/vcu/detail.action?docID=1108978.

10. Batlle D, Boobés K, Manjee KG. The colon as the potassium target: Entering the colonic age of hyperkalemia treatment? *EBioMedicine*. 2015;2(11):1562–1563. doi:10.1016/j.ebiom.2015.10.027.
11. Aronson PS, Giebisch G. Effects of pH on potassium: New explanations for old observations. *J Am Soc Nephrol*. 2011;22(11):1981–1989. doi:10.1681/ASN.2011040414.
12. Adrogué HJ. Sodium and potassium in the pathogenesis of hypertension. *N Engl J Med*. 2007;356:1966–1978.
13. Castro D, Sharma S. Hypokalemia. In: *StatPearls*. StatPearls Publishing; 2021. Accessed September 24, 2021. http://www.ncbi.nlm.nih.gov/books/NBK482465/.
14. Pepin J, Shields C. Advances in diagnosis and management of hypokalemic and hyperkalemic emergencies. *Emerg Med Pract*. 2012;14(2):1–17; quiz 17-18.
15. Collins AJ, Pitt B, Reaven N, et al. Association of serum potassium with all-cause mortality in patients with and without heart failure, chronic kidney disease, and/or diabetes. *Am J Nephrol*. 2017;46(3):213–221. doi:10.1159/000479802.
16. van Dinter TG, Fuerst FC, Richardson CT, et al. Stimulated active potassium secretion in a patient with colonic pseudo-obstruction: A new mechanism of secretory diarrhea. *Gastroenterology*. 2005;129(4):1268–1273. doi:10.1053/j.gastro.2005.07.029.
17. Gennari FJ. Hypokalemia. *N Engl J Med*. 1998;339:451–458. doi:10.1056/NEJM199808133390707.
18. Huang CL, Kuo E. Mechanism of hypokalemia in magnesium deficiency. *J Am Soc Nephrol*. 2007;18(10):2649–2652. doi:10.1681/ASN.2007070792.
19. Cohn JN, Kowey PR, Whelton PK, Prisant LM. New guidelines for potassium replacement in clinical practice: A contemporary review by the National Council on Potassium in Clinical Practice. *Arch Intern Med*. 2000;160(16):2429. doi:10.1001/archinte.160.16.2429.
20. 2005 American Heart Association Guidelines for Cardiopulmonary Resuscitation and Emergency Cardiovascular Care. Part 10.1: Life-threatening electrolyte abnormalities. *Circulation*. 2005;112(24_supplement). doi:10.1161/CIRCULATIONAHA.105.166563.
21. Nyirenda MJ, Tang JI, Padfield PL, Seckl JR. Hyperkalaemia. *BMJ*. 2009;339(Oct 23 1):b4114–b4114. doi:10.1136/bmj.b4114.
22. Betts KA, Woolley JM, Mu F, McDonald E, Tang W, Wu EQ. The prevalence of hyperkalemia in the United States. *Curr Med Res Opin*. 2018;34(6):971–978. doi:10.1080/03007995.2018.1433141.
23. Kamel KS, Schreiber M, Halperin ML. Renal potassium physiology: Integration of the renal response to dietary potassium depletion. *Kidney Int*. 2018;93(1):41–53. doi:10.1016/j.kint.2017.08.018.
24. Kovesdy CP. Management of hyperkalaemia in chronic kidney disease. *Nat Rev Nephrol*. 2014;10(11):653–662. doi:10.1038/nrneph.2014.168.
25. Li L, Harrison SD, Cope MJ, et al. Mechanism of action and pharmacology of patiromer, a nonabsorbed cross-linked polymer that lowers serum potassium concentration in patients with hyperkalemia. *J Cardiovasc Pharmacol Ther*. 2016;21(5):456–465. doi:10.1177/1074248416629549.
26. Mount D. Disorders of potassium balance. In: Skorecki K, ed. *Brenner and Rector's The Kidney*. 10th ed. Elsevier; 2016:559–600.
27. Weir MR, Rolfe M. Potassium homeostasis and renin-angiotensin-aldosterone system inhibitors. *Clin J Am Soc Nephrol*. 2010;5(3):531–548. doi:10.2215/CJN.07821109.
28. Zannad F, McMurray JJV, Krum H, et al. Eplerenone in patients with systolic heart failure and mild symptoms. *N Engl J Med*. 2011;364(1):11–21. doi:10.1056/NEJMoa1009492.
29. Kerendia® [package insert]. Whippany, NJ: Bayer Healthcare Pharmaceuticals, Inc. 2021.
30. Liu LC, Schutte E, Gansevoort RT, van der Meer P, Voors AA. Finerenone: Third-generation mineralocorticoid receptor antagonist for the treatment of heart failure and diabetic kidney disease. *Expert Opin Investig Drugs*. 2015;24(8):1123–1135. doi:10.1517/13543784.2015.1059819.
31. Rossignol P, Legrand M, Kosiborod M, et al. Emergency management of severe hyperkalemia: Guideline for best practice and opportunities for the future. *Pharmacol Res*. 2016;113:585–591. doi:10.1016/j.phrs.2016.09.039.
32. Farese S, Kruse A, Pasch A, et al. Glycyrrhetinic acid food supplementation lowers serum potassium concentration in chronic hemodialysis patients. *Kidney Int*. 2009;76(8):877–884. doi:10.1038/ki.2009.269.
33. Ferrari P. Licorice: A sweet alternative to prevent hyperkalemia in dialysis patients? *Kidney Int*. 2009;76(8):811–812. doi:10.1038/ki.2009.282.
34. Bagshaw SM, Lamontagne F, Joannidis M, Wald R. When to start renal replacement therapy in critically ill patients with acute kidney injury: Comment on AKIKI and ELAIN. *Crit Care*. 2016;20(1). doi:10.1186/s13054-016-1424-0.
35. Elliott MJ, Ronksley PE, Clase CM, Ahmed SB, Hemmelgarn BR. Management of patients with acute hyperkalemia. *CMAJ Can Med Assoc J*. 2010;182(15):1631–1635. doi:10.1503/cmaj.100461.
36. Scott NL, Klein LR, Cales E, Driver BE. Hypoglycemia as a complication of intravenous insulin to treat hyperkalemia in the emergency department. *Am J Emerg Med*. 2019;37(2):209–213. doi:10.1016/j.ajem.2018.05.016.
37. Wheeler DT, Schafers SJ, Horwedel TA, Deal EN, Tobin GS. Weight-based insulin dosing for acute hyperkalemia results in less hypoglycemia: Hyperkalemia treatment and hypoglycemia. *J Hosp Med*. 2016;11(5):355–357. doi:10.1002/jhm.2545.
38. LaRue HA, Peksa GD, Shah SC. A comparison of insulin doses for the treatment of hyperkalemia in patients with renal insufficiency. *Pharmacother J Hum Pharmacol Drug Ther*. 2017;37(12):1516–1522. doi:10.1002/phar.2038.
39. Garcia J, Pintens M, Morris A, Takamoto P, Baumgartner L, Tasaka CL. Reduced versus conventional dose insulin for hyperkalemia treatment.. *J Pharm Pract*. 2020;33(3):262–266. 10.1177/0897190018799220.
40. Keeney KP, Calhoun C, Jennings L, Weeda ER, Weant KA. Assessment of intravenous insulin dosing strategies for the treatment of acute hyperkalemia in the emergency department. *Am J Emerg Med*. 2020;38(6):1082–1085. doi:10.1016/j.ajem.2019.158374.
41. Drug FDA Safety Communication: FDA recommends separating dosing of potassium-lowering drug sodium polystyrene sulfonate (Kayexalate) from all other oral drugs. FDA. Published February 9, 2019. Accessed September 30, 2021. https://www.fda.gov/drugs/drug-safety-and-availability/fda-drug-safety-communication-fda-recommends-separating-dosing-potassium-lowering-drug-sodium
42. Kayexalate® [package insert]. Bridgewater, NJ: Sanofi-aventis U.S. LLC; 2009.
43. McGowan CE, Saha S, Chu G, Resnick MB, Moss SF. Intestinal necrosis due to sodium polystyrene sulfonate (kayexalate) in sorbitol. *South Med J*. 2009;102(5):493–497. doi:10.1097/SMJ.0b013e31819e8978.
44. Sterns RH, Rojas M, Bernstein P, Chennupati S. Ion-exchange resins for the treatment of hyperkalemia: Are they safe and effective? *J Am Soc Nephrol*. 2010;21(5):733–735. doi:10.1681/ASN.2010010079.
45. Mahoney BA, Smith WA, Lo D, Tsoi K, Tonelli M, Clase C. Emergency interventions for hyperkalaemia. Cochrane Kidney and Transplant Group, ed. *Cochrane Database Syst Rev*. Published online April 20, 2005. doi:10.1002/14651858.CD003235.pub2
46. Fordjour KN, Walton T, Doran JJ. Management of hyperkalemia in hospitalized patients. *Am J Med Sci*. 2014;347(2):93–100. doi:10.1097/MAJ.0b013e318279b105.
47. Peacock WF, Rafique Z, Clark CL, et al. Real world evidence for treatment of hyperkalemia in the Emergency Department (REVEAL–ED): A multicenter, prospective, observational study. *J Emerg Med*. 2018;55(6):741–750. doi:10.1016/j.jemermed.2018.09.007.
48. Phillips CO, Kashani A, Ko DK, Francis G, Krumholz HM. Adverse effects of combination angiotensin ii receptor blockers plus angiotensin-converting enzyme inhibitors for left ventricular dysfunction: A quantitative review of data from randomized clinical trials. *Arch Intern Med*. 2007;167(18):1930. doi:10.1001/archinte.167.18.1930.
49. Bakris GL, Agarwal R, Anker SD, et al. Effect of finerenone on chronic kidney disease outcomes in type 2 diabetes. *N Engl J Med*. 2020;383(23):2219–2229. doi:10.1056/NEJMoa2025845.
50. Pitt B, Filippatos G, Agarwal R, et al. Cardiovascular events with finerenone in kidney disease and type 2 diabetes. *N Engl J Med*. Published online August 28, 2021:NEJMoa2110956. doi:10.1056/NEJMoa2110956.
51. Van Buren PN, Adams-Huet B, Nguyen M, et al. Potassium handling with dual renin-angiotensin system inhibition in diabetic nephropathy. *Clin J Am Soc Nephrol*. 2014;9:295–301. 10.2215/CJN.07460713.
52. Lepage L, Dufour AC, Doiron J, et al. Randomized clinical trial of sodium polystyrene sulfonate for the treatment of mild hyperkalemia in CKD. *Clin J Am Soc Nephrol*. 2015;10(12):2136–2142. doi:10.2215/CJN.03640415.
53. Chernin G, Gal-Oz A, Ben-Assa E, et al. Secondary Prevention of hyperkalemia with sodium polystyrene sulfonate in cardiac and kidney patients on renin-angiotensin-aldosterone system inhibition therapy. *Clin Cardiol*. 2012;35(1):32–36. doi:10.1002/clc.20987.
54. Weir MR, Bakris GL, Bushinsky DA, et al. Patiromer in patients with kidney disease and hyperkalemia receiving RAAS Inhibitors. *N Engl J Med*. 2015;372(3):211–221. doi:10.1056/NEJMoa1410853.
55. Bakris GL, Pitt B, Weir MR, et al. Effect of patiromer on serum potassium level in patients with hyperkalemia and diabetic kidney

disease: The AMETHYST-DN randomized clinical trial. *JAMA*. 2015;314(2):151. doi:10.1001/jama.2015.7446.
56. Veltassa® [package insert]. Redwood City, CA: Relypsa, Inc; 2015.
57. Packham DK, Rasmussen HS, Lavin PT, et al. Sodium zirconium cyclosilicate in hyperkalemia. *N Engl J Med*. 2015;372(3):222–231. 10.1056/NEJMoa1411487.
58. Kosiborod M, Rasmussen HS, Lavin P, et al. Effect of sodium zirconium cyclosilicate on potassium lowering for 28 days among outpatients with hyperkalemia: The HARMONIZE randomized clinical trial. *JAMA*. 2014;312(21):2223. doi:10.1001/jama.2014.15688.
59. Lokelma® [package insert]. Wilmington, DE; AstraZeneca Pharmaceuticals, LP. 2021.
60. Chan L. Normal and abnormal magnesium metabolism. In: Schrier R, ed. *Renal and Electrolyte Disorders*. 8th ed. Lippincott Williams & Wilkins; 2018:225–252.
61. Musso CG. Magnesium metabolism in health and disease. *Int Urol Nephrol*. 2009;41(2):357–362. doi:10.1007/s11255-009-9548-7.
62. Blaine J, Chonchol M, Levi M. Renal control of calcium, phosphate, and magnesium homeostasis. *Clin J Am Soc Nephrol*. 2015;10(7):1257–1272. doi:10.2215/CJN.09750913.
63. Wolf F, Hilewitz A. Hypomagnesaemia in patients hospitalised in internal medicine is associated with increased mortality. *Int J Clin Pract*. 2014;68(1):111–116. doi:10.1111/ijcp.12260.
64. Martin KJ, González EA, Slatopolsky E. Clinical consequences and management of hypomagnesemia. *J Am Soc Nephrol*. 2009;20(11):2291–2295. doi:10.1681/ASN.2007111194.
65. Atsmon J, Dolev E. Drug-induced hypomagnesaemia: Scope and management. *Drug Saf*. 2005;28(9):763–788. doi:10.2165/00002018-200528090-00003.
66. Ayuk J, Gittoes NJL. Treatment of hypomagnesemia. *Am J Kidney Dis*. 2014;63(4):691–695. doi:10.1053/j.ajkd.2013.07.025.
67. Rodriguez-Moran M, Guerrero-Romero F. Oral magnesium supplementation improves insulin sensitivity and metabolic control in type 2 diabetic subjects: A randomized double-blind controlled trial. *Diabetes Care*. 2003;26(4):1147–1152. doi:10.2337/diacare.26.4.1147.
68. Pham PCT, Pham PMT, Pham SV, Miller JM, Pham PTT. Hypomagnesemia in patients with type 2 diabetes. *Clin J Am Soc Nephrol*. 2007;2(2):366–373. doi:10.2215/CJN.02960906.
69. Jahnen-Dechent W, Ketteler M. Magnesium basics. *Clin Kidney J*. 2012;5(Suppl 1):i3–i14. doi:10.1093/ndtplus/sfr163.

71

Acid–Base Disorders

Anne M. Tucker and Tami N. Johnson

KEY CONCEPTS

1. The lung plays a central role in acid–base homeostatic regulation through an increase or decrease in respiration to regulate the partial pressure of CO_2 in the blood (PCO_2); an increased respiratory rate (RR) eliminates more CO_2, reduces the PCO_2 in the blood, and results in a reduced carbonic acid concentration and increased pH; the opposite occurs with decreased respiration.
2. The kidney also plays a central role in the regulation of acid–base homeostasis through the excretion or reabsorption of filtered bicarbonate (HCO_3^-), the excretion of metabolic fixed acids, and the generation of new HCO_3^-.
3. Each acid–base disturbance has a compensatory response that attempts to correct the HCO_3^--to-$PaCO_2$ ratio toward normal and mitigate the change in pH. The respiratory compensatory response to metabolic disturbances is initiated rapidly, whereas the metabolic compensatory response to respiratory disturbances occurs more slowly.
4. Metabolic acidosis and metabolic alkalosis are generated by a primary change in the serum bicarbonate concentration. In metabolic acidosis, bicarbonate is lost or a nonvolatile acid is gained, whereas metabolic alkalosis is characterized by a gain in bicarbonate or a loss of nonvolatile acid.
5. Arterial blood gases (ABGs), along with serum electrolytes, physical findings, medical and medication history, and the clinical condition of the patient, are the primary tools to determine the cause of an acid–base disorder and to design and monitor a course of therapy.
6. Renal tubular acidosis (RTA) refers to a group of disorders characterized by impaired tubular renal acid handling despite normal or near-normal glomerular filtration rates. These patients often present with hyperchloremic metabolic acidosis.
7. Primary therapy of most acid–base disorders must include treatment or removal of the underlying cause, not just correction of the pH and electrolyte disturbances.
8. Potassium supplementation is always necessary for patients with chronic metabolic acidosis, as the bicarbonaturia resulting from alkali therapy increases renal potassium wasting.
9. Effective treatment of the underlying cause of some organic acidoses (eg, ketoacidosis) can result in bicarbonate regeneration within hours thus mitigating the need for alkali therapy.
10. A patient's response to volume replacement can be predicted by the urine chloride concentration and permits the differential diagnosis of metabolic alkalosis.
11. Loss of gastric acid from vomiting or nasogastric suctioning may lead to hypochloremia and hyperbicarbonatemia and may often lead to a metabolic alkalosis.
12. Aggressive loop diuretic therapy can produce a metabolic alkalosis, and the accompanying hypokalemia.
13. Management of metabolic alkalosis due to excessive renal acid excretion usually consists of treatment of the underlying cause of mineralocorticoid excess. In patients in whom the mineralocorticoid excess cannot be corrected, chronic pharmacologic therapy may be required.
14. In most cases of acute respiratory acidosis, such as following cardiopulmonary arrest, sodium bicarbonate therapy is not indicated and can be detrimental. Blood gas analysis and the clinical status of the patient should guide therapy.

BEYOND THE BOOK

Watch the video entitled "Acid–Base Balance & Blood Gas Interpretation" in the 2019 National Council Licensure Examination (NCLEX) Review [available at https://youtu.be/kh62SRovgrl]. This 10-minute video provides a brief overview of acid–base balance, disturbances, compensation, and interpretation. This video is useful to enhance student understanding regarding the assessment of acid–base disorders in the patient care process.

INTRODUCTION

Acid–base disorders are common and often serious disturbances that can result in significant morbidity and mortality. This chapter reviews the mechanisms responsible for the maintenance of acid–base balance and the laboratory analyses that aid clinicians in their assessment of acid–base disorders. The pathophysiology of the four primary acid–base disturbances is presented, evidence-based therapeutic options are reviewed, and management guidelines to optimize the outcome of patients with one of these disorders are presented. Given that medications are a frequent cause of acid–base abnormalities and that acid–base abnormalities are often preventable, clinicians must anticipate medication-related problems to avoid or minimize the clinical consequences of acid–base disorders, and when necessary, design appropriate treatment regimens.

ACID–BASE CHEMISTRY

An acid (in this equation, hydrochloric acid) is a substance that can *donate* protons (hydrogen ion [H^+]):

$$\text{(Acid) HCl} \rightarrow H^+ + \text{Chlorideion } (Cl^-)$$

TABLE 71-1 Acid–Base Pairs

Carbonic acid/bicarbonate	H_2CO_3/HCO_3^-
Monobasic/dibasic phosphate	H_2PO_4/HPO_4^-
Ammonium/ammonia	NH_4^+/NH_3
Lactic acid/lactate	$H_6C_3O_2/H_5C_3O_2^-$

A base (in this equation, ammonia [NH_3]) is a substance that can *accept* protons (hydrogen ion [H^+]):

$$\text{(Ammonia)}NH_3 + H^+ \rightarrow NH_4^+\text{(base)}$$

The acid–base pairs commonly encountered in clinical practice are listed in Table 71-1.

The acidity of body fluids is quantified in terms of the hydrogen ion concentration. By convention, the degree of acidity is expressed as pH, or the negative logarithm (base 10) of the hydrogen ion concentration. Thus, hydrogen ion concentration and pH are inversely related. Normally, the pH of blood is maintained at 7.4 ([H^+] of 4×10^{-8} M) with a range of 7.35 to 7.45. A pH of less than 6.7 ([H^+] of 2×10^{-7} M), representing a fivefold increase in hydrogen ion concentration, or greater than 7.7 ([H^+] of 2×10^{-8} M), representing a 50% decrease in hydrogen ion concentration, is considered incompatible with life.

The hydrogen ion concentration in blood may not be indicative of that in other body compartments. For example, the pH within cells, within the cerebrospinal fluid, or on the surface of bone can all be altered without causing an alteration in blood pH.[1] Recognizing this caveat, the acid–base status of the body is usually analyzed based on measurement of blood pH. Alterations in blood pH serve as the basis for the diagnosis of acid–base disorders.

The dissociation of acid–base pairs is an equilibrium reaction. This allows the relationship between hydrogen ion concentration or pH and the relative concentrations of the acid and base to be described mathematically in terms of the dissociation constant for the acid–base buffer pair. When expressed as a logarithmic relationship, where p*K* is the negative logarithm of the dissociation constant *K*, this is known as the Henderson–Hasselbalch equation:

$$pH = pK + \log([\text{base}]/[\text{acid}])$$

BUFFERS

The ability of a weak acid and its corresponding anion (base) to resist change in the pH of a solution with the addition of a strong acid or base is referred to as *buffering*. An acid–base pair is most efficient in functioning as a buffer at a pH close to its p*K*. The principal extracellular buffer is the carbonic acid/bicarbonate (H_2CO_3/HCO_3^-) system. Other physiologic buffers include plasma proteins, hemoglobin, and phosphates. The complex buffering of biologic fluids can be analyzed based on a single buffer pair because the isohydric principle requires that all buffer systems remain in chemical equilibrium.

The carbonic acid/bicarbonate buffer system plays a unique role in acid–base homeostasis. In addition to being the most abundant extracellular buffer, the components of this buffer pair exist under dynamic regulation by the body. In the presence of carbonic anhydrase, carbonic acid, [H_2CO_3], is in equilibrium with carbon dioxide (CO_2) gas. Changes in pulmonary ventilation that alter the partial pressure of CO_2 (PCO_2) in the blood regulate the carbonic acid level in the blood. Conversely, the bicarbonate concentration is independently regulated by the kidney. Because the p*K* for the carbonic acid/bicarbonate system is 6.1, the relationship between pH, carbonic acid, and bicarbonate concentrations can be described by the Henderson–Hasselbalch equation. The concentration of carbonic acid is directly proportional to the amount of CO_2 dissolved in blood, which is equal to the product of PCO_2 and its solubility in physiologic fluids ($PCO_2 \times 0.03$ for PCO_2 expressed in mm Hg or $PCO_2 \times 0.226$ for PCO_2 expressed in kPa). This term can, therefore, be substituted into the equation below in place of [H_2CO_3].

$$pH = 6.1 + \log([HCO_3^-]/[H_2CO_3])$$

$$pH = 6.1 + \log([HCO_3^-]/[PCO_2 \times 0.03]) \text{ for } PCO_2 \text{ in mm Hg}$$

or

$$pH = 6.1 + \log([HCO_3^-]/[PCO_2 \times 0.226]) \text{ for } PCO_2 \text{ in kPa}$$

Thus, hydrogen ion concentration and pH are determined not by the absolute amounts of bicarbonate and PCO_2 present but by their ratio.[2] Under normal physiologic conditions, the kidneys maintain the serum bicarbonate at approximately 24 mEq/L (mmol/L), whereas the lungs maintain the PCO_2 at approximately 40 mm Hg (5.3 kPa). The normal physiologic pH is thus 7.4:

$$pH = 6.1 + \log[24/(0.03 \times 40)] \text{ (or } pH = 6.1 + \log[24/0.226 \times 5.3])$$
$$pH = 6.1 + 1.3 = 7.4$$

If, in response to an acid load, the serum bicarbonate concentration decreases to 12 mEq/L (mmol/L), then the predicted pH would be:

$$[HCO_3^-] = 12 \text{ mEq/L (mmol/L)}$$

$$PCO_2 = 40 \text{ mm Hg (5.3 kPa)}$$

$$pH = 6.1 + \log[12/0.03 \times 40] \text{ or}$$

$$pH = 6.1 + \log([12/(0.226 \times 5.3)])$$

$$pH = 6.1 + 1.0 = 7.1$$

However, the normal respiratory response to an acid load is hyperventilation. As a result, if the PCO_2 decreased to approximately 26 mm Hg (3.5 kPa), then the change in pH would be less:

$$[HCO_3^-] = 12 \text{ mEq/L (mmol/L)}$$

$$PCO_2 = 26 \text{ mm Hg (3.5 kPa)}$$

$$pH = 6.1 + \log[12/0.03 \times 26]$$

$$\text{or } pH = 6.1 + \log[12/(0.226 \times 3.5)]$$

$$pH = 6.1 + 1.19 = 7.29$$

Thus, the physiologic regulation of both PCO_2 and [HCO_3^-] permits the carbonic acid/bicarbonate system to provide more effective buffering of the extracellular fluids (ECFs) than could be achieved on the basis of chemical buffering alone.

REGULATION OF ACID–BASE HOMEOSTASIS

Cellular metabolism results in the production of large quantities of hydrogen that need to be excreted to maintain acid–base balance. In addition, small amounts of acid and alkali are also presented to the body through the diet. The bulk of acid production is in the form of CO_2, with the average adult producing approximately 15,000 mmol of CO_2 each day from the catabolism of carbohydrate, protein, and fat.[2] When respiratory function is normal, the amount of CO_2 produced metabolically is equal to the amount lost by respiration, and the blood CO_2 concentration remains constant.

Digestion of dietary substances and tissue metabolism also result in the production of nonvolatile acids. These acids are derived primarily from the sulfur-containing amino acids cysteine and methionine, as well as from ingested sulfur. In addition, phosphates are generated from the metabolism of proteins and phospholipids.

Neutral substances such as glucose can also be incompletely metabolized to intermediates, such as lactic and pyruvic acid, and fatty acids can be incompletely metabolized to acetoacetic acid and β-hydroxybutyric acid. These dietary and metabolic fixed acids are excreted primarily by the kidney to maintain acid–base homeostasis. On average, daily fixed acid excretion is approximately 0.8-1 mEq/kg/day (mmol/kg/day).[3]

Three processes, each of which varies in its onset, collectively maintain acid–base balance: extracellular buffering, ventilatory regulation of carbon dioxide elimination, and kidney regulation of hydrogen ion and bicarbonate excretion. Extracellular buffering occurs rapidly and is the body's first defense against a sudden increase in hydrogen ion concentration. Hyperventilation then results in a decrease in PCO_2, returning blood pH toward normal. Finally, over a period of day(s), the kidney will excrete the excess hydrogen ion and acid–base balance will return to normal.

Extracellular Buffering

The body's buffering system can be divided into three components: bicarbonate/carbonic acid, proteins, and phosphates. The bicarbonate/carbonic acid buffer system is the most abundant of the body's buffers making it the first line of the defense of changes in pH, because (a) there is more bicarbonate present in the ECF than any other buffer component; (b) the supply of CO_2 is unlimited; and (c) the acidity of ECF can be regulated by controlling either the bicarbonate concentration or the PCO_2.

Carbonic acid represents the respiratory component of the buffer pair because its blood concentration is directly proportional to the PCO_2, which is determined by ventilation. Bicarbonate represents the metabolic component because the kidney may alter its concentration by reabsorption, generating new bicarbonate, or altering elimination.[2] The bicarbonate buffer system easily adapts to changes in acid–base status by alterations in ventilatory elimination of acid (PCO_2) and/or renal elimination of base (HCO_3^-).

The phosphate buffer system consists of serum inorganic phosphate (3.5-5 mg/dL [1.13-1.62 mmol/L]), intracellular organic phosphate, and calcium phosphate in bone. Extracellular phosphate is present only in low concentrations, so its usefulness as a buffer is limited; however, as an intracellular buffer, phosphate is more useful. Calcium phosphate in bone is relatively inaccessible as a buffer, but prolonged metabolic acidosis will result in the release of phosphate from bone.

Intracellular and extracellular proteins also act as buffering systems. The charged side chains of amino acids provide the buffering action. Because the concentration of protein is much greater intracellularly than extracellularly, protein is much more important as an intracellular buffer.

Respiratory Regulation

1 The second process involved in maintenance of acid–base homeostasis is ventilatory regulation of CO_2 elimination. Both the rate and depth of ventilation can be varied to allow for excretion of CO_2 generated by diet and tissue metabolism. Medullary chemoreceptors in the brainstem sense changes in PCO_2 and pH and modulate the control of breathing. Increasing minute ventilation (the total amount of air exhaled over a 1-minute period), by increasing RR and/or tidal volume (the amount of air exhaled in one breath), will increase CO_2 excretion and decrease the blood PCO_2. Conversely, decreasing minute ventilation decreases CO_2 excretion and increases blood PCO_2. This system rapidly adjusts to changes in acid–base balance.[4]

Kidney Regulation

2 Bicarbonate is freely filtered at the glomerulus because it is a small ion. The bicarbonate load delivered to the nephron is approximately 4,500 mEq/day (mmol/day).[2] To maintain acid–base balance, this entire filtered bicarbonate load must be reabsorbed. Bicarbonate reabsorption occurs primarily in the proximal tubule (Fig. 71-1). In the tubular lumen, filtered bicarbonate combines with hydrogen ion, secreted by the apical sodium ion (Na^+)–H^+-exchanger, to form carbonic acid. The carbonic acid is rapidly broken down to CO_2 and water by carbonic anhydrase, an enzyme located on the luminal surface of the brush border membrane. The CO_2 then diffuses into the proximal tubular cell, where it reforms carbonic acid in the presence of intracellular carbonic anhydrase. The carbonic acid dissociates to form hydrogen ions that can again be secreted into the tubular lumen, and bicarbonate that exits the cell across the basolateral membrane and enters the peritubular capillary.

Excretion of metabolic fixed acids and generation of new HCO_3^- are achieved in nearly equal parts by renal ammoniagenesis and distal tubular hydrogen ion secretion. Ammoniagenesis plays a critical role in acid–base homeostasis, with ammonium (NH_4^+) excretion comprising approximately 50% of renal net acid excretion. Ammonium is generated from the deamination of glutamine in the proximal tubule. For each ammonium ion excreted in the urine, one bicarbonate ion is regenerated and returned to the circulation.[2]

Distal tubular hydrogen ion secretion accounts for the remaining 50% of net acid excretion. Although the distal tubule consists of multiple distinct functional segments and cell types, the carbonic anhydrase-containing intercalated cells are primarily responsible for acid–base transport. Specifically, type A intercalated cells function as hydrogen ion secreting cells (Fig. 71-2). In these cells, CO_2 combines with water in the presence of intracellular carbonic anhydrase to form carbonic acid, which dissociates to H^+ and HCO_3^-. The H^+ is actively transported into the tubular lumen by a H^+–adenosine triphosphatase. The bicarbonate exits the cell across the basolateral membrane and enters the circulation.[2]

ACID–BASE DISTURBANCES

3 4 Alterations in blood pH are designated by the suffix "-emia"; *acidemia* is an arterial blood pH less than 7.35 and *alkalemia* is an arterial blood pH more than 7.45. The pathophysiologic processes that result in alterations in blood pH are designated by the suffix "-osis." These disturbances are classified as either metabolic or respiratory in origin. In metabolic acid–base disorders, the primary disturbance is in the plasma bicarbonate concentration. Metabolic acidosis is characterized by a decrease in the plasma bicarbonate concentration, whereas in metabolic alkalosis the plasma bicarbonate concentration is increased. Respiratory acid–base disorders are caused by alterations in alveolar ventilation that produce corresponding changes in the partial pressure of carbon dioxide from arterial blood ($PaCO_2$). In respiratory acidosis, the $PaCO_2$ is elevated; in respiratory alkalosis, it is decreased. Each disturbance has a compensatory (secondary) response that attempts to correct the HCO_3^--to-$PaCO_2$ ratio toward normal and mitigate the change in pH (Table 71-2). Although the time course of the respiratory compensatory response to metabolic disturbances is rapid, the metabolic compensation for respiratory disturbances is slow. As a result, respiratory disturbances are characterized as acute (minutes to hours in duration), indicating that there has not been sufficient time for metabolic compensation, or chronic (days), indicating that sufficient time for metabolic compensation has elapsed.

CLINICAL ASSESSMENT OF ACID–BASE STATUS

A blood gas is measured to determine not only a patient's acid–base status but also their oxygenation. Under normal circumstances, the pH difference between arterial and mixed venous blood is not

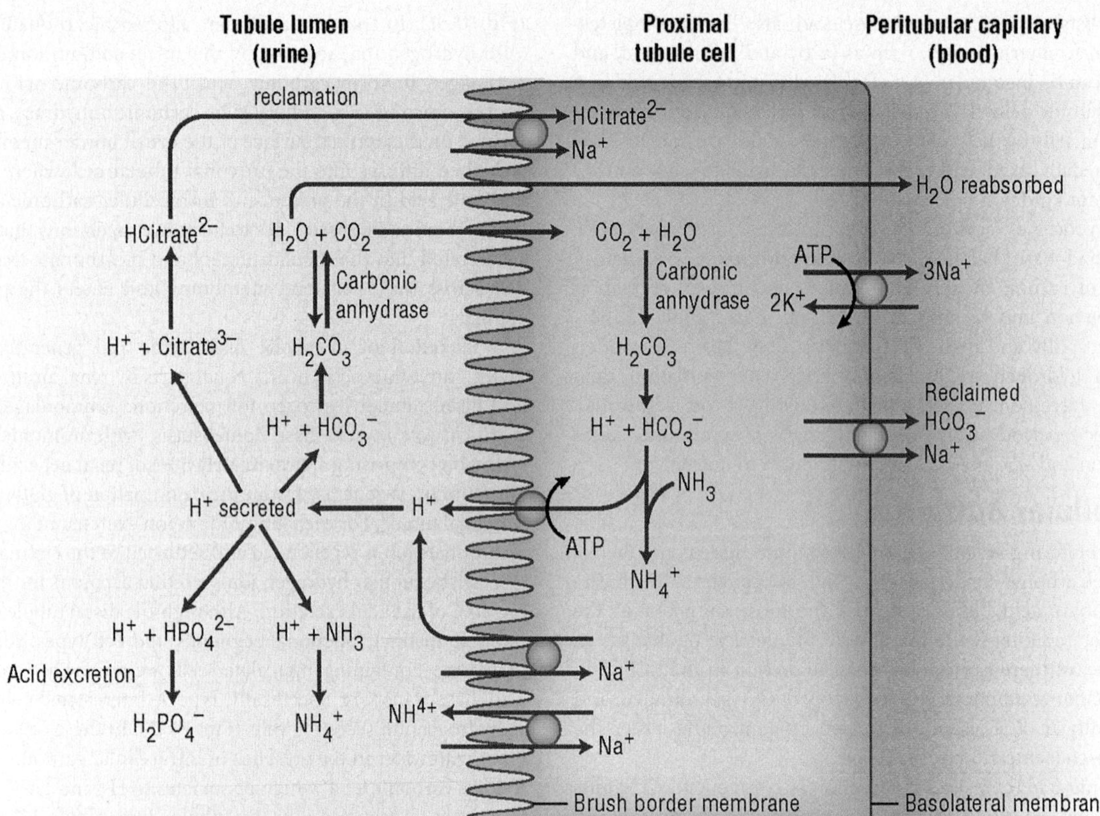

FIGURE 71-1 Proximal tubular bicarbonate reabsorption and renal acid secretion. The diagram shows the cellular processes involved in bicarbonate (HCO_3^-) reabsorption and renal acid (H^+) secretion in the lumen of proximal tubule lumen (left), proximal tubular cell (in the middle), and peritubular capillary (on the right). In the tubular lumen, filtered HCO_3^- combines with a H^+ secreted by an apical sodium ion (Na^+)–H^+ exchanger to form carbonic acid (H_2CO_3). Carbonic anhydrase located on the luminal surface of the brush border membrane rapidly breaks down H_2CO_3 to carbon dioxide (CO_2) and water (H_2O). The H_2O is absorbed from the tubular lumen into the cell and then into the peritubular capillary. The CO_2 then diffuses into the proximal tubular cell, where it reforms H_2CO_3 in the presence of intracellular carbonic anhydrase. Within the tubular cell, H_2CO_3 dissociates into H^+ and HCO_3^-. Ammonium ion (NH_4^+) is also produced and excreted into the tubular lumen. The HCO_3^- exits the tubular cell across the basolateral membrane into the peritubular capillary along with Na^+. The H^+ is secreted back into the tubular lumen where it is used to generate additional HCO_3^- through the above process and facilitate urinary acid secretion through formation of NH_4^+ and dihydrogen phosphate ion ($H_2PO_4^-$). The secreted H^+ may also titrate citrate^{3-} to form HCitrate^{2-} in the tubular lumen which is equivalent to reabsorption of alkali when transported into the tubular cell.

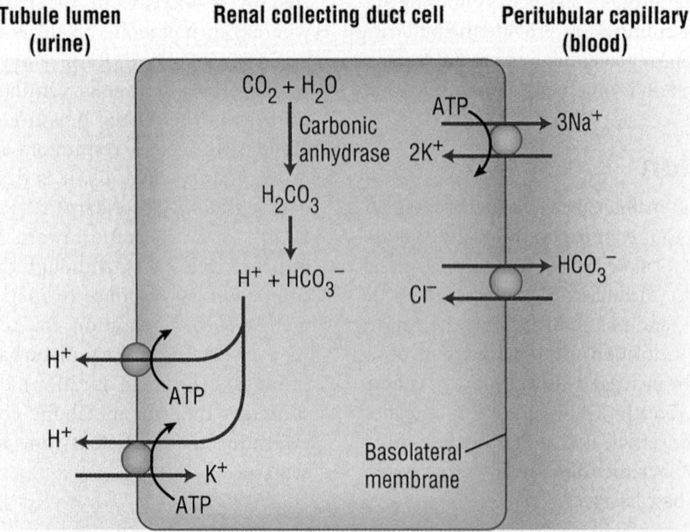

FIGURE 71-2 Collecting duct acid excretion. The diagram shows the cellular processes involved in acid excretion in the lumen of the collecting duct of the nephron (left), renal collecting duct cell (in the middle), and peritubular capillary (on the right). Hydrogen ion (H^+) and bicarbonate (HCO_3^-) are generated intracellularly from carbon dioxide (CO_2) and water (H_2O) in the presence of intracellular carbonic anhydrase. The H^+ is actively secreted into the tubular lumen for excretion by H^+–adenosine triphosphatase located in the apical (luminal) membrane. The HCO_3^- exits the renal collecting duct cell across the basolateral membrane and enters the peritubular capillary as chloride ion (Cl^-) enters the cell.

TABLE 71-2 Interpretation of Simple Acid–Base Disorders

Acid–Base Disorder	pH	Primary Disturbances	Compensation
Acidosis			
Respiratory	Decrease	Increase $PaCO_2$	Increase HCO_3^-
Metabolic	Decrease	Decrease HCO_3^-	Decrease $PaCO_2$
Alkalosis			
Respiratory	Increase	Decrease $PaCO_2$	Decrease HCO_3^-
Metabolic	Increase	Increase HCO_3^-	Increase $PaCO_2$

TABLE 71-3 Normal Blood Gas Values

	Arterial Blood	Mixed Venous Blood
pH	7.40 (7.35-7.45)	7.38 (7.33-7.43)
PO_2	80-100 mm Hg (10.6-13.3 kPa)	35-40 mm Hg (4.7-5.3 kPa)
SaO_2	95% (0.95)	70-75% (0.70-0.75)
PCO_2	35-45 mm Hg (4.7-6.0 kPa)	45-51 mm Hg (6.0-6.8 kPa)
HCO_3^-	22-26 mEq/L (mmol/L)	24-28 mEq/L (mmol/L)

HCO_3^-, bicarbonate; PCO_2, partial pressure of carbon dioxide; PO_2, partial pressure of oxygen; SaO_2, saturation of arterial oxygen.

clinically significant. However, the oxygenation difference between arterial and mixed venous blood is always substantial. Arterial samples are designated with the letter "a" (eg, partial pressure of oxygen from arterial blood [PaO_2] and $PaCO_2$), whereas mixed venous samples are labeled with the letter "v" or not labeled (eg, partial pressure of oxygen from venous blood [PvO_2] and partial pressure of carbon dioxide from venous blood [$PvCO_2$]). The normal values for arterial and venous blood gases are shown in Table 71-3. Arterial blood reflects how well the blood is being oxygenated by the lungs (an accurate measurement of PaO_2), whereas venous blood reflects how much oxygen tissues are using. Arterial blood rather than venous blood should be used whenever possible because venous blood obtained from an extremity can provide misleading information. If metabolism in the extremity is altered by hypoperfusion, exercise, infection, or some other cause, the difference in the amount of dissolved oxygen between arterial and venous blood can be dramatic. The venous pH and PCO_2 during cardiopulmonary resuscitation might be significantly lower and higher, respectively, than the arterial pH and arterial PCO_2. This indicates a severe tissue acidosis from CO_2 accumulation caused by hypoperfusion.

Analysis of Arterial Blood Gas Data

5 ABGs provide an assessment of the patient's acid–base status.[4] Low pH values (less than 7.35) indicate an acidemia, whereas high pH values (more than 7.45) indicate an alkalemia (Fig. 71-3). In a metabolic acidosis, the pH is decreased in association with a decreased serum bicarbonate concentration and a compensatory decrease in $PaCO_2$. In a respiratory acidosis while the pH is decreased, the $PaCO_2$ is elevated. The serum bicarbonate concentration is variable, depending on whether it is an acute disturbance (minimal increase in serum bicarbonate) or a chronic respiratory acidosis (substantial increase in serum bicarbonate). In a metabolic alkalosis, the pH is elevated in association with an increased bicarbonate concentration and a compensatory increase in $PaCO_2$. In a respiratory alkalosis, while the pH is also elevated, the $PaCO_2$ is decreased. As with respiratory acidosis, the metabolic compensation is variable: a minimal decrease in serum bicarbonate is often noted in acute respiratory alkalosis, while a larger decrease in [HCO_3^-] is common with chronic respiratory alkalosis. Although each measurement has a normal range (see Table 71-3), it is often easiest to consider the midpoint of each range as the normal value. This would correlate to a pH of 7.4, $PaCO_2$ of 40 mm Hg (5.3 kPa), and HCO_3^- of 24 mEq/L (mmol/L). Steps in acid–base interpretation, using this physiologic approach, are described in Table 71-4. While beyond the scope of this chapter, two other approaches to assess acid–base status (ie, the physicochemical [Stewart's] approach and the base excess approach) are sometimes used in clinical practice.[5,6]

When ABGs differ significantly from those expected on the basis of the patient's clinical condition and previous laboratory determinations, additional venous blood samples should be drawn to assess plasma electrolyte concentrations. The bicarbonate calculated from the patient's $PaCO_2$ and pH of the blood gas should be compared with the measured total CO_2 content (the amount of CO_2 gas extractable from plasma, consisting of HCO_3^-, H_2CO_3, and

TABLE 71-4 Steps in Acid–Base Diagnosis

1. Obtain ABG and electrolyte panel simultaneously
2. Compare [HCO_3^-] on ABG and electrolyte panel to verify accuracy
3. Calculate SAG (corrected for albumin when appropriate)
4. Is acidemia (pH <7.35) or alkalemia (pH >7.45) present?
5. Is the primary abnormality respiratory (alteration in $PaCO_2$) or metabolic (alteration in HCO_3^-)?
6. Estimate compensatory response (Table 71-7)
7. Compare change in [Cl^-] with change in [Na^+]
8. Compare the relative change of HCO_3^- and SAG to rule out mixed disorder(s)

[Cl^-], chloride ion; [Na^+], sodium ion.

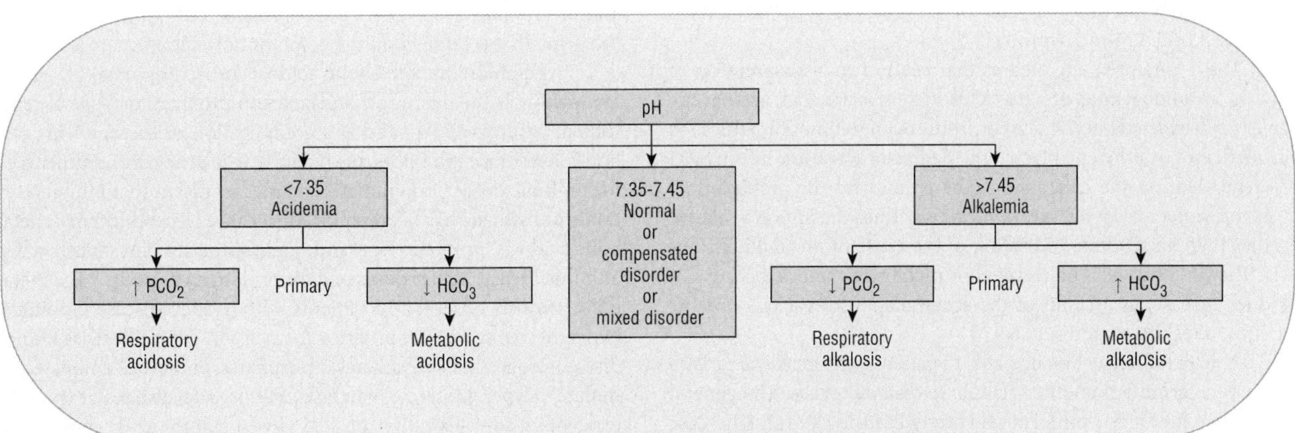

FIGURE 71-3 Analysis of arterial blood gases. (HCO_3^-, bicarbonate; PCO_2, partial pressure of carbon dioxide.)

PCO_2). Ordinarily, the blood gas bicarbonate value is approximately 1 to 2 mEq/L (mmol/L) less than the total CO_2 content.[7] If these values do not correspond, the results should be interpreted with caution because the difference can reflect an error in the blood collection or storage of the sample, or in the calibration of the blood gas analyzer.

METABOLIC ACID–BASE DISORDERS

Metabolic Acidosis

Metabolic acidosis is characterized by a decrease in pH as the result of a primary decrease in serum bicarbonate concentration.

Pathophysiology

Metabolic acidosis can result from the buffering (consumption of HCO_3^-) of an exogenous acid, an organic acid accumulating because of a metabolic disturbance (eg, lactic acid or ketoacids), or the progressive accumulation of endogenous acids secondary to impaired kidney function (eg, phosphates and sulfates).[8] The serum HCO_3^- can also be decreased as the result of a loss of bicarbonate-rich body fluids (eg, diarrhea, biliary drainage, or pancreatic fistula) or occur secondary to the rapid administration of non-alkali–containing IV fluids (dilutional acidosis).[8]

The SAG, as defined below, can be used to determine whether an organic or mineral acidosis is present.

$$SAG = [Na^+] - [Cl^-] - [HCO_3^-]$$

To maintain electroneutrality, the total concentration of cations in the serum must equal the total concentration of anions.

$$[Na^+] + [UCs] = ([Cl^-] + [HCO_3^-]) + [UAs]$$

The cation concentration is equal to the sodium concentration plus that of "unmeasured" cations (UCs), predominantly magnesium, calcium, and potassium. The anion concentration is equal to the concentrations of chloride, bicarbonate, and "unmeasured" anions (UAs), including proteins, sulfates, phosphates, and organic anions. Therefore, as the result of the combination of the two equations above, the SAG can be expressed as:

$$SAG = [UAs] - [UCs]$$

The normal SAG is approximately 10 mEq/L (mmol/L), with a range of 8 to 12 mEq/L (mmol/L). Differences exist in SAG based on clinical laboratories; therefore, the clinician should identify the normal SAG where practicing.[7] Increases in the anion gap (AG) to values of greater than or equal to 20 mEq/L (mmol/L) are indicative of the accumulation of UAs in ECF. The SAG calculation assumes normal serum albumin. In cases of hypoalbuminemia, the SAG may be underestimated. For every decrease in serum albumin by 1 g/dL (10 g/L) below the normal value of 4.5 g/dL (45 g/L), the SAG is decreased by 2.5 mEq/L (mmol/L).[7]

These UAs are generated as the result of the consumption of HCO_3^- by endogenous organic acids such as lactic acid, acetoacetic acid, or β-hydroxybutyric acid or from the ingestion of toxins such as methanol or ethylene glycol. The degree of elevation in the SAG is dependent on the clearance of the anion, and the multiple factors that influence HCO_3^- concentrations. Thus, the SAG is a relative rather than an absolute indication of the cause of metabolic acidosis. The SAG can also be elevated in metabolic acidosis because of kidney disease, as a result of the accumulation of various organic anions, phosphates, and sulfates.

A delta ratio may be calculated in patients with an elevated SAG to help determine if another acid–base disorder exists. The general rule is that for every 1 mmol of acid present causing a 1 mEq increase in SAG, the serum bicarbonate should drop by 1 mEq leading to a delta gap of 1. A delta ratio equal to 1 indicates an uncomplicated or pure elevated SAG metabolic acidosis. A delta ratio less than 1 indicates a mixed elevated SAG and non-SAG metabolic acidosis. A delta ratio greater than 1 indicates an elevated SAG metabolic acidosis and metabolic alkalosis.[9]

TABLE 71-5 Common Causes of Metabolic Acidosis

Increased Serum Anion Gap	Normal Serum Anion Gap/ Hyperchloremic States
Ketoacidosis	Acid ingestion/administration
Alcoholic	(ammonium chloride, hydrochloric acid)
Diabetic	GI bicarbonate loss
Starvation	Diarrhea, high output ileostomy
Kidney disease	External pancreatic or small bowel drainage (fistula)
AKI	Ureteroenterostomy (urinary diversion)
CKD	Calcium chloride (acidifying agent)
Lactic acidosis (see Table 71-7)	Magnesium sulfate (diarrhea)
5-Oxyprolinemia (acetaminophen)	Cholestyramine (bile acid diarrhea)
Toxins/overdoses	Excessive administration of chloride salts (eg, sodium chloride, PN)
Ethylene glycol	Renal bicarbonate loss
Methanol	Adrenal insufficiency
Propyl alcohol	Carbonic anhydrase inhibitors (eg, acetazolamide, topiramate)
Propylene glycol	Hypoaldosteronism
Salicylate	RTA (see Table 71-6)

ACE, angiotensin-converting enzyme; NSAIDs, nonsteroidal anti-inflammatory drugs; PN, parenteral nutrition; RTA, renal tubular acidosis.

In hyperchloremic metabolic acidosis, bicarbonate losses from the ECF are replaced by chloride, and the SAG remains normal. This decrease in bicarbonate may be due to gastrointestinal (GI) tract losses, dilution of bicarbonate in the ECF as a result of the addition of sodium chloride solutions or chloride-containing acids. Common causes of metabolic acidosis with an increased or a normal SAG are listed in Table 71-5.

Hyperchloremic Metabolic Acidosis

Hyperchloremic metabolic acidosis can result from increased GI bicarbonate loss, renal bicarbonate wasting, impaired renal acid excretion, exogenous acid gain, topiramate, or chloride-containing IV fluids.[8] GI disorders such as diarrhea, biliary, or pancreatic drainage through either a surgical drain or fistula can result in the loss of large volumes of bicarbonate-containing fluids. Severe diarrhea, the most common cause of hyperchloremic metabolic acidosis, can lead to significant bicarbonate losses as increased GI motility precludes absorption of bicarbonate in the GI tract. Patients who have undergone ureteral diversion into the sigmoid colon or isolated ileal loop can also develop a hyperchloremic metabolic acidosis. This is the result of a net loss of bicarbonate, given that chloride is reabsorbed, and bicarbonate is secreted by GI epithelial cells in the presence of the urine that is retained in the colon or bowel loop.

Hyperchloremic metabolic acidosis caused by renal bicarbonate wasting is the defining disturbance in proximal or Type II renal tubular acidosis (RTA) and is a complication of therapy with carbonic anhydrase inhibitors, particularly when they are administered for multiple doses.[8] Topiramate, an anticonvulsant that inhibits carbonic anhydrase, has been reported to cause hyperchloremic metabolic acidosis, proximal RTA and nephrolithiasis, particularly when administered at higher doses and for prolonged periods.[10] The metabolic acidosis observed in patients with kidney disease is initially hyperchloremic but can progress to an anion-gap acidosis as kidney disease progresses and sulfates, phosphates, and other anions accumulate.[7] Hyperchloremic metabolic acidosis can also result from the exogenous administration of acid (hydrochloric acid, ammonium chloride) or the unbuffered administration of acid salts from the amino acids in parenteral nutrition.[11]

TABLE 71-6 Renal Tubular Acidosis

	Type I	Type II	Type IV
Location	Distal tubules	Proximal tubules	Adrenal/Distal tubules
Primary defect	Impaired urinary H^+ secretion	Decreased urinary HCO_3^- reabsorption	Aldosterone deficiency or resistance
Acidosis	Yes (severe)	Yes	Yes (mild)
UAG	Positive	Negative	Positive
Urine pH	>5.5	<5.5	<5.5
Serum potassium	Low	Low/normal	High
Etiology*	Heredity Autoimmune diseases Primary biliary cirrhosis Rheumatoid arthritis Sjögren syndrome SLE Thyroiditis Hypercalcemia Medications Amphotericin B Cisplatin Ifosfamide Lithium Pentamidine Trimethoprim	Heredity Amyloidosis Fanconi Syndrome Medications Acetazolamide Aminoglycosides Cisplatin Foscarnet Ifosfamide 6-Mercaptopurine Tetracyclines (expired) Topiramate Valproate Multiple myeloma Nephrotic syndrome Sjögren syndrome Toxic metal exposure	Heredity Adrenal insufficiency, primary Autoimmune adrenalitis Adrenal suppression 21-hydroxylase deficiency Adrenal insufficiency, secondary ACEI/ARB/renin inhibitors CKD Diabetes mellitus type 2 Hypertension Hypothalamic-pituitary disease Aldosterone resistance Aldosterone antagonists NSAIDs Potassium sparing diuretics Trimethoprim Chronic interstitial nephropathy (nephritis, obstructive uropathy, HIV nephropathy) General distal tubule defect Sickle cell nephropathy SLE Amyloidosis Renal transplant rejection Chronic cyclosporine toxicity

*Not a comprehensive list, but includes common clinically important disease associations and medications; ACE, angiotensin-converting enzyme; ARB, angiotensin II receptor blocker; CKD, chronic kidney disease; NSAID, nonsteroidal anti-inflammatory drug; SLE, systematic lupus erythematosus.

Data from References 7, 12, and 13.

Renal Tubular Acidosis

6 Renal tubular disorders can involve the proximal tubule, with a resultant failure to reabsorb filtered bicarbonate, or affect acid excretion in the distal tubule. The distal RTAs are the most common and are all characterized by impaired net acid excretion. The distal RTAs are subdivided into those that are associated with hypokalemia (type I) and those associated with hyperkalemia (type IV). Type II represents proximal RTA. Type III is extremely rare and will not be discussed. Common causes of RTAs are presented in Table 71-6.

Patients with classic distal (type I) RTA have impaired hydrogen ion secretion and are unable to excrete the daily acid load necessary to maintain acid–base balance.[12,13] These patients are unable to maximally acidify their urine (ie, attain urine pH less than 5.5), even in the face of an acid challenge. Type I RTA may be the result of a primary tubular defect or develop secondary to a wide variety of medications (eg, amphotericin B, ifosfamide, lithium) and disorders including hypercalcemia, and autoimmune disorders such as systemic lupus erythematosus.[7,12,13] The primary form of this disorder usually occurs in children and can result in severe acidosis, slowed growth, nephrocalcinosis, and kidney stones. In adults, clinical complications include osteomalacia, nephrocalcinosis, and recurrent kidney stones.

Proximal (type II) RTA is characterized by defects in proximal tubular reabsorption of bicarbonate. Normally, 80% to 85% of filtered bicarbonate is reabsorbed in the proximal tubule.[7,14] Defects in proximal tubular bicarbonate reabsorption result in increased delivery of bicarbonate to the distal nephron, which has a limited capacity for bicarbonate reabsorption. As a result, at a normal serum bicarbonate concentration, the filtered bicarbonate load is incompletely reabsorbed, and is lost in the urine. Thus, patients with proximal RTA present with a chronic, nonprogressive hyperchloremic metabolic acidosis. These patients are able to acidify their urine in response to an acid load but develop bicarbonaturia at a reduced serum bicarbonate concentration following bicarbonate loading. The impaired bicarbonate reabsorption results in salt wasting and secondary hyperaldosteronism. Hypokalemia, which can be severe, usually develops as a result of the hyperaldosteronism and bicarbonaturia.[7,14] Proximal RTA usually presents as an acquired disorder, secondary to carbonic anhydrase inhibitor therapy, a variety of diseases (eg, amyloidosis, multiple myeloma, nephrotic syndrome) or exposure to toxins (eg, lead, cadmium, mercury, expired tetracyclines).

The hyperkalemic distal (type IV) RTAs are a heterogeneous group of disorders characterized by hypoaldosteronism or generalized distal tubule defects. The most common form of type IV RTA is hyporeninemic hypoaldosteronism. This syndrome is most commonly associated with diabetic nephropathy, but can also be seen in a variety of other disorders, including chronic interstitial nephritis, sickle-cell disease, human immunodeficiency virus (HIV) nephropathy, and obstructive uropathy.[7,12] The clinical presentation of this syndrome is often exacerbated by medications that can interfere with the renin–angiotensin–aldosterone system, such as angiotensin-converting enzyme (ACE) inhibitors, angiotensin receptor blockers, renin inhibitors, and nonsteroidal anti-inflammatory drugs (NSAIDs). Patients with this form of RTA are able to maximally acidify their urine (urine pH less than 5.5). The primary defect in acid excretion is impaired ammoniagenesis caused by decreased kidney function. Treatment to control the hyperkalemia is usually sufficient to reverse the metabolic acidosis, and mineralocorticoid replacement is frequently unnecessary.

Hyperkalemic distal (type IV) RTA resulting from generalized distal tubule defects is less common than hyporeninemic hypoaldosteronism but is more common than classic distal (type I) RTA. Patients with this defect have impaired tubular potassium secretion in addition to impaired urinary acidification (urine pH more than 5.5, despite acidemia or acid loading). Urinary obstruction is the most frequent cause of this disorder, but it can also be associated with sickle-cell nephropathy, systemic lupus erythematosus, HIV nephropathy, analgesic misuse nephropathy, amyloidosis, kidney transplant rejection, and chronic cyclosporine nephrotoxicity.

Elevated Anion Gap Metabolic Acidosis

Metabolic acidosis with an increased SAG commonly results from increased endogenous organic acid production.[15] In lactic acidosis, lactic acid accumulates as a by-product of anaerobic metabolism.[16] Accumulation of the ketoacids β-hydroxybutyric acid and acetoacetic acid defines the ketoacidosis of uncontrolled diabetes mellitus (see Chapter 94, Diabetes Mellitus), alcohol intoxication (see Chapter 55, Portal Hypertension and Cirrhosis, and Chapter 86, Substance Use Disorders II), and starvation (see Chapter e83, Eating Disorders) (Table 71-5).[17] Toxic ingestions of methanol and ethylene glycol are also associated with high anion gap metabolic acidosis and can be differentiated from other causes of SAG by the presence of an elevated osmolar gap. An elevated osmolar gap is considered when the measured serum osmolality is more than 10 mOsm/kg (mmol/kg) greater than the calculated serum osmolality.[7] In advanced kidney disease, accumulation of phosphate, sulfate, and organic anions is responsible for the increased SAG, which is usually less than 24 mEq/L (mmol/L).[2] The severe metabolic acidosis seen in myoglobinuric acute kidney injury (AKI) as a result of rhabdomyolysis may be caused by the metabolism of large amounts of sulfur-containing amino acids released from myoglobin. The mechanisms responsible for the development of acidosis in these settings are diverse.

The presence of mild elevations in the SAG cannot be automatically attributed to the presence of a high SAG metabolic acidosis. Elevations in the SAG are commonly seen in hospitalized patients, especially those who are critically ill.[18] A variety of factors can contribute to this nonspecific elevation in the SAG, including the presence of alkalemia, which increases the anionic charge of albumin and other plasma proteins. The usefulness of the SAG as a marker of acid–base status is dependent on proper interpretation of a patient's clinical status. Despite these limitations, when the SAG is greater than or equal to 20 mEq/L (mmol/L), it is generally considered a high anion gap or a significant organic acidosis.

Lactic Acidosis Serum lactate levels are often elevated in acutely ill patients and can be used as a marker for severity of illness and response to therapy.[19] Serum lactate levels are considered normal in healthy subjects at approximately 1 mEq/L (mmol/L).[16] Hyperlactatemia is defined as a serum lactate greater than 2 mmol/L with lactic acidosis considered when serum lactate levels are greater than 4 mmol/L with concomitant acidosis.[19] Lactic acid is the end product of anaerobic metabolism of glucose (glycolysis).[13] In normal individuals, lactic acid derived from pyruvate enters the circulation in small amounts and is promptly removed by the liver. In the liver, and to a lesser extent in the kidney, lactic acid is reoxidized to pyruvic acid, which is then metabolized to CO_2 and H_2O.

Classically, lactic acidosis has been differentiated into disorders associated with tissue hypoxia (type A lactic acidosis) and disorders associated with deranged oxidative metabolism (type B lactic acidosis), although the distinction between them is blurred (Table 71-7).[16,19] Metabolic disturbances can result in increased tissue pyruvate production or impaired utilization, with proportional increases in lactate concentrations. Increased lactate production is more commonly associated with alterations in tissue redox state, resulting in preferential conversion of pyruvate to lactate. During anaerobic metabolism, reduced nicotinamide adenine dinucleotide accumulates, driving the conversion of pyruvate to lactate and increasing the lactate-to-pyruvate ratio. States of enhanced metabolic activity (eg, grand mal seizures, strenuous exercise, hyperthermia), decreased tissue oxygen delivery (eg, severe anemia, hypoxia, circulatory shock, carbon monoxide poisoning), or impaired oxygen utilization (eg, cyanide toxicity) are all associated with lactic acidosis. Impaired hepatic clearance of lactate, as seen in hypoperfusion states, liver failure, and alcohol intoxication, can also result in lactic acidosis.

Cardiovascular and septic shock, with resultant tissue hypoperfusion, are the most common causes of lactic acidosis.[16] Poor tissue perfusion and hypoxia influence enzymatic pyruvate and lactate metabolism to stimulate anaerobic glycolysis and to decrease lactate utilization. This leads to hyperlactatemia and lactic acidosis. The mortality rate of this type of lactic acidosis can be 50% or greater and correlates with the degree of hyperlactatemia.[20]

Lactic acidosis associated with liver disease, toxins, and congenital enzyme deficiency can be caused by deranged oxidative metabolism or impaired lactate clearance.[19] The exact role of diabetes mellitus in the induction of lactic acidosis is not clear. It may involve a decrease in pyruvate dehydrogenase activity, the enzyme responsible for pyruvate metabolism. Lactic acidosis in neoplastic disease is uncommon and reported mostly in patients with myeloproliferative disorders. Leukocytes and neoplastic cells in general have high rates of glycolysis. In the case of a large tumor or tightly packed bone marrow, oxygenation can be decreased, favoring the accumulation of lactate. Lactic acidosis has been reported in patients with massive liver tumors, and it has been postulated that the liver uptake of lactate is decreased in these patients. Lactic acidosis associated with

TABLE 71-7 Causes of Lactic Acidosis

Type A (hypoxia)	Type B (metabolic derangement)
Carbon monoxide poisoning	D-lactic acidosis
Increased oxygen demands	Diabetes mellitus
Hyperthermia	Inborn errors of metabolism and mitochondrial myopathies
Seizures	Medications/Toxins
Shivering	Alcohols
Vigorous exercise	Ethanol
Regional tissue ischemia	Ethylene glycol
Severe anemia	Methanol
Severe hypoxemia	Propofol (prolonged, high dose infusions)
Shock	Propylene glycol (IV formulations of lorazepam, pentobarbital, phenytoin, trimethoprim/sulfamethoxazole)
Cardiogenic	Beta-adrenergic agonists (albuterol, epinephrine)
Hemorrhagic	Cyanide (sodium nitroprusside)
Hypovolemic	Entecavir
Septic	Isoniazid
	Iron
	Linezolid
	Metformin
	NRTIs (abacavir, lamivudine, stavudine, tenofovir)
	Ombitasvir, paritaprevir, ritonavir, dasabuvir (Viekira Pak®)
	Phentermine-topiramate (Qsymia®)
	Salicylates
	Telbivudine
	Theophylline
	Systemic disease
	Malignancy
	Liver failure
	Thiamine deficiency

seizures is usually transient and occurs because of excessive muscle activity.[16,19]

A number of medications have been associated with the development of lactic acidosis. Metformin (0.03 cases per 1,000 person-years) remains the most common medication associated with lactic acidosis.[21] The primary suspected mechanism for metformin-induced lactic acidosis is inhibition of liver gluconeogenesis as the result of its inhibitory effects on pyruvate carboxylase, which is necessary for the conversion of pyruvate to glucose. Other possible pathways for metformin-associated lactic acidosis include a decrease in both hepatic intracellular pH and cardiac output, an increase in lactate production in the gut, and increased renal loss of bicarbonate. Risk factors for metformin-induced lactic acidosis include impaired kidney function, liver disease, dehydration, advanced age, excessive alcohol use, concomitant carbonic anhydrase inhibitor use, and supratherapeutic dosing.[19,22] Metformin should be discontinued during periods of tissue hypoxia (eg, myocardial infarction, sepsis), at the time of or before iodinated contrast imaging procedures in patients with eGFR 30 to 60 mL/min/1.73 m^2, withheld on the day of surgery and during periods of restricted food intake.[23,24] Metformin should only be reinstituted when the patient's kidney function is stable, and the patient is tolerating adequate oral diet.

The older nucleoside-analog reverse transcriptase inhibitors (NRTIs), particularly stavudine, have been associated with lactic acidosis (3.9 cases per 1,000 person-years) in patients with hepatic steatosis.[25] The proposed mechanism of NRTI-induced lactic acidosis is the inhibition of the enzyme DNA polymerase gamma that is responsible for mitochondrial DNA synthesis.[26] Lactic acidosis has been rarely reported with tenofovir, lamivudine, abacavir, and entecavir.

Linezolid impairs mitochondrial function and has been rarely reported to cause lactic acidosis, usually after prolonged (more than or equal to 4 weeks) therapy.[27] The weight loss combination medication phentermine-topiramate (Qsymia®) has been reported to cause lactic acidosis.[28] Use of the Viekira Pak® (ombitasvir, paritaprevir, ritonavir, dasabuvir) may cause lactic acidosis in patients without severe liver dysfunction when used to treat hepatitis C.[29]

Propylene glycol is commonly used as a solubilizing agent in IV medications (eg, lorazepam, pentobarbital, phenytoin, trimethoprim/sulfamethoxazole) and is predominantly metabolized to lactic acid via the hepatic enzyme alcohol dehydrogenase.[30-32] The administration of large doses of propylene glycol, particularly to patients with impaired kidney or liver function, can lead to a lactic acidosis with an osmolar gap. Thus, serial measurement of the osmolar gap can be used to detect propylene glycol accumulation.[30,31]

The association between propofol and lactic acidosis was initially described in children.[33] This association is now recognized in adults and has come to be known as the propofol-related infusion syndrome. In addition to lactic acidosis, cardiac failure, rhabdomyolysis, and AKI have been observed primarily because of uncoupling of oxidative phosphorylation and impaired oxidation of free fatty acids. To minimize the risk of propofol infusion syndrome, it is recommended not to exceed 4 mg/kg/hour for more than 48 hours unless the perceived benefit exceeds the risk.[33]

Clinical Presentation

Chronic metabolic acidosis is usually not associated with severe acidemia and is relatively asymptomatic. The major manifestations are bone demineralization with growth failure and short stature in children and both osteomalacia and osteopenia in adults.[6,28] Chronic metabolic acidosis is also associated with nonspecific symptoms including anorexia, nausea, weight loss, and muscle weakness.

Severe metabolic acidosis is usually associated with acute processes. The manifestations of severe acidemia (pH less than 7.20) involve the cardiovascular, respiratory, and central nervous system (CNS). Hyperventilation is often the first sign of metabolic acidosis. At a pH of 7.2, pulmonary ventilation increases approximately fourfold, and an eightfold increase has been noted at a pH of 7.[34,35] Respiratory compensation can occur as Kussmaul respirations—the deep, rapid respirations seen commonly in patients with diabetic ketoacidosis. In extremely severe acidosis (pH less than 6.8), CNS function is disrupted to such a degree that the respiratory center is depressed.

CNS depression correlates more closely with spinal fluid pH than with blood pH. For this reason, neurologic symptoms tend to occur more frequently and to a greater degree in patients with respiratory acidosis because the CO_2 accumulated in the respiratory form readily crosses the blood–brain barrier to cause acidosis in the CNS.[4] Because of the slow penetration of administered bicarbonate into the CNS, the CNS pH fails to normalize as rapidly as blood pH. Therefore, patients continue to hyperventilate because of sustained CNS acidity, and severe respiratory alkalosis can occur. Sustained lowering of the $PaCO_2$ within 12 to 36 hours is to be anticipated during the correction of any metabolic acidosis.[4]

Systemic acidosis can cause peripheral arteriolar dilatation, characterized by flushing, a rapid HR, and wide pulse pressure. Initially, cardiac output can be increased, but as acidosis becomes more severe, myocardial contractility becomes impaired, and cardiac output decreases. The effects of vagal stimulation are also enhanced at reduced pH levels, likely a consequence of inhibition of acetylcholinesterase. This increases the danger of vagally mediated bradycardia and heart block during acidosis.[36]

GI symptoms of metabolic acidosis include loss of appetite, nausea, and vomiting. Severe acidosis (pH less than 7.1) interferes with carbohydrate metabolism and insulin utilization, and results in hyperglycemia. Metabolic acidosis alters potassium homeostasis and contributes to the development of hyperkalemia. The magnitude of the effect on serum potassium depends on the type of acidosis: Acidosis caused by mineral acids (eg, hydrochloric acid) is associated with a greater change in potassium levels than acidosis caused by organic acids (eg, lactic acidosis), in which the increase in potassium attributable to the acidosis is minimal.[37]

Compensation

The patient's primary means to compensate for metabolic acidosis is to increase carbon dioxide excretion by increasing the RR. This results in a decrease in $PaCO_2$. This ventilatory compensation results from stimulation of the respiratory center by changes in cerebral bicarbonate concentration and pH.[4,38] For every 1 mEq/L (mmol/L) decrease in bicarbonate concentration below the average of 24, the $PaCO_2$ decreases by approximately 1 to 1.5 mm Hg (0.13-0.20 kPa) from the normal value of 40 mm Hg (5.3 kPa). General guidelines for the assessment and interpretation of acid–base disorders based on observed compensatory responses are presented in Table 71-8.[7]

The anticipated $PaCO_2$ associated with a given bicarbonate concentration for patients with uncomplicated metabolic acidosis can also be calculated using the Winters' formula[7]:

$$PaCO_2 = (1.5 \times [HCO_3^-] + 8) \pm 2 \text{ for } PaCO_2 \text{ in mm Hg}$$

$$(PaCO_2 = (0.2 \times [HCO_3^-] + 1.1) \pm 0.3 \text{ for } PaCO_2 \text{ in kPa})$$

For example, 95% of patients with a plasma bicarbonate of 16 mEq/L (mmol/L) should have an arterial PCO_2 of 30 to 34 mm Hg (4.0-4.5 kPa). An observed arterial PCO_2 within this range is consistent with physiologic respiratory compensation for a metabolic acidosis and suggests that there is no respiratory disturbance. In contrast, if the PCO_2 is less than 30 mm Hg (4.0 kPa), a superimposed respiratory alkalosis can be present, whereas if the PCO_2 is greater than 34 mm Hg (4.5 kPa), a superimposed respiratory acidosis is likely present.

CLINICAL PRESENTATION Metabolic Acidosis

General

- The patient usually is relatively asymptomatic if the acidosis is acute and mild. In those with severe acidemia (pH less than 7.20), the cardiovascular, respiratory, and CNS systems can be affected.

Symptoms

- The patient may complain of loss of appetite, nausea, and vomiting.

Signs

- Cardiac: Flushing, a rapid HR, wide pulse pressure, and an increase in cardiac output can be seen initially. This can be followed by a reduction in cardiac output, BP, and liver and kidney blood flow.
- Cerebral: Obtundation or coma.
- Metabolic: Insulin resistance; increased protein degradation; increased metabolic demands.
- GI: Nausea, vomiting, loss of appetite.
- Respiratory: Dyspnea, hyperventilation with deep, rapid respirations is seen in those with severe acidosis.
- Chronic acidemia causes bone demineralization with the development of growth failure and short stature in children and osteomalacia and osteopenia in adults.

Laboratory Tests

- Serum CO_2 is low. Hyperglycemia and hyperkalemia are common. Patients with a pH of less than 7.2 are deemed to have a severe acidosis.

TABLE 71-8 Guidelines for Interpretation of Acid–Base Disorders Based on Compensatory Responses

Acidosis	Compensation
Metabolic	$PaCO_2$ (in mm Hg) should decrease by 1.25 times the fall in plasma [HCO_3^-] (in mEq/L or mmol/L)
Acute respiratory	Plasma [HCO_3^-] should increase by 0.1 times the increase in $PaCO_2$ (in mm Hg)
Chronic respiratory	Plasma [HCO_3^-] should increase by 0.4 times the increase in $PaCO_2$ (in mm Hg)
Alkalosis	**Compensation**
Metabolic	$PaCO_2$ (in mm Hg) should increase by 0.6 times the rise in plasma [HCO_3^-] (in mEq/L or mmol/L)
Acute respiratory	Plasma [HCO_3^-] should decrease by 0.2 times the decrease in $PaCO_2$ (in mm Hg), but usually not to <18 mEq/L (mmol/L)
Chronic respiratory	Plasma [HCO_3^-] should fall by 0.4 times the decrease in $PaCO_2$ (in mm Hg), but usually not to <14 mEq/L (mmol/L)

HCO_3^-, bicarbonate; $PaCO_2$, partial pressure of carbon dioxide from arterial blood; multiply values expressed in kPa by 7.519 to convert to mm Hg.

Data from Reference 7.

TREATMENT OF METABOLIC ACIDOSIS

7 Asymptomatic patients with mild to moderate degrees of acidemia (plasma bicarbonate of 12-20 mEq/L [mmol/L]; pH 7.2-7.4) do not require emergent therapy. They can usually be managed with gradual correction of the acidemia, over a period of days to weeks, using oral sodium bicarbonate or other alkali preparations (Table 71-9). In all forms of chronic metabolic acidosis, primary therapy should be directed at treating the underlying disease state. GI pathology should be treated to reduce ongoing bicarbonate losses, and factors that exacerbate RTA should be treated. If acidemia persists, alkali therapy should be instituted with the goal of normalization of blood pH. The loading dose (LD) of alkali to initially correct the acidemia can be calculated as follows:

$$\text{LD(mEq or mmol/L)} = (V_D \times BW) \times (\text{desired } [HCO_3^-] - \text{current } [HCO_3^-])$$

where V_D is the volume of distribution of bicarbonate (0.5 L/kg) and BW is body weight in kg.[8,39]

Thus, for a 60-kg patient with a serum bicarbonate of 15 mEq/L (mmol/L), the LD is calculated:

$$\text{LD (mEq)} = (0.5 \text{ L/kg} \times 60 \text{ kg}) \times (24 \text{ mEq/L} - 15 \text{ mEqL})$$
$$\text{LD} = 30 \text{ L} \times 9 \text{ mEq/L}$$
$$\text{LD} = 270 \text{ mEq}$$

The calculated LD of alkali should be administered over several days to avoid volume overload from the accompanying sodium load. For this scenario, a regimen of 60 to 70 mEq (mmol) three times a day for 3 to 5 days should result in an increase in HCO_3^- levels toward normal. In addition to the calculated LD, supplemental alkali must also be provided to replace ongoing losses, which can be approximated to be 2 mEq/kg (mmol/kg) per day or 40 mEq (mmol) three times a day. In patients with associated volume depletion, bicarbonate replacement can be provided simultaneously with volume resuscitation by substituting bicarbonate for chloride in IV crystalloid solutions.

In patients with chronic metabolic acidosis because of GI bicarbonate losses, maintenance therapy should provide enough alkali to replace ongoing bicarbonate losses. The magnitude of this replacement is variable and can be substantial (more than 10 mEq/kg [mmol/kg] per day). In addition, associated losses of other electrolytes, such as potassium and magnesium, may need to be replaced (see Chapter 70, Potassium and Magnesium Homeostasis).

Proximal (type II) RTA is a bicarbonate-wasting disorder that requires the administration of large maintenance doses of alkali (10-15 mEq/kg [mmol/kg] per day). As alkali replacement raises the serum bicarbonate concentration toward normal, the proximal tubule's capacity to reabsorb bicarbonate is overwhelmed, and renal bicarbonate wasting increases. In children, aggressive therapy of proximal RTA is necessary to avoid growth retardation and osteopenia. Because this is generally a mild, nonprogressive acidosis in adults, the benefit of alkali therapy is frequently outweighed by the risks of increased potassium wasting. In patients with classic distal (type I) RTA, maintenance therapy usually requires only enough alkali to buffer the amount of acid generated from dietary intake and metabolism. This usually approximates 1 to 3 mEq/kg/day (mmol/kg/day).

8 After initial potassium deficits are replaced, ongoing potassium supplementation may not be required, as renal potassium

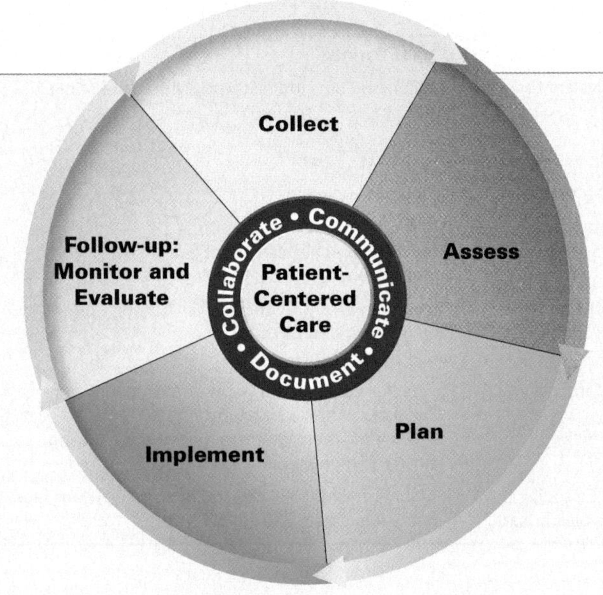

Patient Care Process for Acid–Base Disorders

Collect

- Patient characteristics (eg, age, sex, pregnant)
- Patient medical history (eg, prior acid–base disorder, chronic lung or kidney disease, diabetes mellitus)
- Current medications, including intravenous (IV) fluids (see Tables 71-5, 71-6, 71-7, 71-11, 71-12, 71-13, and 71-14)
- Social history (alcohol use, potential for toxic ingestion)
- Objective data
  - Blood pressure (BP), heart rate (HR), RR, height, weight, oxygen saturation
  - Labs including arterial blood gases (ABG), serum electrolytes (including serum CO_2), serum creatinine (SCr), serum osmolality, serum lactate, blood glucose, urine chloride
  - Current fraction of inspired oxygen (FiO_2)

Assess

- [HCO_3^-] on ABG and electrolyte panel to verify accuracy
- Serum anion gap (SAG)
- Presence of acidemia (pH less than 7.35) or alkalemia (pH greater than 7.45) (see Figure 71-3 and Table 71-4)
- Presence of respiratory disturbance (alteration in $PaCO_2$) or metabolic disturbance (alteration in HCO_3^-)
- Compensatory response (Table 71-8)
- Change in [Cl^-] with change in [Na^+]
- Presence of elevated SAG metabolic acidosis (Tables 71-6 and 71-7)
  - Presence of elevated serum osmolar gap and/or serum lactate
- Presence of metabolic alkalosis (Table 71-11)
  - Presence of urine chloride less than 10 mEq/L (mmol/L) or greater than 20 mEq/L (mmol/L)
- Presence of respiratory acid–base disorder (see Tables 71-12, 71-13, 71-14)

Plan*

- Identification and removal (when possible) of potential cause(s) for the acid–base disorder
- Fluid, electrolyte, or medication therapy (see Tables 71-9 and 71-10, and Figure 71-4)

  Monitoring parameters may include a repeat RR, oxygen saturation, ABG, and serum electrolytes; repeat SCr, serum osmolality, serum lactate, blood glucose, and/or urine chloride
- Referrals to other providers when appropriate (eg, nephrologist, pulmonologist)

Implement*

- Patient education (eg, purpose of treatment, dietary and lifestyle modification, medication-specific information, medication administration instructions) when the acid–base disorder is chronic
- Schedule follow-up when appropriate

Follow-up: Monitor and Evaluate

- Resolution of acid–base disorder symptoms
- Presence of adverse medication reactions (if acid–base disorder treated with medication)
- Patient adherence to treatment plan using multiple sources of information

**Collaborate with patient, caregivers, and other healthcare professionals.*

losses decrease following initiation of appropriate alkali therapy. The use of potassium alkali salts can, however, be desirable in patients with associated nephrolithiasis, because sodium salts can increase urinary calcium excretion.

The metabolic acidosis associated with hyperkalemic distal (type IV) RTA with hyporeninemic-hypoaldosteronism that is often seen in patients with diabetes mellitus can be corrected by the treatment of hyperkalemia alone (see Chapter 70). The use of supplemental alkali (1-2 mEq/kg [mmol/kg] per day) to increase sodium intake and stimulate distal tubular potassium secretion can be beneficial. Some patients may require the administration of pharmacologic amounts of fludrocortisone.[8] Type IV RTA resulting from a generalized distal tubular disorder often responds to low doses of alkali (1.5-2.0 mEq/kg [mmol/kg] per day).[12,14] Corrections of the acidosis along with modest dietary potassium restriction (to 1 mEq/kg [mmol/kg] per day) will often result in the maintenance of serum potassium concentrations of 5 mEq/L (mmol/L) or less.

Veverimer

Veverimer is an investigational medication designed to be used in the treatment of metabolic acidosis of chronic kidney disease (CKD). It is a non-absorbable polymer designed to bind hydrogen chloride in the GI tract with subsequent removal in the feces.[40] Every hydrogen ion bound results in HCO_3^- entering the blood, thus producing an increase in serum HCO_3^- without administering sodium, a mechanism thought to be potentially useful in sodium retentive patients.[41] No changes in fluid or serum concentrations of sodium, potassium, calcium, magnesium, and phosphate have been observed in patients treated with veverimer.[41,42] Adverse medication reactions are primarily GI including nontreatment limiting diarrhea (most

TABLE 71-9 Therapeutic Alternatives for Oral Alkali Replacement

Product	Milliequivalents of Alkali	Dosage Form(s)
Sodium citrate/citric acid	1 mL contains 1 mEq sodium and is equivalent to 1 mEq bicarbonate	Solution, sodium citrate 500 mg, citric acid 334 mg per 5 mL
Sodium bicarbonate	3.9 mEq bicarbonate per tablet (325 mg) 7.8 mEq bicarbonate per tablet (650 mg) 60 mEq bicarbonate per teaspoon (5 g per teaspoon)	Tablet, 325 mg Tablet, 650 mg Baking soda powder
Potassium citrate	Each tablet contains 5, 10, or 15 mEq potassium and delivers approximately 5, 10, or 15 mEq bicarbonate	Tablet Extended Release, 5 mEq Tablet Extended Release, 10 mEq Tablet Extended Release, 15 mEq
Potassium bicarbonate/potassium citrate	Each tablet contains 10, 20, or 25 mEq potassium and delivers approximately 10, 20, or 25 mEq bicarbonate	Tablet Effervescent, 10 mEq Tablet Effervescent, 20 mEq Tablet Effervescent, 25 mEq
Potassium citrate/citric acid	Each packet contains 30 mEq potassium and delivers approximately 30 mEq bicarbonate Each mL contains 2 mEq potassium and delivers approximately 2 mEq bicarbonate	Powder for solution, potassium citrate monohydrate 3,300 mg, citric acid monohydrate 1,002 mg per packet Solution, potassium citrate monohydrate 1,100 mg, citric acid monohydrate 334 mg per 5 mL
Sodium citrate/potassium citrate/citric acid	1 mL contains 1 mEq potassium and 1 mEq sodium ion, and delivers approximately 2 mEq bicarbonate	Solution, citric acid 334 mg, sodium citrate 500 mg, and potassium citrate 550 mg per 5 mL

common), flatulence, nausea, and constipation.[42] Administration is orally as a suspension in water. Dosing has not been fully elucidated but the Phase 3, 40-week study used a dose of 6 grams daily.[42] Veverimer has not yet been approved by the FDA.

Acute Severe Metabolic Acidosis

9 The management of life-threatening acute metabolic acidosis (plasma bicarbonate of 8 mEq/L [mmol/L] and pH less than 7.20) is dependent on the underlying cause and the patient's cardiovascular status. In some cases, patients will require emergent hemodialysis therapy (see Chapter 64). Patients with hyperchloremic acidosis (eg, diarrhea-induced) are unable to regenerate bicarbonate, and the generation of new bicarbonate by the kidneys can require several days before one can observe a meaningful change in their status. Thus, IV alkali therapy is often required for these patients.

Although conventional wisdom recommends the use of alkali replacement in patients with severe acidemia, studies have not demonstrated that its administration improves patient outcomes.[16,39,43] Alkali therapies may either improve or worsen clinically relevant endpoints such as [H^+], $PaCO_2$, lactate concentrations, and cardiac output. The specific patient populations most likely to benefit or be harmed from alkalinizing therapy are presented in Table 71-10.

TABLE 71-10 Patient Populations Likely to Benefit or Suffer from Alkalinizing Therapy

Patients with Potential for Benefit	Patients with Potential for Harm
Distal (type I) renal tubular acidosis	Hypernatremia
Severe hyperchloremic metabolic acidosis secondary to diarrhea or surgical diversion	Hypervolemia
Specific poisonings and intoxications (eg, salicylate overdose with metabolic acidosis)	AKI
	Chronic heart failure
	Pulmonary disease resulting in decreased ventilation
	Acute lung injury where a lung protective ventilation strategy is used
	Diabetic ketoacidosis

There are several therapeutic alternatives available for the acute correction of severe metabolic acidosis. Sodium acetate, sodium citrate, and sodium lactate are unreliable sources of alkali because their alkalinizing effect is dependent on their oxidative conversion to bicarbonate by the liver. This process is often impaired in critically ill patients, especially those with hepatic disease or circulatory failure. Although sodium bicarbonate is the most widely used IV alkalotic agent, it is frequently ineffective and can actually be deleterious, especially in patients with lactic acidosis.[16,39,44] Among the two remaining alternatives, dichloroacetate (DCA) is investigational and not available in most clinical settings. Tromethamine, or THAM, is a carbon dioxide–consuming, commercially available solution that buffers respiratory as well as metabolic acids but was discontinued by its sole US manufacturer in 2016.

Sodium Bicarbonate

While sodium bicarbonate administration provides fluid and electrolyte replacement and increases arterial pH, it does not improve cardiac function, organ perfusion, or intracellular pH.[17,39,44,45] In patients with AKI, sodium bicarbonate may reduce mortality at 28 days.[43] However, additional research is required to further evaluate the role of sodium bicarbonate in patients with severe metabolic acidemia and AKI given the potential role of renal replacement therapy in this setting. In addition, sodium bicarbonate administration can have paradoxical adverse effects on intracellular pH. When bicarbonate is given by IV infusion, the carbon dioxide generated diffuses more readily than bicarbonate across cell membranes and into cerebrospinal fluid. Therefore, the intracellular pH can be decreased by administration of bicarbonate.[8,43]

Excessive sodium bicarbonate administration can result in (a) a shift of the oxyhemoglobin saturation curve to the left, thereby impairing oxygen release from hemoglobin to tissues; (b) sodium and water overload, with subsequent pulmonary congestion and hypernatremia; (c) paradoxical tissue acidosis as a result of the production of CO_2 that freely diffuses into myocardial and cerebral cells; and (d) decreased ionized calcium with a resultant decrease in myocardial contractility.[8,39] If there is an endogenous source of bicarbonate, such as can occur in the case of ketoacidosis or lactic acidosis, a bicarbonate "overshoot" can develop because the ketoacids (acetoacetic acid and β-hydroxybutyric acid) or lactic acid are converted in the liver to bicarbonate once the underlying cause of acidosis is corrected. Alkalosis can also result if too much sodium bicarbonate is administered too quickly.[8,39]

If IV sodium bicarbonate is used, one must be mindful that the goals are to increase, not normalize, pH (to approximately 7.2) and plasma bicarbonate (to 8-10 mEq/L [mmol/L]). There is no calculative method that will assure attainment of these goals with a given dose of sodium bicarbonate because of the multiplicity of competing processes that can affect acid–base status (eg, vomiting, potential increases in endogenous acid production, and kidney disease) and the marked variability in the volume of distribution of bicarbonate (50% of BW in patients with mild acidosis to approximately 100% in those with severe acidosis).[8,46] The dose of sodium bicarbonate may be calculated using a distribution volume of 50% of BW for all patients to avoid overtreatment.[8] The total dose calculated as described previously in the RTA section should be administered as an infusion over one-half to several hours. Follow-up monitoring of ABGs, beginning no sooner than 30 minutes after the end of the infusion, should be used to guide further therapeutic decisions.[46]

Bicarbonate therapy is generally not necessary for patients with cardiac arrest, even if the initial arrest was unmonitored. The American Heart Association Advanced Cardiac Life Support (ACLS) guidelines state the routine use of sodium bicarbonate is not recommended for patients in cardiac arrest, but may be useful in patients with life-threatening hyperkalemia.[47] The initial dose of sodium bicarbonate in this situation is (1 mEq/kg [mmol/kg]) administered by rapid, direct IV injection.[47] Subsequent doses of sodium bicarbonate should be based on measurements of arterial blood pH and $PaCO_2$ given the propensity for it to cause alkalemia.[46]

Tromethamine

THAM, no longer available in the United States, is a highly alkaline, sodium-free organic amine that acts as a proton acceptor to prevent or correct acidosis.[8,48] THAM combines with hydrogen ions from carbonic acid to form bicarbonate and a cationic buffer, and also acts as an osmotic diuretic to increase urine flow, urine pH, and the excretion of fixed acids, CO_2, and electrolytes.[7,48] It should be administered via a central line and used with extreme caution in patients with severe liver or kidney failure.

Dichloroacetate

DCA, another investigational agent, facilitates aerobic lactate metabolism by stimulating the activity of lactate dehydrogenase, thus reversing hyperlactatemia and elevating blood pH.[49-51] DCA does not improve hemodynamic parameters or clinical outcomes compared to conventional management.[49-51] DCA can cause mild drowsiness and peripheral neuropathy that is reversible upon discontinuation.[51] The future role of DCA in the management of metabolic acidosis, particularly lactic acidosis, remains to be clarified.[16]

Metabolic Alkalosis

Pathophysiology

Metabolic alkalosis is a simple acid–base disorder that presents as alkalemia (increased arterial pH) with an increase in plasma bicarbonate. Metabolic alkalosis is predominantly maintained because of an abnormality in kidney function and does not occur or cannot be corrected in a matter of hours. Normally, the kidneys are capable of excreting all of the excess bicarbonate presented to them, even during periods of increased bicarbonate loads.[2] As the serum bicarbonate concentration increases, the filtered bicarbonate load exceeds the maximal rate for bicarbonate reabsorption, and the excess bicarbonate is excreted in the urine. Thus, evaluation of patients with metabolic alkalosis must consider two separate issues: (a) the initial process that generates the metabolic alkalosis; and (b) alterations in kidney function that maintain the alkalemia state.[52]

10 The generation of metabolic alkalosis can result from reduced renal bicarbonate excretion, excessive losses of hydrogen ions from the kidneys or stomach, or from a gain secondary to the ingestion or administration of bicarbonate-rich fluids.[52,53] In general, these mechanisms can be divided into volume-mediated processes (sodium chloride–responsive), volume-independent processes (sodium chloride–resistant), or not classified by either (Table 71-11).[7,53] Patients with a sodium chloride–responsive metabolic alkalosis will have a urinary chloride concentration less than 10 mEq/L (mmol/L) and patients with a sodium chloride–resistant alkalosis will have a urinary chloride concentration greater than 20 mEq/L (mmol/L).[7]

TABLE 71-11 Causes of Metabolic Alkalosis

Sodium chloride–responsive (urinary chloride concentration <10 mEq/L [mmol/L])
GI disorders
Vomiting
Gastric drainage
Villous adenoma of the colon
Chloride diarrhea
Diuretic therapy (distant)
Correction of chronic hypercapnia
Cystic fibrosis
Excessive bicarbonate therapy of an organic acidosis
Mild/moderate potassium deficiency
Sodium chloride–resistant (urinary chloride concentration >20 mEq/L [mmol/L])
Excess mineralocorticoid activity
Hyperaldosteronism
Cushing syndrome
Bartter syndrome (sodium transport defect in loop of Henle)
Gitelman syndrome (sodium transport defect in collecting duct)
Excessive black licorice intake
Profound potassium depletion
Magnesium deficiency
Liddle syndrome (enhanced sodium reabsorption in collecting duct)
Diuretic therapy (recent)
Estrogen therapy
Unclassified
Alkali administration
Milk-alkali syndrome
Massive blood or plasma protein fraction transfusion
Nonparathyroid hypercalcemia
Carbohydrate refeeding after starvation
Large doses of penicillin

Sodium Chloride Responsive 11 Gastric juice, rich in chloride and hydrogen ions, is secreted at a rate of less than 50 mL/hr in the basal state, but can increase up to fivefold with stimulation. In the gastric parietal cells, the hydrogen ion and bicarbonate are generated from CO_2 and water.[1] The hydrogen ion is secreted into gastric fluid, and the bicarbonate is retained in the ECF. Normally, an amount of bicarbonate equal to the bicarbonate generated in the stomach is eliminated in the alkaline pancreatic and small-bowel secretions, maintaining hydrogen ion balance. With vomiting and nasogastric suctioning, the hydrogen ion is lost externally and metabolic alkalosis results. Diarrhea, as seen with secretory villous adenomas and other secretory diarrheas, often results in excessive GI losses of chloride-rich, bicarbonate-poor fluid, and thus leads to the generation of metabolic alkalosis.

12 Diuretic agents acting on the thick ascending limb of the loop of Henle (eg, furosemide, bumetanide, and torsemide) and distal convoluted tubule (eg, thiazides) have most commonly been associated with the generation of metabolic alkalosis.[1,54] These agents promote the excretion of sodium and potassium almost exclusively in association with chloride, without a proportionate increase in bicarbonate excretion. Collecting duct hydrogen ion secretion is stimulated directly by the increased luminal flow rate and sodium delivery, and indirectly by intravascular volume contraction, which results in secondary hyperaldosteronism. Renal ammoniagenesis can also be stimulated by concomitant hypokalemia, further augmenting net acid excretion.

Sodium Chloride Resistant Mineralocorticoid excess plays a significant role in the maintenance of metabolic alkalosis given that it stimulates collecting duct hydrogen ion secretion. Elevated mineralocorticoid levels directly stimulate collecting duct hydrogen ion secretion, indirectly increase ammoniagenesis by causing hypokalemia, and is associated with both acute and chronic causes including profound potassium deficiency, magnesium deficiency, and estrogen therapy.[1,7,54]

Unclassified Metabolic alkalosis can also be generated by the gain of exogenous alkali. This is a result of bicarbonate administration or from the infusion of organic anions that are metabolized to bicarbonate, such as acetate, lactate, and citrate. The milk-alkali syndrome was historically a common cause of metabolic alkalosis in patients with peptic ulcer disease secondary to the ingestion of large quantities of milk products and antacids. Administration of high doses of penicillins (eg, ticarcillin) can produce metabolic alkalosis because they act as nonreabsorbable anions, which enhances the secretion of potassium and hydrogen ions and results in hypokalemia and metabolic alkalosis.[55]

Clinical Presentation

There are no unique signs or symptoms associated with mild-to-moderate metabolic alkalosis, but patients may complain of symptoms related to the underlying cause of the disorder (eg, muscle weakness with hypokalemia or postural dizziness with volume depletion).[52,56] They may have a history of vomiting, gastric drainage, or diuretic use, all of which contribute to the development of metabolic alkalosis. Severe alkalemia (blood pH greater than 7.55) has been associated with cardiac arrhythmias, particularly in patients with heart disease, hyperventilation, and hypoxemia.[56] Neuromuscular irritability can be present, with signs of tetany or hyperactive reflexes, possibly caused by the decreased ionized calcium concentration that occurs secondary to the increase in pH. This decrease in ionized calcium may be caused by a conformational change in the albumin molecules to which the calcium is bound, resulting in increased binding, or by decreased competition from hydrogen ions for binding sites on the albumin molecule. Mental confusion, muscle cramping, and paresthesia can also occur.[52] Lastly, patients will be more difficult to liberate from mechanical ventilation.

Compensation

The respiratory response to metabolic alkalosis is hypoventilation, which results in an increased $PaCO_2$. Respiratory compensation is initiated within hours when the central and peripheral chemoreceptors sense an increase in pH. The $PaCO_2$ increases 6 to 7 mm Hg (0.8-0.9 kPa) for each 10 mEq/L (mmol/L) increase in bicarbonate, up to a $PaCO_2$ of approximately 50 to 60 mm Hg (6.7-8.0 kPa) (see Table 71-8) before hypoxia sensors react to prevent further hypoventilation.[7] If the $PaCO_2$ is normal or less than normal, one should consider the presence of a superimposed respiratory alkalosis, which can be secondary to fever, gram-negative sepsis, or pain.

TREATMENT OF METABOLIC ALKALOSIS

Treatment of metabolic alkalosis should be aimed at correcting the factor(s) responsible for the maintenance of the alkalosis.[56] For example, vomiting should be treated with antiemetics; gastric losses of hydrogen ions during nasogastric suction can be modulated by giving histamine blockers such as famotidine or proton pump inhibitors such as omeprazole, and reducing or discontinuing diuretic therapy.[56,57] Metabolic alkalosis will persist until the renal mechanism responsible for maintaining the disorder is corrected, despite the fact that the original cause of the elevated plasma bicarbonate may have resolved. For example, hypovolemia should be treated with sodium chloride to allow excretion of bicarbonate by the kidney. However, patients with severely compromised cardiovascular function may not be able to tolerate this therapeutic approach. In situations such as this and/or the presence of life-threatening alkalosis, a reduction in pH by controlled hypoventilation sometimes using inspired CO_2 with supplemental oxygen to prevent hypoxia has been used. Dialysis using a low bicarbonate dialysate is also indicated in such patients.[7,58] Therapy for metabolic alkalosis can be conceptualized on the basis of the sodium chloride responsiveness of the disorders (Fig. 71-4).

Sodium Chloride–Responsive Metabolic Alkalosis

Sodium chloride–responsive disorders usually result from volume depletion and chloride loss, which can accompany severe vomiting, prolonged nasogastric suction, and diuretic therapy. Initially, therapy is directed at expanding intravascular volume and replenishing chloride stores. Sodium chloride- and potassium chloride–containing solutions should be administered to patients who can tolerate the volume load.[52] Patients with metabolic alkalosis who are volume overloaded or intolerant to volume administration because of chronic heart failure can benefit from the carbonic anhydrase inhibitor acetazolamide. This agent inhibits the action of carbonic anhydrase, thereby inhibiting renal bicarbonate reabsorption. Unfortunately, it also increases the renal losses of potassium and phosphate. Administration of acetazolamide (250-375 mg once or twice daily) can promote a sufficient bicarbonate diuresis and return the pH toward normal.[52,59] Among mechanically ventilated chronic obstructive pulmonary disease patients having metabolic alkalosis, administration of acetazolamide 500 to 1,000 mg twice daily (initiated within 48 hours of ICU admission and continued to ICU discharge) appears to reduce the degree of alkalosis while not affecting duration of mechanical ventilation or any other clinically relevant outcome.[60]

Hemodialysis using a low-bicarbonate dialysate can be used for the rapid correction of severe (pH greater than 7.55) metabolic alkalosis.[7,58] Acidifying agents including hydrochloric acid, ammonium chloride, and arginine monohydrochloride can also be used in such situations; however, availability limits their use as first line.[61,62] In general, this management is reserved for patients who are unresponsive to conventional fluid and electrolyte management or who are unable to tolerate the requisite volume load because of decompensated heart failure or advanced kidney disease.[58]

Hydrochloric Acid

Hydrochloric acid is usually infused IV via a large central vein as a 0.1 to 0.25 N HCl solution in either 5% dextrose or normal saline, although sterile water has also been used. Extemporaneously prepared solutions can be made by adding 100 to 250 mEq (mmol) of HCl through a 0.22-mm filter into a glass container of saline or dextrose. The rate of infusion should be 100 to 125 mL/hr (10-25 mEq/h [mmol/h]). A severe transient respiratory acidosis can occur if the hydrochloric acid is infused too quickly because of a slower reduction of the elevated bicarbonate concentration in the cerebrospinal fluid than in the ECF. Improvement is usually seen within 24 hours of initiating therapy. To prevent overcorrection, the infusion should be stopped when the arterial pH decreases to 7.5.[7,61] ABGs and serum electrolytes should be drawn every 4 to 8 hours to evaluate and adjust therapy.

The dose of hydrochloric acid can be based on an estimate of the total body chloride deficit[61]:

$$\text{Dose HCl (in mEq or mmol)} = [0.2\ \text{L/kg} \times \text{BW (in kg)}] \times [103 - \text{observed serum chloride}]$$

where the estimated chloride space is 0.2 times the BW, and the average serum chloride is 103 mEq/L (mmol/L). Alternatively, the dose can be calculated based on the estimated base deficit[8,63]:

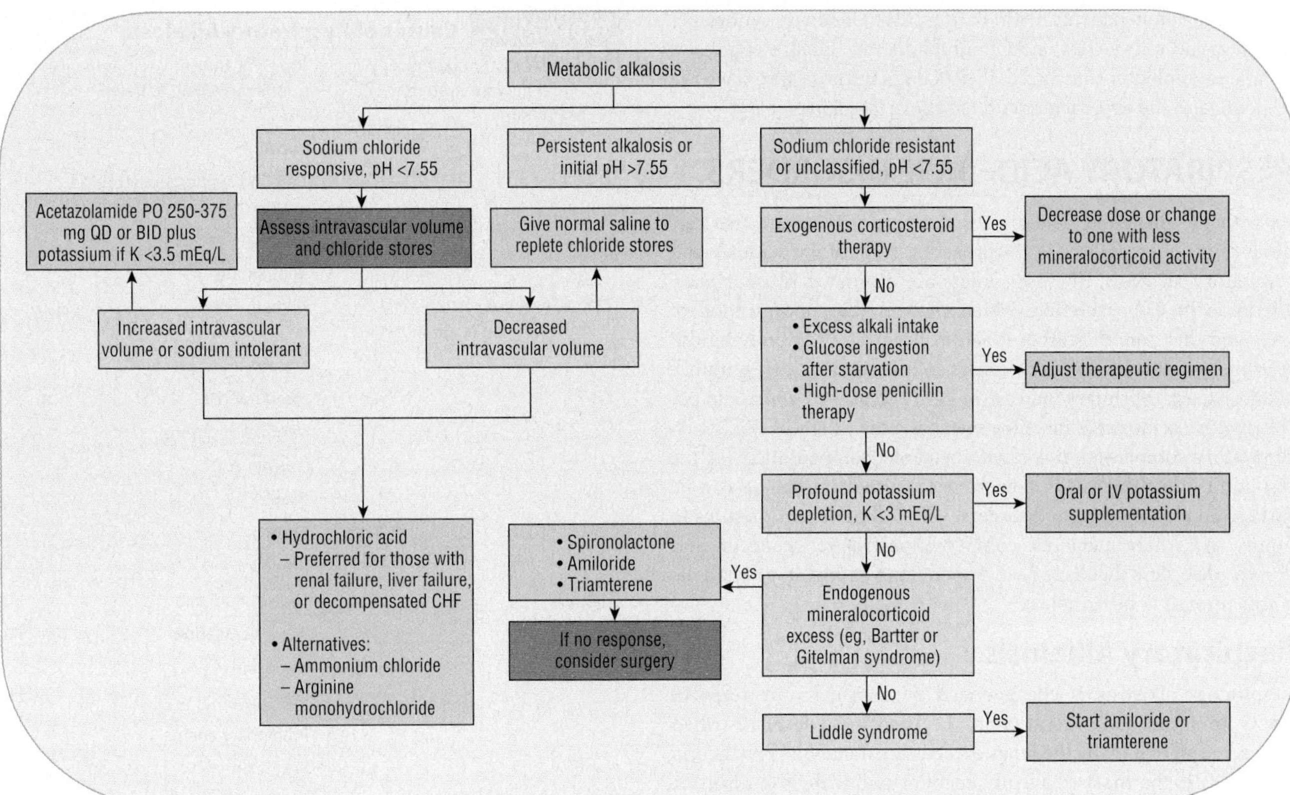

FIGURE 71-4 Treatment algorithm for patients with primary metabolic alkalosis. (BID, twice daily; CHF, chronic heart failure; K, potassium [serum potassium in mEq/L is numerically equivalent to mmol/L]; PO, orally; QD, every day.)

$$\text{Dose HCl (in mEq or mmol)} = [0.5\ \text{L/kg} \times \text{BW (in kg)}] \times (\text{desired}[HCO_3^-] - \text{observed}[HCO_3^-])$$

Ammonium Chloride

Ammonium chloride has a limited role in the treatment of metabolic alkalosis. The liver converts ammonium chloride (NH_4Cl) to urea and free hydrochloric acid[64]:

$$2NH_4Cl + 2HCO_3^- \rightarrow CO(NH_2)_2 - CO_2 + 3H_2O + 2Cl^-$$

The dose of ammonium chloride can be calculated based on the chloride deficit using the same method as for HCl and assuming that 20 g ammonium chloride will provide 374 mEq (mmol) of H^+. However, only one-half of the calculated dose of ammonium chloride should be administered to avoid ammonia toxicity. Ammonium chloride is available as a 26.75% solution containing 100 mEq (mmol) of H^+ in 20 mL, which should be further diluted prior to administration. A dilute solution can be prepared by adding 20 mL of ammonium chloride to 500 mL of normal saline and infusing the solution at a rate of no more than 1 mEq/min (mmol/min). Improvement in metabolic status is usually seen within 24 hours. CNS toxicity, marked by confusion, irritability, seizures, and coma, has been associated with more rapid rates of administration. Ammonium chloride must be administered cautiously to patients with impaired kidney or hepatic function. In patients with impaired hepatic function, decreased conversion of ammonia to urea can result in increased ammonia levels and worsened encephalopathy. In patients with kidney disease, the increased urea synthesis can exacerbate uremic symptoms.[63,64]

Arginine Monohydrochloride

Although not FDA-approved, arginine monohydrochloride at a dose of 10 g/hr given IV has been used to treat metabolic alkalosis. Like ammonium chloride, arginine must undergo metabolism by the liver to produce hydrogen ions, with a conversion of 100 g to 475 mEq (mmol) of H^+. Unlike ammonium chloride, arginine combines with ammonia in the body to synthesize urea; thus, it can be used in patients with relative hepatic insufficiency. Patients with kidney disease should not receive arginine monohydrochloride because it can significantly elevate blood urea nitrogen and is associated with severe hyperkalemia.[64,65] The increase in potassium is caused by arginine-induced shifts of potassium from the intracellular to the extracellular space.

Sodium Chloride–Resistant Metabolic Alkalosis

13 Management of these disorders usually consists of treatment of the underlying cause of the mineralocorticoid excess. For patients taking a corticosteroid, a dosage reduction or a switch to a corticosteroid with less mineralocorticoid activity (eg, methylprednisolone) should be considered. Patients with an endogenous source of excess mineralocorticoid activity can require surgery or the administration of spironolactone, amiloride, or triamterene.[2,52]

Spironolactone is a competitive antagonist of the mineralocorticoid receptor. Amiloride and triamterene are potassium-sparing diuretics that inhibit the epithelial sodium channel in the distal convoluted tubule and collecting duct. All three agents inhibit aldosterone-stimulated sodium reabsorption in the collecting duct. In addition, spironolactone directly inhibits aldosterone stimulation of the hydrogen ion secretory pump. Thus, most patients with mineralocorticoid excess, including Bartter and Gitelman syndromes, respond to therapy with these agents.[7] Liddle syndrome, which is a form of pseudohypoaldosteronism caused by overactivity of the epithelial sodium channel, is not responsive to spironolactone but can be treated with either amiloride or triamterene.[52] Although experience is limited, some patients with Bartter and Gitelman syndromes may respond to NSAIDs or ACE inhibitors.[7,66,67] Finally, aggressive potassium repletion can correct the alkalosis in those who have not responded to the approaches outlined above (see Chapter 70).

RESPIRATORY ACID–BASE DISORDERS

As with the metabolic acid–base disturbances, there are two cardinal respiratory acid–base disturbances: respiratory acidosis and respiratory alkalosis. These disorders are generated by a primary alteration in CO_2 excretion, which changes the concentration of CO_2, and therefore the carbonic acid concentration in body fluids.[4] A primary reduction in $PaCO_2$ causes an increase in pH (respiratory alkalosis), and a primary increase in $PaCO_2$ causes a decrease in pH (respiratory acidosis). Unlike the metabolic disturbances, for which respiratory compensation is rapid, metabolic compensation for the respiratory disturbances is slow. Hence, these disturbances can be further divided into acute disorders, with a duration of minutes to hours, and where metabolic compensation has yet to occur, and chronic disorders that have been present long enough for metabolic compensation to be complete.

Respiratory Alkalosis

Respiratory alkalosis is characterized by a primary decrease in $PaCO_2$ that leads to an elevation in pH. The $PaCO_2$ decreases when the excretion of CO_2 by the lungs exceeds the metabolic production of CO_2. It is the most frequently encountered acid–base disorder, occurring physiologically in normal pregnancy and in persons living at high altitudes.[68] Respiratory alkalosis also occurs frequently among hospitalized patients (Table 71-12).[68,69]

TABLE 71-12 Causes of Respiratory Alkalosis

Medications (stimulation of central nervous system respiration)	Xanthine derivatives (theophylline, aminophylline, caffeine)
	Nicotine
	Catecholamines (epinephrine, norepinephrine, dopamine)
	Salicylate overdose
	Topiramate
Central nervous system stimulation of respiration	Brain tumors
	Encephalitis, meningitis
	Head trauma
	Vascular accidents
	Anxiety
	Pain
	Fever
	Pregnancy
Hypoxia	High altitudes
	Hyperventilation
	Hypoxemia
	Pneumonia
	Pulmonary edema
	Severe anemia
Peripheral stimulation of respiration	Pulmonary embolus
	Asthma
Other	Thyrotoxicosis
	Cirrhosis

Pathophysiology

A decrease in $PaCO_2$ occurs when ventilatory excretion exceeds metabolic production. Because endogenous production of CO_2 is relatively constant, negative CO_2 balance is primarily caused by an increase in ventilatory excretion of CO_2 (hyperventilation). The metabolic production of CO_2, however, can be increased during periods of stress or with excess carbohydrate administration (eg, parenteral nutrition). Hyperventilation can develop from an increase in neurochemical stimulation via either central or peripheral mechanisms, or by the result of voluntary or mechanical (iatrogenic) hyperventilation.

A decrease in $PaCO_2$ can occur in patients with cardiogenic, hypovolemic, or septic shock because oxygen delivery to the carotid and aortic chemoreceptors is reduced. This relative deficit in PaO_2 stimulates an increase in ventilation. The hyperventilation in sepsis is also mediated via a central mechanism. Hyperventilation-induced respiratory alkalosis with an elevation in cardiac index and hypotension without peripheral vasoconstriction can therefore be an early sign of sepsis.

Clinical Presentation

Although most patients are asymptomatic, respiratory alkalosis can cause adverse neuromuscular, cardiovascular, and GI effects.[68] During periods of decreased $PaCO_2$, there is a decrease in cerebral blood flow, which can be responsible for symptoms of light-headedness, confusion, decreased intellectual functioning, syncope, and seizures. Nausea and vomiting can occur, probably as a result of cerebral hypoxia. In severe respiratory alkalosis, cardiac arrhythmias can occur because of sensitization of the myocardium to the arrhythmogenic effects of circulating catecholamines.[70] Acute respiratory alkalosis has no effect on BP or cardiac output in awake individuals. Anesthetized patients, however, can experience a decrease in both cardiac output and BP, possibly owing to the lack of a tachycardic response.[68]

The concentration of serum electrolytes can also be altered secondary to the development of respiratory alkalosis.[7] The serum chloride concentration is usually slightly increased, and serum potassium concentration can be slightly decreased. Clinically significant hypokalemia can be a consequence of extreme respiratory alkalosis, although the effect is usually very small or negligible.[71] Serum phosphorus concentration can decrease by as much as 1.5 to 2 mg/dL (0.48-0.65 mmol/L) because of the shift of inorganic phosphate into cells. Reductions in the blood ionized calcium concentration can be partially responsible for symptoms such as muscle cramps and tetany. Approximately 40% of calcium is bound to albumin, and an increase in pH results in an increase in binding.[72]

Compensation

The initial response of the body to acute respiratory alkalosis is chemical buffering: hydrogen ions are released from the body's buffers—intracellular proteins, phosphates, and hemoglobin—and titrate down the serum bicarbonate concentration. This process occurs within minutes. Acutely, the bicarbonate concentration can be decreased by a maximum of 3 mEq/L (mmol/L) for each 10-mm Hg (1.3 kPa) decrease in $PaCO_2$ (see Table 71-8).[7] When only physicochemical buffering has occurred, the disturbance is referred to as acute respiratory alkalosis.

Metabolic compensation occurs when respiratory alkalosis persists for more than 6 to 12 hours. In response to the alkalemia, proximal tubular bicarbonate reabsorption is inhibited, and the serum bicarbonate concentration decreases. Renal compensation is usually complete within 1 to 2 days. The renal bicarbonaturia as well as decreased NH_4^+ and titratable acid excretion are direct effects of the reduced $PaCO_2$ and pH on renal reabsorption of chloride and bicarbonate.[2,73] The acuity of the respiratory alkalosis can be assessed on the basis of the degree of renal compensation (see Table 71-8). In fully compensated respiratory alkalosis, the bicarbonate concentration decreases by 4 mEq/L (mmol/L) below 24 for each

CLINICAL PRESENTATION Respiratory Alkalosis

General

- The patient is usually asymptomatic if the condition is chronic and mild.

Symptoms

- The patient may complain of light-headedness, confusion, muscle cramps and tetany, and decreased intellectual functioning.
- Nausea and vomiting can occur, probably as a result of cerebral hypoxia.

Signs

- In severe respiratory alkalosis, pH is more than 7.55.

Laboratory Tests

- Serum chloride concentration is usually slightly increased. Serum ionized calcium through increased calcium binding to albumin, potassium, and phosphorus concentration can be decreased.

10-mm Hg (1.3 kPa) drop in $PaCO_2$. For example, a sustained decrease in $PaCO_2$ of 20 mm Hg (2.7 kPa) will lower serum bicarbonate from 24 to 16 mEq/L (mmol/L) with a resultant pH of 7.46. Bicarbonate concentrations differing from those anticipated using the preceding guidelines suggest a mixed acid–base disorder.

TREATMENT OF RESPIRATORY ALKALOSIS

Because most patients with respiratory alkalosis, especially chronic cases, have few or no symptoms and pH alterations are usually mild (pH not exceeding 7.5), treatment is often not required.[70] The first consideration in the treatment of acute respiratory alkalosis with pH more than 7.5 is the identification and correction of the underlying cause. Relief of pain, correction of hypovolemia with IV fluids, treatment of fever or infection, treatment of salicylate overdose, and other direct measures can prove effective. A rebreathing device, such as a paper bag, can be useful in controlling hyperventilation in patients with the anxiety/hyperventilation syndrome. Oxygen therapy should be initiated in patients with severe hypoxemia.[68,70] Patients with life-threatening alkalosis (pH more than 7.55), particularly if it is a mixed respiratory and metabolic condition, tend to have complications, such as arrhythmias or seizures, which can require mechanical ventilation with sedation and/or paralysis to control hyperventilation.[64,68]

Respiratory alkalosis in patients receiving mechanical ventilation is usually iatrogenic. It can often be corrected by decreasing either the set RR or tidal volume, although other measures can also be employed. The use of a capnograph and spirometer in the breathing circuit enables a more precise adjustment of the ventilator settings. Another method of treating respiratory alkalosis is to increase the amount of dead space in the ventilator circuit by placing a known length of tubing between the artificial airway and the "T" piece of the ventilator. This results in "rebreathing" of expired gas, and therefore an increase in the inspired carbon dioxide concentration, which should increase the carbon dioxide tension of the patient, correcting the respiratory alkalosis. In patients breathing more rapidly than the ventilator settings, sedation with or without paralysis can be employed.

Respiratory Acidosis

Pathophysiology

Respiratory acidosis occurs when the lungs fail to excrete CO_2 resulting in a lower pH. This can be the result of conditions that centrally inhibit the respiratory center, diseases that interfere with pulmonary perfusion or neuromuscular function, and intrinsic airway or parenchymal pulmonary disease (Table 71-13).[68,69] Acute respiratory acidosis with hypoxemia, hypercarbia, and acidosis is life threatening. Those disorders that produce an increase in $PaCO_2$ and hypoxemia to a degree compatible with life (eg, chronic obstructive pulmonary disease), with or without oxygen therapy, can result in

TABLE 71-13 Causes of Acute Respiratory Acidosis

Airway and pulmonary abnormalities	Acute airway obstruction
	Acute asthma exacerbation
	Acute cardiogenic pulmonary edema
	Acute respiratory distress syndrome
	Aspiration
	Chronic obstructive pulmonary disease exacerbation
	Obesity hypoventilation syndrome
	Laryngeal spasms
	Obstructive sleep apnea
	Pneumonia
	Pneumothorax
	Smoke inhalation
	Trauma
Central	Anesthetics (bupivacaine, mepivacaine)
	Meningitis
	Neuromuscular blockers (succinylcholine, vecuronium, cisatracurium, rocuronium, pancuronium)
	Opioids (fentanyl, hydromorphone, morphine, oxycodone, codeine)
	Sedatives (alprazolam, diazepam, lorazepam, propofol)
	Status epilepticus
	Stroke
Mechanical ventilator	Inadequate frequency or tidal volume setting
	Large dead space
	Ventilator malfunction
Metabolic	Overfeeding
Neuromuscular abnormalities	Brainstem or cervical cord injury
	Guillain-Barre syndrome
	Myasthenia gravis
Perfusion abnormalities	Cardiac arrest
	Massive pulmonary embolus

CLINICAL PRESENTATION Respiratory Acidosis

General

- The patient is usually symptomatic.

Symptoms

- The patient may complain of confusion or difficulty thinking and headache.

Signs

- In severe respiratory acidosis.
- Cardiac: Increased cardiac output if moderate that decreases if severe. Refractory hypotension can be present in some patients.
- CNS: Abnormal behavior, seizures, stupor, and coma. Papilledema, focal paresis, and abnormal reflexes can also be present.

Laboratory Tests

- Serum potassium concentration can be modestly increased. Hypercapnia can be moderate ($PaCO_2$ of 50-55 mm Hg [6.7-7.3 kPa]) to severe ($PaCO_2$ of more than 80 mm Hg [10.6 kPa]). Hypoxia (PaO_2 is less than 70 mm Hg [9.3 kPa]) is often present.

TABLE 71-14 Causes of Chronic Respiratory Acidosis

Airway abnormalities	Airway stenosis
Metabolic	Chronic overfeeding
Neuromuscular abnormalities/disorders	Amyotrophic lateral sclerosis
	Brainstem lesions
	Critical illness myopathies
	Diaphragmatic paralysis
	Extreme obesity (Pickwickian syndrome)
	Myasthenia gravis
	Multiple sclerosis
	Poliomyelitis
	Primary alveolar hypoventilation syndrome
	Tumors
Pulmonary abnormalities/disorders	Bronchitis
	Chronic obstructive pulmonary disease
	Chronic pulmonary embolism
	Emphysema
	Extreme obesity
	Fibrothorax
	Kyphoscoliosis
	Pulmonary fibrosis

chronic respiratory acidosis (Table 71-14).[68,69] These patients can function normally without noticeable neurologic defects with higher than normal range $PaCO_2$ concentrations, provided that adequate oxygenation is maintained.

Clinical Presentation

Respiratory acidosis can produce neurologic symptoms, including altered mental status, abnormal behavior, seizures, stupor, and coma. Hypercapnia can mimic stroke or CNS tumors by producing headache, papilledema, focal paresis, and abnormal reflexes. These CNS symptoms are attributable to the vasodilator effects of CO_2 in the brain that result in an increase in cerebral blood flow.[2] The CNS response to hypercapnia is extremely variable between patients and is most influenced by the acuity of presentation. Given that chronic hypercapnia blunts the usual respiratory stimulus of an elevated $PaCO_2$, hypoxemia rather than hypercapnia provides the primary ventilatory stimulus in patients with severe chronic respiratory acidosis.[18]

The degree to which cardiac contractility and HR are altered depends on the severity of the acidosis and the rapidity with which it develops. Modest acute hypercapnia ($PaCO_2$ of 50-55 mm Hg [6.7-7.3 kPa]) stimulates a stress-like response, with elevated catecholamines and corticosteroid hormone levels, and can result in increased cardiac output and pulmonary artery pressure. As the severity increases, cardiac output declines and vascular resistance decreases leading to refractory hypotension in some patients.[68]

In respiratory acidosis, the serum potassium concentration increases modestly secondary to cellular shifts. The increases are less than those seen with inorganic metabolic acidosis and are difficult to predict for individual patients.[71]

Compensation

The body responds to acute respiratory acidosis with chemical buffering. The increase in $PaCO_2$ results in increased carbonic acid levels. The carbonic acid dissociates, releasing hydrogen ions, which are buffered by non-bicarbonate buffers (ie, proteins, phosphate, and hemoglobin) and bicarbonate. Thus, based on physicochemical factors, increases in $PaCO_2$ raise the serum bicarbonate concentration. In general, in acute respiratory acidosis, the bicarbonate concentration increases by 1 mEq/L (mmol/L) above 24 for each 10 mm Hg (1.3 kPa) increase in $PaCO_2$ above 40 mm Hg (5.3 kPa) (see Table 71-8).[7]

Metabolic compensation occurs when respiratory acidosis is prolonged beyond 12 to 24 hours. In response to hypercapnia and acidemia, proximal tubular bicarbonate reabsorption, ammoniagenesis, and distal tubular hydrogen secretion are enhanced, resulting in an increase in the serum bicarbonate concentration that raises the pH toward normal. Renal compensation for chronic hypercapnia generally results in the plasma bicarbonate concentration increasing by 4 mEq/L (mmol/L) above 24 for each 10 mm Hg (1.3 kPa) increase in $PaCO_2$ above 40 mm Hg (5.3 kPa) (see Table 71-8).[7] The new steady state in acid–base values is generally achieved within 5 days of the onset of hypercapnia in dogs; the time interval necessary for compensation in humans has not been established.[74]

TREATMENT OF RESPIRATORY ACIDOSIS

The treatment of respiratory acidosis is dependent on the chronicity of the patient's condition. Respiratory decompensation in patients with chronic elevations in $PaCO_2$ is frequently seen in those with acute infections and those recently started on narcotic analgesics or oxygen therapy. Aggressive treatment of these conditions can offer considerable benefit and should be initiated. Furthermore, tranquilizers and sedatives should be avoided and supplemental oxygen, if used, should be minimized.[68]

Acute Respiratory Acidosis

When carbon dioxide excretion is severely impaired ($PaCO_2$ more than 80 mm Hg [10.6 kPa]) and/or life-threatening, hypoxia is present (PaO_2 less than 40 mm Hg [5.3 kPa]); the immediate therapeutic goal is to provide adequate oxygenation. Under these circumstances, hypoxia, not acidemia, is the principal threat to life. A patent airway needs to be established, which can necessitate intubation. Excessive secretions must be cleared from the airway and oxygen administered to restore adequate oxygenation. Mechanical ventilation is usually required.

14 The underlying cause of the acidosis should be treated aggressively (ie, bronchodilators for treatment of severe bronchospasm; narcotic or benzodiazepine antagonists to reverse the deleterious effects of these agents on the respiratory center). Bicarbonate administration is rarely necessary in the treatment of respiratory acidosis. Furthermore, rapid correction of acidosis with bicarbonate can eliminate the patient's respiratory drive or precipitate metabolic alkalosis. Cautious use of alkali (bicarbonate) can restore the responsiveness of bronchial muscles to β-adrenergic agonists and thus can be beneficial for those patients with severe bronchospasm.[74] ABGs should be monitored closely to ensure that the respiratory acidosis is resolving without creating a metabolic alkalosis as the result of compensatory elevation in HCO_3^- and decrease in $PaCO_2$. ABGs should be obtained every 2 to 4 hours during the acute phase and less frequently (every 12-24 hours) as the acidosis improves.

Acute Respiratory Acidosis in a Compensated Chronic Respiratory Acidotic Patient

Patients with a history of chronic respiratory acidosis (eg, those with chronic obstructive pulmonary disease) can experience an acute worsening of their respiratory acidosis. This can result in severe life-threatening hypoxemia. As with acute respiratory acidosis, the goals of therapy are maintenance of a patent airway and adequate oxygenation. Individuals with chronic respiratory acidosis are routinely able to tolerate a low PaO_2 and an elevated $PaCO_2$ because of compensation (increased number of red blood cells, hemoglobin content, and 2,3-diphosphoglycerate). The drive to breathe in these patients is dependent on hypoxemia rather than hypercarbia. Administration of oxygen to a patient with chronic respiratory acidosis can eliminate this drive to breathe and result in the syndrome of carbon dioxide narcosis. In this case, if the PaO_2 is 50 mm Hg (6.7 kPa), no oxygen treatment is necessary. If the PaO_2 is less than 50 mm Hg (6.7 kPa), oxygen therapy should be initiated carefully using a controlled flow of oxygen.[68]

ABGs should be checked periodically to ensure adequate oxygenation. If the $PaCO_2$ increases during oxygen therapy, it can be a sign of impending carbon dioxide narcosis and oxygen therapy may need to be discontinued. The underlying cause of the acute exacerbation should be aggressively managed. Pulmonary infections should be treated with the appropriate antibiotics and bronchodilators administered as necessary. Excess secretions should be cleared from the airway to allow proper gas exchange. This can involve increasing oral fluid intake to decrease the viscosity of secretions, deep breathing, and postural drainage, suction, or bronchoscopy.

MIXED ACID–BASE DISORDERS

Diagnosis

The diagnosis of a mixed disorder depends on an understanding of the appropriate quantitative response of the compensatory mechanisms for each of the simple acid–base disturbances.[38,75] To diagnose mixed disorders, one must know how each of the four simple disorders alters pH, $PaCO_2$, and (HCO_3^-) (see Table 71-8). If a given set of blood gases does not decrease within the range of expected responses for a simple acid–base disturbance, a mixed disorder should be suspected. In addition to laboratory information, a thorough history and physical examination of the patient will often lead to the diagnosis, even before the laboratory data are available. Examples of common mixed disturbances follow.

Mixed Respiratory Acidosis and Metabolic Acidosis

A mixed respiratory and metabolic acidosis disturbance is characterized by a failure of compensation. The respiratory disorder prevents the compensatory decrease in $PaCO_2$ expected in the defense against metabolic acidosis. The metabolic disorder prevents the buffering and renal mechanisms from raising the bicarbonate concentration as expected in the defense against respiratory acidosis. In the absence of these compensatory mechanisms, the pH decreases markedly.

Mixed respiratory and metabolic acidosis may develop in patients with cardiorespiratory arrest, in those with chronic lung disease who are in shock, and in metabolic acidosis patients who develop respiratory failure. When treating this mixed disorder, clinicians need to respond to both the respiratory and metabolic acidosis. Improved oxygen delivery must be initiated to improve hypercarbia and hypoxia. Mechanical ventilation may be needed to reduce $PaCO_2$. During the initial stage of therapy, appropriate amounts of alkali should be given to reverse the metabolic acidosis (see section "Treatment," for "Metabolic Acidosis").

Mixed Respiratory Alkalosis and Metabolic Alkalosis

The combination of respiratory and metabolic alkalosis is the most common mixed acid–base disorder. This mixed disorder occurs frequently in critically ill surgical patients with respiratory alkalosis caused by mechanical ventilation, hypoxia, sepsis, hypotension, neurologic damage, pain, or medications, and with metabolic alkalosis caused by vomiting or nasogastric suctioning and massive blood transfusions. It can also occur in patients with hepatic cirrhosis who hyperventilate, receive diuretics, or vomit, as well as in patients with chronic respiratory acidosis and an elevated plasma bicarbonate concentration who are placed on mechanical ventilation and undergo a rapid decrease in $PaCO_2$.

The renal excretion of bicarbonate that usually occurs as compensation for the respiratory alkalosis is prevented by the complicating metabolic alkalosis. Likewise, the retention of $PaCO_2$ expected to compensate for metabolic alkalosis is prevented by the primary respiratory alkalosis. The failure of compensation that occurs with mixed respiratory and metabolic alkalosis can result in a severe alkalemia.

Administration of sodium chloride and potassium chloride solutions will help correct the metabolic component of a mixed respiratory and metabolic alkalosis, and adjustment of the ventilator and/or treatment of an underlying process that is causing hyperventilation can correct or ameliorate the respiratory component of this mixed disorder.

Mixed Metabolic Acidosis and Respiratory Alkalosis

This mixed disorder is often seen in patients with advanced liver disease, salicylate intoxication, and pulmonary-renal syndromes. The respiratory alkalosis will decrease the $PaCO_2$ beyond the appropriate range for the respiratory compensation usually seen with metabolic acidosis. The plasma bicarbonate concentration also decreases below the level expected in compensation for a simple respiratory alkalosis. In a sense, the defense of pH for either disorder alone is enhanced; thus, the pH can be normal or close to normal, with a low $PaCO_2$ and a low (HCO_3^-). Treatment of this disorder should be directed at the underlying cause. Because of the enhanced compensation, the pH is usually closer to normal than in either of the two simple disorders.

Mixed Metabolic Alkalosis and Respiratory Acidosis

This mixed disorder often occurs in patients with chronic obstructive pulmonary disease and chronic respiratory acidosis who are treated with salt restriction, diuretics, and possibly glucocorticoids. When diuretics are initiated, the plasma bicarbonate may increase because of increased renal bicarbonate generation and reabsorption, providing mechanisms for both generating and maintaining metabolic alkalosis. The elevated pH diminishes respiratory drive and may therefore worsen the respiratory acidosis.

Although the pH may not deviate significantly from normal, treatment may need to be initiated to maintain PaO_2 and $PaCO_2$ at acceptable levels. Because it is often difficult to correctly identify this mixed disorder, it is helpful to observe the patient's response to discontinuation of diuretics and administration of sodium and potassium chloride.[38] The $PaCO_2$ will normalize if the patient has a simple metabolic alkalosis, but it will be minimally affected in the setting of a mixed disorder. Treatment should be aimed at decreasing the plasma bicarbonate with sodium and potassium chloride therapy, thereby allowing the renal excretion of retained bicarbonate from the diuretic-induced metabolic alkalosis. This therapy should be used cautiously to avoid exacerbating any underlying chronic heart failure.

CONCLUSION

Acid–base disorders are a common and widespread problem, and clinicians can play a key role in identifying, preventing, and properly treating them. Acid–base disorders do not occur only in the intensive care unit setting. Patients in ambulatory and extended care settings have many chronic conditions and medication therapies that commonly affect acid–base balance. Thus, clinicians in all practice settings should strive to identify patients at high risk for developing medication-related problems that affect acid–base balance and to undertake appropriate prevention and treatment measures to improve the quality of life of their patients.

ABBREVIATIONS

AKI	acute kidney injury
ABG	arterial blood gas
BP	blood pressure
BW	body weight
CKD	chronic kidney disease
CNS	central nervous system
DCA	dichloroacetate
ECF	extracellular fluid
GI	gastrointestinal
HR	heart rate
H^+	hydrogen ion
HCO_3^-	bicarbonate
H_2CO_3	carbonic acid
HIV	human immunodeficiency virus
IV	intravenous
NH_4^+	ammonium
$PaCO_2$	partial pressure of carbon dioxide from arterial blood
PaO_2	partial pressure of oxygen from arterial blood
PCO_2	partial pressure carbon dioxide in the blood
pH	the negative logarithm (base 10) of the hydrogen ion concentration
p*K*	the negative logarithm of the dissociation constant
$PvCO_2$	partial pressure of carbon dioxide from venous blood
PvO_2	partial pressure of oxygen from venous blood
RTA	renal tubular acidosis
RR	respiratory rate
SAG	serum anion gap
SCr	serum creatinine
THAM	tromethamine (Tris[hydroxymethyl]-aminomethane)
UAs	unmeasured anions
UCs	unmeasured cations

REFERENCES

1. Seifter JL, Chang HY. Extracellular acid-base balance and ion transport between body fluid compartments. *Physiology (Bethesda)* 2017;32(5):367–379. doi: 10.1152/physiol.00007.2017.
2. Hamm LL, Nakhoul N, Hering-Smith KS. Acid-base homeostasis. *Clin J Am Soc Nephrol* 2015;10(12):2232–2242. doi: 10.2215/cjn.07400715.
3. Dhondup T, Qian Q. Acid-base and electrolyte disorders in patients with and without chronic kidney disease: An update. *Kidney Dis (Basel)* 2017;3(4):136–148. doi: 10.1159/000479968.
4. Berend K, de Vries AP, Gans RO. Physiological approach to assessment of acid-base disturbances. *N Engl J Med* 2014;371(15):1434–1445. doi: 10.1056/NEJMra1003327.
5. Adrogué HJ, Madias NE. Assessing acid-base status: Physiologic versus physicochemical approach. *Am J Kidney Dis* 2016;68(5):793–802. doi: 10.1053/j.ajkd.2016.04.023.
6. Berend K. Diagnostic use of base excess in acid-base disorders. *N Engl J Med* 2018;378(15):1419–1428. doi: 10.1056/NEJMra1711860.
7. Yu ASL, Chertow GM, Luyckx VrA, et al. *Brenner & Rector's The kidney* 11th ed. Philadelphia, PA: Elsevier; 2019.
8. Kraut JA, Madias NE. Metabolic acidosis: Pathophysiology, diagnosis and management. *Nat Rev Nephrol* 2010;6(5):274–285. doi: 10.1038/nrneph.2010.33.
9. Seifter JL. Anion-gap metabolic acidemia: Case-based analyses. *Eur J Clin Nutr* 2020;74(Suppl 1):83–86. doi: 10.1038/s41430-020-0685-5.
10. Gupta S, Gao JJ, Emmett M, et al. Topiramate and metabolic acidosis: An evolving story. *Hosp Pract* 2017;45(5):192–195. doi: 10.1080/21548331.2017.1370969.
11. Dounousi E, Zikou X, Koulouras V, et al. Metabolic acidosis during parenteral nutrition: Pathophysiological mechanisms. *Indian J Crit Care Med* 2015;19(5):270–274. doi: 10.4103/0972-5229.156473.
12. Rodríguez Soriano J. Renal tubular acidosis: The clinical entity. *J Am Soc Nephrol* 2002;13(8):2160–2170. doi: 10.1097/01.asn.0000023430.92674.e5.
13. Yaxley J, Pirrone C. Review of the diagnostic evaluation of renal tubular acidosis. *Ochsner J* 2016;16(4):525–530.
14. Reddy P. Clinical approach to renal tubular acidosis in adult patients. *Int J Clin Pract* 2011;65(3):350–360. doi: 10.1111/j.1742-1241.2009.02311.x.
15. Kraut JA, Nagami GT. The serum anion gap in the evaluation of acid-base disorders: What are its limitations and can its effectiveness be improved? *Clin J Am Soc Nephrol* 2013;8(11):2018–2024. doi: 10.2215/cjn.04040413.
16. Kraut JA, Madias NE. Lactic acidosis. *N Engl J Med* 2014;371(24):2309–2319. doi: 10.1056/NEJMra1309483.
17. Kamel KS, Halperin ML. Acid-base problems in diabetic ketoacidosis. *N Engl J Med* 2015;372(6):546–554. doi: 10.1056/NEJMra1207788.
18. Al-Jaghbeer M, Kellum JA. Acid-base disturbances in intensive care patients: Etiology, pathophysiology and treatment. *Nephrol Dial Transplant* 2015;30(7):1104–1111. doi: 10.1093/ndt/gfu289.
19. Andersen LW, Mackenhauer J, Roberts JC, et al. Etiology and therapeutic approach to elevated lactate levels. *Mayo Clin Proc* 2013;88(10):1127–1140. doi: 10.1016/j.mayocp.2013.06.012.
20. Kimmoun A, Novy E, Auchet T, et al. Hemodynamic consequences of severe lactic acidosis in shock states: From bench to bedside. *Crit Care* 2015;19(1):175. doi: 10.1186/s13054-015-0896-7.
21. Moioli A, Maresca B, Manzione A, et al. Metformin associated lactic acidosis (MALA): Clinical profiling and management. *J Nephrol* 2016;29(6):783–789. doi: 10.1007/s40620-016-0267-8.
22. Glucophage and Glucophage XR (metformin HCL tablets and extended-release tablets). Package insert. Bristol-Myers Squibb Company; 2018.

23. American Diabetes Association. Microvascular Complications and Foot Care: Standards of Medical Care in Diabetes—2020. *Diabetes Care* 2020;43(Suppl 1):S135–S151. doi: 10.2337/dc20-S011.
24. American Diabetes Association. Diabetes Care in the Hospital: Standards of Medical Care in Diabetes—2020. *Diabetes Care* 2020;43(Suppl 1):S193–S202. doi: 10.2337/dc20-S015.
25. Margolis AM, Heverling H, Pham PA, et al. A review of the toxicity of HIV medications. *J Med Toxicol* 2014;10(1):26–39. doi: 10.1007/s13181-013-0325-8.
26. Pham AQ, Xu LH, Moe OW. Drug-induced metabolic acidosis. *F1000Res* 2015;4. doi: 10.12688/f1000research.7006.1.
27. Kishor K, Dhasmana N, Kamble SS, et al. Linezolid induced adverse drug reactions: An update. *Curr Drug Metab* 2015;16(7):553–559. doi: 10.2174/1389200216666151001121004.
28. Woloshin S, Schwartz LM. The new weight-loss drugs, lorcaserin and phentermine-topiramate: Slim pickings? *JAMA Intern Med* 2014;174(4):615–619. doi: 10.1001/jamainternmed.2013.14629.
29. Oberg CL, Hiensch RJ, Poor HD. Ombitasvir-paritaprevir-ritonavir-dasabuvir (Viekira Pak)-induced lactic acidosis. *Crit Care Med* 2017;45(3):e321–e325. doi: 10.1097/ccm.0000000000002086.
30. Horinek EL, Kiser TH, Fish DN, et al. Propylene glycol accumulation in critically ill patients receiving continuous intravenous lorazepam infusions. *Ann Pharmacother* 2009;43(12):1964–1971. doi: 10.1345/aph.1M313.
31. Pillai U, Hothi JC, Bhat ZY. Severe propylene glycol toxicity secondary to use of anti-epileptics. *Am J Ther* 2014;21(4):e106–e109. doi: 10.1097/MJT.0b013e31824c407d.
32. Bulathsinghala M, Keefer K, Van de Louw A. Trimethoprim/sulfamethoxazole-induced severe lactic acidosis: A case report and review of the literature. *Medicine (Baltimore)* 2016;95(17):e3478. doi: 10.1097/md.0000000000003478.
33. Mirrakhimov AE, Voore P, Halytskyy O, Khan M, Ali AM. Propofol infusion syndrome in adults: A clinical update. *Crit Care Res Pract* 2015;2015:260385. doi: 10.1155/2015/260385.
34. Albert MS, Dell RB, Winters RW. Quantitative displacement of acid-base equilibrium in metabolic acidosis. *Ann Intern Med* 1967;66(2):312–322. doi: 10.7326/0003-4819-66-2-312.
35. Adrogué HJ. Mixed acid-base disturbances. *J Nephrol.* 2006;19(Suppl 9):S97–S103.
36. Nisbet AM, Burton FL, Walker NL, et al. Acidosis slows electrical conduction through the atrio-ventricular node. *Front Physiol* 2014;5:233. doi: 10.3389/fphys.2014.00233.
37. Palmer BF, Clegg DJ. Physiology and pathophysiology of potassium homeostasis. *Adv Physiol Educ* 2016;40(4):480–490. doi: 10.1152/advan.00121.2016.
38. Garrubba C, Truscott J. A clinical approach to acid-base conundrums. *JAAPA.* 2016;29(4):1–5. doi: 10.1097/01.Jaa.0000481405.96291.79.
39. Velissaris D, Karamouzos V, Ktenopoulos N, et al. The use of sodium bicarbonate in the treatment of acidosis in sepsis: A literature update on a long term debate. *Crit Care Res Pract* 2015;2015:605830. doi: 10.1155/2015/605830.
40. Adrogué HJ, Madias NE. Veverimer: An emerging potential treatment option for managing the metabolic acidosis of CKD. *Am J Kidney Dis* 2020;76(6):861–867. doi: 10.1053/j.ajkd.2020.07.019.
41. Bushinsky DA, Hostetter T, Klaerner G, et al. Randomized, controlled trial of TRC101 to increase serum bicarbonate in patients with CKD. *Clin J Am Soc Nephrol* 2018;13(1):26–35. doi: 10.2215/cjn.07300717.
42. Wesson DE, Mathur V, Tangri N, et al. Long-term safety and efficacy of veverimer in patients with metabolic acidosis in chronic kidney disease: A multicentre, randomised, blinded, placebo-controlled, 40-week extension. *Lancet.* 2019;394(10196):396–406. doi: 10.1016/s0140-6736(19)31388-1.
43. Jaber S, Paugam C, Futier E, et al. Sodium bicarbonate therapy for patients with severe metabolic acidaemia in the intensive care unit (BICAR-ICU): A multicentre, open-label, randomised controlled, phase 3 trial. *Lancet* 2018;392(10141):31–40. doi: 10.1016/S0140-6736(18)31080-8.
44. Kim HJ, Son YK, An WS. Effect of sodium bicarbonate administration on mortality in patients with lactic acidosis: A retrospective analysis. *PLoS One* 2013;8(6):e65283. doi: 10.1371/journal.pone.0065283.
45. Adrogué HJ, Rashad MN, Gorin AB, et al. Assessing acid-base status in circulatory failure. Differences between arterial and central venous blood. *N Engl J Med* 1989;320(20):1312–1316. doi: 10.1056/nejm198905183202004.
46. Ghauri SK, Javaeed A, Mustafa KJ, et al. Bicarbonate therapy for critically ill patients with metabolic acidosis: A systematic review. *Cureus* 2019;11(3):e4297. doi: 10.7759/cureus.4297.
47. Panchal AR, Bartos JA, Cabañas JG, et al. Part 3: Adult basic and advanced life support: 2020 American Heart Association Guidelines for Cardiopulmonary Resuscitation and Emergency Cardiovascular Care. *Circulation* 2020;142(16_suppl_2):S366–S468. doi: 10.1161/CIR.0000000000000916.
48. Hoste EA, Colpaert K, Vanholder RC, et al. Sodium bicarbonate versus THAM in ICU patients with mild metabolic acidosis. *J Nephrol.* 2005;18(3):303–307.
49. Stacpoole PW, Nagaraja NV, Hutson AD. Efficacy of dichloroacetate as a lactate-lowering drug. *J Clin Pharmacol.* 2003;43(7):683–691.
50. Stacpoole PW, Wright EC, Baumgartner TG, et al. A controlled clinical trial of dichloroacetate for treatment of lactic acidosis in adults. *N Engl J Med* 1992;327(22):1564–1569. doi: 10.1056/nejm199211263272204.
51. James MO, Jahn SC, Zhong G, et al. Therapeutic applications of dichloroacetate and the role of glutathione transferase zeta-1. *Pharmacol Ther* 2017;170:166–180. doi: 10.1016/j.pharmthera.2016.10.018.
52. Soifer JT, Kim HT. Approach to metabolic alkalosis. *Emerg Med Clin North Am* 2014;32(2):453–463. doi: 10.1016/j.emc.2014.01.005.
53. Gennari FJ. Pathophysiology of metabolic alkalosis: A new classification based on the centrality of stimulated collecting duct ion transport. *Am J Kidney Dis* 2011;58(4):626–636. doi: 10.1053/j.ajkd.2011.06.004.
54. Miltiadous G, Mikhailidis DP, Elisaf M. Acid-base and electrolyte abnormalities observed in patients receiving cardiovascular drugs. *J Cardiovasc Pharmacol Ther* 2003;8(4):267–276. doi: 10.1177/107424840300800404.
55. Kitterer D, Schwab M, Alscher MD, et al. Drug-induced acid-base disorders. *Pediatr Nephrol* 2015;30(9):1407–1423. doi: 10.1007/s00467-014-2958-5.
56. Kreü S, Jazrawi A, Miller J, et al. Alkalosis in critically Ill patients with severe sepsis and septic shock. *PLoS One* 2017;12(1):e0168563. doi: 10.1371/journal.pone.0168563.
57. Scarpignato C, Gatta L, Zullo A, et al. Effective and safe proton pump inhibitor therapy in acid-related diseases: A position paper addressing benefits and potential harms of acid suppression. *BMC Medicine.* 2016;14(1):179. 10.1186/s12916-016-0718-z.
58. Huber L, Gennari FJ. Severe metabolic alkalosis in a hemodialysis patient. *Am J Kidney Dis* 2011;58(1):144–149. doi: 10.1053/j.ajkd.2011.03.016.
59. Van Berkel MA, Elefritz JL. Evaluating off-label uses of acetazolamide. *Am J Health Syst Pharm* 2018;75(8):524–531. doi: 10.2146/ajhp170279.
60. Faisy C, Meziani F, Planquette B, et al. Effect of acetazolamide vs placebo on duration of invasive mechanical ventilation among patients with chronic obstructive pulmonary disease: A randomized clinical trial. *JAMA* 2016;315(5):480–488. doi: 10.1001/jama.2016.0019.
61. Guffey JD, Haas CE, Crowley A, et al. Hydrochloric acid infusion for the treatment of metabolic alkalosis in surgical intensive care unit patients. *Ann Pharmacother* 2018;52(6):522–526. doi: 10.1177/1060028018754389.
62. Sierra CM, Hernandez EA, Parbuoni KA. Use of arginine hydrochloride in the treatment of metabolic alkalosis or hypochloremia in pediatric patients. *J Pediatr Pharmacol Ther* 2018;23(2):111–118. doi: 10.5863/1551-6776-23.2.111.
63. Martin WJ, Matzke GR. Treating severe metabolic alkalosis. *Clin Pharm.* 1982;1(1):42–48.
64. Adrogué HJ, Madias NE. Management of life-threatening acid-base disorders. Second of two parts. *N Engl J Med* 1998;338(2):107–111. doi: 10.1056/nejm199801083380207.
65. Heble DE Jr., Oschman A, Sandritter TL. Comparison of arginine hydrochloride and acetazolamide for the correction of metabolic alkalosis in pediatric patients. *Am J Ther* 2016;23(6):e1469–e1473. doi: 10.1097/mjt.0000000000000147.
66. Hené RJ, Koomans HA, Dorhout Mees EJ, et al. Correction of hypokalemia in Bartter's syndrome by enalapril. *Am J Kidney Dis* 1987;9(3):200–205. doi: 10.1016/s0272-6386(87)80055-0.
67. Vinci JM, Gill JR Jr., Bowden RE, et al. The kallikrein-kinin system in Bartter's syndrome and its response to prostaglandin synthetase inhibition. *J Clin Invest* 1978;61(6):1671–1682. doi: 10.1172/jci109088.
68. Adrogué HJ, Madias NE. Respiratory acidosis, respiratory alkalosis, and mixed disorders. In: Feehally J, Floege J, Tonelli M, Johnson RJ, eds. *Comprehensive Clinical Nephrology.* 6th ed. Edinburgh: Elsevier; 2019: 170–183.
69. Langer T, Caironi P. *Oxford Textbook of Critical Care.* Pathophysiology and therapeutic strategy of respiratory alkalosis: Oxford University Press; 2016.
70. Foster GT, Vaziri ND, Sassoon CS. Respiratory alkalosis. *Respir Care.* 2001;46(4):384–391.

71. Aronson PS, Giebisch G. Effects of pH on potassium: New explanations for old observations. *J Am Soc Nephrol* 2011;22(11):1981–1989. doi: 10.1681/asn.2011040414.
72. Dimeski G, Treacy O. The influence of albumin and pH on total and ionized calcium and magnesium. *Point of Care* 2018;17(4):123–126. doi: 10.1097/poc.0000000000000173.
73. Gomez H, Kellum JA. Understanding acid base disorders. *Crit Care Clin* 2015;31(4):849–860. doi: 10.1016/j.ccc.2015.06.016.
74. Adrogué HJ, Madias NE. Alkali therapy for respiratory acidosis: A medical controversy. *Am J Kidney Dis* 2020;75(2):265–271. doi: 10.1053/j.ajkd.2019.05.029.
75. Seifter JL. Integration of acid-base and electrolyte disorders. *N Engl J Med* 2014;371(19):1821–1831. doi: 10.1056/NEJMra1215672.

Evaluation of Neurological Illness

e72

Melody Ryan and Stephen J. Ryan

KEY CONCEPTS

1. Accurate diagnosis of neurological disorders leads to effective pharmacotherapy.
2. The clinical neurologic history and examination are the cornerstones of neurologic diagnosis and management.
3. History and examination should be modified for the pediatric patient as appropriate.
4. The neurologic history and examination are directed at localizing the disease process to derive a differential diagnosis.
5. After forming the differential diagnosis, appropriate testing helps pinpoint the correct diagnosis.
6. Accurate diagnosis leads to appropriate therapy and management of neurologic conditions.
7. Specific neurologic history and examination are useful for monitoring and evaluating the pharmacotherapeutic plan.
8. Lumbar puncture (LP) should only be performed when it can be done safely. Relative contraindications may include increased intercranial pressure, mass lesions, papilledema, and coagulopathies.

BEYOND THE BOOK

Watch the video entitled "The Neurologic Screening Exam" in AccessPharmacy by Daniel H. Lowenstein. https://accesspharmacy.mhmedical.com/MultimediaPlayer.aspx?MultimediaID=12986884

This 9-minute video provides a brief overview of the neurologic examination including all five components. This visual depiction will aid in student understanding of the examination. The information collected in the neurologic examination is used in the COLLECT and FOLLOW-UP steps in the patient care process.

INTRODUCTION

1 2 Accurate diagnosis of neurological disorders leads to effective pharmacotherapy. This diagnosis is built upon history, a detailed neurological examination, and appropriate testing. To contribute most effectively to the care of patients with neurologic illness, one must understand the tools used in the diagnosis and management of these patients. In addition, clinicians must be able to gather their own data through patient history and targeted neurologic examination to ensure optimal pharmacotherapy. Despite technological advances and development of sensitive diagnostic tests, the clinical neurologic history and examination are still the cornerstones of diagnosis and management.[1]

SIGNS AND SYMPTOMS OF NEUROLOGIC DISORDERS

As in all of medicine, obtaining an accurate and complete history is of utmost importance in the evaluation of neurologic diseases. In many instances, the differential diagnosis can be made on the basis of the history, and the neurologic examination can be tailored to optimally evaluate the patient and confirm the diagnosis.[1] Open-ended questions allow the patient to provide the salient history without leading the patient toward preconceived diagnoses. Obtaining an accurate history may be difficult because a number of neurologic diseases potentially affect communication and memory. The details obtained from family or other observers support and further expand patient reported history; additionally, family medical history can be helpful in diagnosis.[1] Through patient history, one can determine the main symptoms, location, onset (acute, subacute, or chronic), progression over time (maximal at onset or steadily gaining intensity), and associated illnesses or risk factors for neurologic disease.[2] The history should also identify factors that might precipitate or ameliorate the symptoms.[2] Each patient complaint should be thoroughly investigated while taking the history. See Table e72-1 for questions to assist the clinician in obtaining the neurologic history.

Special attention should be given to the medication history including current medications, doses, dosing schedule (times, relationship to other medications and meals), duration, and adherence. Adverse effects should be recorded in detail. Past and recently discontinued medications as well as any medications used previously, including reasons for discontinuation, to treat the main complaints are important. Clinicians should also consider if the patient's symptoms may be medication-induced.

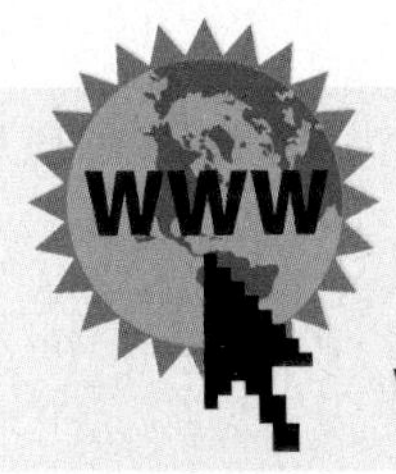

The complete chapter, learning objectives, and other resources can be found at **www.pharmacotherapyonline.com.**

73 Alzheimer Disease

Ericka L. Crouse, Kristin M. Zimmerman, Emily P. Peron, Lana J. Sargent, and Sarah E. Hobgood

KEY CONCEPTS

1. Alzheimer disease (AD) is the most common cause of dementia, the prevalence of which increases with each decade of life.
2. The etiology of AD is unknown, and current pharmacotherapy neither cures nor arrests its pathophysiology.
3. Amyloid plaques and neurofibrillary tangles (NFTs) are the pathologic hallmarks of AD; however, the definitive cause of this disease is yet to be determined.
4. AD affects multiple areas of cognition and is characterized by a gradual onset with a slow, progressive decline.
5. A thorough physical examination (including a neurologic examination), as well as laboratory and imaging studies, are required to rule out other disorders and diagnose AD before considering pharmacotherapy.
6. Pharmacotherapy for AD focuses on impacting three domains: (1) cognition, (2) neuropsychiatric symptoms, and (3) functional ability.
7. Nonmedication therapy and social support for the patient and family are the primary treatment interventions for AD.
8. Cholinesterase inhibitors and memantine are used to treat cognitive symptoms of AD, whereas immunotherapies may have the potential to be disease-modifying.
9. Aducanumab, an amyloid beta-directed antibody, was Food and Drug Administration (FDA)-approved in 2021 for AD via accelerated approval. Three other agents have been granted breakthrough therapy designation and are continuing to be evaluated.
10. Appropriate management of vascular disease risk factors may reduce the risk for developing AD and may prevent the worsening of dementia in people with AD.
11. A thorough behavioral assessment with careful examination of environmental factors should be conducted, and a plan put in place before initiating medication therapy for behavioral symptoms.

BEYOND THE BOOK

Visit the Mini-Cog website at http://mini-cog.com. At the top of the screen select from the "Mini-Cog Versions" drop-down menu the "Standardized Mini-Cog Instrument" tab:

1. Review the three-step process and scoring guidelines. You do not need to print this document, as you can simply draw a circle on a blank piece of paper for your partner to use while you take notes on a separate piece of paper.
2. Work with a classmate to practice administering the Mini-Cog to each other and scoring it accordingly.
3. If you get stuck or are not sure how to score an item, return to the "Mini-Cog Versions" drop-down menu and select "Administering the Mini-Cog" and/or "Scoring the Mini-Cog."
4. You may have questions after working through this exercise, perhaps related to test logistics or next steps. If that is the case, consider returning to the "Mini-Cog Versions" drop-down menu and visiting the "FAQs" page.

This activity is intended to increase your familiarity with a brief, freely available dementia screening tool that is often used in clinical settings and as part of the Medicare Annual Wellness Visit. The Mini-Cog can be administered by any health professional or trained lay health worker.

INTRODUCTION

I now begin the journey that will lead me into the sunset of my life.

—Ronald Reagan

Dementia is an umbrella term used to define the loss of cognitive functioning—thinking, remembering, and reasoning—and behavioral abilities that interferes with a person's daily life and activities. Mild cognitive impairment (MCI) often proceeds dementia, but not all cases progress to dementia. There are a variety of diseases and pathologies that cause dementia, with Alzheimer disease (AD), which is a gradually progressive dementia affecting cognition, behavior, and functional status, being the most common. The exact pathophysiologic mechanisms underlying AD are not entirely known, and no cure exists.[1] Although medications may reduce AD symptoms for a time, the disease is eventually fatal.

Alzheimer disease profoundly affects the family as well as the patient. The need for supervision and assistance increases until the late stages of the disease, when people with AD become totally dependent on a caregiver for all basic needs. To address the growing AD crisis facing the United States, the first national strategic plan, the National Alzheimer's Plan, was released in 2012 with the goal of coordinating efforts across the federal government to prevent and treat AD, increase public awareness, and improve the quality of care and support for patients and their caregivers.[2] The US Department of Health and Human Services has since updated this strategic plan to include a timeline for achieving its goal to "develop effective prevention and treatment modalities by 2025."[2]

TABLE 73-1 Common Types of Dementia

Alzheimer disease
Vascular dementia
Dementia with Lewy bodies
Mixed dementia
Others (eg, Parkinson disease dementia, Frontotemporal dementia, Huntington disease, Creutzfeldt–Jakob disease)
Potentially reversible causes of cognitive dysfunction (eg, normal pressure hydrocephalus, thyroid dysfunction, vitamin B_{12} deficiency, delirium, depression, Wernicke–Korsakoff syndrome, infectious and autoimmune encephalitis)

Data from References 2 and 5.

EPIDEMIOLOGY

1 AD is the most common cause of dementia, accounting for 60% to 80% of cases, although multiple etiologies can result in dementia (Table 73-1).[3,4] This chapter focuses exclusively on dementia of the Alzheimer type. However, the reader is encouraged to use the nonpharmacologic approaches and management of behavioral problems outlined in this chapter as a general treatment approach for other types of dementia that may share similar features with AD.

Approximately 6.2 million adults age 65 years and older in the United States have AD, and by the year 2050, this number is projected to double.[3] Factors determining age of onset and rate of progression remain largely undefined. Onset can be as early as age 30 years, resulting in the arbitrary age classifications of early-onset (younger than age 65 years) AD (EOAD) and late-onset (age 65 years and older) AD (LOAD).[3] Though increasing age is the greatest risk factor for AD, AD is not a normal part of aging.

In people age 65 years and older, survival following AD diagnosis is typically 4 to 8 years but may be as long as 20 years.[3] AD is the fifth leading cause of death for those age 65 years and older in the United States; however, death among people with AD is often not a direct result of the disease but rather the functional impairments that accompany it.[3] Among the most common causes of death in people with AD is pneumonia, possibly resulting from swallowing difficulties and immobility in the terminal stage of the disease.[3] Those diagnosed with AD spend, on average, more years in the most severe stage of the disease than any other stage, and much of this time is spent in a nursing home.[3]

ETIOLOGY

Genetics

2 The exact etiology of AD is unknown; however, several genetic and environmental factors have been explored as potential causes. Genetic factors have been linked to both EOAD and LOAD, although dominantly inherited forms of AD account for less than 1% of cases.[6] More than half of early-onset, dominantly inherited cases of AD can be attributed to alterations on chromosomes 1, 14, or 21. These alterations largely impact the processing of a large membrane protein called amyloid precursor protein (APP). APP is typically broken down by three major secretase enzymes—α-, β-, and γ-secretase—into nonpathologic fragments as well as potentially pathologic 38 to 43 peptide-long β-amyloid peptide (Aβ) fragments. Of these enzymes, α-secretase is responsible for ensuring that APP is broken down into nonpathologic fragments. Relative alterations in the activity of β- and/or γ-secretase may prove pathologic.[7] As a result, these enzymes may be considered potential therapeutic targets.

Rare, autosomal dominant forms of EOAD have been found in *APP* and the presenilin genes (*PSEN1* and *PSEN2*). Scientists have identified more than 160 mutations in *PSEN1* and *PSEN2*, and these mutations result in increased activity of γ-secretase, which may yield larger and more harmful Aβ fragments.[8,9] The *APP* is encoded on chromosome 21. Only a small number of EOAD cases have been associated with mutations in the *APP* gene, resulting in overproduction of Aβ or an increase in the proportion of Aβ ending at peptide 42.[8,9] Presence of these mutations, however, is often indicative of disease development.

Genetic susceptibility to LOAD is primarily linked to the apolipoprotein E (*APOE*) genotype. Hypothetically, *APOE* (a cholesterol transport gene) may be implicated in the pathogenesis of the disease. There are three major subtypes or alleles of *APOE*—**2*, **3*, and **4*. Inheritance of the *APOE*4* allele accounts for much of the genetic risk in LOAD.[10] The mechanism through which *APOE*4* confers an increased risk is unknown, although *APOE*4* is associated with factors that may contribute to AD pathology, such as abnormalities in mitochondria, cytoskeletal dysfunction, and low glucose usage.[11] The risk for AD is two- to threefold higher in individuals with one *APOE*4* allele and 12-fold higher in individuals with two *APOE*4* alleles compared to those with no *APOE*4* alleles.[11] Moreover, onset of symptoms occurs at a relatively younger age as compared with people having no *APOE*4* alleles or only one copy of *APOE*4* in their genotype.[11] The prevalence of individuals who carry two copies of the *APOE*4* alleles is only 2%, while the prevalence of those carrying one allele is 25%. The *APOE*4* allele is not diagnostic of AD, essential for disease presence, or indicative of future disease development. Additionally, the association between *APOE* genotype and AD differs based on ancestral background.[12]

Additional genetic explanatory factors continue to be investigated with a focus on differences in race and ethnicity. Genome-wide association studies (GWAS) have been done on large cohorts of healthy individuals and those with AD, which has led to the identification of more genetic variants. One with the highest post-GWAS research success is the ATP-binding cassette transporter A7, *ABCA7* gene.[13] Both *APOE* and *ABCA7* are involved in lipid metabolism and are the strongest heritable contributors for genetic risk.[14] Important research continues to explore the effects of genetic variations on cognitive function within diverse populations.

Environmental and Other Factors

A number of factors are associated with an increased risk of AD, including age, decreased reserve capacity of the brain (eg, reduced brain size, low educational level, reduced mental and physical activity), head injury, Down syndrome, depression, MCI, and risk factors for vascular disease (eg, hypercholesterolemia, hypertension, atherosclerosis, coronary heart disease, smoking, elevated homocysteine, obesity, metabolic syndrome, diabetes).[3,4,15] Whether these vascular risk factors are true causal risk factors for AD contributing to AD pathology, or whether they result in cerebrovascular pathology that, in turn, contributes to the symptoms of AD, remains to be established. The incidence of AD rises with increasing age, and AD may develop in individuals over the course of decades, suggesting that AD is a disease that likely develops throughout adulthood.[3] Of note, more females than males have AD.[3] While this may largely be a factor of females living longer than males, hypothetically, males who live to be older than 65 years may have better cardiovascular risk profiles than females of the same age; this is commonly referred to as "survival bias."[3] An analysis of the complex interactions between age, sex, vascular health, and AD is beyond the scope of this chapter.

PATHOPHYSIOLOGY

3 The signature lesions in AD include amyloid plaques and neurofibrillary tangles (NFTs) located in the cortical areas and medial temporal lobe structures of the brain.[1,15,16] Along with these lesions, degeneration of neurons and synapses as well as

cortical atrophy occurs. It is unclear if or how these lesions are definitively implicated in the development of AD symptoms. This is particularly true as plaques and NFTs may also be present in other diseases, even in normal aging. Importantly, however, AD-affected subjects appear to have a higher burden of plaques and NFTs in their younger years compared to age-matched controls. Several mechanisms have been proposed to explain changes in the brain that result in symptoms of AD, including misfolding of proteins (Aβ aggregation and deposition leading to the formation of plaques and tangles), synaptic failure and depletion of neurotrophin and neurotransmitters, and mitochondrial dysfunction (oxidative stress, impaired insulin signaling in the brain, vascular injury, inflammatory processes, loss of calcium regulation, and defects in cholesterol metabolism).[1,10,16]

Amyloid Cascade Hypothesis

Cleavage of APP via β- and γ-secretase produces Aβ fragments that are 36 to 43 amino acids in length. Amyloid clearance pathways include degradation by enzymes such as neprilysin-1, phagocytosis by glial cells, or transportation into the vasculature. If not cleared, these soluble, monomeric Aβ fragments can aggregate. These aggregations can include soluble but toxic oligomers or protofibrils, or less soluble, larger, extracellular fibrils and plaques.[17,18] While less common than other Aβ peptides, $Aβ_{42}$ is prone to aggregation and plaque formation.[1,19] Amyloid can also aggregate in the perivascular space between neurons and vessels, as well as vascular smooth muscle and basement cell membranes, contributing to cerebrovascular damage.[17,18]

The amyloid cascade hypothesis states that there is an imbalance between the production and clearance of Aβ peptides resulting in their accumulation and aggregation, insoluble extracellular plaque formation, and ultimately the development of AD.[1,17,19] More recent versions of the amyloid cascade hypothesis assume that soluble oligomer and protofibril forms of Aβ that are not sequestered in plaques actually drive the disease by binding to cell surface receptors, metals, and cellular membranes.[1,17,19] Additionally, it is unknown whether the presence of Aβ in any of these forms is the primary pathology responsible for AD development, or whether these changes are a marker of an alternate pathology. If treatments that reduce Aβ production or remove brain Aβ fail to arrest disease progression in those with early or prodromal disease, it would argue amyloidosis is not the primary pathology in most individuals with AD.

Neurofibrillary Tangles

At the same time Aβ was being identified in plaques, other researchers found that NFTs are common in the cells of the hippocampus and cerebral cortex (regions implicated in AD symptoms) in people with AD. These NFTs are composed of abnormally hyperphosphorylated tau protein. Tau protein provides structural support to microtubules, the cell's transportation, and skeletal support system.[4] When tau filaments undergo abnormal phosphorylation at a specific site, they cannot bind effectively to microtubules, and the microtubules collapse. Without an intact system of microtubules, the cell cannot function properly and eventually dies. Hypothetically, soluble forms of Aβ may trigger initial tau phosphorylation. In general, NFT density correlates with severity of dementia; however, NFTs are found in other dementing illnesses besides AD and may represent a common method by which various inciting factors culminate in cell death.[16,17,20]

Inflammatory Mediators

Inflammatory or immunologic paradigms are additional hypotheses relevant to AD neurodegeneration.[1] Inflammatory/immunologic hypotheses argue that although Aβ may have direct neurotoxicity, at least some of Aβ toxicity might actually be an indirect consequence of an immune response mediated by Aβ protofibril–induced microglia activation and astrocyte recruitment. This inflammatory response may represent an attempt to clear amyloid; however, it is also associated with release of cytokines, nitric oxide, other radical species, and complement factors that can both injure neurons and promote ongoing inflammation.[1] Indeed, levels of multiple cytokines and chemokines are elevated in AD brains, and certain proinflammatory gene polymorphisms are reported to be associated with AD.[1,21]

Cholinergic Hypothesis

Multiple neuronal pathways are destroyed in AD and neuronal damage can be seen in conjunction with plaque structures.[1,16] Widespread cell dysfunction or degeneration results in a variety of neurotransmitter deficits, with cholinergic abnormalities being among the most prominent.[1,10] Loss of cholinergic activity correlates with AD severity. In the late stage of AD, the number of cholinergic neurons is reduced, and there is loss of nicotinic receptors in the hippocampus and cortex. Presynaptic nicotinic receptors control the release of acetylcholine as well as other neurotransmitters important for memory and mood, including glutamate, serotonin, and norepinephrine.[1,10]

The discovery of vast cholinergic cell loss led to the development of a cholinergic hypothesis of AD which targeted cholinergic cell loss as the source of memory and cognitive impairment in AD. Consequently, increasing cholinergic function would improve symptoms of memory loss. This approach is flawed because cholinergic cell loss is a secondary consequence of AD pathology, not the disease-producing event, and cholinergic neurons are only one of many neuronal pathways destroyed in AD. Simple addition of acetylcholine cannot compensate for the loss of neurons, receptors, and other neurotransmitters lost during the course of the illness. Thus, cholinergic therapies are used to minimize or improve symptoms through augmentation of cholinergic neurotransmission at remaining synapses.

Other Neurotransmitter Abnormalities

Although the cholinergic system has received particular attention in AD pharmaceutical research, deficits also exist in other neuronal pathways. For example, serotonergic neurons of the raphe nuclei and noradrenergic cells of the locus coeruleus are lost, while activity of dopamine-metabolizing monoamine oxidase type B is increased. In addition, abnormalities appear in glutamate pathways of the cortex and limbic structures, where a loss of neurons leads to a focus on excitotoxicity models as possible contributing factors to AD pathology.

Glutamate is the major excitatory neurotransmitter in the cortex and hippocampus. Many neuronal pathways essential to learning and memory use glutamate as a neurotransmitter, including the pyramidal neurons (a layer of neurons with long axons carrying information out of the cortex), hippocampus, and entorhinal cortex. Glutamate and other excitatory amino acid neurotransmitters have been implicated as potential neurotoxins in AD.[16] Dysregulated glutamate activity is thought to be one of the primary mediators of neuronal injury after stroke or acute brain injury. Although intimately involved in cell injury, the role of excitatory amino acids in AD is yet unclear; however, blockade of *N*-methyl-D-aspartate (NMDA) receptors decreases activity of glutamate in the synapse and may hypothetically lessen the degree of cellular injury in AD.

Apolipoprotein E

The fat-soluble transporter *APOE* is synthesized in the liver, central nervous system, and cerebrospinal fluid (CSF). It is responsible for transporting cholesterol in the blood and through the brain and interacts with Aβ in almost all pathways, including in its neuronal, glial, and vascular clearance. It is carried by low-density lipoprotein into neurons where it also binds to NFTs. The *APOE*4* allele, previously discussed under genetics, is associated with both modified clearance and increased deposition of Aβ in AD. It is also thought to act as an accelerating modulator in vascular dementia. The *APOE*4* allele is considered a strong risk factor for both EOAD and LOAD, whereas *APOE*2* is associated with a lower risk, and *APOE*3* a protective effect.[18,22]

Brain Vascular Disease and High Cholesterol

There is growing evidence of a causal association between cardiovascular disease and its risk factors and the incidence of AD. Cardiovascular risk factors that are also risk factors for dementia include hypertension, hypercholesterolemia, and diabetes.[23] For a given amount of AD pathology, vascular disease in the brain may compound the degree of cognitive impairment observed.[19] Vascular disease may accelerate amyloid deposition and reduce clearance of Aβ from the brain.[24] Presence of cardiovascular risk factors in midlife is strongly associated with development of AD in late life.[24] Midlife hypertension is adversely associated with AD, while late life hypertension may be inversely associated. Blood pressure decreases in the years leading up to clinical onset of dementia, conceivably because of reductions in physical activity and body weight.[24]

Mechanistically, the increased risk of AD seen among people with prediabetes and diabetes may be a result of microvascular damage or direct neurotoxicity related to increased glucose and insulin levels.[24] Disturbances in insulin-signaling pathways, both in the periphery and the brain, have been linked to AD. Insulin may also regulate the metabolism of Aβ and tau protein.[25]

Research has found multiple links between cholesterol and AD. Elevated cholesterol levels in brain neurons may alter membrane functioning and result in the cascade leading to plaque formation and AD.

Other Mechanisms

Other hypotheses proposed to explain AD pathogenesis include oxidative stress, mitochondrial dysfunction, and loss of estrogen. Each of these mechanisms may contribute to AD pathogenesis, but the extent of their contribution is uncertain. There is a growing body of evidence regarding the role of oxidative stress and the accumulation of free radicals in the brains of people with AD.[4] Some epidemiologic studies suggest vitamin E, and possibly the combination of vitamin E and vitamin C, may reduce AD risk, while others do not.[26] Mitochondrial dysfunction may result in disruption of energy metabolism in the neuron.[1,15] The role of estrogen in cognitive aging and dementia continues to be an active area of investigation. Despite convincing evidence that estrogens affect the brain in ways that would be expected to improve cognitive aging and reduce the risk of AD, the results of clinical studies have been largely disappointing.[27]

A single common mechanism for developing AD does not exist. Regardless of the etiology, however, the features remain the same: degeneration of neurons in higher brain areas; accumulation of NFTs and amyloid plaques; profound destruction of cholinergic pathways; and an insidious dementia, slowly progressive until death.

CLINICAL PRESENTATION

4 In the absence of abrupt changes in cognition or function, the onset of AD can be almost imperceptible. There are often pathologic changes related to AD long before symptoms emerge, and further deficits occur progressively over time, affecting multiple areas of cognition and function.[3,15] Figure 73-1 depicts the transition from preclinical AD to dementia of the Alzheimer type. Early disease may be characterized by changes in learning and memory, planning and organization, and mood. If these deficits do not impact patient function, the patient may be considered to have MCI. Approximately 15% of patients with MCI will develop dementia after 2 years.[3] Within 5 years, approximately one-third will develop dementia of the Alzheimer's type.[3] Patients with MCI may or may not experience further decline that impairs function and transition to dementia. These patients represent a critical juncture in evaluation, management, and potential mitigation of further cognitive decline.[3]

As pathology progresses, patients may experience further decline in these domains, as well as changes in personality, judgment, speech, and spatial orientation that begin to impact function. In the late stages of dementia, functional decline may be associated with gait changes, swallowing difficulties, and incontinence symptoms; behavioral changes may also result. For treatment and assessment purposes, it is helpful to divide AD symptoms into two basic categories: cognitive symptoms and neuropsychiatric (behavioral) symptoms. Cognitive symptoms are present throughout the illness, whereas behavioral symptoms are less predictable. Table 73-2 and Fig. 73-1 summarize the stages of AD.

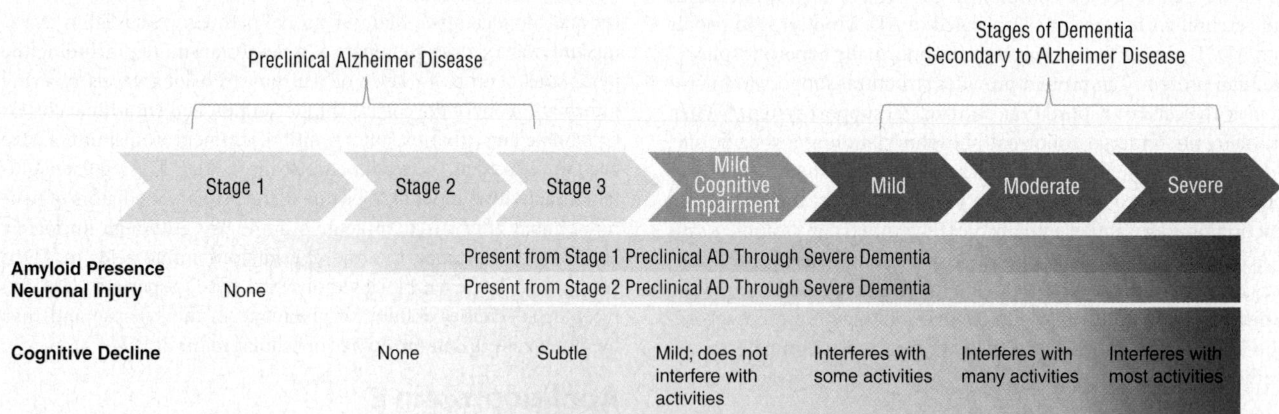

FIGURE 73-1 The continuum of Alzheimer disease: Progression of pathophysiology and clinical symptoms of AD. (*Data from References 162 and 163.*)

CLINICAL PRESENTATION Alzheimer Disease

General

- The patient may have vague memory complaints initially, or the patient's friends or family may report that the patient is "forgetful." Cognitive decline is typically gradual over the course of illness. Behavioral disturbances may be present in moderate stages. Loss of daily function such as dressing, bathing, and toileting is common in advanced stages.

Symptoms

Cognitive

- Memory loss (poor recall and losing items)
- Aphasia (circumlocution and anomia)
- Apraxia
- Agnosia
- Disorientation (impaired perception of time and unable to recognize familiar people)
- Impaired executive function

Neuropsychiatric

- Depression, psychotic symptoms (hallucinations and delusions)
- Behavioral disturbances (physical and verbal aggression, motor hyperactivity, uncooperativeness, wandering, repetitive mannerisms and activities, and combativeness)

Functional

- Inability to care for self (dressing, bathing, toileting, and eating)

TABLE 73-2 Stages of Alzheimer Disease

Mild (MMSE score 26–21)	Patient has difficulty remembering recent events. Ability to manage finances, prepare food, and carry out other household activities declines. May get lost while driving. Begins to withdraw from difficult tasks and to give up hobbies. May deny memory problems.
Moderate (MMSE score 20–10)	Patient requires assistance with activities of daily living. Frequently disoriented with regard to time (date, year, and season). Recall of recent events is severely impaired. May forget some details of past life events and names of family and friends. Functioning may fluctuate from day to day. Patient generally denies problems. May become suspicious or tearful. Loses ability to drive safely. Agitation, paranoia, and delusions are common.
Severe (MMSE score 9–0)	Patient loses ability to speak, walk, and feed self. Incontinent of urine and feces. Requires care 24 hours a day, 7 days a week.

MMSE, Mini-Mental State Examination.

Data from References 5 and 28.

Diagnosis

According to the 2021 World Alzheimer Report, dementia is often underdetected, underdiagnosed, and subsequently undertreated and undermanaged.[29] Up to 75% of individuals seen in a primary care setting are not given an AD diagnosis.[30] Reasons for this include lack of awareness by patients or their family and friends that the early decline may be associated with AD, or limitations due to clinician awareness, training, and/or time.[30] Despite the phenomenon of underdiagnosis, the US Preventive Services Task Force concluded that there are insufficient data to recommend for or against routine cognitive screening in the absence of symptoms as the benefits may not outweigh the risks, as evidence does not suggest that screening impacts decision making.[30] However, screening for cognitive impairment is a required element of the Medicare Annual Wellness Visit.[31,32] Screening should always occur in the presence of symptoms recognized by the patient, family, or clinician. Discussing the diagnosis of dementia is potentially distressing for patients and their loved ones, especially during initial discussions. Most people, however, prefer to be told about a dementia diagnosis, as it allows them to appropriately plan and access necessary support and treatment services in the meantime.[5]

The Mini-Mental State Examination (MMSE) is a 30-point assessment tool for AD frequently cited in the literature and employed in practice; because of its copyrighted status; however, the MMSE must either be administered from memory or paid for by the user. Similarly, the Montreal Cognitive Assessment became proprietary in 2019, and users must now be trained and certified.[33] Alternatives include the Mini-Cog and the Saint Louis University Mental Status Exam.[34] Each of these tools varies in their characteristics, including sensitivity and specificity, for identifying an underlying dementia.

The only way to confirm a clinical diagnosis of AD is through direct examination of brain tissue at autopsy or biopsy. Several criteria have been used in clinical practice and research for the detection and diagnosis of dementia, including the *Diagnostic and Statistical Manual of Mental Disorders*, Fifth Edition (*DSM-5*) criteria,[35] the Agency for Healthcare Research and Quality guidelines,[36] the American Academy of Neurology guidelines,[37] the National Institute of Neurological Disorders and Stroke criteria,[38] and the National Institute of Neurological and Communicative Disorders and Stroke (NINCDS) and the Alzheimer's Disease and Related Disorders Association (ADRDA) criteria.[39] The *DSM-5* has subsumed the terminology dementia under major neurocognitive disorder; however, the term *dementia* is still often used in clinical practice.[35]

In 2011, revisions to the NINCDS-ADRDA criteria for the clinical diagnosis of AD were recommended by the National Institute on Aging (NIA) and the Alzheimer's Association (AA).[40] The new NIA-AA criteria view AD as a spectrum beginning with a preclinical phase progressing to increasingly severe clinical stages of AD, as depicted in Fig. 73-1. Three workgroups formulated diagnostic criteria for the dementia phase[41]; the symptomatic, predementia phase (MCI)[42]; and the asymptomatic, preclinical phase of AD.[45] The preclinical phase has been further broken down into three stages—stage 1 (asymptomatic cerebral amyloidosis), stage 2 (asymptomatic amyloidosis plus neurodegeneration), and stage 3 (amyloidosis plus neurodegeneration plus subtle cognitive/behavioral decline).[43] In 2018, the American Academy of Neurology updated their practice guideline for MCI.[43,44] Commonalities between guidance documents include the association of impairments in multiple cognitive domains and functional impairment with a clinical diagnosis of AD.

AD remains primarily a clinical diagnosis, but this will likely change as brain imaging, CSF testing, and other AD biomarkers supporting definitive diagnosis become increasingly available for routine clinical use. The patient's examination should suggest that cognitive decline from a previously higher baseline has occurred.

The history should corroborate this finding and further indicate that cognitive decline has reached the point where changes in social or occupational functioning are present. It is possible to administer full neuropsychiatric testing—a battery of sophisticated exams that defines cognitive domain strengths and weaknesses and enables a neuroanatomic localization of the observed deficits. When approached in this way, neuropsychiatric testing can indicate a pattern of cognitive decline that is consistent with AD and assist with rendering a diagnosis that is as much a diagnosis of inclusion as it is of exclusion. Neuropsychiatric testing is considered optional but can prove quite useful for the diagnosis of AD, as well as differentiating types of cognitive impairment.

Objectively defining social or occupational dysfunction can prove tricky in the older patient who may be retired, lead a socially restricted lifestyle, or experience frailty. For such patients, the minimal requirement is to establish a negative impact on day-to-day life. Early on, this usually involves a change in instrumental activities of daily living (eg, handling finances and organizing medications) rather than basic activities of daily living (eg, hygiene and dressing). Some AD subspecialists use a detailed, standardized, semistructured interview of a nonpatient informant such as a caregiver as the most critical piece of the diagnostic evaluation.[45]

5 For people who meet criteria for dementia (whether the underlying cause is ultimately suspected to be AD or not), current recommendations from the American Academy of Neurology include a serologic evaluation that includes blood cell counts, serum electrolytes, liver function tests, a test of thyroid function, and a vitamin B_{12} level to rule out other causes of cognitive decline.[37] When circumstances suggest AD is not the leading entity on the differential diagnosis, other neurologic tests such as CSF analysis or electroencephalogram can occasionally be justified.

Guidelines recommend that structural imaging (noncontrast-enhanced computed tomography [or CT] or magnetic resonance imaging [MRI]) be performed in the evaluation of people with suspected dementia.[46] These tests may identify structural abnormalities consistent with AD or other pathology, such as brain atrophy, vascular damage, or tumors. Efforts to define the role of other AD diagnostic tests are ongoing.

Use of preclinical indicators typically reserved for the research setting, such as functional imaging, CSF biomarkers, and genetic tests, may become increasingly important with the emergence of potentially disease-modifying agents. Positron emission tomography, or PET, scanning may be used to identify a pattern of neurodegeneration consistent with AD. Such neurodegeneration may be evidenced by reduced uptake of a glucose tracer, indicating hypometabolism, or by modified uptake of an amyloid- or tau-specific tracer, indicating the presence of CNS pathology.[47] Radiologic tracers specific to amyloid plaques (Pittsburgh compound B [PiB], florbetapir F18, florbetaben F18, and flutemetamol F18) often used in research may be used to identify individuals with early disease; however, without widespread access, clinical utility is limited. Additionally, the diagnostic accuracy of PET scanning alone still lags behind that of the clinical examination and history.[43] The presence of amyloid and tau within the CSF may also be utilized to identify patients with early stages of AD, but similar access and interpretation barriers exist.[48] Likewise, *APOE* genotyping is not clinically recommended now, as presence of an *APOE*4* allele alone does not cause AD.[49] While *APOE* genotyping by itself is insufficient to make a diagnosis of AD, demonstrating an *APOE*4* allele in a suspected patient increases the specificity of the diagnosis. Unless the person developed dementia before the age of 60 years and also had a parent who developed AD before the age of 60 years, *PSEN1*, *PSEN2*, or APP genotyping is usually not indicated. Unclear benefits, potential harms, and ethical concerns limit testing for genetic causes of dementia as a part of routine diagnosis and should only be completed with informed consent following genetic counseling.[49]

Mild Cognitive Impairment

Aging is associated with changes in cognitive function. Importantly, MCI constitutes a syndromic designation that categorizes people with cognitive complaints insufficient to warrant a dementia diagnosis. The NIA-AA criteria specifically address the diagnosis of MCI.[42,44,50] Approximately 15% of patients with MCI will develop dementia after 2 years.[3,50] While clinicians may be seeing the initial manifestation of a progressive, degenerative dementia that will eventually meet AD diagnostic criteria, not everyone meeting MCI criteria will develop AD.[42,44] When a diagnosis of MCI is made, routine cognitive screening should be done to monitor for further cognitive loss.

TREATMENT

Desired Outcome

6 Approved and investigative pharmacologic therapies have generally failed to demonstrate a reduced risk of progression to dementia, including when used in early MCI.[44,51] As such, the primary goal of treatment in AD is to symptomatically treat cognitive difficulties and preserve patient function for as long as possible. Secondary goals include managing psychiatric and behavioral sequelae. Current AD treatments do not seem to prolong life, cure AD, or halt or reverse the pathophysiologic processes of the disorder.[45]

General Approach to Treatment

Prior to initiating treatment for AD, a thorough medication review should be completed, as many medications can contribute to cognitive impairment in vulnerable individuals, but certain classes are more commonly implicated. Benzodiazepines and other sedative hypnotics, anticholinergics, and antipsychotics have been associated with cognitive impairment.[52] In addition, H_2-receptor antagonists, corticosteroids, and opioids like meperidine have been implicated in cases of delirium or acute cognitive change.[52] Because medication use is a reversible cause of cognitive symptomatology, medication review and management are essential.

Clinical trials demonstrate modest benefits of early and continuous treatment with cholinesterase inhibitors with the addition of memantine in moderate-to-severe disease.[53] Following this approach, along with a symptomatic approach to address behavioral symptoms as they arise, allows for maximal maintenance of cognition and activities of daily living. Considering the Food and Drug Administration (FDA) evaluation of potentially disease-modifying immunotherapies for use in MCI and early AD, it remains to be seen how the place in therapy of cholinesterase inhibitors and/or memantine will change, if at all. Patient and family education at the time of diagnosis, including discussion of the course of illness, realistic expectations of treatment, and the importance of legal and financial planning are essential to appropriate treatment.

Dosing recommendations for patients with renal or hepatic dysfunction or low body weight are detailed in Table 73-3. It is important to consider that most people with AD are older adults and therefore may be taking multiple medications for other acute and chronic health conditions.[54] The benefits of medication therapy for AD and other comorbid medical conditions must be weighed against each medication's time-to-benefit and potential for adverse events.

Nonpharmacologic Therapy

7 Evidence has been insufficient to warrant the routine use of nonpharmacologic interventions to prevent or delay the development of dementia or AD. There has been promising evidence; however, that promotion of a healthy lifestyle in mid-life may help modify potential risk factors for LOAD.[64-68] A 2018 meta-analysis found exercise training may delay cognitive decline in persons at risk for AD.[68]

TABLE 73-3 Dosing of Medications Used for Cognitive Symptoms

Medication	Brand Name	Initial Dose	Usual Range	Specific populations	Other
Cholinesterase Inhibitors					
Donepezil	Aricept, Aricept ODT, Adlarity transdermal	5 mg daily in the evening (oral)[a] 5 mg/day (transdermal patch) applied weekly	5-10 mg daily in mild-to-moderate AD 10-23 mg daily in moderate-to-severe AD	No dosage adjustments recommended	Available as: tablet, ODT, oral solution, transdermal patch Can be taken with or without food Incidence of GI adverse effects (including weight loss) are higher with 23 mg daily dose Therapy interruptions require retitration of dose Store transdermal patch in fridge
Rivastigmine	Exelon, Exelon Patch	1.5 mg twice daily (capsule, oral solution) 4.6 mg/day (transdermal patch)	3-6 mg twice daily (capsule, oral solution) 9.5-13.3 mg/day (transdermal patch)	Capsule,oral solution: Renal impairment, hepatic impairment, or low body weight (<50 kg [<110 lb]): may be able to only tolerate lower doses Transdermal patch: Mild-to-moderate hepatic impairment or low body weight: consider maximum daily dose of 4.6 mg every 24 hours	Available as: capsule, oral solution, transdermal patch Therapy interruptions require retitration of dose Take with meals Also indicated for mild-to-moderate dementia associated with Parkinson disease Use of multiple transdermal patches at the same time is associated with hospitalization and death
Galantamine	Razadyne, Razadyne ER	4 mg twice daily (tablet, oral solution) 8 mg daily in the morning (extended-release capsule)	8-12 mg twice a day (tablet, oral solution) 16-24 mg daily (extended-release capsule)	Moderate renal or hepatic impairment: maximum daily dose of 16 mg Severe renal or hepatic impairment: not recommended	Available as: tablet, oral solution, extended-release capsule Recommended to take with meals
***N*-methyl-D-aspartate (NMDA) Receptor Antagonist**					
Memantine	Namenda, Namenda XR	5 mg daily (tablet, oral solution) 7 mg daily (extended-release capsule)	10 mg twice daily (tablet, oral solution) 28 mg daily (extended-release capsule)	Severe renal impairment: recommended maintenance dose of 5 mg twice daily (tablet, oral solution) or 14 mg daily (extended-release capsule) Severe hepatic impairment: administer with caution	Available as: tablet, oral solution, extended-release capsule Therapy interruptions require retitration of dose Can be taken with or without food Can open capsule and sprinkle contents on applesauce for ease of administration
Cholinesterase Inhibitor + NMDA Receptor Antagonist					
Memantine + Donepezil	Namzaric	7 mg/10 mg daily (if patient is stabilized on donepezil and not currently on memantine) 28 mg/10 mg daily (if patient is stabilized on memantine and donepezil)	28 mg/10 mg daily	Severe renal impairment: 14 mg/10 mg daily	Available as: memantine extended-release and donepezil capsule Can be taken with or without food Can open capsule and sprinkle contents on applesauce for ease of administration
Anti-amyloid Monoclonal Antibody					
Aducanumab-avwa	Aduhelm	1 mg/kg intravenous solution	Titrated up to 10 mg/kg intravenous once every 4 weeks	No dosage adjustments recommended	Available as 170 mg/1.7 mL and 300 mg/3 mL single-dose vials Must be diluted in 100 mL of 0.9% NaCl and administered over ~ 1 hour

[a]In cases of insomnia or vivid dreams, may dose in the morning. ODT, orally disintegrating tablet. ER and XR, extended release; NaCl, sodium chloride; GI, gastrointestinal.

Data from References 55-63.

Specifically the World Health Organization (WHO) recommends weekly moderate-intensity aerobic exercise (at least 150 minutes) to help preserve functioning and reduce risk.[68]

AD has a profound effect on both the patient and family. Use of nonpharmacologic interventions is the current primary strategy for management of AD, and medications should be used in the context

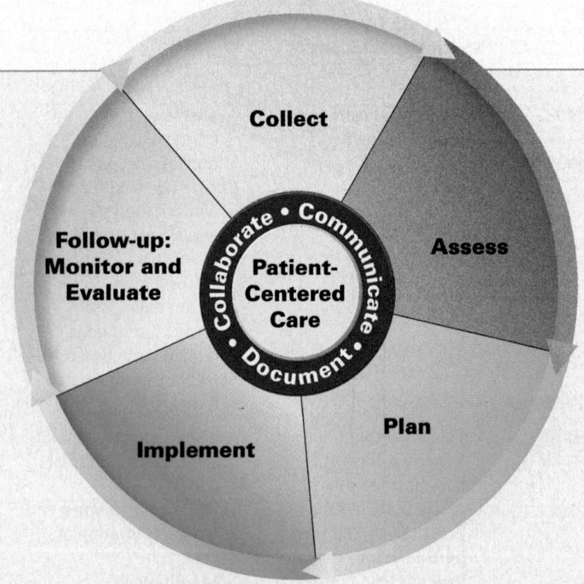

Patient Care Process for Alzheimer Disease

The image shows the five fundamental steps included in The Pharmacist's Care Process endorsed by the Joint Commission for Pharmacy Practitioners (2014). The tagline of this process reads collaborate, communicate, and document. The five fundamental steps listed here are collect, assess, plan, implement, and follow-up: monitor and evaluate. All these steps are listed in a circular block diagram.

Collect

- Patient characteristics (eg, age, sex, race)
- Patient history (eg, past medical, family, and social history)
- Collateral information from family, friends, and caregivers
- Current medications including medications that may cause or worsen cognitive, neuropsychiatric, and/or functional symptoms (see list of common offending agents, in "Assess")
- Assessments for cognitive, neuropsychiatric, and functional symptoms; for example:
  - Mini-Mental State Examination or Montreal Cognitive Assessment (cognition)
  - Neuropsychiatric Inventory (behavioral disturbances)
  - Bristol Activities of Daily Living Scale (function)
- Laboratory data
  - Comprehensive metabolic panel, including electrolytes, glucose, and liver function tests
  - Complete blood cell count
  - Serum B_{12}, homocysteine, and/or methylmalonic acid testing
  - Thyroid function tests
  - Rapid plasma reagin and human immunodeficiency virus testing
  - Urinalysis and/or chest x-ray
- Other Diagnostic Tests
  - CT or MRI scans

Assess

- Risk factors for AD (eg, age, family history, low education level, smoking)
- Cognitive symptoms (eg, memory loss, aphasia, apraxia, agnosia, disorientation, impaired executive function)
- Neuropsychiatric symptoms (eg, depression, psychotic symptoms, behavioral disturbances)
- Functional symptoms (eg, inability to care for self), including patient's ability to manage and self-administer their own medications
- Medications that may cause or worsen cognitive, neuropsychiatric, and/or functional symptoms; for example:
  - Benzodiazepines and other sedative hypnotics
  - Anticholinergics
  - Opioid analgesics
  - Antipsychotics
  - Antiseizure medications
  - Skeletal muscle relaxants
- Labs, diseases, or syndromes that may cause or worsen cognitive, neuropsychiatric, and/or functional symptoms; for example:
  - Alcohol or substance use
  - Depression
  - B_{12} or folate deficiency
  - Hyperhomocysteinemia
  - Hypothyroidism and hyperthyroidism
  - Electrolyte disturbances (eg, hyponatremia)
  - Glucose abnormalities (eg, hypoglycemia)
  - Infectious processes (eg, tertiary syphilis, human immunodeficiency virus, urinary tract infection)
  - Complete blood count to rule out anemia or infection
  - Vision, hearing, or other sensory impairments
  - Other common types of dementia in late life (see Table 73-1)
- Stages of AD (see Table 73-2 and Fig. 73-1)
- Appropriateness of current living situation (eg, independent living, assisted living, nursing home)
- Appropriateness and effectiveness of current medication regimen

Plan*

- Tailored lifestyle modifications (eg, diet, physical activity) for management of brain vascular health
- Medication therapy regimen for cognitive symptoms (if appropriate) including specific medication(s), dose, route, frequency, and intended duration; specify the continuation and discontinuation of existing therapies (see Tables 73-3 and 73-6)
- Monitoring parameters including efficacy, safety (medication-specific potential adverse reactions), and time frame (see Tables 73-7)
- Patient, family, and caregiver education (eg, risks vs benefits of treatment, expected outcomes, medication therapy selection)
- Referrals to other health professionals (eg, social work, psychology, occupational therapy) when appropriate

Implement*

- Provide patient, family, and caregiver education regarding all elements of treatment plan
- Provide caregiver access to local and national resources (see Table 73-5)

(continued)

- Provide family and caregiver education regarding basic principles of care for the patient with AD (see Table 73-4)
- Schedule follow-up

Follow-up: Monitor and Evaluate

- Presence of adverse effects related to medications for cognitive symptoms
- Disease progression, including incidence or worsening of neuropsychiatric symptoms of dementia in accordance with standard assessment tools (see list of commonly used assessments, in "Collect")
- Patient adherence to treatment plan using multiple sources of information
- Patient, family, and caregiver expectations

*Collaborate with patients, caregivers, and other healthcare professionals.

TABLE 73-4 Basic Principles of Care for the Person with Alzheimer Disease

1. Consider vision, hearing, or other sensory impairments
2. Find optimal level of autonomy and adjust expectations for patient performance over time
3. Avoid confrontation. Remain calm, firm, and supportive if the patient becomes upset. Validate their feelings
4. Maintain a consistent, structured environment with stimulation level appropriate for the individual patient
5. Provide frequent reminders, explanations, and orientation cues; employ guiding, demonstration, and reinforcement
6. Reduce choices, keep requests and demands of the patient simple, and avoid complex tasks that lead to frustration
7. Bring sudden declines in function and the emergence of new symptoms to professional attention
8. Redirect to an enjoyable activity

Data from References 2, 49, 72, and 73.

TABLE 73-5 Resources for Caregivers of Persons with Alzheimer Disease

The following organizations provide educational literature and information on diagnosis, treatment, social support, and ongoing research in Alzheimer disease:

- US Administration for Community Living, National Family Caregiver Support Program http://acl.gov/programs/support-caregivers/national-family-caregiver-support-program
- National Institute on Aging (NIA) Alzheimer's Disease Education & Referral Center (ADEAR) http://www.nia.nih.gov/health/about-adear-center
- Alzheimer's Association (AA) http://www.alz.org
- Alzforum http://www.alzforum.org
- Caregiver Action Network http://caregiveraction.org
- Family Caregiver Alliance http://www.caregiver.org

of multimodal interventions. Neuropsychiatric symptoms (also referred to as behavioral and psychological symptoms of dementia [BPSD]) are among the most challenging and distressing symptoms of the disease and may be the determining factor in a family's decision to seek institutional care. Symptoms such as sleep disturbances, wandering, urinary incontinence, agitation, and aggression in patients with dementia are best managed using behavioral interventions rather than medications whenever possible.[53,69]

Upon initial diagnosis, the patient and caregiver should be educated on the course of illness, prognosis, available treatments, legal decisions, and quality of life issues. Caregiving strategies, including stress-management techniques and support group options, should also be discussed. Caregiver education and support programs improve caregiver skill, knowledge, confidence, and quality of life, and even delay time to nursing home placement for their loved one.[70,71] Table 73-4 lists basic principles of care for people with AD.

The general approach to nonpharmacologic strategies for BPSD is to identify the symptom, determine causative factors, and adapt the caregiving environment to remedy the situation.[3] Environmental triggers may include noise, glare, and too much background distraction, including television. Personal discomfort may also trigger behaviors, so it is important to monitor for pain, hunger, thirst, constipation, full bladder, fatigue, infections, skin irritation, personal care, comfortable temperature, fears, and frustrations.[69,71,73] Medical comorbidity is a major source of functional and cognitive impairment in people with AD, so general health maintenance is necessary.[3] Interventions should redirect the patient's attention rather than be confrontational and should specifically address known triggers. Creating a calm environment and removing stressors and triggers is key. Other nonpharmacologic approaches include exercise, light therapy, music therapy, reminiscence therapy, aroma therapy, relaxation techniques, validation therapy, massage and touch therapy, and multisensory stimulation.[71,73] Caregivers should be referred to support services for assistance in developing nonpharmacologic strategies for managing difficult behaviors.

The caregiver must be prepared to face the changes in life that will occur, and acceptance rarely comes easily. Denial on the part of the patient and rationalization on the part of the family are common. The clinician should encourage the family to address legal and financial matters and designate a durable power of attorney for execution of financial and medical decisions once the patient can no longer make those decisions or is deemed incompetent. The caregiver will need to identify resources to provide respite services as they will need time for rest, relaxation, and the conduct of personal business. Eventually, they will need to face critical and difficult questions with respect to institutionalization. Local and national resources, such as the Alzheimer's Association, can provide detailed information regarding support services. Table 73-5 lists this and other referral sources for caregivers. Education, communication, and planning are key nonpharmacologic components of caring for a person with AD. Preparation in the early stages of illness may lessen some caregiver stress as the disease progresses.

Pharmacologic Therapy

Pharmacotherapy for Cognitive Symptoms

8 Table 73-6 presents pharmacologic treatment recommendations for managing cognitive symptoms in AD. Current guidelines recommend initiation of cholinesterase inhibitors for AD with no preference for a specific agent.[53,74] Galantamine and oral rivastigmine are FDA-approved in mild-to-moderate AD. Donepezil and transdermal rivastigmine are FDA-approved in mild, moderate, and severe disease. Despite inconclusive evidence for early intervention, cholinesterase inhibitors are commonly prescribed off-label prior to formal diagnosis of AD. Memantine is indicated for moderate-to-severe AD, as current evidence does not support its use in earlier disease stages.[53,74] Additional benefit may be achieved when memantine

TABLE 73-6 Pharmacologic Treatment Options for Cognitive Symptoms in Alzheimer Disease

- In MCI due to AD, consider therapy with an anti-amyloid mAb (aducanumab), then titrate to recommended maintenance dose as tolerated
- In mild-to-moderate AD, consider therapy with a cholinesterase inhibitor (donepezil, rivastigmine, or galantamine) or aducanumab then titrate to recommended maintenance dose as tolerated
- In moderate-to-severe AD, consider adding antiglutamatergic therapy (memantine), then titrate to recommended maintenance dose as tolerated; alternatively, consider memantine or cholinesterase inhibitor therapy alone
- Behavioral symptoms may require additional pharmacologic approaches

Data from Reference 74.

is added to cholinesterase inhibitor therapy in moderate-to-severe AD; however, the data is conflicting.[53,74] There is no evidence supporting combination therapy of more than one cholinesterase inhibitor. Cholinesterase inhibitors have not demonstrated efficacy for use in MCI.[44,51] At present, anti-amyloid monoclonal antibodies are the only drug class indicated for use in patients with MCI due to AD.[59,60]

8 **Cholinesterase Inhibitors** In the early 1980s, researchers began to examine means to enhance cholinergic activity in people with AD by inhibiting the hydrolysis of acetylcholine through reversible cholinesterase inhibition. Tacrine was the first such medication to be examined in a systematic fashion and is no longer available in the US market, having been replaced by safer, more tolerable cholinesterase inhibitors. The newer cholinesterase inhibitors donepezil, rivastigmine, and galantamine show similar modest symptomatic improvements in cognitive, global, and functional outcomes in people with mild-to-moderate AD, and duration of benefit varies from 3 to 24 months.[75,76] One open-label extension study of galantamine showed benefit beyond the 24-month mark.[77]

The mechanism of action differs slightly between medications in this class.[78] Donepezil specifically and reversibly inhibits acetylcholinesterase. Rivastigmine is a pseudo-irreversible inhibitor of both butyrylcholinesterase (an "overflow" enzyme to acetylcholinesterase) and acetylcholinesterase. Galantamine is a selective, competitive, reversible acetylcholinesterase inhibitor that also enhances the action of acetylcholine on nicotinic receptors. The clinical relevance of these differences is unknown.

Choice of cholinesterase inhibitor therapy for an individual patient is based primarily on ease of use, patient preference, cost, and safety issues, such as potential for interactions. Pharmacokinetic properties should also be considered, as rivastigmine and galantamine have short half-lives (1.5 and 7 hours, respectively) compared to donepezil (70 hours). If rivastigmine or galantamine treatment is interrupted for several days or longer, the patient should be restarted at the lowest dose and titrated up to the current dose. This is true for all formulations of cholinesterase inhibitors, including the rivastigmine transdermal patch.[55-57] Dosing strategies for cholinesterase inhibitors and memantine are summarized in Table 73-3.

Adverse medication reactions and corresponding monitoring parameters are described in Table 73-7. Cholinesterase inhibitors have similar, pro-cholinergic adverse reaction profiles, and are generally well tolerated. The most frequent adverse reactions associated with these agents are mild-to-moderate gastrointestinal (GI) symptoms (eg, nausea, vomiting, and diarrhea) that may impact appetite and weight.[79] Gradual dose titration over several weeks to months can improve tolerability.[34] Alternatives to the immediate-release dosage form are available for patients who have complex dosing regimens, tolerability issues, or difficulty swallowing, though cost may be an issue. Bradycardia has been noted to be a potentially dose-limiting adverse effect for the class and use is contraindicated in patients with a heart rate below 50 beats per minute. When this is a concern, consideration should be given to reducing other heart rate–limiting medications (eg, beta-blockers) where appropriate. In patients who report pro-cholinergic increases in urinary frequency, concurrent use of anticholinergic medications with cholinesterase inhibitors should be avoided and nonpharmacologic interventions employed, if possible.[80] Patients and caregivers should be cautioned against abrupt discontinuation of cholinesterase inhibitor therapy, as this can lead to worsening cognition and behavior in some people with AD.[81] Cholinesterase inhibitors may have some potential to cause seizures; however, they may also be related to AD.[55-57]

The use of high-dose donepezil (23 mg) may be associated with an improvement in cognitive measures; however, some may consider this clinically insignificant.[82] Additionally, this dose is associated with a threefold increased risk of GI effects and a near doubling in the rate of treatment withdrawal, leading to it not being routinely prescribed in clinical practice.

Depending on individual patient response, tolerability, and preference, switching to an alternate dosage form or alternative cholinesterase inhibitor may be necessary during the course of AD treatment. Manufacturer recommendations for this practice are specified in the prescribing information, but the optimal procedure for switching between agents remains uncertain. When switching from one cholinesterase inhibitor to another due to intolerance, a washout period is recommended. Length of the washout period may vary based on pharmacokinetics and time to adverse reaction resolution.[83] Some patients who fail to respond to donepezil, rivastigmine, or galantamine may respond when switched to a different medication with some clinicians preferring an overnight switch to minimize the potential for clinical deterioration.[83] Importantly, loss of benefit over time may not be an appropriate reason to switch cholinesterase inhibitors, as the progressive nature of AD is likely to become more noticeable over time.[83] Indeed, initiation of memantine may be a more appropriate next step as patients progress in their disease course.[49]

In natural disease progression studies, scores on the Alzheimer's Disease Assessment Scale—Cognitive Subscale (ADAS-cog) worsen (increase) by an average of five or fewer points over 1 year in mild dementia and 7 to 11 points annually in moderate dementia. Based on these findings, the consensus is that a four-point change in the ADAS-cog (a scale that ranges from 0-70) represents a clinically significant change.[53] Therefore, if a pharmacotherapeutic agent improves (decreases) the ADAS-cog score by four points, one could think of this as having delayed progression of disease symptoms by 6 months. The usefulness of the ADAS-cog in clinical practice is limited because of the administration time. Therefore, it is much more practical to assess changes in disease severity using the MMSE or other assessment tools. An untreated person with AD has an average decline of two to four points in MMSE score per year. Successful treatment would reflect a decline of less than two points a year. It is reasonable to change to a different cholinesterase inhibitor if the decline in MMSE score is greater than two to four points after 1 year with the initial agent.[83]

8 **Antiglutamatergic Therapy** Memantine is the only NMDA receptor antagonist available for AD. Glutamate is an excitatory neurotransmitter in the brain implicated in long-term potentiation, a neuronal mechanism important for learning and memory.[49] Blocking NMDA receptors can mitigate excitotoxic neurotoxicity and potentially provide neuroprotection (as has been suggested in animal models); however, there is no clinical evidence to indicate that memantine confers neuroprotection in AD.[84]

Memantine is indicated for use in moderate-to-severe AD.[61] Its use has been studied in people with moderate and severe AD as monotherapy and in combination with donepezil with favorable results on cognition and function.[74] To date, studies of memantine

TABLE 73-7 Monitoring Medication Therapy for Cognitive Symptoms

Medication	Adverse Medication Reaction	Monitoring Parameter	Comments
Cholinesterase inhibitors	Dizziness, syncope, bradycardia, atrial arrhythmias, sinoatrial and atrioventricular block, myocardial infarction	Report of dizziness or falls, pulse, blood pressure, and postural blood pressure change	Dizziness is usually mild, transient, and not related to cardiovascular problems Routine pulse checks at baseline, monthly during dose titration, and every 6 months thereafter
	Nausea, vomiting, diarrhea, anorexia, weight loss	Weight and GI complaints	Take with food to decrease GI upset Usually transient, dose-related GI adverse effects seen with medication initiation, dose titration, or medication switch Frail patients or those with low body weight may be more likely to experience GI adverse effects and significant weight loss, particularly when rivastigmine is prescribed or when titrating to donepezil 23 mg GI adverse effects less prominent with transdermal vs oral rivastigmine
	Peptic ulcer disease, GI bleeding	Signs or symptoms of active or occult GI bleeding	Of particular concern for patients at increased risk of developing ulcers, such as those with a history of ulcer disease or concurrently taking NSAIDs
	Insomnia, vivid/abnormal dreams, nightmares	Complaints of sleep disturbances, daytime drowsiness	Donepezil can be taken in the morning to decrease risk of sleep disturbances
Galantamine	Serious skin reactions (Stevens-Johnson syndrome and acute generalized exanthematous pustulosis)	Appearance of skin rash	Discontinue galantamine at first sign of skin rash, unless clearly not medication-related If signs/symptoms are suggestive of a serious reaction, consider alternative treatment and do not rechallenge
Rivastigmine	Allergic dermatitis	Application site reaction spread beyond patch size, evidence of a more intense local reaction (increasing erythema, edema, papules, vesicles), and persistence of symptoms for more than 48 hours after patch removal	Discontinue rivastigmine if evidence of disseminated allergic dermatitis appears Patients sensitized by exposure to the transdermal patch may not be able to take rivastigmine by mouth either; allergy testing and close medical supervision recommended
Memantine	Headache, confusion, dizziness, hallucinations	Report of dizziness or falls, hallucinations	Confusion may be observed during dose titration and is usually transient
	Constipation	GI complaints	Memantine may mitigate GI adverse effects associated with cholinesterase inhibitor therapy
Aducanumab	Amyloid-related imaging abnormalities (ARIA)	MRI at baseline and prior to 7th and 12th infusions or if a patient experiences symptoms suggestive of ARIA to identify brain edema, microhemorrhage, superficial siderosis Symptoms of headache, confusion, dizziness, visual disturbances, and nausea	Vigilance for ARIA and focal neurologic changes are recommended during the first 8 doses, especially during dose titration
	Hypersensitivity reactions	Angioedema and urticaria (rare)	Discontinue infusion at first sign of hypersensitivity reaction

ARIA, amyloid-related imaging abnormalities; GI, gastrointestinal; NSAIDs, nonsteroidal anti-inflammatory drugs.

Data from References 53, 55-57, 61, 62, and 82.

alone and in combination with cholinesterase inhibitors in mild AD have provided insufficient evidence to support an indication for mild AD.[74]

In tablet or oral solution form, memantine should be initiated at 5 mg once a day and titrated weekly in 5 mg intervals to the target maintenance dose of 10 mg twice daily. The extended-release capsule form of memantine is to be initiated at 7 mg daily and titrated weekly up to a maximum of 28 mg daily. Dose titration is achieved in 7 mg intervals with at least 1 week between dose adjustments. Dosing of 5 mg twice daily (tablet and oral solution) or 14 mg daily (extended-release capsule) is recommended in patients with severe renal impairment (creatinine clearance of 5-29 mL/min [0.08-0.49 mL/s]).[61,62]

Memantine has been well tolerated in randomized clinical trials (RCTs). Common adverse events include headache, constipation, confusion, and dizziness. Post-marketing cases of treatment emergent agitation have been reported as well. It has 100% bioavailability regardless of administration with or without food and protein binding is relatively low (45%). Memantine is not metabolized by the liver, does not inhibit cytochrome P450 activity, and is primarily excreted unchanged in the urine with a half-life of 60 to 80 hours.[61,62]

Role of Combination Therapy

Combination therapy with memantine added to a cholinesterase inhibitor is generally prescribed for people with moderate-to-severe AD, as the medication classes have different mechanisms of action. This practice slows cognitive and functional decline to a significant degree compared to cholinesterase inhibitor monotherapy or no treatment.[85] One trial randomized people with moderate-to-severe AD already receiving stable donepezil treatment to either memantine or placebo. At the end of 6 months, participants randomized to receive memantine and donepezil had significantly better outcomes in measures of cognition, function, behavior, and global status than those continued on donepezil monotherapy. This group also had a lower rate of discontinuation due to adverse events.[86] Based on data from this study and others, memantine may have a role in mitigating GI adverse events associated with cholinesterase inhibitors.

In 2014, a combination product containing memantine extended-release and donepezil was approved by the FDA for moderate-to-severe AD in patients already stabilized on memantine and donepezil.[63] As medication effectiveness was based on bioequivalence with the two active ingredients, the package insert separately lists the most common adverse effects of each and not in combination. This product comes in four fixed dose strengths, and dosage reduction is recommended in the case of severe renal impairment. No dosage adjustments are needed in patients with mild or moderate renal or hepatic impairment and it has not been studied in patients with severe hepatic impairment.

Anti-amyloid Monoclonal Antibody

Disease-modifying immunotherapies have long been of interest in pharmacotherapy development; however, both active and passive immunotherapies against amyloid have historically failed to modify disease course. Additionally, they have resulted in serious adverse events, including brain edema and meningitis, thought to be related to transient increases in vascular amyloid secondary to the clearance and removal of vascular amyloid resulting in cerebral edema or microhemorrhage.[18,19,87,88] Hypothetically, agent selectivity and early disease course intervention may optimize success and mitigate such adverse events. The available and investigational agents vary in their mechanism (active vs passive), amyloid target (eg, more pathological oligomeric vs potentially protective monomeric amyloid, soluble vs insoluble amyloid, amyloid amino acid residue) and binding conformations.[87-91] Although active immunotherapies remain in development, passive immunotherapies have been a large part of the pipeline owing to their ability to provide a more predictable and controlled response.

Four humanized, immunoglobulin G1 monoclonal antibodies have been designated as AD breakthrough therapies by the FDA (ie, aducanumab, lecanemab, donanemab, and gantenerumab), where preliminary evidence indicates substantial improvement over existing therapies on significant endpoints.[92-95] One of these agents, aducanumab, was controversially approved under this accelerated pathway for use in MCI due to AD and mild AD. Three clinical trials evaluated the safety and efficacy of aducanumab in this population. While all three trials had reductions in biomarker-indicated pathology such as presence of amyloid or tau in a dose and time-dependent manner, two trials were ended early for presumed clinical futility. A later re-analysis of the data found a significant reduction in cognitive, functional, and behavioral decline in only one trial. Under the accelerated pathway, continued approval of aducanumab is likely to be contingent upon verification of clinical benefit in confirmatory trials underway.[92,93] Phase III trials of donanemab, lecanemab, and gantenerumab are ongoing.[96]

Aducanumab binds to aggregated forms of amyloid in the brain, including oligomer and fibril formations and is reported to preferentially bind perivascular amyloid, which has been hypothesized to reduce the likelihood of cerebral edema or microhemorrhage. It is administered as an infusion delivered every 4 weeks which is titrated to a maintenance dose of 10 mg/kg to reduce the likelihood of CNS adverse effects. It is broken down via endogenous pathways to yield a half-life of approximately 25 days, reaching steady-state before the fifth dose.[59,60]

In addition to infusion-related reactions such as urticaria and angioedema, aducanumab may cause cerebral edema and microhemorrhage. Such CNS-related adverse effects may result in further cognitive decline, focal neurologic changes, and a theoretical increase in risk of intracranial hemorrhage.[59,60] Carriers of *APOE*4* may be at greater risk for these CNS effects owing to a greater burden of vascular amyloid.[97] Screening for baseline cerebrovascular risk and frequent imaging can mitigate these CNS-related effects. Patients at risk for CNS adverse events include those taking anticoagulants and those with underlying cerebrovascular disease. Baseline and monitoring MRI should be conducted to identify patients at risk for these adverse effects, and the development of amyloid-related imaging abnormalities (ARIA) that evidence cerebral edema (ARIA-e) and microhemorrhage (ARIA-h) (see Table 73-7) with treatment. If severe ARIA-h is identified, patients may continue treatment if clinical evaluation and MRI imaging demonstrate stabilization; otherwise therapy should be discontinued. Patients should also be monitored for the development of focal neurologic symptoms. Patients with uncontrolled seizure disorder should be excluded from treatment due to the risk of focal neurologic adverse events.[59,60]

The potential degree and duration of clinical benefit of anti-amyloid antibodies remains largely unclear. The unknown durability of effect and adverse effect profile, combined with the possible decline in self-management capacity to meet the administration and monitoring requirements, render their place in therapy questionable. It is largely unknown what impact therapeutic discontinuation will have on overall progression. In addition, there are access gaps related to reimbursement for medication and ancillary services, as well as the health system resources needed to safely administer and monitor medication use.[98,99] As a result, the Institute for Clinical and Economic review has rated the comparable cost effectiveness of this medication as "insufficient" to demonstrate a net health benefit for patients with MCI due to AD or mild AD.[98]

Effect of Current Treatments on Neurodegenerative Processes

AD is a progressive disorder and affected individuals typically experience some degree of cognitive decline and histologic change for years (if not decades) before a diagnosis is made. Therefore, the ideal treatment will be one that not only reverses symptoms by enhancing cognitive function (a symptomatic treatment) but also arrests the neurodegeneration-relevant molecular processes that underlie cognitive decline (a disease-modifying treatment).

Clinical trials for AD prompt consideration of whether positive outcomes suggest either a symptomatic or disease-modifying effect. Any rapid performance improvement in cognitive ability, activities of daily living, or behavioral end points is indicative of a symptomatic effect. All cholinesterase inhibitor agents and memantine demonstrate this pattern, and aducanumab suggests a similar effect. Arrest of decline or a sustained reduction in the slope of decline would argue the presence of a disease-modifying effect; however, it has not been possible to unequivocally demonstrate this in trials of the approved treatments. Long-duration, double-blind, placebo-controlled trials to evaluate whether available agents have disease-modifying effects are difficult to perform, because doing so would require continuing a placebo arm over an extended period, well beyond demonstration of symptomatic benefit. Also, subject attrition over an extended study would complicate both intent-to-treat and observed case analyses.

With cholinesterase inhibitors and memantine, pivotal placebo-controlled trials were followed by open-label extension studies, lasting as long as 5 years. As part of these studies, decline in the treatment group was compared with "projected" placebo groups based on continued follow-up of the placebo groups included in the 6-month randomized phase of the efficacy study, as well as natural history cohorts from the pre-cholinesterase inhibitor therapy era. Although analyses of this sort conclude that, for up to at least 5 years, people receiving treatment exceed their projected nontreatment cognitive performance, no convincing evidence of a disease-modifying effect emerges.[100-103]

Barriers to Clinical Effectiveness Research

Disagreement exists about how best to determine effectiveness of AD treatments. Selection of qualitative vs quantitative assessment may bias a clinician's impression of response as subtle changes are often detected only by psychometric testing. As no standard has been suggested to define the effectiveness of AD medications, great variation exists between clinicians, and the duration of treatment. Realistic expectations for success may include slowed decline in behavioral, functional, and cognitive abilities and delayed long-term care placement.[104] An initial dramatic improvement in symptoms is unlikely but may be reported by a minority of patients or their caregivers.

Unfortunately, clinical trials have failed to provide answers to key questions in treating people with AD and challenges associated with population heterogeneity and difficulties inherent to the diagnosis, make interpretation of therapeutic response difficult.[105] For example, individuals given a diagnosis for AD often lack the hallmark pathologies (ie, amyloid plaques and NFTs) on postmortem examination. Similarly, clinical trials of potentially disease modifying agents have failed to produce reliable results, indicating that disease stage and preclinical diagnosis may be of increasing importance. Additionally, because of overlap between AD and other dementing illness, trials including those diagnosed with AD may in fact include patients with a heterogenous, mixed profile of dementia. Further, as individuals who fail to display the clinical symptoms of the disease may still be developing the underlying pathologies, there may be contamination of control groups. Each of these factors may present a challenge to the internal validity of clinical trials.

Guidance in extrapolating data related to changes in cognition is needed so a reasonable duration of clinical treatment with pharmacotherapy can be determined. One concern is that those who respond to treatment may lose the benefits of that treatment once the medication is stopped.[106] Gaps in treatment have been linked with worse cognitive outcomes in clinical trial extension studies; however, there is no increased risk of institutionalization or death associated with gaps in cholinesterase inhibitor therapy.[107,108] Regardless, dosing regimens should be simplified and patient and caregiver preferences considered in an effort to improve medication adherence and persistence.

9 Management of Brain Vascular Health

Guidelines for the care of people with AD support the management of vascular brain disease and its associated risk factors as part of treatment.[49] There is a link between AD and cardiovascular disease, including heart failure, atrial fibrillation, and coronary artery disease, and a growing body of evidence that brain vascular disease plays a role in the progression of dementia.[21] Management of brain vascular disease includes monitoring blood pressure, glucose, and cholesterol, and initiation of appropriate interventions.[109-111]

The WHO and Alzheimer's Disease International encourage primary prevention through public health campaigns targeting smoking, underactivity, midlife obesity, midlife hypertension, and diabetes.[112] Adherence to the Mediterranean Diet, Dietary Approaches to Stop Hypertension (DASH) diet, or combination Mediterranean-DASH Intervention for Neurodegenerative Delay (MIND) diet may reduce the risk of cognitive impairment or decline.[24,113] Physical activity is an important component of vascular brain health and is associated with a reduced risk of cognitive impairment.[24,68,114] However, most positive trial findings have been from cognitively healthy older adults.[24,113] While appropriate management of vascular disease risk factors may reduce the risk for developing AD, insufficient evidence exists to draw definitive conclusions on the association between risk factor modification and risk of AD.[24,109]

Other Potential Treatment Approaches

Estrogen Estrogen replacement has been studied extensively for the treatment and prevention for AD with most, but not all, retrospective epidemiologic studies showing a lower incidence of AD with estrogen replacement therapy after menopause. Prospective clinical trials have not supported the use of estrogen as a treatment for cognitive decline, and longer trials tend to suggest harm. The evidence does not support the use of estrogen to treat or prevent dementia.[27] Although phytoestrogens found in soy-containing foods and soy-derived dietary supplements have been suggested for the treatment or prevention of dementia, there are no clinical trials supporting such use.[27]

Anti-inflammatory Agents Retrospective epidemiologic studies suggest a protective effect against AD in patients who have taken nonsteroidal anti-inflammatory drugs (NSAIDs); however, the benefits of anti-inflammatory agents have been less compelling in prospective clinical studies. In fact, there is no significant cognitive benefit in persons with AD treated with NSAIDs, aspirin, or steroids.[115] Due to lack of compelling data and a significant incidence of adverse effects, particularly gastritis and the possibility of GI bleeds, these agents are not recommended for general use in the treatment or prevention of AD.[115]

Lipid-Lowering Agents Four RCTs of statin therapy, given to older individuals at risk for vascular disease, indicated no significant benefit of statin therapy for probable or possible AD.[116] Cognitive impairment has been recognized as a rare adverse event associated with statin therapy.[117] More research is needed to understand the complex relationship between cholesterol, statin therapy, and cognitive functioning but for now, these agents should be reserved for patients who have other indications for their use.

Dietary Supplements Many nutraceuticals, herbal products, medical foods, and other dietary supplements have been promoted for the prevention and treatment of AD, and available evidence has been reviewed.[118-120] While a detailed discussion of their use is beyond the scope of this chapter, the more commonly used supplements are as follows.

Vitamin E Supplementation Based on pathophysiologic theories involving oxidative stress and the accumulation of free radicals in AD, significant interest has evolved regarding the use of antioxidants in the treatment of AD. Two RCTs have evaluated the effects of vitamin E supplementation (1,000 IU twice daily) in people with AD. The first studied people with moderate AD for 2 years and had a significant delay in the time to institutionalization in the treatment group compared to placebo.[121] The second studied the efficacy of α-tocopherol, memantine, or their combination in people with mild-to-moderate AD taking an acetylcholinesterase inhibitor (mean follow-up time of 2.3 years) and showed a reduced annual rate of decline in activities of daily living in those treated with vitamin E, but no cognitive benefits were seen.[122] No significant adverse effects were reported between treatment groups in either study; however, according to a meta-analysis high-dose vitamin E increases mortality.[123] In addition, vitamin E had no benefit in people with MCI in the progression to AD,[124] or in preventing dementia in asymptomatic older males.[125] Considering these findings, there is insufficient evidence to recommend vitamin E supplementation for the treatment or prevention of AD.[126]

Vitamin B Supplementation Elevated serum homocysteine is associated with cognitive decline and supplementation with B vitamins (folic acid along with B_{12} and/or B_6) has been explored to reduce homocysteine levels in older adults with dementia. Clinical trials consistently demonstrate reduced homocysteine levels in the intervention groups receiving vitamin B supplementation, but without significant difference in MMSE scores between control and intervention groups. In other words, reduced homocysteine levels have not translated into improved cognitive outcomes for people with AD thus far.[127]

Ginkgo biloba *Ginkgo biloba* for the prevention and treatment of AD has been extensively studied given its potential to increase blood flow, decrease blood viscosity, antagonize platelet-activating factor receptors, increase anoxia tolerance, inhibit monoamine oxidase, and serve as an antioxidant. Active ingredients in *Ginkgo biloba* include flavonoids, *Ginkgo* flavone glycosides, and bioflavonoids. Most studies reporting benefit in people with cognitive impairment or dementia have studied a standardized extract, EGb 761, in doses of 240 mg/day for 22 to 26 weeks.[128] The clinical significance of the modest benefits detected is unclear, and direct comparisons to cholinesterase inhibitors or memantine are lacking. A large trial of *Ginkgo biloba* 120 mg twice a day did not reduce the overall incidence rate of either dementia or AD in older adults with normal cognition or MCI.[129] In another large trial the long-term use of *Ginkgo biloba* extract did not reduce the risk of progression to AD among older adults suffering from memory complaints compared with placebo.[130] Adverse medication effects reported from EGb 761 studies were typically mild, including nausea, vomiting, diarrhea, headaches, dizziness, palpitations, restlessness, and weakness. Because EGb also has a potent antiplatelet effect, it should be avoided by individuals taking anticoagulant or antiplatelet therapies and should be used cautiously in patients taking NSAIDs.[128,131]

Apoaequorin Prevagen® (apoaequorin) has been postulated to impact cognition by modulating calcium homeostasis and secondary messaging; however, the manufacturer data has not been peer reviewed and only focuses on single domains of cognition. Additionally, a simulation of the gastric environment found that 90% of this compound is broken down within 30 seconds. As the compound is large in size, it is not clear whether there is a mechanism for absorption or ability to cross the blood brain barrier.[132]

Medical Foods Several medical foods have been studied for the treatment of MCI or AD, but there is little evidence of benefit to date. Medical foods constitute a unique category that consists of ingestible entities intended for the treatment of diseases that have "specific nutritional requirements" and for which the medical food may manipulate disease-relevant pathophysiology. Medical foods are intended to be used under the supervision of a physician. The most commonly used for people with mild-to-moderate AD are Axona, Souvenaid®, and CerefolinNAC®.[133]

Axona (caprylidene) is a mixture of medium-chain fatty acids, consisting primarily of the C8 fatty acid caprylic acid.[134] Caprylidene is converted by the liver to a ketone body, β-hydroxybutyrate, which crosses the blood–brain barrier and can be used as an alternative fuel to glucose in the brain. Support for caprylidene efficacy in AD comes from a single clinical trial in which subjects randomized to 40 mg/day of caprylidene for 45 days performed relatively better on the ADAS-cog than did subjects randomized to a placebo; however, this benefit was entirely driven by subjects without the *APOE*4* allele.[135] In general, adverse effects were mild, with GI-related effects being the most common. Coconut oil is a source of caprylic acid but may not contain sufficient quantities to meet the needs of a person with AD; however, it continues to be used by some patients as a less expensive alternative to caprylidene.[134]

Souvenaid is a mixture of omega-3 fatty acids (eicosapentaenoic and docosahexaenoic acids), uridine monophosphate, phospholipids, B complex vitamins (B_6, B_{12}, and folate), choline, vitamin E, and selenium.[136] A systematic review and meta-analysis of three RCTs comparing Souvenaid to placebo found no significant differences in cognition, function, or behavior, although one study showed improvement in verbal recall in people with mild AD in the Souvenaid treatment group.[136] No serious adverse events were reported in the clinical studies.

CerefolinNAC® contains vitamin B_{12}, L-methylfolate, and N-acetylcysteine, and its use targets the association of hyperhomocysteinemia with MCI and progression to dementia. A small prospective case-control study of people with AD and hyperhomocysteinemia suggested longer CerefolinNAC® treatment duration, milder baseline severity, and greater magnitude of homocysteine reduction from baseline were all significant predictors of slowed cognitive decline, when compared to AD subjects with normal homocysteine levels not receiving CerefolinNAC®.[137] Randomized controlled trials are needed to confirm these findings; however, to date, there is insufficient evidence to recommend medical foods for the treatment of AD.

Omega-3 Fatty Acids Arguments that omega-3 fatty acids found in fish oil, such as docosahexaenoic acid and eicosapentaenoic acid, could benefit individuals with AD have existed for some years. A recent Cochrane review found no evidence of significant adverse effects, but also no benefit on cognition, function, dementia severity, or quality of life in people with AD.[138] There is insufficient evidence now to recommend omega-3 fatty acids for the treatment of AD.

Medications and Treatment Strategies in Development

New medication development is focused on disease-modifying and prevention strategies and has fallen broadly into several categories: treatments designed to reduce levels of brain Aβ or manipulate its configuration, treatments targeting tau protein, anti-inflammatory approaches (eg, cytokines, microglial cells), and therapies targeting glutaminergic and cholinergic response (eg, sigma receptors, AMPA-kines). Interest in targeting early, prodromal AD has also risen. The NIA-AA Research Framework provides guidance for biomarker testing to capture such early disease which relies on assessment of three criteria: (1) presence of neurodegeneration, (2) presence of amyloid, or (3) presence of tau in the brain using specific imaging of CSF sampling techniques.[44,139,140]

Although many potential new medications have advanced to early clinical studies, no new agents had entered the market since 2004, until the approval of aducanumab. While progress has been made in developing novel biomarkers and improving RCT designs, results remain disappointing.[25,59,60,94,95] One reason for the failure of so many AD therapies may be that current strategies do not target the pathways that ultimately result in AD. Another reason may be that medications are being initiated when the disease has already progressed too far to be reversed.[25] Focus on the amyloid hypothesis of AD, and to a lesser extent on tau, may have led to discounting other treatment approaches. AD is likely a multifactorial condition, which suggests that a single approach will not prevent or treat AD in all patients. Some of the potential targets of interest going forward include dysfunction of neuronal networks, inflammation, infectious agents such as herpes virus or prions, accumulation of neurotoxic proteins related to sleep deprivation and blood–brain barrier dysfunction, mitochondrial dysfunction, environmental factors, and conditions affecting brain vascular health including diabetes, obesity, hypertension, and hypercholesterolemia.[25] There is also a great deal of attention to identify AD biomarkers and recommendations are likely to evolve over time as we better understand the underlying disease pathophysiology and predictors of patient response. Regardless, now there are no specific recommendations regarding the choice of medication, dosing regimen, or treatment duration for cognitive agents (ie, cholinesterase inhibitors and memantine) based on genotype or other biomarkers.

Given the exponentially increasing number of individuals and families facing the diagnosis of AD, government leaders of G7 countries have strategized to drive innovation and improve the quality of life for people affected by AD, by establishing a goal to find a cure or disease-modifying therapy by 2025.[141] This effort resulted in more research directed toward achieving this goal. Furthermore, the National Institutes of Health, FDA, pharmaceutical companies, and nonprofit organizations joined together to form the "Accelerating

Medicines Partnership" to create networks, share data, and manage RCTs.[142]

Pharmacotherapy of Neuropsychiatric Symptoms

Most patients with AD manifest neuropsychiatric symptoms (also referred to as BPSD) at some point in the illness.[143-145] These symptoms can be roughly divided into four categories: (1) psychotic; (2) hyperactive (eg, inappropriate or disruptive behavior); (3) affective (eg, depression); and (4) apathy.[143,144] Effective management of BPSD is important because symptoms are distressing to both the patient and caregiver, necessitate increased caregiver supervision and patience. Escalating and cahlenging BPSD is a leading reason for nursing home placement.

10 Strategies for treatment of BPSD should include nonpharmacologic interventions first, followed by pharmacologic interventions when necessary. Behaviors, such as agitation, aggression, delusions, hallucinations, repetitive vocalizations, and wandering, may be caused by medications, medical illness (eg, pain, constipation, dehydration, infection), environmental precipitants, physical/verbal abuse, or unmet physical and psychological needs. Correcting possible underlying causes before initiating medication therapy is critical.[145,146] The need for medications may arise when neuropsychiatric symptoms are of sufficient severity to cause significant distress to the patient or caregiver, interfere with function or cause disability, impede delivery of necessary care, or pose a danger to self or others and have not responded to nonpharmacologic interventions.[53,112,145-147] The balance between potential risks and expected benefits of the intended medication must be acceptable to the patient or surrogate decision maker. Medications should be used cautiously, with adequate monitoring for effectiveness and adverse events.

Despite the high prevalence of neuropsychiatric symptoms in AD, relatively little research has been conducted, and no medication is approved by the FDA for the treatment of BPSD; however, clinical trials are ongoing.[140] Considering limited clinical data, treatment is primarily empiric, with adverse effect profiles used as a guide in selecting the appropriate treatment. For instance, psychotropic medications with anticholinergic effects should be avoided because they may worsen cognition and interfere with cholinesterase inhibitor therapy.

General guidelines governing pharmacologic therapy for BPSD can be summarized as follows: reserve for situations where nonpharmacologic therapies failed, use reduced doses, monitor closely, titrate dosage slowly, minimize duration of therapy, attempt tapers, and document carefully. Treatment should be considered temporary.[146] Caregivers may have unrealistic expectations regarding the effects of these medications, and the anticipated benefits and risks should be clearly explained. Disruptive behaviors and delusions wax and wane with disease progression, and some behaviors (eg, wandering, hoarding, screaming, repetitive behaviors) lack evidence of a medication response.[148] Attempts to slowly taper and discontinue medication should be undertaken regularly in minimally symptomatic patients, as behaviors often fluctuate, changing in character and intensity over time, and the medication may no longer be providing a benefit.[145,146]

Cholinesterase Inhibitors and Memantine Cholinesterase inhibitors and memantine may be beneficial in both managing BPSD and reducing their incidence.[144] While cholinesterase inhibitors may improve apathy, depression, tension, and irritability in mild-to-moderate dementia, they do not appear to significantly reduce acute agitation.[144] Memantine may show modest benefit for mitigating agitation, aggression, delusions, and hallucinations; however, recent trials of memantine specifically evaluating its effect on treating agitation in people with AD found no benefit.[144] These benefits should be considered along with cognitive benefits in treatment decisions and weighed against their adverse effects. Long-term effects on behavior have not been demonstrated and further research is needed.

Antidepressants Antidepressants may be prescribed for BPSD to help manage depression, anxiety, apathy, as well as agitation and aggression. Depressive symptoms and anxiety are common in people with AD. Apathy is seen in 48% to 92% of individuals with dementia, and clinically significant depression occurs in approximately 32% with mild dementia, 23% with moderate disease, and 18% in the severe stage of the dementia.[149] Results of trials studying the efficacy of antidepressants in treating depression in people with AD are conflicting,[145] and improvement among participants receiving placebo is also common. In practice, treatment with selective serotonin reuptake inhibitors (SSRIs) is initiated most commonly in people with AD, based on adverse effect profile, risk of interactions, and evidence of efficacy.[145] Among the SSRIs, the best evidence exists for sertraline and citalopram.[72,145] Serotonergic function may also play a role in some of the other BPSD of AD, such as agitation, and some studies support the use of SSRIs in managing these behaviors, even in the absence of depression.[145] Clinical trials are needed to compare the efficacy of SSRIs to second-generation antipsychotics (SGAs). Tricyclic antidepressants should generally be avoided because of their anticholinergic activity.[144] Chapter 88 has a more complete discussion of treatment of depression.

Antipsychotics Antipsychotics are used in the management of neuropsychiatric symptoms in AD despite efforts by the Centers for Medicare and Medicaid Services and other groups to reduce their use in nursing homes.[150] No antipsychotic has gained FDA approval for management of BPSD in AD. There is modestly convincing evidence that certain SGAs provide some benefit for particular neuropsychiatric symptoms with the most studied being aripiprazole, risperidone, olanzapine, and quetiapine. More than 20 RCTs have evaluated SGAs for BPSD, with more than 5,000 patients participating and treatment durations of 6 to 26 weeks for most trials.[151] A meta-analysis of 16 trials demonstrated the efficacy of aripiprazole, risperidone, olanzapine, and quetiapine over placebo; however, they were associated with a higher risk of adverse medication reactions. The investigators concluded the increased risk of adverse reactions and mortality may offset the benefit. An outpatient RCT of 421 people with AD and psychosis, aggression, or agitation randomized to receive olanzapine, quetiapine, risperidone, or placebo for up to 36 weeks found no significant differences among treatments in time to treatment discontinuation or improvement based on the Clinical Global Impression–Change (CGI-C) response. The investigators concluded that adverse medication reactions may offset the therapeutic advantages of SGAs for treatment of psychosis, aggression, or agitation in people with AD.[152]

Adverse medication reactions are common with first-generation antipsychotics (FGAs) and SGAs in people with AD and include somnolence, extrapyramidal symptoms, abnormal gait, cerebrovascular events, and increased risk of death.[154,151] Compared to SGAs, FGAs are associated with more severe extrapyramidal effects and hypotension. In 2005, the FDA mandated the addition of a boxed warning to all SGAs due to increased risk of mortality in older adults with dementia-related psychosis; this warning was expanded in 2008 to include all FGAs as well.[153] Mortality was mostly cardiovascular (eg, sudden death, heart failure) or infectious (eg, pneumonia) in nature. In 2011, the Office of Inspector General released a report which described that the majority (83%) of SGA prescription claims were for nursing home residents without FDA-approved indications.[154] In 2012, the Centers for Medicare and Medicaid Services launched the National Partnership to Improve Dementia Care in Nursing Homes to improve quality of care for nursing home residents with dementia. Although the percentage of residents receiving antipsychotic therapy has since decreased, from 23.9% in 2011 to 14.5% in 2020, about one in six people living in nursing homes are receiving antipsychotic medications.[150,155]

There is a modest expectation of treatment benefit and a potential for significant harm associated with antipsychotic use in people with AD. Individual risk and benefit must be considered and discussed with family and caregivers when initiating therapy. Prescribing of antipsychotics in AD should be restricted to patients with severe symptoms not responding to other measures, and treatment should be tapered as early as possible.[146,147] Doses should be initiated at one-third to one-half of the usual adult starting dose (or with smallest available tablet strength), and target doses are much lower than those for other indications.[146] The American Psychiatric Association (APA) guidelines recommend tapering and discontinuing the antipsychotic after 4 weeks at an adequate dose if no clinical benefit is seen. If benefit is seen, an attempt to taper should be made 4 months after initiation, to reduce risk of harm as original need for the medication may change.[146] A meta-analysis of RCTs of antipsychotic discontinuation showed no significant increase in BPSD severity upon discontinuation compared to the continuation group.[156] For patients continued on antipsychotics, monitor for tardive dyskinesia and metabolic effects. Chapter 87, "Schizophrenia" includes a more detailed discussion of antipsychotic monitoring.

Miscellaneous Therapies Because antipsychotic and antidepressant therapies have only modest efficacy and pose the potential for undesirable adverse effects, medications traditionally used to treat disruptive behaviors and aggression in other psychiatric and neurologic disorders have been suggested as potential alternatives. These alternatives include benzodiazepines and antiseizure medications.[145]

Benzodiazepines have been used to treat anxiety, agitation, and aggression, but the benefit is unclear especially given the risk of sedation, falls, impaired cognition, respiratory depression, and paradoxical disinhibition.[144] Evidence for their use in BPSD is lacking. Antiseizure medications used as "mood stabilizers" such as carbamazepine, lamotrigine, gabapentin, and pregabalin may have some benefit but evidence is limited or conflicting.[157] Adverse effects and interactions of carbamazepine often outweigh benefits. Valproic acid is no longer recommended as a result of an association of mood stabilizers with severe adverse reactions in patients with BPSD.[143,144] In general sedative hypnotics including benzodiazepines and benzodiazepine receptor agonists (eg, zolpidem) should be avoided as the risk of harm (eg, sedation, falls) outweighs the benefit.[52] Melatonin and ramelteon have been used for circadian rhythm disturbances. More recently, suvorexant, an orexin antagonist, was studied for insomnia in patients with mild-to-moderate AD showing improvement in total sleep time and wake after sleep onset. Somnolence and falls occurred in the suvorexant treated groups.[158]

Neuropsychiatric symptoms are often the most difficult aspect of AD for the caregiver. When nonpharmacologic approaches fail, selected antipsychotics and antidepressants may be useful for effective management of behavioral, psychotic, and depressive symptoms, thereby easing caregiver burden and allowing the patient to spend additional time at home. All too often, however, nonpharmacologic measures are not implemented appropriately, and medication overuse is an ongoing problem. Adverse events remain an important concern in this population as well.

EVALUATION OF THERAPEUTIC OUTCOMES

An evaluation of therapeutic outcomes in the person with AD begins with a thorough assessment at baseline and a clear definition of therapeutic goals. Cognitive status, functional performance, mood, and behavior all need to be evaluated before initiation of medication therapy. The clinician should interview both the patient and the caregiver to assess response to medication therapy. In evaluating response to cognitive agents, the clinician should ask questions about the patient's ability to perform daily functional tasks, mood and behavior, and memory and orientation. Objective assessments (eg, MMSE for cognition, Bristol Activities of Daily Living Scale for function, Neuropsychiatric Inventory for behavioral disturbances) can be used to quantify changes over time.[159]

Because target neuropsychiatric symptoms of dementia may manifest differently, a detailed list of target symptoms should be documented in the pharmacotherapy plan to aid in monitoring. These could include, for example, "striking at spouse because patient believes they are an impostor" or "verbal threats and refusal to allow clothes to be changed," as opposed to documenting vague symptoms, such as "aggression" or "delusions." To make an accurate assessment of depression, multiple symptoms (eg, sleep, appetite, activity, interest levels) need to be considered in addition to the patient's stated mood. As noted above, the failure of pharmacologic modalities to impact these target symptoms should result in discontinuation. If responses are seen, tapering and subsequent monitoring for recurrence should be undertaken.

The patient should be observed carefully for potential adverse effects of medication therapy, including the specific adverse effect and how it is being assessed. Consensus on the frequency of monitoring is lacking, but patients should generally be monitored for adverse events within 2 to 4 weeks of initiation of therapy, for therapeutic effect in 8 to 12 weeks, and at least every 3 to 6 months thereafter.[160] The effects of cognitive agents will not necessarily be obvious, and a treatment period of several months to a year may be necessary before it can be determined whether therapy is beneficial. Cognitive effects of the medication are often noticed only as a plateauing during treatment or as deterioration following medication discontinuation. In general, cognitive agents should be continued if the patient is demonstrating no change in clinical status. If there is doubt, the medication can be slowly tapered and discontinued, and the patient monitored off the medication for 4 to 6 weeks to determine the need for continued therapy. Medication deprescribing for people with AD is aided by the availability of deprescribing guidelines and algorithms for antipsychotics, cholinesterase inhibitors, and memantine.[161] The question of when, if ever, to stop medication therapy for AD remains controversial. Treatment benefits are not always evident, and fear of deterioration can lead to patients being prescribed medication therapy for AD from the time of their diagnosis until death. Some clinicians recommend withdrawing medication therapy if the patient significantly deteriorates in cognition or function, while others wait until the patient has lost all cognitive and functional abilities. Tolerability, cost, and patient and family preferences factor heavily into medication therapy discontinuation decisions. If cholinesterase inhibitors are discontinued and cognition worsens or behavioral issues emerge, the medications can be reinitiated.

CONCLUSION

Ultimately, AD, as with other dementias, is a complex condition to evaluate and manage. Clinicians are encouraged to work interprofessionally and collaborate closely with patients and their families to minimize stigma, identify therapeutic goals, and address concerns as they arise.

ABBREVIATIONS

AA	Alzheimer's Association
Aβ	β-Amyloid peptide
AD	Alzheimer disease
ADAS-cog	Alzheimer's Disease Assessment Scale—Cognitive Subscale
ADRDA	Alzheimer's Disease and Related Disorders Association
AHRQ	Agency for Healthcare Research and Quality
APOE	apolipoprotein E
APP	amyloid precursor protein

ARIA	amyloid-related imaging abnormalities
BPSD	behavioral and psychological symptoms of dementia
CGI-C	Clinical Global Impression–Change
CSF	cerebrospinal fluid
CT	computed tomography
DASH	Dietary Approaches to Stop Hypertension
DSM-5	*Diagnostic and Statistical Manual of Mental Disorders, Fifth Edition*
EOAD	early onset Alzheimer disease
FDA	Food and Drug Administration
FGA	first-generation antipsychotics
GI	gastrointestinal
LOAD	late onset Alzheimer disease
MCI	mild cognitive impairment
MIND	Mediterranean-DASH Intervention for Neurodegenerative Delay
MMSE	Mini-Mental State Examination
MRI	magnetic resonance imaging
NFT	neurofibrillary tangle
NIA	National Institute on Aging
NINCDS	National Institute of Neurological and Communicative Disorders and Stroke
NMDA	*N*-methyl-D-aspartate
NSAID	nonsteroidal anti-inflammatory drug
PET	positron emission tomography
PSEN	presenilin genes
RCT	randomized clinical trial
SGA	second-generation antipsychotic
SSRI	selective serotonin reuptake inhibitor

REFERENCES

1. Kumar A, Singh A, Ekavali. A review on Alzheimer's disease pathophysiology and its management: An update. *Pharmacol Rep.* 2015;67(2):195–203.
2. U.S. Department of Health and Human Services. National Plan to Address Alzheimer's Disease. Available at https://aspe.hhs.gov/collaborations-committees-advisory-groups/napa/napa-documents/napa-national-plans. Last accessed August 25, 2022.
   Alzheimer's Association. 2021 Alzheimer's disease facts and figures. *Alzheimers Dement.* 2021;17(3):327–406.
4. Jiang T, Yu JT, Tian Y, Tan L. Epidemiology and etiology of Alzheimer's disease: From genetic to non-genetic factors. *Curr Alzheimer Res.* 2013;10(8):852–867.
5. Robinson L, Tang E, Taylor J-P. Dementia: Timely diagnosis and early intervention. *BMJ.* 2015;350:h3029.
6. Bertram L, Tanzi RE. The genetics of Alzheimer's disease. *Prog Mol Biol Transl Sci.* 2012;107:79–100.
7. Macleod R, Hillert E-K, Cameron RT, Baillie GS. The role and therapeutic targeting of α-, β- and γ-secretase in Alzheimer's disease. *Future Sci OA.* 2015;1(3):FS011.
8. Vilatela MEA, López-López M, Yescas-Gómez P. Genetics of Alzheimer's disease. *Arch Med Res.* 2012;43(8):622–631.
9. Kelleher RJ III, Shen J. Presenilin-1 mutations and Alzheimer's disease. *Proc Natl Acad Sci U S A.* 2017;114(4):629–631.
10. Hampel H, Mesulam M-M, Cuello AC, et al. The cholinergic system in the pathophysiology and treatment of Alzheimer's disease. *Brain.* 2018;141(7):1917–1933.
11. Michaelson DM. APOE ε4: The most prevalent yet understudied risk factor for Alzheimer's disease. *Alzheimers Dement.* 2014;10(6):861–868.
12. Hohman TJ, Cooke-Bailey JN, Reitz C, et al. Global and local ancestry in African-Americans: Implications for Alzheimer's disease risk. *Alzheimers Dement.* 2016;12(3):233–243. doi: 10.1016/j.jalz.2015.02.012.
13. De Roeck A, Van Broeckhoven C, Sleegers K. The role of ABCA7 in Alzheimer's disease: Evidence from genomics, transcriptomics and methylomics. *Acta Neuropathol.* 2019;138(2):201–220. doi: 10.1007/s00401-019-01994-1.
14. Reitz C, Jun G, Naj A, et al. Variants in the ATP-binding cassette transporter (ABCA7), apolipoprotein E ε4, and the risk of late-onset Alzheimer disease in African Americans. *JAMA.* 2013;309(14):1483–1492. doi: 10.1001/jama.2013.2973.
15. Galvin JE, Sadowsky CH. Practical guidelines for the recognition and diagnosis of dementia. *J Am Board Fam Med.* 2012;25(3):367–382.
16. Spires-Jones TL, Hyman BT. The intersection of amyloid beta and tau at synapses in Alzheimer's disease. *Neuron.* 2014;82(4):756–771.
17. Chen GF, Xu TH, Yan Y, et al. Amyloid beta: Structure, biology and structure-based therapeutic development. *Acta Pharmacol Sin.* 2017;38(9):1205–1235. doi: 10.1038/aps.2017.28.
18. Long JM, Holtzman DM. Alzheimer disease: An update on pathobiology and treatment strategies. *Cell.* 2019;179(2):312–339. doi: 10.1016/j.cell.2019.09.001.
19. Prins ND. Immunotherapy against amyloid-β in Alzheimer's disease: An overview. In: Ingelsson M, Lannfelt L, eds. *Immunotherapy and Biomarkers in Neurodegenerative Disorders Methods in Pharmacology and Toxicology.* New York, NY: Humana Press; 2016;3–17.
20. Takeda S. Progression of Alzheimer's disease, tau propagation, and its modifiable risk factors. *Neurosci Res.* 2019;141:36–42. doi: 10.1016/j.neures.2018.08.005.
21. Tublin JM, Adelstein JM, del Monte F, et al. Getting to the heart of Alzheimer's disease. *Circ Res.* 2019;124(1):142–149.
22. Breijyeh Z, Karaman R. Comprehensive review on Alzheimer's disease: Causes and treatment. *Molecules.* 2020;25(24):5789. doi: 10.3390/molecules25245789.
23. O'Brien JT, Markus HS. Vascular risk factors and Alzheimer's disease. *BMC Med.* 2014;12:218.
24. de Bruijn RFAG, Ikram MA. Cardiovascular risk factors and future risk of Alzheimer's disease. *BMC Med.* 2014;12:130.
25. Mullane K, Williams M. Alzheimer's disease (AD) therapeutics – 1: Repeated clinical failures continue to question the amyloid hypothesis of AD and the current understanding of AD causality. *Biochem Pharmacol.* 2018;158:359–375.
26. Forbes SC, Holroyd-Leduc JM, Poulin MJ, Hogan DB. Effect of nutrients, dietary supplements and vitamins on cognition: A systematic review and meta-analysis of randomized controlled trials. *Can Geriatr J.* 2015;18(4):231–245.
27. Henderson VW. Alzheimer's disease: Review of hormone therapy trials and implications for treatment and prevention after menopause. *J Steroid Biochem Mol Biol.* 2014;142:99–106.
28. Folstein MF, Folstein SE, McHugh PR. "Mini-mental state". A practical method for grading the cognitive state of patients for the clinician. *J Psychiatr Res.* 1975;12(3):189–198.
29. Gauthier S, Rosa-Neto P, Morais J, Webster C. *World Alzheimer Report 2021: Journey through the diagnosis of dementia.* London, England: Alzheimer's Disease International. Available at: https://www.alzint.org/u/World-Alzheimer-Report-2021.pdf. Last accessed August 25, 2022.
30. Moyer VA. Screening for cognitive impairment in older adults: U.S. Preventive Services Task Force recommendation statement. *Ann Intern Med.* 2014;160(11):791–797.
31. Cordell CB, Borson S, Boustani M, et al. Alzheimer's Association recommendations for operationalizing the detection of cognitive impairment during the Medicare annual wellness visit in a primary care setting. *Alzheimers Dement.* 2013;9(2):141–150.
32. Colburn JL, Nothelle S. The Medicare annual wellness visit. *Clin Geriatr Med.* 2018;34(1):1–10. doi: 10.1016/j.cger.2017.09.001.
33. MoCA Cognitive Assessment. Available at: mocatest.org. Last accessed November 9, 2021.
34. Rabins PV, Blass DM. In the clinic. Dementia. *Ann Intern Med.* 2014;161(3):ITC1–ITC16.
35. Association AP. *Diagnostic and Statistical Manual of Mental Disorders (DSM-5).* 5th ed. Washington, DC: American Psychiatric Association; 2013.
36. Agency for Health Care Policy and Research. *Diagnosis and Treatment of Clinical Alzheimer's-Type Dementia: As Systematic Review.* Rockville, MD: Agency for Health Care Policy and Research; 2020.
37. Knopman DS, DeKosky ST, Cummings JL, et al. Practice parameter: Diagnosis of dementia (an evidence-based review). Report of the Quality Standards Subcommittee of the American Academy of Neurology. *Neurology.* 2001;56(9):1143–1153.
38. Román GC, Tatemichi TK, Erkinjuntti T, et al. Vascular dementia: Diagnostic criteria for research studies. Report of the NINDS-AIREN International Workshop. *Neurology.* 1993;43(2):250–260.
39. McKhann G, Drachman D, Folstein M, et al. Clinical diagnosis of Alzheimer's disease: Report of the NINCDS-ADRDA Work Group

under the auspices of Department of Health and Human Services Task Force on Alzheimer's Disease. *Neurology.* 1984;34(7):939–944.

40. Jack CR, Albert MS, Knopman DS, et al. Introduction to the recommendations from the National Institute on Aging-Alzheimer's Association workgroups on diagnostic guidelines for Alzheimer's disease. *Alzheimers Dement.* 2011;7(3):257–262.
41. McKhann GM, Knopman DS, Chertkow H, et al. The diagnosis of dementia due to Alzheimer's disease: Recommendations from the National Institute on Aging-Alzheimer's Association workgroups on diagnostic guidelines for Alzheimer's disease. *Alzheimers Dement.* 2011;7(3):263–269.
42. Albert MS, DeKosky ST, Dickson D, et al. The diagnosis of mild cognitive impairment due to Alzheimer's disease: Recommendations from the National Institute on Aging-Alzheimer's Association workgroups on diagnostic guidelines for Alzheimer's disease. *Alzheimers Dement.* 2011;7(3):270–279.
43. Sperling RA, Aisen PS, Beckett LA, et al. Toward defining the preclinical stages of Alzheimer's disease: Recommendations from the National Institute on Aging-Alzheimer's Association workgroups on diagnostic guidelines for Alzheimer's disease. *Alzheimers Dement.* 2011;7(3):280–292.
44. Petersen RC, Lopez O, Armstrong MJ, et al. Practice guideline update summary: Mild cognitive impairment. Report of the Guideline Development, Dissemination, and Implementation Subcommittee of the American Academy of Neurology. *Neurology.* 2018;90(3):126–135.
45. Fillenbaum GG, Peterson B, Morris JC. Estimating the validity of the clinical Dementia Rating Scale: The CERAD experience. Consortium to Establish a Registry for Alzheimer's Disease. *Aging (Milano).* 1996;8(6):379–385.
46. Harper L, Barkhof F, Scheltens P, et al. An algorithmic approach to structural imaging in dementia. *J Neurol Neurosurg Psychiatry.* 2014;85(6):692–698.
47. Jack CR, Bennett DA, Blennow K, et al. NIA-AA Research Framework: Toward a biological definition of Alzheimer's disease. *Alzheimers Dement.* 2018;14(4):535–562.
48. Horgan D, Nobili F, Teunissen C, et al. Biomarker testing: Piercing the fog of Alzheimer's and related dementia. *Biomed Hub.* 2020;5(3): 19–40. doi: 10.1159/000511233.
49. Livingston G, Sommerlad A, Orgeta V, et al. Dementia prevention, intervention, and care. *Lancet.* 2017;390(10113):2673–2734.
50. Geda YE. Mild cognitive impairment in older adults. *Curr Psychiatry Rep.* 2012;14(4):320–327.
51. Matsunaga S, Fujishiro H, Takechi H. Efficacy and safety of cholinesterase inhibitors for mild cognitive impairment: A systematic review and meta-analysis. *J Alzheimers Dis.* 2019;71(2):513–523. doi: 10.3233/JAD-190546.
52. 2019 American Geriatrics Society Beers Criteria® Update Expert Panel. American Geriatrics Society 2019 Updated AGS Beers Criteria® for potentially inappropriate medication use in older adults. *J Am Geriatr Soc.* 2019;(4):674–694.
53. Sadowsky CH, Galvin JE. Guidelines for the management of cognitive and behavioral problems in dementia. *J Am Board Fam Med.* 2012;25(3):350–366. doi: 10.3122/jabfm.2012.03.100183.
54. Parsons C. Polypharmacy and inappropriate medication use in patients with dementia: An under-researched problem. *Ther Adv Drug Saf.* 2017;8(1):31–46.
55. Razadyne (galantamine hydrobromide). Titusville, NJ: Janssen Pharmaceuticals; 2021. Package insert.
56. *Exelon (rivastigmine tartrate).* East Hanover, NJ: Novartis Pharmaceuticals; 2021. Package insert.
57. *Exelon Patch (rivastigmine transdermal system).* East Hanover, NJ: Novartis Pharmaceuticals; 2021. Package insert.
58. *Aricept (donepezil hydrochloride).* Woodcliff Lake, NJ: Eisai; 2018. Package insert.
59. Aducanumab (*Aduhelm*). for Alzheimer's disease. *Med Lett Drugs Ther.* 2021;*63*(1628):105–106.
60. Aducanumab-avwa (Aduhelm). Cambridge, MA: Biogen and Eisai; 2021. Package insert.
61. *Namenda (memantine hydrochloride).* Madison, NJ: Allergan, Inc.; 2019. Package insert.
62. *Namenda XR (memantine hydrochloride).* Madison, NJ: Allergan, Inc.; 2019. Package insert.
63. Namzaric capsules (memantine hydrochloride extended release and donepezil hydrochloride). Madison, NJ: Allergan, Inc.; 2019. Package insert.
64. Ed. Downey A, Stroud C, Landis S, Leshner AI. *Preventing Cognitive Decline and Dementia: A Way Forward.* Washington, DC: National Academy of Sciences; 2017.
65. Deckers K, van Boxtel MP, Schiepers OJ, et al. Target risk factors for dementia prevention: A systematic review and Delphi consensus study on the evidence from observational studies. *Int J Geriatr Psychiatry.* 2015;30(3):234–246. 10.1002/gps.4245 25504093.
66. Vos SJB, van Boxtel MPJ, Schiepers OJG, et al. Modifiable risk factors for prevention of dementia in midlife, late life and the oldest-old: Validation of the LIBRA Index. *J Alzheimers Dis.* 2017;58(2):537–547. doi: 10.3233/JAD-161208.
67. Livingston G, Huntley J, Sommerlad A, et al. Dementia prevention, intervention, and care: 2020 report of the Lancet Commission. *Lancet.* 2020;396(10248):413–446. doi: 10.1016/S0140-6736(20)30367-6.
68. Panza GA, Taylor BA, MacDonald HV, et al. Can exercise improve cognitive symptoms of Alzheimer's disease? *J Am Geriatr Soc.* 2018;66(3):487–495. doi: 10.1111/jgs.15241.
69. Gitlin LN, Kales HC, Lyketsos CG. Nonpharmacologic management of behavioral symptoms in dementia. *JAMA.* 2012;308(19): 2020–2029.
70. Mittelman MS, Bartels SJ. Translating research into practice: Case study of a community-based dementia caregiver intervention. *Health Aff (Millwood).* 2014;33(4):587–595.
71. Caspar S, Davis ED, Douziech A, et al. Nonpharmacological management of behavioral and psychological symptoms of dementia: What works, in what circumstances, and why? *Innov Aging.* 2018;2(1):igy001. doi: 10.1093/geroni/igy001.
72. Alzheimer's Association. Challenging Behaviors. Available at: http://www.alz.org/national/documents/statements_antipsychotics.pdf. Last accessed August 29, 2022.
73. Catic AG. Nonpharmacologic management of behavioral and psychological symptoms of dementia in long-term care residents. *Ann Long-Term Care.* 2015;23(11):23–30.
74. Rabins PV, Rovner BW, Rummans T, et al. GuidelineWatch (October 2014): Practice Guideline for the Treatment of Patients with Alzheimer's Disease and Other Dementias. Available at: http://psychiatryonline.org/pb/assets/raw/sitewide/practice_guidelines/guidelines/alzheimerwatch.pdf. Last accessed August 29, 2022.
75. Birks JS, Grimley Evans J. Rivastigmine for Alzheimer's disease. *Cochrane Database Syst Rev.* 2015;9:CD001191.
76. Buckley JS, Salpeter SR. A risk-benefit assessment of dementia medications: Systematic review of the evidence. *Drugs Aging.* 2015;32(6):453–467.
77. Raskind MA, Peskind ER, Truyen L, et al. The cognitive benefits of galantamine are sustained for at least 36 months: A long-term extension trial. *Arch Neurol.* 2004;61(2):252–256.
78. Masters CL, Bateman R, Blennow K, et al. Alzheimer's disease. *Nat Rev Dis Primers.* 2015;1:15056.
79. Lin JS, O'Connor E, Rossom RC, et al. *Screening for Cognitive Impairment in Older Adults: An Evidence Update for the U.S. Preventive Services Task Force.* Rockville, MD: Agency for Healthcare Research and Quality; 2013.
80. Triantafylidis LK, Clemons JS, Peron EP, et al. Brain over bladder: A systematic review of dual cholinesterase inhibitor and urinary anticholinergic use. *Drugs and Aging.* 2018;35(1):27–41.
81. Bidzan L, Bidzan M. Withdrawal syndrome after donepezil cessation in a patient with dementia. *Neurol Sci.* 2012;33(6):1459–1461.
82. Schwartz LM, Woloshin S. How the FDA forgot the evidence: The case of donepezil 23 mg. *BMJ.* 2012;344:e1086.
83. Massoud F, Desmarais JE, Gauthier S. Switching cholinesterase inhibitors in older adults with dementia. *Int Psychogeriatr.* 2011;23(3):372–378.
84. Fonseca-Santos B, Gremião MPD, Chorilli M. Nanotechnology-based drug delivery systems for the treatment of Alzheimer's disease. *Int J Nanomedicine.* 2015;10:4981–5003.
85. Deardorff WJ, Feen E, Grossberg GT. The use of cholinesterase inhibitors across all stages of Alzheimer's disease. *Drugs Aging.* 2015;32(7):537–547.
86. Tariot PN, Farlow MR, Grossberg GT, et al. Memantine treatment in patients with moderate to severe Alzheimer disease already receiving donepezil: A randomized controlled trial. *JAMA.* 2004;291(3):317–324.
87. Barrera-Ocampo A, Lopera F. Amyloid-beta immunotherapy: The hope for Alzheimer disease? *Colomb Med (Cali).* 2016;47(4):203–212.
88. Suzuki K, Iwata A, Iwatsubo T. The past, present, and future of disease-modifying therapies for Alzheimer's disease. *Proc Jpn Acad Ser B Phys Biol Sci.* 2017;93(10):757–771. doi: 10.2183/pjab.93.048.
89. Sumner IL, Edwards RA, Asuni AA, et al. Antibody engineering for optimized immunotherapy in Alzheimer's disease. *Front Neurosci.* 2018;12:254–254. doi: 10.3389/fnins.2018.00254.
90. Zhao J, Nussinov R, Ma B. Mechanisms of recognition of amyloid-β (Aβ) monomer, oligomer, and fibril by homologous antibodies. *J Biol Chem.* 2017;292(44):18325–18343. doi: 10.1074/jbc.M117.801514.

91. Vander Zanden CM, Chi EY. Passive immunotherapies targeting amyloid beta and tau oligomers in Alzheimer's disease. *J Pharm Sci.* 2020;109(1):68–73. doi: 10.1016/j.xphs.2019.10.024.
92. Schneider L. A resurrection of aducanumab for Alzheimer's disease. *Lancet Neurol.* 2020;19(2):111–112. doi: 10.1016/S1474-4422(19)30480-6.
93. Knopman DS, Jones DT, Greicius MD. Failure to demonstrate efficacy of aducanumab: An analysis of the EMERGE and ENGAGE trials as reported by Biogen, December 2019. *Alzheimers Dement.* 2021;17(4):696–701. doi: 10.1002/alz.12213.
94. Ernst J. FDA grants two antibodies breakthrough therapy designation for Alzheimer's disease. Healio. June 24, 2021. Available at: https://www.healio.com/news/neurology/20210624/fda-grants-lecanemab-breakthrough-therapy-designation-for-treatment-of-alzheimers-disease. Last accessed November 11, 2021.
95. Inacio P. FDA grants breakthrough therapy designation to gantenerumab. Alzheimer's News Today. October 12, 2021. Available at: https://alzheimersnewstoday.com/2021/10/12/gantenerumab-alzheimers-named-fda-breakthrough-therapy/. Last accessed November 11, 2021.
96. Tolar M, Abushakra S, Hey JA, et al. Aducanumab, gantenerumab, BAN2401, and ALZ-801-the first wave of amyloid-targeting drugs for Alzheimer's disease with potential for near term approval. *Alzheimers Res Ther.* 2020;12(1):95–95. doi: 10.1186/s13195-020-00663-w.
97. Pankiewicz JE, Sadowski MJ. APOE genotype and Alzheimer's immunotherapy. *Oncotarget.* 2017;8(25):39941–39942. doi: 10.18632/oncotarget.17990.
98. Lin GA, Whittington MD, Synnott PG, et al. Aducanumab for Alzheimer's disease: Effectiveness and Value. Institute for Clinical and Economic Review. August 5, 2021. Available at: https://icer.org/wp-content/uploads/2020/10/ICER_ALZ_Final_Report_080521.pdf. Last accessed October 25, 2021.
99. Canevelli M, Rossi PD, Astrone P, et al. "Real world" eligibility for aducanumab. *J Am Geriatr Soc.* 2021;69(10):2995–2998. doi: 10.1111/jgs.17390.
100. Rogers SL, Doody RS, Pratt RD, Ieni JR. Long-term efficacy and safety of donepezil in the treatment of Alzheimer's disease: Final analysis of a US multicentre open-label study. *Eur Neuropsychopharmacol.* 2000;10(3):195–203.
101. Farlow MR, Lilly ML, ENA713 B352 Study Group. Rivastigmine: An open-label, observational study of safety and effectiveness in treating patients with Alzheimer's disease for up to 5 years. *BMC Geriatr.* 2005;5:3.
102. Reisberg B, Doody R, Stöffler A, et al. A 24-week open-label extension study of memantine in moderate to severe Alzheimer disease. *Arch Neurol.* 2006;63(1):49–54.
103. Doody RS, Geldmacher DS, Gordon B, et al. Open-label, multicenter, phase 3 extension study of the safety and efficacy of donepezil in patients with Alzheimer disease. *Arch Neurol.* 2001;58(3):427–433.
104. Howard R, McShane R, Lindesay J, et al. Nursing home placement in the donepezil and memantine in moderate to severe Alzheimer's disease (DOMINO-AD) trial: Secondary and post-hoc analyses. *Lancet Neurol.* 2015;14(12):1171–1181.
105. Ryan J, Fransquet P, Wrigglesworth J, Lacaze P. Phenotypic heterogeneity in dementia: A challenge for epidemiology and biomarker studies. *Front Public Health.* 2018;6:181.
106. Rainer M, Mucke HA, Krüger-Rainer C, et al. Cognitive relapse after discontinuation of drug therapy in Alzheimer's disease: Cholinesterase inhibitors versus nootropics. *J Neural Transm.* 2001;108(11):1327–1333.
107. Gaudig M, Richarz U, Han J, et al. Effects of galantamine in Alzheimer's disease: Double-blind withdrawal studies evaluating sustained versus interrupted treatment. *Curr Alzheimer Res.* 2011;8(7):771–780.
108. Pariente A, Fourrier-Réglat A, Bazin F, et al. Effect of treatment gaps in elderly patients with dementia treated with cholinesterase inhibitors. *Neurology.* 2012;78(13):957–963.
109. Dichgans M, Leys D. Vascular cognitive impairment. *Circ Res.* 2017;120(3):573–591.
110. Mongkhon P, Naser AY, Fanning L, et al. Oral anticoagulants and risk of dementia: A systematic review and meta-analysis of observational studies and randomized controlled trials. *Neurosci Biobehav Rev.* 2019;96:1–9.
111. Zonneveld TP, Richard E, Vergouwen MDI, et al. Blood pressure-lowering treatment for preventing recurrent stroke, major vascular events, and dementia in patients with a history of stroke or transient ischaemic attack. *Cochrane Database Syst Rev.* 2018;7:CD007858.
112. World Health Organization and Alzheimer's Disease International. Dementia: A Public Health Priority. Geneva, Switzerland: World Health Organization. Available at: http://apps.who.int/iris/bitstream/10665/75263/1/9789241564458_eng.pdf. Last accessed August 29, 2022.
113. Anstey KJ, Eramudugolla R, Hosking DE, et al. Bridging the translation gap: From dementia risk assessment to advice on risk reduction. *J Prev Alzheimers Dis.* 2015;2(3):189–198.
114. Jeremy Y, Maaike A, Jennifer R, Naji T. Aerobic exercise to improve cognitive function in older people without known cognitive impairment. *Cochrane Database Syst Rev.* 2015;4:CD005381.
115. Jaturapatporn D, Isaac MG, McCleery J, Tabet N. Aspirin, steroidal and non-steroidal anti-inflammatory drugs for the treatment of Alzheimer's disease. *Cochrane Database Syst Rev.* 2012;2:CD006378.
116. McGuinness B, Craig D, Bullock R, et al. Statins for the treatment of dementia. *Cochrane Database Syst Rev.* 2014;7:CD007514.
117. Schultz BG, Patten DK, Berlau DJ. The role of statins in both cognitive impairment and protection against dementia: A tale of two mechanisms. *Transl Neurodegener.* 2018;7:1–11.
118. Butler M, Nelson VA, Davila H, et al. Over-the-counter supplement interventions to prevent cognitive decline, mild cognitive impairment, and clinical Alzheimer-type dementia. *Ann Intern Med.* 2018;168(1):52–62.
119. Spence J, Chintapenta M, Kwon HI, Blaszczyk AT. A brief review of three common supplements used in Alzheimer's disease. *Consult Pharm.* 2017;32(7):412–414.
120. Libro R, Giacoppo S, Rajan TS, et al. Natural phytochemicals in the treatment and prevention of dementia: An overview. *Molecules.* 2016;21(4):518.
121. Sano M, Ernesto C, Thomas RG, et al. A controlled trial of selegiline, alpha-tocopherol, or both as treatment for Alzheimer's disease. *N Engl J Med.* 1997;336(17):1216–1222.
122. Dysken MW, Sano M, Asthana S, et al. Effect of vitamin E and memantine on functional decline in Alzheimer disease: The TEAM-AD VA cooperative randomized trial. *J Am Med Assoc.* 2014;311(1):33–44.
123. Miller ER, Pastor-Barriuso R, Dalal D, et al. Meta-analysis: High-dosage vitamin E supplementation may increase all-cause mortality. *Ann Intern Med.* 2005;142(1):37–46.
124. Petersen RC, Thomas RG, Grundman M, et al. Vitamin E and donepezil for the treatment of mild cognitive impairment. *N Engl J Med.* 2005;352(23):2379–2388.
125. Kryscio RJ, Abner EL, Caban-Holt A, et al. Association of antioxidant supplement use and dementia in the prevention of Alzheimer's disease by vitamin E and selenium trial (PREADViSE). *JAMA Neurol.* 2017;74(5):567–573.
126. Farina N, Llewellyn D, Isaac MGEKN, Tabet N. Vitamin E for Alzheimer's dementia and mild cognitive impairment. *Cochrane Database Syst Rev.* 2017;4:CD002854.
127. Zhang DM, Ye JX, Mu JS, Cui XP. Efficacy of vitamin B supplementation on cognition in elderly patients with cognitive-related diseases: A systematic review and meta-analysis. *J Geriatr Psychiatry Neurol.* 2017;30(1):50–59.
128. Yuan Q, Wang CW, Shi J, Lin ZX. Effects of Ginkgo biloba on dementia: An overview of systematic reviews. *J Ethnopharmacol.* 2017;195:1–9.
129. DeKosky ST, Williamson JD, Fitzpatrick AL, et al. Ginkgo biloba for prevention of dementia: A randomized controlled trial. *JAMA.* 2008;300(19):2253–2262.
130. Vellas B, Coley N, Ousset PJ, et al. Long-term use of standardised Ginkgo biloba extract for the prevention of Alzheimer's disease (GuidAge): A randomised placebo-controlled trial. *Lancet Neurol.* 2012;11(10):851–859.
131. Stoddard GJ, Archer M, Shane-McWhorter L, et al. Ginkgo and warfarin interaction in a large Veterans Administration population. *AMIA Annu Symp Proc.* 2015;2015:1174–1183.
132. Apoaequorin (Prevagen) Natural Medicines database. Apoaequorin [monograph]. Available at: http://naturalmedicines.therapeuticresearch.com.
133. Food and Drug Administration. Frequently Asked Questions About Medical Foods; Second Edition. Available at: https://www.fda.gov/files/food/published/Guidance-for-Industry--Frequently-Asked-Questions-About-Medical-Foods--Second-Edition-%28PDF%29.pdf. Last accessed August 29, 2022.
134. Chintapenta M, Spence J, Kwon HI, Blaszczyk AT. A brief review of caprylidene (Axona) and coconut oil as alternative fuels in the fight against Alzheimer's disease. *Consult Pharm.* 2017;32(12):748–751.
135. Henderson ST, Vogel JL, Barr LJ, et al. Study of the ketogenic agent AC-1202 in mild to moderate Alzheimer's disease: A randomized, double-blind, placebo-controlled, multicenter trial. *Nutr Metab (Lond).* 2009;6:31.

136. Onakpoya IJ, Heneghan CJ. The efficacy of supplementation with the novel medical food, Souvenaid, in patients with Alzheimer's disease: A systematic review and meta-analysis of randomized clinical trials. *Nutr Neurosci.* 2017;20(4):119–227.
137. Hara J, Shankle WR, Barrentine LW, Curole MV. Novel therapy of hyperhomocysteinemia in mild cognitive impairment, Alzheimer's disease, and other dementing disorders. *J Nutr Heal Aging.* 2016;20(8):825–834.
138. Phillips P. Omega 3 fatty acids for the treatment of dementia: A Cochrane review summary. *Int J Nurs Stud.* 2017;67:83–84.
139. Petersen RC, Aisen P, Boeve BF, et al. Mild cognitive impairment due to Alzheimer disease in the community. *Ann Neurol.* 2013;74(2):199–208. doi: 10.1002/ana.23931.
140. US National Library of Medicine. Available at: Clinicaltrials.gov.
141. Pickett J, Bird C, Ballard C, et al. A roadmap to advance dementia research in prevention, diagnosis, intervention, and care by 2025. *Int J Geriatr Psychiatry.* 2018;33(7):900–906.
142. National Institutes of Health. Alzheimer's Disease. Available at: http://www.nih.gov/research-training/accelerating-medicines-partnership-amp/alzheimers-disease. Last accessed August 29, 2022.
143. Masopust J, Protopopová D, Vališ M, et al. Treatment of behavioral and psychological symptoms of dementias with psychopharmaceuticals: A review. *Neuropsychiatr Dis Treat.* 2018;14:1211–1220.
144. Tible OP, Riese F, Savaskan E, von Gunten A. Best practice in the management of behavioural and psychological symptoms of dementia. *Ther Adv Neurol Disord.* 2017;10(8):297–309.
145. Kales HC, Gitlin LN, Lyketsos CG. Assessment and management of behavioral and psychological symptoms of dementia. *BMJ.* 2015;350:h369.
146. Reus VI, Fochtmann LJ, Eyler AE, et al. The American Psychiatric Association practice guideline on the use of antipsychotics to treat agitation or psychosis in patients with dementia. *Am J Psychiatry.* 2016;173(5):543–546.
147. Ngo J, Holroyd-Leduc JM. Systematic review of recent dementia practice guidelines. *Age Ageing.* 2015;44(1):25–33.
148. Cohen-Mansfield J, Jensen B, Resnick B, Norris M. Knowledge of and attitudes toward nonpharmacological interventions for treatment of behavior symptoms associated with dementia: A comparison of physicians, psychologists, and nurse practitioners. *Gerontologist.* 2012;52(1):34–45.
149. Desai AK, Schwartz L, Grossberg GT. Behavioral disturbance in dementia. *Curr Psychiatry Rep.* 2012;14(4):298–309.
150. Crystal S, Jarrín OF, Rosenthal M, et al. National partnership to improve dementia care in nursing homes campaign: State and facility strategies, impact, and antipsychotic reduction outcomes. Innovation in Aging. 2020;4(3):1-13. doi:10.1093/geroni/igaa018.
151. Ma H, Huang Y, Cong Z, et al. The efficacy and safety of atypical antipsychotics for the treatment of dementia: A meta-analysis of randomized placebo-controlled trials. *J Alzheimers Dis.* 2014;42(3):915–937.
152. Schneider LS, Tariot PN, Dagerman KS, et al. Effectiveness of atypical antipsychotic drugs in patients with Alzheimer's disease. *N Engl J Med.* 2006;355(15):1525–1538.
153. Food and Drug Administration Information for Healthcare Professionals: Conventional Antipsychotics. Available at: https://wayback.archive-it.org/7993/20170722190727/https://www.fda.gov/Drugs/DrugSafety/PostmarketDrugSafetyInformationforPatientsandProviders/ucm124830.htm. Last accessed August 29, 2022.
154. Levinson DR. Medicare atypical antipsychotic drug claims for elderly nursing home residents. Available at: http://oig.hhs.gov/oei/reports/oei-07-08-00150.pdf. Last accessed August 29, 2022.
155. Centers for Medicare & Medicaid Services. National Partnership to Improve Dementia Care in Nursing Homes: Antipsychotic Medication Use Data Report (April 2021). Available at: https://www.cms.gov/files/document/antipsychotic-medication-use-data-report-2020q4-updated-07302021.pdf. Last accessed August 29, 2022.
156. Pan YJ, Wu CS, Gau SS, et al. Antipsychotic discontinuation in patients with dementia: A systematic review and meta-analysis of published randomized controlled studies. *Dement Geriatr Cogn Disord.* 2014;37(3-4):125–140.
157. Supasitthumrong T, Bolea-Alamanac BM, Asmer S, et al. Gabapentin and pregabalin to treat aggressivity in dementia: A systematic review and illustrative case report. *Br J Clin Pharmacol.* 2019;(4):690–703.
158. Belsomra (suvorexant). Whitehouse Station, NJ. Merck Sharp and Dohme Corp. 2021. Package insert.
159. Sheehan B. Assessment scales in dementia. *Ther Adv Neurol Disord.* 2012;5(6):349–358.
160. Kim LD, Factora RM. Alzheimer dementia: Starting, stopping drug therapy. *Cleve Clin J Med.* 2018;85(3):209–214.
161. Deprescribing.org. Available at: http://deprescribing.org/resources/deprescribing-guidelines-algorithms/. Last accessed September 3, 2021. Deprescribing Guidelines and Algorithms.
162. 2021 Alzheimer's Disease Facts and Figures, Special Report: Race, Ethnicity and Alzheimer's in America. Alzheimer's Association. Available at: https://www.alz.org/media/documents/alzheimers-facts-and-figures.pdf. Last accessed February 22, 2022.
163. Lazarczyk MJ, Bouras C, Hot PR, et al. Preclinical Alzheimer disease: Identification of cases at risk among cognitively intact older individuals. *BMC Medicine.* 2012;10:127.

Multiple Sclerosis

Jacquelyn L. Bainbridge, Augusto Miravelle, Pei Shieen Wong, Matthew J. Makelky Sr., and Sarah Rajkovic

74

KEY CONCEPTS

1. Multiple sclerosis (MS) etiology is unknown, but it appears to be autoimmune in nature. Currently, there is no cure.
2. Multiple sclerosis is characterized by central nervous system (CNS) demyelination and axonal damage.
3. Multiple sclerosis is classified into several categories, differentiated by disease progression over time, clinical presentation, and response to therapy.
4. Studies only support one Food and Drug Administration (FDA)-approved disease-modifying therapy (DMT), ocrelizumab (Ocrevus), in patients with progressive forms of the illness. However, information derived from multiple studies suggests younger patients with progressive disease and those with either superimposed acute relapses or enhancing lesions on magnetic resonance imaging (MRI) scans may benefit from some of the presently used DMTs.
5. MS diagnosis is made primarily based on clinical symptoms and examination but does require evidence of dissemination of lesions over time in multiple parts of the CNS and/or optic nerve. Additional diagnostic criteria include use of MRI, spinal fluid evaluation, and evoked potentials to aid in the diagnosis.
6. Exacerbations or relapses of MS can be disabling and are treated with high-dose glucocorticoids, such as intravenous (IV) methylprednisolone. The onset of clinical response is typically within 3 to 5 days.
7. Treatment of relapsing-remitting multiple sclerosis (RRMS) with the DMTs interferon-β (IFN-β) (Avonex, Betaseron, Rebif, Extavia), glatiramer acetate (Copaxone), natalizumab (Tysabri), ocrelizumab (Ocrevus), mitoxantrone (Novantrone), fingolimod (Gilenya), siponimod (Mayzent), ozanimod (Zeposia), ponesimod (Ponvory), teriflunomide (Aubagio), dimethyl fumarate (Tecfidera), diroximel fumarate (Vumerity), monomethyl fumarate (Bafiertam), cladribine (Mavenclad), Ofatumumab (Kesimpta), and alemtuzumab (Lemtrada) can reduce the annual relapse rate, lessen relapse severity, slow progression of MRI changes, and slow progression of disability and cognitive decline. In addition, DMTs have been shown to reduce the likelihood of developing a second attack after a first clinically isolated syndrome (CIS) consistent with MS.
8. In most cases, treatment with DMTs should begin promptly after the diagnosis of RRMS or after a CIS if the brain MRI suggests a high risk of further attacks. Natalizumab, and other choices associated with problematic adverse events, should be reserved for those patients who have failed one or more standard therapies and those with poor prognostic signs.
9. The definition of "treatment inadequacy" for RRMS remains unclear, and therapy changes after "treatment failure" should be individualized.
10. Patients suffering with MS frequently have spasticity, bladder dysfunction, fatigue, neuropathic pain, cognitive dysfunction, and depressive symptoms that may require treatment. Providers must counsel patients that DMTs will not relieve these symptoms and that depression is common and can pose the risk of suicide.

BEYOND THE BOOK

Create a table that lists the current FDA-approved multiple sclerosis (MS) therapies for relapsing-remitting MS (RRMS), primary progressive MS (PPMS), clinically isolated syndrome (CIS), and secondary progressive MS (SPMS). Include the mechanism of action (MOA) and how you believe this helps reduce MS symptoms. This activity will get you familiar with MS medications and how they are used in practice for differing forms of the disease.

When treating MS there are many different approaches to the intensity of treatment. What are the risks and benefits of starting a patient on self-injected interferon therapy versus infused immunotherapy? Compare and contrast the decrease in MS symptoms and relapses with these therapies in respect to the adverse medication reactions seen with the same therapies. What adverse medication reactions are more common as years on treatment accumulate?

INTRODUCTION

Multiple sclerosis (MS) is a central nervous system (CNS) inflammatory disease that affects approximately 1 in 450 per 100,000 females and fewer males in the United States.[1] The term "multiple sclerosis" refers to two characteristics of the disease: multiple neurologic symptoms that accrue over time and characteristic plaques or sclerosed areas seen in numerous areas of the brain and spinal cord.

1 MS was first described more than 140 years ago, but the cause remains a mystery, and a cure is still unavailable. However, many recent advances in disease treatment and complication management have improved the quality of life of affected individuals.

EPIDEMIOLOGY

MS affects approximately 2.3 million people worldwide[2] and is usually diagnosed between 15 and 50 years of age, with a peak incidence occurring in the fourth decade. However, MS can occur in young children and significantly in older adults. While females are afflicted more than males by a ratio of 2.8:1, males usually develop the first signs of MS at a later age and are more likely to develop a progressive form of the disease. The rising incidence of MS in females may be associated with urbanization.[2] Additionally, MS occurs more frequently in Whites of Scandinavian ancestry compared to other ethnic groups.[3]

The factors most important in determining disease risk are geography, environmental influences, age, and genetics (discussed under etiology).[1,4-7] In general, MS is more prevalent above the 37th parallel, although recent studies suggest a waning latitude gradient as demonstrated by a substantial increase in Mediterranean regions. An inverse relationship between MS risk and 25-hydroxyvitamin D levels has been proposed.[8]

ETIOLOGY

The exact cause of MS is unknown but is thought to develop in genetically susceptible individuals exposed to random events and environmental factors that trigger immune-mediated CNS damage. Genetic variation accounts for approximately 30% of the overall disease risk, and more than 100 distinct genetic regions are associated with MS, collectively explaining about one-third of its genetic component.

The familial recurrence rate of MS is approximately 5%, with siblings being the most commonly reported relationship,[6] and monozygotic twins displaying a concordance rate of roughly 25%. Genes that lie within the major histocompatibility complex (MHC), on the sixth chromosome,[1,6] as well as interleukin-2α (IL-2α) and interleukin-7α (IL-7α) receptor genes have been associated with disease risk.[9-11] A genetic-environmental interaction is also reported for the human leukocyte antigen (*HLA*) *DRB1*1501* variant.[12] African Americans are less likely to be diagnosed with MS compared with Whites. However, emerging evidence suggests they are more likely to have a severe disease course and respond less to interferon (IFN) therapy.[13,14] A locus on chromosome 1 may be associated with increased susceptibility in African Americans.[15]

While genetics plays a role in overall disease risk, nongenetic factors such as geography, vitamin D deficiency, smoking, high dietary sodium, circadian disruption, human cytomegalovirus (CMV), the Epstein–Barr virus (EBV), and human herpesvirus-6 have been implicated in MS variably. In genetically susceptible individuals who live in a high-risk area for at least 2 years before age 15, the risk of MS is high, especially if exposed to an environmental factor. However, if they move from a high- to a low-risk area before age 15, they can acquire the low-risk status, while moving after age 15 can result in persistence of the high-risk status.[6] Smoking cigarettes has been associated with both an increased risk of developing MS and more severe progression of disability.[11,16] Excess body weight is also associated with a higher risk of developing MS.[17]

Although clear associations have not been identified, certain viruses might participate in the pathogenesis of MS by initiating or activating autoreactive immune cells in genetically susceptible individuals, leading to subsequent demyelination. Evidence supporting a viral etiology includes increased immunoglobulin G (IgG) synthesis in the CNS and increased viral antibody titers. Epidemiologic studies also indicate pathogen exposure in childhood, suggesting "viral" infections may precipitate exacerbations. In addition, data from both humans and experimental animal models suggest that viral infections with incubation periods cause disease with prolonged myelin destruction and a relapsing-remitting course.[1,18] The greatest evidence supports EBV, as autoreactive T cells could be activated by EBV through molecular mimicry due to sequence similarities between EBV and self-peptides. Other potential mechanisms of demyelination include enhanced breakdown and presentation of self-antigens, expression of viral superantigens, or bystander activation.[19] Antibody titers to Epstein–Barr nuclear antigen (EBNA) complex are higher in patients with MS versus controls and are associated with disease risk depending on sample collection time. Antibodies to specific epitopes within EBNA-1 can result in a 24-fold increased disease risk.[19] In addition, anti-EBNA titers are associated with RRMS, conversion of CIS to clinically definite multiple sclerosis (CDMS, confirmed diagnosis of MS), and with MRI measures such as gadolinium-enhancing lesions, change in T2-lesion volume, as well as the EDSS. Anti-EBNA and anti-vascular cell adhesion (anti-VCA) titers are also associated with gray matter atrophy in MS.[20] Evidence of active EBV infection, which in time resolves, may lead to EBV-infected B cells being present in postmortem brain tissue of patients diagnosed with MS [21]; however, these findings have not been implicated.[22] Given all of this, most data suggest that EBV exposure is associated with MS development but does not support the concept of active EBV or aborting infection as directly causing MS.

PATHOPHYSIOLOGY

An important prominent feature of early-stage MS is immune cell infiltration from the periphery to the CNS, as immune cells enter the CNS parenchyma by crossing the blood–brain barrier, the subarachnoid space, or the choroid plexus across the blood-cerebrospinal fluid (CSF) barrier. Other proposed mechanisms include the "inside out" model where disease progression is a neurodegenerative process, similar to primary-progressive multiple sclerosis (PPMS) and secondary-progressive multiple sclerosis (SPMS), where the antigenic constituents are released from the CNS into the periphery, causing the inflammatory response.

2 Once in the CNS, immune cells promote neurodegeneration by stripping the myelin sheath surrounding CNS axons through an inflammatory, perivenular infiltrate consisting of T and B lymphocytes, macrophages, antibodies, and complement.[18] Demyelination renders axons susceptible to damage, which becomes irreversible when they are severed. Irreversible axonal damage correlates with disability and can be visualized as hypointense lesions, or "black holes," on T1-weighted MRI.[23,24]

Peripheral immune cells, along with activated CNS-resident microglia and astrocytes, promote demyelination and oligodendrocyte, and neuroaxonal injury. This is mediated through direct cell contact and the actions of soluble inflammatory and neurotoxic mediators; however, the exact trigger for T-cell activation in the periphery remains unclear, but T cells in MS patients recognize myelin basic protein (MBP), proteolipid protein, myelin oligodendrocyte glycoprotein, and myelin-associated glycoprotein. T-helper subtypes can be either pathogenic or protective in MS. One theory holds that specific T-cell subsets are not terminally differentiated but instead engender a level of plasticity that allows for their conversion from pathogenic to protective and vice versa under certain conditions (Fig. 74-1).[25]

A new concept of T-cell entry into the CNS suggests that the initial lymphocyte invasion may proceed through the ventricles toward the choroid plexus along a gradient that attracts activated Th17 (T-helper) cells.[26] The actual mediator of myelin and axonal destruction has not been established but may reflect a combination of macrophages, antibodies, destructive cytokines, and reactive oxygen intermediates. In patients with stable or mild disease, an increase in the number of cells that express messenger RNA (mRNA) for transforming growth factor-β (TGF-β) and interleukin-10 (IL-10) has been found compared with patients with severe disease. Conversely, a reduction in the number of T-regulatory (Treg) cells, which exhibit suppressor activity, is also associated with active MS and can be found in patients with progressive disease. It should be noted that ratios between various T cells (Treg ratios) do not always correlate with disease activity and that experimental evidence associates high 25-hydroxyvitamin D levels with improved Treg function, favoring the Th2 phenotype in the Th1/Th2 balance.[27] Finally, an immunological hallmark of MS is the intrathecal synthesis of multiple

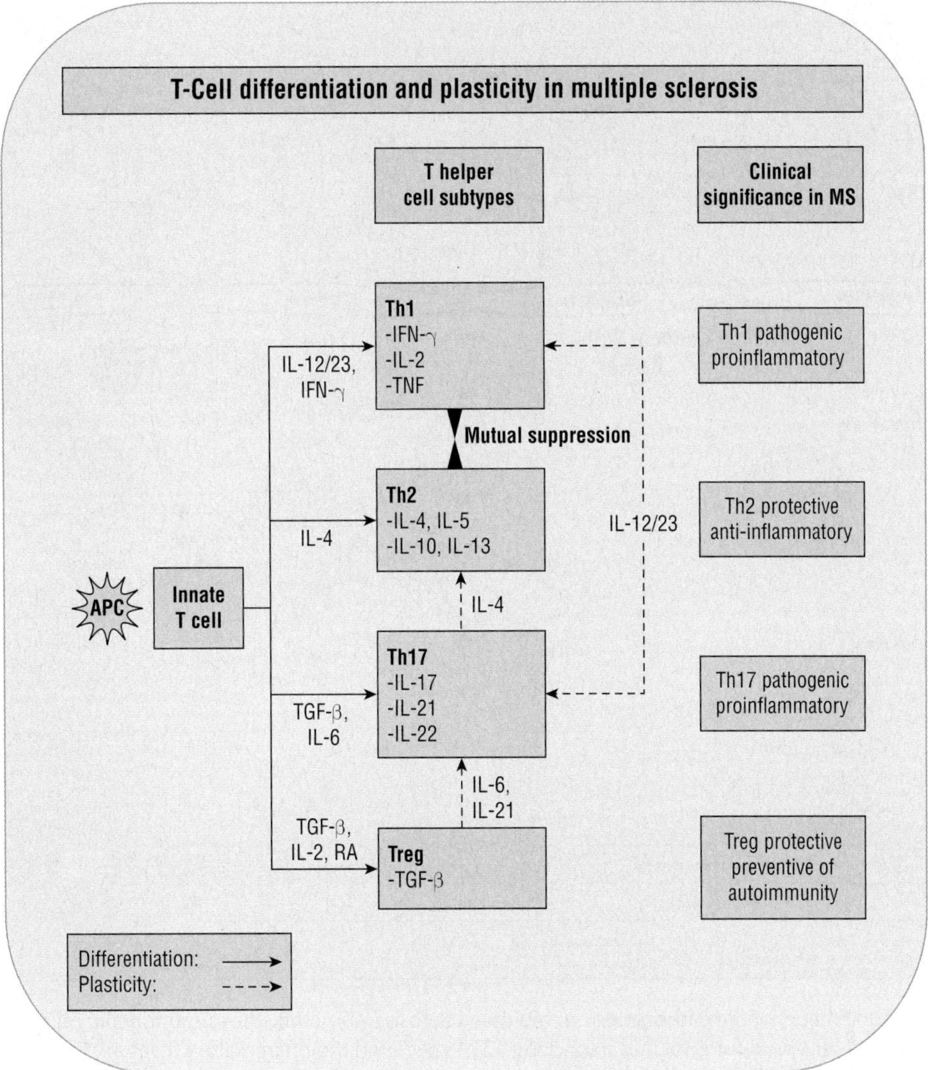

FIGURE 74-1 Upon interaction with an antigen-laden APC and specific cytokines, the innate T cells undergo differentiation into a few lineages (subtypes). Four subtypes significant for MS pathophysiology are illustrated here (Th1, Th2, Th17, and Treg). Th1 and Th17 are proinflammatory, Th2 is anti-inflammatory, and Treg is regulatory. Th1 and Th2 are mutually suppressive and are relatively stable differentiated subtypes. In contrast, Th17 and Treg subtypes exhibit "plasticity" in that they can undergo phenotypic conversion to another T-cell subtype (Th1 or Th2) in the presence of specific cytokine conditions. This plasticity of Th17 and Treg is the immunologic basis for development of therapeutic agents to favor the production of suitable Th subtypes for combating microbial invasion and also concurrently achieving neurocellular recovery after an infection.[25] (APC, antigen presenting cell; Th, T-helper cell.)

immunoglobulin clones with uncertainty regarding the antigen(s) against which they are directed.[28] Therefore, the complex interplay of various cells, antibodies, and cytokines remains to be elucidated.

It is well accepted that MS lesions are heterogeneous, which may be due to differences in the stage of evolution of the lesions over time, differences in underlying immunopathogenesis, or a combination. Acute lesions show demyelination and axonal destruction with lymphocytic activity consistent with an inflammatory state. In contrast, chronic lesions display less inflammatory lymphocytes with active remyelination.[18] As the disease progresses, immune cell infiltration wanes, perhaps due to adaptive immune cell exhaustion from chronic antigen exposure. However, chronic CNS-intrinsic inflammation and neurodegeneration continue independent of peripheral immune activation. Consequently, meningeal tertiary lymphoid-like structures, which have been documented explicitly in secondary progressive disease, may contribute to late-stage inflammation in patients with this form of MS. In general, the relapsing phases of MS are more inflammatory[29] compared to the progressive forms of MS, where you see more neurodegeneration leading to long-term disability.

Although traditional descriptions focus on the white matter as the sole location of MS lesions, recent studies have identified cortical and subcortical gray matter lesions both pathologically[30] and radiographically.[31] In addition, a subset of patients with progressive MS are noted to have abnormalities consistent with B-cell follicles in the meninges.[32]

Just as the full dimensions of the neuropathology are uncertain, so is the pathogenesis of the MS lesion. However, substantial evidence suggests an autoimmune process directed against myelin and oligodendrocytes, the cells that make myelin[18] (Fig. 74-2).

3 The clinical presentation of MS is extremely variable among patients and over time and is impacted by multiple external factors. The signs and symptoms are divided into three categories. Primary symptoms are a direct consequence of conduction disturbances

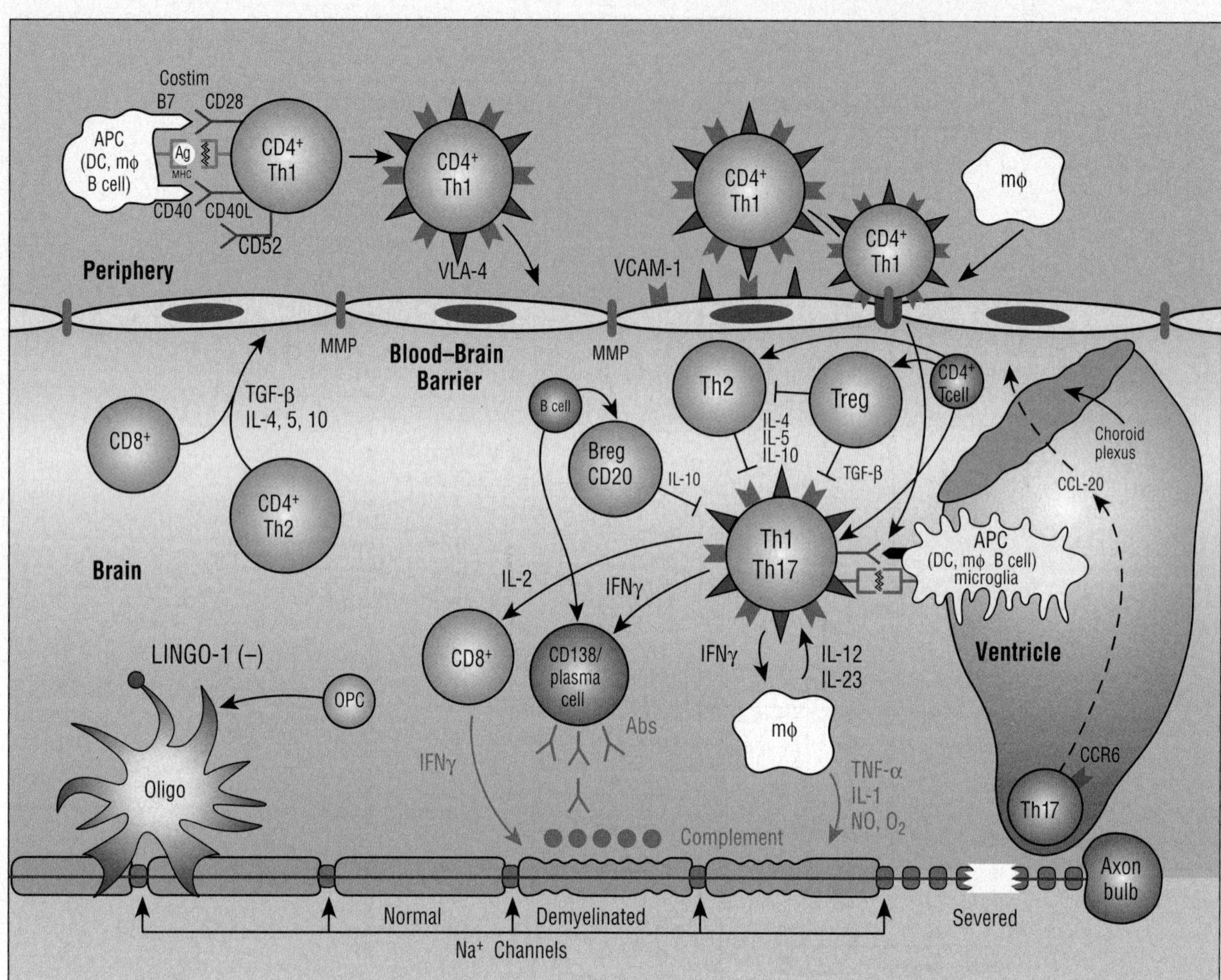

FIGURE 74-2 Autoimmune theory of the pathogenesis of multiple sclerosis (MS). In MS, the immunogenic cells tend to be more myelin-reactive, and these T cells produce cytokines mimicking a Th1-mediated proinflammatory reaction. T-helper cells (CD4$^+$) appear to be critical initiators of myelin destruction in MS. These autoreactive CD4$^+$ cells, especially of the T-helper cell type 1 (Th1) subtype, are activated in the periphery, perhaps following a viral infection. The activation of T- and B-cells requires two signals. The first signal is the interaction between MHC and APC (macrophage, dendritic cell, and B cell). The second signal consists of the binding between B7 on the APC and CD28 on the T cell for T-cell activation. Similarly, CD40 expressed on APCs and CD40L expressed on T cells interact with signaling the proliferation of B cells within the blood—brain barrier following the entry to T cells. The T cells in the periphery express adhesion molecules on their surfaces that allow them to attach and roll along the endothelial cells that constitute the blood—brain barrier. The activated T cells also produce MMP that help create openings in the blood—brain barrier, allowing entry of the activated T cells past the blood—brain barrier and into the CNS. Once inside the CNS, the T cells produce proinflammatory cytokines, especially interleukins (ILs) 1, 2, 12, 17, and 23, tumor necrosis factor-α (TNF-α), and interferon-γ (INF-γ), which further create openings in the blood—brain barrier, allowing entry of B cells, complement, macrophages, and antibodies. The T cells also interact within the CNS with the resident microglia, astrocytes, and macrophages, further enhancing the production of proinflammatory cytokines and other potential mediators of CNS damage, including reactive oxygen intermediates and nitric oxide. The role of modulating, or downregulating, cytokines such as IL-4, IL-5, IL-10, and transforming growth factor-β (TGF-β) also has been described. These cytokines are the products of CD4$^+$, CD8$^+$, and Th1 cells.[9] New pathogenic mechanisms involve, but are not limited to, receptor-ligand–mediated T-cell entry via choroid plexus (CCR6-CCL20 axis),[26] coupling of key receptor-ligands for inhibition of myelination/demyelination (LINGO-1/NOGO66/p75 or TROY complex, Jagged-Notch signaling). (Ag, antigens; APC, antigen presenting cell; DC, dendrite cell; IgG, immunoglobulin G; MΦ, macrophage; Na$^+$, sodium ion; MMP, matrix metalloproteinases; MHC, major histocompatibility complex; OPC, oligodendrocyte precursor cell; VLA, very late antigen; VCAM, vascular cell adhesion molecule.)

produced by demyelination and axonal damage and reflect the damaged CNS area. Secondary symptoms are complications resulting from primary symptoms; for example, urinary retention, a primary symptom, can lead to frequent urinary tract infections (UTIs), a secondary symptom. Lastly, tertiary symptoms relate to the effect of the disease on the patient's everyday life.[33]

The clinical course of CDMS is classified into three categories: (1) RRMS, (2) SPMS, and (3) PPMS.[34] At symptom onset, about 85% of patients have relapses/exacerbations, with new symptoms lasting at least 24 hours and separated from other new symptoms by at least 30 days, followed by complete or incomplete remission. Exacerbations are referred to as relapses or attacks. This course is called RRMS, which is characterized by CNS inflammation. The first clinical presentation of RRMS is typically CIS, which is not a definite form of MS. During the RRMS phase, new brain MRI lesions correlate with clinical attacks, but typically, there are more new MRI

CLINICAL PRESENTATION Multiple Sclerosis

General

- Most patients with MS present with nonspecific complaints.

Primary Symptoms/Signs

- Visual complaints/optic neuritis
- Gait problems and falls
- Paresthesias
- Pain
- Spasticity
- Weakness
- Ataxia
- Speech difficulty
- Psychological changes
- Cognitive changes
- Fatigue
- Bowel/bladder dysfunction
- Sexual dysfunction
- Tremor

Laboratory Tests

- MS is a diagnosis of exclusion
- MRI
- CSF studies
- Evoked potentials

Secondary Symptoms

- Recurrent UTIs
- Urinary calculi
- Decubiti and osteomyelitis
- Osteoporosis
- Respiratory infections
- Poor nutrition
- Depression

Tertiary Symptoms

- Financial problems
- Personal/social problems
- Vocational problems
- Emotional problem

lesions than new clinical symptoms. In RRMS patients, attack frequency tends to decrease over time and becomes independent of the development of progressive disabilities.[35] Neurologic recovery following an exacerbation is often quite good early in the disease course, but recovery following repeated relapses is not as complete. A new concept of a radiologically isolated syndrome (RIS) refers to individuals who have an MRI scan done for other reasons (eg, headache) and have radiological signs suggestive of MS. This is not a form of definite MS; however, over time, a percentage of these patients convert to RRMS.[36] When to start DMT remains unclear and varies by practice.

Approximately 10% to 20% of RRMS patients have a benign course (a retrospective diagnosis), characterized by few relapses that are often sensory in nature with minimal disability over time. Most RRMS patients (not with benign disease) eventually enter a progressive phase, referred to as SPMS, in which attacks and remissions are challenging to identify. Disability tends to accumulate more significantly during this phase of the illness. Additionally, new brain MRI lesions, especially those only seen with contrast media, are less common, and brain atrophy and T1 holes increase.[37]

4 Approximately 15% of patients never have discrete phases of attacks and remissions but rather have progressive disease from the outset, known as PPMS. These patients will have symptoms, especially spastic paraparesis, that may or may not worsen rapidly over time and accrue progressively more disability. Patients with PPMS are often diagnosed at later ages, with the number of males roughly equal to females. In general, PPMS patients tend to have a worse prognosis than those initially presenting with RRMS, although progression is variable.[38] A significant portion of patients with PPMS do not receive benefits from studied therapies, although ocrelizumab (Ocrevus) is FDA-approved for PPMS.[39] Both PPMS and SPMS are characterized as neurodegenerative processes. Previously, a small percentage of patients were classified as having a mixture of both progression and relapses, referred to as progressive-relapsing multiple sclerosis (PRMS), but since they are generally treated as relapsing patients, this nomenclature is no longer used.

The most widely used clinical rating scale is the EDSS, which uses a numerical value ranging from 0 (no disability) to 10 (death) to evaluate neurologic functions.[40] However, this scale is relatively insensitive to clinical changes not involving impairment of ambulation, such as fatigue, cognition, and affect. Other tools, such as the multiple sclerosis functional composite (MSFC), are being evaluated as a more sensitive measure for changes in MS-related disability over time.[41] Increasingly, MRI is used as an index of both disease activity and progression[18] with new lesions appearance or changes in lesion number, size, and volume used as outcome measures in research studies. Optical coherence tomography measures the retinal neural fiber layer thickness and may also be a measurable sign of pathological progression over time.[42]

The unpredictable nature of MS makes it impossible to anticipate exacerbations. However, certain factors, including infections, heat (including fever), sleep deprivation, stress, malnutrition, anemia, concurrent organ dysfunction, exertion, and childbirth, may aggravate symptoms or lead to an attack. Interestingly, patients experience a significant reduction in relapses during the third trimester of pregnancy, followed by a relative increase postpartum.[43]

Between 60% and 80% of individuals diagnosed with MS have been reported to be sensitive to environmental heat, as temperature influences nerve impulses that are blocked or slowed down in a damaged nerve. Clinically, increased body temperature might worsen previous neurological deficits, including fatigue and decreased muscular endurance. Blurred vision, known as Uhthoff's phenomenon, is caused by increased body temperature due to physical exercise or physical restraint; however, these signs and symptoms improve or disappear after temperature normalization.

Multiple sclerosis does not directly diminish life expectancy. However, the development of secondary complications such as pneumonia or septicemia (secondary to aspiration in those with swallowing difficulties, decubitus ulcers, or UTIs), or rapid progression of primary lesions affecting respiratory function, can lead to a shorter than expected life span. Most life span decreases are seen in patients with rapidly progressive disease. Suicide rates in MS patients have been reported to be significantly higher than that seen in the general population.[44] The clinical and demographic factors used to predict prognosis are listed in Table 74-6.[7,42]

Diagnosis

5 Multiple sclerosis is a diagnosis of exclusion as symptoms can frequently be attributed to other neurologic diseases, just as many syndromes can mimic MS. The diagnosis remains primarily a clinical one that requires demonstration of "lesions separated in space and time." This terminology refers to the occurrence of at least two episodes of neurologic disturbance, which reflect specific sites of CNS damage that cannot be explained by other mechanisms.[47] The McDonald criteria, established by an international panel of MS experts,[47] allow for three diagnostic categories which include (1) MS, (2) possible MS (for those individuals at high risk of developing MS), and (3) not MS. These criteria aid in earlier diagnosis compared to older criteria,[45] as they may be somewhat more sensitive and equally specific.[46,48,49] Key to diagnosis is an MRI which is endorsed by the American Association of Neurology consensus panel.[50] In addition to brain MRI lesions, CSF abnormalities, and visual-evoked potential (VEP), studies may be substitutes for clinical lesions in defining "separated in space and time." The 2017 updated McDonald criteria allow for an earlier diagnosis in patients with CIS to establish "dissemination in space and time" with a single MRI.[47] Therefore, patients only need to have lesions in different CNS areas with at least one enhancing lesion that correlates with clinical symptomatology to fulfill these criteria and be diagnosed with CDMS. As an example, several immunotherapies are US FDA-approved for use after a single attack (CIS) of demyelination in the context of an appropriately abnormal brain MRI.

Laboratory Studies

To date, there are no tests specific for MS but rather, evidence is gathered through (1) MRI of the brain and spine,[50,51] (2) CSF evaluation examining for increased oligoclonal bands and increased IgG, (3) evoked potentials,[45,47] and (4) optic coherence tomography.[52] These should all be used in conjunction with the physical examination and history in establishing the diagnosis. Of these tests, MRI is the most valuable diagnostic tool as the brain and spine images reflect damage characteristic of MS plaques in multiple areas of the CNS. Therefore, MRI is the preferred technique for establishing a diagnosis, prognosis, and determining disease progression. Optic neuritis, a lesion or lesions on the optic nerve, is a common first symptom of MS. A more significant number of T2-weighted lesions (called *T2 burden of disease*) on MRI following optic neuritis or CIS appears to correlate with the development of disability and progression to CDMS.[51] Through the use of the contrast agent gadolinium, new lesions and disruptions of the blood–brain barrier can be determined and are associated with early conversion to CDMS in CIS patients.[51,53] However, these gadolinium-enhanced lesions do not correlate well with disability progression when examined over time, while brain atrophy, even early in the course of the illness, probably correlates better.[50]

Differential Diagnosis

Because many disorders can mimic MS, most patients are first screened with blood tests for rheumatologic, collagen-vascular, infectious, and sometimes inherited metabolic diseases. Additionally, electromyography may help in diagnosing amyotrophic lateral sclerosis and neuropathies.

Magnetic resonance imaging is used to rule out tumors and cervical spondylosis and may also lead to MS evaluations for many patients with little or no clinical history of MS. While some patients may have MRI scans suggestive of MS (so-called RIS), most have nonspecific scans with identifiable causes for their symptoms, including age greater than 50 years, hypertension, and migraine.[54] The use of established criteria for distinguishing MS lesions from other etiologies enhances diagnostic accuracy.

TREATMENT

Treatment of MS falls into three broad categories: (1) treatment of exacerbations, (2) disease-modifying therapies (DMTs), and (3) symptomatic therapies. While treatment of exacerbations will shorten the duration and possibly decrease the severity of the attack, the DMTs can alter the course of the illness and diminish progressive disability over time; however, symptomatic disease management is of utmost importance to maintain quality of life. Although different treatment modalities have been studied in the last 30 years, older trials are flawed, and as such, there are no universally accepted treatment algorithms for MS. In 2018 the American Academy of Neurology (AAN) released DMT practice guidelines for adult MS. One potential algorithm for the immunotherapy of CDMS is shown in Fig. 74-3.[55] The Consortium of Multiple Sclerosis Centers also put out guidelines on treatment selection based on patient-specific factors.[56] However, treatment recommendations often vary among clinicians and centers, and decisions are frequently based on the wishes and goals of individual patients.

Desired Outcomes

The main treatment goals are to improve the overall quality of life, maintain employment, and minimize long-term disability for MS patients. Disease-related treatment goals include reducing exacerbations or relapses, decreasing the number of white matter lesions and black holes on MRI, averting brain atrophy, and ultimately halting disease progression. Both treatment and disease-related goals can be obtained with early disease recognition and immediate utilization of FDA-approved DMTs.

General Approach to Treatment

The severity of symptoms at initial presentation will determine whether an induction or escalation algorithm is assigned to an individual patient. When currently available FDA-approved medications do not alter natural disease progression, investigational agents or non–FDA-approved medications, such as rituximab, may be used. The use of escalation approaches early in the disease course with safer yet partially effective medications is thought to be helpful.

MS unfortunately often affects individuals in their most productive years of life. Therefore, practitioners must help patients set realistic expectations over their lifetime by developing long-term treatment and management plans. Throughout this illness, patients are likely to acquire secondary and tertiary MS symptoms. In clinical trials, high nonadherence rates are a factor in treatment failure. Nonadherence may occur due to perceived lack of treatment benefit, cost, adverse effects, depression occurrence, complicated dosing, and/or undesirable routes of administration (eg, subcutaneous, intramuscular injection, intravenous [IV]). Figure 74-3 represents a clinical algorithm for the treatment of MS.[55]

Nonpharmacologic Therapy

Medications are the primary mainstay of MS treatment. Still, patients may find occupational therapy beneficial to improve the activities of daily living or learn new techniques or tools to accomplish these tasks and remain active. Furthermore, physical therapy may improve muscle strength to improve their gait and balance, and stretching exercises reduce muscle spasms or help mobility through aids such as canes or walkers.

Pharmacologic Therapy

Treatment of Exacerbation

6 Exacerbations are the hallmark of early RRMS. Although recovery after relapses is generally complete, continued relapses over time may be associated with a substantial accumulation of

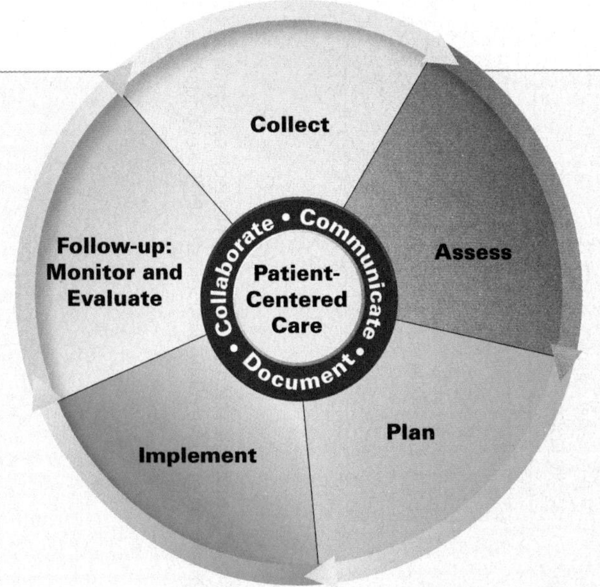

Patient Care Process for Multiple Sclerosis

The image shows the five fundamental steps included in The Pharmacist's Care Process endorsed by the Joint Commission for Pharmacy Practitioners (2014). The tagline of this process reads collaborate, communicate, and document. The five fundamental steps listed here are collect, assess, plan, implement, and follow-up: monitor and evaluate. All these steps are listed in a circular block diagram.

Collect

- Patient-specific demographics such as age, race, gender, geographical places of residence before or after the age of 15, current smoking level and history, family history of MS, and previous infection with certain viruses
- Laboratory values such as vitamin D, liver function tests, complete metabolic panel, and complete blood count (CBC)
- Magnetic resonance imaging (MRI) of the brain and spinal cord with and without contrast
- Lumbar puncture for oligoclonal bands
- Visual-evoked potential results
- Optical coherence tomography (OCT)
- Current diagnosis and date of initial diagnosis and current and past medications

Assess

- Clinical classification of MS (RRMS, SPMS, or PPMS)
- Disease progression using the Expanded Disability Status Scale (EDSS), and MRI results
- Total number of disease exacerbations or relapses
- Duration of therapy and dose for current and past medications, adverse medication reactions experienced during treatment, and medication adherence

Plan*

- Choose a therapy that has the best risk versus benefit profile for use in the specific form of MS diagnosed, as well as patient-specific characterizations and previous treatment history (Tables 74-1 to 74-3)
- Choose a therapy with the best adherence profile (twice yearly infusion vs three times weekly injectable), and more tolerable adverse medication reactions based on stratified risk factors (JC virus)
- Create a patient-specific monitoring plan based on the therapy chosen (Table 74-2)
- Identify the presence of secondary symptoms requiring pharmacologic management (Table 74-4)

Implement*

- Start primary MS therapy as soon as possible to decrease the chance for disease progression during treatment changes
- Figure 74-3 represents a potential algorithm for MS treatment
- Add pharmacologic treatment for secondary symptoms when appropriate
- Discuss with patients the role of complementary and alternative therapies (Table 74-5)

Follow-up: Monitor and Evaluate

- Safety of current DMT at each visit to ensure the current treatment is best for the specific patient
- Monitor for common adverse medication reactions with each specific DMT (Table 74-2) or any adverse medication reactions that are new once therapy is initiated or changed
- Treatment response (reduction in primary, secondary, and tertiary symptoms of MS) or the occurrence of exacerbations and relapses
- Yearly change in brain lesions via MRI
- Change in daily functioning using the EDSS and other clinical factors used to predict MS prognosis (Table 74-6)

**Collaborate with patients, caregivers, and other healthcare professionals.*

disability. Frequent relapses (more than three relapses per year in the first 2 years after diagnosis) have shown a consistent positive correlation with developing neurological disability later. However, mild exacerbations that do not produce functional decline may not require treatment. Therefore, decisions to treat relapses are usually substantiated by patient expectations, prior experience with corticosteroids, and predicted course of recovery. Accepted treatment indications for relapses that are (1) mono- or polysymptomatic presentations; (2) relapses that localize to the optic nerve, spinal cord, or brainstem; (3) those with functional limitations that affect activities of daily living; and (4) symptoms that worsen over a 2-week period. An IV injection of high-dose corticosteroids such as methylprednisolone is recommended by the AAN when functional ability is affected.[55] While corticosteroid mechanism of action in MS is unknown, they may improve recovery by decreasing edema in the area of demyelination. In particular intravenous methylprednisolone can shorten the exacerbation duration and also potentially delay repeat attacks for up to 2 years after optic neuritis,[55] although it does not definitively affect disease progression.[57]

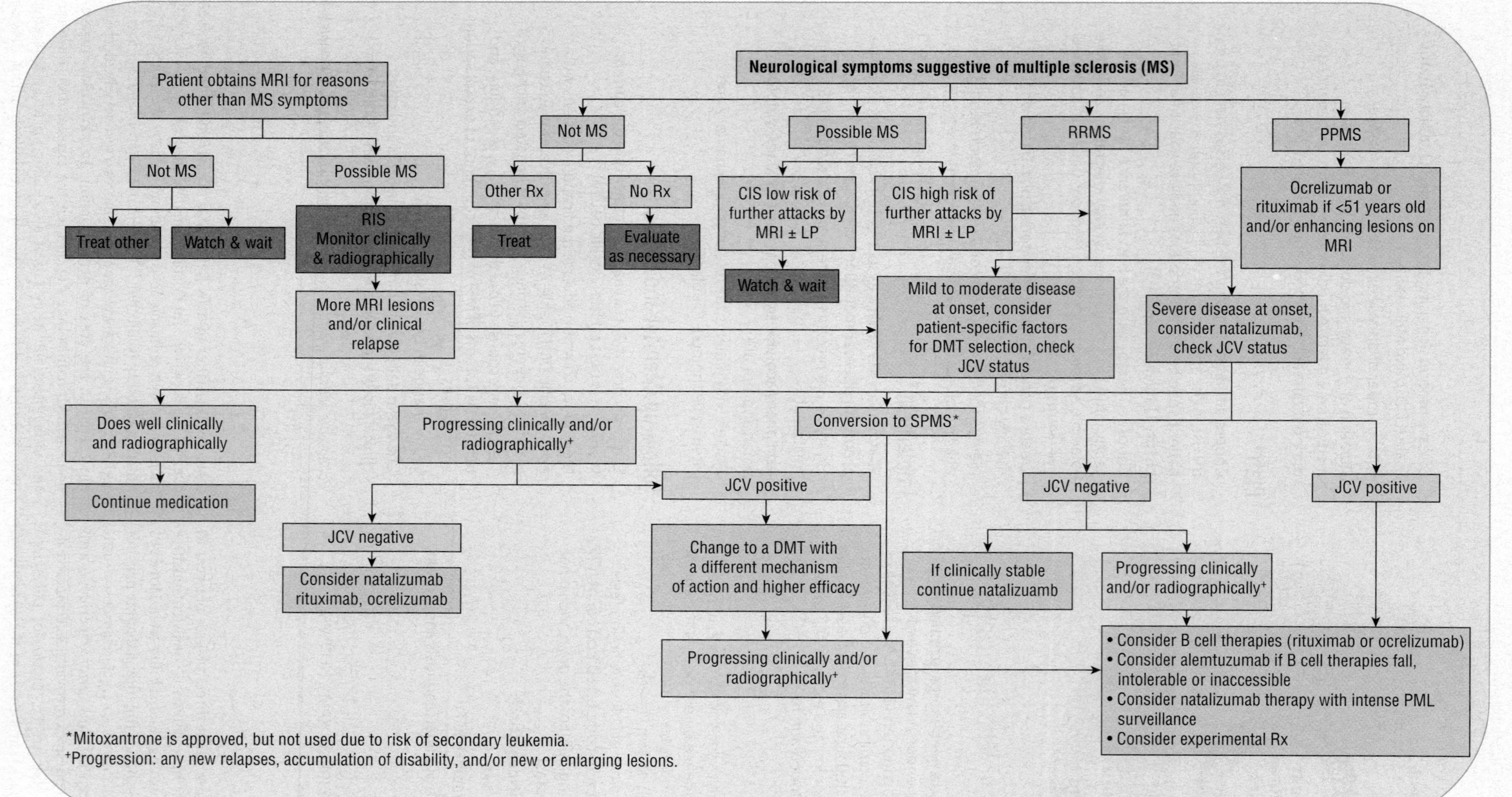

FIGURE 74-3 Algorithm for management of clinically definite multiple sclerosis. (MRI, magnetic resonance imaging; LP, lumbar puncture; MS, multiple sclerosis; CIS, clinically isolated syndrome; JCV, John Cunningham virus, PML, progressive multifocal leukoencephalopathy; RRMS, relapsing-remitting multiple sclerosis; PPMS, primary progressive multiple sclerosis; SPMS, secondary progressive multiple sclerosis; Rx, prescription medication; DMT, disease modifying therapy.)
Adapted from References 55 and 56.

According to clinical response, methylprednisolone doses range from 500 to 1,000 mg/day, given IV for 3 to (rarely) 10 days. In initiated within 2 weeks of symptom onset, the functional recovery after an exacerbation is more rapid, with improvement usually beginning after 3 to 5 days. Short-term steroid use is often accompanied by sleep disturbance, a metallic taste in the mouth, and rarely gastrointestinal (GI) upset. Patients with diabetes mellitus or a predilection to diabetes mellitus may have significant elevations of blood sugar, requiring the use of insulin. Intravenous methylprednisolone therapy is associated with acne and fungal infections, mood alteration, and, rarely, GI hemorrhage (especially in hospitalized patients or in those taking aspirin) when administered for longer durations. Equipotent doses of oral prednisone or dexamethasone can be substituted for IV methylprednisolone, although dexamethasone use is not well supported in the literature. Although adrenocorticotropic hormone (ACTH) is the only FDA-approved agent for MS exacerbation treatment, it is rarely used due to cost and availability.

A small number who experience a relapse of MS will have more severe attacks, manifested by hemiplegia, paraplegia, or quadriplegia. If improvement with aggressive steroid therapy is not seen, plasma exchange (PLEX) every other day for seven treatments can be beneficial for approximately 40% of patients, or intravenous immunoglobulin can be given.

A "pseudoexacerbation" must be ruled out before exacerbation treatment is initiated or DMTs are altered. Within this context, a "pseudoexacerbattion" occurs when symptoms occur for less than 24 hours or are precipitated by something other than the natural course of the disease, such as heat, infections (eg, UTIs), or stress (emotional or physical).

Disease-Modifying Therapy

Table 74-1 shows the indications and dosing of DMTs. Medications used to treat MS are either immunomodulatory (ie, alter the immune signals without cytotoxic effect or bone marrow suppression) or immunosuppressive (ie, alter the immune system through a direct cytotoxic activity or bone marrow suppression). These drugs, however, have a higher risk-to-benefit ratio based on their safety profile when used later on in therapy.[29] The current FDA-approved first-generation therapies are self-injected medications that decrease annualized relapse rate by about 30% and decrease the formation of new white matter lesions. These include four interferon (IFN) formulations and glatiramer acetate (a non-IFN). The first-generation DMTs are not immediately effective for symptoms, but rather their efficacy may be seen approximately 1 to 2 years after starting therapy. In addition to the first-generation DMTs, the FDA has also approved ocrelizumab, natalizumab, mitoxantrone, fingolimod, siponimod, ozanimod, ponesimod, teriflunomide, dimethyl fumarate, diroximel fumarate, monomethyl fumarate, cladribine, ofatumumab, and alemtuzumab for the treatment of relapsing forms of MS. Ocrelizumab is also FDA-approved for PPMS, and mitoxantrone has an additional FDA indication for progressive or worsening MS. These therapies are considered specialty medications and are only available through specialty pharmacies at a yearly cost of upwards of $100,000. This cost does not include nursing, pharmacy, and technical fees, especially for the infusion medications that require administration in an outpatient facility under medical supervision.

8 In some patients with poor prognostic factors and poor clinical presentation, ocrelizumab, natalizumab, fingolimod, teriflunomide, and dimethyl fumarate may be prescribed as initially instead of starting a first-generation DMT associated with less serious side-effect risk. This practice would be considered an induction therapy, where all therapeutic efforts concentrate in the early phases of the disease.

The efficacy of the DMTs may vary considerably between individual patients and for any given patient at different time points. Moreover, patients may have different adverse medication effects or risk tolerance and preferences regarding the administration route. Therefore, access to the full range of therapeutic options is critical for decision making between patients and their clinicians. Table 74-2 outlines adverse medication reactions and monitoring parameters of DMTs.

Interferon-β_{1b} and Interferon-β_{1a} IFN-β_{1b} (Betaseron, Extavia) was the first agent proven to favorably alter the natural course of the illness (Table 74-7).[57] Although its mechanism of action is unknown, it does exert immunomodulating properties, including augmentation of suppressor cell function, reduced IFN-γ secretion by activated lymphocytes, its macrophage-activating effect, and its ability to downregulate the expression of IFN-γ-induced class II MHC gene products on antigen-presenting glial cells. Additionally, IFN suppresses T-cell proliferation and may decrease blood–brain barrier permeability by reducing matrix metalloproteinases.[57] IFN-β also increases the production of regulatory CD56 (bright) natural killer cells and Treg cells.[60] In general, all IFNs exert these actions in the periphery and at the blood–brain barrier level.

IFN-β_{1b} is a nonglycosylated synthetic analog of recombinant IFN-β produced in *Escherichia coli*. It is administered subcutaneously every other day at a dose of 250 mcg (8 million international units). Clinical trials have demonstrated that at these doses, IFN-β_{1b} significantly reduces the annual relapse rate and MRI burden of disease compared with placebo; however, no significant differences between the IFN and placebo were noted with respect to clinical disability.[60] Betaseron is packaged in partially premixed syringes that do not require refrigeration and can be used with an autoinjector. In 2009, Extavia was approved; however, this is the same medicinal product as Betaseron.

IFN-β_{1a} (Avonex, Rebif) is a natural-sequence glycosylated IFN produced in Chinese hamster ovary cells. Avonex is administered as a 30-mcg dose (6 million international units) intramuscularly once weekly and Rebif is given as either 22 or 44 mcg subcutaneously three times weekly. Both are supplied in a 0.5-mL prefilled syringe which should be refrigerated but is stable at room temperature for 30 days. Rebif may have lower immunogenicity and a slightly better side-effect profile than Avonex.[61]

Patients receiving IFN-β_{1a} (Avonex) for 2 years demonstrated statistically significant reductions in annual relapse rates (by approximately one-third), as well as disease progression (defined as a confirmed decrease of one point on the EDSS), compared to placebo.[61] Patients receiving Avonex had significantly fewer new enhancing lesions on MRI compared with placebo, and similar results were seen with the higher dose of (44 mcg) of Rebif.[61] Other studies reveal Avonex's significant effects on slowing brain atrophy[62] and the progression of cognitive decline.[63] Therefore, these observations show that IFN-β possesses significant disease-modifying activity.

Pegylated IFN-β_{1a} (Plegridy) is FDA-approved for relapsing forms of MS. The attachment of polyethylene glycol (PEG) polymer chains to the interferon molecules result in a longer half-life and allows for less frequent dosing, as it is given by subcutaneous injections once every 2 weeks. Plegridy is associated with a significant reduction in annualized relapse rates (35.6%), new MRI lesions, risk of disability progression compared to placebo.[64]

All of the IFNs have similar adverse medication reactions, and CBCs, platelets, and LFTs should be documented at baseline, after 1 month of therapy, every 3 months for 1 year, and every 6 months thereafter. A small percentage of patients develop depressed blood cell counts that usually respond to therapy discontinuation. Transient

TABLE 74-1 Disease-Modifying Therapy

Medication	Brand Name	Indication	Initial Dose	Usual Dose	Comment
First-generation agents					
Self-injectables					
Interferon-β_{1a}	Avonex	Relapsing forms of MS	30 mcg (6 million IU) IM once weekly	30 mcg IM once weekly	Considered low potency interferon
	Rebif	Relapsing forms of MS	22 mcg SQ three times a week	22 or 44 mcg SQ three times a week	Considered a high potency interferon
Interferon-β_{1b}	Betaseron, Extavia	Relapsing forms of MS	250 mcg (8 million IU) SQ every other day	250 mcg SQ every other day	Betaseron/Extavia is considered a high potency interferon Pregnancy category C
Pegylated Interferon-β_{1a}	Plegridy	RRMS	6.3 mcg SQ day 1, then 94 mcg SQ on day 15, then 125 mcg SQ on day 29, then 125 mcg SQ every 14 days	125 mg SQ every 14 days	Can pre-medicate or concurrently use an antipyretic/analgesic for flu-like symptoms. Pregnancy category C
Glatiramer acetate	Copaxone, Glatopa	CIS, RRMS	20 mg SQ once daily or 40 mg SQ three times a week	20 mg SQ once daily or 40 mg SQ three times a week	Glatopa is the generic version of Copaxone. Pregnancy category B
IV infusion					
Mitoxantrone	Novantrone	SPMS and worsening RRMS	12 mg/m² IV every 3 months	12 mg/m² IV every 3 months	Lifetime dose should not exceed 140 mg/m². Pregnancy category D
Second-generation agents					
Oral					
Fingolimod	Gilenya	Relapsing forms of MS, in patients 10 years and older	Adult: 0.5 mg orally once daily. Pediatric: <40 kg 0.25 mg orally once daily, >40 kg 0.5 mg orally once daily	Adult: 0.5 mg orally once daily. Pediatric: <40 kg 0.25 mg orally once daily, >40 kg 0.5 mg orally once daily	Medication Guide required Pregnancy category C
Siponimod	Mayzent	Relapsing forms of MS	CYP2C9 *1/*1, *1/*2, *2/*2: 0.25 mg once daily on days 1 and 2, then 0.5 mg once daily on day 3, then 0.75 mg once daily on day 4, then 1.25 mg once daily on day 5. CYP2C9 *1/*3, *2/*3: 0.25 mg once daily on days 1 and 2, then 0.5 mg once daily on day 3, then 0.75 mg once daily on day 4	CYP2C9 *1/*1, *1/*2, *2/*2: 2 mg once daily beginning on day 6. CYP2C9 *1/*3, *2/*3: 1 mg once daily beginning on day 5	Medication Guide required. May cause fetal harm. CYP2C9 genotype testing required prior to initiating dose
Ozanimod	Zeposia	Relapsing forms of MS	0.23 mg once daily on days 1-4, then 0.46 mg once daily on days 5-7	0.92 mg once daily beginning on day 8	Medication Guide required. May cause fetal harm
Ponesimod	Ponvory	Relapsing forms of MS	2 mg on days 1 and 2, 3 mg on days 3 and 4, 4 mg on days 5 and 6, 5 mg on day 7, 6 mg on day 8, 7 mg on day 9, 8 mg on day 10, 9 mg on day 11, 10 mg on days 12-14	20 mg on day 15 and thereafter	Medication Guide required. May cause fetal harm
Dimethyl fumarate	Tecfidera	Relapsing forms of MS	120 mg delayed release twice daily for 7 days	240 mg delayed release twice daily	Pregnancy category C
Diroximel fumarate	Vumerity	Relapsing forms of MS	231 mg twice daily for 7 days	462 mg twice daily	May cause fetal harm based on animal data
Monomethyl fumarate	Bafiertam	Relapsing forms of MS	95 mg twice daily for 7 days	190 mg twice daily	May cause fetal harm based on animal data
Teriflunomide	Aubagio	Relapsing forms of MS	7 mg orally once daily	7 or 14 mg orally once daily	Cholestyramine and charcoal accelerate teriflunomide elimination. Pregnancy category X
Cladribine	Mavenclad	RRMS and active SPMS	3.5 mg/kg over 2-year treatment course, administered as 1.75 mg/kg in each year. Divide the 1.75 mg/kg dose over 2 cycles, each cycle lasting 4 to 5 consecutive days; do not administer more than 20 mg/day. In the first-year treatment course, initiate the first cycle at any time; administer the second cycle 23 to 27 days after the last dose of the first cycle	Second-year treatment course: Initiate the first cycle ≥43 weeks after the last dose of the first year's second cycle. Administer the second cycle 23 to 27 days after the last dose of the second year's first cycle. Following 2 years of treatment, do not administer oral cladribine during the next 2 years	Medication Guide required Contraindicated for use in females and males of reproductive potential. Lymphocytes must be within normal limits before initiating first treatment course and >800 cells/mm³ (0.8 x10⁹/L) before the second treatment course

(continued)

TABLE 74-1 Disease-Modifying Therapy *(Continued)*

Medication	Brand Name	Indication	Initial Dose	Usual Dose	Comment
IV infusion					
Natalizumab	Tysabri	Relapsing forms of MS	300 mg IV every 4 weeks	300 mg IV every 4 weeks	REMS Program required. Pregnancy category C
Alemtuzumab	Lemtrada	RRMS	First treatment course: 12 mg/day IV for 5 consecutive days (60 mg total dose)	Second treatment course: 12 mg/day IV for 3 consecutive days (36 mg total dose) administered 12 months after first treatment course	REMS Program required. Pregnancy category C. May pre-medicate with 1,000 mg methylprednisolone (or equivalent) immediately prior to infusion for first 3 days. Also, administer herpes viral prophylaxis starting on first day of treatment and continued for at least 2 months after completion of treatment or until $CD4^+$ count is at least 200 cells/mm^3 (0.2×10^9/L), whichever occurs last
Ocrelizumab	Ocrevus	Relapsing forms of MS and PPMS	First treatment course: 300 mg IV followed by 300 mg IV 2 weeks later. Start infusion at 30 mL/hr, then increase by 30 mL/hr every 30 minutes as tolerated to a maximum of 180 mL/hr for a duration of 2.5 hours or longer	Maintenance treatment (given 6 months after the end of first treatment, and every 6 months thereafter): 600 mg IV starting at 40 mL/hr and increased by 40 mL/hr every 30 minutes as tolerated to a maximum rate of 200 mL/hr for a duration of 3.5 hours or longer	REMS Program required. Fetal risk cannot be ruled out. Premedication: antihistamine 30 to 60 minutes prior to infusion and 100 mg methylprednisolone or equivalent corticosteroid 30 minutes prior to infusion. Can also consider and antipyretic. Observe patient for at least 1 hour post infusion
Self-injectable					
Ofatumumab	Kesimpta	Relapsing forms of MS	20 mg once weekly for 3 doses (weeks 0, 1, 2)	20 mg once monthly starting at week 4	Medication Guide required. Single-dose prefilled syringe pen. Based on animal data, may cause fetal harm

CIS, clinically isolated syndrome; IM, intramuscular; PRMS, primary relapsing multiple sclerosis; REMS, Risk Evaluation and Mitigation Strategy; RRMS, relapsing-remitting multiple sclerosis; SPMS, secondary progressive multiple sclerosis; SQ, subcutaneous; IU, international units..

Data from References 58 and 59.

TABLE 74-2 Adverse Medication Reactions and Monitoring Parameters

Medication	Adverse Medication Reaction	Monitoring Parameter	Comments
Interferon-β_{1a}	Depression, flu-like symptoms, leukopenia, injection site reactions	Electrolytes, CBC, LFTs, thyroid function, LVEF, depression LFTs at baseline, 1 month, and every 3 months for a year, and every 6 months thereafter	Avoid use in untreated severe depression
Interferon-β_{1b}	Depression, injection site reactions, leukopenia, flu-like symptoms	Electrolytes, CBC, LFTs, thyroid function, depression	Avoid use in untreated severe depression. More frequent injection site reactions reported
Glatiramer acetate	Injection site reactions, infection, hypersensitivity, chest tightness, urticaria	MRI, tissue necrosis, postinjection reaction	Chest tightness, urticaria can occur at any dose
Mitoxantrone	Bone marrow suppression, neutropenia, cardiotoxicity, AML, nausea, vomiting, diarrhea, alopecia	CBC, ECG, LVEF, LFTs	Secondary leukemia. Lifetime maximum dose due to cardiac toxicity
Fingolimod	Lymphocytopenia, macular retinal edema, AV block, infection, headache	CBC, ECG, varicella zoster antibody, blood pressure, ophthalmic examination, LFTs	Requires first dose observation. Contraindicated in patients receiving Class I and III antiarrhythmic medications and those with recent cardiac diseases*, second- and third-degree AV block. Ketoconazole increases serum concentrations (3A4 inhibition). Vaccine efficacy may be decreased
Siponimod	Infections, macular edema, bradyarrhythmia and atrioventricular conduction delays, decreased pulmonary function, liver injury, increased blood pressure	CBC, ECG, varicella zoster antibody, blood pressure, ophthalmic examination, LFTs	Requires CYP2C9 genomic testing. Contraindicated in *3/*3 genotype. Medication interactions with 2C9 and 3A4 inhibitors and inducers

(continued)

TABLE 74-2 Adverse Medication Reactions and Monitoring Parameters (*Continued*)

Medication	Adverse Medication Reaction	Monitoring Parameter	Comments
Ozanimod	Infections (URTI), AV block, bradycardia, hepatotoxicity, increased blood pressure, lymphopenia, macular edema, neurotoxicity, PML, decreased pulmonary function, varicella zoster infections	CBC, ECG, varicella zoster antibody, blood pressure, ophthalmic examination, LFTs	Medication interactions with strong CYP2C8 inhibitors and inducers and BCRP inhibitors. Avoid use of live attenuated vaccines during and for up to 3 months after treatment
Ponesimod	Infections, bradyarrhythmia and atrioventricular conduction delays, pulmonary function, liver injury, increased blood pressure, cutaneous malignancies, macular edema	CBC, ECG, LFTs, ophthalmic examination, varicella zoster antibody	Contraindicated in patients with recent cardiac diseases*, second- and third-degree AV block, sick sinus syndrome, or sino-atrial block unless patient has functioning pacemaker. Four-hour observation monitoring for patients with certain preexisting cardiac conditions
Dimethyl fumarate	Flushing, rash, pruritus, GI discomfort, lymphocytopenia, increased LFTs, albuminuria, PML	CBC, LFTs, MRI	Taking with food decreases incidence of flushing
Diroximel fumarate	Flushing, GI upset, hepatotoxicity, infections, lymphopenia, PML	CBC, LFTs, MRI	Less GI adverse events compared to dimethyl fumarate and may be better tolerated
Monomethyl fumarate	Flushing, GI upset, hepatotoxicity, infections, lymphopenia, PML	CBC, LFTs, MRI	Less GI adverse events compared to dimethyl fumarate and may be better tolerated
Teriflunomide	Steven-Johnson syndrome, liver failure, neutropenia, respiratory infection, activation of TB, alopecia, neuropathy	CBD, LFTs, blood pressure, pregnancy, TB test	Contraindicated in severe hepatic impairment. Possibility of TB reactivation. Active metabolite of leflunomide
Cladribine	Bone marrow suppression, cardiotoxicity, hepatotoxicity, infection, malignancy, neurotoxicity, PML, renal toxicity, hypersensitivity, headache	CBC before starting, 2 and 6 months after the first course of each cycle and periodically. HIV, HBV, HCV, TB screening, VZV antibody, pregnancy test, LFTs, MRI, PML, infection	Contraindicated with current malignancy, HIV infection or active chronic infections, pregnancy and lactation
Natalizumab	PML, depression, fatigue, respiratory infection, arthralgia, hepatotoxicity	JCV antibody, infection, MRI, LFTs, hypersensitivity reactions,	Risk of PML. Risk of IRIS when discontinued due to PML
Alemtuzumab	Infusion reactions, infections (nasophyaryngitis, UTI, URI, herpes viral infections), autoimmune disorders, thyroid disorders, immune-mediated thrombocytopenic purpura, goodpasture syndrome	CBC, thyroid function, antibodies to varicella zoster virus, HPV screening, serum creatinine, TB prior to treatment, infusion reactions, skin exams, urinalysis	Contraindicated with HIV infection. Birth control should be used during treatment and for 4 months after each treatment course. Nursing is not recommended during treatment and for 4 months following each treatment course
Ocrelizumab	Infusion reactions, nasopharyngitis, upper respiratory tract infection, headache, urinary tract infection, herpes virus–related infections, neoplasms	MRI, active infection before infusion, infusion reactions during and after infusion, skin infections	Live vaccines are not recommended during treatment and after treatment until B-cell repletion, administer all live vaccines 6 weeks before treatment. Evaluate for hepatitis B infection before first dose. Avoid pregnancy during treatment and for 6 months after stopping treatment
Ofatumumab	Infections, injection site reactions, reduction in immunoglobulins, headache	HBV screen, serum immunoglobulins, CBC, PML, MRI	Contraindicated in active HBV infection. Immunize at least 4 weeks prior to initiation for live or live-attenuated vaccines and 2 weeks prior for inactivated vaccines

*Cardiac disease including myocardial infarction, unstable angina, stroke, transient ischemic attack, and heart failure NYHA Class III/IV.

AML, acute myeloid leukemia; CBC, complete blood count; ECG, electrocardiogram; LVEF, left ventricular ejection fraction; IRIS, immune reconstitution inflammatory syndrome; PML, progressive multifocal leukoencephalopathy; LFT, liver function test.

elevations in liver enzymes can also be seen, which respond to treatment discontinuation. However, rare cases of liver failure requiring transplantation have been reported, which have resulted in package insert modifications for all IFN-β products to reflect this risk. Other more common adverse effects include injection-site redness and swelling, menstrual irregularities, and rarely injection-site necrosis. Injection-site reactions with IFN-β_{1b} are probably worse and can occur at any time. They can be lessened by rotating the injection site, using an autoinjector, using topical lidocaine, or applying ice before and after the injection. In addition, injecting the medications at body temperature (place under armpits to warm) will decrease injection-site pain.

Flu-like symptoms (eg, fever, chills, and myalgias) are seen in most patients and typically occur up to 24 hours after injection. These symptoms usually abate within 1 to 3 months after starting the injections; however, for some patients, they may persist. To alleviate these flu-like symptoms, patients may try taking the injection at bedtime to sleep through the most bothersome symptoms. They may also use a nonsteroidal anti-inflammatory agent or acetaminophen before and regularly for 24 hours after IFN-β administration. Using one-quarter or one-half the standard dose, with an increase to the full dosage over 1 to 2 months, is also beneficial in reducing flu-like adverse medication reactions.[65] Lastly, a short burst of oral prednisone can alleviate some adverse effects as this may suppress the transient immune activation that can occur following the introduction of IFN-β.[65]

Less common adverse medication reactions include transient shortness of breath or tachycardia, thyroid dysfunction, and neutralizing antibodies. All the IFNs, but especially IFN-β_{1b}, can produce depressive symptoms. Therefore, clinicians must monitor all patients carefully depressive symptoms and monitor closely for suicide risk. Most patients will not see MS symptom improvement when taking IFNs, and many will experience adverse medication reactions; thus, adherence is a significant issue.

Finally, safety data on IFN-β in pregnancy and lactation is lacking, and abortifacient activity in primates has been noted. Until adequate safety data are available, individuals who are biologically female and are able to get pregnant should be counseled to use appropriate contraception while using these products.

Glatiramer Acetate (Copaxone) Glatiramer acetate (formerly known as copolymer-1) is a synthetic polypeptide consisting of L-alanine, L-glutamic acid, L-lysine, and L-tyrosine. Its precise mechanism of action is unknown, but it appears to mimic the antigenic properties of myelin basic protein (MBP).[66] This agent may act directly to MHC class II receptors and inhibit the binding of MBP peptides to T-cell receptor complexes.[66] Glatiramer acetate induces Th2 (anti-inflammatory) lymphocytes in experimental allergic encephalomyelitis,[66] which is thought to contribute to "bystander" suppression at the site of the MS lesion, resulting in reduced inflammation, demyelination, and axonal damage.[57] However, it may also suppress T-cell activation and recent studies suggest it has a neuroprotective effect by inducing brain-derived neurotrophic factor.[67]

Given subcutaneously, as a daily 20-mg or three times weekly 40-mg dose, glatiramer acetate, or its generic biosimilar, Glatopa appear to have a relatively mild adverse effect profile with mild injection site pain and pruritus being most common. Approximately 10% of patients experience a one-time transient reaction consisting of chest tightness, flushing, and dyspnea beginning several minutes after injection and usually lasting no longer than 20 minutes. This postinjection reaction occurs with any dose and is not limited to the first injection. If patients have no history or evidence of coronary artery disease, they may be assured these reactions are almost always self-limited and benign.

Glatiramer acetate has demonstrated significant reductions in mean annual relapse rate (approximately 29%), comparable with the IFNs and may slow the progression of disability in patients with RRMS.[65] It also delays the development of T1 holes on brain MRIs.[68] Long-term uncontrolled data show that it remains safe and effective for over 10 years.[69] Glatiramer acetate needs to be stored in the refrigerator but can be kept at room temperature for up to 1 week.

The FDA-approved Copaxone for the treatment of RRMS based on a placebo-controlled trial in treatment-naive patients that demonstrated significant reductions in mean annual relapse rate (approximately 34%), number of new T1 and T2 lesions, and similar safety profiles.[70] Recent studies show favorable adverse medication effects and convenience profiles, with comparable efficacy when patients were switched from glatiramer acetate 20 mg daily to 40 mg three times weekly.[71]

Natalizumab (Tysabri) Natalizumab is a partially humanized monoclonal antibody directed at the cell surface adhesion molecule $\alpha_4\beta$-integrin (also known as very-late antigen 1, VLA-1). It works by attaching to VLA-1 and blocking its ability to interact with its ligand on CNS endothelium vascular cell adhesion molecule 1 (VCAM-1), resulting in activated lymphocytes that are denied entry past the blood–brain barrier.

Natalizumab significantly reduces the number of new gadolinium-enhancing lesions by more than 90%, diminished relapses by 60%.[72] Compared to placebo, natalizumab also significantly delayed disability progression.[73] When added to IFN-β_{1a} (Avonex), natalizumab reduced relapse rates by more than 50% and gadolinium-enhancing lesions by 84%, compared to patients who continued with IFN-β_{1a} alone.[74] In these trials, natalizumab was infused IV every four weeks and was relatively well tolerated, although approximately 1% of patients developed infusion reactions, and 6% developed neutralizing antibodies that diminished the efficacy of the medication.

Natalizumab is FDA-approved for use in relapsing forms of MS. Shortly after its approval, three patients were reported to have contracted progressive multifocal leukoencephalopathy (PML), a rare brain infection most commonly seen in patients with human immunodeficiency virus.[75-77] In response, the FDA issued a black-box warning about PML and required enrollment in a Risk Evaluation and Mitigation Strategy (REMS) program called TOUCH. While the estimated risk for PML is low, it is high compared to other MS treatments.[78] As of December 2017, natalizumab is correlated to 756 PML cases, with three factors impacting the overall risk; (1) duration of treatment (24 months or longer); (2) prior use of immunosuppressive therapies (mycophenolate mofetil, alemtuzumab, efalizumab, and rituximab); and (3) a history of anti-John Cunningham virus (JCV) antibodies.[79,80] Current recommendations are to screen patients at baseline and every 6 months with a JCV test while receiving natalizumab.[81] A two-step enzyme-linked immunosorbent assay (ELISA, STRATIFY TEST) is available for the qualitative detection of serum antibodies to the JCV, offering a false-negative rate of 2.5%.[79,80]

For those patients developing PML, a plasma exchange (PLEX) can help rapidly clear the medication from the blood.[82] An acute syndrome, referred to as immune reconstitution inflammatory syndrome (IRIS), is associated with acute neurological deterioration after PLEX, requiring high-dose steroids.[83] Natalizumab is generally reserved for patients with highly active disease or those who have not responded to more well-tolerated agents, given its risk profile.

Sphingosine-1-Phosphate Receptor Agonists (Fingolimod, Siponimod, Ozanimod, Ponesimod) Fingolimod (Gilenya) was the first oral DMT approved for MS. It mechanistically acts as a sphingosine 1-phosphate (S1P) receptor agonist and exhibits its immunosuppressant properties by sequestering circulating lymphocytes into secondary lymphoid organs. Additionally, fingolimod also reduces the infiltration of T lymphocytes and macrophages into the CNS, resulting in neuroprotective effects. In clinical trials, it decreased annualized relapse rates by approximately 52% compared to IFN-β_{1a}, and 92% of patients were free of gadolinium-enhancing lesions after 7 years of continuous therapy. However, this data was obtained using the 1.25 mg dose, which is different from the FDA-approved dose of 0.5 mg once daily. Fingolimod is the first DMT to have a pediatric indication for children age 10 years and older. Siponimod (Mayzent) and Ozanimod (Zeposia) bind to S1P receptors 1 and 5 with higher affinity and Ponesimod (Ponvory) binds to the S1P receptor only, which makes these agents more selective than fingolimod, which binds to receptors 1, 3, 4, and 5.

Fingolimod is associated with pronounced first-dose bradycardia. Other rarer adverse medication reactions include bradyarrhythmia or atrioventricular block, infections, macular edema, a decrease in forced expiratory volume over 1 second in patients with previously compromised lung function, liver enzyme elevation, sustained 1 to 2 mm Hg increases in systolic and diastolic blood pressure, and lymphoma. All patients starting fingolimod should be monitored for signs of bradycardia for 6 hours after the first dose, including hourly pulse and blood pressure measurement. Additionally, ECG monitoring should start before dosing and continue until the end of the observation period or until all symptoms resolve. For patients at higher risk, this monitoring should continue longer than 6 hours, and in some cases, continue overnight. A new 6-hour observation period is required for patients who have discontinued and wish to restart therapy; however, this requirement varies depending on the days of missed treatment. Furthermore, extended monitoring is recommended for patients with certain preexisting conditions such as QT prolongation or those receiving concomitant medications that slow the heart rate or atrioventricular conduction, cause QT interval prolongation, or have a known risk for torsades. The following class Ia and class III antiarrhythmic agents are contraindicated for concurrent use with fingolimod: quinidine, procainamide, disopyramide, amiodarone, bretylium, sotalol, ibutilide, azimilide, dofetilide, and dronedarone.[84] As of March 2018, PML has also been reported with fingolimod use in eight patients, which was seen after 3 years of exposure, and independent of natalizumab treatment.[78] Similar adverse events have been experienced in the pediatric population.

Since siponimod, ozanimod, and ponesimod bind more selectively to the S1P receptor, their labeling only requires first-dose observation for high-risk groups.[85,86] Additionally, ponesimod is a 4-hour first-dose observation compared to a 6-hour observation period.[87] Upon starting therapy, a slow titration is required for all three agents. However, siponimod also requires CYP2C9 genotype testing to determine dose adjustments or contraindications. For CYP2C9 genotypes *1/*1, *1/*2, or *2/*2, associated with normal metabolism, no dose adjustments are required. For CYP2C9 genotypes *1/*3 or *2/*3, associated with intermediate metabolism, a dose reduction is necessary, and siponimod is contraindicated for use in patients with a CYP2C9 *3/*3 genotype associated with poor metabolizer status.[85]

Additional monitoring recommendations for S1P receptor modulator use include baseline CBCs, LFTs, ophthalmologic examinations, and ECG in patients with known heart problems. Importantly, ketoconazole can increase the area under the curve of fingolimod by 70%. For patients requiring live vaccine administration (ie, Zostavax, Flumist, Measles, Mumps, and Rubella [MMR], Yellow Fever [YF-VAX]), consider doing so prior to starting fingolimod or waiting two months after discontinuation. Ozanimod should not be coadministered with CYP2C8 inhibitors, BCRP inhibitors, or strong CYP2C8 inducers.[86] Ponesimod leaves the blood in about 1 week if treatment needs to be stopped for any reason. This provides for flexibility if a patient needs vaccines, desires to start family planning, or has any infections that need to be addressed.[87]

Teriflunomide (Aubagio) Teriflunomide is an oral immunomodulatory agent, the FDA approved for the treatment of relapsing forms of MS. The medication works by inhibiting dihydroorotate dehydrogenase to prevent the proliferation of peripheral lymphocytes (T and B cells). The reduction of activated lymphocytes within the CNS reduces inflammation and demyelination in patients with MS. Teriflunomide is the active metabolite of leflunomide, an agent approved for treating rheumatoid arthritis, and is dosed as 7 or 14 mg orally once daily.

In CDMS patients, teriflunomide (7- or 14-mg dose) resulted in a 31% reduction in annualized relapse rates and unique active lesions per MRI scan compared to placebo.[88] Disability progression was also reduced by almost 30% for those receiving 14 mg of teriflunomide daily.[89]

Although teriflunomide is not metabolized by CYP450 enzymes, it inhibits CYP2C8 and induces CYP1A2. This medication is also a substrate for the breast cancer–resistant protein (BCRP); therefore, inhibitors of BCRP (eg, cyclosporine) may increase serum concentrations of teriflunomide. Additionally, teriflunomide inhibits other organic anion transporters such as OATP1B1 and OAT3; however, the significance of these medication interactions is unknown at this time. Concomitant use of warfarin and teriflunomide resulted in a 25% decrease in the international normalized ratio (INR), necessitating close monitoring. When coadministered with estradiol and levonorgestrel, the mean maximum serum concentration and area under the curve are increased.

Terifluonomide's most common adverse effects are increases in LFTs, alopecia, nausea, diarrhea, influenza, headache, and paresthesia. Recommended monitoring includes monthly LFTs for the first 6 months due to teriflunomide's black-box warning related to hepatotoxicity risk. Additionally, teriflunomide also has a black-box warning for teratogenicity, as animal studies linked oral teriflunomide with fetal malformations and embryo lethality in female rats, as well as reduced sperm count in male rats. Therefore, teriflunomide is contraindicated in pregnancy and in individuals of childbearing potential not using reliable contraception. During therapy or within 2 years after discontinuation, patients who become pregnant should enroll in the Aubagio Pregnancy Registry and consider a cholestyramine washout. Additionally, males may also consider a cholestyramine washout to reduce serum medication levels should their partner's pregnancy be desired, as this medication may remain in the blood for up to 2 years after discontinuation. Teriflunomide may activate tuberculosis, so a negative skin test or treatment of the disease must be documented prior to starting therapy.

Dimethyl Fumarate (Tecfidera), Diroximel Fumarate (Vumerity), and Monomethyl Fumarate (Bafiertam) Dimethyl fumarate, diroximel fumarate, and monomethyl fumarate true mechanism of action is unknown; however, they are in vitro nicotinic acid receptor agonists and in vivo activators of the nuclear factor (erythroid-derived 2)-like 2 (Nrf2) pathway that is involved in the cellular response to oxidative stress. Dimethyl fumarate and diroximel fumarate are both converted to the same active metabolite, monomethyl fumarate. These three DMTs are FDA-approved for relapsing forms of MS, including CIS, relapsing-remitting disease, and active secondary progressive disease in adults.

Esterases metabolize dimethyl fumarate in the GI tract, blood, and tissues with no known medication interactions. It is initially dosed at 120 mg (delayed release) orally twice daily. After 7 days, the dose is increased to 240 mg (delayed release) orally twice daily. Dimethyl fumarate decreases the annualized relapse rate by 44% to 52%.[90,91] Laboratory monitoring includes a CBC before starting therapy, 6 months later, and then annually. Adverse medication reactions include lymphocytopenia (2%-6%), increased LFTs, and flushing (40%), which are reduced by food intake and dissipate over 1 month. Four cases of PML are attributed to dimethyl fumarate use as of March 2018.[78] Rash, abdominal pain, diarrhea, nausea, and vomiting have also been reported, which decrease over 1 month and respond to symptomatic treatment; however, slowing the dose-escalation may reduce GI adverse medication reactions risk. Dimethyl fumarate has a pregnancy Category C classification.

Diroximel fumarate is dosed at 231 mg twice daily orally, increased to a maintenance dose of 462 mg (administered as two 231 mg capsules) twice daily after 7 days.[92] Monomethyl fumarate is dosed at 95 mg twice daily orally, increased to maintenance dose of 190 mg (administered as two 95 mg capsules) twice daily after 7 days.[93] Flushing associated with these agents can be reduced by coadministration with food or with 325 mg of a non-enteric-coated aspirin 30 minutes before dosing.[93] Both diroximel fumerate and monomethyl fumarate carry the same monitoring and laboratory recommendations as dimethyl fumarate, including PML risk. These agents also have a lower incidence of gastrointestinal symptoms compared to dimethyl fumarate.[94,95]

Cladribine (Mavenclad) Cladribine is an oral DMT whose mechanism is thought to impair DNA synthesis, resulting in dose-dependent depletion of both B- and T-lymphocytes. It is a prodrug, activated through phosphorylation to 2-chlorodeoxyadenosine triphosphate (Cd-ATP). It is indicated to treat relapsing forms of MS to include relapsing-remitting disease and active secondary progressive disease in adults. Cladribine has been shown to significantly reduce the annualized relapse rate as 81% of patients in clinical trials did not replase. Additionally, cladribine reduces the time to 3-month confirmed EDSS progression and the median number of active T1 Gd+ lesions and active T2 lesions compared to placebo.[96]

It is administered in two treatment courses, which occur approximately 1 year apart from each other, and consist of two cycles of treatment for a total of four doses over 2 years. The maximum lifetime dose of cladribine is 3.5 mg per kg bodyweight which is 1.75 mg per kg per treatment course. The first treatment course has two cycles, the first dose is started anytime, and the second dose is administered 23-27 days after the first dose of the first course. The second-year treatment course is started approximately 1 year after the start of the first course, and the final dose of treatment should be administered 23 to 27 days after the first dose of the second-year course.[97]

Adverse medication reactions from treatment include increased risk of infection (including Tb, hepatitis B or C, shingles, and PML), liver injury, and heart failure. Cladribine requires a medication guide due to its adverse medication effect profile and increased risk of malignancies and teratogenicity. Treatment monitoring includes cancer screening, CBC, infection screening (including MRI for PML), and liver enzyme tests. It is not indicated for the treatment of CIS due to its severe adverse medication reactions, and therefore should be saved for use in patients who have had an inadequate response or cannot tolerate other DMTs.[97]

Alemtuzumab (Lemtrada) Alemtuzumab is a humanized monoclonal antibody against CD52, a glycosylphosphatidylinositol-anchored protein consisting of 12 amino acids expressed at high levels on T and B lymphocytes, and to a lesser extent on monocytes, macrophages, and eosinophil granulocytes. Within a few minutes after infusion, alemtuzumab leads to depletion of CD52 positive cells through antibody-dependent cell-mediated cytolysis and complement-dependent cytolysis.

Alemtuzumab is FDA-approved for the therapy of RRMS. Compared to IFN-β_{1a} therapy alemtuzumab demonstrated a 50% reduction in relapses and a significant reduction in the 6-month accumulation of disability.[98,99] Additionally, MRI measures also proved alemtuzumab's superiority with significantly less gadolinium-enhancing lesions, new or enlarging T2 lesions, and brain atrophy.[98] Lastly, significantly more alemtuzumab than IFN-β_{1a}–treated patients were free of any clinical and MRI disease activity. Currently, alemtuzumab therapy is approved for two courses of treatment administered a year apart. In the first course, 12 mg is infused for 5 consecutive days and then for 3 days in the second course.

Alemtuzumab's high efficacy parallels its considerable high risk of infusion-associated reactions (IARs), affecting over 90% of patients.[100] Concomitant corticosteroids, antihistamines, and antipyretic medications can help avoid IARs. Other adverse medication reactions are commonly mild to moderate and consist of headache, rash, pyrexia, and nausea. Respiratory tract and UTIs are also common. During the clinical studies, the incidence of herpes infections led to the recommendation that prophylactic acyclovir treatment be implemented 0 to 4 weeks after alemtuzumab infusion to reduce infection rates significantly. Moreover, there are single case reports of spirochetal gingivitis, pyogenic granuloma, esophageal candidiasis, tuberculosis, and listeria meningitis. Thus, it is best to avoid unpasteurized cheeses while taking this medication.[100] PML has also been reported after the second alemtuzumab cycle; therefore, monitoring is warranted for all patients.[101]

Additional risks seen with alemtuzumab use include secondary autoimmune disease occurring in approximately 30% to 40% of patients, predominantly impairing thyroid function and manifesting as hyperthyroidism, hypothyroidism, goiter, and thyroiditis. There is also a small but serious risk of immune thrombocytopenia (ITP) that can occur post-alemtuzumab administration. Lastly, glomerulonephritis and single cases of autoimmune neutropenia, hemolytic anemia, and type 1 diabetes have been reported.[100] Therefore, extensive monitoring and early intervention allow for appropriate risk management.

Ofatumumab (Kesimpta) Ofatumumab is a recombinant human monoclonal immunoglobulin G1 antibody that binds to CD20 expressed B-cells resulting in antibody-dependent cellular cytolysis and complement-mediated lysis. It is indicated for the treatment of relapsing forms of MS, including CIS, RRMS, and active SPMS in adults. Ofatumumab is the only once weekly subcutaneous injection DMT intended for self-administration.

Clinical studies have shown that Ofatumumab results in a significantly lowered annualized relapse rate versus teriflunomide. It also reduces the risk of 3-month confirmed disability progression and the number of T1 Gd+ lesions and T2 lesions. These effects were also seen in subgroup analyses defined by sex, age, body weight, prior nonsteroid MS therapy, and baseline disability and disease activity.[102,103]

The initial dose is 20 mg given at weeks 0, 1, and 2, followed by 20 mg given once a month starting at week 4. Ofatumumab should be given subcutaneously in the abdomen, thigh, or outer upper arm, avoiding any moles, scars, stretch marks, or other irritated or tender skin. The first injection should be administered under the supervision of a healthcare professional. It is available as a Sensoready® pen and prefilled syringes, which are onetime use only. These preparations should be stored in the refrigerator and allowed to reach room temperature for about 15 to 30 minutes prior to administration.

Prior to the first dose, hepatitis B screening and serum immunoglobulins should be performed, as well as the administration of all live or live-attenuated vaccines. The most common adverse medication reactions include upper respiratory tract infection and headache. Other warnings include increased risk of infections (including PML), injection-related reactions, reduction in immunoglobulins, and fetal risk. For these reasons, ofatumumab has a Medication Guide.

Mitoxantrone (Novantrone) Mitoxantrone, a member of the anthracenedione family, is approved by the FDA for reducing neurologic disability and the frequency of clinical relapses in patients with SPMS (chronic) or worsening RRMS.[104] Based on the clinical trials to date, the best MRI outcomes were seen in relapsing patients.[105] Additionally, clinical trials specifically documenting its effects on slowing MS progression in patients with SPMS have not been done.[104,105] Thus, support for the use of mitoxantrone in this context is lacking.[106]

Mitoxantrone is administered as a brief (5- to 15-minute) IV infusion dosed at 12 mg/m^2 every 3 months with a maximum allowable lifetime cumulative dose of 140 mg/m^2. Evaluations of left ventricular ejection fraction and ECG are required prior to each dose, and if signs or symptoms of congestive heart failure develop, they should be reexamined. Other potential adverse medication reactions include nausea, alopecia, menstrual disorder, amenorrhea, upper respiratory tract infection, UTIs, and leukemia. Mitoxantrone's role in the treatment of MS remains unclear due to the cardiac toxicity that limits its long-term use. More recent estimates also suggest the risk of leukemia may be as high as 1 in 145 patients, which has significantly decreased interest in its use for MS patients.[106]

Rituximab (Rituxan) and Ocrelizumab (Ocrevus) Pharmacologically rituximab is a chimeric monoclonal antibody that targets the CD20 antigen on B cells. It is currently not FDA-approved for the treatment of RRMS and PPMS, but is often used off-label for this indication. In one retrospective observational study, its use demonstrated decreased in annualized relapse rate in RRMS and PPMS patients, while the EDSS remained unchanged.[107] Therefore, patients with PPMS who are less than 51 years old and have at least one gadolinium-enhancing lesion may benefit from rituximab therapy when given an infusion twice yearly.[107] The most common adverse reactions seen in this study were mild infusion-related reactions.

Ocrelizumab is a humanized version of the rituximab monoclonal antibody, and theoretically, it has lower autoantibodies formation and infusion reactions than its chimeric counterpart. Its mechanism of action is unknown but is presumed to involve CD20 binding, a cell surface antigen present on pre-B and mature B lymphocytes. Blocking CD20 effectively suppresses immune responses through depletion of CD20-expressing B cells.[39] It is the first medication FDA-approved for PPMS, and relapsing forms of MS.

Ocrelizumab has been associated with lower rates of disease activity and progression compared to interferon β_{1a} over the period of 96 weeks.[108] Its efficacy in PPMS patients was shown by approximately an 18% to 25% risk reduction in all study endpoints (ie, confirmed disability progression, timed 25-ft walk test [~7.5 m] performance, total volume of T2-weighted lesion, and decreased change in brain volume).[39]

Ocrelizumab's adverse events included infusion reactions necessitating subsequent dosing reductions, upper respiratory tract infections, and oral herpes activation. Neoplasms were also more common in the ocrelizumab group than placebo, with four patients receiving ocrelizumab developing breast cancer and three with basal cell carcinoma. Cervical adenocarcinoma in situ and basal cell carcinoma were the two neoplasms seen in the placebo group. This imbalance warrants ongoing evaluation in the context of the epidemiology of neoplasms in the MS population and the long-term experience with this and other CD20 treatments.[39] There have been a handful of cases with patients developing PML on ocrelizumab, but since all had natalizumab as prior therapy, they are considered carryover cases. In 2019, there was one case of a 78-year-old patient who developed PML on ocrelizumab and no prior DMT therapy, but other risk factors likely played a role in increasing this patient's risk. Regardless, monitoring for PML in all patients is recommended.

Ocrelizumab is given as a two-dose series via peripheral infusion, beginning with 300 mg given on day one and followed by another 300 mg on day 14. Subsequent doses of 600 mg are then given in 6-month intervals. Infusion rates are started at 30 mL/hr (for 300 mg in 250-mL bag starting doses) or 40 mL/hr (for 600 mg in 500-mL bag maintenance dose), which is stepped up based on patient tolerance, similar to rituximab. Monitor for infusion reactions throughout and up to 1 hour after infusion completion. The maximum infusion rate for the 300 mg is 180 mL/hr and 200 mL/hr for the 600-mg dose. Before ocrelizumab treatment starts, patients should be screened for hepatitis B, and for active infections before each infusion.[109]

TABLE 74-3 Key Recommendations on Treatment and Access Considerations

- Initiating therapy with an FDA-approved DMT is recommended as soon as possible following a definite diagnosis of relapsing MS. It can also be considered for selected patients with a first clinical attack consistent with MS where other potential causes have been excluded, as well as for patients with progressive MS with clinical relapses and/or inflammatory activity.
- Choice of initial or alternative DMT is complex and should be collaboratively done by the treating clinician and the patient.
- Clinicians should evaluate barriers to treatment adherence and counsel patients on its importance.
- Continue therapy indefinitely unless there is a clear lack of benefit, intolerable adverse medication reactions, inadequate patient adherence, new data that reveal other reasons for cessation, or a better therapy becomes available.
- The absence of relapses while on treatment should not justify treatment discontinuation. When switching DMTs due to suboptimal response, choose an agent with an alternative mechanism of action.
- For patients with highly active MS, clinicians should prescribe alemtuzumab, fingolimod, or natalizumab.
- Natalizumab can be initiated in patients with MS and positive anti-JCV antibody indexes above 0.9 only when there is a reasonable benefit outweighing the severe but low risk of PML.
- Ocrelizumab can be offered to patients with PPMS when the risks of treatment does not outweigh the benefits.
- Clinicians should counsel female patients to stop their DMT before conception for planned pregnancies. If accidental exposure occurs, clinicians should discontinue DMTs during pregnancy. They should not be initiated during pregnancy unless the risk of MS activity outweighs the DMT risk.
- Due to the significant variability in therapeutic response, contraindications, risk tolerance, and treatment adherence seen in the MS population, patient and clinician access to all available therapies is necessary as this may influence decisions regarding the route of administration and/or adverse medication effect tolerance.
- Patient access to medication should not be limited by the frequency of relapses, age or other personal characteristics, or level of disability. Therapy should not be withheld to allow for determination of coverage by payers, as this puts the patient at increased risk for recurrent disease activity.

Data from References 58 and 111.

Remaining Questions for Disease-Modifying Therapy

9 Despite the results from well-conducted clinical trials, several relevant treatment issues remain including; (1) when to begin therapy, (2) which agent to initiate, and (3) when to switch and stop therapies. The AAN has developed evidence-based guidelines regarding DMT use in MS. Key recommendations regarding initiating, switching, and stopping DMTs are summarized in Table 74-3.[55,110]

Decisions about medication use for MS include determining the illness severity, medication efficacy and adverse medication effect risks, and costs related to the therapy. These medications slow the course of the illness but do not suppress it completely, and in some individuals, no apparent benefit is reported. The vast majority of untreated patients will have progressive disease over time, and even in acute lesions, there is significant axonal damage that is essentially irreversible. MRI data show that 80% to 90% of all new enhancing lesions are asymptomatic, suggesting that a "quiet" clinical course does not necessarily mean there is not an ongoing disease activity that ultimately will lead to cognitive deficits and progressive spastic paraparesis.

Very early therapy is effective. In patients with CIS and two or more T2 lesions on brain MRI (ie, at high risk for developing CDMS), placebo-controlled studies with all three of the IFN agents and glatiramer acetate have shown significant delay in a second attack and positive outcomes on a variety of MRI measures.[57,110] Currently, the FDA has approved IFN-β_{1b}, IFN-β_{1a} (Avonex), glatiramer acetate, and some of the newer DMTs for use in CIS patients with abnormal MRIs consistent with demyelination. The AAN and CMSC recommend that patients with relapsing disease should be initiated on an FDA-approved DMT as soon as possible following diagnosis.[55,56,110]

Which DMT to use in which patient is the second major issue as there has not been a single, randomized study comparing DMTs in similar patient populations at the same time.[112] In the case of the first-generation self-injectables (see Table 74-2), results from pivotal placebo-controlled trials were more similar than different, including a nearly identical one-third reduction in relapse rate for all four medications over 2 years. A small number of studies suggest that frequent administration of IFN at higher doses may be more efficacious than lower dose, less frequent administration.[113,114] Other studies argue against this,[111,115] and some note no outcome differences between standard and double dose IFN-β_{1b} and glatiramer acetate,[115,116] or between IFN-β_{1a} (Rebif) and glatiramer acetate.[117]

Further complicating this issue is our understanding of the clinical differences between IFN products and the development of neutralizing antibodies. Between 30% to 40% of patients receiving IFN-β_{1b} develop antibodies directed against the medication; however, the exacerbation rate in these patients was similar to that seen in placebo-treated patients.[118] Neutralizing antibodies can occur as early as 3 to 6 months into IFN-β_{1b} treatment and as late as 18 months, as this product is the most antigenic.[119] Additionally neutralizing antibodies were found in 22% of early trials with IFN-β_{1a} (Avonex), but later studies report an incidence of 2% to 5%. This difference may be due to a formulation change making the product less antigenic.[111,117] Percentages of antibody formation for Rebif (approximately 12%) are intermediate. They may occur in the first 9 to 15 months of treatment, similar to Avonex.[118,119] Approximately 6% of patients treated with natalizumab show neutralizing antibodies that seem to diminish efficacy.[74] The long-term clinical significance of these findings is not completely clear, although data confirms a negative relationship between neutralizing antibodies and relapses, MRI lesions, and disability progression.[119-122] It is unknown if these antibodies cross-react between products, the duration of time in which they can be detected, and the impact corticosteroids have on their formation. Consensus guidelines outline when to test for neutralizing antibodies, which assay to use, or what titer cutoff to apply to patients in clinical settings exist.[123]

8 DMTs have been used to treat MS for more than two decades; however, patients continue to have more relapses, MRI lesions, disabilities, and ongoing disease progression to SPMS.[124] Although there is no accepted definition of treatment inadequacy, the Canadian Multiple Sclerosis Research Council has suggested a relatively simple approach that incorporates the elements of relapse rate, new MRI lesions, and change on the EDSS.[125] First, if significant and persistent IFN antibodies develop, switching to a non-IFN antibody (glatiramer acetate, natalizumab, ocrelizumab, fingolimod, siponimod, ozanimod, ponesimod, teriflunomide, dimethyl fumarate, diroximel fumarate, monomethyl fumarate, ofatumumab, mitoxantrone, or possibly rituximab[126]) is reasonable. A second option is the addition of an immunosuppressant, such as monthly methylprednisolone,[127] azathioprine, methotrexate, or mycophenolate. As noted earlier, natalizumab added to IFN-β_{1a} produces rare cases of PML, and should not be used clinically. Interestingly, the addition of a statin, specifically atorvastatin, into a beta-interferon agent may worsen MS,[128] although more research is needed.

Symptomatic Management

10 Many MS symptoms either do not require pharmacologic management or are nonresponsive. This section addresses the primary symptoms for which pharmacologic management may be beneficial (Table 74-4).[33,129-132]

Gait Difficulties and Spasticity Gait problems can be caused by spasticity, weakness, ataxia, defective proprioception, or a combination of these factors. Spasticity is commonly encountered and tends to affect the legs more markedly than the arms, which can result in falls. As spasticity often presents late in the disease, the increased muscle tone of a spastic limb often lends pseudo-strength to patients with underlying weakness. While spasticity is amenable to pharmacologic intervention, muscle relaxants must not decrease muscle tone to the extent that ambulation is hindered.[33,130] Baclofen (Lioresal), a short-acting γ-aminobutyric acid (GABA) analog, is the preferred agent for spasticity and is started at 10 mg three times daily which is then titrated upward to achieve the desired response. Most patients respond with dosages between 40 and 80 mg/day, although some require dosages higher than the maximum recommended daily dose of 80 mg.[33,130] Due to oral baclofen's relatively short duration of action, continuous intrathecal administration of Gablofen may be used for patients unable to tolerate or unresponsive to oral therapy. Baclofen should not be abruptly discontinued to avoid seizures.[130]

Another effective agent for spasticity is tizanidine (Zanaflex), a short-acting, α-adrenergic agonist that acts in the CNS by increasing the presynaptic inhibition of motor neurons. Its efficacy is comparable to baclofen.[116] Starting at a dosage of 4 mg at bedtime, slowly titrated up over 2 to 4 weeks based on clinical response. The effective dosages range from 2 to 36 mg/day. Sedation, dizziness, and dry mouth are commonly reported adverse effects, but hypotension, as well as rare but severe hepatotoxicity, can occur. Tizanidine can be added to baclofen in small dosages, sometimes resulting in smaller doses of each medication and better outcomes.

In patients unable to tolerate baclofen or tizanidine, diazepam (Valium; 2-10 mg/day), clonazepam (Klonopin; 1-3 mg/day), or dantrolene sodium (Dantrium; 100-400 mg/day) may be alternatives; however, they generally are less effective. Mild spasticity may respond to gabapentin (Neurontin; 1,800-3,600 mg/day) or tiagabine (Gabitril; 8-56 mg/day) may be useful but adverse medication reactions can prohibit their use. Pregabalin (Lyrica; 75-300 mg/day) has similar features as gabapentin but is approximately three times more potent and does not saturate the GI tract L-transporter system, so it may prove helpful in treating spasticity.

Botulinum toxin type A (Botox) is effective in alleviating spasticity.[33] The amount required to exert a pharmacological effect is often too excessive to use safely in the larger muscles; therefore, its use is best limited to smaller areas of focal muscle spasm.

An alternative approach for gait disruptions are K^+ channel blockers such as 4-aminopyridine (4-AP), which can potentiate synaptic transmission and increase muscle twitch tension. Similar to 4-AP, dalfampridine (Ampyra; 20 mg/day) can improve walking speed in patients with MS.[131,132,137,138] In other countries, dalfampridine is referred to as fampridine.[138] Common adverse medication reactions of dalfampridine include UTIs, insomnia, dizziness, headaches, and balance disorders. This agent is associated with the risk of seizures, particularly when the maximum dose of 10 mg twice daily is exceeded. It is contraindicated in patients with a seizure history, and an REMS program is used to manage these risks. It is essential

TABLE 74-4 Treatment of Select Primary MS Symptoms

Spasticity	Bladder Symptoms	Sensory Symptoms	Fatigue
Baclofen	Propantheline	Carbamazepine	Amantadine
Dantrolene	Oxybutynin	Phenytoin	Antidepressants
Diazepam	Dicyclomine	Amitriptyline or other TCAs	Modafinil
Clonazepam	DDAVP	Gabapentin	Methylphenidate
Tizanidine	Self-catheterization	Lamotrigine	Dextroamphetamine
Tiagabine	Imipramine or amitriptyline	Pregabalin	Armodafinil
Gabapentin	Prazosin or terazosin	Duloxetine	Fluoxetine
Pregabalin	Botulinum toxin type A		
Botulinum toxin type A	Solifenacin		
Dalfampridine	Darifenacin		
	Trospium		
	Hyoscyamine		
	Mirabegron		
	Tamsulosin		
	Tolerodine		

DDAVP, desmopressin acetate; TCA, tricyclic antidepressant.

Data from References 28, 131, and 133–136.

to educate patients not to take products containing 4-AP with dalfampridine, as therapeutically, it is a comparable extended-release product, which also means the medication should not be chewed, crushed, or cut. If a dose is missed, patients should take it immediately, take their dose upon recognition and never double the dosage due to seizure risk.

Tremor Cerebellar symptoms such as tremor can be troubling and difficult to control. Helpful medications include propranolol, primidone, and isoniazid.

Bowel and Bladder Symptoms Incontinence, urgency, frequency, and nocturia, are indications of a hyperreflexic bladder (ie, inability to store urine) and are common complaints. A number of anticholinergic agents, including tricyclic antidepressants, are used to treat mild symptoms. Still, with all anticholinergic agents, great care must be used to avoid falls and decreased cognition. Antimuscarinic agents can also treat incontinence. In patients with significant sphincter detrusor dyssynergia, oral α-adrenergic blockers or intramuscular botulinum toxin type A may relax the internal sphincter (see Chapter 105, "Urinary Incontinence").

Intermittent self-catheterization and the Credé maneuver, with or without a concomitant anticholinergic agent, are recommended for large postvoid residual volumes (more than 100 mL) or when the urinary problem is hyporeflexic in nature (failure to empty). Cholinergic agents like bethanechol may also be used for a hyporeflexive bladder. Treatment is important as large post-void residual volumes increase UTI risk, and therefore, urinary acidifiers such as vitamin C or antiseptics such as methenamine mandelate may be used to prevent infections. Antibiotics used for UTI prophylaxis include sulfamethoxazole/trimethoprim, cephalexin, cinoxacin, and nitrofurantoin.

Constipation is the most common bowel complaint seen in patients with MS, as many medications (eg, opioids, anticholinergics) and voluntary water restriction in those patients with urinary urgency and incontinence may contribute to its risk. Increases in dietary fiber and hydration may alleviate this problem, but laxatives or enemas may be necessary (see Chapter 36, "Chronic Heart Failure").

Major Depression Depressive symptoms and major depressive disorder are common in patients with MS. The risk of suicide may be increased markedly.[137] Patients should be monitored closely for symptomatology and treated accordingly (see Chapter 88, "Depressive Disorders"). IFN products and natalizumab should be used cautiously in patients with significant depressive symptoms.

Sensory Symptoms Numbness and paresthesia are frequent sensory complaints related to MS, but usually do not require treatment. However, some patients may develop acute or chronic pain syndromes[130] such as trigeminal neuralgia and painful dysesthesias, for which treatment is necessary (see Chapter 79, "Pain Management").

Sexual Dysfunction Sexual dysfunction in both men and females is common and counseling should be offered to both partners. Phosphodiesterase inhibitors or Alprostadil, a prostaglandin E1, can be very effective for erectile dysfunction (see Chapter 103, "Erectile Dysfunction"). Sildenafil (Viagra) is currently being studied in females with MS and sexual dysfunction. Bupropion (Wellbutrin) is the preferable antidepressant in patients for whom sexual dysfunction is a concern, due to its lower incidence of sexual adverse medication reactions.

Fatigue Fatigue, a common complaint in MS patients, can be severely disabling, but often overlooked. Typically, it presents in the mid-to-late afternoon and can increase with heat exposure, exertion, concurrent infection, spasticity, weakness, and depression. Amantadine hydrochloride (100 mg twice daily) may offer significant relief.[33,129] Methylphenidate (Ritalin), dextroamphetamine (Dexedrine, Adderall), and related products are used commonly. Modafinil (Provigil), 200 to 400 mg daily, may be helpful for MS-related fatigue. Its *R*-enantiomer, armodafinil (Nuvigil), is dosed at 150 mg or 250 mg daily, reaches peak concentrations more quickly, and has potentially fewer adverse medication reactions than modafinil. In patients suffering from both depressive symptoms and fatigue, a more activating antidepressant such as fluoxetine may be employed.

Cognition Cognitive dysfunction affects up to 50% or more of patients and manifests itself as word-finding difficulties and problems with concentration and short-term memory. Carefully review the patient's current medications before adding pharmacotherapy for cognitive dysfunction, as there are reports that statins and long-term proton-pump inhibitors can cause memory concerns. Cognitive dysfunction can be treated with stimulants or cholinesterase inhibitors if appropriate.

Pseudobulbar Palsy Pseudobulbar palsy is a condition caused by progressive degeneration of the corticobulbar tract in patients with MS. Symptoms include dysarthria, dysphonia, dysphagia, and sudden, inappropriate, uncontrollable, emotional outbursts such as crying or laughing. A combination product of dextromethorphan and quinidine 20 mg/10 mg (Nuedexta) is used for its treatment; however, its mechanism of action is unknown. It is dosed as one capsule daily for 1 week, followed by one capsule twice daily. The quinidine included in this product inhibits the CYP2D6 enzyme leading to an increased dextromethorphan serum concentrations.

Complementary and Alternative Therapies for MS

Approximately 33% to 80% of patients with MS use complementary and alternative medicine (CAM) therapies.[133] These include the use of diet and dietary supplements such as vitamins, minerals, and herbs. Antioxidant supplements vitamin A, C, E, α-lipoic acid, coenzyme Q10, grape seed, pine bark extracts, mangosteen, and acai have suggestive benefits. However, for patients with MS, the antioxidant supplements hold a theoretical risk given their ability to stimulate the immune system (T cells and macrophages). Thus, their use may worsen or exacerbate their disease by counteracting the effects of immunomodulators. Other immune-stimulating supplements such as garlic, ginseng (Asian and Siberian), Echinacea, cat's claw, astragalus, alfalfa, and stinging nettle should be used with caution.[134]

Table 74-5 outlines updated AAN evidence-based CAM recommendations in MS.[133] The safety of these therapies when used in combination with DMTs has not been studied. Nor has information about medication interactions, however, healthcare providers can provide objective information regarding CAM use in MS and can assist their patients in making decisions.[122] A few of the CAM therapies listed below have been given Level A recommendations, meaning their use has been established but for most a Level B recommendation has been given, meaning they are probably effective.[122]

Vaccine Recommendations

Avoid live vaccine administration in any patients with MS receiving DMTs due to immunosuppression and the potential for the live virus vaccines to increase MS disease activity. Vaccines considered safe include the human papillomavirus, tetanus, rabies, and inactivated polio.[56] A yearly flu shot is recommended for all patients with MS, including those receiving any DMTs, while the intranasal influenza vaccine FluMist, a live-attenuated vaccine, is not. It is unknown if the intranasal influenza vaccine directly interacts with DMTs.[132] An exception to this rule applies to patients taking fingolimod, and alemtuzumab, who are negative for varicella-zoster antibodies. They should receive the non-live virus immunization at least 2 months

TABLE 74-5 American Academy of Neurology Evidence-Based Recommendations on CAM Therapies in MS

CAM Therapy	Type of MS	Symptoms and Reported Use	Effective	Ineffective	Recommendation Level
Oral cannabis extract	RRMS, SPMS, PPMS, MSU	Symptoms of spasticity and pain	x		A
	RRMS, SPMS, PPMS	Signs of Spasticity (short term), tremor (short term)		x	B
	MSU	Signs and symptoms of spasticity (long term)	x		C
	RRMS, SPMS, PPMS, MSU	Bladder symptoms, urge incontinence			U
Synthetic THC	RRMS, SPMS, PPMS	Symptoms of spasticity, pain	x		B
	RRMS, SPMS, PPMS	Signs of spasticity (short term), tremor (short term)		x	B
	MSU	Signs and symptoms of spasticity (long term)	x		C
	RRMS, SPMS, PPMS, MSU	Bladder symptoms, urge incontinence, central neuropathic pain			U
Sativex oromucosal spray	MSU	Symptoms of spasticity, pain, urinary frequency	x		B
		Signs of spasticity, incontinence episodes		x	B
		Tremor		x	C
		Anxiety/sleep, cognition, QOL, fatigue			U
Smoked cannabis	RRMS, SPMS, MSU	Spasticity, pain, balance and posture, cognition			U
Ginkgo biloba	RRMS, SPMS, PPMS	Fatigue	x		C
		Cognitive function		x	A
Lofepramine plus phenylalanine with B_{12} (Cari Loder regimen)	RRMS, SPMS, PPMS	Disability, symptoms, depression, fatigue		x	C
Reflexology	MSU	Paresthesia	x		C
		Pain, HRGOL, disability, spasticity, fatigue, cognition, bowel/bladder function, depression, anxiety, insomnia			U
Bee venom	RRMS, SPMS	MRI lesion number and volume, relapses, disability, fatigue, HRQOL		x	C
Magnetic therapy	RRMS, SPMS, PPMS	Fatigue	x	x	B
		Depression			B
Low-fat diet with omega-3 supplementation	RRMS	Relapses, disability, MRI lesions, fatigue, QOL		x	B

CAM, complementary and alternative medicine; HRQOL, health-related QOL; MS, multiple sclerosis; MSU, MS type unspecified; PCE, oral cannabis extract; PPMS, primary progressive MS; QOL, quality of life; RRMS, relapsing-remitting MS; SPMS, secondary progressive MS; THC, tetrahydrocannabinol; A, established as effective or ineffective; B, probably effective or ineffective; C, possibly effective or ineffective; U, insufficient evidence to determine effectiveness or ineffectiveness.

Data from Reference 139.

before beginning treatment to allow time to mount an antibody response prior to immunosuppression. For unvaccinated patients at high risk for hepatitis B exposure, this vaccine should be given prior to ocrelizumab doses. This vaccine is not necessary for patients at low risk for exposure.[56]

EVALUATION OF THERAPEUTIC OUTCOMES

For those with acute MS exacerbations, treatment response is commonly seen within days. However, the clinician and patient should recognize that short-term (days to weeks), little or no apparent benefit may be noted when using a DMT. Therefore, therapeutic outcome evaluation is conducted over months to years by monitoring MS exacerbations, hospitalizations, disease progression, and disability measured using scales such as EDSS. Patients should be given realistic goals and treatment expectations to maximize medication adherence, in addition to being fully counseled regarding adverse effects. They should also be encouraged to participate in the evaluation of therapeutic response and actively encouraged to adhere to their prescribed regimens. If nonadherence is suspected, an investigation into barriers, such as injection fatigue or intolerable adverse medication reactions, should be done. Discussion around medication cost and/or switching agents to one that may provide increased adherence should also be done.

Each DMTs has specific safety monitoring recommendations to follow. Specific safety monitoring parameters for the newer DMTs can be found in Table 74-2. In general, patients on any DMT should receive regular laboratory monitoring and close observation, including regular neurologic examinations, frequent evaluation for adverse effects, and/or changes in disability. Natalizumab and alemtuzumab have REMS programs, and fingolimod, siponimod, ozanimod, ponesimod, and cladribine have Medication Guides to monitor safety.

TABLE 74-6 Prognostic Indicators in Multiple Sclerosis

Indicator	Favorable Prognosis	Unfavorable Prognosis
Age at onset	<40 years	>40 years
Gender	Female	Male
Initial symptoms	Optic neuritis or sensory symptoms	Motor or cerebellar symptoms; polysymptomatic
Disability	Late	Early
Attack frequency in early disease	Low	High
Course of disease	Relapsing/remitting	Progressive
Recovery after the first event	Good	Poor
T2 lesions	Low load	High load
T1 black hole lesions	Low rate	High rate
Growth of lesions	Slow	Rapid
Locations of lesions	Single	Multiple

Data from References 45 and 46.

Healthcare providers should follow the requirements of these programs. Laboratory monitoring for IFN therapy should include a CBC, platelet count, and LFTs completed at baseline, every 3 months for 1 year, and every 6 months after that. However, glatiramer acetate requires no specific laboratory monitoring. Teriflunomide requires a transaminase, bilirubin, CBC, tuberculin skin test, and blood pressure before therapy is started. Additionally, alanine aminotransferase should be monitored every 6 months after starting treatment. Patients on teriflunomide should be evaluated for renal failure and increased serum potassium as needed. Dimethyl fumarate requires a CBC prior to beginning therapy, within 6 months after treatment initiation, followed by annually. During these times, LFTs should also be monitored for patients on dimethyl fumarate.

CONCLUSION

The diagnosis and treatment of MS can be difficult, and until recently, treatment was particular to the MS center or treating neurologist. The AAN has the most updated guidelines for DMTs for adults with multiple sclerosis.[55] These focus on shared patient-centered decision making, where the patient is given general information about dosing schedule, route of administration, and adverse medication reactions for their specific disease presentation. The team works with the patient to make treatment decisions on how to best help the patient manage their illness, working to improve primary, secondary, and tertiary disease outcomes. More aggressive treatment with alemtuzumab, fingolimod, or natalizumab is required for people with highly active MS, and with ocrelizumab for patients with PPMS where the benefits outweigh the risks.[55] The most severe adverse effect associated with MS treatments is PML, and guidelines for natalizumab, fingolimod, rituximab, ocrelizumab, and dimethyl fumarate specifically note that patients should be counseled on this adverse effect. By moving to a patient-centered MS care approach, disease outcomes (due to increased adherence) and treatment satisfaction should improve as it is only through collaboration as a care team that we will be able to combat this debilitating disease.

ACKNOWLEDGMENTS

The authors acknowledge Felecia Hart, Golda Wang, and Joan Kaufman, an illustrator, for their contributions to this chapter.

TABLE 74-7 Evidenced-Based Recommendations for Disease-Modifying Treatment of Multiple Sclerosis

Recommendations	Recommendation Grades*
Interferon-β	
• Interferon-β has been shown to reduce attack rates in patients with MS or those with CIS who are at high risk of developing MS	A-I
• It is appropriate to consider IFN-β for any patient with clinically definite MS or who already has RRMS or SPMS and is still experiencing relapses	A-I
• The effectiveness of IFN-β in patients with SPMS but without relapses is uncertain	U-I
• Route of administration of IFN-β products is probably not clinically important with regards to efficacy; however, the side-effect profile does differ	B-II
• Rate of production of neutralizing antibodies is probably less with IFN-β_{1a} than with IFN-β_{1b}	B-I
• Presence of neutralizing antibodies may be associated with a reduction in the clinical effectiveness of IFN-β treatment	C-I
Glatiramer acetate	
• Glatiramer acetate has been shown to reduce the attack rate in patients with RRMS	A-I
• Treatment with glatiramer acetate may slow sustained disability progression in RRMS	C-I
Mitoxantrone	
• Mitoxantrone probably reduces the attack rate in patients with relapsing forms of MS	B-II, III
• Mitoxantrone may have a beneficial effect on disease progression in MS	C-II, III
Natalizumab	
• Natalizumab decreases clinical relapse rate, gadolinium-enhancing lesions, and new T2 lesions	A-I
• Natalizumab in RRMS positively changes measures of disease severity such as EDSS progression rate and changes lesions on MRI in RRMS	A-I
Ocrelizumab	
• Ocrelizumab in PPMS is shown to decrease confirmed disability progression, lessen worsening of timed 25-ft (~7.5-m) walk, decrease T2-weighted MRI lesions volume by 3.5%, and percentage of brain volume loss by 0.90%	A-I
• Ocrelizumab in RRMS positively changes measures of disease severity such as EDSS progression rate and changes lesions on MRI in RRMS	A-I

*Strength of recommendations: A: established; B: probable; C: possible; U: inadequate data to support recommendation.

CIS, clinically isolated syndrome; RCT, randomized controlled trial; RRMS, relapsing-remitting multiple sclerosis; SPMS, secondary-progressive multiple sclerosis.

Quality of evidence: Class I, evidence from one or more prospective, randomized, controlled clinical trial; Class II, evidence from cohort or RCT not meeting criteria for class I; Class III, evidence from other controlled trials; Class IV, evidence from uncontrolled studies, case reports, case series, or expert opinion.

Data from References 60 and 62.

ABBREVIATIONS

AAN	American Academy of Neurology
ACTH	adrenocorticotropic hormone
ADCC	antibody-dependent cell-mediated cytolysis
4-AP	4-aminopyridine
BCRP	breast cancer-resistant protein
CAM	complementary and alternative medicine
CBC	complete blood count

CDMS	clinically definite multiple sclerosis
CIS	clinically isolated syndrome
CNS	central nervous system
CSF	cerebrospinal fluid
DMT	disease-modifying therapy
EBNA	Epstein-Barr nuclear antigen
EBV	Epstein-Barr virus
ECG	electrocardiogram
EDSS	expanded disability status scale
GI	gastrointestinal
HLA	human leukocyte antigen
IAR	infusion-associated reaction
IFN	interferon
IgG	immunoglobulin G
IL	interleukin
INR	international normalized ratio
IRIS	immune reconstitution inflammatory syndrome
ITP	immune thrombocytopenia
IV	intravenous
JCV	John Cunningham virus
LFT	liver function test
MBP	myelin basic protein
MHC	major histocompatibility complex
MRI	magnetic resonance imaging
MS	multiple sclerosis
MSFC	multiple sclerosis functional composite
PEG	polyethylene glycol
PLEX	plasma exchange
PML	progressive multifocal leukoencephalopathy
PPMS	primary-progressive multiple sclerosis
PRMS	progressive-relapsing multiple sclerosis
REMS	Risk Evaluation and Mitigation Strategy
RRMS	relapsing-remitting multiple sclerosis
SPMS	secondary-progressive multiple sclerosis
TGF	transforming growth factor
Th	T-helper cells
THC	tetrahydrocannabinol
Treg	T-regulatory cells
UTI	urinary tract infection
VCA	vascular cell adhesion
VCAM	vascular cell adhesion molecule
VEP	visual-evoked potential
VLA-1	very-late antigen 1

REFERENCES

1. Wallin MT, Culpepper WJ, Campbell JD et al. The prevalence of MS in the United States: A population-based estimate using health claims data. *Neurol.* 2019;92(10):e1029–e1040.
2. National MS Society https://www.nationalmssociety.org/NationalMSSociety/media/MSNationalFiles/Brochures/Brochure-Just-the-Facts.pdf. Accessed October 9, 2020.2018. Available at: Multiple Sclerosis: Just the Facts.
3. Munger KL, Levin LI, Hollis BW. Serum 25-hydroxyvitamin D levels and risk of multiple sclerosis. *JAMA.* 2006;296:2832–2838.
4. Goodin DS. The causal cascade to multiple sclerosis: A model for MS pathogenesis. *PLoS One.* 2009;4:e4565.
5. Oksenberg JR, Baranzini SE, Sawcer S, Hauser SL. The genetics of multiple sclerosis: SNPs to pathways to pathogenesis. *Nat Rev Genet.* 2008;9:516–526.
6. Ebers GC. Environmental factors and multiple sclerosis. *Lancet Neurol.* 2008;7:268–277.
7. Healy BC, Ali EN, Guttmann CRG, et al. Smoking and disease progression in multiple sclerosis. *Arch Neurol.* 2009;66:858–864.
8. Kotzamani D, Panou T, Mastorodemos V, et al. Rising incidence of multiple sclerosis in females associated with urbanization. *Neurology.* 2012;78(22):1728–1735.
9. D'Netto MJ, Ward H, Morrison KM, et al. Risk alleles for multiple sclerosis in multiplex families. *Neurology.* 2009;72:1984–1988.
10. Maier LM, Lowe CE, Cooper J, et al. IL2RA genetic heterogeneity in multiple sclerosis and type 1 diabetes susceptibility and soluble interleukin-2 receptor production. *PLoS Genet.* 2009;5:e1000322.
11. Hafler DA, Compston A, Sawcer S, et al. Risk alleles for multiple sclerosis identified by a genomewide study. *N Engl J Med.* 2007;357:851–862.
12. Sundstrom P, Nystrom M, Ruuth K, et al. Antibodies to specific EBNA-1 domains and HLA DRB1*1501 interact as risk factors for multiple sclerosis. *J Neuroimmunol.* 2009;215(1-2):102–107.
13. Cree BA, Khan O, Bourdette D, et al. Clinical characteristics of African Americans versus Caucasian Americans with multiple sclerosis. *Neurology.* 2004;63:2039–2045.
14. Cree BA, Al-Sabbagh A, Bennett R, et al. Response to interferon beta-1a treatment in African American multiple sclerosis patients. *Arch Neurol.* 2005;62:1681–1683.
15. Reich D, Patterson N, DeJager PL, et al. A whole-genome admixture scan finds a candidate locus for multiple sclerosis susceptibility. *Nat Genet.* 2005;37:1113–1118.
16. Hedstrom AK, Baarnhielm M, Olsson T, Alfredsson L. Tobacco smoking, not Swedish snuff use, increases the risk of multiple sclerosis. *Neurology.* 2009;73(9):696–701.
17. Munger KL, Chitnis T, Ascherio A. Body size and risk of MS in two cohorts of US women. *Neurology.* 2009;73(19):1543–1550.
18. Frohman EM, Racke MK, Raine CS. Multiple sclerosis—the plaque and its pathogenesis. *N Engl J Med.* 2006;354:942–955.
19. Owens GP, Bennett JL. Trigger, pathogen, or bystander: The complex nexus linking Epstein–Barr virus and multiple sclerosis. *Mult Scler.* 2012;18(9):1204–1248.
20. Zivadinov R, Zorzon M, Weinstock-Guttman B, et al. Epstein–Barr virus is associated with grey matter atrophy in multiple sclerosis. *J Neurol Neurosurg Psychiatry.* 2009;80(6):620–625.
21. Serafini B, Rosicarelli B, Franciotta D, et al. Dysregulated Epstein-Barr virus infection in the multiple sclerosis brain. *J Exp Med.* 2007;204:2899–2912.
22. Willis SN, Stadelmann C, Rodig SJ, et al. Epstein–Barr virus infection is not a characteristic feature of multiple sclerosis brain. *Brain.* 2009;132:3318–3328.
23. Trapp BD, Peterson J, Ransohoff RM, et al. Axonal transection in the lesions of multiple sclerosis. *N Engl J Med.* 1998;338:278–285.
24. Truyen L, van Wuesberghe JHTM, Barkof F, et al. Accumulation of hypointense lesions ("black holes") on T1 spin echo MRI correlates with disease progression in multiple sclerosis. *Neurology.* 1996;47:1469–1476.
25. Zhou L, Chong MM, Littman DR. Plasticity of CD4+ T-cell lineage differentiation. *Immunity.* 2009;30(5):646–655.
26. Reboldi A, Coisne C, Baumjohann D, et al. C-C chemokine receptor 6-regulated entry of TH-17 cells into the CNS through the choroid plexus is required for the initiation of EAE. *Nat Immunol.* 2009;10(5):514–523.
27. Smolders J, Thewissen M, Peelan E, et al. Vitamin D status is positively correlated with regulatory T cell function in patients with multiple sclerosis. *PLoS One.* 2009;4:e6635.
28. Owens GP, Bennett JL, Lassmann H, et al. Antibodies produced by clonally expanded plasma cells in multiple sclerosis cerebrospinal fluid. *Ann Neurol.* 2009;65:639–649.
29. Pirko I, Lucchinetti CF, Sriram S, Bakshi R. Gray matter involvement in multiple sclerosis. *Neurology.* 2007;68:634–642.
30. Zivadinov R, Minagar A. Evidence for gray matter pathology in multiple sclerosis: A neuroimaging approach. *J Neurol Sci.* 2009;282:1–4.
31. Magliozzi R, Howell O, Vora A, et al. Meningeal B-cell follicles in secondary progressive multiple sclerosis associate with early onset of disease and severe cortical pathology. *Brain.* 2007;130:1089–1104.
32. Kinkel PR, Miravalle A. Current guidelines and standard treatments of RR-MS. 2011. Addressing unmet medical needs in relapsing-remitting multiple sclerosis. Available at http://www.futuremedicine.com. Accessed October 9, 2020.
33. Schapiro RT. Managing symptoms of multiple sclerosis. *Neurol Clin.* 2005;23:177–187.
34. Lublin FD, Reingold SC, Cohen JA, et al. Defining the clinical course of multiple sclerosis. *Neurology.* 2014;83:278–286.
35. Confavreux C, Vukusic S. Natural history of multiple sclerosis: A unifying concept. *Brain.* 2006;129(3):606–616.
36. Lebrun C, Bensa C, Debouverie M, et al. Association between clinical conversion to multiple sclerosis in radiologically isolated syndrome and magnetic resonance imaging, cerebrospinal fluid, and visual evoked potential: Follow-up of 70 patients. *Arch Neurol.* 2009;66:841–846.
37. Zivadinov R, Zorzon M. Is gadolinium enhancement predictive of the development of brain atrophy in multiple sclerosis? A review of the literature. *J Neuroimaging.* 2002;12:302–309.

38. Tremlett H, Paty D, Devonshire V. The natural history of primary progressive MS in British Columbia, Canada. *Neurology.* 2005;65:1919–1923.
39. Montalban X, Hauser SL, Kappos L, et al. Ocrelizumab versus placebo in primary progressive multiple sclerosis. *N Engl J Med.* 2017;376(3):209–220.
40. Kurtzke JF. Rating neurologic impairment in multiple sclerosis: An expanded disability status scale (EDSS). *Neurology.* 1983;33:1444–1452.
41. Rudick RA, Cutter G, Reingold S. The multiple sclerosis functional composite: A new clinical outcome measure for multiple sclerosis trials. *Mult Scler.* 2002;8:359–365.
42. Gordon-Lipkin E, Chodkowski B, Reich DS, et al. Retinal nerve fiber layer is associated with brain atrophy in multiple sclerosis. *Neurology.* 2007;69:1603–1609.
43. Lee M, O'Brien P. Pregnancy and multiple sclerosis. *J Neurol Neurosurg Psychiatry.* 2008;79:1308–1311.
44. Sadovnick AD, Eisen K, Ebers GC, Paty DW. Cause of death in patients attending multiple sclerosis clinics. *Neurology.* 1991;41:1193–1196.
45. Polman CH, Reingold SC, Edan G, et al. Diagnostic criteria for multiple sclerosis: 2005 revisions to the "McDonald Criteria". *Ann Neurol.* 2005;58:840–846.
46. Dalton C, Brex P, Miszkiel K, et al. New T2 lesions enable an earlier diagnosis of multiple sclerosis in clinically isolated syndromes. *Ann Neurol.* 2003;53:673–676.
47. Thompson AJ, Banwell BL, Barkhof F, et al. Diagnosis of multiple sclerosis: 2017 revisions of the McDonald criteria. *Lancet Neurol.* 2018;17(2):162–173.
48. Swanton JK, Rovira A, Tintore M, et al. MRI criteria for multiple sclerosis in patients presenting with clinically isolated syndromes: A multicentre retrospective study. *Lancet Neurol.* 2007;6:677–686.
49. Lo CP, Kao HW, Chen SY, et al. Prediction of conversion from clinically isolated syndrome to clinically definite multiple sclerosis according to baseline MRI findings: A comparison of revised McDonald criteria and Swanton modified criteria. *J Neurol Neurosurg Psychiatry.* 2009;80:1107–1109.
50. Fisher E, Rudick R, Simon J, et al. Eight-year follow-up study of brain atrophy in patients with MS. *Neurology.* 2002;59:1412–1420.
51. Frohman EM, Goodin DS, Calabresi PA, et al. The utility of MRI in suspected MS. Report of the Therapeutics and Technology Assessment Subcommittee of the American Academy of Neurology. *Neurology.* 2003;61:1332–1338.
52. Galetta KM, Calabresi PA, Frohman EM, Balcer LJ. Optical coherence tomograph (OCT): Imaging the visual pathway as a model for neurodegeneration. *Neurotherapeutics.* 2011;8(1):117–132.
53. Berger T, Rubner P, Schautzer F, et al. Antimyelin antibodies as a predictor of clinically definite multiple sclerosis after a first demyelinating event. *N Engl J Med.* 2003;349:139–145.
54. Zivadinov R, Rudick RA, De Masi R, et al. Effects of IV methylprednisolone on brain atrophy in relapsing-remitting MS. *Neurology.* 2001;57:1239–1247.
55. Rae-Grant A, Day GS, Marrie RA, et al. Practice guideline recommendations summary: Disease-modifying therapies for adults with multiple sclerosis: Report of the Guideline Development, Dissemination, and Implementation Subcommittee of the American Academy of Neurology. *Neurology.* 2018;90(17):777–788.
56. CMSC DMT Guideline Writing Group. CMSC Practical Guidelines for the Selection of Disease-Modifying Therapies in Multiple Sclerosis. Released February 28, 2019. Accessed October 9, 2020.
57. Carmosino MJ, Brousseau KM, Arciniegas DB, et al. Initial evaluations for multiple sclerosis in a university multiple sclerosis center: Outcomes and role of magnetic resonance imaging in referral. *Arch Neurol.* 2005;62:585–590.
58. Fisniku LK, Brex PA, Altmann DR, et al. Disability and T2 MRI lesions: A 20-year follow-up of patients with relapse onset of multiple sclerosis. *Brain.* 2008;131(Pt3):808–817.
59. Confavreux C, Vukusic S. Accumulation of irreversible disability in multiple sclerosis from epidemiology to treatment. *Clin Neurol Neurosurg.* 2006;108(3):327–332.
60. Vandebark AA, Huan J, Agotsch M, et al. Interferon-beta-1a increases CD56 (bright) natural killer cells and CD4+CD25+ Foxp3 expression in subjects with multiple sclerosis. *J Neuroimmunol.* 2009;215:125–128.
61. Giovannoni G, Barbarash O, Casset-Semanaz F, et al. Safety and immunogenicity of a new formulation of interferon beta-1a (Rebif New Formulation) in a Phase IIIb study in patients with relapsing multiple sclerosis: 96-week results. *Mult Scler.* 2009;15:219–228.
62. Simon JH, Jacobs L, Campion M, et al. A longitudinal study of brain atrophy in relapsing MS. *Neurology.* 1999;58:139–145.
63. Fischer JS, Priore RL, Jacobs LD, et al. Neuropsychological effects of interferon-β-la in relapsing multiple sclerosis. *Ann Neurol.* 2000;48:885–892.
64. Calabresi PA, Kieseier BC, Arnold DL, et al. Pegylated interferon beta-1a for relapsing-remitting multiple sclerosis (ADVANCE): A randomized, phase 3 double-blind study. *Lancet Neurol.* 2014;13:657–665.
65. Frohman E, Phillips T, Kokel K, et al. Disease-modifying therapy in multiple sclerosis: Strategies for optimizing management. *Neurology.* 2002;8:227–236.
66. Racke MK, Lovett-Racke AE, Karandikar NJ. The mechanism of action of glatiramer acetate treatment in multiple sclerosis. *Neurology.* 2010;74(suppl 1):S25–S30.
67. Azoulay D, Vachapova V, Shihman B, et al. Lower brain-derived neurotrophic factor in serum of relapsing remitting MS. Reversal by glatiramer acetate. *J Neuroimmunol.* 2005;167:215–218.
68. Fillippi M, Rovaris M, Rocca MA, et al. Glatiramer acetate reduces the proportion of new MS lesions evolving into "black holes". *Neurology.* 2001;57:731–733.
69. Ford CC, Johnson KP, Lisak RP, et al. A prospective open-label study of glatiramer acetate: Over a decade of continuous use in multiple sclerosis patients. *Mult Scler.* 2006;12:309–320.
70. Khan O, Rieckmann P, Boyko A, et al. Three times weekly glatiramer acetate in relapsing-remitting multiple sclerosis. *Ann Neurol.* 2013;73:705–713.
71. Wolinsky JS, Borresen TE, Dietrich DW, et al. GLACIER: An open-label, randomized, multicenter study to assess the safety and tolerability of glatiramer acetate 40 mg three times weekly verus 20 mg daily in patients with relapsing-remitting multiple sclerosis. *Mult Scler Relat Disord.* 2015;4:370–376.
72. Miller DH, Khan OA, Sheremata WA, et al. A controlled trial of natalizumab for relapsing multiple sclerosis. *N Engl J Med.* 2003;348:15–23.
73. Polman CH, O'Conor PW, Havrdova E, et al. A randomized, placebo-controlled trial of natalizumab for relapsing multiple sclerosis (AFFIRM). *N Engl J Med.* 2006;354:899–910.
74. Rudick RA, Stuart WH, Calabresi PA, et al. Natalizumab plus interferon beta-1a for relapsing multiple sclerosis (SENTINEL). *N Engl J Med.* 2006;354:911–923.
75. Kleinschmidt-DeMasters BK, Tyler KL. Progressive multifocal leukoencephalopathy complicating treatment with natalizumab and interferon beta-1a for multiple-sclerosis. *N Engl J Med.* 2005;353:369–374.
76. Langer-Gould A, Atlas SW, Green AJ, et al. Progressive multifocal leukoencephalopathy in a patient treated with natalizumab. *N Engl J Med.* 2005;353:375–381.
77. Van Assche G, Van Ranst M, Sclot R, et al. Progressive multifocal leukoencephalopathy after natalizumab therapy for Crohn's disease. *N Engl J Med.* 2005;353:362–368.
78. Berger JR. Classifying PML risk with disease modifying therapies. *Mult Scler Relat Disord.* 2017;12:59–63.
79. Gorelik L, Lerner M, Bixler S, et al. Anti-JC virus antibodies: Implications for PML risk stratification. *Ann Neurol.* 2010;68:295–303.
80. Bozic C, Richman S, Plavina T, et al. Anti-John Cunningham virus antibody prevalence in multiple sclerosis patients: Baseline results of STRATIFY-1. *Ann Neurol.* 2011;70(5):742–750.
81. Sadiq SA, Puccio LM, Brydon EW. JCV detection in multiple sclerosis patients treated with natalizumab. *J Neurol.* 2010;257:954–958.
82. Khatri BO, Man S, Giovannoni G, et al. Effect of plasma exchange in accelerating natalizumab clearance and restoring leukocyte function. *Neurology.* 2009;72:402–409.
83. Lindå H, von Heijne A, Major EO, et al. Progressive multifocal leukoencephalopathy after natalizumab monotherapy. *N Engl J Med.* 2009;361:1081–1087.
84. U.S. Food and Drug Administration. FDA Drug Safety Communication: Revised recommendations for cardiovascular monitoring and use of multiple sclerosis drug Gilenya fingolimod. FDA 2013. Available at http://www.fda.gov/Drugs/DrugSafety/ucm303192.htm. Accessed October 9, 2020.
85. Siponimod [package insert]. East Hanover, NJ: Novartis Pharmaceuticals Corporation; 2019.
86. Ozanimod [package insert]. Summit, NJ: Celgene Corporation; 2020.
87. Ponesimod [package insert]. Titusville, NJ: Janssen Pharmaceuticals Inc.; 2021.
88. O'Connor P, Wolinsky JS, Confavreux C, et al. Randomized trial of oral teriflunomide for relapsing multiple sclerosis. *N Engl J Med.* 2011;365(14):1293–1303.

89. O'Connor PW, Li D, Freedman MS, et al. A Phase II study of the safety and efficacy of teriflunomide in multiple sclerosis with relapses. *Neurology*. 2006;66(6):894–900.
90. Kita M, Fox RJ, Phillips JT, et al. Effects of BG-12 (dimethyl fumarate) on health-related quality of life in patients with relapsing-remitting multiple sclerosis: Findings from the CONFIRM study. *Mult Scler.* 2014;20(2):253–257.
91. Gold R, Kappos L, Arnold DL, et al. Placebo-controlled phase 3 study of oral BG-12 for relapsing multiple sclerosis. *N Engl J Med.* 2012;367(12):1098–1107.
92. Vumerity [package insert]. Waltham, MA: Alkermes, Inc.; 2019.
93. Bafiertam [package insert]. High Point, NC: Banner Life Sciences LLC.; 2020.
94. Wynn D, Lategan TW, Sprague TN, et al. Monomethyl fumarate has better gastrointestinal tolerability profile compared with dimethyl fumarate. *Mult Scler Rel Dis.* 2020;45:102335.
95. Wundes A, Wolinsky JS, Wray S, et al. Improved gastrointestinal tolerability profile with diroximel fumarate compared to dimethyl fumarate in relapsing MS patients. *Neurol.* 2020;94(15):994.
96. Giovannoni G. Cladribine to treat relapsing forms of multiple sclerosis. *Neurotherap.* 2017;14(4):874–887.
97. Mavenclad [package insert]. Rockland, MA: EMD Serono, Inc.; 2019.
98. Cohen JA, Coles AJ, Arnold DL, et al. Alemtuzumab versus interferon β 1a as first-line treatment for patients with relapsing-remitting multiple sclerosis: A randomised controlled phase 3 trial. *Lancet.* 2012;380:1819–1828.
99. Coles AJ, Twyman CL, Arnold DL, et al. Alemtuzumab for patients with relapsing multiple sclerosis after disease-modifying therapy: A randomised controlled phase 3 trial. *Lancet.* 2012;380:1829–1839.
100. Havrdova E, Horakova D, Kovarova I. Alemtuzumab in the treatment of multiple sclerosis: Key clinical trial results and considerations for use. *Ther Adv Neurol Disord.* 2015;8:31–45.
101. Gerevini S, Capra R, Bertoli D, et al. Immune profiling of a patient with alemtuzumab-associated progressive multifocal leukoencephalopathy. *Mult Scler.* 2019;25(8):1196–1201.
102. Kesimpta [package insert]. East Hanover, NJ: Novartis Pharmaceuticals Corporation; 2020.
103. Hauser SL, Bar-Or A, Cohen JA, et al. Ofatumumab versus teriflunomide in multiple sclerosis. *N Engl J Med.* 2020;383(6):546–557.
104. Hartung HP, Gonsette R, Konig N, et al. Mitoxantrone in progressive multiple sclerosis, a placebo-controlled, double-blind, randomized, multicentre trial. *Lancet.* 2002;360:2018–2025.
105. Krapf H, Morrissey SP, Zenker O, et al. Effect of mitoxantrone on MRI in progressive MS. Results of the MIMS trial. *Neurology.* 2005;65:690–695.
106. Martinelli V, Bellantonio P, Bergamaschi R, et al. Incidence of acute leukaemia in multiple sclerosis patients treated with mitoxandrone: A multicentre retrospective Italian study. *Neurology.* 2009;73:330–333.
107. Yamout BI, El-Ayoubi NK, Nicolas J, et al. Safety and efficacy of rituximab in multiple sclerosis: A retrospective observational study. *J Immun Res.* 2018; 9084759: 1–9.
108. Memon AB, Javed A, Caon C, et al. Long-term safety of rituximab induced peripheral B-cell depletion in autoimmune neurological diseases. *PLoS One.* 2018;13(1):e0190425.
109. Ocrevus [package insert]. San Francisco, CA: Genentech, Inc.; March 2017.
110. Costello K, Halper J, Kalb R, et al. The use of disease-modifying therapies in multiple sclerosis: A consensus paper by the multiple sclerosis coalition. Available at https://ms-coalition.org/the-use-of-disease-modifying-therapies-in-multiple-sclerosis-updated/. Accessed October 29, 2020.
111. Clanet M, Radue E, Kappos L, et al. A randomized, double-blind, dose-comparison study of weekly interferon-β-1a in relapsing MS. *Neurology.* 2002;59:1507–1517.
112. Vartanian T. An examination of the results of the EVIDENCE, INCOMIN, and phase III studies of interferon beta products in the treatment of multiple sclerosis. *Clin Ther.* 2003;1:105–118.
113. Durelli L, Verdun E, Bergui M, et al. Every-other-day interferon-β-1b versus once-weekly interferon-β-1a for multiple sclerosis: Results of a 2-year prospective randomized multicentre study (INCOMIN). *Lancet.* 2002;359:1453–1460.
114. Panitch H, Goodin D, Francis G, et al. Randomized, comparative study of interferon-β-1a treatment regimens in MS. The EVIDENCE Trial. *Neurology.* 2002;59:1496–1506.
115. Koch-Henriksen N, Sorensen PS, Christensen T, et al. A randomized study of two interferon-beta treatments in relapsing-remitting multiple sclerosis. *Neurology.* 2006;66:1056–1060.
116. O'Connor P, Filippi M, Arnason B, et al. 250 mcg or 500 mcg interferon beta-1b versus 20 mg glatiramer acetate in relapsing-remitting multiple sclerosis: A prospective, randomised, multicentre study. *Lancet Neurol.* 2009;8:889–897.
117. Mikol DD, Barkhof F, Chang P, et al. Comparison of subcutaneous interferon beta-1a with glatiramer acetate in patients with relapsing multiple sclerosis (the Rebif vs. Glatiramer Acetate in Relapsing MS Disease [REGARD] study): A multicentre, randomised, parallel, open-label trial. *Lancet Neurol.* 2008;7:903–914.
118. Namaka M, Pollitt-Smith M, Gupta A, et al. The clinical importance of neutralizing antibodies in relapsing-remitting multiple sclerosis. *Curr Med Res Opin.* 2006;22:223–239.
119. Bertolotto A. Neutralizing antibodies to interferon beta: Implications for the management of multiple sclerosis. *Curr Opin Neurol.* 2004;17:241–246.
120. Francis GS, Rice GP, Alsop JC, et al. Interferon beta 1a in MS: Results following development of neutralizing antibodies in PRISMS. *Neurology.* 2005;65:48–55.
121. Kappos L, Clanet M, Sandberg-Wollheim M, et al. Neutralizing antibodies and efficacy of interferon beta-1a: A 4-year controlled study. *Neurology.* 2005;65:40–47.
122. Giovannoni G, Goodman A. Neutralizing anti-IFN-beta antibodies: How much more evidence do we need to use them in practice? *Neurology.* 2005;65:6–8.
123. Goodin DS, Frohman EM, Hurwitz B, et al. Neutralizing antibodies to interferon beta: Assessment of their clinical and radiographic impact: An evidence report. *Neurology.* 2007;67:977–984.
124. Freedman MS, Kappos L, Polman CH, et al. Betaseron in newly emerging multiple sclerosis for initial treatment (BENEFIT): Clinical outcomes. *Neurology.* 2006;(suppl 2):A61.
125. Kappos L, Polman C, Pozzilli C, et al. Final analysis of the European multicenter trial on IFNβ-1b in secondary-progressive MS. *Neurology.* 2001;57:1969–1975.
126. Hauser SL, Waubant E, Arnold DL, et al. B-cell depletion with rituximab in relapsing-remitting multiple sclerosis. *N Engl J Med.* 2008;358:676–688.
127. Sorensen PS, Mellgren SI, Svenningsson A, et al. NORDIC trial of oral methylprednisolone as add-on therapy to interferon beta-1a for treatment of relapsing-remitting multiple sclerosis (NORMIMS study): A randomised, placebo-controlled trial. *Lancet Neurol.* 2009;8:519–529.
128. Birnbaum G, Cree B, Altafullah I, et al. Combining beta interferon and atorvastatin may increase disease activity in multiple sclerosis. *Neurology.* 2008;71:1390–1395.
129. Freedman MS, Patry DG, Grand'Maison F, et al. Treatment optimization in multiple sclerosis. *Can J Neurol Sci.* 2004;31:157–168.
130. Mitchell G. Update on multiple sclerosis therapy. *Med Clin North Am.* 1993;77:231–249.
131. Goodman AD, Brown TR, Krupp LB, et al. Sustained-release oral fampridine in multiple sclerosis: A randomised, double-blind, controlled trial. *Lancet.* 2009;373:732–738.
132. Fox RJ, Bacon TE, Chamot E, et al. Advanced symptom management in multiple sclerosis. *Neurodegener Dis Manag.* 2015;5(6 Suppl):3–10.
133. Yadav V, Bever C Jr, Bowen J, et al. Summary of evidence-based guideline—complementary and alternative medicine in multiple sclerosis: Report of the guideline development subcommittee of the American Academy of Neurology. *Neurology.* 2014;82:1083–1092.
134. Bowling AC. *Optimal Health with Multiple Sclerosis: A Guide to Integrating Lifestyle, Alternative, and Conventional Medicine.* New York, NY: Demos; 2014.
135. Zivadinov R, Weinstock-Guttman B, Hashmi K, et al. Smoking is associated with increased lesion volumes and brain atrophy in multiple sclerosis. *Neurology.* 2009;73(7):504–510.
136. Levin LI, Munger KL, Rubertone MV, et al. Temporal relationship between elevation of Epstein–Barr virus antibody titers and initial onset of neurological symptoms in multiple sclerosis. *JAMA.* 2005;293:2496–2500.
137. Stenager EN, Stenager E, Koch Henriksen N, et al. Suicide and multiple sclerosis: An epidemiological investigation. *J Neurol Neurosurg Psychiatry.* 1992;55:542–545.
138. Egeberg M, Oh CY, Bainbridge JL. Clinical overview of dalfampridine: The agent with a novel mechanism of action to help with gait disturbances. *Clinical Therapeutics.* 2012;34:2185–2194.
139. Goodin DS, Cohen BA, O'Connor P, et al. Assessment—the use of natalizumab (Tysabri) for the treatment of multiple sclerosis (an evidence-based review): Report of the Therapeutics and Technology Assessment Subcommittee of the American Academy of Neurology. *Neurology.* 2008;71(10):766–773.

Epilepsy

75

Viet-Huong V. Nguyen, Sunita Dergalust, and Edward Chang

KEY CONCEPTS

1. The goal of pharmacotherapy is seizure freedom with minimal adverse effects. Between 60% and 80% of patients can achieve this.
2. Accurate classification and diagnosis of seizure type/epilepsy syndrome, including where seizures begin, is critical to selection of appropriate pharmacotherapy.
3. Besides seizure type, antiseizure medication (ASM) selection depends on patient characteristics such as age, sex, ethnicity, susceptibility to adverse medication effects, comorbid conditions, ability to adhere with the prescribed regimen, presence or absence of insurance coverage, and need for therapeutic levels to be reached quickly.
4. Pharmacotherapy for epilepsy is highly individualized and requires dose titration to optimize therapy (maximal seizure control with minimal or no adverse medication effects).
5. If the therapeutic goal is not achieved with monotherapy, a second ASM, preferably with a different mechanism of action, can be added. The patient's ASM can also be switched to an alternative single agent.
6. Patients who do not respond to pharmacotherapy should be referred to a comprehensive epilepsy center to determine if nonpharmacologic treatments such as surgery are potential options.
7. In general, first-generation ASMs are very efficacious but have complex pharmacokinetics, multiple medication interactions, and an increased incidence of adverse effects, which make them more complicated to manage than either the second- or third-generation ASMs.
8. Second-generation ASMs have unique mechanisms of action and are as efficacious as first- and third-generation ASMs with better tolerability. They are generally considered first-line epilepsy pharmacotherapy.
9. Third-generation ASMs should be reserved for failure of other agents due to cost and limited long-term experience.
10. 20% to 35% of patients will have unsatisfactory control with ASMs and will be considered to be treatment-resistant.

BEYOND THE BOOK

Use the following webpage (Epipick.org) to help identify the possible epilepsy types. This resource will also help you select appropriate medications for your patient based on patient-specific characteristics and comorbidities.

Use the following link (https://https://www.ilae.org/) to get acquainted with the International League Against Epilepsy (ILAE), a world association of health professionals and scientists working together to understand, diagnose, and treat patients with epilepsy. Of particular interest may be the section on education which provides links to infographics and videos as well as the section on guidelines, which provides current practice guidelines, reports, and position papers.

INTRODUCTION

Epilepsy is a common neurologic condition in which a person is prone to recurrent epileptic seizures. There are many types of epilepsies characterized by different seizure types, ranging in severity and etiologies. While the specific pathophysiologic mechanisms behind different epilepsies are complex, the general pathophysiologic process underlying all epilepsies is disturbed regulation of electrical activity in the brain resulting in synchronized and excessive neuronal discharge.

Beyond seizures, people with epilepsy face many challenges, including increased risk of neurodevelopmental delay, cognitive impairment, comorbid depression, and anxiety. Furthermore, patients with epilepsy may face educational and vocational challenges, have difficulties with independent living, and be victims of stigma and common public misunderstanding. The International League Against Epilepsy (ILAE) defines epilepsy not only as "a disorder of the brain characterized by an enduring predisposition to generate epileptic seizures" but also by "the neurobiologic, cognitive, psychological, and social consequences of this condition."[1] Clinicians treating epilepsy must address these common psychosocial issues and comorbidities. Pharmacotherapy should be selected not only to reduce the frequency of seizures as much as possible, but also to minimize adverse medication reactions, address coexisting health and social conditions, and enhance overall quality-of-life (QOL) for patients.

EPIDEMIOLOGY

Epilepsy is the fourth most common neurologic disorder globally and in the United States; only following stroke, migraine, and Alzheimer's disease. In the United States, approximately 3.4 million people suffer from epilepsy with a prevalence of 1.2%. While epilepsy is a chronic disease that can present at all ages, the highest number of new epilepsy cases (incidence) will occur in childhood and the older adult population. Among children, epilepsy has the highest incidence in children under 5 years of age with most new cases occurring under 2 years of age. In older populations, the high frequency of epilepsy is now garnering attention as 1.5% of people older than 65 are affected by epilepsy in the United States.[2,3]

The majority of patients with epilepsy has a good prognosis and will be able to attain seizure freedom. However, the mortality rate of patients with epilepsy is two to three times that of the general population and life expectancy may be reduced.[4] Increased mortality has been attributed to a wide variety of causes including sudden unexplained death in epilepsy (SUDEP).[5] While the exact mechanisms underlying SUDEP are unclear, recent research suggests there may be a cardio-respiratory mechanism involved.[5] Although it is rare in patients with well-controlled epilepsy, SUDEP accounts for up to 15% of all epilepsy-related deaths, with a lifetime risk of 4.6% to 8%.[5]

All individuals with epilepsy experience seizures; however, not all individuals who experience seizures will be diagnosed with epilepsy. Some seizures are provoked and occur as a result of systemic, toxic, or metabolic insults such as substance use; alcohol, barbiturate, or benzodiazepine withdrawal; or acute neurologic (eg, brain hemorrhage) or systemic illnesses (eg, hypocalcemia, hypoglycemia, uremia, and eclampsia). Furthermore, some patients will have seizures only associated with fever (eg, febrile seizures). In all of these situations, seizure occurrence does not generally constitute epilepsy, but rather are a symptom of the provoking insult. Once the provoking insult is removed or treated, there is not "an enduring predisposition to generate epileptic seizures." Each year, 120 per 100,000 people in the United States will be evaluated for a newly recognized seizure (provoked or unprovoked), but only 40 to 70 cases per 100,000 will be diagnosed with epilepsy. At least 10% of the general population will have at least one seizure from *any* cause in their lifetime.[2,3]

ETIOLOGY

Hundreds of medical conditions can cause epilepsy, ranging from genetic predisposition to acquired injury (eg, stroke or traumatic brain injury). The most common causes vary depending on the population of interest. For instance, childhood-onset epilepsy is predominantly caused by genetic and/or developmental structural abnormalities, while epilepsy with an onset at older age is most often caused by acquired structural injury (eg, stroke or traumatic brain injury). Therefore, epilepsy etiologies can be generally classified into six categories reviewed here: (1) genetic; (2) structural; (3) infectious; (4) metabolic; (5) immune; and (6) unknown.[6] It is important to note that these categories are not mutually exclusive.

Genetic Etiology

Epilepsies with genetic etiology usually present in infancy or childhood with examples being (1) Dravet syndrome associated with mutations in sodium channel, voltage-gated, type I alpha subunit (SCN1A), (2) childhood absence epilepsy (CAE) associated with many different mutations in T-type Ca^{2+} channels and GABA-receptor subunits, and (3) Juvenile Myoclonic Epilepsy (JME) associated with many different mutations including those in the EF-hand containing protein-1 (EFHC1) and intestinal cell kinase (ICK).[7–11] Prior to 2010, genetic epilepsies were labeled as primary generalized epilepsy or idiopathic generalized epilepsy (IGE), as no clear structural brain abnormalities were found to be responsible for the epilepsy.[6] However, as most of these disorders have abnormalities at the molecular level they are now also called genetic generalized epilepsies.[6] Genetic etiologies usually pass from generation to generation but can also arise from sporadic mutations, and cannot be acquired after birth.

Structural Etiology

Structural etiologies refer to abnormalities visible on structural neuroimaging, and are either acquired or of genetic origin.[6] Common epilepsies caused by structural abnormalities include cortical dysplasia, mesial temporal lobe epilepsy, and posttraumatic epilepsy. In general, cortical dysplasia is a common cause of childhood onset medication-resistant epilepsy and is a result of disruptions in neuronal migration, proliferation, and differentiation during brain development, leading to disorganization of the normal structure of the cerebral cortex in certain brain areas. In general, mesial temporal lobe epilepsy is a common type of adult-onset epilepsy responsible for many of the medication-resistant epilepsies seen in tertiary care epilepsy clinics. In this structural form of epilepsy, sclerosis occurs in the hippocampus, the main structure of the mesial temporal lobe, and is characterized by glial scarring, reduced hippocampal volume as seen on magnetic resonance imaging (MRI), and decreased cellular density as seen on biopsy.[12] In contrast, traumatic brain injury epilepsy results from blunt force injury or stroke that causes structural lesions in the brain.[6]

Infectious Etiology

Infections are the most common epilepsy etiology worldwide[6] and typically occurs when a patient develops epilepsy as the sequelae of an infection, not when a patient experiences seizures in the setting of acute infection such as meningitis or encephalitis. In developing countries, the most common acquired infectious epilepsy is from neurocysticercosis, a parasitic infection of the brain that results from ingestion of pork tapeworm eggs, causing subsequent structural injury that promotes the development of epilepsy.[6]

Metabolic, Immune, and Unknown Etiology

Both the metabolic and immune etiologies of epilepsy are less common, although they are increasingly being recognized and understood.[6] An interesting metabolic etiology is Lafora disease, which is associated with abnormal glycogen metabolism and subsequent development of insoluble glycogen inclusion bodies resulting in epilepsy.[13] Immune epilepsies include anti-*N*-methyl-D-aspartate (anti-NMDA) receptor encephalitis which causes autoimmune-mediated central nervous system (CNS) inflammation and resulting epilepsy.[6] While both of these etiologies carry specific treatment implications, treatment implications are evolving. Patients can also present with unprovoked seizures that do not have an identifiable cause, and thus by definition have epilepsy of unknown cause.[6] While standard epilepsy workup procedures need to be followed, it is possible that these epilepsies may be due to an as-yet-unidentified gene or may be the consequence of an as-yet-unrecognized-structural or metabolic disorder.

Risk Factors and Seizure Triggers

While certain risk factors may suggest a predisposition to epilepsy, they are not necessarily causative, as known epilepsy risk factors include premature birth with small gestational weight, perinatal injury (eg, anoxia), history of alcohol withdrawal seizures, history of febrile seizures, and family history of seizures.[14] While the presence of such risk factors aid in establishing the diagnosis of epilepsy and may help in identifying the underlying epilepsy etiology, they may not explain the mechanistic cause of seizures.

Many factors trigger seizures in susceptible individuals, with two of the best known seizure triggers being hyperventilation and photostimulation (eg, flashing lights or rapidly changing or alternating images) in certain genetic epilepsies including juvenile myoclonic epilepsy and childhood absence epilepsy. Additional triggers include physical and emotional stress, sleep deprivation, sensory stimuli, and hormonal changes occurring around the time of menses, puberty, or pregnancy, as all of these have been associated with the onset of or an increased frequency of seizures. Lastly, medications such as theophylline, high-dose phenothiazines, antidepressants (especially bupropion), alcohol, and substance use have all been associated with lowering seizure threshold and provoking seizures in patients with epilepsy.[15]

PATHOPHYSIOLOGY

The underlying general pathophysiologic process for all epilepsies is neuronal hyperexcitability and hypersynchronization. Initially during a seizure, a small number of hyperexcitable neurons fire abnormally in synchrony resulting in breakdown of normal membrane conductances and inhibitory synaptic currents. This allows the excess excitability to spread, either locally to produce a focal seizure, or the seizure is propagated by physiologic pathways and networks to involve more remote areas, or more widely to produce a generalized seizure.[16]

In general, neuronal hyperexcitability occurs because there is an enhanced predisposition of a neuron to depolarize and discharge when stimulated. While this may occur as the result of multiple mechanisms, alterations in the number, type, and biophysical properties of voltage- or ligand-gated K^+, Na^+, Ca^{2+}, and Cl^- ion channels in neuronal membranes are thought to play a significant role.[17] In fact, many of the available antiseizure medications (ASMs) have mechanisms of actions that act on these specific ion channels, highlighting the importance of these channels in promoting hyperexcitability. Carbamazepine and phenytoin reduce neuronal excitability by binding sodium channels in their inactive state and slowing channel recovery from inactivation, thereby preventing hyperexcitable neurons from rapidly and repetitively firing; this also blocks firing in a use-dependent fashion.[18,19] Benzodiazepines, in contrast, bind to the gamma subunit of the $GABA_A$ receptor leading to an increase in chloride ion conductance and inhibition of action potentials.[20] Mutations within these ion channels have been associated with multiple different epilepsies.[11] While the exact nature of these alterations has not been fully elucidated, these genetic alterations may result in differences between the various genetic epilepsies.

Other mechanisms of epileptogenesis, which may play roles in hyperexcitability, are related to alterations in vesicle trafficking and neurotransmitter release. For instance, synaptic vesicle protein 2A ($SV2_A$), a protein responsible for the fusion of vesicles to the membrane, is upregulated in certain models of epilepsy, and is the target of the second- and third-generation ASMs, levetiracetam and brivaracetam, respectively.[21] Alterations in neurotransmitter uptake and metabolism may also play a role in the pathogenesis of epilepsy.[22] An example of this comes from vigabatrin, which is an irreversible inhibitor of γ-aminobutyric acid transaminase (GABA-T).[23] As this enzyme is responsible for the metabolism of the inhibitory neurotransmitter GABA, this medication is thought to increase GABA through GABA-T inhibition.[23]

Additionally, there are many other possible hyperexcitability promoting mechanisms that may be important in the pathophysiology of epilepsy, including possible biochemical modifications of receptors, modulation of second messaging systems and gene expression, and changes in extracellular ion concentrations.[22] Hyperexcitability that results in increased firing of random individual neurons does not result in epileptic seizures, as synchronization of excessive neuronal firing is required.[24] The intrinsic organization of local circuits of certain cerebral structures including the hippocampus, the neocortex, and the thalamus contributes to synchronization and promotes generation of epileptiform activity. That is why many epileptic networks originate in these specific brain regions.[24,25] Modifications in the ratio and function of inhibitory circuits in these structures play an important role in promoting epileptogenesis, as a large number of these neurons are interconnected and can become simultaneously inhibited, and then synchronously excited. Although under normal circumstances, these neurons are asynchronous, it is believed that under abnormal circumstances, they become synchronous and act as pacemakers promoting epileptiform activity. Sprouting and reorganization of neuronal projections in abnormal tissue or after neuronal injury (eg, head trauma or stroke) may also lead to increased connectivity between neurons and a chronic susceptibility to seizures.[24] Therefore, both excitation and inhibitory connections lie at the heart of the pathophysiologic mechanisms behind epileptogenicity.

CLINICAL PRESENTATION

An epileptic seizure is defined as a transient occurrence of signs and/or symptoms due to abnormal excessive or synchronous neuronal activity in the brain.[3] They can manifest physically in a variety of ways and can range from intense involuntary repetitive muscular contractions (eg, convulsions) to subtle alterations in sensation or consciousness. The new basic seizure classification is based on three key features: (1) where in the brain the seizure originates; (2) the individual's level of awareness during a seizure; and (3) other seizure features.[26]

1 Seizures can be classified into an initial three categories depending on how they begin in the brain (eg, onset): (1) focal seizures (previously called partial seizures) that start in a network of cells on one side of the brain; (2) generalized seizures (previously called primary generalized) that start in a bilaterally distributed network (eg, a network encompassing both sides of the brain); and (3) unknown onset which can later be recategorized when it becomes clear how seizures begin in a particular individual's brain.[26] Understanding seizure onset is important, as it has significant treatment and prognostic implications affecting choice of seizure medication and eligibility for epilepsy surgery. Examples of this include patients with generalized-onset seizures who may have a seizure exacerbation when treated with certain ASMs (eg, treating childhood absence epilepsy with carbamazepine)[27] or patients with medication-resistant focal-onset seizures who may be good candidates for surgical resection, while those with generalized-onset seizures are not.

Focal Seizures

In general, focal seizures may be characterized by whether the patient retains awareness of themselves and their environment including external stimuli (eg, being asked questions) during the seizure, even if immobile and unable to talk or respond. When awareness is retained the seizure is termed a "focal aware seizure" corresponding to what has historically been termed "simple partial seizure." A focal impaired awareness seizure corresponds to the prior term "complex partial seizure" and is an appropriate classification if the person has impaired awareness at any time during the seizure (eg, they are aware in the beginning but lose awareness at the end, or if they have a vague idea of what is occurring and know that someone is speaking to them but respond inappropriately).[26]

Focal seizures can be further subgrouped by earliest most prominent motor sign (eg, automatisms, clonic, myoclonic) or nonmotor sign (eg, autonomic or sensory symptoms) at seizure onset. If motor signs are present, then some type of movement will occur during the seizure such as twitching and jerking (eg, myoclonus), stiffening (tonic contraction), or automatic movements (automatisms) such as smacking lips, rubbing hands, and picking at clothes. Nonmotor signs include changes in sensation, emotions, thinking, or experience. The symptoms felt by the individual at the very beginning of a seizure is sometimes called an aura, although this term is now discouraged. Motor or nonmotor symptoms that may appear at onset are listed in Fig. 75-1.[26]

Focal seizures may propagate beyond one brain hemisphere to also involve the contralateral hemisphere. This seizure type is called "focal to bilateral tonic–clonic" and is a special seizure type which previously was called "partial onset with secondary generalization" or "secondarily generalized tonic–clonic (GTC) seizure." The term "to bilateral" is preferred to distinguish this focal-onset seizure from a generalized-onset seizure. During this type of seizure, the person usually becomes unconscious and displays bilateral convulsive features such as tonic–clonic motor features.[26,28]

Focal aware seizures may manifest clinically in a variety of ways and can vary depending on where the abnormal firing occurs. For

CLINICAL PRESENTATION Epilepsy

Focal Aware Seizures

- Patients retain awareness of themselves and their environment including external stimuli.

Focal Impaired Awareness Seizure

- Patient has impaired awareness at any time during the seizure
- May be able to respond to questions during the seizure, but inappropriate response
- May not recall actions after event

Motor signs

- Automatisms: automatic behaviors like lip smacking, chewing, picking at clothing
- Atonic: loss of tone, going limp
- Clonic: rhythmic jerking or twitching of arm, shoulder, face, or leg
- Spasm: trunk flexion
- Hyperkinetic: thrashing/pedaling
- Myoclonic: arrhythmic jerking of arm, shoulder, face, or leg
- Tonic: extension or flexion postures

Nonmotor signs

- Autonomic: flushing, sweating, piloerection, salivation, pallor
- Behavior arrest: pausing, freezing, activity arrest
- Cognitive: language problems, thinking problems, memory phenomenon, and feelings of familiarity (déjà vu) or unfamiliarity (jamais vu)
- Emotion: feelings of fear, depression, joy, anger, extreme aberration of behavior
- Sensory: numbness, tingling, sounds (ringing/buzzing), smells, tastes, visions (hallucinations), vertigo

Focal to Bilateral Tonic–Clonic

- Focal seizure with impaired awareness which progresses to bilateral convulsive features such as with tonic–clonic motor features

Generalized Onset

- Impaired awareness

Motor signs (more common symptoms described below only)

- Tonic–clonic: sudden sharp tonic stiffening of muscles with a subsequent period of clonic movements such as rhythmic jerking of arms and legs (previously called "grand mal")
- Clonic: rhythmic jerking or twitching of arm, shoulder, face, or leg
- Myoclonic: arrhythmic jerking of arm, shoulder, face, or leg
- Atonic: loss of tone, going limp
- Epileptic spasms: trunk flexion

Nonmotor/absence (more common symptoms described below only)

- Typical: sudden arrest of behavior, blank stare with brief upward rotation of the eyes lasting 2 to 30 seconds
- Eyelid myoclonia: lid jerks

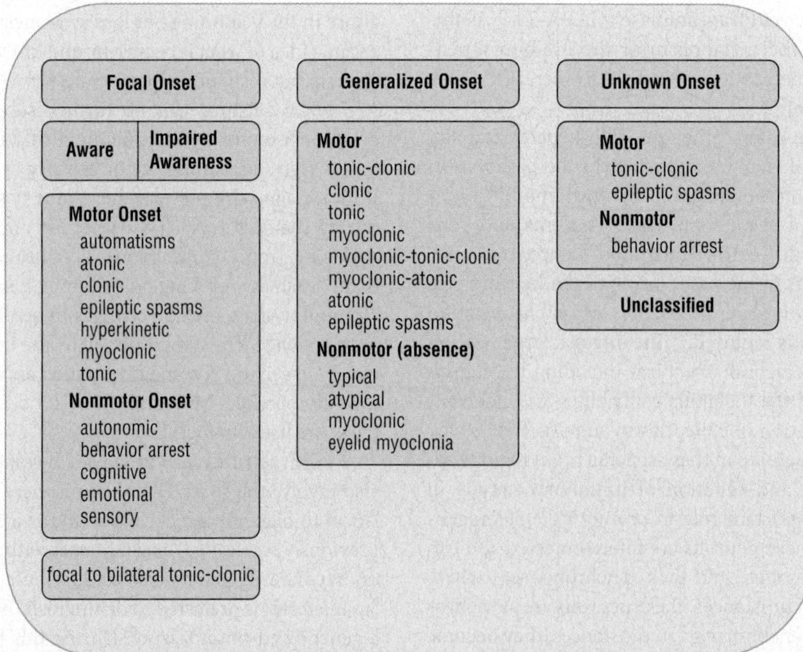

FIGURE 75-1 ILAE 2017 Classification of seizure types—expanded version. (*Reprinted, with permission, from Fisher RS, Cross JH, French JA, et al. Operational classification of seizure types by the International League Against Epilepsy: Position paper of the ILAE Commission for Classification and Terminology. Epilepsia. 2017;58(4):522–530.*)

example, seizures manifesting as abnormal movements such as clonic movements (eg, twitching or jerking) of the arm, shoulder, face, or leg indicate seizure activity in motor pathways. Feelings of numbness or tingling indicate sensory or somatosensory involvement and may indicate parietal lobe involvement. Sensory symptoms can also include feelings of fear, depression, joy, anger, or memory phenomena such as feelings of familiarity (déjà vu) or unfamiliarity (jamais vu) that may indicate temporal lobe seizure activity. Visual disturbances or hallucinations may indicate seizure activity involving the occipital lobe, while ringing or buzzing sounds in the ears may indicate seizure activity in auditory areas of the brain. Autonomic symptoms such as sweating, salivation, or pallor indicate seizure activity in autonomic areas of the brain.[28,29]

Focal impaired awareness seizures may manifest with any of the signs and symptoms described for focal aware seizures except that the patient does not retain awareness. They may still be able to perform routine tasks such as walking, but such movements are not purposeful or planned and after the event is over they may not recall their actions. The patient may be able to respond to questions during the seizure, although they may not respond appropriately. The degree of alteration in awareness and responsiveness may be so subtle that witnesses may not recognize that anything is overtly wrong. For example, they may simply display behavioral arrest and stare off into space for a minute. They may also display subtle automatisms such as lip smacking, chewing, or picking at their clothing without purpose. On the other hand, some patients may display extreme aberrations of behavior, and some are even mistakenly diagnosed as having psychotic episodes. After the seizure (postictal period), the patient may display altered consciousness, drowsiness, confusion, or even paranoia for a variable period of time and frequently go into a deep sleep.[28,29]

Generalized-Onset Seizures

Generalized-onset seizures start in a network that is bilaterally distributed to both brain hemispheres and have previously been referred to as primary generalized seizures. These types of seizures involve impaired awareness and are divided into motor and nonmotor (eg, absence) seizures. Generalized "absence" seizures are not synonymous with an "absent stare" which typically accompanies the behavioral arrest that occurs in other seizure types.[26]

Generalized-onset seizures can have a variety of motor symptoms with the major motor category being tonic–clonic. These generalized-onset tonic–clonic seizures were previously called "grand mal" seizures. During these seizures the patient experiences loss of consciousness, followed by a sudden sharp tonic contraction (stiffening) of muscles with a subsequent period of rigidity and clonic movements, oftentimes described as jerking of the arms and legs. During the seizure, the patient may cry or moan, due to muscles in the larynx being activated or they may lose sphincter control with bladder and/or bowel incontinence or bite their tongue. Postictally, after consciousness is regained, the patient may experience confusion, drowsiness, lack of coordination, soreness throughout the body, and amnesia for the event.[28,29]

It is important to remember that bilateral tonic–clonic seizures can also result from focal propagation to contralateral hemispheres and that these seizures must be differentiated from generalized-onset tonic–clonic seizures. Generalized manifestations of seizures can be asymmetrical or symmetrical, rendering the distinction from focal-onset seizures difficult, but certain distinguishing features such as very early motor or nonmotor signs that may be characteristic of focal-onset seizures, and characteristic findings on EEG aid in distinguishing between the two. Other forms of generalized motor seizures may happen but the generalized tonic–clonic (GTC) seizure is most common and most distinct.[6,28]

In contrast to other motor seizure categories in which there is a sudden onset of increased tone, a sudden loss of muscle tone occurs in *atonic seizures*. Atonic seizures are not preceded by myoclonic or tonic features and can be very brief. They may present as a head drop, the dropping of a limb, or a slumping to the ground (due to loss of postural tone). These patients often wear protective headware to prevent trauma and atonic seizures are one hallmark of Lennox–Gastaut syndrome.[6,28]

Typical generalized nonmotor seizures, aka "absence" seizures, can manifest as typical absence seizures, atypical absence, absence seizures with myoclonia, or absence seizures with eyelid myoclonia. Most commonly, typical absence seizures manifest as a sudden onset interruption of ongoing activities, a blank stare, and possibly a brief upward rotation of the eyes indicating the abrupt onset and offset of impaired consciousness. The staring and behavioral arrest lasts 2 to 30 seconds during which time the patient is unaware of the environment and unresponsive. The patient has neither a warning that the seizure is going to occur, nor does the patient have postictal confusion or lethargy after the seizures. After cessation of the seizure, the patient will often return to the previous activity as if nothing had happened. These absence seizures generally occur in young children through adolescence. It is important to differentiate these seizures from focal unaware seizures; in general, absence-type seizures are much briefer than the staring spells associated with focal unaware seizures and have minimal postictal manifestations.[6,28,29]

Seizures of Unknown Onset

Seizures of unknown onset are classified based on presence of motor or nonmotor features; however, in some cases it may be impossible to classify a seizure at all. Although this should be a rare occurrence, in such cases this seizure would be an unclassified seizure.[26]

Classification of Epilepsies and Epilepsy Syndromes

A seizure is only a symptom that occurs within epilepsy; therefore, seizure classification is distinct from but related to the classification of epilepsies and epilepsy syndromes. The starting point of epilepsy classification is identification of the seizure type, understanding that some patients may have multiple different seizure types. After seizure types are determined, the epilepsy should be classified into one of four categories: (1) focal epilepsy in which a patient only has focal-onset seizures; (2) generalized epilepsy in which a patient displays evidence of only generalized-onset seizures; (3) combined generalized and focal epilepsy; and (4) unknown in which the epilepsy type is unknown (see Fig. 75-2).[6]

After establishing the epilepsy type, an epilepsy syndrome should be determined if possible. In general, while knowing the etiology and specific comorbid characteristics of a patient with epilepsy is important during seizure and epilepsy classification, these parameters can be unknown and are not necessary. However, when determining epilepsy syndromes (the most specific level of epilepsy classification possible), knowing definitive etiology and specific comorbid characteristics is critical (see Fig. 75-2). Epilepsy syndromes are characterized by a known etiology and by a cluster of signs and symptoms including distinctive comorbidities such as intellectual and psychiatric dysfunction that customarily occur together. Other signs and symptoms include type of seizure, specific electroencephalogram (EEG) findings, specific imaging features, anatomy, precipitating factors, age of onset, severity, chronicity, and diurnal and circadian cycling.[6] Common epilepsy syndromes include childhood absence epilepsy (CAE), juvenile absence epilepsy (JAE), and juvenile myoclonic epilepsy (JME).[6] They are often grouped together and called the idiopathic generalized epilepsies (IGEs) or the genetic generalized epilepsies (GGEs). Other well-recognized syndromes are West syndrome, Lennox–Gastaut syndrome (LGS), and Dravet syndrome.[6]

Diagnosis

Epilepsy is a clinical diagnosis, meaning that it is made on the basis of medical signs and patient-reported symptoms, rather than any one diagnostic test. A person is considered to have epilepsy if they meet any

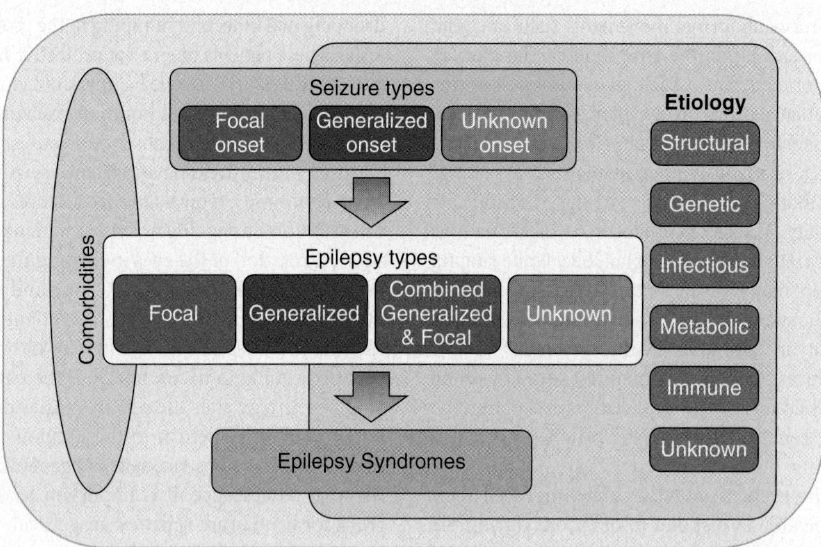

FIGURE 75-2 ILAE framework for classification of the epilepsies. *(Reprinted, with permission, from Scheffer IE, Berkovic S, Capovilla G, et al. ILAE classification of the epilepsies: Position paper of the ILAE Commission for Classification and Terminology. Epilepsia. 2017;58(4):512–521.)*

of the following conditions: (1) at least two unprovoked (or reflex) seizures occurring greater than 24 hours apart; (2) one unprovoked (or reflex) seizure and a probability of further seizures similar to the general recurrence risk (at least 60%) after two unprovoked seizures, occurring over the next 10 years; or (3) diagnosis of an epilepsy syndrome.[30]

Accurate diagnosis also depends on the neurologic examination and diagnostic techniques such as EEG and brain imaging. The neurologic examination is generally nonfocal, and focal findings may suggest a nonepilepsy diagnosis or help identify an epilepsy etiology (eg, stroke). The EEG can identify abnormal brain wave patterns that are associated with certain seizure types and epilepsy syndromes and is one of the most common and important diagnostic tests that can be performed for a patient with epilepsy. However, an abnormal epileptiform EEG is found in only approximately 50% of the patients who have epilepsy and sometimes several EEGs must be obtained before convincing epileptiformver activity is detected. Video EEG is the gold standard for diagnosing epilepsy and involves hospital admission to facilitate recording video and continuous EEG monitoring until the patient has a typical event. However, this is not the standard for most patients and is generally reserved for cases unresponsive to medication or difficult to characterize.[31,32]

Brain imaging with either a computed tomography scan (CT) or MRI can detect structural lesions that aid in the diagnosis of seizures and epilepsy types. A CT is commonly performed in patients who present after their first seizure, as a way to evaluate for a brain tumor, cerebral bleeding, or gross anatomical injury. An MRI is preferred for validation of an epilepsy diagnosis as it is the preferred imaging technique to identify more subtle structural abnormalities (eg, sclerosis in the mesial temporal lobes and traumatic brain injury).[32]

There are no diagnostic laboratory tests for epilepsy; however, in some cases, particularly following generalized convulsive seizures, serum prolactin levels obtained within 10 to 20 minutes can be transiently elevated.[33] Other laboratory tests can be done to rule out treatable causes of seizures (eg, hypoglycemia, altered electrolyte concentrations, infections) that do not represent epilepsy.

TREATMENT

Desired Outcomes

1 ASM therapy is the mainstay of epilepsy treatment; however, all available ASMs are symptomatic treatments which only prevent seizures from occurring. None have been proven to have any disease modifying or antiepileptogenic properties and no ASMs are curative. Surgery is the only possibly curative therapy and only a select number of patients qualify for surgery (see section "Nonpharmacologic Therapy"). Therefore, the majority of patients with epilepsy will be on life-long ASM therapy. The goal of ASM therapy is eliminating the occurrence of seizures within the shortest possible duration of time and with minimal impact on QOL. In most patients the desired outcome is complete seizure freedom with little to no medication adverse effects. However, in 20% to 35% of patients, complete seizure freedom may not be possible[34] and more obtainable goals that balance seizure control with patient-specific QOL factors and wishes (eg, decrease in the number of seizures with minimized adverse effects) should be established.

General Approach to Treatment

When a patient presents after a single isolated seizure, one of three treatment decisions can be made: (1) treat, (2) possibly treat, or (3) do not treat, with the ultimate decision being based on the probability of the patient having a second seizure. The probability of recurrent seizures is higher if certain findings are present, including brain imaging abnormalities (eg, stroke, trauma, CNS infection, cerebral palsy, and other cognitive developmental disabilities), EEG with epileptiform abnormalities (characterized by spikes or sharp waves), or a nocturnal seizure.[35] For patients with any of the above findings present, the probability of seizure recurrence may be 2 to 2.5 times that of those without those findings.[35] The decision on whether to start ASM therapy after a single seizure depends on clinician judgment and available clinical evidence. Some clinicians choose to start ASM treatment after one seizure with a definite abnormal MRI or epileptiform EEG while others do not initiate treatment until a second seizure has occurred. In general, patients who have had two or more unprovoked seizures should be started on ASMs.[30,35]

2 Once the decision to initiate therapy has been determined, accurate identification of seizure type and epilepsy diagnosis is critical for treatment, as an ASM must be effective for the specific seizure type and epilepsy, or epilepsy syndrome, being treated. For instance, if a patient is diagnosed with the epilepsy syndrome, childhood absence epilepsy (CAE), then an ASM that is effective for that syndrome (eg, ethosuximide) should be selected, and an ASM that may exacerbate that syndrome (eg, phenytoin or carbamazepine) should be avoided. Only after an accurate diagnosis is obtained, can a care plan, including selection and/or optimization of ASM therapy, be developed.[27]

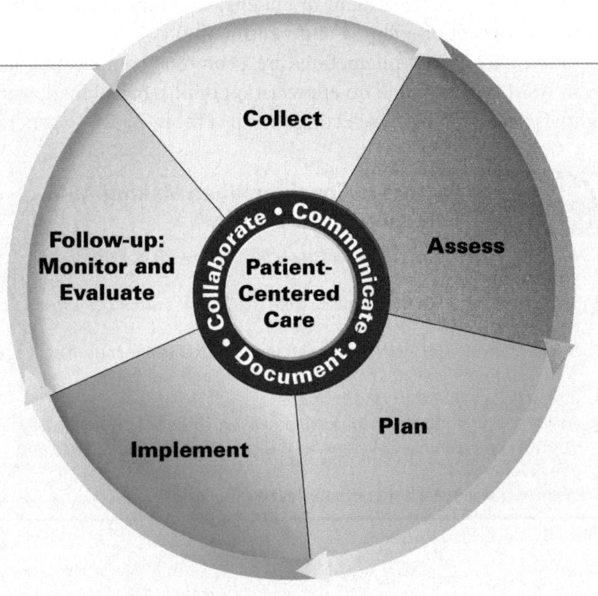

Patient Care Process for Epilepsy

The image shows the five fundamental steps included in The Pharmacist's Care Process endorsed by the Joint Commission for Pharmacy Practitioners (2014). The tagline of this process reads collaborate, communicate, and document. The five fundamental steps listed here are collect, assess, plan, implement, and follow-up: monitor and evaluate. All these steps are listed in a circular block diagram.

Collect

- Patient-specific demographics (eg, age, race, sex, pregnancy status, and desire for pregnancy)
- A detailed description of seizure semiology from the patient and a witness of the seizure, including the following:
  - o Degree of mental status impairment during the event
  - o Presence of ictal motor, sensory, autonomic, or other features at onset of the seizure (Fig. 75-1)
  - o Tongue biting, cheek biting, and bladder or bowel incontinence during the seizures
  - o Seizure time course and any postictal phenomena (eg, fatigue, headaches, confusion, and psychosis)
- Frequency of seizure events and any precipitating factors
- Information on comorbid medical psychiatric, and neurodevelopmental conditions including depression, anxiety, and learning and development conditions
- Family history of epilepsy, risk factors for epilepsy including injury at birth, history of meningitis or encephalitis, history of traumatic brain injury
- Current and past medications including antiseizure medications (ASMs)
- Duration of past ASM therapy and response to each ASM (eg, decrease or increase in seizure frequency and adverse medication reactions experienced)
- Allergies to medications including ASMs
- Laboratory values for electrolytes and glucose to rule out provoked seizures, baseline test for renal function, liver function, and complete blood count (CBC)
- Magnetic resonance imaging (MRI) of brain without contrast
- Electroencephalogram (EEG)

Assess

- Seizure, epilepsy, and epilepsy syndrome classification (Figs. 75-1 and 75-2)
- Duration of therapy on current ASM regimen
- Seizure freedom on current ASMs or current seizure frequency if not seizure-free (Fig. 75-3)
- Adverse medication reactions experienced on current ASMs (Fig. 75-3)
- Factors for optimal ASM selection including patient-specific factors (Table 75-1)
- Other quality-of-life factors

Plan*

- Determine need for monotherapy (usually at initiation of therapy) or polytherapy (usually after failure of first or second ASM) (Fig. 75-3)
- Select an ASM that has efficacy for the specific seizure type, epilepsy, or epilepsy syndrome (Table 75-5)
- Considering patient-specific factors, select an ASM with:
  - o Most tolerable adverse medication reaction profile (Table 75-5)
  - o Least incidence of interactions with other medications (Tables 75-3 and 75-5)
  - o Least complicated ASM pharmacokinetics (Table 75-2)
  - o Utility in treating the patients' other comorbid conditions (Table 75-5)
- Create a patient-specific monitoring plan based on the therapy chosen

Implement*

- Identify initial dose and maintenance dose (Table 75-4) along with appropriate formulation (Table 75-5) and dosage size (eg, 25 mg tablets, 100 mg capsules, 250 mg/5 mL oral solution, 1,500 mg/100 mL of diluted solution for intravenous injection) to meet the patients' needs
- Counsel patient on dose, dose formulation, and how to titrate appropriately
- Provide patient with seizure and adverse medication reaction diary and counsel patient and family on how to record in the diary
- Ensure completion of prior authorizations for insurance coverage as needed
- Ensure prescription is provided on appropriate controlled substance prescription form as needed for any scheduled preparations (Table 75-5)

Follow-up: Monitor and Evaluate

- Treatment response including increase or decrease in seizure frequency and changes in seizure semiology
- Laboratory assessments including CBC, chemistries, liver function tests, and ASM serum concentrations if needed
- Monitor for common dose-related, rare idiosyncratic, and long-term adverse medication reactions
- Monitor for other comorbid conditions such as depression, anxiety, suicidal ideation, and social adjustment
- Monitor for learning and development issues in children
- Monitor seizure triggers
- Monitor adherence

Collaborate with patient, caregivers, and other healthcare professionals.

3 During ASM selection, several possible first-choice agents are identified based on the type of epilepsy, and then narrowed down to an ideal single medication based on patient-specific characteristics including age, sex, susceptibility to adverse effects, comorbid medical conditions, interactions with other medications, ability to adhere to a prescribed regimen, and cost of therapy/insurance coverage (Table 75-1). Patient-specific characteristics must be taken into consideration as individuals may be better suited to receive one ASM over another. For instance, children may be more susceptible to neuropsychiatric adverse effects and ASMs with those effects should be avoided. Females with childbearing potential should not be on ASMs with unacceptable teratogenicity, and ASMs with adverse cognitive effects should be avoided in older adults as they may be more susceptible. On the other hand, patients with comorbid conditions, such as migraine headache, bipolar disorder, or neuropathy, may benefit from the use of particular ASMs that can also treat those comorbid conditions (eg, topiramate for the treatment of epilepsy and migraine, lamotrigine for the treatment of epilepsy and bipolar, pregabalin for the treatment of epilepsy and neuropathy).

Pharmacokinetic interactions are a common complicating factor in ASM selection and an appreciation of pharmacokinetic variability is necessary when selecting therapy (Table 75-2). In general,

TABLE 75-1 Factors to Consider When Making ASM Selection

1. ASM efficacy for the specific seizure type, epilepsy, or epilepsy syndrome
2. Selection of an ASM that can also treat the patient's other comorbid conditions
3. Selection of an ASM with the most tolerable adverse effect profile, considering patient-specific factors including age and sex
4. Interactions with other medications
5. Ability to adhere to a prescribed regimen (eg, three or four times daily dosing) and insurance coverage, as this can affect ASM adherence and effectiveness
6. Need to quickly reach therapeutic levels

TABLE 75-2 Antiseizure Medication Pharmacokinetic Data

ASM	$t_{1/2}$ (Hours)	Time to Steady State (Days)	Unchanged (%)	V_D (L/kg)	Clinically Important Metabolite	Protein Binding (%)
First Generation						
Carbamazepine	12-17 34 (10,11-epoxide)	21-35 for completion of autoinduction	3	0.8-2	10,11-epoxide	76
Clonazepam	30-40	3-10	2	3.2	No	85
Ethosuximide	17-56	7-10	10-20	0.6-0.7	No	22
Phenobarbital	53-180	12-24	25-50	0.5-1	No	50
Phenytoin	22	7-10	unknown	0.5-1	No	90
Primidone	7-22 10-25 (PEMA) 75-126 (PB)	2-4	<1	0.4-1	Phenylethylmelanomide (PEMA); Phenobarbital (PB)	34
Valproic acid	9-16	2-4	<3	0.14-0.23	No	90
Second Generation						
Felbamate	16-22	3-4	40-50	0.73-0.85	No	25
Gabapentin	5-7	1-2	100	58 L	No	<3
Lamotrigine	12-60	3-15	10	0.9-1.3	No	55
Levetiracetam	6-8	2	66	0.7	No	<10
Oxcarbazepine	2 9 (MHD)	2-3	2	49 L	10-monohydroxy-carbazepine (MHD)	40
Tiagabine	7-9	2	2		No	96
Topiramate	21	4	70	0.6-0.8	No	15-41
Zonisamide	63	14	35	1.45	No	40
Third Generation						
Brivaracetam	9		<10	0.5	No	40
Cenobamate	50-60	14	6.8	40-50 L	No	60
Eslicarbazepine	13-20	4-5	67	0.87	S-licarbazepine; oxcarbazepine	<40
Lacosamide	13	3	40	0.6	No	<15
Perampanel	105	14-21	74-80	77 L	No	96
Pregabalin	6	1-2	90	0.5	No	0
Third Generation Approved for Specific Epilepsy Syndromes						
Cannabadiol	56-61	7	Minor	20,963-42,849 L	7-OH cannabadiol	>94
Clobazam	36-42	7-14	2	100 L	N-desmethylclobazam	80-90
Fenfluramine	20		<25	11.9	norfenfluramine	50
Rufinamide	6-10		<2	50 L	No	34
Stiripentol	4.5-13	Varies	0.1	Related to body weight	No	99
Vigabatrin	5-11		80	1.1	No	0

ASM, antiseizure medication; MHD, monohydroxycarbazepine derivative; PEMA, phenylethylmelanomide; PB, phenobarbital; V_D, volume of distribution.

Data from References 17–20, 23, and 36–56.

TABLE 75-3 Antiseizure Medication Elimination Pathways and Major Effects on Hepatic Enzymes

Antiepileptic Medications	Major Hepatic Enzymes	Renal Elimination (%)	Induces	Inhibits
First Generation				
Carbamazepine	CYP3A4	3	CYP1A2; CYP2B6; CYP2C9/19; CYP3A; GT	None
Clonazepam	CYP3A	2	None	None
Ethosuximide	CYP3A4; CYP2E1	10-20	None	None
Phenobarbital	CYP2C9; CYP2C19	25	CYP 3A4/2C9/2C19/1A2; GT	None
Phenytoin	CYP2C9; CYP2C19	unknown	CYP3A; CYP2C; GT	
Primidone		<1		
Valproate	GT; β-oxidation	<3	None	CYP2C9; GT epoxide hydrolase
Second Generation				
Felbamate	CYP3A4; CYP2E1; other	50	CYP3A4	CYP2C19; β-oxidation
Gabapentin	None	Almost completely	None	None
Lamotrigine	GT	10	GT	None
Levetiracetam	None (undergoes nonhepatic hydrolysis)	66	None	None
Oxcarbazepine (MHD is the active metabolite.)	Cytosolic system	<1 (27 as MHD)	CYP3A4; CYP3A5; GT	CYP2C19
Tiagabine	CYP3A4; CYP1A2; CYP2D6; CYP2C19	2	None	None
Topiramate	Not known	70	CYP3A (dose dependent)	CYP2C19
Zonisamide	CYP3A4	35	None	None
Third Generation				
Brivaracetam	CYP2C19	<10	None	CYP2C19 (weak), GT epoxide hydrolase
Cenobamate	UGT2B7/B4; CYP2E1; CYP2A6; CYP2B6; CYP2C19; CYP3A4/5	6.4	CYP2B6; CYP2C8; CYP3A4	CYP 2B6; CYP2C19; CYP3A
Eslicarbazepine	Undergoes hydrolysis	67	GT (mild)	CYP2C19
Lacosamide	CYP2C9/19; CYP3A4	40	None	CYP2C19
Perampanel	CYP3A4/5; CYP1A2; CYP2B6	Undefined	CYP3A4/5; CYP2B6; GT	CYPA3A4/5; CYP2C8; GT
Pregabalin	None	100	None	None
Third Generation with Indications for Specific Epilepsy Syndromes				
Cannabadiol	CYP2C19; CYP3A4; GT	Minor	CYP1A2; CYP2B6; GT	CYP2C8/9/19
Clobazam	CYP3A4; CYP2C19; CYP2B6	2	CYP3A4 (weak)	CYP2C9
Fenfluramine	CYP1A2; CYP2B6; CYP2D6	<25	None	None
Rufinamide	Hydrolysis	2	CYP3A4 (weak)	CYP2E1 (weak)
Stiripentol	CYP1A2; CYP2C19; CYP3A4	0.1	CYP1A2; CYP2B6; CYP3A4	CYP1A2, CYP2B6; CYP3A4; CYP 2C8/19
Vigabatrin	None	Almost completely	CYP2C9	None

CYP, cytochrome P450 isoenzyme system; GT, glucuronyltransferase; MHD, monohydroxy derivative, 10-OH-carbazepine.

Data from References 17–20, 23, and 36–56.

ASM interactions can occur in any of the pharmacokinetic processes (eg, absorption, distribution, metabolism, or elimination); however, their effects on metabolic pathways are particularly complex and significantly affect management. Knowledge of ASM metabolic pathways as well as induction or inhibitory effects on liver enzymes (Table 75-3) can aid in ASM optimization. Caution should be used when ASMs are added to or withdrawn from a drug regimen.

When selecting ASM therapy, a patient's ability to adhere to a prescribed regimen and their insurance coverage are of extreme importance, as these factors can impact outcomes. For instance, a prescribed regimen requiring multiple daily doses may result in nonadherence for a patient who finds it difficult to remember to take medicines leading to decreased seizure control. Switching to an alternative with fewer daily doses may improve outcomes in that case. Similarly, an ASM that is not covered by insurance or is expensive may also promote nonadherence or adversely affect the patient by causing financial hardship. Ultimately, ASM effectiveness results from the interaction of all of these specific factors.

Optimizing Dose

4 Once an ASM has been selected, it should be initiated at an appropriate starting dose, and gradually titrated up to a therapeutic maintenance dose based on individual ASM recommendations (Table 75-4). Titration to an adequate therapeutic dose usually occurs over a few weeks and is necessary to allow the patient to slowly adjust to dose-related adverse effects. Some individuals, such as older adults who are sensitive to falls, sedation, and other neurocognitive adverse effects, need to have lower doses started and titrated more slowly. In such cases, titration can last over many weeks or months and may have a lower goal dose. In patients with multiple recent seizures,

TABLE 75-4 Antiseizure Medication Dosing and Target Serum Concentration Ranges

Generic Medication Name (Brand Name)	Initial Total Daily Dose (TTD)	Usual Effective TDD Range	FDA-Recommended Max TDD	Target Serum Concentration Range	Dosing Notes
First Generation					
Carbamazepine (Tegretol, Tegretol XR)	400 mg (>12 yrs) 200 mg (6-12 yrs) 10-20 mg/kg (<6 yrs)	400-1,200 mg (>12 yrs) 200-1,000 mg (6-12 yrs) 10-35 mg/kg (<6 yrs)	1,600 mg (>12 yrs) 1,000 mg (6-12 yrs) 35 mg/kg (<6 yrs)	4-12 mcg/mL (mg/L; 17-51 μmol/L)	Doses higher than FDA-recommended max have been used in clinical practice.
Clonazepam (Klonopin)	Up to 1.5 mg (≥18 yrs) 0.01-0.03 mg/kg (<10 yrs or <30 kg)	1-8 mg (≥18 yrs) 0.01-0.05 mg/kg (<10 yrs or <30 kg)	20 mg (≥18 yrs) 0.05 mg/kg (<10 yrs or <30 kg)	20-70 ng/mL (mcg/L; 63-222 nmol/L)	Initial adult TDD may be up to 1.5 mg/day although lower TDD is typically initiated (eg, 0.5-1 mg/day).
Ethosuximide (Zarontin)	500 mg (≥6 yrs) 250 mg (3-6 yrs)	500-1,500 mg (≥6 yrs) 20 mg/kg (3-6 yrs)	1,500 mg (All ages)	40-100 mcg/mL (mg/L; 283-708 μmol/L)	FDA-recommended maximum TDD is not explicitly identified, but doses ≥1,500 mg should only be used with strict monitoring.
Phenobarbital (Various)	300 mg (≥18 yrs) 5 mg/kg (<18 yrs) (15-20 mg/kg LD)	300-600 mg (≥18 yrs) 4-8 mg/kg (<18 yrs)	600 mg (≥18 yrs) 300 mg (<18 yrs)	10-40 mcg/mL (mg/L; 43-172 μmol/L)	FDA-recommended doses are not available but usual dose ranges and max doses listed here are commonly used in practice.
Phenytoin (Dilantin)	300 mg (≥18 yrs) 5 mg/kg (<18 yrs) (15-20 mg/kg LD)	300-600 mg (≥18 yrs) 4-8 mg/kg (<18 yrs)	600 mg (≥18 yrs) 300 mg (<18 yrs)	Total: 10-20 mcg/mL (mg/L; 40-79 μmol/L) Unbound: 0.5-3 mcg/mL (mg/L; 2-12 μmol/L)	Patients >6 yrs may require the minimum adult TDD of 300 mg; 600 mg is the maximum recommended TDD in adults; however, higher TDD may be used in practice if serum levels are still within therapeutic range.
Primidone (Mysoline)	100-125 mg (≥8 yrs)	750-1,000 mg (≥8 yrs)	2,000 mg (≥8 yrs)	5-10 mcg/mL (mg/L; 23-46 μmol/L)	
Valproic acid, Divalproex, Valproate (Depakene, Depakote DR, Depakote ER, Depacon)	10-15 mg/kg (≥10 yrs)	20-30 mg/kg (≥10 yrs)	60 mg/kg (≥10 yrs)	50-100 mcg/mL (mg/L; 347-693 μmol/L)	
Second Generation					
Felbamate (Felbatol)	1,200 mg (≥14 yrs) 15 mg/kg (2-14 yrs)	1200-3,600 mg (≥14 yrs) 15-45 mg/kg (2-14 yrs)	3,600 mg (≥14 yrs) 45 mg/kg (2-14 yrs)	30-60 mcg/mL (mg/L; 126-252 μmol/L)	Pediatric dosing listed is for LGS.
Gabapentin (Neurontin)	300-900 mg (≥12 yrs) 10-15 mg/kg (3-11 yrs)	900-1,800 mg (≥12 yrs) 25-40 mg/kg (3-11 yrs)	3,600 mg (≥12 yrs) 50 mg/kg (3-11 yrs)	2-20 mcg/mL (mg/L; 12-117 μmol/L)	In patients 12 yrs, TDDs up to 3,600 mg/day have been tolerated for short durations; TDDs up to 4,800 mg/day have been described in the literature.
Lamotrigine (Lamictal, Lamictal XR)	25 mg (>12 years) 0.3 mg/kg (2-12 yrs)	225-375 mg (>12 yrs) 4.5-7.5 mg/kg (2-12 yrs)	500 mg (>12 yrs) 300 mg (2-12 yrs)	4-20 mcg/mL (mg/L; 16-78 μmol/L)	Dosing recommendations differ if on VPA, CBZ, PB, PHT, PRM, or VPA; refer to PI for specific dose recommendations for patients on those concomitant ASMs.
Levetiracetam (Keppra, Keppra XR)	1,000 mg (≥16 yrs) 20 mg/kg (6-15 yrs) Varies by age (<6 yrs)	2,000-3,000 mg (≥16 yrs) 20-60 mg/kg (6-15 yrs) Varies by age (<6 yrs)	3,000 mg (≥16 yrs) 60 mg/kg (6-15 yrs) Varies by age (<6 yrs)	12-46 mcg/mL (mg/L; 70-270 μmol/L)	Refer to PI for specific age-based dose recommendations for <6 yrs; XR formulation is only approved for ages >/12 years; an initial TDD of 500 mg can be used for older patients; FDA-approved maximum doses are listed although higher doses have been used in clinical practice.

TABLE 75-4 Antiseizure Medication Dosing and Target Serum Concentration Ranges

Generic Medication Name (Brand Name)	Initial Total Daily Dose (TTD)	Usual Effective TDD Range	FDA-Recommended Max TDD	Target Serum Concentration Range	Dosing Notes
Oxcarbazepine (Trileptal, Oxtellar XR)	600 mg (>17 yrs) 8-10 mg/kg-max 600 mg (2-16 yrs)	1,200-2,400 mg (>17 yrs) 900-1,800 mg (2-16 yrs)	2,400 mg (>17 yrs) Varies by age (2-16 yrs)	3-35 mcg/mL (MHD) (mg/L; 12-138 μmol/L)	Pediatric dosing listed varies based on weight, refer to PI for specific weigh-based dose recommendations; XR formulation is approved for ages 6 and older.
Tiagabine (Gabitril)	4 mg if on other ASMs that are inducers and <4 mg if not on inducers (≥12 yrs)	32-56 mg if on other ASMs that are inducers and <32-56 mg if not on inducers (≥12 yrs)	56 mg if on other ASMs that are inducers and <56 mg if not on inducers (≥12 yrs)	0.02-0.2 mcg/mL (mg/L; 0.05-0.5 μmol/L)	Not FDA approved in patients under 12 years
Topiramate (Topamax, Trokendi XR)	25-50 mg (≥10 yrs) 25 mg (2-9 yrs)	200-400 mg (≥ 10 yrs) 150-400 mg based on weight (2-9 yrs)	400 mg (≥10 yrs) Varies based on weight (2-9 yrs)	5-20 mcg/mL (mg/L; 15-59 μmol/L)	Pediatric listed dosing varies based on weight; refer to PI for specific weight-based dose recommendations; XR formulation approved for ages 6 and up; maximum recommended TDD is 400 mg; however, up to 1,600 mg has been described for specific situations (eg, status epilepticus).
Zonisamide (Zonegran)	100 mg (>16 yrs)	200-400 mg (>16 yrs)	600 mg (>16 yrs)	10-40 mcg/mL (mg/L; 47-188 μmol/L)	FDA approved pediatric dosing recommendations not available.
Third Generation					
Brivaracetam (Briviact)	100 mg (≥16 yrs) 50-100 mg if >50 kg or 1-3 mg/kg if <50 kg (1 mo – 15 yrs)	100-200 mg (≥16 yrs) 50-200 mg if >50 kg or 1-6 mg/kg if < 50 kg (1 mo – 15 yrs)	200 mg (≥16 yrs) Varies based on weight (1 mo-15 yrs)	Not defined	Pediatric dosing listed for patients <50 kg varies based on weight; refer to PI for specific weight-based dose recommendations.
Cenobamate (Xcopri)	12.5 mg (≥18 yrs)	200-400 mg (≥18 yrs)	400 mg (≥18 yrs)	Not defined	Not FDA approved in pediatrics.
Eslicarbazepine (Aptiom)	400 mg (≥18 yrs) 200-400 mg (4-17 yrs)	800-1,600 mg (≥18 yrs) 400-1,200 mg (4-17 yrs)	1,600 mg (≥18 yrs) 1,200 mg (4-17 yrs)	Not defined	Pediatric dosing listed is weight-based; refer to PI for specific weight-based dose recommendations.
Lacosamide (Vimpat)	100-200 mg (>17 yrs) 100 mg if >50 kg and 2 mg/kg if <50 kg (4-17 yrs)	200-400 mg (>17 yrs) 200-400 mg if >50 kg or 4-8 mg/kg if <50 kg (4-17 yrs)	400 mg (>17 yrs) 400 mg if >50 kg or 8 mg/kg if <50 kg (4-17 yrs)	Not defined	Dosing listed is for focal onset and generalized onset tonic–clonic seizures
Perampanel (Fycompa)	2 mg	8-12 mg	12 mg	Not defined	Dosing listed is for patients >4 yrs with focal onset seizures or >12 yrs with generalized onset tonic–clonic seizures.
Pregabalin (Lyrica)	150 mg (≥17 yrs) 2.5 mg/kg if >30 kg and 3.5 mg/kg between 11-29 kg (4-17 yrs)	150-600 mg (≥17 yrs) 2.5-10 mg/kg if >30 kg and 3.5-14 mg/kg between 11-29 kg (4-17 yrs)	600 mg (≥17 yrs) 600 mg if >30 kg and 14 mg/kg between 11 and 29 kg (4-17 yrs)	Not defined	
Third Generation with Indications for Specific Epilepsy Syndromes					
Cannabadiol (Epidiolex)	5 mg/kg (≥2 yrs)	10-20 mg/kg (≥2 yrs)	20 mg/kg (≥2 yrs)	Not defined	Dosing listed is for Dravet Syndrome and LGS.
Clobazam (Onfi)	5 mg if ≤30 kg and 10 mg if >30 kg (≥2 yrs)	5-20 mg if ≤30 kg and 10-40 mg if >30 kg (≥2 yrs)	20 mg if <30 kg and 40 mg if >30 kg (≥2 yrs)	0.03-0.3 ng/mL (mcg/L; 0.1-1.0 nmol/L)	Dosing listed is for LGS.

(Continued)

TABLE 75-4 Antiseizure Medication Dosing and Target Serum Concentration Ranges (*Continued*)

Generic Medication Name (Brand Name)	Initial Total Daily Dose (TTD)	Usual Effective TDD Range	FDA-Recommended Max TDD	Target Serum Concentration Range	Dosing Notes
Fenfluramine (Fintepla)	0.2 mg/kg if not on STP and 0.1 mg/kg if on STP and CLB (≥2 yrs)	0.35 mg/kg if not on STP and 0.2 mg/kg/day if on STP and CLB (≥2 yrs)	26 mg if not on STP and 17 mg if on STP and CLB (≥2 yrs)	Not defined	Dosing listed is for Dravet Syndrome.
Rufinamide (Banzel)	400-800 mg (≥17 yrs) 10 mg/kg (1-16 yrs)	1,600-3,200 mg (≥17 yrs) 10-45 mg/kg (1-16 yrs)	3,200 mg (≥17 yrs) 3,200 mg (1-16 yrs)	Not defined	Dosing listed is for LGS. FDA labeling states the efficacy of TDD <3,200 mg is unknown; however, doses <3,200 mg are commonly used in clinical practice.
Stiripentol (Diacomit)	50 mg/kg (≥2 yrs)	50 mg/kg (≥2 yrs)	3,000 mg (≥2 yrs)	4-22 mg/L (mcg/mL; 17-94 μmol/L)	Dosing listed is for patients with Dravet Syndrome who are also on CLB. STP should only be used in combination therapy with CLB.
Vigabatrin (Sabril)	1,000 mg (≥17 yrs) 350-500 mg depending on weight (2-16 yrs) 50 mg/kg (Infants)	1,000-3,000 mg (≥17 yrs) 1,050-2,000 mg depending on weight (2-16 yrs) 50-150 mg/kg (Infants)	3,000 mg (≥17 yrs) Varies by weight (2-16 yrs) 150 mg/kg (Infants)	0.8-36 mcg/mL (mg/L; 6-279 μmol/L)	Infant dosing listed is for infantile spasms; adult and non-infant pediatric dosing listed is for refractory focal seizures.

CLB, clobazam; CBZ, carbamazepine; DR, delayed-release; FDA, Food and Drug Administration; ER, extended-release; LD, loading dose; LGS, Lennox-Gastaut Syndrome; MHD, 10-monohydroxycarbazepine derivative; PB, phenobarbital; PHT, phenytoin; PI, prescribing information; PRM, primidone; STP, Stiripentol; TDD, total daily dose; yrs, years; VPA, valproate; XR, extended release.

Data from References 17-20, 23, and 36-56.

a therapeutic dose needs to be reached much more quickly, and a rapid titration over days instead of weeks is appropriate. For such patients, loading doses, either administered orally or intravenously, may be indicated. When used in this manner, it is important to select ASMs that can be administered safely as loading doses, as medications like lamotrigine and carbamazepine require slow titration and should not be used in patients who require loading to reach therapeutic levels quickly (Table 75-4).

Determining the optimal therapeutic dose for an individual takes into account treatment response and adverse medication reactions. If the patient is seizure free with no adverse reactions at a minimal therapeutic dose, then an optimal dose has been achieved and no further increases is necessary. If the patient continues to have seizures at a minimal or moderate-therapeutic dose, further titration to a maximum dose may be needed for optimal seizure control. If the patient continues to have seizures at a maximum dose, or if the patient experiences intolerable adverse reactions at any dose, adding a second ASM and then tapering and discontinuing the ineffective or intolerable first ASM is appropriate. Selecting an ASM with a different mechanism of action than the first intolerable or ineffective ASM may increase the likelihood of success with the second ASM, although there is no clear evidence to support this.[57]

5 In general, ASM monotherapy is preferred. However, if the patient continues to have seizures after switching to a second ASM as monotherapy at a therapeutic dose, dual ASM therapy may be necessary, and an adjunctive ASM should be gradually added. Selection of an adjunctive ASM with a different or complementary mechanism of action is recommended and is the basis behind rational polytherapy, although there is no clear evidence in humans to support this practice.[57] For individuals who continue to have seizures on dual ASM therapy, polytherapy with three or more agents can be considered. A suggested algorithm for a general approach to the use of ASM monotherapy and polytherapy in the treatment of epilepsy is shown in Fig. 75-3.

Nonpharmacologic Therapy

Pharmacologic therapy with ASMs is the mainstay of treatment for patients with epilepsy. However, approximately 20% to 35% of patients will not achieve adequate seizure control and seizures may be considered medication-resistant.[34] Nonpharmacologic therapies are available for these medication-resistant seizures, as well as for individuals with medication-responsive seizures in whom the benefits of nonpharmacologic therapies outweigh its risk. Nonpharmacologic therapy for epilepsy includes diet, vagus nerve stimulation (VNS), and surgery among other modalities.

The ketogenic diet, devised in the 1920s, is high in fat and low in carbohydrates and protein, which leads to a shift in metabolism resulting in acidosis and ketosis. As protein and calorie intake are set at levels that will meet requirements for growth, most of the calories provided come in the form of heavy cream and butter, although medium-chain triglycerides can be substituted for the dietary fats. Furthermore, no sugar is allowed, the overall fluids are controlled, and vitamins and minerals are supplemented. Given these restrictions, it requires strict control and parental adherence, as this diet is often used in childhood forms of epilepsy. Although some centers find the diet useful for medically refractory patients, particularly those with certain etiologies such as glucose transporter 1 (GLUT1) deficiency, others have found that it is poorly tolerated. Long-term effects include kidney stones, increased bone fractures, and adverse growth effects.[58] An international consensus statement has offered recommendations for employing various forms of the ketogenic diet which may be more tolerable, including the use of the modified Atkins diet and the Low Glycemic Index treatment.[59]

A VNS is an Food and Drug Administration (FDA)-approved implanted medical device that is used as adjunctive therapy in reducing the frequency of seizures in adults and adolescents older than 12 years of age with focal seizures refractory to ASMs. It is

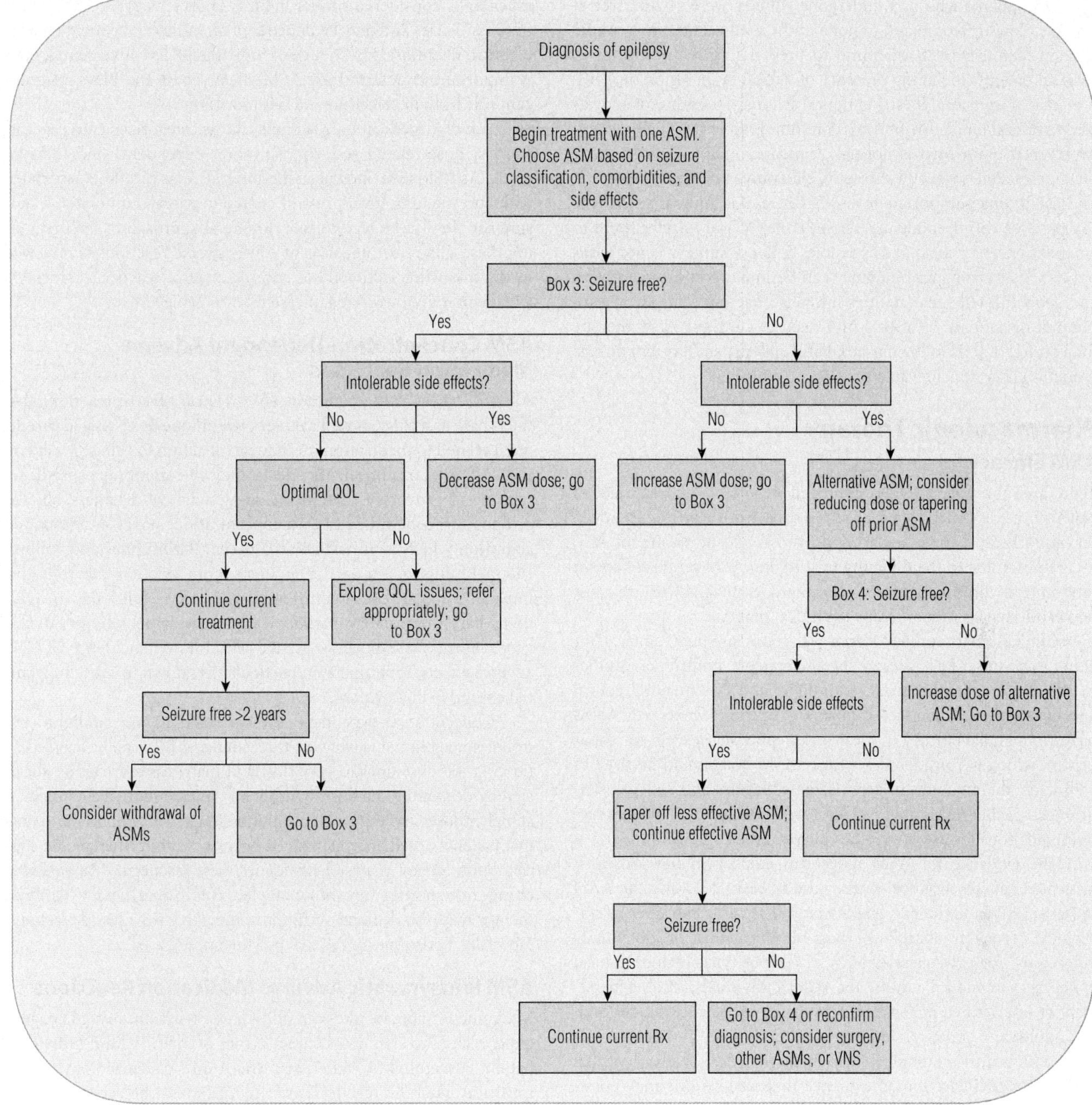

FIGURE 75-3 An algorithm for ASM therapy. (ASM, antiseizure medication; VNS, vagal nerve stimulation.)

also used off-label in the treatment of refractory primary generalized epilepsy. The mechanisms behind VNS's antiseizure actions are unknown. Human clinical studies have shown that VNS changes the cerebrospinal fluid (CSF) concentration of inhibitory and stimulatory neurotransmitters and activates specific areas of the brain that generate or regulate cortical seizure activity through increased blood flow. There is experimental evidence to suggest that the antiseizure effect of VNS is mediated by the locus coeruleus.[60]

The VNS is relatively safe and may have a positive effect on mood and behavior, often independent of seizure reduction.[61] The most common adverse reactions associated with stimulation are hoarseness, voice alteration, increased cough, pharyngitis, dyspnea, dyspepsia, and nausea. Serious adverse reactions reported include infection, nerve paralysis, hypoesthesia, facial paresis, left vocal cord paralysis, left facial paralysis, left recurrent laryngeal nerve injury, urinary retention, and low-grade fever. In the VNS studies, the percentage of patients who achieved a 50% or greater reduction in their seizure frequency (responders) ranged from 23% to 50% at 3 months.[62,63] The effects of VNS are not noted immediately, are more long term, and are also unlikely to lead to seizure freedom but may allow for reduced seizure frequency and reduced medication burden.

6 Surgery is the treatment of choice in select patients with refractory focal epilepsy, especially those with seizures originating from the temporal lobe. A randomized controlled trial, focusing on temporal lobe epilepsy, found that 58% of patients who underwent surgery were seizure free at 1 year compared to 8% of patients who did not undergo surgery.[64] A second randomized controlled study, to evaluate the efficacy of early surgery versus continued medical management in patients who had failed two ASM trials, showed that

11 of 15 patients who had undergone surgery were seizure free at 2-year follow-up, compared to none in the medical therapy group.[65] Certain factors have been found to predict positive outcomes in surgical patients including presence of a focal brain lesion on MRI, presence of unilateral mesial temporal sclerosis, presence of a localized temporal lobe positron emission tomography (PET) abnormality (even if brain MRI is normal), concordant EEG data showing location of ictal onset and shorter preoperative seizure duration.[66-68] The last finding is important to emphasize, as it is imperative to identify patients with treatment-resistant epilepsy and to refer them to an epilepsy center as soon as possible. Epilepsy surgery is not without risk, as learning and memory can be impaired postoperatively, and general intellectual abilities have also been affected in a small number of patients.[68] Patients may need to continue ASM therapy for a period of time following successful epilepsy surgery, but dosage reduction may be achievable.

Pharmacologic Therapy

ASM Efficacy

There are more than 27 FDA-approved ASMs for the treatment of epilepsy in the United States. Only a subset of these are approved for monotherapy, and many are approved as add-on treatment only, in large part due to the difficulty in studying ASM monotherapy in randomized clinical trials. As such, many clinicians will use most ASMs off-label as monotherapy in clinical practice.

Clinical trials for ASM approval focus on their efficacy for either focal-onset epilepsies or specific epilepsy syndromes. Studies to directly compare the efficacy of individual ASMs are not practical and have not been conducted for many of these agents. All ASMs have comparable efficacy in focal-onset epilepsies, except for gabapentin, which is considered a weaker ASM and should be used as adjunctive therapy only. In generalized epilepsies and epilepsy syndromes, specific ASMs are FDA-approved (Table 75-5) or have recommendations for use in specific epilepsy types.

The evidence for ASM long-term efficacy in new-onset or untreated epilepsy was reviewed by the ILAE in 2013 and the AAN in 2018. Based on evidence, ASMs were labeled as "established as efficacious," "probably efficacious," "possibly efficacious," or "potentially efficacious" for new-onset epilepsy of various types including focal epilepsies in children, adults, and older individuals; focal, generalized, or unclassified epilepsy with tonic–clonic seizures in children and adults; and epilepsy syndromes like CAE, JME, and benign epilepsy with centro-temporal spikes (BECT).[27] Additionally, the ILAE and AAN identified limited evidence that some ASMs may possibly precipitate or aggravate certain seizure types, and, therefore, it is suggested that they should be used with caution in those patients (eg, carbamazepine and phenytoin in generalized onset tonic–clonic seizure types or carbamazepine, gabapentin, oxcarbazepine, phenytoin, tiagabine, and vigabatrin among others in patients with CAE or JME).[27] Despite the availability of ILAE and AAN recommendations summarizing ASM efficacy, based on the best available evidence in both new-onset and refractory epilepsy, there continues to be limited evidence to definitively guide pharmacotherapy decisions for refractory epilepsy.[73,74] Therefore, after assessing the evidence for ASM efficacy for a particular epilepsy or seizure type, pharmacotherapy decisions are guided by patient-specific factors, tolerability, risk for medication adverse reactions, and medication interactions (Tables 75-1 to 75-4).

ASM Effectiveness

In general, ASM "efficacy" is a measure of the ability of an ASM to prevent seizures or reduce their frequency in "ideal" circumstances. In contrast, ASM "effectiveness" is a more pragmatic measure of ASM benefit in "real-world" clinical setting and takes into account tolerability and their adverse reaction profiles. While ASM "efficacy" is generally considered similar in focal-onset epilepsies, ASM "effectiveness" varies and may be dependent on individual patient characteristics. Therefore, knowledge of individual ASM adverse reactions is important in determining ASM effectiveness and plays a significant role in their selection and optimization.

Adverse medication reactions can be categorized into two categories, dose-related (eg, concentration dependent) and idiosyncratic. As ASMs are often used life-long, adverse reactions associated with chronic long-term use and related to overall cumulative exposure should also be recognized. A general approach to understanding these different categories of ASM adverse reactions is reviewed in the following sections. For specific adverse reactions associated with each individual ASM, please refer to Table 75-5.

ASM Concentration-Dependent Adverse Medication Reactions

All ASMs have some common dose-related adverse reactions that they share as a class, as well as their own unique dose-related profile, often related to medication mechanism of action. As all ASMs act on the CNS to exert antiseizure effects, they all commonly cause dose-related CNS adverse reactions including sedation, dizziness, blurred or double vision, difficulty with concentration, ataxia, and impaired cognition which is of particular concern. Barbiturates and sodium channel inhibitors in particular cause more sedation and cognitive impairment than other commonly used ASMs (although in children, barbiturates may paradoxically cause hyperactivity). While newer agents have been associated with a lower incidence of CNS adverse effects, topiramate, in particular, is known to cause substantial cognitive impairment.[75]

Concentration-dependent adverse reactions are common and troublesome but not usually life-threatening, as they can be avoided by titrating the dose upward very slowly in many cases or can be alleviated by decreasing the dose.[76] Although they are more likely to occur at higher doses and higher concentration ranges, it is important to note that patients dosed and maintained below or within "therapeutic concentration ranges" may still experience these reactions.[77] Patients who change from polytherapy with multiple agents to dual therapy or monotherapy may also demonstrate improvement in CNS adverse reactions, especially if principles of rational polytherapy are used.

ASM Idiosyncratic Adverse Medication Reactions

More uncommon are idiosyncratic adverse reactions, which are generally related to chemical characteristics of the ASM and individual patient susceptibility, rather than the ASM's pharmacology. While most idiosyncratic reactions are mild, they can be serious, potentially life threatening, and can affect virtually any organ, although the skin, liver, and blood cells are most commonly affected. The most widely recognized idiosyncratic reactions associated with ASMs are rashes, which are more common with particular ASMs (eg, carbamazepine, phenytoin, phenobarbital, and lamotrigine) but may occur with any. While these rashes are often mild, some can progress to severe life-threatening rashes including Steven–Johnsons syndrome (SJS) or toxic epidermal necrolysis (TEN). Hepatitis or blood dyscrasias have also occurred with many ASMs and can progress to acute hepatic failure or fatal aplastic anemia such as those rare cases reported with felbamate. Additionally, ASM treatment itself may sometimes worsen seizures as a paradoxical toxic effect of the medication.[75,76]

A warning on suicidal behavior and ideation also accompanies all ASMs. This is based on pooled analyses of almost 200 placebo-controlled trials of 11 different ASMs showing that patients randomized to an ASM had approximately twice the risk of suicidal thinking or behavior compared to patients randomized to placebo. While the estimated incidence of suicidal ideation was low, less than 0.5% of patients on ASMs, this was greater than the 0.24% of patients on placebo. While some believed that this risk is nonsignificant,

TABLE 75-5 Antiseizure Medications (ASMs)

ASM and Available Formulations	Postulated Mechanism of Action (MOA)/Indication	Advantages/Disadvantages	Interactions	Adverse Medication Reactions
First-Generation ASMs				
Carbamazepine (CBZ) Chewable tablet, ER tablet, liquid suspension	**MOA**: Enhances fast inactivation of voltage-gated sodium channels	**Advantages**: Useful in comorbid bipolar disorder and trigeminal neuralgia	**Effect of CBZ on ASMs**: CBZ is potent inducer of CYP3A4, CYP1A2, CYP2B6, CYP2C9/19; CBZ decreases or possibly decreases levels of brivaracetam, clonazepam, eslicarbazepine, ethosuximide, felbamate, lacosamide, lamotrigine, oxcarbazepine, perampanel, phenytoin, rufinamide, stiripentol tiagabine, topiramate, valproate, zonisamide	**BOXED WARNING**: Increased risk of SJS/TEN with HLA-B*1502 allele; aplastic anemia and agranulocytosis **Common**: CNS effects including diplopia, dizziness, drowsiness; unsteadiness, lethargy; hyponatremia from SIADH
	Indication: Monotherapy/adjunctive therapy for focal onset, TC, and mixed seizure types except for absence seizures	**Disadvantages**: Avoid in absence epilepsy as it worsens other seizure types in those patient; screening required for those at increased risk SJS/TEN in HLA-B*1502 and HLA-A*3101 allele (eg, specific Asian groups); avoid if prior rash with other ASMs due to possible cross-reaction auto-inducer; active metabolite carbamazepine 10,11 epoxide contributes to idiosyncratic adverse reactions; avoid in patients with history of bone marrow depression or sensitivity to tricyclic compounds; cannot use within 14 days of MAO inhibitor; can cause fetal harm	**Effect of ASMs on CBZ**: Cenobamate, eslicarbazepine, felbamate, phenobarbital, phenytoin, primidone, rufinamide may decrease CBZ levels; brivaracetam, felbamate, valproate may increase carbamazepine-10,11 epoxide levels; vigabatrin may increase CBZ levels	**Serious but rare**: Other blood dyscrasias including thrombocytopenia, leukopenia; DRESS; increased intraocular pressure; cardiovascular effects including 2nd and 3rd degree AV heart block; hepatotoxicity
			Others (partial list): CYP3A4 inhibitors/inducers may increase/decrease CBZ levels; CBZ may decrease levels of hormonal contraceptives; do not administer with other liquid agents due to possibility of precipitate occurrence	**Long term**: Hyponatremia from SIADH; metabolic bone disease including osteoporosis, osteopenia, osteomalacia
Clonazepam (Schedule IV) Tablet, ODT	**MOA**: Binds $GABA_A$ receptor and potentiates GABA by modulating chloride conductance	**Advantages**: Useful when there is a need for a benzodiazepine with long half-life	**Effect of clonazepam on ASMs**: Clonazepam may affect levels of phenytoin	**BOXED WARNING**: Concomitant use with opioids may result in profound sedation, respiratory depression, coma, and death **Common**: CNS effects including impairment of cognitive and motor performance due to sedation and ataxia; behavior problems; paradoxical reactions such as agitation, irritability, aggression, anxiety, anger, nightmares, hallucinations and psychoses

(Continued)

TABLE 75-5 Antiseizure Medications (ASMs) (*Continued*)

ASM and Available Formulations	Postulated Mechanism of Action (MOA)/Indication	Advantages/Disadvantages	Interactions	Adverse Medication Reactions
	Indication: Monotherapy/adjunctive therapy for LGS (petit mal variant), akinetic, myoclonic, and absence seizures	**Disadvantages**: May increase TC seizures when used in mixed seizure types; tolerance and dependence may occur; risk of respiratory depression which is increased when used with other CNS depressants including opioids; contraindicated in acute narrow angle glaucoma and severe hepatic impairment; metabolites may accumulate with impaired renal function and may require dose adjustment; some loss of effect may occur after 3 months; withdrawal symptoms including status epilepticus may occur after discontinuation; may increase hypersalivation; no adequate data in pregnancy—may cause fetal harm	**Effect of ASMs on clonazepam**: Carbamazepine, lamotrigine, phenobarbital, phenytoin may decrease clonazepam levels; vigabatrin increases clonazepam, clonazepam may be affected by other enzyme inducing or enzyme-inhibiting ASMs **Other (partial list)**: Use with opioids increases risk of respiratory depression	**Serious but rare**: Respiratory depression; hepatomegaly; muscle weakness **Long term**: Physiologic dependence; hair loss; hirsutism; ankle and facial edema
Ethosuximide (ETX) Capsule, liquid solution	**MOA**: Inhibition of T-type calcium channels	**Advantages**: Medication of choice for absence seizures	**Effect of ETX on ASMs**: ETX may affect levels of carbamazepine, phenobarbital, phenytoin, primidone, valproate	**Common**: GI distress including nausea/vomiting, cramps diarrhea; epigastric and abdominal pain; anorexia and weight loss; CNS effects including lethargy, fatigue, drowsiness, dizziness, ataxia
	Indication: Monotherapy and adjunctive therapy for absence seizures in patients ≥3 years of age	**Disadvantages**: May worsen generalized TC seizures and other seizure types when used alone in mixed types of epilepsy; contraindicated in those with allergies to succinimides; may cause fetal harm; use with caution in hepatic/renal dysfunction	**Effect of ASMs on ETX**: Valproate may increase or decrease ETX levels	**Serious but rare**: Blood dyscrasias including leukopenia, agranulocytosis, pancytopenia, eosinophilia; rash including SJS; DRESS; hepatic/renal dysfunction; lupus erythematosus; psychiatric abnormalities including night terrors and paranoid psychosis **Long-term**: Behavioral changes
Phenobarbital (PB) (Schedule III) Tablet, elixir, injectable solution	**MOA**: Binds $GABA_A$ receptor and potentiates GABA by modulating chloride conductance	**Advantages**: Easily available world-wide; extensive knowledge and experience with PHB use despite not being FDA-approved as PHB developed in early 1900s prior to establishment of FDA and current regulatory practices	**Effect of PB on ASMs**: PB is inducer of CYP1A2, CYP2C9, CYP2C19, CYP3A4. PB may decrease levels of carbamazepine, eslicarbazepine, ethosuximide, felbamate, lacosamide, lamotrigine, oxcarbazepine, perampanel, phenytoin, rufinamide, stiripentol, tiagabine, topiramate, valproate, zonisamide	**Common**: CNS effects including residual sedation or "hangover," impaired cognition, drowsiness, dizziness, vertigo, ataxia, headache, sleep disturbance; paroxysmal effects including excitement, irritability and hyperactivity in older adults and children; GI effects including epigastric pain, nausea, vomiting, diarrhea, and constipation
	Indication: Not FDA-approved; used for focal onset and generalized seizures	**Disadvantages**: Tolerance and dependence may occur; slow taper needed when discontinuing after prolonged use; use with other CNS depressants may produce additive CNS effects; may cause respiratory depression; can cause fetal harm	**Effect of ASMs on PB**: Cenobamate, felbamate, rufinamide, valproate may increase PB levels; phenytoin may increase or decrease PB levels	**Serious but rare**: Respiratory depression and apnea; rash (SJS, TEN); cardiac effects including bradycardia, hypotension with IV administration, syncope; hepatotoxicity; megaloblastic anemia; apnea and hypoventilation
			Other (partial list): PB may decrease levels of oral contraceptives	**Long term**: Behavioral changes; connective tissue disorder; intellectual blunting; metabolic bone disease (Rickets, osteopenia, osteoporosis, osteomalacia); folate deficiency (with megaloblastic anemia)

TABLE 75-5 Antiseizure Medications (ASMs)

ASM and Available Formulations	Postulated Mechanism of Action (MOA)/Indication	Advantages/Disadvantages	Interactions	Adverse Medication Reactions
Phenytoin (PHT) ER capsule; liquid suspension; injectable; chewable tablet (Fosphenytoin, a prodrug desterified by esterases in the blood to phenytoin, also available as injectable solution only)	**MOA**: Enhances fast inactivation of voltage-gated sodium channels; inhibits persistent sodium current (I_{NAP}) and increases threshold for action potential firing	**Advantages**: May be orally or intravenously loaded in patients who require rapid steady-state serum levels; ER formulation useful in nonadherence as dosed once daily	**Effect of PHT on ASMs**: PHT may decreases levels of brivaracetam, carbamazepine, cenobamate, clonazepam, eslicarbazepine, felbamate, ethosuximide, felbamate, lacosamide, lamotrigine, oxcarbazepine, perampanel, rufinamide, stiripentol, tiagabine, topiramate, valproate, zonisamide	**Common**: CNS effects including ataxia, nystagmus, slurred speech, decreased coordination, mental confusion, dizziness, insomnia, transient nervousness, headaches
	Indication: Monotherapy/adjunctive therapy for focal onset psychomotor seizures and TC seizures; prevention or treatment of seizures during or after neurosurgery, severe TBI, status epilepticus	**Disadvantages**: May aggravate seizures in patients with absence seizures; can increase blood sugar levels in diabetes; HLA-B*1502 may be a risk factor for the development of SJS/TEN in patients of Asian ancestry; CYP2C9*3 carriers may increase development of SCARS; monitoring of free phenytoin levels required in renal, hepatic impairment, hypoalbuminemia, and pregnancy; compromised absorption with concomitant tube feeds; dose adjustments required to switch between free acid and sodium salt formulations; phenytoin dose adjustments needed in older adults due to decreased clearance; may exacerbate porphyria	**Effect of ASMs on PHT**: Carbamazepine, eslicarbazepine, vigabatrin may decrease PHT levels; brivaracetam, cenobamate, ethosuximide, felbamate, methsuximide, oxcarbazepine, rufinamide, topiramate may increase PHT levels; phenobarbital, valproate may increase or decrease PHT levels	**Serious but rare**: Blood dyscrasias including thrombocytopenia, leukopenia, granulocytopenia, agranulocytosis, pancytopenia; lymphadenopathy; rash (SJS/TEN/SCARS); DRESS; hepatotoxicity; angioedema; bradycardia/cardiac arrest; purple glove syndrome with IV administration
			Other (partial list): PHT can substantially reduce delavirdine concentrations and cause loss of virologic response and resistance; may decrease contraceptive levels, may increase/decrease PT/INR when given with warfarin	**Long term**: Connective tissue changes including skin thickening, gingival hyperplasia, coarsening of facial features, enlargement of lips; hirsutism; metabolic bone disease (osteoporosis, osteopenia, osteomalacia); peripheral neuropathy; cerebellar atrophy; folate deficiency (with megaloblastic anemia)
Primidone (PRM) Tablet	**MOA**: Prodrug converted to active metabolite phenylethylmalonamide-amide (PEMA) and phenobarbital with same mechanism of action	**Advantages**: Useful in patients with essential tremor	**Effect of PRM on ASMs**: PRM may decrease levels of carbamazepine, eslicarbazepine, ethosuximide, felbamate, lacosamide, lamotrigine, oxcarbazepine, perampanel, phenytoin, rufinamide, stiripentol, tiagabine, topiramate, valproate, zonisamide	**Common**: CNS effects including ataxia, vertigo, nystagmus, diplopia, drowsiness, fatigue; GI effects including nausea/vomiting, anorexia, fatigue; emotional disturbances including hyperirritability **Serious but rare**: Blood dyscrasias including granulocytopenia, agranulocytosis; rash (SJS, TEN); liver dysfunction
	Indication: Monotherapy/adjunctive therapy for focal onset and TC seizures	**Disadvantages**: Contraindicated in porphyria	**Effect of ASMs on PRM**: Valproate may increase PRM levels; phenytoin may increase or decrease PRM levels; carbamazepine, eslicarbazepine may affect levels	**Long term**: Behavioral changes; intellectual blunting; connective tissue disorder; metabolic bone disease (rickets, osteomalacia); folate deficiency (with megaloblastic anemia)

(Continued)

TABLE 75-5 Antiseizure Medications (ASMs) (*Continued*)

ASM and Available Formulations	Postulated Mechanism of Action (MOA)/Indication	Advantages/Disadvantages	Interactions	Adverse Medication Reactions
Valproate (VPA) Divalproex DR sprinkle capsule and tablet, Divalproex ER 24-hour tablet, valproic acid IR capsule, valproate sodium injectable solution	**MOA**: Likely potentiates GABAergic transmission among multiple other unknown mechanisms	**Advantages**: Useful in comorbid bipolar disorder and migraine; commonly used in all age groups including ages <10 years	**Effect of VPA on ASMs**: VPA may increase levels of eslicarbazepine, ethosuximide, felbamate, lamotrigine, oxcarbazepine, phenytoin, phenobarbital, rufinamide, tiagabine, topiramate, zonisamide **Effect of ASMs on VPA**: Carbamazepine, phenobarbital, phenytoin, primidone may decrease VPA levels; felbamate may increase VPA levels	**BOXED WARNING**: Hepatotoxicity especially for children <2 years of age and with mitochondrial disorders; fetal risk including neural tube defects, other major malformations, and decreased IQ; pancreatitis including fatal hemorrhagic pancreatitis **Common**: GI effects including abdominal pain/GI upset (worse with valproic acid IR), constipation, diarrhea, anorexia, increased appetite, weight gain, nausea/vomiting; CNS effects including blurred vision, ataxia, dizziness, headache, insomnia, nystagmus, somnolence, thinking abnormal, tremor; dose-dependent thrombocytopenia (>100 mg/mL)
	Indication: Monotherapy/adjunctive therapy for focal onset and multiple seizure types for patients ≥10 years of age; monotherapy/adjunctive therapy for absence seizures in patients ≥10 years of age	**Disadvantages**: Contraindicated in significant hepatic dysfunction, mitochondrial disorders caused by DNA polymerase γ (POLG) mutations, urea cycle disorders; use with caution in pancreatitis, bleeding and other hematopoietic disorders; risk of hyperammonemia with and without encephalopathy associated with concomitant topiramate use; pregnancy category D—contraindicated in women of childbearing potential and pregnancy category X for pregnant patients treated for migraine prophylaxis		**Serious but rare**: Hyperammonemia with and without encephalopathy; hypothermia with and without hyperammonemia; DRESS; bleeding and other hematopoietic disorders
			Other (partial list): Estrogen OCP may affect VPA levels	**Long-term**: Hair and nail changes including alopecia, hirsutism, hair texture and color changes, nail and nail bed disorders; irregular menses and polycystic ovary-like syndrome; weight gain; cerebral pseudoatrophy; osteoporosis and osteopenia
Second-Generation ASMs				
Felbamate (FBM) Tablet, liquid suspension	**MOA**: Antagonizes NMDA glutamate receptor; binds weakly to $GABA_A$ receptor and possibly augments GABAergic transmission	**Advantages**: May be useful in refractory epilepsy	**Effect of FBM on ASMs**: FBM may decrease carbamazepine levels; FBM may increase carbamazepine-epoxide, phenobarbital, phenytoin, valproate levels	**BOXED WARNING**: Irreversible fatal aplastic anemia aplastic anemia with greater risk in females, or history of cytopenia, ASM allergy or significant toxicity, viral infection, and/or immunologic problems with reported onset between 5-30 weeks; acute liver failure with reported onset occurring in 5 weeks **Common**: GI effects including anorexia, vomiting, nausea; CNS effects including insomnia, headache, dizziness, somnolence
	Indication: Monotherapy/adjunctive therapy for focal onset seizures with and without TC seizures in patients ≥14 years; adjunctive therapy for focal onset and generalized seizures associated with LGS in patients aged 2-14	**Disadvantages**: For severe refractory epilepsy ONLY; contraindicated in patients with hepatic dysfunction, history of blood dyscrasias; use with caution in patients with renal dysfunction; available only through special access program; pregnancy category C	**Effect of ASMs on FBM**: Carbamazepine, phenobarbital, phenytoin, primidone may decrease FBM levels; valproate does not affect FBM levels to a clinically significant degree	

TABLE 75-5 Antiseizure Medications (ASMs)

ASM and Available Formulations	Postulated Mechanism of Action (MOA)/Indication	Advantages/Disadvantages	Interactions	Adverse Medication Reactions
			Other (partial list): Estrogen OCP levels not affected	
Gabapentin (GBP) Tablet, capsule, oral solution	**MOA**: Binds to presynaptic $\alpha_2\delta$ subunit of calcium channels with unknown antiseizure effect	**Advantages**: Useful in post-herpetic neuralgia, chronic pain, and neuropathy; few interactions	**Effect of GBP on ASMs**: No significant effects	**Common**: CNS effects including somnolence, dizziness, ataxia, fatigue, nystagmus; peripheral edema and weight gain; GI effects including nausea/vomiting
	Indication: Adjunctive therapy for focal onset seizures with and without TC seizures in patients ≥3 years	**Disadvantages**: Considered weakly efficacious; potential abuse when taken with opioids; withdrawal reaction characterized by anxiety, insomnia, nausea, sweating, and increased pain; absorption may be impaired for single oral doses >1,200 mg; no adequate data in pregnancy—may cause fetal harm	**Effect of ASMs on GBP**: No significant effects	**Serious but rare**: Anaphylaxis, angioedema, DRESS; neuropsychiatric symptoms in children 3 to 12 years of age **Long-term**: Weight gain, peripheral edema
Lamotrigine (LTG) Tablet, chewable tablet,[a] ODT,[a] XR tablet[a]	**MOA**: Enhances fast inactivation of voltage-gated sodium channels	**Advantages**: Useful in bipolar disease; XR useful in non-adherence as dosed once daily	**Effect of LTG on ASMs**: No significant effects	**BOXED WARNING**: Rash including SJS, TEN with increased risk if given with valproate, exceeding recommended initial dose or dose escalation
	Indication: Adjunctive therapy in focal onset and TC seizures, generalized seizures of LGS in patients ≥2 years of age; monotherapy in patients with focal-onset seizures ≥16 years of age	**Disadvantages**: Slow titration required to avoid rash including SJS; rash more likely to occur if patient with prior rash to other ASM and concomitant use of valproic acid; rash incidence higher in children; may exacerbate myoclonus; dosage adjustment required in patients with moderate and severe liver impairment; no adequate data in pregnancy—may cause fetal harm	**Effect of ASMs on LTG**: Carbamazepine, cenobamate, oxcarbazepine, phenytoin, phenobarbital, primidone, rufinamide may decrease LTG levels; Cannabidiol increases LTG and valproate increases LTG levels by 2×	**Common**: CNS effects including dizziness, headache, diplopia, ataxia, blurred vision, somnolence, tremor; GI effects including nausea/vomiting, abdominal pain, diarrhea; other effects including rhinitis, pharyngitis, infection, fever; rash
			Other (partial list): Estrogen OCPs may decrease LTG by 50%	**Serious but rare**: DRESS; blood dyscrasias; hemophagocytic lymphohistiocytosis (HLH). Rash usually appears after 3-4 weeks of therapy and is typically generalized, erythematous, and morbilliform but can progress to SJS
Levetiracetam (LEV) Tablet, XR tablet,[a] injectable solution	**MOA**: Binds to and selectively inhibits synaptic vesicle $SV2_A$ protein thereby preventing neurotransmitter release	**Advantages**: Minimal interactions; XR useful in nonadherence as dosed once daily	**Effect of LEV on ASMs**: No significant effects	**Common**: CNS effects including somnolence, fatigue; behavior effects including aggression, agitation, anger, anxiety, apathy, depersonalization, depression, emotional lability, hostility, irritability **Serious but rare**: Psychosis, hallucinations
	Indication: Adjunctive therapy for focal onset seizures in patients >1 month, myoclonic seizures in patients with JME ≥12 years of age, and generalized TC seizures in patients ≥6 years of age with generalized epilepsy	**Disadvantages**: May worsen depression, PTSD, anxiety, thought disorders; must dose adjust in dialysis/renal failure; pregnancy category C	**Effect of ASMs on LEV**: No significant effects	
Oxcarbazepine (OXC) Tablet, tablet ER,[a] liquid suspension[a]	**MOA**: Enhances fast inactivation of voltage-gated sodium channels	**Advantages**: Useful in bipolar disorder; ER useful in non-adherence as dosed once daily	**Effects of OXC on ASMs**: OXC is inhibitor of CYP2C19 and inducer of CYP3A4/5; OXC may decrease lamotrigine levels through UGT induction and decrease perampane levels; OXC may increase phenytoin levels	**Common**: CNS effects including dizziness, somnolence, diplopia, fatigue, ataxia, abnormal vision, headache, nystagmus, tremor; GI effects including nausea, vomiting; hyponatremia due to SIADH; rash

(Continued)

TABLE 75-5 Antiseizure Medications (ASMs) (*Continued*)

ASM and Available Formulations	Postulated Mechanism of Action (MOA)/Indication	Advantages/Disadvantages	Interactions	Adverse Medication Reactions
	Indication: Monotherapy/adjunctive therapy for focal onset seizures in patients ≥4 years of age; adjunctive therapy for focal onset seizures in patients ≥2 years of age	**Disadvantages**: Higher incidence of hyponatremia, (as high as 25%); HLA-B*1502 in Asians may increase SJS or TEN risk; may require slower titration in renal impairment; active MHD metabolite may decrease in pregnancy; no adequate data in pregnant patients—may cause fetal harm	**Effect of ASMs on OXC**: Carbamazepine, phenobarbital, phenytoin, primidone may decrease levels of OXC active metabolites; valproate may increase levels of OXC **Other (partial list)**: OXC may decrease estrogen OCP levels	**Serious but rare**: SJS, TEN; DRESS; blood dyscrasias
Tiagabine (TGB) Tablet	**MOA**: Inhibitor of GABA reuptake transporter GAT1	**Advantages**: None noted	**Effect of TGB on ASMs**: TGB may decrease VPA levels by 10%	**Common**: CNS effects including dizziness, lightheadedness, somnolence, thinking abnormal; behavior effects including asthenia, lack of energy, nervousness, irritability, difficulty with concentration or attention; GI effects including abdominal pain, nausea, and vomiting
	Indication: Adjunctive therapy for focal onset seizures in patients ≥12 years of age	**Disadvantages**: Has been associated with new onset seizure, status epilepticus, and exacerbation of EEG abnormalities in those with existing epilepsy; dosage reduction may be necessary in patients with liver disease; pregnancy category C	**Effects of ASMs on TGB**: Carbamazepine, phenobarbital, phenytoin, primidone increases TGB clearance by 60% and may decrease TGB levels; valproate may increase TGB levels by 40%	**Serious but rare**: Increase in generalized seizures and non-convulsive SE in patients with refractory epilepsy; occurrence of seizures and SE in patients without epilepsy; moderately severe to incapacitating generalized weakness; exacerbation of EEG abnormalities; rash including SJS **Long-term**: Possibility of long-term ophthalmologic effects
Topiramate (TPM) Sprinkle capsule, tablet, ER capsule	**MOA**: Antagonizes voltage-gated sodium channel; binds to $GABA_A$ receptor and augments GABAergic transmission, antagonizes AMPA/kainate glutamate receptor, weak carbonic anhydrase inhibitor	**Advantages**: Useful in comorbid migraine and obesity; ER useful in non-adherence as dosed once daily	**Effect of TPM on ASMs**: TPM is weak inhibitor of CYP2C19 and inducer of CYP3A4; TPM may increase or decrease ASMs metabolized by CYP2C19 and 3A4 including felbamate and topiramate	**Common**: CNS effects including fatigue, difficulty concentrating, confusion, language problems, tremor, paresthesias; behavioral effects including nervousness, anxiety
	Indication: Monotherapy/adjunctive therapy for focal onset seizures or primary generalized TC seizures in patients ≥2 years of age; adjunctive therapy for patients with LGS ≥2 years of age	**Disadvantages**: Avoid in patients with preexisting cognitive issues; renally dose adjust with CrCl <70 mL/min (1.17 mL/s); can cause fetal harm	**Effect of ASMs on TPM**: Carbamazepine, phenobarbital, phenytoin, primidone may decrease TPM levels; valproate may increase TPM levels **Other (partial list)**: TPM at higher doses may decrease estrogen OCP levels	**Serious but rare**: Renal stones, glaucoma, hypo/hyperthermia, oligohidrosis, metabolic acidosis, SJS, TEN, and hyperammonemia with and without encephalopathy when used with valproate **Long term**: Weight loss; renal stones; metabolic acidosis
Zonisamide (ZON) Capsule	**MOA**: Enhances fast inactivation of voltage-gated sodium channels; inhibits T-type calcium channels; weak carbonic anhydrase inhibitor	**Advantages**: Useful in tremor; useful in nonadherence as dosed once daily	**Effect of ZON on ASMs**: No significant DDIs	**Common**: CNS effects including sedation, ataxia, confusion, depression, difficulty concentrating, word-finding difficulties
	Indication: Adjunctive therapy for focal onset seizures in adults	**Disadvantages**: Contraindicated in those with sulfa allergy; dose efficacy may plateau at 400 mg; should not be used in renal failure due to increases in SCr and BUN and possible effects on GFR; pregnancy category C	**Effect of ASMs on ZON**: CYP3A4 inhibitors or inducers may alter ZON levels; carbamazepine, phenobarbital, phenytoin, valproate may decrease ZON levels	**Serious but rare**: Oligohidrosis and hyperthermia; renal stones; metabolic acidosis; rash (SJS, TEN); DRESS; fulminant hepatic necrosis; blood dyscrasias **Long term**: Weight loss; renal stones; metabolic acidosis

TABLE 75-5 Antiseizure Medications (ASMs)

ASM and Available Formulations	Postulated Mechanism of Action (MOA)/Indication	Advantages/Disadvantages	Interactions	Adverse Medication Reactions
Third-Generation ASMs				
Brivaracetam (BRV, Schedule V) Tablet, oral solution, injectable solution	**MOA**: Binds to and selectively inhibits synaptic vesicle $SV2_A$ protein thereby preventing neurotransmitter release	**Advantages**: Can consider converting well-controlled patients from levetiracetam if intolerable psychiatric adverse reactions	**Effect of BRV on ASMs**: BRV may increase carbamazepine metabolite; BRV may increase phenytoin levels; no added therapeutic benefit when given with levetiracetam	**Common**: CNS effects including sedation, fatigue, ataxia, nystagmus; behavioral effects including irritability, aggressive behavior, anxiety, agitation, restlessness, tearfulness, apathy, altered mood, mood swings, hyperactivity, adjustment disorder; GI effects including nausea, vomiting
	Indication: Monotherapy/adjunctive therapy for focal onset seizures in patients ≥1 month of age; injection solution approved for ≥16 years of age	**Disadvantages**: Dosage adjustments required in hepatic impairment; no adequate data in pregnancy—may cause fetal harm	**Effect of ASMs on BRV**: CYP2C19 inhibitors may alter BRV levels **Other (partial list)**: rifampin will reduce BRV levels	**Serious but rare**: Angioedema; bronchospasm; decreased neutrophils; psychosis and depression; hematologic abnormalities including leukopenia and neutropenia
Cenobamate (CBM, Schedule V) Tablet	**MOA**: Inhibition of voltage-gated sodium channels; positive allosteric modulator of $GABA_A$ ion channel	**Advantages**: None	**Effect of CBM on ASMs**: CBM is a CYP2C19, CYP2B6, CYP3A inhibitor and may increase substrate levels; CBM is a CY2B6, CYPC8, CYP3A4 inducer and may decrease substrate levels; CBM may increase phenytoin, phenobarbital, clobazam concentrations; CBM may decrease lamotrigine, carbamazepine concentrations; CBM does not affect valproic acid, levetiracetam, or lacosamide	**Common**: CNS effects including somnolence, dizziness, fatigue, diplopia, headache; dizziness and disturbance in gait and coordination; cognitive dysfunction including memory impairment, disturbance in attention, confusional state, slowness of thought; vision changes including diplopia, blurred vision, and impaired vision; laboratory abnormalities including hepatic transaminases, potassium elevation
	Indication: Monotherapy/adjunctive therapy for focal-onset seizures in adults	**Disadvantages**: Must be slowly titrated q2weeks to avoid DRESS; contraindicated in Familial Short QT syndrome; caution when administering with other medications that shorten QT interval; use with caution and dose reduce in hepatic and renal impairment; use not recommended in end-stage hepatic or renal disease; no adequate data in pregnancy—may cause fetal harm	**Effect of ASMs on CBM**: Phenytoin may decrease CBM; valproate, phenobarbital, carbamazepine do not significantly impact CBM **Other (partial list)**: CBM may decrease estrogen OCP levels; additive risk with other medications that shorten the QT interval; use with CNS depressants increases CNS toxicity	**Serious but rare**: DRESS with fast titration (weekly intervals); QT interval shortening; appendicitis
Eslicarbazepine (ESL) Tablet	**MOA**: Selectively enhances fast inactivation of voltage-gated sodium channels	**Advantages**: Useful in non-adherence as dosed once daily	**Effect of ESL on ASMs**: Inhibitor of CYP2C19; ESL may affect carbamazepine, perampanel, phenytoin, phenobarbital, primidone levels	**Common**: CNS effects including dizziness, somnolence, nausea, headache, diplopia, fatigue, vertigo, ataxia, blurred vision, tremor; hyponatremia due to SIADH; rash
	Indication: Monotherapy or adjunctive therapy for focal onset seizures in patients ≥4 years of age	**Disadvantages**: Avoid in severe hepatic impairment; dose adjustment in renal failure; avoid concomitant use with carbamazepine and oxcarbazepine; no adequate data in pregnancy—may cause fetal harm	**Effect of ASMs on ESL**: Carbamazepine, phenobarbital, primidone, and phenytoin may decrease ESL levels **Other (partial list)**: ESL decreases estrogen OCP levels	**Serious but rare**: SJS; anaphylaxis, angioedema, DRESS; cardiac effects including prolonged PR interval, AV block; hepatotoxicity; blood dyscrasias **Long-term**: Hyponatremia

(Continued)

TABLE 75-5 Antiseizure Medications (ASMs) (*Continued*)

ASM and Available Formulations	Postulated Mechanism of Action (MOA)/Indication	Advantages/Disadvantages	Interactions	Adverse Medication Reactions
Lacosamide (LCM) (Schedule V) Tablet, oral solution, injectable solution	**MOA**: Selectively enhances slow inactivation of voltage-gated sodium channels	**Advantages**: Minimal interactions	**Effect of LCM on ASMs**: LCM is a potential CYP2C19 inhibitor but no clinically significant effects of LCM on other ASMs have been observed **Effect of ASMs on LCM**: LCM is a substrate of CYP3A4, CYP2C9, and CYP2C19; carbamazepine, phenytoin, phenobarbital, primidone may decrease LCM levels by 15-20%	**Common**: CNS effects including diplopia, headache, nausea, somnolence, dizziness, ataxia; GI effects including constipation, diarrhea, nausea, vomiting, dyspepsia, dry mouth, oral hypoesthesia/paresthesia; laboratory abnormalities including LFT elevations
	Indication: Monotherapy/adjunctive therapy for focal onset seizures in patients ≥4 years of age	**Disadvantages**: Avoid in 3rd degree heart block; must obtain ECG prior to intravenous infusion; use with caution in patients with underlying proarrhythmic conditions or on concomitant medications that affect cardiac conduction; not recommended in severe hepatic impairment; requires dose adjustment in renal impairment; oral solution contains phenylalanine and is a risk in patients with phenylketonuria no adequate data in pregnancy—may cause fetal harm	**Other (partial list)**: LCM may increase levels of strong CYP3A4 or CYP2C9 inhibitors in renal or hepatically impaired patients; risk of cardiac abnormalities increased with concomitant medications that affect cardiac conduction	**Serious but rare**: Cardiac effects including AV conduction abnormalities, prolonged PR interval, atrial arrhythmias, syncope (especially in patients with diabetes); DRESS and hypersensitivity reactions; blood abnormalities including neutropenia and anemia
Perampanel (PER) (Schedule III) Tablet, oral suspension	**MOA**: Selectively and noncompetitively antagonizes AMPA glutamate receptor on post-synaptic neuron	**Advantages**: Useful in mixed seizure types; useful in non-adherence as dosed once daily	**Effect of PER on ASMs**: PER is a modest enzyme inducer at high doses	**BOXED WARNING**: Aggression, hostility, irritability, anger, and homicidal ideation
	Indication: Monotherapy for focal onset seizures in patients ≥4 years of age; adjunctive therapy for TC seizures in patients ≥12 years of age	**Disadvantages**: Avoid in active psychosis or unstable recurrent affective disorders with significant hostility or aggressive behavior; avoid in severe hepatic/renal impairment or hemodialysis; no adequate data in pregnancy—may cause fetal harm	**Effect of ASMs on PER**: Carbamazepine, eslicarbazepine, oxcarbazepine, phenobarbital, phenytoin, primidone, topiramate decrease PER levels; valproate has no effect on PER levels **Other (partial list)**: PER decreases estrogen OCP levels	**Common**: CNS effects including dizziness, somnolence, fatigue, falls, vertigo, ataxia, headache, confusion; GI effects including nausea, weight gain, vomiting, abdominal pain; behavioral effects including irritability anxiety; weight gain; falls sometimes leading to serious head injuries **Serious but rare**: DRESS
Pregabalin (PGB) (Schedule V) Capsule, tablet CR, oral solution	**MOA**: Binds to presynaptic $\alpha_2\delta$ subunit of calcium channels	**Advantages**: Useful in patients with diabetic peripheral neuropathy, postherpetic neuralgia, fibromyalgia, neuropathic pain with spinal cord injury; minimal DDIs due to renal excretion	**Effect of PGB on ASMs**: No significant effects	**Common**: CNS effects including dizziness, somnolence, blurred vision, difficulty with concentration and attention; dry mouth; edema and weight gain
	Indication: Adjunctive therapy for focal onset seizures in patients ≥4 years of age	**Disadvantages**: Caution in preexisting cognitive disorders; no adequate data in pregnancy—may cause fetal harm	**Effect of ASMs on PGB**: No significant effects	**Serious**: Potential for misuse when taken with opiates **Long term**: Weight gain
Third-Generation ASMs with FDA Approval for Specific Epilepsy Syndrome Indications				
Cannabidiol (CBD, Schedule V) Oral solution	**MOA**: Unknown, does not act on cannabinoid receptors	**Advantages**: Useful for refractory seizures in LGS and Dravet Syndrome	**Effect of CBD on ASMs**: CBD increases lamotrigine levels; CBD increase levels of clobazam active metabolite by 3×	**Common**: CNS effects including somnolence, fatigue, malaise, asthenia; sleep disorders including insomnia, poor quality sleep; GI effects including decreased appetite; diarrhea; transaminase elevations

TABLE 75-5 Antiseizure Medications (ASMs)

ASM and Available Formulations	Postulated Mechanism of Action (MOA)/Indication	Advantages/Disadvantages	Interactions	Adverse Medication Reactions
	Indication: Monotherapy/adjunctive therapy for patients with LGS and Dravet Syndrome, ≥2 years of age	**Disadvantages**: Avoid in patients with hypersensitivity reactions to cannabis, THC; liver function and bilirubin monitoring before and at 1, 3, and 6 months of treatment specially if given with valproate; no adequate data in pregnant woman—may cause fetal harm	**Effect of ASMs on CBD**: CYP3A4 and CYP2C19 inhibitors will increase CBD levels; CYP3A4 and CYP2C19 inducers will decrease CBD levels	**Serious but rare**: Hepatotoxicity; hypoxia; respiratory failure
Clobazam (CLB, Schedule IV) Tablet, oral suspension	**MOA**: Binds $GABA_A$ receptor and potentiates GABA by modulating chloride conductance	**Advantages**: Despite FDA approval for LGS only, may be useful in all types of epilepsy; less sedating benzodiazepine	**Effect of CLB on ASMs**: CLB is inhibitor of CYP2C9 and inducer of CYP3A4; CLB may affect levels of CYP2C9, CYP3A4 substrates	**BOXED WARNING**: Concomitant use with opioids increases risk of death **Common**: CNS effects including somnolence, sedation, lethargy; pyrexia; constipation; drooling
	Indication: Adjunctive therapy for patients with LGS ≥2 years of age	**Disadvantages**: Monitor patients with history of substance use; use with other CNS depressant may produce additive CNS effects; may cause respiratory depression, coma, and death; no adequate data in pregnant patients—may cause fetal harm	**Effect of ASMs on CLB**: Carbamazepine, felbamate, phenobarbital, phenytoin, primidone may decrease CLB levels; cannabidiol, cenobamate, stiripentol increase CLB levels **Other (partial list)**: CLB decreases estrogen OCP levels	**Rare but serious**: Rash (SJS, TEN); anemia; liver enzyme elevations; respiratory depression
Fenfluramine (FEN, Schedule IV) Oral solution	**MOA**: Increases extracellular serotonin through actions on serotonin transporter protein, agonist at serotonin $5HT_2$ receptors	**Advantages**: Useful for refractory seizures in Dravet Syndrome	**Effect of FEN on ASMs**: No significant effects **Effect of ASMs on FEN**: CYP1A2, 2B6 inducers will decrease FEN; stiripentol + clobazam will increase FEN concentrations (max daily dose of FEN is reduced to 17 mg); cyproheptadine and potent 5-HT serotonin receptor binding agents may decrease efficacy of FEN **Other (partial list)**: Rifampin will decrease FEN, strong CYP1A2 and CYP2B6 inducers will decrease FEN	**BOXED WARNING**: Risk of valvular heart disease and pulmonary arterial hypertension; echocardiograms required before, during, and after treatment **Common**: GI effects like decreased appetite/weight, vomiting, diarrhea, constipation; CNS effects like somnolence, sedation, lethargy; fatigue, malaise, asthenia; ataxia, balance disorder, gait disturbance; blood pressure increase; salivary effects like drooling, hypersecretion; pyrexia; falls; status epilepticus; abnormal echocardiogram **Rare but serious**: increased blood pressure including hypertensive crisis; risk of valvular disease and pulmonary arterial hypertension; mydriasis precipitating acute angle closure glaucoma
	Indication: Treatment of seizures associated with Dravet Syndrome in patients ≥2 of age	**Disadvantages**: Contraindicated within 13 days of MAO inhibitors due to risk of serotonin syndrome; may increase blood pressure; not recommended in severe hepatic or renal impairment; available only through FINETPLA REMS; no adequate data in pregnancy—may cause fetal harm		
Rufinamide (RFN) Tablet, oral suspension	**MOA**: Selectively enhances fast inactivation of voltage-gated sodium channels	**Advantages**: useful for refractory seizures in LGS	**Effect of RFN on ASMs**: RFN is weak inhibitor of CYP2E1 and weak inducer of CYP3A4; RFN modestly decreases levels of carbamazepine, lamotrigine; RFN increases levels of phenobarbital, phenytoin	**Common**: CNS effects including somnolence, fatigue, coordination abnormalities, dizziness, gait disturbances, ataxia; GI effects including nausea
	Indication: Adjunctive therapy for patients with LGS ≥1 year of age	**Disadvantages**: Contraindicated in severe liver impairment or in familial short QT syndrome; use caution with other drugs that shorten QT interval; no adequate data in pregnancy—may cause fetal harm	**Effect of ASMs on RFN**: Carbamazepine, phenobarbital, phenytoin decrease RFN levels by 19%-46%; valproate increases RFN levels up to 70% **Other (partial list)**: RFN decreases estrogen OCP levels	**Rare but serious**: DRESS; rash (SJS); status epilepticus; leukopenia; QT interval shortening

(Continued)

TABLE 75-5 Antiseizure Medications (ASMs) (*Continued*)

ASM and Available Formulations	Postulated Mechanism of Action (MOA)/Indication	Advantages/Disadvantages	Interactions	Adverse Medication Reactions
Stiripentol (STP), capsule	**MOA**: Possibly acts on $GABA_A$ receptor and may also inhibit CYP450 to increase blood levels of clobazam and its active metabolite	**Advantages**: Useful for refractory seizures in Dravet Syndrome	**Effect of STP on ASMs**: STP is inhibitor and inducer of CYP1A2, 2B6, 3A4 and possible inhibitor of CYP2C8, 2C19, P-gp transporter, BCRP transporter; STP increases clobazam concentration 2-fold and clobazam active metabolite 5-fold (must decrease clobazam dosage when used together)	**Common**: Somnolence, decreased appetite/weight, agitation, ataxia, hypotonia, nausea, tremor, dysarthria, insomnia
	Indication: Adjunctive therapy with clobazam for seizure associated with Dravet Syndrome in patients ≥2 (no evidence for monotherapy)	**Disadvantages**: Must be used as adjunctive therapy with clobazam; hematologic testing is required prior to first dose and q6months after due to risk of neutropenia and thrombocytopenia; powder formulation contains phenylalanine and is a risk in patients with phenylketonuria; not recommended in moderate or severe hepatic or renal impairment; no adequate data in pregnancy—may cause fetal harm	**Effect of ASMs on STP**: STP is substrate of CYP1A2, CYP2C19, CYP3A4 and phenytoin, phenobarbital, carbamazepine may decrease stiripentol levels	**Rare but serious**: Neutropenia and thrombocytopenia; monitor
Vigabatrin (VGB) Tablet, powder packet	**MOA**: Binds to and irreversibly inhibits GABA transaminase	**Advantages**: Useful in infantile spasms for whom potential benefit outweighs risk of vision loss; renally cleared and has less DDIs than other ASMs	**Effect of VGB on ASMs**: VGB is inducer of CYP2C9; VGB decreases levels of phenytoin by 20%; VGB possibly increases levels of carbamazepine by 10%; VGB increases C_{max} of clonazepam	**BOXED WARNING**: Progressive and permanent bilateral peripheral visual loss including tunnel vision and decrease in visual acuity **Common**: CNS effects including fatigue, somnolence, nystagmus, tremor, blurred vision, memory impairment, abnormal coordination, confusion; weight gain; edema; peripheral neuropathy; laboratory abnormalities including decreases in ALT/AST in pediatric patients; aggression; infection including upper respiratory tract infection, bronchitis, ear infection, and acute otitis media constriction; vision loss
	Indication: Adjunctive therapy for refractory focal onset seizures in patients ≥2 years of age (not indicated as first-line); monotherapy for infantile spasms in patients 1 month to 2 years of age	**Disadvantages**: Permanent vision loss in most patients after a certain duration of exposure requiring eye exams Q3 months; requires REMS program registration; no adequate data in pregnancy—may cause fetal harm	**Effect of ASMs on VGB**: Carbamazepine, primidone, valproate have no effect on VGB **Other (partial list)**: Unlikely to affect estrogen OCP levels	**Serious but rare**: Seizure exacerbation, particularly absence and myoclonic seizures in patients with generalized epilepsies; anemia; onset of vision loss is unpredictable and can occur after weeks, months, or years with risk increasing in a dose-related and life exposure–related manner; abnormal MRI signal changes in infants treated for infantile spasms strongly suggestive of intramyelinic edema in select brain areas

[a]All ASMs may increase the risk of suicidal thoughts or behavior and patients treated with an ASM should be monitored for the emergence or worsening of depression, suicidal thoughts or behavior, or any unusual changes in mood or behavior.

AMPA, A-Amino-3-Hydroxy-5-Methyl-4-Isoxazolepropionic Acid; ASM, antiseizure medication; AV, atrioventricular; BUN, blood urea nitrogen; C_{max}, maximum concentration; CNS, central nervous system; CR, controlled-release; CrCl, creatinine clearance; CYP, cytochrome p450 isoenzyme system; DDI, drug-drug interaction; DR, delayed-release; DRESS, drug rash with eosinophilia and systemic symptoms; EEG, electroencephalogram; FDA, Food and Drug Administration; ER, extended-release; GABA, gamma-aminobutyric acid; GAT1, GABA transporter type 1; GI, gastrointestinal; GFR, glomerular filtration rate; HLA, human leukocyte antigen; IQ, intelligence quotient; IR, immediate release; IV, intravenous; LGS, Lennox–Gastaut syndrome; OCP, oral contraceptives; ODT, orally dissolving tablet; PTSD, posttraumatic stress disorder; SJS, Steven–Johnson syndrome; TEN, toxic epidermal necrolysis; TBI, traumatic brain injury; TC, tonic–clonic; UGT, UDP-glucuronosyltransferase; XR, extended-release.

Data from References 17-20, 23, 36-56, 69, and 88-90.

responsible providers must carefully assess this risk when evaluating their patients for ASM therapy, especially as depression and anxiety are common comorbid conditions in epilepsy. Patients and caregivers should be informed that ASMs may increase the risk of suicidal thoughts and should be advised to be on the alert for any unusual changes in mood or behavior.[76]

Adverse ASM Reactions Associated with Chronic Therapy

Antiseizure medications are often used life-long and one adverse reaction of chronic ASM therapy is osteomalacia and osteoporosis.[78,79] The effects on bone can range from asymptomatic high-turnover disease with findings of normal bone mineral density, to markedly decreased bone mineral density sufficient to warrant the diagnosis of osteoporosis. It has been hypothesized that mechanistically certain ASMs, including phenytoin, phenobarbital, carbamazepine, oxcarbazepine, felbamate, and valproate, may interfere with vitamin D metabolism to cause this adverse reaction.[80] It is unknown whether other ASMs also cause osteomalacia and/or osteoporosis, but patients receiving chronic therapy should receive supplemental vitamin D and calcium, as well as bone mineral density testing if other risk factors for osteoporosis are present.

Antiseizure Medications

Of the ASMs available, their mechanisms of action fall into five broad categories: (1) modification of ionic conductance (eg, sodium channel inhibition, calcium channel inhibition); (2) enhancement of GABAergic (inhibitory) neurotransmission (eg, $GABA_A$-receptor agonism, inhibition of GABA metabolism/reuptake); (3) suppression of excitatory (usually glutamergic) neurotransmission (eg, inhibition of kainate/α-amino-3-hydroxy-5-methylisoxazole-4-propionic acid [AMPA] receptor, inhibition of *N*-methyl D-aspartate [NMDA] receptor; (4) modulation of neurotransmitter release (eg, SV2A binding); and lastly (5) other unique or unknown mechanisms.[69] While it is useful to know mechanism of action for rational therapy and polytherapy, it is easiest to organize the ASMs into three generations which are not determined by structure or mechanism of action but by the time period in which they were FDA-approved. Each of the three generations of ASMs has specific characteristics that should be considered during selection of initial and subsequent ASM therapy. The following section is meant to highlight these major characteristics. Certain unique characteristics of specific medications within each class are also highlighted. For more specific information on pharmacokinetics, dosing, FDA-approved indication, preferred use in therapy, medication interactions, and adverse medication effects, see Tables 75-2 to 75-5. For additional detailed information on each ASM, the reader is referred to the individual FDA-approved ASM package inserts.

First-Generation ASMs

7 The first-generation ASMs, approved by the FDA from 1908 to 1978, are (1) carbamazepine, (2) clonazepam, (3) ethosuximide, (4) phenobarbital, (5) phenytoin (and its esterified prodrug fosphenytoin), (6) primidone, and (7) valproate. Valproate is available as valproic acid and divalproex, which is a specific formulation of valproate composed of sodium valproate and valproic acid in a 1:1 molar relationship. Within the gastrointestinal track, divalproex dissociates to valproate as the active form.[69] The ASMs within this class, while considered to be among the most efficacious in controlling seizures, have complex pharmacokinetics, multiple interactions, and an increased incidence of adverse reactions that, in general, make them more complicated to manage than either the second- or third-generation ASMs.

Mechanisms of Action With the exception of ethosuximide, all the first-generation ASMs have mechanisms of action that act either to primarily promote GABAergic activity or to inhibit sodium channels. The GABAergic first-generation ASMs include the barbiturate phenobarbital, primidone which is a prodrug metabolized to phenobarbital, and the benzodiazepine clonazepam which is a full $GABA_A$-receptor agonist.[20,37,69] Pharmacologically, these GABAerigic ASMs bind to sites at the $GABA_A$ receptor as agonists, increasing chloride channel opening and promoting hyperpolarization, which results in cells that are less susceptible to electrical impuses.[20,37,69] In contrast, phenytoin and carbamazepine bind to voltage-gated sodium channels in their inactive form preventing repetitive and sustained firing of sodium-dependent action potentials and stabilizing the threshold against hyperexcitability.[18,19,69] Because they bind the inactive form of the sodium channel, these agents cause a voltage-dependent and use-dependent block, which may preferentially target hyperexcitable areas that fire frequently.[18,19,69] Lastly, ethosuximide has a unique mechanism of action within this class and inhibits t-type calcium channels in cells of the thalamus and the cortex, preventing the abnormal firing of these cells that occur in absence epilepsies.[38,69]

Pharmacokinetics First-generation ASMs have complex pharmacokinetics, especially phenytoin, with 90% of total phenytoin being protein bound in individuals with normal protein status and 10% being unbound as free phenytoin. Only unbound free phenytoin is pharmacologically active.[19] Reference ranges for total and free phenytoin levels were created with this ratio in mind, with a total phenytoin level in the therapeutic range of 10 to 20 mg/L (mcg/mL; 40-79 μmol/L) corresponding to a pharmacologically active free phenytoin level of 1 to 2 mg/L (mcg/mL; 4-8 μmol/L). Both total phenytoin and free phenytoin levels are routinely used in practice to guide therapy and it is important to understand what phenytoin level is being used to accurately interpret the true level of pharmacologically active medication. In patients with low protein status (eg, hypoalbuminemia, end-stage renal disease, critically ill patients), total serum phenytoin levels in the 10 to 20 mg/L (mcg/mL; 40-79 μmol/L) range no longer correspond to an active free phenytoin level of 1 to 2 mg/L (mcg/mL; 4-8 μmol/L) and does not reflect the true level of pharmacologically active phenytoin.[81] Monitoring of free phenytoin levels better reflect the true therapeutic levels in patients with hypoalbuminemia. However, free phenytoin levels, while commonly ordered, are not rapidly available through many laboratories (eg, results may take days to weeks). Valproate is also extensively bound to albumin, and due to saturable binding, the valproate free fraction will increase as the total serum concentration increases.[39] Similar to phenytoin therapeutic monitoring, the total valproate levels may not represent the amount of free medication available to exert a pharmacologic effect. However, free valproate levels are not commonly ordered, and only total valproate levels are generally available. Therefore, it is also important to know the patient's serum albumin level and protein status to aid in interpretation of total phenytoin and valproate serum levels.[39,81] This is especially true with phenytoin as various correction equations can be used to aid in interpreting total serum phenytoin levels in patients with low protein status, including the Winter–Tozer equation.[81] Valproate levels are not routinely corrected for low protein status in clinical practice, although it is still important to be aware of its possible effect. Carbamazepine, ethosuximide, and phenobarbital are also highly protein bound, but this has less of a clinically meaningful impact in practice.[18,37,38]

Phenytoin is metabolized in the liver by CYP450 enzymes and displays Michaelis–Menten pharmacokinetics.[36] At daily doses ≤300 mg, phenytoin's metabolism is generally linear in most patients. However, at doses ≥300 mg daily, it may saturate its metabolizing enzymes and a small change in dose can result in a disproportionally large increase in serum concentrations, potentially leading to toxicity.[19,36] This can also occur at low serum concentrations in some patients. Therefore, at phenytoin doses ≥300 mg, it is recommended to increase by 30-mg increments instead of 100-mg increments.

Carbamazepine, ethosuximide, phenobarbital, and valproate are also hepatically metabolized by CYP450 enzymes but in general display linear pharmacokinetics at clinically relevant doses.[18,37-39] An exception to this is ethosuximide which displays some evidence of nonlinear kinetics at higher concentrations.[38] Carbamazepine is a particularly strong inducer of CYP metabolism and induces its own metabolism in a process known as autoinduction, where its half-life starts decreasing 3 to 5 days after therapy initiation with autoinduction being complete within 21 to 28 days.[18,36] Importantly, the reversal of autoinduction is rapid upon carbamazepine discontinuation.

Carbamazepine, ethosuximide, phenobarbital, phenytoin, and valproate all have narrow therapeutic ranges and require monitoring of serum concentrations (see Table 75-4 for target therapeutic ranges of specific ASMs and section "Evaluation of Therapeutic Outcomes" for role of serum concentration monitoring).[36]

Medication Interactions As all of the first-generation ASMs undergo CYP450 hepatic metabolism, they also have significant interactions. In particular, carbamazepine, phenobarbital, and phenytoin are substrates and inducers of many CYP enzymes. As such, they will affect each other's metabolism if used in combination and may result in decreased levels of one or the other medication. They also affect metabolism of all other ASMs and medications that go through similar CYP450 pathways (Table 75-4) and vice versa.[18,19,36,37]

Enzyme-inducing ASMs may also induce uridine 5′-diphospho-glucuronosyltransferase (UGT) metabolism and have significant interactions with medications that undergo UGT metabolism, like lamotrigine, a second-generation ASM that undergoes UGT1A4 metabolism.[18,19,36,37]

Valproate on the other hand is an inhibitor of CYP450 and UGT metabolism and inhibits the metabolism of the first-generation ASMs as well as other ASMs and medications that go through similar CYP450 and UGT pathways. In particular, valproate decreases the clearance of phenobarbital and lamotrigine by 30% to 50% and can lead to phenobarbital and lamotrigine toxicity.[36,39]

First-generation enzyme-inducing ASMs may cause increased clearance of oral contraceptives (OCs) compromising their efficacy. The enzyme inhibitor, valproate, does not cause OC failure but OCs may cause increased valproate metabolism and subsequent increased risk in seizures. Therefore, in a patient of childbearing age with epilepsy, education around these interactions is a must.[18,19,37,39]

Adverse Medication Reactions The first-generation ASMs are, in general, associated with a higher incidence of dose-related and idiosyncratic adverse reactions including neurotoxic effects, hepatotoxicity, and SJS/TEN. There are also a number of unique adverse effects associated with first-generation ASMs that are of particular note such as hyponatremia with carbamazepine, hyperactivity with phenobarbital in children, and gingival hyperplasia and osteoporosis with chronic use of phenytoin.[18,40,49] Valproate especially has a number of unique adverse effects including concentration-dependent thrombocytopenia at serum levels above 100 mg/L (mcg/mL; 693 μmol/L), hyperammonemia related to carnitine deficiency that may or may not lead to encephalopathy, idiosyncratic pancreatitis, and well-known teratogenicity.[39,82] Adverse effects of first-generation ASMs are listed in Table 75-5.

Advantages and Disadvantages First-generation ASMs are very efficacious in epilepsy. Valproate, in particular, is considered a broad-spectrum ASM and is useful in both focal-onset and generalized-onset seizures as well as various epilepsy syndromes.[27,73,74] Phenobarbital has been in use for the longest period of time and is readily available worldwide. Carbamazepine and phenytoin are very efficacious in focal-onset seizures and have known efficacy in controlling tonic–clonic seizures but may exacerbate other generalized seizures and should be used with caution in generalized-onset epilepsy, especially generalized atypical absence.[18,19,27,73,74] Valproate and carbamazepine are also useful in multiple other comorbid conditions including migraine and bipolar disorder.[18,39] Despite their known advantages, however, first-generation ASMs should generally be considered after second-generation ASMs have failed, due to the greater tolerability, fewer medication interactions, and generic availability of the second-generation ASMs. The exception to this rule is ethosuximide, which is the medication of first choice for treatment of absence seizures but has limited use in other epilepsies.[36,83]

Second-Generation ASMs

The second-generation ASMs were developed with knowledge regarding the limitations of the first-generation ASMs and were FDA-approved from 1993 to 2000. Included in this class are (1) felbamate, (2) gabapentin, (3) lamotrigine, (4) levetiracetam, (5) oxcarbazepine, (6) tiagabine, (7) topiramate, and (8) zonisamide. In general, these medications are considered to have similar efficacy in controlling seizures as first-generation ASMs, have relatively simple pharmacokinetics with fewer interactions, and have an overall lower incidence of adverse effects.

Mechanisms of Action 8 The second-generation ASMs have mechanisms of action that include enhancement of GABAergic activity (eg, tiagabine) and sodium channel inhibition (eg, lamotrigine, oxcarbazepine, zonisamide) but also expand beyond that.[69] Notably, ASMs with novel mechanisms of action that were introduced within this generation include felbamate that modulates excitatory neurotransmission via inhibition of the *N*-methyl D-aspartate (NMDA) glutamate receptor, topiramate that inhibits the kainate/α-amino-3-hydroxy-5-methylisoxazole-4-propionic acid (AMPA) glutamate receptor,[40,50] and levetiracetam that may modulate both glutamergic and GABAergic neurotransmission through modulation of presynaptic neurotransmitter release via inhibition of SV2A protein, considered the master regulator molecule of neurotransmitter release.[49,69] For the other medications in this class, their therapeutic effects are seen through novel mechanisms that have not been fully elucidated (eg, gabapentin that binds to presynaptic $\alpha_2\delta$ subunit of calcium channels, possibly resulting in decreased release of the excitatory neurotransmitters glutamate, noradrenaline, substance P, and calcitonin gene-related peptide).[41] Furthermore, topiramate and zonisamide are also carbonic anhydrase inhibitors, which can modulate the bicarbonate gradient in the brain and possibly affects GABAA receptor function, although whether or not this impacts antiseizure activity is unknown.[42,50] Additionally, during this time period, a second-generation structurally related derivative of carbamazepine, oxcarbazepine, was also introduced that exhibits a similar mechanism of action, but with an improved pharmacokinetic and adverse reaction profile.[43]

Pharmacokinetics The second-generation ASMs also have pharmacokinetics that are less complex than first-generation ASMs. In general, they are not significantly protein bound and are well absorbed with good bioavailability, although of note, gabapentin relies on the L-amino acid carrier protein in the gut and the CNS to be actively transported across those membranes. As binding is saturable, this causes a dose-dependent bioavailability, with decreasing bioavailability with increasing dose, as the transporter is believed to be saturated at doses ≤1,200 mg per single dose.[41,84]

Unlike the first-generation ASMs which are all hepatically metabolized, two second-generation ASMs, gabapentin and levetiracetam, are primarily renally eliminated and dosage adjustments may be necessary in patients with significantly impaired renal function.[41,49] Additionally, topiramate is approximately 60% renally eliminated and should be dose adjusted in patients with renal impairment, although topiramate also undergoes CYP3A4 metabolism.[50] As for the remaining second-generation ASMs, felbamate, lamotrigine, oxcarbazepine, tiagabine, and zonisamide are all hepatically metabolized.[40,42-45] In contrast to carbamazepine, oxcarbazepine does not undergo autoinduction and also has an active metabolite (a monohydroxy derivative [MHD], 10-OH-carbazepine) that is inactivated by glucuronidation and eliminated by the kidneys. As such, oxcarbazepine may also require dosage reduction with significant renal impairment.[43]

Medication Interactions Since gabapentin and levetiracetam do not undergo any appreciable hepatic metabolism, they display minimal medication interactions.[41,49] Felbamate, oxcarbazepine, tiagabine, zonisamide, and topiramate at higher doses are all hepatically metabolized and while there are some pharmacokinetic effects on the CYP450 pathways,[40,42,43,45,50] these effects are generally much less significant than those of the first-generation ASMs. Specifically, felbamate may induce or inhibit the metabolism of first-generation ASMs (or vice versa).[36,40] Oxcarbazepine inhibits CYP2C19 and induces CYP3A4/5, therefore, causing interactions with first-generation ASMs metabolized by these pathways, although to a lesser extent than its precursor carbamazepine. Additionally, oxcarbazepine may also reduce lamotrigine levels through a suggested induction of UGT enzymes, again to a lesser extent than its precursor carbamazepine.[36,43] Similarly topiramate is a weak inhibitor of CYP2C19 and an inducer of CYP3A4, therefore interacting with the first-generation ASMs as well as other medications that are metabolized by these pathways.[36,50]

Of the second-generation ASMs, lamotrigine has the most substantial interactions, which in some cases can be rather significant. Given valproate's enzyme-inhibiting properties, valproate can substantially inhibit the metabolism of lamotrigine, while carbamazepine, phenobarbital, phenytoin can substantially increase the metabolism of lamotrigine due to enzyme induction. As such, detailed dose and titration recommendations are available in the situation for when lamotrigine is used in combination with these ASMs. It is important to follow dose titration recommendations for lamotrigine carefully, as too rapid dose titrations increase the risk for rash including SJS. Of note, lamotrigine itself does not inhibit liver enzymes and, therefore, has a low potential for pharmacokinetic interactions with other medications.[36,44]

Oxcarbazepine and topiramate both can interact with ethinyl estradiol and cause contraceptive failure, although topiramate doses ≤200 mg/day are unlikely to alter oral contraceptive pharmacokinetics.[43,50] The potential of lamotrigine to affect OC metabolism is minimal, but OCs can affect lamotrigine metabolism[44] as concomitant OCs lead to induction of lamotrigine glucuronidation by ethinyl estradiol. Once the OCs are withdrawn, significant increases in lamotrigine levels can be seen, including during the week of hormone withdrawal as part of various cyclic oral contraceptive treatments.[85]

In contrast to the first-generation ASMs, the second-generation ASMs have wide therapeutic ranges. While serum levels of second-generation ASMs are available through most laboratories, they are not routinely monitored, and levels may take many weeks to come back (see Table 75-3 for target therapeutic ranges of specific ASMs). One may monitor plasma levels of oxcarbazepine's active metabolite (MHD), which is more clinically significant than measuring oxcarbazepine levels directly. The therapeutic range for MHD is between 15 and 35 mcg/mL (mg/L; 59 to 138 μmol/L).[36]

Adverse Medication Reactions The second-generation ASMs are associated with a lower incidence of dose-related CNS adverse reactions and are considered to be better tolerated than the first-generation ASMs. The exceptions are topiramate, which is associated with word-finding difficulties and cognitive slowing, and zonisamide which is a sodium channel inhibitor and associated with increased sedation and cognitive slowing. These neurotoxic effects are more common with rapid titration and high doses.[86,87]

Despite being better tolerated overall, there are a number of unique and severe adverse reactions associated with individual second-generation ASMs that must be considered when selecting therapy. The most severe of these is associated with felbamate which may potentially cause fatal idiosyncratic reactions including acute liver failure (1 in 10,000 patients), with reported onset between 68 and 354 days of therapy, and aplastic anemia (1 in 3,000 patients), with greater risk being seen in females, those with a history of cytopenia, prior ASM allergy or significant ASM toxicity, viral infection, and/or immunologic problems.[40] Tiagabine has been associated with new-onset seizures and status epilepticus.[45] Lamotrigine can cause rash, usually appearing after 3 to 4 weeks of therapy, and is typically generalized, erythematous, and morbilliform, but can progress to SJS. Rashes are more likely to occur if the patient has had a prior rash to another ASM[88] and risk factors for more serious rashes include concomitant use of valproic acid and situations where high initial doses or rapid dosage escalation is used. When dosed appropriately, the incidence of rash is similar to that of carbamazepine and phenytoin. The incidence of lamotrigine rash is higher in children than in adults.[89]

Of more moderate severity, topiramate and zonisamide are uniquely associated with kidney stones which can occur in 1.5% to 4% of patients who should be encouraged to maintain adequate fluid intake for the prevention of this adverse effect. Topiramate and zonisamide can also cause metabolic acidosis especially in patients with renal disease, severe respiratory disorders, diarrhea, surgery, and in patients on the ketogenic diet.[42,50]

Levetiracetam is well-recognized for causing irritability in many patients, which may be lessened with dose reduction.[49] Similarly, in patients receiving gabapentin for pain, abrupt discontinuation is associated with a withdrawal reaction characterized by anxiety, insomnia, nausea, sweating, and increased pain.[41]

Oxcarbazepine generally causes fewer adverse effects than the first-generation carbamazepine, but may have a higher incidence of hyponatremia, reported in as high as 25% of patients.[83] This adverse event occurs more often in older adult patients and in patients receiving concomitant sodium-depleting medications such as diuretics and is not very common in children. The incidence of rash with oxcarbazepine is less compared to carbamazepine, although approximately 25% to 30% of patients who develop a rash with carbamazepine also experience a similar reaction with oxcarbazepine.[43]

Advantages and Disadvantages As previously stated, the second-generation ASMs are considered to be similar in efficacy to first-generation ASMs, but with better tolerability and fewer medication interactions. Levetiracetam, in particular, is considered a useful broad-spectrum ASM with little, if any, CNS adverse effects besides irritability. It is routinely used as first-line monotherapy to treat focal-onset epilepsy and to a lesser extent myoclonic seizures of JME and primary generalized seizures.[36,49] However, increasing recognition of the unusually high prevalence of irritability and impact on QOL is limiting more widespread use of levetiracetam.

Lamotrigine is also efficacious in many epilepsy types, and, besides rash, is generally well tolerated with minimal CNS adverse effects, especially in older adults patients who may experience less cognitive adverse effects with lamotrigine than with other ASMs.[90] However, its use is mainly limited by the need for slow titration to avoid rash (especially if the patient is on valproate) and it is not a good agent for patients who need to reach therapeutic ASM levels quickly.[44] Both lamotrigine and oxcarbazepine may be a good ASM for patients with comorbid bipolar disorder, with oxcarbazepine not requiring very slow dose titration.[36,43,44] (See Chapter 89 for more information on the role of these ASMs for bipolar disorder.)

Topiramate and zonisamide are efficacious agents but due to their effects on cognition are sometimes considered after other ASMs. Topiramate additionally requires a very slow titration due to its CNS adverse reactions, further limiting its use. On the other hand, topiramate is usually considered earlier in therapy for those patients with epilepsy who also have comorbid migraines or those who have a wish to lose weight as it has some efficacy in this regard. Similarly, zonisamide is considered earlier in therapy for those patients who have issues with medication adherence as it is dosed once daily and has one of the longest half-lives of all the ASMs.[36,42,50]

Gabapentin is oftentimes considered a poorly efficacious ASM that may even exacerbate generalized-onset seizures and should be avoided in generalized-onset epilepsies.[27,73,74] However, it is well tolerated and widely used as adjunctive therapy in focal-onset epilepsy mostly for its benefit in comorbid conditions such as neuropathic pain and not necessarily for its efficacy in controlling seizures.[41] Tiagabine and felbamate have serious adverse reactions and are generally reserved for use only after failure of other ASMs, which is unfortunate as felbamate is broad spectrum (eg, can be used in focal-onset epilepsies and generalized-onset epilepsy syndromes like Lennox–Gastaut syndrome [LGS]) and is an effective ASM.[40] Furthermore, because of the risk of fatal aplastic anemia and liver failure, the use of felbamate requires signed written consent.[40]

Third-Generation ASMs

The third-generation ASMs were FDA-approved from 2004 to 2020 and agents in this generation can be further subcategorized into those that are approved for typical seizure indications and ASMs that are approved for specific epilepsy syndromes. The third-generation ASMs approved for typical seizure indications include (1) brivaracetam, (2) cenobamate, (3) eslicarbazepine, (4) lacosamide, (5) perampanel, and (7) pregabalin. The ASMs that are approved for specific epilepsy syndromes include (1) cannabidiol for LGS and Dravet Syndrome, (2) clobazam for LGS, (3) rufinamide for LGS, (4) stiripentol for Dravet Syndrome, and (5) vigabatrin for focal onset seizures as well as infantile spasms. (Note, topiramate, a second-generation ASM is also approved for LGS as well as focal onset or primary generalized seizures.) While many of the ASMs were approved for very specific indications only, they are often used off-label in refractory epilepsy after failure of other first-line ASMs.

Mechanisms of Action Similar to the first-generation ASMs, many of the medications within this classification pharmacologically exert their effects through sodium channel inhibition and GABAergic mechanisms, as these continue to be proven to be efficacious in preventing seizures. Of the third-generation ASMs noted above, eslicarbazepine, lacosamide, and rufinamide are third-generation sodium channel inhibitors.[46,53,56] Eslicarbazepine is a derivative of carbamazepine that has a 5- to 15-fold lower affinity for the resting state of sodium channels than that of carbamazepine or oxcarbazepine, leading to a selectivity for neurons that are firing (typically seen in epilepsy).[46,69] Eslicarbazepine is postulated to inhibit sodium channels, through enhancement of slow inactivation, similar to lacosamide, another third-generation sodium channel inhibitor. Rufinamide, on the other hand, prolongs the inactivation phase of sodium channels similar to phenytoin and carbamazepine.[53,56,69]

Third-generation GABAergic ASMs also include vigabatrin, clobazam, and stiripentol. Vigabatrin is an amino acid that is a structural analog of GABA and is a selective, irreversible inhibitor of GABA-transaminase, the enzyme that degrades GABA.[23] Clobazam is a 1,5-chlorinated benzodiazepine derivative (structurally different from the 1,4 benzodiazepine clonazepam) that binds the $GABA_A$ receptor at the benzodiazepine site as an agonist and enhances inhibitory chloride ion transmission promoting hyperpolarization of the neuron. However, it demonstrates lower affinity for the $GABA_A$ subunits that facilitate sedation, thereby reducing the incidence of this particular adverse effect.[52] Additionally, unlike traditional benzodiazepines which are nonselective full receptor agonists, clobazam is believed to be only a partial agonist.[52,69] Stirpipentol is believed to possibly act on $GABA_A$ receptors and may also inhibit CYP450 enzymes to increase blood levels of clobazam and its active metabolite.[70] Cenobamate is one of the newest ASMs and combines the two most common mechanisms of ASMs as it is believed to inhibit volgatge-gated sodium channels as well as being an allosteric modulator of the $GABA_A$ ion channel.[71]

In addition to these, two other derivatives of second-generation ASMs have also been introduced. The first agent is pregabalin, a derivative of gabapentin which pharmacologically works in a similar fashion by binding to presynaptic $\alpha_2\delta$ subunit of calcium channels.[55] The second agent is brivaracetam, a more selective derivative of levetiracetam that has a 15- to 30-fold higher affinity for SV2A, and binds SV2A to modulate neurotransmitter release and glutamergic and GABAergic transmission.[51,69]

Three new third-generation ASMs with novel mechanisms of action have also been introduced. Perampanel is a highly selective noncompetitive AMPA-type glutamate receptor antagonist,[54] and cannabadiol is purified derivative of cannabis whose exact antiseizure mechanism is unknown.[47] Fenfluramine's exact antiseizure mechanism is also unknown but it is known to increase extracellular serotonin through actions on serotonin transporter protein, and is an agonist at serotonin 5HT receptors and has efficacy in Dravet Syndrome.[72]

Pharmacokinetics The third-generation ASMs have variable pharmacokinetic profiles which are unique to the individual agent and while some have simple pharmacokinetics, others have more complex pharmacokinetics almost similar to that of the first-generation ASMs.

Pregabalin and vigabatrin are the third-generation ASMs with the simplest pharmacokinetics (ie, good absorption, low protein binding, uncomplicated metabolism, linear elimination kinetics) and are the only two in this generation that are renally cleared.[23,36,55] Rufinamide, while hepatically metabolized, also displays simple pharmacokinetics, undergoing biotransformation via a carboxylesterase-mediated hydrolysis with no involvement of the CYP450 and UGT system.[36,56] Eslicarbazepine, despite being a prodrug that requires hydrolytic first-pass metabolism in the liver to form its active metabolite S-licarbazepine, also has relatively simple pharmacokinetics. After first-pass, eslicarbazepine is subsequently glucuronidated and renally excreted, requiring dosage adjustment in renal impairment but surprisingly not requiring adjustment in hepatic impairment.[36,46] Lacosamide is 40% renally eliminated and 60% hepatically metabolized by CYP3A4, CYP2C9, and CYP2C19, requiring dose adjustment in renal and hepatic impairment, but otherwise displays relatively simple pharmacokinetics.[36,53]

The third-generation agents with more complex pharmacokinetic profiles are brivaracetam, clobazam, and perampanel. Brivaracetam is metabolized by CYP2C19, and CYP2C19 poor and fast metabolizers may display altered brivaracetam pharmacokinetics. Brivaracetam dosage adjustment is required in all stages of hepatic impairment.[36,51] Clobazam is metabolized in the liver by CYP3A4 and CYP2C19 to a primary active metabolite *N*-desmethylclobazam which is then metabolized by CYP2C19. As such, its pharmacokinetics are also affected by CYP2C19 polymorphic variants and it also requires dosage adjustment in hepatic impairment.[36,52] Perampanel is highly protein bound (96%-96%) and eliminated primarily via CYP3A4 metabolism to an inactive metabolite with an elimination half-life of about 100 hours. Its use is not recommended in severe renal or hepatic impairment.[36,54]

Fenfluramine is complicated because it goes through hepatic metabolism by CYP1A2, CYP2B6, CYP2D6 with minor involvement of a few other CYPs to an active metabolite norfenfluramine which is then inactivated. Similarily stiripentol is also metabolized by CYP1A2, CYP2C19, and 3A4.[70,72] Of note, eslicarbazepine and perampanel are the two ASMs in this generation that have long half-lives and are dosed once-a-day. Monitoring of third-generation ASM serum concentrations is not routinely done and therapeutic ranges have not been clearly identified for some of these agents.[36]

Medication Interactions As previously stated pregabalin does not undergo hepatic metabolism and, similar to its precursor gabapentin, has little to no interactions.[36,55] Vigabatrin, while not hepatically metabolized, is an inducer of CYP2C9 and has been noted to have slight effects on CYP2C9 substrates (eg, decreases phenytoin plasma levels by approximately 20% and possibly increases serum carbamazepine by 10%).[23,36]

Third-generation ASMs with fewer interactions are lacosamide, rufinamide, and fenfluramine. Lacosamide levels may be increased if used in combination with strong inhibitors of CYP3A4, CYP2C9, but most of these interactions are clinically insignificant.[36,53] Lacosamide is also a substrate of CYP2C19 and its blood levels can be modestly decreased (~15%-20%) by enzyme-inducing ASMs.[36,53] Rufinamide, a weak inhibitor of CYP2E1 and a weak inducer of CYP3A4, may modestly affect the clearance of carbamazepine, lamotrigine, phenobarbital, and phenytoin and vice versa.[36,56] Additionally, concurrent use of rufinamide and OCs may result in reduced OCs efficacy while lacosamide does not reduce OC levels.[53,56] In regards to fenfluramine, stiripentol and clobazam combination act upon fenfluramine to increase its levels and other potent serotonin receptor binding agents may decrease its efficacy. However, fenfluramine does not generally act upon other ASMs and therefore has fewer interactions.[72]

Third-generation ASMs with more significant interactions include brivaracetam, clobazam, eslicarbazepine, and perampanel. Brivaracetam is a CYP2C19 substrate, and carbamazepine, phenobarbital, and phenytoin decrease its levels. Brivaracetam in turn may increase levels of the carbamazepine-epoxide metabolite and phenytoin levels but does not interact with lamotrigine, levetiracetam, oxcarbazepine, topiramate, valproate, or OCs to a significant extent.[51] Clobazam is a CYP3A4 and CYP2C19 substrate and its levels may be affected by CYP3A4- and CYP2C19-inducing and -inhibiting medications such as felbamate and the first-generation ASMs, respectively.[36,52] Additionally, clobazam inhibits CYP2D6 and may affect the metabolism of other medications that use this pathway as well as lowering the serum levels of some OCs due to its weak induction effect on CYP3A4.[52] Like carbamazepine, eslicarbazepine is affected by CYP2C19 inducers and can itself inhibit CYP2C19 and affect plasma concentration of medications metabolized by this enzyme. However, similar to oxcarbazepine, the effects of eslicarbazepine are less significant than carbamazepine. Eslicarbazepine can also induce CYP3A4 affecting medications that are metabolized by this isoenzyme and may also lower OC levels.[36,46] Stiripentol is an inducer and inhibitor of multiple CYP enzymes and may also possibly be an inhibitor of the P-glycoprotein (Pgp) and breast cancer resistance protein (BCRP) transporters.[70] Of the third-generation ASMs, perampanel has the most potential for interactions as its serum levels are decreased by enzyme-inducing ASMs, it displays modest enzyme-inducing properties of its own at the high end of its dose range (12 mg/day), and it may lower OC levels.[36,54]

Adverse Medication Reactions Third-generation ASMs have adverse reactions which are unique to the individual ASM, with some having minimal adverse effects, while others are known for specific serious effects. As the third-generation agents are the most recently FDA-approved ASMs, we have the least long-term experience with their use clinically; therefore, long-term and rare adverse effects may emerge as we gain more experience with them in a large population.

Among this generation, brivaracetam, lacosamide, and pregabalin are generally well tolerated, although we have the least experience with brivaracetam. In general, lacosamide's primary adverse reactions are CNS; however, these occur at a lower incidence than other ASMs and are more common in patients receiving concomitant treatment with other sodium channel inhibitors. Additionally, lacosamide is also associated with a lengthening of the PR interval which is not clinically significant unless used in combination with another ASM that lengthens the PR interval.[53] Pregabalin has an adverse effect profile that is notable for sedation and weight gain.[55]

Similarly, clobazam also is not commonly associated with any serious adverse reactions beyond CNS effects, but as a benzodiazepine, abrupt discontinuation may cause a withdrawal syndrome which could include seizures, psychosis, hallucinations, behavioral disorder, tremor, anxiety, dysphoria, and insomnia.[52]

In contrast, eslicarbazepine, rufinamide, and perampanel have more serious adverse reactions. Eslicarbazepine as a sodium channel inhibitor is associated with CNS effects and hyponatremia, although the occurrence of hyponatremia with this agent is less common than with carbamazepine and oxcarbazepine.[46] Eslicarbazepine like its earlier counterparts may still be associated with rash including SJS and TEN, hepatotoxicity, and hematologic adverse reactions. As rufinamide is also a sodium channel inhibitor, it is also associated with increased CNS effects as well as some rare and serious adverse reactions including an increased incidence of seizures and precipitation of status epilepticus. Additionally, multiorgan hypersensitivity has occurred within 4 weeks of starting treatment with rufinamide in patients younger than 12 years of age.[56] Aggression is a major common adverse reaction with perampanel and there is a FDA-boxed warning pertaining to monitoring of psychiatric, behavioral, mood, or personality changes which may be life-threatening.[54] Cenobamate mostly has CNS adverse reactions but there is also a risk of drug reactions with eosinophilia and systemic symptoms (DRESS) with fast titration; therefore, the dosage should be increased no faster than every two weeks. Additionally cenobamate is associated with QT interval shortening and a rate of appendicitis which was higher than in the normal population. Stiripentol may cause neutropenia and thrombocytopenia which necessitates frequent monitoring of blood counts including prior to the first dose and every 6 months during and 6 months after discontinuing. Fenfluramine which was previously used as a weight-loss medication has known cardiac effects at higher doses and has a boxed warning regarding risk of valvular heart disease and pulmonary arterial hypertension, which requires echocardiograms before, during, and after treatment.[70-72]

Vigabatrin has the most serious adverse effects in this generation, as it may cause progressive, irreversible, bilateral concentric visual field constriction in a high percentage of patients. It may also reduce visual acuity in a dose-related and life exposure–related manner. Vigabatrin also may aggravate seizures, particularly absence and myoclonic seizures in patients with generalized epilepsies, and patients with history of depression, psychosis, or behavioral disturbances may be at greater risk to develop psychiatric effects with vigabatrin use.[23,91] Furthermore, in up to 11% of patients (up to age 3 years) treated with high doses of this medication for infantile spasms, MRI findings have been strongly suggestive of intramyelinic edema in select brain areas. While these findings appear to be reversible, their significance is unclear.[23,91]

Advantages and Disadvantages Cannabadiol, fenfluramine, rufinamide, stiripentol, and vigabatrin have all been approved for specific epilepsy syndromes (Dravet syndrome and LGS, LGS, and infantile spasms, respectively) and in general should be considered for those indications.[23,47,56]

9 In regards to focal-onset epilepsies, third-generation ASMs have been used in clinical practice for the treatment of these epilepsies and probably have similar efficacy to the first- or second-generation ASMs. However, most third generations are not available in generic form now (except for pregabalin) and are less cost-effective than other ASMs. Therefore, third-generation ASMs should be reserved for use after failure of other agents.

Of the third-generation ASMs, lacosamide has become an ASM of choice among many providers, due to its ease of use, including the availability of intravenous loading and lack of medication interactions. However, there is no strong evidence to support this practice and lacosamide is only available as a brand product. Therefore, due to its cost, lacosamide should be reserved as second-line or third-line therapy after failure of other equally efficacious, less expensive ASMs.

Among the third-generation ASMs, clobazam may have the broadest use, as clobazam is believed to be efficacious in a wide variety of epilepsies including focal-onset and primary generalized epilepsies (despite having FDA approval only for LGS seizures) and perampanel is broadly approved for focal-onset seizure with or without secondary generalization as well as for primary GTC seizures.[52,54] Perampanel use, however, is somewhat limited by the appearance of aggression in some patients.[54]

Lastly, all ASMs in this generation except for eslicarbazepine, rufinamide, and vigabatrin are controlled substances making prescribing and access more difficult for these ASMs.[46,47,51-56] While vigabatrin is not a controlled substance, access is still restricted as all providers must be certified in the Vigabatrin Risk Evaluation and Mitigation Strategy (REMS) Program in order to prescribe it.[23]

Therapeutic Considerations in Older Adults and Young

The most important aspect of ASM therapy is tailoring the choice of medication to the individual patient using knowledge of an individual ASM's pharmacodynamic and pharmacokinetic profile and its known advantages and disadvantages combined with knowledge of patient-specific factors including seizure type(s), age, sex, concomitant medical problems (including hepatic function, renal function), and interactions with concurrent medications.

In general, older adults are more often on many different medications which may contribute to increased sensitivity to neurocognitive effects. Additionally, this population may be more prone to the increased possibility of interactions with ASMs that affect the CYP450 system (eg, carbamazepine, phenytoin, and valproate); therefore, a thorough review of all medications is necessary prior to starting or modifying treatment. Hypoalbuminemia is also common in older adults, and highly albumin-bound ASMs (eg, phenytoin and valproate) should be closely monitored.[77] As patients age, they can also experience changes in body mass, such as an increase in fat to lean body mass or decrease in body water, which can affect volume of distribution and elimination half-life.[77] In addition, the older adults may have compromised renal or hepatic function that require ASM dosage adjustment.[77] Lamotrigine is often considered the medication of choice in older adults with focal-onset seizures, as results from a Department of Veterans Affairs cooperative trial found that it had equal efficacy to carbamazepine and gabapentin and was better tolerated than carbamazepine.[90]

For neonates and infants, an increase in the total body water to fat ratio and a decrease in serum albumin and α-acid glycoprotein can result in volume of distribution changes that affect ASM elimination half-life. Additionally, infants up to the age of 3 years have decreased renal elimination of ASMs, with neonates being the most affected. Hepatic activity is also reduced in neonates and infants, but by age 2 to 3 years, hepatic activity becomes more robust than that seen in adults. Therefore, whereas neonates and infants require lower doses of ASMs, children require higher doses than that seen in adults. Therapeutic medication monitoring becomes especially important in the young, even though the definitions of therapeutic blood levels are less certain in these patients than in adults.[77]

Therapeutic Considerations in Females (and Males)

Estrogen and progesterone are among the many hormones that can influence brain electrical excitability, as estrogen has a slight proconvulsant effect, whereas progesterone exerts a mild antiseizure effect.[15] In some individuals, vulnerability to seizures is highest just before and during the menstrual flow (catamenial seizures) and at the time of ovulation, which is believed to be due to a slight increase in estrogen relative to progesterone, or due to progesterone withdrawal and changes in the estrogen-to-progesterone ratio.[15] The risk of catamenial seizures is estimated be anywhere from 10% to 70% in females with epilepsy.[15] In these individuals, conventional ASMs should be used as primary agents, but intermittent supplementation with higher dose of ASM or benzodiazepines should be considered. Acetazolamide has also been used during catamenial periods, but with variable and limited success, and hormonal therapy with progestational agents, particularly cyclic natural progesterone therapy, may be effective in certain subsets of patients.[92]

At menopause, seizures often improve in frequency, particularly in individuals with a catamenial seizure pattern. However, for patients requiring hormone replacement therapy, it has been reported that conjugated equine estrogens plus 2.5 mg of medroxyprogesterone acetate may increase the frequency of epileptic seizures. Therefore, a hormone replacement therapy that consists of just a single estrogenic compound, such as 17-β-estradiol, along with a natural progesterone, may be recommended for individuals with disruptive menopausal symptoms.[93]

Antiseizure medications may also have an effect on endogenous and exogenous hormones. As previously stated, enzyme-inducing ASMs increase the metabolism of estrogen, progesterone, and testosterone and increase production of sex hormone-binding globulin, leading to decreases in the free fraction of these hormones endogenously. These alterations lead to disturbances in the regulation of the hypothalamic–pituitary–adrenal axis and contribute to reproductive endocrine disorders including menstrual irregularity, infertility, sexual dysfunction, and in some patients polycystic ovary syndrome (PCOS).[94] Valproate, in particular, may affect sex hormone concentrations causing hyperandrogenism and polycystic changes, especially in individuals who have gained weight or those who start valproic acid prior to age 20.[94] Exogenously, enzyme-inducing ASMs can cause treatment failures in individuals taking OCs, as discussed in the prior sections, due to increased metabolism of ethinyl estradiol and progestin. Medroxyprogesterone depot injections and hormone-releasing intrauterine systems, on the other hand, are not similarly affected by ASMs, and it is unclear if there is an effect of ASMs on the transdermal contraceptive patch or the emergency contraceptive pill. A supplemental or alternative form of birth control (eg, IUD) is advised if breakthrough bleeding occurs in individuals taking certain types of ASMs (eg, enzyme-inducing ASMs) and OCs, and it has been suggested that they use twice the normal dose of emergency contraception.[95]

Data suggests that males with epilepsy have reduced fertility, and that carbamazepine, oxcarbazepine, and valproic acid are associated with sperm abnormalities. In addition, valproic acid seems to cause testicular atrophy resulting in reduced testosterone volume, whereas levetiracetam slightly increases serum testosterone. Various ASMs have also been anecdotally reported to affect libido and sexual function in both males and females.[95]

Therapeutic Considerations for Pregnancy and Lactation

Pregnancy and epilepsy is a particularly complex topic. The goal of treatment in pregnant patients with epilepsy is to achieve the best possible control of seizure with minimal adverse effects for the pregnant individual and the child. Epilepsy-related complications during pregnancy include possible changes in seizure frequency, fluctuating ASM plasma levels, and possible teratogenic effects of ASMs.[96,97]

Despite multiple reports of both increased and decreased seizure frequency during pregnancy, a recent practice parameter update issued by the American Academy of Neurology (AAN) found that there was inconclusive evidence to support that pregnancy was associated with changes in seizure frequency. What was concluded, however, was that patients with epilepsy who were seizure free for at least 9 months to 1 year prior to pregnancy had a very high probability (84%-92%) of remaining seizure free during pregnancy.[96] However, if seizures are increasing during pregnancy, it is important to inquire about nonadherence in a normally adherent patient, as they may be concerned about the potential adverse medication effects on the developing fetus.[98]

Fluctuations in ASM concentration may be caused by physiologic changes that occur during pregnancy including reduced gastric motility, nausea and vomiting, increased medication distribution, increased renal elimination, altered hepatic enzyme activity as well as changes in protein binding.[95] Physiologic changes, such as changes in protein binding, can begin as early as the first 10 weeks of pregnancy, and may not normalize until 4 weeks postpartum (eg, protein binding of carbamazepine, phenobarbital, and phenytoin). Fluctuations in ASM plasma concentrations due to increased ASM clearance have been found to be true for lamotrigine, carbamazepine, phenytoin, oxcarbazepine, and levetiracetam.[96] Clinical consequences of ASM fluctuations are variable and some patients will not experience increased seizure frequency despite fluctuating levels. Patients on lamotrigine, however, have been found to undergo a 40% decrease in the ratio of plasma lamotrigine concentration to dose, resulting in deterioration of seizure control in approximately 75% of pregnant patients.[95] It is therefore recommended that ASM levels, particularly lamotrigine levels, be monitored closely during pregnancy, and that dosage increases occur over the course of the pregnancy if needed. This should be followed up with a rapid decrease in the postpartum period. Fluctuations have also been reported for phenobarbital, valproic acid, primidone, and ethosuximide, although strong evidence for this is lacking.[96]

Adverse pregnancy outcomes associated with ASM use include an increased risk of major congenital malformations (MCMs) compared to pregnant persons without epilepsy.[97] This risk is believed to be due to ASM exposure and not seizures, as infants born to patients with epilepsy who do not take ASMs have the same risk of birth defects as infants born to seizure-free individuals (2%-3%).[98] The most concerning effects are found with the use of valproic acid which is associated with a risk of MCMs that is 3.5 to 4 times that of offspring from patients without epilepsy, especially if taken during the first trimester of pregnancy.[97,99] Furthermore there is an increased risk of neurodevelopmental deficits, including effects on cognition, in children exposed to valproic acid *in utero*.[97,99] These effects are dose-dependent, and the risk of MCM significantly increases at 600 mg/day, with the greatest risk observed at doses that exceed 1,000 mg/day.[99] However, individual susceptibility is genetically determined, and teratogenicity can occur at much lower doses in some persons. Due to these findings, it is recommended that valproate should not be used in pregnant individuals or in female patients of childbearing potential with epilepsy and that withdrawal of valproate or switching to an alternative treatment should be considered.

Data on teratogenic risk with the newer agents are limited, although topiramate was reclassified from pregnancy category C to D due to an increased association with cleft palate (it may also have a negative effect on birth weight and cause increases in hypospadias).[50] In general, higher ASM doses, higher ASM serum concentrations, polytherapy (especially polytherapy with valproate), and a family history of birth defects increase the teratogenic risk of ASMs.[97] As such, the risk of birth defects is believed to have gone down with decreasing doses and decreasing use of polytherapy.

Deciding on the most effective single-medication treatment prior to conception is vitally important. Teratogenic effects of ASM must always be considered when choosing ASMs for patients of reproductive age, even when the plans are not to become pregnant, as many unplanned pregnancies occur and MCMs generally occur early in pregnancy before the patient is aware of their pregnancy. With proper counseling and management, more than 90% of these pregnancies will still have satisfactory outcomes. Updated practice parameters are available to aid in the selection of ASMs in pregnancy and the counseling and management of pregnant patients with epilepsy.[96,97,99]

Teratogenic effects may possibly be prevented by adequate folate intake. Although data are insufficient to show that folate is effective in preventing MCM in patients with epilepsy, there is no evidence of harm. Therefore, the AAN recommends that all females of childbearing potential, take folic acid prior to conception and during pregnancy. The AAN cites insufficient data to support a specific dose but prenatal vitamins containing folic acid 0.4 to 5 mg/day can be recommended.[100] Folate doses in the high range should be used in individuals with a history of a previous pregnancy with a neural tube defect or in those taking valproic acid. Additionally, some ASMs may possibly cause neonatal hemorrhagic disorder and there is a lack of strong evidence to determine if prenatal vitamin K supplementation can reduce this complication. However, vitamin K 10 mg/day is often administered orally to the pregnant person during the last month of pregnancy and/or administered parenterally to the newborn at delivery.[101]

Some ASMs pass into human milk and those with less protein binding will accumulate more. Treatment with ASMs is not necessarily a reason to discourage breastfeeding, although ASM concentrations are measurable in infants fed human milk. In fact, an argument could be made that since ASMs should rarely be discontinued abruptly, providing human milk after birth allows for a downward titration of a medication that the baby was exposed to for the past 9 months. Infants born to patients taking any ASM (particularly barbiturates or benzodiazepines) should be closely observed for signs of excess sedation, irritability, or poor feeding.[101,102] In general, FDA labeling of ASMs including valproate state that the developmental and health benefits of human milk should be considered along with the patient's underlying seizure disorder, their clinical need for that ASM, and any potential adverse effects from the ASM on the infant fed human milk. Additionally, FDA labeling states caution should be exercised when an ASM is administered to an individual providing human milk to an infant.

Therapeutic Considerations in Patients of Asian and South Asian Decent

A common idiosyncratic effect of ASMs is rash. However, in some cases, the rash can quickly progress to SJS, TEN, or DRESS, which are severe and life-threatening conditions. There is a strong association between the presence of an inherited variant of the *HLA-B* gene, *HLA-B*1502*, in these populations, and the risk of developing SJS/TEN with carbamazepine phenytoin, and oxcarbazepine.[18,19,43] The frequency of HLA-B*15:02 is highest in East Asian (6.9%), Oceanian (5.4%), and South/Central Asian (4.6%) populations, although of note, while it is present, it is less frequent in Japan (<1%) and Korea (<2.5%). The variant is largely absent in individuals not of Asian origin. Testing for HLA B*1502 is recommended for patients with ancestry from genetically at-risk. If the genetic testing is positive, these ASMs should generally be avoided. In addition, the *HLA* genotype *HLA-A*3101* is associated with multiple carbamazepine-induced cutaneous reactions in Chinese, Japanese, and European populations and carbamazepine should be avoided in patients with that genotype.[18] Many *HLA-B*1502*-positive and *HLA-A*3101*-positive patients treated with ASMs will not develop SJS/TEN or other hypersensitivity reactions, and these reactions can still occur infrequently in *HLA-B*1502*-negative and *HLA-A*3101*-negative patients of any ethnicity. Of those who do experience SJS/TEN with carbamazepine, 90% will have this reaction within the first few months of treatment.[18]

EVALUATION OF THERAPEUTIC OUTCOMES

The goal of therapy for all ASMs is seizure freedom or reduction in seizure frequency, while minimizing adverse medication reactions. Determining clinical response to treatment involves identifying the number and type of seizures and adverse medication reactions during the monitoring and follow-up phase of treatment. Providing the patient with a seizure and adverse reactions diary will assist in this effort as the severity and frequency of seizures should be monitored by the patient and the family and recorded in the seizure diary. External factors such as seizure triggers can also influence seizure frequency. Therefore, patients should be educated that seizure triggers should be identified and documented because avoiding them may have a significant impact on seizure control. Additionally, although seizures tend to be stereotyped within an individual, the clinical presentation of the seizure may change over time or with treatment and this should be documented. During all follow-up visits, the seizure diary should be reviewed with both patients and family to determine whether patients are truly seizure free.

Patients should also be monitored for all ASM adverse reactions and assessed for dose-related CNS effects (eg, drowsiness, fatigue, dizziness, blurry vision, and incoordination). Such adverse reactions are common, especially when initiating ASM therapy as well as with polytherapy. If possible, CNS adverse reactions should be avoided, either by dose reduction of monotherapy, reduction or elimination of polytherapy, or substituting for a better tolerated ASM.

Patients should also be assessed for idiosyncratic adverse reactions which usually require withdrawal in an affected patient, including serious rash (ie, SJS, TEN), hematologic dyscrasias, electrolyte abnormalities (eg, hyponatremia), and hepatotoxicity. Laboratory assessment, including complete blood cell (CBC) counts, chemistries, and liver function tests, should be performed at baseline and after initiation of ASMs to monitor for idiosyncratic adverse reactions. Other specific laboratory tests can be performed if there is clinical suspicion of adverse reactions (eg, measuring ammonia levels in a patient with suspected hyperammonemic encephalopathy from valproic acid). Acute organ failure due to an idiosyncratic reaction, when it occurs, generally occurs within the first 6 months of ASM therapy,[103] although there is a delay between treatment initiation and the onset of symptoms. There is also a more rapid onset if a patient who has had an idiosyncratic reaction to a specific ASM is rechallenged.[103]

Patients on chronic ASM therapy should be monitored for long-term medication adverse effects. Specifically, for those patients on chronic ASMs known to cause osteoporosis (eg, phenytoin and phenobarbital), bone density loss can be measured via bone-density scanning (eg, DEXA) after many years of treatment. Gums should be visually inspected for gingival hyperplasia at follow-up (eg, phenytoin) and patients should also be instructed to have regular and thorough dental care.

Medication adherence should also be monitored and when seizures are not controlled, medication nonadherence must always be considered, as it is the single most common reason for treatment failure. It is estimated that up to 60% of patients with epilepsy are nonadherent.[104] The rate of nonadherence is increased by the complexity of the regimen and by doses taken three and four times a day.[104] Frequent uncontrolled seizures can also predispose a patient to nonadherence secondary to confusion over whether the medication was taken. Nonadherence is not influenced by age, sex, psychomotor development, or seizure type.[104]

Obtaining serum concentrations of ASMs is a method by which to optimize therapy for an individual patient, but is not a therapeutic end point in itself. A patient's clinical response is more important than the actual serum medication concentration as seizure control can occur before the "minimum" of the published therapeutic range is achieved, and adverse medication effects can appear before the "maximum" of the range is achieved. Some patients may need and tolerate concentrations beyond the maximum. Clinicians should define a therapeutic range for an individual patient as the concentration below which there are adverse effects and above which the patient experiences seizures. Then serum levels can be useful to document lack of efficacy, loss of efficacy, and to determine how much room there is to increase a dose based on expected toxicity. Serum levels can also be particularly useful to determine nonadherence and should be checked if there are questions. Depending on the ASM, serum levels can also be useful in patients with significant renal and/or hepatic disease, patients taking multiple agents, and individuals who are pregnant or taking OCs.[36,77]

Patients should also be monitored long term for comorbid conditions, social adjustment (including QOL assessments), and medication interactions. Periodic screening for comorbid neuropsychiatric disorders, such as depression, suicidal ideation, and anxiety, is also important. Screening for learning and development issues in children is also imperative as neurodevelopmental comorbidities commonly coexist with epilepsy and may be associated with use of ASMs.[2]

Overall treatment outcomes are increasingly focusing on obtaining an optimal QOL for the patient and the AAN has developed quality performance measures for the clinician that define a high quality of care of these patients. Among those performance measures, it is important to remember to counsel patients about ASM adverse reactions and initiate a discussion about depression. Additionally, factors that can impact QOL in patients with epilepsy which should be addressed include issues about driving, economic security, forming relationships, and epilepsy safety such as precautions when swimming, social isolation, and social stigma.[2,32]

10 After the initiation of treatment, approximately 65% of patients treated for new-onset epilepsy can be expected to be maintained on one ASM and may be seizure free.[34] The percentage of patients who are seizure free on one ASM varies by seizure type. After 12 months of treatment, the percentage who are seizure free is highest for those who have only GTC seizures (48%-55%), lowest for those who have only focal seizures (23%-26%), and intermediate for those with mixed seizure types (25%-32%).[102,105]

Polytherapy with two or more ASMs is appropriate for patients who cannot achieve seizure freedom on ASM monotherapy. Of the 35% of patients with unsatisfactory control on monotherapy, 10% will be well controlled with a two-ASM treatment. Of the remaining patients, 20% will continue to have unsatisfactory control despite greater than two-ASM treatment and are deemed to be medication resistant.[34] The ILAE consensus definition for medication-resistant epilepsy includes lack of seizure freedom from at least two adequate trials of an ASM as monotherapy or polytherapy, which were appropriately chosen and used.[103] Those who have unsatisfactory control despite multiple ASM treatment may be candidates for the ketogenic diet, a vagal nerve stimulator, and/or surgery, which is especially encouraged for those who are good surgical candidates. In fact, the AAN has included assessment about patient knowledge and referral to surgery in their quality performance measures.[32]

For a patient with long-standing epilepsy, adequacy of their current medication regimen, whether they are seizure free or not, should be routinely evaluated. Reevaluate goals when necessary, especially in those 20% to 35% of patients where seizure freedom cannot be achieved, as obtainable goals which balance seizure control with patient-specific QOL factors[2,32] and wishes (eg, decrease in the number of seizures with minimized medication adverse effects) should be established. Patient education and assurance of patient understanding of the goals is also an essential part of the care plan.

For some patients who have not experienced seizures for many years and who are deemed to have a low risk of recurrence, ASM withdrawal may be considered. The AAN has issued guidelines for discontinuing ASMs in seizure-free patients.[106] After assessing the risks and benefits to both the patient and society, ASM withdrawal can be considered in a patient meeting the following profile: seizure free for 2 to 5 years, a history of a single type of focal seizure or primary generalized seizures, a normal neurologic exam and normal IQ, and an EEG that has normalized with treatment.[107,108] When these factors are present, the relapse rate at 1 year is expected to be 35% and 29% at 2 years.[109] For those patients who relapse after withdrawal, ASMs can be restarted; while seizure freedom can be regained for most patients who restart ASMs, it does not happen for all.[110] Factors associated with a poor prognosis in discontinuing ASMs, despite a seizure-free interval, include a history of a high frequency of seizures, repeated episodes of status epilepticus, a combination of seizure types, and development of abnormal mental functioning.[107,108]

CONCLUSION

Epilepsy is a group of diseases that present with variable signs and symptoms and is a major burden in terms of QOL, morbidity, and risk of premature mortality from SUDEP, especially in those who continue to have seizures. Pharmacologic management of epilepsy consists of symptomatic treatment only. The mainstay of pharmacologic therapy is ASMs, with a goal of suppression of seizure occurrence. Over the years, over two dozen ASMs with various mechanisms of action, pharmacokinetics, adverse effect profiles, and interaction profiles have become available for the treatment of epilepsy. When selecting ASM therapy, efficacy must be balanced with ASM adverse effects and cost and take into consideration patient-specific factors including age, sex, susceptibility to adverse effects, concomitant medications, and ability to adhere with selected regimen. Suppression of seizures can be achieved with ASM monotherapy or polytherapy in up to two-thirds of all patients with epilepsy but do not alter long-term prognosis. In patients with medication-resistant epilepsy, nonpharmacologic options such as ketogenic diet, vagal nerve stimulation, and epilepsy surgery should be considered. Epilepsy surgery is the most effective way to achieve long-term seizure freedom, but is an option for only a few people with medication-resistant epilepsy. With improved understanding of epilepsy pathophysiology and pathogenesis, better, disease modifying, and curative pharmacological treatments may become available.

ABBREVIATIONS

AAN	American Academy of Neurology
AES	American Epilepsy Society
AMPA	α-amino-3-hydroxy-5-methylisoxazole-4-propionic acid
ASM	antiseizure medication
AUC	area under the medication concentration time curve
BECT	benign epilepsy with centro-temporal spikes
CAE	childhood absence epilepsy
C_{max}	maximal blood medication concentration
CT	computed tomography
DEXA	dual energy x-ray absorptiometry
DRESS	drug reactions with eosinophilia and systemic symptoms
EEG	electroencephalogram
EFHC1	EF-hand containing protein-1
GABA	γ-aminobutyric acid
GTC	generalized tonic–clonic
IGE	idiopathic generalized epilepsy
ILAE	International League Against Epilepsy
LGS	Lennox–Gastaut syndrome
JME	juvenile myoclonic epilepsy
MCMs	major congenital malformations
MRI	magnetic resonance imaging
NMDA	*N*-methyl-D-aspartate
OC	oral contraceptive
PCOS	polycystic ovary syndrome
QOL	quality of life
REMS	risk evaluation and mitigation strategy
SCARs	severe cutaneous adverse reactions
SE	status epilepticus
SJS	Steven–Johnsons syndrome
SP	simple partial
SUDEP	sudden unexplained death in epilepsy
TEN	toxic epidermal necrolysis
T_{max}	time to maximal blood medication concentration
VNS	vagus nerve stimulation
WBC	white blood cell

REFERENCES

1. Fisher RS, van Emde Boas W, Blume W, et al. Epileptic seizures and epilepsy: Definitions proposed by the international league against Epilepsy (ILAE) and the International Bureau for Epilepsy (IBE). *Epilepsia.* 2005;46(4):470–472.
2. England MJ, Liverman CT, Schultz AM, et al. A summary of the Institute of Medicine report: Epilepsy across the spectrum. Promoting health and understanding. *Epilepsy Behav.* 2012;25(2):266–276.
3. Zack MM, Kobau R. National and State Estimates of the Numbers of Adults and Children with Active Epilepsy—United States, 2015. *MMWR Morb Mortal Wkly Rep.* 2017;66:821–825.
4. Forsgren L, Hauser WA, Olafsson E, et al. Mortality of epilepsy in developed countries: A review. *Epilepsia.* 2005;46(suppl 11):18–27.
5. DiGiorgio CM, Curtis A, Hertling D. Sudden unexpected death in epilepsy: Risk factors, biomarkers, and prevention. *Acta Neurol Scan.* 2018;15:1–11.
6. Scheffer IE, Berkovic S, Capovilla G, et al. ILAE classification of the epilepsies: Position paper of the ILAE Commission for Classification and Terminology. *Epilepsia.* 2017;58(4):512–521.
7. Nieh SE, Sherr EH. Epileptic encephalopathies: New genes and new pathways. *Neurotherapeutics.* 2014;11:796–806.
8. Tanaka M, Olsen RW, Medina MT, et al. Hyperglycosylation and reduced GABA currents of mutated GABRB3 polypeptide in remitting childhood absence epilepsy. *Am J Hum Genet.* 2008;82(6):1249–1261.
9. Suzuki T, Delgado-Escueta AV, Aguan K, et al. Mutations in EFHC1 cause juvenile myoclonic epilepsy. *Nat Genet.* 2004;36(8):842–849.
10. Bailey JN, de Nijs L, Bai D, et al. Variant intestinal cell-kinase in juvenile myoclonic epilepsy. *N Engl J Med.* 2018;378:1018–1028.
11. Wei F, Yan L, Su T, et al. Ion channel genes and epilepsy: Functional alteration, pathogenic potential, and mechanism of epilepsy. *Neurosci Bull.* 2017;33(4):455–477.
12. Malmgren K, Thom M. Hippocampal sclerosis—origins and imaging. *Epilepsia.* 2012;53(S4):19–33.
13. Minassian BA, Lee JR, Herbrick J-A, et al. Mutations in a gene encoding a novel protein tyrosine phosphatase causes progressive myoclonus epilepsy. *Nature Genet.* 1998;20:171–174.
14. Hesdorffer DC. Risk factors. In: Engel J, Pedley TA, eds. *Epilepsy: A Comprehensive Text Book.* 2nd ed. Philadelphia, PA: Lippincott Williams & Wilkins; 2008;57–63.
15. Jallon P, Zifkin BF. Seizure precipitants. In: Engel J, Pedley TA, eds. *Epilepsy: A Comprehensive Text Book.* 2nd ed. Philadelphia, PA: Lippincott Williams & Wilkins; 2008;77–80.
16. Goldberg EM, Coulter DA. Mechanisms of epileptogenesis: A convergence on neural circuit dysfunction. *Nat Rev Neurosci.* 2013;14(5):337–349.
17. Engel J. *Seizures and Epilepsy.* 2nd ed. New York: Oxford University Press; 2013:56–72.
18. Tegretol [package insert]. East Hanover, NJ: Novartis Pharmaceuticals Corporation; March 2018.
19. Dilantin [package insert]. New York, NY: Parke-Davis; January 2009.
20. Klonopin [package insert]. South San Francisco, CA: Genentech; October 2013.

21. Rogawski MA, Bazil CW. New molecular targets for antiepileptic drugs: α2δ, SV2A, and Kv7/KCNQ/M potassium channels. *Curr Neurol Neurosci Rep.* 2008;8(4):345–352.
22. Thijs RD, Surges R, Obrien T, Sander JW. Epilepsy in adults. *Lancet.* 2019;393(10172):689–701.
23. Sabril [package insert]. Deerfield, Il: Lundbeck; February 2018.
24. Engel J. Mechanisms of neuronal excitation and synchronization: Neuronal networks. *Seizures and Epilepsy.* 2nd ed. New York, NY: Oxford University Press; 2013;73–81.
25. Huguenard JR, McCormick DA. Thalamic synchrony and dynamic regulation of global forebrain oscillations. *Trends Neurosc.* 2007;30:350–356.
26. Fisher RS, Cross JH, French JA, et al. Operational classification of seizure types by the International League Against Epilepsy: Position paper of the ILAE Commission for Classification and Terminology. *Epilepsia.* 2017;58(4):522–530.
27. Glauser T, Ben-Menachem E, Bourgeois B, et al. Updated ILAE evidence review of antiepileptic drug efficacy and effectiveness as initial monotherapy for epileptic seizures and syndromes. *Epilepsia.* 2013;54(3):551–563.
28. Noachtar S, Peters AS. Semiology of epileptic seizures: A critical review. *Epilepsy Behav.* 2009;15(1):2–9.
29. Foldvary-Schaefer N, Unnwongse K. Localizing and lateralizing features of auras and seizures. *Epilepsy Behav.* 2011;20(2):160–166.
30. Fisher RS, Acevedo C, Arzimanoglou A, et al. A practical clinical definition of epilepsy. *Epilepsia.* 2014;55(4):475–482.
31. Bouma HK, Labos C, Gore GC, et al. The diagnostic accuracy of routine electroencephalography after a first unprovoked seizure. *Eur J Neurol.* 2016;23(3):455–463.
32. Fountain NB, Van Ness PC, Swain-Eng R, et al. Quality improvement in neurology: AAN epilepsy quality measures: Report of the Quality Measurement and Reporting Subcommittee of the American Academy of Neurology. *Neurology.* 2011;76(1):94–99.
33. Chen DK, So YT, Fisher RS. Use of serum prolactin in diagnosing epileptic seizures. Report of the Therapeutic and Technology Assessment Subcommittee of the American Academy of Neurology. *Neurology.* 2005;65:668–675.
34. Kwan P, Brodie MJ. Early identification of refractory epilepsy. *N Engl J Med.* 2000;342:314–319.
35. Krumholz A, Wiebe S, Gronseth GS, et al. Evidence-based guideline: Management of an unprovoked first seizure in adults. *Neurology.* 2015;84:1705–1712.
36. Patsalos PN, Spencer EP, Berry DJ. Therapeutic drug monitoring of antiepileptic drugs in epilepsy: A 2018 update. *Ther Drug Monit.* 2018;40(5):526–548.
37. Phenobarbital [package insert]. Boucherville, QC, Canada: Sandoz Canada Inc.; February 2015.
38. Zarontin [package insert]. New York, NY: Parke-Davis; April 2009.
39. Depakote ER [package insert]. Chicago, IL: Abbott Laboratories; October 2011.
40. Felbatol [package insert]. Somerset, NJ: Meda Pharmaceuticals; August 2012.
41. Neurontin [package insert]. New York, NY: Parke-Davis; February 2018.
42. Zonegran [package insert]. Teaneck, NJ: Eisai Inc.; 2006.
43. Trileptal [package insert]. East Hanover, NJ: Novartis Pharmaceuticals Inc.; March 2018.
44. Lamictal [package insert]. Research Triangle Park, NC: GlaxoSmithKline; July 2018.
45. Gabitril [package insert]. Frazer, PA: Cephalon; April 2009.
46. Aptiom [package insert]. Marlborough, MA: Sunovion Pharmaceuicals Inc.; September 2017.
47. Epidiolex [package insert]. Carlsbad, CA: Greenwich Biosciences; September 2018.
48. Mysoline [package insert]. Aliso Viejo, CA: Valeant Pharmaceuticals; 2009.
49. Keppra [package insert]. Smyrna, GA: UCB Inc.; October 2017.
50. Topamax [package insert]. Titusville, NJ: Jannsen Pharmaceuticals; June 2018.
51. Briviact [package insert]. Smyrna, GA: UCB Inc.; May 2018.
52. Onfi [package insert]. Deerfield, Il: Lundbeck; June 2018.
53. Vimpat [package insert]. Smyrna, GA: UCB Inc.; November 2018.
54. Fycompa [package insert]. Woodcliff Lake, NJ: Eisai Inc.; September 2018.
55. Lyrica [package insert]. New York, NY: Parke-Davis; May 2018.
56. Banzel [package insert]. Woodcliff Lake, NJ: Eisai Inc.; June 2015.
57. Brigo F, Ausserer H, Tezzon F, et al. When one plus one makes three: The quest for rational antiepileptic polytherapy with supraadditive anticonvulsant efficacy. *Epilepsy Behav.* 2013;27(3):439–442.
58. Groesbeck DK, Blum RM, Kossoff EH. Long-term use of the ketogenic diet: Outcomes of 28 children with over 6 years diet duration. *Neurology.* 2006;66(suppl 2):A41.
59. Dossoff EH, Zupec-Kania BA, Amark PE, et al. Optimal clinical management of children receiving the ketogenic diet: Recommendations of the International Ketogenic Diet Study Group. *Epilepsia.* 2009;50:304–317.
60. Krahl SE, Clark KB, Smith DC, et al. Locus coeruleus lesions suppress the seizure-attenuating effects of vagus nerve stimulation. *Epilepsia.* 1998;39:709–714.
61. Shuchman M. Approving the vagus-nerve stimulator for depression. *N Engl J Med.* 2007;356:1604–1607.
62. Salinsky MC, Uthman BM, Ristanovic RK, et al. Vagus nerve stimulation for the treatment of medically intractable seizures: Results of a 1 year open extension trial. *Arch Neurol.* 1996;53:1176–1180.
63. Handforth A, Degiorgio CM, Schachter SC, et al. Vagus nerve stimulation therapy for partial-onset seizures: A randomized active controlled trial. *Neurology.* 1998;51(1):48–55.
64. Wiebe S, Blume WT, Girvin JP, et al. Effectiveness and efficiency of surgery for Temporal Lobe Epilepsy Study Group: A randomized, controlled trial of surgery for temporal-lobe epilepsy. *N Engl J Med.* 2001;345(5):311–318.
65. Engel J, McDermott MP, Wiebe S, et al. Early surgical therapy for drug-resistant temporal lobe epilepsy. *JAMA.* 2012;307:922–930.
66. TI Jeong SW, Lee SK, Hong KS, et al. Prognostic factors for the surgery for mesial temporal lobe epilepsy: Longitudinal analysis. *Epilepsia.* 2005;46(8):1273–1279.
67. Janszky J, Janszky I, Schulz R, et al. Temporal lobe epilepsy with hippocampal sclerosis: Predictors for long-term surgical outcome. *Brain.* 2005;128(Pt 2):395–404.
68. Jeha LE, Najm IM, Bingaman WE, et al. Predictors of outcome after temporal lobectomy for the treatment of intractable epilepsy. *Neurology.* 2006;66(12):1938–1940.
69. Rogawski MA, Loscher W, Rho JM. Mechanism of action of antiseizure drugs and the ketogenic diet. *Cold Spring Harb Perspect Med.* 2016;6:a022780.
70. Diacomit [package insert]. Beauvais, France: Biobodex; August 2018.
71. Xcopri [package insert]. Paramus, NJ: SK Life Science; April 2021.
72. Fintepla [package insert]. Emeryville, CA: Zogenix; June 2020.
73. Kanner AM, Ashman E, Gloss D, et al. Practice guideline update summary: Efficacy and tolerability of the new antiepileptic drugs I: Treatment of new-onset epilepsy: Report of the American Epilepsy Society and the Guideline Development, Dissemination, and Implementation Subcommittee of the American Academy of Neurology. *Epilepsy Curr.* 2018;18(4):260–268.
74. Kanner AM, Ashman E, Gloss D, et al. Practice guideline update summary: Efficacy and tolerability of the new antiepileptic drugs I: Treatment-resistant epilepsy: Report of the American Epilepsy Society and the Guideline Development, Dissemination, and Implementation Subcommittee of the American Academy of Neurology. *Epilepsy Curr.* 2018;18(4):269–278.
75. Perucca P, Gilliam FG. Adverse effects of antiepileptic drugs. *Lancet.* 2012;11:792–802.
76. EK St Louis. Minimizing AED adverse effects: Improving quality of life in the interictal state in epilepsy care. *Curr Neuropharmacol.* 2009;7(2):106–114.
77. Patsalos PN, Berry DJ, Bourgeois BFD, et al. Antiepileptic drugs—best practice guidelines for therapeutic drug monitoring: A position paper by the Subcommission on Therapeutic Drug Monitoring, ILAE Commission on Therapeutic Strategies. *Epilepsia.* 2008;49:1239–1276.
78. Pack AM, Morrell MJ, McMahon DJ, et al. Bone health in young women with epilepsy after one year of antiepileptic drug monotherapy. *Neurology.* 2008;70:1586–1593.
79. Lado F, Spiegel R, Masur JH, et al. Value of routine screening for bone demineralization in an urban population of patients with epilepsy. *Epilepsy Res.* 2008;78:155–160.
80. Wang Z, Lin YS, Zheng XE, et al. An inducible cytochrome P4503A4-dependent vit D catabolic pathway. *Mol Pharmacol.* 2012;81:498–509.
81. Anderson GD, Pak C, Doane KW, et al. Revised Winter-Tozer equation for normalized phenytoin concentrations in trauma and elderly patients with hypoalbuminemia. *Ann Pharmacother.* 1997;31:279–284.
82. Jentink J, Loane MA, Dolk H, et al. Valproic acid monotherapy in pregnancy and major congenital malformations. *N Engl J Med.* 2010;362:2185–2193.
83. Berghuis B, van der Palen J, de Haan GJ, et al. Carbamazepine- and oxcarbazepine-induced hyponatremia in people with epilepsy. *Epilepsia.* 2017;58(7):1227–1233.

84. Luer MS, Hamani C, Dujovny M, et al. Saturable transport of gabapentin at the blood-brain barrier. *Neurol Res.* 1999;21:559–562.
85. Christensen J, Petrenaite V, Atterman J, et al. Oral contraceptives induce lamotrigine metabolism: Evidence from a double-blind, placebo-controlled trial. *Epilepsia.* 2007;48:484–489.
86. Shorvon SD. Safety of topiramate: Adverse events and relationship to dosing. *Epilepsia.* 1996;37(S2):S18–S22.
87. Mula M, Trimble M, Thompson P, et al. Topiramate and word-finding difficulties in patients with epilepsy. *Neurology.* 2003;60:1104–1107.
88. Hirsch LJ, Weintraub DB, Buchsbaum R, et al. Predictors of lamotrigine-associated rash. *Epilepsia.* 2006;47:318–322.
89. Messenheimer JA. Rash in adult and pediatric patients treated with lamotrigine. *Can J Neurol Sci.* 1998;25:S14–S18.
90. Rowan AJ, Ramsay ER, Collins JF, et al. New onset geriatric epilepsy: A randomized study of gabapentin, lamotrigine, and carbamazepine. *Neurology.* 2005;64:1868–1873.
91. Foorozan R. Vigabatrin: Lessons learned from the United States experience. *J Neuroopthalmol.* 2018;38(4):442–450.
92. Herzog AG. Progesterone therapy in women with epilepsy: A 3-year follow-up. *Neurology.* 1999;52(9):1917–1918.
93. Harden CL, Pulver MC, Ravdin L, et al. The effect of menopause and perimenopause on the course of epilepsy. *Epilepsia.* 1999;40(10):1403–1407.
94. Verrotti A, D'Egidio C, Mohn A, et al. Antiepileptic drug, sex hormones, and PCOS. *Epilepsia.* 2011;52:199–211.
95. Savers A, Harden CL. Gender issues for drug treatment. In: Engel J, Pedley TA, eds. *Epilepsy: A Comprehensive Text Book.* 2nd ed. Philadelphia, PA: Lippincott Williams & Wilkins; 2008;1263–1269.
96. Harden CL, Hopp J, Ting TY, et al. Practice parameter update: Management issues for women with epilepsy—focus on pregnancy (an evidence-based review): Obstetrical complications and change in seizure frequency. *Neurology.* 2009;73:126–132.
97. Harden CL, Meador KJ, Pennell PB, et al. Management issues for women with epilepsy—Focus on pregnancy (an evidence-based review): II. Teratogenesis and perinatal outcomes. *Neurology.* 2009;50:1237–1246.
98. Williams J, Myson V, Steward S, et al. Self discontinuation of AEDs in pregnancy: Detection by hair analysis. *Epilepsia.* 2002;43(8):824–831.
99. Tomson T, Marson A, Boon P, et al. Valproate in the treatment of epilepsy in girls and women of childbearing potential. *Epilepsia.* 2015;56(7):1006–1019.
100. Meador KJ, Pennell PB, May RC, et al. Fetal loss and malformations in the MONEAD study of pregnant women with epilepsy. *Neurology.* 2020;94(14):e1502–e1511. 10.1212/WNL.0000000000008687 31806691.
101. Harden CL, Pennell PB, Koppel BS, et al. Management issues for women with epilepsy—Focus on pregnancy (an evidence-based review): III. Vitamin K, folic acid, blood levels, and breast-feeding: Report of the Quality Standards Subcommittee and Therapeutics and Technology Assessment Subcommittee of the American Academy of Neurology and the American Epilepsy Society. *Epilepsia.* 2009;50:1247–1255.
102. Meador KJ, Baker GA, Browning N, et al. Effects of breastfeeding in children of women taking antiepileptic drugs. *Neurology.* 2010;75:1954–1960.
103. Dreifuss FE, Langer DH, Moline KA, et al. Valproic acid hepatic fatalities-experience since 1984. *Neurology.* 1989;39:201–207.
104. Garnet WR. Antiepileptic drug treatment: Outcomes and adherence. *Pharmacotherapy.* 2000;20:191s–199s.
105. Mattson RH, Cramer JA, Collins JF. Prognosis for total control of complex partial and secondarily generalized tonic-clonic seizures. Department of Veterans Affairs Epilepsy Cooperative Studies No. 118 and No. 264. *Neurology.* 1996;46:68–76.
106. Practice parameter: A guideline for discontinuing antiepileptic drugs in seizure-free patients—summary statement. Report of the Quality Standards Subcommittee of the American Academy of Neurology. *Neurology.* 1996;47(2):600–602.
107. Anderson T, Brathen G, Person A, et al. A comparison between one and three years of treatment in uncomplicated childhood epilepsy: A prospective study. The EEG as a predictor of outcome after withdrawal of treatment. *Epilepsia.* 1997;38:228–232.
108. Chadwick D, Taylor J, Johnson T. Outcomes after seizure recurrence in people with well-controlled epilepsy and the factors that influence it. The MRC antiepileptic drug withdrawal group. *Epilepsia.* 1996;37:1043–1050.
109. Berg AT, Shinnar S. Relapse following discontinuation of antiepileptic drugs: A meta-analysis. *Neurology.* 1994;44:601–608.
110. Kwan P, Arzimanoglou A, Berg AT, et al. Definition of drug resistant epilepsy: Consensus proposal by the ad hoc Task Force of the ILAE Commission on Therapeutic Strategies. *Epilepsia.* 2010;51(6):1069–1077.

76

Status Epilepticus

Elizabeth A. Hall, Stephanie J. Phelps, and James W. Wheless

KEY CONCEPTS

1. Status epilepticus (SE) is a neurologic emergency that may be associated with significant morbidity and mortality.
2. Generalized convulsive status epilepticus (GCSE) is defined as any recurrent or continuous seizure activity lasting longer than 30 minutes in which the patient does not regain baseline mental status. Any seizure that does not stop within 5 minutes should be treated aggressively as impending SE.
3. There are two types of SE, GCSE and nonconvulsive status epilepticus (NCSE). GCSE is the most common type and is divided into four stages: (1) impending, (2) established, (3) refractory, and (4) super-refractory.
4. The pathophysiology of GCSE is unknown; however, experimental models show a dramatic decrease in γ-aminobutyric acid (GABA)–mediated inhibitory synaptic transmission and that glutamatergic excitatory synaptic transmission sustains the seizures.
5. During prolonged GCSE, $GABA_A$ receptors move from the synaptic membrane into the cytoplasm, becoming functionally inactive. Receptor loss on the synaptic surface may result in time-dependent benzodiazepine pharmacoresistance. Glutamatergic *N*-methyl-D-aspartate (NMDA) receptors also increase in number and activity, suggesting a role for ketamine.
6. Treatment is done to prevent or decrease morbidity and mortality of prolonged seizures. Pharmacologic treatment needs to be rapid and aimed at terminating both electrical and clinical seizures. The probability of poorer outcomes increases with an increased length of electroclinical seizure activity.
7. IV lorazepam is the preferred benzodiazepine for initial treatment of GCSE given its efficacy and long duration of action in the central nervous system (CNS), although IM midazolam, IV lorazepam, IV diazepam, and IV phenobarbital effectively terminate seizures lasting at least 5 minutes. Midazolam is the preferred benzodiazepine for IM and intranasal administration in patients without an established IV.
8. The hydantoins (ie, phenytoin, fosphenytoin) continue to be the long-acting antiseizure medications used most frequently, although this is changing. The comparative efficacy of these two antiseizure medications is still unknown; however, fosphenytoin is better tolerated and hence preferred. Either should be given concurrently with benzodiazepines.
9. The second antiseizure medication administered is less effective than the first "standard" antiseizure medication in both adults and pediatric patients. The third antiseizure medication may be significantly less effective.
10. If GCSE is not controlled by two antiseizure medications (a benzodiazepine and a standard antiseizure medication), it is considered refractory. In these cases, anesthetic doses of midazolam, pentobarbital, or propofol may be used and monitored with a continuous electroencephalogram (EEG).

BEYOND THE BOOK

Case Question: An order is written for a 15-mg PE/kg fosphenytoin loading dose for a 60-kg patient. The dose is added to 50 mL of an appropriate fluid and is given at the maximum administration rate. There are questions about the rate settings for the infusion device (mL/min) and how long it will take to infuse the dose. Complete the following table.

	Parenterally Administered Product							
Product information	**Phenytoin**	**Fosphenytoin**	**Valproate**	**Levetiracetam**	**Phenobarbital**	**Diazepam**	**Lorazepam**	**Midazolam**
Refrigeration required yes/no								
Pharmaceutical Vehicle—Propylene glycol: yes/no								
pH of product								
Maximum infusion rate								
Compatible admixture solution(s)*								
IM administration, yes/no								
Cardiac monitoring required								
Reference range (mg/L)								

Solution to be infused, not reconstituted

INTRODUCTION

1 2 Status epilepticus (SE) is a common neurologic emergency associated with brain damage and death. The Commission on Classification and Terminology and the Commission on Epidemiology of the International League Against Epilepsy (ILAE) defines SE as a situation where there is a failure of the mechanisms responsible for seizure termination and prevention of prolonged seizures. There are two operational dimensions to this new definition. First, the length of the seizure and the time point beyond which the seizure is regarded as "continuous seizure activity"; usually 5 minutes. Second is the time of ongoing seizure activity, after which there is a risk of long-term consequences (30 minutes). Both time points are based on animal experiments and clinical research; hence, they should be considered current best estimates.[1] The traditional definition defines SE as (a) any seizure lasting longer than 30 minutes whether or not consciousness is impaired or (b) recurrent seizures without an intervening period of consciousness between seizures.[2] Clinically, this definition is limited, as the average seizure is less than 2 minutes in length and only 40% of seizures lasting 10 to 29 minutes cease without treatment.[3] Pharmacoresistance and mortality significantly increase with prolonged seizure duration. Therefore, aggressive treatment of seizures lasting 5 or more minutes is strongly recommended. It is important to note that SE can present in several forms (Table 76-1), including generalized convulsive status epilepticus (GCSE) and nonconvulsive status epilepticus (NCSE).

Nonconvulsive status epilepticus accounts for up to 20% of all SE cases. It has variable and subtle clinical symptoms, such as cognitive impairment, automatisms, and/or behavioral changes, which make diagnosis challenging.[4] Electroencephalogram (EEG) is an important diagnostic and management tool. A benzodiazepine is the medication of choice for initial treatment, and intravenous (IV) phenytoin, valproic acid, or levetiracetam may be used as second-line.[4] In refractory cases, non-anesthetic antiseizure medication (ASMs), such as lacosamide and topiramate, are typically preferable to IV anesthetic medications, such as midazolam, propofol, and barbiturates.[4]

3 GCSE is the most common and severe form of SE. It is characterized by repeated primary or secondary generalized seizures involving both hemispheres of the brain which result in a loss of consciousness, and a persistent postictal state. GCSE can be divided into four phases: (1) stabilization, (2) initial therapy, (3) secondary therapy, and (4) third therapy (Table 76-2).[5]

EPIDEMIOLOGY

The worldwide incidence of GCSE varies considerably and has ranged from 5.1 to 41 per 100,000, with the incidence being highest in developing countries.[6] GCSE does not have a predilection for gender,[6] and occurs more frequently in nonwhites across all ages.[7] The incidence is highest in those less than 2 years of age[8] and older than 60 years of age.[6] Economic income may contribute

TABLE 76-1 International Classification of Status Epilepticus

Convulsive		Nonconvulsive	
International	**Traditional Terminology**	**International**	**Traditional Terminology**
Generalized SE • Tonic-Clonic[a,b] • Tonic[c] • Clonic[c] • Myoclonic[b] • *Erratic*[d]	Grand mal, epilepticus convulsivus	Absence[c]	Petit mal, spike-and-wave stupor, spike-and-slow-wave or 3/s spike-and-wave, epileptic fugue, epilepsiaminora continua, epileptic twilight, minor SE
Secondary generalized SE[a,b] • Tonic • Partial seizures with secondary generalization		Partial SE[a,b] Simple partial Somatomotor Dysphasic Other types Complex partial	Focal motor, focal sensory, epilepsiapartialis continua, adversive SE Elementary Temporal lobe, psychomotor, epileptic fugue state, prolonged epileptic stupor, prolonged epileptic confusional state, continuous epileptic twilight state

SE, status epilepticus.

[a]Most common in older children.

[b]Most common in adolescents and adults.

[c]Most common in infants and young children.

[d]Most common in neonates.

TABLE 76-2 Generalized Convulsive Status Epilepticus

Phase	Time	Stage	Definition
Stabilization phase	0-5 minutes		An acute condition characterized by convulsive seizures. This may include pre-hospitalization or emergency room care
Initial-therapy phase	0-20 minutes	Impending GCSE	
Second-therapy phase	20-40 minutes	Established GCSE	An acute condition characterized by continuous seizures for at least 20 minutes, or by 20 minutes of intermittent seizures without full recovery of consciousness between events
Third-therapy phase	40-60 minutes	Refractory GCSE	An acute condition characterized by continuous seizures despite initial treatment with two ASMs
	>24 hours	Super-refractory	An acute condition characterized by seizures that continue 24 hours or longer after the administration of anesthesia, including cases in which SE recurs on reduction or withdrawal of anesthesia

ASM, antiseizure medication; GCSE, generalized convulsive status epilepticus; SE, status epilepticus.

to a difference in overall incidence.[6] Most GCSE occurs in individuals with no history of epilepsy; however, approximately 5% of adults and 10% to 25% of children with epilepsy will develop GCSE.

ETIOLOGY

Precipitating events for GCSE vary and generally reflect different populations and referral patterns. Most episodes in individuals with epilepsy occur because of acute antiseizure medication withdrawal, a metabolic disorder or concurrent illness, or a preexisting neurologic disease progression. Common etiologies and mortality rates are shown in Table 76-3.[7,9] Precipitating events are divided into those with or without neurologic structural lesions or those with a precipitating injury or insult. Cases with structural lesions or those with a specific neurologic insult are associated with a poor prognosis.

There are significant differences in pediatric and adult etiologies (see Table 76-3). During their first few weeks of life, infants born to mothers with substance uses can develop medication withdrawal seizures. Other neonates can develop GCSE due to a pyridoxine deficiency, which should resolve after IV pyridoxine (100 mg). In young children, the cause is often a nonspecific illness such as fever and/or a viral illness; however, in those less than one, acute encephalopathy and metabolic disorders are major causes of GCSE. In adults, the most frequent precipitating events are cerebrovascular disease, rapid antiseizure medication withdrawal, and low antiseizure medication serum concentrations. Cerebrovascular disease is the leading cause in those who have their first seizures after age 60. Prescription, OTC, herbal, and unhealthy substance use should be considered in anyone with new-onset GCSE.

TABLE 76-3 Etiology and Mortality for Pediatric and Adult Cases of Status Epilepticus

Etiology	Mortality Number of Cases (%) $n = 200$ Cases of Pediatric SE	Mortality Number of Cases (%) $n = 512$ Cases of Adult SE
Type I (No Structural Lesion)		
Infection	55 (5)	6 (35)
CNS infection	11 (0)	2 (20)
Metabolic	20 (5)	12 (36)
Low ASM levels	16 (0)	24 (7)
Alcohol	0 (0)	13 (8)
Idiopathic	6 (0)	13 (18)
Type II (Structural Lesion)		
Anoxia/hypoxia	27 (13)	14 (65)
CNS tumor	3 (50)	5 (22)
CVA	5 (0)	26 (27)
Substance overdose	5 (0)	3 (23)
Hemorrhage	5 (11)	4 (35)
Trauma	13 (0)	3 (23)
Remote causes[a]	33 (5)	7 (13)

ASM, antiseizure medication; CVA, cerebrovascular accident; SE, status epilepticus.

Percentages do not add up to 100% because some patients have multiple etiologies.

[a]More than half of the remote causes were congenital malformations and CVA in pediatric and adult patients, respectively.

Data from References 7 and 9.

PATHOPHYSIOLOGY

Seizures occur when excitatory neurotransmission overcomes inhibitory impulses in one or more brain regions. After a single, brief, generalized tonic-clonic seizure (less than 5 minutes), the seizure threshold is significantly elevated. And the brain's inhibitory mechanisms restore the balance of normal neurotransmission and prevent runaway excitation. In GCSE, the mechanisms that control normal brain homeostasis fail, which results in seizures occurring in close succession. In a different scenario, the magnitude of the proconvulsant stimulus is severe, and the compensatory mechanisms can be overwhelmed. In both instances, the mechanisms behind these failures are unknown, and the seizures become self-sustaining.

4 Cellurarly, it appears that an imbalance between excitatory (eg, glutamate, calcium, sodium, substance P, and neurokinin B) and inhibitory neurotransmission (eg, γ-aminobutyric acid [GABA], adenosine, potassium, neuropeptide Y, opioid peptides, and galanin) results in a seizure.[10] More specifically, $GABA_A$-mediated inhibition becomes less effective, while at the same time, glutamate's excitatory actions become enhanced. Thus, these mechanisms influence how GCSE progresses to refractory disease and impacts decisions related to sequencing antiseizure medications.

Most research has focused on gated ion channels; however, GCSE is largely caused by glutamate acting on postsynaptic *N*-methyl-D-aspartate (NMDA) and α-amino-3-hydroxy-5-methyl-isoxazole-4-propionate (AMPA)/kainate receptors.[10] During GCSE, NMDA subunits are recruited to the synaptic membrane, where they form additional proconvulsant receptors. Glutamate's activation of NMDA and AMPA receptors causes gated calcium and sodium channels to open, leading to neuronal depolarization.[11] Sustained depolarization may maintain GCSE and eventually cause neuronal death through calcium-, free radical–, and kinase-mediated events.[12] Although medications acting as NMDA and AMPA receptor antagonists seem attractive, glutamate is likely not the sole mechanism for sustaining GCSE, and these other mechanisms become increasingly crucial as seizure duration increases.

5 Within minutes of repetitive seizures, receptor trafficking occurs (eg, metabotropic GABA and glutamate receptors), as the $GABA_A$ postsynaptic receptors control chloride channels to produce hyperpolarization (inhibition) of the postsynaptic cell membrane.[11] These receptors have binding sites for GABA and select antiseizure medications (eg, phenobarbital and benzodiazepines) enhance $GABA_A$-mediated chloride inhibitory currents. It was previously thought that decreased presynaptic GABA led to prolonged seizures; however, it is currently held that GABA concentrations increase during the early phases of GCSE and continue to be elevated during late GCSE. During prolonged seizures, postsynaptic $GABA_A$ receptors experience endocytosis as the receptors move from the synaptic membrane into the cytoplasm. This results in a decrease in the number of γ_2 and β_{2-3} subunits that are functionally active, decreasing response to both endogenous GABA and GABA agonists.[10] The γ_2 subunit is associated with benzodiazepine effectiveness; hence, a loss of these on the synaptic surface would result in time-dependent pharmacoresistance to a benzodiazepine. Clinically, benzodiazepine relative potencies can be reduced up to 20-fold if seizures persist for more than 30 minutes.[11] For this reason, a benzodiazepine should always be combined with another medication that acts differently. A similar phenomenon occurs with sodium channel antagonists (phenytoin); however, the magnitude of resistance is less.

As GCSE persists, complex pathophysiologic and biochemical changes lead to systemic alterations, progression of motor phenomena, and development of specific EEG findings.[12] Although these systemic complications affect the prognosis of GCSE, a prolonged seizure can destroy neurons independent of these events.[11] In fact, the systemic effects of induced seizures in animals can be blocked, but the damage to the neocortex, cerebellum, and hippocampus persists. Two distinct and predictable phases have been identified. Phase I occurs during the first 30 minutes of seizure activity, and phase II immediately follows.[12]

During phase I, each seizure markedly increases plasma epinephrine, norepinephrine, and steroid concentrations, resulting in hypertension, tachycardia, and cardiac arrhythmias. Within minutes, arterial systolic pressures can rise to above 200 mm Hg, and heart rate can increase by 83 beats per minute.[12] Mean arterial pressure does not fall below 60 mm Hg (8.0 kPa); hence, cerebral perfusion pressure is not compromised. In animals, cerebral blood flow is also increased, thereby protecting neurons from hypoxic injury.

In the presence of a hypoxic myocardium, seizure-induced increases in sympathetic and parasympathetic stimulation of the heart can result in ventricular arrhythmias.[12] Autonomic neuron stimulation can cause a release of insulin and glucagon. Concurrently, circulating catecholamines cause an elevation of hepatic cyclic adenosine monophosphate, producing glycogenolysis. Although the patient can be hyperglycemic initially, serum glucose begins to fall.[12]

Seizure-induced muscular contractions and hypoxia cause lactic acid release, producing severe acidosis accompanied by hypotension and shock. Muscle contractions can contribute to severe rhabdomyolysis with secondary hyperkalemia and acute tubular necrosis. The airway can be obstructed, causing cyanosis or hypoxia. Additionally, an increase in salivation and tracheal and pulmonary secretions can cause aspiration pneumonia. Although transient pleocytosis can develop, it should not be attributed to SE until infectious causes have been eliminated. Between seizures, the EEG slows, and blood pressure normalizes, and although metabolic demands increase, the brain can compensate adequately.

When seizures exceed 30 minutes (phase II), the EEG ictal discharge and clonic motor activity become continuous, and the patient begins to decompensate.[12] Despite elevated levels of catecholamines, the patient can become hypotensive. During this time, cerebral blood flow autoregulation becomes dependent on mean arterial pressure and begins to fail. Excessive oxygen and glucose consumption continues; however, compensatory mechanisms are no longer able to meet demands.

During phase II, the serum glucose concentration may be normal or decreased. Profound hypoglycemia, secondary to hyperinsulinemia, can occur in those with hepatic dysfunction or reduced glycogen stores.[12] Hyperthermia and respiratory deterioration with hypoxia and ventilatory failure can develop, and there may be increased sweating and salivation. Metabolic and biochemical complications, including respiratory and metabolic acidosis, hyperkalemia, hyponatremia, and azotemia, may develop.

Morbidity and Mortality

Generalized convulsive status epilepticus is harmful to the brain. While most contend that the GCSE is responsible for the damage, it is unknown if the morbidity results from the underlying etiology or the GCSE. Regardless of the inducing stimulus, neuronal damage in animal models is evident following 30 to 60 minutes of GCSE, and most progress to develop epilepsy following a prolonged seizure. Interestingly, inhibiting the seizure-induced neuronal damage does not prevent the development of epilepsy, suggesting the seizures themselves may be harmful. It is hard to establish a relationship between GCSE and long-term outcomes because it is difficult to weigh the effects of seizure type, etiology, duration, concurrent physiologic events, and therapy or lack thereof. It has been shown that patients with a history of prolonged febrile seizures who later developed epilepsy share similar histopathologic changes (ie, hippocampal sclerosis) to those found in animal models of GCSE. In these cases, the period between the initial GCSE and the first epileptic seizure may be months to decades, suggesting a possible link between GCSE and the development of epilepsy. Importantly, studies of GCSE show that currently available antiseizure medications do not reproducibly prevent the development of epilepsy following prolonged seizures (ie, they are antiseizure medications and not antiepileptogenic).[13]

Patients who develop epilepsy following prolonged GCSE are less likely to experience remission of their seizures and may have decreased cognitive and memory function, mental impairment, or neurologic deficits when compared to those who develop epilepsy and subsequently have GCSE. Most studies have found that younger children, older patients, and those with preexisting epilepsy have a higher propensity for sequelae. Unless accompanied by an underlying neurologic abnormality, febrile SE is less likely to be associated with sequelae.

The overall worldwide case fatality rate of GCSE is 14.9%,[6] with the highest rate in those >60 years of age (24.9%), and in those with refractory GCSE (33.3%). Estimated mortality in the United States following GCSE ranges between 22,000 and 42,000 individuals per year, with rates lowest in children. The duration of seizure also impacts mortality. A 22% 1-year mortality rate has been seen for patients with refractory GCSE compared to 36% for those with super-refractory GCSE.[14] When compared with other populations, neonates have higher mortality and more neurologic sequelae.

Table 76-3 summarizes the etiology and corresponding GCSE mortality rates.[7,9] Interestingly, the mortality associated with many etiologies is significantly greater in adults than in children. Unresponsive patients may die from GCSE, but more frequently, they die from the acute illnesses that precipitated the GCSE. For example, patients with serious CNS structural changes (eg, hemorrhage and stroke) have a poorer prognosis than those with no structural lesion.

The outcome is affected by the time between the onset of GCSE and the initiation of treatment. Additionally, mortality significantly increases with increased seizure duration (eg, 2.6% for seizures 10-29 minutes, 19% for seizures lasting greater than 30 minutes, and 32% for seizures lasting greater than 60 minutes).[3,9] While mortality has decreased over the past decade, this probably reflects recognition of the need to initiate sequenced therapy using large doses of antiseizure medication as soon as possible.

CLINICAL PRESENTATION

Accurate diagnosis requires observation, physical examination, laboratory assessment, EEG, and neurologic imaging. The nature and duration of the seizure should be obtained, but a diagnosis of GCSE should not be made until a seizure is observed by a clinician. Most patients have an altered consciousness, ranging from obtundation to marked lethargy and somnolence with pronounced eyes-open unresponsiveness and waxy rigidity. Motor features can include muscle contractions, extensor or flexor posturing, and spasms. Over time, the clinical manifestations become less apparent. This has significant ramifications as seizures appear to terminate without treatment or with ineffective therapy.

In addition to assessing language and cognitive abilities, the physical and neurological examinations should assess motor, sensory, and reflex abnormalities, pupillary response, asymmetry, and posturing. The patient should also be examined for secondary injuries (eg, tongue lacerations, shoulder dislocations, and head and facial trauma).

Laboratory tests are essential to the diagnosis of various etiologies. Hypoglycemia, hyponatremia, hypernatremia, hypomagnesemia, hypocalcemia, and renal failure all can cause seizures. A urine toxicology screen can help eliminate unhealthy substance use or overdose. Serum medication concentration(s) should be obtained for chronic antiseizure medications, as low concentrations can reflect partial adherence or rapid medication withdrawal. Although a baseline serum antiseizure medication concentration helps determine if a specific antiseizure medication loading dose is required, the time needed to perform the test makes this impractical. Assessment of other laboratory parameters that affect antiseizure medication dosing also can be helpful (eg, hematology and chemistries to include albumin, renal function, and hepatic function). An EEG is a valuable diagnostic tool,

CLINICAL PRESENTATION Status Epilepticus

Symptoms

- Impaired consciousness (eg, lethargy to coma)
- Disorientation once GCSE is controlled
- Pain associated with injuries (eg, tongue lacerations, shoulder dislocations, back pain, myalgias, headache, and head trauma)

Early Signs

- Generalized convulsions
- Acute injuries or CNS insults that cause extensor or flexor posturing
- Hypothermia or fever suggestive of intercurrent illnesses (eg, sepsis or meningitis)
- Incontinence
- Normal blood pressure or hypotension and respiratory compromise

Late Signs

- Clinical seizures may or may not be apparent
- Pulmonary edema with respiratory failure
- Cardiac failure (dysrhythmias, arrest, and cardiogenic shock)
- Hypotension or hypertension
- Disseminated intravascular coagulation, multisystem organ failure
- Rhabdomyolysis
- Hyperpyrexia

Initial Laboratory Tests

- Complete blood count (CBC) with differential
- Serum chemistry profile (eg, electrolytes, calcium, magnesium, glucose, serum creatinine, alanine aminotransferase [ALT], and aspartate aminotransferase [AST])
- Urine toxicology/alcohol screen
- Blood cultures
- Arterial blood gas to assess for metabolic and respiratory acidosis, oxygenation
- Serum medication concentration if previous antiseizure medication(s) are suspected or known

Other Diagnostic Tests

- Spinal tap if CNS infection suspected
- EEG should be obtained on presentation and once clinical seizures are controlled
- CT with and without contrast
- MRI
- Radiograph if indicated to diagnose fractures

particularly in prolonged GCSE in whom clinically apparent seizures are not always evident. The initiation of antiseizure medication therapy should not be delayed while awaiting testing or results.

Once seizures have stopped, it is essential to determine if the patient is febrile or has a systemic or CNS infection. Many physiologic consequences of GCSE (eg, leukocytosis, pleocytosis, and hyperthermia) produce symptoms that can be confused with other conditions. If a CNS infection is suspected, a lumbar puncture should be performed, and empiric antibiotics started. If vascular, neoplastic, or infectious etiologies are suspected, computed tomography (CT) or magnetic resonance imaging (MRI) should be obtained once the seizures are controlled.

TREATMENT

Various treatments are available for the management of GCSE. These range from rescue medications to abort the impending SE, to the use of pharmacologic and nonpharmacologic therapies for GCSE and refractory/resistant SE. The field has recently begun to shift terminology away from the disease focused terms (eg, antiepileptic medication) to the more function focused terms (eg, antiseizure medication). This shift is being done since many of these medications have no impact on the underlying disease, but in fact suppress seizures.[60]

Desired Outcomes

6 The short-term desired outcomes include: (a) immediate termination of all clinical and electrical seizure activity, (b) no clinically significant adverse effects, and (c) lack of recurrent seizure activity. The long-term outcomes involve minimizing or avoiding pharmacoresistant epilepsy and/or the development of neurologic sequelae that significantly impact the quality of life.

Nonpharmacologic Therapy

Stabilization Phase

Most of the treatment for GCSE consists of pharmacologic therapy in addition to supportive care. The time of seizure onset should be noted, and vital signs should be assessed. An adequate and protected airway should be established, ventilation should be maintained, and oxygen should be administered (Fig. 76-1). Intravenous access should be established, and hyperthermia, if present, should be aggressively treated (eg, rectal or IV acetaminophen and cooling blanket). Febrile GCSE is common in pediatrics, and normalization of body temperature helps minimize neurologic morbidity.

Laboratory studies including serum glucose and electrolyte levels (including calcium and magnesium), complete blood count, and renal and hepatic function tests should be performed. Antiseizure medication serum concentration should be obtained as needed, and a urine toxicology screen should be performed if there is a suspicion of ingestion.

Although hypoglycemia rarely causes GCSE, adults and children (ages 2 years and older) with a blood glucose less than 60 mg/dL (3.3 mmol/L) should receive 50 mL of a 50% dextrose solution and 1 mL/kg of a 25% dextrose solution, respectively.[2] Because Wernicke's encephalopathy can develop in patients with an alcohol use disorder, adults should receive IV thiamine (100 mg) before glucose administration. Serum glucose concentration should be determined to assess the need for further supplementation. Children younger than 12 to 18 months of age should receive pyridoxine (Vitamin B_6) until metabolic causes are ruled out.

If an infection is suspected, blood cultures, lumbar puncture, and a urinalysis may be needed. Antibiotic administration does

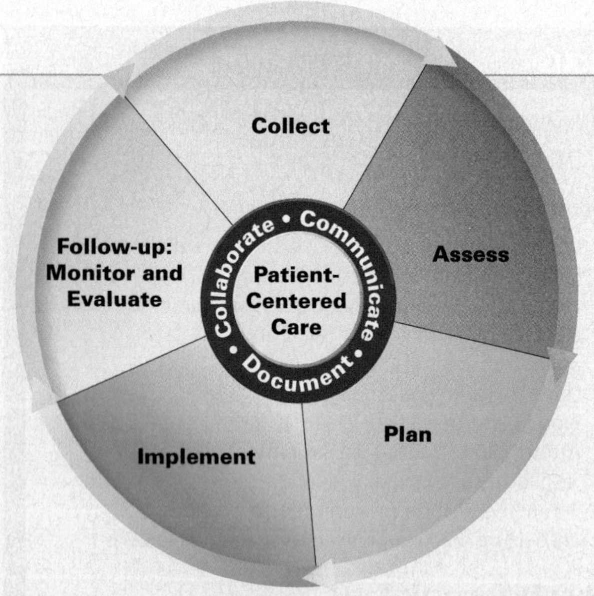

Patient Care Process for Status Epilepticus

The image shows the five fundamental steps included in The Pharmacist's Care Process endorsed by the Joint Commission for Pharmacy Practitioners (2014). The tagline of this process reads collaborate, communicate, and document. The five fundamental steps listed here are collect, assess, plan, implement, and follow-up: monitor and evaluate. All these steps are listed in a circular block diagram.

Collect *(some items may be deferred to a later time due to time constraints associated with a medical emergency)*

- Patient characteristics (eg, age, weight, height)
- Time of seizure onset and duration of seizure activity (see Table 76-2)
- Past medical history (eg, known epilepsy and type or prior seizure, medication-allergies) (see Table 76-1)
- Social history (eg, ethanol use, unhealthy substance use, ketogenic diet)
- Complete a medication history of current prescription, over-the-counter (OTC) medications, herbals products, and dietary supplements, including any recently started or stopped medications (prescription or nonprescription)
- Information (eg, agent, route, dose, response) regarding antiseizure medications administered immediately prior to emergency department/hospitalization
- Objective data
  - Temperature, blood pressure, heart rate, respiratory rate, oxygen (O_2) saturation, arterial blood gases
  - Serum chemistries (eg, electrolytes, glucose, magnesium, renal/hepatic function studies); complete blood count (CBC) with differential and blood/urine cultures; urine toxicology screen; and serum antiseizure medication concentrations
  - Electroencephalogram (EEG), computed tomography (CT), magnetic resonance imaging (MRI) as needed

Assess

- If appropriate, assess medication adherence to antiseizure medications prior to admission and correct delivery of antiseizure medications during hospitalization
- Evaluate the appropriateness, effectiveness, and safety of all chronic or acute prescription and nonprescription medications. Check serum medication concentration for an "effective" or "safe" concentration (see Table 76-4)
- Airway (arterial blood gases, respiratory rate [RR]) and cardiac (blood pressure [BP], heart rate [HR]) stability
- Temperature for the presence of fever
- Possible seizure etiologies (eg, known epilepsy, febrile, infectious, head trauma/cerebral vascular accident [CVA], substance-associated, low antiseizure medication serum concentrations) (see Table 76-3)
- Presence of seizure provoking factors (eg, ethanol, unhealthy substance use, adverse medication/herbal effect, medication interactions, low or elevated antiseizure medication serum concentration) (see Table 76-3)
- Duration of seizure activity and characteristics of the seizure (see Table 76-2)
- Available laboratory studies
- Need for adjusted dosing based on organ function (eg, liver, kidney function), serum albumin, weight

Plan*

- Management of nonepileptic causes for seizure (eg, opioid overdose, electrolytes imbalance) (see Table 76-3 and Fig. 76-1)
- Management of impending seizure activity (initial phase) including agent, dose, route, and method of administration, including the option for alternative agents and need for a second dose (see Table 76-2 and Fig. 76-1)
- Need for concurrent pharmacotherapy including thiamine and glucose, pyridoxine, antipyretic, and empiric antibiotics (see Fig. 76-1)
- First-line antiseizure medication regimens for the second phase (established stage), including agent, dose, method of administration, and frequency, including the option for a second dose if needed (see Tables 76-2 and 76-4 and Fig. 76-1)
- Anesthetic medications for the third phase (refractory GCSE stage) including agent, dosage, method of administration accompanied by a plan to titrate and withdraw therapy (see Tables 76-2 and 76-6 and Fig. 76-1)
- Monitor for effectiveness and safety of antiseizure medications including serum concentration and medication interactions during the management of GCSE (see Table 76-5)
- Pharmacotherapy in transfer to a nonintensive care unit setting or discharge home, including the transition to oral therapy and subsequent monitoring of serum antiseizure medication concentrations (see Table 76-4)
- Rescue therapies in the home environment, including need, agent, dose, method of administration, and plan should first dose fail. Need for cardiopulmonary resuscitation (CPR) training
- Patient and/or legal guardian medication education at discharge, including correct use of rescue therapies

Implement*

- Ensure all medications are ordered, that the dosage is appropriate, and discontinued as appropriate, during the patient's transition from home to the emergency department (ED), ED to hospitalization, and home (see Tables 76-4 and 76-6)

(Continued)

- Ensure all medications are dispensed as prescribed (see Tables 76-4 and 76-6)
- Ensure all antiseizure medications are administered and monitored correctly (see Table 76-5)

Follow-up: Monitor and Evaluate

- Antiseizure medication effectiveness in stopping clinical and electrical seizure activity
- Presence of adverse medication reactions or medication interactions (see Table 76-5)
- Therapeutic medication monitoring performed as needed with subsequent interpretation

*Collaborate with patient, caregivers, and other healthcare professionals.

not need to wait until after the lumbar puncture if the patient is medically unstable. Patients with persistent GCSE should also have frequent arterial blood gas determinations to assess for metabolic acidosis, which should be treated with sodium bicarbonate if the pH is less than 7.2. Assisted ventilation can correct respiratory acidosis.

Because electrical seizures may persist in the absence of overt clinical motor manifestations, an EEG should be performed in patients who continue to have altered consciousness after clinical control of their seizures. Patients with persistent GCSE should also have continuous EEG monitoring.

Ketogenic Diet

A small number of reports have shown that an orally or intravenously administered ketogenic diet in a 4:1 ratio of fat to combined protein and carbohydrate can be used in severe cases of super-refractory SE.[15,16] Before initiating this diet, metabolic disorders as a possible etiology should be eliminated. Close monitoring of total daily fluid, ketosis, and potential complications is essential. If metabolic acidosis develops, treatment to maintain serum bicarbonate levels greater than 18 to 20 mEq/L (mmol/L) is recommended.[15]

Vagus Nerve Stimulation

Acute placement of a vagus nerve stimulator has been used in both pediatric and adult patients with refractory SE. Its use for refractory SE is not recommended currently, as grade D evidence suggests improvement in generalized refractory SE.[17]

Pharmacologic Therapy

Initial-Therapy Phase (5-20 Minutes)

When a seizure does not stop within 5 minutes, or when doubt exists regarding the diagnosis, patients should be treated as if they have GCSE (see Fig. 76-1), and initial therapies used. The benzodiazepines are the most common class of antiseizure medications used for GCSE initial treatment. Only two[18,19] and three[18,20,21] Class 1 studies have evaluated the benzodiazepines in children and adults, respectively.

The benzodiazepines are considered effective initial therapy in most patients. Evidence-based guidelines recommend the initial use of IM midazolam, IV lorazepam, or IV diazepam (see Fig. 76-1) in adults and IV lorazepam or IV diazepam in children.[5] Intramuscular midazolam is preferred if IV access is not available; however, generally, one or two IV doses will terminate seizures within 2 to 3 minutes. All benzodiazepines are effective; therefore, preference is determined by pharmacokinetic differences, route of administration, pharmacoeconomics, adverse-effect profile, and current availability.

Diazepam is highly lipophilic with a large volume of distribution (1-2 L/kg). Although it distributes into the brain within seconds, it rapidly redistributes into fat, causing its CNS half-life to be less than 1 hour and its duration of effect to be less than 30 minutes. The rapid decrease in brain concentration, along with pharmacoresistance, can cause seizure recurrence; hence, a longer-acting antiseizure medication (eg, phenytoin, levetiracetam, or valproate) should be given immediately after diazepam. Table 76-4 outlines dosing.

(7) Most practitioners consider IV lorazepam to be the benzodiazepine of choice for initial therapy of GCSE. A Cochrane Database Review concluded that it is as effective and safer than diazepam in children.[21] Another Cochrane Database Review that included pediatric and adult data noted no difference in death, requirements for ventilator support, or adverse effects between the two agents; however, when compared to diazepam, there was a significantly lower risk of persistent seizures with lorazepam.[22]

Lorazepam is less lipid soluble than diazepam and takes longer to achieve peak concentrations in the brain; however, its minimal redistribution into fat results in a longer CNS duration of action, providing seizure protection for up to 24 hours. It also has a higher-affinity binding to the benzodiazepine receptor compared to diazepam.

Patients chronically on a benzodiazepine (eg, clobazam and clonazepam) might develop tolerance and require large doses. Diazepam and lorazepam contain propylene glycol, which can cause dysrhythmia and hypotension if administered too rapidly (Table 76-5). They also cause vein irritation; therefore, the parenteral product should be diluted with an equal volume of compatible diluent before administration. Because of slow and erratic absorption, standard parenteral formulations should not be given IM.

Unfortunately, there is insufficient data comparing IV lorazepam to IV midazolam in GCSE. Midazolam has an extremely short half-life, and maintenance doses must be given by continuous infusion (see Table 76-4). Because of its increased solubility, midazolam has a more reliable IM absorption than either diazepam or lorazepam. A Class 1 study showed that IM midazolam, as first-line treatment given by medical personnel in the prehospital setting, was superior to IV lorazepam for cessation of seizures. This practice reduced intensive care unit (ICU) admission and subsequent hospitalization, with no differences in recurrent seizures or adverse effects.[18]

Intranasal (IN) midazolam and per rectum (PR) diazepam are increasingly used in out-of-hospital management and emergency department settings. However, evidenced-based guidelines indicate they and buccal midazolam are just probably effective.[5] Recent studies have focused on aborting impending SE via transmucosal benzodiazepine delivery (eg, PR, IN, and buccal) when IV and/or IM administration may be difficult or impossible (eg, home setting, extended care, and paramedic). Rectal absorption of diazepam is rapid but varies significantly (50%-100%) due to first-pass metabolism and can be challenging to administer at home. Buccal and sublingual routes bypass gastric and hepatic first-pass metabolism, but bioavailability can be incomplete as the medication is often swallowed. Buccal administration is easily accomplished, and the volume of fluid is small enough (eg, 2-5 mL) that aspiration is unlikely. While successful sublingual administration is unlikely due to muscular contractions of the jaw and clenching of teeth, non-IV midazolam is as effective as PR diazepam for termination of early SE in children.[23]

Intranasally administered midazolam readily crosses the nasal mucosa and the blood-brain barrier to produce a rapid rise in both serum and cerebrospinal fluid concentrations.[2] In fact, serum

PREHOSPITAL CARE
- Monitor vital signs (HR, RR)
- PR or IN diazepam (0.2-0.5 mg/kg)
- Consider IN midazolam (0.15-0.3 mg/kg) or IM midazolam (0.2 mg/kg up to 10 mg)
- Transport to hospital if seizures persist

INITIAL HOSPITAL CARE
- Time from seizure onset
- Assess and control airway and cardiac function; pulse oximetry
- 100% oxygen
- Place IV catheter; intraosseous if unable to place IV and patient is younger than 6 years
- Begin IV fluids; blood pressure support as needed
- Thiamine 100 mg (adult)
- Pyridoxine 50-100 mg (infant)
- Glucose (adult: 50 mL of 50%; children: 1mL/kg of 10%) if serum glucose is <60 mg/dL (<3.3 mmol/L)
- Naloxone 0.1 mg/kg for suspected narcotic overdose
- Antibiotics if infection suspected
- Treat hyperthermia

LABORATORY STUDIES
- CBC with differential
- Serum chemistry profile (eg, electrolytes, glucose, renal/hepatic function, calcium, magnesium)
- Arterial blood gas
- Blood cultures
- Serum anticonvulsant concentration
- Urine drug/alcohol screen
- EEG as needed

IMPENDING GSCE (0-30 minutes)
- IV lorazepam (0.1 mg/kg over 30-60 seconds up to 6 mg) may repeat in 5 minutes if no response or IN midazolam (0.15-0.3 mg/kg up to 10 mg) or IM midazolam (0.2 mg/kg up to 10 mg)
- Additional therapies may not be required if seizure stops

ESTABLISHED GSCE (30-60 minutes)
First-line
Phenytoin (IV): 18-20 mg/kg over 20 minutes (<1 mg/kg/min; max 50 mg/min); may give an additional 5 mg/kg as needed[a] or Fosphenytoin (IV or IM): 18-20 mg PE/kg (<3 mg PE/kg/min; max <150 mg PE/min)[a]
Valproate (IV): 25-30 mg/kg over 5-15 minutes (<3 mg/kg/min up to 200 mg/min) followed by an infusion of 1 mg/kg/h
Levetiracetam (IV): 40-60 mg/kg, maximum 3,000 mg (administer 2-5 mg/kg/min)
Second-line
Phenobarbital (IV): 15-20 mg/kg over 20 minutes (<100 mg/min)[a]
Third-line
Lacosamide (IV): 50-400 mg; 200 mg given over 15 minutes

REFRACTORY GSCE (>120 minutes)
Implement continuous EEG monitoring
Assure patient is normovolemic
Assure cerebral perfusion pressure is >70 mm Hg (>9.3 kPa)
Administer volume as stated above and then begin vasopressors to achieve adequate mean arterial pressure (>120 mm Hg [>16.0 kPa])
Continuous ECG monitoring if on propofol
First-line
- Midazolam: 0.2-0.4 mg/kg bolus at a rate of 2 mg/min followed by 0.05-2 mg/kg/h
- Pentobarbital: 10-20 mg/kg bolus at a rate of ≤50 mg/min followed by 1-5 mg/kg/h
- Propofol: 1-2 mg/kg bolus followed by <4 mg/kg/h in children; larger dose may be used in adults

SUPER-REFRACTORY GSCE (>24 hours)
Implement continuous EEG monitoring
Assure patient is normovolemic
Assure cerebral perfusion pressure is >70 mm Hg (>9.3 kPa)
Administer volume as stated above and then begin vasopressors to achieve adequate mean arterial pressure (>120 mm Hg [>16.0 kPa])

- Ketamine
- Hypothermia
- Lidocaine
- Topiramate
- Inhaled Anesthetics
- Immunomodulating therapies
- Ketogenic diet
- Vagus Nerve Stimulator

FIGURE 76-1 Algorithm for the treatment of GCSE. (BP, blood pressure; CBC, complete blood count; CI, continuous infusion; D12.5W, 12.5% Dextrose in water; D25W, 25% Dextrose in water; D50W, 50% Dextrose in water; EEG, electroencephalogram; GCSE, generalized convulsive status epilepticus; HR, heart rate; IN, intranasal; PE, phenytoin equivalents; PR, per rectum; RR, respiratory rate)
[a] Because variability exists in dosing, monitor serum concentration.

TABLE 76-4 Dosing of Medications Used in the Initial and Established Treatment of GCSE

Medication (Route)	Brand Name	Initial Dose (Maximum Dose)	Maintenance Dose	Comments
Diazepam (IV)	Valium plus generic			
Adult		0.25 mg/kg[a,b,c] (20 mg)	Not used	Given IV at a rate not to exceed 5 mg/min
Pediatric		0.25-0.5 mg/kg[a,c] (20 mg)	Not used	
Fosphenytoin (IV)	Cerebyx plus generic			
Adult		20-25 mg PE/kg	4-5 mg PE/kg/day	Given IV at a rate not to exceed 150 mg PE/min in adults and 3 mg PE/kg/min in pediatric patients
Pediatric		20-25 mg PE/kg	5-10 mg PE/kg/day	
Lacosamide (IV)	Vimpat			
Adult		200-400 mg	200-400 mg/day, given twice a day	Administer IV over 15 minutes
Pediatric		6-10 mg/kg (400 mg)	6-12 mg/kg/day, given twice a day	
Levetiracetam (IV)	Keppra plus generics			
Adult		2,000-3,000 mg	1,000 mg thrice a day	Given IV over 5-10 minutes
Pediatric		40-60 mg/kg (3,000 mg)	40-60 mg/kg/day, given twice or thrice a day	
Lorazepam (IV)	Ativan plus generic			
Adult		4 mg[b,c] (6 mg)	Not used	Given IV at a rate not to exceed 2 mg/min in adult and pediatric patients
Pediatric		0.1 mg/kg[a,c] (6 mg)	Not used	
Midazolam (IV, IM)	Versed plus generic			
Adult		200 mcg/kg[a,d] (10 mg)	50-500 mcg/kg/hr[e]	Given IV at a rate 0.5-1 mg/min in adults and over 2-3 minutes in pediatric patients
Pediatric		150 mcg/kg[a,d] (10 mg)	60-120 mcg/kg/hr[e]	
Phenobarbital (IV)	Generic			
Adult		10-20 mg/kg[e]	1-4 mg/kg/day[e]	Given IV at a rate not to exceed 100 mg/min in adults and 30 mg/min in pediatric patients
Pediatric		15-20 mg/kg[e]	3-5 mg/kg/day[e]	
Phenytoin (IV)	Dilantin plus generic			
Adult		20-25 mg/kg[f]	4-5 mg/kg/day[e]	Given IV at a rate not to exceed 50 mg/min[g] in adults and 3 mg/kg/min (max 50 mg/min) in pediatric patients
Pediatric		20-25 mg/kg[f]	5-10 mg/kg/day[e]	
Valproate (IV)	Depacon plus generic			
Adult		15-30 mg/kg (3,000 mg)	1-4 mg/kg/hr[e]	Administer at 3 mg/kg/min; and follow by a continuous or intermittent infusion; larger doses may be required in those on hepatic enzyme inducers, monitor serum concentrations
Pediatric		20-25 mg/kg (3,000 mg)	1-4 mg/kg/hr[e], or give every 4-6 hours	

GCSE, generalized convulsive status epilepticus; PE, phenytoin equivalents.

[a]Doses can be repeated every 10 to 15 minutes until the maximum dosage is given.

[b]Initial doses in the older patients are 2 to 5 mg.

[c]Larger doses can be required if patients chronically on a benzodiazepine (eg, clonazepam).

[d]Can be given by the intramuscular, rectal, or buccal routes.

[e]Titrate dose as needed.

[f]Administer additional loading dose based on serum concentration.

[g]The rate should not exceed 25 mg/min in older patients and those with known atherosclerotic cardiovascular disease.

concentrations are comparable to those noted following IV injection. When compared to PR diazepam, all studies have concluded that IN midazolam results in higher serum concentrations, faster onset of action, more effective seizure control, and fewer adverse effects.[24] A commercially available, FDA-approved product for IN administration of midazolam became available in 2019, and a diazepam nasal spray product was approved in early 2020.[25-27]

Benzodiazepines are the first-line treatment for seizure emergencies; however, they are frequently underdosed, particularly in the out of hospital setting. A study including 1,170 benzodiazepine doses found that only 14.3% of midazolam and 23.9% of lorazepam doses met guideline recommendations.[28] Now that several benzodiazepine options are available for out-of-hospital treatment of seizure emergencies, it is critical to ensure that adequate doses are being prescribed and administered.

Guidelines also recommend IV phenobarbital as an alternative first-line agent in adults.[5] It is an effective and well-tolerated initial therapy in adults if benzodiazepines are not an option. Although evidence-based studies establish IV phenobarbital use, its slower administration rate than benzodiazepines relegates it to alternative initial therapy. Phenobarbital has biphasic distribution into body organs, and during phase I, it distributes into highly vascular organs but not the brain. Except for fat, phenobarbital distributes throughout the body during phase II; hence, lean body mass should be used in calculating doses in obese patients. Although the highest brain concentrations occur 12 to 60 minutes after an IV dose, seizures are controlled within minutes of the loading dose.[20]

The loading and maintenance dose for phenobarbital are given in Table 76-4. When necessary, larger loading doses (30 mg/kg) have been used in neonates without adverse effects. Phenobarbital exhibits first-order linear pharmacokinetics, and there is no maximum dose beyond which further doses are likely to be ineffective. For this reason, if the initial loading dose does not stop the seizures within 20 to 30 minutes,

TABLE 76-5 Adverse Medication Reactions and Monitoring of Patients Receiving Medications for GCSE

Medication	Adverse Medication Reaction	Monitoring Parameters	Comments
Diazepam	Hypotension and cardiac arrhythmias	Vital signs and ECG during administration	Propylene glycol causes hypotension and cardiac arrhythmias when administered too rapidly; hypotension may occur with large doses
Fosphenytoin	Hypotension and cardiac arrhythmias; paresthesia, pruritus	Vital signs and ECG during administration	Hypotension is less than that noted with phenytoin, as this product does not contain propylene glycol; pruritus generally involves the face and groin areas, is dose and rate related, and subsides 5-10 minutes after infusion
Lacosamide	Prolonged PR interval	ECG	
Levetiracetam	Somnolence, behavioral abnormalities	Mental status	
Lidocaine	Fasciculations, visual disturbances, tinnitus, seizures		Occur at serum concentrations between 6 and 8 mg/L (26-34 μmol/L); seizures >8 mg/L (34 μmol/L)
Lorazepam	Apnea, hypotension, bradycardia, cardiac arrest, respiratory depression, metabolic acidosis, and renal toxicity	Vital signs and ECG during administration; HCO_3 and serum creatinine; cumulative dose of propylene glycol	Accumulation of propylene glycol during prolong continuous infusions may cause acidosis
Midazolam	Apnea, hypotension, sedation	Vital signs and ECG	
Pentobarbital	Hypotension	Vital signs and ECG during administration	Rate of infusion should be slower or dopamine should be added if hypotension occurs
Phenytoin	Hypotension and cardiac arrhythmia; nystagmus	Vital signs and ECG during administration	Propylene glycol causes hypotension and cardiac arrhythmias when administered too rapidly. Large loading doses are generally not given to older individuals with preexisting cardiac disease or in critically ill patients with marginal blood pressure. The infusion rate should be slowed if the QT interval widens or if hypotension or arrhythmias develop; horizontal nystagmus suggests serum concentration above the reference range and toxicity; if a serum phenytoin concentration validates this, the dose should be decreased
Phenobarbital	Hypotension, respiratory, and CNS depression	Vital signs and mental status; EEG if used in anesthesia doses	Contains propylene glycol; if hypotension occurs, slow the rate of administration or begin dopamine; apnea and hypopnea can be more profound in patients treated initially with benzodiazepines
Propofol	Progressive metabolic acidosis, hemodynamic instability, and bradyarrhythmias	Vital signs, ECG, osmolar gap; EEG if used in anesthesia doses	Referred to as propofol-related infusion syndrome, which can be fatal
Topiramate	Metabolic acidosis	Acid-base status (serum bicarbonate)	Extremely rare

CNS, central nervous system; ECG, electrocardiogram; EEG, electroencephalogram.

an option would be to give an additional dose (10-20 mg/kg) or move to anesthetic agents.[29] Once GCSE is controlled, start the maintenance dose within 12 to 24 hours. Although injectable phenobarbital contains propylene glycol, it can be given more rapidly than phenytoin (see Table 76-4). While it can be safely administered IM, its rate of absorption is too slow to be effective.[2]

Although rare, brief cardiorespiratory depression can necessitate assisted ventilation or require intubation (see Table 76-5). This is especially true if a benzodiazepine is used concomitantly with a barbiturate. The rate of respiratory depression in patients with GCSE who received benzodiazepines is lower than that reported in a similar population treated with placebo.[5] Importantly, there was no difference in cardiorespiratory adverse events in adults who are given either a benzodiazepine or phenobarbital.[20] Hypotension secondary to a reduction in vasomotor tone can occur following large doses of either a benzodiazepine or barbiturate.[2]

Second-Therapy Phase: Established GSCE (20-40 Minutes)

8 9 Second-phase antiseizure medications (eg, hydantoin, valproate, phenobarbital, levetiracetam, or lacosamide) may not be needed if seizures stop after administering initial therapies. The choice of which long-acting, second-line agent to give is controversial as there is no evidence to base a preferred option. When given, an agent should be administered immediately after a benzodiazepine. Dosing can be found in Table 76-4.

A hydantoin is one of three second-line agents that can be used when GCSE is unresponsive to benzodiazepine treatment or continues to occur after successful benzodiazepine treatment.[5] However, data supports a higher rate of seizure cessation and fewer adverse events with levetiracetam versus phenytoin.[30] When used by itself, phenytoin is inferior to lorazepam, phenobarbital, or diazepam plus phenytoin at stopping GCSE within 20 minutes of infusion.[20,31] While the most recent guidelines advocate for a hydantoin,[5] which are frequently used in practice, questions remain regarding if a hydantoin should be administered alone, in larger doses, or at all when seizures recur following benzodiazepine administration.

Phenytoin has a long half-life (20-36 hours) and causes less respiratory depression and less sedation than benzodiazepines or phenobarbital. However, it cannot be delivered rapidly enough to be considered a first-line single agent.[2] Injectable phenytoin should be diluted to greater than or equal to 5 mg/mL in normal saline; otherwise, microcrystals will precipitate if it is mixed in a glucose-containing solution. The vehicle (40% propylene glycol) can cause administration-related hypotension and cardiac arrhythmias (see Table 76-5). For this reason, the maximum rate of infusion is limited (see Table 76-4).

Table 76-4 includes suggested IV loading doses. A loading dose reduction is recommended for older patients, and a larger loading dose is required in obese individuals. If the patient has been on phenytoin prior to admission and the serum concentration is known, consider using this information in determining a loading dose. Although some advocate administering an additional 5 mg/kg dose in those with unresponsive GCSE, there is no evidence supporting this practice. Importantly this can cause concentrations to exceed the reference range and produce toxicity. In addition, because phenytoin has poor lipid solubility and enters the brain slowly, it can take up to 60 minutes before the pharmacodynamic effect is apparent. This delay is significant when considering administration of a second loading dose, as therapeutic serum concentrations, 10 to 20 mg/L (40-79 μmol/L), generally do not persist more than 24 hours; hence, maintenance doses (see Table 76-4) should be started within 12 to 24 hours of the loading dose.

Phenytoin has an alkaline pH, which may cause pain and burning during infusion. Phlebitis can occur during chronic infusion and tissue necrosis is likely on infiltration. Intramuscular administration of phenytoin is not recommended because absorption is delayed, erratic, and can crystallize in tissue. Although oral loading doses have been used in patients not actively seizing, it may take 4 to 12 hours before adequate serum concentrations are obtained. Thus, this practice is not recommended.

Fosphenytoin is considered by many to be the hydantoin of choice[5] as it is a water-soluble phosphate ester that has no known pharmacologic activity, and after IV or IM dosing is converted rapidly (7-15 minutes) and completely (100%) to phenytoin by blood and tissue phosphatases. The conversion delay was a concern initially; however, this time is offset by high protein binding, saturable binding at high concentrations, and the rapid rate of infusion. Since it does not contain propylene glycol, it is compatible with most common IV fluids. It should be dosed using phenytoin equivalents (PE), thereby obviating the need for interconversion between phenytoin and fosphenytoin. The loading dose and rates of administration of fosphenytoin can be found in Table 76-4. Because of delays in achieving adequate phenytoin serum concentrations, a loading dose should not be given IM unless IV access is impossible.

Fosphenytoin serum concentrations have no value, and therefore, serum phenytoin concentrations should be used for therapeutic medication monitoring with the desired serum concentration range being the same as phenytoin. However, fosphenytoin cross-reacts with some phenytoin immunoassays causing an overestimation of phenytoin concentration; hence, levels should not be obtained for at least 2 hours after IV, and 4 hours after IM administration.

Alternatively, the current guidelines also recommend a single dose of IV valproate or IV levetiracetam as acceptable first-line agents, if a benzodiazepine fails to control seizures after 20 minutes, or if seizures recur following a benzodiazepine and/or a hydantoin use.[5] Intravenous valproate and continuous infusion diazepam are comparable in GCSE.[32,33] One meta-analysis noted that valproate controlled refractory SE sooner than diazepam. However, there was no difference within 30 minutes of administration.[34] There was also no difference in control of GCSE between valproate and phenytoin.[27] A second meta-analysis noted that there is sufficient evidence to use valproate as first-line therapy in those with SE refractory to benzodiazepines.[35] Three randomized controlled trials have investigated the efficacy of levetiracetam[36-38] or valproate[36] versus fosphenytoin or phenytoin. One of these found that levetiracetam was not superior to phenytoin,[38] one concluded levetiracetam may be a reasonable alternative to phenytoin,[37] and one found that levetiracetam, fosphenytoin, and valproate all had similar safety and efficacy as a second-line GCSE agents.[36]

Several loading and continuous-infusion doses for valproate (see Table 76-4) have been used in adult and pediatric patients. Current guidelines recommend 40 mg/kg up to 3,000 mg as a single dose.[5] Although the manufacturer originally recommended IV valproate be given no faster than 20 mg/min, much faster rates have been studied (40 mg/min; 2-10 mg/kg/min) and are used for load dose administration. One study suggested the need to consider the effects of enzyme-inducing antiseizure medications when dosing and recommended that the continuous-infusion rate be determined by the presence of concurrent antiseizure medications (no inducers present, 1 mg/kg/hr; one or more inducers [eg, phenytoin and phenobarbital], 2 mg/kg/hr; and inducers and pentobarbital coma, 4 mg/kg/hr).[39] In general, IV valproate is well tolerated with no respiratory depression. Hemodynamic instability is extremely rare; however, vital signs should be monitored closely during the loading dose for hypotension.

Evidence for the use of IV levetiracetam is limited; however, evidence exists to support it as first-line therapy in those refractory to benzodiazepines.[40] Historically, it was used in cases of super-refractory SE, but it is being used earlier due to medication shortages that have made traditional medications unavailable. It is as effective as IV lorazepam in aborting seizures and preventing recurrence,[41-43] and compared to phenytoin is equally effective at terminating seizures and preventing recurrence at 24 hours.[43] Levetiracetam is not hepatically metabolized and is minimally protein bound, making medication interactions unlikely. Doses for IV levetiracetam are noted in Table 76-4 and are infused over about 5 minutes. Although guidelines recommend a maximum single dose of 4,500 mg,[5] most clinicians use 3,000 mg/day.

Despite being recommended as an alternative first-line agent for initial therapy, recent guidelines recommend phenobarbital as an alternative agent when a hydantoin, valproic acid, or levetiracetam is not available or has failed. Before moving to third-therapy phase, all agents noted in phase II should be administered as single doses, and not multiple mini-boluses, given at maximally tolerated doses.

Third-Therapy Phase: Refractory GCSE (40-60 Minutes)

10 When adequate doses of a benzodiazepine and a single dose of a second antiseizure medication (hydantoin, valproate, levetiracetam and/or barbiturate) fail, the condition is termed *refractory*.[5] After initial control, seizures can recur in 6% to 19% of patients. Approximately 10% to 15% of patients will develop refractory GCSE, and about 30% whose seizures are "clinically" controlled will have persistent electrical manifestations after antiseizure medication administration. When a patient develops refractory GCSE, an intense search should be performed for an acute or progressive cause.

While the goal is to stop electrical epileptiform activity, there is no consensus regarding the agent of choice, sequencing of therapy, or treatment of refractory GCSE.[44] Historically, one would recommend a repeat dose of a second-therapy phase; however, practitioners are increasingly using an anesthetic agent and not another traditional antiseizure medication due to the low probability that an additional traditional antiseizure medication will interrupt the established GCSE. There is a clear consensus that if a repeat dose of a traditional antiseizure medication fails, anesthetizing the patient to suppress cerebral ictal discharges should occur.[5] An anesthetic dose of midazolam, pentobarbital, or propofol may be indicated. Doses for these agents can be found in Table 76-5. Although it is likely that the patient is already being mechanically ventilated, intubation and respiratory support are mandatory during the use of anesthetic agents, along with continuous EEG monitoring.

While HLA-B*1502 has been associated with severe skin reactions in patients receiving phenytoin, this is applicable to chronic and not acute, single dose therapy. Recently, CYP2C variants that included CYP2C9*3, which reduce medication clearance, were identified as important genetic factors associated with phenytoin-related severe cutaneous adverse reactions.[45] Medication resistance factors have also been identified in surgically removed human epileptogenic tissue, as multimedication resistance proteins (P-glycoprotein) are localized to endothelial cells in brain capillaries and associated astroglia. Since multimedication resistance factors are localized to abnormal tissues, they appear to have little or no effect on systemic pharmacokinetic parameters of a medication. Still, they may affect local medication distribution within the target epileptogenic areas. If a role in refractory human epilepsy is confirmed, medication s that inhibit P-glycoprotein (eg, verapamil) may prove useful. However, the role of multimedication-resistant proteins in the treatment of seizure emergencies is not clear.

Benzodiazepines

During prolonged seizures, the number of γ_2 and $\beta_{2\text{-}3}$ subunits on the $GABA_A$ receptors decrease as the receptors move from the synaptic membrane into the cytoplasm. This move makes them functionally inactive, which may decrease the effectiveness of both endogenous GABA and GABA agonists resulting in time-dependent pharmacoresistance. Following GCSE that persists for more than 30 minutes, the relative potencies of benzodiazepines can be reduced up to 20-fold. For this reason, some believe that anesthetic doses of midazolam should be the first-line agent in refractory GCSE. If a benzodiazepine is used, it should always be combined with another medication that acts at a different site. Table 76-6 shows the loading and maintenance doses of midazolam.[32] Most patients respond to these doses within an hour. Although studies used seizure termination on EEG as the endpoint for success, EEG burst suppression is rarely achieved with the recommended doses of midazolam. Tachyphylaxis rapidly develops within 24 to 48 hours; hence, the dose is often increased to prevent seizure relapse.[2]

There is no specific protocol for tapering midazolam, but some suggest a seizure-free period of 24 to 48 hours before decreasing by 1 to 2 mcg/kg/min every 15 minutes.[2] Maintaining the patient's phenytoin and phenobarbital serum concentration(s) above 20 mg/L (79 μmol/L) and 40 mg/L (172 μmol/L), respectively, enhances successful discontinuation.

Because of midazolam's short half-life, patients can return to consciousness more rapidly compared to those receiving larger doses of more sedating antiseizure medications (eg, phenytoin and phenobarbital). Generally, continuous-infusion midazolam has been well tolerated, with few cases of hypotension and respiratory depression. If hypotension and poikilothermia occur, they can require supportive therapies. When adverse effects do occur, patients recover quickly; however, the use of large doses has caused a "midazolam infusion syndrome" in adults, which is characterized by delayed arousal (ie, hours to days) following midazolam discontinuation. This has tempered its use in adults; however, its use has continued as an important agent in pediatrics. The availability of a pharmacological antidote for benzodiazepines, flumazenil, enhances the safe use of midazolam.

Pentobarbital

Use of a short-acting barbiturate is another anesthesia option (ie, pentobarbital or thiopental). These agents are preferred because they allow a more rapid reversal of coma. Although barbiturates are used frequently, there are no controlled trials to support this practice. In refractory GCSE, overall response rates are significantly greater in those treated with pentobarbital compared to midazolam or propofol.[46] The recurrence of seizures is also less frequent with pentobarbital and propofol. The reported mortality rates are similar for the three medications, but significant hypotension was more common with pentobarbital.

Several sources note that the initial loading dose of pentobarbital is 5 mg/kg; however, this dose is inadequate to achieve the serum concentrations (40 mg/L; 172 μmoL/L) necessary to induce an isoelectric EEG (see Table 76-6). Although the duration of barbiturate coma in most studies has been 2 to 3 days, it has been used safely for 53 days in an 18-year-old patient.[47] To avoid complications (eg, pneumonia and pulmonary edema), pentobarbital should be discontinued as soon as possible. The risk of seizure recurrence is minimized if other antiseizure medications are therapeutic before pentobarbital is withdrawn. Because pentobarbital is a potent hepatic enzyme inducer, higher maintenance doses of most concurrent antiseizure medications will be needed. Adverse medication reactions should be carefully monitored as de-induction occurs and antiseizure medication concentrations increase, which can occur up to a month after pentobarbital's discontinuation.

Propofol

Propofol is also a viable first-line alternative in phase III. It is extremely lipid soluble and has a large volume of distribution, a very rapid onset of action, and an extremely short half-life that promotes easy titration and rapid awakening on medication discontinuation. Although several studies have compared propofol and barbiturates, most studies were underpowered; however, its efficacy appears to be comparable to midazolam for refractory GCSE.[46,48] Propofol is given as a loading dose followed by a continuous infusion. The loading dose can be repeated every 3 to 5 minutes until the desired clinical response is obtained; however, the dose should be reduced once EEG burst suppression is achieved.

Adverse medication reactions can be found in Table 76-5. Prolonged infusions greater than 4 mg/kg/hr are associated with propofol-related infusion syndrome (PRIS), which may be more common in children and limits its use in this population.[49,50] Signs and symptoms of PRIS include progressive metabolic acidosis, hemodynamic instability, and bradyarrhythmias that are refractory to aggressive pharmacological treatments. It may occur with or without the presence of hepatomegaly, rhabdomyolysis, or lipemia. A retrospective case series of 41 patients with refractory GCSE noted that 10% had sudden unexplained cardiorespiratory arrests, and 35% had non-life-threatening features of PRIS.[50] Propofol may be proconvulsant in some patients as involuntary myoclonic movements have been reported.

Vital signs should be carefully monitored, and a continuous electrocardiogram (ECG) should be assessed for dysrhythmias. Guidelines proposing laboratory monitoring do not exist, but it would seem advisable to assess serum lactic acid, serum triglycerides, serum creatinine, creatine kinase, and hepatic enzymes in patients receiving doses larger than 4 mg/kg/hr and/or those receiving therapy for more than 48 hours.

The role and position of other antiseizure medications in refractory GCSE remains unclear, and shortages often complicate the selection of a second-phase antiseizure medication. The literature supports the use of lacosamide and topiramate's efficacy in refractory GCSE, although these data come from case reports or case series. Two reviews have noted there is insufficient evidence to support the routine use of lacosamide in benzodiazepine-resistant GCSE.[40,51,52] Topiramate has been given orally in adults and in children with GCSE and should be implemented at full therapeutic doses, divided three times a day (see Table 76-6).[2,53] To administer nasogastrically, the tablets should be crushed, mixed with water, and administered via syringe. The response tends to be delayed hours to days. Once seizures are controlled, the dose should be tapered to a standard age/weight–appropriate maintenance dosage. Aggressive implementation of large topiramate doses may cause hyperchloremic, non-anion gap metabolic acidosis due to inhibition of type II and IV carbonic anhydrase enzymes. This is not dose related, as it has been noted following small doses, as well as overdoses. If metabolic acidosis occurs, treat with citrates to maintain serum bicarbonate of at least 20 mEq/L (mmol/L).[2]

Super-Refractory GCSE (>24 Hours)

Persistent GCSE or recurring seizures after anesthetic medications have failed are challenging. Therefore, agents with a broad range of pharmacologic mechanisms may be tried, such as ketamine,

TABLE 76-6 Dosing of Medications Used to Treat Refractory or Super-Refractory GCSE

Medication (Brand Name)	Initial Dose (Maximum Dose)	Maintenance Dose	Comments
Ketamine (generics)			
Adult	1-4 mg	1-5 mg/kg/hr	
Pediatric	0.5-2 mg/kg	1-10 mg/kg/hr	
Lacosamide (Vimpat)			
Adult	200-400 mg	200 mg bid	Administer IV over 15 minutes, monitor serum concentrations
Pediatric	6-10 mg/kg (400 mg)	6-12 mg/kg/day, given twice a day	
Lidocaine (generics)			
Adult	50-100 mg	1.5-3.5 mg/kg/hr	Administer IV in ≤2 minutes
Pediatric	1 mg/kg (maximum 3-5 mg/kg in the first hour)	1.2-3 mg/kg/hr	
Midazolam (Versed plus generic)			
Adult	200 mcg/kg[a]	50-500 mcg/kg/hr[b]	Initial dose may be given IM; administer IV over 0.5-1 mg/min; continuous-infusion rate should be increased every 15 minutes in those who do not respond and should be guided by EEG response; development of tachyphylaxis can require frequent increases in dose; decrease dose by 1 mcg/kg/min every 2 hours once GCSE is controlled
Pediatric	150 mcg/kg[a]	60-120 mcg/kg/hr[b]	
Pentobarbital (generics)			
Adult	10-20 mg/kg	1-5 mg/kg/hr[b]	Over 1-2 hours, the rate of infusion should be slowed or dopamine should be added if hypotension occurs; gradually titrate dose upward until there is evidence of burst suppression on EEG (ie, isoelectric EEG) or prohibitive adverse effects occur. Twelve hours after a burst suppression is obtained, the rate should be titrated downward every 2-4 hours
Pediatric	15-20 mg/kg	1-5 mg/kg/hr[b]	
Propofol (Diprivan plus generic)			
Adult	2 mg/kg	5-10 mg/kg/hr[b]	Over 10 seconds in adults and 20-30 seconds in pediatric patients
Pediatric	3 mg/kg	2-4 mg/kg/hr[c]	
Topiramate (Topamax plus generic)			
Adult	300-500 mg	400-1,600 mg/day	Given orally in divided dose every 12 hours. Doses as large as 25 mg/kg/day for 2-5 days have been used in children. Monitor serum bicarbonate levels and serum concentrations
Pediatric	5-15 mg/kg (400 mg)	5-10 mg/kg/day, given thrice a day	

EEG, electroencephalogram; GCSE, generalized convulsive status epilepticus; IM, intramuscular; IV, intravenous.

[a]Doses can be repeated twice at 10-15 minute intervals until the maximum dosage is given.

[b]Titrate dose as needed.

[c]Generally recommended not to exceed a dose of 4 mg/kg/hr and a duration of 48 hours.

a noncompetitive antagonist of NMDA receptors. During prolonged seizures, the number and activity of GABA receptors gradually decrease; thus, the commonly used first-line and second-line antiseizure medications slowly fail. Simultaneously, the number and activity of glutamatergic NMDA receptors increase, often causing refractory status epilepticus (RSE). A summary of the findings regarding ketamine use in RSE was recently published.[2,54] Additionally, others have proposed an expert consensus-based treatment protocol for its use.[55] Overall, ketamine appears to be a reasonable agent to consider in refractory GCSE that has failed general anesthesia, especially in those with cardiac instability. Ketamine doses can be found in Table 76-6. An advantage of ketamine is its ability to maintain arterial blood pressure, pulse rate, and cardiac output. Adverse events noted include hallucinations upon awakening, increased salivation, and increased intraocular and intracranial pressure.

Currently, weak evidence supports the use of lidocaine in super-refractory GCSE, although clinically it has been used when other agents fail.[56] When administered intravenously (see Table 76-6) it has a rapid onset of action. The therapeutic reference range for GCSE has not been established. However, the reference serum concentration range for the antiarrhythmic effects of lidocaine is 2 to 6 mg/L (8.5-26 μmol/L). Serum lidocaine concentrations and ECG should be monitored to avoid medication accumulation and toxicity (see Table 76-5).

Inhaled anesthetics are currently not used until other approaches fail. A few studies have used inhaled anesthetics (particularly isoflurane) for the treatment of refractory SE.[15,57] Halothane, isoflurane, and other inhaled anesthetics can produce EEG suppression. These agents are challenging to deliver outside the operating room and require an anesthesiologist; however, they offer no proven advantages over traditional antiseizure medications (eg, barbiturate coma or continuous-infusion benzodiazepine), and can increase intracranial pressure. If used, dosing is titrated to obtain EEG burst suppression, and although required concentrations are variable, isoflurane generally stops seizure at concentrations of 0.5% to 3%. It is important to note that these concentrations are not ordinarily associated with hemodynamic effects; however, isoflurane can induce hypotension. Therefore, close hemodynamic monitoring is necessary, and the administration of isotonic fluids and vasopressors as needed.

Data that suggest the development of super-refractory GCSE may be due to antibodies directed against the voltage-gated potassium channels and the NMDA receptor. However, the use of immunomodulating therapies (eg, corticosteroids and IV immune globulin) is based solely upon animal data.[15] Additionally, mounting evidence suggests that inflammation plays a role in epileptogenesis, particularly the activation of select inflammatory signaling pathways (eg, interleukin-1 receptor/toll-like receptor [IL-1R/TLR]). Steroids may also decrease blood-brain barrier opening and reverse GABAergic inhibition and affect NMDA and voltage-gated potassium channels. Although little evidence supports the use of steroids, in the absence of contraindications, a trial of large doses of steroids that IVIG follows should be considered. Typically, patients are given methylprednisolone 15 mg/kg/day every 6 hours, up to 1 g/day, for 3 days. Patients who respond should continue long-term steroids, IV immunoglobulins, and other immunomodulatory agents such as cyclophosphamide or rituximab.[58]

Controlled mild hypothermia reduces excitatory transmission, epileptic discharges, reduces brain edema, cerebral metabolic rate, oxygen utilization, and ATP consumption. Few studies have assessed the efficacy or safety of hypothermia in refractory GCSE and a meta-analysis suggested that only level D evidence supports the use of hypothermia in refractory SE.[59] Despite an absence of medical evidence, there has been a resurgence in the use of hypothermia, especially its use early on in super-refractory GCSE. When used, a core body temperature of about 32°C to 34°C is targeted for at least 24 to 48 hours. It may or may not be given in combination with barbiturate anesthetics,[15] but is often used concurrently with ketamine. Cardiovascular and coagulation parameters, biochemistry and acid-base balance, and serum lactate should all be monitored. Hypothermia may significantly reduce the clearance of several medications, including anesthetics and antiseizure medications, resulting in a need for monitoring of serum concentrations.[2]

EVALUATION OF THERAPEUTIC OUTCOMES

Initial success for GCSE is defined as termination of all clinical and electrical seizure activity, but ultimate success is measured by the patient's subsequent quality of life. The morbidity and mortality associated with GCSE are primarily affected by the underlying etiology; however, morbidity and mortality can be minimized by the rapid implementation of a rational therapeutic plan. The EEG is a vital tool that not only allows practitioners to determine when abnormal electrical activity has been aborted but also can assist in determining which antiseizure medication was effective. Because many antiseizure medications affect the cardiorespiratory system, vital signs (eg, heart rate, respiratory rate, and blood pressure) must be monitored during medication loading and infusion. Finally, the infusion site must be assessed for any evidence of infiltration before and during the administration of phenytoin. Information regarding the patient's past medical and medication history and imaging studies (eg, MRI) can also help determine if there is a defined etiology for the original episode of GCSE. This information can then be used to guide future medication therapy and help determine if the patient is at risk for a poor outcome.

CONCLUSION

GCSE is a medical emergency that requires all healthcare professionals to be knowledgeable about the phases of the disorder, the therapies that align with each phase, and secondary complications that need to be addressed. This requires clinicians to have a working knowledge of the Patient Care Process used for status epilepticus and understand what evidence-based information exists to select therapies. Additionally, knowing and identifying any provoking factors and/or various etiologies important in prevention and treatment is an integral part of care. Finally, it is also essential that outpatient therapies be aggressively used to abort impending SE.

ABBREVIATIONS

AMPA	α-amino-3-hydroxy-5-methyl-isoxazole-4-propionate
ASM	antiseizure medication
CNS	central nervous system
CT	computed tomography
ECG	electrocardiogram
EEG	electroencephalogram, electroencephalography
GABA	γ-aminobutyric acid
GCSE	generalized convulsive status epilepticus
ICU	intensive care unit
IL-1R/TLR	interleukin-1 receptor/toll-like receptor
ILAE	International League Against Epilepsy
IM	intramuscular
IN	intranasal
IV	intravenous
MRI	magnetic resonance imaging
NCSE	nonconvulsive status epilepticus
NMDA	*N*-methyl-D-aspartate
PE	phenytoin equivalents
PRIS	propofol-related infusion syndrome
RSE	refractory status epilepticus
SE	status epilepticus

REFERENCES

1. Trinka E, Cock H, Hesdorffer D, et al. A definition and classification of status epilepticus—Report of the ILAE Task Force on Classification of Status Epilepticus. *Epilepsia*. 2015;56(10):1515–1523.
2. Alford EL, Wheless JW, Phelps SJ. Treatment of generalized convulsive status epilepticus in pediatric patients. *J Pediatr Pharmacol Ther.* 2015;20(4):260–289.
3. DeLorenzo RJ, Garnett LK, Towne AR, et al. Comparison of status epilepticus with prolonged seizure episodes lasting from 10 to 29 minutes. *Epilepsia*. 1999;40(2):164–169.
4. Sutter R, Semmlack S, Kaplan PW. Nonconvulsive status epilepticus in adults—Insights into the invisible. *Nat Rev Neurol.* 2016;12(5):281–293.
5. Glauser T, Shinnar S, Gloss D, et al. Evidence-based guideline: Treatment of convulsive status epilepticus in children and adults: Report of the Guideline Committee of the American Epilepsy Society. *Epilepsy Curr.* 2016;16(1):48–61.
6. Lv RJ, Wang Q, Cui T, et al. Status epilepticus-related etiology, incidence and mortality: A meta-analysis. *Epilepsy Res.* 2017;136:12–17.
7. DeLorenzo RJ, Pellock JM, Towne AR, et al. Epidemiology of status epilepticus. *J Clin Neurophysiol.* 1995;12(4):316–325.
8. Gurcharran K, Grinspan ZM. The burden of pediatric status epilepticus: Epidemiology, morbidity, mortality, and costs. *Seizure*. 2019;68:3–8.
9. DeLorenzo RJ, Towne AR, Pellock JM, et al. Status epilepticus in children, adults, and the elderly. *Epilepsia*. 1992;33(Suppl 4):S15–S25.
10. Wasterlain CG, Chen JW. Mechanistic and pharmacologic aspects of status epilepticus and its treatment with new antiepileptic drugs. *Epilepsia*. 2008;49(Suppl 9):63–73.
11. Pitkänen A, Nehlig A, Brooks-Kayal AR, et al. Issues related to development of antiepileptogenic therapies. *Epilepsia*. 2013;54(Suppl 4)(0 4):35–43.
12. Lothman E. The biochemical basis and pathophysiology of status epilepticus. *Neurology*. 1990;40(5 Suppl 2):13–23.
13. Temkin NR. Antiepileptogenesis and seizure prevention trials with antiepileptic drugs: Meta-analysis of controlled trials. *Epilepsia*. 2001;42(4):515–524.
14. Kantanen AM, Reinikainen M, Parviainen I, et al. Incidence and mortality of super-refractory status epilepticus in adults. *Epilepsy Behav.* 2015;49:131–134.
15. Wheless JW. Treatment of refractory convulsive status epilepticus in children: Other therapies. *Semin Pediatr Neurol.* 2010;17(3):190–194.

16. McDonald TJW, Cervenka MC. Ketogenic diet therapies for seizures and status epilepticus. *Semin Neurol.* 2020;40(6):719–729.
17. Dibué-Adjei M, Brigo F, Yamamoto T, et al. Vagus nerve stimulation in refractory and super-refractory status epilepticus—A systematic review. *Brain Stimulation.* 2019;12(5):1101–1110.
18. Silbergleit R, Durkalski V, Lowenstein D, et al. Intramuscular versus intravenous therapy for prehospital status epilepticus. *N Engl J Med.* 2012;366(7):591–600.
19. Chamberlain JM, Okada P, Holsti M, et al. Lorazepam vs diazepam for pediatric status epilepticus: A randomized clinical trial. *JAMA.* 2014;311(16):1652–1660.
20. Treiman DM, Meyers PD, Walton NY, et al. A comparison of four treatments for generalized convulsive status epilepticus. Veterans Affairs Status Epilepticus Cooperative Study Group. *N Engl J Med.* 1998;339(12):792–798.
21. Alldredge BK, Gelb AM, Isaacs SM, et al. A comparison of lorazepam, diazepam, and placebo for the treatment of out-of-hospital status epilepticus. *N Engl J Med.* 2001;345(9):631–637.
22. Prasad M, Krishnan PR, Sequeira R, et al. Anticonvulsant therapy for status epilepticus. *Cochrane Database Syst Rev.* 2014;2014(9):Cd003723.
23. Brigo F, Nardone R, Tezzon F, et al. Nonintravenous midazolam versus intravenous or rectal diazepam for the treatment of early status epilepticus: A systematic review with meta-analysis. *Epilepsy Behav.* 2015;49:325–336.
24. Hogan RE, Gidal BE, Koplowitz B, et al. Bioavailability and safety of diazepam intranasal solution compared to oral and rectal diazepam in healthy volunteers. *Epilepsia.* 2020;61(3):455–464.
25. Detyniecki K, Van Ess PJ, Sequeira DJ, et al. Safety and efficacy of midazolam nasal spray in the outpatient treatment of patients with seizure clusters: A randomized, double-blind, placebo-controlled trial. *Epilepsia.* 2019;60(9):1797–1808.
26. Hogan RE, Tarquinio D, Sperling MR, et al. Pharmacokinetics and safety of VALTOCO (NRL-1; diazepam nasal spray) in patients with epilepsy during seizure (ictal/peri-ictal) and nonseizure (interictal) conditions: A phase 1, open-label study. *Epilepsia.* 2020;61(5):935–943.
27. Spencer DC, Sinha SR, Choi EJ, et al. Safety and efficacy of midazolam nasal spray for the treatment of intermittent bouts of increased seizure activity in the epilepsy monitoring unit: A double-blind, randomized, placebo-controlled trial. *Epilepsia.* 2020;61(11):2415–2425.
28. Sathe AG, Underwood E, Coles LD, et al. Patterns of benzodiazepine underdosing in the Established Status Epilepticus Treatment Trial. *Epilepsia.* 2021;62(3):795–806.
29. Crawford TO, Mitchell WG, Fishman LS, et al. Very-high-dose phenobarbital for refractory status epilepticus in children. *Neurology.* 1988;38(7):1035–1040.
30. Xue T, Wei L, Shen X, et al. Levetiracetam versus phenytoin for the pharmacotherapy of benzodiazepine-refractory status epilepticus: A systematic review and meta-analysis of randomized controlled trials. *CNS Drugs.* 2020;34(12):1205–1215.
31. Shaner DM, McCurdy SA, Herring MO, et al. Treatment of status epilepticus: A prospective comparison of diazepam and phenytoin versus phenobarbital and optional phenytoin. *Neurology.* 1988;38(2):202–207.
32. Abend NS, Dlugos DJ. Treatment of refractory status epilepticus: Literature review and a proposed protocol. *Pediatr Neurol.* 2008;38(6):377–390.
33. Chen WB, Gao R, Su YY, et al. Valproate versus diazepam for generalized convulsive status epilepticus: A pilot study. *Eur J Neurol.* 2011;18(12):1391–1396.
34. Mehta V, Singhi P, Singhi S. Intravenous sodium valproate versus diazepam infusion for the control of refractory status epilepticus in children: A randomized controlled trial. *J Child Neurol.* 2007;22(10):1191–1197.
35. Liu X, Wu Y, Chen Z, et al. A systematic review of randomized controlled trials on the theraputic effect of intravenous sodium valproate in status epilepticus. *Int J Neurosci.* 2012;122(6):277–283.
36. Kapur J, Elm J, Chamberlain JM, et al. Randomized trial of three anticonvulsant medications for status epilepticus. *N Engl J Med.* 2019;381(22):2103–2113.
37. Lyttle MD, Rainford NEA, Gamble C, et al. Levetiracetam versus phenytoin for second-line treatment of paediatric convulsive status epilepticus (EcLiPSE): A multicentre, open-label, randomised trial. *Lancet.* 2019;393(10186):2125–2134.
38. Dalziel SR, Borland ML, Furyk J, et al. Levetiracetam versus phenytoin for second-line treatment of convulsive status epilepticus in children (ConSEPT): An open-label, multicentre, randomised controlled trial. *Lancet.* 2019;393(10186):2135–2145.
39. Hovinga CA, Chicella MF, Rose DF, et al. Use of intravenous valproate in three pediatric patients with nonconvulsive or convulsive status epilepticus. *Ann Pharmacother.* 1999;33(5):579–584.
40. Yasiry Z, Shorvon SD. The relative effectiveness of five antiepileptic drugs in treatment of benzodiazepine-resistant convulsive status epilepticus: A meta-analysis of published studies. *Seizure.* 2014;23(3):167–174.
41. Rossetti AO, Bromfield EB. Determinants of success in the use of oral levetiracetam in status epilepticus. *Epilepsy Behav.* 2006;8(3):651–654.
42. Misra UK, Kalita J, Maurya PK. Levetiracetam versus lorazepam in status epilepticus: A randomized, open labeled pilot study. *J Neurol.* 2012;259(4):645–648.
43. Chakravarthi S, Goyal MK, Modi M, et al. Levetiracetam versus phenytoin in management of status epilepticus. *J Clin Neurosci.* 2015;22(6):959–963.
44. Vossler DG, Bainbridge JL, Boggs JG, et al. Treatment of refractory convulsive status epilepticus: A comprehensive review by the American Epilepsy Society Treatments Committee. *Epilepsy Curr.* 2020;20(5):245–264.
45. Chung WH, Chang WC, Lee YS, et al. Genetic variants associated with phenytoin-related severe cutaneous adverse reactions. *JAMA.* 2014;312(5):525–534.
46. Claassen J, Hirsch LJ, Emerson RG, et al. Continuous EEG monitoring and midazolam infusion for refractory nonconvulsive status epilepticus. *Neurology.* 2001;57(6):1036–1042.
47. Mirski MA, Williams MA, Hanley DF. Prolonged pentobarbital and phenobarbital coma for refractory generalized status epilepticus. *Crit Care Med.* 1995;23(2):400–404.
48. Brown LA, Levin GM. Role of propofol in refractory status epilepticus. *Ann Pharmacother.* 1998;32(10):1053–1059.
49. Timpe EM, Eichner SF, Phelps SJ. Propofol-related infusion syndrome in critically ill pediatric patients: Coincidence, association, or causation? *J Pediatr Pharmacol Ther.* 2006;11(1):17–42.
50. Iyer VN, Hoel R, Rabinstein AA. Propofol infusion syndrome in patients with refractory status epilepticus: An 11-year clinical experience. *Crit Care Med.* 2009;37(12):3024–3030.
51. Beuchat I, Novy J, Rossetti AO. Newer antiepileptic drugs for status epilepticus in adults: What's the evidence? *CNS Drugs.* 2018;32(3):259–267.
52. Paquette V, Culley C, Greanya ED, et al. Lacosamide as adjunctive therapy in refractory epilepsy in adults: A systematic review. *Seizure.* 2015;25:1–17.
53. Shelton CM, Alford EL, Storgion S, et al. Enteral topiramate in a pediatric patient with refractory status epilepticus: A case report and review of the literature. *J Pediatr Pharmacol Ther.* 2014;19(4):317–324.
54. Dorandeu F, Dhote F, Barbier L, et al. Treatment of status epilepticus with ketamine, are we there yet? *CNS Neurosci Ther.* 2013;19(6):411–427.
55. Gomes D, Pimentel J, Bentes C, et al. Consensus protocol for the treatment of super-refractory status epilepticus. *Acta Med Port.* 2018;31(10):598–605.
56. Zeiler FA, Zeiler KJ, Kazina CJ, et al. Lidocaine for status epilepticus in adults. *Seizure.* 2015;31:41–48.
57. Zeiler FA, Zeiler KJ, Teitelbaum J, et al. Modern inhalational anesthetics for refractory status epilepticus. *Can J Neurol Sci.* 2015;42(2):106–115.
58. Vasquez A, Farias-Moeller R, Tatum W. Pediatric refractory and super-refractory status epilepticus. *Seizure.* 2019;68:62–71.
59. Bennett AE, Hoesch RE, DeWitt LD, et al. Therapeutic hypothermia for status epilepticus: A report, historical perspective, and review. *Clin Neurol Neurosurg.* 2014;126:103–109.
60. French JA, Perucca E. Time to start calling things by their own names? The case for antiseizure medicines. *Epilepsy Curr.* 2020;20:69–72.

Acute Management of the Brain Injury Patient

77

Bradley A. Boucher and G. Christopher Wood

KEY CONCEPTS

1. Cerebral ischemia is the key pathophysiologic event that triggers secondary neuronal injury following severe traumatic brain injury (TBI). Intracellular calcium accumulation is postulated to be a central pathophysiologic process in amplifying and perpetuating secondary neuronal injury via inhibition of cellular respiration and enzyme activation.
2. *Guidelines for the Management of Severe Brain Injury*, 4th edition, published by the Brain Trauma Foundation (BTF)/ American Association of Neurological Surgeons (AANS), serves as the foundation on which clinical decisions in managing adult neurotrauma patients are based; comparable guidelines for infants, children, and adolescents have also been published.
3. Correcting and preventing early hypotension (systolic blood pressure [SBP] less than 100-110 mm Hg depending on age) with an SBP goal of 120 to 140 mm Hg and reversal of hypoxemia are primary goals during the initial resuscitative and intensive care of patients with severe TBI.
4. Nonpharmacologic management of intracranial hypertension includes raising the head of the bed 30°, and ventricular drainage if an extraventricular drain (EVD) is present.
5. The principal monitoring parameter for patients with severe TBI within the intensive care environment is increased intracranial pressure (ICP). Cerebral perfusion pressure (CPP) is also a critical monitoring parameter and should be maintained between 60 and 70 mm Hg (8.0 and 9.3 kPa) (greater than 40 and 50 mm Hg [5.3 and 6.7 kPa] in pediatric patients) through the use of fluids, vasopressors, and/or ICP normalization therapy.
6. Nonspecific pharmacologic management of intracranial hypertension should include analgesics, sedatives, and antipyretics; paralytics may be advantageous under selected circumstances.
7. Specific pharmacologic management of intracranial hypertension includes mannitol, hypertonic saline, furosemide, and high-dose pentobarbital. Neither routine use of corticosteroids nor aggressive hyperventilation (ie, $PaCO_2$ less than 25 mm Hg [3.3 kPa]) should be used in the management of intracranial hypertension.
8. Numerous investigational strategies targeted at limiting injury and/or stimulating axonal repair following severe TBI have been employed; however, no proven therapeutic benefits have been identified.
9. Use of phenytoin (alternatively levetiracetam) for the prophylaxis of posttraumatic seizures generally should be discontinued after 7 days if no seizures are observed.

BEYOND THE BOOK

Watch the video entitled "Overview of Traumatic Brain Injury (TBI)" (https://www.youtube.com/watch?v=TOWBMM7WKL4) presented by Dr. Christopher Wolf and moderated by Brent Ghan at the University of Missouri School of the Health Professions. This 7.5-minute video provides a general overview of human brain anatomy and physiology and a succinct introduction to the more detailed pathophysiology outlined in the chapter and a context for understanding TBI pharmacologic and nonpharmacologic management. This includes TBI pathophysiology including cerebral contusions, diffuse axonal injury, secondary brain injury, in addition to TBI recovery.

INTRODUCTION

TBI is one of the leading causes of death and disability in the United States.[1] A focus on TBI prevention, improved acute care, and rehabilitation remain national priorities. This chapter summarizes TBI epidemiology and pathophysiology, and highlights the major guidelines and systematic literature reviews pertaining to the severe TBI management.

EPIDEMIOLOGY

Approximately 2.87 million persons sustain a TBI each year in the United States equating to one occurring nearly every 11 seconds.[1] Among these individuals, over 288,000 require hospital admission, and over 56,000 die annually.[1] Importantly, an estimated 5.3 million Americans live with disabilities resulting from their TBI, highlighting the enormous physical and emotional toll of this healthcare problem.[2] The economic effects of acute neurotrauma are also enormous, with estimates of direct and indirect spending on patients requiring hospitalization reaching $76.5 billion in the United States in 2010.[2] Economic costs to society from lost productivity are also massive, especially considering the young age of many patients with TBI.[2] Falls are the leading cause of unintentional TBI (48%), while TBI-related hospitalizations and deaths vary based on age.[1,2] For example, death rates from TBI after a fall are highest in patients aged 65 years or older while motor vehicle crashes are the leading cause of death in persons aged 15 to 34 years and adults over 75 years.[1]

PRIMARY AND SECONDARY BRAIN INJURY PATHOPHYSIOLOGY

The neurologic sequelae of brain trauma can occur instantaneously as a consequence of the primary injury or can result from secondary injuries that follow within minutes, hours, or days after the initial injury.[3] Primary injury involves the external transfer of kinetic energy to various structural components of the brain (eg, neurons, nerve synapses, glial cells, axons, and cerebral blood vessels). The biomechanical forces responsible for primary brain injury can be classified broadly as contact (eg, blunt-object blow, penetrating-missile injuries) and acceleration/deceleration (eg, instantaneous brain movements following motor vehicle accidents).[3] Contact forces to the head commonly result in skull fractures, brain contusions, and/or hemorrhages. Primary brain injuries are categorized further as focal (eg, contusions, hematomas) or diffuse,[3,4] with the latter usually being associated with shearing or stretch forces, which primarily affect axons within the brain (ie, diffuse axonal injury).[4] The type of primary injury (ie, focal vs diffuse) is a major factor as to which of the secondary injury mechanisms discussed below will predominate following a TBI; however, many patients, especially those involved in high-speed accidents, sustain both types of injury.[3,4]

1 A complex sequence of pathophysiologic events precipitated by primary brain injury may seriously disrupt the normal central nervous system (CNS) balance between oxygen supply and demand resulting in a metabolic crisis.[5,6] Hypotension during the early posttraumatic period is a major contributor to this imbalance and a primary determinant of outcome. The end result of this imbalance is cerebral ischemia, the key pathophysiologic event triggering secondary injury.[5] Figure 77-1 is a simplified schematic of the processes that constitute secondary brain injury and their various interrelationships. The brain is particularly susceptible to ischemia because of its normally high resting energy requirement and its limited capacity to store oxygen, glucose, and adenosine triphosphate (ATP). These phenomena can result in imbalances in cerebral oxygen delivery (CDO_2) and cerebral metabolic rate of oxygen consumption ($CMRO_2$), processes that are closely autoregulated under normal circumstances.[5] Factors that can diminish cerebral oxygen supply following brain injury include cerebral edema, expanding mass lesions (eg, epidural, subdural, and intracerebral hematomas), cerebral vasospasm, and loss of vasoregulatory control. Vasogenic cerebral edema can develop as a consequence of cerebral capillary endothelial damage and disruption of the blood–brain barrier.[6] Cytotoxic cerebral edema is a consequence of loss of cell wall integrity that accompanies ischemia or hypoxia with accumulation of lactic acid secondary to anaerobic metabolism.[7] With cytotoxic and vasogenic edema comes expansion of the intracellular and extracellular fluid spaces, respectively. Increased intracranial pressure (ICP) is the most detrimental consequence of cerebral edema formation, which occurs as the brain tissue volume increases within the nondistensible skull. A significant ICP increase may further compromise cerebral blood flow (CBF) and extend cytotoxic edema. Hence, increased ICP can be self-perpetuating unless reversed. Hypoxemia can further exacerbate local decreases in cerebral oxygen supply following acute respiratory failure and systemic hypotension. Metabolic demand also can increase following neurotrauma secondary to seizures, agitation, and temperature elevation.

Two distinctive end points along the spectrum of secondary neuronal injury are: (a) energy-independent cellular necrosis characterized by membrane cell lysis, edema, and inflammation, and (b) energy-independent apoptosis leading to cell shrinkage and cell membrane dissolution.[7] Apoptosis, which is also known as programmed cell death, requires a cascade of intracellular events for cell death completion with ionic homeostasis loss being postulated as a key event in fostering secondary brain injury following

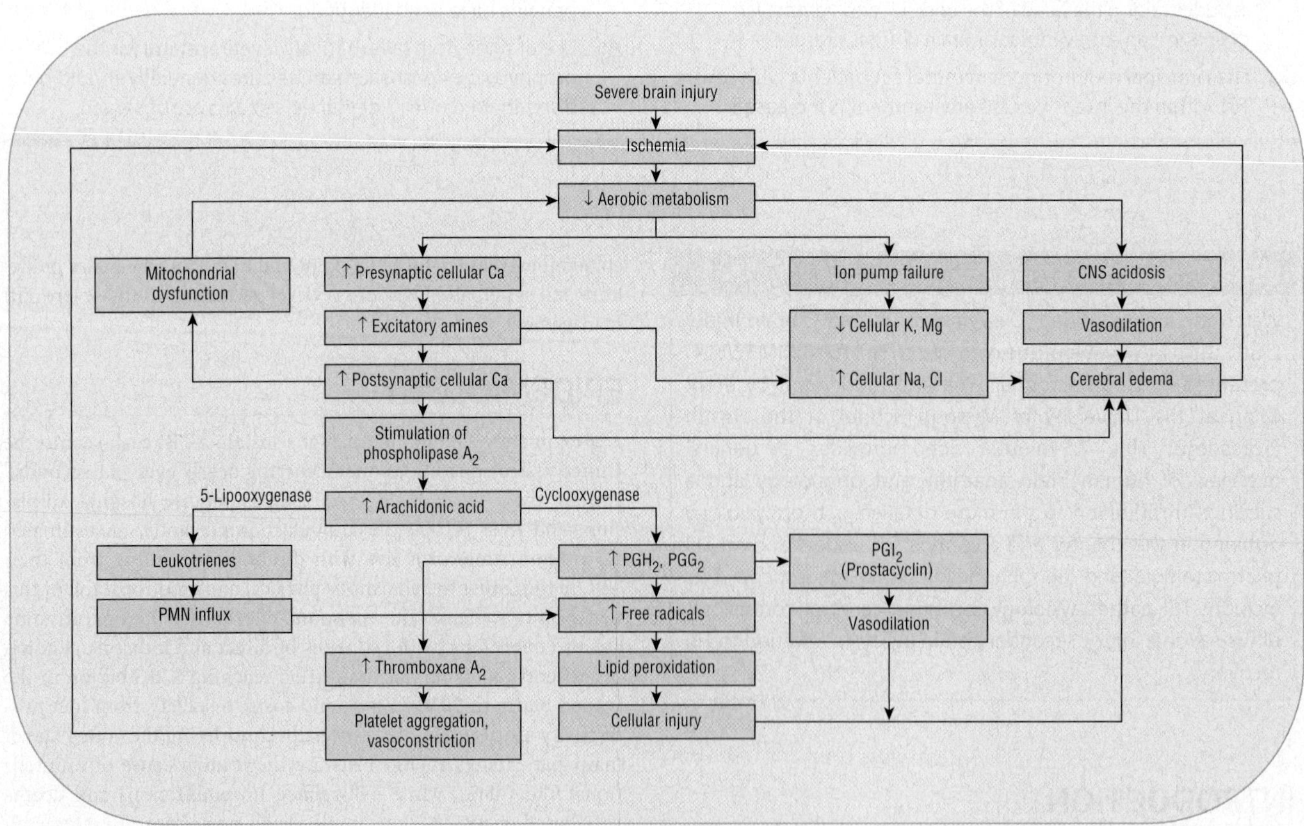

FIGURE 77-1 Schematic illustration of the cascade of biochemical events proposed to occur following severe neurotrauma (secondary brain injury). (Ca, calcium; Cl, chloride; CNS, central nervous system; K, potassium; Mg, magnesium; Na, sodium; PMN, polymorphonucleocyte; PGH_2, prostaglandin H_2; PGG_2, prostaglandin PGG_2; PGI_2, prostaglandin PGI_2.)

cerebral ischemia.[7] In this process, cellular influx of sodium, chloride, magnesium, and water occurs with a corresponding efflux of potassium secondary to cytotoxic edema and Na^+-K^+-ATPase pump dysfunction. Calcium influx into the presynaptic terminal ends of damaged neurons is mediated by N-type voltage-sensitive calcium channels and is postulated to stimulate excessive release of the excitatory amines glutamate and aspartate from the affected neurons. These amines then accumulate in the neuronal synaptic cleft in the presence of cellular energy failure, resulting in ongoing stimulation of postsynaptic cells, which extend neurotoxicity and cell death. The influx of calcium and additional sodium is stimulated by activation of ionophore receptors including the *N*-methyl-D-aspartate (NMDA) receptor.[7] Calcium influx and its intracellular accumulation initiate a number of events that amplify and perpetuate secondary neuronal injury as well as mitochondrial dysfunction, which further inhibits cellular respiration, a process already affected by ischemic and/or hypoxic insults.[5,7] A second major deleterious effect of calcium is activation of autodestructive enzymes, including phospholipases, endonucleases, and proteases, such as the caspase family of enzymes.[7] The effect of phospholipase A_2 stimulation includes formation of several arachidonic acid metabolites derived from membrane lipids (eg, thromboxane A_2, prostaglandins, and leukotrienes) that facilitate lipid peroxidation and reactive oxygen species formation.[5,7] This event occurs early after injury (eg, before hospitalization), which may limit the effectiveness of exogenously administered antioxidants. Cell-mediated injury involving inflammatory mediators (eg, proinflammatory cytokines) and nitric oxide activation is another possible mechanism involved in secondary neuronal injury,[6,7] implicating polymorphonuclear neutrophils, platelets, endothelial cells, and macrophages. However, activation of some inflammatory mediators may actually be beneficial, such that the relative balance of the mediators rather than absolute concentrations may be the most significant pathophysiologic factor following TBI. Stimulation of platelet aggregation, vasodilation, and vasoconstriction also may occur.[5]

The Glasgow Coma Scale (GCS) was designed nearly 50 years ago and is still the most widely used system to grade the arousal and functional capacity of the cerebral cortex,[3] as it defines the level of consciousness according to eye opening, motor response, and verbal response (Table 77-1). A GCS score of 15 corresponds to a normal neurologic

TABLE 77-1 Glasgow Coma Scale

Response	Score
Eyes	
• Open spontaneously	4
• To verbal command	3
• To pain	2
• No response	1
Best motor response	
• To verbal command	6
• Obeys	
• To painful stimulus (pressure to nailbeds)	
• Localizes pain	5
• Flexion, withdrawal	4
• Flexion, abnormal (decorticate rigidity)	3
• Extension (decerebrate rigidity)	2
• No response	1
Best verbal response	
(Arouse patient with painful stimulus if necessary)	
Oriented and converses	5
Disoriented and converses	4
Inappropriate words	3
Incomprehensible sounds	2
No response	1
Total	3-15

CLINICAL PRESENTATION ACUTE BRAIN INJURY

General

- Level of consciousness on admission ranges from completely unresponsive to awake and alert (ie, Glasgow Coma Scale 3-15 [Table 77-1]).

Symptoms

- Posttraumatic amnesia (eg, greater than 1 hour), increasing dizziness, a moderate-to-severe headache, nausea/vomiting, limb weakness, or paresthesia may indicate more severe injury.

Signs

- Cerebrospinal fluid (CSF) otorrhea or rhinorrhea, seizures, or unequal or unreactive pupils may indicate more severe injury.
- A rapid deterioration in mental status strongly suggests the presence of an expanding lesion within the skull.
- Severe TBI may be accompanied by significant alterations or instability in vital signs, including abnormal breathing patterns (eg, apnea, Cheyne–Stokes respiration, tachypnea), hypertension, or bradycardia.

Laboratory Tests

- Arterial blood gases (ABGs) indicating hypoxia (ie, decreased PaO_2) or hypercapnia (ie, increased $PaCO_2$) may indicate compromised ventilation.
- Blood ethanol concentration and/or urine toxicology results indicates that substance intoxication may be affecting the patient's mental status in addition to the TBI.
- Electrolyte disturbances can cause alterations in mental status, and their effects may interfere with assessment of the patient's neurological status.

Other Diagnostic Tests

- CT scan of the head is an important diagnostic tool for detecting the presence of mass lesions and structural signs of edema (eg, midline shift, compressed ventricles).

examination based on eye, motor, and verbal responses. Scores from 3 to 8 correspond to severe brain injury, while scores from 9 to 12 and 13 to 15 is consistent with moderate, and mild or minor brain injury, respectively.[3] Always consider the impact of ethanol or substance intoxication, hypotension, hypoxia, postictal state, hypoglycemia, electrolyte imbalances, or hypothermia on altering the neurologic examination when administering this scale. Opiates, sedatives, and neuromuscular blockers should not be administered until the initial examination is complete, if at all possible, as they affect the neurologic examination. Simple, rapidly attainable clinical variables that are predictive of poor outcomes include extremes of age, presence of hypotension, hypoxia and/or coagulopathy, increased ICP, decreased GCS score (especially the motor score), and pupillary changes.[8]

TREATMENT

Desired Outcomes

The overall goal in TBI management is reduction in morbidity and mortality, and optimization of long-term functional outcome for patients. This requires careful attention to the following short-term therapeutic goals: (a) establishment of an adequate airway and maintenance of ventilation and circulation during the initial period of resuscitation and evaluation, (b) maintenance of balance between CDO_2 and $CMRO_2$, (c) prevention or attenuation of secondary neuronal injury, and (d) prevention and/or treatment of associated medical complications.

General Approach to Treatment

2 The Brain Trauma Foundation (BTF) has developed an extensive document entitled *Guidelines for the Management of Severe Brain Injury* as a joint initiative with the Guidelines Committee of the American Association of Neurological Surgeons (AANS), the Joint Section on Neurotrauma and Critical Care of the AANS, and the Congress of Neurological Surgeons.[9] This document presently constitutes the most widely accepted evidence-based standards, guidelines, and options for the care of patients with severe TBI in the United States.[10] Recommendations are reported as Level I (high quality of evidence), Level II (moderate quality of evidence), or Level III (low quality of evidence). Data show that compliance with the BTF/AANS guidelines results in improved patient outcomes relative to mortality, functional outcome scores, length of hospitalization, and cost. Additionally, guidelines addressing prehospital TBI management[11] and surgical management[12] have also been published, as have TBI management guidelines for infants, children, and adolescents.[13] The recommendations emanating from the published BTF/AANS guidelines on TBI management and various published systematic reviews will be highlighted throughout the remaining portion of this chapter. Recommendations from the BTF/AANS guidelines should serve as the foundation on which all clinical decisions in managing severe TBI are based. Nonetheless, it should be noted that the majority of the guidelines are based on Class II evidence (primarily prospective clinical trials) and Class III evidence (primarily retrospective clinical trials) as few Class I evidence studies (ie, prospective, randomized, controlled trials) are available for treatment of TBI. The pharmacologic management of TBI is summarized in Table 77-2. Recommendations provided in this chapter pertain to adults and children unless specifically noted to the contrary.

TABLE 77-2 Pharmacologic Management of TBI

Hyperosmolar therapy
Mannitol effectiveness in lowering ICP is uncertain (no recommendation level due to insufficient evidence).
Hypertonic saline effectiveness in lowering ICP is uncertain (no recommendation level due to insufficient evidence).
Deep venous thrombosis prophylaxis
LMWH or low-dose unfractionated heparin may be used in combination with mechanical prophylaxis. However, there is an increased risk of expansion of intracranial hemorrhage (Recommendation level III).
Anesthetics, analgesics, and sedatives
Prophylactic administration of barbiturates to reduce burst suppression ECG is not recommended (Recommendation level II B).
High-dose barbiturate administration is recommended to control elevated ICP refractory to maximum standard medical and surgical treatment in adults. Hemodynamic stability is essential before and after barbiturate therapy (Recommendation level II B).
Propofol is recommended for the control of ICP, but not for improvement in mortality or 6-month outcomes. High-dose propofol can produce significant morbidity (Recommendation level II B).
Antiseizure prophylaxis
Prophylactic use of phenytoin or valproate is not recommended for preventing late PTS (occurring later than 7 days) (Recommendation level II A).
Phenytoin is recommended to decrease the incidence of early PTS (within 7 days of injury) (Recommendation level II A).
Levetiracetam cannot be recommended over phenytoin regarding efficacy in preventing early PTS and toxicity. (No recommendation based on insufficient evidence.)
Corticosteroids
The use of steroids is not recommended for improving outcome or reducing ICP in patients with TBI. In patients with moderate or severe TBI, high-dose methylprednisolone is associated with increased mortality and is contraindicated (Recommendation level I).

ECG, electrocardiogram; LMWH, low-molecular-weight heparin; PTS, posttraumatic seizures; TBI, traumatic brain injury. Level I: Recommendation based on a high-quality body of evidence. Level II A: Recommendation based on a moderate-level quality of evidence. Level II B: Recommendation based on a low-quality body of evidence (direct evidence but overall low quality). Level III: Recommendation based on a low-quality body of evidence.

Data from Reference 9.

Pharmacologic Therapy

Initial Resuscitation

3 4 The first priority in the unconscious patient is airway establishment that facilitates adequate oxygenation and prevents aspiration.[14] Thereafter, restoration and maintenance of systolic blood pressure (SBP) between 120 and 140 mm Hg is desired since having an admission SBP outside this range is associated with increased mortality.[15] More specifically correcting and preventing early hypotension (goal SBP >100 mm Hg for patients ages 50 to 69 years or >110 mm Hg for patients ages 15 to 49 or over 70 years) is critical as it is among the most powerful predictors of outcome.[9] Isotonic saline (0.9% normal saline) and lactated Ringer's solution have been traditionally used as initial resuscitation fluids of choice in patients with TBI. While some clinicians believe that hypertonic saline (eg, 3% or 7.5% saline) is beneficial in this situation, clinical studies yield equivocal results relative to their superiority over isotonic solutions.[16] Regardless, no clear consensus exists as to the optimal initial resuscitation fluid. Furthermore, the volume of crystalloids administered requires careful monitoring considering there are data associating lower volumes with improved survival.[17] While colloids may be considered an alternative to crystolloid therapy, strong recommendation against their use was made within a consensus statement regarding fluid therapy in neurointensive care patients.[18]

Vasopressors and inotropic agents may be needed to maintain an adequate mean arterial pressure (MAP) if hypotension persists after adequate restoration of intravascular volume. Nonpharmacologic management of intracranial hypertension includes raising the head of the bed 30°, and ventricular drainage if an extraventricular drain (EVD) is present. Figure 77-2 is an algorithm summarizing treatment priorities in the initial management of acute TBI.

Postresuscitative Care

Following successful resuscitation, priorities shift toward diagnostic evaluation of intracranial and extracranial injuries, and emergent surgical intervention as needed. In many patients, evacuation

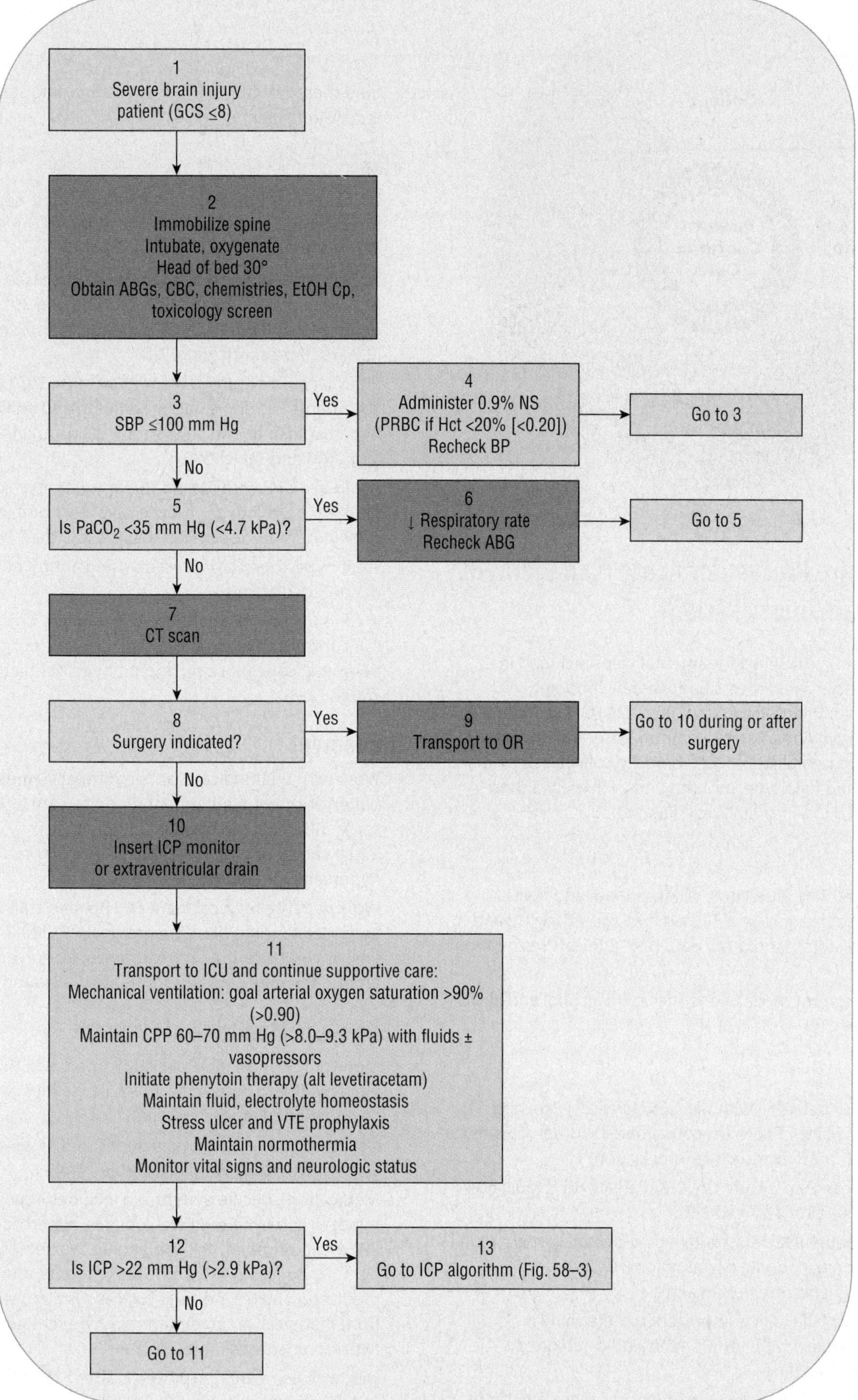

FIGURE 77-2 Algorithm for the acute management of the patient with a TBI. (BP, blood pressure; CBC, complete blood count; CPP, cerebral perfusion pressure; CT, computed tomography; EtOH Cp, ethanol plasma concentration; Hct, hematocrit; ICU, intensive care unit; NS, normal saline; OR, operating room; $PaCO_2$, partial pressure of arterial blood carbon dioxide; PRBC, packed red blood cells.) *(Reprinted, with permission, from Management of Acute Traumatic Brain. In: Richardson M, Chant C, Chessman KH, et al., eds.* Pharmacotherapy Self-Assessment Program, *7th ed. Neurology and Psychiatry. Lenexa, KS: American College of Clinical Pharmacy, 2012:143.)*

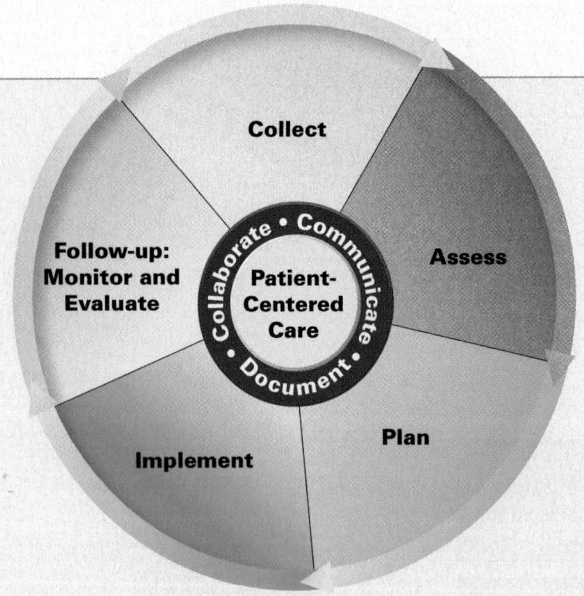

Patient Care Process for Acute Management of the Brain Injury Patient

The image shows the five fundamental steps included in The Pharmacist's Care Process endorsed by the Joint Commission for Pharmacy Practitioners (2014). The tagline of this process reads collaborate, communicate, and document. The five fundamental steps listed here are collect, assess, plan, implement, and follow-up: monitor and evaluate. All these steps are listed in a circular block diagram.

Collect

- GCS (Table 77-1), vital signs, physical exam and head computed tomography (CT) scan findings, ABGs, ICP and CPP (if available), laboratory data (see "Clinical Presentation" section)
- Prior and current medications, including alcohol and illicit substances

Assess

- Consistency between with the GCS/physical exam and injuries on head CT scan (ie, could there be other reasons for the neurologic deficit such as intoxication)
- ICP (goal less than 22 mm Hg [2.9 kPa]) and CPP (goal 60-70 mm Hg [8.0-9.3 kPa]) (Fig. 77-2)
- Need for general ICU supportive care including: mechanical ventilation/appropriate oxygenation, stress ulcer prophylaxis, and sedation/analgesia
- For VTE prophylaxis, it is important to determine if pharmacologic prophylaxis is contraindicated due to intracranial bleeding
- Need for other supportive care measures more specific to TBI including: spine immobilization, seizure prophylaxis, avoiding fever and excessive hyperglycemia, appropriate fluid therapy with a goal of euvolemia, and starting early enteral nutrition

Plan*

- Unless contraindicated, initiate appropriate supportive care measures for the issues outlined above in the Assess section (Fig. 77-2)
- Nonpharmacologic management of increased ICP with first-line options (eg, raise head of the bed 30°, open extraventricular drain if ICP is greater than 22 mm Hg [2.9 kPa, if present]) (Fig. 77-2)
- Pharmacologic management of increased ICP with first-line agents (eg, short-acting sedation and analgesia, and hyperosmolar agents [hypertonic saline, mannitol]) (Fig. 77-3 and Table 77-2)
- Avoid low CPP with IV fluid therapy, possible administration of blood products, or vasopressors (eg, norepinephrine, phenylephrine, dopamine) if SBP is less than 100 mm Hg
- Treat hyperthermia, if present, using antipyretic agents and/or cooling blankets
- If ICP is uncontrolled after optimizing first-line options for ICP control, move to second-line options (eg, pentobarbital, neuromuscular blocking agents, hyperventilation) (Table 77-3)

Implement*

- Work with the medical team on mutually agreeable and patient-centered implementation of treatments where some differences in opinion and practice may exist (eg, initial choice of sedatives, antiseizure medications, or hyperosmolar agents)
- Work with the medical team and nursing staff to implement an understanding of treatment goals (ie, ICP and CPP), as well as clear priorities in treatment selection and escalation among the many options for treating elevated ICP

Follow-up: Monitor and Evaluate

- Monitor ICP and CPP, especially response to therapies for elevated ICP to determine which modalities work best in each patient (Fig. 77-3)
- Other routine monitoring includes GCS, fluid/electrolyte status, ABGs, and vital signs (Table 77-4)
- Medication-specific monitoring includes issues such as: hypotension from sedatives/opiates, hypertriglyceridemia or PRIS from propofol, risk of bleeding/worsening intracranial hemorrhage from VTE prophylaxis agents, antiseizure medication adverse events such as rash, acute kidney injury from mannitol, or hypernatremia/hyperchloremia from hypertonic saline (Table 77-3)
- Discontinue seizure prophylaxis after 7 days if no seizures occur in the hospital (Table 77-2)

Collaborate with patient, caregivers, and other healthcare professionals.

of intracranial hematomas (ie, epidural, subdural, and intracerebral hematomas) is essential to control ICP and improve outcome. Elevation of depressed skull fractures and debridement of penetrating wound tracts are other important emergent surgical procedures. Decompressive craniectomies (ie, removal of a variable amount of skull bone) with or without temporal or frontal lobectomy may be considered in patients with increases in ICP refractory to more conservative measures.[5] In the largest randomized study to date, patients with TBI and refractory elevated ICPs undergoing decompressive craniectomy had significantly improved survival but higher rates of vegetative state and disability compared with medical therapy.[19] Thus, decompressive surgery's role in adult patients with TBI and refractory ICP remains controversial in light of these quality of life data outcomes.

Continuous ICP monitoring (eg, EVD and/or intraparenchymal fiberoptic catheter) has been the mainstay of ICP monitoring and treatment for decades in patients with severe TBI. Extraventricular drains have a therapeutic advantage over the alternatives but are associated with higher complication rates and can be difficult to place in the setting of the swollen brain. Specifically, while CSF can be drained using this device as a means to lower ICP, the most recent BTF/AANS guidelines have softened the indications for ICP monitoring based on data suggesting that invasive monitoring may lack superiority over clinical/radiologic monitoring; challenging the traditional paradigm.[9,20] If continuous ICP monitoring is employed, the goal should be to treat any ICP values above 22 mm Hg (2.9 kPa) since values above this level are associated with increased mortality.[9]

Yet another approach to ICP monitoring or no ICP monitoring is multimodality neuromonitoring (MMM).[21] This practice involves using advanced technologies such as cerebral microdialysis, CBF, brain tissue oxygenation, electroencephalography (EEG), near-infrared spectroscopy, pressure reactivity, and/or transcranial doppler (TCD) monitoring in combination. Although this practice assesses a wide array of cerebral metabolic, oxygen, and cerebrovascular measurements, MMM use is limited to institutions that are equipped to perform such measurements and have individuals capable of utilizing these data to guide expeditious therapy.[22] Furthermore, each of the MMM techniques either alone or in combination with conventional ICP monitoring has limitations and/or potential risks. As such, BTF/AANS guidelines only recommend considering jugular venous oxygen saturation monitoring as a potential advanced monitoring modality to improve outcome in patients with TBI.[9] Biochemical markers (eg, S-100 calcium-binding protein B, neuron-specific enolase, glial fibrillary acid protein, serum substance P[23]) may also have utility in diagnosing and monitoring patients with TBI. However, their role has yet to be defined as each have assorted limitations.[24]

5 Another important monitoring parameter within the intensive care environment is the cerebral perfusion pressure (CPP), which is the difference between MAP and ICP (ie, CPP = MAP − ICP). Maintenance of an acceptable CPP is postulated to be critical in reducing cerebral ischemia and secondary injury. The BTF/AANS guidelines recommend maintaining a CPP range between 60 and 70 mm Hg (8.0 and 9.3 kPa).[9] It is also recommended that aggressive attempts to maintain CPP greater than 70 mm Hg (9.3 kPa) in adults should be avoided due to the risk of the acute respiratory distress syndrome. In children, the recommended CPP goal is between 40 and 50 mm Hg (5.3 and 6.7 kPa). While using a fixed target range is the most common approach for monitoring CPP, the concept of individualizing the CPP target range to restore cerebral vasoreactivity has been advocated.[23,25]

In order to achieve the goal CPP, the MAP may need to be increased either through the use of fluids and/or vasopressors, and/or by lowering elevated ICP. In general the goal of volume expansion should be euvolemia to avoid a hypoosmolar state and negative fluid balance.[26] If the hemoglobin is below 7 g/dL (70 g/L; 4.34 mmol/L), transfusion of packed red blood cells (PRBCs) is indicated. Liberal transfusions should be avoided since using a target goal of 10 g/dL (100 g/L; 6.21 mmol/L) is associated with a higher incidence of thromboembolic events without neurologic outcome improvement based on a randomized trial.[27] More data are needed before these findings can be applied to all patients with TBI. Furthermore, erythropoietin use was not associated with an improved neurologic outcome in the same trial.[27] Volume status should be targeted to a central venous pressure of 7 to 12 cm H_2O (0.7-1.2 kPa) if invasive monitoring is employed. After euvolemia is achieved, the patient's head should also be elevated by 30° to promote venous drainage and decrease ICP.[9] If intravascular volume restoration is inadequate in elevating MAP to an acceptable level, hypertension should be induced using vasopressors (eg, norepinephrine, phenylephrine, dopamine)[9] and patients should be monitored for renal dysfunction, lactic acidosis, and signs of peripheral ischemia when they are used, especially in large doses.

Anesthetics, Analgesics, and Sedatives

6 Analgesics and sedatives have an important primary role in the management of intracranial hypertension (Fig. 77-3 and Table 77-3) that are directly related to the association of pain, agitation, excessive muscle movement, and resisting mechanical ventilation with transient increases in ICP. Paralytics are a secondary option in refractory patients or during stimulatory procedures in patients with elevated ICP.[28] There is no strong evidence that one agent is superior to another in affecting patient outcomes with severe TBI[29] as their effects on ICP, CPP, and MAP are variable.[29] Morphine sulfate is the most commonly used analgesic and sedative in this setting[9,29] and bolus doses of opiates may increase ICP by increasing CBF.[29] While continuous infusions of fentanyl and sufentanil are gaining in popularity, their use also may be associated with mild elevations in ICP.[9,29] Propofol has become the sedative of choice in the treatment of patients with TBI among many clinicians because of its ease of titration, rapidly reversible effects on discontinuation, and possible neuroprotective effects.[9] Although it is used for sedation in infants and children who are mechanically ventilated in the intensive care unit (ICU) setting, the Food and Drug Administration (FDA) requires that the manufacturer labeling contains specific information that it is not approved for sedation of pediatric patients admitted to an ICU. Propofol's biggest safety concerns is the propofol infusion syndrome (PRIS) characterized by hyperkalemia, hepatomegaly, lipemia, metabolic acidosis, myocardial failure, rhabdomyolysis, renal failure, and death in some cases.[30] While initially reported in children, PRIS can also occur in adults; therefore, doses greater than 5 mg/kg/hr and infusions exceeding 48 hours should be used with extreme caution.[30] Triglyceride concentrations also should be monitored in patients receiving prolonged propofol infusions and/or high dosages considering its lipid emulsion formulation and the potential for inducing hypertriglyceridemia under these conditions. Furthermore, evidence of neurotoxicity from animal studies has raised concerns regarding use of this sedative in patients with TBI.[30] Alternative sedatives include short-acting benzodiazepines (eg, midazolam), especially if there is a reasonable suspicion of alcohol withdrawal as the underlying etiology of the agitation,[31] and intermittent low-dose pentobarbital, ketamine,[32] dexmedetomidine,[33,34] or etomidate (particularly useful in rapid-induction anesthesia). The potential for these agents to decrease MAP and CPP must be monitored closely.[29,30,33] Additionally, the cumulative sedative effects of longer-acting medications, especially benzodiazepines, must be taken into account. The use of any sedative or paralytic agent also must be weighed against its potential to obscure the neurologic examination of the patient.

7 High-dose barbiturate therapy (ie, barbiturate coma) has been used for decades in the management of increased ICP despite a lack of evidence documenting beneficial effects on patient morbidity and mortality.[34] Nonetheless, BTF/AANS and pediatric guidelines recommend that high-dose barbiturate therapy be considered in hemodynamically stable patients with severe TBI refractory to maximal medical ICP-lowering therapy and decompressive surgery.[9,13] Prophylactic use of barbiturates is not advocated in light of insufficient evidence supporting this practice and the potential for adverse events (eg, hypotension).[9,13,34] The mechanism responsible for the cerebral protective effects of barbiturates is generally attributed to suppression of cerebral metabolism, thereby cerebral

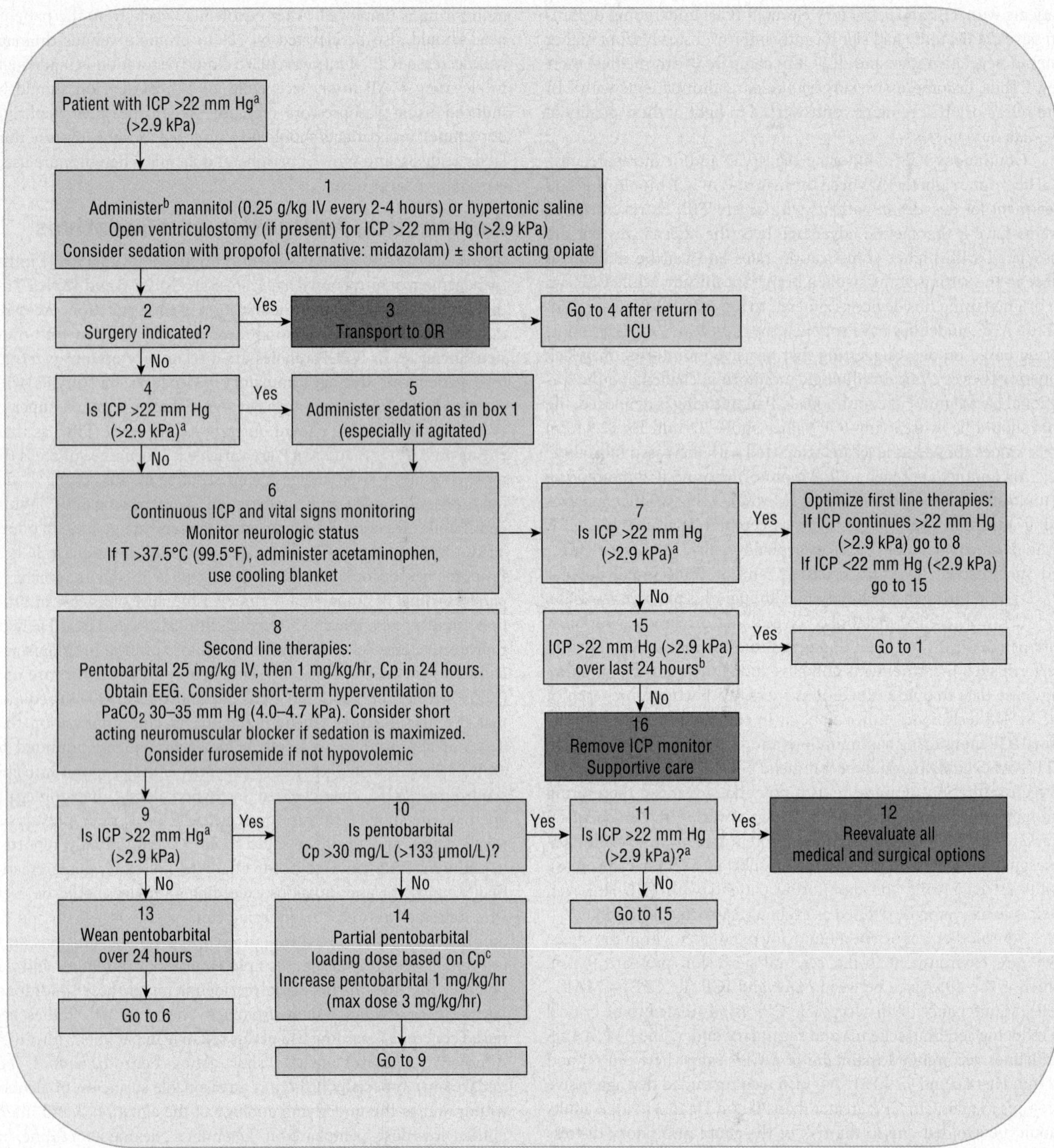

FIGURE 77-3 Algorithm for the management of increased ICP. (Cp, plasma concentration; EEG, electroencephalogram; ICU, intensive care unit; OR, operating room; $PaCO_2$, partial pressure of arterial blood carbon dioxide.) (*Reprinted, with permission, from Management of acute trauma. In: Richardson M, Chant C, Chessman KH, et al., eds. Pharmacotherapy Self-Assessment Program, 7th ed. Neurology and Psychiatry. Lenexa, KS: American College of Clinical Pharmacy, 2012:144.*)

metabolic demands and CBV.[34] Prior to inducing a barbiturate coma, the patient with severe TBI must be mechanically ventilated with continuous monitoring of arterial blood pressure, electrocardiogram (ECG), and ICP. Pentobarbital is the most commonly used barbiturate for this indication, although thiopental also has been used. Pentobarbital should be administered as an IV loading infusion totaling 25 mg/kg (ie, 10 mg/kg over 30 minutes and then 5 mg/kg/hr for 3 hours), followed by a maintenance infusion of 1 to 2 mg/kg/hr.[9,34] If the SBP falls during the loading or maintenance infusions, the rate should be slowed temporarily and blood pressure support initiated. The goal of a barbiturate coma is to maintain ICP and CPP at the previously discussed target thresholds, as well as EEG burst suppression.[9,34] Although there is a poor correlation between serum pentobarbital serum concentrations and outcomes, the goal is to achieve steady-state concentrations between 30 and 40 mg/L (133 and 178 μmol/L).[34] Initiation of barbiturate therapy withdrawal can occur when ICP has been controlled satisfactorily for 24 to 48 hours and should be tapered over 24 to 72 hours to prevent ICP spikes.

Adverse events associated with high-dose barbiturate therapy involve primarily the cardiovascular system. Hypotension caused by peripheral vasodilation may occur in one of every four patients, necessitating decreasing the barbiturate dose or the administration of

TABLE 77-3 Medication Dosing and Monitoring in Patients with TBI

Medication (Brand Name)	Adverse Medication Reactions	Monitoring Parameters	Dosage	Comments
Levetiracetam (Keppra)	CNS changes	Seizures, SCr	500-1,000 mg IV Q12 hr (during first 14 days)	Caution in patients with renal dysfunction If used for active seizures: increase to 1,000 mg every 12 hours after 14 days, then to 1,500 mg every 12 hours after 28 days
Mannitol (Generic)	Hypotension, renal dysfunction, hyperosmolality	ICP, CPP, BP, serum osmolality, Na, UO, SCr	0.25-1 g/kg IV every 2-4 hours	Avoid in patients with renal failure or CHF
Pentobarbital (Nembutal)	Hypotension, GI hypomotility, induction of hepatic medication metabolism	ICP, CPP, BP, EEG, GI function	10 mg/kg IV over 30 minutes, then 5 mg/kg over 3 hours, then 1 mg/kg/hr	Administer via central line. General dose range for infusion is 1-3 mg/kg/hr
Phenytoin (Dilantin)	Hypotension, dysrhythmias, nystagmus, ataxia, mental status changes, exfoliative dermatitis	Seizures, BP, ECG, phenytoin concentrations, skin	15-20 mg/kg IV over 60 minutes, then 5 mg/kg/day divided every 8 hours or every 12 hours	Administer <50 mg/min; use central line if available Round loading doses up to nearest 250 mg, round maintenance doses up to nearest 25 mg Trauma patients often require higher doses (ie, >6 mg/kg/day) to achieve therapeutic concentrations
Propofol (Diprivan)	Hypotension, hyperkalemia, metabolic, acidosis, rhabdomyolysis, renal failure, hepatomegaly, lipemia	ICP, CPP, BP, SCr, K, arterial pH, triglycerides, lactate	General range: 0.5-3 mg/kg/hr titrated to desired effect	Avoid doses greater than 5 mg/kg/hr or prolonged infusions; not approved for use in children

BP, blood pressure; CHF, congestive heart failure; GI, gastrointestinal; K, potassium; Na, sodium; SCr, serum creatinine; UO, urine output.

fluids and vasopressors to maintain blood pressure.[34] Gastrointestinal (GI) effects of barbiturates include decreased GI muscular tone and decreased amplitude of contraction; however, on emergence from coma, there may be a period of GI hypermotility. Care should be taken to avoid extravasation of barbiturate solutions because severe tissue damage may occur. Therefore, barbiturates should be administered by continuous infusion through a central line dedicated for this purpose. The potential for barbiturates to induce the hepatic medication metabolism of concurrent medications should be also considered. Lastly, the potential for prolonged interference with the neurologic examination of patients with TBI must be considered prior to the initiation of high-dose barbiturate therapy.

Corticosteroids

7 Although corticosteroids are effective in preventing or reducing cerebral edema in patients with nontraumatic conditions that produce vasogenic edema, studies in patients with TBI have not demonstrated their ability to lower ICP or improve outcomes.[9,13] Specifically, corticosteroid use following TBI has been associated with increased mortality and complications including GI bleeding, glucose intolerance, electrolyte abnormalities, and infection. The largest investigation to date, known as the Corticosteroid Randomization After Significant Head Injury (CRASH) study, indicated a higher risk of death within 2 weeks of enrollment (relative risk 1.18) in those receiving corticosteroids compared with those receiving placebo.[35] Based on this and several other major randomized trials, the BTF/AANS adult and pediatric guidelines recommend not to use high-dose corticosteroids in patients with moderate-to-severe TBI.[9,13]

Hyperventilation

7 The practice of prolonged aggressive hyperventilation ($PaCO_2$ less than 25 mm Hg [3.3 kPa]) to decrease ICP is no longer recommended[8] as this practice is not associated with improved outcomes. As such, BTF/AANS has removed this intervention as a temporizing measure in managing patients with TBI with elevated ICP from their guidelines.[9]

Hypothermia

Therapeutic hypothermia has been an attractive strategy for attempting to minimize secondary brain injury after TBI for decades. The mechanism underlying its protective effect is likely multifactorial, although a reduction in $CMRO_2$ is most frequently cited as the basis of any therapeutic benefits. Although early studies suggested its benefit for patients with TBI, as well as other patient populations with brain ischemia (eg, cardiac arrest patients), large clinical trials data of prophylactic hypothermia have not demonstrated improved outcomes, but rather may in fact indicate poorer outcomes.[9,36-39] Its potential adverse effects include coagulation disturbances, infectious complications, and cardiac arrhythmias. Thus, prophylactic therapeutic hypothermia is not recommended as a routine neuroprotective strategy,[9] except for perhaps patients with TBI with refractory ICP elevations. However, its use in this case is also unclear at best.[40]

Osmotic Agents

7 Although a number of osmotic diuretics (eg, urea, glycerol) can be used to decrease ICP, mannitol is the most widely employed.[9,41] Despite the common practice of administering mannitol to patients with suspected or actual increases in ICP following brain injury, clinical trials comparing its effects against placebo have not been performed.[42] Based on this lack of evidence, the BTF/AANS guidelines removed the previous recommendation regarding mannitol's effectiveness for control of increased ICP.[9]

Mannitol's beneficial effects likely relate to (a) an immediate plasma-expanding effect that reduces blood viscosity and increases CBF, and (b) establishment of an osmotic concentration gradient across an intact blood–brain barrier that decreases ICP as water diffuses from the brain into the intravascular compartment.[9] Recommended doses typically range from 0.25 to 1 g/kg IV every 2 to 4 hours with higher doses being used in emergency situations and the lower dose for a maintenance regimen.[43] Increased ICP is reduced within minutes following mannitol administration with a maximum effect within 20 to 60 minutes.[43] To maximize benefit and minimize adverse events, it has been suggested that mannitol be administered as a bolus and not as a continuous infusion in this setting.

Several adverse effects are associated with mannitol.[43] In addition to hypotension resulting from its diuretic effect, a reversible acute renal dysfunction may occur in patients with previously normal renal function after long-term, large-dose administration. Patients particularly susceptible are those with advanced age and preexisting renal dysfunction which is based on data in patients with intracranial hemorrhage.[44] As such, mannitol should be avoided in patients with acute kidney injury or chronic kidney diseases. Acute exacerbation of underlying congestive heart failure and pulmonary edema also may occur following rapid intravascular volume expansion and furosemide is recommended as an alternative diuretic for lowering ICP in these latter patient groups.

While hypertonic saline solutions have been advocated by some as a resuscitative fluid following TBI, solutions ranging from concentrations of 3% to 20% have also been used to acutely lower increased ICP.[43] Doses range from approximately 150 mL of 3% saline solution to 75 mL of 7.5% saline solution to 30 mL of 23.4% saline solution boluses.[43] Saline concentrations greater than 3% should be administered via a central venous catheter.[43] Not only do hypertonic saline solutions create an osmotic gradient in favor of reducing cerebral edema, but they may also have beneficial vasoregulatory, immunologic, and neurochemical effects as well.[45] Plasma expansion may also lead to an increase in CBF. However, the 2016 BTF guidelines do not recommend hypertonic saline due to a lack of supporting evidence[9] consistent with a systematic review which found no mortality benefit or beneficial effect on ICP compared with other ICP-lowering agents.[45] In most of these studies, the goal of therapy was to treat an elevated ICP; however, for some the goal was to increase the serum sodium regardless of ICP. If used in this way, hypertonic saline should target serum sodium concentration less than 160 mEq/L (mmol/L) since additional benefit is unlikely at higher concentrations.[43]

Investigational Therapy

8 The steady decrease in morbidity and mortality following severe neurotrauma over the past several decades can be attributed largely to the use of conventional treatment strategies to expeditiously and aggressively manage events resulting in secondary injury (ie, ischemia, hypoxia, increased ICP). Numerous neuroprotective agents targeting specific pathophysiologic processes that are theorized to occur following severe TBI have been investigated over the past three decades in an attempt to further enhance the prospects for a meaningful recovery. Prominent among these strategies have been attempts to modulate calcium influx through the administration of calcium antagonists,[46] glutamate antagonists including magnesium, and the use of antioxidants/free radical scavengers.[47,48] Inhibitors of inflammatory mediators have also been considered as potential neuroprotective agents.[48] Unfortunately, none of these agents to date has demonstrated a significant reduction in morbidity or mortality following severe TBI in clinical trials. There was immense enthusiasm for progesterone as a neuroprotective agent based on two moderately sized clinical studies that demonstrated improved outcome following acute TBI.[49] However, two subsequent large randomized, placebo controlled, prospective trials of progesterone in patients with acute TBI were halted early due to lack of functional outcomes improvement.[50,51] In contrast, interest continues to exist for the pleiotropic cytokine, erythropoietin, as a neuroprotective agent independent of its ability to increase hemoglobin concentrations[47] despite data indicating equivocal results relative to improvement in neurologic outcomes and survival benefits.[52] Other agents that may have beneficial effects in TBI based on limited clinical or epidemiologic data include 3-Hydroxy-3-methylglutaryl-coenzyme A (HMG-CoA) reductase inhibitors and sympatholytics such as β-blockers.[53] While two meta-analysis of β-blockers use in patients with TBI demonstrated mortality benefits,[54,55] their usage was associated with increased infection rates, ICU length of stay, and overall hospitalization days.[55] Thus, evaluation of the benefit to risk ratio for this medication class will require additional prospective, randomized, clinical trials in patients with TBI. Miscellaneous agents and therapies being considered as viable neuroprotective agents based on clinical and/or experimental TBI studies include growth hormone, cyclosporine, nitric oxide synthase inhibitor, minocycline, hyperbaric oxygen, and CNS bone marrow stromal cell transplantation.[53] Others have proposed that stimulation of axonal repair processes versus limiting injury may be the most fruitful neuroprotective pathway for future investigations.[47]

The concept of administering commercially available CNS-active agents for nonapproved indications in patients with TBI should presently be considered investigational. Examples include the use of CNS stimulants in the management and rehabilitation of patients with TBI as data supporting this approach are equivocal.[47] Another example is the use of Parkinson's disease medications (eg, amantadine, bromocriptine, carbidopa/levodopa) in patients with severe TBI in an attempt to enhance dopamine release and inhibit reuptake within the injured region of the brain.[56] While intuitively appealing, use of psychoactive agents to improve CNS sequalae should be administered cautiously since large, well-controlled studies with a wide array of agents are lacking. Additionally, the timing for administration of these medications is controversial and the potential for cardiovascular adverse effects in the face of uncertain benefit would suggest that these medications should be reserved for the postacute phase of treatment (ie, weeks to months postinjury).

Acknowledging the complexities surrounding acute TBI, a broad-based, multidisciplinary approach is undoubtedly needed before breakthrough therapies are identified for this multifaceted, catastrophic condition. Examples of these types of initiatives include the International Mission on Prognosis and Clinical Trial Design (IMPACT) study group,[58] and the BRAIN Initiative—Brain Research Through Advancing Neurotechnologies, which is a Presidential and National Institutes of Health focused program aimed at revolutionizing understanding of the human brain launched in 2014.[59]

Treatment and Prophylaxis of Complications

In addition to specific management of TBI problems such as intracranial hypertension, the potential for secondary complications must also be considered as a wide variety of complications occur in more than 20% of patients with TBI and are associated with increased mortality and length of stay.[60] Development and implementation of clinical pathways for consistency of care, and clinical investigation of neuroprotective agents are important in advancing TBI treatment in the future.

Posttraumatic Seizures

9 It is generally agreed that adult patients who experience one or more seizures following a moderate-to-severe TBI should receive antiseizure medication therapy to avoid increases in $CMRO_2$ that occur with the onset of subsequent seizures and to prevent the development of (sometimes subclinical) status epilepticus associated with increased mortality.[9] Initial therapy should consist of incremental IV doses of diazepam (5-40 mg adults, 0.1-0.5 mg/kg infants and children) or lorazepam (2-8 mg adults, 0.03-0.1 mg/kg infants and children) to terminate any active seizure activity, followed by IV phenytoin to prevent seizure recurrence. Phenytoin dosing regimens for adults and pediatric patients include an IV loading dose of 15 to 20 mg/kg and 10 to 15 mg/kg, respectively, followed by a maintenance dose of 5 mg/kg/day divided into two or three daily doses. Alternatively, fosphenytoin, a water-soluble phosphate ester

of phenytoin, can be administered IV or intramuscularly using the same doses, specified as phenytoin equivalents (PE). The merits of preventive antiseizure medication therapy in patients who have not had a seizure postinjury historically is controversial. Risk factors for early posttraumatic seizures (less than 7 days after injury) include a GCS score of less than 10, a cortical contusion, a depressed skull fracture, a subdural hematoma, an epidural hematoma, an intracerebral hematoma, a penetrating head wound, or a seizure within the first 24 hours of injury.[9] In a landmark randomized, placebo-controlled study, the incidence of early posttraumatic seizures in patients receiving placebo was 14.2% compared with 3.6% in patients receiving phenytoin without a significant increase in medication-related adverse events.[61] Thus, phenytoin should be used to prevent seizures in adult and pediatric patients with TBI for the first 7 days after injury[9,13] despite newer data suggesting that phenytoin may not decrease early posttraumatic seizures and may diminish functional outcome after blunt TBI,[62] which is fueling debate challenging this longstanding practice.[63] Valproate therapy is not recommended for patients with TBI, based on a trend for higher mortality compared to short-term phenytoin therapy.[61] Levetiracetam is a potentially attractive option; however, it should be used cautiously as large randomized clinical trials of its use has not been conducted in patients with TBI. Nevertheless, two meta-analyses found no difference in the rate of early posttraumatic seizures between levetiracetam and phenytoin,[64,65] and levetiracetam may have a superior safety profile based on one of these evaluations.[65] In a survey of nearly 70 neurotrauma centers in Europe, levetiracetam has become the antiseizure medication of choice over phenytoin in patients with TBI.[66] If used in TBI patients, the potential for increased levetiracetam systemic clearance should be considered when dosing this agent.[67] The benefits of prophylactic antiseizure medications beyond 7 days have not been demonstrated, and thus their use for this indication is not recommended.[9,13] Unfortunately, despite reducing the incidence of early seizures following brain injury, no beneficial effects have been documented for antiseizure medications on patient mortality or long-term disability.[9]

Supportive Care

While normalizing ICP and maintaining an adequate CPP are the highest priorities in preventing secondary injury following severe TBI, attention also must be given to preventing and/or treating systemic and extracranial complications. One such complication is systemic hypertension, which can be treated using antihypertensives including IV labetalol, nicardipine, and enaliprilat.

Fluid and electrolyte management is another important area of focus in the critically ill patient with a TBI, as common electrolyte disturbances, that should be monitored and treated aggressively; it includes hyponatremia, hypomagnesemia, hypokalemia, and hypophosphatemia.

Furthermore, aggressive nutritional support should be initiated, as early feeding of patients with TBI (ie, by 7 days) may be associated with a trend toward better outcomes in terms of survival and disability.[9,68] Early enteral nutrition, in particular, is associated with better survival and outcome compared with matched controls not receiving early enteral nutrition.[69]

Hyperglycemia (glucose greater than or equal to 160 mg/dL [8.9 mmol/L]) is also common in patients with TBI and is associated with worse outcomes.[70] Thus, intensive insulin therapy versus conventional glucose control should not be used since it is associated with adverse effects on brain glucose metabolism with little to no gain in neurological outcome.[70]

Infectious complications commonly encountered in patients with severe TBI include nosocomial pneumonia, sepsis, urinary tract infections, and meningitis. Treatment of these potentially devastating infections should be aggressive, with careful attention being paid to antibiotic blood–brain barrier penetration for intracranial infections.

Hyperthermia should also be avoided in patients with TBI because patients with elevated temperatures have poorer outcomes than normothermic patients.[71] Hence, aggressive maintenance of a core temperature of less than 37.5°C (99.5°F) using acetaminophen, nonsteroidal anti-inflammatory drugs (NSAIDs), and cooling blankets is indicated for patients following severe TBI.

Other important therapeutic interventions include acute gastritis prophylaxis, and prevention of decubiti and contractures. Prevention of thromboembolic events is extremely important in the supportive care in TBI patients since they are high risk of developing this complication.[72] This can be accomplished with the use of intermittent pneumatic compression devices (preferred) or graduated compression stockings initially. Thereafter, the decision to start systemic therapy (eg, low-molecular-weight heparin or unfractionated heparin) depends on multiple factors. A noteworthy study revealed better survival and lower thromboembolic complications in patients with TBI receiving LMWH compared with those receiving unfractionated heparin.[73] Generally, patients who had relatively minor bleeding or no bleeding on the initial CT scan and good ICP control can have pharmacological prophylaxis started within 24 to 48 hours postinjury.[74,75] Patients at moderate-to-high risk of intracranial hemorrhage postinjury can safely receive pharmacologic prophylaxis within the first 72 hours postinjury without a corresponding increase in intracranial hemorrhage compared with patients receiving prophylaxis greater than 72 hours after their TBI.[75] Regardless of initiation time, prophylaxis is continued until patients are ambulatory. Systemic anticoagulation must be used with caution in patients with more severe intracerebral hemorrhage, or in patients who may need to undergo craniotomy early in their course.[9] Monitoring for a coagulopathy is important as the incidence is greater than 30%, and coagulopathy is associated with a significantly longer ICU length of stay and an almost 10-fold increase in mortality.[75] A low platelet count was the strongest predictor of intracranial bleeding progression compared with other coagulation tests in patients with TBI based on a retrospective study.[76] Reversal of coagulopathy with recombinant factor VIIa in critically ill trauma patients with TBI was popular among some practitioners despite lacking an approved indication or large clinical trials demonstrating its safety and efficacy in patients with TBI.[77] However, tranexamic acid is a less expensive hemostatic alternative to recombinant factor VIIa. A randomized, placebo-control trial involving over 12,000 TBI patients known as CRASH-3 revealed that patients with a GCS greater than 3, who received tranexamic acid within 3 hours of injury had a significant decrease in overall mortality by 1.5% compared to patients receiving placebo. The reduced mortality occurred without a difference in adverse events (ie, vascular occlusive events or seizures).[78] However, the mortality benefit was not significant in patients with severe TBI suggesting that it may be more effective in mild-to-moderate TBI as outlined in a meta-analysis.[78,79] Based on these findings, it is unclear if tranexamic acid administration will become the standard of care in non-severe TBI patients.

One of the most common general pharmacokinetic challenges seen in patients with TBI is a larger volume of distribution and more rapid hepatic clearance of medications compared to most other patient populations. These pharmacokinetic changes often make phenytoin optimization and, less commonly, pentobarbital optimization difficult. As such, phenytoin and pentobarbital recommended dosing are weight based, and in the case of phenytoin, usually higher than the 300 mg/day dose commonly seen in ambulatory patients. Augmented renal clearance has also been documented in critically ill patients including patients with TBI affecting medications that are renally eliminated.[80] Furthermore, there can be wide interpatient pharmacodynamic variability in the efficacy of pharmacologic and nonpharmacologic interventions for ICP control. For some patients, there is a high degree of trial and error to find the best combination of interventions that are effective and not contraindicated based on other factors.

TABLE 77-4 Evaluation of Therapeutic Outcomes

General	GCS: Record hourly initially, decrease frequency as neurologic status stabilizes Vital signs (BP, HR, RR, temperature): Record hourly initially, decrease frequency as neurologic status stabilizes UO: Record hourly initially, decrease frequency as neurologic status stabilizes Arterial oxygen saturation: Continuously while in ICU
Risk of increased ICP	ICP: Record hourly, decrease frequency as ICP stabilizes <22 mm Hg (2.9 kPa) (usually not until 48-72 hours postinjury at a minimum) CPP: Record hourly, decrease frequency as CPP stabilizes in the desired range[a]
Laboratory tests	Ethanol concentration and urine toxicology results: On admission ABGs: Daily at a minimum while intubated, repeated as needed based on pulmonary instability requiring ventilator setting changes CBC: Daily while in ICU Serum electrolytes (Na, K, Cl): Daily while in ICU. Serum sodium and osmolality may be monitored as frequently as every 6 hours if osmotherapy (mannitol, furosemide, hypertonic saline) is being used Minerals (Mg, Ca, P): Daily initially until concentrations stable
Radiologic procedures	CT scan: Postresuscitation initially with repeat scan(s) as needed based on degree of neurologic instability (eg, decrease in GCS) or initial CT appearance

BP, blood pressure; Ca, calcium; CBC, complete blood count; Cl, chloride; CT, computed tomography; HR, heart rate; K, potassium; Mg, magnesium; Na, sodium; P, phosphorus; RR, respiratory rate; UO, urine output.

[a]Continuous monitoring mandated initially if technologically feasible.

Clinical Pathways/Guideline Implementation

Use of clinical pathways and formal TBI management guidelines/standardized protocols have been demonstrated to improve TBI patient mortality in studies focused on intracranial hypertension.[81,82] Aggressive ICP monitoring has been associated with improved outcomes in patients with moderate-to-severe TBI as well.[83] Furthermore, a cost–benefit analysis revealed that adoption of the BTF/ASSN guidelines resulted in more than 3,600 lives saved among adult patients with severe TBI admitted annually to US hospitals as the proportion of patients having a good outcome based on their Glasgow Outcome Scale (GOS) was estimated to increase from 35% to 66%. This resulted in an overall estimated annual total cost savings exceeding $4 billion.[84] Unfortunately, improved outcomes are not universally reported as there is a wide guideline compliance variability despite the BTF/AANS guidelines availability for over two decades.[10,85] Regardless, few practitioners would dispute the overall importance of integrating current evidence-based management guidelines into clinical practice as a means to optimize care and improve the functional outcome of patients.[48,86]

EVALUATION OF THERAPEUTIC OUTCOMES

The evaluation of therapeutic outcomes is summarized in Table 77-4. Patients with severe TBI initially require ICU monitoring with the goals of maintaining or reestablishing neurologic and systemic homeostasis, as well as readily detecting any neurologic deterioration. This requires frequent evaluation of the patient's neurologic status (eg, GCS), measurement of vital signs, urine output, and arterial oxygen saturation, and ICP in patients with an ICP monitor in place. Careful attention must be paid to the potential development of various electrolyte, mineral, and acid–base disturbances; coagulopathies; and infections by obtaining appropriate laboratory tests on a daily basis initially. The intensity of monitoring will be a function of the relative degree of patient's neurologic and hemodynamic stability in the hours and days following the neurologic insult. Lastly, radiologic tests (eg, CT scans) are essential not only for the initial diagnostic evaluation, but also as means to evaluate the etiology for any subsequent neurologic deterioration.

CONCLUSION

Traumatic brain injuries are exceedingly common and often associated with devastating consequences in both morbidity and mortality. Unraveling the complex pathophysiology of secondary injury following severe TBI has failed to yield major advances to attenuate or reverse these consequences to date. Furthermore, review of several traditional treatment modalities has resulted in recommendations against their use. Adherence to best management practices relative to aggressive treatment of increased ICP, supportive care, and prevention of complications offers victims of severe TBI a promise of improved outcomes. Commitment to this condition at the national level may be the turning point to breakthrough therapies of the future.

ABBREVIATIONS

AANS	American Association of Neurological Surgeons
ABG	arterial blood gas
ATP	adenosine triphosphate
BTF	Brain Trauma Foundation
CBF	cerebral blood flow
CBV	cerebral blood volume
CDO_2	cerebral oxygen delivery
$CMRO_2$	cerebral oxygen consumption
CPP	cerebral perfusion pressure
CSF	cerebrospinal fluid
CT	computed tomography
ECG	electrocardiogram
EEG	electroencephalography
EVD	extraventricular drain
FDA	Food and Drug Administration
GCS	Glasgow Coma Scale
GI	gastrointestinal
GOS	Glasgow Outcome Scale
HMG	3-hydroxy-3-methylglutaryl
ICP	intracranial pressure
ICU	intensive care unit
MAP	mean arterial pressure
NMDA	*N*-methyl-D-aspartate
NSAID	nonsteroidal anti-inflammatory drug
$PbrO_2$	brain tissue oxygen

PRIS	propofol infusion syndrome
PRBCs	packed red blood cells
SBP	systolic blood pressure
$SjvO_2$	jugular venous oxygen saturation
TBI	traumatic brain injury
TCD	transcranial Doppler

REFERENCES

1. CDC. TBI: Get the Facts. https://www.cdc.gov/traumaticbraininjury/get_the_facts.html2021 [cited 2021 March 18, 2021].
2. CDC. CDC grand rounds: Reducing severe traumatic brain injury in the United States. *MMWR Morb Mortal Wkly Rep.* 2013;62(27):549–552.
3. Capizzi A, Woo J, Verduzco-Gutierrez M. Traumatic brain injury: An overview of epidemiology, pathophysiology, and medical management. *Med Clin North Am.* 2020;104(2):213–238. doi:10.1016/j.mcna.2019.11.001.
4. McGinn MJ, Povlishock JT. Pathophysiology of traumatic brain injury. *Neurosurg Clin N Am.* 2016;27(4):397–407. doi:10.1016/j.nec.2016.06.002.
5. Algattas H, Huang JH. Traumatic brain injury pathophysiology and treatments: Early, intermediate, and late phases post-injury. *Int J Mol Sci.* 2014;15(1):309–341. doi:10.3390/ijms15010309.
6. Hinson HE, Rowell S, Schreiber M. Clinical evidence of inflammation driving secondary brain injury: A systematic review. *J Trauma Acute Care Surg.* 2015;78(1):184–191. doi:10.1097/TA.0000000000000468.
7. Quillinan N, Herson PS, Traystman RJ. Neuropathophysiology of brain injury. *Anesthesiol Clin.* 2016;34(3):453–464. doi:10.1016/j.anclin.2016.04.011.
8. Souter MJ, Blissitt PA, Blosser S, et al. Recommendations for the critical care management of devastating brain injury: Prognostication, psychosocial, and ethical management: A position statement for healthcare professionals from the neurocritical care society. *Neurocrit Care.* 2015;23(1):4–13. doi:10.1007/s12028-015-0137-6.
9. Carney N, Totten AM, O'Reilly C, et al. Guidelines for the management of severe traumatic brain injury, fourth edition. *Neurosurgery.* 2017;80(1):6–15. doi:10.1227/NEU.0000000000001432.
10. Khormi YH, Gosadi I, Campbell S, et al. Adherence to Brain Trauma Foundation guidelines for management of traumatic brain injury patients and its effect on outcomes: Systematic review. *J Neurotrauma.* 2018;35(13):1407–1418. doi:10.1089/neu.2017.5345.
11. Gabriel EJ, Ghajar J, Jagoda A, et al. Guidelines for prehospital management of traumatic brain injury. *J Neurotrauma.* 2002;19(1):111–174.
12. Bullock MR, Chesnut R, Ghajar J, et al. Guidelines for the surgical management of traumatic brain injury. *Neurosurgery.* 2006;58(3):S21–S62.
13. Kochanek PM, Tasker RC, Carney N, et al. Guidelines for the management of pediatric severe traumatic brain injury, third edition: Update of the Brain Trauma Foundation Guidelines. *Pediatr Crit Care Med.* 2019;20(3S Suppl 1):S1–S82. doi:10.1097/PCC.0000000000001735.
14. Spaite DW, Bobrow BJ, Keim SM, et al. Association of statewide implementation of the prehospital traumatic brain injury treatment guidelines with patient survival following traumatic brain injury: The excellence in prehospital injury care (EPIC) study. *JAMA Surg.* 2019;154(7):e191152. doi:10.1001/jamasurg.2019.1152.
15. Fuller G, Hasler RM, Mealing N, et al. The association between admission systolic blood pressure and mortality in significant traumatic brain injury: A multi-centre cohort study. *Injury.* 2014;45(3):612–617. doi:10.1016/j.injury.2013.09.008.
16. Gantner D, Moore EM, Cooper DJ. Intravenous fluids in traumatic brain injury: What's the solution? *Curr Opin Crit Care.* 2014;20(4):385–389. doi:10.1097/MCC.0000000000000114.
17. Ko A, Harada MY, Barmparas G, et al. Limit crystalloid resuscitation after traumatic brain injury. *Am Surg.* 2017;83(12):1447–1452.
18. Oddo M, Poole D, Helbok R, et al. Fluid therapy in neurointensive care patients: ESICM consensus and clinical practice recommendations. *Intensive Care Med.* 2018;44(4):449–463. doi:10.1007/s00134-018-5086-z.
19. Hutchinson PJ, Kolias AG, Timofeev IS, et al. Trial of decompressive craniectomy for traumatic intracranial hypertension. *N Engl J Med.* 2016;375(12):1119–1130. doi:10.1056/NEJMoa1605215.
20. Chesnut RM, Temkin N, Carney N, et al. A trial of intracranial-pressure monitoring in traumatic brain injury. *N Engl J Med.* 2012;367(26):2471–2481. doi:10.1056/NEJMoa1207363.
21. Davanzo JR, Sieg EP, Zacko JC, Timmons SD. Use of multimodaility neuromonitoring in the management of traumatic brain injury. In: Timmons SD, ed. *Controversies in Severe Traumatic Brain Injury Management.* Cham, Switzerland: Springer; 2018:17–28.
22. Lazaridis C, Goldenberg FD. Intracranial pressure in taumatic brain injury: From thresholds to heuristics. *Crit Care Med.* 2020;48(8):1210–1213. doi:10.1097/CCM.0000000000004383.
23. Lorente L, Martin MM, Almeida T, et al. Serum substance P levels are associated with severity and mortality in patients with severe traumatic brain injury. *Crit Care.* 2015;19:192. doi:10.1186/s13054-015-0911-z.
24. Neher MD, Keene CN, Rich MC, et al. Serum biomarkers for traumatic brain injury. *South Med J.* 2014;107(4):248–255. doi:10.1097/SMJ.0000000000000086.
25. Petkus V, Preiksaitis A, Krakauskaite S, et al. Benefit on optimal cerebral perfusion pressure targeted treatment for traumatic brain injury patients. *J Crit Care.* 2017;41:49–55. doi:10.1016/j.jcrc.2017.04.029.
26. van der Jagt M. Fluid management of the neurological patient: A concise review. *Crit Care.* 2016;20(1):126. doi:10.1186/s13054-016-1309-2.
27. Robertson CS, Hannay HJ, Yamal JM, et al. Effect of erythropoietin and transfusion threshold on neurological recovery after traumatic brain injury: A randomized clinical trial. *JAMA.* 2014;312(1):36–47. doi:10.1001/jama.2014.6490.
28. Sanfilippo F, Santonocito C, Veenith T, et al. The role of neuromuscular blockade in patients with traumatic brain injury: A systematic review. *Neurocrit Care.* 2015;22(2):325–334. doi:10.1007/s12028-014-0061-1.
29. Oddo M, Crippa IA, Mehta S, et al. Optimizing sedation in patients with acute brain injury. *Crit Care.* 2016;20(1):128. doi:10.1186/s13054-016-1294-5.
30. Boucher BA. What is the optimal sedative regimen in severe traumatic brain injury patients. In: Timmons SD, ed. *Controversies in Severe Traumatic Brain Injury Management.* Cham, Switzerland: Springer; 2018:47–60.
31. Gu JW, Yang T, Kuang YQ, et al. Comparison of the safety and efficacy of propofol with midazolam for sedation of patients with severe traumatic brain injury: A meta-analysis. *J Crit Care.* 2014;29(2):287–290. doi:10.1016/j.jcrc.2013.10.021.
32. Zeiler FA, Teitelbaum J, West M, Gillman LM. The ketamine effect on ICP in traumatic brain injury. *Neurocrit Care.* 2014;21(1):163–173. doi:10.1007/s12028-013-9950-y.
33. Humble SS, Wilson LD, Leath TC, et al. ICU sedation with dexmedetomidine after severe traumatic brain injury. *Brain Inj.* 2016;30(10):1266–1270. doi:10.1080/02699052.2016.1187289.
34. Roberts I, Sydenham E. Barbiturates for acute traumatic brain injury. *Cochrane Database Syst Rev.* 2012;12:CD000033. doi:10.1002/14651858.CD000033.pub2.
35. Roberts I, Yates D, Sandercock P, et al. Effect of intravenous corticosteroids on death within 14 days in 10008 adults with clinically significant head injury (MRC CRASH trial): Randomised placebo-controlled trial. *Lancet.* 2004;364(9442):1321–1328.
36. Watson HI, Shepherd AA, Rhodes JKJ, Andrews PJD. Revisited: A systematic review of therapeutic hypothermia for adult patients following traumatic brain injury. *Crit Care Med.* 2018;46(6):972–979. doi:10.1097/CCM.0000000000003125.
37. Crompton EM, Lubomirova I, Cotlarciuc I, et al. Meta-analysis of therapeutic hypothermia for traumatic brain injury in adult and pediatric patients. *Crit Care Med.* 2017;45(4):575–583. doi:10.1097/CCM.0000000000002205.
38. Lewis SR, Evans DJ, Butler AR, et al. Hypothermia for traumatic brain injury. *Cochrane Database Syst Rev.* 2017;9:CD001048. doi:10.1002/14651858.CD001048.pub5.
39. Andrews PJ, Sinclair HL, Rodriguez A, et al. Hypothermia for intracranial hypertension after traumatic brain injury. *N Engl J Med.* 2015;373(25):2403–2412. doi:10.1056/NEJMoa1507581.
40. Lazaridis C, Robertson CS. Hypothermia for increased intracranial pressure: Is it dead? *Curr Neurol Neurosci Rep.* 2016;16(9):78. doi:10.1007/s11910-016-0681-2.
41. Gu J, Huang H, Huang Y, et al. Hypertonic saline or mannitol for treating elevated intracranial pressure in traumatic brain injury: A meta-analysis of randomized controlled trials. *Neurosurg Rev.* 2019;42(2):499–509. doi:10.1007/s10143-018-0991-8.
42. Zhang W, Neal J, Lin L, et al. Mannitol in critical care and surgery over 50+ years: A systematic review of randomized controlled trials and complications with meta-analysis. *J Neurosurg Anesthesiol.* 2019;31(3):273–284. doi:10.1097/ANA.0000000000000520.
43. Ropper AH. Hyperosmolar therapy for raised intracranial pressure. *N Engl J Med.* 2012;367(8):746–752. doi:10.1056/NEJMct1206321.

44. Kim MY, Park JH, Kang NR, et al. Increased risk of acute kidney injury associated with higher infusion rate of mannitol in patients with intracranial hemorrhage. *J Neurosurg.* 2014;120(6):1340–1348. doi:10.3171/2013.12.JNS13888.
45. Chen H, Song Z, Dennis JA. Hypertonic saline versus other intracranial pressure-lowering agents for people with acute traumatic brain injury. *Cochrane Database Syst Rev.* 2020;1:CD010904. doi:10.1002/14651858.CD010904.pub3.
46. Xu GZ, Wang MD, Liu KG, et al. A meta-analysis of treating acute traumatic brain injury with calcium channel blockers. *Brain Res Bull.* 2013;99:41–47. doi:10.1016/j.brainresbull.2013.09.011.
47. Diaz-Arrastia R, Kochanek PM, Bergold P, et al. Pharmacotherapy of traumatic brain injury: State of the science and the road forward: Report of the Department of Defense Neurotrauma Pharmacology Workgroup. *J Neurotrauma.* 2014;31(2):135–158. doi:10.1089/neu.2013.3019.
48. Hawryluk GW, Bullock MR. Past, present, and future of traumatic brain injury research. *Neurosurg Clin N Am.* 2016;27(4):375–396. doi:10.1016/j.nec.2016.05.002.
49. Ma J, Huang S, Qin S, et al. Progesterone for acute traumatic brain injury. *Cochrane Database Syst Rev.* 2016;12:CD008409. doi:10.1002/14651858.CD008409.pub4.
50. Skolnick BE, Maas AI, Narayan RK, et al. A clinical trial of progesterone for severe traumatic brain injury. *N Engl J Med.* 2014;371(26):2467–2476. doi:10.1056/NEJMoa1411090.
51. Wright DW, Yeatts SD, Silbergleit R, et al. Very early administration of progesterone for acute traumatic brain injury. *N Engl J Med.* 2014;371(26):2457–2466. doi:10.1056/NEJMoa1404304.
52. Menon DK, Maas AI. EPO in traumatic brain injury: Two strikes but not out? *Lancet.* 2015;386(10012):2452–2454. doi:10.1016/S0140-6736(15)00387-6.
53. Gruenbaum SE, Zlotnik A, Gruenbaum BF, et al. Pharmacologic neuroprotection for functional outcomes after traumatic brain injury: A systematic review of the clinical literature. *CNS Drugs.* 2016;30(9): 791–806. doi:10.1007/s40263-016-0355-2.
54. Alali AS, Mukherjee K, McCredie VA, et al. Beta-blockers and traumatic brain injury: A systematic review, meta-analysis, and Eastern Association for the Surgery of Trauma Guideline. *Ann Surg.* 2017;266(6):952–961. doi:10.1097/SLA.0000000000002286.
55. Chen Z, Tang L, Xu X, et al. Therapeutic effect of beta-blocker in patients with traumatic brain injury: A systematic review and meta-analysis. *J Crit Care.* 2017;41:240–246. doi:10.1016/j.jcrc.2017.05.035.
56. Bhatnagar S, Iaccarino MA, Zafonte R. Pharmacotherapy in rehabilitation of post-acute traumatic brain injury. *Brain Res.* 2016;1640(Pt A):164–179. doi:10.1016/j.brainres.2016.01.021.
57. Davanso JR, Timmons SD. Use of consciousness-enhancing medications in the traumatic brain injury patient. In: Timmons SD, ed. *Controversies in Severe Traumatic Brain Injury Management.* Cham, Switzerland: Springer; 2018:179–190.
58. Maas AI, Murray GD, Roozenbeek B, et al. Advancing care for traumatic brain injury: Findings from the IMPACT studies and perspectives on future research. *Lancet Neurol.* 2013;12(12):1200–1210. doi:10.1016/S1474-4422(13)70234-5.
59. National Institutes of Health. BRAIN Initiative; 2014 [cited 2018 March 8, 2018]. http://www.braininitiative.nih.gov.
60. Omar M, Moore L, Lauzier F, et al. Complications following hospital admission for traumatic brain injury: A multicenter cohort study. *J Crit Care.* 2017;41:1–8. doi:10.1016/j.jcrc.2017.04.031.
61. Zimmermann LL, Diaz-Arrastia R, Vespa PM. Seizures and the role of anticonvulsants after traumatic brain injury. *Neurosurg Clin N Am.* 2016;27(4):499–508. doi:10.1016/j.nec.2016.06.001.
62. Bhullar IS, Johnson D, Paul JP, et al. More harm than good: Antiseizure prophylaxis after traumatic brain injury does not decrease seizure rates but may inhibit functional recovery. *J Trauma Acute Care Surg.* 2014;76(1):54–60. doi:10.1097/TA.0b013e3182aafd15.
63. Verduzco-Gutierrez M, Reddy CC, O'Dell MW. Is there a need for early seizure prophylaxis after traumatic brain injury? *PM R.* 2016;8(2):169–175. doi:10.1016/j.pmrj.2016.01.005.
64. Khan NR, Van Landingham MA, Fierst TM, et al. Should levetiracetam or phenytoin be used for posttraumatic seizure prophylaxis? A systematic review of the literature and meta-analysis. *Neurosurgery.* 2016;79(6):775–782. doi:10.1227/NEU.0000000000001445.
65. Xu JC, Shen J, Shao WZ, et al. The safety and efficacy of levetiracetam versus phenytoin for seizure prophylaxis after traumatic brain injury: A systematic review and meta-analysis. *Brain Inj.* 2016;30(9):1054–1061. doi:10.3109/02699052.2016.1170882.
66. Huijben JA, Volovici V, Cnossen MC, et al. Variation in general supportive and preventive intensive care management of traumatic brain injury: A survey in 66 neurotrauma centers participating in the Collaborative European NeuroTrauma Effectiveness Research in Traumatic Brain Injury (CENTER-TBI) study. *Crit Care.* 2018;22(1):90. doi:10.1186/s13054-018-2000-6.
67. Spencer DD, Jacobi J, Juenke JM, et al. Steady-state pharmacokinetics of intravenous levetiracetam in neurocritical care patients. *Pharmacotherapy.* 2011;31(10):934–941. doi:10.1592/phco.31.10.934.
68. Chapple LA, Chapman MJ, Lange K, et al. Nutrition support practices in critically ill head-injured patients: A global perspective. *Crit Care.* 2016;20:6. doi:10.1186/s13054-015-1177-1.
69. Patal R, Rosenthal G. Nutrition: Time to revisit. In: Timmons SD, ed. *Controversies in Severe Traumatic Brain Injury Management.* Cham, Switzerland: Springer; 2018:99–105.
70. Hermanides J, Plummer MP, Finnis M, et al. Glycaemic control targets after traumatic brain injury: A systematic review and meta-analysis. *Crit Care.* 2018;22(1):11. doi:10.1186/s13054-017-1883-y.
71. Bohman LE, Levine JM. Fever and therapeutic normothermia in severe brain injury: An update. *Curr Opin Crit Care.* 2014;20(2):182–188. doi:10.1097/MCC.0000000000000070.
72. Skrifvars MB, Bailey M, Presneill J, et al. Venous thromboembolic events in critically ill traumatic brain injury patients. *Intensive Care Med.* 2017;43(3):419–428. doi:10.1007/s00134-016-4655-2.
73. Benjamin E, Recinos G, Aiolfi A, et al. Pharmacological thromboembolic prophylaxis in traumatic brain injuries: Low molecular weight heparin is superior to unfractionated heparin. *Ann Surg.* 2017;266(3):463–469. doi:10.1097/SLA.0000000000002359.
74. Abdel-Aziz H, Dunham CM, Malik RJ, Hileman BM. Timing for deep vein thrombosis chemoprophylaxis in traumatic brain injury: An evidence-based review. *Crit Care.* 2015;19:96. doi:10.1186/s13054-015-0814-z.
75. Spano PJ, 2nd, Shaikh S, Boneva D, et al. Anticoagulant chemoprophylaxis in patients with traumatic brain injuries: A systematic review. *J Trauma Acute Care Surg.* 2020;88(3):454–460. doi:10.1097/TA.0000000000002580.
76. Joseph B, Aziz H, Zangbar B, et al. Acquired coagulopathy of traumatic brain injury defined by routine laboratory tests: Which laboratory values matter? *J Trauma Acute Care Surg.* 2014;76(1):121–125. doi:10.1097/TA.0b013e3182a9cc95.
77. Yuan Q, Wu X, Du ZY, et al. Low-dose recombinant factor VIIa for reversing coagulopathy in patients with isolated traumatic brain injury. *J Crit Care.* 2015;30(1):116–120. doi:10.1016/j.jcrc.2014.07.009.
78. Crash-trial collaborators. Effects of tranexamic acid on death, disability, vascular occlusive events and other morbidities in patients with acute traumatic brain injury (CRASH-3): A randomised, placebo-controlled trial. *Lancet.* 2019;394(10210):1713–1723. doi:10.1016/S0140-6736(19)32233-0.
79. Yokobori S, Yatabe T, Kondo Y, et al. Efficacy and safety of tranexamic acid administration in traumatic brain injury patients: A systematic review and meta-analysis. *J Intensive Care.* 2020;8:46. doi:10.1186/s40560-020-00460-5.
80. Udy AA, Jarrett P, Lassig-Smith M, et al. Augmented renal clearance in traumatic brain injury: A single-center observational study of atrial natriuretic peptide, cardiac output, and creatinine clearance. *J Neurotrauma.* 2017;34(1):137–144. doi:10.1089/neu.2015.4328.
81. Gerber LM, Chiu YL, Carney N, et al. Marked reduction in mortality in patients with severe traumatic brain injury. *J Neurosurg.* 2013;119(6):1583–1590. doi:10.3171/2013.8.JNS13276.
82. McCredie VA, Alali AS, Scales DC, et al. Impact of ICU structure and processes of care on outcomes after severe traumatic brain injury: A multicenter cohort study. *Crit Care Med.* 2018;46(7):1139–1149. doi: 10.1097/CCM.0000000000003149.
83. Cnossen MC, Polinder S, Andriessen TM, et al. Causes and consequences of treatment variation in moderate and severe traumatic brain injury: A multicenter study. *Crit Care Med.* 2017;45(4):660–669. doi:10.1097/CCM.0000000000002263.
84. Faul M, Wald MM, Rutland-Brown W, et al. Using a cost-benefit analysis to estimate outcomes of a clinical treatment guideline: Testing the Brain Trauma Foundation guidelines for the treatment of severe traumatic brain injury. *J Trauma.* 2007;63(6):1271–1278. doi: 10.1097/TA.0b013e3181493080.
85. Dawes AJ, Sacks GD, Cryer HG, et al. Compliance with evidence-based guidelines and interhospital variation in mortality for patients with severe traumatic brain injury. *JAMA Surg.* 2015;150(10):965–972. doi:10.1001/jamasurg.2015.1678.
86. Cnossen MC, Scholten AC, Lingsma HF, et al. Adherence to guidelines in adult patients with traumatic brain injury: A living systematic review. *J Neurotrauma.* 2016;33. doi: 10.1089/neu.2015.4121.

78

Parkinson Disease

Jessa M. Koch, Khashayar Dashtipour, and Jack J. Chen

KEY CONCEPTS

1. To optimize long-term therapeutic outcomes, minimize adverse effects, and improve quality of life for individuals with idiopathic Parkinson disease (PD), clinicians need to (1) continually access motor and nonmotor symptoms, (2) thoughtfully consider initial and adjunctive therapies, and (3) continually adjust medication dosages throughout the course of this illness.
2. In general, treatment should be initiated when the disease begins to interfere with activities of daily living, employment, or quality of life.
3. Surgery is an option for patients who require additional symptomatic relief or control of motor complications.
4. Anticholinergic medication can be useful for mild symptoms of PD but, due to adverse medication effects, it should be used with caution in older patients and those with pre-existing cognitive difficulties.
5. Monotherapy with amantadine or the irreversible monoamine oxidase type B (MAO-B) inhibitors provide symptomatic benefit, but less than that of dopamine agonists or carbidopa/levodopa (L-dopa).
6. Carbidopa/L-dopa is the most effective medication for symptomatic treatment.
7. Most patients treated with carbidopa/L-dopa will develop motor complications (eg, fluctuations and dyskinesias).
8. MAO-B inhibitors (irreversible and reversible), catechol-*O*-methyltransferase (COMT) inhibitors, and adenosine A2 receptor antagonists are useful add-on therapies to attenuate motor fluctuations in patients treated with carbidopa/L-dopa.
9. Amantadine is a useful add-on agent to attenuate dyskinesias.
10. Dopamine agonists are effective and, compared to L-dopa, associated with less risk of developing motor complications. They do, however, carry a greater risk for psychiatric symptoms, such as hallucinations and impulse control disorders.

BEYOND THE BOOK

Refer to Chapter 69: Parkinson Disease: Slow and Shaky Level III in *Pharmacotherapy Casebook: A Patient-Focused Approach* and read the initial patient presentation to answer the following questions.

(1) What medications may be considered for treatment of this patient's uncontrolled PD? List the different medication options along with specific treatment considerations for this particular patient such as adverse effects, tolerability concerns, etc.

(2) This patient shares that they just saw a commercial for a new medication for Parkinson disease, opicapone, and wants to know if this would be an option right now. Explain why opicapone would not be an initial medication choice for this patient.

(3) Upon closer evaluation of the patient case, you notice that there is no history of past medications this patient has used. You would like to get this information to assess for medication-induced parkinsonism. Create a list of medications that can cause parkinsonian symptoms, and the mechanism by which they can induce symptoms.

INTRODUCTION

The presence of bradykinesia (slowness of movements) along with tremor at rest, rigidity, and postural instability (instability of balance) is considered the hallmark motor features of idiopathic Parkinson disease (PD), a disorder of the extrapyramidal system. These clinical features of PD were adeptly described in 1817 by James Parkinson.[1]

EPIDEMIOLOGY

Up to 1 million individuals in the United States have PD, and this is only projected to increase over time.[2] The overall incidence rate of PD (ie, number of persons newly diagnosed with PD per year) is age- and sex-dependent. For individuals between the ages of 40 and 49 years, there are approximately 3 per 100,000 persons diagnosed with PD. However, for females in the ninth decade of life (ie, 80-89 years), the prevalence is 10 per 100,000 persons compared to males with an incidence of 250 per 100,000 persons.[3] The usual age at the time of diagnosis ranges between 55 and 65 years, and overall, PD affects less than 0.5% of people in their 60s and 2.5% of those older than 80 years.[4]

ETIOLOGY

Parkinson disease occurs sporadically, and the true etiology is unknown. However, the etiopathogenesis of PD likely involves environmental and genetic factors.[5] At the cellular level, degeneration of dopaminergic neurons (axons and soma) projecting from the substantia nigra pars compacta (SNc) to the striatum (caudate nucleus and putamen) is a hallmark of PD.[6] Additionally, neurons in autonomic ganglia, enteric nervous system, limbic system, olfactory bulb, spinal cord, and neocortex are affected. The underlying mechanisms are interconnected and multifaceted with the involvement of toxic biochemical reactions (excitotoxicity, nitric oxide toxicity, oxidative stress), abnormal cellular and cell death signaling pathways (apoptosis, inflammation), dysfunctional organelles (lysosomes, mitochondria), and dysfunctional protein degradation systems (autophagy, ubiquitin proteasomal system) resulting in cytoplasmic protein (α-synuclein) accumulation.[7] Several of these mechanisms result in excessive production of free radicals which exert stress on cells by damaging membranes and organelles. The SNc and the striatum are regions characterized by high levels of oxidative stress due to dopamine degradation and the Fenton reaction (Fig. 78-1).[8] Normally, intrinsic antioxidants (eg, glutathione) buffer against oxidative stress, but in PD, this buffer might be impaired or overwhelmed. Pathologic findings reveal a correlation between the extent of nigrostriatal dopamine loss and the severity of certain PD motor features (eg, bradykinesia and rigidity). At the time of PD onset, the estimated loss of SNc neurons and striatal dopamine content are 30% and 50%, respectively.[9] The loss of striatal dopamine exceeds the loss of SNc cell bodies because cellular degeneration begins in the distal presynaptic axon terminals and proceeds over time toward the cell body/soma (ie, "dying back" axonopathy).[9]

Aging, genetic constitution, lifestyle, and environmental factors likely increase an individual's risk for PD.[7,10] Epidemiologic research links environmental factors (eg, chronic exposure to pesticides), with an elevated risk. Cigarette smoking and caffeine consumption are consistently associated with a lower risk.[11,12] Genetic polymorphisms and epigenetics also modify an individual's risk for PD.[5,7,13] It is known that pesticide exposure and genetic forms of PD (eg, leucine-rich repeat kinase 2 [LRRK2], parkin, and PTEN-induced putative kinase 1 [PINK1]) are associated with mitochondrial dysfunction and oxidative stress.[7]

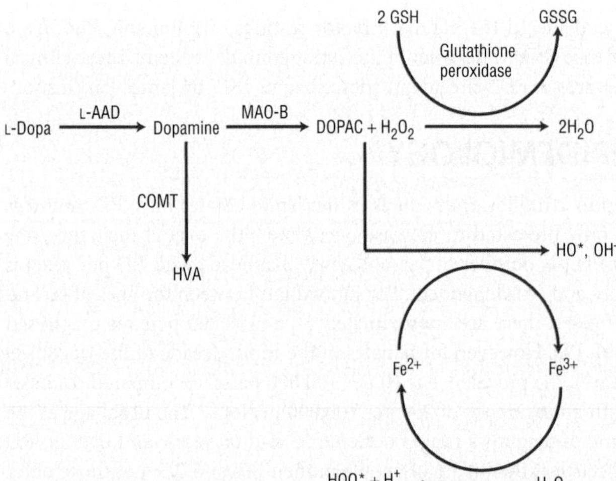

FIGURE 78-1 Dopamine metabolism results in hydrogen peroxide (H_2O_2) formation. In the Fenton reaction, H_2O_2 accepts an electron from ferrous iron (Fe^{2+}) to produce ferric iron (Fe^{3+}) and the hydroxyl radical (HO*). Fe^{3+} is reduced back to Fe^{2+} by another molecule of H_2O_2, forming a hydroperoxyl radical (HOO*). The radicals damage cell membranes and organelles (eg, mitochondria) and also induce apoptotic signaling. (COMT, catechol-*O*-methyltransferase; DOPAC, 3,4-dihydroxyphenylacetic acid; GSH, glutathione; GSSG, glutathione disulfide; H^+, proton; H_2O, water; HVA, homovanillic acid; L-AAD, L-aromatic amino acid decarboxylase; OH^-, the hydroxide ion; MAO-B, monoamine oxidase B).

PATHOPHYSIOLOGY

A function of the basal ganglia (composed of subcortical structures including the substantia nigra, striatum, globus pallidus, and subthalamic nucleus [STN]) is to regulate voluntary movement. These subcortical structures exist in duplicate, with one structure on each side of the midline. The substantia nigra consists of two parts: the SNc and pars reticulata (SNr). Neuronal projections from the SNc to the striatum are referred to as the *nigrostriatal pathway*. The striatum conveys signals to the SNr, via the dopamine$_1$ (D_1) direct and the dopamine$_2$ (D_2) indirect pathways (Fig. 78-2A). The SNr (which is closely linked to the globus pallidus interna [GPi]) receives signals from the striatum and conveys final processed signals to the thalamus, which serves as the "gateway" to the motor cortex. When examining the basal ganglia circuitry, it is important to note that striatal D_1 receptors are coupled to adenylate cyclase and mediate postsynaptic depolarization; thus, D_1 receptor activation results in stimulation of the striatal GABAergic neurons.[14,15] Increased activity of the direct pathway results in increased movement. In contrast, striatal D_2 receptors are coupled to a guanosine triphosphate-binding

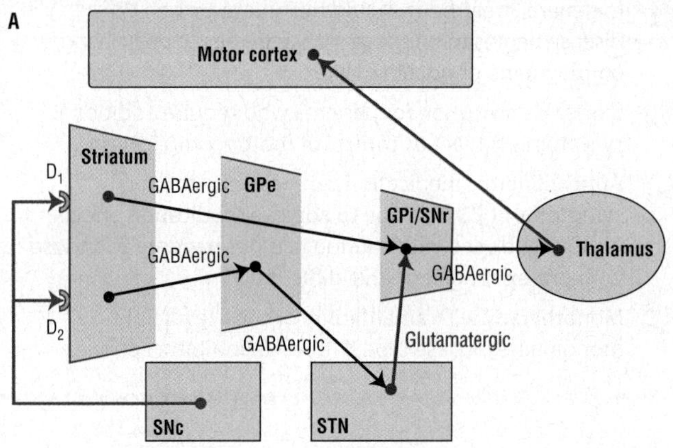

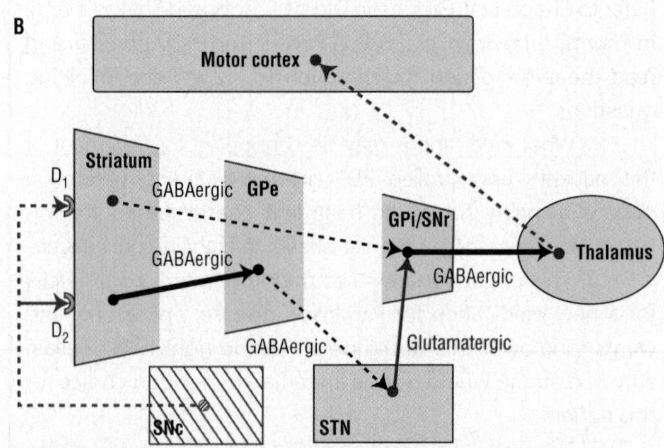

FIGURE 78-2 (*A*) Dopaminergic pathways of the basal ganglia–thalamocortical circuit. Activation of D_1 and D_2 receptors results in depolarization and hyperpolarization, respectively, of postsynaptic neurons. (Red dots and lines represent excitatory input; black dots and lines represent inhibitory input.) (*B*) In Parkinson's disease, degeneration of presynaptic nigrostriatal neurons results in inhibition of the thalamocortical circuit and reduced signaling to the motor cortex. (*Dashed lines* represent reduction of neurotransmitter activity; GPe, globus pallidus externa; GPi, globus pallidus interna; SNc, substantia nigra pars compacta; SNr, substantia nigra pars reticulata; STN, subthalamic nucleus.)

CLINICAL PRESENTATION Idiopathic PD

General Features

- The patient exhibits bradykinesia (slowness of movements) and at least one of the following: resting tremor, rigidity, or postural instability. Asymmetry of motor features is supportive.

Motor Symptoms

- The patient experiences hypokinetic movements, decreased manual dexterity, difficulty arising from a seated position, diminished arm swing during ambulation, dysarthria (slurred speech), dysphagia (difficulty with swallowing), festinating gait (tendency to pass from a walking to a running pace), flexed posture, "freezing" at initiation of movement, hypomimia (reduced facial animation), hypophonia (reduced voice volume), and micrographia (Fig. 78-3).

Autonomic and Sensory Symptoms

- The patient experiences bladder dysfunction, constipation, diaphoresis, fatigue, olfactory impairment, orthostatic intolerance, pain, paresthesia, paroxysmal vascular flushing, seborrhea, sexual dysfunction, and sialorrhea (drooling).

Mental Status Changes

- The patient experiences anxiety, apathy, bradyphrenia (slowness of thought processes), cognitive impairment, depression, and hallucinosis/psychosis.

Sleep Disturbances

- The patient experiences excessive daytime sleepiness, insomnia, obstructive sleep apnea, and rapid eye movement (REM) sleep behavior disorder.

Laboratory Tests

- No laboratory tests are available to diagnose PD.

Other Diagnostic Tests

- Genetic testing is not routinely helpful.
- Neuroimaging may be useful for excluding other diagnoses.
- Medication history should be obtained to rule out medication-induced parkinsonism.

protein and mediate postsynaptic hyperpolarization; thus, D_2 receptor activation results in inhibition of striatal GABAergic neurons, and a net reduction in movement.[14] Additionally, adenosine A2A receptors (A2AR) are located in the striatopallidal GABAergic neurons within this indirect pathway.[15] In PD, reduced dopaminergic activation of D_1 and D_2 receptors and the sequential downstream effect on signaling pathways result in a net inhibitory tone on the thalamus (Fig. 78-2B). Dopaminergic therapies help restore functional activity within the D_1 and D_2 pathways with the latter primarily responsible for mediating clinical improvements. Antagonism of A2ARs (ie, inhibition of the indirect pathway) can result in prolongation of dopaminergic action in PD and is the mechanism of action behind the non-dopaminergic treatment option, istradefylline.[15,16]

Within the SNc, histopathologic features of PD are (1) depigmentation of dopamine-producing neurons (ie, loss of SNc neurons) and (2) presence of Lewy bodies (cytoplasmic filamentous aggregates composed of the protein α-synuclein) in the remaining neurons.[6] Lewy bodies appear in association with adjacent gliosis (ie, a response of glial cells to injury), and the formation and spread of Lewy pathology is proposed to occur in stages. In the premotor stage of PD, Lewy bodies are found in the medulla oblongata, locus coeruleus, raphe nuclei, enteric nervous system, and olfactory bulb. This provides anatomic correlates to observations that mood (eg, anxiety, depression) and peripheral symptoms (eg, constipation, impaired olfaction) are present in premotor stages of PD. Lewy pathology develops peripherally in the enteric nervous system and olfactory system and may spread anterogradely or retrogradely to the brain.[17] With the development of Lewy pathology in the midbrain (particularly the SNc), motor features begin to emerge. In advanced stages, Lewy pathology spreads to the cortex, and this may correlate with cognitive and additional behavior changes. Recent investigations have shown that α-synuclein pathology can propagate into adjacent healthy neurons in a nontoxic infectious manner that results in subsequent neuronal toxicity.[3,18]

The synaptic organization of the basal ganglia also involves a variety of other neurotransmitters and neuromodulators, including acetylcholine, adenosine, enkephalins, γ-aminobutyric acid (GABA), glutamate, serotonin, and substance P. The potential role for medication modulation of these other neurotransmitters and receptor types is an active area of research and novel therapeutic discovery.[19]

Atypical parkinsonian disorders such as multiple system atrophy and progressive supranuclear palsy are characterized by damage to postsynaptic striatal neurons and dopamine receptors. Therefore, dopaminergic therapies are less efficacious in atypical parkinsonism.

The clinical diagnosis of PD is based on the presence of bradykinesia and at least one of three other features: muscular rigidity, resting tremor, and/or postural instability (Table 78-1).[20] Asymmetry of motor features is a supportive finding. It is important to note that tremor is not always present at the time of diagnosis, and postural instability typically occurs in later stages of PD. Overall, a diagnosis of PD can be made with a high level of confidence in a patient who has bradykinesia (along with rest tremor and/or rigidity), prominent asymmetry, and a good response to dopaminergic therapy. For the diagnosis of PD, other conditions must be reasonably excluded (see Table 78-1). Medication-induced parkinsonism can mimic PD and is the second most common form of parkinsonism.[21] It is important to assess for recent use of medications, especially medications that block D_2 receptors, such as antipsychotics (eg, haloperidol), metoclopramide, or phenothiazine antiemetics (eg, prochlorperazine).[21] Neurologic conditions that can be mistaken for PD include atypical parkinsonisms and tremor disorders (eg, dystonic tremor, essential tremor). Because the management and prognosis of PD differ from these other conditions, obtaining an accurate diagnosis is important. When the diagnosis is in doubt, referral to a movement disorders specialist is recommended. Currently, efforts are underway to develop and validate diagnostic tools based on personalized clinical, laboratory, imaging, and genomics data.

TABLE 78-1 Diagnostic Criteria and Differential Diagnosis for Parkinson Disease

Parkinson Disease

- Step 1: Presence of bradykinesia and at least one of the following: resting tremor, rigidity, or postural instability
- Step 2: Exclude other types of parkinsonism or tremor disorders (see "Differential Diagnosis" below)
- Step 3: Presence of at least three supportive positive criteria:
  - Asymmetry of motor signs/symptoms
  - Unilateral onset
  - Progressive disorder
  - Resting tremor
  - Excellent response to carbidopa/L-dopa
  - L-dopa response for 5 years or longer
  - Presence of L-dopa dyskinesias

Differential Diagnosis

- Essential tremor
- Pharmacotoxicity (medication-induced)
  - Antiemetics (eg, metoclopramide, prochlorperazine)
  - Antipsychotics (eg, chlorpromazine, fluphenazine, haloperidol, olanzapine, risperidone, thioridazine)
  - Other medications (α-methyldopa, cinnarizine, flunarizine, tetrabenazine)
- Environmental toxicity (eg, manganese, organophosphates)
- Infections (eg, human immunodeficiency virus, subacute sclerosing panencephalitis)
- Metabolic disorder (eg, hypothyroidism, parathyroid abnormalities)
- Neoplasms, strokes, traumatic lesions involving the nigrostriatal pathways
- Normal-pressure hydrocephalus
- Parkinsonism with other neuronal system degenerations
  - Corticobasal ganglionic degeneration
- Multiple-system atrophies
- Progressive supranuclear palsy
- Familial (hereditary) parkinsonism
  - Autosomal dominant
  - α-Synuclein gene mutation (*PARK1* and *PARK4*)
  - L-responsive dystonia
  - Leucine-rich repeat kinase 2 (LRRK2) mutation
  - Rapid-onset dystonia parkinsonism (DYT12)
  - Spinocerebellar ataxias (SCA2, SCA3)
- Autosomal recessive
  - Wilson disease
  - Young-onset parkinsonism (DJ-1, parkin, PINK1)
- X-linked recessive
  - Fragile X tremor/ataxia syndrome (FXTAS)
  - Lubag (DYT3 or Filipino dystonia parkinsonism)

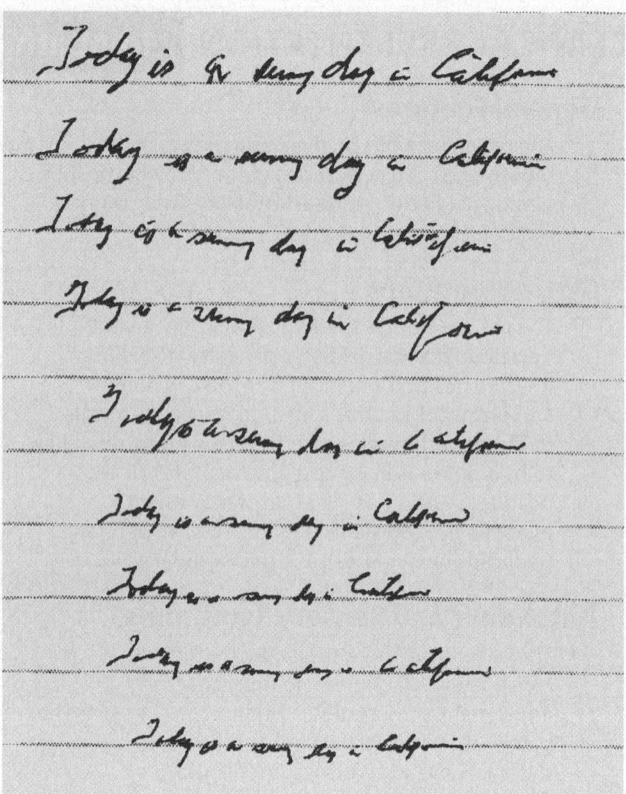

FIGURE 78-3 Example of micrographia in a patient with Parkinson disease. As the sentence "Today is a sunny day in California" is repeatedly handwritten, progressive diminution of letter size occurs (micrographia). The height of each lined row is approximately 5/16 in. (8 mm).

Parkinson disease develops insidiously and progressively worsens over many years. Tremor of an upper extremity occurring at rest (and occasionally an action or postural tremor) is often the sole presenting complaint. However, only two-thirds of patients with PD have tremor on diagnosis, and some never develop this sign. Tremor in PD is present most commonly in the hands, sometimes with a characteristic pill-rolling motion. Less commonly, tremor may involve the jaw or legs. Like other motor features of PD, resting tremor often begins unilaterally and becomes bilateral with disease progression. Stressful or emotional (either negative or positive) situations often increase the tremor amplitude and severity. Usually, tremor is absent during sleep. Although resting tremor is visibly noticeable in PD and may cause social embarrassment for the patient, it often is the least physically disabling of the motor features.

Rigidity is the increased muscular resistance to passive range of motion and most commonly affects the upper and lower extremities and occasionally the neck. If tremor is present in the affected extremity, the rigidity is associated with a cogwheel or ratchet-like quality upon examination. Facial muscles also are affected, resulting in hypomimia that may be erroneously interpreted as apathy, depression, or unfriendliness.

Hypokinesia is a decreased movement and often described as either bradykinesia (slowness of movement) or akinesia (absence of movement). Movement in PD is often slow throughout an intended action and difficulty with the initiation of movement also occurs. A progressive slowing and decline in dexterity may impair tasks such as hand clapping, finger tapping, and handwriting (Fig. 78-3). Intermittent immobility or akinesia (freezing) is another common characteristic. Freezing is especially likely to occur in situations such as when walking through a narrow doorway or initiating a turn.

The clinical diagnosis of PD relies on motor findings; however, neuroimaging along with nonmotor markers (eg, REM sleep behavior disorder, olfactory impairment) may someday aid in the detection of PD in premotor or prodromal stages (ie, before onset of motor impairment).[22]

Postural instability, most common in advanced stages of PD, is one of the most disabling problems of PD because it increases the fall risk and is least amenable to pharmacotherapy.[23] Testing for impaired postural responses by means of the pull test (in which a patient is unable to recover balance after sudden backward displacement at the shoulders) can help identify the risk for falling. Many patients with impaired postural responses also have tendencies for propulsive gait with difficulty halting their steps while in motion (festination) and freezing, which also increases the risk of falling.

Nonmotor symptoms are common in PD and must be identified, assessed, managed, and monitored (Table 78-2). These include anxiety, cognitive impairment, constipation, daytime sleepiness, depression, drooling, dysphagia, falling, fatigue, impulsivity,

TABLE 78-2 Nonmotor Symptoms and Possible Treatments

Symptoms	Possible Treatments
Anxiety	Cognitive behavioral therapy, selective serotonin reuptake inhibitors, serotonin-norepinephrine reuptake inhibitors, minimize "off" times
Cognitive impairment	Eliminate anticholinergic agents, add cholinesterase inhibitor
Constipation	Fiber, hydration, exercise, laxatives, stool softeners
Daytime sleepiness	Proper nighttime sleep hygiene, reduce dose of dopaminergic medications, eliminate anticholinergic agents if possible, referral to sleep specialist to rule outsleep apnea and sleep disorders
Depression	Selective serotonin reuptake inhibitor, serotonin norepinephrine reuptake inhibitor, cognitive behavioral therapy
Drooling	Local injection of botulinum toxin, atropine sublingual drop, glycopyrrolate, ipratropium sublingual spray
Dysphagia	Referral to speech therapist, dysphagia diet, avoid anticholinergic medications, manage dry mouth
Fatigue	Caffeine, armodafinil, modafinil, proper nighttime sleep hygiene, referral to sleep specialist to rule out sleep disorder
Falling	Assess for orthostatic hypotension, referral to physical therapy, assistance with ambulation, minimize risk for bone fractures, treat osteoporosis
Hallucinations/ psychosis	Dose reduction and/or elimination of adjunctive medications, especially anticholinergic agents; consider addition of pimavanserin, quetiapine or clozapine; Note: pimavanserin is FDA-approved for psychosis in PD
Impulse control disorder	Discontinue dopamine agonist or add clozapine, quetiapine, or naltrexone
Insomnia	Cognitive behavioral therapy-insomnia; nonbenzodiazepine $GABA_A$ agonists, trazodone
Orthostatic hypotension	Reduce dose of alpha-blockers, dopamine agonist, diuretics, and/or vasodilators, abdominal compression, add salt and water to diet, water boluses, fludrocortisone, midodrine, droxidopa, pyridostigmine
Overactive bladder	Behavioral therapies (eg, bladder training, fluid management, pelvic floor muscle exercises), antimuscarinic agents, mirabegron, intradetrusor injections of botulinum toxin
Pain	Treatment as per type of pain (eg, dystonic, musculoskeletal, neuropathic), minimize "off" times, appropriate referral to orthopedics, physical therapy, pain specialist, rheumatology
REM sleep behavior disorder	Clonazepam, melatonin
Restless legs syndrome	Dopamine agonist at bedtime; gabapentin

FDA, Food and Drug Administration; GABA, γ-aminobutyric acid; PD, Parkinson disease; REM, rapid eye movement.

insomnia, orthostatic hypotension, overactive bladder, pain, hallucinations/psychosis, REM sleep behavior disorder, and restless legs syndrome.[24] As a component of managing these nonmotor symptoms, it is important to maintain continuous surveillance of prescription and nonprescription medications for potential adverse effects that can exacerbate, mimic, or precipitate nonmotor symptoms. If feasible, any identified offending medication should be deprescribed.

TREATMENT

Desired Outcomes

To date, no treatments effectively change the course of PD by slowing or halting its progression (disease modification).[25] Therefore, the goal for management is to improve motor and nonmotor symptoms so that patients are able to maintain the best possible quality of life.[26] Specific objectives to consider when selecting an intervention include preserving the ability to perform activities of daily living, employment, improvement of mobility, minimization of adverse effects, treatment complications, putative disease modification, and improvement of nonmotor features. To accomplish some of these objectives, consultation with a team of specialists is helpful (eg, movement disorders, pharmacotherapy, physical therapy, psychiatry, and sleep medicine).

General Approach to Treatment

1 2 To optimize long-term therapeutic outcomes, minimize adverse effects, and improve quality of life for individuals with PD, clinicians need to (1) continually access motor and nonmotor symptoms, (2) thoughtfully consider initial and adjunctive therapies, and (3) continually adjust medication dosages throughout the course of this illness. Figure 78-4 illustrates a general treatment approach for early and advanced PD. Table 78-3 summarizes antiparkinsonian medications and dosing, and Table 78-4 summarizes monitoring parameters for potential adverse reactions, and Table 78-5 indicates place in therapy for antiparkinsonian medications (ie, monotherapy, adjunctive). Treatment guidelines and monographs are updated frequently to keep up with new information and changes in treatment paradigms.[24,27-30] Additionally, general guidelines and recommendations for geriatric health maintenance and disease prevention (eg, bone health, routine vaccinations, vitamin and mineral supplementations) should also be observed.

When deciding on therapy for a patient, the following patient-specific factors should be taken into account: age; comorbidities; severity of functional impairment; nonmotor symptoms; patient preferences, therapeutic goals, and outcomes; employment status; medication tolerability; presence of cognitive impairment or motor complications; need for skilled assistance; and health-related economics.[30] The lowest dose of antiparkinsonian medication that provides satisfactory symptomatic results should be used, and for patients already on carbidopa/levodopa (L-dopa), optimization of the regimen should be attempted before adding adjunctive agents (see Table 78-5 for which agents may be used as monotherapy, on demand therapy, and adjunctive therapy). With the increasing motor disability, emergence of medication adverse effects, and changes in severity of nonmotor symptoms, therapy adjustments (eg, dose reductions, medication addition, or discontinuation) are expected, and desired therapeutic endpoints should be routinely reassessed. There are no pharmacogenomic parameters used to guide PD pharmacotherapy.

For mild functional impairment, initial monotherapy may be initiated with an MAO-B inhibitor, such as rasagiline, with the addition of other therapeutic agents as PD motor symptoms progressively worsen. Dopamine agonist monotherapy provides greater symptomatic benefit for patients with mild-to-moderate impairment. However, dopamine agonists are less well tolerated, especially in older patients and for those who are cognitively impaired, intolerant of dopamine agonists, or experiencing moderate or severe functional impairment, carbidopa/L-dopa is preferred.[28-30] Ultimately, all patients will require the use of carbidopa/L-dopa either as monotherapy or in combination with other agents. With the development of motor fluctuations, patients should administer carbidopa/L-dopa more frequently or addition of a catechol-O-methyltransferase (COMT) inhibitor, MAO-B inhibitor, A2AR antagonist, or

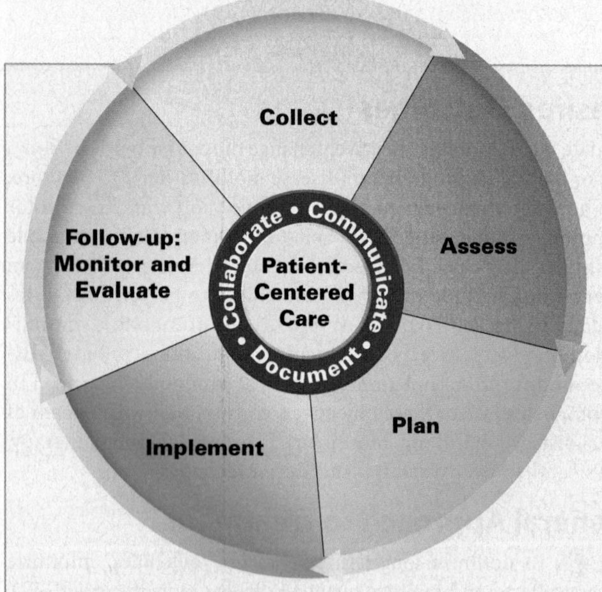

Patient Care Process for Parkinson Disease

The image shows the five fundamental steps included in The Pharmacist's Care Process endorsed by the Joint Commission for Pharmacy Practitioners (2014). The tagline of this process reads collaborate, communicate, and document. The five fundamental steps listed here are collect, assess, plan, implement, and follow-up: monitor and evaluate. All these steps are listed in a circular block diagram.

Collect

- Patient characteristics (eg, age, race, sex, hand dominance)
- Patient history (past medical, family, social—dietary habits, alcohol and tobacco use)
- Motor and nonmotor symptoms (see Tables 78-1 and 78-2)
- Current medications, prior medication use for PD and response to prior medications (eg, effectiveness, adverse effects), prior use of dopamine receptor blockers
- Objective data
    - Height, weight
    - Blood pressure and orthostatic blood pressure
    - Labs (eg, serum creatinine [Scr], liver function tests [LFTs])
    - Other diagnostic tests when indicated (eg, neuroimaging)

Assess

- Past and current use of medications associated with medication-induced parkinsonism (eg, antipsychotics, metoclopramide, tetrabenazine)
- Difficulties with performing activities of daily living
- Gait difficulties and fall risk
- Motor or nonmotor symptoms that are most troublesome for the patient
- Appropriateness, effectiveness, and adverse effects of current medications for the motor and nonmotor symptoms of PD
- Presence of motor complications (eg, motor fluctuations, dyskinesias, freezing)

Plan*

- Tailored lifestyle modifications (eg, exercise)
- Pharmacotherapy regimen including specific medications for PD, dose, route, frequency, and duration; specify the continuation and discontinuation of existing therapies (see Table 78-3)
- Monitoring parameters including efficacy (eg, symptom improvement) and tolerability medication-specific adverse effects (see Table 78-4), and time frame
- Patient education (eg, purpose of treatment, lifestyle modification, pharmacotherapy, adverse effects)
- Self-monitoring of symptoms—where and how to record results
- Referrals to other providers when appropriate (eg, physician, physical therapy, speech therapy)

Implement*

- Provide patient education regarding all elements of treatment plan
- Use motivational interviewing and coaching strategies to maximize adherence
- Schedule follow-up

Follow-up: Monitor and Evaluate

- Symptom relief goal attainment
- Presence of adverse effects
- Occurrence of motor complications, falls, and development/progression of nonmotor symptoms
- Patient adherence to treatment plan using multiple sources of information

Collaborate with patient, caregivers, and other healthcare professionals.

dopamine agonist to the carbidopa/L-dopa regimen should be considered. For management of carbidopa/L-dopa–induced peak-dose dyskinesias, a reduction in L-dopa dose and/or addition of amantadine should be considered. Surgery is considered only in patients who need more symptomatic control or who are experiencing severe motor complications despite pharmacologically optimized therapy.

Ultimately, the treatment plan must evolve as the disease progresses and must include consideration of short-term symptomatic relief as well as long-term effects. Patient education should be communicated with realistic optimism. For example, although there is no cure for PD, medications that can provide relief of symptoms. Nonpharmacologic interventions such as exercise should be encouraged, and problematic nonmotor features of PD should always be addressed.

Nonpharmacologic Therapy

A number of nonpharmacological modalities may help improve motor and non-motor symptoms of PD in combination with

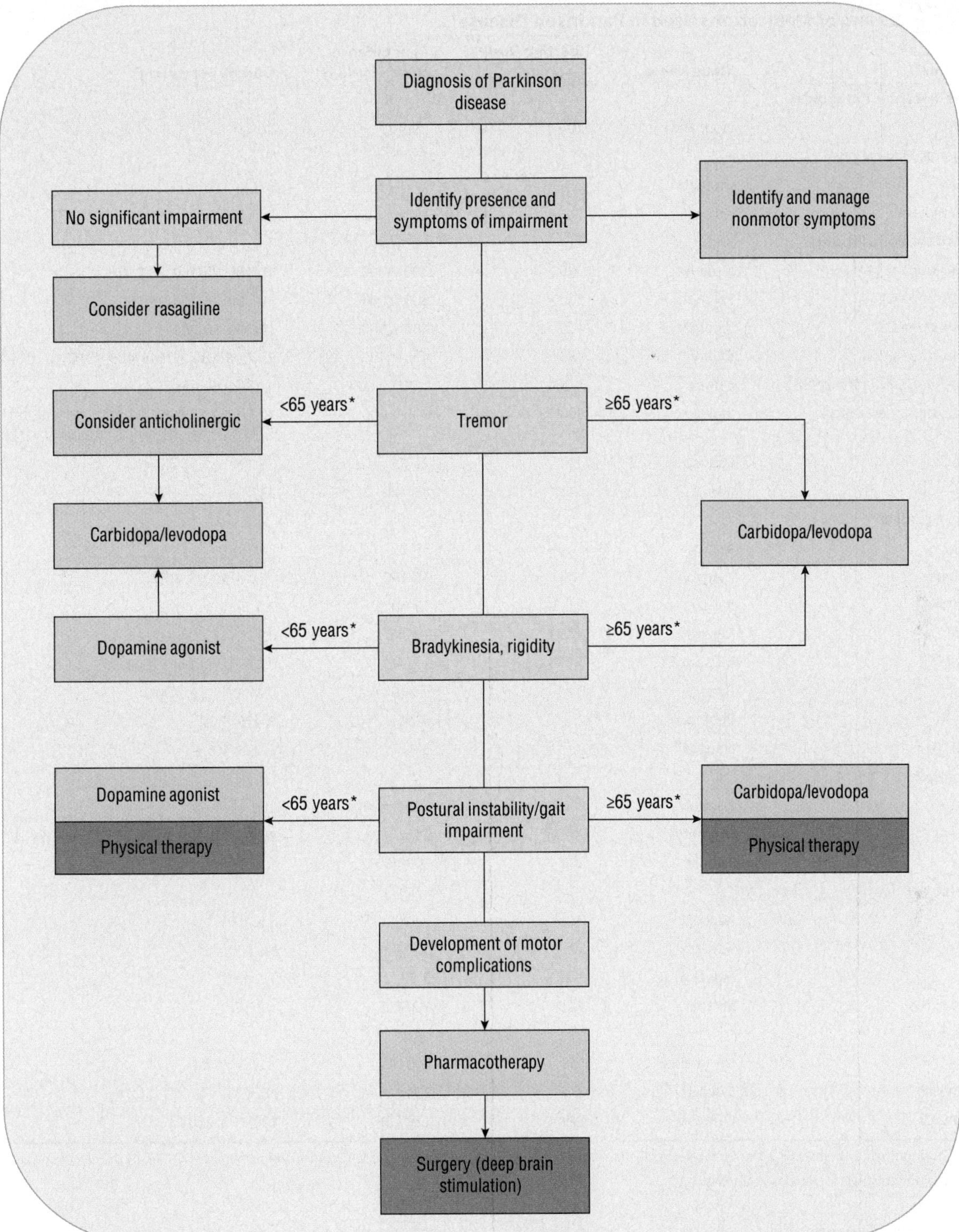

FIGURE 78-4 General approach to the management of early to advanced Parkinson disease. (*Age is not the sole determinant for medication choice. Other factors such as cognitive function and overall medication tolerability, especially in older patients should be considered.)

appropriate pharmacotherapy. Exercise, physiotherapy, yoga, Tai Chi, and dance have evidence to support improvement in PD symptoms.[32] A specific form of physiotherapy that patients with PD may particularly benefit from is the Lee Silvermann Voice Treatment-BIG Therapy. This therapy focuses on increasing the amplitude of movements by focusing on proprioception using sensory cues.[33]

Surgical Therapy

3 Surgery should be considered an adjunct to pharmacotherapy when patients are experiencing frequent motor fluctuations or disabling dyskinesia or tremor despite an optimized medical regimen. There are several patient-selection criteria for surgery, including a diagnosis of L-dopa–responsive PD and absence of cognitive impairment. Anatomic targets include the thalamus, GPi, and the STN. Bilateral, chronic, high-frequency electrical stimulation, also known as deep-brain stimulation (DBS), is the preferred surgical modality.[34]

In DBS surgery, a battery-powered neurostimulator is implanted subcutaneously below the clavicle and provides constant electrical stimulation, via electrode wires, to the targeted brain structure.

TABLE 78-3 Dosing of Medications Used in Parkinson Disease[a]

Generic Name	Trade Name	Starting Dose[b] (mg/day)	Maintenance Dose[b] (mg/day)	Dosage Forms (mg)
Adenosine-Receptor Antagonist				
Istradefylline	Nourianz	20	20-40	20, 40
Anticholinergic Medications				
Benztropine	Cogentin	0.5-1	1-6	0.5, 1, 2
Trihexyphenidyl	Artane	1-2	6-15	2, 5, 2/5 mL
Carbidopa/Levodopa Products				
Carbidopa/L-dopa	Sinemet	300[c]	300-2,000[c]	10/100, 25/100, 25/250
Carbidopa/L-dopa ODT	Parcopa	300[c]	300-2,000[c]	10/100, 25/100, 25/250
Carbidopa/L-dopa CR	Sinemet CR	400[c]	400-2,000[c]	25/100, 50/200
Carbidopa/L-dopa IR/ER	Rytary	435[c]	435-2,450[c]	23.75/95, 36.25/145, 48.75/195, 61.25/245[d]
Carbidopa/L-dopa enteral suspension	Duopa	1,000[c]	1,000-2,000[c]	4.63/20 per mL
Carbidopa/L-dopa/entacapone	Stalevo	600[e]	600-1,600[e]	12.5/50/200, 18.75/75/200, 25/100/200, 31.25/125/200, 37.5/150/200, 50/200/200
Carbidopa	Lodosyn	25	25-75	25
Levodopa	Inbrija	84	84-420	42[f]
Dopamine Agonists				
Apomorphine	Apokyn	1-3	3-12	30/3 mL[g]
Apomorphine	Kynmobi	10	10-150	10, 15, 20, 25, 30[h]
Bromocriptine	Parlodel	2.5-5	15-40	2.5, 5
Pramipexole	Mirapex	0.125	1.5-4.5	0.125, 0.25, 0.5, 0.75, 1, 1.5
Pramipexole ER	Mirapex ER	0.375	1.5-4.5	0.375, 0.75, 1.5, 2.25, 3, 3.75, 4.5
Ropinirole	Requip	0.75	9-24	0.25, 0.5, 1, 2, 3, 4, 5
Ropinirole XL	Requip XL	2	8-24	2, 4, 6, 8, 12
Rotigotine	Neupro	2	2-8	1, 2, 3, 4, 6, 8
COMT Inhibitors				
Entacapone	Comtan	200-600	200-1,600	200
Opicapone	Ongentys	25-50	50	25, 50
Tolcapone	Tasmar	300	300-600	100, 200
MAO-B Inhibitors				
Rasagiline	Azilect	0.5-1	0.5-1	0.5, 1
Safinamide	Xadago	50	50-100	50, 100
Selegiline	Eldepryl	5-10	5-10	5
Selegiline ODT	Zelapar	1.25	1.25-2.5	1.25, 2.5
Miscellaneous				
Amantadine	Symmetrel	100	200-300	100, 50/5 mL
Amantadine ER	Gocovri	137	274	68.5, 137
Amantadine ER	Osmolex	129	129-258	129, 193, 258

COMT, catechol-*O*-methyltransferase; CR, controlled-release; IR, immediate-release; ER, extended-release; MAO, monoamine oxidase; ODT, orally disintegrating tablet.

[a]Marketed in the United States for Parkinson disease.

[b]Dosages may vary.

[c]Dosages expressed as L-dopa component.

[d]Dosages of Rytary were developed to avoid confusion with other oral carbidopa/L-dopa products that contain L-dopa in multiples of 50 mg.

[e]Dosages expressed as entacapone component.

[f]Capsule containing levodopa dry powder for inhalation.

[g]Sterile solution of subcutaneous injection with supplied pen injector.

[h]Sublingual film of apomorphine.

Data from Reference 31.

Thalamic DBS is effective for suppressing tremor (specifically arm tremor), but it does not significantly improve the other parkinsonian features (bradykinesia, rigidity, motor fluctuations, or dyskinesias). Both STN and GPi DBS are associated with improvements in tremor, rigidity, bradykinesia, motor fluctuations, dyskinesia, and activities of daily living; however, STN DBS allows for greater reduction in medications.[35] As with pharmacotherapy, DBS uncommonly improves gait or postural instability.

DBS procedures require routine adjustment of the electrical stimulation parameters (eg, voltage, frequency, and pulse width) to achieve optimal control while minimizing adverse effects. The electrical stimulation parameters (or "electrical dosage") are adjusted via a programmable handheld device to meet each patient's needs and are performed by physicians as well as other trained individuals, including nurse practitioners and clinical pharmacists.

TABLE 78-4 Monitoring of Potential Adverse Reactions to Pharmacotherapy for Parkinson Disease

Generic Name	Adverse Medication Reaction	Monitoring Parameter	Comments
Amantadine	Confusion Livedo reticularis	Mental status; renal function Lower extremity examination; ankle edema	Reduce dosage; adjust dose for renal impairment Reversible upon medication discontinuation
	Livedo reticularis	Lower extremity examination; ankle edema	Reversible upon medication discontinuation
Benztropine and Trihexyphenidyl	Anticholinergic effects, confusion, drowsiness	Dry mouth, mental status, constipation, urinary retention, vision	Reduce dosage; avoid in elderly and in those with a history of constipation, memory impairment, urinary retention
Carbidopa/L-dopa	Drowsiness Dyskinesias Nausea	Mental status Abnormal involuntary movements Nausea	Reduce dose Reduce dose; add amantadine Take with food (eg, nonprotein snack)
Istradefylline	Insomnia, dizziness, nausea, constipation	Sleep, nausea, bowel movements	Take in the morning Take with food
COMT Inhibitors			
Entacapone	Augmentation of L-dopa adverse effects; also diarrhea	See carbidopa/L-dopa; also bowel movements	Reduce dose of L-dopa; antidiarrheal agents
Opicapone	Augmentation of L-dopa adverse effects, constipation	Mental status, abnormal involuntary movements, bowel movements	Reduce dose of L-dopa
Tolcapone	See entacapone; also liver toxicity	See carbidopa/L-dopa; also ALT/AST	See carbidopa/L-dopa; also at start of therapy and for every dose increase, ALT and AST levels at baseline and every 2-4 weeks for the first 6 months of therapy; afterward monitor based on clinical judgment
Dopamine Agonists			
Apomorphine	Drowsiness Nausea Orthostatic hypotension	Mental status Nausea Blood pressure, dizziness upon standing	Reduce dose Premedicate with trimethobenzamide Reduce dose
Bromocriptine	See pramipexole; also pulmonary fibrosis	Mental status; also chest radiograph	Reduce dose; chest radiograph at baseline and once yearly
Pramipexole and Ropinirole	Confusion Drowsiness Edema Hallucinations/delusions Impulsivity Nausea Orthostatic hypotension	Mental status Lower extremity swelling Behavior, mental status Nausea Blood pressure, dizziness upon standing	Reduce dose Reduce dose or discontinue medication Reduce dose or discontinue medication Titrate dose upward slowly; take with food
Rotigotine	See pramipexole; also skin irritation at site of patch application	See pramipexole; also skin examination	See pramipexole; rotate patch application site
MAO-B Inhibitors			
Rasagiline	Nausea	Nausea	Take with food
Safinamide	Nausea Elevation in blood pressure Insomnia	Nausea Blood pressure Sleep	Take with food Monitor blood pressure if have a history of uncontrolled hypertension Take in the morning
Selegiline	Agitation/confusion Insomnia Hallucinations Orthostatic hypotension	Mental status Sleep Behavior, mental status Blood pressure, dizziness upon standing	Reduce dose Administer dose earlier in day Reduce dose Reduce dose

ALT, alanine aminotransferase; AST, aspartate aminotransferase; COMT, catechol-*O*-methyltransferase; MAO, monoamine oxidase.

Pharmacologic Therapy

Anticholinergic Medications

4 Dopamine provides negative feedback to acetylcholine neurons in the striatum; therefore, degeneration of nigrostriatal dopamine neurons affects striatal cholinergic interneuron activity. Recent research investigated the effect of dopamine loss on the striatal interneurons in mice models. Initially, the striatal interneurons decreased acetylcholine production slightly, but with the even greater loss of dopamine (which occurs throughout the progression of PD), the balance among the two neurotransmitters shifted to greater acetylcholine levels.[36] This increased cholinergic activity is believed to contribute to the tremor of PD. The anticholinergic medications (eg, benztropine and trihexyphenidyl) are considered effective against tremor, but no more so than dopaminergic agents.[28] Sometimes dystonic symptoms associated with PD are also improved by anticholinergic agents. Use of anticholinergic agents is limited due to the development of intolerable anticholinergic adverse effects (see Table 78-4), necessitating medication discontinuation. Younger patients are better able to tolerate anticholinergic adverse effects, whereas this medication class is avoided in patients with advanced age, pre-existing cognitive deficits, and dysphagia.[37,38]

Amantadine

5 Although amantadine can be used as monotherapy for the management of tremor, rigidity, and bradykinesia, it is most often used

TABLE 78-5 Summary of Medications for Parkinson Disease Regarding Type: Monotherapy, Adjunctive, and/or On-Demand Options Summary of Medications for Parkinson Disease Regarding Type: Monotherapy, Adjunctive, and/or On-Demand Options

Medication	Class	Monotherapy	Adjunctive	On-Demand
Amantadine	NMDA receptor antagonist	X (rarely)	X	
Apomorphine	Dopamine agonist			X
Benztropine	Anticholinergic	X	X	
Carbidopa	Decarboxylase inhibitor		X[a]	
Entacapone	COMT inhibitor		X[a]	
Istradefylline	Adenosine-receptor antagonist		X	
Levodopa	Dopamine precursor	X	X	X
Opicapone	COMT inhibitor		X[a]	
Pramipexole	Dopamine agonist	X	X	
Rasagiline	MAO-B inhibitor	X	X	
Ropinirole	Dopamine agonist	X	X	
Rotigotine	Dopamine agonist	X	X	
Safinamide	MAO-B inhibitor	X	X	
Selegeline	MAO-B inhibitor		X	
Tolcapone	COMT inhibitor		X[a]	
Trihexyphenidyl	Anticholinergic	X	X	

Of note, table is based upon FDA-approved indications. Some agents may be used off-label as monotherapy/adjunct.
[a]Must be used in combination with Levodopa.

adjunctively for management of L-dopa–induced dyskinesia and in patients experiencing "off" episodes[28,29,39] (Table 78-3). The precise mechanism of action of amantadine for management of PD is unknown, but enhancement of dopamine release from presynaptic terminals and inhibition of glutamatergic *N*-methyl-D-aspartate (NMDA) receptors are implicated.[40] The antidyskinetic properties of amantadine are presumed to be mediated by antiglutamate properties which, in the setting of dyskinesias, dominate over dopaminergic properties. There are currently three different formulations of amantadine available for use; an immediate release (IR) formulation and two different extended release (ER) products. Amantadine immediate-release is typically administered 300 mg/day in divided doses, whereas the extended-release formulations allow for once a day dosing (see Table 78-3).[41] Amantadine is eliminated renally, and a reduced dose should be administered when renal dysfunction is present (eg, amantadine immediate-release 100 mg/day with creatinine clearances of 30-50 mL/min [0.50-0.84 mL/s], 100 mg every other day for creatinine clearances of 15-29 mL/min [0.25-0.49 mL/s], and 200 mg every 7 days for creatinine clearances of less than 15 mL/min [0.25 mL/s], and patients on hemodialysis).[42]

Adverse effects of amantadine include confusion, dizziness, dry mouth, and hallucinations with elderly patients being particularly prone to develop confusion.[43,44] Not uncommonly, amantadine may cause livedo reticularis, a reversible condition characterized by diffuse mottling of the skin affecting the upper or lower extremities and often accompanied by lower-extremity edema (see Table 78-4).[45,46]

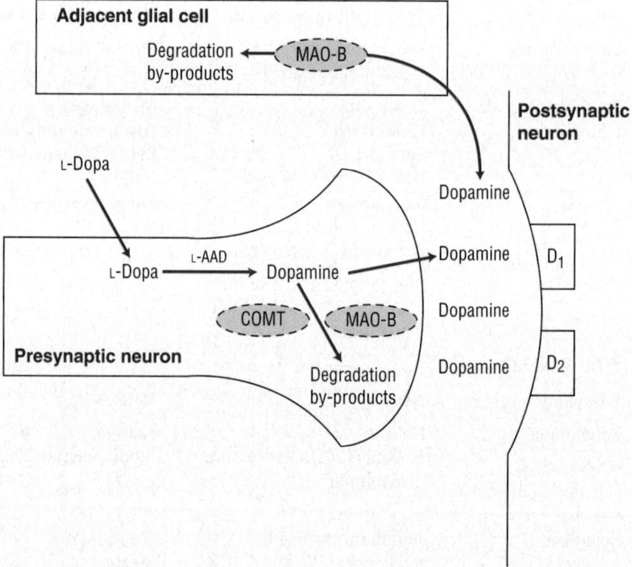

FIGURE 78-5 Dopamine synthesis and metabolism within the striatal neurons. See also Fig. 78-1 for additional details. (COMT, catechol-*O*-methyltransferase; D_1-D_2, dopamine receptors; L-AAD, L-aromatic amino acid decarboxylase; L-Dopa, levodopa; MAO-B, monoamine oxidase B.)

Carbidopa/L-Dopa

6 L-Dopa is the immediate precursor of dopamine and, in combination with a peripherally acting L-amino acid decarboxylase inhibitor (carbidopa or benserazide), remains the most effective medication for the symptomatic treatment of PD.[28,29] In the United States, L-dopa is combined with carbidopa as L-dopa crosses the blood–brain barrier, whereas carbidopa does not, and the carbidopa then reduces the unwanted peripheral conversion of L-dopa to dopamine. As a result, increased amounts of L-dopa are transported into the brain, and the peripheral adverse effects of dopamine, such as nausea, are reduced. In the SNc, L-dopa is converted to dopamine by the enzyme L-amino acid decarboxylase and inactivated by the enzymes MAO and COMT (Figs. 78-1 and 78-5).

6 Regardless of what the initial therapeutic agent is, ultimately all patients with PD will require L-dopa. Regarding carbidopa, about 75 mg/day is required to sufficiently inhibit the peripheral activity of L-amino acid decarboxylase, but some patients require more.[47] Therefore, the usual initial maintenance carbidopa/L-dopa regimen is 25/100 mg three times daily. As the motor features of PD become progressively more severe, use of higher dosages is required. There is no maximum allowable total daily L-dopa dose; however, in patients

with severe PD, the usual maximal dose tolerated is approximately 1,000 to 1,500 mg/day. Slow buildup of dose (eg, increments of 100 mg L-dopa per week) can help minimize treatment-emergent adverse effects, such as drowsiness and nausea (see Table 78-4).

Various formulations of carbidopa/L-dopa are available (see Table 78-3). For patients with difficulty swallowing intact tablets, an orally disintegrating tablet (ODT) preparation of carbidopa/L-dopa is available, and while this formulation rapidly dissolves on contact with saliva, the carbidopa/L-dopa does not undergo transmucosal absorption, and the dissolved medication in saliva must be swallowed for absorption in the proximal duodenum. Additionally, carbidopa/L-dopa is available in an oral capsule formulation containing immediate-release (IR) and extended-release (ER) beads (ie, Rytary) which can be sprinkled on food (eg, apple sauce).

Pharmacokinetics There is marked intra- and intersubject variability in the time to peak plasma concentrations after oral carbidopa/L-dopa. This may in part be attributed to differences in gastric emptying as L-dopa is absorbed in the proximal duodenum by a saturable large neutral amino acid transport system.[48] Therefore, competition for this transporter by large dietary, or pharmaceutical, neutral amino acids (eg, leucine, phenylalanine) may result in reduced L-dopa bioavailability. However, for patients with early PD, this interaction is generally not significant.

L-Dopa is not bound to plasma proteins and is actively transported across the blood–brain barrier by the large neutral amino acid transporter system. In advanced PD, special diets involving protein restriction may improve L-dopa responsiveness and are sometimes implemented. A metabolite of L-dopa, 3-*O*-methyldopa also competes for transport, but it is not clear how this affects L-dopa clinical response.

When peripheral decarboxylation of L-dopa is inhibited by carbidopa, 3-*O*-methylation (via COMT) becomes the predominant catabolic pathway. The elimination half-life of L-dopa is about 1 hour, and this is extended to about 1.5 hours with the addition of carbidopa. With the addition of a COMT inhibitor such as entacapone to carbidopa/L-dopa, the elimination half-life is extended to about 2 to 2.5 hours.

The controlled-release (ie, Sinemet CR) and IR/ER carbidopa/L-dopa formulations (ie, Rytary) are 70% and 75% bioavailable, respectively, compared to standard IR carbidopa/L-dopa.[49] Manufacturer-provided dosage conversion recommendations are available to guide dosing conversions between carbidopa/L-dopa formulations.

7 Motor Complications of L-Dopa Long-term L-dopa therapy is associated with a variety of motor complications, of which end-of-dose "wearing off" (motor fluctuations) and L-dopa peak-dose dyskinesias are the two most encountered.[50] These motor complications can become disabling and a challenge to manage. Risk factors associated with the development of motor complications include higher dosages of L-dopa and a younger age of PD onset.[51,52] The 5-year cumulative incidence of motor complications is about 50% in a medication naïve population.[53] Table 78-6 lists the common motor complications associated with long-term treatment with L-dopa and suggested initial management strategies. Initiating therapy with the controlled release (CR) form of carbidopa/L-dopa (ie, Sinemet CR) does not reduce the development of motor complications compared with IR carbidopa/L-dopa.[28]

7 End-of-Dose "Wearing Off" The terms "off" and "on" refer to periods of poor movement (ie, return of tremor, rigidity, or slowness) and good movement, respectively. End-of-dose "wearing off" prior to the next dose of medication is a common type of response fluctuation. This phenomenon is related to the increasing loss of neuronal storage capability for dopamine as well as the short half-life of L-dopa.[54] Initially, exogenous L-dopa is taken up by the remaining

TABLE 78-6 Common Motor Complications and Possible Initial Treatments

Effects	Possible Treatments
End-of-dose "wearing off" (motor fluctuation)	Increase frequency of carbidopa/L-dopa doses; add either COMT inhibitor or MAO-B inhibitor or dopamine agonist; add or switch to extended-release carbidopa/L-dopa (ie, Rytary); use L-dopa inhalation or apomorphine subcutaneous or sublingual
"Delayed on" or "no on" response	Give carbidopa/L-dopa on empty stomach; use carbidopa/L-dopa ODT; avoid carbidopa/L-dopa SR; use apomorphine subcutaneous or sublingual or L-dopa inhalation
Start hesitation ("freezing")	Increase carbidopa/L-dopa dose; add a dopamine agonist or MAO-B inhibitor; utilize physical therapy along with assistive walking devices or sensory cues (eg, rhythmic commands, stepping over objects)
Peak-dose dyskinesia	Provide smaller doses of carbidopa/L-dopa at the same or increased dosing frequency; reduce dose of adjunctive dopamine agonist; add amantadine

COMT, catechol-*O*-methyltransferase; MAO, monoamine oxidase; ODT, orally disintegrating tablet; SR, sustained release.

SNc neurons, converted to dopamine and stored in synaptic vesicles. With progressive loss of SNc neurons and storage capacity, patients become more dependent on exogenous carbidopa/L-dopa. Hence, the peripheral pharmacokinetic properties of L-dopa increasingly become the determinant of central dopamine synthesis. With advancing PD, the duration of action of a single carbidopa/L-dopa dose progressively shortens and in some cases may produce benefits for as little as 1 hour. As a result, carbidopa/L-dopa needs to be given more frequently, although other options are also available (see Table 78-6). In particular, the addition of the COMT inhibitor entacapone or an MAO-B inhibitor (ie, rasagiline, safinamide), or zonisamide (off-label use in the United States) extends the action of L-dopa and should be considered.[28] A dopamine agonist (eg, pramipexole, ropinirole, or rotigotine) can also be added to a carbidopa/L-dopa regimen for the management of "wearing off." The older CR L-dopa product (ie, Sinemet CR) has been investigated for the management of motor fluctuations, but the evidence is not compelling.[28] A newer IR/ER carbidopa/L-dopa formulation (ie, Rytary) contains beads that dissolve at different rates. Following administration, therapeutic L-dopa levels are rapidly achieved and are maintained for 4 to 5 hours providing efficacy for the management of motor fluctuations.[55] Clinical trials are currently underway investigating another IR/ER carbidopa/L-dopa formulation, which aims to further a steadier L-dopa level.[56]

Carbidopa/L-dopa enteral suspension is effective and safe for patients with advanced PD experiencing persistent, on/off fluctuations.[57] This enteral suspension is contained within a medication cassette reservoir and infusion into the small intestine is achieved by a portable pump device which requires placement of a percutaneous endoscopic gastrostomy tube along with a jejunal extension, through the abdominal wall. The medication infusion typically runs for 16 continuous hours per day and is turned off at night.

Less-invasive deliveries of carbidopa/L-dopa to minimize motor fluctuations are currently being investigated in clinical trials. ND0612 is a self-administered subcutaneous infusion of carbidopa/L-dopa currently in phase III trials. ABBV-951 is another subcutaneous infusion of carbidopa/L-dopa also in phase III clinical trials.[58]

For rapid relief of acute off episodes, apomorphine (available as either a subcutaneously or sublingually administered short-acting dopamine agonist) or a L-dopa dry powder for inhalation may be administered as needed.[59,60] Although not commonly performed, sipping small amounts of carbidopa/L-dopa solution frequently throughout the day is also a method for managing on/off fluctuations. A solution that is stable for 72 hours at room temperature can be prepared by adding 10 crushed tablets of carbidopa/L-dopa 10/100 (or 25/100) mg and 2 g crystalline ascorbic acid to 1 L of water.[61]

Often though, off episodes occur during the night, and patients will awaken in an off state because of an overnight decline of medication levels. Therefore, bedtime administration of a dopamine agonist or a medication formulation that provides sustained medication levels overnight (eg, carbidopa/L-dopa CR or IR/ER, ropinirole XL, pramipexole ER, rotigotine transdermal patch) can help reduce nocturnal off episodes and improve functioning upon awakening.

Nonadherence to medications also contributes to the frequency of off episodes. Therefore, engaging and supporting patients and caregivers in overcoming barriers to medication adherence is important.

"Delayed-On" or "No-On" Response "Delayed-on" or "no-on" responses describe a delayed or absent onset of medication effect to individual doses of carbidopa/L-dopa which can be a result of delayed gastric emptying or decreased duodenum absorption. To overcome this effect, chewing a tablet or crushing it and then drinking a full glass of water or using the ODT formulation on an empty stomach can help mitigate effects of delayed gastric emptying. Alternatively, the use of the inhaled L-dopa bypasses the gastrointestinal (GI) tract to provide systemic absorption and help induce "on" time for patients.[62] Additionally, subcutaneously or sublingually administered apomorphine may be used as on-demand therapy for delayed-on or no-on periods.[62]

Freezing "Freezing," or a sudden, episodic akinesia (lack of movement) of the lower extremities, is an event described by patients as a feeling where their "feet suddenly feel stuck to the floor" during ambulation or they have difficulty initiating steps (start hesitation) or turns (turn hesitation). As freezing often is exacerbated by anxiety or when perceived obstacles (eg, doorways, turnstiles) are encountered, this event may interfere with ambulation and increase the risk of falls. In addition to optimal pharmacological management, physical therapy and use of assistive walking devices and sensory cues aid in the reduction of "freezing" episodes.[63]

9 **Dykinesias** Another complication of L-dopa therapy is "on" period dyskinesias that are involuntary choreiform movements usually involving the neck, trunk, and lower/upper extremities. Dyskinesias are specific to L-dopa therapy and if patients report "shakiness," it is important to clarify if they are referring to tremor or dyskinesias. To help differentiate the two, it is important to note that dyskinesias are usually associated with peak striatal dopamine levels (peak-dose dyskinesia) and, simplistically, can be thought of as too much movement secondary to extension of the L-dopa pharmacologic effect.[64] Lowering the dose of carbidopa/L-dopa to counteract dyskinesias should be attempted. However, the use of a lower dose may result in suboptimal control of parkinsonian features; thus, necessitating addition of another antiparkinsonian agent (eg, dopamine agonist). Another strategy is to lower the individual dose of L-dopa, but administer more frequently. Glutamate overactivity may also be involved, as suggested by the dyskinesia improvement observed with amantadine (NMDA-receptor antagonist) and other antiglutamate ligands.[65] Less commonly, dyskinesias also can develop during the rise and fall of L-dopa effects (the dyskinesia–improvement–dyskinesia or diphasic pattern of response). For severe dyskinesias (despite pharmacologically optimized therapy), surgery should be considered.

"Off-Period" Dystonia In PD, dystonias are sustained muscle contractions that can occur and more commonly affect a distal lower extremity (eg, clenching of toes or involuntary turning of a foot). Dystonias often occur in the early morning hours, due to waning medication levels, and improve with the first carbidopa/L-dopa dose of the day. Remedies for early morning dystonia include bedtime administration of a long-acting dopamine agonist, long-acting carbidopa/L-dopa, or baclofen. Additionally, focal injections of botulinum toxin type A or B are effective for persistent focal dystonias, which can also occur as L-dopa peak dose effect; therefore, additional management of this specific adverse event is similar to that of dyskinesias.[66]

Adenosine Receptor Antagonist One of the newest FDA-approved agents for the adjunctive treatment of PD is the xanthine derivative, istradefylline, an adenosine A2AR antagonist. This non-dopaminergic medication is theorized to exert its effect by antagonizing the adenosine A2AR in the indirect movement pathway.[16] Patients with PD have been found to have an increase in adenosine A2ARs.[67] Adenosine increases the activation of the indirect pathway, further inhibiting movement. Antagonizing the A2AR therefore allows for decreased activation of the indirect pathway and may allow for an increase in movement.

Istradefylline is currently approved as an adjunctive treatment to L-dopa for patients with "off" episodes. It is generally well tolerated with the most common adverse effects including insomnia, hallucination, nausea, and constipation. The pharmacokinetics of istradefylline include metabolism primarily by cytochrome P450 (CYP450) CYP1A1 and CYP3A4 with an elimination half-life of approximately 80 hours.[68] It is recommended to avoid use in the presence of a strong CYP3A4 inducer and to reduce the dose when co-administered with a strong CYP3A4 inhibitor. The recommended starting dose is 20 mg daily, which can be increased to 40 mg daily. In patients who smoke more than 20 cigarettes a day (or equivalent tobacco product), the recommended dose is 40 mg per day.[68]

Monoamine Oxidase B Inhibitors

5 Three selective MAO-B inhibitors (rasagiline, safinamide, selegiline) are available for management of PD (see Table 78-3). The selective inhibition of MAO-B in the brain interferes with the degradation of dopamine and results in prolonged dopaminergic activity. Rasagiline and selegiline contain a propargylamine moiety, which is essential for conferring irreversible inhibition of MAO-B, in contrast to safinamide, which is a reversible MAO-B inhibitor.[69] At therapeutic doses, all three agents preferentially inhibit MAO-B over MAO-A.

A common concern with use of these agents is the potential for interactions with medications that possess serotonergic activity. Concomitant use of MAO-B inhibitors with meperidine and other selected opioid analgesics is contraindicated because of a small risk of serotonin syndrome. However, serotonergic antidepressants can be used concomitantly when clinically warranted, as these are not contraindicated.[70]

MAO-B inhibitors have also been investigated for neuroprotective properties (clinically referred to as *disease modification*). MAO-B inhibitors possess antiapoptotic properties, and MAO-B inhibition diverts dopamine degradation to an alternate route (ie, COMT) that does not generate free radicals (see Figs. 78-1 and 78-5).[71] To date, clinical studies to demonstrate disease modification with MAO-B inhibitors have yielded inconclusive results.[72-74]

5 8 Selegiline, also known as L-deprenyl, is marketed for extending L-dopa effects and is typically administered 5 mg twice daily. Selegiline is also available as an ODT formulation administered 1.25 to 2.5 mg once daily, and a transdermal formulation which is not indicated for PD. As monotherapy in early PD, selegiline provides modest improvements in motor function.[74] In advanced PD, adjunctive use of selegiline can provide up to 1 hour of extra "on" time for patients with "wearing off," although the data

are inconsistent,[28] which may be explained, in part, by the poor and erratic bioavailability of selegiline.

As an amphetamine pharmacophore, selegiline undergoes first-pass hepatic metabolism, predominantly via CYP2B6 and 2C19, to end products of L-methamphetamine and L-amphetamine.[75] Adverse effects of selegiline are minimal but can include agitation, insomnia (especially if administered at bedtime), hallucinations, and orthostatic hypotension (see Table 78-4). Selegiline also increases the peak effects of L-dopa and can worsen pre-existing dyskinesias or psychiatric symptoms such as delusions. With the selegiline ODT formulation, first-pass hepatic metabolism is bypassed as a consequence of transmucosal absorption; hence, bioavailability is improved and formation of amphetamine metabolites is reduced.

5 8 Rasagiline is a second-generation, irreversible, selective MAO-B inhibitor administered at 0.5 or 1 mg once daily, which is effective as monotherapy in early PD. It is also effective as add-on therapy for managing motor fluctuations in advanced PD with efficacy similar to that of entacapone, offering approximately 1 hour of extra "on" time during the day.[28] Rasagiline is well tolerated with minimal GI or neuropsychiatric adverse effects and is metabolized by CYP1A2 to aminoindan, which is inactive and devoid of amphetamine-like properties.[76]

5 8 Safinamide is a reversible, selective MAO-B inhibitor administered at 50 or 100 mg once daily indicated as add-on therapy to carbidopa/L-dopa for managing motor fluctuations and provides up to 1 hour of extra "on" time during the day.[28] Nondopaminergic effects include state-dependent inhibition of voltage-gated sodium channels and modulation of release of glutamate.[77] However, the extent to which these properties of safinamide contribute to the overall medication effect is unclear. Safinamide is well tolerated with minimal GI or neuropsychiatric adverse effects and is predominantly metabolized by nonmicrosomal enzymes (cytosolic amidases) to inactive metabolites which are excreted renally.[77]

Catechol-*O*-Methyltransferase Inhibitors

8 Three COMT inhibitors, entacapone, opicapone, and tolcapone, have been developed to extend the effects of L-dopa and are indicated for managing "wearing off". Mechanistically, all reduce the peripheral conversion of L-dopa to dopamine, thus enhancing central L-dopa bioavailability. Consequently, in the absence of L-dopa, they have no effect on PD symptoms. COMT inhibitors increase L-dopa area under the curve by approximately 35% and, for patients with "wearing off," can increase "on" time by about 1 to 2 hours.[28,78]

Tolcapone inhibits both peripheral and central COMT, but its use is limited by reports of fatal hepatotoxicity, such that strict monitoring of hepatic function, especially during the first 6 months of therapy, is required (see Table 78-4). Because of this risk, it is reserved for patients with fluctuations that are not responding to other therapies.[79]

Entacapone has a shorter half-life than tolcapone, and 200 mg needs to be given with each dose of carbidopa/L-dopa up to a maximum of eight times per day. A triple-combination product of carbidopa/L-dopa/entacapone offers convenience for some patients (ie, fewer tablets to administer). Unlike tolcapone, entacapone is not associated with hepatotoxicity; therefore, it is considered efficacious and clinically useful as adjunctive therapy to manage motor fluctuations.[28]

Opicapone is a third-generation COMT inhibitor that selectively blocks the peripheral conversion of L-dopa. Its long duration of action compared to entacapone and tolcapone allows for once-a-day dosing.[80] Opicapone 50 mg once daily at bedtime is the recommended dose for most patients and 25 mg daily for patients with moderate hepatic impairment. The mean "off" time reduction in clinical trials for opicapone has been greater than that for entacapone, suggesting a more robust clinical response.[81]

With all agents, augmentation of dopaminergic adverse effects may occur and generally are manageable by reduction of the carbidopa/L-dopa dosage. Patients should be advised that other adverse effects include brownish-orange urinary discoloration and diarrhea occurring weeks to months after treatment initiation may occur with the use of entacapone or tolcapone.

Dopamine Agonists

Dopamine agonists fall into two pharmacologic subtypes: ergot-derived agonists (bromocriptine) and the non-ergot agonists (apomorphine, pramipexole, ropinirole, and rotigotine).[82] Non-ergot agonists have a better safety profile and are more commonly used than the ergot-derived agonists. Pharmacologically dopamine agonists stimulate dopamine receptors (eg, D_1, D_2, D_3) and are useful as monotherapy in mild-to-moderate PD and also as adjuncts to carbidopa/L-dopa therapy to reduce "off" time in patients with motor fluctuations.[28]

10 Compared with long-term carbidopa/L-dopa therapy, dopamine agonist significantly reduce the risk of developing motor complications.[83,84] For younger patients, who are more likely to develop motor complications, dopamine agonists are preferred over carbidopa/L-dopa. For older patients, dopamine agonists should be used conservatively due to greater likelihood for the development of intolerable adverse effects and for patients with cognitive problems or dementia, dopamine agonists should be avoided.

Common adverse effects of dopamine agonists include nausea, confusion, drowsiness, hallucinations, lower-extremity edema, and orthostatic hypotension (see Table 78-4).[85] When initiating therapy, a slow dose titration is required to minimize development of adverse effects, particularly nausea. The addition of a dopamine agonist to carbidopa/L-dopa therapy also can induce dyskinesias, especially in patients with pre-existing dyskinesias. Less common but serious adverse effects include impulsive and compulsive behaviors (eg, pathologic gambling or shopping; paraphilia), delusions/psychosis, and sleep attacks (sudden, unexpected episodes of sleep). Hallucinations and delusion should be managed using a systematic approach that starts with dose reduction or discontinuation of the dopamine agonist, and if needed, addition of a second-generation antipsychotic medication such as clozapine, pimavanserin, or quetiapine.[24,30,86] Of these, only pimavanserin is FDA-approved for psychosis in PD. Involvement of caregivers in surveillance for potential adverse effects of dopamine agonists, particularly development of delusions, hallucinations, and impulsive behaviors, facilitates earlier detection and management.

Apomorphine is an aporphine alkaloid originally derived from morphine that lacks narcotic properties.[59] It exhibits poor oral bioavailability due to extensive hepatic first-pass metabolism and is administered either sublingually or subcutaneously. Apomorphine is indicated for patients with advanced PD who are experiencing intermittent "off" episodes despite optimized therapy. Upon subcutaneous administration, apomorphine produces an "on" response within 20 minutes. The effective dose ranges from 2 to 6 mg per injection. Sites of injection (abdomen, upper arm, and upper thigh) should be rotated to avoid development of subcutaneous nodules. The elimination half-life for subcutaneous apomorphine is approximately 40 minutes, and the duration of benefit can be up to 100 minutes.[87] In comparison, the sublingual dosage form of apomorphine typically takes about 30 to 60 minutes to produce therapeutic effects and benefits can last up to 90 minutes.[88,89] Patients may take anywhere from 10 to 30 mg per dose, not to exceed five treatments per day. The half-life for the sublingual formulation is about 90 minutes. Nausea and vomiting are common adverse effects for both formulations, and prior to the initiation of apomorphine, patients should be premedicated with the antiemetic, trimethobenzamide. Of note, apomorphine delivered continuously via a subcutaneous infusion for patients with advanced PD and motor fluctuations is currently being studied in clinical trials in the United States. This delivery of apomorphine is currently an approved therapy in Europe.[90]

Pramipexole is initiated at a dose of 0.125 mg three times a day and increased every 5 to 7 days, as tolerated, to a maximum of 1.5 mg three times a day.[91] An extended-release pramipexole formulation is also available. Immediate-release ropinirole is initiated at 0.25 mg three times a day and increased by 0.25 mg three times a day on a weekly basis to a maximum of 24 mg/day.[92] An extended-release ropinirole formulation also is available. Pramipexole is renally excreted with an 8- to 12-hour half-life. The initial dosage must be adjusted in renal insufficiency (0.125 mg twice daily for creatinine clearances of 35-59 mL/min [0.58-0.99 mL/s], 0.125 mg once daily for creatinine clearances of 15-34 mL/min [0.25-0.57 mL/s]).[91]

Ropinirole has a 6-hour half-life and is metabolized by CYP1A2; therefore, potent inhibitors (eg, fluoroquinolone antibiotics) and inducers (eg, cigarette smoking) of this enzyme likely will lead to alterations in its clearance.[92]

Rotigotine transdermal patch is initiated at 2 mg once daily and increased weekly by 2 mg increments to achieve the desired therapeutic effect. The rotigotine transdermal patch provides continuous release of medication over a 24-hour period.[93] The patch application sites should be rotated to minimize skin irritation and rash. Rotigotine disposition is not affected by hepatic or renal impairment, and CYP-mediated interactions are not significant.

EVALUATION OF THERAPEUTIC OUTCOMES

1 Comprehensive medication management with optimization of medications related to PD improves patient outcomes.[94-97] Routine evaluation and monitoring of motor and nonmotor symptoms should occur every 3 to 6 months for patients on a stable treatment regimen. With the changes in pharmacotherapy (eg, medication addition, discontinuation, dose change), follow-up monitoring for efficacy and adverse effects should occur within 1 or 2 weeks and may occur via telephone.[98] Table 78-7 lists the monitoring parameters for PD therapy. Patient and caregiver satisfaction is an important component of evaluating therapeutic outcomes. Toward this end, establishing appropriate treatment expectations is important. Patients and caregivers should be educated that symptoms of PD often progresses with time, and adjustments to the medication regimen will be required to manage motor and nonmotor features. Additionally, some symptoms do not respond to pharmacotherapy (eg, freezing, gait, and postural instability). Assessment of the patient's general level of functioning, including activities of daily living and mobility, is important to determine when medication adjustments or physical therapy interventions are needed. It is also important to be aware of and adhere to the general guidelines and recommendations for geriatric health maintenance and disease prevention (eg, bone health, routine vaccinations, and vitamin and mineral supplementations).

Patients and caregivers can participate in treatment by recording medication administration times as well as the duration of "on and off" times that can be reviewed at each visit. Periodic review of all prescription and nonprescription medications that the patient is taking should be performed to identify medication therapy problems such as the use of medications with adverse effects that can exacerbate PD motor and nonmotor features. For example, D_2 blockers (such as metoclopramide and firstgeneration antipsychotics) can worsen motor features and should be avoided. If the patient reports memory problems, medications with anticholinergic properties should be avoided.

Nonmotor symptoms must be identified, assessed, managed, and monitored. These include anxiety, cognitive impairment, constipation, daytime sleepiness, depression, dro oling, dysphagia, fatigue, falls, hallucinations/psychosis, impulsivity, insomnia, orthostatic hypotension, overactive bladder, pain, REM sleep behavior disorder, and restless legs syndrome. Screening for anxiety or depressive disorders will help determine if antidepressant or antianxiety therapy is needed.[99] If falling is a problem, it is important to investigate whether falls are secondary to insufficient motor control, orthostatic hypotension, or medication adverse effects, such as dizziness. The former may necessitate an increase in dose of antiparkinsonian agents, and the latter two conditions, a reduction in medication dosage. Physical therapy is also helpful for strengthening ambulation and balance skills to minimize falls. The patient should be questioned about any difficulties with their antiparkinsonian medications, including presence of adverse effects. Recommendations always should be made in view of the patient's perception of the severity of symptoms and effect on quality of life.

TABLE 78-7 Monitoring Parkinson Disease Therapy

1. Monitor medication administration times. Educate the patient that immediate-release carbidopa/L-dopa is absorbed best on an empty stomach but is commonly taken with food (preferably nonprotein snack) to minimize nausea. Avoid administration of conventional selegiline in the late afternoon or evening to minimize insomnia.
2. Monitor to ensure that the patient and/or caregivers understand the prescribed medication regimen. For example, they should understand that catechol-*O*-methyltransferase inhibitors work by enhancing the effect of L-dopa and that the patient should not discontinue medication without notifying the clinician.
3. Monitor and inquire specifically about dose-by-dose effects of medication, including response to doses of medication and the presence of dyskinesias, "wearing-off" effects, dizziness, nausea, orthostasis, or visual hallucinations. Offer suggestions to help alleviate these or encourage the patient to discuss them with the clinician.
4. Monitor caregiver involvement and facilitation for early detection of abnormal behaviors, dyskinesias, falls, hallucinations, impulsivity, memory problems, mood changes, and sleep disorders.
5. Monitor for nonadherence and, if present, inquire for possible reasons (eg, dosing convenience, financial issues, and adverse effects) and offer suggestions.
6. Monitor for presence of medications that can exacerbate idiopathic Parkinson disease motor features (eg, D_2-receptor blockers).
7. Monitor for presence of medications that can exacerbate nonmotor symptoms. Evaluate whether the presence of an anticholinergic agent is causing confusion or cognitive impairment.

CONCLUSION

Despite many advances in neuroscience, a definitive cause of PD remains unknown. Each of the available therapies provide various degrees of symptomatic benefit, and the choice of agent is patient specific. The appropriate pharmacotherapy can significantly improve a patient's quality of life and functional status. The goal of management remains maintaining acceptable functional control with minimal treatment emergent motor and nonmotor complications. Thoughtful consideration for choice of initial and adjunctive therapy is critical for optimizing short- and long-term outcomes.

ABBREVIATIONS

COMT	catechol-*O*-methyltransferase
CR	controlled release
CYP450	cytochrome P450
D_1	dopamine receptor subtype 1
D_2	dopamine receptor subtype 2
DBS	deep-brain stimulation
ER	extended release
GABA	γ-aminobutyric acid
GI	gastrointestinal
GPi	globus pallidus interna
IR	immediate release

L-dopa	levodopa
MAO	monoamine oxidase
NMDA	*N*-methyl-D-aspartate
ODT	orally disintegrating tablet
PD	Parkinson disease
REM	rapid eye movement
SNc	substantia nigra pars compacta
SNr	substantia nigra pars reticulate
STN	subthalamic nucleus

REFERENCES

1. Parkinson J. *An Essay on the Shaking Palsy.* London: Sherwood, Neely, and Jones; 1817:1–66.
2. Marras C, Beck JC, Bower JH, et al. Prevalence of Parkinson's disease across North America. *NPJ Parkinsons Dis.* 2018;410.1038/s41531-018-0058-0.
3. Hirsch L, Jette N, Frolkis A, et al. The incidence of Parkinson's disease: A systematic review and meta-analysis. *Neuroepidemiology* 2016;46:292–300. 10.1159/000445751.
4. Pringsheim T, Jette N, Frolkis A, et al. The prevalence of Parkinson's disease: A systematic review and meta-analysis. *Mov Disord.* 2014;29:1583–1590.
5. Dashtipour K. Do genetic factors protect against Parkinson's disease? What I can learn from my healthy grandma. *Med Hypotheses.* 2014;83:637–639.
6. Jellinger KA. The pathomechanisms underlying Parkinson's disease. *Expert Rev Neurother.* 2014;14:199–215.
7. Jankovic J, Tan EK. Parkinson's disease: Etiopathogenesis and treatment. *J Neurol, Neurosur Psychiatr.* 2020;91:795–808. 10.1136/jnnp-2019-322338.
8. Trist BG, Hare DJ, Double KL. Oxidative stress in the aging substantia nigra and the etiology of Parkinson's disease. *Aging Cell.* 2019;1810.1111/acel.13031.
9. Tagliaferro P, Burke R E. Retrograde axonal degeneration in Parkinson disease. *J Parkinsons Dis.* 2016;6:1–15. 10.3233/jpd-150769.
10. Ascherio AA, Schwarzschild MA. The epidemiology of Parkinson's disease: Risk factors and prevention. *Lancet Neurol.* 2016;15(12):1257–1272. 10.1016/S1474-4422(16)30230-7 27751556.
11. Gallo V, Vineis P, Cancellieri M, et al. Exploring causality of the association between smoking and Parkinson's disease. *Int J Epidemiol.* 2018;48(3)10.1093/ije/dyy230.
12. Hong CT, Chan L, Bai C-H. The Effect of caffeine on the risk and progression of Parkinson's disease: A meta-analysis. *Nutrients.* 2020;12:1860. 10.3390/nu12061860.
13. Simon DK, Tanner CM, Brundin P. Parkinson disease epidemiology, pathology, genetics, and pathophysiology. *Clin Geriatr Med.* 2020;36(1):1–12. 10.1016/j.cger.2019.08.002 31733690.
14. Smith Y, Bevan MD, Shink E, Bolam JP. Microcircuitry of the direct and indirect pathways of the basal ganglia. *Neuroscience.* 1998;86:353–387.
15. Kulisevsky J, Poyurovsky M. Adenosine A_{2A}-receptor antagonism and pathophysiology of Parkinson's disease and drug-induced movement disorders. *Eur Neurol.* 2012;67:4–11. 10.1159/000331768.
16. Jenner P, Mori A, Aradi SD, et al. Istradefylline—a first generation adenosine A2A antagonist for the treatment of Parkinson's disease. *Expert Rev Neurother.* 2021;21:317–333. 10.1080/14737175.2021.1880896.
17. Peelaerts W, Bousset L, Van der Perren A, et al. α-Synuclein strains cause distinct synucleinopathies after local and systemic administration. *Nature.* 2015;522(7556):340–344. 10.1038/nature14547 26061766.
18. McCann H, Cartwright H, Halliday GM. Neuropathology of α-synuclein propagation and braak hypothesis. *Mov Disord.* 2016;31:152–160.
19. Stayte S, Vissel B. Advances in non-dopaminergic treatments for Parkinson's disease. *Front Neurosci.* 2014;8:113.
20. Postuma RB, Berg D, Stern M, et al. MDS clinical diagnostic criteria for Parkinson's disease. *Mov Disord.* 2015;30:1591–1601.
21. de Germay S, Montastruc F, Carvajal A, et al. Drug-induced parkinsonism: Revisiting the epidemiology using the WHO pharmacovigilance database. *Parkinsonism Relat Disord.* 2020;70:55–59. 10.1016/j.parkreldis.2019.12.011.
22. Jennings D, Siderowf A, Stern M, et al. Conversion to Parkinson disease in the PARS hyposmic and dopamine transporter–deficit prodromal cohort. *JAMA Neurol.* 2017;74:933. 10.1001/jamaneurol.2017.0985.
23. Debû B, De Oliveira Godeiro C, Lino JC, et al. Managing gait, balance, and posture in Parkinson's disease. *Curr Neurol Neurosci Rep.* 2018;1810.1007/s11910-018-0828-4.
24. Seppi K, Ray Chaudhuri K, Coelho M, et al. Update on treatments for nonmotor symptoms of Parkinson's disease—An evidence-based medicine review. *Mov. Disord.* 2019;34:180–198. 10.1002/mds.27602.
25. Lang AE., Espay AJ. Disease modification in Parkinson's disease: Current approaches, challenges, and future considerations. *Mov. Disord.* 2018;33:660–677. 10.1002/mds.27360.
26. Chen JJ, Swope DM Pharmacotherapy for Parkinson's disease. *Pharmacotherapy.* 2007;27:161S–173S. 10.1592/phco.27.12part2.161s.
27. Pringsheim T, Day GS, Smith DB, et al. Dopaminergic therapy for motor symptoms in early Parkinson disease practice guideline summary: A report of the AAN Guideline Subcommittee. *Neurology.* 2021;97(20):942–957. 10.1212/WNL.0000000000012868 34782410.
28. Fox SH., Katzenschlager R, Lim S-Y, et al. International Parkinson and movement disorder society evidence-based medicine review: Update on treatments for the motor symptoms of Parkinson's disease. *Mov. Disord.* 2018;33:1248–1266. 10.1002/mds.27372.
29. Fox SH, Katzenschlager R, Lim S-Y, et al. The movement disorder society evidence-based medicine review update: Treatments for the motor symptoms of Parkinson's disease. *Mov. Disord.* 2011;26:S2–S41. 10.1002/mds.23829.
30. National Institute for Health and Care Excellence Parkinson's disease in adults. NICE Guideline[NG71]. https://www.nice.org.uk/guiance/ng71. July 2017.
31. Lexicomp online [online database] Hudson, Ohio: Wolters Kluwer Clinical Drug Information Inc. https://online-lexi-com.catalog.llu.edu.
32. Peterka M, Odorfer T, Schwab M, et al. LSVT-BIG therapy in Parkinson's disease: Physiological evidence for proprioceptive recalibration. *BMC Neurol.* 2020;2010.1186/s12883-020-01858-2.
33. Dong J, Cui Y, Li S, et al. Current pharmaceutical treatments and alternative therapies of Parkinson's disease. *Curr Neuropharmacol.* 2016;14:339–355. 10.2174/1570159x14666151120123025.
34. Peterka M, Odorfer T, Schwab M, et al. LSVT-BIG therapy in Parkinson's disease: Physiological evidence for proprioceptive recalibration. *BMC Neurol.* 2020;20(1):276–276. 10.1186/s12883-020-01858-2 32652957.
35. Larson Paul S. Deep brain stimulation for movement disorders. *Neurotherapeutics.* 2014;11:465–474. 10.1007/s13311-014-0274-1.
36. Rughani A, Schwalb JM, Sidiropoulos C, et al. Congress of Neurological Surgeons Systematic Review and Evidence-Based Guideline on Subthalamic Nucleus and Globus Pallidus Internus Deep Brain Stimulation for the treatment of patients with Parkinson's disease: Executive summary. *Neurosurgery.* 2018;82:753–756. 10.1093/neuros/nyy037.
37. McKinley JW., Shi Z, Kawikova I, et al. Dopamine deficiency reduces striatal cholinergic interneuron function in models of Parkinson's disease. *Neuron.* 2019;103:1056–1072.e6. 10.1016/j.neuron.2019.06.013.
38. Poewe W, Mahlknecht P. Pharmacologic treatment of motor symptoms associated with Parkinson disease. *Neurologic Clinics.* 2020;38:255–267. 10.1016/j.ncl.2019.12.002.
39. American Geriatrics Society 2019 Updated AGS Beers Criteria® for Potentially inappropriate medication use in older adults. *J Am Geriatr Soc.* 2019;67:674–694. 10.1111/jgs.15767.
40. Elmer LW, Juncos JL, Singer C, et al. Pooled analyses of Phase III studies of ADS-5102 (Amantadine) extended-release capsules for dyskinesia in Parkinson's disease. *CNS Drugs.* 2018;32:387–398. 10.1007/s40263-018-0498-4.
41. Müller T, Kuhn W, Möhr J-D. Evaluating ADS5102 (amantadine) for the treatment of Parkinson's disease patients with dyskinesia. *Expert Opin Pharmacother.* 2019;20:1181–1187. 10.1080/14656566.2019.1612365.
42. Hauser RA, Pahwa R, Wargin WA, et al. Pharmacokinetics of ADS-5102 (Amantadine) extended release capsules administered once daily at bedtime for the treatment of dyskinesia. *Clin Pharmacokinet.* 2018;58:77–88. 10.1007/s40262-018-0663-4.
43. Symmetrel [prescribing information] Endo Pharmaceuticals Inc. Chadds Ford, PA; 2009.
44. Pahwa R, Tanner CM, Hauser RA, et al. Amantadine extended release for levodopa-induced dyskinesia in Parkinson's disease (EASED Study). *Mov Disord.* 2015;30:788–795. 10.1002/mds.26159.
45. Perez-Lloret S, Rascol O. Efficacy and safety of amantadine for the treatment of L-DOPA-induced dyskinesia. *J. Neural Transm.* 2018;125:1237–1250. 10.1007/s00702-018-1869-1.
46. Shealy CN, Weeth JB, Mercier D Livedo reticularis in patients with parkinsonism receiving amantadine. *JAMA.* 1970;212(9):1522–1523.

47. Quaresma MV, Gomes ACD, Serruya A, et al. Amantadine-induced livedo reticularis—Case report. *Anais Brasileiros de Dermatologia.* 2015;90:745–747. 10.1590/abd1806-4841.20153394.
48. Hoehn MM. Increased dosage of carbidopa in patients with Parkinson's disease receiving low doses of levodopa. *Arch Neurol.* 1980;37:146. 10.1001/archneur.1980.00500520044006.
49. LeWitt PA. Levodopa therapy for Parkinson's disease: Pharmacokinetics and pharmacodynamics. *Mov Disord.* 2014;30:64–72. 10.1002/mds.26082.
50. Urso D, Chaudhuri KR, Qamar MA, et al. Improving the delivery of levodopa in Parkinson's Disease: A review of approved and emerging therapies. *CNS Drugs.* 2020;34:1149–1163. 10.1007/s40263-020-00769-7.
51. Kadastik-Eerme L, Taba N, Asser T, et al. Factors associated with motor complications in Parkinson's disease. *Brain Behav.* 2017;7:e00837. 10.1002/brb3.837.
52. Fahn S, Oakes D, Shoulson I, et al. Levodopa and the progression of Parkinson's disease. *N. Engl. J. Med.* 2004;351:2498–2508. 10.1056/nejmoa033447.
53. Olanow CW, Stocchi F. Levodopa: A new look at an old friend. *Mov Disord.* 2017;33:859–866. 10.1002/mds.27216.
54. Bjornestad A, Forsaa EB, Pedersen KF, et al. Risk and course of motor complications in a population-based incident Parkinson's disease cohort. *Parkinsonism Relat Disord.* 2016;22:48–53. 10.1016/j.parkreldis.2015.11.007.
55. Freitas M, Hess C, Fox S. Motor complications of dopaminergic medications in Parkinson's disease. *Semin Neurol.* 2017;37:147–157. 10.1055/s-0037-1602423.
56. Hauser RA, Hsu A, Kell S, et al. Extended-release carbidopa-levodopa (IPX066) compared with immediate-release carbidopa-levodopa in patients with Parkinson's disease and motor fluctuations: A phase 3 randomised, double-blind trial. *Lancet Neurol.* 2013;12:346–356. 10.1016/s1474-4422(13)70025-5.
57. Modi NB, Mittur A, Dinh P, et al. Pharmacodynamics, efficacy, and safety of IPX203 in Parkinson disease patients with motor fluctuations. *Clin Neuropharmacol.* 2019;42:149–156. 10.1097/wnf.0000000000000354.
58. Olanow CW, Kieburtz K, Odin P, et al. Continuous intrajejunal infusion of levodopa-carbidopa intestinal gel for patients with advanced Parkinson's disease: A randomised, controlled, double-blind, double-dummy study. *Lancet Neurol.* 2014;13:141–149. 10.1016/s1474-4422(13)70293-x.
59. Prakash N, McFarthing K, Simuni T. Clinical trial highlights—Infusion therapies. *J Parkinsons Dis.* 2020;10:5–17. 10.3233/jpd-199005.
60. Chen JJ, Obering C. A review of intermittent subcutaneous apomorphineinjections for the rescue management of motor fluctuations associated with advanced Parkinson's disease. *Clin Ther.* 2005;27:1710–1724. 10.1016/j.clinthera.2005.11.016.
61. LeWitt PA, Hauser RA, Pahwa R, et al. Safety and efficacy of CVT-301 (levodopa inhalation powder) on motor function during off periods in patients with Parkinson's disease: A randomised, double-blind, placebo-controlled phase 3 trial. *Lancet Neurol.* 2019;18:145–154. 10.1016/s1474-4422(18)30405-8.
62. Pappert Eric J, Buhrfiend C, Lipton JW, et al. Levodopa stability in solution: Time course, environmental effects, and practical recommendations for clinical use. *Mov Disord.* 1996;11:24–26. 10.1002/mds.870110106.
63. Olanow CW, Poewe W, Rascol O, et al. On-demand therapy for off episodes in Parkinson's disease. *Mov Disord.* 2021;36:2244–2253. 10.1002/mds.28726.
64. Gao C, Liu J, Tan Y, et al. Freezing of gait in Parkinson's disease: Pathophysiology, risk factors and treatments. *Trans Neurodegen.* 2020;910.1186/s40035-020-00191-5.
65. Tran TN, Vo Trang NN, Frei K, et al. Levodopa-induced dyskinesia: Clinical features, incidence, and risk factors. *J Neural Transm.* 2018;125:1109–1117. 10.1007/s00702-018-1900-6.
66. Dragašević-Mišković N, Petrović I, Stanković I, et al. Chemical management of levodopa-induced dyskinesia in Parkinson's disease patients. *Expert Opin Pharmacother.* 2018;20:219–230. 10.1080/14656566.2018.1543407.
67. Calabresi P, Standaert DG. Dystonia and levodopa-induced dyskinesias in Parkinson's disease: Is there a connection? *Neurobiol Dis.* 2019;132:104579. 10.1016/j.nbd.2019.104579.
68. Ishibashi K, Miura Y, Wagatsuma K, et al. Occupancy of adenosine A2A receptors by istradefylline in patients with Parkinson's disease using 11C-preladenant PET. *Neuropharmacology.* 2018;143:106–112. 10.1016/j.neuropharm.2018.09.036.
69. Nourianz. [Prescribing Information]. Kyowa Kirin Inc. Bedminster, NJ; 2020.
70. Finberg JPM. Inhibitors of MAO-B and COMT: Their effects on brain dopamine levels and uses in Parkinson's disease. *J Neural Transm.* 2018;126:433–448. 10.1007/s00702-018-1952-7.
71. Panisset M, Chen JJ, Rhyee SH, et al. Serotonin Toxicity Association with Concomitant Antidepressants and Rasagiline Treatment: Retrospective Study (STACCATO). *Pharmacother: J Human Pharmacol Drug Therapy.* 2014;34:1250–1258. 10.1002/phar.1500.
72. Szökő É, Tábi T, Riederer P, et al. Pharmacological aspects of the neuroprotective effects of irreversible MAO-B inhibitors, selegiline and rasagiline, in Parkinson's disease. *J Neural Transm.* 2018;125:1735–1749. 10.1007/s00702-018-1853-9.
73. Olanow CW, Rascol O, Hauser R, et al. A double-blind, delayed-start trial of rasagiline in Parkinson's disease. *New Eng J Med.* 2009;361:1268–1278. 10.1056/nejmoa0809335.
74. Parkinson Study Group. A controlled, randomized, delayed-start study of rasagiline in early Parkinson disease. *Arch Neurol.* 2004;61:561. 10.1001/archneur.61.4.561.
75. Parkinson Study Group. Effects of tocopherol and deprenyl on the progression of disability in early Parkinson's disease. *New Eng J Med.* 1993;328:176–183. 10.1056/nejm199301213280305.
76. Tábi T, Vécsei L, Youdim M, et al. Selegiline: A molecule with innovative potential. *J Neural Transm.* 2019;127:831–842. 10.1007/s00702-019-02082-0.
77. Chen J, Swope D, Dashtipour K. Comprehensive review of rasagiline, a second-generation monoamine oxidase inhibitor, for the treatment of Parkinson's disease. *Clin Ther.* 2007;29:1825–1849. 10.1016/j.clinthera.2007.09.021.
78. deSouza RM, Schapira A. Safinamide for the treatment of Parkinson's disease. *Expert Opin Pharmacother.* 2017;18:937–943. 10.1080/14656566.2017.1329819.
79. Ferreira JJ, Lees A, Rocha J-F, et al. Long-term efficacy of opicapone in fluctuating Parkinson's disease patients: A pooled analysis of data from two phase 3 clinical trials and their open-label extensions. *Eur J Neurol.* 2019;26:953–960. 10.1111/ene.13914.
80. Tasmar [Prescribing Information]. Valeant Pharmaceuticals North America LLC. Bridgewater, NJ; 2013.
81. Fabbri M, Ferreira J, Lees A, et al. Opicapone for the treatment of Parkinson's disease: A review of a new licensed medicine. *Mov Disord.* 2018;33:1528–1539. 10.1002/mds.27475.
82. Lees A, Ferreira J, Rascol O, et al. Opicapone as Adjunct to levodopa therapy in patients with Parkinson disease and motor fluctuations. *JAMA Neurol.* 2017;74:197. 10.1001/jamaneurol.2016.4703.
83. Blandini F, Armentero M-T. Dopamine receptor agonists for Parkinson's disease. *Expert Opin Investig Drugs.* 2013;23:387–410. 10.1517/13543784.2014.869209.
84. Rascol O, Brooks DJ, Korczyn AD, et al. A five-year study of the incidence of dyskinesia in patients with early Parkinson's disease who were treated with ropinirole or levodopa. *N Engl J Med.* 2000;342: 1484–1491. 10.1056/nejm200005183422004.
85. Holloway RG, Shoulson I, Fahn S, et al. Pramipexole vs levodopa as initial treatment for Parkinson disease. *Arch Neurol.* 2004;6110.1001/archneur.61.7.1044.
86. Borovac JA. Side effects of a dopamine agonist therapy for Parkinson's disease: A mini-review of clinical pharmacology. *Yale J Biol Med.* 2016;89(1):37–47.
87. Chen JJ. Treatment of psychotic symptoms in patients with Parkinson disease. *Ment Health Clin.* 2017;7:262–270. 10.9740/mhc.2017.11.262.
88. Carbone F, Djamshidian A, Seppi K, et al. Apomorphine for Parkinson's disease: Efficacy and safety of current and new formulations. *CNS Drugs.* 2019;33:905–918. 10.1007/s40263-019-00661-z.
89. Kynmobi [Prescribing Information]. Sunovion Pharmaceuticals Inc. Marlborough, MA; 2020.
90. Olanow CW, Factor SA, Espay AJ, et al. Apomorphine sublingual film for off episodes in Parkinson's disease: A randomised, double-blind, placebo-controlled phase 3 study. *Lancet Neurol.* 2020;19:135–144. 10.1016/s1474-4422(19)30396-5.
91. Katzenschlager R, Poewe W, Rascol O, et al. Apomorphine subcutaneous infusion in patients with Parkinson's disease with persistent motor fluctuations (TOLEDO): A multicentre, double-blind, randomised, placebo-controlled trial. *Lancet Neurol.* 2018;17:749–759. 10.1016/s1474-4422(18)30239-4.
92. Mirapex. [Prescribing Information]. Boehringer Ingelheim. Ridgefield, CT. 2007.
93. Requip. [Prescribing information]. GlaxoSmithKline. Research Triangle Park, NC. 2007.

94. Chen JJ, Swope DM, Dashtipour K, et al. Transdermal rotigotine: A clinically innovative dopamine-receptor agonist for the management of Parkinson's disease. *Pharmacotherapy.* 2009;29:1452–1467. 10.1592/phco.29.12.1452.
95. Patel Tejal, Chang Feng Practice recommendations for Parkinson's disease. *Canadian Pharmacists Journal/Revue des Pharmaciens du Canada.* 2015;148:142–149. 10.1177/1715163515578146.
96. Henrichsmann M, Hempel G. Impact of medication therapy management in patients with Parkinson's disease. *International Journal of Clinical Pharmacy.* 2015;38:54–60. 10.1007/s11096-015-0206-0.
97. Foppa AA, Chemello C, Vargas-Peláez CM, et al. Medication therapy management service for patients with Parkinson's disease: A before-and-after study. *Neurol Ther.* 2016;5:85–99. 10.1007/s40120-016-0046-4.
98. Stefan TC, Elharar N, Garcia G. Implementation and evaluation of Parkinson disease management in an outpatient clinical pharmacist–run neurology telephone clinic. *Ment Health Clin.* 2018;8:159–162. 10.9740/mhc.2018.05.159.
99. Stuijt C, Karapinar-Çarkit F, van den Bemt B, et al. Effect of pharmacist-led interventions on (non)motor symptoms, medication-related problems, and quality of life in Parkinson disease patients: A pilot study. *Clin Neuropharmacol.* 2018;41:14–19. 10.1097/wnf.0000000000000260.

79

Pain Management

Christopher M. Herndon, Courtney M. Kominek, and Amanda M. Mullins

KEY CONCEPTS

1. Understanding the pathogenesis of pain should guide treatment and patient education.
2. Whenever possible ask patients if they have pain to identify the source of pain and to assess the characteristics of the pain.
3. The etiology of pain may not always be identifiable.
4. A multidisciplinary approach that includes incorporation of nonpharmacologic strategies for pain management should be undertaken.
5. Chronic pain treatment should focus on self-management strategies and focus on active rather than passive approaches.
6. Selection of nonopioids and opioids should be based on the characteristics and type of pain as well as individual patient factors.
7. Oral or topical analgesics are preferred over other dosage forms whenever feasible, but it is important to adjust the route of administration based on the patient's needs.
8. Patients taking analgesics should be monitored for response (analgesia, functionality, quality-of-life) and medication adverse effects.
9. Doses must be individualized for each patient and administered for an adequate duration of time. Around-the-clock regimens should be considered for acute and chronic pain. As-needed regimens should be used for breakthrough pain or when acute pain displays wide variability and/or has subsided greatly.
10. Consider a trial of opioids in those with severe pain who have failed nonpharmacologic and nonopioid treatment only when the anticipated benefits are expected to outweigh the risks.
11. Use risk mitigation strategies such as informed consent/patient agreements, urine toxicology monitoring, opioid overdose education and naloxone distribution (OEND), and prescription drug monitoring programs (PDMP) checks when necessary.

BEYOND THE BOOK

Watch the following videos on YouTube to learn more about this topic:

Understanding pain and what to do about it in less than 5 minutes—presented by Painaustralia

URL: https://tinyurl.com/yxjyltp6

Tame the beast: It's time to rethink persistent pain—Lorimer Moseley, David Moen, Sam Chisholm

URL: https://tinyurl.com/y2nbtbb2

The mystery of chronic pain—Elliot Krane

URL: https://www.ted.com/talks/elliot_krane_the_mystery_of_chronic_pain?language=en

INTRODUCTION

If we know that pain and suffering can be alleviated, and do nothing about it, then we ourselves, become the tormentors.

—Primo Levi[1]

Humans have always known and sought relief from pain.[2] Today, pain's impact on society is still great, and pain remains a primary reason why patients seek medical advice.[3] In general, pain is defined as: "an unpleasant sensory and emotional experience associated with actual or potential tissue damage or described in terms of such damage."[4] However, as pain is subjective, many clinicians define pain as "whatever the patient says it is."

Regrettably, many healthcare providers do not receive adequate training in pain management. Therefore, understanding its pathophysiology and maintaining a thorough understanding of both nonpharmacologic and pharmacologic treatment modalities are important factors in addressing pain control.

EPIDEMIOLOGY

Data collected by the National Health Interview Survey suggest that greater than 50 million persons in the United States live with chronic pain.[5] Of whom, 7.5% report "high impact pain," which is considered chronic pain that limits life or work activities on most days or every day.[5] In 1 year, an estimated 25 million Americans will experience acute pain due to injury or surgery, and one-third will experience severe chronic pain at some point in their lives.[3] Unfortunately, despite much public attention, pain often remains inadequately or inappropriately treated.[6,7]

PATHOPHYSIOLOGY

1 Pain pathophysiology involves complex interactions between neural and immune networks within the peripheral and central nervous system (CNS) in response to afferent sensory stimuli that produce the conscious experience we know as pain. It can be physiologic and protective (adaptive) or pathophysiologic and harmful (maladaptive).[8] Pain is a complex interaction between biological processes (nociception) impacted by individual psychological and social determinates.

Adaptive Pain

The pain experienced from noxious stimuli involving temperature extremes, mechanical trauma, or chemical irritation is called nociceptive pain which is a primitive evolutionary mechanism to protect our body from actual or potential tissue injury. Pain that occurs as a result of unavoidable tissue damage (trauma or surgery) creates sensitization at and adjacent to the site of tissue injury. This process also engages the immune system and is called inflammatory pain. Nociceptive and inflammatory pains are both adaptive and protective. The physiological processing of pain occurs within a neurotransmission circuit via a number of steps known as transduction, conduction, transmission, modulation, and perception.[8]

Transduction

The first step leading to the sensation of pain is stimulation of specialized nerve fiber receptors known as *nociceptors*. These high-threshold receptors are found in both somatic and visceral structures and help to discriminate between noxious and innocuous stimuli. Nociceptors are activated and subsequently sensitized by mechanical, thermal, and chemical stimuli.[8] The underlying mechanism of these noxious stimuli, which in and of themselves may sensitize/stimulate the receptor, may be the release/activation of numerous cytokines and chemokines that sensitize and/or activate the nociceptors (Fig. 79-1).[8-10]

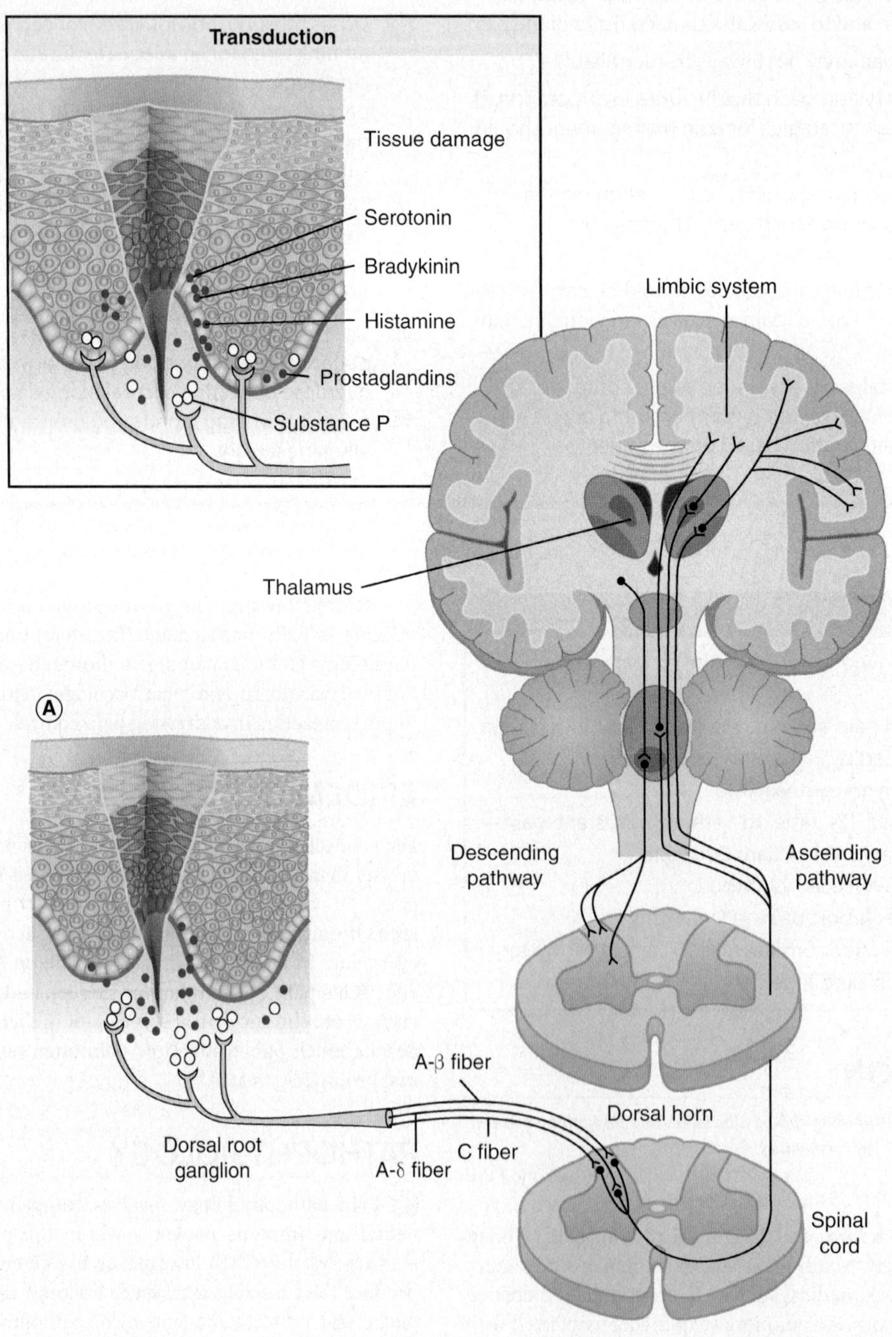

FIGURE 79-1 Schematic representation of nociceptive pain. *(Reprinted from Pasero C, R. Neurophysiology of pain and analgesia and the pathophysiology of neuropathic pain. In: McCaffery M, Pasero C, eds.* Pain Assessment and Pharmacologic Management. *St. Louis, MO: Mosby; 2011:1–12.)*

Conduction

Nociceptor activation leads to the conversion of a chemical signal into an electrical signal through voltage-gated sodium channels, which produce the generation of action potentials that are conducted along primary afferent A-δ and C-polymodal nerve fibers to the dorsal horn of the spinal cord.[11,12] Stimulation of large-diameter, sparsely myelinated A-δ fibers evokes sharp, well-localized pain, whereas stimulation of unmyelinated, small-diameter C fibers produces aching, poorly localized pain.[13]

Transmission

These afferent, nociceptive pain fibers synapse in various layers (laminae) of the spinal cord's dorsal horn and convert the electrical signal back into a chemical signal by releasing excitatory neurotransmitters, such as glutamate and substance P. The N-type voltage-gated calcium channels regulate the release of these excitatory neurotransmitters. The complex array of events that influence pain can be explained in part by the interactions between neuroreceptors and neurotransmitters that take place in this synapse. Pain signals reach the brain through a host of ascending spinal cord pathways, which include the neo- and paleospinothalamic tract.[13] Other sensory information is also carried along these pathways. Thus, pain is influenced by many factors supplemental to nociception, which prevents simple schematic representation. The thalamus acts as a relay station within the brain, as these pathways ascend and pass the impulses to higher cortical structures where pain can be processed further.[13]

Modulation

The brain and spinal cord modulate pain through a number of intricate processes, and transmission may be facilitated by neurotransmitters such as glutamate or substance P to make the signals stronger and the pain more intense. Alternatively, the signal can be attenuated/inhibited by descending pathways that consist of endogenous opioids (eg, enkephalins and β-endorphins), γ-aminobutyric acid (GABA), norepinephrine, or serotonin.[14-16] Like exogenous opioids, endogenous peptides bind to opioid receptor sites and modulate the transmission of pain impulses.[14] Other receptor types, such as the glutamate receptor, also can influence this system. Blockade of one such receptor, *N*-methyl-D-aspartate (NMDA), may increase the mu (μ)-receptors' responsiveness to opiates.[17]

Perception

The complex interplay between ascending excitatory and descending inhibitory pathways is thought to culminate in a conscious experience that takes place in higher cortical structures. While not well understood, cognitive and behavioral functions can modify pain; thus, relaxation, distraction, meditation, and guided mental imagery may strongly influence pain perception and decrease pain.[18,19] In contrast, conditions such as depression or anxiety often worsen pain.[20]

Impact of Immune System on Pain Signaling

A two-way communication exists between neurons and immune cells within the CNS, especially astrocytes and microglia which are the equivalent of a macrophage within the CNS.[17,21] Their activation within the CNS in response to peripheral and central nerve injury leads to a complex cascade of events responsible for the ongoing pain seen in neuropathic pain conditions. Activated microglia may also play a role in the development of opioid tolerance and opioid-induced hyperalgesia. Evidence is emerging that the interface between immune cells and neurons in the CNS plays a significant role in the maintenance of chronic pain and may offer attractive new potential therapeutic targets.[22]

Maladaptive (Pathologic) Pain

1 Pathophysiologic pain is distinctly different from nociceptive pain, in that it becomes disengaged from noxious stimuli or healing and often is described in terms of chronic pain. This type of pain is a result of damage or abnormal functioning of the peripheral nervous system (PNS) and/or CNS.[17] Maladaptive pain can be neuropathic, in which there is ongoing peripheral nerve injury (eg, postherpetic neuralgia, painful diabetic neuropathy, or chemotherapy-induced neuropathy), or in the CNS (eg, following an ischemic stroke or with multiple sclerosis). Maladaptive pain may also be centralized, where no nerve injury or inflammation exists, but a centrally mediated disturbance in pain processing within the CNS leads to pain hypersensitivity and subsequently spontaneous pain. Classic examples are fibromyalgia, irritable bowel syndrome, temporomandibular joint disorder, and myofascial pain syndrome. Chronic pain states are often mixed with all three mechanisms (nociceptive, neuropathic, and centralized) simultaneously.[23] These pain syndromes are frequently challenging to diagnose and difficult to treat. In addition, the pain reported is often not commensurate with physical exam findings or imaging results, which may result in undertreatment and ultimately inadequate pain relief.

The mechanism responsible for pain of this nature may be the nervous system's dynamic nature. Nerve damage or certain disease states may cause both peripheral (eg, alteration in nociceptive nerve fiber sensitivity, alteration of sodium channels, collateral sprouting of nerve fibers) and central (eg, hyperexcitability of central neurons or central sensitization, NMDA-glutamate receptor activation, central disinhibition) changes in neurotransmission leading to increased pain.[14,17] Pain circuits may rewire themselves both anatomically and biochemically (often referred to as neural plasticity), and this produces a mismatch between pain stimulation and inhibition, potentially resulting in a progressive increase in the discharge of dorsal horn neurons.[24] The end result is chronic pain, where patients may present with episodic or continuous pain transmission (often described as burning, tingling, shock-like, or shooting), exaggerated painful response to normally noxious stimuli (hyperalgesia), and/or painful response to normally non-noxious stimuli (allodynia).[13,25,26] This change over time may help explain why this type of pain often manifests long after the injury or when no actual injury is identified.

CLASSIFICATION OF PAIN

1 2 3 It is helpful in guiding the assessment and treatment of pain to classify or subdivide the presenting symptoms by the type of pain (eg, nociceptive, neuropathic, inflammatory), by pain intensity (eg, mild, moderate, or severe), or most commonly by duration of pain (eg, acute, subacute, or chronic pain).

Acute Pain

2 3 Acute pain is a beneficial physiologic process, serving its adaptive purpose by warning individuals of disease states and potentially harmful situations. Unfortunately, severe, unremitting, under-treated acute pain, when it outlives its biologic usefulness, can produce many deleterious effects. Aside from unnecessary suffering, poorly treated acute pain also increases one's risk for the development of chronic pain syndromes.[27] Acute pain is typically short in duration, lasting less than 30 days and is often due to an identifiable cause and is usually nociceptive in nature with common causes including surgery, acute illness, trauma, labor, medical procedures, and cancer or cancer treatment.[28]

Chronic Pain

5 Under normal conditions, acute pain subsides quickly as the healing process decreases the pain-producing stimuli; however, in some instances, pain persists for months to years, leading to a chronic pathologic pain state with features quite different from those of acute pain (Table 79-1).[28,29] In many cases, the exact etiology of

TABLE 79-1 Characteristics of Acute and Chronic Pain

Characteristics	Acute Pain	Chronic Pain
Relief of pain	Highly desirable	Highly desirable
Dependence and tolerance to medication	Unusual	Common
Psychological component	Usually not present	Often a major problem
Organic cause	Common	May not be present
Environmental/family issues	Small	Significant
Insomnia	Unusual	Common component
Treatment goal	Cure	Functionality
Depression	Uncommon	Common

Data from References 28 and 29.

pain may not be identifiable; therefore, chronic pain can be classified as either being associated with cancer (cancer pain) or from noncancer etiologies (chronic noncancer pain). Chronic noncancer pain is often a result of changes to nerve function and transmission, thus making treatment more challenging.[30]

Cancer Pain

1 2 4 Pain associated with potentially life-threatening conditions is often called malignant pain or cancer pain.[32] This type of pain includes both chronic and acute (eg, breakthrough pain) components and often has multiple etiologies. This pain may be caused by the disease itself (eg, tumor invasion, organ obstruction), associated with treatment (eg, anticancer, radiation, and surgical incisions), or as a result of diagnostic procedures (eg, biopsy).[32] Breakthrough cancer pain may be *idiopathic* (no known precipitating factors), *incident* (due to a predictable cause), or *end of dose failure* (predictable worsening of pain at the end of an analgesic's pharmacodynamic efficacy).[33] Regardless of duration of pain, or suspected underlying etiology, a standardized approach to evaluation of a pain complaint is imperative. Cancer pain crises, frequently considered an acute pain overlaying an ongoing chronic pain, should be considered a medical emergency. Additional information about cancer pain can be found in Chapter 150, "Supportive Care."

CLINICAL PRESENTATION

2 4 A patient-oriented approach is essential, and symptom assessment methods for pain should not differ from those used in other conditions.[34] Therefore, a comprehensive history and physical

CLINICAL PRESENTATION Acute and Chronic Pain

Acute Pain

General

- Look for obvious distress (eg, trauma). In infants, presentation may include changes in feeding habits, increased fussiness, or being inconsolable. Those with dementia may exhibit changes in eating habits, increased agitation, or calling out. Attention also must be given to mental/emotional factors that alter the pain threshold. Anxiety, depression, fatigue, anger, and fear are noted to lower this threshold, whereas rest, mood elevation, sympathy, distraction, and understanding raise the pain threshold symptoms.
- Can be described as sharp, dull, shock-like, tingling, shooting, radiating, fluctuating in intensity, and varying in location (these occur in a timely relationship with obvious noxious stimuli).

Signs

- Hypertension, tachycardia, diaphoresis, mydriasis, and pallor, but these signs are *not diagnostic*.
- In some cases, there are no obvious physical signs.
- Comorbid conditions usually not present.
- Outcome of treatment generally predictable.

Laboratory Tests

- Pain is always subjective.
- There are no specific laboratory tests for pain.
- Pain is best diagnosed based on patient description and history.

Chronic Pain

General

- Can appear to have no noticeable suffering. Attention also must be given to mental/emotional factors that alter the pain threshold, similar to acute pain.

Symptoms

- Can be described as sharp, dull, shock-like, tingling, shooting, radiating, fluctuating in intensity, and varying in location (these often occur *without* a temporal relationship with obvious noxious stimuli).
- Over time, the pain stimulus may cause symptoms that completely change (eg, sharp to dull, obvious to vague).

Signs

- Hypertension, tachycardia, diaphoresis, mydriasis, and pallor are seldom present.
- In most cases, there are *no* obvious signs.
- Comorbid conditions are often present (eg, insomnia, depression, and anxiety).
- Outcome of treatment is often unpredictable.

Laboratory Tests

- Pain is always subjective.
- Pain is best diagnosed based on patient description and history.
- There are *no* specific laboratory tests for pain; however, history and/or diagnostic proof of past trauma (eg, computed tomography) may be helpful in diagnosing etiology. General labs that may be considered include vitamin D, thyroid-stimulating hormone (generalized or widespread pain), and B12 (neuropathic pain).

Data from Reference 28.

examination is imperative to evaluate underlying diseases and possible other contributing factors.[28] This includes asking if the patient has pain and identifying the source of pain when possible; however, the absence of a discreet etiology should not preclude appropriate treatment.[28] A baseline characterization of pain should be obtained using a symptom assessment mnemonic (eg, OLDCARTS, SOCRATES, SCHOLAR-MAC, or PQRST).[31] Ongoing assessment should occur using a consistent and validated method (ie, Wong Baker Faces Scale, Brief Pain Inventory, Numeric Rating Scale, or Pain-Enjoyment-General Activity Scale).[35]

TREATMENT

Achieving desired pain management outcomes includes both nonpharmacologic and pharmacologic strategies.

Desired Outcomes

4 5 The primary goal of pain treatment depends on the type of pain present and should be tailored to individual patients and circumstances (see "Patient Care Process" section). For example, a desired outcome in the acute postoperative setting may be to achieve a level of pain relief that allows the patient to attain certain functional goals, such as deep breathing or participation in physical therapy. In comparison, the goals in chronic noncancer pain may be to improve or maintain the patient's level of functioning, decrease pain perception, reduce medication use when possible, improve the patient's quality of life, and minimize the adverse effects of analgesics.[33]

Nonpharmacologic Therapy

2 3 5 The use of nonpharmacologic therapies should always be considered first-line therapy, either alone or in combination with appropriate analgesics. It is important to target all aspects of the biopsychosocial model when treating pain. Collaborating with other professions who are trained to provide nonpharmacologic approaches is essential. In addition, focusing on active therapies over passive therapies is encouraged. The evidence basis for many of the nonpharmacologic approaches is in evolution, and the results of these approaches can have varied efficacy based on the skill of the individual applying the modality as well as the type of pain being treated.

A variety of nonpharmacologic approaches are available. These include physical therapy, manipulation, formal exercise programs, weight loss, and diet changes (Table 79-2).[36-39] There are numerous complementary and integrative approaches with evidence in pain treatment that include acupuncture, Tai chi, yoga, mindfulness, meditation, relaxation, and biofeedback.[40,41] Complementary and integrative approaches to the treatment of chronic pain are outlined in Table 79-3.[40]

5 Simple interventions (eg, education or introductory information about expected discomfort or pain after certain procedures) reduce patient distress and help reduce post-procedure pain.[43] Psychological techniques (eg, cognitive-behavioral therapy, relaxation training, mindfulness-based stress reduction) are effective in reducing pain-related disability and improving global functioning in patients with numerous types of chronic pain.[40,44] Multidisciplinary rehabilitation programs with both psychological and physical components improve pain, function, and disability.[39,42]

Electroanalgesia involves the application of electrical stimulation to various locations and range from noninvasive (eg, transcutaneous or percutaneous electrical nerve stimulation) to highly invasive (implanted spinal cord stimulation).[39,45] Transcutaneous electrical nerve stimulation (TENS) may reduce pain by enhancing natural descending inhibitory pathways within the CNS. The frequency of the electrical stimulation delivered, presence or absence of systemic analgesics, and the type of underlying pain may affect the overall efficacy of this treatment.[46] Although data are conflicting on the efficacy of TENS, with its low risk for adverse effects, it remains a practical option.[45,47]

TABLE 79-2 Nonpharmacologic Approaches to the Treatment of Pain

- Exercise
- Physical therapy
- Diet
  - Anti-inflammatory
  - Elimination
- Weight loss
- Electroanalgesia: application of electrical stimulation to various areas that range from noninvasive to highly invasive
  - Noninvasive: transcutaneous electrical nerve stimulation (TENS)
  - Minimally invasive: percutaneous electrical nerve stimulation (PENS)
  - Highly invasive: spinal cord stimulation (SCS)
- Interventional approaches
- Cognitive behavioral therapy for chronic pain
- Multidisciplinary rehabilitation programs

Data from References 38, 41 and 42.

Pharmacologic Therapy

Appropriate Patient Selection

6 7 8 9 Pharmacologic treatment is often considered the cornerstone of pain management. The potential for benefit with each pharmacologic option, as well as the risk of adverse effects, must be assessed at baseline and periodically when determining the optimal therapeutic plan for an individual patient. The potential for benefit with each pharmacologic option, as well as the risk of adverse effects, must be assessed at baseline and periodically.

Patient Selection Considerations in Acute or Cancer Pain

9 10 11 The World Health Organization (WHO) recommends a three-step ladder approach using the nonopioids as initial treatment and escalating treatment to either "weak" or "strong" opioids based on pain intensity ratings (ie, mild, moderate, or severe).[52] Patient-specific factors, for example, renal or liver dysfunction that would potentially limit treatment with many nonopioid therapies, may lead clinicians to initiate therapy with an opioid to optimize pain relief while minimizing adverse effects. Acute cancer pain crises should be considered a medical emergency and specifics regarding its treatment are included in Chapter 150, "Supportive Care." Inadequate analgesia, opioid-related adverse effects, or loss of an administration route may require rotation to another opioid analgesic. The process for equianalgesic opioid rotation is provided in Table 79-4.[53]

Patient Selection Considerations in Chronic Noncancer Pain

3 4 5 7 8 9 10 11 In all cases of chronic noncancer pain, an integrated systematic approach with a strong emphasis on patient–clinician relationships is essential. Patients and clinicians must realize that optimal treatment may take months or even years to achieve. Opioids are often a treatment of last resort in chronic noncancer pain and initiated as a time-limited trial to assess improvement in the patient's function, while overall tolerability is evaluated. Although long-term opioid therapy can be effective for individual patients in carefully considered situations, limited data exist to support such practice.[37,54] Chronic opioid therapy in this setting requires careful patient selection with judicious attention to risk factors (eg, person or family history of substance use disorder, younger age, male gender, and certain co-occurring mental health conditions) to evaluate the balance between potential benefit of therapy and the potential risks in the individual patient.

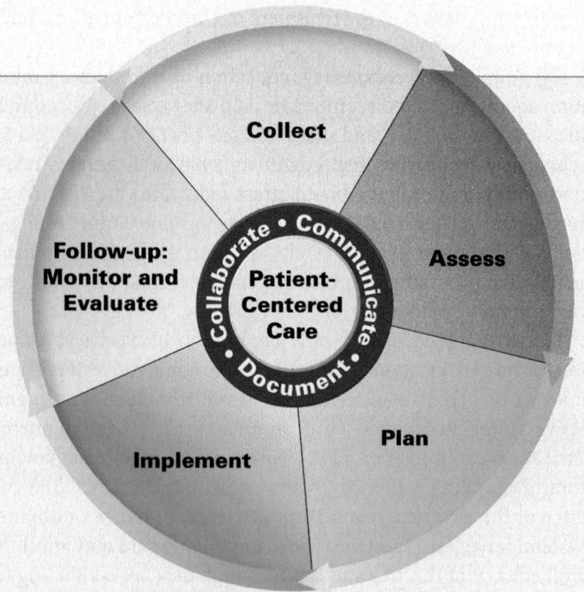

Patient Care Process for Pain Management

The image shows the five fundamental steps included in the patient care process for the treatment of pain. The tagline of this process reads collaborate, communicate, and document. The five fundamental steps listed here are collect, assess, plan, implement, and follow-up: monitor and evaluate. All these steps are listed in a circular block diagram.

Collect

- Patient-specific characteristics (eg, age, gender, pregnancy status, race, and ethnicity)
- Pain and symptom-specific history (eg, onset, location, duration, characteristics, aggravating factors, alleviating factors, timing, severity, and impact on activities of daily living)
- Patient history including current and past medications, nonpharmacologic trials, allergies or medication intolerance, and pertinent social history (eg, tobacco, alcohol, or other substance use)
- Family history focusing on symptoms (ie, Rheumatoid arthritis) and social behavior (ie, substance use)
- Objective data including vitals, pertinent labs, targeted physical exam, and urine toxicology results

Assess

- Presence of co-occurring mental health conditions (ie, substance use disorder, depression, anxiety, or bipolar disorder) which may guide treatment decisions
- Data from prescription drug monitoring programs (PDMP), urine toxicology results, and validated risk screening or assessment tools
- Relative or absolute contraindications to the use of opioids, acetaminophen, antidepressants, antiseizure medications, nonsteroidal anti-inflammatory drugs (NSAIDs), or skeletal muscle relaxants
- Chronicity of pain symptom (eg, acute or chronic), likely etiology (eg, neuropathic, musculoskeletal, or visceral), and severity
- Patient willingness to engage in nonpharmacologic treatment modalities (eg, physical therapy, counseling, acupuncture, nerve blocks, or surgical interventions)

Plan*

- Patient and symptom-specific lifestyle modification (eg, weight loss, smoking cessation, self-pacing, and pain-trigger avoidance; see Table 79-2)
- Nonpharmacologic treatment modalities (see Table 79-3)
- Pharmacotherapy regimen including dose, route, frequency, and duration (see Table 79-4)
- Pharmacotherapy efficacy (analgesic and functional improvement), toxicity, and ongoing appropriateness using tools such as urine toxicology results, PDMP data, and risk assessment tools (see Table 79-6)
- Patient education on safe use, storage, disposal, and risk mitigation following formal Risk Evaluation and Mitigation Strategies when available (see Table 79-7)

Implement*

- Educate patient and/or caregiver regarding all elements of disease process and treatment plan, ensuring patient and/or caregiver understanding
- Informed consent, including pain or treatment agreements when necessary
- Schedule timely follow-up as guided by best practices in medication monitoring, following all appropriate regulations

Follow-up: Monitor and Evaluate

- Attainment of treatment goals (eg, improved activity, improved sleep, improved work attendance)
- Presence of adverse effects
- Completion of validated ongoing risk assessment tools
- Frequent review of PDMP as clinically indicated and/or legally required
- Patient adherence to all facets of treatment plan, including nonpharmacologic modalities

Collaborate with patient, caregivers, and other healthcare professionals.

Nonopioid Analgesics

Acetaminophen and Nonsteroidal Anti-inflammatory Drugs

5 6 7 Analgesics should be initiated with the most effective agent having the fewest potential adverse effects. Acetaminophen and nonsteroidal anti-inflammatory drugs (NSAIDs) are often preferred first-line therapies in the treatment of mild-to-moderate pain, although the efficacy of acetaminophen has been called into question (Table 79-8).[55,56] The exact mechanism of acetaminophen is not completely understood but likely involves central prostaglandin modulation.[57] The NSAIDs inhibit formation of varying prostaglandins produced in response to noxious stimuli, thereby decreasing neuronal pain transmission received by the CNS.[40] While acetaminophen is still considered a first-line therapy for some mild pain conditions, in some pain-related disease states, such as osteoarthritis,

TABLE 79-3 Complementary and Integrative Approaches for Chronic Pain

Intervention	Description	Evidence	Safety
Tai Chi	Low impact Mind body exercise Started in China as a martial art Slow mindful movement with attention to breathing and relaxation	Osteoarthritis Chronic low back pain (CLBP) Fibromyalgia	Minor musculoskeletal aches and pains
Yoga	From India Blend of meditation, breathing, and physical postures	Osteoarthritis Rheumatoid Arthritis Kyphosis Fibromyalgia Low back pain (LBP) Neck pain	Similar to musculoskeletal pain associated with physical therapy (PT) Discuss with provider/yoga instructor if glaucoma or osteoporosis
Acupuncture	Stimulation of certain points of the body typically with the insertion of needles into the skin East Asian	*Acute:* Post-surgical pain (reduces opioid dose) Migraine Acute/subacute LBP Ankle sprain *Chronic:* CLBP Osteoarthritis (knee, hip, general) Temporomandibular disorder (TMD) Headache Migraine Neck pain Shoulder pain Peripheral neuropathy (diabetic, HIV, Bell's palsy, Carpal Tunnel Syndrome [CTS]) Fibromyalgia	Low risk for adverse effects Minor: itching, relaxation, tired Rare: pneumothorax, infections (associated with poor training)
Massage	Soft tissue manipulation	*Acute:* Postoperative pain *Chronic:* CLBP Neck and shoulder pain Osteoarthritis Heel pain Epicondylitis Fibromyalgia	Low risk for adverse effects
Mindfulness, meditation, and relaxation	A variety of mind-body practices to capitalize on body's own calming response through reducing blood pressure and slower breathing. Examples: mindfulness-based stress reduction (MBSR), cognitive behavioral therapy (CBT), pain-coping skills training (PCST), diaphragmatic breathing, progressive muscle relaxation, hypnosis, acceptance and commitment therapy, music therapy, guided imagery	*Acute:* Burn patients (music therapy) Acute/procedural pain (music therapy, hypnosis, guided imagery) *Chronic:* LBP (MBSR, CBT) Chronic pain (music therapy, CBT, guided imagery, ACT, progressive relaxation) Headache (mindfulness and relaxation, MBSR) Fibromyalgia (relaxation, guided imagery) Knee pain (PCST) Osteoarthritis (PCST, guided imagery) Rheumatoid arthritis (PCST, guided imagery) Diabetic neuropathy (mindfulness/meditation) TMD (relaxation)	Rare adverse reactions (psychiatric patients, epilepsy, hx of trauma)
Biofeedback	Mind-body practice in which patients are connected to a device that measures their bodily functions (BP, HR, RR) and use the information to alter thoughts and behaviors	Tension/migraine headache CLBP Fibromyalgia Shoulder pain	No to low risk of adverse reactions
Manipulation	Treatment of spine and other joints	Osteoarthritis (hip, knee, ankle, plantar fasciitis, ankle, shoulder, epicondylitis) LBP CTS TMD	Musculoskeletal aches and pains Uncommon serious adverse reactions (cervical artery dissection, stroke, neck injury)

Data from References 38, 40 and 48-51.

NSAIDs, either oral or topical, may be preferred.[58,59] In addition, NSAIDs are recommended after nonpharmacologic therapy failure for acute, subacute, and chronic low back pain.[60]

6 7 8 Studies comparing the efficacy of individual NSAIDs have failed to identify differences in efficacy. Therefore, the choice of a particular agent often depends on availability, cost, pharmacokinetics, pharmacologic characteristics, and the adverse effects. Because of the large interpatient variability in response to individual NSAIDs, it is considered rational therapy to switch to another member of this class if there is inadequate response after a sufficient therapeutic trial of any single agent.[53] The duration of a sufficient trial has not been well defined; however, typically, an

TABLE 79-4 Steps for Equianalgesic Opioid Calculation

Step 1. Use the equianalgesic dose chart in Table 79-5 for a first estimate of the dose of the new medication that is equianalgesic to the old medication.

Step 2. Record the total dose of each opioid given during the past 24 hours. If both parenteral and oral doses of the same opioid were given, calculate a separate total for each.

Step 3. Divide each 24-hour total by the equianalgesic dose in Table 79-5 for that opioid and route, converting the dose into equianalgesic dose units. Add the equianalgesic dose units for all medications and routes (ie, some clinicians prefer to convert all opioid doses to "oral morphine equivalents" prior to calculating new target dose).

Step 4. Estimate the dose of the new medication by multiplying the sum obtained in Step 3 by the equianalgesic dose for the new medication and route.

Step 5. Modify the initial estimate based on the clinical situation and the specific medications involved. Factors that enter into this process include the following:

a. Effective analgesia, intolerable adverse effects: calculate the dose of the new opioid as outlined in Steps 1 to 4. Reduce target dose by 25% to 50% to account for lack of cross-tolerance between various opioids.

b. Ineffective analgesia, no intolerable adverse effects: calculate the dose of the new opioid as outlined in Steps 1 to 4. Reduction in target dose outlined in (a) may be disregarded depending on clinical situation and patient-specific variables. Those with severe pain on regularly scheduled opioids for >5 days may have their dose increased by 30% to 50% or an increase equal to the use of supplemental PRN medication per day averaged over the previous 2 to 3 days. Consider more conservative increases (ie, 10%-20%) in the first few days of therapy in those who have less severe pain or who are frail. Dose increases are safest after steady-state has been approached (typically 5-6 half-lives).

Step 6. Should PRN dosing of an immediate release medication be necessary for breakthrough pain, provide 10% to 15% of total daily dose of new opioid every 3 to 4 hours depending on individual opioid's duration of analgesia.

Step 7. Reassess the patient frequently following opioid rotation (48-72 hours following dose change).

Data from Reference 53.

NSAID should be continued for a minimum of 1 month prior to evaluating the need to switch agents. Chronic use of NSAIDs may result in serious gastrointestinal (GI), renal, and cardiac toxicity and to a lesser extent liver toxicity. Topical NSAIDs may offer similar efficacy as oral NSAIDs with improved safety and tolerability in the treatment of small or superficial joint arthritis.[62] Appropriate patient selection for NSAID therapy is critical to ensure optimal benefit while minimizing potential adverse effects. Several NSAIDs are subject to pharmacogenomic variants.[63]

Co-Analgesics

5 6 7 Co-analgesics represent a diverse group of pharmacologic agents with individual characteristics that make them useful in the management of pain, but these agents typically are not classified as analgesics. Chronic pain that has a neuropathic component (eg, diabetic neuropathy) often requires co-analgesic therapy. Antiseizure medications (eg, gabapentin, pregabalin, which may decrease neuronal excitability), tricyclic antidepressants and serotonin and norepinephrine reuptake inhibitor antidepressants (eg, duloxetine, venlafaxine—which block the reuptake of serotonin and norepinephrine, thus enhancing pain inhibition), and topically applied local anesthetics (which decrease nerve stimulation) all have demonstrated efficacy in managing various chronic pain conditions.[64]

6 7 8 **Antiseizure Medications** The antiseizure medications frequently employed for pain are presented in Table 79-9.[65-72] Carbamazepine and oxcarbazepine block voltage-gated sodium channels and potentiate the effects of GABA and are considered the agents of choice for trigeminal neuralgia according to multiple guidelines.[64,66,73,74] The primary metabolic pathway for carbamazepine is CYP3A4. The active metabolite, carbamazepine 10,11-epoxide, auto-induces its own metabolism, making titration difficult. Carbamazepine is associated with many medication interactions through induction of CYP3A4, CYP1A2, CYP2B6, CYP2C9, and CYP2C19. Common adverse effects during initiation include dizziness, drowsiness, unsteadiness, nausea, and vomiting and can be avoided with low starting doses. There are rare cases of aplastic anemia and agranulocytosis associated with carbamazepine use, so a complete blood count (CBC) should be monitored during therapy. Hyponatremia is also reported, which requires regular monitoring of sodium.[75] Cardiovascular effects include hyper/hypotension, congestive heart failure, edema, arrhythmias, and atrioventricular block. Hepatic enzymes should be monitored periodically during the treatment for potential elevation.[76]

Oxcarbazepine is the keto derivative of carbamazepine and is metabolized to an active metabolite, 10-monohydroxy oxcarbazepine, which does not undergo Phase I metabolism in the liver. This is advantageous for oxcarbazepine with reduced medications interactions and adverse effects compared to carbamazepine.[76] The most common adverse effects include dizziness, somnolence, diplopia, fatigue, nausea, vomiting, ataxia, abnormal vision, headache, nystagmus, tremor, and abnormal gait. Other adverse effects include hyponatremia, angioedema or anaphylactic reactions, pancytopenia, agranulocytosis, and leukopenia.[75] In addition to its role in trigeminal neuralgia, the National Institute for Health and Care Excellence (NICE) guidelines list oxcarbazepine for the treatment of neuropathic pain in a specialist setting as fourth-line treatment.[64,74,77]

Gabapentinoids, including gabapentin and pregabalin, are common antiseizure medications used in the treatment of neuropathic pain. There are numerous formulations available with varying indications that may include diabetic peripheral neuropathy (DPN), postherpetic neuralgia (PHN), fibromyalgia, neuropathic pain associated with spinal cord injury (SCI), and restless legs syndrome (RLS). Based on several neuropathic pain treatment guidelines, gabapentinoids are considered first-line medications for the treatment of neuropathic pain.[64-67,74] Other roles for gabapentinoids include perioperative pain management as a part of a multimodal approach or "enhanced recovery after surgery" (ERAS) protocols. These agents, however, were not included in the ERAS Society guidelines due to inconclusive evidence.[78] In general, evidence has not supported the use of gabapentinoids for the prevention of chronic post-surgical pain.[78,79] There are negative findings for pregabalin in acute and chronic sciatica as well as gabapentin and pregabalin for nonspecific low back pain.[80,81]

Gabapentinoids do not, as their name may suggest, alter GABA binding, uptake, metabolism, or degradation though their pharmacology does lead to GABA-mimetic effects. Primary pharmacodynamic effects are due to the inhibition of voltage-gated calcium channels specifically by binding to the presynaptic $\alpha 2\delta$ subunit. This results in decreased release of excitatory neurotransmitters glutamate, norepinephrine, and substance P.[70]

Common adverse medication effects, namely dizziness and sedation, can be mitigated with slow dose titration. Gabapentinoids may lead to peripheral edema and weight gain which may be dose-limiting adverse effects. All antiseizure medications have been associated with increased risk for suicidal thoughts and behavior. There have been increasing reports of unhealthy gabapentinoid use, which has resulted in some states classifying them as controlled substances and including them in their PDMPs.[82,83] Gabapentionoids are cleared renally and have recommended renal dose adjustments as well as supplemental doses after hemodialysis.[84]

Several neuropathic pain guidelines place lamotrigine as a fourth-line agent or medication for use in a specialist setting.[64,66,74] The mechanism of action of lamotrigine is not entirely known but thought to be related to the inhibition of voltage-gated sodium channels. One of the main concerns with the use of lamotrigine is the

TABLE 79-5 Opioid Analgesics

Class and Generic Name (Brand Name)	Chemical Source	Metabolic Pathway/Metabolites	Route[a]	Equianalgesic Dose in Adults (mg)	Approximate Onset (min)/ Half-Life (h)[b]
Phenanthrenes (morphine-like agonists)					
Morphine (numerous)	Naturally occurring	Phase II via glucuronidation/M3G[c] (inactive) and M6G[d] (active)	IM/IV	10	10-20/2
			PO	25	30-40/2
Hydromorphone (Dilaudid, Exalgo, various)	Semisynthetic	Phase II via glucuronidation/H3G (active)[e], H6G[f]	IM/IV	1.5	10-20/2-3
			PO	7.5	
Oxymorphone (Numorphan, Opana)	Semisynthetic	Phase II via glucuronidation/O3G (inactive)[g]	IM/IV	1	10-20/2-3
			PO	10	
Levorphanol (various)	Semisynthetic	Phase II via glucuronidation/ levorphanol-3-glucuronide (inactive)	PO	Variable	10-20/12-16
Codeine (various)	Naturally occurring	CYP2D6/morphine (active), Phase II glucuronidation/codeine-6-glucuronide (unknown), CYP3A4/norcodeine (inactive)	PO	15-30[h]	10-30/3
Hydrocodone (available as combination, single entity extended release—Hysingla ER[i], Zohydro ER)	Semisynthetic	CYP3A4/norhydrocodone (inactive); CYP2D6/ hydromorphone (active)	PO	5-10[h]	30-60/4
Oxycodone (OxyContin, Xtampza)[i]	Semisynthetic	CYP3A4/noroxycodone (active), CYP2D6/oxymorphone (active)	PO	15-30[j]	30-60/2-3
Phenylpiperidines (meperidine-like agonists)					
Meperidine (Demerol, various)	Synthetic	Phase II hydrolysis/meperidinic acid, CYP2B6, CYP3A4, & CYP2C19/normeperidine	IM/IV	75	10-20/3-5
			PO	300[j]; not recommended	
Fentanyl (Sublimaze, Duragesic, Lazanda, Abstral, Fentora, Subsys, OTFC, various)	Synthetic	CYP3A4/norfentanyl (inactive)	IM/IV	0.125[k]	7-15/3-4
			Transdermal, Buccal, transmucosal, sublingual, nasal, nebulized	Variable[l]	
Sufentanil (Sufenta, Dsuvia, various)	Synthetic	CYP3A4/norsufentanil (inactive)	IV/SL	0.030 (SL only)	30/2.5
Diphenylheptanes (methadone-like agonists)					
Methadone (Dolophine, various)	Synthetic	CYP3A4, CYP2B6, CYP2C19, CYP2C9, CYP2D6/EDDP (inactive)[m]	IM/IV	Variable[n] (acute)	
			PO	Variable[n] (acute)	30-60/12-190
Centrally Acting Agents					
Tramadol (Ultram, ConZip, various)	Synthetic	CYP3A4/nortramadol (inactive), CYP2D6/*O*-desmethyltramadol (active)	PO	50-100[g,o,p]	<60/5-7
Tapentadol (Nucynta)	Synthetic	Phase II glucuronidation/ tapentadol-o-glucuronide (inactive), CYP2C9 and CYP2C19/*N*-desmethyltapentadol (inactive), CYP2D6/hydroxytapentadol	PO	50-10[h,o,p]	Within 60/4
Agonist–antagonist derivatives					
Pentazocine (Talwin, various)	Synthetic	Liver/Alcoholic and carboxylic acid derivatives (inactive), pentazocine glucuronide (inactive)	IM	Not recommended	
			PO	50[h]	15-30/2-3

(continued)

TABLE 79-5 Opioid Analgesics (*Continued*)

Class and Generic Name (Brand Name)	Chemical Source	Metabolic Pathway/Metabolites	Route[a]	Equianalgesic Dose in Adults (mg)	Approximate Onset (min)/ Half-Life (h)[b]
Butorphanol (Stadol, various)	Synthetic	CYP3A4/hydroxybutorphanol (active), norbutorphanol (inactive)	IM/IV	2	10-20/3-4
			Intranasal	1[h] (one spray)	
Nalbuphine (Nubain, various)	Synthetic	CYP3A4 CYP2C19/nornalbuphine, 6-ketonalbuphine	IM/IV	10	<15/5
Buprenorphine (Buprenex, Butrans, Suboxone, Belbuca, Subutex, various)	Synthetic	CYP3A4/norbuprenorphine (active)	IM/IV	0.3	10-20/2-3
			Transdermal	Variable	
			Sublingual	Variable	

[a]The IM route should be avoided whenever possible—produces significant pain with administration and rate and extent of absorption is highly variable. If IV route is unavailable then administer subcutaneously (SC).

[b]ER/LA formulations may vary greatly in terms of onset and duration of analgesia. The reader should consult individual prescribing labels.

[c]Morphine-3-glucuronide (accumulates in renal failure).

[d]Morphine-6-glucuronide (accumulates in renal failure).

[e]Hydromorphone-3-glucuronide (accumulates in renal failure).

[f]Hydromorphone-6-glucuronide.

[g]Oxymorphone-3-glucuronide.

[h]Starting dose only (equianalgesia not shown).

[i]FDA approved as unhealthy use deterrent formulation.

[j]Starting doses lower (oxycodone 5-10 mg, meperidine 50-150 mg).

[k]Equivalent PO morphine dose = variable.

[l]For breakthrough pain only. Equianalgesic dose conversion should be avoided for Transmucosal Immediate Release Fentanyl (TIRF) products.

[m]2-ethylidene-1,5-dimethyl-3,3-diphenylpyrrolidene (EDDP).

[n]The equianalgesic dose of methadone when compared with other opioids will decrease progressively the higher the previous opioid dose. Caution should be exercised when initiating in opioid naïve patients.

[o]First day of dosing may administer second dose 1 hour after first dose.

[p]Onset of action may differ for long-acting formulations. Ceiling dose recommendations exist and may differ from immediate release dosing recommendations.

IM, intramuscular; IV, intravenous; PO, oral.

Data from References 53 and 61 and individual product package inserts.

TABLE 79-6 Major Adverse Effects of the Opioid Analgesics

Effect	Manifestation
Mood changes	Dysphoria, euphoria
Somnolence	Sedation, inability to concentrate
Stimulation of chemoreceptor trigger zone	Nausea, vomiting
Respiratory depression	Decreased respiratory rate, periodic breathing, oxygen desaturation
Decreased gastrointestinal motility	Constipation
Increase in sphincter tone	Biliary spasm, urinary retention (varies among agents)
Histamine release	Urticaria, pruritus, rarely exacerbation of asthma due to bronchospasm (varies among agents)
Tolerance	Larger doses for same effect
Physical dependence	Withdrawal symptoms upon abrupt discontinuation
Hypogonadism	Fatigue, depression, loss of analgesia, sexual dysfunction, amenorrhea
Sleep	Disrupts sleep–wake cycle, causes dose-dependent rapid eye movement (REM) suppression

Data from References 53 and 61.

possibility of life-threatening rash. To minimize the risk of a rash, the dose is titrated slowly (ie, every 2 weeks). If any signs of rash appear, lamotrigine should be discontinued immediately, although other fatal or life-threatening hypersensitivity reactions can occur as lamotrigine is also associated with blood dyscrasias and aseptic meningitis. More common adverse effects include dizziness, nausea, headache, insomnia, somnolence, fatigue, rhinitis, abdominal pain, diplopia, ataxia, and blurred vision. Utilizing lamotrigine is further complicated by the potential for multiple medication interactions.

For neuropathic pain, topiramate is listed as a fourth-line agent by the Canadian Pain Society guideline and for use in specialist settings by the NICE guidelines.[66,74] Additionally, topiramate has been evaluated for radicular low back pain in two small studies with conflicting data on benefits versus risk.[85,86] It has four components to its proposed mechanism of action including inhibition of voltage-gated sodium channels, increased effects of $GABA_A$ receptors, blocking AMPA/kainate subtype of glutamate receptors, and inhibiting the carbonic anhydrase enzyme. Topiramate has numerous warnings and precautions including secondary angle closure glaucoma, metabolic acidosis, hyperammonemia/encephalopathy, kidney stones, oligohidrosis, hypo/hyperthermia, and cognitive dysfunction. Renal dose adjustments are recommended with a creatinine clearance (CrCl) <70 mL/min (1.17 mL/s), and topiramate is removed via hemodialysis, so supplemental doses are needed. Dose-related adverse effects include paresthesia, fatigue, nausea, anorexia, dizziness, difficulty with memory, diarrhea, weight loss, concentration/attention problems, and somnolence.

TABLE 79-7 Key Recommendations of the Centers for Disease Control and Prevention Guideline for Prescribing Opioids for Chronic Pain

1. Nonpharmacologic and nonopioid modalities are preferred.
2. If opioid analgesia is warranted, establish realistic treatment goals.
3. Discuss the known risks and realistic benefits of opioid analgesics prior to initiation.
4. Immediate-release opioids are preferred over controlled release or long-acting (CR/LA) opioid formulations.
5. Use the lowest effective dose of opioid possible. Use caution at any dosage, and carefully reassess evidence of benefit versus risk when exceeding ≥50 MME/day and avoid increasing dose ≥90 MME/day without careful justification.
6. Opioid analgesia should be used for the shortest duration possible. In most cases, 3 days is sufficient for acute pain. More than 7 days will rarely be required for most acute pain indications.
7. Clinicians should regularly evaluate the benefits and harms of ongoing opioid analgesia within 1 to 4 weeks of initiation and at least every 3 months when ongoing opioid therapy is required. Consider taper and discontinuation when harm risk outweighs benefit potential.
8. Careful evaluation of opioid overdose risk should be assessed frequently, and naloxone co-prescribed at opioid doses of ≥50 MME/day or when patients are exposed to concurrent opioid and benzodiazepines.
9. Prescription drug monitoring programs should be reviewed at opioid initiation and periodically, ranging from every prescription to at least every 3 months.
10. Clinicians should use urine toxicology results prior to initiating opioid therapy and periodically when ongoing therapy is warranted.
11. Concurrent prescribing of opioid analgesics and benzodiazepines should be avoided when possible.
12. When opioid use disorder is recognized or suspected, clinicians should offer evidence-based treatment such as pharmacotherapy (ie, methadone or buprenorphine/naloxone) in combination with behavioral therapies.

MME, morphine milligram equivalent; CR, controlled release; LA, long acting.

Data from Reference 37.

Antidepressants

6 7 8 Select antidepressants have long been used for their antinociceptive effects (Table 79-10).[61,65,87] In general, the tricyclic antidepressants (TCAs) are often used for the treatment of neuropathic pain. According to the Canadian Pain Society, the Neuropathic Pain Special Interest (NeuPSIG) from the International Association of the Study of Pain, and the European Federation for Neurological Societies (EFNS), TCAs are first-line options for neuropathic pain.[63-65] The NICE guidelines list amitriptyline as a first-line option for neuropathic pain.[64-66] Interestingly, the American Diabetes Association does not list TCAs as first-line because they are not FDA-approved for this indication.[67] Other evidence-based uses of TCAs include low back pain, fibromyalgia, and migraine prophylaxis.[69]

TCAs exert their effects through inhibition of serotonin and norepinephrine reuptake that enhances the descending inhibitory pain pathway, often at doses significantly less than used for the treatment of depression.[69] Additionally, TCAs interact with and inhibit acetylcholine muscarinic receptors, alpha-adrenergic receptors, histamine-1 receptors, and voltage-gated sodium channels, all of which contribute to their many adverse effects.[88,89] Notably, TCAs can be divided into two different subgroups—tertiary amines (eg, amitriptyline and imipramine) and secondary amines (eg, nortriptyline and desipramine) with the tertiary amines being metabolized to secondary amines. Secondary amines interact with fewer receptors associated with adverse effects and provide similar analgesic efficacy.[70] TCAs are also impacted by pharmacogenomic variants though existing guidelines focus on the role of TCAs for depression with a small section discussing neuropathic pain (see Personalized Pharmacotherapy section).[90]

The major downfall with TCAs is their adverse-effect profile, as they are associated with slowed cardiac conduction, QTc prolongation, arrhythmias, tachycardia, and orthostatic hypotension. Doses

TABLE 79-8 Nonopioid Analgesics

Class and Generic Name (Brand Name)	Approximate Half-Life (h)	Usual Dosage Range (mg)	Maximal Dose (mg/day)
Salicylates			
Acetylsalicylic acid[a]—aspirin (various)	0.25	325-1,000 every 4-6 hours	4,000
Diflunisal (Dolobid, various)	8-12	500-1,000 initial 250-500 every 8-12 hours	1,500
Salsalate (various)	1	1,000 every 12 hours or 500 every 6 hours	3,000
***Para*-aminophenol**			
Acetaminophen[a] (Oral: Tylenol, various; Parenteral: Ofirmev)	2-3	325-1,000 every 4-6 hours	4,000[b] Dosing for peds lower based on weight
Fenamates			
Meclofenamate (various)	0.8-3.3	50-100 every 4-6 hours	400
Mefenamic acid (Ponstel)	2	Initial 500, 250 every 6 hours (max. 7 days)	1,000[c]
Pyranocarboxylic acid			
Etodolac (various) (immediate release)	7.3	200-400 every 6-8 hours	1,000-1,200 with extended-release product
Acetic acid			
Diclofenac potassium (Cataflam, various, Flector [patch] Voltaren Gel, Pennsaid [solution])	1.9	In some patients, initial 100, 50, 3 times per day Patch available: to be applied twice daily to painful area (intact skin only), gel and solution dosing joint specific	150[d]
Propionic acids			
Ibuprofen[a] (Motrin, Caldolor, various)	2-2.5	200-400 every 4-6 hours injectable, 400-800 every 6 hours (infused over 30 minutes)	3,200,[e] 2,400,[e] 1,200[f]
Fenoprofen (Nalfon, various)	3	200 every 4-6 hours	3,200
Ketoprofen (various)	2	25-50 every 6-8 hours	300 200 with extended-release product

(continued)

TABLE 79-8 Nonopioid Analgesics (*Continued*)

Class and Generic Name (Brand Name)	Approximate Half-Life (h)	Usual Dosage Range (mg)	Maximal Dose (mg/day)
Naproxen (Naprosyn, Anaprox, various)	12-17	500 initial 500 every 12 hours or 250 every 6-8 hours	1,000[c]
Naproxen sodium[a] (Aleve, various, combined with esomeprazole [Vimovo])	12-17	In some patients, 440 initial[f] 220 every 8-12 hours[f]	660[f]
Pyrrolizine carboxylic acid			
Ketorolac–parenteral (Toradol, various)	5-6	30[g]-60 (single IM dose only) 15[g]-30 (single IV dose only) 10[g]-30 every 6 hours (IV dose) (max. 5 days)	30[g]–60 15[g]–30 60[g]-120
Ketorolac—oral, indicated for continuation with parenteral only (various)	5-6	10 every 4-6 hours (max. 5 days, which includes parenteral doses)	40
Ketorolac—nasal spray, indicated for acute, moderate to moderately severe pain		1 spray (15.75 mg) in each nostril every 6-8 hours in adults <65 years of age and weight ≥50 kg 1 spray (15.75 mg) in one nostril every 6-8 hours in adults >65 years of age or weight <50 kg	126
Pyrazols			
Celecoxib (Celebrex)	11	Initial 400 followed by another 200 on first day, then 200 twice daily (note some recommend maintenance doses of 200 mg/day due to cardiovascular concerns)	400

[a]Available both as an over-the-counter preparation and as a prescription medication.

[b]Food and Drug Administration maximum dose. OTC maximum dose 3,000 mg daily. Lower with weight-based dosing in pediatric patients.

[c]Up to 1,250 mg on the first day.

[d]Up to 200 mg on the first day.

[e]Some individuals may respond better to 3,200 mg as opposed to 2,400 mg, although well-controlled trials show no better response; consider risk versus benefits when using 3,200 mg/day.

[f]Over-the-counter dose.

[g]Dose for older patients and those under 50 kg (110 lb).

FDA, Food and Drug Administration; h, hours; IM, intramuscular; IV, intravenous; ND, no data.

Data from References 53 and 61.

TABLE 79-9 Co-Analgesics: Antiseizure Medications

Medication	Mechanism of Action	Role	Dosing	Notes
Carbamazepine and carbamazepine XR	Inhibits voltage-gated sodium channels, potentiate GABA	Trigeminal neuralgia Neuropathic pain	Initial dose: 100 mg PO BID Titrate dose by 100 mg PO BID Target dose: 300–900 mg/day Maximum dose: 1,200 mg/day	Significant medication interactions Monitor CBC, LFTs, sodium level Recommended testing *HLA-B*15:02*[a] *HLA-A*31:02* in patients with Asian ancestry Therapeutic medication levels only indicated for high-dose therapy to avoid toxicity. No correlation between analgesia and serum medication concentration
Gabapentin	Inhibition α2δ subunit of the voltage-gated calcium channel leading to decreased release of excitatory neurotransmitters including glutamate, norepinephrine, and substance P	PHN[a] Neuropathic pain Perioperative pain	100-300 mg steps Increase every 3-5 days as tolerated by 100-300 mg increments	Median dose for response 1,600-2,400 mg/day Risk for substance use disorder Requires renal dose adjustment
Gabapentin (Gralise)	Refer to gabapentin	PHN[a]	Take once daily with evening meal Day 1: 300 mg Day 2: 600 mg Day 3-6: 900 mg Days 7-10: 1,200 mg Days 11-14: 1,500 mg Day 15: 1,800 mg Maximum dose: 1,800 mg/day	Refer to gabapentin

(*continued*)

TABLE 79-9 Co-Analgesics: Antiseizure Medications (*Continued*)

Medication	Mechanism of Action	Role	Dosing	Notes
Gabapentin enacarbil	Refer to gabapentin	PHN[a] Restless leg syndrome (RLS)[a]	Initial dose: 600 mg PO QAM × 3 days Titrate dose: 600 mg PO BID Maximum dose: 1,200 mg/day	Refer to gabapentin
Lamotrigine	Inhibits sodium channels	Neuropathic pain (fourth-line Canadian NP guidelines, specialist setting NICE guidelines)	Initial 25 mg PO daily Titrate q2weeks to 50 mg/day, 100 mg/day, and 200 mg/day Maximum dose: 400 mg/day	Stevens–Johnson syndrome
Oxcarbazepine	Inhibits sodium channels	Trigeminal neuralgia (EFNS) Neuropathic pain (specialist setting NICE guidelines)	Initial: 150 mg PO BID Titrate by 300 mg q3 days Target dose: 300-600 mg BID Max dose: 1,800 mg/day	Improved tolerability and less medication interactions compared to CBZ Pharmacogenomic testing recommended in Asian patients due to *HLA-B*15:02* variant
Oxcarbazepine XR	Refer to oxcarbazepine	(See above under oxcarbazepine)	Initial dose: 600 mg PO daily Titrate by 600 mg/day weekly Maximum: 2,400 mg/day	Refer to oxcarbazepine
Pregabalin	Refer to gabapentin	DPN[a] Fibromyalgia[a] Neuropathic pain associated with spinal cord injury[a] Neuropathic pain PHN[a] Perioperative pain	Initial dose: 150 mg/day in two or three divided doses Titrate dose by 300 mg/day at 1 week Maximum dose: varies by indication. Overall 600 mg/day	Refer to gabapentin
Pregabalin CR	Refer to gabapentin	DPN[a] PHN[a]	Initial dose: 165 mg daily Maximum dose: 330 mg/day (DPN) or 330-660 mg/day (PHN)	Refer to gabapentin
Topiramate and Topiramate XR	Inhibits voltage-gated sodium channels, AMPA/kainite subtype of glutamate receptor, and carbonic anhydrase; increases activity of GABA-A receptor	Alcohol use disorder Migraine prophylaxis Neuropathic pain (fourth-line Canadian NP guidelines, specialist setting NICE guidelines)	Initial dose: 25 mg PO daily × 1 week Titrate by 25-50 mg week Target dose: 50 mg PO BID (migraine ppx) or 200-400 mg/day neuropathic pain	Monitor serum bicarbonate and renal function Increase risk for kidney stones Weight loss Decreased sweating/hyperthermia Hyperammonemia Paresthesias Cognitive dulling

[a]FDA-approved indication.

All anticonvulsants associated with increased risk for suicidal thoughts and behaviors.

Data from References 61 and 65.

of TCAs in excess of 100 mg/day have been associated with sudden cardiac death.[91] There are varying recommendations regarding electrocardiogram monitoring with TCAs but may be appropriate in patients greater than or equal to 40 to 50 years of age prior to starting and periodically during continued use.[70,91] Anticholinergic effects are another major issue with TCAs and often preclude their use in patients with benign prostatic hypertrophy, glaucoma, or cognitive impairment. Sedative effects, owing to their inhibition of histamine receptors, may be unwanted in some patients, though desired in patients with insomnia; thus, TCAs are typically given at bedtime.

Duloxetine, venlafaxine, and milnacipran are serotonin norepinephrine reuptake inhibitors (SNRIs) that are either FDA-approved or have evidence to support their use in various chronic pain syndromes. Similar to TCAs, SNRIs inhibit the reuptake of serotonin and norepinephrine and modulate the descending pain pathway. Though a mental health diagnosis is not needed for analgesic benefit, SNRIs may be particularly useful in those with mental health comorbidities as doses used for pain are frequently similar to those used for mental health conditions. In addition to major depressive disorder (MDD) and generalized anxiety disorder (GAD), duloxetine is FDA-approved for fibromyalgia, chronic musculoskeletal pain (low back pain and osteoarthritis), and diabetic peripheral neuropathic pain. The American College of Physicians' guideline for low back pain recommends duloxetine as a second-line medication for those that fail nonpharmacological approaches and NSAIDs.[60] Venlafaxine is not FDA-approved for any pain diagnoses; however, there is evidence supporting the use of venlafaxine for neuropathic pain, low back pain, fibromyalgia, migraine prophylaxis, and tension-type headache prophylaxis.[68,92-96] Duloxetine and venlafaxine are considered first-line options for neuropathic pain according to several neuropathic pain guidelines.[64-67,73] Milnacipran is FDA-approved for fibromyalgia syndrome only.[97]

More likely adverse effects of SNRIs include nausea, somnolence, dry mouth, anorexia, erectile dysfunction, and constipation. Seizures, hyponatremia, and worsening of acute angle closure glaucoma may also occur. Because SNRIs impact norepinephrine, transient elevations in blood pressure should be anticipated. Therefore, it is important to ensure optimal blood pressure control prior to initiation and ongoing monitoring during therapy. In addition, venlafaxine has been associated with QTc prolongation, so caution is advised in those with cardiovascular disease or risk factors for QTc prolongation.[98] There are no agreed upon recommendations for QTc monitoring with venlafaxine. All SNRIs have liver and renal considerations; however, the specific criteria vary among the different SNRIs. Furthermore, SNRIs interfere with platelet aggregation and increase risk for bleeding, particularly

TABLE 79-10 Co-Analgesics: Antidepressants

Medication	Mechanism of Action (MOA)	Role	Dosing	Notes
Tricyclic antidepressants (TCA)				
Amitriptyline Desipramine Imipramine Nortriptyline	Inhibit reuptake serotonin and norepinephrine which in turn inhibit descending pain pathway Analgesic effects independent of antidepressant effects and lower doses needed for analgesic effects compared to MDD doses	Fibromyalgia Low back pain Migraine prophylaxis Neuropathic pain	Initial: 10-25 mg PO QHS Titrate by 10-25 mg q3-7 days Maximum: 150 mg	Secondary amines (desipramine, nortriptyline) less anticholinergic activity = less ADE Multiple cardiac AME (including QTc prolongation, orthostatic hypotension, arrhythmias, tachycardia) Doses >100 mg/day associated with sudden cardiac death Lowers seizure threshold Impacted by Pharmacogenomics
Serotonin norepinephrine reuptake inhibitors (SNRI)				
Duloxetine	Inhibits reuptake serotonin and norepinephrine which in turn inhibits descending pain pathway Analgesic effects independent of antidepressant effects	Chronic musculoskeletal pain (low back pain [LBP], osteoarthritis)[a] Diabetic peripheral neuropathy (DPN)[a] Fibromyalgia[a] Chemotherapy-induced neuropathic pain (CINP)	Initial: 30 mg PO daily × 1 week (2 weeks if an older patient) Target dose: 60 mg PO daily Maximum dose: 120 mg/day though limited evidence for doses >60 mg providing additional benefit in pain	Avoid eGFR <30 mL/min (0.50 mL/s) Avoid chronic liver disease or cirrhosis Hypertension Hyponatremia Increased risk of bleeding (GI and CNS)
Milnacipran	Inhibits reuptake serotonin and norepinephrine which in turn inhibits descending pain pathway Analgesic effects independent of antidepressant effects	Fibromyalgia[a]	Day 1: 12.5 mg PO daily Days 2-3: 12.5 mg PO BID Days 4-7: 25 mg PO BID Then increase to 50 mg PO BID Target dose: 100 mg/day Maximum dose: 200 mg/day	Avoid eGFR <30 mL/min (0.50 mL/s) Caution with severe hepatic impairment Increase risk for bleeding
Venlafaxine	Inhibits reuptake serotonin and norepinephrine which in turn inhibits descending pain pathway Analgesic effects independent of antidepressant effects	CINP DPN Fibromyalgia LBP Migraine prophylaxis Painful polyneuropathy Tension-type headache	Initial: venlafaxine SA 37.5 mg PO daily Titrate: by no more than 75 mg/day q4 days Maximum dose: 225 mg/day	Higher doses needed to achieve SNRI effect Dose adjustments with renal/hepatic impairment Hypertension Hyponatremia QTc prolongation Increased bleeding risk

[a]FDA-approved indication(s).

AME, adverse medication effect.

Data from References 61, 65 and 87.

when combined with NSAIDs, anticoagulants, or corticosteroids. This risk of gastrointestinal bleeding can be reduced with concomitant proton pump inhibitors use.[99]

Skeletal Muscle Relaxants

6 7 8 Skeletal muscle relaxants (SMRs) are composed of antispasmodic and antispasticity medications (Table 79-11).[61,100-104] Diazepam and Tizanidine have properties of both categories. Spasticity and spasms have several differences including etiology, symptoms, and causes.[105]

Spasticity involves an upper motor neuron disorder.[105] Symptoms include stiffness, hypertonicity, and hyperreflexia.[105] Causes of spasticity include multiple sclerosis, cerebral palsy, spinal cord injury, traumatic brain injury, and post-stroke syndrome.[105] Medications used for spasticity include baclofen, dantrolene, diazepam, and tizanidine.

Baclofen is similar in structure to GABA and binds to $GABA_B$ receptors. These receptors are coupled to Ca^{2+} and K^+ channels located pre- and postsynaptically. Essentially this leads to reduction in the release of excitatory glutamate and increases presynaptic inhibition. Additionally, baclofen may reduce the release of substance P. Sedation, dizziness, weakness, and nausea are possible adverse effects, with the most concerning being associated with baclofen as hallucinations or seizures may occur during withdrawal with abrupt discontinuation. Therefore, baclofen must be tapered slowly.[105] Baclofen also requires dose adjustment for decreased renal function.[106]

Diazepam is not often used for non-cancer pain because of its sedative effects and potential for physical dependence. Its mechanism of action involves binding to $GABA_A$ resulting in increased chloride conductance which subsequently leads to presynaptic inhibition of the spinal cord. Abrupt discontinuation of diazepam can lead to a withdrawal syndrome, namely seizures. Diazepam has a long half-life (20-50 hours for parent and up to 100 for active metabolites) which is problematic especially for older patients. Avoid the use of diazepam in patients with renal or hepatic impairment.[105]

Similar to diazepam, tizanidine has both antispasticity and antispasmodic uses and is a centrally acting α_2-agonist. Presynaptically, tizanidine inhibits the release of excitatory neurotransmitters that leads to a reduction in postsynaptic activation of the upper motor neuron. In addition, tizanidine leads to the potentiation of glycine. Not surprisingly, because of its α_2-agonist activity, hypotension can occur and rebound hypertension seen with abrupt discontinuation. Other significant issues with tizanidine include sedation

TABLE 79-11 Skeletal Muscle Relaxants

Medication	Role	Mechanism of Action	Dosing	Notes
Baclofen	Antispasticity	Related to GABA, works at spinal cord, inhibits polysynaptic and monosynaptic reflexes	Initial: 5 mg PO TID Titrate: q3 days to effect Maximum: 80 mg/day	Withdrawal syndrome (hallucinations, seizures) Respiratory depression Requires renal dose adjustment
Carisoprodol	Antispasmodic/ antispasticity	Centrally acting, changing interneuronal activity in descending reticular formation and spinal cord Meprobamate (primary metabolite) leads to barbiturate effects at $GABA_A$	250-300 mg four times daily	Meprobamate (a barbiturate) is primary metabolite and has physical dependence potential Schedule IV controlled substance Withdrawal syndrome Respiratory depression with opioids, benzodiazepines, or barbituates Metabolized by CYP2C19 which has genetic variabilities
Chlorzoxazone	Antispasmodic	Works in spinal cord and subcortical areas of brain by inhibiting multisynaptic reflex arcs	Initial: 250-500 mg three to four times daily Maximum dose: 750 mg three to four times daily	Rare hepatotoxicity Urine discoloration Respiratory depression when combined with opioids, benzodiazepines, or barbiturates
Cyclobenzaprine	Antispasmodic	Structurally related to TCAs, sedative effects, works at brainstem level, decreases excitability of alpha and gamma motor neurons	Initial: 5 mg PO TID Titrate: increase to 7.5-10 mg TID × 2-3 weeks Older patients: 5 mg dose with less frequent doses Doses used in fibromyalgia 10 mg QAM, 20 mg QHS	Anticholinergic effects Avoid in older patients Caution in patients with cardiac conduction/arrhythmias Avoid closed angle glaucoma Hepatic dose adjustments
Diazepam	Antispasmodic/ antispasticity	Postsynaptic inhibition of GABA neurons in spinal cord	Adults: 2-10 mg three to four times daily	Long half-life Avoid in older patients and those renal/ hepatic impairment Withdrawal with abrupt discontinuation
Methocarbamol	Antispasmodic	Unknown, sedative properties	Initial: 1,500 mg PO four times daily × 2-3 day Then: 750-1,000 mg PO four times daily	Urine discoloration Respiratory depression with opioids, benzodiazepines, or barbiturates
Metaxalone	Antispasmodic	Unknown, sedative properties	800 mg PO three to four times daily	Respiratory depression when used with opioids, benzodiazepines, or barbiturates Contraindicated in severe liver/renal impairment
Orphenadrine	Antispasmodic	Unknown, suspect analgesic and anticholinergic effects, H_1 receptor antagonist, NMDA receptor antagonist	100 mg PO BID	Anticholinergic effects Rare aplastic anemia
Tizanidine	Antispasmodic/ antispasticity	Centrally acting α-2 agonist, inhibits presynaptic motor neurons, decreases polysynaptic reflex and abnormal contraction of opposing muscle groups	Initial: 4 mg Titrate by 2-4 mg q6-8 h Maximum: 36 mg/day	Hypotension Hepatotoxicity Tablets and capsules not bioequivalent Withdrawal syndrome with abrupt discontinuation

Data from References 61 and 105.

and elevation in hepatic enzymes requiring periodic monitoring. Tizanidine is metabolized by CYP1A2 and is contraindicated in combination with ciprofloxacin or fluvoxamine.[105,107]

Spasms are involuntary contractions of the muscle and antispasmodics treat musculoskeletal conditions and symptoms like jerks, twitches, and cramps.[105,107] Associated causes include musculoskeletal pain, fibromyalgia, mechanical low back pain, sciatica, disc herniation, and myofascial pain.[105] Skeletal muscle relaxants or NSAIDs are recommended as pharmacologic treatment for patients with acute or subacute low back pain.[60] While studies suggest SMRs are associated with a small increase in pain relief, there is no evidence to support improvement in function with SMRs.[60] Importantly, SMRs should be used short-term. If used long-term, SMRs may increase the risk for adverse effects and polypharmacy, particularly in older patients, as many appear (like other medications used to manage pain) on the Beer's List of Potentially Inappropriate Medications for Use in the Elderly from the American Geriatrics Society.[108,109] Antispasmodics include carisoprodol, chlorzoxazone, cyclobenzaprine, diazepam, metaxalone, methocarbamol, orphenadrine, and tizanidine.

Carisoprodol is a Schedule IV controlled substance and is metabolized via CYP2C19 to meprobamate, a barbiturate. Because of its barbiturate activity, carisoprodol has the potential for physical dependence. It is centrally acting and changes interneuronal activity in the descending reticular formation and spinal cord. Meprobamate has activity at $GABA_A$ receptors, and withdrawal can occur with abrupt discontinuation. Furthermore, respiratory depression can occur when combined with opioids, benzodiazepines, or barbiturates.[105,107]

Chlorzoxazone blocks multisynaptic reflex arcs in the spinal cord and subcortical areas of the brain. Sedation is a common effect and rare adverse effects include hepatotoxicity or GI bleeding. If used chronically, hepatic transaminase monitoring is recommended. Urine discoloration may be experienced and respiratory depression may occur when combined with opioids, benzodiazepines, or barbiturates.[105,107]

Structurally, cyclobenzaprine is similar to the TCAs. It is thought to exert its effects through decreasing the excitability of alpha and gamma motor neurons while also leading to CNS depression through the brain stem. Anticholinergic adverse effects are common and should be used with caution in those with cardiac arrhythmias or conduction disturbances. Cyclobenzaprine should be avoided in those with acute narrow angle glaucoma and those of older age. With mild hepatic impairment, dose adjustments are recommended and cyclobenzaprine should be avoided in those with moderate-to-severe hepatic impairment.[105,107]

The mechanism of action of metaxalone is unclear as it has no activity on skeletal muscle or nerve fibers. Thus, it is suspected that its effects are primarily due to CNS depression. Metaxalone is metabolized through multiple CYP enzymes including CYP1A2, CYP2D6, CYP2E1, and CYP3A4. In those with severe renal or hepatic impairment, metaxalone should be avoided. Rare adverse effects of metaxalone include leukopenia, hemolytic anemia, or hepatic transaminase elevation. Again, respiratory depression can occur when combined with opioids, benzodiazepines, or barbiturates.[105,107]

Similar to metaxalone, the mechanism of action of methocarbamol is unknown and suspected to be associated with its sedative properties. Respiratory depression can occur when used concomitantly with other medications. Urine discoloration (brown, green, black) is also possible.[105,107]

Orphenadrine is structurally related to diphenhydramine and possesses comparatively higher anticholinergic effects. Yet again, the mechanism of action is not completely elucidated and conjectured due to its sedative and anticholinergic effects. Orphenadrine also inhibits histamine-1 and NMDA receptors. With orphenadrine, GI irritation may occur and there is a rare incidence of aplastic anemia. It should be avoided in those with glaucoma, myasthenia gravis, or cardiospasm. Because of the anticholinergic effects, it should be avoided in older patients. It has a relatively long half-life ranging from 13 to 20 hours. Its CNS depressant effects are magnified when used with other CNS depressants.[105,107]

Topicals

6 7 8 9 The advantages of topicals include addressing local symptoms while minimizing systemic exposure and risk for adverse effects (Table 77-10).[110,111] According to the NICE osteoarthritis guidelines, topical NSAIDs should be considered for knee or hand OA before a trial of oral NSAIDs.[112] The American College of Rheumatology (ACR) guidelines for hand, hip, and knee OA also strongly recommend topical NSAIDs for knee OA and conditionally for hand OA. Additionally, topical capsaicin may be considered as an adjunct to core treatments for hand and knee osteoarthritis according to the NICE guidelines although ACR conditionally recommends against capsaicin in hand OA, while recommending conditionally for capsaicin use in knee OA.[58,112] Capsaicin appears in several neuropathic pain guidelines as either second-line, third-line, or fourth-line for various peripheral neuropathic pain syndromes.[64-66,74] Capsaicin activates transient receptor potential vanilloid 1 (TRPV1) channels. There are various over-the-counter and prescription strength products available. Burning may occur with initial application and that this decreases over time with repeated, scheduled use. Capsaicin is not recommended for "as needed" use as repeated application is needed to desensitize C-fibers. The capsaicin 8% patch is FDA-approved for several neuropathic pain syndromes and is to be administered under the direct supervision of a physician. There are specific administration directions in the packaging information including pretreatment of the area with topical anesthetic. Topical medications should not be applied to open skin. The NICE guidelines recommend against the use of rubefacients for osteoarthritis.[112] Lidocaine is also used topically and works by inhibiting voltage-gated sodium channels. For PHN, one guideline places lidocaine as a first-line option and may even be preferred over other first-line options in older patients when CNS adverse effects are of concern.[63] Other guidelines list topical lidocaine as second-line or fourth-line options for neuropathic pain.[65,66] Table 79-16 includes commonly used topical analgesics.

Emerging Agents

Two agents have received widespread attention for their potential analgesic benefit, namely cannabis and ketamine. Medical cannabis has been studied primarily in neuropathic pain conditions with equivocal results. Route of administration, dose, and monitoring recommendations are still unclear. More importantly, research on the specific cannabinoids and terpenes present in many of the *cannabis* strains is required considering the widely variable pharmacologic profiles of these substances.[113,114] The non-psychoactive cannabinoid, *cannabidiol* (CBD) may have a significant role in the treatment of chronic pain, although its utility in the absence of delta-9-tetrahydrocannabinol (THC) is unclear.[115,116]

Ketamine, a non-competitive NMDA glutamate receptor antagonist, is typically used for procedural sedation and for induction of anesthesia. Given its potent glutamate antagonism, its use has gained popularity among pain specialists for maladaptive pain syndromes, such as Complex Regional Pain Syndrome (CRPS). Guidelines for the use of ketamine as an adjunct analgesic in acute pain are available, but appropriate dose, duration, and patient selection for chronic pain are still unclear.[117] Use of this agent should be supervised by clinicians experienced in its use.

Opioid Agents

1 7 8 9 10 11 Opioids are often the next step in the management of acute pain and cancer-related chronic pain (see Chapter 150 for use in cancer pain). This medication class may also be an effective treatment option in the management of chronic noncancer pain; however, this continues to be controversial. When a trial of opioids is warranted, it should follow a complete assessment of the pain complaint, an assessment of the patient's functionality goals, and risk factors for opioid use disorder or overdose.[118]

Opioid choice should be based on patient acceptance, analgesic effectiveness, as well as pharmacokinetic, pharmacodynamic, and adverse-effect profiles with the attributes provided in Tables 79-5 and 79-12.[53,61]

The pharmacologic activity of opioids depends on their affinity for and action at one or more central and peripheral opiate receptors. These g-protein coupled receptors include mu (MOR), kappa (KOR), delta (DOR), and noceptin (OLR-1), which have variable physiologic effects. Therapeutic activities and adverse effects for this medication class range from those exhibited by the MOR agonists (eg, morphine) to those seen with the nonselective antagonists (eg, naloxone). Partial MOR agonists (eg, buprenorphine) and mixed MOR antagonists/KOR agonists (eg, nalbuphine) compete with agonists for opiate receptor sites. Depending on the inherent agonist and antagonist properties, these medications may precipitate opioid withdrawal and pain crisis if initiated in patients with physical MOR dependence or tolerance.[120] Additionally, patients stable on a partial or mixed MOR agonists may exhibit an attenuated response to pure MOR agonists when administered for pain. Efficacy and adverse effects also may further differ among opioid agents because of receptor subtype variability and partially explain why some patients respond differently to certain opioids, specifically MOR agonists.[121] Opioid antagonists may act centrally (eg, naloxone or naltrexone) or be limited to peripheral action only (eg, alyimopan, naloxegol, methylnaltrexone, or naldemedine) (Table 79-13).[61,122]

TABLE 79-12 Dosing Guidelines

Agent(s)	Doses (Use Lowest Effective Dose, Titrate Up or Down Based on Patient Response, Opioid-Tolerant Patients May Need Dose Modification)	Notes
Morphine	PO 5-30 mg every 4 hours[a]	Medication of choice in severe pain
	IM 5-20 mg every 4 hours[a]	Use immediate-release product with SR product to control breakthrough pain in cancer patients
	IV 5-15 mg every 4 hours[a]	Typical patient-controlled analgesia IV dose is 1 mg with a 10-minute lock-out interval
	SR 15-30 mg every 12 hours (may need to be every 8 hours in some patients)	Every 24-hour products available
	Rectal 10-20 mg every 4 hours[a]	
Hydromorphone	PO 2-4 mg every 4-6 hours[a]	Use in severe pain
	XR 8 mg to 64 mg every 24 hours	More potent than morphine; otherwise, no advantages
	IM 1-2 mg every 4-6 hours[a]	
	IV 0.5-2 mg every 4 hours[a]	Typical patient-controlled analgesia IV dose is 0.2 mg with a 10-minute lock-out interval
	Rectal 3 mg every 6-8 hours[a]	Every 24-hour product (Exalgo) available
Oxymorphone	IM 1-1.5 mg every 4-6 hours[a]	Use in severe pain
	IV 0.5 mg every 4-6 hours[a]	No advantages over morphine
	PO immediate-release 5-10 mg every 4-6 hours[a]	Use immediate-release product with controlled-release product to control breakthrough pain in cancer or chronic pain patients
	PO extended-release 5-10 mg every 12 hours[a]	Manufacturer recommends 5 mg every 12 hours in opioid-naïve patients
		Take ER on empty stomach
Levorphanol	PO 2-3 mg every 6-8 hours[a] (Levo-Dromoran)	Use in severe pain
	PO 2 mg every 3-6 hours[a] (Levorphanol Tartrate)	Extended half-life useful in cancer patients
	IM 1-2 mg every 6-8 hours[a]	In chronic pain, wait 3 days between dosage adjustments
	IV 1 mg every 3-6 hours[a]	
Codeine	PO 15-60 mg every 4-6 hours[a]	Use in mild-to-moderate pain
	IM 15-60 mg every 4-6 hours[a]	Weak analgesic; analgesic prodrug
Hydrocodone	PO 5-10 mg every 4-6 hours[a]	Use in moderate/severe pain
Oxycodone	PO 5-15 mg every 4-6 hours[a]	Use in moderate/severe pain
	Controlled release 10-20 mg every 12 hours	
		Use immediate-release product with controlled-release product to control breakthrough pain in cancer or chronic pain patients
		CR reformulated to deter unhealthy use
Meperidine	IM 50-150 mg every 3-4 hours[a]	Use in severe pain
	IV 5-10 mg every 5 minutes prn[a]	Oral not recommended
		Do not use in renal failure
		May precipitate tremors, myoclonus, and seizures
		Monoamine oxidase inhibitors can induce hyperpyrexia and/or seizures or opioid overdose symptoms
Fentanyl	IV 25-50 mcg/hours	Used in severe pain
	IM 50-100 mcg every 1-2 hours[a]	Do not use transdermal in acute pain
	Transdermal 25 mcg/hr every 72 hours	Transmucosal for breakthrough cancer pain in patients already receiving or tolerant to opioids
	Transmucosal (Actiq/OTFC Lozenge and Onsolis buccal film) 200 mcg may repeat × 1, 30 minutes after first dose is started, then titrate	Always start with lowest dose despite daily opioid intake; product-specific titration recommendations exist
	Transmucosal (Fentora Buccal Tablet) 100 mcg, may repeat × 1, 30 minutes after first dose is started, then titrate	
	Intranasal (Lazanda Spray) 100 mcg (one spray) in one nostril. Wait 2 hours prior to redosing	
	Sublingual (Subsys Spray) 100 mcg (1 spray). Wait 4 hours prior to redosing	

(continued)

TABLE 79-12 Dosing Guidelines (*Continued*)

Agent(s)	Doses (Use Lowest Effective Dose, Titrate Up or Down Based on Patient Response, Opioid-Tolerant Patients May Need Dose Modification)	Notes
	Sublingual (Abstral Tablet) 100 mcg tablets placed sublingually. Must wait 2 hours prior to redosing	
Methadone	PO 2.5-10 mg every 8-12 hours[a]	Effective in severe chronic pain
	IM 2.5-10 mg every 8-12 hours[a]	
		Some chronic pain patients can be dosed every 12 hours
		Equianalgesic dose of methadone when compared with other opioids will decrease progressively the higher the previous opioid dose. Avoid dose titrations more frequently than weekly in chronic pain maintenance
Pentazocine	PO 50-100 mg every 3-4 hours[b] (max. 600 mg daily, for those 50 mg tablet containing 0.5 mg of naloxone)	Second-line agent for moderate-to-severe pain; may precipitate withdrawal in patients with physical opioid dependence; parenteral doses not recommended
	PO 25 mg every 4 hours[b] (max. 150 mg daily, for those 25 mg tablet containing 325 mg of acetaminophen)	
Butorphanol	IM 1-4 mg every 3-4 hours[b]	Second-line agent for moderate-to-severe pain
	IV 0.5-2 mg every 3-4 hours[b]	May precipitate withdrawal in patients with physical opioid dependence
	Intranasal 1 mg (1 spray) every 3-4 hours[b]	
	If inadequate relief after initial spray, may repeat in other nostril × 1 in 60-90 minutes	
	Max. 2 sprays (one per nostril) every 3-4 hours[2]	
Nalbuphine	IM/IV 10 mg every 3-6 hours[b] (max. 20 mg dose, 160 mg daily)	Second-line agent for moderate-to-severe pain; may precipitate withdrawal in patients with physical opioid dependence
		Used frequently in low doses to treat/prevent opioid-induced pruritus
Buprenorphine	IM 0.3 mg every 6 hours[b]	Second-line agent for moderate-to-severe pain
	Slow IV 0.3 mg every 6 hours[b]	May precipitate withdrawal in patients with physical opioid dependence
		Transdermal delivery systems (5, 7.5, 10, 15, 20 mcg/hr) available for every 7 day administration. Detailed manufacturer dosing conversion recommendations exist
		Buccal delivery system (75, 150, 300, 450, 600, 750, and 900 mcg) available. Detailed manufacturer dosing conversion recommendations exist
		Naloxone may not be effective in reversing respiratory depression
Tramadol	PO 50-100 mg every 4-6 hours[a]	Maximum dose for nonextended-release, 400 mg/24 hr; maximum for extended release, 300 mg/24 hr
	If rapid onset not required, start 25 mg/day and titrate over several days	Decrease dose in patient with renal impairment and in older patients
	Extended release PO 100 mg every 24 hours	
Tapentadol	PO 50-100 mg every 4-6 hours[a]	First day of therapy may administer second dose after the first within 1 hour maximum dose first day 700 mg, max. dose thereafter 600 mg (maximum dose for CR 500 mg)

[a]May start with an around-the-clock regimen and switch to prn if/when the painful signal subsides or is episodic.

[b]May reach a ceiling analgesic effect.

HCL, hydrochloride; IM, intramuscular; IV, intravenous; NSAID, nonsteroidal anti-inflammatory drug; PO, oral; prn, as needed; SR, sustained release; OTFC, Oral transmucosal fentanyl citrate; CR, controlled release; XR, extended release; mcg, microgram; mg, milligram.

Data from References 53, 61, and 119.

The effects of the opioid analgesics are relatively selective and, at normal therapeutic concentrations, do not affect other sensory modalities.[9,120] While sensations of touch and proprioception are preserved, undesirable adverse effects may increase as the dose is escalated (Table 79-6).[9,120] Frequently, when opioids are administered, pain is not eliminated, but its unpleasantness is decreased. Patients report that although their pain is still present, it no longer bothers them.

8 9 Opioids share related pharmacologic attributes and exert a profound effect on the CNS and GI tract. Mood changes, sedation, nausea, vomiting, decreased GI motility, constipation, respiratory depression, physical dependence, pruritus, and tolerance are evident in varying degrees with all agents.[120] Tolerance to adverse effects (except to constipation) often develops over time. Some differences exist between the opioids in regards to incidence of adverse effects, which may assist in selection of the most appropriate agent.

7 8 9 The route of administration depends on individual patient needs, with the oral route being preferred. However, the onset of analgesic effect for oral medications is approximately 45 minutes, and the peak effect usually occurs 1 to 2 hours after administration.[9,53] This delay must be considered when immediate relief is needed in the management of acute pain (ie, postsurgical or

TABLE 79-13 Central and Peripheral Opioid Antagonists

Generic Name (Brand Name)	Activity	Role	Route	Dose in Adults (mg)	Special Considerations
Naldemedine (Symproic)	Peripheral	CNMP[a], OIC[b]	PO	0.2 mg qday	Avoid with severe hepatic impairment
Naloxone	Central	Opioid reversal	IV, IM, IN	0.4-2 mg[e]	Onset 1-2 (IV) minutes, 2-5
(Narcan, various)	Peripheral	Cancer and CNMP[a] OIC[b]	SC (both), PO	Variable	(IM) minutes
Methylnaltrexone	Central	AUD,[c]	(CNMP)	12 mg Qday-Q12 (PO)	Half-life 0.5-1.3 h
(Relistor)	Peripheral	OUD[d]	PO, IM	380 mg q4weeks (IM)	Renal dose adjustments
Naltrexone	Peripheral	Postoperative ileus	PO	12 mg PO 30 minutes-	Opioid free for 7-10 days
(ReVia, Vivitrol)		CNMP[a], OIC[b]	PO	5 hours before surgery	before initiation
Alvimopan				then 12 mg PO BID	Limited to 15 doses
(Entereg)				starting day after surgery	Renal dose adjustments
Naloxegol				for maximum of 7 days	Avoid with moderate 3A4
(Movantik)				12.5-25mg qday	inhibitors
				1 hour before, 2 hours after	
				a meal	

[a]Chronic nonmalignant pain.

[b]Opioid-induced constipation.

[c]Alcohol use disorder.

[d]Opioid use disorder.

[e]Starting doses to be used in cases of opioid overdose.

Data from individual package inserts.

cancer breakthrough). Therefore, in some scenarios, such as acute severe pain (eg, pain crisis) or when the patient is unable to take oral medications, alternative routes of therapy, such as intravenous (IV) administration, may be preferred.[33] The relative potency, defined by the equianalgesic dose, of opioids differs greatly (Table 79-5). Equianalgesic dose tables are often based on single-dose studies without regard for patient variability and should be used only as a guide, with further dose titration frequently required.[53,119]

Although true opioid allergies are rare, Table 79-5 can also be used when treating a patient who has a documented hypersensitivity to opioids. Differing chemical classes of opioids may theoretically provide some reduction in cross-reactivity when hypersensitivity is of concern. Most reactions, such as pruritus or rash, are either related to associated histamine release from cutaneous mast cells or activation of central MOR receptors and not a true allergic or immunoglobulin-E (IgE) or T-cell response.[123-125] Although caution is always advised, a decrease in potential cross-sensitivity is thought to exist when moving from one opioid structural class to another.[124] The classes are phenanthrenes (morphine-like agonists), benzomorphans (pentazocine), phenylpiperidines (fentanyl-like agonists), and diphenylheptanes (methadone-like agonists). When considering hypersensitivity cross-reactivity, the mixed agonist–antagonist and partial agonist class acts much like the morphine-like agonists.[125]

8 9 In the initial stages of acute pain, analgesics should be given around the clock. This should commence after administering a typical starting dose and titrating up or down, depending on the patient's degree of pain and demonstrated adverse effects (eg, sedation). As-needed schedules may produce wide swings in analgesic plasma concentrations resulting in alternating states of uncontrolled pain and sedation. This may initiate a vicious cycle where increasing amounts of pain medications are needed for relief. As the pain improves and the need for medication decreases, as-needed schedules may be appropriate, which may also be useful in patients who present with pain that is intermittent or sporadic in nature. When opioids are used in the management of chronic noncancer pain, around-the-clock administration schedules can be considered. While rare, as-needed immediate-release opioids may be used in conjunction with ER/LA opioids for times when patients experience significant breakthrough pain (Fig. 79-2). This practice is more common in treatment pain associated with cancer or its treatment.

7 Continuous IV infusion of opioids should be reserved for opioid-tolerant patients.[126,127] An alternative method is patient-controlled analgesia (PCA), which is a technique by which patients can self-administer a preset dose of an IV opioid via a pump electronically interfaced with a timing device. Compared with traditional as-needed opioid dosing, PCA yields better pain control, improved patient satisfaction, and relatively few differences in adverse effects.[126,128]

Administration of opioids directly into the CNS (eg, epidural and intrathecal/subarachnoid routes) may also be used by anesthesiology pain consult services in the control of acute, chronic noncancer, and cancer pain and is useful in more difficult to control pain states (Table 79-14).[129,130]

8 Due to reports of respiratory depression, pruritus, nausea, vomiting, urinary retention, and hypotension, these methods of analgesia require careful monitoring and are best used by experienced practitioners. Respiratory depression is of concern and can occur within minutes after intrathecal fentanyl or manifest as late as 19 hours after a single dose of intrathecal morphine. Guidelines mandate respiratory monitoring for at least 24 hours after a single dose of intrathecal or epidural morphine with standing orders for naloxone (opioid antagonist) for full or partial reversal.[126,127] Analgesia and adverse effects are evident at even lower doses when opioids are administered intrathecally instead of epidurally. This form of analgesia is often administered as a continuous-infusion and/or on a patient-controlled basis. When given simultaneously with intrathecal or epidural local anesthetics such as bupivacaine, opioid analgesics have been proven relatively safe and effective. All agents administered directly into the CNS should be preservative free.

Full Mu Opioid Receptor Agonists

6 10 Despite the availability of several newer agents, morphine remains the prototype opiate analgesic. As new opioid and nonopioid compounds are developed, their efficacy and adverse-effect profiles are typically compared against morphine as the standard. Using equianalgesic tables, clinicians often refer to "oral morphine equivalents" when describing efficacy or risk of harms of other opioids.[37,119] Many clinicians consider morphine the first-line agent when treating moderate-to-severe pain due to its relative low cost, broad clinical experience, and abundant dosage forms/strengths.

Adverse effects can be numerous, particularly when morphine is first initiated or when doses are significantly increased. Morphine causes nausea and vomiting through direct stimulation of the chemoreceptor trigger zone, decreased peristalsis, and a vestibular mechanism.[120] Opioid-induced nausea typically subsides over time with continued dosing, although this adverse effect may be incredibly

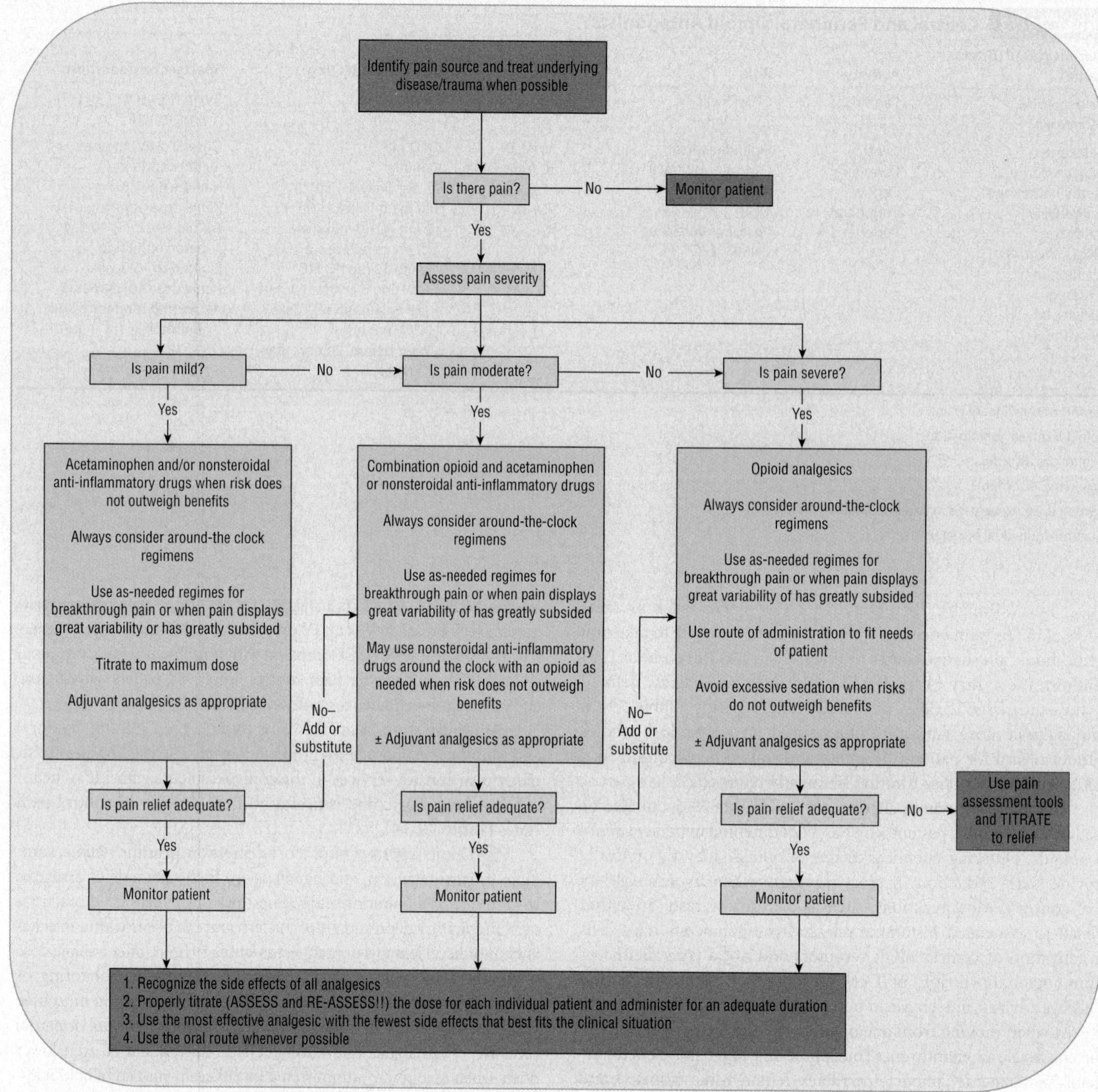

FIGURE 79-2 Algorithm for acute pain. *(Adapted from Omnicare, Inc., Acute Pain Pathway.)*

TABLE 79-14 Intraspinal Opioids

Agent	Single Dose (mg)	Onset of Pain Relief (min)	Duration of Pain Relief (hr)	Continual Infusion Dose (mg/hr)
Epidural route				
Morphine	1-6	30	6-24	0.1-1
Hydromorphone	0.8-1.5	5-8	4-8	0.1-0.3
Fentanyl	0.025-0.1	5	2-8	0.025-0.1
Sufentanil	0.01-0.06	5	2-4	0.01-0.05
Subarachnoid route				
Morphine	0.1-0.3	15	8-34	–
Fentanyl	0.005-0.025	5	3-6	–

Doses above should not be interpreted as equianalgesic doses for conversion to or from the specific opioid or route of administration.

Data from References 53, 61, and 130.

troublesome to patients, especially following surgery.[131] As doses of morphine are increased, the respiratory center becomes less responsive to carbon dioxide, causing progressive respiratory depression.[9] This effect is more pronounced with concurrent administration with other respiratory depressants.[132] Respiratory depression often manifests as a decrease in respiratory rate (although minute volume and tidal exchange also are affected).[120] End-tidal capnography has become commonplace as a means to monitor opioid-induced respiratory depression, especially in those at increased risk.[133]

10 11 Opioid-induced respiratory depression can be rapidly reversed by the opioid antagonist, naloxone.[120] In patients with underlying pulmonary dysfunction or sleep disordered breathing, caution must be exercised when opioids are used, as these patients are already using compensatory breathing mechanisms and are at risk for further respiratory compromise.[134] Caution is also urged when combining opiate analgesics with alcohol or other CNS depressants (ie, benzodiazepines, SMRs, and sleep hypnotics), because this combination is potentially harmful and possibly lethal.[37]

Therapeutic doses of morphine have minimal effects on blood pressure, cardiac rate, or cardiac rhythm when patients are supine; however, morphine does produce venous and arteriolar vessel dilation, potentially resulting in orthostatic hypotension, and hypovolemic patients may be more susceptible to morphine-induced cardiovascular changes (eg, decreases in blood pressure).[9] Because morphine prompts a decrease in myocardial oxygen demand in ischemic cardiac patients, it is often used to treat pain associated with myocardial infarction, although this practice has been called into question due to the potential for increased mortality.[135]

Morphine decreases the propulsive contractions of the GI tract resulting in constipation. Morphine-induced spasms of the sphincter of Oddi have also been observed; however, the clinical significance of this is unclear. Urinary retention is another significant adverse effect of morphine and should be routinely assessed. Morphine-induced histamine release often manifests as pruritus and may even exacerbate bronchospasm in patients with a history of asthma.[53] Therapeutic doses of morphine are not contraindicated in head injury, but medication-induced respiratory depression can increase intracranial pressure. Thus, caution is advised in head trauma patients who are not mechanically ventilated because morphine may increase intracranial pressures and cloud the neurologic examination results.[120]

Morphine is metabolized to morphine-3-glucuronide (M3G) and morphine-6-glucuronide (M6G). Whereas M6G contributes to analgesia, M3G may contribute to unwanted neurologic adverse effects. The metabolites are renally cleared and can accumulate in patients with renal impairment, contributing to greater adverse effects.[120] Most clinicians recommend avoiding morphine in renally compromised patients (ie, creatinine clearance ≤30 mL/minute [0.50 mL/s]). Morphine also inhibits the release of gonadotropin-releasing hormone from the hypothalamus, thus decreasing plasma testosterone and cortisol (opioid-induced hypogonadism). Male patients may present with symptoms of erectile dysfunction, decreased libido, and decreased analgesic efficacy. Females may experience alopecia, amenorrhea, and depressed mood, as well as decreased analgesic efficacy. Recommendations for clinical replacement of these hormones in patients using chronic opioid therapy are not well defined.[136] While the clinical meaning has not clearly been elucidated, morphine and other opioids, depending on the situation being used, may either enhance or inhibit the immune system.[53,120]

Hydromorphone is more potent than morphine, but its overall pharmacologic profile is similar. Some clinicians believe hydromorphone is associated with fewer adverse effects, especially pruritus, compared with other opioids. However, the research is limited and does not conclusively demonstrate this difference. Oxymorphone is available both orally and parenterally, although it offers no pharmacologic advantage over morphine. Levorphanol has an extended half-life and purported NMDA glutamate receptor activity, but its overall therapeutic effects are similar to the other agents in this class and cost is frequently a barrier to its use.[137,138]

Codeine is a commonly used opioid for the treatment of mild-to-moderate pain. It often is combined with other analgesic products (eg, acetaminophen). Unfortunately, it has the propensity to produce the adverse effects as morphine. Due to the risk of toxicity in patients with rapid metabolizer phenotypes, the FDA recommends against codeine's use in children and, in particular, infants being fed human milk.[139] Hydrocodone is perhaps the most commonly prescribed opioid in the United States and is available orally as immediate-release combined with nonopioid analgesics, as well as extended-release formulations. Its pharmacologic properties are similar to those of morphine. Oxycodone is a useful oral analgesic for moderate-to-severe pain. This is especially true when the product is used in combination with nonopioids. Although oxycodone shares basic morphine characteristics, the availability of an immediate-release and controlled-release oral dosage form also makes it very useful in chronic pain as well as cancer pain. Oliceridine, a novel opioid analgesic medication approved for IV use for moderate-severe pain, is classified as a biased opioid agonist. It displays selective mu opioid receptor agonism and is structurally dissimilar from other opioid analgesics. Oliceridine is associated with fewer tolerability concerns than traditional opioids; however, more literature is needed to support this claim. The prototype phenylpiperidine, meperidine, has a pharmacologic profile comparable with that of morphine; however, it is not as potent and has a shorter analgesic duration. Meperidine offers no analgesic advantage over morphine, has greater toxicity (CNS hyperirritability caused by its renally eliminated metabolite normeperidine), and should be limited in use, especially in older patients, those with renal dysfunction, or for prolonged treatment durations.[53,140]

Fentanyl is a synthetic opioid structurally related to meperidine but is significantly more potent and faster acting. It can be administered parenterally, transmucosally, sublingually, intranasally, and transdermally.[9,120] Numerous fentanyl-like agents exist including remifentanil, alfentanil, and sufentanil. Remifentanil and alfentanil are limited to use as part of general anesthesia, whereas sufentanil can be used for acute pain as a sublingual tablet in medically supervised settings.[141]

Methadone is a useful analgesic due to its oral efficacy, extended duration of action, and low cost. Properties unique to methadone, compared with other opioids, include the s-isomer's ability to antagonize NMDA receptors, agonist effects at the kappa and delta opioid receptor, as well as the blockade of serotonin and norepinephrine reuptake.[120,142] These properties may prove useful in the treatment of neuropathic and chronic pain. However, few trials have thoroughly evaluated methadone's risks versus benefits.[142,143] Epidemiologic studies suggest an increased number of methadone-related deaths, and cardiac arrhythmias have been associated with this medication, particularly at higher doses or when used concurrently with other agents that prolong QTc intervals.[132] Recommendations exist for specific echocardiogram monitoring for methadone.[143] The equianalgesic dose of methadone may decrease with higher doses of the comparator opioid, complicating conversions from other opioids to methadone. Methadone should not be titrated more frequently than every 5 to 7 days due to its unpredictable potency and variable half-live.[143] Thus, given the risks, methadone should be reserved to specialists with experience in its use.

Mixed Opioid Agonist–Antagonists

This analgesic class produces analgesia and has the potential for less respiratory depression than opioid agonists as they exert their analgesic activity via the KOR and either block or act as partial agonists at the MOR.[120] Agents in this class are considered to less physical dependence than morphine, but psychotomimetic responses (eg, hallucinations and dysphoria), limited analgesic effect, and a potential to initiate withdrawal in opioid-dependent populations have precluded their widespread clinical use. Both butorphanol and nalbuphine are available parenterally, with butorphanol also available as an intra-nasal spray. Nalbuphine is gaining popularity as a treatment for MOR agonist–associated pruritus.[144]

Buprenorphine is a pharmacologically complex opioid, which exhibits KOR antagonism, and several MOR-related actions, including partial agonism. Buprenorphine also displays agonist properties at the opioid receptor-like 1 (ORL-1) receptor which may have clinical ramifications in prevention of tolerance, euphoria/reward, and hyperalgesia.[145] Buprenorphine is available as a sublingual tablet, a buccal film, a once-weekly transdermal patch, or in combination with naloxone as a sublingual film or sublingual tablet. While buprenorphine's use for opioid use disorder previously required a special DEA license to prescribe, practitioners may now bypass this training requirement and obtain a waiver under the Controlled Substances Act by submitting a letter of intent to the Substance Abuse and Mental Health Services Administration (SAMHSA). The decrease in requirements for prescribing buprenorphine for OUD expands access to treatment.[146]

Central-Acting Opioids

Tramadol and tapentadol are the only centrally acting opioids available in the United States. Tramadol binds to MOR receptors and inhibits the reuptake of serotonin, and to a lesser extent, norepinephrine.[147] Tapentadol also binds the MOR receptor, but inhibits largely norepinephrine reuptake. Tramadol is indicated for the relief of moderate to moderately severe pain, while tapentadol is indicated for moderate-to-severe acute pain and diabetic peripheral neuropathy.

Both tramadol and tapentadol have adverse-effect profiles similar to that of the previously mentioned opioid analgesics (eg, dizziness, nausea, somnolence, and constipation). Tapentadol has not been systematically evaluated in patients with seizures, and it should be used with caution. Seizure risk, as well as risk of hypoglycemia and hyponatremia, may be elevated in patients taking tramadol.[147,148] Tramadol may have a place in treating patients with chronic pain, especially neuropathic pain, while tapentadol may be useful in the management of acute pain and the controlled release product may have a role in chronic pain treatment (eg, diabetes-related nerve pain).[149,150] Tapentadol is also associated with less physical dependence over time when compared with morphine and pentazocin.[151]

Opioid Antagonists

11 The opioid antagonist naloxone binds competitively to opioid receptors but does not produce an analgesic or opioid adverse effect response. Therefore, it is used most often to reverse the toxic effects of agonist- and agonist–antagonist-derived opioids. Other opioid antagonists exist, including naltrexone, naloxegol, naldemedine, and methylnaltrexone. Naltrexone's use is primarily limited to substance use disorder treatment, while naloxegol, naldemedine, and methylnaltrexone are peripherally acting only and used for opioid-induced constipation.[122]

11 With the growing prevalence of heroin and fentanyl analogs overdoses, healthcare providers are increasingly being called upon to assist in the prevention of these deaths. Many states have legislation in place that allow pharmacists to provide expanded access to naloxone which may be administered intranasally in addition to the traditional intravenous or intramuscular formations.[152] Further discussion of naloxone education, administration, and monitoring is provided in Chapter 85, "Substance-Related Disorders: Overview and Depressants, Stimulants, and Hallucinogens."

Tolerance, Hyperalgesia, Physical Dependence, and Opioid Use Disorder

1 2 3 4 11 A barrier that consistently causes clinicians to misjudge and mistreat pain is the misunderstanding of opioid tolerance, hyperalgesia, and physical dependence. Tolerance is the reduction of medication effect over time as a result of exposure to the agent.[120] It develops at different rates and with great patient variability. However, with stable disease, opioid doses may stabilize over time. Hyperalgesia is an increased sensitivity to pain. Opioids have been implicated in contributing to this phenomenon and can be seen with rapid opioid escalation or high-dose administration.[153] The mechanism or true clinical impact of this phenomenon is not understood.

Opioid physical dependence is characterized by an abstinence syndrome following administration of an antagonist medication or abrupt dose reduction or discontinuation of an opioid.[120,121] Clinicians must understand that physical dependence and tolerance are not equivalent to substance use disorder, and with chronic opioid use, physical dependence is expected.[121]

A baseline assessment and ongoing evaluation of patient behaviors is critical to mitigate risks of chronic opioid therapy and to balance effective pain management and patient safety.[154,155] Risk for opioid use disorder is associated with a family history of a substance use disorder, and/or underlying psychiatric diagnoses. Modifications to the treatment plan, which should be stratified based on patient risk, include baseline and random urine toxicology results, patient–provider treatment agreements, pill counts, a smaller prescription supply, and regular assessment of use behaviors. Table 79-7 outlines the CDC's guidelines to assist clincians.[156] Combining these approaches with regular and ongoing assessments of pain and functionality may result in improved outcomes. Chapter e84, "Introduction to Substance Use Disorders" contains additional information.

Multimodal Therapy

4 5 6 Commonly, multimodal therapy may be employed to optimize either acute or chronic pain management. Multimodal therapy is the concomitant use of different therapeutic interventions with the intent of obtaining additive therapeutic effects. Multimodal analgesia, one type of multimodal therapy, includes combining medications from different analgesic classes (eg, combination therapy with opioids and nonopioids or co-analgesics).[9,121] This often results in analgesia superior to that produced by either agent alone. Multimodal analgesia may also permit the use of lower doses and provide a more favorable adverse-effect profile, for example when NSAIDs are prescribed with opioids yielding an "opioid sparing" effect.

Regional Analgesia

7 9 Regional analgesia with properly administered local anesthetics can provide relief of both acute and chronic pain (Table 79-15).[130,157,158] These agents can be positioned by injection (eg, in joints, in the epidural or intrathecal space, along nerve roots, or in a nerve plexus) or topically. Lidocaine in the form of a patch has proven effective in treating focal neuropathic pain.[65] Regional nerve blocks with local anesthetics may effectively relieve pain. Although rare, elevated plasma concentrations of local anesthetics can cause CNS-excitation and depression, including dizziness, tinnitus, drowsiness, disorientation, muscle twitching, seizures, and respiratory arrest.[157] This syndrome is called LAST (local anesthetic systemic toxicity).[159] Cardiovascular adverse effects include myocardial depression, hypotension, decreased cardiac output, heart block, bradycardia, arrhythmias, and cardiac arrest. Disadvantages of such methods include the

TABLE 79-15 Local Anesthetics[a]

Agent (Brand Name)	Onset (min)	Duration (h)
Esters		
Procaine (Novocain, various)	2-5	0.25-1
Chloroprocaine (Nesacaine, various)	6-12	0.5
Tetracaine (Pontocaine)	≤15	2-3
Amides		
Mepivacaine (Polocaine, various)	3-5	0.75-1.5
Bupivacaine (Marcaine, various)	5	2-4
Bupivacaine liposomal (Exparel—wound infiltration only)	variable	24 local 96 systemic
Lidocaine (Xylocaine, various)	<2	0.5-1
Prilocaine (Citanest)	<2	1-2
Ropivacaine[b] (Naropin)	10-30	0.5-6

[a]Unless otherwise indicated, values are for infiltrative anesthesia.

[b]Epidural administration.

Data from Reference 61.

TABLE 79-16 Topical Analgesics

Medication	Uses	Mechanism of Action	Dosing	Notes
Capsaicin cream (various)	Temporary relief of minor aches and pains of muscles and joints Localized neuropathic pain	Transient receptor potential vanilloid 1 (TRPV1) receptor agonist	Apply 3-4 times daily	Continue scheduled use for 2-4 weeks for best results
Capsaicin 8% patch (Qutenza)	PHN, DPN	Transient receptor potential vanilloid 1 (TRPV1) receptor agonist	Apply 1-4 patches to affected area for 60 minutes (PHN) or 30 minutes (DPN) Cleansing gel must be used on application site following patch removal Repeat no more frequently than q3 months Max: 4 patches	Administer under supervision of physician Specific administration directions in packaging information Apply topical anesthetic before applying Monitor blood pressure due to transient increase in blood pressure during application
Diclofenac 1% gel (Voltaren)	Pain of osteoarthritis of joints amenable to topical treatment (knees, hands)	Nonsteroid anti-inflammatory drugs (NSAIDs)	Lower extremities: 4 g QID, max 16 g/day Upper extremities: 2 g QID, max 8 g/day Total dose maximum: 32 g/day	Same black box warnings as PO NSAIDs despite low systemic bioavailability (6% of systemic exposure from oral diclofenac) Use dosing card to measure amount
Diclofenac epolamine 1.3% patch (Flector)	Topical treatment of acute pain due to minor strains, sprains, and contusions	NSAIDs	1 patch to most painful area BID	Systemic effects were <1% after 4 days of repeated dosing
Diclofenac topical solution (Pennsaid)	Pain from osteoarthritis of the knee	NSAIDs	1.5%: 40 drops to each affected knee 4 times daily. Apply 10 drops at a time 2%: 2 pumps (40 mg) on each painful knee BID	Same black box warnings as PO NSAIDs
Lidocaine gel/ointment/patch (various)	Neuropathic pain	Sodium channel blocker	Cream/ointment: Apply to affected area 3 times daily Patch: apply 1 patch to affected area up to 12 h	Apply to intact skin only
Lidocaine 5% patch (Lidoderm, also available in 4% over the counter)	PHN	Sodium channel blocker	Apply 1-3 patches to site of pain for 12 h Maximum: 3 patches	May cut lidocaine patches Apply to intact skin only Severe hepatic impairment increases risk of adverse effects
Menthol/methyl salicylate (various)	Minor aches and pains of muscles and joints (simple backache, arthritis, strains, bruises, sprains)	Rubefacient	Apply topically 3-4 times a day to affected area	
Trolamine salicylate cream 10% (various)	Aches and pains of muscles and joints (arthritis, simple backache, bruises, sprains, strains)	Rubefacient	Apply topically 3-4 times a day to affected area	Do not apply to damaged skin

Data from Reference 61.

need for skillful technical application, need for frequent administration, and highly specialized follow-up procedures.

SPECIAL POPULATIONS

6 9 Some patients are at a higher risk for under-treatment because of potential inability to communicate or rate their pain (eg, infants, noncommunicative adults, or those with dementia). It is in these cases that parent or caregiver input becomes paramount to identify changes in behavior, which might suggest pain (eg, fussy, inconsolable, changes in eating patterns, crying out, or agitation). When patients cannot verbalize their pain (eg, coma), monitoring behaviors (eg, agitation) and physiologic signs and symptoms (eg, heart rate) are appropriate. Validated pain assessment tools are available to assist the clinician in approaching patients who are unable to readily communicate the severity of their pain.[160]

In addition, those living with chronic, debilitating, and life-threatening illnesses need specialized pain control and care that is palliative in nature.[158] Although care must be taken in these populations to ensure that proper individualized treatment plans follow accepted guidelines, the key concepts in pain management as outlined in this chapter are the guiding tenets in maximizing pain control.[161,162]

PERSONALIZED PHARMACOTHERAPY

6 8 9 Pharmacogenomics is one factor that can impact medication response, and pharmacogenomic differences can contribute both to a lack of response (analgesia) and toxicity (adverse effects).[163] Guidance is available for prescribing and dosing certain NSAIDs, opioids, and antidepressants that are used in pain management when pharmacogenomic information is available.[63,90,164] However, guidance is not available on when to use pharmacogenomic testing in pain management as it is not a routine practice. Pharmacogenomic testing may be considered in polypharmacy, high-risk patients, potential for significant adverse effects, and medications with specific dosing considerations.[165,166]

Several NSAIDs are metabolized by CYP2C9 and impacted by pharmacogenomic variability. NSAIDs involved include celecoxib, flurbiprofen, ibuprofen, meloxicam, and piroxicam. Those that are intermediate or poor metabolizers of CYP2C9 are at increased risk of adverse effects due to reduced metabolism. Dosing recommendations vary depending on the phenotype, from use of standard doses to initiation at lower doses or use of alternate NSAIDs not metabolized through CYP2C9 like aspirin, ketorolac, naproxen, or sulindac.[63]

Tricyclic antidepressants are metabolized by CYP2D6 and CYP2C19. While CPIC guidelines exist for TCAs, they are geared toward TCA use in the management of depression, not pain. Since TCAs, when used in pain management, are used at lower doses than used for depression, those that are poor or intermediate CYP2D6 or CYP2C19 metabolizers are less likely to encounter adverse effects, so dose adjustments are not recommended. However, if higher doses of amitriptyline are used for managing pain than the recommendations for depression should be considered.[90]

Other antidepressants used in the management of pain are either partially or significantly metabolized by CYP2D6 though have less clear pharmacogenomic guidance. Duloxetine is metabolized more so by CYP1A2, with some contribution by CYP2D6 to hydroxy metabolites. Venlafaxine is metabolized by CYP2D6 to O-desmethylvenlafaxine. Guidance from the Royal Dutch Association for the Advancement of Pharmacy does not recommend any dose adjustments for duloxetine based on pharmacogenomics as it is not a gene-drug interaction.[167] For venlafaxine in intermediate and poor CYP2D6 metabolizers, there is unclear information if there is an increased risk of adverse effects and thus no firm guidance on how to adjust the dose is provided; alternate recommendations include the use of an alternate antidepressants not impacted by CYP2D6.[168] In CYP2D6 ultrarapid metabolizers, the dose of venlafaxine can be increased by 150% the standard dose; however, if dose adjustment is not effective or leads to adverse effects, then venlafaxine should be avoided.

For patients of Asian ancestry, the FDA recommends testing for *HLA-B*15.02* and HLA-A*31.01 prior to initiation of carbamazepine and *HLA-B*15.02* before starting oxcarbazepine due to the increased risk for life-threatening dermatologic reactions including Steven–Johnson Syndrome (SJS)/toxic epidermal necrolysis (TEN), drug reaction with eosinophilia and systemic symptoms (DRESS), and maculopapular exanthema (MPE). Those with *HLA-B*15.02* and/or *HLA-A*31.01* positive genotyping should not be started on carbamazepine or if *HLA-B*15.02* do not initiate oxcarbazepine if naïve. Severe dermatologic reactions usually occur within the first 3 months, so if a patient used carbamazepine for 3 months without issue, it can be considered in those that are *HLA-B*15.02* positive or *HLA-A*31.01* positive.[164]

CPIC guidelines cover CYP2D6, mu opioid-receptor-1 (OPRM1), and catechol-o-methyltransferase (COMT) consideration with specific opioids.[169] Codeine and tramadol are both metabolized by CYP2D6 to active metabolites which are responsible for their analgesic and adverse effects. In CYP2D6 rapid metabolizers, codeine and tramadol should be avoided due to increased formation of their active forms contributing to significant adverse effects including respiratory depression. For CYP2D6 poor metabolizers, codeine and tramadol should be avoided to the potential for lack of analgesic benefit. Hydrocodone has less evidence supporting need for dose adjustment in CYP2D6 ultrarapid metabolizers compared to codeine and tramadol. There is some evidence showing decreased metabolism of hydrocodone to hydromorphone in CYP2D6 poor metabolizers but no specific dose adjustments are recommended. Oxycodone and methadone are not thought to be impacted significant by CYP2D6, so no recommendations are provided.

In some cases, genotype results may further help explain cases where patients require higher doses to achieve adequate analgesia. For example, data suggest that variants in opioid-receptor subtypes, specifically MOR-1 (OPRM1 gene), may predict efficacy and dosing requirements for some opioids such as morphine or hydromorphone.[170-172] CPIC does not provide recommendations based on COMT or OPRM1 genotypes.[169]

Use of pharmacogenomic testing results may be beneficial in the accurate interpretation of urine toxicology test results when assessing adherence to chronic opioid therapy. For instance, results from a urine toxicology report reveal only parent medication and no expected metabolites, which may be explained by medication interactions, CYP poor metabolizer phenotype, or diversion (pill shaving).

For more information regarding specific medication gene pairs related to pharmacogenomics, CPIC provides evidence-based peer-reviewed guidelines on interpretation of these testing results (www.cpicpgx.org).

EVALUATION OF THERAPEUTIC OUTCOMES

8 Consistent monitoring for effectiveness (eg, pain relief, adequate functionality) and adverse effects (eg, sedation) is critical in optimizing therapeutic outcomes. Numerous validated scoring tools exist (eg, numeric rating scale, visual analog scale); however, the tools need to be appropriate for the type of pain being evaluated, used consistently, and with good clinical judgment.[28,34] Pain management efficacy, any change in pain, and medication adverse effects (eg, opioid-induced sedation or constipation) must be assessed and reassessed on a regular basis. Frequency of reassessment should be dictated by the medication's route of administration, duration of action, various pharmacokinetic factors, or other concomitant therapies. Postoperative pain and acute exacerbation of cancer pain may need to be assessed hourly or even more frequently, whereas chronic noncancer pain may require only daily or less frequent assessment. Pain intensity assessment is vital in acute pain, whereas functionality becomes more of an issue in chronic pain. Quality of life must be assessed on a regular basis in all patients. Many advocate for using the five "A's" (analgesia, activity, aberrant drug behavior, adverse effects, affect) as key assessment measures for any patient with chronic pain.

Often, objective signs are lacking for pain evaluation. Acute pain may result in increased sympathetic tone (eg, hypertension, tachycardia, and tachypnea); however, this response is usually diminished as acute pain progresses to chronic pain. The clinician must rely on the patient's description of their pain.

8 9 All opioids can cause constipation. The best management of constipation is prevention and patients should be counseled on the proper intake of fluids and fiber. A stimulant laxative with or without a stool softener should be added with chronic opioid use. For constipation that doesn't respond to standard bowel regimens, peripherally acting mu-opioid receptor antagonists (PAMORAs) are available for treating opioid-induced constipation. All CNS depressants (eg, alcohol, benzodiazepines) amplify CNS depression when used with opioid analgesics, and use of these combinations should be discouraged when possible. When the combinations are used, patients should be monitored closely.

CONCLUSION

Pain represents a significant source of disability as well as health-care resource utilization. A thorough understanding of pain pathogenesis is imperative for clinicians involved in its treatment. Multidisciplinary and multimodal approaches to pain management must be considered with nonpharmacological and nonopioid modalities preferred as first-line treatments. Opioid analgesics are important analgesic alternatives and should be considered after careful patient selection. Monitoring for the occurrence of a substance use disorder while these agents are employed is essential. Adverse effects of all pharmacologic therapy for pain require judicious anticipation and treatment (Fig. 79-2).

ABBREVIATIONS

ASAM	American Society of Addiction Medicine
CNS	central nervous system
COX-2	cyclooxygenase-2

CPIC	Clinical Pharmacogenomics Implementation Consortium
CYP	cytochrome P450
DOR	delta opioid receptor
GABA	γ-aminobutyric acid
GI	gastrointestinal
IgE	immunoglobulin E
IM	intramuscular
IV	intravenous
KOR	kappa opioid receptor
M3G	morphine-3-glucuronide
M6G	morphine-6-glucuronide
MOR	mu-opioid receptor
NMDA	*N*-methyl-D-aspartate
NSAIDs	nonsteroidal anti-inflammatory drugs
OPRM1	opioid receptor, mu-1 gene subtype
ORL-1	opioid receptor-like receptor (nociceptin receptor)
PCA	patient-controlled analgesia
PNS	peripheral nervous system
SAMHSA	Substance Abuse and Mental Health Services Administration
TENS	transcutaneous electrical nerve stimulation
WHO	World Health Organization

REFERENCES

1. Bennett DS, Breakthrough pain: Treatment rationale with opioids. Available at: http://www.medscape.org/viewarticle/461612. Accessed January 6, 2019.
2. Stimmel B. *Pain, Analgesia, and Addiction: The Pharmacology of Pain.* New York, NY: Raven Press; 1983.
3. Blackwell DL, Lucas JW, Clarke TC. Summary health statistics for U.S. adults: National health interview survey, 2012. *Vital Heal Stat 10.* 2014;(260):1–161. Accessed October 4, 2018. http://www.ncbi.nlm.nih.gov/pubmed/24819891.
4. Raja SN, Carr DB, Cohen M, et al. The revised International Association for the Study of Pain definition of pain: Concepts, challenges, and compromises. *Pain.* 2020;161(9):1976–1982. 10.1097/j.pain.0000000000001939 32694387.
5. Dahlhamer J, Lucas J, Zelaya C, et al. Prevalence of chronic pain and high-impact chronic pain among adults - United States, 2016. *MMWR Morb Mortal Wkly Rep.* 2018;67(36):1001–1006. 10.15585/mmwr.mm6736a2 30212442.
6. Humble SR, Dalton AJ, Li L. A systematic review of therapeutic interventions to reduce acute and chronic post-surgical pain after amputation, thoracotomy or mastectomy. *Eur J Pain.* 2015;19(4):451–465. doi:10.1002 / ejp.567.
7. Webster LR, Fine PG. Approaches to improve pain relief while minimizing opioid abuse liability. *J Pain.* 2010;11(7):602–611. doi:10.1016 / j.jpain.2010.02.008.
8. Woolf CJ. What is this thing called pain? *J Clin Invest.* 2010;120(11):3742–3744. doi:10.1172 / JCI45178.
9. Pasero C, Quinn TE, Portenoy RD. Physiology and pharmacology of opioids analgesics. In: McCafferty M, Pasero C, eds. *Pain Assessment and Pharmacologic Management.* St Louis: Mosby; 2011:283–300.
10. McEntire DM, Kirkpatrick DR, Dueck NP, et al. Pain transduction: A pharmacologic perspective. *Expert Rev Clin Pharmacol.* 2016;9(8):1069–1080. doi.10.1080/17512433.2016.1183481.
11. Dubin AE, Patapoutian A. Nociceptors: The sensors of the pain pathway. *J Clin Invest.* 2010;120(11):3760–3772. doi:10.1172/JCI42843.
12. Cummins TR, Sheets PL, Waxman SG. The roles of sodium channels in nociception: Implications for mechanisms of pain. *Pain.* 2007;131(3):243–257. doi:10.1016/j.pain.2007.07.026.
13. Fong A, Schug SA. Pathophysiology of pain: A practical primer. *Plast Reconstr Surg.* 2014;134(4 suppl 2):8S–14S. doi.10.1097/PRS.0000000000000682.
14. Pasero C. Neurophysiology of pain and analgesia and the pathophysiology of neuropathic pain. In: McCaffery M, Pasero C, eds. *Pain Assessment and Pharmacologic Management.* St. Louis, MO: Mosby; 2011:1–12.
15. Randich A, Ness T. Modulation of spinal nociceptive processing. In: Fishman SM, Ballantyne JC, Rathmell JP, eds. *Bonica's Pain Management.* Baltimore, MD: Wolters Kluwer Health; 2010.
16. Palazzo E, Luongo L, Novellis V, et al. The role of cannabinoid receptors in the descending modulation of pain. *Pharmaceuticals (Basel).* 2010;3(8):2661–2673. 10.3390/ph3082661 27713370.
17. Woolf CJ. Central sensitization: Implications for the diagnosis and treatment of pain. *Pain.* 2011;152(suppl):S2–S15. doi:10.1016/j.pain.2010.09.030.
18. Uman LS, Birnie KA, Noel M, et al. Psychological interventions for needle-related procedural pain and distress in children and adolescents. *Cochrane Database Syst Rev.* 2013;(10):CD005179–. 10.1002/14651858.CD005179.pub3 24108531.
19. Wetherell JL, Afari N, Rutledge T, et al. A randomized, controlled trial of acceptance and commitment therapy and cognitive-behavioral therapy for chronic pain. *Pain.* 2011;152(9):2098–2107. 10.1016/j.pain.2011.05.016 21683527.
20. Tsatali M, Papaliagkas V, Damigos D, Mavreas V, Gouva M, Tsolaki M. Depression and anxiety levels increase chronic musculoskeletal pain in patients with Alzheimer's disease. *Curr Alzheimer Res.* 2014;11(6):574–579. doi:10.2174/1567205011666140618103406.
21. Scholz J, Woolf CJ. The neuropathic pain triad: Neurons, immune cells and glia. *Nat Neurosci.* 2007;10(11):1361–1368. doi.10.1038 / nn1992.
22. Grace PM, Hutchinson MR, Maier SF, Watkins LR. Pathological pain and the neuroimmune interface. *Nat Rev Immunol.* 2014;14(4):217–231. doi:10.1038 / nri3621.
23. Clauw DJ. Fibromyalgia. *J Am Med Assoc.* 2014;311(15):1547. doi:10.1001 / jama.2014.3266.
24. Apkarian OF, Baliki MN, Farmer MA. Predicting transition to chronic pain. *Curr Opin Neurol.* 2013;26(4):360–367. doi:10.1097 / WCO.0b013e32836336ad.
25. Gold MS, Gebhart GF. Peripheral pain mechanisms and nociceptor sensitization. In: Fishman SM, Ballantyne JC, Rathmell JP, eds. *Bonica's Pain Management.* Baltimore, MD: Wolters Kluwer Health; 2010;24–34.
26. Apkarian AV. Pain and brain changes. In: Benzon HT, Rathmell JP, Wu CL, eds. *Raj's Practical Management of Pain.* Philadelphia, PA: Mosby; 2008:151–173.
27. Hanley MA, Jensen MP, Smith DG, Ehde DM, Edwards WT, Robinson LR. Preamputation pain and acute pain predict chronic pain after lower extremity amputation. *J Pain.* 2007;8(2):102–109. doi:10.1016 / j.jpain.2006.06.004.
28. McCaffery M, Herr K, Pasero C. Assessment. In: Pasero C, McCaffery M, eds. *Pain Assessment and Pharmacologic Management.* St. Louis, MO: Mosby Elsevier; 2011.
29. Twycross RG. Pain and analgesics. *Curr Med Res Opin.* 1978;5(7):497–505. doi:10.1185/03007997809108992.
30. Latremoliere A, Woolf CJ. Central sensitization: A generator of pain hypersensitivity by central neural plasticity. *J Pain.* 2009;10(9):895–926. doi:10.1016 / J.JPAIN.2009.06.012.
31. Clayton HA, Reschak GL, Gaynor HE, Creamer JL. A novel program to assess and manage pain. *Medsurg Nurs.* 2000;9(6):317–321. http://www.ncbi.nlm.nih.gov/pubmed/11904868.
32. Swarm RA, Abernethy AP, Anghelescu DL, et al. Adult cancer pain. *J Natl Compr Canc Netw.* 2013;11(8):992–1022. http://www.ncbi.nlm.nih.gov/pubmed/23946177. Accessed October 9, 2018.
33. Swarm RA, Paice JA, Anghelescu DL, et al. *NCCN Clinical Practice Guidelines in Oncology: Adult Cancer Pain.* 2018. https://www.nccn.org/professionals/physician_gls/PDF/pain.pdf.
34. Breivik H, Borchgrevink PC, Allen SM, et al. Assessment of pain. *Br J Anaesth.* 2008;101(1):17–24. doi:10.1093 / bja / aen103.
35. Krebs EE, Lorenz KA, Bair MJ, et al. Development and initial validation of the PEG: A three-item scale assessing pain intensity and interference. *J Gen Intern Med.* 2009;24(6):733–738. doi.10.1007/s11606-009-0981-1.
36. Chou R, Qaseem A, Snow V, et al. Diagnosis and treatment of low back pain: A joint clinical practice guideline from the American College of Physicians and the American Pain Society. *Ann Intern Med.* 2007;147(7):478–491. http://www.ncbi.nlm.nih.gov/pubmed/17909209.
37. Dowell D, Haegerich TM, Chou R. CDC guideline for prescribing opioids for chronic pain: United States. *JAMA.* 2016;315(15):1624–1645. doi.10.1001 / jama.2016.1464.
38. Bonakdar RA, Sukiennik AW, eds. *Integrative Pain Management.* Oxford: Oxford University Press; 2016. 10.1093 / with / 9780199315246.001.0001.
39. Skelly AC, Chou R, Dettori JR, et al. Noninvasive nonpharmacological treatment for chronic pain: A systematic review. Comparative Effectiveness Review No. 209. (Prepared by the Pacific Northwest Evidence-based Practice Center under Contract No. 290-2015-00009-I.) AHRQ Publication No 18-EHC013-EF. Rockville, MD: Agency for Healthcare Research and Quality; June 2018. Posted final reports are located on the Effective Health Care Program search page. doi: https://doi.org/10.23970/AHRQEPCCER20. https://effectivehealthcare.ahrq.gov/products/nonpharma-treatment-pain/research-2018.

40. Tick H, Nielsen A, Pelletier KR, et al. Evidence-based nonpharmacologic strategies for comprehensive pain care. *Explore.* 2018;14(3):177–211. doi.10.1016/j.explore.2018.02.001.
41. Chou R, Deyo R, Friedly J, et al. Nonpharmacologic therapies for low back pain: A systematic review for an American college of physicians clinical practice guideline. *Ann Intern Med.* 2017;166(7):493–505. 10.7326/M16-2459 28192793.
42. Kamper SJ, Apeldoorn AT, Chiarotto A, et al. Multidisciplinary biopsychosocial rehabilitation for chronic low back pain: Cochrane systematic review and meta-analysis. *BMJ.* 2015;350:h444–h444. 10.1136/bmj.h444 25694111.
43. O'Donnell KF. Preoperative pain management education: A quality improvement project. *J PeriAnesthesia Nurs.* 2015;30(3):221–227. doi:10.1016/j.jopan.2015.01.013.
44. Darnall BD. Minimize opioids by optimizing pain psychology. *Pain Manag.* 2014;4(4):251–253. doi:10.2217/pmt.14.18.
45. Johnson MI, Jones G. Transcutaneous electrical nerve stimulation: Current status of evidence. *Pain Manag.* 2017;7:1–4, 10.2217/pmt-2016-0030.
46. Vance CG, Dailey DL, Rachel BA, Devour KA. Using TENS for pain control: The state of the evidence. *Pain Manag.* 2014;4(3):197–209. doi.10.2217/pmt.14.13.
47. Wu LC, Weng PW, Chen CH, et al. Literature review and meta-analysis of transcutaneous electrical nerve stimulation in treating chronic back pain. *Reg Anesth Pain Med.* 2018;43(4):425–433. 10.1097/AAP.0000000000000740 29394211.
48. Lee C, Crawford C, Hickey A. Active self-care therapies for pain (PACT) Working Group. Mind–body therapies for the self-management of chronic pain symptoms. *Pain Med.* 2014;15(S1):S21–S39. doi.10.1111 / pme.12383.
49. Kligler B, Teets R, Quick M. Complementary/integrative therapies that work: A review of the evidence. *Am Fam Physician.* 2016;94(5):369–374. http://www.ncbi.nlm.nih.gov/pubmed/27583423. Accessed November 6, 2018.
50. Solloway MR, Taylor SL, Shekelle PG, et al. An evidence map of the effect of Tai Chi on health outcomes. *Syst Rev.* 2016;5(1):126. doi:10.1186 / s13643-016-0300-y.
51. NCCIH, Pain: Considering Complementary Approaches. Accessed October 26, 2021. https://files.nccih.nih.gov/s3fs-public/Pain-eBook-2019_06_508.pdf.
52. *WHO Guidelines for the Pharmacological and Radiotherapeutic Management of Cancer Pain in Adults and Adolescents.* WHO; 2018. doi: 10.4135/9781446222126.n9.
53. Herndon C, Arnstein P, Darnall B, et al. *Principles of Analgesic Use.* 7th ed. Chicago: American Pain Society; 2016. https://www.amazon.com/Principles-Analgesic-Use-7th-APS/dp/B071WG3PSW. Accessed October 1, 2018.
54. Chou R, Deyo R, Devine B, et al. Evidence Report/Technology Assessment Number 218. *Agency Healthc Res Qual.* 2014. doi:10.23970 / AHRQEPCERTA218.
55. Moore RAA, Derry S, Wiffel PJJ, Straube S, Aldington DJJ. Overview review: Comparative efficacy of oral ibuprofen and paracetamol (acetaminophen) across acute and chronic pain conditions. *Eur J Pain.* 2014;19(9):1213–1223. doi:10.1002 / ejp.649.
56. Machado GC, Maher CG, Ferreira PH, et al. Efficacy and safety of paracetamol for spinal pain and osteoarthritis: Systematic review and meta-analysis of randomised placebo controlled trials. *BMJ.* 2015;350:h1225. Accessed October 9, 2018. http://www.ncbi.nlm.nih.gov/pubmed/25828856.
57. Aronoff D, Oates J, Boutaud O. New insights into the mechanism of action of acetaminophen: Its clinical pharmacologic characteristics reflect its inhibition of the two prostaglandin H2 synthases. *Clin Pharmacol Ther.* 2006;79(1):9–19. doi:10.1016/j.clpt.2005.09.009.
58. Kolasinski SL, Neogi T, Hochberg MC, et al. 2019 American College of Rheumatology/Arthritis Foundation Guideline for the Management of Osteoarthritis of the Hand, Hip, and Knee. *Arthritis Care Res (Hoboken).* 2020;72(2):149–162. 10.1002/acr.24131 31908149.
59. Bannuru RR, Osani MC, Vaysbrot EE, et al. OARSI guidelines for the non-surgical management of knee, hip, and polyarticular osteoarthritis. *Osteoarthritis Cartilage.* 2019;27(11):1578–1589. 10.1016/j.joca.2019.06.011 31278997.
60. Qaseem A, Wilt TJ, McLean RM, Forciea MA. Noninvasive treatments for acute, subacute, and chronic low back pain: A clinical practice guideline from the American College of Physicians. *Ann Intern Med.* 2017;166(7):514–530. doi:10.7326/M16-2367.
61. Lexicomp. Lexicomp Online; 2018. Available at: online.lexi.com.
62. Rannou F, Pelletier JP, Martel-Pelletier J. Efficacy and safety of topical NSAIDs in the management of osteoarthritis: Evidence from real-life setting trials and surveys. *Semin Arthritis Rheum.* 2016;45(4 Suppl):S18–21. 10.1016/j.semarthrit.2015.11.007 26806189.
63. Theken KN, Lee CR, Gong L, et al. Clinical Pharmacogenetics Implementation Consortium Guideline (CPIC) for CYP2C9 and nonsteroidal anti-inflammatory drugs. *Clin Pharmacol Ther.* 2020;108(2):191–200. 10.1002/cpt.1830 32189324.
64. Attal N, Cruccu G, Baron R, et al. EFNS guidelines on the pharmacological treatment of neuropathic pain: 2010 revision. *Eur J Neurol.* 2010;17(9):1113–E88. doi:10.1111/j.1468-1331.2010.02999.x.
65. Finnerup NB, Attal N, Haroutounian S, et al. Pharmacotherapy for neuropathic pain in adults: A systematic review and meta-analysis. *Lancet Neurol.* 2015;14(2):162–173. doi.10.1016/S1474-4422(14)70251-0.
66. Moulin D, Boulanger A, Clark AJ, et al. Pharmacological management of chronic neuropathic pain: Revised consensus statement from the Canadian Pain Society. *Pain Res Manag.* 2014;19(6):328–335.
67. Pop-Busui R, Boulton Ajm, Feldman EL, et al. Diabetic neuropathy: A position statement by the American Diabetes Association. *Diabetes Care.* 2016;40(January):136–154. 10.2337/dc16-2042.
68. Waldfogel JM, Nesbit SM, et al. Pharmacotherapy for diabetic peripheral neuropathy pain and quality of life. *Neurology.* 2017;88(29):1958–1967. doi:10.1212 / WNL.0000000000003882.
69. Dharmshaktu P, Tayal V, Kalra BS. Efficacy of antidepressants as analgesics: A review. *J Clin Pharmacol.* 2012;52(1):6–17. doi:10.1177/0091270010394852.
70. Dworkin RH, O'Connor AB, Backonja M, et al. Pharmacologic management of neuropathic pain: Evidence-based recommendations. *Pain.* 2007;132(3):237–251. doi:10.1016/j.pain.2007.08.033.
71. Wiffen PJ, Derry S, Moore RA, Kalso EA, et al. Carbamazepine for chronic neuropathic pain and fibromyalgia in adults. *Cochrane Database Syst Rev.* 20144):CD005451–CD005451. 10.1002/14651858.CD005451.pub3 24719027.
72. Wiffen PJ, Derry S, Moore RA. Lamotrigine for acute and chronic pain. *Cochrane Database Syst Rev.* 20112):CD006044–CD006044. 10.1002/14651858.CD006044.pub3 21328280.
73. Gronseth G, Cruccu G, Alksne J, et al. Practice parameter: The diagnostic evaluation and treatment of trigeminal neuralgia. *Neurology.* 2008;71:1183–1190.
74. National Institute for Health and Care Excellence. Neuropathic pain – pharmacological management. The pharmacological management of neuropathic pain in adults in non-specialist settings. NICE clinical guideline 173. *Natl Inst Heal Care Excell.* 2013.
75. Berghuis B, de Haan G-J, van den Broek MPH, Sander JW, Lindhout D, Koeleman BPC. Epidemiology, pathophysiology and putative genetic basis of carbamazepine- and oxcarbazepine-induced hyponatremia. *Eur J Neurol.* 2016;23(9):1393–1399. doi:10.1111/ene.13069.
76. Al-Quliti KW. Update on neuropathic pain treatment for trigeminal neuralgia: The pharmacological and surgical options. *Neurosciences.* 2015. doi:10.17712/nsj.2015.2.20140501.
77. Zhou M, Chen N, He L, Yang M, Zhu C, Wu F. Oxcarbazepine for neuropathic pain. *Cochrane Database Syst Rev.* 2013;12(3):CD007963. doi:10.1002/14651858.CD007963.pub2.
78. Verret M, Lauzier F, Zarychanski R, et al. Perioperative use of gabapentinoids for the management of postoperative acute pain: A systematic review and meta-analysis. *Anesthesiology.* 2020(133): 265–279, 10.1097/ALN.0000000000003428
79. Martinez V, Pichard X, Fletcher D. Perioperative pregabalin administration does not prevent chronic postoperative pain: Systematic review with a meta-analysis of randomized trials. *Pain.* 2017;158(5):775–783. doi:10.1097/j.pain.0000000000000838.
80. Shanthanna H, Gilron I, Rajarathinam M, et al. Benefits and safety of gabapentinoids in chronic low back pain: A systematic review and meta-analysis of randomized controlled trials. *PLoS Med.* 2017;14(8):e1002369. doi:10.1371/journal.pmed.1002369.
81. Mathieson S, Maher CG, McLachlan AJ, et al. Trial of pregabalin for acute and chronic sciatica. *N Engl J Med.* 2017;376(12):1111–1120. doi.10.1056/NEJMoa1614292.
82. Schifano F. Misuse and abuse of pregabalin and gabapentin: Cause for concern? *CNS Drugs.* 2014;28(6):491–496. doi:10.1007/s40263-014-0164-4.
83. Evoy KE, Morrison MD, Saklad SR. Abuse and misuse of pregabalin and gabapentin. *Drugs.* 2017;77(4):403–426. doi:10.1007/s40265-017-0700-x.
84. Koncicki HM, Unruh M, Schell JO. Pain management in CKD: A guide for nephrology providers. *Am J Kidney Dis.* 2017;69(3):451–460. doi:10.1053/j.ajkd.2016.08.039.
85. Khoromi S, Patsalides A, Parada S, Salehi V, Meegan JM, Max MB. Topiramate in chronic lumbar radicular pain. *J Pain.* 2005;6(12):829–836. doi:10.1016/j.jpain.2005.08.002.
86. Muehlbacher M, Nickel MK, Kettler C, et al. Topiramate in treatment of patients with chronic low back pain: A randomized, double-blind, placebo-controlled study. *Clin J Pain.* 2006;22(6):526–531. doi.10.1097/.ajp.0000192516.58578.a4.

87. Macfarlane GJ, Kronisch C, Dean LE, et al. EULAR revised recommendations for the management of fibromyalgia. *Ann Rheum Dis.* 2017;76(2):318–328. doi.10.1136/annrheumdis-2016-209724.
88. DeBattista C. Antidepressant agents. In: Katzung B, ed. *Basic and Clinical Pharmacology.* 14th ed. New York, NY: 2017.
89. Teter C, Kando J, Wells B.Major depressive disorders. In: DiPiro J, Talbert R, Yee G, Matzke G, Wells B, Posey L, eds. *Pharmacotherapy: A Pathophysiologic Approach.* 10th ed. New York, NY: McGraw-Hill; 2016.
90. Hicks JK, Sangkuhl K, Swen JJ, et al. Clinical pharmacogenetics implementation consortium guideline (CPIC) for CYP2D6 and CYP2C19 genotypes and dosing of tricyclic antidepressants: 2016 update. *Clin Pharmacol Ther.* 2017;102(1):37–44. 10.1002/cpt.597 27997040.
91. Gelenberg AJ, Marlene Freeman CP, Markowitz JC, et al. *Practice Guideline for the Treatment of Patients with Major Depressive Disorder Third Edition Work Group on Major Depressive Disorder.* 2010. http://www.psychiatryonline.com/pracGuide/pracGuideTopic_7.aspx.
92. Kus T, Aktas G, Alpak G, et al. Efficacy of venlafaxine for the relief of taxane and oxaliplatin-induced acute neurotoxicity: A single-center retrospective case–control study. *Support Care Cancer.* 2016;24(5):2085–2091. doi:10.1007/s00520-015-3009-x.
93. Rej S, Dew MA, Karp JF. Treating concurrent chronic low back pain and depression with low-dose venlafaxine: An initial identification of "easy-to-use" clinical predictors of early response. *Pain Med (United States).* 2014;15(7):1154–1162. doi:10.1111/pme.12456.
94. O'Connor AB, Dworkin RH. Treatment of neuropathic pain: An overview of recent guidelines. *Am J Med.* 2009;122(10 Suppl):S22–S32. doi:10.1016/j.amjmed.2009.04.007.
95. Bendtsen L, Evers S, Linde M, Mitsikostas DD, Sandrini G, Schoenen J. EFNS guideline on the treatment of tension-type headache: Report of an EFNS task force. *Eur J Neurol.* 2010;17(11):1318–1325. doi.10.1111/j.1468-1331.2010.03070.x.
96. Silberstein SD, Holland S, Freitag F, Dodick DW, Argoff C, Ashman E. Evidence-based guideline update: Pharmacologic treatment for episodic migraine prevention in adults report of the quality standards subcommittee of the American Academy of Neurology and the American Headache Society. *Neurology.* 2012;78(17):1337–1345. doi:10.1212/WNL.0b013e3182535d20.
97. Sansone RA, Sansone LA. Serotonin norepinephrine reuptake inhibitors: A pharmacological comparison. *Innov Clin Neurosci.* 2014;11(3-4):37–42. Accessed September 25, 2018. http://www.ncbi.nlm.nih.gov/pubmed/24800132.
98. Herndon C, Lider J, Daniels A. Ask the expert: QT interval and antidepressants. *Pract Pain Manag.* 2015;15(10):1–3. https://www.practicalpainmanagement.com/treatments/pharmacological/non-opioids/qt-intervals-antidepressants. Accessed October 20, 2018.
99. Bixby AL, VandenBerg A, Bostwick JR. Clinical management of bleeding risk with antidepressants. *Ann Pharmacother.* 2019;53(2):186–194. 10.1177/1060028018794005 30081645.
100. Heetla HW, Staal MJ, Proost JH, Van Laar T. Clinical relevance of pharmacological and physiological data in intrathecal baclofen therapy. *Arch Phys Med Rehabil.* 2014;95(11):2199–2206. doi:10.1016/j.apmr.2014.04.030.
101. van Tulder MW, Touray T, Furlan AD, Solway S, Bouter LM. Muscle relaxants for non-specific low back pain. *Cochrane Database Syst Rev.* 2003;(2):Cd004252. doi:10.1002/14651858.cd004252.
102. Beebe FA, Barkin RL, Barkin S. A clinical and pharmacologic review of skeletal muscle relaxants for musculoskeletal conditions. *Am J Ther.* 2005;12(2):151–171. doi:10.1097/01.mjt.0000134786.50087.d8.
103. Witenko C, Moorman-li R, Motycka C, et al. Considerations for muscle relaxants in low back pain. *Pharm Ther.* 2014;39(6):427–435.
104. Malanga GA, Gwynn MW, Smith R, Miller D. Tizanidine is effective in the treatment of myofascial pain syndrome. *Pain Physician.* 2002;5(4):422–432. http://www.ncbi.nlm.nih.gov/entrez/query.fcgi?cmd=Retrieve&db=PubMed&dopt=Citation&list_uids=16886022.
105. See S, Ginzburg R. Skeletal muscle relaxants. *Pharmacotherapy.* 2008;28(2):207–213.
106. Vlavonou R, Perreault MM, Barrière O, et al. Pharmacokinetic characterization of baclofen in patients with chronic kidney disease: Dose adjustment recommendations. *J Clin Pharmacol.* 2014;54(5):584–592. doi.10.1002/jcph.247.
107. Fudin J, Raouf M. A review of skeletal muscle relaxants for pain management. *Pract Pain Manag.* 2017;16(5):1–4.
108. Raouf M, Fudin J. A review of skeletal muscle relaxants for pain management. *Pract Pain Manag.* 2016.
109. By the 2019 American Geriatrics Society Beers Criteria® Update Expert Panel. American Geriatrics Society 2019 Updated AGS Beers Criteria® for potentially inappropriate medication use in older adults. *J Am Geriatr Soc.* January 2019. doi.10.1111/jgs.15767.
110. Argoff CE. Topical analgesics in the management of acute and chronic pain. *Mayo Clin Proc.* 2013;88(2):195–205. doi:10.1016/j.mayocp.2012.11.015.
111. Derry S, Wiffen PJ, Kalso EA, et al. Topical analgesics for acute and chronic pain in adults: An overview of Cochrane reviews. *Cochrane Database Syst Rev.* 2017;5:CD008609. doi.10.1002/14651858.CD008609.pub2.
112. Management of osteoarthritis: NICE Pathways. National Institute for Health and Care Excellence; 2015. Available at: https://pathways.nice.org.uk/pathways/osteoarthritis#path=view%3A/pathways/osteoarthritis/management-of-osteoarthritis.xml&content=view-node%3Anodes-pharmacological-treatments. Accessed November 6, 2018.
113. McCormick M. *The Health Effects of Cannabis and Cannabinoids*; 2017. doi:10.17226/24625.
114. Whiting PF, Wolff RF, Deshpande S, et al. Cannabinoids for medical use: A systematic review and meta-analysis. *J Am Med Assoc.* 2015;313(24):2456–2473. doi.10.1001/jama.2015.6358.
115. Baron EP. Medicinal properties of cannabinoids, terpenes, and flavonoids in cannabis, and benefits in migraine, headache, and pain: An update on current evidence and cannabis science. *Headache J Head Face Pain.* 2018;58(7):1139–1186. doi:10.1111/head.13345.
116. VanDolah HJ, Bauer BA, Mauck KF. Clinicians' guide to cannabidiol and hemp oils. *Mayo Clin Proc.* 2019;94(9):1840–1851. 10.1016/j.mayocp.2019.01.003 31447137.
117. Cohen SP, Bhatia A, Buvanendran A, et al. Consensus guidelines on the use of intravenous ketamine infusions for chronic pain from the American Society of Regional Anesthesia and Pain Medicine, the American Academy of Pain Medicine, and the American Society of Anesthesiologists. *Reg Anesth Pain Med.* 2018;43(5):521–546. doi.10.1097/AAP.0000000000000808.
118. Nuckols TK, Anderson L, Popescu I, et al. Opioid prescribing: A systematic review and critical appraisal of guidelines for chronic pain. *Ann Intern Med.* 2013;160(1):38–47. doi.10.7326/0003-4819-160-1-201401070-00732.
119. McPherson ML. *Demystifying Opioid Conversion Calculations.* 2nd ed. Bethesda, MD: American Society of Health-System Pharmacists; 2018.
120. Yaksh TL, Wallace MS. Opioids, analgesia, and pain management. In: Brunton LL, Chabner BA, Knollman BC, eds. *The Pharmacological Basis of Therapeutics.* 13th ed. New York, NY: McGraw-Hill; 2018;355–386.
121. Pasternak GW. Molecular insights into mu opioid pharmacology: From the clinic to the bench. *Clin J Pain.* 2010;26(suppl 10):S3–S9. doi:10.1097/AJP.0b013e3181c49d2e.
122. Crockett S, Greer K, Heidelbaugh J, Falck-Ytter Y, Hanson B, Sultan S. American Gastroenterological Association Institute guideline on the medical management of opioid-induced constipation. *Gastroenterology.* 2018. [epub ahea:1-9. doi.10.1053/j.gastro.2015.11.008.
123. Topaz M, Seger DL, Lai K, et al. High override rate for opioid drug-allergy interaction alerts: Current trends and recommendations for future. *Stud Health Technol Inform.* 2015;216:242–246. http://www.ncbi.nlm.nih.gov/pubmed/26262047. Accessed October 11, 2018.
124. DeDea L. Prescribing opioids safely in patients with an opiate allergy. *JAAPA.* 2012;25(1):17. http://www.ncbi.nlm.nih.gov/pubmed/22384750. Accessed October 11, 2018.
125. Woodall HE, Chiu A, Weissman DE. Opioid Allergic Reactions #175. *J Palliat Med.* 2008;11(10):1340–1342. doi:10.1089/jpm.2008.9817.
126. Chou R, Gordon DB, De Leon-casasola OA, et al. Management of postoperative pain: A clinical practice guideline from the American Pain Society, the American Society of Regional Anesthesia and Pain Medicine, and the American Society of Anesthesiologists' Committee on Regional Anesthesia. *J Pain.* 2016;17(2):131–157. doi.10.1016/j.jpain.2015.12.008.
127. American Society of Anesthesiologists Task Force on Acute Pain Management. Practice guidelines for acute pain management in the perioperative setting: An updated report by the American Society of Anesthesiologists Task Force on Acute Pain Management. *Anesthesiology.* 2012;116(2):248–273. doi.10.1097/ALN.0b013e31823c1030.
128. McNicol ED, Ferguson MC, Hudcova J. Patient controlled opioid analgesia versus non-patient controlled opioid analgesia for postoperative pain. *Cochrane Database Syst Rev.* 2015;(6):CD003348. doi:10.1002/14651858.CD003348.pub3.
129. Bujedo BM, Santos SG, Azpiazu AU, et al. A review of epidural and intrathecal opioids used in the management of postoperative pain. *J Opioid Manag.* 2012;8(3):177–192. doi:10.5055/jom.2012.0114.

130. Ghafoor V, Epshteyn M, Carlson G, Terhaar D, Charry O, Phelps P. Intrathecal drug therapy for long-term pain management. *Am J Health Syst Pharm.* 2007;64:2447–2461. doi:10.2146/ajhp060204.
131. Jokinen J, Smith AF, Roewer N, Eberhart LH, Kranke P. Management of postoperative nausea and vomiting: How to deal with refractory PONV. *Anesth Clin.* 2012;30(3):481–493. doi.10.1016/j.anclin.2012.07.003.
132. Chou R, Weimer MB, Dana T. Methadone overdose and cardiac arrhythmia potential: Findings from a review of the evidence for an American Pain Society and College on Problems of Drug Dependence clinical practice guideline. *J Pain.* 2014;15(4):338–365. doi.10.1016/j.jpain.2014.01.495.
133. Conway A, Douglas C, Sutherland J. Capnography monitoring during procedural sedation and analgesia: A systematic review protocol. *Syst Rev.* 2015;4(1):92. doi.10.1186/s13643-015-0085-4.
134. Zedler B, Xie L, Wang L, et al. Development of a Risk Index for serious prescription opioid-induced respiratory depression or overdose in Veterans' Health Administration patients. *Pain Med.* 2015;16(8):1566–1579. doi.10.1111/pme.12777.
135. Meine TJ, Roe MT, Chen AY, et al. Association of intravenous morphine use and outcomes in acute coronary syndromes: Results from the CRUSADE Quality Improvement Initiative. *Am Heart J.* 2005;149(6):1043–1049. doi.10.1016/j.ahj.2005.02.010.
136. Coluzzi F, Billeci D, Maggi M, et al. Testosterone deficiency in non-cancer opioid-treated patients. *J Endocrinol Invest.* 2018;41(12):1377–1388. 10.1007/s40618-018-0964-3 30343356.
137. McNulty JP. Chronic pain: Levorphanol, methadone, and the N-methyl-D-aspartate receptor. *J Palliat Med.* 2009;12(9):765–766. doi.10.1089/jpm.2009.0105.
138. Prommer E. Levorphanol: Revisiting an underutilized analgesic. *Palliat Care.* 2014;8:7–10. doi.10.4137/PCRT.S13489.
139. Drug Safety and Availability—FDA Drug Safety Communication: FDA restricts use of prescription codeine pain and cough medicines and tramadol pain medicines in children; recommends against use in breastfeeding women. Available at: https://www.fda.gov/Drugs/DrugSafety/ucm549679.htm. Accessed November 6, 2018.
140. Latta KS, Ginsberg B, Barkin RL. Meperidine: A critical review. *Am J Ther.* 2002;9(1):53–68. Accessed October 11, 2018. http://www.ncbi.nlm.nih.gov/pubmed/11782820.
141. Reardon CE, Kane-Gill SL, Smithburger PL, et al. Sufentanil sublingual tablet: A new option for acute pain management. *Ann Pharmacother.* 2019;53(12):1220–1226. 10.1177/1060028019863144 31280585.
142. Chou R, Deyo R, Devine B, et al. *The Effectiveness and Risks of Long-Term Opioid Treatment of Chronic Pain.* Agency for Healthcare Research Quality; 2014. http://www.effectivehealthcare.ahrq.gov/.
143. Chou R, Cruciani RA, Fiellin DA, et al. Methadone safety: A clinical practice guideline from the American Pain Society and College on Problems of Drug Dependence, in collaboration with the Heart Rhythm Society. *J Pain.* 2014;15(4):321–337. doi.10.1016/j.jpain.2014.01.494.
144. Somrat C, Oranuch K, Ketchada U, Siriprapa S, Thipawan R. Optimal dose of nalbuphine for treatment of intrathecal-morphine induced pruritus after caesarean section. *J Obstet Gynaecol Res.* 1999;25(3):209–213. http://www.ncbi.nlm.nih.gov/pubmed/10467795. Accessed October 11, 2018.
145. Davis MP. Twelve reasons for considering buprenorphine as a frontline analgesic in the management of pain. *J Support Oncol.* 2012;10(6):209–219. doi:10.1016/j.suponc.2012.05.002.
146. Weeks WB, O'Connell MJ. Buprenorphine waivers for physicians. *Health Aff.* 2015;34(8):1428–1428. doi:10.1377/hlthaff.2015.0762.
147. Young JWS, Juurlink DN. Tramadol. *CMAJ.* 2013;185(8):E352. doi:10.1503/cmaj.121592.
148. Nelson LS, Juurlink DN. Tramadol and hypoglycemia: One more thing to worry about. *JAMA Intern Med.* 2015;175(2):194–195. doi.10.1001/jamainternmed.2014.5260.
149. Elling C, Galic M, Steigerwald I. Tapentadol prolonged release in the treatment of neuropathic pain related to diabetic polyneuropathy. *Lancet Neurol.* 2015;14(7):684–685. doi:10.1016/S1474-4422(15)00059-9.
150. Russell IJ, Kamin M, Bennett RM, Schnitzer TJ, Green JA, Katz WA. Efficacy of tramadol in treatment of pain in fibromyalgia. *J Clin Rheumatol.* 2000;6(5):250–257. http://www.ncbi.nlm.nih.gov/pubmed/19078481. Accessed October 11, 2018.
151. Ahsan MZ, Zhao MJ, Shoaib RM, et al. Comparative study of dezocine, pentazocine and tapentadol on antinociception and physical dependence. *Life Sci.* 2021;285:119996–119996. 10.1016/j.lfs.2021.119996 34597607.
152. Coe MA, Walsh SL. Distribution of naloxone for overdose prevention to chronic pain patients. *Prev Med.* 2015;80:41–43. doi:10.1016/j.ypmed.2015.05.016.
153. Chen L, Sein M, Vo T, et al. Clinical interpretation of opioid tolerance versus opioid-induced hyperalgesia. *J Opioid Manag.* 2014;10(6):383–393. doi:10.5055/jom.2014.0235.
154. ASAM. Public policy statement: Definition of addiction; 2011. Available at: https://www.asam.org/resources/definition-of-addiction. Accessed September 24, 2015.
155. *Standards of Care for the Addiction Specialist Physician.* Chevy Chase, MD: 2013. http://www.asam.org/docs/default-source/practice-support/quality-improvement/asam-standards-of-care.pdf?sfvrsn=10.
156. CDC guideline for prescribing opioids for chronic pain—United States, 2016. Regulatory Alert FDA Warning/Regulatory Alert Recommendations. *Morb Mortal Wkly Rep.* 2016;65(1).
157. Mitra R, Jones S. Adjuvant analgesics in cancer pain: A review. *Am J Hosp Palliat Med.* 2012;29(1):70–79. doi.10.1177/1049909111413256.
158. Melton S, Spencer S. Regional anesthesia techniques for acute pain management. In: Fishman SM, Ballantyne JC, Rathmell JP, eds. *Bonica's Pain Management.* Baltimore, MD: Lippincott, Williams & Wilkins; 2010;723–754.
159. Goyal R, Shukla RN. Local anesthetic systemic toxicity (LAST): Should we not be concerned? *Med J Armed Forces India.* 2012. doi.10.1016/j.mjafi.2012.02.011.
160. Zieliński J, Morawska-Kochman M, Zatoński T. Pain assessment and management in children in the postoperative period: A review of the most commonly used postoperative pain assessment tools, new diagnostic methods and the latest guidelines for postoperative pain therapy in children. *Adv Clin Exp Med.* 2020;29(3):365–374. 10.17219/acem/112600 32129952.
161. Dans M, Smith T, Back A, et al. *NCCN Guidelines Index Table of Contents Discussion NCCN Guidelines Version 1. 2018 Panel Members Palliative Care.* 2018. https://www.nccn.org/professionals/physician_gls/PDF/palliative.pdf.
162. American Geriatrics Society Panel on Pharmacological Management of Persistent Pain in Older Persons, AGS. Pharmacological management of persistent pain in older persons. *J Am Geriatr Soc.* 2009;57(8):1331–1346. doi:10.1111/j.1532-5415.2009.02376.x.
163. Nerenz RD, Tsongalis GJ. Pharmacogenetics of opioid use and implications for pain management. *J Appl Lab Med.* 2018;2(4):622–632. 10.1373/jalm.2017.023150 33636885.
164. Phillips EJ, Sukasem C, Whirl-Carrillo M, et al. Clinical Pharmacogenetics Implementation Consortium Guideline for HLA Genotype and Use of Carbamazepine and Oxcarbazepine: 2017 Update. *Clin Pharmacol Ther.* 2018;103(4):574–581. 10.1002/cpt.1004 29392710.
165. Nicholson WT, Formea CM, Matey ET, et al. Considerations when applying pharmacogenomics to your practice. *Mayo Clin Proc.* 2021;96(1):218–230. 10.1016/j.mayocp.2020.03.011 33308868.
166. Keeling NJ, Rosenthal MM, West-Strum D, et al. Preemptive pharmacogenetic testing: Exploring the knowledge and perspectives of US payers. *Genet Med.* 2019;21(5):1224–1232. 10.1038/gim.2017.181 31048813.
167. PharmGKB. Duloxetine. https://www.pharmgkb.org/chemical/PA10066/prescribingInfo. Accessed November 5, 2021.
168. PharmGKB. Venlafaxine. https://www.pharmgkb.org/chemical/PA451866/prescribingInfo. Accessed November 5, 2021.
169. Crews KR, Gaedigk A, Dunnenberger HM, et al. Clinical Pharmacogenetics Implementation Consortium Guidelines for cytochrome P450 2D6 genotype and codeine therapy: 2014 update. *Clin Pharmacol Ther.* 2014;95(4):376–382. doi.10.1038/clpt.2013.254.
170. Verbeurgt P, Mamiya T, Oesterheld J. How common are drug and gene interactions? Prevalence in a sample of 1143 patients with *CYP2C9, CYP2C19* and *CYP2D6* genotyping. *Pharmacogenomics.* 2014;15(5):655–665. doi:10.2217/pgs.14.6.
171. Boswell MV, Stauble ME, Loyd GE, et al. The role of hydromorphone and OPRM1 in postoperative pain relief with hydrocodone. *Pain Physician.* 2013;16(3):E227–E235. http://www.ncbi.nlm.nih.gov/pubmed/23703421. Accessed October 12, 2018.
172. Ofoegbu A, B Ettienne E. Pharmacogenomics and morphine. *J Clin Pharmacol.* 2021;61(9):1149–1155. 10.1002/jcph.1873 33847389.

80

Headache Disorders

Kimberly B. Tallian and Natalie T. Heinrich

KEY CONCEPTS

1. Acute migraine therapies should provide consistent, rapid relief, and enable the individual to resume normal activities at home, school, or work.
2. The selection of initial treatment is based on headache-related disability, symptom severity, and preference for the individual with migraine.
3. Strict adherence to maximum daily and weekly doses of anti-migraine medication is essential.
4. Preventive therapy should be considered for recurring migraine attacks that produce significant disability; frequent attacks requiring symptomatic medication more than twice per week; symptomatic therapies that are ineffective, contraindicated, or produce serious adverse effects; and uncommon migraine variants that cause profound disruption and/or risk of neurologic injury.
5. The selection of an agent for headache prophylaxis should be based on individual response, tolerability, convenience of the medication formulation, and coexisting conditions.
6. Each prophylactic medication should be given an adequate therapeutic trial (usually 6 months) to judge its maximal efficacy.
7. A general wellness program that considers headache triggers should be included in the management plan.
8. After an effective abortive agent and dose have been identified, subsequent treatments should begin with that same regimen.

BEYOND THE BOOK

Read the article by Vandenbussche N, Laterza D, Lisicki M, et al.[23]

Review other existing literature related to whether medication-overuse headache is a distinct entity. Summarize two key points on both the pro and con sides of the issue. Be prepared to discuss or debate in class. (Note to instructors: It would be a good opportunity to assign teams and have an in-class discussion or formal debate.)

INTRODUCTION

Headache is among the top five principal reasons adults 18 to 44 years of age visit US emergency departments and are one of the most common complaints encountered by healthcare practitioners.[1] They can be symptomatic of a distinct pathologic process or can occur without an underlying cause. In 2018, the International Headache Society (IHS) updated its classification system and diagnostic criteria for headache disorders, cranial neuralgias, and facial pain.[2] The IHS classification provides more precise definitions and standardized nomenclature for both the primary (migraine, tension-type, and cluster headache) and secondary (symptomatic of organic disease) headache disorders. These criteria are designed to facilitate headache diagnosis in clinical practice, as well as being used for research. This chapter focuses on the management of primary headache disorders.

Most recurrent headaches result from a benign chronic primary headache disorder, with the most common being tension-type and migraine headache.[3] The peak prevalence for these headaches occurs during the most productive years of life (18-54 years of age).[4] Despite this and their associated disability, most headache sufferers do not obtain appropriate medical care for their headaches.[4,5] While most are benign, some headaches are symptomatic of a serious underlying medical condition, such as an infection, cerebral hemorrhage, or brain mass lesion. Therefore, a thorough evaluation of the headache history is essential to establish an accurate headache diagnosis and identify individuals who can benefit from these specific therapeutic options. In addition, advances in the field's understanding of the diagnosis and pathophysiologic mechanisms of the primary headache disorders, particularly migraine, have led to the development of medications that provide rapid relief from moderate to severe attacks.

MIGRAINE HEADACHE

Epidemiology

Approximately 20.7% of females and 9.7% of males in the United States experience one or more migraine headaches per year. While the prevalence of migraine varies by age and sex, the epidemiologic profile has remained stable over the past 8 years. Sex differences in migraine prevalence have been linked to menstruation, but these differences persist beyond menopause. Prevalence is highest in both males and females between the ages of 18 and 44 years and is inversely related to income and educational attainment. In the American Migraine Prevalence and Prevention Study, 93% of those with migraine reported some headache-related disability, and 54% were severely disabled or needed bed rest during an attack.[4,5] The economic burden of migraine is substantial as are the indirect costs from work-related disability and losses in productivity.[6,7] Several neurologic, psychiatric, and cardiovascular disorders, including stroke, epilepsy, major depression, sleep apnea, obesity, and anxiety, and other pain disorders, show increased comorbidity with migraine.[8,9] Whether this relationship is causal or representative of a common pathophysiologic mechanism is unknown.

Etiology

The etiology of migraine is not entirely understood. Most clinicians now believe that the pathogenesis of migraine may be related to complex dysfunctions in neuronal and broad sensory processing.[2,8,9] However, earlier theories included hypotheses involving intracerebral arterial vasoconstriction, reactive extracranial vasodilation, in addition to neurovascular mechanisms.

The pain and symptoms of migraine are a combination of altered perceptions resulting from neural suppression and activation of subcortical structures and trigeminal systems. Migraine pain is believed to result from activity within the trigeminovascular system, a network of visceral afferent fibers that arises from the trigeminal ganglia and projects peripherally to innervate the pain-sensitive intracranial extracerebral blood vessels, dura mater, and large venous sinuses[10] (Fig. 80-1). These fibers also project centrally, terminating in the trigeminal nucleus caudalis in the brain stem and upper cervical spinal cord, and, thus, provide a pathway for nociceptive transmission from meningeal blood vessels into higher centers of the central nervous system (CNS). Activation of trigeminal sensory nerves triggers the release of vasoactive neuropeptides, including calcitonin gene-related peptide (CGRP), neurokinin A, and substance P, from perivascular axons. The released neuropeptides interact with dural blood vessels to promote vasodilation and dural plasma extravasation, resulting in neurogenic inflammation. Orthodromic conduction along trigeminovascular fibers transmits pain impulses to the trigeminal nucleus caudalis, where information is relayed further to higher cortical pain centers. Continued afferent input can result in sensitization of these central sensory neurons, producing a hyperalgesic state that responds to previously innocuous stimuli and maintains the headache.[9,10]

Aura occurs in a subgroup of individuals with migraines and other primary headache disorders. The neurologic changes of the aura parallel those that occur during cortical spreading depression, a neuronal event characterized by a wave of depressed electrical activity that advances across the brain cortex, causing inflammation and activation of the trigeminal nucleus caudalis. This neuronal event occurs at a rate consistent with the spread of aura symptoms.[2,9] It is not clear whether this cortical spreading depression and the aura are the substrate of pain or trigger the presentation of migraine.[9,11]

Pathophysiology

Genetic factors play an important role in susceptibility to migraine attacks. Studies in monozygotic twins suggest a 50% heritability of migraine with a multifactorial polygenic basis.[11] Although it is possible for any individual to experience a migraine attack, their abnormal recurrence can result in a diagnosis of migraine. Attack occurrence and frequency are governed by CNS sensitivity to migraine specific triggers or environmental factors. Individuals with migraine appear to have a lowered threshold of response to specific environmental circumstances resulting from genetic factors governing the balance of CNS excitation and inhibition at various levels. Thus, triggering factors modulate the genetic set point that predisposes to migraine headache.[9,11] The hyperresponsiveness of the individual's brain may be the result of an inherited abnormality in calcium and/or sodium channels and sodium/potassium pumps that regulate cortical excitability through serotonin (5-hydroxytryptamine [5-HT]) and other neurotransmitter releases. Increased levels of excitatory amino acids such as glutamate and/or alterations in extracellular levels of potassium also can affect the migraine threshold, resulting in the initiation and propagation of the phenomenon of cortical spreading depression.[11]

Serotonin (5-HT) is an important mediator of migraine headache and specific 5-HT receptor subfamilies are involved in the pathophysiology and treatment of migraine headache.[9,12] Acute antimigraine medications such as the ergot alkaloids and triptan derivatives are agonists of vascular and neuronal 5-HT_1 receptor subtypes, resulting in vasoconstriction of meningeal blood vessels, inhibition of vasoactive neuropeptide release and pain signal transmission.[12,13] Specifically, triptans bind nonspecifically to 5-$HT_{1B/D}$ receptors with variable 5-HT_{1F} receptor affinity, resulting in direct vascular vasoconstriction. In contrast, the ditans selectively bind to 5-HT_{1F} receptors without vasoconstrictive effects.[14] During a headache, CGRP

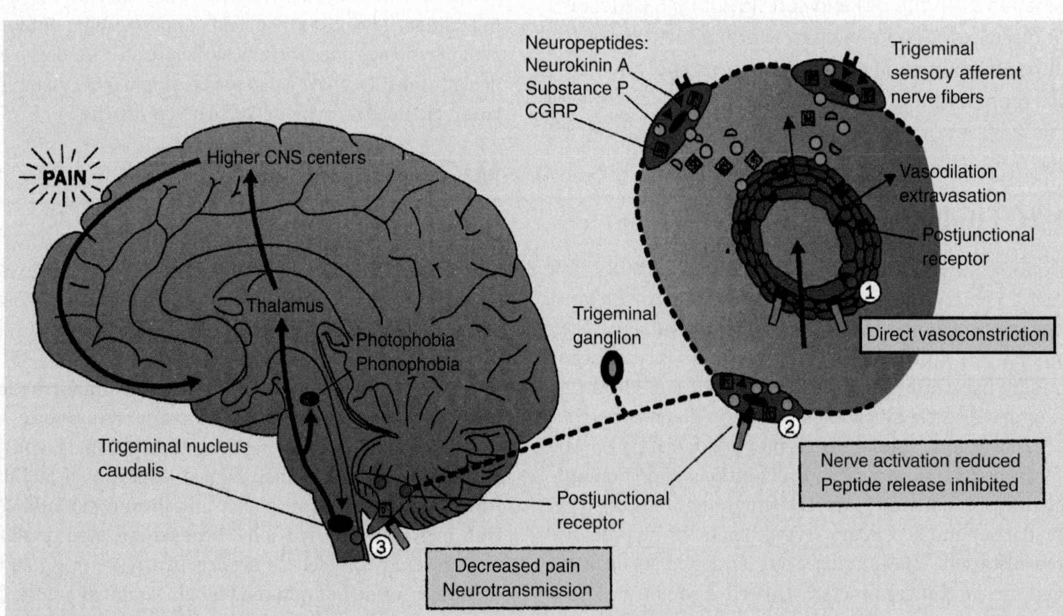

FIGURE 80-1 The pathophysiology of migraine headache. Vasodilation of intracranial extracerebral blood vessels (possibly the result of an imbalance in the brainstem) results in the activation of the perivascular trigeminal nerves that release vasoactive neuropeptides to promote neurogenic inflammation. Central pain transmission may activate other brainstem nuclei, resulting in associated symptoms (nausea, vomiting, photophobia, and phonophobia). The antimigraine effects of the 5-$HT_{1B/ID}$ receptor agonists are highlighted at areas 1, 2, and 3. (CGRP, calcitonin gene-related peptide.) *(Reprinted from Ferrari MD. Migraine.* Lancet. *1998 Apr 4;351(9108):1043-51.)*

CLINICAL PRESENTATION Migraine Headache

General

- Common, recurrent, severe headache
- Interferes with normal functioning
- Divided into two major subtypes
  - Migraine without aura
  - Migraine with aura

Symptoms

- Recurring episodes of throbbing head pain, frequently unilateral, lasting from 4 to 72 hours if left untreated
- Headaches can be severe and associated with nausea, vomiting, as well as sensitivity to light, sound, and/or movement, but not all symptoms are present in every attack
- Diagnostic alarms from evaluation include:
  - Acute onset of the "first" or "worst" headache ever
  - Accelerating pattern of headache following subacute onset
  - Onset of headache after age 50 years
  - Headache associated with systemic illness (eg, fever, nausea, vomiting, stiff neck, and rash)
  - Headache with focal neurologic symptoms or papilledema
  - New-onset headache in an individual with cancer or human immunodeficiency virus infection

Signs

- A stable pattern, absence of daily headache
- Positive family history for migraine
- Normal neurologic examination
- Food and menstruation may serve as triggers
- Improvement in headache with sleep
- Aura can signal the migraine headache but is not required for diagnosis

Laboratory Tests

- No one test can diagnose migraine headaches
- Possible tests to consider are:
  - Serum chemistries
  - Urine toxicology profiles
  - Thyroid function tests
  - Lyme disease studies
  - Complete blood count
  - Antinuclear antibody titer
  - Erythrocyte sedimentation rate
  - Antiphospholipid antibody titer

Diagnostic Tests

- General medical and neurologic physical examination
- Vital signs (fever, hypertension)
- Funduscopy (papilledema, hemorrhage, and exudates)
- Palpation and auscultation of the head and neck (sinus tenderness, hardened or tender temporal arteries, trigger points, temporomandibular joint tenderness, bruits, nuchal rigidity, and cervical spine tenderness)
- Neurologic examination (identify abnormalities or deficits in mental status, cranial nerves, deep tendon reflexes, motor strength, coordination, gait, and cerebellar function)
- Consider neuroimaging studies in individuals with abnormal neurologic examination findings of unknown etiology and those with additional risk factors warranting imaging

is released by the trigeminal ganglion in response to vasoconstriction resulting in dilation and maintenance of cerebral blood flow.[15] By blocking CGRP release, migraine attacks can be either acutely aborted or prevented by antimigraine medications. Other medications used for migraine prophylaxis also modulate neurotransmitter systems[16] consistent with the current understanding of migraine pathophysiology and neurovascular disorders.

Clinical Presentation

The migraine attack is divided into several phases. *Premonitory symptoms* are experienced by up to 77% of those with migraine headaches in the hours or days before the onset of headache.[2,7] Premonitory symptoms vary widely among individuals with migraine but usually are consistent within an individual. Neurologic symptoms (eg, allodynia, phonophobia, photophobia, hyperosmia, and difficulty concentrating) are common, but psychological (eg, anxiety, depression, euphoria, irritability, drowsiness, fatigue, hyperactivity, and restlessness), autonomic (eg, polyuria, diarrhea, and constipation), and constitutional (eg, stiff neck, yawning, thirst, food cravings, and anorexia) symptoms also are reported.[2,7] The previously popular terms *prodrome* and *warning symptoms* should generally be avoided because these are often used mistakenly to include aura.[2]

The migraine *aura*, a complex of positive and negative focal neurologic symptoms that precedes or accompanies an attack, is experienced by approximately 25% of those with migraine headaches on some occasions.[2,9] The aura typically evolves over 5 minutes or longer and lasts less than 60 minutes. Headache usually occurs within the end 60 minutes of the aura; however, sometimes aura symptoms begin at the onset of headache or during the attack. The aura is most often visual and frequently affects half the visual field.[2] Visual auras vary in their complexity and can include both positive (scintillations, photopsia, teichopsia, or fortification spectrum) and negative (scotoma and hemianopsia) features. Sensory and motor aura symptoms, such as paresthesias or numbness involving the arms and face, dysphasia or aphasia, weakness, and hemiparesis, also are reported.[2,9]

Migraine *headache* pain is usually gradual in onset, peaking in intensity over a period of minutes to hours and lasting between 4 and 72 hours. Pain can occur anywhere in the face or head but most often involves the frontotemporal region. The headache is typically unilateral and throbbing or pulsating in nature; however, pain can be bilateral at onset or become generalized during the course of an attack.[2,9] Gastrointestinal (GI) symptoms almost invariably accompany the headache. During an attack, individuals with migraine frequently experience nausea and emesis sometimes occurs. Other systemic symptoms associated with the headache phase can include anorexia, food cravings, constipation, diarrhea, abdominal cramps, nasal stuffiness, blurred vision, diaphoresis, facial pallor, and localized facial, scalp, or periorbital edema. Sensory hyperacuity, manifested as photophobia, phonophobia, or osmophobia, is reported frequently. Because headache pain usually is aggravated by physical activity, most individuals with migraine headache seek a dark, quiet room for rest and relief. Impaired concentration, depression, irritability, fatigue, or anxiety often accompanies the headache. Once headache pain wanes, individuals may experience a postdrome or *resolution phase* characterized by feeling tired, exhausted, irritable, or listless. Impaired concentration may continue, as well as scalp tenderness or mood changes. Some individuals experience depression and malaise, whereas others can feel unusually refreshed or euphoric.[2,9,17]

Diagnosis of migraine can be refined based on the frequency of monthly migraine days (MMDs) and monthly headache days (MHDs). Individuals with fewer than 15 MMDs or MHDs have episodic migraine, whereas chronic migraine is diagnosed in those with at least 15 MHDs for at least 3 months, of which at least eight are MMDs.[2,18]

Although headaches have many potential causes, most are considered primary headache disorders. A comprehensive headache history is the most essential element in establishing the clinical diagnosis of migraine.[2,8] This history should include age at onset, attack frequency and timing, duration of attacks, precipitating or aggravating factors, ameliorating factors, description of neurologic symptoms, characteristics of the headache pain (quality, intensity, location, and radiation), associated signs and symptoms, treatment history, family and social history, and the impact of headaches on daily life.

Secondary headaches can be identified or excluded based on the headache history, as well as the results of general medical and neurologic examinations. Diagnostic and laboratory testing also can be warranted in the setting of suspicious headache features or an abnormal examination. Routine neuroimaging (computed tomography or magnetic resonance imaging) is generally not indicated in individuals with migraines and a normal neurologic examination but should be considered in individuals with an unexplained abnormal neurologic examination or an atypical headache history. Because migraine headaches usually begin by the second or third decade of life, those beginning after age 50 suggest an organic etiology such as a mass lesion, cerebrovascular disease, or temporal arteritis.[2,3,9] Table 80-1 lists the IHS diagnostic criteria for migraine with and without aura.[2]

TABLE 80-1 IHS Diagnostic Criteria for Migraine

Migraine without aura

At least five attacks

Headache attack lasts 4-72 hours (untreated or unsuccessfully treated)

Headache has at least two of the following characteristics:

- Unilateral location pulsating quality
- Moderate or severe intensity
- Aggravation by or avoidance of routine physical activity (ie, walking or climbing stairs)

During headache at least one of the following:

- Nausea, vomiting, or both
- Photophobia and phonophobia
- Not attributed to another disorder

Migraine with aura (classic migraine)

At least two attacks

Migraine aura fulfills criteria for typical aura, hemiplegic migraine, retinal migraine, or brainstem aura

Not attributed to another disorder

Typical aura

Fully reversible visual, sensory, or speech symptoms (or any combination) but no motor weakness

Homonymous or bilateral visual symptoms including positive features (eg, flickering lights, spot, lines) or negative features (eg, loss of vision) or unilateral sensory symptoms including positive features (eg, pins and needles) or negative features (ie, numbness), or any combination

At least two of the following:

- At least one symptom that develops gradually over a minimum of 5 minutes or different symptoms that occur in succession or both
- Each symptom lasts for at least 5 minutes and for no longer than 60 minutes
- Headache that meets criteria for migraine without aura begins during the aura or follows aura within 60 minutes

Adapted from Parisi P, Belcastro V, Verrotti A, et al. "Ictal epileptic headache" and the revised International Headache Classification (ICHD-3) published in Cephalalgia 2018, vol. 38(1) 1-211: Not just a matter of definition!

TABLE 80-2 Goals of Therapy in Migraine Management

Goals of migraine prevention
Reduce migraine frequency, severity, and disability
Reduce reliance on poorly tolerated, ineffective, or unwanted acute pharmacotherapies
Improve quality of life
Prevent headache
Avoid escalation of headache medication use
Educate and enable individuals to manage their disease
Reduce headache-related distress and psychological symptoms
Goals of acute migraine treatment
Treat migraine attacks rapidly and consistently without recurrence
Restore the individual's ability to function
Minimize the use of backup and rescue medications[a]
Optimize self-care for overall management
Be cost-effective in overall management
Cause minimal or no adverse effects

[a]Rescue medications are defined as medications used at home when other treatments fail that permit the individual to get relief without a visit to the physician's office or emergency department.

Data from References 12, 18, and 19.

TREATMENT

Desired Outcome

1 Clinicians who care for individuals with migraine must appreciate the impact of this painful and debilitating disorder on the life of the individual, the individual's family, and the individual's employer. Treatment strategies must address both immediate and long-term goals. Acute migraine therapies should provide consistent, rapid relief and enable the individual to resume normal activities at home, school, or work. Recurrence of symptoms and treatment-related adverse effects should be minimal. Ideally, individuals should be able to manage their own headaches effectively without a medical visit. In addition, individuals should take an active role in the creation of a long-term formal management plan. An individualized approach to treatment can result in a reduction in attack frequency and severity; therefore, minimizing headache-related disability and emotional distress and improving the individual's quality of life. Goals of long-term and acute treatment of migraine are listed in Table 80-2.[13,18,19]

General Approach to Treatment

2 Nonpharmacologic and pharmacologic interventions are available for migraine management; however, medication therapy is the treatment mainstay for most individuals. Pharmacotherapeutic management can be acute (ie, symptomatic or abortive) or preventive (ie, prophylactic). Therapy decisions should consider the individual's response to specific medications, their tolerability, and coexisting illnesses that limit treatment choices. Abortive or acute therapies can be migraine-specific (eg, ergots, triptans, and CGRP antagonists) or nonspecific (eg, analgesics, antiemetics, NSAIDs, and corticosteroids). Most effective at relieving pain and associated

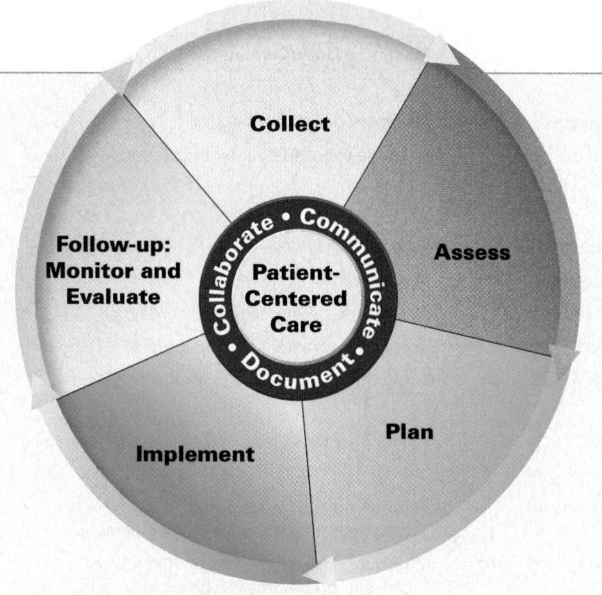

Patient Care Process for Headache Disorders

Collect

Subjective and Objective Data
- Presence of other symptoms
  - Nausea
  - Vomiting
  - Sensitivity to light, sound, and/or movement
- Identification of triggers or aura (Table 80-5)
- Patient characteristics (eg, age, sex, pregnant)
- Patient medical history (personal and family)
- Social history (smoking, diet, physical activity)
- Description of migraine/headache pain (including frequency and location)
- Presence of diagnostic alarms (see CLINICAL PRESENTATION)

Medication History

- Current use, dosage, and frequency of medications (especially over-the-counter aspirin/nonsteroidal anti-inflammatory drug [NSAID] use, herbal products, and dietary supplements) (Tables 80-3 and 80-4)

Diagnostic Tests

- Consider neuroimaging studies in individuals with abnormal neurologic examination findings of unknown etiology and in those with additional risk factors warranting imaging
- Physical Exam
- Neurological Exam
- Diagnostic abnormalities (Table 80-1)
  - Vital signs (fever, hypertension)
  - Funduscopy (papilledema, hemorrhage, and exudates)
  - Palpation and auscultation of the head and neck (sinus tenderness, hardened or tender temporal arteries, trigger points, temporomandibular joint tenderness, bruits, nuchal rigidity, and cervical spine tenderness)
  - Deficits in mental status, cranial nerves, deep tendon reflexes, motor strength, coordination, gait, and cerebellar function

Assess

Initial Assessment
- Type of headache, acute or chronic[2]
- Other contributing factors (eg, presence of anxiety, depression, or medication overuse)

Medication Assessment
- Evaluate the need for therapy
- Evaluate current therapy for appropriateness, response, adverse effects, and medication adherence
- Evaluate other therapy options (compare/contrast based on safety, efficacy, and cost/coverage by insurance)

Plan*

- Acute medication therapy regimen if needed (symptomatic or abortive)
- Establish individualized treatment plan for long term
  - Nonspecific agents for mild-to-moderate attacks
  - Reserve migraine-specific agents for more severe attacks
  - Use of prophylactic agents
- Identify goals of treatment and monitoring parameters (Tables 80-2 to 80-4)
- Patient education (avoidance of triggers, headache diary and patient adherence)
- Referrals to other providers when appropriate (eg, secondary headache, psychiatry)

Implement*

- Provide patient education regarding all elements of treatment plan
- Patient education on the risk of medication, as well as caffeine overuse and limits
- Use motivational interviewing and coaching strategies to maximize adherence
- Schedule follow-up, sooner if an individual is unable to perform daily activities

Follow-up: Monitor and Evaluate*

- Strive for resolution of pain (Table 80-2)
- Aim for absence of adverse effects
- Reduce headache frequency, severity, and associated-disability
- Improve quality of life
- Optimize self-care and management

**Collaborate with patients, caregiver(s), and other healthcare professionals.*

symptoms when administered at the onset of migraine[12,13,16,18-20] (Table 80-3). An initial treatment based on headache-related disability and symptom severity is the preferred treatment strategy.[12,20] Because attack severity varies in individuals, individuals may be advised to use nonspecific agents for mild-to-moderate headaches not causing disability, while reserving migraine-specific medications for more severe attacks. The gastric stasis or nausea and vomiting that accompany migraine may compromise the absorption

TABLE 80-3 Dosing of Self-Administered Acute Migraine Therapies[a]

Medication	Dose	Maximum Dose/Comments
Analgesics		
Acetaminophen[a] (Tylenol)	500-1,000 mg every 4-6 hours as needed	Maximum daily dose is 4 g
Acetaminophen 250 mg/aspirin 250 mg/caffeine 65 mg[a] (Excedrin Migraine)	Two tablets every 6 hours as needed	Available over-the-counter as Excedrin Migraine
Nonsteroidal anti-inflammatory drugs		
Aspirin[a]	500-1,000 mg every 4-6 hours as needed	Maximum daily dose is 4 g
Ibuprofen[a] (Advil, Motrin)	400-800 mg every 4-6 hours as needed	Maximum daily dose is 3.2 g
Naproxen sodium[a] (Aleve, Anaprox)	220-550 mg every 8-12 hours as needed	Avoid doses greater than 1.375 g/day
Diclofenac potassium[a] (Cataflam, Cambia)	50-100 mg every 8 hours as needed	Avoid doses greater than 150 mg/day
Ketorolac nasal (Sprix)	31.5 mg (one spray each nostril) every 6-8 hours as needed	Maximum daily dose is 126 mg/day × 5 days
Ketorolac IM[b]	30-60 mg every 6 hours as needed	Maximum daily dose is 120 mg/day × 5 days
Ergotamine tartrate		
Oral tablet (1 mg) with caffeine 100 mg[b] (Cafergot)	2 mg at onset; can repeat 1-2 mg every 30 minutes as needed	Maximum dose is 6 mg/day or 10 mg/week; consider pretreatment with an antiemetic
Sublingual tablet (2 mg) (Ergomar)	2 mg at onset; can repeat 2 mg every 30 minutes as needed	Maximum dose is 4 mg/day or 10 mg/week; consider pretreatment with an antiemetic
Rectal suppository (2 mg) with caffeine 100 mg[b] (Cafergot, Migergot)	Insert half to one suppository at onset; can repeat after 1 hour if needed	Maximum dose is 4 mg/day or 10 mg/week; consider pretreatment with an antiemetic
Dihydroergotamine		
Injection 1 mg/mL (D.H.E. 45)[b]	0.25-1 mg (IM, IV, or subcutaneous) at onset; can repeat every hour as needed	Maximum dose is 3 mg/day or 6 mg/week
Nasal spray 4 mg/mL[a] (Migranal, Trudhesa)	One spray (0.5 mg) in each nostril at onset; can repeat sequence 15 minutes later (total dose is 2 mg or four sprays) (Migranal) 0.725 mg (one spray) in each nostril, may repeat once in 1 hour (Trudhesa)	Maximum dose is 3 mg/day or 6 mg/week; prime sprayer four times before using; do not tilt head back or inhale through nose while spraying; discard open ampules after 8 hours (Migranal) Two (four sprays)/day or three (six sprays)/week (Trudhesa)
Triptans		
Sumatriptan[a]		
Injection (Imitrex, Zembrace Symtouch)	1-6 mg subcutaneous at onset; can repeat after 1 hour if needed	Maximum daily dose is 12 mg
Oral tablets (Imitrex)	25, 50, 85, or 100 mg at onset; can repeat after 2 hours if needed	Maximum daily dose is 200 mg; combination product with naproxen, 85/500 mg
Nasal spray (Imitrex)	5 or 20 mg at onset; can repeat after 2 hours if needed	Maximum daily dose is 40 mg
Nasal spray (Tosymra)	10 mg intranasally at onset; can repeat after 1 hour if needed	Maximum daily dose is 30 mg
Nasal powder (Onzetra Xsail)	22 mg (one 11-mg nosepiece in each nostril) at onset; can repeat after 2 hours if needed	Maximum daily dose is 44 mg (four nosepieces, 11 mg each)
Transdermal (Zecuity)	Apply 6.5 mg patch to upper arm or thigh over 4 hours; can apply second patch after 2 hours	Maximum daily dose is two patches
Zolmitriptan[a]		
Oral tablets/ODT (Zomig, Zomig-ZMT)	1.25, 2.5, or 5 mg at onset; can repeat after 2 hours if needed	Maximum daily dose is 10 mg; do not divide ODT dosage form
Nasal spray (Zomig)	2.5 or 5 mg intranasally at onset; can repeat after 2 hours if needed	Maximum daily dose is 10 mg
Naratriptan[a] (Amerge)	1 or 2.5 mg at onset; can repeat after 4 hours if needed	Maximum daily dose is 5 mg
Rizatriptan[a] oral tablets/ODT (Maxalt, Maxalt-MLT)	5 or 10 mg at onset; can repeat after 2 hours if needed	Maximum daily dose is 30 mg; use 5 mg dose (15 mg/day maximum) in individuals on propranolol
Almotriptan[a] (Axert)	6.25 or 12.5 mg at onset; can repeat after 2 hours if needed	Maximum daily dose is 25 mg
Frovatriptan[a] (Frova)	2.5 or 5 mg at onset; can repeat in 2 hours if needed	Maximum daily dose is 7.5 mg
Eletriptan[a] (Relpax)	20 or 40 mg at onset; can repeat after 2 hours if needed	Maximum daily dose is 80 mg
Ditans		
Lasmiditan (Reyvow)	50, 100, or 200 mg at onset	Maximum of one dose per 24 hours; safety of treating more than four migraine attacks in a 30-day period has not been established

(continued)

TABLE 80-3 Dosing of Self-Administered Acute Migraine Therapies[a] (*Continued*)

Medication	Dose	Maximum Dose/Comments
CGRP Antagonists		
Ubrogepant (Ubrelvy)	50 or 100 mg at onset; can repeat after 2 hours if needed	Maximum daily dose is 200 mg; safety of treating more than eight migraine attacks in a 30-day period has not been established
Rimegepant (Nurtec ODT)	75 mg at onset	Maximum of one dose per 24 hours; take on an empty stomach
Anti-emetics/Miscellaneous		
Acetaminophen, Isometheptene, and Dichloralphenazone (generic Midrin)	Two capsules to start followed by one capsule every hour until relief is obtained	Maximum five capsules/12 hours
Metoclopramide[b] (Reglan)	10 mg every 4-6 mg hours as needed	Maximum daily dose is 40 mg (also available as ODT)
Metoclopramide[a] and Aspirin[a]	10 mg (metoclopramide) and 1,000 mg (aspirin) every 4-6 hours as needed	Maximum daily dose is 40 mg (metoclopramide) + 4 g (aspirin)
Prochlorperazine[b] (Compazine)	5-10 mg orally 3-4 times daily as needed or 25 mg via rectal suppository up to twice daily as needed	Maximum daily dose is 40 mg for oral and 50 mg for suppository
Promethazine (Phenergan)	25 mg oral or via rectal suppository every 4-6 hours as needed	Maximum daily dose is 100 mg

[a]Level A—established efficacy (≥2 Class I studies).

[b]Level B—probably effective (1 Class I or 2 Class II studies). IM, intramuscular; IV, intravenous; ODT, orally disintegrating tablet.

Data from References 12, 19, and 20.

and efficacy of orally administered medications. Pretreatment with antiemetic agents or use of non-oral formulations (eg, suppositories, nasal sprays, or injections) is advisable when nausea and vomiting are severe.[12,20]

3 The frequent or excessive use of acute migraine medications can also result in *medication-overuse headache* (or *rebound headache*), characterized by increased headache frequency and medication consumption.[2,21] This syndrome evolves as a self-sustaining headache-medication cycle in which the headache returns as the medication wears off, leading to more medication consumption for relief. The headache history often reflects the gradual onset of an atypical daily or near-daily headache with superimposed episodic migraine attacks. Medication overuse is one of the most common causes of chronic daily headache.[21-23] Agents most commonly implicated include simple and combination analgesics and opiates, and triptans.[21-23] Discontinuation of the offending agent leads to a gradual decrease in headache frequency and severity and a return of the original headache characteristics. Although detoxification can be accomplished on an outpatient basis, hospitalization may be necessary for refractory rebound headache and other withdrawal symptoms (eg, nausea, vomiting, asthenia, restlessness, and agitation).[21,22] Regulation of nociceptive systems and renewed responsiveness to therapy usually occur within 2 months of medication withdrawal.[2] Most experts recommend individuals limit triptan, ergotamine, and ditan use to fewer than 10 days per month, or 2 days per week. Exceptions include limiting aspirin, acetaminophen, and NSAIDs to 15 days or less per month with recommended.[2,6,24] Those with chronic migraine may be instructed to restrict all abortive therapy to fewer than 10 days per month. Additionally, they may be advised to limit the time period in which one or more medications are regularly taken to less than 3 months to avoid the development of medication-overuse headache. One exception to this recommendation is with the CGRP antagonists, which have not caused medication-overuse headache.[25]

4 5 6 Preventive migraine therapies are administered daily on a routine basis to reduce the frequency, severity, and duration of attacks and improve responsiveness to symptomatic migraine therapies[26,27] (Table 80-4). Preventive therapy should be considered in the setting of recurring migraine attacks that produce significant disability despite acute therapy; for frequent attacks occurring more than twice per week with the risk of developing medication-overuse headache; for symptomatic therapies that are ineffective or contraindicated, or produce serious adverse effects; or for uncommon migraine variants that cause profound disruption and/or risk of permanent neurologic injury (eg, hemiplegic migraine, basilar migraine, and migraine with prolonged aura); and individual preference to limit the number of attacks.[18,24] Preventive therapy may also be administered preemptively or intermittently when headaches recur in a predictable pattern (eg, exercise-induced migraine or menstrual migraine).[18] The various agents used for migraine prophylaxis are reviewed. Only propranolol, timolol, divalproex sodium, topiramate, erenumab-aooe, fremanezumab-vfrm, galcanezumab-gnlm, eptinezumab-jjmr, atogepant, and rimegepant are currently FDA approved, although other agents have established or have probable efficacy for this indication.[28] Guidelines identify which agents might be effective, but the preference for one therapy over another is not advised due to lack of established results. Thus, the agent selection is based on adverse effect profiles and the individual's coexisting/comorbid conditions.[18,26,27] A therapeutic trial of 2 to 3 months is necessary to achieve clinical benefit, but reductions in attack frequency can be evident by the first month with maximal benefits observed within 6 months.[16,18,26] Medication therapy should be initiated with low doses and gradually increased to therapeutic effect or intolerable adverse effects. Doses for migraine prophylaxis are often lower than those necessary for other indications.[18,27] Overuse of acute headache medications will interfere with preventative treatment effects.[2,18] Prophylactic treatment usually is continued for at least 6 to 12 months after the frequency and severity of headaches have diminished. After that time, based on discussions with the individual, gradual tapering or discontinuation may be reasonable.[16,24-26] Many individuals with migraine headache experience fewer and less severe attacks for lengthy periods following discontinuation of prophylactic medications or taper to a lower dose. Figures 80-2 and 80-3 identify treatment and management algorithms for migraine headache.

Nonpharmacologic Therapy

7 Nonpharmacologic therapy of acute migraine headache is limited but can include application of ice to the head and periods of rest or sleep, usually in a dark, quiet environment. Preventative measures

TABLE 80-4 Dosing of Prophylactic Migraine Therapies

Medication	Initial Dose	Usual Range	Comments
β-Adrenergic antagonists			
Atenolol[a] (Tenormin)	25-50 mg/day	50-200 mg/day	
Metoprolol[b] (Toprol, Toprol XL)	25-100 mg/day in divided doses	100-200 mg/day in divided doses	Dose short-acting two to four times a day and extended-release one to two times a day
Nadolol[a] (Corgard)	40-80 mg/day	80-240 mg/day	
Propranolol[b] (Inderal, Inderal LA)	40 mg/day in divided doses	40-160 mg/day in divided doses	Dose short-acting two to three times a day and extended-release one to two times a day
Timolol[b] (Blocadren)	20 mg/day in divided doses	20-60 mg/day in divided doses	
Antidepressants			
Amitriptyline[a] (Elavil)	10 mg at bedtime	20-50 mg at bedtime	
Venlafaxine[a] (Effexor, Effexor-XR)	37.5 mg/day	75-150 mg/day	Dose short-acting two times a day and extended-release once daily
Antiseizure Medications			
Topiramate[b] (Topamax)	12.5-25 mg/day	50-200 mg/day in divided doses or only at bedtime	Increase by 12.5-25 mg/week
Valproic acid/divalproex sodium[b] (Depakene, Depakote, Depakote ER)	250-500 mg/day in divided doses, or daily for extended release	500-1,500 mg/day	Dose short-acting two times a day and extended-release once daily; monitor levels if compliance is an issue
CGRP Antagonists (Anti-CGRP Antibodies)			
Erenumab-aooe (Aimovig)	70 mg subcutaneously monthly	70-140 mg subcutaneously every month	
Fremanezumab-vfrm (Ajovy)	225 mg subcutaneously monthly or 675 mg subcutaneously every 3 months	225 mg subcutaneously monthly or 675 mg subcutaneously every 3 months	
Galcanezumab-gnlm (Emgality)	240 mg subcutaneous loading dose, followed by 120 mg subcutaneously monthly	120 mg subcutaneously every month	
Eptinezumab-jjmr (Vyepti)	100 mg via IV infusion over 30 minutes every 3 months	100-300 mg IV infusion over 30 minutes every 3 months	
CGRP Antagonists ("gepants")			
Atogepant (Quilpta)	10 mg/day	60 mg/day	Taken with or without food
Rimegepant (Nurtec ODT)	75 mg every other day	75 mg/day	No titration required and taken on an empty stomach
Nonsteroidal anti-inflammatory drugs – *For prevention of menstrual migraine only*			
Ibuprofen[a] (Motrin)	200 mg/day in three to four divided doses	200-800 mg/day in three to four divided doses (maximum daily dose is 3,200 mg)	Use intermittently only; daily or prolonged use may lead to medication-overuse headaches
Ketoprofen[a] (Orudis)	150 mg/day in divided doses	150 mg/day in divided doses	Use intermittently only; daily or prolonged use may lead to medication-overuse headaches
Naproxen sodium[a] (Aleve, Anaprox)	550 mg/day in divided doses	550-1,100 mg/day in divided doses	Use intermittently only; daily or prolonged use may lead to medication-overuse headaches
Triptans – *For prevention of menstrual migraine only*			
Frovatriptan[b] (Frova)	2.5 mg/day or 5 mg/day in divided doses; start 6 days prior to anticipated start of menstruation	5 mg/day in divided doses	Use intermittently only; daily or prolonged use may lead to medication-overuse headaches
Naratriptan[a] (Amerge)	2 mg/day in divided doses; start 6 days prior to anticipated start of menstruation	2 mg/day in divided doses	Use intermittently only; daily or prolonged use may lead to medication-overuse headaches
Zolmitriptan[a] (Zomig)	5-7.5 mg/day in divided doses; start 6 days prior to anticipated start of menstruation	5-7.5 mg/day in divided doses	Use intermittently only; daily or prolonged use may lead to medication-overuse headaches
Miscellaneous			
Histamine[a] (Histatrol)	1-10 ng 2 times/week	Same as initial dose	May cause transient itching and burning at injection site
Magnesium[a]	400 mg/day	800 mg/day in divided doses	May be more helpful in migraine with aura and menstrual migraine

(continued)

TABLE 80-4 Dosing of Prophylactic Migraine Therapies (*Continued*)

Medication	Initial Dose	Usual Range	Comments
MIG-99[a] (feverfew)	10-100 mg/day in divided doses	Same as initial dose	Withdrawal may be associated with increased headaches
Petasites[b]	100-150 mg/day in divided doses	150 mg/day in divided doses	Use only commercial preparations, plant is carcinogenic
Riboflavin[a]	400 mg/day in divided doses	400 mg/day in divided doses	Benefit only after 3 months

[a]Level B—probably effective (1 Class I or 2 Class II studies).

[b]Level A—established efficacy (≥2 Class I studies).

Data from References 26, 28, and 29.

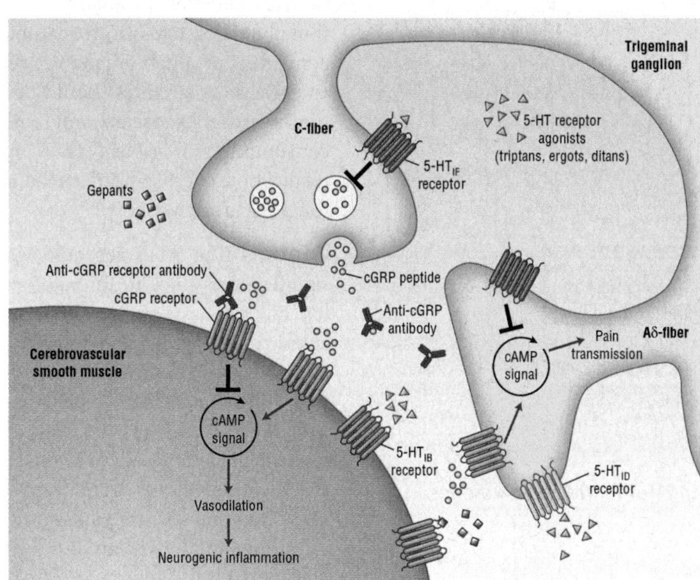

FIGURE 80-2 Mechanism of action of migraine medications. Nerve activity in the trigeminovascular pain pathway leads to the release of neuropeptides (ie, CGRP) and neurotransmitters (ie, serotonin and glutamate) that can hyperexcite neurons. CGRP release leads to activation of cyclic adenosine monophosphate (cAMP) signaling, which results in vasodilation of cerebrovascular smooth muscle, as well as pain signaling via Aδ fibers. Thus, injectable CGRP antagonists known as anti-CGRP antibodies bind to the CGRP receptor or CGRP ligand to block the effects of CGRP on vasodilation and neurogenic inflammation. Similarly, oral CGRP antagonists ("gepants") also inhibit the action of CGRP at the receptor. Serotonin (or serotonin agonist) binding to 5-HT receptors can inhibit presynaptic vesicular release of CGRP and inhibit postsynaptic cAMP signaling cascades.

typically suggest individuals identify and avoid individual factors or triggers that consistently provoke migraine attacks, although some triggers are not modifiable[2,3,18,24,30] (Table 80-5). Changes in estrogen levels associated with menarche, menstruation, pregnancy, menopause, oral contraceptive use, and other hormone therapies can trigger, intensify, or alleviate migraine.[3,31] A headache diary that records the frequency, severity, and duration of attacks can facilitate identification of migraine triggers. In appropriate situations, some individuals may learn to cope with triggers after a process of controlled exposure and approach/confront strategies.[32] Individuals also can benefit from wellness programs that include regular sleep, exercise, and eating habits, smoking cessation, and limited caffeine intake. Behavioral interventions, such as acupuncture, relaxation therapy, biofeedback (often used in combination with relaxation therapy), neuromodulation devices that use currents or magnets to modulate or change brain activity such as Cefaly® and Nerivio®, and cognitive therapy, are preventive treatment options for individuals who prefer non-medication therapy or when symptomatic therapies are poorly tolerated, contraindicated, or ineffective.[18,30,33,34] A multimodal approach with non-pharmacologic interventions has Level A evidence for migraine management and should be recommended to individuals.

Pharmacologic Therapy

Abortive Treatments

Analgesics and NSAIDs Simple analgesics and NSAIDs are effective medications for managing many migraine attacks (see Table 80-3). They offer a reasonable first-line choice for mild-to-moderate migraine attacks or severe attacks that have been responsive to similar NSAIDs or nonopiate analgesics in the past. Of the NSAIDs, aspirin, diclofenac, ibuprofen, naproxen sodium, and the combination of acetaminophen plus aspirin and caffeine have established efficacy in controlled clinical trials.[12,19,20] Oral acetaminophen alone also has efficacy for non-incapacitating migraine attacks.[19] The comparable efficacy of NSAIDs and triptans in acute migraine is known, although comparisons with other therapeutic classes are limited. Baseline headache intensity does not predict aspirin or other NSAID therapy success or failure.[2,36] No studies have compared the relative efficacy of different NSAIDs.[12,20]

NSAIDs prevent neurogenically mediated inflammation in the trigeminovascular system through the inhibition of prostaglandin synthesis. Metoclopramide can speed the absorption of analgesics and alleviate migraine-related nausea and vomiting.[37] Moreover, when metoclopramide is combined with aspirin, the combination

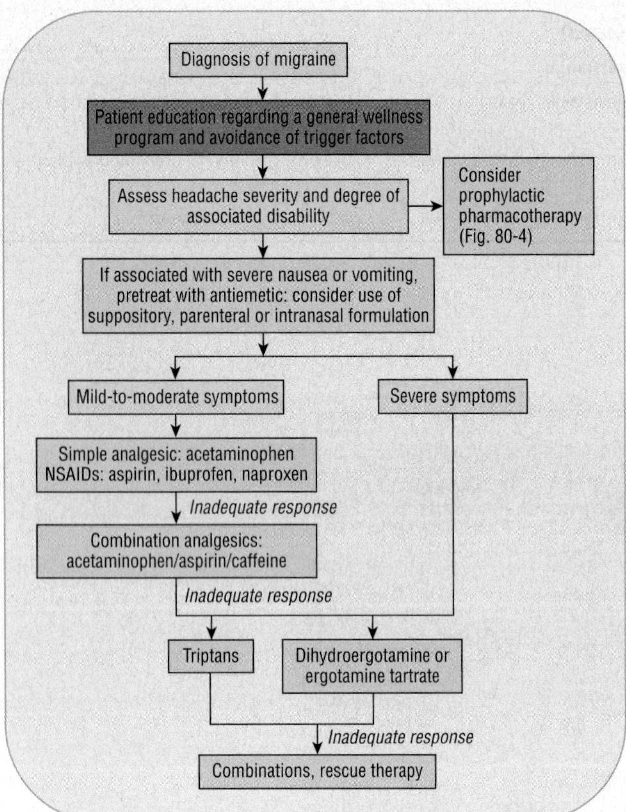

FIGURE 80-3 Treatment algorithm for migraine headaches.

TABLE 80-5 Commonly Reported Triggers of Migraine

Food triggers
Alcohol
Caffeine (greater than 200 mg/day)/caffeine withdrawal
Chocolate
Fermented and pickled foods
Monosodium glutamate (eg, in Chinese food, seasoned salt, and instant foods)
Nitrate-containing foods (eg, processed meats)
Saccharin/aspartame (eg, diet foods or diet sodas)
Tyramine-containing foods
Environmental triggers
Glare or flickering lights
High altitude
Loud noises
Strong smells and fumes
Tobacco smoke
Weather changes*
Behavioral–physiologic triggers
Excess or insufficient sleep
Fatigue
Menstruation, menopause*
Sexual activity
Skipped meals/fasting*
Strenuous physical activity (eg, prolonged overexertion)
Stress or poststress*

*Not easily modified triggers.

Data from References 9, 30, and 35.

has similar efficacy to sumatriptan and is an alternative for individuals where triptans are contraindicated.[12,13] Suppository analgesic preparations are an option when nausea and vomiting are severe.[20] Acute NSAID therapy is associated with GI (eg, dyspepsia, nausea, vomiting, and diarrhea) and CNS (eg, somnolence, dizziness) adverse effects. These agents should be avoided or used cautiously in individuals with previous ulcer disease, renal disease, severe cardiovascular disease, or hypersensitivity to aspirin.[12,20]

The nonprescription combination of acetaminophen, aspirin, and caffeine was approved for migraine treatment in the United States given its efficacy in relieving pain and associated symptoms.[19,20] Aspirin and acetaminophen are also available in prescription combination products containing a short-acting barbiturate (butalbital) or narcotic (codeine). While butalbital or butalbital-containing products are possibly effective for acute migraine, these analgesics or narcotics should be limited due to overuse, medication-overuse headache, and withdrawal concerns.[19–21] Frequent consumption of aspirin or acetaminophen alone can result in medication-overuse headache, and combination analgesics appear to pose a greater risk.[21]

Triptans The 5-HT receptor agonists, or triptans, represented a significant advance in migraine pharmacotherapy. The first member of this class, sumatriptan, and the second-generation agents zolmitriptan, naratriptan, rizatriptan, almotriptan, frovatriptan, and eletriptan are selective agonists of the 5-HT_{1B} and 5-HT_{1D} receptors. With these agents, relief from migraine headache results from three key actions: (1) normalization of dilated intracranial arteries through enhanced vasoconstriction, (2) inhibition of vasoactive peptide release from perivascular trigeminal neurons, and (3) inhibition of transmission through second-order neurons ascending to the thalamus.[12,20] The triptans all have established efficacy and are appropriate first-line therapy for mild to severe migraine. They are also used for rescue therapy when nonspecific medications are ineffective.[19,20]

Sumatriptan, the most extensively studied acute therapy, is available for subcutaneous, oral, and intranasal administration. Subcutaneous sumatriptan is consistently superior to placebo in alleviating migraine headache and associated symptoms, with relief reported in 70% of individuals at 2 hours.[19] It also has a more rapid onset of action when compared with the oral formulation and is packaged as an autoinjector device for self-administration. Intranasal sumatriptan provides a faster onset of effect than the oral formulation and produces similar response rates in placebo-controlled studies.[12,20]

Triptan selection is based on headache characteristics, convenience of dosing, and the individual's preference. At all marketed doses, oral triptans are effective and generally well tolerated[20] and differ in their pharmacokinetic and pharmacodynamic profiles (Table 80-6). In general, they can be divided into those with a faster onset and higher efficacy and those with a slower onset and lower efficacy. A meta-analysis summarizes the efficacy and tolerability of the oral triptans across published and unpublished studies. Using 100 mg of sumatriptan as the reference dose and based on 2-hour response rates, most of the triptans show similar therapeutic gains at manufacturer recommended doses. Exceptions to this were frovatriptan and naratriptan with lower efficacy. These agents also have the longest half-lives, the slowest onset of action, and less headache recurrence, making them more suitable for individuals who have migraine attacks with slow onset and longer duration. Faster-acting triptans are more efficacious when a rapid onset is necessary. Subcutaneous, intranasal, or orally dissolving tablets may be useful in individuals with prominent early nausea or vomiting or those who have difficulty in swallowing tablets. Most individuals prefer oral formulations even though oral absorption can be delayed during attacks.[12,20]

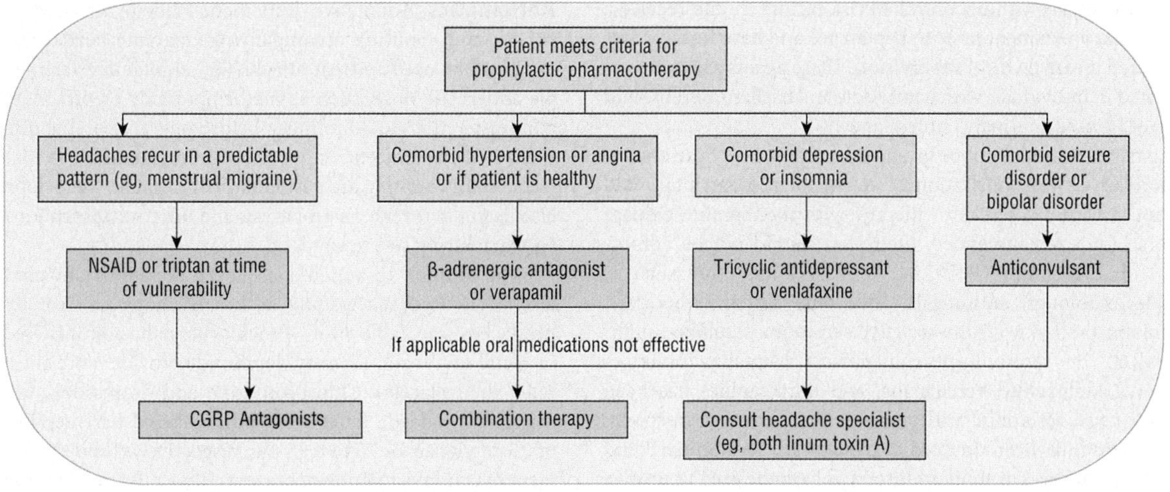

FIGURE 80-4 Treatment algorithm for prophylactic management of migraine headaches. (NSAID, nonsteroidal anti-inflammatory drug).

TABLE 80-6 Pharmacokinetic Characteristics of Triptans

Medication	Half-Life (hours)	Time to Maximal Concentration (t_{max})	Bioavailability (%)	Elimination
Almotriptan	3-4	1.4-3.8 hours	80	MAO-A, CYP3A4, CYP2D6
Eletriptan	4-5	1-2 hours	50	CYP3A4
Frovatriptan	25	2-4 hours	24-30	Mostly unchanged, CYP1A2
Naratriptan	5-6	2-3 hours	63-74	Largely unchanged, CYP450 (various isoenzymes); primary sulfa medication
Rizatriptan	2-3		45	MAO-A
Oral tablets		1-1.2 hours		
Disintegrating		1.6-2.5 hours		
Sumatriptan	2			MAO-A; primary sulfa medication
Subcutaneous injection		12-15 minutes	97	
Oral tablets		2.5 hours	14	
Nasal spray		10 minutes	17	
Nasal powder		45 minutes		
Patch		1.1 hours	45	
Zolmitriptan	3		40-48	CYP1A2, MAO-A
Oral		2 hours		
Disintegrating		3.3 hours		
Nasal		4 hours		

CYP, cytochrome P450; MAO-A, monoamine oxidase type A.
Data from References 12, e13, and 37–40.

8 Triptan clinical response can vary considerably among individuals and responses cannot be predicted. If one triptan fails, an individual can be switched successfully to another.[12,13] After an effective agent and dose are identified, subsequent treatments with that same regimen should begin. Combination therapy may improve response rates and diminish migraine recurrence. A proprietary single tablet formulation of sumatriptan 85 mg plus naproxen 500 mg was more effective in clinical trials for headache relief and sustained pain-free response than either agent as monotherapy.[19,20]

Triptan adverse effects are common but are usually mild to moderate in nature, of short duration, and common among the class; including paresthesias, fatigue, dizziness, flushing, warm sensations, and somnolence. Local adverse effects are reported with the subcutaneous (minor injection site reactions) and intranasal (taste perversion, nasal discomfort) routes. Up to 25% of individuals report "triptan sensations," including tightness, pressure, heaviness, or pain in the chest, neck, or throat. The mechanism of these symptoms is unknown, but a cardiac source seems unlikely in most individuals; however, all triptans are partial agonists of human 5-HT coronary artery receptors in vitro, resulting in a small but significant vasoconstrictor response. Other adverse cardiac events are rare, with only isolated cases of myocardial infarction and coronary vasospasm with ischemia reported. The triptans are contraindicated in individuals with a history of ischemic heart disease (eg, angina pectoris, Prinzmetal's angina, or previous myocardial infarction), uncontrolled hypertension, and cerebrovascular disease. Individuals at risk for unrecognized coronary artery disease should use triptans with caution. Postmenopausal females, males older than 40 years of age, and individuals with uncontrolled risk factors should receive a cardiovascular assessment prior to triptan use and have initial doses administered under medical supervision. These agents are also contraindicated in individuals with hemiplegic and basilar migraine and should not be used routinely in pregnancy.[20,23]

The triptans should not be given within 24 hours of the ergotamine derivatives. Administration of sumatriptan, rizatriptan, and zolmitriptan within 2 weeks of therapy with monoamine oxidase inhibitors is not recommended. Eletriptan should not be administered with cytochrome P4503A4 (CYP3A4) inhibitors such as macrolide antibiotics, antifungals, and some antiviral therapies. Concomitant therapy with the selective serotonin reuptake inhibitors (SSRIs) or serotonin-norepinephrine reuptake inhibitors (SNRIs) (eg, duloxetine, venlafaxine, and mirtazapine) has been reported to cause serotonin syndrome based on several case reports. This interaction has been doubted as triptans are serotonin 1B and 1D agonists, whereas serotonin syndrome is hypothesized to involve 2A and 1A receptors.[41] Regulatory agencies, including the FDA, caution against concurrent administration, although it appears the likelihood of CNS adverse events is extremely low. The potential risk of these combinations should be carefully considered and discussed with the individual.[12,13,20] Frequent use of the triptans has been associated with the development of medication-overuse headache.[6,21]

Ergot Alkaloids and Derivatives Ergotamine tartrate and dihydroergotamine can treat moderate-to-severe migraine attacks (see Table 80-4). These medications are nonselective 5-HT_1 receptor agonists that constrict intracranial blood vessels, centrally inhibit the trigeminovascular system, and prevent neurogenic inflammation development.[12,13] These agents also have agonist activity at dopaminergic receptors. Venous and arterial constriction occur with therapeutic doses, but ergotamine tartrate exerts more potent arterial effects than dihydroergotamine.[12,20]

The oral and rectal preparations of ergotamine tartrate containing caffeine, to enhance absorption and potentiate analgesia, are probably effective.[19] The dosage should be strictly titrated to establish an effective subnauseating dose for future attacks. The efficacy of ergotamine alone in migraine is inconsistent, despite its clinical use for decades.[12,20]

Dihydroergotamine is probably effective and available for intranasal and parenteral administration by the IM, subcutaneous and IV routes.[13,19,20] Parenteral dihydroergotamine was previously used as an inpatient or emergency department treatment for moderate-to-severe migraine or intractable headache, but individuals can be trained to self-administer either IM or subcutaneously. Clinical studies support the nasal spray and pulmonary inhaler (still in development) as effective.[13,19]

Nausea and vomiting resulting from chemoreceptor trigger zone stimulation are among the most common ergotamine derivative adverse effects. Pretreatment with an antiemetic agent should be considered with ergotamine and IV dihydroergotamine therapy. Other common adverse effects include abdominal pain, weakness, fatigue, paresthesias, muscle pain, diarrhea, and chest tightness. Rarely, symptoms of severe peripheral ischemia (ergotism), including cold, numb, painful extremities, continuous paresthesias, diminished peripheral pulses, and claudication, can result from their vasoconstrictor effects. Gangrenous extremities, myocardial infarction, hepatic necrosis, and bowel and brain ischemia have also been reported; however, dihydroergotamine is rarely associated with such adverse effects. Triptans and ergot derivatives should not be used within 24 hours of each other,[12,20] and they are contraindicated in individuals with renal or hepatic failure; coronary, cerebral, or peripheral vascular disease; uncontrolled hypertension; and sepsis; or in individuals who are pregnant or nursing. Dihydroergotamine does not appear to cause rebound headache, but dosage restrictions for ergotamine tartrate should be strictly observed to prevent this complication.[20]

Antiemetics Adjunctive antiemetic therapy is useful for the nausea and vomiting accompanying migraine headaches and the medications used to treat attacks (eg, ergotamine tartrate). A single antiemetic dose, such as metoclopramide or prochlorperazine, administered 15 to 30 minutes before migraine oral abortive treatment is often sufficient. Suppository preparations are available when nausea and vomiting are particularly prominent. Metoclopramide is also useful to reverse gastroparesis and improve absorption from the GI tract during severe attacks.[12]

In addition to antiemetic effects, dopamine antagonists have also been used successfully as monotherapy to treat intractable headaches (see Table 80-4). Prochlorperazine administered IV, IM, or rectal routes and IV metoclopramide provide more effective pain relief than placebo. Chlorpromazine and droperidol also provide migraine headache relief when administered parenterally at doses of 0.1 mg/kg and 2.75 to 8.25 mg, respectively. Their precise mechanism of action is unknown; however, they offer an alternative to the narcotic analgesics for refractory migraine treatment. Drowsiness and dizziness were reported occasionally, and extrapyramidal adverse effects were reported infrequently in migraine trials. Most of these medications have a risk for QT prolongation and torsades de pointes.[12,19,20]

Ditans Lasmiditan is in a new class of abortive migraine medications known as "ditans." Unlike the triptan mechanism of agonists at 5-HT_{1B} and 5-HT_{1D}, lasmiditan is a highly selective 5-HT_{1F} agonist whereby vasoconstrictive activity is minimized.[41] Ditans act by blocking both neurogenic inflammation in the dura and stimulation of the trigeminal nucleus caudalis. In clinical trials, all doses of lasmiditan were significantly superior to placebo both for headache-free days and improvement in most bothersome symptoms (eg, nausea, phonophobia, or photophobia) 2 hours post-dose, for individuals with three to eight migraine attacks per month.[42,43] Common adverse effects reported in 2% of individuals or more were dizziness, paresthesia, sedation, and nausea/vomiting. Lasmiditan is associated with significant driving impairment where sleepiness has been reported after each dose. This adverse effect has prompted specific labeling warnings and precautions regarding not driving a motor vehicle or operating heavy machinery for at least 8 hours following each dose.

CGRP Antagonists ("gepants") Two small-molecule CGRP antagonists, ubrogepant and rimegepant, which are also known as "gepants," have been FDA approved for the acute treatment of migraine. During a migraine attack, CGRP levels rise resulting in vasodilation and neurogenic inflammation.[44,45] Thus, the blockade of CGRP receptors has become a breakthrough treatment for individuals with migraines. The clinical data regarding the efficacy of these medications is similar to triptans and lasmiditan, though they tend to have improved tolerability, and in contrast to triptans, the presence or history of cardiovascular disease is not a contraindication. Furthermore, medication overuse headache does not occur as a result of gepant use.[46]

The primary outcomes evaluated in clinical trials for these agents were pain freedom and reduction in most bothersome symptoms, two hours after dosing. Using these outcomes, ubrogepant (50-mg and 100-mg doses) and rimegepant (75-mg dose) have efficacy in pain freedom and freedom from most bothersome symptoms (photophobia, phonophobia, or nausea) at two hours. The incidence of adverse effects was very low (less than 5%) but included nausea for rimegepant and nausea, xerostomia, and somnolence for ubrogepant. Rimegepant is a relatively long-acting acute medication with a half-life of 11 hours, and thus, it is not recommended to repeat a dose within 24 hours. Ubrogepant has a shorter half-life of 5 to 7 hours, and the dose can be repeated two hours after the initial administration. These two medications have significant medication interactions, and concomitant use with strong CYP3A4 inhibitors,

P-gp inhibitors, and BCRP inhibitors should be avoided; otherwise, dose adjustments may need to be made. Additionally, these agents should be avoided in severe renal or hepatic impairment and dose adjustments may need to be made in mild to moderate renal or hepatic impairment.

Opiate Analgesics There is inadequate evidence supporting narcotic analgesic use (ie, parenteral butorphanol, meperidine, methadone, and tramadol or oral codeine) in the treatment of acute migraine. However, oral codeine or tramadol combinations with acetaminophen are probably effective and butorphanol nasal spray has established efficacy.[19] Opiates have no vasopressor or anti-inflammatory effects and can cause central sensitization, increasing the risk of medication-overuse headache and interfering with the efficacy of other treatments even with intermittent use.[12,19,21] These agents should generally be reserved for individuals with moderate-to-severe infrequent headaches in whom conventional therapies are contraindicated, or as "rescue medication" after individuals have failed to respond to conventional therapies. Opioid therapy should be supervised closely because of the risk of sedation and the potential for unhealthy use.[12,20]

Miscellaneous Nonspecific Medications Corticosteroids can be considered rescue therapy for status migrainous (a severe, continuous migraine that can last up to 1 week) or to reduce migraine recurrence. Intravenous (IV) dexamethasone at a 4- to 16-mg dose has been used as an adjunct to abortive therapy, although evidence is incomplete.[19,20] IV valproate 400 to 1,000 mg also plays a role in moderate or severe intensity headaches, although data to support this is limited. When used the majority of individuals report improvement after one dose. Lastly, magnesium sulfate 1,000 to 2,000 mg IV (in migraine with aura) and generic isometheptene combinations are probably effective. A more defined role for these agents in migraine management must be established.[19]

Prophylactic Pharmacologic Therapy

Antiseizure Medications Antiseizure medications have emerged as important therapeutic options for migraine prophylaxis with valproate, divalproex, and topiramate all having established efficacy.[25] The beneficial effects of these agents are likely due to multiple mechanisms of action, including enhancement of γ-aminobutyric acid–mediated inhibition, modulation of the excitatory neurotransmitter glutamate, and inhibition of sodium and calcium ion channel activity. Antiseizure medications are particularly useful in individuals with migraine and comorbid seizures, anxiety disorder, or bipolar illness.[18,26,47,48] The use of sodium valproate and divalproex sodium (a 1:1 molar combination of valproate sodium and valproic acid) is effective based on multiple placebo-controlled studies. In most headache prophylaxis trials, there were no significant differences in treatment-emergent adverse effects between these agents and placebo. Nausea and vomiting are the most common early adverse effects but are self-limited and appear to be less common with divalproex sodium and gradual dose titration. Alopecia, tremor, asthenia, somnolence, and weight gain are also complaints.[18,26] The extended-release formulation of divalproex sodium is administered once daily and is better tolerated than the enteric-coated formulation. Hepatotoxicity is the most serious adverse effect associated with valproate, but the risk appears to be low in individuals with migraine headache (eg, individuals older than 10 years of age who are receiving monotherapy and have no underlying metabolic or neurologic disorder). Baseline liver function tests should be obtained, but routine follow-up is not necessary for asymptomatic adults on monotherapy. Regular follow-up is needed for dosage adjustments and adverse effect monitoring. Valproate when used for migraine prophylaxis, is contraindicated in pregnant individuals due to potential teratogenicity and for individuals with a history of pancreatitis or chronic liver disease.[18,26]

Topiramate is the most extensively studied antiseizure medication for migraine prophylaxis. Its efficacy shows improvements in health-related quality of life such as daily work, home, and social activities.. To minimize adverse effects, topiramate should be initiated at a low dose and slowly titrated upward. The benefits of topiramate are observed as early as 2 weeks after therapy initiation, with significant reductions in migraine frequency within the first month. Approximately half of the individuals treated to target doses are responders, defined as a 50% or greater reduction in mean headache frequency. Treatment-emergent adverse events include paresthesia, fatigue, anorexia, diarrhea, weight loss, hypesthesia, difficulty with memory, language problems, taste perversion, and nausea. Paresthesia, the most common adverse event, occurs in about half of the individuals at target doses. Weight loss, occurring in 9% to 12% of individuals, is a unique adverse effect, as weight gain is a common reason to discontinue other preventive medications. Topiramate should be used with caution or avoided in individuals with a history of kidney stones or cognitive impairment.[18,26]

Carbamazepine is possibly effective for migraine phophylasis and gabapentin has modest impact.[49] Lamotrigine is classified as possibly or probably ineffective.[26]

Additional information regarding all antiseizure medications can be found in Chapter 75, "Epilepsy."

Antidepressants The beneficial effects of antidepressants in migraine are independent of their antidepressant activity and may be related to downregulation of central 5-HT_2 receptors resulting in increased levels of synaptic norepinephrine, and enhanced endogenous opioid receptor actions.[9] The tricyclic antidepressant (TCA) amitriptyline and SNRI venlafaxine have demonstrated efficacy in placebo-controlled and comparative studies and are classified as probably effective for migraine prophylaxis (see Table 80-4).[18,26] Use of other antidepressants is based primarily on clinical and anecdotal experience. There is neither support nor refusal regarding the efficacy of other antidepressants, such as protriptyline, fluoxetine, or fluvoxamine, for migraine prophylaxis.[26]

Anticholinergic adverse effects are common with the TCAs and limit their use in individuals with benign prostatic hyperplasia and glaucoma. Evening doses are preferred because of associated sedation. Increased appetite and weight gain can also occur. Orthostatic hypotension and slowed atrioventricular conduction are also occasionally reported.[18,26] Venlafaxine's most common adverse effects are nausea, vomiting, and drowsiness. Again, the potential risk of 5-HT syndrome should be considered in individuals using SSRIs or SNRIs along with a triptan.[20,26] Additional information about the adverse effects of antidepressants can be found in Chapter 88.

β-Adrenergic Antagonists β-Adrenergic antagonists are among the most widely used medications for migraine prophylaxis. Metoprolol, propranolol, and timolol have established efficacy and reduce the frequency of attacks by half in more than 50% of individuals.[18,26] Atenolol and nadolol are probably effective, while nebivolol and pindolol are possibly effective (see Table 80-5).[25] Because the individual agent's relative efficacy has not been established, β-blocker selection can be based on β-selectivity, formulation, and tolerability. β-Blockers may raise the migraine threshold by modulating adrenergic or serotonergic neurotransmission in cortical or subcortical pathways, although their precise mechanism is unknown. Although not first-line treatment for hypertension, β-blockers may be useful along with other therapy in individuals with comorbid hypertension or angina. Adverse effects can include drowsiness, fatigue, sleep disturbances, vivid dreams, memory disturbance, depression, impotence, bradycardia, and hypotension. The β-blockers should be used with caution in individuals with congestive heart failure, peripheral vascular disease, atrioventricular conduction disturbances, asthma, depression, and diabetes.[18,26]

CGRP Antagonists (Anti-CGRP Antibodies) Inhibition of the CGRP receptor is the newest target in the prophylaxis of migraine.[9,18,46,47] Several anti-CGRP receptor monoclonal antibodies have been FDA approved in recent years such as erenumab-aooe, fremanezumab-vfrm, galcanezumab-gnlm, and eptinezumab-jjmr. While erenumab targets the CGRP receptor, the others target the CGRP ligand. These biologic agents have efficacy, safety, and tolerability for the prevention of episodic and chronic migraine.[17] Erenumab, fremanezumab, and galcanezumab are all administered as monthly subcutaneous injections and fremanezumab has a quarterly (every 3 months) dosing option. Eptinezumab is a quarterly IV infusion. The lack of hepatic metabolism or renal clearance for these agents avoids medication interactions with this medication class. Injection site reactions are the most common adverse event for all of the subcutaneous agents. For erenumab worsening of pre-exisitng hypertension can occur within 7 day of initiation and constipation has been reported in less than 5% of users. For eptinezumab, nasopharyngitis is reported in less than 10% of individuals and hypersensitivity is reported in less than 3%. The cost of these biological medications is higher than the oral preventive medications, and it is recommended that they are reserved for individuals who have been unable to tolerate or who did not respond to at least two of the preventive oral medications with highest level of evidence (topiramate, divalproex/valproate sodium, beta blockers, tricyclic antidepressants, or venlafaxine/duloxetine).

CGRP Antagonists ("gepants") Unlike the large-molecule, injectable, preventative monoclonal antibodies, the "gepants" are small-molecule agents that block the ability of CGRP to bind to the CGRP docking station, which prevents prolonged migraine attacks. There are two "gepants," atogepant and rimegepant, that are FDA approved for preventative treatment of episodic migraine headaches in adults.

Atogepant (placebo, 10 mg daily, 30 mg daily, 60 mg daily) was evaluated in two, 12-week, multicenter, randomized, placebo-controlled trials for episodic migraine headache prevention.[50,51] IA decrease of approximately 4 mean migraine days a month over a 12-week period for atogepant was seen compared with a decrease of approximately 2.5 days in the placebo group. Fatigue, nausea, and constipation appeared to increase at the higher doses, and some adverse effects were noted at about 2% compared with a placebo. No liver abnormalities above the placebo rate were seen.[51] Like rimegepant and ubrogepant, atogepant has significant medication interactions, and concomitant use with strong CYP3A4 inhibitors, strong as well as moderate CYP3A4 inducers, and OATP inhibitors should be avoided; otherwise, dose adjustments may be needed. Additionally, atogepant should be avoided in severe renal or hepatic impairment. Rimegepant (75 mg every other day) was used in the prevention of episodic migraine headache for over 12 weeks in a multicenter, randomized, placebo-controlled study. Overall the difference in the reduction of migraine days was 0.8 days per month with rimegepant versus placebo.[52] Two percent of adverse medication effects associated with rimegepant included nasopharyngitis, nausea, urinary tract infection, and upper respiratory tract infection were mild to moderate in severity. Adverse rimegepant effects include reversible alanine aminotransferase or aspartate aminotransferase greater than three times the upper limit of normal, reversible asymptomatic elevation of aminotransferases with alanine aminotransferase greater than 10 times the upper limit of normal, and hereditary liver disorder related where bilirubin levels greater than two times the upper limit of normal.

Nonsteroidal Anti-Inflammatory Drugs NSAIDs are modestly effective for reducing the frequency, severity, and duration of migraine attacks, but potential GI and renal toxicity limit the daily or prolonged use of these agents. Consequently, NSAIDs have been used intermittently to prevent headaches recurring in a predictable pattern, such as menstrual migraine. NSAID administration in the perimenstrual period can be beneficial in females with true menstrual migraine. They should be initiated up to 1 week prior to the expected onset of headache and continued for no more than 10 days.[27] If long-term NSAID therapy is initiated, renal function and occult blood loss should be monitored. The evidence for efficacy is strongest for naproxen and weakest for aspirin.[27,32]

Triptans Triptans are also useful for the prevention of menstrual migraine. Frovatriptan has established efficacy, while naratriptan and zolmitriptan are probably effective. These agents are usually started 1 or 2 days before the expected onset of headache and continued during the period of vulnerability.[27,32] Regulatory authorities are currently deliberating a separate indication for pure menstrual migraine.[26]

Miscellaneous Prophylactic Agents At least two placebo-controlled studies show that petasites, an extract from the butterbur plant *Petasites hybridus*, is an effective preventive treatment for migraine.[18,29] There is a probable efficacy of riboflavin (vitamin B2) 400 mg daily in migraine prophylaxis, based on double-blind, placebo-controlled study. Riboflavin is well tolerated and associated with a 50% or greater improvement in attack frequency in most individuals. However, these benefits were only significant after 3 months.[18,29] The relatively stable extract of feverfew (*Tanacetum parthenium*), MIG-99, is the most studied herbal preparation for migraine prevention and it reduces migraine frequency by almost two attacks per month and is classified as probably effective.[18,29] As CNS levels of magnesium are significantly low during migraine attacks, magnesium supplementation may be particularly effective for prevention of menstrual migraine.[31] The evaluation of various formulations of magnesium has yielded mixed results, but there is probable efficacy.[18,29] Subcutaneous histamine has been compared with placebo, sodium valproate, and topiramate, with favorable results indicating probable efficacy in improving headache frequency, duration, and intensity. Transient burning and itching at the injection site were the only reported adverse effects with histamine administration.[29]

Other agents are also possibly effective for migraine prevention.[26,29] The angiotensin-converting enzyme inhibitor lisinopril and the angiotensin II receptor blocker candesartan provided effective migraine prophylaxis in recent clinical trials.[18,26] Clonidine and guanfacine also have possible efficacy, although adverse effects limit their use.[26] Coenzyme Q10 was effective for migraine prevention and well-tolerated in a small, randomized, double-blind, controlled study.[18,29] Cyproheptadine (4 mg/day) was as effective as propranolol (80 mg/day) in reducing migraine frequency, duration, and severity, while the combination was more effective in attack frequency reduction.[26,29]

The calcium channel blockers, primarily verapamil, have been widely used for preventive treatment, although the results of their use is inadequate or conflicting.[18,26] Extensive clinical experience and verapamil's ease of use suggest a possible role in migraine prevention. Adverse effects include constipation, hypotension, bradycardia, atrioventricular block, and exacerbation of congestive heart failure.[26]

Localized injections of botulinum toxin type A have been used for various conditions and pain syndromes, including chronic migraines. This agent is FDA approved for individuals who have 15 or more headache days per month lasting 4 or more hours daily. The American Academy of Neurology concludes that a 6-week trial of botulinum toxin is effective as a second-line agent after inadequate response or adverse effects to at least two of the following agents: topiramate, divalproex sodium/valproate sodium, beta-blocker, tricyclic antidepressant, or SNRI.[18]

TENSION-TYPE HEADACHE

Epidemiology

Tension-type headache is the most common type of primary headache, with an estimated 1-year prevalence of 38% to 86%.[3,53] It peaks in the fourth decade of life and is higher among females; however, the incidence decreases with age.[32] Although most individuals with tension-type headaches experience some degree of functional impairment during their attacks, few seek medical attention, likely because they have intermittent attacks. These headaches are classified as either episodic (infrequent or frequent) or chronic based on the frequency and duration of the attacks.[2] Infrequent episodic tension-type headache (defined as fewer than one episode per month) is experienced by 64% of sufferers, while 22% have a frequent episodic tension-type headache for about 1-14 days per month). The prevalence of chronic tension-type headache (defined as 15 or more days/month, perhaps without recognizable episodes) is estimated at 0.9% to 2.2%.[2,53] Risk factors associated with a poor outcome include coexisting migraine, depression, anxiety, poor stress management, and the presence of chronic tension-type headache.[55]

Pathophysiology

Although tension-type headache is the most common type of headache, it is the least studied primary headache disorder, and there is limited understanding of key pathophysiologic concepts.[2,53] Migraine and tension-type headaches represent a continuum of headache severity with similarities in mechanisms and pathophysiology. However, tension-type headache has been recognized as a distinct disorder.[2,53] The mechanism of pain in chronic tension-type headache is thought to originate from myofascial factors and peripheral sensitization of nociceptors. Central mechanisms also are involved, with heightened sensitivity of CNS pain pathways.[53] Mental stress, nonphysiologic motor stress, a local myofascial release of irritants, or a combination of these may be the initiating stimulus. Following activation of supraspinal pain perception structures, a self-limiting headache results in most individuals owing to central modulation of the incoming peripheral stimuli. Chronic tension-type headache can evolve from episodic headaches in predisposed individuals due to changes in central circuits and nociceptive processing along the brain stem reflex pathway and subsequent CNS sensitization.[53] Other pathophysiologic mechanisms also contribute to the development of tension-type headache.

Clinical Presentation

Premonitory symptoms and aura are absent with this headache, and the pain usually is mild to moderate in intensity. It is often is described as bilateral dull, nonpulsatile tightness, or pressure classically described as having a "hatband" pattern.[2,53] Associated symptoms generally are absent, but mild photophobia or phonophobia may be reported. The disability associated with tension-type headache is typically minor compared to migraine headaches, and routine physical activity does not affect severity.[2,49] Palpation of the pericranial or cervical muscles can reveal tender spots or localized nodules in some individuals.[2]

TREATMENT

Desired Outcomes

While pain relief and prevention of further headaches are the main desired outcomes of treatment, the vast majority of episodic tension-type headache sufferers self-medicate with nonprescription medications and do not consult a healthcare professional. Although pharmacologic and nonpharmacologic treatments are available, simple analgesics and NSAIDs are the mainstay of acute therapy. Most agents used for tension-type headache have not been studied in controlled clinical trials.[54]

Nonpharmacologic Therapy

Psychophysiologic therapy and physical therapy have been used in their management. Behavioral treatments can consist of cognitive-behavioral therapy (ie, stress management), relaxation training, and biofeedback.[55] These therapies (alone or in combination with pharmacotherapy) can result in a 33% to 64% reduction in headache activity. Relaxation training combined with biofeedback is more effective than other behavioral therapy options.[55] The effect of physical therapeutic options, such as heat or cold packs, ultrasound, electrical nerve stimulation, stretching, exercise, massage, acupuncture, manipulations, ergonomic instruction, and trigger point injections or occipital nerve blocks, is somewhat inconsistent. However, individuals may benefit from selected modalities in reducing the frequency of tension-type headache or during an acute episode.[54,55]

Pharmacologic Therapy

Simple analgesics (alone or in combination with caffeine) and NSAIDs are effective for the acute treatment of most mild-to-moderate tension-type headaches. Acetaminophen, aspirin, diclofenac, ibuprofen, naproxen, ketoprofen, and ketorolac have efficacy in placebo-controlled and comparative studies.[54] Failure of nonprescription agents can warrant therapy with prescription medications. The combination of aspirin or acetaminophen with butalbital or, rarely, codeine can be effective options in selected individuals; however, use of butalbital and codeine combinations should be avoided when possible owing to the high potential for overuse and unhealthy use.

Acute medications should be taken for episodic tension-type headache no more than 10 days a month for butalbital-containing or combination analgesics, or 15 days a month for NSAIDs. This practice helps prevent the development of medication-overuse or chronic tension-type headache.[54] The efficacy of muscle relaxants in episodic tension-type headache management is not known.[2,54] Preventive treatment is appropriate for most individuals with chronic tension-type headache and should be considered in those whose episodic headache occur more than twice per week, last more than 3 to 4 hours, or their severity results in medication overuse or substantial disability.[55]

Preventive treatment for tension-type headaches is similar to migraine headaches. The TCAs are prescribed most often for prophylaxis, but other medications can also be selected after considering comorbid medical conditions and medication adverse effect profiles. In general, the SSRIs are only effective in individuals with tension-type headache and depression, and limited studies support the mirtazapine and venlafaxine use in individuals with chronic tension-type headache without depression.[55] Topiramate, gabapentin, and tizanidine may have benefits in chronic tension-type headache; however, randomized clinical trials need to be done. Lidocaine trigger point injections may reduce headache frequency for frequent episodic or chronic tension-type headache. Injection of botulinum toxin into pericranial muscles has inconsistent efficacy in the prophylaxis, and because of this, it is of uncertain benefit.[55]

CLUSTER HEADACHE

Epidemiology

Cluster headache is the most severe of the primary headache disorders and is characterized by attacks of excruciating, unilateral head pain that occur in series lasting for weeks or months. These cluster periods are separated by remission periods, usually lasting months or years.[2,56] These headaches can be episodic or chronic[2] and are relatively uncommon among the primary headache disorders. However, the exact prevalence is uncertain. Estimates from pooled population studies show a lifetime prevalence of 124 per 100,000 or 0.12%.[56,57] The male-to-female ratio for cluster headache is approximately 4:1 with onset typically in the second to third decade of life. Up to 85% of individuals with cluster headaches are tobacco smokers or have a smoking history. Tobacco cessation, however, does not seem to improve the course of headaches. Recent genetic epidemiologic surveys support a predisposition for cluster headache in certain families.[56-58]

Pathophysiology

The etiologic and pathophysiologic mechanisms of these headaches are not entirely understood. Neuroimaging studies performed during acute attacks show activation of the ipsilateral hypothalamic gray area, implicating the hypothalamus as a modulator. The hypothalamus secondarily activates trigeminal-autonomic reflexes, leading to the ipsilateral pain and cranial autonomic features characteristic of cluster headache.[56-58] The cyclic and circadian rhythmicity of attacks also implicates pathogenesis of hypothalamic dysfunction.[57,58] Cluster headache may result from inflammation of the nerves traversing the cavernous sinus resulting in injury to sympathetic fibers of the internal carotid artery.[57]

Clinical Presentation

One hallmark of cluster headaches is the circadian rhythm of painful attacks. Episodic cluster headaches are the most common cluster headache subtype, occurring in up to 90% of individuals.[57] These episodic attacks occur daily for a week to several months, followed by long pain-free intervals. Headache remission averages 2 years in length but can range from 2 months to 20 years in duration. Approximately 15% of individuals have chronic symptoms with attacks recurring for over 1 year without remission or with remission periods lasting less than 1month.[56,57]

Cluster headache attacks occur commonly at night and frequently in the spring and fall. These attacks occur suddenly and pain peaks quickly after onset. The pain is excruciating, penetrating, and of a boring (ie, deep, non-pulsating, behind the eye) intensity in orbital, supraorbital, and temporal unilateral locations. They generally lasts 15 to 180 minutes and are accompanied by cranial autonomic symptoms such as conjunctival injection, lacrimation, nasal stuffiness, rhinorrhea, eyelid edema, facial sweating, and miosis/ptosis. Most sufferers also describe restlessness or agitation; however, all of these symptoms resolve when the headache ceases. While individuals with migraine retreat to a quiet, dark room, individuals with cluster headache generally sit and rock or pace about the room clutching their head. Auras are not present and during the cluster period, attacks occur from once every other day to eight times per day.[56,57] Specific diagnostic criteria for cluster headaches are provided within the IHS classification system.[2]

TREATMENT

Desired Outcomes

As in migraine, therapy for cluster headaches involves both abortive and prophylactic therapy with the overall desired outcomes being resolution or prevention of pain and disability. Abortive therapy is directed at managing the acute attack, whereas prophylactic therapies are started early in the cluster period in an attempt to induce remission. Individuals with chronic cluster headache can require prophylactic medications indefinitely.

Abortive Therapy

Oxygen The standard acute treatment of cluster headache is inhalation of 100% oxygen by a nonbreather facial mask at a rate of at least 12 to 15 L/min, with effects usually starting 15 to 20 minutes after treatment.[58-61] Repeat or frequent administration over a short period of time should be avoided, as overuse may increase the frequency or merely delay rather than abort the attack in some individuals.[59,60] No adverse effects have been reported with the use of oxygen, but caution should be used for those who smoke or have chronic obstructive pulmonary disease.

Triptans The quick onset of subcutaneous and intranasal triptans makes them safe and effective abortive agents for cluster headaches. Subcutaneous sumatriptan (6 mg) is the most effective agent, whereas nasal sprays, which are less effective than subcutaneous administration, may be better tolerated in some individuals. Adverse events reported with triptan use in individuals with cluster headache are similar to those seen in individuals with migraine. Orally administered triptans have limited use in cluster attacks because of their relatively slow onset of action; oral zolmitriptan (10 mg), however, was modestly effective in individuals with episodic cluster headache.[55]

Ergotamine Derivatives All forms of ergotamine have been used in cluster headaches, although no controlled clinical trials support their use.[38,39] In clinical use, IV dihydroergotamine may be given as a bolus followed by repeated administration over several days to break the cycle of frequent attacks. In addition, ergotamine tartrate has provided effective relief from cluster headache attacks when administered sublingually.[59] Dosing guidelines are similar to those for migraine headache therapy.

Prophylactic Therapy

Verapamil The preferred first-line treatment for cluster headaches prevention is verapamil, a calcium channel blocker with antianginal and antiarrhythmic properties.[58,60,61] Its beneficial effects often appear within 2 to 3 weeks of therapy, starting with a dose of 240 mg/day, titrated to a target dose of 360 to 960 mg/day. Rarely, individuals with refractory cluster headaches require doses as high as 1,200 mg/day. In such individuals, an electrocardiogram should be obtained as the dose is increased, due to concerns for bradycardia or heart block.[59,61]

Galcanezumab Galcanezumab is a monoclonal antibody that binds to the CGRP ligand that FDA approved for episodic cluster headache. It has a modest benefit in reducing the number of cluster headaches per week for one to three weeks for individuals with episodic cluster headaches in a randomized controlled trial. Galcanezumab is dosed subcutaneously (300 mg) at the onset of the cluster period, and then continued monthly until the end of the cluster period. It should be reserved for individuals with prior episodic cluster headache periods lasting longer than 1 month when first-line preventive medications are ineffective, poorly tolerated, or contraindicated. It was well tolerated with injection site reaction (less than 10%) being the most frequently reported adverse event.[62]

Lithium Lithium carbonate is effective for episodic and chronic cluster headache attacks and can be used when other medications are ineffective or contraindicated. A positive response is seen in up to 78% of individuals with chronic cluster headache and in up to 63% of individuals with episodic cluster headache. The usual dose is 600 to 1,200 mg/day, with a suggested starting dose of 300 mg twice daily. Lithium levels should be monitored and maintained between 0.4 and 1.2 mEq/L (mmol/L).[59]

Major adverse effects include tremors, thyroid, and renal dysfunction, and rarely cardiac arrhythmias. Liver, thyroid, and renal function must be carefully monitored during therapy. Lithium should be administered with caution to individuals with significant renal or cardiovascular disease, dehydration, pregnancy, or concomitant diuretic or NSAID use.[59,61] Additional details regarding lithium administration can be found in Chapter 86, "Substance Use Disorders II: Alcohol Nicotine and Caffeine."

Corticosteroids Corticosteroids can be used effectively for inducing cluster headache remission, although clinical trial data are lacking.[59] Therapy is initiated as 60 to 100 mg/day prednisone for 5 days and then tapered by approximately 10 mg/day. Long-term use is generally not recommended to avoid steroid-induced complications, and headaches can recur when therapy is tapered or discontinued.[59,61]

Miscellaneous Agents Other therapies used in the acute management of cluster headache include intranasal lidocaine and subcutaneous octreotide. There is limited support for the use of topiramate, divalproex sodium, melatonin, indomethacin, long-acting triptans, and intranasal capsaicin for cluster headache prevention.[59-61]

For individuals refractory to pharmacologic therapy, neurosurgical interventions to relieve debilitating chronic cluster headaches may be considered.[59] Neurostimulation has gained attention in the last several years, and vagal nerve stimulation and sphenopalatine stimulation have positive results in small clinical trials.[58,59,63]

EVALUATION OF THERAPEUTIC OUTCOMES

Pharmacologic treatment should occur with medications that have the highest level of efficacy and management should be individualized based on the individual's clinical presentation and medical history, using the lowest effective doses titrated to clinical benefit and absence of adverse events. Avoid medications that increase headache frequency or severity. Nonpharmacologic or nonprescription treatments for headache management can be used either before or concurrently with other pharmacologic therapy. However, individuals may not know how to use these products optimally and often need instructions and dosing limits.

Analgesics and NSAIDs are considered the medications of choice for infrequent mild-to-moderate and severe attacks. The triptans or dihydroergotamine can be used if initial therapies prove ineffective or as first-line therapy in moderate-to-severe migraine headache. Abortive therapy should be instituted early in the course of the attack to optimize efficacy and minimize migraine-related pain and disability. Preventive therapy should be considered for recurring migraine attacks that produce significant disability or frequent attacks requiring symptomatic medication more than twice per week. Additionally, preventative therapy should be considered if symptomatic therapies that are ineffective or contraindicated or produce serious adverse effects and in the case of uncommon migraine variants that cause risk of neurologic injury. The efficacy of any prescribed prophylactic regimen should be periodically assessed for efficacy and adverse effects. Therapeutic interventions require an adequate trial to achieve clinical benefit, and maximal benefit may not be seen for 6 months or more. A prolonged headache-free interval could allow for gradual dosage reduction and discontinuation of therapy.

Monitor individuals for headache frequency, intensity, and duration, as well as any change in the headache pattern. To this end, they should be encouraged to keep a headache diary, documenting the frequency, severity, and duration of attacks and response to medication and potential trigger factors. Careful monitoring is essential to initiate the most appropriate pharmacotherapy, document therapeutic successes and failures, identify medication contraindications, and prevent or minimize adverse events. Individuals using acute therapies should be monitored for prescription and nonprescription medication use frequency to identify potential medication-overuse headache.

Although migraine is widely recognized as a disease that exacts an enormous toll on the sufferer, healthcare providers often do not recognize the degree and scope of functional impairment imposed on the individual. Approximately one out of every six healthcare visits for migraine occurs in the emergency department, although management in this setting is often suboptimal. The use of opioids for the acute migraine treatment in the emergency department is increasing, and the likelihood of unnecessary radiation exposure is greater.[5] Although most episodic migraine sufferers take medications for their headaches, only two-thirds of individuals who have been diagnosed consult with a healthcare provider regarding use of migraine-specific treatments. Just 11% of those eligible for medications to prevent migraines currently use them, although approximately 38% would benefit from prophylaxis.[14] Patient counseling is necessary to allow for proper medication use (eg, self-injection with sumatriptan), to encourage medication use early in the headache cycle, and enhance individual compliance. Strict adherence to dosing guidelines should be stressed to minimize potential toxicity. Patterns of abortive medication use should be documented to establish the need for prophylactic therapy. Prophylactic therapies also should be monitored closely (every 3-6 months until stable) for adverse reactions, abortive therapy needs, adequate dosing, and compliance. Since many individuals with migraine who receive inadequate care experience substantial levels of pain and disability, improvement in migraine diagnosis, care, and treatment potentially could result in lower direct and indirect disease costs. Consultation with other healthcare practitioners should be encouraged when changes in headache patterns or medication use occur.

CONCLUSION

Even though headache disorders result from neuronal dysfunction, the precise etiology and nature of the dysfunction are unknown. Serotonergic neurotransmission and the trigeminovascular system appear to play important roles. A careful individual workup, including patient history, physical examination, and appropriate laboratory tests, should identify most headache individuals with major disease. Various strategies can help manage migraine, tension-type, and cluster headaches to suppress acute attacks and prevent recurrences. Continuing research in existing and newly identified pathways will better define pathophysiologic mechanisms and aid the search for less toxic and more efficacious pharmacologic agents.

ABBREVIATIONS

5-HT	5-hydroxytryptamine
CGRP	calcitonin gene-related peptide
CNS	central nervous system
CYP	Cytochrome P450
FDA	Food and Drug Administration
GABA	γ-aminobutyric acid
GI	gastrointestinal
5-HT	serotonin, 5-hydroxytryptamine
IHS	International Headache Society
IM	intramuscular
IV	intravenous
MHD	monthly headache days
MMD	monthly migraine days
NSAIDs	nonsteroidal anti-inflammatory drugs
OATP	organic anion transporting polypeptides
ODT	orally disintegrating tablet
OTC	over the counter
SNRI	serotonin-norepinephrine reuptake inhibitor
SSRI	selective serotonin reuptake inhibitor
TCA	tricyclic antidepressant

REFERENCES

1. Weiss AJ, Wier LM, Stocks C, Blanchard J. Overview of emergency department visits in the United States, 2011. Statistical Brief #174. June 2014. Agency for Health Care Policy and Research, Rockville, MD. Available at: http://www.hcup-us.ahrq.gov/reports/statbriefs/sb174-Emergency-Department-Visits-Overview.pdf. Accessed August 9, 2015.

2. Headache Classification Committee of the International Headache Society. The international classification of headache disorders, 3rd ed. *Cephalalgia.* 2018;38(1):1–211.
3. Wootton RJ, Wippold FJ, Whealy MA. Evaluation of headache in adults. *UpToDate.* 2020;21:1–23. Available at: www.uptodate.com. Accessed January 1, 2021.
4. Smitherman TA, Burch RC, Sheikh H, Loder E. The prevalence, impact, and treatment of migraine and severe headaches in the United States: A review of statistics from national surveillance studies. *Headache.* 2013;53:427–436.
5. Burch RC, Rizzoli P, Loder E. The prevalence and burden of migraine and severe headache in the United States: Figures and trends from government health surveillance studies. *Headache.* 2018;58(4):496–505.
6. Steiner TJ, Birbeck GL, Jensen RH, et al. Headache disorders are third cause of disability worldwide. *J Headache Pain.* 2015;16:58.
7. Messali A, Sanderson J, Blumenfeld AM, et al. Direct and indirect costs of chronic and episodic migraine in the United States: A web-based survey. *Headache.* 2016;56:306–322.
8. Charles A. Migraine. *N Engl J Med.* 2017;377:553–561.
9. Cutrer FM. Pathophysiology, clinical manifestations, and diagnosis of migraine in adults. *UpToDate.* 2020;33:1–35. Available at: www.uptodate.com. Accessed January 1, 2021.
10. Ferrari MD. Migraine. *Lancet.* 1998;351:1043–1051.
11. Silberstein SD, Dodick DW. Migraine genetics: Part II. *Headache.* 2013;53:1218–1229.
12. Ong JJY, De Felice M. Migraine treatment: Current acute medications and their potential mechanisms of action. *Neurotherapeutics.* 2018;15:274–290.
13. Da Silva AN, Tepper SJ. Acute treatment of migraines. *CNS Drugs.* 2012;10:823–839.
14. Oswald JC, Schuster NM. Lasmiditan for the treatment of acute migraine: A review and potential role in clinical practice. *J Pain Res.* 2018;11:2221–2227.
15. Edvinsson L, Goadsby PJ. Discovery of CGRP in relation to migraine. *Cephalalgia.* 2019;39(3):331–332.
16. Lipton RB, Silberstein SD. Episodic and chronic migraine headache: Breaking down barriers to optimal treatment and prevention. *Headache.* 2015;S2:103–122.
17. Bose P, Goadsby PJ. The migraine postdrome. *Curr Opin Neurol.* 2016;29:299–301.
18. American Headache Society (AHS). AHS Consensus Statement: The AHS position statement on integrating new migraine treatments into clinical practice. *Headache.* 2019;59:1–18.
19. Marmura MJ, Silberstein SD, Schwedt TJ. The acute treatment of migraine in adults: The American Headache Society evidence assessment of migraine pharmacotherapies. *Headache.* 2015;55:3–20.
20. Smith JH. Acute treatment of migraine in adults. *UpToDate.* 2020;51:1–43. Available at: www.uptodate.com. Accessed October 18, 2021.
21. Garza I, Schwedt TJ. Medication overuse headache: Etiology, clinical features, and diagnosis. *UpToDate.* 2020;11:1–18. Available at: www.uptodate.com. Accessed January 1, 2021.
22. Garza I, Schwedt TJ. Medication overuse headache: Treatment and prognosis. *UpToDate.* 2020;14:1–23. Available at: www.uptodate.com. Accessed October 18, 2021.
23. Vandenbussche N, Laterza D, Lisicki M, et al. Medication-overuse headache: A widely recognized entity amidst ongoing debate. *J Headache Pain.* 2018;19(1):50.
24. MacGregor EA. Migraine. *Ann Intern Med.* 2013;159:ITC51.
25. Navratilova E, Behravesh S, Oyarzo J, et al. Ubrogepant does not induce latent sensitization in a preclinical model of medication overuse headache. *Cephalalgia.* 2020;40(9):892–902.
26. Silberstein SD, Holland S, Freitag F, et al. Evidence-based guideline update: Pharmacological treatment for episodic migraine prevention in adults: Report of the Quality Standards Subcommittee of the American Academy of Neurology and the American Headache Society. *Neurology.* 2012;78:1337–1345.
27. Rizzoli P. Preventive pharmacotherapy in migraine. *Headache.* 2014;54:364–369.
28. American Headache Society Position Statement on Integrating New Migraine Treatment into Clinical Practice. *Headache.* 2019;59(1):1–18.
29. Holland S, Silberstein SD, Freitag F, et al. Evidence-based guideline update: NSAIDs and other complementary treatments for episodic migraine prevention in adults: Report of the Quality Standards Subcommittee of the American Academy of Neurology and the American Headache Society. *Neurology.* 2012;78:1346–1353.
30. Marmura MJ. Triggers, projectors, and predictors in episodic migraine. *Curr Pain Headache Rep.* 2018;22(12):1–9.
31. O'Neal MA. Estrogen-associated migraine, including menstrual migraine. *UpToDate.* 2020;26:1–24. Available at: www.uptodate.com. Accessed October 18, 2021.
32. Martin PR. Behavioral management of the triggers of recurrent headache: A randomized controlled trial. *Behav Res Ther.* 2014;61:1–11.
33. Schiapparelli P, Allais G, Castagnoli Gabellari I, et al. Non-pharmacological approach to migraine prophylaxis: part II. *Neurol Sci.* 2010;31(suppl 1):S137–S139.
34. Puledda F, Shields K. Non-pharmacological approaches for migraine. *Neurotherapeutics.* 2018;15(2):336–345.
35. Finkle AG, Yerry JA, Mann D. Dietary considerations in migraine management: Does a consistent diet improve migraine? *Curr Pain Headache Rep.* 2013;17(11):373.
36. Lampl C, Voelker M, Steiner TJ. Aspirin is first-line treatment for migraine and episodic tension-type headache regardless of headache intensity. *Headache.* 2012;52:48–56.
37. Kirthi V, Derry S, Moore RA et al. Aspirin with or without an antiemetic for acute migraine headaches in adults. *Cochrane Database Syst Rev.* 2010;14(4):CD008041.
38. Triptans. Micromedex Solutions. Truven Health Analytics, Inc. Ann Arbor, MI. Available at: http://www.micromedexsolutions.com. Accessed October 18, 2021.
39. Cortelli P, Allais G, Benedetto C. Overview of triptans in the treatment of acute migraine. *Eur Neurol Rev.* 2017:12(2):71–77.
40. Ansari H, Ziad S. Drug-drug interactions in headache medicine. *Headache.* 2016;56(7):1241–1248.
41. Orlova Y, Rizzoli P, Loder E. Association of co-prescription of triptan antimigraine drug and selective norepinephrine reuptake inhibitor antidepressants with serotonin syndrome. *JAMA Neurol.* 2018;75(5):566–572.
42. Clemow DB, Johnson KW, Hochstetler HM, et al. Lasmiditan mechanism of action: Review of a selective 5-HT1F agonist. *J Headache Pain.* 2020;21(71):1–13.
43. Kuca B, Silberstein SD, Wietecha L, et al. Lasmiditan is an effective acute treatment for migraine: A phase 3 randomized study. *Neurology.* 2018;19(24):e2222–e2232.
44. Goadsby PJ, Wietecha LA, Dennehy EB, et al. Phase 3 randomized, placebo-controlled, double-blind study of lasmiditan for acute treatment of migraine. *Brain.* 2019;142(7):1894–1904.
45. Deem M, Correnti E, Kamm P, et al. Blocking CGRP in migraine patients: A review of pros and cons. *J Headache Pain.* 2017;18(96):1–9.
46. Tepper SJ. History and review of anti-calcitonin gene related peptide (CGRP) therapies: From translational research to treatment. *Headache.* 2018;58(Suppl 3):238–275.
47. Moreno-Ajona D, Chan C, Villar-Martinez MD, et al. Targeting CGRP and 5-HT1F receptors for the acute therapy of migraine: A literature review. *Headache.* 2019;59(Suppl 2):3–19.
48. Minen MT, Begasse De Dhaem O, Kroon Van Diest A, et al. Migraine and its psychiatric comorbidities. *J Neurol Neurosurg Psychiatry.* 2016;87:741–749.
49. Perloff MD, Berlin RK, Gillette M et al. Gabapentin in headache disorders: What is the evidence? *Pain Medicine.* 2016;17:162–171.
50. Ailani J, Lipton RB, Goadsby PJ et al. Atogepant for the preventative treatment of migraine. *N Eng L Med.* 2021;385:695–706.
51. Schwedt TJ, Lipton RB, Ailani J et al. Time course of efficacy of atogepant for the preventative treatment of migraine: Results from the randomized, double-blind ADVANCE trial. *Cephalalgia.* 2021;0(0):1–9.
52. Croop R, Lipton RB, Kudrow D et al. Oral rimegepant for preventative treatment of migraine: A phase 2/3, randomised, double-blind, placebo-controlled trial. *Lancet.* 2021;397(51):1–10.
53. Taylor FR. Tension-type headache in adults: Pathophysiology, clinical features, and diagnosis. *UpToDate.* 2020;14:1–25. Available at: www.uptodate.com. Accessed October 18, 2021.
54. Taylor FR. Tension-type headache in adults: Acute treatment. *UpToDate.* 2020;14:1–15. Available at: www.uptodate.com. Accessed October 18, 2021.
55. Taylor FR. Tension-type headache in adults: Preventive treatment. *UpToDate.* 2020;15:1–19. Available at: www.uptodate.com. Accessed October 18, 2021.
56. Nesbitt AD, Goadsy PJ. Cluster headache. *BMJ.* 2012;344:e2407.
57. May A. Cluster headache: Epidemiology, clinical features, and diagnosis. *UpToDate.* 2020;11:1–17. Available at: www.uptodate.com. Accessed October 18, 2021.
58. Hoffman J, May A. Diagnosis, pathophysiology, and management of cluster headache. *Lancet Neurol.* 2018;17:75–83.

59. May A. Cluster headache: Treatment and prognosis. *UpToDate*. 2020;31:1–24. Available at: www.uptodate.com. Accessed October 18, 2021.
60. Martelletti P. Cluster headache management and beyond. *Expert Opin Pharmacother.* 2015;16(10):1411–1415.
61. Tfelt-Hansen PC, Jensen RH. Management of cluster headache. *CNS Drugs*. 2012;26(7):571–580.
62. Goadsby PJ, Dodick DW, Leone M et al. Trial of galacanezumab in prevention of episode cluster headache. *N Engl J Med.* 2019;381(2):132–141.
63. Wolter T, Kaube H. Neurostimulation for chronic cluster headache. *Ther Adv Neurol Disord.* 2012;5(3):175–180.

Evaluation of Psychiatric Illness

e81

Mark E. Schneiderhan, Leigh Anne Nelson, Jeffrey R. Bishop, and Steven J. Bauer

KEY CONCEPTS

1. Patients with psychiatric conditions are treated in all healthcare settings. All clinicians should apply the basic principles of the psychiatric assessment to provide the best care.
2. The *Diagnostic and Statistical Manual of Mental Disorders,* Fifth Edition (*DSM-5*) and the Pocket Guide to the *DSM-5 Diagnostic Exam* provides clinicians with a standardized approach for the initial assessment and follow-up of patients with psychiatric conditions.
3. The World Health Organization's International Classification of Diseases and Related Health Problems (ICD) classification is currently used in all patient care settings for billing purposes.
4. Clinicians should be prepared to gather both psychiatric and physical health histories from their patients. Obtaining a release of information (ROI) from patients to communicate with other healthcare providers or significant others is often necessary when sharing protected health information (PHI).
5. Patient interviews should be conducted in an atmosphere that ensures the comfort and privacy of both the patient and the clinician. Effective listening skills and the application of open-ended questions are essential in the interview process and for building a therapeutic relationship. Motivational interviewing can empower patients to participate and help design achievable treatment goals.
6. If a patient is in crisis, the clinician may feel some apprehension about asking certain assessment questions. Knowing what specific questions to ask can help facilitate inquiry about sensitive areas, such as delusional thinking and suicidality.
7. Current and past medication histories, including allergies, adverse effects, and clinical response, are cornerstones of effective medication management. The medication history should be assessed for safety (eg, contraindications and medication interactions), tolerability (eg, adverse effects), efficacy (eg, response of target symptoms and adequate dosage and duration), and adherence (eg, affordability and the ability to take medications as prescribed).
8. Baseline mental status examination (MSE), psychiatric rating scales, and psychological/neuropsychological tests are useful tools in diagnosing and monitoring the severity of symptoms and response to treatments of psychiatric disorders.
9. Although there are no diagnostic tests for psychiatric disorders, physical and laboratory assessments can help rule out substances, medications, or medical conditions that may produce similar or overlapping symptoms.
10. Psychiatric rating scales, cognitive testing, and psychological testing provide objective measures of psychiatric symptoms, adverse effects, memory, and intellectual capacity and are often used in research and clinical settings.

BEYOND THE BOOK

Watch the following videos to learn about the mental status examination (MSE) and build your knowledge of the MSE which is an assessment commonly used in psychiatry. The "Objective" component of the S.O.A.P. acronym S (Subjective), O (Objective), A (Assessment), and P (Plan) is used to describe the physical examination in the field of medicine. In contrast, psychiatry uses the MSE as the "Objective" component to describe the patient's appearance, concentration, thoughts, and feelings. Understanding the MSE can help you identify target symptoms for psychiatric pharmacotherapy. Try completing a practice MSE on a simulated patient.

Psychiatric history and MSE tutorial:
http://www.youtube.com/watch?v=U5KwDgWX8L8
(This video describes the MSE.)

Video demonstrating components of the MSE link: http://www.youtube.com/watch?v=1HbgPhq3MzA

(This video gives examples of the MSE and offers the opportunity to complete a practice MSE.)

Self-evaluation questions:

1. When would you administer an MSE? What type of information do you get from the MSE?
2. How would you use the information obtained from the MSE to care for a patient with psychiatric illness?
3. What is the difference between the MSE and the mini-mental state examination (MMSE)?

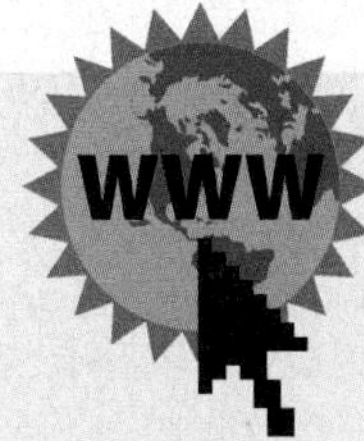

The complete chapter, learning objectives, and other resources can be found at **www.pharmacotherapyonline.com.**

82

Attention Deficit Hyperactivity Disorder

Danielle L. Stutzman, Julie A. Dopheide, and Steven Pliszka

KEY CONCEPTS

1. Untreated or ineffectively treated childhood attention deficit/hyperactivity disorder (ADHD) can lead to poor school performance, poor socialization, and increased risk for traffic accidents, psychiatric comorbidities, unemployment, and involvement with the criminal legal system during adolescence and adulthood.
2. ADHD is 74% genetic in origin and is associated with decreased brain volume, a delay in cortical maturation, and possible dysregulation of the "default mode network," a brain system that regulates attention, prioritization of information, memory, and impulse control.
3. To meet *DSM-5* diagnostic criteria for ADHD, symptoms of inattention or hyperactivity-impulsivity, separately or all together, must be present during childhood and cause functional impairment in two different settings for 6 months. Adult-onset ADHD requires further study.
4. Physical, mental health, and psychiatric comorbidities must be assessed, prior to initiating pharmacotherapy, and the goals of treatment must be set.
5. Preschoolers, school-age children, adolescents, and adults with ADHD all can benefit from nonpharmacologic interventions that include a healthy diet, education on ADHD, and potentially effective educational, cognitive, and behavioral treatments.
6. The stimulants are the most effective pharmacologic treatment option for all ages with a rapid therapeutic effect, typically within 1 or 2 hours of an effective dose. Methylphenidate is recommended as first-line for children and adolescents while amphetamines are first-line treatment for adults based on efficacy and tolerability.
7. Alpha-2 adrenergic agonists such as extended-release preparations of guanfacine and clonidine are less effective than stimulants as monotherapy and are used in combination with stimulants or as monotherapy in youth to improve symptom control, particularly oppositional behaviors and insomnia.
8. When ADHD coexists with other neuropsychiatric conditions, such as anxiety disorders, major depression, autism spectrum disorder (ASD), or Tourette disorder, it is optimal to treat the most functionally impairing disorder first (whether it is ADHD or the co-occurring condition) and then treat the second disorder.
9. When ADHD coexists with bipolar disorder, it is necessary to first stabilize the mood with lithium, an antiseizure medication (or mood stabilizer), or a second generation antipsychotic before adding an ADHD-specific medication such as a stimulant.
10. Atomoxetine is a good option to manage ADHD symptoms in adolescents or adults with substance use disorders or when stimulants are intolerable. It has a delayed onset of effect (2–4 weeks) and has no potential for physical dependence. Viloxazine has similarities with delayed onset and also lacks physical dependence potential, but it requires further study compared to atomoxetine and stimulants to fully assess its place in therapy.

BEYOND THE BOOK

Watch the approximately 7-minute video (Video link) by an ADHD researcher and a child psychiatrist, Dr. Steven R. Pliszka, as he provides an example of a typical interview with a child undergoing evaluation for ADHD and he discusses the clinical assessment of ADHD. An ADHD diagnostic rating tool is used to collect and document information from the child utilized in the diagnostic assessment. Versions of validated diagnostic rating tools for parents and teachers are routinely utilized for diagnostic formulation as well. The video is useful to enhance student understanding regarding the COLLECT and ASSESS steps in the patient care process for managing ADHD.

INTRODUCTION

Once considered primarily a childhood disorder, attention deficit/hyperactivity disorder (ADHD) is now known to persist into adolescence for 75% and into adulthood for approximately 50% of individuals.[1,2] The American Academy of Pediatrics (AAP) considers ADHD a chronic condition that requires ongoing management.[3-5] ADHD has been correlated with neuroanatomical and functional brain changes that functionally result in inattention, impulsivity, and hyperactivity.[6,7] It is unusual for an individual to display signs of the disorder in all settings or even in the same setting at all times; however, there is a persistent pattern of symptoms that continues for 6 months or more.[1,7] Co-occurring anxiety, mood disorders, learning disabilities, medical conditions, and substance use disorders (SUDs) must be considered during assessment and treatment. Behavioral interventions and medications are effective for all ages, but there are special treatment plan considerations when developing and monitoring each age group.[3-5,8]

(1) The psychiatric assessment of a child requires obtaining information from the child, parents, caregivers, and teachers.[1,5,9] Treating children with psychotropic medications requires a different approach than treating adults. Children undergo neurologic, physiologic, and psychosocial changes throughout development. Age-related pharmacodynamic and pharmacokinetic differences

can alter drug disposition and response. Psychotropic medication treatment of children is intended to control symptoms or behaviors that impair learning and development.[1,5,9] Children may not be able to articulate symptom response or adverse effects of a medication. Adolescents and adults with ADHD may not have been diagnosed and treated during childhood, putting them at greater risk for the psychosocial consequences of ADHD, including unemployment, unstable relationships, substance abuse, and incarceration.[1,2,5,10,11]

EPIDEMIOLOGY

ADHD is the most well-known and researched neurodevelopmental disorder of childhood and occurs in approximately 5% to 10% of children and approximately 2.5% to 5% of adults.[12-14] Non-Hispanic Caucasian and African-American children are more likely diagnosed with ADHD compared with children of Hispanic or Asian descent according to CDC and National Children's Health survey data.[12,15] It is more prevalent in males than females with a ratio of 2:1 in children and 1.6:1 in adults.[1] In 2016, 6.1 million children in the United States or 9.4% of those aged 2 to 17 years were diagnosed with ADHD: almost twice the actual rate according to worldwide prevalence studies and the *Diagnostic and Statistical Manual of Mental Disorders* (*DSM-5*).[1,5,16] Methodological inconsistencies in diagnostic assessments likely contribute to increasing diagnosis and differences in prevalence rates internationally. Investigators evaluating 135 ADHD prevalence studies representing seven regions (North America, South America, Europe, Asia, Africa, Oceania, and the Middle East) found when consistent diagnostic criteria from the *DSM-5* are applied, the prevalence of ADHD for children and adolescents is similar among countries globally, at approximately 5.5%.[5,13,14,16] There is increasing concern among healthcare professionals and the public regarding the overdiagnosis of ADHD leading to stigmatization and potentially inappropriate treatment.[5]

Increasing rates of ADHD diagnosis in the United States is likely a factor associated with the observed increased prescribing of ADHD medications. In 2016, the US Centers for Disease Control (CDC.gov) reported that 2 million of the 6.1 million children with ADHD were first diagnosed at 2 to 5 years of age.[12,16] Of concern is the mode of treatment for these toddlers, as CDC data showed three out of four 2- to 5-year-olds with ADHD were prescribed medications and only one out of two were prescribed behavioral interventions. The AAP recommends a 6-month trial of behavioral classroom interventions and parent training in behavioral management prior to pharmacotherapy in children less than 6 years old.[12,16] In addition to young children, adolescents and young adults are increasingly being diagnosed with ADHD. A large US pharmacy benefits management company, Express Script's, analysis of pharmacy claims representing 400,000 privately insured individuals younger than 65 years, showed that ADHD medication use increased by 35.5% for all age groups between 2008 and 2012. In addition, while the number of adults using ADHD medications was up 53.4% from 2008 to 2012, children still received a higher percentage of ADHD prescriptions compared to adults and 80% of these were stimulants.[17] In 2015, 4% of privately insured females ages 15 to 44 filled a prescription for an ADHD medication, most often a stimulant such as amphetamine salts or methylphenidate. This represents a 344% increase in ADHD medication prescribing in 2015 compared to 2003. Over the same time period, filled prescriptions for nonstimulant ADHD medications did not increase.[18]

Therefore, healthcare professionals and teachers should recommend a thorough assessment of ADHD by an experienced clinician using standardized criteria and investigating all possible causes of inattention, impulsivity, and hyperactivity in order to avoid overdiagnosis and potentially inappropriate treatment.

ETIOLOGY AND PATHOPHYSIOLOGY

2 There has been substantial progress in understanding the role of both genetics and the environment, as well as their interaction, in the pathophysiology of ADHD. An extensive review of twin studies over the past 40 years has shown that the heritability of ADHD (the amount of variance in ADHD symptoms attributable to genetics) averages around 74%.[19] The most extensive genome-wide association study (GWAS) to date was a meta-analysis of 12 studies comparing 20,183 persons with ADHD and 35,191 controls.[20] This study discovered 12 regions that achieved genome-wide significance with *none* of the genes identified in previous candidate gene studies (ie, dopamine transporter) being significant.[19] It remains to be seen exactly how the newly identified genes might be involved in ADHD. Despite the size of the study, all 12 loci identified accounted for only 22% of the genetic variance as the remaining ~50% of the heritability is "missing."[19]

Some of the missing heritability may occur because patients have copies or deletions in the genome that cover multiple genes called copy number variants (CNVs). Current CNV studies have implicated a number of systems in ADHD: cholinergic receptors and genes for central nervous system (CNS) development[21] and an area of chromosome 15q13.[22] The CNVs affecting the metabotropic glutamatergic receptor 5 gene were enriched in cohorts of patients with ADHD relative to controls.[23]

Increasingly, there is clear evidence that genes involved in ADHD are also involved in other major psychiatric disorders, including schizophrenia, and affective (mood) disorders.[25] A significant genetic correlation has been found between ADHD and autism spectrum disorder (ASD) in a large GWAS of individuals with ASD.[26] Thus, genes for neurodevelopmental disorders are not specific to ADHD and may show considerable pleiotropy (one gene influences two or more seemingly unrelated phenotypic traits).[27]

Since gene by environment interaction may also be important, it is critical to examine environmental factors. Twin studies can estimate the amount of variance related to the environment and further subdivide environmental effects into "shared" (an event both twins experience, such as neighborhood) and "non-shared" (one twin has a head injury, the other does not). Surprisingly, shared environmental factors do not appear to have a relationship to ADHD symptoms.[28] In an Australian population-based control study, over 12,000 children with ADHD were compared to over 30,000 controls on maternal, pregnancy, and birth data.[29] Mothers of children with ADHD were significantly more likely to be younger, single, or to have smoked in pregnancy. Additionally, they had a higher level of induced labor, preterm labor, preeclampsia, or early term delivery. Antidepressant use in pregnancy is not related to ADHD,[30] and in an extensive review of prenatal factors in ADHD, Sciberras et al.[31] noted that carefully done prospective studies are needed to determine causality of these factors.

2 Genetics and environment work together to shape the brain, and there is an emerging picture of differences in brain structure, function, and connectivity that occur across the life span in individuals with ADHD. Cortical surface area is reduced in ADHD versus controls in both childhood and adulthood; in addition, the age of peak thickness occurs later in ADHD, with the most pronounced delay occurring in the prefrontal cortex.[32] Cortical thickness is also reduced in children with ADHD relative to controls, but when adults with ADHD remit, their cortical thickness is not different from controls.[33] There is evidence that the continued use of stimulants for the treatment of ADHD is associated with greater normalization of cortical thickness.[34] Reduced cerebellar volume is the most pronounced difference in ADHD versus controls.[35] The ENIGMA ADHD study obtained structural MRI in 1,713 individuals with ADHD and 1,529 controls, both children and adults.[36] Subcortical structures (accumbens, amygdala, caudate, hippocampus, and putamen) were reduced

in those with ADHD relative to controls, with effect sizes of around 0.2. Effects were larger in children than adults. In totality, the structural imaging data suggest ADHD is caused by a wide scale process affecting many regions of the brain.

2 Functional MRI has shown that the brains of children with ADHD fail to activate a network of regions involved in attention and impulse control relative to controls.[37] During inhibitory tasks, children with ADHD fail to activate the right inferior frontal cortex and anterior cingulate cortex. When performing attention tasks, children with ADHD have reduced activation in the basal ganglia, prefrontal cortex, and parietal lobe, while they have increased activation of cuneus. There is increasing interest in the role of the default mode network (DMN) in many psychiatric disorders.[38] The DMN consists of the medial prefrontal cortex, medial parietal lobe, or precuneus, as well as the posterior cingulate. These areas are active during the "resting state" when attention is not engaged; this system is actively suppressed during active attention. A lack of connectivity between the prefrontal cortex and precuneus is associated with failure of suppression of the DMN, causing lapses in attention and inhibitory control. Multiple studies have shown that both children and adults diagnosed with ADHD, DMN activity is not appropriately connected to the attention/control areas compared to controls.[38-40] Treatment with stimulants normalizes DMN activity.[39] Functional MRI can be used to assess general connectivity between a large number of brain regions. A major review showed that children with ADHD have stronger short-range connections (particularly with limbic areas) than controls, but reduced number of long-range connections in the attention and control systems of the brain.[41]

Overall, ADHD is a complex neurodevelopmental disorder involving an array of genetic and environmental risk factors, many of which are shared with other psychiatric disorders. Clinicians can help families to better understand ADHD and minimize its negative impact on outcomes. More background information regarding pharmacogenomics can be found in Chapter e6, "Pharmacogenetics."

CLINICAL PRESENTATION

3 The AAP guideline for the diagnosis, evaluation, and treatment of ADHD in children and adolescents recommends an evaluation for any child between ages 4 and 18 years who presents with academic or behavioral problems and symptoms of inattention, hyperactivity, or impulsivity.[3] The *DSM-5* diagnosis in children 4 to 12 years old only requires at least six symptoms of inattention or hyperactivity and impulsivity causing impairment in more than one major setting (eg, home, school) for 6 months and an onset of symptoms before age 12. Only five symptoms are required for older adolescents and adults (age 17 and over).[1] Validated rating scales, such as the Connors Rating Scales—revised (CRS-revised) and the Vanderbilt ADHD diagnostic scale, are recommended for objective symptom ratings from parents and teachers in different age groups. (See Chapter e81 for more information.)[3-5] To make a diagnosis of ADHD, the clinician should rule out alternative causes of symptoms (eg, learning disability, situational stressor) and assess for other conditions that may coexist with ADHD including oppositional defiant and conduct disorders (CDs), Tourette disorder, ASD, and sleep and mood disorders.[1,3-5,42]

Preschoolers (3 to 5 Years)

Preschool-age onset of ADHD may be more likely in children with multiple risk factors including maternal smoking, lead exposure, iron deficiency, developmental delay, ASD, intellectual disability, or genetic loading.[43,44] The *DSM-5* diagnostic criteria for ADHD can be applied to preschool-age children, although it may be difficult to document symptoms in multiple settings with different caregivers if the child does

CLINICAL PRESENTATION ADHD

General

- Onset of symptoms must be before 12 years of age

Symptoms

- *Inattention:*
  - Often fails to give close attention to details or makes careless mistakes in schoolwork, at work, or during other activities (eg, overlooks or misses details, or work is inaccurate)
  - Often has difficulty sustaining attention in play activities or tasks (eg, has difficulty remaining focused during lectures, conversations, or lengthy reading)
  - Often has difficulty organizing tasks and activities (eg, poor time management, disorganized work, fails to meet deadlines)
  - Avoids tasks that require sustained mental effort (eg, schoolwork, reviewing lengthy papers, or preparing reports)
  - Often does not seem to listen when spoken to directly (eg, mind seems to wander)
  - Often does not follow through on instructions and fails to finish schoolwork, chores, or duties in the workplace
  - Is easily distracted by extraneous stimuli (may include unrelated thoughts)
  - Is often forgetful in daily activities (eg, doing chores, returning calls, paying bills)
  - Loses things necessary for activities (eg, school materials, keys, wallet)
- *Hyperactivity and impulsivity:*
  - Often fidgets with hands or feet or squirms in seat
  - Often leaves seat when remaining seated is expected
  - Often runs about or climbs excessively at inappropriate times (in adolescents or adults may be limited to feeling restless)
  - Often has difficulty playing quietly
  - Often blurts out answers before a question is completed (also finishes the sentences of others; cannot wait for turn in conversation)
  - Often interrupts or intrudes on others; may take over what others are doing
- Six or more symptoms must be present for at least 6 months; significant impairment must be seen in two or more settings (eg, home and school); symptoms must be documented by parent, teacher, and clinician. Only five symptoms are required in older adolescents and adults (17 years of age and older)

Data from Reference 166.

not attend preschool.[1,3,12,44] Enrollment in a qualified preschool and a parent training program is often recommended. Both can help parents develop reasonable expectations for their child's development and foster the development of management skills for problem behaviors while diagnostic assessment is underway.

School Age (6 to 11 Years)

Most cases of ADHD are first realized during ages 6 to 9 years, with the child having difficulty academically and/or socially in school and at home. Most children have combined inattentive and hyperactive or impulsive symptoms that cause functional impairment. This period is crucial to the child's success in school, socialization, and the development of his or her sense of self; therefore, accurate diagnosis and treatment are critical. Comorbid oppositional defiant disorder (ODD), CD, and aggression are indicators that the child is at greater risk for issues with the criminal legal system and an SUD in adolescence.[8,10,45] This is the most well-studied age group, with strong data showing benefits of recognition and treatment with behavioral interventions and medications.[4,5]

Adolescents (12 to 18 Years)

Hyperactivity decreases in adolescents, and inattention and impulsivity are the more prominent. There may be fewer numbers of symptoms of ADHD in adolescence, but the symptoms present cause significant functional impairment.[1,8,10] Adolescents with ADHD are increasingly identified as "moody" or having a temper. They are easily overwhelmed by demands and may avoid tasks or approach multiple tasks in a disorganized manner.[8] Decision making is impaired (eg, discontinues ADHD treatment despite functional impairment) and decisions are made based on peer approval.[8] Higher rates of delinquency, substance and alcohol use, and psychiatric comorbidity have been documented in adolescents with ADHD compared with those without ADHD.[3,4,10,11,46] Assessment for substance use and risk of diversion must be considered before starting stimulant medication.[8,46] Speeding and increased motor vehicle accidents occur at higher rates in teens with ADHD compared to those without the disorder.[8,47]

Adults

The presence of multiple comorbid conditions, particularly CD or mood disorder, can increase the likelihood of ADHD chronicity into adulthood. *DSM-5* criteria for ADHD in childhood and adolescence also apply to adults. Inattentive symptoms are the most common and functionally impairing in adults, but hyperactive/restless and impulsive symptoms such as being overly talkative, impatient, and intrusive are experienced by many and are associated with higher rates of bipolar disorder and psychosis.[1,2,10,11,48] Cognitive deficits (eg, executive functioning, working memory, task prioritization, lower IQ) have been documented in adults with ADHD in addition to a greater risk for unstable relationships, unemployment, psychiatric hospitalization, and interaction with the criminal legal system compared with those without ADHD.[2,10,11,48] In 2017, the World Health Organization published a six-item questionnaire to update the Adult ADHD Self-Report Scale (ASRS) with *DSM-5* diagnostic criteria. This validated screening tool can be used as a first step to a more thorough diagnosis with an experienced clinician.[2,49] Gathering collateral information from family and friends is recommended to either support or refute the diagnosis.

Adult-Onset ADHD

Adult-onset ADHD is increasingly recognized although still controversial. A Brazilian study evaluated 5,249 youth in 1993 at age 11 and found 393 (8.9%) met criteria for ADHD. Evaluation of the group in 2015 at age 18 to 19 years revealed 492 (12.2%) youth who had no symptoms in childhood, now meeting criteria for ADHD.[50] Interestingly, the childhood-onset group was predominantly male and the young adult-onset group was predominantly female. Both groups had increased levels of impairment (eg, comorbidities, involved with the criminal justice system, suicide attempts) compared to those without ADHD. United Kingdom investigators studied 2,040 twins longitudinally between 1994 and 2015. In adulthood, 166 met criteria for ADHD and 111 of whom (67%) had no symptoms during childhood.[51] Adult-onset ADHD raises many questions about potential causes (eg, cannabis use, alcohol use, chronic anxiety), diagnostic categorization, and treatment. Is young adult-onset ADHD a different brain disorder with similar symptoms to childhood-onset ADHD; is the course different? More research is needed.

Complex ADHD

A person is said to have "Complex ADHD" when there is moderate-to-severe functional impairment, diagnostic uncertainty, coexisting conditions (eg, neurodevelopmental, mental health, medical, or psychosocial factors adversely affecting health and development), inadequate response to treatment or when functionally impairing symptoms present before age 4, or after age 12. The Society for Developmental and Behavioral Pediatrics developed this designation to encourage expert evaluation and treatment of these individuals beyond usual care.[52]

TREATMENT

Stimulants are considered first-line therapy in most cases of ADHD; however, age, comorbid conditions, and patient/family preference impact treatment plan development. Pharmacotherapy should be considered whenever a thorough diagnostic assessment results in an ADHD diagnosis. ADHD-specific educational, cognitive, and behavioral interventions are recognized as necessary components of an overall treatment plan aimed at symptom relief and optimal functioning. Several studies show combining medications with behavioral interventions produces the greatest symptom relief and the best outcomes.[2-4,17,53]

Desired Outcomes

4 Specific goals of treatment or desired outcomes must be identified (eg, able to sit in chair for 20 minutes, completes homework assignments, or no longer blurts out comments in class without being called upon).[3,42] For adults, the desired outcome may be to read an entire newspaper before starting another project, improving safety while driving or successfully completing tasks on time at school or at work.[2,8,48]

Treatment for ADHD may decrease the rate of some serious injuries in youth. Investigators evaluated a large German healthcare database (reflecting 20% of the population) and found that in children with ADHD aged 3 to 17 years, treated with a stimulant or atomoxetine, there was no difference in overall injury rates requiring hospital admission compared to untreated children; however, there was a 34% decrease in severe brain injury in the treated group.[54] Similarly, an international review and meta-analysis of about 13,000 youth found that pharmacologic treatment in pediatric patients with ADHD likely has a protective effect, with a 10% reduction in the incidence of any unintentional injury. Of note, traumatic brain injury was excluded as an endpoint, given the potential to increase a patient's likelihood for being diagnosed with ADHD.[55]

Improvement in academic performance and on-task behavior in the classroom has been associated with stimulant treatment of ADHD.[56] A study of 930 young adults with ADHD found that treatment with pharmacotherapy (eg, stimulants and atomoxetine) was associated with significantly improved scores on higher education

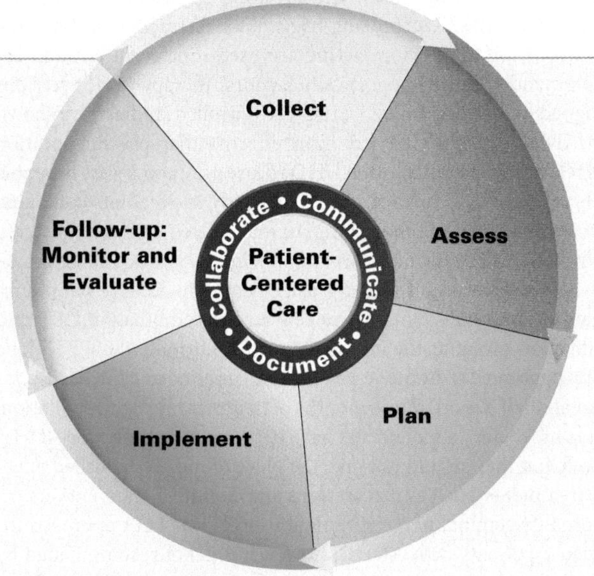

Patient Care Process for Attention Deficit/ Hyperactivity Disorder (ADHD)

Collect

- Patient characteristics (eg, age, gender, sex, pregnancy status)
- Social and family history (eg, foster care, single parent home, extended family involvement; marital status for adults)
- Substance use history (eg, cigarettes, cannabis, alcohol, methamphetamine, hallucinogens, cocaine, opioids, kratom, salvia)
- Dietary issues (eg, "picky" eater, gluten-sensitive, food allergies)
- Sleep patterns (eg, latency, duration, restless legs)
- Current medications including OTCs, herbal products, dietary supplements, and prior medications for ADHD
- Cardiovascular health history (eg, history of sudden death in family)
- Goals of treatment (eg, finish homework assignments or work projects, prevent injury, await turn in lines, positive peer/family interactions)
- Information on past and current co-occurring neuropsychiatric conditions (eg, Tourette disorder, CD, bipolar disorder, ASD, epilepsy)
- Objective data
  - Measure symptoms of ADHD with validated rating scales for children or adolescents (eg, Conners, Vanderbilt) and ADHD self-rating questionnaire for adults
  - Gather information on symptoms in multiple settings (eg, school, work, home)
  - Blood pressure (BP), heart rate (HR), respiratory rate (RR), height, weight, body mass index (BMI), growth chart data on percentiles based on general pediatric population
  - Labs including liver function tests (LFTs), electrolytes, renal function, fasting lipid panel, and HgA1c, thyroid tests if co-occurring anxiety or mood symptoms, ECG and/or echocardiogram if history reveals significant cardiovascular disease or sudden unexplained death in family member, and pregnancy status in females

Assess

- Number and predominance of symptoms (eg, are inattentive symptoms the only significant symptom?)
- Severity of symptoms (eg, hyperactivity, impulsivity, and inattention) and associated functional impairment
- Presence and severity of co-occurring conditions (eg, Tourette disorder, CD, bipolar disorder, ASD)
- Presence of active SUD in patient and family members
- Presence of adverse reactions from current medications (Tables 80-3 and 80-4)
- Ability/willingness to participate in nonpharmacologic treatment including psychosocial, cognitive, and behavioral interventions
- Identify barriers to adherence to pharmacotherapeutic interventions and participation in ongoing treatment (eg, cost, frequency of medication administration throughout the day, transportation challenges to follow-up appointments)

Plan*

- Medication therapy regimen including specific medication(s), dose, route, frequency, and duration (Tables 80-2 through 80-4 and Fig. 82-1)
- Monitoring parameters including efficacy (eg, decreased symptoms on rating scales) and safety (eg, heart rate, blood pressure, abnormal involuntary movements); frequency and timing of follow-up (Tables 80-3 and 80-4)
- Patient education (eg, purpose of treatment, dietary and lifestyle modification, medication-specific information, medication administration)
- Referrals to other providers when appropriate (eg, pediatrician, dietician)

Implement*

- Provide patient, parent, caregiver(s), teacher, partner education regarding all elements of treatment plan; education should be delivered in multiple forms (Table 82-1)
- Use motivational interviewing and coaching strategies to maximize adherence
- Schedule follow-up appointment for monitoring and pharmacotherapy dosage adjustment (Tables 80-1 through 80-3)

Follow-up: Monitor and Evaluate

- Significant improvement in ADHD symptoms (eg, inattention, hyperactivity, impulsivity)
- Presence of adverse effects (eg, insomnia/sedation, appetite change, increased or decreased HR)
- Presence of significant medication interactions (eg, fluoxetine and atomoxetine, or paroxetine and amphetamine salts)
- Patient adherence to treatment plan using multiple sources of information
- Re-evaluate dosage and tolerability every 1 to 3 months

**Collaborate with patient, caregiver(s), and other healthcare professionals.*

entrance exams compared to never-medicated peers.[57] Review of the Icelandic Medicines Registry and the Database of National Scholastic Examinations revealed that delayed initiation of pharmacologic treatment may be associated with academic decline among youth age 9 to 12 years, particularly in math.[58] Additionally, other studies have demonstrated improvement in math productivity, accuracy, and reading speed with methylphenidate treatment, although academic improvements were thought to be small compared to overall symptom improvement.[59]

Nonpharmacologic Therapy

Educational, Psychosocial, Cognitive, and Behavioral Interventions

5 Education that ADHD is a biologic disorder with brain-derived causes is essential for destigmatizing ADHD and improving treatment acceptance. Parent training and behavioral interventions such as positive rewards for good behavior and structured limit setting are recommended as first-line interventions before medication trials in preschoolers (3- to 5-year-olds) with ADHD. Behavioral interventions for ADHD are described in Table 82-1. It is crucial to get parents, teachers, and clinicians involved to coordinate care and provide consistent behavioral management for the child at home and at school. Although methylphenidate has been found safe and effective for ADHD in 4- and 5-year-olds, behavioral interventions are recommended first by most clinicians and guidelines.[3,60] School-age children (6-11 years) also benefit from these behavioral interventions in addition to strategies, such as breaking up homework assignments into shorter, manageable segments. Although it varies by state, children and adolescents with ADHD may qualify for an individualized educational program (IEP) that allows for more time to take an exam, preferred seating, and modified work assignments.[3,4,45] It is noteworthy that most studies comparing behavioral intervention with stimulant therapy in youth found a much stronger effect on ADHD core symptoms from stimulants.[4,5,7,61] Combined behavioral and stimulant therapy resulted in greater improvements on academic and conduct measures in some studies with greater parent and teacher satisfaction ratings. Lower doses of stimulant were effective when behavioral interventions were administered according to several studies.[4,62]

5 Recommended behavioral interventions for adolescents and adults include keeping an external organizer (eg, smart phone, notebook with "to-do" lists) and breaking up activities into short, manageable tasks. Recognizing triggers for distraction and making a point of thinking before acting are useful interventions and are recommended during cognitive behavioral therapy (CBT) sessions designed to manage adult ADHD.[53,63] Controlled studies have shown that ADHD-specific CBT was more effective than psychoeducation and relaxation in adults with ADHD whose symptoms were only partially responsive to medication.[63] One study in 88 adults compared 12 weekly sessions (1.5 hour long) of manualized CBT administered with a long-acting formulation of methylphenidate or amphetamine salts to CBT alone and found greater benefit in ADHD symptoms, organizational skills, and self-esteem in the combination CBT and medication group at the end of 12 weeks. Of note, the CBT alone group continued to improve according to unblinded clinician assessment and self-report after 6 months of treatment.[53] Yoga, meditation, and some dietary supplements have been recommended for ADHD as well, but they should not take the place of more established effective treatments, such as medications and cognitive interventions.[61,64] External trigeminal nerve stimulation (eTNS) is FDA approved for pediatric patients with ADHD; however, it is not recommended by the AAP guidelines given lack of long-term safety and efficacy data.[3]

TABLE 82-1 Cognitive, Behavioral, and Psychosocial Interventions for ADHD

Age	Description of Intervention	Typical Outcomes
Preschool and school age	Parent and family education on ADHD	Improved parental understanding and satisfaction
	Parent/caregiver training on behavioral management	Improved compliance with parental commands
	Classroom management instruction for teachers	Improved teacher satisfaction
Adolescent	Breakup homework assignments into manageable segments. Structured schedule; organizer	Completion of assignments improves; improved self-esteem and sense of self
Adolescent and adult	ADHD-specific cognitive behavioral therapy	Improved productivity and vocational success
	Metacognitive therapy	Improved relationships

ADHD, attention deficit/hyperactivity disorder.

Data from References 3, 5, 42, 53, 60, 61, and 63.

Dietary Interventions

Extensive research has evaluated dietary interventions for ADHD, primarily in children with some adolescent data. Omega-3 fatty acids are the most studied dietary intervention for ADHD. While studies have demonstrated variable impact on core ADHD symptoms, omega-3 supplementation is generally well tolerated and has demonstrated and effect size of approximately 0.3.[65] High eicosapentaenoic acid (EPA) to docosahexaenoic acid (DHA) ration may be associated with the largest effect.[65]

When iron and zinc are supplemented in youth with known deficiencies, the therapeutic benefit of stimulant therapy can be enhanced, frequently allowing lower effective doses.[66-68] Vitamin D may also improve symptoms of ADHD, particularly in youth with deficiencies according to a randomized double-blind trial in 96 children of mean age 9 years old.[69]

The role of gingko biloba, Memoemet syrup, and other complementary and alternative products has also been evaluated, with variable efficacy and tolerability.[5] While some evidence is promising, ongoing evaluations are needed before recommending these products, given variability in study design (eg, use of concomitant pharmacotherapy, rating scales to assess symptom improvement, and variability among products used). While it has been anecdotally suggested that cannabidiol oil is beneficial for ADHD, it has not been rigorously studied for core symptoms and is not recommended.[3]

Although scientific evidence is lacking, there is a universal belief among families that the avoidance of sugar and artificial sweeteners improves ADHD symptoms. The attention paid to sugar avoidance and healthy diet is the more likely reason for improved behavior. An overall healthy diet with the proper balance of protein, fresh produce, and fiber is recommended.[12,17,61,66]

Pharmacologic Therapy

Figure 82-1 is an algorithm for medication selection in the treatment of ADHD.

Several studies demonstrate the superiority of stimulants over other pharmacotherapies and behavioral interventions in alleviating core symptoms of ADHD in schoolage children, adolescents, and adults.[5,17,60] Although the United Kingdom's 2018 National Institute for Health and Care Excellence (NICE) guidelines recommend considering medication as early as 5 years of age, the clinician needs to weigh the risks of starting medication at an early age against the harm of delaying diagnosis and treatment.[3,4,42,44] Clinicians should educate all parents and caregivers regarding realistic expectations of medication therapy, goals of treatment, and the need for adverse

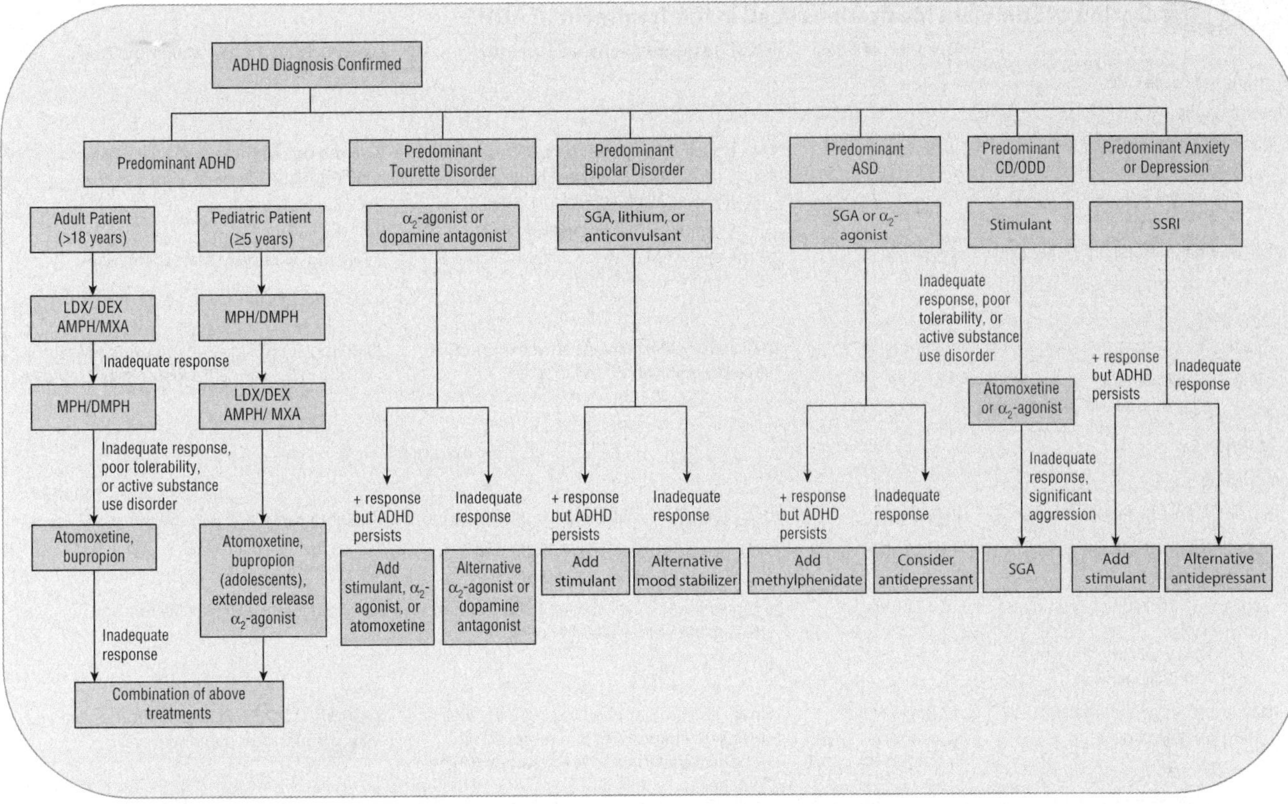

FIGURE 82-1 Algorithm for medication selection in the management of attention deficit/hyperactivity disorder (ADHD). Treat predominant disorder first, reassess, and consider alternative or adjunct medications for optimal symptom control. (AMPH, amphetamine; DEX, dextroamphetamine; DMPH, dexmethylphenidate; LDX, lisdexamfetamine; MPH, methylphenidate; MXA, mixed amphetamine salts; SSRI, selective serotonin reuptake inhibitor; TCA, tricyclic antidepressant.)
(Data from References 2, 5, 45, 60, and 70–77.)

effect monitoring in children. Adolescents and adults should be actively engaged in shared decision making regarding medication therapy and monitoring in an attempt to improve treatment persistence. Studies show higher rates of medication non-adherence in adolescents (50%) and adults (30%) compared to children (10–30%).[8] Preventing misuse and diversion of stimulants through frequent communication with patients and family, the use of a controlled substance agreement, and by tracking state-wide prescription medication monitoring databases is recommended.[2]

Stimulants

Stimulants are broadly divided into two main chemical classes: methylphenidate (includes dexmethylphenidate) and amphetamines (includes dextroamphetamine and mixed amphetamine salts). Methylphenidate and amphetamines block presynaptic dopamine and norepinephrine reuptake; amphetamines also increase dopamine release.[7,78] Both medications inhibit monoamine oxidase (MAO), amphetamines more potently than methylphenidate.[78] Because different stimulants work through slightly different mechanisms, the lack of response to one chemical class of stimulant (eg, methylphenidate or dexmethylphenidate) does not preclude response to another class (eg, mixed amphetamine salts, dextroamphetamine, or lisdexamfetamine).[7]

6 Stimulants are the most effective medication treatment options, with a pooled average effect size of 0.7 to 1.0. This is in contrast to nonstimulant medication treatment options such as guanfacine, clonidine, and atomoxetine whose effect sizes range from 0.35 to 0.7 signifying lower efficacy.[4,71,74] A systematic review and meta-analysis of 133 double-blind randomized controlled trials (81 in children and adolescents [$n = 11{,}018$], 51 in adults [$n = 5{,}362$], 1 in both) was conducted to assess the efficacy and tolerability of ADHD pharmacotherapy over 12 weeks in different age groups. Overall, the analysis showed stimulants were more effective than nonstimulant medications in all ages; however, stimulants were not as effective in adults compared to children and adolescents.[71]

Among children and adolescents, all approved ADHD medications were superior to placebo (clinician report), with amphetamines superior to methylphenidate, modafinil, atomoxetine, and guanfacine. Methylphenidate was superior to atomoxetine. Per teacher report, only methylphenidate and modafinil were superior to placebo. Guanfacine and amphetamines were less well tolerated than placebo, with amphetamines demonstrating a significant increase in systolic blood pressure and weight loss among children and adolescents, more than methylphenidate.

Because the largest analysis of clinical trial data showed overall better tolerability with methylphenidate in children and adolescents compared to amphetamine compounds, many clinicians recommend methylphenidate first-line in younger age groups. Nonetheless, amphetamine may be used first-line if patient and clinician prefer it.

In contrast to recommendations for pediatric patients, an amphetamine compound is preferred over methylphenidate as a first-line medication for adults based on the analysis of 12-week trials showing greater efficacy and acceptable tolerability of amphetamine compounds in adults versus pediatric patients.[71] In adults, amphetamines, methylphenidate, bupropion, and atomoxetine were superior to both placebo and modafinil. Modafinil did not demonstrate superiority in adults. With the exception of bupropion, all agents in adults were less well tolerated than placebo.[71]

Stimulant dosing should be titrated for maximum individual efficacy and minimum adverse medication reactions[4,5,7,42] (Table 82-2).

TABLE 82-2 Dosing of Stimulant Medications Used in the Treatment of ADHD

Stimulant	Duration of Effect	Initial Dose and Available Strengths	Usual Dosing Range; Maximum Dose
Methylphenidate C-II[a]			
Short-acting IR			
Ritalin, methylin, generics[b]	3-5 hours	5 mg two or three times daily; increase by 5-10 or 20 mg/day at weekly intervals; available as 5, 10, and 20 mg tablets; 5 mg/mL and 10 mg/5 mL solution	5-20 mg two or three times daily; Max: 60 mg/day
Dexmethylphenidate (Focalin) C-II	3-5 hours	2.5 mg every AM or twice daily; available as 2.5, 5, and 10 mg tablets	2.5-10 mg twice daily; Max: 20 mg/day
Intermediate-acting			
Ritalin SR[b] Methylphenidate SR[b] Metadate ER[b] Methylin ER[b]	3-8 hours	20 mg every AM; increase at weekly intervals; available only as 20 mg tablets	20-40 mg every AM or 40 mg every AM and 20 mg in the early afternoon; Max: 60 mg/day
Long-acting			
Ritalin LA 50% IR, 50% ER beads[b]	8-10 hours	20 mg every AM; available as 10, 20, and 30 mg	20-60 mg every AM; Max: 60 mg/day
Metadate CD 30% IR, 70% ER beads[b]	10-12 hours	20 mg every AM; available as 20, 30, and 40 mg	
Concerta (OROS controlled-release delivery)[b] *ER inner compartments coated with IR methylphenidate*	10-12 hours	18 mg every AM; available as 18, 27, 36, and 54 mg; 90% bioavailability of IR	27-72 mg every AM; Max: 72 mg/day
Daytrana methylphenidate transdermal system[b]	12 hours when worn for 9 hours	10 mg (12.5 cm^2) applied to clean, dry area on hip each morning and removed after 9 hours; available as 10, 15, 20, and 30 mg patches	10-30 mg (12.5-37.5 cm^2). Medication active for 3 hours after patch removal
Aptensio XR 40% IR, 60% ER	10-12 hours	10 mg; available as 10, 20, 30, 40, 50, and 60 mg capsules	10-60 mg every AM; Max: 60 mg/day
Cotempla XR-ODT 25% IR, 75% ER[b]	10-12 hours	17.3 mg every AM; available as 8.6, 17.3, 25.9 mg oral disintegrating tablets	17.3-51.8 mg every AM; Max: 51.8 mg/day
Quillivant extended-release suspension 20% IR/80% ER[b] *Must be reconstituted by pharmacist to 25 mg/5 mL concentration. Stable for 4 months after reconstituted*	10-12 hours	10-20 mg in AM; available as 25 mg/5 mL suspension *Only studied in 6- to 12-year-olds*	20-60 mg every AM; Max: 60 mg/day
QuilliChew ER 30% IR, 70% ER	10-12 hours	10-20 mg in AM; available as 20, 30, and 40 mg tablets	
Jornay PM[b] delayed-release, extended-release formulation *(administer at bedtime)*		20 mg in PM; available as 20, 40, 60, 80, and 100 mg capsules	20 mg every evening between 7 and 9 PM; Max: 100 mg/day
Adhansia XR 20% IR, 80% ER	12-16 hours	25 mg every AM; available as 25, 35, 45, 55, 70, and 85 mg capsules	25-85 mg every AM; Max: 70 (child) 85 (adult) mg/day
Focalin (dexmethylphenidate) XR 50% IR, 50% ER beads[b]	10-12 hours	5 mg every AM; available as 5, 10, 15, 25, 30, 35, and 40 mg capsules	5-40 mg every AM; Max: 30 mg/day (children and adolescents); Max 40 mg/day (adults)
Serdexmethylphenidate (SDX)/dexmethylphenidate (Azstarys) 70% SDX, 30% IR dMPH	10-12 hours	39.2/7.8 mg every AM; available as 26.1/5.2, 39.2/7.8, 52.3/10.4 mg capsules (SDX/dMTP)	26.1/5.2–52.3/10.4 mg every AM; Max 52.3/10.4 mg/day
Mixed Amphetamine Salts C-II			
Short-acting IR			
Adderall, mixed amphetamine generics[c] *(dextroamphetamine and levoamphetamine 3:1 ratio)*	4-6 hours	2.5-5 mg every AM to twice daily; available as 5, 10, 7.5, 12.5, 15, 20, 30 mg tablets	5-40 mg every AM or divided 2.5-20 mg twice daily; Max: 40 mg/day
Amphetamine C-II (dextroamphetamine and levoamphetamine ratio 1:1)[c] (Evekeo)	4-6 hours	2.5-5 mg every AM to twice daily; available as 5 and 10 mg tablets	5-40 mg every AM or divided 2.5-20 mg twice daily; Max: 40 mg/day
Long-acting			
Long-acting XR (Adzenys XR-ODT) dextroamphetamine and levoamphetamine ratio 3:1[d] 3.1 mg Adzenys ODT ~5 mg of Adderall XR	10-12 hours	3.1-9.4 mg every AM; available as 3.1, 6.3, 9.4, 12.5, 15.7, 18.8, extended-release oral disintegrating tablets	3.1-18.8 mg every AM; Max: 18.8 mg/day
Mydayis (triple-bead formulation of mixed amphetamine salts)[e]	12-16 hours	12.5-25 mg every AM; available as 12.5, 25, 37.5, 50, extended-release capsules	12.5-50 mg every AM; Max: 50 mg/day (adults), 25 mg/day (pediatrics)
Adzenys ER-oral suspension[d]	10-12 hours	1.25 mg/mL oral suspension	6.3-18.8 mg every AM; Max: 18.8 mg/day

(Continued)

TABLE 82-2 Dosing of Stimulant Medications Used in the Treatment of ADHD (*Continued*)

Stimulant	Duration of Effect	Initial Dose and Available Strengths	Usual Dosing Range; Maximum Dose
Dyanavel XR 2.5 mg/mL Dextroamphetamine and levoamphetamine ratio 3.2:1[d]	10-12 hours	2.5 mg/1 mL oral suspension 2.5 mg of suspension ~4 mg of mixed amphetamine salts	5-20 mg every AM; Max: 20 mg/day
Xelstrym dextroamphetamine transdermal system	12 hours when worn for 9 hours	4.5 mg (4.76 cm^2) applied to clean, dry area on hip, upper arm, chest, upper back or flank and remove after 9 hours. Available as 4.5, 9, 13.5, 18 mg patches	13.5-18 mg (14.29-19.05 cm^2); Max:18 mg (19.05cm^2). Medication active for 3 hours after patch removal
Mixed amphetamine salts C-II Extended-release capsule (Adderall XR) dextroamphetamine and levoamphetamine ratio 3:1[d]	10-12 hours	5-10 mg every am; available as 5, 10, 20, 30 mg extended-release capsule	5-30 mg every AM; Max: 30 mg/day
Dextroamphetamine C-II			
Short-acting			
Dextroamphetamine generics[c] Dexedrine, Zenzedi[c]	3-5 hours	2.5 mg every AM to two or three times daily; available as 2.5, 5, 7.5, 10, 15, 20, and 30 mg tablets and 5 mg/5 mL solution	5-20 mg twice daily; Max: 40 mg/day
Intermediate-acting			
Dexedrine Spansule[d]	5-8 hours	5 mg every AM; available as 5 and 10 mg	5-30 mg every AM or 5-15 mg twice daily; maximum: 40 mg/day
Long-acting			
Lisdexamfetamine (Vyvanse)[d] (prodrug converted to dextroamphetamine)	10-12 hours	30 mg every AM; available as 20, 30, 40, 50, 60 capsules and chewable tablets and 70 mc capsules	Start at low end; titrate weekly to response; give in AM; Slower onset compared with other dextroamphetamine products

ER, extended release; IR, immediate release; OROS, osmotically released oral delivery system; ODT, orally disintegrating tablet; SR, sustained release; XR, extended release.

[a]The Drug Enforcement Administration label C-II, schedule II refers to significant abuse potential.

[b]Methylphenidate and dexmethylphenidate products are FDA approved in ≥6 years old.

[c]Immediate-release amphetamine and dextroamphetamine products are FDA approved in ≥3 years old.

[d]Extended-release amphetamine and dextroamphetamine products are FDA approved in ≥6 years old.

[e]Extended-release amphetamine products (immediate-release bead, small intestine dissolution bead, large intestine dissolution bead) are FDA approved in ≥13 years old.

Data from References 74, 79–81 and stimulant product package inserts or Daily Med.

Stimulants are available in diverse formulations (immediate release, delayed release, extended release, liquids, orally disintegrating tablets [ODTs] and patches) to allow for individualization based on a child's ability to swallow solid formulations and to individualize the duration of symptom control. Once-daily stimulant formulations are the preferred treatment for ADHD in most individuals due to convenience and better medication adherence.[5,74,81] Immediate-release formulations have the advantage of lower cost, less insomnia, and potentially fewer growth effects versus extended-release products; however, they also carry a higher risk of diversion and abuse.[2,45,74]

Administration of stimulant medications with food can delay the absorption and subsequently delay the onset of therapeutic effect by 30 minutes to 1 hour for immediate-release preparations and 1 to 2 hours for extended-release preparations.[74,81] Total bioavailability of stimulant can be decreased by 10% to 30% with coadministration of food, more so for beaded formulations of extended-release stimulant compared with osmotic controlled-release oral delivery system (OROS) methylphenidate or lisdexamfetamine.[17,74,81]

With immediate-release stimulants, most patients require a two or three times daily dosing schedule because of the short half-lives and duration of action of these medications (2-4 hours for methylpheniwate and dexmethylphenidate and ~4 to 6 hours for dextroamphetamine or mixed amphetamine salts).[4,7] Medication response is maximal during the absorption phase, is evident in 15 to 30 minutes, and lasts 2 to 6 hours.[4,7]

Drug delivery systems of once-daily products (amphetamine aspartate, amphetamine sulfate, dextroamphetamine sulfate, and dextroamphetamine saccharate [Adderall XR]; methylphenidate [Concerta]; methylphenidate [Daytrana]; dexmethylphenidate [Focalin XR]; methylphenidate [Metadate CD]; and methylphenidate long-acting [Ritalin LA]) provide 8 to 12 hours of symptom control.[74,80] Concerta uses an oral OROS, whereas other oral preparations use combinations of immediate-release and extended-release beads.[74,80] Concerta is a nondeformable tablet, and it should not be given to children with gastrointestinal (GI) narrowing because of the risk of obstruction. Mydayis, a long-acting mixed amphetamine salt, provides up to 16 hours of symptom control in adolescents and adults via pH-dependent, triple bead technology.[79,82] Adhansia XR is an extended release methylphenidate capsule with a duration of action up to 16 hours.[80] A novel evening-dosed delayed-release/extended-release methylphenidate product (Jornay PM) has demonstrated improvement in early morning functional impairment among youth with ADHD. DELXIS technology utilizes a dual-layer (outer delayed-release, inner extended-release layer) microbead delivery system that surrounds an inner methylphenidate loaded core.[81,83,84]

Aztarys is a novel long-acting product composed of 30% immediate release dexmethylphenidate and 70% serdexmethylphenidate, a prodrug of dexmethylphenidate. A long-acting effect is produced through gradual bioactivation of serdexmethylphenidate to dexmethylphenidate in the lower GI tract.[85]

For patients with trouble swallowing pills, several alternative stimulant formulations are available. Methylphenidate transdermal system provides up to 12 hours of symptom control when worn for 9 hours.[74,80] Dyanavel XR, an extended-release amphetamine oral suspension, utilizes ion exchange chemistry (LiquiXR™ technology) to provide continuous release of amphetamine throughout the day.[86] Adzenys ER oral suspension (MXA) is a long-acting mixed amphetamine salt that has demonstrated efficacy in youth 6 to 17 years of age.[87] Cotempla XR-ODT (methylphenidate) and Adzenys XR-ODT MXA should also be considered for youth with trouble swallowing pills. Both products utilize micro-particle technology and have effects for 10 to 12 hours.[87,88] Lisdexamfetamine is a prodrug conjugated to an amino acid that requires cleavage during metabolism to the active dextroamphetamine. It has a longer time to onset of

TABLE 82-3 Stimulant Adverse Medication Reactions and Their Management

Adverse Reaction	Recommendation/Management Strategy
Common	
Reduced appetite, weight loss	Give high-calorie meal when stimulant effects are low (at breakfast or at bedtime) or consider cyproheptadine at bedtime
Stomach ache	Administer stimulant on a full stomach; lower dose if possible
Insomnia	Give dose earlier in the day; lower the last dose of the day or give it earlier; consider a sedating medication at bedtime (guanfacine, clonidine, melatonin, or cyproheptadine)
Headache	Divide dose, give with food, or give an analgesic (eg, acetaminophen or ibuprofen)
Rebound symptoms	Consider longer-acting stimulant trial, atomoxetine, or antidepressant
Irritability/jitteriness	Assess for comorbid condition (eg, bipolar disorder); reduce dosage; consider mood stabilizer or second-generation antipsychotic
Uncommon to Rare	
Dysphoria	Reduce dosage; reassess diagnosis; consider alternative therapy
Skin discoloration (chemical leukoderma)	Counsel regarding risk before using methylphenidate patch
Zombie-like state	Reduce dosage or change stimulant medication
Tics or abnormal movements	Reduce dosage; consider alternative medication
Priapism (painful erection)	Obtain medical assistance immediately; consider alternative treatment
Hypertension, pulse fluctuations	Reduce dosage; change medication
Hallucinations	Discontinue stimulant; reassess diagnosis; mood stabilizer and/or antipsychotic may be needed
Peripheral vasculopathy, including Raynaud's phenomenon	Obtain medical assistance if severe digital changes observed; consider reducing dosage or alternative medication

Data from References 45, 60, 71, 74, and 89-92.

effect (~2 hours) but provides 10 to 12 hours of symptom control. As a prodrug, it has lower risk for misuse compared to other long-acting amphetamines where beads may be crushed or snorted. NICE guidelines recommend it as a preferred long-acting amphetamine formulation due to the extent of evidence for efficacy and safety in children, adolescents, and adults, and a lower misuse risk.[74,80]

Adverse Effects The most common adverse effects of stimulants and their management strategies are listed in Table 82-3.[45,89] At least 15 cases of priapism (painful prolonged erection), associated with stimulant use, have been reported to the FDA in males with a mean age of 12.5 years. A few cases of priapism have been reported with atomoxetine, and all cases require immediate medical attention.[45,90] The FDA has received at least 51 reports of skin discoloration associated with the methylphenidate transdermal system, also known as chemical leukoderma, that may not be reversible.[74]

Psychiatric, cardiac, and growth effects of stimulants have been extensively studied with key data and recommendations in the sections below.

Psychiatric Although considered rare, the FDA has added warnings to the labeling of all ADHD medications (ie, stimulants, atomoxetine, α_2-adrenergic agonists) regarding three broad categories of psychiatric adverse effects: psychosis, mood disturbance (ie, irritability, lability, or depression), and severe anxiety or panic attacks. Treatment-emergent psychosis is estimated to occur in approximately 1.5% of youth with ADHD treated with stimulant medications based on placebo-controlled trials.[45] Hallucinations involving visual or tactile sensations of insects, snakes, or worms were typical in children, with adolescents and adults experiencing hallucinations and delusions.[93] Multimodal Treatment Study of Children with ADHD (MTA), analyzing available data on the emergence of psychosis in 509 youth diagnosed with ADHD at age 7 to 9 years, showed that 5.1% reported psychosis which was not statistically different than 3.9% of the 276 local normal controls who reported psychosis over the same 10-year follow-up period. Therefore, investigators did not correlate stimulant use or an ADHD diagnosis in either group with the emergence of psychosis, but frequent cannabis use was associated with increased risk of psychosis in both groups.[94]

Sadness from stimulants may in part be genetically mediated, as an association was found in 77 youth taking immediate-release methylphenidate and two single nucleotide polymorphisms (SNPS) in the gene encoding for carboxylesterase (CES1), which may impact stimulant metabolism.[95] There is also evidence to suggest that preschool-aged youth are more susceptible to sadness, irritability, and mood lability with stimulant treatment compared with adolescents and adults.[3,45,89]

Literature reviews describe treatment-emergent mania and psychosis with atomoxetine, primarily in those with underlying bipolar disorder or depression. Labeling for atomoxetine includes a warning of increased suicidality largely because of its mechanism of action that is similar to antidepressants. A worldwide analysis of clinical trial and post-marketing data show no increase in suicidality (hazard ratio of 0.96).[96] Both stimulants and atomoxetine/viloxazine have the potential to cause or exacerbate mania, anxiety, panic attacks, or depression. In addition, stimulants and atomoxetine should not be given to manage attention in individuals with a primary psychotic illness such as schizophrenia or schizoaffective disorder due to the high risk of worsening psychosis.[45,96] Clonidine and guanfacine are much less likely than stimulants or atomoxetine to cause psychosis, mania, or anxiety, but treatment-emergent psychosis, irritability, depression, and nightmares have been reported.[97] When psychiatric adverse effects occur, dose reduction or cessation of therapy and supportive treatment is recommended.[45]

Cardiac Stimulants, atomoxetine, viloxazine, and α_2-adrenergic agonists have well-described cardiac and cardiovascular adverse reactions that are not significant for most youth, but can be intolerable in some, particularly in those with existing cardiac/cardiovascular disease.[45,98] Clinical trial data show that children who take stimulants for ADHD can have an increased heart rate by 3 to 10 beats/min and/or increased systolic or diastolic blood pressure by 2 to 14 mm Hg.[45,98] To explore the extent of cardiac adverse reactions more thoroughly, investigators used ECG and echocardiography to evaluate cardiac function in 58 children (ages 6-18 years old) with ADHD diagnosed, for at least 6 months, who were taking OROS methylphenidate (mean dose 39.40 mg or 0.93 mg/kg/day) and compared them to 58 matched control group children diagnosed with ADHD but not yet started on medication. Overall no significant differences were found in terms of blood pressure or ECG findings including QTc measurements; however, youth taking methylphenidate had lower E'septal values on echocardiography.[99] This difference was considered within normal limits and not indicative of cardiac dysfunction.

Clinical trial and post-marketing surveillance data shows atomoxetine treatment has been associated with increased heart rate at an average of approximately 5 beats/min and increased systolic or diastolic blood pressure of approximately 12 mm Hg. An Eli Lilly cardiovascular safety review showed 8% to 10% of patients taking atomoxetine had more significant increases in pulse at greater than or equal to 20 bpm and increase in systolic and/or diastolic blood pressure of greater than 15 to 20 mm Hg.[96] Clinical trial data demonstrate viloxazine treatment is associated with a greater than or equal to 20 beats/min increase in heart rate and greater than or equal to 15 mm Hg increase in diastolic blood pressure. Heart rate and blood pressure should be monitored prior to the initiation of treatment, following dose increases, and throughout treatment.[100] Clonidine and guanfacine may cause dose-related bradycardia and lowered blood pressure in youth, which may prevent upward titration in addition to modest widening of the QTc interval (5-7 msec) that warrants monitoring, particularly if the child takes another agent known to prolong QTc such as an antidepressant or antipsychotic.[45,97]

A 9.5-year prospective cohort study of children with ADHD found that, although rare, adverse cardiovascular events were twice as likely to occur in stimulant users as in nonusers.[101] There were 111 cardiovascular events in the 8,300 children with ADHD included in this analysis with hypertension, heart disease not otherwise specified, and cardiovascular disease not otherwise specified comprising 62% of adverse cardiac events, while arrhythmias comprised 23%, and cardiac arrest accounted for less than 1%.[45] The same investigators looked at national rates of stimulant use ($n = 714{,}258$) and found 1.8 times greater risk of cardiovascular events in those taking stimulants with greater risk seen with higher doses compared with lower doses.[101]

Overall, stimulant products should be used with caution in pediatrics and in adults with known structural cardiac abnormalities. The American Heart Association recommends careful screening of all children and adolescents prior to initiating pharmacologic therapy for ADHD, including a medical and family history and physical examination.[45] Before starting pharmacotherapy for ADHD in youth or adults, the clinician should consider a baseline electrocardiogram (ECG) and consultation with a cardiologist if past medical history or family history suggests cardiovascular disease.[3,98,99]

Growth The impact of ADHD medications on growth has been investigated extensively over the past 40 years as dose-dependent growth deficits of 1 to 1.4 cm/year have been observed with short-term stimulant treatment, mainly in the first 2 years. Weight deficits are more prominent with a mean 3 kg (6.6 lbs) weight decrease in the first year of treatment and 1.2 kg (2.6 lbs) weight decrease in the second year of treatment according to the MTA data.[102] Long-term studies on stimulants have reported divergent effects on growth, with many studies showing no clinically significant height deficits by adulthood. MTA study investigators assessed the largest cohort of children with ADHD ranging from 7-9 years old to 25 years old ($n = 515$) and compared them to classmates without ADHD ($n = 258$). These authors reported an overall adult height deficit of 4.7 cm among those consistently taking stimulant medication compared to those not taking a stimulant. Growth deficits were less when stimulants were taken inconsistently. Those taking stimulants consistently were 2.36 cm ± 1.13 cm shorter than those in the "inconsistent" group. Proposed mechanisms of stimulant effects on growth include alterations in growth hormone or growth factor, decreased thyroxine secretion, and suppression of appetite leading to reduced caloric intake.[45,102]

If symptoms can be managed with medication during weekends or summers, a medication-free trial may be considered every year.[45] Time off stimulant lessens stimulant growth suppressant effects, but evidence is lacking to firmly determine the impact of medication holidays on growth.[5,102] Consideration must be given to the risks of untreated ADHD symptoms on learning, socialization, and self-image while off stimulant therapy when determining the frequency and duration of the medication-free trial.[7,103] Medication dosage often varies from year to year, largely because of age-related pharmacokinetic changes. As a child develops, hepatic metabolism slows, and volume of distribution increases.[7]

Other Cases of stimulant-induced peripheral vasculopathy, including Raynaud's phenomenon, have been reported and are related to the peripheral release of catecholamines, resulting in vasoconstriction. Symptoms are typically intermittent and mild but can include digital ulceration and/or soft tissue breakdown. A retrospective, case–control study demonstrated that among children treated with stimulants, there was a significant association between the development of Raynaud's phenomenon and past or current use of stimulants.[104] This risk is dose-dependent, with symptoms typically resolving after dose reduction or discontinuation of the medication.[92,105] Additionally, there is a case report of dose-dependent Raynaud's phenomenon with atomoxetine use.[106] Close monitoring for digital changes is necessary during treatment with stimulants, α_2-adrenergic agonists, and atomoxetine/viloxazine. Rheumatology consultation may be required for some individuals.

Nonstimulants

Compared to the simulants, nonstimulant medications used for the treatment of ADHD are less effective alternatives than simulants in both children and adolescents. However, for most of these agents, the FDA has approved them both as monotherapy and as adjuncts to stimulants in children and adolescents for improving overall response and for managing behavioral symptoms and insomnia associated with ADHD. Some have also received FDA for the treatment of ADHD in adults. Potential advantages of non-simulants relative to stimulants include reduced potential for physical dependence or misuse, less potential for growth effects, and less sleep disturbance.[45] See Table 82-4 for dosing. Antipsychotic use is primarily for symptoms related to comorbid aggression, mood disorders, tics, or irritability associated with ASD and not for the core symptoms of ADHD.

Atomoxetine Atomoxetine is a selective norepinephrine reuptake inhibitor that should be taken in divided doses in the morning or late afternoon by children for improved tolerability.[108] Adults can take it once daily, usually in the morning.[108,112] Placebo-controlled, short-term trials (6-12 weeks) have shown that atomoxetine is effective in reducing ADHD symptoms in children, teens, and adults, and long-term studies show ongoing benefit and safety for children and adolescent responders out to 4 years.[96,97,109,112] A controlled trial comparing atomoxetine, OROS methylphenidate, and placebo over 6 weeks in 6- to 16-year-old patients showed that both medications were significantly better than placebo at improving ADHD symptoms, but OROS methylphenidate was superior to atomoxetine.[108,112] There was evidence for a preferential response to atomoxetine over stimulants in some individuals.[108]

Atomoxetine has a significantly slower onset of therapeutic effect than stimulants (2-4 weeks vs 1-2 hours with an effective stimulant dose), and full benefit may not be seen for 6 to 12 weeks.[108,109] The practice of combining atomoxetine with a stimulant in partially responsive patients is based on limited data from open trials and case series describing fewer late-day rebound effects and better sleep when atomoxetine is given in the evening; however, the adverse effects are additive.[108,109]

Possible adverse effects of atomoxetine and their management are similar to those of stimulants, including upset stomach and psychiatric and cardiac adverse effects (see Table 82-4 and "Psychiatric" and "Cardiac" sections). Although atomoxetine has less potential for growth suppression compared with stimulants, it has a greater risk of fatigue, sedation, and dizziness compared with stimulants or bupropion. Studies show that adults experience overall similar adverse effects as youth but they are less likely to report decreased appetite and are more likely to report urinary hesitation/retention and sexual adverse reactions (decreased libido and erectile disturbances) compared to youth.[109] Unlike stimulants, atomoxetine labeling includes a bolded warning of

TABLE 82-4 Dosing and Adverse Medication Reaction Monitoring of Nonstimulant Medications Often Used in ADHD

	Dosing Range and Titration Schedule	Adverse Reaction Monitoring
Serotonin norepinephrine reuptake inhibitors		
Atomoxetine (Strattera)	≤70 kg (154 lb): start at 0.3-0.5 mg/kg every AM or twice daily, maximum: 1.4 mg/kg/day; ≥70 kg (154 lb): start at 40 mg every AM or divided twice daily, maximum: 100 mg/day	Nausea, anorexia, ↑ blood pressure, ↑ pulse, insomnia, fatigue, sedation, severe liver injury (rare), suicidality
Viloxazine (Qelbree)	6-11 years: start at 100 mg/day. 12-17 years: start at 200 mg/day. Titrate in 100 mg increments/week, maximum: 400 mg/day	Nausea, vomiting, decreased appetite, sedation, insomnia, irritability, ↑ blood pressure, ↑ pulse, suicidality
Bupropion (Wellbutrin SR, XL)	50-300 mg/day; 3 mg/kg/day by end of week 1; can increase to 6 mg/kg/day or maximum of 300 mg/day as tolerated	Nausea, insomnia, rash, tics; dose-related risk of seizures
Antipsychotics (for comorbid aggression, mood disorders, tics, or irritability associated with ASD)		
Aripiprazole (Abilify)	2-5 mg daily; can titrate weekly as tolerated to response (usual range: 5-20 mg/day)	Nausea, restlessness, insomnia extrapyramidal symptoms, dizziness, sedation
Haloperidol[a] (Haldol)	0.5-1 mg twice daily; can titrate every 3-4 days as tolerated to response (usual range: 0.5-5 mg/day)	Extrapyramidal symptoms, dizziness, ↑ serum prolactin, sedation
Olanzapine[a] (Zyprexa)	2.5-5 mg every day; can titrate every 3-4 days as tolerated to response (usual range: 7.5-15 mg/day)	Sedation, severe weight gain, restlessness, extrapyramidal symptoms Diabetes, marked hyperlipidemia (never a first-line treatment)
Quetiapine[a] (Seroquel)	25-50 mg twice daily; can titrate every 3-4 days as tolerated to response (usual range: 200–600 mg/day)	Sedation, dizziness, weight gain, diabetes, hyperlipidemia
Risperidone[a] (Risperdal)	0.25-0.5 mg twice daily; can titrate every 3-4 days as tolerated to response (1-4 mg/day)	Extrapyramidal symptoms, dizziness, ↑ serum prolactin, decreased skeletal bone mass, hepatotoxicity, weight gain Diabetes, hyperlipidemia
Ziprasidone[a] (Geodon)	10-20 mg twice daily; can titrate every 3-4 days as tolerated to response (usual range: 40-160 mg/day)	Nausea, restlessness, insomnia extrapyramidal symptoms, sedation, QTc prolongation
Others		
Bupropion (Wellbutrin SR, XL)	50-300 mg/day; 3 mg/kg/day by end of week 1; can increase to 6 mg/kg/day or maximum of 300 mg/day as tolerated	Nausea, insomnia, rash, tics; dose-related risk of seizures
Alpha-2 adrenergic agonists		
Clonidine (Catapres) or clonidine extended-release XR (Kapvay)	0.05 mg two or four times daily; can increase as tolerated to 0.1-0.4 mg/day. For XR, give 0.1 mg at bedtime; may increase by 0.1 mg weekly; maximum: 0.4 mg/day given twice a day if dose >0.2 mg/day	Sedation, dizziness, heart block (check ECG), constipation, headache, upper abdominal pain
Guanfacine (Tenex) or guanfacine extended-release XR (Intuniv)	0.5 once or twice daily; can increase as tolerated to 1-4 mg/day; Max: 4 mg/day in children/adolescents For XR, give 1 mg in the AM; titrate weekly to response; Max: 4 mg/day in children; 7 mg/day in adolescents	Same as above with potentially lower risk of sedation. Effective dose higher in heavier children

[a]Short-term use (1-4 months) only for severe aggression associated with ADHD; may be longer if comorbidity such as bipolar disorder, Tourette disorder, or autism spectrum disorder.

ADHD, attention deficit/hyperactivity disorder; ASD, autism spectrum disorder; ECG, electrocardiogram; SR, sustained release; XL, extended length.

Data from References 42, 45, 97, 100, 105, and 107.

potential severe liver injury based on two cases (one adult, one child) of hepatic injury leading to transplant. A comprehensive safety review over 10 years described 133 cases of liver injury "possibly" related to atomoxetine, with liver functioning returning to normal after atomoxetine discontinuation. Although hepatotoxicity is considered rare, patients and families should be counseled to report signs of liver injury including dark urine, jaundice, or right upper quadrant pain.[96,109]

Viloxazine Viloxazine is a selective norepinephrine reuptake inhibitor, FDA approved for patients 6 to 17 years with ADHD. Compared to atomoxetine, viloxazine is a less potent inhibitor of the norepinephrine transporter. In addition to norepinephrine reuptake inhibition, viloxazine increases 5-HT levels in the prefrontal cortex via modulation of serotonin receptors.[110] Viloxazine extended release capsules are administered once daily in the morning and can be opened and sprinkled onto applesauce.[100]

Improvement in ADHD symptoms was apparent at week 1 in clinical trials, suggesting a possible quicker onset of effect compared to atomoxetine.[111-113] Given viloxazine's unique mechanism of action, there is interest in evaluating its role for comorbid depressive and anxiety symptoms.[110] Notably, viloxazine is a strong CYP1A2 inhibitor.[100]

The most common adverse effects associated with viloxazine include somnolence, decreased appetite, nausea/vomiting, insomnia, and irritability.[100] Changes in heart rate and blood pressure should be monitored after initiation and as the dose is titrated (see Table 80-4 and "Cardiac" section). Viloxazine, like atomoxetine, has a boxed warning for emergence of suicidal thoughts and behavior.[100]

α_2-Adrenergic Agonists Guanfacine and clonidine are central α_2-adrenergic agonists, acting both presynaptically to inhibit norepinephrine release and postsynaptically to increase blood flow in the prefrontal cortex, which enhance working memory and executive functioning. Pharmacologically, both of these medications affect a multitude of neurotransmitter systems, including catecholamine, indolamine, and α_2-adrenergic receptors on parasympathetic neurons, opioids, imidazole, and amino acid systems.[78,97]

(7) Guanfacine has a longer elimination half-life and duration of action (18 hours) compared with clonidine (12 hours), and its greater selectivity for the α_{2a}-adrenergic receptor, compared with clonidine, imparts less sedation and dizziness.[97] Clonidine and guanfacine are not as effective as stimulants for monotherapy treatment (effect size 0.22-0.58 vs 0.8-1.2 for stimulants).[97] In addition to being approved as monotherapy, extended-release clonidine and guanfacine are FDA approved

as adjuncts to stimulants in children and adolescents. Therefore, both are prescribed frequently as adjuncts to reduce disruptive behavior, control aggression, or improve sleep in youth.[5,97] Neither has been studied sufficiently for ADHD in adults.

Guanfacine XR can be given once daily during monotherapy while clonidine XR should be given twice daily for optimal symptom coverage. Both are considered acceptable second-line agents for children and adolescents unresponsive to or unable to tolerate stomach upset or insomnia with stimulant medications. Extended-release guanfacine and clonidine are more sedating than stimulants or atomoxetine; therefore, sleepiness during the school day requires careful monitoring.[97] Immediate-release α_2-adrenergic agonists are increasingly used to treat symptoms of ADHD in adolescents within the criminal legal system and adults due to no risk of physical dependence and potential benefits in controlling aggression and impulsivity, but this practice requires further study.[114]

The most common adverse medication reactions of clonidine and guanfacine are dose-dependent sedation, hypotension, and constipation.[4,5,97] The sedation seen with treatment usually subsides after 2 to 3 weeks of therapy.[97] Clinical trials show a mean decrease of 3 to 5 mm Hg in blood pressure with mean heart rate decrease of 3 to 5 beats/min. Both heart block and sudden death have been reported rarely with α_2-adrenergic agonists, and further analysis revealed that these events occurred in the context of polypharmacy and/or congenital heart malformation. Regardless, prescreening for existing cardiac problems and increased monitoring when combining medications is warranted.[45,97] Peripheral vasculopathies are well documented with α_2-adrenergic agonists, given their effects on peripheral catecholamine release; however, close monitoring and consideration of a rheumatology referral is warranted should these adverse events occur.[92,105]

Bupropion Bupropion, a monocyclic antidepressant, is a weak dopamine and norepinephrine reuptake inhibitor with no significant direct effect on serotonin or MAO. Its active metabolites augment noradrenergic and dopaminergic function. While not FDA approved for the treatment of ADHD, investigations with bupropion in children and adolescents demonstrated efficacy greater than placebo in two controlled trials and efficacy comparable with methylphenidate in two separate controlled trials ($n = 18$ and $n = 44$).[114] Bupropion has been found beneficial for adolescents with depression and ADHD and causes less appetite suppression and weight loss compared with stimulants, but it has a greater risk of seizures.[114] An analysis of data evaluating bupropion for ADHD in adults show it is significantly more effective than placebo and modafinil but less effective than methylphenidate or amphetamine salts.[71]

Bupropion's adverse effects include nausea, which can resolve over time or with slower dosage titration, and rash, which can require discontinuation of therapy if severe (see Table 82-4). Due to an elevated risk of seizures, bupropion should not be used in patients with a seizure or eating disorder. Additionally, it can cause or exacerbate tics and should be dosed early in the day to minimize the risk of insomnia.[114]

Lithium and Valproate Lithium or valproate can be used to control aggression and explosive behavior in patients with a co-diagnosis of ODD or CD, or those who are not responsive or are only partially responsive to treatment with a stimulant. Given the symptoms heterogeneity and overlap between some mental illnesses, some patients actually have childhood-onset bipolar disorder or combined ADHD–bipolar disorder.[77] Limited data show lithium is ineffective for ADHD alone but it is more likely effective when bipolar disorder coexists with ADHD.[77] Valproate is the most well-studied antiseizure medication (ASM) for aggression associated with ADHD. Dosing starts in low divided doses with titration over 1 to 2 weeks to therapeutic response.[115] See Chapter 75, "Epilepsy," for a more extensive discussion regarding adverse events for ASMs and Chapter 89, "Bipolar Disorder," for lithium.

Antipsychotics First-generation antipsychotics such as chlorpromazine and haloperidol can improve symptoms of hyperactivity and impulsivity in children with ADHD, but their negative effects on learning, cognitive functioning, and the significant risk of extrapyramidal adverse reactions (eg, dystonia and tardive dyskinesia) limit their usefulness.[107]

Second-generation antipsychotics such as risperidone, olanzapine, quetiapine, ziprasidone, and aripiprazole have been used to control severe aggression in refractory cases of ADHD, particularly if CD or bipolar disorder coexists.[9,115] In general, the second-generation antipsychotics pose a lower risk of extrapyramidal adverse reactions compared with conventional agents, but they can cause metabolic adverse reactions such as hyperlipidemia, hyperglycemia, and weight gain in addition to hyperprolactinemia.[107] Ziprasidone has the lowest risk of metabolic adverse reactions among these second-generation antipsychotics. Risperidone is the most well studied for aggression associated with ADHD,[70] but because it has the most potent dopamine antagonism and poses the highest risk of hyperprolactinemia and associated early puberty, gynecomastia, galactorrhea, amenorrhea, and decreased bone density.[70,107,116] Aripiprazole is least likely to elevate prolactin due to its dopamine agonist effects.[107] See Chapter 87, "Schizophrenia," for a more thorough discussion regarding the antipsychotics and their adverse effects.

Comorbidity and Polytherapy in ADHD

8 As previously stated, individuals with ADHD often present with comorbid conditions (Fig. 82-1), which may make polytherapy attractive or necessary. But this can complicate monitoring of therapy, because if multiple medications are started simultaneously, it is impossible to determine the impact of each medication. In general, the predominance and urgency of symptoms guide the medication selection process. For example, if a child presents as severely anxious or depressed with associated attentional problems, then an antidepressant should be initiated first with monitoring to determine if attentional symptoms improve.[4,76] When a child presents with severe ADHD and associated anxiety or depression, a stimulant should be initiated to treat the more severe ADHD. If ADHD symptoms improve significantly, but anxiety or depression persists, then an antidepressant can be added.[4,76] Studies show that stimulants do not routinely make anxiety disorders worse, but they might not improve symptoms either.[7,76]

Bipolar Disorder

9 Childhood bipolar disorder may be difficult to distinguish from ADHD because inattention, hyperactivity, and impulsivity are common with both conditions. When ADHD is diagnosed in an individual with bipolar disorder, the mood must be stabilized first with lithium, an ASM, or a second generation antipsychotic before considering an ADHD-specific treatment.[77,115]

Autism Spectrum Disorders

Autism spectrum disorders are estimated to occur in 20% to 50% of youth with ADHD and 30% to 80% of youth with ASD exhibit symptoms of inattention.[117] Impairments can range from mild to severe with poor language development, poor social skills, sensory over-responsivity, emotional dysregulation, inattention, impulsivity, irritability, oppositional behavior, and aggression.[117] There are few studies to guide treatment of ADHD in individuals with ASD. A Cochrane review of four US randomized controlled trials involving 113 youth with ASD and ADHD treated with methylphenidate for 4 to 6 weeks demonstrated short-term benefit for hyperactivity and possibly inattention in children who could tolerate methylphenidate. Of note, youth who could not tolerate a test-dose were excluded, and there was no evidence that methylphenidate was helpful for social interaction or stereotypical behaviors.[118]

Available evidence shows that stimulants can be an effective treatment strategy in pediatric patients with ASD, but are less effective and less well tolerated for managing ADHD in youth with more severe forms of ASD or with comorbid intellectual disability.[117-119] Atomoxetine was only slightly better than placebo in managing ADHD symptoms in children with ASD according to a 8-week controlled trial that included 97 children between the ages of 6 and 17 years.[72] Clonidine and guanfacine have small, uncontrolled studies only showing benefit in improving attention and decreasing aggressive/impulsive behavior in children with ASD.[117]

The AAP ASD guidelines recommend starting with a low-dose stimulant and monitoring carefully for worsening stereotypies, obsessional symptoms, sleep difficulties, poor appetite, depressive symptoms, social withdrawal, irritability, or the emergence of seizures.[119] If the stimulant is ineffective or poorly tolerated guidelines recommend atomoxetine, particularly if comorbid social anxiety, or an α_2-adrenergic agonist.[117]

Seizure Disorders

Patients with ADHD are two to three times more likely to experience seizures than age-matched peers, and ADHD is the most common comorbidity in youth with epilepsy.[120] While some reviews have demonstrated seizure aggravation and EEG changes related to stimulant treatment, most studies show methylphenidate is safe and effective for managing ADHD in youth with epilepsy.[120-122] A retrospective review of 18,000 Medicaid-enrolled youth with epilepsy and ADHD treated with a stimulant did not demonstrate an increased risk for seizure-related hospitalizations among current or former stimulant users.[123] Given the risk for stimulants to lower the seizure threshold, all individuals should be stabilized and seizure-free on an ASM prior to initiation of the stimulant.[76,123,124] Notably, valproate use may worsen attentional issues in children with ADHD. Additionally, antiseizure medication polytherapy may be associated with an increase in behavioral problems, although this may be attributed to more severe underlying neurologic symptoms.[120] If new or worsening seizures are suspected, discontinuation of the stimulant should be considered and cautiously reintroduced once stabilized.[60] The impact of atomoxetine, viloxazine, clonidine, and guanfacine on seizure frequency requires further study.[120,124] Bupropion use is contraindicated in patients with a seizure disorder.

Substance Use Disorders

The prevalence of SUD in adults with ADHD is estimated nine times higher than in those without ADHD.[125] Genetics, age (14- to 25-year-olds), psychosocial factors, and comorbidities all influence one's risk for SUDs,[46,126] with ADHD itself being a known risk factor for the development of an SUD. Among individuals with ADHD, persistent symptoms, a diagnosis later in adolescence or adulthood, and co-occurring diagnoses of ODD/CD are known predictors of developing an SUD.[127] A large Danish population-based cohort study (N = 13,116) investigated risk factors for SUD development among individuals with ADHD. Results indicated that age greater than or equal to 13 years at first ADHD diagnosis (OR = 3.28) and comorbid ODD/CD (OR = 2.87) were most strongly associated with SUD development. Male sex and parental factors (eg, SUD, psychiatric condition, low paternal income and education) were also identified risk factors.[127]

A review of 27 longitudinal studies that followed children with and without ADHD into adolescence or adulthood found that compared with control subjects without ADHD, children with ADHD were (1) nearly three times more likely to report nicotine use in adolescence/adulthood, (2) almost two times more likely to meet diagnostic criteria for alcohol use disorder, (3) approximately 1.5 times more likely to meet criteria for cannabis use disorder, (4) twice as likely to develop cocaine use disorder, and (5) more than 2.5 times more likely to develop an SUD overall.[10,126] Observational follow-up of the MTA has provided additional information regarding long-term substance use in children with ADHD. As reported on the Substance Use Questionnaire (SUQ), youth with ADHD compared to their peers were more likely to use cannabis weekly (32.8% vs 21.3%) and cigarettes daily (35.9% vs 17.5%) as adults. Additionally, early substance use, specifically the use of alcohol, cigarettes, and cannabis, was more common in the ADHD group compared to peers.[10] This highlights the need for early substance use screening in adolescence, particularly among those with ADHD.[10]

10 Caregivers frequently express concern that treating their child with a stimulant, particularly early treatment, may increase the risk of substance use. Follow-up studies show that stimulant therapy for ADHD neither increases nor decreases the risk of subsequent SUDs.[10,46] There is evidence that individuals initiating treatment early (before age 8) are less likely to use substances than those who have delayed onset of treatment. Behavioral therapy may also confer some protection against substance use and issues with the criminal legal system.[10,46,126] Atomoxetine, an α_2-adrenergic agonist, or bupropion is the preferred agent for individuals with ADHD and active SUDs.

Furthermore, other comorbid conditions including depression, anxiety, low self-esteem, CD, ODD, and antisocial personality disorder all increase the risk for developing an SUD in an individual with ADHD.[10,126,127] These comorbidities also increase the risk for issues with the criminal legal system that can prevent treatment and lead to ongoing SUDs. As youth with ADHD transition to adolescence, parents and clinicians should pay attention to whether the teen could be at risk for an SUD or misuse of their prescribed medications.[126,128,129]

Several studies have evaluated protective factors against substance use and issues with the criminal legal system for youth both with and without ADHD. These studies found that a quality parent–youth relationship, involving good communication, regular time together, consistent rules, and sharing of information (eg, how the child or adolescent spends free time and who their friends are) can be effective in deterring alcohol and substance use in youth with or without ADHD.[46,126] Youth support groups at high schools, such as the Gay/Straight Alliance (GSA), are credited with assisting schools with achieving lower rates of substance use and the misuse of the prescribed ADHD medications compared with schools without GSAs.[128]

Eating Disorders

All patients with ADHD should be screened for eating disorders given inattention and impulsivity associated with ADHD increase the risk of aberrant eating behavior and obesity. Inattentive symptoms can lead to mindless eating when not hungry, or impulsive, out of control eating aimed at emotional regulation.[130,131] A meta-analysis of 728,136 participants, 48,161 with ADHD (46,115 children; 2,046 adults), and 679,975 comparison subjects (616,228 children; 63,747 adults) showed that the pooled prevalence of obesity was increased by about 70% in adults with ADHD and 40% in children with ADHD. A genetic association has been found with non-restricting eating disorders such as bulimia nervosa and binge eating disorder, particularly in females.[132] Lisdexamfetamine is an FDA-approved effective treatment for both ADHD and binge eating disorder in adults.[133,134]

Oppositional Defiant and Conduct Disorders

Oppositional defiant disorder and CD occur in 30% to 60% of youth diagnosed with ADHD and are commonly associated with severe aggression and functional impairment.[135] Causes of ODD, CD, and associated severe aggression in youth with ADHD are multifactorial and include psychosocial adversity factors (eg, maternal mental disorder, paternal criminality, violence in the home), learning disability, disruptive mood dysregulation disorder (DMDD), or bipolar disorder.[135-137] Experts consider psychosocial interventions that include parent training and support for the child's family an essential part of the treatment plan for youth with ADHD, co-occurring with ODD or CD.[5,42,60,137-141]

Effective treatment of ADHD and CD/ODD is critical in the reduction of a wide range of psychosocial consequences (eg, substance use, violence, unemployment). Evidence-based guidelines recommend stimulants as first-line treatment for oppositional behavior, conduct problems, and aggression in youth with ADHD and comorbid CD/ODD.[138-140] Optimization of stimulant monotherapy (particularly methylphenidates) has demonstrated rapid, long-lasting improvements in emotion dysregulation, aggression, and ADHD symptoms.[142-144] A 2-year follow-up study of youth ($n = 33{,}835$) with ADHD found that patients with higher rates of adherence to stimulants or atomoxetine were less likely to eventually develop CD/ODD compared to those with poorer adherence, suggesting a possible protective effect of medication treatment.[145]

Studies in adolescents and adults with ADHD show that doses of stimulant above the recommended daily maximum are frequently needed for optimal symptom control prompting the American Academy of Child and Adolescent Psychiatry to publish an "off-label maximum dosage of 100 mg/day for methylphenidate and 60 mg/day for dextroamphetamine and mixed amphetamine salts." These dosage ranges appear in the academy's practice parameter on the treatment of ADHD.[42]

A head-to-head, randomized, 24-week open-label trial among youth treated with atomoxetine ($n = 80$) or OROS-methylphenidate ($n = 80$) demonstrated improvement in emotional/behavioral/externalizing problems in youth, with greater improvement in aggressive behavior and conduct problems in the OROS-methylphenidate group.[146] Treatment guidelines recommend that atomoxetine be considered in individuals who do not respond to or poorly tolerate stimulants.[138-140] Clonidine and guanfacine can be considered as monotherapy or add-on to stimulant treatment, but evidence to support their use is much lower quality.[138,139]

Unfortunately, optimizing ADHD-specific medications such as stimulant or atomoxetine is not universally effective for aggression and over half of youth with ADHD and ODD/CD need more than one medication for optimal symptom control.[70] The treatment of severe childhood aggression (TOSCA) study included 168 youth with ADHD and either ODD or CD (mean age of 9 years) and showed that adding risperidone 1 to 3 mg daily to parent training, behavioral therapy, and optimized stimulant resulted in moderate improvement in aggression. A 52-week follow-up of study participants demonstrated an overall benefit for youth who remained on medication, with the risperidone augmented-group demonstrating a small added benefit (improved CGI-S scores). This warrants close evaluation considering the long-term use of risperidone was associated with significant increased risk for weight gain and increased serum prolactin.[147] Overall, guidelines recommend that risperidone should be considered as a short-term treatment for severe aggression and/or explosive anger if not effectively managed by traditional ADHD medications.[138,139]

Aggression

Aggressive behavior is a common reason children present to higher levels of psychiatric care and is most prevalent in children with ADHD, often combined with ODD, CD, or DMDD.[148,149] Stimulants are typically considered first line for co-occurring aggression and ADHD, with some pediatric patients requiring adjunct pharmacologic treatment (eg, second-generation antipsychotic, mood stabilizer).[149] A randomized, controlled trial including 6- to 12-year-olds ($N = 175$) with ADHD, a disruptive disorder, significant aggression, and prior stimulant treatment demonstrated significant reduction in aggression (63% experienced remission) with rapid symptom-guided stimulant titration. This suggests that quick optimization of stimulant treatment and concurrent behavioral therapy may minimize the need for additional medications. For those who do not experience a significant reduction in aggression, adjunctive medications like risperidone and valproate may be helpful but are associated with risk (eg, weight gain).[149]

Tourette Disorder

ADHD occurs in 50% to 60% of youth with chronic tics or Tourette disorder, and 20% of children with ADHD go on to develop chronic tics or Tourette disorder.[72,73,91] Experts cautioned that stimulants should not be first-line treatments for ADHD in youth with tic disorders due to the stimulant's ability to increase central dopaminergic and noradrenergic activity, potentially exacerbating tics. However, a meta-analysis of 22 placebo-controlled trials involving 2,385 children with ADHD and Tourette disorder showed that stimulants were not more likely to worsen tics than placebo, and the association between stimulants and new-onset tics was more coincidental than a cause-and-effect relationship.[91] Additionally the timing of tic development in the context of ADHD may have led clinicians to inappropriately attribute new onset tics to stimulant treatment, as epidemiologic studies show that when ADHD and Tourette co-occur, symptoms of ADHD are present 2 to 3 years before tics emerge. Tourette disorder is known for fluctuating symptom severity with tics worsening and remitting in an unpredictable pattern, further diminishing the ability to accurately attribute tic causality.[75,91] When a stimulant trial is necessary to manage functionally impairing ADHD in a person with Tourette disorder, methylphenidate is recommended due to better evidence for effectiveness and tolerability in this population.[150]

A double-blind, placebo-controlled trial compared methylphenidate or clonidine monotherapy with the combination of methylphenidate and clonidine in patients with ADHD and Tourette disorder. Combination therapy demonstrated the greatest benefit in reducing symptoms of ADHD and tics, and clonidine appeared most helpful for impulsivity and hyperactivity, whereas methylphenidate was most helpful for inattention.[75,91] All treatments were well tolerated, but sedation was common (28%) in those receiving clonidine.[75]

Furthermore, guanfacine was administered to 34 children (mean age 10.4 years), with ADHD and tic disorder during an 8-week, placebo-controlled trial at a dose of 1.5 to 3 mg/day. Tic severity decreased by 31% in the guanfacine group compared with 0% in the placebo group.[75] There was a mean improvement of 37% on the teacher-rated ADHD scale compared with 8% improvement with placebo. Therefore, as previously stated, clonidine or guanfacine alone is a less effective alternative to stimulants in the treatment of children with ADHD and this holds true for those with comorbid Tourette disorder.

Atomoxetine appears to be an effective treatment for ADHD and tics in pediatric patients with comorbid Tourette syndrome or chronic motor tic disorder. For this study, 148 children and adolescents were randomized to atomoxetine (0.5-1.5 mg/kg/day) or placebo for up to 18 weeks of treatment. Overall, atomoxetine resulted in improvements in the severity of ADHD (effect size = 0.6) and tics (effect size = 0.3).[109]

Individuals with Tourette disorder and ADHD are more prone to disruptive behaviors including poor frustration tolerance, aggression, and impulsivity, often requiring behavioral interventions and medications that may include second-generation antipsychotics.[75] Second-generation antipsychotics such as risperidone, aripiprazole, and ziprasidone have evidence from controlled trials to support their use in managing motor and vocal tics associated with Tourette disorder; however, aripiprazole is the only agent FDA approved for managing Tourette disorder.[75] See Chapter 87 for more information about antipsychotics.

Personalized Pharmacotherapy

There are many things to consider when making therapeutic decisions in patients with ADHD such as age, comorbidities, tolerability, potential for medication interactions, and patient preference. In addition, there may be pharmacokinetic and pharmacogenomic factors to consider when personalizing pharmacotherapy. In looking specifically at pharmacogenomics, the functional activity of cytochrome P450 (CYP) 2D6, norepinephrine and dopamine transporters (SLC6A2, SLC6A3), catechol-*o*-methyltransferase (COMT), dopamine receptor (DRD4), carboxylesterases (CES1), and α_2-adrenergic receptor (ADRA2A) has been evaluated as a predictive tool for ADHD medication response and tolerability.[151-155] As the pharmacogenomics of ADHD treatments is a rapidly evolving field, an evidence-based resource available to decipher this work is provided by the Clinical Pharmacogenomics Implementation Consortium (CPIC, www.cpicpgx.org) or the Pharmacogenomics Research Network (PGRN, www.pharmgkb.org).[156] Specifically, the CPIC website contains evidence-based expert guidelines for interpretation of specific gene drug pairs, which may be used when testing is completed. It is important to note that CPIC does not recommend testing, but rather aims to serve as a reference for when testing results are available.

A CPIC guideline is available to guide dosing of atomoxetine based on CYP2D6 genotype in pediatric patients.[157] Exposure to atomoxetine increases 10-fold among CYP2D6 poor metabolizers and has a longer half-life, 20 hours compared to 5 hours, resulting in increased total plasma exposure compared to normal metabolizers.[157] Some studies have shown that CYP2D6 poor metabolizers may experience more insomnia, weight loss, increased heart rate and blood pressure, constipation, and depression associated with atomoxetine treatment compared to normal metabolizers.[158-160] Additionally, poor metabolizers may demonstrate greater therapeutic benefit due to increased exposure to the medication.[155,158] The CPIC guideline provides specific recommendations for starting doses based on CYP2D6 genotype and atomoxetine peak plasma concentrations and the manufacturer recommends dose adjustments based on genotype and concomitant treatment with potent CYP2D6 inhibitors.[157,160,161]

As methylphenidate is de-esterified by CES1 prior to elimination, it is less likely to have metabolic drug interactions compared with mixed amphetamine salts.[162] Sex influences the absorption of methylphenidate, with males having increased bioavailability compared with females.[7] Variability in dosage requirements for amphetamine salts, atomoxetine, and bupropion can be due to interindividual variability in plasma concentration achieved at a given dose. As all are metabolized via CYP2D6, the bioavailability and half-life of CYP2D6 substrates can be four to eight times greater in those taking a CYP2D6 inhibitor (eg, bupropion, fluoxetine, or paroxetine).[158-160]

While the routine use of pharmacogenomic testing is not recommended prior to initiation of ADHD medication, consideration should be made in particular clinical scenarios: (a) prior to the initiation of atomoxetine in pediatric patients with previous poor response/tolerability to other substrates of CYP2D6 and/or who are particularly sensitive to changes in HR/BP; (b) poor tolerability to atomoxetine/stimulants at starting doses; (c) individuals presenting with several psychiatric comorbidities and a history of psychotropic medication poor response/tolerability; and (d) family history of poor medication tolerability.

EVALUATION OF THERAPEUTIC OUTCOMES

Careful documentation of baseline symptoms and complaints over a 1-month pre-medication period is essential to the evaluation of therapeutic and adverse outcomes. Investigation regarding family history of psychiatric disorders and cardiac disease is essential to determine risk for related adverse medication reactions and to implement appropriate monitoring.[45,60] Baseline symptoms can be measured using videotapes, clinician rating scales (eg, ADHD Rating Scale IV, Vanderbilt ADHD Diagnostic Scale), or both. In addition, height, weight, and eating and sleeping patterns should be recorded at baseline and every 3 months.[5,42,45,60]

After the initiation and titration of any medication treatment, it is necessary that caregivers, teachers, and clinicians assess the overall functioning of the child or adult using standardized rating scales to determine if significant therapeutic benefit justifies continuing medication.[4,42] Therapeutic effects of the stimulants include decreased motor activity and impulsivity and increased attention span.[4,7,42] This suggests that stimulants are indicated for ADHD symptoms and not for primary learning disorders. The benefits of medication therapy must outweigh the potential for adverse effects to justify continued treatment.[4,42]

There is a lack of standardized assessment tools for adults; however, the adult ADHD screening tool can be useful.[49] Short-term studies (1 year or less) in adults with ADHD show that treatment with stimulants improves subjective quality of life. Long-term studies are needed to better assess the risk versus benefit of stimulant therapy on psychosocial and health outcomes.[163]

Atomoxetine, α_2-adrenergic agonists, and bupropion also require monitoring to detect changes in appetite, weight, and sleep patterns, as well as pulse and blood pressure. A therapeutic trial of atomoxetine or bupropion consists of 6 weeks at maximum tolerated doses unless response occurs at a lower dose.[4,42] Atomoxetine's full therapeutic benefit may continue to build over weeks to months, but if there is no significant benefit in the initial 6 weeks, it is unlikely that atomoxetine will be effective; therefore, it can be tapered off.[109]

When guanfacine or clonidine is given, careful clinical monitoring for fatigue, dizziness, and autonomic changes (eg, blood pressure and pulse) is recommended.[45,97] The American Heart Association has stated that ECG monitoring is not required for α_2-adrenergic agonists treatment in children, although many clinicians continue to assess for ECG changes, particularly if there is a family history of cardiac disease, if the patient is taking other agents that impact cardiac function, or if clinical symptoms warrant.[45] When discontinuing treatment, clonidine and guanfacine should be withdrawn slowly (0.05 mg clonidine/0.5 mg guanfacine reductions every 3-7 days) to prevent rebound hypertension or behavioral dyscontrol.[97,164] A therapeutic trial requires 1 to 2 months to assess therapeutic response, although increased sleep usually occurs immediately.[97,164]

Evaluation of therapeutic outcomes is particularly important when antipsychotics are used in youth as the US Office of Inspector General's peer review of psychiatrists found quality of care concerns in 67% of 475 medical records of youth receiving antipsychotics through Medicaid.[165] Among the biggest problems were lack of appropriate indications and lack of appropriate monitoring to ensure safety. Baseline weight, lipids, and fasting glucose should be monitored every 6 months in addition to the need to monitor for extrapyramidal symptoms and hyperprolactinemia.[9,107,165]

CONCLUSION

ADHD is a heritable, well-studied brain disorder that can present at any age, with or without co-occurring conditions. It is best treated with a combination of psychosocial, educational, cognitive-behavioral, and pharmacologic interventions. Treatments should be selected based on age, co-occurring conditions, and patient/family preference.

ABBREVIATIONS

AAP	American Academy of Pediatrics
ADHD	attention deficit/hyperactivity disorder
ASD	autism spectrum disorder
CBT	cognitive behavioral therapy
CD	conduct disorder

CNS	central nervous system
CNV	copy number variants
CRS-revised	Conners' Rating Scales—revised
CYP	cytochrome P450
DMDD	disruptive mood dysregulation disorder
DSM-5	*Diagnostic and Statistical Manual of Mental Disorders, Fifth Edition*
ECG	electrocardiogram
FDA	Food and Drug Administration
GI	gastrointestinal
IEP	individualized educational program
MAO	monoamine oxidase
MTA	Multimodal Treatment Study of Children with ADHD
NICE	National Institute for Health and Care Excellence
NIH	National Institute of Health
NNT	number needed to treat
ODD	oppositional defiant disorder
ODT	orally disintegrating tablet
OROS	osmotically released oral delivery system
SSRI	selective serotonin reuptake inhibitor
SR	sustained release
TOSCA	Treatment of Severe Childhood Aggression Study
TCA	tricyclic antidepressant

REFERENCES

1. American Psychiatric Association. *Diagnostic and Statistical Manual of Mental Disorders.* Fifth Edition (*DSM-5*). Arlington, VA: American Psychiatric Publishing; 2013.
2. Fields SA, Williams MJ, Hassig MB. Adult ADHD: Addressing a unique set of challenges. *J Fam Pract.* 2017;66(2):68–74.
3. Wolraich ML, Hagan JF Jr, Allan C, et al; Subcommittee on Children and Adolescents with Attention-deficit/Hyperactive Disorder. Clinical practice guideline for the diagnosis, evaluation, and treatment of attention-deficit/hyperactivity disorder in children and adolescents. *Pediatrics.* 2019;144(4):e20192528.
4. American Academy of Pediatrics (AAP) Algorithm Pediatrics. Supplemental information: Implementing the key action statements: An algorithm and explanation for process of care for the evaluation, diagnosis, treatment, and monitoring ADHD in children and adolescents. *Pediatrics.* 2011;(suppl):S11–S21.
5. Kemper AR, Maslow GR, Hill S, et al. Attention Deficit Hyperactivity Disorder: Diagnosis and Treatment in Children and Adolescents. Comparative Effectiveness Review No. 203. (Prepared by the Duke University Evidence-based Practice Center under Contract No. 290-2015-00004-I.) AHRQ Publication No. 18-EHC005-EF. Rockville, MD: Agency for Healthcare Research and Quality; January 2018. Posted final reports are located on the Effective Health Care Program.
6. Friedman LA, Rapoport JL. Brain development in ADHD. *Curr Opin Neurobiol.* 2015;30:106–111.
7. Pliszka SR. Psychostimulants. In: Rosenberg DR, West GS, eds. *Pharmacotherapy of Child and Adolescent Psychiatric Disorders.* Sussex, UK: Wiley-Blackwell; 2012;65–104.
8. Chan E, Fogler JM, Hammerness PG. Treatment of ADHD in adolescents: A systematic review. *JAMA.* 2016;315(18):1997–2008.
9. Texas Department of Family and Protective Services Web site. 2016. Psychotropic Medications. A Guide to Medical Services at CPS. (Utilization parameters for children and youth in foster care.) Available at: https://www.dfps.state.tx.us/Child_Protection/Medical_Services/documents/reports/2016-03_Psychotropic_Medication_Utilization_Parameters_for_Foster_Children.pdf. Accessed October 2018.
10. Molina BSG, Howard AL, Swanson JM, et al. Substance use through adolescence into early adulthood after childhood-diagnosed ADHD: Findings from the MTA longitudinal study. *J Child Psychol Psychiatry.* 2018;59(6):692–702.
11. Young S, Moss D, Sedgwick O, et al. A meta-analysis of the prevalence of attention deficit hyperactivity disorder in incarcerated populations. *Psychol Med.* 2014;45:247–258.
12. Danielson ML, Bitsko RH, Ghandour RM, Holbrook JR, Kogan MD, Blumberg SJ. Prevalence of parent-reported ADHD diagnosis and associated treatment among U.S. children and adolescents, 2016. *J Clin Child Adolesc Psychol.* 2018;47(2):199–212.
13. Polanczyk G, Willcutt EG, Salum GA, et al. ADHD prevalence estimates across three decades: An updated systematic review and meta-regression analysis. *Int J Epidemiol.* 2014;43(2):434–442.
14. Visser SN, Danielson MLL, Bitsko RH, et al. Trends in the parent-report of health care provider-diagnosed and medicated ADHD: United States, 2003–2011. *J Am Acad Child Adolesc Psychiatry.* 2014;53(1):34–46.
15. Bloom B, Jones LI, Freeman G. Summary health statistics for U.S. children: National Health Interview Survey, 2012. National Center for Health Statistics. Vital Health Stat 10 (258). 2013.
16. Centers for Disease Control and Prevention. "Prevalence of ADHD in Young Children" May 2016 posting; Available at: www.cdc.gov/vitalsigns/adhd data. Accessed November 12, 2018.
17. Austerman J, Muzina DJ. US Medication Trends for ADHD: An Express Scripts Report. Available at: http://lab.express-scripts.com/publications/turning-attention-to-adhd-report. March 2014. Accessed August 28, 2015.
18. Anderson KN, Ailes EC, Danielson M, et al. Attention-deficit/hyperactivity disorder medication prescription claims among privately insured women aged 15–44 years—United States, 2003–2015. *Morbidity and Mortality Weekly Report.* 2018;67(2):66–70.
19. Faraone SV, Larsson H. Genetics of attention deficit hyperactivity disorder. *Mol Psychiatry.* 2018. doi:10.1038/s41380-018-0070-0. [Epub ahead of print]
20. Demontis D, Walters RK, Martin J, et al. Discovery of the first genome-wide significant risk loci for attention deficit/hyperactivity disorder. *Nat Genet.* 2018. doi:10.1038/s41588-018-0269-7. [Epub ahead of print]
21. Stergiakouli E, Hamshere M, Holmans P, et al. Investigating the contribution of common genetic variants to the risk and pathogenesis of ADHD. *Am J Psychiatry.* 2012;169:186–194.
22. Scerif G, Baker K. Annual research review: Rare genotypes and childhood psychopathology—Uncovering diverse developmental mechanisms of ADHD risk. *J Child Psychol Psychiatry.* 2015;56:251–73.
23. Elia J, Glessner JT, Wang K, et al. Genome-wide copy number variation study associates metabotropic glutamate receptor gene networks with attention deficit hyperactivity disorder. *Nat Genet.* 2012;44:78–84.
24. Elia J, Ungal G, Kao C, et al. Fasoracetam in adolescents with ADHD and glutamatergic gene network variants disrupting mGluR neurotransmitter signaling. *Nat Commun.* 2018;9:4.
25. Lee SH, Ripke S, et al. Cross-Disorder Group of the Psychiatric Genomics C. Genetic relationship between five psychiatric disorders estimated from genome-wide SNPs. *Nat Genet.* 2013;45:984–994.
26. Grove J, Ripke S, Als TD, et al. Common risk variants identified in autism spectrum disorder. bioRxiv2017.
27. Thapar A. Discoveries on the genetics of ADHD in the 21st century: New findings and their implications. *Am J Psychiatry.* 2018;175:943–950.
28. Barkley RA. Etiologies of ADHD. In: Barkley RA, ed. *Attention-Deficit Hyperactivity Disorder: A Handbook for Diagnosis & Treatment.* 4th ed. New York: The Guilford Press; 2014:356–90.
29. Silva D, Colvin L, Hagemann E, Bower C. Environmental risk factors by gender associated with attention-deficit/hyperactivity disorder. *Pediatrics.* 2014;133:e14–22.
30. Laugesen K, Olsen MS, Telen Andersen AB, et al. In utero exposure to antidepressant drugs and risk of attention deficit hyperactivity disorder: A nationwide Danish cohort study. *BMJ Open.* 2013;3:e003507.
31. Sciberras E, Mulraney M, Silva D, Coghill D. Prenatal risk factors and the etiology of ADHD-review of existing evidence. *Current Psychiatry Reports.* 2017;19:1.
32. Shaw P, Malek M, Watson B, Sharp W, Evans A, Greenstein D. Development of cortical surface area and gyrification in attention-deficit/hyperactivity disorder. *Biol Psychiatry.* 2012;72:191–197.
33. Shaw P, Malek M, Watson B, Greenstein D, de Rossi P, Sharp W. Trajectories of cerebral cortical development in childhood and adolescence and adult attention-deficit/hyperactivity disorder. *Biol Psychiatry.* 2013;74:599–606.
34. Shaw P, Sharp WS, Morrison M, et al. Psychostimulant treatment and the developing cortex in attention deficit hyperactivity disorder. *Am J Psychiatry.* 2009;166:58–63.
35. Valera EM, Faraone SV, Murray KE, Seidman LJ. Meta-analysis of structural imaging findings in attention-deficit/hyperactivity disorder. *Biological Psychiatry.* 2007;61:1361–1369.
36. Hoogman M, Bralten J, Hibar DP, et al. Subcortical brain volume differences in participants with attention deficit hyperactivity disorder

in children and adults: A cross-sectional mega-analysis. *Lancet Psychiatry.* 2017;4:310–319.
37. Hart H, Radua J, Nakao T, et al. Meta-analysis of functional magnetic resonance imaging studies of inhibition and attention in attention-deficit/hyperactivity disorder: Exploring task-specific, stimulant medication, and age effects. *JAMA Psychiatry.* 2013;70:185–198.
38. Castellanos FX, Aoki Y. Intrinsic functional connectivity in attention-deficit/hyperactivity disorder: A science in development. *Biol Psychiatry Cogn Neurosci Neuroimaging.* 2016;1:253–261.
39. Liddle EB, Hollis C, Batty MJ, et al. Task-related default mode network modulation and inhibitory control in ADHD: Effects of motivation and methylphenidate. *Journal of Child Psychology & Psychiatry.* 2011;52:761–771.
40. Sripada C, Kessler D, Fang Y, et al. Disrupted network architecture of the resting brain in attention-deficit/hyperactivity disorder. *Hum Brain Mapp.* 2014.
41. Tomasi D, Volkow ND. Abnormal functional connectivity in children with attention-deficit/hyperactivity disorder. *Biological Psychiatry.* 2012;71:443–450.
42. Pliszka SR, Bernet W, Bukstein O, et al. American Academy of Child and Adolescent Psychiatry Work Group on Quality Issues. Practice parameter for the assessment and treatment of children and adolescents with ADHD. *J Am Acad Child Adolesc Psychiatry.* 2007;46:894–921.
43. Ghuman JK, Aman MG, Lecavalier L, et al. Randomized, placebo-controlled, crossover study methyphenidate for attention deficit/hyperactivity disorder symptoms in preschoolers with developmental disorders. *J Child Adolesc Psychopharmacol.* 2009;19(4):329–339.
44. Kaplan A, Adesman A. Clinical diagnosis and management of ADHD in preschool children. *Curr Opin Pediatr.* 2011;23:684–692.
45. Schneider BN, Enenbach M. Managing the risks of ADHD treatments. *Curr Psychiatry Rep.* 2014;16(10):479. doi:10.1007/s11920-014-0479-3.
46. Molina BS, Pelham WE Jr. Attention-deficit/hyperactivity disorder and risk of substance use disorder: developmental considerations, potential pathways, and opportunities for research. *Annu Rev Clin Psychol.* 2014;10:607–639.
47. Surman CBH, Fried R, Rhodewalt, Boland H. Do pharmaceuticals improve driving in individuals with ADHD? *CNS Drugs.* 2017;31:857–866.
48. Hechtman L, Swanson J, Sibley MH, et al. Functional adult outcomes 16 years after childhood diagnosis of ADHD: MTA results. *J Am Acad Child Adolesc Psych.* 2016;55(11):945–952.
49. Ustun B, Adler LA, Rudin C, et al. The World Health Organization Attention-deficit hyperactivity disorder self-report screening scale for DSM-5. *JAMA.* 2017;74(5):520–526.
50. Caye A, Rocha TB, Anselmi L, Murray J, et al. Attention-deficit/hyperactivity disorder trajectories from childhood to young adulthood: Evidence from a birth cohort supporting a late-onset syndrome. *JAMA Psychiatry.* 2016;73(7):705–712. doi:10.1001/jamapsychiatry.2016.0383.
51. Agnew-Blais JC, Polanczyk GV, Danese A, et al. Evaluation of the persistence, remission, and emergence of attention-deficit/hyperactivity disorder in young adulthood. *JAMA Psychiatry.* 2016;73(7):713–720. doi:10.1001/jamapsychiatry.2016.0465.
52. Barbaresi WJ, Campbell L, Diekroger EA, et al. Society for Developmental and Behavioral Pediatrics Clinical Practice Guideline for the Assessment and Treatment of Children and Adolescents with Complex Attention-Deficit/Hyperactivity Disorder. *J Dev Behav Pediatr.* 2020;41 (Suppl 2S):S35–S57. 10.1097/DBP.0000000000000770 31996577.
53. Cherkasova MV, French LR, Syer CA, et al. Efficacy of cognitive behavioral therapy with and without medication for adults with ADHD: A randomized clinical trial. *J Attent Disorders.* 2016;1–15.
54. Mickolajycyk R, Horn J, Biomath D, et al. Injury prevention by medication among children with ADHD: A case only study. *JAMA Peds.* 2015;169(4):391–395.
55. Ruiz-Goikoetxea M, Cortese S, Aznarez-Sanado M, et al. Risk of unintentional injuries in children and adolescents with ADHD and the impact of ADHD medications: A systematic review and meta-analysis. *Neurosci Biobehav Rev.* 2018;84:63–71.
56. Prasad V, Brogan E, Mulvaney C, et al. How effective are drug treatments for children with ADHD at improving on-task behaviour and academic achievement in the school classroom? A systematic review and meta-analysis. *Eur Child Adolesc Psychiatry.* 2013;22(4):203–16.
57. Lu Y, Sjölander A, Cederlöf M, et al. Association between medication use and performance on higher education entrance tests in individuals with Attention-Deficit/Hyperactivity Disorder. *JAMA Psychiatry.* 2017;74(8):815–822. doi:10.1001/jamapsychiatry.2017.1472.
58. Zoëga H, Rothman KJ, Huybrechts KF, et al. A population-based study of stimulant drug treatment of ADHD and academic progress in children. *Pediatrics.* 2012;130(1):e53–62.
59. Kortekaas-Rijlaarsdam AF, Luman M, Sonuga-Barke E, Oosterlaan J. Does methylphenidate improve academic performance? A systematic review and meta-analysis. *Eur Child Adolesc Psychiatry.* 2018. doi:10.1007/s00787-018-1106-3. [Epub ahead of print]
60. ADHD Diagnosis and Management: National Institute for Health and Care Excellence (NICE) Guidelines, published in March 2018. Available at: https://www.nice.org.uk/guidance/ng87. Accessed November 2018.
61. Goode AP, Coeytaux RR, Maslow GR, et al. Nonpharmacologic treatments for attention-deficit/hyperactivity disorder: A systematic review. *Pediatrics.* 2018;141(6).
62. Pelham WE, Burrows-MacLean, Gnagy EM, et al. A dose-ranging study of behavioral and pharmacological treatment in social settings for children with ADHD. *J Abnorm Child Psychol.* 2014;42:1009–1031.
63. Watson SM, Richels C, Michalek AP, Raymer A. Psychosocial treatments for ADHD: A systemic appraisal of the evidence. *J Atten Disord.* 2015;19(1):3–10.
64. Bader A, Adesman A. Complementary and alternative therapies for children and adolescents with ADHD. *Curr Opin Pediatr.* 2012;24(6):760–769.
65. Chang JP, Su KP, Mondelli V, et al. Omega-3 polyunsaturated fatty acids in youths with attention deficit hyperactivity disorder: A systematic review and meta-analysis of clinical trials and biological studies. *Neuropsychopharmacology.* 2018;43(3):534–545. 10.1038/npp.2017.160 28741625.
66. Millichap JG, Yee MM. The diet factor in attention deficit hyperactivity disorder. *Pediatrics.* 2012;129:330–337.
67. Turner CA, Xie D, Zimmerman BM, Carlarge CA. Iron status in toddlerhood predicts sensitivity to psychostimulants in children. *J Atten Disord.* 2012;16(4):295–303.
68. Tseng PT, Cheng YS, Yen CF, et al. Peripheral iron levels in children with attention-deficit hyperactivity disorder: A systematic review and meta-analysis. *Sci Rep.* 2018;8(1):788. doi:10.1038/s41598-017-19096-x.
69. Dehbokri N, Noorazar G, Ghaffari A, et al. Effect of vitamin D treatment in children with attention-deficit hyperactivity disorder. *World J Pediatr.* 2019;15(1):78–84. 10.1007/s12519-018-0209-8 30456564.
70. Aman MG, Bukstein OG, Gadow KD, et al. What does risperidone add to parent training and stimulant for severe aggression in child ADHD? *J Am Acad Child Adolesc Psychiatry.* 2014;53(1):47–60.
71. Cortese S, Adamo N, Del Giovane C, et al. Comparative efficacy and tolerability of medications for ADHD in children, adolescents, and adults: A systematic review and network meta-analysis. *Lancet Psych.* 2018;5:727–738.
72. Harfterkamp M, van de Loo-Neus G, Minderaa RB, et al. A randomized double-blind study of atomoxetine versus placebo for attention-deficit/hyperactivity disorder symptoms in children with autism spectrum disorder. *J Am Acad Child Adolesc Psychiatry.* 2012;51(7):733–741.
73. Hirschtritt ME, Lee PC, Pauls DL, et al. Tourette Syndrome Association International Consortium for Genetics. Lifetime prevalence, age of risk, and genetic relationships of comorbid psychiatric disorders in Tourette syndrome. *JAMA Psychiatry.* 2015;72(4):325–33.
74. Mattingly GW, Wilson J, Rostain AL. A clinician's guide to ADHD treatment options. *Postgrad Med.* 2017;129(7):657–666. doi:10.1080/00325481.2017.1354648.
75. Murphy TK, Lewin AB, Storch EA, et al. Practice parameter for the assessment and treatment of children and adolescents with tic disorders. *J Am Acad Child Adolesc Psychiatry.* 2013;52(12):1341–1359.
76. Naguy A. Psychopharmacotherapy of attention deficit-hyperactivity disorder in children with comorbid conditions. *Pediatr Neurol.* 2018;82:7–12. doi:10.1016/j.pediatrneurol.2017.09.010.
77. Pataki C, Carlson GA. The comorbidity of ADHD and bipolar disorder: Any less confusion? *Curr Psychiatry Rep.* 2013;15(7):372. doi:10.1007/s11920-013-0372-5.
78. Wilens TE. Mechanism of agents used for ADHD. *J Clin Psychiatry.* 2006;67(suppl 8):32–37.
79. Brams M, Childress AC, Greenbaum M, et al. SHP465 mixed amphetamine salts in the treatment of attention-deficit/hyperactivity disorder in children and adolescents: Results of a randomized, double-blind placebo-controlled study. *J Child Adolesc Psychopharmacol.* 2018;28(1):19–28. doi:10.1089/cap.2017.0053.
80. Steingard R, Taskiren S, Connor DF. New formulations of stimulants: An update for clinicians. *J Child and Adolesc Psychopharmacol.* 2019;29(5):324–339.
81. Pliszka SR, Wilens TE, Bostrom S, et al. Efficacy and safety of HLD200, delayed-release and extended-release methylphenidate, in children with attention-deficit/hyperactivity disorder. *J Child Adolesc Psychopharmacol.* 2017;27(6):474–482. doi:10.1089/cap.2017.0084.

82. Mydayis package insert. Available at: http://pi.shirecontent.com/PI/PDFs/Mydayis_USA_ENG.pdf, Shire, Lexington MA, U.S. Inc. Accessed November 29, 2018.
83. Childress A, Mehrotra S, Gobburu J, et al. Single-dose pharmacokinetics of HLD200, a delayed-release and extended-release methylphenidate formulation, in healthy adults and in adolescents and children with attention-deficit/hyperactivity disorder. *J Child Adolesc Psychopharmacol.* 2018;28(1):10–18. doi:10.1089/cap.2017.0044.
84. Jornay PM package insert. Available at: https://www.accessdata.fda.gov/drugsatfda_docs/label/2018/209311s000lbl.pdf, Ironshore Pharmaceuticals, Toronto Canada. Accessed November 29, 2018.
85. Aztarys package insert. Available at: https://corium.com/products/AZSTARYS/AZSTARYS_PI_ENGLISH_US.pdf, Corium, Grand Rapids MI. Accessed October 30, 2021.
86. Dyanavel XR package insert. Available at: http://dyanavelxr.com/pdfs/pi.pdf, Tris Pharma, Inc, Monomouth Junction, NJ. Accessed November 29, 2018.
87. Adzenys XR-ODT package insert. Available at: http://www.neostxcontent.com/Labeling/Adzenys/Adzenys_PI.pdf, Neos Therapeutics, Grand Prairie TX, U.S. LLC. Accessed November 29, 2018.
88. Cotempla XR-ODT package insert. Available at: http://www.neostxcontent.com/Labeling/Cotempla/Cotempla_PI.pdf, Neos Therapeutics, Grand Prairie TX, U.S. LLC. Accessed November 29, 2018.
89. Clavenna A, Bonati M. Safety of medicines used for ADHD in children. *Arch Dis Child.* 2014;99:866–872.
90. Eiland LS, Bell EA, Erramouspe J. Priapism associated with the use of stimulant medications and atomoxetine for ADHD in children. *Ann Pharmacother.* 2014;48(10):1350–1355.
91. Cohen SC, Mulqueen JM, Ferracioli-Oda E, et al. Meta-analysis: Risk of tics associated with psychostimulant use in randomized placebo-controlled trials. *J Am Acad Child Adolesc Psychiatry.* 2015;54(9):728–736.
92. Khouri C, Blaise S, Carpentier P, et al. Drug-induced Raynaud's phenomenon: Beyond β-adrenoceptor blockers. *Br J Clin Pharmacol.* 2016;82(1):6–16. doi:10.1111/bcp.12912.
93. Kraemer M, Uekerman J, Wiltfang J, et al. Methylphenidate-induced psychosis in adult ADHD: Report of 3 new cases and review of the literature. *Clin Neuropharmacol.* 2010;33(4):204–206.
94. Vitiello B, Perez Algorta G, Arnold LE, et al. Psychotic symptoms in attention-deficit/hyperactivity disorder: An analysis of the MTA database. *J Am Acad Child Adolesc Psychiatry.* 2017;56(4):336–343. doi:10.1016/j.jaac.2017.01.016.
95. Johnson KA, Barry E, Lambert D, et al. Methylphenidate side effect profile is influenced by genetic variation in the ADHD-Associated CES1 Gene. *J Child Adolesc Psychopharmacol.* 2013;23(10):655–664.
96. Reed VA, Buitelaar JK, Anand E, et al. The safety of atomoxetine for the treatment of children and adolescents with ADHD: A comprehensive review of over a decade of research. *CNS Drugs.* 2016;30:603–628.
97. Hirota T, Schwartz S, Correll CU. Alpha-2 agonists for attention-deficit/hyperactivity disorder in youth: A systematic review and meta-analysis of monotherapy and add-on trials to stimulant therapy. *J Am Acad Child Adolesc Psychiatry.* 2014;53(2):153–173.
98. Berger S. Attention deficit hyperactivity disorder medications in children with heart disease. *Curr Opin Pediatr.* 2016;28(5):607–612.
99. Kara T, Mihcioglu M, Yilmaz S, Akaltun I. Effects of long-term use of prescription methylphenidate on myocardial performance in children with ADHD: A tissue Doppler imaging study. *J Child Adolesc Psychopharmacol.* 2018 (ahead of print). doi:10.1089/cap.2018.0052.
100. Qelbree package insert. Available at: https://www.supernus.com/sites/default/files/Qelbree-Prescribing-Info.pdf, Supernus Pharmaceuticals Inc, Rockville MD, Accessed October 30, 2021.
101. Dalsgaard S, Kvist AP, Leckman JF, et al. Cardiovascular safety of stimulants in children with ADHD: A nationwide prospective cohort study. *J Child Adolescent Psychopharmacology.* 2014;24(6):302–310.
102. Richardson E, Seibert T, Uli NK. Growth perturbations from stimulant medications and inhaled corticosteroids. *Transl Pediatr.* 2017;6(4):237–247. doi:10.21037/tp.2017.09.14.
103. Díez-Suárez A, Vallejo-Valdivielso M, Marín-Méndez JJ, et al. Weight, height, and body mass index in patients with attention-deficit/hyperactivity disorder treated with methylphenidate. *J Child Adolesc Psychopharmacol.* 2017;27(8):723–730. doi:10.1089/cap.2016.0150.
104. Goldman W, Seltzer R, Reuman P. Association between treatment with central nervous system stimulants and Raynaud's syndrome in children: A retrospective case-control study of rheumatology patients. *Arthritis Rheum.* 2008;58(2):563–566. doi:10.1002/art.23301.
105. Bayram Ö, Hergüner S. OROS-methylphenidate-induced Raynaud's phenomenon: A dose-related side effect. *J Child Adolesc Psychopharmacol.* 2015;25(6):521–522. doi:10.1089/cap.2015.0033.
106. Gökçen C, Kutuk MO, Coşkun Ş. Dose-dependent Raynaud's phenomenon developing from use of atomoxetine in a girl. *J Child Adolesc Psychopharmacol.* 2013;23(6):428–430. doi:10.1089/cap.2012.0131.
107. Seida JC, Schouten JR, Boylan K, et al. Antipsychotics for children and young adults: A comparative effectiveness review. *Pediatrics.* 2012;129:e771–e784.
108. Newcorn JH, Kratochvil CJ, Allen RJ, et al. Atomoxetine and osmotically released methylphenidate for the treatment of ADHD: Acute comparison and differential response. *Am J Psych.* 2008;165:721–730. 2008;165:721-730.
109. Savill NC, Buitelaar JK, Anand E, et al. The efficacy of atomoxetine for the treatment of children and adolescents with attention-deficit/hyperactivity disorder: A comprehensive review of over a decade of clinical research. *CNS Drugs.* 2015;29(2):131–151.
110. Yu C, Garcia-Olivares J, Candler S, et al. New insights into the mechanism of action of viloxazine: Serotonin and norepinephrine modulating properties. *J Exp Pharmacol.* 2020;12:285–300. 10.2147/JEP.S256586 32943948.
111. Johnson JK, Liranso T, Saylor K, et al. A phase II double-blind, placebo-controlled, efficacy and safety study of SPN-812 (extended-release viloxazine) in children with ADHD. *J Atten Disord.* 2020;24(2):348–358. 10.1177/1087054719836159 30924702.
112. Nasser A, Liranso T, Adewole T, et al. A Phase III, randomized, placebo-controlled trial to assess the efficacy and safety of once-daily SPN-812 (viloxazine extended-release) in the treatment of attention-deficit/hyperactivity disorder in school-age children. *Clin Ther.* 2020;42(8):1452–1466. 10.1016/j.clinthera.2020.05.021 32723670.
113. Nasser A, Hull JT, Liranso T, et al. The effect of viloxazine extended-release capsules on functional impairments associated with attention-deficit/hyperactivity disorder (ADHD) in children and adolescents in four Phase 3 placebo-controlled trials. *Neuropsychiatr Dis Treat* 2021;17:1751–1762. 10.2147/NDT.S312011 34113106.
114. Ng QX. A systematic review of the use of Bupropion for attention-deficit/hyperactivity disorder in children and adolescents. *J Child Adolesc Psychopharmacol.* 2017;27(2):112–116. doi:10.1089/cap.2016.0124.
115. Carlson GA, Klein DN. How to understand divergent views on bipolar disorder in youth. *Annu Rev Clin Psychology.* 2014;10:529–551.
116. Calarge CA, Burns TL, Schlechte JA, et al. Longitudinal examination of the skeletal effects of selective serotonin reuptake inhibitors and risperidone. *J Clin Psychiatry.* 2015;76(5):607–613.
117. Dopheide JA. Autism spectrum disorder. In: Eiland LS, Todd TJ, eds. *Advanced Pediatric Therapeutics: Pediatric Pharmacy Advocacy Group.* Memphis, TN: Allen Press Copyright; 2015;1–8.
118. Sturman N, Deckx L, van Driel ML. Methylphenidate for children and adolescents with autism spectrum disorder. *Cochrane Database Syst Rev.* 2017;11:CD011144. doi:10.1002/14651858.CD011144.pub2.
119. Hyman SL, Levy SE, Myers SM. Identification, evaluation, and management of children with autism spectrum disorder. *Pediatrics.* 2020;145(110)1542/peds.2019-3447 31843864.
120. Auvin S, Wirrell E, Donald KA, et al. Systematic review of the screening, diagnosis, and management of ADHD in children with epilepsy. Consensus paper of the Task Force on Comorbidities of the ILAE Pediatric Commission. *Epilepsia.* 2018;59(10):1867–1880. 10.1111/epi.14549 30178479.
121. Park J, Choi HW, Yum MS, et al. Relationship between aggravation of seizures and methylphenidate treatment in subjects with ADHD and epilepsy. *J Child Adolesc Psychopharmacol.* 2018;28(8):1–10.
122. Ravi M, Ickowicz A. Epilepsy, attention-deficit/hyperactivity disorder and methylphenidate: Critical examination of guiding evidence. *J Can Acad Child Adolesc Psychiatry.* 2016;25:50–58.
123. Liu X, Carney PR, Bussing R, et al. Stimulants do not increase the risk of seizure-related hospitalizations in children with epilepsy. *J Child Adolesc Psychopharmacol.* 2018;28(2):111–116.
124. Verrotti A, Moavero R, Panzarino G, et al. The challenge of pharmacotherapy in children and adolescents with epilepsy-ADHD comorbidity. *Clin Drug Investig.* 2018;38(1):1–8. doi:10.1007/s40261-017-0585-1.
125. Chen Q, Hartman CA, Haavik J, et al. Common psychiatric and metabolic comorbidity of adult attention-deficit/hyperactivity disorder: A population-based cross-sectional study. *PLoS One.* 2018;13(9):e0204516–e0204516. 10.1371/journal.pone.0204516 30256837.
126. Harstad E, Levy S. Committee on substance abuse: Attention-deficit/hyperactivity disorder and substance abuse. *Pediatrics.* 2014;134(1):e293–e301. doi:10.1542/peds.2014-0992.
127. Wimberley T, Agerbo E, Horsdal HT, et al. Genetic liability to ADHD and substance use disorders in individuals with ADHD. *Addiction.* 2020;115(7):1368–1377. 10.1111/add.14910 31803957.

128. Heck NC, Livingston NA, Flentje A, et al. Reducing risk for illicit drug use and prescription drug misuse: High school gay-straight alliances and lesbian, gay, bisexual, and transgender youth. *Addict Behav.* 2014;39(4):824–828.
129. Rabiner DL. Stimulant prescription cautions: Addressing misuse, diversion and malingering. *Curr Psychiatry Rep.* 2013;15(7):375.
130. Cortese S, Moreira-Maia CR, St Fleur D, et al. Association between ADHD and obesity: A systematic review and meta-analysis. *Am J Psychiatry.* 2016;173(1):34–43. 10.1176/appi.ajp.2015.15020266 26315982.
131. Kooij JJ. 2016 ADHD and obesity. *Am J Psychiatry*. 173, 1-2. 10.1176/appi.ajp.2015.15101315.
132. Yao S, Kuja-Halkola R, Martin J, et al. Associations between attention-deficit/hyperactivity disorder and various eating disorders: A Swedish Nationwide population study using multiple genetically informative approaches. *Biol Psychiatry.* 2019;86(8):577–586. 10.1016/j.biopsych.2019.04.036 31301758.
133. Hudson James I, McElroy Susan L, Ferreira-Cornwell M. Celeste, et al. Efficacy of lisdexamfetamine in adults with moderate to severe binge-eating disorder. *JAMA Psychiatry.* 2017;74:903. 10.1001/jamapsychiatry.2017.1889.
134. Kornstein SG, Bliss C, Kando J, et al. Clinical characteristics and treatment response to lisdexamfetamine dimesylate versus placebo in adults with binge eating disorder: Analysis by gender and age. *J Clin Psychiatry.* 2019;80(2).10.4088/JCP.18m12378 30817099.
135. Findling RL, McBurnett K, White C, Youcha S. Guanfacine extended release adjunctive to a psychostimulant in the treatment of comorbid oppositional symptoms in children and adolescents with attention-deficit/hyperactivity disorder. *J Child Adolesc Psychopharmacol.* 2014;24(5):245–52.
136. Bayard F, Nymberg Thunell C, Abé C, et al. Distinct brain structure and behavior related to ADHD and conduct disorder traits. *Mol Psychiatry*. 2018. doi:10.1038/s41380-018-0202-6. [Epub ahead of print].
137. Blader JC, Pliszka SR, Kafantaris V, et al. Prevalence and treatment outcomes of persistent negative mood among children with attention-deficit/hyperactivity disorder and aggressive behavior. *J Child Adolesc Psychopharmacol.* 2016;26(2):164–73. doi:10.1089/cap.2015.0112.
138. Gorman DA, Gardner DM, Murphy AL, et al. Canadian guidelines on pharmacotherapy for disruptive and aggressive behaviour in children and adolescents with attention-deficit hyperactivity disorder, oppositional defiant disorder, or conduct disorder. *Can J Psychiatry.* 2015;60(2):62–76.
139. Lillig M. Conduct disorder: Recognition and management. *Am Fam Physician.* 2018;98(10):584–592.
140. Pringsheim T, Hirsch L, Gardner D, Gorman DA. The pharmacological management of oppositional behaviour, conduct problems, and aggression in children and adolescents with attention-deficit hyperactivity disorder, oppositional defiant disorder, and conduct disorder: A systematic review and meta-analysis. Part 1: psychostimulants, alpha-2 agonists, and atomoxetine. *Can J Psychiatry.* 2015;60(2):42–51.
141. Pappadopulos E, Macintyre Ii JC, Crismon ML, et al. Treatment recommendations for the use of antipsychotics for aggressive youth (TRAAY). Part II. *J Am Acad Child Adolesc Psychiatry.* 2003;42(2):145–61.
142. Dougherty DM, Olvera RL, Acheson A, et al. Acute effects of methylphenidate on impulsivity and attentional behavior among adolescents comorbid for ADHD and conduct disorder. *J Adolesc.* 2016;53:222–230. doi:10.1016/j.adolescence.2016.10.013.
143. Kutlu A, Akyol Ardic U, Ercan ES. Effect of methylphenidate on emotional dysregulation in children with attention-deficit/hyperactivity disorder + oppositional defiant disorder/conduct disorder. *J Clin Psychopharmacol.* 2017;37(2):220–225. doi:10.1097/JCP.0000000000000668.
144. Masi G, Manfredi A, Nieri G, et al. A naturalistic comparison of methylphenidate and risperidone monotherapy in drug-naive youth with attention-deficit/hyperactivity disorder comorbid with oppositional defiant disorder and aggression. *J Clin Psychopharmacol.* 2017;37(5):590–594. doi:10.1097/JCP.0000000000000747.
145. Wang LJ, Lee SY, Chou MC, et al. Impact of drug adherence on oppositional defiant disorder and conduct disorder among patients with attention-deficit/hyperactivity disorder. *J Clin Psychiatry.* 2018;79(5): pii. 17m11784.doi:10.4088/JCP.17m11784.
146. Shih HH, Shang CY, Gau SS. Comparative efficacy of methylphenidate and atomoxetine on emotional and behavioral problems in youths with attention-deficit/hyperactivity disorder. *J Child Adolesc Psychopharmacol.* 2018. doi:10.1089/cap.2018.0076. [Epub ahead of print] PubMed PMID: 30457349.
147. Gadow KD, Brown NV, Arnold LE, et al. Severely aggressive children receiving stimulant medication versus stimulant and risperidone: 12-month follow-up of the TOSCA trial. *J Am Acad Child Adolesc Psychiatry.* 2016;55(6):469–478. doi:10.1016/j.jaac.2016.03.014.
148. Merikangas KR, He JP, Burstein M, et al. Service utilization for lifetime mental disorders in U.S. adolescents: Results of the National Comorbidity Survey-Adolescent Supplement (NCS-A). *J Am Acad Child Adolesc Psychiatry.* 2011;50(1):32–45. 10.1016/j.jaac.2010.10.006 21156268.
149. Blader JC, Pliszka SR, Kafantaris V, et al. Stepped treatment for attention-deficit/hyperactivity disorder and aggressive behavior: A randomized, controlled trial of adjunctive risperidone, divalproex sodium, or placebo after stimulant medication optimization. *J Am Acad Child Adolesc Psychiatry.* 2021;60(2):236–251. 10.1016/j.jaac.2019.12.009 32007604.
150. Shaw ZA, Coffey BJ Tics and Tourette syndrome. *Psychiatr Clin North Am.* 2014;37(3):269–286. 10.1016/j.psc.2014.05.001 25150562.
151. Bonvicini C, Faraone SV, Scassellati C. Attention-deficit hyperactivity disorder in adults: A systematic review and meta-analysis of genetic, pharmacogenetic and biochemical studies. *Mol Psychiatry.* 2016;21(7):872–884. doi:10.1038/mp.2016.74.
152. Levy F. Applications of pharmacogenetics in children with attention-deficit/hyperactivity disorder. *Pharmgenomics Pers Med.* 2014;7:349–356.
153. Myer NM, Boland JR, Faraone SV. Pharmacogenetics predictors of methylphenidate efficacy in childhood ADHD. *Mol Psychiatry.* 2018;23(9):1–8.
154. Unal D, Unal MF, Alikasifoglu M, Cetinkaya A. Genetic variations in attention deficit hyperactivity disorder subtypes and treatment resistant cases. *Psychiatry Investig.* 2016;13(4):427–433.
155. Wehry AM, Ramsey L, Dulemba SE, et al. Pharmacogenomic testing in child and adolescent psychiatry: An evidence-based review. *Curr Probl Pediatr Adolesc Health Care.* 2018;48(2):40–49.
156. Clinical Pharmacogenetics Implementation Consortium. CPIC guidelines. Available at: https://cpicpgx.org/. Accessed December 29, 2018.
157. Brown JT, Bishop JR, Sangkuhl K, et al. Clinical Pharmacogenetics Implementation Consortium Guideline for Cytochrome P450 (CYP)2D6 Genotype and Atomoxetine Therapy. *Clin Pharmacol Ther.* 2019;106(1):94–102. 10.1002/cpt.1409 30801677.
158. Brown JT, Bishop JR. Atomoxetine pharmacogenetics: Associations with pharmacokinetics, treatment response and tolerability. *Pharmacogenomics.* 2015;16(13):1513–1520. doi:10.2217/PGS.15.93.
159. Fijal BA, Guo Y, Li SG, Ahl J, et al. CYP2D6 predicted metabolizer status and safety in adult patients with attention-deficit hyperactivity disorder participating in a large placebo-controlled atomoxetine maintenance of response clinical trial. *J Clin Pharmacol.* 2015;55(10):1167–1174.
160. Yu G, Li GF, Markowitz JS. Atomoxetine: A review of its pharmacokinetics and pharmacogenomics relative to drug disposition. *J Child Adolesc Psychopharmacol.* 2016;26(4):314–326.
161. Atomoxetine package insert. Available at: https://pi.lilly.com/us/strattera-pi.pdf, Eli Lilly, Indianapolis IN, U.S. Inc. Accessed November 29, 2018.
162. Stevens T, Sangkuhl K, Brown JT, et al. PharmGKB summary: Methylphenidate pathway, pharmacokinetics/pharmacodynamics. *Pharmacogenet Genomics.* 2019;29(6):136–154. 10.1097/FPC.0000000000000376 30950912.
163. Surman CBH, Hammerness PG, Pion K, et al. Do stimulants improve functioning in adults with ADHD: A review of the literature. *European Neuropsychopharmacology.* 2013;23:528–533.
164. Faraone SV, McBurnett K, Sallee FR, et al. Guanfacine extended release: A novel treatment for ADHD in children and adolescents. *Clin Therapeutics.* 2013;35(11):1778–1793.
165. Department of Health and Human Services (HHS), Office of Inspector General. *Second-Generation Antipsychotic Drug Use among Medicaid-Enrolled Children: Quality of Care Concerns.* HHS Web site. Available at: https://oig.hhs.gov/oei/reports/oei-07-12-00320.pdf. Accessed November 15, 2018.
166. American Psychiatric Association. Disorders usually first evident in infancy, childhood or adolescence. In: *Diagnostic and Statistical Manual of Mental Disorders*, Fifth Edition. Arlington, VA, American Psychiatric Association, 2013:59–66.

e83

Eating Disorders

Steven C. Stoner, Valerie L. Ruehter, and Melissa C. Palmer

KEY CONCEPTS

1. Eating disorders are more commonly recognized than years past although patients are likely to not seek help and medication treatment options are limited.
2. Symptoms common to eating disorders include excessive intake of calorie-laden food over a short period of time (eg, binge eating or bingeing), and inappropriate compensatory behaviors to expend calories such as self-induced vomiting, the overuse of laxatives, diuretics, enemas, fasting, or excessive exercise (eg, purging behaviors).
3. Shifting between different eating disorder diagnostic categories is possible, especially if treatment does not result in symptom remission.
4. Psychiatric comorbidities are common with all forms of eating disorders. The differential diagnosis should generally include evaluation for depression, schizophrenia, generalized anxiety, obsessive-compulsive disorder (OCD), and personality disorders.
5. Calories must be gradually introduced during caloric restoration to prevent the potentially fatal complication known as refeeding syndrome. Failure to restore calories quickly enough may result in an unfeeding syndrome.
6. Clinicians must monitor closely for suicidality and educate individuals appropriately, similar to patients with major depressive disorder taking antidepressants, as mortality from suicide is not uncommon.
7. The treatment approach for anorexia nervosa (AN) includes a minimum of 6 months of psychotherapy, preferably cognitive behavioral therapy (CBT), in adults and family-based therapy in children. There are no FDA-approved agents for the treatment of AN.
8. Despite limited data, antidepressants in combination with nonpharmacologic treatment are the preferred pharmacotherapy for the acute and maintenance phases of bulimia nervosa (BN). Fluoxetine is the only FDA-approved medication to treat adult BN.
9. Use of selective serotonin reuptake inhibitors (SSRIs) and topiramate for the treatment of binge-eating disorder (BED) along with CBT and interpersonal psychotherapy (IPT) is supported by the literature. Lisdexamfetamine is the sole FDA-approved agent for BED.
10. It is important to transition patients being treated for AN gradually to outpatient care as there is a high risk of relapse within the first 60 days of inpatient refeeding.

BEYOND THE BOOK

Watch the video entitled "After Anorexia: Life's too short to weigh your cornflakes" (https://www.youtube.com/watch?v=gZpcTVqpaPw) a TEDx Talk from Catherine Pawley, a patient recovering from anorexia. In this 8-minute video you will hear a brief overview of one person's experience with anorexia nervosa and will enhance understanding of the symptoms and emotional challenges associated with eating disorders. This video will also enhance understanding regarding the COLLECT and ASSESS part of the Patient Care Process.

INTRODUCTION

Eating disorders are widely accepted as serious mental illnesses. The spectrum of eating disorders encompasses several complex diseases, with most sharing the pathologic feature of overvaluation of body shape and weight. Eating disorders arise from the complex interaction between environmental, societal, developmental, psychosocial, genetic, and biologic factors. About 5 to 10 million females and 1 million males in the United States alone have an eating disorder. The urbanization of society, social pressure, and obsession with perfection and being thin have led to an increasing prevalence of eating disorders, with a median age of onset between 18 and 21 years, though estimates in adolescent studies suggest median ages of onset between 12 and 13 years.[1,2] Anorexia nervosa (AN), bulimia nervosa (BN), and binge-eating disorder (BED) are the most prevalent forms of eating disorders.[3]

1 Despite an improved understanding of these cognitively and emotionally disabling, and potentially fatal disorders, treatment remains difficult. Patients with eating disorders often demonstrate social difficulties prior to the onset of illness.[4] Pharmacologic intervention is a small part of a comprehensive treatment plan that emphasizes psychotherapy to address some of the social challenges, notably cognitive behavioral therapy (CBT) in adults and family therapy in younger patients.

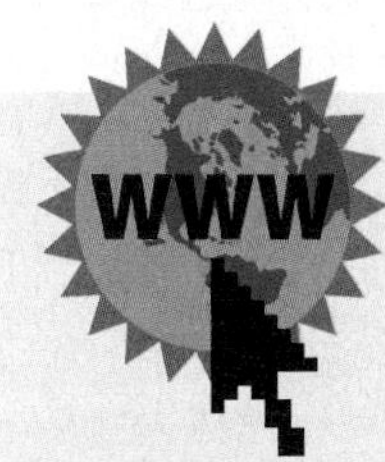

The complete chapter, learning objectives, and other resources can be found at **www.pharmacotherapyonline.com.**

Introduction to Substance Use Disorders

e84

Jessica L. Moreno, Patrick Leffers, and Vicki L. Ellingrod

KEY CONCEPTS

1. Substance use disorders (SUDs), including those pertaining to prescription medications, affect the health and well-being of millions of Americans.
2. Patients with SUDs are treated in all healthcare settings.
3. The use of prescription medications other than as prescribed, alone is estimated to cost more than 750 billion dollars annually.
4. There are several national efforts ongoing to monitor substance use trends in adults and children.
5. The etiology for SUDs is unknown, as there is no way to predict why some individuals exposed to substances develop a SUD, while others may not. It is felt that SUDs occur when some patients with genetic, psychological, and environmental risk factors are exposed to certain substances.
6. The *DSM-5* has established nine types of substance-related disorders including alcohol, cannabis, hallucinogens, inhalants, opioids, sedatives/hypnotics/anxiolytics, stimulants (ie, cocaine, amphetamine substances), tobacco, and caffeine.
7. The diagnosis of SUD is based on a set of behaviors related to that substance which fall into four categories including impaired control, social impairment, risky use, and pharmacological indicators.
8. The current *DSM-5* stratifies substance-related disorders into two groups: SUDs and substance-induced disorders (eg, intoxication, withdrawal, or medication-induced mental issues).[1]
9. The American Society of Addiction Medicine (ASAM) has endorsed recommendations of the Descriptive and Diagnostic Terminology Action Group (DDTAG) to clarify SUD-related terms.
10. Validated scales and screening tools provide objective measures of SUDs and are often used in research and clinical settings.
11. Treatment of SUDs focuses on a holistic biopsychosocial approach, to provide a recovery that allows the patient to live a full life as they manage symptoms and decrease risk of relapse.
12. Terminology surrounding SUDs is evolving. All healthcare providers should strive to use terms and language that are patient-oriented, medically precise, and without stigma.

BEYOND THE BOOK

Review the General Interviewing Guidelines provided by the National Institute on Drug Abuse (NIDA) at

General Interviewing Guidelines

https://https://www.drugabuse.gov/sites/default/files/general_interviewing_guidelines4-28-06.pdf

Watch the following video of a patient interview and note how you could improve the interaction for the patient and the interviewer.

https://https://www.youtube.com/watch?v=_VlvanBFkvl

INTRODUCTION

Psychoactive substance use dates back to prehistoric times where humans in the Neolithic era (8,500-4,000 BC) were found to use mood altering plants and fruits.[2] Thus, SUDs are not new; however, the types of substance used have evolved from the naturally occurring sources such as opium, alcohol, cannabis, peyote, psychedelic mushrooms, and coca leaves to synthetic or manufactured products. In fact, illicitly manufactured fentanyl (IMF) products fueled the third phase of the overdose crisis and have contributed to unprecedented overdose deaths across the United States.[3]

1 Society's views on what are considered non-socially acceptable drugs have also changed with time. Alcohol, nicotine, and caffeine are three prime examples substances considered by most to be socially acceptable. Much of this is due to a prohibitionist approach the United States has taken against most other drugs, which cannot be separated from the county's sordid past with racism such that drugs more often used by people of color have been, and continue to be, more heavily policed.[4] Even though alcohol and nicotine tend to be more socially acceptable substances, their use imposes an enormous social and economic cost on our society. The World Health Organization (WHO) estimates that in 2016, there were more than 3 million deaths worldwide attributed alcohol consumption with the majority being males. Additionally, it is estimated that more than 2.4 million individuals with an alcohol use disorder (AUD) also have another SUD.[5]

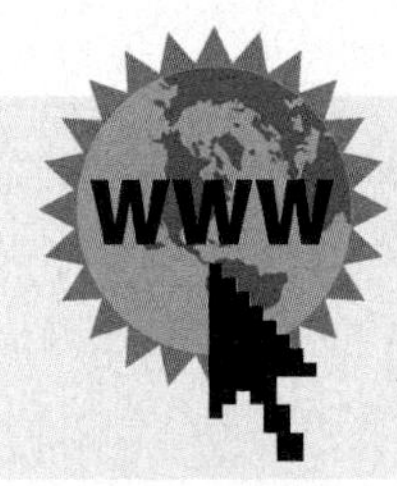

The complete chapter, learning objectives, and other resources can be found at **www.pharmacotherapyonline.com.**

Substance Use Disorders I: Opioids, Cannabis, and Stimulants

85

Patrick Leffers, Brittany N. Johnson, and Patrick Aaronson

KEY CONCEPTS

1 The financial impact of the opioid crises is estimated to have totaled $504 billion in 2015, which accounted for approximately 2.8% of the gross domestic product (GDP).

2 Opioids accounted for over 70% of all overdose deaths in 2019. The Centers for Disease Control and Prevention (CDC) estimates each day at least 136 people in the United States die from an opioid overdose.

3 Between 2006 and 2012, opioid prescribing in the United States steadily increased with a peak annual opioid prescription count of 255 million prescriptions.

4 Opioid overdoses involving prescription opioids, synthetic opioids, and heroin have continued to increase while healthcare professionals, legislators, and the community have worked together to reverse this trend, by focusing on prevention, treatment, recovery, and enforcement.

5 The pathophysiology of opioid use disorder, as with other substance use disorders (SUDs), centers around the reward centers and mechanisms in the brain.

6 Opioid use disorder (OUD) is a chronic often relapsing condition. Viewing OUD as a disorder and providing medications for the treatment of OUD, patient education, and support have been shown to decrease the risk of accidental overdose or full relapse into opioid use.

7 There are three Food and Drug Administration (FDA)–approved medications used in OUD: buprenorphine, methadone, and naltrexone. All three medications have demonstrated superiority for substance use disorder over no treatment. Pharmacotherapy in combination with psychosocial therapy has been found to be more effective than either treatment alone.

8 Patients who achieve clinical stability have longer acting options that may improve adherence and quality of life.

9 While not a treatment for OUD, naloxone is an integral treatment option that has been shown to save lives. Naloxone is a mu-opioid receptor antagonist that can be used in the reversal of an opioid overdose. It can be administered by multiple routes and is available without a prescription in many states. Healthcare providers play an important educational role on the importance of naloxone use in an opioid overdose situation.

10 Benzodiazepine prescribing has increased by over 65% from 1996 to 2013 and continues to climb. Overdose rates have increased over sevenfold from 2002 to 2019, the peak occurring in 2017.

11 Symptomatic and supportive care is the standard of care for benzodiazepine intoxication. Flumazenil is an antagonizing antidote that can be considered in select overdose situations. Treatment of benzodiazepine withdrawal is similar to treatment of alcohol withdrawal.

12 Stimulants including cocaine, methamphetamines, and newer derivatives continue to pose a significant issue to the population. Treatment of acute intoxication from these agents centers on supporting vital functions, while treatment for chronic use is less well described for such stimulants.

13 Expanded legalization of cannabis by individual states has brought an increase in chronic use. Emerging evidence supports the occurrence of an associated syndrome of effects known as cannabinoid use disorder (CUD). Treatment of CUD is in its infancy.

14 Cannabinoid hyperemesis syndrome (CHS) is a syndrome of cyclical vomiting in individuals with habitual use of cannabis that abates after discontinuation of use. The pathophysiology underlying CHS is not completely elucidated.

15 Many individuals who experience CHS report that hot showers improve symptoms, but that the benefit is short-lived. If intravenous fluids and traditional antiemetics are unsuccessful, other treatment options that are less established have been reported. Dopamine antagonists like haloperidol have been used successfully as well as topical capsaicin products.

BEYOND THE BOOK

Watch the video entitled "Opioid Overdose-Administration of Naloxone" by NIH Pain Consortium Centers of Excellence in Pain Education at Saint Louis University Edwardsville. This brief video provides an overview of the three FDA-approved naloxone delivery methods for the treatment of opioid overdose.

https://tinyurl.com/slvh6fx

Determine if your state has approved use of cannabis for medical purposes and/or legalized recreational use. Determine if your state's governing board has issued a statement or policy about medical cannabis. Think about how your health system is affected by these state laws.

INTRODUCTION: OPIOIDS

In 1889, the Boston Medical and Surgical Journal published a piece by J.F. Adams, M.D., addressing the unique and indispensable place opium holds in the pharmacopeia. "While surpassing other remedies in its beneficent effects, it is alike remarkable in its power to harm. Hence, its medical use requires a degree of caution not less than that with which a surgeon handles a scalpel." Adams goes on to highlight his concerns with opioid use (eg, risk of overdose, significant side effect profile, and risk of dependence) advocating for judicious stewardship of these agents.[1] Negating Adams' previous concerns was a 1980 single paragraph letter to the Editor of the *New England Journal of Medicine* reporting the risk of physical dependence was rare in patients without a history.[2] A bibliometric analysis identified 600 citations of this letter occurring between 1981 and 2017. Interestingly, the majority of these citations occurred after the FDA approval of OxyContin© (extended-release oxycodone hydrochloride) in 1995.[3] OxyContin® promotion was done by targeting primary care providers claiming it was less addictive than traditional opioids. While this marketing sparked an exponential increase in prescribing, an intense morphine-like high could still be experienced when it was crushed and injected, snorted, or swallowed. This promotion of opioid prescribing and availability was further perpetuated in late 1990s by professional organizations (eg, American Pain Society, American Academy of Pain Medicine, and the American Geriatrics Society) who endorsed the use of opioids in chronic non-malignant pain.[4] In the early 2000s, the Joint Commission linked healthcare quality and patient satisfaction with pain control which prompted providers to take action in addressing patient-reported pain scores. The overall result from this series of overlapping events was increased opioid prescribing, increased non-medical use of prescription opioids, and an increase in opioid-related deaths.

In an attempt to regain equilibrium, national and global health organizations allocated efforts and resources to addressing what was now a public health issue. Clinical guidelines and safety measures regarding controlled substance prescribing, prescription drug monitoring programs, education on proper storage and disposal of opioids, and take-home naloxone were expanded.[5] While these actions resulted in decreased opioid prescribing beginning in 2006, opioid-related overdose deaths continued to increase. An epidemic once fueled by the use of pharmaceutical opioids is now overshadowed by illicit manufactured fentanyl (IMF), fentanyl analogs, and heroin use. Thus, diluting the previous progress made by organizations such as the Centers for Disease Control and Prevention (CDC), the National Institute on Drug Abuse (NIDA), and the FDA. As a result, OUD continues to plague individuals, their families, and their communities.[6]

Like the disease itself, solutions related to extinguishing the opioid epidemic are multifaceted and multifarious in nature. Confronting this epidemic begins with addressing the social stigma of SUDs, increasing patient access to treatment, and ensuring provider comfort with prescribing treatment. Enlisting the help of communities through education on proper storage and disposal of opioids, as well as training on the use of the rescue medication naloxone[7] will be essential in reducing opioid-related deaths. These interventions will be costly, but they are needed to mitigate the cost of the ongoing crisis.

1 The council of economic advisers, an agency to the executive office of the president estimates the financial impact of the opioid crises (both fatality- and non-fatality–related costs) to have totaled $504 billion in 2015, a figure which accounts for approximately 2.8% of the gross domestic product (GDP) that year.[8]

Epidemiology

Despite the focus on prescription opiates, the opioid issue continues to worsen. Between 1999 and 2019, the number of overdose deaths in the United States more than quadrupled. 2 Opioids accounted for over 70% of all overdose deaths in 2019 and the CDC now estimates each day at least 136 people in the United States die from an opioid overdose.[9,10] These overdoses often involve poly-substance use making it difficult to interpret and classify mortality data. Over the last 20 years, the United States has seen three different waves of opioid overdose-related deaths. The first wave started in 1999 with prescription opioids (eg, natural opioids, semi-synthetic opioids, and methadone) and continued to rise as the second wave began in 2010 marked by a substantial increase in heroin overdoses. In 2013, a third wave created an exponential rise in synthetic opioid overdoses predominantly driven by IMF compounds in cocaine, heroin, and counterfeit pharmaceuticals.[9,10]

SUD is associated with comorbidities such as cardiovascular disease, stroke, cancer, lung disease, hepatitis, and infection with the human immunodeficiency virus. These healthcare issues occur without regard to the amount or frequency of substance use by an individual. The interplay between mental health and co-occurring SUD has yet to be fully elucidated. However, the National Survey of Drug Use and Health (NSDUH)[11] indicates an association between the two, with 397,000 adolescents aged 12 to 17 reporting major depressive episodes plus SUD. Along with 9.5 million reporting having both a mental illness and SUD. The impact of this disease combination is known to further inhibit functional ability, reduce treatment success rates, increase risk of homelessness, suicidality, incarceration, morbidity, mortality, and healthcare costs when compared to individuals with a single diagnosis. While current guidelines support addressing both disorders congruently, only 1.3% of adolescents with SUD and major depressive disorder (MDD) and 7.8% of adults with SUD and acute mental health issues received concomitant treatment in 2019.[11]

The Opioid Epidemic

3 Opioid prescribing in the United States steadily increased beginning in 2006 and peaked in 2012 with 255 million prescriptions dispensed annually. Between 2012 and 2019 the rate of opioid prescribing was nearly cut in half going from 81.3 prescriptions per 100 people to 46.7 per 100 in 2019.[12] However, in 2017 over 17% of the US population still had at least one opioid prescription filled. The greater than 19% decrease in prescribing may be attributable to a combination of factors including increased regulatory oversight, enhanced awareness of opioid-related risks, educational initiatives, and new legislative efforts to improve the prescribing and dispensing of controlled substances.

A large contributor to oversight improvement came with the implementation of statewide prescription drug monitoring programs (PDMPs), which are now operational in 49 of 50 states.[13] The PDMPs are electronic systems used for tracking controlled substance prescriptions with the intent to prevent diversion (eg, patients obtaining opioids from multiple providers) and improving patient safety, while still maintaining access.[14] Pharmacies are required to report dispensing information routinely to the program in the states that participate and over 40 states also require healthcare practitioners to access this database prior to prescribing a controlled substance. Specific requirements vary by state; however, interstate communication between programs has also become common. In an effort to optimize the use of PDMPs, some states have allowed incorporation of the PDMPs into the electronic health record (EHR) systems, decreased barriers to the registration process, and the ability for prescribers to assign delegates to review the PDMP under their license.[14]

Another measure focused on promoting opioid safety and reducing related harms (eg, OUD, overdose) included the CDC's 2016 publication of a Guideline for Prescribing Opioids for Chronic Pain.[15] This document provides recommendations for primary care physicians treating adults with chronic non-malignant pain in the outpatient setting (eg, excluding malignant pain, palliative care, and end-of life care). This guideline intended to (1) improve safety and effectiveness of long-term opioid therapy and pain treatment, (2) reduce the risks associated with opioid therapy, and (3) improve communication. The publication outlines three major areas of clinical consideration: (1) determining when to initiate or continue opioids for chronic pain; (2) opioid selection, dosage, duration, follow-up, and discontinuation; (3) assessing risk and addressing harms of opioid use (see Chapter 78, Table 85-1).[15] While this guidance was originally labeled as "voluntary," many states, organizations, and third-party payers have adopted them as their foundation for policy development and legislative change related to opioid prescribing.

Implementation inconsistencies surrounding the application of these recommendations in clinical practice has remained a point of controversy. Examples of these inconsistencies include reports of applying the guidelines to patients outside of the primary care setting (eg, patients with cancer, sickle cell disease, or recent surgery), imposing opioid prescribing limitations (eg, quantity, dosage, or duration), and tapering or discontinuing opioids without patient involvement, or adequate preparation.[16] In response to a consensus panel which outlined these challenges, the CDC issued clarification reiterating the importance of implementing the guidelines as they were intended and stressed that treatment be individualized to each patient.[17]

The FDA also launched a broad campaign in partnership with the Department of Health and Human Services (HHS), the National Academy of Medicine (NAM), and the National Institute of Health (NIH) to develop a systematic framework for the review of opioid medications that addresses their potential public health consequences (eg, long-term risk of addiction, diversion risk, and adverse effect profiles), and to expedite the approval pipeline for non-opioid analgesics and use deterrent formulations.[18] Several opioids with use-deterrent labeling and formulations have come to market since, which are designed to make it more difficult to administer

TABLE 85-1 Differences Between the Medications Used to Treat OUD

	Methadone	Extended-Release Injectable Naltrexone (XR-NTX)	Buprenorphine
Pharmacology in OUD	Full opioid agonist at mu-opioid receptor with long half-life to allow for once daily dosing for OUD	Antagonist at mu-opioid receptor (*note:* does not provide analgesia)	Partial agonist at mu-opioid receptor with long half-life (up to 36 hours via sublingual administration); blocks intoxicating effects of other opioids
Phase of treatment in OUD; effect	Medically supervised withdrawal, maintenance; reduces or eliminates withdrawal symptoms and cravings to use opioids, blocks or blunts the effects of illicit opioids	Prevention of relapse to opioid dependence following medically supervised withdrawal; reduces or eliminates cravings to use opioids and blunts or blocks the effects of opioids	Medically supervised withdrawal, maintenance; reduces or eliminates withdrawal symptoms and cravings to use opioids and blocks or blunts the effects of opioids
Route of administration	Provided orally once daily: Commonly given as liquid concentrate in treatment programs, but current guidelines also allow use of solid oral-dosage forms	IM extended-release (depot naltrexone) (*note:* oral not as effective and its use is not common in the treatment of OUD due to insufficient evidence of efficacy and poor medication adherence)	Sublingual, buccal tablet, buccal film Other routes of administration available after meeting specific criteria: subdermal implant, subcutaneous extended-release injection
Restrictions for prescribing each product	CII; patient must meet Federal Opioid-Treatment Program standards; can be used in hospital settings for OUD treatment	Not a controlled substance but requires a prescription. All naltrexone products can be prescribed by general practitioners and in OUD treatment	CIII; requires waiver to prescribe outside of a treatment program. Prescribers will receive a separate DEA number with a "X" upon meeting requirements of DATA 2000. They may prescribe for up to 275 individuals. To confirm practitioner verification: https://www.samhsa.gov/bupe/lookup-form Implant: Prescribers must be certified in buprenorphine REMS program to insert/remove implants Subcutaneous: Healthcare settings and pharmacies must be certified in the Sublocade REMS program and the medication is only dispensed directly to a provider for administration
Patients that are commonly considered for this type of therapy	Patients with OUD; physically dependent on opioids and meet federal OTP admission criteria	Patients with OUD; those who are abstinent from short-acting opioids for 7-10 days and long-acting opioids 10-14 days	Patients with OUD; physically dependent on opioids
Major side effects	Constipation, vomiting, dizziness, sedation, QTc prolongation, respiratory depression (risk is highest during methadone initiation, dose titration or with concurrent benzodiazepines or alcohol use)	Injection site pain and tenderness, risk of injection site induration, toothache, LFT elevation, insomnia, nasopharyngitis	Constipation, vomiting, dizziness, sedation, insomnia, blurred vision, respiratory depression (highest risk with concurrent use of CNS depressants including benzodiazepines); sublingual buprenorphine/naloxone sublingual and buccal film: oral hypoesthesia, oral mucosal erythema, glossodynia

CII, Schedule II Prescription; CIII, Schedule III Prescription; Federal Drug Addiction Treatment Act (DATA 2000); IM, Intramuscular; LFT, Liver Function Test.

Data from Reference 5.

the product via intravenous injection, nasal snorting, or chewing. Unfortunately, despite preliminary enthusiasm, conflicting evidence exists regarding the ability of these formulations to substantially reduce opioid use, OUD, overdose or death.[19] Further post-marketing analysis of these agents will add to the current body of evidence in determining the impact of these formulations on adverse events. Another measure to reduce opioid-related deaths by the FDA was the expansion of boxed warnings on benzodiazepines, opioid analgesics, and opioid-containing cough medicines notifying patients and their caregivers of the increased risk associated when opioids and benzodiazepines are taken concurrently.[20]

In 2018, the Risk Evaluation and Mitigation Strategy (REMS) program was expanded to include both short-acting and long-acting opioid formulations. Included with this was a requirement that training be available to all healthcare practitioners involved in pain management. The Opioid REMS Education Blueprint for Health Care Providers delivers education on pain assessment and management strategies for providers managing acute or chronic pain in the primary care setting to reduce inappropriate prescribing and adverse outcomes, while continuing to maintain access to pain medications.[21] For those healthcare practitioners still in training, the Association of American Medical Colleges continues to advance educational content related to pain assessment and management, SUDs, and responsible opioid prescribing.[22]

In 2018, the Substance Use Disorder Prevention That Promotes Opioid Recovery and Treatment (SUPPORT) for Patient and Communities Act[23] was enacted to focus on prevention, treatment, recovery, and enforcement to help of combat the opioid epidemic. This bill has many policy changes but major policy changes include the following:

- Remove restrictions on medications used for the treatment of OUD and expand prescribing rights of these agents to select physician extenders.
- Direct Center for Medicare and Medicaid Services (CMS) to look for further options in providing telehealth services for SUDs for Medicaid and Medicare patients.
- Expand existing programs allowing more first responders to carry and use naloxone.
- Allow more federal agencies to pursue expanded research projects related to pain, substance use, and risk for addiction.
- Adjust Medicare and Medicaid processes to limit overprescribing of opioids and allow expansion of substance use treatments including adjusting restrictions to improve access to care.
- Authorize SAMHSA[24] grant programs for "Comprehensive Opioid Recovery Centers" for communities.
- Improve initiatives for education and awareness for healthcare providers on proper pain treatment.
- Improve coordination between federal agencies to test, detect, and stop substances often used at the border.
- Increase penalties for medication manufacturers and distributers related to overprescribing of opioid.
- Create incentive programs for students to pursue a career in the SUD treatment field.

Since 2018, several additional bills introduced to congress have focused on reducing barriers to the prescribing and dispensing of buprenorphine for the treatment of OUD. Accompanying these is a proposal for a national education campaign encouraging practitioners to integrate SUD treatment into practice.[25]

Etiology

Overall, the true etiology behind OUD is still unknown, as there is no way to predict why some individuals exposed to an opioid develop an OUD, while others may not. In general, it is felt that there needs to be a triad of the right patient, with the right genetic risk factors, being exposed to the right substances in order for an OUD to occur.

4 The high bioavailability, near immediate onset of action, and increased potency of IMF and its respective analogs is thought to play a causal role in overdose fatalities.[10] This postulation is affirmed by the 1,040% increase in synthetic-opioid–related deaths observed from 2013 to 2019. Death rates related to prescription opioids, and heroin correspondingly have continued to rise in the presence of synthetic opioids. These combined upward trends imply that medication-related overdoses are continuing to intensify across the United States.[26]

Pathophysiology

5 Understanding of OUD pathophysiology is growing and, like with other SUDs, focuses on the reward center and mechanism in the brain. Substances or activities that release dopamine (DA) in the nucleus accumbens (NAc) have been clearly linked to disordered use. The current understanding is that the rapid release of DA following an opioid reaches the NAc to stimulate D1 receptors which in turn activates cyclic AMP (cAMP). This leads to the downstream effects such as euphoria and pleasure. This feeling conditions the person to associate using the substance and their surrounding environment and situation with the euphoric and pleasurable sensations. Receptors for *N*-methyl-D-aspartate (NMDA) and α-amino-3-hydroxy-5-methyl-4-isoxazolepropionic acid (AMPA) in the synapse are also conditioned by the DA release to increase glutamate signaling. These changes further modify the interconnected neural loops that lead to habit formation and disordered response to opioids. While DA and glutamate are direct signals in this system, emerging evidence seems to implicate indirect signaling via γ-aminobutyric acid (GABA), serotonin, acetylcholine, endogenous opioids, and endogenous cannabinoid compounds.[27]

CLINICAL PRESENTATION

After repeated exposure to opioids, the nervous system adapts by creating a level of tolerance. When this repeated exposure is removed a hyper-excitable state results. Opioid withdrawal presents with similar signs and symptoms no matter the agent(s) used. Onset, duration, and severity of withdrawal may differ depending on the pharmacokinetics of the opioid agent, chronicity of use, and dosage consumed. Opioid withdrawal itself is not life-threatening; however, consequences of withdrawal can be significant. Patients can experience uncontrolled pain, miscarriages, premature delivery, and increased risk of suicide due to psychological distress. To avoid needless suffering during the withdrawal period supportive therapies (eg, clonidine, buprenorphine) can be implemented as appropriate to mitigate severity of discomfort. To assess withdrawal severity several validated assessment tools are available (eg, COWS, OOWS). Frequent reassessment will be prudent, as the onset, duration, and peak effects of withdrawal are dependent on the substance involved. Typically, withdrawal symptoms begin within 8 to 24 hours for opioids with a short half-life (eg, heroin), and can last up to 7 to 10 days. For agents with a long half-life (eg, methadone), symptoms can begin as early as 24 hours following the last dose but takes up to 96 hours to peak with gradual reduction of symptoms over 2 weeks or longer. The post-acute phase of withdrawal can last for weeks, months, or even longer leading to symptoms such as opioid craving and a negative affect including symptoms such as fear and irritability. It is also important to remember patients who have withdrawn from opioids will have a reduced opioid tolerance that could increase the risk of opioid overdose.[30]

Methadone

In 2014, methadone accounted for one in four prescription opioid-related deaths despite only accounting for 1% of all opioids

CLINICAL PRESENTATION Acute Opioid Withdrawal and Intoxication

See Chapter e84, "Introduction to Substance Use Disorders" for complete *DSM-5* diagnostic criteria.

General

- Opioid withdrawal presents with similar signs and symptoms across the agents in the class.
- Onset, duration, and severity of withdrawal may differ depending on the opioid agent, chronicity of use, and dosage consumed.
- Onset of the acute phase of withdrawal ranges from 8 to 24 hours for short-acting opioids and 36 to 72 hours for long-acting opioids.
- The duration of withdrawal ranges from days to weeks for short-acting and long-acting opioids, respectively.
- Similarly, duration and severity of opioid intoxication is dependent on the agent, dosage, and frequency of use.

Symptoms

- Opioid intoxication: euphoria, dysphoria, apathy, lethargy, somnolence, and impaired motor skills. Individual agents may also have idiosyncratic presentations (eg, seizures with tramadol, QTc prolongation with methadone).
- Opioid withdrawal: insomnia, muscle or bone aches, abdominal cramps, vomiting, diarrhea, and anxiety or agitation. The Clinical Opiate Withdrawal Scale (COWS) or the Objective Opioid Withdrawal Scale (OOWS) are clinician-rated assessment tools used to trend the severity of opioid withdrawal symptoms and medication efficacy.

Signs

- Opioid intoxication: miotic pupils, drooping eyelids, scratching due to histamine release, decreased respiratory drive, pulmonary edema, loss of consciousness, and death.
- Opioid withdrawal: tachycardia, hypertension, hyperthermia, abnormally heightened reflexes, lacrimation, increased respiratory rate, restlessness, tremor, nausea/vomiting, diarrhea, irritability/anxiety, rhinorrhea, yawning, insomnia, dilated pupils, gooseflesh, and perspiration.

Laboratory Tests

- A comprehensive metabolic panel, complete blood count, urine toxicology screen, physical exam, electrocardiogram (EKG), and pregnancy screening will help guide medication selection for management of withdrawal symptoms and identification of potential medications for OUD treatment.
- For suspected opioid intoxication, blood gas, pulse oximetry, and capnography assist in monitoring for opioid-induced respiratory depression and can be used as appropriate.
- Abnormal findings may require further evaluation or referral.

Management

- To avoid needless suffering during opioid withdrawal, clinicians should attempt to manage patients in discomfort with supportive therapies.
- Patients presenting with acute opioid intoxication may require naloxone administered intermittently or in more severe cases as an intravenous infusion.

Data from References 28, 29, 31, and 32.

prescribed.[31] Methadone has pharmacologic properties that are unique among opioids, and a lack of knowledge by practitioners and patients regarding these unique properties is thought to contribute to methadone-related deaths. Methadone's elimination half-life (15-60 hours; some reports as long as 120 hours) is longer than its duration of analgesic action (4-8 hours) and its full analgesic effect is usually not achieved for 3 to 5 days.[32] Doses should not be increased more frequently than every 5 to 7 days according to recent guidelines.[32] Fatal errors have been reported during conversion from other opioid agonists to methadone, as it has wide variability in equianalgesic dosing compared to other opioids. Therefore, vigilance is necessary during treatment initiation, during conversion between opioids, and during dose adjustments. Medications administered concomitantly with methadone should be evaluated for potential interactions, as methadone has many. Due to its association with prolongation of the QTc interval (in the most severe cases leading to torsades de pointes) it is prudent to monitor a patient's ECG prior to initiation and after significant dose adjustments of methadone.

Heroin

Heroin, also known as diacetylmorphine, is a serious threat to the United States and its use has increased since 2007. Since 2016 the number of heroin-related deaths has trended down, but in 2019, an estimated 14,019 Americans died from heroin-related overdoses. It remains to be seen if this is a temporary plateauing of annual deaths or the beginning of a more prolonged decrease. Overdose deaths involving co-ingestion of psychostimulants (primarily methamphetamine or derivatives) and opioids has continued to increase since 2016, which may also be contributing to the reduced mortality.[28]

The main factors associated with increases in heroin use are increased availability, low cost, and increased purity.[28,29] The DEA expects that high-purity heroin, commonly referred to as white powder heroin, will continue to be available in the United States. Now exacerbating the overdose deaths is heroin laced or adulterated with fentanyl and related derivatives that are 50 to 100 times more potent than heroin. There are conflicting opinions about whether policy changes implemented to reduce nonmedical prescription opioid use had unintended consequences by increasing the use of heroin in the United States. Opioid prescribing policies could help decrease heroin overdose deaths.[33]

Heroin is hydrolyzed to 6-acetyl morphine and subsequently morphine. It acts as an agonist at opioid receptors including the mu, kappa, and delta receptors. Administration can occur via multiple routes including intranasal, intravenous, subcutaneous, intramuscular routes, or smoking. Heroin is very lipophilic and crosses the blood brain barrier (BBB) quickly which leads to very rapid absorption and arrival at the site of action; 5 to 10 minutes when administered subcutaneously, 3 to 5 minutes intranasally and intramuscularly, and <1 minute when administered intravenously.[34] Although the initial half-life is approximately 8 hours, the ultimate duration of effect from heroin is dependent on the person's history with the medication and how it is administered. The oral route is typically not preferred due to first pass metabolism to morphine which leads to less rapid onset of action.[34]

As tolerance develops, the half-life decreases leading to earlier withdrawal symptoms including dilated pupils, hostility, sweating, vomiting, diarrhea, yawning, and piloerection. Those that use heroin increase doses and rates of administration to avoid these withdrawal symptoms, which increases their overdose risk. Symptoms of heroin use include sedation, decreased respiration, apnea, cardiac arrest, and death without medical treatment such as administration of naloxone.[35] Testing for heroin in urine, blood, or other biological samples is difficult due to the very short half-life of intact heroin (2-6 minutes). Unfortunately, the next metabolite, 6-acetylmorphine (6-AM) is only present in urine and blood for approximately 6 to 25 minutes before it is hydrolyzed to morphine and other metabolites. As morphine and other metabolites can be detected on a urine screen after heroin use, as well as after use of certain prescription opioids, results from urine screens are often misinterpreted and require confirmatory secondary testing and a thorough clinical evaluation.[35,36]

Fentanyl

Fentanyl is a synthetic short-acting opioid analgesic, that is 50 to 100 times more potent than morphine and is approved for managing acute or chronic pain, as well as pain associated with advanced cancer. Although pharmaceutical fentanyl can be diverted for use, most cases of fentanyl-related morbidity and mortality have been linked to illicitly manufactured fentanyl and fentanyl analogs (IMF). Since 2015, there have been almost yearly CDC public health fentanyl advisories including a public health advisory regarding increased fentanyl-related overdose deaths, a warning that fentanyl was found in counterfeit pills in the United States, and a report regarding the rise in fentanyl analogs contributing to opioid overdose deaths.[37]

Generally, the IMF products are sold via illicit markets, with individuals seeking them out for their heroin-like effect. Additionally these illegal products are often mixed with heroin and cocaine and marketed as an oral opioid or benzodiazepine.[37] Deaths from counterfeit opioids and benzodiazepine pills laced with fentanyl have been reported and are believed to be contributing to the increased overdose rates. A CDC analysis from 31 states and Washington DC from 2015 to 2016 showed that overdose death rates increased by 21.5%, and the death rates from synthetic opioids (presumed to be IMF) more than doubled. The death rates for heroin, cocaine, and psychostimulants also increased by 19.5%, 52.4%, and 33.3%, respectively, and the CDC attributes a portion of rate increases to the presence of IMF in the respective products.[38]

Other Opioid-Related Substances

Intoxication from the OTC cough suppressant, dextromethorphan[39] occurs from consuming large doses of liquid cough syrup that is known as "robodosing" or "robotripping" and those who use the cough syrup in this manner are sometimes called "syrup heads."[39] Additionally, "skittles" is a term used to describe use of other cough and cold remedies because they look similar to the popular candy. As dextromethorphan is an opioid analog, large doses can create a depressant and sometimes profound hallucinogenic effect, and since it is available OTC it is easily procured by adolescents.[39]

Loperamide is also another dangerous example of OTC medication that is often used. Pharmacologically this medication acts as an intestinal mu-opioid agonist that works locally for the short-term treatment of diarrhea. When used in this fashion, at normal recommended doses, it does not cross the blood brain barrier and will not have any CNS effects.[40] When taken at high doses, or with concomitant medications that inhibit the P-glycoprotein efflux transporter, CNS effects can be seen.

TREATMENT

Desired Outcomes

6 As with any use disorder the desired treatment outcomes for OUD are reduction in use of the substance, reduction in substance-induced disorders, and prevention of death from the substance. The course and prognosis of OUD is variable. Getting patients to stop misusing can be quite difficult, and many patients return to opioid use even after treatment. It has been reported that as many as 40% to 60% of treated patients with an SUD will relapse within 1 year.[41] However, many patients can achieve recovery with proper treatment and continued care in counseling programs or 12-step programs such as Narcotics Anonymous. It is important to note that the treatment of OUD is a chronic condition that needs proper medical treatment and appropriate follow-up, as relapses are common. Therefore, providing medication for long-term maintenance decreases the risk of an accidental overdose or full relapse into opioid use. Continued patient education and support is vital to helping patients continue their set treatment goals.

Pharmacologic Therapy

A variety of treatment regimens are used for patients during the acute opioid withdrawal phase. Initiating buprenorphine in the emergency room for patients who present with opioid withdrawal symptoms has become a treatment option. The reader is directed to Cisewski et al.[42] for a detailed review outlining the process for establishing this stepwise treatment practice.

Methadone has also been used as a long-acting opioid option to aid in treatment of withdrawal symptoms.[43] The use of clonidine, an alpha-2 agonist, has commonly been used to attenuate withdrawal symptoms such as anxiety, tachycardia, hypertension, chills, and piloerection. Patients must be monitored for side effects including hypotension, dizziness, and sedation following administration of clonidine.[43] Lofexidine, also an alpha-2 agonist, has been found to be more effective than placebo in managing withdrawal from methadone or heroin and has demonstrated a better safety profile compared to clonidine.[43,44] Replacement of fluids due to losses from perspiration, vomiting, and diarrhea is crucial during withdrawal and other patient-specific supportive care measures should be provided until the patient stabilizes. Ongoing follow-up is important since post-acute withdrawal can continue for an extended period of time. This can increase risk of relapse and heighten the risk of overdose.

7 Although OUD can range from mild to severe, it often requires continual care including patient-centered care involving mental health services, medical services, counseling, and the use of medications for treatment. The three FDA-approved medications used in OUD include methadone, buprenorphine, and naltrexone that work by blunting or blocking the effects of opioids and reducing or eliminating craving. All three agents have demonstrated superiority over no treatment in reducing opioid use,[30,45,46] and methadone and buprenorphine decrease the risk of overdose deaths. All of these medications have unique characteristics that healthcare providers must be aware of, including differences in mechanism of action, routes of administration, and side effects. It is also important to understand in what phase of treatment each of these agents is used, and the regulations associated with their use (Table 85-1).

Methadone Methadone is a mu-opioid agonist that suppresses withdrawal symptoms and controls the craving for opioids in

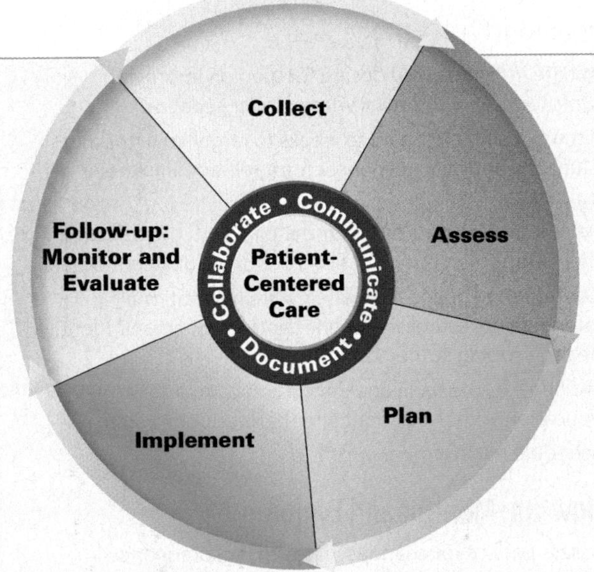

Patient Care Process for Opioid Use Disorder (OUD)

The image shows the five fundamental steps included in The Pharmacist's Care Process endorsed by the Joint Commission for Pharmacy Practitioners (2014). The tagline of this process reads collaborate, communicate, and document. The five fundamental steps listed here are collect, assess, plan, implement, and follow-up: monitor and evaluate. All these steps are listed in a circular block diagram.

Collect

Objective Data

- Patient characteristics (eg, age, sex, pregnancy status)
- Blood pressure (BP), heart rate (HR), respiratory rate (RR), height, weight
- Prescription drug monitoring program (PDMP) data
- Practitioner observed pill counts
- Labs including urine or oral fluid drug testing, pregnancy test, liver function tests (LFTs), Hepatitis B and C serology, Human Immunodeficiency Virus (HIV) serology

Medication history

- Current medications including herbal products, dietary supplements, over-the-counter (OTC) medications, nonprescribed medications, prescription medications, illicit substances
- Known medication allergies or intolerances

Past medical history

- Past or current co-occurring illnesses (physical and mental), injuries, surgeries, and hospitalizations
- General state of current physical and mental health (eg, good, fair, poor, concern for suicidal ideation)

Social and environmental history

- Substance use (eg, tobacco/ethanol use, substance use, prescribed and/or non-prescribed medication use)
- Opioid use history (eg, age of first use, frequency and recentness of use, routes of use, overdose history, medication and drug mixing, withdrawal, tolerance, history of treatment for substance use disorder [SUD])
- Problems resulting from substance use
- Participation in high-risk activities for contracting sexually transmitted infections (STIs)
- Living environment and transportation resources
- Current support systems (eg, family, friends, group therapy)
- Family history of SUD (eg, parents, siblings, partners)
- Childhood or adolescent abuse (eg, emotional, sexual, physical, verbal)

Assess

Signs of opioid intoxication or withdrawal

- Physical
  - Dental caries, perforated septum, skin abscesses, needle track marks, swollen extremities, withdrawal (eg, goose bumps, nausea, abdominal cramps, tearing, yawning, runny nose, yawning) or intoxication (eg, drooping eyelids, constricted pupils, reduced respirations, itching, head nodding)
- Neurological
  - Dilated or constricted pupils, slurred or rapid speech, agitation, insomnia, falling asleep at inappropriate times, unstable gait
- Psychiatric and Behavioral
  - Depression, anxiety, low self-worth, mental health disorders, feelings of hopelessness or loss of control, resentment
  - Use of other substances, conduct disorders, impulsivity, alienation from others, involvement with the criminal justice system
- Risk stratification
  - Assess patients for alcohol, tobacco, substance use, and substance use disorders
  - Screening tools and symptom surveys may aid in determining opioid risk (eg, Pain Medication Questionnaire, Opioid Risk Tool, Current Opioid Misuse Measure), opioid withdrawal (eg, Clinical Opioid Withdrawal Scale, Objective Opioid Withdrawal Scale), alcohol use disorder (alcohol use disorder identification test), and respiratory depression (Risk Index for Overdose or Serious Opioid-Induced Respiratory Depression).
  - The *Diagnostic and Statistical Manual of Mental Disorders, 5th Edition* (*DSM-5*) criteria for diagnosis of SUD should be established by a provider prior to proceeding forward with treatment.
- Evaluate patient readiness
  - Highlight consequences that may motivate positive change
  - Identify patients' reasons to start treatment (eg, people, quality of life, self)
  - Determine the patients' preferred treatment setting (eg, opioid treatment programs, outpatient office visits with a prescriber)

(Continued)

- Discuss potential barriers for patient access to treatment for OUD, mental health support, and laboratory tests for monitoring

Plan*

- Engage the patient in shared decision making regarding the risks and benefits of using medications to treatment of OUD, including alternative treatments
- Review medication options for the treatment of OUD (Tables 85-1, 85-2, and 85-3)
- Design a medication therapy regimen (eg, specific medication(s), dose, route, frequency, and anticipated duration of therapy (Tables 85-1, 85-2, 85-3, and 85-5)
- Communicate monitoring parameters including efficacy (eg, cravings, relapse, and withdrawal symptoms) and safety (eg, medication interactions, adverse medication effects); frequency and timing of follow-up
- Educate patients about their diagnosis, medication, and expectations (eg, purpose of treatment, possible adverse medication effects, importance of proper storage of medication, naloxone education, risk of overdose with discontinuation of treatment and return to substance use, notify other providers they are on this medication) (Table 85-4)
- Refer patient to other providers when appropriate (eg, behavioral health specialist, social worker)

Implement*

- Initiate individualized dosing focused on improving symptoms of withdrawal without over-sedation
- Titrate dosing over days to weeks to target cravings and blunt the euphoric responses from self-administered illicit opioids
- Review all elements of treatment plan with the patient and their support system (eg, friends, family, significant others)
- Continue to engage the patient with motivational interviewing, establish patient-centered goals and identify healthy coping strategies
- Provide a home naloxone device and complete proper education with the patient and their support system
- Schedule patient follow-up visit

Follow-up: Monitor and Evaluate

- Assess patient for changes in health (eg, pregnancy, pulmonary disease, hepatitis) and medications, including those non-prescribed substances, prescribed medications, OTC, or herbals)
- Reevaluate medication therapy daily to weekly until stable
- Continue random drug testing, and monitoring for medication-related adverse medication effects

**Collaborate with patient, caregivers, and other healthcare professionals.*

maintenance therapy. Controlled trials have shown that methadone use in patients with OUD is superior to placebo and has demonstrated a reduction of mortality, incidence of HIV infection, and criminality.[10] Recommended once daily dosing of methadone on the first day of treatment for patients tolerant to opioids can range from 10 to 30 mg, depending on the patient's use pattern. The patient should be reassessed in 2 to 4 hours after this initial dose for signs of sedation or symptoms of withdrawal. Additional monitoring and/or treatment can continue if needed during the first day based on the initial response. Although rare, if the dose does exceed 30 mg on the first day of treatment, monitoring for over-sedation should occur for multiple days.[30] In patients who are older than 60 years of age, have identified medication interactions, or have other medical conditions that can lead to increased risk of hypoxia, it is recommended to limit the initial maximum methadone daily dosing to 10 to 20 mg. Dosing ranges for stabilization that eliminate withdrawal and craving, block euphoric effects of illicit opioids, and that are not normally associated with sedation are commonly between 60 and 120 mg administered once a day for most patients but this can vary considerably.[30] Titrating the methadone dose must be individualized and based on a full assessment of the patient. Due to its long half-life and extended time to reach steady state, daily dose adjustments should not occur, as they can result in over-sedation and possible increased risk of toxicity. It is recommended that dose adjustments of 5 to 10 mg should occur gradually, with each adjustment occurring no sooner than every 4 to 7 days based on clinical response. This will allow for achievement of steady state and account for the other numerous factors that can impact serum levels.[30,32] Concerns with methadone include medication interactions due to the variety of concomitant cytochrome P450 (CYP 450) inducers that can reduce methadone levels. Concomitant use of alcohol or benzodiazepines can lead to overdose and use should be assessed. Additionally, the risk of QT prolongation is increased with methadone use, especially when given with other medications that also prolong the QT interval. The use of methadone for the treatment of OUD is only approved through the opioid treatment programs controlled by the DEA and SAMHSA. However, methadone for the treatment of OUD may be provided to patients during a hospital admission for the treatment of other health conditions such as pain. Patients who as part of an opioid treatment program most often receive it on a daily basis with daily onsite administration; however, some patients are allowed to take doses at home if they meet a list of criteria set by federal regulations.[47]

Naltrexone Naltrexone is a mu-opioid antagonist available as both an oral tablet and an extended-release injectable formulation for the treatment of OUD.[48,49] It is important to note that while the oral tablet has not been found to be any more effective than placebo in a meta-analysis of 13 studies,[50] naltrexone reduces opioid use and retained treatment participation compared to placebo.[45]

To use the oral formulation, patients need to have confirmation of being opioid free for 7 to 10 days as assessed through the use of a urine drug screen or naloxone challenge. The initial dose given is 25 mg once daily and if no symptoms of withdrawal are demonstrated, this can be increased to the target dose of 50 mg once daily.[48] Extended-release injectable naltrexone (Vivitrol®) is FDA-approved for use following opioid detoxification to help prevent relapse.[49] It is important to review all medication-associated adverse effects with patients, including education on the length of time naltrexone is active and their vulnerability to opioid effects at the end of a dosing interval, after a missed dose, or with treatment discontinuation. Patients should be informed to contact their provider if any excessive swelling, bruising, or pruritus occurs at the injection site since this could be a sign of improper subcutaneous injection and may require medical treatment. The REMS information highlights the risk of severe injection site reactions and provides education for healthcare providers including proper techniques to reduce severe injection site reactions as well as important counseling points to use with patients to identify any signs or symptoms of injection site reactions.[49] Naltrexone is not a controlled substance and is not included in the opioid treatment program regulations, but it does require a prescription and a monthly medical office visit. The use of extended-release injectable naltrexone should be part of a comprehensive patient program that includes psychological counseling and support.

Buprenorphine Buprenorphine is a partial mu-receptor agonist that is very lipophilic and available as buprenorphine alone or in combination with naloxone. These products have been shown in numerous studies and clinical trials to be effective treatment options for OUD both in reducing opioid use and treatment retention.[47] It is now recommended by the Best Practice Guidelines (TIP 63) expert panel[30] and the Department of Veterans Affairs Guidelines[51] that FDA-approved buprenorphine formulations should be offered to patients with OUD who are appropriate candidates. As buprenorphine is a partial mu-receptor agonist, it does provide some intrinsic pain control. Additionally, due to the partial agonist activity, it also has a ceiling effect for respiratory depression, except when combined with CNS depressants such as benzodiazepines or alcohol, where there have been reports of increased risk of respiratory depression. Furthermore, due to the partial agonist activity, any full agonist activity will be blunted, such as that provided from heroin or other opioids. This effect will be prolonged due to the long half-life and prolonged receptor dissociation properties of buprenorphine.[52] At the time of this writing there are buprenorphine/naloxone sublingual tablets and films, buprenorphine/naloxone buccal films, buprenorphine implants, buprenorphine tablets, and a buprenorphine extended-release injection.[52] Newer products have greater bioavailability compared to previous products, making product selection and conversion between buprenorphine products an important consideration for healthcare providers (Tables 85-2 and 85-3).[52,53]

8 Patients who achieve clinical stability have longer acting options that may improve adherence and improve quality of life (Table 85-3). Buprenorphine is a Schedule III controlled substance with specific prescribing restrictions. Table 85-1 outlines some of these restrictions. Recent legislation has extended regulations to allow physician assistants, nurse practitioners, clinical nurse specialists, certified nurse midwives, and certified registered nurse anesthetists to prescribe buprenorphine. This practice varies by state based on laws and regulations, therefore each state licensing board should be consulted for the most up to date laws and regulations.

Prior to prescribing buprenorphine, a full assessment including reviewing the PDMP database and a full medication review should be completed. Care should be taken to screen for medication interactions including HIV medications, benzodiazepines, CNS depressants, and CYP 450 inducers/inhibitors. Additionally, a urine drug screen, informed consent, and treatment agreement should be completed. Comprehensive patient education is very important to help improve adherence to the treatment plan and improve patient safety (Table 85-4).

When the patient presents to begin buprenorphine, it is important for the clinician to assess the patient carefully for signs of sedation or intoxication since buprenorphine should not be started under these circumstances. As the patient should be present in the beginning stages of withdrawal to start buprenorphine, a validated assessment scale, such as the Clinical Opiate Withdrawal Scale (COWS), can be used for assessment. It is recommended that treatment start with a COWS score of 12 or higher for the first dose, based on buprenorphine REMS.[30]

Medically supervised withdrawal with buprenorphine consists of an induction phase and a dose-reduction phase, followed by maintenance.[30] Best practice guidelines are periodically issued for treatment of OUDs. The TIP 40[52] (entitled "The Guideline for the Use of Buprenorphine in the Treatment of Opioid Addiction") provides consensus- and evidence-based guidance on the use of buprenorphine and the TIP 63 provides similar guidelines as outlined below for buprenorphine treatment.[30] Induction is the first stage of buprenorphine treatment and involves helping patients begin the process of switching from the used opioid to buprenorphine. The goal of this phase is to find the minimum dose of buprenorphine at which the patient discontinues or markedly diminishes use of other opioids and experiences no withdrawal symptoms, minimal or no adverse medication effects, and no craving for the used substance. This phase is commonly initiated in the physician office when the patient is in mild to moderate withdrawal with the last dose of opioid use occurring 6 to 12 hours prior for heroin or short-acting opioids. For longer-acting opioids such as methadone, it is recommended to wait 24 to 72 hours after the last dose. Patients are typically monitored in the office at approximately 2-hour intervals after the first dose of buprenorphine with continued dose titration until the withdrawal symptoms are eliminated. Guidelines recommend weekly follow-up until the patient is stable and then monthly follow-up can be considered.[52] Although office-based induction has traditionally been recommended, home induction is an alternative growing in use.[30] The American Society of Addiction Medicine

TABLE 85-2 Oral Buprenorphine Products Used in Treatment of Opioid Use Disorder

	Buprenorphine Tablet	Suboxone SL Tablet	Zubsolv SL Tablet	Suboxone SL Film	Bunavail Buccal Film
Strengths of products commercially available/Routes of Administration	**Sublingual Tablet:** 2 mg 8 mg	**Sublingual Tablet:** 2/0.5 mg 8/2 m g	**Sublingual Tablet:** 0.7/0.18 mg 1.4/0.36 mg 2.9/0.71 mg 5.7/1.4 mg 8.6/2.1 mg 11.4/2.9 mg	**Sublingual or Buccal Film:** 2-0.5 mg 4-1 mg 8-2 mg 12-3 mg	**Buccal Film:** 2.1-0.3 mg 4.2-0.7 mg 6.3-1 mg
Recommended Once-Daily Target Maintenance Dose and Dosing Ranges	**Target Maintenance Dose:** 16 mg **Dosing Range:** 4-24 mg[a]	**Target Maintenance Dose:** 16/4 mg **Dosing Range:** 4/1 to 24/6 mg[a]	**Target Maintenance Dose:** 11.4/2.9 mg **Dosing Range:** 2.9/0.71 to 17.2/4.2 mg[b]	**Target Maintenance Dose:** 16/4 mg **Dosing Range:** 4/1 to 24/6 mg[a]	**Target Maintenance Dose:** 8.4/1.4 mg **Dosing Range:** 2.1/0.3 to 12.6/2.1 mg

SL, sublingual.

[a]Doses higher than 24/6 mg do not offer any further benefit.

[b]Doses higher than 17.2/4.2 mg do not offer any added benefit.

Note: Refer to individual product dosing information when switching formulations due to possible bioequivalence variability. Monitoring is recommended following a switch in products due to possible variation in response to different formulations.

Data from References 32, 54-57, 63, and 64.

TABLE 85-3 Patient Education Points for Buprenorphine Treatment

Prior to starting buprenorphine therapy and repeated at induction

- **Communication with prescriber:** Tell your prescribers all medications including over-the-counter (OTC), herbal, creams, injections, inhalants, street medications, etc. that you are currently taking. This is important so your healthcare team is aware of what is in your body and if there are any chances of a dangerous medication interactions. Additionally, it is important to tell all of your prescriber and healthcare team you are taking buprenorphine, especially if you are being treated for pain.
- **Goals of therapy:** The goal of your first week of treatment is to improve withdrawal symptoms without causing any over-sedation (making you too tired or feeling over medicated). It is important to notify your prescriber if you are feeling overly tired/sedated or euphoric within 1 to 4 hours of your dose. Dose adjustments might occur initially and it will take a little time for the buprenorphine to become stable in your system. The goals of therapy include finding the right dose to eliminate withdrawal, decrease or even eliminate cravings for opioids, and block the effects of other opioids without severe adverse medication effects.
- **Product use:**
  - Buprenorphine products (tablets, sublingual film, and buccal film) are not equivalent. If you have to transition to a new buprenorphine product, a dose adjustment might be required.
  - Take your dose at regular intervals and only as prescribed.
  - If you miss a dose, take the dose as soon as possible. If it is almost time for the next dose, do not double your dose, take only the dose that is prescribed.
  - Leave medication in packaging until you are ready to use.
  - Do not swallow sublingual tablets or film. This can lead to a decreased effect of buprenorphine that can lead to withdrawal symptoms.
    - Sublingual tablets:
      1. Place tablets under tongue and allow the tablet to fully dissolve which can take several minutes.
      2. If your dose requires multiple tablets, all tablets can be placed under the tongue at one time. If this is uncomfortable, only place two tablets under the tongue at a time.
    - Sublingual film:
      1. Drink water prior to placing the film to help the film dissolve easily.
      2. Place film under the tongue, to the left or right of the center of the tongue, and allow to completely dissolve
      3. If you are prescribed 2 films at a time, place the second film on the opposite side of the tongue. Do not allow the films to touch.
      4. If you are prescribed more than 2 films at a time, wait until previous films have dissolved and repeat the process.
    - Buccal film:
      1. Wet the inside of your cheek with your tongue or rinse with water prior to placing film.
      2. Hold the film by the edges with two fingers and place on inside of cheek until fully dissolved that can take up to 30 minutes.
      3. If you are prescribed two films, place the second film inside the opposite cheek.
      4. Do not adjust the film placement or touch the film, do not chew or swallow the film.
      5. Do not drink or eat until the film has completely dissolved.
- **Common adverse medication effects:** These do not happen all of the time and do not happen to everyone. If you are experiencing any of these adverse medication effects please tell your healthcare team immediately. Do not stop taking buprenorphine without first speaking to your prescriber. The most common adverse medication effects that have been experienced include headache, nausea, constipation, abdominal pain, insomnia, sweating, and a possible feeling of weakness or lack of energy.
- **Precautions and warnings:**
  - Using benzodiazepines or alcohol while taking buprenorphine is very dangerous and can lead to increased risk of overdose and possibly death.
  - Using tobacco products prior to using buprenorphine has been shown to decrease the absorption of buprenorphine decreasing its effectiveness.
  - Long-term buprenorphine maintenance is recommended in many cases. If you stop buprenorphine, there is a high risk of overdose if you return to misusing opioids.
  - Buprenorphine is an opioid that can cause physical dependence. Do not stop taking buprenorphine without consulting your prescriber. If you stop buprenorphine abruptly, you could experience withdrawal symptoms.
  - All medications, including buprenorphine, should be stored in a secure area, preferably in a locked cabinet or safe. It is important to keep medication away from children.
  - It is recommended that you do not drive, operate heavy machinery, or perform any dangerous activities until you are fully aware of how this medication affects you.
  - If you feel you have taken too much buprenorphine, you will need emergency medical attention immediately. Some possible signs include dizziness, confusion, unsteady or faint, slowed reflexes, or breathing slower.
  - Do not inject these products. Serious life-threatening infections could occur. Additionally, serious withdrawal reactions can also occur upon injecting many of these buprenorphine products.
- **Pregnancy:** It is very important to inform your healthcare team if you become pregnant.
- **Counseling options:** Recovery resources and counseling resources are available for you and your family. We can give you further information on this when you are ready.

Maintenance

- **Adherence assessment:** If any discrepancies arise, initiate discussion to identify reasons for discrepancies.
  - Complete pill/film count.
  - Review Prescription Drug Monitoring Program.
  - Confirm current buprenorphine dose.
  - Review results of urine drug analysis.
- **Treatment assessment and counseling:**
  - Review treatment goals and assess progress.
  - Review and assess benefits and risks of continuing buprenorphine treatment.
  - Discuss participation in counseling or encourage counseling if not receiving counseling.

Data from References 30, 43, and 58.

National Practice Guidelines recommends that both the patient and prescriber have prior experience with the medications used to treat OUD, in order to consider this option.[52,60]

The stabilization phase begins when a patient is experiencing no withdrawal symptoms, is experiencing minimal or no adverse medication effects, and no longer has uncontrollable cravings for opioid agonists. Buprenorphine dosage adjustments may be necessary during early stabilization, and frequent contact with the patient increases the likelihood of compliance. Ongoing psychological evaluation for mental health or psychological issues is recommended so proper medical assistance can be provided immediately if needed.[30]

Maintenance is the longest phase of treatment as this period may be indefinite and longer treatment has been associated with

TABLE 85-4 Extended-Release Products Approved by FDA for Opioid Use Disorder

Medication	Trade Name	Dose	Comments
Naltrexone Tablets	Revia	Following 7-10 day opioid-free period for short-acting opioids or 10-14 day opioid-free period for long-acting opioids: begin with dose of 25 mg daily with food. If no signs of withdrawal, increase dose to 50 mg PO daily.	• Should be part of a comprehensive treatment plan that includes psychosocial support • Although specific dosage adjustments are not available for patient with hepatic dysfunction, reports of elevated LFTs have been reported; use with caution • Use with caution in patients with renal impairment, although data is limited, naltrexone and active metabolite are renally excreted
Naltrexone XR Injection	Vivitrol	Following 7-10 day opioid-free period for short-acting opioids or 10-14 day opioid-free period for long-acting opioids: 380-mg IM in gluteal area alternating buttocks; every 4 weeks or once a month.	• Must be administered by a healthcare provider • Must use manufacture provided needle and assess body size of patient at each visit so proper needle size is used • Monitor injection site closely for any signs of abnormal pain and contact healthcare provider immediately if this occurs • Dose adjustment is required in mild or moderate hepatic impairment. No data available in severe hepatic impairment • No dose adjustments in mild renal impairment; use caution in patients with moderate-to-severe renal impairment; naltrexone and active metabolite are renally excreted

Buprenorphine	Probuphine	Four implants are inserted subdermally in the inner side of the upper arm and should remain in place for 6 months.	• Patients must meet specific criteria for use of Probuphine:
			  • Only indicated for patients who are opioid tolerant
			  • Demonstrates clinical stability on transmucosal buprenorphie with Subutex or Suboxone 8 mg/day or less (or transmucosal equivalent) for 3 months or longer without requiring supplemental dose adjustments
			• Probuphine must be inserted or removed within a facility and by a certified provider who has completed the required live training
			• It is recommended to not prescribe prn transmucosal buprenorphine products. If patient is requesting these products, reassessment is indicated
			• Moderate-to-severe hepatic impairment: use not recommended
			• Limited data in renal impairment, currently no dosage adjustments listed

Buprenorphine	Sublocade	For patients who have achieved clinical stability on equivalent of 8-24 mg of a transmucosal buprenorphine product daily. *Available in two extended-release solutions:* • *100 mg/0.5 mL* • *300 mg/1.5 mL* Directions: Inject 300 mg subcutaneously once a month in abdominal area for 2 months, then decrease dose to 100 mg once monthly in abdominal area.	• Must be administered by a healthcare provider • Steady state occurs after 4-6 months; after discontinuation of detectable buprenorphine levels could occur 12 months or longer; urine and plasma concentration correlations are not known • Injections must occur at least 26 days apart. Follow all manufacturers' direction for preparation and injection • Do not give the injection at the belt or waistband area where pressure will occur • It is important to counsel the patient that there will be a small bump at the injection site that will decrease in size over the next several weeks. It is important not to rub or massage this area. • If needed, the most recently injected depot can be removed within the 14 days of injection under local anesthesia. • Doses can be adjusted back to 300 mg monthly for patients in which benefits exceed risks. • Examine injection site each month for evidence of tampering • Moderate-to-severe hepatic impairment: use not recommended • Limited data in renal impairment, currently no dosage adjustments listed

mg, milligram; IM, intramuscularly; mL, milliliters.

Data from References 5, 51, 58, and 59.

positive treatment outcomes.[61] During the maintenance phase, attention must be focused on the psychosocial and family issues that have been identified during the course of treatment that contribute to a patient's OUD.[61] Other issues related to OUD that need to be addressed during maintenance treatment include, but are not limited to, psychiatric comorbidity, consequences of drug use, family support issues, structuring of time in prosocial activities, employment and financial issues, legal consequences of medication use, and the use of other substances. Ongoing monitoring will continue to include urine drug tests, and patient education regarding this aspect is important so there is understanding that this testing is used more to help them meet treatment goals and not as a tool for punishment.[30]

Naloxone 9 Naloxone is a key strategy in reducing opioid-related deaths,[62] as patients who are being treated for OUD, or who are not taking medications for OUD but are at high risk of returning to opioid use, are at substantial risk of overdose. It is imperative that patients and their caregivers are educated on the availability of naloxone and the proper use of this agent. Pharmacologically, naloxone hydrochloride is a competitive mu-opioid receptor antagonist that can be used in the reversal of an opioid overdose. It can be administered through a variety of routes including intravenous (IV), intramuscular (IM), subcutaneous, intraosseous, (IO), and intranasal (IN).[63] The onset of action when delivered via intravenous route can be as fast as 60 seconds, but is approximately 2 to 5 minutes when delivered IN.[63] The duration of effect is dependent upon the dose and the specific opioid naloxone is reversing. It is important for interested parties to know that if a long-acting opioid such as methadone is involved, the patient could show decompensation after initial improvement due to the long half-life of methadone and comparatively short half-life of naloxone.

The FDA has approved two devices to deliver naloxone that can be administered by nonmedical bystanders: the intramuscular autoinjector Evzio® and an intranasal delivery device, Narcan®. A third option readily available prior to these new devices, the generic injectable naloxone solution used with a mucosal atomization device, is used in the community setting, although it is not approved by the FDA. For this device, extra education is necessary on how to connect the components and then administer the 1-mg dose per

TABLE 85-5 Naloxone Delivery Options

	Intramuscular Injection	Auto-Injector (Evzio)	Nasal Spray (Narcan)	Intranasal Spray (Atomizer)
Description of device or what is provided	Two single use 0.4-mg/mL naloxone vials Two single use 3-mL syringe 23-25 gauge 1-1.5 in. needles	One box 2-mg/0.4-mL prefilled auto injector that include 2 devices and a trainer devices	One box that contains two 4-mg/0.1-mL intranasal devices	2-mg/2-mL prefilled naloxone needleless syringe Two mucosal atomizer devices
Directions for use	Inject 1-mL intramuscularly in shoulder or thigh upon signs of opioid overdose. Call 911 immediately. May repeat once more in 2-3 minutes if inadequate response.	Apply one auto-injector to the outer thigh by depressing and holding for 5 seconds. The voice automation will direct the patient with this device. Call 911. May repeat once more in 2-3 minutes if inadequate response.	Use full contents of nasal spray in one nostril upon signs of opioid overdose. Call 911. May repeat once more in 2-3 minutes if inadequate response using the other nostril.	Spray one-half of contents of syringe into each nostril upon signs of opioid overdose. Call 911. May repeat once more in 2-3 minutes if inadequate response.

Naloxone pearls:

- Naloxone has not been shown to cause severe effects or adverse medication effects if administered to patients who are currently not taking opioids.
- Naloxone should be given if the patient is intoxicated by a combination of products since the naloxone will still work for the opioid but not for other products such as benzodiazepines or alcohol.

Naloxone counseling topics that should be covered:

- Overdose recognition, response, prevention
- Importance of seeking emergency medical care
- Proper device use and counseling of family members and caregivers
- Proper storage, shelf life. Periodically check expiration date
- Potential adverse medication effects associated with naloxone
- Availability of substance use disorder treatment program

General opioid safety counseling:

- Take medication only prescribed for you, only take prescribed doses
- Do not mix opioids with alcohol or sleeping pills
- Always store all medications in a locked and secure place
- Dispose of unused medications appropriately
- Do not use opioids/medications in seclusion. Never buy opioids/medications from unknown source
- Do not restart opioid at same dose if there is a period of abstinence. Overdose is possible due to lower tolerance

Data from References 63-65.

nostril.[63] Table 85-5 includes more information about naloxone delivery options and counseling information.

Inadequate response to less sensitive opioids such as buprenorphine, fentanyl, or other synthetic opioids may be seen with take-home naloxone (THN).[62,64] Higher doses of naloxone may be needed in such a scenario; therefore, it is vital that emergency services are contacted to provide ongoing care.[62,65] However, the THN products might provide time for arrival of medical professionals and/or transportation to medical facilities for more definitive treatment.

Controversy exists regarding concerns that distribution of naloxone may increase drug use, as some authors feel naloxone has contributed by "providing a safety net that encourages riskier use."[66] However, data from communities that have implemented overdose programs prior to this report have documented a decrease in overdose death rates. In fact, overdose education and naloxone distribution (OEND) programs in the community have been occurring since 1996, and this practice was embraced by the World Health Organization (WHO) guidelines which recommend that anyone who might witness an overdose have access to naloxone and proper training.[66]

As the number of opioid overdoses has continued to increase, CDC guidelines have recommended increasing use of THN. In fact, improving access has become a goal of many states through expanding those able to distribute naloxone or simplifying the process of obtaining the naloxone. Additionally, improved education of healthcare providers and the community as a whole has also been a primary goal.[67]

Opioid Use Disorder in Pregnancy As the rates of opioid use in the United States have increased, the number of pregnant women diagnosed with OUD has increased substantially.[68] The occurrence of opioid use during pregnancy results in an increased risk of preterm labor, neonatal abstinence syndrome, and maternal mortality. The CDC reported the rate of OUDs in women at delivery has more than quadrupled between 1999 and 2014.[68] Current recommendations for a pregnant woman with an OUD requesting treatment includes methadone or buprenorphine, and behavioral interventions. Now, the safety of extended-release injectable naltrexone is still under study. For patients taking naltrexone, it is recommended that it be converted to buprenorphine or methadone during the pregnancy.[69] More specifics regarding treatment in this population can be obtained from recently released guidance documents for healthcare providers entitled "Clinical Guidance for Treating Pregnant and Parenting Women with Opioid Use Disorder and Their Infants."[69]

Key to the success of OUD treatments in this population is patient education, which should include topics such as the risks and benefits of the chosen medication. During this discussion, it is important to stress to the patient there are some disagreements on the risks associated with these medications. Now, research efforts have not linked buprenorphine or methadone use with an increased risk of birth defects and or issues with long-term neurodevelopment.[69] Other important topics to discuss with the patient include risk of neonatal abstinence syndrome and details associated with this syndrome, as well as important strategies for improving the patient's health and the pregnancy. Due to the large number of pregnant women presenting with OUDs, all healthcare providers should look for substance use behaviors in their pregnant patients, and if identified, provide a referral for therapy as quickly as possible to improve the outcome for both the mother and the baby.[69]

INTRODUCTION: BENZODIAZEPINES AND OTHER SEDATIVE-HYPNOTICS

Benzodiazepines, while not first-line treatment options, are commonly prescribed for anxiety, muscle spasms, and insomnia in a variety of practices. While their therapeutic use can be quite helpful to patients, similar to opioids, their CNS effects can make them substances commonly misused.

Epidemiology

10 Benzodiazepine prescribing has increased by over 65% from 1996 to 2013 and continues to climb. Overdose rates have increased over sevenfold from 2002 to 2019, the peak occurring in 2017.[28] When benzodiazepines are given concomitantly with an opioid, the combination can lead to increased CNS effects such as dizziness and sedation but also deadly respiratory depression. A cohort study that included over 2 million opioid prescriptions in 1 year demonstrated 80% of these were co-prescribed with a benzodiazepine and the rates of overdose deaths in this group were 10 times higher than opioid analgesics alone.[70] In 2016, the FDA announced a class-wide medication labeling change for both opioids and benzodiazepines requiring both classes to include black box warning indicating that concurrent use could cause sedation, respiratory depression, coma, and death.[71] Additionally, the CDC Guidelines for prescribing opioids for chronic pain recommends avoiding concurrent benzodiazepine and opioid prescriptions whenever possible highlighting the dangers of using this combination.[15]

Etiology

Pharmacologically, the benzodiazepines increase the affinity of gamma amino butyric acid (GABA) for its receptor and augment GABA-mediated inhibitory signaling. This occurs by targeting the $GABA_A$ receptor that has multiple subunits. Activation of these subunits leads to an increase in frequency of ion channel opening that leads to an influx of chloride ions and membrane hyperpolarization.[72] Benzodiazepines vary in pharmacokinetic properties, with additional details being found in Chapters 90 and 91.

A class of medications related to the benzodiazepines include eszopiclone, zaleplon, and zolpidem, which are prescribed for insomnia, and commonly known as the Z-hypnotics. While pharmacologically they may differ from benzodiazepines, tolerance and withdrawal have been reported with their use and they should be used with caution.[73] Additionally, this class of medication is required by the FDA to include labeling that warns of a variety of psychological and behavioral adverse medication effects that include sleep driving. Depression and suicidal thoughts have also been linked to these products, although this has been seen mainly in patients taking both sedatives and hypnotics concurrently.[73]

Pathophysiology

Benzodiazepines have been shown to cause release of dopamine in the mesolimbic region of the brain, which is a hallmark of substances that can lead to use disorders.[73] Additionally, benzodiazepines have demonstrated an ability to activate dopaminergic neurons in the ventral tegmental area through $GABA_A$ interactions involving interneurons in the region. These two neuronal pathways within the addiction centers of the brain explain their potential for developing disordered use of this medication class. Due to their use liability, patients cannot be switched from one benzodiazepine to another in hopes of decreasing this behavior pattern. Additionally, long-term use of even therapeutic doses of these agents can cause physical dependence and withdrawal symptoms after abrupt discontinuation, including seizures. In general, shorter-acting benzodiazepines have higher risk of use potential due to the immediate "rush" or "high" feeling. Gradual tapering (4 weeks or longer) of dosage is also associated with less withdrawal and rebound anxiety than abrupt discontinuation.[73]

TREATMENT

Desired Outcomes

Similar to the desired outcomes for individuals misusing opioids, the overall goals of treatment are to reduce dependency, the incidence of substance-induced disorders, and death.

Non-pharmacological management as a primary treatment for benzodiazepine intoxication or withdrawal is not indicated. Rather, direct pharmacologic care of an individual intoxicated with a benzodiaepines includes the use of supportive care. For patients undergoing benzodiazepine withdrawal, supportive care should be provided in combination with pharmacologic therapy.

CLINICAL PRESENTATION Benzodiazepine Intoxication and Withdrawal

General

- The intoxicated patient may be in acute distress during overdoses or when benzodiazepines are combined with alcohol.
- Patients in withdrawal may be in acute distress and should be treated with a benzodiazepine taper to prevent seizures.

Symptoms

- Symptoms of intoxication may include memory impairment, drowsiness, visual disturbances, confusion, and gastrointestinal disturbances. Patient may appear intoxicated, with slurred speech, poor coordination, swaying, and bloodshot eyes, with or without the odor of alcohol.
- Symptoms of withdrawal can include agitation and restlessness, confusion, anxiety, sleep disturbances, dizziness, flu-like symptoms, impaired memory and concentration, irritability, nausea and vomiting, nightmares, visual disturbances, convulsions, hallucinations, and psychosis.

Signs

- Hypotension or nystagmus may be observed and urinary retention may occur.
- Nervousness, sweating, trembling, hypertension, tachycardia, weakness, tremors, and seizures are examples of possible signs in acute withdrawal.

Laboratory Tests

- Qualitative testing to confirm presence of benzodiazepines is useful for diagnostic purposes, but quantitative plasma concentrations are usually not clinically useful due to the length of time required for results to be obtained at most institutions.

Pharmacologic Therapy for Benzodiazepine Intoxication and Withdrawal

11 Symptomatic and supportive care is the standard of care for benzodiazepine intoxication. Management primarily includes support of bodily functions to allow for metabolism and excretion of the medication from the system. For individuals that use short-term, withdrawal is not expected and thus flumazenil can be considered. Flumazenil reverses the intoxicating effects of benzodiazepines and Z-hypnotics by competitively inhibiting the GABA/benzodiazepine receptor complex. However, caution should be exercised as indiscriminate use can potentiate seizures in those that have used benzodiazepines chronically and those who have co-ingested a seizure-potentiating substance (eg, bupropion, tricyclic antidepressants, and lithium). The dosing scheme is to give 0.2 mg of flumazenil IV, then 0.3-mg IV if there is an insufficient response, then repeated doses of 0.5-mg IV up to a maximum of 3 mg.[74]

Treatment of benzodiazepine withdrawal is very similar to the treatment of alcohol withdrawal. The major differences in management is the length of treatment.[73] The duration of withdrawal symptoms in patients physically dependent on benzodiazepines can be variable due to multiple factors including benzodiazepine dose, duration of use, duration of taper, and pharmacokinetic half-life.[75] Current recommendations suggest a gradual taper extending over 4 to 8 weeks and sometimes longer depending on the duration of use. It is recommended to reduce the daily dose approximately 10% to 25% every 2 weeks to decrease the risk of severe withdrawal reactions and seizures.[73] If a patient is taking multiple benzodiazepines, it is recommended to convert the patient to an equivalent single dose of diazepam, given its long half-life, and begin the taper as directed. There is limited evidence for converting a patient from a single short half-life benzodiazepine to a long half-life benzodiazepine so this practice is generally not recommended. With all benzodiazepines, protracted minor abstinence symptoms—such as anxiety, insomnia, irritability, sensitivity to light and sound, and muscle spasms—can remain for several weeks or longer in patients with a history of long-term exposure. This can occur even after the acute phase of benzodiazepine withdrawal is complete.[76] Additional information on benzodiazepine tapers can be found in Chapter 90.

INTRODUCTION: STIMULANTS, HALLUCINOGENS, AND CANNABINOIDS

12 Acute intoxication with stimulants, hallucinogens, cannabinoids, and other mind-altering substances continues to be a relevant issue around the world. Improved outcomes are achieved through prompt recognition of symptoms and supportive care. At the time of writing, no antidotes or targeted therapies are available for these agents. Active monitoring and management of vital organ function is often sufficient for a positive outcome. Chronic use disorder and withdrawal from these agents are complex disease states that can require inpatient monitoring. No medication-assisted therapy is available for the treatment of chronic use involving these agents. Data involving successful treatment of SUDs involving stimulants, cannabinoids, and cathinones is in its infancy. It likely requires outpatient follow-up and psychosocial intervention for long-term sustained recovery.

Stimulants

The physiologic and psychologic effects of amphetamines and other stimulants are qualitatively similar, as they diminish fatigue, increase alertness, and suppress appetite. In higher doses stimulants can lead to behavioral changes, perception disturbances, and frank psychosis. Pharmacologically, amphetamines increase the activity of catecholamine neurotransmitters (eg, norepinephrine and dopamine) by stimulating release, decreasing reuptake into the neuron through blocking of vesicular monoamine transporters (VMAT2), and by inhibiting the degradation via monoamine oxidase (MAO). Stimulants improve mood, self-confidence, energy levels, alertness, concentration, and physical performance. Negative consequences of stimulant use range from headache, palpitations, hypertension, tachycardia, dizziness, anxiety and insomnia to confusion, agitation, paranoia, convulsions, and delirium.

Methamphetamine

The pathophysiology of methamphetamine use disorder (MUD) results from dopamine, serotonin, norepinephrine, and epinephrine release from the synaptic vesicle into the cytosol.[77] Dopamine is also increased through several mechanisms such as the inhibition of monoamine oxidase and increase in tyrosine hydroxylase activity. However, excessive dopamine can also increase reactive oxygen species that lead to cell structure damage. With this damage, the brain's metabolic state is altered through acidification of the microenvironment, and dysregulation of cell signaling via reactive oxygen species. This mirrors degenerative central nervous system diseases. The resultant neuronal and microglia cellular dysregulation is associated with dysfunctional neural processing, altered reward motivation, and reduced prefrontal control. Through this, the imbalance in the orbitofrontal cortex of the brain leads to cognitive deterioration affecting valuation and decision making. This results in poor task performance, and inattention, which facilitates continued-seeking behavior. Mortality from MUD is commonly associated with cerebrovascular disease such as stroke, and cardiovascular disease such as cardiac collapse.[77] Because methamphetamine elevates mood, people who experiment with it tend to use it with increasing frequency and in increasing doses, despite their original intent.[78]

Methamphetamine is used orally, intranasally, rectally, intravenously, and by smoking. Immediately after inhalation or intravenous injection, the individual using methamphetamine experiences an intense sensation, called a "rush" or "flash," that lasts only a few minutes and is described as extremely pleasurable. The timing and intensity of the "rush" that accompanies methamphetamine use results from the release of high levels of dopamine in the brain, but this depends in part on the method of administration. Specifically, the effect is almost instantaneous when smoked or injected, whereas it takes approximately 5 minutes after snorting or 20 minutes after oral ingestion.[79] The duration of effect is about 12 hours per administration but can be altered by route of administration and individual characteristics.[78]

Methamphetamine-induced caries, or "meth mouth," is a characteristic pattern of dental decay commonly observed in patients that smoke methamphetamine. Prolonged use of methamphetamine can result in a tolerance for the medication and increased use at higher dosage levels, creating dependence. Such continual use of the medication with little or no sleep may lead to an extremely irritable and paranoid state. Discontinuing use of methamphetamine often results in a state of depression, as well as fatigue, anergia, and some types of cognitive impairment that can last from 2 days to several months.[79]

Healthcare providers working in the retail setting, such as pharmacists, should be wary of persons wishing to purchase large quantities of products containing nonprescription sympathomimetic products such as pseudoephedrine, as this is a key ingredient for methamphetamine production. As a precaution, federal legislation now limits the quantities that can be purchased, along with mandating pseudoephedrine-containing products be kept behind a counter, and suitable identification be shown before purchasing.

Cocaine

Cocaine is perhaps the most behaviorally reinforcing of all used substances. It acts as a local anesthetic through inhibition of voltage-gated sodium channels when topically applied. Cocaine also acts as a sympathetic nervous system stimulator through α- and β-adrenergic stimulation which can precipitate chest pain and myocardial infarction. In the CNS, the stimulant and euphoric effects occur through inhibition of dopamine and norepinephrine reuptake. The excess dopamine in the ventral tegmental area (VTA) leads to the psychostimulant properties, contributes to psychotic behavior, and portends a high rate of addiction.[80]

For many years, cocaine has been administered as the hydrochloride salt form, usually by insufflation, but also by injection. Conversion to the cocaine base, also known as "crack" or "rock," allows for smoke inhalation. This is generally a more inexpensive form and thus more widely available. The time to peak concentration is rapid for all routes but is fastest by intravenous injection (instantaneous), then smoking (6 minutes), and then finally nasal insufflation (45 minutes).[80] Smoking the drug leads to almost instant absorption and intense euphoria. The high from insufflating is more prolonged lasting 15 to 30 minutes, whereas the high from smoking rapidly dissipates lasting only 5 to 10 minutes. Cocaine is metabolized and eliminated rapidly, with a half-life of approximately 1 hour contributing to its very short duration of effect.[81] Therefore, the rapid onset and short duration combined provide a powerful incentive for repeated use of the drug. The primary cocaine metabolite (benzoylecgonine) may be detected for up to 5 days in a urine sample with little cross-reactivity.[82] Increased use can reduce the period of stimulation and an appreciable tolerance to the high can develop. Many individuals that use cocaine report failing to achieve as much pleasure as they did from their first exposure with continued use which may lead to intense drug-use cycling, sometimes lasting days, characterized by rapidly repeating doses of cocaine until their money or supply is exhausted.

Other patterns of use such as consumption of alcohol along with cocaine are common and add to the toxicity. Such drug use would seem counterintuitive based on the counteracting effects of the two substances; however, in the presence of alcohol, cocaine is metabolized to cocaethylene, a longer-acting but

CLINICAL PRESENTATION Cocaine Intoxication and Withdrawal

General

- In overdoses, cocaine is a CNS and cardiac stimulant.
- Cocaine-related deaths are often a result of cardiac arrest or seizures followed by respiratory arrest.

Symptoms

- Symptoms of intoxication include motor agitation, elation, euphoria, hypervigilance, sweating, nausea, and vomiting.
- Symptoms of withdrawal include fatigue, sleep disturbances, nightmares, depression, and changes in appetite.

Signs

- Tachycardia, mydriasis, and elevated blood pressure may be observed with overdose.
- Cardiac abnormalities (eg, arrhythmias, infarction) and respiratory depression may be observed with overdose.
- Bradyarrhythmias and tremors may be observed in acute withdrawal.

Laboratory Tests

- Qualitative urine screening tests are available; however, they do not change clinical treatment significantly.

Other Diagnostic Tests

- Markers of organ dysfunction may be ordered as clinically indicated.

CLINICAL PRESENTATION Amphetamine Intoxication and Withdrawal

General

- Amphetamine intoxication is an acute condition that may result in death. Pharmacotherapy may be indicated for symptomatic control of agitation, psychosis, and seizures.
- Patients may experience withdrawal symptoms for several days but are usually not in acute distress. Treatment of withdrawal is supportive in nature.

Symptoms

- Amphetamine intoxication may present as increased wakefulness, increased physical activity, decreased appetite, increased respiration, hyperthermia, and euphoria. Other CNS effects include irritability, insomnia, confusion, tremors, convulsions, anxiety, paranoia, chest pain, and aggressiveness. Hyperthermia and convulsions can result in death.
- Depression, altered mental status, substance craving, dyssomnia, and fatigue are all symptoms of withdrawal.

Signs

- Patients with amphetamine intoxication may present with tachycardia, hypertension, seizures, or stroke.

Laboratory Tests

- A qualitative urine screening can identify patients who have been exposed to amphetamines. However, false positives are common and the diagnostic benefit is limited.

potent psychoactive compound compared to the parent drug. The risk of death from cocaethylene is greater than from cocaine alone and this combination is one of the most common among individuals who come to hospital emergency departments with acute substance abuse problems.[81]

Ecstasy

There are several dozen analogs of amphetamine and methamphetamine that are mildly hallucinogenic. Two methamphetamine analogs of most concern are 3,4-methylenedioxyamphetamine and especially 3,4-methylenedioxymethamphetamine (MDMA, Ecstasy or Molly). Ecstasy usually refers to a tablet or pill formulation, whereas Molly is most often a powdered form that can be insufflated or smoked. Trends in MDMA use have been declining since its peak in 2001; however, the annual prevalence of use has held steady.[11]

Individuals that use MDMA report feelings of trust and empathy with others, decreased inhibition when socializing, and enhanced proprioception in addition to stimulating effects that MDMA shares with amphetamines. These effects are due to the preferential selectivity of MDMA for serotonergic over dopaminergic neurotransmission.[83] In addition to these positively reinforcing effects, MDMA use can result in negative effects such as panic, anxiety, depression, paranoid thinking, and psychosis. Physical symptoms include muscle tension, nausea, blurred vision, faintness, chills, and sweating, as well as vomiting, hyperthermia, dehydration, tremors, insomnia, and convulsions. Furthermore, MDMA also increases heart rate and blood pressure due to its structural similarities with amphetamines.[84]

In general, those that use MDMA perceive it to be a harmless drug, based in part on the fact that the risk of death is low compared with other drugs such as heroin and cocaine. However, mounting evidence points to MDMA's neurotoxic effects, involving a complex and incompletely understood mechanism. Mechanistically MDMA has been shown to destroy serotonergic neurons in animals, but further research is needed to understand the mechanism behind this loss of serotonin following MDMA exposure.[84] Recent publication of small studies exploring ecstasy being used therapeutically further complicates the assessment of MDMA's risks and benefits, as preliminary studies have been conducted in posttraumatic stress disorder (PTSD), anxiety disorders, and social anxiety in autism. It should be noted that most of these studies also include psychotherapy as part of the treatment regimen.[85,86]

Hallucinogens

The drugs commonly classified as hallucinogens are lysergic acid diethylamide (LSD), psilocybin, dimethyltryptamine (DMT), mescaline, phencyclidine (PCP), ketamine, and other related compounds. Approximately 1.4 million people aged 12 or older are estimated to be currently using hallucinogens, with variability seen in each age ranging from 0.6%, 1.7%, and 0.3% for adolescents, young adults, and adults, respectively.[11] These statistics may not include ketamine use as this was recently added to the NSDUH Survey. Pharmacologically, LSD and related drugs stimulate both presynaptic (5-HT_{1A} and 5-HT_{1B}) and postsynaptic (5-HT_2) serotonin receptors in the brain, which functionally can cause either agonist or antagonist effects on serotonin activity. Precisely how the hallucinogens exert their effects remains unclear. Overall, LSD is an extraordinarily potent compound, producing observable CNS effects at doses as low as 25 mcg. For an in-depth review of the history, current status, and future uses of LSD, the reader is directed to a review by Smith and colleagues.[87]

Cannabinoids

Cannabis use is common in the United States. Despite a multitude of states passing laws allowing medical use and recreational use, cannabis is still an illegal substance according to federal law. In addition, increased media attention surrounding potential medical uses has also contributed to the public's evolving beliefs surrounding its use. In 2019, an estimated 48 million (a steady increase since 2002) Americans aged 12 or older used cannabis which corresponds to 17.5% of this population.[11] This use is likely to increase for the foreseeable future making abuse and subsequent treatment an increasingly important topic for healthcare providers. Cannabinoids are the active compounds within most available products or preparations. One chemical component of cannabis is δ-9-tetrahydrocannabinol (THC) which interacts with the two cannabinoid receptors within the CNS to cause its euphoric and psychoactive effects. Cannabidiol (CBD) does not have psychoactive effects. Epidiolex™ is a CBD preparation, FDA approved to treat Lennox-Gastaut syndrome and Dravet syndrome, two disorders that leave the afflicted with refractory seizures.[88]

As a group, cannabinoids interact with two subsets of cannabinoid receptors in the body: cannabinoid receptor 1 (CB1) and cannabinoid receptor 2 (CB2). Anandamide and 2-arachidonoylglycerol are the endogenous complements to the CB receptors, although their effects have not been completely described. The CB1 receptors are found in presynaptic neurons of the prefrontal cortex and in the hippocampus, and the CB2 receptors are located in smaller numbers in the prefrontal cortex, hippocampus, and hypothalamus. However, they are thought to play a much larger role in systemic effects of cannabinoids due to their abundance in the immune, peripheral nervous, and gastrointestinal systems.[89] Since THC is a partial agonist at CB1 and CB2 receptors, it is thought to create its psychoactive effects through CB1 receptors. In contrast, CBD binds less tightly with CB receptors and may interact with other receptors within and outside of the CNS.[90] Although the knowledge base surrounding the pharmacology and pharmacodynamics of cannabinoids is rapidly expanding, the current knowledge regarding their therapeutic effects is relatively incomplete compared to other FDA-approved medications. While cannabis is most commonly smoked, it can be ingested orally with THC and CBD extracts now being incorporated into many other usable forms including edible candies/snacks and vaporizable liquids that can be more palatable for new, young, or those not experienced in using cannabis. Cannabinoid pharmacokinetic properties are not well characterized, but they do show highly variable effects that are greatly affected by route of use. After inhalation of smoke or vapors, peak blood concentrations occur in about 10 minutes and although bioavailability is higher through inhalation relative to oral ingestion, many factors can affect this. Both THC and CBD are poorly bioavailable due to extensive first-pass metabolism by the liver; therefore, peak concentrations occur at about 2 hours when taken via the oral route. The terminal half-life of THC and CBD after a single use is about 24 hours; however, in those that use chronically, the terminal half-life is highly altered due to accumulation and subsequent redistribution from fatty tissues after chronic use.[90]

Cannabis use disorder (CUD) is loss of control over use, repeated failures to quit, and continuous usage despite negative consequences. The pathophysiology of CUD lies in chronic neuroadaptation over time. The primary euphoric psychoactive component of cannabis THC targets the body's natural endogenous endocannabinoid system leading to downregulation in those that use chronically. This downregulation results in alterations to the processes that regulate cognition, emotional processing, stress sensitivity, and reward goal directed behavior occurs. Additionally, THC-induced alterations modify synaptic plasticity, specifically leading to a reduction in synapses of the hippocampal neurons.[91]

13 According to the *DSM-5*, CUD leads to significant social impairment and or psychological distress in spite of negative personal consequences.[92] It is often associated with multiple failed attempts at

halting cannabis use, with the rate of occurrence in North America being estimated to be as high as 749 in 100,000.[93] Although CUD has quite a high incidence, its detection and treatment are limited in part by beliefs that cannabis is safe and natural.[91] Abrupt discontinuation of cannabis use can elicit a withdrawal syndrome including anxiety, dysphoria, sleep changes, irritability, and anorexia. Although not life threatening, these withdrawal symptoms can make permanent discontinuation difficult. Treatment of CUD most often centers around psychosocial interventions such as cognitive behavioral therapy (CBT), motivational enhancement therapy (MET), or a combination there of. Both CBT and MET have been shown to decrease the number of days of cannabis use, and improve the severity of CUD. Additionally, CBT has been shown to increase abstinence rates where MET has yet to show this effect in clinical studies. Regardless, the combination of CBT and MET is synergistic.[91] Attempts at using pharmacotherapeutic agents to alleviate CUD have been mostly unsuccessful with escitalopram, fluoxetine, bupropion, nefazodone, venlafaxine, valproate, baclofen, modafinil, atomoxetine, buspirone, and naltrexone all proving ineffective. However, several therapeutic candidates have met with some success. Cannabinoid receptor agonists including dronabinol, nabilone (a synthetic THC analogue), and nabiximols (Sativex, a combination THC/CBD product) have had varying degrees of success in improving withdrawal symptoms in CUD. One small study found gabapentin was effective in decreasing cannabis use in addition to abating withdrawal symptoms. N-Acetylcysteine, a cysteine precursor thought to affect glutamate transmission, decreased rates of cannabis use in adolescents. However, follow-up studies in adults did not confirm these results. Regardless these studies should be interpreted and extrapolated cautiously due to the low number of patients involved.[91]

Synthetic Cannabinoids

A growing collection of synthetically derived cannabinoids are being misused for their psychoactive effects. Following identification of THC in 1964, and the endogenous cannabinoid receptors in the 1980s, there was a pharmaceutical effort to synthesize cannabinoid receptor agonists for potential therapeutic indications like nausea and pain. However, the vast majority of these efforts never reached commercial fruition, and they have begun showing up in the illicit market. To increase their attractiveness, they are often brightly packaged and given colorful names such as "K2," "Spice," "Aroma," "Mr. Smiley," "Zohai," "Eclipse," "Black Mamba," "Red X Dawn," "Blaze," and "Dream." Due to unclear laws regarding their legality, these products had been readily available at gas stations and convenience stores. However, since being listed as a schedule I controlled substance, the overt availability has decreased but they are still readily available.[94] Some synthetic cannabinoids produce a combination of intended effects, as well as unintended adverse effects, that resemble intoxication from THC. However, synthetic cannabinoids appear to be more potent than natural cannabinoids, and may interact with CB receptors for longer than THC. Symptoms of synthetic cannabinoid toxicity are similar to the euphoric and psychoactive effects of THC. The adverse effects of synthetic cannabinoids include severe agitation, anxiety, nausea, vomiting, tachycardia, elevated blood pressure, tremors, seizures, hallucinations, paranoid behavior, and nonresponsiveness. These effects are likely due to complex CB1 receptor interactions, direct and indirect, with dopaminergic, serotonergic, and glutaminergic pathways within the parts of the brain linked to psychosis.[95] However, it must not be forgotten that most reported adverse experiences with synthetic cannabinoids are troubled by incomplete knowledge of the specific cannabinoid product used, as well as adulteration with other substances.

Cannabis Hyperemesis Syndrome

14 Cannabinoid hyperemesis syndrome (CHS) is a syndrome of cyclical vomiting in individuals with habitual use of cannabis that abates after discontinuation of use. Although first officially recognized in 2004, the syndrome has likely existed much longer. The pathophysiology underlying CHS is not completely elucidated and several hypotheses are being explored. Since cannabinoids are used therapeutically to treat chemotherapy associated nausea and vomiting, current hypotheses indicate that pathway signaling may be altered in a way that leads to excessive nausea and vomiting. Cannabinoids are also known to alter gastrointestinal hormones, potentially leading to aberrant GI function such as emesis. Other potential explanations include non-THC metabolite interactions, genetic variations in metabolism of cannabinoids, and vasodilation of splanchnic vascular beds.[96] Overall, CHS can be difficult to diagnose as nausea and vomiting are symptoms of many issues, and patients may not be forthcoming with their cannabis use due to its questionable legality. One interesting symptom, that often sets CHS apart from other causes of severe vomiting, is that CHS sufferers often report relief from hot baths or showers.

A systematic review found that CHS is diagnosed in males with greater frequency. The median age when cannabis use started was 16 years and the median age when symptoms developed was 24 years. The fact there is a long pattern of use before CHS develops which makes it harder to diagnose as both the person using as well as the clinician are likely to consider more recent changes or developments over chronic use. In the same review, all people diagnosed with CHS self-identified as using it at least weekly and a large majority (~75%) used daily. There are no consensus diagnostic criteria now.[96] Treatment of CHS is also far from standardized due to an incomplete delineation of causative mechanism. Abstinence from cannabis is the most effective treatment option, but takes several days to weeks for the cyclic vomiting to abate. While the use of hot bathing is effective for some people, its benefit is short-lived and it is not a sustainable treatment modality.[97] If intravenous fluids and traditional antiemetics are unsuccessful at improving CHS symptoms, other treatment options that are less established have been reported. Dopamine antagonists like haloperidol have been used successfully in small case reports.[98] A growing number of case reports have shown some benefit with topical capsaicin application which is thought to interact with the transient receptor potential cation channel subfamily V member 1 or vanilloid receptor 1 (TRVP1 or VR1) to improve nausea and vomiting, although the mechanism isn't clearly understood.[96,97,99,100] The incidence of CHS is likely to increase as the availability of cannabis use increases and the potency of THC-containing products increases.

EVALUATION OF THERAPEUTIC OUTCOMES

There are a range of situations and substances where patients can present in regards to substance use. When considering overall therapeutic outcomes, each treatment must be evaluated to determine its efficacy and safety as there are a variety of factors that must be considered based on the current stage of therapy and the patient's specific treatment goals. Each of the medications used in the acute or the chronic setting have unique qualities that must be evaluated for each individual patient. Consistent monitoring for efficacy and appropriateness through treatment is critical. Monitoring for withdrawal reactions utilizing proper assessment scales (ie, COWS) can aid in evaluating the patient appropriately. When developing the treatment plans, the unique adverse effect profiles and medication and drug-interaction concerns for the selected treatment regimen must be considered. Data from urine drug screens and profiles from the Prescription Drug Monitoring Program (PDMP) can also help provide critical information on the full clinical picture for each patient. Patient education must occur throughout treatment to ensure proper medication administration and safety as therapy continues. SUD is a chronic disorder that will need not only pharmacological treatment but also ongoing psychosocial and educational support. It is important for healthcare providers working in this setting, to partner closely with the patient to continue setting appropriate goals in order to achieve favorable treatment outcomes.

CONCLUSION

OUD along with other SUDs continue to be escalating health problem in the United States. The true scope of the problem has only recently been explored. Management of OUD and SUD, whether through pharmacotherapy or behavioral therapy, is a rapidly progressing field. Healthcare providers can help in all aspects of tackling this problem, from identifying those with SUD, directing pharmacotherapy, assisting with treatment, and patient education using a patient-centered model.

ABBREVIATIONS

5-HT	5-hydroxytryptamine
6-AM	6-acetylmorphine
AMPA	α-amino-3-hydroxy-5-methyl-4-isoxazolepropionic acid
ASAM	The American Society of Addiction Medicine
BBB	blood brain barrier
BP	blood pressure
cAMP	cyclic adenosine monophosphate
CB1 and CB2	cannabinoid receptor 1 and 2
CBD	cannabidiol
CBT	cognitive behavioral therapy
CDC	Centers for Disease Control and Prevention
CHS	cannabinoid hyperemesis syndrome
CMS	Centers for Medicare & Medicaid Services
CNS	central nervous system
COWS	Clinical Opiate Withdrawal Scale
CUD	cannabis use disorder
CYP450	cytochrome P450 isoenzyme
DA	dopamine
DEA	Drug Enforcement Administration
DMT	dimethyltryptamine
DSM-5	*Diagnostic and Statistical Manual of Mental Disorders, Fifth Edition*
FDA	Food and Drug Administration
GABA	γ-aminobutyric acid
GDP	gross domestic product
GI	gastrointestinal
HHS	Department of Health and Human Services
HIV	human immunodeficiency virus
HR	heart rate
IM	intramuscular
IMF	illicitly manufactured fentanyl
IN	intranasal
IO	intraosseous
IV	intravenous
LFT	liver function test
MAO	monoamine oxidase
MDD	major depressive disorder
MDMA	3,4-methylenedioxymethamphetamine
MET	motivation enhancement therapy
MME	morphine milligram equivalents
MUD	methamphetamine use disorder
NAc	nucleus accumbens
NAM	National Academy of Medicine
NIDA	National Institute on Drug Abuse
NIH	National Institute of Health
NMDA	*N*-methyl-D-aspartate
NSDUH	National Survey on Drug Use and Health
OEND	overdose education and naloxone distribution
OTC	over-the-counter
OTP	opioid-treatment programs
OUD	opioid use disorder
PCP	phencyclidine
REMS	Risk Evaluation and Mitigation Strategy
SAMHSA	Substance Abuse and Mental Health Services Administration
SCr	serum creatinine
STI	sexually transmitted infection
SUD	substance use disorder
THC	δ-9-tetrahydrocannabinol
THN	take home naloxone
TIPS	Treatment Improvement Protocols
TJC	The Joint Commission
TRVP1 or VR1	transient receptor potential cation channel subfamily V member 1 or vanilloid receptor 1
VMAT2	vesicular monoamine transporter
VTA	ventral tegmental area
WHO	World Health Organization
XR-NTX	extended-release injectable naltrexone

REFERENCES

1. Adams JFA. Substitutes for Opium in Chronic Diseases. *NEJM.* (121):351–356. Oct 1889. doi:10.1056/NEJM188910101211502.
2. Jick H, Miettinen OS, Shapiro S, et al. Comprehensive drug surveillance. *JAMA.* 1970;213:1445–1460.
3. Leung PTM, Macdonald EM, Stanbrook MB, Dhalla IA, Juurlink DN. A 1980 letter on the risk of opioid addiction. *N Engl J Med.* 2017 Jun 1;376(22):2194–2195. 10.1056/NEJMc1700150.
4. The management of chronic pain in older persons: AGS Panel on Chronic Pain in Older Persons. American Geriatrics Society. *J Am Geriatr Soc.* 1998May;46(5):635–651. 10.1111/j.1532-5415.1998.tb01084.x. Erratum in: *J Am Gerriatr Soc.* 1998 Jul;46(7):913.
5. Vadivelu N, Kai AM, Kodumudi V, et al. The opioid crisis: A comprehensive overview. *Curr Pain Headache Rep.* 2018;22:16. https://doi.org/10.1007/s11916-018-0670-z.
6. The Surgeon General's Report on Alcohol, Drugs, and Health. Available at: https://addiction.surgeongeneral.gov/. Accessed April 2021.
7. Lyden J, Binswanger IA. The United States opioid epidemic. *Semin Perinatol.* 2019Apr;43(3):123–131. 10.1053/j.semperi.2019.01.001. Epub 2019 Jan 14.
8. The Council of Economic Advisers. The Underestimated Cost of the Opioid Crises. Nov. 2017. Accessed Mar 2021.
9. Centers for Disease Control and Prevention. 2019 Annual Surveillance Report of Drug-Related Risks and Outcomes—United States. Surveillance Special Report. Centers for Disease Control and Prevention, U.S. Department of Health and Human Services. Published November 1, 2019. Available at: https://www.cdc.gov/drugoverdose/pdf/pubs/2019-cdc-drug-surveillance-report.pdf. Accessed March 2021.
10. CDC Drug Overdose Deaths. Available at: https://www.cdc.gov/drugoverdose/epidemic/index.html. Accessed March 2021.
11. Substance Abuse and Mental Health Services Administration. Key substance use and mental health indicators in the United States: Results from the 2019 National Survey on Drug Use and Health (HHS Publication No. PEP20-07-01-001, NSDUH Series H-55). 2020. Rockville, MD: Center for Behavioral Health Statistics and Quality, Substance Abuse and Mental Health Services Administration. Retrieved from https://www.samhsa.gov/data/ Accessed February 11, 2021.
12. US Prescribing Rate Maps December 7, 2020. Available at: https://www.cdc.gov/drugoverdose/maps/rxrate-maps.html. Accessed May 2021.
13. When are prescribers required to use prescription drug monitoring programs? PEW. Available at: http://www.pewtrusts.org/en/research-and-analysis/data-visualizations/2018/when-are-prescribers-required-to-use-prescription-drug-monitoring-programs. Accessed March 2021.
14. CDC Prescription Drug Monitoring Programs (PDMPs). June 2020. Available at: https://www.cdc.gov/drugoverdose/pdmp/states.html. Accessed March 2021.

15. Dowell D, Haegerich TM, Chou R. CDC Guideline for Prescribing Opioids for Chronic Pain—United States, 2016. *MMWR Recomm Rep*. 2016;65(No. RR-1):1–49. doi:http://dx.doi.org/10.15585/mmwr.rr6501e1.
16. Kroenke K, Alford DP, Argoff C, et al. Challenges with implementing the Centers for Disease Control and Prevention opioid guideline: A consensus panel report. *Pain Medicine*. 2019.
17. Dowell D, Haegerich T, Chou R. No shortcuts to safer opioid prescribing. *N Engl J Med*. 2019 Jun 13;380(24):2285–2287. 10.1056/NEJMp1904190. Epub 2019 Apr 24.
18. Califf RM, Woodcock J, Ostroff S. Proactive response to prescription opioid abuse. *N Engl J Med*. 2016;374:1480–1485. doi:10.1056/NEJMsr1601307.
19. Litman R. Abuse-deterrent opioid formulations. *Anesthesiology*. 2018;128:1015–1025. https://doi.org/10.1097/ALN.0000000000002031.
20. The US Food and Drug Administration. New Safety Measures Announced for Opioid Analgesics, Prescription Opioid Cough Products, and Benzodiazepines. Available at: https://www.fda.gov/drugs/information-drug-class/new-safety-measures-announced-opioid-analgesics-prescription-opioid-cough-products-and. Accessed April 2021.
21. FDA Opioid Analgesic Risk Evaluation and Mitigation Strategy (REMS). Available at: https://www.fda.gov/drugs/information-drug-class/opioid-analgesic-risk-evaluation-and-mitigation-strategy-rems. Accessed April 2021.
22. Association of American Medical Colleges. Academic Medicines Response to the Opioid Crises. Available at: https://www.aamc.org/news-insights/opioids. Accessed April 2021.
23. H.R. 6 The Substance Use-Disorder Prevention the Promotes Opioid Recovery and Treatment for Patients and Community (SUPPORT) Act. Available at: https://www.congress.gov/bill/115th-congress/house-bill/6. Accessed April 2021.
24. Substance Abuse and Mental Health Services. Detoxification and Substance Abuse Treatment: A Treatment Improvement Protocol (TIP 45). Available at: https://store.samhsa.gov/sites/default/files/d7/priv/sma15-4131.pdf. Accessed April 2021.
25. US Congress, HR 1394, S.445, HR 2482 https://www.congress.gov/search?q={%22source%22:%22legislation%22,%22search%22:%22buprenorphine%22}&searchResultViewType=expanded. Accessed May 2021.
26. O'Donnell JK, Halpin J, Mattson CL, et al. Deaths Involving Fentanyl, Fentanyl Analogs, and U-47700—10 States, July–December 2016. *MMWR Morb Mortal Wkly Rep*. 2017; 66:1197–1202. doi:http://dx.doi.org/10.15585/mmwr.mm6643e1.
27. Naloxone Hydrochloride Injection, USP Package Insert. Vizient, Inc. Last updated April 2018. Available at: http://labeling.pfizer.com/ShowLabeling.aspx?id=4541. Accessed January 13, 2019.
28. National Institute on Drug Abuse Overdose Death Rates. https://www.drugabuse.gov/drug-topics/trends-statistics/overdose-death-rates. Accessed May 2021.
29. 2018 National Drug Threat Assessment October 2018 DEA-DCT-DIR-032-18. Available at: https://www.dea.gov/sites/default/files/2018-11/DIR-032-18%202018%20NDTA%20final%20low%20resolution.pdf. Accessed May 2021.
30. Substance Abuse and Mental Health Services Administration. Medications for Opioid Use Disorder. Treatment Improvement Protocol (TIP) Series 63, Full Document. HHS Publication No. (SMA) 18-5063FULLDOC. Rockville, MD: Substance Abuse and Mental Health Services Administration, 2020. Available at: https://store.samhsa.gov/product/TIP-63-Medications-for-Opioid-Use-Disorder-Full-Document/PEP20-02-01-006; https://store.samhsa.gov/product/TIP-63-Medications-for-Opioid-Use-Disorder-Full-Document/PEP20-02-01-006.
31. Faul M, Bohm M, Alexander C. Methadone prescribing and overdose and the association with Medicaid preferred drug list policies—United States, 2007–2014. *MMWR Morb Mortal Wkly Rep*. 2017;66:320–323. http://dx.doi.org/10.15585/mmwr.mm6612a2.
32. Chou R, Cruciani R, Fiellin D, et al. Methadone safety: A clinical practice guideline from the American pain society and college on problems of drug dependence, in collaboration with the heart rhythm society. *The Journal of Pain*. 2014;15(4):321–337.
33. Dowell D, Zhang K, Noonan RK, et al. Mandatory provider review and pain clinic laws reduce the amounts of opioids prescribed and overdose death rates. *Health Aff (Mill-Wood)*. 2016;35(10):1876–1883.
34. Huecker MR, Marraffa J. Heroin. [Updated 2017 Jun 26]. In: StatPearls [Internet]. Treasure Island (FL): StatPearls Publishing; 2018. Available at: https://www.ncbi.nlm.nih.gov/books/NBK441876/. Accessed October 18, 2018.
35. Oelhaf RC, Bhimji SS. Heroin Toxicity. [Updated 2018 Sep 8]. In: StatPearls [Internet]. Treasure Island (FL): StatPearls Publishing; 2018. Available at: https://www.ncbi.nlm.nih.gov/books/NBK430736/. Accessed October 15, 2018.
36. Ellis A, McGwin G, Davis G, et al. Identifying cases of heroin toxicity where 6-acetylmorphine (6-AM) is not detected by toxicological analysis. *Forensic Sci Med Pathol*. 2016;12:243–247.
37. O'Donnell J, Gladden RM, Mattson CL, Kariisa M. Notes from the Field: Overdose Deaths with Carfentanil and Other Fentanyl Analogs Detected—10 States, July 2016–June 2017. *MMWR Morb Mortal Wkly Rep*. 2018;67:767–768.
38. The United States' Center for Disease Control. U.S. drug overdose deaths continue to rise, increases fueled by synthetic opioids. Available at: https://www.cdc.gov/media/releases/2018/p0329-drug-overdose-deaths.html. Press release March 29, 2018. Accessed September 4, 2018.
39. Reissig CJ, Carter LP, Johnson MW, et al. High doses of dextromethorphan, an NMDA antagonist, produce effects similar to classic hallucinogens. *Psychopharmacology (Berl)*. 2012;223(1):115.
40. Miller H, Panahi L, Tapia D, et al. Loperamide misuse and abuse. *J Am Pharm Assoc*. 2017;57:S45S50.
41. Substance Abuse and Mental Health Services Administration, Office of Applied Studies. Treatment Episode Data Set (TEDS): 2005. Discharges from Substance Abuse Treatment Services, DASIS Series: S-41, DHHS Publication No. (SMA) 08-4314, Rockville, MD, 2008. Accessed September 27, 2018.
42. Cisewski DH, Santos C, Koyfman A, Long B. Approach to buprenorphine use for opioid withdrawal treatment in the emergency setting. *Am J Emerg Med*. 2019;37(1):143–150. Accessed November 23, 2018. https://doi.org/10.1016/j.ajem.2018.10.013.
43. *Guidelines for the Psychosocially Assisted Pharmacological Treatment of Opioid Dependence*. Geneva: World Health Organization; 2009. https://www.ncbi.nlm.nih.gov/books/NBK143185. Accessed October 1, 2018.
44. Gowing L, Farrell M, Ali R, White JM. Alpha2-adrenergic agonists for the management of opioid withdrawal. *Cochrane Database Syst Rev*. 2016;(5):CD002024. doi:10.1002/14651858.CD002024.pub5.
45. Krupitsky E, Nunes EV, Ling W, Illeperuma A, Gastfriend DR, Silverman BL. Injectable extended-release naltrexone for opioid dependence: A double-blind placebo controlled, multicenter randomised trial. *Lancet*. 2011;377:1506–1513.
46. Mattick RP, Breen C, Kimber J, Davoli M. Buprenorphine maintenance versus placebo or methadone maintenance for opioid dependence. *Cochrane Database Syst Rev*. 2014;(2):CD002207. doi:10.1002/14651858.CD002207.pub4.
47. Substance Abuse and Mental Health Services Administration. Sublingual and Transmucosal Buprenorphine for Opioid Use Disorder: Review and Update. Advisory, Volume 15, Issue 1. 2016. Available at: https://store.samhsa.gov/system/files/sma16-4938.pdf. Accessed October 11, 2018.
48. Gold Standard, Inc. Buprenorphine. Clinical Pharmacology [database online]. Available at: http://www.clinicalpharmacology.com. Accessed October 11, 2018.
49. Gold Standard, Inc. Naltrexone. Clinical Pharmacology [database online]. Available at: http://www.clinicalpharmacology.com. Accessed October 11, 2018.
50. Sublocade Medication Guide. Last Updated November 2017. Available at: https://www.accessdata.fda.gov/drugsatfda_docs/label/2017/209819s000lbl.pdf. Accessed October 11, 2018.
51. VA/DoD clinical practice guideline for the management of substance use disorders. Available at: https://www.healthquality.va.gov/guidelines/MH/sud/VADODSUDCPGRevised22216.pdf. Accessed September 27, 2018.
52. TIP 40 Center for Substance Abuse Treatment. Clinical Guidelines for the Use of Buprenorphine in the Treatment of Opioid Addiction. Treatment Improvement Protocol (TIP) Series 40. Rockville, MD: Substance Abuse and Mental Health Services Administration; 2004. DHHS Publication No. (SMA) 04-3939. Available at: http://www.ncbi.nlm.nih.gov/bookshelf/br.fcgi?book=hssamhsatip&part=A72248. Accessed October 25, 2018.
53. Volkow ND, Blanco C. The changing opioid crisis: Development, challenges and opportunities. *Mol Psychiatry*. 2021 January;26(1):218–233. doi:10.1038/s41380-020-0661-4.
54. Buprenorphine, USP Package Insert. Boehringer Ingelheim, Inc. Available at: https://docs.boehringer-ingelheim.com/Prescribing%20Information/PIs/Roxane/Buprenorphine%20HCl%20Sublingual%20Tabs/10004964_01%20Buprenorphine%20HCl%20Sublingual%20Tabs.pdf. Accessed June 2022.
55. Suboxone USP Package Insert. Indivior Inc. Available at: https://www.suboxone.com/pdfs/prescribing-information.pdf. Accessed June 2022.

56. Zubsolv USP Package Insert, Orexo Inc. Available at: https://www.zubsolv.com/prescribinginformation. Accessed June 2022.
57. Bunavil USP Package Insert, BioDelivery Sciences International, Inc. Available at: https://www.accessdata.fda.gov/drugsatfda_docs/label/2014/205637s000lbl.pdf. Accessed June 2022.
58. Revia package insert Duramed Pharmaceuticals last updated October 2013. Available at: https://www.accessdata.fda.gov/drugsatfda_docs/label/2013/018932s017lbl.pdf. Accessed October 7, 2018.
59. Vivitrol (extended release naltrexone) prescription drug label. U.S. National Library of Medicine. Available at: https://dailymed.nlm.nih.gov/dailymed/drugInfo.cfm?setid=cd11c435-b0f0-4bb9-ae78-60f101f3703f. December 2015. Accessed September 27, 2018.
60. American Society of Addiction Medicine, The ASAM National Practice Guideline for the Use of Medications in the Treatment of Addiction Involving Opioid Use. 2015. Available at: https://www.asam.org/docs/default-source/practice-support/guidelines-and-consensus-docs/asam-national-practice-guideline-supplement.pdf. Accessed September 25, 2018.
61. Weinsteine Z, Kim H, Chen D, et al. Long-term retention in office based opioid treatment with buprenorphine. *J Subst Abuse Treat.* 2017;74:65–70.
62. Doleac JL, Mukherjee A. The Moral Hazard of Lifesaving Innovations: Naloxone Access, Opioid Abuse, and Crime. Available at: http://dx.doi.org/10.2139/ssrn.3135264. Accessed November 11, 2018.
63. Naloxone Hydrochloride Injection, USP Package Insert. Vizient, Inc. Last updated April 2018. Available at: http://labeling.pfizer.com/ShowLabeling.aspx?id=4541. Accessed May 2021.
64. Lim J, Bratberg J, Corey D, et al. Prescribe to prevent: Overdose prevention and naloxone rescue kits for prescribers and pharmacists. *J Addict Med.* 2016;10(5):300–310.
65. Keck Graduate Institute School of Pharmacy. Opioid Safety: Focus on Furnishing Naloxone. A Guide for California Community Pharmacists. Claremont, CA. August 2018. Available at: http://prescribetoprevent.org/wp2015/wp-content/uploads/OpioidSafetyFocusOnNaloxone-Pharmacists-June2018-links.pdf. Accessed October 23, 2018.
66. McDonald R, Campbell N, Strang J. Twenty years of take-home naloxone for the prevention of overdose deaths from heroin and other opioids—Conception and maturation. *Drug Alcohol Depend.* 2017;178:176–187.
67. National Alliance for Model State Drug Laws. Naloxone Access Statutes. Available at: http://www.namsdl.org/library/06A653E3-E04E-9112-0CBB0B0FA325DC79/. Accessed October 5, 2018.
68. Haight SC, Ko JY, Tong VT, Bohm MK, Callaghan WM. Opioid Use Disorder Documented at Delivery Hospitalization—United States, 1999–2014. *MMWR Morb Mortal Wkly Rep.* 2018;67:845849. doi:http://dx.doi.org/10.15585/mmwr.mm6731a1.
69. Substance Abuse and Mental Health Services Administration. Clinical Guidance for Treating Pregnant and Parenting Women With Opioid Use Disorder and Their Infants. HHS Publication No. (SMA) 18-5054. Rockville, MD: Substance Abuse and Mental Health Services Administration, 2018.
70. Dasgupta N, Funk M, Proescholdbell S, et al. Cohort study of the impact of high-dose opioid analgesics on overdose mortality. *Pain Med.* 2016;17:85–98.
71. FDA Drug Safety Communication: FDA warns about serious risks and death when combining opioid pain or cough medicines with benzodiazepines; requires its strongest warning. Available at: https://www.fda.gov/Drugs/DrugSafety/ucm518473.htm. Accessed May 2021.
72. Allain F, Minogianis EA, Roberts DCS, Samaha AN. How fast and how often: The pharmacokinetics of drug use are decisive in addiction. *Neurosci Biobehav Rev.* 2015;56:166–179. doi:10.1016/j.neubiorev.2015.06.012.
73. Soyka M. Treatment of benzodiazepine dependence. *N Engl J Med.* 2017;376:1147–1157.
74. Flumazenil Package Insert. Roche Laboratories Inc. Last Updated February 2007. Available at: https://www.accessdata.fda.gov/drugsatfda_docs/label/2007/020073s016lbl.pdf. Accessed January 15, 2019.
75. Lader M, Kyriacou A. Withdrawing benzodiazepines in patients with anxiety disorders. *Curr Psychiatry Rep.* 2016;18:8.
76. Puening S, Wilson M, Nordstrom K. Psychiatric emergencies for clinicians: Emergency department management of benzodiazepine withdrawal. *J Emerg Med.* 2017;52(1):66–69.
77. Paulus MP, Stewart JL. Neurobiology, clinical presentation, and treatment of methamphetamine use disorder. *JAMA Psychiatry.* 2020; 77(9): 959–965.
78. AA. DARK side of amphetamine and analogues: Pharmacology, syndromic manifestation, and management of amphetamine addiction. *ACS Chem Neurosci.* 2018;9(10):2299–2303. doi:10.1021/acschemneuro.8b00137.
79. Radfar SR, Rawson RA. Current research on methamphetamine: Epidemiology, medical and psychiatric effects, treatment, and harm reduction efforts. *Addict Health.* 2014;6(3-4):146–154.
80. Drake LR, Scott PJ. DARK classics in chemical neuroscience: Cocaine. *ACS Chem Neurosci.* 2018;9(10):2358–2372. doi:10.1021/acschemneuro.8b00117.
81. Allain F, Minogianis EA, Roberts DCS, Samaha AN. How fast and how often: The pharmacokinetics of drug use are decisive in addiction. *Neurosci Biobehav Rev.* 2015;56:166–179. doi:10.1016/j.neubiorev.2015.06.012.
82. https://www.mayocliniclabs.com/test-info/drug-book/cocaine-metabolite.html. Accessed February 11, 2021.
83. Dolan SB, Chen Z, Huang R, Gatch M. "Ecstasy" to addiction: Mechanisms and reinforcing effects of three synthetic cathinone analogs of MDMA. *Neuropharmacology.* 2018;133:171–180.
84. Parrott AC. MDMA, serotonergic neurotoxicity, and the diverse functional deficits of recreational "Ecstasy" users. *Neurosci Biobehav Rev.* 2013;37(8):1466–1484. doi:10.1016/j.neubiorev.2013.04.016.
85. Yazar-Klosinski BB, Mithoefer MC. Potential psychiatric uses for MDMA. *Clin Pharm and Ther.* 2017;101:194–196.
86. Feduccia AA, Holland J, Mithoefer MC. Progress and promise for the MDMA drug development program. *Psychopharmacology.* 2018;235:561–571.
87. Smith DE, Raswyck GE, Davidson LD. From Hofmann to the Haight Ashbury, and into the future: The past and potential of lysergic acid diethylamide. *J Psychoactive Drugs.* 2014;46(1):310.
88. Epidiolex package insert Greenwich Biosciences last updated June 2018. Available at: https://www.accessdata.fda.gov/drugsatfda_docs/label/2018/210365lbl.pdf.
89. Fantegrossi WE, Wilson CD, Berquist MD. Propsychotic effects of synthetic cannabinoids: Interactions with central dopamine, serotonin, and glutamate systems. *Drug Metabolism Reviews.* 2018;50(1):65–73. doi:10.1080/03602532.2018.1428343.
90. Lucas CJ, Galettis P, Schneider J. The pharmacokinetics and the pharmacodynamics of cannabinoids. *Br J Clin Pharmacol.* 2018;84(11):2477–2482. doi:10.1111/bcp.13710.
91. Ferland, JN, Hurd YL. Deconstructing the neurobiology of cannabis use disorder. *Nature Neuroscience.* 2020;23:600–610.
92. American Psychiatric Association. *Statistical Manual of Mental Disorders.* 5th ed. Arlington, VA: American Psychiatric Association. Accessed April 2021. Available at: https://dsm.psychiatryonline.org/doi/full/10.1176/appi.books.9780890425596.dsm16.
93. Peacock A, Leung J, Larney S, et al. Global statistics on alcohol, tobacco and illicit drug use: 2017 Status report. *Addiction.* 2017;113:1905–1926.
94. Johnston LD, Miech RA, O'Malley PM, Bachman JG, Schulenberg JE, Patrick ME. *Monitoring the Future National Survey Results On Drug Use: 1975–2017: Overview, Key Findings on Adolescent Drug Use.* Ann Arbor, MI: Institute for Social Research, The University of Michigan; 2018. Accessed October 1, 2018. http://monitoringthefuture.org/pubs/monographs/mtf-overview2017.pdf.
95. Fantegrossi WE, Wilson CD, Berquist MD. Propsychotic effects of synthetic cannabinoids: Interactions with central dopamine, serotonin, and glutamate systems. *Drug Metabolism Reviews.* 2018;50(1):6573. doi:10.1080/03602532.2018.1428343.
96. Sorensen CJ, DeSanto K, Borgelt L, et al. Cannabinoid hyperemesis syndrome: Diagnosis, pathophysiology, and treatment—A systematic review. *J Med Toxicol.* 2017;13:71–87. doi:10.1007/s13181-016-0595-z.
97. Richards JR, Lapoint JM, Burillo-Putze G. Cannabinoid hyperemesis syndrome: Potential mechanisms for the benefit of capsaicin and hot water hydrotherapy in treatment. *Clinical Toxicology.* 2018;56(1):15–24. doi:10.1080/15563650.2017.1349910.
98. Inayat F, Virk H, Ullah W, et al. Is haloperidol the wonder drug for cannabinoid hyperemesis syndrome? *BMJ Case Rep.* 2017;2017:pii: bcr2016218239. doi:10.1136/bcr-2016-218239.
99. Dezieck L, Hafez Z, Conicella A, et al. Resolution of cannabis hyperemesis syndrome with topical capsaicin in the emergency department: A case series. *Clinical Toxicol.* 2017;55(8):908–913. doi:10.1080/15563650.2017.1324166.
100. Graham J, Barberio M, Wang GS. Capsaicin cream for treatment of cannabinoid hyperemesis syndrome in adolescents: A case series. *Pediatrics.* 2017;140(6):pii: e20163795. doi:10.1542/peds.2016-3795.

Substance Use Disorders II: Alcohol, Nicotine, and Caffeine

86

Lori H. Dupree and Robin Moorman Li

KEY CONCEPTS

1. Globally, more than 3 million people, predominantly males, died in 2016 from alcohol consumption, which represents 1 in 20 deaths.
2. Studies have identified genotypic and functional phenotypic variants that either serve to protect or predispose individuals toward developing an alcohol use disorder.
3. The metabolism of alcohol follows zero-order kinetics, except at very high and very low blood concentrations. This has important implications for the time course for the effects of alcohol.
4. Disulfiram, naltrexone, extended-release naltrexone, and acamprosate are FDA-approved for the treatment of alcohol use disorder. Their clinical utility to improve sustained abstinence and reduce heavy drinking remains controversial.
5. Tobacco is the most preventable cause of death in the United States.
6. Clinicians should ask all individuals about tobacco use, advise on how to stop using tobacco products, and provide pharmacotherapy and behavioral treatment options to aid in smoking cessation.
7. All forms of nicotine replacement therapy are effective in reducing the amount smoked and achieving abstinence.
8. Varenicline has similar efficacy to the nicotine patch and may be more efficacious than all other single nicotine replacement therapies (NRTs). It is approved for up to 6 months of maintenance therapy by the Food and Drug Administration (FDA).
9. As many as one in five adults consume doses of caffeine generally considered large enough to cause clinical symptoms.
10. Energy drinks continue to be popular, particularly among adolescents and emerging adults. Concerns have been raised regarding the safety of these products.

BEYOND THE BOOK

Alcohol Use Disorder

Watch this five-minute video titled "Brief intervention: Steve," which provides an example of an outpatient clinician making an intervention on an individual with unhealthy alcohol use. This video enhances understanding of how the AUDIT tool can help collect information during an interview and how motivational interviewing can effectively help individuals realize their problem and develop a plan of action.

https://tinyurl.com/y5xvt3u3

1. The patient in the video scored in Zone 2 of the AUDIT questionnaire. Describe how you would interpret those results.
2. Motivational interviewing is a counseling approach where clinicians use a patient-centered stance in combination with techniques to help patients explore and resolve their own mixed feelings about changing unhealthy behaviors.

   The principles of motivational interviewing include:

   - Expressing empathy—building rapport and engaging the patient by seeking to understand his/her perspective
   - Developing discrepancy—determining the patient's perception of how well current behaviors match desired behaviors
   - Rolling with resistance—letting the patient make the arguments for a change instead of the clinician arguing for change
   - Supporting self-efficacy—using reflective statements to restate the patient's belief which he/she verbalized to be able to change a specific behavior

   In the video, which principle(s) of motivational interviewing did the clinician utilize when interviewing the patient?

Smoking Cessation

1. Review the brief case provided.
2. Watch the 3-minute video titled, "The 5As in Practice: Role Play of a Brief Intervention," which provides an example of the 5As in smoking cessation used in the clinic setting.

https://tinyurl.com/y437notb

1. List treatment recommendations that could be considered for this patient's case. Further instructions provided with the table.

Case:

A 43-year-old patient presented to primary care 2 weeks ago for treatment for a chronic productive cough. During this visit, a smoking cessation discussion was captured (see video above), and it was determined they would begin the nicotine patches in 1 week. They are now returning 2 weeks later reporting an adverse reaction to the patch adhesive. They have called the quitline once but would like some other recommendations from you in regard to strategies for smoking cessation as well. What would you recommend?

PMH:

Asthma

Allergies:

PCN

Adhesive (just added today to medical record from experience from nicotine patches)

Completing the table below will help complete the Implement section of the PPCP

Goals of therapy		
	Recommendation #1	Recommendation #2
Medication(s)		
Name, dose, route, etc.		
Rationale for recommended action		
Pros		
Cons		
Possible adverse effects		
Other concerns		
Behavior intervention recommendations		

INTRODUCTION—ALCOHOL

1 Alcohol, nicotine, and caffeine are considered to be socially acceptable substances, yet they impose enormous social and economic costs on our society. The World Health Organization (WHO) estimates that in 2016, there were more than 3 million people worldwide who died from alcohol consumption with the majority being males. Long-term unhealthy alcohol use often leads to chronic disease, and a causal relationship has been established between unhealthy use and at least 200 types of chronic disease or injury worldwide (eg, cancers, liver disease, cardiovascular disease, seizures, homicide, HIV/AIDS, and motor vehicle accidents).[1] Nationally, alcohol contributes to approximately 18.5% of emergency department visits, and more than 95,000 people die annually from alcohol-related causes. This makes alcohol one of the leading causes of preventable death in the United States.[2]

EPIDEMIOLOGY

According to the National Survey on Drug Use and Health (NSDUH), 139.7 million Americans over age 12 reported current alcohol use, with 11.5% reporting heavy alcohol use. Additionally, 47.1% report binge alcohol use, defined as consuming five drinks or more on the same occasion on at least 1 day in the past 30 days for males and four drinks or more on the same occasion on at least 1 day in the past 30 days for females.[3] Furthermore, 1.2% reported heavy alcohol use, defined as binge drinking on 5 days or more in the past 30 days. It is estimated that 1 in 10 adolescents between the ages of 12 and 17 years are current alcohol users, which equates to 2.3 million young adults in one month.[3] Although, over the last 5 years, there has been an overall decline in alcohol use in this age group, within this specific age range, there are over 208,000 adolescents who are currently heavy alcohol users. In contrast, the estimates of heavy alcohol users in 2019 decreased to 2.8 million for individuals between the ages of 18 and 25, and 13 million for those 26 years and older.[3]

2 The disease concept of addiction, using alcoholism as a model, states that individuals who suffer from the disease do not choose to contract the disease any more than someone who suffers from heart disease or diabetes mellitus chooses to contract that illness. Alcohol use disorder (AUD) is a chronic disease characterized by problematic and uncontrolled drinking and is diagnosed based on DSM-5 criteria, which requires 2 of the 11 criteria to be met during a 12-month period. The DSM-5 criteria ask 11 questions about the amount of alcohol use, the effects of alcohol use both personally and professionally, and any presence of withdrawal symptoms in the past year. Severity is determined based on the number of criteria met and subsequently classified as mild (2-3 symptoms), moderate (4-5 symptoms), or severe (6 or more symptoms).[4,5] See Chapter e84, "Introduction to Substance Use Disorders," for more information.

It has long been recognized that unhealthy alcohol use is heritable, as 50% of first-degree relatives of people with AUD become alcohol-dependent themselves.[6–8] Similarly, twin and adoption studies have had comparable results.[8] Additional research continues to identify common and rare genetic variations leading to not only variations in responses to alcohol but also the response to the pharmacological treatment of AUDs. Prospective data are lacking to determine the effects of genetic polymorphisms on individual responses of medications to treat AUD.[6,7] Large-scale pharmacoepidemiologic studies have further elucidated the environmental risk factors associated with either protective effects or predisposition toward unhealthy alcohol use (Table 86-1).[9]

ETIOLOGY

Alcohol is a central nervous system (CNS) depressant that acts in a dose-dependent fashion, producing sedation that progresses to sleep, unconsciousness, coma, and finally fatal respiratory depression potentially leading to cardiovascular collapse. Alcohol affects endogenous opiates and several neurotransmitter systems in the brain, including γ-aminobutyric acid (GABA), glutamate, serotonin, and dopamine.

TABLE 86-1 Genotypic, Phenotypic, and Environmental Factors That Increase Alcohol-Use Disorder Risk

Susceptibility Genes	Phenotype	Environment
Regions on chromosomes 1 and 4 that code for the following receptors:	Personality traits that include:	Religious background
$GABA_A$	Novelty seeking	Urban residence (vs rural)
Serotonin 1B	Impulsivity	History of sexual abuse
DRD4	Aggression	Being single
Neuropeptide Y	Depression	Having deceased parents
	Early Exposure	
	Maximum number of alcoholic drinks consumed per day	
Gene that codes for:		
ADH1B		
ALDH2		
5HTTLPR		

ADH1B, alcohol dehydrogenase 1B; ALDH2, aldehyde dehydrogenase 2; DRD4, type 4 dopamine receptor gene; GABA, γ-aminobutyric acid; 5HTTLPR, 5 hydroxytryptamine transporter.

Data from References 6, 7, and 9.

Alcohol is available in a variety of concentrations in various alcoholic beverages. There is approximately 14 g of alcohol in a 12-oz (355 mL) can of beer (approximately 5%), in 5 oz (148 mL) of nonfortified wine (approximately 12%), or in one shot (1.5 oz [44 mL]) of 80-proof whiskey (40%).[8,11] Full consumption of this amount will cause an increase in blood alcohol level of approximately 20 to 25 mg/dL (4.3 to 5.4 mmol/L) in a healthy 70-kg (154 lb) male, although this varies with the time frame of alcohol consumption, the type of alcoholic beverage, whether food is consumed co-currently, and many other patient-specific variables. The lethal dose of alcohol in humans is variable, but deaths generally occur when blood alcohol levels are greater than 400 to 500 mg/dL (87-109 mmol/L).[12]

PATHOPHYSIOLOGY

Approximately 20% of alcohol is absorbed through the stomach, with the remaining through the small intestine. Absorption begins in the stomach within 5 to 10 minutes of oral ingestion, with the onset of clinical effects following fairly rapidly. Peak serum concentrations of alcohol are usually achieved 30 to 90 minutes after finishing the last drink, although this depends on the type of alcoholic beverage, type and timing of food consumption, and other factors.[11,13]

More than 90% of alcohol in the plasma is metabolized in the liver by three enzyme systems that operate within the hepatocyte. The first system is metabolism to acetaldehyde by alcohol dehydrogenase (ADH) in the liver cell. In turn, acetaldehyde is metabolized to carbon dioxide and water by the enzyme aldehyde dehydrogenase (ALDH). A second pathway for oxidation of alcohol uses catalase, an enzyme located in the peroxisomes and microsomes. The third enzyme system, the microsomal alcohol oxidase system, has a role in the oxidation of alcohol to acetaldehyde. These last two mechanisms are of lesser importance than the alcohol dehydrogenase–aldehyde dehydrogenase system.[13,14] Beyond these, the remainder of alcohol is excreted by the lungs, and in urine and sweat.

3 The elimination of alcohol generally follows zero-order pharmacokinetics, where the concentration of alcohol in the blood decreases at a constant amount per unit of time. This can, in fact, be an oversimplification because at very high or very low concentrations elimination can follow first-order pharmacokinetics, where a constant percentage of alcohol is eliminated per unit of time. Blood alcohol concentration (BAC) measures the amount of alcohol present in the blood, and as BAC rises, the alcohol can result in different levels of impairment (Table 86-2) and the relationship between alcohol consumption and BAC is variable. On average, the BAC is lowered from 15 to 22.2 mg/dL (3.3-4.8 mmol/L) per hour in the nontolerant individual, assuming that the individual is in the post-absorptive state. In healthy males and females, alcohol has a volume of distribution of 0.7 and 0.6 L/kg, which corresponds closely with total body water.[15]

CLINICAL PRESENTATION

Screening for Alcohol Use Disorder

The CAGE questionnaire is a mnemonic for four questions: (a) Have you ever felt the need to cut down on your drinking? (b) Have people annoyed you by criticizing your drinking? (c) Have you ever felt bad or guilty about your drinking? (d) Have you ever had a drink the first thing in the morning to steady your nerves or get rid of a hangover ("eye opener")? This commonly used tool can be used for detecting individuals more likely to be misusing alcohol and therefore at greater risk for alcohol withdrawal. Each question is scored as 0 for a "no" answer and 1 for a "yes" answer. A positive response, a total of 2 or more to these four questions, suggests an increased likelihood of unhealthy alcohol use with an average sensitivity of 0.71 (71%) and an average specificity of 0.90 (90%).[17]

The Alcohol Use Disorders Identification Test (AUDIT) is a validated 10-question screening tool originally developed to screen for alcohol use disorder and the amount and frequency of alcohol consumption in adults in the primary care setting. This screening tool can be completed by the patient or can be completed via an interview with a healthcare provider. Each question is scored from 0 to 4. Out of a possible score of 40, scores greater than 8 indicate harmful or hazardous drinking. Scores higher than 13 for females and 15 for males necessitate further evaluation for alcohol use disorder.[18] The AUDIT tool, as well as a short version of AUDIT (AUDIT-C), has been used within a broad range of patient populations and is an appropriate first step in identifying those struggling with unhealthy alcohol use. However, a new adaptation of the AUDIT, the USAUDIT, was adapted to US standard drink size and hazardous drinking guidelines and has been developed to more accurately detect drinking in excess of recommended levels.[18]

Acute Effects of Alcohol

At lower serum concentrations, euphoria and disinhibition may be noted. Additionally, slurred speech, altered perception of the environment, impaired judgment, ataxia, incoordination, nystagmus, and hyperreflexia may occur. As plasma levels increase, combative and destructive behavior may occur. With higher levels still, somnolence and respiratory depression may ensue.[16] The typical effects of various BACs are shown in Table 86-2, although effects vary from individual to individual.

Alcohol Poisoning

Acute alcohol poisoning, also commonly referred to as alcohol overdose, usually occurs with the rapid consumption of large quantities of alcoholic beverages. With sustained drinking of moderate alcohol amounts, the user passes out before a toxic dose can be ingested, and/or the person vomits to rid the stomach of its toxic reservoir. With rapid drinking, the person may fall asleep or pass out without vomiting, allowing continued alcohol absorption from the gastrointestinal (GI) tract until fatal BACs are achieved.[16]

Laboratory Studies

In the emergency room, a BAC should be ordered in any patient in whom alcohol ingestion is suspected, regardless of the presenting complaint. For clinical purposes, most laboratories report BAC in units of mg/dL or mmol/L. In legal cases, results are reported in percentage (grams of ethyl alcohol per 100 mL of whole blood). Along with a BAC, a complete blood count should be ordered to assess

CLINICAL PRESENTATION Alcohol Withdrawal

General

- Acute alcohol detoxification and withdrawal after chronic unhealthy alcohol use is a serious condition that can require hospitalization and adjunctive pharmacotherapy.
- At a very high BAC, death is possible.

Symptoms

- The intoxicated individual can present with slurred speech and ataxia. The patient can be sedated or unconscious.
- As BACs decrease rapidly, nausea, vomiting, tremors, and hallucinations can ensue. Delirium tremens (DT) and seizures are the most severe symptoms.
- An evaluation should be completed using the Clinical Institute Withdrawal Assessment for Alcohol, revised (CIWA-Ar), a 10-item scale to document and score the patient's baseline symptoms (nausea and vomiting, tremors, paroxysmal sweats, anxiety, tactile/auditory/visual disturbances, headache, agitation, orientation and clouding of sensorium).

Signs

- The intoxicated individual can present with nystagmus.
- In withdrawal, the individual can present with tachycardia, diaphoresis, hypertension, and/or hyperthermia.

Laboratory Tests

- In the emergency department, a BAC should be ordered when alcohol ingestion is suspected. A whole blood alcohol level of 150 mg/dL (33 mmol/L) reported in the hospital corresponds to 0.15% BAC obtained by law enforcement.
- Order a complete blood count to assess for anemia, a complete metabolic panel to assess electrolytes, glucose, renal, and liver function, and serum magnesium.
- A complete toxicologic screen to rule out the presence of other substances can be useful.

Other Diagnostic Tests

- Differentiate acute alcohol intoxication from other medical illnesses (eg, head trauma).
- Order computed tomography (CT) on any patient with focal neurologic findings, failure to improve, new-onset seizures, or mental status out of proportion to the degree of intoxication.

TABLE 86-2 Specific Effects of Alcohol Related to Blood Alcohol Concentration

BAC (%)* (mmol/L)	Type of Impairment	Effect(s)
0.0-0.05 (0-11)	Mild	Mild speech/memory/attention/coordination/balance impairment, relaxation, sleepiness
0.06-0.15 (12-34)	Increased	Impaired speech/memory/attention/coordination/balance, risk of aggression, significantly impaired driving skills, increased risk of injury to self and others, moderate memory impairment
0.16-0.30 (35-65)	Severe	Impaired speech/memory/attention/coordination/reaction time, balance significantly impaired, driving skills dangerously impaired, judgment and decision making dangerously impaired, blackouts, vomiting, and signs of alcohol poisoning common, loss of consciousness
0.31-0.45 (66-98)	Life-threatening	Loss of consciousness, danger of life-threatening alcohol poisoning, significant risk of death

*Grams of ethyl alcohol per 100 mL of whole blood.

BAC, blood alcohol concentration.

Data from Reference 22.

for anemia and a complete metabolic panel plus serum magnesium should be ordered to assess electrolytes, glucose, and renal and liver function. If the diagnosis is unclear, if the intoxication seems atypical, or when there is suspicion of multiple substance ingestions, a complete toxicologic screen may be useful to rule out other substances.[19]

TREATMENT

Desired Outcomes

While alcohol withdrawal most likely occurs in the face of alcohol use disorder, it is necessary to treat acute withdrawal symptoms (or prevent them from occurring) before other alcohol use disorder treatments are started. The goals for alcohol-dependent persons trying to decrease or discontinue alcohol intake include (a) the prevention and treatment of withdrawal symptoms (including withdrawal seizures and DT) and medical or psychiatric complications, (b) long-term abstinence after detoxification, and (c) entry into ongoing medical and unhealthy alcohol use treatment.[20]

Nonpharmacologic Therapy

Due to the severity of signs and symptoms and associated morbidity and mortality with alcohol withdrawal, nonpharmacologic therapy is not recommended. Patients with alcohol withdrawal require a coordinated approach in a monitored setting with the use of inpatient, outpatient, and rehabilitation services.[19]

Pharmacologic Therapy

A baseline assessment using a validated tool, such as the Clinical Institute Withdrawal Assessment for Alcohol, revised (CIWA-Ar), should be completed.[21] Symptom-triggered treatment with a benzodiazepine is the current standard of care in alcohol detoxification to assess severity and avoid progression to more severe withdrawal stages. All benzodiazepines appear to be similarly efficacious in reducing the signs and symptoms of withdrawal. However, there are pharmacokinetic differences (ie, onset of action, duration, metabolism) between benzodiazepines, in addition to route of administration and cost, that guide pharmacotherapy decisions.[19,22,23]

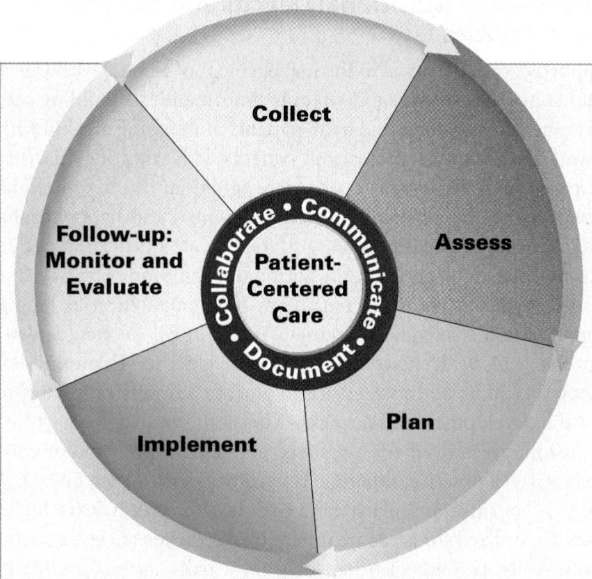

Patient Care Process for Alcohol Use Disorder

The image shows the five fundamental steps included in The Pharmacist's Care Process endorsed by the Joint Commission for Pharmacy Practitioners (2014). The tagline of this process reads collaborate, communicate, and document. The five fundamental steps listed here are collect, assess, plan, implement, and follow-up: monitor and evaluate. All these steps are listed in a circular block diagram.

Collect

- Patient characteristics (eg, age, sex, pregnant)
- Patient medical history (personal and family)
- Social history (eg, tobacco/alcohol use) and dietary habits
- Utilize CAGE questionnaire or Alcohol Use Disorders Identification Test (AUDIT) to assess for alcohol use disorder
- Current medications including prescription, over-the-counter (OTC), herbal products, dietary supplements
- Objective data
  - Blood pressure (BP), heart rate (HR), respiratory rate (RR), height, weight, O_2-saturation
  - Labs including serum creatinine (SCr), liver function tests (LFTs)

Assess

- Hemodynamic instability (eg, systolic BP <90 mm Hg, HR >110 bpm, O_2-sat <90% (0.90), RR >20) to assess for signs of acute alcohol withdrawal
- Utilize motivational interviewing to assess the individual's readiness to quit
- Ability/willingness to pay for pharmacotherapy options for Alcohol Use Disorder (AUD), and abstain from alcohol with disulfiram and avoid opiates with naltrexone
- Ability/willingness to obtain laboratory monitoring tests (eg, SCr [eg, naltrexone, acamprosate], LFTs [ie, disulfiram])
- Emotional status (eg, presence of anxiety, depression)

Plan*

- Pharmacotherapy regimen including specific AUD agent, dose, route, frequency, and duration (see Table 86-5)
- Monitoring parameters including efficacy (eg, decrease in craving, adherence) and safety (eg, adverse effects specific to selected agent, SCr, LFTs); frequency and timing of follow-up
- Patient education (eg, purpose of treatment, medication-specific information, importance of adherence)
- Self-monitoring for adverse effects from pharmacotherapy treatment
- Referrals to other providers when appropriate (eg, behavioral health; highly recommended but not required for pharmacotherapy treatment)

Implement*

- Provide patient education regarding all elements of treatment plan
- Utilize motivational interviewing and coaching strategies to maximize adherence
- Schedule follow-up (eg, adherence assessment, SCr [eg, naltrexone, acamprosate], LFTs [eg, disulfiram])

Follow-up: Monitor and Evaluate

- Presence of adverse effects (eg, medication specific)
- Individual adherence to treatment plan using multiple sources of information
- Reevaluate duration of therapy initially with frequent follow-up and then lengthen follow-up to every 1 to 2 months

**Collaborate with patient, caregivers, and other healthcare professionals.*

Benzodiazepines are first-line treatment and the standard of care, given their documented efficacy in reducing the signs and symptoms of withdrawal.[23] Other agents with activity on the GABA system have been evaluated in the treatment of alcohol withdrawal. A Cochrane review[24] of the efficacy and safety of pharmacological options in treating alcohol withdrawal syndrome included a total of 7,333 patients. The medications evaluated included benzodiazepines, baclofen, antiseizure medications (ie, phenobarbital, valproic acid, carbamazepine, gabapentin, topiramate), and psychotropic analgesic nitrous oxide (PAN), along with gamma-hydroxybutyrate. Efficacy was determined based on the impact on alcohol withdrawal seizures. Benzodiazepines were more efficacious when compared to both placebo (RR 0.16; 95% CI 0.04-0.69) and antipsychotics (RR 0.24; 95% CI 0.07–0.88). Within the benzodiazepine class comparison, there was a trend toward better efficacy with chlordiazepoxide; however, no benzodiazepine was shown to be superior.[24] Phenobarbital, with a rapid onset of action and a long half-life, is the most commonly used alternative to benzodiazepines in alcohol withdrawal, demonstrating efficacy and safety with monitoring when used alone or in combination with benzodiazepines.[19,23]

Treatment Regimens

Front-Loading Therapy

One initial approach to managing alcohol withdrawal includes using an initial high dose of a long-acting benzodiazepine, such as diazepam 10 to 20 mg or chlordiazepoxide 100 mg, and administered in repeated doses every 1 to 2 hours until the patient is sedated. Adequate sedation is usually obtained after three doses. Front-loading therapy is recommended when the CIWA-Ar score is 19 or above. Patients must be closely monitored under clinical supervision for benzodiazepine toxicity, such as excessive sedation, respiratory depression, and delirium. This approach should be used with extreme caution in older patients or in those with liver disease since the elimination rate will be extended, leading to an increased risk of toxicity.[22,23]

Symptom-Triggered Therapy

With symptom-triggered therapy, medication is given only when the patient has symptoms and the CIWA-Ar score is 8 or above. Various benzodiazepines have been used in this therapy, including diazepam, chlordiazepoxide, oxazepam, and lorazepam. Agent choice depends on the patient's age, liver function, available dosage forms, the hospital's formulary, and cost. The patient is then reassessed hourly utilizing the CIWA-Ar. If the score remains above 8, they continue to receive a dose of the selected benzodiazepine. If the score is lower than 8 and the patient appears stable, the time frame for assessment and treatment can extend to 4 to 8 hours (Table 86-3). When used in the inpatient setting, this standard of care results in a shorter treatment duration and reduced risk for over-sedation, which allows the clinician to focus on specific therapy for alcohol use disorder. This approach is also appropriate for the outpatient setting if monitoring of signs and symptoms can be reliably performed by the patient or caregiver.[23,25]

Fixed-Dose Therapy

Although benzodiazepines given regularly at fixed dosing intervals and subsequently tapered off have been highly effective for alcohol withdrawal, additional medication may be needed for breakthrough withdrawal symptoms. With this approach, monitoring for excessive sedation and respiratory depression is still important. Due to the administration of medication regardless of symptoms, fixed-dose therapy could be preferred in patients with a history of seizures or DT, although there is a lack of evidence to determine superiority over symptom-triggered therapy.[19,23]

Treatment of Severe Alcohol Withdrawal

The progression of symptoms to include seizures and/or DT describes severe alcohol withdrawal, where patients are often refractory to benzodiazepines and require aggressive treatment in a closely monitored setting. For hospitalized patients, the Prediction of Alcohol Withdrawal Severity Scale (PAWSS) can be used to assess the risk of developing severe or complicated alcohol withdrawal. The PAWSS tool is a questionnaire that incorporates patient responses and clinical evidence to assess severity, with a score of 4 or greater pointing toward a high risk of moderate to severe alcohol withdrawal. For patients with severe alcohol withdrawal (CIWA-Ar greater than 19), front-loading therapy with a benzodiazepine is recommended as a first-line treatment followed by phenobarbital. With close monitoring, phenobarbital can be utilized as either adjunctive therapy for patients not responding to high doses of benzodiazepines or alternative therapy if benzodiazepines are contraindicated.[19,25,26]

Alcohol withdrawal seizures do not require treatment with an antiseizure medication, such as phenytoin, unless they progress to status epilepticus or unless there is an underlying concomitant seizure disorder. In general, patients experiencing seizures, and/or experiencing resistant alcohol withdrawal, should be treated supportively under institutional/hospital-specific protocols. These patients should be closely monitored in an intensive care unit in case intubation and mechanical ventilation become necessary. For those requiring escalating doses of benzodiazepines, adjunctive therapy options to manage refractory withdrawal symptoms might include propofol with mechanical ventilation, dexmedetomidine, or ketamine.[19,25,26]

Treatment of Nutritional Deficits and Electrolyte Abnormalities

Supportive care is critical in the management of alcohol withdrawal. Fluid status, electrolyte, and vitamin abnormalities should be carefully assessed and corrected in all patients undergoing alcohol withdrawal. Hydration is necessary in patients with vomiting, diarrhea, increased body temperature, or severe agitation. Electrolyte imbalances, such as hypokalemia, hypomagnesemia, and hypophosphatemia, can often be seen because of inadequate nutrition and fluid volume related to antidiuretic hormone inhibition. Hypokalemia can be corrected with oral potassium supplementation as long as renal function is adequate. Thiamine (vitamin B1) is often depleted and can lead to decreased absorption of glucose. Thiamine deficiency should be addressed prior to glucose administration to prevent the development of Wernicke–Korsakoff syndrome (eg, mental confusion, eye movement disorders, and ataxia [poor motor coordination]). In practice, thiamine is usually given 100 mg once daily orally, IV, or intramuscularly for 3 to 5 days for prophylaxis; higher doses are utilized for acute treatment of Wernicke's encephalopathy. Additionally, patients also benefit from a daily multivitamin with folate due to poor nutritional status (see Table 86-3).[23,26]

Alcohol hypoglycemia was first described 60 years ago and usually occurs in the absence of overt liver disease. It is more likely to occur if the patient is fasting, exercising, or is sensitive to alcohol, and it is less likely if the patient is obese. Mechanistically, this occurs as alcohol directly interferes with hepatic gluconeogenesis, but not glycogenolysis. The energy required for alcohol metabolism is diverted away from the energy needed to take up lactate and pyruvate—substrates for gluconeogenesis. So, those who drink alcohol can become hypoglycemic once glycogen stores are depleted. Neurologic symptoms of hypoglycemia can be confused with alcohol intoxication, and in the inpatient setting, blood glucose should be monitored regularly.[28]

In general, alcohol withdrawal treatment can take place in hospitals, inpatient detoxification units, or outpatient settings. Only patients with mild-to-moderate symptoms should be considered for outpatient treatment, and it is a good idea to have a responsible, non-using person available to help the patient monitor symptoms and administer medications. Patients with a strong craving for alcohol, who concurrently use other substances, who have severe psychiatric problems (ie, suicidal ideations, psychosis), and/or who have a history of seizures or DT, are not good candidates for outpatient treatment. Pharmacologic agents used in the treatment of alcohol withdrawal are summarized in Table 86-4.[23,27,29]

Treatment of Alcohol Use Disorder

Nonpharmacologic Therapy

In alcohol use disorder, psychosocial interventions proven to be beneficial include motivational enhancement therapy, family therapies, cognitive behavioral therapy, behavioral approaches, and 12-step programs, such as Alcoholics Anonymous. The combination of a psychosocial intervention and pharmacologic therapy for alcohol use disorder can help reduce the frequency of drinking and the risk of binge drinking.[30]

Pharmacologic Therapy

4 In the United States, disulfiram, naltrexone, once-monthly injectable extended-release naltrexone, and acamprosate are the only four medications FDA approved for the treatment of alcohol use disorder. Disulfiram acts as a deterrent to the resumption of drinking, and naltrexone is a competitive opioid antagonist that has been shown to reduce cravings for alcohol. Acamprosate is a GABAergic agonist that modulates alcohol cravings (Table 86-4). Other medications, including nalmefene, baclofen, bupropion, various serotonergic

TABLE 86-3 Dosing and Monitoring of Pharmacologic Agents Used in the Treatment of Alcohol Withdrawal

Agent/Route	Dosage Range Per Day (Unless Otherwise Noted)	Indication	Monitoring	Duration of Dosing	Level of Evidence for Efficacy*
Multivitamin oral/IV	1 tablet	Malnutrition	Diet	At least until eating a balanced diet at caloric goal	B3
Thiamine oral/IV	100 mg	Deficiency	CBC, WBC, nystagmus	Empiric for 5 days. More if evidence of deficiency	B2
Crystalloid fluids IV (NS or D5-0.45 NS with 20 mEq [mmol] of KCl per liter)	50-100 mL/hour	Dehydration	Weight, electrolytes urine output, nystagmus if dextrose	Until intake and outputs stabilize and oral intake is adequate	A3
Clonidine oral (Catapres)	0.05-0.3 mg Consider dose reduction in older individuals	Autonomic tone rebound and hyperactivity, hypertensive urgency	Shaking, tremor, sweating, blood pressure	3 days or less	B2
Clonidine transdermal (Catapres-TTS)	TTS-1 to TTS-3 Consider dose reduction in older individuals	Autonomic tone rebound and hyperactivity	Shaking, tremor, sweating, blood pressure	1 week or less. One patch only	B3
Haloperidol oral/IV (Haldol)	2.5 to 5 mg every 2-4 hours	Agitation unresponsive to benzodiazepines, hallucinations (tactile, visual, auditory, or otherwise), or delusions	Subjective response plus rating scale (CIWA-AR or equivalent), ECG	Individual doses as needed	B1
Antipsychotics, second generation		Agitation unresponsive to benzodiazepines, hallucinations, or delusions in patients intolerant of first-generation antipsychotics	Subjective response plus rating scale (CIWA-AR or equivalent)	Individual doses as needed in addition to scheduled antipsychotic	C3
Quetiapine oral (Seroquel)	25-200 mg; dosage adjustment is necessary in hepatic impairment				
Aripiprazole oral (Abilify)	5-15 mg				
Benzodiazepines					
Lorazepam oral/IV/IM (Ativan)	0.5-8 mg	Tremor, anxiety, diaphoresis, tachypnea, dysphoria, seizures	Subjective response plus rating scale (CIWA-AR or equivalent)	Individual doses as needed. Underdosing is more common than overdosing	A2
Chlordiazepoxide oral (Librium)	25-300 mg				
Diazepam oral/IV/IM (Valium)	5-40 mg				
Oxazepam oral (Serax)	15-30 mg				
Dexmedetomidine IV (Precedex)	0.2 mcg/kg/hr, titrate based on response	Adjunct to BZD for autonomic hyperactivity, sympathetic symptom control	Tremor, blood pressure, heart rate	5 days or less	B2
Phenobarbital oral/IV (Luminal)	30-260 mg	Adjunct to BZD, promotes BZD binding to $GABA_A$ receptor	Sedation, respiratory depression, blood pressure	5 days or less	B2
Alcohol oral/IV		Prevent withdrawal	Subjective signs of withdrawal	Wide variation	C3

*Strength of recommendations, evidence to support recommendation: A, good; B, moderate; C, poor.

Quality of evidence: (1) evidence from more than one properly randomized controlled trial; (2) evidence from more than one well-designed clinical trial with randomization, from cohort or case-control analytic studies or multiple time series, or dramatic results from uncontrolled experiments; and (3) evidence from opinions of respected authorities, based on clinical experience, descriptive studies, or reports of expert communities.

CBC, complete blood count; CIWA-Ar, Clinical Institute Withdrawal Assessment for Alcohol, revised; D5, dextrose 5%; ECG, electrocardiogram; KCl, potassium chloride; NS, normal saline; WBC, white blood cell count.

Data from References 19, 26, and 27.

agents (including selective serotonin reuptake inhibitors and serotonin-3 [5-HT3] receptor antagonists), topiramate, gabapentin, and varenicline, have also been used off-label in the United States or abroad for alcohol use disorder. A Cochrane review[31] of 25 trials with 2,641 patients evaluated a variety of antiseizure medications, including gabapentin, topiramate, oxcarbazepine, valproate, levetiracetam, pregabalin, zonisamide, and carbamazepine, to determine efficacy in the treatment of alcohol use disorder. Overall, these agents did perform better than placebo when comparing the number of drinks per day and average heavy drinking days, but there was insufficient evidence that these agents resulted in increased alcohol abstinence rates. The conclusion was there is insufficient evidence of efficacy to support the use of antiseizure medications in alcohol use disorder.[31] A recent meta-analysis of seven randomized controlled trials found that topiramate had moderate benefits on the number of abstinence days and frequency of heavy drinking. Of the antiseizure medications, topiramate appears to decrease alcohol consumption and is increasingly prescribed off-label as a treatment of AUD.[32]

For moderate-to-severe AUD, the American Psychiatric Association's (APA) practice guideline recommends (1) naltrexone or acamprosate to reduce alcohol consumption or achieve abstinence or (2) disulfiram for patients who have not responded to naltrexone and acamprosate and who understand the potential adverse effects with concurrent alcohol intake. Additionally, the APA also recommends gabapentin or topiramate in moderate-to-severe AUD, for patients who prefer one of these medications or who are intolerant of or who have not responded to the FDA-approved agents.[33]

Disulfiram Disulfiram was the first FDA-approved medication for alcohol use disorder. It deters a patient from drinking by producing an aversive reaction if alcohol is consumed; otherwise, it has minimal effects. Pharmacologically, it inhibits aldehyde dehydrogenase in the biochemical pathway for alcohol metabolism, allowing acetaldehyde to accumulate. If a patient consumes alcohol within 12 to 24 hours of taking disulfiram, the resulting increase in acetaldehyde causes severe facial flushing, throbbing headache, nausea and vomiting, chest pain, palpitations, tachycardia, weakness, dizziness, blurred vision, confusion, and hypotension, referred to as a "disulfiram reaction." In severe (rare) cases, the reaction can lead to myocardial infarction, congestive heart failure, cardiac arrhythmia, respiratory depression, convulsions, and death, particularly in vulnerable individuals. When disulfiram is prescribed, abstinence from alcohol is a critical component of patient education and supervision is recommended to promote adherence.[20,33] Evidence in a meta-analysis of 22 randomized trials found that, in 17 open-labeled studies, disulfiram was associated with a higher abstinence benefit compared with controls; blinded studies did not demonstrate a benefit.[34]

Naltrexone Naltrexone, a potent opiate antagonist, is available for the treatment of unhealthy opioid use as it blocks the effects of exogenous opioids (for more details, see Chapter 85, "Substance Use Disorders I: Opioids, Cannabis, and Stimulants"). It is also FDA-approved for the treatment of unhealthy alcohol use, and it is thought to attenuate the reinforcing effects of alcohol. Those who consume alcohol while taking naltrexone report feeling less intoxicated and having fewer alcohol cravings.[4,29] Evidence suggests that genetics play a role in the clinical response to naltrexone, and its efficacy varies greatly among individuals. In previous preliminary studies, the Asn40Asp (118A>G, A355G, rs1799971) polymorphism in the μ-opioid receptor gene (*OPRM1*) demonstrated an increased response to naltrexone with lower rates of relapse to heavy drinking; however, a recent controlled clinical trial disputed these results,[35] and further studies are ongoing.

Naltrexone administration does not induce alcohol withdrawal; however, it should not be given to patients currently receiving opiates because it will block their therapeutic effects and can precipitate severe opioid withdrawal syndrome. Naltrexone should be used with caution in patients with moderate-to-severe renal impairment and baseline liver function tests (LFTs) are recommended. Current evidence supports the tolerability of naltrexone in high-risk patients with hepatitis C and human immunodeficiency virus (HIV). When initiating naltrexone, the patient should not be in acute alcohol withdrawal and should be involved in psychosocial treatment.[33,36] A review of 50 randomized controlled studies,[37] which included 7,793 patients, found that oral naltrexone decreased drinking days by 4% and decreased the risk of heavy drinking by 83% compared to placebo. The most common adverse effects were nausea and daytime sedation. The usual starting dose of oral naltrexone is 50 mg/day, but doses of 100 mg/day have been used.[37]

In April 2006, the FDA approved Vivitrol, a once-monthly intramuscular naltrexone formulation, given at a dose of 380 mg that can be administered in an outpatient setting.[36]

Extended-release formulations reduce the likelihood of forgetting or choosing not to take the medication, ensuring medication adherence for the next month. However, the cost is considerably higher than the oral formulation.[36]

The extended-release form of naltrexone may be more beneficial in reducing heavy drinking rather than abstinence. In a recent meta-analysis of seven randomized, double-blind trials, all requiring abstinence before treatment, extended-release naltrexone resulted in two fewer drinking days and one to two fewer heavy drinking days per month compared to placebo. Larger reductions in heavy drinking were reported in trials that did not require abstinence prior to study enrollment and that lasted longer than 3 months.[38]

Acamprosate Acamprosate is a glutamate modulator at the *N*-methyl-D-aspartate receptor that reduces alcohol craving. Individuals treated with acamprosate are more successful in maintaining abstinence from alcohol versus placebo. Acamprosate is well tolerated, with GI adverse effects being the most common. It is not metabolized through the liver but is excreted through the kidneys and should be used with caution in individuals with severe renal dysfunction by making appropriate dose adjustments.[29,33]

A Cochrane review of 24 randomized controlled trials with 6,915 participants[39] found that acamprosate significantly reduced the risk of any drinking and significantly increased the cumulative abstinence duration (mean difference 10.94 days) compared to placebo. Diarrhea was the only adverse effect more frequently reported with acamprosate than placebo.

Table 86-4 includes the dosing information for acamprosate and other options used in treating alcohol use disorder.[20,29,30] When selecting a medication for an individual patient, factors such as ease of administration, available formulations, renal or hepatic disease, pregnancy, adverse effects, presence of co-occurring conditions, or specific symptoms of AUD should guide medication therapy decisions. Duration of treatment is dependent on several patient-specific factors, such as clinical response, tolerability, patient preference, history of relapses, and severity of the disorder.[23]

EVALUATION OF THERAPEUTIC OUTCOMES

Considering the increasing rates of alcohol use and the variable effects of alcohol from individual to individual, screening tools such as the CAGE questionnaire and AUDIT are instrumental in detecting unhealthy alcohol use and identifying those at risk for alcohol withdrawal. Treating alcohol withdrawal takes precedence over the treatment of alcohol use disorder. The assessment of alcohol withdrawal begins with utilizing the CIWA-Ar to assess withdrawal symptom severity before initiating pharmacologic therapy with benzodiazepines. Close monitoring is essential to avoid progression to severe withdrawal, which includes seizures and/or DT.

For alcohol use disorder, both psychosocial interventions and pharmacologic therapy can be beneficial to reduce drinking frequency. Four agents have FDA approval for the treatment of alcohol use disorder. Careful consideration of patient-specific factors needs to be done, as each agent works pharmacologically different to reduce cravings (acamprosate and extended-release naltrexone) or act as a deterrent to the resumption of drinking (disulfiram). Patient counseling on potential adverse effects followed by close monitoring and follow-up are necessary to assess response to therapy and promote adherence.

INTRODUCTION—NICOTINE

5 Annually, approximately 480,000 deaths in the United States are attributable to tobacco use, making smoking the leading cause of preventable death and disease in the United States.[40-42] Adverse health effects of tobacco use impact almost every organ in the body and can result in an increased risk of cancer, respiratory disease, and cardiovascular disease, as well as negatively impacting the immune

TABLE 86-4 Dosing and Monitoring of Pharmacologic Agents Used in the Treatment of Unhealthy Alcohol Use

Medication	Dosage Range Per Day	Indication	Monitoring	Level of Evidence for Efficacy*
Disulfiram (Antabuse)	125-500 mg; use with caution in patients with hepatic disease or insufficiency	Deterrence	Facial flushing, liver enzymes	B2
Acamprosate (Campral)	999-1,998 mg and higher (333 mg tablets) Dosage adjustment necessary in renal impairment	Craving	Patient-reported craving, renal function	A1
Naltrexone (ReVia)	50-100 mg; dosage adjustment may be needed in renal and liver impairment	Craving	Patient-reported craving, liver enzymes	A1
Naltrexone (Vivitrol)	380 mg intramuscularly once every 4 weeks	Craving	Patient-reported craving, liver enzymes, injection site reactions	B2
Antiseizure Medications (eg, topiramate [Topamax], carbamazepine [Tegretol], valproic acid [Depakote], gabapentin [Neurontin], oxcarbazepine [Trileptal])	Seizure disorder doses	Craving	Patient-reported craving, plasma medication levels	B2
Antidepressants (eg, fluoxetine [Prozac], amitriptyline [Elavil], citalopram [Celexa], sertraline [Zoloft])	Depression doses	Craving, depression, anxiety	Patient-reported craving	B2

*Strength of recommendations: A, B, and C, good, moderate, and poor evidence to support recommendation, respectively.

Quality of evidence: (1) evidence from more than one properly randomized controlled trial; (2) evidence from more than one well-designed clinical trial with randomization, from cohort or case-control analytic studies or multiple time series, or dramatic results from uncontrolled experiments; and (3) evidence from opinions of respected authorities, based on clinical experience, descriptive studies, or reports of expert communities.

Data from References 23, 29, and 30.

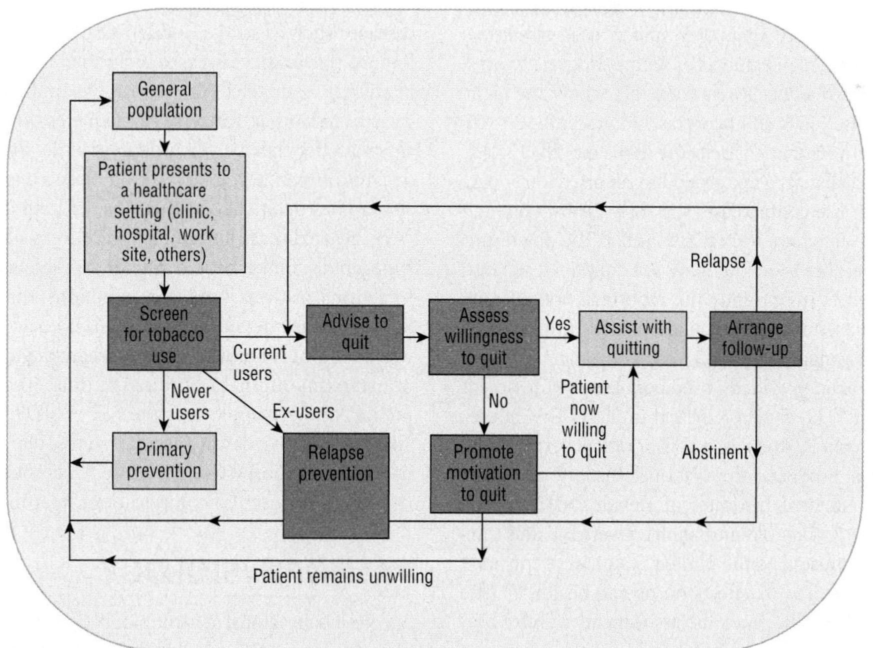

FIGURE 86-1 Model for treatment of tobacco use and use disorder.

system and reproductive health. Over 16 million Americans currently suffer from diseases directly related to smoking.[41,43]

The number of individuals who smoke cigarettes has continued to decline over the years. In 2019, the National Health Interview Survey reported 14% or 34.1 million of adults smoked cigarettes, which is reduced from the 42% reported in 1964, when the first Surgeon General's report on smoking was released.[44]

Although smoking cigarettes is still the most popular method of tobacco exposure,[10] a small percentage of individuals use alternative forms of nicotine products such as cigars (3.6%), pipes (1%), smokeless tobacco (2.4%), and e-cigarettes (4.5%).[44] It is important to recognize the downward trend in the percent of individuals who smoke cigarettes is not uniform across all populations in the United States. In order to reduce the disparities seen in tobacco use, continued education for healthcare providers is needed. Behavioral and pharmacotherapy interventions have proven effective and these are supported by the clinical guidelines for tobacco use and use disorder as outlined in Fig. 86-1.[10]

There have been numerous approaches to smoking cessation, including a focus on sales, marketing, and manufacturing of all tobacco products marketed in the United States that are now regulated by the FDA. Federal tobacco excise taxes have increased, and states have also added cigarette excise tax rates. Additionally, many states have enacted comprehensive smoke-free laws, and further opportunities for access to smoking cessation pharmacotherapy and counseling are available through the Affordable Care Act.[41,45]

National telephone quitlines, smoking cessation counseling services, and mass media campaigns have been utilized to improve smoking cessation rates. "Tips from Former Smokers" was a successful federally funded national mass media antismoking campaign,[46,47] and various Internet and mobile phone text messaging programs have been developed over the years. The QuitGuide Mobile App is a free app released by Smokefree.gov, which provides resources to track craving patterns and motivation, and monitors progress as milestones are achieved.[48] Despite the proven effectiveness of pharmacological and counseling services to aid in sustained smoking cessation, cigarette smoking continues to be the leading cause of preventable morbidity and mortality in the United States.[41]

EPIDEMIOLOGY

The National Survey on Drug Use and Health (NSDUH) reported in 2017 that an estimated 58.1 million people (21.1%) had exposure to a tobacco product at least once in the month prior to being interviewed. Additionally, 45.9 million of the US population age 12 and older currently smoke cigarettes, defined as smoking at least a part of the cigarette. Of these, 58.4% were daily smokers (26.8 million) and 40.5% (10.8 million) reported smoking a pack or more of cigarettes per day.[3] In addition, 11.7 million smoked cigars, 8.5 million used smokeless tobacco, and 1.9 million smoked pipe tobacco.[3] Comparing age groups, data from 2019 demonstrated adults 26 years and older have the highest rate of daily cigarette use (62.5%). In contrast, adolescents 12 to 17 years of age reported the lowest daily cigarette use in the month (13.2%). This data from 2019 shows that each age group has reported lower percentages of daily cigarette use compared to the early 2000s, although the percentages in recent years have been fairly similar. The downward trend over the last two decades is encouraging but continued tobacco cessation education is needed. Importantly, this report has not included vaping of nicotine products; however, tracking of trends in the use of nicotine vaping products is ongoing.[3]

Additional data has been provided in the Population Assessment of Tobacco and Health (PATH) Study launched in 2011. This household-based longitudinal cohort study is a collaboration between the FDA Center for Tobacco Products, the National Institute on Drug Abuse (NIDA) and the National Institutes of Health (NIH), which include youths age 12 to 17 years old and adults. Overall 45,000 current tobacco users and nonusers in the United States were included to help evaluate tobacco use and its effects on overall health.[49,50] The PATH study differs from NSDUH since the assessment includes biomarker collection, a detailed assessment of tobacco-use behaviors, and further detailed examination of specific tobacco products to distinguish between them and ensure clarity in usage patterns.[51] The goals of this study are to determine what products are commonly used including the use of e-cigarettes; factors associated with susceptibility of use; evaluate patterns of use; review the overall health impacts associated with smoking, smoking cessation, and relapse; and identifying any racial/ethnic, gender, and age differences in use.[51]

The Wave 1 data, collected from September 2013 through December 2014, indicated that more than 25% of adults used one type of tobacco product during this time period. Approximately 9% of youth used a tobacco product in the last 30 days, and 1.6% of these were daily users of tobacco. Forty percent of the respondents indicated they were using multiple tobacco products at the same time, with the most common combination being cigarettes and e-cigarettes together. The PATH Study also found that in adults, tobacco use is higher in males, members of racial minority groups, and individuals who have lower household incomes or lower education levels.[51]

However, tobacco-related health disparities (TRHD) have been identified in many patient populations.[52] In addition to those reported in the PATH study, individuals with mental health conditions, and substance use disorders also have higher rates of tobacco use.[10] Additionally, certain geographic locations in the United States have been identified as having a higher prevalence of cigarette smoking, including the Midwest and South compared to the Northeast and West. The prevalence of cigarette smoking is higher in the lesbian, gay, bisexual, transgender, and queer (LGBTQ+) population in both adults and youth. Further study on tobacco-related health disparities is needed to continue to develop guidelines and policies on how to effectively identify and reduce disparities, inequities, and inequalities to improve overall care and continue to improve the tobacco cessation rates.[41]

Economic Impact of Smoking

The yearly direct healthcare expenditures associated with smoking for adults is estimated at nearly $170 billion for direct medical care and $156 billion in indirect costs, such as lost productivity.[43,53] Included in these costs are the estimated $39 billion annually for Medicaid patients. This number is significant, as this small subset of the population has higher smoking rates compared to privately insured patients.[54]

Health Risks of Smoking

Cigarette smoking greatly increases the risk of (a) cardiovascular diseases such as stroke, sudden death, and heart attack; (b) nonmalignant respiratory diseases including emphysema, asthma, chronic bronchitis, and chronic obstructive pulmonary disease; (c) lung cancer and other cancers, (d) diabetes, and (e) harmful effects to reproductive health, including erectile dysfunction.[40,43] Exposure to environmental tobacco smoke (*passive exposure and secondhand smoke*) has been cited as the cause of lung cancer, stroke, and coronary heart disease in adults.[55] Children who are exposed to environmental smoke have a higher risk of heart disease, respiratory infections, asthma, and ear infections than those not exposed.[55] Sudden infant death syndrome (SIDS) occurs more often in infants whose mothers smoked during pregnancy compared to offspring of nonsmoking mothers. Studies continue to determine how environmental smoke can increase the risk of SIDS. Additionally, long-term adverse negative cardiovascular consequences have been identified in children exposed to environmental smoke leading to an increased risk of cardiovascular complications later in life.[56]

PATHOPHYSIOLOGY

Nicotine is an agonist at nicotinic acetylcholine receptors (nAchRs) with pharmacologic effects highly dependent on dose. These effects include central and peripheral nervous system stimulation and depression, respiratory stimulation, skeletal muscle relaxation, catecholamine release by the adrenal medulla, peripheral vasoconstriction, and increased blood pressure, heart rate, cardiac output, and oxygen consumption. Cigarette smoking or low doses of nicotine produce an increased alertness and increased cognitive functioning by stimulating the cerebral cortex. At higher doses, nicotine stimulates dopamine within the "reward" center in the brain's limbic system.[57] When nicotine is ingested, a feeling of pleasure and relaxation can occur. Repetitive exposure to nicotine leads to neuroadaptation, which builds tolerance to the initial effects. An accumulation of nicotine in the body leads to a more substantial withdrawal reaction if cessation is attempted. Common symptoms experienced during withdrawal can include anxiety, difficulty concentrating, irritability, and strong cravings for tobacco.[58] Onset of these withdrawal symptoms usually occurs within 24 hours and can last for days, weeks, or longer. Additionally, some might experience a state of malaise or inability to experience pleasure during this nicotine withdrawal period. These types of reactions have been termed "hedonic dysregulation" and can be rapidly reversed with nicotine readministration.[59] This powerful force of nicotine effects leading to physical dependence is one reason smokers attempting smoking cessation have a high rate of relapse, and only 3% remain abstinent 6 months following the quit date.[60]

The genetics associated with nicotine addiction is very complex and continues to be studied with great interest. Progress continues to be made in understanding the human genome and identifying more specific markers for various diseases. Many phenotypes and corresponding genes have been identified as markers, which include the genetic markers, nicotinic cholinergic receptor alpha5 subunit (CHRNA5) and cytochrome P450 2A6 (CYP2A6), and the metabolic marker, nicotine metabolism ratio (NMR). All three of these have been found to have a relationship with smoking behavior, including nicotine physical dependence and cigarettes per day. Additionally, the CHRNA5-CHRNA3-CHRNB4 locus has been found to predict lung cancer, chronic obstructive pulmonary disease (COPD), coronary artery disease, and mortality.[61,62] Having the ability to identify patients at higher risk can improve chances of diagnosing cancer earlier in the disease process so treatment can begin sooner and improve prognosis.[61]

Studies continue to evaluate the effects of polymorphisms on various genes and the effect this has on the efficacy of pharmacotherapy treatment options in order to offer options for more personalized treatment in the future.[62] Genetic variability in nicotine metabolism continues to be evaluated since variations in CYP2A6 lead to different rates of nicotine physical dependence and responses to NRT.[61] Further understanding of these variations will continue to prove helpful in creating a personalized pharmacotherapy plan to improve smoking cessation rates.

TREATMENT

Desired Outcomes

Ideally, the desired outcome is for all tobacco users to quit, and that young people never take up the habit. Unfortunately, this is unlikely to happen. The Healthy People 2030 target has set a goal prevalence of tobacco use at less than or equal to 16.2% in adults 18 years and older. This is a realistic and believed to be an achievable goal since the National Health Interview Survey 2018 figures have reported at 20.1% of adults use any tobacco product, as well as continued declines in the percent of the adult population who smoke cigarettes.[44,63]

Nicotine Physical Dependence: Recognition of Behavior

6 The United States Preventive Services Task Force (USPSTF) released the "Interventions for Tobacco Smoking Cessation in Adults, Including Pregnant Persons in 2021."[10] This recommendation stresses that all healthcare providers should ask each adult about tobacco use, advise any adult using tobacco to stop using, and provide behavioral inventions and pharmacotherapy options to aid in smoking cessation (Fig. 86-2). These recommendations also included pregnant individuals and are summarized in Table 86-5. Additional information regarding the challenges of pharmacotherapy treatment options for smoking cessation in pregnant persons is also available.[10]

A well-established method of assessing an individual's smoking status utilizes the 5As as follows[10]:

1. **A**sk about tobacco use
2. **A**dvise the person to quit through clear individualized messages

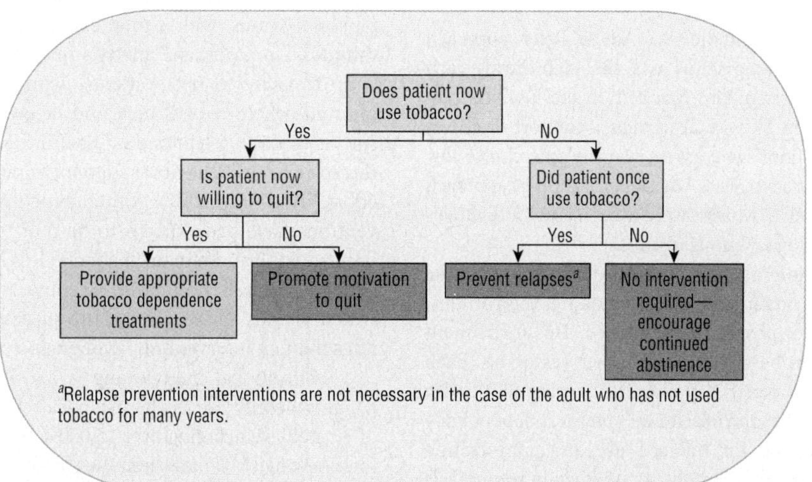

FIGURE 86-2 Algorithm for treating tobacco use.

CLINICAL PRESENTATION Nicotine Withdrawal

General

- The patient may experience anxiety, but may not be in acute distress. Symptoms can wax and wane over time.

Symptoms

- The patient may complain of cravings, difficulty concentrating, frustration, irritability, and impatience. Hostility, insomnia, and restlessness can also occur.
- Increased skin temperature can be present.

TABLE 86-5 Summary US Preventive Services Task Force (USPSTF) Interventions for Tobacco Smoking Cessation in Adults, Including Pregnant Persons

Population	Adults >18 Years Old (Nonpregnant)	Pregnant Persons >18 Years Old
Assessment	Screen for all tobacco Consider the following approaches: • 5As • Ask Assist Refer • Use smoking status as a vital sign	Screen for all tobacco Consider the following approaches: • 5As • Ask Assist Refer • Use smoking status as a vial sign • Consider using a multiple choice question approach during assessment to improve comfort level
Behavioral interventions	• In person behavioral support and counseling >4 sessions which each session averaging 90-300 minutes (group/individual option) • Efficacy improves with 8 sessions or more • Telephone counseling/mobile phone–based interventions (>3 sessions)	• Counseling • Self help materials • Feedback • Health education • Incentives • Social support
Pharmacotherapy	• NRT • Bupropion SR • Varenicline • +/− Behavioral interventions • Combination of NRT (long acting + short acting NRT demonstrated higher efficacy vs single NRT approach)	• Inadequate evidence due to lack of studies to determine benefit vs risk
Comments on benefits and harms	Conclusion from USPSTF; behavioral interventions and +/− pharmacotherapy interventions with FDA-approved pharmacotherapy agents for smoking cessation demonstrated substantial benefit	Conclusion from USPSTF; behavioral interventions demonstrated substantial benefit for perinatal outcome and improved smoking abstinence
Electronic nicotine delivery systems (electronic cigarettes)	Evidence on the use of ENDS for tobacco cessation is insufficient, benefit vs risk cannot be determined	Evidence on the use of ENDS for tobacco cessation is insufficient, benefit vs risk cannot be determined

ENDS, Electronic Nicotine Delivery Systems; FDA, Food and Drug Administration; NRT, Nicotine Replacement Therapy.

Data from Reference 10.

3. **A**ssess the person's willingness to quit
4. **A**ssist in quitting
5. **A**rrange follow-up and support

Other approaches recommend using the "Ask, Advise, Refer" approach or recording the patient's smoking status as a vital sign during each appointment. The USPSTF statement expanded on the 5As and recommended that for pregnant individuals a higher comfort level was demonstrated if these questions were asked in a multiple-choice format instead of open-ended questions.[10] Additionally, another approach includes the "Ask, Advise, Refer," which can be used to assist individuals in obtaining access to smoking cessation services.

The Fagerström test for nicotine physical dependence can be used to help identify how much someone is smoking, the compulsion to use, and the level of physical dependence. This instrument includes questions that can be answered as either yes or no. Each question answered as yes is worth 1 point. The scoring is 0 to 10; the higher the score, the higher the individual's physical dependency to nicotine.[64] When assessing for tobacco use and approaching tobacco cessation counseling, there might be times when someone is not ready to consider an attempt tobacco cessation. A motivational intervention to consider is the 5Rs.[65]

- Relevance: Discuss possible reasons why tobacco cessation is personally relevant.
- Risks: Explore the individual's views of potential risks and negative consequences of tobacco use.
- Rewards: Explore what positive benefits could result in tobacco cessation.
- Roadblocks: Encourage the individual to identify and voice potential benefits of tobacco cessation.
- Repetition: Commit to address tobacco cessation during each interaction and continue to encourage those who have previously failed attempts.

Nonpharmacologic Therapy

The USPSTF statement emphasized the importance of counseling sessions and highlighted the goal of reaching at least four in-person sessions, with a total contact time ranging from 90 to 300 minutes.[10] A Cochrane analysis reviewed 65 trials, which included approximately 23,000 patients, who received a combination of pharmacotherapy treatment and behavioral support either in person or through telephone interaction. This review determined that the addition of behavioral support improves the smoking cessation efforts by 10% to 20%.[66] Although comprehensive behavioral interventions have been shown to be more effective in helping people quit smoking and remain abstinent, less intensive treatments may be beneficial as well. Even minimal contacts lasting less than 3 minutes, which include the 5As, are more successful in increasing cessation rates than an intervention involving no contact.[41]

Motivational interviewing is a collaborative approach to help patients identify barriers for making a behavior change. A meta-analysis of 37 studies, including over 15,000 smokers undergoing motivational interviewing (MI) compared the efficacy of both intensive MI and less intensive MI to no treatment, other smoking cessation treatments, and other types of smoking cessation treatments. Overall, MI is moderately effective in increasing the chances of long-term smoking cessation when utilized with other smoking cessation treatment approaches and when compared to other treatment approaches without the MI approach. However, there was insufficient evidence to determine if MI improves smoking cessation when compared with no treatment. Further research is needed to continue to evaluate the efficacy of MI.[67]

Additionally, other forms of interventions are effective in improving smoking cessation rates. Telephone-based quitlines, which are operated by the National Cancer Institute and offered in all 50 states, the District of Columbia, Puerto Rico, and Guam via 1-800-QUIT-NOW, provide various options, such as recorded messages, counseling services, mailed materials, counselor follow-up services, and access to pharmacotherapy options for smoking cessation.[68] Along with continued support and monitoring of state quitlines, the Centers for Disease Control and Prevention (CDC) has now established the National Quitline Data Warehouse (NQDW) for continual evaluation and support of services.[69] The use of technology to further enhance counseling opportunities has also increased over the years, including websites, text messaging, social networking, and smartphone applications. A systematic review and meta-analysis evaluated 26 manuscripts that included over 33,000 smokers who received text messages for smoking cessation. Overall patients receiving the text messages were much more likely to achieve smoking cessation by 50% to 60%.[70]

Furthermore, while counseling alone can be effective, its efficacy is further augmented by the addition of pharmacotherapy, with NRT also being effective independent of counseling services.[10] The combination of pharmacotherapy and behavioral interventions were evaluated in different subpopulations, including ethnic minorities and patients suffering from mental health conditions. No evidence was found suggesting there was a difference in risk or benefit of this treatment approach within these populations.[41]

Pharmacologic Therapy

Pharmacologic therapy helps facilitate the process of tobacco cessation by the following mechanisms[71]:

1. "Reducing nicotine withdrawal symptoms"
2. "Reducing the rewarding effects of nicotine from smoking by blocking or desensitizing nicotine receptors"
3. "Providing an alternative source of nicotine with the desired pharmacologic effect previously provided by nicotine from cigarettes"

All patients attempting to quit should be encouraged to use effective pharmacotherapy agents for smoking cessation except in the presence of special circumstances or contraindications. For pregnant individuals, the USPSTF statement recommends that clinicians weigh the benefits and the harms associated with pharmacotherapy interventions and treat each patient on an individual basis.[10] Current recommendations list seven first-line agents including the NRT medications, sustained release bupropion hydrochloride, and varenicline tartrate as treatment options.[10,41] First-line therapy options in smoking cessation are summarized in Table 86-6.[41,72-79]

Nicotine Replacement Therapy

7 Nicotine replacement therapy provides lower peak levels and lower levels of nicotine concentrations compared to cigarettes, leading to reductions in the reinforcing effects of smoking. Another benefit of NRT includes the decrease and eventual elimination of exposure to the harmful substances included in cigarettes.[80] Individuals have easy access to many of these products since five of these are available over-the-counter, with only the nasal inhaler

TABLE 86-6 First-Line Pharmacotherapy Treatment Options for Smoking Cessation

Medication	Dosing (For individuals 18 years or older. For those <18 years, discuss with a prescriber before use)	Duration	Comments/Monitoring Parameters
Nicotine Replacement Therapies (NRTs)			

Nicotine patch	Based on cigarettes smoked per day:
	>10 cigs/day:
	Step 1: 21 mg/day: Weeks 1-6
	Step 2: 14 mg/day: Weeks 7-8
	Step 3: 7 mg/day: Weeks 9-10
	<10 cigs/day:
	Step 2: 14 mg/day: 6 Weeks
	Step 3: 7 mg/day: 2 Weeks
		8-10 weeks	• Patch can be worn for up to 24 hours per day
			  • If patient has sleep disturbances, remove patch at night and place one patch in morning (~16 hours per day)
			  • If waking up with cravings, patch should be worn for 24 hours
			• Recommended to place patch on stop day. However, if patient smokes with patch on, there is no major risk
			• Place a new patch on each day, hold patch on for 10 seconds to help adherence
			• Rotate patches to avoid skin irritation
			• Do not cut patches, do not wear patches for greater than 24 hours, do not use more than one patch at a time

Nicotine gum	1st cigarette ≤30 minutes after waking: 4 mg
	1st cigarette ≥30 minutes after waking: 2 mg
	Weeks 1-6: 1 piece of gum every 1-2 hours prn
	Weeks 7-9: 1 piece every 2-4 hours prn
	Weeks 10-12: 1 piece every 4-8 hours prn
	Then stop
	Do not exceed 24 pieces/day
		12 weeks	• Continuous use can lead to adverse effects (pyrosis, nausea, hiccups)
			• 4 mg strength has shown to be more efficacious in heavy smokers over 6-week time period
			• If patient uses with a cigarette, there is no major risk
			• Counseling on proper use of gum:
			  • Do not eat or drink 15 minutes before or during use of gum
			  • Chew each piece slowly
			  • Park between cheek and gum after a peppery sensation becomes apparent
			  • Repeat process until peppery sensation does not reoccur (approximately 30 minutes)
			  • Use alternate sides of mouth when using chew and park method
			  • Use at least 9 pieces of gum per day for first 6 weeks to improve cessation

Lozenge available as Nicorette lozenge or Nicorette mini lozenge	1st cigarette ≤30 minutes after waking: 4 mg
	1st cigarette ≥30 minutes after waking: 2 mg
	Weeks 1-6: 1 lozenge by mouth every 1-2 hours prn
	Weeks 7-9: 1 lozenge by mouth every 2-4 hours prn
	Weeks 10-12: 1 lozenge by mouth every 4-8 hours prn
	Then stop
	Do not exceed 5 lozenges in 6 hours or 20 lozenges/day
		12 weeks	• Counseling points
			  • Do not eat or drink anything 15 minutes prior to or during lozenge use
			  • Allow the lozenge to dissolve slowly, approximately 20-30 minutes
			  • Nicotine release could create a tingling or warm sensation
			  • Do not chew or swallow the lozenge
			  • Periodically rotate the lozenge to different areas of the mouth
			  • Use at least 9 lozenges per day for first 6 weeks to improve cessation

(continued)

TABLE 86-6 First-Line Pharmacotherapy Treatment Options for Smoking Cessation (*Continued*)

Medication	Dosing (For individuals 18 years or older. For those <18 years, discuss with a prescriber before use)	Duration	Comments/Monitoring Parameters

Nicotine oral inhaler + cartridge plus mouthpiece (Nicotrol)	10 mg nicotine/cartridge; supplies 80 puffs
	1. Stop smoking completely before use
	2. Initial dose: 1 cartridge every 1-2 hours
	3. Begin gradual reduction of device after 3 months of use
	4. Gradual dose taper over 6-12 weeks
		6 months	• Patients should stop smoking prior to starting this product
			• Most successful patients in trials; use ranged from 6-16 cartridges per day, 20 minutes continuous puffing
			• Recommended duration of treatment: 3 months with subsequent weaning with gradual reduction over 6-12 weeks
			• Treatment longer than 6 months has not been studied
			• Precautions: patients with asthma, chronic pulmonary disease, history of recent myocardial infarction, serious arrhythmias, or worsening angina
			• Counseling:
			  • Insert cartridge into mouthpiece and inhale medication quickly by puffing on mouthpiece for continuously for 20 minutes or four 5 minute sessions
			  • Deep inhalation is not necessary when using this product
			  • Change cartridge when nicotine taste is no longer detected
			  • Dosing is individualized; initially it is recommended to use at least 6 cartridges per day for 3-6 weeks. Do not exceed 16 cartridges per day

Nicotine metered nasal spray (Nicotrol NS)	Availed in 10 mg/mL bottle 1 spray (0.5 mg nicotine/spray) into each nostril 1-2 times each hour when craving cigarette
	Max dose:
	10 sprays per hour
	(max of 80 sprays per day)
		3-6 months	• Two sprays is considered 1 dose
			• Treatment duration is 3 months; safety beyond 6 months has not been studied
			• Counseling:
			  • Breathe normally while administering spray, do not sniff or inhale deeply while administering spray
			  • Wait at least 2-3 minutes before blowing nose after using product
			  • For best results, use at least 16 sprays per day which has been found as the minimum effective dose
			  • Pregnancy category D

Non-Nicotine Replacement Options			

Bupropion (Zyban)	150 mg by mouth daily × 3 days then 150 mg by mouth twice daily (dosing interval should be >8 hours)	3-6 months	• Do not exceed 300 mg/day
			• Recommend initiating therapy 1-2 weeks prior to set "quit" day
			• Tapering is not needed with discontinuing agent
			• Black box warning for neuropsychiatric warning and suicide warnings removed in 2016; downgraded to warning
			• Pregnancy category: C, excreted into breastmilk
			• Monitor patients with renal/hepatic impairment
			• Counseling points:
			  • May cause dry mouth
			  • May cause insomnia, avoid bedtime dosing
			  • May help with post-cessation weight gain
			  • Recommended dosing interval: more than 8 hours when taking twice daily

Varenicline (Chantix)	Start with dose titration:
	Days 1-3: 0.5 mg by mouth once daily
	Days 3-7: 0.5 mg by mouth twice daily
	Week 2 until end of treatment: 1 mg by mouth twice daily
		12 weeks; an additional 12-week course may be used in select patients	• Take with food and a full glass of water
			• Quit day can be flexible with four options:
			  • Start varenicline 1 week after quit day
			  • Start varenicline and establish quit day between days 8 and 35
			  • Start varenicline and gradually reduce smoking with goal of cessation by week 12 of therapy
			• If patient has difficulty with cessation, taper smoking by 50% each month with a goal of smoking abstinence in 12 weeks, continue varenicline for another 12 weeks for a full 24-week therapy
			• Maintenance up to 6 months therapy is approved
			• Renal impairment dosing for CrCl ≤30 mL/min (0.5 mL/s)
			• No dosing adjustment needed in hepatic impairment
			• Neuropsychiatric adverse events: black box warning removed in December 2016, warning remains
			• Counseling Points:
			  • Varenicline works in two ways by reliving symptoms of nicotine withdrawal and blocking rewards of smoking
			  • Most common adverse medication effects: nausea, sleep problems, constipation, gas, vomiting
			  • Consider dose reduction if experiencing insomnia

Data from References 41, 72–79.

and the nasal spray currently being prescription products. A recent review showed that all the commercially available forms of NRT (eg, chewing gum, transdermal patches, nasal spray, lozenge, inhalers, and tablets) were effective for smoking cessation, increased the quit rate by 50% to 60%, and were tolerated with very limited reports of serious adverse events.[81] Combinations of these agents have been demonstrated in multiple studies and meta-analyses to improve abstinence rates in comparison to monotherapy.[10,82]

In some smoking cessation protocols, it is suggested that NRT use begins on the patient's defined quit day. However, other recommendations have suggested patients utilize the preloading approach with NRT in which patients start NRT prior to setting the quit date. It is thought the use of NRT with smoking will reduce the satisfaction associated with smoking and break the reward pattern associated with smoking. This approach can allow the patient to set the quit date when comfortable. A recent Cochrane review for 9 studies with over 4,000 patients demonstrated there is moderate evidence to support this approach in improving quit rates (RR 1.25, 95%, CI 1.08-1.44).[82]

Nicotine Gum

Nicotine gum offers a rapid onset and short duration of effect that can be very beneficial since the amount of nicotine and the timing can be controlled by the patient. The recommended dosing is based on the "time to first cigarette" (TTFC), which indicates the response to the nicotine deprivation.[83] The FDA has approved the nicotine starting doses of 4 mg for patients who experience TTFC less than 30 minutes and 2 mg for patients who experience the TTFC greater than 30 minutes.[84] Recent studies have demonstrated utilization of the 4-mg dose will increase the chances of achieving smoking cessation compared to the use of the 2-mg gum in highly dependent smokers.[82] The gum should be chewed slowly until a peppery or minty taste emerges and then "parked" between the cheek and gums to facilitate nicotine absorption through the oral mucosa. Acidic beverages (eg, coffee, juices, or soft drinks) interfere with the buccal absorption of nicotine, so eating and drinking anything except water should be avoided for 15 minutes before and during chewing. Instructions to chew the gum on a fixed schedule (at least one piece every 1-2 hours) for at least 1 to 3 months can be more beneficial than ad libitum use.[78] Generally, the gum should be used for up to 12 weeks with no more than 24 pieces chewed per day.[78]

Nicotine Lozenge

The nicotine lozenge is available as a 2-mg or 4-mg dose, with the lower amount recommended for patients who normally smoke their first cigarette later than 30 minutes after awakening, and the higher dose being reserved for smokers who smoke within 30 minutes of waking. It is recommended that no more than 20 lozenges should be used in 1 day, for up to 12 weeks. The most common adverse effect of the lozenge is nausea. As with the nicotine gum, acidic beverages (eg, coffee, juices, or soft drinks) interfere with the buccal absorption of nicotine, so eating and drinking anything except water should be avoided for 15 minutes before and during use of the lozenge.[75]

Nicotine Patch

The nicotine patch is available as a nonprescription medication and is the NRT option with the highest rate of adherence.[71] This nicotine product provides a steady amount of transdermal nicotine for 16 to 24 hours based on the selected product. The patch is available in three strengths and package labeling suggests individuals who smoke more than 10 cigarettes per day start with the 21-mg patch and those who smoke less than 10 cigarettes per day start with the 14-mg patch. This initial regimen will be worn for 4 to 6 weeks and then a tapering regimen will begin which includes reducing the patch strength approximately every 2 weeks.[41,77] The patch can be used up to 8 to 10 weeks per the labeling guidelines. Patients who experience sleep disruption should remove the 24-hour patch prior to bedtime or use the 16-hour patch. The patient should place a new patch on a relatively hairless location, typically between the neck and waist. The site of application should be changed daily to diminish any skin irritation from the patch adhesive. There are no restrictions on activity while using the patch.[41,77]

The patient should be told that using the patch results in less desire to smoke and provides an opportunity for a new nonsmoker to reduce their hand-mouth habit without being burdened by craving. The patient should understand that with smoking, there are naturally peaks and valleys in the amount of nicotine in the bloodstream. However, with the patch, there is a steady gradual rise in the blood nicotine concentration that levels off and remains constant for much of the day, and then gradually decreases while the person is asleep.[41] A recent Cochrane review concluded that in individuals who smoke more than 15 cigarettes per day, the 21-mg nicotine patches resulted in a higher quit rate compared to the lower 14-mg nicotine patches.[81] Combining the nicotine patch with an oral formulation, such as the nicotine gum which allows ad libitum nicotine delivery, can improve overall cessation without significant increased risk for harm.[41] In fact, various studies have evaluated combination NRTs and based on high certainty evidence, the use of a nicotine patch can be used with the nicotine gum, lozenge, or nasal spray on an as-needed basis to improve the long-term quit rate compared to NRT monotherapy.[82] However, it is important to also incorporate behavioral strategies with pharmacotherapy as recommended by current guidelines.[41,79,85]

Nicotine Nasal Spray

Nicotine nasal spray is available exclusively as a prescription medication and differs from the other short-acting NRTs due to the higher peak and trough concentrations, as it is more rapidly absorbed and eliminated than other forms.[85] A dose of nicotine nasal spray consists of one 0.5 mg delivery to each nostril (1 mg total). Initial dosing should be one to two doses per hour, increasing as needed for symptom relief. The minimum recommended treatment is 8 doses per day, with a maximum limit of 40 doses per day (five doses per hour). Recommended duration of therapy is 3 months. Individuals should not sniff, swallow, or inhale through the nose while administering doses because this increases irritating adverse effects.[74]

Nicotine Oral Inhaler

The nicotine oral inhaler consists of a mouthpiece and a plastic cartridge placed into the inhaler, which delivers 4 mg or 10 mg of nicotine, through vapor inhalation. Approximately 2 mg is systemically absorbed mainly in the throat and upper airway.[71,72] It is suggested that the individual actively puff on the inhaler for 5 minutes at a time and adjust use based on effect, as the cartridge can be used for up to 20 minutes of active puffing. The recommended initial dosing is 6 to 16 cartridges per day for up to 12 weeks of therapy. Tapering of the product should start 6 weeks after initiation.[72] As the inhaler resembles a cigarette, it also provides the sensory stimulation to help decrease some of the cue-induced cravings by alleviating the hand-mouth habit.[41,71,85] However, there are some concerns this inhaler may do the opposite and possibly reinforce smoking habits.[85]

Instructing Patients in the Use of NRT

Compliance with NRT improves when individuals are presented a clear rationale for its use and realistic expectations about response. It should be explained that nicotine is responsible for physical dependence and that discontinuation causes cigarette craving, tension, irritability, sadness, problems with sleep, and difficulty concentrating. The NRT products help reduce these physical symptoms so individuals can modify behavioral and psychological aspects associated with smoking.[71] The products have relatively few adverse effects; however, nausea and light-headedness are possible symptoms of nicotine overdose that warrant a dose reduction.[10,82]

Duration

Initially, when NRT products were approved by the FDA, they were approved for 8 to 12 weeks of therapy. However, more recent practice is to inform those who commit to quitting smoking than using NRT for up to 3 months is common. Additionally, some individuals will experience severe withdrawal even beyond this time period, and thus long-term use of NRT might be indicated. The long-term use of NRT 6 months or longer has not been linked to any safety concerns,[41,71] although there is still insufficient efficacy data based on a meta-analysis and further research is needed.[41,86]

Electronic Nicotine Delivery Systems

Electronic nicotine delivery systems (ENDS) (also known as e-cigarettes or electronic cigarettes, or vaping devices) are designed to deliver a propylene glycol or glycerin product with a combination of nicotine, flavorings, and/or other chemicals through an aerosol. The device usually includes a battery, a heating coil, an atomizer, a cartridge, which contains the e-liquid (also called "juice"), and a mouthpiece. The range of nicotine delivered to the user can vary according to the product type and brand, and is available in first-, second-, third-, and fourth-generation models, with some products not containing any nicotine at all.[87] The first-generation devices are disposable and resemble a cigarette, and the second-generation products are tank devices that can be recharged. Pod/pod mods are the third-generation products that allow for high levels of nicotine and are refillable, and the fourth-generation products are vape pens that are battery operated and can be refilled.[88] It has been suggested that using the ENDS products instead of smoking traditional cigarettes can eliminate the exposure to most of the toxins commonly seen in traditional cigarettes. However, no e-cigarette has been approved by the FDA as a cessation aid. A Cochrane review of 56 studies with over 12,000 currently smoking adults evaluated the use of quit rates with e-cigarette use compared to the quit rates of e-cigarettes without nicotine or traditional smoking cessation pharmacotherapy options including NRT, varenicline, and behavioral support. Overall there is moderate evidence supporting e-cigarettes as effective in achieving smoking cessation for 6 months or longer. There is some data to indicate e-cigarettes could be more effective than traditional smoking cessation treatments.[89] Adverse effects associated with e-cigarettes were limited and included coughing, throat and mouth irritation, and headache; all of which resolved with continuous exposure to the e-cigarettes. However, it was emphasized that more studies are needed since the overall evidence is low and concern over long-term health effects of e-cigarettes continues.[89] Thus, although ENDS may offer a possible benefit during the smoking cessation process, their use is controversial as the potential harms associated with their use are still being evaluated and studied.[41,71] E-cigarette use for smoking cessation has also been evaluated for use in pregnant individuals.[10] Although it has been well established that the exposure to toxins is much lower when using an e-cigarette compared to cigarette smoke, there are no long-term safety studies in humans to determine if e-cigarettes are safer than traditional cigarettes.[41,90]

In the fall of 2019, a severe lung illness related to use of e-cigarettes and vaping, referred to as "E-cigarette or Vaping use-Associated Lung Injury" (EVALI) was reported. By February 2020, over 2,800 patients were hospitalized, and 68 patients died. Most cases were linked to THC-containing products (82%), but some cases were linked to nicotine-only products. The EVALI outbreak was linked to an additive, vitamin E acetate, in predominately THC-containing products. A public awareness campaign was launched to educate the public on the risk associated with vaping THC or using THC-containing e-cigarettes. Additionally, vitamin E acetate was removed from products and law enforcement worked to remove illicit products from the market. Although these actions have decreased the number of EVALI cases reported, the CDC has stressed that there is insufficient evidence to rule out other chemicals as the cause of EVALI and further research is needed.[91]

The e-cigarettes have proven to be very appealing children, adolescents, and young adults due to the variety of devices, high concentration of nicotine, flavor-based products, and wide promotion of these products on social media.[41] Based on the data from the 2020 National Youth Tobacco Survey (NYTS), e-cigarettes use among middle school and high school students steadily increased from 2011 to an epidemic level peak in 2019, where 10.5% (1.24 million) of middle students and 27.5% (4.11 million) of high school students reported e-cigarette use.[92] Data from 2020 demonstrated a decrease in use among both age groups, where 4.7% of middle students (555,000) and 19.6% of high school students (3.02 million) reported current use of electronic cigarettes.[92] To improve regulation of these products, the Deeming Rule expanded the FDA's regulatory authority to include manufacture, import, packaging, labeling, advertising, promotion, sale, and distribution of all tobacco products, including ENDS. This prohibited the sale of ENDS products to youth under 18 years of age, banning their sale in most vending machines (only allowed in adult-only facilities), or providing free samples. Manufacturers now have to receive marketing authorization from the FDA, and health warnings on ENDS and other tobacco products are now required.[93] Furthermore, vape shops that mix e-liquid must comply with the same legal requirements as tobacco manufacturers. In December 2019, the Federal Food, Drug, and Cosmetic Act was amended via the Tobacco 21 legislation to raise the federal minimum age of sale of tobacco products, including e-cigarettes, from the age of 18 to 21.[93] All 50 states and territories have now also restricted the sale of e-cigarettes to individuals 21 years of age and older.[94] The FDA additionally issued an enforcement policy focusing on the flavor-based e-cigarette products that appeal to adolescents.[93] Despite changes in regulations, these products are still very popular in the United States. The FDA continues to promote education campaigns, such as "The Real Cost" Youth E-Cigarette Prevention Campaign, which is aimed at youth who have experience with using ENDS or are considering trying these devices. Regardless, work continues in an effort to reduce the toxicity of the tobacco products, find ways to make products less appealing and less addictive, and improve the child-resistant packaging.[95]

The level of harm and/or risk associated with secondary passive exposure to ENDS aerosol is an ongoing debate, as passive exposure to the vapor emitted from the ENDS user could be hazardous based on a systematic review of 16 studies.[96] Data show e-cigarette vapor could expose bystanders to chemicals, including nicotine, glycine, formaldehyde, acetaldehyde, and propylene glycol, leading to an impact on indoor air quality. This risk, however, was noted to be lower than that associated with passive exposure from conventional cigarettes.[96] To limit second-hand exposure, many states have extended indoor smoking bans to include ENDS, although the laws for each state vary considerably.[94] The level of carcinogen and toxicant delivered to the user of the ENDS has been raised as a safety concern and due to the large variations in delivery devices and fluctuations in the amount of product a user will receive, it is difficult to study. While additional concerns have been raised regarding ENDS and toxic substances, the toxic levels of ENDS are estimated to be 1/4th to 1/95th the levels of the traditional cigarette.[97] Continued research is needed to evaluate the efficacy of e-cigarette use in regards to its role in helping with smoking cessation, youth exposure, and overall safety of this delivery system. Based on the current available evidence, USPSTF continues to recommend behavioral counseling and pharmacotherapy in nonpregnant adults and utilization of only behavioral counseling in pregnant individuals.[10]

Non-Nicotine Options

Bupropion (Zyban) Pharmacologically, bupropion inhibits neuronal reuptake of norepinephrine and dopamine and potentiates their effects. Although its precise mechanism in smoking cessation is not well understood, bupropion's dopaminergic effects help reduce nicotine craving as dopamine neurotransmission is key to the brain's reward system.[71]

Bupropion SR is marked under the brand name Zyban and has been shown to be an effective treatment option for smoking cessation, although the brand product Wellbutrin contains the same pharmacological product.[76] A recent meta-analysis involving 155 trials showed that bupropion significantly increased the incidence of long-term cessation when used as a sole agent in 45 separate trials.[98] Other trials using bupropion as an add-on agent with NRT did not show bupropion had an additional benefit in improving cessation rates.[98] For smoking cessation, the manufacturer recommends a dosage of 150 mg once daily for 3 days and then twice daily (dosing should be at least 8 hours apart) for 7 to 12 weeks or longer, with or without NRT. Patients are instructed to initiate bupropion 1 week prior to the scheduled quit date and are encouraged to use counseling and support services along with the medication.[41] For maintenance therapy, consider bupropion SR 150 mg twice daily for up to 6 months.[71]

Contraindications to bupropion use include current or past seizure disorders, a history of monoamine oxidase inhibitor use over the last 14 days, and a history of anorexia nervosa or bulimia. Along with multiple other precautions listed in the product labeling, current alcohol use and use of medications that lower seizure threshold (eg, antidepressants and antipsychotics) are possible concerns when using this medication.[76] In 2009, the FDA required bupropion manufacturers to add new boxed warnings and to develop a medication guide highlighting the risk of serious neuropsychiatric symptoms in patients using this product. Possible symptoms include depressed mood, agitation, anxiety, hostility, changes in behavior, suicidal thoughts and behavior, and attempted suicide. However, in 2016 following a FDA-requested clinical trial review, the FDA announced the removal of the Black Box Warning and the Risk Evaluation and Mitigation Strategies (REMS) requirement for bupropion although continued to caution that the risk of mental health adverse effects are still possible, particularly in patients with a past history of mental health disorders or currently being treated for anxiety, depression, or schizophrenia.[41,99] The risk of adverse effects is higher with bupropion compared to placebo, including a higher rate of psychiatric adverse effects compared to placebo, leading to a higher number of discontinuation of treatment compared to placebo.[98]

Varenicline (Chantix) 8 Pharmacologically, varenicline is a partial agonist that binds selectively to α_4-β_2-nicotinic acetylcholine receptors (nAChRs) with a greater affinity than nicotine. When bound to the receptor, the medication blocks nicotine binding and also evokes a response, but to a lesser degree than nicotine.[73] Clinically, varenicline acts at sites in the nicotine-affected brain in two ways: by providing nicotine effects to ease withdrawal symptoms and by blocking the effects of nicotine from cigarettes if smoking is resumed. Additionally, varenicline has been found to have full agonist, although less potent, activity at α_7 and α_4-β_2 nAChRs and a full agonist at serotonin 3 receptor (5-HT_3).[100] A systematic review of 39 trials showed a two- to threefold increased likelihood of long-term smoking cessation with varenicline compared with no NRT treatment (placebo).[101] Data from the trials included in this review also suggested that varenicline could have a role in relapse prevention and that it demonstrated better results compared to bupropion and NRT. These results were also seen in the largest randomized controlled trial for smoking cessation to date, the Evaluating Adverse Events in a Global Smoking Cessation Study (EAGLES) trial, which showed that varenicline is more efficacious than all other single NRTs, except for similar efficacy to the nicotine patch.[102]

The recommended dosage for varenicline is 0.5 mg daily for 3 days, increased to 0.5 mg twice daily for 3 days, and then increased to 1 mg twice daily for a standard 12-week treatment. It is suggested the quit date should be set for 1 week after initiating varenicline, but studies have shown allowing a flexible quit date is efficacious and safe. If abstinence has not been achieved after the 12-week treatment, then a second 12-week treatment may be prescribed.[103] Preloading varenicline for 4 weeks prior to the designated stop date has also demonstrated some higher response rates and can be considered as a treatment option.[104,105] Additionally, continuing varenicline as maintenance therapy for 6 months has been shown to decrease the risk of relapse.[41]

Common adverse effects associated with varenicline are nausea, vomiting, and insomnia. Over the years there have been concerns of neuropsychiatric adverse effects including suicidal thoughts, depression, and psychosis, leading to the black box warning. The previously mentioned EAGLES trial[102] also included a composite measure of neuropsychiatric symptoms as a primary safety endpoint and indicated there was no evidence of a significant increase in neuropsychiatric adverse effects which could be attributed to varenicline or bupropion. Specifically, in the individuals with psychiatric histories, moderate-to-severe neuropsychiatric symptoms were reported for varenicline (6.5%), bupropion (6.7%), nicotine patch (5.2%), and placebo (4.9%). In comparison, for patients without psychiatric histories, moderate-to-severe neuropsychiatric symptoms were reported as 1.3% to 2.5% of those enrolled in the trial. Overall, the risk differences reported for varenicline and bupropion versus placebo or the nicotine patch were nonsignificant. Following review of the trial results, the FDA announced the removal of the black box warning for varenicline and bupropion. In addition, a statement was included confirming bupropion, varenicline, and nicotine replacement patches are all more efficacious in smoking cessation compared to placebo regardless of mental illness history.[102] The most recent FDA Drug Safety communication indicates that although the risks of direct adverse effects from varenicline are lower than previously thought, the risk is still possible, especially in patients diagnosed with a mental illnesses, including schizophrenia, depression, or anxiety.[99] Cardiovascular safety concerns have also been raised regarding varenicline over the years and, to date, the results of various studies are still conflicting. In 2012, the FDA released a safety review update on the risk of cardiovascular adverse events indicating there is a higher risk of cardiovascular risks associated with varenicline.[106] However, results from the EAGLES extension trial, which was specifically designed to evaluate cardiovascular safety data, concluded there was no evidence of any cardiovascular adverse effects associated with these medications.[107]

Combination Therapy

Strong evidence exists for NRT combination therapy utilizing a short-acting form of NRT in combination with a nicotine patch based on a meta-analysis (RR 1.34; 95% CI: 1.18-1.48).[82] Additionally, a small systematic review and meta-analysis of three randomized controlled trials with 904 patients found that combining varenicline with NRT is more effective than varenicline alone. Individuals treated with both the nicotine patch and varenicline had similar adverse events to monotherapy except for skin reactions from the nicotine patch. Although the results for this study were positive for the combination, there were limited numbers of studies included in this analysis, so larger controlled clinical trials are needed.[108] Utilizing bupropion plus NRT has been shown to be more effective than bupropion monotherapy.[109] A meta-analysis evaluating the effectiveness of combining varenicline and bupropion in heavy smokers has demonstrated efficacy at 6 months but sustained cessation was not observed at 12 months. Increased reports of adverse effects including insomnia and anxiety were reported with the combination compared to varenicline monotherapy.[110]

Second-Line Medications

Second-line medications are therapeutic options for treating tobacco use, but have a more limited role than first-line medications because (a) the FDA has not approved them for smoking cessation and (b) there are more concerns about potential adverse medication effects than with first-line medications.[41] Although these second-line medications have shown some efficacy for smoking cessation, they should only be considered for use on a case-by-case basis after first-line treatments have been used or considered.

Clonidine

Results from a meta-analysis of six trials showed that clonidine increased smoking cessation rates by 9%.[111] The main significant adverse effect reported with its use is hypotension, particularly postural hypotension; thus, blood pressure should be monitored.[111] Additional adverse effects include dry mouth, drowsiness, dizziness, and sedation. Overall, clonidine can be considered a second-line, off label, agent for smoking cessation.

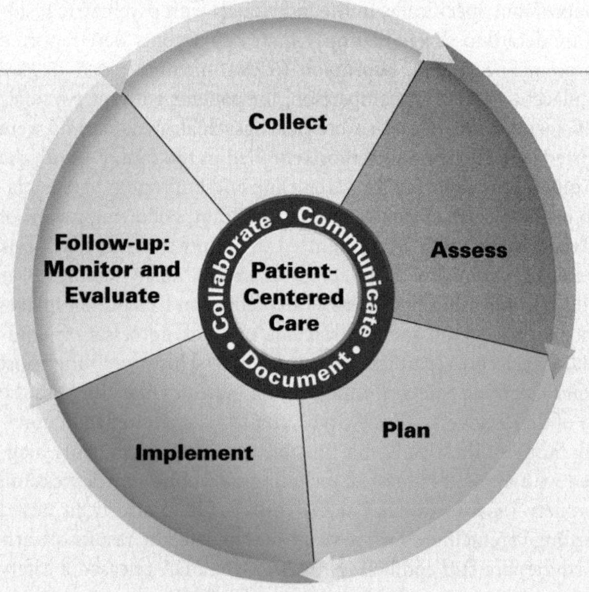

Patient Care Process for Smoking Cessation

The image shows the five fundamental steps included in The Pharmacist's Care Process endorsed by the Joint Commission for Pharmacy Practitioners (2014). The tagline of this process reads collaborate, communicate, and document. The five fundamental steps listed here are collect, assess, plan, implement, and follow-up: monitor and evaluate. All these steps are listed in a circular block diagram.

Collect

- Patient characteristics (eg, age, sex, pregnant)
- Patient medical history (personal and family)
- Social history (eg, tobacco/ethanol use) and dietary habits
- Smoking history (eg, current triggers, last cessation attempt, pharmacotherapy trials used in cessation, individual's level of interest for cessation at this time)
- Current medications including prescription, OTC use, herbal products, dietary supplements
- Objective data
    - Blood pressure (BP), heart rate (HR), respiratory rate (RR), height, weight, O_2-saturation
    - Labs including serum creatinine (SCr), liver function tests (LFTs)

Assess

- Hemodynamic stability (eg, systolic BP >90 mm Hg, HR <110 bpm, O_2-sat >90% (0.90), RR >20)
- Utilize motivational interviewing to assess readiness to quit
- Ability/willingness to pay for pharmacotherapy options and/or behavioral treatment for smoking cessation
- Ability/willingness to obtain laboratory monitoring tests (eg, LFTs [ie, bupropion], SCr [ie, varenicline])
- Emotional status (eg, presence of anxiety, depression)

Plan*

- Medication therapy regimen including specific nicotine replacement therapy (NRT), non-NRT, dose, route, frequency, and duration (see Tables 86-5 and 86-7)
- Monitoring parameters including efficacy (eg, decreases in craving, smoking) and safety (eg, adverse medication effects specific to selected agent); frequency and timing of follow-up
- Patient education (eg, purpose of treatment, lifestyle modification, medication-specific information, medication administration technique; see Table 86-7)
- Self-monitoring for adverse medication effects from pharmacotherapy treatment
- Referrals to other providers when appropriate (eg, behavioral health; highly recommended but not required for pharmacotherapy treatment)

Implement*

- Provide patient education regarding all elements of treatment plan
- Use motivational interviewing and coaching strategies to maximize adherence
- Set quit date if appropriate for this patient at this time (if appropriate)
- Schedule follow-up (eg, adherence assessment)

Follow-up: Monitor and Evaluate*

- Quit date set
- Presence of adverse effects (eg, medication specific)
- Individual adherence to treatment plan using multiple sources of information
- Reevaluate duration of therapy initially with frequent follow-up and then lengthen follow-up to every 1 to 2 months

**Collaborate with patient, caregivers, and other healthcare professionals.*

Nortriptyline

Nortriptyline is also considered to be efficacious as a second-line agent for smoking cessation. When used for this indication, therapy is initiated 10 to 28 days before the quit date to allow for steady state to be reached at the target dose. Trials have initiated treatment at a dose of 25 mg/day, increasing gradually to a target dose of 75 to 100 mg/day.[111] Treatment duration used in smoking cessation trials have been approximately 12 weeks. A meta-analysis of 6 trials with 975 patients showed that nortriptyline as a sole agent is efficacious for smoking cessation when compared to placebo but is less efficacious when compared to varenicline.[98,112] Adding nortriptyline as an adjuvant to NRT did not prove to be an additional benefit in four trials which included over 1,600 patients.[112] Most commonly reported adverse effects included sedation, dry mouth, blurred vision, urinary retention, light-headedness, and tremor.[113]

EVALUATION OF THERAPEUTIC OUTCOMES

Assisting a patient for tobacco cessation is a process that could take an extended period of time with extensive education and continual monitoring being vital to this process. The most effective treatment strategy for smoking cessation is a combination of behavioral and pharmacological treatment and frequent monitoring of both early on in the process is recommended. There are seven pharmacological treatment options and agent selection will be determined by a variety of factors. Patient counseling on selected pharmacotherapy options and common adverse effects is vital to ensure proper use and maximum efficacy. Frequent reassessment should occur to monitor overall treatment efficacy and to evaluate breakthrough cravings, withdrawal symptoms, and relapses. Dose adjustments should be made accordingly and individuals should be monitored closely and asked to immediately report any adverse effects to ensure proper adherence and prevent relapse.

INTRODUCTION—CAFFEINE

9 Caffeine is the most widely used psychoactive substance in the world, with approximately 90% of adults in the United States regularly consuming behaviorally active doses,[114] which result in psychoactive or stimulating responses including an increased sense of well-being, concentration, energy, alertness, and sociability. Caffeine is generally recognized as safe by the FDA for use in cola-type beverages as long as levels do not exceed 0.02% (200 parts per million), which is 30 to 40 mg of caffeine in a 12-oz (355 mL) serving.[115] A systematic review of data regarding potential adverse effects associated with caffeine found up to 400 mg caffeine per day in healthy adults was not associated with cardiovascular, behavioral, reproductive, or developmental adverse effects.[116] The FDA has cited that 400 mg per day, which is approximately four to five cups of coffee, is generally considered safe for adults.[114] However, in the United States, children consume an average 37.3 mg of caffeine per day.[117] Doses of 100 to 400 mg of caffeine have been reported to result in stimulant-related effects, such as jitteriness in children and adolescents. The American Academy of Pediatrics discourages children and adolescents consuming stimulants or caffeine due to the possible negative impact on sleep and blood pressure.[118] There is limited knowledge of caffeine effects on cognitive development and further study is necessary to determine the proper levels of safe consumption for this patient population.[115,117] Although, in general, caffeine consumption in reasonable amounts has been considered fairly safe, there are situations in which problems arise. Caffeinism has been associated with a daily caffeine intake of 1,000 to 1,500 mg. This term was coined to describe the clinical syndrome produced by acute or chronic unhealthy use of caffeine, which is usually characterized by central nervous system and peripheral manifestations, most notably, anxiety, psychomotor alterations, sleep disturbances, mood changes, and psychophysiological complaints.[119]

Pharmacologically, the risk of developing meaningful clinical manifestations from caffeine becomes high when intake exceeds 500 mg/day.[120] It could be assumed this level of caffeine might not be reached when traditionally drinking coffee. This helps explain why, up until recently, deaths from acute ingestions of caffeine were virtually nonexistent. However, pure caffeine powder and liquid formulations are available via the Internet and just small doses could be toxic. One teaspoonful of highly concentrated powder is estimated to be equivalent to 28 cups of coffee (approximately 3,200 mg caffeine) and just one-half cup of highly concentrated liquid is equivalent to approximately 20 cups of coffee (approximately 2,000 mg caffeine).[121] A 200 mg caffeine dose of pure caffeine powder is considered 1/16 teaspoon, where the caffeine liquid is 2.5 teaspoonfulls.[122] Due to the concerns of safety and reported deaths associated with concentrated caffeine products, the FDA has provided guidance documents to companies manufacturing, marketing, and distributing these products. Subsequent warning letters have been sent to all identified and who continue to sell illegal caffeine products.[122]

Caffeine in general has been proposed as a model of substance use despite the fact that its sale is largely unrestricted and that heavy consumption of caffeine-containing beverages is not considered to be problematic. The following information represents a broad overview of physical dependence, withdrawal, and tolerance. Interested readers are encouraged to consult Meredith et al. and Sweeny et al. for further information.[123,124]

EPIDEMIOLOGY

Recently, data from the National Health and Nutrition Examination Survey (NHANES) 2007-2012 was evaluated regarding caffeine consumption through caffeinated beverages, foods, and energy drinks in adults 19 years of age and older. Approximately 90% of individuals in the United States consume caffeine daily, predominantly through caffeinated beverages (98%). The most common being coffee (64%), with tea and soft drinks being less popular (16% and 18%, respectively). Caffeine intake averaged 169 mg/day and mostly was consumed in the morning hours. Older adults, ages 75 to 79, consumed a greater amount of caffeine (153 mg/day) compared to younger adults ages 20 to 24 who averaged 107 mg/day. Caffeine intake varied with ethnicity, where non-Hispanic black individuals averaged the lowest caffeine consumption (80 mg/day) and non-Hispanic white individuals had the highest consumption averaging 194 mg/day.[114] Intake among children, adolescents, and young adults is prevalent from foods and beverages based on the 2011-2012 NHANES data. The average caffeine intake increased with age where 4- to 8-year-olds averaged 15 mg/day, 9- to 13-year-olds averaged 26 mg/day, and 14- to 19-year-olds averaged 61 mg/day.[125]

10 Energy drinks containing caffeine also include a variety of other products, such as taurine, vitamins, minerals, electrolytes, and sugar. These products are sold under brand names such as Red Bull, Monster Energy, Rockstar, and Bang Energy and are promoted to increase energy, enhance alertness, and physical performance. They continue to gain popularity among adolescents and emerging adults.

CLINICAL PRESENTATION Caffeine Intoxication

General

- The individual may not be in acute distress.

Symptoms

- The individual may complain of nausea, vomiting, diarrhea, and psychomotor agitation, and can appear restless, nervous, and excited.

Signs

- The individual can present with facial flushing, diuresis, and muscle twitching.
- Tachycardia or cardiac arrhythmias can also occur.

Laboratory Tests

- Caffeine serum concentrations are rarely used clinically.

CLINICAL PRESENTATION Caffeine Withdrawal

General

- The individual may not be in acute distress.

Symptoms

- Complaints of headache, nausea, vomiting, drowsiness, poor concentration, and depressed mood may be seen which are adversely affecting overall social/occupational functioning and/or leading to distress.

Laboratory Tests

- Caffeine serum concentrations are rarely used clinically.

Data from the 2003-2016 NHANES demonstrated an increase in consumption of energy drinks among a wide range of individuals, including adolescents (12-19 years old), young adults (20-39 years old), and middle-aged adults (40-59 years old). However, further analysis of the data did indicate that there could be a small decline in use patterns within the younger age groups, including adolescents and young adults, and an upward trend for middle-aged adults.[126] It is reported, aside from multivitamins, that these products are the most popular dietary supplement for young adults.[127] There are two types of products on the market based on volume. One product is similar to a soft drink, for example, Red Bull (8.4 oz [250 mL]) which contains 80 mg of caffeine, although other products can contain higher amounts of caffeine depending on the size of the container. The second product is a smaller volume product referred to as an "energy shot," which provides a range of 200 to 300 mg of caffeine in a 2- to 3-ounce product. Additionally, these products also commonly contain other products such as B vitamins, creatine, and CoQ10.[128]

Over the years, there have been many questions regarding the safety of these products and emergency room visits attributed to these energy drinks doubled from 2007 to 2011, with 58% of visits involving energy drinks alone and 42% including energy drinks with other substances including alcohol, marijuana, and/or stimulants.[129] Each year, the most common age group seen in the emergency room due to energy drink consumption included patients ages 18-25. However, energy drink–related emergency visits in patients older than 40 years of age have increased over 279%.[129] A recent study evaluated adverse event reports associated with energy drinks alone and in combination with other substances from 2008 to 2015. During this time period, a total of 13,179 reports were received on single product energy drinks and 1,084 reports on energy drinks combined with other substances.[130] A variety of health complications have been associated with their use in the adolescent population, including insomnia, arrhythmias, high blood pressure, agitation, anxiety, and migraines.[131] Energy drink consumption has also been associated with a higher rate of unhealthy alcohol and substance use.[132]

PATHOPHYSIOLOGY

Caffeine is rapidly and completely absorbed from the GI tract, reaching a peak blood level within 30 to 60 minutes after oral ingestion. It easily crosses the blood–brain barrier, and levels achieved in the brain are proportional to the dose administered.[133] Caffeine is metabolized by cytochrome P450 1A2 (CYP1A2) and has a half-life of approximately 4 to 5 hours in healthy nonsmoking adults. Fast metabolizers of CYP1A2 include heavy caffeine users, children less than 12 years old, and individuals who smoke cigarettes. Individuals in later stages of pregnancy are slower metabolizers of caffeine, as are those with liver dysfunction.[119,133] Overdoses of caffeine are now more common due to the wide availability of energy drinks. Caffeine increases the heart rate and force of cardiac contractions, and also has a strong diuretic effect. Due to the stimulating properties of caffeine, nervousness, agitation, and insomnia may occur with more serious reactions including cardiac arrhythmias, hypotension, and seizures.[116,119] The key factor promoting caffeine use and dosage increases can be the substance's reinforcing effect on pleasure and reward centers of the brain. Caffeine's pharmacologic actions appear comparable (although less potent) to those of other stimulants, such as amphetamines and cocaine.[134]

CLINICAL PRESENTATION

The *DSM-5* has four caffeine-related diagnoses, including caffeine intoxication, caffeine withdrawal, other caffeine-induced disorders, which include both caffeine-induced sleep and anxiety disorders, and unspecified caffeine-related disorder. Each of these diagnoses could include symptoms which might be attributed to caffeine use, but do not fit in any other category. The *DSM-5* does not currently list a diagnosis of caffeine use disorder, but it has been identified as an area that needs further research to determine if it should become an official diagnosis.[5]

The diagnostic criteria for caffeine intoxication include recent consumption of caffeine normally exceeding 250 mg and five or more symptoms during, or shortly after, consumption of caffeine. The symptoms of caffeine intoxication will usually decrease over 24 hours as the caffeine is eliminated from the body; however, consumption of very high doses of caffeine could be dangerous and require immediate medical attention.[5]

Caffeine withdrawal is a DSM-5 diagnosis, which occurs after the abrupt cessation of chronic caffeine use and can occur even with low doses of caffeine. The diagnosis of caffeine withdrawal requires three of the five listed symptoms, including headache (most common), marked fatigue or drowsiness, altered mood (depressed, irritable, and dysphoric), difficulty concentrating, or flu-like symptoms, including nausea, vomiting, and muscle pain/stiffness. The extent and severity of withdrawal can vary individually but normally will be more severe with higher chronic doses of caffeine (Table 86-7).[5]

TABLE 86-7 *DSM-5* Diagnostic Criteria for Caffeine Withdrawal

Criteria
Prolonged daily use of caffeine
Abrupt cessation or decrease use in caffeine leading to at least three of the following symptoms after 24 hours of cessation • Concentration problems • Mood changes: dysphoric mood, depressed mood, irritability • Dramatic fatigue or drowsiness • Headache • Flu-like symptoms • Nausea • Vomiting • Muscle pain/stiffness
Symptoms negatively impact areas of functioning such as social or occupational aspects of life.
The symptoms experienced cannot be explained by other concurrent medical conditions.

Data from Reference 5.

Effect on Sleep

Caffeine is commonly used to improve alertness and improve performance during times of sleep deprivation at doses of 75 to 150 mg. Sleep disruption can occur with caffeine consumptions ranging from 200 to 600 mg.[119] Caffeine's disruptive effects following a fixed dose of 400 mg provided 0, 3, and 6 hours prior to the usual bedtime has been associated with sleep disruption at all administration time periods.[135] However, any sleep disruption is likely to resolve 8 hours after caffeine consumption.[119]

Caffeine During Pregnancy

Over the years, there has been much discussion regarding the safety of caffeine intake during pregnancy and possible risks to the developing fetus. A systematic review of 380 studies published in 2017 evaluated data from 2001 through June 2015 and determined daily consumption of up to 300 mg of caffeine per day in a healthy pregnant individuals was not associated with any adverse health outcomes or developmental effects.[116] A narrative review which evaluated 42 original observational studies and 14 meta-analysis evaluating maternal consumption of caffeine during pregnancy reported increased negative outcomes during pregnancy including miscarriage, stillbirth, low birthweight/small gestational age. Additionally, increased risk of childhood leukemia as well as childhood overweight/obesity were identified in these studies.[136] Safe levels of caffeine consumption were recommended in this review; however, the author recommended based on this evidence, pregnant individuals should consider avoiding all caffeine consumption.[136] Currently, American College of Gynecology suggests limiting caffeine consumption to less than 200 mg per day and reports this level of caffeine intake has not been identified as a major contributing factor to miscarriage and preterm birth. Further information on the effect of caffeine intake on intrauterine growth was undetermined.[137] The March of Dimes also advises pregnant individuals to limit their caffeine intake to less than 200 mg/day.[138] Data will continue to be collected and evaluated to determine safe levels of caffeine consumption in pregnancy.

TREATMENT

Desired Outcomes

Many people drink coffee, tea, and other caffeinated beverages without problems. When adverse health effects occur (eg, insomnia, headaches, anxiety, and palpitations), it may be necessary to cut down on the amount of caffeine ingested or to eliminate it altogether to achieve elimination of these symptoms.

Nonpharmacologic Therapy

The primary treatment of caffeinism is reducing or discontinuing the use of the substance. For some it may be necessary to wean off the substance gradually because a rapid reduction in consumption can lead to adverse reactions, such as irritability, headaches, fatigue, flu-like symptoms, difficulty concentrating, and reduction in alertness.[123,124] The gradual reduction in caffeine intake over multiple days can reduce the risk of common withdrawal reactions.[139] For cases of extreme caffeine toxicity and withdrawal, necessary supportive measures should be instituted to prevent short- and or long-term sequelae.[118]

EVALUATION OF THERAPEUTIC OUTCOMES

Identifying the treatment goals associated with the individual's current caffeine consumption and addressing these goals will be the primary focus in evaluating therapeutic outcomes. When an individual is working to reduce or discontinue caffeine, frequent reassessment should occur to monitor the individual for symptoms of caffeine withdrawal and educate on possible effects of withdrawal. If effects of withdrawal are experienced, appropriate adjustments should be made to improve reaching treatment goals.

CONCLUSION

Alcohol, nicotine, and caffeine are considered by most to be socially acceptable substances, yet they impose an enormous social and economic cost on our society. It is vital that all healthcare professionals continue to educate individuals on the healthcare risks of each of these substances to decrease the negative impact that can occur with their chronic use.

ABBREVIATIONS

ADH	alcohol dehydrogenase
ALDH	aldehyde dehydrogenase
AUD	alcohol use disorder
AUDIT	Alcohol Use Disorders Identification Test
AUDIT-C	Alcohol Use Disorders Identification Test—Consumption questions
BAC	blood alcohol concentration
BP	blood pressure
CHRNA5	cholinergic receptor alpha5 subunit
CIWA-Ar	Clinical Institute Withdrawal Assessment for Alcohol, revised
CNS	central nervous system
COPD	chronic obstructive pulmonary disease
CT	computed tomography
CUD	caffeine use disorder
CYP	cytochrome P450
DSM-5	*Diagnostic and Statistical Manual of Mental Disorders, Fifth Edition*
DT	delirium tremens
EAGLES	Evaluating Adverse Events in a Global Smoking Cessation Study
ENDS	electronic nicotine delivery systems
EVALI	e-cigarette or vaping use-associated lung injury
FDA	Food and Drug Administration
GABA	γ-aminobutyric acid
GI	gastrointestinal
5-HT_3	serotonin-3 receptor
HIV	human immunodeficiency virus
HR	heart rate
IM	intramuscular
IV	intravenous
LFTs	liver function tests
LGBTQ+	lesbian, gay, bisexual, transgender, queer (or sometimes questioning), and others
MI	motivational interviewing
nAChRs	α4-β2-nicotinic acetylcholine receptors
NHANES	National Health and Nutrition Examination Survey
NIH	National Institute of Health
NIDA	National Institute on Drug Abuse
NMR	nicotine metabolic ratio
NQDW	National Quitline Data Warehouse
NRT	nicotine replacement therapy
NSDUH	National Survey on Drug Use and Health
NYTS	National Youth Tobacco Survey
O_2	oxygen
OPRM1	μ-opioid receptor gene

OTC	over the counter
PAN	psychotropic analgesic nitrous oxide
PATH	Population Assessment of Tobacco and Health
PAWSS	Prediction of Alcohol Withdrawal Severity Scale
REMS	risk evaluation and mitigation strategies
RR	respiratory rate
SCr	serum creatinine
SIDS	sudden infant death syndrome
SR	sustained release
THC	tetrahydrocannabinol
TRHD	tobacco-related health disparities
TTFC	time to first cigarette
USAUDIT	United States Alcohol Use Disorders Identification Test
USPSTF	United States Preventive Services Task Force
WHO	World Health Organization

REFERENCES

1. World Health Organization Department of Mental Health and Substance Abuse. *Global Status Report on Alcohol and Health 2018.* Geneva: World Health Organization; 2018. License: CC BY-NC-SA 3.0IGO. http://www.who.int/substance_abuse/publications/global_alcohol_report/en/.
2. NIAAA. Alcohol facts and statistics. 2021. https://www.niaaa.nih.gov/publications/brochures-and-fact-sheets/alcohol-facts-and-statistics. Accessed July 9, 2021.
3. Substance Abuse and Mental Health Services Administration. *Key substance use and mental health indicators in the United States: Results from the 2017 National Survey on Drug Use and Health (HHS Publication No. SMA 18-5068, NSDUH Series H-53).* Rockville, MD: Center for Behavioral Health Statistics and Quality, Substance Abuse and Mental Health Services Administration; 2018. https://www.samhsa.gov/data. Accessed September 28, 2018.
4. NIDA. Drug Abuse and Addiction: One of America's Most Challenging Public Health Problems. National Institute on Drug Abuse website. https://archives.drugabuse.gov/publications/drug-abuse-addiction-one-americas-most-challenging-public-health-problems. June 1, 2005. Accessed July 22, 2021.
5. American Psychiatric Association. *Diagnostic and Statistical Manual of Mental Disorders, 5th ed, DSM-5.* Arlington, VA: American Psychiatric Association; 2013.
6. Enoch M. Genetic influences on the development of alcoholism. *Curr Psychiatry Resp.* 2013;15(11):412. doi:10.1007/s11920-013-0412-1.
7. Edenberg HJ, Foroud T. Genetics and alcoholism. *Nat Rev Gastroenterol Hepatol.* 2013;10(8):487–494. 10.1038/nrgastro.2013.86 23712313.
8. Verhulst B, Neale M, Kendler K. The heritability of alcohol use disorders: A meta-analysis of twin and adoption studies. *Psychologic Med.* 2015;54:1061–1072.
9. Agrawal A, Verweij KJ, Gillespie NA, et al. The genetics of addiction—a translational perspective. *Transl Psychiatry.* 2012;2:e140. doi:10.1038/tp.2012.54.
10. Krist AH, Davidson KW, Mangione CM, et al. Interventions for tobacco smoking cessation in adults, including pregnant persons: US Preventive Services Task Force Recommendation Statement. *JAMA.* 2021;325(3):265–279. 10.1001/jama.2020.25019 33464343.
11. Chan L, Anderson G. Pharmacokinetic and pharmacodynamics drug interactions with ethanol (alcohol). *Clin Pharmacokinet.* 2014;53:1115–1136.
12. Perry PJ, Doroudgar S, Van Dyke P. Ethanol forensic toxicology. *J Am Acad Psychiatry Law.* 2017;45:429–438.
13. Cedarbaum AI. Alcohol metabolism. *Clin Liver Dis.* 2012;16:667–685.
14. Nassir F, Ibdah J. Role of mitochondria in alcoholic liver disease. *World J Gastroenterol.* 2014;20(9):2136–2142.
15. Jones AW. Pharmacokinetics of ethanol—Issues of forensic importance. *Forensic Sci Rev.* 2011;23:91–136.
16. Understanding the dangers of alcohol overdose. National Institute on Alcohol Abuse and Alcoholism. Updated May 2021. https://www.niaaa.nih.gov/publications/brochures-and-fact-sheets/understanding-dangers-of-alcohol-overdose. Accessed July 30, 2021.
17. Dhalla S, Kopec JA. The CAGE questionnaire for alcohol misuse: A review of reliability and validity studies. *Clin Invest Med.* 2007;30:33–41.
18. Babor TF, Higgins-Biddle JC, Saunders JB, Monteiro MG. *AUDIT: The Alcohol Use Disorders Identification Test: Guidelines for Use in Primary Care.* 2nd ed. Geneva: World Health Organization; 2001.
19. Wolf C, Curry A, Nacht J, et al. Management of alcohol withdrawal in the emergency department: Current perspectives. *Open Access Emerg Med.* 2020;12:53–65. 10.2147/OAEM.S235288 32256131.
20. Holt SR, Tobin DG. Pharmacotherapy of alcohol use disorder. *Med Clin N Am.* 2018;102:653–666.
21. Sulivan JT, Sykora K, Schneiderman J, et al. Assessment of alcohol withdrawal: The revised clinical institute withdrawal assessment for alcohol scale (CIWA-Ar). *Br J Addict.* 1989;84:1353–1357.
22. Carlson RW, Kumar NN, Wong-McKinstry E, et al. Alcohol withdrawal syndrome. *Crit Care Clin.* 2012;28:549–585.
23. Lindsay DL, Freedman K, Jarvis M, et al. Executive Summary of the American Society of Addiction Medicine (ASAM) Clinical Practice Guideline on Alcohol Withdrawal Management. *J Addict Med.* 2020;14(5):376–392. 10.1097/ADM.0000000000000732 32909985.
24. Amato L, Minozzi S, Davoli M. Efficacy and safety of pharmacological interventions for the treatment of the alcohol withdrawal syndrome. *Cochrane Database Syst Rev.* 2011;(6):CD008537. doi:10.1002/14651858.CD008537.pub2.
25. Mirijello A, D'Angelo C, Ferruli A, et al. Identification and management of alcohol withdrawal syndrome. *Drugs.* 2015;75:353–365.
26. Schmidt KJ, Doshi MR, Holzhausen JM, et al. Treatment of severe alcohol withdrawal. *Ann Pharmacother.* 2016;50:389–401.
27. Muncie HL, Yasinian Y, Oge' L. Outpatient management of alcohol withdrawal syndrome. *Am Fam Physician.* 2013;88(9):589–595.
28. Marks V, Teale JD. Drug-induced hypoglycemia. *Endocrinol Metab Clin North Am.* 1999;28:555–577.
29. Fairbanks J, Umbreit A, Kolla BP, et al. Evidence-based pharmacotherapies for alcohol use disorder: Clinical pearls. *Mayo Clin Proc.* 2020;95(9):1964–1977. 10.1016/j.mayocp.2020.01.030 32446635.
30. Kranzler HR, Soyka M. Diagnosis and pharmacotherapy of alcohol use disorder: A review. *JAMA.* 2018:320:815–824.
31. Pani PP, Trogu E, Pacini M, Maremmani I. Anticonvulsants for alcohol dependence. *Cochrane Database Syst Rev.* 2014;(2):CD008544. doi:10.1002/14651858.CD008544.pub2.
32. Blodgett JC, Del Re AC, Maisel NC, et al. A meta-analysis of topiramate's effects for individuals with alcohol use disorders. *Alcohol Clin Exp Res.* 2014;38:1481–1488.
33. Reus VI, Fochtmann LJ, Bukstein O, et al. The American Psychiatric Association practice guideline for the pharmacological treatment of patients with alcohol use disorder. *Am J Psychiatry.* 2018;175:86–90.
34. Skinner MD, Lahmek P, Pham H, et al. Disulfiram efficacy in the treatment of alcohol dependence: A meta-analysis. *PLoS One.* 2014;9(2):e87366.
35. Oslin D, Leong S, Lynch K, et al. Naltrexone vs. Placebo for the treatment of alcohol dependence. *JAMA Psychiatry.* 2015;72(5):430–437.
36. Sudakin D. Naltrexone: Not just for opioids anymore. *J Med Toxicol.* 2016;12:71–75.
37. Rosner S, Hackl-Herwerth A, Leucht S, et al. Opioid antagonists for alcohol dependence. *Cochrane Reviews.* 2010;(12):CD001867. doi:10.1002/14651858.
38. Murphy CE 4th, Wang RC, Montoy JC, Whittaker E, Raven M, et al. Effect of extended-release naltrexone on alcohol consumption: A systematic review and meta-analysis. *Addiction.* 202110.1111/add.15572 34033183.
39. Rösner S, Hackl-Herrwerth A, Leucht S, et al. Acamprosate for alcohol dependence. *Cochrane Database Syst Rev.* 2010;(9):CD004332.
40. US Department of Health and Human Services. *The Health Consequences of Smoking—50 Years of Progress: A Report of the Surgeon General.* Atlanta: US Department of Health and Human Services, Centers for Disease Control and Prevention, National Center for Chronic Disease Prevention and Health Promotion, Office on Smoking and Health; 2014. https://www.surgeongeneral.gov/library/reports/50-years-of-progress/full-report.pdf. Accessed October 21, 2018.
41. U.S. Department of Health and Human Services. Smoking cessation: A report of the Surgeon General. U.S. Department of Health and Human Services. Centers for Disease Control and Prevention, National Center for Chronic Disease Prevention and Health Promotion, Office on Smoking and Health. https://www.cdc.gov/tobacco/data_statistics/sgr/2020-smoking-cessation/index.html#full-report. Updated January 23, 2020. Accessed May 10, 2021.
42. Cornelius ME, Wang TW, Jamal A, et al. Tobacco product use among adults—United States, 2019. *MMWR Morb Mortal Wkly Rep.* 2020;69(46):1736–1742. 10.15585/mmwr.mm6946a4 33211681.

43. CDC: Smoking & tobacco statistics: https://www.cdc.gov/tobacco/data_statistics/fact_sheets/fast_facts/index.htm. Accessed May 10, 2021.
44. National Center for Health Statistics. Survey description, National Health Interview Survey, 2019. Hyattsville, MD: US Department of Health and Human Services, CDC, National Center for Health Statistics; 2020. ftp://ftp.cdc.gov/pub/Health_Statistics/NCHS/Dataset_Documentation/NHIS/2019/srvydesc-508.pdfpdf icon. Accessed May 10, 2021.
45. Young-Wolff KC, Klebaner D, Campbell CI, et al. Association of the Affordable Care Act With Smoking and Tobacco Treatment Utilization Among Adults Newly Enrolled in Health Care. *Med Care.* 2017;55(5):535–541. 10.1097/MLR.0000000000000712 28288073.
46. Murphy-Hoefer R, Davis KC, Beistle D, King BA, Duke J, Rodes R, et al. Impact of the tips from former smokers campaign on population-level smoking cessation, 2012–2015. *Prev Chronic Dis.* 2018;15:180051. http://dx.doi.org/10.5888/pcd15.180051.
47. Shrestha SS, Davis K, Mann N, et al. Cost Effectiveness of the Tips From Former Smokers® Campaign—U.S., 2012–2018. *Am J Prev Med.* 2021;60(3):406–410. 10.1016/j.amepre.2020.10.009 33455819.
48. CDC Tips From Former Smokers. FREE QuitGuide Mobile App. Available at: https://www.cdc.gov/tobacco/campaign/tips/quit-smoking/mobile-quit-guide/index.html?s_cid=OSH_tips_D9405. Accessed November 2, 2018.
49. Hyland A, Kasza KA, Borek N, et al. Overview of tobacco use transitions for population health. *Tob Control.* 2020;29(Suppl 3):s134–s138. 10.1136/tobaccocontrol-2019-055367 32321846.
50. Stanton CA, Sharma E, Seaman EL, et al. Initiation of any tobacco and five tobacco products across 3 years among youth, young adults and adults in the USA: Findings from the PATH Study Waves 1-3 (2013–2016). *Tob Control.* 2020;29(Suppl 3):s178–s190. 10.1136/tobaccocontrol-2019-055573 32321852.
51. Kasza K, Ambrose B, Conway K, et al. Tobacco-product use by adults and youths in the United States in 2013 and 2014. *NEJM.* 2017;376(4):342–353.
52. U.S. National Cancer Institute. A Socioecological Approach to Addressing Tobacco Related Health Disparities. National Cancer Institute Tobacco Control Monograph 22. NIH Publication No. 17-CA-8035A. Bethesda, MD: U.S. Department of Health and Human Services, National Institutes of Health, National Cancer Institute; 2017.
53. Xu X, Bishop EE, Kennedy SM, Simpson SA, Pechacek TF. Annual healthcare spending attributable to cigarette smoking: An update. *Am J Prev Med.* 2015;48(3):326–333. Epub 2014/12/17. pmid:25498551; PubMed Central PMCID: PMCPmc4603661.
54. DiGiulio A, Jump Z, Yu A, et al. State Medicaid coverage for tobacco cessation treatments and barriers to accessing treatments—United States, 2015–2017. *Morbidity and Mortality Weekly Report.* 2018;67(13):390–395.
55. Saccone N, Baurley J, Bergen A, et al. The value of biosamples in smoking cessation trials: A review of genetic, metabolomic, and epigenetic findings. nicotine & tobacco. *Nicotine Tob Res.* 2018;20(4):403–413. 30521502.
56. Raghuveer G, White DA, Hayman LL, Woo JG, Villafane J, Celermajer D, Ward KD, de Ferranti SD, Zachariah J. Cardiovascular consequences of childhood secondhand tobacco smoke exposure: Prevailing evidence, burden, and racial and socioeconomic disparities: A scientific statement from the American Heart Association. *Circulation.* 2016;134(16):e336–e359. 10.1161/CIR.0000000000000443 27619923.
57. Balfour DJ. Neuroplasticity within the mesoaccumbens dopamine system and its role in tobacco dependence. *Curr Drug Targets CNS Neurol Disord.* 2002;1(4):413–421. 10.2174/1568007023339076 12769613.
58. Benowitz N. Nicotine addiction. *NEJM.* 2010;362:2295–2303.
59. Benowitz NL. Clinical pharmacology of nicotine implications for understanding, preventing, and treating tobacco addiction. *Clin Pharmacol Ther.* 2008;83:531–541.
60. Benowitz N. Pharmacology of nicotine: Addiction, smoking-induced disease, and therapeutics. *Annu Rev Pharmacol Toxicol.* 2009;49:57–71.
61. Chen LS, Horton A, Bierut L. Pathways to precision medicine in smoking cessation treatments. *Neuroscience Letters.* 2018;669:83–92.
62. Icick R, Forget B, Cloëz-Tayarani I, et al. Genetic susceptibility to nicotine addiction: Advances and shortcomings in our understanding of the CHRNA5/A3/B4 gene cluster contribution. *Neuropharmacology.* 2020;177:108234–108234. 10.1016/j.neuropharm.2020.108234 32738310.
63. U.S. Department of Health and Human Services Healthy People 2030. https://health.gov/healthypeople/objectives-and-data/browse-objectives/tobacco-use/reduce-current-tobacco-use-adults-tu-01/data. Accessed May 20, 2021.
64. NIDA CTN Common Data Elements: Instrument: Fagerstrom Test for Nicotine Dependence (FTND). https://cde.drugabuse.gov/instrument/d7c0b0f5-b865-e4de-e040-bb89ad43202b. Accessed May 20, 2021.
65. Patients Not Ready To Make A Quit Attempt Now (The "5 R's"). Content last reviewed December 2012. Agency for Healthcare Research and Quality, Rockville, MD. https://www.ahrq.gov/prevention/guidelines/tobacco/5rs.html. Accessed May 10, 2021.
66. Hartmann-Boyce J, Hong B, Livingstone-Banks J, et al. Additional behavioural support as an adjunct to pharmacotherapy for smoking cessation. *Cochrane Database Syst Rev.* 2019;6:CD009670–CD009670. 10.1002/14651858.CD009670.pub4 31166007.
67. Lindson-Hawley N, Thompson TP, Begh R. Motivational interviewing for smoking cessation. *Cochrane Database Syst Rev.* 2015;(3):CD006936.
68. Centers for Disease Control and Prevention. Frequency Asked Questions about 1-800-QUIT-NOW and National Network of Tobacco Cessation Quitlines. (n.d.). Available at: https://www.cdc.gov/tobacco/quit_smoking/cessation/pdfs/1800quitnow_faq.pdf. Accessed October 2, 2018.
69. Centers for Disease Control and Prevention. Smoking and Tobacco Use. https://www.cdc.gov/tobacco/quit_smoking/cessation/faq-about-1-800-quit-now/. Accessed May 20, 2021.
70. Whittaker R, McRobbie H, Bullen C, et al. Mobile phone text messaging and app-based interventions for smoking cessation. *Cochrane Database Syst Rev.* 2019;10:CD006611–CD006611. 10.1002/14651858.CD006611.pub5 31638271.
71. Prochaska JJ, Benowitz NL. Current advances in research in treatment and recovery: Nicotine addiction. *Sci Adv.* 2019;5(10):eaay9763–eaay9763. 10.1126/sciadv.aay9763 31663029.
72. Nicotrol Inhaler package insert. Pfizer. Last revised December 2008. Available at: https://www.pfizer.com/files/products/uspi_nicotrol_inhaler.pdf. Accessed October 11, 2018.
73. Varenicline Package insert. Pfizer. Last revised June 2018. Available at: http://labeling.pfizer.com/showlabeling.aspx?id=557. Accessed October 11, 2018.
74. Nicotrol Nasal Spray package insert. *Pfizer.* Last revised January 2010. Available at: https://www.pfizer.com/files/products/uspi_nicotrol.pdf. Accessed October 11, 2018.
75. Nicorette Lozenge labeling information. Available at: https://www.accessdata.fda.gov/drugsatfda_docs/label/2013/022360Orig1s007lbl.pdf. Accessed October 11, 2018.
76. Bupropion package insert. Last revised May 2017. GlaxoSmithKline. Available at: https://www.gsksource.com/pharma/content/dam/GlaxoSmithKline/US/en/Prescribing_Information/Zyban/pdf/ZYBAN-PI-MG.PDF. Accessed October 11, 2018.
77. Nicoderm CQ Nicotine patch extended release package insert. Last revised May 2016. GlaxoSmithKline. Available at: https://dailymed.nlm.nih.gov/dailymed/drugInfo.cfm?setid=93b2d1b9-83c1-40b5-b6af-90c38c8d6cef. Accessed October 11, 2018.
78. Nicorette Gum labeling information. Available at: https://www.accessdata.fda.gov/drugsatfda_docs/label/2013/022360Orig1s007lbl.pdf. Accessed October 11, 2018.
79. Barua RS, Rigotti NA, Benowitz NL, et al. 2018 ACC Expert Consensus Decision Pathway on Tobacco Cessation Treatment: A Report of the American College of Cardiology Task Force on Clinical Expert Consensus Documents. *J Am Coll Cardiol.* 2018;72(25):3332–3365. 10.1016/j.jacc.2018.10.027 30527452.
80. Prochaska J, Benowitz N. The past, present, and future of nicotine addiction therapy. *Annu Rev Med.* 2016;67:467–468.
81. Hartmann-Boyce J, Chepkin SC, Ye W, Bullen C, Lancaster T. Nicotine replacement therapy versus control for smoking cessation. *Cochrane Database of Systematic Reviews.* 2018;(5):CD000146. doi:10.1002/14651858.CD000146.pub5.
82. Lindson N, Chepkin SC, Ye W, et al. Different doses, durations and modes of delivery of nicotine replacement therapy for smoking cessation. *Cochrane Database Syst Rev.* 2019;4:CD013308–CD013308. 10.1002/14651858.CD013308 30997928.
83. Branstetter SA, Muscat JE, Mercincavage M. Time to first cigarette: A potential clinical screening tool for nicotine dependence. *J Addict Med.* 2020;14(5):409–414. 10.1097/ADM.0000000000000610 31972768.
84. Shiffman S, Sembower M, Rohay J, et al. Assigning dose of nicotine gum by time to first cigarette. *Nicotine & Tobacco Research.* 2013; 15(2):407–412.
85. Hsia S, Myers M, Chen T. Combinations nicotine replacement therapy: Strategies for initiation and tapering. *Preventative Medicine.* 2017;97:45–49.
86. Livingstone-Banks J, Norris E, Hartmann-Boyce J, et al. Relapse prevention interventions for smoking cessation. *Cochrane Database Syst Rev.* 2019;2:CD003999–CD003999. 10.1002/14651858.CD003999.pub5 30758045.

87. Williams M, Talbot P. Design features in multiple Generations of Electronic Cigarette Atomizers. *Int J Environ Res Public Health.* 2019;16(1610.3390/ijerph16162904 31416115.
88. Substance Abuse and Mental Health Services Administration (SAMHSA): Reducing Vaping Among Youth and Young Adults. SAMHSA Publication No. PEP20-06-01-003. Rockville, MD: National Mental Health and Substance Use Policy Laboratory, Substance Abuse and Mental Health Services Administration, 2020. https://doi.org/10.4135/9781452240121.n378.
89. Hartmann-Boyce J, McRobbie H, Bullen C, Begh R, Stead LF, Hajek P. Electronic cigarettes for smoking cessation. *Cochrane Database of Systematic Reviews.* 2016;(9):CD010216. doi:10.1002/14651858.CD010216.pub3.
90. Gotts JE, Jordt SE, McConnell R, et al. What are the respiratory effects of e-cigarettes? *BMJ.* 2019;366:l5275–l5275. 10.1136/bmj.l5275 31570493.
91. CDC Smoking & Tobacco Use. Outbreak of Lung Injury Associated with the Use of E-Cigarette, or Vaping, Products. https://www.cdc.gov/tobacco/basic_information/e-cigarettes/severe-lung-disease.html. Accessed May 23, 2021.
92. Wang TW, Neff LJ, Park-Lee E, et al. E-cigarette Use Among Middle and High School Students - United States, 2020. *MMWR Morb Mortal Wkly Rep* 2020;69(37):1310–1312. 10.15585/mmwr.mm6937e1 32941408.
93. U.S. Food and Drug Administration Vaporizers, E-Cigarettes, and other Electronic Nicotine Delivery Systems (ENDS). https://www.fda.gov/tobacco-products/products-ingredients-components/vaporizers-e-cigarettes-and-other-electronic-nicotine-delivery-systems-ends. Accessed May 23, 2021.
94. CDC State Tobacco Activities Tracking and Evaluation (STATE) System. STATE System E-Cigarette Fact Sheet. https://www.cdc.gov/statesystem/factsheets/ecigarette/ECigarette.html#. Accessed May 23, 2021.
95. FDA. The Real Cost Campaign. https://www.fda.gov/tobacco-products/public-health-education/real-cost-campaign. Accessed May 23, 2021.
96. Hess IM, Lachireddy K, Capon A. A systematic review of the health risks from passive exposure to electronic cigarette vapor. *Public Health Res Pract.* 2016;26(2):e2621617. doi:10.17061/phrp2621617.
97. Glasser A, Collins L, Pearson J. Overview of electronic delivery systems: a systematic review. *Am J Prev Med.* 2017;52(2):e33–e66.
98. Howes S, Hartmann-Boyce J, Livingstone-Banks J, Hong B, Lindson N, et al. Antidepressants for smoking cessation. *Cochrane Database Syst Rev* 2020;4:CD000031–CD000031. 10.1002/14651858.CD000031.pub5 32319681.
99. FDA Drug Safety Communication: Accessed May 23, 2001. Available at: https://www.fda.gov/Drugs/DrugSafety/ucm532221.htm?source=govdelivery&utm_medium=email&utm_source=govdelivery. Accessed May 23, 2021.FDA revises description of mental health side effects of the stop-smoking medicines Chantix (varenicline) and Zyban (bupropion) to reflect clinical trial findings
100. Gomez-Coronado N, Walker A, Berk M, et al. Current and emerging pharmacotherapies for cessation of tobacco smoking. *Pharmacotherapy.* 2018;38(2):235–258.
101. Cahill K, Lindson-Hawley N, Thomas KH, Fanshawe TR, Lancaster T. Nicotine receptor partial agonists for smoking cessation. *Cochrane Database of Systematic Reviews.* 2016;(5):CD006103. doi:10.1002/14651858.CD006103.pub7.
102. Anthenelli R, Benowitz N, West R, et al. Neuropsychiatric safety and efficacy of varenicline, bupropion, and nicotine patch in smokers with and without psychiatric disorders (EAGLES): A double-blind, randomized, placebo-controlled clinical trial. *The Lancet.* 2016;387:2507-2520.
103. Rennard S, Hughes J, Cinciripini P, et al. A randomized placebo-controlled trial of varenicline for smoking cessation allowing flexible quite dates. *Nicotine Tob Res.* 2012;14(3):343–350.
104. Hajek P, McRobbie HJ, Myers KE, et al. Use of varenicline for 4 weeks before quitting smoking: decrease in ad lib smoking and increase in smoking cessation rates. *Arch Intern Med* 2011;171(8):770–7. 10.1001/archinternmed.2011.138 21518946.
105. Tonstad S, Arons C, Rollema H, et al. Varenicline: mode of action, efficacy, safety and accumulated experience salient for clinical populations. *Curr Med Res Opin* 2020;36(5):713–730. 10.1080/03007995.2020.1729708 32050807.
106. FDA Drug Safety Communication: Safety review update of Chantix (varenicline) and risk of cardiovascular adverse events. Available at: #professionals findings https://www.fda.gov/Drugs/DrugSafety/ucm330367.htm #professionals findings https://www.fda.gov/Drugs/DrugSafety/ucm532221.htm. Accessed May 23, 2021.
107. Benowitz N, Pipe A, West R, et al. Cardiovascular safety of varenicline, bupropion, and nicotine patch in smokers a randomized clinical trial. *JAMA Intern Med.* 2018;178(5):622–631.
108. Chang P, Chiang C, Ho W, et al. Combination therapy of varenicline with nicotine replacement therapy is better than varenicline alone: A systematic review and meta-analysis of randomized controlled trials. *BMC Public Health.* 2015;15:689. doi:10.1186/s12889-015-2055-0.
109. Stead LF, Perera R, Bullen C, et al. Nicotine replacement therapy for smoking cessation. *Cochrane Database Syst Rev.* 2012;(11):CD000146.
110. Zhong Z, Zhao S, Zhao Y, et al. Combination therapy of varenicline and bupropion in smoking cessation: A meta-analysis of the randomized controlled trials. *Compr Psychiatry* 2019;95:152125–152125. 10.1016/j.comppsych.2019.152125 31669972.
111. Cahill K, Stevens S, Perera R, Lancaster T. Pharmacological interventions for smoking cessation: An overview and network meta-analysis. *Cochrane Database of Systematic Reviews.* 2013;(5):CD009329. doi:10.1002/14651858.CD009329.pub2.
112. Hughes JR, Stead LF. Antidepressants for smoking cessation. *Cochrane Database Syst Rev.* 2014;(1):CD000031.
113. Pamelor Package Insert Mallinckrodt. Last revised May 2007. https://www.accessdata.fda.gov/drugsatfda_docs/label/2007/018013s58lbl.pdf. Accessed May 25, 2021.
114. Lieberman HR, Agarwal S, Fulgoni VL 3rd Daily Patterns of Caffeine Intake and the Association of Intake with Multiple Sociodemographic and Lifestyle Factors in US Adults Based on the NHANES 2007-2012 Surveys. *J Acad Nutr Diet* 2019;119(1):106–114. 10.1016/j.jand.2018.08.152 30446428.
115. Spilling the beans: How much caffeine is too much. Food and Drug Administration. https://www.fda.gov/consumers/consumer-updates/spilling-beans-how-much-caffeine-too-much. Accessed May 25, 2021.
116. Wikoff D, Welsh B, Henderson R, Brorby G, et al. Systematic review of the potential adverse effects of caffeine consumption in health adults, pregnant women, adolescents, and children. *Food and Chemical Toxicology.* 2017;109:585–648.
117. Zhang H, Lee ZX, Qiu A Caffeine intake and cognitive functions in children. *Psychopharmacology (Berl)* 2020;237(10):3109–3116. 10.1007/s00213-020-05596-8 32601990.
118. Sojar SH, Shrier LA, Ziemnik RE, et al. Symptoms Attributed to Consumption of Caffeinated Beverages in Adolescents. *J Caffeine Res* 2015;5(4):187–191. 10.1089/jcr.2015.0006 26649254.
119. Doepker C, Lieberman H, Smith AP, et al. Caffeine: Friend or Foe? *Annu Rev Food Sci Tech-nol.* 2016;7:117–137.
120. Willson C The clinical toxicology of caffeine: A review and case study. *Toxicol Rep* 2018;5:1140–1152. 10.1016/j.toxrep.2018.11.002 30505695.
121. FDA Pure and Highly Concentrated Caffeine. https://www.fda.gov/food/dietary-supplement-products-ingredients/pure-and-highly-concentrated-caffeine. Accessed June 3, 2021.
122. FDA warns companies to stop selling dangerous and illegal pure and highly concentrated caffeine products. https://www.fda.gov/news-events/press-announcements/fda-warns-companies-stop-selling-dangerous-and-illegal-pure-and-highly-concentrated-caffeine. Accessed June 3, 2021.
123. Meredith SE, Juliano LM, Hughes JR, et al. 2013 Caffeine Use Disorder: A Comprehensive Review and Research Agenda., J Caffeine Res, 3, 114-130, 10.1089/jcr.2013.0016
124. Sweeney MM, Weaver DC, Vincent KB, et al. Prevalence and Correlates of Caffeine Use Disorder Symptoms Among a United States Sample. *J Caffeine Adenosine Res* 2020;10(1):4–11. 10.1089/caff.2019.0020 32181442.
125. Drewnowski A, Rehm CD Sources of Caffeine in Diets of US Children and Adults: Trends by Beverage Type and Purchase Location. *Nutrients* 2016;8(3):154–154. 10.3390/nu8030154 26978391.
126. Vercammen KA, Koma JW, Bleich SN Trends in Energy Drink Consumption Among U.S. Adolescents and Adults, 2003-2016. *Am J Prev Med* 2019;56(6):827–833. 10.1016/j.amepre.2018.12.007 31005465.
127. NIH National Center for Complementary and Integrative Health: Energy Drinks. Available at: https://nccih.nih.gov/health/energy-drinks. Accessed September 23, 2018.
128. Caffeine informer Top Selling Energy Drink Brands. https://www.caffeineinformer.com/the-15-top-energy-drink-brands. Accessed June 4, 2021.
129. Mattson ME. Update on Emergency Department Visits Involving Energy Drinks: A Continuing Public Health Concern. January 10, 2013. In: The CBHSQ Report. Rockville (MD): Substance Abuse and Mental Health Services Administration (US). Available at: https://www.ncbi.nlm.nih.gov/books/NBK384664/. Accessed October 2, 20018.

130. Markon AO, Jones OE, Punzalan CM, et al. Caffeinated energy drinks: adverse event reports to the US Food and Drug Administration and the National Poison Data System, 2008 to 2015. *Public Health Nutr* 2019;22(14):2531–2542. 10.1017/S1368980019001605 31317857.

131. De Sanctis V, Soliman N, Soliman AT, et al. Caffeinated energy drink consumption among adolescents and potential health consequences associated with their use: A significant public health hazard. *Acta Biomed.* 2017;88(2):222–231. 10.23750/abm.v88i2.6664 28845841.

132. Chrysant SG, Chrysant GS. Cardiovascular complications from consumption of high energy drinks: Recent evidence. *J Hum Hypertens.* 2015;29(2):71–76. 10.1038/jhh.2014.47 24943288.

133. Benowitz N. Clinical pharmacology of caffeine. *Ann Rev Med.* 1990;41:277–288.

134. Ferré S. Mechanisms of the psychostimulant effects of caffeine: Implications for substance use disorders. *Psychopharmacology (Berl).* 2016;233(10):1963–1979. 10.1007/s00213-016-4212-2 26786412.

135. Drake C, Roehrs T, Shambroom J, et al. Caffeine effects on sleep taken 0, 3, or 6 hours before going to bed. *J Clin Sleep Med.* 2013;9(11):1195–1200. 10.5664/jcsm.3170 24235903.

136. James JE. Maternal caffeine consumption and pregnancy outcomes: A narrative review with implications for advice to mothers and mothers-to-be. *BMJ Evid Based Med.* 2021;26(3):114–115. 10.1136/bmjebm-2020-111432 32843532.

137. ACOG Committee Opinion No. 462: Moderate caffeine consumption during pregnancy. *Obstet Gynecol.* 2010;116(2 Pt 1):467–468. 10.1097/AOG.0b013e3181eeb2a1 20664420.

138. March of Dimes. Caffeine in pregnancy. https://www.marchofdimes.org/pregnancy/caffeine-in-pregnancy.aspx. Accessed June 3, 2021.

139. van Dam RM, Hu FB, Willett WC. Coffee, caffeine, and health. *N Engl J Med.* 2020;383(4):369–378. 10.1056/NEJMra1816604 32706535.

87

Schizophrenia

M. Lynn Crismon, Tawny L. Smith, and Peter F. Buckley

KEY CONCEPTS

1. Although dysfunction in multiple neurotransmitters is involved in schizophrenia, the etiology is likely mediated by multiple subcellular processes that are influenced by different genetic polymorphisms.
2. The clinical presentation of schizophrenia is characterized by positive symptoms, negative symptoms, and impairment in cognitive functioning.
3. Comprehensive care for individuals with schizophrenia must occur in the context of a multidisciplinary mental healthcare environment that offers comprehensive psychosocial services in addition to psychotropic medication management.
4. A thorough patient evaluation (eg, history, mental status examination, physical examination, psychiatric diagnostic interview, and laboratory analysis) should occur to establish a diagnosis of schizophrenia and to identify potential co-occurring disorders, including substance use disorders and general medical disorders.
5. Given that it is challenging to differentiate among antipsychotics based on efficacy, adverse medication reaction profiles become important in choosing an antipsychotic for an individual patient.
6. Pharmacotherapy guidelines should emphasize antipsychotic monotherapies that optimize benefit-to-risk ratios before progressing to medications with greater adverse reaction risks. Combination regimens should only be used in the most treatment-resistant patients.
7. Adequate time on a given medication at a therapeutic dose is the most important variable in predicting medication response.
8. Long-term maintenance antipsychotic treatment is necessary for most patients with schizophrenia in order to prevent relapse.
9. Thorough patient and family psychoeducation should be implemented, utilizing motivational interviewing methods that focus on patient-driven outcomes in an effort to allow patients to achieve life goals.
10. Pharmacotherapy decisions should be guided by systematic monitoring of patient symptoms, preferably with the use of brief symptom rating scales and systematic assessment of potential adverse effects.

BEYOND THE BOOK

Watch the approximately 9-minute video on YouTube, "Four Patients with Schizophrenia."

For each of the patients, list the symptoms that are associated with schizophrenia. Use Table 87-11 as a reference, and for each patient list those symptoms that are present on the Brief Positive and Negative Symptom Scales. The intent of this learning activity is to help you identify symptoms associated with schizophrenia and identify symptoms that can be used to monitor response to pharmacotherapy.

INTRODUCTION

Schizophrenia is one of the most complex and challenging psychiatric disorders as it represents a heterogeneous syndrome of disorganized and bizarre thoughts, delusions, hallucinations, inappropriate affect, and impaired psychosocial functioning. From the time that Kraepelin first described dementia praecox in 1896 until publication of the *Diagnostic and Statistical Manual of Mental Disorders, Fifth Edition* (*DSM-5*) in 2013, the description of this illness has continuously evolved.[1] Scientific advances that increase our knowledge of central nervous system (CNS) physiology, pathophysiology, and genetics will likely improve our understanding of schizophrenia in the future.

EPIDEMIOLOGY

The lifetime prevalence of schizophrenia ranges from 0.28% to 0.6%[2] with the worldwide prevalence being similar among most cultures. Schizophrenia most commonly has its onset in late adolescence or early adulthood and rarely occurs before adolescence or after the age of 40 years. Although the prevalence of schizophrenia is equal between the sexes, the onset of illness tends to be earlier in males as they typically have their first episode during their early 20s, whereas with females it is usually during their late 20s.[1]

ETIOLOGY

Although the etiology of schizophrenia is unknown, research has demonstrated various abnormalities in brain structure and function.[3] However, these changes are not consistent among all individuals with schizophrenia. The cause of schizophrenia is likely multifactorial, that is, multiple pathophysiologic abnormalities can play a role in producing the similar but varying clinical phenotypes we refer to as schizophrenia.

A neurodevelopmental model, formed from the study of brains from individuals diagnosed with schizophrenia, has been evoked as one possible explanation for its etiology.[3,4] Although many different avenues of research have been undertaken, most find that biological and functional abnormalities in cell shape, position, symmetry, and connectivity have been associated with development of abnormal brain circuits that lead to the symptoms seen in schizophrenia.[4] The changes seen as part of this research are consistent with a cell migration abnormality during the second trimester of pregnancy, and some studies associate upper respiratory infections during the second trimester of pregnancy with a higher incidence of schizophrenia.[4] Other studies associate low birth weight (LBW; less than 2.5 kg [5.5 lb]), obstetric complications, or neonatal hypoxia with schizophrenia.[4] Theories of maternal stress have been developed which may be related to aberrations in circulating glucocorticoids in utero as a risk factor for schizophrenia.[4] Although imaging studies show decreased cortical thickness and increased ventricular size in the brains of many patients with schizophrenia, this occurs in the absence of widespread changes in the glial cells (or gliosis).[4] One hypothesis for these changes is that obstetric complications and hypoxia, in combination with a genetic predisposition, could activate a glutamatergic cascade resulting in increased neuronal pruning. Genes controlling *N*-methyl-D-aspartate (NMDA) receptor activity are hypothesized to be part of this process, as dendrite pruning, which is part of normal neurodevelopmental process, is higher in individuals with schizophrenia. As synaptic pruning predominantly involves glutamatergic dendrites, hypoxia or other prenatal insults can result in fewer basal neurons overall, and glutamatergic activation can exaggerate the pruning process.[3,4] Furthermore, a relationship has been documented between autoimmune encephalitis and psychosis, which is based upon glutamate receptor autoantibodies. This is important as studies have shown an increased susceptibility to immune/autoimmune disorders in schizophrenia, as well as abnormalities of autoantibodies and cytokine functioning.[5] Although this etiology is felt to be uncommon, it serves as a model for the heuristic immune hypothesis of schizophrenia, which also emphasizes integration of mental and physical well-being.[5] A plethora of diverse findings point to immune dysfunction in schizophrenia.

Numerous studies have shown neuropsychological abnormalities, impairment in reaching normal motor milestones and abnormal movements, in young children who later develop schizophrenia.[4] These abnormalities in brain function occur long before the onset of psychotic symptomatology and provide empirical evidence for schizophrenia being a neurodevelopmental disorder.[2] Furthermore, brain imaging studies show deteriorative brain changes in patients with frequent relapses,[4,6] with these changes being most pronounced among adolescents with early onset schizophrenia.[4,7] Therefore, continued pathophysiological changes, secondary to the original neurodevelopmental insult, may lead to the first psychotic episode, and brain morphology resembling neurodegeneration.[3,4,7]

Although the risk of developing schizophrenia is estimated as 0.28% to 0.6% worldwide, the risk is approximately 3% if a second-degree relative has the illness and 10% if there is a first-degree relative.[4] If both parents have schizophrenia, the risk of schizophrenia, to the offspring, increases to approximately 40%. Dizygotic twins report a 12% to 14% risk if one twin has the illness, with this increasing to 48% for monozygotic twins.[4] Furthermore, in siblings the onset of illness tends to occur at the same age in each, and adoption studies indicate that environmental changes during the child's developmental stages do not alter their genetic risk, both of which give less credence to the possibility of an environmental precipitant.

1 Numerous approaches have been utilized to study the genetics of neurodevelopment and schizophrenia risk, but one single genetic risk factor has not been found.[7] Genome-wide association studies (GWAS) have identified over 120 genetic small-effect loci that account for a small percent of the risk.[3,7] Of major interest is the finding that polymorphisms of the complement component 4 (*C4*) genes on chromosome 6 may be implicated in the abnormal dendritic pruning seen in individuals with schizophrenia.[8] Additionally, schizophrenia risk has been increasingly linked to about a dozen recurrent copy number variants (CNV) that have high penetrance; however, cumulatively they likely account for no more than 1% to 2% of all cases.[3,7] Genetic risk has also been attributed to the synaptic protein neurexin 1 (NRXN1) and neuregulin 1 (NRG1) which, in particular, may increase the risk of developing the first psychotic episode for those who are already at high risk.[3] MicroRNAs (mRNA), which are small noncoding RNAs critical to neurodevelopment and regulation of adult neuronal processes, have also been linked to schizophrenia risk and are being actively explored.[3]

There is an overlap—both clinically and biologically—between schizophrenia and mood disorders with single nucleotide polymorphisms (SNPs) from chromosomes 3, 10, and 12 being common across schizophrenia, bipolar disorder, and major depression. Two of these SNPs were at loci related to the pathophysiology of calcium-channels.[3,7] Some of the CMVs identified for schizophrenia risk have also been associated with autism spectrum disorder, intellectual disability, and attention-deficit hyperactivity disorder.[7] Thus, several genetic and biological studies now suggest a greater shared genetic—and neurobiological—basis across psychiatric disorders so that the idea of schizophrenia being a distinct "condition" is increasingly being challenged.

PATHOPHYSIOLOGY

Studies have found consistent decreases in gray matter in multiple brain areas, including the frontal lobes, cingulate gyri, and medial temporal regions among others. A longitudinal study of high-risk youth showed a substantially greater decrease in gray matter in high-risk youth who progressed to psychosis than in high-risk youth who did not progress to psychosis or in normal controls.[9] Additionally, increases in ventricular size, as well as decreased white matter in the corpus callosum, have been observed.[9] Changes in hippocampal volume may correspond with impairment in neuropsychological testing.[4,6] It is felt then, that rather than a decrease in the number of neurons in affected brain areas, a decrease in axonal and dendritic communications between cells can result in a loss of connectivity impacting neuronal adaptivity and CNS homeostasis,[4,6] which are likely consistent with the evidence for abnormal neuronal pruning.[2] Intense research efforts have been made to explore and link brain imaging and other biomarkers to disease expression and progression, in an effort to arrive at clinically relevant biomarkers that could aid treatment of schizophrenia—just as has occurred in cancer and other medical conditions.

1 Historically, schizophrenia has been attributed to dopamine (DA) receptor defects, but increasingly subcortical dopaminergic dysregulation, including increased DA synthesis and release have been observed.[10] While presynaptic changes in dopaminergic neurons occur and are consistent with the neurodevelopmental model that has been proposed,[3,6] numerous positron emission tomography (PET) studies have shown brain abnormalities including increased glucose metabolism in the caudate nucleus and decreased blood flow and glucose metabolism in the frontal lobe and left temporal lobe.[4] These findings may indicate dopaminergic hyperactivity in the head of the caudate nucleus and dopaminergic hypofunction in the frontotemporal regions, which may be confirmed by alterations in dopamine-2 (D_2) receptor densities.[4,6] However, increases in presynaptic DA synthesis and release into the striatum may only translate into a small increase in $D_{2/3}$ receptor availability.[11]

Additionally, PET studies assessing dopamine-1 (D_1) receptor function suggest that subpopulations of patients with schizophrenia may have decreased densities of D_1 receptors in the caudate nucleus and the prefrontal cortex, in addition to the D_2 receptors. Clinically this may lead to hypofrontality within the prefrontal cortex, which can be associated with a lack of volition and cognitive dysfunction, core features of schizophrenia. It is unknown whether these changes represent a primary event or secondary processes related to other pathophysiologic abnormalities in schizophrenia. Because of the heterogeneity in the clinical presentation of schizophrenia, the DA hypothesis may be more applicable to individuals who respond to antipsychotic treatment, with multiple different etiologies possibly being responsible for causing schizophrenia.[4,6] While attempts have been made to develop relationships between these abnormal findings and behavioral symptoms present in patients with schizophrenia, the positive symptoms of schizophrenia are possibly more closely associated with DA-receptor hyperactivity in the mesocaudate, whereas negative symptoms and cognitive impairment are most closely related to DA-receptor hypofunction in the prefrontal cortex. As the presynaptic D_1 receptors in the prefrontal cortex are thought to be involved in modulating glutamatergic activity, this hypofunctionality can impact working memory in individuals with schizophrenia.[4,6]

One can examine different neurotransmitter alterations in the context of different proposed phases of schizophrenia.[12] The Predrome Phase typically occurs before an individual is diagnosed with schizophrenia. This phase can last weeks to years where clinically high-risk individuals are thought to exhibit glutamategic synaptic dysfunction that results in a glutamate signaling defect, leading to some affective and/or psychotic symptoms. Partial compensation by gamma-aminobutyric acid (GABA) downregulation and synaptic proliferation are associated with the Prodromal Phase. This deficit in GABA is felt to result in less inhibition of excitatory circuits, producing dopaminergic dysfunction, the onset of psychosis, and the Syndrome Phase, with the degree of dopamine dysfunction associated with more severe disease.[6] During the Syndrome Phase, most individuals are officially diagnosed with schizophrenia. In the last phase, the Chronic Phase, years of chronic schizophrenia symptoms and treatments are thought to be associated with the loss of gray matter compounding the synaptic deficits.[12]

As the glutamatergic system is one of the most widespread excitatory neurotransmitter systems in the brain, hypo- or hyperactive alterations in function can result in toxic neuronal reactions.[12] Dopaminergic innervation from glutamate in the ventral striatum decreases the limbic system's inhibitory activity (perhaps through GABA interneurons) and thus increases arousal. The corticostriatal glutamate pathways have the opposite effect, whereas inhibiting dopaminergic function from the ventral striatum allows increased inhibitory activity in the limbic system. Due to the interaction between glutamatergic and dopaminergic tracts, as well as through GABA interneurons, glutamatergic deficiency produces symptoms similar to those of dopaminergic hyperactivity and possibly those seen in schizophrenia. Therefore, alterations in the interactions between dopamine and glutamate due to NMDA hypofunction have been associated with the latent clinical expression of psychotic symptoms in late adolescence or early adulthood.

Schizophrenia is a complex disorder, and multiple etiologies likely exist. Based on current knowledge, it is naïve to think that any one proposed etiology or one dysfunction in neurotransmission can adequately explain the genesis of this complex disease. Moreover, ongoing research into distinct biomarkers for schizophrenia, as well as the promise of stem cell research to disentangle the pathobiology of this enigmatic disorder, will also help identify phenotypes and help to determine the boundaries between psychosis and mood disorders.[3,7,11,13]

CLINICAL PRESENTATION

The clinical presentation of functional psychosis seen with schizophrenia is highly variable. Despite numerous attempts to portray a stereotype in movies and on television, the stereotypic person with schizophrenia essentially does not exist, and schizophrenia is not a "split personality." It is a chronic disorder of thought and affect with the individual having a significant disturbance in interpersonal relationships and ability to function in society.

2 The first psychotic episode can be sudden in onset with few premorbid symptoms, or more commonly is preceded by withdrawn, suspicious, peculiar behavior, termed schizoid. During acute psychotic episodes, the patient loses touch with reality, and in a sense, the brain creates a false reality to replace it. Acute psychotic symptoms can include hallucinations (especially hearing voices), delusions (fixed false beliefs), and ideas of influence (beliefs that one's actions are controlled by external influences). Thought processes are disconnected (loose associations), the patient may not be able to carry on logical conversation (alogia), and can have simultaneous contradictory thoughts (ambivalence). The patient's affect can be flat (no emotional expression), or it can be inappropriate and labile. The patient is often withdrawn and inwardly directed (autism). Uncooperativeness, hostility, and verbal or physical aggression can be seen because of the patient's misperception of reality. Self-care skills are impaired, and patients may be dirty and unkempt with generally poor hygiene during acute episodes. Sleep and appetite are often disturbed. When the acute psychotic episode remits, the patient typically has residual features, which is an important point in differentiating schizophrenia from other psychotic disorders. Although residual symptoms and their severity vary, patients can have difficulty with anxiety management, suspiciousness, and lack of volition, motivation, insight, and judgment. They often have difficulty living independently, and because of poor anxiety management and suspiciousness, they are frequently withdrawn socially, and have difficulty forming close relationships with others. Impaired volition and motivation contribute to poor self-care skills and make it difficult for the patient with schizophrenia to maintain employment.

Patients with schizophrenia frequently experience a lack of historicity, or difficulty in learning from their experiences, resulting in them repeatedly making the same mistakes in social conduct and situations requiring judgment. They have difficulty understanding the importance of treatment, including medications, in maintaining their ability to function. Therefore, they tend to discontinue treatments, increasing the risk of relapse and rehospitalization.

The co-occurrence of substance use disorder (SUD) (predominantly alcohol or polysubstance—alcohol, cannabis, and cocaine) in patients with schizophrenia is very common and is another frequent reason for relapse and hospitalization.[1] This effect can be caused by direct toxic effects of these substances on the brain,[14] but is also caused by the medication nonadherence that is associated with substance use. Some substances—most notably heavy cannabis use during adolescence—have been associated with a higher prevalence of schizophrenia, as cannabis use raises the risk of schizophrenia four- to sixfold.[15]

Although the course of schizophrenia is variable, the long-term prognosis for many patients is poor. It is marked by intermittent acute psychotic episodes and impaired psychosocial functioning between acute episodes, with most of the deterioration in psychosocial functioning occurring within 5 years after the first psychotic episode.[16] By late life, the patient can appear "burned out," that is, they cease to have acute psychotic episodes, but residual symptoms persist (the chronic phase). In a subpopulation of patients, probably 5% to 15%, psychotic symptoms are nearly continuous, and response to antipsychotics is poor.[16]

Schizophrenia is a chronic disorder, and the patient's history must be carefully assessed for dysfunction that has persisted for longer than 6 months. After their first episode, patients with schizophrenia rarely have a level of adaptive functioning as high as before the onset of the disorder. *The Diagnostic and Statistical Manual of Mental Disorders, Fifth Edition* (*DSM-5*) should be consulted for the

CLINICAL PRESENTATION Schizophrenia and Symptoms Clusters

Positive Symptoms

- Suspiciousness
- Unusual thought content (delusions)
- Hallucinations
- Conceptual disorganization

Negative Symptoms

- Affective flattening
- Alogia
- Anhedonia
- Avolition

Cognitive Symptoms

- Impaired attention
- Impaired working memory
- Impaired executive function

complete criteria for a diagnosis of schizophrenia.[1] The *DSM-5* also asks the clinician to specify the episode severity for schizophrenia after having the diagnosis for at least 1 year and whether the patient is presenting with catatonia.[1]

The *DSM-5* classifies the symptoms of schizophrenia into two categories: positive and negative; however, greater emphasis is now being placed on a third symptom category, cognitive dysfunction.[1,16] The areas of cognition found to be abnormal in schizophrenia include attention, working memory, and executive function. Positive symptoms have traditionally attracted the most attention and are the ones most improved by antipsychotics. However, negative symptoms and impairment in cognition are more closely associated with poor psychosocial function.

Along with these characteristic features of schizophrenia, many patients also have comorbid psychiatric and general medical disorders.[2,16] These include depression, anxiety disorders, SUD, and general medical disorders such as respiratory disorders, cardiovascular disorders, and metabolic disturbances. These comorbidities substantially complicate the clinical presentation and course of schizophrenia.

Symptom complexes are correlated with prognosis, cognitive functioning, structural abnormalities in the brain, and response to antipsychotic medications. Negative symptoms and cognitive impairment are more closely associated with prefrontal lobe dysfunction and positive symptoms with temporolimbic abnormalities. As many patients demonstrate both positive and negative symptoms, those with negative symptoms frequently have more antecedent cognitive dysfunction, poor premorbid adjustment, low level of educational achievement, and a poorer overall prognosis.[1,16]

TREATMENT

Desired Outcome

3 Pharmacotherapy is a mainstay of treatment in schizophrenia, as it is impossible to effectively implement psychosocial rehabilitation programs without antipsychotic treatment in most patients.[14] The most current treatment guidelines for schizophrenia espouse 24 recommendations, three of which relate to overall assessment and treatment planning, 11 of which cover medication treatments, and the remaining 10 focus on psychosocial approaches to care (Table 87-1). A pharmacotherapeutic treatment plan should be developed that delineates medication-related aspects of therapy. Most deterioration in psychosocial functioning occurs during the first 5 years after the initial psychotic episode, and treatment should be particularly assertive during this period.[16] The individualized treatment plan created for each patient should have explicit end points defined, including realistic goals for the target symptoms most likely to respond, and the relative time course for response.[17] Other desired outcomes include avoiding unwanted adverse medication reactions, integrating the

TABLE 87-1 Guidelines for the Care of Patients with Schizophrenia

Patients have a comprehensive initial assessment
Initial assessment includes a quantitative measure of symptoms—functioning
Treatment planning includes evidence based pharmacologic and nonpharmacologic treatments
Patients receive antipsychotic medications for treatment, evaluating both efficacy and safety
Patients whose illness has improved with medication receive continued antipsychotic treatment
Patients with treatment resistant schizophrenia receive clozapine
Patients with persistent suicidality/risk of suicidality despite other treatments receive clozapine
*Patients with aggression that persists despite other treatments receive clozapine
*Patients with preference and/or history of inadequate medication noncompliance receive long-acting injectable antipsychotic medication
Patients with antipsychotic-induced dystonia receive an anticholinergic medicine
*Patients with antipsychotic-induced parkinson symptoms have their medication dosage reduced or switched to another antipsychotic or receive an anticholinergic medication
*Patients with antipsychotic induced akathisia have their medication dosage reduced, switch to another antipsychotic, or receive either a benzodiazepine or beta blocker
Patients with at least moderate tardive dyskinesia that is antipsychotic induced receive a vesicular monoamine transporter 2 (VMAT2) reversible inhibitor
Patients with first episode psychosis are treated in a comprehensive program
Patients receive cognitive behavioral therapy
Patients receive psychoeducation
Patients receive supported employment opportunities
Patients with social complications contributing to recurrent relapses receive assertive community treatment
*Patients with family contact receive family supportive activities
*Patients receive recovery-based activities
*Patients receive cognitive remediation
*Patients with focus on social performances receive social skills training
*Patients receive supportive psychotherapy

** Recommended or suggested by the American Psychiatric Association (APA). Data from References 18 and 20-22.*

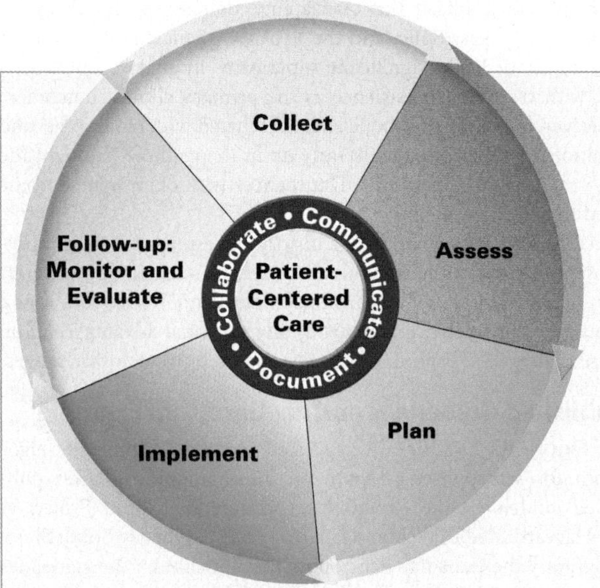

Patient Care Process for Schizophrenia

The image shows the five fundamental steps included in The Patient Care Process endorsed by the Joint Commission for Pharmacy Practitioners (2014). The tagline of this process reads collaborate, communicate, and document. The five fundamental steps listed here are collect, assess, plan, implement, and follow-up: monitor and evaluate. All these steps are listed in a circular block diagram.

Collect

- Patient characteristics (eg, age, race, sex, gender identity, pregnancy status)
- Patient history (past mental and medical, medication adherence, family, social—diet, alcohol and substance use, tobacco use)
- Mental status exam
- Medications (current and past)
- Objective data
- Brief Positive and Negative Symptom Scales (see Table 87-11)
- Blood pressure (BP), heart rate (HR), height, weight, and body mass index (BMI) (see Table 87-12)
- Labs: Hemoglobin A1c (HgA1c), lipids, other tests if indicated (see Table 87-12)

Assess

- Patient's concerns and attitudes toward treatment, medication adherence (see Table 87-5)
- Symptom severity and the extent that treatment goals have been met
- Do any co-occurring disorders (mental, substance use disorder, medical) need to be addressed?
- Are patient's psychosocial needs being met? (see Table 87-2)
- Adverse medication reactions (see Tables 87-7 and 87-12)
- Potential for medication interactions (see Tables 87-9 and 87-10)
- Appropriateness and effectiveness of current psychotropic regimen

Plan*

- Actively engage patient in care plan
- Medication therapy regimen (egspecify the continuation and discontinuation of existing therapies) (see Fig. 87-1 and Tables 87-3, 87-4, and 87-6)
- Monitoring parameters including efficacy and time frame (see Tables 87-11 and 87-12)
- Patient education (eg, medication, life style management)
- Referrals to other providers as appropriate (eg, physician, psychologist, social worker)

Implement*

- Provide patient education regarding all elements of treatment plan
- Use motivational interviewing and coaching strategies to maximize adherence
- Schedule follow-up

Follow-up: Monitor and Evaluate*

- Determine symptom attainment (see Table 87-11)
- Presence of adverse effects (see Table 87-12)
- Presence of medication interactions (see Tables 87-9 and 87-10)
- Need for psychosocial interventions
- Patient adherence to treatment plan using multiple sources of information

**Collaborate with patient, caregivers, and other healthcare professionals.*

patient back into the community, increasing adaptive functioning to the extent possible, and preventing relapse.

Nonpharmacologic Therapy

Psychosocial rehabilitation programs focused on improving patients' adaptive functioning are the mainstay of non-medication treatment for schizophrenia. These programs include case management, psychoeducation, targeted cognitive therapy, basic living skills, social skills training, basic education, work programs, supported housing, and financial support. In particular, programs aimed at supportive employment and housing are effective and considered "best practices." Those that involve families in the care and life of the patient have been shown to decrease rehospitalization and improve functioning in the community. For particularly low-functioning patients, assertive intervention programs, referred to as *active community treatment* (ACT), are effective in improving patients' functional outcomes. These ACT teams are available on a 24-hour basis and work in the patient's home and/or place of employment to provide comprehensive treatment, including medication, crisis intervention, daily living skills, and supported employment and housing.[18] Pharmacotherapy cannot be successful without proper attention to these other aspects of care, as people with schizophrenia need comprehensive care, with coordination of services across psychiatric, SUD, medical, social, and rehabilitative services. In the United States, care coordination is often insufficient, putting patients at risk to "fall through the cracks." Some countries have implemented more robust primary and secondary preventative approaches, highlighting early identification, ease of access to care, and staging of disease management.[19] The National Institute of Mental Health (NIMH) Recovery After Initial Schizophrenia Episode (RAISE) study found that four core interventions ("personalized medication management, family psychoeducation, resilience-focused individual therapy, and supported employment and education") significantly improved the quality of life over a 24-month period for individuals with early schizophrenia as compared to usual community care.[20]

The patient-centered approach to the recovery-based system of care is growing, where the person's lifetime aspirations and goals become the center of care, rather than symptom reduction being the primary focus. This recovery-based approach recognizes the strengths and resilience of people with schizophrenia, and acknowledges how people with schizophrenia can be a support to others who are living with the illness.[20] It is important to frame clinical decision making in the context of a mutual process involving patient and clinician. Psychosocial/cognitive behavioral strategies can help some patients, and emerging computer-based therapies and social media–related approaches may be helpful. Cognitive remediation—which uses computer-based cognitive retraining techniques—has been shown to be of benefit.[21] Social media and mobile technology strategies may be harnessed to improve communications, medication adherence, and potentially detect early warning signs of impending relapse in patients with schizophrenia.

Pharmacologic Therapy

4 The importance of an initial accurate diagnostic assessment cannot be overemphasized. A thorough mental status examination (MSE), psychiatric diagnostic interview, physical and neurologic examination, complete family and social history, and laboratory workup must be performed to confirm the diagnosis and exclude general medical or substance-induced causes of psychosis. Laboratory tests, biologic markers, and commonly available brain imaging techniques do not assist in the diagnosis of schizophrenia or selection of medication. A pretreatment patient workup not only is important in excluding other pathology but also serves as a baseline for monitoring potential adverse medication reactions, and should include vital signs, complete blood count, electrolytes, hepatic function, renal function, electrocardiogram (ECG), fasting serum glucose, hemoglobin A1c, serum lipids, thyroid function, and urine drug screen.

5 Both first-generation antipsychotics (FGAs, also known as traditional) and second-generation antipsychotics (SGAs, also known as atypical) are used in the treatment of schizophrenia,[14,23] with no absolute criterion distinguishing between the two. As compared with FGAs, SGAs appear to have the ability to produce antipsychotic response with fewer occurring extrapyramidal symptoms (EPS). Other attributes that have been ascribed to some SGAs include enhanced efficacy (particularly for negative symptoms and cognition), near absence of propensity to cause tardive dyskinesia, and lack of effect on serum prolactin.[24] To date, only clozapine truly fulfills all of these criteria, with other SGAs having some of these attributes.[24] Therefore, the major factor used in practice when distinguishing among antipsychotics is adverse effects.[22-24] While the SGAs have a lower risk of neurologic adverse reactions, particularly effects on movement, this is offset by increased risk of metabolic syndrome with some SGAs, including weight gain, hyperlipidemias, and diabetes mellitus. Adverse medication reaction profiles differ among antipsychotics, and this information should be used in combination with individual patient characteristics when choosing a medication for an individual patient.

Results from the Clinical Antipsychotic Trials of Intervention Effectiveness (CATIE) study, primarily in patients with chronic schizophrenia, indicate that olanzapine, compared with quetiapine, risperidone, ziprasidone, and the FGA perphenazine, had modest but not statistically significant superiority in maintenance therapy with treatment persistence as the primary clinical outcome.[17] However, increased metabolic effects occurred with olanzapine, and additional studies of patients early on in their illness highlight the high rate of cardiometabolic disturbances with olanzapine and the need to tailor treatment.[25]

Previous patient or family history of response to an antipsychotic is helpful in the selection of an agent. Acquisition cost varies significantly among different antipsychotics and dosage forms, and should be considered in context of any potential advantages of an agent. Table 87-2 lists antipsychotics and their usual dosage ranges.

Published Guidelines and an Algorithm Example

6 Figure 87-1 outlines a suggested pharmacotherapeutic algorithm for schizophrenia, based on information from four published guidelines, the Psychopharmacology Algorithm Project at the Harvard Medical School Department of Psychiatry South Shore Program,[23] the Canadian Schizophrenia Guidelines,[22] the guidelines from the World Federation of Biological Psychiatry, and the APA Guidelines.[14,22,24]

Stage 1A of the treatment algorithm applies to those patients experiencing their first acute episode of schizophrenia. Use of SGAs during the first acute episode may result in greater treatment retention and effectiveness in preventing a second psychotic episode compared to FGAs. In addition, SGAs carry a reduced risk of EPS.[24] Among the SGAs, aripiprazole, olanzapine, quetiapine, risperidone, and ziprasidone have evidence of efficacy in first-episode patients, with lurasidone showing efficacy in adolescents with schizophrenia, but most were not treatment naive.[23,34] Despite its efficacy, olanzapine is not recommended in first episode because of weight gain and adverse metabolic effects.[23,24]

Since quetiapine is associated with less time to rehospitalization compared to other SGAs and causes greater weight gain, some guidelines do not recommend it in stage 1A.[23] This leaves aripiprazole, risperidone, and ziprasidone as the evidence-based options in first-episode patients (stage 1A).[23] Of these, aripiprazole and ziprasidone produce the least weight gain. However, few head-to-head clinical trials have been conducted, and the level of evidence is not sufficiently high to recommend these as the only preferred agents in first episode.[14,22] The 2021 APA Guidelines do not provide any preference among initial antipsychotic selection. Because first-episode patients demonstrate greater sensitivity to adverse medication reactions, antipsychotic dosing should be initiated at the lower end of the dose range.[20,22,23]

In first-episode patients, long-acting risperidone injectable was more effective than oral risperidone in preventing relapse over a 1-year period.[35] The relapse rate was six times higher in the oral risperidone group than with the long-acting injectable (LAI); therefore, risperidone LAI can be considered as a treatment option for first-episode patients. If this medication is used, patients should first be stabilized on oral risperidone. It is critical that enriched psychosocial programs be implemented along with appropriate pharmacotherapy.

Stage 1B addresses pharmacotherapy for a patient who was previously treated with an antipsychotic, and treatment is being restarted because the patient stopped taking the medication. If during the initial antipsychotic trial, the patient experienced a robust improvement in symptoms, good tolerability, and is positive about taking this antipsychotic again, then that medication can be restarted. If a different medication is needed, one from stage 2 should be used. Stage 2 addresses pharmacotherapy in a patient who had inadequate clinical improvement with the antipsychotic used in stage 1A or 1B, or the patient responded but subsequently had a relapse while taking the medication. Stage 2 recommends

TABLE 87-2 Available Antipsychotics and Dosage Ranges

Generic Name	Trade Name	Starting Dose (mg/day)	Usual Dosage Range (mg/day)	Comments
First-Generation Antipsychotics				
Chlorpromazine	Thorazine	50-150	300-1,000	Most weight gain among FGAs
Fluphenazine	Prolixin	5	5-20	
Haloperidol	Haldol	2-5	2-20	Higher dropout rate in first episode
Loxapine	Loxitane	20	50-150	
Loxapine inhaled	Adasuve	10	10	Maximum 10 mg per 24 hours. Approved REMS program only
Perphenazine	Trilafon	4-24	16-64	
Thioridazine	Mellaril	50-150	100-800	Significant QTc prolongation
Thiothixene	Navane	4-10	4-50	
Trifluoperazine	Stelazine	2-5	5-40	
Second-Generation Antipsychotics				
Aripiprazole	Abilify	5-15	15-30	
Asenapine	Saphris	5	10-20	Sublingual only, no food or drink for 10 minutes after administration
Brexpiprazole	Rexulti	1	2-4	
Cariprazine	Vraylar	1.5	1.5-6	Due to long half-life, steady state is not reached for several weeks
Clozapine	Clozaril	25	100-800	REMS program. Check plasma level before exceeding 600 mg
Iloperidone	Fanapt	1-2	6-24	Care with dosing in CYP2D6 slow metabolizers
Lumateperone	Caplyta	42	42	Bioavailability increased by 9% when administered with high fat meal
Lurasidone	Latuda	20-40	40-120	Take with food; ≥350 calories (1,460 Joules)
Olanzapine	Zyprexa	5-10	10-20	Avoid in first episode because of weight gain
Paliperidone	Invega	3-6	3-12	Bioavailability increased when administered with food
Quetiapine	Seroquel	50	300-800	
Quetiapine XR	Seroquel XR	300 mg	400-800	
Risperidone	Risperdal	1-2	2-8	
Ziprasidone	Geodon	40	80-160	Take with food, ≥500 calories (2,100 Joules)

REMS: Risk Evaluation and Mitigation Strategy. XR: extended release.

Note: In first-episode patients, starting dose and target dose should generally be 50% of the usual dose range. See Long-Acting Injectable Antipsychotics in text for dosing of these agents.

Data from References 24 and 26-33.

antipsychotic monotherapy with an FGA or SGA not used in stage 1 or stage 1B.[14,22-24] Because of safety concerns and the need for white blood cell (WBC) monitoring, clozapine is not generally recommended at stage 2.[14,22,23] However, clozapine has superior efficacy in decreasing suicidal behavior, and it should be considered at stage 2 for the patient with suicidal thoughts.[22,23] Clozapine can also be considered at stage 2 in patients with a history of violence or comorbid substance use disorder.[22,23,36] If a patient has an unacceptable adverse medication reaction with the antipsychotic used during stage 1A, stage 1B, or stage 2, then an alternate antipsychotic for that stage should be chosen.

Long-acting injectable antipsychotics (LAIAs) should be considered as an option at stage 2. The use of LAIAs should be discussed with the patient as a life style choice, and their use should not be reserved for patients with poor medication adherence. In fact, if a patient prefers receiving a LAIA, it should be considered as an option at Stages 1A, 1B, and 2.[22-24] If there is good documentation of poor symptom improvement with two different antipsychotic trials at appropriate dose and duration, then pharmacotherapy should be initiated with the stage 3 recommended treatment clozapine.[22-24] In stage 4, minimal evidence exists for any treatment option for patients who do not have adequate symptom improvement with clozapine. The Harvard Department of Psychiatry South Shore algorithms present various treatment options for such patients; however, none of these options have conclusive evidence.[23] It is important to note that the use of antipsychotic combinations is controversial, as limited evidence supports increased efficacy for antipsychotic polypharmacy, despite this practice being somewhat common.[22,23] The APA Guidelines state that electroconvulsive therapy (ECT) combined with an antipsychotic may be useful in some patients with treatment resistance.[22]

Predictors of Response

Obtaining a thorough medication history is important, and previous treatment response should help guide antipsychotic selection, in that either a good prior response favors the use of the same agent or a negative prior response suggests the selection of a dissimilar medication. Substance use can influence psychiatric presentation and needs to be considered when making decisions regarding a patient's diagnosis or antipsychotic response. Amphetamines and other CNS stimulants, cocaine, corticosteroids, digitalis glycosides, indomethacin, cannabis, pentazocine, phencyclidine, other medications, and substances can induce psychosis in susceptible individuals or exacerbate psychosis in patients with preexisting psychiatric

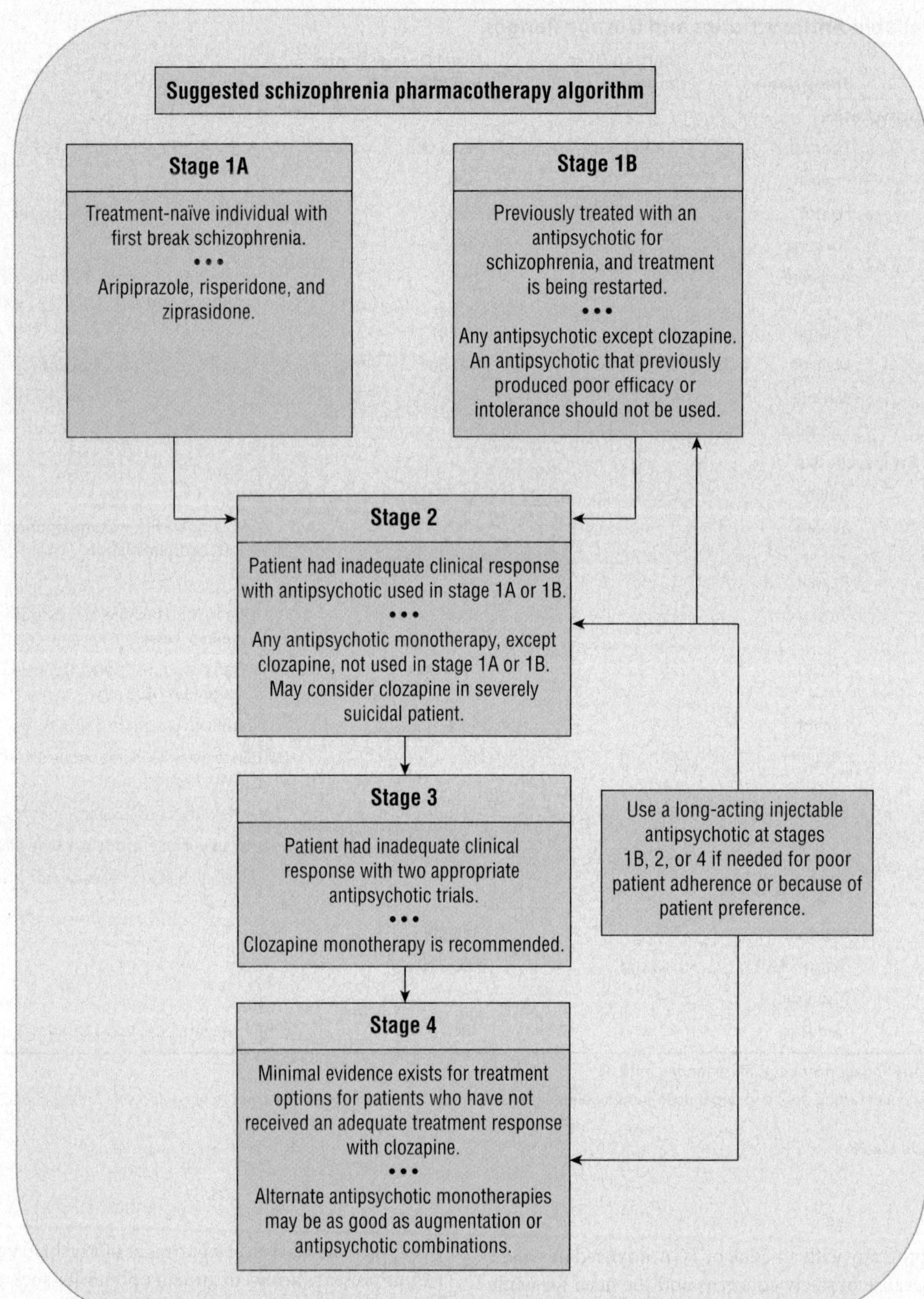

FIGURE 87-1 Suggested pharmacotherapy algorithm for treatment of schizophrenia. Schizophrenia should be treated in the context of an interprofessional model that addresses the psychosocial needs of the patient, necessary psychiatric pharmacotherapy, psychiatric co-occurring mental disorders, treatment adherence, and any medical problems the patient may have. (See the text for a description of the algorithm stages.)

illness.[1,16,22,23] Patients with schizophrenia who use alcohol or other substances usually have a poor response to medications and a poor overall prognosis. Furthermore, alcohol, cannabis, caffeine, and nicotine use may potentially interact with antipsychotics.

Individual predictors of patient response have been either proposed or identified. Acute onset of symptoms and short duration of illness, presence of acute stressors or precipitating factors, later age of onset, family history of affective illness, and good premorbid adjustment as reflected in stable interpersonal relationships or employment are all predictors of good response.[14]

Although controversial, affective symptoms can correlate with an overall good response, while negative symptoms and neuropsychological deficits related to cognition and neurologic soft signs can correlate with poor antipsychotic response.[14,16,22,23] Subjective positive patient response within the first 48 hours after FGA administration can be associated with medication responsiveness,[37] whereas an initial dysphoric response, demonstrated by stating a dislike of the medication, feeling worse or "zombie-like," anxiety or akathisia-like symptoms, is associated with poor medication response, adverse effects, and nonadherence.

The importance of developing a therapeutic alliance between the patient and the clinician cannot be underestimated (see Chapter e81, "Evaluation of Psychiatric Illness"). Patients who form positive therapeutic alliances are more likely to be adherent with all aspects of therapy, experience a better outcome at 2 years, and require lower antipsychotic doses.[20] However, a certain minority of patients fail to benefit from antipsychotic therapy, and their psychosocial functioning can worsen with antipsychotic continuation.

Initial Treatment in an Acute Psychotic Episode

The goals during the first 7 days of treatment should be decreased agitation, hostility, combativeness, anxiety, tension, and aggression, and normalization of sleep and eating patterns. The usual recommendation is to initiate therapy and to titrate the dose over the first few days to an average effective dose, unless the patient's physiologic status or history indicates that this dose can result in unacceptable adverse medication reactions. Because of strong alpha-1 (α_1) receptor antagonism and resulting risk of hypotension, iloperidone and clozapine should be titrated more slowly than other SGAs. Rapid titration to high doses is not recommended. Table 87-2 lists the usual dosage range, with an average dose typically being midrange.[14,22-24] Because patients with first-episode psychosis have an increased sensitivity to adverse medication reactions, particularly EPS, typical dosing ranges are approximately 50% of the doses used in chronically ill individuals.[22,23] If "cheeking" of medication is suspected (where the patient places the medication in their cheek and then spits it out later), liquid formulations and orally disintegrating tablets are available for some antipsychotics. If a patient has no improvement after 2 weeks at a therapeutic dose, then later clinical response is unlikely, and moving to the next treatment stage of the algorithm is recommended.[38]

Although some clinicians believe that larger daily doses are necessary in patients with more severe symptoms, data do not support this practice. Some symptoms, such as agitation, tension, aggression, and increased motor activity, may respond more quickly, but adverse medication reactions can be more common with higher doses. However, interindividual differences in dosage and response do occur. In patients with partial response who are tolerating the chosen antipsychotic, it may be reasonable to titrate above the usual dose range. However, this tactic should be time-limited (ie, 2-4 weeks), and if the patient does not achieve further improvement, either the dose should be decreased or an alternative treatment strategy should be tried. As previously stated, rapid titration of antipsychotic dosage is not indicated[14,22-24]; however, intramuscular (IM) antipsychotic administration (eg, haloperidol 2-5 mg IM, olanzapine 2.5-10 mg IM, or ziprasidone 10-20 mg IM) can be used to assist in calming a patient with severe agitation. Clinically, agitation can manifest as loud, physically or verbally threatening behavior, motor hyperactivity, or physical aggression. Although use of IM antipsychotics can assist in calming a patient with acute agitation due to psychosis, it does not improve the rate of remission, time to remission, or the length of hospitalization. Haloperidol (an FGA) given IM for treatment of acute aggression is associated with a higher incidence of EPS than IM SGAs. If the patient is receiving an antipsychotic within the usual therapeutic range, the use of lorazepam 2 mg IM as needed in combination with the maintenance antipsychotic is a rational alternative for treatment of aggression. Hypotension, respiratory depression, CNS depression, and death have been reported with injectable lorazepam in combination with either olanzapine or clozapine; thus, injectable lorazepam is not recommended in combination with either of these medications.[24]

Inhaled loxapine powder is Food and Drug Administration (FDA)-approved for treatment of acute agitation associated with schizophrenia or bipolar disorder. Because of the risk of bronchospasm, pulmonary distress, and pulmonary arrest, the medication can only be administered in a healthcare facility through the FDA-approved Risk Evaluation and Mitigation Strategy (REMS). Before administration, patients must be screened for a history of asthma, chronic obstructive pulmonary disease, or other lung disease associated with bronchospasm, and use is limited to one 10 mg inhaled dose per 24-hour period.[26] Whether inhaled loxapine offers any therapeutic advantages in acute agitation compared with other antipsychotics is unknown, and patients must be sufficiently cooperative to inhale it appropriately.

Stabilization Therapy

7 Symptom improvement may occur over 6 to 12 weeks with appropriate medication therapy and comprehensive treatment. During the first 2 to 3 weeks, goals should include increased socialization and improvement in self-care habits and mood. Improvement in any formal thought disorder should follow and may take an additional 6 to 8 weeks. Patients who are early in the course of their illness tend to experience a more rapid resolution of symptoms than individuals who are more chronically ill. In general, if a patient has shown no improvement after 2 weeks of treatment at therapeutic doses, or has achieved only a partial decrease in positive symptoms within 8 to 12 weeks at adequate doses, then the next algorithm stage should be considered. In more chronically ill patients, symptoms may continue to improve over 3 to 4 months. Quantifying symptom change using a brief symptom rating scale can be helpful in monitoring treatment and making decisions. An optimum target medication dose should be estimated in the initial treatment plan. If the patient begins to show adequate response at a dose, then the patient should remain at this dosage if symptoms continue to improve. In general, adequate time on a therapeutic antipsychotic dose is the most important factor in predicting medication response. However, if necessary, dose titration can continue within the therapeutic range every 1 or 2 weeks if the patient has no adverse medication reactions.

Before changing medications in a patient with poor response, the following should be considered: Were the initial target symptoms indicative of schizophrenia or did they represent manifestations of a different diagnosis, a long-standing behavioral problem, a substance use disorder, or a general medical condition? Is the patient adherent with pharmacotherapy? Are the persistent symptoms poorly responsive to antipsychotics (eg, impaired insight or judgment, or fixed delusions)? How does the patient's current status compare with response during previous exacerbations? Would this patient potentially benefit from advancing to a different treatment stage (Fig. 87-1)? Does this patient have treatment-resistant schizophrenia?

The conclusion that the patient with a partial response has achieved as much symptomatic improvement as possible is one that must be made with great care as treatment goals must be realistic. Medications are effective in decreasing many of the symptoms of schizophrenia (and are thus referred to as palliative), but they are not curative, and not all symptoms may abate. Although one should aim to achieve full remission to minimal residual positive symptoms, it is still unclear what a realistic goal is regarding maximum improvement in negative symptoms.

It is important to screen patients for co-occurring psychiatric disorders, and their presence can become more apparent during the stabilization or maintenance phases of treatment. Examples include substance use disorders, depression, obsessive-compulsive disorder, and panic disorder. As co-occurring disorders will limit symptom and functional improvement and increase the risk of relapse. It is critical that treatment for the co-occurring disorder be implemented in combination with evidence-based treatment for schizophrenia.

Maintenance Treatment

Maintenance medication therapy prevents relapse, as shown in numerous double-blind studies, which is a major goal of treatment.[14,22-24] The average relapse rate after 1 year is 18% to 32% with active medication (including some patients with nonadherence) versus 60% to 80% for placebo.[14,22-24]

8 After treatment of the first psychotic episode in a patient with schizophrenia, medication should be continued for at least 18 months after remission.[14,22-24] Many experts recommend that patients with robust medication response be treated for at least 5 years; however, in chronically ill individuals, continuous or lifetime pharmacotherapy is necessary in most patients to prevent relapse. This practice should be approached with the lowest effective antipsychotic dose that is tolerated by the patient.[14,22-24]

Antipsychotics should be tapered slowly before discontinuation as abrupt discontinuation, especially with clozapine, can result in withdrawal symptoms, felt to be a manifestation of rebound cholinergic outflow. Insomnia, nightmares, headaches, gastrointestinal symptoms (eg, abdominal cramps, stomach pain, nausea, vomiting, and diarrhea), restlessness, increased salivation, and sweating are reported. Although available evidence does not indicate a best way to switch from one antipsychotic to another, it is often recommended to taper and discontinue the first antipsychotic over at least 1 to 2 weeks while the second antipsychotic is initiated and the dose titrated.[24] Tapering needs to occur more slowly with clozapine.[38]

Long-Acting Injectable Antipsychotics

Early studies did not consistently demonstrate an advantage of LAIAs over oral agents. However, studies, designed to reflect real-world practices, have more consistently demonstrated an advantage in reduced hospitalizations and relapse prevention in patients with schizophrenia, findings that were confirmed in a meta-analysis.[39,40] Despite the potential advantages, the use of LAIAs is relatively low compared with oral antipsychotics, and in most Western countries use falls below 20%.[41] Barriers to LAIA use may be clinician or patient driven and include: biases and attitudes, limited insurance coverage, or lack of experience with LAIAs.[42] Traditionally, LAIAs have been primarily used later in the course of treatment and in patients who are unreliable in taking oral medication. It has been suggested to offer LAIAs to patients as a treatment option earlier in their disease before they develop a pattern of nonadherence.[41,42] For example, they can be presented to a patient as a life style option, in which the patient does not need to take a medication daily.[22] Normalizing the use of LAIAs, providing appropriate education to families and patients on LAIAs, utilizing motivational interview techniques, and offering it as an early treatment option may aid in improving LAIA acceptability with patients.[39]

Treatment nonadherence rates as high as 60% in patients with schizophrenia can lead to negative clinical outcomes.[41] Nonadherence can be due to several factors including cognitive impairment, persistent symptoms, substance use, or lack of insight. However, before declaring a patient as nonadherent, it should be determined whether the patient is experiencing adverse medication reactions. If so, an alternative medication with better tolerability should be considered before initiating a LAIA. The patient's motivation for treatment is a major factor influencing outcome.

There are 10 LAIAs available for use in the United States: risperidone (two different formulations), paliperidone palmitate (three formulations), aripiprazole (monohydrate and lauroxil), olanzapine pamoate, haloperidol decanoate, and fluphenazine decanoate. Conversion from an oral antipsychotic to a LAIA should start with stabilization on an oral dosage form of the same agent for a short trial (4-14 days) to determine whether the patient tolerates the medication without significant adverse medication reactions, especially if the patient has no previous exposure to the oral agent.[39]

With risperidone microspheres (Consta), measurable serum concentrations are not seen until approximately 3 weeks after single-dose administration. Thus, it is important that the oral antipsychotic be administered for at least 3 weeks after the first injection. The recommended starting dose with risperidone microspheres is 25 mg. Clinical experience suggests that titration to doses greater than or equal to 37.5 mg per injection may be necessary for maintenance treatment; however, efficacy was demonstrated with doses of 25 to 50 mg IM every 2 weeks. Dose adjustments are recommended to be made no more often than once every 4 weeks.[43] Doses above 50 mg every 2 weeks are not recommended, as research indicates no greater clinical efficacy but more EPS.[25] With risperidone extended-release injectable suspension (PERSERIS), dosing is 90 or 120 mg once monthly, no oral overlap or loading dose is necessary, and it is the only LAIA that is administered subcutaneously in the abdomen.[44]

Paliperidone palmitate (Invega Sustenna) has the advantage of easy conversion from oral paliperidone to IM treatment, as there is no need for oral overlap, and this formulation offers once-monthly injections with the option to convert to 3-month or 6-month formulations.[43] It is initiated with 234 mg on day 1 and 156 mg a week later (+/− 4 days) with deltoid administration for the first two doses as gluteal absorption results in 28% lower C_{max}. The 1-month paliperidone palmitate (1MPP) IM doses are then titrated according to response within a range of 39 to 234 mg and can be injected into either the deltoid or gluteal muscle.[43] If a patient's oral paliperidone is established prior to converting to the 1MPP, the maintenance dose required for similar paliperidone exposure is outlined in Table 87-5.[45]

A 3-month paliperidone palmitate (3MPP, Invega Trinza) and 6-month paliperidone palmitate (6MPP, Invega Hafyera) LAIA are approved for the management of schizophrenia, with both formulations being found to significantly delay time to relapse compared with placebo. The 3MPP and 6MPP provide the longest dosing interval available, but require patients to be treated for at least 4 months with 1MPP prior to 3MPP initiation. Those who have received at least one dose of the 3MPP may be converted to the 6MPP. The first 3MPP dose is based on the previous 1 month injection dose, and the first 6MPP dose is based on either the 1- or 3-month injection dose, as shown in Table 87-3.[46]

Olanzapine pamoate monohydrate is a LAIA administered every 2 or 4 weeks that does not require oral overlap. It is recommended for deep gluteal injection, and the initial injectable dose varies from 210 to 405 mg depending on the oral olanzapine daily maintenance dose and the frequency of injectable administration.[43,50] A disadvantage to olanzapine pamoate is its association with post-injection delirium/sedation syndrome (PDSS) occurring in <2% of patients.[50] The symptoms of PDSS are similar to those of an oral olanzapine overdose and include delirium, ataxia, confusion, heavy sedation, or altered levels of consciousness. Although PDSS can occur with any dose and at any time during treatment, most cases have occurred within the first three injections.[51] The most likely explanation for the occurrence of PDSS is an accidental intravascular injection resulting in the medication dissolving more rapidly and sharp increases in plasma levels.[51,52] The product labeling contains an FDA-boxed warning regarding PDSS, and olanzapine pamoate is subject to a REMS with the FDA labeling limiting the availability of olanzapine LAIA to a restricted distribution program. The injection must be administered in a registered healthcare facility, and the patient must be observed by a health professional for at least 3 hours after administration and must not drive or operate machinery that day.[50]

Aripiprazole monohydrate LAIA (Abilify Maintena) is administered as a single intramuscular injection in the gluteal or deltoid muscle once a month at a starting and maintenance dose of 400 mg. If the patient does not tolerate the 400 mg dose, the next injection can be reduced to 300 mg. After the first injection of aripiprazole monohydrate LAIA, a 14-day overlap with oral aripiprazole (10-20 mg/day) or any other antipsychotic is recommended.[43] Aripiprazole lauroxil LAIA (Aristada) is administered as a single intramuscular injection in the deltoid (441 mg only) or gluteal (441, 662, or 882 mg, once a month). The 882 mg dose can be administered every 6 weeks and the 1,084 mg every 2 months. Aripiprazole lauroxil has the advantage of having initiation dosing available (Aristada Initio)[47];

TABLE 87-3 Summary of Available Long-Acting Injectable Antipsychotics (LAIAs)

Medication Name	Fluphenazine Decanoate	Haloperidol Decanoate	Risperidone (Risperdal Consta)	Risperidone (PERSERIS)	Paliperidone Palmitate (Invega Sustenna) (1MPP)	Paliperidone Palmitate (Invega Trinza) (3MPP)	Paliperidone Palmitate (Invega Hafyera) (6MPP)	Olanzapine Pamoate (Zyprexa Relprevv)	Aripiprazole Monohydrate (Abilify Maintena)	Aripiprazole (Lauroxil Aristada)
Dose Range (mg)	12.5-100	20-450	12.5-50	90-120	39-234	273-819	1,092-1,560	150-405	300-400	441-882[b]
PO Overlap	None	4 weeks (none if loading); use PO dose patient was taking prior to injection	3 weeks after first injection: use PO dose patient was taking prior to injection	None	None	None	None	None	2 weeks PO dose ranges from 10 to 20 mg/day	21 days PO overlap after first injection
Recommended maximum dose	100 mg every 2-3 weeks	450 mg every 4 weeks	50 mg every 2 weeks	120 mg monthly	234 mg every 4 weeks	819 mg every 3 months	1,560 mg every 6 months	300 mg every 2 weeks or 405 mg every 4 weeks	400 mg monthly	882 mg monthly
Initiation or Loading	Can Load	Can Load	None	None	Initiation required	None required, dose based on last Invega Sustenna dose: If 78 mg give 273 mg If 117 mg give 410 mg If 156 mg give 546 mg If 234 mg give 819 mg	None required, dose used depends on last Invega Sustenna or Trinza dose For Invega Sustenna: If 156 mg give 1,092 mg If 234 mg give 1,560 mg For Invega Trinza: If 546 mg give 1,092 mg If 819 mg give 1,560 mg	Initiation required	None	None required, dose based on PO dose: If 10 mg/day give 441 mg If 15 mg/day give 662 mg If 20 mg give 882 mg
Time to peak	8-24 hours	4-11 days	4-5 weeks	4-6 hr	13 days	30-33 days	29-32 days	<1 week	5-7 days	5-6 days
T_{ss}	2-3 months	2-3 months	6-8 weeks	60 days	7-11 months	Continues steady state	Continues steady state	3 months	3-4 months	4 months
Half-life	14 ± 2[a] days	21 days	3-6 days	9-11 days	25-49 days	84-89 days (deltoid) 118-139 days (gluteal)	148-159 days	30 days	30-47 days	29-35 days

(continued)

TABLE 87-3 Summary of Available Long-Acting Injectable Antipsychotics (LAIAs) (*Continued*)

Medication Name		Fluphenazine Decanoate	Haloperidol Decanoate	Risperidone (Risperdal Consta)	Risperidone (PERSERIS)	Paliperidone Palmitate (Invega Sustenna) (1MPP)	Paliperidone Palmitate (Invega Trinza) (3MPP)	Paliperidone Palmitate (Invega Hafyera) (6MPP)	Olanzapine Pamoate (Zyprexa Relprevv)	Aripiprazole Monohydrate (Abilify Maintena)	Aripiprazole (Lauroxil Aristada)
Injection Site	Gluteal	Yes	Yes	Yes	Abdominal only	Yes after 2nd dose	Yes	Yes	Yes	Yes	Yes
	Deltoid	Yes	Yes	Yes		Yes	Yes	No	No	No	Yes, but only 441 mg dose
Injection Method/ Technique		Z-Track	Z-Track			Subcutaneous Injection					
Notes				A starting dose of 12.5 mg is recommended in patients with hepatic or renal impairment	90 mg = 3 mg PO Risperidone 120 mg = 4 mg PO Risperidone	Avoid use in patients with moderate-to-severe renal impairment (CrCl <50 mL/min [0.83 mL/s])	Requires at least a 4-month trial with 1MPP. Not recommended in patients with moderate or severe renal impairment (CrCl <50 mL/min [0.83 mL/s])	Requires at least a 4 month trial with 1MPP or at least 1 cycle of 3MPP. Not recommended in patients with moderate or severe renal impairment (CrCl <50 mL/min [0.83 mL/s])	Monitor for PDSS Subject to REMS	Maintenance dose reduced to 300 mg if patient experiences adverse events. Dose adjustment needed in CYP2D6 slow metabolizers. Avoid use in patients taking CYP 3A4 inhibitors >14 days	May require 2 week PO trial to establish efficacy before initiating LAIA Avoid use of strong CYP2D6 and 3A4 inhibitors for 662 and 882 mg dose, no adjustment needed for 441 mg dose

CrCl, creatine clearance; IM, intramuscular; LAIA, long-acting injectable; PO, oral; Tss, time to steady state.

[a]Based on multiple-dose data. Single-dose data indicate a β-half-life of 6-10 days.

[b]Additional dosing regimens include extended intervals up to 1,064 mg every 8 weeks; loading protocol with Aristada Initio 675 mg + maintenance Aristada dose + PO 30 mg ×1 dose does not require PO overlap.

Data from References 38, 43, and 45-52.

however, if Aristada Initio is not utilized, oral overlap is required for 3 weeks with this LAIA formulation.[52]

For the FGA fluphenazine decanoate, the simplest dosing conversion method recommends 1.25 times the oral fluphenazine daily dose for stabilized patients, rounding to the nearest 12.5 mg interval, which is administered in weekly doses for the first 4 to 6 weeks; or 1.6 times the oral daily dose given weekly for the first 4 weeks for more acutely ill patients.[48] Subsequently, fluphenazine decanoate can be administered once every 2 to 3 weeks. Although oral fluphenazine can be overlapped for 1 week, the dose should be reduced by half with the first injection to reduce the risk of EPS.[48] For haloperidol decanoate, the first dose should be 10 to 20 times the oral haloperidol daily dose. In patients who are at high risk of relapse, and are tolerant to oral haloperidol, a loading dose of 20 times the oral dose can be considered.[48] In patients naïve to haloperidol decanoate, the initial injection is limited to 100 mg followed by the remaining balance of the first monthly dose given 3 to 7 days later.[43] Overlap with oral haloperidol overlap is not necessary if the patient receives a loading dose, but is recommended for the first month if a loading dose strategy is not utilized. The maintenance dose is typically 10 to 15 times the oral dose once monthly. Table 87-3 provides a summary of the LAIAs.

Methods to Enhance Patient Adherence

Treatment nonadherence rates are as high as 60% in patients with schizophrenia, which can lead to negative clinical outcomes.[41] If nonadherence is suspected, the clinician should ask in a nonjudgmental manner if the patient is having any difficulty taking their medication and then the reason for nonadherence should be determined. If nonadherence is occurring because of adverse effects, then a medication with a more favorable tolerability profile should be considered. Suspected nonadherence can also be assessed by obtaining an antipsychotic serum concentration.[53]

Maintaining appropriate medication adherence is often challenging for individuals with chronic illnesses and partial adherence is a reality and should be expected to be the norm.[24] Individuals with serious psychiatric disorders have higher nonadherence rates than those with general medical disorders, with the following explanations provided: denial of illness, lack of insight, grandiosity or paranoia, no perceived need for medication, perceived lack of input into choice of medication or dosage, adverse medication reactions, misperceived "allergies," too many medications prescribed, or too many doses prescribed daily (see Table 87-4). It is estimated that half of patients with schizophrenia or schizoaffective disorder take their medication less than 70% of the time.[24] Discussions regarding this topic should be approached in a positive, nonjudgmental manner, with the clinician actively engaging the patient in care and using motivational interviewing techniques as mechanisms to enhance therapeutic alliance and patient adherence.

TABLE 87-4 Nonadherence with Antipsychotic Medications Is a Multidimensional Dilemma

Patient Factors	Medication Factors	Other Factors
Lack of insight	Efficacy	Family perspectives
Paranoia	Adverse medication reactions	Cultural influences
Attitude to ward medications	Mode of delivery/ ingestion	Clinician perspectives and influences
Prior experiences	Cost	Insurance coverage
Perception of efficacy of medication	Availability	Cost of care
Comorbid substance use disorder		Medication access and support
		Mental illness stigma

Data from References 54 and 55.

(9) Numerous different methods have been used to improve treatment adherence of patients with schizophrenia. Interventions that provide continuous focus on adherence and that are of long duration have shown benefit. These should incorporate problem-solving techniques and be accompanied by technical learning aids. As previously noted, programs need to include a focus on patient-driven outcomes, and not just medication adherence, and interventions should include efforts to allow patients to achieve life goals and function. This requires that programs be tailored to the needs of individual patients.[54] Psychoeducation strategies should include motivational interviewing techniques in individual counseling as well as group activities.

Compliance therapy, targeted cognitive behavioral therapy focusing on medication adherence, can improve patient adherence, but the success seen in early studies has not been consistently replicated.[54]

Groups facilitated by trained individuals who have the illness are thought to be more effective in enhancing awareness and acceptance of schizophrenia and necessary treatment, than groups led only by professionals. Active involvement of family members further increases the likelihood of patient adherence with treatment. In addition to programs provided by community mental health centers, support groups operated by consumer groups such as the National Alliance on Mental Illness (NAMI) are available for patients and their families in most urban areas. In the hospital, self-medication administration can reinforce the patient's perception of his or her active role in treatment. When patients miss outpatient appointments, active outreach interventions must be implemented to enhance patient engagement in treatment.[54]

The LAIAs have been a mainstay of treatment for people who are nonadherent with taking oral medications. However, for various reasons, they are used in only a relatively small subset of patients, and many patients simply do not like getting injections. Abilify MyCite, an FDA-approved technology, includes a biosensor inside the aripiprazole tablet; after the medication is ingested, the coating is degraded and a specific patch worn by the patient picks up a biosensor signal from the formulation.[49] Data are then transferred to a smart phone application and can be shared by the patient with the treating clinician via the Internet. It is not clear whether this technology improves patient adherence in a population that is often suspicious and paranoid. Regardless, a great deal of education is necessary to make sure that the patient knows how to use the technology and to assure that the patient wears the patch and uses the smart phone application correctly.

Management of Treatment-Resistant Schizophrenia

In general, "treatment resistant" describes a patient who has had inadequate symptom response from multiple antipsychotic trials.[22-24,53] The clinical definition of treatment resistance requires persistent symptoms of at least moderate severity, despite treatment with two different antipsychotics at adequate dosage for at least 6 weeks, each with good treatment adherence.[53] Between 10% and 30% of patients receive minimal symptomatic improvement after multiple antipsychotic monotherapy trials.[22-24] An additional 30% to 60% of patients have partial but inadequate improvement in symptoms or unacceptable adverse medication reactions associated with antipsychotic use. In patients not responding to two or more pharmacotherapy trials, a treatment-refractory evaluation should be performed to reexamine diagnosis, substance use, medication adherence, and psychosocial stressors. Targeted cognitive behavioral therapy or other psychosocial augmentation strategies should be considered.[22,23] While clozapine remains the treatment of choice for treatment-resistant schizophrenia, its use has declined over time in favor of sequential treatment trials of SGAs. This is problematic and trainees need exposure to initiating clozapine therapy, given the low likelihood of later use in clinical practice without this experience.

Clozapine Only clozapine has shown superiority over other antipsychotics in randomized clinical trials for the management of treatment-resistant schizophrenia as most other SGAs have either not been studied in this patient population, or have been evaluated in small open trials. In a seminal study, clozapine was effective in approximately 30% of patients with treatment-resistant schizophrenia, compared with only 4% treated with a combination of chlorpromazine and the anticholinergic benztropine.[56] Other candidates for clozapine include those patients with severe suicidality, aggressive behavior, or those who cannot tolerate neurologic adverse medication reactions from conservative doses of other antipsychotics.

Symptomatic improvement with clozapine in the treatment-refractory patient often occurs slowly, and as many as 60% of patients continue to improve if clozapine is used for up to 6 months. This, in combination with clozapine's tolerability profile, provides sufficient information to conclude that clozapine is not a panacea for schizophrenia. Polydipsia and hyponatremia (psychogenic water drinking) is are a frequent problems among treatment-refractory patients, and clozapine reportedly decreases water drinking and increases serum sodium in such patients.[23,24]

Because of the risk of orthostatic hypotension, clozapine is usually titrated more slowly than other antipsychotics, particularly on an outpatient basis. If a 12.5-mg test dose does not produce hypotension, then clozapine 25 mg at bedtime is recommended, increased to 25 mg twice a day after 3 days, and then increased in 25 to 50 mg/day increments every 3 days until a dose of at least 300 mg/day is reached. If tolerated, a minimum trial should be 3 months with a clozapine serum concentration of at least 350 ng/mL (mcg/L; 1.07 μmol/L). Because high doses are associated with significantly increased adverse medication reactions, including seizures, a clozapine serum concentration is recommended before exceeding 600 mg/day.[24] If the clozapine serum concentration is greater than 350 ng/mL (mcg/L; 1.07 μmol/L), then further dosage increases are not indicated.[53]

Augmentation and Combination Strategies Limited empirical evidence exists to guide treatment decisions for patients who do not respond to clozapine.[22-24] Current strategies include augmentation with a non-antipsychotic medication in patients with poor or partial response, or combination treatment using two antipsychotics simultaneously.

In a small, single blind, randomized trial, 50% of patients demonstrated clinically significant improvement in symptoms with electroconvulsive therapy (ECT) augmentation of clozapine, compared with no responders in the clozapine monotherapy group. When the patients in the clozapine monotherapy group received ECT, 47% demonstrated clinically significant improvement.[23]

Mood stabilizers are frequently used as an augmentation strategy, and while lithium does not enhance the antipsychotic effect, it may improve labile affect and agitated behavior in select patients.[23] Enzyme induction with carbamazepine can cause a decrease in antipsychotic serum concentrations and potentially worsen psychotic symptoms in some patients.[23,57]

Only limited data are available to support antidepressant augmentation of antipsychotics.[22-24] However, consistently positive results have been reported when using selective serotonin reuptake inhibitors (SSRIs) to treat obsessive-compulsive symptoms that worsen or arise during clozapine treatment.

Combining an FGA with an SGA and combining different SGAs have been suggested as intervention strategies for treatment-resistant patients. Pharmacodynamically, there is limited rationale to explain how combinations of antipsychotics would produce enhanced efficacy, but increased adverse medication reactions, particularly increased EPS, metabolic effects, and hyperprolactinemia, are possible results.[22] The evidence to support antipsychotic combinations is scant. However, a large Finnish database study, using patients as their own controls, found that clozapine plus aripiprazole had a lower rehospitalization rate than any other monotherapy or combination antipsychotic treatment.[58] This observational study was not in patients identified as treatment resistant. Regardless, this topic remains highly contentious, and clinicians' practice is often not aligned with available evidence. Moreover, the availability of new treatment options can result in combination therapies being tried with antipsychotics with insufficient scientific evidence. This approach further complicates the application of systematic, evidence-based treatments for schizophrenia. In general, a series of antipsychotic monotherapy courses, including clozapine, are preferred over antipsychotic combinations.[22] However, when clozapine fails to produce desired outcomes, a time-limited combination trial is sometimes considered (eg, maximum 12 weeks) with the patient carefully evaluated using standardized rating scales to assess symptomatology.[23] If no apparent improvement is observed, then one of the medications should be tapered and discontinued. However, if the patient has a partial response (greater than or equal to 20% improvement in positive symptoms) after 12 weeks with combination treatment, medications should be titrated to doses at the upper end of the therapeutic range, and treatment should continue for an additional 12 weeks before a change in treatment is considered.

Violence in Schizophrenia

Most people with schizophrenia do not exhibit violent behavior; however, they are more likely to be violent than the general population. The rate of violence in people with schizophrenia is 9.9% compared with 1.6% in the general population.[36] Risk factors for violence include those associated with violence in the general population (eg, childhood trauma and exposure to violence, alcohol and substance use disorders, psychopathy, and access to firearms) and (to lesser extent) psychotic symptoms.[36] Most of the risk of violence is associated with co-occurring substance use disorders.[36] Patients are at risk to become violent when they relapse and so keeping patients clinically stable is a major consideration. Clozapine has been found to be superior to other antipsychotics in decreasing aggressive and violent behavior.[36] Some states have outpatient commitment laws where patients at risk of violence are "forced" to get ongoing care, and if they default, they are sent back to the hospital. Patients who are dangerous are invariably managed either in the legal system itself or legally as "forensic" patients where they are held by court order in a psychiatric facility.

Antipsychotic Mechanism of Action

The exact mechanism of actions of antipsychotics are unknown. Antipsychotics is are classified into three different categories: (a) typical (traditional or FGAs) (high D_2 antagonism and low serotonin-2 receptor [$5\text{-}HT_{2A}$] antagonism); (b) atypical (SGAs) (moderate-to-high D_2 antagonism and high $5\text{-}HT_{2A}$ antagonism); and (c) atypical clozapine-like (low D_2 antagonism and high $5\text{-}HT_{2A}$ antagonism).[59] With the exception of aripiprazole and brexpiprazole, all current SGAs have a greater affinity for $5\text{-}HT_{2A}$ receptors than D_2 receptors, and brexpiprazole shows stronger antagonism of the $5\text{-}HT_{2A}$ receptor than aripiprazole.[59,60] Brexpiprazole also demonstrates higher affinity for the serotonin-1A ($5\text{-}HT_{1A}$) receptor compared to aripiprazole but with less intrinsic D_2 activity than aripiprazole.[60]

Prospective studies of antipsychotic receptor binding in humans have used PET scans to examine neurotransmitter receptor binding 12 hours post-dose in small numbers of individuals at steady-state concentrations. It has been proposed that at least 60% to 65% D_2 receptor occupation is necessary to decrease positive psychotic symptoms, whereas blockade of approximately 77% or more of D_2 receptors is associated with EPS.[59] Table 87-5 outlines the relative differences in receptor binding for various agents. In general, all FGAs are DA receptor antagonists with high affinity for D_2 receptors, and during chronic treatment, between 70% and 90% of D_2 receptors in the striatum are usually occupied. In

TABLE 87-5 Relative Neuroreceptor Binding Affinities of Select Antipsychotics

	Aripiprazole	Asenapine	Chlorpromazine	Clozapine	Haloperidol	Iloperidone	Lumateperone	Lurasidone	Olanzapine	Paliperidone	Quetiapine	Risperidone	Ziprasidone
D_1	-	++	+	+	+				++	+	-	+	+
D_2	++++	+++	+++	+	++++	+++	++	+++	++	+++	+	+++	+++
D_3	++	+++	+++	+	+++	+++	++		+	++	-	++	++
D_4	+	+++	+++	++	+++	++			++	-	-	-	++
$5\text{-}HT_{1A}$	++	++	-	-	-	++		+	-	-	-	-	+++
$5\text{-}HT_{1D}$	+			-	-				-	+	-	+	+++
$5\text{-}HT_{2A}$	+++	+++	++	+++	+	++++	++++	+++	+++	+++	++	++++	++++
$5\text{-}HT_{2C}$	+	++++	++	++	-	++	+		++	+	-	++	++++
$5\text{-}HT_6$	+	+++	++	++	-	++			++	-	-	-	+
$5\text{-}HT_7$	++	+++	++	++	-			++++	-	++	-	+++	++
α	+	+++	++++	+++	+++	++++	++	+	++	+++	+++	+++	++
α	+	++	+	+	-	++		+	+	++	-	++	-
H_1	+	++	++++	+++	-	++	-	-	+++	-	++	-	-
m_1	++	-		++++	-	-	+/-	-	+++	-	++	-	-

Relative neuroreceptor binding affinities of select antipsychotics.

(-) = minimal or none; (+) = low; (++) = moderate; (+++) = high; (++++) = very high

Data from References 61 and 62.

contrast, during clozapine treatment only 38% to 47% of D_2 receptors are occupied, even with high doses. Newer SGAs have variable D_2 binding. Low D_2 binding seen with the SGAs, can be directly associated with how rapidly the antipsychotic disassociates from the D_2 receptor.[59] This transient blockade of DA receptors may be adequate to produce antipsychotic effect, but longer term D_2 blockade is required for production of EPS and sustained hyperprolactinemia. Aripiprazole and brexpiprazole are partial agonists at D_2 receptors, and represent a further elaboration of the DA hypothesis of antipsychotic action.[59,60]

Iloperidone's pharmacology is different in that it has high affinity for D_2, dopamine-3 (D_3), and 5-HT_{2A} receptors, and moderate affinity for dopamine-4 (D_4), serotonin-6 (5-HT_6), serotonin-7 (5-HT_7), and α_1-receptors.[27] Asenapine has high affinity for 5-HT_{2A} and D_2 receptors as well as for α_1- and histamine-1 receptors with D_2 occupancy approximating 80% with a sublingual dose of 5 to 10 mg twice daily.[28] Cariprazine has high affinity for D_2 and D_3 receptors as a partial agonist, with the D_3 potency being significantly greater than D_2. It is also a partial agonist at 5-HT_{1A} receptors and an antagonist at serotonin-1B (5-HT_{1B}) receptors.[29] Therefore, given all of these different mechanisms of action, our understanding of the manner in which they produce a clinical profile is still in its infancy.

With low-dose risperidone (2-5 mg/day), D_2 binding ranges from 60% to 79%, but with doses greater than 6 mg daily, binding commonly exceeds the 77% threshold associated with the development of EPS. Risperidone 2 mg/day produces 5-HT_{2A} binding greater than 70%, and with 4 mg/day it is nearly 100%.[59] Olanzapine 10 to 20 mg/day produces D_2 binding ranging from 71% to 80%, whereas at 30 to 40 mg/day, it ranges from 83% to 88%. Ziprasidone has the highest 5-HT_{2A}-to-D_2 affinity ratio of any of the currently available antipsychotics. It is also a potent serotonin-1A (5-HT_{1A}) agonist.[59]

Quetiapine has the lowest D_2 binding. At doses of 300 to 600 mg/day, 12-hour post-dose D_2 binding ranges from 0% to 27%. Even at quetiapine 800 mg/day, only 30% of D_2 receptors are occupied. At these same daily doses, 45% to 90% of 5-HT_{2A} receptors are occupied. However, when quetiapine D_2 binding is examined 2 to 3 hours post-dose, 58% and 64% of receptors were occupied with 400 and 450 mg, respectively.

Lumateperone is a moderate antagonist at both D_1 and D_2 receptors and a potent antagonist at 5-HT_{2A} receptors. In individuals with schizophrenia, lumateperone occupied approximately 42% of D^2 receptors. It is also a presynaptic DA agonist and a 5-HT reuptake inhibitor. It indirectly modulates glutamatergic activity resulting in increased NMDA and AMPA activity.[33,62]

The primary therapeutic effects of antipsychotics are thought to occur in the limbic system, including the ventral striatum, whereas EPS are thought to be related to DA blockade in the dorsal striatum. For SGAs, 5-HT_{2A} antagonism in combination with modest D_2 blockade leads to release of DA in the prefrontal cortex, and this is one explanation for the decrease in negative symptoms and improvement in cognition reported with these antipsychotics.[48] Medications that are not D_2 antagonists are currently in clinical trials for the treatment of schizophrenia. If these medications are approved by the FDA, they may have a significant effect on how we look at antipsychotic mechanisms of action and efficacy.

As discussed, antipsychotics vary in their effects on other neurotransmitter receptor systems.[59] Although the significance of these different mechanisms on efficacy is unclear, they do potentially explain differences in adverse medication reaction profiles. These differences in pharmacodynamics profiles point out that the SGAs are not alike, and patients obtaining an inadequate clinical response (either efficacy or adverse medication reactions) with one antipsychotic may have a superior response/tolerability on an alternate medication. Thus, serial SGA monotherapy trials should be tried in patients receiving a suboptimal clinical response (see Fig. 87-1).

Pharmacokinetics

As a class, antipsychotics are highly lipophilic and highly bound to membranes and plasma proteins. They distribute readily into most tissues with a high blood supply and can accumulate in tissues; therefore, they have large volumes of distribution.[63] Most antipsychotics are largely metabolized, primarily through the cytochrome P450 (CYP) pathways in the liver, except for ziprasidone, which is largely metabolized by aldehyde oxidase. Fluphenazine and perphenazine are metabolized through CYP2D6, and thus are susceptible to pharmacogenetically regulated metabolism.[64] This is also one of the major pathways for the metabolism of aripiprazole, brexpiprazole, haloperidol, iloperidone, and risperidone.[64] Thirty percent to 35% of people of African and Asian descent are slow to intermediate CYP2D6 metabolizers, and approximately 0% to 5% of African American, 1% of Asian, and 5% to 10% of White populations are poor metabolizers.[65] In addition, some people of Swedish descent and up to 30% of those from Northern Africa may be ultra-rapid CYP2D6 metabolizers.[66] Genetic variation within CYP1A2 can potentially result in a decrease in the metabolic rate of clozapine, whereas smoking may increase clozapine and olanzapine metabolism due to the effect of cigarette smoke inducing CYP1A2 linked to a specific genotype.[64,65] Pharmacogenomics should be considered when dosing and monitoring the clinical effects of antipsychotics.[64-66] Additional resources related to specific gene and drug pairs for pharmacogenomics information can be obtained at the Clinical Pharmacogenomics Implementation Consortium (CPIC) Website (www.cipicpgx.org). Table 87-6 outlines the prominent metabolic pathways of selected antipsychotics.

Asenapine is unique in that it has less than 2% bioavailability after oral administration, but has a bioavailability of approximately 35% sublingually—the FDA-approved route of administration. Eating and drinking within 10 minutes after sublingual administration will reduce bioavailability, and bioavailability decreases with single doses above 10 mg.[28,66]

Most antipsychotics have long elimination half-lives, generally 24 hours or more, with the exception of quetiapine and ziprasidone, which have short half-lives.[63,66] Among the SGAs, only clozapine has an established therapeutic serum concentration, with efficacy being associated with a clozapine plasma concentration greater than 350 ng/mL (mcg/L; 1.07 μmol/L).[63] Whether a potential maximum therapeutic clozapine serum concentration exists is unknown. Clozapine serum concentration should be obtained before exceeding 600 mg daily, in patients who develop unusual or severe adverse medication reactions, in patients who are taking concomitant medications that can cause medication interactions, in patients who have age or pathophysiologic changes suggesting a change in pharmacokinetics, or for assessment of patient adherence.[63,66]

Adverse Medication Reactions

5 Table 87-7 presents the relative risk of common categories of antipsychotic adverse medication reactions, which are discussed below with respect to organ system affected. A general approach to monitoring and assessing adverse medication reactions requires prospective monitoring by clinicians, preferably using a thorough review of systems approach. Patient-oriented self-rated scales can be helpful, as many patients with schizophrenia do not readily endorse adverse medication reactions.

As mentioned previously, adverse medication reactions are one of the primary predictors of patient nonadherence. With the variety of antipsychotics available, using an alternative should be considered to improve patient outcomes in those who endorse poorly tolerated adverse medication reactions. As we learn more about relative risks (eg, metabolic, QTc prolongation, and EPS), it will be necessary to regularly reconsider which antipsychotics should be considered first-line treatment alternatives.

TABLE 87-6 Pharmacokinetic Parameters of Selected Antipsychotics

Medication	Bioavailability (%)	Half-Life	Major Metabolic Pathways	Active Metabolites
Selected First-Generation Antipsychotics (FGAs)				
Chlorpromazine	10-30	8-35 hr	FMO3, CYP3A4	7-Hydroxy, others
Haloperidol	40-70	12-36 hr	**CYP2D6**, CYP1A2, CYP3A4	Reduced haloperidol
Perphenazine	20-25	8.1-12.3 hr	**CYP2D6**	7-OH-perphenazine
Second-Generation Antipsychotics (SGAs)				
Aripiprazole	87	48-68 hr	**CYP2D6, CYP3A4**	Dehydroaripiprazole
Asenapine	<2 orally 35 SL Nonlinear	13-39 hr	**CYP1A2, UGT1A4**, CYP2D6, CYP3A4	None known
Brexpiprazole	95	91 hr	**CYP2D6, CYP3A4**	DM-3411
Cariprazine		2-4 days, DDCAR 1-3 weeks	**CYP3A4**, CYP2D6	Desmethyl cariprazine (DCAR), Didesmethyl cariprazine (DDCAR)
Clozapine	12-81	11-105 hr	**CYP1A2, CYPD6, CYP3A4**	Desmethylclozapine
Iloperidone	96	18-33 hr	**CYP2D6, CYP3A4**	P88
Lumateperone	4.4	13-21 hr	**CYP3A4**, CYP1A2, CYP2C8, Aldoketoreductase 1C1, UGT1A1, UGT1A4, UGT 2B15	IC200131, IC200161, IC200565
Lurasidone	10-20	18 hr	**CYP3A4**, CYP1A2	ID-14233 and ID-14326
Olanzapine	80	20-70 hr	CYP1A2, CYP3A4, FMO3	*N*-Glucuronide; 2-OH-methyl; 4-*N*-oxide
Paliperidone ER	28	23 hr	Renal unchanged (59%) CYP3A4 and multiple pathways	None known
Quetiapine	9 ± 4	6.88 hr	**CYP3A4**, CYP3A5	N-desalkylquetiapine
Quetiapine XR		7 hr	**CYP3A4**, CYP3A5	N-desalkylquetiapine
Risperidone	68	3-24 hr	**CYP2D6**, CYP3A4	9-OH-risperidone
Ziprasidone	59	4-10 hr	Aldehyde oxidase, CYP3A4, CYP1A2	None

UGT, UDP glucuronosyltransferases genes; FMO3, flavin containing monooxygenase 3 gene; SL, sublingual.

[a]**Bold** print indicates major pathway.

Data from References 27-29, 33, 60, and 63-67.

TABLE 87-7 Relative Incidence of Adverse Medication Reactions from Commonly Used Antipsychotics[a,b]

	Sedation	EPS	Anticholinergic	Orthostasis	Weight Gain	Prolactin
Aripiprazole	+	+[c]	+	+	+	±
Asenapine	++	+/++	+	+	++	+
Brexpiprazole	+	+	±	+	+	+
Cariprazine	±	+/++[c]	+	+	+	+
Chlorpromazine	+++	+++	++++	++++	++	++
Clozapine	++++	+	++++	++++	++++	±
Fluphenazine	+	++++	+	+	+	+++
Haloperidol	++	++++	+	+	+	+++
Iloperidone	+	±	+++	+++	+++	+
Lumateperone	+	±	+	+	+	+
Lurasidone	++	+/++[c]	+	+	+	++
Olanzapine	++	++	+++	++	++++	+
Paliperidone	+	++	+	+	++	++++
Perphenazine	+	++++	+	+	+	+++
Quetiapine	+++	+	++++	++	+++	+
Risperidone	++	++	+	++	++	++++
Thioridazine	++	+++	++++	++++	+	+++
Thiothixene	++	++++	+	+	+	+++
Ziprasidone	++	++	+	+	+	+

EPS, extrapyramidal side effects—includes dystonias, parkinsonism, akathisia, and tardive dyskinesia.

Relative side effect risk: ±, negligible; +, low; ++, moderate; +++, moderately high; ++++, high.

[a]Adverse medication reactions shown are relative risk based on doses within the recommended therapeutic range.

[b]Individual patient risk varies depending on patient-specific factors.

[c]Primarily akathisia.

Endocrine System Within the hypothalamic tuberoinfundibular tract, DA blockade results in increased prolactin levels with hyperprolactinemia occurring in up to 71% of patients diagnosed with schizophrenia and treated with antipsychotics.[68] While US-based studies show no sex difference in the incidence of antipsychotic-induced hyperprolactinemia, UK-based studies suggest females are twice as likely to experience antipsychotic-induced hyperprolactinemia than males (52% vs 26%, respectively).[68,69] The major symptoms associated with hyperprolactinemia are gynecomastia, galactorrhea, menstrual irregularities, infertility, and sexual dysfunction. Although the clinical significance is unclear, chronic hyperprolactinemia has been associated with decreased bone mineral density, which may put patients at higher risk of osteoporosis.[70] Tolerance does not appear to develop to antipsychotic-induced hyperprolactinemia.[71] In general, FGAs are associated with higher rates of hyperprolactinemia than SGAs, the exceptions being risperidone and paliperidone which have reported rates exceeding 70%.[68,69,71] As they have poor penetration of the blood-brain barrier, their greater presence at D_2 receptors in the pituitary gland may be contributing to this adverse effect.[68,69,71] On the other hand, a D_2 partial agonist, aripiprazole is more prolactin sparing and other newer antipsychotics including asenapine, iloperidone, lurasidone, brexpiprazole, cariprazine, and lumateprone have not been shown to induce clinically meaningful changes in prolactin levels.[27,28,30,68,72,73]

If a patient experiences symptomatic hyperprolactinemia, switching to an agent that has minimal sustained effect on prolactin is a reasonable treatment option, as is attempting to lower the antipsychotic dose. However, both interventions run the risk of relapse. Augmentation with aripiprazole 5 to 30 mg daily may help reduce risperidone-induced hyperprolactinemia.[74] However, there have also been case series reporting symptom exacerbation with the addition of aripiprazole and, in general, antipsychotic polypharmacy is discouraged.[68] Dopamine agonists, bromocriptine, cabergoline, and pramipexole have been shown to decrease prolactin, but this approach is not recommended due to the lack of controlled trials, as well as reports of psychosis exacerbation.[68] For females with schizophrenia who suffer from amenorrhea due to antipsychotic-induced hyperprolactinemia, metformin 750 to 1,500 mg/day has been shown to restore menstrual function, with associated reduction in prolactin level.[75] While this is a potentially appealing intervention, especially in patients who are gaining weight and at risk for Type 2 diabetes mellitus (T2DM), additional evidence is needed before recommending metformin as a first-line intervention for females with antipsychotic-induced hyperprolactinemia.[75]

Weight gain is frequently reported in both adults and children receiving antipsychotics,[76,77] and is often seen within the first 12 weeks of antipsychotic initiation, with the rate of weight gain decreasing over time.[76,77] The risk of cardiovascular-related mortality is higher in individuals with schizophrenia,[78] and this is further aggravated by medication-related weight gain and the high prevalence of smoking. Additionally, obesity is a risk factor for diabetes mellitus.[78,79] Weight gain during treatment is concerning for patients and a reason for poor medication adherence.[55] Clozapine and olanzapine have the highest rates of antipsychotic-induced weight gain (AIWG), with olanzapine being the most studied and likely producing the highest risk. Mid-risk antipsychotics include asenapine, iloperidone, paliperidone, quetiapine, and risperidone. Aripiprazole, lurasidone, and ziprasidone are associated with the lowest risk of AIWG.[28,30,72,76] Newer agents, brexpiprazole, cariprazine and lumateperone, also appear to have low risk of AIWG, similar to aripiprazole.[31,33,73]

Although the exact mechanism for AWIG uncertain, it has been associated with antihistaminic effects, antimuscarinic effects, adrenaline alpha-1, and blockade of 5-HT_{2C} receptors.[77] However, dietary factors and activity levels can play a significant role in this population, as well as nourishment after a period of poor self-care. The risk of weight gain may be greater in patients with their first psychotic episode and those who are underweight at baseline.

Several different genetic variations have been associated with predisposition for AIWG. The 5-HT_{2c} gene and its relationship to AIWG is the most extensively studied polymorphism.[64,80] A meta-analysis of all genetic studies looking at the C–759T promoter region polymorphism of the $5\text{-}HT_{2C}$ receptor gene confirmed the relationship with AIWG. While the C allele is the major allele in the population, the meta-analysis found that T allele is protective against AIWG.[80] In this same meta-analysis, polymorphisms of dopamine receptor D_2 (*D2*), alpha-2 adrenergic receptor (α_2), and melanocortin-4 receptor (*MC4R*) genes were also found to be associated with AIWG. Insulin-induced gene 2 (*INSIG2*) and Guanine Nucleotide Binding Protein (*GNB3*) had smaller effect sizes, but were also found to be associated with AIWG. Polymorphisms in leptin and leptin receptor genes, methylenetetrahydrofolate reductase (*MTHFR*), and brain-derived neurotrophic factor (*BDNF*) gene have been genetic targets; however, results are inconsistent regarding a potential relationship between these polymorphisms and AIWG.[64,80,81] In general, AIWG is most likely polygenic and impacted by environmental factors.

The combination of olanzapine and samidorphan was FDA-approved for use in schizophrenia and bipolar disorder in May 2021. The addition of samidorphan, a functional opioid antagonist, to olanzapine is a novel approach to attenuate olanzapine-induced weight gain. In a 24-week Phase 3 trial, the olanzapine/samidorphan combination resulted in significantly less weight gain compared to olanzapine monotherapy, with the mean increase in weight of 3.18 kg (7.01 lb) and 5.08 kg (11.2 lb), respectively.[82] Additionally, significantly fewer subjects in the combination group had >7% weight gain as compared to olanzapine monotherapy (27.5% vs 42.7%, respectively). Unfortunately, the olanzapine/samidorphan combination did not result in any metabolic benefit when compared to olanzapine monotherapy.[82]

Several other approaches have been recommended to address weight gain. Switching the antipsychotic to another agent with less weight gain liability is one choice, and an American Diabetes Association consensus task force recommends consideration of a change in antipsychotic if a patient gains more than 5% of baseline body weight after starting the medication.[83] Metformin is effective in treating AIWG with a meta-analysis indicating an average of a 3.17 kg (6.99 lb) weight loss compared with placebo.[84] Dietary restriction, exercise, and behavior modification programs are reported to be successful. Both the Reducing Weight and Diabetes Risk in an Underserved Population (STRIDE) and the Randomized Trial of Achieving Healthy Lifestyles in Psychiatric Rehabilitation (ACHIEVE) clinical trials showed behavioral weight loss interventions resulted in significant weight loss in patients with mental illness receiving antipsychotics. The STRIDE study also showed reductions in fasting glucose over 6- and 12-month periods using such interventions.[80,85,86]

The Improving Metabolic Parameters in Antipsychotic Child Treatment (IMPACT) trial is the only randomized trial to compare different strategies to address overweight/obese youth who had experienced significant weight gain on antipsychotics.[87] All groups received health lifestyle education and were randomized to either the addition of metformin, a switch to aripiprazole, or continueing their baseline antipsychotic. In this 24-week trial, the additional of metformin or a switch to aripiprazole resulted in a decrease in BMI z-score where continued antipsychotic resulted in an increase.[87]

Patients with schizophrenia have a twofold higher prevalence of T2DM compared with the general population.[78] While the illness itself contributes to elevated risk, antipsychotics are a major contributing factor, with individuals exposed to antipsychotics having higher rates of T2DM than those unexposed.[78,79] The exact mechanism by which antipsychotics elevate the risk of T2DM is unknown.

While weight gain seen with antipsychotics can lead to insulin resistance and elevated risk of T2DM, a systematic review of antipsychotic-associated diabetic ketoacidosis (DKA) found that weight gain was only associated with roughly half of the included cases, and DKA was often the first indicator of a diabetes diagnosis. The SGAs can rapidly and directly influence glucose metabolism independent of AIWG and adiposity.[88] Antipsychotics also may directly cause T2DM through increased insulin resistance or impaired β-cell function or a combination of the two.[79] The greatest increase in glucose impairment typically occurs during the first 14 weeks of treatment,[85] and for clozapine, olanzapine, quetiapine, and risperidone nearly 60% of new-onset diabetes occurred within the first 6 months of treatment initiation.[83,85]

The FDA-approved product labeling for all SGAs reflects the increased risk of diabetes mellitus in patients taking these medications, but risk varies based on the antipsychotic. Clozapine and olanzapine have the highest risk of new-onset diabetes followed by quetiapine and risperidone, while the risk appears lowest with ziprasidone and aripiprazole.[83,85] Although inadequate data are available for asenapine, iloperidone, lurasidone, brexpiprazole, cariprazine, and lumateperone, their risk also appears low.[33,89] Olanzapine is not recommended as a first-line antipsychotic option due to its metabolic risks[14,22,23]; therefore, designing care models and standards for managing diabetes in patients with schizophrenia is important in addressing this major health problem.

Cardiovascular System

Orthostatic Hypotension Orthostatic hypotension, thought to be caused by α-adrenergic blockade, is a common adverse reaction of antipsychotics.[90] Clozapine and quetiapine had the highest incidence of orthostatic hypotension in the CATIE study, and iloperidone appears to have the highest risk among newer SGAs.[90] Orthostatic hypotension can occur in any patient, but patients with diabetes and preexisting cardiovascular disease and older adults are particularly predisposed. Other risk factors may include dehydration, presence of alcohol associated neuropathy and antipsychotic combination treatment.[90,91] Patients should be advised to avoid sudden positional changes to allow for adaptation. Tolerance to orthostatic hypotension may occur within 2 to 3 months. If not, lower doses or a change to an antipsychotic with less α-blockade can be attempted. Fluid resuscitation or increasing salt intake may also help minimize orthostatic blood pressure changes.[90,91]

Electrocardiographic Changes The electrocardiographic (ECG) changes seen with antipsychotics include increased heart rate (through sinus tachycardia from anticholinergic effects, or reflex tachycardia from α-adrenergic blockade), flattened T waves, ST segment depression, and prolongation of QT and PR intervals. The most clinically important of these potential changes is prolongation of the QTc interval, which has been associated with ventricular arrhythmias, including torsade de pointes syndrome. This is thought to occur as a result of blockade of the cardiac delayed potassium rectifier channel as well as impairment in autonomic function.[89,91] Among the antipsychotics, thioridazine is most likely to cause these changes and has been shown to prolong the QTc an average of about 30 msec, which is over 20 msec longer than haloperidol, risperidone, olanzapine, or quetiapine, and 15 msec longer than ziprasidone.[92] Thioridazine's effect on QTc prolongation is dose related, and has led to a boxed warning in the FDA-approved product labeling. A comprehensive review was not able to stratify the degree of QTc prolongation of nine different SGAs.[93] Iloperidone, however, is subject to pharmacogenomic differences in metabolism, and there may be an increased risk of QTc prolongation in CYP2D6 poor metabolizers.[27] High IV doses of haloperidol elevate the risk for QTc prolongation, resulting in a boxed warning in the FDA-approved labeling.[94] Although the precise point at which QTc prolongation becomes clinically dangerous is unclear, the risk for arrhythmia escalates when the QTc interval exceeds 500 msec, or is 60 msec above the baseline QTc.[93,94] Accordingly, it has been recommended to discontinue a medication associated with QTc prolongation if the interval consistently exceeds 500 msec. QTc intervals greater than or equal to 450 msec and/or a 30 msec increase in QTc interval from baseline may be predictors of a medication's risk to cause torsades.[93]

While QTc prolongation may predict torsade de pointes, it rarely happens in the absence of other risks factors, including patients greater than 60 years, female gender, those with preexisting cardiac or cerebrovascular disease (including bradycardia, second- or third-degree AV block, and congenital long QTc syndrome), hepatic impairment, hypokalemia, hypomagnesemia, concomitant medications that prolong the QTc interval, metabolic inhibition by another medication, or preexisting QTc prolongation.[93,94] For patients over the age of 50 years of age, a pretreatment ECG is recommended, as are baseline serum potassium and magnesium levels.

Myocarditis and Cardiomyopathy Myocarditis is an infrequent and dose independent adverse effect that is most likely to occur with clozapine, but has been reported with quetiapine,[90] and possibly with olanzapine.[95] Eighty-seven percent of clozapine-induced myocarditis cases occur within the first 4 weeks of treatment, but cases as late as 22 weeks have been reported.[89,96] Symptoms of clozapine-induced myocarditis can be nonspecific and include: flu-like symptoms (eg, fever, myalgias), respiratory (eg, dyspnea, cough, orthopnea), and cardiac (persistent tachycardia, chest pain, syncope) symptoms. Myocarditis is considered a life-threatening event and therefore early detection is essential. While the incidence of clozapine-induced myocarditis may be as high as 3%, and the mortality rate upwards of 10% to 30%, there are no mandatory monitoring parameters.[96] Recommended laboratory monitoring has been proposed with baseline and weekly monitoring of C-Reactive Protein (CRP) for the first 4 weeks, while troponin (I or T) and B-type natriuretic peptide monitoring has also been suggested. A baseline echocardiogram (ECHO) is recommended and repeated if myocarditis is suspected. Both CRP elevations above 100 mg/L and troponin greater than two times the upper limit of normal have been shown to be highly sensitive in detecting clozapine-induced myocarditis. Clozapine rechallenge after the occurrence of myocarditis is debated, and only a few cases have been reported. The decision to rechallenge should only be made in patients where the clinical value greatly outweighs the potential risk, and only after full resolution of the myocarditis and no signs of permanent cardiac damage. A rechallenge should be conducted in a hospital where close monitoring can occur, as myocarditis recurrence during rechallenge has been reported.[96]

Cardiomyopathy, a potentially life-threatening adverse effect, can also be seen with clozapine, which typically presents later during treatment than myocarditis, with an average time of onset of 14 months.[96,97] The current incidence of cardiomyopathy is estimated to be 0.02% to 0.1%, but this adverse effect may be under-reported,[97] as shortness of breath, palpitations, and fatigue are the most frequently reported symptoms. The diagnosis of cardiomyopathy is typically made with an ECHO with a reduction in ejection fraction (EF) being the most consistent finding. For patients with an EF less than 25%, lower recovery and higher mortality rates have been seen, whereas those with an EF greater than 40% typically fully recover.[97] In suspected cases of clozapine-induced cardiomyopathy, clozapine should be discontinued, and a rechallenge is not recommended.[98]

Sudden Cardiac Death The risk of sudden cardiac death (SCD) with use of FGAs and SGAs is reported to be twice that of nonusers, with risk increasing with escalated dose.[89,90] Fifteen cases of SCD may occur per 10,000 years of antipsychotic exposure.[89,90] There is insufficient evidence to confer a greater risk with one class of antipsychotics over another.[89,90] A case-crossover study involving over 17,000 patients showed that antipsychotic use was associated with a

1.53-fold increase in ventricular arrhythmia or SCD. The magnitude of effect was greatest among patients who received antipsychotics for a short term (less than 28 days).[99] Nonetheless, prospectively designed studies are needed to confirm dose-dependency with antipsychotic-associated cardiovascular sudden death, and whether risk is different among antipsychotics.

Lipid Changes Treatment with at least some SGAs and phenothiazines is associated with elevated serum triglycerides and cholesterol. Among the SGAs, olanzapine, clozapine, and quetiapine have the highest risk for dyslipidemia, with elevations in serum triglycerides being the most frequently reported abnormality.[28,30] Increased appetite and subsequent weight increase can negatively affect lipids. Independent of weight gain, antipsychotic effects on apolipoprotein B, lipoprotein oxidation, and elevations in sterol regulatory element binding protein-controlled gene expression are among possible mechanisms by which lipid changes may occur with antipsychotics.[100] As previously discussed, olanzapine is associated with greater and significant adverse effects on metabolic parameters, including lipids, blood glucose, and body weight as compared with other antipsychotics in the CATIE trial.[17]

The occurrence of weight gain, diabetes, and lipid abnormalities during antipsychotic therapy is consistent with the development of metabolic syndrome, and cohorts of patients with schizophrenia have shown elevated prevalence of metabolic syndrome as compared with general population cohorts. Prevalence rates of metabolic syndrome in US populations treated with antipsychotics range from 28% to 60%, with 40.9% reported in the prospectively designed CATIE trial.[101]

Metabolic syndrome consists of raised triglycerides (greater than or equal to 150 mg/dL [1.70 mmol/L]), low HDL cholesterol (less than or equal to 40 mg/dL [1.03 mmol/L] for males, less than or equal to 50 mg/dL [1.29 mmol/L] for females), elevated fasting glucose (greater than or equal to 100 mg/dL [5.6 mmol/L]), blood pressure elevation (greater than or equal to 130/85 mm Hg), and weight gain (abdominal circumference greater than 102 cm [40 in.] for males, greater than 89 cm [35 in.] in females).[102] A diagnosis of metabolic syndrome can be made in individuals who meet at least three of these criteria. Therefore, these abnormalities dictate an important role for general health screening and monitoring in patients with schizophrenia, and prompt intervention when such abnormalities occur. The propensity of individual antipsychotics to produce metabolic disturbances should be considered in the context of individual patient risk factors at the time of medication selection.

Thromboembolism Compared to the general population, the risk of venous thromboembolism (VTE) is twofold higher in individuals with schizophrenia. Sedentary lifestyle, smoking, and metabolic syndrome are all potential explanations for the higher incidence. Increased rates have also been reported in stuporous catatonia and prolonged physical restraints. Additionally, both FGAs and SGAs have been associated with elevating the risk of VTE. The risk may be highest within the first 30 days of antipsychotic exposure and with higher doses. Although the mechanism for increased VTE risk is unknown, increased sedative adverse medication reactions, metabolic effects, antipsychotic effect on platelet aggregation, and hyperprolactinemia indirectly increasing venous stasis have been proposed.[103] The QThrombosis (https://qthrombosis.org/) is a validated VTE risk calculator that includes antipsychotics in the risk assessment model.[104] This tool may be helpful in identifying patients at elevated risk for VTE and can easily be implemented in clinic practice.

Anticholinergic Effects Patients receiving antipsychotics or antipsychotics in combination with anticholinergics can experience anticholinergic adverse reactions (eg, dry mouth, constipation, tachycardia, blurred vision, inhibition or impairment of ejaculation, urinary retention, or impaired memory). These adverse medication reactions are particularly seen with low-potency FGAs, and in older adult patients who are especially sensitive to these effects. Of the SGAs, clozapine and olanzapine have moderately high rates of anticholinergic effects. Constipation, caused by slowed peristaltic movement and decreased intestinal fluid content, should be closely monitored and treated, especially in older adults. Paralytic ileus and necrotizing enterocolitis can also occur.[89,90]

Central Nervous System

Extrapyramidal System Extrapyramidal symptoms (EPS) is an umbrella term used to describe antipsychotic-induced movement symptoms due to excess dopamine blockade in the nigrostriatal pathway. These symptoms include: dystonia, akathisia, parkinsonism, and tardive dyskinesia, which are explained in detail below.

Dystonia Dystonia is a state of abnormal tonicity, sometimes described simplistically as a severe "muscle spasm.[105] More accurately, dystonias are prolonged tonic contractions, with a rapid onset, usually within 24 to 96 hours of initiating or increasing the dose of an antipsychotic.[106] Types of dystonic reactions include trismus, glossospasm, tongue protrusion, pharyngeal–laryngeal spasms, blepharospasm, oculogyric crisis, torticollis, and retrocollis, but can occur with any skeletal muscle group. They can be life-threatening, as in the case of pharyngeal–laryngeal dystonias, and can contribute significantly to patient medication nonadherence. Dystonic reactions occur primarily with high potency FGAs and are greatly reduced with SGAs. Risk factors for dystonia include younger patients, male sex, the use of high-potency agents, rapid titration, and high dosage. The overall incidence from the 1960s to the mid-1970s ranged from 2.3% to 10%, but as higher-potency traditional antipsychotics became more widely used, the rate increased to as high as 64%.

Intramuscular or IV anticholinergics (Table 87-8) are the treatment of choice for dystonias, with benzodiazepines being a second-line option.[106] Benztropine 2 mg or diphenhydramine 50 mg can be given IM or IV, whereas diazepam 5 to 10 mg by slow IV push or lorazepam 1 to 2 mg intramuscularly are treatment alternatives. Relief from the dystonia is typically seen within 15 to 20 minutes of an IM injection or within 5 minutes of IV administration.

TABLE 87-8 Agents Used to Treat Extrapyramidal Symptoms

Generic Name	Equivalent Dose (mg)	Daily Dosage Range (mg)
Antimuscarinic		
Benztropine[a]	1	1-8[b]
Biperiden[a]	2	2-8
Trihexyphenidyl	2	2-15
Antihistamine		
Diphenhydramine[a]	50	50-400
Dopamine Agonist		
Amantadine	NA	100-400
Benzodiazepine		
Lorazepam[a]	NA	1-8
Diazepam	NA	2-20
Clonazepam	NA	2-8
β-Blocker		
Propranolol	NA	20-160

NA, Not applicable.

[a]Injectable dosage form can be given intramuscularly for relief of acute dystonia.

[b]In treatment-refractory cases, dosage can be titrated to 12 mg/day with careful monitoring; nonlinear pharmacokinetics have been reported.

The antipsychotic can be continued, with concomitant short-term use of an oral anticholinergic, which is then subsequently tapered and stopped. In general, prophylactic anticholinergic medications are not recommended routinely. However, prophylaxis is reasonable when using high-potency FGAs (eg, haloperidol or fluphenazine) in young males and in patients with a history of dystonia.[105] Dystonias can also be minimized by the use of lower initial FGA doses or the use of SGAs. Anticholinergics are good choices for prophylaxis, whereas amantadine has not been proven effective for this purpose.

Akathisia Akathisia is defined as the inability to sit still and having functional motor restlessness. The most accurate diagnosis is made by combining subjective patient reports with objective observations (pacing, shifting, shuffling, or tapping feet). Subjectively, patients may describe a feeling of inner restlessness or disquiet or a compulsion to move or remain in constant motion that provides some relief. Akathisia occurs in 20% to 40% of patients treated with high-potency FGAs[105,107] and is frequently accompanied by dysphoria. In severe cases, akathisia may be mistaken for aggression and if left untreated, has been linked to insomnia, increased suicidality, and development of tardive dyskinesia.[107]

Akathisia generally appears early in antipsychotic treatment, but can be chronic if not appropriately addressed.[107] Risk of akathisia is greater when the antipsychotic dose is increased rapidly or multiple antipsychotics are used, as well as in antipsychotic naïve individuals.[107] Traditionally, a reduction in antipsychotic dosage has been considered the best intervention; however, this might not be a realistic goal in a patient with acute psychosis. A logical alternative is to switch to an antipsychotic with a lower risk of akathisia, or an antipsychotic the patient previously tolerated. Akathisia can occasionally occur with SGAs, particularly aripiprazole, cariprazine, lurasidone, or risperidone. Iloperidone, quetiapine, and clozapine appear to have the lowest risk of producing akathisia.[72,107]

Unlike acute dystonias, akathisia responds poorly to anticholinergics[107]; therefore, benzodiazepines have been used for treatment of akathisia, but the high prevalence of co-occurring substance use disorders in schizophrenia discourages their use.[107] The β-blockers (eg, propranolol in doses up to 160 mg daily) are effective and have the most evidence.[105,107] Additionally, 5-HT_2 receptor antagonists may be protective against akathisia and may be used for its management. Examples of such agents include mirtazapine, trazodone, and cyproheptadine, with mirtazapine having the most data to support its use.[105,107]

Parkinson Symptoms Antipsychotic-induced parkinson symptoms resemble idiopathic Parkinson disease with symptom onset typically within 1 to 2 weeks after antipsychotic initiation or a dose increase. For some it may be delayed with 50% to 75% of cases occurring within a month and 90% within 3 months.[105,106] A patient with antipsychotic-induced parkinson symptoms can present with any of four cardinal symptoms: (a) akinesia, bradykinesia, or decreased motor activity including difficulty initiating movement, as well as extreme slowness, mask-like facial expression, micrographia, slowed speech, and decreased arm swing; (b) tremor that is predominant at rest and decreases with movement, and known as the pill-rolling type, usually involves the fingers and hands, although tremors can also be seen in the arms, legs, neck, head, and chin; (c) cogwheel rigidity, seen as the patient's limbs yielding in jerky, ratchet-like fashion when passively moved by the examiner; and (d) postural abnormalities and instability manifested as stooped posture, difficulty in maintaining stability when changing body position, and a gait that ranges from slow and shuffling to festinating. Fatigue and weakness can be noted, as well as oral abnormalities including dysphagia, dysarthria, and abnormal palmomental and glabellar reflexes. The overall incidence of FGA-induced parkinson symptoms ranges from 15.4% to 36%, depending on the medication and dose, and akinesia alone can be seen in 59% of patients on high-potency FGAs. The risk of parkinson symptoms with SGAs is low. A secondary data analysis from the CATIE study did not find marked differences in rates of EPS between perphenazine and SGAs, suggesting that a less potent FGA at modest doses may present a similar risk of parkinson symptoms as SGAs.[108] Other risk factors for the development of parkinson symptoms include increasing age and possibly female sex.

The efficacy of anticholinergic medications in treating antipsychotic-induced parkinson symptoms is well established,[105,106] although diphenhydramine produces more sedation than the other agents. Table 87-7 outlines the dosing of these medications. Symptoms typically begin to resolve within 3 to 4 days after initiation of treatment, but a minimum of at least 2 weeks of treatment is normally required for full response. Amantadine may be as efficacious for parkinson symptoms as anticholinergics, but with significantly less impact on cognition.[105,106] Prophylactic use of these agents against parkinson symptoms is less convincing compared with dystonias, and is unnecessary when using SGAs.[105,106] The long-term treatment of parkinson symptoms with antiparkinson medication is somewhat controversial. An attempt should be made to taper and discontinue these agents in 6 weeks to 3 months after symptom resolution. If symptoms reappear, then switching to an SGA should be considered. Quetiapine, aripiprazole, brexpiprazole, iloperidone, asenapine, lumateperone, and clozapine are reasonable alternatives in a patient experiencing EPS with other SGAs.[33,72,109]

Tardive Dyskinesia Tardive dyskinesia (TD) is a syndrome characterized by abnormal involuntary hyperkinetic movements occurring late in onset in relation to initiation of antipsychotic therapy. The classic description of tardive dyskinesia is an insidious onset of oral or orofacial movements often associated with lip smacking or tongue thrusting as the disorder progresses, which can interfere with the patient's ability to chew, speak, or swallow. Other facial movements include frequent blinking, brow arching, grimacing, and upward deviation of the eyes. Involvement of the extremities sometimes occurs, and may involve any skeletal muscle group. Orofacial movements are more common in older patients, whereas the truncal axial movements are classically reported in young adults. Movements can worsen with stress, decrease with sedation, and disappear during sleep. Concentration on motor tasks or attempts to suppress the movements can increase them.[110]

Early signs of tardive dyskinesia can be reversible but if allowed to persist, can become irreversible, even with medication discontinuation. The exact time point in which TD becomes irreversible is unknown, which underscores the importance of early detection.[106] When the antipsychotic dose is decreased or tapered and discontinued, worsening of abnormal movements may occur, followed by possible slow improvement after months or years if the patient remains on lower doses or discontinues treatment. Younger age correlates with a greater chance of reversing TD.[106] No standardized diagnostic criteria for tardive dyskinesia are available. Abnormal involuntary movements can be detected early through physical assessment and the use of rating scales. Available rating scales include the Abnormal Involuntary Movement Scale (AIMS) and the Dyskinesia Identification System: Condensed User Scale (DISCUS).[109] Neither scale is diagnostic (see Chapter e81).

One of the greatest risk factors for TD is older age, with patients over 65 having a two-to-fivefold higher incidence of TD than younger adults.[111] Other possible risk factors include history of acute EPS, poor antipsychotic medication response, diagnosis of organic mental disorders, diabetes mellitus, mood disorders, female sex, use of anticholinergics, current and cumulative antipsychotic doses, and duration of antipsychotic exposure.[110] Additionally, genetic variation within CYP2D6, vesicular monoamine transporter-2 (VMAT2) gene, and D_2 receptor gene have been suggested as being associated with increased risk.[112] A systematic review of 12 studies lasting 1 year or more found the overall risk of TD with SGAs to be approximately 2.9% per year in adults under 65 years of age as compared with 7.7% for FGAs.[113] These results were confirmed with a meta-analysis which indicated that olanzapine and aripiprazole may have a small advantage over other non-clozapine SGAs.[114] Tardive dyskinesia is not always permanent, with spontaneous remission of symptoms observed in 25% of patients after 5 years of continued treatment[24]; however, overall morbidity and mortality are greater in tardive dyskinesia patients.

Prevention of TD is important, as treatment of the movements once they occur is difficult. One of the more compelling arguments for the first-line use of SGAs is their lower risk of TD.[24] Therefore, regular neurologic examinations (AIMS or other scales) should be performed at baseline, and APA guidelines recommend TD monitoring at least every 6 months for those at high risk and every 12 months for all others.[22] At the first sign of TD, the need for continuing antipsychotic treatment should be assessed, and if the patient is taking an FGA and continuing treatment is indicated, the medication should be switched to an SGA.

The VMAT2 inhibitors deutetrabenazine and valbenazine are FDA-approved medications for the treatment of TD. Both are considered first-line interventions, as they produced clinically significant decreases in AIMS scores in both short- and long-term trials.[115] However, when valbenazine treatment is discontinued, TD symptoms can rapidly return toward pretreatment levels within 4 weeks after discontinuation.[116]

Deutetrabenzine should be initiated at 6 mg twice daily with food, with weekly dose increases of 6 mg up to a maximum dose of 48 mg per day. It is primarily metabolized via CYP2D6 and a maximum daily dose of 36 mg is recommended with concomitant strong CYP2D6 inhibitors or in CYP2D6 poor metabolizers.[103] It is contraindicated in individuals with severe hepatic impairment or those taking a monoamine oxidase inhibitor. Valbenazine is initiated at 40 mg once daily and increased to 80 mg after 1 week. This medication is not recommended for use in combination with strong CYP3A4 inducers, and a maximum daily dose of 40 mg is recommended when used with CYP3A4 strong inhibitors. Use in individuals with severe renal impairment is not recommended. Labeling for both deutetrabenzine and valbenazine includes warnings about suicidality, depression, and QTc prolongation.[115,116]

Numerous other medications have been used to treat tardive dyskinesia. In two controlled trials lasting 22 to 52 weeks, clozapine decreased abnormal involuntary movement[24]; therefore, switching to clozapine has been recommended as a treatment for moderate-to-severe TD.[14,22-24] A 2013 guideline developed by the American Academy of Neurology (AAN) recommended short-term treatment of TD with either clonazepam (up to 4.5 mg daily) or ginkgo biloba extract 240 mg daily based upon randomized clinical trial data. However, long-term treatment data are lacking.[117] The AAN guideline was developed before the availability of the two VMAT2 inhibitors. However, in patients who do not have access to these agents, or do not tolerate or respond with their use, clonazepam or ginkgo biloba can be considered.[115]

Seizures An increased risk of medication-induced seizures can occur in patients receiving antipsychotics as these agents decrease the seizure threshold. However, this risk is greater if the following predisposing factors are present: preexisting seizure disorder, history of medication-induced seizure, abnormal electroencephalogram (EEG), and preexisting CNS pathology or head trauma. Seizures are more closely associated with high plasma concentrations, rapid dosage titration, and treatment initiation. The exact mechanism is unknown, but involvement of D_2 and D_s receptors has been proposed.[90] When an isolated seizure occurs, a dosage reduction of the antipsychotic is first recommended, and routine prophylactic use of antiseizure medication is not recommended. Although spontaneously occurring seizures have been reported with most antipsychotics, the highest potential risk for an antipsychotic-related seizure is with clozapine or chlorpromazine. If a change in antipsychotic therapy is required because of a medication-induced seizure, aripiprazole, risperidone, thioridazine, haloperidol, pimozide, trifluoperazine, and fluphenazine are associated with the lowest potential.[90]

Thermoregulation Poikilothermia, the body temperature adjusting to the ambient temperature, can be a serious adverse reaction in temperature extremes.[118] Hyperpyrexia can be a danger in hot weather or during exercise. Additionally, inhibition of sweating, a result of anticholinergic properties impairing the peripheral mechanisms of heat dissipation can contribute to this problem, which in its severest form can lead to heat stroke. Hypothermia is a risk in cold temperatures, particularly in older adults. All patients receiving antipsychotics should be educated about these potential problems. Thermoregulatory problems are reportedly more common with the use of low-potency FGAs, but can occur with the more anticholinergic SGAs.

Neuroleptic Malignant Syndrome Neuroleptic malignant syndrome (NMS) occurs in <1% of patients and is reported with both FGAs and SGAs, with the highest incidence occurring with high-potency FGAs.[90] High antipsychotic doses, rapid parenteral administration, use of multiple antipsychotics, previous history of NMS, dehydration, physical restraints, and older age all increase the risk.[90] Symptoms are most likely to occur within the first week of antipsychotic initiation and develop rapidly over the course of 24 to 72 hours. The mortality rates associated with NMS is high at approximately 10%, with premorbid dehydration elevating the risk of mortality.

Possible mechanisms of NMS include disruption of the central thermoregulatory processes or excess production of heat secondary to skeletal muscle contractions, including the involvement of proinflammatory cytokines. Regardless of the mechanism, the differential diagnoses for NMS include: heat stroke, lethal catatonia, malignant hyperthermia, anticholinergic toxicity, and serotonin toxicity. The cardinal signs and symptoms of NMS are body temperature exceeding 38°C (100.4°F) on at least two occasions, mental status changes, autonomic instability (tachycardia, blood pressure, diaphoresis, tachypnea, or urinary or fecal incontinence), and rigidity.[119] Laboratory evaluation, although nonspecific, frequently shows leukocytosis with or without a left shift, and increases in creatine kinase, aspartate aminotransferase, alanine aminotransferase, lactate dehydrogenase, and myoglobinuria.[118,119] Importantly, NMS treatment should begin with antipsychotic discontinuation and supportive care (eg, IV fluid hydration and benzodiazepines). Dantrolene, bromocriptine, or amantadine may be useful in severe cases as all three agents have reports of reduced time to clinical improvement and reduction in mortality rates.[118]

Many patients with schizophrenia, despite having had NMS, will require future antipsychotic pharmacotherapy. The literature suggests that the risk of rechallenge is acceptable in most patients, provided that the patient is observed for an extended period of time (2 weeks or more is suggested) without antipsychotics, that there is careful monitoring, slow dose titration, and that the patient is maintained on the lowest possible dose.[118,119] A different antipsychotic, an SGA or a low-potency FGA, should be used for rechallenge following an episode of NMS.

Psychiatric Adverse Medication Reactions Aripiprazole has been associated with impulse control disorders, including pathological gambling, uncontrolled sexual urges, uncontrolled spending, binge or compulsive eating, and other intense urges. This led to an FDA safety announcement in 2016 and subsequent update to the warnings in the package labeling for all aripiprazole products.[120] Mechanistically the D_2 partial agonist activity and possible D_3 receptor activity seen with aripiprazole have been implicated as potential pathways for these reactions.[120] Clinicians are encouraged to monitor for changes in impulse control behaviors and reduce the dose or stop aripiprazole should urges develop or worsen.

Ophthalmologic Effects Anticholinergic effects of antipsychotics or concomitant antiparkinson medications can exacerbate narrow-angle (angle-closure) glaucoma. Therefore, antipsychotics with low anticholinergic effects should be used in such individuals, and they should be appropriately monitored.[121]

Opaque deposits in the cornea and lens can occur with chronic phenothiazine treatment, with this adverse event occurring most frequently with chlorpromazine. Although visual acuity is not usually affected, periodic ophthalmologic examinations are frequently recommended in patients receiving long-term treatment with phenothiazines, as fully formed cataracts are possible.[121]

Because of cataract development and lenticular changes in animals, baseline and periodic eye examinations are recommended in quetiapine product labeling. However, the effect of quetiapine on lens opacity was found to be no different than risperidone in a 2-year comparative trial.[122] Lastly, retinitis pigmentosa can result from use of thioridazine doses greater than 800 mg daily, due to melanin deposits that can result in permanent visual impairment or blindness.

Genitourinary System Urinary hesitancy and retention, secondary to antipsychotic anticholinergic effects are reported with low-potency FGAs and with clozapine; those with benign prostatic hypertrophy are especially prone to this effect.[90] Reducing the antipsychotic dose or switching to an antipsychotic with less anticholinergic activity may help. Alternatively, bethanecol can be used to treat antipsychotic-induced urinary hesitancy and retention.

Urinary incontinence is thought to be caused by α-blockade, and among the SGAs, it appears to be particularly problematic with clozapine.[90] The incidence has been reported to be as high as 44%, and it can be persistent in 25% of patients. Female sex and previous urinary incontinence can be risk factors for developing incontinence.[90]

Although inadequately studied, multiple mechanisms are likely responsible for sexual dysfunction seen with antipsychotic use, including dopaminergic blockade, hyperprolactinemia, histaminergic blockade, anticholinergic effects, and α-adrenergic blockade. However, unmedicated individuals with schizophrenia also report decreased libido. Most, but not all, studies show a relationship between hyperprolactinemia and sexual dysfunction, including decreased libido, erectile dysfunction, difficulty achieving orgasm, and ejaculatory abnormalities. Risperidone and paliperidone produce at least as much sexual dysfunction as FGAs, while other SGAs, with weak effects on prolactin, produce less sexual dysfunction. Patients experiencing sexual dysfunction with FGAs or risperidone or paliperidone should be switched to an SGA with less effect on prolactin.[123]

Priapism, a sustained and painful erection that is unprovoked and persists for longer than an hour, is increasingly reported with antipsychotic medication use. This is believed to occur because of α_1-adrenergic receptor blockade, leading to intracavernosal blood stasis.[124] This can evolve into a urologic emergency, due to the ischemic nature of the priapism, and as such patients experiencing this adverse event require emergency treatment. If left untreated, priapism may lead to permanent impotence.

Hematologic System Transient leukopenia can occur during initial treatment with antipsychotics; however, it typically does not progress to be clinically significant.[125] Agranulocytosis reportedly occurs in 0.01% of patients receiving FGAs, and more frequently with chlorpromazine and thioridazine. The three antipsychotics with the highest relative risk for neutropenia in rank order are clozapine, chlorpromazine, and olanzapine.[125] The onset is usually within the first 8 weeks of therapy. If the absolute neutrophil count (ANC) is less than 500/μL (0.5×10^9/L), the antipsychotic should be discontinued and the ANC monitored closely until it returns to normal and the patient monitored for the development of secondary infections. Agranulocytosis can initially manifest as a local infection, with sore throat, leukoplakia, erythema, and ulcerations of the pharynx. These symptoms in any patient receiving antipsychotics should signal the immediate need for an ANC. Additionally, isolated rare cases of thrombocytopenia and eosinophilia have been reported.

Agranulocytosis with clozapine has significantly inhibited use of this agent, and it is only available in the United States through the Clozapine REMS Program.[32] The risk of developing neutropenia or agranulocytosis with clozapine is approximately 3% and 0.8%, respectively,[124] and most cases occur between 6 weeks and 6 months. The baseline ANC must be at least 1,500/μL (1.5×10^9/L) to start clozapine, and weekly ANC monitoring for the first 6 months of therapy is mandated in the FDA-approved product labeling. After this time, if the patient's ANC remains greater than 1,500/μL (1.5×10^9/L), the labeling allows monitoring to be decreased to every 2 weeks for the next 6 months. After this, monitoring can be decreased to monthly if all ANCs remain greater than 1,500/μL (1.5×10^9/L). If at any time the ANC drops to less than 500/μL (0.5×10^9/L), clozapine must be discontinued and the ANC monitored daily until it is greater than 1,500/μL (1.5×10^9/L). The FDA-approved product labeling should be consulted for more detailed information regarding ANC monitoring, including monitoring for mild and moderate leukopenia and recommendations for patients with benign ethnic neutropenia.[32]

Dermatologic System Allergic reactions are rare and usually occur within 8 weeks of initiating therapy, manifesting as maculopapular, erythematous, pruritic rashes that are evident on the face, neck, trunk, or extremities. Contact dermatitis, including the oral mucosa, has been reported in patients and medical personnel exposed to FGA liquid formulations. The risk of oral mucosal reactions can be decreased by mixing the FGA concentrate in a sufficient quantity of a nonacidic liquid and swallowing it quickly. Care should be taken in the handling and preparation of liquid FGAs. Ziprasidone's FDA-approved label contains a warning regarding the risk of a rare but fatal skin reaction called *Drug Reaction with Eosinophilia and Systemic Symptoms* (DRESS).[126]

Phenothiazines can absorb ultraviolet light, resulting in the formation of free radicals, which can have damaging effects on the skin. All antipsychotics can cause photosensitivity resulting in erythema and sunburn; therefore, exposure to sunlight should be limited, and patients should be educated about the use of a maximally blocking sunscreen, hats, protective clothing, and sunglasses.[125]

Blue-gray or purplish skin coloration in areas exposed to sunlight occurs in patients receiving higher doses of low-potency phenothiazines during long-term administration, especially with chlorpromazine. This adverse event commonly occurs with concurrent corneal or lens pigmentation.

Miscellaneous Adverse Effects Clozapine-induced sialorrhea (drooling), which is typically prominent at night,[125] affects up to 54% of patients receiving clozapine. The mechanism behind this drooling is unclear; however, two theories exist. The first involves muscarinic receptor activity and clozapine's imbalanced binding affinity to this receptor. The other involves clozapine's α-antagonist activity at the salivary glands leaving unopposed beta-receptor stimulation and hence hyper-salivation.[125] Anticholinergics such as benztropine and atropine, and α-agonists such as clonidine have been used to treat clozapine-related sialorrhea.[127]

Use in Pregnancy and Lactation

The reproductive health of females with schizophrenia has historically received little attention from clinicians or researchers, partly due to reports of lower fertility rates in individuals with schizophrenia. However, with the introduction of more prolactin sparing SGAs (exceptions being risperidone and paliperidone), fertility rates in schizophrenia are increasing.[128] While data on the safety of antipsychotic medication use during pregnancy and lactation are limited, greater than 50% of individuals with schizophrenia who discontinue their medication will experience relapse.[129] Additionally, pregnant individuals with untreated schizophrenia are more likely to use alcohol, tobacco and other substances and are less likely to engage in prenatal care visits.[127] Therefore, these factors may put pregnant individuals and their offspring at greater risk, outweighing any potential risks associated with antipsychotic use.

The risk of teratogenesis with FGAs has not been sufficiently studied, and a specific pattern of teratogenicity has not been found.[130,131] The use of phenothiazines and low dose haloperidol to treat hyperemesis gravidarum provides additional reassurance that FGAs are not major teratogens.[132] Haloperidol is the best studied FGA with approximately 400 reported exposures.[127] With regard to labor and delivery complications, one small study found greater than a twofold elevated risk of preterm birth in pregnant individuals with schizophrenia taking FGAs as compared with those not taking antipsychotics, but did not find an association between FGA exposure and low birth weight or small for gestational age.[133] A major limitation in interpreting this study are the confounding variables such as disease severity, concurrent substance use or other concurrent medications that were not addressed.

Data regarding the safety of SGAs in pregnancy are rapidly increasing but also limited. All SGAs cross the blood-placenta barrier, but to varying degrees. In one study sample, the highest rates of transfer were for olanzapine (72.1%), followed by haloperidol (65.5%) and risperidone (49.2%), with quetiapine being the lowest (24.1%).[134] Among the SGAs, safety data are most abundant for olanzapine, quetiapine, aripiprazole, and risperidone. As a class, SGAs are not thought to be major teratogens. Results from the largest database study to date (9,258 pregnant females with SGA exposure in the first trimester) suggest that the SGAs aripiprazole, olanzapine, quetiapine, risperidone, and ziprasidone collectively do not increase the risk of congenital malformations or cardiac malformation. This finding held true when evaluating each agent individually, except for a small, but statistically significant increase of congenital malformations with risperidone (RR, 1.26; 95% CI, 1.02-1.56).[135-138] A meta-analysis of 12 studies (which did not include the previous study) found a greater risk of congenital malformations with SGA exposure in early pregnancy, but no specific abnormality was identified. In this same study, an increased risk of preterm birth was present in the SGA-treated group. However, healthy females composed the control group in these studies, and the underlying disease state being treated with an SGA is an important confounder.[139] Data on pregnancy exposure with the newer SGAs (eg, asenapine, lurasidone, brexpiprazole, lumateperone, and cariprazine) are minimal or absent. While large, well-controlled studies are still needed to determine the safety of all SGAs during pregnancy, the British Association for Psychopharmacology Consensus Guidelines do not currently consider them major teratogens.[127]

The potential for antipsychotic-related postnatal and gestational complications is of interest. Weight gain associated with SGAs and the potential risk of gestational diabetes should be considered in medication selection. A systematic review that included 10 studies did not find an association between SGAs collectively and gestational diabetes.[140] A retrospective cohort study reported an increased risk of gestational diabetes in individuals who continued quetiapine or olanzapine during the first 20 weeks of pregnancy versus those who discontinued those agents.[141] An increased risk was not observed with risperidone, aripiprazole, or ziprasidone which indicates that risk may differ among SGAs.[127] An increased risk of hypertension in individuals taking antipsychotics during pregnancy as well as venous thromboembolism have also been reported.[128]

Risk of neonatal EPS is increased with in utero exposure to FGAs, with effects in the infant lasting for 3 to 12 months after birth. In 2011, the FDA issued a safety announcement informing healthcare professionals that the pregnancy section of medication labels had been updated for the entire antipsychotic class, highlighting the potential risk for EPS and withdrawal symptoms in newborns exposed to antipsychotics in utero during the third trimester.[142] Symptoms of neonatal withdrawal reported to the FDA included agitation, hypertonia, hypotonia, tremor, somnolence, respiratory distress, and feeding disorder.

To date, little is known about in utero exposure to antipsychotics and neurodevelopmental teratology with most data being derived from case reports and case-series. One case-control study (n=76) reported a transient delay in cognitive, motor, social-emotional, and adaptive behavior in SGA-exposed infants at 2 months of age that resolved by 12 months.[143] One prospective study reported in utero exposure to antipsychotics (n =22) was associated with lower neuromotor screening measures at 6 months of age compared to either antidepressant-exposed infants or no psychotropic exposure.[144] A population-based cohort study of 411,251 children did not find an elevated risk of autism spectrum disorder or attention deficit hyperactivity disorder with in utero exposure to SGAs.[145]

For many individuals with schizophrenia, discontinuing the antipsychotic during pregnancy may not be recommended, despite the lack of safety data. The risk of antipsychotic use must be weighed against the benefits of pharmacotherapy in pregnant individuals experiencing disorganized thoughts, delusions about change in body image or pregnancy, or who are unable to engage in prenatal care.[133] A national pregnancy exposure registry monitors pregnancy outcomes in those exposed to SGAs during pregnancy. Clinicians are encouraged to report SGA use in pregnancy through the registry to assist in gathering safety information. This registry can be accessed at: http://womensmentalhealth.org/clinical-and-research-programs/pregnancyregistry/atypicalantipsychotic.

Data regarding the antipsychotics and human milk are even more limited than their use during pregnancy. Olanzapine is the most studied antipsychotic in lactation (n = 170 exposures), followed by quetiapine (n = 14), risperidone (n = 8), and aripiprazole (n = 4). Overall, olanzapine and quetiapine have reported relative infant doses (RIDs) of less than 2%, meaning that with continued exposure to human milk, infants would only be exposed to 2% of maternal dosage overall.[146] Risperidone (+ 9-OH-risperidone) and aripiprazole have reports of slightly higher RID ranges (2.8-9.1 and 0.7-8.3, respectively).[146] Of note, treatment with aripiprazole may lead to reduced milk production as a result of reduced prolactin release.[147] Breastfeeding while on clozapine is not recommended due to the risk of severe neutropenia and seizures in the infant.[127] For all of the FGAs, the overall RID is thought to be less than 10%, which is a common threshold indicating that these medications are safe when feeding infants human milk.

Data evaluating long-term outcomes in infants exposed to antipsychotics through human milk are minimal to absent. The coadministration of chlorpromazine and haloperidol is reported to result in developmental delays at 12 to 18 months of age; however, these were not controlled studies.[127] Although most antipsychotics are not contraindicated in lactation, the lowest antipsychotic dosage should be used, and the infant carefully monitored for antipsychotic adverse events such as EPS, sedation, seizures, and developmental delays.[127,146,147] Additional studies evaluating short- and long-term adverse effects, including developmental outcomes, of infants exposed to antipsychotics via human milk are warranted.

Medication Interactions

Most medication interactions occur because of pharmacodynamic or pharmacokinetic interactions (Tables 87-9 and 87-10). Common examples of pharmacodynamic interactions resulting in enhanced effect include the excess sedation that can occur when antipsychotics are used concomitantly with other medications that have sedative adverse effects. Additive antimuscarinic effects can also be seen when antipsychotics are used with other medications possessing antimuscarinic effects, potentially resulting in urinary retention, constipation, blurred vision, or other anticholinergic adverse effects.[148] Both combined sedative and anticholinergic effects from multiple medications can result in impaired cognition or delirium, particularly in older adults and other patients predisposed to such problems.[148] Patients are more likely to experience symptomatic orthostatic hypotension when an antipsychotic is used with other medications that cause orthostasis. Metoclopramide, a DA antagonist, is prescribed for treating esophageal reflux or gastroparesis, and patients may be more likely to experience akathisia and other EPS (including TD) if it is used concomitantly with antipsychotics.[149] Although some selective serotonin reuptake inhibitors (SSRIs) can interact with antipsychotics through enzyme inhibition, they can also interact through pharmacodynamic mechanisms. Since 5-HT_2 receptors are present on the presynaptic dopaminergic neuron, their activation leads to decreased DA release from the presynaptic terminal. Increased availability of 5-HT through the SSRI's effect can activate these receptors, which in turn results in decreased DA release, and adds to the dopaminolytic effects of antipsychotics.[57] In the absence of enzyme inhibition, SSRIs can still precipitate akathisia or EPS when added to a patient stabilized on an antipsychotic. Several cases of serotonin syndrome have been reported with SGAs used in combination with serotonergic agents, such as SSRIs or tramadol.[57] Another potentially dangerous interaction can occur when medications that slow myocardial conduction, and thus prolong the QTc interval, are used in combination with antipsychotics having the same effect.[57] Careful monitoring should occur with medications that prolong the QTc interval, as well as when antipsychotics with this effect are combined with diuretics.[57]

Food enhances the absorption of both ziprasidone and lurasidone, with the product labels noting a greater than twofold increase in bioavailability when the agents are given with food (Table 87-10). The exact mechanism for the impact of food on absorption is not fully understood[30,150] but simply doubling the dose in a fasted state will not necessarily double the level.[150] Therefore, ziprasidone requires administration with a 500 kcal (2,100 kJ) meal and 350 kcals (1,460 kJ) with lurasidone.[30,150] Asenapine, on the other hand, requires that food and drink be avoided for at least 10 minutes after administration to reduce the chance of the patient swallowing the medication instead of allowing for sublingual absorption, which as previously discussed, impacts bioavailability.[28,66]

Asenapine inhibits CYP2D6, and is the only SGA that has been shown to significantly affect the pharmacokinetics of other

TABLE 87-9 Common Potential Pharmacodynamic Interactions with Antipsychotic Medications

Mechanism of Interaction	Examples of Interacting Drugs or Other Substances		Clinical Effect
Muscarinic receptor blockade	Anticholinergics Benztropine Diphenhydramine Trihexyphenidyl		Increased risk of anticholinergic adverse reactions
Additive or synergistic sedation	*Sedatives* Benzodiazepines Concomitant AP Diphenhydramine Melatonin and melatonin agonists Mirtazapine Trazodone TCAs Hypnotics Opiates	*Anticholinergics* Benztropine Diphenhydramine Trihexyphenidyl Mirtazapine	Increased risk of sedation Lethargy Impaired cognition Impaired psychomotor activity Risk of accidents
DA antagonist use for different indication	Metoclopramide		Increased risk of EPS
Cardiovascular interactions			
QTc prolongation	Amitriptyline Clomipramine Imipramine Citalopram Fluorquinolone antibiotics	Procainamide Quinidine	Increased risk of ECG changes and dysrhythmias
Electrolyte changes	Diuretics		Increased risk of ECG changes and dysrhythmias
Stimulation of presynaptic 5-HT receptors on DA neuron	SSRIs		Increased EPS
Sympatholytics: α-blockade decreases NE release	Clonidine Methyldopa Prazosin Nitric oxide containing products		Increased hypotension
Increased DA receptor binding	Antipsychotics		Increased adverse medication reactions particularly EPS

DA, dopamine; ECG, electrocardiogram; EPS, extrapyramidal symptoms; 5-HT, serotonin; SSRI, serotonin selective reuptake inhibitor; TCAs, tricyclic antidepressants; NE, norepinephrine.

Data from References 27-30, 32, 37, 148, and 149.

TABLE 87-10 Common Potential Pharmacokinetic Interactions with Antipsychotic Medications

Substrate Antipsychotic and Mechanism of Interaction	Interacting Medication or Substance			Clinical Effect
Aripiprazole, brexpiprazole, cariprazine, and iloperidone				
Inhibition of AP metabolism (CYP2D6, CYP3A4)	*Antidepressants* Bupropion Clomipramine Doxepin Duloxetine Fluoxetine Fluvoxamine Paroxetine Sertraline *HIV protease inhibitors* Indinavir Nelfinavir Ritonavir	*Anti-infectives* Ciprofloxacin Clarithromycin Erythromycin Fluconazole Ketoconazole Itraconazole *Antipsychotics* Asenapine Chlorpromazine Haloperidol Perphenazine Thioridazine	*Miscellaneous* Chlorpheniramine Cimetidine Cocaine Diltiazem Diphenhydramine Cimetidine Grapefruit juice Hydroxyzine Methadone Quinidine Ticlopidine Verapamil	Increased AP effect and risk of adverse medication reactions
Induction of AP metabolism	*Antiseizure Medications* Carbamazepine Oxcarbazepine Phenobarbital Phenytoin	*Anti-infectives* Rifampin *Miscellaneous* Glucocorticoids Modafinil	*Herbals* St. John's wort	Decreased AP effect
Asenapine				
Inhibition of AP metabolism (CYP1A2)	*Antidepressants* Fluvoxamine	*Anti-infectives* Ciprofloxacin Fluroquinolones	*Miscellaneous* Amidarone Cimetidine	Increased AP effect and risk of adverse medication reactions
Induction of AP metabolism	*Anti-infectives* Nafcillin	*Miscellaneous* Broccoli Brussels sprouts Chargrilled meat Smoking tobacco	*Miscellaneous* Insulin Modafinil Omeprazole	Decreased AP effect
NOTE: Eating food or drinking liquids within 10 minutes of asenapine sublingual administration will decrease bioavailability				
Clozapine				
Inhibition of AP metabolism (CYP3A4, CYP1A2, CYP2D6)	*Antidepressants* Fluoxetine Fluvoxamine *HIV protease inhibitors* Indinavir Nelfinavir Ritonavir	*Anti-infectives* Ciprofloxacin Clarithromycin Erythromycin Fluconazole Fluroquinolones Ketoconazole Itraconazole Nafcillin	*Miscellaneous* Amidarone Cimetidine Diltiazem Grapefruit juice Haloperidol Ticlopidine Verapamil Cimetidine	Increased AP effect and risk of adverse medication reactions
Induction of AP metabolism	*Antiseizure Medications* Carbamazepine Phenobarbital Phenytoin	*Miscellaneous* Glucocorticoids Insulin Modafinil Omeprazole Smoking tobacco	*Herbals* St. John's wort *Anti-infectives* Rifampin	Decreased AP effect
Haloperidol				
Inhibition of AP metabolism (CYP2D6, CYP3A4, CYP1A2)	*Antidepressants* Bupropion Doxepin Duloxetine Fluoxetine Fluvoxamine Paroxetine Sertraline *HIV protease inhibitors* Indinavir Nelfinavir Ritonavir Sequinavir	*Anti-infectives* Ciprofloxacin Clarithromycin Erythromycin Fluoconazole Fluoroquinolones Ketoconazole Itraconazole *Antipsychotics* Chlorpromazine Perphenazine	*Miscellaneous* Amiodarone Chlorpheniramine Cimetidine Diltiazem Diphenhydramine Quinidine Diphenhydramine Cimetidine Grapefruit juice Hydroxyzine Methadone Quinidine Verapamil	Increased AP effect and risk of adverse medication reactions

(continued)

TABLE 87-10 Common Potential Pharmacokinetic Interactions with Antipsychotic Medications (*Continued*)

Substrate Antipsychotic and Mechanism of Interaction	Interacting Medication or Substance			Clinical Effect
Induction of AP metabolism	*Antiseizure Medications* Carbamazepine Oxcarbazepine Phenobarbital Phenytoin	*Anti-infectives* Nafcillin Rifampin Miscellaneous Broccoli Brussels sprouts Chargrilled meat Glucocorticoids Insulin Modafinil Omeprazole	*Herbals* St. John's wort Tobacco smoking	Decreased AP effect
Olanzapine				
Inhibition of AP metabolism (CYP3A4 and CYP1A2)	*Antidepressants* Fluoxetine Fluvoxamine *HIV protease inhibitors* Indinavir Nelfinavir Ritonavir	*Anti-infectives* Ciprofloxacin Clarithromycin Erythromycin Fluconazole Fluoroquinolones Ketoconazole Itraconazole	*Miscellaneous* Amiodarone Cimetidine Diltiazem Cimetidine Grapefruit juice Verapamil	Increased AP effect and risk of adverse medication reactions
Induction of AP metabolism	*Antiseizure Medications* Carbamazepine Oxcarbazepine Phenobarbital Phenytoin *Anti-infectives* Nafcillin Rifampin	*Miscellaneous* Broccoli Brussels sprouts Chargrilled meat Glucocorticoids Insulin Modafinil Omeprazole	*Herbals* St. John's wort Smoking tobacco *HIV protease inhibitors* Efavirenz Nevirapine	Decreased AP effect
Paliperidone				
The bioavailability of paliperidone is significantly increased when it is taken with food. Although this could increase paliperidone effect, including adverse effects, the clinical significance is undetermined. Only potent CYP3A4 (eg, carbamazepine, rifampin, St. John's wort) inducers appear to increase paliperidone metabolism and affect dose requirements.				
Lurasidone, lumateperone, and quetiapine				
Inhibition of AP metabolism (CYP3A4)	*Antidepressants* Fluoxetine Fluvoxamine Nefazodone *HIV protease inhibitors* Indinavir Nelfinavir Ritonavir Sequinavir	*Anti-infectives* Ciprofloxacin Clarithromycin Erythromycin Fluconazole Ketoconazole Itraconazole	*Miscellaneous* Amiodarone Cimetidine Diltiazem Grapefruit juice Verapamil	Increased AP effect and risk of adverse medication reactions
Induction of AP metabolism	*Antiseizure Medications* Carbamazepine Oxcarbazepine Phenobarbital Phenytoin	*Anti-infectives* Rifampin *Miscellaneous* Glucocorticoids Modafinil	*Herbals* St. John's wort *HIV protease inhibitors* Efavirenz Nevirapine	Decreased AP effect
NOTE: Lurasidone AUC and Cmax increase by two- and threefold when given with at least 350 calories (1,460 J) of food regardless of fat content. NOTE: Lumateperone is metabolized through multiple different pathways, but interactions have been found with moderate to potent CYP3A4 inhibitors and a CYP3A4 inducer.				
Perphenazine and risperidone				
Inhibition of AP metabolism (CYP2D6)	*Antidepressants* Bupropion Clomipramine Doxepin Duloxetine Fluoxetine Paroxetine Sertraline *Antipsychotics* Chlorpromazine Haloperidol (reduced haloperidol) Perphenazine	*Miscellaneous* Amiodarone Cimetidine Chlorpheniramine Cocaine Diphenhydramine Cimetidine Hydroxyzine Methadone Quinidine		Increased AP effect and risk of adverse medication reactions

(*continued*)

TABLE 87-10 Common Potential Pharmacokinetic Interactions with Antipsychotic Medications (*Continued*)

Substrate Antipsychotic and Mechanism of Interaction	Interacting Medication or Substance		Clinical Effect
Induction of AP metabolism (via CYP3A34, a minor pathway for risperidone)	*Miscellaneous* Dexamethasone	*Anti-infectives* Rifampin	Decreased AP effect
NOTE: Because risperidone's metabolite formed through CYP2D6 metabolism is active (paliperidone), the clinical significance of pharmacokinetic interactions with risperidone is unclear.			
Ziprasidone			
The bioavailability of ziprasidone is increased twofold when it is taken with food. Consistent administration with food is recommended.			

AP, antipsychotic; AUC, Area Under the Curve; Cmax, maximum plasma concentration.

Data from References 27-33, 57, and 148-150.

medications.[28] Table 87-6 lists the known major pathways involved in the metabolism of SGAs. Risperidone is largely metabolized by CYP2D6 to its active metabolite, 9-OH-risperidone (paliperidone), which is thought to have a similar pharmacodynamic profile.[57] Although paliperidone is primarily eliminated renally unchanged, potent inducers of CYP3A4 can cause a potential need for dosage adjustment.[57,66] For asenapine, CYP1A2 is the primary isoenzyme responsible for metabolism with CYP3A4 also being a significant pathway.[57,66]

Based on current information, inhibitors of CYP1A2 have the greatest potential for causing interactions with clozapine and olanzapine, and some concern with asenapine.[57] Examples include cimetidine, fluvoxamine, and fluoroquinolone antibiotics (ie, ciprofloxacin) to varying degrees. To date, however, no serious inhibition interactions have been reported with olanzapine, which may be a result of olanzapine's wide therapeutic index; however, carbamazepine has been reported to increase olanzapine elimination by as much as 50%.[57] Cigarette smoking is a potent inducer of CYP1A2, and one would expect lower mean olanzapine serum concentrations in smokers compared with those in nonsmokers.

Because of the risk of seizures with higher clozapine tissue concentrations, interactions that inhibit clozapine's metabolism are potentially significant. In particular, fluvoxamine increases clozapine serum concentrations by an average of two- to threefold and up to fivefold.[57] Ciprofloxacin, other fluroquinolones, fluoxetine, and erythromycin can also increase clozapine serum concentrations.[57] As smoking has been associated with a 33% to 55% increase in clozapine clearance,[57] smoking cessation can result in increased clozapine serum concentration that may increase the risk of seizures.[66] Carbamazepine can also induce clozapine metabolism and lead to lower serum concentrations.[57]

A study with the potent CYP3A4 inhibitor ketoconazole showed minimal effects on ziprasidone single-dose pharmacokinetics, with only a 33% mean increase in the ziprasidone area under the time-versus-concentration curve.[57] These results are consistent with data suggesting that aldehyde oxidase is the major metabolic pathway for ziprasidone, with only 30% to 35% being metabolized by CYP3A4.[57]

Modest elevations of aripiprazole serum concentrations occur in the presence of ketoconazole or quinidine, which inhibit CYP3A4 and 2D6, respectively. Ketoconazole has a profound effect on decreasing lurasidone metabolism, and it is recommended that they not be used concomitantly.[30,57] Carbamazepine has been reported to decrease aripiprazole serum concentrations.[57]

Since iloperidone is metabolized through CYP2D6 and 3A4, its clearance can be impaired by inhibitors of these pathways. These types of interactions have the potential to be clinically significant. For example, it is recommended that the iloperidone dose be decreased by 50% when used with CYP2D6 inhibitors such as fluoxetine or paroxetine.[27,57]

Multiple enzymes are responsible for the metabolism of lumateperone. AKR1C1 is the predominant enzyme metabolizing lumateperone to the alcohol metabolite IC200131.[151] Multiple other enzymes are involved in its metabolism including CYP3A4. Dosage adjustments should occur in patients taking moderate to strong CYP3A4 inhibitors or inducers.[33]

Personalized Pharmacotherapy

Pharmacotherapy must be individualized for each person with schizophrenia. Apart from iloperidone, no laboratory tests are generally available that will predict a patient's response to treatment. Past response to treatment, potential adverse effects, patient personal preference, and medication price are the primary variables that should be used in selecting an antipsychotic that is included in stages 1A, 1B, or 2 of the treatment algorithm. In the CATIE study, the number one reason for medication discontinuation was the patient not wanting to take that medication any more, and the second most common reason was adverse effects.[17] These two factors should be carefully considered in antipsychotic selection and medication dosage must be individualized within the usual dose ranges. Careful consideration must also be given to concomitant medications that may interact with the antipsychotic and necessitate a change in dosage.

Preliminary data suggest a relationship between different genetic markers and clinical improvement as well as QTc prolongation in patients treated with iloperidone.[27,64] Substantial interest exists regarding the potential utility of pharmacogenetic monitoring in the pharmacotherapy of schizophrenia. Increasing relationships are being identified between specific genetic variation in relation to both the pharmacodynamics and pharmacokinetics of different antipsychotics. However, no convincing data have demonstrated that clinical outcomes are superior when using routine pharmacogenetic monitoring in the pharmacotherapy of schizophrenia, nor have cost-effectiveness studies of its use been performed.[64,65] Although promising for the future, routine pharmacogenetic monitoring in all patients with schizophrenia is not currently recommended. However, it may be useful in select patients. For example, if a patient appears particularly sensitive to developing EPS when treated with antipsychotics metabolized through CYP2D6, it might be useful to perform pharmacogenetic testing to determine whether the patient is a poor CYP2D6 metabolizer. If so, antipsychotics metabolized through

CYP2D6 should be used at lower doses, or the patient switched to an antipsychotic not metabolized by CYP2D6.[64] Clinicians should consult accepted guidelines, such as those by the Clinical Pharmacogenetics Implementation Consortium (https://cpicpgx.org/), before utilizing pharmacogenetic data.[67]

Given that no antipsychotic has proven superiority regarding efficacy in the treatment of schizophrenia (with the exception of clozapine in treatment resistance), cost should be a factor in antipsychotic selection. Many antipsychotics have generic equivalents available, and this should be a factor in selecting an antipsychotic (Table 87-9).

Evaluation of Therapeutic Outcomes

10 Assessment of response has traditionally been done subjectively or empirically (a relative sense of how the clinician feels the patient is doing). A formal mental status exam (MSE) is used to structure the patient interview and focus on items related to appearance, mood, sensorium, intellectual functioning, and thought processes. However, the MSE is neither specific nor quantitative for the measurement of medication response. Clinicians should be trained to use simple, standardized psychiatric rating scales to assist in objectively rating patient medication responses.[152] The Brief Psychiatric Rating Scale (BPRS) and the Positive and Negative Syndrome Scale (PANSS) were developed for use in clinical trials as research tools to quantify symptom improvement seen with antipsychotic treatment (see Chapter e81). Objectively, a numeric indicator (eg, 20%, 30%, or 40% reduction in BPRS score) has been used to quantify overall symptom reduction and classify patients according to different degrees of response. However, these types of rating scales are too long and unwieldy to be routinely used within the time constraints of most clinical practices. Symptom scales used in clinical practice must be sufficiently brief to be used during an ordinary clinic visit (eg, 15-30 minutes) while measuring both positive and negative symptoms, and being sufficiently representative of overall symptomatology. The four-item Positive Symptom Rating Scale (PSRS) and the four-item Brief Negative Symptom Assessment (BNSA) are brief scales that meet such criteria (Table 87-11).[152] A brief rating scale of positive symptoms, such as the PSRS, should be used at baseline before starting pharmacotherapy, and at each time response to pharmacotherapy is assessed.

Similarly, the pharmacotherapeutic plan should include specific monitoring parameters for adverse medication reactions (Table 87-12). The plan should include how the potential reactions will be evaluated, and the frequency of assessment. Given the risk of weight gain, diabetes, and lipid abnormalities associated with many of the SGAs, a consensus task force led by the American Diabetes Association recommends the following baseline parameters before beginning antipsychotics: family history, weight, height, BMI, waist circumference, blood pressure, fasting plasma glucose, and fasting lipid profile.[83] They also recommend follow-up monitoring of these parameters after beginning or changing SGAs. Weight should be monitored monthly for the first 3 months and quarterly thereafter. The other parameters should be assessed at the end of 3 months, and if normal, then at least annually. Self-assessments can be a useful adjunct in treating the patient. Although the patient with schizophrenia may not always be accurate in evaluating symptom severity, the use of patient self-assessments increases patient engagement in care, enhances therapeutic alliance, and gives the clinician an opportunity to identify misconceptions the patient may have regarding symptoms associated with the illness, adverse medication reactions, and the like.[55] Traditionally, clinicians have often accepted partial symptom response in schizophrenia as success, and have not been aggressive in attempting to achieve greater symptomatic remission. The advent of multiple different SGAs with varying tolerability profiles should encourage clinicians to be more assertive in attempting to achieve symptom remission. This is consistent with an increasing focus on remission as a goal of treatment and the evolving emphasis on consumerism in the care of patients with severe mental illness.[54]

CONCLUSION

Schizophrenia is a neurodevelopmental disorder whose etiology is currently unknown. A multitude of medications, primarily working through dopamine, serotonin, and glutamatergic antagonism, have been developed to treat symptoms associated with this syndrome. Although there is no cure for schizophrenia, lifelong antipsychotic use combined with comprehensive psychosocial services can allow many of these individuals to function. However, medication adherence can be challenging, and the use of long-acting injectable antipsychotics combined with psychosocial services designed to address

TABLE 87-11 Brief Clinical Assessments for Monitoring Antipsychotic Response in Schizophrenia

Four-Item Positive Symptom Rating Scale (PSRS)								
Use each item's anchor points to rate the patient								
1. Suspiciousness	NA	1	2	3	4	5	6	7
2. Unusual thought content	NA	1	2	3	4	5	6	7
3. Hallucinations	NA	1	2	3	4	5	6	7
4. Conceptual disorganization	NA	1	2	3	4	5	6	7
Each item is scored from 1 (not present) to 7 (extremely severe)	SCORE:							
Brief Negative Symptom Assessment (BNSA)								
Use each item's anchor points to rate the patient								
1. Prolonged time to respond	1	2	3	4	5	6		
2. Emotion: Unchanging facial expression, blank, expressionless face	1	2	3	4	5	6		
3. Reduced social drive	1	2	3	4	5	6		
4. Poor grooming and hygiene	1	2	3	4	5	6		
Each item is scored from 1 (normal) to 6 (severe)	SCORE:							

[a]NA, not able to be assessed.

Data from Reference 152.

TABLE 87-12 Antipsychotic Adverse Reactions and Monitoring Parameters

Adverse Reaction	Monitoring Parameter	Frequency	Comments
Adverse Reaction Monitoring Parameters for All Antipsychotic Medications			
Akathisia	Ask about restlessness or anxiety. Observe patient for restlessness. Barnes Akathisia Scale can also be used	Every visit	
Anticholinergic adverse effects	Ask patient about constipation, blurry vision, urinary retention, or unusual dry mouth	Every visit	
Glucose intolerance	FBS or HbA1c	At baseline, after 3 months, and if normal, then annually	
Hyperlipidemia	Lipid profile	At baseline, after 3 months, and if normal, then annually	
Orthostatic hypotension	Ask patient about dizziness on standing. If present, check BP and HR in sitting and standing positions	Every visit	The degree of orthostatic change in BP to produce symptoms varies. In general, a BP change of 20 mm Hg or more is significant
Hyperprolactinemia	In females, ask about expression of milk from the breast and menstrual irregularities. In males, ask about breast enlargement or expression of milk from nipples. If symptoms present, check serum prolactin level	Every visit	In the absence of symptoms, there is no need to monitor serum prolactin
Sedation	Ask patient about unusual sedation or sleepiness	Every visit	
Sexual dysfunction	Ask patient about decreased sexual desire, difficulty being aroused, or problems with orgasm	Every visit	Patients with schizophrenia have more sexual dysfunction than the normal population. Compare symptoms with medication-free state
Tardive dyskinesia	Standardized rating scale such as the AIMS or the DISCUS	At baseline, and then every 6 months for FGAs and every 12 months for SGAs	
Weight gain	Measure body weight, BMI, and waist circumference	BMI every visit for 6 months and at least quarterly thereafter	Waist circumference is the single best predictor of cardiac morbidity
Adverse Reaction Monitoring Parameters for Specific Antipsychotics			
Agranulocytosis	Absolute neutrophil counts (ANC)	At baseline, weekly for 6 months, then every 2 weeks for 6 months, and then monthly	Clozapine only
Sialorrhea or excess drooling	Ask patient about problems with excess drooling, waking in the morning with a wet ring on his or her pillow. Visual observation of the patient for drooling	Every visit	Clozapine only
Bronchospasm, respiratory distress, respiratory depression, respiratory arrest	Before administration, patients must be screened for a history of asthma, chronic obstructive pulmonary disease, or other lung disease associated with bronchospasm. Monitor patient every 15 minutes for a minimum of 1 hour after medication administration for signs and symptoms of bronchospasm (ie, vital signs and chest auscultation). Only one 10-mg dose can be given every 24 hours	Every dose administration	Inhaled loxapine only. Can only be administered in approved healthcare facilities registered in REMS program
Post injection sedation/delirium syndrome	Observation of the patient for at least 3 hours after medication administration. Monitor for possible sedation, altered level of consciousness, coma, delirium, confusion, disorientation, agitation, anxiety, or other cognitive impairment	Every dose administration	Long-acting olanzapine pamoate monohydrate only. Can only be administered in approved healthcare facilities registered in REMS program

FBS, fasting blood sugar; AIMS, Abnormal Involuntary Movement Scale; DISCUS, dyskinesia identification system condensed user scale; FGA, first-generation antipsychotic; SGA, second-generation antipsychotic.

engagement with treatment can promote adherence. Antipsychotic medications have a multitude of potential adverse reactions, and prudent monitoring is necessary. As the common core symptoms associated with schizophrenia (positive, negative, and cognitive) vary among person to person, continual evaluation of therapeutic outcomes focusing on overall functioning and quality of life is necessary.

ABBREVIATIONS

α_1	alpha one adrenergic receptor
α_2	alpha two adrenergic receptor
AAN	American Academy of Neurology
ACHIEVE	Randomized Trial of Achieving Healthy Lifestyles in Psychiatric Rehabilitation

ACT	active community treatment
ADTA2A	adrenoreceptor alpha-2a
AIMS	Abnormal Involuntary Movement Scale
AIWG	antipsychotic-induced weight gain
ANC	absolute neutrophil count
AP	antipsychotic
APA	American Psychiatric Association
ASD	autism spectrum disorder
AUC	area under the curve
β_2	beta-2 adrenergic receptor
BDNF	brain-derived neurotrophic factor
BLM	buccal–lingual–masticatory
BMI	body mass index
BP	blood pressure
BNSA	Brief Negative Symptom Assessment
BPRS	Brief Psychiatric Rating Scale
C4	complement component 4 genes
CACN1A2	voltage-dependent calcium channel 1A2
CATIE	Clinical Antipsychotic Trials of Intervention Effectiveness
CK	creatine kinase
CNS	central nervous system
CNV	copy number variant
C_{max}	maximum plasma concentration
CRP	C-reactive protein
CYP	cytochrome P450
D_1	dopamine-1 receptor
D_2	dopamine-2 receptor
D_3	dopamine-3 receptor
D_4	dopamine-4 receptor
DA	dopamine
DISCUS	Dyskinesia Identification System: Condensed User Scale
DKA	diabetic ketoacidosis
DRESS	Drug Reaction with Eosinophilia and Systemic Symptoms
DSM-5	*Diagnostic and Statistical Manual of Mental Disorders, Fifth Edition*
ECG	electrocardiogram or electrocardiographic
ECHO	echocardiogram
ECT	electroconvulsive therapy
EEG	electroencephalogram
EF	ejection fraction
EPS	extrapyramidal side effect
FBS	fasting blood sugar
FDA	Food and Drug Administration
FGA	first-generation antipsychotic
FMO3	flavin containing monooxygenase 3 gene
GABA	gamma-aminobutyric acid
GNB3	guanine nucleotide binding protein
GWAS	genome-wide association studies
HgA1c	hemoglobin A1c
5-HT	serotonin or 5-hydroxytryptamine
5-HT_{1A}	serotonin-1A receptor
5-HT_2	serotonin-2 receptor
5-HT_{2A}	serotonin-2A receptor
5-HT_{2C}	serotonin-2C receptor
5-HT_6	serotonin-6 receptor
5-HT_7	serotonin-7 receptor
HR	heart rate
ICD	impulse control disorder
IM	intramuscular
INSIG2	insulin-induced gene 2
IV	intravenous
LAIA	long-acting injectable antipsychotic
LBW	low birth weight
MC4R	melanocortin-4-receptor
1MPP	1-month paliperidone palmitate (Invega Sustenna)
3MPP	3-month paliperidone palmitate (Invega Trinza)
mRNA	microribonucleic acid
MTHFR	methylenetetrahydrofolate reductase
MSE	mental status examination
NAMI	National Alliance on Mental Illness
NE	norepinephrine
NIMH	National Institute of Mental Health
NMDA	*N*-methyl-D-aspartate
NMS	neuroleptic malignant syndrome
NRG1	neuregulin 1
NRXN1	synaptic protein neurexin 1
PANSS	Positive and Negative Symptom Scale
PDSS	post injection delirium/sedation syndrome
PET	positron emission tomography
PORT	Patient Outcomes Research Team
PSRS	Positive Symptom Rating Scale
RAISE	Recovery After Initial Schizophrenia Episode
REMS	Risk Evaluation and Mitigation Strategy
RID	relative infant dose
RNA	ribonucleic acid
SCD	sudden cardiac death
SEs	side effects
SGA	second-generation antipsychotic
SNP	single nucleotide polymorphism
SSRI	selective serotonin reuptake inhibitor
STRIDE	Reducing Weight and Diabetes Risk in an Underserved Population
T2DM	type 2 diabetes mellitus
TCA	tricyclic antidepressant
TD	tardive dyskinesia
UK	United Kingdom
VMAT2	vesicular monoamine transporter-2
VTE	venous thromboembolism
WBC	white blood cell

REFERENCES

1. American Psychiatric Association. Schizophrenia spectrum and other psychotic disorders. In: *Diagnostic and Statistical Manual of Mental Disorders*. 5th ed. Arlington, VA: American Psychiatric Association; 2013:87–122.
2. Charlson FJ, Ferrari AJ, Santomauro DF, et al. Global epidemiology and burden of schizophrenia: findings from the global burden of disease study 2016. *Schizophr Bull*. 2018;44:1195–1203.
3. Milan ML, Andrieux A, Bartzokis G, et al. Altering the course of schizophrenia: progress and perspectives. *Nat Rev Drug Discov*. 2016;15:485–515.
4. Price AJ, Jaffe AE, Weinberger DR. Cortical cellular diversity and development in schizophrenia. *Mol Psychiatry*. 2021;26(1):203–217. 10.1038/s41380-020-0775-8 32404946.
5. Dalmau J, Graus F. Antibody-mediated encephalitis. *N Engl J Med*. 2018;378:840–851.
6. Howes OD, Murray RM. Schizophrenia: an integrated sociodevelopmental cognitive model. *Lancet*. 2014;383:1677–1687.
7. Arsalan A, Kowalec K. Genetic architecture of schizophrenia: a review of major advancements. *Psychol Med*. 2021;51(13):2168–2177. 10.1017/S0033291720005334 33550997.
8. Sekar A, Bialas AR, de Rivera H, et al. Schizophrenia risk from complex variation of complement component 4. *Nature*. 2016;530:177–183. doi: 10.1038/nature16549.
9. Cannon TD, Chung Y, He G, et al. North American Prodrome Longitudinal Study Consortium. Progressive reduction in cortical thickness as psychosis develops: a multisite longitudinal neuroimaging study of youth at elevated clinical risk. *Biol Psychiatry*. 2015;77(2):147–157.

10. McCutcheon RA, Reis Marques T, Howes OD. Schizophrenia—an overview. *JAMA Psychiatry*. 2020;77(2):201–210. 10.1001/jamapsychiatry.2019.3360 31664453.
11. Howes OD, Kambeitz J, Kim E, et al. The nature of dopamine dysfunction in schizophrenia and what this means for treatment. *Arch Gen Psychiatry*. 2012;69:776–786.
12. Krystal JH, Anticevic A. Toward illness phase-specific pharmacotherapy for schizophrenia. *Biol Psychiatry*. 2015;78:738–740.
13. Wright R, Rethelyi JM, Gage FG. Enhancing induced pluripotent stem cell models of schizophrenia. *JAMA Psychiatry*. 2014;71(3):334–335.
14. Hasan A, Palkai P, Wobrock T, et al. World Federation of Societies of Biological Psychiatry (WFSBP) guidelines for biological treatment of schizophrenia—short version for primary care. *Int J Psychiatry Clin Pract*. 2017;21:82–90.
15. Evins AE, Green AI, Kane JM, Murray RM. Does using marijuana increase the risk for developing schizophrenia? *J Clin Psychiatry*. 2013;74:e08. doi: 10.4088/JCP.12012tx2c.
16. Lieberman JA, First MB. Psychotic disorders. *New Engl J Med*. 2018;379:270–180.
17. Lieberman JA, Stroup S. The NIMH-CATIE schizophrenia study: what did we learn? *Am J Psychiatry*. 2011;168:770–775.
18. Addington D, Anderson E, Kelly M, et al. Canadian practice guidelines for comprehensive community treatment for schizophrenia and schizophrenia spectrum disorder. *Can J Psychiatry*. 2017;62:662–672.
19. McGorry PD. The next stage for diagnosis: validity through utility. *World Psychiatry*. 2013;12(3):213–214.
20. Kane JM, Robinson DG, Schooler NR, et al. Comprehensive versus usual community care for first-episode psychosis: 2-year outcomes from the NIMH RAISE early treatment program. *Am J Psychiatry*. 2015;173:362–372. doi: 10.1176/appi.ajp.2015.15050632.
21. Saperstein AM, Kurtz MM. Current trends in the empirical study of cognitive remediation for schizophrenia. *Can J Psychiatry*. 2013;58(6):311–318.
22. Keepers GA, Fochtmann LJ, Anzia JM, et al. The American Psychiatric Association Practice Guideline for the Treatment of Patients with Schizophrenia. *Focus (Am Psychiatr Publ)*. 2020;18(4):493–497. 10.1176/appi.focus.18402 33343262.
23. Osser DN, Jalali-Roudsari M, Manschreck T. Schizophrenia. Psychopharmacology algorithms, from the Psychopharmacology Algorithm Project at the Harvard Medical School Dept. of Psychiatry, South Shore Program. Available at: http://psychopharm.mobi/algo_live/. Accessed December 26, 2018.
24. Hazari N, Kate N, Grover S, et al. Clozapine and tardive movement disorders: a review. *Asian J Psychiatr*. 2013;6(6):439–51. 10.1016/j.ajp.2013.08.067 24309853.
25. Correll CU, Robinson DG, Schooler NR, et al. Cardiometabolic risk in patients with first-episode schizophrenia spectrum disorders: baseline results from the RAISE-ETP Study. *JAMA Psychiatry*. 2014;71(12):1350–1363.
26. de Berardis D, Fornaro M, Orsolini L, et al. The role of inhaled loxapine in the treatment of acute agitation in patients with psychiatric disorders: a clinical review. *Int J Molo Sci*. 2017;18:349. doi: 10.3390/ijms18020349.
27. Citrome L. Iloperidone for schizophrenia: a review of the efficacy and safety profile for this newly commercialized second-generation antipsychotic. *Int J Clin Pract*. 2009;63:1237–1248.
28. Citrome L. Asenapine for schizophrenia and bipolar disorder: a review of the efficacy and safety profile for this newly approved sublingually absorbed second-generation antipsychotic. *Int J Clin Pract*. 2009;63:1762–1784.
29. McCormack PL. Cariprazine: first global approval. *Drugs*. 2015;75:2035–2043.
30. Citrome L. Lurasidone for schizophrenia: a review of the efficacy and safety profile for this newly approved second-generation antipsychotic. *Int J Clin Pract*. 2011;65:189–210.
31. Frankel JS, Schwartz TL. Brexpiprazole and cariprazine: distinguishing two new antipsychotics from the original dopamine stabilizer aripiprazole. *Ther Adv Psychopharmacol*. 2017;7:29–41. doi: 10.1177/2045125316672136.
32. Prescribing information. *Clozaril*. Rosemont, PA: HLS Therapeutics (USA), Inc. HLS Therapeutics, Inc.; 2017.
33. Greenwood J, Acharya RB, Marcellus V, et al. Lumateperone: a novel antipsychotic for schizophrenia. *Ann Pharmacother*. 2021;55(1):98–104. 10.1177/1060028020936597 32590907.
34. Goldman R, Loebel A, Cucchiaro J, et al. Efficacy and safety of lurasidone in adolescents with schizophrenia: a 6-week, randomized placebo-controlled study. *J Child Adolesc Psychopharmacol*. 2017;27:516–525.
35. Subotnik KL, Casaus LR, Ventura J, et al. Long-acting injectable risperidone for relapse prevention and control of breakthrough symptoms after a recent first episode of schizophrenia. *JAMA Psychiatry*. 2015;72:822–829.
36. Patchan K, Vyas G, Hackman AL, et al. Clozapine in reducing aggression and violence in forensic populations. *Psychiatr Q*. 2018;89:157–168.
37. Van Putten T, Marder SR. Behavioral toxicity of antipsychotic drugs. *J Clin Psychiatry*. 1987;48(suppl 9):13–19.
38. Samara MT, Leucht C, Leeflang MM, et al. Early improvement as a predictor of later response to antipsychotics in schizophrenia: a diagnostic test review. *Am J Psychiatry*. 2015;172:617–629.
39. Sajatovic M, Ross R, Legacy SN, et al. Initiating/maintaining long-acting injectable antipsychotics in schizophrenia/schizoaffective or bipolar disorder—expert consensus survey part 2. *Neuropsychiatr Dis Treat*. 2018;14:1475–1492.
40. Kishimoto T, Hagi K, Kurokawa S, et al. Long-acting injectable versus oral antipsychotics for the maintenance treatment of schizophrenia: a systematic review and comparative meta-analysis of randomised, cohort, and pre-post studies. *Lancet Psychiatry*. 2021;8(5):387–404. 10.1016/S2215-0366(21)00039-0 33862018.
41. Parellada E, Bioque M. Barriers to the use of long-acting injectable antipsychotics in the management of schizophrenia. *CNS Drugs*. 2016;30:689–701.
42. Buckley PF. Treatment-resistant schizophrenia. *Focus (Am Psychiatr Publ)*. 2020;18(4):364–367. 10.1176/appi.focus.20200025 33343247.
43. Citrome L. New second-generation long-acting injectable antipsychotics for the treatment of schizophrenia. *Expert Rev Neurother*. 2013;13:767–783.
44. Prescribing information. *PERSERIS*. North Chesterfield, VA: Indivior Inc.; 2018.
45. Prescribing information. *INVEGA SUSTENNA*. Titusville, NJ: Janssen Pharmaceuticals Inc.; 2017.
46. Prescribing information. *Invega Trinza*. Titusville, NJ: Janssen Pharmaceuticals Inc.; 2018.
47. Prescribing information. *Aristada Initio*. Waltham, MA: Alkermes, Inc.; 2018.
48. Meyer JM. Understanding the depot antipsychotics: sn illustrated guide to kinetics. *CNS Spectrums*. 2013;18:58–68.
49. Prescribing information. *ABILIFT MYCITE*. Rockville, MD: Otsuka America Pharmaceutical Inc.; 2017.
50. Prescribing information. *Zyprexa Relprevv*. Indianapolis, IN: Lilly USA; 2018.
51. Samalin L, Garay R, Ameg A, Llorca PM. Olanzapine pamoate for the treatment of schizophrenia: an safety evaluation. *Expert Opin Drug Saf*. 2016;15(3):403–411. doi: 10.1517/14740338.2016.1141893.
52. Jann MW, Penzak SR. Long-acting injectable second-generation antipsychotics: an update and comparison between agents. *CNS Drugs*. 2018;32:241–257. https://doi.org/10.1007/s40263-018-0508-6.
53. Howes OD, McCutcheon R, Agid O, de Bartolomeis A, et al. Treatment resistant schizophrenia: treatment response and resistance in psychosis (TRRIP) working groups consensus guidelines on diagnosis and terminology. *Am J Psychiatry*. 2017;174(3):216–229.
54. Barkhof E, Meijer CJ, de Sonneville LMJ, et al. Interventions to improve adherence to antipsychotic medications in patients with schizophrenia—a review of the past decade. *Eur Psychiatry*. 2012;27:9–18.
55. Velligan DI, Weiden PJ, Sajatovic M, et al. The expert consensus guideline series: adherence problems in patients with serious and persistent mental illness. *J Clin Psychiatry*. 2009;70:1–48.
56. Kane J, Honigfeld G, Singer J, et al. Clozapine for the treatment-resistant schizophrenic: a double-blind comparison with chlorpromazine. *Arch Gen Psychiatry*. 1988;45:789–796.
57. Kennedy WK, Jann MW, Kutscher EC. Clinically significant drug interactions with atypical antipsychotics. *CNS Drugs*. 2013;27:1021–1048.
58. Tiihonen J, Taipale H, Mehtälä J, et al. Association of antipsychotic polypharmacy vs monotherapy with psychiatric rehospitalization among adults with schizophrenia. *JAMA Psychiatry*. 2019;76(5):499–507. 10.1001/jamapsychiatry.2018.4320 30785608.
59. Miyamoto S, Miyake N, Jarskog LF, Fleischhacker WW, Lieberman JA. Pharmacological treatment of schizophrenia: a critical review of the pharmacology and clinical effects of current and future therapeutic agents. *Mol Psychiatry*. 2012;17:1206–1227.
60. Maeda K, Sugino H, Akazawa H, et al. Brexpiprazole I: in vitro and in vivo characterization of a novel serotonin-dopamine activity modulator. *J Pharmacol Exp Ther*. 2014;350:589–604.
61. Nucifora FC, Miohaljevic M, Lee BJ, Sawa A. Clozapine as a model for antipsychotic development. *Neurotherapeutics*. 2017;14:750–761.

62. Snyder GL, Vanover KE, Davis RE, et al. A review of the pharmacology and clinical profile of lumateperone for the treatment of schizophrenia. *Adv Pharmacol.* 2021;90:253–276. 10.1016/bs.apha.2020.09.001 33706936.
63. Mauri MC, Volonteri LS, Colasanti A, et al. Clinical pharmacokinetics of atypical antipsychotics: a critical review of the relationship between plasma concentrations and clinical response. *Clin Pharmacokinet.* 2007;46:359–388.
64. Eum S, Lee AM, Bishop JR. Pharmacogenetic tests for antipsychotic medications: clinical implications and considerations. *Dialogues Clin Neurosci.* 2016;18:323–337.
65. Pouget JG, Shams TA, Tiwari AK, Muller DJ. Pharmacogenetics and outcome with antipsychotic drugs. *Dialogues Clin Neurosci.* 2014;16:555–566.
66. Preskorn SH. Clinically important differences in the pharmacokinetics of the ten newer atypical antipsychotics: Part 2. Metabolism and elimination. *J Psychiatr Pract.* 2012;18:361–368.
67. Clinical Pharmacogenetics Implementation Consortium. Available at: https://cpicpgx.org/. Accessed December 1, 2018.
68. Tewksbury A, Olander A. Management of antipsychotic induced hyperprolactinemia. *Ment Health Clin.* 2016;6(4):185–190. doi: 10.9740/mhc.2016.7.185.
69. Wong-Anuchit C. Clinical management of antipsychotic-induced hyperprolactinemia. *Perspect Psychiatr Care.* 2015;52:145–152. doi: 10.1111/ppc.12111.
70. Kinon BJ, Liu-Seifert H, Stauffer VL, Jacob J. Bone loss associated with hyperprolactinemia in schizophrenia. *Clin Schizophr Relat Psychoses.* 2013;7:114–123.
71. Peuskens J, Pani L, Detraux J, De Hert M. The effects of novel and newly approved antipsychotics on serum prolactin levels: a comprehensive review. *CNS Drugs.* 2014;28:421–453.
72. Huhn M, Nikolakopoulou A, Schneider-Thoma J, et al. Comparative efficacy and tolerability of 32 oral antipsychotics for the acute treatment of adults with multi-episode schizophrenia: a systematic review and network meta-analysis. *Lancet.* 2019;394(10202):939–951. 10.1016/S0140-6736(19)31135-3 31303314.
73. Kane JM, Durgam S, Satlin A, et al. Safety and tolerability of lumateperone for the treatment of schizophrenia: a pooled analysis of late-phase placebo- and active-controlled clinical trials. *Int Clin Psychopharmacol.* 2021;36(5):244–250. 10.1097/YIC.0000000000000371 34054112.
74. Meng M, Li W, Zhang S, et al. Using aripiprazole to reduce antipsychotic-induced hyperprolactinemia: meta-analysis of currently available randomized controlled trials. *Shanghai Arch Psychiatry.* 2015;27(1):4–17.
75. Bo QJ, Wang ZM, Li XB, Ma X, Wang CY, de Leon J. Adjunctive metformin for antipsychotic-induced hyperprolactinemia: a systematic review. *Psychiatr Res.* 2016;237:257–263.
76. Musil R, Obermeier M, Russ P, Haerle M. Weight gain and antipsychotics: a drug safety review. *Expert Opin Drug Saf.* 2015;14(1):73–96.
77. Jeon SW, Kim YK. Unresolved issues for utilization of atypical antipsychotics in schizophrenia: antipsychotic polypharmacy and metabolic syndrome. *Int J Mol Sci.* 2017;18(10):E2174. doi: 10.3390/ijms18102174.9e.
78. Reynolds GP, McGowan OO. Mechanism underlying metabolic disturbances associated with psychosis and antipsychotic drug treatment. *J Psychopharmacol.* 2017;31(11):1430–1436. doi: 10.1177/0269881117722987.
79. Whicher CA, Price H, Holt RIG. Mechanisms in endocrinology: antipsychotic medication and diabetes and impaired glucose regulation. *Eur J Endocrinol.* 2018;178(6):R245–R258. doi: 10.1530/EJE-18-0022.
80. Shams TA, Muller DJ. Antipsychotic induced weight gain: genetics, epigenetics and biomarkers reviewed. *Curr Psychiatry Rep.* 2014;16:473–481. doi: 10.1007/s11920-014-0473-9.
81. Zhang JP, Lencz T, Zhang RX, et al. Pharmacogenetic associations of antipsychotic drug-related weight gain: a systematic review and meta-analysis. *Schizophr Bull.* 2016;42(6):1415–1437. doi: 10.1093/schlbulk/sbw058.
82. Correll CU, Newcomer JW, Silverman B, et al. Effects of olanzapine combined with samidorphan on weight gain in schizophrenia: a 24-week phase 3 study. *Am J Psychiatry.* 2020;177(12):1168–1178. 10.1176/appi.ajp.2020.19121279 32791894.
83. American Diabetes Association. Consensus development conference on antipsychotic drugs and obesity and diabetes. *Diabetes Care.* 2004;27:596–601.
84. Mizuno Y, Suzuki T, Nakagawa A, et al. Pharmacological strategies to counteract antipsychotic-induced weight gain and metabolic adverse effects in schizophrenia: a systematic review and meta-analysis. *Schizophr Bull.* 2014;1385–13403.
85. Wani RA, Dar MA, Margoob MA, Rather YH, Haq I, Shah MS. Diabetes mellitus and impaired glucose tolerance in patients with schizophrenia, before and after antipsychotic treatment. *J Neurosci Rural Pract.* 2015;6(1):17–22.
86. Green CA, Yarborough BJ, Leo MC, et al. The STRIDE weight loss and lifestyle intervention for individuals taking antipsychotic medications: a randomized trial. *Am J Psychiatry.* 2015;172(1):71–81.
87. Correll CU, Sikich L, Reeves G, et al. Metformin add-on vs. antipsychotic switch vs. continued antipsychotic treatment plus healthy lifestyle education in overweight or obese youth with severe mental illness: results from the IMPACT trial. *World Psychiatry.* 2020;19(1):69–80. 10.1002/wps.20714 31922663.
88. Koalchuk C, Castenllani L, Chintoh A, Remington G, Giacca A, Hahn M. Antipsychotics and glucose metabolism: how brain and body collide. *Am J Physiol Endocrino Metab.* 2018. doi: 10.1152/ajpendo.00164.2018.
89. Orsolini L, Tomasetti C, Valchera A, et al. An update of the safety of clinically used atypical antipsychotics. *Expert Opin Drug Saf.* 2016;15(10):1329–1347. doi: 10.1080/14740338.2016.1201475.
90. Solmi M, Murru A, Pacciarotti I, et al. Safety, tolerability and risks associated with first- and second-generation antipsychotics: a state-of-the-art review. *Ther Clin Risk Manag.* 2017;13:757–777.
91. Leung JY, Barr AM, Procyshyn RM, Honer WG, Pang CC. Cardiovascular side-effects of antipsychotic drugs: the role of the autonomic nervous system. *Pharmacol Ther.* 2012;135(2):113–122.
92. Harrigan EP, Miceli JJ, Anziano R, et al. A randomized evaluation of the effects of six antipsychotic agents on QTc, in the absence and presence of metabolic inhibition. *J Clin Psychopharmacol.* 2004;24:62–69.
93. Hasnain M, Vieweg WVR. QTc interval prolongation and torsades de pointes associated with second generation antipsychotics and antidepressants: a comprehensive review. *CNS Drugs.* 2014;28:887–920.
94. Wenzel-Seifert K, Wittmann M, Haen E. QTc prolongation by psychotropic drugs and the risk of torsade de pointes. *Dtsch Arztebl Int.* 2011;108:687–693.
95. Vang T, Rosenzweig M, Bruhn CH, et al. Eosinophilic myocarditis during treatment with olanzapine: report of two possible cases. *BMC Psychiatry.* 2016;16:70. doi: 10.1186/s12888-016-0776-y.
96. Curto M, Girardi N, Lionetto L, Ciavarella GM, Ferracuti S, Balderssarini RJ. Systematic review of clozapine cardiotoxicity. *Curr Psychiatry Rep.* 2016;18:68. doi: 10.1007/s11920-0704-3.
97. Alawani M, Wasywich C, Cicovic A, Kenedi C. A systematic review of clozapine induced cardiomyopathy. *Int J Cardiol.* 2014;176:315–320.
98. Nielsen J, Correll CU, Manu P, Kane JM. Termination of clozapine due to medical reasons: when is it warranted and how can it be avoided? *J Clin Psychiatry.* 2013;74:603–613.
99. Wu CS, Tsai YT, Tsai HJ. Antipsychotic drugs and the risk of ventricular arrhythmia and/or sudden cardiac death: a nationwide case-crossover study. *J Am Heart Assoc.* 2015;4(2). pii: e001568. doi: 10.1161/JAHA.114.001568.
100. Ballon JS, Pajvani UB, Mayer LES, et al. Pathophysiology of drug induced weight gain and metabolic effects: findings from an RCT in healthy volunteers treated with olanzapine, iloperidone, or placebo. *Psychopharmacol.* 2018;32:533–540. doi: 10.1177/0269881118754708.
101. McEvoy JP, Meyer JM, Goff DC, et al. Prevalence of the metabolic syndrome in patients with schizophrenia: baseline results from the Clinical Antipsychotic Trials of Intervention Effectiveness (CATIE) schizophrenia trial and comparison with national estimates from NHANES III. *Schizophr Res.* 2005;80(1):19–32.
102. Monteleone P, Martiadis V, Maj M. Management of schizophrenia with obesity, metabolic and endocrinological disorders. *Psychiatr Clin North Am.* 2009;32:775–794.
103. Hsu WY, Lane HY, Lin CL, Kao CH. A population-based cohort study on deep vein thrombosis and pulmonary embolism among schizophrenia patients. *Schizophr Res.* 2015;162(1-3):248–252. doi: 10.1016/j.schres.2015.01.012.
104. Hippisley-Cox J, Coupland C. Development and validation of risk prediction algorithm (QThrombosis) to estimate future risk of venous thromboembolism: prospective cohort study. *BMJ.* 2011;343:d4656. doi: https://doi.org/10.1136/bmj.d4656.
105. Burkhard PR. Acute and subacute drug-induced movement disorders. *Parkinsonism Relat Disord.* 2014;20S1:S108–S112.
106. Caroff SN, Campbell EC. Drug-induced extrapyramidal syndromes: implications for contemporary practice. *Psychiatr Clin North Am.* 2016;39(3):391–411. doi: 10.1016/j.psc.2016.04.003.
107. Pringsheim T, Gardner D, Addington D, et al. Assessment and treatment of antipsychotic-induced akathisia. *Can J Psychiatry.* 2018. doi: 10.1177/0706743718760288.

108. Peluso M, Lewis S, Barnes T, et al. Extrapyramidal motor side-effects of first and second-generation antipsychotic drugs. *Br J Psychiatry.* 2012;200:387–392.
109. Sprague RL, Kalachnik JE. Reliability, validity, and a total score cutoff for the Dyskinesia Identification System Condensed User Scale (DISCUS) with mentally ill and mentally retarded populations. *Psychopharmacol Bull.* 1991;27:51–58.
110. Ricciardi L, Pringsheim T, Barnes TRE. Treatment recommendations for tardive dyskinesia. *Can J Psychiatry.* 2019;64(6):388–399. 10.1177/0706743719828968 30791698.
111. Solmi M, Pigato G, Kane JM, Correll CU. Clinical risk factors for the development of tardive dyskinesia. *J Neurol Sci.* 2018;389:21–27. doi: 10.1016/j.jns.2018.02.012.
112. Zai CC, Maes MS, Tiwari AK, Zai GC, Remington G, Kennedy JL. Genetics of tardive dyskinesia: promising leads and ways forward. *J Neurol Sci.* 2018;389:28–34. doi: 10.1016/j.jns.2018.02.011.
113. Correll CU, Schenk EM. Tardive dyskinesia and new antipsychotics. *Curr Opin Psychiatry.* 2008;21:151–156.
114. Carbon M, Kane JM, Leucht S, Correll CU. Tardive dyskinesia risk with first-generation and second-generation antipsychotics in comparative randomized controlled trials: a meta-analysis. *World Psychiatry.* 2018;17:330–340. doi:10.1002/wps.20579.
115. Bhidayasiri R, Jitkritsadakul O, Friedman JH, Fahn S. Updating the recommendations for treatment of tardive syndromes: a systematic review of new evidence and practical treatment algorithm. *J Neurol Sci.* 2018;389:67–75. 10.1016/j.jns.2018.02.010 29454493.
116. Correll CU, Josiassen RC, Liang GS, Burke J, O'Brien CF. Efficacy of valbenazine (NBI-98854) in treating subjects with tardive dyskinesia and mood disorder. *Psychopharmacol Bull.* 2017;47:53–60.
117. Bhidayasiri R, Fahn S, Gronseth GS, et al. Evidence-based guideline: Treatment of tardive syndromes—report of the guideline development subcommittee of the American Academy of Neurology. *Neurology.* 2013;81:463–469.
118. Wilson MP, Vilke GM, Hayden SR, Nordstrom K. Psychiatric emergencies for clinicians: emergency department management of neuroleptic malignant syndrome. *J Emerg Med.* 2016;51:66–69.
119. Gurrera RJ, Caroff SN, Cohen A, et al. An international consensus study of neuroleptic malignant syndrome diagnostic criteria using the Delphi method. *J Clin Psychiatry.* 2011;72:1222–1228.
120. Citrome L. Agitation in schizophrenia: origins and evidence-based treatment. *Curr Opin Psychiatry.* 2021;34(3):216–221. 10.1097/YCO.0000000000000685 33395103.
121. Li J, Tripathi RC, Tripathi BJ. Drug-induced ocular disorders. *Drug Saf.* 2008;31:127–141.
122. Laties AM, Flach AJ, Baldycheva I, et al. Cataractogenic potential of quetiapine versus risperidone in long-term treatment of patients with schizophrenia or schizoaffective disorder: a randomized open-label, ophthalmologist-masked, flexible-dose, non-inferiority trial. *J Psychopharmacol.* 2015;29:69–79.
123. Rettenbacher MA, Hofer A, Ebenbichler C, et al. Prolactin levels and sexual adverse effects in patients with schizophrenia during antipsychotic treatment. *J Clin Psychopharmacol.* 2010;30:711–715.
124. Andersohn F, Schmedt N, Weinmann S, et al. Priapism associated with antipsychotics: role of alpha1 adrenoceptor affinity. *J Clin Psychopharmacol.* 2010;30:68–71.
125. Hasan A, Falkai P, Wobrock T, et al. World Federation of Societies of Biological Psychiatry (WFSBP) guidelines for biological treatment of schizophrenia, part 2: update 2012 on the long-term treatment of schizophrenia and management of antipsychotic induced side effects. *World J Biol Psychiatry.* 2013;14:2–44.
126. FDA Drug Safety Communication: FDA reporting mental health drug ziprasidone (Geodon) associated with rare but potentially fatal skin reactions: 2014. Available at: http://www.fda.gov/Drugs/DrugSafety/ucm426391.htm. Accessed June 1, 2015.
127. Ben-Sheetrit J, Huller-Harari L, Rasner M, et al. Psychiatric disorders and compliance with prenatal care: a 10-year retrospective cohort compared to controls. *Eur Psychiatry.* 2018;49:23–29. 10.1016/j.eurpsy.2017.11.011 29353177.
128. Vigod SN, Seeman MV, Ray JG, et al. Temporal trends in general and age-specific fertility rates among women with schizophrenia (1996–2009): a population-based study in Ontario, Canada. *Schizophr Res.* 2012;139:169–175.
129. Damkier P, Videnbech P. The safety of second-generation antipsychotics during pregnancy: a clinically focused review. *CNS Drugs.* 2018;32:351–366.
130. Einarson A, Boskovic R. Use and safety of antipsychotic drugs during pregnancy. *J Psychiatr Pract.* 2009;15(3):183–92. 10.1097/01.pra.0000351878.45260.94 19461391.
131. Huybrechts KF, Hernández-Díaz S, Patorno E, et al. Antipsychotic use in pregnancy and the risk for congenital malformations. *JAMA Psychiatry.* 2016;73(9):938–46. 10.1001/jamapsychiatry.2016.1520 27540849.
132. Arsenault MY, Lane CA, MacKinnon CJ, et al. The management of nausea and vomiting of pregnancy. *J Obstet Gynaecol Can.* 2002;24(817–831); quiz 832-3.
133. Lin HC, Chen IJ, Chen YH, et al. Maternal schizophrenia and pregnancy outcome: does the use of antipsychotics make a difference? *Schizophr Res.* 2010;116(1):55–60.
134. Newport DJ, Calamaras MR, DeVane CL, et al. Atypical antipsychotic administration during late pregnancy: placental passage and obstetrical outcomes. *Am J Psychiatry.* 2007;164(8):1214–1220. 10.1176/appi.ajp.2007.06111886 17671284.
135. Huybrechts KF, Hernandez-Diaz S, Patorno E, et al. Antipsychotic use in pregnancy and the risk for congenital malformations. *JAMA Psychiatry.* 2016;73:938–946. doi: 10.1001/jamapsychiatry.2016.1520.
136. Coughlin CG, Blackwell KA, Bartley C, et al. Obstetric and neonatal outcomes after antipsychotic medication exposure in pregnancy. *Obstet Gynecol.* 2015;125(5):1224–1235. 10.1097/AOG.0000000000000759 25932852.
137. Ellfolk M, Leinonen MK, Gissler M, et al. Second-generation antipsychotic use during pregnancy and risk of congenital malformations. *Eur J Clin Pharmacol.* 2021;77(11):1737–1745. 10.1007/s00228-021-03169-y 34100993.
138. Viguera AC, Freeman MP, Góez-Mogollón L, et al. Reproductive safety of second-generation antipsychotics: updated data from the Massachusetts General Hospital National Pregnancy Registry for Atypical Antipsychotics. *J Clin Psychiatry.* 2021;82(4):20m13745. 10.4088/JCP.20m13745. PMID: 34352165.
139. Terrana N, Koren G, Pivovarov J, Etwel F, Nulman I. Pregnancy outcomes following in utero exposure to second-generation antipsychotics: a systematic review and meta-analysis. *J Clin Psychopharmacol.* 2015;35:559–565.
140. Uguz F. Antipsychotic use during pregnancy and the risk of gestational diabetes mellitus: a systematic review. *J Clin Psychopharmacol.* 2019;39(2):162–167. 10.1097/JCP.0000000000001002 30624301.
141. Park Y, Hernandez-Diaz S, Bateman BT, et al. Continuation of atypical antipsychotic medication during early pregnancy and the risk of gestational diabetes. *Am J Psychiatry.* 2018;175:564–874. doi: 10.1176/appi.ajp.2018.17040393.
142. FDA Drug Safety Communication: Antipsychotic drug labels updated on use during pregnancy and risk of abnormal muscle movements and withdrawal symptoms in newborns. U.S. Food and Drug Administration, February 22, 2011. Available at: http://www.fda.gov/Drugs/DrugSafety/ucm243903.htm. Accessed September 9, 2018.
143. Peng M, Gao K, Ding Y, et al. Effects of prenatal exposure to atypical antipsychotics on postnatal development and growth of infants: a case-controlled, prospective study. *Psychopharmacology (Berl).* 2013;228(4):577–84. 10.1007/s00213-013-3060-6 23559219.
144. Johnson KC, LaPrairie JL, Brennan PA, et al. Prenatal antipsychotic exposure and neuromotor performance during infancy. *Arch Gen Psychiatry.* 2012;69(8):787–794. 10.1001/archgenpsychiatry.2012.160 22474072.
145. Wang Z, Chan AYL, Coghill D, et al. Association between prenatal exposure to antipsychotics and attention-deficit/hyperactivity disorder, autism spectrum disorder, preterm birth, and small for gestational age. *JAMA Intern Med.* 2021;181(10):1332–1340. 10.1001/jamainternmed.2021.4571 34398171.
146. Uguz F. Second generation antipsychotics during the lactation period. A comparative systematic review on infant safety. *J Clin Psychopharmcol.* 2016;36:244–252.
147. Cuomo A, Goracci A, Fagiolini A. Aripiprazole use during pregnancy, peripartum and lactation. A systematic literature search and review to inform clinical practice. *J Affect Disord.* 2018;228:229–237.
148. Ereshefsky L. Drug–drug interactions with the use of psychotropic medications. *CNS Spectr.* 2009;14(suppl 8):1–8.
149. Gaertner J, Ruberg K, Schlesiger G, Frechan S, Voltz R. Drug interactions in palliative care—it's more than cytochrome P450. *Palliat Med.* 2012;26:813–825.
150. Citrome L. Using oral ziprasidone effectively: the food effect and dose-response. *Adv Ther.* 2009;26(8):739–748.
151. Center for Drug Evaluation and Research.Administrative and correspondence documents. https://www.accessdata.fda.gov/drugsatfda_docs/nda/2019/209500Orig1s000OtherR.pdf. Accessed December 20, 2021.
152. Velligan DI, Lopez L, Castillo DA, et al. Interrater reliability of using brief standardized outcome measures in a community mental health setting. *Psychiatr Serv.* 2011;62:558–560.

88

Depressive Disorders

Amy M. VandenBerg

KEY CONCEPTS

1. Multiple guidelines are available to guide the treatment of major depressive disorder (MDD), including medication management. Clinicians treating individuals with MDD should be familiar with key tenets of these guidelines.
2. Other potential causes of symptoms such as medical conditions, medications, and other substances must first be ruled out when evaluating a patient for a diagnosis of MDD.
3. The goals of treatment for MDD are the resolution of current symptoms (ie, remission) and the prevention of further episodes of depression (ie, relapse or recurrence).
4. When counseling patients with MDD who are receiving traditional antidepressant medications, the patient should be informed that transient adverse medication reactions might occur initially, while the symptoms of depression may take 2 to 4 weeks to improve and up to 3 months for full resolution. Adherence to the treatment plan is essential for a successful outcome, and tools to help increase medication adherence should be discussed with each patient.
5. Since available antidepressants are considered equally efficacious for MDD, factors such as comorbid medical conditions, age, adverse effect profile, and past history of response are used to guide medication selection.
6. When determining if a particular medication is ineffective for a patient, it is essential to evaluate the dose and duration of treatment as well as patient adherence to the medication.
7. Novel antidepressants that target GABA and glutamate systems may have a more rapid and transient effect on symptoms. They are typically used in conjunction with traditional antidepressants for refractory symptoms.
8. Pharmacogenetic tests are now commercially available. Resources are available to guide their use when clinicians are presented with testing results as it relates to antidepressant treatment of MDD.
9. When evaluating antidepressant response, the clinician must consider quality-of-life issues, such as social, and occupational functioning in addition to target signs and symptoms. The tolerability of the agent should also be assessed due to the occurrence of adverse medication reactions that may lead to medication nonadherence. This is especially important in cases of recurrent episodes and long-term medication management.

BEYOND THE BOOK

Watch the TED talk entitled Depression the Secret We Share by Andrew Solomon. This talk provides an engaging patient perspective on the experience of depression including Solomon's own experiences and that of others he interviewed.

Alternatively, watch "Pharmacology – Antidepressants – SSRIs, SNRIs, TCAs, MAOIs, lithium (Made Easy)" at https://www.youtube.com/watch?v=T25jvLC6X0w. This 19-minute video provides a brief visual narrated overview of the monoamine theory of depression and mechanisms of commonly used antidepressant medications.

INTRODUCTION

Major depressive disorder (MDD) is diagnosed when an individual experiences one or more major depressive episodes without a history of mania or hypomania. A major depressive episode and MDD are defined by the criteria listed in the *Diagnostic and Statistical Manual of Mental Disorders, Fifth Edition* (*DSM-5*).[1] Depression is associated with significant functional disability, morbidity, and mortality. Antidepressants, such as the selective serotonin reuptake inhibitors (SSRIs), are equally effective and better tolerated than older agents, such as the tricyclic antidepressants (TCAs) and the monoamine oxidase inhibitors (MAOIs). While depressive episodes also occur in bipolar disorder, this chapter focuses exclusively on the diagnosis and treatment of MDD.

1 Three key evidence-based guidelines on the assessment and management of MDD are available to assist the clinician. The American Psychiatric Association *Practice Guideline for the Treatment of Patients with Major Depressive Disorder*, Third Edition (2010) (available at www.psych.org) is a practical guide to the management of MDD based on both available data and clinical consensus.[2] The updated British Association of Psychopharmacology (BAP) *evidence-based guidelines for treating depressive disorders with antidepressants* (2015) provide recommendations for antidepressant treatment of MDD.[3] Finally, the Canadian Network for Mood and Anxiety Treatments (CANMAT) 2016 *Clinical Guidelines for the management of adults with major depressive disorder* outline evidence-based pharmacological treatments for MDD.[4] These three guidelines have many similarities in recommendations.

EPIDEMIOLOGY

While the actual prevalence of depressive disorders, including undiagnosed cases, is unknown, the estimated rate has increased over the past 25 years, with additional increases since 2020.[5-8] Overall, the lifetime prevalence of depression is estimated at 7% to 15% with rate in females 1.5- to 2.5-fold higher than males.[2,3] In looking at non-sex factors, the prevalence of depression is highest in those less than

60 years of age, within non-White populations, and in individuals at high poverty levels compared to White populations over the age of 60 without poverty.[9] Intersectionality, or the study of how different social classes intersect, and its relationship to depression epidemiology is becoming a high priority field of study. Adolescent depression is increasingly common with an annual prevalence (2015) of 19.4% in females and 6.4% in males between 12 and 17 years of age (up from 13.1% and 4.5%, respectively, in 2004).[2,10] In addition, transgender and non-gender conforming individuals are also at risk for increased mental health issues. In particular adolescents in these groups with poor social support report a higher degree of suicidal ideation and attempts.[11]

Depressive disorders and suicide tend to occur within families. Approximately 8% to 18% of patients with MDD have at least one first-degree relative (father, mother, brother, or sister) with a history of depression, compared with 5.6% of those without depression.[12] First-degree relatives of patients with depression are 1.5 to 3 times more likely to develop depression than those without the family history.[4,12] The heritability of liability for MDD has been estimated at 37%, with the remaining 63% of the variance in liability due to individual-specific environment (eg, high stress, trauma).[12] Therefore, MDD is relatively common, and occurs more frequently in females than in males, and prevalence is influenced by both genetic and environmental factors.

ETIOLOGY

The etiology of depressive disorders is too complex to be explained by a single social, developmental, or biologic theory. Several factors appear to work together to cause or precipitate depressive disorders. Interactions between important factors such as individual's sex, gender identity, race, ethnicity, culture, social status, genetics, and environment are at the heart of understanding the role of intersectionality on the etiology of depression.

PATHOPHYSIOLOGY

The monoamine hypothesis that depression is caused by decreased brain levels of serotonin (5-HT), dopamine (DA), and norepinephrine (NE) has been supported for over 50 years. However, the actual chemical basis for depression remains elusive.[13] This biogenic amine hypothesis evolved as a result of several observations made in the early 1950s that the antihypertensive medication reserpine depleted neuronal storage of NE, 5-HT, and DA and produced clinically significant depression in 15% or more of patients.[14] Subsequently, the hypothesis was supported by the mechanism(s) of antidepressant medications. Additionally, recurrence of depression has been induced by acute depletion of tryptophan (precursor of 5-HT) and 5-HT metabolite levels in cerebrospinal fluid are lower in some patients with MDD.[15] Evidence reveals the complexities of the monoamine systems in the brain. These systems are mediated by gamma aminobutyric acid (GABA), neuroactive steroids, endogenous opioids, and nutritional imbalances.[16-22] For the purposes of this chapter, the focus of medication mechanism of action will be the monoamine hypothesis unless otherwise specified (Figs. 88-1 and 88-2).

Monoamine systems do not function independently, but serve as feedback mechanisms for each other. Therefore, a medication that preferentially enhances NE transmission may secondarily alter both 5-HT and DA activity.[23,24]

Although increase in synaptic monoamines (eg, NE, DA, and 5-HT) occurs rapidly after initiation of an antidepressant, the clinical effects (ie, measurable symptom improvement) are generally delayed by weeks.[15,23] This delay may be the result of a cascade of events from receptor occupancy to gene transcription, downregulation of presynaptic feedback mechanisms, and secondary effects on other neurotransmitter symptoms or neuroplasticity.[13,15,25] This led

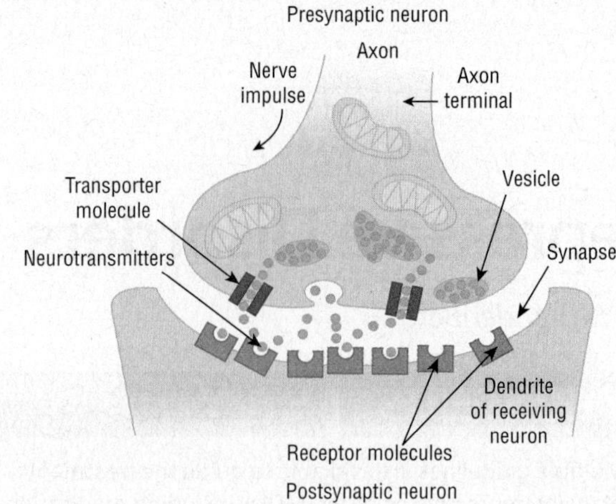

FIGURE 88-1 Monoamine neurotransmitter (NT) regulation at the neuronal level. NTs carry messages between cells. Each NT generally binds to a specific receptor, and this coupling initiates a cascade of events. NTs are reabsorbed back into nerve cells by reuptake pumps (ie, transporter molecules) at which point they may be recycled for later use or broken down by enzymes. For their primary mechanism of action, most antidepressants are thought to inhibit the transporter molecules and allow more NT to remain in the synapse. *(Reprinted from Mind Over Matter: The Brain's Response to Drugs—Teacher's Guide Revision. NIH Publication No. 05-3592. Office of Science Policy and Communications, National Institutes of Health. Revised May 2005. https://teens.drugabuse.gov/sites/default/files/moms-combined_0.pdf.)*

researchers to focus on the adaptive changes induced by antidepressants. In the mid-1970s, chronic, but not acute, administration of antidepressants to animals caused desensitization of NE-stimulated cyclic adenosine monophosphate synthesis. In fact, for most antidepressants, downregulation of β-adrenergic receptors accompanies this desensitization.[26,27] Studies of many antidepressants have demonstrated that either desensitization or downregulation of NE receptors corresponds the time course for antidepressant effects.[27] Other studies have revealed desensitization of presynaptic 5-HT_{1A} autoreceptors following chronic administration of antidepressants.[15] These theories based on changes in receptor sensitivity provide a cogent explanation for the delayed onset of therapeutic response with antidepressant medications. The dysregulation hypothesis incorporates the diversity of antidepressant activity with the adaptive changes occurring in receptor sensitization over several weeks. In this theory, emphasis is placed on a failure of homeostatic regulation of NT systems rather than on absolute increases or decreases in their activities. According to this hypothesis, effective antidepressant agents restore efficient regulation to the dysregulated NT system.[13]

Traditional explanations of the biologic basis of depressive disorders have focused largely on NE and 5-HT. However, most of the evidence that coalesced into the biogenic amine hypothesis of depression does not clearly distinguish between NE and DA. There is an abundance of evidence suggesting that DA transmission is decreased in depression, and agents that increase dopaminergic transmission have been found to be effective antidepressants.[23] Specifically, increased DA transmission in the mesolimbic pathway accounts for at least part of the mechanism of action of antidepressant medications.[23] The mechanisms by which antidepressant medications alter DA transmission remain unclear, but may be mediated either directly by dopaminergic changes or indirectly by primary actions at NE or 5-HT terminals. The complexity of the interaction between 5-HT, NE, and DA is gaining greater appreciation, but a more in-depth understanding of the precise mechanism is needed. The

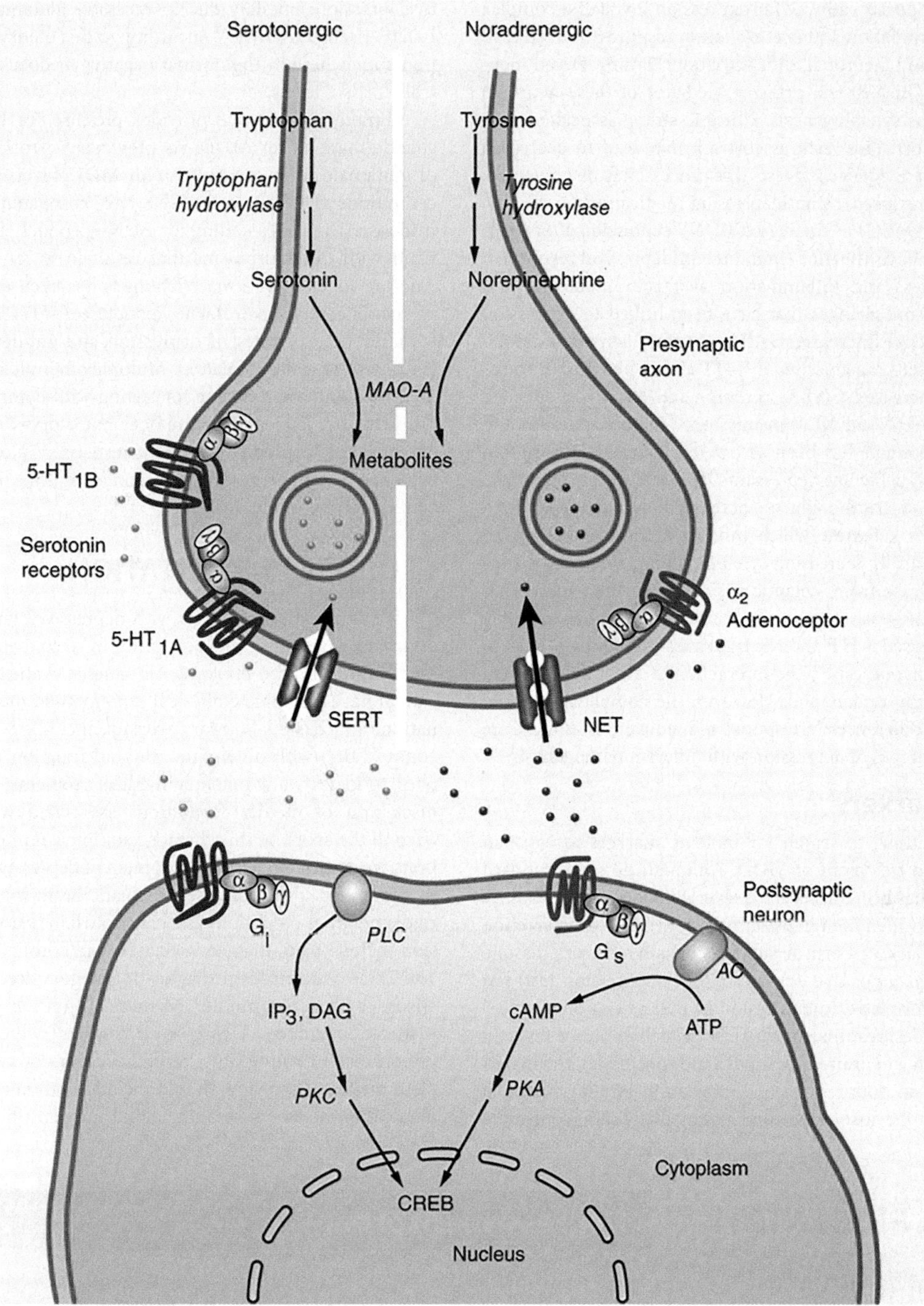

FIGURE 88-2 The presynaptic regulation and postsynaptic actions of serotonin and norepinephrine are multifaceted and many of the steps have been implicated in the pathophysiology of depression. Currently available oral antidepressants have mechanisms focused on presynaptic regulation. Most first-line antidepressants target serotonin and/or norepinephrine transporters which are responsible for "reuptake" of the neurotransmitters into presynaptic neurons (hence, selective serotonin reuptake inhibitors or serotonin and norepinephrine reuptake inhibitors). Polymorphisms in these transporters have been associated with depression and may impact efficacy of medications that target the transporters. Other medication targets include MAO, 5HT1A receptors (vilazodone, vortioxetine), and α2 receptors (mirtazapine). Due to the complexity of these systems, there are numerous other targets at various stages of investigation. *(Reproduced, with permission, from DeBattista C. Antidepressant Agents. Katzung BG, ed. Basic & Clinical Pharmacology. 15th ed. New York, NY: McGraw-Hill; 2021.)*

availability of dopaminergic-based first-line and augmentation antidepressant strategies (eg, bupropion, high-dose venlafaxine, second-generation antipsychotics) may help answer remaining questions.

Neuroactive steroids are a growing area of research in depression as a link between the progesterone metabolite, allopregnanolone, and depression has been found. Allopregnanolone release is increased in the setting of acute stress and may serve a neuroprotective role. However, with chronic stress and MDD central nervous system (CNS) concentrations of allopregnanolone may decrease. Rapid decline in allopregnanolone levels in the postpartum period has been associated with postpartum depression.[28] Furthermore, certain antidepressants have been shown to increase cerebral spinal fluid (CSF) levels of allopregnanolone proportional to depressive symptom response.[18]

Another proposed pathway for depression involves a complex interplay of inflammation and overexcitation resulting in decreased neuroplasticity and neuronal differentiation. Brain-derived neurotrophic factor (BDNF) is a primary mediator of these neuronal changes as well as synaptogenesis. Chronic stress, associated with increased glucocorticoids such as cortisol, may lead to decreased BDNF expression. Evidence suggests this process may be prevented, or possibly even reversed, by antidepressant medications or electroconvulsive therapy (ECT).[29] Increased BDNF expression after treatment initiation follows timeline similar to antidepressant response.[29]

Chronic stress and inflammation also alter glutamate and GABA transmission, changes that have been linked to depression and decreased BDNF. Increased $GABA_A$ receptor activity is associated with decreased transmission of 5-HT and increased NE transmission while increased $GABA_B$ receptor activation is associated with decreased 5-HT and NE transmission.[24] Increased serum and extrasynaptic glutamate has been associated with MDD symptom severity. Many available antidepressants decrease serum glutamate concentrations and are thought to increase BDNF activity.[16,29] An example of this is ketamine which inhibits extrasynaptic NMDA receptors, theoretically increasing synaptic glutamate activity, triggering BDNF release from synaptic vesicles.[30] Further, BDNF has been shown to decrease expression of $GABA_A$ receptors possibly resulting in increased 5-HT and NE transmission linking it back to the monoamine hypothesis.[29] The interaction of all of these related systems is not fully understood. However, the complexities could partially explain differences in response to medications as there are likely distinct subtypes of depression with different pathogenesis.

Biologic Markers

Investigators continue to search for biologic markers to assist in the diagnosis and treatment of MDD. Although no gold-standard biologic marker has been discovered, several biologic abnormalities have been variably identified in patients with MDD. Hypersecretion of cortisol or a lack of cortisol suppression after dexamethasone administration (ie, a positive dexamethasone suppression test) has been positively correlated to depression as well as risk of suicide.[31] Although the widespread use of this test has fallen out of favor in recent decades (due to limited sensitivity and specificity), the inability of the brain to suppress the hypothalamic–pituitary–adrenal (HPA) axis and the associated stress response could contribute to depression, possibly due to excessive glutamate and decreased BDNF discussed above.[31] According to this theory, there is a disruption somewhere in the normal negative feedback system that controls cortisol levels.

Emerging evidence provides promise for both biologic and genetic markers for MDD. As previously mentioned serum levels of glutamate have correlated with MDD severity and rising concentrations of BDNF in the CNS have correlated to antidepressant response. The genes coding for BDNF production have been identified with polymorphisms that result in lower levels of BDNF.[29] Another focus of pharmacogenomics has been on polymorphisms of methylenetetrahydrofolate reductase (*MTHFR*) as they relate to differences in rates of depression and antidepressant response (inconsistent results to date).[32] Multiple other phenotypes have been identified and are available for testing with commercially available products, but evidence to date does not support routine testing for diagnosis or to predict treatment response.[33] Nor is there enough evidence to support testing CNS concentrations of BDNF or serum concentrations of glutamate.

CLINICAL PRESENTATION

2 When a patient presents with depressive symptoms, it is necessary to investigate the possibility of a contributing medical or medication-induced etiology. All patients evaluated for depression should have a complete physical examination, mental status examination, and basic laboratory workup, including a complete blood count (CBC) with differential, thyroid function tests, and electrolytes, to identify any potential medical problems. While a complete discussion of medical conditions associated with depression is beyond the scope of this chapter, multiple common medical conditions are associated with development of depressive symptoms, such as stroke, Parkinson disease, traumatic brain injury, and hypothyroidism. Other conditions associated with increased risk for depression include pain, diabetes, seizures, and coronary artery disease.[36] The *DSM-5* describes a diagnostic category for both "Depressive Disorder Due to Another Medical Condition" and "Substance/Medication-Induced Depressive Disorder,"[1] which emphasizes the importance of ruling out alternative causes of symptoms. A complete medication review should include both current and previous medications to assess for both helpful and contributing medications.

CLINICAL PRESENTATION Depressive Disorder

Emotional Symptoms

- Diminished ability to experience pleasure
- Loss of interest and pleasure in usual activities, hobbies, or work (anhedonia)
- Pessimism, hopelessness regarding feeling better
- Anxiety
- Voices (eg, auditory hallucinations) saying negative comments or suggesting suicide

Physical Symptoms

- Chronic fatigue resulting in decreased ability to attend to daily tasks (eg, bathing, grooming)
- Fatigue does not improve with rest and is often associated with pain, headache
- Changes in sleep (eg, early morning awakening, difficulty falling asleep, frequent awakening or increased sleep with associated fatigue)[34]
- Appetite changes (eg, most common decreased appetite and unintentional weight loss; increased appetite/weight gain atypical)[34,35]
- Gastrointestinal disturbances, genitourinary issues, cardiovascular complaints (eg, palpitations), loss of libido

Cognitive Symptoms[35]

- Decreased concentration or slowed thinking
- Poor memory for recent events (especially older adults)
- Confused or indecisive

Psychomotor Disturbances

- Slow physical movements, speech and thought processes (psychomotor retardation)
- Restlessness (eg, pacing, wringing of hands), outbursts of anxiety or agitation (eg, crying or yelling); together known as psychomotor agitation

TABLE 88-1 Select Medications Associated with Depressive Symptoms

Medication Class	Individual Agents	Comments
Acne treatment	Isotretinoin	• REMS program iPledge recommends monitoring psychiatric symptoms
Antiseizure medications	All FDA-approved antiseizure medications (including clorazepate and clonazepam)	• Specific warning added to labeling under Warnings and Precautions regarding increased risk of suicidal thoughts or behavior • Not all agents with warning have demonstrated increased risk • Controversial
Cardiovascular medications	Reserpine	• Rarely used due to historical reports of depression due to depletion of monoamines
	Angiotensin receptor blockers β-Blockers Calcium channel blockers Clonidine Methyldopa	• Conflicting data for most agents • β-Blockers classically linked to depression; however, most evidence supports only physical symptoms of fatigue and low energy • Link between cardiovascular disease and depression must be considered
Central nervous system agents	Deutetrabenazine Tetrabenazine Valbenazine	• Deplete synaptic monoamines via decreasing vesicular transport in presynaptic neurons • Deutetrabenazine and tetrabenazine have boxed warning for depression and suicidality
Hormonal therapy	Gonadotropin-releasing hormone Oral contraceptives	• Linked to alterations in progesterone and estrogens and possible link to monoamine oxidase activity
	Steroids (eg, prednisone)	• Possible association with inflammation and HPA axis changes in depression
Immunologic agents	Interferons	• Labeled warning
Smoking cessation medications	Varenicline	• Reports to FDA MedWatch after release • Large postmarketing study does not support increased risk

REMS, Risk Evaluation and Mitigation Strategy; FDA, Food and Drug Administration.

Data from References 2 and 37–44.

TABLE 88-2 Diagnostic Criteria for Major Depressive Episode

S	Suicidal ideation with or without plan, suicide attempt; recurrent thoughts of death
I	Interest—loss of interest or pleasure in activities; anhedonia
G	Guilt—inappropriate or excessive in nature; feelings of worthlessness
E	Energy decreased
C	Concentration decreased; difficulty making decisions
A	Appetite changes; typically decreased; resulting in 5% change in weight from baseline
P	Psychomotor agitation or retardation
S	Sleep impairment; typically insomnia but may be hypersomnia

- At least five symptoms must be consistently present over a 2-week period.
- Symptoms must include depressed mood or anhedonia.
- Symptoms must cause substantial distress or impairment in functioning.
- Other medical conditions or substance use do not account for symptoms.

Data from Reference 1.

Additionally, consider the contribution of substance withdrawal (eg, cocaine, cannabis, or alcohol) to depressive symptoms. Table 88-1 lists medications commonly associated with causing or exacerbating depressive symptoms.[37-44]

Once other medical-, medication-, or substance-related causes of symptoms have been ruled out, the patient should be evaluated for MDD. According to the *DSM-5*, a single major depressive episode is characterized by five (or more) of the symptoms described in Table 88-2.[1] At least one of the symptoms is depressed mood (often an irritable mood in children or adolescents) or loss of interest or pleasure in nearly all activities.[1] These symptoms must have been present nearly every day for at least 2 weeks and must represent a change from the patient's previous level of functioning. The diagnostic code for MDD is determined by whether this is a single or recurrent depressive episode, current severity, presence of psychotic features, and remission status. The diagnosis can be followed by specifiers that apply to the current episode. The possible specifiers include anxious distress, mixed features (ie, presence of manic/hypomanic features), melancholic features, atypical features, mood-congruent or incongruent psychotic features, catatonia, peripartum onset, and seasonal pattern. The clinician must consider presenting symptoms, their duration, and the patient's current level of social, occupational, or other important areas of functioning. Significant stressors or life events may trigger depression in some individuals; however, not all patients will have a clear precipitant.[1]

Depression Rating Scales

Instruments to assess the severity of depressive symptoms can be used for both clinical and research purposes. For example, the Montgomery-Åsberg Depression Rating Scale (MADRS) is a clinician-administered scale that is commonly used in clinical trials given its sensitivity to change.[45] Some depression rating scales are self-administered such as the Beck Depression Inventory (BDI) that takes only 5 to 10 minutes to complete by the respondent.[46] The PHQ-9 is another brief scale that has been validated for use.[47] For a more detailed explanation of these instruments, as well as other rating scales and evaluation approaches, refer to Chapter e81.

Emotional Symptoms

A major depressive episode is characterized by a persistent, diminished ability to experience pleasure, and as such a loss of interest and pleasure in usual activities, hobbies, or work is common. Patients appear sad or depressed, and they are often pessimistic and believe that nothing will help them feel better. The occurrence of guilty feelings that are unrealistic is common, and these may reach delusional levels where patients feel that they deserve punishment and may view their present illness as a punishment. A patient suffering from

MDD with psychotic features may hear voices, usually auditory hallucinations saying that they are a bad person or should try to die by suicide. Depression with psychotic features may require hospitalization, especially if the patient becomes a danger to self or others. Additionally, anxiety symptoms are present in almost 90% of outpatients with depression, which may have treatment implications.

Additional Symptoms of Depression

Physical symptoms, rather than emotional symptoms, often motivate patients, especially older adults, to seek medical attention. Chronic fatigue, with a decreased ability to perform normal daily tasks is a common presenting symptom. The fatigue seen in patients with depression often appears worse in the morning, does not improve with rest, and is frequently accompanied by pain, especially headache.

Sleep disturbances generally present as early morning awakening with difficulty returning to sleep. This may coexist with difficulty falling asleep and frequent nighttime awakening, daytime exhaustion or fatigue. Hypersomnia (increased sleep) is less common. Recognition and management of sleep disturbances among patients with depression are crucial, as approximately 60% to 90% of patients experiencing MDD report sleep disturbances.[34]

Appetite disturbances, specifically decreased appetite, often result in substantial weight loss, especially in older adults.[34,35] Some patients lose 2 lb (0.9 kg) or more per week without dieting. Other patients may overeat and gain weight, although they typically do not enjoy eating.

Patients may present with a variety of other symptoms such as gastrointestinal (GI) issues (eg, pain, nausea, diarrhea, constipation), genitourinary issues (eg, incontinence, pain), cardiovascular complaints (eg, palpitations), cognitive impairment (especially older adults), or muscle fatigue. Lastly, patients frequently present with a loss of sexual interest or libido.

In addition to physical symptoms patients with MDD frequently experience cognitive and psychomotor disturbances noted in the Clinical Presentation box.

Suicide Risk Evaluation and Management

As of 2018, the Centers for Disease Control and Prevention listed death by suicide as the tenth leading cause of death among Americans and the second leading cause of death among 10- to 44-year-olds.[6] Suicide rates increased between 6% and 58% in 49 of 50 states between 1999 and 2016 and the rates in adolescents in particular are rising in the face of the COVID pandemic.[8,48] All patients diagnosed with MDD should be assessed for suicidal thoughts and factors associated with increased risk for suicide including other psychiatric disorders, substance use disorders, adolescents and younger adults, physical illness, recent stressful life event, childhood trauma, hopelessness, and male gender.[49] Those with a higher level of risk often have high degree of suicidal intent and describe more specific plans, in particular, plans that are violent and irreversible.[49] The risk of death by suicide in those recovering from MDD may increase as they develop the energy and capacity to act on a plan made earlier in a course of illness. Despite factors to help identify those at greatest risk, it remains very difficult to predict suicidality in any given individual. Therefore, when suicidal intent is suspected, it is important to ask, "Are you thinking about harming or killing yourself?" (See Chapter e81 for more information.) If the risk is significant, the patient must be referred immediately to an appropriate healthcare professional. Certain depression rating scales, such as the MADRS and PHQ-9 discussed above, include questions that target suicidality, which may help identify those patients at risk. Additionally, the Columbia-Suicide Severity Rating Scale is widely accepted in clinical practice as a validated assessment of suicide risk.[50]

In September 2004, the FDA required manufacturers of antidepressants to add a boxed warning stating that all antidepressants increase the risk of suicidal thinking and behavior in short-term studies in children and adolescents with depressive disorders. These risks have become a new source of concern among those treating their patients with antidepressants. In order to help deal with the confusion these warnings have caused, experts have recommended the following[51]:

1. It is especially important to closely monitor patients for suicidal ideation and behavior at the beginning of treatment and among younger patients.
2. Discuss the possibility that adverse medication reactions may occur, including behavioral agitation or anger, and encourage patients to seek help should this occur.
3. Deal with the subject of suicide directly.

Withholding antidepressant treatment may not decrease the risk of suicide and may actually increase the risk. Furthermore, it may be that longer-term medication is needed for any protective effects against suicidality.[51]

In May 2007, the FDA expanded the boxed warning regarding suicidality to include young adults 18 to 24 years of age, during the initial stages of treatment. The warning also applies to any medication with either monotherapy or adjunct treatment of depression as an FDA-approved indication even if not classified as an "antidepressant" (eg, aripiprazole, quetiapine).

Assessment of actual suicide risk has proven to be difficult as there are differences in coding of events in clinical trials and complete case data from trials is often not available. Additionally, there appears to be an increased risk of suicidality in the 30 days after antidepressant discontinuation, which is not routinely evaluated in clinical trials.[52] An increased risk of suicidality in children and adolescents has been found in multiple studies and this population should be evaluated carefully upon initiation or discontinuation of antidepressant treatment. The complex relationships between antidepressant use and suicidality will continue to be explored with the hopes of more unequivocal recommendations.

TREATMENT

Desired Outcomes

3 The goal of treating depression is resolution of depressive symptoms and return to previous level functioning. Initial treatment may occur in the hospital or in outpatient treatment settings. Hospitalization is more likely when there is a high risk of suicide, poor physical health, limited social support or psychotic symptoms. Response, typically defined as 50% decrease in symptoms and is achieved in 40% to 50% of patients 8 to 12 weeks after medication initiation. Remission (absence of symptoms) is achieved in 25% to 30% of patients within 8 to 12 weeks after medication initiation.[3]

General Approach to Treatment

There are three treatment phases for patients with MDD: (a) the *acute* phase lasting approximately 6 to 12 weeks in which the goal is remission; (b) the *continuation* phase lasting 4 to 9 months after remission is achieved, in which the goal is to eliminate residual symptoms or prevent relapse (ie, return of symptoms within 6 months of remission); and (c) the *maintenance* phase lasting at least 12 to 36 months in which the goal is to prevent recurrence (ie, a separate episode of depression).[2,53] The duration of antidepressant therapy depends on the risk of recurrence which increases with each depressive episode. Some guidelines recommend lifelong maintenance therapy for persons at greatest risk for recurrence (younger than 40 years of age with two or more prior episodes or any age with three or more prior episodes).[2] An alternative guideline is to treat for at least 2 years in

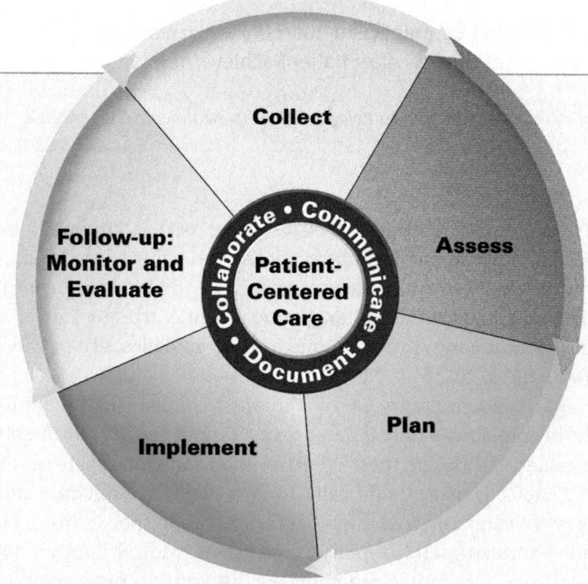

Patient Care Process for Major Depressive Disorder

The image shows the five fundamental steps included in The Pharmacist's Care Process endorsed by the Joint Commission for Pharmacy Practitioners (2014). The tagline of this process reads collaborate, communicate, and document. The five fundamental steps listed here are collect, assess, plan, implement, and follow-up: monitor and evaluate. All these steps are listed in a circular block diagram.

Collect

- Patient characteristics (eg, age, sex, gender identity, race, pregnancy status)
- Current and past medical/psychiatric history (including information on first-degree family members)
- Past medication history, including medications not tolerated and any medication allergies (also collect on first-degree family members)
- Social history (eg, tobacco, ethanol, and other substance use as well as social supports and/or stressors)
- Current medications including over-the-counter (OTC), herbal products, dietary supplements, and medical or recreational cannabis use
- Objective data
  - Blood pressure, heart rate, weight
  - Labs including thyroid function tests, serum creatinine, complete blood count (CBC), liver function tests, urine toxicology screen, blood alcohol level, medication serum concentrations, and pharmacogenomics testing if available
  - Reported symptoms of depression or other rating scale assessment (eg, Patient Health Questionnaire 9 [PHQ-9], Beck Depression inventory [BDI]) (Tables 88-1 and 88-2 and Chapter e81, "Evaluation of Psychiatric Illness")

Assess

- Suicidality (eg, Columbia-Suicide Severity Scale)
- Severity of illness/need for hospitalization
- Impact of substance use on symptoms and whether a substance use disorder is contributing to symptoms
- Presence of physical conditions that may overlap with depression symptoms (eg, pain resulting in insomnia or limited activity, gastrointestinal symptoms resulting in weight loss) or medications that may be contributing to depressive symptoms (Table 88-1)
- Past response and adherence (personal or family) to antidepressant medications
- Ability/willingness to follow up with psychiatry services including antidepressant medication management, cognitive behavioral therapy (CBT), outpatient groups
- Barriers to participation in medication management or CBT
- Barriers to adjunctive treatments (eg, exercise, stretching, yoga)
- Pharmacogenomics testing results

Plan*

- Medication therapy regimen including specific agent(s), dose, frequency, and titration plan if applicable (Table 88-3)
- Monitoring parameters including efficacy (looking for some improvement in 2-4 weeks), safety (change in suicidality), and adverse medication reactions (may be seen in first 1-2 weeks of treatment) (Table 88-11)
- Patient education (eg, purpose of treatment, medication-specific information, medication adherence, and review of laboratory/pharmacogenomics results)
- Patient education regarding self-monitoring, when to call the clinic with questions or concerns, and when to seek emergency medical attention (eg, suicidality)
- Obtain release of information to gather collateral information (eg, family members, therapists, medical providers)
- Nonpharmacological interventions (eg, diet, exercise, mindfulness)
- Make referrals to other providers when appropriate (eg, neurologist, pain specialist, substance use disorder treatment)
- Potential for medication interactions (Tables 88-5, 88-9, and 88-10)

Implement*

- Provide patient education regarding all elements of the treatment plan
- Use motivational interviewing and coaching to maximize adherence
- Schedule follow-up to monitor and assess medication effectiveness (eg, PHQ-9, BDI) and adherence to treatment plan, including therapeutic medication monitoring when appropriate.

Follow-up: Monitor and Evaluate

- Resolution of depressive symptoms using standardized rating scales
- Presence of adverse medication reactions (Table 88-11)
- Laboratory follow-up when indicated (eg, sodium, liver function tests)
- Patient adherence to treatment plan based in multiple sources of information (eg, medication refill records, patient/caregiver report)

(continued)

- Consider scheduling early or more frequent (every 1-2 weeks) follow-up visits after initiating therapy to monitor response and behavioral risks such as suicidality. Reevaluate initial response at 2 to 4 weeks and again at 8 to 12 weeks.

Reevaluate treatment plan quarterly and reevaluate duration of therapy after patient achieves remission.

Collaborate with patient, caregivers, and other healthcare professionals.

patients considered to be at high risk for relapse.[3] The decision as to "when" and "how" to taper/discontinue an antidepressant regimen is always going to depend on patient- and medication-specific variables. Both SSRIs and SNRIs have an idiosyncratic discontinuation syndrome that may occur; therefore, it is recommended to slowly taper these agents over weeks to months to minimize. However, a slow taper is not always effective in preventing discontinuation symptoms.[54]

4 Educating the patient and their support system (eg, family and friends) regarding the delay in antidepressant effects and the importance of medication adherence should occur before and during the entire course of treatment. The treatment of MDD generally includes both nonpharmacologic and pharmacologic strategies.

Nonpharmacologic Therapy

In addition to pharmacologic interventions, psychotherapy ("talk therapy") should be employed whenever the patient is able and willing to participate. Traditionally, psychotherapy alone is recommended only for mild to moderately severe cases of MDD. However, evidence supports the benefit of cognitive behavioral therapy (CBT) for even severe MDD.[55] Psychotherapy should not be the primary treatment modality for patients with psychotic features. The effects of psychotherapy and antidepressant medications are considered to be additive, thus combined treatment may be advantageous for patients with partial responses to either treatment alone and for those with a chronic course of illness. In practice, CBT as primary treatment is limited significantly by cost and logistics (eg, need for more frequent appointments and time off work). Additionally, many insurance plans do not adequately cover the cost of psychotherapy, the availability of providers may be limited in certain areas, and patients may be more reluctant to spend the time in therapy versus taking medication. In the Sequenced Treatment Alternatives to Relieve Depression study (STAR*D), evaluation of the psychotherapy arm was limited by low participation rates.[56]

Electroconvulsive therapy (ECT) is a safe and effective treatment for severe MDD. Ideally it is used when a rapid response is needed (eg, severe suicidality, nutritional deficiency, catatonic symptoms), risks of other treatments outweigh potential benefits, symptoms refractory to two antidepressant trials, or there is history of good response to ECT, and the patient expresses a preference for ECT. Another nonpharmacologic approach is repetitive transcranial magnetic stimulation (rTMS), which has demonstrated efficacy in treating MDD symptoms without the anesthesia required for ECT.[57]

The health benefits of physical activity have long been recognized for many medical conditions, and data suggest benefits in depressed patients. The Treatment with Exercise Augmentation for Depression (TREAD) study demonstrated that 16 kcal (67 kJ) per kilogram per week (KKW) exercise was associated with greater MDD remission rates compared with 4 KKW, when both were used as augmentation to an SSRI.[58] According to APA Task Force, integrating exercise into the MDD treatment plan is medically appropriate and confers many well-accepted health benefits.[59]

Pharmacologic Therapy

Antidepressants are considered first-line treatment for a moderate-to-severe depressive episode.[2-4] They can be classified in several ways, including by chemical structure and the presumed mechanism of antidepressant activity. Although the link between the presumed mechanism of action and antidepressant response is tenuous, this classification has the advantage of being based on established pharmacology and clearly explains some of the common, but expected, adverse medication reactions. The knowledgeable clinician can use these antidepressant properties to tailor treatment to individual patient needs optimizing treatment outcomes. Currently available antidepressants, including dosing guidance, are provided in Table 88-3.[2,3,53,60-62]

5 Antidepressants are of *equivalent efficacy* when administered in comparable doses. Because one cannot predict which antidepressant will be the most effective in an individual patient, the initial choice is made empirically. Factors that often influence antidepressant choice include the patient's history of response, history of familial antidepressant response, concurrent medical illnesses and medications, presenting symptoms (eg, insomnia vs hypersomnia), potential for medication interactions, adverse medication reactions, patient preference, and medication cost. Although the precise pathophysiology of MDD remains elusive, clinicians can now select from multiple approved medications with different mechanisms of action (Tables 88-3 and 88-8).[2-4,63] Failure to respond to one antidepressant class or one antidepressant agent within a class does not predict a failed response to another class or another agent within the same class (Fig. 88-3). Approximately 50% to 60% of patients with MDD improve with acute medication therapy, compared with about 30% to 40% who improve with placebo.[3,64]

Selective Serotonin Reuptake Inhibitors

The efficacy of SSRIs is superior to placebo and comparable to other antidepressant classes in treating patients with MDD.[2,53] They are generally chosen as *first-line* due to relative safety in overdose and improved tolerability over TCAs and MAOIs. The decision of which SSRI to use is typically based on the nuances of each medication, such as differences in interaction profile and pharmacokinetic (PK) parameters (eg, half-life). These concepts will be discussed in greater detail later in this chapter. The STAR*D trial demonstrated that nonresponse to one SSRI does not predict nonresponse to an alternative SSRI and a recent meta-analysis found no differences in efficacy between agents.[56,65]

The SSRIs, as the name implies, have a low affinity for other receptors including alpha$_1$-adrenergic ($\alpha 1$), histaminic (H1), and muscarinic (M1) receptors. Given this pharmacology, they are associated with lower rates of orthostatic hypotension, sedation, weight gain, and anticholinergic effects compared to TCAs.[2-4,63] The most common dose-dependent tolerability issues with SSRI use, which generally are mild and limited to 1 to 2 weeks after initiation or dose increases, are GI symptoms (eg, nausea, vomiting, and diarrhea), anxiety, and headache.[66] Both somnolence and insomnia have been reported with all SSRIs.[67] Additionally the SSRIs may cause clinically relevant impairment in all three stages of the human sexual response (arousal, libido, orgasm)[68]; however, it is important to note that depression itself may be associated with sexual dysfunction. A discontinuation or withdrawal syndrome may occur if SSRIs are abruptly discontinued (see details below with SNRIs). Paroxetine has more anticholinergic and antihistaminergic activity that has been linked with increased sedation and weight gain compared to other SSRIs.[2-4,63] The FDA released a safety announcement linking citalopram to a dose-dependent increase in QT interval, with recommended, age-dependent dose limits.[69] There has since been controversy regarding this safety warning and potential unintended consequences (eg, underdosing, discontinuation leading to

TABLE 88-3 Adult Dosing Guidance for Currently Available Antidepressant Medications

Medication (Brand Name)	Initial Dose (mg/day)	Usual Dosage Range (mg/day)	Comments (eg, Maximum Daily Dosage, Suggested Therapeutic Plasma Concentration)
Selective Serotonin Reuptake Inhibitors (SSRIs)			
Patients with significant anxiety should start with lower initial dose to improve tolerability; however, target dose does not differ.			
Citalopram (Celexa)	10-20	20-40	Doses >40 mg/day not recommended due to QTc prolongation risk; maximum 20 mg/day for CYP2C19 poor metabolizers, coadministration with CYP2C19 inhibitors or patients older than 60 years of age
Escitalopram (Lexapro)	5-10	10-20	Maximum 20 mg/day; dose may be increased to maximum daily dose after 1 week
Fluoxetine (Prozac)	10-20	20-60	Maximum 80 mg/day; dose may be increased in 20-mg increments
Fluvoxamine (Luvox)	25-50	50-300	Maximum 300 mg/day; daily doses >100-mg total dose should be divided twice daily, with the larger dose given at night Maximum 300 mg/day (ER formulation)
Paroxetine (Paxil)	10-20	20-50	Maximum 50 mg/day (IR formulation); titrate 10 mg/day increments weekly Maximum 62.5 mg/day (CR formulation); titrate 12.5 mg/day increments weekly
Sertraline (Zoloft)	25-50	50-200	Maximum 200 mg/day; titrate 25 mg/day increments weekly
Serotonin–Norepinephrine Reuptake Inhibitors (SNRIs)			
Newer-generation SNRIs			
Desvenlafaxine (Pristiq)	50	100	Doses up to 400 mg/day have been studied; however, tolerability decreases with doses >50 mg. Dose reductions or discontinuation may be required if sustained hypertension occurs
Duloxetine (Cymbalta)	30	30-90	Maximum 120 mg/day (given once or twice daily); doses >60 mg/day not shown to provide increased efficacy for the treatment of MDD
Venlafaxine (Effexor)	37.5-75	75-225	Maximum 375 mg/day (IR); maximum 225 mg/day (ER); may increase in increments up to 75 mg/day at a minimum of every 4 days. Dose reductions or discontinuation may be required if sustained hypertension occurs
Levomilnacipran (Fetzima)	20	40-120	Initial dose (20 mg) for 2 days before dose increases is recommended at intervals of 2 or more days. Dose adjustment or discontinuation may be required if sustained elevated heart rate or hypertension occurs
Tricyclic antidepressants (TCAs)			
Amitriptyline (Elavil)	25	100-200	Maximum 300 mg/day for MDD; as single daily dose at bedtime or divided doses; therapeutic serum level 80-200 ng/mL (mcg/L; ~300-740 nmol/L); parent medication plus metabolite (nortriptyline)
Desipramine (Norpramin)	25	100-200	Maximum 300 mg/day; suggested therapeutic concentration range for combined imipramine + desipramine: 100-300 ng/mL (mcg/L; ~370-1,100 nmol/L)
Doxepin (Sinequan)	25	100-200	Maximum 300 mg/day as a single daily dose at bedtime (if tolerated) or in divided doses; a single dose should not exceed 150 mg
Imipramine (Tofranil)	25	100-200	Maximum 300 mg/day as single daily dose at bedtime (if tolerated) or divided doses; suggested therapeutic concentration range for combined imipramine + desipramine: 150-300 ng/mL (mcg/L; ~550-1,100 nmol/L)
Nortriptyline (Pamelor)	25	50-150	Maximum 150 mg/day as single daily dose (if tolerated) or divided doses; therapeutic serum level 50-150 ng/mL (mcg/L; 190-570 nmol/L)
Norepinephrine and Dopamine Reuptake Inhibitor (NDRI)			
Bupropion (Wellbutrin)	150 (75 mg given twice daily)	150-450	Maximum 450 mg/day (IR, ER), 400 mg/day (SR); ER dosed once daily; SR dosed once or twice daily; IR may be dosed up to three times daily. Adhering to labeled maximum daily and maximum single doses minimizes effect on seizure threshold
Mixed Serotonergic Effects (Mixed 5-HT)			
Nefazodone (Serzone)	100	200-400	Maximum 600 mg/day; daily doses should be divided twice daily; boxed warning hepatotoxicity
Trazodone (Desyrel)	50	150-300	Maximum 600 mg/day
Vilazodone (Viibryd)	10	20-40	Target dose 20-40 mg/day unless coadministered with CYP3A4 inhibitor (dose not to exceed 20 mg/day). Dose titration: 10 mg/day for 7 days, 20 mg/day for 7 days, and then may increase to 40 mg/day. Dose must be taken with food to ensure adequate absorption
Vortioxetine (Trintellix)	10	20	Maximum 20 mg/day
Serotonin and α_2-Adrenergic Antagonist			
Mirtazapine (Remeron)	15	15-45	Maximum 45 mg/day
Monoamine Oxidase Inhibitors (MAOIs)			
Phenelzine (Nardil)	15	30-90	Maximum 90 mg/day; divided dosing; increase by 15 mg at 1- to 3-week intervals
Selegiline (transdermal) (Emsam)	6	6-12	Not to exceed 12 mg/24 hours; dose may be increased by 3 mg/day increments every 2 weeks; site of application should be rotated

(continued)

TABLE 88-3 Adult Dosing Guidance for Currently Available Antidepressant Medications (*Continued*)

Medication (Brand Name)	Initial Dose (mg/day)	Usual Dosage Range (mg/day)	Comments (eg, Maximum Daily Dosage, Suggested Therapeutic Plasma Concentration)
Tranylcypromine (Parnate)	10 10-20	20-40 30-60	Maximum 60 mg/day; divided dosing; increase by 10 mg at 1- to 3-week intervals
Isocarboxazid (Marplan)	10-20	30-60	Maximum 60 mg/day; divided dosing
Second-generation Antipsychotics (SGA) as Augmentation (5HT$_{2A}$ and D$_2$ modulators)			
Aripiprazole (Abilify)	2	2-15	FDA-approved for augmentation; CANMAT Level 1 evidence, 1st line
Brexpiprazole (Rexulti)	1	1-3	Not FDA-approved for augmentation; CANMAT Level 1 evidence, 2nd line
Olanzapine (Zyprexa)	2.5	2.5-10	Not FDA-approved for augmentation; CANMAT Level 1 evidence, 2nd line
Olanzapine/ fluoxetine (Symbyax)	3/25	6-12/25-50	FDA-approved for treatment-resistant depression
Quetiapine (Seroquel)	50	150-300	FDA-approved for augmentation; CANMAT Level 1 evidence, 1st line
Risperidone (Risperdal)	1	1-3	Not FDA-approved for augmentation; CANMAT Level 1 evidence, 1st line
Alternative Augmentation Agents (Not FDA-Approved for Antidepressant Augmentation)			
Buspirone (Buspar)	10	10-60	Divided dosing 2 to 3 times daily 5HT1A partial agonist
Lithium	300	600-1,200	Dose based on therapeutic levels (target 0.6-1 mEq/L [mmol/L]) Mechanism in depression not fully understood
Triiodothyronine (Cytomel)	0.025	0.025-0.05	Once daily dosing; monitor free T3 levels

CANMAT, Canadian Network for Mood and Anxiety Treatments; CR, continuous release; ER, extended release; IR, immediate release; MDD, major depressive disorder; SR, sustained release.

Data from References 2, 3, 53, and 60-62.

relapse).[69,70] Dose-dependent increase in QT interval may also be associated with escitalopram; however, clinical significance of the QT increase is questionable with both agents.[69]

Serotonin–Norepinephrine Reuptake Inhibitors (SNRIs)

Tricyclic Antidepressants Although TCAs are effective in treating MDD, use has diminished greatly due to the availability of equally effective therapies that are better tolerated and much safer in overdose. All TCAs potentiate the activity of NE and 5-HT by blocking their reuptake. However, the potency and selectivity of TCAs for the inhibition of NE and 5-HT reuptake vary greatly among these agents (see Table 88-4). Nortriptyline is most commonly used and may be selected in patients with comorbid migraine headaches, neuropathic pain, or fibromyalgia.

The TCAs affect other neurotransmitters and produce a wide range of pharmacologic actions, including several unwanted, but expected, adverse medication reactions. The most commonly occurring dose-related adverse reactions are anticholinergic in nature and include dry mouth, constipation, blurred vision, urinary retention, dizziness, and tachycardia (see Table 88-8). In older adult patients or with very high doses, memory impairment or delirium may occur.[71] Although some tolerance does develop, these reactions have the potential to impact patient adherence, particularly in older adults and those receiving long-term maintenance therapy. Additional tolerability issues that decrease TCA adherence include weight gain and sexual dysfunction.[71]

Orthostatic hypotension is a common, dose-related reaction attributed to the affinity of the TCAs for α_1 receptors.[63] In patients with history of myocardial infarction, TCAs should be avoided due to risk of severe arrhythmias (QTc prolongation, torsades de pointes) thought to be associated with their class IA antiarrhythmic effects.[72] Additionally, TCAs can cause cardiac conduction delays, may induce heart block in patients with a preexisting conduction disorder, and overdose is associated with severe arrhythmias.[71] Desipramine's prescribing information reflects an increased risk of death in patients receiving the medication who have a *family history* of sudden cardiac death, cardiac dysrhythmias, and cardiac conduction disturbances. More on this reaction can be found at the FDA's MedWatch Website. Caution should be exercised when prescribing these agents, especially in higher doses, to patients with clinically significant cardiac disease, and to patients with a family history of a cardiac event.

Newer-Generation SNRIs Venlafaxine and its primary active metabolite, desvenlafaxine, inhibit 5-HT reuptake at low doses, and NE reuptake at higher doses, whereas duloxetine equally inhibits both 5-HT and NE reuptake inhibition across all doses. This difference in receptor binding has not been associated with significant differences in efficacy. According to some studies, the SNRIs may be associated with higher rates of response and remission than other antidepressants; however, most of these studies involved venlafaxine, and not all studies support this conclusion.[65] The BAP guidelines discuss the possibility of a slight efficacy advantage (ie, lower number needed to treat; NNT) for venlafaxine (as well as escitalopram and sertraline) compared to other antidepressants.[3]

The most recent SNRI to be FDA-approved for MDD is levomilnacipran. This is a single-isomer, extended-release formulation of milnacipran which is FDA-approved only for the treatment of fibromyalgia. It is too soon to determine its place in therapy for MDD; however, pharmacologically it is relatively unique among the SNRIs given its greater potency at inhibiting NE reuptake compared to 5-HT reuptake.[63,73] One NE selective reuptake inhibitor, reboxetine, available in non-US markets, was not FDA-approved due to poor tolerability and lack of efficacy.

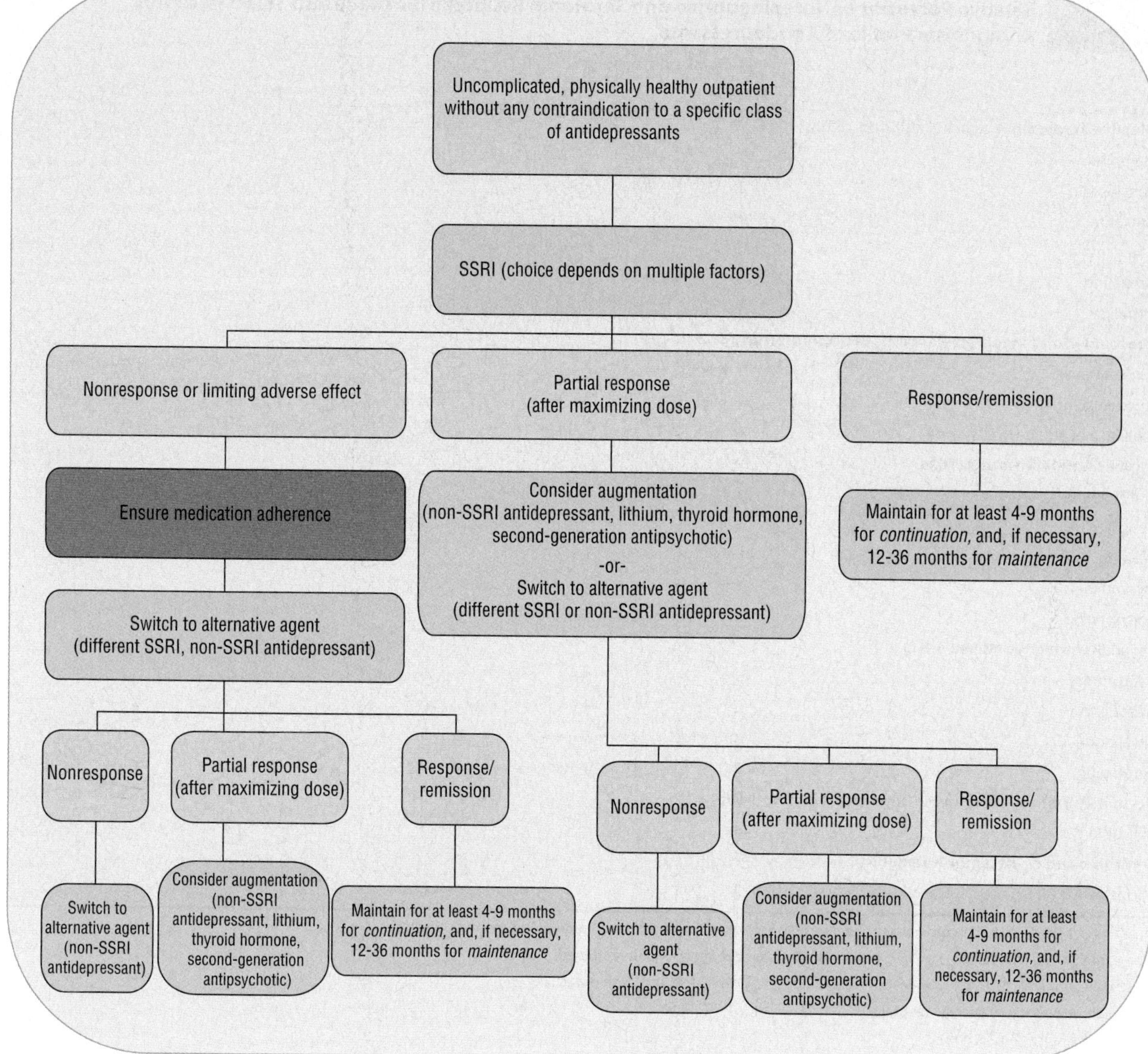

FIGURE 88-3 Suggested algorithm for treatment of uncomplicated MDD. (SSRI, selective serotonin reuptake inhibitor.) Note: Both the British Association of Pharmacology (BAP) guidelines and the STAR*D trial suggest that switching and augmentation strategies are supported by stronger evidence compared to dose increases (among poor antidepressant responders).

The most commonly reported tolerability issues with SNRIs, similar to those of SSRIs, may be dose-related and include nausea, sexual dysfunction, and activation.[2-4] Hyperhidrosis (excessive sweating) occurs primarily with SNRIs. Dose-related increases in blood pressure have been reported more with venlafaxine and levomilnacipran but may also occur with duloxetine and desvenlafaxine.[2] Blood pressure should be monitored at baseline and regularly during therapy, especially after dose increases. The discontinuation or withdrawal syndrome that can occur when treatment is stopped appears to be more severe with SNRIs than SSRIs. Common withdrawal symptoms include headache, fatigue, sweating, musculoskeletal pain, electric shock sensations, and anxiety. While slowly tapering off the medication may help to reduce the risk of the withdrawal syndrome, it may not fully prevent.[54] Duloxetine has also been associated with idiosyncratic hepatotoxicity (1 per 100,000 case exposures) with enzyme elevations more than three times upper limit of normal in 1% of patients, but does not carry the boxed warning associated with nefazodone.[74]

Mixed Serotonergic Medications (Mixed 5-HT)

Trazodone and nefazodone have dual actions on serotonergic neurons, acting as both postsynaptic 5-HT_2 antagonists and presynaptic 5-HT reuptake inhibitors. They may also enhance 5-HT_{1A}-mediated neurotransmission.[63] Trazodone blocks α_1 and H1 receptors leading to adverse reactions (eg, dizziness and sedation) that limit its use as an antidepressant. Use of nefazodone declined after reports of hepatotoxicity and the FDA-approved labeling includes a boxed warning describing rare cases of fulminant liver failure (1 case per 300,000 treatment years) and hepatic impairment (29 cases per 100,000 treatment years).[74] Trazodone and nefazodone are effective agents in treating MDD; however, both carry risks that limit their usefulness. Immediate-release trazodone is most often used adjunctively (in low

TABLE 88-4 Relative Potencies of Norepinephrine and Serotonin Reuptake Blockade and Select Receptor Antagonism Profile of Antidepressants

	Reuptake Antagonism				
	NE	**5-HT**	**M1**	**H1**	**α1**
Selective Serotonin Reuptake Inhibitors (SSRIs)					
Citalopram	0	++++	0	+	0
Escitalopram	0	++++	0	0	0
Fluoxetine	+	++++	0	0	0
Fluvoxamine	0	++++	0	0	0
Paroxetine	++	++++	++	+	0
Sertraline	0	++++	0	0	+
Serotonin–Norepinephrine Reuptake Inhibitors (SNRIs)					
Duloxetine	+++	++++	0	0	0
Levomilnacipran	++++	+++	+	0	0
Venlafaxine[a] and desvenlafaxine	+++	++++	0	0	0
Tricyclic Antidepressants (TCAs)					
Amitriptyline	++	++++	++++	++++	+++
Desipramine	++++	++	+	++	++
Doxepin	++	++	+++	++++	+++
Imipramine	++	++++	+++	++++	+++
Nortriptyline	++++	++	++	+++	++
Mixed Serotonergic (Mixed 5-HT)					
Nefazodone	0	++	0	+++	+++
Trazodone	0	++	0	++	+++
Vilazodone	0	++++	0	+	0
Vortioxetine	0	++++	0	+	0
Norepinephrine and Dopamine Reuptake Inhibitor (NDRI)					
Bupropion[b]	+	0	+	0	0
Serotonin and α_2-Receptor Antagonist					
Mirtazapine	0	0	0	+++	+

M1, antimuscarinic/anticholinergic adverse reactions; H1, antihistamine, sedation; α1 antiadrenergic, hypotension.

++++, high; +++, moderate; ++, low; +, very low; 0, absent or not adequately studied.

[a]Venlafaxine: primarily 5-HT at lower doses, NE at higher doses, and DA at very high doses.

[b]Bupropion: also blocks dopamine reuptake.

Data from References 2-4, 53, and 63.

doses) with other antidepressants to treat insomnia associated with MDD.[67]

Trazodone and nefazodone have minimal anticholinergic effects and comparatively less 5-HT agonist adverse reactions (eg, sexual dysfunction), but they can cause orthostatic hypotension. Sedation, cognitive slowing, and dizziness are the most frequent dose-limiting adverse reactions associated with trazodone, although the dosage used for the treatment of depression is significantly higher than the dosage often used for the treatment of insomnia (25-200 mg).[4,67] Common adverse medication reactions associated with nefazodone include light-headedness, dizziness, orthostatic hypotension, and somnolence. Nefazodone treatment should not be initiated in individuals with active liver disease or with elevated baseline serum transaminases. A rare but potentially serious adverse reaction of trazodone is priapism, which is reported to occur in approximately 1 in 6,000 male patients. Some cases have required surgical intervention (1 in 23,000), and permanent impotence may result.[75] There have been no reports of priapism associated with nefazodone use in males, but there is a published case report of nefazodone-induced clitoral priapism.[75]

Vilazodone and vortioxetine are combination SSRI and 5-HT_{1A} presynaptic receptor partial agonists approved for the treatment of MDD.[73] Presynaptic 5-HT_{1A} partial agonism has previously been hypothesized as a mechanism for SSRI augmentation with pindolol, which has preferential antagonism at the presynaptic 5-HT_{1A} receptor.[76] The primary dose-limiting adverse reaction of these two newer agents is nausea. Vortioxetine additionally antagonizes 5-HT_3 which is proposed to mitigate some of the nausea, and is also a partial agonist at 5-HT_{1B}, and an antagonist at 5-HT_{1D} and 5-HT_7 receptors.[62] Preliminary data support a linkage between the 5-HT_7 receptor antagonism and lack of cognitive slowing and potential for improved cognitive symptoms with vortioxetine in patients with MDD.

Vilazodone and vortioxetine are both associated with significant dose-related GI tolerability issues (eg, diarrhea and nausea), dizziness, insomnia, and decreased libido (particularly among males) when compared to placebo.[73] Rates of sexual dysfunction appear to be lower than with SSRIs; however, in some trials comparator agents known to cause sexual dysfunction (eg, duloxetine) also had lower rates of sexual dysfunction.[62,73]

Norepinephrine and Dopamine Reuptake Inhibitor (NDRI)

Bupropion has no appreciable effect on the 5-HT reuptake, and inhibits both the NE and DA reuptake making it one of the most activating antidepressants.[63] This can be particularly helpful for decreased motivation, low energy, and fatigue, which are common symptoms in older adult patients. It is also FDA-approved for smoking cessation and in a combination product with naltrexone for weight loss.

Adverse medication reactions associated with bupropion include nausea, vomiting, tremor, insomnia, and dry mouth. The occurrence of seizures in patients taking bupropion appears to be strongly dose-related, and may be increased by predisposing factors such as history of prior seizure activity, severe alcohol withdrawal, head trauma, or CNS tumor. Bupropion use is contraindicated in patients with eating disorders such as bulimia and anorexia. In addition to risk for further appetite suppression, these patients are prone to electrolyte abnormalities and are therefore at higher risk for seizure activity. At daily doses of 450 mg (the FDA-approved maximum dose) or less, the incidence of seizures is 0.4%, which is similar to reported rates for clomipramine, desipramine, and citalopram.[77] Bupropion is associated with minimal sexual dysfunction compared with the SSRIs and may actually improve SSRI-induced sexual dysfunction when used as adjunctive treatment.[78]

Serotonin and α_2-Adrenergic Receptor Antagonists

Mirtazapine enhances central noradrenergic and serotonergic activity through the antagonism of central presynaptic α_2-adrenergic autoreceptors and heteroreceptors.[79] Furthermore, it antagonizes postsynaptic 5-HT_2, 5-HT_3, and H1 receptors resulting in anxiolytic, anti-nausea, and sedative effects, respectively.

The most common adverse medication reactions of mirtazapine are somnolence, weight gain (>7%), likely due to relatively strong antihistaminergic properties.[67] Mirtazapine is associated with minimal sexual dysfunction.

Monoamine Oxidase Inhibitors

Monoamine oxidase inhibitors increase the concentrations of NE, 5-HT, and DA within the neuronal synapse through inhibition of the MAO enzymes. The MAOIs isocarboxazid, phenelzine, and tranylcypromine are nonselective inhibitors of MAO-A and MAO-B. A selegiline transdermal patch allows inhibition of MAO-A and MAO-B in the brain, yet has reduced effects on MAO-A in the gut.[80]

The most common adverse reaction of oral MAOIs is postural hypotension, which is more likely to occur with phenelzine and may be minimized with divided doses. Other common adverse reactions include weight gain and sexual dysfunction (eg, decreased libido and anorgasmia).[2] Phenelzine has mild-to-moderate sedating effects, while tranylcypromine and selegiline may exert a stimulating effect and insomnia due to amphetamine-like metabolites.[61]

Hypertensive crisis, which is a potentially serious and life-threatening but rare adverse reaction, may occur when MAOIs are taken concurrently with foods containing tyramine. Tyramine is usually metabolized by MAO-A in the gut and not absorbed into systemic circulation where it acts as a potent vasoconstrictor. Oral MAOIs block gut MAO-A resulting in absorption of tyramine. In patients on MAOIs, 10 mg of tyramine can cause marked hypertension and severe headache, and 25 mg can result in hypertensive crisis, whereas the average adult can tolerate over 500 mg of tyramine without a significant impact on blood pressure.[61,81] This may also occur when MAOIs are co-ingested with medications that increase norepinephrine (eg, decongestants, stimulants, SNRIs). Symptoms of hypertensive crisis include occipital headache, stiff neck, nausea, vomiting, sweating, and sharply elevated blood pressure which may culminate in cerebrovascular accident and death. For details regarding management of hypertensive emergencies, refer to Chapter 30, "Hypertension." The other significant risk of MAOIs is serotonin syndrome with concurrent use of other medications that increase serotonin (eg, antidepressants other than MAOIs). Education of patients taking MAOIs regarding dietary and medication restrictions is extremely important. Examples of potentially high tyramine foods and medications that should be avoided or used with caution are provided in Table 88-5.[61,81]

Second-Generation Antipsychotics

The second-generation antipsychotics (SGAs) aripiprazole, brexpiprazole, and quetiapine have been FDA-approved for augmentation of antidepressant treatment. The combination of olanzapine/fluoxetine is FDA-approved for treatment refractory depression. Additionally, cariprazine, olanzapine, and risperidone have been studied and are recommended in some treatment guidelines for refractory symptoms.[3,4] The specific mechanisms for these medications in MDD is not fully understood, but is thought to involve modulation of 5-HT and DA activity as they have variable activity at 5-HT_{1A}, 5-HT_{2A}, D_2, and D_3 receptors.[60] While these medications may be useful in the treatment of depression they are associated with the risk of metabolic complications and movement disorders. As discussed in detail in Chapter 87, "Schizophrenia," patients taking SGAs must have baseline and follow-up monitoring of metabolic parameters

TABLE 88-5 Dietary and Medication Restrictions for Patients Taking Monoamine Oxidase Inhibitors[a]

Foods to Avoid Completely	Approximate Tyramine Content (mg) per Ounce	
Aged cheeses (eg, cheddar, blue, Swiss, Camembert)	25-45	
Chicken liver	60	
Dry aged meats (eg, mortadella, salami, prosciutto)	2-45	
Fava beans	Unknown	
Kim chee	Unknown	
Red wine	Variable	
Sauerkraut	1-3	
Smoked or pickled fish (eg, lox, caviar, pickled herring)	0-80	
Soy sauce, fermented soy, miso	Varies	
Tap beer	20-40	
Yeast extract	2-60	
Foods to Eat in Moderation		
American cheese, Parmesan cheese	<2	
Canned, filtered beer	<2 per 12 oz (355 mL)	
Havarti, brie	Thought to be low	
Pepperoni	<2	
Pizza (large commercial chains generally safe; avoid gourmet with aged cheeses and meats)	2 slices	
White wine	<1 per 4 oz (120 mL)	
Foods Without Restrictions		
Fresh dairy products (cottage cheese, cream cheese, fresh milk, ice cream, ricotta, sour cream, yogurt)		
Fresh meats (including fresh sausage)		
Processed meats (eg, lunch meat, hot dogs, ham)		
Spirits (eg, bourbon, gin, rum, vodka)		
Yeast bread products		
Medications to Avoid Completely		
Antidepressants[a]	Dopamine	Methylphenidate
Amphetamines	Ephedrine	Reserpine
Appetite suppressants	Epinephrine	Sympathomimetics
Asthma inhalants	Guanethidine	
Buspirone	Levodopa	Tramadol
Carbamazepine	Local anesthetics[b]	Tryptophan
Decongestants	Meperidine	
Dextromethorphan	Methyldopa	

[a]Tricyclic antidepressants may be used with caution by experienced clinicians in treatment-refractory populations.

[b]Those containing sympathomimetic vasoconstrictors.

Data from References 61 and 81.

(weight, glucose, lipids, blood pressure) due to the risk of metabolic syndrome. Additionally, patients should be assessed for treatment emergent extrapyramidal symptoms (eg, parkinsonism, akathisia, dystonia). See Chapter 87 for greater detail.

New/Investigational Agents with Novel Mechanisms

Medications with novel mechanisms have transitioned from proof of concept research to formal clinical trials and, in some cases, FDA approval (see Table 88-10). As mentioned above, while these agents do not directly alter activity of monoamines, they likely alter activity of monoamines as a secondary effect.

Ketamine, an older anesthetic agent, has increasingly been studied and used in the past decade for treatment resistant depression (TRD). Ketamine modulates glutamate activity via extrasynaptic *N*-methyl-*D*-aspartate (NMDA) receptor antagonism that is thought to increase synaptic glutamate activity resulting in increased BDNF activity and synaptogenesis.[30] Though not FDA-approved for MDD, ketamine has demonstrated rapid antidepressant effects in sub-anesthetic intravenous doses (typically 0.5 mg/kg) for TRD in multiple studies.[19] Esketamine, the single *s*-isomer of ketamine, has a higher affinity for the NMDA receptor than the *r*-isomer.[82] An intranasal formulation of esketamine was FDA-approved for TRD in 2019. The intranasal formulation overcomes some of the barriers associated with intravenous ketamine use, but has logistical barriers of its own. It requires supervised, in-clinic self-administration with two to six intranasal sprays per session and 2 hours of in-clinic observation after administration. In trials, patients received doses twice weekly for 4 weeks and variable dosing thereafter.[83] Overall both ketamine and esketamine appear to be relatively well tolerated at the doses used in clinical trials; however, transient psychotomimetic/dissociative effects and blood pressure elevation (10-20 mm Hg) occurred at higher rates than placebo with both agents.[19,83]

Based on research involving endogenous allopregnanolone levels and depression, specifically alterations in pregnancy and postpartum, brexanolone (exogenous allopregnanolone) was developed and FDA-approved for the indication of postpartum depression in 2019. Administration involves a 60-hour stepped dose, intravenous infusion. First-pass metabolism precludes oral administration. Brexanolone is thought to exert antidepressant effect by allosteric modulation of $GABA_A$ receptors, which may increase 5HT and NE transmission.[24,84] The most common adverse medication reactions in brexanolone trials were headache, dizziness, and somnolence. In up to 4% of patients, the infusion was stopped due to excessive sedation or loss of consciousness.[84] It has a mandatory Risk Evaluation and Mitigation Strategies (REMS) program with Elements to Ensure Safe Use (ETASU). Analogues of brexanolone with oral bioavailability, including zuranolone, are in development but not yet FDA-approved (Table 88-6).

Additional Adverse Events

Serotonin Syndrome Any antidepressant that increases serotonergic neurotransmission can be associated with serotonin syndrome (SS), especially in situations where interactions increase release or duration of serotonin activity. The typical triad of symptoms seen in SS includes mental status changes, autonomic instability, and neuromuscular abnormalities (eg, hyperreflexia, myoclonus) which can be lethal.[86] As SS is primarily a diagnosis of exclusion, other causes of symptoms including neuroleptic malignant syndrome, anticholinergic toxicity, and malignant hyperthermia must be ruled out, with particular attention being paid to concurrent medications to guide differential diagnosis. Prompt medical attention is needed for any patient suspected of having SS syndrome, to discontinue all potentially causative agents, manage blood pressure and heart rate and maintain hydration.

TABLE 88-6 Novel Antidepressants

Medication	Administration	Comments
Ketamine[a] 10 mg/mL, 50 mg/mL, and 100 mg/mL Diluted for infusion	*Not FDA-approved for MDD* *Based on clinical trials* Most common dose: 0.5 mg/kg IV infusion Dose range: 0.1-1 mg/kg IV infusion Frequency: Ranges from single dose up to 3 doses per week × 2-6 weeks	Sub-anesthetic dose Optimal duration of treatment not established Requires IV access Lower rate of dissociation compared with anesthetic doses of ketamine Limited sites of care May not be covered by insurance
Esketamine (Spravato) 28 mg per nasal spray device (14 mg per spray)	*FDA-approved indications: Treatment resistant depression* One spray per nostril (28 mg) Repeat in 5 minutes for 56 mg and again in 5 minutes for 84 mg 2×/week for 4 weeks then weekly for 4 weeks then every 1-2 weeks *MDD with suicidality* 84 mg 2×/week for 4 weeks	Sub-anesthetic dose Optimal duration of treatment not established Requires in office administration and observation post-dose Rate of dissociative symptoms comparable to low dose IV ketamine Limited sites of care Costly SPRAVATO REMS program: sedation, dissociation, use and misuse
Brexanolone (Zulresso) 100 mg/20 mL	*FDA-approved for postpartum depression only* Single 60-hr stepped infusion 0 to 4 hr 30 mcg/kg/hr 4 to 24 hr 60 mcg/kg/hr 24 to 52 hr 90 mcg/kg/hr 52 to 56 hr 60 mcg/kg/hr 56 to 60 hr 30 mcg/kg/hr	Requires hospitalization ZULRESSO REMS program: excessive sedation and sudden loss of consciousness Effect past 30 days not established Limited sites of care Costly: ~$30,000 per infusion

[a]Not FDA-approved for treatment of MDD.

IV, intravenous; REMS, Risk Evaluation and Mitigation Strategy.

Data from References 60, 84, and 85.

Pharmacokinetics and Pharmacodynamics of Antidepressants

The PK of the antidepressants is summarized in Table 88-7.[60,73,87] The diversity of SSRIs is evident not only in their chemical structures but also in their PK profiles as the unique PK attributes of each SSRI can be used to guide treatment. For example, the long half-life of fluoxetine and its active metabolite norfluoxetine may be beneficial in instances of partial nonadherence. Conversely, caution must be taken to monitor for medication interactions prior to combining another medication with fluoxetine, fluvoxamine, or paroxetine.

Bioavailability is low (30%-70%) for most TCAs as a result of first-pass metabolism, which shows great interindividual variation.[89]

TABLE 88-7 Pharmacokinetic Properties of Antidepressants

Generic Name	Elimination Half-Life[a]	Plasma Protein Binding (%)	Clinically Important Metabolites
Selective Serotonin Reuptake Inhibitors (SSRIs)			
Citalopram	33 hr	80	None
Escitalopram	27-32 hr	56	None
Fluoxetine	4-6 days[b]	94	Norfluoxetine[c]
Fluvoxamine	15-26 hr	77	None
Paroxetine	24-31 hr	95	None
Sertraline	27 hr	99[d]	None
Serotonin–Norepinephrine Reuptake Inhibitors (SNRIs)			
Desvenlafaxine	11 hr	30	None
Duloxetine	12 hr	90	None
Levomilnacipran	12 hr	22	None
Venlafaxine	5 hr	27-30	*O*-Desmethyl-venlafaxine
TCAs			
Amitriptyline	9-46 hr	90-97	Nortriptyline
Desipramine	11-46 hr	73-92	2-Hydroxy-desipramine
Doxepin	8-36 hr	68-82	Desmethyl-doxepin
Imipramine	6-34 hr	63-96	Desipramine
Nortriptyline	16-88 hr	87-95	10-Hydroxy-nortriptyline
Mixed Serotonergic (Mixed 5-HT)			
Nefazodone	2-4 hr	99	*meta*-Chlorophenyl-piperazine
Trazodone	6-11 hr	92	*meta*-Chlorophenyl-piperazine
Vilazodone	25 hr	>95	
Vortioxetine	66 hr	98	
Norepinephrine/Dopamine Reuptake Inhibitor (NDRI)			
Bupropion	10-21 hr	82-88	Hydroxy-bupropion Threohydro-bupropion Erythrohydro-bupropion
Serotonin and α_2–Adrenergic Antagonists			
Mirtazapine	20-40 hr	85	None

[a]Biologic half-life in slowest phase of elimination.

[b]Four to 6 days with chronic dosing; norfluoxetine, 4 to 16 days.

[c]Take with food to increase area under the curve concentrations by greater than 60%.

[d]Increases 30% to 40% when taken with food.

Data from References 60, 73, and 87.

The TCAs have a large volume of distribution and concentrate in brain and cardiac tissue in laboratory animals. They are bound extensively and strongly to plasma albumin, erythrocytes, α_1-acid glycoprotein, and lipoprotein.[89] The major metabolic pathways are demethylation, aromatic and aliphatic hydroxylation, and glucuronide conjugation, although enterohepatic cycling has been described.[89] Normally, the PK of TCAs is linear within the usual dosage range; however, the elimination half-lives can vary greatly among individual patients, which may be related to pharmacogenomic variability, primarily within CYP2D6 and CYP2C19.[89]

Venlafaxine is metabolized to an active metabolite, *O*-desmethylvenlafaxine, which contributes to the overall pharmacologic effect, and is also FDA-approved as an antidepressant (desvenlafaxine). Immediate release (IR) venlafaxine is generally dosed twice daily to avoid end of dose discontinuation symptoms, while extended release venlafaxine and desvenlafaxine have a longer duration of action and can be dosed once daily.[60] Bupropion is metabolized to multiple active metabolites (Table 88-7), and there are three formulations of bupropion hydrochloride (immediate release, sustained release, and extended release), which are equivalent on a total daily dose basis as well as a bupropion hydrobromide formulation that can be converted to equivalent hydrochloride doses.[90] The bupropion peak plasma concentrations are lower for the sustained-release formulation, which are believed to contribute to a lower seizure risk.[90] Mirtazapine undergoes biotransformation to several metabolites[91,92]; however, it is primarily eliminated unchanged in the urine. The mirtazapine metabolites are present at such low plasma concentrations they minimally contribute to the overall pharmacologic profile. Levomilnacipran is primarily metabolized via CYP3A4 with renal elimination of over 50% of the dose.[60]

Brexanolone undergoes extensive first-pass metabolism and is only available in intravenous formulation.[80] Ketamine (IV) and esketamine (nasal) undergo extensive oxidative metabolism and have elimination half-lives of approximately 2 hours and 7 to 12 hours, respectively.

An important PK difference between oral selegiline (FDA-approved only for Parkinson disease) and transdermal selegiline impacts their pharmacodynamic profiles. Oral selegiline undergoes extensive first-pass metabolism resulting in bioavailability of 4% versus 73% for the transdermal formulation.[80] At the low CNS concentrations achieved with the oral formulation, selegiline selectively inhibits MAO-B resulting in increased DA levels (hence, the use for Parkinson disease). Nonselective inhibition of both MAO-A (resulting in increased NE and 5HT levels) and MAO-B, which is thought to be important to achieve an antidepressant effect, occurs at the higher CNS concentrations only achieved with the transdermal formulation.[80]

Antidepressant Altered Pharmacokinetics Antidepressants may have significantly altered PK in patients with hepatic or renal disease; however, the data regarding the altered PK parameters are often derived from small, single-dose studies. Changes are variably reported as decreased clearance, increased area under the curve (AUC) or increased half-life.[91,92] In patients with chronic liver disease, clearance may be decreased 30% (citalopram, mirtazapine) to over 70% (duloxetine, sertraline) and half-life may be increased twofold (citalopram, paroxetine) to threefold (duloxetine, fluoxetine). The AUC of TCAs and bupropion have been reported to increase threefold in cirrhosis.[92] Duloxetine is not recommended in patients with significant hepatic impairment.

Renal impairment and end-stage renal disease (ESRD) do not significantly alter antidepressant PK, with notable exceptions. The half-life of citalopram, escitalopram, and paroxetine may increase 30% to 40%.[91] The AUC of bupropion desvenlafaxine, duloxetine, mirtazapine, and venlafaxine may increase twofold.[91] Duloxetine labeling recommends against use in patients with estimated glomerular filtration rate (eGFR) <30 mL/min/1.73 m^2.[91] Bupropion metabolites have also demonstrated accumulation in ESRD. Renal failure does not alter nortriptyline metabolism, but the 10-hydroxy metabolite may accumulate, and protein binding may be diminished, with resulting enhanced sensitivity to the medication.[89]

In patients with significant renal or hepatic impairment, it is reasonable to initiate treatment with 50% lower dose and titrate to 50% to 75% of maximum dose based on tolerability and response. Patients should be monitored for electrolyte abnormalities and low platelets that can increase risk of arrhythmias and bleeding. Additionally, lower doses and cautious monitoring are prudent when patients are on concomitant medications with overlapping toxicity profiles.

Plasma Concentration and Clinical Response For the newer antidepressants, a strong correlation between plasma concentration and clinical response or tolerability has not been established, while this has been established for some TCAs (eg, amitriptyline, nortriptyline, desipramine, and imipramine). However, the best established therapeutic range is for nortriptyline (50-150 ng/mL [mcg/L; 190-570 nmol/L]),[89] which appears to demonstrate a curvilinear plasma concentration-response relationship.

Clinical response, not plasma concentration, should dictate dosage adjustments, as some patients with plasma concentrations outside the suggested therapeutic range respond to treatment, whereas others are nonresponsive even with "therapeutic" plasma concentration.

Plasma Concentration Monitoring Because of interindividual variations in plasma concentrations achieved by a given dose, interpretation of plasma concentrations can be very difficult for the TCAs.[89] Although plasma concentration monitoring is not performed routinely, some indications include inadequate response, relapse, serious or persistent adverse medication reactions, use of higher-than-standard doses, suspected toxicity, older adult patients, pregnant patients, cardiac disease, suspected nonadherence, and suspected PK interactions. If plasma concentration monitoring is used to detect nonadherence, a cutoff as low as 30 ng/mL (mcg/L; ~110 nmol/L) for the TCAs has been suggested to avoid confusion with low bioavailability or unusually rapid metabolism. Blood samples for plasma concentration determinations should be obtained at steady state, usually after a minimum of 1 week at constant dosage. Sampling should be performed during the elimination phase, usually in the morning, 12 hours after the last dose. Samples collected in this manner are comparable for patients on once-, twice-, or thrice-daily regimens.[89]

TABLE 88-8 Antidepressants and Cytochrome (CYP) P450 Enzyme Inhibitory Potential

	CYP Enzyme Inhibition			
Medication	**1A2**	**2C**	**2D6**	**3A4**
Bupropion	0	0	+++	0
Citalopram	0	0	+	NA
Duloxetine	0	0	+++	0
Escitalopram	0	0	+	0
Fluoxetine	0	++	++++	++
Fluvoxamine	++++	++	0	+++
Mirtazapine	0	0	0	0
Nefazodone	0	0	0	++++
Paroxetine	0	0	++++	0
Sertraline	0	++	+	+
(des)-Venlafaxine	0	0	0/+	0
Vilazodone	0	0	0	0
Vortioxetine	0	0	0	0

++++, high; +++, moderate; ++, low; +, very low; 0, absent.

Data from References 60 and 88.

Medication Interactions

Interactions fall into two broad categories: PK and PD medication interactions, with the PK interactions being the most common. Antidepressants are primarily substrates for cytochrome P450 enzymes and variably act as inhibitors of the enzymes (see Table 88-8).[60,88]

Pharmacokinetic Interactions Interactions may occur when an antidepressant is coadministered with another medication metabolized through the cytochrome P450 system. Two of the cytochrome P450 system isoenzymes, CYP2D6 and CYP3A4, are responsible for the metabolism of most currently marketed medications.[88] The ability of an antidepressant to inhibit the activity of these enzymes will be a significant contributory factor in determining its capability to cause a PK interaction when administered concomitantly. Table 88-8 shows the cytochrome P450 enzyme inhibitory potential of antidepressant agents. Patients taking substrates of these enzymes should be monitored closely if started on an antidepressant with inhibitory potential. Select examples can be found in Table 88-9.

Because the TCAs are metabolized in the liver through the cytochrome P450 system, they may interact with other medications that modify hepatic enzyme activity or hepatic blood flow. TCAs are also extensively protein bound, which can result in interactions through displacement from protein-binding sites. Many commonly used medications can interact when given concurrently with TCAs.

As nefazodone use has been severely limited due to its potential to induce liver toxicity, and trazodone is primarily used as a non-FDA-approved hypnotic at low doses, neither of these agents is likely to be involved in clinically significant medication interactions. However, nefazodone is a potent inhibitor of CYP3A4.[88] Vilazodone is primarily metabolized via CYP3A4 and vortioxetine is primarily metabolized via CYP2D6 and both require dose adjustment with inhibitors.[60,62]

Pharmacodynamic Medication Interactions Certain PD medication interactions that may occur with antidepressants are concerning and require close monitoring. For example, concurrent use of serotonergic antidepressants with other medications that augment serotonergic function can increase the risk of SS with some combinations conferring a higher risk than others.[86]

TABLE 88-9 Select Pharmacokinetic Interactions of Antidepressants

Antidepressant	Interacting Medication/Medication Class	Effect
Selective Serotonin Reuptake Inhibitors		
Citalopram and escitalopram	Omeprazole	Increased concentrations of citalopram and escitalopram
Fluoxetine	Alprazolam	Increased concentrations and half-life of alprazolam; increased psychomotor impairment
	Antipsychotics (eg, aripiprazole, haloperidol)	Increased antipsychotic concentrations; increased extrapyramidal symptoms
	β-Adrenergic blockers	Increased metoprolol concentrations; increased bradycardia; possible heart block
	Carbamazepine	Increased concentrations of carbamazepine; symptoms of carbamazepine toxicity
	Phenytoin	Increased concentrations of phenytoin; symptoms of phenytoin toxicity
	Tamoxifen	Decreased conversion of tamoxifen to active metabolites
	TCAs	Markedly increased TCA concentrations; symptoms of TCA toxicity
	Thioridazine	Thioridazine C_{max} increased; prolonged QTc interval
Fluvoxamine	Alosetron	Increased alosetron AUC (sixfold) and half-life (threefold)
	Alprazolam	Increased AUC of alprazolam by 96%, increased alprazolam half-life by 71%; increased psychomotor impairment
	β-Adrenergic blockers	Fivefold increase in propranolol concentration; bradycardia and hypotension
	Carbamazepine	Increased concentrations of carbamazepine; symptoms of carbamazepine toxicity
	Clozapine	Increased clozapine concentrations; increased risk for seizures and orthostatic hypotension
	Diltiazem	Bradycardia
	Methadone	Increased methadone plasma concentrations; symptoms of methadone toxicity
	Ramelteon	Increased AUC (190-fold) and C_{max} (70-fold)
	TCAs	Increased TCA concentration; symptoms of TCA toxicity
	Theophylline and caffeine	Increased concentrations of theophylline or caffeine; symptoms of theophylline or caffeine toxicity
	Thioridazine	Thioridazine C_{max} increased; prolonged QTc interval
	Warfarin	Increased effect of warfarin
Paroxetine	Antipsychotics (eg, aripiprazole, haloperidol)	Increased antipsychotic concentrations; increased CNS and extrapyramidal symptoms
	β-Adrenergic blockers	Increased metoprolol concentrations; increased bradycardia; possible heart block
	Tamoxifen	Decreased conversion of tamoxifen to active metabolites
	TCAs	Markedly increased TCA concentrations; symptoms of TCA toxicity
	Thioridazine	Thioridazine C_{max} increased; prolonged QTc interval
Sertraline	Methadone	Increased methadone levels
Serotonin–Norepinephrine Reuptake Inhibitors		
Venlafaxine and desvenlafaxine	CYP3A4 inhibitors	May increase levels of venlafaxine and *O*-desmethylvenlafaxine especially in CYP2D6 poor metabolizers
Duloxetine	Metoprolol	May increase metoprolol levels twofold
	Tamoxifen	Decreased conversion of tamoxifen to active metabolites
	Thioridazine	Thioridazine C_{max} increased; prolonged QTc interval
Levomilnacipran	CYP3A4 inhibitors	Clinically relevant increases in levomilnacipran concentrations may occur
Mixed Serotonergic (Mixed 5-HT)		
Vilazodone	CYP3A4 inhibitors	Maximum vilazodone dose 20 mg with coadministration of potent CYP3A4 inhibitor
Vortioxetine	CYP2D6 inhibitors	May need to reduce vortioxetine dose by half with coadministration of potent CYP2D6 inhibitor
Serotonin and α-2-Adrenergic Antagonist		
Mirtazapine	Carbamazepine	Mirtazapine concentration decreased (60%)
Norepinephrine and Dopamine Reuptake Inhibitor		
Bupropion	Tamoxifen	Decreased conversion of tamoxifen to active metabolites

AUC, area under the time concentration curve; C_{max}, maximum concentration; MAOI, monoamine oxidase inhibitor.

Note: Any medication that augments serotonergic function may impact bleeding risk and should be used with caution in patients receiving NSAIDs or other medications with hematologic effects.

Data from References 2, 60, 73, and 88.

Tramadol presents as an example of a PK interaction increasing the risk of a PD interaction. When tramadol is coadministered with strong CYP2D6 inhibitors, the decrease in metabolism may result in higher levels of tramadol, which also exhibits SNRI effects. Therefore, high doses of the combination have been reported to cause serotonin syndrome.[86,93]

See Table 88-10 for key examples of PD interactions.[60,86,93-96]

TABLE 88-10 Select Pharmacodynamic Medication Interactions of Antidepressants

Medication/ Medication Class	Antidepressants/ Antidepressant Class	Effect and Management
NSAIDs Aspirin Anticoagulants Antiplatelet agents	SSRIs, SNRIs, TCAs, trazodone, vilazodone, vortioxetine	• FDA warning for increased risk of bleeding • Number needed to harm with NSAIDs = 82 vs >700 with SSRI alone • Assess for baseline bleeding risk and monitor closely • Educate at risk patients regarding signs of bleeding • Consider histamine-2 (H_2) antagonist in high-risk patients
Triptans	MAOIs, SSRIs, and SNRIs	• FDA warning in labeling • Very low risk • Monitor for signs of serotonin syndrome when frequent high doses are used • Triptan toxicity possible when almotriptan, rizatriptan, sumatriptan, or zolmitriptan are combined with MAO inhibitors
Linezolid	All serotonergic antidepressants	• Linezolid is weak, reversible, nonselective, MAOI • FDA labeling recommends against use with other MAOIs and recommends discontinuing antidepressants if linezolid is started • Actual rate of serotonin syndrome with combination reported at <1% • Abrupt discontinuation of antidepressants can have negative consequences • If linezolid is indicated and patient is already on an antidepressant, monitor for signs of serotonin syndrome upon initiating combination • If patient is on short course of linezolid and in need of treatment for depression, consider postponing antidepressant initiation until course is complete
Tramadol	Bupropion, duloxetine, fluoxetine, paroxetine	• Decreased metabolism results in increased SNRI activity of tramadol • Rare cases of high dose tramadol combined with CYP2D6 inhibitors resulting in serotonin syndrome have been reported • Monitor for increased signs of serotonin syndrome and decreased analgesic response when combination is used

Data from References 60, 86, and 93-96.

There are two types of PD medication interactions that may occur between antidepressant medications and NSAIDs. An increased risk for abnormal bleeding (eg, upper GI and intracranial hemorrhage) associated with combined antidepressants and NSAID use is a potentially very serious pharmacodynamic interaction.[94] This interaction is likely mediated by serotonergic mechanisms that occur at the platelet level. Additionally, NSAIDs may lessen the efficacy of SSRIs; however, the evidence is insufficient to draw firm conclusions.[95] However, given the volume of prescriptions for both NSAIDs and SSRIs, this is an area of pharmacotherapy that certainly deserves further research and thoughtful prescribing practices.

Lastly, refer to the section "Monoamine Oxidase Inhibitors" above and Table 88-5 regarding the hypertensive crisis that may result following coadministration of MAOIs and other medications that increase vasopressor response (eg, amphetamines). Notably, MAOIs and TCAs have been coadministered safely in TRD patients with apparent increased efficacy compared with monotherapy; however, severe reactions (eg, hypertensive crisis) and fatalities have occurred.[2,89] Therefore, this combination should be used sparingly by experienced clinicians and monitored extremely carefully.

Alternative Pharmacotherapy

The APA Task Force on Complementary and Alternative Medicine (CAM) as well as CANMAT guidelines include evidence-based and consensus-based recommendations on the use of CAM for the treatment of MDD.[59,97] While these recommendations are not the focus of this chapter, clinicians treating patients with MDD should be cognizant of them.

Omega-3 Fatty Acids Eicosapentaenoic acid (EPA) and docosahexaenoic acid (DHA) omega-3 fatty acids are generally low-risk and demonstrate variable benefit as augmentation in the treatment of MDD. Use of EPA alone or the combination of EPA/DHA is likely more effective than DHA alone. As these agents may increase bleeding risk, their use should be carefully considered in patients taking SSRIs and other concomitant medications associated with bleeding risk (eg, NSAIDs, anticoagulants).

St. John's Wort There is a lack of consensus regarding St. John's wort for the treatment of MDD. Furthermore, St. John's wort induces hepatic metabolic enzymes and is associated with significant interactions. The APA Task Force conservatively states that St. John's wort may be reasonable for some individuals with mild-to-moderate MDD while CANMAT considers it to have level 1 evidence as first-line therapy for mild-to-moderate MDD.[2,4] Further, the BAP guidelines state a "standardized" preparation of St. John's wort "could be considered" in patients with mild-to-moderate MDD, if other first-line medications are not an option.[3]

S-Adenosyl-L-Methionine (SAMe) The use of SAMe received a favorable review by the APA Task Force. However, the final consensus was that more rigorous studies need to confirm the efficacy of SAMe for treating MDD. The CANMAT guidelines consider SAMe as a second-line augmentation strategy while the BAP guidelines state that evidence is developing for use of SAMe as an augmentation strategy in the treatment of MDD.[3]

Folate The three compounds in this category are (a) folic acid, (b) folinic acid, and (c) 5-methyltetrahydrofolate (5-MTHF) as these compounds are involved in the synthesis of key neurotransmitters such as 5-HT. The APA Task Force states that augmentation with these compounds is reasonable, but more work is needed to clarify which subgroup of patients may achieve the greatest response.[59] For example, in one study, only females responded to folic acid augmentation of fluoxetine treatment. Regardless, CANMAT guidelines consider folate supplementation a third-line augmentation strategy.[4]

Special Populations

Older Adult Patients Depression in older adults is a major public health problem as many older adult patients with depression are inadequately treated, or have their depression missed or mistaken for another disorder, such as dementia. In these patients, depressed mood, the typical signature symptom of depression, may be less prominent than other depressive symptoms such as loss of appetite, cognitive impairment, sleeplessness, anergia, and anhedonia. Previous research supports that somatic (physical) complaints (eg, pain, fatigue, gastrointestinal symptoms) present more frequently in older adults with depression. However, there are many confounders that may account for this (eg, higher rates of physical illness).[34] Appropriate recognition and treatment of depression in older adults is extremely important as individuals 65 years of age and older have a high rate of suicidality. Increased suicide attempts in older adults with depression have been associated with access to firearms, diminished cognitive functioning, sleep disruptions, poor social interactions, and inattention among primary caregivers.[98]

Before initiating antidepressant treatment, a complete physical examination should be performed. When prescribed antidepressants, older adults may be either overtreated or under-treated. Overtreatment occurs when age-related PK and PD factors are overlooked and under-treatment results from an overly conservative approach as a result of the patient's advanced age or concurrent medical problems. In older adults, SSRIs are usually selected as first-line treatment, and this may enable the clinician to avoid some of the problematic intolerances commonly associated with TCAs (eg, sedative, anticholinergic, and cardiovascular adverse reactions). Furthermore, there is evidence to suggest that the long-term use of antidepressants such as SSRIs in older adults, administered with either psychotherapy or clinical management, may prevent a depressive relapse.[34,35] Hyponatremia is more common in elderly females, especially in those taking concomitant diuretics. Mirtazapine has been shown to be an effective antidepressant in adults older than 65 years of age and better tolerated than the SSRI paroxetine. Furthermore, secondary measures of anxiety and sleep were improved following mirtazapine administration.[99] In addition to sleep benefits, mirtazapine can be helpful in improving appetite which is commonly diminished in older adults with depression. For those patients whose depressive symptoms include lack of overall energy, use of bupropion may capitalize on the stimulant effect of this medication. Regardless of the specific antidepressant chosen, the effect sizes for antidepressants as a pharmacological class, compared to placebo, may be smaller in older adult patients than in younger adult populations.[3]

Pediatric Patients Accumulating evidence indicates that childhood depression occurs quite commonly and symptoms of depression in the young may vary from accepted diagnostic criteria to include several nonspecific symptoms such as boredom, anxiety, somatic complaints (eg, stomach ache), and impulsivity.[100]

Data collected under controlled conditions that support the efficacy of antidepressants in children and adolescents are sparse, and only fluoxetine and escitalopram are FDA-approved for depression in patients younger than 18 years of age, although other antidepressants (eg, sertraline) have been studied in this population.[100] The Treatment of Adolescent Depression Study (TADS) found that the combination of fluoxetine and CBT was superior to fluoxetine monotherapy or CBT alone in adolescents 12 to 17 years of age.[101] The Treatment of Resistant Depression in Adolescents (TORDIA) study switched adolescents 12 to 18 years of age with SSRI-resistant depression to venlafaxine or sertraline with or without CBT after nonresponse to antidepressant. Overall this study found no difference in outcomes between the two medications and also found no difference in outcomes when CBT was added to medication.[102] Additionally, the Adolescent Depression Antidepressant and Psychotherapy Trial (ADAPT) did not find a benefit of adding CBT to SSRI therapy in adolescents 11 to 17 years of age.[103]

The use of antidepressants in children and adolescents was complicated when the FDA issued a boxed warning in the product labeling for antidepressant medications warning clinicians and patients of the increased risk for suicidal ideation and behavior when antidepressants are used in this population. Results of subsequent studies attempting to elucidate the risk of antidepressants in young patients have varied. A meta-analysis of published and unpublished clinical trials supported an increased risk; however, the study was impeded by limited data access. In contrast, several retrospective longitudinal reviews of antidepressant use in children refute the increased risk of suicide attempts or deaths.[104] Furthermore, studies demonstrated a decreased rate of prescribing antidepressants and an increase in deaths by suicide after the warning appeared in labeling.[105]

The treatment of depression in children remains challenging, as depression can be difficult to diagnose and, once identified, treat. Furthermore, differences in efficacy between medication and placebo may be small and not significant in children below the age of 13 years.[3] However, antidepressants (in particular, the SSRIs) remain viable treatment options when prescribed and monitored appropriately.

Pregnant and Lactating Patients The crucial decision as to whether to use antidepressants during pregnancy continues to be debated and must always include a risk-benefit analysis based upon the available evidence at the time of treatment. Approximately 14% of pregnant individuals develop clinically significant depression during pregnancy.[106] Furthermore, it has been documented that those who discontinued antidepressant therapy before or during pregnancy were five times more likely to have a relapse than those who continued treatment.[107] While numerous studies, reviews, and meta-analyses have been published over the last decade, the absolute risk of antidepressants in pregnancy is still not clear due to methodological issues and confounding factors (eg, prenatal care, continued depressive symptoms during treatment, medical and psychiatric comorbidities, and substance use).[108] An approximate 25% relative increase in congenital heart defects associated with SSRIs is the most consistent finding; however, the increase in risk ranges from 10% to a twofold increase across studies.[108] Other findings have included increased risk of low birth weight and newborn respiratory distress.[106] An oft-cited study reported a sixfold greater likelihood of persistent pulmonary hypertension of newborn infants exposed to an SSRI after the 20th week of gestation; however, the degree of this risk has been debated.[109] These are selected examples of studies assessing both risks and benefits of antidepressants in pregnancy. A full exploration of the conflicting literature on this topic is beyond the scope of this chapter.

Four therapeutic principles have been proposed to guide the clinician in treating pregnant individuals or individuals who desire pregnancy: (a) Pregnancy does not protect against the occurrence of depression, and the likelihood of relapse is very high in untreated individuals with recurrent illness. (b) Depression during pregnancy adversely affects child development, and prenatal depression may adversely affect the offspring. (c) When attempting to balance benefit and risk, transient postnatal behavioral abnormalities in the offspring of pregnant individuals receiving pharmacotherapy must not be assumed to portend long-term compromise. (d) SSRIs, the most commonly used and best-tolerated treatment for depression, carry a small but significant risk for a serious medical consequence.[110]

The APA and the American College of Obstetricians and Gynecologists have a report discussing the treatment of depression during pregnancy. One of the prominent conclusions of this report was that *both* antidepressant treatment and untreated depression have been associated with potential problems during pregnancy. However, studies to date have not been able to adequately control for all the necessary variables involved in birth outcomes (eg, maternal depressive disorder) and more work needs to be done.[111]

In summary, the risks and benefits of medication therapy during pregnancy must always be weighed, and concerns about the risks of untreated depression during pregnancy should be considered. These include the possibility of low birth weight secondary to poor pregnancy weight gain, suicidality, potential for hospitalization, potential for relationship discord, inability to engage in appropriate obstetric care, and difficulty caring for other children. Several different approaches exist for dealing with pregnancy and antidepressant use. First, discontinuation of an antidepressant before conception is an option for individuals who are stable and appear likely to remain well while not taking antidepressant medication (eg, no history of recurrence upon discontinuation, no history of severe symptoms or suicidality, stable psychosocial supports). Second, continuation of the antidepressant until conception may be reasonable and one with the lowest risk for the fetus should be chosen in individuals of child bearing potential or those trying to conceive. For those who have a history of depressive relapse after medication discontinuation, the antidepressant should be continued throughout pregnancy. There is a great deal of uncertainty regarding long-term antidepressant exposure in infants exposed through human milk due to the lack of data. However, sertraline is recommended and appears in relatively low concentrations in human milk and in samples taken from infants.[112] The risks of not treating depression in a patient who is pregnant or providing milk to an infant should not be underestimated or minimized. Additional information can be found in Chapter 99, "Pregnancy and Lactation."

Relative Resistance and Treatment-Resistant Depression

The majority of patients with TRD likely have had inadequate (low dose, short duration) therapy (relative resistance). This theory is supported by data from the National Institute of Mental Health (NIMH) Sequenced Treatment Alternatives to Relieve Depression (STAR*D) study, which is generally considered to be one of the premier antidepressant trials among patients with depressive disorders.[56,113] According to this study, one in three patients with depression who previously did not achieve remission with an antidepressant (citalopram) became symptom free with an additional medication (bupropion SR or buspirone) and one in four achieved remission after switching to a different antidepressant (bupropion SR, sertraline, or venlafaxine XR). Furthermore, patients can be switched to another medication within the same class.[114] For example, patients in the STAR*D study not responding to an initial SSRI were shown to be as likely to respond to another SSRI as they were to a medication from a different class.[115] Other key findings of STAR*D include the importance of maximizing dose (higher doses associated with higher remission rates) and adequate trial duration of at least 8 to 12 weeks before deeming a medication ineffective.[56] The BAP guidelines place a higher level of confidence in both augmentation and switching strategies, compared to dosage increase approaches.[3]

Although several different definitions for TRD have been proposed, the most widely accepted is depression that has not achieved remission after two optimal antidepressant trials, which represents more than 40% of patients with MDD treated with antidepressants.[115] Three pharmacologic approaches that have been used with success for TRD include the following:

1. The current antidepressant may be stopped and another agent initiated (ie, switching). For example, the STAR*D trial compared switching to mirtazapine (up to 60 mg/day) versus nortriptyline (up to 200 mg/day) after two consecutive ineffective medication treatments.[115] In the mirtazapine group, 12.3% of patients met the remission criterion of a score of 7 or less on the Hamilton Rating Scale for Depression (HAM-D), while 19.8% of nortriptyline patients met this criterion at the end of 14 weeks.
2. The current antidepressant can be augmented by the addition of another agent such as lithium, or another antidepressant (ie, combination antidepressant treatment). For example, the STAR*D trial evaluated the addition of lithium or triiodothyronine (T_3) to current antidepressant treatment. After approximately 10 weeks, T_3 augmentation resulted in higher remission rates (24.7%) compared with lithium (15.9%). However, the differences between these two augmentation strategies were modest and not statistically significant.[116] Although T3 and lithium demonstrated similar remission rates in this seminal trial, the BAP guidelines provide a stronger recommendation rating for lithium (ie, "A") compared to T3-based approaches (ie, "B").[116] In contrast, the CANMAT guidelines consider both agents second-line for augmentation with level 2 evidence.[4]
3. The use of SGAs to augment the antidepressant response is increasing. Aripiprazole, brexpiprazole, and quetiapine are FDA-approved for adjunctive treatment for MDD. Aripiprazole and quetiapine have been recommended as first-line agents to augment an antidepressant medication.[4] In a predominantly male population in the Veterans Health Administration, augmentation with aripiprazole was found to be more effective than switching to bupropion but no different from bupropion augmentation.[117]

The APA practice guideline for the treatment of patients with MDD offers direction for managing patients whose symptoms are refractory to medications. These guidelines advise that if patients are still symptomatic after 6 to 8 weeks of medication, a reappraisal of the treatment regimen should be considered.[2] Those with partial response should consider changing the dose, augmenting the antidepressant, or adding psychotherapy or ECT. For those with no response, options include changing to a different antidepressant or adding psychotherapy or ECT. Again, the BAP guidelines suggest that stronger evidence exists for switching or augmentation strategies compared to dose increases in patients with inadequate antidepressant response.[3] Comorbid medical or psychiatric conditions should be identified and treated because they may complicate treatment.

6 Before changing a patient's treatment, the clinician is advised to evaluate the adequacy of the medication dosage and adherence with the prescribed regimen. Issues to be addressed in assessing the patient who has not responded to treatment include the following:

1. Is the diagnosis correct?
2. Does the patient have a psychotic depression?
3. Has the patient received an adequate dose and adequate duration of treatment?
4. Do adverse medication reactions preclude adequate dosing?
5. Is patient adherence to the prescribed regimen appropriate?
6. Was a stepwise approach to treatment used?
7. Was treatment outcome adequately measured?
8. Is there a coexisting or preexisting medical or psychiatric disorder?
9. Are there other factors that interfere with treatment?

Personalized Pharmacotherapy

7 Pharmacogenetic (PGx) applications in psychiatry have been explored for some time. Multiple commercially available PGx tests are now available and in patients who present with the testing already completed or for whom a test is ordered, evidence-based guidelines

produced by the Clinical Pharmacogenomics Implementation Consortium (CPIC) can help determine test interpretation (www.cpic.org). CPIC does not specifically recommend testing in patients, but rather serves as a resource for clinicians who are presented with PGx testing results and are looking for assistance in their interpretation. Therefore, while this testing may, one day, be routinely used to guide pharmacotherapy, it is not utilized routinely in practice for several reasons.[118] Included on several of the commercially available test are genes associated with PK parameters that have long been one of the primary considerations when choosing among the antidepressants, particularly within a medication class.[2] For example, PK parameters help the clinician choose a particular SSRI (eg, longer fluoxetine half-life for partial nonadherence). The data regarding the interpretation of PGx testing results for the PK genes is more concrete than that associated with PD genes.

A clinician can use other aspects of a medication's pharmacological profile to tailor the treatment to a particular patient. For example, antidepressants can generally be classified as either activating or sedating based upon their mechanism of action, and this is often a major consideration in antidepressant choice. Medications that promote noradrenergic activity (eg, bupropion, venlafaxine) or serotonin (eg, SSRIs) may be activating upon initiation and therefore poor choices for a patient suffering from significant insomnia. In contrast, mirtazapine and trazodone have been shown to improve sleep, likely due to antagonism of H_1 and 5-HT_{2A} receptors.[67] Furthermore, doxepin is FDA-approved (in lower doses compared to those used for depression) as pharmacotherapy for primary insomnia.[60]

EVALUATION OF THERAPEUTIC OUTCOMES

8 Several monitoring parameters, in addition to plasma or serum concentrations, are useful in managing patients (Tables 88-3 and 88-11).[2,60] Patients must be monitored for adverse medication reactions, such as sedation and anticholinergic effects, and for remission of previously documented target symptoms. The presence of adverse medication reactions does not necessarily indicate adequate or excessive dosage. In addition, changes in social and occupational functioning should be assessed. Patients receiving SNRIs should have their blood pressure monitored at regular intervals. Patients older than 40 years of age should receive a pretreatment ECG before starting TCA therapy, and follow-up ECGs should be performed periodically to assess for arrhythmias. Patients should be monitored for the emergence of suicidal ideation after initiation or discontinuation of any antidepressant, especially if other risk factors for death by suicide (eg, sleep disturbances) are present. If significant activation or insomnia occurs upon antidepressant initiation, a short-term anxiolytic or hypnotic may be appropriate.[67] Weight gain and sexual dysfunction, common adverse reactions associated with most antidepressants, may increase nonadherence and should be monitored and discussed with the patient (Table 88-11).

In addition to the clinical interview, psychometric rating instruments (such as those highlighted earlier in this chapter and in Chapter e81) allow for rapid and reliable measurement of the nature

TABLE 88-11 Adverse Medication Reactions and Monitoring Parameters Associated with Select Antidepressants

Medication	Adverse Medication Reaction	Monitoring	Comments
Antidepressants from Each Pharmacologic Class			
Common to all antidepressants			
	Suicidality	Behavioral changes Mental status	(US boxed warning) for all antidepressants; caregivers should be alerted to monitor for acute changes in behavior (especially early in treatment)
Selective Serotonin Reuptake Inhibitors (SSRIs)			
Common to all			
	Anxiety or nervousness	Assess severity and impact on patient functioning and quality of life	Most prominent on initial treatment; lower initial doses recommended in patients with prominent anxiety
	Hyponatremia	Serum sodium	More likely in older adult females; sodium may decrease within 72 hours of initiating antidepressant
	Nausea	Frequency and severity	May improve with slower dose titration
	Sleep changes (insomnia and somnolence)	Sleep patterns	Among SSRI class: fluoxetine may be more activating; paroxetine may be more sedating
	Sexual dysfunction	Assess severity and impact on patient functioning and quality of life	Spontaneous self-reporting may be low; clinician should assess symptoms; reversible on medication discontinuation
SSRI-Specific			
Citalopram (possibly escitalopram)	QTc interval prolongation	Electrocardiogram; electrolytes (eg, potassium, magnesium)	Caution use in "at-risk" patients (eg, electrolyte disturbance); discontinue if QTc persistently >500 ms or increased >50 ms over baseline
Paroxetine	Anticholinergic effects	Symptoms: dry mouth, constipation, urinary retention, mental status	Avoid in older adults
Serotonin–Norepinephrine Reuptake Inhibitors (SNRIs)			
Common to all			
	Cardiovascular changes	Increases in blood pressure; heart rate	Possibly less likely with duloxetine; may need to lower/discontinue dose
	Insomnia	Sleep patterns	Possibly less likely with duloxetine
	Nausea	Frequency and severity	May improve with slower dose titration

(continued)

TABLE 88-11 Adverse Medication Reactions and Monitoring Parameters Associated with Select Antidepressants (*Continued*)

Medication	Adverse Medication Reaction	Monitoring	Comments
	Sexual dysfunction	Assess severity and impact on patient functioning and quality of life	Spontaneous self-reporting may be low; clinicians should assess symptoms; reversible on medication discontinuation
	Sweating	Frequency and severity	May require change in therapy
SNRI-Specific			
Desvenlafaxine	Dose-related hyperlipidemia	Lipid profile	Elevations in total cholesterol, low-density lipoproteins, and triglycerides
Duloxetine	Liver toxicity	Liver function tests	May be transient upon initiation or sustained
Mixed Serotonergic Effects (Mixed 5-HT)			
Nefazodone	Liver toxicity	Liver function tests	Nefazodone boxed warning in the United States for hepatotoxicity
Trazodone	Orthostatic hypotension	Blood pressure, pulse	May be more severe as compared with other antidepressants; rate-limiting adverse medication reactions
	Priapism	Patient report of sexual dysfunction, especially painful erection	Patient should seek medical attention for prolonged erection (ie, >4 hr)
Vilazodone and vortioxetine	Nausea	Frequency and severity	Most common dose limiting adverse reaction
Serotonin and α_2–Adrenergic Antagonist			
Mirtazapine	Weight gain	Body weight	Frequently occurring and significant (>7% over baseline) weight gain among adults; diet mediated
Norepinephrine and Dopamine Reuptake Inhibitor (NDRI)			
Bupropion	Seizure activity	Electroencephalogram if indicated	See Table 88-3 for proper dosing, which can help decrease seizure risk; caution use in patients with eating disorders or alcohol use disorders

Data from References 2, 60, 62, 73, 74, and 80.

and severity of depressive and associated symptoms. It is helpful to administer the rating scales prior to treatment, 2 to 4 weeks and 8 to 12 weeks after initiation of therapy, and periodically thereafter. It is important to note that lack of robust response at 2 to 4 weeks does not necessarily predict lack of response at 8 to 12 weeks.[56] Interviewing a family member or friend (with the patient's permission) regarding symptoms and daily functioning also can assist in assessment of progress, as they may notice symptom improvements before the patient. Patients should be monitored at more frequent intervals early in treatment, particularly for suicidality. Monitoring is then continued at regular intervals throughout the continuation and maintenance phases of treatment and assessing for reemergence of target symptoms continued for several months after antidepressant therapy is discontinued.

Finally, one useful set of criteria that can be used with a variety of psychometric scales uses the following definitions: (a) *nonresponse* is less than a 25% decrease in baseline symptoms, (b) *partial response* is a 26% to 49% decrease in baseline symptoms, and (c) *partial remission or response* is greater than a 50% decrease in baseline symptoms.[53] Consistent with other recommendations, *remission* is a return to baseline functioning with no symptoms present.[2]

CONCLUSION

Depression is a highly pervasive and complex disease state that can be impacted by comorbid medical and psychiatric conditions, psychosocial factors, as well as medications. While the precise pathophysiology of MDD is still elusive, antidepressant medications have directly targeted monoamine systems for the past half-century, and our understanding is evolving to include other complementary mechanisms. Additionally, research is revealing more about the complexity of the disease and the impact of genetic polymorphisms (both on pathophysiology and impact on pharmacotherapy outcomes). Individual patient characteristics should be considered when selecting antidepressant therapy and monitoring treatment. The goals of treatment should include remission (complete resolution of symptoms) and improved functioning.

ABBREVIATIONS

AHRQ	Agency for Healthcare Research and Quality
APA	American Psychiatric Association
BAP	British Association of Psychopharmacology
BDI	Beck Depression Inventory
BDNF	brain-derived neurotrophic factor
CAM	complementary and alternative medicine
DA	dopamine
DHA	docosahexaenoic acid
DSM-5	*Diagnostic and Statistical Manual of Mental Disorders,* Fifth Edition
ECG	electrocardiogram
ECT	electroconvulsive therapy
EPA	eicosapentaenoic acid
5-HT	serotonin
GI	gastrointestinal
HAM-D	Hamilton Rating Scale for Depression
HPA	hypothalamic–pituitary–adrenal
KKW	kilocalories per kilogram per week
5-MTHF	5-methyltetrahydrofolate
MADRS	Montgomery-Åsberg Depression Rating Scale

MAOI	monoamine oxidase inhibitor
MDD	major depressive disorder
NDRI	norepinephrine and dopamine reuptake inhibitor
NE	norepinephrine
NIMH	National Institute of Mental Health
NT	neurotransmitter
PD	pharmacodynamic
PK	pharmacokinetic
rTMS	repetitive transcranial magnetic stimulation
SAMe	*S*-adenosyl-L-methionine
SNRI	serotonin–norepinephrine reuptake inhibitor
SS	serotonin syndrome
SSRI	selective serotonin reuptake inhibitor
STAR*D	Sequenced Treatment Alternatives to Relieve Depression
T_3	triiodothyronine
TADS	Treatment for Adolescents with Depression Study
TCA	tricyclic antidepressant
TORDIA	Treatment of Resistant Depression in Adolescents
TRD	treatment resistant depression
TREAD	Treatment with Exercise Augmentation for Depression

REFERENCES

1. American Psychiatric Association. *Diagnostic and Statistical Manual of Mental Disorders.* 5th ed. Arlington, VA: American Psychiatric Association; 2013.
2. American Psychiatric Association. *Practice Guideline for the Treatment of Patients With Major Depressive Disorder.* 3rd ed. Arlington, VA: American Psychiatric Association; 2010.
3. Cleare A, Pariante CM, Young AH, et al. Evidence-based guidelines for treating depressive disorders with antidepressants: A revision of the 2008 British Association for Psychopharmacology guidelines. *J Psychopharmacol.* 2015;29(5):459–525.
4. Kennedy SH, Lam RW, McIntyre RS, et al. Canadian network for mood and anxiety treatments (CANMAT) 2016 clinical guidelines for the management of adults with major depressive disorder: Section 3. Pharmacological treatments. *Can J Psych.* 2016;61(9):540–560.
5. Iranpour S, Sabour S, Koohi F, Saadati HM, et al. The trend and pattern of depression prevalence in the U.S.: Data from National Health and Nutrition Examination Survey (NHANES) 2005 to 2016. *J Affect Disord.* 2022;298(Pt A):508–515. 10.1016/j.jad.2021.11.027 34785265.
6. Centers for Disease Control and Prevention. National VitalStatistics Report. 2017, May 17; 70(4) Available at: https://www.cdc.gov/nchs/data/nvsr70/nvsr70-04-508.pdf. Accessed October 7, 2021.
7. Global prevalence and burden of depressive and anxiety disorders in 204 countries and territories in 2020 due to the COVID-19 pandemic. *Lancet.* 2021;398(10312):1700–1712. 10.1016/S0140-6736(21)02143-7 34634250.
8. Centers for Disease Control and Prevention. Vital Signs: Suicide rising across the US. Available at: https://www.cdc.gov/vitalsigns/suicide/index.html. Accessed November 27, 2018.
9. Substance Abuse and Mental Health Services Administration. 2017 National Survey on Drug Use and Health: Major Depressive Episode in the Past Year. Available at: https://www.samhsa.gov/data/report/2017-nsduh-annual-national-report. Accessed Novemeber 27, 2018.
10. Weissman MM, Gershon ES, Kidd KK, et al. Psychiatric disorders in the relatives of probands with affective disorders. The Yale University—National Institute of Mental Health Collaborative Study. *Arch Gen Psychiatry.* 1984;41(1):13–21.
11. Stewart SL, Van Dyke JN, Poss JW. Examining the mental health presentations of treatment-seeking Transgender and Gender Nonconforming (TGNC) Youth. *Child Psychiatry Hum Dev.* 202110.1007/s10578-021-01289-1 34860314.
12. Sullivan PF, Neale MC, Kendler KS. Genetic epidemiology of major depression: Review and meta-analysis. *Am J Psychiatry.* 2000;157(10):1552–1562.
13. Belmaker RH, Agam G. Mechanisms of disease major depressive disorder. *N Engl J Med.* 2008;358:55–68.
14. Baumeister AA, Hawkins MF, Uzelac SM. The myth of reserpine-induced depression: Role in the historical development of the monoamine hypothesis. *J Hist Neurosci.* 2003;12(2):207–220.
15. Yohn CN, Gergues MM, Samuels BA. The role of 5-HT receptors in depression. *Mol Brain.* 2017;10(1):1–12.
16. Pehrson AL, Sanchez C. Altered γ-aminobutryic acid neurotransmission in major depressive disorder: A critical review of the supporting evidence and the influence of serotonergic antidepressants. *Drug Des Devel Ther.* 2015;9:603–624.
17. Taylor GT, Manzella F. Kappa opioids, salvinorin A and major depressive disorder. *Curr Neuropharmacol.* 2016;14(2):165–176.
18. Schüle C, Nothdurfter C, Rupprecht R. The role of alloprenganolone in depression and anxiety. *Prog Neurobiol.* 2014;113:79–87.
19. Newport DJ, Carpenter LL, McDonald WM. Ketamine and other NMDA antagonists: Early clinical trials and possible mechanisms in depression. *Am J Psychiatry.* 2015;172:950–966.
20. Koopman M, El Aidy S; MIDtrauma consortium. Depressed gut? The microbiota-diet-inflammation trialogue in depression. *Curr Opin Psychiatry.* 2017;30(5):369–377.
21. Bender A, Hagan K, Kinston N. The association of folate and depression: A meta-analysis. *J Psychiatr Res.* 2017;95:9–18.
22. Farioli-Vecchioli S, Sacchetti S, di Robilant NV, et al. The role of physical exercise and omega-3 fatty acids in depressive illness in the elderly. *Curr Neuropharmacol.* 2018;16(3):308–326.
23. Dunlop BW, Nemeroff CB. The role of dopamine in the pathophysiology of depression. *Arch Gen Psychiatry.* 2007;64:327–337.
24. Taylor C, Fricker AD, Devi L, et al. Mechanisms of action of antidepressants: From neurotransmitter systems to signaling pathways. *Cell Signal.* 2005;17(5):549–557.
25. Niciu MJ, Ionescu DF, Mathews DC, et al. Second messenger/signal transduction pathways in major mood disorders—moving from membrane to mechanism of action, part I: Major depressive disorder. *CNS Spectrums.* 2013;18:231–241.
26. Feighner JP. Mechanism of action of antidepressant medications. *J Clin Psychiatry.* 1999;60(suppl 4):S4–S11; discussion 12–13.
27. Rivero G, Gabilondo AM, García-Sevilla JA, et al. Increased α2- and β1-adrenoreceptor densities in post-mortem brain of subjects with depression: Differential effect of antidepressant treatment. *J Affective Disorders.* 2014;167:343–350.
28. Kanes S, Colquhoun H, Gunduz-Bruce H, et al. Brexanolone (SAGE-547 injection) in post-partum depression: A randomised controlled trial. *Lancet.* 2017;390:480–489.
29. Björkholm C, Monteggia LM. BDNF: A key transducer of antidepressant effects. *Neuropharmacology.* 2016;102:72–79.
30. Strasburger SE, Bhimani PM, Kaabe JH, et al. What is the mechanism of ketamine's rapid-onset antidepressant effect? A concise overview of the surprisingly large number of possibilities. *J Clin Pharm Ther.* 2017;42(2):147–154.
31. Coryell W, Schlesser M. The dexamethasone suppression test and suicide prediction. *Am J Psychiatry.* 2001;158(5):748–753.
32. Wan L, Yuhong L, Zhang Z, et al. Methylenetetrahydrofolate reductase and psychiatric diseases. *Transl Psychiatry.* 2018;8:242.
33. Bousman CA, Dunlop BW. Genotype, phenotype, and medication recommendation agreement among commercial pharmacogenetic-based decision support tools. *Pharmacogenomics J.* 2018;18(5):613–622.
34. Haigh E, Bogucki O, Sigmon S, et al. Depression among older adults: A 20-year update on five common myths and misconceptions. *Am J Geriatr Psychiatry.* 2018;26(1):107–122.
35. Kok RM, Reynolds CF. Management of depression in older adults: A review. *JAMA.* 2017;317(20):2114–2122.
36. Voinov B, Richie WD, Bailey RK. Depression and chronic diseases: It is time for a synergistic mental health and primary care approach. *Prim Care Companion CNS Disord.* 2013;15(2):pii: PCC.
37. Qato DM, Ozenberger K, Olfson M. Prevalence of prescription medications with depression as a potential adverse effect among adults in the United States. *JAMA.* 2018;319(22):2289–2298.
38. Gorton HC, Webb RT, Kapur N, et al. Non-psychotropic medication and risk of suicide or attempted suicide: A systematic review. *BMJ.* 2016;6:e009074.
39. Gibbons RD, Mann JJ. Varenicline, smoking cessation, and neuropsychiatric adverse events. *Am J Psychiatry.* 2013;170(12):1460–1467.
40. Risk evaluation and mitigation strategy (REMS) The iPLEDGE Program. Available at https://www.fda.gov/downloads/Drugs/DrugSafety/PostmarketDrugSafetyInformationforPatientsandProviders/UCM234639.pdf. Accessed November 20, 2018.
41. Hesdorffer DC, Kanner AM. The FDA alert on suicidality and antiepileptic drugs: Fire or false alarm? *Epilepsia.* 2009;50(5):978–986.

42. Skovlund CW, Mørch LS, Kessing LV, et al. Association of hormonal contraception with depression. *JAMA Psychiatry.* 2016;73(11):1154–1162.
43. Solmi M, Pigato G, Kane JM, et al. Treatment of tardive dyskinesia with VMAT-2 inhibitors: A systematic review and meta-analysis of randomized controlled trials. *Drug Des Devel Ther.* 2018;12:1215–1238.
44. Ranchord AM, Spertus JA, Buchanan DM, et al. Initiation of β-blocker therapy and depression after acute myocardial infarction. *Am Heart J.* 2016;174:37–42.
45. Montgomery SA, Asberg M. A new depression scale designed to be sensitive to change. *Br J Psychiatry.* 1979;134:382–389.
46. Beck AT, Ward CH, Mock J, Erbaugh J. An inventory for measuring depression. *Arch Gen Psychiatry.* 1961;4:561–571.
47. Kroenke K, Spitzer RL, Williams JB. The PHQ-9: Validity of a brief depression severity measure. *J Gen Intern Med.* 2001;16(9):606–613.
48. Hill RM, Rufino K, Kurian S, et al. Suicide ideation and attempts in a pediatric emergency department before and during COVID-19. *Pediatrics.* 2021;147(310.1542/peds.2020-029280 33328339.
49. Jacobs DG, Baldessarini RJ, Fawcett JA, et al. Practice guidelines for the assessment and treatment of patients with suicidal behaviors. *Am J Psychiatry.* 2003;160(11 suppl):S1–S60.
50. Posner K, Brown GK, Stanley B, et al. The Columbia-Suicide Severity Rating Scale: Initial validity and internal consistency findings from three multisite studies with adolescents and adults. *Am J Psychiatry.* 2011;168(12):1266–1277.
51. Fawcett JA, Baldessarini RJ, Coryell WH, et al. Defining and managing suicidal risk in patients taking psychotropic medications. *J Clin Psychiatry.* 2009;70(6):782–789.
52. Sharma T, Guski LW, Freund N, et al. Suicidality and aggression during antidepressant treatment: Systematic review and meta-analyses based on clinical study reports. *BMJ.* 2016;352:i65.
53. Mann JJ. The medical management of depression. *N Engl J Med.* 2005;353(17):1819–1834.
54. Fava GA, Benasi G, Lucente M. Withdrawal symptoms after serotonin-noradrenalin reuptake inhibitor discontinuation: Systematic review. *Psychother Psychosom.* 2018;87:195–203.
55. Weitz ES, Hollon SD, Twisk J, et al. Baseline depression severity as moderator of depression outcomes between cognitive behavioral therapy vs pharmacotherapy: An individual patient data meta-analysis. *JAMA Psychiatry.* 2015;72(11):1102–1109.
56. Gaynes BN, Rush AJ, Trivedi MH, et al. The STAR*D study: Treating depression in the real world. *Cleve Clin J Med.* 2008;75(1):57–66.
57. Brunoni AR, Chaimani A, Moffa AH, et al. Repetitive transcranial magnetic stimulation for the acute treatment of major depressive episodes: A systematic review with network meta-analysis. *JAMA Psychiatry.* 2017;74(2):143–153.
58. Trivedi MH. The link between depression and physical symptoms. *Prim Care Companion J Clin Psychiatry.* 2004;6(suppl 1):S12–S16.
59. Freeman MP, Fava M, Lake J, et al. Complementary and alternative medicine in major depressive disorder: The American Psychiatric Association Task Force report. *J Clin Psychiatry.* 2010;71(6):669–681.
60. Lexicomp Online. Lexi-Comp, Inc (Copyright 1978–2018). Available at: http://online.lexi.com. Accessed November 15, 2021.
61. Wimbiscus M, Kostenko O, Malone D. MAO inhibitors: Risks, benefits, and lore. *Cleve Clin J Med.* 2010:77(12):859–882.
62. Al-Sukhni M, Maruschak NA, McIntyre RS. Vortioxetine: A review of efficacy, safety and tolerability with a focus on cognitive symptoms in major depressive disorder. *Expert Opin Drug Saf.* 2015;14(8):1291–1304.
63. O'Donnell JM, Bies RR, Shelton RC. Drug therapy of depression and anxiety disorders. In: Brunton LL, Hilal-Dandan R, Knollmann BC, eds. *Goodman & Gilman: The Pharmacological Basis of Therapeutics.* 13th ed. McGraw Hill Education; 2018.
64. Walsh BT, Seidman SN, Sysko R, Gould M. Placebo response in studies of major depression: Variable, substantial, and growing. *JAMA.* 2002;287(14):1840–1847.
65. Cipriani A, Forukawa TA, Salanti G, et al. Comparative efficacy and acceptability of 21 antidepressant drugs for the acute treatment of adults with major depressive disorder: A systematic review and network meta-analysis. *Lancet.* 2018;391:1357–1366.
66. Goldstein BJ, Goodnick PJ. Selective serotonin reuptake inhibitors in the treatment of affective disorders—III. Tolerability, safety and pharmacoeconomics. *J Psychopharmacol.* 1998;12(3 suppl B):S55–S87.
67. Wichniak A, Wierzbicka A, Walecka M, et al. Effect of antidepressants on sleep. *Curr Psychiatry.* 2017;19:63.
68. La Torre A, Giupponi G, Duffy D, Conca A. Sexual dysfunction related to psychotropic drugs: A critical review—part I: Antidepressants. *PharmacoPsychiatry.* 2013;46(5):191–199.
69. Howland RH. A critical evaluation of the cardiac toxicity of citalopram part 1. *J Psychosocial Nursing.* 2011;49(11):13–16.
70. Rector TS, Adabag S, Cunningham F, et al. Outcomes of citalopram dosage risk mitigation in a veteran population. *Am J Psychiatry.* 2016;173:896–902.
71. Settle EC. Antidepressant drugs: Disturbing and potentially dangerous adverse effects. *J Clin Psychiatry.* 1998;59(Suppl 16):S25–S30.
72. Glassman AH, Roose SP, Bigger JT. The safety of tricyclic antidepressants in cardiac patients risk benefit reconsidered. *JAMA.* 1993;269(20):2673–2675.
73. McIntyre RS. The role of new antidepressants in clinical practice in Canada: A brief review of vortioxetine, levomilnacipran ER, and vilazodone. *Neuropsychiatr Dis Treat.* 2017;13:2913–2919.
74. Sedky K, Nazir R, Joshi A. Which psychotropic medications induce hepatotoxicity. *Gen Hosp Psychiatry.* 2012;34:53–61.
75. Stimmel GL, Gutierrez MA. Counseling patients about sexual issues. *Pharmacotherapy.* 2006;26(11):1608–1615.
76. Rabiner EA, Gunn RN, Castro ME, et al. β-Blocker binding to human 5-HT_{1A} receptors *in vivo* and *in vitro*: Implications for antidepressant therapy. *Neuropsychopharmacol.* 2000;23:285–293.
77. Steinert T, Fröscher W. Epileptic seizures under antidepressive drug treatment: Systematic review. *Pharmacopsychiatry.* 2018;51:121–135.
78. Taylor MJ, Rudkin L, Bullemor-Day P, Lubin J, Chukwujekwu C, Hawton K, et al. Strategies for managing sexual dysfunction induced by antidepressant medication. *Cochrane Database Syst Rev.* 20135):CD003382–CD003382. 10.1002/14651858.CD003382.pub3 23728643.
79. Gorman JM. Mirtazapine: Clinical overview. *J Clin Psychiatry.* 1999;60(suppl 17):S9–S13.
80. Azzaro AJ, Ziemnia J, Kemper E, et al. Pharmacokinetics and absolute bioavailability of selegiline following treatment of healthy subjects with selegiline transdermal system (6 mg/24 h): A comparison with oral selegiline capsules. *J Clin Pharmacol.* 2007;47:1256–1267.
81. Shulman KI, Walker SE, MacKenzie S, et al. Dietary restriction, tyramine and the use of monoamine oxidase inhibitors. *J Clin Psychopharmacol.* 1989;9:397–402.
82. Daly EJ, Singh JB, Fedgchin M, et al. Efficacy and safety of intranasal esketamine adjunctive to oral antidepressant therapy in treatment-resistant depression: A randomized clinical trial. *JAMA Psychiatry.* 2018;75(2):139–148.
83. Canuso CM, Singh JB, Fedgchin M, et al. Efficacy and safety of intranasal esketamine for the rapid reduction of symptoms of depression and suicidality in patients at imminent risk for suicide: Results of a double-blind, randomized, placebo-controlled study. *Am J Psychiatry.*2018;175(7):620–630.
84. Walkery A, Leader LD, Cooke E, VandenBerg A, et al. Review of allopregnanolone agonist therapy for the treatment of depressive disorders. *Drug Des Devel Ther.* 2021;15:3017–3026. 10.2147/DDDT.S240856 34267503.
85. Bahji A, Vazquez GH, Zarate CA Jr. Comparative efficacy of racemic ketamine and esketamine for depression: A systematic review and meta-analysis. *J Affect Disord.* 2021;278:542–555. 10.1016/j.jad.2020.09.071 33022440.
86. Boyer EW, Shannon M. The serotonin syndrome. *N Engl J Med.* 2005;352(11):1112–1120.
87. DeVane CL. Metabolism and pharmacokinetics of selective serotonin reuptake inhibitors. *Cell Mol Neurobiol.* 1999;19(4):443–466.
88. Drug interactions Flockhart Table. Available at https://drug-interactions.medicine/iu.edu/MainTable.aspx. Accessed November 15, 2021.
89. Wells BG. Tricyclic antidepressants. In: Taylor WJ, Caviness MHD, eds.Taylor WJ, Caviness MHD, eds. *A Textbook for the Clinical Application of Therapeutic Drug Monitoring.* Irving, TX: Abbott Laboratories; 1986:449–465.
90. Jefferson JW, Pradko JF, Muir KT. Bupropion for major depressive disorder: Pharmacokinetic and formulation considerations. *Clin Ther.* 2005;27(11):1685–1695.
91. Mullish BH, Kabir MS, Thursz MR, et al. Review article: Depression and the use of antidepressants in patients with chronic liver disease or liver transplantation. *Ailment Pharmacol Ther.* 2014;40:880–892.
92. Eyler RF, Unruh ML, Quinn DK, et al. Psychotherapeutic agents in end-stage renal disease. *Semin Dial.* 2015;28(4):417–426.
93. Rickli A, Liakoni E, Hoener MC, et al. Opioid-induced inhibition of the human 5-HT and noradrenaline transporters *in vitro*: Link to clinical reports of serotonin syndrome. *Br J Pharmacol.* 2018;175(3):532–543.
94. Bixby AL, VandenBerg A, Bostwick JR. Clinical management of bleeding risk with antidepressants. *Ann Pharmacother.* 2018; [Epub ahead of print].

95. Köhler O, Petersen L, Mors O, et al. Inflammation and depression: Combined use of selective serotonin reuptake inhibitors and NSAIDs or paracetamol and psychiatric outcomes. 2015;5(8):e00338.
96. Lorenz RA, VandenBerg AM, Canepa EA. Serotonergic antidepressants and linezolid: A retrospective chart review and presentation of cases. *Int J Psychiatry Med.* 2008;38(1):81–90.
97. Ravindran AV, Balneaves LG, Faulkner G, et al. Canadian network for mood and anxiety treatments (CANMAT) 2016 clinical guidelines for the management of adults with major depressive disorder. Section 5. Complementary and alternative medicine treatments. *Can J Psychiatry.* 2016;61(9):576–587.
98. Turvey CL, Conwell Y, Jones MP, et al. Risk factors for late-life suicide: A prospective, community-based study. *Am J Geriatr Psychiatry.* 2002;10(4):398–406.
99. Schatzberg AG, Kremer C, Rodriguez HE, et al. Double-blind, randomized comparison of mirtazapine and paroxetine in elderly depressed patients. *Am J Geriatr Psychiatry.* 2002;10(5):541–550.
100. Mullen S. Major depressive disorder in children and adolescents. *Ment Health Clin.* 2018;8(6):275–283.
101. March J, Silva S, Petrycki S, et al. Fluoxetine, cognitive-behavioral therapy, and their combination for adolescents with depression: Treatment for adolescents with depression study (TADS) randomized controlled trial. *JAMA.* 2004;292(7):807–820.
102. Emslie GJ, Mayes T, Porta G, et al. Treatment of resistant depression in adolescents (TORDIA): Week 24 outcomes. *Am J Psychiatry.* 2010;167:782–791.
103. Goodyer I, Dubicka B, Wilkinson P, et al. A randomised controlled trial of cognitive behaviour therapy in adolescents with major depression treated by selective serotonin reuptake inhibitors. The ADAPT trial. *Health Technol Assess.* 2008;12(14):iii–iv,ix-60.
104. Gibbons RD, Brown CH, Hur K, et al. Suicidal thoughts and behavior with antidepressant treatment. *Arch Gen Psychiatry.* 2012;69(6):580–587.
105. Gibbons RD, Brown CH, Hur K, et al. Early evidence on the effects of regulators' suicidality warnings on SSRI prescriptions and suicide in children and adolescents. *Am J Psychiatry.* 2007;164:1356–1363.
106. Oberlander TF, Warburton W, Misri S, et al. Neonatal outcomes after prenatal exposure to selective serotonin reuptake inhibitor antidepressants and maternal depression using population-based linked health data. *Arch Gen Psychiatry.* 2006;63(8):898–906.
107. Cohen LS, Altshuler LL, Harlow BL, et al. Relapse of major depression during pregnancy in women who maintain or discontinue antidepressant treatment. *JAMA.* 2006;295(5):499–507.
108. Gao SY, Wu QJ, Zhang TN, et al. Selective serotonin reuptake inhibitor use during early pregnancy and congenital malformations: A systematic review and meta-analysis of cohort studies of more than 9 million births. *BMC Medicine.* 2018;16:205.
109. Chambers CD, Hernandez-Diaz S, Van Marter LJ, et al. Selective serotonin-reuptake inhibitors and risk of persistent pulmonary hypertension of the newborn. *N Engl J Med.* 2006;354(6):579–587.
110. Rubinow DR. Antidepressant treatment during pregnancy: Between Scylla and Charybdis. *Am J Psychiatry.* 2006;163(6):954–956.
111. Yonkers KA, Wisner KL, Stewart DE, et al. The management of depression during pregnancy: A report from the American Psychiatric Association and the American College of Obstetricians and Gynecologists. *Gen Hosp Psychiatry.* 2009;31(5):403–413.
112. Freeman MP. Breastfeeding and antidepressants: Clinical dilemmas and expert perspectives. *J Clin Psychiatry.* 2009;70(2):291–292.
113. Trivedi MH, Rush AJ, Wisniewski SR, et al. Evaluation of outcomes with citalopram for depression using measurement-based care in STAR*D: Implications for clinical practice. *Am J Psych.* 2006;163:28–40.
114. Rush AJ, Trivedi MH, Wisniewski SR, et al. Bupropion-SR, sertraline, or venlafaxine-XR after failure of SSRIs for depression. *N Engl J Med.* 2006;354(12):1231–1242.
115. Fava M, Rush AJ, Wisniewski SR, et al. A comparison of mirtazapine and nortriptyline following two consecutive failed medication treatments for depressed outpatients: A STAR*D report. *Am J Psychiatry.* 2006;163(7):1161–1172.
116. Nierenberg AA, Fava M, Trivedi MH, et al. A comparison of lithium and T(3) augmentation following two failed medication treatments for depression: A STAR*D report. *Am J Psychiatry.* 2006;163(9):1519–1530.
117. Mohamed S, Johnson GR, Chen P, et al. Effect of antidepressant switching vs augmentation on remission among patients with major depressive disorder unresponsive to antidepressant treatment. The VAST-D randomized clinical trial. *JAMA.* 2018;318:132–145.
118. Rosenblat JD, Lee Y, McIntyre RS. Does pharmacogenomics testing improve clinical outcomes for major depressive disorder. A systematic review of clinical trials and cost-effectiveness studies. *J Clin Psychiatry.* 2017;78(6):720–729.

89

Bipolar Disorder

Jordan C. Haygood and Shannon J. Drayton

KEY CONCEPTS

1. Bipolar disorder is a cyclic mental illness with recurrent mood episodes that occur over a person's lifetime. The symptoms, course, severity, and response to treatment differ among individuals.
2. Bipolar disorder is likely caused by genetic factors, environmental triggers, and the dysregulation of neurotransmitters, neurohormones, and second messenger systems in the brain.
3. Clinicians should obtain a detailed history, including medical history and substance use history, to expedite the diagnosis and treatment of bipolar disorder.
4. Bipolar disorder is a complex psychiatric illness with significant morbidity and mortality. Suicidal thoughts and behaviors are common in individuals with bipolar disorder and need to be managed with medical and therapeutic interventions.
5. The goal of therapy for bipolar disorder should be to improve an individual's functioning by reducing mood episodes. This is accomplished by maximizing adherence to therapy and limiting medication adverse effects.
6. Patients and family members should be educated about bipolar disorder and treatments. Long-term monitoring and adherence to treatment are primary factors in achieving disease stabilization.
7. Lithium, valproate, and second-generation antipsychotics are the mainstays of treatment for different phases of bipolar disorder, acting as primary mood stabilizers. When individuals with bipolar disorder present with an acute mood episode (eg, depressed episode, manic episode or mixed state) despite a primary mood stabilizer, adjunctive medications are considered to target the specific mood state or subtype. These medications can often be tapered once the acute episode has resolved and euthymia is reached. Baseline and follow-up laboratory tests are required for most medications used for bipolar disorder to monitor for adverse effects.
8. Some individuals can be stabilized on one mood stabilizer, but others may require combination therapies or adjunctive agents during an acute mood episode. Adjunctive agents should be tapered and discontinued when the acute mood episode remits and the patient is stabilized, if possible. These agents may include benzodiazepines, additional mood stabilizers, antipsychotics, and/or antidepressants.

BEYOND THE BOOK

Introductory Video About Bipolar Disorder: Use the link below to view the video titled, "Mental Illness in Stressful Times—An Asian American Family's Story" on the National Institute of Mental Health website. This 6-minute video provides a glimpse into one family's experience with bipolar disorder. The viewing of this video is intended to stimulate deeper thinking about social implications of bipolar disorder and to provoke an appreciation of the hardships and successes that patients with the disorder may face.

Link to video: https://www.nimh.nih.gov/news/media/2016/mental-illness-in-stressful-times-an-asian-american-familys-story.shtml

INTRODUCTION

1 Bipolar disorder is a common, chronic, and often severe cyclic mood disorder characterized by recurrent fluctuations in mood, energy, and behavior.[1,2] It differs from recurrent major depression, or unipolar depression, in that a manic or hypomanic episode occurs during the course of the illness (see section "Clinical Presentation and Diagnosis").[1] Bipolar disorder is a lifelong illness with a variable course and requires both non-pharmacologic and pharmacologic treatments for mood stabilization.[1,2]

EPIDEMIOLOGY

The lifetime prevalence of bipolar disorder in the United States is 4.4% with 1% of patients meeting criteria for bipolar I, 1.1% for bipolar II, and 2.4% of patients with subthreshold bipolar disorder (ie, cyclothymia, unspecified bipolar disorder).[3] Similar rates of bipolar I disorder are seen in males and females.[4] Symptom onset for depression, mania, or hypomania in bipolar disorder typically occurs in late adolescence or early adulthood, with approximately one-third to two-thirds of patients diagnosed with bipolar disorder experiencing their first episode as a child or adolescent.[2] Depression and mixed presentations may occur more frequently in females.[2,5]

ETIOLOGY AND PATHOPHYSIOLOGY

2 The exact etiology of bipolar disorder is unknown but is thought to be influenced by a complex of developmental, genetic, neurobiologic, and psychological factors.[4,6] Many theories have been proposed regarding the pathophysiology of mood disorders. Family, twin, and adoption studies report an increased lifetime prevalence risk of having mood disorders among first-degree relatives of patients with bipolar disorder.[7] Genetic linkage studies suggest that multiple gene loci, such as Calcium Channel, Cardiac Dihydropyridine-Sensitive, Alpha-1 Subunit

(*CACNA1C*), and Ankyrin 3 (*ANK3*), may be involved in the heredity of mood disorders.[6] Additionally, recent studies have uncovered that there may be genetic differences driving the manifestations of the bipolar disorder subtypes.[8] Neuroimaging studies indicate that several anatomic regions, primarily the amygdala within the limbic system and the prefrontal cortex, may contribute to functional abnormalities in patients with bipolar disorder.[9] It is suspected that altered synaptic and circuit functioning account for mood and cognitive changes seen in bipolar disorder, rather than the dysfunction of individual neurotransmitters.[9] Environmental or psychological stressors, immunologic factors, and sleep dysregulation are also associated with bipolar disorder and can negatively influence the course of illness.[4,10,11]

CLINICAL PRESENTATION AND DIAGNOSIS

Bipolar disorder is a cyclic mood disorder where patients sequentially experience different types of episodes with or without a period of normal mood (euthymia) between episodes. Individuals with bipolar disorder can have mood fluctuations that continue for months, or after one episode, they can sometimes go years without the recurrence of any type of mood episode. 1 The essential feature of bipolar spectrum disorders is a history of mania or hypomania that is not caused by any other medical conditions, substances, or psychiatric disorders.[1] The *Diagnostic and Statistical Manual of Mental Disorders, Fifth Edition* (*DSM-5*) of the American Psychiatric Association (APA) details the present understanding of mood disorders.[1] Bipolar disorder is divided into five subtypes based on the identification of specific mood episodes: bipolar I, bipolar II, cyclothymic disorder, other specified bipolar and related disorder, and unspecified bipolar and related disorder.[1] Table 89-1 defines the mood disorders by type of episode. Specifiers (ie, hypomanic or major depressive episode) can be added to bipolar I and II to reflect the most recent mood state. Comorbid conditions associated with bipolar disorder include, but are not limited to, unhealthy substance use, personality disorders, anxiety disorders, eating disorders, and a higher incidence of several medical conditions.[1,2,4]

Diagnostic Difficulty

Episodes of mania or depression may be induced or caused by medical illness, medications, or substance intoxication or withdrawal (refer to Table 89-2 for causes of mania[13-21] and Chapter 88, "Depressive Disorders" for causes of depression). The timely diagnosis and treatment of bipolar disorder may be difficult due to frequent episodes of depression, comorbid conditions, and lack of treatment during periods of elevated mood. A complete medical, psychiatric, and medication history; physical examination; and laboratory testing are important tools to rule out any organic causes of mania or depression.[22] An accurate diagnosis is critical as some psychiatric and neurologic disorders present with mania-like or depressive-like symptoms.[2] Bipolar disorder commonly co-occurs with substance use disorders and may be difficult to diagnose in the presence of cocaine use or other illicit substances (eg, psychostimulants, bath salts, synthetic cannabinoids).[2] When making the diagnosis of new-onset bipolar disorder, particularly in an older population, clinicians should be aware of secondary causes of mania and depression that may impact the treatment.[23,24]

Schizoaffective disorder, which is essentially a mix between schizophrenia and bipolar disorder or unipolar depression, also presents similarly to bipolar disorder. Patients with schizoaffective

TABLE 89-1 Mood Disorders Defined by Episodes

Disorder Subtype	Episode(s)[a]
Major depressive disorder, single episode	Major depressive episode
Major depressive disorder, recurrent	Two or more major depressive episodes
Bipolar I disorder[b]	Manic episode ± major depressive or hypomanic episode
Bipolar II disorder[c]	Major depressive episode + hypomanic episode
Persistent depressive disorder (Dysthymia)	Depressed mood most days for at least 2 years (1 year in children and adolescents)
Cyclothymic disorder[d]	Chronic fluctuations between subsyndromal depressive and hypomanic episodes (2 years for adults and 1 year for children and adolescents)
Unspecified bipolar and related disorder	Mood states do not meet full criteria for any specific disorder in the bipolar and related disorders class

[a]The length and severity of a mood episode and the interval between episodes vary from patient to patient. Manic episodes are usually shorter and end more abruptly than major depressive episodes, and even with treatment episodes may last upwards of 3 months and 5 months, respectively. The average length of untreated manic episodes ranges from 4 to 13 months. Episodes can occur regularly (at the same time or season of the year) and often cluster at 12-month intervals. Females have more depressive episodes than manic episodes, whereas males have a more even distribution of episodes.

[b]For bipolar I disorder, 90% of individuals who experience a manic episode later have multiple recurrent major depressive, manic, or hypomanic episodes alternating with a normal mood state.

[c]Approximately 5% to 15% of patients with bipolar II disorder will develop a manic episode over a 5-year period. If a manic episode develops in a patient with bipolar II disorder, the diagnosis is changed to bipolar I disorder.

[d]Patients with cyclothymic disorder have a 15% to 50% risk of later developing a bipolar I or II disorder.

Data from References 1 and 12.

TABLE 89-2 Secondary Causes of Mania

Medical conditions that induce mania

- CNS disorders (eg, brain tumor, strokes, head injuries, subdural hematoma, multiple sclerosis, systemic lupus erythematosus, temporal lobe seizures, Huntington's disease)
- Infections (eg, encephalitis, neurosyphilis, sepsis, human immunodeficiency virus)
- Electrolyte or metabolic abnormalities (eg, calcium or sodium fluctuations, hyperglycemia, or hypoglycemia)
- Endocrine or hormonal dysregulation (eg, Addison's disease, Cushing disease, hyperthyroidism or hypothyroidism, menstruation-related, or pregnancy-related or perimenopausal mood disorders)

Medications or drugs that induce mania

- Alcohol intoxication
- Drug withdrawal states (eg, alcohol, α_2-adrenergic agonists, antidepressants, barbiturates, benzodiazepines, opiates)
- Antidepressants (eg, MAOIs, TCAs, 5-HT and/or NE and/or DA reuptake inhibitors, 5-HT antagonists)
- DA-augmenting agents (CNS stimulants: amphetamines, cocaine, sympathomimetics; DA agonists, releasers, and reuptake inhibitors)
- Hallucinogens (eg, LSD, PCP)
- Cannabis intoxication precipitates psychosis, paranoid thoughts, anxiety, and restlessness
- NE-augmenting agents (eg, α_2-adrenergic antagonists, β-agonists, NE reuptake inhibitors)
- Steroids (eg, anabolic, adrenocorticotropic hormone, corticosteroids)
- Thyroid preparations
- Xanthines (eg, caffeine, theophylline)
- Non-prescription weight loss agents and decongestants (eg, ephedra, pseudoephedrine)
- Herbal products (eg, St. John wort)

Somatic therapies that induce mania

- Bright light therapy
- Deep brain stimulation
- Sleep deprivation

CNS, central nervous system; DA, dopamine; 5-HT, serotonin; LSD, lysergic acid diethylamide; MAOI, monoamine oxidase inhibitor; NE, norepinephrine; PCP, phencyclidine; TCA, tricyclic antidepressant.

Data from References 1, 4, and 13–21.

CLINICAL PRESENTATION Major Depressive Disorder[a]

DSM-5 Criteria[b]

At least 2-week period of either depressed mood or loss of interest or pleasure in normal activities, associated with at least five of the following symptoms:

- Depressed, sad mood in adults, can be irritable mood in children
- Decreased interest and pleasure in normal activities
- Decreased or increased appetite, weight loss or weight gain
- Insomnia or hypersomnia
- Psychomotor retardation or agitation
- Decreased energy or fatigue
- Feelings of excessive guilt or worthlessness
- Impaired concentration or indecisiveness
- Recurrent thoughts of death, suicidal thoughts, or attempts

Mania[a]

DSM-5 Criteria[b]

At least 1-week period of abnormally and persistently elevated mood (eg, expansive or irritable) and energy, associated with at least three of the following symptoms (four if the mood is only irritable):

- Inflated self-esteem (grandiosity)
- Decreased need for sleep
- Increased talking (pressure of speech)
- Racing thoughts (flight of ideas)
- Distractibility (poor attention)
- Increased goal-directed activity (socially, at work, or sexually) or psychomotor agitation
- Excessive involvement in activities that are pleasurable but have a high risk for serious consequences (buying sprees, sexual indiscretions, poor judgment in business ventures)

Hypomania[a]

DSM-5 Criteria[b]

At least 4 days of abnormally and persistently elevated mood (eg, expansive or irritable) and energy, associated with at least three of the following symptoms listed under Mania above (four if the mood is only irritable)

[a]Impairment in social or occupational functioning; may include need for hospitalization because of potential self-harm, harm to others, or psychotic symptoms.

[b]The disorder is not caused by a medical condition (eg, hypothyroidism) or substance-induced disorder (eg, antidepressant treatment, other medications), or a substance use disorder. Numerous specifiers are available to further characterize episodes (eg, with mixed features, with anxious distress, with rapid cycling, with melancholic features).

Data from Reference 1.

disorder have mood episodes, but a primary distinguishing factor from bipolar disorder is the occurrence of psychosis between mood episodes during periods of euthymic mood.[1,2] Clinicians must rely on the longitudinal history provided by collateral historians who know the patient well to determine if the patient experiences psychosis between mood episodes. It can be difficult for clinicians to obtain a full psychiatric history on individuals presenting with manic or psychotic symptoms, thus making schizoaffective disorder difficult to differentiate from bipolar disorder.[2] Schizoaffective disorder, bipolar type is best treated with antipsychotics with or without a mood stabilizer as maintenance therapy.

Course of Illness

3 Bipolar disorder is frequently not recognized or treated for many years because of its initial fluctuating course with subsyndromal symptoms of depression, irritability, and hypomania that build up gradually in intensity. Though the overall average age of onset falls within the early 20s, patients typically experience delays averaging 8 years after the index mood episode until appropriate medication initiation.[2,25] This delay confers a risk of poor social functioning, increased hospitalizations, and a greater likelihood of lifetime suicide attempts.[26] Onset of illness in early childhood, as opposed to onset in early adulthood, tends to be associated with longer delay to treatment initiation, increased mood episodes, rapid cycling, and comorbid psychiatric conditions as well as a stronger family history of mood disorders.[27,28] Gender differences may influence the course of illness, tolerability of medication, and response to treatment. Females are more likely to have increased depressive symptoms, older age of onset, better adherence, complex management in pregnancy, and higher association with physical illness such as thyroid abnormalities. In males, there may be increased incidence of mania and substance use/misuse.[29]

The kindling theory is used to explain how bipolar disorder can progress over one's life and why preventive treatment is imperative. Without effective treatment, episodes can become more frequent, severe, and refractory to treatment.[4,10,30,31,44] Usually, there is a period of euthymia between episodes, but approximately 20% to 30% of patients with bipolar I disorder and 15% with bipolar II disorder have no inter-episode period of euthymia because of mood lability, residual subsyndromal mood symptoms, or a direct switch to the opposite polarity.[1]

Rapid cycling is defined as four or more mood episodes per year and is more common in females and has a lifetime prevalence as high as 25% to 43% in all patients with bipolar disorder.[2,32] Frequent and severe episodes of depression are the most common hallmark of rapid cycling. The use of alcohol, stimulants, and antidepressants, as well as sleep deprivation, hypothyroidism, and seasonal changes, can play a role in rapid cycling.[2,32] Seasonal patterns of mania in the summer and depression during the winter have been observed. Patients with rapid cycling have a poorer long-term prognosis and often require combination therapies.[1,2]

Fluctuations in hormones and neurotransmitters during the luteal phase of the menstrual cycle, postpartum period, and perimenopause, starting ~10 years before menopause, can precipitate mood changes and increase mood cycling.[1,2] Evidence supports that females with a history of premenstrual dysphoric disorder (PMDD) diagnosed with bipolar disorder display higher rates of rapid cycling and a greater number of mood episodes.[33] Females with bipolar disorder are at greater risk for relapse into mania or depression during the postpartum period.[2] If a severe mood episode occurs postpartum, there is an increased risk for recurrences during subsequent postpartum periods.[2]

Bipolar disorder is associated with several comorbid psychiatric diagnoses most commonly substance use disorders, anxiety disorders, personality disorders, and impulse control disorders that require careful treatment considerations. Often times, medications utilized to stabilize mood may also be effective in managing comorbidities. Conversely, certain treatment options for comorbidities such as anxiety disorders may further destabilize patients if adequate treatment for mood stability is not first employed. A hierarchical approach should be taken when managing comorbid psychiatric diagnoses.[2]

Alcohol and other substance use or misuse is common among patients with bipolar disorder and can have a significant impact on the age of onset, course of the illness, and response to treatment.[2] Substance use disorders have been reported in 33% to 45% of individuals with bipolar disorder.[34,35] Those with substance use disorders are more likely to have an earlier onset of their illness, mixed states, higher rates of relapse, poorer response to treatment, comorbid personality disorders, increased suicide risk, and more psychiatric hospitalizations.[2] When individuals with bipolar disorder use substances such as alcohol, cannabis, or cocaine during episodes, it can result in further impairment of judgment, poor impulse control, treatment non-adherence, and a worsening of the clinical course. Alcohol and other substance use should be addressed as early as possible in the individual's clinical course to improve outcomes.[2]

4 For those living with bipolar disorder, approximately one-half of their lifetime is spent with syndromal and subsyndromal symptoms, particularly those with depressive episodes.[2] More than one-half (55%-65%) of patients with bipolar I have some degree of functional disability after the onset of their illness, and approximately 10% to 20% of patients with bipolar disorder have severe impairment in their psychosocial and occupational functioning.[1,22,36] Functional impairment is often more pronounced in patients with depression, a greater number of previous episodes, a longer duration of illness, and lower cognition. In a 1-year longitudinal study in 258 patients with bipolar disorder, two-thirds had four or more mood episodes a year despite comprehensive pharmacologic treatment, and approximately 33.2% of the year was spent being depressed compared with 10.8% of the time in the mania phase.[36]

Compared with the general population, individuals with bipolar disorder have a two-fold higher mortality rate.[37] Suicide attempts occur in one-third to one-half of individuals with bipolar disorder, and approximately 6% to 7% of individuals with bipolar I disorder die by suicide.[2,38] Roughly 43% of patients with bipolar disorder worldwide report suicidal ideation. Many factors are associated with suicide attempts including female sex, depression as a current or more recent episode, previous attempts, and comorbid substance use disorder.[2]

The best predictor for the level of functioning during a person's lifetime is adherence with medication treatment. Medication non-adherence is estimated to occur in 20% to 60% of patients secondary to multiple factors including intolerance of adverse medication effects.[39] Due to failure to recognize the disorder, reluctance to acknowledge it, or poor adherence with treatment, an estimated two-thirds of patients with bipolar disorder do not receive appropriate treatment. Non-adherence with pharmacologic treatment and substance use are major factors in relapse and hospitalizations.[2]

TREATMENT

Desired Outcomes

5 The desired outcome in treating bipolar disorder is to effectively resolve acute manic, hypomanic, and depressive episodes, as well as prevent further episodes, maintain healthy functioning, promote treatment adherence, and minimize medication adverse effects.[2,4] The general principles and goals for the management of bipolar disorder are listed in Table 89-3.

TABLE 89-3 General Principles for the Management of Bipolar Disorder

Goals of treatment

- Eliminate mood episode with complete remission of symptoms (ie, acute treatment)
- Prevent recurrences or relapses of mood episodes (ie, continuation phase treatment)
- Return to baseline psychosocial functioning
- Maximize adherence with therapy
- Minimize adverse effects
- Use medications with the best tolerability and fewest drug interactions
- Minimize polypharmacy when possible
- Treat comorbid substance use and use disorders
- Eliminate alcohol, cannabis, cocaine, amphetamines, and hallucinogens
- Minimize nicotine use and stop caffeine intake at least 8 hours prior to bedtime
- Avoid stressors or substances that precipitate an acute episode

Data from References 2 and 4.

General Approach to Treatment

6 Treatment of bipolar disorder must be individualized because the clinical presentation, severity, and frequency of episodes vary widely among patients. Treatment approach should include both non-pharmacologic and pharmacologic strategies.[2] Patients and family members should be educated about bipolar disorder (eg, symptoms, causes, and course) and treatment options. Long-term adherence to treatment is the most important factor in achieving stabilization of the disorder.

7 The treatment of bipolar disorder can vary depending on the type of episode the patient is experiencing. Once diagnosed with bipolar disorder, patients should remain on a mood stabilizer (eg, lithium, valproate, or a second-generation antipsychotic) for their lifetime. During acute episodes, medications can be added and then tapered once the patient is stabilized and euthymic. For example, when treating a patient for mania with psychotic features, the patient should be on a mood stabilizer and an antipsychotic. If an antipsychotic is the patient's currently prescribed maintenance therapy, the dose should be increased or perhaps the medication should be changed altogether if the patient's mood becomes manic. If treating a patient for a severe depressive episode, a clinician may need to maximize the dose of the mood stabilizer or add another medication (eg, quetiapine) with efficacy in that polarity.

Non-pharmacologic Therapy

The basics of non-pharmacologic approaches should address issues of adequate nutrition, sleep, exercise, and stress reduction.[2] Sleep deprivation, high stress, and dietary deficiencies in essential amino acids, fatty acids, vitamins, and minerals can exacerbate mood episodes and result in worse outcomes.[2,40,41] Psychological interventions are aimed at providing individuals with self-management skills and tools for mood regulation. Adjunctive psychosocial interventions are useful for acute depressive episodes and in maintenance and relapse prevention.[2] Evidence-based approaches include: cognitive behavioral therapy (CBT), interpersonal and social rhythm therapy, group psychoeducation, family-focused therapy, and enhanced relapse prevention/individual psychoeducation.[2] Common features of these approaches are providing education about the condition, identifying prodromal warning signs, and developing coping strategies and crisis plans.[2]

Pharmacologic Therapy

7 Pharmacotherapy is crucial for acute and maintenance treatments of bipolar disorder and includes lithium, valproate, carbamazepine, lamotrigine, first-generation antipsychotics (FGAs), second-generation antipsychotics (SGAs), and adjunctive agents such as antidepressants and benzodiazepines. General treatment guidelines for the acute treatment of mood episodes in patients with bipolar I disorder are listed in Table 89-4.[2,22]

TABLE 89-4 Algorithm and Guidelines for the Acute Treatment of Mood Episodes in Patients with Bipolar I Disorder

Acute Manic or Mixed Episode		**Acute Depressive Episode**	
General Guidelines		**General Guidelines**	
Assess for secondary causes of mania or mixed states (eg, alcohol or drug use) Discontinue antidepressants Taper off stimulants and caffeine if possible Treat substance use Encourage good nutrition with regular protein and essential fatty acid intake, exercise, adequate sleep, stress reduction, and psychosocial therapy		Assess for secondary causes of depression (eg, alcohol or drug use) Taper off antipsychotics, benzodiazepines, or sedative–hypnotic agents if possible Treat substance use/misuse Encourage good nutrition with regular protein and essential fatty acid intake, exercise, adequate sleep, stress reduction, and psychosocial therapy	
Hypomania	**Mania**	**Mild-to-Moderate Depressive Episode**	**Severe Depressive Episode**
First, optimize current mood stabilizer if non-adherence is suspected or initiate mood-stabilizing medication: lithium,[a] valproate,[a] carbamazepine,[a] or SGAs Consider adding a benzodiazepine (eg, lorazepam or clonazepam) for short-term adjunctive treatment of agitation or insomnia if needed Oxcarbazepine is an alternative medication treatment option **Second**, if response is inadequate, consider a two-drug combination: Lithium[a] **plus** an antiseizure medication or an SGA, or antiseizure medication **plus** an antiseizure medication or SGA	**First**, optimize the previously prescribed mood stabilizer or medication regimen if non-adherence suspected or initiate new mood-stabilizing two- or three-drug combinations (lithium,[a] valproate,[a] or SGA) **plus** a benzodiazepine (eg, lorazepam or clonazepam) and/or antipsychotic for short-term adjunctive treatment of agitation or insomnia; lorazepam is recommended for catatonia Do not combine antipsychotics Alternative options: carbamazepine[a]; if patient does not respond or tolerate, consider oxcarbazepine **Second**, if response is inadequate, consider a three-drug combination: Lithium[a] **plus** an antiseizure medication **plus** an antipsychotic, or antiseizure medication **plus** an antiseizure medication **plus** an antipsychotic **Third**, if response is inadequate, consider ECT for mania with psychosis or catatonia[b] or add clozapine for treatment-refractory illness	**First**, initiate and/ or optimize mood-stabilizing medication: lithium,[a] quetiapine, lurasidone Alternative antiseizure medications: lamotrigine,[c] valproate[a] Alternative antipsychotics: fluoxetine/olanzapine combination, cariprazine, lumateperone	**First**, optimize current mood stabilizer if non-adherence is suspected or initiate a new mood-stabilizing medication: lithium,[a] quetiapine, or lurasidone Alternative fluoxetine/olanzapine combination If psychosis is present, optimize current antipsychotic or initiate in combination with above Alternative antipsychotics: cariprazine, lumateperone Do not combine antipsychotics Alternative antiseizure medications: lamotrigine,[c] valproate[a] **Second**, if response is inadequate, consider carbamazepine[a] or adding antidepressant[d] **Third**, if response is inadequate, consider a three-drug combination: Lithium **plus** lamotrigine[c] **plus** an antidepressant[d] Lithium **plus** quetiapine **plus** antidepressant[d] **Fourth**, if response is inadequate, consider ECT for treatment-refractory illness and depression with psychosis or catatonia[b]

ECT, electroconvulsive therapy; SGA, second-generation antipsychotic.

[a]Use standard therapeutic serum concentration ranges if clinically indicated; if partial response or breakthrough episode, adjust dose to achieve higher serum concentrations without causing intolerable adverse effects; lithium, SGAs, and/or lamotrigine are preferred over valproate and carbamazepine for bipolar depression.

[b]ECT is used for severe mania or depression during pregnancy and for mixed episodes; prior to treatment, antiseizure medication, lithium, and benzodiazepines should be tapered off to maximize therapy and minimize adverse effects.

[c]Lamotrigine is not approved for the acute treatment of depression, and the dose must be started low and slowly titrated up to decrease adverse effects if used for maintenance therapy. Lamotrigine may be initiated during acute treatment with plans to transition to this medication for long-term maintenance. A drug interaction and a severe dermatologic rash can occur when lamotrigine is combined with valproate (ie, lamotrigine doses must be halved from standard dosing titration).

[d]Controversy exists concerning the use of antidepressants, and they are often considered third line in treating acute bipolar depression, except in patients with no recent history of severe acute mania or potentially in bipolar II patients.

Data from References 2, 22, and 47.

Product information, dosing, and administration of agents used in the treatment of bipolar disorder are found in Table 89-5.

7 The term *mood stabilizer* is often used to describe the class of medications used for stabilizing the patient's mood and as maintenance therapy for the prevention of mood fluctuations (eg, mania or depression). However, this term may not be accurate, as some medications are more effective for acute mania, some for the depressive episode, and others for the maintenance phase. Table 89-5 provides the US Food and Drug Administration (FDA) approval status for medications used.

Combination therapies (eg, lithium plus valproate or carbamazepine, lithium, or valproate plus an SGA) can provide better acute response and long-term prevention of relapse and recurrence than monotherapy in some patients with bipolar disorder.[48] The majority of patients hospitalized for an acute episode will be initiated on combination therapy, and after acute symptoms resolve, the medication regimen should be simplified as much as possible.

Several guidelines and algorithms have been published regarding bipolar disorder treatment, based on the best available data and expert consensus. The Canadian Network for Mood and Anxiety Treatments (CANMAT) and International Society for Bipolar Disorders (ISBD) published updated treatment guidelines in 2018.[2] In addition, an international task force of the World Federation of Societies of Biological Psychiatry (WFSBP) has published guidelines for maintenance of mania, depression, and mixed episodes.[49-52]

An example treatment algorithm for acute mood episodes in adult patients with bipolar I disorder is listed in Table 89-4. The selection of treatment for acute mood episodes (eg, mania or depression) and for maintenance treatment should be individualized. Treatment plans should be based on patient-specific characteristics, comorbid psychiatric and medical conditions, consideration of drug interactions, and avoidance of adverse effects.[2]

Lithium

Lithium was first used in 1949 as a treatment for mania and was approved in 1972 in the United States for the treatment of acute mania and for maintenance therapy. Despite numerous investigations into the biologic and clinical properties of lithium, there is no unified theory for its mechanism of action[42]; however, it is thought to modulate neurotransmission at both the neuronal and intracellular levels, and chronic administration may modulate gene expression and have neuroprotective effects.[53] Lithium is a monovalent cation

TABLE 89-5 Products, Dosage and Administration, and Clinical Use of Agents Used in the Treatment of Bipolar Disorder

Drug (Brand Name)	Initial Dosing	Usual Dosing; Special Population Dosing	Comments
Lithium salts			
Lithium carbonate (Eskalith)[a,b] (Eskalith CR) (Lithobid) Lithium citrate (Cibalith-S)[a,b]	300 mg twice daily	900-2,400 mg/day in two to four divided doses, preferably with meals Renal impairment: lower doses required with frequent serum monitoring. There is wide variation in the dosage needed to achieve therapeutic response. Trough serum lithium concentration (ie, 0.6-1.2 mEq/L [mmol/L] for maintenance therapy and 0.8-1.2 mEq/L [mmol/L] for acute mood episodes taken 12 hours after the last dose)	Use alone or in combination with other medications (eg, valproate, carbamazepine, antipsychotics) for the acute treatment of mania and for maintenance treatment
Antiseizure medications			
Divalproex sodium (Depakote)[a] (Depakote ER) Valproic acid[a] (Depakene) Valproate sodium (Depacon)	250-500 mg twice daily A loading dose of divalproex (20-30 mg/kg/day) can be given	750-3,000 mg/day (20-60 mg/kg/day) given once daily or in divided doses Titrate to clinical response Dose adjustment needed with hepatic impairment	Use alone or in combination with other medications (eg, lithium, carbamazepine, antipsychotics) for the acute treatment of mania and for maintenance treatment Use caution when combining with lamotrigine because of potential drug interaction
Lamotrigine (Lamictal)[b]	25 mg daily	50-400 mg/day in divided doses. Dosage should be slowly increased (eg, 25 mg/day for 2 weeks, then 50 mg/day for weeks 3 and 4, and then 50-mg/day increments at weekly intervals up to 200 mg/day) Dose adjustment needed with hepatic impairment	Use alone or in combination with other medications (eg, lithium, carbamazepine) for long-term maintenance treatment for bipolar I disorder
Carbamazepine (Equetro)[a] (Tegretol) (Epitol) (Tegretol-XR) (Carbatrol)	200 mg twice daily	200-1,800 mg/day in two to four divided doses Titrate to clinical response Dose adjustment needed with hepatic impairment	Use alone or in combination with other medications (eg, lithium, valproate, antipsychotics) for the acute and long-term maintenance treatment of mania or mixed episodes for bipolar I disorder. APA guidelines recommend reserving it for patients who were unable to tolerate or who have inadequate response to lithium or valproate Extended-release tablets should be swallowed whole and not be broken or chewed "Carbatrol" capsules can be opened and contents sprinkled over food
Oxcarbazepine (Trileptal)	300 mg twice daily	300-1,200 mg/day in two divided doses Titrate based on clinical response Dose adjustment required with severe renal impairment	Use after patients have failed treatment with carbamazepine or have intolerable adverse medication effects May have fewer adverse effects and be better tolerated than carbamazepine
Second-generation antipsychotics			
Aripiprazole (Abilify)[a,b] (Abilify Maintena)[b]	10-15 mg daily	10-30 mg/day once daily	
Asenapine (Saphris)[b]	5-10 mg twice daily sublingually	5-10 mg twice daily sublingually	
Cariprazine (Vraylar)[a]	1.5 mg daily	3-6 mg daily	
Lumateperone (Caplyta)[c]	42 mg daily	42 mg daily	
Lurasidone (Latuda)[c]	20 mg daily	20-120 mg daily with food	
Olanzapine (Zyprexa)[a,b] (Zyprexa Zydis)	2.5-5 mg twice daily	5-20 mg/day once daily or in divided doses	
Olanzapine and fluoxetine (Symbyax)[c]	6 mg olanzapine and 25 mg fluoxetine daily	6-12 mg olanzapine and 25-50 mg fluoxetine daily	
Quetiapine (Seroquel)[a,b]	50 mg twice daily	50-800 mg/day in divided doses or once daily when stabilized	
Risperidone (Risperdal)[a] (Risperdal M-Tab) (Risperdal Consta)[b]	0.5-1 mg twice daily	0.5-6 mg/day once daily or in divided doses	
Ziprasidone (Geodon)[a]	40-60 mg twice daily	40-160 mg/day in divided doses	

(continued)

TABLE 89-5 Products, Dosage and Administration, and Clinical Use of Agents Used in the Treatment of Bipolar Disorder (*Continued*)

Drug (Brand Name)	Initial Dosing	Usual Dosing; Special Population Dosing	Comments
Benzodiazepines			
Various	Dosage should be slowly adjusted up and down according to response and adverse effects	Use in combination with other medications (eg, antipsychotics, lithium, valproate) for the acute treatment of mania or mixed episodes Use as a short-term adjunctive sedative–hypnotic agent	

[a]FDA-approved for acute mania.

[b]FDA-approved for maintenance.

[c]FDA-approved for acute bipolar depression.

FDA-approved agents may be used as monotherapy in various phases of the illness as noted in table footnotes.

Data from References 42 and 47.

that is rapidly absorbed and widely distributed with no protein binding. It is also not metabolized and is excreted unchanged in the urine and other body fluids.[42]

Efficacy Lithium is considered a first-line agent for acute mania and maintenance treatment of bipolar I and II disorders.[2] Early placebo-controlled studies with lithium reported up to a 78% response rate in aborting an acute manic or hypomanic episode, but more recent studies suggest a slower onset of action and more moderate effectiveness when compared with other agents.[54,55]

Recent treatment guidelines recommend lithium as a second-line agent for acute bipolar II depression based on conflicting efficacy in clinical studies comparing lithium alone to various alternative treatments or placebo.[2] In placebo-controlled studies in bipolar depression, lithium has been found to have efficacy, but there can be a 6- to 8-week delay for its antidepressant effects.[55] A potential rationale for lithium's reduced efficacy in certain trials may be subtherapeutic serum levels in the lithium treatment arm.[2] Lithium also produces antisuicidal actions in patients with bipolar disorder which has been demonstrated consistently in clinical studies.[56] Relapse can be reduced with the combination of lithium and other medications such as valproate, carbamazepine, lamotrigine, and antipsychotics.[55] Abrupt discontinuation or non-adherence with lithium therapy can increase the risk of relapse.[55]

Adverse Effects Adverse effects related to lithium use can be divided into three categories: those that occur early in therapy but are generally innocuous and transient, those that are not dose related occurring with long-term treatment, and toxic effects that occur with high serum concentrations.[42]

Initial gastrointestinal (GI) and central nervous system (CNS) adverse effects are often dose related and are worse at peak serum concentrations, approximately 1-2 hours post-dose. GI side effects are often associated with lithium initiation and may include anorexia, nausea, vomiting, abdominal pain, and diarrhea.[57] Standard approaches for minimizing adverse effects include lowering the dose, taking doses with food, using extended-release products, and trying once-daily dosing at bedtime.[57] Diarrhea can sometimes be managed by switching from tablet or capsule formulation to liquid formulation.[57] Diarrhea produced by lithium is commonly an osmotic diarrhea, and therefore switching to a formulation that clears the gut quickly can ameliorate symptoms.

A benign fine hand tremor can be evident in many patients while a course hand tremor may be a sign of toxicity.[2,54] Strategies to reduce the fine tremor include standard approaches (eg, switch to long-acting preparation, lower dose if possible) or adding a β-adrenergic antagonist (eg, propranolol 20-120 mg/day).[57]

Polydipsia with polyuria associated with or without nephrogenic diabetes insipidus (DI) can occur in patients treated with lithium. About 20% to 40% of patients will develop nephrogenic DI soon after treatment initiation.[2] Patients who develop uncontrolled nephrogenic DI may experience fluid and electrolyte disturbances.[58] Nephrogenic DI will persist in about 10% to 25% of patients on continued treatment and typically is reversible with discontinuation of lithium.[42] Other nonspecific renal effects may be seen with lithium treatment, including proteinuria, distal renal tubular acidosis, and reduced glomerular filtration rate.[58]

Both overt (8%-19%) and subclinical (23%) hypothyroidism can occur in patients treated with lithium, occurring more frequently in females than males.[54,57] Supplemental exogenous thyroid hormone (ie, levothyroxine) can be added to the patients' regimen. If lithium is discontinued, the need for the exogenous thyroid hormone should be reassessed because hypothyroidism can be reversible.[2]

Lithium can cause a variety of benign and reversible cardiac effects, particularly T-wave depression in up to 16% to 33% of patients, atrioventricular block, and bradycardia.[42,59] If a patient has significant preexisting cardiac disease, consultation with a cardiologist and an electrocardiogram (ECG) is recommended at baseline and during lithium therapy.[25]

Other adverse effects associated with lithium include acne and folliculitis, reversible leukocytosis, and weight gain.[42] Approximately 20% of patients gain greater than 10 kg [22 lbs] which can be related to fluid retention, the consumption of high-calorie beverages as a result of polydipsia, or a decreased metabolic rate because of hypothyroidism.[60]

Toxicity Lithium is an extremely toxic medication if accidentally or intentionally taken in overdose. Lithium toxicity usually occurs with serum levels greater than 1.5 mEq/L (mmol/L), but older patients may experience toxicity at lower levels.[42] Severe lithium intoxication occurs when concentrations are higher than 2 mEq/L (mmol/L), and there is a worsening in several key adverse medication effects: *GI* (eg, vomiting, diarrhea, or incontinence), *coordination* (eg, fine to coarse hand tremor, unstable gait, slurred speech, and muscle twitching), and *cognition* (eg, poor concentration, drowsiness, disorientation, confusion, apathy, and coma).[4,54] There have been several reports of seizures, cardiac dysrhythmias, permanent neurologic impairments with ataxia and memory deficits, and kidney damage with reduced glomerular filtration rate after lithium intoxication.[54]

Situations that predispose patients to lithium toxicity include sodium restriction, dehydration, vomiting, diarrhea, older than 50 years, heart failure, cirrhosis, and drug interactions that decrease lithium clearance. Heavy exercise, sauna baths, hot weather, and fever can promote sodium loss.[61,62] Patients should be cautioned to maintain adequate sodium and fluid intake (2.5-3 qt [~2.5-3 L] per day of fluids) and to avoid the excessive use of alcohol, coffee, tea, cola, and other caffeine-containing beverages.

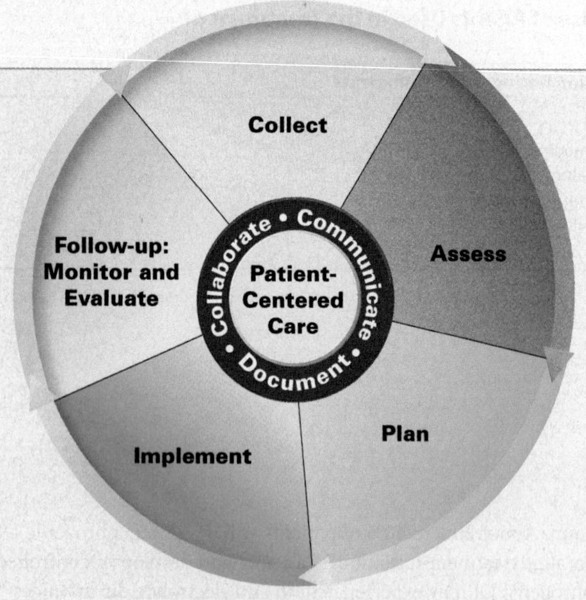

Patient Care Process for Bipolar Disorder

Collect

- Patient characteristics (eg, age, race, sex, pregnancy status)
- Patient psychiatric, medical, social, and family history
- Current medications and prior medication use
- Current and past sleep habits/patterns
- Objective data
  - o Blood pressure, heart rate, height, weight, and body mass index (BMI)
  - o Laboratory test (eg, serum electrolytes, serum creatine [SCr], liver function tests [LFTs], thyroid stimulating hormone [TSH], urine drug screen [UDS], pregnancy test)
  - o Rating scale scores (eg, Young Mania Rating Scale [YMRS], Hamilton Depression Rating Scale (HDRS or HAM-D), Patient Health Questionnaire 9 [PHQ-9])

Assess

- Presence of hypomania, mania, or depression
- Adherence to medication regimen
- Appropriateness, tolerability, and effectiveness of current medication regimen
- Serum concentration of medication if appropriate (eg, lithium)
- Current medications and/or substances that may contribute to or worsen mania or depression
- Suicidality
- Current sleep patterns
- If no response to current medication regimen, reassess diagnosis

Plan*

- If exhibiting euthymia, continue current regimen if appropriate
- If exhibiting mania symptoms, immediately discontinue antidepressants, optimize regimen, and consider the short-term use of benzodiazepine (see Table 89-4)
- If exhibiting depressive symptoms, optimize regimen and consider adding an antipsychotic (ie, quetiapine, cariprazine, or lurasidone) (see Table 89-4)
- Lifestyle modifications (eg, nutrition, sleep, exercise, stress and substance use reduction)
- Monitor for efficacy and safety of medications (see Table 89-6)
- Treat comorbid psychiatric disease states
- Patient education (eg, purpose of treatment, lifestyle modification, drug therapy)
- Self-monitoring for new mood episodes (eg, daily mood chart) and sleep patterns
- Referrals to other providers when appropriate (eg, psychologist, psychiatrist, primary care)

Implement*

- Provide education to patients and their families regarding all elements of treatment plan
- Use motivational interviewing and coaching strategies to maximize adherence
- Schedule follow-up visits

Follow-up: Monitor and Evaluate

- Patient's psychiatric status (eg, rating scale) and safety (eg, suicidality)
- Mood episodes: Document symptoms on a daily mood chart including life stressors, type of episode, length of episode, and treatment outcome. Monthly and yearly life charts are valuable for documenting patterns of mood cycles
- Suicidal ideation or attempts: 6% to 7% of patients with bipolar I disorder die by suicide. Suicide attempts are primarily associated with depressive episodes, mixed episodes with severe depression, or presence of psychosis
- Presence of medication-associated adverse effects should be managed rapidly and vigorously to avoid non-adherence (eg, weight gain, sedation)
- Laboratory tests (see Table 89-6)
- Patient adherence to treatment plan using multiple sources of information and presence of residual symptoms (eg, missing doses of medications is a primary reason for non-response and recurrence of episodes)

**Collaborate with patient, caregivers, and other healthcare professionals.*

If lithium toxicity is suspected, the person should go to an emergency room to be monitored, and lithium should be discontinued.[22] Gastric lavage and IV fluids may be needed, and the patient should be monitored for fluid balance, renal/electrolyte status, and neurologic changes. Activated charcoal is not useful in the setting of lithium toxicity due to its electrically charged nature. Serial serum concentrations should be obtained as renal excretion of lithium may reach a ceiling.[57] Intensive care unit measures should be considered in patients experiencing severe symptoms of toxicity including dysrhythmias, obtundation, or complex fluid/electrolyte imbalances. Hemodialysis may be considered in lithium-naïve patients who may be presenting in an acute overdose situation when lithium concentrations equal or exceed 4 mEq/L (mmol/L) regardless of clinical status or in patients previously taking lithium when lithium concentrations are 2.5 mEq/L (mmol/L) or greater and moderate-to-severe neurologic toxicity, or as clinically indicated.[63] If hemodialysis is initiated, it should be continued until the lithium concentration is below 1 mEq/L (mmol/L) with levels being taken 8 hours after the last dialysis to account for lithium redistribution leading to additional increases in serum levels.

Chronic lithium toxicity may be uncommonly associated with interstitial nephris. Patients exposed to elevated serum levels of lithium and longer-term use may be at risk.[58] Risk of chronic kidney disease is low and mimic that which is seen in the general population.[64]

Drug-Drug Interactions Thiazide diuretics, non-steroidal anti-inflammatory drugs, cyclooxygenase-2 inhibitors, angiotensin-converting enzyme inhibitors, and salt-restricted diets can elevate lithium levels.[42] Neurotoxicity can occur when lithium is combined with antipsychotics, metronidazole, methyldopa, and phenytoin.[42] Combining lithium with non-dihydropyridine calcium channel blockers is not recommended because of reports of altered lithium levels and neurotoxicity.[42] Analgesics such as acetaminophen or aspirin and loop diuretics are less likely to interfere with lithium clearance. Caffeine and theophylline can enhance the renal elimination of lithium. Because lithium has no effect on hepatic metabolizing enzymes, it has fewer drug-drug interactions compared with carbamazepine, oxcarbazepine, and valproate.

Dosing and Administration Lithium dosing depends on the patient's age and weight, tolerance to adverse effects, and the acuity of the illness. Lithium therapy is usually initiated with low-to-moderate doses (600 mg/day) for prophylaxis and higher doses (900-1,200 mg/day) for acute mania, using a two-to-three-times daily dosing regimen.[42] The dose should be adjusted based on the steady-state serum concentration and clinical picture of the patient. Immediate-release lithium preparations should be given in two or three divided daily doses, whereas extended-release products can be given once or twice daily. In clinical practice many clinicians dose the immediate-release and extended-release preparations once daily. It is best to initially begin a patient on divided dosing, but once stabilized many patients are able to switch to once-daily dosing without decompensating.[54,65]

Lithium levels should be monitored for efficacy and to guide dosing. In general, lithium serum concentrations should be maintained between 0.6 and 1 mEq/L (mmol/L) for maintenance therapy.[2,55] Lithium levels are considered to be at steady-state at approximately day 5, and serum samples should be drawn 12 hours post dose. When being used acutely, some clinicians may order lithium levels prior to reaching steady-state to more closely monitor the therapy. Once a desired serum concentration has been achieved, levels should be redrawn in 2 weeks. Maintenance lithium serum concentrations are usually measured every 3 months but can be adjusted to every 6 months for stabilized patients, or more frequently if clinically indicated (eg, patients with frequent mood episodes).[2] Lithium clearance rates increase by 50% to 100% during pregnancy and return to normal postpartum. Thus, lithium levels should be determined monthly during pregnancy and weekly the month before delivery. At delivery, rapid fluid changes can significantly increase lithium levels; thus, a reduction to pre-pregnancy lithium doses and adequate hydration are recommended.[22]

The recommended guidelines for baseline and routine laboratory testing for lithium are listed in Table 89-6. A therapeutic trial for outpatients should last a minimum of 4 to 6 weeks with lithium serum concentrations of 0.6 to 1.2 mEq/L (mmol/L). Antidepressant efficacy may take longer. Acutely manic patients can require serum concentrations of 1 to 1.2 mEq/L (mmol/L), and some need up to 1.5 mEq/L (mmol/L) to achieve a therapeutic response. Although serum concentrations less than 0.6 mEq/L (mmol/L) may be associated with higher rates of relapse, some patients can do well at 0.4 to 0.7 mEq/L (mmol/L).[55] For prevention of relapse in older patients, serum concentrations of 0.4 to 0.6 mEq/L (mmol/L) are recommended because of increased sensitivity to adverse effects with up to 0.8 mEq/L (mmol/L) being beneficial for acute episodes.[2]

Antiseizure Medications

Antiseizure medications are widely prescribed for the treatment of bipolar disorder with varying degrees of evidence. Divalproex sodium (also known as sodium valproate) was marketed in 1995 and is FDA-approved only for the treatment of acute manic or mixed episodes. However, it is commonly used in clinical practice as maintenance monotherapy for bipolar disorder. Limited data support its use in acute bipolar depression.[2] Carbamazepine is commonly used for both acute and maintenance therapy with the only formulation approved in the United States for bipolar disorder being extended-release carbamazepine, although other formulations can be used. Some data support the use of oxcarbazepine, a 10-keto analog of carbamazepine, in the treatment of bipolar disorder. However, it is not approved for the treatment of bipolar disorder in the United States. Valproate, carbamazepine, and oxcarbazepine all have a wide range of neurologic, GI, electrolyte, and hematologic adverse effects that require regular assessment and routine blood work.[43,45,46] Lamotrigine is FDA-approved for the maintenance treatment of bipolar I disorder. This medication is most effective in the prevention of relapse of depression.[2]

Sodium Valproate and Valproic Acid Valproate has antimigraine, mood-stabilizing, and antiaggressive effects.[45] In 1995, the enteric-coated formulation divalproex sodium (sodium valproate) was approved for the acute treatment of mania. Data have shown valproate to be more effective than placebo for acute mania and perhaps as effective as lithium and olanzapine.[68] In addition, valproate can potentially be more effective than lithium in certain subtypes of bipolar disorder (eg, multiple prior episodes, mixed features, comorbid substance use disorder).[2] Valproate reduces or prevents recurrent manic, depressive, and mixed episodes.[2]

Giving lithium, carbamazepine, antipsychotics, or benzodiazepines with valproate can augment its antimanic effects. The addition of valproate to lithium can have synergistic effects in patients who are treatment-refractory and have specifiers of rapid cycling or mixed features, and the combination has demonstrated efficacy in maintenance therapy for bipolar I disorder. Combinations of valproate and carbamazepine can have synergistic effects, but the potential drug interactions make serum level monitoring of both agents essential.[2] Adding adjunctive SGAs to valproate can be effective for breakthrough mania if there is incomplete or partial response to monotherapy, or for quicker time to treatment response. Clozapine, olanzapine, and quetiapine can increase the risk of sedation and weight gain when combined with valproate. The combination of valproate and lamotrigine can be effective, but valproate reduces the clearance of lamotrigine leading to increased risk of serious rashes, ataxia, tremor, sedation, and fatigue.[45]

Adverse Effects The most frequent dose-related adverse effects with valproate are GI complaints (eg, anorexia, nausea, indigestion, vomiting, mild diarrhea, and flatulence), fine hand tremors, and sedation.[45] The GI complaints are usually transient, but they can be minimized by giving the medication with food, using lower initial doses with gradual increases, or switching to divalproex sodium extended-release tablets.[2] Dose reduction or the addition of a β-blocker can alleviate tremors, and giving the total daily dose at bedtime can minimize daytime sedation.[22]

Other adverse effects of valproate include ataxia, lethargy, alopecia, changes in the texture or color of hair, pruritus, prolonged bleeding because of inhibition of platelet aggregation, transient increases in liver enzymes, and hyperammonemia.[45] Increased appetite and propensity for significant weight gain is associated with long-term therapy, and should be considered prior to combining with agents

TABLE 89-6 Guidelines for Baseline and Routine Laboratory Tests and Monitoring for Patients with Bipolar Disorder Taking Mood Stabilizers

	Baseline: Physical Examination and General Chemistry[a]	Hematologic Tests[b]		Metabolic Tests[c]		Liver Function Tests[d]		Renal Function Tests[e]		Thyroid Function Tests[f]		Serum Electrolytes[g]		Dermatologic[h]		Pharmacogenomic Testing
	Baseline	Baseline	6-12 months	Baseline	6-12 months	Baseline	6-12 months	Baseline	6-12 months	Baseline	6-12 months	Baseline	6-12 months	Baseline	6-12 months	Baseline
SGAs[i]	X			X	X											
Carbamazepine[j]	X	X	X			X	X	X				X	X	X	X	X
Lamotrigine[k]	X													X	X	
Lithium[l]	X	X	X	X	X			X	X	X	X	X	X	X	X	
Oxcarbazepine[m]	X											X	X			X
Valproate[n]	X	X	X	X	X	X	X							X	X	

SGAs, second-generation antipsychotics.

[a]Screen for substance use and pregnancy.

[b]Complete blood cell count (CBC) with differential and platelets.

[c]Fasting glucose, lipid panel, and weight.

[d]Lactate dehydrogenase, aspartate aminotransferase, alanine aminotransferase, total bilirubin, and alkaline phosphatase.

[e]Serum creatinine, blood urea nitrogen, urinalysis, urine osmolality, and specific gravity.

[f]Triiodothyronine, total thyroxine, thyroxine uptake, and thyroid-stimulating hormone.

[g]Serum sodium.

[h]Rashes, hair thinning, and alopecia.

[i]Second-generation antipsychotics: Monitor for increased appetite with weight gain (primarily in patients with initial low or normal body mass index); monitor closely if rapid or significant weight gain occurs during early therapy; cases of hyperlipidemia and diabetes reported.

[j]Carbamazepine: Manufacturer recommends CBC and platelets (and possibly reticulocyte counts and serum iron) at baseline and that subsequent monitoring be individualized by the clinician (eg, CBC, platelet counts, and liver function tests every 2 weeks during the first 2 months of treatment, and then every 3 months if normal). Monitor more closely if patient exhibits hematologic or hepatic abnormalities or if the patient is receiving a myelotoxic drug; discontinue if platelets are <100,000/mm^3 (100×10^9/L), if white blood cell (WBC) count is <3,000/mm^3 (3×10^9/L), or if there is evidence of bone marrow suppression or liver dysfunction. Serum electrolyte levels should be monitored in older patients or those at risk for hyponatremia. Carbamazepine interferes with some pregnancy tests.

[k]Lamotrigine: If renal or hepatic impairment, monitor closely and adjust dosage according to manufacturer's guidelines. Serious dermatologic reactions have occurred within 2 to 8 weeks of initiating treatment and are more likely to occur in patients receiving concomitant valproate, with rapid dosage escalation, or using doses exceeding the recommended titration schedule.

[l]Lithium: Obtain baseline electrocardiogram for patients older than 40 years or if preexisting cardiac disease (benign, reversible T-wave depression can occur). Renal function tests should be obtained every 2 to 3 months during the first 6 months, and then every 6 to 12 months; if impaired renal function, monitor 24-hour urine volume and creatinine every 3 months; if urine volume>3 L/day, monitor urinalysis, osmolality, and specific gravity every 3 months. Thyroid function tests should be obtained once or twice during the first 6 months, and then every 6 to 12 months; monitor for signs and symptoms of hypothyroidism; if supplemental thyroid therapy is required, monitor thyroid function tests and adjust thyroid dose every 1 to 2 months until thyroid function indices are within normal range, and then monitor every 3 to 6 months.

[m]Oxcarbazepine: Hyponatremia (serum sodium concentrations <125 mEq/L [mmol/L]) has been reported and occurs more frequently during the first 3 months of therapy; serum sodium concentrations should be monitored in patients receiving drugs that lower serum sodium concentrations (eg, diuretics or drugs that cause inappropriate antidiuretic hormone secretion) or in patients with symptoms of hyponatremia (eg, confusion, headache, lethargy, malaise). Hypersensitivity reactions have occurred in approximately 25% to 30% of patients with a history of carbamazepine hypersensitivity and require immediate discontinuation.

[n]Valproate: Weight gain reported in patients with low or normal body mass index. Monitor platelets and liver function during first 3 to 6 months if evidence of increased bruising or bleeding. Monitor closely if patients exhibit hematologic or hepatic abnormalities or in patients receiving drugs that affect coagulation, such as aspirin or warfarin; discontinue if platelets are <100,000/mm^3 (100×10^9/L) or if prolonged bleeding time. Pancreatitis, hyperammonemic encephalopathy, polycystic ovary syndrome, increased testosterone, and menstrual irregularities have been reported; not recommended during first trimester of pregnancy due to risk of neural tube defects.

Data from References 42–47, 66, and 67.

that also cause weight gain (eg, SGAs). Thrombocytopenia can occur at higher doses, and patients should be monitored for bleeding and bruising. Lowering the valproate dose can restore platelet counts to normal levels.[22] Fatal necrotizing hepatitis is a rare idiosyncratic, non–dose-related adverse effect that has occurred in children with epilepsy receiving multiple antiseizure drugs.[45] A life-threatening hemorrhagic pancreatitis has been reported in both children and adults.[45] An in-depth discussion of adverse effects can be found in Chapter 75, "Epilepsy."

Drug-Drug Interactions A summary of drug-drug interactions for valproate can be found in Chapter 75.

Dosing and Administration For healthy inpatient adults with acute mania, the initial starting dosage of valproate is typically 20 mg/kg/day in divided doses over 12 hours.[45] The daily dose is adjusted by 250 to 500 mg every 1 to 3 days based on clinical response and tolerability. Maximum recommended dosing is 60 mg/kg/day (see Table 89-5).[45] For outpatients experiencing hypomania or euthymia, or for older patients, the initial starting dose is generally lower (5-10 mg/kg/day in divided doses) and gradually titrated to avoid adverse effects. Once an optimal dose has been achieved, the total daily dose can be continued in two divided doses or given once at bedtime if tolerated.[45] Extended-release divalproex can be administered once daily, but bioavailability can be 15% lower than that of immediate- and delayed-release products, thus requiring slightly higher doses.[45,69] In clinical practice, patients with bipolar disorder who are stable can be switched between formulations without having to change the dose. This is not the case for patients with seizure disorders.

Recommended baseline and routine laboratory tests for patients taking valproate are listed in Table 89-6. Although therapeutic serum concentrations of valproic acid have not been established in bipolar disorder, most clinicians use the antiseizure therapeutic serum range of 50 to 125 mcg/mL (mg/L; 347-866 μmol/L) taken 12 hours after the last dose.[2,45] Levels greater than 94.1 mcg/mL (mg/L; 652 μmol/L) have been found to have greater efficacy for bipolar mania.[70] Patients with cyclothymia or mild bipolar II disorder can have a therapeutic response to lower doses and serum levels, whereas some patients with a more severe form of bipolar disorder can require up to 150 mcg/mL (mg/L; 1,040 μmol/L). Serum valproic acid levels are most useful when assessing for adherence and toxicity.[2]

Carbamazepine Carbamazepine, an iminostilbene derivative, is structurally related to tricyclic antidepressants (TCAs).[46] It is not a first-line agent for bipolar disorder and is generally reserved for use after treatment failure with lithium or divalproex sodium due to its drug interactions and other safety concerns.[2] Data supporting the use of carbamazepine for bipolar depression are lacking and are not strong for the routine use of carbamazepine in maintenance treatment.[2] Patients with a history of head trauma, anxiety, or a substance use disorder may respond to treatment with carbamazepine. The combination of carbamazepine with lithium, valproate, or antipsychotics is often used for treatment-resistant patients experiencing a manic episode.[2]

Adverse Effects A summary of adverse effects for carbamazepine can be found in Chapter 75. Acute overdoses are potentially lethal, and serum levels above 15 mcg/mL (mg/L; 63 μmol/L) are associated with ataxia, choreiform movements, diplopia, nystagmus, cardiac conduction changes, seizures, and coma.[22] Gastric decontamination, hemoperfusion, ECG monitoring, and symptomatic treatment are recommended for the management of carbamazepine toxicity.[22,71] New information is quickly evolving in the area of pharmacogenomics that may help clinicians individualize treatment for patients with bipolar disorder. Pharmacogenetic testing is available to determine if patients are poor or rapid metabolizers of cytochrome P450 2D6 and 2C19, as well as other important pharmacogenomic variants, thus predicting an individual's potential to respond to particular therapies as well as help to tailor dosing regimens in an effort to reduce adverse effects. The use of commercially available testing panels is controversial; however, the Clinical Pharmacogenomic Implementation Consortium (CPIC), funded by the National Institutes of Health, has resources to guide clinicians in the use of this information (http://cpicpgx.org/). For carbamazepine in particular, a boxed warning is located in the FDA package insert recommending genetic testing for the human leukocyte antigen (HLA) allele, HLA-B 1502, in patients of Asian ancestry to help detect a higher risk of Stevens–Johnson syndrome and toxic epidermal necrolysis.[46] Similar considerations should be made for patients prior to prescribing oxcarbazepine based on manufacturer's labeling.[43]

Drug-Drug Interactions There are numerous drug-drug interactions that clinicians must consider when prescribing carbamazepine as it significantly induces the hepatic cytochrome P450 isoenzyme 3A4 and to a lesser degree 1A2, 2C9/10, and 2D6, thus increasing the metabolism of many medications (eg, quetiapine, lurasidone).[46] Individuals taking oral contraceptives who receive carbamazepine should be counseled to use alternatives such as intrauterine devices or depot medroxyprogesterone acetate in addition to barrier methods of birth control.[72]

Carbamazepine is metabolized to an active 10,11-epoxide metabolite; thus, medications that inhibit 3A4 isoenzymes can result in carbamazepine toxicity (eg, valproate, diltiazem, fluconazole, ketoconazole, nefazodone, verapamil).[46] Combining clozapine and carbamazepine is not recommended because of decreased clozapine concentrations and the possibility of bone marrow suppression with both agents.[46]

Dosing and Administration During an acute manic episode in most hospitalized patients, carbamazepine can be started at 400 to 600 mg/day in divided doses with meals and increased by 200 mg/day every 2 to 4 days up to a usual range of 1,200 to 1,600 mg/day.[46] In outpatients, the initial dose of carbamazepine should be lower, and in all patients, the dose should be titrated gradually until response is achieved or there is evidence of toxicity. Conversely, some patients may require up to 1,600 to 1,800 mg/day.[46] Many patients are able to tolerate once-daily dosing of carbamazepine once their mood episode has stabilized. During the first month of therapy, serum concentrations of carbamazepine may be affected due to autoinduction of the cytochrome P450 3A4 isoenzyme.[46]

Carbamazepine serum levels are usually obtained every 1 to 2 weeks during the first 2 months and then every 6 to 12 months during maintenance therapy.[2,46] Trough serum levels should be drawn 10 to 12 hours after the dose at least 2 to 5 days after a dosage change.[46] Although there is no correlation between carbamazepine serum concentrations and degree of mania or depressive symptom response, most clinicians attempt to maintain levels between 6 and 10 mcg/mL (mg/L; 25 and 42 μmol/L). However, some treatment-resistant patients can require serum concentrations of 12 to 14 mcg/mL (mg/L; 51-59 μmol/L). Recommended baseline and routine laboratory tests for carbamazepine are listed in Table 89-6.

Oxcarbazepine There are currently less data supporting the use of oxcarbazepine than carbamazepine in the treatment of bipolar disorder. Guidelines typically recommend oxcarbazepine as a third-line treatment option for bipolar mania, and it is not recommended for the treatment of bipolar depression.[2]

Adverse Effects Severe and sometimes life-threatening dermatologic reactions (eg, Stevens–Johnson syndrome) have been reported; therefore, oxcarbazepine should be discontinued at the first sign of a skin reaction.[43] Risk of this adverse effect may be greater in patients with specific genetic markers similar to carbamazepine. Other adverse effects may include impaired cognitive or psychomotor performance, somnolence or fatigue, and coordination difficulties.[43]

Incidence of hyponatremia with oxcarbazepine is greater than that seen with carbamazepine, ranging from 0.14% to 73.3% versus 4.8% to 31.3%, respectively, in clinical studies depending on study design and serum sodium cut offs.[74] An in-depth discussion of adverse effects can be found in Chapter 75, "Epilepsy."

Drug-Drug Interactions Oxcarbazepine, a cytochrome P450 2C19 enzyme inhibitor and a 3A4/5 enzyme inducer, has the potential for causing drug interactions.[43] It induces the metabolism of oral contraceptives; thus, alternative contraceptive measures are required.[72] Additional drug interactions can be found in Chapter 75.

Dosing and Administration Initial dosing usually follows that of epilepsy at 150 to 300 mg twice daily, with daily doses being increased by 300 to 600 mg every 3 to 6 days up to 1,200 mg/day in divided doses (with or without food).[43]

Lamotrigine Lamotrigine is effective for the maintenance treatment of bipolar I disorder in adult patients.[2,22] Doses of 200 mg/day are more effective than lower doses, and there are no advantages to using 400 mg/day.[75] Lamotrigine has mood-stabilizing effects; it may have augmenting properties when combined with lithium or valproate and have low rates of switching patients to mania.[2] There are case reports of possible lamotrigine-induced mania when added to lithium, carbamazepine, and valproate.[76] In each of these cases, the patients had depressive mood symptoms or rapid mood changes requiring additional therapy.[76] Although lamotrigine is not effective for acute mania when compared with standard mood stabilizers, it may be beneficial as maintenance therapy of treatment-resistant bipolar I and II disorders.[2] It may also be effective for acute bipolar depression[2,77] and is most effective for the prevention of bipolar depression; therefore, clinically, it is often used in the treatment of patients with bipolar II.

Adverse Effects Common adverse effects include headache, nausea, dizziness, ataxia, diplopia, drowsiness, tremor, rash, and pruritus.[44] Approximately 10% of individuals treated with lamotrigine will develop a non-serious rash.[2] Although most rashes are self-limiting and resolve with continued treatment, some progress to life-threatening conditions such as Stevens–Johnson syndrome. The incidence of rash is greatest with co-administration of valproate, with higher than recommended initial doses, and with rapid dose escalation.[2,44] Patients should be warned about the rash and the need for discontinuing lamotrigine and seeking medical attention if the rash is diffuse, involves mucosal membranes, and is accompanied by a fever or sore throat. For an in-depth discussion of the adverse effects of lamotrigine, see Chapter 75.

Drug-Drug Interactions Valproate decreases the clearance of lamotrigine (ie, more than doubles the half-life), and lamotrigine must be administered at a reduced dosage of approximately half the standard dose.[44] For an in-depth discussion of drug-drug interactions with lamotrigine, see Chapter 75.

Dosing and Administration For the maintenance treatment of bipolar disorder, the usual dosage range of lamotrigine is 50 to 300 mg/day. The target dose is generally 200 mg/day (100 mg/day in combination with valproate and 400 mg/day in combination with carbamazepine).[44] For patients not taking medications that affect lamotrigine clearance, the dose is 25 mg/day for the first 2 weeks of therapy, 50 mg/day for weeks 3 and 4, 100 mg/day for week 5, and 200 mg/day for week 6 and beyond.[44] Patients who stop lamotrigine therapy for more than a few days should be restarted on a low dose and titrated every 2 weeks back to their maintenance dose.[44]

Antipsychotics

FGAs and SGAs such as aripiprazole, asenapine, haloperidol, olanzapine, quetiapine, risperidone, and ziprasidone are effective as monotherapy or adjunctive therapy in the treatment of acute mania.[2] Controlled studies in acute mania with lithium or valproate plus an antipsychotic suggest greater efficacy with combination therapies compared to these agents alone.[2,22] The FGAs (eg, chlorpromazine and haloperidol) are effective in acute mania, particularly those with psychosis and psychomotor agitation,[2,22] while the SGAs have demonstrated similar efficacy for the treatment of acute mania associated with agitation, aggression, and psychosis.[2]

Treating acute bipolar depression is challenging, and some antipsychotics may play a useful role. Multiple large randomized controlled trials support the use of quetiapine and lurasidone as a monotherapy and adjunctive treatment options for bipolar depression.[2] Data also support the use of combined fluoxetine/olanzapine in treating bipolar depression.[2] Newer SGAs, cariprazine and lumateperone, have also gained FDA approval for bipolar depression (monotherapy for bipolar I, monotherapy or adjunct for bipolar I and bipolar II, respectively).

Oral aripiprazole, olanzapine, sublingual asenapine, and long-acting risperidone are effective and FDA approved as monotherapy options for maintenance treatment in bipolar disorder.[2,47] Long-acting injectable FGAs (eg, haloperidol decanoate, fluphenazine decanoate) can have a place in maintenance treatment of bipolar disorder for patients who are non-adherent or treatment-resistant.[2] Clozapine adjunct and monotherapy has acute and long-term mood-stabilizing effects in refractory bipolar disorder but requires regular white blood cell monitoring for agranulocytosis.[2] The long-term safety of antipsychotics as monotherapy or as adjunctive therapy for bipolar maintenance treatment should be evaluated with ongoing assessment of utility.[2] Refer to Table 89-5 for antipsychotic specific indications. Metabolic syndrome is comorbid in 20%-65% of patients with bipolar disorder; therefore, the risks versus benefits must be weighed due to the long-term metabolic and endocrine adverse effects (eg, weight gain, type 2 diabetes, hyperlipidemia, hyperprolactinemia) in addition to tardive dyskinesia that antipsychotics may cause.[2,78]

Adverse Effects A summary of adverse effects for antipsychotics can be found in Chapter 87, "Schizophrenia."

Drug-Drug Interactions A summary of drug interactions with antipsychotics can be found in Chapter 87.

Dosing and Administration For acute mania, higher initial doses of antipsychotics may be required (eg, olanzapine 20 mg/day in hospitalized patients). Once the acute mania is controlled (usually within 7-28 days), the antipsychotic can be gradually tapered and discontinued, and the patient maintained on the mood stabilizer monotherapy as appropriate.

Monitoring 7 Recommendations for baseline and routine laboratory testing for patients receiving antipsychotics are found in Table 89-6.

Alternative Medication Treatments

8 Some patients can be stabilized on one mood stabilizer, but others may require combination therapies or adjunctive agents during an acute mood episode. If possible, adjunctive agents should be tapered and discontinued when the acute mood episode remits and the patient is stabilized.

Benzodiazepines Benzodiazepines such as clonazepam and lorazepam may be used as an alternative to or in combination with antipsychotics when patients are experiencing acute mania, agitation, anxiety, panic, and insomnia, or cannot take mood stabilizers (eg, during the first trimester of pregnancy).[2] Risk versus benefit should be carefully weighed in patients with a history of substance use disorders and/or acute risk for suicide.[2] Lorazepam is available for intramuscular injection and is useful in the acute management of agitation. Benzodiazepines cause minimal adverse effects compared with antipsychotics, and at higher doses, rapidly reduce symptoms in patients experiencing agitation. They can cause CNS depression, sedation, cognitive and motor impairment, dependence, and withdrawal reactions. When no longer required, benzodiazepines should be gradually tapered and discontinued to avoid withdrawal symptoms.

Antidepressants For many years, antidepressants were recommended as adjunctive therapy for acute bipolar depression. Data from the Systematic Treatment Enhancement Program for Bipolar Disorder (STEP-BD) suggest that adjunctive antidepressants may be no better than placebo for acute bipolar depression when combined with mood stabilizers.[79] A meta-analysis of six trials identified a small treatment effect on clinician-rated depressive symptoms when antidepressants such as selective serotonin reuptake inhibitors (SSRIs) and bupropion were added to lithium, antiseizure drugs, or SGAs.[2,80] The concern of mood switching (ie, rapidly switching from depression to mania or hypomania) with the use of antidepressants is valid, although not common. Data show that the rate of mood switch with dual-acting agents (eg, TCAs or venlafaxine) is higher, and thus, these agents should be used with caution.[81] Additionally, the type of bipolar disorder may play a role in increased risk of mood switching, in that patients with bipolar I may carry a greater risk.[81] Controversy exists concerning the use of antidepressants, and many clinicians and treatment guidelines consider them to be second or third line in treating acute bipolar depression and should be avoided or used with extreme caution in patients with a history of antidepressant-induced mania/hypomania, mixed features, or recent rapid cycling.[2] Generally before initiating therapy with an antidepressant, it is important to ensure that the patient is on a therapeutic dosage or serum level of a primary mood stabilizer (eg, lithium, antiseizure medications, or antipsychotics).[2] Patients who have a history of mania after a depressive episode should be treated cautiously with antidepressants.[22] For more information, see Chapter 88 for comparisons among antidepressants.

Special Populations

The approach for treating bipolar disorder in special populations can vary among clinicians. Patients with comorbid medical conditions or concomitant substance use, those older than 65 or younger than 18 years, and pregnant individuals can require different treatment approaches.

Bipolar Disorder in Pregnancy

Comprehensive management during pregnancy is important to decrease the risk of birth defects, perinatal complications and mortality, preterm birth, low birth weight, low Apgar scores, and adverse neurodevelopmental effects.[2,82] Pharmacotherapy during pregnancy is complicated, and the risk-to-benefit ratio must be weighed. Clinicians should always use the lowest effective dose of any medication during pregnancy. Monotherapy should also be considered in order to decrease the risk to the pregnant individual and child. Contraception and pre-conception counseling should be a part of the patient education plan for individuals of child-bearing age diagnosed with bipolar disorder, who are able to become pregnant.[2] Education should include information regarding the risk of medications for the fetus, the impact of pregnancy on bipolar illness and vice versa. Additionally, consideration into contraceptive methods should take into account that antiseizure drugs such as carbamazepine and lamotrigine may have pharmacokinetic interactions with oral contraceptives.[2]

When lithium is given during the first trimester, the prevalence of Ebstein's anomaly is estimated between 1 and 10:1,000 and the risk of neural tube defects is 13:1,000.[82] Though newer data may suggest that the absolute risk of cardiac abnormalities may be small, lithium use is generally not recommended in the first trimester of pregnancy unless the benefit outweighs the risk.[2,83,84] Lithium freely crosses the placenta and is found in equal concentrations in the fetal and pregnant person's blood.[42] When lithium is used during pregnancy, it should be tapered down to the lowest effective dose necessary to decrease the risk of relapse. Lithium can cause perinatal complications in the infant such as hypotonia, jaundice, cyanosis, and lethargy.[82] Dose adjustments and close monitoring of serum levels will be needed due to changes in glomerular filtration rates and renal perfusion rates during pregnancy and immediately after delivery.[57,82] Milk concentrations of lithium range from 30% to 50% of the parent's serum concentration, and serum concentrations in the nursing infant are 10% to 50% of the adult's; thus, nursing is usually discouraged.[42,57]

Neural tube defects cause the most concern for clinicians treating pregnant patients during their first trimester. Data from the North American Antiepileptic Drug Pregnancy Registry show the risk of neural tube defects is about 0.12% for non-exposed babies.[85] Carbamazepine's risk of neural tube defects is estimated to be 3%.[85] Carbamazepine is excreted in breast milk with a milk-to-plasma ratio of ~0.4.[46] Craniofacial abnormalities, developmental delays, microcephaly, and other abnormalities are also of concern when using antiseizure drugs. For pregnant patients treated with lamotrigine, the risk of neural tube defects is estimated to be 2%, but data for lamotrigine are limited compared with those for some older antiseizure drugs.[85] If the pregnant individual requires lamotrigine while nursing, infants should be monitored as infant concentrations can reflect 18% to 50% of the parent's serum concentration.[86,87] Valproate is usually not recommended during the first trimester of pregnancy because the risk of neural tube defects is estimated to be 4%.[85] Australian registry data in patients with epilepsy show dose-related teratogenicity with doses greater than 1,100 mg/day of valproate.[88] Additionally, data from the North American Antiepileptic Drug Pregnancy Registry showed that the median daily dose for first trimester exposure in babies born without malformations was 750 mg.[85] Fetal valproate syndrome is characterized by abnormalities such as facial clefts, cardiac and limb defects, and abnormal facial features.[86] The risks versus benefits of using valproate during pregnancy must be discussed with the patient.[2] Administration of folate can reduce the risk of neural tube defects. Individuals of child-bearing age, able to become pregnant receiving valproate and those currently pregnant should receive folic acid supplementation; however, there is not a consensus on the recommended folic acid dose to use. Valproate is excreted into human milk in low concentrations and is considered to be compatible with nursing.[45] One case report of thrombocytopenia and anemia from valproate exposure has been reported in a nursing infant.[45] If the nursing parent receives valproate, the infant should have identical laboratory monitoring.

Caution should be used when prescribing antipsychotics during pregnancy. FGAs have been prescribed for many years in pregnancy and data show little teratogenic risk, but the data are not without question.[89] Data on the SGAs are limited, and clinicians should consider the potential risk of gestational diabetes.[89] Extrapyramidal symptoms, neonatal withdrawal, and sedation should also be considered when using both FGAs and SGAs during the third trimester of pregnancy.[89] There is still a paucity of human data with antipsychotics, and therefore, risk-to-benefit ratio must be weighed.

Child and Adolescent Bipolar Disorder

Approximately one-third to two-thirds of patients diagnosed with bipolar disorder experience their first episode as a child or adolescent; however, there are few controlled studies in this population.[2] Little is known about the long-term efficacy and safety of specific agents or combination therapies in this population.[90] Lithium is the only medication approved as a mood stabilizer for children and adolescents and its efficacy in pediatric manic or mixed states has been documented in one double-blind placebo-controlled trial as well as an open-label trial.[90] Age restrictions vary by formulation, with immediate-release lithium being approved in children age 7 years and older for acute manic or mixed episodes and maintenance treatment, and extended-release being approved in children aged 12 years and older for acute manic and mixed episodes.[42]

Valproate and carbamazepine are utilized in pediatric patients based on experience in adults.[2,90]

Aripiprazole and risperidone are FDA-approved for bipolar mania or mixed states in patients aged 10 to 17 years.[90] Quetiapine and quetiapine XR are approved as monotherapy or adjunct to lithium or divalproex in patients aged 10 to 17 years during a manic or mixed episode, but did not show efficacy in two double-blind, placebo-controlled studies in children and adolescents with bipolar depression.[2,90] Olanzapine is approved for use in patients with manic or mixed episodes aged 13 to 17 years as well as for monotherapy maintenance treatment in this subset of patients.[67] Ziprasidone has supporting data for its use in pediatric acute mania but does not have FDA approval.[6] Lurasidone's approval includes monotherapy treatment of bipolar depression in children 10 years of age and older.[91] Long-term data are still needed and recommendations on the treatment of pediatric bipolar depression and maintenance treatment are lacking due to insufficient data.[2] Additionally, children and adolescents treated with SGAs are more susceptible to metabolic effects of these medications, requiring close attention to diet and physical exercise.[2]

Bipolar Disorder Management in Individuals with Comorbidities

Patients with bipolar illness are more likely to have medical comorbidities than the general population complicating the management of bipolar disorder in older adults who average three to four medical comorbidities (eg, hypertension, diabetes).[2] Older adults may be more susceptible to mood stabilizer and antipsychotic adverse effects. Anticholinergic burden of medications should be considered when prescribing.[2] Specific for lithium and aging, reductions in renal clearance may significantly increase the elimination half-life in older patients requiring more frequent renal monitoring.[42] The elimination of valproate has been reported to also decrease with age and has been associated with motor side effects and metabolic effects in older patients.[2,45] The efficacy and tolerability of lithium and divalproex sodium for acute manic, hypomanic, or mixed episodes in patients age 60 years and older have been studied in one randomized double-blind trial.[92] Both medications were efficacious at serum concentrations between 0.8 and 0.99 mEq/L (mmol/L) for lithium and 80 to 99 mcg/mL (mg/L; 555-686 μmol/L) for divalproex, though greater reduction in manic symptoms was seen with lithium at the expense of tremor.[92]

EVALUATION OF THERAPEUTIC OUTCOMES

The establishment and maintenance of a therapeutic alliance between the patient and clinician is essential in monitoring a patient's psychiatric status and safety; enhancing treatment adherence; promoting good nutrition, sleep, and exercise; identifying stressors; recognizing new mood episodes; and minimizing adverse reactions and drug interactions.[2] Patients who have a partial response or non-response to established bipolar therapies should be reassessed for an accurate diagnosis, concomitant medical or psychiatric conditions, adherence with treatment (including serum levels if appropriate), and medications or substances that exacerbate mood symptoms. Nonadherence to medication treatment, delusional symptoms, alcohol or substance use, rapid cycling, or mixed states are often associated with poorer treatment outcomes.

CONCLUSION

The diagnosis and treatment of bipolar disorder can be complicated. Once an accurate diagnosis is made, clinicians must collaborate with patients and follow the patient-centered model to select the best treatment regimen. Clinicians must educate patients to be diligent in self-monitoring of their disease and the reporting of medications adverse effects. Adherence with medications is a key component in treatment. Clinicians must realize that there are various options for treating each phase of bipolar disorder and selection of the correct medication is essential to achieve optimal patient outcomes.

ABBREVIATIONS

5-HT	serotonin
ANK3	Ankyrin 3
APA	American Psychiatric Association
BMI	body mass index
CACNA1C	Calcium Voltage-Gated Channel Subunit Alpha1 C
CANMAT	Canadian Network for Mood and Anxiety Treatments
CBC	complete blood count
CBT	cognitive behavioral therapy
CNS	central nervous system
CPIC	Clinical Pharmacogenomic Implementation Consortium
DA	dopamine
DI	diabetes insipidus
DSM-5	*Diagnostic and Statistical Manual of Mental Disorders, Fifth Edition*
ECG	electrocardiogram
ECT	electroconvulsive therapy
FDA	Food and Drug Administration
FGAs	first-generation antipsychotics
GI	gastrointestinal
HAM-D or HDRS	Hamilton Depression Rating Scale
HLA	human leukocyte antigen
ISBD	International Society for Bipolar Disorders
LFTs	liver function tests
LSD	lysergic acid diethylamide
MAOI	monoamine oxidase inhibitor
NE	norepinephrine
PCP	phencyclidine
PHQ-9	Patient Health Questionnaire 9
PMDD	premenstrual dysphoric disorder
Scr	serum creatinine
SGAs	second-generation antipsychotics
SSRI	selective serotonin reuptake inhibitor
STEP-BD	Systematic Treatment Enhancement Program for Bipolar Disorder
TCA	tricyclic antidepressant
TSH	thyroid stimulating hormone
UDS	urine drug screen
WFSBP	World Federation of Societies of Biological Psychiatry
YMRS	Young Mania Rating Scale

REFERENCES

1. American Psychiatric Association. Available at: http://dsm.psychiatryonline.org/book.aspx?bookid=556. DSM-5 Task Force Diagnostic and Statistical Manual of Mental Disorders DSM-5: American Psychiatric Association; 2013. http://dsmpsychiatryonlineorg/book.aspx?bookid=556.
2. Yatham LN, Kennedy SH, Parikh SV. Canadian Network for Mood and Anxiety Treatments (CANMAT) and International Society for Bipolar Disorders (ISBD) 2018 guidelines for the management of patients with bipolar disorder. *Bipolar Disord.* 2018;20(2):97–170. Epub 2018/03/15. doi: 10.1111/bdi.12609. PubMed PMID: 29536616; PubMed Central PMCID: PMCPMC5947163.
3. Merikangas KR, Jin R, He JP, et al. Prevalence and correlates of bipolar spectrum disorder in the world mental health survey initiative. *Arch*

Gen Psychiatry 2011;68(3):241–51. Epub 2011/03/09. doi: 10.1001/archgenpsychiatry.2011.12. PubMed PMID: 21383262; PubMed Central PMCID: PMCPMC3486639.

4. Carvalho AF, Firth J, Vieta E. Bipolar disorder. *N Engl J Med.* 2020;383(1):58–66. Epub 2020/07/02. doi: 10.1056/NEJMra1906193. PubMed PMID: 32609982.
5. Sole E, Garriga M, Valenti M, et al. Mixed features in bipolar disorder. *CNS Spectr.* 2017;22(2):134–40. Epub 2016/12/30. doi: 10.1017/S1092852916000869. PubMed PMID: 28031070.
6. Harrison PJ, Geddes JR, Tunbridge EM. The emerging neurobiology of bipolar disorder. *Trends Neurosci.* 2018;41(1):18–30. Epub 2017/11/25. doi: 10.1016/j.tins.2017.10.006. PubMed PMID: 29169634; PubMed Central PMCID: PMCPMC5755726.
7. Craddock N, Sklar P. Genetics of bipolar disorder. *Lancet.* 2013;381(9878):1654–62. Epub 2013/05/15. doi: 10.1016/s0140-6736(13)60855-7. PubMed PMID: 23663951.
8. Charney AW, Ruderfer DM, Stahl EA, et al. Evidence for genetic heterogeneity between clinical subtypes of bipolar disorder. *Transl Psychiatry* 2017;7(1):e993. Epub 2017/01/11. doi: 10.1038/tp.2016.242. PubMed PMID: 28072414; PubMed Central PMCID: PMCPMC5545718.
9. Acuff HE, Versace A, Bertocci MA, et al. Association of neuroimaging measures of emotion processing and regulation neural circuitries with symptoms of bipolar disorder in offspring at risk for bipolar disorder. *JAMA Psychiatry* 2018;75(12):1241–51. Epub 2018/09/08. doi: 10.1001/jamapsychiatry.2018.2318. PubMed PMID: 30193355; PubMed Central PMCID: PMCPMC6528787.
10. Aldinger F, Schulze TG. Environmental factors, life events, and trauma in the course of bipolar disorder. *Psychiatry Clin Neurosci.* 2017;71(1):6–17. Epub 2016/08/09. doi: 10.1111/pcn.12433. PubMed PMID: 27500795; PubMed Central PMCID: PMCPMC7167807.
11. Takaesu Y. Circadian rhythm in bipolar disorder: a review of the literature. *Psychiatry Clin Neurosci.* 2018;72(9):673–82. Epub 2018/06/06. doi: 10.1111/pcn.12688. PubMed PMID: 29869403.
12. Tondo L, Vazquez GH, Baldessarini RJ. Depression and mania in bipolar disorder. *Curr Neuropharmacol.* 2017;15(3):353–8. Epub 2017/05/16. doi: 10.2174/1570159X14666160606210811. PubMed PMID: 28503106; PubMed Central PMCID: PMCPMC5405618.
13. Ceide ME, Rosenberg PB. Brief manic episode after rituximab treatment of limbic encephalitis. *J Neuropsychiatry Clin Neurosci.* 2011;23(4):E8. Epub 2012/01/11. doi: 10.1176/jnp.23.4.jnpe8. PubMed PMID: 22231352.
14. Dias RS, Lafer B, Russo C, et al. Longitudinal follow-up of bipolar disorder in women with premenstrual exacerbation: findings from STEP-BD. *Am J Psychiatry* 2011;168(4):386–94. Epub 2011/02/18. doi: 10.1176/appi.ajp.2010.09121816. PubMed PMID: 21324951.
15. Goldsmith M, Singh M, Chang K. Antidepressants and psychostimulants in pediatric populations: is there an association with mania? *Paediatr Drugs.* 2011;13(4):225–43. Epub 2011/06/23. doi: 10.2165/11591660-000000000-00000. PubMed PMID: 21692547; PubMed Central PMCID: PMCPMC3394932.
16. Habek M, Brinar M, Brinar VV, et al. Psychiatric manifestations of multiple sclerosis and acute disseminated encephalomyelitis. *Clin Neurol Neurosurg.* 2006;108(3):290–4. Epub 2005/12/21. doi: 10.1016/j.clineuro.2005.11.024. PubMed PMID: 16364539.
17. Navinés R, Castellví P, Solà R, et al. Peginterferon- and ribavirin-induced bipolar episode successfully treated with lamotrigine without discontinuation of antiviral therapy. *Gen Hosp Psychiatry* 2008;30(4):387–9. Epub 2008/07/01. doi: 10.1016/j.genhosppsych.2007.12.010. PubMed PMID: 18585548.
18. Plante DT, Winkelman JW. Sleep disturbance in bipolar disorder: therapeutic implications. *Am J Psychiatry* 2008;165(7):830–43. Epub 2008/05/17. doi: 10.1176/appi.ajp.2008.08010077. PubMed PMID: 18483132.
19. Santos CO, Caeiro L, Ferro JM, et al. Mania and stroke: a systematic review. *Cerebrovasc Dis.* 2011;32(1):11–21. Epub 2011/05/18. doi: 10.1159/000327032. PubMed PMID: 21576938.
20. Spiegel DR, Weller AL, Pennell K, et al. The successful treatment of mania due to acquired immunodeficiency syndrome using ziprasidone: a case series. *J Neuropsychiatry Clin Neurosci.* 2010;22(1):111–4. Epub 2010/02/18. doi: 10.1176/jnp.2010.22.1.111. PubMed PMID: 20160218.
21. Valenti M, Pacchiarotti I, Bonnin CM, et al. Risk factors for antidepressant-related switch to mania. *J Clin Psychiatry* 2012;73(2):e271–6. Epub 2012/03/10. doi: 10.4088/JCP.11m07166. PubMed PMID: 22401488.
22. American Psychiatric Association. Practice guideline for the treatment of patients with bipolar disorder (revision). *Am J Psychiatry* 2002;159(4 Suppl):1–50. Epub 2002/04/18. PubMed PMID: 11958165.
23. Brooks JO, 3rd, Hoblyn JC. Secondary mania in older adults. *Am J Psychiatry* 2005;162(11):2033–8. Epub 2005/11/03. doi: 10.1176/appi.ajp.162.11.2033. PubMed PMID: 16263839.
24. Sami M, Khan H, Nilforooshan R. Late onset mania as an organic syndrome: a review of case reports in the literature. *J Affect Disord.* 2015;188:226–31. Epub 2015/09/15. doi: 10.1016/j.jad.2015.08.027. PubMed PMID: 26368947.
25. National Collaborating Centre for Mental Health (UK). Bipolar Disorder: The NICE Guideline on the Assessment and Management of Bipolar Disorder in Adults, Children and Young People in Primary and Secondary Care (Updated 2020). 2014. (number 40)
26. Conus P, Macneil C, McGorry PD. Public health significance of bipolar disorder: implications for early intervention and prevention. *Bipolar Disord.* 2014;16(5):548–56. Epub 2013/10/17. doi: 10.1111/bdi.12137. PubMed PMID: 24127825.
27. Frías Á, Palma C, Farriols N. Comorbidity in pediatric bipolar disorder: prevalence, clinical impact, etiology and treatment. *J Affect Disord.* 2015;174:378–89. Epub 2014/12/30. doi: 10.1016/j.jad.2014.12.008. PubMed PMID: 25545605.
28. Joslyn C, Hawes DJ, Hunt C, et al. Is age of onset associated with severity, prognosis, and clinical features in bipolar disorder? A meta-analytic review. *Bipolar Disord.* 2016;18(5):389–403. Epub 2016/08/18. doi: 10.1111/bdi.12419. PubMed PMID: 27530107.
29. Vega P, Barbeito S, Ruiz de Azúa S, et al. Bipolar disorder differences between genders: special considerations for women. *Women's Health* (Lond). 2011;7(6):663–74; quiz 75-6. Epub 2011/11/02. doi: 10.2217/whe.11.71. PubMed PMID: 22040208.
30. Kemner SM, Mesman E, Nolen WA, et al. The role of life events and psychological factors in the onset of first and recurrent mood episodes in bipolar offspring: results from the Dutch Bipolar Offspring Study. *Psychol Med.* 2015;45(12):2571–81. Epub 2015/04/14. doi: 10.1017/s0033291715000495. PubMed PMID: 25865058.
31. Kemner SM, van Haren NE, Bootsman F, et al. The influence of life events on first and recurrent admissions in bipolar disorder. *Int J Bipolar Disord.* 2015;3:6. Epub 2015/02/27. doi: 10.1186/s40345-015-0022-4. PubMed PMID: 25717427; PubMed Central PMCID: PMCPMC4339321.
32. Carvalho AF, Dimellis D, Gonda X, et al. Rapid cycling in bipolar disorder: a systematic review. *J Clin Psychiatry* 2014;75(6):e578–86. Epub 2014/07/09. doi: 10.4088/JCP.13r08905. PubMed PMID: 25004199.
33. Slyepchenko A, Frey BN, Lafer B, et al. Increased illness burden in women with comorbid bipolar and premenstrual dysphoric disorder: data from 1 099 women from STEP-BD study. *Acta Psychiatr Scand.* 2017;136(5):473–82. Epub 2017/08/29. doi: 10.1111/acps.12797. PubMed PMID: 28846801; PubMed Central PMCID: PMCPMC5630503.
34. Hunt GE, Malhi GS, Cleary M, et al. Prevalence of comorbid bipolar and substance use disorders in clinical settings, 1990-2015: systematic review and meta-analysis. *J Affect Disord.* 2016;206:331–49. Epub 2016/10/25. doi: 10.1016/j.jad.2016.07.011. PubMed PMID: 27476137.
35. Hunt GE, Malhi GS, Cleary M, et al. Comorbidity of bipolar and substance use disorders in national surveys of general populations, 1990-2015: systematic review and meta-analysis. *J Affect Disord.* 2016;206:321–30. Epub 2016/10/25. doi: 10.1016/j.jad.2016.06.051. PubMed PMID: 27426694.
36. Post RM, Denicoff KD, Leverich GS, et al. Morbidity in 258 bipolar outpatients followed for 1 year with daily prospective ratings on the NIMH life chart method. *J Clin Psychiatry* 2003;64(6):680–90; quiz 738-9. Epub 2003/06/26. doi: 10.4088/jcp.v64n0610. PubMed PMID: 12823083.
37. Walker ER, McGee RE, Druss BG. Mortality in mental disorders and global disease burden implications: a systematic review and meta-analysis. *JAMA Psychiatry* 2015;72(4):334–41. Epub 2015/02/12. doi: 10.1001/jamapsychiatry.2014.2502. PubMed PMID: 25671328; PubMed Central PMCID: PMCPMC4461039.
38. Miller JN, Black DW. Bipolar disorder and suicide: a review. *Curr Psychiatry Rep.* 2020;22(2):6. Epub 2020/01/20. doi: 10.1007/s11920-020-1130-0. PubMed PMID: 31955273.
39. Jawad I, Watson S, Haddad PM, et al. Medication nonadherence in bipolar disorder: a narrative review. *Ther Adv Psychopharmacol.* 2018;8(12):349–63. Epub 2018/12/14. doi: 10.1177/2045125318804364. PubMed PMID: 30524703; PubMed Central PMCID: PMCPMC6278745.
40. Beyer JL, Payne ME. Nutrition and bipolar depression. *Psychiatr Clin North Am.* 2016;39(1):75–86. Epub 2016/02/16. doi: 10.1016/j.psc.2015.10.003. PubMed PMID: 26876319.
41. Bauer IE, Galvez JF, Hamilton JE, et al. Lifestyle interventions targeting dietary habits and exercise in bipolar disorder: a systematic

review. *J Psychiatr Res.* 2016;74:1–7. Epub 2016/01/03. doi: 10.1016/j.jpsychires.2015.12.006. PubMed PMID: 26724541; PubMed Central PMCID: PMCPMC4744495.
42. Lexicomp Online. Lithium. Hudson, OH: Lexi-Comp, Inc.
43. Lexicomp Online. Oxcarbazepine. Hudson, OH: Lexi-Comp, Inc.
44. Lexicomp Online. Lamotrigine. Hudson, OH: Lexi-Comp, Inc.
45. Lexicomp Online. Valproic acid and derivatives. Hudson, OH: Lexi-Comp, Inc.
46. Lexicomp Online. Carbamazepine. Hudson, OH: Lexi-Comp, Inc.
47. Lexicomp Online. Lexi-Drugs. Hudson, OH: Lexi-Comp, Inc.
48. Buoli M, Serati M, Altamura AC. Is the combination of a mood stabilizer plus an antipsychotic more effective than mono-therapies in long-term treatment of bipolar disorder? A systematic review. *J Affect Disord.* 2014;152-154:12–8. Epub 2013/09/18. doi: 10.1016/j.jad.2013.08.024. PubMed PMID: 24041717.
49. Grunze H, Vieta E, Goodwin GM, et al. The World Federation of Societies of Biological Psychiatry (WFSBP) Guidelines for the Biological Treatment of Bipolar Disorders: Acute and long-term treatment of mixed states in bipolar disorder. *World J Biol Psychiatry* 2018;19(1):2–58. Epub 2017/11/04. doi: 10.1080/15622975.2017.1384850. PubMed PMID: 29098925.
50. Grunze H, Vieta E, Goodwin GM, et al. The World Federation of Societies of Biological Psychiatry (WFSBP) guidelines for the biological treatment of bipolar disorders: update 2009 on the treatment of acute mania. *World J Biol Psychiatry* 2009;10(2):85–116. Epub 2009/04/07. doi: 10.1080/15622970902823202. PubMed PMID: 19347775.
51. Grunze H, Vieta E, Goodwin GM, et al. The World Federation of Societies of Biological Psychiatry (WFSBP) Guidelines for the Biological Treatment of Bipolar Disorders: Update 2010 on the treatment of acute bipolar depression. *World J Biol Psychiatry* 2010;11(2):81–109. Epub 2010/02/13. doi: 10.3109/15622970903555881. PubMed PMID: 20148751.
52. Grunze H, Vieta E, Goodwin GM, et al. The World Federation of Societies of Biological Psychiatry (WFSBP) guidelines for the biological treatment of bipolar disorders: update 2012 on the long-term treatment of bipolar disorder. *World J Biol Psychiatry* 2013;14(3):154–219. Epub 2013/03/14. doi: 10.3109/15622975.2013.770551. PubMed PMID: 23480132.
53. Malhi GS, Tanious M, Das P, et al. Potential mechanisms of action of lithium in bipolar disorder. *Current Understanding* 2013;27(2):135–53. Epub 2013/02/02. doi: 10.1007/s40263-013-0039-0. PubMed PMID: 23371914 CNS Drugs.
54. Won E, Kim YK. An oldie but goodie: lithium in the treatment of bipolar disorder through neuroprotective and neurotrophic mechanisms. *Int J Mol Sci.* 2017;18(12). Epub 2017/12/14. doi: 10.3390/ijms18122679. PubMed PMID: 29232923; PubMed Central PMCID: PMCPMC5751281.
55. Curran G, Ravindran A. Lithium for bipolar disorder: a review of the recent literature. *Expert Rev Neurother.* 2014;14(9):1079–98. Epub 2014/08/19. doi: 10.1586/14737175.2014.947965. PubMed PMID: 25130062.
56. Smith KA, Cipriani A. Lithium and suicide in mood disorders: updated meta-review of the scientific literature. *Bipolar Disord.* 2017;19(7):575–86. Epub 2017/09/13. doi: 10.1111/bdi.12543. PubMed PMID: 28895269.
57. Grandjean EM, Aubry JM. Lithium: updated human knowledge using an evidence-based approach: part III: clinical safety. *CNS Drugs.* 2009;23(5):397–418. Epub 2009/05/21. doi: 10.2165/00023210-200923050-00004. PubMed PMID: 19453201.
58. Gong R, Wang P, Dworkin L. What we need to know about the effect of lithium on the kidney. *Am J Physiol Renal Physiol.* 2016;311(6):F1168–F71. Epub 2016/04/29. doi: 10.1152/ajprenal.00145.2016. PubMed PMID: 27122541; PubMed Central PMCID: PMCPMC5210210.
59. Mehta N, Vannozzi R. Lithium-induced electrocardiographic changes: a complete review. *Clin Cardiol.* 2017;40(12):1363–7. Epub 2017/12/17. doi: 10.1002/clc.22822. PubMed PMID: 29247520; PubMed Central PMCID: PMCPMC6490621.
60. Gitlin M. Lithium side effects and toxicity: prevalence and management strategies. *Int J Bipolar Disord.* 2016;4(1):27. Epub 2016/12/03. doi: 10.1186/s40345-016-0068-y. PubMed PMID: 27900734; PubMed Central PMCID: PMCPMC5164879.
61. Heath LJ, Billups SJ, Gaughan KM, et al. Risk factors for utilization of acute care services for lithium toxicity. *Psychiatr Serv.* 2018;69(6):671–6. Epub 2018/04/03. doi: 10.1176/appi.ps.201700346. PubMed PMID: 29606078.
62. Hedya S, Avula A, Swoboda H. *Lithium Toxicity*. Treasure Island, FL: StatPearls Publishing.; 2021.
63. Baird-Gunning J, Lea-Henry T, Hoegberg LCG, et al. Lithium poisoning. *J Intensive Care Med.* 2017;32(4):249–63. Epub 2016/08/16. doi: 10.1177/0885066616651582. PubMed PMID: 27516079.
64. Bendz H, Schon S, Attman PO, et al. Renal failure occurs in chronic lithium treatment but is uncommon. *Kidney Int.* 2010;77(3):219–24. Epub 2009/11/27. doi: 10.1038/ki.2009.433. PubMed PMID: 19940841.
65. Malhi GS, Tanious M. Optimal frequency of lithium administration in the treatment of bipolar disorder: clinical and dosing considerations. *CNS Drugs.* 2011;25(4):289–98. Epub 2011/03/24. doi: 10.2165/11586970-000000000-00000. PubMed PMID: 21425882.
66. American Diabetes A, American Psychiatric A, American Association of Clinical E. Consensus development conference on antipsychotic drugs and obesity and diabetes. *J Clin Psychiatry* 2004;65(2):267–72. Epub 2004/03/09. doi: 10.4088/jcp.v65n0219. PubMed PMID: 15003083.
67. Lexicomp Online. Olanzapine. Hudson, OH: Lexi-Comp, Inc.
68. Jochim J, Rifkin-Zybutz RP, Geddes J, et al. Valproate for acute mania. *Cochrane Database Syst Rev.* 2019;10:CD004052. Epub 2019/10/18. doi: 10.1002/14651858.CD004052.pub2. PubMed PMID: 31621892; PubMed Central PMCID: PMCPMC6953329.
69. American Psychiatric Association. Practice guideline for the treatment of patients with bipolar disorder. *Am J Psychiatry* 1994;151(12 Suppl):1–36. Epub 1994/12/01. doi: 10.1176/ajp.151.12.1. PubMed PMID: 7977902.
70. Allen MH, Hirschfeld RM, Wozniak PJ, et al. Linear relationship of valproate serum concentration to response and optimal serum levels for acute mania. *Am J Psychiatry* 2006;163(2):272–5. Epub 2006/02/02. doi: 10.1176/appi.ajp.163.2.272. PubMed PMID: 16449481.
71. Al Khalili Y, Sekhon S, Jain S. Carbamazepine Toxicity. 2021. In: StatPearls [Internet]. Treasure Island (FL): StatPearls Publishing Copyright © 2021, StatPearls Publishing LLC.
72. Tepper NK CK, Cox S, Whiteman MK, et al., US Medical Eligibility Criteria for Contraceptive Use; US Medical Eligibility Criteria for Contraceptive Use. 2016; http://dx.doi.org/10.15585/mmwr.rr6503a1 65:1104.
73. Zaccara G, Perucca E. Interactions between antiepileptic drugs, and between antiepileptic drugs and other drugs. *Epileptic Disord.* 2014;16(4):409–31. Epub 2014/12/18. doi: 10.1684/epd.2014.0714. PubMed PMID: 25515681.
74. Lu X, Wang X. Hyponatremia induced by antiepileptic drugs in patients with epilepsy. *Expert Opin Drug Saf.* 2017;16(1):77–87. Epub 2016/10/16. doi: 10.1080/14740338.2017.1248399. PubMed PMID: 27737595.
75. Calabrese JR, Bowden CL, Sachs G, et al. A placebo-controlled 18-month trial of lamotrigine and lithium maintenance treatment in recently depressed patients with bipolar I disorder. *J Clin Psychiatry* 2003;64(9):1013–24. Epub 2003/11/25. doi: 10.4088/jcp.v64n0906. PubMed PMID: 14628976.
76. Raskin S, Teitelbaum A, Zislin J, et al. Adjunctive lamotrigine as a possible mania inducer in bipolar patients. *Am J Psychiatry* 2006;163(1):159–60. Epub 2006/01/05. doi: 10.1176/appi.ajp.163.1.159-a. PubMed PMID: 16390907.
77. Calabrese JR, Huffman RF, White RL, et al. Lamotrigine in the acute treatment of bipolar depression: results of five double-blind, placebo-controlled clinical trials. *Bipolar Disord.* 2008;10(2):323–33. Epub 2008/02/15. doi: 10.1111/j.1399-5618.2007.00500.x. PubMed PMID: 18271912.
78. de Almeida KM, Moreira CL, Lafer B. Metabolic syndrome and bipolar disorder: what should psychiatrists know? *CNS Neurosci Ther.* 2012;18(2):160–6. Epub 2011/11/11. doi: 10.1111/j.1755-5949.2011.00240.x. PubMed PMID: 22070636; PubMed Central PMCID: PMCPMC6493593.
79. Sachs GS, Nierenberg AA, Calabrese JR, et al. Effectiveness of adjunctive antidepressant treatment for bipolar depression. *N Engl J Med.* 2007;356(17):1711–22. Epub 2007/03/30. doi: 10.1056/NEJMoa064135. PubMed PMID: 17392295.
80. McGirr A, Vöhringer PA, Ghaemi SN, et al. Safety and efficacy of adjunctive second-generation antidepressant therapy with a mood stabiliser or an atypical antipsychotic in acute bipolar depression: a systematic review and meta-analysis of randomised placebo-controlled trials. *The Lancet Psychiatry* 2016;3(12):1138–46. 10.1016/s2215-0366(16)30264-4.
81. Pacchiarotti I, Bond DJ, Baldessarini RJ, et al. The International Society for Bipolar Disorders (ISBD) task force report on antidepressant use in bipolar disorders. *Am J Psychiatry* 2013;170(11):1249–62. Epub 2013/09/14. doi: 10.1176/appi.ajp.2013.13020185. PubMed PMID: 24030475; PubMed Central PMCID: PMCPMC4091043.

82. Gentile S. Lithium in pregnancy: the need to treat, the duty to ensure safety. *Expert Opin Drug Saf.* 2012;11(3):425–37. Epub 2012/03/10. doi: 10.1517/14740338.2012.670419. PubMed PMID: 22400907.
83. Patorno E, Huybrechts KF, Bateman BT, et al. Lithium use in pregnancy and the risk of cardiac malformations. *N Engl J Med.* 2017;376(23):2245–54. Epub 2017/06/08. doi: 10.1056/NEJMoa1612222. PubMed PMID: 28591541; PubMed Central PMCID: PMCPMC5667676.
84. Fornaro M, Maritan E, Ferranti R, et al. Lithium exposure during pregnancy and the postpartum period: a systematic review and meta-analysis of safety and efficacy outcomes. *Am J Psychiatry* 2020;177(1):76–92. Epub 2019/10/19. doi: 10.1176/appi.ajp.2019.19030228. PubMed PMID: 31623458.
85. Hernández-Díaz S, Smith CR, Shen A, et al. Comparative safety of antiepileptic drugs during pregnancy. *Neurology* 2012;78(21):1692–9. Epub 2012/05/04. doi: 10.1212/WNL.0b013e3182574f39. PubMed PMID: 22551726.
86. Khan SJ, Fersh ME, Ernst C, et al. Bipolar disorder in pregnancy and postpartum: principles of management. *Curr Psychiatry Rep.* 2016;18(2):13. Epub 2016/01/20. doi: 10.1007/s11920-015-0658-x. PubMed PMID: 26781551.
87. LactMed. Lamotrigine. Bethesda, MD: National Library of Medicine; 2006.
88. Vajda FJ, Hitchcock A, Graham J, et al. The Australian Register of Antiepileptic Drugs in Pregnancy: the first 1002 pregnancies. *Aust N Z J Obstet Gynaecol.* 2007;47(6):468–74. Epub 2007/11/10. doi: 10.1111/j.1479-828X.2007.00781.x. PubMed PMID: 17991111.
89. Galbally M, Snellen M, Power J. Antipsychotic drugs in pregnancy: a review of their maternal and fetal effects. *Ther Adv Drug Saf.* 2014;5(2):100–9. Epub 2014/08/02. doi: 10.1177/2042098614522682. PubMed PMID: 25083265; PubMed Central PMCID: PMCPMC4110873.
90. Stepanova E, Findling RL. Psychopharmacology of bipolar disorders in children and adolescents. *Pediatr Clin North Am.* 2017;64(6):1209–22. Epub 2017/11/28. doi: 10.1016/j.pcl.2017.08.002. PubMed PMID: 29173781.
91. Lexicomp Online. Lurasidone. Hudson, OH: Lexi-Comp, Inc.
92. Young RC, Mulsant BH, Sajatovic M, et al. GERI-BD: A randomized double-blind controlled trial of lithium and divalproex in the treatment of mania in older patients with bipolar disorder. *Am J Psychiatry* 2017;174(11):1086–93. Epub 2017/11/02. doi: 10.1176/appi.ajp.2017.15050657. PubMed PMID: 29088928; PubMed Central PMCID: PMCPMC6214451.

Generalized Anxiety Disorder, Panic Disorder, and Social Anxiety Disorder

90

Sarah T. Melton and Cynthia K. Kirkwood

KEY CONCEPTS

1. Anxiety disorders are among the most common psychiatric disorders and are underdiagnosed and undertreated.
2. The long-term goal in treatment of generalized anxiety disorder (GAD) is remission with minimal or no anxiety symptoms and no functional impairment.
3. Antidepressants are the agents of choice for the management of GAD.
4. In GAD, antidepressants have a lag time of 2 to 4 weeks or longer before antianxiety effects occur.
5. When monitoring the effectiveness of antidepressants in panic disorder, it is important to allow an adequate amount of time (8-12 weeks) to achieve full therapeutic response.
6. The optimal duration of panic therapy is unknown; 12 to 24 months of pharmacotherapy is recommended before gradual medication discontinuation over 4 to 6 months is attempted.
7. Social anxiety disorder (SAD) is a chronic long-term illness requiring extended therapy. After improvement, a 6- to 12-month or longer medication maintenance period is recommended before considering treatment discontinuation.
8. The selective serotonin reuptake inhibitors or venlafaxine are considered first-line pharmacotherapy for SAD.
9. An adequate trial of antidepressants in SAD lasts at least 8 weeks, and maximal benefit may not be seen until 12 weeks.
10. In SAD, the three principal domains in which improvement should be observed are symptoms, functionality, and well-being.

BEYOND THE BOOK

Visit the National Institute of Mental Health (NIMH) website for Anxiety Disorders (https://www.nimh.nih.gov/health/topics/anxiety-disorders/index.shtml) and review the patient brochures for generalized anxiety disorder and panic disorder. Compare and contrast the signs and symptoms and the available treatment options for these two anxiety disorders. This activity will help you to differentiate the clinical presentation of each disorder and assist you with the ASSESS portion of the "Patient Care Process."

Complete the case "Bundle of Nerves" in Pharmacotherapy Casebook: A Patient-Focused Approach. This activity will help you to practice the ASSESS, PLAN, and MONITOR portions of the "Patient Care Process."

INTRODUCTION

Anxiety is an emotional state commonly caused by the perception of real or perceived danger that threatens the security of an individual. It allows a person to prepare for or react to environmental changes. Everyone experiences a certain amount of nervousness and apprehension when faced with a stressful situation. This is an adaptive response and is transient in nature.

Anxiety can produce uncomfortable and potentially debilitating psychological (eg, worry or feeling of threat) and physiologic arousal (eg, tachycardia or shortness of breath) if it becomes excessive. Some individuals experience persistent, severe anxiety symptoms and possess irrational fears that significantly impair normal daily functioning. These persons often suffer from an anxiety disorder.[1]

(1) Anxiety disorders are among the most frequent psychiatric disorders encountered in clinical practice and are often underdiagnosed and undertreated.[2] Healthcare professionals often mistake anxiety disorders for physical illnesses, and less than one-third of patients receive appropriate treatment.[2] Failure to diagnose and manage anxiety disorders results in negative outcomes including overuse of healthcare resources, increased risk for suicide, and substance use disorders (SUDs).[3] Individuals with anxiety disorders develop cardiovascular, cerebrovascular, gastrointestinal (GI), and respiratory disorders at a significantly higher rate than the general population.[3]

To treat anxiety appropriately, the clinician must make a reliable diagnosis. Understanding the distinction between short-term symptoms of anxiety and anxiety disorders is essential. Common or situational anxiety is a normal response to a stressful circumstance. Although symptoms can be severe, they are temporary and usually last no more than 2 or 3 weeks. In this situation, short-term, "as-needed" treatment with an anxiolytic agent such as a benzodiazepine is common and can provide some symptomatic relief; prolonged medication therapy is not recommended for situational anxiety.[4]

EPIDEMIOLOGY

Anxiety disorders, as a group, are the most commonly occurring psychiatric disorders as approximately 34% of the population are affected by an anxiety disorder during their lifetime.[5] According to the National Comorbidity Survey Replication which assessed the prevalence, severity, and comorbidity estimates of mental disorders in the United States, the most recent 1-year prevalence rate for anxiety disorders was 21.3% in persons aged 18 years and older. Specific phobias were the most common anxiety disorder, with a 12-month prevalence of 10.1%. The 1-year prevalence of generalized anxiety disorder (GAD) was 2.9%, panic disorder was 3.1%, and social anxiety disorder (SAD) was 8.0%.[5]

In general, anxiety disorders are a group of heterogeneous illnesses that develop before age 30 years and are more common in females, individuals with social issues, and those with a family history of anxiety and depression. Patients often develop another anxiety disorder, major depression, or SUDs.[1,2] The clinical picture of mixed anxiety and depression is much more common than an isolated anxiety disorder.[6,7]

ETIOLOGY

The differential diagnosis of anxiety disorders includes medical and psychiatric illnesses and certain medications or substances.[6,7] Hypotheses on the etiology of anxiety disorders are based on interactions between a combination of factors including vulnerability (eg, genetic predisposition and early childhood adversity) and stress (eg, occupational and traumatic experience). The vulnerability may be associated with genetic factors and neurobiologic adaptations of the central nervous system (CNS).[8]

Medical Diseases Associated with Anxiety

Anxiety symptoms are an inherent part of the initial clinical presentation of several diseases, which complicates the distinction between anxiety disorders and medical disorders.[4,7] Furthermore, anxiety disorders are associated with chronic medical illness, low levels of physical health-related quality of life (QOL), and physical disability.[2] If anxiety symptoms are secondary to a medical illness, they usually will subside as the medical situation stabilizes. However, the knowledge that one has a physical illness can trigger anxious feelings and further complicate therapy. Persistent anxiety subsequent to a physical illness requires further assessment for an anxiety disorder. Common somatic symptoms of anxiety that frequently present in medical disorders include abdominal pain, palpitations, tachycardia, sweating, flushing, tremor, chest pain or tightness, and shortness of breath. Although less specific, symptoms of muscle tension, headache, and fatigue are also common manifestations of anxiety. Medical disorders most closely associated with anxiety are listed in Table 90-1.

Psychiatric Diseases Associated with Anxiety

Anxiety can be a presenting feature of several major psychiatric illnesses. Anxiety symptoms are extremely common in patients with mood disorders, schizophrenia, dementia, and SUDs. Most patients with psychiatric illness will have two or more concurrent (comorbid) psychiatric disorders within their lifetime.[5] It is important to diagnose and treat all comorbid psychiatric conditions in patients with anxiety disorders.

Medication- and Substance-Induced Anxiety

Medications and substances are a common cause of anxiety symptoms (Table 90-2). While anxiety occurs during the use of CNS-stimulants in a dose-dependent manner, ingestion of minimal amounts can result in marked anxiety, including panic attacks, in some individuals. The onset of medication-induced anxiety is usually rapid after the initiation of therapy. A thorough medication history evaluating for a recently initiated medication or dosage change as well as unhealthy substance use is important to rule out a medication- or unhealthy substance-induced etiology for the anxiety.

Anxiety occurs occasionally during the use of CNS depressants, especially in children and older adults; however, anxiety symptoms are more common as complications of withdrawal after the abrupt discontinuation of these agents.[6]

PATHOPHYSIOLOGY

The modulation of normal and pathologic anxiety states is associated with multiple regions of the brain and abnormal function in several neurotransmitter systems, including norepinephrine (NE), γ-aminobutyric acid (GABA), serotonin (5-HT), dopamine (DA), corticotropin-releasing factor (CRF), and cholecystokinin.[9] Neuroanatomic models of fear (ie, the response to danger) and anxiety (ie, the feeling of fear that is disproportionate to the actual threat) include some key brain areas. The amygdala, a temporal lobe structure, plays a critical role in the assessment of fear stimuli and learned response to fear.[9,10] The locus ceruleus (LC), located in the brain stem, is the primary NE-containing site, with widespread projections to areas responsible for implementing fear responses (eg, vagus, lateral, and paraventricular hypothalamus). The hippocampus is integral in the consolidation of traumatic memory and contextual fear conditioning. The hypothalamus is the principal area for integrating neuroendocrine and autonomic responses to a threat.[9] Recent reviews of potential biomarkers for anxiety disorders in neurochemistry, genetics, and neuroimaging report insufficient evidence of specific biomarkers for diagnosis and treatment response.[11,12]

Neurochemical Theories

Noradrenergic Model

The basic premise of the noradrenergic theory is that the autonomic nervous system of patients with anxiety disorders is hypersensitive

TABLE 90-1 Common Medical Illnesses Associated with Anxiety Symptoms

Cardiovascular
- Angina, arrhythmias, cardiomyopathy, congestive heart failure, hypertension, ischemic heart disease, mitral valve prolapse, myocardial infarction

Endocrine and metabolic
- Cushing disease, diabetes, hyperparathyroidism, hyperthyroidism, hypothyroidism, hypoglycemia, hyponatremia, hyperkalemia, pheochromocytoma, vitamin B_{12} or folate deficiencies

Gastrointestinal
- Crohn's disease, irritable bowel syndrome, ulcerative colitis, peptic ulcer disease

Neurologic
- Migraine, seizures, stroke, neoplasms, poor pain control

Respiratory system
- Asthma, chronic obstructive pulmonary disease, pulmonary embolism, pneumonia

Others
- Anemias, cancer, systemic lupus erythematosus, vestibular dysfunction

Data from References 3, 6, and 7.

TABLE 90-2 Medications and Substances Associated with Anxiety Symptoms

Antiseizure medications: Carbamazepine, phenytoin
Antidepressants: Bupropion, selective serotonin reuptake inhibitors, serotonin–norepinephrine reuptake inhibitors
Antihypertensives: Clonidine, felodipine
Antibiotics: Quinolones, isoniazid
Bronchodilators: Albuterol, theophylline
Corticosteroids: Prednisone
Dopamine agonists: Amantadine, levodopa
Herbals: Ginseng, ephedra
Unhealthy substance use: Ecstasy, cannabis, cocaine
Nonsteroidal anti-inflammatory medications: Ibuprofen, indomethacin
Stimulants: Amphetamines, caffeine, methylphenidate, nicotine
Sympathomimetics: Pseudoephedrine, phenylephrine
Thyroid hormones: Levothyroxine
Toxicity: Anticholinergics, antihistamines, digoxin

Data from References 1 and 4.

and overreacts to various stimuli. Many patients with anxiety disorders clearly display symptoms of peripheral autonomic hyperactivity. In response to threat or fearful situations, the LC serves as an alarm center, activating NE release and stimulating the sympathetic and parasympathetic nervous systems. Chronic central noradrenergic overactivity downregulates α_2-adrenoreceptors in patients with GAD. This receptor is hypersensitive in some patients with panic disorder.[9] By administering medications that have a relatively specific effect on the LC, researchers have further explored the NE theory of anxiety and panic disorder. Medications with anxiogenic effects (eg, yohimbine [an α_2-adrenergic receptor antagonist]) stimulate LC firing and increase noradrenergic activity. The resultant NE release in turn increases glutamate release (an excitatory neurotransmitter).[9] This produces subjective feelings of anxiety and can precipitate a panic attack in those with panic disorder, but not in normal volunteers.[9] Medications with anxiolytic or antipanic effects (eg, benzodiazepines and antidepressants) inhibit LC firing, decrease noradrenergic activity, and block the effects of anxiogenic agents.[9]

GABA-Receptor Model

The major inhibitory neurotransmitter in the CNS, GABA has a strong regulatory or inhibitory effect on the 5-HT, NE, and DA systems. There are two superfamilies of GABA-protein receptors: $GABA_A$ and $GABA_B$. Medications that reduce anxiety and produce sedation target the $GABA_A$ receptor. The $GABA_A$ receptors are ligand-gated ion channels composed of five protein subunits. Several classes of subunits (ie, $\alpha_{1\text{-}6}$, $\beta_{1\text{-}3}$, $\gamma_{1\text{-}3}$, δ, ε, θ, π, $\rho_{1\text{-}3}$) surround a central pore, and the receptor is connected to the cytoskeleton.[13] When GABA binds to the $GABA_A$ receptor, neuronal excitability is reduced. Benzodiazepine ligands enhance the inhibitory effects of GABA.[13] The $GABA_B$ receptor is a G-protein–coupled receptor postulated to be involved in the presynaptic inhibition of GABA release[9,13]

The specific role of the GABA receptors in anxiety disorders has not been established. The number of $GABA_A$ receptors can change with alterations in the environment (eg, chronic stress), and the subunit expression can be altered by hormonal changes.[13] Reductions in benzodiazepine binding and GABA concentrations in the brain are reported in patients with panic disorder.[11]

Serotonin Model

Although there are data suggesting that the 5-HT system is dysregulated in patients with anxiety disorders, definitive evidence that shows a clear abnormality in 5-HT function is lacking. In general, 5-HT is primarily an inhibitory neurotransmitter that is used by neurons originating in the raphe nuclei of the brain stem and projecting diffusely throughout the brain (eg, cortex, amygdala, hippocampus, and limbic system). Abnormalities in serotonergic functioning through release and uptake at the presynaptic autoreceptors ($5\text{-}HT_{1A/1D}$), the serotonin-reuptake transporter (SERT), or effect of 5-HT at the postsynaptic receptors (eg, $5\text{-}HT_{1A}$, $5\text{-}HT_{2A}$, and $5\text{-}HT_{2C}$) may play a role in anxiety disorders.[9,11] Greater 5-HT function may facilitate avoidance behavior; however, reducing 5-HT may increase aggression.[9] Greater 5-HT activity reduces NE activity in the LC, inhibits defense/escape response via the periaqueductal gray (PAG) region, and reduces hypothalamic release of CRF. The selective serotonin reuptake inhibitors (SSRIs) acutely increase 5-HT levels by blocking the SERT to increase the amount of 5-HT available postsynaptically and are efficacious in blocking the manifestations of panic and anxiety.[9]

Low 5-HT activity may lead to a dysregulation of other neurotransmitters. Both the NE and 5-HT systems are closely linked, and interactions between the two are reciprocal and vary. As NE may act at presynaptic 5-HT terminals to decrease 5-HT release, its activity at postsynaptic receptors can cause increased 5-HT release.

Buspirone is a selective $5\text{-}HT_{1A}$ partial agonist that is effective for GAD but not for panic disorder.[14] Because the selective $5\text{-}HT_{1A}$ partial agonists reduce serotonergic activity, GAD symptoms may reflect excessive 5-HT transmission or overactivity of the stimulatory 5-HT pathways. There is circumstantial evidence for the involvement of serotonergic and dopaminergic systems in the pathophysiology of generalized SAD.[15]

Neuroimaging Studies

Functional neuroimaging studies support the crucial role of the amygdala, anterior cingulate cortex (ACC), ventromedial prefrontal cortex, and insula in the pathophysiology of anxiety.[8,11] In GAD there is an abnormal increase in the brain's fear circuitry, as well as decreased activity in the prefrontal cortex, which appears to have a compensatory role in reducing GAD symptoms.[16] Patients with panic have abnormalities of midbrain structures, including the PAG. Neuroimaging studies have shown activation of insula and upper brain stem (including the PAG), as well as deactivation of the ACC during experimental panic attacks.[10] Patients with SAD have greater activity than matched comparison subjects in the amygdala and insula, structures linked to negative emotional responses.[11] Both pharmacotherapy and psychotherapy decrease cerebral blood flow in the amygdala, hippocampus, and surrounding cortical areas in patients with SAD.[8,11]

CLINICAL PRESENTATION

The *Diagnostic and Statistical Manual of Mental Disorders, Fifth Edition (DSM-5)* classifies anxiety disorders into categories including GAD, panic disorder, agoraphobia, SAD, specific phobia, and separation anxiety disorder.[1] The characteristic features of these illnesses are anxiety and avoidance behavior. Anxiety symptoms must cause significant distress and impairment in social, occupational, or other areas of functioning, and should not be secondary to a medication or unhealthy substance use or a general medical disorder or occur solely as part of another psychiatric disorder.[1] The anxiety-related

CLINICAL PRESENTATION Generalized Anxiety Disorder

Psychological and Cognitive Symptoms

- Excessive anxiety
- Worries that are difficult to control
- Feeling keyed up or on edge
- Trouble concentrating or mind going blank

Physical Symptoms

- Restlessness
- Fatigue
- Muscle tension
- Sleep disturbance
- Irritability

Data from References 1, 2, and 3.

CLINICAL PRESENTATION Panic Attack

Psychological Symptoms

- Depersonalization (being detached from oneself)
- Derealization (feelings of being detached from one's environment)
- Fear of losing control, going crazy, or dying

Physical Symptoms

- Abdominal distress
- Chest pain or discomfort
- Chills
- Dizziness or light-headedness
- Feeling of choking
- Heat sensations
- Nausea
- Palpitations
- Paresthesias
- Sensations of shortness of breath or smothering
- Sweating
- Tachycardia
- Trembling or shaking

Data from References 1, 2, and 3.

syndromes, posttraumatic stress disorder, and obsessive-compulsive disorder are discussed in Chapter 91 "Posttraumatic Stress Disorder and Obsessive-Compulsive Disorder."

Generalized Anxiety Disorder

The diagnostic criteria for GAD require persistent symptoms for most days for at least 6 months.[1] The essential feature of GAD is unrealistic or excessive anxiety and worry about a number of events or activities.[1] The anxiety or apprehensive expectation is accompanied by at least three psychological or physical symptoms. Anxiety and worry are not confined to features of another psychiatric illness (eg, having a panic attack, being embarrassed in public).[1]

The onset, course of illness, and comorbid conditions of GAD are important considerations. While GAD has a gradual onset with an average age of 21 years, there is a bimodal distribution. Onset occurs earlier when GAD is the primary presentation and later when GAD is secondary. In general, GAD can be exacerbated or precipitated in later life by severe psychological stressors. Most patients present between the ages of 35 and 45 years, with females twice as likely to have GAD as males. The course of the illness is chronic (ie, episodes can last for a decade or longer) and there is a high percentage of relapse with low overall rates of recovery.[1] Patients report substantial interference with their lives and have a high probability of seeking treatment. Lifetime comorbidity with another psychiatric disorder occurs in 90% of patients with GAD, with depression in over 50%.[17]

Panic Disorder

Panic disorder begins as a series of unexpected (spontaneous) panic attacks involving an abrupt surge of intense fear or intense discomfort. The unexpected panic attacks are followed by at least 1 month of persistent concern about having another panic attack, worry about the possible consequences of the panic attack, or a significant maladaptive change in behavior related to the attacks.[1] During an attack, patients describe at least four psychological and physical symptoms. Panic attacks usually last no more than 20 to 30 minutes, with the peak intensity of symptoms within the first 10 minutes. Often patients seek help at a physician's office or emergency department, only to have their symptoms resolve before or on arrival. Because panic symptoms mimic those of several medical conditions, patients often are misdiagnosed, and multiple referrals are common.[1]

Up to 50% of patients develop agoraphobia secondary to the panic attacks.[1] Agoraphobia is marked fear or anxiety about being in at least two situations in which escape might be difficult or where help might not be available in the event of developing panic-like symptoms.[1] As a result, patients often avoid specific situations (eg, using public transportation, being in open or enclosed places, being in a crowd or being outside of the home alone) in which they fear a panic attack might occur.[1]

Complications of panic disorder include depression (10%-65% have major depressive disorder), alcohol use disorder, and high use of health services and emergency rooms.[1] Patients with panic disorder have a high lifetime risk for suicide attempts compared with the general population.[1] The usual course is chronic but waxing and waning.

Social Anxiety Disorder

Social anxiety disorder is characterized by marked fear about one or more social situations in which the individual is exposed to possible scrutiny by others. Exposure to the feared circumstance usually provokes an immediate situation-related panic attack. Blushing is the principal physical indicator and distinguishes SAD from other anxiety disorders. The fear and anxiety are out of proportion to the actual threat posed by the social situation and is persistent, typically lasting for 6 months or longer.[1] If the fear is restricted to speaking or performing in public, the SAD is specified as performance only.

The mean age of onset of SAD is during the mid-teens with rates slightly higher among females than males and more frequent in younger cohorts. It is a chronic disorder with a mean duration of 20 years.[1] People with SAD can be reluctant to seek professional help despite the existence of beneficial treatments because consultation with a clinician is perceived as a feared social interaction.[18]

Differentiating SAD from other anxiety disorders can be difficult. Panic attacks occur in both SAD and panic disorder, but the distinction between the two is the rationale behind the fear, whereas fear of anxiety symptoms is characteristic of panic disorder and fear of embarrassment from social interaction typifies SAD.[1] A majority of patients with SAD eventually develop a concurrent mood, anxiety, or SUD.[18]

Specific Phobia

Specific phobia is marked and persistent fear of a circumscribed object or situation (eg, insects or heights). Apart from contact with the feared object or situation, the patient is usually free of symptoms. Most persons simply avoid the feared object and adjust to certain restrictions on their activities.[1]

CLINICAL PRESENTATION Social Anxiety Disorder

Fears of Being

- Scrutinized by others
- Negatively evaluated (ie, humiliated, embarrassed, or rejected)

Some Feared Situations

- Eating or writing in front of others
- Interacting with authority figures
- Speaking in public
- Talking with strangers
- Use of public toilets

Symptoms of Anxiety

- Blushing
- "Butterflies in the stomach"
- Diarrhea
- Stumbling over words
- Sweating
- Tachycardia
- Trembling

Specifier

Performance; applies only if the fear is restricted to speaking or performing in public.

Data from References 1 and 18.

TREATMENT—GENERALIZED ANXIETY DISORDER

Desired Outcomes

2 The goals of therapy in the acute management of GAD are to reduce the severity and duration of the anxiety symptoms and to improve overall functioning. The long-term goal in GAD is remission with minimal or no anxiety symptoms, no functional impairment, and increased QOL.[17] Prevention of recurrence is another long-term consideration.

General Approach

Once GAD is diagnosed, a patient-specific treatment plan, which usually consists of both psychotherapy and pharmacotherapy, is developed. The plan depends on the severity and chronicity of symptoms, age, medication history, and comorbid medical and psychiatric conditions.[19] Factors such as anticipated adverse medication reactions, history of prior response in the patient or family member, patient preference, and cost should be considered when treatment is initiated. Psychotherapy is the least invasive and safest treatment modality. Antianxiety medication is indicated for patients experiencing symptoms severe enough to produce functional disability. Table 90-3 lists medication choices for GAD, panic disorder, and SAD.

The need for treatment is determined by patient-specific factors including severity and duration of symptoms, degree of disability, and the presence of coexisting disorders (ie, mood or other anxiety disorders). The patient should be assessed for response to or intolerance of previous treatment approaches. The selection of a specific treatment modality should be based on concurrent medical conditions, contraindications, patient's preference of treatment, and the availability of potential treatment options. The clinician should consider Food and Drug Administration (FDA) warnings (eg, QTc prolongation for citalopram and hydroxyzine, teratogenicity with paroxetine) and potential for adverse events with medical disease (eg, anticholinergic effects and weight gain with paroxetine in patients with diabetes, obesity, or benign prostatic hyperplasia) when selecting an agent. Increased risk of suicidality should be considered in patients taking antidepressants who are younger than 25 years of age. All patients should receive education that includes information about GAD, treatment choices, and resources for support in the community. The patient should be an integral part of decision making and should be informed about effectiveness, common adverse medication reactions, duration of treatment, costs associated with treatment, and what to expect when treatment is discontinued.[2]

TABLE 90-3 Medication Choices for Anxiety Disorders

Anxiety Disorder	First-Line Medications	Second-Line Medications	Alternatives
Generalized anxiety disorder	Duloxetine Escitalopram Paroxetine Sertraline Venlafaxine XR	Benzodiazepines Buspirone Imipramine Pregabalin	Hydroxyzine Quetiapine
Panic disorder	SSRIs Venlafaxine XR	Alprazolam Citalopram Clomipramine Clonazepam Imipramine	Phenelzine
Social anxiety disorder	Escitalopram Fluvoxamine CR Paroxetine Sertraline Venlafaxine XR	Clonazepam Citalopram	Gabapentin Phenelzine Pregabalin

CR, controlled-release; SSRI, selective serotonin reuptake inhibitor; XR, extended-release.

Data from References 2, 20, and 21.

Nonpharmacologic Therapy

Nonpharmacologic treatment modalities in GAD include psychoeducation, short-term counseling, stress management, psychotherapy, mindfulness-based therapy, or exercise. Psychoeducation includes information on the etiology and management of GAD (eg, Anxiety and Depression Association of America, www.adaa.org). For all anxiety and psychiatric disorders, peer-to-peer support obtained through the National Alliance for Mental Illness (NAMI) can be helpful (https://www.nami.org/Support-Education/Mental-Health-Education/NAMI-Peer-to-Peer). Patients with anxiety should be instructed to avoid caffeine, nicotine, nonprescription stimulants, diet pills, and excessive use of alcohol. Most patients with GAD require psychological therapy, alone or in combination with antianxiety medications, to overcome fears and to learn to manage their anxiety and worry.[22] Cognitive behavioral therapy (CBT) is the most effective psychological therapy in individuals with GAD. In general, CBT for GAD includes self-monitoring of worry, cognitive

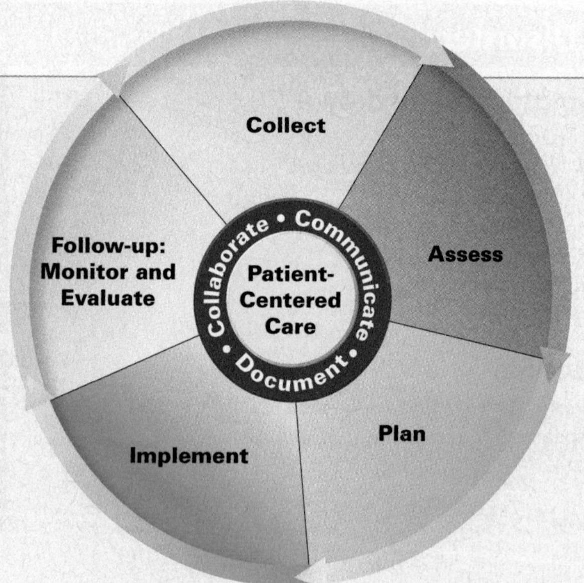

Patient Care Process for Anxiety Disorders

The image shows the five fundamental steps included in The Pharmacist's Care Process endorsed by the Joint Commission for Pharmacy Practitioners (2014). The tagline of this process reads collaborate, communicate, and document. The five fundamental steps listed here are collect, assess, plan, implement, and follow-up: monitor and evaluate. All these steps are listed in a circular block diagram.

Collect

- Patient characteristics (eg, age, sex, pregnancy)
- Patient medical history (personal and family)
- Patient psychiatric history (personal and family)
- Social history (eg, caffeine, nicotine, ethanol, or other substance use including route of administration)
- Current medications including over-the-counter (OTC), herbal products, dietary supplements, and prior psychiatric medication use
- Mental status examination
- Objective data
    - Blood pressure (BP), heart rate (HR), respiratory rate (RR), height, and weight
    - Labs including thyroid stimulating hormone (TSH)
    - Urinalysis including urine medications testing
    - Generalized Anxiety Disorder 7-Item Scale, Hamilton Anxiety Disorder Rating Scale (HAM-A), Sheehan Disability Scale, and Patient Health Questionnaire-9 (PHQ-9)

Assess

- Presence of generalized anxiety disorder, panic disorder, or social anxiety disorder
- Presence of comorbid depression or substance use disorder
- Ability/willingness to begin nonpharmacologic treatments, including availability in geographic region
- Ability/willingness to begin pharmacologic treatment
- Ability/willingness to afford nonpharmacologic and/or pharmacologic treatment(s)
- Support of family members/caregivers for treatment

Plan*

- Pharmacotherapy regimen including specific medication(s), dose, route, frequency, and duration (see Fig. 90-1, and Tables 90-4, 90-5, 90-8, and 90-9)
- Monitoring parameters including efficacy (eg, rating scales, quality of life)
- Patient education (eg, disease, life style changes, medication adherence, when to expect medication to begin working, possible adverse reactions, expected duration of therapy, when to contact healthcare professional)
- Self-monitoring for resolution of anxiety symptoms

Implement*

- Provide patient education regarding all aspects of treatment plan
- Use motivational interviewing and coaching strategies to maximize adherence
- Schedule follow-up

Follow-up: Monitor and Evaluate

- Resolution of anxiety symptoms
- Presence of adverse medication reactions (eg, sedation, psychomotor impairment, nausea, headaches, weight gain, sexual dysfunction)
- Psychiatric rating scale results
- Patient adherence to treatment plan using multiple sources of information
- Re-evaluate in 2 weeks until stable, then every 3 months

**Collaborate with patient, caregivers, and other healthcare professionals.*

restructuring, relaxation training, and rehearsal of coping skills.[22] Psychotherapy or medication alone has comparable efficacy in acute treatment.[21] The relapse rate with CBT is less than with other types of psychological modalities.[21] Controlled trials comparing the efficacy of combining medication and psychotherapy over long-term treatment are lacking.[21] Advantages of CBT over pharmacotherapy include patient preference and lack of troubling adverse medication reactions. However, CBT is not widely available, requires specialized training, and entails weekly sessions for an extended time period (ie, 12-16 weeks).[23] Other options include group therapy (8-12 sessions) and computer-based therapy.[23]

Pharmacologic Therapy

The benzodiazepines are the most effective and commonly prescribed medications for the rapid relief of acute anxiety symptoms (Table 90-4). All benzodiazepines are equally effective anxiolytics, and consideration of pharmacokinetic properties and the patient's clinical situation will assist in the selection of the most appropriate agent.[17]

As antidepressants lack the physical dependence and adverse medication reactions seen with benzodiazepines, they have emerged as the treatment of choice for the management of chronic anxiety, especially in the presence of comorbid depressive symptoms. Buspirone is

TABLE 90-4 Benzodiazepine Antianxiety Agents

Medication	Brand Name	Approved Dosage Range (mg/day)	Maximum Dosage for Geriatric Patients (mg/day)	Approximate Equivalent Dose (mg)	Comments
Alprazolam[a]	Xanax	0.75-4	2	0.5	Associated with interdose rebound anxiety
	Xanax XR	1-10[b]			
Chlordiazepoxide[a]	Librium	25-400	40	10	
Clonazepam[a]	Klonopin	1-4[b]	3	0.25-0.5	
	Klonopin Wafer[c]				
Clorazepate[a]	Tranxene	7.5-60	30	7.5	
Diazepam[a]	Valium	2-40	20	5	
Lorazepam[a]	Ativan	0.5-10	3	1	Preferred in older adults
Oxazepam[a]	Serax	30-120	60	30	Preferred in older adults

XR, extended-release.

[a]Available generically.

[b]Panic disorder dose.

[c]Orally disintegrating formulation.

Data from References 24-26.

TABLE 90-5 Nonbenzodiazepine Antianxiety Agents for Generalized Anxiety Disorder

Medication	Brand Name	Initial Dose	Usual Range (mg/day)[a]	Comments
Antidepressants				
Duloxetine	Cymbalta	30 or 60 mg/day	60-120	FDA-approved; available generically
Escitalopram	Lexapro	10 mg/day	10-20	FDA-approved; available generically
Imipramine	Tofranil	50 mg/day	75-200	Available generically
Paroxetine	Paxil	20 mg/day	20-50	FDA-approved; available generically; avoid in pregnancy
	Pexeva			
Sertraline	Zoloft	50 mg/day	50-200	Available generically
Venlafaxine XR	Effexor XR	37.5 or 75 mg/day	75-225[b]	FDA-approved; available generically
Vilazodone	Viibryd	10 mg/day	20-40[b]	During concomitant use of a strong CYP3A4 inhibitor (eg, itraconazole, clarithromycin, voriconazole), dose should not exceed 20 mg once daily
Vortioxetine	Trintellix	5 mg/day	5-20	
Azapirone				
Buspirone	BuSpar	7.5 mg twice daily	15-60[b]	FDA-approved; available generically
Diphenylmethane				
Hydroxyzine	Vistaril	25 or 50 mg four times daily	200-400	FDA-approved; approved in children for anxiety and tension in divided daily doses of 50-100 mg; available generically
Antiseizure Medications				
Pregabalin	Lyrica	50 mg three times daily	150-600	Dosage adjustment required in renal impairment; available generically
Second-generation antipsychotic				
Quetiapine XR	Seroquel XR	50 mg at bedtime	150-300	Available generically

XR, extended-release.

[a]Older adult patients are usually treated with approximately one-half of the dose listed.

[b]No dosage adjustment is required in older adult patients.

Data from References 3 and 27-34.

an additional anxiolytic option (Table 90-5) in patients without comorbid depression or other anxiety disorders. Because of the high risk of adverse reactions and toxicity, barbiturates, antipsychotics, antipsychotic–antidepressant combinations, and antihistamines generally are not indicated in the treatment of GAD.[3] It is important to note that the benzodiazepines are more effective in treating the somatic and autonomic symptoms of GAD as opposed to the psychological symptoms (eg, apprehension and worry), which are reduced by antidepressants.[3]

The most recent evidence-based treatment guidelines come from the World Federation of Societies of Biological Psychiatry, the National Institute for Health and Clinical Evidence, and British Association for Psychopharmacology.[3,21,22] A descriptive flowchart with recommendations based on levels of evidence from the International Psychopharmacology Algorithm Project for the psychosocial and pharmacologic management of GAD is shown in Fig. 90-1.[35]

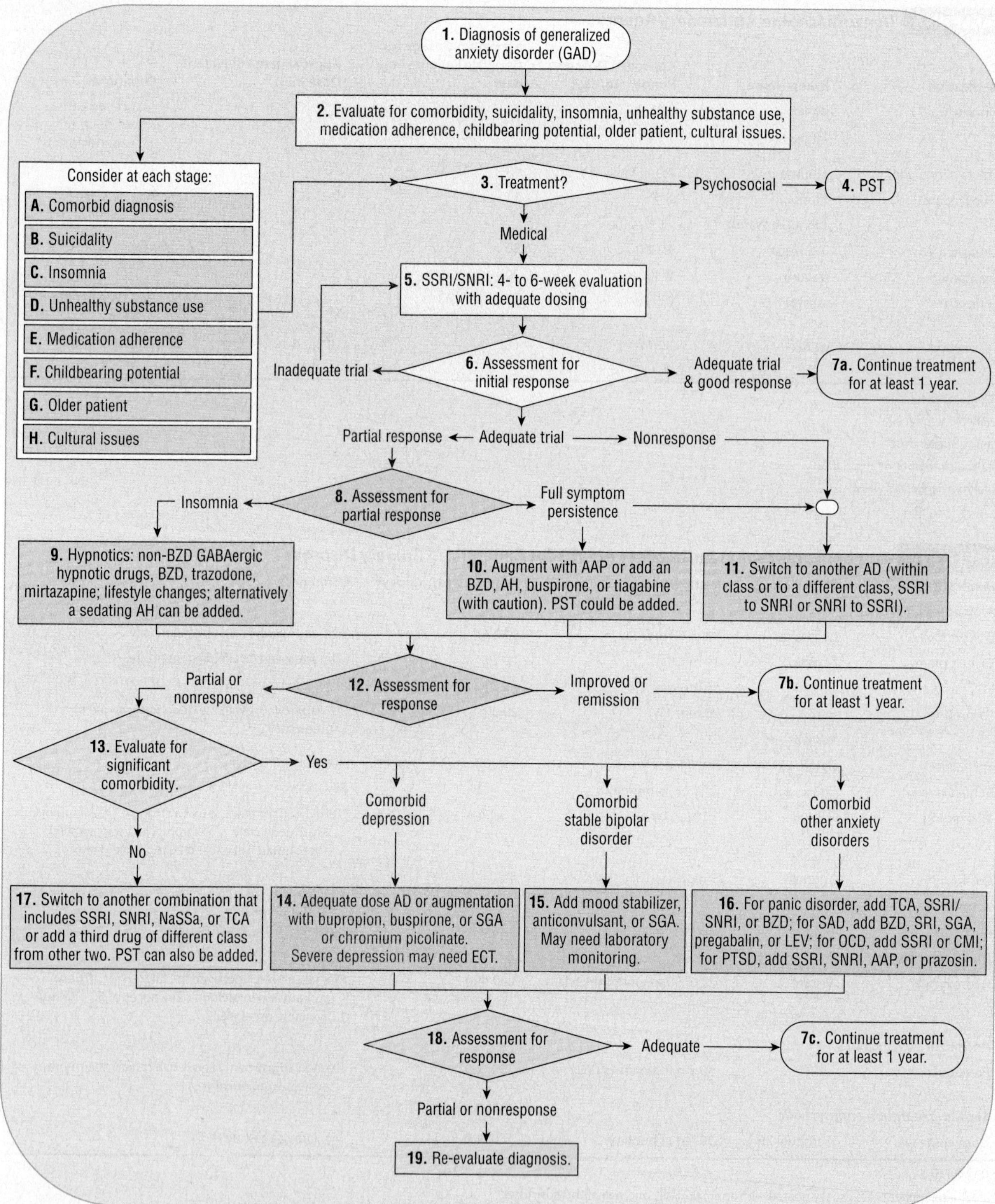

FIGURE 90-1 International Psychopharmacology Algorithm Project (IPAP) generalized anxiety disorder (GAD) algorithm flowchart. Yellow, first-line treatment (nodes 2, 3, 5, 6); green, second-line treatment (nodes 8-12); blue, third-line treatment, no comorbidity (nodes 13, 17, 18, 19); orange, third-line treatment, with comorbidity (nodes 14-16); light green, assessment and evaluation. Levels of evidence used in development of the flowchart were: 1, more than one placebo-controlled trial with sample sizes over 30; 2, one placebo-controlled trial (or active vs active medication comparison) with sample size of 30 or greater; 3, one or small ($n < 30$) placebo-controlled trial; 4, case reports or open-label trials; and 5, expert consensus without published evidence. (AD, antidepressant; AH, antihistamine; BZD, benzodiazepine; CMI, clomipramine; ECT, electroconvulsive therapy; GAD, generalized anxiety disorder; LEV, levetiracetam; NaSSa, noradrenergic and selective serotonergic antidepressant; PST, psychosocial treatment; SAD, social anxiety disorder; SGA, second-generation antipsychotic; SNRI, serotonin-norepinephrine reuptake inhibitor; SRI, serotonin reuptake inhibitor; SSRI, selective serotonin reuptake inhibitor; TCA, tricyclic antidepressant.) *(Reprinted from The International Psychopharmacology Algorithm Project. IPAP–Generalized Anxiety Disorder Algorithm. http://www.ipap.org/gad/index.php. Accessed November 11, 2021.)*

Antidepressant Therapy

3 Antidepressants are considered first-line agents in the management of GAD. Venlafaxine extended-release, duloxetine, paroxetine, and escitalopram are all FDA-approved antidepressants for GAD (see Table 90-5). Imipramine is considered a second-line agent, despite its efficacy, because of higher toxicity and adverse effect rates.[3]

4 The antianxiety response of antidepressants is delayed by 2 to 4 weeks or longer.[3,17] The pharmacology, pharmacokinetics, and medications interactions of the antidepressants are reviewed in Chapter 88, "Depressive Disorders."

Efficacy Antidepressants are effective in the acute and long-term management of GAD. Data support the use of the SSRIs (eg, escitalopram, paroxetine, sertraline), and the serotonin–norepinephrine reuptake inhibitors (SNRIs) (eg, venlafaxine extended-release and duloxetine), for acute therapy (8- to 12-week trials) with response rates between 60% and 68%, and remission rates of approximately 30%.[3,21] Venlafaxine, escitalopram, paroxetine, duloxetine, and quetiapine may be the most likely to achieve remission of GAD symptoms; however, sertraline was the best tolerated.[36]

Mechanism of Action The mechanism of action for antidepressants in anxiety disorders is not fully understood. Antidepressants may modulate receptor activation of neuronal signal transduction pathways connected to the neurotransmitters 5-HT, DA, and NE. In an animal model of anxiety, a number of candidate genes were identified that were normalized by fluoxetine treatment selectively in the hypothalamus.[37] By activating stress-adapting pathways, SSRIs and SNRIs reduce the somatic anxiety symptoms and the general distress experienced by patients.

Adverse Medication Reactions The adverse reactions of medications used to treat anxiety disorders are provided in Table 90-6. In general, SSRIs and SNRIs are well tolerated, with GI adverse medication reactions and sleep disturbances being the most commonly reported. Headaches and diaphoresis occur early in treatment and are often transient, whereas weight gain and sexual dysfunction may continue in long-term treatment. The use of tricyclic antidepressants (TCAs) in clinical practice is limited by troublesome adverse reactions (eg, sedation, anticholinergic effects, and weight gain) in some patients as well as the risk of toxicity in overdose.

Dosing and Administration The antidepressants can be dosed once daily (see Table 90-5). Importantly, most patients require small initial daily doses for the first week or so of therapy to limit the development of transient increased anxiety, also known as jitteriness syndrome. The dose should then be slowly titrated to effect in order to reduce the occurrence of this excess anxiety. Patient education on this particular point in starting medications is critical to assure early treatment discontinuation does not occur, as this increase in anxiety will dissipate with time and a slow titration regimen.

Benzodiazepine Therapy

Although all benzodiazepines possess anxiolytic properties, only seven of the currently marketed agents have FDA approval for the treatment of GAD (see Table 90-4) as estazolam, flurazepam, temazepam, quazepam, and triazolam are marketed as sedative–hypnotic agents. Clonazepam is marketed as an antipanic agent and an antiseizure medication,[38] and midazolam and remimazolam are labeled for preoperative sedation. Alprazolam is indicated for the treatment of panic disorder with or without agoraphobia, as well as GAD.[39] Clobazam is indicated for adjunctive treatment of seizures in Lennox–Gastaut syndrome.[26]

Pharmacology and Mechanism of Action The GABA-receptor model of anxiety theorizes that benzodiazepines ameliorate anxiety through potentiation of the inhibitory activity of GABA.[40] Pharmacologically benzodiazepines bind on the $GABA_A$ receptor at the α_1, α_2, α_3, and α_5 subunits in combination with a β subunit and the γ_2 subunit.[41] The anxiolytic effects of benzodiazepines are mediated at the α_2 site, while sedative effects result from binding at the α_1 subunit. The binding sites of GABA and benzodiazepines are at the receptor interfaces of α/β and α/γ_2, respectively. The GABA receptor controls tonic inhibition to reduce neuronal excitability[40]; however, other neurotransmitters (eg, 5-HT, NE, and DA) may also be involved in benzodiazepine activity.

Pharmacokinetics Wide differences in milligram potency exist between the benzodiazepines; however, when appropriately dosed, all agents have similar anxiolytic and sedative–hypnotic activity. The variations in lipid solubility between compounds influence their pharmacokinetic properties. Knowledge of the different pharmacokinetic and pharmacodynamic properties can assist in choosing an appropriate anxiolytic (Table 90-7). After a single dose, the onset, intensity, and duration of pharmacologic effects are important factors to consider when using benzodiazepines for the short-term, intermittent, or as-needed treatment of anxiety. Knowledge of a medication's pharmacokinetic properties, along with specific factors such as metabolic pathways (including active metabolites), lipophilicity, and protein binding can aid in selecting therapy.

The primary determinant of a medication's onset of effect after a single oral dose is the rate of absorption. Because of high lipophilicity, diazepam and clorazepate are absorbed rapidly and distributed quickly into the CNS. Therefore, the onset of anxiolytic effect occurs within 30 to 60 minutes, which results in a rapid and intense relief of anxiety. High lipophilicity also increases the extent of medication redistribution into the periphery, particularly adipose tissue, resulting in a shorter duration of effect after a single dose than is suggested by single-dose elimination half-life studies.[41] Clinically, patients can perceive a rapid onset of action, or "rush," which can be euphoric and contribute to misuse, while others may experience an unpleasant feeling of drowsiness or loss of control.

Compared with diazepam, lorazepam and oxazepam are relatively less lipophilic and have a slower absorption and onset of effect. These benzodiazepines have smaller volumes of distribution and a resulting longer duration of action.[41]

Parenteral administration via the intramuscular route should be avoided with diazepam secondary to variability in the rate and extent of medication absorption. Intramuscular lorazepam provides rapid, reliable, and complete absorption.

After multiple dosing, the rate and extent of medication accumulation are functions of the medication's elimination half-life in relation to dosing intervals, clearance, and formation of active metabolites. Differences in clinical effects that occur during and after repeated dosages are related in part to variability in metabolism and metabolite accumulation.[41]

The benzodiazepines undergo two primary metabolic processes, hepatic oxidation (catalyzed by mainly cytochrome P450 [CYP] 3A4/5, as well as CYP2C19) and glucuronide conjugation. With the exception of lorazepam and oxazepam (which are conjugated only) and clonazepam (which undergoes nitroreduction through N-acetyltransferase-2 [NAT2]), all benzodiazepines are oxidized first and then conjugated and excreted renally.[42] Diazepam's metabolism specifically is also catalyzed by CYP2C19. Oxidation can be impaired in patients with liver disease, in older adults, and in those who simultaneously use medications that inhibit oxidation resulting in higher levels of the parent medication and/or an active metabolite.

Many benzodiazepines are converted to desmethyldiazepam (DMDZ), an active metabolite with a long elimination half-life (see Table 90-7) which is further oxidized to oxazepam and then conjugated and excreted. After multiple dosing, accumulation of DMDZ occurs, therapeutically providing a long-lasting antianxiety

TABLE 90-6 Monitoring of Adverse Reactions Associated with Medications Used for Anxiety Disorders

Medication Class/ Medication	Adverse Medication Reaction	Monitoring Parameter	Comments
SSRIs			
	Jitteriness syndrome	Patient interview	
	Suicidality	Patient interview	Monitor weekly in first few weeks in patients with comorbid depression and patients under age 25
	Nausea, diarrhea	Patient interview	Typically transient
	Headache	Patient interview	Typically transient
	Weight gain	Body weight, BMI, waist circumference	Paroxetine may be more likely to cause weight gain
	Sexual dysfunction	Patient interview	Significant reason for nonadherence
	Hyponatremia	Basic metabolic panel	Monitor at baseline and periodically thereafter. More frequent monitoring required in high-risk groups, especially older adults (>65 years)
	Thrombocytopenia	Complete blood count	Reported with citalopram
	Teratogenicity	Pregnancy test at baseline	Avoid paroxetine in pregnancy
	QT prolongation	ECG	Before starting citalopram, consider ECG and measurement of QT interval in patients with cardiac disease
	Discontinuation syndrome	Patient interview	Avoid abrupt discontinuation in all but fluoxetine
SNRIs			
	Jitteriness syndrome	Patient interview	
	Suicidality	Patient interview	Monitor weekly in first few weeks in patients with comorbid depression and patients under age 25
	Nausea, diarrhea	Patient interview	Typically transient
	Headache	Patient interview	Typically transient
	Elevated blood pressure	Blood pressure	Monitor blood pressure on initiation and regularly during treatment
	Sexual dysfunction	Patient interview	Significant reason for nonadherence
	Discontinuation syndrome	Patient interview	Avoid abrupt discontinuation
TCAs			
	Jitteriness syndrome	Patient interview	
	Suicidality	Patient interview	Monitor weekly in first few weeks in patients with comorbid depression and patients under age 25
	Anticholinergic effects	Patient interview	Contraindicated with narrow-angle glaucoma, prostatic hypertrophy, and urinary retention
	Weight gain	Body weight, BMI, waist circumference	
	Sexual dysfunction	Patient interview	Significant reason for nonadherence
	Sedation	Patient interview	Administer dosage at bedtime when feasible
	Arrhythmia	ECG	At baseline and periodically in children and patients >40 years of age
	Orthostatic hypotension	Blood pressure with position changes	
	Cholinergic rebound	Patient interview	Avoid abrupt discontinuation; taper doses
Benzodiazepines			
	Drowsiness, fatigue	Patient interview	Avoid operating large machinery; tolerance to sedation develops after repeated dosing
	Anterograde amnesia and memory impairment	Patient interview	Risk of anterograde amnesia is worsened with concomitant intake of alcohol
	Use disorder	Patient interview; prescription monitoring program	Monitor for early refills or escalation of dosage
	Withdrawal symptoms	Physical examination; patient interview	Taper doses on discontinuation
	Respiratory depression	Respiratory rate	Avoid administering with other CNS depressants (ie, opioids, alcohol)
	Psychomotor impairment	Physical examination	Increased risk of falls
	Paradoxical disinhibition	Physical examination; family report	Increase in anxiety, irritability, or agitation may be seen in older adults or children
Other Medications			
Buspirone	Nausea, abdominal pain	Patient interview	Typically transient
	Drowsiness, dizziness	Patient interview	Typically transient

(continued)

TABLE 90-6 Monitoring of Adverse Reactions Associated with Medications Used for Anxiety Disorders ***(Continued)***

Medication Class/ Medication	Adverse Medication Reaction	Monitoring Parameter	Comments
Phenelzine	Jitteriness syndrome	Patient interview	
	Suicidality	Patient interview	Monitor weekly in first few weeks in patients with comorbid depression and patients under age 25
	Hypertensive crisis	Blood pressure	Tyramine-free diet and avoidance of medications interactions required
	Orthostatic hypotension	Blood pressure with position changes	
Pregabalin	Dizziness, somnolence	Patient interview	
	Peripheral edema	Physical examination	
	Thrombocytopenia	Complete blood count	
	Weight gain	Body weight	
Quetiapine	Sedation	Patient interview	
	Metabolic syndrome	Body weight, BMI, waist circumference, fasting lipids and glucose	Fasting labs at baseline and then periodically
	Akathisia	Patient interview	
	Tardive dyskinesia	Abnormal Involuntary Movement Scale	
	Orthostatic hypotension	Blood pressure with position changes	

BMI, body mass index; ECG, electrocardiogram; SNRI, serotonin–norepinephrine reuptake inhibitor; SSRIs, selective serotonin reuptake inhibitors; TCAs, tricyclic antidepressants.

TABLE 90-7 Pharmacokinetics of Benzodiazepine Antianxiety Agents

Medication	Time to Peak Plasma Level (Hours)	Elimination Half-Life, Parent (Hours)	Metabolic Pathway	Clinically Significant Metabolites	Protein Binding (%)
Alprazolam	1-2	12-15	Oxidation	—	80
Chlordiazepoxide	1-4	5-30	*N*-Dealkylation Oxidation	Desmethyl chlordiazepoxide Demoxepam DMDZ[a]	96
Clonazepam	1-4	30-40	Nitroreduction	—	85
Clorazepate	1-2	Promedication	Oxidation	DMDZ	97
Diazepam	0.5-2	20-80	Oxidation	DMDZ Oxazepam	98
Lorazepam	2-4	10-20	Conjugation	—	85
Oxazepam	2-4	5-20	Conjugation	—	97

[a]Desmethyldiazepam (DMDZ) half-life 50-100 hours.

Data from References 26 and 41.

effect. Furthermore, if oxidation of DMDZ is impaired, its half-life is prolonged, and further medication accumulation can result with repeated dosing.

Clorazepate is a promedication and possesses no anxiolytic effects until metabolized to DMDZ. Before absorption, clorazepate is metabolized rapidly in the stomach through a pH-dependent process under acidic conditions.

Benzodiazepines with shorter half-lives (eg, alprazolam, lorazepam, and oxazepam) reach steady-state plasma concentrations rapidly, and accumulation after repeated dosing is minimal. Oxazepam and lorazepam have no active metabolites.

Benzodiazepine protein binding is extensive, especially for the agents with a long elimination half-life. After a single dose of a benzodiazepine with a long elimination half-life, the expected duration of clinical activity may not parallel the medication's pharmacokinetic half-life because of medication redistribution.[41] After multiple dosing, medications with long elimination half-lives and active metabolites require 1 to 2 weeks to reach steady state.

Efficacy In clinical trials of benzodiazepines, 65% to 75% of patients with GAD showed a marked to moderate response, with most of the improvement occurring in the first 2 weeks of therapy.[21,22] Benzodiazepines are more effective on the somatic symptoms of anxiety and fail to obviate the cognitive or psychological symptoms (eg, worry) as mentioned previously.

Adverse Medication Reactions The most common adverse reactions associated with benzodiazepine therapy involve CNS depression (see Table 90-6). This is manifested clinically as drowsiness, sedation, psychomotor impairment, and ataxia.[43] A transient mild drowsiness is experienced commonly by patients during the first few days of treatment; however, tolerance often develops. Disorientation, depression, confusion, irritability, aggression, and excitement are reported.[42]

Impairment of memory and recall also can occur during benzodiazepine treatment. The memory loss induced typically is limited to events occurring after medication ingestion (anterograde amnesia).[42] Anterograde amnesia is secondary to disordered consolidation processes that store information and is not impairment in the perception or retrieval of information.[3] Benzodiazepines with high affinity for binding to the benzodiazepine receptor (eg, alprazolam) appear to possess a higher potential for amnesia.[42]

Physical Dependence, Withdrawal, and Tolerance Two serious complications of benzodiazepine therapy are the potential for unhealthy use and development of physical dependence. Benzodiazepine misuse is rare in the general population; however, individuals with a history of multiple substance use (eg, alcohol or sedatives) are at the greatest risk for developing a sedative, hypnotic, or anxiolytic use disorder.[42]

Because of the chronicity of illness, persons with GAD and panic disorder are at high risk of developing physical dependence to benzodiazepines which is a physiologic phenomenon demonstrated by the appearance of a predictable abstinence syndrome (withdrawal symptoms) on abrupt discontinuation of therapy.[42,43] Withdrawal symptoms can result because of the sudden dissociation of a benzodiazepine from its receptor site. After abrupt discontinuation, an acute decrease in GABA neurotransmission results, producing a less inhibited CNS.

Benzodiazepine Discontinuation After benzodiazepine therapy is discontinued suddenly, several events can occur. Rebound anxiety represents an immediate, but transient return of original symptoms, at an increased intensity compared with baseline. In contrast, anxiety recurrence or relapse is the return of original symptoms with similar intensity as before treatment.

Withdrawal symptoms are the emergence of new symptoms and a worsening of preexisting symptoms after benzodiazepine discontinuation. Symptoms can persist for days to weeks and resolve gradually over months. In some patients it may be difficult to distinguish benzodiazepine withdrawal or rebound symptoms from the recurrence, or relapse of the underlying anxiety disorder.

Common symptoms of benzodiazepine withdrawal include anxiety, insomnia, restlessness, muscle tension, and irritability. Less frequently occurring symptoms are nausea, malaise, coryza, blurred vision, diaphoresis, nightmares, depression, hyperreflexia, and ataxia. Tinnitus, confusion, paranoid delusions, hallucinations, and seizures occur rarely. Withdrawal seizures typically occur approximately 1 week after discontinuation for agents with a long elimination half-life. For agents with a short elimination half-life, withdrawal seizures can occur with both therapeutic and high doses of benzodiazepines use and usually within 3 days of medication discontinuation. Each patient who has abruptly stopped a benzodiazepine or has experienced seizures should be individually approached because high benzodiazepine doses, a long duration of therapy, and concurrent ingestion of substances or medications that lower the seizure threshold are all risk factors.

Furthermore, similar to withdrawal seizures, the onset of generalized withdrawal symptoms in patients ingesting benzodiazepines with short elimination half-lives occurs much earlier (within 24-48 hours) than in those taking benzodiazepines with long elimination half-lives (within 3-8 days). Other factors associated with an increased incidence and severity of benzodiazepine withdrawal include high doses and long-term benzodiazepine therapy.[42,43]

A strategy to minimize the severity of benzodiazepine withdrawal is a 25% dosage reduction per week if therapy had exceeded 8 weeks.[43] The rate can be decreased to 25% every 2 weeks if withdrawal symptoms emerge near the end of the dosage taper. Long-term use of benzodiazepines (ie, 1 year or longer) requires a 2- to 4-month slow taper. Tapering will not eliminate the emergence of withdrawal symptoms entirely but will prevent severe withdrawal. Slow medication taper is extremely important for the medications with a short elimination half-life because some individuals have greater difficulty with discontinuation. Withdrawal symptoms with short half-life benzodiazepines were no more severe than with longer half-life agents; therefore, switching from a short- to long-acting benzodiazepine before gradual taper is not supported. Adjunctive use of pregabalin can help reduce withdrawal severity during the benzodiazepine taper.[44] A combination of psychotherapy interventions (including CBT) with tapering protocols resulted in superior discontinuation outcomes.[45] Patients should avoid the intake of alcohol and stimulants during the withdrawal process. Although tolerance develops to the sedative, muscle relaxant, and antiseizure activities, the benzodiazepines do not appear to lose anxiolytic or antipanic efficacy. However, the anxiolytic efficacy of benzodiazepines in long-term clinical trials (greater than 6-8 months of chronic use) has not been documented.[3,21,22]

Medication Interactions Medication interactions with the benzodiazepines generally fall into two categories: pharmacodynamic and pharmacokinetic. Simultaneous use of alcohol and a benzodiazepine results in additive CNS depressant effects. In addition, concurrent use of a benzodiazepine and other medications/substances with CNS depressant properties (eg, opioids, antipsychotics, and antihistamines) can potentiate the adverse sedative effects. When ingested alone in an overdose attempt, benzodiazepines are rarely life-threatening. However, the combination of benzodiazepines with alcohol or other CNS depressant agents is potentially fatal.

Concurrent use of medications that inhibit CYP3A4 (eg, ketoconazole, nefazodone, and ritonavir) can increase the blood levels of alprazolam and diazepam. Medications that induce cytochrome CYP3A4 (eg, carbamazepine, St. John's wort) can reduce benzodiazepine levels. Medications that inhibit or induce CYP2C19 (eg, fluoxetine, fluvoxamine, omeprazole) or *N*-acetyltransferase 2 activity can alter diazepam and clonazepam metabolism, respectively. Consult a medications interaction website (http://www.factsandcomparisons.com/facts-comparisons-online.aspx) for further information.

Dosing and Administration Benzodiazepine dosage requirements vary widely among patients and must be individualized. Therapy should be initiated using low doses (eg, alprazolam 0.25 mg three times a day or equivalent doses of other benzodiazepines) and titrated upward to relieve anxiety symptoms and avoid adverse events. After an initial treatment response is achieved, agents with long elimination half-lives can be dosed at bedtime. Dosage adjustments should be made weekly. Three to 4 weeks of a daily dose at the maximum dose constitutes an adequate clinical trial (see Table 90-4).[2,21,22]

The duration of benzodiazepine therapy for the acute management of anxiety should be limited to 2 to 4 weeks. In general, benzodiazepines should be used with a regular dosing regimen and not on an as-needed basis when used for the treatment of an anxiety disorder.[3] Only in the treatment of short-term distress (eg, air travel, dental phobia) as-needed use may be justified.[3] Individuals with persistent symptoms should be managed with antidepressants because of the risk of dependence with continued benzodiazepine therapy.

Patient education should include the anticipated length of medication therapy, potential adverse reactions, and consequences of the ingestion of alcohol and other CNS depressants. Patients should understand that benzodiazepines provide symptomatic relief but do not solve underlying psychological problems. Patients should be instructed not to decrease or discontinue benzodiazepine usage without contacting their prescriber.

Buspirone Therapy

Buspirone is a nonbenzodiazepine anxiolytic that lacks antiseizure, muscle relaxant, hypnotic, motor impairment, and physical dependence properties. It is considered to be a second-line agent for GAD because of inconsistent reports of efficacy (particularly long term), delayed onset of effect (ie, 2 weeks or longer), and lack of efficacy for other potential, concurrent, depressive, and anxiety disorders.[2]

Unlike benzodiazepines, buspirone is effective for the psychological symptoms of anxiety.[2]

Pharmacology and Mechanism of Action Buspirone's anxiolytic mechanism of action is unknown. It may exert its anxiolytic effect through partial agonist activity at the 5-HT_{1A} presynaptic receptors, thus reducing the firing of 5-HT neurons.[41]

Pharmacokinetics After an oral dose, buspirone is absorbed rapidly and completely, and undergoes extensive first-pass metabolism. The mean elimination half-life is 2.5 hours, and it must be dosed two to three times daily, which adversely affects medication adherence.[41]

Adverse Medication Reactions Includes dizziness, nausea, and headaches[41] (see Table 90-6).

Interactions Medications that inhibit CYP3A4 (eg, verapamil, itraconazole, fluvoxamine) can increase buspirone levels, and rifampin caused a 10-fold reduction in buspirone levels. Buspirone reportedly elevates blood pressure in patients taking a monoamine oxidase inhibitor (MAOI).

Dosing and Administration The dose of buspirone can be titrated in increments of 5 mg/day every 2 to 3 days as needed.[41] The onset of improvement in psychological symptoms precedes the relief of somatic symptoms; maximum therapeutic benefit might not be evident for 4 to 6 weeks.

Buspirone is a treatment option for patients with GAD, particularly for those with uncomplicated GAD, in patients who fail other anxiolytic therapies, or in patients with SUDs. It is not useful in clinical situations requiring immediate anxiolysis or for situations requiring as-needed anxiolytic therapy.[41] Buspirone may have less efficacy in patients who have previously used benzodiazepines, as it does not provide the same rapid relief of symptoms.[2]

Alternative Medication Treatments

Hydroxyzine, pregabalin, and second-generation antipsychotics (SGAs) are alternative treatments in GAD.[21,27] The effectiveness of hydroxyzine as an antianxiety agent for long-term use (ie, more than 4 months) has not been assessed by systematic clinical studies.[34] Hydroxyzine is commonly used in the primary care setting, but it is considered to be a second-line agent because of adverse medication reactions and lack of efficacy for comorbid disorders.[3] Pregabalin binds to the $\alpha_2\delta$ subunit of voltage-gated calcium channels to reduce nerve terminal calcium influx and acts on "hyperexcited" neurons. The anxiolytic effects produced by pregabalin compare to lorazepam and alprazolam with fewer dropouts in acute efficacy trials.[46] Quetiapine extended-release 150 mg/day monotherapy was superior to placebo in three studies and was as effective as paroxetine 20 mg/day and escitalopram 10 mg/day but with an earlier onset of action.[27] In a 52-week treatment of GAD, quetiapine extended-release was superior to placebo in the prevention of anxiety relapse.[27] Notably, quetiapine is not FDA-approved for GAD, and the long-term risks and benefits of SGAs in the treatment of GAD are unclear.[27] Despite some evidence of efficacy, support for the use of kava kava for GAD has been blunted by ongoing safety concerns following numerous reports of liver toxicity.[47] Although valerian, St. John's wort, and passionflower have been used to manage GAD, there is insufficient evidence of their effectiveness and safety.[47]

Special Populations

The management of anxiety in patients with SUDs, pregnant individuals, children, older adult patients, and those patients with adherence problems requires special consideration in the choice of anxiolytic. Patients with GAD may use alcohol, cannabis, or other substances to manage anxiety. The symptoms of GAD are similar to those of withdrawal, and it is difficult to confirm the diagnosis of GAD until after abstinence is obtained; therefore, benzodiazepine therapy should be avoided in this population if possible.

Pregnancy Anxiety that occurs during pregnancy and the postpartum period potentially may pose significant risk to the child. Clinical practice guidelines for anxiety disorders recommend use of fluoxetine, sertraline, or citalopram; however, jitteriness, myoclonus, and irritability in the neonate and premature infant have been reported.[48] Paroxetine should be avoided in pregnant individuals because of risk of cardiovascular malformations.[30]

Cleft lip, cleft palate, and other teratogenic effects are associated with benzodiazepine use, but a causal relationship is inconclusive. Clinicians should avoid benzodiazepine use during the first trimester or using the agent as monotherapy. In addition, efforts should be made to use the lowest dosage for the shortest period of time and divide the total daily dosage into two or three doses to prevent high peak plasma levels.[48] Benzodiazepine risks for the child during the third trimester include sedation, withdrawal symptoms, and "floppy baby syndrome" (eg, hypotonia, low Apgar scores, hypothermia). Alprazolam should be avoided during pregnancy because of neonatal withdrawal. Should benzodiazepines be required during pregnancy, the preferred agents are diazepam and chlordiazepoxide[49]; however, the antidepressants are favored for GAD during pregnancy based on safety considerations. Diazepam and clonazepam should not be used by individuals providing human milk to infants due to risk of sedation, lethargy, and weight loss seen for the child.[49]

Children and Adolescents There are few controlled clinical trials of medications in children and adolescents with GAD. Use of CBT alone or in conjunction with antidepressants can have long-term benefits.[50] Randomized controlled trials of fluvoxamine, fluoxetine, sertraline, duloxetine, and venlafaxine extended-release indicate short-term efficacy[50]; however, irritability and oppositional behavior was reported with clonazepam.[50] No antidepressant is FDA-indicated for GAD in children or adolescents. Increased monitoring for behavioral changes with benzodiazepines and suicide-related adverse effects with antidepressants is necessary if these agents are prescribed.

Hepatic Disease and Older Adult Patients Patients with hepatic disease are at risk for medication accumulation and subsequent complications. In particular, duloxetine use should be avoided in patients with hepatic insufficiency.[28] Accumulation of benzodiazepines can result in older adults secondary to a decreased capacity for oxidation and alterations in the volume of distribution. Therefore, intermediate- or short-acting benzodiazepines without active metabolites are preferred for chronic use. Older adult patients are also sensitive to the CNS adverse medication reactions of benzodiazepines (regardless of half-life), and their use is associated with a high frequency of falls and hip fractures. Recent studies of buspirone, duloxetine, escitalopram, sertraline, venlafaxine, and pregabalin showed efficacy in older adult patients with GAD.[2,51,52]

Evaluation of Therapeutic Outcomes

Initially, patients with GAD should be monitored once every 2 weeks for a reduction in the frequency, duration, and severity of anxiety symptoms and improvement in functioning.[2] The clinician should assess the patient for response to treatment by asking about specific target symptoms of anxiety and emergence of adverse events. Ideally, the patient should have no or minimal anxiety or depressive symptoms and no functional impairment. Use of an objective measurement of remission of GAD (eg, Hamilton Rating Scale for Anxiety score less than or equal to 7 and a Sheehan Disability Scale score less than or equal to 1 on each item) can assist in the evaluation of medication response.[2] The Generalized Anxiety Disorder 7-Item Scale is a patient-rated scale that can be used for screening and monitoring improvement of symptoms.[23] See Chapter e81, "Evaluation of Psychiatric Illness" for more information about assessments for anxiety disorders.

The definition of treatment resistance is defined as a poor, partial, or lack of response with at least two antidepressants from different classes. Treatment strategies for patients who do not achieve an appropriate response with a first-line agent include increasing the dose of the SSRI/SNRI, changing to a different agent in the same class, changing to a different agent from a different class, or augmentation of therapy. At any point of nonresponse or loss of previous response, the clinician should assess for (a) symptoms (eg, psychotic symptoms) that may suggest a need for additional medications or (b) reasons for treatment nonadherence (eg, adverse medication reactions, cost of medications, limited understanding of the illness or treatments). Patients should also be assessed for concurrent SUD, concurrent illnesses, and suicidal thoughts. Once a patient has responded to pharmacotherapy, the regimen should be continued for at least 1 year.[22,35] Early discontinuation is associated with a greater risk of relapse.[22]

TREATMENT—PANIC DISORDER

Desired Outcomes

The goal of therapy in panic disorder is remission. Patients should be free of panic attacks, have no or minimal anticipatory anxiety and agoraphobic avoidance, and have no functional impairment.[20]

General Approach

Therapeutic options include single or combined pharmacologic agents, concurrent psychotherapy, or psychotherapy followed by pharmacotherapy. Most patients without agoraphobic avoidance will improve with pharmacotherapy alone; however, if avoidance is present, CBT is typically initiated concurrently. With all effective pharmacotherapy, resolution of agoraphobic avoidance tends to occur slowly. A meta-analysis comparing the use of SSRIs and venlafaxine in panic disorder showed response to be similar among treatments.[53] Adding psychosocial treatment to pharmacotherapy may improve long-term outcomes by reducing the likelihood of relapse when pharmacotherapy is stopped.[20]

Considerations that guide selection of the treatment modality for panic disorder include patient preference, treatment history, the presence of co-occurring medical or other psychiatric conditions, cost, and treatment availability. Psychosocial treatment in the form of CBT is recommended for patients who prefer nonpharmacologic therapy and who are able to invest the effort and time to attend weekly sessions and between-session homework exercises. Pharmacotherapy with a first-line agent is recommended for patients who prefer medications or who do not have access to or resources to engage in CBT. Combination with psychotherapy and pharmacotherapy is appropriate for patients who have failed monotherapy with medication or CBT.

Providing education about the disorder may relieve some of the symptoms of panic by helping the patient to realize that the symptoms are neither life-threatening nor uncommon. Patients should be informed regarding the lag time before a therapeutic response will occur and any problematic adverse medication reactions that might affect early adherence or result in premature treatment discontinuation (eg, jitteriness syndrome). Many patients are reluctant to take medications for fear that their illness will worsen or that they will become physically dependent. Adverse events are often perceived as a worsening of the illness and can contribute to nonadherence or prevent necessary dosage increases. A strong therapeutic alliance between the clinician and the patient is important in supporting the patient through the aspects of the treatment that may provoke anxiety.

Nonpharmacologic Therapy

Patients should be educated to avoid agents that can precipitate panic attacks, including caffeine, nicotine, alcohol, other substances, and nonprescription stimulants.[1,20] Daily smoking increases risk for panic attacks and may be a causal or exacerbating factor in some individuals with panic disorder.[20] Aerobic exercise (eg, walking for 60 minutes or running for 20-30 minutes 4 day/week) may benefit patients with panic disorder.[22] Participation in CBT is associated with short-term improvement in 80% to 90% of patients and 6-month improvement in 75% of patients. A CBT course for panic disorder is 16 to 20 hours in length conducted over a period of 4 months.[22] Bibliotherapy (the use of self-help books), exercise, and Internet-based CBT are other options.[20]

Pharmacologic Therapy

Panic disorder is treated effectively with several medications including SSRIs, the SNRI venlafaxine, imipramine, and the benzodiazepines alprazolam and clonazepam[20,22] (Table 90-8). Alprazolam, clonazepam, fluoxetine, paroxetine, sertraline, and venlafaxine are all approved for this indication. In general, SSRIs are the first-line agents because of their tolerability and efficacy in acute and long-term studies[2,20]; however, the benzodiazepines are the most commonly used medications for panic disorder.[20] In a meta-analysis of the pharmacotherapy of panic disorder, the following antidepressants were significantly superior to placebo with the following *increasing* order of effectiveness: citalopram, sertraline, paroxetine, fluoxetine, and venlafaxine for panic symptoms and paroxetine, fluoxetine, fluvoxamine, citalopram, venlafaxine, and mirtazapine for overall anxiety symptoms.[53] Imipramine is effective for panic disorder; however, it is considered to be a second-line agent because of the significant cardiovascular and anticholinergic adverse medication reactions associated with its use. Five practice guidelines are published,[2,3,20-22] and Fig. 90-2 is an algorithm for the pharmacologic therapy of panic disorder.

Benzodiazepines are considered second-line agents, and because of the risk of physical dependence should be used only after several trials of antidepressants have failed.[2,20] Additionally because of the potential emergence of depressive symptoms during treatment, benzodiazepines should not be used as monotherapy in a patient who is clinically depressed or has a history of depression. The short-term (4-6 weeks) addition of alprazolam or clonazepam to antidepressants may produce a more rapid therapeutic response, with discontinuation of the benzodiazepine by week 7 of therapy.[2] However, in patients whose illness is complicated by a history of alcohol or unhealthy substance use, benzodiazepine use should be avoided.[20]

Selective Serotonin Reuptake Inhibitors

5 **Efficacy** All SSRIs may be effective in panic disorder.[20] The percentage of patients who become panic-free ranges between 60% and 80%.[20] The antipanic effect of SSRIs is delayed for at least 4 weeks, and some patients do not respond for 8 to 12 weeks.[20]

Adverse Medication Reactions Typical antidepressant doses of SSRIs can cause insomnia, jitteriness, restlessness, and agitation, and lead to medication discontinuation in patients with panic disorder, similar to the effects previously described. Table 90-6 includes additional adverse medication reactions associated with SSRI use in panic disorder.

Dosing and Administration Low initial doses of SSRIs are recommended (see Table 90-8) to avoid stimulatory adverse medication reactions (eg, insomnia or nervousness), and should be maintained for the first week of therapy. However, doses at the upper end of the dosing range can be necessary to achieve response after careful titration.[22,54]

Serotonin–Norepinephrine Reuptake Inhibitors

Efficacy Venlafaxine extended-release 75 to 150 mg/day is superior to placebo in the proportion of patients becoming free from full-symptom panic attacks. Other data support the efficacy of venlafaxine in reducing the severity of anticipatory anxiety, fear,

TABLE 90-8 Medications Used in the Treatment of Panic Disorder

Class/Generic Name	Brand Name	Starting Dose	Antipanic Dosage Range (mg)	Comments
SSRIs				
Citalopram	Celexa	10 mg/day	20-40	Dosage used in clinical trials; maximum dose limited by QT prolongation; available generically
Escitalopram	Lexapro	5 mg/day	10-20	Dosage used in clinical trials; available generically
Fluoxetine	Prozac	5 mg/day	10-30	Available generically
Fluvoxamine	Luvox	25 mg/day	100-300	Available generically
Paroxetine	Paxil	10 mg/day	20-60	FDA-approved; available generically
	Pexeva			
	Paxil CR	12.5 mg/day	25-75	
Sertraline	Zoloft	25 mg/day	50-200	FDA-approved; available generically
SNRI				
Venlafaxine XR	Effexor XR	37.5 mg/day	75-225	FDA-approved; available generically
Benzodiazepines				
Alprazolam	Xanax	0.25 mg three times a day	4-10	FDA-approved; available generically
	Xanax XR	0.5-1 mg/day	1-10	
Clonazepam	Klonopin	0.25 mg once or twice per day	1-4	FDA-approved; available generically
Diazepam	Valium	2-5 mg three times a day	5-20	Dosage used in clinical trials; available generically
Lorazepam	Ativan	0.5-1 mg three times a day	2-8	Dosage used in clinical trials; available generically
TCA				
Imipramine	Tofranil	10 mg/day	75-250	Dosage used in clinical trials; available generically
MAOI				
Phenelzine	Nardil	15 mg/day	45-90	Dosage used in clinical trials; available generically

CR, controlled release; MAOI, monoamine oxidase inhibitor; SNRI, serotonin–norepinephrine reuptake inhibitor; SSRIs, selective serotonin reuptake inhibitors; TCA, tricyclic antidepressant; XR, extended-release.

Data from References 3, 20, and 54.

and avoidance.[54] Venlafaxine is similar in efficacy to paroxetine in patients with panic disorder and superior to placebo in a relapse prevention study.[54]

Adverse Medication Reactions The most common for venlafaxine extended-release in clinical trials of panic disorder were nausea, dry mouth, constipation, anorexia, insomnia, somnolence, tremors, sweating, and sexual dysfunction.[20]

Dosing and Administration The dosage of venlafaxine extended-release is 37.5 mg/day for the first 3 to 7 days, and then increased to a minimum of 75 mg/day (Table 90-8). Increasing the dose to 150 mg/day after initial nonresponse or partial response is recommended. A dose-response relationship was not evident in clinical trials.[31]

Tricyclic Antidepressants

Efficacy Imipramine is the most studied TCA, alleviating panic attacks in 75% of patients. It effectively blocks panic attacks within at least 4 weeks. However, maximal improvement (including antiphobic response) does not occur until 8 to 12 weeks.[20]

Adverse Medication Reactions See Table 90-6. Up to 40% of patients experience stimulant-like effects, including anxiety, insomnia, and jitteriness.[20] These adverse medication reactions often affect patient adherence, result in premature treatment discontinuation, prevent medication dosage increases, and interfere with the overall treatment outcome.

Other problems with TCA use in panic disorder are well documented and include anticholinergic effects, orthostatic hypotension, delayed onset of antipanic effects, and toxicity in overdose.[20] Approximately 25% of patients reportedly discontinue treatment because of adverse medication reactions especially weight gain.[20]

Dosing and Administration When using imipramine, treatment should be slowly increased by 10 mg every 2 to 4 days as tolerated (Table 90-8).

Benzodiazepines

Efficacy The high-potency benzodiazepines clonazepam and alprazolam are the preferred agents for the treatment of panic disorder.[20,22] Alprazolam provides rapid relief for patients in distress, but because of its short half-life, multiple daily dosing is required and often results in profound withdrawal symptoms with missed doses.[20] Additionally diazepam and lorazepam, when taken in sufficiently high doses, are possibly effective in treating panic disorder.[20] Therapeutic response to benzodiazepines occurs in 1 to 2 weeks, and relapse rates of 50% or higher are common despite slow medication tapering during discontinuation of therapy.[43]

Adverse Medication Reactions Patient acceptance of benzodiazepines is usually not a problem, and except for sedation, adverse medication reactions are rarely reported (see Table 90-6).

Dosing and Administration Doses of clonazepam can be increased by 0.25 or 0.5 mg every 3 days to 4 mg/day if needed,[39] and alprazolam can be slowly increased over several weeks to reach an ideal dose. The duration of action of immediate-release alprazolam can be as little as 4 to 6 hours which may result in breakthrough symptoms; use of the extended-release alprazolam or clonazepam will avoid this problem. Most patients require 3 to 6 mg/day of

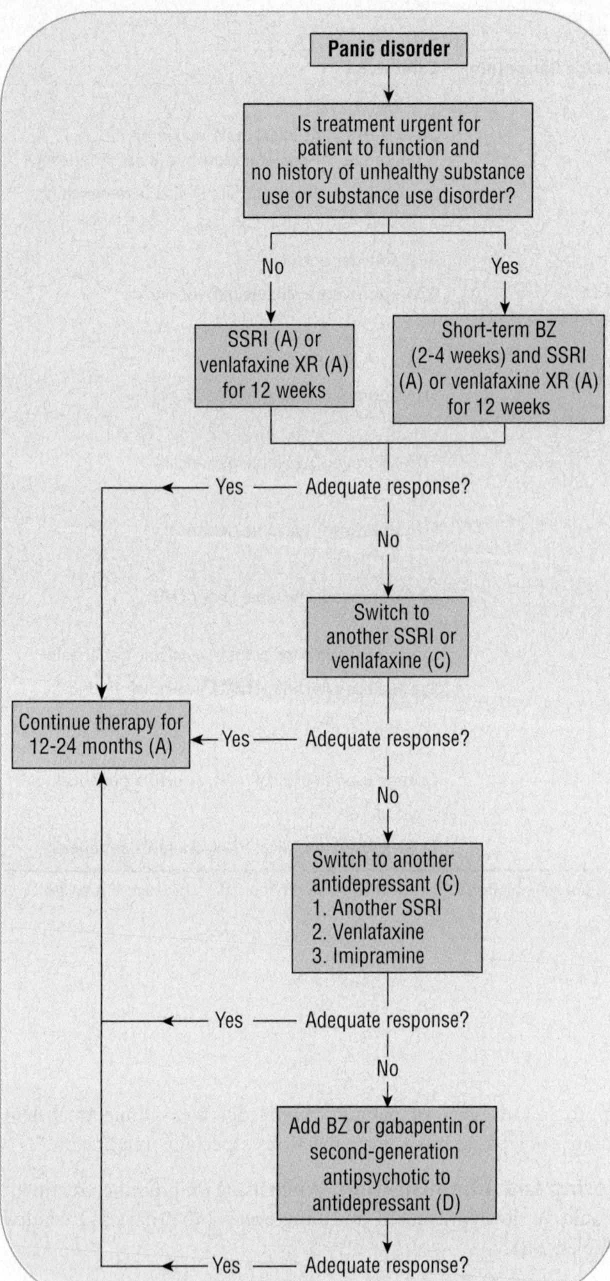

FIGURE 90-2 Algorithm for the pharmacotherapy of panic disorder. Strength of recommendations: A, directly based on category I evidence (ie, meta-analysis of randomized controlled trials [RCT] or at least one RCT); C, directly based on category III evidence (ie, nonexperimental descriptive studies); D, directly based on category IV evidence (ie, expert committee reports or opinions and/or clinical experience of respected authorities). (BZ, benzodiazepine; SSRI, selective serotonin reuptake inhibitor.) *(Adapted from References 20 and 22.)*

alprazolam, and some need higher doses to obtain a full therapeutic (antipanic and antiphobic) response.

Alternative Medication Treatments

Buspirone, trazodone, bupropion, antipsychotics, antihistamines, and β-blockers are ineffective in panic disorder.[2,3,20-22] The majority of studies assessing the efficacy of MAOIs in treating panic disorder were open-labeled and lacked adequate sample sizes. Therefore, MAOIs are reserved for the most refractory or difficult patients.[20]

Phases of Therapy

Acute Phase The main goal of therapy in the acute phase is reduction of symptoms (eg, resolution of panic attacks, reduction in anxiety and phobic fears, resumption of the patient's usual activities).[20,21] The duration of this phase is generally 1 to 3 months depending on the choice of medication. Therapy should be altered if there is no response after 6 to 8 weeks of an adequate dose.

The guiding principle for SSRIs and SNRIs in panic disorder is to start with low doses (approximately one-fourth to one-half of the starting doses for depression), use an adequate dose, and treat for about 12 weeks.[20,21] Adverse medication reactions often from too high an initial dose, can prevent achievement of an optimal dosage, compromise treatment response, contribute to patient nonadherence, and lead to premature treatment discontinuation.

The duration of the acute phase with benzodiazepines is approximately 1 month because response is rapid. A regular dosing schedule rather than an "as-needed" schedule is preferred for patients with panic disorder who are taking benzodiazepines, where the goal is to prevent panic attacks rather than reduce symptoms once an attack has already occurred.[20]

Maintenance Phase and Discontinuation 6 The optimal length of therapy is unknown; however, the total duration of therapy appears to be 12 to 24 months before medication discontinuation over 4 to 6 months is attempted.[20] The dose used in the acute phase is continued into the maintenance phase.[20] When medications are discontinued too early, a high rate of relapse occurs; thus, longer periods of treatment are associated with a more sustained response. Reinstitution of medication usually results in renewed clinical response.[20] Pharmacotherapy, even of a long duration, might not prevent relapse, and many patients require long-term maintenance therapy.

The most important determinant of adherence with maintenance therapy is the tolerability of adverse events.[20] Some adverse events that are experienced short term become unbearable during long-term management (eg, sexual dysfunction and weight gain). All TCAs, SSRIs (except fluoxetine), and venlafaxine can be associated with discontinuation symptoms, which can present as flu-like symptoms.

The primary risk of long-term benzodiazepine use is the development of physical dependence and withdrawal symptoms upon discontinuation. Misuse of benzodiazepines usually is confined to patients with a personal or family history of substance or alcohol use disorders.[43,44] The approach to benzodiazepine discontinuation involves a slow and gradual tapering of the dose because withdrawal symptoms and rebound anxiety may occur during discontinuation. Benzodiazepines should be tapered very slowly in patients with panic disorder over 2 to 4 months at rates no higher than 10% of the dose per week.[20,43] Patients receiving benzodiazepines and antidepressants should be told not to decrease or discontinue therapy unless authorized by their clinician.[20]

Treatment Refractory Symptoms

Common reasons for nonresponse to treatment are comorbid psychiatric disorders, rapid dosage increases with resulting intolerable adverse medication reactions and underdosage.[20] All standard treatments should be tried before using augmentation strategies. In patients with a partial response to one agent, a low dose of another antipanic agent (eg, a TCA, benzodiazepine, or an SSRI) can be added.[20]

Special Populations

Older adult patients with panic disorder have fewer, less intense symptoms and avoidant behavior than younger patients.[20] Youth often present with fear that they are dying or being smothered, and agoraphobia can be manifested as a fear of leaving home.[1] Overall, CBT is effective in both populations. If pharmacotherapy is used, antidepressants, especially the SSRIs, are preferred for management of panic disorder, and benzodiazepines are second-line agents because of potential problems with disinhibition in these two populations. The course of panic disorder may be highly variable during pregnancy and the postpartum period. It is unclear whether uncontrolled symptoms of panic disorder affect the course or outcome of pregnancy.[20] Little evidence exists on the use of psychosocial interventions for individuals with panic disorder who are pregnant, lactating, or planning to become pregnant. Nonpharmacologic interventions should be considered as first-line treatment in these patients. Pharmacotherapy may also be indicated but requires careful evaluation of the potential benefits and risks.[20]

EVALUATION OF THERAPEUTIC OUTCOMES

During the first few weeks of the acute phase of therapy, patients with panic disorder should be seen every 1 to 2 weeks when starting a new medication, and then every 2 to 4 weeks to adjust medication dosages based on improvement in panic symptoms and to monitor for adverse events.[20,22] After the dose is stabilized and symptoms have decreased, visits every 2 months should suffice.[21] The patient should be counseled to maintain a diary to record the date, time, frequency, duration, and intensity of panic episodes, level of anticipatory anxiety or agoraphobic avoidance, and the severity of distress and impairment related to the panic disorder. Treatment outcomes can be assessed objectively by use of the Panic Disorder Severity Scale. Remission is defined as equal to or less than 3 with no or mild agoraphobic avoidance, anxiety, disability, or depressive symptoms. Treatment response is indicated by a 40% or greater reduction in overall score.[2]

At scheduled visits, the clinician can inquire about the level of disability experienced by the patient and have the patient complete the Sheehan Disability Scale (with a goal of less than or equal to 1 point on each item). See Chapter e81 for additional assessments that can be used to evaluate therapeutic outcomes for anxiety disorders. During medication discontinuation, the frequency of appointments should be increased to evaluate for emergence of potential withdrawal symptoms and monitor for relapse.

TREATMENT—SOCIAL ANXIETY DISORDER

Desired Outcomes

The goals of therapy in the acute phase of treatment are to reduce physiologic symptoms of anxiety (eg, tachycardia, flushing, and sweating), social anxiety, and phobic avoidance. The duration of this phase is 4 to 12 weeks, depending on the medication therapy.

The goals of therapy in the continuation phase (3-6 months) are to extend the therapeutic benefits, especially the patient's ability to participate in social activities, and improve QOL. Although the primary goal of treatment is to reduce anxiety symptoms to manageable levels, even modest reductions in avoidance and discomfort can be highly valued by patients.[18]

7 At least a 6- to 12-month medication maintenance period is recommended to maintain improvement and decrease the rate of relapse.[2,3,21] Situations suggesting a possible need for long-term treatment include the presence of unresolved symptoms or comorbidity, an early onset of disease, and a prior history of relapse.[18] The long-term goal in the treatment of SAD is remission with the disappearance of the core symptoms of social anxiety, little or no anxiety, and no functional impairment or concurrent depressive symptoms.[18,55]

General Approach

Patients with SAD should be identified early and treated aggressively.[18] Obstacles to effective treatment include patient avoidance of therapy secondary to fear and shame, treatment directed toward somatic symptoms or concurrent conditions, and financial barriers.[18] Patients with SAD often respond more slowly and less completely than patients with other anxiety disorders. Therefore, it is important to set reasonable expectations for response to therapy. Consideration of current symptoms, prior treatments, concurrent conditions, and history of SUD guides treatment selection.

Both CBT and pharmacotherapy are effective in the treatment of SAD.[2,18,55,56] Pharmacotherapy is often the most practical choice because CBT might not be available in medically underserved areas. Acute treatment outcomes for CBT and pharmacotherapy are equivalent.[2,3,18] Pharmacotherapy is superior in reducing subjective general anxiety acutely, although CBT has a greater likelihood of maintaining response after termination.[18,55,56]

There are no data to predict which patients will respond best to pharmacotherapy, CBT, or a combination, or maintain gains after discontinuing pharmacotherapy. The only significant indication of treatment response in pharmacotherapy is duration of treatment.[55-58] Some patients elect lifelong therapy, and many are reluctant to attempt medication discontinuation because of fear of relapse.

Despite the availability of effective treatments for social anxiety, most adults in the United States with social anxiety do not receive mental health care for their symptoms. Often the symptoms that patients desire to relieve interfere with the ability to seek treatment. Patients often feel embarrassed of what others might think or say about them. It is important to develop an alliance with the patient and offer reassurance throughout the treatment process.

Certain complications may influence the choice of first-line pharmacotherapy. Comorbid depression or suicidal ideation requires careful evaluation and close monitoring. Patients with comorbid SUD on presentation may require postponing pharmacotherapy until after detoxification and avoidance of use of benzodiazepines as part of treatment.

Patient-specific education about treatment is important. Patients should be instructed about the gradual onset of effect, when to expect full therapeutic benefit, and that long-term therapy is required. When pharmacotherapy is discontinued, the dosage needs to be gradually decreased over several months, and the patient should be seen more frequently to monitor for signs and symptoms of relapse or withdrawal.

Although pharmacotherapy usually leads to improvement in social and occupational functioning, most patients do not achieve a full remission. Many patients require additional treatment, often in the form of CBT.

Nonpharmacologic Therapy

Patients should be educated about SAD and support groups. Self-help group programs that focus on effective communication can benefit people with anxiety involving public speaking. The peer-to-peer support groups provided by NAMI can be another resource for patients with SAD.

In general, CBT consists of exposure therapy, cognitive restructuring, relaxation training techniques, and social skills training.[2,3,18,21,56] Through CBT, patients learn to overcome anxiety in social situations and alter the beliefs and responses that maintain this anxiety, with therapy usually lasting several months and is often conducted in groups.[18,57]

Pharmacologic Therapy

Antidepressant Therapy

8 The SSRIs and venlafaxine are beneficial for patients with concurrent depression and are safe when used in patients with an SUD. Paroxetine, sertraline, fluvoxamine extended-release, and venlafaxine extended-release are approved for the treatment of SAD and are considered first-line agents because of efficacy and tolerability (Table 90-9). Controlled trials comparing different

TABLE 90-9 Medications Used in the Treatment of Social Anxiety Disorder

Medication	Brand Name	Initial Dose	Usual Range (mg/day)	Comments
SSRIs				
Citalopram	Celexa	20 mg/day	20-40	Dosage used in clinical trials; maximum dose of 40 mg limited by QT prolongation; available generically
Escitalopram	Lexapro	5 mg/day	10-20	Dosage used in clinical trials; available generically
Fluvoxamine CR	Luvox CR	100 mg	100-300	FDA-approved; available generically
Paroxetine	Paxil	10 mg/day	10-60	FDA-approved; available generically
Paroxetine CR	Paxil CR	12.5 mg/day	12.5-37.5	FDA-approved; available generically
Sertraline	Zoloft	25-50 mg/day	50-200	FDA-approved; available generically
SNRI				
Venlafaxine XR	Effexor XR	75 mg/day	75-225	FDA-approved; available generically
Benzodiazepine				
Clonazepam	Klonopin	0.25 mg/day	1-4	Dosage used in clinical trials; used as augmenting agent; available generically
MAOI				
Phenelzine	Nardil	15 mg at bedtime	60-90	Dosage used in clinical trials; available generically
Alternative Agents				
Buspirone	BuSpar	10 mg twice per day	45-60	Dosage used in clinical trials; used as augmenting agent; available generically
Gabapentin	Neurontin	100 mg three times a day	900-3,600	Dosage used in clinical trials; dosage adjustment required in renal impairment; available generically
Pregabalin	Lyrica	100 mg three times a day	600	Dosage used in clinical trials; dosage adjustment required in renal impairment; available generically
Quetiapine	Seroquel	25 mg at bedtime	25-400	Dosage used in clinical trials; available generically

CR, controlled-release; MAOI, monoamine oxidase inhibitor; SNRI, serotonin–norepinephrine reuptake inhibitor; SSRIs, selective serotonin reuptake inhibitors; XR, extended-release.

Data from References 2, 3, 21, 29, and 55.

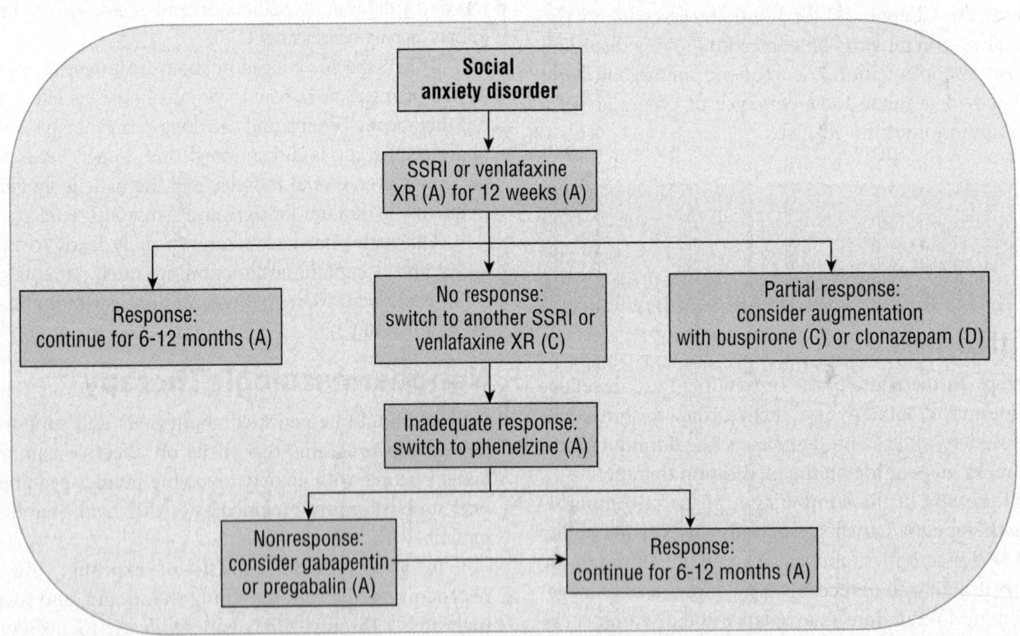

FIGURE 90-3 Algorithm for the pharmacotherapy of social anxiety disorder. Strength of recommendations: A, directly based on category I evidence (ie, meta-analysis of randomized controlled trials [RCT] or at least one RCT); C, directly based on category III evidence (ie, nonexperimental descriptive studies); D, directly based on category IV evidence (ie, expert committee reports or opinions and/or clinical experience of respected authorities). SSRI, selective serotonin reuptake inhibitor. *(Adapted from References 2, 3, 21, and 55.)*

SSRIs, or SSRIs and an SNRI, demonstrated equivalent efficacy between agents.[55-57] The TCAs are not effective in SAD.[2,21] Evidence-based guidelines for the treatment of SAD were published by the Canadian Psychiatric Association, World Federation of Societies of Biological Psychiatry, the National Institute for Health and Care Excellence, and the British Association for Psychopharmacology.[2,3,18,21] An algorithm for the pharmacotherapy of SAD appears in Fig. 90-3.

Selective Serotonin Reuptake Inhibitors

Efficacy Large trials of escitalopram, fluvoxamine (immediate- and controlled-release), paroxetine, sertraline, and venlafaxine extended-release have shown efficacy and tolerability. Results of studies with fluoxetine have been inconsistent. The onset of effect with SSRIs is delayed 4 to 8 weeks, and maximum benefit is often not observed until 12 weeks or longer. Large relapse prevention trials with escitalopram, paroxetine, and sertraline demonstrated relapse rates of 4% to 14% with continued medication treatment, compared with 36% to 39% with placebo.[55,57]

Dosing and Administration The SSRIs should be initiated at doses similar to those used for the treatment of depression and administered as a single daily dose (see Table 90-9). If the patient suffers from comorbid panic disorder, the SSRI dose should be started at one-fourth or one-half of the dose. The dose-response curve for SSRIs tends to be relatively flat, but individual patients can require higher doses. Increase the dose as tolerated in patients who have not responded after 4 weeks of therapy.[55-58] When discontinuing an SSRI, the dosage should be tapered monthly (ie, decreasing sertraline by 50 mg or paroxetine by 10 mg) to reduce the risk of relapse and discontinuation symptoms.

Venlafaxine

Efficacy The efficacy of venlafaxine extended-release was established in four double-blind, parallel-group, 12-week, multicenter, placebo-controlled, flexible-dose studies and one double-blind, parallel-group, 6-month, placebo-controlled, fixed/flexible-dose study.[31] Efficacy was assessed with the Liebowitz Social Anxiety Scale (LSAS). In these five trials, venlafaxine extended-release was significantly more effective than placebo on change from baseline to end point on the LSAS total score.[31]

Adverse Medication Reactions Include anorexia, dry mouth, nausea, insomnia, and sexual dysfunction (see Table 90-6).

Dosing and Administration Additional therapeutic benefits of venlafaxine extended-release above 75 mg/day have not been shown.[31] Venlafaxine should be tapered slowly (ie, decreasing by 37.5 mg/month) to decrease the risk of relapse during discontinuation.

Alternative Agents

Benzodiazepines Benzodiazepines are commonly used in the treatment of patients who cannot tolerate or fail to respond to antidepressants. They are not considered first-line therapy for SAD because of concerns over the adverse medication reactions potential for physical dependence, the possibility of rebound anxiety, and ineffectiveness in the treatment of depression. Clonazepam is the most extensively studied benzodiazepine for the treatment of generalized SAD.[55-58]

If clonazepam is prescribed, the acute phase of therapy is about 1 month. Patients should be instructed not to decrease or discontinue clonazepam without consulting their clinician because of the risks of rebound anxiety and withdrawal symptoms. Clonazepam should be gradually tapered at a rate not to exceed 0.25 mg every 2 weeks.

Antiseizure Medications Gabapentin and pregabalin were effective in controlled trials, whereas levetiracetam was ineffective.[55-59]

β-Blockers β-Blockers decrease the perception of anxiety by blunting the peripheral autonomic symptoms of arousal (eg, rapid heart rate, sweating, blushing, and tremor), and they are often used to decrease anxiety in performance-related situations.[55] For patients with performance anxiety, 10 to 80 mg of propranolol or 25 to 100 mg of atenolol can be taken 1 hour before a performance as needed. A test dose should be taken at home before the presentation to assure that β-blockade is sufficient and there are no adverse events. Controlled trials with β-blockers do not support daily use in SAD.[18]

Treatment Refractory Symptoms

9 An adequate antidepressant trial usually consists of 8 to 12 weeks (at maximum dosages).[55-58] Subsequent options include a trial of a second SSRI or venlafaxine extended-release. Some patients experience clinical benefit during the first 4 weeks of therapy.[55-58] If nonresponsiveness continues, a trial of an alternative agent is warranted.

There are little data on the choice of treatments if there is a partial response to antidepressant therapy in SAD. Published studies offer preliminary support for the combination of an SSRI with a benzodiazepine, gabapentin, or pregabalin.[55-58]

Second-generation antipsychotics and MAOIs are options in treatment-resistant SAD. Quetiapine monotherapy showed a large effect size on the Social Phobia Inventory when compared with placebo.[55-58] Although phenelzine is effective in 77% of patients with SAD,[2,18] dietary restrictions, potential interactions, and adverse medication reactions (eg, weight gain and hypertensive crisis) have limited its use. If a patient is switched from another antidepressant to phenelzine, an appropriate washout period should be followed. See Chapter 88 for more detail.

Special Populations

SAD can present in children of preschool to elementary school age. If the disorder is not treated, it can persist into adulthood and increase the risk of depression and SUD. Both CBT and social skills training are effective nonpharmacologic therapies in children.[55-58] Placebo-controlled and open-label trials have provided evidence of efficacy of pharmacotherapy with an SSRI or SNRI in children between ages 6 and 17 years.[2,18,55-58] Children and adolescents prescribed an SSRI or SNRI for social anxiety (or for other purposes) should be closely monitored for increased risk of suicidal ideation. Headache, nausea, drowsiness, insomnia, jitteriness, and stomachaches were reported in children receiving antidepressants.[55-58]

Benzodiazepines should be reserved as the last-line agents in children with SAD.[18,50] If prescribed, they should be used for the shortest time period possible. The adverse medication reactions of benzodiazepines in children include drowsiness, oppositional behavior, disinhibition, and fatigue.

Approximately one-fifth of patients with SAD also suffer from an alcohol use disorder, as many people with SAD report that they use alcohol to cope with anxiety. Paroxetine significantly reduced social anxiety and the frequency and severity of alcohol use in patients with SAD and an alcohol use disorder.[60] Neither MAOIs nor benzodiazepines are appropriate therapy for patients with SAD and alcohol use disorder as SSRIs are the medications of choice.

Evaluation of Therapeutic Outcomes

10 The pharmacotherapy of SAD can be monitored in three principal domains: SAD symptoms (eg, fears and physical symptoms), functionality, and well-being or overall improvement.[24,25,58] Response to pharmacotherapy in SAD is defined as a stable, clinically meaningful improvement, where patients no longer have the full range of symptoms but typically continue to experience more than minimal symptoms.[24,25,58]

During the acute phase of treatment, patients should be seen weekly while the medication dosage is titrated. Once the patient responds and the dosage is stabilized, the patient can be seen monthly. Many patients report improvement during the first 4 weeks of therapy, but more than one-quarter of those who do not have a response at week 8 may have a response at 12 weeks. At each visit, the patient should be asked about adverse medication reactions and improvement in symptoms. The patient should be instructed to keep a diary to record fear levels, physical symptoms, cognitions, and anxious behaviors in actual exposures to social situations. The LSAS is a clinician-rated scale of clinical severity which can be used to assess change in SAD for monitoring response.[61] Patients can use the Social Phobia Inventory for self-assessment of SAD symptoms.[58,61] Full remission is defined as a complete resolution of symptoms across the three SAD domains that is maintained for 3 months or an LSAS score of less than or equal to 30 points.[55]

TREATMENT—SPECIFIC PHOBIA

Specific phobia is considered unresponsive to pharmacotherapy, although highly responsive to CBT. The use of benzodiazepines or paroxetine in patients who failed CBT is supported by limited data. Benzodiazepines can be detrimental in patients with specific phobias treated with CBT.[21]

CONCLUSION

Anxiety disorders are common in the population and occur concurrently with other psychiatric disorders. The proper management of anxiety disorders begins with the correct diagnosis as not all patients should receive antianxiety agents. Nonpharmacologic interventions often are effective alone or when combined with pharmacotherapy.

There are several subtypes of anxiety disorders, and the diagnosis determines the type of medication and nonpharmacologic intervention selected. Although benzodiazepines remain the medications of choice for situational anxiety, antidepressants have emerged as first-line therapy for GAD, panic disorder, and SAD. Benzodiazepines are reserved for use in situations requiring immediate anxiety relief during the first 2 to 4 weeks of therapy with a long-term agent such as an antidepressant. Antidepressants, including the SSRIs and SNRIs, and the benzodiazepines clonazepam and alprazolam are used extensively in patients with GAD, panic disorder, and SAD.

The long-term goal of therapy for GAD, panic disorder, and SAD is remission of core anxiety symptoms with no impairment in functionality, minimal anxiety, and no depressive symptoms. Augmentation with antiseizure medications and SGAs shows some promise in treatment-resistant cases.

ABBREVIATIONS

ACC	anterior cingulate cortex
CBT	cognitive behavioral therapy
CNS	central nervous system
CRF	corticotropin-releasing factor
DA	dopamine
DMDZ	desmethyldiazepam
GABA	γ-aminobutyric acid
GAD	generalized anxiety disorder
GI	gastrointestinal
HAM-A	Hamilton Anxiety Rating Scale
5-HT	serotonin
LC	locus ceruleus
LSAS	Liebowitz Social Anxiety Scale
NAMI	National Alliance for Mental Illness
MAOI	monoamine oxidase inhibitor
NE	norepinephrine
PAG	periaqueductal gray
PHQ-9	Patient Health Questionnaire-9
QOL	quality of life
SAD	social anxiety disorder
SERT	serotonin reuptake transporter
SGA	second-generation antipsychotic
SNRI	serotonin–norepinephrine reuptake inhibitor
SSRI	selective serotonin reuptake inhibitor
SUD	substance use disorder
TCA	tricyclic antidepressant

REFERENCES

1. American Psychiatric Association. *Diagnostic and Statistical Manual of Mental Disorders.* 5th ed. Washington, DC: American Psychiatric Association; 2013:189–233.
2. Katzman MA, Bleau P, Blier P, et al. Canadian clinical practice guidelines for the management of anxiety, posttraumatic stress and obsessive-compulsive disorders. *BMC Psychiatry.* 2014; 14(suppl 1):S1.
3. Bandelow B, Sher L, Bunevicius R, et al. Guidelines for the pharmacological treatment of anxiety disorders, obsessive-compulsive disorder and posttraumatic stress disorder in primary care. *Int J Psychiatry Clin Pract.* 2012;16:77–84.
4. Roy-Byrne P. Treatment-refractory anxiety; definition, risk factors, and treatment challenges. *Dialogues Clin Neurosci.* 2015;17(2):191–206.
5. Bandelow B, Michaelis S. Epidemiology of anxiety disorders in the 21st century. *Dialogues Clin Neurosci.* 2015;17(3):327–335.
6. DeMartini J, Patel G, Fancher TL. Generalized anxiety disorder. *Ann Intern Med.* 2019;170(7):ITC49–ITC64. 10.7326/AITC201904020 30934083.
7. Niles AN, Dour H, Stanton AL, et al. Anxiety and depressive symptoms and medical illness among adults with anxiety disorders. *Psychosom Res.* 2015;78(2):109–115.
8. Craske MG, Stein MB, Elay TC, et al. Anxiety disorders. *Nat Rev Dis Primers.* 2017;3:17024. doi:10.1038/nrdp.2017.24.
9. Martin EI, Ressler KJ, Binder E, et al. The neurobiology of anxiety disorders: brain imaging, genetics, and psychoneuroendocrinology. *Psychiatr Clin North Am.* 2009;32:549–575.
10. LeDoux JE, Pine DS. Using neuroscience to help understand fear and anxiety: a two-system framework. *Am J Psychiatry.* 2016;173(11):1083–1093.
11. Bandelow B, Baldwin D, Abelli M, et al. Biological markers for anxiety disorders, OCD and PTSD: a consensus statement. Part I: neuroimaging and genetics. *World J Biol Psychiatry.* 2017;17(5):321–365.
12. Bandelow B, Baldwin D, Abelli M, et al. Biological markers for anxiety disorders, OCD and PTSD: a consensus statement. Part II: neurochemistry, neurophysiology and neurocognition. *World J Biol Psychiatry.* 2017;18(3):162–214.
13. Nuss P. Anxiety disorders and GABA neurotransmission: a disturbance of modulation. *Neuropsychiatr Dis Treat.* 2015;11:165–175.
14. Imai H, Tajika A, Chen P, et al. Azapirones versus placebo for panic disorder in adults. *Cochrane Database Syst Rev.* 2014;(9):CD010828. doi:0.1002/14651858.CD010828.pub2.
15. Warwick JM, Carey PD, Cassimjee N, et al. Dopamine transporter binding in social anxiety disorder: the effect of treatment with escitalopram. *Metab Brain Dis.* 2012;27(2):151–158.
16. Maron E, Nutt D. Biological markers of generalized anxiety disorder. *Dialogues Clin Neurosci.* 2017;19:147–157.
17. Reinhold JA, Rickel K. Pharmacological treatment for generalized anxiety disorder in adults: an update. *Expert Opin Pharmacother.* 2015;16(11):1669–1681.
18. National Institute for Health and Care Excellence: Guidance. Social anxiety disorder: recognition, assessment and treatment. NICE Clinical Guideline 159. May 2013. Available at: http://www.nice.org.uk/guidance/cg159. Accessed November 11, 2021.
19. Abejuela HR, Osser DN. The psychopharmacology algorithm project at the Harvard South Shore Program: an algorithm for generalized anxiety disorder. *Harv Rev Psychiatry.* 2016;24(4):243–256.
20. American Psychiatric Association. *Practice Guideline for the Treatment of Patients with Panic Disorder.* Arlington, VA: American Psychiatric Association; 2009. http://www.psychiatryonline.com/pracGuide/pracGuideTopic_9.aspx. Accessed November 11, 2021. Accessed December 19, 2018.
21. Baldwin DS, Anderson IM, Nutt DJ, et al. Evidence-based pharmacological treatment of anxiety disorders, post-traumatic stress disorder and obsessive-compulsive disorder: a revision of the 2005 guidelines from the British Association for Pharmacology. *J Psychopharmacol.* 2014;28(5):403–439.
22. National Institute for Health and Care Excellence. Generalised anxiety disorder and panic disorder (with or without agoraphobia) in adults. Management in primary, secondary, and community care. NICE Clinical Guideline 113. January 2011. Available at: http://www.nice.org.uk/guidance/cg113. Accessed November 11, 2021.
23. Stein MB, Sareen J. Generalized anxiety disorder. *N Engl J Med.* 2015;373:2059–2068.
24. Bostwick JR, Cusher MI, Yasugi S. Benzodiazepines: a versatile clinical tool. *Current Psychiatry.* 2012;11(4):55–64.
25. PL Detail-Document, Benzodiazepine Toolbox. Pharmacist's Letter/Prescriber's Letter. August 2014.
26. Benzodiazepines. Facts and Comparisons® eAnswers (Online). Wolters Kluwer Health Inc., 2018. Available at: http://www.wolterskluwercdi.com/facts-comparisons-online/. Accessed November 11, 2021.

27. Hershenberg R, Gros DF, Brawman-Mintzer O. Role of atypical antipsychotics in the treatment of generalized anxiety disorder. *CNS Drugs.* 2014;28(6):519–533.
28. Cymbalta [package insert]. Indianapolis, IN: Eli Lily and Company; December 2017.
29. Lexapro [package insert]. Madison NJ: Allergan Allergan; September 2021.
30. Paxil [package insert]. Weston, FL: Apotex Corporation; October 2021.
31. Effexor XR [package insert]. Philadelphia, PA: Wyeth Pharmaceuticals Inc, a subsidiary of Pfizer Inc.; July 2021.
32. Gommoll C, Forero G, Mathews M, et al. Vilazodone in patients with generalized anxiety disorder: a double-blind, randomized, placebo-controlled, flexible-dose study. *Int Clin Psychopharmacol.* 2015;30(6):297–306.
33. Pae CU, Wang SM, Han C, et al. Vortioxetine, a multimodal antidepressant for generalized anxiety disorder: a systematic review and meta-analysis. *J Psychiatr Res.* 2015;64:88–98.
34. Vistaril [package insert]. New York, NY: Pfizer Labs; June 2020.
35. The International Psychopharmacology Algorithm Project. IPAP—Generalized Anxiety Disorder Algorithm. Available at: http://www.ipap.org/gad/index.php. Accessed November 11, 2021.
36. Kong W, Deng H, Wan J, et al. Comparative remission rates and tolerability of drugs for generalised anxiety disorder: a systematic review and network meta-analysis of double-blind randomized controlled trials. *Front Pharmacol.* 2020;11:580858–580858. 10.3389/fphar.2020.580858 33343351.
37. David DJ, Samuels BA, Rainer Q, et al. Neurogenesis-dependent and independent effects of fluoxetine in an animal model of anxiety/depression. *Neuron.* 2009;62(4):479–493.
38. Klonopin [package insert]. San Francisco, CA: Genentech Inc; February 2021.
39. Xanax XR [package insert]. New York, NY: Pharmacia and Upjohn Company Inc; March 2021.
40. Chen X, van Gerven J, Cohen A, Jacobs G Human pharmacology of positive GABA-A subtype-selective receptor modulators for the treatment of anxiety. *Acta Pharmacol Sin.* 2019;40(5):571–582. 10.1038/s41401-018-0185-5 30518829.
41. Labbate LA, Fava M, Rosenbaum JF, Arana GW. *Handbook of Psychiatric Therapy.* 6th ed. Philadelphia, PA: Lippincott Williams & Wilkins; 2010:163–192.
42. Lader M. Benzodiazepine harm: how can it be reduced? *Br J Clin Pharmacol.* 2014;77(2):295–301.
43. Gold J, Ward K. Pharmacist Toolkit: Benzodiazepine Taper. College of Psychiatric and Neurologic Pharmacists 2018. Available at: https://cpnp.org/guideline/benzo. Accessed November 11, 2021.
44. Caniff K, Telega E, Bostwick JR, Gardner KN. Pregabalin as adjunctive therapy in benzodiazepine discontinuation. *Am J Health Syst Pharm.* 2018;75(2):67–71. 10.2146/ajhp160712 29317396.
45. Canadian Agency for Drugs and Technologies in Health. Discontinuation strategies for patients with long-term benzodiazepine use: A review of clinical evidence and guidelines. Ottawa (ON); July 2015. Available at: http://www.ncbi.nlm.nih.gov/pubmedhealth/PMH0078914/pdf/PubMedHealth_PMH0078914.pdf. Accessed November 11, 2021.
46. Generoso MB, Trevizol AP, Kasper S, et al. Pregabalin for generalized anxiety disorder: an updated systematic review and meta-analysis. *Int Clin Psychopharmacol.* 2017;32:49–55.
47. Sarris J, et al. Herbal medicines in the treatment of psychiatric disorders: 10-year updated review. *Phytother Res.* 2018;32(7):1147–1162. 10.1002/ptr.6055 29575228.
48. McAllister-Williams RH, Baldwin DS, Cantwell R, et al. British Association for Psychopharmacology consensus guidance on the use of psychotropic medication preconception, in pregnancy and postpartum 2017. *J Psychopharmacol.* 2017;31(5):519–552. 10.1177/0269881117699361 28440103.
49. Bellantuono C, Tofani S, Di Sciascio G, Santone G. Benzodiazepine exposure in pregnancy and risk of major malformations: a critical overview. *Gen Hosp Psychiatry.* 2013;35:3–8.
50. Wehry AW, Beesdo-Baum K, Hennelly MM, et al. Assessment and treatment of anxiety disorders in children and adolescents. *Curr Psychiatry Rep.* 2015;17(7):52. doi:10.1007/s11920-015-0591-z.
51. Andreescu C, Varon D. New research on anxiety disorders in the elderly and an update on evidence-based treatments. *Curr Psychiatry Rep.* 2015;17(7):53. doi: 10.1007/s11920-015-0595-8.
52. Karaiskos D, Pappa D, Tzavellas E, et al. Pregabalin augmentation of antidepressants in older patients with comorbid depression and generalized anxiety disorder: an open-label study. *Int J Geriatr Psychiatry.* 2013;28(1):100–105.
53. Andrisano C, Chiesa A, Serretti A. Newer antidepressants and panic disorder: a meta-analysis. *Int Clin Psychopharmacol.* 2012;28:33–45.
54. Du Y, Du B, Diao Y, et al. Comparative efficacy and acceptability of antidepressants and benzodiazepines for the treatment of panic disorder: a systematic review and network meta-analysis. *Asian J Psychiatr.* 2021;60:102664–102664. 10.1016/j.ajp.2021.102664 33965693.
55. Blanco C, Bragdon LB, Schneier FR, et al. The evidence-based pharmacotherapy of social anxiety disorder. *Int J Neuropsychopharmacol.* 2013;16(1):235–249.
56. Leichsenring F, Leweke F. Social anxiety disorder. *N Engl J Med.* 2017;376:2255–2264.
57. Pelissolo A, Abou Kassm S, Delhay L. Therapeutic strategies for social anxiety disorder: where are we now? *Expert Rev Neurother.* 2019;19(12):1179–1189. 10.1080/14737175.2019.1666713 31502896.
58. Dalrymple KL. Issues and controversies surrounding the diagnosis and treatment of social anxiety disorder. *Expert Rev Neurother.* 2012;2(8):993–1008.
59. Kawalec P, Cierniak A, Pilc A, et al. Pregabalin for the treatment of social anxiety disorder. *Expert Opin Investig Drugs.* 2015;24(4):585–594.
60. Ipser JC, Wilson D, Akindipe TO, et al. Pharmacotherapy for anxiety and comorbid alcohol use disorders. *Cochrane Database Syst Rev.* 2015;1:CD007505.
61. Osório Fde L, Crippa JA, Loureiro SR. Instruments for the assessment of social anxiety disorder: validation studies. *World J Psychiatry.* 2012;2(5):83–5. 10.5498/wjp.v2.i5.83 24175172.

Posttraumatic Stress Disorder and Obsessive-Compulsive Disorder

91

Kristen N. Gardner, Jolene R. Bostwick, and Ericka L. Crouse

KEY CONCEPTS

1. Trauma-focused cognitive behavioral therapy (CBT) and eye movement desensitization and reprocessing are the most effective nonpharmacologic methods to reduce symptoms of posttraumatic stress disorder (PTSD).
2. The selective serotonin reuptake inhibitors (SSRIs) and venlafaxine at moderate to high dose are considered first-line treatments for PTSD.
3. An adequate trial of SSRIs in PTSD is 8 to 12 weeks.
4. Patients with PTSD who respond to pharmacotherapy should continue treatment for at least 12 months.
5. CBT with behavioral techniques (eg, exposure and response prevention [ERP]) is the most common initial nonpharmacologic treatment of choice in obsessive-compulsive disorder (OCD).
6. Moderate-to-high dose SSRIs are the medication of choice for the treatment of OCD.
7. Clomipramine, a tricyclic antidepressant (TCA) with strong serotonin (5-HT) reuptake inhibition, is a second-line treatment option for OCD.
8. An adequate antidepressant trial for OCD treatment is 8 to 12 weeks.
9. Augmentation of SSRI treatment of OCD with low-to-moderate doses of antipsychotics may be helpful.
10. Medication taper can be considered after 1 to 2 years of treatment in patients with OCD.

BEYOND THE BOOK

PTSD

Prior to class visit the website PTSD: National Center for PTSD on the US Department of Veterans Affairs website at: www.ptsd.va.gov. Expand the section "Understand PTSD" then "Types of Trauma" to review one or two types of trauma (eg, war and combat, violence and abuse, disaster and terrorism).

On the left-hand side menu, visit the section "For Providers" and complete the following steps:

1. Click on Assessment
2. Click on Adult Self-Report
3. Review the following screening tools: The PTSD Checklist for *DSM-5* (PCL-5)
4. Work with a friend or partner to role play and practice administering the PCL-5

This activity is intended to build your awareness of different types of traumas that patients may experience as well as familiarize yourself with the types of symptoms that patients are screened for when considering a diagnosis of PTSD.

OCD

Identify a mobile-app that may help manage OCD and related symptoms (eg, nOCD, GGOC, Headspace). Evaluate the mobile-app from the perspective of a patient with OCD and write a brief review for this application (eg, a single paragraph). Consider the following questions (you do not need to address each item):

- What symptom(s) is this mobile-app intended to help?
- How interactive is the mobile-app in giving feedback to the end user?
- Can the mobile-app be personalized for the end user?
- Do you foresee the mobile-app content and delivery methods accomplishing its purpose?
- Is there scientific research that demonstrates its effectiveness?
- Describe the patient population for which this mobile-app is best suited.

This activity is intended to build your awareness of the growing interest and use of mobile health technology devices to empower patients in self-management of their mental health.

INTRODUCTION

Traumatic or stressful events (eg, wars, terrorist attacks, natural disasters, pandemics, robbery, physical or sexual assault) can lead to development of posttraumatic stress disorder (PTSD).[1] Initially diagnosed in veterans of war, PTSD is now acknowledged as a significant psychiatric illness in the civilian population and among deployed service personnel of the Afghanistan and Iraq campaigns in whom the suicide rate has escalated.[1,2] In clinical practice, PTSD continues to be poorly recognized and diagnosed.[3] Because of its co-occurrence (greater than 50%) with anxiety disorders, depression, substance use, and traumatic brain injury, the overlapping symptoms can lead to diagnostic uncertainty.[3] PTSD has been shown to increase the risk of lifetime suicide attempt.[3-7] Advances in the science and treatment of PTSD can assist clinicians in all fields to screen for a history of trauma and effectively manage PTSD.

Intrusive obsessive thoughts and compulsive ritualistic behaviors characterize obsessive-compulsive disorder (OCD),[1] with symptoms potentially being severe enough that they impair functioning in social, family, and work settings, and decrease overall quality of life (QOL). Comorbid depression is common with OCD, with approximately 40% of patients having a history of major depression during their lifetime.[6] A diagnosis of OCD is also associated with an increased risk of suicide, with a mean of 13.4% (range 1%-46.3%) of patients reporting a previous history of suicide attempt. Increased understanding of symptom dimensions and treatment response can improve QOL in patients suffering from OCD.

EPIDEMIOLOGY

Within the US population, the estimated lifetime prevalence of PTSD is 8.7%,[1] whereas the lifetime prevalence of OCD has been estimated at 2.3%.[8]

PTSD is associated with the incidence of trauma,[1] with the most frequently reported traumatic events in the United States being assault (physical and sexual) with a 52% lifetime prevalence and accidents or fires with a 50% lifetime prevalence.[3] The conditional probability of developing PTSD differs between sex and type of trauma. The probability of developing PTSD for males and females after rape is 65% and 46%, after physical assault 2% and 22%, and after an accident are 6% and 9%, respectively.[7,9] Prevalence of PTSD is consistently higher among females (10.4%-12.3%) than males (5%).[7] Gender roles, genetic predispositions as well as hormonal influences may put females at higher risk of PTSD.[10] While the age of onset and course of PTSD are variable, it is important to note that PTSD can occur at any age, but most cases occur before the age of 40 years. The presentation is also not predictable, because symptoms are impacted by the duration and intensity of the trauma, the presence of other psychiatric disorders, and early posttrauma interventions.[3] Genetic factors can increase vulnerability to PTSD if an individual is exposed to a traumatic event. Lastly, veterans and those whose jobs increase the risk of traumatic exposure (eg, firefighters, first responders, police) have higher rates of PTSD.[1,3]

The epidemiology of OCD is also influenced by age and sex. The age of onset has a bimodal distribution peaking in late childhood/early adolescence and then again in early adulthood.[11,12] In males, the onset of illness is more frequently seen during childhood/adolescence versus early adulthood in females. The annual US prevalence of OCD is greater in females (1.8%) versus males (0.5%).[7] Patients with childhood-onset OCD often have concurrent ADHD and tic disorders, whereas mood disorders, other anxiety disorders, and obsessive-compulsive personality disorder are common comorbidities in adult-onset OCD.[1] Greater than 50% of patients with Tourette Syndrome have OCD symptoms, and around 30% will eventually be diagnosed with OCD.[13] Patients with eating disorders have a wide range of reported comorbid OCD.[14] Heredity is stronger when there is an early age of onset or comorbidity with tic disorder.[1] The average delay in time to appropriate treatment for OCD following symptom onset is nearly 8 to 10 years[12] as OCD is a disorder that is poorly recognized and patients often do not seek treatment until late during illness.

ETIOLOGY

The exact etiologies of PTSD and OCD are unknown; however, it is likely that abnormalities in several areas of brain functioning interact to cause these chronic disorders. Genetics may play a role in PTSD and OCD expression, but environmental factors are also involved. A number of genetic markers for PTSD are under evaluation, including genes associated with the hypothalamic-pituitary-adrenal (HPA) axis (eg, FKBP5), the amygdala-medial prefrontal cortex (mPFC)-hippocampus circuit, and the serotonin transporter.[15-18] Given the heterogeneity and individual differences in course and presentation of PTSD, recent studies have focused on gene by environment (G x E).[16,18] There is increasing evidence of immune dysregulation in PTSD, but it is unknown if it is a predisposing factor versus comorbidity related.[18] The behaviors in OCD are also heterogeneous, suggesting OCD is a polygenic disorder.[13,19-21] Potential genes include those affecting serotonin (5-HT), dopamine (DA), and glutamate.[13] An association with the D_2 receptor gene has been identified in OCD with tics and other potential genes associated with OCD include 5-HT transporter and receptors (eg, 5-HT_{1D} beta, 5-HT_{2A}, and 5-HT_{2C}). Research on the role of glutamate in OCD has identified genes of interest including glutamate-related synapse (*SAPAP/DLGAP*); glutamate transporter (*SLC1A1*); and N-methyl-D-aspartate (NMDA) receptor genes (*GRIN2B* and *GRIK*).[13,19,20] Twin studies found higher concordance rates in monozygotic versus dizygotic twins, suggesting an approximate 48% OCD heritability. Some subtypes, such as early-onset OCD with tics, may have higher heritability.[20,21] Further understanding of the roles genetics and the environment play in the development of PTSD and OCD may impact future treatment strategies and are current research areas.

In children, the occurrence of sudden onset OCD and chronic tic disorder following a streptococcal infection has been reported and previously labeled Pediatric Autoimmune Neuropsychiatric Disorders Associated with Streptococcal Infections (PANDAS).[20,21] Controversy currently exists as to whether PANDAS should be characterized as a subtype of OCD. Although most patients with OCD do not have a streptococcal etiology, an accurate medical history regarding onset of illness is imperative because specific treatment strategies are indicated. More recently, PANDAS has been broadened to pediatric acute-onset neuropsychiatric syndrome, or PANS, to include OCD symptoms that start after nonstreptococcal infections.

Substance/medication-induced OCD has been described with stimulants including cocaine, amphetamines, and methylphenidate. Furthermore, cases of OCD-like behaviors (eg, pathologic gambling) have been described with dopamine agonists (eg, ropinirole, pramipexole).[13]

PATHOPHYSIOLOGY

Research findings in the areas of neuroendocrinology, neurobiology, and neuroimaging have advanced theories on the pathophysiology of OCD, and PTSD. Neuroendocrine changes in the HPA axis are implicated in the pathophysiology of PTSD. The neurobiology of PTSD focuses on alterations in fear learning, threat detection, executive function, and emotional regulation, as well as contextual processing.[3] Dysfunction in the cortico-striato-thalamo-cortical (CSTC) circuit is implicated in OCD.[20,21] As reviewed in Chapter 90, "Generalized Anxiety Disorder, Panic, and Social Anxiety Disorders," data from neurochemical and neuroimaging studies indicate that the modulation of normal and pathologic anxiety states is associated with multiple regions of the brain (eg, amygdala, hippocampus, thalamus, and prefrontal cortex).[3] Abnormal function in several neurotransmitter systems, including norepinephrine (NE), γ-aminobutyric acid (GABA), glutamate, DA, and 5-HT, may affect the manifestations of OCD and PTSD.[16,22,23]

Neuroendocrine Theories

Neuroendocrine studies provide data that abnormalities occurring pretrauma, during trauma, and posttrauma contribute to PTSD. Trauma exposure is linked to abnormal HPA activity and cortisol patterns.[24] Normally the immediate reaction to stress occurs as an automatic response from the amygdala to the sympathetic and parasympathetic systems and the HPA axis.[22] The release of corticotropin-releasing factor (CRF) stimulates cortisol secretion from the adrenal gland and both catecholamines and cortisol levels rise in tandem. Cortisol then reduces the stress response by tempering the sympathetic reaction through negative feedback on the pituitary and hypothalamus[22] with both systems returning to normal after a few hours.

Data implicate a role for the neuropeptides CRF and neuropeptide Y (NPY) in PTSD, as patients with PTSD have a hypersecretion of CRF but demonstrate subnormal levels of cortisol at the time of trauma and then chronically.[22] Lower plasma cortisol concentrations were associated with greater severity of PTSD symptoms in nonmilitary patients[23] and dysregulation of the HPA axis is postulated to be a risk factor for eventual development of PTSD.[22] The NPY system is a mediator between exposure to stress and development of resilient versus maladaptive responses and the role of NPY in improving resilience is a continued area of research interest.[25]

Neurochemical Theories

Several neurotransmitters may be involved in the pathophysiology of PTSD as 5-HT, NE, and glutamate are associated with the processing of emotional and somatic contents of memories in the amygdala.[23] Alterations in these neurotransmitters are linked to alterations in amygdala activity.[3] The amygdala is involved in processing emotions, and acquiring, expressing, and regulating fear and traumatic memories, including fear conditioning.[24] The medial prefrontal cortex (mPFC) and hippocampus are involved in contextual processing. The noradrenergic theory posits that the autonomic nervous system of patients with anxiety is hypersensitive and overreacts to stimuli. The alarm center, the locus ceruleus, releases NE to stimulate the sympathetic and parasympathetic nervous systems. Hyperactive noradrenergic signaling in patients with PTSD is a consistent research finding and includes increased 24-hour catecholamine excretion.[23] Glutamate signaling abnormalities may result in distortion of amygdala-dependent emotional processing under stress.[22,23] Dysregulation of the processing of sensory input and memories may contribute to the dissociative and hypervigilant symptoms in PTSD. Abnormalities of GABA inhibition may lead to increased awareness or response to stress, as seen in PTSD.[26]

Both 5-HT and DA are implicated in the pathogenesis of OCD. Selective and potent serotonin reuptake inhibitors have consistently been shown effective for symptoms of the illness,[27] especially at higher doses. The most commonly studied serotonin receptors in OCD are 5-HT_{2A}, 5-HT_{1B}, and 5-HT_{2C}.[28] Dopamine dysregulation may also contribute to some forms of OCD, as neurologic symptoms (eg, tics) are part of the clinical presentation in some patients with OCD and Tourette Syndrome, a disorder of DA function.[1,13] Additionally use of dopamine agonists can worsen OCD symptoms, whereas augmentation with antipsychotics may improve symptoms in patients with OCD who are partially responsive to selective serotonin reuptake inhibitors (SSRIs).[13] More recently glutamate has become another neurotransmitter of interest in OCD, especially in genetic research.[19]

Neuroimaging Studies

Neuroimaging studies suggest that certain areas of the brain are altered by psychological trauma. In PTSD, most functional neuroimaging studies have involved the amygdala, mPFC, dorsal anterior cingulate cortex (dACC), insula, and hippocampus.[3] Findings of increased activation of the amygdala after trauma-related imagery, sounds, or smells indicate that this structure plays a role in the persistence of traumatic memory.[29] Decreased amygdala activation is correlated with resilience to PTSD and response to CBT. Historically, studies have suggested patients with PTSD have reduced amygdala volume; however, a recent study suggested instead that smaller amygdala volume is related to exposure to trauma and not necessarily PTSD.[24] Hypofunctioning of the mPFC is theorized to prevent extinction of fear in patients with PTSD, and is associated with impairments in extinction recall, abnormalities in processing contextual information, and impairments in safety-signal learning.[3] Hyperresponsivity of the dACC, amygdala, and the insula may correlate with impaired response to emotional or salient stimuli or impaired threat detection. Not all magnetic resonance imaging (MRI) studies show reduced hippocampal volume in PTSD; however, reduced hippocampal volume has been linked to reexperiencing symptoms in PTSD.[24] In twin studies, the unaffected twin of patients with PTSD also demonstrated smaller hippocampi compared with twins without PTSD that may suggest that lower hippocampal volumes are likely a precursor associated with vulnerability for subsequent PTSD development.[22]

Neuroimaging studies consistently show evidence that dysfunction in the CSTC circuit, which regulates self-control, is associated with OCD.[13,19-21] The role of neuromodulation treatment in OCD supports the CSTC model.[21] Positron emission tomography (PET) and single-photon emission computed tomography (SPECT) studies in OCD have shown increased activity in the anterior cingulate cortices, and different patterns of activation in the caudate.[11] Evidence suggests that lower pretreatment activity in the orbitofrontal cortex predicts a better response to SSRIs and improved fluvoxamine response has been correlated with abnormalities in the posterior cingulate cortex.

CLINICAL PRESENTATION

The *Diagnostic and Statistical Manual of Mental Disorders, Fifth Edition* (*DSM-5*) made several changes to the classification of anxiety and related disorders[1] with individual chapters for anxiety disorders, trauma- and stressor-related disorders, and obsessive-compulsive and related disorders. Generalized anxiety disorder, panic disorder, and social anxiety disorder are discussed in Chapter 90.

Posttraumatic Stress Disorder

Exposure to a traumatic event is required for a diagnosis of PTSD[1] in that the person must have witnessed, experienced, or been confronted with a situation that involved definite or threatened death or serious injury, sexual violence, or possible harm to self or others. Some examples of traumatic events include physical attacks by an intimate partner, severe traffic accidents, military combat, natural disasters, being held hostage, child sexual abuse, witnessing a murder or injury of another, and learning of a traumatic event that happened to a close family member or friend. While systematic reviews have yet to be conducted, the impact of the coronavirus (COVID-19) pandemic on PTSD has been published across populations, including healthcare workers experiencing PTSD and young adults with worsening PTSD symptoms.[30,31]

The resulting PTSD symptoms include persistent reexperiencing of the traumatic event, avoidance of stimuli associated with the trauma, numbing of general responsiveness, and persistent symptoms of hyperarousal.[1] Patients must have at least one intrusion symptom, at least one symptom of avoidance of stimuli associated with the trauma, at least two symptoms of negative alterations in cognition and mood, and at least two symptoms of increased arousal. Symptoms from each category need to be present for longer than 1 month and cause significant distress or impairment in functioning. Most persons diagnosed with PTSD also meet criteria for another psychiatric disorder, most commonly mood, anxiety, and substance use disorders.[1,4,32]

Anxiety and dissociative symptoms (eg, absence of emotional responsiveness, derealization, inability to recall important features of the trauma) emerging within 1 month after exposure to a traumatic stressor are classified as Acute Stress Disorder (ASD).[1] Symptoms of ASD are experienced during or immediately after the trauma,

CLINICAL PRESENTATION Posttraumatic Stress Disorder

Intrusion Symptoms

- Recurrent, intrusive distressing memories of the trauma
- Recurrent, disturbing dreams of the event
- Feeling that the traumatic event is recurring (eg, dissociative flashbacks)
- Physiologic reaction to or psychological distress from reminders of the trauma

Avoidance Symptoms

- Avoidance of conversations, thoughts, or feelings about the trauma
- Avoidance of people, places, or activities that are reminders of the event

Persistent Negative Alterations in Thinking and Mood

- Inability to recall an important aspect of the trauma
- Estrangement from others
- Restricted affect
- Negative beliefs about oneself
- Distorted beliefs causing one to blame others or themselves for the trauma
- Negative mood state

Hyperarousal Symptoms

- Decreased concentration
- Easily startled
- Self-destructive behavior
- Hypervigilance
- Insomnia
- Irritability or anger outbursts

Specifiers

- Dissociative symptoms: depersonalization or derealization
- With delayed expression: full criteria are not met until at least 6 months posttrauma

Data from References 1 and 32.

last for at least 3 days, and resolve within 1 month. The severity and course of illness is fluctuating and often worsens, with life stressors.

Obsessive-Compulsive Disorder

The diagnostic criteria for OCD require the presence of obsessions and/or compulsions that are severe enough to cause marked distress, to be time-consuming (occupy more than 1 hr/day), or cause significant impairment in social or occupational functioning.[1] An obsession is a recurrent, persistent idea, thought, impulse, or image that is experienced as intrusive and inappropriate and produces marked anxiety. A compulsion is defined as a repetitive behavior or act generally performed in response to an obsession. While it is most common for patients to have both obsessions and compulsions, some may only have one or the other. Diagnostically, the compulsive behavior is not pleasurable and is designed to prevent discomfort or the occurrence of a dreaded event that is often unknown and part of the obsession. Therefore, compulsive behaviors are usually performed according to certain rules or in a stereotyped fashion. Common symptom dimensions involve cleaning (eg, contamination obsessions and cleaning compulsions), symmetry (eg, symmetry obsessions and ordering or arranging compulsions), forbidden or taboo thoughts (eg, violent, sexual, or religious obsessions and related compulsions), and harm (eg, fears of causing harm or superstitions and related compulsions).[1,12] For example, patients obsessed with the fear of causing harm (eg, inadvertently hitting a pedestrian), may cause them marked distress and lead to repetitive checking (eg, driving past crosswalks to check for injured pedestrians).[12]

There are two specifiers for OCD related to the degree of insight and the presence of tic-related symptoms.[1] While individuals vary widely in their insight into the irrationality of their obsessive-compulsive symptoms, most will have good or fair insight. The addition of an insight specifier allows the diagnosis to include individuals with poor to absent insight such as those with comorbid psychosis.[12] Individuals with tic-related OCD appear to differ from

CLINICAL PRESENTATION Obsessive-Compulsive Disorder

Obsessions

- Repetitive thoughts (eg, feeling contaminated by germs, fears of harming others)
- Repetitive images (eg, recurrent sexually explicit pictures)
- Repetitive urges (eg, need for symmetry or putting things in specific order)

Compulsions

- Repetitive activities (eg, hand washing, need to ask, need to confess)
- Repetitive mental acts (eg, counting excessively, repeating words silently, praying)

Specifiers

- Insight: good or fair insight, poor insight, or absent insight/delusional beliefs
- Related to a tic disorder

Data from References 1 and 12.

those with non-tic-related OCD in terms of etiology, illness course, symptom presentation, comorbidities, heredity, and pharmacotherapy response.[1]

The diversity of OCD symptoms can obscure an accurate diagnosis as patients often present in a seemingly incongruous manner to non-mental health clinicians for other complaints—dermatologists for eczema or chapped skin, pediatricians for parental concerns over a child's compulsive hand washing, neurologists for tics, or dentists for gum lesions from compulsive teeth brushing.[12] Because patients recognize their compulsive behavior as illogical or irrational, they also can become extremely adept at denying symptoms, disguising their rituals, and concealing their illness from friends and family.[1]

It is important to note that OCD is a chronic illness in most patients, with symptom severity varying in intensity over time,[12] resulting in a significantly impaired QOL.

TREATMENT

Posttraumatic Stress Disorder

Desired Outcomes

The short-term goal of therapy in the management of PTSD is a reduction in core symptoms (eg, intrusive reexperiencing, avoidance, and hyperarousal). Additional goals include improvement in disability, concurrent psychiatric conditions, resilience, and QOL with the long-term goal of PTSD remission.

General Approach to Treatment

In general, individuals who seek treatment acutely after a trauma and are in intense distress should receive therapy based on their presenting symptoms (eg, a nonbenzodiazepine hypnotic for difficulty sleeping). Short courses of exposure-based, trauma-focused cognitive behavioral therapy (TFCBT) can be helpful to prevent chronic PTSD in patients with ASD or acute PTSD.[4] If symptoms (eg, hyperarousal, avoidance, dissociation, sleep difficulties, or depressed mood) persist for 3 to 4 weeks and the patient experiences marked social, occupational, and/or interpersonal impairment, they can be treated with pharmacotherapy, psychotherapy, or both. Many patients with PTSD will improve substantially with pharmacotherapy but retain some symptoms. Treatment regimens usually combine psychoeducation, psychosocial support and/or treatment, and pharmacotherapy; however, newer guidelines specifically emphasize the utility of individual trauma-focused psychotherapies.[3,5,33,34]

Nonpharmacologic Therapy

Psychotherapy can be used when a patient suffers from mild symptoms, in patients who prefer not to use medications, or in conjunction with medication in patients with severe symptoms to improve response.[5,35] Notably, current clinical practice guidelines emphasize the role of trauma-focused psychotherapy as the preferred treatment approach.[5,33,34] Patients who have experienced trauma should be educated that they can experience anxiety, depression, nightmares, and even flashbacks as a reaction to the event. Brief courses of individual trauma-focused psychotherapy, focusing on exposure or cognitive restructuring, near the traumatic event resulted in lower rates of PTSD 3 and 6 months later. Single-session critical incident stress debriefing has not shown to be effective in preventing development of PTSD and may cause harm.[3,5] Involving the patient in the selection of preferred treatment, especially in those that prefer prolonged exposure therapy, has demonstrated improved health-related QOL.[36]

1 Psychotherapies for treating PTSD include prolonged exposure, TFCBT, cognitive processing therapy (CPT), eye movement desensitization and reprocessing (EMDR), and psychoeducation.[4,5,35] The unique treatment EMDR involves the process of patients imagining exposure to the traumatic event, while simultaneously engaging in bilateral eye movements to assist with processing of this event, along with relaxation.[4] The cognitive and behavioral approaches of TFCBT and EMDR are more effective than stress management or group therapy to reduce symptoms of PTSD. Psychoeducation includes information about the disease state, treatment options, and avoidance of excessive use of alcohol and other used substances. Evidence suggests insomnia associated with PTSD benefits from CBT.[5] Novel nonpharmacologic approaches (eg, interpersonal psychotherapy, narrative exposure therapy, written narrative exposure, imagery, transcranial magnetic stimulation [TMS], neurofeedback, acupuncture, yoga, emotional freedom technique, virtual reality exposure, somatic experiencing, mindfulness therapies, and delivery methods [eg, telemedicine and other technology-based treatments]) are under study.[3,5,37]

Pharmacologic Therapy

2 Antidepressants are the major pharmacotherapeutic treatment for PTSD, in addition to also being effective for concurrent depression and anxiety disorders. SSRIs and venlafaxine are the first-line pharmacotherapy of PTSD[4-6,32,33,38,39,42,57]; however, the tricyclic antidepressants (TCAs) and monoamine oxidase inhibitors (MAOIs) can also be effective despite their less favorable side-effect profiles (Table 91-1). Both sertraline and paroxetine are approved for the acute treatment of PTSD,[40,41] and sertraline is approved for the long-term (eg, 52 weeks) management of PTSD.[41] A number of medications can be used as augmentation (eg, antiadrenergic agents, second-generation antipsychotics, and antiseizure medications).[4,5,42] Benzodiazepines are not effective for PTSD.[5,32-34,39] A number of

TABLE 91-1 Dosing of Antidepressants in the Treatment of PTSD

Medication	Brand Name	Initial Dose	Usual Range (mg/day)	Comments
SSRIs				
Fluoxetine	Prozac	10 mg daily	10-80[a]	
Paroxetine	Paxil, Pexeva	10-20 mg daily	20-50	Maximum dose is 60 mg daily[a]
Sertraline	Zoloft®	25 mg daily	50-100	Maximum dose is 200 mg daily[b]
Other Agents				
Amitriptyline	Elavil	25 or 50 mg daily	75-200[a]	
Imipramine	Tofranil	25 or 50 mg daily	75-200[a]	
Mirtazapine	Remeron	15 mg every night	30-60[a]	
Nefazodone	n/a	25-100 mg twice daily	150-600[a]	Product has a black box warning for hepatotoxicity
Phenelzine	Nardil	15 or 30 mg every night	45-90[a]	
Venlafaxine extended-release	Effexor XR	37.5 mg daily	75-225[a]	

[a]Dosage used in clinical trials but not FDA-approved.

[b]Dosage is FDA-approved.

PTSD, posttraumatic stress disorder; SSRIs, selective serotonin reuptake inhibitors; n/a, not applicable.

Data from References 5, 32, 30 and 41.

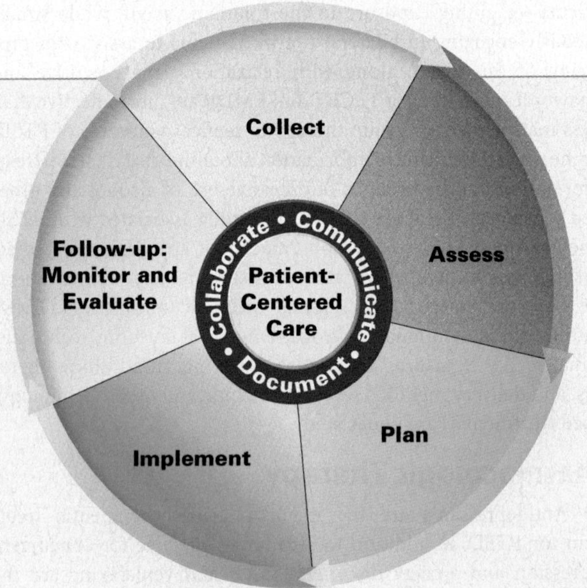

Patient Care Process for Posttraumatic Stress Disorder and Obsessive-Compulsive Disorder

The image shows the five fundamental steps included in patient care process posttraumatic stress disorder and obsessive-compulsive disorder. The tagline of this process reads collaborate, communicate, and document. The five fundamental steps listed here are collect, assess, plan, implement, and follow-up: monitor and evaluate. All these steps are listed in a circular block diagram.

Collect

- Patient characteristics (eg, age, sex, pregnancy status)
- Patient medical history (personal and family, include first-degree relatives' response to medication)
- Social history (eg, tobacco use/ethanol use/substance use/sexual activity)
- Current medications including OTC use, herbal products, dietary supplements, and prior psychiatric medication use
- Patient health preferences, beliefs, and treatment goals
- Objective data
  - Blood pressure (BP), heart rate (HR), respiratory rate (RR), height, weight
  - Lipid panel and A1c or fasting blood sugar if starting antipsychotic therapy
  - Electrocardiogram (ECG) if starting a tricyclic antidepressant (TCA) in a patient with cardiovascular disease, patient <18 or >40 years of page, or with other risk factors for QT prolongation (eg, electrolyte abnormalities, concomitant medications with the potential to prolong the QT)
  - Validated rating scale score (eg, Clinician Administered PTSD Scale [CAPS] or Yale-Brown Obsessive-Compulsive Scale [Y-BOCS])
  - Results of any pharmacogenomics testing

Assess

- Target symptoms (eg, intrusion, avoidance, reactivity, mood/cognition for PTSD and obsessions and/or compulsions for OCD) using CAPS, Y-BOCS, or other rating scale assessments
- Functional impairment/quality of life
- Sleep hygiene
- Psychotic symptoms
- Engagement in psychotherapy
- Medication adherence
- Ability/willingness to utilize and pay for pharmacotherapy or engage in psychotherapy
- Ability/willingness to return to clinic for continued regular symptom assessment
- Need to alter treatment plans due to results of pharmacogenomics testing

Plan*

- Pharmacotherapy regimen including specific medication, dose, route, frequency, onset of action, and duration (see Fig. 91-1, Tables 91-1 through 91-4)
- Monitoring parameters including efficacy (eg, rating scale score, sleep, other symptoms such as irritability, functional impairment, symptom diary) and safety (eg, suicidal ideation, adverse effects including insomnia, worsening anxiety or depression, gastrointestinal distress, sexual dysfunction, agitation); frequency and timing of follow-up
- Patient education (eg, purpose of treatment, lifestyle modification, onset of action, treatment duration, medication specific information, medication administration technique; see Fig. 91-1 and Tables 91-2, 91-3, and 91-5)
- Self-monitoring for changes in PTSD/OCD symptoms, when to seek emergency medical attention
- Referrals to other providers when appropriate (eg, substance use treatment)

Implement*

- Provide patient education regarding all elements of treatment plan
- Use motivational interviewing and coaching strategies to maximize adherence
- Schedule follow-up (eg, CAPS/Y-BOCS or other rating scale assessments, adherence assessment, adverse effect assessment)
- Engage caregiver/family in treatment plan, if possible, and with patient permission

Follow-up: Monitor and Evaluate

- Improvement in rating scale scores of PTSD/OCD symptoms
- Presence of medication related adverse effects (eg, sexual dysfunction, insomnia)
- Patient adherence to treatment plan using multiple sources of information
- Reevaluate sleep hygiene
- Reevaluate effectiveness of psychotherapy
- Assess risk for suicidality

Collaborate with patient, caregivers, and other healthcare professionals.

TABLE 91-2 Summary of Key Points in Treatment Guidelines for PTSD

Recommendations	Comments
First-Line Treatments	
SSRIs: Fluoxetine, paroxetine, sertraline SNRIs: Venlafaxine	At 4 weeks if there is partial response, continue for another 4 weeks. At 8 weeks, if no improvement, increase dose to maximum tolerated or switch to another first-line treatment
Second-Line Treatments	
TCAs: Amitriptyline, imipramine	The risk of adverse effects and potential for fatalities in a TCA overdose are higher than with SSRIs or SNRIs
Mirtazapine	
Augmentation with prazosin for sleep/nightmares	Not recommended in the VA guidelines ***for use in veteran population***
Third-Line treatments	
Augmentation with antiseizure medications or second-generation antipsychotics	The VA guidelines recommend against using risperidone as an augmenting agent secondary to metabolic adverse effects. There is insufficient evidence to support routine use of other second-generation antipsychotics or antiseizure medications
MAOIs: Phenelzine	Potential adverse effects and dietary restrictions limit use
Nefazodone	Risk for hepatotoxicity limits use

PTSD, posttraumatic stress disorder; SNRIs, serotonin–norepinephrine reuptake inhibitors; SSRIs, selective serotonin reuptake inhibitors; TCA, tricyclic antidepressant; VA, Veterans Affairs.

Data from References 4, 5 and 39.

treatment guidelines are published,[4,5,32-34,42] with Table 91-2 providing a summary of key points from the treatment guidelines for PTSD. An algorithm for the treatment of PTSD appears in Fig. 91-1.

Selective Serotonin Reuptake Inhibitors

The SSRIs pharmacologically enhance serotonergic functioning and large prospective guidelines document the efficacy and consistently recommend use of fluoxetine, sertraline, and paroxetine in the acute management of PTSD.[5,32-34,36,39] While a meta-analysis found that SSRIs were significantly better than placebo for the treatment of PTSD, the overall effect size was small.[43] Adverse reactions reported in patients with PTSD treated with SSRIs include gastrointestinal symptoms, sexual dysfunction, insomnia, and agitation. Additionally, long-term use of SSRIs (durations of 9-12 months) has been shown to be effective in preventing relapse.[4,42]

Other Antidepressants

The serotonin–norepinephrine reuptake inhibitor (SNRI) venlafaxine has shown efficacy in PTSD. In a 12-week, placebo-controlled trial comparing venlafaxine extended-release and sertraline, venlafaxine was effective in reducing the avoidance/numbing and hyperarousal clusters of PTSD, whereas sertraline improved all PTSD symptom clusters.[44] The remission rates for venlafaxine extended-release were 30.2% after 12 weeks[44] and 50.1% after 6 months.[45] In one retrospective study, when compared with fluoxetine, sertraline, paroxetine, and topiramate, venlafaxine demonstrated higher 12-week acute phase remission rates, though additional studies are needed.[46]

Other antidepressants have been studied in controlled trials with mirtazapine considered a second-line agent in one guideline,[4] while others highlight insufficient data to recommend use.[5,32,37,42] Specifically, one recent prospective, placebo-controlled trial found mirtazapine did not reduce PTSD, depression, or insomnia symptoms among male combat veterans.[47] The TCAs amitriptyline and imipramine are considered second-line agents, whereas phenelzine and nefazodone are considered third-line antidepressants if therapeutic trials of SSRIs or venlafaxine have failed. Potential adverse effects or risks associated with these agents (eg, daytime drowsiness and toxicity in overdose with TCAs; dietary restrictions and potential medication interactions with MAOIs; or risk of liver failure with nefazodone) limit their use clinically.[4,5,35,42] Bupropion is not recommended in patients with PTSD due to poor quality of evidence, but this agent may be considered as a third-line option.[4,5,32]

Alternative Medication Treatments

Second-generation antipsychotics, α_1-adrenergic receptor antagonists, and antiseizure medications can be used as augmenting agents for persistent PTSD symptoms, in cases of partial response to SSRI therapy after 4 to 6 weeks, or for comorbidities.[4,32,39,42,48] Data on the efficacy of second-generation antipsychotics are conflicting with one study showing quetiapine monotherapy was generally well tolerated and associated with improvements in overall symptomology, reexperiencing, and hyperarousal.[49] Further, guidelines suggest second-generation antipsychotics may be useful in targeting intrusive symptoms,[4] whereas others advise against use due to insufficient evidence[5,32] or use with caution.[33] Any potential benefit must be considered in the context of risks, including metabolic complications. One meta-analysis supports risperidone use among the second-generation antipsychotics,[50] while other recent guidelines advise against use of any second-generation antipsychotic for PTSD due to limited evidence and adverse effect profile.[5,32]

Prazosin (an α_1-adrenergic receptor antagonist) can be useful in some patients with PTSD, with earlier studies showing that it may decrease nightmares and symptoms of hyperarousal, increase total sleep time and sleep quality, and improve core PTSD symptoms. When used for PTSD the daily doses start at 1 mg and may be increased as tolerated to 25 mg.[51] Its presumed mechanism of action is reduction of noradrenergic transmission.[51] In a more recent study, use of prazosin among veterans with chronic PTSD did not improve nightmares or sleep quality compared to placebo, though the study population may have selected patients who were less likely to respond to prazosin.[52] In light of this data, newer Veterans Administration guidelines cite prazosin effects to be similar to placebo and state there is insufficient evidence to recommend use of this agent in this population,[5] whereas other studies and guidelines continue to support prazosin use, when indicated.[53,54] Other pharmacologic options for persistent sleep disturbances are limited. Medications with sedative properties (eg, nefazodone, imipramine, mirtazapine, phenelzine, or second-generation antipsychotics) may be considered depending upon individual comorbidities.[5,39] Other therapies that may be useful for PTSD-related nightmares are discussed in the American Academy of Sleep Medicine Position Paper.[55]

Antiseizure medications can assist in reducing impulsive anger and can also be used in patients with comorbid bipolar disorder; however, the use of an antiseizure medication is not recommended as monotherapy. Some data support efficacy of lamotrigine and topiramate, though overall data with antiseizure medications are inconsistent.[4,5,32,39]

Dosage and Administration

3 Acute Phase Symptoms of PTSD respond slowly to pharmacotherapy, and some patients never experience full resolution; therefore, SSRIs should be started 3 to 4 weeks after exposure to a trauma in patients with no improvement in their acute stress response. The initiation of an SSRI should be at a low dose with gradual titration upward as tolerated to moderate to high doses. Eight to 12 weeks is an appropriate duration of antidepressant therapy to determine response.[4,38,42]

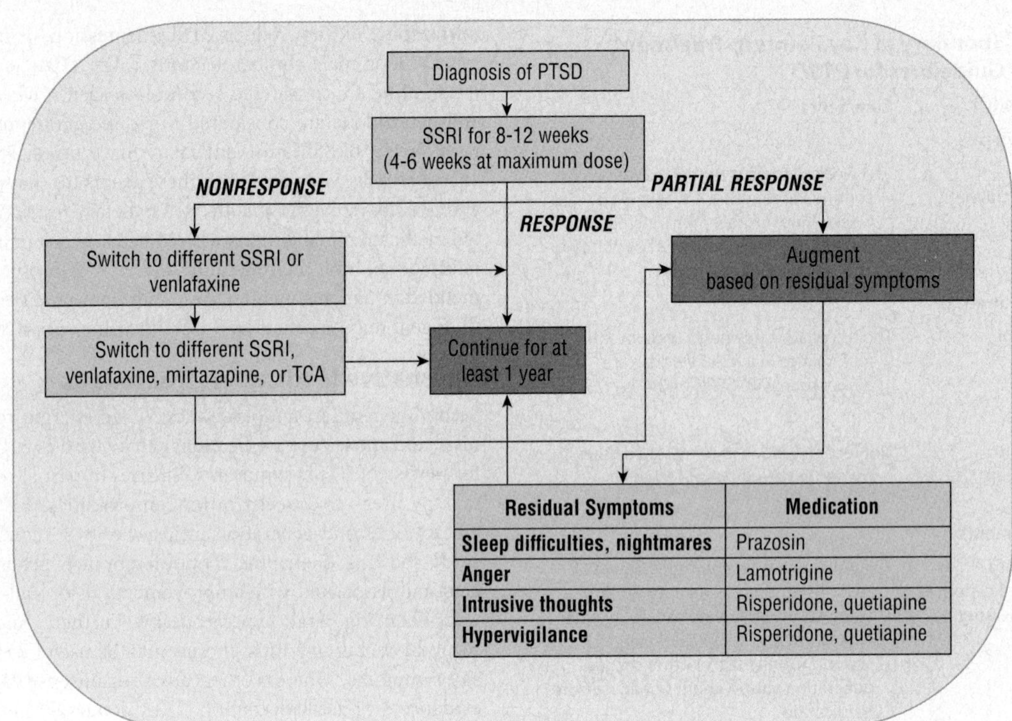

FIGURE 91-1 Algorithm for the pharmacotherapy of posttraumatic stress disorder (PTSD). (SSRI, selective serotonin reuptake inhibitor; TCA, tricyclic antidepressant.) *(Data from References 38 and 39.)*

Continuation Phase Many patients undergo psychotherapy during the continuation phase of therapy, and medication dosages can vary as patients deal with past traumatic experiences. During this phase, symptoms continue to improve. Six-month relapse prevention trials in patients responsive to fluoxetine or sertraline indicate low rates of relapse with SSRI therapy compared with placebo.[42]

4 **Maintenance and Discontinuation** Patients with PTSD who respond to pharmacotherapy should continue treatment for at least 12 months.[4,38,42,56] If residual symptoms persist, medication therapy should be continued. The decision about when to discontinue therapy is based on response, relapse prevalence, presence of ongoing stresses, adverse effects, and patient preference. Once the decision is made to discontinue therapy, the medications should be withdrawn and tapered slowly over a period of at least 1 month to reduce the potential for relapse.

Special Populations

Adults are not the only population susceptible to PTSD, as children who experience stress and trauma (eg, sexual or physical abuse or loss of a parent) are predisposed to develop mood and anxiety disorders. For this patient population, SSRIs are the initial pharmacologic agents of choice[57]; however, psychotherapy (eg, TFCBT) is also a treatment option and studies are ongoing to assess the comparative efficacy and acceptance of psychotherapies for PTSD among children and adolescents.[58,59]

Patients with PTSD and co-occurring unhealthy substance use disorders also warrant careful consideration given the greater risk for attempted suicide.[60] Guidelines suggest this population may benefit from concurrent treatment of both PTSD and substance use disorder and trauma-focused therapies have demonstrated improvement in PTSD symptoms in this population.

Choosing Pharmacotherapy

The choice of pharmacotherapy should be individualized to the patient's presenting symptoms. Selection of SSRI or venlafaxine monotherapy is based on the patient's history of prior response, safety, and side-effect tolerability and is largely a trial-and-error process.[61] When selecting an agent, the clinician should consider the potential for adverse consequences in patients with comorbid conditions (eg, anticholinergic effects and weight gain with paroxetine in patients with benign prostatic hypertrophy or obesity) or adverse effects (eg, insomnia with fluoxetine in patients with sleep difficulties). Increased risk of suicidality should be considered in patients taking antidepressants who are under 25 years of age.

Currently there are no guidelines or articles that specifically address the use of pharmacogenomics testing in PTSD.[43] However, there are data that can help guide medication selection based on specific gene medication pairs for many of the antidepressants used in treating PTSD.[61] The Clinical Pharmacogenomics Implementation Consortium (CPIC) is a valuable resource for understanding dosing recommendations for these various medication and gene combinations.[62]

EVALUATION OF THERAPEUTIC OUTCOMES

During the acute phase of therapy, patients should be seen frequently. During months 3 to 6 of therapy, the patient can usually be seen monthly, and in months 6 to 12, visits can usually be extended to every 2 months. On each visit the patient should be asked about previously identified PTSD target symptoms as well as other symptoms including insomnia, suicidal ideation, anger outbursts, irritability, psychosis, ongoing trauma, and disability. The Clinician-Administered PTSD Scale (CAPS) can be used by the clinician to assess symptom severity at each visit.[5] Remission in patients with PTSD is defined as a 70% or greater reduction in symptoms. A 50% or greater reduction in symptoms is considered adequate response, while a 25% to 50% reduction in symptoms is considered partial response. Before deciding that a patient is not responsive to pharmacotherapy, the clinician should ensure patient adherence and that the medication trial has been adequate in both dose and duration.

Many patients with PTSD are sensitive to the adverse effects of medications and should be monitored carefully for adverse reactions that can delay dose escalation or cause the patient distress. See Chapter 88 for details on monitoring antidepressants. Routine assessment of the metabolic profile is necessary if a second-generation antipsychotic is used concurrently (see Chapter 87).[4,33] When pharmacotherapy is discontinued, patients should be seen more frequently and monitored carefully for signs of relapse or withdrawal.

TREATMENT

Obsessive Compulsive Disorder

Desired Outcomes

Major goals of therapy for OCD include reduction in the frequency and severity of obsessive thoughts and time spent performing compulsive acts.[63] Treatment for OCD generally does not eliminate obsessions or compulsions, but patients can feel remarkably improved with partial resolution of symptoms. Patients typically experience waxing and waning symptoms with only 20% going on to achieve full remission.[1] Optimal treatment increases psychosocial and occupational functioning and improves overall QOL.[63] Efforts should be made to minimize adverse medication events and prevent interactions.

General Approach to Treatment

It is important at the outset of therapy to identify and document the specific target symptoms for pharmacotherapy. Rating scales can be used to measure symptom severity at baseline and during treatment to ascertain the degree of improvement. The Yale-Brown Obsessive-Compulsive Scale (Y-BOCS) is the most widely used clinician-administered OCD rating scale. A QOL scale can assist the clinician in identifying other areas to target for treatment (eg, depression and reduced physical well-being).[63,64]

The FDA has approved five antidepressants for the management of OCD: clomipramine, fluoxetine, fluvoxamine, paroxetine, and sertraline. First-line therapy for OCD includes CBT alone, SSRI monotherapy, or the combination of CBT and an SSRI.[63,64] The choice of therapy is based on clinical judgment, symptom severity, and patient preferences[63]; however, CBT has been largely found to be more effective compared to SSRI monotherapy.[65,66] Patients unable to participate in CBT or with a prior history of medication therapy response should be treated with SSRI monotherapy.[63] Combined CBT and SSRIs is recommended in patients who do not respond to SSRI monotherapy or in those with severe OCD. If a combination of CBT and an SSRI at maximum tolerated dose is unsuccessful, subsequent management options include intensifying CBT, switching to an alternate SSRI, switching to clomipramine, or augmenting with either clomipramine or an antipsychotic.[12,27]

Table 91-3 provides a summary of key points from the treatment guidelines for OCD. Although some OCD symptoms can improve over the first 2 to 6 weeks of therapy, an adequate trial is considered 8 to 12 weeks.[12,26,67]

Nonpharmacologic Therapy

5 Cognitive behavioral therapy with behavioral techniques (eg, exposure and response prevention [ERP]) is the most common initial nonpharmacologic treatment of choice in OCD and is largely considered to be more efficacious than pharmacotherapy.[12,36,66,68] It is preferred for motivated patients, particularly children and adolescents, with both mild OCD symptoms and psychiatric comorbidities, and in those with a desire to avoid medications.[11,12,63,68] Additionally, CBT offers flexibility in dosing (eg, weekly or intensively) and format (eg, individual, group, with or without family involvement).[12,68] Furthermore, family psychoeducation to minimize family accommodation (eg, adaptation of family routines that facilitate ritualistic compulsions) should be integrated into treatment plans to minimize the patient's functional impairment, family conflict/distress, and disruptive behavior to facilitate improved treatment response.[69]

Other nonpharmacologic options for OCD include neuromodulatory approaches (eg, deep brain stimulation [DBS], TMS, and electroconvulsive therapy [ECT]) and ablative neurosurgery for severely symptomatic patients as a treatment of last resort.[12,27] DBS is FDA-approved as a humanitarian device for severe, treatment-resistant

TABLE 91-3 Summary of Key Points in Treatment Guidelines for OCD

Recommendation	Comments
First-Line Treatments	
CBT alone	13-20 sessions
SSRI alone	8-12 weeks, at least 4-6 weeks at maximum tolerated dose
CBT + SSRI	If monotherapy with CBT or SSRI alone does not provide adequate response, combination therapy with CBT + SSRI should be tried before augmentation with another pharmacologic agent
Second-Line Treatments	
Switch to another SSRI or clomipramine	
Augmentation with antipsychotic	Aripiprazole and risperidone are preferred second-generation antipsychotics for OCD treatment
Switch to venlafaxine	
Third-Line Treatments	
Switch to another antipsychotic augmenting agent	
Switch to duloxetine or mirtazapine	
Augmentation of SSRI with clomipramine	Citalopram, escitalopram, and sertraline have less risk to cause clinically significant medication interactions with clomipramine
Maintenance and Discontinuation Phase	
After 1-2 years, gradual taper over several months	
Periodic CBT booster sessions for 3-6 months	

CBT, cognitive behavioral therapy; OCD, obsessive-compulsive disorder; SSRI, selective serotonin reuptake inhibitor.

Data from References 4 and 63.

OCD.[64] Despite the FDA clearing one TMS device for treatment of OCD, the significant heterogeneity across published study designs and outcomes calls for careful interpretation and application.[70] Preliminary data regarding ECT are promising but still inconclusive to support routine use.[27] While these alternatives may be effective in some patients, uncertainties regarding optimal stimulation site and settings for these neuromodulatory approaches likely contribute to heterogeneity in outcomes.

Pharmacologic Therapy

6 7 As a class, SSRIs are the medications of choice for patients with OCD,[63] and while not all are FDA-approved, citalopram and escitalopram have also shown efficacy in reduction of OCD symptoms.[12,66] Clomipramine, a TCA with strong 5-HT reuptake inhibition, is a second-line treatment option.[71] Benzodiazepines should not be used to treat OCD-related obsessions and compulsions.[27,63]

Antidepressant Medications

Current evidence indicates that 5-HT is important for the antiobsessional effects of these medications.[72] Pharmacologically, SSRIs and clomipramine inhibit 5-HT reuptake into the presynaptic neuron, making more 5-HT available to postsynaptic receptors and reducing formation of the 5-HT metabolite 5-hydroxyindoleacetic acid. Although other nonclomipramine TCAs (eg, amitriptyline, imipramine, and nortriptyline) inhibit 5-HT reuptake, they are less potent and selective. Prolonged exposure to increased amounts of 5-HT after chronic antidepressant treatment (2-3 weeks) leads to altered responsiveness of postsynaptic 5-HT receptors or presynaptic autoregulatory receptors that govern 5-HT release in specific brain regions. An improvement in obsessional symptoms may correlate with plasma concentrations of clomipramine but not desmethylclomipramine, the metabolite of clomipramine with less selectivity for 5-HT reuptake inhibition.[73]

Most experts agree that SSRIs are better tolerated than clomipramine.[12] Table 91-5 details the monitoring of SSRI and clomipramine pharmacotherapy in patients with OCD. Clomipramine is more likely to cause sedation, anticholinergic side effects and weight gain, however, is less likely than SSRIs to cause insomnia, akathisia, nausea, and diarrhea. Regardless of the specific medication used, antidepressant side effects can be dose related and worse with faster dose escalation.

The SSRIs are effective in the treatment of OCD with almost half (40%-60%) of patients achieving a response.[12] Well-designed trials comparing these medications with placebo in head-to-head comparative trials, and meta-analyses have established that fluoxetine, fluvoxamine, paroxetine, sertraline, citalopram, and escitalopram are equally effective.[27,66] However, the literature is conflicting as to whether clomipramine is more effective than the SSRIs.[12,27,66]

Venlafaxine and duloxetine, 5-HT and NE reuptake inhibitors, and mirtazapine may also be effective for OCD.[27] Therefore, these antidepressants can be considered second- or third-line therapy options.[4] See Table 91-3.

Pharmacokinetics Clomipramine is rapidly absorbed after oral administration[71] with maximum plasma concentrations occurring within 2 to 6 hours. Clomipramine is highly protein-bound (97%) in the blood and has a half-life of 19 to 37 hours. It is metabolized to an active metabolite, desmethylclomipramine, which inhibits NE reuptake. See Table 91-4 for information on monitoring clomipramine plasma levels. The pharmacokinetics of SSRIs is discussed in Chapter 88. It is important to note that since clomipramine and the SSRIs are extensively metabolized in the liver, patients with significant liver disease should be prescribed these medications cautiously and in lower doses than those without liver disease. Additionally, increased plasma concentrations of paroxetine occur in subjects with renal impairment necessitating a reduced initial dose.[40] For older patients, little information is available regarding pharmacokinetic changes; therefore, medication selection should be based on history of response and adverse effect profile, with treatment initiated at low dose, which is then increased slowly, with vigilant monitoring for adverse effects.[38,63]

Adverse Effects When selecting pharmacotherapy, the clinician should consider medication specific adverse effects such as QTc prolongation risk with citalopram and escitalopram; anticholinergic effects and weight gain risk (eg, with paroxetine in patients with benign prostatic hypertrophy or obesity); insomnia risk with fluoxetine in patients with sleep difficulties; increased risk of suicidality in patients under 25 years of age taking antidepressants; and medication interaction risk for which citalopram, escitalopram, and sertraline have the least potential for cytochrome P450 (CYP450) isoenzyme inhibition (see Chapter 88).[27]

Risks to consider with clomipramine include lethality in overdose in patients with suicidal ideation; and anticholinergic effects in patients with constipation, narrow-angle glaucoma, or urinary hesitancy.[71] Clomipramine use is associated with the risk of QTc

TABLE 91-4 Adult Dosing of Serotonin Reuptake Inhibitors in the Treatment of OCD

Medication	Brand Name	Initial Dose	Usual Range	Comments
Citalopram[a]	Celexa	20 mg daily	20-40 mg daily	Maximum dose is 40 mg in adults daily to prevent QTc prolongation; maximum dose of 20 mg daily in older patients, CYP2C19 poor metabolizers, or use with concurrent moderate-to-strong CYP2C19 inhibitors (eg, cimetidine, omeprazole)
Clomipramine	Anafranil	25 mg daily	100-250 mg daily	Doses up to 300 mg daily may be needed in some patients. Steady-state trough plasma levels (clomipramine and desmethylclomipramine) should be <500 ng/mL (mcg/L; ~1.7 μmol/L) to minimize risk of conduction delays and seizures
Escitalopram[a]	Lexapro	10 mg daily	10-20 mg daily	Doses up to 40 mg may be needed in some patients
Fluoxetine	Prozac	20 mg daily	40-60 mg daily	Doses of 80 mg or higher may be needed in some patients
Fluvoxamine	Luvox Luvox CR	50 mg daily 100 mg bedtime	100-300 mg daily 100-300 mg daily	
Paroxetine	Paxil, Paxil CR, Pexeva	20 mg daily	40-60 mg daily	Higher doses may be needed in some patients
Sertraline	Zoloft	50 mg daily	50-200 mg daily	Higher doses may be needed in some patients

OCD, obsessive-compulsive disorder.

[a]Not FDA-approved for treatment of obsessive-compulsive disorder. Optimal dosing guidelines are not well established.

Data from References 12, 38, 40, 41, 71, and 75.

prolongation when used alone and in combination with other agents that prolong the QTc interval.[71,74] Clomipramine should also be used with caution in patients with a history of cardiovascular disease or conduction abnormalities. Because of sedative and anticholinergic side effects, clomipramine is not usually chosen as first-line therapy for older patients with OCD.[63] The use of antidepressants in older individuals is discussed in Chapter 88.

Dosage and Administration

8 Table 91-4 summarizes dosing guidelines for SSRIs and clomipramine. The SSRI dose to achieve response in OCD is often higher than doses used in other indications.[63,64] Data from fixed-dose studies in adults indicate that higher SSRI doses are more efficacious than lower doses, although there is a higher adverse effect burden.[27] However, there are no fixed dose studies to guide clinicians on how high to increase the clomipramine dose. If there is inadequate response to an average antidepressant dose, then it should be incrementally increased to the maximum dose within 5 to 9 weeks from the start of treatment. If there is an inadequate response after 4 to 6 weeks at the maximum dose, then another antidepressant should be tried.[63] Eight to 12 weeks is considered an adequate antidepressant trial for OCD treatment before changing to another agent.

Alternative Medication Treatments

9 **Augmentation with Antipsychotics** Augmentation of SSRI treatment with low-to-moderate doses of antipsychotics may be helpful,[12,27,76] and should be considered for patients with tic-related OCD, comorbid psychosis, and treatment-refractory symptoms. One-third of patients with treatment-refractory OCD respond to antipsychotic augmentation.[27] A recent meta-analysis found greater effect sizes for aripiprazole, haloperidol, and risperidone, whereas olanzapine, paliperidone, and quetiapine failed to differentiate from placebo; however, quetiapine and olanzapine have been associated with at least one positive result from a randomized controlled trial.[77] First-generation antipsychotics, such as haloperidol, are less preferred given risk of extrapyramidal symptoms. As the long-term use of second-generation antipsychotic augmentation results in higher rates of adverse effects (eg, weight gain, increased blood glucose, lipid abnormalities), treatment should be discontinued if no benefits have been observed after 6 to 10 weeks.[27] Monitoring of antipsychotics can be found in Chapter 87.

Novel Augmentation Strategies While augmentation with antipsychotics has the most evidence,[76] recent studies have examined novel augmentation approaches using glutamatergic agents (eg, *N*-acetylcysteine, lamotrigine, memantine, minocycline, riluzole, and topiramate) and ondansetron with initial promising results.[12,77] Some experts may prefer a trial of glutamatergic agents relative to antipsychotics to avoid antipsychotic-related adverse effects. Using D-cycloserine to augment ERP in patients with refractory OCD has had mixed results; further research is needed to identify patient and treatment characteristics that may differentially moderate response.[78]

Special Populations

Pregnancy OCD may be triggered during the peripartum or postpartum period.[20] Risk–benefit analysis should be made by practitioners when deciding to use pharmacotherapy options during pregnancy.[63,79] The use of antidepressants in pregnancy and lactation is discussed in Chapter 88 and the use of antipsychotics in pregnancy and lactation is discussed in Chapter 87. Chapter 99 also discusses pregnancy and lactation in general.

Children and Adolescents Younger patients exhibit poorer insight regarding obsessions, have more obsessions involving fear of harm and separation, and possess more rituals involving family members. Similar to adult OCD, CBT including ERP and family members and/or SSRI treatment are considered first-line for pediatric patients depending on illness and patient characteristics.[65,69,74] For mild-to-moderate pediatric OCD, CBT is superior to pharmacotherapy.[65]

Both childhood and adult OCD appear to respond similarly to antidepressant therapy with approximately at 50% response rate being seen during the initial SSRI trial in children. Clomipramine, fluvoxamine, sertraline, paroxetine, and fluoxetine are approved by the FDA for the treatment of OCD in children and adolescents.[63] Importantly, in children, the specific adverse effects of SSRI therapy more likely to occur compared to adults include treatment-emergent suicidal ideation, behavioral activation, and mania. In fact, all antidepressants now include a boxed warning regarding risk for suicide in patients 24 years and younger.[69,76] The risk of suicidality in youth is discussed in Chapter 88. Augmentation of SSRIs with antipsychotics or clomipramine is not well studied in pediatric patients but can be considered for treatment-refractory illness after failed SSRI augmentation with CBT, based on expert opinion and guideline recommendations.[69,74]

Antidepressant Dosing in Children Pediatric patients often require smaller initial doses of medications (eg, fluoxetine 10 mg daily) compared to adults (eg, fluoxetine 20 mg daily). The starting dose of clomipramine in children is 25 mg daily in divided doses[71] with dose escalations occurring over the first 2 weeks up to 3 mg/kg or 100 mg, whichever is smaller. Over the next several weeks, the dose can be increased up to 3 mg/kg with a maximum of 200 mg daily given once daily at bedtime.

Choosing Pharmacotherapy

The choice of an SSRI for the treatment of OCD is based on history of prior response, safety, and adverse effect tolerability of the patient (see Table 91-5). While all SSRIs are considered equally efficacious, a patient may respond better to one agent over another.[63,66] Therefore, antidepressant treatment decisions should consider patient specific factors, such as previous treatment, family history of medication response, patient preference, and insurance coverage of medications. Currently, there are no guidelines that specifically address the use of pharmacogenomics testing in OCD. However, there are data that can help guide medication selection based on specific gene medication pairs for many of the antidepressants used in treating OCD. A valuable resource for understanding dosing recommendations for these various medication and gene combinations is CPIC.[62] Use of these guidelines, along with any testing interpretation results, may help reduce the risk of antidepressant specific adverse events, potentially, facilitating successful treatment.

EVALUATION OF THERAPEUTIC OUTCOMES

Target symptoms of OCD should be monitored closely with degree of response being used to indicate a need to modify dosage, change medication, or augment therapy. Rating scales can be used to monitor symptom response to therapy for OCD (eg, Y-BOCS) and changes in QOL.[27,63] Response is often defined by an improvement of 25% to 35% in baseline symptoms, whereas remission is defined as a total Y-BOCS score less than 16 (out of a total score of 40), both of which still indicate substantial symptomatology.[27] The clinician should inquire about and address problematic adverse effects, including the emergence of suicidal ideation, reported by the patient, and the amount of time the patient spends obsessing and performing compulsions (see Table 91-5).[63] Additionally, changes in social and occupational functioning should be assessed.

10 After patients have responded in the acute phase of treatment, treatment gains are maintained with maintenance-phase

TABLE 91-5 Monitoring of Patients Being Treated for OCD

Medication	Adverse Medication Effects	Monitoring Consideration
Clomipramine	Dry mouth, constipation, nausea, dyspepsia, anorexia, somnolence, tremors, dizziness, nervousness	Assess at every visit, however, tolerance to these adverse events should occur in 2 weeks after treatment is started or a dosage increase is made. New onset adverse events may occur due to medication interactions
	Seizures	Assess if new onset seizures have occurred at each visit
	Orthostatic hypotension, tachycardia, ECG changes	Obtain baseline ECG and vital signs in pediatric patients, patients >40 years, those with cardiovascular disease, or those with other risk factors for QTc prolongation (eg, electrolyte abnormalities, concomitant QTc prolonging medications)
	Suicidality	Obtain at every visit. Highest risk is in patients ≤24 years
	Agranulocytosis, leukopenia	Obtain CBC with differential if patient complains of sore throat, fever
	Weight gain	Obtain vitals (including height and weight) and assess at each visit
SSRIs	Nausea, vomiting, diarrhea, sexual dysfunction, headache, insomnia	Should be assessed at every visit, but generally these adverse events and mild and short-lived. They may reoccur due to a new medication interaction
	Anxiety and agitation	Assess at each visit. May occur in some patients early in treatment
	Discontinuation syndrome	Slowly taper medication to reduce the occurrence of this adverse event. Patient education is key in recognizing its occurrence
	Suicidality	Assess at every visit. Highest risk is in patients ≤24 years
	QTc prolongation	Obtain baseline ECG and electrolytes. Of most concern with citalopram doses over 40 mg daily in adults and 20 mg daily in older patients or in those with risk factors >60 years old, female sex, cardiovascular disease, hypokalemia, hypomagnesemia, or concurrent use of medications or substances that prolong QTc

strategies.[63] Monthly follow-up visits are recommended for at least 3 to 6 months, and a medication taper can be considered after 1 to 2 years of treatment depending on relapse prevalence, medication adverse effects, and patient preferences.[39,63,74] Treatment discontinuation results in higher relapse rates compared with treatment continuation[56] and medication should not be rapidly discontinued. Booster CBT sessions can reduce the risk of relapse when medication is withdrawn.[63] When making the decision to withdraw medication therapy, the dosage can be decreased by 10% to 25% every 1 to 2 months with careful observation for symptom relapse. However, most patients require lifelong medication therapy given chronicity of symptoms.[56]

CONCLUSION

Beginning with the *DSM-5*, both PTSD and OCD related disorders were removed from the anxiety disorder classification. Neurobiological changes in the HPA axis and the CSTC circuit are largely implicated in PTSD and OCD, respectively. The age of onset of PTSD is variable since it depends on trauma or stressful event exposure though it typically occurs before age 40 years while OCD has a bimodal age of onset peaking in late childhood/adolescence and in early adulthood. Both conditions have effective nonpharmacological methods to reduce symptoms including trauma focused therapy, EMDR for PTSD, and CBT with ERP in OCD. The SSRIs are first-line treatment for both conditions; however, moderate-to-high dose SSRIs are typically needed in OCD treatment. The use of antipsychotics in PTSD is controversial, whereas there is a clearer role for antipsychotic augmentation in OCD treatment. Pharmacotherapy should be continued for at least 1 year in PTSD and 1 to 2 years in OCD.

ABBREVIATIONS

5-HT	serotonin
ASD	acute stress disorder
CAPS	Clinician-Administered Posttraumatic Stress Disorder Scale
CBT	cognitive behavioral therapy
CPIC	Clinical Pharmacogenomics Implementation Consortium
CRF	corticotropin-releasing factor
CSTC	cortico-striatal-thalamo-cortical
CYP450	cytochrome P450 isoenzyme
DA	dopamine
dACC	dorsal anterior cingulate cortex
DBS	deep brain stimulation
EMDR	eye movement desensitization and reprocessing
ERP	exposure and response prevention
GABA	γ-aminobutyric acid
HPA	hypothalamic-pituitary-adrenal
MAOI	monoamine oxidase inhibitor
MRI	magnetic resonance imaging
NE	norepinephrine
NMDA	N-methyl-D-aspartate
NPY	neuropeptide Y
OCD	obsessive-compulsive disorder
PANDAS	pediatric autoimmune neuropsychiatric disorder associated with streptococcal infection
PCL-5	PTSD Checklist for *DSM-5*
PET	positron emission tomography
PTSD	posttraumatic stress disorder
QOL	quality of life
SNP	single nucleotide polymorphism
SNRI	serotonin–norepinephrine reuptake inhibitor
SPECT	single-photon emission computed tomography
SSRI	selective serotonin reuptake inhibitor
TCA	tricyclic antidepressant
TFCBT	trauma-focused cognitive behavioral therapy
TMS	transcranial magnetic stimulation
mPFC	medial prefrontal cortex
Y-BOCS	Yale-Brown Obsessive-Compulsive Scale

REFERENCES

1. American Psychiatric Association. *Diagnostic and Statistical Manual of Mental Disorders*. 5th ed. Arlington, VA: American Psychiatric Association; 2013.
2. Sher L, Braquehais M, Casas M. Posttraumatic stress disorder, depression, and suicide in veterans. *Cleve Clin J Med*. 2012;79(2):92–97.
3. Shalev A, Liberzon I, Marmar C. Post-traumatic stress disorder. *N Engl J Med*. 2017;376:2459–2469.

4. Katzman MA, Bleau P, Blier P, et al. Canadian clinical practice guidelines for the management of anxiety, posttraumatic stress and obsessive-compulsive disorders. *BMC Psychiatry*. 2014;14(suppl 1):S1.
5. Veterans Health Administration, Department of Defense. VA/DoD clinical practice guideline for the management of post-traumatic stress disorder and acute stress disorder. Washington, DC: Veterans Health Administration, Department of Defense; 2017 June. Available at: https://www.healthquality.va.gov/guidelines/MH/ptsd/VADoDPTSDCPGFinal.pdf. Accessibility verified April 9, 2018.
6. De La Vega D, Giner L, Courtet P. Suicidality in subjects with anxiety or obsessive-compulsive and related disorders: Recent advances. *Curr Psychiatry Rep*. 2018;20(4):26.
7. Gradus JL. Prevalence and prognosis of stress disorders: A review of the epidemiologic literature. *Clin Epid*. 2017;9:251–260.
8. National Institute of Mental Health. Obsessive-compulsive disorder among adults. Available at https://www.nimh.nih.gov/health/statistics/obsessive-compulsive-disorder-ocd.shtml. Accessed June 20, 2018.
9. Shalev A, Liberzon I, Marmar C. Post-traumatic stress disorder. *N Engl J Med*. 2017;376:2459–2469.
10. Christiansen DM, Berke ET. Gender- and sex-based contributors to sex differences in PTSD. *Curr Psychiatr Rep*. 2020;22(4):19.
11. Richter PMA, Ramos RT. Obsessive-compulsive disorder. *Continuum (Minneap Minn)*. 2018;24(3):828–844.
12. Hirschtritt ME, Bloch MH, Mathews CA. Obsessive-compulsive disorder: advances in diagnosis and treatment. *JAMA*. 2017;317(13):1358–1367.
13. Bokor G, Anderson PD. Obsessive-compulsive disorder. *J Pharm Pract*. 2014;27(2):116–130.
14. Mandelli L, Draghetti S, Albert U, et al. Rates of comorbid obsessive-compulsive disorder in eating disorders: A meta-analysis of the literature. *J Affect Disord*. 2020;927–939.
15. Logue MW, Smith AK, Baldwin C, et al. An analysis of gene expression in PTSD implicates genes involved in the glucocorticoid receptor pathway and neural responses to stress. *Psychoneuroendocrinology*. 2015;57:1–13.
16. Guillen-Burgos HF, Gutierrez-Ruiz K. Genetic advances in post-traumatic stress disorder. *Rev Colomb Psiquiat*. 2018;647(2):108–118.
17. Navarro-Mateu F, Escamez T, Koenen KC, et al. Meta-analysis of the 5-HTTLPR polymorphisms in post-traumatic stress disorder. *PLoS One*. 2013;8:e66227.
18. Daskalakis NP, Rijal CM, King C, et al. Recent genetics and epigenetics approaches to PTSD. *Curr Psychiatry Rep*. 2018:20(5):30.
19. Rajendram R, Kronenberg S, Burton CL, Arnold PD. Glutamate genetics in obsessive-compulsive disorder: A review. *J Can Acad Child Adolesc Psychiatry*. 2017;26(3):205–213.
20. Stein DJ, Costa DLC, Lochner C, et al. Obsessive-compulsive disorder. *Nat Rev Dis Primers*. 2020;5(1):52.
21. Goodman WK, Storch EA, Sheth SA. Harmonizing the neurobiology and treatment of obsessive-compulsive disorder. *Am J Psychiatry*. 2021;178(1):17–29.
22. Sherin JE, Nemeroff CB. Posttraumatic stress disorder: The neurobiological impact of psychological trauma. *Dialogues Clin Neurosci*. 2011;13:263–278.
23. Martin EI, Ressler KJ, Binder E, Nemeroff CB. The neurobiology of anxiety disorders: Brain imaging, genetics and psychoneuroendocrinology. *Psychiatr Clin North Am*. 2009;32:549–575.
24. Fragkaki I, Thomaes K, Sijbrandij M. Posttraumatic stress disorder under ongoing threat: A review of neurobiological and neuroendocrine findings. *Eur J Psychotraumatology*. 2016;9:30915.
25. Kautz M, Charney DS, Murrough JW. Neuropeptide Y, resilience, and PTSD therapeutics. *Neurosci Lett*. 2017;649:164–169.
26. Issari Y, Jakubovski E, Bartley CA, et al. Early onset of response with selective serotonin reuptake inhibitors in obsessive-compulsive disorder: A meta-analysis. *J Clin Psychiatry*. 2016;77(5):e605–e611.
27. Fineberg N, Reghuneudanan S, Simpson HB, et al. Obsessive-compulsive disorder (OCD): Practice strategies for pharmacologic and somatic treatment in adults. *Psychiatry Res*. 2015;227:114–125.
28. Sinopoli VM, Burton CL, Kronenberg S, et al. A review of the role of serotonin system genes in obsessive-compulsive disorder. *Neurosci Biobehav Rev*. 2017;80:372–381.
29. Shin LM, Liberzon I. The neurocircuitry of fear, stress and anxiety disorders. *Neuropsychopharmacology*. 2010;35:169–191.
30. Carmassi C, Foghi C, Dell'Oste V, et al. PTSD symptoms in healthcare workers facing the three coronavirus outbreaks: What can we expect after the COVID-19 pandemic. *Psychiatry Res*. 2020;292:113312.
31. Liu CH, Zhang E, Wong GTF, Hyun S, Hahm HC. Factors associated with depression, anxiety, and PTSD symptomatology during the COVID-19 pandemic: Clinical implications for U.S. young adult mental health. *Psychiatry Res*. 2020;290:113172.
32. Hoffman V, Middleton JC, Feltner C, Gaynes BN, Weber RP, Bann C, Viswanathan M, Lohr KN, Baker C, Green J. Psychological and Pharmacological Treatments for Adults With Posttraumatic Stress Disorder: A Systematic Review Update. Comparative Effectiveness Review No. 207. (Prepared by the RTI International-University of North Carolina at Chapel Hill Evidence-based Practice Center under Contract No. 290-2015-00011-I for AHRQ and PCORI.) AHRQ Publication No. 18-EHC011-EF. PCORI Publication No. 2018-SR-01. Rockville, MD: Agency for Healthcare Research and Quality; May 2018. Posted final reports are located on the Effective Health Care Program search page.
33. National Institute for Health and Care Excellence. Post-traumatic stress disorder (NICE Quality Standard NG116), 2018. Available at: https://www.nice.org.uk/guidance/ng116/evidence/f-pharmacological-interventions-for-the-prevention-and-treatment-of-ptsd-in-adults-pdf-6602621010. Accessed August 2, 2021.
34. American Psychological Association. Clinical practice guideline for the treatment of PTSD. 2017. Available at: https://www.apa.org/ptsd-guideline/ptsd.pdf. Accessed August 2, 2021.
35. Charney ME, Hellberg SN, Bui E, Simon NM. Evidenced-based treatment of posttraumatic stress disorder: An updated review of validated psychotherapeutic and pharmacological approaches. *Harv Rev of Psychiatry*. 2018;26(3):99–115.
36. Le QA, Doctor JN, Zoellner LA, Feeny NC. Effects of treatment, choice, and preference on health-related quality-of-life outcomes in patients with posttraumatic stress disorder (PTSD). *Qual Life Res*. 2018;27(6):1555–1562.
37. Posttraumatic Stress Disorder Prevention and Treatment Guidelines: Methodology and Recommendations. International Society for Traumatic Stress Studies. 2019. Available at: https://istss.org/getattachment/Treating-Trauma/New-ISTSS-Prevention-and-Treatment-Guidelines/ISTSS_PreventionTreatmentGuidelines_FNL-March-19-2019.pdf.aspx. Accessed August 2, 2021.
38. Bandelow B, Sher L, Bunevicius R, et al. Guidelines for the pharmacological treatment of anxiety disorders, obsessive-compulsive disorder, and post-traumatic stress disorder in primary care. *Int J Psychiatry Clin Pract*. 2012;16:77–84.
39. Ipser JC, Stein DJ. Evidence-based pharmacotherapy of post-traumatic stress disorder. *Int J Neuropsychopharmacol*. 2012;15(6):825–840.
40. Paxil [package insert]. Research Triangle Park, NC: GlaxoSmithKline; October 2016.
41. Zoloft [package insert]. New York, NY: Pfizer Inc.; January 2018.
42. Baldwin DS, Anderson IM, Nutt DJ, et al. Evidence-based pharmacological treatment of anxiety disorders, post-traumatic stress disorder and obsessive-compulsive disorder: A revision of the 2005 guidelines from the British Association of Psychopharmacology. *J Psychopharmacol*. 2014;28(5):403–439.
43. Hoskins M, Pearce J, Bethell A, et al. Pharmacotherapy for posttraumatic stress disorder: Systematic review and meta-analysis. *BJP*. 2015;206:93–100.
44. Davidson J, Rothbaum BO, Tucker P, et al. Venlafaxine extended release in posttraumatic stress disorder: A sertraline- and placebo-controlled study. *J Clin Psychopharmacol*. 2006;26:259–267.
45. Davidson J, Baldwin D, Stein DJ, et al. Treatment of posttraumatic stress disorder with venlafaxine extended release: A 6-month randomized controlled trial. *Arch Gen Psychiatry*. 2006;63:1158–1165.
46. Shiner B, Leonard CE, Gui J, et al. Comparing medications for DSM-5 PTSD in routine VA practice. *J Clin Psychiatry*. 2020;81(6):20m13244.
47. Davis LL, Pilkinton P, Lin C, Parker P, Estes S, Bartolucci A. A randomized, placebo-controlled trial of mirtazapine for the treatment of posttraumatic stress disorder in veterans. *J Clin Psychiatry*. 2020;81(6):20m13267. Published 2020 Oct 20.
48. Huang Z-D, Zhao Y-F, Li S, et al. Comparative efficacy and acceptability of pharmaceutical management for adults with post-traumatic stress disorder: A systematic review and meta-analysis. *Front Pharmacol*. 2020;11:559.
49. Villarreal G, Hamner MB, Cañive JM, et al. Efficacy of quetiapine monotherapy in posttraumatic stress disorder: A randomized, placebo-controlled trial. *Am J Psychiatry*. 2016;173(12):1205–1212.
50. Cipriani A, Williams T, Nikolakopoulou A, et al. Comparative efficacy and acceptability of pharmacological treatments for post-traumatic stress disorder in adults: A network meta-analysis. *Psychol Med*. 2018;48(12):1975–1984.
51. Singh B, Hughes AJ, Mehta G, Erwin PJ, Parsaik AK. Efficacy of prazosin in posttraumatic stress disorder: A systematic review and

meta-analysis. *Prim Care Companion CNS Disord.* 2016;18(4). doi:10.4088/PCC.16r01943.
52. Raskind MA, Peskind ER, Chow B, et al. Trial of prazosin for post-traumatic stress disorder in military veterans. *N Engl J Med.* 2018;378(6):507–517.
53. Zhang Y, Ren R, Sanford LD, et al. The effects of prazosin on sleep disturbances in post-traumatic stress disorder: A systematic review and meta-analysis. *Sleep Med.* 2020;67:225–231.
54. Reist C, Streja E, Tang CC, Shapiro B, Mintz J, Hollifield M. Prazosin for treatment of post-traumatic stress disorder: A systematic review and meta-analysis [published online ahead of print, 2020 May 4]. *CNS Spectr.* 2020;1–7.
55. Morgenthaler TI, Auerbach S, Casey KR, Kristo D, Maganti R, Ramar K, Zak R, Kartje R. Position paper for the treatment of nightmare disorder in adults: An American Academy of Sleep Medicine position paper. *Clin Sleep Med.* 2018;14(6):1041–1055.
56. Batelaan NM, Bosman RC, Muntingh A, Scholten WD, Huijbregts KM, van Balkom AJLM. Risk of relapse after antidepressant discontinuation in anxiety disorders, obsessive-compulsive disorder, and post-traumatic stress disorder: Systematic review and meta-analysis of relapse prevention trials. *BMJ.* 2017;358:j3927.
57. Ipser JC, Stein DJ, Hawkridge S, Hoppe L. Pharmacotherapy for anxiety disorders in children and adolescents. *Cochrane Database Syst Rev.* 2009;3:CD005170. doi:10.1002/14651858.CD005170.pub2.
58. Keeshin BR, Strawn JR. Psychological and pharmacologic treatment of youth with posttraumatic stress disorder: An evidence-based review. *Child Adolesc Psychiatr Clin N Am.* 2014;23:399–411.
59. Zhang Y, Zhou X, Yang L, et al. Comparative efficacy and acceptability of psychotherapies for post-traumatic stress disorder in children and adolescents: Study protocol for a systematic review and network meta-analysis. *BMJ Open.* 2018;8(3):e020198.
60. Norman SB, Haller M, Hamblen JL, Soutwick SM, Pietrzak RH. The burden of co-occurring alcohol use disorder and PTSD in US Military veterans: Comorbidities, functioning, and suicidality. *Psychol Addict Behav.* 2018;32(2):224–229.
61. Miller MW. Leveraging genetics to enhance the efficacy of PTSD pharmacotherapies. *Neurosci Lett.* 2018 April 22. pii: S0304-3940(18)303021. doi:10.1016/j.neulet.2018.04.039. [Epub ahead of print].
62. Clinical pharmacogenetics implementation consortium. Available at: https://cpicpgx.org/. Last accessed, August 10, 2018.
63. American Psychiatric Association. *Practice Guideline for the Treatment of Patients with Obsessive-Compulsive Disorder.* Arlington, VA: American Psychiatric Association; 2007. Available at: http://psychiatryonline.org/pb/assets/raw/sitewide/practice_guidelines/guidelines/ocd.pdf. Accessed, July 6, 2018.
64. American Psychiatric Association. Guideline Watch (2013): Practice Guideline for the Treatment of Patients with Obsessive-Compulsive Disorder. Available at: http://psychiatryonline.org/pb/assets/raw/sitewide/practice_guidelines/guidelines/ocd-watch.pdf. Accessed, July 6, 2018.
65. Öst LG, Riise EN, Wergeland GJ, et al. Cognitive behavioral and pharmacological treatments of OCD in children: A systematic review and meta-analysis. *J Anxiety Disord.* 2016;43:58–69.
66. Skapinakis P, Caldwell DM, Hollingworth W, et al. Pharmacological and psychotherapeutic interventions for management of obsessive-compulsive disorder in adults: A systematic review and network meta-analysis. *Lancet Psychiatry.* 2016;3:730–739.
67. Varigonda AL, Jakubovski E, Bloch MH. Systematic review and meta-analysis: Early treatment response of selective serotonin reuptake inhibitors and clomipramine in pediatric obsessive-compulsive disorder. *J Am Acad Child Adolesc Psychiatry.* 2016;55(10):851–859.
68. Lewin AB, Wu MS, McGuire JF, Storch EA. Cognitive behavior therapy for obsessive-compulsive and related disorder. *Psychiatr Clin N Am.* 2014;37:415–445.
69. Bloch MH, Storch EA. Assessment and management of treatment-refractory obsessive-compulsive disorder in children. *J Am Acad Child Adolesc Psychiatry.* 2015;54(4):251–262.
70. Lusicic A, Schruers KRJ, Pallanti S, Castle D. Transcranial magnetic stimulation in the treatment of obsessive-compulsive disorder: Current perspective. *Neuropsych Dis Treat.* 2018;14:1721–1736.
71. Anafranil [package insert]. Hazelwood, MO: Mallinckrodt Inc; February 2018.
72. Nestadt G, Grados M, Samuels JF. Genetics of OCD. *Psychiatr Clin North Am.* 2010;33(1):141–158.
73. Marcourakis T, Bernik MA, Lotufo NF, et al. Clomipramine demethylation rate is important on the outcome of obsessive-compulsive disorder treatment. *Int Clin Psychopharmacol.* 2015;30(1):43–48.
74. Geller DA, March J. Practice parameter for the assessment and treatment of children and adolescents with obsessive-compulsive disorder. *J Am Acad Child Adolesc Psychiatry.* 2012;51(1):98–113.
75. Balant-Gorgia AE, Gex-Fabry M, Balant LP. Clinical pharmacokinetics of clomipramine. *Clin Pharmacokinet.* 1991;20(6):447–462.
76. Dold M, Aigner M, Lazenberger R, Kasper S. Antipsychotic augmentation of serotonin-reuptake inhibitors in treatment-resistant obsessive-compulsive disorder: An update meta-analysis of double-blind, randomized, placebo-controlled trials. *Int J Neuropsychopharmacol.* 2015;18(9):1–11.
77. Marinova Z, Chuang D, Fineberg N. Glutamate-modulating drugs as a potential therapeutic strategy in obsessive-compulsive disorder. *Current Neuropharmacology.* 2017;15:977–995.
78. Mataix-Cols D, Fernandez de la Cruz L, Monzani B, et al. D-cycloserine augmentation of exposure-based cognitive behavior therapy for anxiety, obsessive-compulsive disorder, and posttraumatic stress disorders: A systematic review and meta-analysis of individual participant data. *JAMA Psychiatry.* 2017;74(5):501–510.
79. Uguz F. Pharmacotherapy of obsessive-compulsive disorder during pregnancy: A clinical approach. *Rev Bras Psiquiatr.* 2015;37(4):334–342.

92

Sleep Disorders

John M. Dopp and Bradley G. Phillips

KEY CONCEPTS

1. Common causes of insomnia include concomitant mental illness, significant psychosocial stressors, alcohol use, caffeine intake, and nicotine use.
2. Good sleep hygiene, including relaxing before bedtime, exercising regularly, establishing a regular bedtime and wake-up time, and discontinuing alcohol, caffeine, and nicotine, alone and in combination with pharmacotherapy, should be part of patient education and treatments for insomnia.
3. Long-acting benzodiazepines should be avoided in older individuals.
4. Benzodiazepine receptor agonist tolerance and physical dependence are avoided by using low-dose therapy for the shortest possible duration.
5. Obstructive sleep apnea may be an independent risk factor for the development of hypertension. When hypertension is present, it is often refractory to pharmacotherapy until sleep-disordered breathing is alleviated.
6. Nasal continuous positive airway pressure is the first-line therapy for obstructive sleep apnea, and weight loss should be encouraged in all obese patients.
7. Pharmacologic management of narcolepsy is focused on two primary areas: treatment of excessive daytime sleepiness and rapid eye movement (REM) sleep abnormalities.
8. Short-acting benzodiazepine receptor agonists, ramelteon, or melatonin taken at appropriate target bedtimes for east or west travel reduce jet lag and shorten sleep latency.
9. The alpha-2-delta ligands, gabapentin, gabapentin enacarbil, and pregabalin, are standard therapy for chronic restless legs syndrome and have not caused symptom augmentation during chronic therapy.

BEYOND THE BOOK

Construct a table of medications used for insomnia, list the half-lives of their parent compound, and whether they are used for difficulty initiating or maintaining sleep.

Medication	Parent Medication Half-Life (hours)	Insomnia Use
Amitriptyline	15	Difficulty maintaining sleep
Zaleplon	1	Difficulty initiating sleep

INTRODUCTION

Approximately 70 million Americans suffer with a sleep-related problem, and as many as 60% of those experience a chronic disorder.[1] More than 80% of patients aged 65 years and older report a sleep-related disturbance.[1]

Sleep Cycles

Sleep is divided into two phases: nonrapid eye movement (NREM) sleep and rapid eye movement (REM) sleep. Each night humans typically experience four to six cycles of NREM and REM sleep, with each cycle lasting between 70 and 120 minutes.[2] There are three stages of NREM sleep. Healthy sleep will typically progress through the three stages of NREM sleep prior to the first REM period. From wakefulness, sleep typically progresses quickly through stages 1 and 2. Stage 1 of NREM sleep is the stage between wakefulness and sleep, and individuals describe this experience as being awake, being drowsy, or being asleep. During stage 3 NREM, both metabolic activity and brain waves slow. This slow-wave sleep occurs most frequently early in the sleep period. Stage 3 sleep is called *delta sleep*, as the sleep is characterized by high amplitude and slow activity waves known as delta waves (0.5–3 Hz) with no eye movements and low tonic muscle activity.

REM sleep involves a dramatic physiologic change from NREM sleep to a state in which the brain becomes electrically and metabolically activated.[2] REM occurs in bursts and is accompanied by a 62% to 173% increase in cerebral blood flow, generalized muscle atonia, bursts of bilateral REMs, poikilothermia, dreaming, and fluctuations in respiratory and cardiac rate.[2] REM cycles tend to lengthen in the later stages of the sleep cycle.[2]

Circadian Rhythm

At birth, human infants spend up to 20 hours a day sleeping with differentiation between REM and NREM sleep occurring at 3 to 6 months of age and the ultradian sleep–wake rhythm changing to a circadian pattern by age 3. Key to this is the suprachiasmatic nucleus of the brain which serves as the biologic clock and paces the circadian rhythm; although the length of a day is 24 hours, in environments devoid of light cues, the sleep–wake cycle lasts about 25 hours.[3] Through development from childhood into adolescence, the amount of nightly delta sleep declines and amount of REM sleep increases. In midlife, however, there is a gradual decline in sleep efficiency and sleep time,[2] and older persons have lighter and more fragmented sleep, with intermittent arousals, shifts in the sleep stages, and a gradual reduction of slow-wave sleep.

Neurochemistry

The neurochemistry of sleep is complex, as sleep cannot be localized to either a specific area of the brain or a specific neurotransmitter.

Overall, NREM sleep appears to be controlled by the basal forebrain, the lower brain stem to the thalamus, and hypothalamus with numerous neurotransmitters mediating NREM sleep, including γ-aminobutyric acid (GABA) and adenosine.[3] In contrast, REM sleep appears to be turned on by cholinergic cells in the mesencephalic, medullary, and pontine gigantocellular regions and turned off by the dorsal raphe nucleus, the locus coeruleus, and the nucleus parabrachialis lateralis, the latter two of which are primarily noradrenergic. The ascending reticular activating system and the posterior hypothalamus also facilitate arousal and wakefulness[4] through neurotransmitters such as dopamine, which has an alerting effect.[5] Additional neurochemicals involved in wakefulness include norepinephrine and acetylcholine in the cortex, and histamine and neuropeptides such as substance P and corticotropin-releasing factor in the hypothalamus.[5,6]

Polysomnography

Polysomnography (PSG) is the primary method used to assess and record variables that characterize sleep and aid in diagnosis of sleep disorders. As part of this assessment, sleep is typically measured and observed in sleep laboratories using an electroencephalogram, electrooculograms of each eye, electrocardiogram, electromyogram, air thermistors, abdominal and thoracic strain belts, and oxygen saturation monitor. Variables obtained during PSG include sleep onset, arousals, sleep stages, eye movements, leg and jaw movements, arrhythmias, airflow during sleep, respiratory effort, and oxygen desaturations. Additionally, home sleep monitoring that measures variables such as electrocardiogram, oxygen saturation, airflow, and respiratory effort is increasingly used to diagnose sleep apnea.

Classification of Sleep Disorders

The *Diagnostic and Statistical Manual of Mental Disorders, Fifth Edition (DSM-5)* classifies sleep–wake disorders into 10 categories: (1) insomnia disorder, (2) hypersomnolence disorder, (3) narcolepsy, (4) breathing-related sleep disorders, (5) circadian rhythm sleep disorders, (6) non-REM sleep arousal disorders, (7) nightmare disorder, (8) REM sleep behavior disorder, (9) restless legs syndrome (RLS), and (10) substance- or medication-induced sleep disorder.[7]

INSOMNIA

Insomnia is one of the most common complaints in general medical practice[8] as it frequently causes distress, due to the fear or a feeling of not being able to fall asleep at bedtime, leading to impaired work-related productivity because of daytime fatigue or drowsiness. Therefore, insomnia disorder is subjectively characterized as trouble initiating sleep, maintaining sleep or waking up early with inability to fall back asleep, that is associated with daytime consequences (insomnia not attributed to environment or limited opportunity for sleep).[7-9] Insomnia is classified as chronic when it has a duration of at least three months, occurring at least three times per week.[7,9]

Primary insomnia usually begins in early or middle adulthood and is rare in childhood or adolescence. Short-term insomnia occurs in 33% to 50% of the adult population,[8] with a year prevalence study of insomnia in the United States reporting that one-third of the individuals surveyed complained of insomnia and 17% reported that the symptoms were serious.[1] Conservative estimates of chronic insomnia range from 9% to 12% in adulthood and up to 20% in older individuals.[1,10] Although young adults are more likely to complain that they have difficulty falling asleep, middle-aged and older adults are more likely to complain that they have middle-of-the-night awakening or early morning awakening. Females complain of insomnia twice as frequently as males and individuals who are older, unemployed, separated, or widowed, and those with a lower socioeconomic status report a significantly higher incidence of insomnia than the general population. Forty per cent of individuals with insomnia also have a concurrent psychiatric disorder (eg, anxiety, depression, or substance use disorder),[11] and a significant percentage of those with insomnia use nonprescription medications or alcohol to self-treat.

TABLE 92-1 Common Etiologies of Insomnia

Situational
• Work or financial stress, major life events, interpersonal conflicts
• Jet lag or shift work
Medical
• Cardiovascular (eg, angina, arrhythmias, heart failure)
• Respiratory (eg, asthma, sleep apnea)
• Chronic pain
• Endocrine disorders (eg, diabetes, hyperthyroidism)
• Gastrointestinal (eg, gastroesophageal reflux disease, ulcers)
• Neurologic (eg, delirium, epilepsy, Parkinson disease)
• Pregnancy
Psychiatric
• Mood disorders (eg, depression, mania)
• Anxiety disorders (eg, generalized anxiety disorder, obsessive-compulsive disorder)
• Substance use disorders (eg, alcohol or sedative-hypnotic withdrawal)
Pharmacologically induced
• Antiseizure medications
• Central adrenergic blockers
• Diuretics
• Selective serotonin reuptake inhibitors
• Steroids
• Stimulants

Clinical Presentation

Insomnia is considered to be an endogenous disorder caused by either a neurochemical or a structural disorder affecting the sleep–wake cycle. Individuals with primary insomnia can be light sleepers who are easily aroused by noise, temperature, or anxiety. Primary insomnia is a "hyperarousal state," in that insomnia patients have increased metabolic rates compared with controls and thus take longer to fall asleep.[2] Comorbid or secondary insomnia is frequently a symptom or manifestation of another medical disorder. Evaluation of individuals with complaints of transient or short-term insomnia should focus on recent stressors, such as a separation, a death in the family, a job change, or college exams.

1 Chronic insomnia is frequently comorbid with psychiatric or medical conditions. A complete diagnostic examination should be completed in these individuals and should include routine laboratory tests, physical and mental status examinations, as well as ruling out any medication- or substance-related causes.[12] Other sleep disorders that can have a similar presentation should be ruled out, including restless legs syndrome (RLS) periodic limb movement disorder, and sleep apnea. Common causes of insomnia are listed in Table 92-1.

TREATMENT

Desired Outcomes

The goals of treatment for insomnia are to correct the underlying sleep complaint, consolidate sleep, improve daytime functioning and sleepiness, and avoid adverse effects from selected therapies. Pharmacotherapy should be used in the lowest possible dose, for the shortest possible time period.

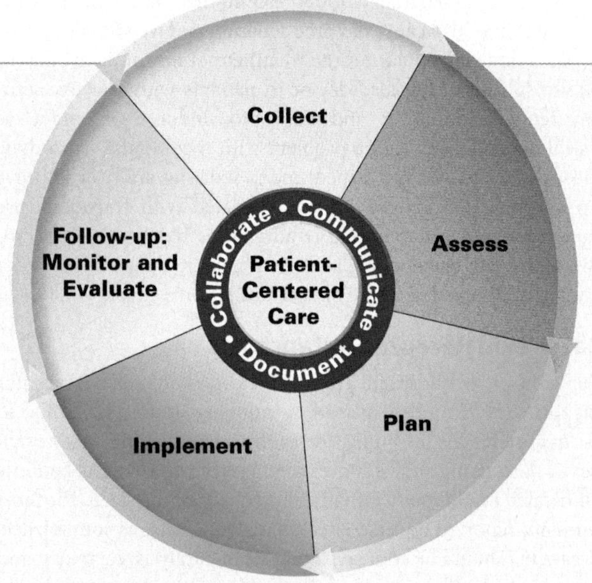

Patient Care Process for Sleep–Wake Disorders

The image shows the five fundamental steps included in The Pharmacist's Care Process endorsed by the Joint Commission for Pharmacy Practitioners (2014). The tagline of this process reads collaborate, communicate, and document. The five fundamental steps listed here are collect, assess, plan, implement, and follow-up: monitor and evaluate. All these steps are listed in a circular block diagram.

Collect

- Patient characteristics (eg, age, sex, concomitant medical conditions, environmental or social stressors)
- Information about nighttime sleep complaints and daytime consequences from patient and bed partner
- Detailed medication history of prescription, over the counter (OTC), and complementary/alternative medication use
- Subjective and objective data about daytime sleepiness, sleep quality, limb movements, snoring, witnessed apneas, and parasomnias
- Information about sleep routine, sleep hygiene, and social history (eg, caffeine, alcohol, and tobacco use)
- Results from sleep testing (if available)

Assess

- Evaluate if individual environmental or social issues are contributing to sleep difficulties.
- Assess medications to determine if any may be contributing to sleep and/or daytime complaints.
- Assess any laboratory or sleep study test results that aid in assessment/treatment of sleep complaints (eg, serum ferritin, TSH, and so on).
- Concomitant mental illness or other medical conditions that should be addressed as part of sleep evaluation (eg, presence of anxiety, depression, chronic pain).

Plan*

- Optimize sleep hygiene and related behaviors (Tables 92-1 and 92-2) that may influence sleep and daytime symptoms.
- For insomnia, if sedative-hypnotic therapy is prescribed, match the agent's duration of action to sleep complaint (eg, short-duration agents for difficulty initiating sleep and moderate duration agents for difficulty maintaining sleep) (Table 92-3).
- Ensure that lowest doses of medication are used, but if response is inadequate, consider increasing dose or adding complementary medication.
- For narcolepsy or sleepiness disorders, consider use of long-acting stimulants to increase wakefulness throughout the day. Add as needed short-acting stimulants for late afternoon or evening periods requiring wakefulness (Table 92-4).

Implement*

- Provide patient education regarding all elements of treatment plan.
- Use motivational interviewing and coaching strategies to maximize adherence.
- Answer patient questions about medications and potential adverse effects.

Follow-up: Monitor and Evaluate

- Evaluate improvement in the specific sleep complaint (eg, how has therapy affected sleep latency or sleep maintenance?).
- Monitor daytime sleepiness, sleep diaries, and diaries of sleep events (eg, periodic limb movements of sleep [PLMS], hallucinations, snoring, apneas, and so on) and monitor cataplexy and other daytime symptoms to determine if therapy is effective.
- Make appropriate changes to therapy to address inadequately controlled symptoms and reported adverse effects (Tables 92-4 and 92-5).

**Collaborate with patients, caregivers, and other healthcare professionals.*

General Approach to Treatment

Therapeutic management of insomnia is initially based on whether the individual has experienced a short-term or chronic sleep disturbance. Clinical history should assess the onset, duration, and frequency of the symptoms; effect on daytime functioning; sleep hygiene habits; and history of previous symptoms or treatment.[13] Management of all patients with insomnia should include identifying and correcting the cause, patient education on sleep hygiene, and stress management. Any unnecessary pharmacotherapy that may worsen insomnia should be eliminated.[10] Short-term insomnia, which generally occurs as a result of acute stressors, is expected to resolve quickly and should be treated with good sleep hygiene and careful use of sedative-hypnotics.[11,13] Chronic insomnia requires careful assessment for possible underlying medical causes, nonpharmacologic approaches, and careful use of sedative-hypnotics.[12]

Nonpharmacologic Therapy

2 In many cases, insomnia can be treated without sedative-hypnotics. Education about normal sleep and habits for good sleep hygiene is important for all patients with insomnia. Nonpharmacologic interventions for insomnia frequently consist of short-term cognitive behavioral therapies, most commonly stimulus control therapy, sleep restriction, relaxation therapy, cognitive therapy, paradoxical intention, biofeedback, and education on good sleep hygiene (Table 92-2).[10,14] In patients aged 55 years and older, cognitive behavioral therapy may be more effective than pharmacologic therapy at improving certain measures of insomnia.[15,16]

Pharmacologic Therapy

Antihistamines

Antihistamines exhibit sedating properties and are included in many nonprescription sleep agents. They are effective in the treatment of mild insomnia and generally safe.[13] Diphenhydramine and doxylamine are available in OTC formulations. However, patients quickly experience tolerance to sedative effects, and increasing the dose will not produce a linear increase in response. Antihistamines are considered to be less effective than benzodiazepines, and they have the disadvantages of anticholinergic adverse effects, which are especially troublesome in older individuals.[13,17]

Sedating Antidepressants

For patients with nonrestorative sleep who should not receive benzodiazepines, antidepressants may be an alternative treatment, especially those who have depression, pain, or a history of, or at risk for a substance use disorder. Using antidepressants for insomnia without depression is common but not well studied, and the doses used for treating insomnia are not effective antidepressant doses.[9,13,14] However, low-dose doxepin (3-6 mg) is FDA-approved for the treatment of sleep maintenance insomnia. Other sedating antidepressants such as amitriptyline, doxepin, and nortriptyline are effective in inducing sleep continuity, although daytime sedation and adverse effects can be significant.[9,13] Anticholinergic activity, adrenergic blockade, and cardiac conduction prolongation can be problematic, especially in older individuals and in overdose situations.[9]

TABLE 92-2 Nonpharmacologic Recommendations for Management of Insomnia

Stimulus control procedures

1. Establish regular time to wake up and to go to sleep, including weekends.
2. Sleep only as much as necessary to feel rested.
3. Go to bed only when sleepy. Avoid long periods of wakefulness in bed. Use the bed only for sleep or intimacy; do not read or watch television in bed.
4. Avoid trying to force sleep; if you do not fall asleep within 20-30 minutes, leave the bed and perform a relaxing activity (eg, read, listen to music) until drowsy. Repeat this as often as necessary.
5. Avoid blue spectrum light from television, smart phones, tablets, and other mobile devices.
6. Avoid daytime naps.
7. Schedule worry time during the day. Do not take your troubles to bed.

Sleep hygiene recommendations

1. Exercise routinely (eg, three to four times weekly) but not close to bedtime because this can increase wakefulness.
2. Create a comfortable sleep environment by avoiding temperature extremes, loud noises, and illuminated clocks in the bedroom.
3. Discontinue or reduce the use of alcohol, caffeine, and nicotine.
4. Avoid drinking large quantities of liquids in the evening to prevent nighttime trips to the restroom.
5. Do something relaxing and enjoyable before bedtime.

Mirtazapine is a sedating antidepressant that may help patients sleep, but it may also cause daytime sedation and weight gain.

Trazodone is popular for the treatment of insomnia in patients prone to substance use disorder or in patients with selective serotonin reuptake inhibitor and bupropion-induced insomnia, as physical dependence is not a problem with trazodone.[11] Trazodone in doses of 25 to 100 mg at bedtime is sedating and can improve sleep continuity.[11] Adverse effects associated with trazodone use include carryover sedation and α-adrenergic blockade and orthostasis, which can occur at any age, but it is more dangerous in older individuals. Priapism is a rare but serious adverse effect.[18]

Dual Orexin Receptor Antagonists

Suvorexant and lemborexant are dual orexin A and orexin B receptor antagonists (DORA) that instead of inducing sleepiness, similar to most treatments for insomnia, turns off wake signaling. Suvorexant doses of 10 to 20 mg and lemborexant doses of 5 to 10 mg, at bedtime are indicated for difficulty initiating and maintaining sleep. The most commonly reported adverse effect with DORA use is somnolence, and patients should be counseled that sleep paralysis, cataplexy, and other narcolepsy-like symptoms may rarely occur.[19] Caution should be used in patients with depression as DORA use can worsen mood and trigger thoughts of suicide in a dose-dependent manner.

Melatonin Receptor Agonists

Ramelteon is a melatonin receptor (MT) agonist approved for the treatment of sleep-onset insomnia. It is selective for the MT1 and MT2 melatonin receptors that are thought to regulate the circadian rhythm and sleep onset. The recommended dose is 8 mg taken at bedtime to induce sleep, and although generally well tolerated, the most common adverse events reported are headache, dizziness, and somnolence. Ramelteon is not a controlled substance and can be a viable option for patients with a history of, or at risk for a substance use disorder; however, patients may not feel that it is as effective, as it does not cause the acute drowsiness associated with other insomnia agents. It does, however, effectively treat sleep-onset difficulties in patients with chronic obstructive pulmonary disease and sleep apnea.[20,21]

Miscellaneous

Valerian is a herbal sleep remedy that is purported to effectively treat insomnia but is not recommended by American Academy of Sleep Medicine based on a lack of high quaility evidence supporting its use.[8] The mechanism of action is not fully understood but may involve increasing concentrations of GABA. Doses range from 300 to 600 mg. Although frequently used by patients to help with sleep, melatonin has weak evidence supporting its use for treatment of insomnia.

Benzodiazepine Receptor Agonists

The most commonly used treatments for insomnia have been the benzodiazepine receptor agonists (BZDRAs) which are FDA-labeled for the treatment of insomnia (Table 92-3). The Food and Drug Administration (FDA) requires BZDRA labeling to include a caution regarding anaphylaxis, facial angioedema, and complex sleep behaviors (eg, sleep driving, phone calls, sleep eating, and so on). The BZDRAs consist of the newer nonbenzodiazepine $GABA_A$ agonists and the traditional benzodiazepines. All BZDRAs bind to $GABA_A$ receptors in the brain, resulting in agonist effects on GABAergic transmission and hyperpolarization of neuronal membranes. Traditional benzodiazepines have sedative, anxiolytic, muscle relaxant, and antiseizure medication properties; newer nonbenzodiazepine GABA agonists possess only sedative properties.

Benzodiazepines relieve insomnia by reducing sleep latency and increasing total sleep time by increasing stage 2 sleep while decreasing delta sleep.[11] Benzodiazepine hypnotics should not be prescribed for individuals who are pregnant or who have untreated sleep apnea or a history of substance use disorder, and patients

TABLE 92-3 Pharmacokinetics of Benzodiazepine Receptor Agonists

Generic Name (Brand Name)	t_{max} (hours)[a]	Half-Life[b] (hours)	Daily Dose Range (mg)	Metabolic Pathway	Clinically Significant Metabolites
Estazolam (ProSom)	2	12-15	1-2	Oxidation	–
Eszopiclone (Lunesta)	1-1.5	6	2-3	Oxidation	–
				Demethylation	
Flurazepam (Dalmane)	1	8	15-30	Oxidation	Hydroxyethylflurazepam, flurazepam aldehyde
				N-dealkylation	*N*-desalkylflurazepam[c]
Quazepam (Doral)	2	39	7.5-15	Oxidation, *N*-dealkylation	2-Oxo-quazepam, *N*-desalkylflurazepam[c]
Temazepam (Restoril)	1.5	10-15	15-30	Conjugation	–
Triazolam (Halcion)	1	2	0.125-0.25	Oxidation	–
Zaleplon (Sonata)	1	1	5-10	Oxidation	–
Zolpidem (Ambien; Intermezzo)	1.6	2-2.6	1.75-10[d]	Oxidation	–

[a]Time to peak plasma concentration.

[b]Half-life of parent medication.

[c]*N*-desalkylflurazepam, mean half-life 47 to 100 hours.

[d]Oral and sublingual dosing 5 to 10 mg; sublingual tablets for middle-of-the-night dosing 1.75 to 3.5 mg (1.75 for females, 3.5 for males).

should be instructed to avoid alcohol and other central nervous system (CNS) depressants.

Adverse effects

Adverse effects are dose dependent and vary according to the pharmacokinetics of the individual benzodiazepine. High doses with long or intermediate elimination half-lives have a greater potential for producing daytime sedation, psychomotor incoordination, and cognitive deficits. Most traditional benzodiazepines maintain hypnotic efficacy for 1 month. However, tolerance can develop with time.

Anterograde amnesia, an impairment of memory and recall of events occurring after the dose is taken, has been reported with most BZDRAs, and is more likely to occur with short-acting agents.[11] Additionally, after abrupt discontinuation of BZDRAs, rebound insomnia, characterized by increased wakefulness beyond baseline amounts, may occur and last for a few nights. Therefore, the lowest effective dosage should be used to minimize rebound insomnia and avoid adverse effects on memory.

3 Benzodiazepine half-lives are prolonged in older patients, increasing the potential for medication accumulation and the incidence of CNS adverse effects, including prolonged sedation and cognitive and psychomotor impairment. BZDRAs with long elimination half-lives (eg, flurazepam and quazepam) are generally not first-line agents in older patients. Benzodiazepine use is also associated with increased risk of falls and hip fractures in older individuals, but since insomnia itself increases fall and fracture risk, it is unclear if benzodiazepines increase risk independent of sleep problems.[22]

Nonbenzodiazepine $GABA_A$ Agonists

Zolpidem, zaleplon, and eszopiclone are nonbenzodiazepine hypnotics that selectively bind to $GABA_A$ receptors and effectively induce sleepiness. Zolpidem has a duration of action of 6 to 8 hours[23] and is comparable in efficacy to benzodiazepine hypnotics, in that it is effective in reducing sleep latency and nocturnal awakenings, and increasing total sleep time. It does not have significant effects on next-day psychomotor performance. Sustained-release, sublingual, and reduced-strength (1.75 and 3.5 mg) formulations of zolpidem are available and are used to increase total sleep time, to reduce sleep latency, and for middle-of-the-night rescue dosing, respectively.

Zolpidem is less disruptive of sleep stages than benzodiazepines and adverse effects include drowsiness, amnesia, dizziness, headache, and gastrointestinal complaints, which are dose-related.[23] Sleep eating during zolpidem therapy can result in significant weight gain. The recommended daily dose of zolpidem is 10 mg in male patients, or 5 mg in female patients, older patients, and those with hepatic impairment. Because food decreases its absorption, zolpidem should be taken on an empty stomach.[24]

Zaleplon has a rapid onset of action with a half-life of 1 hour, and is metabolized to inactive metabolites.[25] It is effective in decreasing time to sleep onset but not for reducing nighttime awakening or for increasing total sleep time.[26] Because of its short half-life, zaleplon has no effect on next-day psychomotor performance and can be used as a sleep aid for middle-of-the-night awakenings.[27] The recommended dose is 10 mg in adults and 5 mg in older individuals.[25] The most common adverse effects with zaleplon are dizziness, headache, and somnolence. There are two interactions of note: zaleplon plasma levels increase when combined with cimetidine and decrease with rifampin.[23]

Eszopiclone is effective in reducing time to sleep onset, wake time after sleep onset, and number of awakenings, and increasing total sleep time and sleep quality. Eszopiclone's duration of action is up to 6 hours.[28] It can be a good option for treatment of sleep maintenance insomnia or early morning awakenings. The most common adverse effects with eszopiclone are somnolence, unpleasant taste, headache, and dry mouth.[28] Eszopiclone is labeled for long-term use and may be taken nightly for up to 6 months.[28,29]

In general, nonbenzodiazepine hypnotics seem to be associated with less physical withdrawal, tolerance, and rebound insomnia than benzodiazepine hypnotics. None of the nonbenzodiazepine $GABA_A$ agonists have significant active metabolites.

EVALUATION OF THERAPEUTIC OUTCOMES

An algorithm for the evaluation and treatment of sleep–wake disorders is shown in Fig. 92-1. Patients with short-term or chronic insomnia should be evaluated after 1 week of therapy to assess for medication efficacy, adverse effects, and adherence to nonpharmacologic recommendations. For the treatment of insomnia, the choice of a particular BZDRA can be based on its pharmacokinetic profile. When used as a single dose, the extent of distribution and elimination half-life are important in predicting the duration of action. However, after multiple doses, the elimination half-life and formation of active metabolites determine the extent of medication accumulation and resultant clinical effects.[11] Advanced age, liver

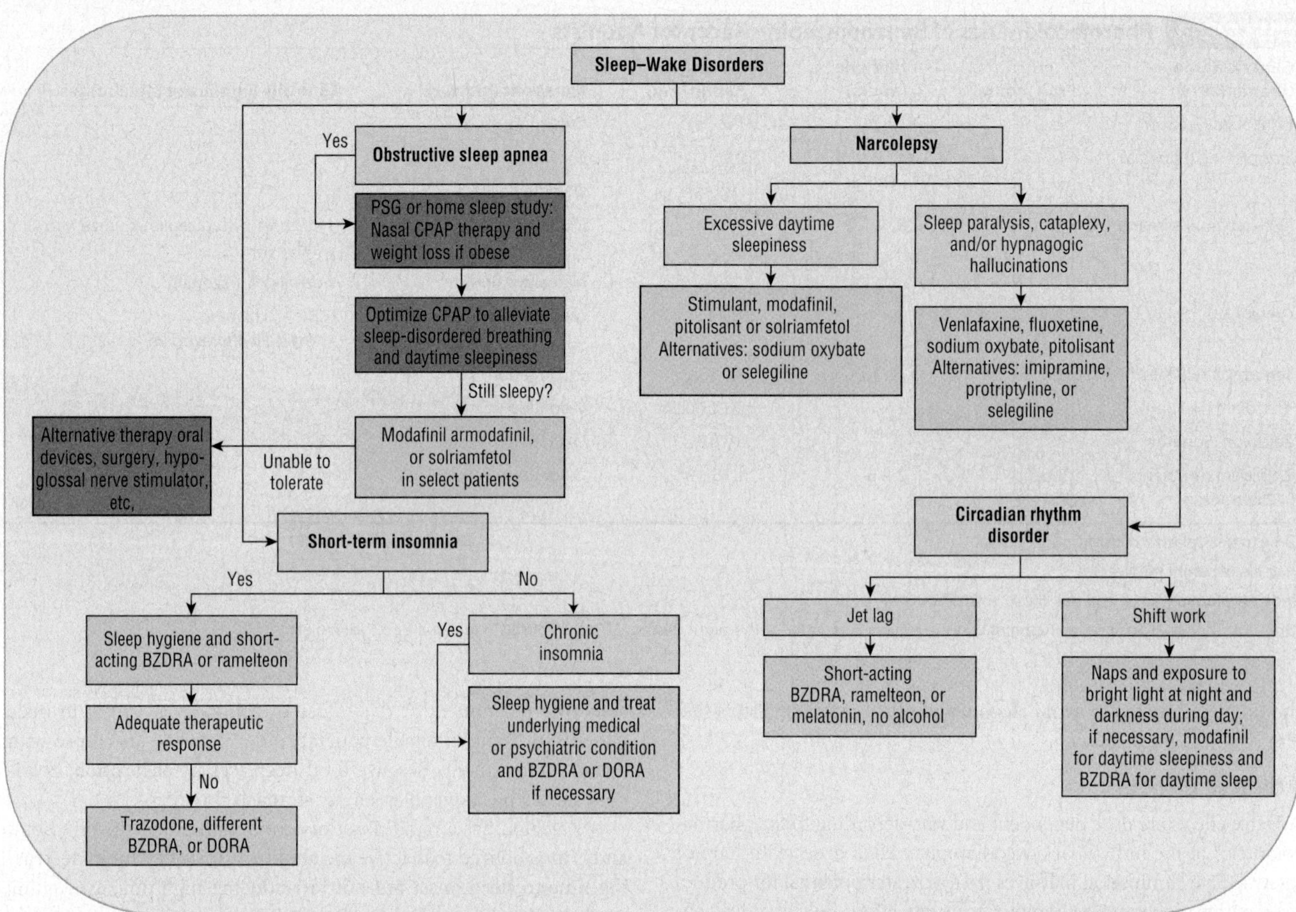

FIGURE 92-1 Algorithm for treatment of sleep and wake disorders. (BZDRA, benzodiazepine receptor agonist; CPAP, continuous positive airway pressure) *(Adapted, with permission, from Reference 70.)*

dysfunction, and medication interactions can prolong medication effects. The pharmacokinetic profiles of BZDRAs are summarized in Table 92-3.

Patients should be instructed to keep a sleep diary that includes daily recording of bedtime, wake time, latency of sleep onset, number and duration of awakenings, medication ingestion, naps, and an index of sleep quality. For patients with chronic insomnia, possible medical, psychiatric, and pharmacologic causes should be identified and managed.[11] Patients with insomnia should receive education about possible medication adverse effects and their management.

4 Clinicians should educate patients about the concepts of tolerance, physical withdrawal, and rebound insomnia. Tolerance and physical dependence can be avoided by using hypnotics at the lowest possible dose, intermittently, and for the shortest duration possible. Patients should also receive instruction about frequency of medication use and the expected duration of therapy to help prevent development of physical dependence. Withdrawal symptoms can be diminished by tapering the dosage gradually.

SLEEP APNEA

Sleep apnea is a common disease, affecting 20 to 25 million Americans. It has a higher prevalence in males, particularly in African American and Hispanic populations.[30,31] It also occurs in children and adolescents. It is characterized by repetitive episodes of cessation of breathing during sleep followed by blood oxygen desaturation and brief arousal from sleep to restart breathing. As a result, individuals with sleep apnea experience fragmented sleep, poor sleep architecture, and periods of apnea and hypopnea. PSG, or a home sleep study, is used to diagnose and quantify sleep apnea as central, obstructive, or mixed. Central sleep apnea (CSA) involves impairment of the respiratory drive, whereas obstructive sleep apnea (OSA) is caused by upper airway collapse and obstruction. Patients with mixed sleep apnea experience both CSA and OSA. The overall severity of sleep apnea is determined by the number of apnea (total cessation of airflow) and hypopnea (partial airway closure with blood oxygen desaturation) episodes documented by PSG, which is expressed as the respiratory disturbance index (RDI). Patients with mild sleep apnea have an RDI of between 5 and 15 episodes/hour, and those with moderate apnea have an RDI between 15 and 30 episodes/hour, whereas individuals with severe OSA exhibit more than 30 episodes/hour.

OSA is associated with a greater risk for motor vehicle accidents, depression, increased cancer risk, stroke, and cardiovascular disease.[32-35] Therefore, alleviation of sleep-disordered breathing may improve patient outcomes, particularly those related to cardiovascular disease.[35]

Obstructive Sleep Apnea

OSA is characterized by partial or complete closure of the upper airway, posterior from the nasal septum to the epiglottis, during inspiration. The reason for the loss of upper airway patency is not fully understood and is likely caused by several competing factors. Anatomical factors including neck obesity, narrow airway, and fixed upper airway lesions (eg, polyps, enlarged tonsils) can narrow the upper airway. The intraluminal negative pressure generated during each inspiration also promotes collapse of the upper airway that competes with dilating forces, primarily the pharyngeal dilator muscle. Acromegaly, amyloidosis, and hypothyroidism as well as neurologic conditions that impair upper airway muscle tone may cause OSA. The hallmarks of OSA are witnessed apneas, gasping, or both. Other recognized signs, symptoms, and considerations of sleep apnea include obesity, snoring, daytime sleepiness, family history, and hypertension.

5 OSA is increasingly linked to cardiovascular and cerebrovascular morbidity and mortality, independent of other risk factors.[35] Individuals with OSA are at risk for developing hypertension, and when hypertension is present, it is often resistant to medication therapy.[36] Alleviation of sleep-disordered breathing with nasal positive airway pressure (PAP) only modestly improves blood pressure (2-3 mmHg), but increased use of PAP correlates with greater blood pressure reductions.[37,38]

Central Sleep Apnea

CSA causes fragmented sleep and consequent daytime somnolence. However, unlike OSA, arousals from sleep are not required to initiate airflow. During PSG, there is an absence of airflow out of the mouth and nose with no activation of the inspiratory muscles. The prevalence of CSA is not well established and is less than OSA. CSA can be idiopathic but more commonly is caused by underlying autonomic nervous system lesions (eg, cervical cordotomy), neurologic diseases (eg, poliomyelitis, encephalitis, and myasthenia gravis), high altitudes, opioid use disorder, and congestive heart failure. For these reasons, potential underlying causes for CSA should be evaluated and treated. For example, worsening CSA in heart failure patients can signal the need to optimize heart failure therapies. Practice parameters for the treatment of CSA have been published by the American Academy of Sleep Medicine.[45]

TREATMENT

Desired Outcomes

In the absence of an underlying cause (eg, hypothyroidism, acromegaly), alleviation of sleep-disordered breathing and prevention of associated complications are the primary goals of treatment. Nonpharmacologic measures are the treatments of choice. There is no medication therapy for OSA. However, medications that worsen sleep should be avoided. Practice parameters for the medical treatment of OSA have been published by the American Academy of Sleep Medicine.[39]

Nonpharmacologic Therapy

6 Positive Airway Pressure

Nasal PAP during sleep is the standard treatment for most patients with OSA. This procedure produces a positive pressure column in the upper airway using room air to maintain patency by using a flexible tube that connects the PAP machine to a mask that covers the nose or nose and mouth.

PAP delivery may be continuous (CPAP), bi-level (providing a reduced applied pressure during expiration), or auto-titrating continuous positive airway pressure therapy (AutoPAP). The AutoPAP machines may be programmed to a pressure range allowing the machine to provide individualized pressure based on breath-to-breath analysis of the necessary pressure to keep the airway open. The CPAP pressure may be identified during PSG as the pressure setting that results in elimination of sleep-disordered breathing up to 20 cm H_2O (2.0 kPa). Alternatively, the CPAP pressure may also be identified as the pressure used by the AutoPAP machine 90% to 95% of the time. Barriers to PAP adherence, such as ill-fitted mask and nasal dryness, can be managed; however, PAP nonadherence for one night results in a complete reversal of the gains made in daytime alertness.[40]

Weight Reduction

Obesity can worsen sleep apnea, and weight management should be implemented for all overweight patients with OSA. Additionally, OSA can predispose patients to weight gain, and in obese patients with mild OSA weight loss alone can be effective.[41] Individuals who are morbidly obese and have severe OSA may consider bariatric surgery for weight loss.

Surgery

Surgical therapy (uvulopalatopharyngoplasty) opens the upper airway by removing the tonsils, trimming and reorienting the posterior and anterior tonsillar pillars, and removing the uvula and posterior portion of the palate. Due to the invasive nature of surgical treatment, this is not a first-line option. In very severe cases, a tracheostomy may be necessary. This procedure can be indicated for select individuals who are morbidly obese, have severe facial skeletal deformity, experience severe drops in oxygen saturation (eg, less than 70% [0.7]), or have significant cardiac arrhythmias associated with their OSA.

Other Therapies

For individuals who experience OSA only during certain sleep positions (eg, when lying on their back), positional therapies can be effective alone, but are usually used in conjunction with PAP therapy. Oral appliances can also be used to advance the lower jawbone and to keep the tongue forward to enlarge the upper airway. Alternatively, hypoglossal nerve stimulators that contract the genioglossus muscle during sleep to maintain airway patency are increasingly being used. These therapies should be considered when PAP therapy cannot be tolerated.[42]

Pharmacologic Therapy

The most important pharmacologic intervention for sleep apnea is the avoidance of all CNS depressants (eg, alcohol, hypnotics) and medications that promote weight gain as both of these worsen OSA. The use of CNS depressants is potentially lethal, as it reduces the brain's reflex ability to cause a mini-arousal and resume breathing. In addition, certain CNS depressants can relax airway muscles, promoting upper airway collapse. Medications that can cause rhinopharyngeal inflammation and cough as an adverse effect of therapy (ie, angiotensin-converting enzyme inhibitor) may also worsen sleep-disordered breathing.

There is no pharmacotherapy for OSA. In clinical trials, serotonergic agents (eg, fluoxetine, paroxetine), tricyclic antidepressants (TCAs) (ie, imipramine, protriptyline), respiratory stimulants (eg, theophylline), medroxyprogesterone, and clonidine have not clinically improved severity of OSA. The effects of antihypertensive agents on sleep apnea are inconsistent and are likely not clinically significant.

Wake-promoting medications (eg, modafinil, armodafinil, and solriamfetol) are FDA-approved to improve wakefulness in patients who have residual excessive daytime sleepiness (EDS) while being treated with PAP. Initiation of therapy should be attempted in patients only after PAP therapy has been optimized to alleviate sleep-disordered breathing and EDS. Wake-promoting medications should be avoided in those with concomitant cardiovascular disease. In patients with concurrent rhinitis, nasal steroids are recommended for use along with PAP therapy.[39]

Medication therapy for CSA is limited and is individualized for each patient, based on underlying etiology. Acetazolamide, which induces a metabolic acidosis that stimulates respiratory drive, and theophylline, which improves severity of CSA, have been studied but have minimal effects on clinical variables.[46,47]

EVALUATION OF THERAPEUTIC OUTCOMES

Individuals with sleep apnea should be evaluated after 1 to 3 months of treatment for improvement in alertness and daytime symptoms (eg, sleepiness, impaired memory, and irritability) and weight

CLINICAL PRESENTATION Narcolepsy

Symptoms

- Patients may complain of EDS and disrupted nighttime sleep; often they have some accompanying REM sleep abnormality, sleep paralysis, cataplexy, and/or hallucinations.

Laboratory Tests

- Although not routinely tested, there is a high incidence of human leukocyte antigen (HLA) haplotypes DR2 and HLA-DQ6/DQB1 in narcolepsy.
- Cerebrospinal fluid (CSF) concentrations of hypocretin-1 can be measured to confirm a diagnosis. CSF concentrations less than 110 pg/mL (ng/L; 31 pmol/L) positively predict narcolepsy.

Other Diagnostic Tests

- Narcolepsy is diagnosed using the multiple sleep latency test (nap test). The patient takes four to five naps in a day, and narcolepsy is diagnosed if the patient falls asleep quickly, within less than 5 minutes, and goes into REM sleep in two of those nap periods.

reduction. Individuals experiencing symptoms (eg, daytime sleepiness, snoring, loss of blood pressure control) despite PAP therapy should have repeat evaluation of sleep apnea severity. Symptoms can recur if patients gain weight, requiring a higher-pressure setting. Conversely, PAP pressure settings can be decreased if weight loss is achieved. Patient adherence to PAP therapy can be monitored by assessing the built-in compliance meter, which is also uploaded to a cloud database that measures the hours used at effective pressure and residual apnea occurrence.

NARCOLEPSY

Narcolepsy, which is a severely debilitating neurologic disease that affects between 0.03% and 0.06% of adult Americans,[43] often goes undiagnosed or misdiagnosed for years. The prevalence is equal or somewhat higher in males compared to females, and it is commonly recognized in the second decade of life and increases in severity through the third and fourth decades.[43] Individuals with narcolepsy complain of EDS, and in the sleep laboratory, exhibit impairment of both the onset and the offset of REM and NREM sleep and have arousals and disturbed sleep during the night.

Narcolepsy is classified as narcolepsy type 1 (narcolepsy with cataplexy) and narcolepsy type 2 (narcolepsy without cataplexy).[9] Four characteristic symptoms differentiate narcolepsy from other sleep disorders and are known as the *narcolepsy tetrad*: EDS, cataplexy, hallucinations, and sleep paralysis. Cataplexy is a sudden bilateral loss of muscle tone of varying severity and duration without the loss of consciousness, which occurs in 60% to 70% of people with narcolepsy.[43] Cataplexy is often precipitated by situations characterized by high emotion (eg, laughter, anger, excitement) and can manifest as subtle changes, such as jaw or head slumping, or severe weakness, such as knee buckling or collapsing to the ground. Cataleptic episodes can be brief, lasting seconds, or can last for several minutes. Sleep paralysis is an episodic loss of voluntary muscle tone that occurs when the individual is falling asleep or waking where they are conscious but not able to move or speak. Hallucinations while falling asleep (ie, hypnagogic) and on awakening (ie, hypnopompic) are brief, dream-like experiences that intrude into wakefulness and are experienced by nearly 60% of patients with narcolepsy. Unfortunately, these symptoms sometimes lead to an incorrect mental illness diagnosis.[43] Mechanistically, cataplexy, sleep paralysis, and hypnagogic hallucinations can be attributed to REM sleep disturbances.[43]

Loss of normal function of the hypocretin-orexin neurotransmitter system plays a central role in the pathophysiology of narcolepsy. Neurons containing hypocretin-orexin are found in the lateral hypothalamus and project to various parts of the brain that are thought to regulate sleep. In 75% of patients with narcolepsy, hypocretin-orexin is undetectable in cerebrospinal fluid.[44,45] Since patients with narcolepsy and cataplexy have low concentrations of hypocretin-1 (less than 110 pg/mL [ng/L; 31 pmol/L]),[9] an autoimmune process may be responsible for the destruction of hypocretin-producing cells.[46,47] Molecular studies of human leukocyte antigens (HLA) have found a high prevalence of the HLA-DR2 and HLA-DQ6/DQB1 haplotypes in patients with narcolepsy.[48] However, the HLA-DR2 haplotype is also common in the non-narcolepsy populations and is not diagnostic.[47] As 3% of patients have a first-degree relative with the disorder, there may also be a genetic component associated with this disease.[44] Lastly, as the onset of this disease occurs in adolescence or adulthood, but not at birth, environmental influences also play a role.

TREATMENT

Desired Outcomes

Nonpharmacologic management of narcolepsy includes counseling the patient and family concerning the illness to alleviate misconceptions around the individual's behavior. Good sleep hygiene should be encouraged, as well as two or more scheduled daytime naps as naps lasting 15 minutes each can help the individual with narcolepsy feel refreshed. The primary objective of pharmacologic treatment of narcolepsy is to reduce symptoms that adversely influence the patient's quality of life and to produce the fullest possible return of normal function for individuals within work, school, home, and social settings.

Pharmacologic Therapy

7 Pharmacologic management of narcolepsy is focused on two primary areas: treatment of EDS and REM sleep abnormalities. Clinical practice guidelines for treatment of narcolepsy in adults were updated and strongly recommend modafinil, pitolisant, sodium oxybate, and solriamfetol for the treatment of narcolepsy. Armodafinil, dextroamphetamine, and methylphenidate are also suggested as second-line options. Medication therapy for narcolepsy is summarized in Table 92-4.

Modafinil, a racemic compound unrelated to psychostimulants, and armodafinil (its active R-isomer) are FDA-approved for treatment of EDS in narcolepsy. The precise mechanism of action of modafinil and armodafinil is not fully understood. Common adverse reactions are usually mild and include headache, nausea, nervousness, anxiety, and insomnia. The dose of modafinil is between 100 and 400 mg/day, and armodafinil doses are between 150 and 250 mg/day.[50] Although both of these agents are effective in treating EDS, they lack efficacy for the treatment of cataplectic symptoms.[51]

TABLE 92-4 Dosing of Medications Used to Treat Narcolepsy

Generic Name	Brand Name	Initial Dose (mg)	Usual Dose (mg)	Comments
Excessive daytime somnolence				
Dextroamphetamine	Dexedrine	5-10	5-60	Concurrent use of amphetamines and acidic foods may reduce amphetamine absorption
Dextroamphetamine/ Amphetamine salts[a]	Adderall	5-20	5-60	See above
Methamphetamine[b]	Desoxyn	5-15	5-15	See above
Lisdexamfetamine	Vyvanse	20-30	20-70	Prodrug of dextroamphetamine
Methylphenidate	Ritalin	10-40	30-80	May increase risk of bleeding with concomitant warfarin therapy
Solriamfetol	Sunosi	75	75-150	Renally eliminated; specific dosing required for renal impairment
Modafinil	Provigil	100-200	200-400	May reduce effectiveness of hormonal contraceptives
Armodafinil	Nuvigil	150	150-250	May reduce effectiveness of hormonal contraceptives
Sodium oxybate[c]	Xyrem	4.5 g/night	4.5-9 g/night	Do not use with other CNS depressants
Pitolisant[c]	Wakix	8.9	17.8-35.6	May reduce effectiveness of hormonal contraceptives
Agents for cataplexy				
Atomoxetine	Strattera	18-100	40-100	Lower doses in CYP2D6 poor metabolizers
Fluoxetine	Prozac	10-20	20-80	Will see cataplexy benefits sooner than antidepressant benefits
Imipramine	Tofranil	50-100	50-250	Anticholinergic adverse effects
Nortriptyline	Aventyl, Pamelor	50-100	50-200	Anticholinergic adverse effects
Protriptyline	Vivactil	5-10	5-30	
Venlafaxine	Effexor	37.5	37.5-225	May increase blood pressure
Selegiline	Eldepryl	5-10	20-40	Doses less than 10 mg/day do not require dietary tyramine restrictions

[a]Dextroamphetamine sulfate, dextroamphetamine saccharate, amphetamine aspartate, and amphetamine sulfate.

[b]Not available in some states.

[c]Also is effective in treating cataplexy.

Data from References 47 and 49.

EDS can also be treated with stimulants to improve alertness and to increase daytime performance. Dextroamphetamine and methylphenidate also have FDA approval for the treatment of narcolepsy. Methamphetamine and mixed amphetamine salts have also been used on an off-label basis. Methylphenidate and amphetamines have a fast onset of action and durations of 6 to 10 and 3 to 4 hours, respectively. The doses of methylphenidate and amphetamine formulations can range from 5 to 60 mg daily.

Stimulants improve alertness and daytime performance, and they can elevate mood and prevent sleep. Adverse medication reactions can include insomnia, hypertension, palpitations, and irritability. Tolerance to long-term stimulant therapy can occur, necessitating dosage increases. Amphetamine use is associated with a greater likelihood of a substance use disorder and tolerance, especially when prescribed in high doses. Lisdexamfetamine is an amphetamine prodrug rapidly absorbed and converted in the body to dextroamphetamine, which has a longer duration of action and less risk of a substance use disorder since it is active only when taken orally.

To individualize treatment of narcolepsy many clinicians prescribe both immediate-release and sustained-release stimulants to increase alertness throughout the day. Sustained-release stimulants are prescribed with scheduled administration times, and immediate-release stimulants can be taken as needed when the patient requires alertness (eg, driving). There are no guidelines that recommend pharmacogenomics testing to predict response to simulant medication when being used for the treatment of sleep disorders.

Solriamfetol, a norepinephrine and dopamine reuptake inhibitor, and pitolisant, a histamine-3 antagonist/inverse agonist, are relatively new medications approved for treatment of EDS in narcolepsy. Pitolisant is also approved for treatment of cataplexy, and because it has a completely different mechanism of action, it may be prescribed with other wake-promoting medications. Solriamfetol improves wakefulness and quality of life in patients with narcolepsy.[49]

The most commonly used treatments for cataplexy are tricyclic antidepressants (TCAs), selective norepinephrine reuptake inhibitors (SNRIs), and selective serotonin reuptake inhibitors (SSRIs). The mechanism of antidepressants in relieving cataplexy, hypnagogic hallucinations, and sleep paralysis is thought to be mediated through blockade of serotonin and norepinephrine reuptake in the locus coeruleus and raphe which subsequently suppresses REM sleep.[52] Imipramine, protriptyline, clomipramine, fluoxetine, and nortriptyline are effective in approximately 80% of patients. Selegiline improves hypersomnolence and cataplexy through REM suppression and an increase in REM latency. Atomoxetine may improve cataplexy and sleepiness in children, but is less effective than other therapies in older teenagers and adults. In contrast to the antidepressants, methylphenidate and amphetamines alone are usually ineffective for complete relief from cataplexy.

Sodium oxybate (γ-hydroxybutyrate, Xyrem) improves symptoms of EDS and decreases episodes of sleep paralysis, cataplexy, and hypnagogic hallucinations. A low sodium formulation (Xywav) was developed and has similar dosing to the traditional formulation.

Nightly administration of sodium oxybate changes sleep architecture to resemble normal sleep. It increases slow-wave sleep, decreases nighttime awakenings, and increases REM efficiency.[53] Sodium oxybate is available only as a liquid and is taken in two doses; one is taken at bedtime and the second dose is taken 2.5 to 4 hours later. Sodium oxybate is a potent sedative-hypnotic and should not be used concomitantly with any other sedating medications. The most common adverse reactions include nausea, somnolence, confusion, dizziness, and incontinence.

EVALUATION OF THERAPEUTIC OUTCOMES

Patients with narcolepsy should keep a diary of the frequency and severity of cataplexy, sleep paralysis, and sleep hallucinations. Patients should be evaluated regularly during medication titrations and then every 6 to 12 months to assess for adverse medication reactions (eg, sleep disturbances, hypertension, and cardiovascular abnormalities). The healthcare provider should consider the benefit-to-risk ratio for the individual patient, the cost of medication, the convenience of administration, and the cost of laboratory tests when selecting narcolepsy therapies.[49] One wake-promoting agent may work better than another in an individual patient. Thus, if one agent is not effective at adequate doses, a trial with another agent should be undertaken.

CIRCADIAN RHYTHM DISORDERS

The sleep–wake cycle is under the circadian control of oscillators and can be disrupted by misalignment between an individual's biologic clock and external demands on the sleep cycle. Circadian rhythm sleep disorders usually present with either insomnia or hypersomnia, depending on the individual's performance requirements. Two commonly occurring circadian rhythm sleep disorders are jet lag and shift work sleep problems.

Jet Lag

Jet lag occurs when a person travels across time zones, and the external environmental time is mismatched with the internal circadian clock. Disturbances in sleep due to jet lag typically last for 2 to 3 days, but can last as long as 7 to 10 days if the time zone changes are greater than 8 hours. Compared with westward travel, eastward travel is associated with a longer duration of jet lag. In addition to decrease in alertness and performance, jet lag can also lead to increased incidence of gastrointestinal disturbances.

8 Treatment of jet lag includes nonpharmacologic approaches alone or in combination with medication therapy. Jet lag can be minimized in coast-to-coast travel in the United States if the duration is less than 7 days and the normal sleep–wake cycle is observed. For travel lasting longer than 7 days, jet lag severity can be lessened by 1- to 2-hour adjustments in sleep and wake times prior to departure to the destination time zone. Appropriate timing of light exposure along with short-acting BZDRAs, ramelteon, and 0.5 to 5 mg melatonin, taken at appropriate target bedtimes for east or west travel, reduce jet lag and shorten sleep latency.[54]

Shift Work Sleep Disorder

Shift workers comprise approximately 20% of the workforce.[55] Night shift work causes a misalignment in the sleep–wake cycle and circadian rhythm that is associated with a decrease in alertness, performance, and quality of daytime sleep. More than 65% of workers on rotating shifts complain of insomnia, compared with only 20% who work one shift.[56] Shift workers ultimately are at risk of developing shift work sleep disorder, which is a complaint of insomnia or excessive sleepiness that occurs because of circadian sleep disruption due to working shifts during normal sleep time.[9,55] Shift workers have a higher injury rate, divorce rate, occurrence of on-the-job sleepiness, and incidence of substance use disorder. They may also be at increased risk of developing peptic ulcers, depression, breast cancer, and sleepiness-related accidents.[55-57] Night shift workers are usually in a state of permanent circadian misalignment because of the tendency to revert to conventional sleep schedules on nonwork days.[56]

Treatment for shift work sleep problems includes optimizing sleep hygiene, extending daytime sleep by sleeping in the afternoon, scheduling a 2- to 3-hour nap on days off from work, or switching to a day shift job. Short-acting BZDRAs, ramelteon, and melatonin can consolidate sleep during day sleep periods and reduce lost sleep time. Modafinil and armodafinil are FDA-approved to improve wakefulness in patients with EDS associated with shift work sleep disorder. Scheduled exposure to bright lights at night and darkness in the daytime improves adaptation to night work and daytime sleep.[56]

Restless Legs Syndrome

RLS, or Willis-Ekbom syndrome, is characterized by paresthesias that are usually felt deep in the calf muscles resulting in the urge to keep limbs in motion. Additionally, these paresthesias can also appear in the thighs and arms. RLS occurs in both sexes, and it occurs more frequently in older individuals. It has been associated with chronic kidney disease and pregnancy. Additionally, RLS can be caused by iron deficiency in the substantia nigra in the CNS[58] and caffeine, stress, alcohol, and fatigue can worsen symptoms. The diagnosis of RLS is based on patient- or partner-reported symptoms and specific diagnostic criteria that include (a) an urge to move the limbs that are usually associated with uncomfortable and unpleasant sensations, (b) symptoms that begin or worsen during rest or inactivity, (c) symptoms that are exclusively present or worse in the evening or night, (d) symptoms that are temporarily relieved by movement, and (e) occurrence of symptoms is not accounted for as symptoms of another medical condition.[59] The discomfort returns when the person tries to sleep, resulting in insomnia. RLS adversely affects work performance, quality of life, and increased risk for cardiovascular disease.[60-62]

Periodic Limb Movements of Sleep

Periodic limb movements of sleep (PLMS) are stereotypic, repetitive, periodic movements of the legs that occur during sleep every 20 to 40 seconds and last 10 minutes to several hours.[66] The movements usually involve the big toe, but the ankle, knee, and hip can also flex. They can be terminated by a violent kick or other body movements. Often patients will be unaware of these movements and only recognize consequent insufficient sleep and morning leg cramps. A bed partner can describe PLMS. PLMS is diagnosed in the sleep laboratory using electromyogram recordings.

PLMS can occur with RLS or alone because of systemic disease (eg, renal failure) or medication therapy.[72] In fact RLS patients commonly have PLMS, while approximately one-third of patients with PLMS have RLS.[66] TCAs, SSRIs, dopaminergic antagonists, xanthines, nicotine, alcohol, and caffeine can all worsen PLMS.

TREATMENT

Pharmacologic Therapy

For treatment of intermittent symptoms, occurring less than 2 days per week, levodopa or benzodiazepines are recommended for as-needed use. However, for chronic, persistent symptoms, alternative therapies are recommended.

9 The alpha-2-delta ligands gabapentin, gabapentin enacarbil, and pregabalin are standard therapy for chronic RLS and have not caused symptom augmentation during chronic therapy. Gabapentin

TABLE 92-5 Monitoring Patients Taking Medications for RLS and PLMS

Medication or Medication Class	Adverse Medication Reaction	Monitoring Parameter	Comments
Dopamine agonists	Compulsive behaviors	Frequency and quantity of eating, gambling, shopping, other reward behaviors	May occur at any time during therapy but is dose-related
Levodopa/Carbidopa	Symptom augmentation	Location and timing of RLS symptoms	Appearance of symptoms in other areas of body and earlier in day
Gabapentin/Pregabalin	Dizziness	Subjective dizziness, falls	-
Sedative-hypnotics (eg, clonazepam, temazepam, zolpidem, and so on)	Carryover sedation	Morning sleepiness, grogginess	More likely to occur with longer duration agents
Opioids (eg, oxycodone, codeine, hydrocodone, and so on)	Tolerance, constipation	Patient RLS symptoms and response to ongoing therapy	-
Oral iron therapy (eg, ferrous sulfate, and so on)	Gastrointestinal upset, constipation	Monitor for constipation	Prophylactic stool softeners may be necessary to reduce risk of constipation

100 to 1,800 mg near bedtime may be especially effective for those with paresthetic or painful RLS symptoms.[63] Gabapentin enacarbil (Horizant) is a gabapentin prodrug that is FDA-approved for the treatment of RLS at a dose of 300 to 600 mg taken at 5 pm. Pregabalin has similar or greater efficacy for RLS compared to dopamine agonists. These medications should have the dose slowly increased to achieve therapeutic effect, as their benefit may not be evident until therapeutic doses are reached. Iron studies should be completed in patients with RLS and iron supplementation initiated in those who are deficient. In patients with ferritin concentrations less than 75 mcg/L (ng/mL) or transferrin saturation less than 20%, iron supplementation improves RLS symptoms.[64,65]

The dopamine agonists ropinirole, pramipexole, and rotigotine are FDA-approved for RLS treatment.[66] Lower doses of dopamine agonists are used when treating RLS compared with Parkinson's disease. Providers should caution patients that compulsive behaviors (eg, gambling, shopping, eating, and so on) and sudden periods of extreme sleepiness may emerge during therapy with dopamine agonists. Due to levodopa's short half-life, it may not provide relief over the entire night. Additionally, dopaminergic agents are associated with a high incidence of symptom augmentation, which is a worsening in symptom severity, increase in symptom distribution, emergence of symptoms earlier in the evening, shortening duration of symptom control, and need for escalating dopaminergic doses to control symptoms. Augmentation can be treated by tapering and discontinuing dopaminergic medications, repleting low body iron stores and switching to alternative medications such as gabapentin. Sedative-hypnotic agents can be effective in patients who have frequent awakenings from their RLS symptoms. Clonazepam at doses ranging from 0.5 to 2 mg has been most frequently studied; however, patients may experience carryover sedation because of its long duration of action. Shorter half-life sedative-hypnotics (eg, zolpidem, zaleplon) can improve sleep and reduce daytime sleepiness without carryover sedation. Opioids such as methadone 5 to 20 mg, and prolonged release oxycodone-naloxone are effective in patients with painful RLS; however, the potential for tolerance and physical dependence on opioid therapy should be considered. Patients with RLS or PLMS should be evaluated regularly to monitor for excessive daytime somnolence, tolerance, efficacy, and adverse effects of the medication. Therapy should be monitored for adverse medication reactions found in Table 92-5.

The treatment approach for PLMS is similar to that of RLS in that if the PLMS do not cause disruptions for the patient or bed partner or daytime symptoms, they may not require treatment. Symptomatic or problematic PLMS should be treated with dopaminergic medications or alpha-2-delta ligands to suppress limb movements or sedative-hypnotics to reduce awakenings and consolidate sleep.

PARASOMNIAS

Parasomnias are abnormal behavior or physiologic events that either occur during sleep or are exaggerated by sleep. Many of these disorders are considered to be disorders of partial arousal from various sleep stages. Parasomnias can be categorized as disorders of arousal (sleepwalking, sleep terrors), sleep–wake transition disorders (sleep-talking), rhythmic movement disorder, REM parasomnias (REM behavior disorder, nightmares), and miscellaneous parasomnias (enuresis, bruxism). Sleepwalking, sleep terrors, and sleep-talking predominantly occur during NREM sleep, whereas others, such as REM behavior disorder, occur during REM sleep.

Sleepwalking and sleep terrors are found normally in children between the ages of 4 and 12 years and usually resolve in adolescence. These disorders are increasingly recognized to also occur in adulthood, and, contrary to previous beliefs, are not related to psychological or psychiatric pathology.[67] In adults, sleep terrors can begin between the ages of 20 and 30 years. Onset of sleepwalking in adults without a childhood history of sleepwalking should prompt a search for a neurologic or substance use disorder.[68] Sleepwalking and sleep terror disorder involve intrusions of wakefulness into NREM sleep during the first third of the night. In sleepwalking, individuals become ambulatory, are difficult to awaken, and are amnestic for the event. Sleep terrors involve intense fear and autonomic arousal. Individuals are difficult to awaken, inconsolable, and amnestic for the event.[68] Patients with REM behavior disorder act out their dreams, often in a violent manner, and are at risk for injury.

Treatment of sleepwalking involves protecting the individual from harm by putting safety latches on doors and windows, removing hazardous objects from bedrooms, and covering glass doors with heavy curtains. In adult patients, benzodiazepines, SSRIs, or TCAs can be beneficial therapies for sleepwalking or other NREM disorders of arousal.[67] Benzodiazepines can also be helpful in curtailing sleep terrors in adults.[68] Nightmares are anxiety-provoking dreams characterized by vivid recall and treatment is directed at reducing stress, anxiety, and sleep deprivation. In extreme cases, low-dose benzodiazepines can be indicated. Clonazepam is the treatment of choice for REM behavior disorder. Melatonin (3-12 mg at bedtime) and pramipexole can also be an effective therapy for REM behavior disorder.[69]

CONCLUSION

Sleep and wake disorders are common but they may be challenging to diagnose since clinical presentation and precise symptoms may be unknown to the individual who is asleep. Practitioners need to perform a sleep history that involves both the patient and their bed-partner. Treatments for sleep and wake disorders are effective, but not curative, and need to be monitored carefully for both safety and efficacy. Practitioners should use the lowest doses of medications for the shortest durations possible, and thoroughly investigate potential underlying causes for sleep and wake disturbances.

ABBREVIATIONS

AutoPAP	auto-titrating positive airway pressure
BZDRA	benzodiazepine receptor agonist
CNS	central nervous system
CPAP	continuous positive airway pressure
CSA	central sleep apnea
DSM-5	*Diagnostic and Statistical Manual of Mental Disorders*, Fifth Edition
DORA	dual orexin receptor antagonist
EDS	excessive daytime sleepiness
GABA	γ-aminobutyric acid
GI	gastrointestinal
HLA	human leukocyte antigen
NREM	nonrapid eye movement
OSA	obstructive sleep apnea
PAP	positive airway pressure
PLMS	periodic limb movements of sleep
PSG	polysomnography
RDI	respiratory disturbance index
REM	rapid eye movement
RLS	restless legs syndrome
SSRI	selective serotonin reuptake inhibitor
TCA	tricyclic antidepressant

REFERENCES

1. Walsh JK, Engelhardt CL. The direct economic costs of insomnia in the United States for 1995. *Sleep*. 1999;22(Supp 2):S386–S393.
2. Neylan TC, Reynolds CF III, Kupfer DJ. Sleep disorders. In: Yudofsky SC, Hales RE, eds. *American Psychiatric Press Textbook of Neuropsychiatry*. 4th ed. Washington, DC: American Psychiatric Press; 2003:975–1000.
3. Benca RM, Cirelli C, Rattenborg NC, Tononi G. Basic science of sleep. In: Sadock BJ, Sadock VA, eds. *Kaplan and Sadock's Comprehensive Textbook of Psychiatry*. 8th ed. Philadelphia, PA: Lippincott Williams & Wilkins; 2005:280–294.
4. Dagan Y, Abadi J. Sleep–wake disorder disability: A lifelong untreatable pathology of the circadian time structure. *Chronobiol Int*. 2001;18(6):1019–1027.
5. Franken P. Long-term versus short-term processes regulating REM sleep. *J Sleep Res*. 2002;11(1):17–28.
6. Stickgold R, Hobson JA, Fosse R, Fosse M. Sleep, learning and dreams: Off-line memory reprocessing. *Science*. 2001;294(5544):1052–1058.
7. American Psychiatric Association. Sleep-wake disorders. In: *Diagnostic and Statistical Manual of Mental Disorders*. 5th ed. 2013. Available at: http://dx.doi.org/10.1176/appi.books.9780890425596.dsm12.
8. Sateia MJ, Buysse DJ, Krystal AD, Neubauer DN, Heald JL. Clinical practice guideline for the pharmacologic treatment of chronic insomnia in adults: An American Academy of Sleep Medicine Clinical Practice Guideline. *J Clin Sleep Med*. 2017;13(2):307–349.
9. American Academy of Sleep Medicine. International Classification of Sleep Disorders, Third Edition: Diagnostic and Coding Manual. Westchester, IL: American Academy of Sleep Medicine; 2014.
10. Chesson AL, Anderson WM, Littner M, et al. Practice parameters for the nonpharmacologic treatment of chronic insomnia. *Sleep*. 1999;22(8):1–6.
11. Kirkwood CK. Management of insomnia. *J Am Pharm Assoc*. 1999;39(5):688–696.
12. Sateia MJ, Doghramji K, Hauri PJ, et al. Evaluation of chronic insomnia. *Sleep*. 2000;23(2):1–39.
13. Lippmann S, Mazour I, Shabab H. Insomnia: Therapeutic approach. *South Med J*. 2001;94:866–874.
14. Vaughn-McCall W. A psychiatric perspective on insomnia. *J Clin Psychiatr*. 2001;62(Suppl 10):27–32.
15. Morgenthaler TI, Kramer M, Alessi C, et al. Practice parameters for the psychological and behavioral treatment of insomnia: An update. An American Academy of Sleep Medicine report. *Sleep*. 2006;29(11):1415–1419.
16. Sivertsen B, Omvik S, Pallesen S, et al. Cognitive behavioral therapy vs zopiclone for treatment of chronic primary insomnia in older adults: A randomized controlled trial. *JAMA*. 2006;295(24):2851–2858.
17. Hauri PJ. Insomnia. *Clin Chest Med*. 1998;19(1):157–168.
18. Trazodone [Product Information]. Weston, FL: Apotex Corp, 2014.
19. Belsomra, suvorexant [Product Information]. Whitehouse Station, NJ: Merck and Co., Inc., 2014.
20. Kryger M, Roth T, Wang-Weigand S, et al. The effects of ramelteon on respiration during sleep in subjects with moderate to severe chronic obstructive pulmonary disease. *Sleep Breath*. 2009;13(1):79–84.
21. Kryger M, Wang-Weigand S, Roth T. Safety of ramelteon in individuals with mild to moderate obstructive sleep apnea. *Sleep Breath*. 2007;11(3):159–164.
22. Stone KL, Ensrud KE, Ancoli-Israel S. Sleep, insomnia and falls in elderly patients. *Sleep Med*. 2008;9(Suppl 1):S18–S22.
23. Terzano MG, Rossi M, Palomba V, et al. New drugs for insomnia: Comparative tolerability of zopiclone, zolpidem and zaleplon. *Drug Saf*. 2003;26(4):261–282.
24. Ambien, zolpidem [product information]. Bridgewater, NJ: Sanofi-Aventis, 2012.
25. Elie R, Ruteher E, Farr IK, et al. Sleep latency is shortened during 4 weeks of treatment with zaleplon, a novel nonbenzodiazepine hypnotic. *J Clin Psychiatry*. 1999;60(8):536–544.
26. Walsh JK, Fry J, Erwin CS, et al. Efficacy and tolerability of 14-day administration of zaleplon 5 mg and 10 mg for the treatment of primary insomnia. *Clin Drug Investig*. 1998;16:347–354.
27. Walsh JK, Pollack CP, Shark MMB, et al. Lack of residual sedation following middle-of-the-night zaleplon administration in sleep maintenance insomnia. *Clin Neuropharmacol*. 2000;23(1):17–21.
28. Lunesta, eszopiclone [product information]. Marlborough, MA: Sunovion, 2010.
29. Krystal AD, Walsh JK, Laska E, et al. Sustained efficacy of eszopiclone over 6 months of nightly treatment: Results of a randomized, double-blind, placebo-controlled study in adults with chronic insomnia. *Sleep*. 2003;26(7):793–797.
30. Young T, Peppard PE, Gottlieb DJ. Epidemiology of obstructive sleep apnea: A population health perspective. *Am J Respir Crit Care Med*. 2002;165(9):1217–1239.
31. Young T, Palta M, Dempsey J, et al. The occurrence of sleep-disordered breathing among middle-aged adults. *N Engl J Med*. 1993;328(17):1230–1235.
32. Peppard PE, Szklo-Coxe M, Hla KM, Young T. Longitudinal association of sleep-related breathing disorder and depression. *Arch Intern Med*. 2006;166(16):1709–1715.
33. Young T, Finn L, Peppard PE, et al. Sleep disordered breathing and mortality: Eighteen-year follow-up of the Wisconsin sleep cohort. *Sleep*. 2008;31(8):1071–1078.
34. Terán-Santos J, Jimenez-Gomez A, Cordero-Guevara J. The association between sleep apnea and the risk of traffic accidents. *N Engl J Med*. 1999;340(11):847–851.
35. Somers VK, White DP, Amin R, et al. Sleep apnea and cardiovascular disease: An American Heart Association/American College of Cardiology Foundation scientific statement from the American Heart Association Council for High Blood Pressure Research Professional Education Committee, Council on Clinical Cardiology, Stroke Council, and Council on Cardiovascular Nursing. *J Am Coll Cardiol*. 2008;52(8):686–717.
36. Calhoun DA, Jones D, Textor S, et al. Resistant hypertension: Diagnosis, evaluation, and treatment: A scientific statement from the American Heart Association Professional Education Committee of the Council for High Blood Pressure Research. *Circulation*. 2008;117(25): e510–e526.
37. Fava C, Dorigoni S, Dalle Vedove F, et al. Effect of CPAP on blood pressure in patients with OSA/hypopnea: A systematic review and meta-analysis. *Chest*. 2014;145(4):762–771.
38. Martinez-Garcia MA, Capote F, Campos-Rodriguez F, et al. Effect of CPAP on blood pressure in patients with obstructive sleep apnea and resistant hypertension: The HIPARCO randomized clinical trial. *JAMA*. 2014;310(22):2407–3415.
39. Morganthaler TI, Kapen S, Lee-Chiong T, et al. Practice parameters for the medical therapy of obstructive sleep apnea. *Sleep*. 2006;29(8):1031–1035.

40. Kribbs NB, Pack AJ, Kline LR, et al. Effects of one night without nasal CPAP treatment on sleep and sleepiness in patients with obstructive sleep apnea. *Am Rev Respir Dis.* 2003;147(5):1162–1168.
41. Peppard PE, Young T, Palta M, et al. Longitudinal study of moderate weight change and sleep-disordered breathing. *JAMA.* 2000;284(23):3015–3021.
42. Ferguson KA, Cartwright R, Rogers R, et al. Oral appliances for snoring and obstructive sleep apnea: A review. *Sleep.* 2006;29(2):244–262.
43. Mitler M, Hayduk R. Benefits and risks of pharmacotherapy for narcolepsy. *Drug Saf.* 2002;25(11):791–809.
44. Nishino S, Ripley B, Overeem S, et al. Low cerebrospinal fluid hypocretin (orexin) and altered energy homeostasis in human narcolepsy. *Ann Neurol.* 2001;50(3):381–388.
45. Thannicakal TC, Moore RY, Nienhuis R, et al. Reduced number of hypocretin neurons in human narcolepsy. *Neuron.* 2000;27(3):469–474.
46. Lin L, Hungs M, Mignot E. Narcolepsy and the HLA region. *J Neuroimmunol.* 2001;117(1-2):9–20.
47. Mignot E, Thorsby E. Narcolepsy and the HLA system [letter]. *N Engl J Med.* 2001;344(9):692.
48. Nakayama J, Miura M, Honda M, et al. Linkage of human narcolepsy with HLA association to chromosome 4p-13-q21. *Genomics.* 2000;65(1):84–86.
49. Maski K, Trotti LM, Kotagal S, et al. Treatment of central disorders of hypersomnolence: An American Academy of Sleep Medicine clinical practice guideline. *J Clin Sleep Med.* 2021;17(9):1881–1893.
50. Robertson P, Hellriegel ET. Clinical pharmacokinetic profile of modafinil. *Clin Pharmacokinet.* 2003;42(2):123–127.
51. Feldman N. Narcolepsy. *South Med J.* 2003;96(3):277–287.
52. Rosenthal MS. Physiology and neurochemistry of sleep. *Am J Pharm Educ.* 1998;62:204–208.
53. Mamelak M, Black J, Montplaisir J, et al. A pilot study of the effects of sodium oxybate on sleep architecture and daytime alertness in narcolepsy. *Sleep.* 2004;27(7):1327–1334.
54. Herxheimer A, Petrie KJ. Cochrane Depression, Anxiety and Neurosis Group. Melatonin for the prevention and treatment of jet lag [systematic review]. *Cochrane Database Syst Rev.* 2005;2.
55. Drake CL, Roehrs T, Richardson G, et al. Shift work sleep disorder: Prevalence and consequences beyond that of symptomatic day workers. *Sleep.* 2004;27(8):1453–1462.
56. Garbarino S, Nobili L, Beelke M, et al. Sleep disorders and daytime sleepiness in state police shiftworkers. *Arch Environ Health.* 2002;57(2):167–175.
57. Knutsson A. Health disorders of shift workers. *Occup Med (Lond).* 2003;53:103–108.
58. Connor JR, Boyer PJ, Menzies SL, et al. Neuropathological examination suggests impaired brain iron acquisition in restless legs syndrome. *Neurology.* 2003;61:304–309.
59. Allen RP, Picchietti DL, Garcia-Borreguero D, et al. Restless legs syndrome/Willis-Ekbom disease diagnostic criteria: Updated International Restless Legs Syndrome Study Group (IRLSSG) consensus criteria—history, rationale, description, and significance. *Sleep Med.* 2014;15(8):860–873.
60. Allen RP, Bharmal M, Calloway M. Prevalence and disease burden of primary restless legs syndrome: Results of a general population survey in the United States. *Mov Disord.* 2011;26(1):114–120.
61. Allen RP, Walters AS, Montplaisir J, et al. Restless legs syndrome prevalence and impact: REST general population study. *Arch Intern Med.* 2005;165(11):1286–1292.
62. Winkelman JW, Finn L, Young T. Prevalence and correlates of restless legs syndrome symptoms in the Wisconsin Sleep Cohort. *Sleep Med.* 2006;7(7):545–552.
63. Garcia-Borreguero D, Larrosa O, de la Llave Y, et al. Treatment of restless legs syndrome with gabapentin: A double-blind, cross-over study. *Neurology.* 2002;59(10):1573–1575.
64. Wang J, O'Reilly B, Venkataraman R, et al. Efficacy of oral iron in patients with restless legs syndrome and low-normal ferritin: A randomized, double-blind, placebo-controlled study. *Sleep Med.* 2009;10(9):973–975.
65. Trenkwalder C, Winkelmann J, Oertel W, et al. Ferric carboxymaltose in patients with restless legs syndrome and nonanemic iron deficiency: A randomized trial. *Mov Disord.* 2017;32(10):1478–1482. doi:10.1002/mds.27040 28643901.
66. Aurora RN, Kristo DA, Bista SR, et al. The treatment of restless legs syndrome and periodic limb movement disorder in adults—An update for 2012: Practice parameters with an evidence-based systematic review and meta-analyses. *Sleep.* 2012;35(8):1039–1062.
67. Mahowald MW, Cramer Bornemann MA. NREM arousal parasomnias. In: Kryger MH, Roth T, Dement WC, eds. *Principles and Practice of Sleep Medicine.* 5th ed. St. Louis, MO: Elsevier Saunders; 2011:1075–1082.
68. Schenck CH, Mahowald MW. Parasomnias managing bizarre sleep-related behavior disorders. *Postgrad Med.* 2000:107(3):145–156.
69. Mahowald MW, Schenck CH. REM sleep parasomnias. In: Kryger MH, Roth T, Dement WC, eds. *Principles and Practice of Sleep Medicine.* 5th ed. St. Louis, MO: Elsevier Saunders; 2011:1083–1097.
70. Jermaine DM. Sleep disorders. In: Carter BL, Angaran DM, Lake KD, Raebel MA, eds. *Pharmacotherapy Self-Assessment Program.* 2nd ed. Kansas City, MO: American College of Clinical Pharmacy; 1995:139–154. Psychiatry Module.
71. Montplaisir J, Nicolas A, Denesle R, Gomez-Mancilla B. Restless legs syndrome improved by pramipexole: A double-blind randomized trial. *Neurology.* 1999;52(5):938–943.
72. Javaheri S. Acetazolamide improves central sleep apnea in heart failure: A double-blind, prospective study. *Am J Respir Crit Care Med.* 2006;173:234–237.
73. Javaheri S, Parker TJ, Wexler L, et al. Effect of theophylline on sleep-disordered breathing in heart failure. *N Engl J Med.* 1996;335:562–567.
74. Aurora RN, Chowdhuri S, Ramar K, et al. The treatment of central sleep apnea syndromes in adults: Practice parameters with an evidence-based literature review and meta-analyses. *Sleep.* 2012;35:17–40.

Developmental Disabilities

e93

Steven R. Erickson

KEY CONCEPTS

1. People with intellectual and developmental disabilities (IDD) have higher incidence of mental illness and challenging behaviors, with dual diagnoses being common.
2. Persons diagnosed with Down syndrome (DS) can be at increased risk for medical and psychiatric comorbidities.
3. People with IDD experience high rates of polypharmacy and polypsychotropic medication use. Assessment should include physical disorders, as well as social and environmental factors complicating their care.
4. People with DS have higher rates of Alzheimer-type dementia. A thorough evaluation is needed to differentiate between depression and Alzheimer disease (AD).
5. Treatment plans for persons with autism spectrum disorder (ASD) focus on increasing social interactions, improving verbal and nonverbal communication, and minimizing the occurrence or impact of ritualistic, repetitive behaviors and other related mood and behavioral challenges (eg, over activity, irritability, and self-injury).
6. Many purported pharmacologic and nonpharmacologic treatments for ASD lack objective evidence-based support.
7. A structured teaching approach focusing on increasing social communication and integration with peers is needed when providing services to persons with ASD.
8. Nonpharmacologic interventions for sleep disturbances in individuals diagnosed with ASD should be implemented prior to pharmacotherapy considerations.
9. Psychopharmacologic treatment planning should include monitoring of objective, measurable medication-responsive target behaviors and assessment of potential adverse effects, which are of critical importance when treating the behavioral challenges of ASD. Furthermore, the response of individuals to pharmacotherapy is highly variable.
10. The use of FDA-approved medication for off-label indications is an acceptable clinical practice if founded on evidence-based research and includes informed consent.

BEYOND THE BOOK

Compare and contrast the Patient Care Process and the assessment and follow-up tools available on the website for "Healthcare for Adults with Intellectual and Developmental Disabilities. Toolkit for Primary Care Providers." https://iddtoolkit.vkcsites.org/

Behavioral Problems and Emotional Concerns-Primary Care Provider Checklist
Psychiatric Symptoms and Behavior Checklist
Psychotropic Medication Checklist
Management Plan

Compare and contrast the criteria for each step of the PCP with those of the Toolkit Behavioral and Mental Health Issues "Behavioral Problems and Emotional Concerns-Provider Checklist," the "Risk Assessment Tools for Adults with IDD in Behavioral Crisis," and the "Psychotropic Medication Checklist." This activity will help you envision the important points to assess when consulting on a patient who has an IDD and challenging behavior.

INTRODUCTION

Developmental disabilities (DD) are chronic disabilities that can be cognitive, physical, or both. They appear before the age of 22 and are likely to be lifelong.[1] Some DDs are largely physical challenges, such as cerebral palsy or seizure disorders, and some individuals may have a condition that includes both a physical and an intellectual disability. Intellectual disability (ID) is a disability characterized by significant limitations in both intellectual functioning and adaptive behavior, which covers many everyday social and practical skills.[2] This chapter will use the term "intellectual or developmental disabilities" (IDD) to refer to people who have conditions associated with DD, ID, or both.

EPIDEMIOLOGY

Down syndrome and autism spectrum disorder are several of the more common diagnoses which make up IDD. About 1.5% to 2.5% of the US population is living with some form of IDD.[3] The actual frequency and per cent of the US population characterized as having IDD varies based on the data source and the definition used. According to the 2010 US Census Bureau, 1.2 million adults (0.5%) had an ID and 944,000 (0.4%) had a DD.[4] Globally, the prevalence of ID is about 1% of the population.[5] People with IDD primarily live in the community in living situations that include living with family (71%), group homes, or in supported living arrangements (eg, living by themselves or with one or two roommates with an aid). Only 13% of adults with IDD live in supervised residential settings.[6]

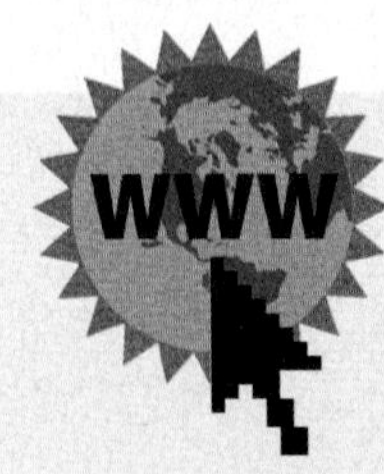

The complete chapter, learning objectives, and other resources can be found at **www.pharmacotherapyonline.com.**

Diabetes Mellitus

94

Jennifer M. Trujillo and Stuart T. Haines

KEY CONCEPTS

1. Diabetes mellitus (DM) is a metabolic disorder. While there are numerous etiological causes, defects in insulin secretion, insulin action (sensitivity), or both lead to elevations in blood glucose as well as altered fat and protein metabolism.
2. DM is a leading cause of eye and kidney disease. Patients with DM are at high risk for CV events, heart failure, and atherosclerotic disease.
3. The two most common classifications of DM are type 1 (absolute insulin deficiency) and type 2 (relative insulin deficiency due to β-cell dysfunction coupled with insulin resistance). They differ in clinical presentation, pathophysiology, and treatment approach.
4. The prevalence of type 2 DM has doubled worldwide over the last 40 years. This has been attributed to an alarming increase in the prevalence of obesity due to diminished physical activity and increased caloric consumption.
5. The diagnosis of diabetes is made using any of the following criteria: (1) fasting plasma glucose (FPG) ≥126 mg/dL (7.0 mmol/L); (2) a hemoglobin A1C (A1C) ≥6.5% (0.065; 48 mmol/mol); (3) a random plasma glucose level ≥200 mg/dL (11.1 mmol/L) coupled with classic symptoms of diabetes; or (4) a 2-hour plasma glucose ≥200 mg/dL (11.1 mmol/L) during a 75-g oral glucose tolerance test (OGTT). A diagnosis using criteria 1-3 requires two abnormal test results from the same sample or in two separate test samples.
6. The goals of therapy in DM are to achieve optimal glycemic control (based on age, comorbid conditions, and patient preferences), reduce the onset and progression of diabetes-related complications, aggressively address CV risk factors, and improve quality of life.
7. Intensive glycemic control prevents the onset and slows the progression of microvascular complications (eg, neuropathy, retinopathy, and nephropathy).
8. Knowledge of the patient's meal patterns and activity levels, as well as the pharmacologic properties of antihyperglycemic agents, is essential to creating an individualized treatment plan that achieves optimal glycemic control, avoids hypoglycemia, and minimizes adverse effects.
9. Metformin is the drug of choice and, in the absence of contraindications or intolerability, should be included in the treatment regimen for most patients with type 2 DM due to its effectiveness, low risk of hypoglycemia, positive or neutral effects on weight, potential positive impact on CV risk, and low cost.
10. Type 2 DM often requires the use of multiple therapeutic agents (combination therapy) including oral and injected antihyperglycemics to achieve and maintain optimal glycemic control. A persistent decline in β-cell function over time often necessitates periodic adjustment and changes in therapy.
11. Insulin therapy is required in type 1 DM. Intensive basal-bolus insulin therapy, either via multiple daily injections of insulin or continuous subcutaneous insulin infusion therapy (aka an insulin pump), in motivated individuals is more likely to achieve optimal glycemic control. Basal-bolus therapy includes a long-acting insulin to address fasting glucose and a rapid-acting insulin for mealtime coverage. The use of adjunctive therapy in combination with insulin in patients with uncontrolled or erratic glucose concentrations may be warranted.
12. Aggressive management of CV risk factors in DM is necessary to reduce the incidence of CV events and death. This includes smoking cessation, use of moderate or high potency statins in most patients with DM, and treatment of hypertension.
13. Good blood pressure control in patients with diabetes lowers not only the risk of retinopathy and nephropathy but also CV events.
14. Strategies to prevent type 1 DM have not yet been successful. For patients at high risk, type 2 DM can be delayed or prevented by engaging in regular aerobic exercise, losing weight, reducing dietary fat, and increasing fiber intake. These lifestyle habits can reduce the risk of type 2 DM by 60%. Although no medication is currently FDA-approved to prevent diabetes, several have been shown to delay diabetes onset in high-risk patients.
15. Repeated inaction by practitioners to intensify treatment when patients are not meeting treatment goals is called therapeutic inertia. Several factors contribute to therapeutic inertia. This is a common problem and among the leading contributors to poor outcomes. Diabetes is a chronic condition that requires periodic medication changes to attain and maintain glycemic goals.
16. Patient self-management, therapeutic lifestyle behaviors, and appropriate medication use are equally important components of each patient's treatment plan. Interprofessional teams including physicians (primary care, endocrinologists, ophthalmologists), dentists, dietitians, nurses, pharmacists, podiatrists, social workers, behavioral health specialists, and certified diabetes care and education specialists (CDCESs) working together can assist persons with DM in achieving optimal health outcomes.

BEYOND THE BOOK

Part 1:

Donna is a 53-year-old woman with a 5-year history of type 2 DM. She also has dyslipidemia and hypertension. She has atherosclerotic cardiovascular disease with two coronary artery stents placed 1 year ago. She has gained 5 lb (2.3 kg) in the last 6 months. She takes metformin 1,000 mg by mouth twice daily for type 2 DM. Her most recent laboratory results include: A1C 8.1% (0.081; 65 mmol/mol), eGFR >60 mL/min/1.73 m^2, UACR 14 mg/g (1.6 mg/mmol). She wants to lose weight and has commercial insurance. The patient's nurse practitioner wrote a prescription for insulin glargine U-100 10 units SC once daily.

Find the current diabetes treatment guidelines from both the American Diabetes Association (ADA) and the American Association of Clinical Endocrinologists/American College of Endocrinology (AACE/ACE). Is this treatment approach in Donna's case consistent with the guidelines? If it is, explain why. If it is not, determine what would be recommended instead and explain why.

Part 2:

Assume that the prescription for insulin glargine is appropriate. Review the following resource on how to inject insulin.

Find two additional resources that you could use when educating Donna on this new prescription. How did you find them? How did you determine the resource was from a reputable and reliable source? What are the key components you should discuss with this patient about the proper use of insulin?

INTRODUCTION

1 2 Diabetes mellitus (DM) is a diverse group of metabolic disorders that all have chronically elevated blood glucose (BG) as their defining feature. In addition to hyperglycemia, DM is associated with abnormal fat and protein metabolism. In the absence of effective treatment, DM can lead to acute complications such as diabetic ketoacidosis (DKA) and hyperosmolar hyperglycemic syndrome (HHS). Chronic hyperglycemia can cause vascular and nerve damage, resulting in microvascular, macrovascular, and neuropathic complications. DM is a worldwide problem, significantly impacting people and healthcare systems in low-, middle-, and high-income countries.[1] More than 442 million adults around the globe are now living with DM, and its prevalence has nearly doubled over the last 30 years. According to the Centers for Disease Control and Prevention, slightly more than 34 million Americans, including 13% of adults, have DM.[2] While 1.5 million new cases of DM are diagnosed in the United States every year, one in four Americans with DM are unaware they have it. While these numbers are startling, the number of adults with prediabetes is far greater—an estimated 88 million in the United States alone. Prediabetes is a condition of abnormal BG that is not sufficiently high to meet the thresholds that define diabetes but often progresses to the diagnosis. The total direct and indirect medical costs for treating people with DM in the United States were $327 billion in 2017.[3] The average person with DM spent $16,750 in 2017 on medical care, an amount that was nearly two-and-half times greater than the amount spent by people without DM. DM is the seventh leading cause of death in the United States and among the principal causes of end-stage kidney disease (ESKD), lower extremity amputations, and blindness. Finally, people with DM are at far greater risk for CV disease (eg, myocardial infarction, ischemic stroke).[2] Optimal management of DM substantially lowers the risk of complications, increases life expectancy, and improves the quality of life.

EPIDEMIOLOGY

3 The vast majority of patients with DM are classified into one of two broad categories: type 1 DM and type 2 DM.[4] Patients with type 1 DM have an absolute insulin deficiency. Patients with type 2 DM have varying degrees of β-cell dysfunction often coupled with insulin resistance. Women who develop diabetes during pregnancy are classified as having gestational diabetes (GDM). Less common types of diabetes are caused by genetic defects, pancreatic destruction, endocrine disorders, and medications. See Table 94-1.

Type 1 DM accounts for 5% to 10% of all cases of DM and is most often due to autoimmune destruction of the pancreatic β-cells.[6] The prevalence of β-cell autoimmunity in a population is directly related to the incidence of type 1 DM. For example, in Sweden and Finland 3% to 4.5% of the population have circulating islet cell autoantibodies (ICAs), and this is associated with the highest incidence of type 1 DM in the world: 22 to 35 per 100,000 people. The worldwide prevalence of type 1 DM is increasing, but the cause is not fully understood.[7]

Markers of β-cell autoimmunity can be found in many adults with diabetes.[6] A variant of type 1 DM is called latent autoimmune diabetes of adults (LADA). These patients often have a poor response to oral agents and require insulin therapy much sooner than most patients with type 2 DM. The cause of idiopathic type 1 DM is unknown, but it is not believed to be from an autoimmune process. Idiopathic type 1 DM is most frequently seen in patients of African and Asian descent. These patients have periods of profound hyperglycemia but only intermittently require insulin therapy.

4 Type 2 DM accounts for 90% to 95% of all cases of DM. The prevalence of type 2 DM in the United States is about 12.1% in adults.[2] The risk of developing type 2 DM increases with age and varies widely among racial and ethnic groups.[8] When compared to people of European ancestry, Native Americans, Latino/Hispanic Americans, African Americans, Asian Americans, and Pacific Islanders are more likely to develop type 2 DM. Whether the observed differences in the prevalence of type 2 DM among ethnic and racial groups is primarily due to genetic factors or social factors, such as lifestyle behaviors and cultural behaviors, is unclear. While the prevalence of type 2 DM increases with age, the disorder is increasingly being diagnosed in adolescence and young adulthood. This is likely due to the increasing incidence of obesity and lack of regular physical activity. Genetics plays an important role in the development of type 2 DM. Most cases of type 2 DM appear to be polygenic.

The incidence of GDM is increasing and, between 2007 and 2010, it was estimated to occur in 9% of all pregnancies in the United States.[9] Most women become normoglycemic after pregnancy; however, up to 50% of these women develop type 2 DM later in life.[10]

Other less common (1%-2%) forms of DM occur through a variety of mechanisms.[4] Maturity-onset diabetes of the young (MODY) and neonatal diabetes are inheritable forms of DM caused by specific single-gene mutations. Endocrine disorders, particularly acromegaly and Cushing syndrome, commonly induce hyperglycemia. Diseases that injure or destroy the pancreas such as cystic fibrosis, pancreatitis, and pancreatic cancer can damage β-cells and impair insulin secretion. Several medications can also contribute to hyperglycemia by either impairing insulin secretion, increasing insulin resistance, or both.[5]

ETIOLOGY AND PATHOPHYSIOLOGY

1 DM is caused by derangements in the secretion of insulin, glucagon, and other hormones and results in abnormal carbohydrate and fat metabolism.[6,8] This is often coupled with insulin resistance,

TABLE 94-1 Classification of Diabetes Mellitus

Type 1 diabetes[a] (immunologically mediated destruction of β-cells leading to absolute insulin deficiency)
Type 2 diabetes (progressive loss of β-cell insulin secretory function accompanied by resistance to insulin action)
Gestational diabetes mellitus
Monogenic defects
Maturity-onset diabetes of the young (MODY) caused by a mutation in GCK, HNF1A, HNF1B, or HNF4A gene
Neonatal diabetes caused by a mutation in KCNJ11, ABCC8, INS, GATA6, EIF2AK3, or FOXP3 gene
Genetic syndromes associated with diabetes
Down syndrome
Hemochromatosis
Klinefelter syndrome
Turner syndrome
Diseases impacting the pancreas leading to diabetes
Cystic fibrosis
Pancreatitis
Pancreatic cancer
Pancreatectomy
Posttransplantation diabetes mellitus
Endocrine diseases frequently associated with diabetes
Acromegaly
Aldosteronoma
Cushing syndrome
Glucagonoma
Hyperthyroidism
Pheochromocytoma
Somatostatinoma
Medication-induced hyperglycemia[5]
Atypical antipsychotics (eg, risperidone, olanzapine)
β-Blockers (eg, propranolol, atenolol)
β-Adrenergic agonists (eg, albuterol)
Calcineurin inhibitors (eg, cyclosporine, tacrolimus)
Diazoxide
Gatifloxacin
Glucocorticoids (eg, dexamethasone, prednisone)
Growth hormone (rhGH)
HMG-CoA reductase inhibitors (eg, atorvastatin, simvastatin)
Niacin/nicotinic acid
Pentamidine
Protease inhibitors (eg, ritonavir, saquinavir)
Thiazide diuretics (eg, chlorthalidone, hydrochlorothiazide)

[a]Patients with any form of diabetes may require insulin treatment at some stage of their disease. Insulin use does not itself classify the type of diabetes.

Data from Reference 4.

particularly in those with type 2 DM. In many cases, the underlying etiology of the disorder is complex and involves multiple mechanisms.

After consuming food, carbohydrate ingestion increases the plasma glucose concentration and stimulates the release of incretin hormones from the gut and insulin release from the pancreatic β-cells.[8] The resultant hyperinsulinemia (1) suppresses hepatic glucose production, (2) suppresses glucagon release, and (3) triggers glucose uptake by peripheral tissues. Upwards of 75% of total body glucose disposal occurs in tissues, including the brain and peripheral nerves, which do not require insulin. Brain glucose uptake occurs at the same rate during fed and fasting periods. The remaining 25% of glucose metabolism takes place in the liver and muscle, tissues that require insulin to promote glucose uptake into the cells. During periods of fasting, approximately 85% of glucose is produced by the liver and the remainder by the kidney.

Although fat tissue is responsible for only a small portion of total body glucose disposal, it plays an important role in glucose homeostasis.[8] Insulin exerts a potent antilipolytic effect, reducing plasma-free fatty acid (FFA) levels. Increased levels of FFAs inhibit the uptake of glucose by muscle and stimulate hepatic gluconeogenesis. Lower FFA concentrations result in increased glucose uptake in muscle and indirectly reduce hepatic glucose production.

Glucagon is produced by pancreatic α cells and is secreted in the fasting state.[8] Glucagon stimulates hepatic glucose production and glycogenolysis. Glucagon and insulin secretion are closely linked. Appropriate secretion of both hormones is needed to keep plasma glucose concentrations within a normal range.

Type 1 Diabetes

Type 1 DM is the result of autoimmune destruction of the β-cells of the pancreas.[6] Given that insulin therapy is required when treating type 1 diabetes, it was previously called insulin-dependent diabetes mellitus, and some references, patients, and providers continue to use this, albeit incorrect, terminology. Type 1 DM is believed to be initiated by exposure to an environmental trigger in a genetically susceptible individual.[11] There is a link between currently known genetic markers for autoimmunity and the development of type 1 DM. However, β-cell autoimmunity develops in less than 10% of the genetically susceptible individuals and progresses to type 1 DM in less than 1%. On the other hand, β-cell autoimmunity, including ICAs, is present at the time of diagnosis in 90% of individuals. Type 1 diabetes most commonly develops in childhood or young adulthood; however, it can occur at any age. Children and adolescents typically have a more rapid rate of β-cell destruction and are more likely to present with DKA. Adults may maintain sufficient insulin secretion to prevent ketoacidosis for many months or years; this slowly progressive form of type 1 DM is sometimes referred to as LADA.

Several genetic polymorphisms have been linked to the development of type 1 DM, including certain human leukocyte antigens (HLA) class II alleles on chromosome 6.[11] Some genetic variants are associated with a higher risk of developing type 1 DM (eg, *DRB1*03-DQB1*0201*, *DRB1*04-DQB1*302*, and *HLA-B*39*) but others appear to be protective (eg, *DRB1*1501-DQA1*0102-DQB1*0602*). Genetic predisposition to the development of type 1 DM has also been associated with certain polymorphisms in the insulin gene region on chromosome 11. Other genes, including PTPN22, IL2RA, and CTLA-4, may also play a role in some individuals. However, it should be noted that genetic markers are present in only 30% to 50% of patients with type 1 DM. Moreover, only 50% of identical twins and approximately 10% of dizygotic twins develop type 1 DM. Thus, genetic mutations alone do not predict or explain the etiology of the disease.

In order for type 1 DM to develop, a genetically susceptible individual must be exposed to a trigger that initiates the autoimmune process and destruction of pancreatic β-cells.[11] See Fig. 94-1. However, it is unknown precisely what the inciting factors are. Several triggers have been implicated, including early exposure to cow's milk, lack of breastfeeding, gut bacteria (ie, intestinal microbiome), and certain viruses (eg, enterovirus and rotavirus). Although vitamin D deficiency is more prevalent in patients who develop type 1 DM, it is unclear if the relationship is causal or merely an association.

The autoimmune process is mediated by macrophages and T lymphocytes with circulating autoantibodies to various β-cell antigens.[11] The most commonly detected antibody associated with type 1 DM is islet cell autoantibodies (ICAs). Other antibodies may

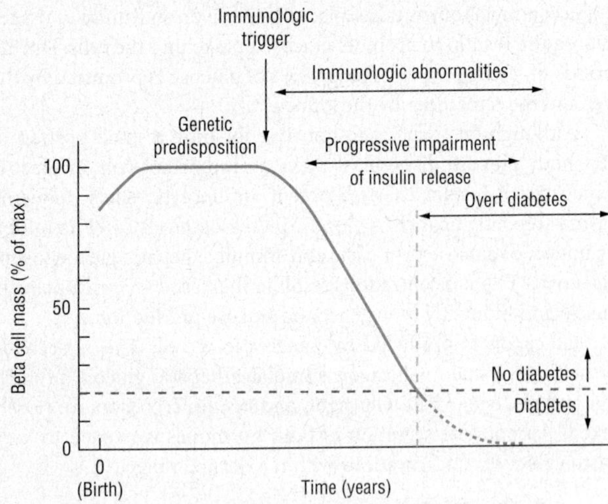

FIGURE 94-1 Clinical course of type 1 diabetes mellitus. *(Adapted from Kaufman ER. Medical Management of Type 1 Diabetes. 6th ed. Alexandria, VA: American Diabetes Association; 2012.)*

TABLE 94-2 Risk Factors for Type 2 Diabetes

Age ≥45 years old
Family history of type 2 DM (ie, parents or siblings with type 2 diabetes)
High-risk racial and ethnic groups (ie, African American, Hispanic/Latino, Native American, Asian American, Native Hawaiian, or Pacific Islander)
Overweight or obese (ie, ≥20% over ideal body weight or body mass index [BMI] ≥25 kg/m^2)
Sedentary lifestyle (ie, limited daily physical activity)
History of impaired glucose tolerance (IGT), impaired fasting glucose (IFG), or elevated A1C
Hypertension (≥140/90 mm Hg in adults or on therapy for hypertension)
Dyslipidemia (high-density lipoprotein [HDL] cholesterol ≤35 mg/dL (0.91 mmol/L) or a triglyceride level ≥250 mg/dL (2.83 mmol/L)
History of GDM or delivery of a baby weighing more than 9 lb (4 kg)
History of vascular disease (eg, myocardial infarction, ischemic stroke, peripheral arterial disease)
Presence of acanthosis nigricans (ie, dark, thick, and velvety skins around the neck or armpits)
Polycystic ovary syndrome

be formed to insulin, glutamic acid decarboxylase 65 (GAD65), insulinoma-associated antigen-2 (IA-2), and zinc transporter 8 (ZnT8). These antibodies are generally considered markers of disease rather than mediators of β-cell destruction. These markers have been used to identify individuals at risk for type 1 DM and may be useful screening tests to initiate disease prevention strategies. Other autoimmune disorders such as Hashimoto's thyroiditis, Graves' disease, Addison's disease, vitiligo, and celiac sprue are more common in patients with type 1 DM.

In many patients who develop type 1 DM, there is a long preclinical period during which markers of autoimmunity can be detected.[11] β-Cell autoimmunity may precede the diagnosis of type 1 DM by up to 13 years. Autoimmunity remits in some individuals and progresses to absolute β-cell failure in others. Hyperglycemia occurs when 60% to 90% of the β-cells have been destroyed. After the initial diagnosis, there is occasionally a period of transient remission called the "honeymoon" phase during which insulin therapy may not be necessary. Eventually, continued β-cell destruction requires lifelong insulin replacement therapy.

Amylin is a hormone that is co-secreted from the pancreatic β-cell with insulin. Amylin is also deficient in patients with type 1 DM secondary to the destruction of β-cells. Amylin suppresses inappropriate glucagon secretion, slows gastric emptying, and centrally mediated satiety.

Type 2 Diabetes

Type 2 DM is the result of β-cell dysfunction coupled with some degree of insulin resistance.[8] Older references as well as some patients and practitioners continue to call this form of DM non-insulin-dependent diabetes or adult-onset diabetes. Both of these descriptors are erroneous because many patients with type 2 DM will require insulin therapy at some point as β-cell function progressively declines. Moreover, type 2 DM can develop in childhood and is increasingly diagnosed during adolescence. Most individuals with type 2 DM are overweight or obese. Abdominal adiposity is a major contributor to insulin resistance. Genetics play a critical role in the development of type 2 DM as there is a strong inheritance pattern. Hundreds of gene mutations have been linked to the development of type 2 DM. The majority of genetic mutations associated with type 2 DM appear to influence the development and function of β-cells, the sensitivity of cells to insulin action, or the development of obesity. However, none of these single-gene mutations have demonstrated a strong association with type 2 DM. Thus, type 2 DM is likely polygenetic, with more than one genetic defect contributing to its pathogenesis and a diverse combination of derangements contributing to its development in different populations.

In patients with type 2 DM, high blood pressure and dyslipidemia, characterized by high-serum triglycerides and low HDL-cholesterol levels, are very frequent comorbid conditions. Elevated serum plasminogen activator inhibitor-1 (PAI-1), which contributes to a hypercoagulable state, is also common. There are multiple risk factors for the development of type 2 DM.[12] See Table 94-2.

Most patients who develop type 2 DM have multiple defects that impact the regulation of plasma glucose: (1) impaired insulin secretion; (2) deficiency and resistance to incretin hormones; (3) insulin resistance involving muscle, liver, and adipocytes; (4) excess glucagon secretion; (5) increased hepatic glucose production; (6) upregulation of the sodium-glucose cotransporter in the kidney; (7) systemic inflammation; and (8) diminished satiety.[8] See Fig. 94-2.

The pancreas in people with normal-functioning β-cells is able to adjust insulin secretion to maintain normal plasma glucose levels. In obese individuals who do not yet have diabetes, insulin increases in proportion to the severity of the insulin resistance, and plasma glucose remains normal. Impaired insulin secretion is therefore requisite for the development of type 2 DM. In the early stages of β-cell dysfunction, first-phase insulin release is deficient, resulting in impaired glucose tolerance (IGT) (Fig. 94-3). First-phase insulin involves the release of stored insulin in the β-cell and acts to "prime" the liver for nutrient intake. Without appropriate first-phase insulin release, second-phase insulin must compensate for the subsequent postprandial carbohydrate load in order to normalize glucose levels. When insulin release is no longer sufficient to normalize plasma glucose, dysglycemia, including prediabetes and diabetes, ensue. In patients with type 2 DM, β-cell mass and function are both reduced. β-Cell failure is progressive, starting years prior to the diagnosis of diabetes. People with type 2 DM lose approximately 5% to 7% of β-cell function per year. Progressive β-cell loss is likely the result of several factors, including (1) glucotoxicity; (2) lipotoxicity; (3) insulin resistance; (4) age; (5) genetics; and (6) incretin deficiency. Glucotoxicity occurs when glucose levels chronically exceed 140 mg/dL (7.8 mmol/L). The β-cell is unable to maintain sufficient

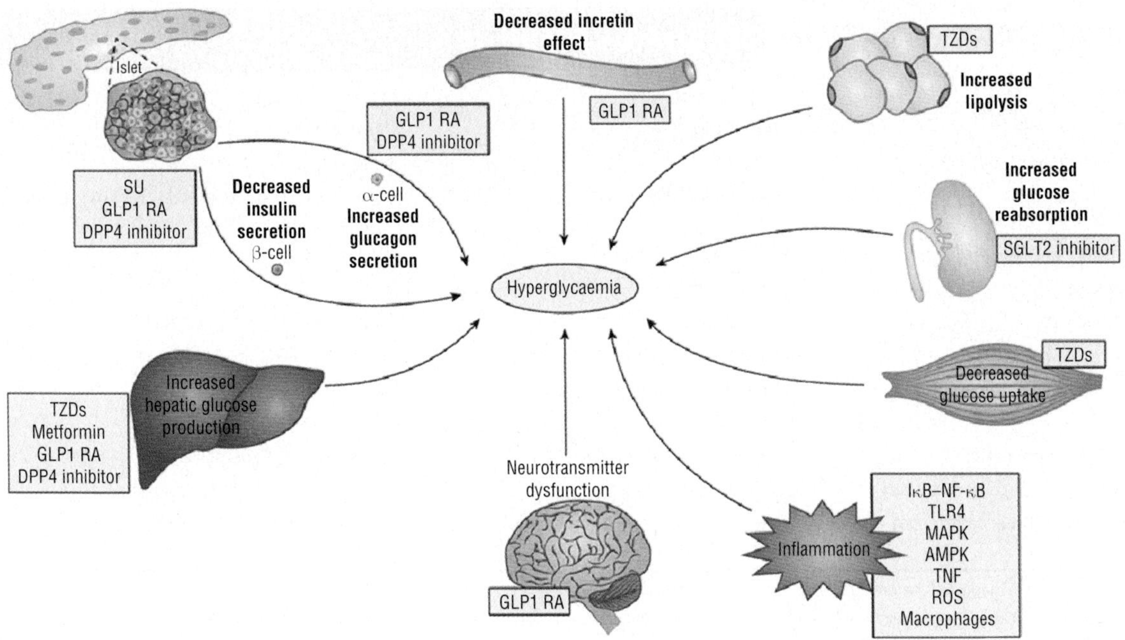

FIGURE 94-2 Pathophysiology of type 2 diabetes mellitus. Multiple defects known as the ominous octet. *(Reproduced, with permission, from Defronzo RA. Banting Lecture. From the triumvirate to the ominous octet: a new paradigm for the treatment of type 2 diabetes mellitus. Diabetes. 2009;58(4):773-95.)*

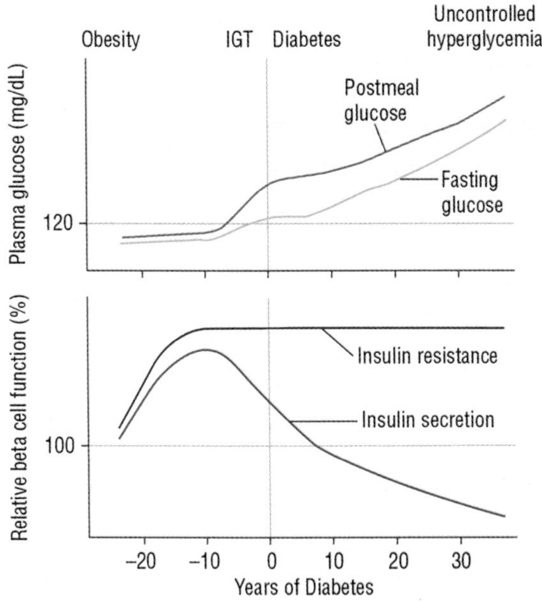

FIGURE 94-3 Natural history of type 2 diabetes. (IGT, impaired glucose tolerance.) For several years prior to the onset of overt hyperglycemia, β-cell dysfunction and the progressive loss of β-cells begins. Moreover, resistance to the action of insulin in muscle and fat tissue is accelerated by weight gain and central adiposity. With increasing insulin resistance and β-cell dysfunction, post-prandial blood glucose concentrations become abnormal. However, fasting blood glucose concentrations typically remain normal or only slightly elevated. As β-cell loss continues, fasting blood glucose readings begin to rise. It is at this point that most patients are diagnosed. Initial treatments improve glycemic control by improving insulin secretion or reducing insulin resistance, or both. Over time, as β-cell loss continues and insulin secretion dwindles to <20% of normal, near-normal blood glucose concentrations cannot be achieved without supplemental insulin therapy. Blood glucose values in mg/dL can be expressed in mmol/L by multiplying by 0.0555.

insulin secretion and, paradoxically, releases less insulin as glucose levels increase.

Gestational Diabetes

GDM develops during pregnancy.[13] If DM is diagnosed prior to pregnancy, this is not GDM, but rather pregnancy with preexisting DM. Hormone changes during pregnancy result in increased insulin resistance, and GDM may ensue if the mother cannot increase insulin secretion to adequately compensate to maintain normoglycemia. Women who develop GDM are predisposed to subsequently developing type 2 DM. GDM and type 2 DM likely share much of the same etiological causes. In most cases, glucose intolerance first appears near the beginning of the third trimester. However, risk assessment and intervention should begin from the first prenatal visit. Detection is important, as therapy will reduce perinatal morbidity and mortality.

Other Types of Diabetes

MODY is characterized by impaired insulin secretion in response to a glucose stimulus with minimal or no insulin resistance.[4] Patients typically exhibit mild hyperglycemia at an early age, and diagnosis is often delayed. The disease is inherited in an autosomal-dominant pattern with at least six different mutations identified to date. MODY 2 and 3 are most common.

The production of mutant insulin molecules has been identified in a few families and also results in abnormal glucose intolerance. Several genetic mutations have been described in the insulin receptor and are associated with insulin resistance. Type A insulin resistance is a clinical syndrome characterized by acanthosis nigricans, virilization in women, polycystic ovaries, and hyperinsulinemia. Anti-insulin receptor antibodies may block the binding of insulin. This has been referred to as type B insulin resistance.

CLINICAL PRESENTATION

The clinical presentation and features of type 1 DM and type 2 DM are different. Although type 1 DM can develop at any age, most patients are diagnosed before the age of 20. Patients with type 1

CLINICAL PRESENTATION Diabetes Mellitus

Characteristic	Type 1 DM	Type 2 DM
Typical age at diagnosis	<20 years[a]	>30 years[b]
Body habitus	Lean (BMI <25 kg/m^2)	Overweight or obese (BMI ≥25 kg/m^2); abdominal obesity and increased waist:hip ratio
Family history of DM in first-degree relatives	Uncommon (<10%)	Common (>80%)
Insulin resistance	Uncommon (occurs if obese)	Very common
Autoantibodies	Usually present	Rarely present
Onset	Abrupt (days/weeks)	Gradual (years)
Symptoms[c]	Common and may be dramatic	Uncommon and often mild
Ketosis	Prone	Rare
Acute complication	Diabetic ketoacidosis (DKA)	Hyperosmolar hyperglycemic state (HHS)
Need for insulin replacement therapy	Immediate	Years after diagnosis
Long-term complications present at diagnosis	Rare—screening for complications unnecessary	Common—screening for complications recommended

[a]While most patients are diagnosed before age 20, type 1 DM can occur at any age.

[b]While most patients are diagnosed after age 30, type 2 DM is increasingly common in obese adolescents and young adults, especially in high-risk populations (eg, Black Americans, Latino/Hispanic Americans, Native Americans).

[c]The classic symptoms of DM include polyuria, polydipsia, polyphagia, weight loss, and fatigue.

DM are often lean or thin at the time of diagnosis. In the absence of an adequate supply of insulin, patients with type 1 DM are prone to developing ketoacidosis and many initially present with DKA. Patients with type 1 DM often have symptoms in the days or weeks preceding the diagnosis. These symptoms often include frequent urination (polyuria) due to an osmotic diuresis from glucosuria, excessive thirst (polydipsia) due to dehydration, increased appetite (polyphagia), and weight loss due to caloric loss. Fatigue and lethargy are also common. The onset of symptoms can be triggered by an infection, trauma, or psychological stress.

In contrast, a majority of patients with type 2 DM are asymptomatic or have only mild fatigue at the time of diagnosis. Many patients are incidentally discovered to have type 2 DM based on the results of a routine laboratory test (eg, plasma glucose or A1C) or development of complications (eg, myocardial infarction, stroke, kidney impairment). Mild hyperglycemia is likely present for many years prior to the diagnosis and thus explains why both microvascular and macrovascular complications are often present at the time of diagnosis. Most patients with type 2 DM are overweight or obese with an elevated waist:hip ratio. Many will report having first-degree relatives with diabetes.

TABLE 94-3 Definitions of Normal and Abnormal Glycemia

Fasting plasma glucose (FPG)	
Normal fasting glucose	70-99 mg/dL (3.9-5.5 mmol/L)
Impaired fasting glucose (IFG)	100-125 mg/dL (5.6-6.9 mmol/L)
Diabetes mellitus	≥126 mg/dL (7.0 mmol/L)
2-hour post-load plasma glucose (oral glucose tolerance test)	
Normal glucose tolerance	<140 mg/dL (7.8 mmol/L)
Impaired glucose tolerance (IGT)	140-199 mg/dL (7.8-11.0 mmol/L)
Diabetes mellitus	≥200 mg/dL (11.1 mmol/L)
Glycosylated hemoglobin (A1C)	
Normal A1C	4-5.6% (0.04-0.056; 20-38 mmol/mol)
Increased risk of diabetes mellitus (Prediabetes)	5.7-6.4% (0.057-0.064; 39-46 mmol/mol)
Diabetes mellitus	≥6.5% (0.065; 48 mmol/mol)

Data from Reference 4.

Diagnosis of Diabetes

5 The diagnosis of diabetes requires the use of glycemic cut points that discriminate patients with normal BG from patients with IFG, IGT, and diabetes (Tables 94-4 and 94-5). The cut points are meant to reflect the level of glucose above which microvascular complications have been shown to increase.[4] Cross-sectional studies have shown a consistent increase in the risk of developing retinopathy at an FPG level above 116 mg/dL (6.4 mmol/L), a 2-hour PPG level above 185 mg/dL (10.3 mmol/L), and an A1C above 6.0% (0.060; 41-42 mmol/mol).

If an NGSP (previously known as the National Glycohemoglobin Standardization Program) method is used, the A1C is the logical test for the diagnosis of diabetes as it measures glycemic exposure over the last 2 to 3 months, in contrast to a single-day, single-point glucose measurement. In addition, patients do not need to fast, and the A1C is a readily available test. An A1C of 6.0% to 6.4% (0.06-0.064;

TABLE 94-4 Criteria for the Diagnosis of Diabetes Mellitus

1. A1C ≥6.5% (0.065; 48 mmol/mol). The test should be performed in a laboratory using a method that is NGSP certified and standardized to the Diabetes Control and Complications Trial (DCCT) assay.[a]
2. Fasting plasma glucose ≥126 mg/dL (7.0 mmol/L). Fasting is defined as no caloric intake for at least 8 hours.[a]
3. Two-hour plasma glucose ≥200 mg/dL (11.1 mmol/L) during an OGTT. The test should be performed as described by the World Health Organization, using a glucose load containing the equivalent of 75 g anhydrous glucose dissolved in water.[a]
4. In a patient with classic symptoms of hyperglycemia or hyperglycemic crisis, a random plasma glucose concentration ≥200 mg/dL (11.1 mmol/L).

[a]In the absence of unequivocal hyperglycemia, a diagnosis requires two abnormal test results from the same sample or in two separate test samples.

Data from Reference 4.

TABLE 94-5 Screening for and Diagnosis of Gestational Diabetes Mellitus (GDM)

1. One-step method (fasting 75-g OGTT)[a]	
One abnormal value is diagnostic of GDM	
Time	**Plasma Glucose**
Fasting	≥92 mg/dL (5.1 mmol/L)
1 hour	≥180 mg/dL (10.0 mmol/L)
2 hours	≥153 mg/dL (8.5 mmol/L)
2. Two-step method	
Step 1: Perform a 50-g OGTT (nonfasting) at 24-28 weeks of gestation in women not previously diagnosed with diabetes	
1 hour	≥140 mg/dL[b] (7.8 mmol/L)
Step 2: If a screening test is positive, perform 100-g OGTT (fasting)	
Two or more abnormal values are diagnostic for GDM	
Fasting	95 mg/dL (5.3 mmol/L)
1 hour	180 mg/dL (10.0 mmol/L)
2 hours	155 mg/dL (8.6 mmol/L)
3 hours	140 mg/dL (7.8 mmol/L)

[a]Should be performed at 24-28 weeks gestation unless the patient has diabetes. The test should be done in the morning after an 8- to 14-hour fast.

[b]The ACOG recommends a lower threshold of 135 mg/dL (7.5 mmol/L) in high-risk ethnic populations with a higher prevalence of GDM; some experts also recommend 130 mg/dL (7.2 mmol/L).

Data from Reference 4.

42-46 mmol/mol) denotes a 10-fold increase in the risk of developing diabetes but does not consistently identify patients with impaired fasting glucose or impaired glucose tolerance. There are slight racial differences in normal A1C levels. One-third fewer individuals with diabetes are identified using the A1C ≥6.5% (0.065; 48 mmol/mol) threshold versus an FPG ≥126 mg/dL (7.0 mmol/L), yet providers may be more likely to diagnose diabetes from an A1C than from an elevated FPG level. While an A1C ≥6.5% (0.065; 48 mmol/mol) is perhaps the most convenient and sensitive method of diagnosing DM, there are three other criteria that can be used to diagnose DM in nonpregnant adults. See Table 94-4. If the patient has symptomatic hyperglycemia and a random plasma glucose ≥200 mg/dL (11.1 mmol/L), reconfirming the diagnosis is not required.

Serial measurements at clinician-defined intervals can help to identify patients moving toward diabetes and those who are stable. Patients who have even minor increases in glucose or A1C values over time should be followed more closely as they are more likely to progress to DM. The A1C measurement can be affected by anemias and several hemoglobinopathies, which would necessitate the use of one of the plasma glucose criteria in these individuals. More information about the A1C assay can be found at the NGSP website: http://www.ngsp.org/interf.asp.

Screening for Diabetes

Given the long-term complications associated with DM and the positive impact that early interventions can have on hyperglycemia and health outcomes, efforts to screen at-risk patients for impaired FPG and the development of diabetes are recommended. Screening begins with identifying patients who are at risk for developing diabetes and, once identified, encouraging patients to obtain an FPG and A1C measurement.

Type 1 Diabetes

The prevalence of type 1 DM is low in the general population. Due to the acute onset of symptoms in most individuals, screening for type 1 DM in asymptomatic children or adults is not recommended.[4] Screening for β-cell autoantibody status in high-risk family members may be appropriate in the context of clinical research trials for the prevention of type 1 DM.

Type 2 Diabetes

The ADA recommends screening for type 2 DM in adults who are overweight (BMI ≥25 kg/m^2 or ≥23 kg/m^2 in Asian-Americans) and have at least one other risk factor for the development of type 2 DM.[4] See Table 94-2. The risk of type 2 DM increases with age, and therefore all adults, even those without risk factors, should be screened every 3 years starting at 35 years old. The recommended screening tests are an FPG, A1C, or 2-hour oral glucose tolerance test (OGTT). The optimal time between screening tests is not known, but it may be prudent to screen patients with multiple risk factors every year.

Children and Adolescents

Despite a lack of clinical evidence to support widespread testing of children for type 2 DM, it is clear that more children and adolescents are developing type 2 DM. The ADA recommends screening overweight (defined as BMI >85th percentile for age and sex, weight for height >85th percentile, or weight >120% of ideal) youths who have at least one of the following risk factors: a family history of type 2 DM in first- and second-degree relatives; Native Americans, African Americans, Hispanic Americans, and Asians/South Pacific Islanders; those with signs or conditions associated with insulin resistance (eg, acanthosis nigricans, hypertension, dyslipidemia); or maternal history of diabetes or GDM during the child's gestation.[4] Screening should be done every 3 years starting at age 10 years or at the onset of puberty if it occurs at a younger age.

Gestational Diabetes

Risk assessment for GDM should occur at the first prenatal visit. Due to the high prevalence of obesity and undiagnosed DM, women with multiple risk factors for type 2 DM should be tested as soon as feasible.[4] All women, even if the initial screen test at the first prenatal visit was negative, should undergo testing between weeks 24 and 28 of gestation. Screening for GDM may be done in one of two ways: (1) a one-step strategy using a fasting 75-g OGTT, or (2) a two-step strategy starting with a nonfasting 50-g glucose load test (GLT). With the standard 75-g OGTT, the diagnosis of GDM is confirmed when fasting, 1-hour, 2-hour, and/or 3-hour glucose values are equal or greater to cutoff values. If a nonfasting 50-g GLT is performed, a fasting 100-g glucose tolerance test must be performed if the 1-hour value is elevated. See Table 94-5.

TREATMENT

General Approach to Treatment

During an initial visit, a thorough medical evaluation should be completed to confirm the diagnosis, classify the type of diabetes, evaluate for any complications or potential comorbid conditions, and review previous treatments and risk factors in established patients. Past medical, family, and social history should be taken as well as medication use, adherence, tolerability, and use of diabetes technology. Screening for psychosocial conditions, self-management education needs, and hypoglycemia should occur. A thorough physical exam (including height, weight, BMI, blood pressure, thyroid palpitation, and foot exam) and laboratory evaluation (including A1C, lipid profile, liver function tests, serum creatinine, and eGFR) should be performed. A 10-year atherosclerotic cardiovascular disease (ASCVD) risk score should also be calculated.[14,15]

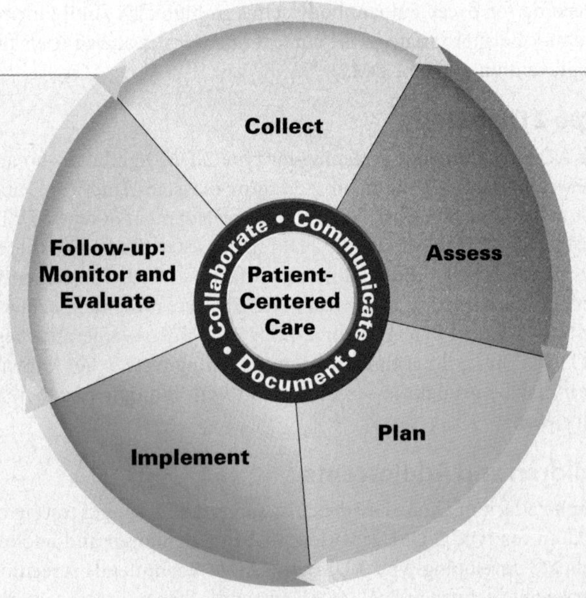

PATIENT CARE PROCESS

Patient Care Process for the Management of Diabetes Mellitus

The image shows the five fundamental steps included in The Pharmacist's Care Process endorsed by the Joint Commission for Pharmacy Practitioners (2014). The tagline of this process reads collaborate, communicate, and document. The five fundamental steps listed here are collect, assess, plan, implement, and follow-up: monitor and evaluate. All these steps are listed in a circular block diagram.

Collect

- Patient characteristics (eg, age, sex, reproductive status)
- Characteristics of diabetes (eg, type, age of onset, initial presentation)
- Microvascular and macrovascular complications
- Hypoglycemia episodes, symptoms, frequency, and suspected cause(s)
- History of diabetic ketoacidosis (DKA) or hyperosmolar hyperglycemic syndrome (HHS)—frequency, severity, and suspected cause(s)
- Patient history (past medical, family, social—dietary habits, weight history, sleep behaviors, physical activity)
- Current medications (including complementary and alternative therapies) and medication-taking behaviors (eg, adherence, injection technique)
- Past diabetes treatments, response to therapy, the reason for discontinuation
- Diabetes and nutritional education (currently enrolled and completed)
- Self-monitoring of blood glucose (BGM) or continuous glucose monitoring (CGM) results and self-management behaviors
- Social and cultural issues—preferences, values, and beliefs; health literacy
- Physical exam: height, weight, BMI, blood pressure, heart rate, comprehensive foot exam
- Labs (eg, glucose, hemoglobin A1c [A1C], serum creatinine [Scr], blood urea nitrogen [BUN], estimated glomerular filtration rate [eGFR], fasting lipid panel [FLP], urine albumin to creatinine ratio [UACR], serum electrolytes)

Assess

- Diagnosis and classification (see Tables 94-1, 94-3, and 94-4)
- Microvascular and macrovascular complications and potential comorbid conditions
- Achievement of A1C and glycemic goals (see Table 94-6)
- Appropriateness, effectiveness, safety/tolerability, treatment burden, cost, and adherence to the current antihyperglycemic regimen
- Achievement of weight, lifestyle, and other behavioral goals
- Achievement of goals for comorbidities (eg, blood pressure, lipids, neuropathic pain)
- Screen for depression, anxiety, disordered eating
- Screen for psychosocial problems and barriers to diabetes self-management

Plan*

- Appropriate A1C and glycemic goals based on age, comorbidities, and other factors (see Table 94-6)
- Tailored lifestyle modifications (eg, diet, exercise, weight management)
- Drug therapy regimen including specific antihyperglycemic agent(s), dose, route, frequency, and duration; specify continuation and discontinuation of existing therapies (see Tables 94-7 to 94-11)
- Monitoring parameters including efficacy (eg, A1C, BGM) safety (medication-specific adverse effects, hypoglycemia), and timeframe (see Table 94-11)
- Patient education (eg, the purpose of treatment, drug administration, dietary and lifestyle modification)
- Referrals to other providers when appropriate (eg, diabetes care and education specialist, registered dietician, eye care professional, podiatrist, mental health professional)

Implement*

- Provide patient education regarding all elements of the treatment plan
- Use motivational interviewing and coaching strategies to maximize adherence
- Schedule follow-up including telehealth visits to monitor and adjust treatment

Follow-up: Monitor and Evaluate

- Determine A1C and glycemic goal attainment
- Identify the presence of medication-related adverse effects (see Table 94-10)
- Assess occurrence/development/progression of diabetes-related complications
- Evaluate patient adherence to treatment plan using multiple sources of information

**Collaborate with patient, caregivers, and other healthcare professionals.*

Goals of Therapy

6 7 The primary goals of therapy for DM are to prevent or delay the progression of long-term micro- and macrovascular complications including retinopathy, neuropathy, diabetic kidney disease, and ASCVD. Additional goals of therapy are to alleviate symptoms of hyperglycemia, minimize hypoglycemia and other adverse effects, minimize treatment burden, and maintain quality of life. This requires glycemic control as well as control of comorbidities and CV risk factors. Glycemic control has well-documented benefits in terms of reducing both short-term and long-term complications associated with DM, but overly intensive control has also led to poor outcomes. Thus, glycemic targets should be individualized for each patient and should be based on balanced considerations of clinical trial evidence and patient-specific factors.[15,16]

Evidence to Support Intensive Glycemic Control

The first trial to definitively prove that good glycemic control could prevent or delay diabetes-related complications was the Diabetes Complications and Control Trial (DCCT).[17] The DCCT enrolled patients with type 1 DM. Patients in the intensive group were treated with intensive basal-bolus insulin therapy (three or more insulin injections per day or insulin pump), with frequent alterations of insulin therapy based on blood glucose monitoring (BGM) results plus frequent contact with a health professional. Patients in the conventional therapy were treated with one or two insulin injections per day. After 6.5 years, retinopathy, neuropathy, and nephropathy were significantly reduced in the intensive group, but symptomatic and severe hypoglycemia was significantly more frequent. Long-term follow-up of the trial participants demonstrated a reduction in macrovascular complications as well as persistent reductions in microvascular complications, even though the difference in A1C values between treatment groups disappeared over time.[18,19]

Another landmark clinical trial, The United Kingdom Prospective Diabetes Study (UKPDS), enrolled more than 5,000 patients with type 2 DM between 1977 and 1991. Patients were followed for an average of 10 years to determine the impact of intensive versus conventional glycemic control on the incidence of long-term complications in patients with newly diagnosed type 2 DM. The results showed that intensive glycemic control (using sulfonylureas and insulin) achieved an A1C of 7.0% (0.070; 53 mmol/mol) compared to 7.9% (63 mmol/mol) in the conventional group. This translated into a modest but significant (12%) reduction in diabetes-related complications, most of which was due to a 25% reduction in microvascular complications.[20] Intensive glucose control using metformin as the initial therapy lowered the risk of diabetes-related complications by 32%, diabetes-related death by 42%, and all-cause mortality by 36% compared to conventional treatment in an overweight cohort of patients.[21] In the long-term UKPDS follow-up study, microvascular benefits of good glycemic control persisted 10 years after the end of the original trial, and a significant long-term reduction in myocardial infarction (MI) and all-cause mortality emerged in the intensive glucose control arm.[22]

Three additional large clinical trials were performed after the UKPDS to compare the effects of different intensities of glycemic control on the risk of macrovascular complications. These studies were done in patients with long-standing type 2 DM who were at high risk for ASCVD. The Action to Control CV Risk in Diabetes (ACCORD) study showed that lower A1C levels (achieved mean A1C 6.4% vs 7.5% [0.064 vs 0.075; 46 vs 58 mmol/mol]) reduced the risk of some microvascular complications but did not reduce the risk of macrovascular complications. The risk of hypoglycemia was significantly higher in the intensive treatment group. Most importantly, this study was stopped early due to an increase in mortality in the intensive treatment arm.[23] The Action in Diabetes and Vascular Disease: Preterax and Diamicron Modified Release Controlled Evaluation (ADVANCE) study similarly showed no significant differences in ASCVD outcomes between two levels of glycemic control (achieved mean A1C 6.3% vs 7.0% [0.063 vs 0.070; 45 vs 53 mmol/mol]) but did show that the more intensive glucose control reduced microvascular complications.[24] The Veterans Affairs Diabetes Trial (VADT) also suggested reduced microvascular complications but no significant reduction in ASCVD outcomes with more intensive glycemic control (6.9% vs 8.5% [0.069 vs 0.085; 52 vs 69 mmol/mol).[25] Based on the results of these studies in aggregate, there appear to be some benefits in terms of microvascular complications but not ASCVD outcomes from intensive glycemic control. However, achieving more stringent glucose targets requires more intensive treatment, which is often more complex and costly, and increases the risk of severe hypoglycemia when insulin therapy is used. The short-term and long-term benefits and risks must be carefully considered when setting intensive glycemic targets.

Glycemic Targets

Based on the clinical evidence that glycemic control reduces microvascular complications and also has long-term benefits in reducing macrovascular complications, several organizations, including the ADA and AACE, recommend surrogate targets for glycemic control. The ADA Standards of Care indicate that an A1C <7% (0.07; 53 mmol/mol) is reasonable for most non-pregnant adults. A fasting or preprandial plasma glucose (FPG) target range of 80 to 130 mg/dL (4.4 and 7.2 mmol/L) and a peak postprandial plasma glucose (PPG) target of <180 mg/dL (10.0 mmol/L) (1-2 hours after the beginning of a meal) correspond with an A1C target <7% (0.07; 53 mmol/mol).[16] The AACE guidelines are more aggressive and indicate that an A1C ≤6.5% (0.065; 48 mmol/mol) is optimal if it can be achieved in a safe and affordable manner. An FPG target of <110 mg/dL (6.1 mmol/L) and a 2-hour PPG target of <140 mg/dL (7.8 mmol/L) correspond with this recommendation (Table 94-6).[26]

Many patients now use a CGM device to assist with glucose management. The use of a CGM can be beneficial for many patients with diabetes and is recommended in patients who use intensive insulin therapy and for those who experience severe or frequent hypoglycemia. A CGM device can report the percentage of time in, above, and below the recommended target ranges and can report the variability of glucose readings. Ideally, the time in range, defined as 70 to 180 mg/dL (3.9 to 10.0 mmol/L), should be at least 70% and the time below range, defined as <70 mg/dL (3.9 mmol/L), should be less than 4%. A CGM device can also report glucose variability, an outcome that is increasingly being recognized as a clinically meaningful outcome beyond A1C. Emerging data indicates that, regardless of A1C, fluctuations in glucose are associated with increased risk of diabetes complications, and A1C alone does not provide the full picture of glycemic control (see Fig. 94-4). Glucose variability is defined as the percent coefficient of variation (%CV) and should be ≤36%.[16] These glucose statistics can be viewed through the ambulatory glucose profile (AGP) report, which also includes a summary glucose profile graph and daily glucose graphs (see Fig. 94-5). The AGP report is a standardized, single-page report that is easy to interpret and provides consistent data regardless of what device is being used.[27]

Glycemic targets must be individualized based on patient-specific factors and the potential risks and benefits of treatment (see Fig. 94-6). Ideally, glycemic targets should be established at the time of diagnosis and should be reviewed and re-evaluated at each visit. When possible, these decisions should be made in collaboration with the patient. Patient or disease factors to consider include treatment-related risks including hypoglycemia and other adverse effects, ability to sense or articulate hypoglycemia symptoms, disease duration, life expectancy, comorbidities, established vascular complications, patient attitude and expected treatment effort, access to CGM or other resources,

TABLE 94-6 Glycemic Target Recommendations in Various Populations

Glycemic targets for most nonpregnant adults with diabetes[a]		
	American Diabetes Association	**American Association of Clinical Endocrinologists**
Glycosylated hemoglobin (A1C)	<7.0% (0.07; 53 mmol/mol)	≤6.5 (0.065; 48 mmol/mol)
Fasting/preprandial plasma glucose (FPG)	80-130 mg/dL (4.4-7.2 mmol/L)	<110 mg/dL (6.1 mmol/L)
Peak postprandial glucose (PPG)	<180 mg/dL (10.0 mmol/L)	<140 mg/dL (7.8 mmol/L)
Time in range (TIR); % of CGM readings and time between 70 and 180 mg/dL (3.9-10.0 mmol/L)	>70%	
Time below range (TBR); % of CGM readings and time <70 mg/dL (3.9 mmol/L)	<4%	
Glycemic variability (% CV)	<36%	
Glycemic targets for adolescents and children		
A1C	<7.0% (0.07; 53 mmol/mol)	
FPG/preprandial glucose	90-130 mg/dL (5.0-7.2 mmol/L)	
Bedtime or overnight glucose	90-150 mg/dL (5.0-8.3 mmol/L)	
Glycemic targets for pregnant women		
A1C	<6.5% (0.065; 48 mmol/mol)	
FPG or premeal glucose	<95 mg/dL (5.3 mmol/L)	
Postprandial glucose (1 hr)	<140 mg/dL (7.8 mmol/L)	
Postprandial glucose (2 hr)	<120 mg/dL (6.7 mmol/L)	

American Diabetes Association glycemic targets for older adults			
Patient characteristics/health status	A1C	FPG or preprandial glucose	Bedtime glucose
Healthy (few coexisting chronic illnesses, intact cognitive and functional status)	<7.0%-7.5% (0.07-0.075; 53-58 mmol/mol)	80-130 mg/dL (4.4-7.2 mmol/L)	80-180 mg/dL (4.4-10 mmol/L)
Complex/intermediate (multiple coexisting chronic illnesses or 2+ instrumental ADL impairments or mild-to-moderate cognitive impairment)	<8.0% (0.080; 64 mmol/mol)	90-150 mg/dL (5.0-8.3 mmol/L)	100-180 mg/dL (5.6-10.0 mmol/L)
Very complex/poor health (LTC or end-stage chronic illnesses or moderate-to-severe cognitive impairment or 2+ ADL dependencies)	Avoid reliance on A1C; avoid hypoglycemia and symptomatic hyperglycemia	100-180 mg/dL (5.6-10.0 mmol/L)	110-200 mg/dL (6.1-11.1 mmol/L)

ADL, activities of daily living; CGM, continuous glucose monitoring; CV, coefficient of variation; LTC, long-term care

[a]Glycemic targets should be individualized. More or less stringent goals may be appropriate for some patients.

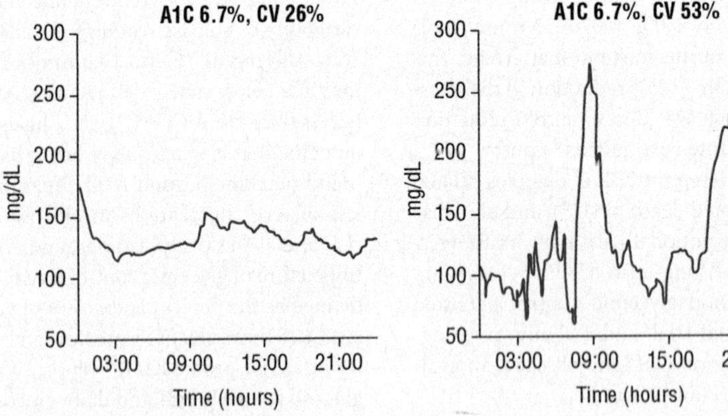

FIGURE 94-4 Glucose variability.

and support system. While an A1C <7% (0.07; 53 mmol/mol) is recommended for most patients, a more stringent goal (such as <6.5% [0.065; 48 mmol/mol]) may be appropriate for some patients if it can be achieved without significant adverse effects, particularly hypoglycemia. Those patients might be younger, with a long life expectancy, with a short duration of diabetes, those treated only with lifestyle modifications or metformin, or those without significant comorbidities. Less stringent goals (such as <8% [0.08; 64 mmol/mol]) may be appropriate for patients who are older or who have a long duration of diabetes, a history of severe hypoglycemia, extensive serious comorbidities, or advanced complications. A higher A1C goal may also be appropriate for a patient in whom it remains difficult to achieve the goal despite appropriate education, monitoring, and drug therapy. For those treated with complex medication regimens, especially those that include insulin, the risk of trying to achieve stringent glycemic goals may outweigh the benefit.

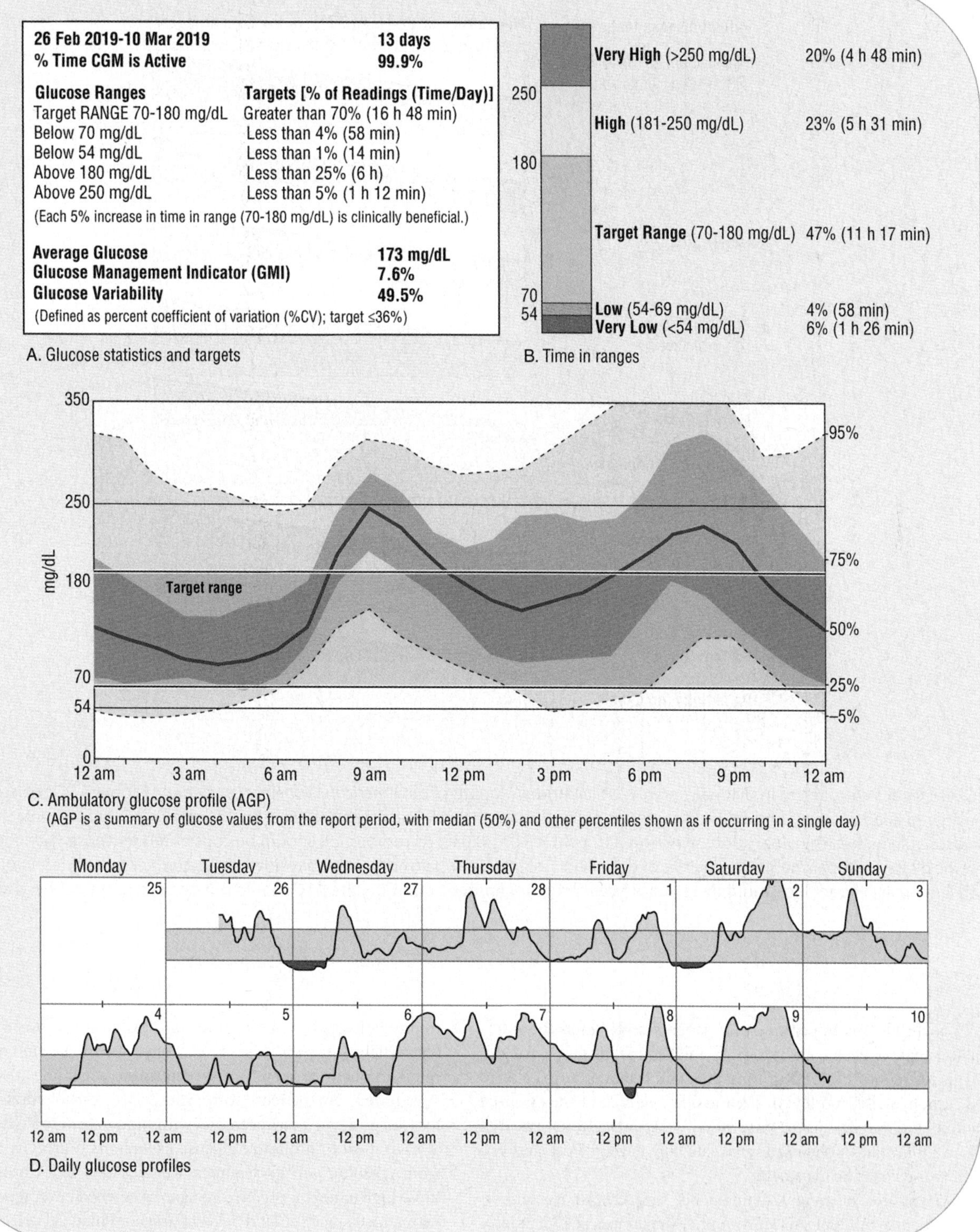

FIGURE 94-5 Ambulatory glucose profile report from a continuous glucose monitoring device.

Nonpharmacologic Therapy

8 Nonpharmacologic therapy such as medical nutrition therapy (MNT), physical activity, glucose monitoring, and diabetes self-management education (DSME) is a cornerstone of treatment for all patients with diabetes.

Medical Nutrition Therapy

MNT is an evidence-based medical approach to treating diabetes through the use of an individually tailored nutrition plan. There is no standardized "diabetes diet," nor is there a single ideal distribution of macronutrients; therefore, meal planning should be

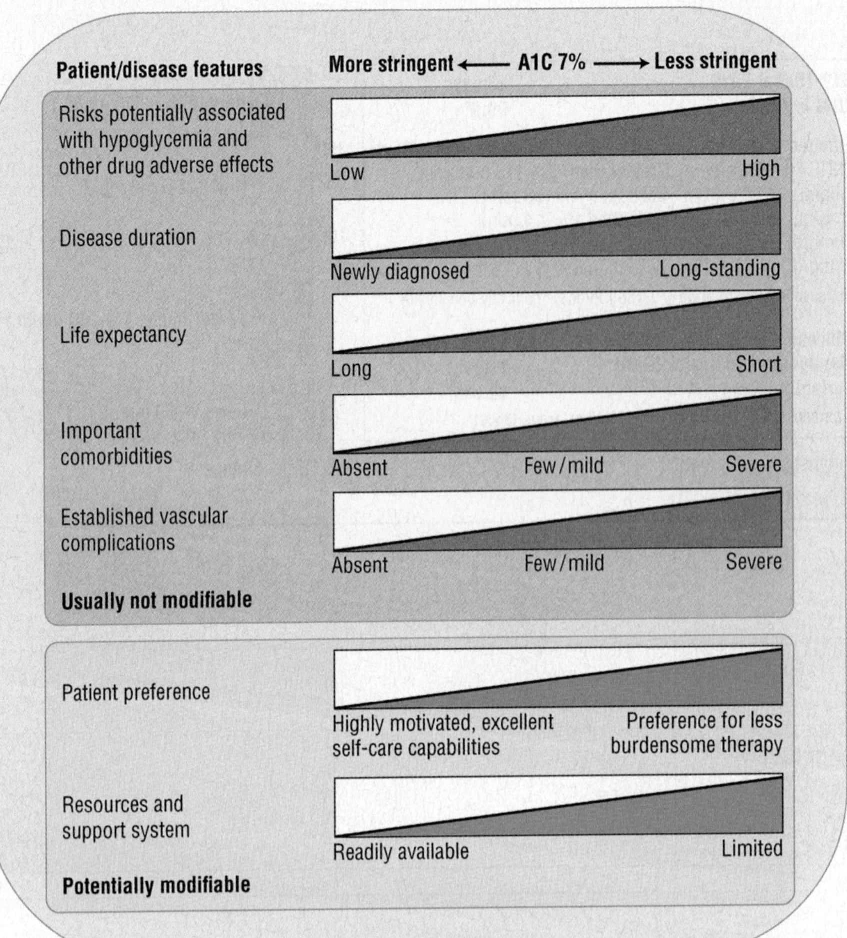

FIGURE 94-6 Approach to individualizing glycemic targets. *(Adapted from American Diabetes Association.)* Higher A1C goals should be considered in adolescents and children as well as patients older than 65 years (Table 94-6).[28] An A1C goal <7.5% (0.075; 58 mmol/mol) is reasonable for healthy older adults, while an A1C goal <8.0% (0.080; 64 mmol/mol) should be considered for those with coexisting chronic diseases, impairments of activities of daily living, cognitive impairment, or who reside in long-term care facilities. In older adults with limited life expectancy, multiple comorbid conditions, or limited cognition, the A1C should not be used to guide therapy.

individualized. It is imperative that patients understand the interrelationships between carbohydrate intake, medications, weight, and glucose control. A healthy meal plan that is moderate in calories and carbohydrates and low in saturated fat, with all of the essential vitamins and minerals, is recommended. A Mediterranean-style diet rich in mono- and polyunsaturated fats may have glucose and CV benefits and could be considered.[29]

Weight loss or weight maintenance is a crucial element in many patients with type 2 DM. An initial weight loss goal of at least 5% should be targeted in all patients who are overweight or obese through calorie restriction. Strategies to reduce calories include reducing portions and frequency of food intake, decreasing the consumption of empty calories, added sugars, and saturated fats, increasing nutrient-dense foods (eg, nonstarchy vegetables), employing low-calorie cooking methods, and tracking calorie intake. Helping the patient adopt healthier eating behaviors that lead to sustained weight loss over time is more important than a specific diet.[29]

Carbohydrate counting is another valuable component of diabetes care. The appropriate amount (grams) and type of carbohydrates are controversial. For individuals with type 1 DM, the focus is more on physiologically regulating insulin administration. For those on fixed doses of mealtime insulin, consistent intake of carbohydrates is recommended to improve glucose control and minimize hypoglycemia. For those on flexible insulin dosing regimens (eg, matching insulin doses to carbohydrate intake amounts), accurate carbohydrate counting to determine mealtime insulin doses is required. For patients with type 2 DM, carbohydrate counting focuses more on a balanced diet with moderate carbohydrate intake at each meal to minimize glucose excursions. Carbohydrate intake from vegetables, fruits, legumes, whole grains, dairy products, and those high in fiber is preferred. Sugar-sweetened beverages and foods with added sugars should be discouraged. Financial constraints and cultural food practices must also be considered. Discourage bedtime and between-meal snacks, set realistic goals, determine what the patient is willing to change, and follow up to see how and whether those changes were implemented.[29]

Physical Activity

Most patients with diabetes benefit from regular physical activity. Aerobic exercise improves insulin sensitivity, modestly improves glycemic control in the majority of individuals, reduces CV risk, contributes to weight loss or maintenance, and improves well-being. Patients should choose activities that they enjoy and are likely to do at regular intervals. Start exercise slowly in previously sedentary patients. It is unclear if asymptomatic patients should be screened for ASCVD prior to beginning an exercise regimen. Screening is reasonable in patients with long-standing disease (more than or equal to 10 years), multiple CV risk factors, microvascular disease (especially kidney disease), or evidence of atherosclerotic disease. If the patient has uncontrolled hypertension, autonomic neuropathy, insensate feet, or proliferative retinopathy, restrictions on recommended activities are recommended. Physical activity goals include at least 150 minutes per week of moderate (50%-70% maximal heart rate) intensity exercise spread over at least 3 days a week with no more than 2 days between activities. In addition, resistance/strength training is recommended at least two times a week as long as the patient does not have proliferative diabetic retinopathy.[29]

Glucose Monitoring

Patients with diabetes should be reassessed every 3 to 6 months (3 months if uncontrolled and 6 months if controlled). An A1C should be drawn, and treatment should be adjusted as needed.[16]

Patients on intensive insulin therapy should BGM at least four times daily, before meals and at bedtime, or should use a CGM device. Patients should also test before exercise, prior to critical tasks such as driving, and if symptoms of hypoglycemia occur. BGM or CGM use is crucial during times of intercurrent illness to detect and prevent acute hyperglycemic complications such as DKA. Patients may also benefit from occasionally testing 2 hours after meals.[16]

Continuous glucose monitors report interstitial glucose levels in real-time and provide insight into glucose trends. Data from these devices can be used for insulin dose calculations, and some are integrated with insulin pumps. CGM use with intensive insulin therapy can reduce A1C, hypoglycemia, and glucose variability. Current guidelines support the use of CGM in patients on intensive insulin therapy. CGM is also recommended in patients with hypoglycemia unawareness to better detect and prevent hypoglycemic events.[76]

Diabetes Self-Management Education and Support (DSME/S)

Consistent, long-term diabetes control requires patients to have a good understanding of their disease and participate in routine self-management strategies to control it. All patients should be offered access to diabetes self-management education and support (DSME/S) programs. There are four critical times to evaluate the need for DSME/S: at diagnosis, annually, when complicating factors arise, and when transitions in care occur.[29] The Association of Diabetes Care and Education Specialists (ADCES) has identified seven self-care behaviors that can be targeted through DSME/S. The behaviors include healthy eating, being active, monitoring, taking medications, problem-solving, reducing risk, and healthy coping.[30] The patient must be involved in the decision-making process and the process must be collaborative. Emphasize that complications can be prevented or minimized with good glycemic control and managing risk factors for ASCVD. Motivational interviewing techniques have been shown to be effective. Briefly, this involves asking open-ended questions that encourage patients to identify and acknowledge barriers that hinder achieving health goals, and then work to address them with the educator's guidance.

Health professionals with formal training and experience in diabetes education can become certified. A certified diabetes care and education specialist (CDCES) must document their experience providing patient education and pass a certification examination. An increasing number of nurses, pharmacists, dietitians, and physicians are becoming a CDCES. Formal diabetes education programs often employ several health professionals including a CDCES. Accredited diabetes education programs can receive payment through Medicare and private health insurance plans. The AADE and ADA accredit diabetes education programs. It must be noted, however, that there are not enough practitioners who hold the CDCES credential to provide education to all patients with diabetes. Therefore, all healthcare professionals must be well-versed in the educational needs related to diet, physical activity, and other self-care behaviors to provide education and reinforcement of these crucial management strategies. Finally, patients should be advised not to smoke, and smoking cessation counseling should be a routine component of diabetes care.

Pharmacologic Therapies

Insulin

Endogenously produced insulin is cleaved from the larger proinsulin peptide in the β-cell to the active peptide of insulin and inactive C-peptide. All commercially available insulin preparations contain only the active insulin peptide and are produced and manufactured exclusively using recombinant DNA technology. "Human" insulins (NPH, regular) are recombinant DNA–derived human insulin, while insulin analogs have had amino acids substitutions in the insulin molecule that change the onset or duration of action. Most insulin products are administered subcutaneously for the chronic management of diabetes, except for inhaled human insulin which is a dry powder of human recombinant DNA regular insulin which is inhaled and absorbed through pulmonary tissue. The main advantage of insulin over other antihyperglycemic agents is that it can achieve a wide range of glucose targets and the dose can be individualized based on glycemic levels. Disadvantages include the risk of hypoglycemia, the need for injection(s), weight gain, and treatment burden.

Insulin is available in several concentrations containing 100 units/mL (U-100), 200 units/mL (U-200), 300 units/mL (U-300), or 500 units/mL (U-500). The most commonly used insulin concentration is U-100. Concentrated insulins containing more than 100 units/mL may be considered for individuals that require larger doses of insulin to control their diabetes.

The pharmacokinetics and pharmacodynamics of insulin products are characterized by the onset, peak, and duration of appearance and action (see Table 94-7). Absorption of insulin from a subcutaneous depot is dependent on several factors, including source of insulin, concentration of insulin, additives to the insulin preparations (eg, zinc and protamine), blood flow to the area (rubbing of injection area, increased skin temperature, and exercise in muscles near the injection site may enhance absorption), and injection site. The abdomen provides the most consistent absorption for insulin.

Basal insulin, also called background insulin, refers to longer-acting insulins that regulate BG levels in between meals by suppressing hepatic glucose production and maintaining near-normal glycemic levels in the fasting state. Bolus insulin refers to short- or rapid-acting insulins that cover meals (also called prandial insulin) or glycemic excursions (also called correction insulin). Basal insulin is the preferred and most convenient initial insulin formulation in patients with type 2 DM while patients with type 1 DM require a combination of basal and bolus insulin to achieve adequate glycemic control.[31,32]

Basal insulin options include NPH, detemir, glargine U-100, glargine U-300, degludec U-100, or degludec U-200. From a pharmacokinetic/pharmacodynamic (PK/PD) perspective, NPH is the least ideal basal insulin as it has a distinct peak and a duration of action much less than 24 hours. While it can be given once daily in some patients with type 2 DM, it usually is dosed twice daily. Detemir also has a peak and often lasts less than 24 hours, but has a more ideal profile compared to NPH. It can be given once daily in some patients but should be dosed twice daily when low doses (less than 0.3 units/kg) are used. Insulin glargine U-100 offers a slightly better profile; it is considered to be peakless and can usually be given once daily. The longer-acting agents (glargine U-300 and degludec) have no peak and a longer duration of action compared to glargine U-100 and detemir. They are given once daily. It is important to consider

TABLE 94-7 Pharmacodynamics of Insulin Preparations

Preparations (U-100 Unless Otherwise Noted)	Onset	Peak[a]	Duration[a]
Ultra-rapid acting			
Insulin aspart (Fiasp)	15-20 min[b]	90-120 min	5-7 hr
Insulin lispro aabc (Lyumjev)	15-17 min[c]	120-174 min	4.6-7.3 hr
Insulin human—inhaled (Afrezza)	12 min	35-55 min	1.5-4.5 hr
Rapid-acting			
Insulin aspart (NovoLog)	10-20 min	30-90 min	3-5 hr
Insulin lispro U-100, U-200 (Humalog, Admelog)			
Insulin glulisine (Apidra)			
Short-acting			
Regular (Humulin R, Novolin R)	30-60 min	2-4 hr	5-8 hr
Intermediate-acting			
NPH (Humulin N, Novolin N)	2-4 hr	4-10 hr	10-24 hr
Regular U-500 (Humulin R 500)	15-30 min	4-8 hr	13-24 hr
Long-acting			
Insulin detemir (Levemir)	1.5-4 hr	6-14[d] hr	16-20 hr
Insulin glargine (Lantus, Basaglar)	2-4 hr	No peak	20-24 hr
Insulin glargine U-300 (Toujeo)	6 hr	No peak	36 hr
Insulin degludec U-100, U-200 (Tresiba)	1 hr	No peak	42 hr
Combination Products			
70% NPH/30% Regular (Humulin 70/30, Novolin 70/30)	30-60 min	Dual	10-16 hr
75% NPL, 25% lispro (Humalog 75/25)	5-15 min		10-16 hr
50% NPL, 50% lispro (Humalog 50/50)	5-15 min		10-16 hr
70% insulin aspart protamine, 30% insulin aspart (Novolog 70/30)	5-15 min		15-18 hr

NPH, neutral protamine Hagedorn; NPL, insulin lispro protamine suspension.

[a]The peak and duration of insulin action are variable, depending on the injection site, duration of diabetes, kidney function, smoking status, and other factors.

[b]Onset of appearance is 2.5 minutes compared to 5.2 minutes for insulin aspart (NovoLog).

[c]Onset of appearance is 1 minute.

[d]Long-acting insulins are considered "peakless," although they have exhibited peak effects during comparative testing.

whether these PK/PD differences translate into clinically meaningful differences in patient outcomes. Clinical trial evidence indicates that all basal insulins can achieve similar A1C reductions if dosed and titrated properly; but the longer-acting basal insulins have a lower risk of hypoglycemia, particularly nocturnal hypoglycemia, and may result in less glucose variability. They do, however, cost more, so the benefits and risks need to be considered on a patient-specific level.

Bolus insulin options include short-acting regular, rapid-acting insulins (aspart, lispro, and glulisine), and ultra-rapid insulins (inhaled human insulin, fast-acting insulin aspart [Fiasp], and insulin lispro aabc [Lyumjev]). Similar to basal insulins, the PK/PD profiles of bolus insulins have improved over time with the rapid-acting insulins offering a faster onset and shorter duration of action compared to regular insulin and the ultra-rapid insulins offering an even faster onset. Rapid and ultra-rapid acting agents may more closely mimic prandial endogenous insulin release. This is likely more relevant to patients with type 1 DM, where therapy is aiming to mimic a functioning pancreas that secretes insulin rapidly after a meal. Rapid-acting insulins have a modestly lower risk of hypoglycemia compared to regular insulin; however, efficacy can be achieved with all prandial insulins and the differences in cost can be substantial. Therefore, when selecting a bolus insulin, a patient-specific evaluation of the benefits and risks should be done.[31,32]

U-500 regular insulin is reserved for use in patients with extreme insulin resistance. It is most often given two or three times a day. To avoid medication errors, it is recommended to prescribe U-500 regular in a pen device or to use U-500 syringes if dispensing U-500 regular in a vial.

Various premixed insulin products, which contain both a basal and a prandial component, are also available and can offer an alternative for patients who require fewer injections or a simpler regimen. However, these products are limited by their fixed mixed formulations which can make tailoring the dosing regimen challenging.

Although endogenous hyperinsulinemia and insulin resistance have been associated with increased CV risk, exogenous insulin therapy has not been associated with increased adverse CV outcomes in several large-scale clinical trials.[17,20,33]

The most common adverse effect reported with insulin is hypoglycemia. It is more common in patients on intensive insulin therapy regimens. Patients with type 1 DM experience more hypoglycemic events when compared to type 2 DM patients who use insulin. In the UKPDS study, the percentage of type 2 DM patients who needed third-party assistance due to a severe hypoglycemic reaction was 2.3%.[20] In the DCCT study, intensive glycemic control increased the risk of severe hypoglycemia threefold when compared to conventional therapy in patients with type 1 DM.[17] Insulin use is associated with an increased risk of hospitalizations in older adults based on public health surveillance data.[34]

Insulin also causes dose-dependent weight gain, which predominantly occurs in truncal fat. Weight gain can be minimized by using physiologic insulin replacement strategies or combining insulin therapy with other medications that mitigate weight gain or promote weight loss.

Insulin can cause injection site reactions including redness, pain, itching, urticaria, edema, and inflammation. Administration of insulin subcutaneously can result in lipoatrophy (depression in the skin) or lipohypertrophy (enlargement or thickening of tissue) in some patients. Lipohypertrophy is caused by repeated injections into the same injection site. Due to insulin's anabolic actions, fat accumulates at the injection site and absorption at this site becomes variable. Lipoatrophy, in contrast, is due to insulin antibodies or allergic-type reactions that destroy the fat at the site of injection. Routinely rotating injection sites prevents these problems from developing and, when lipodystrophy is detected, the injection site should be avoided.

Concerns have been raised about a potential risk of cancer with insulin glargine, but trial results have been conflicting. While some studies using administrative data have found an association between insulin glargine and cancer, other meta-analyses and prospective studies have not.[33]

Inhaled human insulin can cause cough and upper respiratory infections and its use in chronic obstructive pulmonary disease and asthma is contraindicated due to bronchospasm risk. Inhaled insulin use has been associated with a small decline in pulmonary function and patients should have spirometry tests performed at baseline, 6 months, and annually thereafter. If a 20% reduction or greater in forced expiratory volume in 1 second is observed, inhaled insulin should be discontinued.

Insulin is degraded in the liver, muscle, and kidney. Liver deactivation is 20% to 50% in a single passage through the liver. Approximately 15% to 20% of insulin metabolism occurs in the kidney. This may explain the lower insulin dosage requirements and longer duration of activity observed in patients with ESKD.

The dose of insulin must be individualized. In type 1 DM, the average daily requirement for insulin is 0.5 to 0.6 units/kg, with approximately 50% being delivered as basal insulin, and the remaining 50% dedicated to meal coverage. During the honeymoon phase, it may fall to 0.1 to 0.4 units/kg. During acute illness or with ketosis or states of relative insulin resistance, the need for higher dosages is common. In type 2 DM, a higher dosage is required for those patients with significant insulin resistance. Dosages vary widely depending on the degree of insulin resistance and concomitant antihyperglycemic medication use. More specific information on insulin dosing is included in the "General Approach to Hyperglycemia Management" section.

The effectiveness of insulin is highly dependent on its appropriate use. Product selection, education and training, and reinforcement are crucial. Counseling must include proper administration (including dose, injection technique, and timing of injection), glycemic targets, BGM, dose titration or adjustment, storage, and prevention, detection, and treatment of hypoglycemia. Each insulin product is unique in the delivery device used. Some insulin products are available in vials, disposable pen devices, or pen cartridges, but many newer insulins are only available in pen devices. Each pen device product has different quantities, maximum injection doses, storage requirements, and expirations. NPH insulin and all suspension-based insulin preparations should be inverted or rolled gently at least 20 times to fully suspend the insulin prior to each use. Improper mixing of the suspension prior to administration can lead to glycemic variability. Pharmacists should review recent guidelines on proper injection technique and prescribing information for specific products prior to counseling patients and utilize reliable, up-to-date patient education resources to ensure product-specific, accurate counseling information.[35,36]

Biguanides

Metformin is the only biguanide available in the United States. It is oral and available as an immediate-release formulation that is dosed twice daily or an extended-release (XR) formulation that is dosed once or twice daily (Table 94-8). Its benefits in relation to glucose-lowering are complex and not yet fully understood. At the cellular level, metformin activates AMP kinase. Metformin has been shown to decrease hepatic glucose production, yet not all of its effects can be explained by that mechanism and there is increasing evidence of mechanisms in the gut. Additionally, metformin's effects may be partially related to enhanced insulin sensitivity in peripheral (muscle) tissues, which allows for an increased uptake of glucose into muscle cells. Metformin has no direct effect on the β-cell, but insulin concentrations are reduced due to improved insulin sensitivity.[37]

Metformin is generally the initial drug of choice for glucose lowering in patients with type 2 DM due to extensive experience, high efficacy, minimal hypoglycemia risk, positive or neutral effects on weight, potential positive impact on CV risk, manageable side-effect profile, and low cost. Current treatment guidelines recommend initiating metformin as first-line pharmacotherapy unless a contraindication or intolerability exists.[31,32] Metformin consistently reduces A1C levels by 1.5% to 2.0% (0.015 and 0.020; 16 and 22 mmol/mol) and FPG levels by 60 to 80 mg/dL (3.3-4.4 mmol/L) in drug-naïve patients with A1C values of approximately 9% (0.09; 75 mmol/mol). Metformin does not cause weight gain, and may actually lead to a modest (2-3 kg) weight loss. Since metformin does not directly increase insulin secretion from the pancreas, it has a low risk of hypoglycemia. Metformin also has positive effects on several components of the insulin resistance syndrome. Metformin decreases plasma triglycerides and low-density lipoprotein cholesterol (LDL-C) by approximately 8% to 15% and modestly increases high-density lipoprotein cholesterol (HDL-C) by 2%.

Metformin reduced the composite of all diabetes-related endpoints by 32%, diabetes-related death by 42%, and all-cause mortality by 36% in overweight subjects in the UKPDS compared to conventional treatment. Intensive treatment with metformin was also significantly better than intensive treatment with sulfonylureas or insulin at reducing any diabetes-related endpoint, all-cause mortality, and stroke. However, meta-analyses have not confirmed these benefits.[21,38,39] Metformin frequently causes GI side effects, including diarrhea, abdominal discomfort, and/or stomach upset. These side effects are usually dose-dependent, transient, mild in nature, and can be minimized with slow dose titration. Patients should take metformin with or immediately after meals. When initiating therapy, it is important to use a low dose, typically 500 mg given with the largest meal, to minimize GI adverse effects. The dose is then increased in 500 mg increments over several weeks. Approximately 5% to 10% of patients cannot tolerate metformin despite the slow dose titration. Extended-release metformin may lessen some of the GI side effects, but a recent head-to-head comparison of immediate-release versus extended-release metformin found no significant differences in rates of GI adverse effects.[40]

Metformin may cause a metallic taste, due to metformin in salivary secretions and may lower vitamin B_{12} concentrations. Therefore, B_{12} levels or methylmalonic acid should be measured annually or if a deficiency is suspected. Peripheral neuropathy, a microvascular complication that is common in diabetes, could manifest or worsen with B_{12} deficiency. Vitamin B_{12} supplementation by sublingual, oral, or injection easily treats this deficiency.

Rare cases of lactic acidosis have been reported with metformin, usually in the setting of severe illness or acute kidney injury. The risk appears to be exceedingly small but may increase in patients with moderate-to-severe kidney insufficiency or tissue hypoperfusion states such as acute congestive heart failure, excessive alcohol intake, and hepatic impairment. The clinical presentation of lactic acidosis is often nonspecific flu-like symptoms. The diagnosis is therefore made by laboratory confirmation of high lactic acid levels and acidosis.

Metformin can be used in combination with any other antihyperglycemic therapy and is often continued when insulin therapy is initiated. The target dose for metformin is 1,000 mg twice daily or 2,000 mg daily if the extended-release product is used. The minimal effective dose of metformin is 1,000 mg/day (Table 94-8). Approximately 80% of the glycemic-lowering effect may be seen at 1,500 mg daily.

Metformin is renally excreted and accumulates in patients with kidney insufficiency; therefore, metformin is contraindicated in patients with an eGFR <30 mL/min/1.73 m^2 and should be used with caution in patients with milder kidney insufficiency. Initiation of metformin is not recommended in patients with an eGFR 30 to 45 mL/min/1.73 m^2 but can be continued with increased kidney function monitoring; a dose reduction of 50% of maximal dose may be warranted.[41-43] Due to the risk of acute kidney failure when IV contrast dye is used during imaging procedures, metformin therapy should be withheld starting the day of the procedure and resumed 2 to 3 days later, if normal kidney function has been documented. It need not be withheld for days prior to the procedure.

Sodium-Glucose Co-transporter-2 Inhibitors

Four SGLT-2 inhibitors have been approved by the FDA including canagliflozin, dapagliflozin, empagliflozin, and ertugliflozin, all

TABLE 94-8 Dosing Recommendations for Oral Medications Used to Treat Type 2 Diabetes

Generic Name	Starting Dose	Usual Recommended Dose	Maximal Dose (mg/day)	Dosing/Use Based on Kidney Function[a]
Biguanides				
Metformin	500 mg once or twice daily or 850 mg once daily, titrate to target dose as tolerated	1,000 mg twice daily	2,550	Do not initiate if eGFR 30-45; Do not use if eGFR<30
Metformin XR	500 mg to 1,000 mg once daily, titrate to target dose as tolerated	2,000 mg once daily	2,500	Do not initiate if eGFR 30-45; Do not use if eGFR<30
Sodium-glucose co-transporter (SGLT)-2 inhibitors				
Canagliflozin	100 mg once daily	100-300 mg once daily	300	100 mg once daily if eGFR 30-60; Do not initiate if eGFR <30
Dapagliflozin	5 mg once daily[b]	5-10 mg once daily	10	Not recommended for glycemic control if eGFR <45[c]; Do not initiate if eGFR <25
Empagliflozin	10 mg once daily	10-25 mg once daily	25	Not recommended if eGFR <45
Ertugliflozin	5 mg once daily	5-15 mg once daily	15	Do not initiate if eGFR <60; Do not use if eGFR <30
Dipeptidyl peptidase (DPP)-4 inhibitors				
Alogliptin	25 mg once daily	25 mg once daily	25	12.5 mg once daily if CrCl 30-60 mL/min (0.5-1.0 mL/s); 6.25 mg once daily if CrCl <30 mL/min (0.5 mL/s)
Linagliptin	5 mg once daily	5 mg once daily	5	No dose adjustment needed
Saxagliptin	2.5-5 mg once daily	5 mg once daily	5	2.5 mg once daily if eGFR ≤50
Sitagliptin	100 mg once daily	100 mg once daily	100	50 mg once daily if eGFR 30-50 25 mg once daily if eGFR <30
Thiazolidinediones (TZD)				
Pioglitazone	15 mg once daily	30 mg once daily	45	No dose adjustment required
Rosiglitazone	4 mg once daily or in two divided doses	4 mg once daily or in two divided doses	8	No dose adjustment required
Sulfonylureas (first generation)				
Chlorpropamide	250 mg once daily (100 mg once daily in older adults)	100-500 mg once daily	750	Consider alternative agent or initiate conservatively at 100 mg in kidney insufficiency to avoid hypoglycemia
Tolazamide	250 mg once daily (100 mg once daily in older adults or if FPG <200 mg/dL [11.1 mmol/L])	250-500 mg once daily	1,000	Consider alternative agent or initiate conservatively at 100 mg in kidney insufficiency to avoid hypoglycemia
Tolbutamide	1,000-2,000 mg once daily (250-500 mg once daily in older adults)	1,000-2,000 mg once daily	3,000	Consider alternative agent or initiate conservatively in kidney insufficiency to avoid hypoglycemia
Sulfonylureas (second generation)				
Glimepiride	1-2 mg once daily (1 mg once daily in older adults)	4 mg once daily	8	Initiate conservatively at 1 mg in kidney insufficiency to avoid hypoglycemia
Glipizide	5 mg once daily (2.5 mg daily in older adults)	5-10 mg once daily	40	Initiate conservatively at 2.5 mg in kidney insufficiency to avoid hypoglycemia
Glipizide XL	5 mg once daily (2.5 mg once daily in older adults)	5-10 mg once daily	20	Initiate conservatively at 2.5 mg in kidney insufficiency to avoid hypoglycemia
Glyburide	2.5-5 mg once daily (1.25 mg once daily in older adults)	5-10 mg once daily	20	Consider alternative agent or initiate conservatively at 1.25 mg in kidney insufficiency to avoid hypoglycemia
Glyburide micronized	1.5-3 mg once daily (0.75 mg once daily in older adults)	3-6 mg once daily	12	Consider alternative agent or initiate conservatively at 0.75 mg in kidney insufficiency to avoid hypoglycemia
Meglitinides				
Nateglinide	120 mg three times daily before meals	120 mg three times daily before meals	360	No adjustment required
Repaglinide	1-2 mg three times daily before meals (0.5 mg before meals if A1C<8% [0.08; 64 mmol/mol])	2-4 mg three times daily before meals	16	Initiate conservatively at 0.5 mg before meals if CrCl 20-40 mL/min (0.33 to 0.67 mL/s)
α-Glucosidase inhibitors				
Acarbose	25 mg once to three times daily with meals	50 mg once to three times daily with meals	300	Avoid if CrCl <25 mL/min (0.42 mL/s)
Miglitol	25 mg once to three times daily with meals	50 mg once to three times daily with meals	300	Avoid if CrCl <25 mL/min (0.42 mL/s)
Bile acid sequestrants				
Colesevelam	1.875 g twice daily or 3.75 g once daily	1.875 g twice daily or 3.75 g once daily	3.75 g/day	No dose adjustment needed
Dopamine agonists				
Bromocriptine	0.8 mg once daily	1.6-4.8 mg once daily	4.8	No dose adjustment needed

[a]eGFR units: mL/min/1.73 m^2.

[b]For indications other than glycemic control; the recommended starting dose is 10 mg.

[c]For indications other than glycemic control: 10 mg for eGFR >25; if eGFR <25 patients may continue until dialysis but initiation is not recommended.

of which are oral, once-daily products. SGLT-2 inhibitors reduce plasma glucose by preventing the kidneys from reabsorbing glucose back into the bloodstream, leading to increased glucose excretion in the urine. By inhibiting SGLT-2, the renal tubular threshold for glucose reabsorption is lowered and glucosuria occurs at lower levels of plasma glucose concentrations. SGLT-2 inhibition lowers BG through an insulin-independent mechanism and exerts its glucose-lowering effect whenever the plasma glucose is elevated. Thus, SGLT-2 inhibitors can lower both FPG and PPG and are effective even in the absolute absence of insulin. Although SGLT-2 inhibitors block the reabsorption of 90% of the filtered glucose load, which could theoretically result in up to 170-g loss of glucose/day in the urine, urinary glucose excretion (UGE) does not exceed 75 to 85 g/day, because SGLT-1 begins to compensate and can reabsorb up to 30% to 40% of the filtered glucose load, when working at maximal capacity. Thus, when SGLT-2 is inhibited, SGLT-1 instantaneously can augment its reabsorption of glucose and blunt the glucosuric effect of the SGLT-2 inhibitor.

The SGLT-2 inhibitors are considered to have intermediate A1C-lowering efficacy and reduce A1C by 0.5% to 1% (0.005 to 0.01; 6 to 11 mmol/mol). They appear to be more efficacious in patients with higher baseline A1C levels. As eGFR declines, the amount of glucose that reaches the proximal tubule declines; thus, kidney impairment decreases the glucose-lowering efficacy of SGLT-2 inhibitors. Increased UGE leads to the loss of 200 to 300 kcal/day (840 to 1,300 kJ/day), which may contribute to 1 to 5 kg of weight loss. The filtering of more glucose in the urine also causes an osmotic diuresis effect that can result in modest reductions in systolic BP by 3 to 4 mm Hg and diastolic BP by 1 to 2 mm Hg. Because of the insulin-independent mechanism, SGLT-2 inhibitors are unlikely to cause hypoglycemia unless combined with medications such as sulfonylureas, meglitinides, or insulin.

The SGLT-2 inhibitors have additional benefits related to improving CV, HF, and CKD outcomes. Large-scale, CV outcome trials have been completed for empagliflozin, canagliflozin, and dapagliflozin. Both empagliflozin and canagliflozin demonstrated benefit at reducing major adverse CV events (myocardial infarction, stroke, or CV death) in patients with type 2 DM and established CVD or high CV risk.[44-46] Secondary endpoints of HF hospitalizations and worsening nephropathy were also reduced in these studies. Dapagliflozin was noninferior (but not superior) to placebo at reducing major adverse CV events in patients with type 2 DM who had or were at risk for ASCVD. There was a significant reduction in the composite endpoint of heart failure hospitalizations or CV death with dapagliflozin compared to placebo, and a reduction in the progression of kidney disease.[47] Additional outcome trials have provided primary outcomes evidence demonstrating a significant benefit from dapagliflozin and empagliflozin at reducing the risk of worsening heart failure or CV death in patients with heart failure, with or without type 2 DM[48,49] and the benefit from dapagliflozin at reducing the risk of adverse kidney-related outcomes in patients with CKD with or without type 2 DM.[50] There is also primary outcome evidence demonstrating kidney benefit of canagliflozin in patients with CKD and type 2 DM.[51,52] Due to these benefits, the SGLT-2 inhibitors have expanded FDA indications beyond glucose-lowering (Table 94-9).

For glycemic control, the SGLT-2 inhibitors can be added to metformin or used in combination with other second-line agents. They can be used as monotherapy in patients who cannot tolerate or take metformin. They are recommended by the ADA guidelines for many patient populations including those with indicators of high risk or established ASCVD, HF, or CKD. For patients with those comorbidities, SGLT-2 inhibitors should be considered independently of baseline A1C, individualized A1C target, or metformin use. The SGLT-2 inhibitors are also recommended for those with a compelling need to avoid hypoglycemia or a compelling need to avoid weight gain or induce weight loss.

TABLE 94-9 SGLT-2 Inhibitors and GLP-1 Receptor Agonists with FDA Indications Beyond Glycemic Control[a]

Drug Name	FDA Indications Beyond Glycemic Control
SGLT-2 inhibitors	
Canagliflozin	• to reduce the risk of major adverse CV events in adults with type 2 DM and established CVD • to reduce the risk of ESKD, doubling of serum creatinine, CV death, and hospitalization for HF in adults with type 2 DM and diabetic nephropathy with albuminuria
Dapagliflozin	• to reduce the risk of hospitalization for HF in adults with type 2 DM and either established CVD or multiple CV risk factors • to reduce the risk of CV death and hospitalization for HF in adults with HF with reduced ejection fraction (NYHA class II-IV) • to reduce the risk of sustained eGFR decline, ESKD, CV death and hospitalization for HF in adults with CKD at risk of progression
Empagliflozin	• to reduce the risk of CV death in adult patients with type 2 DM and established CVD • to reduce the risk of CV death and hospitalization for heart failure in adults with heart failure
GLP-1 receptor agonists	
Dulaglutide	• to reduce the risk of major adverse CV events in adults with type 2 DM who have established CVD or multiple CV risk factors
Liraglutide	• to reduce the risk of major CV events such as heart attack, stroke, or death in adults with type 2 DM with known heart disease
Semaglutide (SC)	• to reduce the risk of major adverse CV events (CV death, nonfatal myocardial infarction or nonfatal stroke) in adults with type 2 DM and established CVD

[a]Liraglutide and semaglutide (SC) are also indicated for weight loss under different brand names at higher doses.

Excess glucose in the urine is responsible for causing genital mycotic infections, the most common side effect of the SGLT-2 inhibitors. There is also a slightly increased risk of urinary tract infections. Genitourinary (GU) infections occur more frequently in women and uncircumcised men. In clinical trials, GU infections led to discontinuation in less than 1% of patients; most GU infections were treated and patients were able to continue the SGLT-2 therapy. Patients should be educated about the signs and symptoms of GU infections and the importance of proper personal hygiene.

SGLT-2 inhibitors can also cause polyuria, dehydration, dizziness, or hypotension due to the osmotic diuresis effects. Symptomatic hypotension may occur more frequently in patients with low baseline BP or an eGFR less than 60 mL/min/1.73 m^2. Concomitant diuretic use may increase the risk of orthostatic hypotension and electrolyte abnormalities. Patients should be monitored carefully and dose or drug therapy adjustments may be needed. Older adults and patients with stage 4 or 5 CKD are not optimal candidates for SGLT-2 inhibitors. Older adults typically have diminished kidney function and, because they may have poor thirst response, they are predisposed to dehydration. The mechanism of action and osmotic diuresis with SGLT-2 inhibitors may affect several laboratory tests. LDL-C and HDL-C increase slightly with SGLT-2 inhibitors. Hemoconcentration from diuresis can result in a 2% to 3% increase in hematocrit. Urinalysis will always be positive for glucose due to the mechanism of action.

Other safety concerns that have been raised since SGLT-2 inhibitors have come to market include ketoacidosis, amputations, fractures, and Fournier gangrene. Several cases of ketoacidosis have been reported and meta-analyses have shown a small increased risk, although absolute numbers are small. Unlike the typical presentation of DKA, SGLT-2 inhibitor-related ketoacidosis presents uniquely, in that glucose levels typically do not go over 250 mg/dL (13.9 mmol/L) because of the increased UGE. Most cases have been in patients with type 1 DM, thus the SGLT-2 inhibitors are not currently approved by the FDA in this population. Insulin-deficient patients (those with type 1 DM, LADA, or insulin-requiring type 2 DM) are at the highest risk, especially in the setting of decreased insulin use, increased insulin needs (acute illness or infection, surgery, trauma), or low-carbohydrate intake or dehydration. Patients should be well hydrated prior to treatment initiation, temporarily stop the drug if a serious illness is encountered, and should not decrease the insulin dose prospectively when it is initiated.

Canagliflozin was associated with an increased risk of bone fracture and lower-limb amputations in its large CV outcome trial. Many of the fractures were distal fractures of the upper extremities after a fall, and thus may be related to dizziness and orthostatic hypotension. Amputations are more common in patients with peripheral neuropathy, peripheral vascular disease, or prior amputations, so caution should be used in this patient population when considering SGLT-2 inhibitor therapy.

The use of SGLT-2 inhibitors has been associated with Fournier gangrene, a rare urological emergency characterized by necrotizing infection of the external genitalia, perineum, and perianal region. To date, 55 cases have been reported and, thus, causality has not been established.[53]

The SGLT-2 inhibitors should be initiated at a low dose. Volume status, adverse effects, and kidney function should be assessed. The dose may be titrated in patients who are tolerating the drug well and require additional glucose control. Since the glucose-lowering effect of these medications is dependent on kidney function, it is not recommended to start or continue SGLT-2 therapy for the purpose of glucose-lowering when the eGFR is consistently less than 45 mL/min/1.73 m^2, although these medications can be used for alternative indications at lower eGFR levels. Use and dose recommendations vary between agents for patients with kidney dysfunction (Table 94-8).

Glucagon-Like Peptide-1 Receptor Agonists

Currently, seven GLP-1 RAs are available in the United States. Six of these are delivered subcutaneously with dosing schedules ranging from twice daily to once weekly and one is delivered orally once daily (Table 94-10). The class mimics the action of endogenous GLP-1. They stimulate insulin secretion from pancreatic β-cells in a glucose-dependent manner. In addition, during hyperglycemia, GLP-1 RAs reduce inappropriately elevated levels of glucagon, which results in decreased hepatic glucose output. These agents also have a direct effect on the stomach through the autonomic nervous system to slow gastric emptying, thereby reducing meal-related glucose excursions. Additionally, agents that penetrate the blood-brain barrier increase satiety via the central nervous system. These actions result in a reduction in both glucose and weight. GLP-1 RAs also potentially preserve pancreatic β-cell function and protect against cytokine-induced apoptosis. All GLP1 RAs result in pharmacologic levels of GLP-1 activity and are resistant to the rapid degradation by the dipeptidyl peptidase 4 (DPP-4) enzyme.

The A1C-lowering efficacy with GLP-1 RAs is considered high but depends on baseline glycemic control, background therapy, and the specific agent used. GLP-1 RAs can also lead to weight loss. The average weight loss is about 1-3 kg with GLP-1 RAs but is highly dependent on the specific agent and dose used, with clinical trial results varying from an average 0.3 kg weight gain to as much as a 6.5 kg weight loss.

Currently, available GLP-1 RAs include dulaglutide, exenatide, exenatide XR, lixisenatide, liraglutide, and semaglutide (in both an injectable and oral formulation). Multiple differences exist in the characteristics of the individual agents within the class, including molecular structure and size, half-life, duration of action, ability to penetrate different tissue compartments, and homology to native GLP-1, which, in turn, lead to important clinical differences in efficacy, rates of adverse effects, dosing schedules, and impact on glucose profile (Table 94-10). Short-acting agents (exenatide and lixisenatide) predominantly lower PPG levels, likely due to their effect on gastric emptying. Long-acting agents (dulaglutide, liraglutide, exenatide XR, and semaglutide) lower both FPG and PPG, but demonstrate larger effects on FPG levels, due to their longer half-life and resultant suppression of glucagon overnight. Based on several head-to-head trials comparing specific GLP-1 RAs to each other, dulaglutide, liraglutide, and semaglutide have the highest A1C-lowering efficacy while exenatide and lixisenatide have the lowest.[54] Semaglutide appears to have the highest weight loss efficacy, followed by liraglutide, dulaglutide, exenatide, and lixisenatide.[55,56]

The GLP-1 RAs have additional benefits related to improving CV and CKD outcomes. Large-scale CV outcome trials have been completed for dulaglutide, exenatide XR, lixisenatide, liraglutide, and semaglutide (SC). Both lixisenatide and exenatide XR demonstrated CV safety but did not reduce the rate of major adverse CV events (myocardial infarction, stroke, or CV death). Liraglutide, semaglutide, and dulaglutide, however, not only demonstrated CV safety but also demonstrated benefit at reducing the risk of major adverse CV events (myocardial infarction, stroke, or CV death) in patients with type 2 DM and established CVD or high CV risk.[44,57-59] The secondary endpoint of worsening nephropathy was also reduced in these studies. Due to these benefits, the GLP-1 RAs have expanded FDA indications beyond glucose-lowering (Table 94-9).

For glycemic control, the GLP-1 RAs are treatment options at multiple time points in the type 2 DM treatment algorithm and can be used in combination with many other agents including metformin, sulfonylureas, SGLT-2 inhibitors, and basal insulin. They can be used as monotherapy in patients who cannot tolerate or take metformin. They are recommended for many patient populations including those with indicators of high risk or established ASCVD or CKD, and those with a compelling need to avoid hypoglycemia or a compelling need to avoid weight gain or induce weight loss. They should not be used in combination with DPP-4 inhibitors due to the similar mechanisms of action. A significant amount of evidence shows the beneficial effect of the combination of GLP-1 RA and a basal insulin.

The most common adverse effects associated with GLP1-RAs are GI in nature, including nausea, vomiting, and diarrhea. These adverse effects appear to be dose-related so dose titration is recommended. They usually occur early in the treatment course, are typically mild in nature, and transient. Occasionally, the GI side effects are significant enough to require discontinuation. Long-acting preparations tend to have less impact on gastric emptying, and thus a slightly lower risk of nausea, compared to short-acting agents. Patients should be instructed to eat slowly and stop eating when satiated otherwise nausea may worsen or cause vomiting.

GLP-1 RAs enhance insulin secretion in a glucose-dependent manner in response to food intake; thus, the risk of hypoglycemia is low when combined with metformin, DPP-4 inhibitors, SGLT-2 inhibitors, or a TZD. However, when combined with a sulfonylurea or insulin, hypoglycemia may occur.

Antibody formation to GLP-1 RAs may occur, which could potentially attenuate the glycemic-lowering effects. Antibody formation is more likely to occur with exendin-4-based agents (exenatide, exenatide XR, and lixisenatide) than with other agents. Injection site reactions have also been reported in patients taking injectable GLP-1 RAs. These reactions may be more common in patients with high antibody titers. Exenatide XR can also cause injection site nodules, likely due to its formulation. It is encapsulated in microspheres made of a biodegradable polymer, which releases the drug over a sustained

TABLE 94-10 Clinical Comparisons of GLP-1 Receptor Agonists

Generic Name	Primary Glucose Profile Target	Dose/Route	Interval	Dose/Use Based on Kidney Function	Availability, Storage, Preparation
Exenatide	PPG	5-10 mcg SC	Twice daily (within 60 minutes before breakfast and dinner)	Avoid if CrCl[a] <30 (0.5 mL/s); Use caution when initiating or increasing dose if CrCl 30-50 (0.5-0.83 mL/s)	• Multidose pens (5 mcg/dose, 10 mcg/dose, 60 doses per pen) • Pen needles not supplied with pen • Keep refrigerated • After first use, store at room temperature; discard 30 days after first use
Lixisenatide	PPG	10-20 mcg SC	Once daily (1 hr before breakfast)	Limited experience in severe kidney impairment; avoid if eGFR <15[b]	• Multidose pen (10 mcg, 20 mcg, 14 doses per pen) • Pen needles not supplied with pen • Keep refrigerated • After first use, store at room temperature; discard 14 days after first use
Dulaglutide	FPG and PPG	0.75-4.5 mg SC	Once weekly	Use with caution in patients with ESKD	• Single-dose pen (0.75 mg, 1.5 mg, 3.0 mg, 4.5 mg) • Pen needle attached • Keep refrigerated • May store at room temperature for 14 days
Exenatide XR	FPG and PPG	2 mg SC	Once weekly	Limited experience in severe kidney impairment; not recommended if eGFR or CrCl <30 (0.5 mL/s); Use with caution if CrCl 30-50 (0.5-0.83 mL/s)	• Single-dose pen (2 mg) • Pen needle supplied with pen • Keep refrigerated; may store at room temperature for 4 weeks • Store flat in original packaging, protected from light • Remove from refrigerator 15 minutes prior to mixing • Requires reconstitution; administer dose immediately once reconstituted
Liraglutide	FPG and PPG	0.6-1.8 mg SC	Once daily	Limited experience in ESKD	• Multidose pen (6 mg/mL, 3 mL; each pen delivers doses of 0.6, 1.2, or 1.8 mg) • Pen needles not supplied with pen • Keep refrigerated • After first use, store at room temperature; discard 30 days after first use
Semaglutide	FPG and PPG	0.25-1 mg SC	Once weekly	No dose adjustment recommended	• Multidose pen (low dose pen: 1.34 mg/mL, 2 mg/1.5 mL, delivers 0.25 mg or 0.5 mg doses; high-dose pen: 1.34 mg/mL, 4 mg/3 mL, delivers 1 mg dose) • Pen needles supplied with pen • Keep refrigerated • After first use, store at room temperature; discard 56 days after first use
Semaglutide	FPG and PPG	3-14 mg orally	Once daily	No dose adjustment recommended	• Store at room temperature • Should be taken 30 minutes before first food, beverage, or other medication of the day with no more than 4 ounces of water

CrCl, creatinine clearance; eGFR, estimated glomerular filtration rate; ESKD, end-stage kidney disease; FPG, fasting plasma glucose; PPG, postprandial glucose; SC, subcutaneous.

[a]CrCl units: mL/min.

[b]eGFR units: mL/min/1.73 m^2.

time interval. The microspheres can lead to injection site nodules described as pea-sized, hard, subcutaneous, lumps, masses, or induration. Hypersensitivity reactions, including anaphylaxis and angioedema, have also been reported with most GLP-1 RAs.

GLP-1 RAs have been associated with cases of acute pancreatitis, but no causal relationship has been established. While additional study is needed, it should be noted that (1) patients with type 2 DM are at inherently higher risk for developing pancreatitis; (2) GLP-1 RAs may mask the initial signs of pancreatitis, including nausea, vomiting, and abdominal pain; and (3) large studies have not linked GLP-1 RA use to a higher incidence of acute pancreatitis. In a patient with a history of pancreatitis, the benefits must be weighed against the potential risks. A GLP-1 RA should not be used in patients with chronic pancreatitis. If a patient reports abdominal pain, nausea, and repeated vomiting, it is best to discontinue therapy temporarily and confirm that the symptoms are not a sign of a more serious underlying problem. GLP-1 RAs have not been studied in patients with gastroparesis, but since they delay gastric emptying they are not recommended in this patient population.

Long-acting GLP-1 RAs are contraindicated in patients with a history of medullary thyroid carcinoma or multiple endocrine neoplasia type 2 due to a risk of medullary thyroid carcinoma. This contraindication is based on rodent model data that reported a higher risk of C-cell tumors of the thyroid but has not been seen in humans. Rodents may not be the ideal model to study this effect as they express a high number of GLP-1 receptors on thyroid C-cells. The expression of GLP-1 receptors in the thyroid of humans is minimal. Rodents also have a higher baseline prevalence of C-cell tumors compared to humans. There is no contraindication in patients with a history of other types of thyroid cancers.

Most GLP-1 RAs require subcutaneous administration into the abdomen, thigh, or upper arm. Each agent uses a unique injection pen device with unique administration requirements; patients must be instructed on how to use the specific product they have been prescribed. The short-acting agents have specific timing requirements in relation to meals since their mechanisms are more targeted toward slowing gastric emptying postprandially. If the dose of exenatide or lixisenatide is missed, it should not be taken after the meal. The long-acting agents have more flexibility with the timing of doses and can be taken at any time of day, with or without food. Oral semaglutide should be taken 30 minutes before the first food, beverage, or other medication of the day with no more than 4 ounces of water. Most of the GLP-1 RAs (except for exenatide XR) have recommended lower doses when initiating the drug, followed by titration to higher doses if needed for glycemic control. This is to minimize GI adverse effects since the GI adverse effects are dose-related and transient. For the once-weekly agents, steady state is attained at 6 to 8 weeks. For GLP-1 RAs administered weekly, if a dose is missed it should be taken as soon as possible but not within 3 days of the next dose. Use caution when starting or increasing the dose of GLP-1 RAs in patients with kidney insufficiency as there have been case reports of acute kidney injury or worsening kidney function. Most occurred in patients who experienced nausea, vomiting, diarrhea, or dehydration. Exenatide and exenatide XR should be avoided in patients with eGFR<30 mL/min/1.73 m^2, and lixisenatide should be avoided in patients with eGFR <15 mL/min/1.73 m^2.

Dipeptidyl Peptidase-4 Inhibitors

Four DPP-4 inhibitors are approved by the FDA: sitagliptin, saxagliptin, linagliptin, and alogliptin, all of which are oral, once-daily products. These agents inhibit the DPP-4 enzyme responsible for the rapid degradation of GLP-1 and GIP, thereby prolonging the half-life of endogenously produced GLP-1 and GIP. Levels of GLP-1 are deficient in patients with type 2 DM. As these agents block nearly 100% of the DPP-4 enzyme activity for at least 12 hours, normal physiologic, GLP-1 levels are achieved. This leads to an increase in glucose-dependent insulin secretion from the pancreas and a reduction in inappropriate postprandial glucagon secretion, resulting in lower glucose levels without an increase in hypoglycemia when used as monotherapy. These drugs do not alter gastric emptying and do not cause nausea or have significant effects on satiety. DPP-4 inhibitors have a neutral impact on weight.

The DPP-4 inhibitors have moderate glucose-lowering efficacy, with an average reduction in A1C of 0.5% to 0.9% (0.005-0.009; 6-10 mmol/mol) when used at maximum doses. DPP-4 inhibitors have a shallow dose-response curve. There are no clear differences in efficacy between medications within the class. DPP-4 inhibitors are considered second- or third-line therapy in the ADA algorithm, particularly when there is a compelling need to minimize hypoglycemia or weight gain, but they have less A1C-lowering efficacy compared to other medication classes. Potential advantages of the DPP-4 inhibitors include once-daily dosing, oral administration, weight neutrality, low risk of hypoglycemia, and good tolerability. They may be used in older adults with moderate-to-severe kidney insufficiency or those where drug tolerability is a priority. However, their ability to lower BG is modest and they are expensive.

The DPP-4 inhibitors are extremely well-tolerated. Adverse effects are uncommon but could include stuffy, runny nose; headache; or upper respiratory tract infections. Safety concerns that have arisen post-market with the DPP-4 inhibitors include heart failure, pancreatitis, and joint pain. The CV outcome trials with saxagliptin, sitagliptin, linagliptin, and alogliptin all demonstrated the overall CV safety of these agents, with no significant differences in major CV outcomes compared with placebo.[44] However, an increased risk of heart failure hospitalizations with saxagliptin compared with placebo reached statistical significance, and there was a trend toward increased heart failure hospitalizations with alogliptin compared with placebo.[44,60] Because of these findings, prescribing information for both saxagliptin and alogliptin includes information about the increased risk of hospitalization for heart failure, particularly in patients with existing heart or kidney disease. Patients taking these medications should contact their health professional if they develop signs and symptoms of heart failure, and providers should consider discontinuing the medication in patients who develop heart failure.

The FDA has also issued a warning on the risk of severe joint pain with DPP-4 inhibitors. This warning was based on 33 cases between 2006 and 2013. The joint pain occurred between 1 day to years after initial use, and symptoms were relieved after discontinuation of the DPP-4 inhibitor. Patients should not stop taking the drug if symptoms occur but should contact their health professional.

Similar to the GLP-1 RA class, there have been reports of increased risk of pancreatitis with DPP-4 inhibitors, but a causal relationship has not been established and individual, large, prospective studies have not shown an increased risk. A meta-analysis did show a small but statistically significant increased risk of pancreatitis with DPP-4 inhibitor use compared with placebo showing one to two cases of acute pancreatitis for every 1,000 patients treated for 2 years. Thus, pancreatitis appears to be an established yet rare safety concern with these agents.[61] Patients should be informed of the risk and appropriate monitoring should occur if a patient develops signs or symptoms of pancreatitis while taking a DPP-4 inhibitor.

DPP-4 plays an important role in T-cell activation. Theoretically, the inhibition of DPP-4 could be associated with adverse immunologic reactions. To date, however, there has been no evidence of clinically relevant changes in immune function.

There is no need to titrate the dose of DPP-4 inhibitors; however, dose adjustments for kidney function are required for alogliptin, saxagliptin, or sitagliptin (Table 94-8).

Thiazolidinediones

Pioglitazone and rosiglitazone are the two currently FDA-approved TZDs for the treatment of type 2 DM. They are oral agents, dosed once daily (Table 94-8). TZDs work by binding to the peroxisome proliferator activator receptor-γ (PPAR-γ), a nuclear receptor that is predominantly located on fat cells and vascular cells. Activation of PPAR-γ alters the transcription of several genes involved in glucose and lipid metabolism and energy balance. TZDs enhance insulin sensitivity at muscle, liver, and fat tissues. TZDs cause preadipocytes to differentiate into mature fat cells in subcutaneous fat stores. Small fat cells are more sensitive to insulin and more able to store FFAs. This allows a flux of FFAs out of the plasma, visceral fat, and liver into subcutaneous fat, a less insulin-resistant storage tissue. Muscle intracellular fat products, which contribute to insulin resistance, also decline. TZDs also affect adipokines (eg, angiotensinogen, tissue necrosis factor-α, interleukin 6, PAI-1), which can positively affect insulin sensitivity, endothelial function, and inflammation. Of particular note, adiponectin is reduced with obesity and diabetes, but is increased with TZD therapy, which improves endothelial function, insulin sensitivity, and has a potent anti-inflammatory effect.[62]

TZDs are considered second- or third-line agents and can be used in combination with metformin and other commonly prescribed medications for type 2 DM. TZDs have high glycemic-lowering efficacy and reduce A1C values approximately 1.0% to 1.5% (0.010-0.015; 11-22 mmol/mol), FPG levels by 60 to 70 mg/dL (3.3-3.9 mmol/L) at maximal doses, and they have high durability over time. Glycemic-lowering onset is slow and maximal effects may not be seen until 3 to 4 months of therapy. It is important to inform patients of this fact and that they should not stop therapy even if minimal changes in BG levels are initially seen. Pioglitazone consistently decreases plasma triglyceride levels by 10% to 20%, whereas rosiglitazone tends to have a neutral effect. LDL-C concentrations tend to increase with rosiglitazone 5% to 15%, but do not significantly increase with pioglitazone. Both appear to convert small, dense LDL particles, which have been shown to be more atherogenic, to large, buoyant LDL particles, which may be less atherogenic. Both drugs increase HDL, though pioglitazone may raise it more than rosiglitazone. The ADA algorithm recommends TZDs as a potential second-line treatment choice for type 2 DM, particularly when medication cost is a major concern or for those with a compelling need to avoid hypoglycemia. They can be used in combination with metformin and other second-line options.[31,32]

The effects of TZDs on macrovascular complications are controversial and are not similar between rosiglitazone and pioglitazone. A meta-analysis published in 2007 reported higher rates of myocardial infarction (MI) with rosiglitazone compared to placebo or other diabetes medications.[63] This prompted a safety communication from the FDA and prescribing restrictions for the drug. These restrictions were later removed after re-evaluation of the data determined no increased risk. The prospective, multicenter, open-label trial found that rosiglitazone was noninferior to the metformin/sulfonylurea comparator for all CV outcomes except heart failure.[64,65] Alternatively, pioglitazone has been associated with benefits related to macrovascular outcomes. In the PROactive study, 3 years of pioglitazone 45 mg resulted in a significant reduction of the composite of all-cause mortality, nonfatal MI, or stroke in patients with type 2 DM who had previous macrovascular events.[66] Pioglitazone has also been shown to decrease the risk of recurrent strokes, but this was not in a diabetes population.

Adverse effects of TZDs include edema, new-onset or worsening of preexisting heart failure, weight gain, and bone fractures. TZDs cause fluid retention due to peripheral vasodilation and improved insulin sensitization at the kidney with a resultant increase in renal sodium and water retention. Resultant effects include peripheral edema, heart failure, hemodilution of hemoglobin and hematocrit, and weight gain. Peripheral edema is reported in 4% to 5% of patients using TZD monotherapy, but the incidence is significantly increased (more than 15%) when a TZD is used in combination with insulin. TZDs are contraindicated in patients with New York Heart Association Class III and IV heart failure, and great caution should be used in patients with Class I and II heart failure. Edema is dose-related and if not severe, a reduction in the dose may allow the continuation of therapy in the majority of patients. Rarely, TZDs have been reported to worsen macular edema of the eye. Weight gain is also dose-related and is a result of both fluid retention and fat accumulation. Average weight gain varies but a 4-kg weight gain is not uncommon; higher amounts of weight gain may necessitate discontinuation of therapy.

TZDs have also been associated with an increased fracture rate in the upper and lower limbs of postmenopausal women. The risk may relate to TZDs' effect on the pluripotent stem cell and shunting of new cells to fat instead of osteocytes as well as altering osteoblasts/osteoclasts.[67,68] A patient's risk factors for fractures should be considered before selecting a TZD.

TZDs have also been linked to bladder cancer. Bladder tumors have been noted in rodent models using TZDs. Interim analysis of a 10-year observational study with pioglitazone reported an excess of three cases of bladder cancer per 10,000 patient-years of treatment after 5 years of pioglitazone use. Ten-year data using the same database showed no association.[69,70] Other population-based and prospective studies have also reported increased risk with pioglitazone. Excess risk, if present, appears to be mostly in men and smokers, and is dose and duration associated. TZDs should not be used in patients with active bladder cancer and the benefits and risks should be carefully considered before using pioglitazone in patients with a history of bladder cancer.

Premenopausal anovulatory patients may resume ovulation on TZDs due to their insulin-sensitizing effects. Adequate pregnancy and contraception precautions should be explained to all women capable of becoming pregnant.

The recommended starting dosage of pioglitazone is 15 mg once daily and rosiglitazone is 2 mg once daily. Dosages may be increased after 3 to 4 months based on the response to treatment and side effects. The maximum dose and maximum effective dose of pioglitazone is 45 mg and 8 mg once daily for rosiglitazone (Table 94-8). To minimize weight gain and edema, the lowest effective dose should be used. If side effects occur with a higher dose, the dose should be reduced. Lower doses are recommended when used in combination with insulin, and edema and weight gain should be monitored carefully.

Sulfonylureas

Sulfonylureas are oral agents, available in either immediate-release or extended-release formulations, typically dosed once or twice daily (Table 94-8). They enhance insulin secretion by binding to a specific sulfonylurea receptor (SUR1) on pancreatic β-cells. Binding closes an adenosine triphosphate-dependent K^+ channel, leading to decreased potassium efflux and subsequent depolarization of the membrane. Voltage-dependent Ca^{+2} channels open and allow an inward flux of Ca^{+2}. Increases in intracellular Ca^{+2} bind to calmodulin on insulin secretory granules, causing translocation of secretory granules of insulin to the cell surface and resultant exocytosis of the granule of insulin. Elevated secretion of insulin from the pancreas travels via the portal vein and subsequently suppresses hepatic glucose production.

Sulfonylureas are classified as first-generation and second-generation agents. The classification schemes are based on relative potency. First-generation agents (chlorpropamide, tolazamide, and tolbutamide) are lower in potency relative to the second-generation drugs (glyburide, glipizide, and glimepiride), and are rarely used due to a higher risk of adverse effects. When given in equipotent doses, all sulfonylureas are equally effective at lowering BG. On average, glucose-lowering efficacy is considered high with A1C reductions of 1.5% to 2% (0.015 and 0.02; 16 and 22 mmol/mol) and FPG reductions of 60 to 70 mg/dL (3.3-3.9 mmol/L) in drug-naïve patients but is dependent on baseline values and duration of diabetes.

Sulfonylureas are the second most prescribed oral drugs for the treatment of type 2 DM. However, their place in therapy is controversial. Based on their extensive track record of safety and effectiveness, their low cost, and their oral route of administration, many clinicians feel comfortable using them. However, many diabetes experts as well as major organizations that publish guidelines for diabetes management either discourage the use of sulfonylureas or suggest using caution due to the risk of hypoglycemia and weight gain. Soon after sulfonylureas are taken, a robust reduction in A1C is seen, but long-term durability is poor in most patients. Sulfonylureas cause a tachyphylaxis to their insulin secretion effect on the β-cell. In vitro testing of β-cells has reported depolarization of the cell, resulting in its inability to secrete insulin. Whether this effect is reversible is unclear. Clinically, this is recognized by the deterioration of A1C.

Sulfonylureas were used extensively in the UKPDS and ADVANCE trials, which both showed a reduction in microvascular complications in patients targeting a more intensive glycemic goal.[20,24] Results from the University Group Diabetes Program raised early concerns about the CV safety of sulfonylureas, with documented higher rates of coronary artery disease in type 2 DM patients given tolbutamide compared to patients given insulin or placebo. Since then, most evidence suggests that sulfonylurea use does not increase macrovascular outcomes or all-cause mortality compared to other active treatments.[20,24,71,72]

The most common side effect of sulfonylureas is hypoglycemia. Due to its active metabolite, glyburide has a higher risk of hypoglycemia compared to other sulfonylureas while glipizide and glimepiride have lower risks.[72,73] Those who skip meals, exercise vigorously, or lose substantial amounts of weight are more prone to experiencing hypoglycemia. A lower dose should initially be used in high-risk patients, in addition, hypoglycemia on low-dose sulfonylureas may dictate a switch to therapy with a low risk of hypoglycemia. Severe hypoglycemia on sulfonylureas would warrant the same intervention. Because of their risk of hypoglycemia, sulfonylureas should be avoided or used with extreme caution in older adults.[28]

Weight gain is common with sulfonylureas—typically 1 to 2 kg. Whenever possible, clinicians should avoid the use of medications that cause weight gain in patients who are overweight or obese.[74] Many patients report having a sulfa allergy, but cross-reactivity with sulfonylureas is very rare. However, if the patient has a history of anaphylaxis-type reactions to sulfa, it may be best to use a different class of medication.

The starting dose, usual dose, and maximum dose of sulfonylureas are summarized in Table 94-8. Sulfonylureas with long durations of action or those with active metabolites should be avoided in older patients and those with kidney insufficiency due to the high risk of hypoglycemia, an alternative agent should be selected. Within the sulfonylurea class, glipizide may be the safest alternative. The dosage can be titrated as soon as every 2 weeks based on FPG values to achieve glycemic goals. Immediate-release glipizide's maximal dose is 40 mg/day, but its maximally effective dose is about 15 to 20 mg/day. Indeed, the maximally effective dose of sulfonylureas is typically 60% to 75% of the stated maximum dose.[31,75]

α-Glucosidase Inhibitors

Currently, there are two α-glucosidase inhibitors approved by the FDA, acarbose and miglitol, both of which are taken by mouth before meals. α-Glucosidase inhibitors competitively inhibit maltase, isomaltase, sucrase, and glucoamylase in the small intestine, delaying the breakdown of sucrose and complex carbohydrates. There is no malabsorption of these nutrients but merely a delay in their absorption. The net effect of this action is to reduce the PPG rise. Distal intestinal degradation of undigested carbohydrates by the gut flora results in gas, CO_2, and methane, as well as the production of short-chain fatty acids, which may stimulate GLP-1 release from intestinal L-cells.

The A1C-lowering effects of the α-glucosidase inhibitors are modest. PPG concentrations are reduced by 40 to 50 mg/dL (2.2-2.8 mmol/L) while FPG levels are relatively unchanged. Patients near target A1C with near-normal FPG levels but high PPG levels are candidates for therapy. Due to their mechanism, GI side effects, including flatulence, abdominal pain, and diarrhea, are very common and limit their use. Because of the modest A1C effect and the high rates of unpleasant side effects, the ADA does not include the class on their treatment algorithm, but the AACE/ACE algorithm considers them an alternative option that can be used when other medications may be contraindicated or the patient has intolerances. To effectively lower PPG, α-glucosidase inhibitors must be taken three times a day with the first bite of each meal.

Meglitinides

Meglitinides are similar to sulfonylureas, except they have a faster onset and shorter duration of action. By binding to a site adjacent to the sulfonylurea receptor, nateglinide and repaglinide stimulate insulin secretion from the β-cells of the pancreas. As monotherapy, both nateglinide and repaglinide significantly reduce PPG excursions and reduce A1C by approximately 0.8% to 1% (0.008-0.01; 9-11 mmol/mol). Similar to sulfonylureas, the main side effects are hypoglycemia and weight gain. Due to the lack of clinical evidence, their role in therapy is unclear. They are not recommended in the ADA algorithm and are considered a less favorable choice on the AACE/ACE treatment algorithm. Nateglinide or repaglinide should be taken by mouth with each meal, initiated at a low dose, and titrated over time until glycemic control is achieved. These agents may be used in patients with kidney insufficiency and may be a good option for those with erratic meal schedules. Multiple daily dosing may decrease adherence.

Bile Acid Sequestrants

The only bile acid sequestrant approved for the treatment of type 2 DM is colesevelam, an oral once-daily medication. Colesevelam acts in the intestinal lumen to bind bile acid, decreasing the bile acid pool for reabsorption. The role of bile acid sequestrants in the treatment of type 2 DM is unclear. A1C-lowering efficacy is modest. Colesevelam reduces LDL-C cholesterol in patients with type 2 DM by 12% to 16%. Colesevelam is weight neutral and has a low risk of hypoglycemia. Although colesevelam lowers plasma glucose and LDL-C, it has not been proven to prevent CV morbidity or mortality. Patients with type 2 DM who need a small reduction in A1C as well as additional LDL-C lowering may be candidates for this agent.

Dopamine Agonists

While bromocriptine has been used to treat Parkinson's disease and other disorders for decades, a new formulation, bromocriptine mesylate, was FDA-approved for the treatment of type 2 DM. Bromocriptine used for type 2 DM is a quick-release formulation of the dopamine agonist. The exact mechanism by which it improves glycemic control is unknown. Low hypothalamic dopamine levels, especially upon waking are augmented, which may decrease sympathetic tone and output. These effects are speculated to improve hepatic insulin sensitivity and decrease hepatic glucose output. The A1C-lowering efficacy is modest and its role in the treatment of type 2 DM is unclear.

Amylin Analogs

Pramlintide is a synthetic analog of amylin, differing from amylin by three amino acids. It is given subcutaneously before meals and is used in patients currently treated with insulin. Pramlintide mimics the action of amylin, a neurohormone co-secreted from the β-cells with insulin, and regulates glucose by three key mechanisms: reduces glucagon secretion, slows gastric emptying, and increases satiety.

Pramlintide was the first noninsulin agent approved for patients with type 1 DM. Pramlintide is effective at lowering PPG levels and A1C and can be an attractive option for some patients as it can also decrease weight and may allow for lower mealtime insulin doses. Pramlintide lowers A1C by approximately 0.6% (0.006; 7 mmol/mol) and produces an average weight loss of 1.5 kg in patients with type 2 DM. In patients with type 1 DM, the average reduction in A1C was 0.4% to 0.5% (0.004-0.005; 5-6 mmol/mol). Pramlintide is primarily used in patients with type 1 DM as adjunctive therapy in patients who are not achieving PPG goals despite maximizing mealtime insulin doses.

The most common adverse effects associated with pramlintide are GI. Nausea occurs in approximately 20% of patients with type 2 DM and 40% to 50% of patients with type 1 DM. Vomiting or anorexia occurs in approximately 10% of patients. GI adverse effects decrease over time and are dose-related, thus starting with a low dose and slowly titrating as tolerated is recommended. Pramlintide alone does not cause hypoglycemia, but when used in patients on insulin hypoglycemia can occur. To minimize the risk of severe hypoglycemia, the dose of mealtime insulin should be empirically reduced by 30% to 50% when pramlintide is initiated.

Pramlintide dosing is different in patients with type 1 DM and type 2 DM. In type 2 DM, the starting dose is 60 mcg prior to meals and is titrated to the maximally recommended 120-mcg dose as tolerated and warranted based on PPG concentrations. In type 1 DM, dosing starts at 15 mcg prior to meals and can be titrated up in 15-mcg increments to a maximum of 60 mcg prior to each meal, if tolerated.

Treatment—Type 2 Diabetes

Hyperglycemia management in patients with type 2 DM should be patient-centered, using shared decision making and a stepwise approach. The treatment approach should place emphasis on compelling evidence, avoidance of unwanted adverse effects, and minimizing hypoglycemia and weight gain. Management decisions should focus on the impact on comorbidities in addition to the impact on glycemia. Upon diagnosis of type 2 DM, the clinician should assess key patient characteristics including current lifestyle, existing comorbidities, clinical characteristics including A1C, age, weight, presence or absence of symptoms, as well as motivation, cultural preferences, health literacy level, and cost limitations. A patient-specific A1C target should be set and discussed with the patient.

Initial Therapy

Comprehensive lifestyle modifications (medical nutrition therapy [MNT], physical activity, weight loss, smoking cessation, and psychological support) should be implemented at the time of diagnosis and reinforced at every visit since they are the foundational components of diabetes management. To achieve lifestyle modification goals, all patients with type 2 DM should be offered access to ongoing DSME/S programs.

MNT should include improved diet quality and calorie restriction for weight loss or weight maintenance. There is no specific recommended ratio of macronutrients for type 2 DM. Instead, patients should focus on eating patterns that promote foods of demonstrated health benefits and minimize foods of demonstrated harm. All overweight or obese patients should be encouraged to participate in intensive lifestyle management programs to lose weight, with an initial weight loss goal of 5%. Increased physical activity should be encouraged in all patients with type 2 DM to improve glycemic control. Most adults should engage in at least 150 minutes of moderate or vigorous intensity aerobic physical activity spread over the week with no more than 2 consecutive days without activity.[29]

Patients with type 2 DM should consider the quantity, quality, and timing of carbohydrate intake in their diet as a strategy to minimize glucose excursions. Patients should increase carbohydrate intake from vegetables, fruits, legumes, whole grains, and dairy products and should decrease processed foods, refined carbohydrates (ie, foods made with white flour or sugar), or foods/drinks high in added sugar (eg, soda, candy).[29] Quantities of carbohydrates should be considered, although the scientific evidence for specific recommendations is lacking. Education materials often encourage patients to limit daily carbohydrate intake to no more than 60 to 75 g/meal for men or 45 to 60 g/meal for women, and 15 g for snacks. An easier strategy is to limit the grain/starch of the meal to one-quarter of a 9-in. (23 cm) plate. Carbohydrate intake should be spread out across all meals and snacks.

9 In addition to comprehensive lifestyle modification, metformin should be started as first-line therapy in patients who do not have contraindications or tolerability issues. This is based on the efficacy, safety, tolerability, cost, clinical evidence, and extensive experience with this medication. Metformin should be started at a low dose and titrated to the maximum effective dose over time to improve tolerability.[31,32]

If a patient's initial A1C is close to goal (eg, ≤7.5% [0.075; 58 mmol/mol]) and the patient is motivated to initiate lifestyle modifications, the clinician could consider initial treatment with lifestyle alone.[31] Since the effectiveness of most oral medications rarely exceeds a 1% (0.01; 11 mmol/mol) reduction in A1C, the clinician may consider starting two medications (metformin plus a second agent) if a patient's initial A1C is more than 1.5% (0.015; 16 mmol/mol) higher than the target A1C.[32] In addition, there is data to support that initial combination therapy can reduce glucose faster and maintain glycemic control for longer compared to a stepwise approach.[32] Early introduction of basal insulin should be considered in patients with very high A1C levels (>10% [0.10; 86 mmol/mol), those with symptoms of hyperglycemia, or those with evidence of catabolism (eg, weight loss).[32]

To avoid therapeutic inertia, treatment should be reassessed and modified regularly. Patients not meeting their goals should be seen at least every 3 months. Those that are meeting their goals should be seen at least every 6 months. At these points of reassessment, an A1C level should be drawn, medication adherence should be evaluated, and lifestyle recommendations should be reinforced. If glucose targets have not been met, additional therapy should be added.[31,32]

Stepwise Addition of Medications

10 Type 2 DM is a progressive disease, and the majority of patients will eventually require combination therapy. Intensification beyond metformin monotherapy requires careful consideration of patient- and drug-related factors when determining the best regimen for a given patient. Patient-specific factors to consider when selecting a medication include the individualized A1C target and the presence of specific comorbidities (eg, ASCVD, heart failure, CKD, obesity). Drug-specific factors to consider include glucose-lowering efficacy, impact on other comorbidities, impact on weight and hypoglycemia risk, side effect profile, ease of use, and cost (Table 94-11).[31,32]

The first consideration is whether the patient has indicators of high risk or established ASCVD, CKD, or HF. Because of evidence from CV outcome trials, SGLT-2 inhibitors or GLP-1 RAs with proven CV benefit (canagliflozin, empagliflozin, dulaglutide, liraglutide, or SC semaglutide) are recommended as compelling agents to reduce the risk of major adverse CV events in patients with high risk or established ASCVD. If HF coexists, SGLT-2 inhibitors with a proven benefit of reducing HF progression (empagliflozin, canagliflozin, dapagliflozin) are recommended. In patients with CKD, SGLT-2 inhibitors with primary evidence of reducing CKD progression (canagliflozin, dapagliflozin) are preferably recommended. If an SGLT-2 inhibitor is contraindicated or not tolerated, a GLP-1 RA with proven CVD benefit is recommended.[31] TZDs should be avoided in patients with HF. If the A1C target is not achieved after 3 months of dual therapy or if the patient did not tolerate the selected drug, then triple therapy is warranted and a drug from the other class can then be added.[31] These recommendations are independent of baseline A1C, individualized A1C target, or metformin use. In other words, one of these medications should be added irrespective of the need for glucose control and this recommendation is actionable whenever these comorbidities become new clinical considerations regardless of background glucose-lowering medications.

In those without established ASCVD, CKD, or HF, other considerations should be taken into account. If there is a compelling need to minimize weight gain or promote weight loss, GLP-1 RAs or SGLT-2 inhibitors are preferred. GLP-1 RAs have demonstrated varying amounts of weight loss in clinical studies, with the greatest weight loss seen with semaglutide followed by liraglutide, dulaglutide, exenatide, and lixisenatide. If dual therapy does not achieve glycemic control, a drug from the other class can be added. If a GLP-1 RA or an SGLT-2 inhibitor cannot be used, a weight-neutral medication such as a DPP-4 inhibitor can be selected. Sulfonylureas, insulin, and TZDs are not preferred and should be used cautiously due to weight gain. If there is a compelling need to minimize hypoglycemia, DPP-4 inhibitors, GLP-1 RAs, SGLT-2 inhibitors, or TZDs could be added to metformin. If dual therapy does not achieve glycemic control, a drug from a different recommended class can be added. DPP-4 inhibitors and GLP-1 RAs should not be used together due to similar physiologic actions. Basal insulin and sulfonylureas are not preferred in this setting as they increase the risk of hypoglycemia and should be considered only if necessary and used with caution. If

TABLE 94-11 Considerations When Selecting Pharmacotherapy for Type 2 Diabetes

Medication Class	Primary Physiologic Action	A1C Reduction Efficacy	Hypoglycemia Risk[a]	Effect on Weight	ASCVD Effects	Cost	Oral/SC	Adverse Effects and Safety
Metformin	↓ hepatic glucose production	High	No	Neutral	Potential benefit	Low	Oral	GI (diarrhea), B12 deficiency
SUs	↑ insulin secretion	High	Yes	Gain	Neutral	Low	Oral	Hypoglycemia, weight gain
TZDs	↑ insulin sensitivity	High	No	Gain	Potential benefit (pioglitazone)	Low	Oral	Edema, weight gain, risk of heart failure, bone fractures, bladder cancer
DPP-4 inhibitors	↑ insulin secretion (glucose dependent); ↓ glucagon secretion (glucose dependent)	Intermediate	No	Neutral	Neutral	High	Oral	Risk of heart failure, pancreatitis, joint pain
SGLT-2 inhibitors	Blocks glucose reabsorption by the kidney, increasing glucosuria	Intermediate	No	Loss	Benefit[b] (empagliflozin, canagliflozin)	High	Oral	GU infections, risk of volume depletion, hypotension, risk of amputations, bone fractures (canagliflozin), risk of DKA
GLP-1 RAs	↑ insulin secretion (glucose dependent); ↓ glucagon secretion (glucose dependent); slows gastric emptying; ↑ satiety	High	No	Loss	Benefit (liraglutide, semaglutide, dulaglutide)	High	SC/Oral	GI (nausea, vomiting), injection site reactions, risk of thyroid C-cell tumors, pancreatitis, cholelithiasis
Basal insulin	↑ glucose disposal; ↓ hepatic glucose production; suppresses ketogenesis	High	Yes	Gain	Neutral	High	SC	Hypoglycemia, weight gain, injection site reactions

ASCVD, atherosclerotic CV disease; DKA, diabetic ketoacidosis; DKD, diabetic kidney disease; DPP, dipeptidyl peptidase; GI, gastrointestinal; GLP, glucagon-like peptide; GU, genitourinary; RA, receptor agonist; SC, subcutaneous; SGLT, sodium-glucose co-transporter; SU, sulfonylurea; TZD, thiazolidinedione.

[a]When used as monotherapy.

[b]Specific drugs listed as beneficial are based on current available evidence. It is not clear whether the benefit is a class effect.

there is a compelling need to minimize cost, sulfonylureas or TZDs can be considered.[32]

Addition of Injectable Medications

The approach to insulin use in type 2 DM is quite different than in type 1 DM. People with type 1 DM initiate intensive insulin regimens shortly after diagnosis and require basal and prandial insulin to achieve glycemic control. People with type 2 DM can often be managed with oral medications for years before the addition of insulin is needed. Insulin is recommended for patients with extreme (A1C >10% [0.10; 86 mmol/mol]) or symptomatic hyperglycemia. Otherwise, GLP-1 RAs are preferred over insulin as the first injectable agent. GLP-1 RAs have demonstrated equal or superior A1C-lowering efficacy compared to basal insulin and lead to weight loss instead of weight gain with a low risk of hypoglycemia. Most GLP-1 RAs are started at a low dose and titrated slowly to improve tolerability. If additional glucose-lowering is needed after the GLP-1 RA dose has been maximized, basal insulin can be initiated. Switching to a fixed-ratio combination of GLP-1 RA plus basal insulin could be considered as well. Basal insulin is started at a low dose (10 units once daily or 0.1-0.2 units/kg/day) and titrated slowly over time to a target FPG range. Many titration strategies are used in clinical practice. A common method is the 3-0-3 method where the patient checks FPG levels daily for 3 days and calculates the average of those three readings. If the average is greater than 130 mg/dL (7.2 mmol/L), then the patient increases the dose by 3 units. The patient continues this titration until achieving target FPG levels (ie, 80-130 mg/dL [4.4-7.2 mmol/L] for patients targeting an A1C <7% [0.07; 53 mmol/mol]) or until they have reached a basal insulin dose of 0.7-1.0 units/kg/day. If unexplained hypoglycemia occurs, the dose is decreased by 3 units. If the A1C target is not reached by maximally titrating basal insulin, it indicates that PPG levels are likely elevated. Thus, at that point, a medication that lowers PPG can be considered. GLP-1 RAs or SGLT-2 inhibitors should be considered if the patient is not already taking one. Prandial insulin is also an option. A stepwise approach is recommended when initiating prandial insulin; starting with 4 units or 10% of the basal dose with the largest meal of the day. If the A1C is <8% (0.08; 64 mmol/mol), the basal dose can be decreased by the same amount to avoid hypoglycemia. The dose should be titrated over time to achieve target PPG levels <180 mg/dL (10.0 mmol/L). A second or third injection can be added to the other meals if needed. The addition of prandial insulin requires more BGM and patient knowledge and awareness of the relationship between insulin and carbohydrates. It also increases the risk of hypoglycemia and weight gain.[31,32]

It is important to re-evaluate the appropriateness of oral medications when a patient starts injectable agents. GLP-1 RAs can be used in combination with all oral agents except DPP-4 inhibitors. When insulin is started, metformin should be continued. TZDs should be stopped or the dose should be reduced. Sulfonylureas should be stopped or the dose should be reduced, especially if prandial insulin is initiated. SGLT-2 inhibitors can be continued, although the patient should be educated about the risk of DKA, and DPP-4 inhibitors can be continued.[32]

Guideline Recommendations

Several organizations such as the ADA and AACE offer guidance for hyperglycemia management in patients with type 2 diabetes. The ADA and AACE guidelines are similar, in that they both recommend a stepwise approach to treatment, with lifestyle modifications and metformin as first-line therapy, followed by the addition of medications from other classes. They also recommend the use of SGLT-2 inhibitors or GLP-1 RAs in patients with established or high ASCVD risk and/or CKD, independent of glycemic control. The AACE guidelines recommend a more aggressive A1C target (<6.5% [0.065; 48 mmol/mol]) for most patients. Dual therapy is recommended initially for any patient with an A1C >7.5% (0.075; 58 mmol/mol) and insulin is recommended for patients with an A1C >9% (0.09; 75 mmol/mol) with symptoms. Finally, the AACE treatment algorithm lists drugs in order of preference with a focus on minimizing hypoglycemia, weight gain, and other adverse effects.[26]

Treatment—Type 1 Diabetes

11 Due to the absolute deficiency of endogenous insulin in people with type 1 DM, exogenous insulin therapy is a requirement. Achieving adequate glycemic control in type 1 DM usually requires intensive insulin therapy. Intensive insulin regimens are designed to provide insulin in a manner that mimics normal physiologic insulin secretion (Fig. 94-7), with the consistent secretion of basal insulin throughout the day to manage glucose levels overnight and in between meals (ie, basal insulin), and bursts of insulin in response to glucose rises after the ingestion of carbohydrates (ie, prandial insulin).

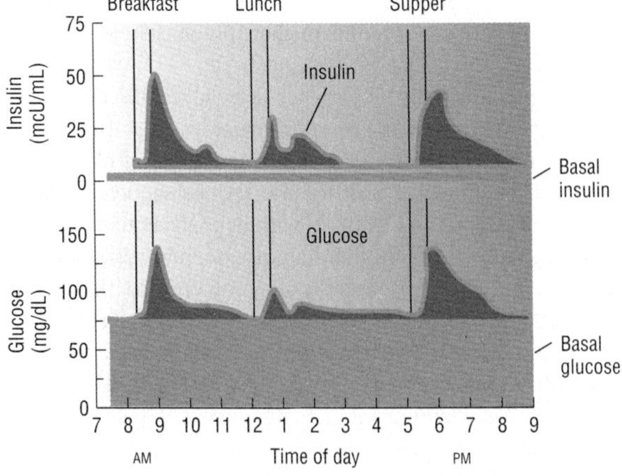

FIGURE 94-7 Relationship between insulin and glucose over the course of a day. Blood glucose values in mg/dL can be expressed in mmol/L by multiplying by 0.0555.

The ADA Standards of Care indicate that most people with type 1 DM should be treated with intensive insulin regimens, either multiple daily injections (MDI) or use of continuous subcutaneous insulin infusion (CSII) via an insulin pump.[31] The choice of which delivery method to use should be tailored to the individualized needs and preferences of the person with type 1 DM. Intensive insulin therapy is complex because it requires multiple injections or pump boluses per day in addition to basal insulin, routine monitoring, and collaborative decision making. The most successful therapy is delivered and adjusted based on changes in nutritional intake, glucose levels, stress, and physical activity.

Examples of intensive insulin regimens are portrayed in Fig. 94-8. A common MDI approach is one injection of long-acting insulin (eg, insulin glargine U-100) to provide the basal

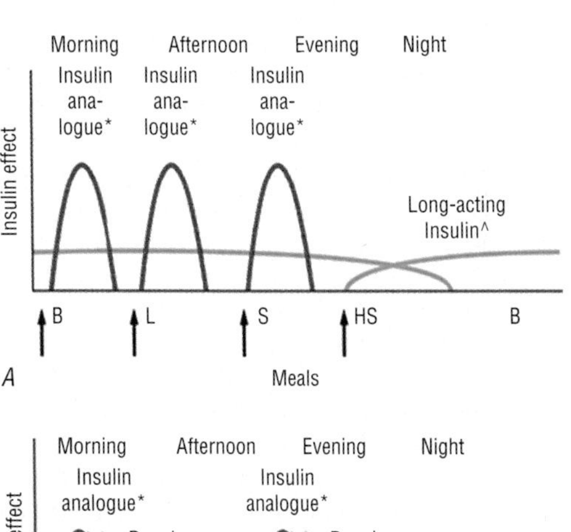

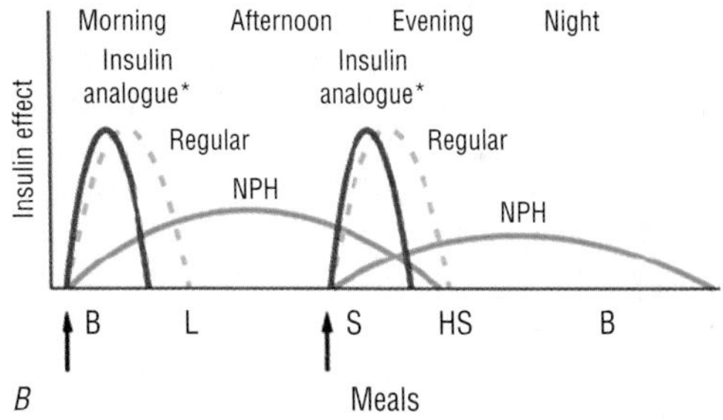

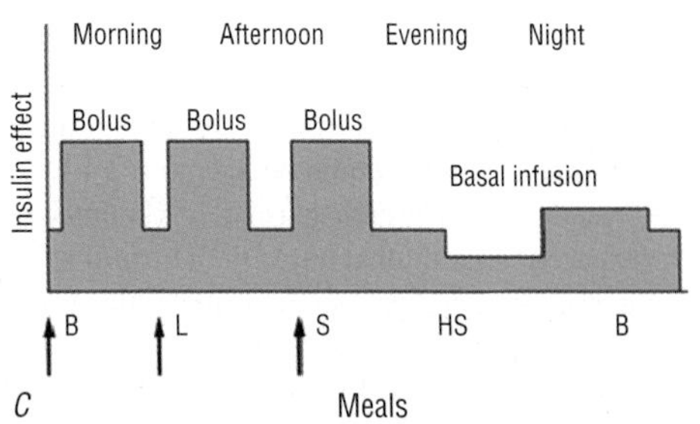

FIGURE 94-8 Common insulin regimens. (A) Multiple-component insulin regimen consisting of one injection of long-acting insulin (^detemir, glargine, degludec) to provide basal glycemic coverage and three injections of rapid-acting insulin (*aspart, lispro, glulisine) to provide glycemic coverage for each meal. (B) Insulin regimen consisting of two injections of intermediate-acting insulin (NPH) and rapid-acting insulin (*aspart, lispro, glulisine [solid red line]), or short-acting regular insulin (green dashed line). Only one formulation of short-acting insulin is used. (C) Insulin administration by an insulin infusion device. The basal insulin rate is decreased during the evening and increased slightly prior to the patient awakening in the morning. Rapid-acting insulin (aspart, lispro, or glulisine) is used in the insulin pump. *(Reproduced, with permission, from Lebovitz HE, ed. Therapy for Diabetes Mellitus and Related Disorders. 4th ed. Alexandria, VA: American Diabetes Association; 2004.)*

component and three injections of rapid-acting insulin (eg, insulin lispro U-100) to provide the prandial component. This regimen utilizes insulin products with more ideal PK properties, but the cost can be prohibitive. A less expensive option consists of two injections of intermediate-acting insulin (eg, NPH insulin) and two injections of short-acting insulin (eg, regular insulin). However, the ADA Standards of Care recommend that most individuals with type 1 DM should use rapid-acting insulins as opposed to regular insulin to reduce the risk of hypoglycemia.[31]

Insulin pump therapy or CSII infuses rapid-acting insulin to cover both the basal and prandial insulin needs. The pump infuses a basal rate constantly throughout the day and allows the patient to give bolus doses using a bolus dose calculator based on current glucose levels, carbohydrate intake, and insulin on board. Insulin pump therapy can provide more precise glucose control and allow more flexibility and fine-tune tailoring. However, CSII requires significant patient education and support and both MDI and CSII can achieve good glycemic control. Insulin pump technology is advancing quickly with new-generation devices entering the market regularly.

When initiating insulin therapy in someone with newly diagnosed type 1 DM, the starting dose is typically 0.4 to 1.0 units/kg/day of total insulin. The total daily dose of insulin is then divided to give 50% as basal insulin and 50% as prandial insulin (distributed across meals). As an example, an 80-kg patient initiated on 0.5 units/kg/day would start with a total daily dose of 40 units. He could be initially prescribed 20 units of a long-acting insulin such as insulin detemir or glargine and 7 units of rapid-acting insulin, such as insulin aspart, lispro, or glulisine, with breakfast, lunch, and dinner. The insulin doses would then be adjusted based on BGM data.

The above example provides a starting point, but there is no one gold standard for starting insulin in patients with type 1 DM. Ideally, patients with type 1 DM should learn how to count carbohydrates so they can match their prandial insulin doses to their carbohydrate intake. Patients should also do BGM before each meal or use CGM to evaluate the insulin regimen and make treatment decisions. Bolus insulin doses can be better individualized by using carbohydrate to insulin ratios (C:I ratios) and correction factors (CF). The C:I ratio is used to estimate how many grams of carbohydrate each unit of rapid-acting insulin will cover. A typical C:I ratio for a patient with type 1 DM is 15:1, meaning that 1 unit of rapid-acting insulin will cover 15 g of ingested carbohydrates. An initial C:I ratio can be estimated by dividing 550 by the total daily dose of insulin the patient is taking. For example, if a patient was taking 40 units of insulin total per day, then his initial C:I ratio would be 550/40 = 14:1.

The CF is used to reduce high glucose levels detected before meals; it is the expected amount that one unit of insulin will decrease the BG under normal circumstances. The initial CF is estimated by dividing 1,650 by the total daily dose. For example, if a patient was taking 40 units of insulin per day, then his CF would be 1,650/40 = 41 (which would likely be rounded to 40 for easier use). Once the patient has a C:I and CF established, he can use these before each meal to calculate a specific premeal dose of rapid-acting insulin. For the example above, if the patient expected to eat 60 g of carbohydrates, had a premeal glucose reading of 200 mg/dL (11.1 mmol/L), and a target glucose of 100 mg/dL (5.6 mmol/L), he would take 7 units of rapid-acting insulin (60/14 = 4.3 units for the carbohydrates and 100/40 = 2.5 units for the correction).

The 550 rule and 1650 rule to calculate the C:I and CF are not well studied, and in clinical practice, some clinicians use 500 instead of 550 and others use 1,500 or 1,800 instead of 1,650. Regardless, these calculations provide an initial C:I and CF values that must be reevaluated and adjusted over time based on glucose monitoring data.

Lifestyle modifications differ between type 1 DM and type 2 DM. Patients with type 2 DM are often encouraged to "count carbs" as a way to prevent glucose excursions after meals. This involves limiting carbohydrates to 45 to 75 g/meal or limiting starches/grains to one-quarter of a 9-in. (23 cm) plate. Patients with type 1 DM count carbs in order to match their prandial insulin dose with their carbohydrate intake using a C:I ratio. To be successful, this requires much more accurate estimations of carbohydrate content than what is needed for type 2 DM management.

Adjunctive Therapy

Pramlintide is an amylin agonist indicated as adjunctive treatment in patients with type 1 DM who are not achieving glycemic targets despite optimization of mealtime insulin. Pramlintide is discussed in more detail earlier in this chapter. In this setting, pramlintide may improve glycemic control and minimize weight gain caused by insulin. However, its use is limited by adverse effects such as nausea and vomiting, modest glucose improvements, increased injections and cost, and increased risk of hypoglycemia. Several other medications have been used off-label and/or are currently being studied as adjunctive therapy in type 1 DM, including the SGLT-2 inhibitors and GLP-1 RAs.

HYPOGLYCEMIA

Hypoglycemia is a common complication of some diabetes medications, including insulin, sulfonylureas, and meglitinides, and a major limiting factor to optimal glycemic control. Hypoglycemia can range in severity and is classified as level 1 (hypoglycemia alert value; ≤70 mg/dL [3.9 mmol/L]) which may not cause symptoms but is sufficiently low that it should be treated with a fast-acting carbohydrate; level 2 (clinically significant hypoglycemia; <54 mg/dL [3.0 mmol/L]) which is sufficiently low to indicate serious, clinically important hypoglycemia; and level 3 (severe hypoglycemia) which is associated with cognitive impairment requiring external assistance for recovery and can be life-threatening.[16] Hypoglycemia is associated with falls, injury, motor vehicle accidents, decreased quality of life, as well as an increased risk of CV events, QT prolongation, arrhythmias, and death. Recurrent hypoglycemia increases the risk of developing dementia, and the degree of cognitive impairment has been associated with the frequency and severity of hypoglycemia. All patients taking medications that can cause hypoglycemia should be educated about the prevention, detection, and treatment of hypoglycemia. BGM is essential to detecting hypoglycemia and taking appropriate action.

Patients can present with a variety of symptoms during an episode of hypoglycemia. Initial autonomic symptoms can include tachycardia, palpitations, sweating, tremors, and hunger. β-Blockers may mask some of these early symptoms. Neuroglycopenic symptoms often occur when the BG is <60 mg/dL (3.3 mmol/L) and can include cognitive impairment, confusion, behavioral changes, anger, irritability, blurred vision, headaches, seizures, and loss of consciousness. It is important for patients to self-monitor their BG when symptoms occur to confirm that the glucose is <70 mg/dL (3.9 mmol/L).

Some patients may experience hypoglycemia unawareness, defined as the asymptomatic onset of hypoglycemia. These patients are unable to detect the early warning symptoms of hypoglycemia and are thus at increased risk for the serious sequelae associated with severe hypoglycemia. Patients with hypoglycemia unawareness are typically those with longstanding disease, more stringent glycemic control, and frequent episodes of hypoglycemia. These patients should check their BG levels prior to any activities that require them to be alert and oriented (eg, driving). CGM can be particularly helpful to identify hypoglycemic events in patients with hypoglycemia unawareness. Also, temporarily raising glucose targets may reverse hypoglycemia unawareness.

Prevention of hypoglycemic events is a critical component of diabetes management. BGM can be helpful but may not be frequent enough to identify hypoglycemia. CGM can be particularly useful in preventing hypoglycemia since it provides the patient with glucose trends which patients can use to adjust their management decisions prior to becoming hypoglycemic. Patients must be educated to understand situations that increase their risk of hypoglycemia, including delaying meals, during or after exercising, or fasting for blood tests or procedures.

Treatment of hypoglycemia dictates the ingestion of carbohydrates. Glucose is preferred. Patients should be counseled to carry a source of fast-acting glucose with them at all times. The "rule of 15" is commonly used to teach patients the proper treatment. First, the patient should perform BGM to confirm a glucose <70 mg/dL (3.9 mmol/L) and then ingest 15 g of fast-acting carbohydrates (1/2 cup [125 mL] of milk, juice, or soda, one tablespoon of honey, hard candy, jelly beans, or glucose tablets or gel equivalent to 15 g of carbohydrates). Foods that include protein or fat should not be used acutely to treat hypoglycemia due to the delayed absorption of glucose. BGM should be repeated in 15 minutes; if the glucose remains <70 mg/dL (3.9 mmol/L), the process should be repeated. Once the BG is normalized, the patient should eat a snack or meal that includes complex carbohydrates and protein to prevent further hypoglycemic episodes.

If the patient is unconscious, IV glucose or glucagon (either via the intramuscular or intranasal route) should be given. Glucagon increases glycogenolysis in the liver and may be given in any situation in which IV glucose cannot be rapidly administered. A glucagon product should be prescribed and readily available to all patients on insulin who have a history of severe hypoglycemia or are at high risk for such events. Family and close friends of the patient should be educated regarding the preparation and administration of glucagon. It can take 10 to 15 minutes for the injection to start raising glucose levels and patients often vomit. It is important to position the patient on the side with the head tilted slightly downward to avoid aspiration. New glucagon products have been recently approved that make glucagon administration easier; a pre-filled syringe that is administered intramuscularly but does not require reconstitution and a dry powder nasal spray that is administered intranasally.

Finally, clinicians should inquire about hypoglycemia at every visit. This involves asking the patient about the frequency, severity, and timing of hypoglycemic events, the need for assistance by a third party, or the need to administer glucagon. Patients experiencing frequent or severe hypoglycemia should have their treatment regimen re-evaluated with a goal of minimizing hypoglycemia.

COMPLICATIONS AND COMORBIDITIES

Achieving good glycemic control is important to reduce the risk of both short-term and long-term complications in patients with type 1 or type 2 DM.[14] Short-term complications include symptoms of excessive urination, fatigue, and weight loss. In patients who are ketosis-prone, sustained elevations of BG above 200 to 300 mg/dL (11.1-16.7 mmol/L) can lead to DKA, a potentially life-threatening condition that often requires hospitalization to receive IV fluids and electrolytes. (See Chapter e95, "Acute Hyperglycemia.") Even in patients who are not prone to ketosis, prolonged periods of poor glycemia can lead to HHS. Poor glycemic control can lead to an increased risk of soft-tissue and urinary tract infections, even in the short term. Long-term complications are the result of vascular and tissue damage. Long-term complications include ASCVD leading to CV events, nephropathy often resulting in kidney insufficiency, retinopathy potentially leading to vision loss, and neuropathy that can cause a wide variety of debilitating symptoms. The combination of vascular damage, peripheral nerve dysfunction, and a diminished immune response significantly increase the risk of toe, foot, and leg amputations in patients with diabetes. Males with diabetes are more prone to developing erectile dysfunction. In short, diabetes can negatively impact nearly every organ system throughout the body, and therefore a very comprehensive approach to patient monitoring is required.

Macrovascular Complications

12 Macrovascular complications are the leading cause of death in people with diabetes. The risk for coronary heart disease (CHD) and ischemic stroke is two to four times greater in patients with diabetes when compared to individuals without diabetes.[51] Moreover, CV disease is the leading cause of mortality in patients with DM. Addressing CV risk factors—lipids, hypertension, smoking cessation, and antiplatelet therapy—will reduce macrovascular events. The ADA recommends low-dose aspirin therapy (75-162 mg daily) in all patients who have established ASCVD. If the patient is allergic to aspirin, clopidogrel may be used. The role of antiplatelet therapy for the primary prevention of a CV event in patients with diabetes is unclear. While low-dose aspirin reduces the risk of vascular events, in adults who do not have established ASCVD the benefits are offset by a higher risk of major bleeding.[77] Some clinical practice guidelines recommend aspirin therapy if the 10-year risk of a CV event is greater than 20% and the patient is at relatively low risk for bleeding complications. In patients who are older than 70 years of age, the risks outweigh the potential benefits of using antiplatelet therapy for the primary prevention of a CV event.

In patients with diabetes and established ASCVD, the use of a GLP-1 RA or an SGLT-2 inhibitor should be strongly considered.[78] Several agents in these two classes of medications have been shown in clinical trials to reduce the risk of major cardiovascular adverse events in patients with a history of coronary artery disease, myocardial infarction, ischemic stroke, or peripheral artery disease and those at very high risk of vascular events with multiple ASCVD risk factors in addition to diabetes. The SGLT-2 inhibitors, specifically empagliflozin, canagliflozin, and dapagliflozin, significantly reduce the risk of hospitalization due to heart failure. Therefore, this class is preferred in patients with preexisting heart failure or those who are at high risk of developing heart failure due to structural heart disease.

Following a myocardial infarction, β-blocker therapy protects patients with diabetes from recurrent CHD events, and the magnitude of benefit is greater than that seen in patients without diabetes.[79] While the adrenergic symptoms produced by hypoglycemia (eg, tachycardia, tremor) can be masked by β-blockers, sweating and neuroglycopenic symptoms are not. Therefore, β-blockers should not be withheld in patients with diabetes if there is a compelling indication to use them.

13 High blood pressure increases the risk of both microvascular and macrovascular complications in patients with DM.[51] The ADA recommends dietary changes, specifically the Dietary Approaches to Stop Hypertension (DASH), and increased physical activity be instituted for all patients whose BP exceeds 120/80 mm Hg. Weight loss is also recommended in those patients who are overweight or obese. Pharmacological therapy, preferably using a class of agents proven to reduce CV event rates, should be instituted if the patient's confirmed office-based BP exceeds 140/90 mm Hg. A combination of two medications should be used if the blood pressure exceeds 160/100 mm Hg. The ADA recommended thresholds and targets for treatment are slightly different than those recommended by the American College of Cardiology/American Heart Association guidelines.[80] While epidemiological data and clinical trials support a blood pressure target of less than 130/80, studies that used intensive BP targets often excluded patients with diabetes.[81] The ACCORD-BP study failed to find a significant benefit when patients with diabetes and ASCVD or multiple CV risk factors were treated to a systolic BP target less than 120 mm Hg when compared to patients treated to a 130 to 140 mm Hg target.[82] The ADA guidelines suggest that a lower target, such as 130/80 mm Hg, is appropriate in patients at high risk of CV events (ie, 10-year ASCVD risk >15%) but does not give this a grade A recommendation due to the lack of high-quality data in patients with diabetes.

Angiotensin converting enzyme (ACE) inhibitors and angiotensin receptor blockers (ARBs) are often used as the initial pharmacological treatment for high blood pressure in patients with diabetes due to their well-documented CV and kidney protective effects.[51] However, thiazide diuretics and CCB have also been shown to improve outcomes in patients with diabetes. Most patients require multiple agents, on average three, to attain the BP goals. Thus, diuretics and calcium channel blockers frequently are used in combination with an ACE inhibitor or ARB. For more information regarding the treatment of hypertension in patients with diabetes, see Chapter 30, "Hypertension."

High-intensity statin therapy is recommended in all patients with diabetes and preexisting ASCVD.[51] In the absence of ASCVD, a moderate-intensity statin should be prescribed to all patients with type 1 or type 2 DM over the age of 40. In patients younger than 40 years of age, moderate-intensity statin therapy may be appropriate if the patient has multiple CV risk factors.[83] The benefits of statins for the primary prevention of CV events in patients with diabetes were established in the Collaborative Atorvastatin Diabetes Study (CARDS).[84] Patients with diabetes and no documented ASCVD were randomized to atorvastatin 10 mg daily or placebo. The trial was stopped early because major CV events were reduced by 37% in the atorvastatin-treated patients. Data from the Heart Protection Study (HPS) also affirm the benefit of statin therapy. Simvastatin 40 mg daily reduced the risk of a major CV event in patients with diabetes by nearly 25% when compared to placebo-treated patients. Statin therapy is recommended regardless of baseline lipid or LDL-C levels. Because statins may cause birth defects, they should only be used in women of childbearing age who do not wish to become pregnant and are using a reliable form of contraception.

After a statin has been initiated for CV risk reduction, markedly elevated triglycerides (≥500 mg/dL [5.65 mmol/L]) may require additional therapy. Patients with marked hypertriglyceridemia are at risk for pancreatitis. In these circumstances, a fibrate (eg, fenofibrate), omega-3 fatty acid, or niacin can be used to reduce serum triglycerides.[85] The routine use of medications to address hypertriglyceridemia in patients with diabetes with baseline elevations less than 500 mg/dL (5.65 mmol/L) is controversial. The Fenofibrate Intervention and Event Lowering in Diabetes (FIELD) was conducted in patients with type 2 DM and failed to show a CV benefit from fenofibrate 200 mg daily when compared to placebo. In a subgroup analysis, subjects without ASCVD at baseline appeared to have a significant reduction in CV events. However, the lipid arm of the ACCORD study also evaluated the use of fenofibrate, and it did not significantly lower CV events. Niacin in combination with a statin failed to improve CV outcomes in patients with diabetes as well.

Peripheral arterial disease is another potential macrovascular complication associated with diabetes, which often contributes to foot ulcers and limb amputation.[51] Claudication and nonhealing foot ulcers are common in patients with type 2 DM. Smoking cessation, statin therapy, good glycemic control, and antiplatelet therapy are important strategies in treating peripheral arterial disease. Cilostazol may be useful in select patients to reduce symptoms. Revascularization surgery can be considered; however, small vessel disease that cannot be bypassed is common in diabetes. If a patient develops foot lesions, early detection, debridement, and appropriate footwear are critical to prevent foot or limb loss. For more advanced lesions, skin grafts, topical wound healing, and hyperbaric treatments may be necessary. Foot examinations during each face-to-face encounter with the patient and a yearly Semmes-Weinstein 10 gram-force monofilament test to assess for loss of protective sensation can be used to identify high-risk patients who need further evaluation, routine podiatric care, and closer follow-up.

Microvascular Complications

Microvascular complications are closely related to glycemic control, and efforts to improve glycemia significantly reduce the risk of developing these complications and slow their progression.[86] Microvascular complications take many forms but most commonly manifest as damage to the kidneys, eyes, and peripheral nerves.

Nephropathy

DM, particularly type 2 DM coupled with hypertension, is among the leading causes of ESKD in the United States.[86] Albuminuria is a marker of kidney damage and a strong predictor of ESKD in patients with type 1 DM. In type 2 DM, the presence of albuminuria is a strong risk factor for macrovascular disease but a weaker predictor for ESKD. The ADA recommends measuring a patient's eGFR and screening for albuminuria at the time of diagnosis and annually thereafter in persons with type 2 DM. In type 1 DM, proteinuria rarely occurs before puberty. Annually screening individuals with type 1 DM should begin with puberty or when the disease duration has been at least 5 years. Patients with a UACR >300 mg/g or an eGFR 30-60 mL/min/1.73 m^2 should be monitored twice annually to guide therapy. There are three methods for assessing albuminuria: (1) a random spot collection, preferably the first-morning void; (2) a 24-hour timed collection; and (3) a timed (eg, 4- or 10-hour overnight) collection. Modestly elevated albuminuria is defined as a ratio of 30 to 299 mg/g (3.4-33.8 mg/mmol) albumin:creatinine and overt albuminuria as a ratio ≥300 mg/g (33.9 mg/mmol). Timed collections are cumbersome to perform but more accurate than a random spot collection. There is significant day-to-day variability in urinary protein excretion. Therefore, unless the results are unequivocally positive, albuminuria should be confirmed on at least two of three samples over 3 to 6 months. Additionally, when assessing urine protein, conditions that may cause transient elevations in urinary protein or albumin excretion should be excluded. These conditions include intense exercise, recent urinary tract infections, hypertension, short-term hyperglycemia, heart failure, and acute febrile illness.

Glucose and blood pressure control are important for preventing and retarding the progression of nephropathy.[86] The SGLT-2 inhibitors, specifically empagliflozin, canagliflozin, and dapagliflozin, significantly reduce the decline in kidney function in patients with CKD, with or without diabetes. Therefore, this class is preferred in the treatment of type 2 DM in patients with CKD, specifically in those with eGFR 30-60 mL/min/1.73 m^2 and a UACR >300 mg/g (33.9 mg/mmol). While the glucose-lowering effects of the SGLT-2 inhibitors are substantially reduced when the patient's eGFR is <45 mL/min/1.73 m^2, the kidney protective effects are not. The GLP-1 RAs also appear to slow the progression of CKD, but these findings have not yet been confirmed in studies specifically designed to determine the impact of GLP-1 RAs on kidney function in patients with CKD.

ACE inhibitors and ARBs have also been shown to slow the progression of kidney disease in patients with diabetes. However, using a combination of agents to block the renin–angiotensin–aldosterone system—for example, using an ACE inhibitor with an ARB, aldosterone receptor blockers, or direct renin inhibitors—has not been shown to improve outcomes but clearly increase the risk of adverse effects. Diuretics frequently are necessary due to the volume-expanded state of patients with CKD and are recommended second-line therapy. The ADA currently recommends a blood pressure goal less than 140/90 mm Hg in patients with nephropathy, but a lower blood pressure target (eg, less than 130/80), if it can be achieved without undue burden or side effects, may be desirable. Three or more antihypertensives are often needed to reach goal blood pressure.

Retinopathy

Diabetic retinopathy is caused by ischemia in the microcirculation in the eye coupled with the inappropriate release of vascular growth factors.[86] Patients with diabetes should have routine dilated eye examinations to fully evaluate the retina. The ADA recommends patients with type 1 DM and patients with established retinopathy be seen by an ophthalmologist or optometrist trained in diabetic eye disease. Early background retinopathy may reverse with improved glycemic control and optimal blood pressure control. More advanced retinopathy will not fully regress with improved glycemia. Aggressive reductions in BG may acutely worsen retinopathy. Laser photocoagulation has markedly improved sight preservation and is recommended in patients with macular edema and proliferative retinopathy. Intravitreal anti-vascular endothelial growth factor (VEGF) therapy has also been shown to be highly effective for sight preservation. Both bevacizumab, used off-label, and ranibizumab are anti-VEGF monoclonal antibodies. Aflibercept is a VEGF decoy receptor. People with diabetes also have a higher rate of cataracts and open-angle glaucoma.

Neuropathy

Neuropathy in people with diabetes can manifest as (1) peripheral neuropathy, (2) autonomic neuropathy, and/or (3) focal neuropathies.[86] Distal, symmetrical, peripheral neuropathy is the most common complication seen in type 2 DM patients in outpatient clinics. Paresthesias, perceived hot or cold, numbness, or pain are the predominant symptoms. The feet are involved far more often than the hands as peripheral nerve damage initially affects longer nerve fibers and progresses proximally. Efforts to improve glycemic control are the primary treatment strategy and may alleviate some of the symptoms. If neuropathy is painful, symptomatic treatments can be used, but they will not change the course of the neuropathy. No medication has been shown to be clearly superior to another for the relief of neuropathic pain, and treatment selection should be based on adverse effects, cost, and convenience. Treatment with low-dose tricyclic antidepressants (preferably nortriptyline or desipramine), duloxetine, gabapentin, pregabalin, venlafaxine, topical capsaicin, and tramadol may be considered. If these are unsuccessful, patients should be referred to a pain clinic or neurologist for further evaluation. Duloxetine and pregabalin are FDA-approved for the treatment of neuropathic pain associated with diabetic peripheral neuropathy. For patients with primarily numbness and minimal or no pain, medications are not effective. However, these patients are at high risk for developing foot ulcerations and should be carefully assessed at every face-to-face visit and preferably followed by a podiatrist.

Autonomic neuropathy impacts the autonomic nerves and can lead to resting tachycardia, orthostatic hypotension, chronic constipation, gastroparesis, erectile dysfunction, anhidrosis, heat intolerance, gustatory sweating, dry skin, and hypoglycemic unawareness.[87] Gastroparesis can be a severe and debilitating complication of DM. Improved glycemic control, discontinuation of medications that slow gastric motility, and the use of metoclopramide or low-dose erythromycin may be helpful. Unfortunately, tachyphylaxis to drug therapies develops within days or weeks. Gastric pacemakers can be considered if symptoms are severe and persistent. Domperidone may also be considered. Although it is not approved for use in the United States, domperidone is available in many other countries and can be requested through the FDA for compassionate use. Diabetic diarrhea most frequently occurs at night. Celiac disease, exocrine insufficiency, and gut bacterial overgrowth should be ruled out. Diabetic diarrhea frequently responds to a 10- to 14-day course of an antibiotic such as doxycycline or metronidazole. In more unresponsive cases, octreotide may be used.

If a patient develops orthostatic hypotension, antihypertensive agents should be discontinued, and dietary sodium intake should be liberalized. Some patients may require pharmacologic treatment for orthostatic hypotension with mineralocorticoids (eg, fludocortisone) or adrenergic agonist agents (eg, midodrine). In severe cases, supine hypertension may be extreme, mandating that the patient sleep in a sitting or semi-recumbent position. Patients with cardiac autonomic neuropathy are at a higher risk for silent MI and sudden cardiac death.

Erectile dysfunction is common in diabetes, and initial treatment should include a trial of one of the phosphodiesterase type 5 inhibitors (eg, sildenafil) prior to referral.[86] People with diabetes often require the highest doses of these medications to achieve an adequate response.

Sudomotor dysfunction may cause reduced sweating and dry, cracked skin. The use of hydrating creams and ointments is needed. Autonomic neuropathy may also result in gustatory sweating after eating. If sweating is excessive, it may be treated with antiperspirants or anticholinergic drugs. Hypoglycemic unawareness requires the patient to avoid hypoglycemia, as the body will slowly increase the glycemic level at which it will activate the autonomic signals.

Focal neuropathies occur most often in older patients with poorly controlled diabetes. Cranial nerve III, IV, and VI neuropathies, as well as Bell's palsy, produce quite dramatic symptoms, but the course is usually self-limited—partial or full recovery occurs in a few weeks to months. Diabetic amyotrophy, which is characterized by proximal thigh muscle pain and weakness, can be very debilitating. Carpal tunnel syndrome, caused by radial nerve entrapment in the wrist, is also more common in people with diabetes, and tarsal tunnel syndrome may cause foot paresthesias.

SPECIAL POPULATIONS

Prediabetes and Preventing Type 2 DM

Prediabetes, as the name implies, is a condition that frequently precedes the development of diabetes.[4] Patients with prediabetes do not have marked elevated BG but rather IFG (100-125 mg/dL [5.6-6.9 mmol/L]) or IGT (140-199 mg/dL [7.8-11.0 mmol/L] 2 hours after ingesting a 75 g carbohydrate load) and often an elevated A1C (5.7%-6.4% [0.057-0.064; 39-46 mmol/mol]). None of these abnormal readings is sufficiently high to meet the diagnostic criteria for diabetes. One in three adults in the United States has prediabetes.[2] Most patients with prediabetes are overweight or obese, and many concurrently have high blood pressure and dyslipidemia. This is an important patient population to identify because they are at high risk of eventually developing type 2 DM.

14 Given that prediabetes often progresses, there has been significant interest in using both nonpharmacologic and pharmacologic means to prevent or delay the onset of type 2 DM. Weight loss, regular aerobic activity, increased fiber intake, and limiting fat consumption are the four lifestyle pillars for both the treatment and prevention of type 2 DM. The Diabetes Prevention Program (DPP) was a landmark clinical trial that demonstrated that modest weight loss and regular physical activity dramatically reduced the risk of developing type 2 DM in patients with IGT.[88] Patients assigned to the lifestyle intervention group walked 30 minutes per day 5 days per week and lost a mean of 8-lb (3.6 kg) over the 2.8-year study. These lifestyle changes resulted in a 58% reduction in the risk of developing type 2 DM when compared to a usual care group (5% per year vs 11% per year). Diet and exercise interventions were effective regardless of age or baseline weight. A third arm of the study randomized patients to receive metformin 850 mg twice daily. The patients in the metformin arm received usual care and did not engage in intensive lifestyle changes. Metformin use leads to, on average, a 4-lb (1.8 kg) weight loss and reduces the risk of developing type 2 DM by 31% when compared to usual care. Younger and overweight individuals who took metformin experienced the greatest reductions. These findings suggest that metformin use may have the greatest impact when prescribed to middle-aged adults who are obese.

Several other medications have also been shown to delay or prevent diabetes. Rosiglitazone and pioglitazone reduce the risk of developing type 2 DM by 60% to 70% in patients with impaired glucose tolerance.[89,90] Acarbose reduced the risk of developing type 2 DM by 25% in the STOP NIDDM study and may be particularly useful in patients who consume a diet high in starchy carbohydrates such as rice. The GLP1-RAs, liraglutide and semaglutide, have also been shown to slow the progression to type 2 DM, reducing the risk by 80% in obese patients taking the medication for weight loss.[91,92] Insulin glargine reduced the risk of developing type 2 DM by approximately 30% in patients with prediabetes. ACEi or ARBs have also been shown to lower the risk of developing type 2 DM by 25% in a pooled analysis of several large CV studies.[93] Given that many patients with prediabetes concurrently have high blood pressure, an ACEi or ARB should be preferentially used in this population to treat hypertension.

Unfortunately, pharmacological methods to "prevent" diabetes do not cure but rather delay the onset of diabetes. No pharmacologic agent is currently FDA-approved for the prevention of type 2 DM. Given its relatively low cost and favorable long-term safety profile, metformin, in conjunction with lifestyle changes, is recommended by the ADA to delay the onset of diabetes in patients with prediabetes, particularly those with a BMI >35 kg/m^2, those aged <60 years, and women with a history of GDM.[94] Liraglutide and once-weekly semaglutide are attractive options for weight loss in obese patients with prediabetes.

Children and Adolescents with Type 2 DM

The incidence and prevalence of type 2 DM are increasing in adolescence.[95] Obesity and physical inactivity are the likely culprits, but innate genetic susceptibility is also an underlying factor. Given that children will potentially live with diabetes for many decades and that the timeline for microvascular complications mimics that of adults with diabetes, extraordinary efforts should be made to assist the child and the family adopt lifestyle changes that normalize BG. The only FDA-approved oral agent for the treatment of type 2 DM in children (10-16 years of age) is metformin, and, similar to adult guidelines, some experts recommend its routine use in the absence of contraindications. Unfortunately, the durability of the response to metformin monotherapy is relatively poor. Liraglutide and exenatide XR have also recently been approved for use in children (10 years of age and older). Sulfonylureas are also commonly used. TZDs improve glycemic control when added to metformin therapy but are not currently FDA-approved for use in children. While the DPP-4 inhibitors are an attractive option because they do not cause hypoglycemia, this class of medications has not been adequately studied in children. Insulin therapy continues to be the standard of care when glycemic goals cannot be achieved or maintained with metformin monotherapy. See Table 94-6 for treatment goals in children and adolescents.

Older Adults

Nearly one in four adults over the age of 65 years has diabetes, and slightly more than half have prediabetes. Older adults, particularly those with functional disability and cognitive impairments, are less able to adopt healthy lifestyle behaviors and more likely to experience adverse effects from medications.[28] The ADA guidelines recommend a patient-centered approach, and there are several factors that should be considered when treating older adults. The number and severity of comorbid conditions, kidney dysfunction, ability to engage in self-care, nutritional status, social support, the risk of falls, and life expectancy should all influence glycemic goals and treatment selection. (See Table 94-6 and Fig. 94-6.) The ADA recommends an A1C goal ≤7.0%-7.5% (0.070-0.075; 53-58 mmol/mol) for otherwise healthy older adults who have intact cognitive function, but a less stringent goal A1C ≤8.0% (0.080; 64 mmol/mol) is reasonable in those with multiple chronic diseases. In patients who have limited life expectancy, significant cognitive impairments, require long-term care, or are unable to engage in activities of daily living, an A1C should not be used as the primary means to guide therapy. Instead, clinicians should use blood glucose monitoring to keep fasting blood glucose between 100 and 180 mg/dL (5.6 and 10.0 mmol/L) in order to avoid hypoglycemia.

Older adults often have altered perceptions of hypoglycemia and may not experience adrenergic symptoms (eg, tremor, jitteriness, palpitations) due to the age-related loss of autonomic nerve function.[28] Thus, neuroglycopenic symptoms (eg, altered mental status, personality changes) may be the first indication the patient's BG is low. For these reasons, over-treatment of DM should be avoided, and de-escalation should be strongly considered should severe or frequent hypoglycemia occur. Older adults in long-term care facilities are particularly vulnerable to hypoglycemia. However, glycemic control should not be relaxed so far as to cause symptoms of hyperglycemia or risk the development of DKA or HHS.

Other therapeutic goals related to the management of blood pressure and dyslipidemia to prevent the development or progression of kidney disease and CV complications should be similarly tailored in older adults based on the patient-specific circumstances.[28] While a decline in kidney function may preclude the use of metformin in some older adults, lower doses may be used if coupled with more frequent monitoring (eg, every 3 months) of kidney function when the eGFR is consistently above 30 mL/min/1.73 m^2.[28] The efficacy of the SGLT-2 inhibitors declines as kidney function declines, thus older adults typically have a diminished response to this class of agents. SGLT-2 inhibitors may also increase the frequency of urination and cause orthostatic blood pressure changes, increasing the risk of falls.

Sulfonylureas, particularly longer-acting agents such as glyburide and chlorpropamide, are more likely to cause hypoglycemia and should be avoided. A higher risk of distal extremity fracture from falls has been documented with canagliflozin as well as the TZDs. The TZDs often cause fluid retention and increase the risk of congestive heart failure. DPP-4 inhibitors are generally well-tolerated and do not cause hypoglycemia. Similarly, α-glucosidase inhibitors are generally safe and may also be used. The GLP-1 RAs and the SGLT-2 inhibitors are unlikely to cause hypoglycemia and produce a modest weight loss, which can be advantageous in overweight individuals. However, older patients may be more prone to GI side effects from GLP-1 RAs. Simple insulin regimens using a single daily basal insulin dose can be used in older adults, especially if tight glycemic control is not the goal. Both the injectable GLP-1 RAs and insulin therapy require the patient to have adequate motor skills and visual acuity to self-administer doses.

Pregnant Women

The prevalence of DM has increased significantly among women during their reproductive years.[13] In women with type 1 or type 2 DM, discussions about family planning and achieving good glycemic control prior to pregnancy are critical. Organogenesis is largely completed within the first 8 weeks of pregnancy—well before good glycemic control can be achieved in the absence of preconception planning. Unfortunately, major congenital malformations due to poor glucose control in the first trimester of pregnancy remain the leading cause of mortality and serious morbidity in infants of mothers with DM. During preconception planning, all drugs should be reviewed for safety. Known teratogens, such as ACE inhibitors and statins, should be stopped and, if treatment is still needed, an appropriate alternative recommended.

GDM is diagnosed during pregnancy, and all women should be screened for GDM between weeks 24 and 28 of the pregnancy. See Table 94-5. The adverse outcomes associated with GDM include birth defects, miscarriage, cesarean section delivery, maternal pre-eclampsia/eclampsia, preterm delivery, neonatal hypoglycemia, shoulder dystocia, birth injury, and hyperbilirubinemia.[13] Medical nutritional therapy to minimize wide fluctuations in BG is of paramount importance. Intensive educational efforts are usually necessary. Pregnant women without DM maintain plasma glucose concentrations between 50 and 130 mg/dL (2.8 and 7.2 mmol/L). Normoglycemia is the goal, and failure to maintain this despite dietary interventions will necessitate medication use. Goals during therapy are to keep fasting glucose less than 95 mg/dL (5.3 mmol/L), and either a 1-hour postprandial plasma glucose levels less than 140 mg/dL (7.8 mmol/L) or 2-hour postprandial plasma glucose levels less than 120 mg/dL (6.7 mmol/L). See Table 94-6. Ketosis should also be avoided as much as possible.

Similarly, in patients who have preexisting type 1 or type 2 DM who become pregnant, premeal, bedtime, and overnight BGM should be less than 95 mg/dL (5.7 mmol/L) with a peak PPG less than 140 mg/dL (7.8 mmol/L). While the A1C during pregnancy should ideally be between 6% and 6.5% (0.06 and 0.065; 42 and 48 mmol/mol), BGM must be used to guide therapy because it provides daily information about glycemic control. In women with type 2 DM controlled by lifestyle modification alone, conversion to insulin is often necessary soon after the pregnancy is confirmed. Patients previously treated with insulin typically need to intensify the regimen to achieve the more stringent therapeutic goals recommended during pregnancy. This may require the use of more complicated regimens coupled with carbohydrate counting and adjustments guided by BGM. While NPH remains the recommended basal insulin to use during pregnancy, insulin detemir appears to be safe. Insulin pump therapy can be considered. In highly motivated patients, CSII can achieve excellent glycemic control and is routinely adjusted throughout the pregnancy.

In women with type 2 DM or GDM, both metformin and glyburide have been studied as alternatives to insulin therapy.[13] Both appear to be effective and safe based on the results of small randomized controlled trials and meta-analyses. However, rare or uncommon adverse fetal events are difficult to discern from these data. Glyburide was not detected in the cord serum of any infant in one study, whereas metformin crosses the placenta. Further study in larger patient populations is needed prior to routinely recommending them, but in patients for whom the complexity of insulin is too difficult or refuses insulin, glyburide or metformin use is justified. Patients with GDM should be evaluated approximately 6 weeks after delivery to ensure that normoglycemia has returned. The lifetime risk for the development of type 2 DM is 30% to 50%, making the periodic screening of women with a history of GDM warranted.

Patients with HIV

Patients living with HIV are at higher risk for developing type 2 DM. This risk may be related to HIV infection, concomitant infections such as hepatitis C, and medications often used to treat HIV and its comorbidities. Pentamidine, used for *Pneumocystis carinii* pneumonia infections, is a β-cell toxin and may cause some patients to develop hypoglycemia from insulin release followed by hyperglycemia. Megestrol, used as an appetite stimulant, can have glucocorticoid-like effects and cause hyperglycemia in some patients. Protease inhibitors, used to treat HIV infection, can worsen insulin sensitivity, decrease the ability of the β-cell to secrete insulin, and worsen lipotoxicity. Long-term use of stavudine also increases the risk of developing diabetes. Redistribution of fat from subcutaneous to the visceral compartment from medications or HIV infection also increases the risk of developing diabetes. Metformin is the drug of choice for HIV patients as weight gain can be minimized. Stavudine, zidovudine, and didanosine may cause lactatemia, especially upon long-term use. It may be advisable to check lactate levels in patients taking these medications prior to metformin use. If lactate levels are greater than two times normal, alternative therapy should be considered. If excess visceral adiposity is noted, a TZD that redistributes fat into subcutaneous adipose tissue and causes visceral fat apoptosis may be considered. Drugs that promote weight loss should also be considered. Significant drug-drug interactions may also be present.

EVALUATION OF PATIENT OUTCOMES

Glycemic control can be measured in several ways.[96] Plasma and BG measurements collected during fasting and postprandial periods can be used to determine the patient's current glycemic status. CGM devices collect glucose monitoring data throughout the day. These tests of glycemia are useful for detecting hypoglycemia, making adjustments in insulin therapy, and determining the patient's glycemic patterns. For those using a CGM, time in range (TIR), time below range, and glycemic variability are useful markers of glycemic control. The A1C is the gold standard for determining overall glycemic control for the previous 2 to 3 months and correlates with the risk of developing many of the long-term complications associated with diabetes. Fructosamine, which measures the amount of glycation on plasma proteins such as albumin, is a test of glycemia that can be useful in patients with altered red blood cell lifespan or a hemoglobinopathy. Fructosamine measures glucose control over the previous 2 to 3 weeks. Unfortunately, fructosamine is not as reliable as the A1C, and the correlation between fructosamine measurements and the risk of complications from diabetes is unknown. Thus, glycemic goals based on fructosamine have not been established.

While these glycemic goals recommended by the ADA and AACE are useful general targets, treatment goals need to be individualized. Less stringent A1C goals are appropriate in patients with a history of severe hypoglycemia, limited life expectancy, advanced micro/macrovascular complications or comorbidities, and in patients who are frail, have dementia, or have limited social or financial resources. Less stringent goals should also be set for younger children. Conversely, more aggressive glycemic goals are appropriate in patients who are young or middle-aged adults, newly diagnosed, and using treatments that are unlikely to cause hypoglycemia.

BGM and CGM are important tools that provide an opportunity to adjust medications, food intake, or physical activity. BGM and CGM improve safety by enabling patients to detect hypoglycemia so that it can be treated. In general, BGM frequency should match how frequently medication changes are needed to achieve glycemic control as well as the risk of hypoglycemia. BGM and CGM empower patients to make day-to-day adjustments in prandial insulin doses and are used to determine if corrective doses of insulin are needed. Even in patients who do not use insulin therapy, BGM and CGM can be useful to see how a change in diet or exercise impacts BG. BGM readings are needed to check the accuracy of some CGM devices. For patients with type 1 DM, CGM is generally preferred, but BGM can be performed four to six times per day—prior to food intake and physical activity as well as at bedtime. The optimal frequency of BGM and the use of CGM in patients with type 2 DM on oral agents is unknown and its role controversial. BGM and CGM in patients with type 2 DM may be useful in patients who are actively using the information to make changes in their lifestyle behaviors and for a few weeks after medication changes.

The use of CGM has become increasingly common and helpful in patients using intensive insulin therapy. CGM measures interstitial glucose, which lags behind fingertip capillary BGM. CGM can be particularly useful in patients with frequent episodes of hypoglycemia, hypoglycemic unawareness, and nocturnal hypoglycemia. CGM can be used to identify glucose patterns and evaluate patients with higher or lower than expected A1C results. Some CGMs must be calibrated using BGM readings after insertion of a new sensor and periodically thereafter. A new sensor must be placed every 7 to 14 days. CGM data can be transmitted to insulin pumps which can then make recommendations to the patient or automatically adjust the insulin doses based on the results. The ADA currently recommends daily use of personal CGM in patients on intensive insulin therapy to lower or maintain A1C levels and/or reduce hypoglycemia.

Alternate site testing for BGM performed on the palm, forearm, or thigh is less painful than obtaining blood samples from fingertip samples, but only some BG test strips are designed for alternative site testing. Alternate sites tend to have fewer nerve endings than fingertips and may be more comfortable for a patient. Glucose readings obtained from alternative sites will lag behind fingertip capillary blood by 20 to 30 minutes. Therefore, alternate site testing is discouraged in any situation where immediate action will be needed based on the glucose reading, such as testing for hypoglycemia or when the BG is changing rapidly, such as after a meal.

Choosing an appropriate meter to perform BGM depends on the patient's dexterity, vision acuity, cost of the meter and strips, and desired features. Insurance coverage often influences meter choice. When a patient first obtains a new glucometer, it is important to demonstrate the testing methods and have the patient perform the technique. Each meter has specifications for hematocrit, elevation, and temperature tolerances for optimal operation.

Medication Adherence and Persistence

Despite the armamentarium of treatment options, a large percentage of patients fail to achieve target A1C and blood glucose levels. One major contributing factor to uncontrolled diabetes is poor medication adherence and persistence. Key contributors to adherence include perceived efficacy, hypoglycemia, weight gain, treatment complexity, convenience, cost, patient beliefs about medications, and trust in the healthcare provider.[97] Therefore, it is crucial to assess adherence and barriers to adherence at every visit and include the patient in the decision-making process. Simplifying the treatment regimen may improve adherence and glycemic control. Fixed-dose combination products may be one way to simplify treatment and have been shown to improve adherence and glycemic control.[98,99]

Therapeutic Inertia

15 Another contributing factor to uncontrolled diabetes is therapeutic inertia, which is the failure to initiate or intensify therapy in a timely manner according to evidence-based clinical guidelines. Several studies have shown that it often takes years before treatment is intensified in patients with uncontrolled diabetes. There are multiple reasons for therapeutic inertia including barriers at the patient, provider, and system level. Given the risk of development or progression of diabetes-related complications during treatment delays, it is vital that clinicians combat therapeutic inertia by routinely monitoring patients with DM and taking action in those who are not achieving therapeutic targets.[100]

CONCLUSION

16 DM is a heterogeneous group of metabolic disorders which all have elevated BG as their defining characteristic. Achieving good glycemic control, although important, is but one ingredient to optimal health outcomes in patients with diabetes. A comprehensive plan of care should include not only pharmacological and nonpharmacological strategies to lower BG but also methods to screen, prevent, and manage microvascular and macrovascular complications. Current Health Plan Employer Data and Information Set (HEDIS), performance measures annually reported by the National Committee for Quality Assurance (NCQA), recognizes that quality care to patients with diabetes must address glycemia, blood pressure control, statin use, and recommended screening exams.[12] Diabetes is a life-long disease, and patients with diabetes need ongoing support through an interprofessional, team-based approach to care. Adjustments to diet, exercise, and pharmacologic therapies are frequently needed. Clinical inertia should be avoided, and treatment intensification should be implemented if treatment goals have not been met. Patients should receive follow-up care every 3 months, but more frequent follow-up may be necessary if treatment changes have been made. The A1C should be measured every 3 to 6 months, even in patients who are stable on a therapeutic regimen and meeting treatment goals. Identifying and mitigating CV risks—particularly high blood pressure, dyslipidemia, and tobacco use—is critical. Blood pressure should be measured at every encounter and, in patients with elevated blood pressure, home blood pressure monitoring is strongly encouraged. A fasting lipid profile should be obtained as part of an initial assessment and to determine if statin therapy has adequately reduced LDL cholesterol. Performing foot examinations at each face-to-face visit and obtaining a dilated eye examination at least once a year are also important. People with diabetes should receive the influenza vaccine every year and the pneumococcal vaccines and the hepatitis B vaccine series per Center for Disease Control and Prevention recommendations. Using an integrated electronic health record, standardized progress notes, and flow sheets can assist the clinician to determine whether the patient has met these standards of care. As with many chronic diseases, adherence to dietary recommendations, physical activity, and medications is a challenge for most patients. Frequent follow-up, patient education, and positive family engagement can help patients with diabetes lead healthier, happier lives.

ABBREVIATIONS

AACE	American Association of Clinical Endocrinologists
AADE	American Association of Diabetes Educators
ADA	American Diabetes Association
A1C	hemoglobin A1C
ASCVD	atherosclerotic cardiovascular disease
BG	blood glucose
BGM	blood glucose monitoring
BP	blood pressure
BMI	body mass index
CDCES	Certified Diabetes Care and Education Specialist
CF	correction factor
CGM	continuous glucose monitor
CHD	coronary heart disease
C:I	carbohydrate to insulin ratio
CKD	chronic kidney disease
CSII	continuous subcutaneous insulin infusion
CV	cardiovascular
CVD	cardiovascular disease
DKA	diabetic ketoacidosis
DPP-4	dipeptidyl peptidase-4
DM	diabetes mellitus
DSME/S	diabetes self-management education/support
eGFR	estimated glomerular filtration rate
ESKD	end-stage kidney disease
FDA	Food and Drug Administration
FFA	free fatty acid
FPG	fasting plasma glucose
GDM	gestational diabetes
GI	gastrointestinal
GIP	glucose-dependent insulinotropic polypeptide
GLP-1	glucagon-like peptide-1
GLP-1 RA	glucagon-like peptide-1 receptor agonist
GU	genitourinary
HDL-C	high-density lipoprotein cholesterol
HF	heart failure
HHS	hyperglycemic hyperosmolar syndrome
ICAs	islet cell autoantibodies
ICU	intensive care unit
IFG	impaired fasting glucose
IGT	impaired glucose tolerance
IV	intravenous
LADA	latent autoimmune disease in adults
LDL-C	low-density lipoprotein cholesterol

MDI	multiple daily injections
MNT	medical nutrition therapy
MODY	mature-onset diabetes in the young
NPH	neutral protamine Hagedorn
OGTT	oral glucose tolerance test
PAI-1	plasminogen activator inhibitor-1
PK/PD	pharmacokinetic/pharmacodynamic
POC	point of care
PPAR-γ	peroxisome proliferator activator receptor-γ
PPG	postprandial glucose
SC	subcutaneous
SGLT-2	sodium-glucose co-transporter 2
SU	sulfonylurea
TZD	thiazolidinedione
UGE	urinary glucose excretion
VAT	visceral adipose tissue
XR	extended-release

REFERENCES

1. World Health Organization. Global report on diabetes. World Health Organization; 2016. Available at: http://www.who.int/iris/handle/10665/204871.
2. Centers for Disease Control and Prevention. National Diabetes Statistics Report, 2020. Estimates of Diabetes and Its Burden in the United States. Atlanta, GA. Available at: https://www.cdc.gov/diabetes/pdfs/data/statistics/national-diabetes-statistics-report.pdf. Accessed June 1, 2021.
3. Economic Costs of Diabetes in the U.S. in 2017. *Diabetes Care.* 2018;41(5):917–928. 10.2337/dci18-0007 29567642.
4. American Diabetes Association. 2. Classification and diagnosis of diabetes: standards of medical care in diabetes-2021. *Diabetes Care.* 2021;44(suppl 1):S15–S33. PMID 33298413
5. Repaske DR. Medication-induced diabetes mellitus. *Pediatr Diabetes.* Sep 2016;17(6):392–397.
6. Atkinson MA, Eisenbarth GS, Michels AW. Type 1 diabetes. *Lancet.* 2014;383(9911):69–82.
7. Mayer-Davis EJ, Lawrence JM, Dabelea D, et al. Search for diabetes in youth study: incidence trends of type 1 and type 2 diabetes among youths, 2002–2012. *New Engl J Med.* 2017;376(15):1419–1429.
8. DeFronzo RA, Ferrannini E, Groop L, et al. Type 2 diabetes mellitus. *Nat Rev Dis Primers.* 2015;1:15019.
9. DeSisto CL, Kim SY, Sharma AJ. Prevalence estimates of gestational diabetes mellitus in the United States, pregnancy risk assessment monitoring system (PRAMS), 2007–2010. *Prev Chronic Dis.* 2014;11:E104.
10. Kampmann U, Madsen LR, Skajaa GO, et al. Gestational diabetes: a clinical update. *World J Diabetes.* 2015;6(8):1065–1072.
11. Van Belle TL, Coppieters KT, Von Herrath MG. Type 1 diabetes: etiology, immunology, and therapeutic strategies. *Physiol Rev.* 2011;91:79–118.
12. American Diabetes Association. 1. Improving care and promoting health in populations: standards of medical care in diabetes—2021. *Diabetes Care.* 2021;44(suppl 1):S7–S14. PMID 33298412
13. American Diabetes Association. 14. Management of diabetes in pregnancy: standards of medical care in diabetes—2021. *Diabetes Care.* 2021;44(suppl 1):S200–S210. PMID 33298415
14. American Diabetes Association. 4. Comprehensive medical evaluation and assessment of comorbidities: standards of medical care in diabetes—2021. *Diabetes Care.* 2021;44(suppl 1):S40–S52.
15. Handelsman Y, Bloomgarden ZT, Grunberger G, et al. American Association of Clinical Endocrinologists and American College of Endocrinology clinical practice guidelines for developing a diabetes mellitus comprehensive care plan—2015. *Endocrine Practice.* 2015;21(suppl 1):187.
16. American Diabetes Association. 6. Glycemic targets: standards of medical care in diabetes—2021. *Diabetes Care.* 2021;44(suppl 1):S73–S84. PMID 33298417
17. Diabetes Control and Complications Trial Research Group. The effect of intensive treatment of diabetes on the development and progression of long-term complications in insulin-dependent diabetes mellitus. *N Engl J Med.* 1993;329:977–986.
18. DCCT/EDIC Study Research Group. Intensive diabetes treatment and cardiovascular disease in patients with type 1 diabetes. *N Engl J Med.* 2005;353:2643–2653.
19. Lachin JM, White NH, Hainsworth DP, et al. Effect of intensive diabetes therapy on the progression of diabetic retinopathy in patients with type 1 diabetes: 18 years of follow-up in the DCCT/EDIC. *Diabetes.* 2015;64:631–642.
20. UK Prospective Diabetes Study (UKPDS) Group. Intensive blood-glucose control with sulphonylureas or insulin compared with conventional treatment and risk of complications in patients with type 2 diabetes (UKPDS 33). *Lancet.* 1998;352:837–853.
21. UK Prospective Diabetes Study (UKPDS) Group. Effect of intensive blood-glucose control with metformin on complications in overweight patients with type 2 diabetes (UKPDS 34). *Lancet.* 1998;352:854–865.
22. Holman RR, Paul SK, Bethel MA, Mathews DR, Neil HAW. 10-year follow-up of intensive glucose control in type 2 diabetes. *N Engl J Med.* 2008;359:1577–1589.
23. The Action to Control Cardiovascular Risk in Diabetes Study Group. Effects of intensive glucose lowering in type 2 diabetes. *N Engl J Med.* 2008;358:2545–2559.
24. The ADVANCE Collaborative Group. Intensive blood glucose control and vascular outcomes in patients with type 2 diabetes. *N Engl J Med.* 2008;358:2560–2572.
25. Duckworth W, Abraira C, Mortiz T, et al. Glucose control and vascular complications in veterans with type 2 diabetes. *N Engl J Med.* 2009;360:111.
26. Garber AJ, Handelsman Y, Grunberger G, et al. Consensus statement by the American Association of Clinical Endocrinologists and American College of Endocrinology on the comprehensive type 2 diabetes management algorithm: 2020 executive summary. *Endocrine Practice.* 2020;26(1):107–139.
27. Battelino T, Danne T, Bergenstal RM, et al. Clinical targets for continuous glucose monitoring data interpretation: recommendations from the International Consensus on Time in Range. *Diabetes Care.* 2019;42(8):1593–1603. PMID 31177185
28. American Diabetes Association. 12. Older adults: standards of medical care in diabetes—2021. *Diabetes Care.* 2021;44(suppl 1):S168–S179. PMID 33298423
29. American Diabetes Association. 5. Facilitating behavior change and well-being to improve health outcomes: standards of medical care in diabetes-2021. *Diabetes Care.* 2021;44(suppl 1):S53–S72. PMID 33298416
30. Beck J, Greenwood DA, Blanton L, et al. National standards for diabetes self-management education and support. *Diabetes Educator.* 2017;43(5):448–464.
31. American Diabetes Association. 9. Pharmacologic approaches to glycemic treatment: standards of medical care in diabetes—2021. *Diabetes Care.* 2021;44(suppl 1):S111–S124. PMID 33298420
32. Davies MJ, D'Alessio DA, Fradkin J, et al. Management of hyperglycemia in type 2 diabetes, 2018. A consensus report by the American Diabetes Association (ADA) and the European Association for the Study of Diabetes (EASD). *Diabetes Care.* Published online Sep; dci180033. Available at: https://doi.org/10.2337/dci18-0033.
33. The ORIGIN trial investigators. Basal insulin and cardiovascular and other outcomes in dysglycemia. *N Engl J Med.* 2012;367:319–328.
34. Budnitz DS, Lovegrove MC, Shehab N, Richards CL. Emergency hospitalizations for adverse drug events in older Americans. *N Engl J Med.* 2011;365:2002–2012.
35. Frid AH, Kreugel G, Grassi G, et al. New insulin delivery recommendations. *Mayo Clin Proc.* 2016;91(9):1231–1255.
36. American Association of Diabetes Educators. Insulin Injection Resources. Available at: https://www.diabeteseducator.org/practice/educator-tools/insulin-injection-resources2. Accessed December 12, 2018.
37. Rena G, Hardie D, Pearson ER. The mechanism of action of metformin. *Diabetologia.* 2017;60(9):1577–1585.
38. Griffin SJ, Leaver JK, Irving GF. Impact of metformin on cardiovascular disease: a meta-analysis of randomized trials among people with type 2 diabetes. *Diabetologia.* 2017;60(9):1620–1629.
39. Maruther NM, Tseng E, Hutfless S, et al. Diabetes medications as monotherapy or metformin-based combination therapy for type 2 diabetes: a systematic review and meta-analysis. *Ann Intern Med.* 2016;164(11):740–751.
40. Aggarwal N, Singla A, Mattheu C, et al. Metformin extended-release versus immediate-release: an international, randomized, double-blind, head-to-head trial in pharmacotherapy-naïve patients with type 2 diabetes. *Diabetes Obes Metab.* 2018;20(2):463–467.

41. Inzucchi SE, Lipska KJ, Mayo H. Metformin in patients with type 2 diabetes and kidney disease: a systematic review. *JAMA.* 2014;312(24):2668–2675.
42. Lipska KJ, Bailey CJ, Inzucchi SE. Use of metformin in the setting of mild-to-moderate renal insufficiency. *Diabetes Care.* 2011;34(6):1431–1437.
43. Lalau JD, Kajbaf F, Bennis Y, et al. Metformin treatment in patients with type 2 diabetes and chronic kidney disease stages 3A, 3B, or 4. *Diabetes Care.* 2018;41(3):547–553.
44. Cefalu WT, Kaul S, Gerstein HC, et al. Cardiovascular outcomes trials in type 2 diabetes: where do we go from here? Reflections from a Diabetes Care editors' expert forum. *Diabetes Care.* 2018;41:14–31.
45. Zinman B, Wanner C, Lachin JM, et al. Empagliflozin, cardiovascular outcomes, and mortality in type 2 diabetes. *N Engl J Med.* 2015;373:2117–2128.
46. Neal B, Perkovic V, Mahaffey KW, et al. Canagliflozin and cardiovascular and renal events in type 2 diabetes. *N Engl J Med.* 2017;377(7):644–657.
47. Wiviott SD, Raz I, Bonaca MP, et al. Dapagliflozin and cardiovascular outcomes in type 2 diabetes. *N Engl J Med.* 2019;380(4):347–357.
48. McMurray JJV, Solomon SD, Inzucchi SE, et al. DAPA-HF Trial Committees and Investigators. Dapagliflozin in patients with heart failure an dreduced ejection fraction. *N Engl J Med.* 2019;381:1995–2008. PMID 31535829
49. Packer M, Anker SD, Butler J, et al. Cardiovascular and renal outcomes with empagliflozin in heart failure. *N Engl J Med.* 2020;383:1413–1424. PMID 32865377
50. Heerspink HJL, Stefansson BV, Correa-Rotter R, et al. Dapagliflozin in patients with chronic kidney disease. *N Engl J Med.* 2020;383:1436–1446. PMID 32970396
51. American Diabetes Association. 10. Cardiovascular disease and risk management: Standards of medical care in diabetes—2021. *Diabetes Care.* 2021;44(suppl 1):S125–S150. PMID 33298421
52. Perkovik V, Jardine MJ, Neal B, et al. Canagliflozin and renal outcomes in type 2 diabetes and nephropathy. *N Engl J Med.* 2019;380:2295–2306. PMID 30990260
53. Bersoff-Matcha SJ, Chamberlain C, Cao C, Kortepeter C, Chong WH. Fournier gangrene associated with sodium-glucose cotransporter-2 inhibitors: a review of spontaneous postmarketing cases. *Ann Intern Med.* 2019;170(11):764–769. 10.7326/M19-0085. PMID 31060053
54. Trujillo JM, Nuffer W, Ellis SL. GLP-1 receptor agonists: a review of head-to-head clinical studies. *Ther Adv Endocrinol Metab.* 2015;6(1):19–28.
55. Trujillo JM, Nuffer W, Smith BA. GLP-1 receptor agonists: an updated review of head-to-head clinical studies. *Ther Adv Endocrinol Metab.* 2021;12:1–15.
56. Wilding JPH, Batterham RL, Calanna S, et al. Once-weekly semaglutide in adults with overweight or obesity. *N Eng J Med.* 2021; 384: 989–1102. PMID 33567185
57. Marso SP, Daniels GH, Brown-Frandsen K, et al. Liraglutide and cardiovascular outcomes in type 2 diabetes. *N Engl J Med.* 2016;375:311–322.
58. Marso SP, Bain SC, Consoli A, et al. Semaglutide and cardiovascular outcomes in patients with type 2 diabetes. *N Engl J Med.* 2016;375:1834–1844.
59. Gerstein HC, Colhoun HM, Dagenais GR, et al. Dulaglutide and cardiovascular outcomes in type 2 diabetes (REWIND): a double-blind, randomized placebo-controlled trial. *Lancet.* 2019;394(10193):121–130. PMID 31159511
60. Nauck MA, Meier JJ, Cavender MA, et al. Cardiovascular actions and clinical outcomes with glucagon-like peptide-1 receptor agonists and dipeptidyl peptidase-4 inhibitors. *Circulation.* 2017;136(9):849–870.
61. Devries JH, Rosenstock J. DPP-4 inhibitor related pancreatitis: rare but real! *Diabetes Care.* 2017;40:161–163.
62. Hauner H. The mode of action of thiazolidinediones. *Diabetes Metab Res Rev.* 2002;18(suppl 2):S10–S15.
63. Nissen SE, Wolski K. Rosiglitazone revisited: an updated meta-analysis of risk for myocardial infarction and cardiovascular mortality. *Arch Intern Med.* 2010;170:1191–1201.
64. Mahaffey KW, Hafley G, Dickerson S, et al. Results of a reevaluation of cardiovascular outcomes in the RECORD trial. *Am Heart J.* 2013;166:240–249.
65. Home PD, Pocock SJ, Beck-Nielsen H, et al. Rosiglitazone evaluated for cardiovascular outcomes in oral agent combination therapy for type 2 diabetes (RECORD): a multicentre, randomised, open-label trial. *Lancet.* 2009;373:2125–2135.
66. Dormandy JA, Charbonnel B, Eckland DJA, et al. Secondary prevention of vascular events in patients with type 2 diabetes in the PROactive study prospective pioglitazone clinical trial in macrovascular events: a randomized controlled trial. *Lancet.* 2005;366:1279–1289.
67. Viscoli CM, Inzucchi SE, Young LH, et al. Pioglitazone and risk for bone fracture: safety data from a randomized clinical trial. *J Clin Endocrinol Metab.* 2017;102(3):914–922.
68. Kahn SE, Zinman B, Lachin JM, et al. Rosiglitazone-associated fractures in type 2 diabetes: an analysis from a diabetes outcome progression trial (ADOPT). *Diabetes Care.* 2008;31(5):845–851.
69. Lewis JD, Ferrara A, Peng T, et al. Risk of bladder cancer among diabetic patients treated with pioglitazone: interim report of a longitudinal cohort study. *Diabetes Care.* 2011;34(4):916–922.
70. Lewis JD, Habel LA, Quesenberry CP, et al. Pioglitazone use and risk of bladder cancer and other common cancers in persons with diabetes. *JAMA.* 2015;314(3):265–277.
71. Meinert CL, Knatterud GL, Prout TE, Klimt CR. A study of the effects of hypoglycemic agents on vascular complications in patients with adult-onset diabetes. II. Mortality results. *Diabetes.* 1970;19(suppl.):789–830.
72. Khunti K, Chatterjee S, Gerstein HC, et al. Do sulfonylureas still have a place in clinical practice? *Lancet Diabetes Endocrinol.* 2018;6(10):821–832.
73. Gangji AS, Cukierman T, Gerstein HC, et al. A systematic review and meta-analysis of hypoglycemia and cardiovascular events: a comparison of glyburide with other secretagogues and with insulin. *Diabetes Care.* 2007;30(2):389–394.
74. American Diabetes Association. 8. Obesity management for the treatment of type 2 diabetes: standards of medical care in diabetes—2021. *Diabetes Care.* 2021;44(suppl 1):S100–S110. PMID 33298419
75. Neumiller JJ, Alicic RZ, Tuttle KR. Therapeutic considerations for antihyperglycemic agents in diabetic kidney disease. *J Am Soc Nephrol.* 2017;28(8):2263–2274.
76. American Diabetes Association. Diabetes technology: standards of medical care in diabetes—2021. *Diabetes Care.* 2021;44(suppl 1):S85–S99. PMID 33298418
77. The ASCEND Study Collaborative Group. Effects of aspirin for primary prevention in persons with diabetes mellitus. *N Engl J Med.* 2018;379:1529–1539.
78. Das SR, Everett BM, Birtcher KK, et al. 2018 ACC expert consensus decision pathway on novel therapies for cardiovascular risk reduction in patients with type 2 diabetes and atherosclerotic cardiovascular disease: a report of the American College of Cardiology Task Force on Expert Consensus Decision Pathways. *J Am Coll Cardiol.* November 2018. doi:10.1016/j.jacc.2018.09.020.
79. Amsterdam EA, Wenger NK, Brindis RG, et al. 2014 AHA/ACC guideline for the management of patients with non-st-elevation acute coronary sydnromes: executive summary. *Circulation.* 2014(130):2354–2394.
80. ACC/AHA/AAPA/ABC/ACPM/AGS/APhA/ASH/ASPC/NMA/PCNA. Guideline for the prevention, detection, evaluation, and management of high blood pressure in adults: a report of the American College of Cardiology/American Heart Association Task Force on Clinical Practice Guidelines. *J Am Coll Cardiol.* 2018;71:e127–e248.
81. The SPRINT Research Group. A randomized trial of intensive versus standard blood-pressure control. *N Engl J Med.* 2015;373:2103–2116.
82. The ACCORD Study Group. Effects of intensive blood-pressure control in type 2 diabetes mellitus. *N Engl J Med.* 2010;362:1575–1585.
83. ACC/AHA/AACVPR/AAPA/ABC/ACPM/ADA/AGS/APhA/ASPC/NLA/PCNA. Guideline on the management of blood cholesterol: a report of the American College of Cardiology Foundation/American Heart Association Task Force on Clinical Practice Guidelines. *J Am Coll Cardiol.* November 10, 2018 [Epub ahead of print].
84. Naeem F, Mckay G, Fisher M. Cardiovascular outcomes trials with statins in diabetes. *Br J Diabetes.* 2018;18:7–13.
85. Pang J, Chan DC, Watts GF. Origin and therapy for hypertriglyceridaemia in type 2 diabetes. *World J Diabetes.* 2014;5(2):165–175.
86. American Diabetes Association. 11. Microvascular complications and foot care: standards of medical care in diabetes—2019. *Diabetes Care.* 2019;42(suppl 1):S124–S138.
87. Verrotti A, Prezioso G, Scattoni R, Chiarelli F. Autonomic neuropathy in diabetes mellitus. *Frontier Endocrinol.* 2014;5:205.
88. Diabetes Prevention Program Group. Reduction in the incidence of type 2 diabetes with lifestyle intervention or metformin. *N Engl J Med.* 2012;346(6):393–403.

89. The DREAM (Diabetes Reduction Assessment with Ramipril and Rosiglitazone Medication) Trial Investigators. Effect of rosiglitazone on the frequency of diabetes in patients with impaired glucose tolerance or impaired fasting glucose: a randomized controlled trial. *Lancet.* 2006;368:1096–1105.
90. DeFronzo RA, Tripathy D, Schwenke DC, et al. Pioglitazone for diabetes prevention in impaired glucose tolerance. *N Engl J Med.* 2011;364(12):1104–1115.
91. le Roux CW, Astrup A, Fujioka K, et al. 3 years of liraglutide versus placebo for type 2 diabetes risk reduction and weight management in individuals with prediabetes: a randomised, double-blind trial. *Lancet.* 2017;389(10077):1399–1409.
92. Wilding JP, Batterham RL, Calanna S, et al. Once-weekly semaglutide in adults with overweight and obesity. *N Eng J Med.* 2021;384(11):989–1002. PMID: 33567185
93. Abuissa H, Jones PG, Marso SP, O'Keefe JH. Angiotensin-converting enzyme inhibitors or angiotensin receptor blockers for prevention of type 2 diabetes: a meta-analysis of randomized clinical trials. *J Am College Cardiol.* 2005;46(5):821–826.
94. American Diabetes Association. 3. Prevention or delay of type 2 diabetes: standards of medical care in diabetes—2019. *Diabetes Care.* 2019;42(suppl 1):S29–S33.
95. American Diabetes Association. 13. Children and adolescents: standards of medical care in diabetes—2019. *Diabetes Care.* 2019;42(suppl 1):S148–S164.
96. Goldstein DE, Little RR, Lorenz RA, et al. Tests of glycemia in diabetes. *Diabetes Care.* 2004;27(7):1761–1773.
97. Polonsky WH, Henry RR. Poor medication adherence in type 2 diabetes: recognizing the scope of the problem and its key contributors. *Patient Prefer Adherence.* 2016;10:1299–1307.
98. Han S, Iglay K, Davies MJ, et al. Glycemic effectiveness and medication adherence with fixed-dose combination or co-administered dual therapy of antihyperglycemic regimens: a meta-analysis. *Curr Med Res Opin.* 2012;28:969–977.
99. Vijayakumar TM, Jayram J, Meghana Cheekireddy V, et al. Safety, efficacy, and bioavailability of fixed-dose combinations in type 2 diabetes mellitus: a systematic updated review. *Curr Ther Res Clin Exp.* 2017:84:49.
100. Khunti K, Gomes MB, Pocock S, et al. Therapeutic inertia in the treatment of hyperglycemia in patients with type 2 diabetes: a systematic review. *Diabetes Obes Metab.* 2018;20:427–437.

e95

Acute Hyperglycemia

Paul M. Szumita, James F. Gilmore, and Jennifer M. Trujillo

KEY CONCEPTS

1. Hyperglycemia is common among patients admitted to the hospital; at least one-third of hospitalized patients experience hyperglycemia.
2. Acute hyperglycemia and hypoglycemia can lead to increases in mortality as well as complications such as surgical site infections and end-organ dysfunction.
3. Hospitalized patients are unstable, as such, a patient's treatment strategies will change as the patient moves through different levels of care.
4. Insulin is the mainstay of therapy in acutely ill patients in the hospital.
5. The three core components of a complete insulin regimen are basal, nutritional, and correctional.
6. Hyperglycemic emergencies require hospitalization and are managed through a multifaceted approach of fluid resuscitation, insulin administration, and electrolyte monitoring/repletion.

BEYOND THE BOOK

Listen to the *Run the List* podcast, Episode 37: Inpatient Diabetes Management. Dr. Nadine Palermo, an endocrinologist and the Associate Director of the Acute Diabetes Care program at Brigham and Women's Hospital, talks with Joyce Zhou (host) and Jakub Glowala (case presenter) to discuss the management of inpatient diabetes patients.

Available at https://www.runthelistpodcast.com/endocrinology/#T2DM-inpatient.

Download the companion PDF available at https://static1.squarespace.com/static/5d2501c14c57720001ff2b07/t/5f10a42db1f8645d718ced26/1594926131571/RTL_Inpatient_DM.pdf

INTRODUCTION

1 Acute hyperglycemia is a common presentation in the ambulatory, emergency department, and inpatient hospital settings. The management of acute hyperglycemia in the emergency department and in the inpatient setting often differs from the management of diabetes in the ambulatory setting. Acute hyperglycemia is also managed differently depending on diagnosis (eg, diabetic ketoacidosis [DKA] or hyperosmolar hyperglycemic state [HHS], or acute stress hyperglycemia) and patient acuity (critically ill, acutely ill, step-down, and transitioning to outpatient). Increases in mortality and morbidity have been observed with hyperglycemia, hypoglycemia, and glycemic variability.[1-4]

2 Controlling blood glucose (BG) during hospitalization has clear benefits, including improved outcomes and decreased length of stay.[4] This chapter will review the causes of dysglycemia in the hospital, as well as recommendations to manage hyperglycemia and prevent negative outcomes. Patients being admitted to the hospital may pass through several phases of care, including the emergency department, general ward, and the intensive care unit (ICU). Each of these phases poses unique challenges, different goals in treatment, and different modalities of therapeutics. This chapter will evaluate medication therapy options for patients in the hospital experiencing acute hyperglycemia, as well as patients experiencing a hyperglycemic emergency such as DKA or HHS. A multidisciplinary effort to identify, treat, and monitor glucose throughout the hospitalization is critical to achieving positive patient outcomes during the hospital stay, safely and efficiently transitioning patients home, and preventing readmission to the ICU or hospital.

EPIDEMIOLOGY

Greater than one-third of patients who are hospitalized experience hyperglycemia.[5,6] Many patients with acute hyperglycemia may not have a diagnosis of diabetes. Patients without a current diagnosis of diabetes may have stress-induced hyperglycemia or previously undiagnosed diabetes and should be evaluated for a diagnosis of diabetes. Routine monitoring of BG is the standard of care in all patients who are admitted to the hospital to identify dysglycemia. Patients with known diabetes should have a hemoglobin A1C (A1C) drawn when admitted if a result is not available from the past 2 to 3 months. Obtaining an A1C should also be done in patients with BG greater than 140 mg/dL (7.8 mmol/L) admitted to the hospital if not performed in the prior 3 months.[4] Obtaining an A1C upon admission is needed to determine whether a patient meets diagnostic criteria for diabetes, which, in turn, will dictate the discharge plan and long-term management strategy beyond the acute hyperglycemia.

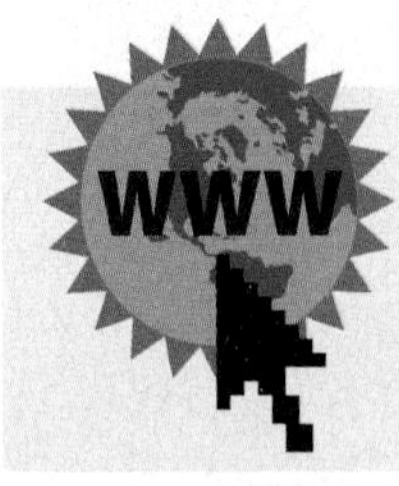

The complete chapter, learning objectives, and other resources can be found at **www.pharmacotherapyonline.com.**

96

Thyroid Disorders

Michael P. Kane and Gary Bakst

KEY CONCEPTS

1. Thyrotoxicosis is most commonly caused by Graves' disease, which is an autoimmune disorder in which thyroid-stimulating antibody (TSAb) directed against the thyrotropin receptor elicits the same biologic response as thyroid-stimulating hormone (TSH).
2. Hyperthyroidism may be treated with antithyroid drugs such as methimazole (MMI) or propylthiouracil (PTU), radioactive iodine (RAI: sodium iodide-131 [^{131}I]), or surgical removal of the thyroid gland; selection of the initial treatment approach is based on patient characteristics such as age, concurrent physiology (eg, pregnancy), comorbidities (eg, chronic obstructive lung disease), and convenience.
3. MMI and PTU reduce the synthesis of thyroid hormones and are similar in efficacy, although their dosing ranges differ by 20-fold. Overall, PTU has a greater incidence of side effects. Agranulocytosis is a rare but severe adverse effect associated with both medications.
4. Response to MMI and PTU is seen in 4 to 6 weeks and therefore β-blocker therapy may be concurrently initiated to reduce adrenergic symptoms. Maximal response is typically seen in 4 to 6 months; treatment usually continues for 1 to 2 years, and therapy is monitored by clinical signs and symptoms and by measuring the serum concentrations of TSH and free thyroxine (FT_4).
5. Adjunctive therapy with β-blockers controls the adrenergic symptoms of thyrotoxicosis but does not correct the underlying disorder; iodine may also be used adjunctively in preparation for surgery and acutely for thyroid storm.
6. Many patients choose to have ablative therapy with ^{131}I rather than undergo repeated courses of MMI or PTU treatment; most patients receiving RAI eventually become hypothyroid and require thyroid hormone supplementation.
7. Hypothyroidism is most often due to an autoimmune disorder known as *Hashimoto's thyroiditis*.
8. The drug of choice for replacement therapy in hypothyroidism is levothyroxine.
9. Studies of combination therapy with levothyroxine and liothyronine have not shown reproducible benefits. This approach to the treatment of hypothyroidism requires further study.
10. Monitoring of levothyroxine replacement therapy is achieved by observing clinical signs and symptoms and by measuring the serum TSH level. An elevated TSH indicates under-replacement; a suppressed TSH indicates over-replacement.

BEYOND THE BOOK

To get a basic understanding of hyperthyroidism and hypothyroidism, visit the Websites of National Institutes of Health and National Institute of Diabetes and Digestive and Kidney Diseases for a quick overview:

https://www.niddk.nih.gov/health-information/endocrine-diseases/hyperthyroidism

https://www.niddk.nih.gov/health-information/endocrine-diseases/hypothyroidism

INTRODUCTION

Thyroid hormones affect the function of virtually every organ system. In a child, thyroid hormone is critical for normal growth and development. In an adult, the major role of thyroid hormone is to maintain metabolic stability. Substantial reservoirs of thyroid hormone in the thyroid gland and blood provide constant thyroid hormone availability. In addition, the hypothalamic-pituitary-thyroid axis is exquisitely sensitive to small changes in circulating thyroid hormone concentrations, and alterations in thyroid hormone secretion maintain peripheral free thyroid hormone levels within a narrow range. Patients seek medical attention for evaluation of symptoms due to abnormal thyroid hormone levels or because of diffuse or nodular thyroid enlargement.

Thyroid Hormone Synthesis

The thyroid hormones thyroxine (T_4) and triiodothyronine (T_3) (Fig. 96-1) are formed within thyroglobulin (TG), a large glycoprotein synthesized in the thyroid cell. Because of the unique tertiary structure of this glycoprotein, iodinated tyrosine residues present in TG are able to bind together to form active thyroid hormones.

Iodide is actively transported through the basolateral membrane via a Na^+/I^- symporter from the extracellular space into the thyroid follicular cell against an electrochemical gradient, driven by the coupled transport of sodium.[1] Structurally related anions such as thiocyanate (SCN^-), perchlorate (ClO_4^-), and pertechnetate (TcO_4^-) are competitive inhibitors of iodine transport.[1] In addition, bromine, fluorine, and, under certain circumstances, lithium block iodide transport into the thyroid (Table 96-1). Inorganic iodide that enters the thyroid follicular cell is ushered through the cell to the apical membrane, where it is transported into the follicular lumen by pendrin, and possibly other transport proteins.[1] Located on the luminal side of the apical membrane, thyroid peroxidase oxidizes iodide and

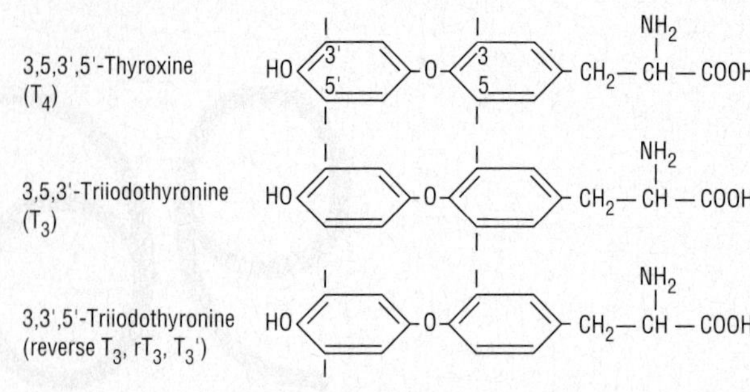

FIGURE 96-1 Structure of thyroid hormones.

TABLE 96-1 Thyroid Hormone Synthesis and Secretion Inhibitors

Mechanism of Action	Substance
Blocks iodide transport into the thyroid	Bromine Fluorine Lithium
Impairs organification and coupling of thyroid hormones	Thionamides Sulfonamide Salicylamide Antipyrine
Inhibits thyroid hormone secretion	Iodide (large doses) Lithium

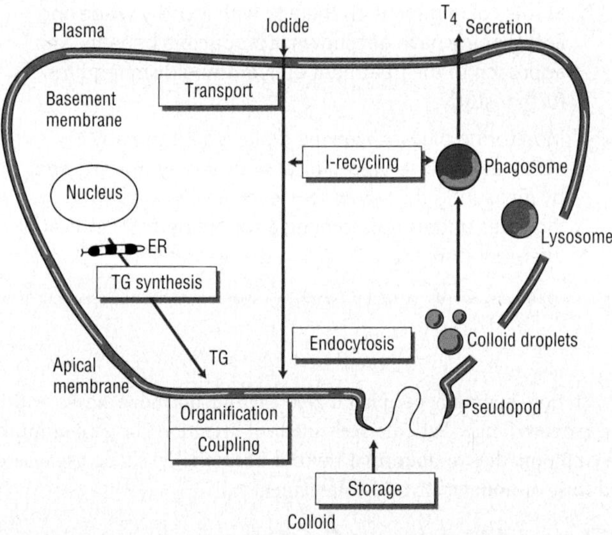

FIGURE 96-2 Thyroid hormone synthesis. Iodide is transported from the plasma, through the cell, to the apical membrane, where it is organified and coupled to the thyroglobulin (TG) synthesized within the thyroid cell. Hormone stored as colloid re-enters the cell through endocytosis and moves back toward the basal membrane, where thyroxine (T_4) is secreted.

covalently binds the organified iodide to tyrosine residues within TG (Fig. 96-2). It is interesting that although salivary glands and the gastric mucosa are able to actively transport iodide, they are unable to effectively incorporate iodide into proteins, given the lack of similar oxidizing machinery.

The iodinated tyrosine residues monoiodotyrosine (MIT) and diiodotyrosine (DIT) combine to form iodothyronines (Fig. 96-3). Thus, two molecules of DIT combine to form T_4, whereas MIT and

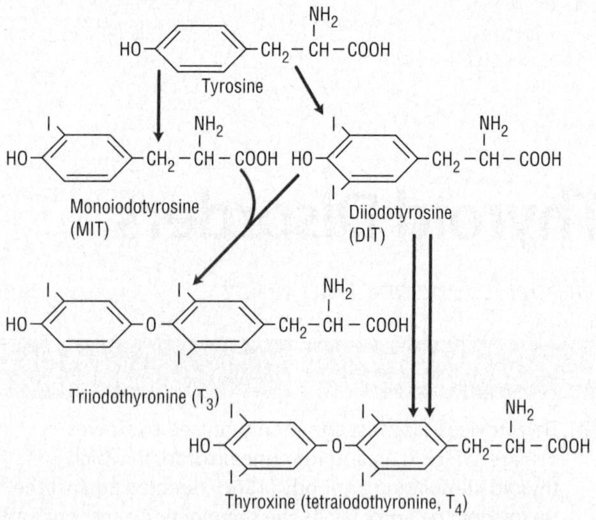

Tyrosine

Monoiodotyrosine (MIT)

Diiodotyrosine (DIT)

Triiodothyronine (T_3)

Thyroxine (tetraiodothyronine, T_4)

FIGURE 96-3 Scheme of coupling reactions. After tyrosine is iodinated to form monoiodotyrosine (MIT) or diiodotyrosine (DIT) (organification of the iodine), MIT and DIT combine to form triiodothyronine (T_3) or two molecules of DIT combine to form thyroxine T_4 (coupling).

DIT constitute T_3. In addition to its role in iodine organification, the hemoprotein thyroid peroxidase also catalyzes the formation of iodothyronines (coupling).

Iodine deficiency causes an increase in the MIT:DIT ratio in TG and leads to a relative increase in the production of T_3:T_4. Because T_3 is more potent than T_4, the increase in T_3 production in iodine-deficient areas may be beneficial. The thionamide drugs used to treat hyperthyroidism inhibit thyroid peroxidase and thus block thyroid hormone synthesis.

Thyroglobulin is stored in the follicular lumen and must reenter the cell, where the process of proteolysis liberates thyroid hormone into the bloodstream. Thyroid follicles active in hormone synthesis are identified histologically by columnar epithelial cells lining a follicular lumen, which is depleted of colloid. Inactive follicles are lined by cuboidal epithelial cells and are replete with colloid. Both iodide and lithium block the release of preformed thyroid hormone, through poorly understood mechanisms.

T_4 and T_3 are transported in the bloodstream primarily by three proteins: (1) thyroxine-binding globulin (TBG), (2) transthyretin (TTR; also known as TBPA, thyroxine-binding prealbumin), and (3) albumin. It is estimated that 99.96% of circulating T_4 and 99.5% of T_3 are bound to these proteins. However, only the unbound (free) thyroid hormone is able to diffuse into the cell, elicit a biologic effect, and regulate thyroid-stimulating hormone (TSH; also known as *thyrotropin*) secretion from the pituitary. Multiple functions have been ascribed to these transport proteins, including (a) assuring minimal urinary loss of iodide, (b) providing a mechanism for uniform tissue distribution of free hormone, and (c) transporting hormone into the central nervous system (CNS).

Whereas T_4 is secreted solely from the thyroid gland, less than 20% of T_3 is produced in the thyroid. The majority of T_3 is formed from the breakdown of T_4 catalyzed by the 5′-monodeiodinase enzymes found in extrathyroidal peripheral tissues. Because the binding affinity of nuclear thyroid hormone receptors (TRs) is 10 to 15 times higher for T_3 than for T_4, the deiodinase enzymes play a pivotal role in determining overall metabolic activity. Three different monodeiodinase enzymes are present in the body. Of the enzymes that catalyze 5′-monodeiodination, type I enzymes are present in peripheral tissues such as the liver and kidney, whereas

TABLE 96-2 Properties of Iodothyronine 5′-Deiodinase Isoforms

Property	Type I	Type II	Type III
Susceptibility to propylthiouracil	High	Low	Low
Tissue localization	Thyroid, liver, kidney	Pituitary, thyroid, CNS, brown adipose tissue	Placenta, developing brain, skin
Preferred substrate	rT_3 and T_3	T_4 and rT_3	T_3 and T_4
Physiologic or pathophysiologic role	Clearance of rT_3 and T_3, the predominant extrathyroidal source of T_3 in hyperthyroidism	Intracellular T_3 production, especially for the brain in hypothyroidism or iodine deficiency, and maintenance of plasma T_3	Clearance of T_3 and T_4
Developmental expression	Expressed latest in development; predominant deiodinase in adult	Expressed second; especially high in brain and brown adipose tissue	Expressed first; high in developing brain; may be important for fetal thyroid hormone metabolism

rT_3, reverse T_3; T_3, triiodothyronine; T_4, thyroxine.

type II enzymes are found in the CNS, pituitary, and thyroid. Type III enzymes, found in the placenta, skin, and developing brain, inactivate T_4 and T_3 by deiodinating the inner ring at the 5 position. The principal characteristics of these enzymes are listed in Table 96-2. T_4 may also be acted on by the enzyme 5′- monodeiodinase to form reverse T_3, but this accounts for a small component of hormone metabolism. Polymorphisms in the deiodinase genes may prove to be of clinical significance. For example, a polymorphism in the type I deiodinase leading to increased activity seems to be associated with an increased circulating ratio of free T_3 to free T_4.[2] Reverse T_3 has no known biological activity. T_3 is removed from the body by deiodinating degradation and through the action of sulfotransferase enzyme systems converting to T_3 sulfate and 3,3-diiodothyronine sulfates, thus facilitating enterohepatic clearance. Thyronamines are derivatives of thyroid hormones that are present in low concentrations in human serum. The most studied thyronamine, 3-iodothyronamine, can theoretically be made from T_4 by decarboxylation and deiodination. Administration of pharmacologic amounts of 3-iodothyronamine to animals has profound effects on temperature regulation and cardiac function and shifts fuel metabolism from carbohydrates to lipids. However, a possible physiologic role for thyronamines has yet to be determined, although altered levels may be associated with some disease states.

Thyroid Hormone Regulation and Action

The growth and function of the thyroid are stimulated by activation of the thyrotropin receptor by TSH.[3] The receptor belongs to the family of G-protein–coupled receptors. The thyrotropin receptor is coupled to the α subunit of the stimulatory guanine-nucleotide–binding protein (Gsα), activating adenylate cyclase and increasing the accumulation of cyclic adenosine monophosphate. Through this mechanism, TSH stimulates the expression of Na^+/I^- symporter, TG, and thyroid peroxidase genes as well as increases apical iodide efflux. Somatic activating mutations in the receptor are commonly seen in autonomously functioning thyroid nodules.[4] Rarely, germline-activating mutations of the TSH receptor have been reported in kindreds with Leclere syndrome, and thyrotoxicosis can result from germline-activating mutations in G-protein signaling in McCune–Albright syndrome. Conversely, thyrotropin resistance results from point mutations that prevent TSH binding, leading to abnormalities in the thyrotropin receptor–adenylate cyclase system and congenital hypothyroidism.[3] Individuals with this abnormality have high levels of TSH but decreased TG levels and a normal or small thyroid gland.

Thyroid hormone nuclear receptors regulate the transcription of target genes in the presence of physiologic concentrations of T_3.[3] Unlike most other nuclear receptors, TRs also actively regulate gene expression in the absence of hormone, typically resulting in an opposite effect. TRs translocate from the cytoplasm to the nucleus, interact in the nucleus with T_3, and target genes and other proteins required for basal and T_3-dependent gene transcription. TRs exist in several isoforms, including TRβ1, TRβ2, and TRα1.[3] Thyroid hormone has different actions in different tissues based on the tissue-specific expression of the different TR isoforms. There is interest in developing thyroid hormone analogs that selectively activate specific TR isoforms. Such agents could theoretically have targeted desirable effects such as stimulating energy expenditure without having adverse effects on other tissues.[5]

The production of thyroid hormone is regulated in two main ways. First, thyroid hormone is regulated by TSH secreted by the anterior pituitary. The secretion of TSH is itself under negative feedback control by the circulating level of free thyroid hormone and the positive influence of hypothalamic thyrotropin-releasing hormone (TRH). Second, extrathyroidal deiodination of T_4 to T_3 is regulated by a variety of factors including nutrition, nonthyroidal hormones, ambient temperatures, drugs, and illness.

HYPERTHYROIDISM AND THYROTOXICOSIS

Thyrotoxicosis results when tissues are exposed to excessive levels of T_4, T_3, or both.[6] Hyperthyroidism, which is one cause of thyrotoxicosis, refers specifically to overproduction of thyroid hormone by the thyroid gland.

EPIDEMIOLOGY—THYROTOXICOSIS

In the National Health and Nutrition Examination Survey (NHANES) III, 0.7% of those surveyed who were not taking thyroid medications and had no history of thyroid disease had subclinical hyperthyroidism (TSH less than 0.1 mIU/L, and T_4 normal), and 0.5% had "clinically significant" hyperthyroidism (TSH less than 0.1 mIU/L, and T_4 more than 13.2 mcg/dL [170 nmol/L]).[7] The prevalence of suppressed TSH values peaks in people aged 20 to 39, declines in those 40 to 79, and increases again in those 80 or older. Abnormal TSH levels were more common among women than among men.

ETIOLOGY AND PATHOPHYSIOLOGY—THYROTOXICOSIS

If the clinical history and examination do not provide pathognomonic clues to the etiology of the patient's thyrotoxicosis, measurement of the radioactive iodine uptake (RAIU) is critical in the evaluation (Table 96-3). The normal 24-hour RAIU ranges from 10% to 30% with some regional variation that is due to differences in iodine intake. An elevated RAIU indicates endogenous hyperthyroidism; that is, the patient's thyroid gland is actively overproducing

TABLE 96-3 Differential Diagnosis of Thyrotoxicosis Based on Radioactive Iodine Uptake (RAIU)

Increased RAIU[a]	Decreased RAIU
TSAb (Graves' disease)	Exogenous sources of thyroid hormone
Multinodular goiter	Medications containing thyroid hormone or iodine
Toxic adenoma	Painless thyroiditis
hCG (trophoblastic diseases)	Subacute thyroiditis
TSH-induced hyperthyroidism	Inflammatory thyroid disease
TSH-secreting tumors	Food sources containing thyroid gland
Selective pituitary resistance to T_4	Ectopic thyroid tissue
Thyroid stimulators other than TSH	Struma ovarii
	Metastatic follicular carcinoma

[a]The RAIU may be decreased if the patient has been recently exposed to excess iodine.

hCG, human chorionic gonadotropin; RAIU, radioactive iodine uptake; TSAb, thyroid-stimulating antibody.

T_4, T_3, or both. Conversely, a low RAIU in the absence of iodine excess indicates that high levels of thyroid hormone are not a consequence of thyroid gland hyperfunction but are likely due to thyroiditis or hormone ingestion. The importance of differentiating endogenous hyperthyroidism from other causes of thyrotoxicosis lies in the widely different prognosis and treatment of the diseases in these two categories. Therapy of thyrotoxicosis associated with thyroid hyperfunction is mainly directed at decreasing the rate of thyroid hormone synthesis, secretion, or both. Such measures are ineffective in treating thyrotoxicosis that is not the result of endogenous hyperthyroidism because hormone synthesis and regulated hormone secretion are already at a minimum.

Causes of Thyrotoxicosis Associated with Suppressed RAIU

Subacute Thyroiditis

Painful subacute (granulomatous or de Quervain) thyroiditis often develops after a viral syndrome, but rarely has a specific virus been identified in thyroid parenchyma. A genetic predisposition exists, with a markedly higher risk for developing subacute thyroiditis for patients with HLA-Bw35. Systemic symptoms often accompany the syndrome, including fever, malaise, and myalgia, in addition to those symptoms due to thyrotoxicosis. Typically, patients complain of severe pain in the thyroid region, which often extends to the ear on the affected side. With time, the pain may migrate from one side of the gland to the other. On physical examination, the thyroid gland is firm and exquisitely tender. Signs of thyrotoxicosis are present.[17]

Thyroid function tests typically run a triphasic course. Initially, serum T_4 levels are elevated due to the release of preformed thyroid hormone from disrupted follicles. The 24-hour RAIU during this time is less than 2% due to thyroid inflammation and TSH suppression by the elevated T_4 level. As the disease progresses, intrathyroidal hormone stores are depleted, and the patient may become mildly hypothyroid with an appropriately elevated TSH level. During the recovery phase, thyroid hormone stores are replenished, and serum TSH concentration gradually returns to normal. Recovery is generally complete within 2 to 6 months. Most patients remain euthyroid, and recurrences of painful thyroiditis are extremely rare. The patient with painful thyroiditis should be reassured that the disease is self-limited and is unlikely to recur. Thyrotoxic symptoms may be relieved with β-blockers. nonsteroidal anti-inflammatory drugs (NSAIDs) will usually relieve the pain. Occasionally, prednisone (30-40 mg daily) must be used to suppress the inflammatory process. Antithyroid drugs (ATD) are not indicated because they will not be effective as they do not decrease the release of preformed thyroid hormone.

Painless Thyroiditis

Painless (silent and lymphocytic) thyroiditis is a common cause of thyrotoxicosis and may represent up to 15% of cases of thyrotoxicosis in North America. When lymphocytic thyroiditis develops during the first 12 months after the end of pregnancy, the condition is also called *postpartum thyroiditis*. The etiology is not fully understood and may be heterogeneous, but evidence indicates that autoimmunity underlies most cases. There is an increased frequency of HLA-DR3 and DR5 in patients with painless thyroiditis; non-endocrine autoimmune diseases are also more common. Histologically, diffuse lymphocytic infiltration is generally identified. The triphasic course of this illness mimics that of subacute thyroiditis. Most patients present with mild thyrotoxic symptoms. Lid retraction and lid lag are present, but exophthalmos is absent. The thyroid gland may be diffusely enlarged, but thyroid tenderness is absent.

The 24-hour RAIU will typically be suppressed to less than 2% during the thyrotoxic phase of painless thyroiditis. Anti-TG and antithyroid peroxidase antibody (anti-TPOAb) levels are elevated in more than 50% of patients. Patients with mild hyperthyroidism and painless thyroiditis should be reassured that they have a self-limited disease, although patients with postpartum thyroiditis may experience a recurrence of the disease with subsequent pregnancies. As with other thyrotoxic syndromes, adrenergic symptoms may be ameliorated with propranolol or metoprolol. ATDs, which inhibit new hormone synthesis, are not indicated because they do not decrease the release of preformed thyroid hormone. A small proportion of patients may have recurrent episodes of thyroiditis or may develop permanent hypothyroidism.[17]

Exogenous Thyroid Hormone

Thyrotoxicosis factitia is hyperthyroidism due to ingestion of thyroid hormone. This category includes hyperthyroidism produced by the intentional ingestion of exogenous thyroid hormone. Obesity is the most common non-thyroidal disorder for which thyroid hormone is inappropriately used, but thyroid hormone has been used for almost every conceivable problem from menstrual irregularities and infertility to hypercholesterolemia and baldness. There is little evidence to suggest that treatment with thyroid hormone is beneficial for any of these conditions in euthyroid individuals.[18] Thyrotoxicosis factitia can also occur when too large a dose of thyroid hormone is used to treat conditions in which it is likely to be beneficial, such as differentiated thyroid carcinoma. In addition to this iatrogenic cause, thyrotoxicosis factitia may occur after accidental pediatric ingestion or pharmacy error. Thyrotoxicosis factitia may also be caused by the purposeful and secretive ingestion of thyroid hormone by patients (usually with a healthcare background) who wish to obtain attention or lose weight.

Thyroid hormone may also be accidentally ingested in food sources. Reports of thyrotoxicosis in Minnesota and Nebraska in the 1980s were attributed to ingestion of ground beef contaminated by bovine thyroid glands. More recently thyrotoxicosis due to porcine thyroid tissue in meat products has been reported in Spain and Uruguay.

Thyrotoxicosis factitia should be suspected in a thyrotoxic patient without evidence of increased hormone production, thyroidal inflammation, or ectopic thyroid tissue. The RAIU is at low levels because the patient's thyroid gland function is suppressed by the exogenous thyroid hormone. Measurement of plasma TG is a valuable laboratory aid in the diagnosis of thyrotoxicosis factitia. TG is normally secreted in small amounts by the thyroid gland; however, when thyroid hormone is taken orally, TG levels tend to be lower than the normal range. In other entities characterized by a low RAIU, such as thyroiditis, leakage of preformed thyroid hormone results in elevated TG levels. If a history of thyroid hormone ingestion is elicited or deduced, exogenous thyroid hormone should be withheld for 4 to 6 weeks, and thyroid function tests should be repeated to ensure a euthyroid state has been restored. Rarely, thyroid hormones may be the drug of abuse and detection is difficult with standard thyroid hormone assays. For example, tiratricol (TRIAC), an endogenous metabolite of T_3 that has been used for weight loss and paradoxically by bodybuilders, will suppress TSH at high doses and may cross-react in many T_3 immunoassays; thus, thyrotoxicosis factitia due to tiratricol abuse may be misinterpreted as T_3 toxicosis, and also lead to serious side effects.

Medications Containing Iodine

Amiodarone may induce thyrotoxicosis (2%–3% of patients), overt hypothyroidism (5% of patients), subclinical hypothyroidism (25% of patients), or euthyroid hyperthyroxinemia, depending on the underlying thyroid function and pathology.[19] Because amiodarone contains 37% iodine by weight, approximately 6 mg/day of iodine is released for each 200 mg of amiodarone, 1,000 times greater than the recommended daily amount of iodine of 150 mcg/day. As a result of this iodine overload, iodine-exacerbated thyroid dysfunction commonly occurs among those patients with preexisting thyroid disease: thyrotoxicosis in patients with hyperthyroidism or euthyroid nodular autonomy and hypothyroidism in patients with autoimmune thyroid disease. In contrast to hyperthyroidism with increased synthesis of thyroid hormone induced by amiodarone (type I), destructive thyroiditis with leakage of TG and thyroid hormones also occurs (type II), typically among individuals with otherwise normal glands. The two types of amiodarone-induced thyrotoxicosis may be differentiated using color-flow Doppler ultrasonography. Such distinction is critically important, given the therapeutic implications of the two syndromes: type I amiodarone-induced hyperthyroidism responds somewhat to thionamides, whereas type II may respond to glucocorticoids.[19] Obviously, RAI therapy is inappropriate in type I due to the drug-induced iodine excess, and in type II due to lack of increased hormone synthesis. The manifestations of amiodarone-induced thyrotoxicosis may be atypical symptoms such as ventricular tachycardia and exacerbation of the underlying chronic obstructive pulmonary disease, both of which are significant, given the severe underlying cardiac pathology that led to the use of amiodarone in the first place. Amiodarone also directly interferes with type I 5′-deiodinase, leading to reduced conversion of T_4 to T_3 and hyperthyroxinemia without thyrotoxicosis.[19]

High intake of biotin can interfere with thyroid hormone assays, leading to false results of thyroid function tests.[20,21] Excess biotin leads to falsely elevated results of TT_4, FT_4, and TT_3 (competitive immunoassays), and to falsely low TSH levels (immunometric or sandwich immunoassays). This is not an issue of endogenous interference but an interference with the assay itself. Biotin doses of greater than 5,000 mcg/day are associated with major interference on immunoassays; in such circumstances, it is recommended patients hold their biotin doses for 24 to 48 hours before laboratory testing.

Thyroid Cancer

In widely metastatic differentiated papillary or follicular carcinomas with relatively well-preserved function, sufficient thyroid hormones can be synthesized and secreted to produce thyrotoxicosis. In most instances, a previous diagnosis of thyroid malignancy has been made. The diagnosis can be confirmed by whole-body ^{131}I scanning. Treatment with ^{131}I is generally effective at ablating functioning thyroid metastases.

Struma Ovarii

Struma ovarii is a teratoma of the ovary that contains differentiated thyroid follicular cells and is capable of making thyroid hormones. This extremely rare cause of thyrotoxicosis is suggested by the absence of thyroid enlargement in a thyrotoxic patient with a suppressed RAIU in the neck and no findings to suggest thyroiditis. The diagnosis is established by localizing functioning thyroid tissue in the ovary with whole-body RAI (sodium iodide-131 [^{131}I]) scanning. Interestingly, struma ovarii not associated with hyperthyroidism is much more common than struma ovarii associated with hyperthyroidism. Because the tissue is neoplastic and potentially malignant, combined surgical and radioiodine treatment of malignant struma ovarii for both monitoring and therapy of relapse is the recommended treatment.

Causes of Thyrotoxicosis Associated with Elevated RAIU

Graves' Disease

1 Graves' disease is an autoimmune syndrome that usually includes hyperthyroidism, diffuse thyroid enlargement, exophthalmos, and, less commonly, pretibial myxedema and thyroid acropachy (Fig. 96-4).[6,9] Graves' disease is the most common cause of hyperthyroidism, with a prevalence estimated to be 3 per 1,000 population in the United States. Hyperthyroidism results from the action of thyroid-stimulating antibodies (TSAbs), which are directed against the thyrotropin receptor on the surface of the thyroid cell. When these immunoglobulins bind to the receptor, they activate downstream G-protein signaling and adenylate cyclase in the same manner as TSH. Autoantibodies that react with orbital muscle and fibroblast tissue in the skin are responsible for the extrathyroidal manifestations of Graves' disease, and these autoantibodies are encoded by the same germline genes that encode for other autoantibodies for striated muscle and thyroid peroxidase. Clinically, the extrathyroidal disorders may not appear at the same time that hyperthyroidism develops.

There is now compelling evidence that heredity predisposes the susceptible individual to the development of clinically overt autoimmune thyroid disease in the setting of appropriate environmental and hormonal triggers. A role for gender in the emergence of Graves' disease is suggested by the fact that hyperthyroidism is approximately eight times more common in women than in men. Other lines of evidence support a role for heredity. First, there is a well-recognized clustering of Graves' disease within some families. Twin studies in Graves' disease have revealed that a monozygotic twin has a 35% likelihood of ultimately developing the disease compared with a 3% likelihood for a dizygotic twin, resulting in an estimation that 79% of the predisposition to Graves' disease is genetic. Second, the occurrence of other autoimmune diseases, including Hashimoto's thyroiditis, is also increased in families of patients with Graves' disease. Third, several studies have demonstrated an increased frequency of certain human leukocyte antigens (HLAs) in patients with Graves' disease. Differing HLA associations have been identified in the various ethnic groups studied. In White patients, for example, the relative risk of Graves' disease in carriers of the HLA-DR3 haplotype is between 2.5 and 5, whereas lesser associations have been reported for HLA-B8 and the HLA-DQA*0501allele. Several gene loci have been associated with autoimmune thyroid diseases such as Graves' disease. It is thought that these susceptibility genes interact with environmental triggers to induce thyroid disease through epigenetic effects.

The thyroid gland is diffusely enlarged in the majority of patients with Graves' disease and is commonly 40 to 60 g (two to three times the normal size). The surface of the gland is either smooth or bosselated, and the consistency varies from soft to firm. For patients with severe disease, a thrill may be felt and a systolic bruit may be heard over the gland, reflecting the increased intraglandular vascularity typical of hyperplasia. Whereas the presence of any of the extrathyroidal manifestations of this syndrome, including

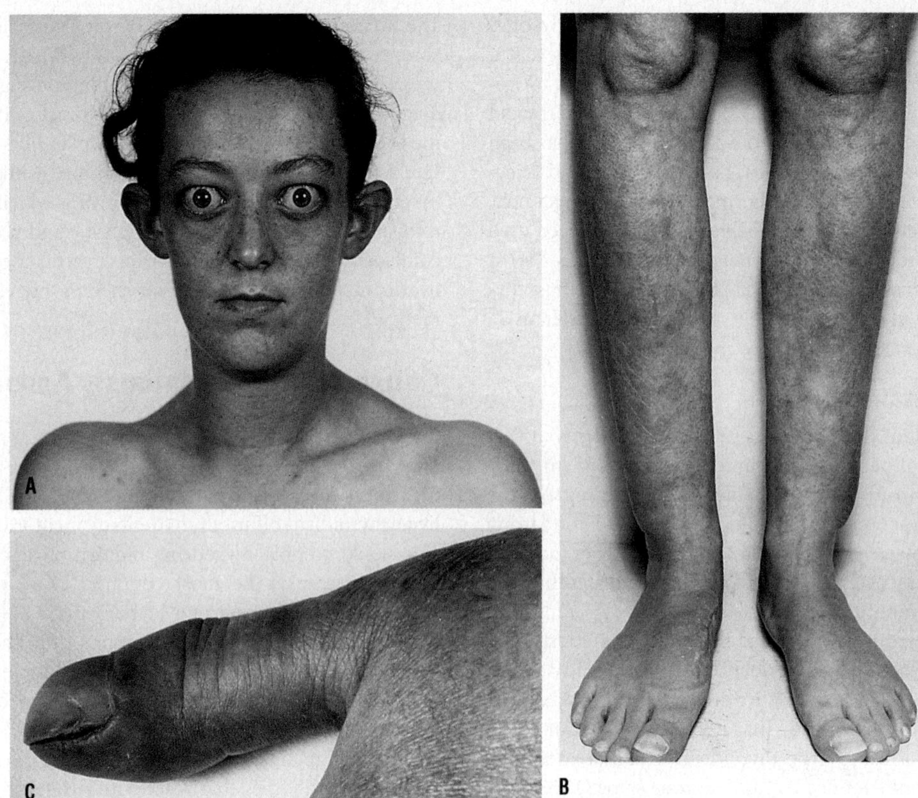

FIGURE 96-4 Features of Graves' disease. (*A*) Facial appearance in Graves' disease; lid retraction, periorbital edema, and proptosis are marked. (*B*) Thyroid dermopathy over the lateral aspects of the shins. (*C*) Thyroid acropachy. *(Reproduced with permission from Fauci AS, Kasper DL, Longo DL, et al., eds. Harrison's Principles of Internal Medicine. 16th ed. New York: McGraw Hill; 2005:2114.)*

exophthalmos, pretibial myxedema, or thyroid acropachy, in a thyrotoxic patient is pathognomonic of Graves' disease, most patients can be diagnosed on the basis of their history and examination of their diffuse goiter (see Fig. 96-4). An important clinical feature of Graves' disease is the occurrence of spontaneous remissions, albeit uncommon. The abnormalities in TSAb production may decrease or disappear over time.

The results of laboratory tests in thyrotoxic Graves' disease include an increase in the overall hormone production rate with a disproportionate increase in T_3 relative to T_4 (Table 96-4). In an occasional patient, the disproportionate overproduction of T_3 is exaggerated, with the result that only the serum T_3 concentration is increased (T_3 toxicosis). The saturation of TBG is increased due to the elevated levels of serum T_4 and T_3. As a result, the concentrations of free T_4 and free T_3 are increased to an even greater extent than are the measured serum total T_4 and T_3 concentrations. The TSH level will be suppressed or undetectable due to negative feedback by elevated levels of thyroid hormone at the pituitary.

For the patient with symptomatic disease, measurement of the serum-free T_4 concentration, total T_4, total T_3, and the TSH value will confirm the diagnosis of thyrotoxicosis. For the patient who is not pregnant or lactating, a 24-hour RAIU should be obtained if there is any diagnostic uncertainty, for example, recent onset of symptoms or other factors suggestive of thyroiditis. An increased RAIU indicates that the thyroid gland is inappropriately utilizing the iodine to produce more thyroid hormone at a time when the patient is thyrotoxic.

Thyrotoxic periodic paralysis is a rare complication of hyperthyroidism most commonly observed in Asian and Hispanic populations.[10] It presents as recurrent proximal muscle flaccidity ranging from mild weakness to total paralysis. The paralysis may be asymmetric and usually involves muscle groups that are strenuously exercised before the attack. Cognition and sensory perception are spared, whereas deep tendon reflexes are markedly diminished. The condition is characterized by hypokalemia and low urinary potassium excretion. Hypokalemia results from a sudden shift of potassium from extracellular to intracellular sites rather than reduced total body potassium. High-carbohydrate loads and exercise provoke the attacks. Treatment includes correcting the hyperthyroid state, potassium administration, spironolactone to conserve potassium, and propranolol to minimize intracellular shifts. Some patients with this condition have a mutation in the inwardly rectifying potassium channel Kir2.6.[11]

TABLE 96-4 Thyroid Function Tests in Different Thyroid Conditions

	Total T_4	Free T_4	Total T_3	TSH
Normal	4.5-10.9 mcg/dL(58-140 nmol/L)	0.8-2.7 ng/dL (10.3-34.7 pmol/L)	60-181 ng/dL (0.92-2.79 nmol/L)	0.5-4.7 mIU/L
Hyperthyroid	↑↑	↑↑	↑↑↑	↓↓[a]
Hypothyroid	↓↓	↓↓	↓	↑↑[a]
Increased TBG	↑	Normal	↑	Normal

[a]Primary thyroid disease.

Toxic Adenoma

An autonomous thyroid nodule is a discrete thyroid mass whose function is independent of pituitary and TSH control. The prevalence of toxic adenoma ranges from about 2% to 9% of thyrotoxic patients and depends on iodine availability and geographic location. Toxic adenomas are benign tumors that produce thyroid

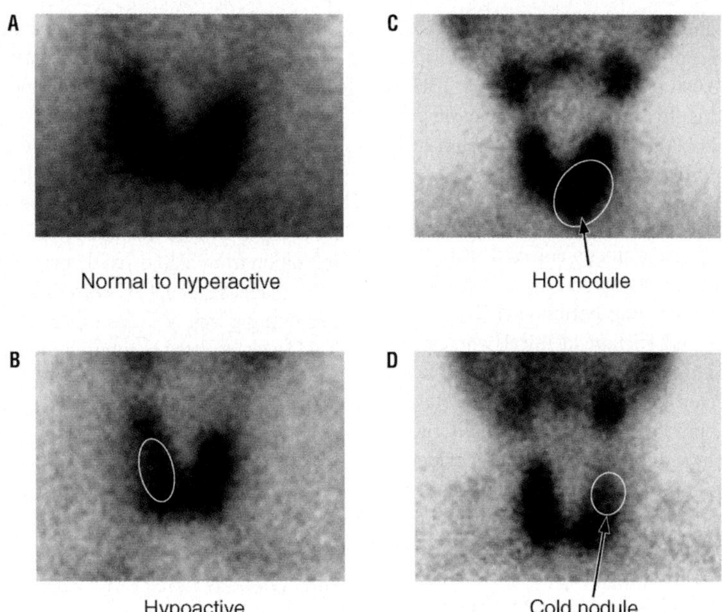

FIGURE 96-5 Radioiodine thyroid scans. (A) Normal or increased thyroid uptake of iodine-125 (^{125}I). (B) Thyroid with a marked decrease in ^{125}I uptake in a large palpable mass. (C) Increased ^{125}I uptake isolated to a single nodule, the "hot nodule." (D) Decreased thyroid ^{125}I uptake in an isolated region, the "cold nodule." *(Reproduced with permission from Molina PE. Endocrine Physiology. 2nd ed. New York: McGraw Hill; 2006:90. Images courtesy of Dr. Luis Linares, Memorial Medical Center, New Orleans, LA.)*

hormones. They arise from gain-of-function somatic mutations of the TSH receptor or, less commonly, the Gsα protein; more than a dozen TSH receptor mutations have been described.[6] These nodules may be referred to as *toxic adenomas*, or "hot" nodules, because of their persistent uptake on a radioiodine thyroid scan, despite suppressed uptake in the surrounding non-nodular gland (Fig. 96-5). The amount of thyroid hormone produced by an autonomous nodule is mass related. Therefore, hyperthyroidism usually occurs with larger nodules (ie, those more than 3 cm in diameter). Older patients (older than 60 years) are more likely (up to 60%) to be thyrotoxic from autonomous nodules than are younger patients (12%). There are many reports of isolated elevation of serum T_3 in patients with autonomously functioning nodules. Therefore, if the T_4 level is normal, a T_3 level must be measured to rule out T_3 toxicosis. If autonomous function is suspected but the TSH is normal, the diagnosis can be confirmed by a failure of the autonomous nodule to decrease its iodine uptake during exogenous T_3 administration sufficient to suppress TSH. Surgical resection, thionamides, percutaneous ethanol injection, and radioactive iodine (RAI) ablation are treatment options, but since thionamides do not halt the proliferative process in the nodule, definitive therapies are recommended. Ethanol ablation may be associated with pain and damage to surrounding extrathyroidal tissues, limiting its acceptance in the United States. It has been hypothesized that sublethal radiation doses received by the surrounding non-nodular thyroid tissue during RAI therapy of toxic nodules may lead to induction of thyroid cancer. However, thyroid cancer has rarely been associated with RAI therapy, and newer studies suggest hyperthyroidism itself, rather than RAI therapy, as being associated with non-thyroid malignancies.[12] There is a modest positive association between the dose of radioactive iodine absorbed into the gland and risk of solid cancer death;[13] however, the same authors later indicated that after controlling for known confounding, there no longer appeared to be a significant association in the risk of solid cancer mortality by treatment group.[14] An autonomously functioning nodule, if not large enough to cause thyrotoxicosis, can often be managed conservatively without therapy.

Multinodular Goiters

In multinodular goiters (MNGs), follicles with autonomous function coexist with normal or even nonfunctioning follicles. The pathogenesis of MNG is thought to be similar to that of toxic adenoma: diffuse hyperplasia caused by goitrogenic stimuli, leading to mutations and clonal expansion of benign neoplasms. The functional status of the nodule(s) depends on the nature of the underlying mutations, whether activating such as TSH receptor mutations or inhibitory such as RAS mutations. Thyrotoxicosis in an MNG occurs when a sufficient mass of autonomous follicles generates enough thyroid hormone to exceed the needs of the patient. It is not surprising that this type of hyperthyroidism develops insidiously over a period of several years and predominantly affects older individuals with long-standing goiters. The patient's complaints of weight loss, depression, anxiety, and insomnia may be attributed to old age. Any unexplained chronic illness in an elderly patient presenting with an MNG calls for the exclusion of hidden (silent) thyrotoxicosis.[15] Current third-generation TSH assays are able to detect subclinical hyperthyroidism.

A thyroid scan will show patchy areas of autonomously functioning thyroid tissue intermixed with hypofunctioning areas. When the patient is euthyroid, therapy is based on the need to reduce goiter size due to mass-related symptoms such as dysphagia. Doses of thyroid hormone sufficient to suppress TSH levels may slow goiter growth or cause some degree of shrinkage, but, in general, suppression therapy for nodular disease is inadequate to address mass effect. The preferred treatment for toxic MNG is RAI or surgery. Surgery is usually selected for younger patients and patients in whom large goiters impinge on vital organs. Alternatively, percutaneous injection of 95% ethanol has also been used to destroy single or multinodular adenomas with a 5-year success rate approaching 80%.

Trophoblastic Diseases Human chorionic gonadotropin (hCG) is a stimulator of the TSH receptor and may cause hyperthyroidism. The basis for the thyrotropic effect of hCG is the structural similarity of hCG to TSH (similar α subunits and unique β subunits). For patients with hyperthyroidism caused by trophoblastic tumors, serum hCG levels usually exceed 300 U/mL (kU/L) and always exceed 100 U/mL (kU/L). The mean peak hCG level in normal pregnancy is 50 U/mL (kU/L). On a molar basis, hCG has only 1/10,000 the activity of pituitary TSH in mouse bioassays. Nevertheless, this thyrotropic activity may be very substantial for patients with trophoblastic tumors, whose serum hCG concentrations may reach 2,000 U/mL (kU/L).

TSH-Induced Hyperthyroidism To better understand these syndromes, we must first review TSH biosynthesis and secretion. TSH is synthesized in the anterior pituitary as separate α- and β-subunit precursors. The α subunits from luteinizing hormone (LH), follicle-stimulating hormone (FSH), hCG, and TSH are identical, whereas the β subunits are unique and confer immunologic and biologic specificity. Free β subunits are devoid of receptor-binding and biologic activity and require combination with an α subunit to express their activity. Criteria for the diagnosis of TSH-induced hyperthyroidism include (a) evidence of peripheral hypermetabolism, (b) diffuse thyroid gland enlargement, (c) elevated free thyroid hormone levels, and (d) elevated or inappropriately "normal" serum immunoreactive TSH concentrations. Because the pituitary gland is extremely sensitive to even minimal elevations of free T_4, a "normal" or elevated TSH level in any thyrotoxic patient indicates the inappropriate production of TSH.

TSH-Secreting Pituitary Adenomas TSH-secreting pituitary tumors occur sporadically and release a biologically active hormone that is unresponsive to normal feedback control.[16] The mean age at diagnosis is around 40 years, with women being diagnosed more than men (8:7). These tumors may co-secrete prolactin or growth hormone; therefore, the patients may present with amenorrhea/galactorrhea or signs of acromegaly. Most patients present with classic symptoms and signs of thyrotoxicosis. Visual field defects may be present due to impingement of the optic chiasm by the tumor. Tumor growth and worsening visual field defects have been reported following antithyroid therapy because lowering of thyroid hormone levels is associated with loss of feedback inhibition from high thyroid hormone levels.

Diagnosis of a TSH-secreting adenoma should be made by demonstrating a lack of TSH response to TRH stimulation, inappropriate TSH levels, elevated α-subunit levels, and radiologic imaging; given the lack of routine availability of TRH, the other three criteria are essential. Note that some small tumors are not identified by MRI. Moreover, 10% of "normal" individuals may have incidental pituitary tumors or other benign focal lesions noted on pituitary imaging.

Transsphenoidal pituitary surgery is the treatment of choice for TSH-secreting adenomas. Pituitary gland irradiation is often given following surgery to prevent tumor recurrence. Dopamine agonists and octreotide have been used to treat tumors, especially those that co-secrete prolactin.

Pituitary Resistance to Thyroid Hormone Resistance to thyroid hormone is a rare condition that can be due to a number of molecular defects, including mutations in the TRβ gene.

CLINICAL PRESENTATION Thyrotoxicosis

General

- Signs and symptoms of thyrotoxicosis affect multiple organ systems. Patients often have symptoms for an extended period before the diagnosis of hyperthyroidism is made.

Symptoms

- The typical clinical manifestations of thyrotoxicosis include nervousness, anxiety, palpitations, emotional lability, easy fatigability, menstrual disturbances, and heat intolerance. A cardinal sign is weight loss despite an increased appetite.
- Elderly patients are more likely to develop atrial fibrillation with thyrotoxicosis than younger patients. The frequency of bowel movements may increase, but frank diarrhea is unusual. For the elderly patient and for the patient with severe disease, anorexia may be present as well. Palpitations are a prominent and distressing symptom, particularly in the patient with preexisting heart disease. Proximal muscle weakness is common and is noted on climbing stairs or in getting up from a sitting position. Women may note their menses are becoming scanty and irregular. Extremely thyrotoxic patients may have tachycardia, heart failure, psychosis, hyperpyrexia, and coma, a presentation described as thyroid storm.[8] Long-term hyperthyroidism may also be associated with a loss of bone mineral density and an increased risk of osteoporosis-related fracture.

Signs

- A variety of physical signs may be observed including warm, smooth, moist skin, exophthalmos (in Graves' disease only), pretibial myxedema (in Graves' disease only), and unusually fine hair. Separation of the end of the fingernails from the nail beds (onycholysis) may be noted. Ocular signs that result from thyrotoxicosis include retraction of the eyelids and lagging of the upper lid behind the globe when the patient looks downward (lid lag). Physical signs of a hyperdynamic circulatory state are common and include tachycardia at rest, a widened pulse pressure, and a systolic ejection murmur. Gynecomastia is sometimes noted in men. Neuromuscular examination often reveals a fine tremor of the protruded tongue and outstretched hands. Deep tendon reflexes are generally hyperactive. Thyromegaly is usually present. Elderly patients may present with the absence of clinical evidence of excess thyroid hormones (palpitations, anxiety, tremor, heat intolerance, and diaphoresis), but instead present with weight loss, apathy, and depression (apathetic hyperthyroidism).

Diagnosis

- Low TSH serum concentration. Elevated free and total T_4 and T_3 serum concentrations, particularly in more severe disease.
- Elevated radioactive iodine uptake (RAIU) by the thyroid gland when the hormone is being overproduced; suppressed RAIU in thyrotoxicosis due to thyroid inflammation (thyroiditis).

Other Tests

- Thyroid-stimulating antibodies (TSAbs)
- TG
- Thyrotropin receptor antibodies

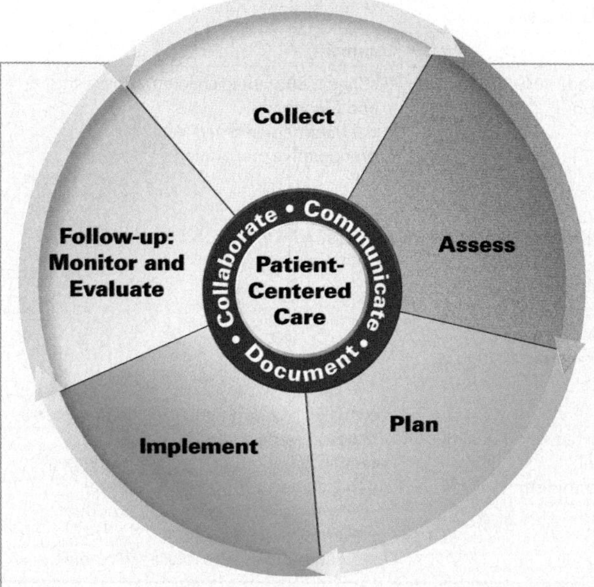

Patient Care Process for the Management of Hyperthyroidism

The image shows the five fundamental steps included in The Pharmacist's Care Process endorsed by the Joint Commission for Pharmacy Practitioners (2014). The tagline of this process reads collaborate, communicate, and document. The five fundamental steps listed here are collect, assess, plan, implement, and follow-up: monitor and evaluate. All these steps are listed in a circular block diagram.

Collect

- Patient characteristics (eg, age, race, sex, pregnancy status)
- Patient history (past medical, family, social) including patient signs and symptoms: warm, smooth, moist skin, palpitations, exophthalmos, pretibial myxedema, and unusually fine hair; anxiety, tremor, heat intolerance, tachycardia, weight loss, and menstrual disturbances (see Clinical Presentation Box)
- Current medications (including over-the-counter [OTC] and herbal medication use)
- Objective data
  - Heart rate, blood pressure (BP), weight, and body mass index (BMI)
  - Labs (eg, FT_4, TT_3, TSH, thyroid-stimulating antibodies; serum electrolytes, Scr, ALT)
  - Other diagnostic tests when indicated (eg, thyroid ultrasound, raidioactive iodine uptake [RAIU] scan)

Assess

- Cause of hyperthyroidism (see Table 96-3)
- Current medications that may contribute to or worsen hyperthyroidism
- Current medications that may interact with antithyroid therapy
- Appropriateness and effectiveness of current antithyroid regimen

Plan*

- Drug therapy regimen including specific antithyroid therapy, dose, and duration (see Table 96-5)
- Monitoring parameters including efficacy (eg, resolution of signs and symptoms) and safety (symptomatic hypothyroidism, adverse effects of medications), laboratory tests (TSH, FT_4, TT_3, LFTs, and CBC), and time frame
- Patient education (eg, purpose of treatment, dietary and lifestyle modification, drug therapy)

Implement*

- Provide patient education regarding all elements of the treatment plan
- Use motivational interviewing and coaching strategies to maximize adherence
- Schedule follow-up

Follow-up: Monitor and Evaluate

- Resolution of signs and symptoms
- Presence of adverse effects
- Patient adherence to treatment plan using multiple sources of information

**Collaborate with patient, caregivers, and other healthcare professionals.*

Pituitary resistance to thyroid hormone (PRTH) refers to selective resistance of the pituitary thyrotrophs to thyroid hormone. As nonpituitary tissues respond normally to thyroid hormone, patients experience the toxic peripheral effects of thyroid hormone excess. About 90% of patients studied have an appropriate increase in TSH in response to TRH; conversely, the TSH will be suppressed by T_3 administration.

Patients with PRTH require treatment to reduce their elevated thyroid hormone levels. Determining the appropriate serum T_4 level is difficult because TSH cannot be used to evaluate the adequacy of therapy. Any reduction in thyroid hormone carries the risk of inducing thyrotroph hyperplasia. Ideally, agents that suppress TSH secretion could be used to treat these individuals. Glucocorticoids, dopaminergic drugs, somatostatin and its analogs, and thyroid hormone analogs with reduced metabolic activity have all been tried, but with relatively little benefit. β-Blocker therapy can also be used. Triiodothyroacetic acid (TRIAC), an agent that is devoid of thyromimetic properties on peripheral tissues, but blocks the secretion of TSH, has been used to treat this condition. However, it is not available in the United States. Given the ability of retinoid X receptor ligands to inhibit TSH production, drugs such as bexarotene may have therapeutic benefit in PRTH.

TREATMENT

Thyrotoxicosis

2 Three common treatment modalities are used in the management of hyperthyroidism: surgery, antithyroid medications, and RAI (Table 96-5).

TABLE 96-5 Treatments for Hyperthyroidism Caused by Graves' Disease

Treatment	Advantages	Disadvantages	Comment
Methimazole (first-line pharmacotherapy) Propylthiouracil (second-line pharmacotherapy)	Noninvasive Low initial cost Low risk of permanent hypothyroidism Possible remissions due to immune effects	Low cure rate (average 40%-50%) Adverse drug reactions Drug compliance	First-line treatment in children, adolescents, and pregnancy Initial treatment in severe cases or preoperative preparation
Radioactive iodine (^{131}I)	Cure of hyperthyroidism Lowest cost, before adjustment for quality of life	Permanent hypothyroidism almost inevitable Might worsen ophthalmopathy Pregnancy must be deferred for 6-12 months; no breast-feeding Small potential risk of exacerbation of hyperthyroidism	Best treatment for toxic nodules and toxic multinodular goiter
Surgery	Rapid, effective treatment, especially in patients with large goiters	Most invasive Least costly in long term after quality-of-life adjustment Permanent hypothyroidism Pain, scar	Potential choice in pregnancy (2nd trimester) if major side effect from ATDs Potential complications (recurrent laryngeal nerve damage, hypoparathyroidism) Useful when coexisting suspicious nodule present Option for patients who refuse radioiodine

Desired Outcomes

The overall therapeutic objectives are to eliminate the excess thyroid hormone and minimize the symptoms and long-term consequences of hyperthyroidism.

General Approach to Treatment

Therapy must be individualized based on the type and severity of hyperthyroidism, patient age and gender, the existence of nonthyroidal conditions, and response to previous therapy.[22,23] For example, patients with swallowing or breathing difficulties due to impingement of the esophagus or trachea are generally taken for surgical removal of the thyroid. Clinical guidelines for the treatment of hyperthyroidism have been published.[6] Selected recommendations from these guidelines are shown in Table 96-6.

Nonpharmacologic Therapy

Surgery should be considered for patients with a large thyroid gland (more than 80 g), severe ophthalmopathy, and a lack of remission on antithyroid drug treatment. In case of cosmetic issues or pressure symptoms, the choice in MNG stands between surgery, which is still the first choice, and radioiodine therapy if uptake is adequate. In addition to surgery, the solitary nodule, whether hot or cold, can be treated with percutaneous ethanol injection therapy. For hot nodules, radioiodine is the therapy of choice.[6] Appropriate preparation of the patient for thyroidectomy includes MMI until the patient is biochemically euthyroid (usually 6-8 weeks), followed by the addition of iodides (500 mg/day) for 10 to 14 days before surgery to decrease the vascularity of the gland. Propranolol for several weeks preoperatively and 7 to 10 days after surgery has also been used to maintain a pulse rate of less than 90 beats/min. Combined pretreatment with propranolol and 10 to 14 days of potassium iodide has also been advocated.

The overall complication rate when surgery is performed for MNG by an experienced endocrine surgeon is low. If subtotal thyroidectomy, or an operation that attempts to maintain euthyroidism, is performed for Graves' disease, there is a risk of recurrence of hyperthyroidism that is directly related to remnant thyroid gland size. Near-total thyroidectomy is generally recognized as the procedure of choice for patients with Graves' disease.[6] The complication rates of surgery for Graves' disease are low when surgery is performed by a high-volume thyroid surgeon. Surgical complications include hypoparathyroidism (up to 2%) and laryngeal nerve injury (up to 1%).

Pharmacologic Therapy

Antithyroid Medications

3 **Thionamide Drugs** Two drugs within this category, MMI and PTU, are approved for the treatment of hyperthyroidism in the United States.[23] They are classified as thioureylenes (thionamides), which incorporate an N–C–S=N group into their ring structures.

Mechanism of Action MMI and PTU share several mechanisms to inhibit the biosynthesis of thyroid hormone.[24] These drugs serve as preferential substrates for the iodinating intermediate of thyroid peroxidase and divert iodine away from potential iodination sites in TG. This prevents subsequent incorporation of iodine into iodotyrosines and ultimately iodothyronine ("organification"). Second, they inhibit the coupling of MIT and DIT to form T_4 and T_3. The coupling reaction may be more sensitive to these drugs than the iodination reaction. Experimentally, these drugs exhibit immunosuppressive effects, although the clinical relevance of this finding is unclear. For patients with Graves' disease, antithyroid drug treatment has been associated with lower TSAb titers and restoration of normal suppressor T-cell function. However, perchlorate (ClO_4^-), which has a different mechanism of action, also decreases TSAbs, suggesting that normalization of the thyroid hormone level may itself improve the abnormal immune function. PTU inhibits the peripheral conversion of T_4 to T_3. This effect is dose-related and occurs within hours of PTU administration. MMI does not have this effect. After several weeks of use, depletion of stored hormone and lack of continuing synthesis of thyroid hormone results in the clinical effects of these drugs.

Pharmacokinetics Both ATDs are well absorbed (80%-95%) from the gastrointestinal tract, with peak serum concentrations about 1 hour after ingestion. The plasma half-life ranges of PTU and MMI are 1 to 2.5 and 6 to 9 hours, respectively, and are not appreciably affected by thyroid status. Urinary excretion is about 35% for PTU and less than 10% for MMI. These drugs are actively concentrated in the thyroid gland, which may account for the disparity between their relatively short plasma half-lives and the effectiveness of once-daily dosing regimens even with PTU. Approximately 60% to 80% of PTU is bound to plasma albumin, whereas MMI is not protein-bound.

TABLE 96-6 Selected Recommendations from the American Thyroid Association Hyperthyroidism Guidelines

Question	Recommendation Strength	Quality of Evidence
How should thyrotoxicosis be evaluated and initially managed?	β-Adrenergic blockade is recommended in all patients with symptomatic thyrotoxicosis, especially elderly patients and thyrotoxic patients with resting heart rates in excess of 90 beats per minute or coexistent cardiovascular disease.	Strong recommendation, moderate quality
If ^{131}I therapy is chosen (*for GD*), how should it be accomplished?	Sufficient radiation should be administered in a single dose (typically 10-15 mCi [370-555 MBq]) to render the patient with GD hypothyroid.	Strong recommendation, moderate quality
If ATDs are chosen as initial management of GD, how should the therapy be managed?	Methimazole should be used in virtually every patient who chooses antithyroid drug therapy for GD, except during the first trimester of pregnancy when propylthiouracil is preferred, in the treatment of thyroid storm, and in patients with minor reactions to methimazole who refuse radioactive iodine therapy or surgery.	Strong recommendation, moderate quality
If ATDs are chosen as initial management of GD, how should patients be monitored?	A differential WBC count should be obtained during febrile illness and at the onset of pharyngitis in all patients taking antithyroid medication.	Strong recommendation, low-quality
If thyroidectomy is chosen for treatment of GD, how should it be accomplished?	If surgery is chosen as the primary therapy for GD, near-total or total thyroidectomy is the procedure of choice.	Strong recommendation, low quality
If thyroidectomy is chosen for treatment of GD, how should it be accomplished?	Patients should be rendered euthyroid prior to the procedure.	Strong recommendation, moderate quality
How should overt hyperthyroidism due to TMNG or TA be managed?	Patients should be treated with RAI therapy or thyroidectomy.	Weak recommendation, moderate quality
How should GD be managed in children and adolescents?	Children with GD should be treated with MMI, RAI therapy, or thyroidectomy. RAI therapy should be avoided in very young children (<5 years). Under age 5, thyroidectomy should be performed.	Strong recommendation, moderate quality
How should hyperthyroidism in pregnancy be managed?	ATD therapy should be used for overt hyperthyroidism due to GD during pregnancy. PTU should be used when ATD therapy is given during the first trimester. MMI should be used when ATD therapy is started after the first trimester.	Strong recommendation, low quality
How should antithyroid treatment be managed during pregnancy?	GD during pregnancy should be treated with the lowest possible dose of ATDs needed to keep the mother's thyroid hormone levels at or slightly above the reference range for total T_4 and T_3 values in pregnancy (1.5 times above nonpregnant reference ranges in the second and third trimesters), and the TSH below the reference range for pregnancy. Similarly, free T_4 levels should be kept at or slightly above the upper limit of the pregnancy trimester reference range for the assay. Thyroid function should be assessed monthly, and the ATD dose adjusted as required.	Strong recommendation, low quality
How should other causes of thyrotoxicosis be managed?	Patients taking medications known to cause thyrotoxicosis, including interferon (IFN)-α, interleukin-2, tyrosine kinase inhibitors, and lithium, should be monitored clinically and biochemically at 6-month intervals for the development of thyroid dysfunction.	Strong recommendation, low quality

GD, Graves' disease; ^{131}I, radioactive I-131; TMNG, toxic multinodular goiter; TA, toxic adenoma; SH, subclinical hyperthyroidism.

Data from Reference 6.

MMI readily crosses the placenta and appears in breast milk. Older studies suggested that PTU crosses the placental membranes only one-tenth as well as MMI; however, these studies were done in the course of therapeutic abortion early in pregnancy. Newer studies show little difference between fetal concentrations of PTU and MMI, and both are associated with elevated TSH in about 20% and low T_4 in about 7% of fetuses.

4 ***Dosing and Administration*** MMI is available as 5 and 10 mg tablets and PTU as 50 mg tablets. MMI is approximately 10 to 20 times more potent than PTU. Initial therapy with MMI is given in two or three divided doses totaling 30 to 60 mg/day. PTU is given in dose ranges from 300 to 600 mg daily, usually in three or four divided doses. Although the traditional recommendation is for divided doses, evidence exists that both drugs can be given as single daily doses. Patients with severe hyperthyroidism may require larger initial doses, and some may respond better at these larger doses if the dose is divided. The maximal blocking doses of MMI and PTU are 120 and 1,200 mg daily, respectively. Once the intrathyroidal pool of thyroid hormone is reduced and new hormone synthesis is sufficiently blocked, clinical improvement should ensue. Usually, within 4 to 8 weeks of initiating therapy, symptoms will diminish and circulating thyroid hormone levels will return to normal. Now, the tapering regimen can be started. Changes in dose for each drug should be made monthly because the endogenously produced T_4 will reach a new steady-state concentration in this interval. Typical ranges of daily maintenance doses for MMI and PTU are 5 to 30 mg and 50 to 300 mg, respectively.

If the objective of therapy is to induce long-term remission in a patient with Graves' Disease, the patient should remain on continuous antithyroid drug therapy for a minimum of 12 to 24 months. Antithyroid drug therapy induces permanent remission rates of 10% to 98%, with an overall average of about 40% to 50%. This is much higher than the remission rate seen with propranolol alone (22%–36%). Patient characteristics for a favorable outcome include older patients (older than 40 years), low T_4:T_3 ratio (less than 20), a small goiter (less than 50 g), short duration of disease (less than 6 months), no previous history of relapse with ATDs, duration of therapy 1 to 2 years or longer, and low TSAb titers at baseline or a reduction with treatment.[24] A 2012 study provides preliminary evidence that a new assay that has better specificity for detection of antibodies that stimulate the TSH receptors, without detecting coexistent blocking antibodies, may be a useful predictor of remission of Graves' disease.[25]

A remission of Graves' hyperthyroidism most often occurs after 4 to 11 years of treatment, with a better prognosis if TSH binding inhibitor immunoglobulin (TBII) activity disappeared within 5 years without TBII fluctuation or enlargement of the goiter. A longer duration until normalization of TBII and higher final thyroid weight were associated with a poor prognosis.[26]

In another study in which patients were treated for their first episodes of Graves' hyperthyroidism, patients were treated for a minimum of 18 to 24 months of methimazole and then randomized to receive an additional 36 to 102 months of treatment or discontinued methimazole. Patients in both treatment groups were followed 48 months after discontinuing methimazole. Patients who received 60 to 120 months of methimazole were significantly more likely to achieve remission compared to patients who received only an 18- to 24-month course of treatment (85% vs 47%).[27]

A systematic review on remission rates in children with Graves' disease found that 23.7% of the participants achieved remission after 1.5 to 2.5 years of treatment and 75% achieved remission after 9 years of treatment. Adverse events occurred in 17.6% of patients but major side effects occurred in only 1.1%. In summary, longer treatment was associated with greater efficacy and is generally well tolerated.[28]

It is important that patients be followed every 6 to 12 months after remission occurs. If a relapse occurs, alternate therapy with RAI is preferred over a second course of ATDs, however, continued long-term low-dose MMI can be considered.[29] Relapses seem to plateau after about 5 years and eventually, 5% to 20% of patients will develop spontaneous hypothyroidism. Some researchers have speculated whether concurrent administration of T_4 with thionamide therapy for thyrotoxicosis and subclinical hyperthyroidism can reduce autoantibodies directed toward the thyroid gland and improve the remission rate. In general, this approach is not recommended because of the higher rates of side effects seen with the larger doses of ATDs needed for this regimen.[6]

Subclinical hyperthyroidism is defined as a serum TSH below the lower limit of the reference range combined with free T_4 and T_3 concentrations that are normal. Subclinical hyperthyroidism is associated with an increased risk of atrial fibrillation and may be associated with increased all-cause mortality. Some studies show an increased risk of hip fractures in postmenopausal women with subclinical hyperthyroidism. Most practitioners agree that the treatment of older patients (greater than 65 years) with TSH values below 0.1 mIU/L is reasonable. In patients who are younger or have TSH values of 0.1 to 0.4 mIU/L a decision whether to treat the patient for mild hyperthyroidism or to monitor thyroid function depends on the patient's cardiovascular risk factors and bone health.[6,30]

Adverse Effects Minor adverse reactions to MMI and PTU have an overall incidence of 5% to 25% depending on the dose and the drug, whereas major adverse effects occur in 1.5% to 4.6% of patients receiving these drugs.[23] Pruritic maculopapular rashes (sometimes associated with vasculitis based on skin biopsy), arthralgias, and fevers occur in up to 5% of patients and may occur at a greater frequency with higher doses and in children. Rashes often disappear spontaneously but, if persistent, may be managed with antihistamines. Under the supervision of an allergist, desensitization to methimazole is an option for treating patients who experience rash or itching from the drug.[31]

One of the most common side effects is a benign transient leukopenia characterized by a WBC count of less than 4,000/mm^3 (4×10^9/L) This condition occurs in up to 12% of adults and 25% of children and sometimes can be confused with mild leukopenia seen in Graves' disease. This mild leukopenia is not a harbinger of the more serious adverse effect of agranulocytosis, so therapy can usually be continued. If a minor adverse reaction occurs with one ATD, the alternate thiourea may be tried, but cross-sensitivity occurs for about 50% of patients.[23]

Agranulocytosis is one of the serious adverse effects of thiourea drug therapy and is characterized by fever, malaise, gingivitis, oropharyngeal infection, and a granulocyte count less than 250/mm^3 (0.250×10^9/L).[23] These drugs are concentrated in granulocytes, and this reaction may represent a direct toxic effect rather than hypersensitivity. This toxic reaction has occurred with both thioureas, and the incidence varies from 0.5% to 6%. It is higher for patients over age 40 receiving an MMI dose greater than 40 mg/day or the equivalent dose of PTU, and is more frequent with initial MMI doses of 30 mg compared with 15 mg. A systematic review and meta-analysis found strong associations of ATD-induced agranulocytosis with HLAB* 27:05, HLA-B*38:02, and HLA-DRB1*08:03 alleles, especially in carbimazole/methimazole-induced agranulocytosis.[32]

Agranulocytosis usually develops in the first 3 months of therapy. Because the onset is sudden, routine WBC count monitoring has not been recommended. Colony-stimulating factors have been used with some success to restore cell counts to normal, but it is unclear how effective this form of therapy is compared with routine supportive care. Peripheral lymphocytes obtained from patients with PTU-induced agranulocytosis undergo a transformation in the presence of other thionamides, suggesting that these severe reactions are immunologically mediated and patients should not receive other thionamides. Aplastic anemia has been reported with MMI and may be associated with an inhibitor to colony-forming units. Once ATDs are discontinued, clinical improvement is seen over several days to weeks. Patients should be counseled to discontinue therapy and contact their physician when flu-like symptoms such as fever, malaise, or a sore throat develops. Treatment of agranulocytosis requires immediate suspension of the ATD and initiation of broad-spectrum antibiotics. Definitive treatment of hyperthyroidism is subsequently required.[33] Clinicians will often concomitantly provide an order for a complete blood cell count (with WBC count differential) when prescribing MMI or PTU therapy. If the patient becomes ill and is unable to reach the provider, the patient can still visit the nearest laboratory to have potential agranulocytosis diagnosed.

Arthralgias and a lupus-like syndrome (sometimes in the absence of antinuclear antibodies) have been reported in 4% to 5% of patients. This generally occurs after 6 months of therapy. Uncommonly, polymyositis, presenting as proximal muscle weakness and elevated creatine phosphokinase, has been reported with PTU administration. Gastrointestinal intolerance is also reported to occur in 4% to 5% of patients. Hypoprothrombinemia is a rare complication of thionamide therapy. Patients who have experienced a major adverse reaction to one thiourea drug should not be converted to the alternate drug because of cross-sensitivity.[6]

In 2019 the European Medicines Agency (EMA) issued a warning and the product labeling for methimazole was changed to include acute pancreatitis as a serious side effect. This decision was based on six case reports of acute pancreatitis in patients treated with methimazole, developing within 90 days of starting the drug. In one study, ongoing use of methimazole was associated with a 56% increase in the risk of being admitted to the hospital for acute pancreatitis, whereas propylthiouracil was not associated with an increased risk.[34]

Hepatotoxicity can be seen with both MMI and PTU, with a prevalence of approximately 1.3%. At moderate doses, some authors have found that initial hepatic enzyme elevations eventually normalize in most patients with continued therapy. PTU-induced subclinical liver injury is common and is usually transient and asymptomatic. Thus, it has generally been thought that therapy with PTU may be continued with caution in the absence of symptoms and hyperbilirubinemia. However, a 1997 literature review documented

49 cases of hepatotoxicity. Twenty-eight cases were associated with PTU use, and 21 cases were associated with MMI use. The hepatotoxicity was associated with seven deaths and three deaths in the PTU and MMI groups, respectively. There did not appear to be a relationship between the dose or duration of thionamide treatment and outcome. During the past 20 years of PTU use in the United States, 22 adults developed severe hepatotoxicity leading to nine deaths and five liver transplants. The risk of this complication was greater in children (1:2,000) than in adults (1:10,000). A recent reanalysis of data reported to the Food and Drug Administration (FDA) from 1982 to 2008 found that toxicity in children was generally related to higher doses of PTU and that toxicity in both children and adults was associated with therapy lasting more than 4 months in duration.[35] Thus, the American Thyroid Association (ATA) and the FDA recommend against the use of PTU as first-line therapy in either adults or children.[6] One of three exceptions includes the first trimester of pregnancy, when the risk of MMI-induced embryopathy may exceed that of PTU-induced hepatotoxicity. Other exceptions include intolerance to MMI and thyroid storm.

Older reports suggested that congenital skin defects (ie, aplasia cutis) may be caused by MMI and carbimazole, although a registry review from the Netherlands could not find an association between maternal use of these drugs and skin defects. Several serious congenital malformations including tracheoesophageal fistulas and choanal atresia have been observed with MMI and carbimazole but not PTU use during pregnancy. PTU has traditionally been considered the drug of choice throughout pregnancy for women with hyperthyroidism, because of concerns about the possible teratogenic effects of MMI. However, currently heightened concerns about the greater risk of hepatotoxicity with PTU when compared to MMI have led to the recommendation that PTU no longer be considered a first-line drug, except during the first trimester of pregnancy. The choice of antithyroid agent during pregnancy has been further complicated by two studies that suggest that fetuses exposed to either MMI or PTU during gestation may increase the risk of drug-induced fetal malformations. A Danish study revealed that 2% to 3% of children exposed to PTU developed birth defects associated with this therapy.[36] In another study, PTU associated birth defects, though less severe than MMI-associated birth defects, occurred with similar incidence in a Korean population.[37] Recommendations regarding the management of thyroid disease during pregnancy recommends using the lowest effective dose of the ATD as possible, targeting maternal serum FT_4/TT_4 at the upper limit or moderately above the reference range and utilizing a team approach with close collaboration among endocrinologists, maternal-fetal medicine specialists, and neonatologists.[38]

While there is debate regarding optimal therapy of Graves' disease, a study assessing the quality of life (QoL) in patients 6 to 10 years after treatment for Graves' disease with RAI, thyroidectomy, or ATDs. Patients treated with RAI had worse thyroid-related and general QoL than patients treated with ATD or thyroidectomy on the majority of QoL scales. However, regardless of treatment modality, patients with GD had worse thyroid-related QoL 6 to 10 years after diagnosis compared to the general population.[39]

Iodides Iodide was the first form of drug therapy for Graves' disease. Its mechanism of action is to acutely block thyroid hormone release, inhibit thyroid hormone biosynthesis by interfering with intrathyroidal iodide utilization (the Wolff–Chaikoff effect), and decrease the size and vascularity of the gland. This early inhibitory effect provides symptom improvement within 2 to 7 days of initiating therapy, and serum T_4 and T_3 concentrations may be reduced for a few weeks. Despite the reduced release of T_4 and T_3, thyroid hormone synthesis continues at an accelerated rate, resulting in a gland rich in stored hormones. The normal and hyperfunctioning thyroid soon escapes from this inhibitory effect within 1 to 2 weeks by decreasing the active transfer of iodide into the gland. Iodides are often used as adjunctive therapy to prepare a patient with Graves' disease for surgery, to acutely inhibit thyroid hormone release and quickly attain the euthyroid state in severely thyrotoxic patients with cardiac decompensation, or to inhibit thyroid hormone release following RAI therapy. However, large doses of iodine may exacerbate hyperthyroidism or indeed precipitate hyperthyroidism in some previously euthyroid individuals (Jod–Basedow disease). This Jod–Basedow phenomenon is most common in iodine-deficient areas, particularly for patients with pre-existing nontoxic goiter. Iodide is contraindicated in toxic MNG as the autonomous tissue utilizes the iodine for subsequent thyroid hormone synthesis. Although it is not the standard of care in the United States, potassium iodide therapy was effective in two-thirds of cases, and induced remission in approximately 40% of the patients in a Japanese study of hyperthyroid patients with thionamide-associated side effects.[40] Because iodide crosses the placenta and may cause hypothyroidism and goiter in the newborn, its use is generally avoided in pregnant women.

Potassium iodide is available either as a saturated solution (SSKI), which contains 38 mg of iodide per drop or as Lugol's solution, which contains 6.3 mg of iodide per drop. The typical starting dose of SSKI is 3 to 10 drops daily (120-400 mg) in water or juice. There is no documented advantage to using doses in excess of 6 to 8 mg/day. When used to prepare a patient for surgery, it should be administered 7 to 14 days preoperatively. As an adjunct to RAI, SSKI should not be used before, but rather 3 to 7 days after RAI treatment, so that the radioactive iodide can concentrate in the thyroid. The most frequent toxic effects with iodide therapy are hypersensitivity reactions (skin rashes, drug fever, rhinitis, and conjunctivitis), salivary gland swelling, "iodism" (metallic taste, burning mouth and throat, sore teeth and gums, symptoms of a head cold, and sometimes stomach upset and diarrhea), and gynecomastia.

Other compounds containing organic iodide have also been used therapeutically for hyperthyroidism. These include various radiologic contrast media that share a triiodoaminobenzene and monoaminobenzene ring with a propionic acid chain (eg, iopanoic acid and sodium ipodate). The effect of these compounds is a result of the iodine content inhibiting thyroid hormone release as well as competitive inhibition of 5′- monodeiodinase conversion related to their structures, which resemble thyroid analogs. Unfortunately, these extremely useful agents are no longer available in the United States.

5 **Adrenergic Blockers** Because many of the manifestations of hyperthyroidism are mediated by β-adrenergic receptors, β-blockers (especially propranolol) have been used widely to ameliorate symptoms such as palpitations, anxiety, tremor, and heat intolerance. Although β-blockers are quite effective for symptom control, they have no effect on the urinary excretion of calcium, phosphorus, hydroxyproline, creatinine, or various amino acids, suggesting a lack of effect on peripheral thyrotoxicosis and protein metabolism. Furthermore, β-blockers neither reduce TSAb nor prevent thyroid storm. Propranolol and nadolol partially block the conversion of T_4 to T_3, but this contribution to the overall therapeutic effect is small in magnitude. Inhibition of conversion of T_4 to T_3 is mediated by D-propranolol, which is devoid of β-blocking activity, and L-propranolol, which is responsible for the antiadrenergic effects, has little effect on the conversion.

β-Blockers are usually used as adjunctive therapy with ATDs, RAI, or iodides when treating Graves' disease or toxic nodules; in preparation for surgery; or in thyroid storm. The only conditions for which β-blockers are primary therapy for thyrotoxicosis are those associated with thyroiditis. The dose of propranolol required to relieve adrenergic symptoms is variable, but an initial dose of 20 to 40 mg four times daily is effective (goal heart rate less than 90 beats/min) for most patients. Younger or more severely toxic patients may require as much as 240 to 480 mg/day because there seems to be an increased clearance rate for these patients. β-Blockers are contraindicated for patients with decompensated heart failure unless it is caused solely by tachycardia (high output failure). Nonselective agents and those lacking intrinsic sympathomimetic activity should be used with caution for patients with asthma and bronchospastic chronic obstructive lung disease. β-Blockers that are cardioselective and have intrinsic sympathomimetic activity may have a slight margin of safety in these situations. Other patients in whom contraindications exist are those with sinus bradycardia, those receiving monoamine oxidase inhibitors or tricyclic antidepressants, and those with spontaneous hypoglycemia. β-Blockers may also prolong gestation and labor during pregnancy. Other side effects include nausea, vomiting, anxiety, insomnia, light-headedness, bradycardia, and hematologic disturbances.

Antiadrenergic agents such as centrally acting sympatholytics and calcium channel antagonists may have some role in the symptomatic treatment of hyperthyroidism. These drugs might be useful when contraindications to β-blockade exist. When compared with nadolol 40 mg twice daily, clonidine 150 mcg twice daily reduced plasma catecholamines, whereas nadolol increased both epinephrine and norepinephrine after 1 week of treatment. Diltiazem 120 mg given every 8 hours reduced heart rate by 17%; fewer ventricular extrasystoles were noted after 10 days of therapy, and diltiazem has been shown to be comparable to propranolol in lowering heart rate and BP.

Therapeutic plasmapheresis is an effective alternative treatment option to prepare for ablative treatment in patients that have side effects or who do not respond adequately to anti-thyroid drugs.[41] In a retrospective study in patients with Graves' disease, amiodarone-induced thyrotoxicosis, or toxic nodular goiter, the median free triiodothyronine (FT_3) fell from 9.9 pg/mL to 4.0 pg/mL (0.15 pmol/L to 0.06 pmol/L) and FT_4 levels fell from 2.9 ng/dL to 1.6 ng/dL (37.3 pmol/L to 20.6 pmol/L). Each apheresis session lasted for 2.5 to 3 hours and was performed daily until normal thyroid function was achieved (median 4, range 1-7 days).

6 **Radioactive Iodine** Although other radioisotopes have been used to ablate thyroid tissue, ^{131}I is considered to be the agent of choice for Graves' disease, toxic autonomous nodules, and toxic MNGs.[6] RAI is administered as a colorless and tasteless liquid that is well absorbed and concentrates in the thyroid. ^{131}I is a β- and γ-emitter with a tissue penetration of 2 mm and a half-life of 8 days. Other organs take up ^{131}I, but the thyroid gland is the only organ in which organification of the absorbed iodine takes place. Initially, RAI disrupts hormone synthesis by incorporating into thyroid hormones and TG. Over a period of weeks, follicles that have taken up RAI and surrounding follicles develop evidence of cellular necrosis, breakdown of follicles, development of bizarre cell forms, nuclear pyknosis, and destruction of small vessels within the gland, leading to edema and fibrosis of the interstitial tissue. Pregnancy is an absolute contraindication to the use of RAI since radiation will be delivered to the fetal tissue, including the fetal thyroid.

β-Blockers may be given any time without compromising RAI therapy, accounting for their role as a mainstay of adjunctive therapy to RAI treatment. If iodides are administered, they should be given 3 to 7 days after RAI to prevent interference with the uptake of RAI in the thyroid gland. Because thyroid hormone levels will transiently increase following RAI treatment due to the release of preformed thyroid hormone, patients with cardiac disease and elderly patients are often treated with thionamides prior to RAI ablation. For patients with underlying cardiac disease, it may be necessary to reinstitute antithyroid drug therapy following RAI ablation. The standard practice is to withdraw the thionamide 4 to 6 days prior to RAI treatment and to reinstitute it 4 days after therapy is concluded. Administering antithyroid drug therapy immediately following RAI treatment may result in a higher rate of posttreatment recurrence or persistent hyperthyroidism. Pretreatment with PTU may lead to higher rates of treatment failure, but this does not appear to be the case with MMI pretreatment. The use of lithium, as adjunctive therapy to RAI therapy, has multiple benefits of increasing the cure rate, shortening the time to cure, and preventing a post-therapy increase in thyroid hormone levels.[42] Lithium is likely to achieve these effects by increasing RAI retention in the thyroid and inhibiting thyroid hormone release from the gland, although it is not commonly used due to its narrow therapeutic index.

Corticosteroid administration will blunt and delay the rise in antibodies to the TSH receptor, TG, and thyroid peroxidase while reducing T_3 and T_4 concentrations following RAI. Theoretically, if a shared thyroidal and orbital antigen is involved in the pathogenesis of Graves' ophthalmopathy, antigen released with RAI treatment could aggravate pre-existing eye disease. There is some disagreement as to what degree of ophthalmopathy should be considered a contraindication to RAI. However, in those with moderate or severe orbitopathy, it seems reasonable to delay RAI until the patient's eye disease has been stable. Traditionally, corticosteroids, radiation therapy, and surgical correction have been the mainstays of therapy for Graves' ophthalmopathy. Rituximab, tocilizumab, and teprotumumabIn have been assessed in RCTs.[43] In 2020, the FDA approved teprotumumab, a monoclonal anti-insulin-like growth factor I receptor antibody for the treatment of thyroid eye disease. Patients completing the eight-infusion treatment course of teprotumumab over 24 weeks demonstrated significant improvement in proptosis, diplopia, quality of life, and Clinical Activity Score.[44] The most commonly reported adverse events with teprotumumab were muscle spasm (18%), hearing loss (10%), and hyperglycemia (8%).

Destruction of the gland attenuates the hyperthyroid state, and hypothyroidism commonly occurs months to years following RAI.[6,24] The goal of therapy is to destroy overactive thyroid cells, and a single dose of 4,000 to 8,000 rad (40 to 80 Gy) results in a euthyroid state in 60% of patients at 6 months or less. The remaining 40% become euthyroid within 1 year, requiring two or more doses. It is advisable that a second dose of RAI be given 6 months after the first RAI treatment if the patient remains hyperthyroid.[6] Variables that predict an unsuccessful outcome of RAI include gender (men are less likely to develop hypothyroidism), race, the size of the thyroid (euthyroidism is less likely in large glands), the severity of disease, and perhaps a higher level of TSAb. Predictors of successful treatment with RAI included higher ablative dose, female gender, lower free T_4 levels at diagnosis, and absence of a palpable goiter.[24] The acute, short-term side effects of ^{131}I therapy are minimal and include mild thyroidal tenderness and dysphagia. Concern about mutations and congenital defects now appears to be unfounded because long-term follow-up studies have not revealed an increased risk for these complications.[45] Although RAI is very effective in the treatment of hyperthyroidism, long-term follow-up from Great Britain suggests that among patients with hyperthyroidism treated with RAI, mortality from all causes and mortality resulting from cardiovascular and cerebrovascular disease and fracture are increased.

A common approach to Graves' hyperthyroidism is to administer a single dose of 5 to 15 mCi (185 to 555 mBq; 80-200 μCi/g of tissue [3.0 to 7.4 mBq/g]). The optimal method for determining ^{131}I treatment doses for Graves' hyperthyroidism is unknown, and techniques have varied from a fixed dose to more elaborate calculations based on gland size, iodine uptake, and iodine turnover.[6] In a trial of 88 patients with Graves' disease, no difference in outcome was seen among high or low, fixed or adjusted doses. Thyroid glands estimated to weigh more than 80 g may require larger doses of RAI. Larger doses are likely to induce hypothyroidism and are seldom given outside the United States due to the imposition of stringent safety restrictions. For example, in the United Kingdom, a nursery school teacher is advised to stay out of school for 3 weeks following a 15 mCi (555 mBq) dose of ^{131}I.

Special Populations

Graves' Disease and Pregnancy

Inappropriate increase in the production of hCG is a cause of abnormal thyroid function tests during the first half of pregnancy, and hCG can cause either subclinical (normal T_4 and suppressed TSH) or overt hyperthyroidism. This is because the homology of hCG and TSH leads to hCG-mediated stimulation through the TSH receptor. At hCG concentrations greater than 400 IU/mL (kIU/L), TSH levels were invariably suppressed and free T_4 levels were generally above the normal range. Most patients with hCG greater than 200 IU/mL (kIU/L) did not have symptoms of hyperthyroidism. The variability of the thyrotropic potency of hCG is believed to depend on its carbohydrate composition.

A very comprehensive guideline has been published by the ATA regarding the management of thyroid disease during pregnancy.[38] Hyperthyroidism during pregnancy is almost solely caused by Graves' disease, with approximately 0.1% to 0.4% of pregnancies affected. Although the increased metabolic rate is usually well tolerated in pregnant women, two symptoms suggestive of hyperthyroidism during pregnancy are failure to gain weight despite a good appetite and persistent tachycardia. There is no increase in maternal mortality or morbidity in well-controlled patients. However, postpartum thyroid storm has been reported in about 20% of untreated individuals. Fetal loss is also more common, due to the fact that spontaneous abortion and premature delivery are more common in untreated pregnant women, as are low-birth-weight infants and eclampsia. Transplacental passage of TSAb may occur, causing fetal as well as neonatal hyperthyroidism. An uncommon cause of hyperthyroidism is molar pregnancy; women present with a large-for-dates uterus and evacuation of the uterus is the preferred management approach.

Because RAI is contraindicated in pregnancy and surgery is usually not recommended (especially during the first trimester), antithyroid drug therapy is usually the treatment of choice for hyperthyroidism. MMI readily crosses the placenta and appears in breast milk.

As previously mentioned, propylthiouracil has been considered the drug of choice during the first trimester of pregnancy, with the lowest possible doses used to maintain the maternal T_4 level in the high-normal range.[38] During this period the risk of MMI-associated embryopathy is believed to outweigh that of PTU-associated hepatotoxicity. To prevent fetal goiter and suppression of fetal thyroid function, PTU is usually prescribed in daily doses of 300 mg or less and tapered to 50 to 150 mg daily after 4 to 6 weeks. PTU doses of less than 200 mg daily are unlikely to produce fetal goiter. During the second and third trimesters, when the critical period of organogenesis is complete, MMI has been thought to be the drug of choice because of the greater risk of hepatotoxicity with PTU.[38] However, it is unclear whether this strategy of switching thionamides, and thus exposing the fetus to both drugs, is the optimum approach.[36] Thionamide doses should be adjusted to maintain free T_4 within 10% of the upper normal limit of the nonpregnant reference range. During the last trimester, TSAbs fall spontaneously, and some patients will go into remission so that ATD doses may be reduced. A rebound in maternal hyperthyroidism occurs in about 10% of women postpartum and may require more intensive treatment than in the last trimester of pregnancy.

Neonatal and Pediatric Hyperthyroidism

Following delivery, some babies of hyperthyroid mothers will be hyperthyroid due to placental transfer of TSAbs, which stimulates thyroid hormone production in utero and postpartum. This is likely if the maternal TSAb titers were quite high. The disease is usually expressed 7 to 10 days postpartum and treatment with ATDs (PTU 5-10 mg/kg/day or MMI 0.5-1 mg/kg/day) may be needed for as long as 8 to 12 weeks until the antibody is cleared (immunoglobulin G half-life is about 2 weeks). Iodide (potassium iodide one drop per day or Lugol's solution one to three drops per day) and sodium ipodate may be used for the first few days to acutely inhibit hormone release.

Childhood hyperthyroidism has classically been managed with either MMI or PTU. Long-term follow-up studies suggest that this form of therapy is quite acceptable, with 25% of a cohort experiencing remission every 2 years. Again, current recommendations suggest using MMI as a first-line agent in both adults and children.[6]

Thyroid Storm

Thyroid storm is a life-threatening medical emergency characterized by decompensated thyrotoxicosis, high fever (often more than 39.4°C [103°F]), tachycardia, tachypnea, dehydration, delirium, coma, nausea, vomiting, and diarrhea.[8] Graves' disease and less commonly toxic nodular goiter are usually the underlying thyrotoxic pathology.

Precipitating factors for thyroid storm include infection, trauma, surgery, RAI treatment, and withdrawal from ATDs. Although the duration of clinical decompensation lasts for an average duration of 72 hours, symptoms may persist up to 8 days. With aggressive treatment, the mortality rate has been lowered to 20%. The following therapeutic measures should be instituted promptly: (a) suppression of thyroid hormone formation and secretion, (b) antiadrenergic therapy, (c) administration of corticosteroids, and (d) treatment of associated complications or coexisting factors that may have precipitated the storm. Specific agents used in thyroid storm are outlined in Table 96-7. PTU in large doses may be the preferred thionamide because, in addition to interfering with the production of thyroid hormones, it also blocks the peripheral conversion of T_4 to T_3. However, β-blockers and corticosteroids will serve the same purpose. A theoretical advantage of MMI is that it has a longer duration of action. If patients are unable to take medications orally, the tablets can be crushed into suspension and instilled by a gastric or rectal tube. Iodides, which rapidly block the release of preformed thyroid hormone, should be administered after thionamide is initiated to inhibit iodide utilization by the overactive gland. If iodide is administered first, it could theoretically provide a substrate to produce even higher levels of thyroid hormone.

Antiadrenergic therapy with the short-acting agent esmolol is preferred, both because it may be used in the patient with pulmonary disease or at risk for cardiac failure and because its effects may be rapidly reversed. Corticosteroids are generally recommended,

TABLE 96-7 Drug Dosages Used in the Management of Thyroid Storm

Drug	Regimen
Propylthiouracil	900-1,200 mg/day orally in four or six divided doses
Methimazole	90-120 mg/day orally in four or six divided doses
Sodium iodide	Up to 2 g/day IV in single or divided doses
Lugol's solution	5-10 drops three times a day in water or juice
Saturated solution of potassium iodide (SSKI)	1-2 drops three times a day in water or juice
Propranolol	40-80 mg every 6 hours
Dexamethasone	5-20 mg/day orally or IV in divided doses
Prednisone	25-100 mg/day orally in divided doses
Methylprednisolone	20-80 mg/day IV in divided doses
Hydrocortisone	100-400 mg/day IV in divided doses

although there is no convincing evidence of adrenocortical insufficiency in thyroid storm, and the benefits derived from steroids may be caused by their antipyretic action and their effect of stabilizing BP.[8] General supportive measures, including acetaminophen as an antipyretic (do not use aspirin or other NSAIDs because they may displace bound thyroid hormone), fluid and electrolyte replacement, sedatives, digitalis, antiarrhythmics, insulin, and antibiotics, should be given as indicated. Plasmapheresis and peritoneal dialysis have been used to remove excess hormone (and to remove thyroid-stimulating immunoglobulins in Graves' disease) when the patient has not responded to more conservative measures, although these measures do not always work.

EVALUATION OF THERAPEUTIC OUTCOMES—THYROTOXICOSIS

After therapy (surgery, thionamides, or RAI) for hyperthyroidism has been initiated, patients should be evaluated on a monthly basis until they reach a euthyroid condition. Clinical signs of continuing thyrotoxicosis (tachycardia, weight loss, and heat intolerance, among others) or the development of hypothyroidism (bradycardia, weight gain, and lethargy, among others) should be noted. β-Blockers may be used to control symptoms of thyrotoxicosis until the definitive treatment has returned the patient to a euthyroid state. If T_4 replacement is initiated, the goal is to maintain both the free T_4 level and the TSH concentration in the normal range. Once a stable dose of T_4 is identified, the patient may be followed up every 6 to 12 months.

A common, potentially confusing clinical situation should be mentioned. Some patients may have TSH concentrations that continue to be suppressed despite having free T_4 concentrations that become normal or low. For patients with long-standing hyperthyroidism, the pituitary thyrotrophs are responsible for making TSH become atrophic. The average amount of time required for these cells to resume normal functioning is 6 to 8 weeks. Therefore, if a thyrotoxic patient has his or her free T_4 concentration lowered rapidly before the thyrotrophs resume normal function, a period of "transient central hypothyroidism" will be observed. In addition, autoimmune mechanisms may also play a role, with a slower TSH recovery in patients with higher titers of thyroid-binding inhibitory immunoglobulins.

CONCLUSION—HYPERTHYROIDISM

Management of hyperthyroidism includes treatment with ATDs, RAI, or thyroidectomy. Optimal treatment is patient-specific, depending on patient clinical presentation, including age, history of arrhythmias or atherosclerotic disease, goiter size, and severity of thyrotoxicosis. ATDs are the primary therapy during pregnancy.

HYPOTHYROIDISM

Hypothyroidism is defined as the clinical and biochemical syndrome resulting from decreased thyroid hormone production.[46] Biochemically, primary hypothyroidism is defined as TSH concentrations above the reference range and FT_4 and/or triiodothyronine levels below the reference range.

EPIDEMIOLOGY—HYPOTHYROIDISM

Overt hypothyroidism occurs in 1.5% to 2% of women and 0.2% of men, and its incidence increases with age. In the Third National Health and Nutrition Examination Survey (NHANES III), levels of serum TSH and total T_4 were measured in a representative sample of adolescents and adults (age 12 or older). Among 16,533 people who neither were taking thyroid medication nor reported histories of thyroid disease, 3.9% had subclinical hypothyroidism (serum TSH more than 4.5 mIU/L, and T_4 normal), and 0.2% had "clinically significant" hypothyroidism (TSH more than 4.5 mIU/L, and T_4 less than 4.5 mcg/dL [58 nmol/L]).[7] Subclinical hypothyroidism is commonly regarded as a sign of impending thyroid failure.

ETIOLOGY AND PATHOPHYSIOLOGY—HYPOTHYROIDISM

The vast majority of patients have primary hypothyroidism due to thyroid gland failure caused by chronic autoimmune thyroiditis. Special populations with higher risk of developing hypothyroidism include postpartum women, individuals with a family history of autoimmune thyroid disorders and patients with previous head and neck or thyroid irradiation or surgery, other autoimmune endocrine conditions (eg, type 1 diabetes mellitus, adrenal insufficiency, and ovarian failure), some other nonendocrine autoimmune disorders (eg, celiac disease, vitiligo, pernicious anemia, Sjögren's syndrome, and multiple sclerosis), primary pulmonary hypertension, and Down's and Turner's syndromes.

Central hypothyroidism is rare and affects both sexes equally. It is more often associated with pituitary than hypothalamic disorders but frequently involves both.[47] Biochemically, central hypothyroidism is defined by low or low-to-normal TSH concentrations and a disproportionately low concentration of FT_4. Secondary hypothyroidism due to pituitary failure is uncommon but should be suspected in a patient with decreased levels of T_4 and inappropriately normal or low TSH levels. Most patients with secondary hypothyroidism due to inadequate TSH production will have clinical signs of more generalized pituitary insufficiency, such as abnormal menses and decreased libido, or evidence of a pituitary adenoma, such as visual field defects, galactorrhea, or acromegaloid features, but isolated TSH deficiency can be congenital or acquired as a result of autoimmune hypophysitis.[48] Generalized (peripheral and central) resistance to thyroid hormone is extremely rare.

Table 96-8 outlines the causes of hypothyroidism. These causes fall into two broad categories involving dysfunction of the thyroid gland (primary hypothyroidism) or dysfunction of the pituitary or hypothalamus (secondary hypothyroidism).

Chronic Autoimmune Thyroiditis

7 Autoimmune thyroiditis (Hashimoto's disease) is the most common cause of spontaneous hypothyroidism in the adult.[46] Patients may present either with goitrous thyroid gland enlargement and mild hypothyroidism or with thyroid gland atrophy and more severe thyroid hormone deficiency. Both forms of autoimmune thyroiditis probably result from cell- and antibody-mediated thyroid injury. The presence of specific defects in suppressor T-lymphocyte function leads to the survival of a randomly mutating clone of helper T lymphocytes, which are directed against normally occurring antigens on the thyroid membrane. Once these T lymphocytes

TABLE 96-8 Causes of Hypothyroidism

Primary hypothyroidism
Hashimoto's disease
Iatrogenic hypothyroidism
Less common:
- Iodine deficiency
- Enzyme defects
- Thyroid hypoplasia
- Goitrogens

Secondary hypothyroidism
Pituitary disease
Hypothalamic disease

CLINICAL PRESENTATION Hypothyroidism

General

- Hypothyroidism can lead to a variety of end-organ effects with a wide range of disease severity, from entirely asymptomatic to coma with multisystem failure. In the adult, manifestations of hypothyroidism are nonspecific. In the child, thyroid hormone deficiency may manifest as delays in growth or intellectual development.
- Thyroid hormone is essential for normal growth and development during embryonic life. Uncorrected thyroid hormone deficiency during fetal and neonatal development results in mental retardation and/or cretinism. Both in children and adults, there is a slowing of physical and mental activity, as well as of cardiovascular, gastrointestinal, and neuromuscular function.

Symptoms

- Common symptoms of hypothyroidism include dry skin, cold intolerance, weight gain, constipation, and weakness.
- Complaints of lethargy, depression, fatigue, exercise intolerance, or loss of ambition and energy are also common but are less specific.
- Muscle cramps, myalgia, and stiffness are frequent complaints of hypothyroid patients.
- Menorrhagia and infertility may present commonly in women.

Signs

- Objective weakness is common, with proximal muscles being affected more than distal muscles. Slow relaxation of deep tendon reflexes is common.
- The most common signs of decreased levels of thyroid hormone include coarse skin and hair, cold or dry skin, periorbital puffiness, and bradycardia.
- Speech is often slow, and the voice may be hoarse.
- Reversible neurologic syndromes such as carpal tunnel syndrome, polyneuropathy, and cerebellar dysfunction may also occur.
- Galactorrhea may be found in women.

Diagnosis

- A rise in the TSH is the first evidence of hypothyroidism in primary hypothyroidism.
- In secondary hypothyroidism in patients with pituitary disease, serum TSH concentrations are generally low or normal. A serum TSH concentration in the normal range is clearly inappropriate if the patient's T_4 is low.
- Many patients will have a free T_4 level within the normal range (compensated or subclinical hypothyroidism), with few, if any, symptoms of hypothyroidism. As the disease progresses, the free T_4 concentration will drop below the normal level. With increased TSH stimulation, thyroidal production will shift toward greater amounts of T_3, and thus T_3 concentrations will often be maintained in the normal range in spite of a low T4. Eventually, free and/or total T_4 and T_3 serum concentrations should be low.

Other Tests

- TPOAbs and anti-TG antibodies are likely to be elevated in autoimmune thyroiditis.

interact with thyroid membrane antigen, B lymphocytes are stimulated to produce thyroid antibodies. Readers are referred to an excellent review regarding biochemical testing in thyroid disorders.[49] Antithyroid peroxidase (antimicrosomal) antibodies are present in virtually all patients with Hashimoto's thyroiditis and appear to be directed against the enzyme thyroid peroxidase. These antibodies are capable of fixing complement and inducing cytotoxic changes in thyroid cells. Antibodies that are capable of stimulating thyroid growth through interaction with the TSH receptor may occasionally be found particularly in goitrous hypothyroidism; conversely, antibodies that inhibit the trophic effects of TSH may be present in the atrophic type.

Iatrogenic Hypothyroidism

Iatrogenic hypothyroidism follows exposure to destructive amounts of radiation (radioiodine or external radiation) or surgery. Hypothyroidism occurs within 3 months to a year after ^{131}I therapy in most patients treated for Graves' disease. Thereafter, it occurs at a rate of approximately 2.5% each year. External radiation therapy to the region of the thyroid using doses of greater than 2,500 centigray (cGy) for therapy of neck carcinoma also causes hypothyroidism. This effect is dose-dependent and more than 50% of patients who receive more than 4,000 cGy to the thyroid bed develop hypothyroidism. Total thyroidectomy causes hypothyroidism within 1 month. Excessive doses of thionamides used to treat hyperthyroidism can also cause iatrogenic hypothyroidism.

Other Causes of Primary Hypothyroidism

Iodine deficiency, enzymatic defects within the thyroid gland, thyroid hypoplasia, and maternal ingestion of goitrogens during fetal development may cause cretinism. Early recognition and treatment of the resultant thyroid hormone deficiency is essential for optimal mental development. Large-scale neonatal screening programs in North America, Europe, Japan, and Australia are now in place. The frequency of congenital hypothyroidism in North America and Europe is 1 per 3,500 to 4,000 live births. In the United States, there are racial differences in the incidence of congenital hypothyroidism, with White patients being affected seven times as frequently as Black patients.

In the adult, hypothyroidism is rarely caused by iodine deficiency and goitrogens. Iodine ingestion in the form of expectorants can lead to hypothyroidism. In sensitive persons (particularly those with autoimmune thyroiditis), the iodide blocks the synthesis of thyroid hormone, leading to increased secretion of TSH and thyroid enlargement. Thus, both iodine excess and iodine deficiency can cause decreased secretion of thyroid hormone. An example of a goitrogen that can induce hypothyroidism is raw bok choy. Several medications can cause hypothyroidism, including lithium,

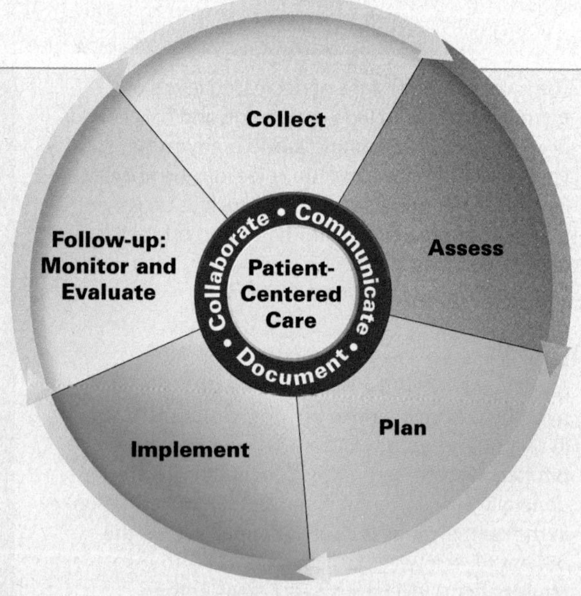

Patient Care Process for the Management of Hypothyroidism

The image shows the five fundamental steps included in The Pharmacist's Care Process endorsed by the Joint Commission for Pharmacy Practitioners (2014). The tagline of this process reads collaborate, communicate, and document. The five fundamental steps listed here are collect, assess, plan, implement, and follow-up: monitor and evaluate. All these steps are listed in a circular block diagram.

Collect

- Patient characteristics (eg, age, race, sex, pregnancy status)
- Patient history (past medical, family, social) including signs and symptoms: coarse skin and hair, cold or dry skin, periorbital puffiness, and bradycardia; cold intolerance, weight gain, constipation, weakness, muscle cramps, myalgia, and galactorrhea (see Clinical Presentation Box)
- Current medications (including OTC and herbal medication use)
- Objective data
  - Heart rate, BP, weight, and BMI
  - Labs (eg, TSH, FT_4, TT_3, anti-TG antibodies, TPO antibodies; serum electrolytes, Scr, ALT)
  - Other diagnostic tests when indicated (eg, thyroid ultrasound, RAIU scan)

Assess

- Cause of hypothyroidism (see Table 96-8)
- Current medications that may contribute to or worsen hypothyroidism
- Current medications that may interact with thyroid hormone replacement therapy
- Appropriateness and effectiveness of current thyroid hormone replacement regimen

Plan*

- Drug therapy regimen including specific thyroid hormone replacement therapy and dose (see Table 96-9)
- Monitoring parameters including efficacy (eg, resolution of signs and symptoms) and safety (arrhythmias, angina, osteoporosis, or symptomatic hyperthyroidism), laboratory data (TSH, FT_4, TT_3), and follow-up monitoring time frame
- Patient education (eg, purpose of treatment, dietary and lifestyle modification, drug therapy)

Implement*

- Provide patient education regarding all elements of the treatment plan
- Use motivational interviewing and coaching strategies to maximize adherence
- Schedule follow-up visits and laboratory tests

Follow-up: Monitor and Evaluate

- Resolution of signs and symptoms
- Presence of adverse effects
- Patient adherence to treatment plan using multiple sources of information

Collaborate with patient, caregivers, and other healthcare professionals.

amiodarone, interferon-α, interleukin-2, tyrosine kinase inhibitors, perchlorate, and checkpoint inhibitors.[50]

Pituitary Disease

TSH is required for normal thyroid secretion. Thyroid atrophy and decreased thyroid secretion follow pituitary failure. Pituitary insufficiency may be caused by the destruction of thyrotrophs by either functioning or nonfunctioning pituitary tumors, surgical therapy, external pituitary radiation, postpartum pituitary necrosis (Sheehan's syndrome), trauma, and infiltrative processes of the pituitary such as metastatic tumors, tuberculosis, histiocytosis, and autoimmune mechanisms.[51] In all these situations, TSH deficiency most often occurs in association with other pituitary hormone deficiencies. The identification of secondary hypothyroidism due to bexarotene use has led to a recognition of the role of rexinoids and retinoids to cause dysregulation of TSH production.[52]

Note that pituitary enlargement in hypothyroidism does not invariably indicate the presence of a primary pituitary tumor. Pituitary enlargement is seen in patients with severe primary hypothyroidism due to compensatory hyperplasia and hypertrophy of the thyrotrophs. With thyroid hormone replacement therapy, serum TSH concentrations decline, indicating that the TSH secretion is not autonomous, and the pituitary resumes a more normal configuration. These patients are easily separated from patients with primary pituitary failure by measuring a TSH level.

Hypothalamic Disease

TRH deficiency also causes a rare form of secondary hypothyroidism (also referred to as tertiary hypothyroidism). In both adults and children, it may occur from cranial irradiation, trauma, infiltrative diseases, or neoplastic diseases.

TREATMENT

Hypothyroidism

Most cases of hypothyroidism result from progressive and permanent damage to the thyroid gland. Replacement of thyroid hormone is the cornerstone of treatment.

Desired Outcomes

The goals of therapy are to restore normal thyroid hormone concentrations in tissue, provide symptomatic relief, prevent neurologic deficits in newborns and children, and reverse the biochemical abnormalities of hypothyroidism.

General Approach to Treatment

8 Levothyroxine (L-thyroxine, T_4) is considered to be the drug of choice for treatment of hypothyroidism (Table 96-9).[18] Other commercially available thyroid preparations can be obtained but are not considered preferred therapy. Available thyroid preparations are synthetic (L-thyroxine, liothyronine, and liotrix) or natural in origin (ie, desiccated thyroid). The preparations containing both T_4 and T_3 (liotrix, desiccated thyroid) have relatively high proportions of T_3 and may cause thyrotoxicosis.[18] Liothyronine is a short-acting preparation that requires dosing multiple times a day in order to achieve stable hormone concentrations. The availability of sensitive and specific assays for total and free hormone levels as well as TSH now allows precise dose titration to make adequate replacement without inadvertent overdose. The response of TSH to TRH had been advocated for use by some in order to "fine tune" thyroid replacement, but this is not necessary if the third-generation chemiluminometric assays for TSH, which have detection limits of about 0.01 mIU/L, are used. Clinical guidelines for the management of hypothyroidism have been published by the ATA and provide specific treatment recommendations and critically examine the use of combination therapy with T_4 and T_3[18] (Table 96-10).

Pharmacologic Therapy

Levothyroxine is the drug of choice for thyroid replacement and suppressive therapy because it is chemically stable, relatively inexpensive, active when orally administered, free of antigenicity, and has uniform potency. Levothyroxine (T_4) administration results in a pool of thyroid hormones that is readily converted to T_3 when needed; in this regard, levothyroxine may be thought of as a prohormone.

Liothyronine (T_3) is chemically pure with a known potency and has a shorter half-life of 1.5 days. Although it can be used diagnostically in the T_3 suppression test, T_3 has some clinical disadvantages, including a higher incidence of cardiac adverse effects, higher cost, and difficulty in monitoring with conventional laboratory tests. If used, T_3 needs to be administered three times a day and it may take a prolonged period of adjustment to achieve stable euthyroidism. Liotrix is a combination of synthetic T_4 and T_3 in a 4:1 ratio. It is chemically stable and pure and has a predictable potency. The major limitations to this product are high cost and lack of therapeutic rationale because most T_3 is peripherally converted from T_4. In addition, the T_4:T_3 ratio is much higher than the 14:1 molar ratio produced by the thyroid gland in humans.

9 The use of combination therapy of levothyroxine and liothyronine remains highly controversial with conflicting results from clinical trials.[53] The American Thyroid Association, British Thyroid Association, and European Thyroid Association reviewed the latest basic science and clinical evidence regarding thyroid hormone combination therapy and published a position statement to guide the design of future clinical trials of T_4/T_3 therapy.[54] A well-designed, adequately powered clinical trial of combination therapy in patients dissatisfied with levothyroxine replacement therapy is anticipated.

A study conducted in rats suggested impairment of type 2 deiodinase activity in the whole body during levothyroxine monotherapy due to deiodinase inactivation, compared with maintenance of deiodinase activity in the hypothalamus.[55] The lesser activation in the hypothalamus leads to efficient T_3 production in the hypothalamus and normalization of TSH before T_3 is normalized in the rest of the body. Accompanying the inactivation of type 2 deiodinase in other tissues, lower serum T_3 and higher T_4/T_3 ratios were seen in rats during monotherapy with L-thyroxine, compared with combination therapy employing a subcutaneous slow-release T_3 pellet. Clinical trials of a slow-release T_3 preparation, other than a pharmacokinetic study of T_3 sulfate in profoundly hypothyroid individuals,[56] has yet to be conducted.

Desiccated thyroid has historically been derived from pig, beef, or sheep thyroid glands, although pigs are currently the usual source. The United States Pharmacopeia requires thyroid USP to contain

TABLE 96-9 Thyroid Preparations Used in the Treatment of Hypothyroidism

Drug (Brand Name)	Dosage Form	Content	Relative Dose	Comments/Equivalency
Thyroid USP (Armour Thyroid, Nature-Throid, Westhroid, WP Thyroid) T_4:T_3 ratio approximately 4.2:1	Doses include 1/4, 1/2, 1, 2, 3, 4, and 5 grain tabletsArmour 1 grain = 60 mg; Nature-Throid and Westhroid, 1 grain = 65 mg.	Desiccated pork thyroid gland	1 grain (equivalent to 74 mcg of T_4)	High T_3:T_4 ratio; inexpensive
Levothyroxine (Euthyrox, Levoxyl, Synthroid,Unithroid,Tirosint, and Tirosint-SOL)	25, 50, 75, 88, 100, 112, 125, 137, 150, 175, 200, 300 mcg tablets Tirosint 13-150 mcg liquid in gelatin capsule Liquid solution: 13, 25, 50, 75, 88, 100, 112, 125, 137, 150, 175, and 200 mcg in unit-dose ampules injection: 200 and 500 mcg per vial	Synthetic T_4	100 mcg	Stable; predictable potency; generics may be bioequivalent; when switching from natural thyroid to L-thyroxine, lower dose by one-half grain; variable absorption between products; half-life = 7 days, so daily dosing; considered to be drug of choice
Liothyronine (Cytomel)	5, 25, and 50 mcg tablets	Synthetic T_3	33 mcg (~equivalent to 100 mcg T_4)	Uniform absorption, rapid onset; half-life = 1.5 days, rapid peak and troughs
Liotrix (Thyrolar)	1/4-, 1/2-, 1-, 2-, and 3-grain tablets	Synthetic T_4:T_3 in 4:1 ratio	Thyrolar 1 = 50 mcg T_4 and 12.5 mcg T_3 (~equivalent to 100 mcg T_4)	Stable; predictable; expensive; risk of T_3 thyrotoxicosis because of high ratio of T_3 relative to T_4

TABLE 96-10 Selected Recommendations from the American Thyroid Association Hypothyroidism Guidelines

Question	Synopsis or Paraphrase of Recommendation	Grading
Is levothyroxine monotherapy considered to be the standard of care for hypothyroidism?	Levothyroxine is recommended as the preparation of choice for the treatment of hypothyroidism due to its efficacy in resolving the symptoms of hypothyroidism.	Strong recommendation, moderate quality
What are the clinical and biochemical goals for levothyroxine replacement in primary hypothyroidism?	Levothyroxine replacement therapy has three main goals. These are (i) to provide resolution of the patients' symptoms and hypothyroid signs, (ii) to achieve normalization of serum thyrotropin, and (iii) to avoid overtreatment.	Strong recommendation, moderate quality
Are there situations in which therapy with levothyroxine dissolved in glycerin and supplied in gelatin capsules may have advantages over standard levothyroxine?	Although there are preliminary small studies suggesting that levothyroxine dissolved in glycerin and supplied in gelatin capsules may be better absorbed than standard levothyroxine, the present lack of controlled long-term outcome studies does not support a recommendation for the use of such preparations in these circumstances.	Weak recommendation, low quality
What factors determine the levothyroxine dose required by a hypothyroid patient for reaching the appropriate serum thyrotropin goal?	When deciding on a starting dose of levothyroxine, the patient's weight, lean body mass, pregnancy status, etiology of hypothyroidism, degree of thyrotropin elevation, age, and general clinical context should all be considered.	Strong recommendation, moderate quality
What is the best approach to initiating and adjusting levothyroxine therapy?	Thyroid hormone therapy should be initiated as an initial full replacement or as a partial replacement with gradual increments in the dose titrated upward using serum thyrotropin as the goal. Dose adjustments should be made, with thyrotropin assessment 4-6 weeks after any dosage change.	Strong recommendation, moderate quality
What approach should be taken in patients treated for hypothyroidism who have normal serum thyrotropin values but still have unresolved symptoms?	A minority of patients with hypothyroidism, but normal serum thyrotropin values, may perceive a suboptimal health status of unclear etiology. Acknowledgment of the patients' symptoms and evaluation for alternative causes is recommended in such cases.	Weak recommendation, low quality
In adults requiring thyroid hormone replacement treatment for primary hypothyroidism, is treatment with thyroid extracts superior to treatment with levothyroxine alone?	We recommend that levothyroxine be considered as routine care for patients with primary hypothyroidism, in preference to use of thyroid extracts. High-quality controlled long-term outcome data are lacking to document the superiority of this treatment compared to levothyroxine therapy.	Strong recommendation, moderate quality
In adults requiring thyroid hormone replacement treatment for primary hypothyroidism, is combination treatment including levothyroxine and liothyronine superior to the use of levothyroxine alone?	There is no consistently strong evidence of superiority of combination therapy over monotherapy with levothyroxine. Therefore, we recommend against the routine use of combination treatment with levothyroxine and liothyronine as a form of thyroid replacement therapy in patients with primary hypothyroidism.	Weak recommendation, moderate quality
In adults requiring thyroid hormone replacement treatment for primary hypothyroidism who feel unwell while taking levothyroxine, is combination treatment including levothyroxine and liothyronine superior to the use of levothyroxine alone?	For patients with primary hypothyroidism who feel unwell on levothyroxine therapy alone, there is currently insufficient evidence to support the routine use of a trial of a combination of levothyroxine and liothyronine therapy outside a formal clinical trial or N-of-1 trial, due to uncertainty in the long-term risk-benefit ratio of the treatment.	Insufficient evidence
Are there data regarding therapy with triiodothyronine alone, either as standard liothyronine or as sustained release triiodothyronine, that support the use of triiodothyronine therapy alone for the treatment of hypothyroidism?	Although short-term outcome data in hypothyroid patients suggest that thrice-daily synthetic liothyronine may be associated with beneficial effects on parameters such as weight and lipids, longer-term controlled clinical trials are needed before considering synthetic liothyronine therapy for routine clinical use.	Strong recommendation, moderate quality

Data from Reference 10.

Strong recommendation: Benefits clearly outweigh risks and burden, or risks and burden clearly outweigh benefits. Weak recommendation: Benefits finely balanced with risks and burden. Quality of evidence: High, moderate, or low.

38 mcg (±15%) of L-thyroxine and 9 mcg (±10%) of liothyronine for each 60 to 65 mg (one grain). Thyroid USP, as an animal protein-derived product, may be antigenic in allergic or sensitive patients. Even though desiccated thyroid is inexpensive, its limitations preclude it from being considered as a drug of choice for hypothyroid patients.

Pharmacokinetics

The half-life of levothyroxine is approximately 7 days. This long half-life is responsible for a stable pool of prohormone and the need for only once-daily dosing with levothyroxine. Older studies with levothyroxine suggested that bioavailability was low and erratic; however, this product has been reformulated, and the average bioavailability improved to approximately 80%. Different levothyroxine preparations contain different excipients such as dyes and fillers. However, because the relationship between T_4 concentration and TSH is not linear, very small changes in T_4 concentration can lead to substantial changes in TSH, which is a more accurate reflection of hormone replacement status. The FDA mandates that L-thyroxine bioequivalency testing be done using normal volunteers (600 mcg in the fasted state) and three baseline free T_4 concentrations be used to correct for endogenous T_4 production. Bioequivalency is based on the area under the curve (AUC) and maximum concentration (C_{max}) of T_4 out to 48 hours. Approximately 70% of the AUC is derived from endogenous production. TSH is not considered, and it is now very clear that T_4 is too insensitive as a measure of bioequivalency.[57] To avoid overtreatment and undertreatment, once a product is selected, switches between levothyroxine products in patients who are stable are not recommended. Several levothyroxine products are available, including AB1, AB2, AB3, and AB4 rated products. This has created several permutations for product interchangeability since no reference drug is mandated in bioequivalency testing.

Adverse Effects

Serious untoward effects are unusual if dosing is appropriate and the patient is carefully monitored during the initial treatment. Suboptimal thyroid hormone therapy including under-replacement and over-replacement is common among patients with hypothyroidism.[58] Levothyroxine replacement in athyreotic hypothyroid patients restores systolic and diastolic left ventricular performance within 2 weeks, and the use of levothyroxine may increase the frequency of atrial premature beats but not necessarily ventricular premature beats. Excessive doses of thyroid hormone may lead to heart failure, atrial fibrillation, angina pectoris, and myocardial infarction; rarely, the latter may be caused by coronary artery spasm. Allergic or idiosyncratic reactions can occur with natural animal-derived products such as desiccated thyroid, but these are extremely rare with the synthetic products used today. The 0.05 mg (50 mcg) Synthroid tablet is the least allergenic (due to a lack of dye and few excipients) and should be tried for the patient suspected to be allergic to thyroid hormone tablets.

Hyper-remodeling of cortical and trabecular bone due to hyperthyroidism leads to reduced bone density and may increase the risk of fracture. Compared with normal controls, excess exogenous thyroid hormone results in histomorphometric and biochemical changes similar to those observed in osteoporosis and untreated hyperthyroidism.[59] The risk for this complication seems to be related to the dose of levothyroxine, patient age, and gender. Markers for bone turnover include urinary *N*-telopeptides, pyridinoline crosslinks of type I collagen, osteocalcin, procollagen type 1 N-terminal propeptide, and bone-specific alkaline phosphatase. When doses of levothyroxine are used to suppress TSH concentrations to below-normal values (eg, less than 0.3 mIU/L) in postmenopausal women, this adverse effect is more likely to be seen. Cortical bone is affected to a greater degree than trabecular bone at suppressive doses of L-thyroxine. In contrast, it appears to be much less likely in men and in premenopausal women. Maintaining the TSH between 0.7 and 1.5 mIU/L does not alter bone mineral density in premenopausal women. Although not all studies have shown consistent results, a cohort study suggests that treatment with L-thyroxine to achieve a normal TSH has no adverse effect on bone density.[60]

Drug-Drug and Drug-Food Interactions

The time to maximal absorption of levothyroxine is about 2 hours and this should be considered when T_4 concentrations are determined. Ingestion of L-thyroxine with food can impair its absorption.[18] This can potentially affect the TSH concentration achieved if levothyroxine timing with respect to food is varied. Mucosal diseases, such as celiac sprue, diabetic diarrhea, and ileal bypass surgery, can also reduce absorption. Cholestyramine, calcium carbonate, sucralfate, aluminum hydroxide, ferrous sulfate, soybean formula, dietary fiber supplements, and espresso coffee may also impair the absorption of levothyroxine from the gastrointestinal tract (reviewed extensively in recent hypothyroidism guidelines[18]). Acid suppression with histamine blockers and proton pump inhibitors may also reduce levothyroxine absorption. Drugs that increase nondeiodinative T_4 clearance include rifampin, carbamazepine, and possibly phenytoin. Selenium deficiency and amiodarone may block the conversion of T_4 to T_3.

Several non-randomized studies have suggested that liquid formulations of levothyroxine or formulations in which the levothyroxine is dissolved in glycerin and encased in a gelatin capsule may circumvent the impaired absorption of levothyroxine that may occur with tablet preparations.[61] For patients receiving enteral feeding, liquid levothyroxine added directly to the feeding tube was associated with a similar serum TSH to that seen in another group of patients in whom the feeding was interrupted in order to administer crushed tablets.[62] The former procedure was found to be more convenient by providers. In a study of patients taking proton pump inhibitors, switching to an oral solution was associated with a decrease in serum TSH from a mean of 5.4 to 1.7 mIU/L, suggesting better absorption of the liquid preparation in these patients.[63] A study of patients with gastritis who had a stable serum TSH while taking levothyroxine tablets and were then switched to a lower dose of levothyroxine gel capsules showed that two-thirds of patients had a similar TSH on the lower dose, again suggesting better absorption of the gel capsule formulation.[64] In a double-blind, randomized, crossover trial of liquid thyroxine in 77 treatment-naive patients with hypothyroidism, no significant differences in thyroid function tests were seen when the liquid preparation was ingested at breakfast or 30 minutes before breakfast.[65] This could provide a solution for patients with difficulties ingesting levothyroxine before breakfast. If the findings of these studies are bolstered by randomized controlled studies in the future, these levothyroxine formulations may prove very convenient for hypothyroid patients. Alternatively, studies in adults with hypothyroidism suggest an equal efficacy of bedtime versus early morning intake of levothyroxine.[66]

10 Dosing and Administration

The average maintenance dose of levothyroxine for most adults is about 125 mcg/day.[53] The replacement dose of levothyroxine is affected by body weight. Estimates of weight-based doses for replacement in hypothyroid patients without any autonomous thyroid function include 1.6 and 1.7 mcg/kg/day, though hypothyroid patients still producing some thyroid hormone will require lower doses.[18] There is, however, a wide range of replacement doses, necessitating individualized therapy and appropriate TSH monitoring to determine an adequate but not excessive dose.

In addition to alleviation of symptoms, the goal of treatment for patients with hypothyroidism is to maintain the patient's TSH within the normal range. Some clinicians are of the opinion that the traditional reference range of approximately 0.5 to 4.5 mIU/L includes at its upper end some individuals who have unrecognized thyroid disease. Thus, some believe that the reference range should be modified downward to 0.5 to 3.5 mIU/L or even 0.5 to 2.5 mIU/L.[67] If this premise is accepted, both the TSH values that trigger L-thyroxine treatment and the TSH treatment goal could potentially be altered. There are cogent arguments on both sides of the issue. Those who suggest maintaining current reference ranges believe that lowering the upper limit of the reference range could result in treating many individuals with thyroid hormone who would not necessarily benefit from such treatment.[68] Those who favor narrowing the reference range suggest that additional patients would, in fact, derive benefit from thyroid hormone treatment.[67] There are calls by some for increasing the thyrotropin reference range specifically among individuals aged 80 years and older.[69] TSH reference ranges also differ for different populations, such as those who are pregnant, specific ethnic groups, and older individuals.[18]

The required dose of levothyroxine is dependent on the patient's age and the presence of associated disorders, as well as the severity and duration of hypothyroidism.[18] Most patients devoid of any thyroid function will require approximately 1.7 mcg/kg/day once they reach steady-state for full replacement. Dose requirement may be better estimated based on ideal body weight, rather than actual body weight. In patients with long-standing disease and older individuals without known cardiac disease, therapy should be initiated with 50 mcg daily of levothyroxine and increased after 1 month. The recommended initial daily dose for older patients with known cardiac disease is 25 mcg daily titrated upward in increments of 25 mcg at monthly intervals to prevent stress on the cardiovascular system. Some patients may experience an exacerbation of angina with higher doses of thyroid hormone. Although TSH is an indicator of under-replacement or over-replacement, clinicians often fail to alter the dose based on TSH values clearly outside of the normal range.

Subclinical hypothyroidism is a laboratory-defined phenomenon in which a patient has an elevated TSH level in the presence of a normal FT_4 level. Patients with subclinical hypothyroidism often complain of symptoms commonly seen in patients with overt hypothyroidism such as cold insensitivity, dry skin, fatigue, constipation, muscle cramps, poor memory, slowed thinking, and depression. However, up to a quarter of people with normal TSH levels report up to two of these symptoms, pointing to the nonspecific nature of these symptoms. An estimated 13 million people in the United States have subclinical hypothyroidism. Subclinical hypothyroidism progresses to overt hypothyroidism in 2% to 5% of patients per year.[70] The risk of progression is significantly greater in individuals with antibodies to thyroid peroxidase (TPO) and in those with higher baseline TSH levels. Levothyroxine therapy was not associated with a significant improvement in hypothyroid symptoms, fatigue, or quality-of-life in patients age 80 years or older with subclinical hypothyroidism.[71] These results argue against the routine use of levothyroxine for the treatment of subclinical hypothyroidism, particularly in the elderly. Thyroid hormone therapy was associated with lowering the mean thyrotropin value into the normal reference range compared with placebo but was not associated with improvements in general quality of life or thyroid-related symptoms.[72] While most patients with subclinical hypothyroidism can be observed without treatment, treatment may be indicated for patients with subclinical hypothyroidism and serum thyrotropin levels of 10 mU/L or higher, or for young and middle-aged individuals with subclinical hypothyroidism and symptoms consistent with mild hypothyroidism.[70]

Once euthyroidism is attained, the daily maintenance dose of levothyroxine does not fluctuate greatly. As patients age, the dosing requirement may be reduced.[18] Third-generation TSH assays improved the accuracy with which thyroid hormone replacement can be monitored. The TSH concentration is the most sensitive and specific monitoring parameter for adjustment of levothyroxine dose. Plasma TSH concentrations begin to fall within hours and are usually normalized within 2 weeks, but they may take up to 6 weeks for some patients, depending on the baseline value. Both TSH and T_4 concentrations are used to monitor therapy, and they should be checked every 6 weeks until a euthyroid state is achieved.[18] Laboratory assessment of thyroid function should be performed approximately 6 weeks after levothyroxine dose initiation or change. This time frame allows achievement of steady-state, as the half-life of levothyroxine is approximately 1 week. Serum T_4 concentrations can be useful in detecting noncompliance, malabsorption, or changes in levothyroxine product bioequivalence, among other things.[73] An elevated TSH concentration indicates insufficient replacement. The appropriate dose maintains the TSH concentration in the normal range. T_4 disposal is accelerated by nephrotic syndrome, other severe systemic illnesses, and several antiseizure medications (phenobarbital, phenytoin, and carbamazepine) and rifampin. Pregnancy increases the T_4 dose requirement for 75% of women, probably because of factors such as increased degradation by the placental deiodinase, increased T_4 pool size, and transfer of T_4 to the fetus. The etiology of hypothyroidism also affects the magnitude of the dosage increase. Initiating postmenopausal hormone replacement therapy increases the dose needed in 35% of women, perhaps due to an increased circulating TBG level. Patient noncompliance with prescribed T_4, the most common cause of inadequate treatment, might be suspected for patients with a dose that is higher than expected, variable thyroid function test results that do not correlate well with prescribed doses, and an elevated serum TSH concentration with serum-free T_4 at the upper end of the normal range, which can suggest improved compliance immediately before testing, with a lag in the thyrotropin response.

For patients with central hypothyroidism caused by hypothalamic or pituitary failure, the serum TSH cannot be used to assess the adequacy of replacement. Alleviation of the clinical syndrome and restoration of serum T_4 to the normal range are the only criteria available for estimating the appropriate replacement dose of L-thyroxine. Keeping free T_4 values in the upper part of the normal laboratory reference range is a reasonable approach, with modification of this goal to the middle of the normal range in older patients or patients with comorbidities. Concurrent use of dopamine, dopaminergic agents (bromocriptine), somatostatin or somatostatin analogs (octreotide), and corticosteroids suppresses TSH concentrations in individuals with primary hypothyroidism and may confound the interpretation of this monitoring parameter.[18]

TSH-suppressive levothyroxine therapy can be given to patients with nodular thyroid disease and diffuse goiter, and to patients with a history of thyroid irradiation. It is also usually given to patients with papillary or follicular thyroid cancer. The rationale for suppression therapy is to reduce TSH secretion, which promotes the growth and function of abnormal thyroid tissue. However, such management, other than for patients with thyroid cancer or with elevated TSH levels, is quite controversial. Some clinicians rarely recommend or use such therapy; others will recommend a trial of levothyroxine as suppressive therapy in some patients. Three meta-analyses concluded that suppressive therapy for nodules was associated with a small decrease in nodule growth, a nonsignificant reduction in nodule growth, and a significant reduction in nodule growth with longer-term treatment. L-Tyroxine may be given in nontoxic MNG to suppress the TSH to low- normal levels of 0.5 to 1 mIU/L if the baseline TSH is more than 1 mIU/L. Goiter size and thyroid volume may be reduced with suppression therapy. Diffuse goiter associated with autoimmune thyroiditis may also be treated with levothyroxine to reduce goiter size and thyroid volume. If suppressive therapy with levothyroxine is pursued, the age, gender, and menopausal status of the patient need to be considered, along with the risk of cardiac arrhythmias and reduced bone mineral density. Levothyroxine suppression therapy is of benefit to all but the lowest-risk thyroid cancer patients and is generally used in the management of patients with differentiated thyroid cancer, with the TSH goal being influenced by the patient's thyroid cancer stage and other risk factors. Current guidelines from the ATA suggest suppressing the TSH to below 0.1 mIU/L in higher-risk patients but keeping TSH around the lower limit of normal (0.1-0.5 mIU/L) in low-risk patients.[74]

Special Populations

Myxedema Coma

Myxedema coma is a rare consequence of decompensated hypothyroidism.[8] Clinical features include hypothermia, advanced stages of hypothyroid symptoms, and altered sensorium ranging from delirium to coma. Mortality rates of 60% to 70% necessitate immediate and aggressive therapy. Traditionally, the initial treatment has been IV bolus levothyroxine 300 to 500 mcg.[18] However, as deiodinase activity is markedly reduced, impairing T_4 to T_3 conversion, initial treatment with IV T_3, or a combination of both hormones, has also been advocated.[8] Glucocorticoid therapy with IV hydrocortisone 100 mg every 8 hours should be given until coexisting adrenal suppression is ruled out.[18] All therapies must be administered parenterally as cessation of gastrointestinal peristalsis occurs, preventing the absorption of orally administered medications. Consciousness, lowered TSH concentrations, and improvement in vital signs are expected within 24 hours. Maintenance doses of levothyroxine are typically 75 to 100 mcg given IV until the patient stabilizes and oral therapy is begun. Supportive therapy must be instituted to maintain adequate ventilation, BP, and body temperature, and ensure euglycemia. Any underlying disorder which may have precipitated the event, such as sepsis or myocardial infarction, obviously must be diagnosed and treated.

Congenital Hypothyroidism

In congenital hypothyroidism, full maintenance therapy should be instituted early to improve the prognosis for mental and physical development. The average maintenance dose in infants and children depends on the age and weight of the child. Several studies demonstrate that aggressive therapy with levothyroxine is important for normal development, and current recommendations are for initiation of therapy as soon as possible after birth at a dose of 10 to 15 mcg/kg/day. This dose is used to keep T_4 concentrations at about 10 mcg/dL (130 nmol/L) within 30 days of starting therapy and is associated with improved IQs. The dose is progressively decreased to a typical adult dose as the child ages, with the adult dose given starting in puberty.

Hypothyroidism During Pregnancy

Hypothyroidism during pregnancy leads to an increased rate of stillbirths and possibly lower neuropsychological scores in infants born of women who received inadequate replacement during pregnancy.[38] Thyroid hormone is necessary for fetal growth and must come from the maternal side during the first 2 months of gestation. Although liothyronine may cross the placental membrane slightly better than levothyroxine, the latter is considered the drug of choice. The objective of treatment is to decrease TSH to normal, based on the normal reference range for pregnancy. Current guidelines suggest a TSH below 2.5 mIU/L during the first trimester and a TSH below 3 mIU/L during the remainder of the pregnancy.[38] Based on elevated TSH levels during pregnancy, the mean dose of levothyroxine had to be increased by 48% to decrease TSH into the normal range. However, in individual women, the dosage increase needed may vary from approximately 10% to 80%. Increased production of binding proteins, a marginal decrease in free hormone concentration, modification of peripheral thyroid hormone metabolism, and increased T_4 metabolism by the fetal-placental unit all may contribute to increased thyroid hormone demand. As these changes regress after delivery, the need for increased levothyroxine will decline.[38] Up to 60% of women need to have levothyroxine dose adjustment during pregnancy. An upward adjustment in the dose will usually be needed by the eighth week of pregnancy. Current guidelines recommend that hypothyroid patients receiving levothyroxine who become pregnant should increase their levothyroxine dose by 20% to 30% (two additional tablets weekly) as soon as they know they are pregnant.[38] After delivery the levothyroxine dose can be reduced based on T_4 concentrations and measurement of TSH, typically about 6 to 8 weeks after delivery. Many patients can return to their pre-pregnancy dose requirement.

EVALUATION OF THERAPEUTIC OUTCOMES—HYPOTHYROIDISM

Patients with idiopathic hypothyroidism and Hashimoto's thyroiditis on optimal thyroid hormone replacement therapy should have TSH and free T_4 serum concentrations in the normal range.[18] Those who are being treated for thyroid cancer should have TSH suppressed to low levels, with the appropriate TSH concentration being determined based on the patient's risk of recurrence or progression, and TG levels should be undetectable.[74] Given the 7-day half-life of T_4 and the potential delayed response of the hypothalamus, the appropriate monitoring interval for follow-up thyroid function testing is no more frequent than every 4 to 6 weeks. The signs and symptoms of hypothyroidism should be improved or absent (see Clinical Presentation of Hypothyroidism discussed earlier), although it may take several months for the full benefit of therapy to manifest.

CONCLUSION

Hypothyroidism is a common disorder but if left untreated it can progress into myxedema coma in the absence of an adequate endogenous thyroid reserve. Levothyroxine is a readily available and highly effective treatment that rapidly reverses the biochemical and clinical abnormalities that characterize hypothyroidism. Serum TSH and thyroid hormone levels are useful measures for adjusting the levothyroxine dose.

ABBREVIATIONS

anti-TPO Ab	anti-thyroid peroxidase antibody
ATD	antithyroid drug
AUC	area under the curve
BMI	body mass index
BP	blood pressure
cGy	centigray
C_{max}	maximum concentration
ClO_4^-	perchlorate
CNS	central nervous system
DIT	diiodotyrosine
FSH	follicle-stimulating hormone
FT_3	free triiodothyronine
FT_4	free thyroxine
$Gs\alpha$	the α subunit of the stimulatory guanine-nucleotide–binding protein
hCG	human chorionic gonadotropin
HLA	human leukocyte antigen
^{131}I	sodium iodide-131
L-thyroxine	levothyroxine
LH	luteinizing hormone
MIT	monoiodotyrosine
MMI	methimazole
MNG	multinodular goiter
NHANES III	Third National Health and Nutrition Examination Survey
OTC	over the counter
PRTH	pituitary resistance to thyroid hormone
PTU	propylthiouracil
RAI	radioactive iodine
RAIU	radioactive iodine uptake
rT_3	reverse triiodothyronine
SCN^-	thiocyanate
SSKI	saturated solution of potassium iodide
T_3	triiodothyronine
T_4	thyroxine
TBG	thyroxine-binding globulin
TBII	TSH binding inhibitor immunoglobulin
TBPA	thyroid-binding prealbumin
TcO_4^-	pertechnetate

TG	thyroglobulin
TPOAb	thyroid peroxidase antibodies
TR	thyroid hormone receptor
TRH	thyrotropin-releasing hormone
TRIAC	triiodothyroacetic acid
TSAb	thyroid-stimulating antibody
TSH	thyroid-stimulating hormone
TT_3	total triiodothyronine
TT_4	total thyroxine
TTR	transthyretin
WBC	white blood cell

REFERENCES

1. Portulano C, Paroder-Belenitsky M, Carrasco N. The Na^+/I^- symporter (NIS): Mechanism and medical impact. *Endocr Rev.* 2014;35:106–149. doi:10.1210/er.2012-1036.
2. Verloop H, Dekkers OM, Peeters RP, et al. Genetics in endocrinology—Genetic variation in deiodinases: A systematic review of potential clinical effects in humans. *Eur J Endocrinol.* 2014;171:R123–R135. doi:10.1530/EJE-14-0302.
3. Mendoza A, Hollenberg AN. New insights into thyroid hormone action. *Pharmacol Ther.* 2017;173:135–145. doi:10.1016/j.pharmthera.2017.02.012.
4. Kleinau G, Biebermann H. Constitutive activities in the thyrotropin receptor: Regulation and significance. *Adv Pharmacol.* 2014;70:81–119. doi:10.1016/B978-0-12-417197-8.00003-1.
5. Mackenzie LS. Thyroid hormone receptor antagonists: From environmental pollution to novel small molecules. *Vitam Horm.* 2018;106:147–162. doi:10.1016/bs.vh.2017.04.004.
6. Ross DS, Burch HB, Cooper DS, et al. 2016 American Thyroid Association Guidelines for diagnosis and management of hyperthyroidism and other causes of thyrotoxicosis. *Thyroid.* 2016;26:1343–421. doi:10.1089/thy.2016.0229.
7. Hollowell JG, Staehling NW, Flanders WD, et al. Serum TSH, T(4), and thyroid antibodies in the United States population (1988 to 1994): National Health and Nutrition Examination Survey (NHANES III). *J Clin Endocrinol Metab.* 2002;87:489–499. doi:10.1210/jcem.87.2.8182.
8. Ylli D, Klubo-Gwiezdzinska J, Wartofsky L. Thyroid emergencies. *Pol Arch Intern Med.* 2019;129:526–534. doi:10.20452/pamw.14876.
9. Burch HB, Cooper DS. A young woman with palpitations, goitre and low thyroid-stimulating hormone. *CMAJ.* 2014;186:289–291. doi:10.1503/cmaj.
10. Chaudhry MA, Wayangankar S. Thyrotoxic periodic paralysis: A concise review of the literature. *Curr Rheumatol Rev.* 2016;12:190–194. doi:10.2174/1573397112666160404124822.
11. Fan C, Kuhn M, Mbiol AP, et al. Kir2.2 p.Thr140Met: a genetic susceptibility to sporadic periodic paralysis. *Acta Myol.* 2018;37:193–203. eCollection 2018 Sep.
12. Ryodi E, Metso S, Jaatinen P, et al. Cancer incidence and mortality in patients treated with RAI or thyroidectomy for hyperthyroidism—A nation-wide cohort study with a long-term follow-up. *J Clin Endocrinol Metab.* 2015;100(10):3710–3717. doi:10.1210/jc.2015-1874.
13. Kitahara CM, Berrington de Gonzalez A, Bouville A, et al. Association of radioactive iodine treatment with cancer mortality in patients with hyperthyroidism. JAMA Intern Med. 2019;179:1034–1042. doi:10.1001/jamainternmed.2019.0981.
14. Kitahara CM, Preston DL, Sosa JA, et al. Association of radioactive iodine, antithyroid drug, and surgical treatments with solid cancer mortality in patients with hyperthyroidism. *JAMA Netw Open.* 2020;3(7):e209660. doi:10.1001/jamanetworkopen.2020.9660.
15. Goichot B, Caron P, Landron F, et al. Clinical presentation of hyperthyroidism in a large representative sample of outpatients in France: Relationships with age, aetiology and hormonal parameters. *Clin Endocrinol (Oxf).* 2016;84:445–451. doi:10.1111/cen.12816.
16. Beck-Peccoz P, Giavoli C, Lania A. A 2019 update on TSH-secreting pituitary adenomas. *Endocrinol Invest.* 2019 Dec;42(12):1401–1406. doi:10.1007/s40618-019-01066-x.
17. Caron P. Thyroiditis and SARS-CoV-2 pandemic: a review. *Endocrine.* 2021 May;72(2):326–331. doi:10.1007/s12020-021-02689-y.
18. Jonklaas J, Bianco AC, Bauer AJ, et al. Guidelines for the treatment of hypothyroidism: Prepared by the American Thyroid Association task force on thyroid hormone replacement. *Thyroid.* 2014;24:1670–1751. doi:10.1089/thy.2014.0028.
19. Ylli D, Wartofsky L, Burman KD. Evaluation and treatment of amiodarone-induced thyroid disorders. *J Clin Endocrinol Metab.* 2021;106:226–236. doi:10.1210/clinem/dgaa68.
20. Barbesino G. Misdiagnosis of Graves' disease with apparent severe hyperthyroidism in a patient taking biotin megadoses. *Thyroid.* 2016;26:860–863. doi:10.1089/thy.2015.0664.
21. Elston MS, Sehgal S, Du Toit S, et al. Factitious Graves' disease due to biotin immunoassay interference: A case and review of the literature. *J Clin Endocrinol Metab.* 2016;101:3251–3255. doi:10.1210/jc.2016-1971.
22. Sundaresh V, Brito JP, Wang Z, et al. Comparative effectiveness of therapies for Graves' hyperthyroidism: A systematic review and network meta-analysis. *J Clin Endocrinol Metab.* 2013;98(9):3671–3677. doi:10.1210/jc.2013-1954.
23. Smith TJ, Hegedüs L. Graves' disease. *N Engl J Med.* 2016;375:1552–1565. doi:10.1056/NEJMra1510030.
24. Burch HB, Cooper DS. Management of Graves' disease: A review. *JAMA.* 2015;314:2544–2554. doi:10.1001/jama.2015.16535.
25. Giuliani C, Cerrone D, Harii N, et al. A TSHR-LH/CGR chimera that measures functional thyroid-stimulating autoantibodies (TSAb) can predict remission or recurrence in Graves' patients undergoing antithyroid drug (ATD) treatment. *J Clin Endocrinol Metab.* 2012;97(7):E1080–E1087. doi:10.1210/jc.2011-2897.
26. Bandai S, Okamura K, Fujikawa M, et al. The long-term follow-up of patients with thionamide-treated Graves' hyperthyroidism. *Endocrine J.* 2019;66:535–545. doi:10.1507/endocrj.EJ18-0418.
27. Azizi F, Amouzegar A, Tohidi M, et al. Increased remission rates after long-term methimazole therapy in patients with Graves' disease: Results of a randomized clinical trial. *Thyroid.* 2019;29:1192–1200. doi:10.1089/thy.2019.0180.
28. van Lieshout JM, Mooij CF, van Trotsenburg ASP, et al. Methimazole-induced remission rates in pediatric Graves' disease: A systematic review. *Eur J Endocrinol.* 2021 Jun 1;EJE-21-0077.R1. doi:10.1530/EJE-21-0077.
29. Kahaly GJ, Bartalena L, Hegedüs L, et al. 2018 European Thyroid Association Guideline for the management of Graves' hyperthyroidism. *Eur Thyroid J.* 2018;7:167–186. doi:10.1159/00049038.
30. Biondi B, Cooper DS. Subclinical hyperthyroidism. *N Engl J Med.* 2018;378:2411–9. doi:10.1056/NEJMcp1709318.
31. Mazhari A, Emanuele MA, Espiritu B. Desensitization to methimazole. *Endocr Pract.* 2021;27(3):185–190. doi 10.1016/j.eprac.2020.10.019.
32. Chen W-T, Chi CC. Associations of HLA genotypes with antithyroid drug-induced agranulocytosis: A systematic review and meta-analysis of pharmacogenomics studies. *Br J Clin Pharmacol.* 2019;85:1878–1887. doi:10.1111/bcp.13989.
33. Vicente N, Cardoso L, Barros L, et al. Antithyroid drug-induced agranulocytosis: State of the art on diagnosis and management. *Drugs R D.* 2017;17:91–96. doi:10.1007/s40268-017-0172-1.
34. Brix TH, Lund LC, Henriksen DP, et al. Methimazole and risk of acute pancreatitis. *Lancet Diabetes Endocrinol.* 2020;8:187–189. doi:10.1016/S2213-8587(20)30025-5.
35. Glinoer D, Cooper DS. The propylthiouracil dilemma. *Curr Opin Endocrinol Diabetes Obes.* 2012;19(5):402–407. doi:10.1097/MED.0b013e3283565b49.
36. Andersen SL, Olsen J, Wu CS, et al. Birth defects after early pregnancy use of antithyroid drugs: A Danish nationwide study. *J Clin Endocrinol Metab.* 2013;98(11):4373–4381. doi:10.1210/jc.2013-2831.
37. Seo GH, Kim TH, Chung JH. Antithyroid drugs and congenital malformations: A nationwide Korean cohort study. *Ann Intern Med.* 2018;168:405–413. doi:10.7326/M17-1398.
38. Alexander EK, Pearce EN, Brent GA, et al. 2017 guidelines of the American Thyroid Association for the diagnosis and management of thyroid disease during pregnancy and the postpartum. *Thyroid.* 2017;27(3):315–389. doi:10.1089/thy.2016.0457.
39. Törring O, Watt T, Sjölin G, et al. Impaired quality of life after radioiodine therapy compared to antithyroid drugs or surgical treatment for Graves' hyperthyroidism: A long-term follow-up with the thyroid-related patient-reported outcome questionnaire and 36-item short form health status survey. *Thyroid.* 2019;29:322–331. doi 10.1089/thy.2018.0315.
40. Okamura K, Sato K, Fujikawa M, et al. *J Clin Endocrinol Metab.* 2014;99:3995–4002. doi:10.1210/jc.2013-4466.
41. Simsir IY, Ozdemir M, Duman S, et al. Therapeutic plasmapheresis in thyrotoxic patients. *Endocrine.* 2018 Oct;62(1):144–148. doi:10.1007/s12020-018-1661-x.

42. Hammond EN, Vangu M-D-T HW. Effect of adjuvant lithium on thyroxine (T4) concentration after radioactive iodine therapy. *Eur J Nucl Med Mol Imaging.* 2016;43:1980–7. doi:10.1007/s00259-016-3388-3.
43. Dosiou C, Kossler AL. Thyroid eye disease: Navigating the new treatment landscape. *J Endocrine Soc.* 2021;5:1–13. doi:10.1210/jendso/bvab034.
44. Douglas RS, Kahaly GJ, Patel A, et al. Teprotumumab for the treatment of active thyroid eye disease. *N Engl J Med.* 2020;382:341–52. doi:10.1056/NEJMoa1910434.
45. Francis N, Francis T, Lazarus JH, et al. Current controversies in the management of Graves' hyperthyroidism. *Expert Rev Endocrinol Metab.* 2020;15:159–169. doi:10.1080/17446651.2020.1754192.
46. Chaker L, Bianco AC, Jonklaas J, et al. Hypothyroidism. *Lancet.* 2017;390(10101):1550–1562. doi:10.1016/S0140-6736(17)30703-1.
47. Beck-Peccoz P, Rodari G, Giavoli C, et al. Central hypothyroidism - a neglected thyroid disorder. *Nat Rev Endocrinol.* 2017;13:588–598. doi:10.1038/nrendo.2017.47.
48. Peters C, van Trotsenburg ASP, Schoenmakers N. Diagnosis of endocrine disease: Congentital hypothyroidism: update and perspectives. *Eur J Endocrinol.* 2018;179:R297–R317. doi:10.1530/EJE-18-0383.
49. Esfandiari NH, Papaleontiou M. Biochemical testing in thyroid disorders. *Endocrinol Metab Clin North Am.* 2017;46:631–648. doi:10.1016/j.ecl.2017.04.002.
50. O'Malley G, Lee HJ, Parekh S, et al. Rapid evolution of thyroid dysfunction in patients treated with nivolumab. *Endocr Pract.* 2017;23:1223–1231. doi:10.4158/EP171832.OR.
51. Yeliosof O, Gangat M. Diagnosis and management of hypopituitarism. *Curr Opin Pediatr.* 2019;31:531–536. doi:10.1097/MOP.0000000000000779.
52. Makita N, Manaka K, Sato J, et al. Bexarotene-induced hypothyroidism: Characteristics and therapeutic strategies. *Clin Endocrinol (Oxf).* 2019;91:195–200. doi:10.1111/cen.13975.
53. Jonklaas J, Cappola AR, Celi FS. Editorial: Combination therapy for hypothyroidism: The journey from bench to bedside. *Front Endocrinol (Lausanne).* 2020;11:422. doi:10.3389/fendo.2020.00422.
54. Jonklaas J, Bianco AC, Cappola AR, et al. Evidence-based use of levothyroxine/liothyronine combinations in treating hypothyroidism: A consensus document. *Thyroid.* 2021;31(2):156–182. doi:10.1089/thy.2020.0720.
55. Werneck de Castro JP, Fonseca TL, Ueta CB, et al. Differences in hypothalamic type 2 deiodinase ubiquitination explain localized sensitivity to thyroxine. *J Clin Invest.* 2015;125(2):769–781. doi:10.1172/JCI77588.
56. Santini F, Giannetti M, Ricco I, et al. Steady-state serum T3 concentrations for 48 hours following the oral administration of a single dose of 3,5,3'-triiodothyronine sulfate (T3S). *Endocr Pract.* 2014;20(7):680–689. doi:10.4158/EP13331.OR.
57. Benvenga S, Carlé A. Levothyroxine formulations: Pharmacological and clinical implications of generic substitution. *Adv Ther.* 2019;36(Suppl 2):S59–S71. doi.org/10.1007/s12325-019-01079-1.
58. Dew R, Okosieme O, Dayan C, et al. Clinical, behavioural and pharmacogenomic factors influencing the response to levothyroxine therapy in patients with primary hypothyroidism-protocol for a systematic review. *Syst Rev.* 2017;6:60. doi:10.1186/s13643-017-0457-z.
59. Williams GR, Bassett JHD. Thyroid diseases and bone health. *J Endocrinol Invest.* 2018;41:99–109. doi:10.1007/s40618-017-0753-4.
60. Schneider R, Schneider M, Reiners C, et al. Effects of levothyroxine on bone mineral density, muscle force, and bone turnover markers: A cohort study. *J Clin Endocrinol Metab.* 2012;97(11):3926–3934. doi:10.1210/jc.2012-2570.
61. Virili C, Trimboli P, Romanelli F, et al. Liquid and softgel levothyroxine use in clinical practice: State of the art. *Endocrine.* 2016;54:3–14. doi:10.1007/s12020-016-1035-1.
62. Pirola I, Daffini L, Gandossi E, et al. Comparison between liquid and tablet levothyroxine formulations in patients treated through enteral feeding tube. *J Endocrinol Invest.* 2014;37:583–587. doi:10.1007/s40618-014-0082-9.
63. Vita R, Saraceno G, Trimarchi F, et al. Switching levothyroxine from the tablet to the oral solution formulation corrects the impaired absorption of levothyroxine induced by proton-pump inhibitors. *J Clin Endocrinol Metab.* 2014;99:4481–4486. doi:10.1210/jc.2014-2684.
64. Santaguida MG, Virili C, Del Duca SC, et al. Thyroxine softgel capsule in patients with gastric-related T4 malabsorption. *Endocrine.* 2015;49(1):51–57. doi:10.1007/s12020-014-0476-7.
65. Fallahi P, Ferrari SM, Antonelli A. Oral l-thyroxine liquid versus tablets in patients with hypothyroidism without malabsorption: A prospective study. *Endocrine.* 2016;52:597–601. doi:10.1007/s12020-015-0836-y.
66. Pang X, Pu T, Xu L, et al. Effect of l-thyroxine administration before breakfast vs at bedtime on hypothyroidism: A meta-analysis. *Clin Endocrinol (Oxf).* 2020;92:475–481. doi:10.1111/cen.14172.
67. Wartofsky L, Dickey RA. The evidence for a narrower thyrotropin reference range is compelling. *J Clin Endocrinol Metab.* 2005;90(9):5483–5488. doi:10.1210/jc.2005-0455.
68. Surks MI, Goswami G, Daniels GH. The thyrotropin reference range should remain unchanged. *J Clin Endocrinol Metabol.* 2005;90(9):5489–5496. doi 10.1210/jc.2005-0170.
69. Cappola AR. The thyrotropin reference range should be changed in older patients. *JAMA.* 2019;322(20):61–62. doi 10.1001/jama.2019.14728.
70. Biondi B, Cappola AR, Cooper DS. Subclinical hypothyroidism: A Review. *JAMA.* 2019;322(2):153–160. doi 10.1001/jama.2019.9052.
71. Mooijaart SP, Du Puy RS, Stott DJ, et al. Association between levothyroxine treatment and thyroid-related symptoms among adults aged 80 years and older with subclinical hypothyroidism. *JAMA.* 2019;322(20):1977–1986. doi:10.1001/jama.2019.17274.
72. Feller M, Snel M, Moutzouri E, et al. Association of thyroid hormone therapy with quality of life and thyroid-related symptoms in patients with subclinical hypothyroidism A systematic review and meta-analysis. *JAMA.* 2018;320:1349–1359. doi:10.1001/jama.2018.13770.
73. Centanni M, Benvenga A, Sachmechi I. Diagnosis and management of treatment-refractory hypothyroidism: An expert consensus report. *J Endocrinol Invest.* 2017;40(12):1289–1301. doi:10.1007/s40618-017-0706-y.
74. Haugen BR, Alexander EK, Bible KC, et al. 2015 American Thyroid Association Management Guidelines for adult patients with thyroid nodules and differentiated thyroid cancer. *Thyroid.* 2016;26(1):1–133. doi 10.1089/thy.2015.0020.

97

Adrenal Gland Disorders

Steven M. Smith, Christopher R. Piszczatoski, and John G. Gums

KEY CONCEPTS

1. Glucocorticoid secretion from the adrenal cortex is stimulated by adrenocorticotropic hormone (ACTH) or corticotropin that is released from the anterior pituitary in response to the hypothalamic-mediated release of corticotropin-releasing hormone (CRH).
2. To ensure the proper treatment of Cushing syndrome requires diagnostic procedures to (1) establish the presence of hypercortisolism and (2) discover the underlying etiology of the disease.
3. The rationale for treating Cushing syndrome is to reduce the morbidity and mortality resulting from disorders such as diabetes mellitus, cardiovascular disease, and electrolyte abnormalities.
4. The treatment of choice for both ACTH-dependent and ACTH-independent Cushing syndrome is surgery. Pharmacologic agents are reserved for adjunctive therapy, refractory cases, or inoperable disease.
5. Pharmacologic agents that may be used to manage the patient with Cushing syndrome include steroidogenesis inhibitors, adrenolytic agents, neuromodulators of ACTH release, and glucocorticoid-receptor blocking agents.
6. Spironolactone, a competitive aldosterone-receptor antagonist, is the drug of choice in bilateral adrenal hyperplasia (BAH)–dependent hyperaldosteronism.
7. Addison disease (primary adrenal insufficiency) is a state of deficiency in cortisol, aldosterone, and various androgens due to the loss of function in all regions of the adrenal cortex.
8. Secondary adrenal insufficiency usually results from exogenous steroid use, leading to hypothalamic–pituitary–adrenal (HPA)–axis suppression followed by a decrease in ACTH release, and low levels of androgens and cortisol.
9. Virilism results from the excessive secretion of androgens from the adrenal gland and often manifests as hirsutism in females.

BEYOND THE BOOK

- Watch the video Primary adrenal insufficiency (Addison disease): pathology, symptoms, diagnosis, treatment by Osmosis.org URL: https://youtu.be/V6XcBp8EV7Q
- Watch the video Cushing syndrome—causes, symptoms, diagnosis, treatment, pathology by Osmosis.org URL: https://youtu.be/ea1sXgd5ui8
- Create a table with mechanisms for drug-induced secondary adrenal insufficiency

INTRODUCTION

The adrenals are small endocrine glands located atop each kidney that produce several hormones that regulate blood pressure, metabolism, immune response, stress response, and other bodily functions. Under- or over-production of these hormones causes a constellation of symptoms and most commonly results in Cushing syndrome (hypercortisolism), Addison's disease (adrenal insufficiency), or hyperaldosteronism. Adrenal disorders affecting the hormone cortisol are rare, typically effecting fewer than 1 person in a thousand. On the other hand, aldosterone-related disorders, particularly hyperaldosteronism, are relatively common. Left untreated, complications from these disorders can include organ damage, physical manifestations, electrolyte abnormalities, cardiovascular crises, and even death. Thus, prompt identification and treatment is critical. Screening and management of these conditions lower the risk of complication, increase life expectancy, and improve quality of life for those affected.[1]

PHYSIOLOGY, ANATOMY, AND BIOCHEMISTRY

The adrenal glands are located on the upper poles of each kidney (Fig. 97-1). On average, each adrenal gland weighs 4 g and is 2 to 3 cm in width and 4 to 6 cm in length. The gland is fed by small arteries from the abdominal aorta and renal and phrenic arteries.

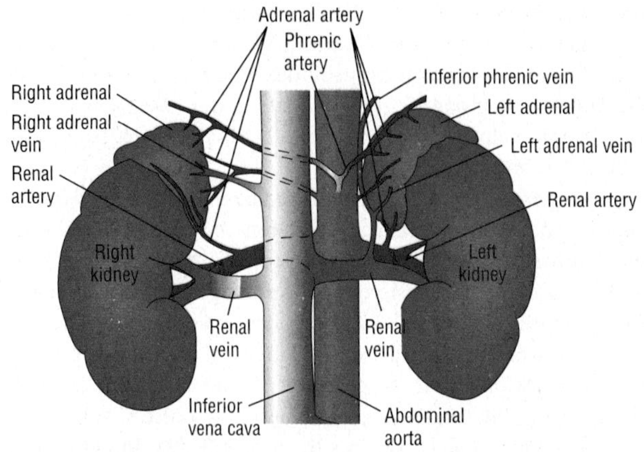

FIGURE 97-1 Anatomy of the adrenal gland.

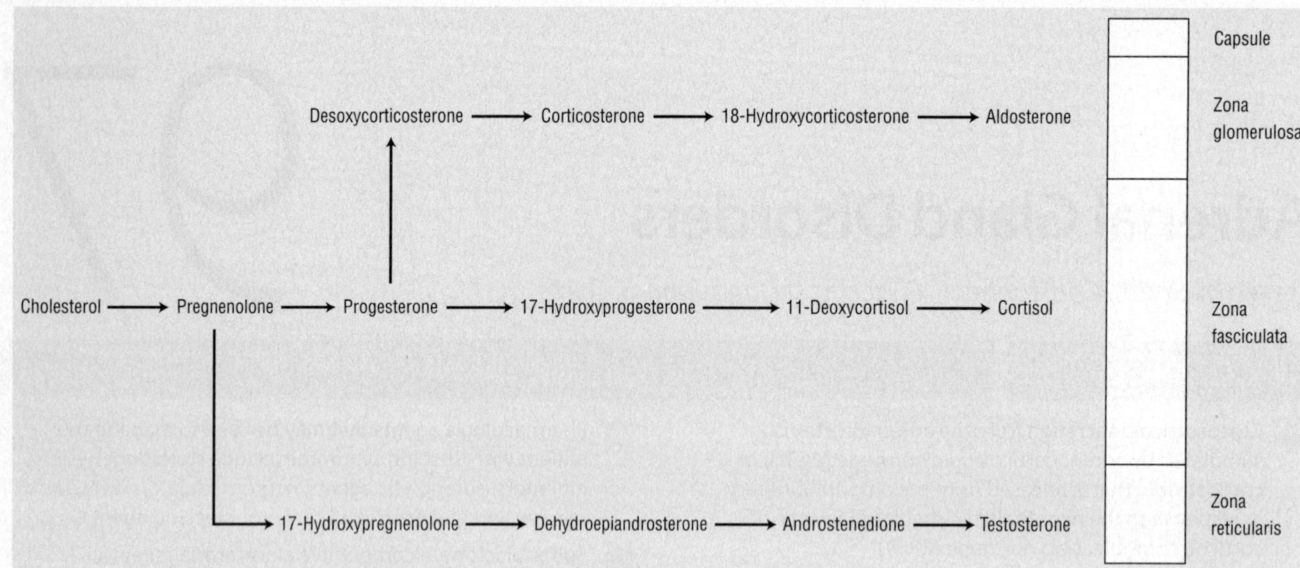

FIGURE 97-2 Hormone synthetic pathways in relation to the zones of the adrenal cortex.

Drainage of the adrenal gland occurs via the renal vein on the left and the inferior vena cava on the right.

The adrenal medulla comprises 10% of the total gland and is responsible for the secretion of catecholamines. The adrenal cortex accounts for the remaining 90% and is responsible for the secretion of three types of hormones (Fig. 97-2) from three separate zones.

The zona glomerulosa accounts for 15% of the total adrenal cortex and is responsible for mineralocorticoid production, of which aldosterone is the principal end product. Aldosterone maintains electrolyte and volume homeostasis by altering potassium and magnesium secretion and renal tubular sodium reabsorption. The zona fasciculata, the middle zone, makes up 60% of the cortex, is high in cholesterol, and is responsible for basal and stimulated glucocorticoid production. Glucocorticoids, mainly cortisol, are responsible for the regulation of fat, carbohydrate, and protein metabolism. The zona reticularis occupies 25% of the adrenal cortex and is responsible for adrenal androgen production. The androgens, testosterone, and estradiol are the major end products and influence the reproductive system in addition to modulating primary and secondary sex characteristics.

Hormone Production and Metabolism

Adrenal steroid hormone synthesis begins with the conversion of cholesterol to pregnenolone by cytochrome P450 (CYP) enzymatic side-chain cleavage (Fig. 97-2). Following this rate-limiting step, pregnenolone is converted to various 19- and 21-carbon steroids, depending on the enzymatic capabilities within each zone of the cortex. Androgenic properties predominate in the 19-carbon steroids, whereas mineralocorticoid and glucocorticoid properties manifest in the 21-carbon steroids.

Aldosterone production is initiated by the 21-hydroxylation of progesterone to form deoxycorticosterone. Subsequently, aldosterone synthase converts deoxycorticosterone to aldosterone through the intermediary, corticosterone. The zona glomerulosa preferentially produces aldosterone for three main reasons. First, the zona glomerulosa lacks 17α-hydroxylase activity and therefore can only convert pregnenolone to progesterone. Second, in contrast to the other zones, cells in the zona glomerulosa possess aldosterone synthase activity, which catalyzes the terminal steps in aldosterone synthesis. Lastly, cells of the zona glomerulosa display a greater number of angiotensin II receptors than cells of the other zones. The binding of angiotensin II to these receptors provides the stimulus for initiating the aldosterone biosynthesis cascade. Thus, aldosterone synthesis is a unique feature of the zona glomerulosa, explaining why aldosterone is not affected during disease processes limited to the zona fasciculata or reticularis.

Cortisol is produced from pregnenolone via four successive hydroxylations. These hydroxylations occur primarily in the zona fasciculata, although the zona reticularis is also capable of producing glucocorticoids.

Androgens, produced primarily in the zona reticularis and less commonly in the zona fasciculata, have a 19-carbon structure and serve as precursors to more potent analogs produced in the periphery. The adrenal gland can synthesize estradiol and estrone from testosterone and androstenedione, respectively; however, the quantities synthesized by the adrenal gland are extremely small. The rates of production for the various steroids produced by the adrenal gland are listed in Table 97-1.

Glucocorticoid metabolism occurs in the liver and is responsible for converting inactive steroids to active metabolites, as well as modifying active steroids to less active or inactive metabolites. Most pharmaceutical steroid products are active; however, in the case of prednisone and cortisone, metabolism is necessary for conversion to the active prednisolone and cortisol, respectively.

Following metabolic conversion, glomerular filtration is primarily responsible for eliminating endogenously produced glucocorticoids. The half-life of cortisol is 70 to 120 minutes, whereas aldosterone exhibits extremely high intrinsic clearance and a half-life of only 15 minutes.

Metabolism and conversion of the various steroids can be altered by a variety of disease states and medicinal compounds. Drugs known to enhance steroid clearance include phenytoin, phenobarbital, rifampin, and mitotane. Likewise, diseases such as hyperthyroidism and renal disease can enhance steroid clearance. In contrast, drugs such as estrogens and estrogen-containing oral contraceptives reduce steroid clearance. Similarly, liver disease, age, pregnancy, hypothyroidism, anorexia nervosa, protein-calorie malnutrition, and renal disease are associated with reduced steroid clearance.

Plasma glucocorticoids are bound to one of three plasma proteins in varying degrees. Corticosteroid-binding globulin (CBG), albumin, and α_1-glycoprotein are capable of binding glucocorticoids,

TABLE 97-1 Rates of Adrenal Production and Plasma Concentrations of Various Steroids

Steroid	24-hour Secretion (mg)	Plasma Concentration
Aldosterone	0.15 (0.42 μmol)	2-9 ng/dL (55-250 pmol/L; supine, normal-sodium diet)
Androstenedione	2.2-2.5 (7.7-8.7 μmol)	50-250 ng/dL (1.7-8.7 nmol/L)
Corticosterone	1-4 (3-12 μmol)	2.4 ± 1.5 ng/dL (69 ± 43 nmol/L; female) 4.2 ± 2.2 ng/dL (121 ± 64 nmol/L; male)
Cortisol	8-25 (22-69 μmol)	0-25 μg/dL (0-690 nmol/L)
11-Deoxycorticosterone	0.60 (1.8 μmol)	2-19 ng/dL (60-575 pmol/L)
11-Deoxycortisol	0.40 (1.2 μmol)	12-158 ng/dL (350-4,560 pmol/L)
Progesterone	0	<20 ng/dL (0.6 nmol/L; female)[a] 300-2,000 ng/dL (9.5-64 nmol/L; female)[b] <20-140 ng/dL (0.6-4.5 nmol/L; male)
Testosterone (total)	0.23 (0.8 μmol; female)	6-86 ng/dL (0.2-3.0 nmol/L; female) 270-1,070 ng/dL (9.4-37 nmol/L; male)

[a]Follicular phase of menstrual cycle.

[b]Luteal phase of menstrual cycle.

Data from Kratz A, Ferraro M, Sluss PM, Lewandrowski KB. Laboratory reference values. N Engl J Med. 2004;351(15):1548-1563.

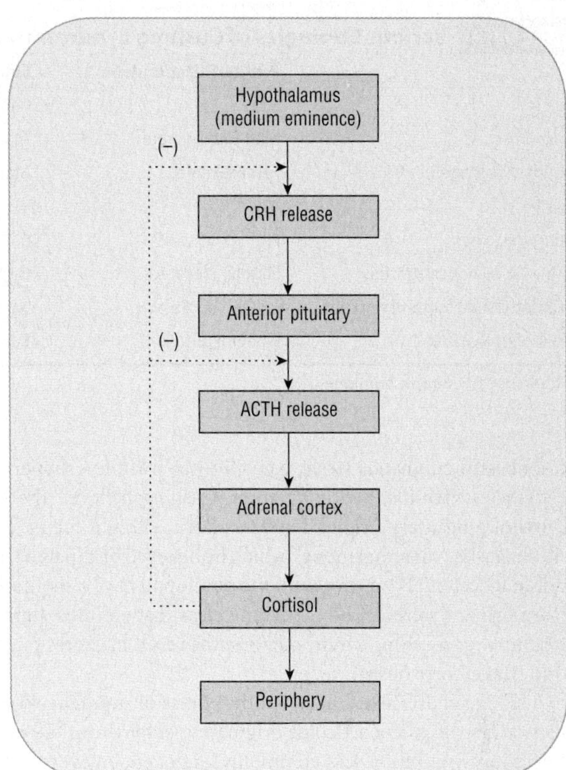

FIGURE 97-3 Negative feedback system involved in the regulation of cortisol secretion under normal conditions. (CRH, corticotropin-releaseing hormone; ACTH, adrenocorticotropic hormone)

with CBG being the principal binding protein. Steroid binding serves as a reservoir for steroids in their inactive state and more than 95% of cortisol is normally bound. Binding to plasma proteins prevents glucocorticoid activity at receptor-activating sites. Therefore, a final but important variable in the altered plasma concentration of free (active) steroids is the concentration of plasma proteins.

Regulation of Hormone Secretion

1 Glucocorticoid secretion is regulated by the pituitary hormone, adrenocorticotropic hormone (ACTH [also known as corticotropin]). Under normal conditions, ACTH is released from the anterior pituitary in response to corticotropin-releasing hormone (CRH), which is secreted by the median eminence of the hypothalamus (Fig. 97-3). Vasopressin and oxytocin have weak ACTH-releasing activity through binding to the inferior V_3 receptor. CRH, in combination with vasopressin and oxytocin, stimulates greater ACTH secretion than each hormone individually.

Additionally, histochemical studies have demonstrated that certain neurotransmitters, such as serotonin and norepinephrine, can stimulate the production of CRH and ACTH. After release, ACTH stimulates the adrenal gland to release cortisol and, to a lesser extent, aldosterone and androgens. The rising cortisol concentration inhibits the secretion of CRH and ACTH through a negative feedback mechanism. In addition, leptin, an adipocyte hormone, has an inhibitory effect on hypothalamic–pituitary–adrenal (HPA) activity.

Adrenal androgens are regulated in a similar fashion to cortisol. When plasma androgen reaches sufficient concentrations, production is terminated via a negative feedback loop. Androgen release is increased during puberty and in women with hirsutism. Adrenal androgen release decreases with age and in fasting states, including anorexia nervosa.

In contrast to cortisol and adrenal androgens, the regulation of aldosterone secretion is considerably more complex. The renin-angiotensin system regulates aldosterone secretion through both intrarenal and extrarenal mechanisms. Renin production and subsequent aldosterone secretion are stimulated by blood pressure-lowering (due to volume depletion), erect posture, salt depletion, β-adrenergic stimulation, and CNS excitation (see Chapter 30, "Hypertension"). Renin production is inhibited by salt loading, angiotensin II, vasopressin, potassium, calcium, blood pressure increases, and a variety of drugs. The renin-mediated production of angiotensin II is the initial stimulus for aldosterone synthesis. Additionally, angiotensin II can be acted on by aminopeptidase and converted to angiotensin III. Both angiotensin II and III are capable of stimulating the zona glomerulosa to secrete aldosterone. Following aldosterone secretion, increases in renal sodium, water retention, and blood pressure occur thereby turning off the stimulus for renin release.

HYPERFUNCTION OF THE ADRENAL GLAND

Adrenal disorders can be categorized as hyperfunction or hypofunction of the adrenal gland. Hyperfunction of the adrenal gland generally involves excess production of adrenal hormones, most notably cortisol, resulting in Cushing syndrome, or aldosterone, resulting in hyperaldosteronism.

Cushing Syndrome

In 1932, Cushing first described a syndrome of pituitary basophilism that attracted national attention. These patients had unexplained

TABLE 97-2 Various Etiologies of Cushing Syndrome and Their Respective Differences

	Pituitary-Dependent	Ectopic ACTH Syndrome	Adrenal Adenoma	Adrenal Carcinoma
Course	Slow	Rapid	Slow	Rapid
Symptoms	Mild to moderate	Atypical	Mild to moderate	Severe
Dominant sex/age	Female/male	Male	None noted	Children
Virilization	+	+	+	+++
Abdominal mass	0	0	0	++
Plasma ACTH concentration	Slightly elevated	High	Low	Low
Dexamethasone suppression test	≥50% suppression	No suppression	No suppression	No suppression
Iodocholesterol scan	Bilateral uptake	Bilateral uptake	Unilateral	None

ACTH, adrenocorticotropic hormone

central obesity, cutaneous striae, osteoporosis, weakness, hypertension, diabetes mellitus, and congestion. Cushing believed the disease was of a pituitary origin. Ten years later, Albright focused his attention on the "sugar hormone," which he believed originated from the adrenal cortex.[2] It was not until the development of a method to measure urinary steroids did it become clear that elevated steroids in patients with Cushing syndrome were the result of excess plasma cortisol (hypercortisolism).

Cushing syndrome results from the effects of supraphysiologic concentrations of glucocorticoids originating either from the exogenous administration or, less commonly, endogenous overproduction by the adrenal glands. Excess glucocorticoids are produced in response to the overproduction of ACTH (ACTH-dependent) or by abnormal adrenocortical tissues (ACTH-independent). ACTH-dependent Cushing syndrome (≈80% of all Cushing syndrome cases) usually originates from an overproduction of ACTH by the pituitary gland. Excessive ACTH chronically stimulates the adrenal glands causing bilateral adrenal hyperplasia (BAH). Approximately 85% of these cases are caused by pituitary adenomas (Cushing disease). Ectopic ACTH-secreting tumors and non-neoplastic corticotropin hypersecretion, possibly secondary to excess CRH production, account for the remainder of ACTH-dependent causes.[3] Ectopic ACTH syndrome refers to excessive ACTH production resulting from an endocrine or nonendocrine tumor, usually of the pancreas, thyroid, or lung. Small-cell carcinoma of the lung will lead to ectopic ACTH secretion in 0.5% to 2% of cases, whereas bronchial carcinoid tumors are usually the most common.[4] Distinguishing between the various etiologies requires a careful history and laboratory work (Table 97-2).

The remaining 20% of Cushing syndrome cases are ACTH-independent and divided almost equally between adrenal adenomas and adrenal carcinomas. In rare cases, macronodular hyperplasia, primary pigmented nodular adrenal disease, or McCune–Albright syndrome is the culprit.[3,5] The majority of adrenal cortex tumors are benign adenomas. Adrenal carcinoma is found more often in children than in adults with Cushing syndrome.

Patients with Cushing syndrome commonly present (>90% of patients) with central obesity and facial rounding. Approximately 50% of patients exhibit some peripheral obesity and fat accumulation. Fat accumulation in the dorsocervical area (buffalo hump) is often associated with weight gain, whereas increased supraclavicular fat pads are more specific for Cushing syndrome. Striae are usually present along the lower abdomen and have a red to purple color. Traditionally, complications caused by high blood pressure have been major contributors to the morbidity and mortality of Cushing syndrome. Hypertension is diagnosed in 75% to 85% of patients, with diastolic blood pressures greater than 119 mm Hg noted in over 20% of patients.[6] Glucose intolerance is present in 60% of patients. Thus, many patients meet diagnostic criteria for the metabolic syndrome and have a corresponding increased risk of coronary heart disease (CHD) and stroke. Screening for Cushing syndrome in this population and in patients with uncontrolled diabetes mellitus has been suggested,[7,8] particularly when these conditions surface at an unusually early age.[9] However, screening all patients with type 2 diabetes is likely not cost-effective.[10]

Iatrogenic (exogenous) causes of Cushing syndrome is the most common etiology. Therefore, all patients exhibiting hypercortisolism should undergo a comprehensive history and evaluation assessing medication use before laboratory testing is performed to identify endogenous sources. Iatrogenic Cushing syndrome can occur from the administration of oral, inhaled, intranasal, intra-articular, and topical glucocorticoids, as well as progestins such as medroxyprogesterone acetate and megestrol acetate.[11] Disease severity correlates with exogenous glucocorticoid potency, dose, frequency, route, and treatment duration. Moreover, patients taking CYP3A4 inhibitors concurrently with a glucocorticoid can be at higher risk of developing iatrogenic Cushing syndrome.[12,13] If exogenous glucocorticoids are being taken, the plasma cortisol concentration can increase, while the corticosterone concentration remains low.[14]

In the absence of any known exogenous causes, the clinician will need to differentiate the syndrome from other causes, such as pseudo-Cushing syndrome, that mimic true Cushing syndrome. Patients with obesity, chronic alcoholism, depression, and acute illness of any type can present with certain features of Cushing syndrome. For example, patients who have major depressive disorder may have urinary steroid abnormalities seen in Cushing syndrome, but do not have the cushingoid appearance. In chronic alcoholism, steroid laboratory panels generally return to baseline after ceasing alcohol intake. And obese patients often will have normal cortisol concentrations for both serum and urinary screening tests. Thus, identifying true cases of Cushing syndrome requires a comprehensive history in combination with laboratory and possibly imaging assessment.

2 The diagnosis of Cushing syndrome involves two steps: (a) establishing the presence of hypercortisolism, which is relatively easy, and (b) determining the etiology, which can be challenging (Fig. 97-4).[5,8,15] The presence of hypercortisolism can be established via one or more of the following tests: 24-hour UFC, midnight plasma cortisol, late-night salivary cortisol, or the low-dose DST (using 1 mg dexamethasone for the overnight test or 0.5 mg/6 hr for the classic 2-day study). However, because these tests cannot determine the etiology of Cushing syndrome, other tests and procedures must be subsequently employed. Such tests can include any of the following: plasma ACTH via immunoradiometric assay (IRMA) or radioimmunoassay (RIA); adrenal vein catheterization; metyrapone stimulation test; adrenal, chest, or abdominal computed tomography (CT); CRH stimulation test; inferior petrosal sinus sampling (IPSS); jugular venous sampling (JVS); cavernous sinus sampling; and pituitary magnetic resonance imaging (MRI). High-dose DST has been used in the past but is no longer recommended due to its poor specificity and limited diagnostic value. Other possible tests and procedures include insulin-induced hypoglycemia, somatostatin receptor

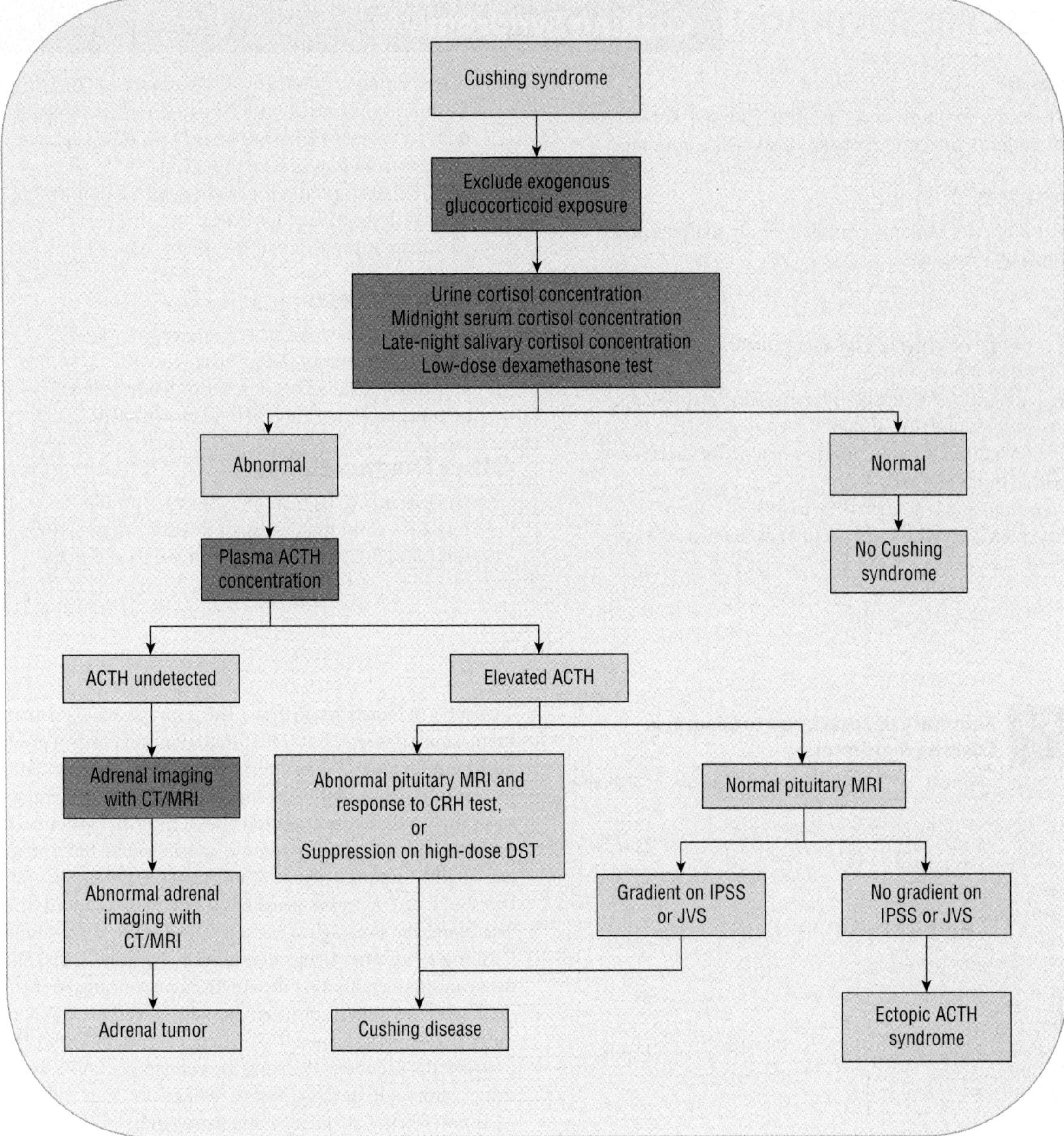

FIGURE 97-4 Algorithm for diagnosing Cushing syndrome. (ACTH, adrenocorticotropic hormone; CRH, corticotropin-releasing hormone; CT, computed tomography; DST, dexamethasone suppression test; IPSS, inferior petrosal sinus sampling; JVS, jugular venous sampling; MRI, magnetic resonance imaging.)

scintigraphy, the desmopressin stimulation test, the naloxone CRH stimulation test, the loperamide test, the hexarelin stimulation test, and radionuclide imaging.[5,6,8,15-20] Table 97-3 summarizes the findings from some of the tests used to diagnose Cushing syndrome.

Elevated UFC concentrations are highly suggestive of Cushing syndrome, especially values fourfold greater than the upper limit of normal.[3,17] In contrast to plasma measurements of cortisol, UFC measures only unbound cortisol. Consequently, the UFC test is unaffected by conditions and medications that alter CBG levels. Normal reference values for UFC are 10 to 60 μg per 24-hour period (30-170 nmol/day). A two- to threefold increase in urine cortisol is not uncommon in the patient with hyperfunction of the adrenal gland. Starvation, hydration from water loading (≥5 L/day), alcoholism, and acute stress are all capable of elevating urine cortisol concentrations. Likewise, elevated UFC results can occur during therapy with carbamazepine, fenofibrate, and topical steroids depending on the type of UFC test. Conversely, renal impairment (creatinine clearance [CrCl] of <60 mL/min [1.0 mL/s]) can falsely lower UFC concentrations. Because other pathologic conditions can increase the amount of free cortisol, additional tests may be warranted to confirm the diagnosis, or the diagnostic evaluation should be repeated when the acute stress has resolved. Of all urinary measures, UFC is the most useful assessment for patients with suspected Cushing syndrome.[8,17,19]

In healthy individuals, cortisol release follows a circadian rhythm whereby serum cortisol concentration peaks around 8:00 am and thereafter declines by 60% to 80%, reaching a nadir between 1:00 and 3:00 am. This rhythm is lost in the patient with Cushing syndrome. Although many patients with Cushing syndrome will have serum cortisol values in the high normal range if the serum is assayed in the morning, only 3.4% will have normal values if measured late at night.[14] Thus, a midnight serum cortisol greater than 7.5 μg/dL (210 nmol/L; >1.8 μg/dL [50 nmol/L] if the patient is sleeping) is a highly sensitive assay for Cushing syndrome. However, this test is cumbersome and rarely recommended because it requires that patients be admitted for more than 48 hours to avoid false-positive

CLINICAL PRESENTATION Cushing Syndrome

General

- The most common findings, which are present in 90% of patients, are central obesity and facial rounding.

Symptoms

- A majority of patients complain of myopathies and muscular weakness.

Signs

- Peripheral obesity and fat accumulation are found in 50% of patients.
- Facial plethora is caused by underlying atrophy of the skin and connective tissue.
- Patients often are described as having moon faces with a buffalo hump.
- Hypertension is seen in 75% to 85% of patients.
- Psychiatric changes can occur in as many as 55% of patients.
- Approximately 50% to 60% of patients will develop Cushing syndrome–induced osteoporosis. Of these, 40% will present with back pain and 20% will have compression fractures of the spine.
- Gonadal dysfunction is common with amenorrhea seen in up to 75% of females.
- Hirsutism is present in 80% of females.

Laboratory Tests

- A midnight plasma cortisol, late-night salivary cortisol, 24-hour urinary free cortisol (UFC), and/or low-dose dexamethasone suppression test (DST) will establish the presence of hypercortisolism.

Other Diagnostic Tests

- The plasma ACTH test, metyrapone stimulation test, CRH stimulation test, or inferior petrosal sinus sampling (IPSS) will help determine the etiology.

TABLE 97-3 Summary of Tests Used to Diagnose Cushing Syndrome

Test	Normal	Hyperplasia	Adenoma	Carcinoma
Plasma				
Cortisol (μg/dL or nmol/L, in brackets; for am/pm)	5-25/5-15 (140-690/140-415)	↑/↑↑	↑↑/↑↑	↑↑↑/↑↑↑
After low-dose DST	↓	↔	↔	↔
After high-dose DST	↓	↓/↔	↔	↔
ACTH (pg/mL or pmol/L, in brackets)	6-76 (1.3-17)	↑↑	↓	↓
Urine				
Cortisol (μg/24 hours or nmol/day, in brackets)	20-90 (55-250)	↑↑	↑↑	↑↑↑
Saliva				
Cortisol (μg/dL or nmol/L), PM)	Assay-dependent	↑↑	↑↑	↑↑↑

Data from Kratz A, Ferraro M, Sluss PM, Lewandrowski KB. Laboratory reference values. N Engl J Med. 2004;351(15):1548–1563.

responses secondary to the stress of hospitalization. An alternative assay is the measurement of late-night salivary cortisol. Salivary cortisol is highly correlated with free serum cortisol and independent of salivary flow rates. Moreover, salivary cortisol concentration reflects changes in serum cortisol within minutes. Salivary cortisol can be considered an acceptable alternative to UFC because of its convenience, stability (1 week), accuracy, and reproducibility. Unfortunately, normal reference ranges are assay-dependent, and cutoff points vary among institutions.[21,22]

In the overnight DST, 1 mg of dexamethasone is administered at 11:00 pm. The following morning at 8:00 am fasting plasma cortisol is obtained for analysis. This supraphysiologic dose of dexamethasone suppresses ACTH stimulation and cortisol production in healthy individuals. In contrast, the negative feedback loop is ineffective in patients with Cushing syndrome who generally exhibit a morning cortisol concentration above 5 μg/dL (140 nmol/L). Some patients with Cushing syndrome administered the overnight DST can slightly suppress cortisol and using a 1.8 μg/dL (50 nmol/L) threshold can increase sensitivity, but with reduced specificity.[23] Therefore, the overnight DST is useful only as a screening tool for Cushing syndrome. Drugs that induce or inhibit CYP3A4 metabolism can significantly alter dexamethasone concentration, increasing the likelihood of false-positive and false-negative DSTs. Concurrent measurements of dexamethasone concentration with cortisol may improve the accuracy of testing for patients on CYP3A4-modifying drugs, although dexamethasone assays are not widely available. Also noteworthy, pregnancy and estrogen use (including oral contraceptives) increase CBG levels and frequently elicit false-positive results.[17] Consequently, UFC testing is preferred over DST in these patient populations.

The first test used to determine the etiology of Cushing syndrome is the plasma ACTH test. Plasma ACTH concentrations can be measured via RIA or IRMA.[16] In ACTH-dependent Cushing syndrome, ACTH can be normal or elevated. Very high levels of ACTH favor ectopic production. In contrast, ACTH values generally are low (<5 pg/mL [1.1 pmol/L]) in ACTH-independent (adrenal) Cushing syndrome. Furthermore, ACTH levels can appear artificially low in some ectopic ACTH-producing tumors because ACTH can be secreted as an active prohormone that is not detected by the assay.

IPSS offers the highest sensitivity and specificity of any test in differentiating the etiology of Cushing syndrome. This technique requires catheterization of both petrosal sinuses with serial measurements of ACTH in each sinus and a peripheral vein after administration of CRH. A central-to-peripheral ACTH gradient is diagnostic for Cushing disease, whereas no gradient indicates ectopic ACTH production. Complications, such as venous thromboembolism, brain stem vascular damage, high cost, and technical expertise can limit the use of this test.[16] JVS uses the same concept as IPSS, is less invasive, and produces fewer complications; however, sensitivity is compromised.

Abnormal adrenal anatomy is effectively identified using high-resolution CT scanning and MRI.[24] Nodules as small as 1 to 1.5 cm on the adrenal cortex are easily identified by CT. With the use of thin-section scanning, nodules as small as 3 to 5 mm can be visualized.[25] Importantly, adrenal incidentalomas (masses observed incidentally on imaging) are prevalent in 5% to 10% of the general population. These masses may be functional (secreting), requiring intervention, or nonfunctional (nonsecreting), requiring only periodic observation. For this reason, abnormal imaging results alone are insufficient to conclusively diagnose adrenal disease. Nonadrenal imaging studies may be useful for identifying ectopic sources of ACTH secretion in patients for whom IPSS has ruled out Cushing disease.

3 If left untreated, Cushing syndrome is associated with high morbidity and mortality due to hypertension, diabetes mellitus, cardiovascular disease, and electrolyte abnormalities. On average, patients with Cushing syndrome live only 4 to 5 years following initial diagnosis. The desired outcomes of treatment are to limit such detrimental outcomes and return the patient to a normal functional state by removing the source of hypercortisolism while minimizing pituitary or adrenal deficiencies.

4 The treatment of choice for both ACTH-dependent and ACTH-independent Cushing syndrome is surgical resection of any offending tumors.[3,15] Pharmacologic treatment options which target the etiology of the disease are generally reserved as second-line treatment for those patients who are not surgical candidates (Table 97-4).[3,26-29] Pharmacotherapy may also be used preoperatively or as adjunctive therapy in the postoperative period awaiting a response. Rarely, pharmacotherapy is used as a palliative treatment when surgery is not indicated.

Non-Pharmacologic Therapy

Pituitary Adenoma The treatment of choice for Cushing disease is transsphenoidal resection of the pituitary tumor.[3,15,29-31] The advantages of this procedure include preservation of pituitary function, low complication rate, and high clinical improvement rate. The overall cure rate of histologically proven microadenomas (tumor diameter <10 mm) approaches 90%, whereas remission rates for macroadenomas (tumor diameter ≥10 mm) generally do not exceed 65%.

For persistent disease following transsphenoidal surgery or when tumor-specific surgery is not possible, several second-line treatment options are available and should be tailored toward the individual patient.[29] In the case of persistent disease following transsphenoidal surgery, repeat surgery may be performed, particularly in patients with evidence of incomplete resection or pituitary lesion on imaging.[29] Although overall remission rates are lower with subsequent procedures, remission can be achieved rapidly when compared to alternative second-line treatments.[29] Alternatively, radiotherapy may be preferred for tumors invading the dura or cavernous sinus because these tumors respond poorly to surgical intervention.[32] Radiotherapy provides clinical improvement in approximately 50% of patients within 3 to 5 years, but increases the risk for pituitary-dependent hormone deficiencies (hypopituitarism).

Adrenal Adenoma Laparoscopic adrenalectomy is often preferred in patients with unilateral adrenal adenomas for whom transsphenoidal surgery and pituitary radiotherapy have failed or cannot be used.[3,15,30] Bilateral adrenalectomy rapidly reverses hypercortisolism. However, patients can develop Nelson syndrome, an aggressive pituitary tumor that secretes high quantities of ACTH, which causes hyperpigmentation. Because Nelson syndrome occurs in as many as 30% of bilateral adrenalectomy cases, patients should undergo regular MRI scans and ACTH level assessments. Additionally, these patients require lifelong glucocorticoid and mineralocorticoid supplementation.

Surgical resection of benign adrenal adenoma is associated with relatively few side effects and a high cure rate (95%). The contralateral gland in the patient with adrenal adenoma is usually atrophic; therefore, steroid replacement is needed both perioperatively and postoperatively. Table 97-5 outlines an approach to steroid replacement for three separate routes of hydrocortisone. Therapy should be continued for 6 to 12 months following surgery. Before replacement therapy is discontinued, recovery of the adrenal axis can be assessed by measuring the morning (8:00 am) cortisol concentration. The cortisol concentration should exceed 20 μg/dL (550 nmol/L) before discontinuing exogenous steroids.[11]

Adrenal Carcinoma Unlike the benign adenoma patient, those with adrenal carcinoma generally have an unfavorable outcome with surgical resection.[15] Often the complete tumor cannot be excised, leaving the patient with some degree of symptoms and extra-adrenal involvement. Radiotherapy can be used if metastases are discovered. In a patient with adrenal carcinoma who is not a surgical candidate, the focus of treatment is on palliative pharmacologic intervention.

Mitotane may be used in inoperable functional and non-functional adrenal carcinoma or as adjuvant therapy in surgical patients with a high risk of relapse and may prolong survival by 2 to 3 years.[33] However, mitotane induces tumor regression in fewer

TABLE 97-4 Possible Treatment Options in Cushing Syndrome Based on Etiology

	Treatment	
Etiology	**Non-pharmacologic**	**Pharmacologic**
Ectopic ACTH syndrome	Surgery, chemotherapy, irradiation	Metyrapone Ketoconazole
Pituitary-dependent	Surgery, irradiation	Mitotane Metyrapone Mifepristone Cabergoline Pasireotide
Adrenal adenoma	Surgery, postoperative replacement	Ketoconazole
Adrenal carcinoma	Surgery	Mitotane

TABLE 97-5 Alternative Steroid Replacement Regimens in the Adrenal Adenoma Patient

	Hydrocortisone Dose (mg)		
Time	**IV**	**IM**	**po**
Operation day	300	50 before surgery and 50 after surgery	
Postoperative day 1	200	50 every 12 hours	
Postoperative day 2	150	50 every 12 hours	
Postoperative day 3	100	50 every 12 hours	
Postoperative day 4		50 every 12 hours	25 every 6 hours
Postoperative day 5		25 every 12 hours	25 every 6 hours[a]
Postoperative day 7			25 every 6 hours
Postoperative days 8-10			25 every 8 hours
Postoperative days 11-20			25 every 12 hours
Postoperative days 21+			20 at 8:00 am
			10 at 4:00 pm

(PO, by mouth/orally)

[a]Add fludrocortisone 0.05-2 mg orally once daily starting on postoperative day 5. Adjust dose based on blood pressure, body weight, and serum electrolytes.

than 20% of patients.[34] Metyrapone and ketoconazole can be given as adjunctive treatment to attempt control of steroid hypersecretion. 5-Fluorouracil also has been used in combination therapy.

Ectopic Adrenocorticotropic Hormone Syndrome In ectopic ACTH syndrome, ACTH-secreting tumors may exist in a variety of sites, including thymic, pulmonary, appendiceal, pancreatic, and thyroid tissues. Locating these sites is often difficult, but essential for determining an appropriate treatment strategy. Surgical resection is the most effective treatment option for these patients, but only approximately 10% to 30% of patients are cured following surgery due to high rates of metastatic disease or occult tumors. The remaining 70% to 90% receive postoperative medication.

Pharmacologic management with steroidogenesis inhibitors is effective in patients with ectopic ACTH syndrome and may be used as primary treatment in patients with occult or metastatic ectopic ACTH syndrome.[29] Mitotane has been used in this setting; however, its side-effect profile generally limits its use. Mifepristone and somatostatin analogs also have been reported to reduce the clinical signs of ectopic ACTH syndrome.[35]

Additional tumor-directed therapy can include systemic chemotherapy, interferon α, chemoembolization, radiofrequency ablation, and radiation therapy.[32] If all else fails, bilateral adrenalectomy can prevent the downstream effects (eg, steroidogenesis) of high levels of tumor ACTH secretion.

Pharmacologic Therapy

5 Pharmacotherapy of Cushing syndrome can be divided into four categories based on the anatomic site of action: (1) steroidogenesis inhibitors, (2) adrenolytic agents, (3) neuromodulators of ACTH release, and (4) glucocorticoid-receptor blocking agents.[26,27] Dosing and monitoring parameters can be found in Table 97-6 and Table 97-7, respectively.[3,28,29]

TABLE 97-6 Drug Dosing in the Treatment of Cushing Syndrome

Drug	Initial Dose	Usual Range	Special Populations	Comments
Cabergoline	0.5 mg once weekly	0.5-7 mg once weekly		Maximum: 7 mg/week
Etomidate	0.03 mg/kg IV bolus	0.1-0.3 mg/kg/hr infusion		Maximum: 0.3 mg/kg/hr infusion; titrate based on serum cortisol concentration
Ketoconazole	200 mg once or twice a day	200-1,200 mg/day, divided twice a day	Contraindicated in patients with hepatic disease	Maximum: 1,600 mg/day; CYP3A4 substrate and inhibitor (strong)
Metyrapone	0.5-1 g/day, divided every 4-6 hours	1-2 g/day, divided every 4-6 hours		Maximum: 6 g/day; CYP3A4 inducer
Mifepristone	300 mg once daily, increased by 300 mg/day every 2-4 weeks	600-1,200 mg/day	Do not exceed 600 mg/day in mild-to-moderate hepatic impairment; avoid in severe hepatic impairment. Do not exceed 600 mg/day in renal impairment	Maximum: 1,200 mg/day not to exceed 20 mg/kg/day
Mitotane	0.5-1 g/day, increased by 0.5-1 g/day every 1-4 weeks	1-4 g/day		Maximum: 12 g/day (most patients unable to tolerate >8 g/day). Take with food to decrease GI effects
Osilodrostat	2 mg twice daily	2-7 mg twice daily	Moderate hepatic impairment: 1 mg twice daily; Severe hepatic impairment: 1 mg once daily in the evening	Comments: Maximum 60 mg/day
Pasireotide	0.6-0.9 mg twice daily	0.3-0.9 mg twice daily	Reduce dose in hepatic impairment	Maximum: 1.8 mg/day

GI, gastrointestinal.

TABLE 97-7 Drug Monitoring in the Treatment of Cushing Syndrome

Drug	Adverse Drug Reaction	Monitoring Parameters	Comments
Cabergoline	Nausea, dizziness, headache, nasal congestion, constipation, psychiatric symptoms, valvulopathy	Echocardiogram	
Etomidate	Sedation, pain at the injection site, hypotension, myoclonus, nausea, vomiting	Frequent sedation scoring initially, serum potassium, serum cortisol	
Ketoconazole	GI upset, dermatologic reactions; elevated hepatic transaminases, hepatotoxicity	Liver function tests, including ALT/AST, total bilirubin, ALP, prothrombin time, and INR testing	Approximately 10% will experience reversible LFT elevations
Metyrapone	Androgenic effects (hirsutism, acne, etc.), blood pressure and electrolyte abnormalities, nausea, vomiting, vertigo, headache, dizziness, abdominal discomfort, allergic rash	Blood pressure, electrolytes	
Mifepristone	Hypokalemia, nausea, fatigue, headache, peripheral edema, dizziness, endometrial hyperplasia	Serum potassium, pregnancy testing, pelvic ultrasound	Abortifacient; rule out pregnancy in women of childbearing potential
Mitotane	GI upset, nausea, diarrhea, lethargy, somnolence, CNS disturbances	UFC and urinary steroid production, serum potassium	GI upset in up to 80%; GI and CNS effects appear to be dose-dependent
Pasireotide	Nausea, diarrhea, cholelithiasis, increased hepatic transaminases, hyperglycemia, sinus bradycardia, QT prolongation	Serum glucose, serum potassium, hemoglobin A1c, liver function tests, UFC, thyroid function, heart rate, ECG	Only available as a subcutaneous injection; expensive

ALP, alkaline phosphatase; ALT, alanine aminotransferase; AST, aspartate aminotransferase; CNS, central nervous system; FDA, Food and Drug Administration; INR, international normalized ratio; LFT, liver function tests; GI, gastrointestinal; ECG, electrocardiogram; UFC, urinary free cortisol.

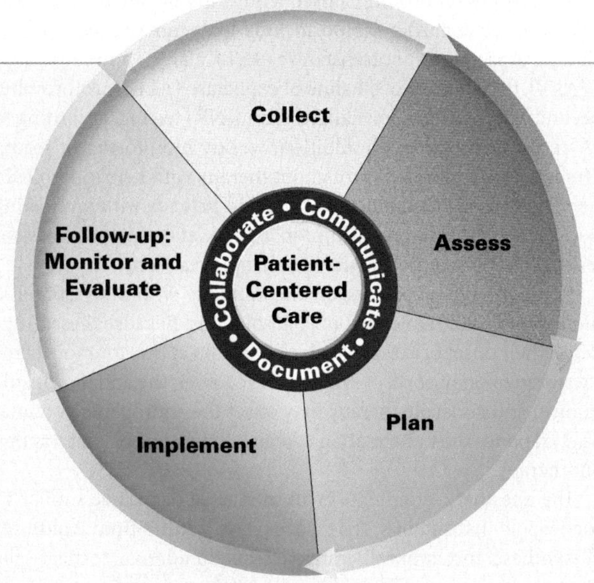

Patient Care Process for Cushing Syndrome

The image shows the five fundamental steps included in The Pharmacist's Care Process endorsed by the Joint Commission for Pharmacy Practitioners (2014). The tagline of this process reads collaborate, communicate, and document. The five fundamental steps listed here are collect, assess, plan, implement, and follow-up: monitor and evaluate. All these steps are listed in a circular block diagram.

Collect

- Patient characteristics (eg, age, sex, pregnant)
- Patient medical history (personal and family)
- Social history (eg, tobacco/ethanol use)
- Iatrogenic causes of Cushing syndrome: current medications including corticosteroids (all routes, past and present), medroxyprogesterone acetate, megestrol acetate, gamma-hydroxybutyic acid, CYP3A4 inhibitors, and inducers
- Objective data
  - Blood pressure, heart rate, body mass index
  - Test for hypercortisolism: 24-hour UFC, midnight plasma cortisol, late-night salivary cortisol, or low-dose DST
  - Follow-up diagnostic tests to differentiate etiologies (see Fig. 97-4)

Assess

- Presence of Cushing syndrome complications:
  - Metabolic: impaired glucose metabolism, dyslipidemia
  - Cardiovascular: hypertension, vascular damage, thrombosis, hypokalemia
  - Immunologic: bacterial, fungal, and viral infections; rebound autoimmunity Musculoskeletal: osteopenia/osteoporosis, myopathy
  - Neuropsychiatric: depression, anxiety, bipolar disorder, lethargy
  - Reproductive: decreased libido, hypogonadism (men), menstrual irregularity (women)
  - Dermatologic: hirsutism, alopecia, hyperhidrosis
- Physical exam: Peripheral obesity, fat accumulation (Buffalo Hump), rounded face (moon face), striae, ecchymosis, hyperpigmentation, acanthosis nigricans, acne, and thin skin
- Current medications that may contribute to or worsen Cushing syndrome
- Results of follow-up diagnostic testing for etiology (see Fig. 97-4 and Tables 97-2 and 97-3)
- Ability/willingness to pursue surgical/chemotherapeutic (if indicated) versus medical management

Plan*

- Ensure proper administration of necessary corticosteroid therapy; discontinue unnecessary corticosteroid therapy, with taper if HPA axis integrity is suspect
- Nondrug options for endogenous Cushing syndrome, depending on etiology: surgery, chemotherapy, irradiation, postoperative steroid replacement (see Table 97-4)
- Steroid replacement regimens postoperatively for patients with adrenal adenomas (see Table 97-5)
- Medical management when surgery is not possible or against patient wishes (see Tables 97-6 and 97-7 for specific drugs, dose, route, frequency, adverse effects, and monitoring parameters)
- Patient education (eg, purpose of treatment, dietary and lifestyle modification, invasive procedures, drug-specific information) and specialist referral when appropriate (eg, endocrinologist)

Implement*

- Provide patient education regarding all elements of the treatment plan
- Use motivational interviewing and coaching strategies to maximize adherence
- Schedule follow-up for monitoring

Follow-up: Monitor and Evaluate

- Clinical response, including resolution of signs/symptoms
- Treatment-emergent adverse effects (eg, adrenal insufficiency [all], medication-specific adverse effects)
- Monitoring parameters including efficacy (eg, UFC) and safety (eg, ECG, liver function, electrolytes, A1c)
- Frequency and timing of follow-up for specific agents (see Table 97-7 and text for agent-specific monitoring)

Collaborate with patient, caregivers, and other healthcare professionals.

Several factors may limit the ability to personalize pharmacotherapy in patients with Cushing syndrome. First, few rigorous studies have compared the various pharmacologic options used in Cushing syndrome. Apart from the benefits seen with pasireotide in patients with modestly elevated UFC and the use of mifepristone in patients with concomitant hyperglycemia, data are limited in terms of clinical predictors of disease response to these agents. Second, virtually nothing is known of the pharmacogenomic predictors of individual patient response in these disease states. Finally, because most agents are used off-label, scarce data exist on agent-specific pharmacokinetic parameters in this patient population.

With these limitations in mind, drug selection is determined according to the etiology of Cushing syndrome, individual patient factors, drug-drug interactions, and cost. Once the etiology has been correctly identified, patient sex and gender should be considered since some pharmacologic options (steroidogenesis inhibitors in particular) used in Cushing syndrome affect the sex hormones. Specifically, metyrapone is a clear second choice in women due to a high incidence of hirsutism, whereas ketoconazole may be a secondary choice in men due to drug-induced gynecomastia and hypogonadism. During pregnancy, metyrapone is commonly used, while mifepristone must be avoided. Additionally, women desiring pregnancy within the next five years should avoid mitotane as this agent is stored in adipose tissue for up to several years following discontinuation. Preexisting medication profiles should also be considered since many of the pharmacologic options can inhibit (eg, ketoconazole) or induce (eg, metyrapone) important CYP isoenzymes such as 3A4.

Ultimately, pharmacotherapy is guided by patient response and several agents may need to be sequentially tried to elicit a substantial response. Combination therapy may be more effective and better tolerated than monotherapy in some patients, but studies involving multi-drug regimens are lacking.

Steroidogenesis Inhibitors

As their name implies, steroidogenesis inhibitors block the production of cortisol. This class includes metyrapone, ketoconazole, etomidate, and osilodrostat. Metyrapone inhibits 11β-hydroxylase, the enzyme responsible for converting 11-deoxycortisol to cortisol. Following administration, a sudden decrease in cortisol concentration occurs within hours and prompts a compensatory rise in plasma ACTH concentrations. As ACTH increases and blockage of cortisol synthesis persists, adrenal steroidogenesis efforts are shunted toward androgen production. Consequently, metyrapone is associated with significant androgenic side effects, including hirsutism and increased acne, making it less ideal for women. In addition, metyrapone blocks aldosterone synthesis and causes the accumulation of aldosterone precursors, which exhibit weak mineralocorticoid activity. Blood pressure and electrolyte perturbations can ensue, depending on the level of circulating 11-deoxycortisol and the degree of aldosterone inhibition. Additional adverse effects, including nausea, vomiting, vertigo, headache, dizziness, abdominal discomfort, and allergic rash, have been reported following administration, but are often signs of overtreatment.[26,27,30]

The imidazole derivative antifungal, ketoconazole, effectively inhibits steroidogenesis via multiple mechanisms when used in large doses. In contrast to the quick onset of metyrapone, the benefits of ketoconazole therapy are achieved only after several weeks of therapy. In addition to lowering serum cortisol levels, ketoconazole exhibits antiandrogenic activity attributable to its inhibition of multiple CYP enzymes as well as 11β-hydroxylase and 17α-hydroxylase.[26] This activity may be beneficial in women with Cushing syndrome but can cause gynecomastia and hypogonadism in men. Sustained therapy with ketoconazole also imparts beneficial effects on serum cholesterol profiles, including lowering total and low-density lipoprotein (LDL) cholesterol levels. Ketoconazole induces a reversible elevation of hepatic transaminases in approximately 10% of patients.[36] However, concerns have been raised over the risk of severe hepatotoxicity associated with ketoconazole use. In July 2013, the US Food and Drug Administration (FDA) significantly changed the labeling of oral ketoconazole, removing various indications for fungal infections and recommending that oral ketoconazole not be used as first-line therapy for fungal infections. Similarly, the European Medicines Agency has recommended the complete removal of oral ketoconazole from European Union markets. These changes were based largely on data in patients with fungal infections, who require lower doses of ketoconazole. However, few data are available on the incidence of severe hepatotoxicity with ketoconazole at the higher doses used in Cushing syndrome. Consequently, monitoring during treatment with ketoconazole should include liver function at baseline, including aspartate aminotransferase (AST), alanine aminotransferase (ALT), total bilirubin, alkaline phosphatase (ALP), prothrombin time, and international normalized ratio (INR) testing, according to FDA recommendations. In addition, weekly monitoring of serum ALT should be continued throughout therapy with ketoconazole. In general, ketoconazole should be avoided in patients with preexisting hepatic disease. Additional common adverse effects include gastrointestinal (GI) discomfort and dermatologic reactions.

Ketoconazole may be used concomitantly with metyrapone to achieve synergistic reductions in cortisol levels. Because these drugs differ in their onset of action, coadministration allows for more complete suppression of cortisol synthesis. Moreover, the antiandrogenic actions of ketoconazole therapy may offset the androgenic potential of metyrapone, thus attenuating a major limitation of metyrapone monotherapy.

The anesthetic etomidate is an imidazole derivative similar to ketoconazole that inhibits 11β-hydroxylase.[26] Inhibition of aldosterone synthase and antiproliferative effects on adrenal cortical cells may also play a role.[37] Etomidate is available only in a parenteral formulation and is therefore limited to patients with acute hypercortisolemia requiring emergency treatment or in preparation for surgery. Low doses of etomidate are often sufficient to suppress cortisol synthesis, thus potentially avoiding some of the adverse effects observed with higher doses used in anesthesia. However, close monitoring is recommended to avoid excess sedation with this agent.[37] Frequent monitoring of serum cortisol is also advised to prevent hypocortisolemia. Replacement corticosteroid doses may be necessary if a complete blockade of cortisol is desired.

Osilodrostat prevents cortisol synthesis via inhibition of 11β-hydroxylase and is indicated for treating patients with Cushing disease who are either not candidates for surgical therapy or in whom symptoms persist after surgery. Osilodrostat is available as an oral tablet administered twice daily, with or without food. Electrolyte imbalances, namely hypokalemia and hypomagnesemia, should be corrected prior to use, and an ECG should be obtained at baseline and again one week after treatment initiation to monitor possible QTc prolongation. Adverse effects are similar to other 11β-hydroxylase inhibitors, including hypocortisolism, QTc prolongation, nausea, and headache.

Adrenolytic Agents

Mitotane is a cytotoxic drug that structurally resembles the insecticide dichlorodiphenyltrichloroethane (DDT). Mitotane inhibits the 11-hydroxylation of 11-desoxycortisol and 11-desoxycorticosterone in the adrenal cortex, resulting in an inhibition of cortisol and corticosterone synthesis. Similar to ketoconazole, mitotane takes weeks to months to exert beneficial effects. Sustained cortisol suppression occurs in most patients (~80%) and may persist following discontinuation of therapy in up to one-third of patients. Because of its cytotoxic nature, mitotane degenerates cells within the zona fasciculata and reticularis, resulting in atrophy of the adrenal cortex. The zona glomerulosa is minimally affected during acute therapy but can be damaged during long-term treatment.[28,29]

Importantly, mitotane can induce significant neurologic and GI side effects and patients should be monitored carefully or hospitalized when initiating therapy. Nausea and diarrhea are common adverse effects that occur at doses greater than 2 g/day and can be avoided by gradually increasing the dose and/or administering the agent with food. Most patients are unable to tolerate doses exceeding 8 g/day. Approximately 80% of patients treated with mitotane develop lethargy and somnolence, and other central nervous system (CNS) adverse drug reactions occur in approximately 40% of patients. Furthermore, significant but reversible hypercholesterolemia and prolongation of bleeding times can result from mitotane use.[26,27] Mitotane increases production of CBG resulting in elevated plasma cortisol measurements; thus, UFC and urinary steroid production should be monitored to assess response to therapy.[26] If necessary, steroid replacement therapy can be given. However, because mitotane also increases extra-adrenal metabolism of exogenously administered corticosteroids (especially hydrocortisone), higher steroid replacement doses may be required. In select patients, supplemental androgen therapy also may be necessary.

Neuromodulatory Agents

Pituitary secretion of ACTH is normally mediated by various neurotransmitters, including serotonin, γ-aminobutyric acid (GABA), acetylcholine, and the catecholamines. Although ACTH-secreting pituitary tumors (Cushing disease) self-regulate ACTH production to some degree, these neurotransmitters are still capable of promoting pituitary ACTH production. Consequently, agents that target these neurotransmitters have been proposed for the treatment of Cushing disease. Such agents include cyproheptadine, ritanserin, ketanserin, bromocriptine, cabergoline, valproic acid, octreotide, lanreotide, pasireotide, rosiglitazone, and tretinoin. However, with the exception of pasireotide, none of these drugs have demonstrated consistent clinical efficacy in the treatment of Cushing disease.

Cyproheptadine, a nonselective serotonin-receptor antagonist and anticholinergic drug, can decrease ACTH secretion in some patients with Cushing disease. However, side effects, including sedation and weight gain, significantly limit the use of this drug. Likewise, selective serotonin type 2-receptor antagonists, including ritanserin and ketanserin, have demonstrated limited efficacy. Owing to their poor efficacy and high relapse rates, these drugs should be avoided except in nonsurgical candidates refractory to more conventional treatments.

Dopamine D_2-receptor agonists, including bromocriptine and cabergoline, initially reduce ACTH secretion in as many as half of all patients with Cushing disease. This action occurs through the activation of inhibitory D_2 receptors that are expressed in approximately 80% of pituitary adenomas.[38] Reductions in ACTH levels are often minor and rarely sustained with long-term bromocriptine therapy. Cabergoline exhibits a higher specificity and affinity for D_2 receptors as well as a prolonged half-life compared with bromocriptine. These differences may explain the greater response rates observed with cabergoline monotherapy; however, a sustained response occurs in only 30% to 40% of patients.[39,40] Although generally well-tolerated, side effects associated with cabergoline include nausea, orthostasis, headache, nasal congestion, constipation, nightmares, vivid dreams, and psychosis. The risk of cabergoline-associated cardiac valvulopathy (observed with higher doses used to treat Parkinson disease) has not been well-studied in lower doses typically used for the treatment of Cushing disease.[41]

The somatostatin analogs octreotide and lanreotide generally are ineffective in reducing ACTH secretion in Cushing disease. These two agents primarily target somatostatin receptor subtype 2 (sst_2), whereas pituitary adenomas predominantly express sst_5. Pasireotide, a somatostatin analog, exhibits a high affinity for sst_1, sst_2, sst_3, and, especially, sst_5 receptor subtypes. In a phase 3 study of 162 adults with Cushing disease and an elevated UFC, pasireotide administered at 600 or 900 μg injected subcutaneously twice daily reduced the median UFC by 50% by month two; levels remained stable for the duration of the 12-month study.[42] Pasireotide is especially effective at normalizing UFC concentrations in patients whose baseline UFC is less than five times the upper limit of normal. Clinical signs and symptoms of Cushing disease are also improved as are blood pressure, weight, LDL cholesterol, and quality of life. Side effects are mostly GI in nature, although 50% to 70% of subjects experience an adverse event related to hyperglycemia; preexisting diabetes mellitus or impaired glucose tolerance increases the risk for these events. Notably, pasireotide increases glycated hemoglobin A1c by an average of 1.4% (0.014; 15 mmol/mol Hb) at 6 months and this effect may be sustained with long-term therapy,[43] likely due to impaired insulin secretion.[44]

Since coexpression of D_2 and sst_5 receptors is common in adrenocorticotropin-secreting adenomas, the combination of pasireotide and cabergoline may produce synergistic effects in reducing cortisol levels.[3] Limited data suggest that step-wise addition of cabergoline and ketoconazole in patients unresponsive to pasireotide may achieve normalization of UFC in the majority of patients; however, additional studies are needed to confirm the efficacy of this combination therapy. Potential drug-drug interactions exist with the combination of pasireotide and ketoconazole, and thus, the combination should be used with caution.[43,45,46]

Glucocorticoid-Receptor Blocking Agents

Mifepristone is a potent progesterone- and glucocorticoid-receptor antagonist that inhibits dexamethasone suppression and increases endogenous cortisol and ACTH levels in normal subjects.[26,30] Clinical experience and trial data in Cushing syndrome suggest that mifepristone is highly effective in reversing the manifestation of hypercortisolism, including hyperglycemia, hypertension, and weight gain.[47] Consequently, mifepristone has an FDA-approved indication for treatment of endogenous Cushing syndrome in patients who have diabetes mellitus or glucose intolerance, and who are not eligible for or have had poor response to surgery. However, because of its novel site of action, mifepristone induces a compensatory rise in ACTH and cortisol. Consequently, efficacy and toxicity monitoring must rely on clinical signs rather than laboratory assessments. Common adverse effects of mifepristone include fatigue, nausea, headache, arthralgia, peripheral edema, endometrial thickening (with or without vaginal bleeding), and significant reductions in serum potassium. Oral potassium supplementation or spironolactone can be effective in mitigating the latter adverse effect, although high doses may be required.[47]

Close monitoring of 24-hour UFC and serum cortisol is essential to detect treatment-induced adrenal insufficiency. Steroid secretion should be monitored with all of these drugs except mifepristone and steroid replacement given as needed. Whatever the choice, pharmacologic therapy in pituitary-dependent disease is mainly centered around patient stabilization prior to surgery or in patients waiting for potential response to other therapies.

Hyperaldosteronism

Excess aldosterone secretion, hyperaldoteronism, can be the result of either primary or secondary causes.[48-51] In primary hyperaldosteronism (PA), the stimulation for aldosterone secretion arises from within the adrenal gland. Conversely, extra-adrenal stimulation is classified as secondary aldosteronism.

Primary Aldosteronism

Etiology The most common causes of PA include BAH (65%) and aldosterone-producing adenoma (APA; otherwise known as Conn syndrome) (30%). Rare causes include unilateral (primary) adrenal hyperplasia, adrenal cortex carcinoma, renin-responsive adrenocortical adenoma, and three forms of familial hyperaldosteronism (FH): FH type I, also known as glucocorticoid-remediable aldosteronism (GRA); FH type II, also known as familial occurrence of adenoma or hyperplasia type II; and FH type III.[48,50,51]

CLINICAL PRESENTATION

PA is present in approximately 10% of patients with hypertension and is a leading cause of secondary hypertension and treatment resistant hypertension. The disease is more common in women than in men, and diagnosis usually occurs between the third and sixth decades of life. Signs and symptoms can include arterial hypertension, which

CLINICAL PRESENTATION Primary Aldosteronism

Symptoms

- Patients may complain of muscle weakness, fatigue, paresthesias, and headache.

Signs

- Hypertension
- Tetany/paralysis
- Polydipsia/nocturnal polyuria

Laboratory Tests

- A plasma-aldosterone-concentration–to–plasma-renin-activity (PAC–to–PRA) ratio or aldosterone-to-renin ratio (ARR) greater than 30 ng/dL per ng/(mL·h) (830 pmol/L per mcg/([L·h]) and a PAC greater than 15 ng/dL (420 pmol/L) is suggestive of PA.
- Common laboratory findings include suppressed PRA, elevated PAC, hypernatremia (>142 mEq/L [mmol/L]), hypokalemia, hypomagnesemia, elevated bicarbonate concentration (>31 mEq/L [mmol/L]), and glucose intolerance.

Confirmatory Tests

- Oral or IV saline loading, fludrocortisone suppression test (FST), and genetic testing

is often moderate to severe and resistant to pharmacologic intervention. Many patients also have hypokalemia (10%-40%), muscle weakness, fatigue, and headache. These features are nonspecific and many patients are asymptomatic. Historically, hypokalemia was considered a requisite feature for PA diagnosis; however, normokalemia exists frequently in patients and does not rule out PA. Unexplained new-onset of atrial fibrillation or other arrhythmias may also be indicative of PA.[52]

Diagnosis

Early diagnosis and treatment of PA are essential as patients with PA are at increased risk of adverse cardiovascular outcomes compared to patients with essential hypertension alone.[53] Diagnostic confirmation of PA is obtainable through screening, confirmatory tests, and subtype differentiation (Fig. 97-5). The discovery of the underlying etiology ensures proper treatment. Table 97-8 lists the various abnormalities that must be ruled out when hyperaldosteronism is suspected.

Initial diagnosis is made by screening patients with suspected PA. Any patient with a blood pressure greater than 150/100 mm Hg measured on three separate days and those meeting the criteria for treatment-resistant hypertension should be screened.[54] Additional patients at risk for PA include those with diuretic-induced hypokalemia, hypertension and adrenal incidentaloma, hypertension and sleep apnea, hypertension and a family history of early-onset hypertension or cerebrovascular accident at an age less than 40 years, and all patients with hypertension and a first-degree relative diagnosed with PA.

Screening for PA is most often done by using the PAC-to-PRA ratio, otherwise known as the ARR. An elevated ARR is highly suggestive of PA; however, an optimal cutoff ratio remains elusive because testing conditions (posture, time, current drug therapy, recent dietary salt intake), patient characteristics, and assay variability can significantly alter test results.[55] ARR cutoffs of 20 to 40 ng/dL per ng/(mL·h) (550 to 1100 pmol/L per [mcg/(L·h]) with an aldosterone concentration greater than 15 ng/dL (420 pmol/L) are used most often.[49,55-57]

Following a positive ARR screening test, confirmatory testing must be performed to exclude false-positive cases. Confirmatory tests include the oral sodium loading test, saline infusion test (SIT), fludrocortisone suppression test (FST), and the captopril challenge test (CCT). Although individual tests can vary in sensitivity, specificity, and reliability, any test can be used depending on patient- and institution-specific considerations. FST generally is considered the most reliable but requires hospitalization. The SIT and CCT are both accurate alternatives to FST. However, a post-CCT evaluation of PAC is recommended to help interpret results of this confirmatory test.[58] Prior to performing these tests, potassium must be normalized and renin-angiotensin-aldosterone system (RAAS) inhibitors should be temporarily discontinued, if possible. Positive tests indicate autonomous aldosterone secretion under inhibitory pressures and are diagnostic for PA. After diagnosis, patients with confirmed PA before age 20 or with a family history of PA or strokes before age 40 should undergo genetic testing for GRA.[55]

Differentiating between an APA and BAH is imperative to formulate a proper treatment plan. Most adenomas are singular and small (<1 cm) and occur more often in the left adrenal gland than the right. Patients with APA generally have more severe hypertension, more profound hypokalemia, and higher plasma and urinary aldosterone concentrations compared with patients with BAH. Adrenal venous sampling (AVS) provides the most accurate means of differentiating unilateral from bilateral forms of PA. However, AVS is expensive, invasive, and often unavailable. CT scanning can detect most adenomas, although an incidentaloma can occasionally cause confusion. If CT scanning is inconclusive, AVS is performed to characterize lateralization.[49,59-61]

The underlying abnormality in BAH remains a mystery, but some investigators believe that a hormone factor stimulates the zona glomerulosa, resulting in increased sensitivity to angiotensin II. In contrast to those with an APA, patients with BAH are able to maintain control of the renin-angiotensin system, with little effect following doses of ACTH.

TREATMENT

6 BAH-Dependent Aldosteronism

Aldosterone-receptor antagonists are the treatment of choice in BAH. Drug dosing and monitoring parameters can be found in Tables 97-9 and 97-10. Spironolactone, a nonselective aldosterone-receptor antagonist, competes with aldosterone for binding at the aldosterone receptor, thus preventing the negative downstream effects of aldosterone-receptor activation. Additionally, spironolactone is capable of inhibiting aldosterone synthesis within the adrenal gland; however, the magnitude of inhibition is relatively small and the effect only occurs above recommended doses.[62] Spironolactone is available in oral form, with most patients responding to doses between 25 and 400 mg/day. The clinician should wait 4 to 8 weeks before reassessing the patient for urinary electrolytes and blood pressure control. Adverse effects of

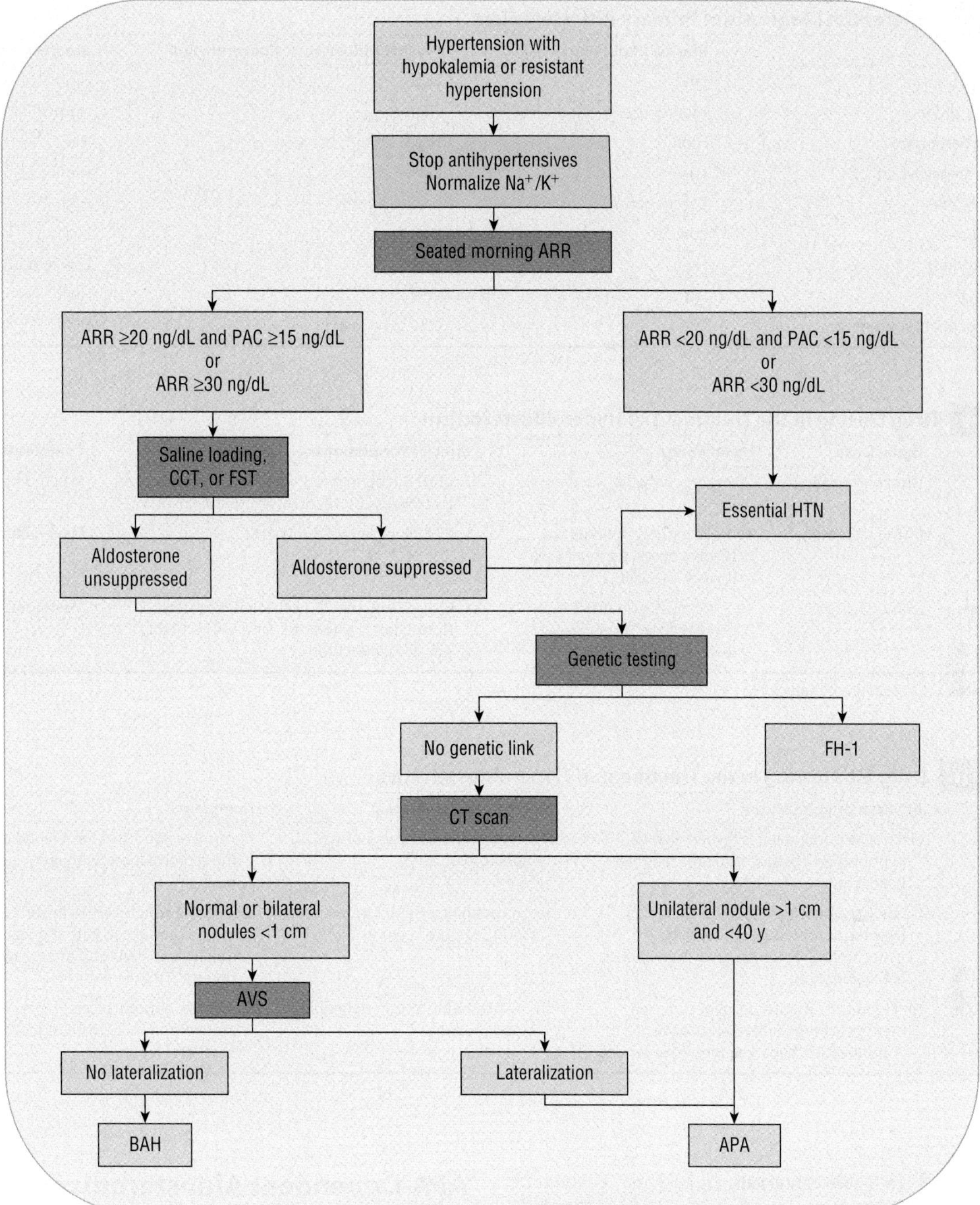

FIGURE 97-5 Algorithm for the diagnosis of primary aldosteronism. (ARR, aldosterone-to-renin ratio expressed in ng/dL per ng/(mL·h); HTN, hypertension; PAC, plasma aldosterone concentration [multiply values by 27.74 for units of pmol/L] FST, fludrocortisone suppression test; FH-1, familial hyperaldosteronism type 1; AVS, adrenal venous sampling; BAH, bilateral adrenal hyperplasia; APA, aldosterone-producing adenoma).

spironolactone are dose-dependent and include GI discomfort, impotence, gynecomastia, menstrual irregularities, and hyperkalemia. Gynecomastia and menstrual irregularities observed with spironolactone therapy arise from activity at androgen and progesterone receptors and inhibition of testosterone biosynthesis. Additionally, because salicylates increase the renal secretion of canrenone, the active metabolite of spironolactone, patients should be advised to avoid concomitant therapy with salicylates. In patients intolerant of spironolactone, alternative options include eplerenone and amiloride.[50,51,63-65]

Eplerenone is a selective aldosterone-receptor antagonist with high affinity for the aldosterone receptor and low affinity for androgen and progesterone receptors. Consequently, eplerenone elicits fewer sex steroid–dependent effects than spironolactone. Randomized controlled trial data have been inconclusive with regard to whether eplerenone achieves similar blood pressure reductions to spironolactone and there are limited long-term data comparing these agents.[66,67] Eplerenone dosing starts at 50 mg daily, with titration to 50 mg twice a day; some patients may require total daily doses as high as 200 to 300 mg.[63] Titration

TABLE 97-8 Differential Diagnosis of Primary Aldosteronism

Disease	Plasma Renin Activity	Plasma Aldosterone Concentration	Blood Pressure
Primary aldosteronism	Low	High	High
Edematous disorders	High	High	Normal
Malignant hypertension	High	High	High
Congenital adrenal hyperplasia	Low	Low	High
Cushing syndrome	Low to normal	Low to normal	High
Liddle syndrome	Low	Low	High
Bartter syndrome	High	High	Low to normal
Licorice ingestion	Low	Low	High
Low-renin essential hypertension	Low	Low to normal	High

TABLE 97-9 Drug Dosing in the Treatment of Hyperaldosteronism

Drug	Initial Dose	Usual Range	Special Populations	Comments
Amiloride	5 mg twice daily	20 mg/day in two divided doses	CrCl 10-50 mL/min (0.17-0.84 mL/s): reduce dose by 50%; CrCl <10 mL/min (0.17 mL/s): CI	Maximum: 30 mg/day
Eplerenone	50 mg once daily	100-300 mg/day in single or divided doses; titrate at 4- to 8-week intervals	CrCl <30 mL/min (0.5 mL/s): CI	Maximum: 300 mg/day
Spironolactone	25 mg once daily	100-400 mg/day in single or divided doses; titrate at 4- to 8-week intervals	CrCl 10-50 mL/min (0.17-0.84 mL/s): extend dosing interval to once daily; CrCl <10 mL/min (0.17 mL/s): CI	Maximum: 400 mg/day

CI, contraindicated; CrCl, creatinine clearance.

TABLE 97-10 Drug Monitoring in the Treatment of Hyperaldosteronism

Drug	Adverse Drug Reaction	Monitoring Parameters	Comments
Amiloride	Electrolyte abnormalities (hyperkalemia), hypotension, nausea, vomiting, diarrhea, headache	Serum creatinine, serum potassium, blood pressure	Electrolyte abnormalities (hyperkalemia) more pronounced with reduced renal function
Eplerenone	Electrolyte abnormalities (hyperkalemia), hypotension, dizziness, headache; gynecomastia and menstrual irregularities are uncommon	Serum creatinine, serum potassium, blood pressure	Electrolyte abnormalities (hyperkalemia) more pronounced with reduced renal function. CYP3A4 substrate; avoid use with potent CYP3A4 inhibitors
Spironolactone	GI discomfort, impotence, gynecomastia, menstrual irregularities, electrolyte abnormalities (hyperkalemia), hypotension	Serum creatinine, serum potassium, blood pressure	Electrolyte abnormalities (hyperkalemia) more pronounced with reduced renal function

should occur at 4- to 8-week intervals. In addition, eplerenone is a substrate of CYP3A4 and should not be taken with potent CYP3A4 inhibitors. Eplerenone is the preferred aldosterone antagonist during pregnancy since spironolactone can cause ambiguous genitalia in a male fetus.[68]

Amiloride, a potassium-sparing diuretic, is dosed at 5 mg twice a day up to 30 mg/day if necessary. Amiloride is less effective than spironolactone and patients often require additional therapy to adequately control blood pressure. Additional second-line options include calcium channel blockers, ACE inhibitors, and diuretics such as chlorthalidone, although all lack outcome data in PA.[61,64] However, some agents (eg, diuretics, calcium channel blockers) can promote a reactive rise in PRA, ultimately leading to increased aldosterone levels and potentially worsening PA. A prudent strategy would be to use these agents only in combination with RAAS inhibitors to mitigate the downstream aldosterone effects of any increase in PRA.

Initiation of these drugs, particularly spironolactone and eplerenone, should be accompanied by close monitoring of blood pressure. Both agents can cause significant reductions in blood pressure and patients may need to reduce the dose or discontinue other antihypertensive drugs in their regimens.

APA-Dependent Aldosteronism

The treatment of choice for APA-dependent aldosteronism remains laparoscopic resection of the adenoma.[69] Nearly 100% of patients show blood pressure improvement and up to 72% are permanently cured.[65,70] Because APAs are small and often occur in multiples, resection should target the entire adrenal gland. In successful cases, blood pressure control is achieved in one to three months. Medical management with an aldosterone receptor antagonist is often effective in this population if surgery is contraindicated. However, medical management may be significantly more expensive than unilateral resection.

Glucocorticoid-Remediable Aldosteronism

Glucocorticoids are very effective in treating GRA.[32] Low doses of long-acting glucocorticoids are used (0.125-0.5 mg/day of dexamethasone or 2.5-5 mg/day of prednisone) because complete suppression of ACTH-stimulated aldosterone release is unnecessary. If blood pressure fails to normalize with glucocorticoid therapy alone, the addition of spironolactone, eplerenone, or amiloride may help control symptoms.[49]

Secondary Aldosteronism

Secondary aldosteronism results from an appropriate response to excessive stimulation of the zona glomerulosa by an extra-adrenal factor, usually the renin-angiotensin system. Excessive potassium intake can promote aldosterone secretion as well as oral contraceptive use, pregnancy (aldosterone secretion 10 times normal by the third trimester), and menses. Congestive heart failure, cirrhosis, renal artery stenosis, and Bartter syndrome also can lead to elevated aldosterone concentrations.

Treatment of secondary aldosteronism is dictated by the etiology. Control or correction of the extra-adrenal stimulation of aldosterone secretion should resolve the disorder. Medical therapy with spironolactone is the mainstay of treatment until an exact etiology can be identified.

HYPOFUNCTION OF THE ADRENAL GLAND

Hypofunction of the adrenal gland can affect any or all adrenal hormones, depending on the etiology of the disorder. However, hypofunction does not always lead to insufficient production of adrenal hormones. Some types of adrenal hypofunction can lead to excess production of certain hormones.

Addison's Disease

7 Primary adrenal insufficiency, or Addison disease, most often involves the destruction of all regions of the adrenal cortex. Deficiencies arise in cortisol, aldosterone, and the various androgens, and levels of CRH and ACTH increase in a compensatory manner. In developed countries, autoimmune dysfunction is responsible for most cases (80%-90%), whereas tuberculosis predominates as the cause in developing countries. Approximately 50% of patients with autoimmune etiologies present with one or more concomitant autoimmune disorders, usually involving other endocrine organs. Autoimmune thyroid disorders (eg, Hashimoto thyroiditis or Graves' disease) are the most common, but the ovaries, pancreas, parathyroid gland, and organs of the GI system can also be affected. This polyglandular failure syndrome, termed autoimmune polyendocrine syndrome (APS), is associated with the idiopathic etiology only and has not been seen with adrenal insufficiency associated with tuberculosis or other invasive diseases. Medications that inhibit cortisol synthesis (ketoconazole) or accelerate cortisol metabolism (phenytoin, rifampin, phenobarbital) can also cause primary adrenal insufficiency.[71]

8 Secondary insufficiency is characterized by reduced glucocorticoid production secondary to decreased ACTH levels. Low levels of ACTH most commonly result from exogenous steroid use, leading to suppression of the HPA axis and decreased release of ACTH, as well as impaired androgen and cortisol production. These effects occur with oral, inhaled, intranasal, and topical glucocorticoid administration.[72-74] Moreover, mirtazapine and progestins, such as medroxyprogesterone acetate and megestrol acetate, have been reported to induce secondary adrenal insufficiency.[75,76] Chronic suppression also can result in atrophy of the anterior pituitary and hypothalamus, impairing recovery of function if the exogenous steroid is reduced. Endogenous secondary insufficiency can occur with tumor development in the hypothalamic-pituitary region. Secondary disease classically presents with normal concentrations of mineralocorticoids since the zona glomerulosa is controlled by the renin-angiotensin system rather than ACTH levels.

Approximately 90% of the adrenal cortex must be destroyed before the symptoms of adrenal insufficiency become clinically manifest.[77] Etiologies for both primary and secondary insufficiency are listed in Table 97-11. Adrenal hemorrhage can result from multiple etiologies including traumatic shock, coagulopathies, ischemic disorders, and other situations of severe stress, but septicemia is the most common. Symptoms include truncal pain, fever, shaking, chills, hypotension preceding shock, anorexia, headache, vertigo, vomiting, rash, psychiatric symptoms, abdominal rigidity or rebound, and death in 6 to 48 hours if not treated. The most common organisms found on autopsy are *Neisseria meningitidis*, *Pseudomonas aeruginosa*, *Streptococcus pneumoniae*, Group A *Streptococcus*, and *Haemophilus influenzae*.[77,78]

TABLE 97-11 Etiologies of Primary and Secondary Adrenal Insufficiency

Primary Insufficiency	Secondary Insufficiency
Slow onset	Craniopharyngioma
Acquired immunodeficiency syndrome	Cure of Cushing syndrome
Adrenomyeloneuropathy	Empty sella syndrome
Adrenoleukodystrophy	Tumors of the third ventricle
Amyloidosis	Histiocytosis
Autoimmune adrenalitis[a]	Hypothalamic tumors
Bilateral adrenalectomy	Hypopituitarism
Congenital adrenal hypoplasia	Long-term corticosteroid administration
Hemochromatosis	Lymphocytic hypophysitis
Isolated glucocorticoid deficiency	Pituitary surgery, radiation, or tumor
Metastatic neoplasia	Sarcoidosis
Systemic fungal, bacterial, or viral infections, tuberculosis[b]	Medications—progestins and glucocorticoid discontinuation
Medications—ketoconazole, etomidate, rifampin, phenytoin, phenobarbital	Postpartum pituitary necrosis Necrotic or bleeding pituitary macroadenoma
Fast onset	
Adrenal thrombosis, hemorrhage, sepsis, trauma, or necrosis	Head trauma, lesions of the pituitary stalk, pituitary or adrenal surgery for Cushing syndrome

[a]Approximately 70% of cases.

[b]Approximately 20% of cases.

CLINICAL PRESENTATION

Diagnosis

Distinguishing Addison disease from secondary insufficiency is difficult; however, the following guidelines may be helpful:

1. Hyperpigmentation, commonly found in areas of skin exposed to increased friction, is seen only in Addison disease because of excess secretion of ACTH and other proopiomelanocortin (POMC) peptides that induce melanocyte-stimulating hormone production. Secondary adrenal insufficiency is fundamentally characterized by deficient ACTH and POMC peptide secretion and a correspondingly low level of melanocyte-stimulating hormone production. In fact, some patients with secondary insufficiency may exhibit pale-colored skin secondary to hypopigmentation.
2. Aldosterone secretion usually is preserved in secondary insufficiency.
3. Weight loss, dehydration, hyponatremia, hyperkalemia, and elevated blood urea nitrogen are common in Addison disease.
4. Addison disease will have an abnormal response to the short corticotropin stimulation test. Plasma ACTH levels

CLINICAL PRESENTATION Adrenal Insufficiency

Symptoms

- Patients commonly complain of weakness, weight loss, GI symptoms, craving for salt, headaches, memory impairment, depression, and postural dizziness.
- Early symptoms of acute adrenal insufficiency also include myalgias, malaise, and anorexia. As the situation progresses, vomiting, fever, hypotension, and shock will develop.

Signs

- Increased pigmentation
- Hypotension (postural)
- Fever
- Decreased body hair
- Vitiligo
- Features of hypopituitarism (amenorrhea and cold intolerance)

Laboratory Tests

- The short cosyntropin stimulation test can be used to assess patients suspected of hypercortisolism.

Other Diagnostic Tests

- Other tests include the insulin hypoglycemia test, the metyrapone test, and the CRH stimulation test.

are usually elevated (400-2,000 pg/mL [88-440 pmol/L]) in primary insufficiency, versus low to normal (5-50 pg/mL [1.1-11 pmol/L]; see Table 97-3) in secondary insufficiency. A normal corticotropin stimulation test does not rule out secondary adrenal insufficiency, particularly in mild cases.

The short corticotropin stimulation test, also known as the cosyntropin stimulation test, can be used to assess patients suspected of hypocortisolism. A 250 μg dose of synthetic ACTH intravenously or intramuscularly to the patient and the serum cortisol is measured at immediately prior to and 30 to 60 minutes after the injection. A resulting cortisol concentration ≥18 μg/dL (500 nmol/L) rules out adrenal insufficiency.[79] Because 250 μg represents a massive supraphysiologic dose, this test can elicit normal, elevated cortisol responses in some cases of mild secondary insufficiency. Thus, some suggest that higher cutoff values (≥22 μg/dL [610 nmol/L]) should be used to prevent false-negative test results.[80] Alternatively, a low-dose corticotropin stimulation test, using 1 μg of synthetic ACTH, can achieve similar results to the standard dose test. Neither test is very effective in ruling out secondary insufficiency.[81] Other tests include the insulin hypoglycemia test, the metyrapone test, and the CRH stimulation test.[71]

The standard cutoffs described above are of limited use in acutely ill patients.[71] Severe infection, trauma, burns, illnesses, or surgery can increase cortisol production by as much as a factor of 6, making the recognition of adrenal insufficiency in this population extremely difficult. In the critically ill, a random cortisol concentration below 15 μg/dL (415 nmol/L) is suggestive of adrenal insufficiency, whereas a concentration greater than 34 μg/dL (940 nmol/L) suggests that adrenal insufficiency is unlikely.[71] For patients who fall between these two values, a poor response to corticotropin (<9 μg/dL [250 nmol/L] increase in plasma cortisol from baseline at 30 or 60 minutes) indicates the possibility of adrenal insufficiency and a need for corticosteroid supplementation.[71] A hypoproteinemic patient (albumin <2.5 g/dL [25 g/L]) will have markedly lower CBG, which can underestimate the actual free fraction of cortisol. These patients may benefit from measurement of free cortisol, although the assay may not be routinely available.[71]

TREATMENT

Treatment of Addison disease must include adequate patient education, so that the patient is aware of treatment complications, the expected outcome, consequences of missed doses, and drug side effects. The agents of choice are hydrocortisone and cortisone acetate administered two or three times daily. The treatment goal is to establish the lowest effective dose mimicking the normal diurnal adrenal rhythm.[79] Twice-daily dosing is usually adequate depending on the agent used. Once-daily prednisolone is an alternative when adherence to a multi-dose regimen is a concern.

Endogenous cortisol production varies between 5 and 10 mg/m²/day.[82] Hence, the classically recommended 12 to 15 mg/m²/day dose for cortisol supplementation will be excessive in most patients. Starting doses to properly mimic endogenous cortisol production are 15 to 25 mg of hydrocortisone daily, which is roughly equal to 20 to 35 mg of cortisone acetate daily, or 3 to 5 mg of prednisolone daily.[71,82] For hydrocortisone or cortisone, the majority of the dose (67%) is given in the morning and the remainder (33%) is given 6 to 8 hours later to duplicate the normal circadian rhythm of cortisol production. Continuous infusion of glucocorticoids delivered via infusion pump may provide a more physiological circadian maintenance of ACTH and cortisol concentration when compared to conventional oral replacement.[83] Since no laboratory test adequately determines the appropriateness of dosing, the patient's symptoms should be monitored every 6 to 8 weeks to assess proper glucocorticoid replacement. Monitoring parameters should include body weight, postural blood pressures, subjective energy levels, and signs of frank glucocorticoid excess.

In primary insufficiency, fludrocortisone acetate can be used to supplement mineralocorticoid loss. For most patients, a dose of 0.05 to 0.2 mg by mouth once a day is adequate to maintain volume status. If parenteral therapy is needed, 2 to 5 mg of deoxycorticosterone trimethylacetate in oil intramuscularly every 3 to 4 weeks can be substituted. Mineralocorticoid replacement attenuates the development of hyperkalemia, and patients on fludrocortisone therapy do not need to restrict salt intake. However, mineralocorticoid replacement may be unnecessary in some primary cases because glucocorticoids, particularly at large doses, also bind to mineralocorticoid receptors. For example, a daily dose of hydrocortisone 40 to 50 mg has similar mineralocorticoid effects to 0.1 mg of fludrocortisone. Adverse effects must be monitored closely and include gastric upset, edema, hypertension, hypokalemia, insomnia, excitability, and diabetes mellitus. In addition, patient weight, blood pressure, and ECG should be monitored regularly.[71]

Most adrenal crises occur secondary to glucocorticoid dose reduction or lack of stress-related dose adjustments. Patients receiving corticosteroid replacement therapy should receive an additional 5 to 10 mg of hydrocortisone shortly before strenuous activities such as exercise.[71] Likewise, during times of severe physical stress such as febrile illnesses or injury, patients should be instructed to double their daily dose until recovery.[71,84] For major trauma, surgery, or in critically ill patients, larger doses—up to 10 times the usual daily dose—may be required.[71] Parenteral therapy should be used for patients experiencing diarrhea or vomiting. In patients with concomitant, newly diagnosed, or uncontrolled hypothyroidism, thyroid replacement should take place only after adequate glucocorticoid replacement as euthyroidism can trigger an adrenal crisis by accelerating cortisol metabolism.[79]

The endpoint of therapy is difficult to assess in most patients, but a reduction in excess pigmentation is a good clinical marker. The development of features of Cushing syndrome indicates excessive replacement. Treatment of secondary adrenal insufficiency is similar to primary disease treatment, except that mineralocorticoid replacement usually is unnecessary. Patient education is paramount with emphasis placed on the medication regimen and adrenal crisis prevention.

Acute Adrenal Insufficiency

Adrenal crisis, or Addisonian crisis, is characterized by an acute adrenocortical insufficiency and represents a true endocrine emergency. Although no universally accepted definition for adrenal crisis exists, major clinical features include volume depletion and hypotension that resolves within one to two hours after parenteral glucocorticoid administration.[85] Anything that increases adrenal requirements dramatically can precipitate an adrenal crisis. Stressful situations, surgery, infection, and trauma all are potential triggering events, especially in the patient with some underlying adrenal or pituitary insufficiency. The most common cause of an adrenal crisis is HPA-axis suppression brought on by abrupt withdrawal of chronic glucocorticoid use.

Treatment of adrenal crisis involves the administration of parenteral glucocorticoids. Hydrocortisone is the agent of choice owing to its combined glucocorticoid and mineralocorticoid activity. Hydrocortisone is initially administered at a dose of 100 mg IV through rapid infusion, followed by 200 mg of hydrocortisone over 24 hours via a continuous infusion or a 50-mg intermittent bolus every 6 hours.[71] Intravenous administration is continued for an additional day at a reduced dose of 100 mg over 24 hours, at which time if the patient is stable, oral hydrocortisone can be administered at a dose of 50 mg every 6 to 8 hours, followed by tapering to the individual's chronic replacement needs. Fluid replacement often is required and can be accomplished with dextrose 5% in normal saline solution (D_5NS) at a rate to support blood pressure. If therapy is needed for hypoglycemia, dextrose 25% in water ($D_{25}W$) can be infused at a dose of 2 to 4 mL/kg (maximum single dose of 25 g dextrose). During initial treatment for adrenal crisis, mineralocorticoid replacement generally is unnecessary because of hydrocortisone's mineralocorticoid activity. If hyperkalemia is present after the hydrocortisone maintenance phase, additional mineralocorticoid supplementation can be achieved with 0.1 mg of fludrocortisone acetate daily.

Patients with adrenal insufficiency should be instructed to carry a card or wear a bracelet or necklace, such as MedicAlert, that contains information about their condition. Additionally, patients should have easy access to injectable hydrocortisone or glucocorticoid suppositories in case of an emergency or during times of physical stress, such as febrile illness or injury.[71]

Hypoaldosteronism

Hypoaldosteronism is rare and usually associated with low-renin status (hyporeninemic hypoaldosteronism), diabetes, complete heart block, or severe postural hypotension, or it can occur postoperatively following tumor removal. Hypoaldosteronism can be part of a multi-hormonal insufficiency or a stand-alone defect. In nonselective hypoaldosteronism, generalized adrenocortical insufficiency is the most likely etiology (see Addison Disease). In selective hypoaldosteronism, insufficient aldosterone levels are precipitated by a specific defect in the stimulation of adrenal aldosterone secretion, with 21-hydroxylase deficiency being the most common. Pseudohypoaldosteronism results from a defect in peripheral aldosterone action, whether from peripheral resistance or a reduced number of functional aldosterone receptors.

Laboratory analysis reveals hyponatremia, hyperkalemia, or both. Patients often will present with hyperchloremic metabolic acidosis. In most cases, the deficiency is in mineralocorticoid production and fludrocortisone given 0.05 to 0.2 mg daily is usually effective. Patients should be monitored for blood pressure response as well as electrolyte status.

Congenital Adrenal Hyperplasia

Because many enzyme systems are needed to complete the complex cholesterol-to-cortisol pathway, enzyme deficiencies can lead to disruptions of the normal cascade of events (see Fig. 97-2). This group of enzyme disorders is collectively referred to as congenital adrenal hyperplasia (CAH) because of the resultant chronic adrenal gland stimulation that occurs following enzyme deficiency.[71,86,87] The most frequent cause of CAH is steroid 21-hydroxylase deficiency, accounting for more than 90% of cases. Any enzyme deficiency is capable of affecting any one or all three of the steroid pathways. Therefore, treatment focuses on the replacement of the deficient hormone, psychological support, and surgical repair of the external genitalia in female patients.[88] Pediatric patients receiving glucocorticoid replacement (eg, with hydrocortisone and fludrocortisone) should be monitored for adverse outcomes, especially incident hypertension and decreased bone mineral density.[89,90] Six of the most common enzyme deficiencies are outlined briefly in Table 97-12.

Adrenal Virilism

9 Virilism, excessive secretion of androgens from the adrenal gland, commonly occurs as a result of congenital enzyme defects. Depending on the enzyme deficiency, patients accumulate excess levels of a variety of androgens, most notably testosterone. The condition affects women more often than men, with hirsutism being the dominant feature. Additional coexisting features can include voice deepening, acne, increased muscle mass, menstrual abnormalities, clitoral enlargement, redistribution of body fat and loss of female body contour, breast atrophy, and hair recession and crown balding.[91]

Treatment of virilism centers on the suppression of the pituitary-adrenal axis with exogenous glucocorticoids. In adults, the usual steroids used are dexamethasone (0.25-0.5 mg), prednisone (2.5-5 mg), or hydrocortisone (10-20 mg).[92]

Hirsutism

Women presenting with hirsutism exhibit excess terminal hair growth in an androgen-dependent distribution. Such growth has obvious cosmetic consequences, but also can adversely affect quality of life and psychological well-being.[93] Most cases of hirsutism occur in women with some degree of excess androgen production. Androgen excess can be derived from either the ovaries or the adrenal glands, or rarely from pituitary disorders. Polycystic ovary syndrome (PCOS) is responsible for most cases of ovarian excess and is the most common cause of hirsutism.[94] CAH accounts for 5% of cases while adrenal and ovarian tumors cause hyperandrogenemia in 0.2% of women.

Cosmetic approaches generally are tried first, with repeated photoepilation offering the greatest long-term success.[95] If these approaches are unsuccessful, subsequent treatment should include pharmacologic intervention. Oral contraceptives are the treatment of choice in most hirsute women, particularly in those requiring concurrent contraception. If oral contraceptives are used, a progestin with low androgen activity (norethindrone, ethynodiol diacetate) or antiandrogenic activity (drospirenone) should be chosen. Other antiandrogens, including spironolactone and finasteride, can supplement or replace oral contraceptive therapy in women who cannot or choose not to conceive. Antiandrogens can take 6 to 12 months to alleviate hirsutism and treatment should be continued for 2 years, followed by a slow dose

TABLE 97-12 Congenital Adrenal Hyperplasia

Enzyme Deficiency (Disorder)	Symptoms	Laboratory Tests	Comments
21-Hydroxylase (nonvirilizing CAH)	Enlarged female genitalia and adrenal gland (caused by cholesterol)	All steroids are low in blood and urine	Poor prognosis for infants
17-Hydroxylase (nonvirilizing CAH)	Hypertension usually present	Low concentrations of cortisol and estrogens	Mineralocorticoid replacement is not necessary
21-Hydroxylase (virilizing CAH)	Pubertal irregularities (acne, early pubic hair, voice lowering, and increased muscularity); mature normally with replacement	High progesterone, renin, 17-hydroxyprogesterone, and ACTH; low cortisol, sodium, and aldosterone	Most common form of CAH (90% of total), incidence of 1:10,000; monitor growth velocity, bone age, renin, and 17-hydroxyprogesterone
11-Hydroxylase (virilizing CAH)	Hypertension secondary to high deoxycortisol and virilism from androgen excess; mistaken for Cushing, but no glucose intolerance	Low plasma cortisone and aldosterone; high ACTH and MSH concentrations	Second most common form of CAH (9% of total), the incidence of 1:100,000; the final step in the biosynthesis of corticosterone and cortisol; found only in the adrenal cortex
3-Hydroxysteroid dehydrogenase (mixed CAH)	Both cortisol and aldosterone deficiencies	Decreased aldosterone, cortisol, estrogens, and androgens; increased pregnenolone and cholesterol	The defect affects both adrenals and gonads
18-Hydroxysteroid dehydrogenase (corticosterone methyloxidase deficiency)	Hypotension	Restricted to zona glomerulosa; sole aldosterone defect; hyponatremia, hyperkalemia, increased renin	Mineralocorticoid replacement without glucocorticoid replacement

MSH, melanocyte-stimulating hormone; CAH, congenital adrenal hyperplasia; ACTH, adrenocorticotropic hormone.

TABLE 97-13 Relative Potencies of Glucocorticoids

Glucocorticoid	Anti-inflammatory Potency	Equivalent Potency (mg)	Approximate Half-Life (min)	Sodium-Retaining Potency
Cortisone	0.8	25	30	2
Hydrocortisone	1	20	90	2
Prednisone	3.5	5	60	1
Prednisolone	4	5	200	1
Triamcinolone	5	4	300	0
Methylprednisolone	5	4	180	0
Betamethasone	25	0.6	100-300	0
Dexamethasone	30	0.75	100-300	0

reduction.[96] Dexamethasone (and other glucocorticoids) can be modestly effective if the androgen source is adrenal, but can induce cushingoid symptoms even at doses of 0.5 mg/day.

Gonadotropin-releasing hormone can be an effective adjunct or alternative to oral contraceptives if the source of androgen is ovarian. However, these products generally are not recommended due to excessive costs, injectable-only routes of administration, and adverse effects resulting from estrogen deficiency. Additionally, insulin sensitizers, such as metformin or thiazolidinediones, can show modest metabolic and glycemic improvement in women with PCOS, but their routine use is not recommended due to their limited impact on hirsutism, acne, and infertility.[94]

Eflornithine hydrochloride, an irreversible ornithine decarboxylase inhibitor, moderately reduces the rate of hair growth but does not remove hair already present. The drug is available as a topical cream applied as a thin layer to the affected area twice daily, at least 8 hours apart. Reduction in unwanted hair can be noted within 6 to 8 weeks with a maximal effect at 8 to 24 weeks; therapy must be continued indefinitely to prevent hair regrowth.[92,96] Skin irritation can occur that resolves on discontinuation.

PRINCIPLES OF GLUCOCORTICOID ADMINISTRATION

The term *glucocorticoid* was initially given to these agents to describe their glucose-regulating properties. However, carbohydrate metabolism is only one of the myriad effects exhibited by steroids. The activity produced by these drugs is a function of the receptor activated (glucocorticoid vs mineralocorticoid), the location of the receptor, as well as the agent and dose prescribed.

The mechanism of action of glucocorticoids is complex and not fully known. The glucocorticoid enters the cell through passive diffusion and binds to its specific receptor. Between 5,000 and 100,000 receptors exist in each cell. Steroids exhibit various binding affinities to the vast number of receptors in almost every tissue and therefore elicit a wide variety of biologic effects.

Following receptor binding, a structural change occurs in the receptor, known as *activation*. After activation, the receptor–steroid complex binds to deoxyribonucleic acid sites in the cell called *glucocorticoid response elements* (GREs). This binding alters nearby gene expression and stimulates or, in some cases, inhibits transcription of specific mRNAs. Consequently, the resulting protein, which produces the stimulatory or inhibitory glucocorticoid action, varies according to the tissue and cell type in which the glucocorticoid receptor exists.

Pharmacokinetic properties of the glucocorticoids vary by agent and route of administration. In general, most orally administered steroids are well absorbed. Water-soluble agents are more rapidly absorbed following intramuscular injection than are lipid-soluble agents. Intravenous administration is recommended when a quick onset of action is needed. A summary of these agents is provided in Table 97-13.

In addition to causing iatrogenic Cushing syndrome, systemic steroids can lead to increased susceptibility to infection,

TABLE 97-14 Appropriate Use of Glucocorticoid Therapy

Monitoring	Glucose concentrations (serum and urine) Electrolytes (serum and urine) Ophthalmologic examinations Stool tests for occult blood loss Growth and development (children and adolescents)
Patient education	Take with food to minimize GI discomfort Never discontinue medication on your own; check with your physician; gradual dose reduction is usually necessary Carry or wear medical identification indicating that you are on long-term glucocorticoid therapy Dosage increases can be necessary at times of increased stress (surgery or emergency treatments) Be aware of potential side effects (ie, visual disturbances, bruising, and delayed wound healing) What to do if you miss a dose: If your dosing schedule is: *Every other day*: Take as soon as possible if remembered that morning. If not remembered until later, skip that day. Take the next morning, and then skip the following day *Every day*: Take as soon as possible, but skip if almost time for the next dose. Never double doses
Recognizing complications	Early in therapy and essentially unavoidable: insomnia, enhanced appetite, weight gain Common in patients with underlying risk factors: hypertension, diabetes mellitus, peptic ulcer disease Long-term intense treatment: cushingoid habitus, hypothalamic pituitary-adrenal suppression, impaired wound healing Delayed and insidious: cataracts, atherosclerosis Rare and unpredictable: psychosis, glaucoma, pancreatitis

Data from References 101 and 102.

osteoporosis, sodium retention with resultant edema, hypokalemia, hypomagnesemia, cataracts, peptic ulcer disease, seizures, and generalized suppression of the HPA axis. Long-term complications tend to be insidious and less likely to respond to steroid withdrawal.

Suppression of the HPA axis is a major concern whenever systemic steroids are tapered or withdrawn. Single doses of glucocorticoids can prevent the axis from responding to major stressors for several hours. In general, steroid administration at a high dose for long periods of time causes suppression of the axis. However, the possibility of suppression occurs any time the patient is exposed to supraphysiologic steroid doses.[11,97] Symptoms of steroid withdrawal resemble those seen in a patient with adrenocortical deficiency.

A variety of recommendations for steroid tapering are available.[11,98-100] In general, patients who have been on long-term steroid therapy will need to be gradually withdrawn toward physiologic doses over months. On average, the normal adult produces approximately 10 to 30 mg of cortisol per day with the peak concentration occurring around 8:00 am. As the steroid or steroid-equivalent dose approaches the 20- to 30-mg level, the taper should be slowed and the patient checked for axis function. The primary modes to test HPA integrity are the ACTH test, either high or low dose, or a morning (8:00 am) serum cortisol. A normal morning serum cortisol (>20 μg/dL [550 nmol/L]) or a normal ACTH test indicates that daily steroid maintenance therapy may be discontinued. If morning serum cortisol is between 3 and 20 μg/dL (85 and 550 nmol/L), the ACTH or CRH stimulation test can be useful in the assessment of pituitary-adrenal function.[11] A morning cortisol less than 3 μg/dL (85 nmol/L) indicates axis suppression and the need for continued replacement therapy. Suppression can persist for up to a year in some patients. Caution should be used to prevent disease exacerbation during the steroid taper and to avoid the need for another course of high-dose steroids.

Alternate-day therapy (ADT) regimens have been promoted as a means to lessen the impact of prolonged steroid administration.[11,100] ADT theoretically minimizes the hypothalamic-pituitary suppression as well as some of the adverse effects seen with once-daily therapy. This hypothetical advantage may be especially pertinent in treating children and young adults, in whom growth suppression is a major concern. ADT is not recommended for initial management, but rather in the management of the stabilized patient who needs long-term therapy. The patient is exposed to "on" and "off" days, with the "on" day dose gradually increased corresponding with a dose reduction in the "off" day dose over a period of 14 days. After 2 weeks, no medication is taken on "off" days. Not all patients will have equivalent disease control on ADT, and it should be avoided in certain indications.[11,100]

EVALUATION OF THERAPEUTIC OUTCOMES

Successful glucocorticoid therapy involves counseling and monitoring the patient, as well as recognizing complications of therapy (Table 97-14). The risk-to-benefit ratio of glucocorticoid administration should always be considered, especially with concurrent disease states such as hypertension, diabetes mellitus, peptic ulcer disease, and uncontrolled systemic infections.

ABBREVIATIONS

ACTH	adrenocorticotropic hormone
ADT	alternate-day therapy
ALP	alkaline phosphatase
ALT	alanine aminotransferase
APA	aldosterone-producing adenoma
APS	autoimmune polyendocrine syndrome
ARR	aldosterone-to-renin ratio
AST	aspartate aminotransferase
AVS	adrenal venous sampling
BAH	bilateral adrenal hyperplasia
CAH	congenital adrenal hyperplasia
CBG	corticosteroid-binding globulin
CCT	captopril challenge test
CHD	coronary heart disease
CNS	central nervous system
CrCl	creatinine clearance
CRH	corticotropin-releasing hormone
CT	computed tomography
CYP	cytochrome P450
D_5NS	dextrose 5% in normal saline solution
$D_{25}W$	dextrose 25% in water
DDT	dichlorodiphenyltrichloroethane
DST	dexamethasone suppression test
ECG	electrocardiogram
FDA	Food and Drug Administration
FH	familial hyperaldosteronism
FST	fludrocortisone suppression test
GABA	γ-aminobutyric acid
GI	gastrointestinal
GRA	glucocorticoid-remediable aldosteronism
GRE	glucocorticoid response element
HPA	hypothalamic–pituitary–adrenal

INR	international normalized ratio
IPSS	inferior petrosal sinus sampling
IRMA	immunoradiometric assay
JVS	jugular venous sampling
LDL	low-density lipoprotein
MRI	magnetic resonance imaging
PA	primary aldosteronism
PAC	plasma aldosterone concentration
PAC-to-PRA	plasma aldosterone concentration–to–plasma renin activity
PCOS	polycystic ovarian syndrome
POMC	proopiomelanocortin
PRA	plasma renin activity
RAAS	renin-angiotensinaldosterone system
RIA	radioimmunoassay
SIT	saline infusion test
sst	somatostatin receptor subtype
UFC	urinary free cortisol

REFERENCES

1. Conn JW. Primary aldosteronism, a new clinical syndrome. *J Lab Clin Med* 1955;45:6–17.
2. Albright F. Cushing syndrome. *Harvey Lect* 1942–1943;38:123–186.
3. Lacroix A, Feelders RA, Stratakis CA, Nieman LK. Cushing syndrome. *Lancet* 2015;386(9996):913–927.
4. Isidori AM, Kaltsas GA, Pozza C, et al. The ectopic adrenocorticotropin syndrome: Clinical features, diagnosis, management, and long-term follow-up. *J Clin Endocrinol Metab* 2006;91:371–377.
5. Boscaro M, Barzon L, Sonino N. The diagnosis of Cushing syndrome: Atypical presentations and laboratory shortcomings. *Arch Intern Med* 2000;160:3045–3053.
6. Arlt W. Disorders of the adrenal cortex. In: Kasper D, Fauci A, Hauser S, Longo D, Jameson J, Loscalzo J.eds. *Harrison's Principles of Internal Medicine*, 19th ed. New York, NY: McGraw-Hill; 2015. http://accessmedicine.mhmedical.com/content.aspx?bookid=1130&Sectionid=79752055.
7. Catargi B, Rigalleau V, Poussin A, et al. Occult Cushing syndrome in type-2 diabetes. *J Clin Endocrinol Metab* 2003;88:5808–5813.
8. Findling JW, Raff H. Screening and diagnosis of Cushing syndrome. *Endocrinol Metab Clin North Am* 2005;34:385–402.
9. Nieman LK, Biller BMK, Findling JW, et al. The diagnosis of Cushing syndrome: An Endocrine Society clinical practice guideline. *J Clin Endocrinol Metab* 2008;93:1526–1540.
10. Terzolo M, Reimondo G, Chiodini I, et al. Screening of Cushing syndrome in outpatients with type 2 diabetes: Results of a prospective multicentric study in Italy. *J Clin Endocrinol Metab* 2012;97:3467–3475. doi:10.1210/jc.2012-1323.
11. Hopkins RL, Leinung MC. Exogenous Cushing syndrome and glucocorticoid withdrawal. *Endocrinol Metab Clin North Am* 2005;34:371–384.
12. Bolland MJ, Bagg W, Thomas MG, et al. Cushing syndrome due to interaction between inhaled corticosteroids and itraconazole. *Ann Pharmacother* 2004;38:46–49.
13. Samaras K, Pett S, Gowers A, et al. Iatrogenic Cushing syndrome with osteoporosis and secondary adrenal failure in human immunodeficiency virus-infected patients receiving inhaled corticosteroids and ritonavir-boosted protease inhibitors: Six cases. *J Clin Endocrinol Metab* 2005;90:4394–4398.
14. Newell-Price J, Trainer P, Besser M, Grossman A. The diagnosis and differential diagnosis of Cushing syndrome and pseudo-Cushing states. *Endocr Rev* 1998;19:647–672.
15. Nieman LK, Ilias I. Evaluation and treatment of Cushing syndrome. *Am J Med* 2005;118:1340–1346.
16. Lindsay JR, Nieman LK. Differential diagnosis and imaging in Cushing syndrome. *Endocrinol Metab Clin North Am* 2005;34:403–421.
17. Arnaldi G, Angeli A, Atkinson AB, et al. Diagnosis and complications of Cushing syndrome: A consensus statement. *J Clin Endocrinol Metab* 2003;88:5593–5602.
18. Jackson RV, Hockings GI, Torpy DJ, et al. New diagnostic tests for Cushing syndrome: Uses of naloxone, vasopressin and alprazolam. *Clin Exp Pharmacol Physiol* 1996;23:579–581.
19. Ambrosi B, Bochicchio D, Colombo P, et al. Loperamide to diagnose Cushing syndrome. *JAMA* 1993;270:2301–2302.
20. Papanicolaou DA, Mullen N, Kyrou I, Nieman LK. Nighttime salivary cortisol: A useful test for the diagnosis of Cushing syndrome. *J Clin Endocrinol Metab* 2002;87:4515–4521.
21. Viardot A, Huber P, Puder JJ, et al. Reproducibility of nighttime salivary cortisol and its use in the diagnosis of hypercortisolism compared with urinary free cortisol and overnight dexamethasone suppression test. *J Clin Endocrinol Metab* 2005;90:5730–5736.
22. Findling JW, Raff H, Aron DC. The low-dose dexamethasone suppression test: A reevaluation in patients with Cushing syndrome. *J Clin Endocrinol Metab* 2004;89:1222–1226.
23. Rockall AG, Babar SA, Sohaib SA, et al. CT and MR imaging of the adrenal glands in ACTH-independent Cushing syndrome. *Radiographics* 2004;24:435–452.
24. Peppercorn PD, Reznek RH. State-of-the-art CT and MRI of the adrenal gland. *Eur Radiol* 1997;7:822–836.
25. Nieman LK. Medical therapy of Cushing disease. *Pituitary* 2002;5:77–82.
26. Labeur M, Arzt E, Stalla GK, Paez-Pereda M. New perspectives in the treatment of Cushing syndrome. *Curr Drug Targets Immune Endocr Metabol Disord* 2004;4:335–342.
27. McEvoy GK ed. *American Hospital Formulary Service (AHFS) Drug Information*. Bethesda, MD: American Society of Health-System Pharmacists; 2015.
28. Nieman LK, Biller BMK, Findling JW, et al. Treatment of Cushing syndrome: An Endocrine Society Clinical Practice Guideline. *J Clin Endorcrinol Metab.* 2015;100:2807–2831.
29. Utz AL, Swearingen B, Biller BM. Pituitary surgery and postoperative management in Cushing disease. *Endocrinol Metab Clin North Am* 2005;34:459–478.
30. Dang CN, Trainer P. Pharmacological management of Cushing syndrome: An update. *Arq Bras Endocrinol Metabol* 2007;51:1339–1348.
31. Biller BMK, Grossman AB, Stewart PM, et al. Treatment of adrenocorticotropin-dependent Cushing syndrome: A consensus statement. *J Clin Endocrinol Metab* 2008;93:2454–2462.
32. Terzolo M, Angeli A, Fassnacht M, et al. Adjuvant mitotane treatment for adrenocortical carcinoma. *N Engl J Med* 2007;356:2372–2380.
33. Veytsman I, Nieman L, Fojo T. Management of endocrine manifestations and the use of mitotane as a chemotherapeutic agent for adrenocortical carcinoma. *J Clin Oncol* 2009;27:4619–4629.
34. Morris D, Grossman A. The medical management of Cushing syndrome. *Ann N Y Acad Sci* 2002;970:119–133.
35. Stowasser M, Gordon RD. Primary aldosteronism: From genesis to genetics. *Trends Endocrinol Metab* 2003;14:310–317.
36. Preda VA, Sen J, Karavitaki N, Grossman AB. Etomidate in the management of hypercortiolaemia in Cushing syndrome: A review. *Eur J Endocronol.* 2012;167:137–143.
37. Pivonello R, Ferone D, de Herder WW, et al. Dopamine receptor expression and function in corticotroph pituitary tumors. *J Clin Endocrinol Metab* 2004;89:2452–2462.
38. Godbout A, Manavela M, Danilowicz K, et al. Cabergoline monotherapy in the long-term treatment of Cushing disease. *Eur J Endocrinol* 2010;163:709–716.
39. Tritos NA, Biller BMK, Swearingen B. Management of Cushing disease. *Nat Rev Endocrinol* 2011;7:279–289.
40. Tritos NA, Biller BM. Medical management of Cushing disease. *J Neurooncol* 2014;117(3):407–414.
41. Colao A, Petersenn S, Newell-Price J, et al. A 12-month phase 3 study of pasireotide in Cushing disease. *N Engl J Med* 2012;366:914–924.
42. Petersenn S, Salgado LR, Schopohl J, et al. Long-term treatment of Cushing's disease with pasireotide: 5-year results from an open-label extension study of a Phase III trial. *Endocrine* 2017;57(1):156–165. doi: 10.1007/s12020-017-1316-3.
43. Guarnotta V, Pizzolanti G, Ciresi A, Giordano C. Insulin sensitivity and secretion and adipokine profile in patients with Cushing's disease treated with pasireotide. *J Endocrinol Invest.* 2018;2:1–1.
44. Feelders RA, de Bruin C, Pereira AM, et al. Pasireotide alone or with cabergoline and ketoconazole in Cushing disease. *N Engl J Med* 2010;362:1846–1848.
45. Nieman LK. Update in the medical therapy of Cushing disease. *Curr Opin Endocrinol Diabetes Obesm* 2013;20:330–334.
46. Fleseriu M, Biller BMK, Findling JW, et al. Mifepristone, a glucocorticoid receptor antagonist, produces clinical and metabolic benefits in patients with Cushing syndrome. *J Clin Endocrinol Metab* 2012;97:2039–2049.

47. Semple PL, Vance ML, Findling J, Laws ER. Transsphenoidal surgery for Cushing disease: Outcome in patients with a normal magnetic resonance imaging scan. *Neurosurgery* 2000;46:553–558.
48. Stowasser M, Gordon RD. Primary aldosteronism. *Best Pract Res Clin Endocrinol Metab* 2003;17:591–605.
49. Wu V, Chao C, Kuo C, et al. Diagnosis and management of primary aldosternoism. *Acta Nephrologica* 2012;26(3):111–120.
50. Chao C, Wu V, Kuo C, et al. Diagnosis and management of primary aldosteronism: An updated review. *Ann Med.* 2013;45:375–383.
51. Monticone S, D'Ascenzo F, Moretti C, et al. Cardiovascular events and target organ damage in primary aldosteronism compared with essential hypertension: A systematic review and meta-analysis. *Lancet Diabetes Endocrinol.* 2018;6(1):41–50. doi: 10.1016/S2213-8587(17)30319-4.
52. Seccia TM, Letizia C, Muiesan ML, Lerco S, Cesari M, Bisogni V, Petramala L, Maiolino G, Volpin R, Rossi GP, et al. Atrial fibrillation as presenting sign of primary aldosteronism: Results of the prospective appraisal on the prevalence of primary aldosteronism in hypertensive (PAPPHY) study. *J Hypertens* 2020;38(2):332–339. 10.1097/HJH.0000000000002250 31834121.
53. Funder JW, Carey RM, Mantero F, et al. The management of primary aldosteronism: Case detection, diagnosis, and treatment: An Endocrine Society Clinical Practice Guidelines. *J Clin Endocrinol Metab* 2016;101(5):1889–1916. doi: 10.1210/jc.2015-4061.
54. Funder JW, Carey RM, Fardella C, et al. Case detection, diagnosis, and treatment of patients with primary aldosteronism: An Endocrine Society Clinical Practice Guideline. *J Clin Endocrinol Metab* 2008;93:3266–3281.
55. Schwartz GL, Turner ST. Screening for primary aldosteronism in essential hypertension: Diagnostic accuracy of the ratio of plasma aldosterone concentration to plasma renin activity. *Clin Chem* 2005;51:386–394.
56. Kumar B, Swee M. Aldosterone-renin ratio in the assessment of primary aldosteronism. *JAMA* 2014;312(2):184–185.
57. Song Y, Yang S, He W, et al. Confirmatory tests for the diagnosis of primary aldosteronism: A prospective diagnostic accuracy study. *Hypertension.* 2018;71(1):118–124. 10.1161/HYPERTENSIONAHA.117.10197.
58. Mulatero P, Dluhy RG, Giacchetti G, et al. Diagnosis of primary aldosteronism: From screening to subtype differentiation. *Trends Endocrinol Metab* 2005;16:114–119.
59. Young WF, Stanson AW, Thompson GB, et al. Role for adrenal venous sampling in primary aldosteronism. *Surgery* 2004;136:1227–1235.
60. Nwariaku FE, Miller BS, Auchus R, et al. Primary hyperaldosteronism: Effect of adrenal vein sampling on surgical outcome. *Arch Surg* 2006;141:497–502.
61. Ye P, Yamashita T, Pollock DM, Rainey WE. Contrasting effects of eplerenone and spironolactone on adrenal cell steroidogenesis. *Horm Metab Res* 2009;41:35–39.
62. Nishizaka MK, Calhoun DA. Primary aldosteronism: Diagnostic and therapeutic considerations. *Curr Cardiol Rep* 2005;7:412–417.
63. Young WF Jr. Primary aldosteronism: Management issues. *Ann N Y Acad Sci* 2002;970:61–76.
64. Young WF. Primary aldosteronism: Treatment options. *Growth Horm IGF Res.* 2003;13:S102–S108.
65. Parthasarathy HK, Menard J, White WB, et al. A double-blind, randomized study comparing the antihypertensive effect of eplerenone and spironolactone in patients with hypertension and evidence of primary aldosteronism. *J Hypertens.* 2011;29:980–990.
66. Karashima S, Yoneda T, Kometani M, et al. Comparison of eplerenone and spironolactone for the treatment of primary aldosteronism. *Hypertens Res.* 2016;39(3):133–137. doi: 10.1038/hr.2015.129.
67. Cabassi A, Rocco R, Berretta R, et al. Eplerenone use in primary aldosteronism during pregnancy. *Hypertension* 2012;49:e18–19.
68. Meria P, Kempf BF, Hermieu JF, et al. Laparoscopic management of primary aldosteronism: Clinical experience with 212 cases. *J Urol* 2003;169:32–35.
69. Meyer A, Brabant G, Behrend M. Long-term follow-up after adrenalectomy for primary aldosteronism. *World J Surg* 2005;29:155–159.
70. Bornstein SR, Allolio B, Arlt W, et al. Diagnosis and treatment of primary adrenal insufficiency: An Endocrine Society Clinical Practice Guideline. *J Clin Endocrinol Metab* 2016;101(2):364–389. doi: 10.1210/jc.2015-1710.
71. Husebye ES, Pearce SH, Krone NP, Kämpe O. Adrenal insufficiency. *Lancet* 2021;397(10274):613–629. 10.1016/S0140-6736(21)00136-7 33484633.
72. Bello CE, Garrett SD. Therapeutic issues in oral glucocorticoid use. *Lippincotts Prim Care Pract* 1999;3:333–341.
73. Sizonenko PC. Effects of inhaled or nasal glucocorticosteroids on adrenal function and growth. *J Pediatr Endocrinol Metab* 2002;15:5–26.
74. Goodman A, Cagliero E. Megestrol-induced clinical adrenal insufficiency. *Eur J Gynaecol Oncol* 2000;21:117–118.
75. Schule C, Baghai T, Bidlingmaier M, et al. Endocrinological effects of mirtazapine in healthy volunteers. *Prog Neuropsychopharmacol Biol Psychiatry* 2002;26:1253–1261.
76. Alevritis EM, Sarubbi FA, Jordan RM, Peiris AN. Infectious cause of adrenal insufficiency. *South Med J* 2003;96:888–890.
77. Torrey SP. Recognition and management of adrenal emergencies. *Emerg Med Clin North Am* 2005;23:687–702.
78. Michels A, Michels N. Addison disease: Early detection and treatment principles. *Am Fam Physician* 2014;89(7):563–568.
79. Oelkers W. The role of high- and low-dose corticotropin tests in the diagnosis of secondary adrenal insufficiency. *Eur J Endocrinol* 1998;139:567–570.
80. Ospina NS, Al Nofal A, Bancos I, et al. ACTH stimulation tests for the diagnosis of adrenal insufficiency: Systematic review and meta-analysis. *J Clin Endocrinol Metab* 2016;101(2):427–434. doi: 10.1210/jc.2015-1700.
81. Crown A, Lightman S. Why is the management of glucocorticoid deficiency still controversial: A review of the literature. *Clin Endocrinol (Oxf)* 2005;63:483–492.
82. Oksnes M, Bjornsdottir S, Isaksson M. Continuous subcutaneous hydrocortisone infusion versus oral hydrocortisone replacement for treatment of Addison's disease: A randomized clinical trial. *J Clin Endocrinol Metab* 2014;99(5):1665–1674.
83. Nieman LK, Turner MC. Addison's disease. *Clin Dermatol.* 2006;24:276–280.
84. Speiser PW, White PC. Congenital adrenal hyperplasia. *N Engl J Med* 2003;349:776–788.
85. Rushworth RL, Torphy DJ, Falhammar H. Adrenal crisis. *N Engl J Med* 2019;381(9):852–861. doi: 10.1056/NEJMra1807486.
86. Forest MG. Recent advances in the diagnosis and management of congenital adrenal hyperplasia due to 21-hydroxylase deficiency. *Hum Reprod Update* 2004;10:469–485.
87. Merke DP, Bornstein SR. Congenital adrenal hyperplasia. *Lancet* 2005;365:2125–2136.
88. Halper A, Sanchez B, Hodges JS, et al. Bone mineral density and body composition in children with congenital adrenal hyperplasia. *Clin Endocrinol (Oxf)* 2018;88(6):813–819. doi: 10.1111/cen.13580.
89. Maccabee-Ryaboy N, Thomas W, Kyllo J, et al. Hypertension in children with congenital adrenal hyperplasia. *Clin Endocrinol (Oxf)* 2016;85(4):528–534. doi: 10.1111/cen.13086.
90. Yildiz BO. Diagnosis of hyperandrogenism: Clinical criteria. *Best Pract Res Clin Endocrinol Metab* 2006;20:167–176.
91. Rosenfield RL. Hirsutism. *N Engl J Med* 2005;353:2578–2588.
92. Koulouri O, Conway GS. Management of hirsutism. *BMJ* 2009;338:823–826.
93. Azziz R. The evaluation and management of hirsutism. *Obstet Gynecol* 2003;101:995–1007.
94. Moghetti P. Treatment of hirsutism and acne in hyperandrogenism. *Best Pract Res Clin Endocrinol Metab* 2006;20:221–234.
95. United States Pharmacopeial Convention Inc. USPDI. *Advice for the Patient: Drug Information in Lay Language*, Vol. II, 19th ed. Taunton, MA: Rand-McNally; 1999:612–616.
96. Boumpas DT, Chrousos GP, Wilder RL, et al. Complications of therapy. In: Boumpas DT, moderator. Glucocorticoid therapy for immune-mediated diseases: Basic and clinical correlates. *Ann Intern Med.* 1993;119:1198–1208.
97. Arvat E, Giordano R, Ramunni J, et al. Adrenocorticotropin and cortisol hyperresponsiveness to hexarelin in patients with Cushing disease bearing a pituitary microadenoma, but not in those with macroadenoma. *J Clin Endocrinol Metab* 1998;83:4207–4211.
98. Martin KA, Chang RJ, Ehrmann DA, et al. Evaluation and treatment of hirsutism in premenopausal women: An Endocrine Society Clinical Practice Guideline. *J Clin Endocrinol Metab* 2008;93:1105–1120.
99. Henzen C, Suter A, Lerch E, et al. Suppression and recovery of adrenal response after short-term, high-dose glucocorticoid treatment. *Lancet* 2000;355:542–545.
100. Krasner AS. Glucocorticoid-induced adrenal insufficiency. *JAMA* 1999;282:671–676.
101. Kountz DS, Clark CL. Safely withdrawing patients from chronic glucocorticoid therapy. *Am Fam Physician* 1997;55:521–552.
102. Baxter JD. Advances in glucocorticoid therapy. *Adv Intern Med* 2000;45:317–349.

Pituitary Gland Disorders

e98

Joseph K. Jordan, Amy Heck Sheehan, and Kashif M. Munir

KEY CONCEPTS

1. Pharmacologic therapy for acromegaly should be considered when surgery and irradiation are contraindicated, when there is a poor likelihood of surgical success, when rapid control of symptoms is needed, or when other treatments have failed to normalize growth hormone (GH) and insulin-like growth factor-1 (IGF-1) serum concentrations.
2. Pharmacotherapy for acromegaly using dopamine agonists has several advantages including oral administration and lower cost when compared to somatostatin analogs and pegvisomant. However, dopamine agonists effectively normalize IGF-1 serum concentrations in only 10% to 30% of patients. Therefore, somatostatin analogs remain the mainstay of therapy.
3. Blood glucose concentrations should be monitored frequently in the early stages of somatostatin analog therapy, especially when using pasireotide.
4. Pegvisomant appears to be the most effective agent for normalizing IGF-1 serum concentrations.
5. Recombinant growth hormone (GH) is currently considered the drug of choice for the treatment of children with growth hormone–deficient short stature. Prompt diagnosis of growth hormone deficiency (GHD) and initiation of replacement therapy with recombinant GH is crucial for optimizing final adult heights.
6. All GH products are equally effective. The recommended initial dose for treatment of GHD short stature in children is 0.16 to 0.24 mg/kg/wk.
7. Pharmacologic agents that antagonize dopamine or increase the release of prolactin can induce hyperprolactinemia. Discontinuation of the offending medication and initiation of an appropriate therapeutic alternative usually normalizes serum prolactin concentrations.
8. Cabergoline is more effective than bromocriptine for the medical management of prolactinomas and offers the advantage of less-frequent dosing and fewer adverse effects.
9. Although currently available data do not suggest that cabergoline has significant teratogenic potential, cabergoline is not recommended for use during pregnancy. Patients receiving cabergoline or bromocriptine who plan to become pregnant should discontinue the medication as soon as pregnancy is detected.
10. Pharmacologic treatment of panhypopituitarism includes the use of glucocorticoids, thyroid hormone, sex steroids, and recombinant GH, when appropriate, as lifelong replacement therapies.

BEYOND THE BOOK

Create a diagram of anterior pituitary hormones, noting the upstream signals (ie, hypothalamic-releasing or inhibiting hormones) and downstream targets of the hormones secreted by the anterior pituitary. When applicable, note inhibitory or excitatory feedback mechanisms in this process.

INTRODUCTION

It wasn't until the 1950s that the physiologic importance of pituitary hormones was understood and the neurohormonal regulation of the pituitary by the hypothalamus described.[1] The pituitary gland plays an essential role in homeostasis, and for this reason, it is often referred to as the *master gland.* The hypothalamus and the pituitary gland are closely connected, and together they provide a means of communication between the brain and many of the body's endocrine organs. The hypothalamus uses input from the central nervous system and metabolic signals from the body to control the secretion of pituitary hormones that regulate growth, thyroid function, adrenal activity, reproduction, lactation, and fluid balance.

ANATOMY AND PHYSIOLOGY

The hypothalamus (Fig. e98-1) is a small region at the base of the brain that receives autonomic nervous input from different areas of the body to regulate limbic functions, food and water intake, body temperature, cardiovascular function, respiratory function, and diurnal rhythms. In addition, the hypothalamus controls the release of hormones from the anterior and posterior regions of the pituitary gland. Neurons in the hypothalamus produce vasopressin and oxytocin and make many hormone-releasing factors that stimulate or inhibit the release of trophic hormones from the anterior pituitary that subsequently stimulate endocrine tissues to grow and release hormones.

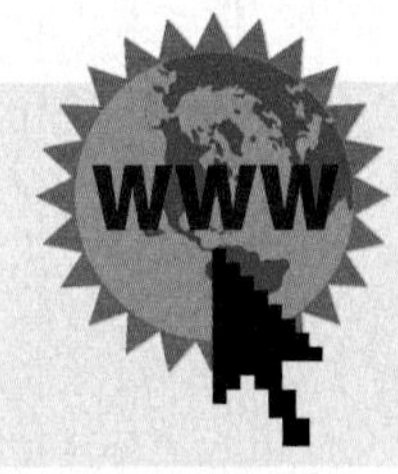

The complete chapter, learning objectives, and other resources can be found at **www.pharmacotherapyonline.com.**

99 Pregnancy and Lactation

Alicia B. Forinash and Kylie N. Barnes

KEY CONCEPTS

1. Complex physiology surrounds the process of fertilization and pregnancy progression.
2. Medication characteristics and physiologic changes modify pharmacokinetics during pregnancy, including changes in absorption, protein binding, distribution, and elimination, requiring individualized pharmacotherapy selection and dosing.
3. Although medication-induced teratogenicity is a serious concern during pregnancy, most medications can be used during pregnancy. Healthcare providers need to evaluate the risk of the medication with the risk of the untreated condition. Informed selection of pharmacotherapy is essential.
4. Healthcare practitioners must know where to find and how to evaluate evidence related to medications used during pregnancy and lactation.
5. Acute pregnancy issues, such as nausea and vomiting, can be treated with nonpharmacologic treatment or carefully selected pharmacotherapy.
6. Some acute and chronic illnesses pose additional risks during pregnancy, requiring treatment with appropriately selected and monitored pharmacotherapies to minimize risk to the fetus and pregnant individual.
7. Management of the pregnant individuals during the peripartum period not only can encompass uncomplicated pregnancies/deliveries, but can also include a wide variety of potential complications that require use of evidence-based treatments to maximize positive outcomes.
8. Understanding the physiology of lactation and pharmacokinetic factors affecting medication distribution, metabolism, and elimination can assist the clinician in selecting appropriate medications during lactation.

BEYOND THE BOOK

Search the Food and Drug Administration (FDA) Website (https://tinyurl.com/2ujhjm) for "Pregnancy and Lactation Labeling Rule." Choose one link to review and then summarize the key points about the new pregnancy and lactation labeling requirements. How do they differ from pregnancy categories? Do pregnancy categories still exist? This activity is useful to enhance understanding about what type of pregnancy and lactation information to expect in medication product labeling.

INTRODUCTION

As medication use in pregnancy and lactation is a controversial and emotionally charged subject, due to medicolegal and ethical implications, it is often a topic underemphasized in the education of health professionals. However, clinicians are responsible for ensuring appropriate therapy before conception, during pregnancy and parturition, and after delivery. Optimal treatments of illnesses during pregnancy sometimes differ from those used in the nonpregnant patient, and active patient participation in this process is essential.

In many cases, medication dosing recommendations for acute or chronic illnesses in pregnant individuals are the same as for the general population. However, some cases require different dosing and selection of medications. Principles of medication use during lactation, although similar, are not the same as those applicable during pregnancy.

Within this chapter, the text has been written to reduce the use of gendered terms to be more inclusive to transgender individuals as recommended by the American College of Obstetricians and Gynecologists (ACOG) and International Lactation Consultants Association (ILCA). Thus, all included gendered terms refer to biological sex and not gender.

PHYSIOLOGY OF PREGNANCY

1 Fertilization and progression of pregnancy are complex, resulting in survival of only approximately 40% to 50% of embryos.[1] Because most losses occur early, usually in the first 2 weeks after fertilization, many individuals do not realize they were pregnant. Spontaneous loss of pregnancy later in gestation (ie, after 12 weeks) accounts for less than 20% of miscarriages.[2]

Fertilization occurs when a sperm attaches to the outer protein layer of the egg, the zona pellucida, and renders the egg nonresponsive to other sperm.[3] The attached sperm releases enzymes that allow the sperm to fully penetrate the zona pellucida and contact the egg's cell membrane. The membranes of the sperm and egg then combine to create a new, single cell called a *zygote*. Male and female chromosomes join in the zygote, fuse to create a single nucleus, and organize for cell division.[2,3]

Fertilization usually occurs in the fallopian tube. The fertilized egg travels down the fallopian tube over 3 to 4 days, with cell division taking place and by day 3, it reaches the uterus. Cell division continues for another 2 to 3 days in the uterine cavity before implantation. Approximately 6 days after fertilization, the cell mass is termed

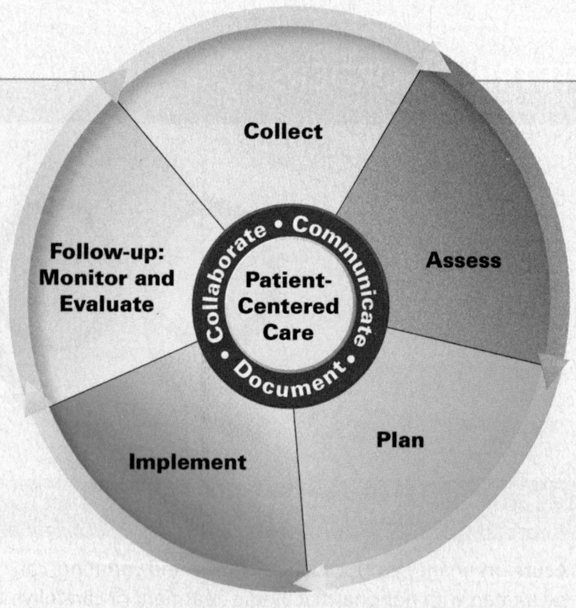

Patient Care Process for the Management of Gestational Diabetes

The image shows the five fundamental steps included in The Pharmacist's Care Process endorsed by the Joint Commission for Pharmacy Practitioners (2014). The tagline of this process reads collaborate, communicate, and document. The five fundamental steps listed here are collect, assess, plan, implement, and follow-up: monitor and evaluate. All these steps are listed in a circular block diagram.

Collect

- Patient characteristics (eg, age, race, gender identity, biological sex, pregnancy status)
- Characteristics of the pregnancy (eg, gestational age, gravidity and parity, weight gain to date)
- Characteristics of previous pregnancy(ies) (eg, prior gestational diabetes, birth weight of previous children, unexplained fetal demise)
- Patient history (past medical, family, social habits, physical activity habits, and dietary discretion)
- Current medications (including complementary or alternative therapies) and adherence to medication schedules
- Social and cultural issues: preferences, values, and beliefs; health literacy
- Physical exam: height, weight, body mass index (BMI), blood pressure, heart rate
- Labs (urine dipstick results for glucose, protein, and albumin)

Assess*

- Risk factors and need for early screening and diagnosis (see Table 99-2)
- Screening and diagnostic testing between 24 and 28 weeks gestation for all; first trimester testing for high-risk patients (see Table 99-2)
- Achievement of target fasting and 1- or 2-hour postprandial glucose goals
- Efficacy and adherence to dietary modifications and current antihyperglycemic regimen and alternative therapies
- Achievement of goals for comorbidities (eg, blood pressure)
- Assess for depression, anxiety regarding treatment, dietary habits
- Screen for psychosocial problems and barriers to diabetes self-management

Plan*

- Set appropriate blood glucose goals based on age, comorbidities, and other factors
- Tailored lifestyle modifications (eg, diet, exercise)
- Medication therapy regimen including specific antihyperglycemic agent(s), dose, route, frequency, and duration
- Monitoring parameters including efficacy (eg, self-monitored blood glucose), safety (medication-specific adverse events, hypoglycemia), and timeframe
- Patient education (eg, potential maternal and fetal adverse events, self-monitoring parameters, risks of uncontrolled blood glucose levels, purpose of treatment, medication administration, dietary and lifestyle modifications)
- Encourage screening at 4-12 weeks postpartum visit and periodically throughout life
- Encourage follow-up with primary care provider postpartum if not already established for continued care

Implement*

- Provide patient education regarding all elements of treatment plan
- Use motivational interviewing and coaching strategies to maximize adherence to the treatment plan
- Schedule follow-up clinic visits to adjust the treatment plan and monitor and evaluate adverse effects

**Collaborate with patient, caregivers, and other healthcare professionals.*

a *blastocyst.* Implantation begins with the blastocyst sloughing the zona pellucida to rest directly on the endometrium, allowing initiation of growth into the endometrial wall. Human chorionic gonadotropin (hCG) becomes detectable in serum or urine by pregnancy testing, as early as 8 or 9 days after ovulation; however, sensitivity may vary by brand of test.[2] By day 10 postfertilization, the blastocyst is implanted under the endometrial surface and receives nutrition from pregnant individual's blood. On the first day of the third week postfertilization, it is called an *embryo.*[4,5]

After the embryonic period (between weeks 2 and 8 postfertilization), the embryo is renamed a *fetus.* Most body structures are formed during the embryonic period, and they continue to grow and mature during the fetal period. The fetal period continues until the pregnancy reaches term, approximately 40 weeks after the last menstrual period.[5]

Gravidity is the number of times that an individual has been pregnant. A multiple birth is counted as a single pregnancy. *Parity* refers to the number of pregnancies exceeding 20 weeks of gestation and relates information regarding the outcome of each pregnancy.

Medical terminology abbreviations are used to indicate an individual's gravidity (G) and parity (P) history. In sequence, the numbers reflect (a) term deliveries, (b) premature deliveries, (c) aborted pregnancies, and (d) number of living children.[2,6] For example, in an individual who has been pregnant four times and has experienced two term deliveries, one premature delivery, one ectopic pregnancy and has three living children their designation would be G_4P_{2113}.

Characteristics of Pregnancy

Pregnancy lasts approximately 280 days (about 40 weeks or 9 months) with the time period being measured from the first day of the last menstrual period to birth. *Gestational age* refers to the age of the embryo or fetus beginning with the first day of the last menstrual period, which is about 2 weeks prior to fertilization.[2] For remainder of the chapter pregnancy information will be described in gestational age. When calculating the estimated due date, add 7 days to the first day of the last menstrual period then subtract 3 months. Pregnancy is divided into three periods of 3 calendar months, each being called a *trimester*.[2] The first trimester occurs between gestational weeks 1 and 13, the second trimester weeks 14 through 27, and the third trimester weeks 28 to 40, or delivery.

Early symptoms of pregnancy include fatigue and increased frequency of urination. After the first or second missed menstrual period, nausea and vomiting can occur. While commonly called *morning sickness*, this is a misnomer as it can happen at any time of the day; however, it usually resolves at 14 to 16 weeks gestation. Pregnant individuals may begin to feel fetal movements in the lower abdomen as early as 13 to 16 weeks gestation, with most individuals feeling movement by 18 to 20 weeks gestation.[7] Signs of pregnancy include cessation of menses, change in cervical mucus consistency, bluish discoloration of the vaginal mucosa, increased skin pigmentation, and anatomic breast changes.[2,6]

Pharmacokinetic Changes During Pregnancy

2 Normal physiologic changes that occur during pregnancy may alter medication effects, resulting in the need to more closely monitor and, sometimes, adjust therapy. Physiologic changes begin in the first trimester and peak during the second trimester. For medications that can be monitored by blood or serum concentration measurements, monitoring should occur throughout pregnancy due to the many changes that occur during this time.

During pregnancy, a pregnant individual's plasma volume, cardiac output, and glomerular filtration each increase (50%, 30%-50%, and 50%-80%, respectively), potentially lowering the concentration of renally eliminated medications.[8] With changes in plasma volume and body weight, the volume of distribution of medications may be affected. Plasma albumin concentration decreases, which increases the volume of distribution of medications that are highly protein bound. However, unbound medications are more rapidly cleared by the liver and kidney during pregnancy, resulting in little change in concentration. Hepatic perfusion also increases, which could theoretically increase the hepatic extraction of medications; activity of metabolic enzymes and drug transporters changes during pregnancy. Activity of cytochrome P450 3A4, 2C9, and 2D6, as well as UGT1A4 are increased while that of 1A2 is decreased.[9,10] Nausea and vomiting, as well as delayed gastric emptying, may also alter the absorption of medications.

Transplacental Medication Transfer

2 Although once thought to be a barrier to medication transfer, the placenta is the organ of exchange between the pregnant individual and fetus for a number of substances, including medications.[12] Most move from the pregnant individual's circulation to the fetal circulation by diffusion.[14] Certain chemical properties impact transplacental medication transfer, such as half-life, lipid solubility, electrical charge, molecular weight, and degree of protein binding of medications. Providers prefer medications with a high molecular weight, shorter half-life, high protein binding, as medications with these properties have a lower potential to cross the placenta.[13,14]

Medications with molecular weight less than 500 Da readily cross the placenta, whereas larger molecules (600-1,000 Da) cross more slowly.[14] Medications with molecular weight greater than 1,000 Da, such as insulin and heparin, usually do not cross the placenta in significant amounts. Lipophilic medications, such as opioids and antibiotics, cross the placenta more easily than do water-soluble medications. A pregnant individual's plasma albumin progressively decreases, which may result in higher concentrations of certain protein-bound medications in the fetus. Fetal pH is slightly more acidic than pregnant individual's pH.[14,15] Once in the fetal circulation, weak bases (eg, bupivicaine) become more ionized leading to ion trapping, higher fetal levels, and are less likely to diffuse back into the pregnant individual's circulation.[14,15]

PHARMACOTHERAPY SELECTION DURING PREGNANCY

3 Many misconceptions exist regarding the association of medications and birth defects. Although some have the potential to cause teratogenic effects, most required by pregnant individuals can be used.

The baseline risk (also known as background risk) for congenital malformations is approximately 3% to 5%.[16] It is imperative when selecting medications to compare the baseline risk to the potential risk of medication exposure. Medication exposure is estimated to account for less than 1% of all birth defects; instead 80% are related to unknown causes, 15% chromosomal causes, 4% genetic causes, and less than 1% from other environmental issues (eg, a pregnant individual's conditions and infections).[2]

Factors such as the stage of pregnancy during exposure, medication route of administration, and dose can also affect outcomes.[12] In the first 4 weeks of gestation, exposure to a teratogen may result in an "all-or-none" phenomenon, which could either destroy the embryo or cause no problems.[17] Organogenesis occurs during the embryonic period when organ systems are developing; therefore, teratogenic exposures may result in structural anomalies. For the remainder of the pregnancy, exposure to teratogens may result in growth restriction, central nervous system (CNS) abnormalities, impaired organ function, and fetal demise. Examples of medications associated with teratogenic effects in the period of organogenesis include some chemotherapy agents (eg, methotrexate and cyclophosphamide), some sex hormones (eg, androgens), lithium, retinoids, thalidomide, warfarin, and certain antiseizure medications. Other medications, such as nonsteroidal anti-inflammatory drugs (NSAIDs) and tetracycline derivatives, are more likely to exhibit effects in the second or third trimester.[2,12]

Medications are often necessary during pregnancy for treatment of acute and chronic conditions. Identifying patterns of medication use before conception, eliminating nonessential medications and discouraging self-medication, minimizing exposure to medications known to be harmful, and adjusting doses are all strategies to optimize the pregnant individual's health while minimizing the risk to the fetus. In summary, a small number of medications have the potential to cause congenital malformations, and many can be avoided during pregnancy. In situations where a medication may be teratogenic but is necessary for the pregnant individual's care, considerations related to route of administration, dosage form, and dosing may lessen the risk.

Methods and Resources for Determining Medication Safety in Pregnancy

4 When assessing the safety of using medications during pregnancy, evaluation of the quality of the evidence is important. Ideally,

safety data from randomized, controlled trials are most desirable, but pregnant individuals are not usually eligible for participation in clinical trials. Other types of data commonly used to estimate the risk associated with medication use during pregnancy include animal studies, case reports, case–control studies, prospective cohort studies, historical cohort studies, and voluntary reporting systems (eg, registries). Information can be found from the FDA (https://www.fda.gov/science-research/womens-health-research/list-pregnancy-exposure-registries) and package inserts, and patients should be encouraged to enroll in medication registries when medications are used throughout pregnancy to increase information on medication exposure.

Animal studies are a required component of medication testing, but extrapolation of the results to humans is not always valid, and 75% of the time animal medication exposure does not demonstrate a similar response in humans. Additionally relying on animal data is often limited due to species differences, issues with poor study methodology, concerns for publication bias, study or data inconsistency, and lack of clinical translation.[18] A prime example of this is thalidomide, which was regarded as safe in some animal models, but proved to have significant teratogenic effects in human offspring.[2,12] The value of case reports is limited because birth defects in the offspring of pregnant individuals who used medication during pregnancy may occur by chance.[12] It is important to also consider other factors that can influence pregnancy outcomes, such as exposure to tobacco, alcohol, recreational substances, environmental factors, and infection or uncontrolled disease states in an pregnant individual, as these factors are not always accounted for in literature and each can impact pregnancy outcomes.[2,12] Case–control studies identify an outcome (congenital anomaly), match subjects with or without that outcome, and report how often exposure to a suspected agent occurred. Recall bias is a concern, with retrospective design, as individuals with an affected pregnancy may be more likely to remember medications used during the pregnancy than those with a routine pregnancy.

Cohort studies that evaluate the intervention (use of a particular medication) in a group of persons and compare outcomes in a similar group of subjects without the intervention are also possible.[1,12] Prospective studies eliminate some of the problems with recall bias, but require time and large numbers of participants and may not adequately account for potential confounding variables. Despite these disadvantages, cohort studies are often used for evaluating the effects of medication exposure on pregnancy outcomes.

Teratology information services provide pregnant individuals and healthcare providers with information about potential exposures during pregnancy. Many also offer additional resources including patient education materials (eg, https://mothertobaby.org/fact-sheets/).[12] These services may publish pooled data to facilitate information sharing about medications used during pregnancy. Some pharmaceutical companies have organized voluntary reporting systems (also called pregnancy registries) for medications used during pregnancy.

4 Computerized databases (eg, LactMed [https://ncbi.nlm.nih.gov/books/NBK501922/), guidelines and textbooks with information regarding medication use during pregnancy and lactation offer valuable assistance.

The FDA approved product-labeling requirements for medications approved after June 20, 2015 include a subsection for pregnancy that provides information about pregnancy exposure registries, a risk summary, clinical considerations, supporting data, lactation, and if there are concerns for reproductive health. Prescription medications approved after June 30, 2001 are required to have updated product labeling to meet the new requirements and use of the new requirements have been phased in gradually. Medications approved before June 30, 2001 do not have to implement the new labeling requirements, but were required to remove the pregnancy category from product labeling. Risk categories remain in product labeling only for over-the-counter (OTC) medications, due to the multiple limitations of the pregnancy risk categories (ie, A, B, C, D, and X) previously used to guide clinicians regarding medication risk during pregnancy.[19]

In summary, determining medication safety during pregnancy is limited by the quality of data and the types of study designs that can be used. While information from product labeling may provide a rough estimate of risks for medication-related adverse fetal outcomes, careful evaluation of other available information sources is necessary to make decisions about medication use in pregnant individuals.

PRECONCEPTION PLANNING

Pregnancy outcomes are influenced by the pregnant individual's health status, lifestyle, and history prior to conception. The goal of preconception care is health promotion, through modification of behavioral, biomedical, and social risks in all individuals of reproductive age able to become pregnant, to ensure optimal health and improve pregnancy outcomes.[20] Almost half of all pregnancies in the United States are unintended. Preconception planning is important, since some behaviors and exposures impart risk to the fetus during the first trimester, often before prenatal care is begun or even before pregnancy is detected. Table 99-1 lists selected preconception risk factors, the potential adverse pregnancy outcomes, and management or prevention options.

The most common major congenital abnormalities are neural tube defects (NTDs), cleft palate and lip, and cardiac anomalies. Each year in the United States approximately 3,000 pregnancies are affected by an NTD.[22,33] Folic acid supplementation in individuals of childbearing potential substantially reduces the incidence of NTDs in their offspring. This is also true in individuals who have previously delivered babies with NTDs, as they occur within the first month of conception due to neural tube closure occurring by gestational week 6. Folic acid supplementation of at least 0.4 mg daily is recommended throughout the reproductive years, since many pregnancies are unplanned and may not be recognized until after the first month.[22,34] Additionally, 4 mg of folic acid per day starting 3 months prior to conception and continued until 12 weeks gestation is recommended for individuals at high risk for neural tube defects, which includes those with a personal, partner, or previous pregnancy history of neural tube defects.[22]

Use of alcohol and substances during pregnancy is also associated with risk (see Table 99-1).[2,12,21-32] In 2012 in the United States, alcohol use, substance use, and cigarette use were reported in 8.5%, 5.9%, and 15.9% of pregnant individuals, respectively.[35] ACOG recommends that patients should be educated about the risks of smoking and potential risks of using nicotine replacement therapy, and patients should be closely monitored while on therapy.[31] Nicotine replacement therapy during pregnancy may help improve cessation rates and theoretically imparts less risk than exposure to the over 4,000 chemicals found in cigarettes.[31,36] Although bupropion is not associated with risk during pregnancy, a Cochrane review found that bupropion did not improve cessation rates in pregnancy.[31,36] Varenicline has limited safety and efficacy data in pregnancy, but available data has not demonstrated teratogenic effects.[31,36]

ACUTE PREGNANCY ISSUES

Pregnancy causes or exacerbates conditions that pregnant individuals commonly experience, including nausea and vomiting, constipation, hemorrhoids, and gastroesophageal reflux. Individuals with pregnancy-influenced gastrointestinal (GI) issues can be treated with lifestyle modification or medications, many of them are nonprescription.

TABLE 99-1 Selected Preconception Risk Factors for Adverse Pregnancy Outcomes

Preconception Risk Factor	Potential Adverse Pregnancy Outcomes	Management or Prevention Options
Use of known teratogens		
• Antiseizure Medications	• Some are known teratogens; causes craniofacial, cardiac, and limb defects[a] • NTD • Fetal hydantoin syndrome	• Optimize to lower risk therapy while maintaining control prior to conception • Avoid valproic acid • use monotherapy if possible • Start folic acid at least 0.4 mg daily preferably at least 1 month prior to conception
• Retinoids	• Spontaneous abortion • Known teratogen; causes CNS, craniofacial, and cardiac defects[a]	• Discontinue at least 1 month (isotretinoin, bexarotene) or 3 years (acitretin) before attempting conception • Enrolled in iPLEDGE (isotretinoin), Education and Pregnancy Prevention for Acitretin (EPPA) or Do Your P.A.R.T. (acitretin). Follow manufacturer recommendations for contraception (isotretinoin, acitretin, bexarotene)
• Warfarin	• Fetal warfarin syndrome	• Switch to nonteratogenic anticoagulant (eg, LMWH) before becoming pregnant • Patients with mechanical valves may remain on warfarin for some or all of the pregnancy
Lifestyle factors		
• Alcohol use	• Fetal alcohol syndrome	• Cease alcohol intake before conception
• Obesity	• Malformations (eg, NTD and orofacial) • Preterm delivery • Spontaneous abortion • Stillbirth • Macrosomia • Impaired growth • Cesarean section	• Weight loss with appropriate nutritional intake before pregnancy
• Tobacco use	• Preterm birth • Low birth weight • Spontaneous abortion • Increased perinatal mortality • Orofacial clefts • Intrauterine growth restriction • Sudden infant death syndrome	• Ideally, cease tobacco use before conception • Individualize approach with nonpharmacologic therapies (including psychosocial and behavioral interventions like CBT, motivational interviewing, and counseling) and can consider NRT products, bupropion, varenicline. Discuss risks and benefits with the patient
• Cannabis use	• Intrauterine fetal demise • Low birth rate[b] • Preterm delivery[b]	• Ask about medical and nonmedical use of marijuana in all patients • Educate about potential risks • Encourage to discontinue use ideally prior to conception

[a]List is not all-inclusive.

[b]When stratified by frequency of use (risk at least weekly use).

CBT, cognitive behavioral therapy; CNS, central nervous system; HTN, hypertension; NRT, nicotine replacement therapy; NTD, neural tube defect; VTE, venous thromboembolism.

Data from References 2-12, and 21-32.

Nausea and Vomiting

5 Nausea and vomiting of pregnancy (NVP) impacts 50% to 80% of pregnant individuals.[37] NVP usually begins between weeks 4 and 6 of gestation and usually resolves by weeks 14 to 16 with peak symptoms occurring between weeks 8 and 12.[2,11] Hyperemesis gravidarum (HG; ie, unrelenting vomiting causing weight loss of more than 5% prepregnancy weight, dehydration, electrolyte imbalance, and ketonuria) occurs in 0.3% to 3% of pregnant individuals.[2,11,37] Healthcare providers should educate patients with NVP on nonpharmacological interventions. Dietary modifications, such as eating frequent, small, bland or dry meals every 1 to 2 hours, consuming crackers before getting out of bed in the morning, snacking on high-protein foods, and eliminating fatty or spicy foods, may be helpful. Applying pressure at acupressure point P6 on the volar aspect of the wrist (between the two tendons on about three fingers below the wrist) may be beneficial. Avoiding triggers such as odor, heat, humidity, noise, and flickering lights may help.[11,37] Additionally, ACOG recommends ginger 250 mg capsules four times daily. If pharmacologic therapy is needed, ACOG recommends pyridoxine 10 to 25 mg with or without doxylamine 12.5 mg up to four times daily, depending on the formulation selected, as the first-line therapy.[37] Immediate release tablets for both agents are available over the counter; however, adverse events such as sedation with doxylamine may limit use. Both extended and delayed release combination tablets are available by prescription, but cost may limit use. If symptoms persist, second line add-on therapies include dimenhydrinate, diphenhydramine, prochlorperazine, and promethazine. Both prochlorperazine and promethazine are available as suppositories if patients are struggling to keep oral products down. For continued symptoms in patients without dehydration, recommended therapies include metoclopramide, ondansetron, and trimethobenzamide as third-line agents.[37] Although metoclopramide has not been associated for a risk of malformations, it carries a boxed warning for tardive dyskinesia.[37,38] Additionally, combination of dopamine antagonist therapies such as metoclopramide and phenothiazines may also increase the risk for extrapyramidal symptoms.[37] Conflicting data exist regarding ondansetron use and the risk for malformations such as cardiovascular defects and oral clefts.[26,37] Ondansetron use prior to 10 weeks gestation should be individualized by patient, after careful consideration of the associated risks and benefits. Additionally, ondansetron use may prolong the QT interval, particularly in patients with underlying cardiac issues, personal or family history of QT prolongation, use with other medications that can prolong the QT, or electrolyte imbalances. In patients with dehydration, intravenous fluids should

be administered, and providers consider intravenous therapy with dimenhydrinate, metoclopramide, ondansetron, or promethazine. Intravenous or intramuscular chlorpromazine or methylprednisolone may be added on for patients with persistent symptoms. Corticosteroids may be effective for HG; use should be reserved until after 10 weeks gestation due to a small increase in the risk of oral clefts.[37]

Constipation and Hemorrhoids

5 Constipation during pregnancy is prevalent, affecting almost 40% of individuals and may contribute to the development or exacerbation of hemorrhoids which are more prevalent in pregnant persons compared with the general population.[11] Nonpharmacologic treatment (ie, high dietary fiber intake, maintaining hydration by increasing water intake, and use of sitz baths) or moderate physical activity should be recommended alone or in combination with medication therapy. Bulk-forming agents (eg, psyllium, methylcellulose, and polycarbophil) are considered appropriate for long-term use because they are not absorbed or associated with an increased risk of malformations. However, they are not always effective, can take several days to work, and can be associated with unpleasant adverse effects including gas, bloating, and cramping. In addition, bulk-forming agents may lack palatability, especially for patients struggling with nausea and vomiting throughout pregnancy. Osmotic laxatives, specifically polyethylene glycol, are commonly utilized throughout pregnancy. Their use has not been associated with adverse effects in pregnancy; however, the patient might experience adverse effects such as bloating and increased flatulence. Polyethylene glycol is the preferred medication for patients with chronic constipation during pregnancy. In addition, stool softeners (eg, docusate) may be also be used and are well tolerated.[11] Stimulant laxatives (ie, senna and bisacodyl) are associated with a fast onset of action, however should be reserved for short-term use. If utilized long-term, use should be limited to 3 days per week.[39] Use of magnesium should be cautioned, as can lead to dehydration secondary to diarrhea, and long-term use may lead to magnesium toxicity. In addition, magnesium may increase the risk for electrolyte imbalances. Castor oil and mineral oil should be avoided because they may cause stimulation of uterine contractions and impairment of fat-soluble vitamin absorption, respectively.[11,26] Data supporting other management options for hemorrhoids during pregnancy are limited. Topical anesthetics, skin protectants, and astringents (eg, witch hazel) can be used for anal irritation and pain. Hydrocortisone may reduce inflammation and pruritis.[40]

Gastroesophageal Reflux Disease

5 Up to 80% of individuals experience gastroesophageal reflux disease during pregnancy.[41] Nonpharmacologic therapy with lifestyle and dietary modifications can be recommended alone or with medication therapy (see Chapter 50, "Gastroesophageal Reflux Disease"). Antacids (eg, aluminum, calcium, magnesium preparations) are commonly used to relieve symptoms. Magnesium trisilicate-based antacids (eg, Gaviscon®) are less preferred because when used in high doses or long-term have been associated with nephrolithiasis, hypotonia, cardiovascular impairment and respiratory disease in the fetus. In addition, sodium bicarbonate-based antacids (eg, Alka-Seltzer®) are generally not recommended in pregnancy due to risk for fluid overload and metabolic alkalosis.[41] Additionally, sucralfate is used along with lifestyle modifications because it has minimal systemic absorption.[39] Histamine-2 receptor antagonist (H_2RAs), most commonly famotidine, can be used for patients unresponsive to lifestyle changes and antacids or sucralfate. Twice daily dosing with H_2RA therapy is commonly used in pregnancy. The use of proton pump inhibitors (PPIs) during pregnancy are generally reserved for patients who fail H_2RA therapy or who required a PPI prior to pregnancy. PPI therapy does not appear to increase the risk of major birth defects; however, most data comes from use of omeprazole.[11,26] Despite previous concerns regarding omeprazole use during pregnancy, a large cohort study evaluating PPI use during pregnancy did not show an increased risk of birth defects in females who took PPIs, including omeprazole.[42] In instances where delayed gastric emptying is contributing to reflux symptoms, metoclopramide may be considered as an add-on therapy to an H_2RA or PPI.

Diabetes in Pregnancy

6 Up to 7% of pregnancies are complicated by any type of diabetes, with gestational diabetes mellitus (GDM) accounting for roughly 86% of cases overall.[44] Diabetes diagnosed prior to pregnancy is commonly referred to as pregestational diabetes, whereas GDM is most commonly diagnosed between 24 to 28 weeks gestation. GDM is a complex condition characterized by the development of carbohydrate intolerance, pancreatic β-cell dysfunction, and insulin resistance that occurs during pregnancy. Diabetes that develops during the first trimester of pregnancy is most commonly type 2 diabetes that has been previously undiagnosed; however, this condition may be type 1 diabetes or GDM. The most common risk factor for developing GDM is a history of GDM in a previous pregnancy. Additional risk factors include: high-risk race (Asian American, American Indian, Pacific Islander, African American, and Latinx populations), BMI greater than or equal to 25 kg/m² (or greater than or equal to 23 kg/m² for Asian individuals), history of diabetes in a first-degree relative, previous birth of an infant weighing 4,000 g (about 9 pounds) or more, physical inactivity, hypertension or on medication for hypertension, polycystic ovary syndrome, high-density lipoprotein cholesterol less than 35 mg/dL (0.91 mmol/L), triglycerides greater than 250 mg/dL (2.83 mmol/L), A1c greater than 5.7% (0.057; 39 mmol/mol) or impaired fasting glucose on previous testing, other clinical indications of insulin resistance such as prepregnancy BMI greater than 40 kg/m² or acanthosis nigricans, and history of cardiovascular disease.[43,44]

Complications During Pregnancy

Poorly controlled diabetes, regardless of type, can increase the risk for fetal malformations, fetal morbidity and mortality, and morbidity for the pregnant individual. The most common fetal complications include macrosomia (birthweight greater than 4,000 g), neonatal hypoglycemia often requiring neonatal intensive care unit stay, hyperbilirubinemia, and birth trauma.[45] In individuals with pregestational diabetes, preconception A1c plays an important role in determining risk for fetal malformations. Patients with a preconception A1c between 5% to 6% (0.05-0.06; or 31-42 mmol/mol) have a fetal malformation rate similar to pregnancies not impacted by diabetes. As a patient's preconception A1c approaches 10% (0.1; 86 mmol/mol) and higher, the fetal malformation rate increases to 20% to 25%. The most commonly observed malformations include cardiac defects, CNS anomalies, and skeletal malformations.[46] An increased risk for long-term complications also exist for the child, and include impaired glucose tolerance, type 2 diabetes, hypertension, obesity, and hyperlipidemia. Risk to the pregnant individual include higher incidence of cesarean delivery, hypertension and preeclampsia, metabolic syndrome, and cardiovascular disease. In addition, individuals with GDM are at a 10-fold increased risk for developing type 2 diabetes later in life, and those with pregestational diabetes are at risk for worsening retinopathy and deteriorating renal function.[43,47]

Screening and Diagnostic Criteria

Due to the risks for both the pregnant individual, fetus, and neonate, the American Diabetes Association (ADA) and American College of Obstetricians and Gynecologists (ACOG) recommend universal screening for GDM in all patients not previously diagnosed with type 1 or 2 diabetes between 24 to 28 weeks' gestation.

TABLE 99-2 Screening and Diagnosis of Gestational Diabetes Mellitus

One-Step Method	
Complete a 75-g oral glucose tolerance test. Plasma glucose is assessed at fasting, and after 1 and 2 hours. The test should be performed in the morning following an overnight fast of at least 8 hours.	GDM diagnosis is confirmed when one or more of the plasma glucose levels are met or exceeded: Fasting: 92 mg/dL (5.1 mmol/L) 1 hour: 180 mg/dL (10.0 mmol/L) 2 hour: 153 mg/dL (8.5 mmol/L)
Two-Step Method	
Step 1: Complete a 50-g oral glucose loading test. This is typically done in a non-fasting state. Plasma glucose is assessed after 1 hour.	If the plasma glucose level is greater than or equal to 140 mg/dL[a] (7.8 mmol/L), the patient moves to step 2.
Step 2: Complete a 100-g oral glucose tolerance test. Plasma glucose is assessed at fasting, after 1, 2, and 3 hours.	GDM diagnosis is confirmed when at least two of the following plasma glucose levels are met or exceeded: Fasting: 95 mg/dL (5.3 mmol/L) 1 hour: 180 mg/dL (10 mmol/L) 2 hour: 155 mg/dL (8.6 mmol/L) 3 hour: 140 mg/dL (7.8 mmol/L)

[a]A lower threshold of 130 or 135 mg/dL (7.2 or 7.5 mmol/L) may be utilized by some providers; ADA recommends 140 mg/dL (7.8 mmol/L).

Data from References 43 and 44.

Individuals considered at an increased risk for GDM as defined previously should be screened in early pregnancy. Generally, screening is recommended at the first pregnancy visit for those at high risk if the patient is able to tolerate screening; however, screening may be delayed in patients with uncontrolled nausea or vomiting. If GDM is not diagnosed with early screening, screening should be completed again between 24 and 28 weeks' gestation.[44] A diagnosis of GDM can be confirmed using two different approaches: a one-step strategy or a two-step strategy (Table 99-2).

Glucose Monitoring

Daily self-monitoring of blood glucose is recommended for all persons with diabetes during pregnancy, including those with GDM. Evidence supporting optimal frequency of glucose monitoring is lacking; however, in general, patients are recommended to test at least four times daily, with some testing up to seven times a day. Common testing times include fasting glucose, one or two hours after each meal, and before bedtime, with postprandial glucose levels being the best indicator of risk of macrosomia and other complications during pregnancy. Additional testing times are commonly recommended for the following scenarios: premeal glucose monitoring in patients using an insulin pump or if insulin doses are based on premeal values, and between 2 and 3 am if nocturnal hypoglycemia is suspected. Regular A1c monitoring is considered a secondary measure of glycemic control during pregnancy and is not routinely utilized for guiding glucose management, however may still be assessed once a trimester. Of note, A1c levels decrease by as much as 0.5% (0.006; 0.6 mmol/mol) during normal pregnancy due to an increase in red blood cell turnover. An A1c target of less than 6% (0.06; 42 mmol/mol) is optimal during pregnancy as it is associated with the lowest risk of large for gestational age infants, preterm delivery, and preeclampsia.[43,44]

Glycemic control can change dramatically during pregnancy and frequent adjustments to management are often needed. Medical nutrition therapy, exercise, and blood glucose monitoring are considered first-line therapies for all with GDM, and as many as 70% to 85% of patients can achieve control with these interventions.[43] Dietary and exercise interventions should be recommended for all patients, but plans are individualized. Refer to the guidelines for specific recommendations.[43,44,46]

Glucose Management

Pharmacotherapy should be initiated when medical nutrition therapy and exercise fail to achieve glucose goals within 1 to 2 weeks after initiation.[44] The general threshold that triggers the need for pharmacologic therapy has not been well established; however, many providers will start therapy if most of the glucose concentrations within the most recent week are elevated above goal. The current ACOG guidelines recommend starting insulin under the following parameters: fasting glucose concentrations consistently greater than 95 mg/dL (5.3 mmol/L), 1-hour postprandial concentrations consistently greater than 140 mg/dL (7.8 mmol/L), or 2-hour postprandial concentrations consistently greater than 120 mg/dL (6.7 mmol/L).[44] Insulin is the recommended first line when medication therapy is needed. If patient refuses insulin or has financial limitations, language barriers, or the provider has significant concerns for routine patient follow-up, oral therapy with metformin or glyburide may be considered.[43,44]

Insulin Both ACOG and ADA recommend insulin as first-line therapy for glucose management during pregnancy. Human insulin does not cross the placenta, whereas animal insulins can cross in insignificant amounts.[26,43] A preferred insulin regimen during pregnancy has not been established.[48] Basal insulin options include insulin NPH, insulin glargine, and insulin detemir. The initial studies of glucose management in GDM used insulin NPH; thus it is the standard to which all other insulins are compared. Insulin glargine and detemir are the most commonly used long-acting insulins for basal insulin coverage during pregnancy.[49,50] Data regarding insulin degludec during pregnancy are limited, although pregnancy outcomes appear to be similar to outcomes with other insulin regimens.[51]

Bolus insulin options include insulin lispro and insulin aspart and both do not cross the placenta and are commonly used during pregnancy. Either insulin lispro or insulin aspart should be used primarily over regular insulin because they are associated with a quicker onset of action which helps prevent hypoglycemia and insulin dosing errors. Data regarding insulin glulisine during pregnancy are limited; however, information available has not shown an increased risk for adverse pregnancy outcomes.[52]

Several daily injections of insulin are often needed during pregnancy to achieve optimal control. The ADA and ACOG do not specify a preferred insulin dosing approach for initiating therapy during pregnancy, nor do they prefer specific insulin. A general weight-based approach suggests starting 0.7 to 1 unit/kg/day of insulin in divided doses.[44] Due to patient variability in dietary intake and increases in insulin resistance that increases throughout pregnancy, insulin doses will likely be titrated often based on the patient's home glucose monitoring.

Metformin Both ADA and ACOG recommend metformin as an alternative agent for lowering blood glucose during pregnancy. Metformin readily crosses the placenta and was previously used frequently during pregnancy. Metformin is associated with a lower risk of neonatal hypoglycemia and lower weight gain in pregnant individuals compared to insulin, which made it a viable oral option for glucose management during pregnancy.[53,54] Data evaluating metformin in combination with insulin during pregnancy found individuals on the combination required less insulin, gained less weight, lower incidence of macrosomia, and had fewer cesarean deliveries compared to insulin alone.[55] In addition, more than 40% of those on metformin monotherapy during pregnancy ultimately require insulin to achieve glycemic control.[44] There are concerns for long-term metabolic changes in offspring exposed to metformin during pregnancy.[56,57] The long-term metabolic impact on metformin use during pregnancy is not well established; however, there are concerns with exposure during pregnancy and additional data are needed to fully assess the long-term safety and efficacy outcomes. Individuals started on metformin during pregnancy should be educated that metformin crosses the placenta and fetal exposure could result in long-term metabolic effects into childhood.

Glyburide Both ADA and ACOG recommend glyburide as an alternative to metformin for lowering blood glucose during pregnancy.[43,44] As a class, sulfonylureas cross the placenta; however, glyburide is the only agent used in pregnancy due to minimal crossing through the placenta. Compared to both insulin and metformin, glyburide is associated with an increased risk of infant macrosomia and neonatal hypoglycemia, even when controlling for similar levels of glycemic control.[44] Observational studies have also reported higher incidence of preeclampsia, hyperbilirubinemia, and stillbirth in patients taking glyburide compared to insulin.[43] In addition, more than 20% of those on glyburide monotherapy during pregnancy ultimately require insulin to achieve glycemia control.[43] Glyburide therapy may be less effective in patients with higher baseline fasting glucose concentrations at diagnosis, and in patients with a history of GDM in a previous pregnancy or when GDM is diagnosed before 26 weeks' gestation.[58]

Postpartum Management and Screening

Insulin resistance begins to decline rapidly postpartum immediately once the placenta is delivered, requiring close glucose monitoring and often aggressive insulin adjustments.[59] During the first one to two weeks postpartum, insulin sensitivity begins to return to prepregnancy levels. Patients with GDM can often discontinue insulin during this time, and patients with type 1 or 2 diabetes often require significant insulin adjustments. Patients should be educated about the increased risk of hypoglycemia, including how to treat hypoglycemia, especially during this time of decreased sleep and when eating schedules can be erratic. Breastfeeding should be encouraged and supported for patients with diabetes during pregnancy.

Although many individuals with GDM return to normal glycemic control shortly after delivery, patients with GDM have a 10-fold increased risk of developing type 2 diabetes in their lifetime.[43] Due to this increased risk, the ADA recommends patients diagnosed with GDM during pregnancy be screened for persistent diabetes between 4 and 12 weeks postpartum most commonly with a 2-hour oral glucose tolerance test.[43] Diagnostic criteria for diagnosing diabetes follow the nonpregnant criteria. If type 2 diabetes is not diagnosed during the postpartum period, periodic screening is recommended every 1 to 3 years with any recommended glycemic test. Lifestyle interventions with a healthier diet and lower weight, and metformin can help prevent or delay the progression to diabetes by 35% to 40%, respectively, over 10 years.[43]

Hypertensive Disorders of Pregnancy

6 Hypertensive disorders of pregnancy (HDP) are one of the most common causes of mortality in pregnancy, as well as perinatally. Four categories of HDP are established: (1) chronic hypertension (HTN) (pre-existing HTN or developing before 20 weeks gestation); (2) gestational HTN (HTN without proteinuria developing after 20 weeks of gestation); and (3) preeclampsia (HTN with proteinuria) with gestational HTN, may present as the first symptoms of HTN disorder during pregnancy; and (4) chronic HTN with superimposed preeclampsia.[60,61] Hypertension in pregnancy is defined as either systolic blood pressure (sBP) above 140 mm Hg or diastolic blood pressure (dBP) above 90 mm Hg based upon two or more measurements at least 4 hours apart.[61] Severe hypertension is diagnosed after two measurements of sBP > 160 mm Hg and/or dBP > 110 mm Hg. The two measurements can be confirmed within a short interval (minutes) in order to start antihypertensive therapy quickly.

Risk factors for development of gestational HTN include nulliparity, individuals with first degree relative with history of gestational HTN (eg, sibling or parent), non-singleton pregnancies, age less than 20 years or older than 40 years, and a history of HTN or kidney disease in a previous pregnancy.[62]

TABLE 99-3 Risk Factors for Preeclampsia

High-Risk Factors	Moderate-Risk Factors
Preeclampsia in a prior pregnancy	Nulliparity
Non-singleton pregnancy	Prepregnancy BMI greater than 30 kg/m^2
Chronic hypertension	Family history of preeclampsia (1st degree relative—parent or sibling)
Pregestational diabetes	Sociodemographic characteristics (eg, African American race, low socioeconomic status)
Renal disease	Age greater than 35 years
Autoimmune disease (eg, systemic lupus erythematosus, antiphospholipid syndrome)	Medical history factors (eg, low birth weight or small for gestational age, previous adverse pregnancy outcome, more than 10-year pregnancy interval)
Combinations of multiple moderate-risk factors	

Data from References 61 and 66.

Preeclampsia is a more complex, multisystem syndrome that complicates up to 8% of pregnancies. Risk factors for development of preeclampsia are detailed in Table 99-3. Preeclampsia can be divided into early onset (prior to 34 weeks or requiring delivery prior to 37 weeks), late onset, or present up to 6 weeks postpartum. Early onset preeclampsia is typically severe in nature and associated with more morbidity for pregnant individuals. Diagnosis of preeclampsia includes elevated blood pressure as with HDP and proteinuria (>300 mg/24 hours or a protein/creatinine ratio of >300 mg/g [30 mg/mmol] are preferred, or urine dipstick of 2+). If proteinuria is not present, new onset of any of the following findings with new onset HTN is indicative of preeclampsia: thrombocytopenia (count less than 100×10^3/L [100×10^9/L]), serum creatinine above 1.1 mg/dL (97 μmol/L) or a doubling of serum creatinine, elevated liver transaminases at least twice the upper limit of normal, pulmonary edema, or new onset headache nonresponsive to analgesics or with visual symptoms.[61] Individuals may also experience chest pain or dyspnea, vomiting, and epigastric pain. Other signs and symptoms of preeclampsia that would warrant delivery include: severe uncontrolled HTN, eclampsia, persistent severe headache, pulmonary edema, placental abruption, disseminated intravascular coagulation, and HELLP syndrome (Hemolysis, Elevated Liver enzymes, Low Platelets) or evidence of adverse fetal effects, such as growth restriction.[61]

Preeclampsia may progress rapidly to eclampsia, which is defined by new-onset tonic-clonic, focal, or multifocal seizures superimposed on preeclampsia. Eclampsia is a medical emergency that can occur antepartum, intrapartum, or postpartum. It is often preceded by a headache, visual changes such as blurred vision or photophobia, or altered mental status; however, it may present with no warning signs or symptoms.[61,63]

Complication of Hypertension

All types of HDP are associated with risks to the fetus and pregnant individuals, with these risks increasing with uncontrolled HTN. Complications for the pregnant individual associated with HDP include preeclampsia, eclampsia, stroke, labor induction, and placental abruption. Fetal complications include intrauterine growth restriction, preterm delivery, low birth weight, and stillbirth. Additionally, chronic HTN is associated with increased risk for additional pregnancy and fetal complications including death, pulmonary edema, renal insufficiency and failure, myocardial infarction, cesarean delivery, postpartum hemorrhage, gestational diabetes, and congenital anomalies (eg, heart defects, hypospadias, esophageal atresia).[60]

Management of Hypertension

There is no consensus on treatment thresholds in individuals with mild hypertension. The ACOG recommends pharmacotherapy be initiated quickly in individuals with acute-onset severe HTN that is confirmed as persistent (lasting more than 15 minutes).[61] Due to a lack of evidence supporting the use of antihypertensive medications in patients with lower blood pressures, pharmacologic therapy is recommended once the patient has persistent blood pressures greater or equal to sBP 160 mm Hg and/or dBP 110 mm Hg. The ACOG recommends providers consider using lower blood pressure thresholds in individuals with comorbidities or underlying impaired renal function, but does not provide a specific threshold. When antihypertensive medications are used, it is recommended to maintain blood pressure levels between sBP 120 mm Hg and 160 mm Hg and dBP between 80 mm Hg and 110 mm Hg. Lowering of blood pressure should occur over a period of hours and aggressive blood pressure lowering should be avoided due to concerns for decreased uteroplacental blood flow.[60]

Treatment of Hypertension

Labetalol and nifedipine are the preferred treatment options for management of HTN during pregnancy. Labetalol is commonly used in practice; however, use may be limited in patients with asthma due to potential for bronchoconstrictive effects. It is also important to monitor the patient for bradycardia. Nifedipine extended-release is also commonly used in practice with twice daily dosing due to increased elimination. Immediate-release formulations are usually reserved for severe or acutely elevated blood pressure levels in hospitalized patients. Methyldopa is rarely used in practice due to lack of efficacy and increased adverse effects (eg, sedation, dizziness). Hydrochlorothiazide is generally considered a second- or third-line agent for HTN during pregnancy due to theoretical concern for fetal growth restriction and oligohydramnios. Clonidine and prazosin have also been used during pregnancy, but use is generally reserved for patients being closely followed by maternal-fetal medicine or cardiology specialist. Atenolol is associated with fetal growth restriction and generally not utilized during pregnancy. Angiotensin-converting enzyme inhibitors, angiotensin receptor blockers, renin inhibitors, and mineralocorticoid receptor antagonists are not recommended.[60]

The urgent need for blood pressure control in the setting of severe HTN is typically managed with intravenous labetalol, intravenous or intramuscular hydralazine, or immediate release oral nifedipine. Second-line treatment options include nicardipine or esmolol infusions. Once the patient's blood pressure is controlled, it is important to initiate oral maintenance therapy to maintain control.[61]

Intravenous magnesium sulfate is recommended in patients with severe HTN with preeclampsia to prevent the progression to eclampsia, and to treat eclamptic seizures. Although the duration of magnesium use varies, the usual duration is throughout active labor and continued for 12 to 24 hours postpartum. Benzodiazepines and phenytoin may be considered as treatment for eclampsia in patients with contraindications to magnesium (eg, myasthenia gravis, moderate-to-severe renal failure) or in settings where magnesium is unavailable.[60]

Low-dose aspirin (81 mg/day) prophylaxis is recommended for patients with one high-risk factor or two or more moderate-risk factors for preeclampsia (Table 99-3) to reduce the risk of preeclampsia.[64] Newer data suggests aspirin doses up to 150 mg may provide more protection; however, because this dose is not available in the United States, providers will often recommend 162 mg daily.[65] The exact mechanism of aspirin in the prevention of preeclampsia is not fully understood. Aspirin should be started between 12 weeks and 28 weeks gestation, ideally before 16 weeks, and continued daily until delivery.[66] In high-risk groups, adding low-dose aspirin in 50 pregnant individuals corresponds to preventing one case of preeclampsia.[39] Aspirin prophylaxis is also associated with a risk reduction for preterm birth, small for gestational age, intrauterine growth restriction, and perinatal mortality.[64]

Thyroid Disorders

6 Universal screening for thyroid disorders during pregnancy is not recommended.[67] During pregnancy, stimulation of the thyroid gland may occur because of hCG's structural similarity to thyroid-stimulating hormone (TSH; thyrotropin). This can occur in the first 12 weeks of gestation. In some individuals, gestational transient thyrotoxicosis (GTT) may result but treatment with antithyroid medication is usually not needed. Occurrence of GTT is often associated with HG and the nausea and vomiting can be treated as for patients without this pseudo-hyperthyroid state.[67]

Hypothyroidism is present in 2 to 10 per 1,000 pregnancies. Untreated hypothyroidism increases the risk of low birth weight, preeclampsia, premature birth, miscarriage, fetal death, and placental abruption; impaired neurological development in the fetus may also occur.[67] Causes of hypothyroidism include autoimmune diseases (eg, Hashimoto's thyroiditis), iodine deficiency (uncommon in the United States), and thyroid dysfunction following surgery or ablative therapy for previous hyperthyroidism.[67,68] If hypothyroidism is present, thyroid replacement should occur with levothyroxine. A reasonable levothyroxine starting dose is 1 to 2 mcg/kg/d or 0.1 mg/day. Individuals receiving thyroid replacement therapy before pregnancy are recommended to receive a 25% dose increase in levothyroxine once the pregnancy is confirmed. Laboratory follow-up of TSH should occur every 4 to 6 weeks during pregnancy to allow for dose titration according to TSH levels of the lower limit of the reference range up to 2.5 mU/L.[67]

Hyperthyroidism affects 0.2 to 0.7% of pregnancies and is associated with spontaneous abortion, fetal death, low birth weight, and medically indicated preterm delivery. Overall, 95% of hyperthyroidism in pregnancy is due to Graves' disease. Therapy includes the thioamides (eg, methimazole and propylthiouracil). Propylthiouracil is the preferred therapy during the first trimester because methimazole is associated with a higher risk for malformations. Although either thioamide can be used for the remainder of the pregnancy, many providers switch to methimazole because propylthiouracil has been associated with clinically significant hepatotoxicity. The risks of uncontrolled hyperthyroidism outweigh the risks of the thioamides. The goal of therapy is to attain free thyroxine concentrations near the upper limit of normal to allow for dose minimization and to limit fetal or neonatal hypothyroidism. Radioiodine is not recommended because of the risk of thyroid damage in the fetus. If adjunctive therapy is needed to treat symptomatic palpitations, propranolol is the preferred agent.[67]

Although not all pregnant individuals experience postpartum thyroiditis similarly, the typical presentation is characterized by transient hyperthyroidism during the first several months postpartum followed by a period of transient hypothyroidism between 4 and 8 months postpartum. Many cases spontaneously return to euthyroidism. The initial hyperthyroid state usually does not require treatment; however, β-blockers can provide symptomatic relief of adrenergic symptoms. Because postpartum thyroiditis is from a destructive inflammation process and not overproduction of thyroid hormone, antithyroid medications are ineffective. Up to one-third of individuals affected by postpartum thyroiditis develop permanent hypothyroidism.[67]

Thromboembolic Disorders

6 Thromboembolism is one of the most common causes of pregnancy-related death in the United States. The risk of developing a venous thromboembolism (VTE) in pregnant or postpartum individuals is increased by fourfold to fivefold over nonpregnant individuals.[69] Low-molecular-weight heparin (LMWH) is recommended over unfractionated heparin and other anticoagulants for both treatment and prophylaxis.[69,70] Warfarin is reserved as a treatment option in patients with a mechanical valve.[69] Warfarin is not universally used because of the risk for multiple malformations, fetal bleeding, and fetal demise.[26,69] The direct oral anticoagulants (eg, dabigatran, rivaroxaban, apixaban, and edoxaban) are not recommended due to limited data.[25,26,69] If a patient is not a candidate for heparin products (eg, heparin induced thrombocytopenia, severe allergic reaction), fondaparinux should be considered.[69] Specific recommendations for using prophylaxis, intermediate, or dose-adjusted therapy can be found in the ACOG practice bulletin.[69] For acute thromboembolism, anticoagulation therapy should be continued throughout pregnancy and for at least 6 weeks after delivery; the minimum total duration should not be less than 3 months.[69]

Recurrent VTE is divided into three categories: low risk, intermediate risk, and high risk of recurrence. Antepartum monitoring is recommended for individuals with a single episode of VTE who have a low risk of recurrence such as those with one transient risk factor (ie, surgery, injury, lengthy travel, or immobility). For intermediate risk (ie, hormone-related, pregnancy-related, or unprovoked VTE) and high risk (ie, more than one unprovoked VTE or continuous risk factors), antepartum therapy with LMWH or heparin plus 6-week postpartum therapy with either LMWH or warfarin is recommended.[69] Specific recommendations for thrombophilias (eg, antiphospholipid antibodies, Factor V Leiden, prothrombin G20201A, protein C and S deficiencies) can be found in the ACOG Practice Bulletin addressing inherited thrombophilias in pregnancy.[70]

Anticoagulation management of individuals with mechanical heart valves during pregnancy is complex and requires a thorough discussion of the risks and benefits to allow for shared decision making. Management options include continuing warfarin throughout the pregnancy if the patient uses less than 5 mg/day, using dose-adjusted LMWH during the first trimester then warfarin during the second and third trimesters, or using dose-adjusted LMWH throughout the pregnancy. Although warfarin is the most effective therapy for patients with mechanical valves, it crosses the placenta and has fetal risks; however, it appears that doses less than 5 mg daily have less risk for malformations than doses greater than 5 mg daily.[25] Additionally, it has been associated with spontaneous abortion, fetal intracranial hemorrhage, neonatal death, and central nervous system defects.[25,26] Both LMWH and heparin therapies do not cross the placenta but may have a higher risk for thromboembolic events. When heparin products are utilized, dose adjustment should be made to achieve a peak anti-Xa at 4 to 6 hours post-dose of 0.8 to 1.2 U/mL (kU/L) or a prothrombin time (aPTT) at least twice the control value, respectively. Additionally, individuals with mechanical heart valves may also receive low-dose aspirin (75-100 mg/daily). Delivery planning is important to optimize therapy to decrease risks for both the patient and fetus, and patients are switched to unfractionated heparin prior to delivery. See the current American College of Cardiology/American Heart Association guidelines for specific recommendations. Individuals with bioprosthetic valves have a lower risk of thromboembolism than those with mechanical valves; however, management of anticoagulation during pregnancy is similar.[25]

Urinary Tract Infection

6 Urinary tract infections (UTIs) are common during pregnancy. Typically, UTIs are characterized as asymptomatic (eg, asymptomatic bacteriuria) or symptomatic (eg, lower [cystitis] or upper [pyelonephritis]). Similar to the nonpregnant population, *Escherichia coli* (*E. coli*) is the most common pathogen found in both asymptomatic bacteriuria and UTIs during pregnancy.[71] Asymptomatic bacteriuria occurs in 2% to 15% of all pregnancies, with most cases occurring during early pregnancy. When asymptomatic bacteriuria is left untreated, it progresses to a symptomatic UTI, including acute pyelonephritis, in 20% to 35% of pregnancies. In addition, it has been associated with increased risk for preterm birth and low birth weight; however, evidence is conflicting.[71]

Multiple organizations based in the United States recommend screening pregnant individuals for asymptomatic bacteriuria, although the timing is not universally agreed upon. The Infectious Diseases Society of American recommends pregnant persons be screened for asymptomatic bacteriuria at least once in early pregnancy (prior to 16 weeks gestation) with a urine culture.[72] Guidelines for rescreening patients with an initial negative culture are unclear and generally not recommended. Use of rapid screening tests, such as dipsticks, should be avoided because of the potential for false-negative results.[71]

Acute cystitis occurs in about 1% to 2% of pregnancies, whereas acute pyelonephritis occurs in up to 2%, with most cases occurring in the second or third trimesters.[72] Acute cystitis has not been associated with an increased risk for preterm delivery, low birth weight, or pyelonephritis, most likely because most pregnant individuals receive treatment for symptomatic UTIs. Pyelonephritis during pregnancy has been associated with preterm birth (primarily between 33 and 36 weeks gestation), anemia in the pregnant individual, sepsis and respiratory distress.[73] Treatment of asymptomatic bacteriuria and acute cystitis is necessary during pregnancy to help prevent progression to pyelonephritis and preterm delivery. The optimal therapy and treatment duration are not well defined. Local antibiograms should be used to direct empiric treatment while also considering medication exposure and safety to the fetus. A short-course therapy for asymptomatic bacteriuria is routinely accepted in practice, with a 3- to 7-day course commonly recommended.[71]

Beta-lactams (including penicillins and cephalosporins) have been widely used to treat asymptomatic bacteriuria and cystitis. Beta-lactams are not known teratogens; however, increasing resistance to ampicillin and amoxicillin limits their use as single agents.[74] Nitrofurantoin is not active against Proteus species and should not be used after week 37 in patients with glucose-6-phosphate dehydrogenase deficiency because of a theoretical risk for hemolytic anemia in the neonate. Sulfa-containing medications can contribute to the development of newborn kernicterus; use should be avoided during the last weeks of gestation. Trimethoprim is a folate antagonist and is relatively contraindicated during the first trimester because of associations with cardiovascular malformations.[74] Regionally, increased rates of resistance to trimethoprim-sulfa may limit its use. Single-dose fosfomycin may be considered, as it successfully treats bacteriuria and acute cystitis; however, use may be limited by lack of insurance formulary coverage.[75] Fluoroquinolones and tetracyclines are contraindicated because of potential associations with impaired cartilage development and deciduous teeth discoloration (if given after 5 months of gestation), respectively.[71]

Prophylactic or suppressive antibiotics may be considered in patients with recurrent cystitis.[75] Hospital admission for parenteral antibiotics is the standard of care for pregnant individuals with pyelonephritis. Intravenous antibiotics are utilized until the patient is afebrile for 24 to 48 hours and symptomatically improving; at that point antibiotic therapy can be converted to an oral regimen. Broad spectrum beta-lactam antibiotics (eg, cefazolin, ceftriaxone, cefuroxime, ampicillin plus gentamicin) are preferred for the initial empiric treatment. Choice between specific agent should be guided by local antibiograms and patient tolerance. Nitrofurantoin and fosfomycin should be avoided because both fail to achieve therapeutic levels outside of the urine. In addition, fluroquinolones and aminoglycosides should be avoided when possible. Outpatient antibiotic therapy can be considered after initial inpatient observation in individuals who are afebrile and less than 24 weeks of gestation. The total duration of antibiotic therapy for acute pyelonephritis may vary by antibiotic reigimen, however in general is recommended for 7 to 14 days.[75]

Sexually Transmitted Infections

6 Sexually transmitted infections (STIs) in pregnant individuals range from infections that may be transmitted across the placenta and infect the infant prenatally (eg, syphilis) to organisms that may be transmitted during birth and cause neonatal infection (eg, Chlamydia trachomatis, Neisseria gonorrhoeae, or herpes simplex virus [HSV]) to infections that pose a threat for preterm labor (eg, bacterial vaginosis). Screening recommendations for STI during pregnancies as well as tests of cure and repeat testing that may be needed for various infections during pregnancy are provided in Table 99-4. Treatment for select STIs is summarized in Table 99-5.[76]

Syphilis

Syphilis is caused by Treponema pallidum and can cause many complications in pregnancy (eg, mucocutaneous lesions, altered mental status, visual and auditory abnormalities, gumma, cranial nerve palsies). Syphillis in a pregnant individual increases the risk for congenital syphilis, and all exposed neonates should be evaluated after birth. Ultrasound monitoring of the fetus to evaluate for congenital syphilis (eg, hepatomegaly, ascites, hydrops, fetal anemia, thickened placenta) should be performed if syphilis is diagnosed in the second half of pregnancy. If these signs are detected, a second dose of penicillin G may be administered for fetal treatment. Penicillin effectively prevents transmission to the fetus and treats the fetus, if already infected. Treatment during the second half of pregnancy may increase the risk for preterm labor and fetal distress because a Jarisch–Herxheimer reaction may occur; however, treatment should not be withheld or delayed.[76]

Chlamydia and Gonorrhea

Infections with both chlamydia and gonorrhea in pregnant individuals are capable of vertical transmission (passing of the infection from the pregnant individual to the neonate) through exposure of the infected cervix during delivery. Perinatal infections of *C. trachomatis* most commonly cause conjunctivitis that develops 5 to 12 days postpartum. A subacute, afebrile pneumonia with an onset at ages 1 to 3 months may occur.[76]

With *N. gonorrhoeae* infections, neonatal symptoms usually manifest within 2 to 5 days after delivery. Milder manifestations include rhinitis, vaginitis, urethritis, and scalp infections at sites where fetal monitoring electrodes were placed. More severe presentations include ophthalmia neonatorum and sepsis. Because untreated ocular infections can lead to perforation of the globe of the eye and blindness, the United States Preventative Services Task Force recommends all neonates receive ocular erythromycin ointment as prophylaxis within 24 hours after delivery.[76]

Bacterial Vaginosis and Trichomoniasis

Bacterial vaginosis and trichomoniasis infections characterized by vaginal discharge. Bacterial vaginosis is not an STI but is more common in sexually active individuals and may increase the risk for other STIs. Bacterial vaginosis results from the lack of normal vaginal flora (ie, *Lactobacillus* species) and replacement with anaerobic bacteria, mycoplasmas, and *Gardnerella vaginalis*. Untreated bacterial vaginosis increases the risk for premature rupture of membranes, preterm labor, preterm birth, intraamniotic infection, and postpartum endometritis.[76]

Trichomoniasis is caused by the protozoa, *Trichomonas vaginalis,* and infection is associated with an increased risk of premature rupture of the membranes, preterm delivery, and low birth weight. Treating the pregnant individual during pregnancy can help prevent neonatal respiratory and genital infections.[76]

Hepatitis Infections

Hepatitis infections may be identified during pregnancy with routine laboratory screening. Patients who have not been vaccinated

TABLE 99-4 STI Recommendations During Pregnancy

STI	When to Screen in Pregnancy	When to Test of Cure After Treatment	When to Repeat Screening
Chlamydia	1st prenatal visit less than 25 years old: all greater than 25 years old: only if increased risk[a] 3rd trimester: if at increased risk[a]	4 weeks after treatment	3 months after treatment
Gonorrhea	1st prenatal visit less than 25 years old: all greater than 25 years old: only if increased risk[a] 3rd trimester: if at increased risk[a]		3 months after treatment
Hepatitis B[b]	All: 1st prenatal visit		
Hepatitis C	All (unless infection rate is less than 0.01%)		
HIV	All: 1st prenatal visit High risk[c]: 3rd trimester (before 36 weeks)		
Syphillis	All: 1st prenatal visit High risk[d]: 28 weeks and delivery	See guidelines for specific recommendations	

[a]Increased risk defined as not monogamous, multiple sexual partners, new sexual partner, or partner with an STI. Additionally, patients should have gonorrhea testing if they are diagnosed with other STIs during pregnancy.

[b]Individuals should be screened with the hepatitis B surface antigen. Individuals at high risk for hepatitis B should be vaccinated.

[c]High risk defined as injection substance users, STI diagnosed in pregnancy, not monogamous, new sexual partner during pregnancy, partner with HIV, receive healthcare in a facility with HIV incidence > 1 per 1,000 individuals per year, incarcerated, live in an area with high HIV rates, signs or symptoms of acute HIV (fever, lymphadenopathy, skin rash, myalgia, arthralgia, headache, oral ulcers, leukopenia, thrombocytopenia, or transaminase elevation).

[d]High risk defined as live in a community with high syphilis rate or at risk for syphilis infection during pregnancy (STI diagnosed in pregnancy, multiple partners, sex in conjunction with substance use or transactional sex, late or absent prenatal care, methamphetamine or heroin use, incarceration of the patient or her partner, unstable housing or homelessness).

STI, sexually transmitted infection.

Data from Reference 76.

TABLE 99-5 Management of Sexually Transmitted Infections in Pregnancy

STI	Recommended Therapy	Alternative Therapy
Bacterial vaginosis	Metronidazole 500 mg by mouth twice daily for 7 days Metronidazole 0.75% gel 5 g intravaginally once daily for 5 days Clindamycin 2% cream 5 g intravaginally at bedtime for 7 days	Clindamycin 300 mg by mouth twice daily for 7 days Clindamycin ovules 100 mg intravaginally at bedtime for 3 days
Chlamydia	Azithromycin 1 g by mouth for 1 dose	Amoxicillin 500 mg by mouth three times a day for 7 days
Genital herpes	Suppression (starting at 36 weeks) Acyclovir 400 mg by mouth three times a day Valacyclovir 500 mg by mouth twice daily	
Gonorrhea	Ceftriaxone 500 mg IM for 1 dose. If chlamydia has not been excluded, treat for chlamydia as well.	Consult with infectious disease specialists or STI clinical expert if patient has a cephalosporin allergy or other reasons to not use the preferred treatment.
Syphilis[a]		
Primary, secondary, early latent	Benzathine penicillin G 2.4 million units IM for 1 dose; a second dose can be given 1 week after initial dose to help reduce the risk for congenital syphilis	
Tertiary[b], late latent[c]	Benzathine penicillin G 2.4 million units IM for 3 doses at 1-week intervals	
Neurosyphilis, ocular syphilis, otosyphilis	Aqueous crystalline penicillin G 3-4 million units IV every 4 hours or 18-24 million units IV continuously for 10-14 days	Procaine penicillin 2.4 million units IM daily for 10-14 days PLUS Probenecid 500 mg by mouth four times daily for 10-14 days
Trichomoniasis	Metronidazole 500 mg by mouth twice daily for 7 days	

[a]Pregnant individuals with history of penicillin allergy should undergo penicillin desensitization as no proven alternatives exist.

[b]With normal cerebrospinal fluid examination.

[c]If a patient misses a dose (ie, greater than 9 days between doses), series needs to be restarted.

CSF, cerebrospinal fluid; g, grams; IM, intramuscular; IV, intravenous; mg, milligrams; STI, sexually transmitted infection.

Data from Reference 76.

for hepatitis A and/or B should be vaccinated during the pregnancy if they are at risk for the infections. Although several newer medications are available for treating hepatitis C infections, no recommendations are available now.[76] If a provider decides to treat during pregnancy, ribavirin-based regimens should be avoided.[26]

Genital Herpes

Neonatal herpes often occurs in infants born to individuals lacking histories of genital herpes. The risk of neonatal transmission is under 1% for those with a history of recurrent herpes at term or those who acquire herpes in the first half of pregnancy, but is 30% to 50% for individuals who initially acquire genital herpes near term. However, because recurrent herpes occurs more commonly than new acquisition during pregnancy, it remains the cause for most cases of neonatal transmission. Prevention strategies include counseling uninfected individuals to avoid intercourse during the third trimester with partners having known or suspected genital herpes infection. Individuals with no history of orolabial herpes should avoid receptive oral sex during the third trimester with partners who have orolabial herpes. Prevention of genital herpes transmission to pregnant individuals using antiviral agents has not been studied.[76]

All patients should be asked about symptoms of genital herpes at the time of delivery and should be examined for lesions. For those who have no symptoms (including prodromal symptoms) or lesions, proceed with vaginal childbirth; however, in those with evidence of an outbreak it is recommended that a cesarean section be performed to decrease the risk of neonatal transmission. Suppression therapy with either acyclovir or valacyclovir starting at 36 weeks decreases recurrence of genital herpes at term, which decreases the need for cesarean delivery.[76,77]

The Centers for Disease Control and Prevention (CDC) and ACOG recommend both medications, but both require more frequent administration during pregnancy due to increased renal elimination.[76,77] Although acyclovir may be less expensive, it needs to be administered three times a day whereas valacyclovir is administered twice daily during pregnancy. Both cost and adherence should be considered for patients.[77] For initial or recurrent episodes, most patients receive oral therapy; IV acyclovir is reserved for severe infections. In those seropositive for HSV but who have not experienced an outbreak, no data suggest a treatment benefit.[76,77]

Human Immunodeficiency Virus Infection

The rate of perinatal HIV transmission is 1% or less in the United States and Europe as a result of national recommendations for universal prenatal HIV counseling and testing, antiretroviral (ARV) therapy use, cesarean delivery if the HIV RNA is greater than 1,000 copies/mL (1×10^6/L) near delivery, infant ARV therapy, and breastfeeding avoidance. The primary goal for HIV-infected individuals is to achieve sustained viral load suppression below the limits of detection before conception as well as throughout pregnancy and remainder of their life. ARV therapy should be started preconception for patients with known HIV, regardless of viral load or CD4 count, for the patient's health and to decrease the risk for perinatal and partner transmission. In patients newly diagnosed with HIV or who have not previously received ARV therapy, pharmacotherapy should be initiated as soon as pregnancy is determined since risk of perinatal transmission is lower with earlier viral suppression, and the regimen can be adjusted if needed after resistance results are available.[78] Recommendations regarding combination ARV therapy change frequently as new data becomes available, and providers should check the most up to date guidelines (https://aidsinfo.nih.gov).

For pregnant individuals with HIV RNA levels above 1,000 copies/mL (1×10^6/L) or unknown who are approaching delivery, a scheduled cesarean section at 38 weeks of gestation is recommended to reduce the risk of perinatal HIV transmission. Scheduled cesarean section is not recommended if HIV RNA levels are 1,000 copies/mL (1×10^6/L) or below because of the low rate of perinatal transmission. If the viral load is greater than 1,000 copies/mL (1×10^6/L) or not known, IV zidovudine should be initiated with a 1-hour loading dose (2 mg/kg) followed by a continuous infusion (1 mg/kg) for 2 hours with a minimum of 3 hours total. Intravenous zidovudine should still be administered in the presence of resistance to zidovudine. Consider administration of IV zidovudine to individuals with a viral load between 50 and 1,000 copies/mL (0.05×10^6 and 1×10^6/L) near delivery. Although there is inadequate information that zidovudine provides additional protection, there may be benefit as there is a slightly higher rate of transmission with a viral load in this range. Patients with a viral load below 50 copies/mL (0.05×10^6/L) near delivery do not require IV zidovudine, but they should continue their ARV therapy. Specific recommendations for different clinical scenarios during antepartum, intrapartum, and postpartum are provided in the clinical guidelines.[78]

Headache

6 Primary headaches (eg, tension and migraine) in pregnant and nonpregnant individuals are the most common types of headache. Hormonal fluctuations, particularly changes in estrogen, can be a trigger for headaches throughout pregnancy. Secondary headaches can also occur, indicating a more serious underlying condition, and include those caused by preeclampsia, stroke, postdural puncture, cerebral angiopathy, and cerebral venous thrombosis. Warning signs for a secondary headache include elevated blood pressure, altered mental status or confusion, fever, seizures, and abnormal findings on neurologic examination.[79]

Pregnant individuals with a history of migraine headaches have an increased risk of developing hypertension, pulmonary embolism, stroke, and myocardial infarction. The risk increases with age, and in overweight individuals. In early pregnancy, migraine frequency typically decreases, with improvement seen in roughly 50% of patients during the first trimester. By the third trimester, 87% of individuals have improved migraine symptoms and frequency. In 3% to 7% of cases, patients will experience new onset migraine headaches during pregnancy, typically developing during the first trimester.[79]

Relaxation therapy, cognitive-behavioral therapy, and biofeedback are all effective nonpharmacologic treatment methods that can be utilized during pregnancy. Sleep hygiene should be encouraged as a poor sleep pattern can increase headache frequency. In addition, maintaining adequate hydration, reducing caffeine intake, and exercise may all benefit as well.[79]

Pharmacologic treatment for migraines typically involves acetaminophen and antiemetics (eg, promethazine, prochlorperazine, and metoclopramide are most commonly used).[79] Opioids have been used but may contribute to migraine-associated nausea and routine use can increase migraine frequency and severity. Long-term use of opioids near the end of pregnancy can cause neonatal opioid withdrawal syndrome. For migraines that are not responsive to other treatments, triptans may be used. Of note, the package insert for sumatriptan indicates pregnancy as a contraindication for use; however, no human data have suggested teratogenicity for any medication in the triptan class.[79] Sumatriptan is the triptan of choice because medication transport across the placenta is small and it has a short elimination half-life of 2 hours. Migraine prophylaxis may be indicated for patients with frequent, disabling headaches to help decrease headache frequency and severity. A few dietary supplements have shown benefit for prophylaxis, and include daily riboflavin, or magnesium supplementation.[79] Ergotamine and dihydroergotamine are contraindicated because of effects on uterine tone.[26] Other typical migraine prophylactic therapy is often evaluated on an individual basis for medication safety and necessity.

Tension headaches are less studied; however, most patients report no change in the frequency or intensity of tension headaches, although remission is possible. Tension headaches are treated similarly, with acetaminophen being the treatment of choice for pain management. The NSAIDs are not recommended for use during pregnancy, particularly in late pregnancy (after 20 weeks gestation) or during labor and delivery, because they inhibit prostaglandin synthesis, which may cause harm including oligohydramnios, prolong labor, or premature closure or constriction of the ductus arteriosus.[26,79,80] Antiemetics may be added in patients experiencing nausea and vomiting. Opioids are rarely used.

Allergic Rhinitis and Asthma

6 Asthma and rhinitis are common chronic illnesses in pregnancy, and asthma affects approximately 4% to 8% of pregnancies.[81] During pregnancy, a third of patients have symptoms that worsen, a third will have symptoms improve, and a third will have symptoms remain unchanged.[82] Diagnosis, goals, and staging of asthma during pregnancy are the same as in nonpregnant individuals, although more frequent follow-up is necessary because of changes in disease severity. Bronchoprovocation should be avoided.[82] Health consequences of poorly controlled asthma include morbidity and mortality, preterm labor, preeclampsia, cesarean delivery, intrauterine growth restriction, premature birth, and low birth weight for infants; therefore, the treatment goal is to achieve and maintain control of asthma symptoms to prevent hypoxic episodes in both the pregnant patient and fetus.[81,82]

Risks of medication use to the fetus are lower than the risks of untreated asthma; therefore, use of medications to achieve and maintain control is warranted.[81,82] Routine pulmonary function evaluation, peak flow testing, and symptom monitoring are recommended during pregnancy because asthma severity can change during pregnancy.[81] Treatment recommendations are divided into multiple steps based on symptom control and follow a stepwise approach. Because inhaled corticosteroid therapy decreases the risk for exacerbations and discontinuation of these medications can significantly increase the risk for an exacerbation, the Global Initiative for Asthma (GINA) guidelines recommend continuing inhaled corticosteroids for individuals who are planning to become or are currently pregnant. Additionally, the GINA guidelines recommend that step down therapy should be a low priority until the patient is postpartum.[82]

Pre-existing or newly developed allergic rhinitis occurs during pregnancy and nasal congestion can be caused by pregnancy because of vascular engorgement in the nasal passages and hormonal effects on mucus secretion. Treatment strategies for allergic rhinitis during pregnancy are similar to those used in nonpregnant individuals and include avoidance of allergens, immunotherapy, and pharmacotherapy. Oral antihistamines and leukotriene receptor antagonists as well as intranasal antihistamines, decongestants (limit duration because of the risk for medication-induced rhinitis), cromones, and corticosteroids can be used. Oral corticosteroids may be considered when needed.[83] Immunotherapy is not contraindicated in pregnancy, however should not be initiated for the first time during pregnancy due to risk for anaphylaxis.[81]

Epilepsy

6 Seizure frequency does not change for most pregnant individuals with epilepsy. Of those who have been seizure free for at least 9 months prior to pregnancy, 84% to 92% will remain seizure free during pregnancy. Studies have demonstrated no change in seizure frequency in 54% to 80% of pregnant individuals with epilepsy, while

decreased seizure frequency occurs in 3% to 24% and increased in approximately 14% to 32%.[84] Seizures may become more frequent because of changes in hormones, sleep deprivation, and medication adherence problems due to perceived teratogenic risk. Another potential cause is changes in free serum concentrations of antiseizure medications resulting from changes in absorption, increased volume of distribution in the pregnant individual, decreased protein binding from hypoalbuminemia, increased hepatic metabolism, and increased renal clearance.[24,85] A patient's clinical condition and serum concentrations, either total or free depending of the medication, should be the basis for dose adjustments, and some experts recommend checking levels preconception and monthly during the pregnancy.[24] The 2009 American Academy of Neurology guidelines recommends checking levels for lamotrigine, carbamazepine, phenytoin, levetiracetam, oxcarbazepine during pregnancy.[86] As more pregnancy evidence is available, additional agents may also benefit evaluating levels during pregnancy. New guidelines are anticipated to be released in 2022.

The risks of uncontrolled seizures to the fetus, particularly tonic-clonic seizures, are considered to be greater than those associated with antiseizure medications. Pregnant individuals with epilepsy are at an increased risk for spontaneous abortion, preeclampsia, pregnancy-induced hypertension, preterm labor and delivery, bleeding complications, death, and cesarean delivery compared to those without epilepsy.[21,24,84] Additionally, focal seizures with loss of consciousness are associated with uterine contractions and fetal heart rate changes whereas frequent tonic-clonic seizures have been associated with decreased neurodevelopment in the child.[24,85] However, major malformations are two to three times more likely to occur in children born to individuals taking antiseizure medications than to those who do not.[61] Teratogenic effects with some antiseizure medications are related to the dose, often with a threshold above which risks increase.[87] Major malformations with valproic acid are dose related and range from 4.7% to 13.8%.[24] Use of valproic acid should be avoided during pregnancy due to high risk of neural tube defects and facial clefts with first trimester exposure, and cognitive teratogenicity with exposure throughout pregnancy. Although many antiepileptic medications are associated with potential risks during pregnancy, including malformations, it is important to consider the benefits of preventing seizures to both the pregnant individual and the fetus. Because some organs form early in gestation, the ideal time to switch to a preferred therapy is prior to pregnancy.[21] Topiramate and zonisamide have been associated with lower birth weights and length.[88]

When possible, antiseizure medication monotherapy is recommended with medication regimen optimization occurring before conception. If gradual medication withdrawal is attempted because of epilepsy remission, it should be fully completed and evaluated before trying to conceive. Medication change to avoid use of valproic acid, phenytoin, carbamazepine, phenobarbital, and polytherapy is suggested during the first trimester; however, if either is used during pregnancy because of treatment failure with other medications, the lowest effective dose should be used.[21,24] All pregnant individuals taking antiseizure medications should receive folic acid supplementation starting before pregnancy and continuing through at least the first trimester. Many experts continue to recommend 4 mg daily dose, but this recommendation is not universal. Because evidence has not definitively shown the efficacy of high dose folic acid supplementation with antiseizure medications, the American Academy of Neurology recommends at least 0.4 mg daily.[86]

Mental Health Conditions

6 Psychiatric illness affects approximately 500,000 pregnancies each year.[89]

Depression occurs in approximately 17% of pregnant individuals. The risks associated with uncontrolled depression or bipolar disorder are similar, and include an increased incidence of low birth weight, decreased fetal growth, and postnatal complications including admission to neonatal intensive care units. In addition to the potential impact of depression during pregnancy on obstetric complications, untreated depression may cause the infant to cry more and be harder to console, and have long-term implications for normal infant development.[88] Symptoms of depression are often overlooked during pregnancy because they overlap with many symptoms of pregnancy (eg, irritable mood, weight loss or gain, appetite and sleep changes, fatigue/loss of energy). There are several survey tools that can be utilized during pregnancy and during the postpartum period to help distinguish depression symptoms from normal symptoms of pregnancy (eg, the Edinburgh Postnatal Depression Scale, Beck Depression Inventory, and Postpartum Depression Screening Scale). All patients should be screened for depression at least once in the peripartum period and at the initial postpartum visit.[90]

Anxiety disorders are also common during pregnancy, impacting an estimated 18% of adults 18 years and old. Anxiety during pregnancy is associated with spontaneous abortions, preterm delivery, and delivery complications including prolonged labor, precipitate labor, fetal distress, and forceps deliveries. Long-term anxiety during pregnancy has been linked to decreased developmental scores and inadaptability, and slowed mental development at 2 years of age. Obsessive-compulsive disorder (OCD) is a type of anxiety disorder. Although the incidence of OCD in pregnancy is unknown, pregnancy has been linked as a potential trigger for OCD symptom onset. In addition, OCD symptoms tend to worsen after delivery.[89]

Up to 70% of individuals with mental health conditions discontinue or refuse treatment because of concerns about teratogenicity.[91] Patients who stop taking antidepressants are more likely to relapse, which can also have implications for the well-being of the fetus. The risks and benefits of mental health medication use during pregnancy and the risks of untreated depression must be discussed with all patients in order to increase understanding. Because most mental health medications are used to treat more than one condition, the reader should refer to Chapters 80-90 for information about treatment of specific mental health diagnoses. In general, monotherapy is preferred over polytherapy even if higher doses are required.[89]

Selective serotonin reuptake inhibitors (SSRIs) are the most commonly used medication for depression and anxiety during pregnancy; however, serotonin-norepinephrine reuptake inhibitors (SNRIs) and atypical antidepressants are also utilized (see Chapter 88, "Depressive Disorders"). Conflicting studies about the risk of cardiac malformations with paroxetine are published in the literature.[26,92] One study found it was associated with doses greater than 25 mg a day.[26] Despite this association, SSRIs as a class are not considered major teratogens, as no consistent information supports an association with structural malformations,[92] and risks with SNRIs are less defined. Use of SSRIs and SNRIs in the latter part of pregnancy is associated with persistent pulmonary hypertension of the newborn and poor neonatal adaptation syndrome which encompasses transient neonatal complications of mild respiratory distress, tachycardia, weak or abnormal cry, poor muscle tone or color, irritability, tremor, jitteriness, lethargy, tachypnea, and rarely seizures. Symptoms are usually mild.[89,93,94] Second-generation antipsychotics are generally well tolerated and effective in managing symptoms of treatment-resistant depression. Second-generation antipsychotics can cause weight gain, gestational diabetes, and metabolic syndrome which have implications for poorer obstetric outcomes (see Chapter 87, "Schizophrenia").[95] In addition, exposure to antipsychotic agents during pregnancy may increase preterm delivery and small for gestational age newborns, although evidence is inconsistent.[96,97] Some providers may also use buspirone for anxiety symptoms. Tricyclic antidepressants were commonly used in pregnancy before the introduction of SSRIs and are not considered major teratogens, although they have also been associated with a neonatal withdrawal syndrome when used late in pregnancy.[89,92]

In general, benzodiazepine use is not recommended during pregnancy. If patients are taking benzodiazepines during pregnancy, the benzodiazepine should not be abruptly discontinued due to risk for withdrawal. Benzodiazepine use in the third trimester can cause infant sedation and withdrawal symptoms (eg, restlessness, hypertonia, hyperreflexia, tremulousness, apnea, diarrhea, and vomiting) lasting up to 3 months postpartum. In addition, floppy baby syndrome is associated with benzodiazepine use before delivery and consists of hypothermia, lethargy, poor muscle tone, feeding difficulties, and poor respiratory effort.[89]

Mood stabilizers, such as lithium, lamotrigine, carbamazepine, and valproic acid, are often used to treat bipolar disorder.[89] The reader can find information related to the safety of antiseizure medications used for mood stabilization in Chapters 75, "Epilepsy" and 89, "Bipolar Disorder." Abrupt discontinuation of lithium therapy during pregnancy is associated with an increased risk for relapse. Lithium use in early pregnancy has also been associated with cardiovascular anomalies, particularly Ebstein's anomaly.[89] The risk of cardiac malformation was only found with doses higher than 900 mg daily.[98] In addition, when lithium is used during pregnancy providers need to be aware of potential changes in lithium levels due to pharmacokinetic changes, dehydration in the pregnant individual, and medication interactions. Because lithium use near term is associated with toxicities in the newborn, it is recommended that lithium is held starting 24 to 48 hours before or at the onset of labor. Once the patient is medically stable after delivery, therapy can be resumed.[26,99] Other reported neonatal adverse effects include floppy baby syndrome, nephrogenic diabetes insipidus, hypoglycemia, cardiac arrhythmias, thyroid dysfunction, polyhydramnios, and premature delivery. Lithium may cause lethargy, hypotonia, hypothermia, cyanosis, and changes in electrocardiogram in infants exposed through human milk. The decision to use lithium during pregnancy should be a shared decision making between the patient and provider, and be based on disease severity, history of illness, and timing of exposure. If breastfeeding, the infant's lithium levels, thyroid function, hydration status, and complete blood count should be monitored.[89]

LABOR AND DELIVERY

Management of the pregnant individuals during the perinatal period often requires medication therapy for pain and for potential complications associated with labor and delivery.

Preterm Labor

7 Preterm birth occurs in approximately 12% of all live deliveries in the United States, and is the leading cause of infant mortality and hospitalization. Preterm labor is generally diagnosed when uterine contractions start before 37 weeks gestation in the presence of changes in cervical dilation and/or effacement, or when the initial presentation includes regular contractions and cervical dilation of at least 2 cm.[100] Risk factors for preterm delivery include previous preterm delivery, history of cervical surgery, short cervical length, infections, vaginal bleeding, UTIs, and periodontal disease. In addition, low prepregnancy weight, smoking, substance use disorders, and shorten interval between pregnancies have all been associated as increased risk factors for preterm delivery.[101]

Historically, nonpharmacologic recommendations have included bed rest, refraining from sexual intercourse and orgasm, and hydration; however, they do not decrease the risk and should not be routinely recommended. Pharmacologic interventions include tocolytic medications to stop uterine contractions, antibiotics to treat potential intrauterine infections, antenatal steroids to help with fetal lung maturation, and magnesium for fetal neuroprotection.[100]

Tocolytic Therapy

7 The purposes of tocolytic therapy are threefold: (a) postpone delivery long enough to allow for the maximum effect of antenatal corticosteroid and magnesium administration; (b) allow for transportation of the pregnant patient to a facility equipped to deal with high-risk deliveries; and (c) prolongation of pregnancy when there are underlying, self-limited conditions that can cause labor, such as pyelonephritis or abdominal surgery, that are unlikely to cause recurrent preterm labor. Tocolytics are generally not utilized before neonatal viability or beyond 34 weeks of gestation.[100]

Four classes of tocolytics are available in the United States: β-adrenergic receptor agonists, magnesium, calcium channel blockers, and NSAIDs. All four therapies prolong pregnancy between 48 hours to 1 week; however, this prolongation is not associated with a significant neonatal benefit. The β-adrenergic receptor agonist, terbutaline, has been used off-label for tocolytic therapy; however, it has been associated with a higher incidence of adverse effects in the pregnant individual, including hyperkalemia, arrhythmias, hyperglycemia, hypotension, and pulmonary edema. In addition, terbutaline has a boxed warning against oral dosing or prolonged parenteral use (beyond 48-72 hours) because of the risk of cardiotoxicity and death in the pregnant patient.[100]

Intravenous magnesium sulfate has been used for tocolysis; however, it is primarily utilized for fetal neuroprotection and reducing the incidence of cerebral palsy. Adverse effects associated with magnesium therapy in the pregnant individual are common and include a general feeling of warmth, flushing, diaphoresis, nausea, loss of deep tendon reflexes, and respiratory depression. If magnesium sulfate is used during preterm labor for fetal neuroprotection and the patient is still experiencing preterm labor, an additional agent should be added for short-term tocolysis.[100]

The calcium channel blocker, nifedipine, is also often used and associated with fewer adverse effects than magnesium or β-adrenergic receptor agonist therapy. Common adverse medication reactions include dizziness, flushing, and hypotension.[100]

The NSAIDs, such as indomethacin, have been used effectively for tocolysis. An increased rate of premature constriction of the ductus arteriosus has been noted in infants with indomethacin use after 32 weeks of gestation and with use exceeding 48 hours. In addition, indomethacin is the preferred tocolytic agent in patients receiving magnesium for neuroprotection prior to 32 weeks gestation, because other agents can cause hypotension when administered concurrently with magnesium.[100]

Other Medication Therapies for Preterm Labor Prevention

7 Intrauterine bacterial infections are a common cause of preterm labor before 32 weeks gestation. Infection and inflammation are thought to be associated with contractions; however, due to lack of evidence for improved outcomes, antibiotics are not routinely recommended for preterm labor. If a patient experiences prelabor rupture of membranes (PROM) before 34 weeks of gestation, prophylactic antibiotics should be initiated to prolong pregnancy, reduce infections in the patient and neonate, and reduce major morbidities including death, respiratory distress syndrome, early sepsis, severe intraventricular hemorrhage, and necrotizing enterocolitis. A 7-day course of broad-spectrum antibiotics should be used with the intent to prolong latency, which is the time from ruptured membranes to delivery. Multiple antibiotic regimens have shown benefit with a common regimen including IV ampicillin and erythromycin for 2 days followed by oral amoxicillin and erythromycin for 5 days. Amoxicillin-clavulanate is not recommended due to increased rates of necrotizing enterocolitis. In patients allergic to β-lactam antibiotics, another agent effective against Group B *Streptococcus* (GBS) may be considered to replace the β-lactam.[100]

Progesterone is also often administered in patients with a history of prior preterm birth. Progesterone use is based upon its effects to diminish cervical ripening (softening of the cervix necessary for cervical dilation before birth), reduce uterine wall contractility, and modulate inflammation. Evidence also supports progesterone supplementation in patients with no prior history of preterm birth who have a singleton pregnancy and a short cervix. Progesterone is not indicated for multiple gestation pregnancies. Progesterone supplementation is offered through either vaginal route or intramuscularly.[101]

Antenatal Corticosteroids

7 The ACOG recommends antenatal corticosteroids for fetal lung maturation to prevent respiratory distress syndrome, intraventricular hemorrhage, necrotizing enterocolitis, and neonatal mortality in infants delivered prematurely.[100] Patients between 24 weeks and 34 weeks gestation who are at risk of preterm birth within the next 7 days, including those with ruptured membranes, are recommended to receive a single course of corticosteroids. When patients present between 23 and 24 weeks gestation, administration of corticosteroids may be considered. Due to the infant's small size and change of survival if delivered before 24 weeks gestation, the family's wishes regarding resuscitation must be carefully considered. In addition, a single course of steroids should be considered in patients presenting in the late preterm period between 34 and 37 weeks gestation who are at risk of delivery and have not previously received corticosteroids. The most common steroid regimens include betamethasone administered intramuscularly as two doses 24 hours apart and dexamethasone as four doses 12 hours apart for 48 hours. A rescue course is often administered to patients who have received a previous corticosteroid course more than 14 days prior who are at risk of delivering before 34 weeks gestation.[100]

Group B *Streptococcus* Infection

7 Between 10% and 30% of pregnant individuals are colonized with GBS, leading to an increased risk for pregnancy loss, premature delivery, and transmission of the bacteria to the infant during delivery. Approximately 50% of patients colonized with GBS will transmit the bacteria to their newborns. The consequences of neonatal infections include death, apnea, and need for blood pressure support and neonatal intensive care.[103]

Universal screening for GBS colonization is recommended between 36 and 38 weeks gestation. Intrapartum antibiotics are given if the patient has GBS colonization, or if they previously gave birth to an infant with invasive GBS disease, or GBS bacteriuria was identified at any time during the pregnancy. If a patient presents in labor and no screening information is available, antibiotics are given for fever greater than or equal to 100.4°F (38°C), amniotic membrane rupture at least 18 hours prior, gestation under 37 weeks, or known positive GBS colonization in previous pregnancy.[103]

Intravenous penicillin given every 4 hours until delivery is the recommended treatment regimen. Alternatively, ampicillin can be given IV, every 4 hours. For patients with a penicillin allergy but not at risk for anaphylaxis, cefazolin IV every 8 hours, is recommended. In patients at high risk for anaphylaxis, clindamycin IV every 8 hours is recommended. For penicillin-allergic patients, GBS cultures should be sent for sensitivities. If resistant to clindamycin or erythromycin, vancomycin IV every 8 hours until delivery is appropriate. A minimum of 4 hours of therapy with a beta-lactam antibiotic is required for adequate prophylaxis.[101]

Cervical Ripening and Labor Induction

7 Cervical ripening is the process of softening and thinning the cervix to facilitate labor. If a patient needs an induction and the cervix is not ready for labor, agents to induce cervical ripening may be utilized.

Nearly 26% of patients undergo labor induction, either elective or medically indicated.[102] The most common indications for induction are post-term pregnancies (beyond 42 weeks) and pregnancy-induced hypertension.[105] Other reasons for induction include fetal growth restriction or compromise, hypertension, premature rupture of membranes with no active onset of labor, and social factors. A number of nonpharmacologic methods are used for cervical ripening including membrane stripping, amniotomy, and nipple stimulation; however, available evidence is inconclusive on the efficacy of these methods.[105]

Prostaglandin E_2 analogs (eg, dinoprostone [Prepidil gel, Cervidil vaginal insert]) are commonly used for cervical ripening. Prepidil 500 mcg is administered intracervically and may be repeated after 6 hours to a maximum of three doses in 24 hours. After administration, the patient remains supine for 30 minutes. Cervidil contains 10 mg dinoprostone with a slower, more constant release of medication compared to the gel. The patient should remain in a recumbent position for 2 hours after placement and the insert should be removed when labor begins or after 12 hours. Fetal heart rate monitoring is recommended with both agents.[105]

Misoprostol, a prostaglandin E1 analog, is an effective and inexpensive medication for cervical ripening and labor induction. Intravaginal administration of misoprostol (oral tablets are split to obtain dose) given every 3 to 6 hours is at least as effective as other prostaglandin agents and results in a shorter time to delivery. Oral misoprostol has been used successfully and results in a quicker onset and shorter duration. Sublingual and buccal routes of misoprostol administration have less information regarding the efficacy compared to other routes. There is little benefit of using misoprostol for longer than 24 hours. The most common adverse effects are uterine hyperstimulation and meconium-stained amniotic fluid. Use of misoprostol is contraindicated in individuals with a previous uterine scar because of its association with uterine rupture, a catastrophic medical event.[105]

Oxytocin is the most commonly used agent for labor induction after cervical ripening. Patients may vary in response and sensitivity to oxytocin, but in theory administration should trigger a response similar to a spontaneous labor. Upon administration, a uterine response begins to occur after 3 to 5 minutes. Patients with a lower BMI, a greater cervical dilation at time of induction, more previous deliveries after 24 weeks gestation, and higher gestational age are more likely to have a successful response to labor induction from oxytocin. Refer to the ACOG practice bulletin for detailed administration information.[105]

Labor Analgesia

7 The first phase of labor occurs from onset of labor to complete cervical dilation, while the second phase of labor is the period of time between complete cervical dilation and delivery. During the first phase of labor, patients perceive visceral pain caused by uterine contractions.[104] Pain in the second phase of labor is somatic pain associated with perineal stretching.[106]

Nonpharmacologic Approaches to Analgesia

Massage, water immersion during the first stage of labor, and acupuncture, relaxation, and hypnotherapy have all been utilized for pain management during pregnancy.[106] In addition, the use of visualization and breathing techniques, yoga postures, massage, acupressure, and facilitated partner support lead to more vaginal deliveries, and have been shown to reduce epidural use and shorten the second stage of labor.[107]

Pharmacologic Approaches to Labor Pain Management

Labor causes considerable pain for many patients. The two main types of pharmacologic approaches in the United States are parenteral opioids and epidural analgesia. Use of nitrous oxide during labor is an alternative for pain management.

Parenteral opioids (eg, fentanyl, morphine, butorphanol) are commonly used to alleviate labor pain. Up to 42% of individuals receive parenteral medications, although there is no consensus that one agent is more effective or safe than another. Overall, though, they are less effective than epidural analgesia, have more adverse effects, and possibly less reliable pain response.[106]

Approximately 60% of pregnant individuals in the United States choose an epidural for pain relief during labor and report better pain relief than with other analgesic modalities.[108] With epidural analgesia, a catheter is introduced into the epidural space, and an opioid and/or an anesthetic (eg, fentanyl and/or bupivacaine) is administered. Combined spinal-epidural analgesia consists of injecting a single opioid bolus into the subarachnoid space to provide instant pain relief with additional use of a local anesthetic epidural. Compared with traditional epidurals, combined spinal-epidural anesthesia has a slightly shorter mean time to onset of effective analgesia.[106] Patient-controlled epidural analgesia results in a lower total dose of local anesthetics used over the course of labor compared with continuous epidural infusions.[106]

Adverse effects of regional anesthesia include hypotension, pruritus, and inability to void. Epidural analgesia is associated with prolongation of the second stages of labor, but it does not lead to higher numbers of instrumental deliveries, cesarean sections (for fetal distress), or fever when compared to intravenous opioid therapy.[108,109] A rare complication of epidural anesthesia is puncture of the subarachnoid space leading to a severe headache, which occurs in approximately 1% of patients. Other complications include hypotension, nausea, vomiting, itching, and urinary retention.[110] Low back pain has not been associated with the use of epidural analgesia.

Nitrous oxide, as a 50% mixture with oxygen, can be employed in patients desiring a non-medicated labor. It is less effective than epidural anesthesia but is quickly reversible and does not limit the patient's mobility.[106]

Postpartum Hemorrhage

7 Postpartum hemorrhage (PPH) in pregnant patients is defined as blood loss of more than 1,000 mL, regardless of vaginal or cesarean delivery, or blood loss with signs and symptoms of hypovolemia within 24 hours after delivery. There are various risk factors for PPH, some of which include prior PPH, incomplete placenta at delivery, a macrosomic fetus or multiple gestation, preeclampsia, operative vaginal delivery, chorioamnionitis, and prolonged or augmented labor.[111]

Administration of oxytocin should be initiated before placental delivery to institute active management of labor after all uncomplicated vaginal deliveries, as this practice results in reduced blood loss, fewer cases of PPH, and a shorter third stage of labor. Other uterotonic agents should be used if an inadequate response is attained with oxytocin alone. Methylergonovine, carboprost, and rectal, sublingual, or oral misoprostol can all be used as second-line agents. None has been shown to be more effective than another. Tranexamic acid, an antifibrinolytic agent, has been shown to reduce deaths from obstetric hemorrhage if given within 3 hours of delivery. A limited amount of evidence has shown a modest decrease in blood loss when tranexamic acid is given prophylactically. If uterotonic medication therapies fail to control the bleeding, a variety of different surgical techniques can be used.[111]

POSTPARTUM ISSUES

Medication Use During Lactation

8 A wide variety of benefits (eg, health, nutritional, immunologic, psychological, economic, developmental, and social) are imparted by breastfeeding, not only to the infants, but also to the family. The American Academy of Pediatrics recommends that infants be given human milk exclusively for 6 months and that this continue until at least 12 months of age while other foods are introduced, provided this is still desired by both the infant and parent.[113] Healthy People 2020 increased its target for breastfeeding to 81.9% for infants ever breastfed, 60.5% for infants at 6 months, and 34.1% for infants at 12 months.[112]

Adequate milk removal from the breast by nursing or pumping is necessary to maintain or increase milk production.[113] Milk supply is adequate when the baby is feeding 8 to 12 times per day, steady weight gain is by day 4/5 after delivery, and has 6 to 8 wet diapers per day; whereas signs of dehydration and low milk supply include jaundice, insufficient number of dry or soiled diapers, lethargy, inconsolability, stools are not bright yellow by day 5, and lack of steady weight gain by day 4.[114] Relactation is the process of increasing the milk supply for those whose milk has not "come in," who have inadequate milk production despite appropriate nursing frequency or pumping, or who have weaned or never breastfed after delivery. Nonpharmacological measures (massage, eating snacks and increasing hydration, looking at a picture of baby when pumping, listening to music, massaging downward toward nipple, applying warmth to the breast, pumping after feeding, decreased time between feeding/pumping, etc.) should be implemented first.[113-116] In fact, individuals producing breastmilk have an increased caloric need of 450 to 500 kcal/day (1.9×10^3 to 2.1×10^3 kJ/d).[112] Additionally, education, especially with a lactation specialist, may be helpful to review positioning, latching, and duration of feedings as pharmacologic and herbal agents efficacy is inconclusive. ACOG and the Academy of Breastfeeding Medicine do not recommend any specific galactogogues or use as a first-line agent due to the inconclusive evidence and potential for adverse events.[113,114] Although metoclopramide and domperidone have both used to increase milk production, both carry risk for the parent and infant. Metoclopramide may increase the risk for GI symptoms, extrapyramidal symptoms, and methemoglobinemia in the infant.[113,117] The FDA recommended against the use of domperidone during lactation because of cardiac arrhythmias, arrest, and sudden death. Because of the cardiac risks, it is not approved for any indication in the United States.[118] In circumstances where a patient has contraindications to breastfeeding, is unable to produce enough milk, or does not desire to breastfeed, formula is an acceptable option to consider for supplemental or full nutrition.

Most medications transfer into breast milk, but breastfeeding may be continued in most circumstances. Healthcare providers should encourage breastfeeding individuals who require medications to continue whenever possible. Passive diffusion is the primary mechanism for medication transfer into breast milk, but other medication-related factors influence medication transfer from parental circulation into breast milk, including (a) degree of protein binding in parental plasma, (b) molecular weight, (c) lipid solubility (and corresponding fat content of milk), (d) plasma concentration in the parent, (e) medication half-life, and (f) medication pH.[119] The degree of protein binding to parent plasma proteins is one of the most significant factors affecting medication transfer to breast milk; highly bound medications transfer in low amounts. Low-molecular-weight medications passively diffuse into breast milk, but larger molecules are not likely to transfer in large amounts. Higher lipid solubility of medications also increases the likelihood of transfer. Colostrum is secreted in the first couple of days after birth and has high quantities of immunoglobulins, parental lymphocytes, and parental macrophages. While greater amounts of medications are present in colostrum, the amount received by the nursing infant is minimal because of the limited volume of colostrum produced. A greater volume of mature milk is produced, but medication transfer into mature milk is lower because of tight cell-to-cell junctions. The higher the concentration of medication in the parent's serum, the higher the concentration in the breast milk. As the medication is metabolized and excreted by the parent, the parent's serum concentration drops, and the medication in the breast milk may redistribute back into the parent's bloodstream. The pH of plasma is 7.4, while the pH of breast milk ranges between 6.8 and 7. Weak bases are not ionized in the parental circulation and easily transfer to breast milk.[119] In the lower pH of breast milk, molecules become ionized and are less likely to diffuse back into parental circulation ("ion trapping"). Likewise, medications with longer half-lives are more likely to maintain higher levels in breast milk, resulting in greater exposure to the infant.

Infant-related factors may also influence the amount of medication ingested through breastfeeding as both the frequency of feedings and the amount of milk ingested are important considerations. Exclusively breastfed infants are more likely to ingest larger amounts of medications than older infants who receive other foods. Medication that are unstable in gastric acid (aminoglycosides, PPIs, and insulin) are less likely to be absorbed by infants.[119] Finally, infants may vary in their ability to metabolize and excrete ingested medication. Premature and full-term infants may not have full renal and liver function.

Strategies for reducing the risk to the infant include selection of medications that would be considered safe for use in the infant. Medications with shorter half-lives accumulate less, and those that are more protein bound do not cross into breast milk as well as those that are less protein bound. When choosing between different pharmacotherapies, medications with lower oral bioavailability and lower lipid solubility may be better choices to reduce infant exposure. If the parent is using a once-daily medication, administration before the infant's longest sleep period may be advised to increase the interval to the next feeding. For medications taken multiple times per day, administration immediately after breastfeeding provides the longest interval for back diffusion of medication from the breast milk to the parent's serum. During short-term medication therapy, the parent can pump and discard milk to preserve their milk-producing capability if the necessary medication is not considered compatible with breastfeeding.[120,121]

Information regarding medication use during breastfeeding is available from expert committees (eg, American Academy of Pediatrics Committee on Drugs) and evidence-based textbooks or databases (eg, LactMed [http://toxnet.nlm.nih.gov/newtoxnet/lactmed.htm]). All may be of assistance in determining safety and appropriate medications to use during breastfeeding.

Mastitis

8 Mastitis is inflammation of the breast that occurs in 3% to 20% of lactating individuals. It can be infectious or noninfectious and the most common cause is milk stasis. Signs and symptoms include breast tenderness, redness, warmth, flulike symptoms, chills, and fever (temperature 101.3°F [38.5°C] or greater). Risk factors for developing mastitis include breast engorgement, infrequent or short duration of feedings, poor attachment or uncoordinated suckling leading to inefficient milk removal, parental or infant illness, rapid weaning, pressure on the breast (eg, tight bra), parental stress and fatigue, plugged milk ducts, oversupply of milk, and cracked nipples.[122]

Penicillin-resistant *Staphylococcus aureus* is the most common bacterial cause of mastitis; *E. coli* and *Streptococcus* have also been implicated.[122] A 10- to 14-day course of antibiotics is usually given for treatment of mastitis; penicillinase-resistant penicillins (eg, dicloxacillin, oxacillin) and alternatively first-generation cephalosporins (eg, cephalexin) are frequently prescribed. Anti-inflammatory medications, such as ibuprofen, may provide some pain relief. Application of heat just prior to feeding may also be helpful along with direct massage of the affected area toward the nipple during feeding as tolerated. Additionally, cold compresses after feedings can be utilized to help decrease pain and edema. Affected individuals should be educated to continue breastfeeding from both breasts throughout treatment and to pump if breasts are not emptied completely with feedings. Feedings should start on the affected breast and occur more frequently.[122]

Postpartum Depression

8 Mood disorders in the postpartum period may include postpartum blues, postpartum depression, and postpartum psychosis.[122] Postpartum blues ("baby blues") is common, usually affecting 15% to 85% of new parents within the first 10 days of delivery, and generally does not require treatment. Symptoms include anxiety, anger, fatigue, insomnia, tearfulness, and sadness. Postpartum psychosis is more severe and can present as mania, psychotic depression, or schizophrenia but is rare, affecting less than 1% of new parents; hospitalization is usually indicated.[123]

Postpartum depression affects up to 13% of individuals, with almost 5% experiencing major depression. Symptoms may develop during pregnancy or up to 6 months after delivery, although the strict definition for major depressive disorder after delivery specifies symptom occurrence within 4 to 6 weeks.[123] Uncontrolled postpartum depression increases the risk for poor parental health, decreased quality of life, risky behaviors, relationship difficulties including bonding with and caring for the infant as well as impact infant physical health, growth, sleep, and development of motor, cognition, language, emotional, social, and behavior skills.[124] Psychotherapy, including interpersonal psychotherapy, cognitive behavioral therapy, and group/family therapy, has been shown to be effective for treatment of postpartum depression.[123]

Some suggest that the benefits of breastfeeding to the infant exceed the risks of antidepressant exposure in patients with postpartum depression. In cases where pharmacotherapy is warranted, selection of medication with low transfer to breast milk is desirable.[120] Sertraline, paroxetine, fluoxetine, and nortriptyline are the most studied in the postpartum period; however, the FDA approved brexanolone for the treatment of postpartum depression (see Chapter 88, "Depressive Disorders"). Given the high unintended pregnancy rate in the United States, some experts would recommend against using paroxetine as this agent has been associated with potential risks in early pregnancy. Given that long-term effects of exposure to antidepressants are largely unknown, monitoring growth and neurodevelopment should be considered for children exposed to antidepressants present in breast milk.[120]

CONCLUSION

Pregnant individuals may experience pregnancy-influenced, acute, and chronic conditions during pregnancy, with some requiring pharmacotherapy. Medication exposure during pregnancy can elicit fear and anxiety since many believe that the risk of birth defects with exposure is high.

Very few medications carry an absolute contraindication for use during pregnancy and providers must weigh the risk of medication exposure with the risk of the untreated disease state using the available evidence and considering timing of exposure. Individuals using medications during pregnancy should be educated using this same approach. In some situations, optimal parental health requires treatment with medications that have been associated with a higher risk of adverse effects to the fetus. The healthcare provider should provide realistic information about the types and likelihood of adverse effects to assist the patient in making the best possible decisions based on the patient's beliefs, concerns, and need for treatment.

Evidence-based resources, databases and reference books related to medication use in pregnancy and lactation, and primary and secondary literature provide healthcare practitioners with access to relevant and current medication information to manage medication therapy needs during pregnancy and lactation. Collaboration among healthcare providers who care for pregnant individuals is essential to seek, evaluate, and present the most up to date and accurate information to their patients.

ABBREVIATIONS

ACOG	American College of Obstetricians and Gynecologists
ADA	American Diabetes Association
ARV	antiretroviral
BMI	body mass index
CDC	Centers for Disease Control and Prevention
CNS	central nervous system
dBP	diastolic blood pressure
FDA	Food and Drug Administration
GINA	Global Initiative for Asthma
GBS	Group B *Streptococcus*
GDM	gestational diabetes mellitus
GI	gastrointestinal
GTT	gestational transient thyrotoxicosis
H_2	histamine-2
hCG	human chorionic gonadotropin
HDP	hypertensive disorders of pregnancy
HELLP	hemolysis, elevated liver enzymes, low platelets
HG	hyperemesis gravidarum
HIV	human immunodeficiency virus
HSV-1	herpes simplex virus 1
HSV-2	herpes simplex virus 2
HTN	hypertension
IADPSG	International Association of Diabetes and Pregnancy Study Groups
LMWH	low-molecular-weight heparin
NSAID	nonsteroidal anti-inflammatory drug
NTD	neural tube defect
NVP	nausea and vomiting of pregnancy
OGTT	oral glucose tolerance test
PID	pelvic inflammatory disease
PPH	postpartum hemorrhage
PPI	proton pump inhibitor
aPPT	Prothrombin time
PROM	prelabor rupture of membranes
PPT	postpartum thyroiditis
PTU	propylthiouracil
RPG	random plasma glucose
sBP	systolic blood pressure
SMBG	self-monitored blood glucose
SNRI	serotonin–norepinephrine reuptake inhibitor
SSRI	selective serotonin reuptake inhibitor
STI	sexually transmitted infection
TENS	transcutaneous electrical nerve stimulation
TSH	thyroid-stimulating hormone
UFH	unfractionated heparin
UTI	urinary tract infection
VTE	venous thromboembolism

REFERENCES

1. Jarvis GE. Early embryo mortality in natural human reproduction: what the data say. *F1000Res.* 2016;5:2765. doi:10.12688/f1000research.8937.2.
2. Cunningham FG, Leveno KJ, Bloom SL, et al. *Williams Obstetrics.* New York: McGraw Hill; 2018.
3. Anifandis G, Messini CI, Dafopoulos K, et al. Sperm contributions to oocyte activation: more that meets the eye. *J Assist Reprod Genet.* 2016;33:313–316. doi:10.1007/s10815-016-0653-0.
4. Implantation and placental development. In: Cunningham F, Leveno KJ, Bloom SL, et al. eds. *Williams Obstetrics.* 25th ed. [electronic version] 2018, *AccessMedicine.* Available at: http://accessmedicine.mhmedical.com/content.aspx?bookid=1918§ionid=185046233. Accessed July 10, 2018.
5. Embryogenesis and fetal development . In: Cunningham F, Leveno KJ, Bloom SL, et al., eds. *Williams Obstetrics.* 25th ed. [electronic version] 2018, *AccessMedicine.* Available at: http://accessmedicine.mhmedical.com/content.aspx?bookid=1918§ionid=141464503. Accessed July 10, 2018.
6. Bernstein HB, VanBuren G. Normal pregnancy and prenatal care. In: DeCherney AH, Nathan L, Laufer N, et al. eds. *CURRENT Diagnosis & Treatment: Obstetrics & Gynecology.* 11th ed. [electronic version] 2013, *AccessMedicine.* Available at: http://accessmedicine.mhmedical.com/content.aspx?bookid=498§ionid=41008595. Accessed July 10, 2018.
7. American Pregnancy Association. First fetal movement: quickening. https://americanpregnancy.org/healthy-pregnancy/pregnancy-health-wellness/first-fetal-movement/. Accessed September 28, 2021.
8. Mastrobattista JM, Monga M. In: Resnik R, Lockwood CJ, Moore TR. eds. *Creasy and Resnik's Maternal Fetal Medicine.* 8th ed. Philadelphia, PA: Elsevier; 2019:141–147.
9. Feghali MN, Mattison DR. Clinical therapeutics in pregnancy. *J Biomed Biotechnol.* 2011;2011:783528. doi:10.1155/2011/783528.
10. Tasnif Y, Morado J, Hebert MF. Pregnancy-related pharmacokinetic changes. *Clin Pharmacol Ther.* 2016;100:53–62.
11. Gomes CF, Sousa M, Lourenco I, et al. Gastrointestinal diseases during pregnancy: what does the gastroenterologist need to know? *Ann Gastroenterol.* 2018;31:385–94. doi:10.20524/aog.2018.0264.
12. Chambers C, Friedman JM. In: Resnik R, Lockwood CJ, Moore TR. eds. *Creasy and Resnik's Maternal Fetal Medicine.* 8th ed. Philadelphia, PA: Elsevier; 2019:539–548.
13. Feghali M, Venkataramanan R, Caritis S. Pharmacokinetics of drugs in pregnancy. *Semin Perinatal.* 2015;39:512–519. doi:10.1053/j.semperi.2015.08.003.
14. Syme MR, Paxton JW, Keelan JA. Drug transfer and metabolism by the human placenta. *Clin Pharmacokinet.* 2004;43:487–514.
15. Kazma JM, van den Anker J, Allegaert K, et al. Anatomical and physiological alternations of pregnancy. *J Pharmacokinet Pharmacodyn.* 2020;47:271–85. doi:10.1007/s10928-020-09677-1.
16. Savitz DA, Hertz-Picciotto I, Poole C, et al. Epidemiologic measures of the course and outcome of pregnancy. *Epidemiol Rev.* 2002;24:91–101. doi:10.1093/epirev/mxf006.
17. Adam MP. The all-or-none phenomenon revisited. *Birth Defects Res A Clin Mol Teratol.* 2012;94:664–669.
18. Ram R. In: Herrmann K, Jayne K. eds. *Animal Experimentation: Working Towards a Paradigm Change.* 22th ed. Leiden: The Netherlands: Koninklijke Brill; Available at: https://brill.com/view/book/edcoll/9789004391192/BP000020.xml?body=pdf-43180. Accessed Oct 1, 2021.
19. Food and Drug Administration. Content and format of labeling for human prescription drug and biological products: requirements for pregnancy and lactation labeling (final rule). *Federal Register.* 2014;79:72064–72103.
20. Callegari LS, Ma EW, Schwarz EB. Preconception care and reproductive planning in primary care. *Med Clin North Am.* 2015;99:663–682.
21. Harden CI, Meador KJ, Pennell PB, et al. Practice parameter update: management issues for women with epilepsy—focus on pregnancy (an evidence-based review): teratogenesis and perinatal outcomes. *Neurology.* 2009;73:133–141.
22. American College of Obstetricians and Gynecologists. Neural tube defects. ACOG practice bulletin No. 187. *Obstet Gynecol.* 2017;130:e279–290. doi:10.1097/AOG.0000000000002412.
23. American College of Obstetricians and Gynecologists. Gynecologic management of adolescents and young women with seizure disorders. ACOG practice bulletin No. 806. *Obstet Gynecol.* 2020;135:e213–220. doi:10.1097/AOG.0000000000003827.
24. Gerard EE, Meador KJ. Managing epilepsy in women. *Continuum.* 2016;22:204–226. doi:10.1212/CON.0000000000000270.
25. Otto CM, Nishimura RA, Bonow RO, et al. 2020 ACC/AHA guideline for the management of patients with valvular heart disease: a report of the American College of Cardiology/American Heart Association Joint Committee on Clinical Practice Guidelines. *Circulation.* 2021;143:e72–227. doi:10.1161/CIR.0000000000000923.
26. Briggs GG, Towers CV, Forinash AB. *A Reference Guide to Drug Use in Pregnancy and Lactation.* 12th ed. Philadelphia, PA: Wolters Kluwer Health; 2021.
27. Bates SM, Middeldorp S, Rodger M, James AH, Greer I. Guidance for the treatment and prevention of obstetric-associated venous thromboembolism. *J Thromb Thrombolysis.* 2016;41:92–128.
28. El-Ibiary SY, Raney EC, Moos MK. The pharmacist's role in promoting preconception health. *J Am Pharm Assoc.* 2014;54:e288. doi:10.1331/JAPhA.2014.13138.
29. Behnke M, Smith VC. Committee on Substance Abuse. Prenatal substance abuse: short- and long- term effects on the exposed fetus. *Pediatrics.* 2013;131:e1009–1024.

30. American College of Obstetricians and Gynecologists. Obesity in pregnancy. ACOG practice bulletin No. 230. *Obstet Gynecol.* 2021;137:e128–144. 10.1097/AOG.0000000000004395.
31. American College of Obstetricians and Gynecologists. Tobacco and nicotine cessation during pregnancy. ACOG committee opinion No. 807. *Obstet Gynecol.* 2020;135:e221–229. 10.1097/AOG.0000000000003825.
32. American College of Obstetricians and Gynecologists. Marijuana use during pregnancy and lactation. Committee opinion No. 722. *Obstet Gynecol.* 2017;130:e205–209. 10.1097/AOG.0000000000002354.
33. Centers for Disease Control and Prevention. Folic acid: birth defects COUNT. Available at: https://www.cdc.gov/ncbddd/birthdefectscount/data.html. Accessed October 1, 2021.
34. Bibbins-Domingo K, Grossman DC, et al. U.S. Preventive Services Task Force. Folic acid supplementation for the prevention of neural tube defects: US Preventive Services Task Force Recommendation Statement. *JAMA.* 2017;317:183–189.
35. Forray A. Substance use during pregnancy. *F1000Research.* 2016;5:887.
36. Claire R, Chamberlain C, Davey MA, et al. Pharmacological interventions for promoting smoking cessation during pregnancy. *Cochrane Database Syst Rev.* 2020;3:CD010078. doi:10.1002/14651858.CD010078.pub3.
37. American College of Obstetricians and Gynecologists. Nausea and vomiting of pregnancy. ACOG practice bulletin No. 189. *Obstet Gynecol.* 2018;131:e15–30. doi:10.1097/AOG.0000000000002604.
38. Package insert. Metoclopramide. Amneal Pharmaceuticals, 2016.
39. Kelly TF, Savides TJ. In: Resnik R, Lockwood CJ, Moore TR, et al. eds. *Creasy and Resnik's Maternal Fetal Medicine.* 8th ed. Philadelphia, PA: Elsevier; 2019;1158–1172.
40. Zielinski R, Searing K, Deibel M. Gastrointestinal distress in pregnancy: Prevalence, assessment, and treatment of 5 common minor discomforts. *J Perinat Neonatal Nurs.* 2015;29:23–31.
41. Thelin CS, Richter JE. Review article: the management of heartburn during pregnancy and lactation. *Aliment Pharmacol Ther.* 2020;51: 421–434. doi:10.1111/apt.15611.
42. Pasternak B, Hviid A. Use of proton-pump inhibitors in early pregnancy and the risk of birth defects. *N Engl J Med.* 2010;363: 2114–2123. doi:10.1056/NEJMoa1002689.
43. American Diabetes Association. Management of diabetes in pregnancy: standards of medical care in diabetes—2021. *Diabetes Care.* 2021;44:S200–210. doi:10.2337/dc21-S014.
44. American College of Obstetricians and Gynecologists. Gestational diabetes mellitus. ACOG practice bulletin No. 190. *Obstet Gynecol.* 2018;131:e49–64. doi:10.1097/AOG.0000000000002501.
45. Kc K, Shakya S, Zhang H. Gestational diabetes mellitus and macrosomia: a literature review. *Ann Nutr Metab.* 2015;66(Suppl 2): 14–20. doi:10.1159/000371628.
46. American College of Obstetricians and Gynecologists. Pregestational diabetes mellitus. ACOG practice bulletin No. 201. *Obstet Gynecol.* 2018;132:e228–248. 10.1097/AOG.0000000000002960.
47. Plows JF, Stanley JL, Baker PN, et al. The pathophysiology of gestational diabetes mellitus. *Int J Mol Sci.* 2018;19:3342. doi:10.3390/ijms19113342.
48. O'Neill SM, Kenny LC, Khashan AS, et al. Different insulin types and regimens for pregnant women with preexisting diabetes. *Cochrane Database Syst Rev.* 2017;2:CD011880. doi:10.1002/14651858.CD011880.pub2.
49. Koren R, Toledano Y, Hod M. The use of insulin detemir during pregnancy: a safety evaluation. *Expert Opin Drug Saf.* 2015;14:593–599. 10.1517/14740338.2015.1013533.
50. Herrera KM, Rosenn BM, Foroutan J, et al. Randomized controlled trial of insulin detemir versus NPH for the treatment of pregnant women with diabetes. *Am J Obstet Gynecol.* 2015;213:426.e1–7. doi:10.1016/j.ajog.2015.06.010.
51. Bonora BM, Avogaro A, Fadini GP. Exposure to insulin degludec during pregnancy: report of a small series and review of the literature. *J Endocrinol Invest.* 2019;42:345–349. 10.1007/s40618-018-0926-9.
52. Doder Z, Vanechanos D, Oster M, et al. Insulin glulisine in pregnancy—experience from clinical trials and post-marketing surveillance. *Eur Endocrinol.* 2015;11:17–20. doi:10.17925/EE.2015.11.01.17.
53. Balsells M, Garcia-Patterson A, Sola I, et al. Glibenclamide, metformin, and insulin for the treatment of gestational diabetes: a systemic review and meta-analysis. *BMJ.* 2015;350:h102. doi:10.1136/bmj.h102.
54. Jiang Y-F, Chen X-Y, Ding T, et al. Comparative efficacy and safety of OADs in management of GDM: network meta-analysis of randomized controlled trials. *J Clin Endocrinol Metab.* 2015;100:2071–2080. 10.1210/jc.2014-4403.
55. Feig DS, Donovan LE, Zinman B, et al. Metformin in women with type 2 diabetes in pregnancy (MiTy): a multicentre, international, randomised, placebo-controlled trial. *Lancet Diabetes Endocrinol.* 2020;8:834–844. doi:10.1016/S2213-8587(20)30310-7.
56. Rowan JA, Rush EC, Plank LD, et al. Metformin in gestational diabetes: the offspring follow-up (MiG TOFU): body composition and metabolic outcomes at 7-9 years of age. *BMJ Open Diabetes Res Care.* 2018;6:e000456. doi:10.1136/bmjdrc-2017-000456.
57. van Weelden W, Wekker V, de Wit L, et al. Long-term effects of oral antidiabetic drugs during pregnancy on offspring: a systemic review and meta-analysis of follow-up studies of RCTs. *Diabetes Ther.* 2018;9:1811–1829. 10.1007/s13300-018-0479-0.
58. Harper LM, Glover AV, Biggio JR, et al. Predicting failure of glyburide therapy in gestational diabetes. *J Perinatol.* 2016;36:347–351. 10.1038/jp.2015.216.
59. Roeder HA, Moore TR, Ramos GA. Changes in postpartum insulin requirements for patients with well-controlled type 1 diabetes. *Am J Perinatol.* 2016;33:683–687. 10.1055/s-0036-1571323.
60. American College of Obstetricians and Gynecologists. Chronic hypertension in pregnancy. ACOG practice bulletin No. 230. *Obstet Gynecol.* 2019;133:e26–e50. doi:10.1097/AOG.0000000000003020.
61. American College of Obstetricians and Gynecologists. Gestational hypertension and preeclampsia. ACOG practice bulletin No. 222. *Obstet Gynecol.* 2020;135:e237–260. 10.1097/AOG.0000000000003891.
62. American Pregnancy Association. Gestational hypertension: Pregnancy induced hypertension (PIH). Available at: https://americanpregnancy.org/pregnancy-complicationsgestational-hypertension/. Accessed August 16, 2021.
63. Leeman L, Dresang LT, Fontaine P. Hypertensive disorders of pregnancy. *Am Fam Physician.* 2016;93:121–127.
64. US Preventive Services Task Force, Davidson KW, Barry MJ, et al. Aspirin use to prevent preeclampsia and related morbidity and mortality: US Preventive Services Task Force recommendation statement. *JAMA.* 2021;326:1186–1191. doi:10.1001/jama.2021.14781.
65. Van Doorn R, Mukhtarova N, Flyke IP, et al. Dose of aspirin to prevent preterm preeclampsia in women with moderate or high-risk factors: a systemic review and meta-analysis. *PLos One.* 2021;16:e0247782. doi:10.1371/journal.pone.0247782.
66. American College of Obstetricians and Gynecologists. Low-dose aspirin use during pregnancy. ACOG committee opinion No. 743. *Obstet Gynecol.* 2018;132:e44–e52. doi:10.1097/AOG.0000000000002708.
67. American College of Obstetricians and Gynecologists. Thyroid disease in pregnancy. ACOG practice bulletin No. 223. *Obstet Gynecol.* 2020;135:e261–e274. doi:10.1097/AOG.0000000000003893.
68. Alexander EK, Pearce EN, Brent GA, et al. 2017 guidelines of the American Thyroid Association for the diagnosis and management of thyroid disease during pregnancy and the postpartum. *Thyroid.* 2017;27:315–89. doi:10.1089/thy.2016.0457.
69. American College of Obstetricians and Gynecologists. Thromboembolism in pregnancy. ACOG practice bulletin No. 196. *Obstet Gynecol.* 2018;132:e1–e17. doi:10.1097/AOG.0000000000002706.
70. American College of Obstetricians and Gynecologists. Inherited thrombophilias in pregnancy. ACOG practice bulletin No. 197. *Obstet Gynecol.* 2018;132:e18–e34. doi:10.1097/AOG.0000000000002703.
71. Smaill FM, Vazquez JC. Antibiotics for asymptomatic bacteriuria in pregnancy. *Cochrane Database Syst Rev.* 2019;2019:CD000490. doi:10.1002/14651858.CD000490.pub4.
72. Nicolle LE, Gupta K, Bradley SF, et al. Clinical practice guideline for the management of asymptomatic bacteruria: 2019 update by the infectious diseases society of America. *Clin Infect Dis.* 2019;68:e83–110. doi:10.1093/cid/ciy1121.
73. Wing DA, Fassett MJ, Getahun D. Acute pyelonephritis in pregnancy: an 18-year retrospective analysis. *Am J Obstet Gynecol.* 2014;210(219):e1–6. doi:10.1016/j.ajog.2013.10.006.
74. Hill JB, Sheffield JS, McIntire DD, et al. Acute pyelonephritis in pregnancy. *Obstet Gynecol.* 2005;105:18–23. doi:10.1097/01.AOG.0000149154.96285.a0.
75. Glaser AP, Schaeffer AJ. Urinary tract infection and bacteriuria in pregnancy. *Urol Clin North Am.* 2015;42:547–560. doi:10.1016/j.ucl.2015.05.004.
76. Workowski KA, Bachmann LH, Chan PA, et al. Sexually transmitted infections treatment guidelines, 2021. *MMWR Recomm Rep.* 2021;70: 1–187. doi:10.15585/mmwr.rr7004a1.
77. American College of Obstetricians and Gynecologists. Management of genital herpes in pregnancy. Practice bulletin No. 220. *Obstet Gynecol.* 2020;135:e193–202. doi:10.1097/AOG.0000000000003840.
78. Panel on treatment of pregnant women with HIV infection and prevention of perinatal transmission. Recommendations for the use of antiretroviral drugs in pregnant women with HIV infection and

interventions to reduce perinatal HIV transmission in the United States. Available at: https://clinicalinfo.hiv.gov/en/guidelines/perinatal/introduction?view=full. Accessed August 13, 2021.
79. Lucas S. Migraine and other headache disorders: ACOG clinical updates in women's health care primary and preventive care review summary volume XVIII, Number 4. *Obstet Gynecol.* 2019;134:211. doi:10.1097/AOG.0000000000003322.
80. Food and Drug Administration. FDA recommends avoiding use of NSAIDs in pregnancy at 20 weeks or later because they can result in low amniotic fluid. Available at: https://www.fda.gov/media/142967/download. Accessed October 1, 2021.
81. American College of Obstetricians and Gynecologists. Asthma in pregnancy. ACOG practice bulletin No. 90. *Obstet Gynecol.* 2008;111:457–464. doi:10.1097/AOG.0b013e3181665ff4.
82. Global initiative for asthma. Global strategy for asthma management and prevention, 2021. www.ginasthma.org. Accessed August 17, 2021.
83. Ridolo E, Caminati M, Martignago I, et al. Allergic rhinitis: Pharmacotherapy in pregnancy and old age. *Expert Rev Clin Pharmacol.* 2016;9:1081–1089. doi:10.1080/17512433.2016.1189324.
84. Harden CI, Hopp J, Ting TY, et al. Practice parameter update: management issues for women with epilepsy—focus on pregnancy (an evidence-based review): obstetrical complications and change in seizure frequency. *Neurology.* 2009;73:126–132. 10.1212/WNL.0b013e3181a6b2f8.
85. Tomson T, Landmark CJ, Battino D. Antiepileptic drug treatment in pregnancy: changes in drug disposition and their clinical implications. *Epilepsia.* 2013;54:405–414. 10.1111/epi.12109.
86. Harden CI, Pennell PB, Koppel BS, et al. Practice parameter update: management issues for women with epilepsy—focus on pregnancy (an evidence based review): vitamin K, folic acid, blood levels, and breastfeeding. *Neurology.* 2009;73:142–149. 10.1212/WNL.0b013e3181a6b325.
87. Tomson T, Battino D, Bonizzoni E, et al. Dose-dependent teratogenicity of valproate in mono- and polytherapy: An observational study. *Neurology.* 2015;85:866–872. doi:10.1212/WNL.0000000000001772.
88. Hernandez-Diaz S, Mittendorf R, Smith CR, et al. Association between topiramate and zonisamide use during pregnancy and low birth weight. *Obstet Gynecol.* 2014;123:21–28.
89. American College of Obstetricians and Gynecologists. Use of psychiatric medications during pregnancy and lactation. ACOG practice bulletin No. 92. *Obstet Gynecol.* 2008;111:1001–1020. 10.1097/AOG.0b013e31816fd910.
90. American College of Obstetricians and Gynecologists. Screening for perinatal depression. Committee opinion No. 630. *Obstet Gynecol.* 2015;125:1268–1271.
91. Gentile S. Drug treatment for mood disorders in pregnancy. *Curr Opin Psychiatry.* 2011;24:34–40.
92. Yonkers KA, Wisner KL, Stewart DE, et al. The management of depression during pregnancy: a report from the American Psychiatric Association and the American College of Obstetricians and Gynecologists. *Obstet Gynecol.* 2009;114:703–713.
93. Ornoy A, Koren G. SSRIs and SNRIs (SRI) in pregnancy: effects on the course of pregnancy and the offspring: how far are we from having all the answers? *Int J Mol Sci.* 2019;20:2379. doi:10.3390/ijms20102370.
94. Ornoy A, Koren G. Selective serotonin reuptake inhibitors during pregnancy: do we have now more definite answers related to prenatal exposure? *Birth Defects Res.* 2017;109:898–908. doi:10.1002/bdr2.1078.
95. Pearlstein T. Use of psychotropic medication during pregnancy and the postpartum period. *Womens Health (Lond).* 2013;9:605–615. 10.2217/whe.13.54.
96. Coughlin CG, Blackwell KA, Bartley C, et al. Obstetric and neonatal outcomes after antipsychotic medication exposure in pregnancy. *Obstet Gynecol.* 2015;125:1224–35. doi:10.1097/AOG.0000000000000759.
97. Wang Z, Chan AYL, Coghill D, et al. Association between prenatal exposure to antipsychotics and attention-deficit/hyperactivity disorder, autism spectrum disorder, preterm birth, and small for gestational age. *JAMA Intern Med.* 2021;e214571. doi:10.1001/jamainternmed.2021.4571.
98. Patorno E, Huybrechts KF, Bateman BT, et al. Lithium use in pregnancy and the risk of cardiac malformations. *N Engl J Med.* 2017;376:2245–2254. 10.1056/NEJM1612222.
99. Hudson (OH): Lexicomp Inc.: 2021 [updated 9 Oct 2021; cited 14 October 2021]. Available at: http://online.lexi.com.http://onlinelexi.com.
100. American College of Obstetricians and Gynecologists. Management of preterm labor. ACOG practice bulletin No. 171. *Obstet Gynecol.* 2016e155–164. 10.1097/AOG.0000000000001711.
101. American College of Obstetrics and Gynecologists. Prediction and prevention of spontaneous preterm birth. ACOG practice bulletin No. 234. *Obstet Gynecol.* 2021;138:e65–90. doi:10.1097/AOG.0000000000004479.
102. American College of Obstetricians and Gynecologists. Prelabor rupture of membranes. ACOG practice bulletin No. 217. *Obstet Gynecol.* 2020;e80–97. doi:10.1097/AOG.0000000000003700.
103. American College of Obstetricians and Gynecologists. Prevention of group B streptococcal early-onset disease in newborns. ACOG committee opinion No. 797. *Obstet Gynecol.* 2020;135:e51–72. doi:10.11097/AOG.0000000000003668.
104. Declercq E, Belanoff C, Iverson R. Maternal perceptions of the experience of attempted labor induction and medically elective inductions: analysis of survey results from listening to mothers in Calfornia. *BMC Pregnancy Childbirth.* 2020;20:458. doi:10.1186/s12884-020-03137-x.
105. American College of Obstetricians and Gynecologists. Induction of labor. ACOG practice bulletin No. 107. *Obstet Gynecol.* 2009;114:386–397. 10.1097/AOG.0b013e3181b4ef5.
106. American College of Obstetricians and Gynecologists. Obstetric analgesia and anesthesia. ACOG practice bulletin No. 209. *Obstet Gynecol.* 2019;133:e208–225. 10.1097/AOG.0000000000003132.
107. Levett KM, Smith CA, Bensoussan A, Dahlen HG. Complementary therapies for labour and birth study: a randomised controlled trial of antenatal integrative medicine for pain management in labour. *BMJ Open.* 2016;6:e010691. doi:10.1136/bmjopen-2015-010691.
108. Koyyalamudi V, Sidhu G, Cornett EM, et al. New labor pain treatment options. *Curr Pain Headache Rep.* 2016;20:11. doi:10.1007/s11916-016-0543-2.
109. Jones L, Othman M, Dowswell T, et al. Pain management for women in labour: an overview of systematic reviews. *Cochrane Database Syst Rev.* 2012;3:CD009234. doi:10.1002/14651858.CD009234.pub2.
110. Anim-Somuah M, Smyth RM, Cyna AM, Cuthbert A. Epidural versus non-epidural or no analgesia for pain management in labour. *Cochrane Database Syst Rev.* 2018;5:CD000331. doi:10.1002/14651858.CD000331.pub4.
111. American College of Obstetricians and Gynecologists. Postpartum hemorrhage. ACOG practice bulletin No. 183. *Obset Gynecol.* 2017;130:e168–186. 10.1097/AOG.0000000000002351.
112. Section on Breastfeeding. Breastfeeding and the use of human milk. *Pediatrics.* 2012;129:e827–e841.
113. Academy of Breastfeeding Medicine Protocol Committee. ABM clinical protocol #9: use of galactogogues in initiating or augmenting the rate of maternal milk secretion. *Breastfeed Med.* 2011;6:41–49. doi:10.1089/bfm.2011.9998.
114. American College of Obstetricians and Gynecologists. Breastfeeding challenges. ACOG committee opinion No. 820. *Obstet Gynecol.* 2021;137:e42–e53. doi:10.1097/AOG.0000000000004253.
115. Novak S. How to increase your breast milk supply. Available at: https://www.whattoexpect.com/poor-milk-supply-breastfeeding.aspx. Accessed September 28, 2021.
116. Children's Health Queensland Hospital and Health Service. Increasing your breast milk supple. Available at: https://www.childrens.health.qld.gov.au/fact-sheet-increasing-your-breast-milk-supply/. Accessed September 28, 2021.
117. Reglan. Prescribing information. ANI Pharmaceuticals, 2017.
118. Food and Drug Administration. FDA talk paper: FDA warns against women using unapproved drug, domperidone, to increase milk production. https://www.fda.gov/drugs/information-drug-class/fda-talk-paper-fda-warns-against-women-using-unapproved-drug-domperidone-increase-milk-production. Accessed October 1, 2021.
119. Rowe H, Baker T, Hale TW. Maternal medication, drug use, and breastfeeding. *Child Adolesc Psychiatr Clin N Am.* 2015;24:1–20. doi:10.1016/j.chc.2014.09.005.
120. Sachs HC; Committee On Drugs. The transfer of drugs and therapeutics into human breast milk: an update on selected topics. *Pediatrics.* 2013;132:e796–809. doi:10.1542/peds.2013-1985.
121. Berlin CM Jr, van den Anker JN. Safety during breastfeeding: drugs, foods, environmental chemicals, and maternal infections. *Semin Fetal Neonatal Med.* 2013;18:13–8. doi:10.1016/j.siny.2012.09.003.
122. Amir LH, Academy of Breastfeeding Medicine Protocol C. ABM clinical protocol #4: Mastitis, revised March 2014. *Breastfeed Med.* 2014;9:239–243. doi:10.1089/bfm.2014.9984.
123. Molyneaux E, Howard LM, McGeown HR, Karia AM, Trevillion K. Antidepressant treatment for postnatal depression. *Cochrane Database Syst Rev.* 2014;9:CD002018. doi:10.1002/14651858.CD002018.pub2.
124. Slomian J, Honvo G, Emonts P, et al. Consequences of maternal postpartum depression: a systematic review of maternal and infant outcomes. *Womens Health (Lond).* 2019;15:1745506519844044. doi:10.1177/1745506519844044.

100 Menstrual-Related Disorders

Kathleen M. Vest and Danielle C. Mayer

KEY CONCEPTS

1. A urine pregnancy test should be one of the first steps in evaluating amenorrhea; however, the majority of primary amenorrhea cases can be attributed to either physical anomalies of the gonads, outflow tract, or anomalies of the hypothalamic–pituitary–ovarian (HPO) axis.
2. For hypoestrogenic conditions associated with primary and secondary amenorrhea, estrogen (with a progestin) is recommended if correction of the underlying cause does not restore menses.
3. Heavy menstrual bleeding (HMB) is generally caused by either uterine structural abnormalities or nonstructural causes.
4. Pregnancy, including intrauterine pregnancy, ectopic pregnancy, and miscarriage, is at the top of the differential diagnosis for any person presenting with heavy menses.
5. The levonorgestrel intrauterine system (IUS) is associated with a 61% lower discontinuation rate and 82% fewer treatment failures when compared to other conventional pharmacotherapies for HMB.
6. Intrauterine devices (IUD) or IUS are considered therapeutic options in a variety of menstruation-related disorders. The American College of Obstetricians and Gynecologists (ACOG) guidelines indicate that both nulliparous and multiparous females at low risk of sexually transmitted diseases are good candidates for IUS use.
7. Abnormal uterine bleeding associated with ovulatory dysfunction (AUB-O) is caused by oligo- or anovulation, leading to irregular, heavy menstrual bleeding due to chronic unopposed estrogen on the endometrium.
8. Polycystic ovary syndrome (PCOS) can present as AUB-O, and symptoms include amenorrhea, oligomenorrhea, intermenstrual bleeding, and HMB. Its exact definition continues to evolve, but it is a disorder of androgen excess accompanied by ovulatory dysfunction and/or polycystic ovarian morphology. Insulin resistance is often present, and PCOS is a risk factor for the metabolic syndrome, type 2 diabetes, dyslipidemia, hypertension, and possibly cardiovascular disease.
9. Combined hormonal contraceptives (CHCs) alone should be recommended for the management of irregular menstrual cycles and clinical hyperandrogenism in adults and adolescents with PCOS.
10. The selective serotonin reuptake inhibitors (SSRIs) are first-line pharmacologic treatment options for premenstrual dysphoric disorder (PMDD).

BEYOND THE BOOK

Watch this video about the Menstrual Cycle.

Alternatively, watch the video entitled "The Menstrual Cycle." This 9-minute video provides an overview of a normal menstrual cycle and its hormonal regulation and is useful to enhance understanding of the pathophysiology of various menstrual disorders.

Guided questions for videos:

1. Describe the major role of the following hormones in regulation of the normal menstrual cycle:
   a. GnRH
   b. LH
   c. FSH
   d. Estrogen
   e. Progesterone
2. What hormone levels are highest and lowest in the follicular phase of the normal menstrual cycle and what outcome occurs as a result?
3. What hormone levels are highest and lowest in the luteal phase of the normal menstrual cycle and what outcome occurs as a result?
4. Describe folliculogenesis. What does this term mean, in what phase of the menstrual cycle does this occur, and what hormones are most active during this process?
5. Describe the corpus luteum. What is it, in what phase of the menstrual cycle does it develop, and what hormones are most active while it is present?
6. Draw the hypothalamus–pituitary–ovarian (HPO) axis and associated hormones. Plot the negative or positive feedback loops that occur in the follicular phase, during ovulation, and in the luteal phase.

INTRODUCTION

Problems related to the menstrual cycle are exceedingly common in females of reproductive age. This chapter discusses the most frequently encountered menstruation-related difficulties: amenorrhea; heavy menstrual bleeding (HMB); premenstrual syndrome (PMS) and premenstrual dysphoric disorder (PMDD), dysmenorrhea, and abnormal uterine bleeding associated with ovulatory dysfunction (AUB-O), including polycystic ovary syndrome (PCOS). The need for effective treatments of these disorders stems from their negative impact on an individual's quality of life, reproductive health, and long-term detrimental health effects, such as increased risk of osteoporosis with amenorrhea and risk of diabetes with PCOS.

Similar to other chapters in this section, general discussions around menstruation-related disorders and their treatment are primarily framed around cisgender women. However, any individual with a female reproductive system may experience issues with menstruation. Therefore, the use of the term female is specifically meant to refer to biology, and this chapter has been written to include transgender individuals.

Before menstrual disorders are discussed, what constitutes a normal menstrual cycle needs to be considered. The American College of Obstetrics and Gynecologists recommends that clinicians ask about an individual's first day of the patient's last menstrual period, as well as the pattern of menses, during every clinical encounter.[1] Identification of menstrual patterns should begin in adolescence, which may improve the early detection of potential health concerns.[1] Before menstrual disorders are discussed, what constitutes a normal menstrual cycle for the individual needs to be considered.

In adolescents, immaturity of the hypothalamic–pituitary–ovarian axis in the early years after menarche may lead to longer cycles due to anovulation.[1] However, 90% of these cycles will be within the range of 21 to 45 days.[1] The following menstrual characteristics and patterns are considered normal:[1]

- Median age of menarche of 12.4 years, and menarche by age 15
- Menstrual cycle interval between 21 and 45 days
- Menstrual flow length 7 days or less
- Menstrual product use between 3 to 6 pads or tampons per day

In adult females not using hormonal contraception, a normal menstrual period lasts between 4.5 and 8 days, and cycle lengths range from 24 to 28 days.[2] Normal variation in cycle length is considered to be 7 to 9 days, depending on a patient's age: 18 to 25 years $\leq$ 9 days, 26 to 41 $\leq$ 7 days, 42 to 45 $\leq$ 9 days.[3] Blood loss between 5 and 80 mL during each period is considered normal.[2]

AMENORRHEA

Epidemiology

Amenorrhea is defined as no menstrual bleeding in a 90-day period,[2] and can be either primary or secondary in nature. Primary amenorrhea is the absence of menses by age 15 years in females who have never menstruated.[4] Secondary amenorrhea is the absence of menses for three cycles or for 6 months in a previously menstruating individual.[4,5]

Primary amenorrhea occurs in less than 0.1% of the general population. Secondary amenorrhea, in comparison, has an incidence of 3% to 4% in the general population and occurs more frequently in individuals younger than 25 years with a history of menstrual irregularities and in those involved in competitive athletics.[6]

Etiology

In two-thirds of females, menses occur generally at 28 + 3 days, and cycle lengths of 18 to 40 days are considered within the normal range.[5] Amenorrhea is not itself a diagnosis, but a sign of a disorder.[5] There are three broad categories of amenorrhea etiology:

- Anatomical causes, including pregnancy and uterine structural abnormalities
- Endocrine disturbances leading to chronic anovulation
- Ovarian insufficiency/failure

1 While a urine pregnancy test is one of the first steps in evaluating amenorrhea, the majority of primary amenorrhea cases can be attributed to either anomalies involving (i) the hypothalamic–pituitary axis resulting in endocrine disturbances, (ii) ovarian function, or (iii) outflow tract.[7] Similarly, greater than 50% of secondary amenorrhea cases are due to the impact of disturbances of the hypothalamic–pituitary–adrenal (HPA) axis or the hypothalamic–pituitary–ovarian (HPO) axis.[6] Therefore, in organizing an approach to diagnosis and treatment, it is helpful to consider the organ systems

CLINICAL PRESENTATION Amenorrhea

General

- Although patients may be concerned about the cessation of menses and implications for fertility, patients are generally not in acute physical distress.

Symptoms

- Patients will note cessation of menses.
- Patients may complain of infertility, vaginal dryness, or decreased libido.

Signs

- Cessation of menses for more than 6 months in individuals with established menstruation, absence of menses by age 16 in the presence of normal secondary sexual development, or absence of menses by age 14 in the absence of normal secondary sexual development.
- Recent significant weight loss or weight gain.
- Presence of acne, hirsutism, hair loss, or acanthosis nigricans may suggest androgen excess.

Laboratory Tests

- Pregnancy test
- Serum FSH and LH
- Thyroid-stimulating hormone
- Prolactin
- If hyperandrogenic state (eg, PCOS) is suspected, consider free and total testosterone, dehydroepiandrosterone, fasting glucose, and fasting lipid panel

Other Diagnostic Tests

- Progesterone challenge to confirm functional anatomy and adequate estrogenization.
- Pelvic ultrasound to evaluate for polycystic ovaries, presence/absence of uterus, and/or structural abnormalities of the reproductive tract organs.

involved in the menstrual cycle, which include the uterus, ovaries, anterior pituitary, and hypothalamus.

Pathophysiology

Ovulation is required for the follicle (an estrogen-secreting body) to become a corpus luteum (a progesterone-secreting body). Without ovulation, the proper sequence of estrogen production, progesterone production, and estrogen/progesterone withdrawal will not occur. This can result in amenorrhea. Anovulation can occur secondary to endocrine disturbances or ovarian insufficiency.

Each organ in the HPO axis, along with the uterus, is of importance in determining amenorrhea's etiology and pathophysiology. Beginning with the uterus/outflow tract and progressing caudally will result in a comprehensive differential diagnosis. However, coexisting physical signs and symptoms, and a thorough history, typically help the clinician prioritize evaluation steps. Table 100-1 lists the pathophysiology of amenorrhea relative to the organ system(s) involved and the specific condition(s) that results in amenorrhea.

Uterus/Outflow Tract

For menstruation to occur, a uterus, functional endometrium, and patent vagina must be present. Several anatomic abnormalities may cause amenorrhea.[7] Congenital anomalies such as imperforate hymen or uterine agenesis may be discovered by physical examination. An acquired condition of the genital tract, such as Asherman's syndrome or cervical stenosis, is more likely in secondary amenorrhea.

Ovaries

Normal ovarian function is critical for menstruation to occur. The ovaries must respond appropriately to follicle-stimulating hormone (FSH) and luteinizing hormone (LH) by secreting estrogen and progesterone in the proper sequence to influence endometrial growth and shedding (Fig. 100-1).

Primary ovarian insufficiency occurs when potentially viable primordial follicles in the ovaries have been depleted.[9] Estrogen production from the remaining ovarian follicles is insufficient to stimulate endometrial growth in the absence of follicles. The etiologies for primary ovarian insufficiency include bilateral oophorectomy,[10]

TABLE 100-1 Pathophysiology of Selected Menstrual Bleeding Disorders

Organ System	Condition	Pathophysiology/Laboratory Findings
Amenorrhea		
Uterus	Asherman's syndrome	Postcurettage/postsurgical uterine adhesions
	Congenital uterine abnormalities	Abnormal uterine development
Ovaries	Turner's syndrome	Lack of ovarian follicles
	Gonadal dysgenesis	Other genetic abnormalities
	Premature ovarian failure	Early loss of follicles
	Chemotherapy/radiation	Gonadal toxins
Anterior pituitary	Pituitary prolactin-secreting adenoma	↑ Prolactin suppresses the HPO axis
	Hypothyroidism	TRH causes ↑ prolactin, other abnormalities
	Medication (antipsychotics, verapamil)	↑ Prolactin suppresses the HPO axis
Hypothalamus	FHA	↓ Pulsatile GnRH secretion in the absence of other abnormalities
	Eating disorder	↓ Pulsatile GnRH secretion, ↓ FSH and LH secondary to weight loss
	Exercise	↓ Pulsatile GnRH secretion, ↓ FSH and LH secondary to low body fat
	Anovulation/PCOS	Asynchronous gonadotropin and estrogen production, abnormal endometrial growth
Abnormal Uterine Bleeding Associated with Ovulatory Dysfunction (AUB-O)		
Physiologic causes	Adolescence	Immaturity of the HPO axis: no LH surge
	Perimenopause	Declining ovarian function
Pathologic causes	Hyperandrogenic anovulation (PCOS)	Hyperandrogenism: high testosterone, high LH, hyperinsulinemia, and insulin resistance
	Hypothalamic dysfunction (physical or emotional stress, exercise, weight loss)	Suppression of pulsatile GnRH secretion and estrogen deficiency: low LH, low FSH
	Hyperprolactinemia (pituitary gland tumor, psychiatric medications)	High prolactin
	Hypothyroidism	High TSH
	Premature ovarian failure	High FSH
Heavy Menstrual Bleeding (HMB)		
Hematologic	von Willebrand disease	Factor VII defect causing impaired platelet adhesion and increased bleeding time
	Idiopathic thrombocytopenic purpura	Decrease in circulating platelets, can be acute or chronic
Hepatic	Cirrhosis	Decreased estrogen metabolism, underlying coagulopathy
Endocrine	Hypothyroidism	Alterations in the HPO axis
Uterine	Fibroids	Alteration of endometrium, changes in uterine contractility
	Adenomyosis	Alteration of endometrium, changes in uterine contractility
	Endometrial polyps	Alteration of endometrium
	Gynecologic cancers	Various dysplastic alterations of endometrium, uterus, cervix

FHA, functional hypothalamic amenorrhea; FSH, follicle-stimulating hormone; GnRH, gonadotropin-releasing hormone; HPO, hypothalamic–pituitary–ovarian axis; LH, luteinizing hormone; PCOS, polycystic ovary syndrome; TSH, thyroid-stimulating hormone; TRH, thyrotropin-releasing hormone.

Data from References 4-9, 12, and 17.

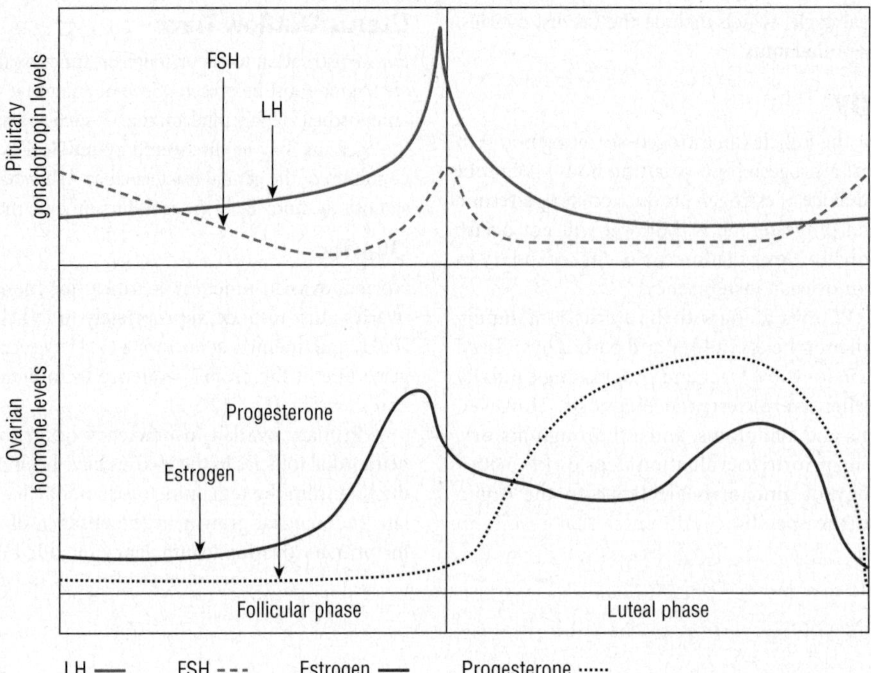

FIGURE 100-1 Hormonal fluctuations with the normal menstrual cycle. (FSH, follicle-stimulating hormone; LH, luteinizing hormone.)

genetic anomalies,[9] autoimmunity, and iatrogenic causes as a result of radiation or chemotherapy.[11] However, in 90% of cases, the cause cannot be identified.[9]

Pituitary Gland

The anterior pituitary gland secretes FSH and LH in sequential fashion in response to hypothalamic stimulation and a complex ovarian feedback mechanism. Normal secretion of FSH and LH is altered by several endocrinologic and iatrogenic conditions, including thyroid disease, hyperprolactinemia, and dopaminergic medication administration.

Hypothalamus

The hypothalamus secretes cyclic gonadotropin-releasing hormone (GnRH), which causes the pituitary to produce FSH and LH. Disrupting this cyclic process interrupts the hormonal cascade that results in normal menstruation. Anorexia nervosa, bulimia, intense exercise, and stress may cause hypothalamic amenorrhea, known as functional hypothalamic amenorrhea (FHA). Further, research has confirmed the role of leptin insufficiency in causing hypogonadotropic hypogonadism leading to hypothalamic amenorrhea.[12]

TREATMENT

Desired Outcomes

In general, the treatment options for amenorrhea depend on its causes. Therapeutic modalities for amenorrhea should ensure the occurrence of normal puberty and restore the menstrual cycle. Treatment goals include bone density preservation, bone loss prevention, and ovulation restoration to improve fertility if desired. Hypoestrogenism may affect quality of life via hot flash induction (premature ovarian failure), dyspareunia, and, in prepubertal females, lack of secondary sexual characteristics and absence of menarche. Treatment is targeted at reversing these effects.

General Approach to Treatment

The overall success of any intervention to treat amenorrhea depends on proper identification of the disorder's underlying cause(s). Once the cause is identified, the appropriate intervention(s) can be made. For patients experiencing amenorrhea secondary to hypoestrogenic states, a diet rich in calcium and vitamin D is essential to minimize any negative impact on bone health.

Nonpharmacologic Therapy

Nonpharmacologic therapy for amenorrhea varies depending upon the underlying cause. Amenorrhea secondary to anorexia may respond to weight gain. In young individuals for whom excessive exercise is an underlying cause, reduction of exercise quantity and intensity are important. Evaluation for a possible eating disorder may be appropriate (see Chapter e83 "Eating Disorders," for more information). Cognitive behavioral therapy has been shown to restore ovarian function in individuals with FHA.[13] In 2017, the Endocrine Society Clinical Practice Guideline recommended a reasonable trial of psychological, nutrition, and/or modified exercise intervention prior to use of pharmacotherapy in patients with FHA.[14] In medication-induced hyperprolactinemia (Table 100-2),[15] the clinician may consider alternative agents that do not inhibit dopamine receptors or increase prolactin levels.

TABLE 100-2 Medications That May Induce Hyperprolactinemia

Medication Class	Agents
First-generation antipsychotics	Phenothiazines (eg, prochlorperazine, chlorpromazine)
	Butyrophenones (eg, haloperidol)
	Thioxanthenes (eg, chlorprothixene)
Second-generation antipsychotics	Risperidone
	Molindone
Antidepressants	Clomipramine
Monoamine oxidase inhibitors	Pargyline
	Clorgyline
Antihypertensives	Verapamil
Gastrointestinal promotility agents	Metoclopramide
	Domperidone

Data from Reference 15.

Pharmacologic Therapy

2 For hypoestrogenic conditions associated with primary or secondary amenorrhea, historically estrogen has been supplemented as an oral contraceptive, conjugated equine estrogen, or estradiol patch, in conjunction with progestin in an attempt to decrease osteoporosis risk. However, data supporting estrogen supplementation in FHA are based on a limited number of studies with small sample size and short follow-ups.[16] Therefore, the primary approach for FHA should be the correction of energy balance to restore HPO axis function.[16] The 2017 Endocrine Society Clinical Practice Guideline for FHA recommends the short-term use of transdermal estradiol with cyclic oral progestins, after an adequate trial of nonpharmacological therapy (eg, psychological and nutritional intervention).[14] Combined hormonal contraceptives (CHC) and synthetic ethinyl estradiol are no longer recommended as first-line agents for patients with FHA.[14] However, CHCs are also useful for pregnancy prevention, treatment of acne, and other conditions in this population.[14] For individuals with primary ovarian insufficiency, a prospective study with estradiol 100 mcg/day transdermal patch suggested improvement in bone mineral density to normal population values.[17] Table 100-3 lists therapeutic agents for amenorrhea treatment, including recommended doses. Figure 100-2 illustrates a treatment algorithm for the management of amenorrhea.

TABLE 100-3 Therapeutic Agents for Selected Menstrual Disorders

Specific Menstrual Disorder(s)	Agent(s)	Brand Name(s)	Usual Recommended Dose
Amenorrhea (primary or secondary)	CEE	Premarin, Cenestin, Enjuvia	0.625-1.25 mg by mouth daily on days 1-25 of the cycle
	Ethinyl estradiol patch	Alora, Climara, Vivelle-Dot	50 mcg/24 hr
	CHC	Various	30-40 mcg formulations
Amenorrhea (secondary)	Oral MPA	Provera	5-10 mg my mouth daily for 5 to 10 days
	Progesterone vaginal gel	Crinone	1.125 g of 4% gel intravaginally every other day for 6 doses; if no response, increase to 8% gel for 6 doses
	Norethindrone	Aygestin	2.5-10mg by mouth daily for 5-10 days
	Micronized progesterone	Prometrium	400mg by mouth daily at bedtime for 10 days
Amenorrhea related to hyperprolactinemia	Bromocriptine	Parlodel, Cycloset	2.5-15 mg daily in 2 to 3 divided doses
	Cabergoline	Dostinex	0.25-2 mg by mouth once weekly or in 2 divided doses
Anovulatory bleeding	CHC	Cyred 28, Emoquette 28, Yasmin 28, Yaz, Beyaz, and others	≤35 mcg ethinyl estradiol
Dysmenorrhea	CHC	Examples include: Norgestrel containing: Cryselle 28, Low-Ogestrel, Levonorgestrel containing: Levora 28, Camrese, Aviane 28, Lessina 28 Other progestins: Sprintec 28, Yasmin 28, Yaz Extended-cycle: Introvale, Setlakin, Seasonique, LoSeasonique	<35 mcg formulations; use of extended-cycle formulations may be beneficial for this indication
	Injectable MPA	Depo-Provera, Depo-SubQ Provera 104	150 mg intramuscularly or 104 mg subcutaneously every 12 weeks
	LNG-IUS	Mirena	20 mcg released daily
	NSAIDs (any are acceptable); the most commonly studied/cited are included in this table	Ibuprofen (Motrin, Advil)	Ibuprofen 800 mg by mouth initially, followed by 400-800 mg every 8 hr as needed
		Naproxen (Naprosyn)	Naproxen 440-550 mg by mouth initially, followed by 220-550 mg every 12 hr as needed
		Mefanamic acid	500 mg by mouth initially, followed by 250 mg every 6 hr as needed
		Celecoxib (Celebrex)	400 mg by mouth initially, followed by 200 mg every 12 hr as needed
Heavy menstrual bleeding	CHC	Various: estradiol valerate/dienogest (Natazia)	1 tablet daily in the order presented in the blister pack
	LNG-IUS	Mirena	20 mcg released daily
	Oral MPA	Provera	5-10 mg by mouth on days 5-26 of the cycle or during the luteal phase
	Tranexamic acid	Lysteda	1,300 mg by mouth every 8 hr once heavy bleeding begins; dose for 4-7 days as needed per cycle
Heavy menstrual bleeding associated with uterine fibroids	Elagolix/estradiol/norethindrone acetate plus elagolix	Oriahnn	Elagolix 300 mg/estradiol 1 mg/norethindrone acetate 0.5 mg in the morning and elagolix 300 mg in the evening for up to 24 months

(continued)

TABLE 100-3 Therapeutic Agents for Selected Menstrual Disorders *(Continued)*

Specific Menstrual Disorder(s)	Agent(s)	Brand Name(s)	Usual Recommended Dose
PCOS-related amenorrhea and/or AUB-O	Injectable MPA, CHC	Depo-Provera, Depo-SubQ Provera 104 Desogestrel containing: Cyred 28, Cred EQ 28 Norgestimate containing: Tri-Lo Sprintec Drospirenone containing: Yasmin 28, Yaz, Beyaz	150 mg intramuscularly or 104 mg subcutaneously every 12 weeks ≤30 mcg ethinyl estradiol with either desogestrel, norgestimate, or drospirenone
	Oral MPA	Provera	10 mg by mouth for 10 days
	Metformin	Glumetza	1,500-2,000 mg by mouth daily
PMDD	Clomipramine	Anafranil	25-75 mg by mouth daily taken either continuously or only during the luteal phase
	Drospirenone	Yasmin 28, Yaz, Beyaz	3 mg (+ ≤30 mcg ethinyl estradiol) by mouth on days 1-21 of the menstrual cycle
	Leuprolide	Lupron Depot	3.75 mg intramuscularly
PMDD	SSRIs	Citalopram, escitalopram, fluoxetine (Sarafem or Prozac), paroxetine, sertraline	Citalopram 10-30 mg; escitalopram 10-20 mg; fluoxetine 10-20 mg; fluvoxamine 50 mg; paroxetine 10-30 mg; sertraline 25-150 mg; all agents are given by mouth daily and can be dosed either continuously or during the luteal phase only
	SNRIs	Venlafaxine (IR and XR), duloxetine	Venlafaxine 50-200 mg, can be dosed continuously or during the luteal phase only; duloxetine 60 mg dosed continuously

CEE, conjugated equine estrogen; LNG-IUS, levonorgestrel intrauterine system; MPA, medroxyprogesterone acetate; NSAID, nonsteroidal anti-inflammatory drug; CHC, combined hormonal contraceptive; PCOS, polycystic ovary syndrome; PMDD, premenstrual dysphoric disorder; SSRI, selective serotonin reuptake inhibitors; SNRI, serotonin–norepinephrine reuptake inhibitors.

Data from References 3, 4, 7, 8, 14, and 18-36.

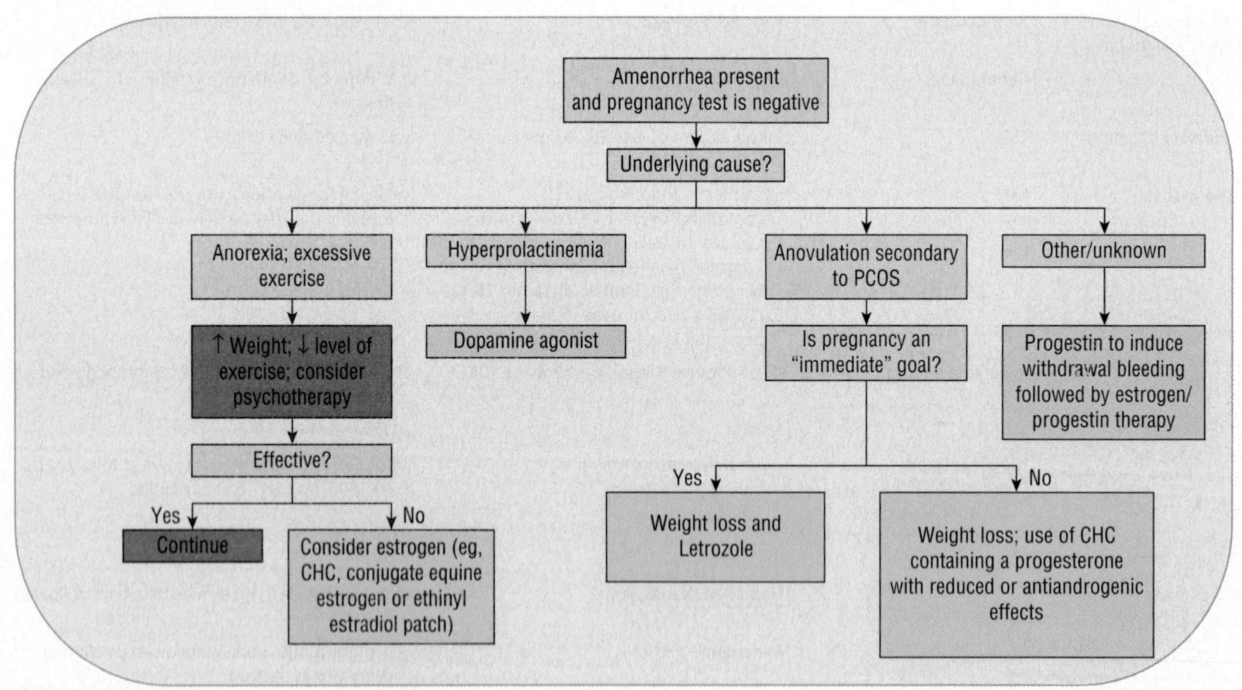

FIGURE 100-2 Treatment algorithm for amenorrhea. (CHC, combined hormonal contraceptive; PCOS, polycystic ovary syndrome.)

When hyperprolactinemia is the cause of amenorrhea, dopamine agonists such as bromocriptine and cabergoline aid in reducing prolactin concentrations and the resumption of menses. Bromocriptine normalizes prolactin levels in 58% of affected patients, while cabergoline has the same effect in 85%.[14]

Progestins induce withdrawal bleeding in those with secondary amenorrhea. Absence of withdrawal bleeding after a progestin challenge may suggest outflow tract obstruction or insufficient endometrial estrogen exposure.[14]

Progestin efficacy for secondary amenorrhea varies by formulation used. Progesterone in oil administered intramuscularly results in withdrawal bleeding in 70% of treated patients, whereas oral medroxyprogesterone acetate (MPA) induces withdrawal bleeding in 95% of treated patients.[37] Table 100-3 identifies the types and doses of progestins used for secondary amenorrhea treatment, and Fig. 100-2 illustrates when to consider progestin use for amenorrhea treatment.

Amenorrhea related to PCOS-induced anovulation is discussed subsequently in the "abnormal uterine bleeding" section.

Adolescents

Amenorrhea in the adolescent population is of concern because developmentally this is the time when peak bone mass is achieved. The cause of amenorrhea, whether primary or secondary, must be promptly identified, as amenorrhea and its related hypoestrogenism negatively affect bone development. In addition to treating or eliminating amenorrhea's underlying cause, ensuring that the patient is receiving adequate amounts of calcium and vitamin D is imperative. Estrogen replacement is important for bone health.

Evaluation of Therapeutic Outcomes

Table 100-4 identifies the mechanisms of action, expected outcomes, and monitoring parameters for pharmacologic agents used for amenorrhea management.

HEAVY MENSTRUAL BLEEDING

Epidemiology

Heavy menstrual bleeding (HMB) is the term now used in place of menorrhagia.[41] The classical definition, however, remains the same: menstrual blood loss greater than 80 mL per cycle or menstrual bleeding lasting greater than 7 days per cycle.[38] This definition has been questioned because of difficulty quantifying menstrual loss in clinical practice. Additionally, many individuals with "heavy menses" but whose blood loss is less than 80 mL merit treatment consideration because of flow containment issues, unpredictably heavy flow days, or other associated symptoms.[23,42] Diagnosis has also been considered based upon the impact of HMB on quality of life and social, professional, familial, or sexual roles.

HMB is one of the most commonly encountered gynecological problems, accounting for 18% to 30% of gynecologic visits.[25] HMB affects an individual's physical, psychological, and social function. The amount of blood loss may make it impractical or embarrassing to leave home for fear of soiling outer garments, leading to decreased work productivity and limited social activities.[25]

Etiology

3 4 The International Federation of Gynecology and Obstetrics Menstrual Disorders Working Group created the PALM-COEIN classification system to define the causes of abnormal uterine bleeding (AUB).[43] The PALM group of classification includes structural causes of AUB: **P**olyp, **A**denomyosis (endometrial tissue within the myometrium), **L**eiomyoma (also known as Fibroids), and **M**alignancy.[43] The COEIN components include nonstructural causes: **C**oagulopathy, **O**vulatory disorders, and **E**ndometrial disorders, **I**atrogenic causes and **N**ot classified.[43] Combined the PALM-COEIN classification also characterizes intermenstrual bleeding as bleeding that occurs between predictable and clearly cyclic menses, while AUB is defined as bleeding that is abnormal in either regularity, timing, or volume.[25,43] Under these definitions, HMB specifically refers to an abnormally excessive volume of menstrual bleeding that affects the individual's quality of life. Causes of HMB may include AUB due to polyps (AUB-P), adenomyosis (AUB-A), leiomyoma (AUB-L), as well as nonstructural causes such as coagulopathy (AUB-C), and endometrial dysfunction (AUB-E).[25] Pregnancy, including intrauterine pregnancy, ectopic pregnancy, and miscarriage, must be at the top of the differential diagnosis list for any patient presenting with heavy menses.[12] Bleeding disorders including von Willebrand disease, symptomatic hemophilia, platelet dysfunction, and Factor VIII and IX deficiencies must also be considered as these were found to exist in 20% of patients with HMB.[19] Hypothyroidism also may be associated with heavy menses.[19,41] Additionally, uterine structural abnormalities, such as polyps, adenomyosis, and leiomyoma, are not uncommon in those with HMB,[25] with fibroids, specifically, being identified in as many as 40% of patients with HMB.[28]

Pathophysiology

HMB may be the result of one of several very diverse causes including hematologic, hepatic, endocrine, and/or uterine disorders. Table 100-1 lists the pathophysiology of HMB relative to the organ system(s) involved and the specific conditions that may result in HMB.

TREATMENT

Desired Outcomes

The primary goal of treatment for HMB is to reduce menstrual flow. Along with this, treatments should be initiated to improve the patient's quality of life, and defer the need for surgical intervention.

General Approach to Treatment

As several treatment options exist for HMB, the choice regarding which specific agent to use depends on the patient's treatment history, concomitant concerns, and the adverse medication effect profile for the various agents.

Nonpharmacologic Therapy

Nonpharmacologic interventions for HMB include surgical procedures generally reserved for patients not responding to pharmacologic treatment. These interventions vary from conservative endometrial ablation to hysterectomy.[25,42]

Pharmacologic Therapy

While surgical treatment may be an option for HMB, effective medical treatments are recommended as the initial treatment choice. Estrogen is the recommended treatment for managing acute severe bleeding episodes in patient's without suspected or known bleeding disorders.[44] Following its initial use to control acute bleeding episodes, therapy continuation may be necessary to prevent future occurrences. Both estrogen-containing CHCs and progestin-only regimens can be used for maintenance therapy.[25] Although it is assumed that all CHCs will reduce menstrual blood loss, the only agent that has been FDA approved is a combination of estradiol valerate and dienogest.[25] Table 100-2 identifies the variety of pharmacologic treatment options and their recommended dosing for HMB management.

Among the agents used to treat HMB, the nonsteroidal anti-inflammatory drugs (NSAIDs) have the advantage of administration only during menses and are associated with a 10% to 51% reduction in blood loss.[25] For individual's desiring to avoid pregnancy, CHC should be considered as a 30% to 60% reduction in menstrual blood loss has been observed.[25] The 1-year continuation rates of CHCs in individuals with HMB range from 72% to 84%.[25] The best studied CHC option for HMB and the only agent approved by the FDA for the indication of HMB is the four-phasic formulation containing estradiol valerate and dienogest.[24,25]

For those with contraindications to CHCs, progestin-only methods induce amenorrhea and reduce menstrual blood loss.[25] Cyclic progesterone therapy for 14 days, administered as oral norethindrone acetate or medroxyprogesterone acetate, reduces

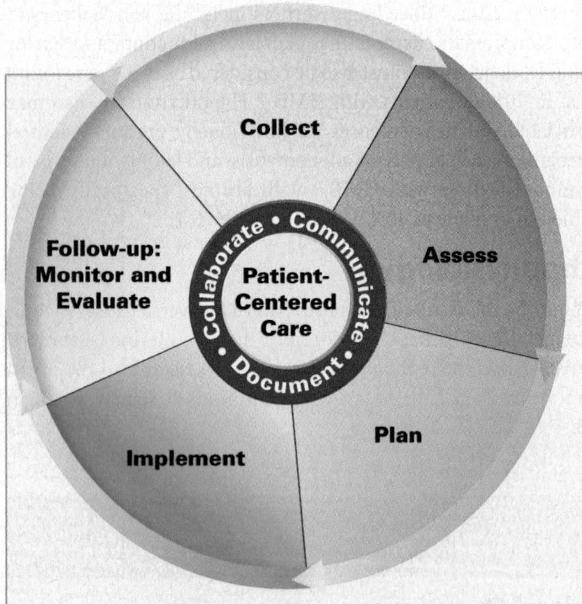

Patient Care Process for Menstruation-Related Disorders

The image shows the five fundamental steps included in The Pharmacist's Care Process endorsed by the Joint Commission for Pharmacy Practitioners (2014). The tagline of this process reads collaborate, communicate, and document. The five fundamental steps listed here are collect, assess, plan, implement, and follow-up: monitor and evaluate. All these steps are listed in a circular block diagram.

Collect

- Patient characteristics (age)
- Patient medical history
    - First day of the last menstrual cycle
    - Age of menarche
    - Cycle length and predictability
    - Number of days of each menstrual cycle, and the number of absorbent products used per day
    - History of current symptoms including relationship with menstrual cycles
    - Menstrual diary and recorded symptoms
- Social history (eg, tobacco/ethanol use), dietary and physical activity habits (especially for those with PCOS)
- Current medications including over-the-counter (OTC) nonsteroidal anti-inflammatory drug (NSAID) use, herbal products, and dietary supplements
- Objective data
    - Blood pressure (BP), heart rate (HR), respiratory rate (RR), height, weight
    - Labs depend on suspected underlying conditions. Common labs include follicle-stimulating hormone (FSH) and thyroid-stimulating hormone (TSH) (see Table 100-1). Total and free testosterone, other androgen precursors, glucose tolerance test, and fasting lipids may be obtained if PCOS is suspected. If anemia associated with heavy menstrual bleeding is suspected, obtain CBC with differential.

Assess

- Presence of severe anemia or acute bleeding that necessitates immediate treatment
- Presence of suicidal ideation associated with premenstrual dysphoric disorder that necessitates immediate psychiatric evaluation and treatment
- Whether the patient desires contraception or is attempting pregnancy
- Comorbid conditions that may affect treatment choice (eg, a nonestrogen-containing regimen should be considered in a patient with a history of deep venous thrombosis, and NSAID should not be an initial choice for a patient with a history of GI bleed)
- Acceptability of available treatment choice to the patient

Plan*

- Pharmacotherapy regimen including specific agent(s), dose, route, frequency, and duration (see Table 100-3)
- Monitoring parameters including efficacy and safety (see Table 100-4)
- Patient education (eg, purpose of treatment, dietary and lifestyle modification, invasive procedures, medication-specific information)
- Referrals to other providers when appropriate (eg, thrombosis specialist to evaluate bleeding disorders, behavioral health, dietician)

Implement*

- Provide patient education regarding all elements of the treatment plan
- Use motivational interviewing and coaching strategies to maximize adherence in lifestyle interventions for individuals with PCOS

Follow-up: Monitor and Evaluate*

- Resolution of symptoms
- Presence of adverse effects
- Patient adherence to treatment plan using multiple sources of information
- Reevaluate therapy as life goals change (eg, changing from desiring contraception to desiring fertility)

Collaborate with patient, caregivers, and other healthcare professionals.

menstrual blood loss in only 2% to 30% of patients.[25] However, when administered as long course (for 21 days, starting on day 5 after onset of menses), they reduce menstrual blood loss in 63% to 78% of patients.[25]

Another progestin-only treatment option for HMB is the levonorgestrel-releasing intrauterine system (LNG-IUS). This is considered the most effective treatment to reduce menstrual flow.[25] In particular, a 70% to 96% reduction in blood loss has been observed with its use,[25] and its use has also resulted in postponing or canceling scheduled endometrial ablation surgery or hysterectomy.[40] Among those using this treatment option, only 9% eventually opted for surgery.[40] Further, its therapeutic

CLINICAL PRESENTATION Heavy Menstrual Bleeding

General

- Patients may or may not be in acute distress.

Symptoms

- Patients may complain of heavy/prolonged menstrual flow. They also may have signs of fatigue and lightheadedness in cases of severe blood loss. These symptoms may or may not occur with dysmenorrhea.

Signs

- Orthostasis, tachycardia, and pallor may be noted in cases of significant anemia or acute blood loss.

Laboratory Tests

- Complete blood count and ferritin levels; hemoglobin and hematocrit results may be low.
- If the history dictates, testing (eg, prothrombin time, activated partial thromboplastin time, international normalized ratio, von Willebrand factor antigen, Factor VIII, factor IX activity) may be performed to identify coagulation disorder(s) as a cause.

Other Diagnostic Tests

- Pelvic ultrasound
- Pelvic magnetic resonance imaging
- Papanicolaou (Pap) smear
- Endometrial biopsy
- Hysteroscopy
- Sonohysterogram

efficacy is similar to endometrial ablation up to 2 years following treatment.[29]

Tranexamic acid is also approved in the United States for primary HMB treatment. Its use is associated with 34% to 56% reduction in menstrual blood loss.[25] Compared to many of the other options, its use may be preferable among those desiring pregnancy or in whom hormonal therapy may not be appropriate.

5 For individuals in whom pregnancy is not an immediate goal, it is reasonable to start with either a CHC or the LNG-IUS. While either choice is acceptable for both nulligravid and multiparous patients who desire a long-term reversible form of contraception, cost-effectiveness data suggest LNG-IUS is the best first-line choice for those desiring contraception.[28,42] Clinical trial data illustrate a higher failure rate with the oral CHCs (32%) compared to the LNG-IUS (11%) as the primary treatment method.[28] When compared to other conventional medical therapies used for HMB, the LNG-IUS is associated with a 61% lower discontinuation rate and 82% fewer treatment failures.[26]

For those who have HMB associated with ovulatory cycles and do not desire hormonal therapy and/or contraception, NSAIDs during menses is a reasonable choice in the absence of any contraindications or GI disorders such as peptic ulcer disease or gastroesophageal reflux disease. This choice is convenient (only taken during menses) and comparatively inexpensive. Given their adverse effects, reduced efficacy compared to the first-line agents, and/or cost, use of oral progesterone, and depot MPA should be reserved. Tranexamic acid is another treatment option that can be taken only during menses.[25] Figure 100-3 presents an algorithm for HMB treatment.

For patients with HMB associated with uterine fibroids a new oral agent, Elagolix/estradiol/norethindrone acetate and elagolix (Oriahnn), was approved in June 2020.[44] Elagolix is a novel non-peptide oral, short-acting gonadotropin-releasing hormone (GnRH) receptor antagonist dosed as one capsule containing elagolix 300 mg, estradiol 1 mg, and norethindrone 0.5 mg in the morning and one capsule containing elagolix 300 mg in the evening.[45,46] Based on data from phase three clinical trials, subgroup analyses, and extension studies, it is reasonable to consider Elagolix/estradiol/norethindrone acetate and elagolix as an oral option for the management of HMB associated with uterine fibroids.[46-48] There are some clinical relevant safety considerations that may limit the use of this agent in some patient populations. One of the primary concerns is the risk of potentially irreversible BMD loss due to estrogen blockade.[45] As a result, use should be limited to 24 months. It is also contraindicated in individuals with existing cardiovascular disease or at high risk of a cardiovascular event.[45] Individuals taking this medication must also utilize non-hormonal contraception for the duration of treatment, as pregnancy is contraindicated with therapy.[45,46]

Special Populations 6 Although it was believed IUS use should be avoided in nulliparous patients, guidelines from the American College of Obstetricians and Gynecologists (ACOG) indicate that both multiparous and nulliparous females (including adolescents) at low risk of sexually transmitted infections are good candidates for intrauterine system (IUS) use.[49] Therefore, any of the treatments discussed (including the LNG-IUS) are options in those presenting with HMB.

Dosage adjustment for tranexamic acid is recommended for reduced renal function. Patients with serum creatinine between 1.4 and 2.8 mg/dL (124 and 252 μmol/L) should receive only 1,300 mg by mouth twice daily; those with serum creatinine between 2.9 and 5.7 mg/dL (253 and 504 μmol/L) should receive 1,300 mg by mouth once daily; those with serum creatinine above 5.7 mg/dL (504 μmol/L) should receive 650 mg by mouth once daily. Additionally, due to its potential to increase the risk for venous thromboembolism, it should be used with extreme caution in individuals with a history of thrombosis and should not be combined with estrogen-containing contraceptives.[25]

Evaluation of Therapeutic Outcomes

Table 100-4 identifies the significant pharmacologic properties of agents used for the management of HMB, the expected outcomes for each agent, and specific monitoring parameters for the treatment modalities used in HMB management.

PREMENSTRUAL SYNDROME AND PREMENSTRUAL DYSPHORIC DISORDER

Epidemiology

Premenstrual syndrome (PMS) is represented by a cyclic pattern of symptoms (Table 100-5) occurring in the late luteal phase of the

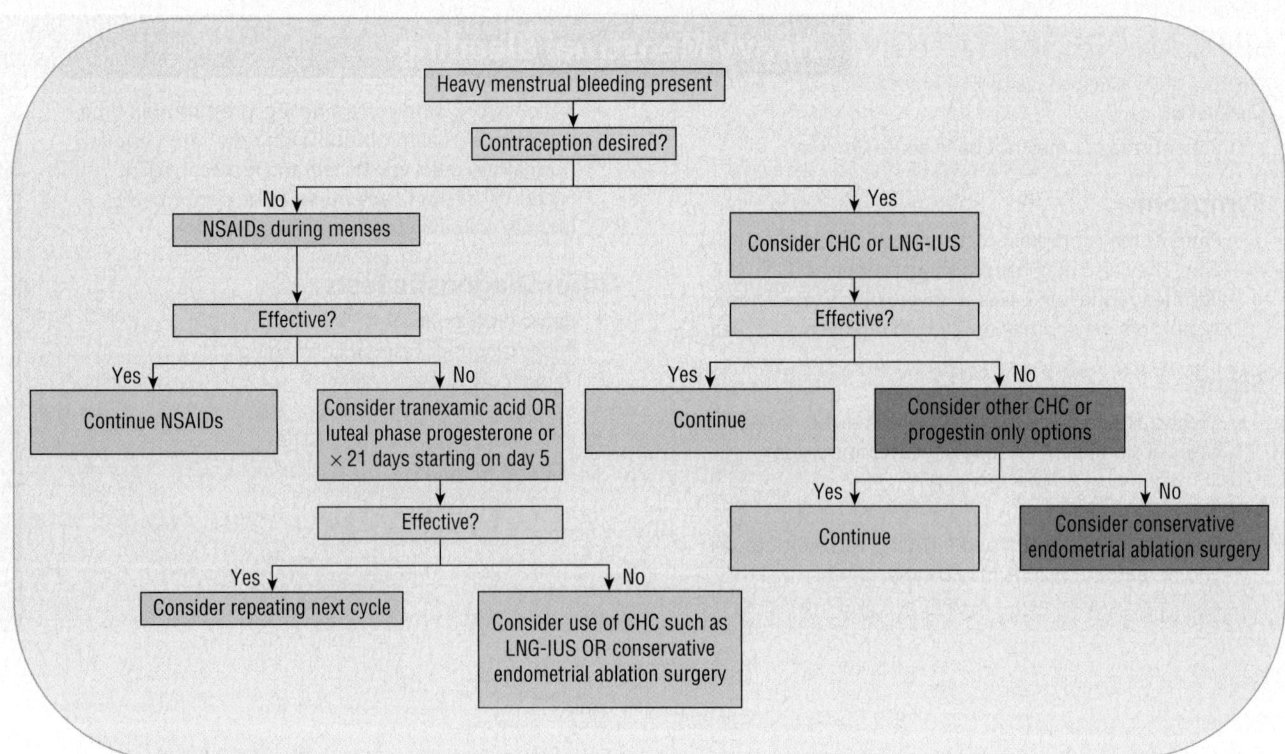

FIGURE 100-3 Treatment algorithm for HMB. (CHC, combined hormonal contraceptive; LNG-IUS, levonorgestrel-releasing intrauterine system; NSAIDs, nonsteroidal anti-inflammatory drugs.)

menstrual cycle that resolve at the onset of menses. Up to 80% of menstruating patients experience PMS symptoms.[31] However, most do not report impairment of their daily activities.[31] There have been over 100 symptoms reported by patients with PMS and they will often present differently, thus requiring an individualized treatment plan. Charting symptoms is helpful for the patient and clinician to identify the symptoms, severity, and patterns in which they occur as well as response to treatment. Diagnosis requires that at least one moderate-to-severe somatic or psychiatric symptom is present in the last week of the luteal phase for at least 3 months.[32,50]

Some patients experience severe mood symptoms known as premenstrual dysphoric disorder (PMDD). This is a mood-related condition recognized by the *Diagnostic and Statistical Manual, 5th edition* (*DSM-5*; see diagnostic criteria) and can have significant impact on a patient's quality of life, productivity and interpersonal relationships. The prevalence of PMDD ranges from 1.3% to 9%.[32,50]

Individuals experiencing PMS and PMDD symptoms miss significantly more work and school compared to those without PMS or PMDD. They also report significant impairment of their ability to participate in social activities, hobbies, and in their relationships with others, as well having a lower health-related quality of life and higher medical expenses.[32]

An exact PMS prevalence is difficult to ascertain, because symptoms and severity tend to fluctuate.

Etiology

While it is unclear why PMS occurs, there are theories. First, it is thought that patients with PMS have an underlying neurological vulnerability to the normal cyclic hormonal fluctuations that occur during the menstrual cycle. When ovulation is suppressed medically or surgically, symptoms usually improve. It is thought that abnormal serotonergic function plays a role with mood related symptoms and cravings as well as PMDD.[51]

Pathophysiology

According to some evidence PMS and PMDD symptoms are related to low levels of the centrally active progesterone metabolite allopregnanolone in the luteal phase and/or lower cortical γ-aminobutyric acid levels in the follicular phase.[51] A number of studies suggest a link between PMS and PMDD and low serotonin levels.[51] Although several cross-cultural studies suggest PMS physical symptoms are consistent across cultures, the negative affective symptoms are part of the negative "menstrual socialization" in western culture.[51]

TREATMENT

Desired Outcome

Treatment of PMS and PMDD attempts to relieve psychiatric and somatic symptoms through ovulation suppression, or through affecting neurotransmitter (eg, serotonin, norepinephrine, or dopamine) concentrations in the brain.[32] Therefore, PMS and PMDD interventions should alleviate the presenting symptoms and subsequently improve quality of life. Table 100-3 lists the various agents used in managing PMS and PMDD and their recommended dosing.

General Approach to Treatment

A treatment modality that is minimally invasive or without systemic effects is desired for initial therapy. Key to the successful choice of pharmacologic therapy for PMS and PMDD is having the patient chart their specific symptoms for at least two menstrual cycles to

CLINICAL PRESENTATION Premenstrual Dysphoric Disorder

A summary of the American Psychiatric Association's *Diagnostic and Statistical Manual of Mental Disorders, Fifth Edition (DSM-5)* criteria for PMDD is as follows[74]:

- Symptoms are temporally associated with the last week of the luteal phase and remit with the onset of menses.
- At least five of the following symptoms are present: affective lability, anger, or irritability often characterized by interpersonal conflicts, markedly depressed mood, anxiety, decreased interest in activities, fatigue, difficulty concentrating, changes in appetite, sleep disturbance, feelings of being overwhelmed, and physical symptoms, such as breast tenderness or bloating.
- One of the symptoms must be affective lability, irritability, markedly depressed mood, or anxiety.
- Symptoms interfere significantly with work and/or social relationships.
- Symptoms are not an exacerbation of another underlying psychiatric disorder.
- The criteria are confirmed prospectively by daily ratings over two menstrual cycles and must have occurred during most menstrual cycles in the past year.

assist in ruling out premenstrual exacerbation of underlying psychiatric disorders.

Nonpharmacological Therapy

Some lifestyle changes for the management of mild-to-moderate premenstrual symptoms include minimizing intake of caffeine, refined sugar, and sodium and increasing exercise.[33] Although exercise appears to improve PMS symptoms, definitive, evidence-based recommendations cannot be made due to methodological limitations of these studies.[33] Vitamin and mineral supplements, such as vitamin B_6 (50-100 mg daily) and calcium carbonate (1,200 mg daily), may help to reduce the physical symptoms associated with PMS; however, clinical trial data is limited and/or mixed precluding a definitive conclusion regarding their use.[33] Cognitive behavioral therapy has also been studied showing moderate efficacy.[33] However, the frequency and duration therapy have not been defined. Nonetheless, acceptance-based cognitive behavior therapy and mindfulness-based exercises may be helpful in reducing symptoms.[32] A Cochrane review of herbal supplements for PMS, including angelica root, bitter orange, dragon's teeth, ginkgo, peppermint, saffron, turmeric, tangerine leaf, and vitex agnus-castus, among others, do not support their use.[52,53] Although acupuncture and acupressure appear to improve physical and psychological symptoms of PMS, evidence was from limited sample sizes and of low quality.[54]

Pharmacologic Therapy

Investigations have focused on the selective serotonin reuptake inhibitors (SSRIs) for this disorder.[34] Studies have revealed positive results relative to most symptoms associated with PMDD. Other agents that have been studied and are alternatives include the selective serotonin–norepinephrine reuptake inhibitor (SNRI) venlafaxine, as well as CHCs and GnRH agonists.

Among SSRIs, data support the use of citalopram, escitalopram, fluoxetine, fluvoxamine, paroxetine, and sertraline for the treatment of severe mood-related symptoms of PMS and PMDD.[32,33] Research evaluating the dosing of these agents continuously or only during the luteal phase (ie, days 14-28 of the menstrual cycle) has illustrated similar efficacy between the two regimens, such that one cannot be recommended over another although more studies directly comparing continuous versus luteal phase administration are needed.[32,33] Treatment decisions will often be based on patient preference as some prefer continuous dosing so they do not have to track their cycle as closely, whereas some prefer just taking the medication during the luteal phase to minimize medication exposure. Interestingly, when used in PMDD, antidepressants tend to be very effective and have a faster onset than what is typically seen in the treatment of major depression. Most medication adverse effects also appear to be similar between continuous and luteal dosing, except decreased libido which occurs at a higher rate with continuous dosing.[33] In addition, abrupt cessation of SSRI at the end of the menstrual cycle is not associated with discontinuation symptoms.[35] All SSRI doses appear to be effective for psychiatric symptoms, and should be titrated to individual patients' symptom improvement and tolerability.[32] The safety of SSRIs use during early pregnancy has been an active area of investigation. In a large-scale analysis, reassuring evidence was provided for some SSRIs, but birth defects (including anencephaly, atrial septal defects, right ventricular outflow tract obstruction, and gastroschisis) can be 2 to 3.5 times more frequent with paroxetine or fluoxetine use in early pregnancy.[55]

The SNRI, venlafaxine, has been studied for PMDD and, similar to the SSRIs, found to result in a 50% or greater improvement in symptoms in 60% of treated patients compared with only 35% in the control group.[33] The norepinephrine and dopamine reuptake inhibitor, bupropion, has not been proven effective for PMS or PMDD.[32]

It is important that concomitant pharmacotherapy be evaluated closely for pharmacokinetic interactions when an SSRI or venlafaxine is prescribed, given the interface of these medications with cytochrome P450 isoenzyme systems. Additional information regarding antidepressant dosing, adverse medication effects, pharmacokinetics, and medication interactions can be found in Chapter 88, "Depressive Disorders."

The use of a monophasic oral CHC containing 20 mcg of ethinyl estradiol and 3 mg of drospirenone, a progesterone with antiandrogenic effects, improves premenstrual symptoms in persons with PMDD, and is FDA approved for this indication.[33] The continuous cycle CHC regimen delivering 90 mcg of levonorgestrel and 20 mcg of ethinyl estradiol daily has also been studied in controlled trials resulting in a 30% to 59% improvement in PMDD symptoms.[36] For PMS symptoms, in a large-scale study, both triphasic and monophasic CHCs led to reduction in physical symptoms but not mood symptoms.[33] Superiority of one CHC relative to another has not been established.

If treatment with the above options is unsuccessful, hormonal treatment with a GnRH agonist, such as leuprolide, can be considered.[33] Leuprolide improves premenstrual emotional symptoms as well as some physical symptoms, such as bloating and breast tenderness. However, its cost, the need for intramuscular administration, and its hypoestrogenism effects (eg, vaginal dryness, hot flashes, and bone demineralization) severely limit its use.[35] Table 100-4 lists the significant pharmacologic properties for agents used to treat PMDD that require monitoring.

TABLE 100-4 Pharmacologic Properties and Monitoring Parameters for Select Agents or Classes of Medications Used in the Management of Menstrual Disorders

Therapeutic Agent or Medication Class	Mechanism of Action/Role in Particular Menstrual Disorders	Adverse Medication Reactions	Monitoring for Expected Outcomes of Specific Menstrual Disorders	Comments
Dopamine agonists (bromocriptine and cabergoline)	Suppresses prolactin production from pituitary tumors such that resumption of normal FSH and LH production occurs	Hypotension, nausea, constipation, anorexia, Raynaud's phenomenon, fatigue, headache	Amenorrhea related to hyperprolactinemia: Baseline and weekly prolactin levels should be measured with dosage increases until resumption of menses is observed. Continue therapy for 6-12 months following return of menses and continued normalization of serum prolactin levels	Inhibits CYP3A4 and is metabolized by CYP3A4 St John's Wort induces CP3A4; coadministration may lead to treatment failure
Tricyclic antidepressants (clomipramine)	PMDD: Exact mechanism unknown	Dry mouth, constipation, fatigue, vertigo, sweating	Reduction in or absence of initial symptoms and improved quality of life within 1-3 menstrual cycles of therapy	
Oral combined hormonal contraception (CHC)	Exogenous estrogen and progesterone that suppresses FSH and LH production and thus inhibits ovulation Can be used to reduce menstrual flow (Heavy menstrual bleeding, dysmenorrhea), and control menstrual cycle (anovulatory bleeding secondary to hypoestrogenism)	Thromboembolism, breast enlargement, breast tenderness, bloating, nausea, GI upset, headache, peripheral edema	Amenorrhea: Resumption of menses within 1-2 months of therapy Anovulatory bleeding: Improvement in pattern of abnormal bleeding within 1-2 months of therapy Dysmenorrhea: Reduction in or absence of pelvic pain within 1-2 months of therapy Heavy menstrual bleeding: Reduction in blood loss with menses over 1-2 months of therapy. Improvement in hemoglobin/hematocrit after 3 months of therapy compared to baseline	St John's Wort contributes to altered menstrual bleeding. Rifampin induces estrogen metabolism, possibly contributing to treatment failure. Sulfa-containing medications may contribute to increased photosensitivity
Conjugated equine estrogen (CEE)	Estrogen replacement for hypoestrogenic states leading to anovulatory bleeding	As noted for oral CHC	Anovulatory bleeding: Improvement in pattern of abnormal bleeding within 1-2 months of therapy	Same as oral CHC
Drospirenone-containing CHCs	Progesterone with antimineralocorticoid and antiandrogenic properties; decreases emotional lability associated with PMDD	As noted for oral CHC; increased risk of hyperkalemia	PCOS-related amenorrhea or anovulatory bleeding: In addition to the improvement in the pattern of abnormal bleeding within 1-2 months of treatment, patients should also experience an improvement in androgen-excess symptoms such as acne/oily skin and hirsutism	Same as oral CHC Coadministration of potassium-sparing diuretics or diets high in potassium may contribute to increased serum potassium concentrations, particularly in patients with renal dysfunction
Ethinyl estradiol transdermal patch	Same as combination oral CHC and CEE	As noted for oral CHC; however, lesser effects on serum cholesterol concentrations because patch avoids first-pass metabolism	Amenorrhea: Resumption of menses within 1-2 months of therapy	Same as oral CHC
Leuprolide	GnRH agent that contributes to suppression of FSH and LH and ultimately a reduction in estrogen and progesterone, inhibiting the normal menstrual cycle/hormonal fluctuations	Hot flashes, night sweats, headache, nausea	PMDD: Improvement in PMDD signs and symptoms within 1-2 months of therapy	
Levonorgestrel intrauterine system (LNG-IUS)	Suppresses FSH and LH and ultimately estrogen and progesterone, inhibiting the usual growth of the endometrium	Irregular menses, amenorrhea	Dysmenorrhea: Reduction in or absence of pelvic pain after 1-2 months of therapy Heavy menstrual bleeding: Reduction in blood loss with menses over 1-2 months of therapy. Improvement in hemoglobin/hematocrit after 3 months of therapy compared to baseline	

(continued)

TABLE 100-4 Pharmacologic Properties and Monitoring Parameters for Select Agents or Classes of Medications Used in the Management of Menstrual Disorders (*Continued*)

Therapeutic Agent or Medication Class	Mechanism of Action/Role in Particular Menstrual Disorders	Adverse Medication Reactions	Monitoring for Expected Outcomes of Specific Menstrual Disorders	Comments
Medroxyprogesterone acetate (MPA) (oral and injectable)	Suppresses FSH and LH and ultimately estrogen and progesterone, inhibiting the usual growth of the endometrium	Edema, anorexia, depression, insomnia, weight gain or loss, increase in serum total and LDL cholesterol, may reduce HDL cholesterol	Dysmenorrhea: Reduction in or absence of pelvic pain after 1-2 months of therapy Heavy menstrual bleeding: Reduction in blood loss with menses over 1-2 months of therapy Improvement in hemoglobin/hematocrit after 3 months of therapy compared to baseline PCOS-related amenorrhea and/or anovulatory bleeding: Resumption of menses over 1-2 courses of therapy	
Metformin	Inhibits hepatic glucose production and increases sensitivity of tissues to insulin, thus reducing insulin resistance	Anorexia, nausea, vomiting, diarrhea, flatulence, lactic acidosis (rare)	PCOS-related amenorrhea and/or anovulatory bleeding: If desired, monitor for ovulation after 3-6 months of therapy	IV contrast dye may increase the risk of lactic acidosis; stop metformin 1 day prior and restart when renal function is normal and stabilized following the IV dye
Nonsteroidal anti-inflammatory drugs (NSAIDs)	Inhibits prostaglandin release that occurs with menses, thus reducing inflammatory response contributing to dysmenorrhea	GI upset, stomach ulcer, nausea, vomiting, heartburn, indigestion, rash, dizziness	Dysmenorrhea: Reduction in or absence of pelvic pain within hours of initiating Heavy menstrual bleeding: Reduction in blood loss with menses over 1-2 months of therapy	
Selective serotonin reuptake inhibitors (SSRIs)	Exact mechanism in PMDD unknown	Sexual dysfunction (reduced libido, anorgasmia), insomnia, sedation, hypersomnia, nausea, diarrhea	Improvement in PMDD signs and symptoms observed within 1-3 months of therapy	
Tranexamic acid	Antifibrinolytic effects by reversibly blocking lysine binding sites on plasminogen, preventing fibrin degradation and a reduction in menstrual blood loss	Nausea, vomiting, diarrhea, dyspepsia	Heavy menstrual bleeding: Reduction in blood loss with menses should be noticeable with the first month of therapy Improvement in hemoglobin/hematocrit after 3 months of therapy compared to baseline	
Venlafaxine	Exact mechanism in PMDD unknown		Improvement in PMDD signs and symptoms observed within 1-3 months of therapy	

CEE, conjugated equine estrogen; FSH, follicle-stimulating hormone; GnRH, gonadotropin-releasing hormone; HDL, high-density lipoprotein; LDL, low-density lipoprotein; LH, luteinizing hormone; LNG-IUS, levonorgestrel intrauterine system; MPA, medroxyprogesterone acetate; NSAID, nonsteroidal anti-inflammatory drug; PMDD, premenstrual dysphoric disorder; SSRI, selective serotonin reuptake inhibitor.

Data from References 8, 10, 11, 18, 23, 26-28, 30-34, and 38-40.

Evaluation of Therapeutic Outcomes

Table 100-4 lists the expected outcomes and specific monitoring parameters for the treatment modalities used in PMDD management.

DYSMENORRHEA

Epidemiology

Dysmenorrhea is one of the most commonly encountered gynecologic complaints and is defined as crampy pelvic pain occurring with or just prior to menses. Primary dysmenorrhea implies pain in the setting of normal pelvic anatomy and physiology, while secondary dysmenorrhea is associated with underlying pelvic pathology.[56,57] Dysmenorrhea prevalence rates vary but range from 16% to 90%, and its presence may be associated with significant interference in work and school attendance.[57] In addition, significant reductions in quality of life and lower overall life satisfaction and contentment ratings have been observed in patients with dysmenorrhea compared to controls.[56] Risk factors include menarche before the age of 12 years, current age less than 30 years, heavy menses, nulliparity, low body mass index, and a history of sexual abuse.[57]

Etiology

For most patients, dysmenorrhea is accompanied by normal ovulatory cycles and normal pelvic anatomy. This is referred to as primary, or functional, dysmenorrhea.[58] Primary dysmenorrhea typically occurs within 6 to 12 months of menarche, when adolescents attain ovulatory cycles.[21] However, in approximately 10% of the adolescents and young adults presenting with painful menses, an underlying anatomic or physiologic cause exists.[57] Comparatively, secondary dysmenorrhea associated with pelvic pathology should be suspected in patients over 30 years of age without a history of dysmenorrhea.[50]

Pathophysiology

The most significant mechanism for primary dysmenorrhea is the release of prostaglandins and leukotrienes into the menstrual fluid, initiating an inflammatory response and vasopressin-mediated vasoconstriction.[19,23] The most common cause of secondary dysmenorrhea is endometriosis. Other causes include current or history of pelvic inflammatory disease, uterine fibroids, Müllerian anomalies, obstructive reproductive tract abnormalities, and adenomyosis leiomyomata.[39,57] Pregnancy and miscarriage must be considered in new-onset dysmenorrhea.

TREATMENT

Desired Outcomes

Initial treatment choice is influenced by whether or not the patient desires pregnancy. Medical management of dysmenorrhea should relieve the pelvic pain, result in reducing lost school and work days, and contribute to an improved quality of life. Table 100-3 identifies the agents used to manage dysmenorrhea and their recommended doses. Figure 100-4 shows a treatment algorithm for dysmenorrhea management. Note that if symptoms persist for 3 to 6 months further work-up for secondary dysmenorrhea is warranted.

General Approach to Treatment

A variety of effective treatment options for dysmenorrhea are available, including nonhormonal and hormonal pharmacologic options and noninvasive nonpharmacologic options. Treatment choice is influenced by the desire for contraception, the patient's level of sexual activity, potential for adverse effects, and cost. For patients suffering from secondary dysmenorrhea due to endometriosis, treatment is directed toward management of symptoms, prevention of disease progression, and protection of future fertility, if desired. Treatment of endometriosis is covered in Chapter 101.

Nonpharmacologic Therapy

Several nonpharmacologic interventions are used for managing dysmenorrhea. Among these, topical heat therapy, exercise, acupuncture, and a low-fat vegetarian diet have been shown to reduce

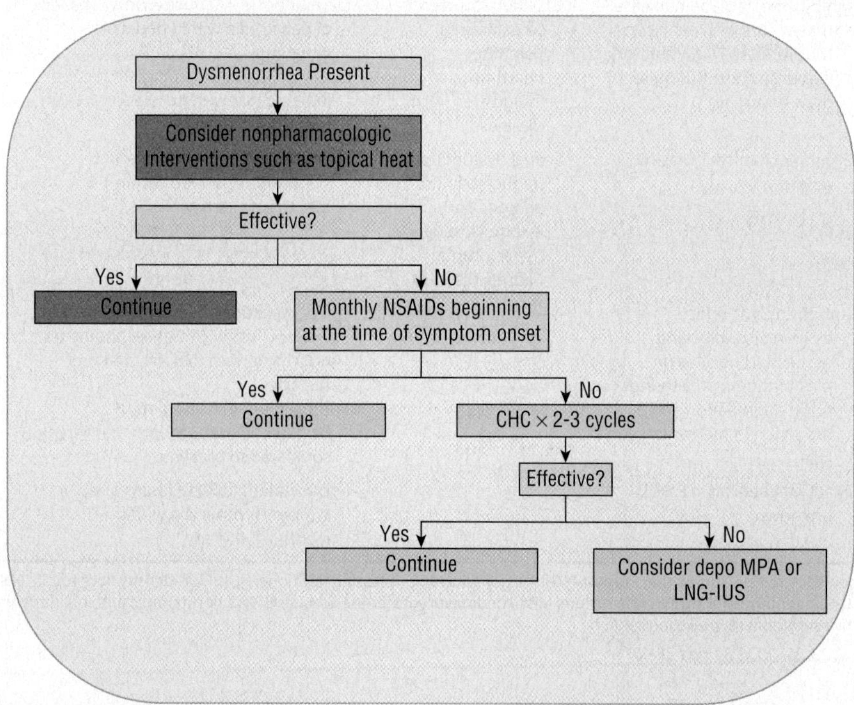

FIGURE 100-4 Treatment algorithm for dysmenorrhea. (LNG-IUS, levonorgestrel-releasing intrauterine system; MPA, medroxyprogesterone acetate; NSAIDs, nonsteroidal anti-inflammatory drugs; CHC, combined hormonal contraceptive.)

TABLE 100-5 Symptoms Often Reported with Premenstrual Syndrome

At least one of the following somatic or affective symptoms should be present during the 5 days before menses in the last three menstrual cycles

Somatic symptoms		Affective symptoms	
Abdominal bloating	Nausea/vomiting	Angry outbursts	Sadness
Breast swelling or tenderness	Acne	Anxiety	Tension
Headache Muscle or joint pain	Pelvic pressure/heaviness	Depression	Tearfulness
Swelling of extremities	Constipation or diarrhea	Difficulty in concentration	Restlessness
Weight gain	Menstrual migraines	Confusion	Loneliness
Fatigue	Appetite changes	Irritability	Food cravings
Dizziness		Social withdrawal	Change in libido
		Forgetfulness	

Data from Reference 32.

CLINICAL PRESENTATION Dysmenorrhea

General

- Patients may or may not be in acute distress, depending on the level of menstrual pain experienced

Symptoms

- Patients complain of crampy pelvic pain beginning shortly before or at the onset of menses. Symptoms typically last from 8 to 72 hours.
- Associated symptoms may include low back pain, headache, diarrhea, fatigue, and/or nausea and vomiting.

Laboratory Tests

- Pelvic examination should be performed to screen for sexually transmitted diseases and/or pelvic inflammatory disease as a cause of the pain in sexually active females.
- Gonorrhea, Chlamydia cultures or polymerase chain reaction, wet mount.

Other Diagnostic Tests

- Transvaginal/pelvic ultrasound can be used to identify potential anatomic abnormalities such as masses/lesions or to detect ovarian cysts and endometriomas.

dysmenorrhea intensity.[57,59,60] Dietary changes may shorten dysmenorrhea duration. Topical heat application via an abdominal patch is as effective as 400 mg of ibuprofen dosed three times daily.[41,61] Because topical heat, exercise, and dietary changes do not impart systemic effects, they are associated with little to no risk compared to the pharmacologic options. Although a variety of dietary supplements, including fenugreek, fish oil, vitamin B_1, ginger, valerian, and zinc sulfate, have been evaluated for dysmenorrhea, a Cochrane analysis concluded that evidence supporting their use is of low or very low quality due to limited sample sizes and methodological concerns.[62] Similarly, although there is some evidence supporting the use of acupuncture and acupressure, a Cochrane analysis also concluded that the quality evidence was low or very low.[60]

Pharmacologic Therapy

Given the role of prostaglandins in dysmenorrhea pathophysiology, NSAIDs are the initial treatment of choice. These agents do not differ in efficacy with the most commonly used agents being naproxen and ibuprofen.

All NSAIDs have a propensity for causing GI distress and ulceration; their administration with food or milk minimizes these effects. In patients who have a history of NSAID-induced gastric effects, the use of celecoxib, a cyclo-oxygenase-2 (COX-2) inhibitor, is an alternative.[23] Increasing fluid intake may also help reduce renal adverse effects.[21] Choice of one agent over another may be based on cost, convenience, and patient preference.[21] All NSAIDs should be dosed on an individual basis and are most effective if started 1 to 2 days prior to the onset of menses and continued through the first 2 to 3 days of menstrual bleeding.[21] According to some research, NSAID therapy should begin at the onset of menses or perhaps even the day before and continued around the clock instead of waiting until symptom onset; however, the data substantiating this are weak.[63] Acetaminophen is inferior to NSAID use in the treatment of this disorder.[23] Opioid should be avoided for dysmenorrhea pain management as adolescents can develop dependence in as few as 7 days, leading to physical withdrawal symptoms.[21] If an NSAID or celecoxib use is contraindicated or not desired, hormonal agents should be considered.

Overall, the CHCs improve dysmenorrhea by inhibiting endometrial tissue proliferation which reduces endometrial-derived prostaglandins and leukotrienes that cause the pelvic pain.[19,21] Significant improvements in mild, moderate, and severe dysmenorrhea have been noted with CHCs. Although one study suggested that a CHC containing a potent progestin (eg, levonorgestrel) may be more beneficial, other studies using CHCs with other progestins suggest that pain reduction is not limited to levonorgestrel-containing regimens.[22] Compared with cyclic regimens, continuous CHC regimens may result in more rapid pain reduction.[21] However, both cyclic and continuous regimens have been used successfully.[21]

Long-acting progesterones, such as depot MPA and the LNG-IUS, can be considered for dysmenorrhea treatment. Their efficacy is secondary to their ability to render most patients amenorrheic within 6 to 12 months of use.[19,22] Because the pelvic pain of dysmenorrhea is related to the prostaglandins released during menses, in the setting of amenorrhea the underlying cause of dysmenorrhea is removed.

Several factors influence the choice of first-line treatment for dysmenorrhea. If contraception is desired, then a hormonal option may be considered taking into account cost, adherence issues, and adverse effects. If contraception is not desired, then NSAID use would be desirable from both cost and convenience standpoints. If NSAIDs are not tolerated, celecoxib could be recommended. In patients for whom hormonal contraception, NSAIDs, or celecoxib are not an option, topical heat should be considered.

Adolescents According to the American College of Obstetricians and Gynecologists, adolescents are particularly at risk of receiving delayed medical care for symptoms of dysmenorrhea.[39] Because NSAIDs impact prostaglandin production specifically, they are recommended as the initial treatment choice for adolescents with primary dysmenorrhea.[39] Adolescent patients are more likely to engage in self-directed treatment use of NSAIDs and, therefore, are at higher risk of sub-therapeutic treatment. Early diagnosis, treatment, and education is essential in this population.[39] In adolescent patients desiring contraception, or in whom NSAIDs do not provide adequate relief, hormonal contraceptives can be used alone, or in combination with NSAIDs.[21] Prolonged use of depot MPA may lead to significant loss of bone mineral density (BMD) loss which may not be completely reversible after depot MPA discontinuation.[22] Adolescence is a critical period for BMD accrual. Hence, depot MPA may not be the first choice in this population.[22] Table 100-4 identifies the significant pharmacologic properties for agents used to treat dysmenorrhea that require monitoring.

Evaluation of Therapeutic Outcomes

Table 100-4 lists the expected outcomes and specific monitoring parameters for the treatment modalities used in the management of dysmenorrhea.

ABNORMAL UTERINE BLEEDING WITH OVULATORY DYSFUNCTION

Epidemiology

7 Abnormal uterine bleeding associated with ovulatory dysfunction (AUB-O) is caused by oligo- or anovulation, leading to irregular, heavy menstrual bleeding due to chronic unopposed estrogen on the endometrium.[18] While it does encompass bleeding patterns such as HMB and amenorrhea, this section will focus specifically on AUB-O as it relates to oligo-anovulation.

The estimated annual prevalence of menstrual irregularities is 53 per 1,000 females.[63] In reproductive-age females, polycystic ovary syndrome (PCOS) is one of the most common causes of AUB-O,[18] with a prevalence range of 8% to 13%.[64] In perimenopausal individuals, bleeding changes are due to normal menopausal transition, with the average age of menopause being 51 years in developed countries. In North America, the mean duration of menopausal transition is 4 years, and during this time period menstrual irregularity is commonly observed.[18]

Etiology

When considering the etiology of AUB-O, the patient's age must be taken into account. As previously discussed, all patients presenting with abnormal bleeding should be evaluated for pregnancy. In adolescents though, anovulation is the most common cause of AUB-O.[18] During the first 12 to 18 months after menarche, immaturity of the HPO axis is frequently the cause of AUB-O.[18] By the third year after the onset of menstruation, 60% to 80% of cycles are regular.[18] If regular menstrual cycles have not been established within 5 years of menarche, further evaluation for the cause, such as PCOS, should be considered.[31] When irregular menses is associated with significant bleeding, an inherited bleeding disorder should be considered as a cause, especially in adolescence.[18] Individuals experiencing AUB-O in their reproductive years should be evaluated for pathologic causes, including PCOS, thyroid dysfunction, hyperprolactinemia, primary pituitary disease, premature ovarian failure, hypothalamic dysfunction, disordered eating, adrenal disease, and androgen-producing tumors.[18] Individuals in their perimenopausal years may experience "physiologic" anovulatory cycles because of intermittently declining estrogen levels. Regardless of age, evaluation for endometrial hyperplasia and/or endometrial cancer should be considered when a patient experiences excessive bleeding with irregular menses.[18] When considering the etiology of AUB-O, more than one condition may coexist (eg, PCOS and hypothyroidism), each contributing to the constellation of symptoms.

Pathophysiology

Normal menstrual cycles occur through a complex interaction of the hypothalamus, pituitary gland, ovaries, and endometrium (see Fig. 100-1). In an ovulatory cycle, the ovary produces a mature, estrogen-secreting follicle in response to FSH release from the pituitary. The endometrium proliferates under the influence of this estrogen production. At a critical level of estrogen concentration, the pituitary responds by producing an "LH surge," which creates a cascade of ovarian events, culminating in ovulation. Upon oocyte release, the follicle becomes a progesterone-producing corpus luteum. The endometrium "organizes" into secretory endometrium in the presence of adequate progesterone, preparing itself for a possible pregnancy. If conception and implantation do not occur, corpus luteum involution causes a decline in estrogen and progesterone leading to predictable, organized menstrual flow as the endometrium sloughs.

If ovulation does not occur, progesterone is not produced, and the endometrium will continue to proliferate in an "unorganized" fashion under the influence of continued estrogen production. Eventually, the endometrium will become so thick that it can no longer be supported by continued estrogen production. This results in unorganized, sporadic sloughing of the endometrium, characteristic of the unpredictable and heavy bleeding associated with AUB-O.

Overall, AUB-O has various etiologies, which will require a careful history and examination along with laboratory assessments to elucidate. For example, in adolescence, HPO axis immaturity contributes to the absence of the LH surge required for ovulation. In patients with anorexia, the hypothalamus loses much of its pulsatile GnRH release, leading to low levels of FSH and LH, and in certain cases enough for estrogen production but not enough to induce ovulation. Oocyte decline and abnormal follicular development contribute to anovulatory cycles common among individuals in the perimenopause transition.[18]

8 In females of reproductive-age, PCOS is one of the most common causes of AUB-O.[18] Generally, PCOS can present as AUB-O, and symptoms include amenorrhea, oligomenorrhea, intermenstrual bleeding, and HMB. Although its exact definition continues to evolve, it is a disorder of androgen excess accompanied by ovulatory dysfunction and/or polycystic ovarian morphology.[65,66] Insulin resistance is often present, and PCOS is a risk factor for metabolic syndrome, type 2 diabetes, dyslipidemia, hypertension, and possibly cardiovascular disease.[31] Besides PCOS, common causes of AUB-O in reproductive-age females include hyperprolactinemia, hypothalamic amenorrhea, also known as hypogonadotropic hypogonadism, primary ovarian insufficiency, and thyroid dysfunction.[18]

The criteria for diagnosing PCOS in adolescents are controversial as the pathologic features used for the diagnosis in adults, specifically acne and irregular menses, may be normal pubertal occurrences. Adolescent hyperandrogenism (as opposed to adult hyperandrogenism) may be a natural consequence of the lack of synchronicity within the HPO axis during prolonged anovulatory cycles that are typical during puberty. Additionally, there is a high background prevalence of polycystic ovarian morphology in this population.[67] Menstrual irregularity for over 2 years and accurate assessment of hyperandrogenic as well as metabolic features, in addition to reduced reliance on ultrasound diagnosis of polycystic ovarian morphology, may be suitable strategies for PCOS diagnosis in the adolescent population.[67] More research is needed to definitively identify the appropriate diagnosis of PCOS among adolescents so that appropriate treatment(s) can be recommended.

TREATMENT

Desired Outcomes

The optimal therapy for AUB-O depends upon the underlying cause(s) and the treatment options for AUB-O are wide and varied. When applicable, control of excessive bleeding in the short term is paramount. Longer-term goals of therapy include restoring the natural cycle of orderly endometrial growth and shedding, preventing endometrial hyperplasia,[18] addressing fertility concerns, decreasing the risk of osteopenia in cases of ovarian insufficiency, and improving the overall quality of life. Table 100-3 identifies the agents used to manage AUB-O and their recommended doses. Medical treatment, as opposed to surgical management, to resolve AUB-O should be initiated, as AUB-O is primarily an endocrinologic abnormality.[18]

Nonpharmacologic Therapy

Nonpharmacologic treatment options for AUB-O depend on the underlying cause. In a female of reproductive age with PCOS, weight loss of 5% to 10% may result in improved menstrual regularity and ovulatory function, reduced hirsutism, increased insulin sensitivity,

CLINICAL PRESENTATION Abnormal Uterine Bleeding with Ovulatory Dysfunction

General

- Patients typically will not be in acute distress.

Symptoms

- Irregular, heavy, or prolonged uterine bleeding
- Perimenopausal symptoms (eg, hot flashes, night sweats, and vaginal dryness) in ovarian insufficiency or menopausal transition

Signs

- Acne, hirsutism, and obesity in PCOS

Laboratory Tests

- Pregnancy testing
- If PCOS is suspected, consider free or total testosterone, fasting glucose, fasting lipid panel
- If perimenopause is suspected, measure FSH
- Thyroid-stimulating hormone

Other Diagnostic Tests

- Endometrial biopsy for patients with risk factors for endometrial hyperplasia or malignancy
- Pelvic ultrasound to evaluate for polycystic ovaries

and improved response to fertility treatments.[30] Further, sustained weight loss has resulted in a return to ovulatory cycles in those without PCOS who experienced anovulatory cycles.[18] In patients with AUB-O who have completed childbearing or who have not responded to medical management, endometrial ablation or resection and hysterectomy are surgical options. In the short term, ablation results in less morbidity and shorter recovery periods compared to other surgical interventions. However, patients should be counseled about the risks regarding the ability to detect and diagnose endometrial cancer in the future.[18] Importantly, procedure choice involves shared decision making with the patient.

Pharmacologic Therapy

Hormonal contraceptives prevent recurrent AUB-O by providing a progestin and suppressing ovarian hormones. The CHCs are also useful for cycle regulation, leading to predictable menstrual cycles. In individuals with contraindication(s) to estrogen or in whom the adverse medication effects are unacceptable, progesterone-only products are an option. They should be strongly considered for patients experiencing HMB associated with anovulatory cycles.[18] Depot and intermittent oral MPA provide endometrial protection through endometrial suppression.[4] Another progesterone option is placement of the LNG-IUS,[18] particularly if pregnancy is not desired. Studied specifically in females over 30 years of age, use of the LNG-IUS resulted in a greater than 95% reduction in menstrual blood loss by 2 years.[68] Patient satisfaction rates were greater than 80%, with 74% agreeing to recommend it to others.[68]

9 For individuals with PCOS who have high androgen levels and its related signs (eg, hirsutism), CHCs also increase sex hormone-binding globulin (SHBG) which binds androgens and reduces their circulating free concentrations. The 2018 international PCOS guideline recommends that CHCs alone should be recommended in adults and adolescents with PCOS for management of irregular menstrual cycles and clinical hyperandrogenism.[30] For patients with PCOS, CHCs containing less than or equal to 35 mcg of ethinyl estradiol and a progesterone that exhibits minimal androgenic effects (eg, norgestimate and desogestrel) or with antiandrogenic effects (eg, drospirenone) may be desirable.

The 2018 international PCOS guidelines also recommend that metformin should be considered in adults and adolescents with PCOS for management of metabolic features when lifestyle changes do not achieve desired goals.[30] Although metformin improves insulin sensitivity, and can reduce circulating androgen concentrations and improve ovulation rates,[31,69] CHCs are more effective in cycle regulation and decreasing androgens. The 2018 international PCOS guidelines recommend that metformin can be used in combination with CHCs for treatment of hyperandrogenic-related alopecia or hirsutism if at least 6 months of CHCs and cosmetic therapy do not adequately improve symptoms.[30] While not typically an issue among the relatively young population of patients treated with metformin for PCOS, one must be cognizant of the risk of lactic acidosis in metformin users with renal impairment. As such, this medication should be avoided in individuals with serum creatinine greater than 1.4 mg/dL (124 μmol/L). In addition, metformin may lead to spontaneous ovulation, and birth control should be advised in patients with PCOS not desiring pregnancy.[30]

Hormonal contraceptives containing antiandrogenic progesterones are very effective for managing the acne and hirsutism that accompany PCOS as they suppress ovarian androgen production and increase SHBG, thus reducing free testosterone concentrations. Controversy regarding their use in PCOS exists secondary to their potential adverse effects on insulin resistance and glucose tolerance.[70] An increase in high-sensitivity C-reactive protein and an increase in homocysteine levels, both indicators of cardiovascular risk, have been observed with the use of CHCs.[58] Another trial found a reduction in brachial artery flow-mediated dilatation and an increase in carotid intima-media thickness, both indicators of endothelial dysfunction, following therapy with oral CHCs containing ethinyl estradiol and cyproterone acetate in patients with PCOS.[71] Additional, longer-term clinical trials will clarify whether the benefits of these agents outweigh the risks. It has been suggested that cardiovascular risk calculators be employed as an adjunct to guidelines suggesting the use of oral CHCs in this patient population.[72]

If the treatment goal is fertility, letrozole should be considered first-line treatment for ovulation induction in individuals with PCOS with anovulatory infertility and no other infertility factors.[30] Letrozole has been found to lead to significantly more ovulatory cycles, pregnancies, and live births compared to clomiphene in patients with PCOS.[73] It is dosed at 2.5 mg daily for 5 days beginning on cycle day 3 after induced withdrawal bleeding with a progesterone such as MPA 10 mg daily orally for 10 days. If ovulation does not occur, doses can be increased in subsequent cycles to a maximum of 7.5 mg daily in up to 5 cycles.[73] As an alternative ovulation induction agent, clomiphene citrate is administered in a similar manner, initiated at 50 mg daily, with dose increase in subsequent cycles to a maximum of 150 mg daily.[73]

Overall, the treatment(s) of choice depends on accurate etiologic diagnosis as well as identification of the desired treatment outcome(s). Hormonal contraceptives are the first-choice treatment in individuals with AUB-O who do not desire pregnancy.[18] In those with PCOS, CHCs are first-line pharmacologic agents for cycle control and minimizing the androgenic signs and symptoms of PCOS, while metformin is primarily used for metabolic improvement when lifestyle interventions do not yield adequate improvements.[30] Letrozole is used for ovulation induction in PCOS.[30] Table 100-4 lists the important pharmacologic properties of agents used to treat AUB-O that require monitoring.

Perimenopause

Anovulatory cycles are fairly common in the perimenarchal reproductive years. Ovulation typically is established 1 year or more following menarche. If excessive bleeding occurs, the patient should be evaluated for bleeding disorders, as HMB since menarche may indicate an undetected coagulopathy.[25] If identified, the specific bleeding disorders should be treated. Acute severe bleeding can be managed with intravenous conjugated equine estrogen, high-dose CHCs, or high-dose oral progestins.[44]

Evaluation of Therapeutic Outcomes

Table 100-4 lists the expected outcomes and specific monitoring parameters for the treatment modalities used to manage AUB-O.

CONCLUSION

Problems related to the menstrual cycle are very common in females of reproductive age. The most frequently encountered menstruation-related difficulties include amenorrhea; heavy menstrual bleeding (HMB); abnormal uterine bleeding associated with ovulatory dysfunction (AUB-O), including polycystic ovary syndrome (PCOS); dysmenorrhea; and premenstrual syndrome (PMS) and premenstrual dysphoric disorder (PMDD). The diagnosis of various menstruation-related disorders begins with a thorough history of the patient's menstrual patterns, co-occurring symptoms. Problems related to the menstrual cycle negatively affect quality of life, reproductive potential, and may have long-term detrimental health effects.

ABBREVIATIONS

ACOG	American College of Obstetricians and Gynecologists
AUB-O	abnormal uterine bleeding with ovulatory dysfunction
CHC	combined hormonal contraception
COX-2	cyclo-oxygenase-2
FHA	functional hypothalamic amenorrhea
FSH	follicle-stimulating hormone
GnRH	gonadotropin-releasing hormone
HC	hormonal contraceptive
HMB	heavy menstrual bleeding
HPA	hypothalamic–pituitary–adrenal
HPO	hypothalamic–pituitary–ovarian
IUSs	Intrauterine systems
hCG	human chorionic gonadotropin
LH	luteinizing hormone
LNG-IUS	levonorgestrel-releasing intrauterine system
MPA	medroxyprogesterone acetate
NSAID	nonsteroidal anti-inflammatory drug
PCOS	polycystic ovary syndrome
PMDD	premenstrual dysphoric disorder
PMS	premenstrual syndrome
SHBG	sex hormone-binding globulin
SNRI	serotonin–norepinephrine reuptake inhibitor
SSRI	selective serotonin reuptake inhibitor

REFERENCES

1. The American College of Obstetricians and Gynecologists' Committee on Adolescent Health Care. Committee opinion 651: Menstruation in girls and adolescents using the menstrual cycle as a vital sign. Obstet Gynecol. Available at: http://www.acog.org/-/media/Committee-Opinions/Committee-on-Adolescent-Health-Care/co651.pdf?dmc=1&ts=20170604T2324312143. Published 2015. Accessed November 21, 2018.
2. Fraser IS, Critchley HOD, Broder M, Munro MG. The FIGO recommendations on terminologies and definitions for normal and abnormal uterine bleeding. *Semin Reprod Med.* 2011;29(5):383–390.
3. Munro MG, Critchley HOD, Fraser IS. The two FIGO systems for normal and abnormal uterine bleeding symptoms and classification of causes of abnormal uterine bleeding in the reproductive years: 2018 revisions. *Int J Gynaecol Obstet.* 2018;143(3):393–408. 10.1002/ijgo.12666 30198563.
4. Klein DA, Poth MA. Amenorrhea: an approach to diagnosis and management. *Am Fam Physician.* 2013;87(11):781–788.
5. Rebar R. Evaluation of amenorrhea, anovulation, and abnormal bleeding [updated 2018 Jan 15]. In: De Groot KJ, Chrousos G, Kungan K, eds. *Endotext [Internet].* South Dartmouth, MA: MDText.com, Inc; 2018.
6. Fourman LT, Fazeli PK. Neuroendocrine causes of amenorrhea: an update. *J Clin Endocrinol Metab.* 2015;100(3):812–824.
7. Marsh CA, Grimstad FW. Primary amenorrhea: diagnosis and management. *Obstet Gynecol Surv.* 2014;69(10):603–612.
8. Arduc A, Gokay F, Isik S, et al. Retrospective comparison of cabergoline and bromocriptine effects in hyperprolactinemia: a single center experience. *J Endocrinol Invest.* 2015;38(4):447–453.
9. Nelson LM. Primary ovarian insufficiency. *N Engl J Med.* 2009;360:606–614.
10. Sullivan SD, Sarrel PM, Nelson LM. Hormone replacement therapy in young women with primary ovarian insufficiency. *Fertil Steril.* 2016;106:1588–1599.
11. Sarrel PM, Sullivan SD, Nelson LM. Hormone replacement therapy in young women with surgical primary ovarian insufficiency and early menopause. *Fertil Steril.* 2016;106(7):1580–1587.
12. Chou SH, Mantzoros C. Role of leptin in human reproductive disorders. *J Endocrinol.* 2014;223(1):T49–T62.
13. Michopoulos V, Mancini F, Loucks TL, Berga SL. Neuroendocrine recovery initiated by cognitive behavioral therapy in women with functional hypothalamic amenorrhea: a randomized, controlled trial. *Fertil Steril.* 2013;99(7):2084–2091.
14. Gordon CM, Ackerman KE, Berga SL, et al. Functional hypothalamic amenorrhea: an Endocrine Society clinical practice guideline. *J Clin Endocrinol Metab.* 2017;102(5):1413–1439.
15. Molitch ME. Medication-induced hyperprolactinemia. *Mayo Clin Proc.* 2005;80(8):1050–1057.
16. Altayar O, Al Nofal A, Carranza Leon BG, Prokop LJ, Wang Z, Murad MH. Treatments to prevent bone loss in functional hypothalamic amenorrhea: a systematic review and meta-analysis. *J Endocr Soc.* 2017;1(5):500–511.
17. Popat VB, Calis KA, Kalantaridou SN, et al. Bone mineral density in young women with primary ovarian insufficiency: results of a three-year randomized controlled trial of physiological transdermal estradiol and testosterone replacement. *J Clin Endocrinol Metab.* 2014;99(9):3418–3426.
18. The American College of Obstetricians and Gynecologists. ACOG Practice Bulletin No. 136. Management of abnormal uterine bleeding associated with ovulatory dysfunction. *Obs Gynecol.* 2013;122(1):176–185.
19. Jamieson MA. Disorders of menstruation in adolescent girls. *Pediatr Clin North Am.* 2015;62(4):943–961.
20. De Souza MJ, Nattiv A, Joy E, et al. 2014 Female Athlete Triad Coalition consensus statement on treatment and return to play of the female athlete triad. *Clin J Sport Med.* 2014;24(2):96–119.
21. The American College of Obstetricians and Gynecologists' Committee on Adolescent Health Care. ACOG Committee Opinion 760: Dysmenorrhea and endometriosis in the adolescent. *Obstet Gynecol.* 2018;132(6):e249–e258.
22. Harel Z. Dysmenorrhea in adolescents and young adults: etiology and management. *Expert Opin Pharmacother.* 2012;13(15):2157–2170.
23. Marjoribanks J, Ayeleke RO, Farquhar C, Proctor M. Nonsteroidal anti-inflammatory drugs for dysmenorrhoea. *Cochrane Database Syst Rev.* 2015;(7):CD001751.
24. LYSTEDA [prescribing information]. Parsippany, NJ: Ferring Pharmaceuticals, Inc; 2016.
25. Sripraserl I, Pakrashi T, Kimble T, Archer DF. Heavy menstrual bleeding diagnosis and medical management. *Contracept Reprod Med.* 2017;2:20.

26. Qiu J, Cheng J, Wang Q, Hua J. Levonorgestrel-releasing intrauterine system versus medical therapy for menorrhagia: a systematic review and meta-analysis. *Med Sci Monit.* 2014;20:1700–1713.
27. Lethaby A, Hussain M, Jr R, Mc R. Progesterone or progestogen-releasing intrauterine systems for heavy menstrual bleeding. *Cochrane Database Syst Rev.* 2015;(4):CD002126.
28. Abu Hashim H. Medical treatment of idiopathic heavy menstrual bleeding. What is new? An evidence based approach. *Arch Gynecol Obstet.* 2013;287(2):251–260.
29. Kaunitz AM, Meredith S, Inki P, Kubba A, Sanchez-Ramos L. Levonorgestrel-releasing intrauterine system and endometrial ablation in heavy menstrual bleeding: a systematic review and meta-analysis. *Obstet Gynecol.* 2009;113(5):1104–1116.
30. Teede HJ, Misso ML, Costello MF, et al. Recommendations from the international evidence-based guideline for the assessment and management of polycystic ovary syndrome. *Fertil Steril.* 2018;110(3):364–379.
31. Setji TL, Brown AJ. Polycystic ovary syndrome: update on diagnosis and treatment. *Am J Med.* 2014;127(10):912–919.
32. Hofmeister S, Bodden S. Premenstrual syndrome and premenstrual dysphoric disorder. *Am Fam Physician.* 2016;94(3):236–240.
33. Maharaj S, Trevino K. A comprehensive review of treatment options for premenstrual syndrome and premenstrual dysphoric disorder. *J Psychiatr Pract.* 2015;21(5):334–350.
34. Marjoribanks J, Brown J, O'Brien PMS, Wyatt K. Selective serotonin reuptake inhibitors for premenstrual syndrome. *Cochrane database Syst Rev.* 2013;(6):CD001396.
35. Yonkers KA, Kornstein SG, Gueorguieva R, Merry B, Steenburgh KV, Altemus M. Symptom-onset dosing of sertraline for the treatment of premenstrual dysphoric disorder: a multi-site, double-blind, randomized, placebo-controlled trial. *JAMA Psychiatry.* 2015;72(10):1037–1044.
36. Freeman EW, Halbreich U, Grubb GS, et al. An overview of four studies of a continuous oral contraceptive (levonorgestrel 90 mcg/ ethinyl estradiol 20 mcg) on premenstrual dysphoric disorder and premenstrual syndrome. *Contraception.* 2012;85(5):437–445.
37. Simon JA. Progestogens in the treatment of secondary amenorrhea. *J Reprod Med.* 1999;44(2 suppl):185–190.
38. Uhm S, Perriera L. Hormonal contraception as treatment for heavy menstrual bleeding: a systematic review. *Clin Obstet Gynecol.* 2014;57(4):694–717.
39. Faje A, Nachtigall L. Current treatment options for hyperprolactinemia. *Expert Opin Pharmacother.* 2013;14(12):1611–1625.
40. Bitzer J, Heikinheimo O, Nelson AL, Calaf-Alsina J, Fraser IS. Medical management of heavy menstrual bleeding: a comprehensive review of the literature. *Obstet Gynecol Surv.* 2015;70(2):115–130.
41. Ray S, Ray A. Non-surgical interventions for treating heavy menstrual bleeding (menorrhagia) in women with bleeding disorders. *Cochrane database Syst Rev.* 2014;(11):CD010338.
42. Heliovaara-Peippo S, Hurskainen R, Teperi J, et al. Quality of life and costs of levonorgestrel-releasing intrauterine system or hysterectomy in the treatment of menorrhagia: a 10-year randomized controlled trial. *Obstet Gynecol Surv.* 2014;69(4):204–205.
43. Munro MG, Critchley HOD, Fraser IS, FIGO Menstrual Disorders Working Group. The FIGO classification of causes of abnormal uterine bleeding in the reproductive years. *Fertil Steril.* 2011;95(7):2204–2208.
44. The American College of Obstetricians and Gynecologists. ACOG Committee on Gynecologic Practice No. 557: Management of acute abnormal uterine bleeding in nonpregnant reproductive-aged women. *Obs Gynecol.* 2013;121(4):891–896.
45. Oriahnn. https://www.oriahnnhcp.com/?cid=ppc_ppd_oriahnn_ggl_br_7096&gclid=CjwKCAiA1uKMBhAGEiwAxzvX99Xp49NKrW2R2YrAyJm1XI3xpscSb5LJkdPhhXdrpk2RM-V_EyJIFxoC9-EQAvD_BwE&gclsrc=aw.ds. North Chicago, Illinois; AbbVie Inc, 2020.
46. Schlaff WD, Ackerman RT, Al-Hendy A, et al. Elagolix for heavy menstrual bleeding in women with uterine fibroids. *N Engl J Med.* 2020;382(4):328–340. 10.1056/NEJMoa1904351 31971678.
47. Al-Hendy A, Bradley L, Owens CD, et al. Predictors of response for elagolix with add-back therapy in women with heavy menstrual bleeding associated with uterine fibroids. *Am J Obstet Gynecol.* 2021;224(1):72.e1–72.e50. 10.1016/j.ajog.2020.07.032 32702363.
48. Simon JA, Al-Hendy A, Archer DF, et al. Elagolix treatment for up to 12 months in women with heavy menstrual bleeding and uterine leiomyomas. *Obstet Gynecol.* 2020;135(6):1313–1326. 10.1097/AOG.0000000000003869 32459423.
49. The American College of Obstetricians and Gynecologists. ACOG Practice Bulletin No. 186. Long-acting reversible contraception: implants and intrauterine devices. *Obstet Gynecol.* 2017;130(5):e251–e269.
50. The American College of Obstetricians and Gynecologists. *Guidelines for Women's Health Care: A Resource Manual.* 4th ed. Washington, D.C.: American College of Obstetricians and Gynecologists; 2014.
51. Matsumoto T, Asakura H, Hayashi T. Biopsychosocial aspects of premenstrual syndrome and premenstrual dysphoric disorder. *Gynecol Endocrinol.* 2013;29(1):67–73.
52. Jang SH, Kim DI, Choi M-S. Effects and treatment methods of acupuncture and herbal medicine for premenstrual syndrome/ premenstrual dysphoric disorder. *BMC Complement Altern Med.* 2014;14:11.
53. Jing Z, Yang X, Ismail KMK, Chen X, Wu T. Chinese herbal medicine for premenstrual syndrome. *Cochrane Database Syst Rev.* 2009;(1):CD006414.
54. Armour M, Ee CC, Hao J, Wilson TM, Yao SS, Smith CA. Acupuncture and acupressure for premenstrual syndrome. *Cochrane Database Syst Rev.* 2018;(8):CD005290.
55. Reefhuis J, Devine O, Friedman JM, Louik C, Honein MA. Specific SSRIs and birth defects: Bayesian analysis to interpret new data in the context of previous reports. *BMJ.* 2015;350:h3190.
56. Iacovides S, Avidon I, Bentley A, Baker FC. Reduced quality of life when experiencing menstrual pain in women with primary dysmenorrhea. *Acta Obstet Gynecol Scand.* 2014;93(2):213–217.
57. Osayande AS, Mehulic S. Diagnosis and initial management of dysmenorrhea. *Am Fam Physician.* 2014;89(5):341–346.
58. Harmanci A, Cinar N, Bayraktar M, Yildiz BO. Oral contraceptive plus antiandrogen therapy and cardiometabolic risk in polycystic ovary syndrome. *Clin Endocrinol (Oxf).* 2013;78(1):120–125.
59. Potur DC, Kömürcü N. The effects of local low-dose heat application on dysmenorrhea. *J Pediatr Adolesc Gynecol.* 2014;27(4):216–221.
60. Smith CA, Armour M, Zhu X, Li X, Lu ZY, Song J. Acupuncture for dysmenorrhoea. *Cochrane Database Syst Rev.* 2016;(4):CD007854.
61. Navvabi Rigi S, Kermansaravi F, Navidian A, et al. Comparing the analgesic effect of heat patch containing iron chip and ibuprofen for primary dysmenorrhea: a randomized controlled trial. *BMC Womens Health.* 2012;12:25.
62. Pattanittum P, Kunyanone N, Brown J, et al. Dietary supplements for dysmenorrhoea. *Cochrane Database Syst Rev.* 2016;(3):CD002124.
63. Kjerulff KH, Erickson BA, Langenberg PW. Chronic gynecological conditions reported by US women: findings from the National Health Interview Survey, 1984 to 1992. *Am J Public Health.* 1996;86(2):195–199.
64. Azziz R, Carmina E, Chen Z, et al. Polycystic ovary syndrome. *Nat Rev Dis Prim.* 2016;2:16057.
65. Legro RS, Arslanian SA, Ehrmann DA, et al. Diagnosis and treatment of polycystic ovary syndrome: an endocrine society clinical practice guideline. *J Clin Endocrinol Metab.* 2013;98(12):4565–4592.
66. Goodman NF, Cobin RH, Futterweit W, Glueck JS, Legro RS, Carmina E. American Association of Clinical Endocrinologists, American College of Endocrinology, and Androgen Excess and PCOS Society disease state clinical review: guide to the best practices in the evaluation and treatment of polycystic ovary syndrome—Part 1. *Endocr Pract.* 2015;21(12):1415–1426.
67. Hardy TSE, Norman RJ. Diagnosis of adolescent polycystic ovary syndrome. *Steroids.* 2013;78(8):751–754.
68. Mansukhani N, Unni J, Verma S, et al. Are women satisfied when using levonorgestrel-releasing intrauterine system for treatment of abnormal uterine bleeding? *J Midlife Health.* 2013;4(1):31.
69. Palomba S, Pasquali R, Orio F, Nestler JE. Clomiphene citrate, metformin or both as first-step approach in treating anovulatory infertility in patients with polycystic ovary syndrome (PCOS): a systematic review of head-to-head randomized controlled studies and meta-analysis. *Clin Endocrinol (Oxf).* 2009;70(2):311–321.
70. Adeniji AA, Essah PA, Nestler JE, Cheang KI. Metabolic effects of a commonly used combined hormonal oral contraceptive in women with and without polycystic ovary syndrome. *J Womens Heal.* 2016;25(6):638–645.
71. Gode F, Karagoz C, Posaci C, et al. Alteration of cardiovascular risk parameters in women with polycystic ovary syndrome who were prescribed to ethinyl estradiol-cyproterone acetate. *Arch Gynecol Obstet.* 2011;284(4):923–929.
72. Beller JP, McCartney CR. Cardiovascular risk and combined oral contraceptives: clinical decisions in settings of uncertainty. *Am J Obstet Gynecol.* 2013;208(1):39–41.
73. Legro RS, Brzyski RG, Diamond MP, et al. Letrozole versus clomiphene for infertility in the polycystic ovary syndrome. *N Engl J Med.* 2014;371(2):119–129.
74. The American Psychiatric Association. *Diagnostic and Statistical Manual of Mental Disorders. Fifth Edition.* In: Washington, DC: American Psychiatric Association; 2013.

101

Endometriosis

Kathleen M. Vest and Sarah E. Lynch

KEY CONCEPTS

1. Endometriosis is a chronic condition in reproductive age females that can cause chronic pelvic pain and infertility.
2. Endometriosis is characterized by endometrial tissue outside the uterus, but the exact pathophysiology and biological mechanisms are multifactorial and still remain unclear.
3. Endometriosis should be suspected in any biological female of reproductive age presenting with recurring pelvic pain or otherwise unexplained infertility. Failure of first-line treatment options like nonsteroidal anti-inflammatory drugs (NSAIDs) or combined hormonal contraceptives (CHCs) to relieve dysmenorrhea is highly suspect of endometriosis.
4. Definitive diagnosis of endometriosis requires direct surgical visualization; however, it is acceptable to empirically treat these symptoms without a definitive diagnosis.
5. Treatment strategies are based on patient symptoms and preferences with regards to desire for pregnancy.
6. Pharmacologic and surgical options are indicated to treat endometriosis-associated pain. Surgery/reproductive technology is the only treatment option for endometriosis-related infertility.
7. Treatment options are not curative of endometriosis and only provide symptom management.
8. First-line pharmacologic options include NSAIDs, CHCs, and progestins. Other options include gonadotropin-releasing hormone (GnRH) agonists, GnRH antagonists, danazol, and aromatase inhibitors.
9. Add-back therapy can be utilized with certain agents to minimize hypoestrogenic adverse events such as bone mineral density (BMD) loss and vasomotor symptoms.

BEYOND THE BOOK

Create a chart comparing and contrasting the use of each class of medications in the following individuals with endometriosis:

- 17-year-old patient with severe dysmenorrhea
- 34-year-old patient with dysmenorrhea despite use of combined oral contraceptive
- 28-year-old patient looking for something to help with pain relief and contraception
- 43-year-old patient with osteoporosis
- 31-year-old patient with no insurance

INTRODUCTION

1 Endometriosis is a common gynecologic condition that affects females during their reproductive years, defined as the growth of endometrial tissue outside the uterus. Clinically, endometriosis can cause several symptoms with the most common being dysmenorrhea, dyspareunia, and infertility. It is usually diagnosed in individuals in their thirties and forties; however, it is also common in adolescent age. Chronic pelvic pain is the most common complaint, especially in adolescents. Patients are often asymptomatic; therefore, it is difficult to confirm the true incidence of endometriosis. Similar to other chapters in this section, general discussions around endometriosis and its treatment are primarily framed around cisgender women. However, any individual with a female reproductive system may experience endometriosis. Therefore, the use of the term *female* is specifically meant to refer to biology, and this chapter has been written to include transgender individuals.

While the pathophysiology of endometriosis is not completely understood, it is believed that retrograde menstrual flow causes several endometriosis symptoms. This backflow of fluid often leads to endometrial deposits in various areas of the genitourinary tract including the bladder, ureter, and ovaries in addition to the gastrointestinal tract. Other theories include hematogenous or lymphatic transport, stem cells from bone marrow, and coelomic metaplasia. Interventions are focused on the desire of the patient to become pregnant, relieve symptoms, or both. Pregnancies are often beneficial for improving symptoms.

EPIDEMIOLOGY

The incidence of endometriosis in the general population is approximately 10%.[1,2] It is a common cause of infertility and chronic pelvic pain and has an incidence of approximately 38% in females with infertility (with some estimates of around 50%); and more than 60% of patients with chronic pelvic pain have a diagnosis of endometriosis (with some reports of 71%-87%).[2] Roughly 1 in 10 females of reproductive age are diagnosed with endometriosis. However, it is probable that approximately 11% of individuals are undiagnosed. There is a strong genetic predisposition, and it has been noted that females with a first-degree relative with endometriosis have a 7- to 10-fold increased risk for developing endometriosis.[2]

ETIOLOGY

Endometriosis is characterized by the growth of endometrial tissue outside of the uterus[1,2]; and while it can be diagnosed in any age, it is most commonly found during the reproductive years. In addition to genetic predisposition, several risk factors have been identified. The risk of endometriosis is higher in those with early menarche (defined as the start of menses at 11 years old or younger), short menstrual cycles (<27 days), and heavy, prolonged menses. The environmental factors play a role in the pathogenesis of endometriosis. For example, dioxins, chemicals that have been found in the environment, have been thought to increase the risk for developing endometriosis or worsening symptoms.[3,4] Multiple parity has been associated with a lower risk of endometriosis and/or improvement in endometriosis symptoms. Additionally, regular exercise of more than 4 hours per week has been associated with a lower risk of the development of endometriosis.[2,5]

In addition to infertility and chronic pain, endometriosis is a major cause of hysterectomy and hospitalization in the United States and can lead to decreased quality of life.

PATHOPHYSIOLOGY

2 While not well understood, the pathophysiology of endometriosis is related to the finding of endometrial implants (the tissue forming the lining of the uterus) outside of the uterus. These implants occur outside of the uterus due to retrograde menstrual flow. Endometrial implants are often found in the peritoneum, ovaries, fallopian tubes, uterus, bladder, ureters, intestines, and rectum.[6,7] The growth of implants is dependent on estrogen, and throughout the menstrual cycle they grow and bleed just as the endometrium thickens and sheds during menstruation. When the implants proliferate, adhesions (collections of scar tissue) can form that can lead to further bleeding, inflammation, and scarring especially prior to and during menses.

While retrograde menstruation can explain the endometrial deposits in the peritoneal cavity, there are also other theories regarding the development of endometriotic implants. Additionally, some have retrograde menstruation, yet do not develop endometriosis. There is a 90% prevalence of retrograde menstruation, yet 10% prevalence of endometriosis.[8] Four well-supported hallmarks of the pathophysiology of endometriosis include genetic predisposition, estrogen dependence, progesterone resistance, and inflammation.[6-10]

In patients with endometriosis, there are alterations in estrogen- and progesterone-dependent processes including inflammatory and immune responses, angiogenesis, and apoptosis. These alterations lead to survival and replenishment of endometriotic tissue. Genetic alterations that have been noted include the upregulation of B-cell lymphoma 2 (*BCL-2*), which is an antiapoptotic gene and is present in both eutopic and ectopic endometrium from patients with endometriosis.[8] An observation in endometriotic tissue showed the increased expression of the aromatase enzyme and decreased expression of 17β-hydroxysteroid dehydrogenase (17β-HSD) type 2, which leads to an increase in the concentration of estradiol. Estradiol stimulates prostaglandin E2 that further can stimulate aromatase activity. Estrogen can stimulate the release of other inflammatory cytokines such as cyclooxygenase 2 (COX-2). Additionally, endometriotic lesions have decreased progesterone receptor expression and an absence of progesterone receptor-B. This can lead to an incomplete transition of endometrium from the luteal phase to the secretory phase of the menstrual cycle. While estradiol tends to have proinflammatory and antiapoptotic effects on endometrial cells, progestins inhibit inflammatory pathways and induce apoptosis in endometriotic cells.

Endometriosis has been considered a pelvic inflammatory condition because the peritoneal fluid tends to contain several inflammatory markers that are believed to contribute to pain, formation of adhesions, tissue fibrosis, and scarring. In patients without endometriosis, the immune system clears refluxed endometrial tissue deposits from the peritoneum. Endometrial lesions can lead to inflammation with the activation of macrophages and proinflammatory cytokines. The peritoneal fluid of patients with endometriosis often contains proinflammatory cytokines such as tumor necrosis factor alpha and interleukins 1, 6, and 8 that lead to prostaglandin induction. There is also an increased density of nerve fibers and a high expression of nerve growth factor in endometriotic lesions which further increases pain. Compression of nerve fibers by endometrial implants along with bleeding from endometrial tissues can increase a patient's pain. Lastly, endometriotic nerve fibers influence dorsal root neurons thereby increasing pain perception.

Infertility and the reason for its development have been less well described, especially in mild cases of endometriosis. In more severe cases, inflammation and anatomic abnormalities such as ovarian cysts and adhesions can lead to blockage of the fallopian tubes and hindrance of oocyte and embryo development. The inflammatory cytokines can lead to damage of sperm DNA and cell membranes and the general inflammation seen may result in adhesions and scarring.[1] Hormonal dysregulation can also lead to irregularities in the menstrual cycle, alterations in endometrial receptivity and implantation, and altered oocyte and embryo quality, or issues with uterotubal transport.[8]

CLINICAL PRESENTATION

Symptoms

3 Endometriosis presents in a variable and unpredictable manner with regard to clinical presentation and clinical course. Dysmenorrhea and infertility are the most commonly reported symptoms in patients; however, several other symptoms are often present, or a patient can remain asymptomatic. Typical symptoms include abdominopelvic pain, dysmenorrhea, and dyspareunia; and those experiencing these classic symptoms are more likely to be diagnosed than those presenting without these symptoms. Deep pain during or after sexual intercourse, period-related or cyclical gastrointestinal symptoms, such as painful bowel movements, menorrhagia, ovulation pain, and chronic fatigue are other possible symptoms. Chronic pelvic pain can vary in severity and may be cyclic or acyclic. Pain can lead to a decreased quality of life depending on the severity; however, some patients may be asymptomatic.[2,6,7]

Signs

Physical examination of a patient with endometriosis often reveals pelvic tenderness, enlarged ovaries, pelvic masses or nodules, uterosacral ligaments, or a fixed, retroverted uterus. These signs are usually most significant during menses, so it is recommended to perform the examination at that time. Imaging studies such as transvaginal ultrasound or magnetic resonance imaging are also used to visualize endometrial lesions. If a patient with suspected endometriosis has normal imaging studies, laparoscopic surgery can be considered to further evaluate the pelvis and endometrial lesions. Lesions can vary in size from small lesions in the ovaries or peritoneum to endometriomas, which are large cysts. The lesions are often described as "powder burn" or "gunshot" lesions; dark brown, black or blue lesions, nodules, and cysts; and blood containing endometriomas are called "chocolate cysts."[11]

Diagnosis

4 The diagnosis of endometriosis can be challenging and may take several years due to variability of symptoms. Additionally, a definitive diagnosis can only be made by histological examination of lesions removed during surgery. Treatment guidelines do discuss

CLINICAL PRESENTATION Endometriosis

Physical Symptoms

- Dysmenorrhea
- Infertility
- Pelvic pain
- Dyspareunia (Deep pain during or after sexual intercourse)
- Menstrual cycle-related or cyclical gastrointestinal symptoms (eg, painful bowel movements)
- Menorrhagia
- Ovulation pain
- Chronic fatigue are other possible symptoms

Other considerations

- Chronic pelvic pain can vary in severity and may be cyclic or acyclic
- Pain can lead to a decreased quality of life depending on the severity
- Some patients may be asymptomatic

Signs: From physical examination of a patient with endometriosis

- Pelvic tenderness
- Enlarged ovaries
- Pelvic masses or nodules
- Uterosacral ligaments
- Fixed, retroverted uterus
- *Note: These signs are usually most significant during menses*

Data from References 2, 6, and 7.

ruling out all causes of pain and providing a nondefinitive diagnosis in patients with chronic pelvic pain. Ultrasonography, magnetic resonance imaging, and computed tomography are often used to assess pelvic or adnexal masses, but have a lower sensitive for investigating endometrial lesions. However, in some cases pelvic and abdominal examinations can be used, especially during menstruation and positive findings include pelvic tenderness, enlarged ovaries, or a fixed, retroverted uterus. Imaging studies can be utilized to determine whether there is endometrial tissue in the bowel, bladder, or ureter. Transvaginal ultrasounds are used to determine if endometrial tissue is infiltrating the rectum. Cancer antigen 125 (CA-125) is a marker for ovarian and endometrial cancer, which has been noted to be elevated in some patients with endometriosis but is not a diagnostic marker.[11] However, for diagnosis of endometriosis, the CA-125 measurement is limited due to the fact that an elevated level is not diagnostic.[2,11]

Disease Staging

In general, endometriosis disease severity can be classified according to the American Society of Reproductive Medicine (ASRM) staging system which ranges from stage I (mild) to stage IV (severe). This system stages endometriosis according to not only anatomic location but also the severity of disease.[2] Although staging of disease can be helpful, it is limited in its clinical utility because it does not predict pregnancy after treatment and does not correlate well with symptoms of pain or dyspareunia.[2] Regardless, staging may be useful in guiding decisions regarding prognosis and treatment for infertility.[2,12]

TABLE 101-1 Evidence-Based Recommendations for Treatment of Endometriosis-Related Pain

Treatment Options	Grade of Recommendation—ESHRE
CHCs	
Oral	B
Vaginal	C
Transdermal	C
Continuous use of CHC	C
Progestins	
Oral	A
Depot	A
LNG-IUS	B
Danazol	A
GnRH Agonist	A
Initiate add-back therapy with GnRH agonist initiation to prevent anti-estrogen adverse effects	A
NSAIDs	GPP
Aromatase inhibitors (in patients in refractory endometriosis, used in combination with oral CHCs, progestins, GnRH agonists)	B
Surgical Treatment	A

ESHRE, European Society of Human Reproduction and Embryology; CHC, combined hormonal contraceptive; LNG-IUS, levonorgestrel-releasing intrauterine system; GnRH, gonadotropin-releasing hormone; NSAID, nonsteroidal anti-inflammatory drug.

A = Meta-analysis or multiple randomized trials (of high quality); B = Meta-analysis or multiple randomized trials of moderate quality, single randomized trial, large nonrandomized trials, or case-control/cohort studies of high quality; C = Single randomized trial, large nonrandomized trial(s), or case-control/cohort studies (of moderate quality); D = Nonanalytic studies or case reports/case series (of high or moderate quality); GPP = Good practice point based on expert opinion.

Data from Reference 12.

TREATMENT

Multiple guidelines and expert opinions exist for the management of endometriosis, with key guidelines coming from organizations such as the American College of Obstetricians and Gynecologists (ACOG), the American Society for Reproductive Medicine, Society of Obstetricians and Gynecologists of Canada, National Institute for Health and Care Excellence,[11] and the European Society of Human Reproduction and Embryology (ESHRE).[12,13] Table 101-1 is a summary of the ESHRE-graded recommendations.

Desired Outcomes

7 5 Endometriosis is not curable with available treatment modalities; therefore, the present available options allow for the management of disease primarily through pain relief and correction of infertility treatment. Patient-specific goals and desired outcomes will vary and should be considered when making a treatment plan, as the individual patient's desires will greatly impact the treatment options available. Reducing pain and improving quality of life can be achieved through pharmacologic options and/or surgery.[2,10,14]

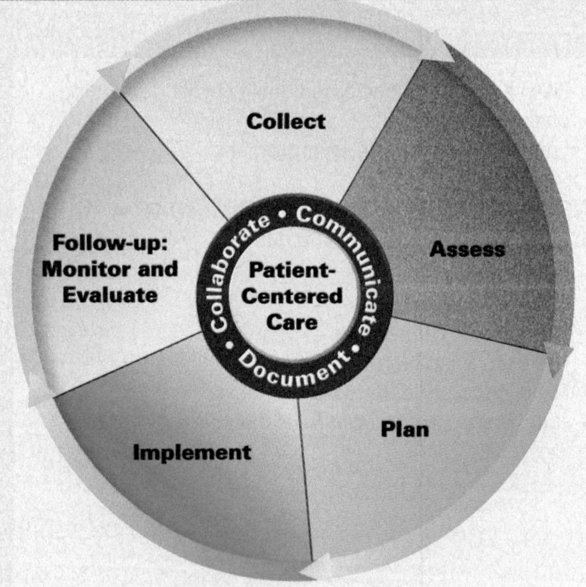

Patient Care Process for Endometriosis

The image shows the five fundamental steps included in The Pharmacist's Care Process endorsed by the Joint Commission for Pharmacy Practitioners (2014). The tagline of this process reads collaborate, communicate, and document. The five fundamental steps listed here are collect, assess, plan, implement, and follow-up: monitor and evaluate. All these steps are listed in a circular block diagram.

Collect

- Patient characteristics (age, race, ethnicity, sex, gender identity, pregnancy status, and interest in becoming pregnant)
- Patient medical history (personal and family)
- Patient's desire and timeline for fertility
- Symptoms (type of pain, location, frequency, cyclic vs acyclic)
- Objective data
  - Imaging procedure results confirming diagnosis of endometriosis (if available)

Assess

- Whether patient is a candidate for pharmacotherapy or surgical procedures
- Patient goals and treatment options (Tables 101-1 and 101-2)
- Presence of contraindications to treatment options
- Ability/willingness to use various formulations such as injections, vaginal ring, transdermal patch, intrauterine device
- Ability/willingness to pay for treatment options
- Likely adherence to options

Plan*

- Pharmacotherapy regimen including specific medication(s), dose, route, frequency, and duration (Table 101-3)
- Monitoring parameters including efficacy and safety (pain relief, adverse medication effects) (Table 101-3)
- Prepare patient education
- Referrals to other providers

Implement*

- Provide patient education regarding all elements of treatment plan
- Use motivational interviewing and coaching strategies to maximize adherence
- Schedule follow-up appointment (typically 2-3 months to determine treatment efficacy)

Follow-up/Monitor

- Resolution of symptoms
- Presence of adverse medication effects (Table 101-3)
- If using GnRH agonists: bone mineral density and serum lipids
- Patient adherence to treatment plan
- Duration of therapy depending on desire to become pregnant or patient entering menopause

**Collaborate with patients, caregivers, and other healthcare professionals.*

Endometriosis-related infertility does not respond to available pharmacologic therapies and requires surgical intervention.[2,10]

General Approach to Treatment

Endometriosis-related pain can be managed with medical treatment, surgical treatment, or both. The best option for an individual patient will depend on their specific goals for treatment. Current medical therapies relieve endometriosis-related pain through induction of a pseudopregnancy or pseudo menopausal state, which reduces painful lesions, but does not improve fertility. Therefore, individuals looking to become pregnant will typically require surgical intervention and may also require the use of assisted reproductive technologies. Pregnancy success rates do increase after surgical procedures, but the exact magnitude is unclear due to the lack of well-designed clinical studies.[2,10,14]

Medical management options include nonsteroidal anti-inflammatory drugs (NSAIDs), combined hormonal contraceptive (CHCs), progestins, gonadotropin-releasing hormone (GnRH) agonists, GnRH antagonists, danazol, and aromatase inhibitors. In general, the NSAIDs, CHCs, and progestins are recommended first line due to their proven success in dysmenorrhea management, tolerability, and cost. The GnRH agonists and danazol are both highly effective but are considered second-line options because of their adverse effect profiles. Aromatase inhibitors are considered last line after failure of other medical or surgical therapies.

The patient's chief complaint, possible adverse effects seen with various pharmacotherapeutic agents, extent of prescription medication coverage, contraindications to treatment, and adherence should all be considered when developing a treatment plan.[2,10,12,15] Information regarding pharmacotherapy options can be seen in Table 101-2. The NSAIDs are appropriate to use in conjunction with each listed treatment option, barring the existence of contraindications to use, as endometriosis treatments are not typically guaranteed to provide full relief of symptoms and may require adjunctive analgesic use.

TABLE 101-2 Evidence-Based Considerations in Endometriosis Treatment

Treatment Considerations	Grade of Recommendation—ESHRE
Empirical treatment of pain (without specific diagnosis) with CHCs or progestins	GPP
Preoperative hormonal treatment should NOT be initiated prior to surgery with the primary goal to improve surgery outcomes	A
Postoperative hormonal treatment should NOT be initiated after surgery with the primary goal to improve surgery outcomes	A
CHCs and LNG-IUS are preferred treatment options for postoperative secondary prevention of dysmenorrhea	A
Operative laparoscopy is the preferred treatment option for patients with infertility secondary to endometriosis who are looking to become pregnant	A
Hysterectomy–oophorectomy may be considered in patients finished with childbearing who have failed more conservative options	GPP

A = Meta-analysis or multiple randomized trials (of high quality); B = Meta-analysis or multiple randomized trials of moderate quality, single randomized trial, large nonrandomized trials, or case-control/cohort studies of high quality; C = Single randomized trial, large nonrandomized trial(s), or case-control/cohort studies (of moderate quality); D = Nonanalytic studies or case reports/case series (of high or moderate quality); GPP = Good practice point based on expert opinion.

Data from Reference 12.

Asymptomatic patients with an incidental diagnosis of endometriosis do not need treatment, but rather can be monitored for the development of pain or infertility and then managed at that point.[12]

Nonpharmacologic Therapy

6 Laparoscopic surgery is used as a diagnostic and therapeutic tool for endometriosis.[2,10,12] As part of this procedure, surgeons remove any visible lesions when performing a diagnostic surgery. Otherwise, individuals may seek surgery if they are infertile or are not responding to available medical treatment options. A hysterectomy–oophorectomy is an option for individuals who do not desire future pregnancy, but, as with other treatment modalities, this surgery does not guarantee full relief of symptoms.[12]

For those undergoing surgery, pre- and posttreatment with hormone therapy does not improve outcomes related to surgery. The ESHRE guidelines separate postsurgical treatment into adjunctive (use for <6 months) and secondary prevention (use for >6 months) categories. These guidelines state that short-term adjunctive hormonal treatment will not improve the surgical outcomes after surgery, but long-term medical treatment may be started postsurgery for purposes of contraception or secondary prevention. Secondary prevention recommendations include using CHCs or the levonorgestrel-releasing intrauterine system (LNG-IUS) for at least 18 to 24 months to prevent recurrence of endometriomas.[12,16,17]

Pharmacologic Therapy

Pharmacologic therapy is typically the first choice for treatment of endometriosis-related pain to minimize risks from multiple surgeries such as scarring and tissue adhesions. First-line treatment options are such because they are equally effective but have an improved tolerability and cost compared to alternative therapy options (Table 101-3).[2,10,12,15]

Medication Treatments of First Choice

8 First-line therapy for endometriosis-associated pain includes oral CHCs, oral progestins (norethindrone acetate or medroxyprogesterone acetate [MPA]), or depot medroxyprogesterone acetate (DMPA). These medications tend to be well-tolerated and are safe for long-term use, which is important because endometriosis symptoms typically return shortly after treatment is discontinued.[2,10,12,15]

Studies demonstrating direct comparisons between these products are lacking, so the decision of which product to use should depend on patient preference, including formulation type, dosing schedule, and potential adverse effects.[2]

Although laparoscopic imaging provides the only definitive diagnosis of endometriosis, these options may be initiated empirically for suspected endometriosis in patients of any age prior to laparoscopy.[2,10,12,15] Response to hormonal treatment does not predict the presence or absence of endometriosis, but use of these options before laparoscopy can avoid an invasive procedure.[12]

Nonsteroidal Anti-inflammatory Drugs Dysmenorrhea is a primary symptomatic feature of endometriosis and NSAIDs are indicated as the first-line treatment of menstrual pain with or without an endometriosis diagnosis. Individuals may initially self-treat with over-the-counter options, such as ibuprofen and naproxen; however, prescription strength versions of these are available as well, and individuals may find they need to use the upper end of the recommended dosing range in order to find relief from pain.[2,10,11]

Combined Hormonal Contraception CHCs are a first-line treatment option for suppression of endometriosis and are widely used due to their efficacy, tolerability, safety profile, and cost.[18] Their exact mechanism of action for endometrial pain relief is unclear because the pathogenesis of endometriosis is unclear. However, there are several widely accepted theories.[18] The CHCs alleviate dysmenorrhea, a common symptom of endometriosis, reduce the growth of endometrial tissue, decrease menstrual flow, and reduce prostaglandin generation.[18] They also downregulate cell proliferation and increase apoptosis in the eutopic endometrium.[18] Secondary benefits of CHCs include menstrual cycle regulation and contraception.

Oral CHCs have efficacy in a small number of observational, placebo-controlled, and active-comparator trials. The majority of studies on CHC efficacy have been for oral products; however, one study proved effectiveness of the CHC patch and vaginal ring, which may have appealing dosing schedules compared to their oral counterparts.[19] The decision between CHCs should be based upon patient preference, including adherence and cost.[2]

The CHCs have traditionally been dosed cyclically, with 3 weeks of active hormone followed by 1 week of placebo, allowing for a withdrawal bleed. However, some individuals prefer the option to dose continuously, either through commercially available "extended cycle" options or by skipping the placebo week of their CHC. The continuous dosing may be more efficacious than cyclic dosing after individuals with recurrent postoperative dysmenorrhea were switched from cyclic to continuous CHC dosing and reported a significant reduction in pain.[20] Other studies have mimicked these results, and the ESHRE guidelines now specifically recommend continuous dosing as an option for patients.[12]

Due to the proposed estrogen dependency of endometriotic lesions, it has been proposed that the estrogen dose in CHCs should be limited to avoid feeding the endometriosis tissue. Even the lowest doses of commercially available CHCs are four to six times the physiologic dose of estrogen; therefore, clinicians should consider initiating patients on CHCs with the lowest effective estrogen dose to limit this possibility.

Progestins Progestins are another first-line option for suppression of endometriosis due to their efficacy in treating dysmenorrhea, the overall tolerability of progestins, and their reasonable price. Progestins suppress growth of endometriotic implants, eventually causing endometriotic atrophy. They have also demonstrated inhibition of

TABLE 101-3 Dosing, Adverse Effects (AE) Monitoring, and Comments

Pharmacotherapy Options	Brand Name	Dosing	Adverse Effects	Monitoring Parameters and Counseling Points
NSAID				
Ibuprofen	Motrin; Advil	200-800 mg orally 3 times daily	Gastrointestinal upset, dizziness, skin rash, tinnitus	Take with food to limit GI upset
Naproxen	Aleve, Naprosyn	200-220 mg orally 2-3 times daily up to 500-550 mg twice daily		Consider monitoring blood pressure if using regularly
Diclofenac	Voltaren	50 mg orally 3 times daily		
CHC				
Various (oral tablet)	Various	1 tablet orally daily	Nausea, vomiting, breast tenderness, weight gain, acne, oily skin, fatigue, breakthrough bleeding, spotting, elevated blood pressure, application site reaction (patch only), vaginal irritation (ring only)	Continuous dosing may improve outcomes
Etonogestrel/ethinyl estradiol (vaginal ring)	NuvaRing	Insert one ring vaginally for 3 weeks and remove for 1 week		Many AEs improve after 2-3 cycles
Norelgestromin/ ethinyl estradiol (transdermal)	Ortho Evra; Xulane	Apply one patch weekly for 3 weeks and remove for 1 week		Measure blood pressure within 3 months of starting new method
Progestin				
Norethindrone (oral tablet)	Aygestin	5 mg orally daily; may titrate to 20 mg daily	Breast tenderness, nausea, peripheral edema, VTE	
MPA (oral tablet)	Provera	30 mg orally daily; may titrate to 60 mg daily	Menstrual irregularities, nausea, peripheral edema, VTE	
DMPA (IM or SubQ)	Depo-Provera IM	150 mg IM every 13 weeks	Menstrual irregularities, weight gain, acne, hirsutism, depression, decreased BMD	BMD testing not recommended
	Depo-SubQ Provera	104 mg SubQ every 12-14 weeks		
LNG-IUS	Mirena	Single insertion for up to 5 years	Menstrual irregularities, insertion-related complications, expulsion, pelvic inflammatory disease	
GnRH Agonist				
Goserelin	Zoladex	3.6 mg monthly SubQ implant	Acne, depression, hot flashes, mood swings, peripheral edema, vaginitis, BMD loss	Use add-back to prevent many AEs
Leuprolide	Leupron Depot	3.75 mg IM monthly or 11.25 mg IM every 3 months	Acne, depression, hot flashes, mood swings, vaginitis, BMD loss, VTE, anaphylaxis, nausea/vomiting, headache, dizziness, triglyceride elevation	Consider BMD testing every 1-2 years and serum lipid levels every 6 months if treatment exceeds 12 months
Naferelin	Naferelin	400 mcg intranasally daily (one spray in one nostril AM and one spray in the opposite nostril PM); may titrate to 800 mcg daily	Acne, headache, hot flash, mood swing, vaginal dryness, BMD loss, VTE	
Triptorelin	Triptorelin	3.75 mg IM monthly	Headache, elevated blood pressure, hot flashes, anaphylaxis, angioedema	
GnRH Antagonist				
Elagolix	Orilissa	150 mg orally once daily or 200 mg orally twice daily	Headache, nausea, anxiety, hot flash, BMD loss, change in lipid levels, insomnia, mood swings, night sweats	
Androgen				
Danazol	Danocrine	100-200 mg orally twice daily; may titrate to 400 mg twice daily	Acne, peripheral edema, hirsutism, lipid abnormalities, weight gain, hepatic dysfunction	Liver function tests and serum cholesterol every 3-6 months
Aromatase Inhibitor				
Anastrozole	Arimidex	1 mg orally daily	Arthralgias, hot flashes, myalgias, nausea, diarrhea, decreased BMD	Use with CHC, progestin, or GnRH agonist
Letrozole	Femara	2.5 mg orally daily		Consider BMD testing every 1-2 years if treatment exceeds 12 months

AEs, adverse effects; BMD, bone mineral density; DMPA, depot medroxyprogesterone acetate; IM, intramuscular; MPA, medroxyprogesterone acetate; SubQ, subcutaneous; VTE, venous thromboembolism.

blood vessel growth and anti-inflammatory action, in addition to their anovulatory effects, all which relieve the dysmenorrhea associated with endometriosis.[21-23]

Progestins may be administered orally (norethindrone acetate or MPA), intramuscularly or subcutaneously (DMPA) or as an LNG-IUS. As with other endometriosis treatment options, studies comparing progestin options directly are limited; therefore, selection should account for the individual's opinion about dosage form, as well as cost and potential adverse effects and risks.[24]

Oral Progestins Oral progestins are widely available as contraceptive and menopausal hormonal replacement products. Importantly, contraceptive progestin products have the added benefit of preventing pregnancy and managing other menstrual-related adverse effects, such as acne.

Injectable Depot Medroxyprogesterone Acetate The downsides to injectable DMPA use include a slow return to fertility and potential bone mineral density (BMD) loss, as DMPA carries a black box warning to avoid use for greater than 2 years due to the risk of potentially irreversible BMD loss. Controversy exists on the potential irreversibility of BMD loss and despite this labeling, the ACOG has stated that clinicians may continue its use beyond 2 years in patients who are responding well.[25] For those who wish to become pregnant shortly after discontinuing treatment, this option may not be preferred because of its associated slow return of normal ovulation. DMPA has a mean conception time of 10 months after discontinuation, compared to other hormonal products that have shorter return to fertility.[26]

Levonorgestrel Intrauterine System Insertion of an LNG-IUS is an option for those seeking long-acting reversible contraceptive benefits in addition to endometriosis pain relief. There are various forms of LNG-IUSs available in the market. Approximately 20% to 30% of patients experience amenorrhea within the first year of using an LNG-IUS, reducing the major symptom of endometriosis, dysmenorrhea.[27] Despite their efficacy at reducing endometriosis-related pain, no LNG-IUSs are Food and Drug Administration (FDA)-approved for the treatment of endometriosis.

The LNG-IUSs do not inhibit ovulation, yielding a potential for the growth of ovarian endometriomas. Other disadvantages of the LNG-IUS include potential difficulty of inserting the device into nulliparous individuals, a 5% expulsion rate, and cost of the procedure.[15]

Alternative Medication Treatments

Other options for treatment of endometriosis pain include GnRH agonists, GnRH antagonists, danazol, and aromatase inhibitors.[2,12,15,28] Treatments fall into this category for several reasons: lack of data supporting their efficacy in treating endometriosis, proven efficacy but intolerable adverse events, or unknown long-term safety.

None of these methods is proven superior over others, so treatment decisions should be made based on patient preference of dosage form and dosing schedule, patient-specific response, potential adverse effects, and medication costs/insurance coverage.[2,10,12,15]

Several of the options in this category can be combined with other medications to limit their adverse effects. For example, GnRH agonists are used with estrogen-progestin products to limit anti-estrogenic adverse effects and aromatase inhibitors are prescribed with CHCs, progestins, or GnRH agonists.

Gonadotropin-Releasing Hormone Agonists The GnRH agonists are highly effective at treating endometriosis-associated pain, but their use is limited by adverse effects and cost. The ACOG guidelines recommend their empiric use in the event of NSAID or contraceptive failure.[2] Pharmacologically the GnRH agonists inhibit follicle-stimulating hormone and luteinizing hormone secretion, which effectively mimics an oophorectomy.

The GnRH agonists create a gonadotropic flare prior to their long-term receptor downregulation, which may increase pain during this period. This can be minimized by initiating therapy during the mid-luteal phase or overlapping therapy with a CHC or progestin for 3 weeks. Pain will recur quickly upon discontinuation, making GnRH agonists a chronic treatment option.[29,30] Although GnRH agonist are approved by the FDA for only 12-month courses of treatment, if a patient responds well to therapy, it is often continued for longer with add-back therapy (subsequently discussed).[2]

Adverse medication effects seen with GnRH agonists are the result of the hypoestrogenic environment and include BMD loss and vasomotor symptoms, such as hot flushes, vaginal dryness, and insomnia. With long-term use (>6 months) BMD loss becomes a major concern. Utilization of add-back therapy minimizes this loss and other adverse events and has demonstrated safety for up to 10 years.[31,32] It is recommended to start add-back therapy on immediate initiation of GnRH agonist treatment.[2,12,15] Monitoring for this class of medications includes physical findings, bone density, and serum lipids.[2]

Add-Back Therapy 9 Add-back regimens may consist of progestins alone, estrogens, and progestins and bisphosphonates and are utilized in combination with GnRH agonists to reduce or eliminate BMD loss and provide symptomatic relief against the anti-estrogenic effects of GnRH agonists. The estrogen-progestin combinations are more effective than progestin monotherapy at protecting for BMD loss.[30,33,34]

Adding estrogen to a GnRH agonist has a potential to negate its anti-estrogenic effects that relieve endometriosis pain. Therefore, the dose of estrogen must be low enough to maintain a serum estrogen level <50 pg/mL (180 pmol/L) in order to prevent growth of new endometrial tissue while preventing anti-estrogenic adverse effects such as BMD loss and vasomotor symptoms. The CHCs should not be used as add-back therapy because they will yield a higher serum level than recommended; therefore, menopausal preparations are typically appropriately dosed to reach this serum level.[15] Examples of regimens studied include oral conjugated equine estrogens 0.625 mg/day plus oral norethindrone acetate 5 mg/day, and transdermal estradiol 25 μg twice weekly plus oral MPA 5 mg/day, and oral estradiol 2 mg/day plus oral norethindrone acetate 1 mg/day.[33]

Gonadotropin-Releasing Hormone Antagonists Elagolix is the only FDA-approved medication indicated to treat endometriosis. It is a member of the class of GnRH antagonists, which competitively inhibit GnRH receptors in the pituitary in order to rapidly decreases circulating estradiol and gonadotropins.[35] GnRH antagonists may represent a class of medications with similar efficacy but better tolerability compared to the GnRH agonists: while effectively downregulating the same hormones as GnRH agonists, the GnRH antagonists differ in their quicker onset and avoidance of a painful gonadotropin flare upon initiation. Elagolix can be dosed to achieve partial or full suppression, which may minimize hypoestrogenic adverse events compared to GnRH agonists. It is not clear whether add-back therapy is appropriate to minimize these adverse events if they do occur.

Adverse effects of elagolix include headache, nausea, anxiety, hot flashes, and some breakthrough bleeding and spotting.[36] Hypoestrogenic effects include hot flashes, increased serum lipid levels, and BMD loss. It is unknown whether the BMD loss is reversible and what the long-term effects of use may be.

Elagolix does not fully suppress ovulation and the effect of GnRH antagonists on pregnancy is unknown now.[36] Individuals are recommended to use contraception to avoid pregnancy while on this class of medications until further information is known.

Androgens Danazol is an androgen that serves as a second-line hormonal treatment option. Danazol inhibits endometrial tissue growth, induces endometrial atrophy, and causes amenorrhea due to the hypo-estrogenic/hypo-progestogenic environment it creates. It is highly effective and was formerly considered the gold standard of endometriosis treatment but is now used in a limited manner because of the androgenic properties of its adverse medication effect profile.[37]

Danazol should not be initiated in individuals with hyperlipidemia or liver disease. Barrier contraception must be used in conjunction with use of this medication due to its teratogenicity. Common adverse medication effects include hirsutism, mood changes, voice deepening, and acne, although some individuals may experience significant weight gain and fluid retention.[37]

Three studies have looked at the use of vaginal danazol formulations in an effort to limit systemic medication exposure and limit androgenic effects. Each study proved improvements in dysmenorrhea, deep dyspareunia, and pelvic pain without systemic adverse effects. The vaginal formulation of danazol is notavailable in the United States.[38-40]

Aromatase Inhibitors Aromatase inhibitors are a more recent addition to the endometriosis-treatment toolkit. While the ACOG guidelines do not support their routine use based on limited data, the ESHRE guidelines support their use in individuals with endometriosis refractory to other medical or surgical treatment.[2,12] This class lowers overall estrogen concentrations by inhibiting aromatase, which is key enzyme in the conversion of adrenal androgens to estrogens. The resultant reduction of estrogen concentrations then diminishes endometrial lesions.

Numerous case reports and studies have looked at aromatase inhibitors in combination with progestins, oral CHCs and GnRH agonists. Based on the results of these studies, there is decreased pain, improved quality of life, and reduced postoperative recurrence of disease in patients refractory to other treatments.[40-44]

As the aromatase inhibitors reduce circulating estrogen levels, long-term use may impact BMD, similar to other pharmacologic therapies. Safety information for this class of medications is mainly from studies in postmenopausal patients with cancer, which differs from the typical female of reproductive age who would be using these agents for endometriosis pain. Limited available data does indicate that the use of progestin monotherapy or CHCs in addition to the aromatase inhibitor would limit BMD loss.[40,41] The progestin and combined oral contraceptives may also limit the follicle-stimulating hormone release, which may lead to chronic ovarian stimulation.[2]

Special Populations

Endometriosis is most commonly diagnosed in individuals in their thirties and forties, but endometriosis is the most common diagnosis in adolescent patients presenting with secondary dysmenorrhea.[15] Endometriosis commonly presents as early stage in adolescents, so physical findings will often be normal and laparoscopic findings may be atypical compared to those seen in older individuals.[15]

Treatment of adolescent patients is similar to adult treatment guidelines, with the most notable difference related to the use of options that affect BMD.[15,28,45] Both DMPA and the GnRH agonists should be used with caution in adolescents due to BMD loss concerns and while they are not completely contraindicated, their use should be held off as long as possible and only started after full consideration of the risk/benefit profile.[45]

Dysmenorrhea in adolescents is typically treated empirically with first-line options including NSAIDs and CHCs. These can be trialed for 3 months to assess pain relief. If pain persists after 3 months, CHCs may be switched from cyclic to continuous dosing to instigate amenorrhea. The next step after failure of this first-line option typically includes consideration of laparoscopic diagnostic/treatment surgery because failure correlates highly to a diagnosis of endometriosis.

The incidence of endometriosis, pelvic pain, and irregular or heavy menses in transgender individuals has not been well characterized. Endometriosis is likely underdiagnosed in this patient group, but based on recent reports up to 50% of transgender men presenting for gender-affirming hysterectomy reported pelvic pain. Of these, one-third had findings of endometriosis including irregular bleeding and/or heavy menses.[46] Treatments such as progestins, oral contraceptives, danazol, and testosterone can sometimes relieve these symptoms.[47] Importantly, endometriosis symptoms can continue to occur despite the use of testosterone for their transition and thus may necessitate additional suppression. More studies are needed to better understand the clinical presentation and optimal treatment for this patient population.

EVALUATION OF THERAPEUTIC OUTCOMES

Outcome monitoring for endometriosis is based upon subjective relief of symptoms. Factors such as size, number, and distribution of endometrial lesions do not correlate to pain symptoms or potential fertility, limiting the use of objective tests to measure response to treatment.

The Endometriosis Treatment Satisfaction Questionnaire is a patient-reported outcome instrument that was developed and validated to measure patient reported pain before and/or during periods, pain during and/or after sex, endometriosis pain, bleeding and spotting, tolerability, and overall satisfaction using a seven-point Likert scale. Another validated tool is the Medical Outcomes Study Questionnaire Short Form 36 Health Survey (SF-36).[2,48,49]

Medical treatment of endometriosis should relieve endometriosis-related pain within 2 months of initiation. If symptoms are not relieved, individuals may try another medical option and/or surgery.

Surgery is frequently required in endometriosis-related infertility. Individuals must allow 6 months postintervention to try to conceive. If pregnancy is not achieved within this time-span, assisted reproductive technologies are the next line in treatment.

CONCLUSION

1 5 7 Endometriosis is a common disease with implications ranging from pain and reduced quality of life to infertility. Treatment modalities are not curative but may be successful at diminishing discomfort and improving quality of life. Treatment plans should be designed while taking into account patient-specific factors and goals.

ABBREVIATIONS

ACOG	American College of Obstetricians and Gynecologists
BMD	bone mineral density
CHC	combined hormonal contraceptive
DMPA	depot medroxyprogesterone acetate
ESHRE	European Society of Human Reproduction and Embryology
GnRH	gonadotropin-releasing hormone
LNG-IUS	levonorgestrel-releasing intrauterine system
MPA	medroxyprogesterone acetate
NSAID	nonsteroidal anti-inflammatory drug
VTE	venous thromboembolism

REFERENCES

1. Bedaiwy MA, Alfaraj S, Yong P, Casper R. New developments in the medical treatment of endometriosis. *Fertil Steril.* 2017;107(3):555–565.
2. Committee on Gynecologic Practice. ACOG Practice Bulletin No. 114: Management of endometriosis. *Obstet Gynecol.* 2010;116(1):223–236.

3. Cano-Sancho G, Ploteau S, Matta K, et al. Human epidemiological evidence about the associations between exposure to organochlorine chemicals and endometriosis: Systematic review and meta-analysis. *Environ Int.* 2019;123:209–223.
4. World Health Organization. Dioxins and their effects on human health. Available at: https://www.who.int/en/news-room/fact-sheets/detail/dioxins-and-their-effects-on-human-health. Accessed December 8, 2018.
5. Signorello LB, Harlow BL, Cramer DW, et al. Epidemiologic determinants of endometriosis: A hospital-based case control study. *Ann Epidemiol.* 1997;7:267–741.
6. Bulun SE. Endometriosis. *N Engl J Med.* 2009;360(3):268–279.
7. American College of Obstetricians and Gynecologists. Endometriosis FAQs. Available at: https://www.acog.org/womens-health/faqs/endometriosis. Accessed November 21, 2018.
8. Jones RK, Searle RF, Bulmer JN. Apoptosis and BCL-2 expression in normal human endometrium, endometriosis and ademomyosis. *Human Reprod.* 1998;13:3496–3502.
9. Peterson CM, Johnstone EB, Hammoud AO, et al. Risk factors associated with endometriosis: Importance of study population for characterizing disease in the ENDO study. *Am J Obstet Gynecol.* 2013;208(6):451.e1–451.e11.
10. Practice Committee of the American Society for Reproductive Medicine. Treatment of pelvic pain associated with endometriosis: A committee opinion. *Fertil Steril.* 2014;101(4):927–935.
11. National Institute for Health and Care Excellence. Endometriosis diagnosis and management. Available at: https://www.nice.org.uk/guidance/ng73. Accessed November 25, 2018.
12. Dunselman GAJ, Vermeulen N, Becker C, et al. ESHRE guideline: Management of women with endometriosis. *Human Reprod.* 2014;29(3):400–412.
13. Hirsch M, Begum M, Paniz É, et al. Diagnosis and management of endometriosis: A systematic review of international and national guidelines. *BJOG Int J Obstet Gyn.* 2017;125(5):556–564.
14. Ziegler D, Borghese B, Chapron C. Endometriosis and infertility: Pathophysiology and management. *Lancet.* 2010;376(9742):730–738.
15. Leyland N, Casper R, Laberge P, Singh SS. Endometriosis: Diagnosis and management. *J Obstet Gynaecol Can.* 2010;32(7 suppl 2):S1–S32.
16. Wu L, Wu Q, Liu L. Oral contraceptive pills for endometriosis after conservative surgery: A systematic review and meta-analysis. *Gynecol Endocrinol.* 2013;29(10):883–890.
17. Tanmahasamut P, Rattanachaiyanont M, Angsuwathana S, et al. Postoperative levonorgestrel-releasing intrauterine system for pelvic endometriosis-related pain. *Obstet Gynecol.* 2012;199(3):519–526.
18. Harada T, Momoeda M, Taketani Y, et al. Low-dose oral contraceptive pill for dysmenorrhea associated with endometriosis: A placebo-controlled, double-blind, randomized trial. *Fertil Steril.* 2008;90(5):1583–1588.
19. Vercellini P, Barbara G, Somigliana E, et al. Comparison of contraceptive ring and patch for the treatment of symptomatic endometriosis. *Fertil Steril.* 2010;93(7):2150–2161.
20. Vercellini P, Frontino G, Giorgi OD, et al. Continuous use of an oral contraceptive for endometriosis-associated recurrent dysmenorrhea that does not respond to a cyclic pill regimen. *Fertil Steril.* 2003;80(3):560–563.
21. Schweppe K-W. Current place of progestins in the treatment of endometriosis-related complaints. *Gynecol Endocrinol.* 2001;15(S6):22–28.
22. Vercellini P, Fedele L, Pietropaolo G, et al. Progestogens for endometriosis: Forward to the past. *Hum Reprod Update.* 2003;9:387–396.
23. Gezer A, Oral E. Progestin therapy in endometriosis. *Women's Health.* 2015;11(5):643–652.
24. Brown J, Kives S, Akhtar M. Progestagens and anti-progestagens for pain associated with endometriosis. *Cochrane Database Syst Rev.* 2012;(3):CD002122. doi: 10.1002/14651858.CD002122.pub2.
25. Committee on Adolescent Health Care, Committee on Gynecologic Practice. Committee Opinion No. 602: Depot medroxyprogesterone acetate and bone effects. *Obstet Gynecol.* 2014;123(6):1398–1402.
26. Hatcher RA, Trussell J, Nelson AL, et al. *Contraceptive Technology.* 21st ed. New York, NY: Ardent Median, Inc.; 2015.
27. Vercellini P, Aimi G, Panazza S, et al. A levonorgestrel-releasing intrauterine system for the treatment of dysmenorrhea associated with endometriosis: A pilot study. *Fertil Steril.* 1999;72(3):505–508.
28. Dovey S, Sanfilippo J. Endometriosis and the adolescent. *Clin Obstet Gynecol.* 2010;53(2):420–428.
29. Surrey ES. Gonadotropin-releasing hormone agonist and add-back therapy: What do the data show? *Curr Opin Obstet Gynecol.* 2010;22(4):283–288.
30. Divasta AD, Feldman HA, Gallagher JS, et al. Hormonal add-back therapy for females treated with gonadotropin-releasing hormone agonist for endometriosis. *Obstet Gynecol.* 2015;126(3):617–627.
31. Bedaiwy MA, Casper RF. Treatment with leuprolide acetate and hormonal add-back for up to 10 years in stage IV endometriosis patients with chronic pelvic pain. *Fertil Steril.* 2006;86(1):220–222.
32. Wu D, Hu M, Hong L, et al. Clinical efficacy of add-back therapy in treatment of endometriosis: A meta-analysis. *Arch Gynecol Obstet.* 2014;290(3):513–523.
33. Farmer JE, Prentice A, Breeze A, et al. Gonadotrophin-releasing hormone analogues for endometriosis: Bone mineral density. *Cochrane Database Syst Rev.* 2003;(4):CD001297.
34. DiVasta AD, Feldman HA, Gallagher JS, et al. The effect of hormonal add-back therapy in adolescents treated with a gonadotropin-releasing hormone (GnRH) agonist for endometriosis: A randomized trial. *J Adolescent Health.* 2015;56(2):S24.
35. Taylor HS. Use of elagolix in gynaecology. *J Obstet Gynaecol Can.* 2018;40(7):931–934.
36. Taylor HS, Giudice LC, Lessey BA, et al. Treatment of endometriosis-associated pain with elagolix, an oral GnRH antagonist. *N Engl J Med.* 2017;377(1):28–40.
37. Barbieri RL, Evans S, Kistner RW. Danazol in the treatment of endometriosis: Analysis of 100 cases with a 4-year follow-up. *Fertility and Sterility.* 1982;37(6):737–746.
38. Razzi S, Luisi S, Calonaci F, et al. Efficacy of vaginal danazol treatment in women with recurrent deeply infiltrating endometriosis. *Fertil Steril.* 2007;88(4):789–794.
39. Bhattacharya SM, Tolasaria A, Khan B. Vaginal danazol for the treatment of endometriosis-related pelvic pain. *Int J Gynaecol Obstet.* 2011;115(3):294–295.
40. Ferrero S, Tramalloni D, Venturini PL, Remorgida V. Vaginal danazol for women with rectovaginal endometriosis and pain symptoms persisting after insertion of a levonorgestrel-releasing intrauterine device. *Int J Gynaecol Obstet.* 2011;113(2):116–119.
41. Pavone ME, Bulun SE. Aromatase inhibitors for the treatment of endometriosis. *Fertil Steril.* 2012;98(6):1370–1379.
42. Abushahin F, Goldman KN, Barbieri E, et al. Aromatase inhibition for refractory endometriosis-related chronic pelvic pain. *Fertil Steril.* 2011;96(4):939–942.
43. Colette S, Donnez J. Are aromatase inhibitors effective in endometriosis treatment? *Expert Opin Investig Drugs.* 2011;20(7):917–931.
44. Nothnick WB. The emerging use of aromatase inhibitors for endometriosis treatment. *Reprod Biol Endocrinol.* 2011;9:87.
45. Stuparich MA, Donnellan NM, Sanfilippo JS. Endometriosis in the adolescent patient. *Semin Reprod Med.* 2017;35(1):102–109.
46. Ferrando CA, Chapman G, Pollard R. Preoperative pain symptoms and the incidence of endometriosis in transgender men undergoing hysterectomy for gender affirmation. *J Minim Invasive Gynecol.* 2021;28(9):1579–1584. 10.1016/j.jmig.2021.01.018 33497725.
47. Shim JY, Laufer MR, Grimstad FW. Dysmenorrhea and endometriosis in transgender adolescents. *J Pediatr Adolesc Gynecol.* 2020;33(5):524–528. doi: 10.1016/j.jpag.2020.06.001 32535219.
48. Deal LS, Williams VS, DiBenedetti DB, Fehnel SE. Development and psychometric evaluation of the endometriosis treatment satisfaction questionnaire. *Qual Life Res.* 2010;19(6):899–905.
49. Stull DE, Wasiak R, Kreif N, et al. Validation of the SF-36 in patients with endometriosis. *Qual Life Res.* 2014;23(1):103–117.

Menopausal Hormone Therapy

102

Devra K. Dang and Judy T. Chen

KEY CONCEPTS

1. The decision to use menopausal hormone therapy (MHT) and the type of formulation used must be individualized based on several factors, including personal preference, age, menopause onset, the severity of menopausal symptoms, and the risks of cardiovascular disease, breast cancer, osteoporotic fracture, and venous thromboembolic events (VTE).
2. Menopausal hormone therapy is the most effective treatment option for alleviating moderate-to-severe vasomotor symptoms.
3. Cardiovascular disease—including coronary artery disease, stroke, and peripheral vascular disease—is the leading cause of death among females, but MHT should not be used for reducing the risk of cardiovascular disease.
4. The risk of breast cancer associated with MHT is associated with the addition of progestogen therapy to estrogen. Use of estrogen alone does not increase the risk of breast cancer.
5. Use of MHT at doses lower than those prescribed prior to the Women's Health Initiative (WHI) study is effective in reducing bone loss and managing menopausal symptoms.
6. Use of transdermal MHT is preferred over oral preparations due to lower risk of thrombosis, and possibly stroke and coronary artery disease.
7. Because of the increased risk of endometrial hyperplasia and endometrial cancer with estrogen monotherapy (ie, unopposed estrogen), use of systemic estrogen in individuals with an intact uterus must always be accompanied by progestogen or tissue-selective estrogen complex (estrogen-bazedoxifene) for endometrial protection.
8. In individuals experiencing postmenopausal symptoms, initiation of systemic estrogen therapy should generally be limited to those younger than 60 years of age or within 10 years of menopause onset.

BEYOND THE BOOK

Create a table that compares and contrasts the three main formulations of estrogen: oral, transdermal, and vaginal. Suggested characteristics for comparison include name, dose, efficacy in treating symptoms of menopause, and common and major adverse effects. Summarize the major advantages and disadvantages of each formulation.

INTRODUCTION

Menopause is the permanent cessation of menses following the loss of ovarian follicular activity. It is a natural life event, not a disease, as all females undergo menopause, and each experiences it differently. Natural menopause occurs in stages including perimenopause (in the 5th decade), menopause, and postmenopause (1 year after menopause and beyond). Induced menopause can be experienced any time before natural menopause with bilateral oophorectomy (removal of both ovaries) or iatrogenic ablation of ovarian function (eg, chemotherapy, pelvic radiation). Symptoms of menopause can vary widely with induced menopause typically causing more severe symptoms. Due to the variability in duration, severity, and presence of menopausal symptoms, treatment should be individualized with treatment goals and decisions established in a shared decision-making process. In general, discussions around menopause and its treatment are primarily framed around cisgender women. However, any individual with a female reproductive system who has not undergone medical interventions may experience menopause. Therefore, the use of the term female is specifically meant to refer to biology, and this chapter has been written to include transgender individuals.

EPIDEMIOLOGY

The median age at the onset of menopause in the United States is 51 years, but can vary widely from 40 to 58 years.[1] An estimated 6,000 individuals in the United States reach menopause each day, and will spend approximately 40% of their lives in postmenopause.[2] By 2025, the number of postmenopausal individuals will be 1.1 billion worldwide.[1] By definition, menopause is a normal physiologic event that occurs after 12 consecutive months of amenorrhea, so the time of the final menses is determined retrospectively.[3] Individuals who have undergone hysterectomy (removal of the uterus) must rely on their symptoms to estimate the actual time of menopause, but typically occurs a few years earlier than natural menopause.

ETIOLOGY

A nomenclature and staging system for the female reproductive aging continuum was developed at the Stages of Reproductive Aging Workshop (STRAW) in 2001 and revised in 2011 with the STRAW+10 staging system, which is now considered to be the gold standard for characterizing reproductive aging.[3] The menopause transition refers to the span of time including menstrual, endocrine, and symptom changes starting with variation in menstrual cycle length and ending with the final menstrual period (FMP). Postmenopause occurs during the years beyond the FMP with stabilization of hormone levels and limited endocrine changes.

PATHOPHYSIOLOGY

A female is born with approximately two million primordial follicles in their ovaries. During a normal reproductive life span, they ovulate fewer than 500 times; therefore, the vast majority of follicles undergo atresia.

The hypothalamic–pituitary–ovarian axis dynamically controls reproductive physiology throughout the reproductive years. The pituitary is regulated by pulsatile secretion of gonadotropin-releasing hormone (GnRH) from the hypothalamus. Follicle-stimulating hormone (FSH) and luteinizing hormone (LH), produced by the pituitary in response to GnRH, regulate ovarian function. These gonadotropins also are influenced by negative feedback from estradiol and progesterone. Ovarian follicular activity is reflected by the circulating concentrations of sex steroids and by peptide hormones including inhibin, activin, and anti-Mullerian hormone (AMH). Overall, AMH is a product of growing ovarian follicles, which is independent of the hypothalamic–pituitary–gonadal axis. It is a principal regulator of early follicular recruitment from the primordial pool such that the concentration of AMH in blood may also reflect the nongrowing follicle population. In general, AMH concentrations decline with age, starting from 21 years and decrease 5.6% annually; subsequently, the AMH level reaches a precipitous drop and becomes unpredictable 3 to 5 years before menopause onset.[4] While AMH levels may predict the median time to menopause, obtaining levels of AMH, FSH, and estradiol may be best reserved for those seeking fertility. The sex steroids include estradiol, produced by the dominant follicle; progesterone, produced by the corpus luteum after maturation of the dominant ovarian follicle; and androgens, primarily testosterone and androstenedione, secreted by the ovarian stroma. These sex steroids are important for the healthy functioning of many organs, including the bones, brain, skin, and reproductive and urogenital tracts as they act primarily by regulating gene expression.

Physiologic changes associated with menopause are caused by loss of ovarian follicular activity. Since ovarian primordial follicle numbers decrease with advancing age, by the time of menopause, few follicles remain in the ovary. Hence, the postmenopausal ovary is no longer the primary site of estradiol or progesterone synthesis as it secretes primarily androstenedione. In contrast to the acute fall in circulating estrogen at the time of menopause, circulating androgens begin to decline in the decade prior to the average age of natural menopause and closely parallels increasing age. Whether the ovary continues to secrete testosterone after menopause remains controversial.

With advancing age and ongoing follicle loss, a progressive rise in circulating FSH and a concomitant decline in ovarian inhibin-B and AMH are observed.[5] The associated decline in inhibin B results in the loss of negative feedback on FSH. Inside the ovary, low levels of AMH serve to facilitate FSH-stimulated follicle growth and estrogen synthesis and secretion. Eventually, these compensatory hormonal mechanisms are no longer adequate with further follicle loss.[5] Low AMH concentrations, measured at any time in the cycle, predicts diminishing ovarian reserve.[6] Clear elevations in serum FSH with declining AMH are seen in accelerated depletion of the resting follicle pool after the age of 35 years.[5] When ovarian function has ceased, serum FSH concentrations are greater than 40 IU/L (mIU/mL). Menopause is characterized by a 15-fold increase in circulating FSH concentrations compared with concentrations of FSH in the follicular phase of the cycle, a 10-fold increase in LH, and a greater than 90% decrease in circulating estradiol concentrations.[5] During the perimenopause, FSH concentrations may rise to the postmenopausal range during some cycles but return to premenopausal levels during subsequent cycles. Thus, high concentrations of FSH should not be used to diagnose or manage menopause in perimenopausal individuals since frequency and severity of menopause do not correlate with FSH or serum estradiol levels and may be misleading.[7,8] There is a reciprocal relationship between declining inhibin B level and increasing FSH levels. The continuous decline in estradiol level may not reach its nadir until 1 to 2 years after the final menstrual period.[5]

CLINICAL PRESENTATION

Perimenopause commences with the onset of menstrual irregularity and ends 12 months after the last menstrual period.[3] Approximately 90% of females have 4 to 8 years of menstrual cycle changes with heavier flow of longer duration before natural menopause occurs.[1] The menstrual cycle irregularity is most often caused by the increased frequency of anovulatory cycles, but may also be due to thyroid abnormalities, hyperprolactinemia, or polycystic ovary syndrome. Symptoms are commonly experienced during perimenopause, which substantially impacts an individual's health and daily function. Vasomotor symptoms (eg, hot flashes and night sweats) develop in up to 80% of individuals and the symptoms on average persist for 7.4 years, with longer duration in those experiencing menopause at an earlier age.[9] However, only less than one-third of individuals seek medical attention for treatment. While the frequency of vasomotor symptoms varies, individuals on average report having 4 to 5 hot flashes per day with some experiencing as many as 20 hot flashes per day. Individuals of different race/ethnicity experience vasomotor symptoms differently, whereas Black individuals had the highest prevalence and longest duration of vasomotor symptoms, followed by Hispanic and White individuals with Asian individuals having the lowest prevalence.[9] Vasomotor symptoms persist for an average of 7.4 years with moderate-to-severe vasomotor symptoms extending in 42% of individuals aged 60 to 65 years.[9,10] Research has shown that 60% of individuals experience moderate hot flashes, 20% experience severe vasomotor symptoms, 68% experience urinary incontinence, 23% experience psychological symptoms (eg, depression), and 42% to 88% experience sexual dysfunction, along with reports of increased sleep disturbances.[10-13] Genitourinary syndrome of menopause (GSM) is a collection of symptoms associated with decreased estrogen and other sex steroids that create changes to the labia, clitoris, vestibule/introitus, vagina, urethra, and bladder.[13] Resulting symptoms include genital dryness, burning, and irritation; sexual symptoms of lubrication difficulty, discomfort or pain, and impaired sexual function; and urinary urgency, dysuria, and recurrent urinary tract infections. Vaginal symptoms occur in 27% to 84% of individuals.[13] While vasomotor symptoms generally improve over time, GSM is usually progressive without effective therapy. The majority of individuals report GSM negatively affect their sexual function and overall quality of life, yet many are not aware these symptoms are related to menopause and therefore these symptoms remain untreated.[12,13]

Perimenopause is associated with a higher vulnerability to depression with the risk increasing from early-to-late perimenopause and decreasing during postmenopause.[14] During the menopausal transition or early postmenopause, individuals are two to four times more likely to experience major depressive episode than in premenopause.[10] Those who experience a major depressive episode during perimenopause often represents a reoccurrence of their major depressive disorder.[14]

In addition to the symptoms of menopause, loss of estrogen production results in significant metabolic changes including effects on body composition, cognition, lipids, vascular function, and bone metabolism. The menopause transition is associated with a significant increase in central abdominal fat leading to an average weight gain during the menopausal transition of 5 lb (2.3 kg); however, this is likely to be related to aging and lifestyle rather than menopause.[1] Skin changes including decreased thickness and elasticity, loss of collagen, and wrinkling, and hair changes including alopecia and hirsutism are also associated with menopause. Poor concentration

CLINICAL PRESENTATION Perimenopause and Menopause

Signs

- Perimenopause: Abnormal uterine bleeding (AUB) as a result of anovulatory cycles (other gynecologic disorders should be excluded)
- Menopause: permanent cessation of menses

Symptoms

- Vasomotor symptoms (hot flashes and night sweats)
- Sleep disturbances
- Mood changes
- New-onset depression
- Problems with concentration and memory
- Arthralgia
- Genitourinary Syndrome of Menopause (GSM): vaginal dryness, burning and irritation of reproductive organs and structures, sexual dysfunction, dysuria, dyspareunia, urinary urgency, recurrent urinary tract infections

Laboratory Tests

- Perimenopause: FSH on day 2 or 3 of the menstrual cycle greater than 10 to 12 IU/L (mIU/mL)
- Menopause: 15-fold increase in FSH (a high FSH is not required to make the diagnosis)

Other Relevant Diagnostic Tests

- Thyroid function tests
- Iron stores
- Serum prolactin
- Lipid profile
- Serum hCG

and memory are common during the menopause transition and early postmenopause.[1] Approximately 60% of individuals report memory performance and processing speed slightly decline during the menopausal transition, characterized by the absence of learning during perimenopause that resolves in postmenopause.[15] While these cognitive symptoms can be affected by other symptoms of menopause such as sleep disturbances, hot flashes, depressed mood, fatigue, and midlife stressors, recent studies have suggested that the decline in cognitive performance is not related to menopause, but rather, is a function of chronological aging.[15]

Abnormal uterine bleeding (AUB) is characterized by a deviation of regularity, frequency, duration, or volume of menstrual fluid typical of a female's menses. In general, AUB may occur during the perimenopausal years because of anovulatory cycles; however, unusual uterine bleeding always merits investigation when it cannot be simply explained by menopausal cyclical irregularity. Hormonal treatment options for AUB include insertion of an intrauterine progestin-only device, systemic progestogen therapy, or the combined oral contraceptive pill unless contraindicated.[1]

TREATMENT

Desired Outcomes

Menopause is a natural life event, not a disease. The primary goals of therapy are to relieve symptoms and improve quality of life while minimizing adverse effects. This can be best achieved by individualizing treatment based on medical, social, and family history as well as the individual's symptoms and quality of life goals.

General Approach to Treatment

In those with mild vasomotor symptoms, nonpharmacologic therapy can be considered, while menopausal hormone therapy (MHT) is the treatment of choice for individuals with moderate-to-severe hot flashes and vulvovaginal symptoms, unless contraindicated (Table 102-1). Topical vaginal products should be reserved for individuals exclusively experiencing vulvovaginal atrophy. Treatment of mild vulvovaginal symptoms should include nonhormonal lubricants and moisturizers. However, for some individuals, these treatments are not effective. Figure 102-1 outlines an algorithm for the general management of menopausal individuals.

1 The decision to use MHT and the type of formulation used must be individualized based on several factors, including personal preference, age, menopause onset, the severity of menopausal symptoms and the risks of cardiovascular disease, breast cancer, osteoporotic fracture, and venous thromboembolic events (VTE). Breast cancer risk is increased with concomitant progestogen use in menopausal individuals with an intact uterus, and VTE may also increase with higher estrogen doses and oral administration.[16]

The duration of therapy also needs to be individualized according to the severity of symptoms, health status, and concerns regarding risks. Approved indications of MHT include treatment of moderate-to-severe vasomotor symptoms, moderate-to-severe vulvovaginal atrophy, and prevention of postmenopausal osteoporosis. For treatment of vasomotor symptoms, systemic MHT is the most effective pharmacologic intervention (Fig. 102-1). For genitourinary syndrome of menopause, such as vaginal dryness, intravaginal products should be considered.[6,13]

Nonpharmacologic Therapy

Mild menopausal symptoms may be managed effectively with lifestyle modifications, including wearing layered clothing that can be removed or added as necessary, lowering room temperature, decreasing intake of hot spicy foods, caffeine, and hot beverages, exercise, and other general good health practices. Some dietary supplements have been promoted as alternatives to MHT with conflicting results.[17]

Pharmacologic Therapy

Pharmacologic therapy is the mainstay of management of menopausal symptoms and includes both hormonal (estrogen with or without progestogen) and nonhormonal medications.

First Choice Treatment

2 Menopausal hormone therapy is the most effective treatment option for alleviating moderate-to-severe vasomotor symptoms. In individuals with an intact uterus, systemic MHT consists of an estrogen plus a progestogen or a tissue-selective estrogen complex (estrogen/bazedoxifene) to prevent endometrial hyperplasia. In those who have undergone hysterectomy, estrogen therapy is given unopposed by a progestogen (ie, as monotherapy). Mild vulvovaginal symptoms may be adequately managed with nonhormonal lubricants and

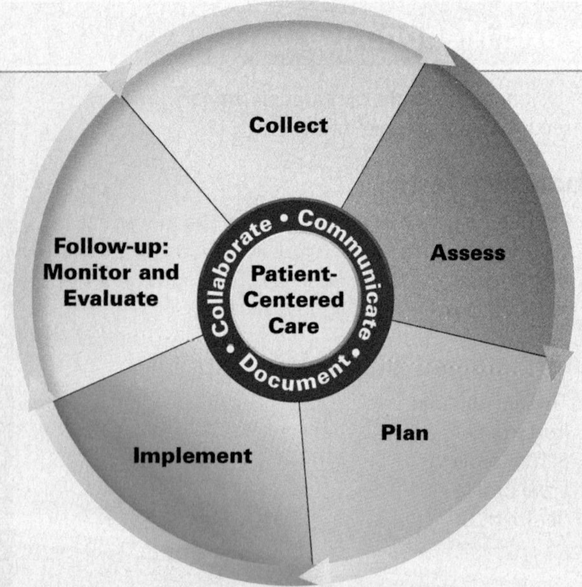

Patient Care Process for Post Menopausal Hormone Therapy

The image shows the five fundamental steps included in The Pharmacist's Care Process endorsed by the Joint Commission for Pharmacy Practitioners (2014). The tagline of this process reads collaborate, communicate, and document. The five fundamental steps listed here are collect, assess, plan, implement, and follow-up: monitor and evaluate. All these steps are listed in a circular block diagram.

Collect

- Patient characteristics: age, race, cis or transgender
- Personal and family medical history: cancer, cardiovascular disease, thromboembolic risks, osteoporosis, date of last menses, menstrual bleeding pattern, diabetes (Table 102-1)
- Gynecological surgical history
- Physical examination: breast and pelvic examination, Papanicolaou (PAP) cervical cytologic examination, mammography, liver function, assessment for gallbladder disease
- Bone mineral density results
- Current medication including prescription, nonprescriptions, and dietary supplements
- Social history: Tobacco use, ethanol use, caffeine use
- Symptoms: hot flashes, night sweats, irregular periods, sleep disturbances, mood changes, thinning of hair, difficulty with concentration or memory, arthralgia, and genitourinary syndrome of menopause (eg, vaginal dryness, burning and irritation of reproductive organs and structures, sexual dysfunction, dysuria, dyspareunia, urinary urgency, recurrent urinary tract infections) (see Clinical Presentation box)
- Signs: Abnormal uterine bleeding, decreased vaginal moisture, vaginal tissue fragility, thinning hair, skin changes (see Clinical Presentation box)
- Labs/Tests: Thyroid function tests, iron stores, serum prolactin, lipid profile, follicle stimulating hormone (FSH) levels
- Patient's expectations, preferences, and goals for therapy (eg, reduce frequency/predictability of menses, symptom relief)

Assess

- Evaluate the individual's menstrual cycle history or menstrual calendar
- Stage of menopausal transition; perimenopause, menopause, postmenopause
- Does the patient still have a uterus intact
- Rule out causes other than the menopausal transition for abnormal uterine bleeding and amenorrhea (eg, pregnancy, hyperprolactinemia, and hyperthyroidism) (see Clinical Presentation box)
- Emotional status (eg, anxiety, depression) (see Clinical Presentation box)
- Define patient's risk for osteoporosis, coronary heart disease, thromboembolic risks, cancer
- Risks and benefits of various therapy options (Table 102-3)
- Insurance coverage and patient's ability to afford treatment options

Plan*

- Nonpharmacologic lifestyle interventions including smoking cessation, dress in layers, weight loss, exercise, limit intake of spicy foods, caffeine, and hot beverages
- Develop a drug therapy regimen (including specific medication, dose, route, frequency, duration) to provide symptom relief, maximize adherence, provide endometrial protection, and minimize long-term risk (Tables 102-3 through 102-7, Table 102-9, and Fig. 102-1)
- Monitoring parameters for efficacy of therapy: reduction in vasomotor symptoms, improvement in genitourinary syndrome of menopause (GSM) signs and symptoms, mood stability, improved sleep (Table 102-8)
- Monitoring parameters for adverse effects: breast tenderness, bloating, premenstrual-like symptoms, mood changes, withdrawal bleeding or abnormal bleeding patterns (Table 102-8)
- Self-monitoring for vasomotor symptoms, GSM signs and symptoms, adverse effects, signs and symptoms of thrombosis

Implement*

- Provide patient education regarding all elements of treatment plan
- Educate patient regarding risks and benefits of treatment options, lifestyle modifications, drug-specific information
- Use motivational interviewing and coaching strategies to maximize adherence
- Schedule follow-up

Follow-up: Monitor and Evaluate

- Resolution of bothersome symptoms
- Presence of adverse effects
- Patient adherence to treatment
- Reevaluate need and continuation of therapy (Table 102-8)

**Collaborate with patient, caregivers, and other healthcare professionals.*

TABLE 102-1 FDA-Labeled Indications and Contraindications for Menopausal Hormone Therapy with Estrogens and Progestins

Indications	
For systemic use	Treatment of moderate-to-severe vasomotor symptoms (ie, moderate-to-severe hot flashes)
For intravaginal use (low systemic exposure)	Treatment of moderate-to-severe symptoms of genitourinary syndrome of menopause (ie, moderate-to-severe vaginal dryness, dyspareunia, and atrophic vaginitis)
Contraindications	
Absolute contraindications	Undiagnosed abnormal genital bleeding Known, suspected, or history of breast cancer Known or suspected estrogen- or progesterone-dependent neoplasia Active deep vein thrombosis, pulmonary embolism, or a history of these conditions Active or recent (eg, within the past year) arterial thromboembolic disease (eg, stroke, myocardial infarction) Liver dysfunction or disease
Relative contraindications	Elevated blood pressure Hypertriglyceridemia Impaired liver function and past history of cholestatic jaundice Hypothyroidism Fluid retention Severe hypocalcemia Ovarian cancer Exacerbation of endometriosis Exacerbation of asthma, diabetes mellitus, migraine, systemic lupus erythematosus, epilepsy, porphyria, and hepatic hemangioma

moisturizers.[13] However, vaginal estrogen therapy (cream, tablet, and ring) may be needed for moderate-to-severe vulvovaginal symptoms. Progestogen therapy for endometrial protection is not recommended with the use of low-dose vaginal estrogens (ie, those with minimal systemic exposure) with the exception of one vaginal ring (Femring®) known to deliver adequate systemic estrogen concentration to treat vasomotor symptoms.[13,18]

A number of national and international guidelines and consensus statements on the management of menopause are available.[6,7,13,17,19-27] The US Preventive Services Task Force also provides a recommendation statement on the use of MHT for the prevention of chronic medical conditions in postmenopausal individuals.[28]

Therapy for Perimenopausal Individuals

Despite a decline in fertility with age, sexually active females may become pregnant during the perimenopausal years. Furthermore, perimenopausal individuals can experience hot flashes despite having menstrual cycles. Combined hormonal contraceptives (containing low-dose estrogen and progestogen) provide contraception and vasomotor symptom relief. Perimenopausal individuals should not use estrogen-containing contraceptives if they smoke or have a history of estrogen-dependent cancer, cardiovascular or cerebrovascular disease, hypertension, diabetes with vascular disease, or risk factors for thromboembolism, liver disease, or migraine headaches. For perimenopausal individuals with AUB due to anovulatory cycles, a progestin-only intrauterine device may be a useful option. Combined hormonal contraceptives provide the additional benefit of reducing the risk of ovarian and endometrial cancer.

Menopausal Hormone Therapy for Vasomotor and Genitourinary Syndrome Symptoms

Menopausal hormone therapy remains the most effective treatment for moderate and severe vasomotor symptoms, impaired sleep quality, and vulvovaginal symptoms of menopause.[1,6,13,20-22]

Vasomotor Symptoms Fewer than 25% of females experience a menopausal transition without symptoms, whereas more than 25% suffer severe menopausal symptoms, most commonly hot flashes and night sweats. The average duration of vasomotor symptoms is 7.4 years with some individuals experiencing symptoms for more than 10 years. Individuals with mild vasomotor symptoms can experience relief by lifestyle modification, and at least 25% of participants of clinical trials reported significant improvement of vasomotor symptoms when taking placebo. The most effective treatment for vasomotor symptoms is MHT.[1,6,20-22] Benefits and risks of MHT should be weighed individually and assessed on an annual basis. Clinicians should select the most appropriate dose, duration, and routes of administration based on patient symptoms and medical history to provide the most benefits.

Genitourinary Syndrome of Menopause The lower genitourinary tract contains a high concentration of estrogen receptors and is particularly vulnerable to estrogen deficiency, resulting in symptoms which progressively worsen over time. Up to 85% of postmenopausal individuals report symptoms of GSM,[13] which results in vaginal dryness, burning, irritation, discomfort, and dyspareunia. Lower urinary tract symptoms include urethritis, recurrent urinary tract infection, urinary urgency, and frequency.

Most individuals with moderate-to-severe vulvovaginal symptoms require local or systemic estrogen therapy for symptom relief. Local (vaginal) estrogen delivery is preferred when vaginal symptoms are the only menopausal symptom complaint, as it minimizes systemic absorption and is more effective than oral estrogen therapy.[6,13] Vaginal estrogen has also been shown to improve atrophic symptoms and vaginal mucosal appearance, decrease vaginal pH, improve vaginal and/or urethral cytology, and reduce the risk of lower urinary tract symptoms and recurrent urinary tract infections possibly by modifying the vaginal flora.[6,13] Local estrogen therapy, but not systemic estrogen treatment, has demonstrated robust evidence for treatment of urinary incontinence in postmenopausal individuals.[29] Moderate-to-severe vulvovaginal symptoms can be treated with a vaginal estrogen cream, tablet, or ring; or with the selective estrogen receptor modulator (SERM) ospemifene given 60 mg orally per day.[13] Current data do support benefit of using combined systemic and vaginal estrogen in individuals suffering from severe GSM.[13] Ospemifene carries similar prescribing precautions as those with estrogens and other estrogen antagonist/antagonists, including increased risk of endometrial cancer. It also has a nearly full estrogen agonist effect in the vaginal epithelium to improve dyspareunia, sexual function, and overall satisfaction in postmenopausal individuals with moderate-to-severe vaginal dryness and has been well tolerated.[13] Individuals with moderate-to-severe dyspareunia can also consider prescription intravaginal dehydroepiandrosterone (DHEA) prasterone.

Dose-related adverse effects of vaginal estrogen include vaginal discharge, vulvovaginal candidiasis, vaginal bleeding, breast pain, and nausea.[13] Current prescribing information for low-dose vaginal estrogen therapy contains precautions similar to systemic hormone therapy (eg, CHD, stroke, VTE, breast, and endometrial cancer); however, these risks are highly unlikely given the minimal systemic absorption and reassuring findings from clinical and observational studies.[13] Concomitant progestogen therapy is unnecessary when low-dose vaginal estrogen is used with the exception of one vaginal ring (Femring) which is known to deliver a systemic concentration of estrogen.[18] Therapeutic response to vaginal estrogen

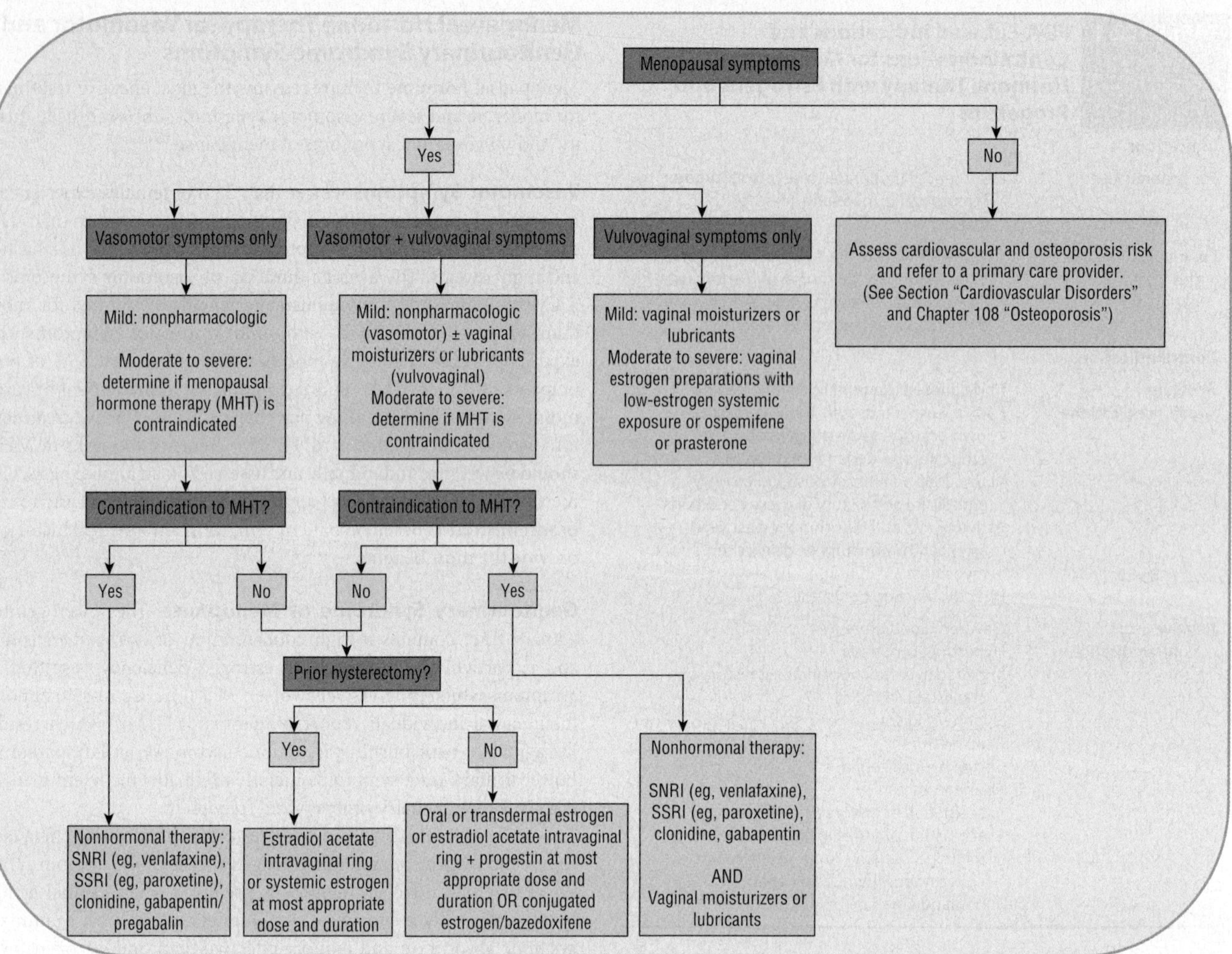

FIGURE 102-1 Algorithm for pharmacologic management of menopausal symptoms. SNRI: serotonin norepinephrine reuptake inhibitor, SSRI: selective serotonin reuptake inhibitor.

therapy is typically attained after 2 weeks of daily estrogen use. For maintenance therapy, the frequency of administration is generally decreased to two to three times weekly.

Vaginal rejuvenation devices using carbon dioxide laser therapy and other energy-based devices to destroy or reshape vagal tissues are marketed to help individuals with variety of symptoms related to menopause such as urinary incontinence, vaginal atrophy, dyspareunia, itchiness, or sexual dysfunction. They are considered a new approach and their use have increased globally despite recent warning posed by the US FDA due to reports of serious risks.[30] Efficacy and long-term safety of these procedures have not yet established and international societies do not endorse its use.[31] Further well-designed clinical trials are needed before definite conclusions can be drawn. Use of only FDA-approved therapies is recommended for individuals suffering from GSM.

Assessing Benefits and Risks of Systemic Menopausal Hormone Therapy

The Women's Health Initiative (WHI) was a randomized, double-blind, placebo-controlled trial launched in 1991 to evaluate the effects of MHT on heart disease, osteoporosis, and cancer. The WHI trial had two arms: the estrogen-plus-progestin arm involving females with an intact uterus and the estrogen-alone arm involving females with a history of hysterectomy.[16] The combined estrogen and progestin arm included 16,608 participants aged 50 to 79 years (mean age, 63 years), and the estrogen-only arm enrolled 10,739 participants aged 50 to 79 years (mean age, 64 years). The primary outcome was incidence of coronary heart disease (CHD) (nonfatal myocardial infarction or CHD death), and the primary safety outcome was invasive breast cancer. A global index was used to summarize the balance of risks and benefits, which included the two primary outcomes plus stroke, pulmonary embolism, endometrial cancer, colorectal cancer, hip fracture, and death due to other causes. The estrogen-plus-progestin arm was terminated prematurely after only 5.2 years (the planned duration was 8.5 years) because the global index statistic supported risks exceeding benefits on the major clinical outcomes. The estrogen-only arm also was terminated early (after 6.8 years) because of excess risk of stroke. Results of the WHI trial are shown in Table 102-2.[16] Upon discontinuation of the trial, participants were asked to discontinue study medication and invited to participate in a follow-up phase of the study that has resulted in multiple ancillary analyses.[14,16,32-38]

Use of MHT has greatly evolved to recognize the need to tailor therapy for individuals based on patient-specific factors (eg, age, risk factors, and goals of therapy). A summary of various clinical considerations described in the 2017 Hormone Therapy Position Statement of the North American Menopause Society is provided in Table 102-3.[1,6,12,17,22,23,28,29]

Furthermore, several national and international organizations have published guidelines or position statements to outline points of consensus regarding the safe and effective use of MHT.[1,6,17,19,20,23-27,39]

TABLE 102-2 Principal Results of the Women's Health Initiative Hormone Therapy Trial

	Estrogen + Progestogen Arm (Median Duration 5.6 Years)			Estrogen-Only Arm (Median Duration 7.2 Years)		
	MHT ($n = 8{,}506$)	Placebo ($n = 8{,}102$)		MHT ($n = 5{,}310$)	Placebo ($n = 5{,}429$)	
Outcome	No. Patients (Annualized %)	No. Patients (Annualized %)	Hazard Ratio (Nominal 95% CI)	No. Patients (Annualized %)	No. Patients (Annualized %)	Hazard Ratio (Nominal 95% CI)
CHD	196 (0.41)	159 (0.35)	1.18 (0.95-1.45)	204 (0.55)	222 (0.58)	0.94 (0.78-1.14)
Stroke	159 (0.33)	109 (0.24)	1.37 (1.07-1.76)	169 (0.45)	130 (0.34)	1.35 (1.07-1.70)
Pulmonary Embolism	87 (0.18)	41 (0.09)	1.98 (1.36-2.87)	52 (0.14)	39 (0.10)	1.35 (0.89-2.05)
Invasive Breast Cancer	206 (0.43)	155 (0.35)	1.24 (1.01-1.53)	104 (0.28)	135 (0.35)	0.79 (0.61-1.02)
Colorectal Cancer	50 (0.10)	75 (0.17)	0.62 (0.43-0.89)	65 (0.17)	58 (0.15)	1.15 (0.81-1.64)
Endometrial Cancer	27 (0.06)	30 (0.07)	0.83 (0.49-1.40)	NA	NA	NA
Hip Fracture	53 (0.11)	75 (0.17)	0.67 (0.47-0.95)	48 (0.13)	74 (0.19)	0.67 (0.46-0.96)
All Cause Mortality	250 (0.52)	238 (0.53)	0.97 (0.81-1.16)	301 (0.80)	299 (0.77)	1.03 (0.88-1.21)
Global Index	876 (1.89)	736 (1.68)	1.12 (1.02-1.24)	753 (2.08)	755 (2.04)	1.03 (0.93-1.13)

CI, confidence interval; MHT, menopausal hormone therapy.

Data from Reference 16.

TABLE 102-3 Summary of North American Menopause Society Position Statement on Menopausal Hormone Therapy

Symptom/Condition	Summary Statement(s)
Vasomotor symptoms	Estrogen therapy (± progestogen) is the most effective therapy, including consequences of vasomotor symptoms such as sleep quality, irritability, difficulty concentrating, and quality of life
Genitourinary syndrome of menopause (GSM)	Estrogen therapy is the most effective treatment for moderate-to-severe GSM symptoms. Local therapy is recommended for sole vaginal symptoms; progestogen generally not indicated for low-dose vaginal estrogen therapy. Individuals at risk of endometrial cancer may warrant endometrial surveillance. No data to support initial use of combined systemic and vaginal estrogen for severe GSM.
Sexual function	Low-dose local estrogen therapy may improve lubrication, blood flow, and vaginal sensation; however, MHT is not recommended as treatment for other problems of sexual function (eg, libido, orgasmic response)
Osteoporosis	Standard-dose MHT reduces postmenopausal osteoporotic fractures (hip, vertebral, and nonvertebral) and many systemic MHT products are approved for prevention of osteoporosis. MHT is not indicated for treatment. Benefits of MHT dissipate when discontinued
Coronary heart disease	Observational and randomized control data are conflicting. Estrogen only therapy may reduce CHD risk when initiated in newly menopausal Individuals (age 50-59 years). Estrogen + progestogen therapy initiated between ages 50 and 59 years or within 10 years of menopause does not increase CHD risk. Individuals initiating therapy after 10 years since menopause have an increased risk of CHD. MHT is not recommended any time for coronary protection
Stroke	Increased risk of ischemic stroke (not hemorrhagic) exists with estrogen only and estrogen + progestogen use
Venous thromboembolism (VTE)	Increased risk of VTE with oral MHT across all ages. Risk increases with personal risk factors including obesity, previous history of VTE, and the presence of Factor V Leiden mutation. The type of progestogen may impact risk. Transdermal formulations have lower VTE risk than oral formulations

CHD, coronary heart disease; MHT, menopausal hormone therapy; VTE, venous thromboembolism.

Data from References 1, 6, 12, 16, 19, and 23.

Overall, consensus recommendations regarding the use of MHT include:

- Menopausal hormone therapy is the most effective treatment for vasomotor symptoms. Healthy, recently menopausal individuals (before the age of 60 years or within 10 years of menopause) have the most favorable benefit-to-risk profile.
- Menopause hormone therapy should not be used for the primary and secondary prevention of CHD at present.
- Estrogen-only therapy may decrease heart disease and all-cause mortality in 50- to 59-year-old individuals with a history of hysterectomy. In this age group, combined estrogen and progestogen therapy shows similar trends for mortality, but no significant difference in CHD.
- Estrogen alone is appropriate for individuals after hysterectomy; additional progestogen is required when a uterus is present.
- Use of MHT should be individualized based on the severity of menopausal symptoms and personal risk factors (eg, age, time since menopause, history of VTE, stroke, ischemic heart disease, osteoporosis risks, and breast cancer).
- Risk of VTE and stroke increases with oral MHT containing estrogen, but the absolute risk is low in individuals below 60 years of age. Based on observational studies, transdermal MHT and low-dose oral estrogen therapy have a lower risk of VTE and stroke compared to standard-dose oral estrogen regimens.
- Menopausal hormone therapy is contraindicated in individuals with a personal history of breast cancer. The risk of

MHT-related breast cancer is associated with the addition of progestogen to estrogen and increases after 5 or more years of continuous combined use. However, the use of estrogen alone decreases rather than increase breast cancer risk.

- Select the most appropriate dose, duration, and routes of administration of hormone therapy to provide the most benefits and adequately manage menopausal symptoms. Duration of therapy should not be discontinued solely based on the patient's age.

Cardiovascular Disease 3 Cardiovascular disease—including coronary artery disease, stroke, and peripheral vascular disease—is the leading cause of death among females, but MHT should not be used for reducing the risk of cardiovascular disease. Menopause is associated with the development of a more adverse lipid profile, and the presence of vasomotor symptoms has been associated with an increased risk of cardiovascular disease.[40]

In the decade prior to the publication of the WHI results in 2002, an expectation of coronary benefit had been a major reason for use of postmenopausal hormones because observational studies indicated that individuals who use MHT have a 35% to 50% lower risk of CHD than nonusers. In addition, previous studies had shown that estrogen exerts protective effects on the cardiovascular system, including lipid-lowering, antioxidant, and vasodilating effects.[41] However, in the 2000s, published results of several randomized clinical trials provided no evidence of cardiovascular disease protection and even some evidence of harm with MHT.[16,34]

The primary findings of the estrogen plus progestogen arm of the WHI trial showed an overall increase in the risk of CHD (HR 1.18, 95% CI: 0.95-1.45) among healthy postmenopausal participants receiving combined estrogen–progestogen MHT compared with those receiving placebo.[16] The primary findings of the estrogen-only arm of the WHI trial show no effect (either increase or decrease) on the risk of CHD in participants taking estrogen alone.[16] Similar patterns of risk and benefits profile of estrogen-alone therapy are seen in individuals with and without bilateral oophorectomy.[6,16] In the extended post-intervention follow-up of 13 years revealed that individuals who initiated MHT 10 or more years after the time of menopause tended to have increased CHD risk compared with those who initiated therapy within 10 years of menopause.[14] Estrogen plus progestogen was associated with a non-significantly elevated CHD events in individuals aged 50 to 59 years, whereas estrogen alone was associated with reduced risk of CHD in those who were younger than 60 years and/or who are within 10 years of menopause onset.[6,16] Older individuals (age 70-79) who are more than 20 years past menopause onset experience highest risk of CHD that is significant compared with placebo group when estrogen plus progestogen therapy is initiated.[6,16] Most individuals who commence estrogen or estrogen plus progestogen therapy do so within the first few years of becoming menopausal.

A randomized controlled study of 1,006 recently menopausal individuals revealed that 10-year MHT was associated with a significantly reduced risk of cardiovascular disease.[42] In addition, studies of recently menopausal individuals showed that the presence and severity of hot flashes are associated with vascular endothelial dysfunction and vascular inflammation (markers of increased risk for CHD); MHT improved both these parameters.[43]

In an attempt to resolve some of the controversies, the Kronos Early Estrogen Prevention Study (KEEPS) randomized 727 recently menopausal participants (mean age 52 years and less than 3 years since FMP) to cyclic progestogen and either oral estrogen (conjugated estrogen 0.45 mg/day), transdermal estrogen (estradiol 50 μg/day), or placebo to examine the rate of atherosclerosis.[43] While KEEPS provided reassurance regarding safety and efficacy of MHT regimen, there was no difference among the study arms on atherosclerotic progression as evidenced by carotid intima-media thickness (CIMT) and coronary artery calcium during 4 years of treatment.[43] However, in the Early versus Late Intervention Trial with Estradiol (ELITE) trial, use of hormone therapy (oral 17β-estradiol 1 mg/day plus progesterone vaginal gel administered sequentially in participants with intact uterus) showed reduced carotid intima-media thickness progression in early postmenopausal individuals who initiated hormone therapy within 6 years of menopause onset, but similar cardioprotective effect was not observed among postmenopausal individuals who initiated hormone therapy 10 years after menopause onset.[44] Posttrial analysis from ELITE further supported that higher plasma estradiol (E2) levels were differentially associated with atherosclerosis progression according to the timing of hormone therapy initiation.[45] While both groups have higher plasma estradiol levels, those in early postmenopause had decreased CIMT progression rate, whereas individuals in late postmenopause had increased CIMT progression rate. While results from the ELITE trial provide preliminary evidence for the "timing hypothesis" or the "window of opportunity" concept that the benefits of hormone therapy are dependent on the timing of initiation and that hormone therapy may be cardioprotective if started around the time of menopause. Therapy may be harmful when initiated in late postmenopausal individuals, and currently available clinical data remain inconsistent and additional research is still needed.[1,46]

With available data, current guidelines caution against initiating or continuing menopausal hormone therapy solely for primary or secondary prevention of cardiovascular disease.[6,28] Use of menopausal hormone therapy is not indicated for individuals with a high risk of CVD.[6] Adherence to a healthful lifestyle (smoking cessation, regular exercise, healthy diet, and body mass index less than 25 kg/m^2) may prevent the onset of cardiovascular disease in postmenopausal individuals.[17] It should be noted that use of vaginal estrogen is not associated with an increased risk of CHD.[32]

Oral estrogen monotherapy have favorable effect on lipoprotein levels, glycemia, insulin, and CVD risks; however, addition of progestogen attenuates some of the beneficial effects of estrogen.[47] In the estrogen plus progestogen arm of the WHI study, the increased risk for stroke (HR 1.37, 95% CI: 1.07-1.76) and pulmonary embolism (HR 1.98, 95% CI: 1.36-2.87) was evident, even during the postintervention phase.[16] Increased risk was observed only for ischemic stroke but not for hemorrhagic stroke. In the estrogen-alone arm of the study, a similar increased risk (HR 1.35, 95% CI: 1.07-1.70) for stroke was observed.[16] After the cessation of treatment, the risks for stroke remain higher compared with placebo groups at 13-year follow-up.[16] The optimal duration of hormone therapy with respect to stroke risk remains to be determined.[48] Oral micronized progesterone seems to have least adverse effects.[49] Transdermal estrogens (<50 μg/day) have improved adverse effect profile than oral estrogens and suggested a lower risk of stroke than oral estrogens.[47,48] It should be noted that use of vaginal estrogen is not associated with an increased risk of stroke.[32]

In the cumulative 18-year follow-up from WHI trials, hormone therapy with combined estrogen–progestogen or estrogen alone have not been shown to increase all-cause mortality including death from CVD, CHD, and stroke.[33] In fact, younger individuals (aged 50-59 years) who initiated estrogen monotherapy for 7.1 years was found to have a significant and sustained beneficial impact on overall mortality.[33] Recent meta-analysis of randomized controlled trials and observation studies support similar findings that menopausal hormone therapy was not associated with increase all-cause death, myocardial infarction, or cardiovascular death but was associated with an increased risk of stroke, venous thromboembolism, and pulmonary embolism which further emphasized that underlying disease and timing of initiation should be carefully considered before starting MHT.[49]

The Endocrine Society clinical practice guideline recommends evaluating an individual's 10-year CVD risk before initiation of MHT using the ACC/AHA Cardiovascular Risk Calculator.[20,50] Regardless of years since menopause onset, the guideline recommends avoiding hormone therapy for symptomatic individuals at high CV risk (>10%) and advocates for the use of nonhormone therapy. For individuals at moderate risk of CVD (5%-10%), use of transdermal estrogen is preferred over oral formulations with oral micronized progesterone in those with an intact uterus.[20]

Venous Thromboembolism In general, VTE, including thrombosis of the deep veins of the legs and embolism to the pulmonary arteries, is uncommon in the general population. Conversely, individuals taking oral estrogen therapy have a twofold increased risk for thromboembolic events, with the highest risk occurring in the first 1 to 2 years of use.[6,16,34] One of the main predictors of future VTE is duration of hormone therapy use.[48] However, individuals with certain risk factors for VTE including those with a Factor V Leiden mutation, protein C and protein S deficiencies, congenital thrombophilic disorders, obesity, and history of previous thromboembolic events are at increased risk with MHT.[6,51] Patients with confirmed COVID-19 infections are also at higher thromboembolic risk and may warrant special management and considerations.[52] Lower doses of estrogen are associated with a decreased risk for thromboembolism as compared with higher doses. Oral administration of estrogen increases the risk of VTE compared to the transdermal route.[6,47,51] There is no indication for thrombophilia screening before initiating MHT. However, MHT should be avoided in individuals at high risk for thromboembolic events. It should be noted that use of vaginal estrogen is not associated with an increased risk of pulmonary embolism or VTE.[32]

Breast Cancer 4 There have been controversies regarding the association between MHT and breast cancer. The risk of breast cancer associated with MHT is associated with the addition of progestogen therapy to estrogen, as use of estrogen alone does not increase the risk of breast cancer. The WHI trial found that combined estrogen plus progestogen oral therapy has an increased risk of invasive breast cancer (HR 1.28, 95% CI: 1.13-1.45) and a trend toward increasing risk with increasing duration of therapy.[36] After discontinuation of estrogen plus progestogen therapy, WHI study results demonstrated a year-to-year reduction in breast cancer risk but elevated risk overall persists more than a decade after discontinuation of hormone therapy (HR 1.23, 95% CI: 0.96-1.59).[36] On the contrary, the estrogen-only arm of the WHI trial found a lower risk for breast cancer (HR 0.78, 95% CI: 0.65-0.93) after more than 20 years of cumulative follow-up, which persisted after treatment discontinuation.[36] This association between estrogen-only therapy and lower incidence of breast cancer was evident in year 5 and subsequently thereafter, the observed benefit was greater among participants without first-degree relative with breast cancer.[36] Furthermore, death from breast cancer was significantly lowered among postmenopausal participants who took estrogen monotherapy compared to placebo (HR 0.60, 95% CI: 0.37-0.97).[35] No significant differences by age, year since menopause, duration of prior hormone use, or gap time (time since menopause to earlier of first hormone therapy use) was observed in regards to breast cancer risks among postmenopausal individuals on hormone treatments.[35] However, younger postmenopausal individuals (aged 50-59 years) who have some years of estrogen deprivation (>5 years) prior to starting hormone therapy have the most favorable health benefits versus risks profile. This is especially evident for breast cancer, whereas post-hysterectomy individuals (aged 50-59 years) having short gap times (<5 years) prior to starting hormone therapy do not show breast cancer risk reduction.[53] Further analysis suggested for younger individuals (aged 50-59 years), that lower breast cancer risk with estrogen-alone therapy, are more closely tied to a large gap time than to prior bilateral oophorectomy status.[54] The benefit of large gap time could possibly be supported by the estrogen-induced apoptosis theory, which suggested that prolonged periods of estrogen deprivation cause breast cancer cells to become vulnerable and undergo apoptotic cell death when exposed to exogenous estrogen.[55,56] Breast cancer risk is similar between low-dose (<0.625 mg) and conventional dose (0.625 mg) of conjugated equine estrogen, but a lower risk of breast cancer is noted with the transdermal formulation.[36]

Addition of progestogens to estrogen may increase breast cancer risk beyond that observed with estrogen alone.[16,17,36] In the estrogen plus progestogen arm of the WHI, the increased breast cancer risk became significant in year 6 and remained significantly thereafter.[36] The breast cancers diagnosed in females in the menopausal hormone therapy group were more likely to be in an advanced stage with lymph node involvement compared with those in the placebo group.[36] Despite increased incidence of breast cancer risk with combined estrogen plus progestogen therapy, no significant increased risk of death from breast cancer was noted during the 20 years of cumulative follow-up (HR 1.35, 95% CI: 0.95-1.95).[36] In fact, a large population-based study found that individuals who received menopausal hormone therapy prior to diagnosis of breast cancer were associated with an improved breast cancer survival with 23% to 43% risk reduction of all-cause, breast cancer and CVD mortality after approximately 18 years of follow-up.[57,58]

While estrogen plus progestogen findings from randomized controlled trials are generally consistent with the observational studies, the findings of estrogen monotherapy on incidence of breast cancer and breast cancer mortality contrast with most prospective observational studies. In a meta-analysis from the Collaborative Group on Hormonal Factors in Breast Cancer, gathered evidence from worldwide epidemiological studies suggested that both hormone therapy regimens (estrogen plus progesterone and estrogen-only) increased incidences of breast cancer.[59] These results are also consistent with increased 20-year breast cancer mortality observed with both menopausal hormone preparations from the Million Women Study.[60] The effect of menopausal hormone therapy on breast cancer remains unsettled with discordance from observational studies and WHI studies despite several proposed explanations attempt to reconcile these discrepancies. The effect of hormone therapy on breast cancer and replications of the findings from WHI studies are needed.

For females in the United States, the lifetime risk of developing breast cancer is approximately one in eight, and the greatest incidence occurs in those older than 60 years.[61] The Endocrine Society clinical practice guideline recommends evaluating breast cancer risk before MHT initiation using either the 5-year risk assessment tool from National Cancer Institute Breast Cancer Risk Assessment Tool (https://bcrisktool.cancer.gov) or the 10-year International Breast Intervention Study calculator (http://ibis.ikonopedia.com).[20] Consideration of individual's underlying breast cancer risk should also be clearly communicated. In general, current guideline cautions against using hormone therapy for individuals in the intermediate-risk category, and advises against using systemic hormone therapy for those in the high-risk category, particularly with a personal history of breast cancer.[6,20] Hormone therapy regimens and formulations differ substantially on their effect on breast cancer risks with continuous combined estrogen-progestogen regimen associated with a threefold increase in breast cancer risks and sequential therapy was only associated with suggestive risk.[62] Furthermore, breast cancer risk varies with the type of progestins used with dydrogesterone (not currently available in the United States) conveying a lower risk than medroxyprogesterone, levonorgesterel, and norethisterone-containing hormone regimens and increase risk with increased duration of use.[63] While use of vaginal estrogen with minimal systemic absorption has not been demonstrated to increase risk of breast cancer, use of low-dose local vaginal estrogen may be considered only after unsuccessful trials of nonhormone therapies in conjunction with consultation with the patient's oncologist.[13]

Endometrial Cancer It is well documented that systemic estrogen alone given to individuals with an intact uterus significantly increases uterine cancer risk.[6,34,58,64] The excess risk increases with dose and duration of estrogen and persists for many years after estrogen replacement is discontinued.[6,20] While estrogen alone is appropriate for individuals after hysterectomy, use of systemic estrogen in patients with an intact uterus must always be accompanied by adequate dose and duration of progestogen for endometrial protection. The protective effect of hormone therapy on the uterus and risk of developing endometrial cancer vary based on the different types and duration of progestogen used.[64] Although results from the WHI trial's postintervention and follow-up phase demonstrated a reduced risk of endometrial cancer with combined oral MHT,[14] for symptomatic individuals with advanced cancer or higher risk for endometrial cancer, use of nonhormone therapies is still recommended and the use of systemic hormone therapy is not recommended.[64] Individuals preferring not to take progestogen may consider tissue-selective estrogen complex (estrogen/bazedoxifene) as an alternative to reduce risk of endometrial hyperplasia. Recent meta-analysis suggested that use of combined estrogen-progestogen therapy and the cyclic regimen do not increase incidence of endometrial cancer reoccurrence in postmenopausal individuals treated with early stages of endometrial cancer, but racial disparities exist on cancer reoccurrence with a much higher risk observed among Black American females.[65] In the presence of insufficient high-quality evidence, further studies are still needed to clarify the long-term impact of hormone therapy in endometrial cancer survivors.[66]

Ovarian Cancer Lifetime risk of ovarian cancer is low (1.7%) and results from the WHI trial suggested that orally administered combined MHT does not increase the risk of ovarian cancer (HR 1.41, 95% CI: 0.75-2.66) with the risk remaining non-significant after 13 years of cumulative follow-up.[6] However, limited observation data have reported inconsistent results.[6] A meta-analysis of 37 observational epidemiological studies suggested that ovarian cancer risks is increased (RR 1.16, 95% CI: 1.06-1.26) in those who received both estrogen monotherapy and estrogen–progestogen therapy.[58] Despite the increased incidences of ovarian cancers with use of menopausal hormone therapy, individuals who received menopausal hormone therapy (either estrogen-only or estrogen–progestogen therapy) prior to diagnosis of ovarian cancer had improved ovarian cancer overall survival.[58,67]

Ultimately, the use of hormone therapy in menopausal ovarian cancer survivors needs to be individualized because ovarian cancers have different histological subtypes and require different considerations balancing the risks of cancer reoccurrence and quality of life is needed.[68] Although the evidence is limited, hormone therapy for ovarian cancer survivor with germ cell tumor or non-serous epithelial ovarian cancer is generally considered safe.[66,68] However, the use of systemic or topical hormone therapy is not recommended for patients with history of ovarian granulosa cell tumor as this cancer subtype is hormonally active and their use warrants careful consideration. Patients should always involve their treating oncologist in decision making regarding the use of hormone therapy. Further data are needed for more rare ovarian tumors such as borderline tumors and sex-cord stromal tumors.[68]

Lung Cancer Estrogen and progesterone receptors are expressed in lung cancer cells. The WHI trial found that combined oral estrogen–progestogen therapy did not increase lung cancer incidence,[16] but significantly increased deaths from lung cancer have been observed in the post-hoc analysis of the WHI intervention, mainly from non-small cell lung cancers in individuals already at elevated risk due to past or current smoking status.[69] The increased risk of lung cancer mortality (RR 1.10, 95% CI: 1.00-1.21) was noted in a recent meta-analysis of three randomized controlled trials in patients who received estrogen–progestogen therapy.[58] In the estrogen-only arm of the WHI trial found no increased risk for lung cancer; however, it should be noted that the WHI was not originally designed to assess the relationship between hormone use and lung cancer.[6] Further studies to explicitly evaluate association between hormone therapy use and lung cancer mortality are warranted.

Osteoporosis Postmenopausal osteoporosis is a serious age-related condition that affects millions of females throughout the world. Menopause is accompanied by accelerated bone loss, and the central role of estrogen deficiency in postmenopausal osteoporosis is well established. The WHI was the first randomized trial to demonstrate that MHT reduces the risk of fractures at the hip, spine, and wrist.[6] Estrogen therapy reduces bone turnover and increases bone density in postmenopausal individuals of all ages. In the WHI, both oral estrogen monotherapy and estrogen-progestogen reduced vertebral, hip, and other fractures. The protective effect persists as long as the treatment is maintained; however, bone protection is quickly lost with cessation of therapy, although there is no evidence of rebound fracture.[6,16] Several oral and transdermal estrogen only and estrogen-progestin combination formulations, as well as the estrogen-bazedoxifene product, are FDA-approved for the prevention of postmenopausal osteoporosis. The standard bone-sparing daily estrogen dose is equivalent to 0.625-mg conjugated equine estrogen (CEE) with lower effect on bone mineral density with lower doses.

In individuals who experience vasomotor symptoms and are younger than 60 years of age or within 10 years of menopause onset, systemic estrogen therapy may be indicated for the prevention of bone loss and osteoporotic fractures.[6] General protective health measures, such as regular weight-bearing exercise and avoidance of detrimental lifestyle habits such as smoking and alcohol abuse, are appropriate for all. Some individuals require calcium supplementation to their usual dietary intake and adequate vitamin D intake and/or supplementation are also needed. Appropriate risk assessment and evaluation is needed to determine appropriate treatment strategies in menopausal individuals. See Chapter 112, "Osteoporosis," for a full discussion of osteoporosis prevention and treatment.

Mood, Cognition, and Dementia Menopausal hormone therapy improves depressive symptoms in symptomatic menopausal individuals, most likely by relieving hot flash and improving sleep. Those with vasomotor symptoms receiving MHT have improved mental health and fewer depressive symptoms compared with receiving placebo. However, MHT may worsen quality of life in individuals without flashes.[70]

More than 33% of females aged 65 years and older will develop dementia during their lifetime.[71] Several observational studies have suggested that estrogen therapy may be protective against Alzheimer disease. The WHI Memory Study (WHIMS, an ancillary study of the WHI trial) evaluated the effect of MHT on dementia and cognition in 4,532 female participants aged 65 to 79 years.[72] The study found that postmenopausal individuals aged 65 years and older taking estrogen plus progestogen therapy had twice the rate of dementia, including Alzheimer disease, than those taking placebo (HR 2.05, 95% CI: 1.21-3.48).[72] In addition, estrogen plus progestogen therapy in these individuals did not prevent mild cognitive impairment, a cognitive and functional state between normal aging and dementia that frequently progresses to dementia.[72] The estrogen-alone arm of the WHI trial showed similar findings.[72,73]

In contrast, the Women's Health Initiative Memory Study of Younger Women (WHIMSY) found that neither estrogen plus progestogen nor estrogen-alone therapy confers any risk or benefit to cognitive function when taken by postmenopausal individuals aged 50 to 55 years old.[74] In another study, the ancillary Cognitive and Affective Study (KEEPS-Cog) of the Kronos Early Estrogen Prevention Cognitive Study (KEEPS) evaluated the effects of up to 4 years of MHT on cognition and mood in recently menopausal participants (mean age 52.6 years and 1.4 years past FMP) with low cardiovascular risk.[75] Specifically, of the 693 participants, 220 were randomized to receive 0.45 mg/day oral CEE plus 200 mg/day micronized progesterone for the first 12 days of each month, 211 were randomized to receive 50 μg/day transdermal estradiol plus 200 mg/day micronized progesterone for the first 12 days of each month, and 262 were randomized to receive placebo pills and patches. After a mean length of follow-up of 2.85 years for cognition outcomes, no treatment-related benefits were observed. After a mean follow-up of 2.76 years regarding mood outcomes, model estimates indicated that those treated with oral CEE showed improvements in depression and anxiety symptoms over the 48 months of treatment, compared to those on placebo.[75]

Diabetes In healthy postmenopausal females, hormone therapy has a beneficial effect on fasting glucose levels in individuals with elevated fasting insulin concentrations.[76] Also, in individuals with coronary artery disease, hormone therapy reduces the incidence of diabetes by 35%.[77] Participants who received estrogen plus progestogen in the WHI trial had a significant 21% reduction (HR, 0.79; 95% CI: 0.67-0.93) in the incidence of type 2 diabetes requiring treatment.[78] These findings provide important insights into the metabolic effects of hormone therapy but are insufficient to recommend the long-term use of hormone therapy in postmenopausal females with diabetes.

Body Weight A meta-analysis of randomized controlled trials showed that unopposed estrogen or estrogen combined with a progestogen has no effect on body weight, suggesting that hormone therapy does not cause weight gain in excess of that normally observed at the time of menopause.[79]

Gallbladder Disease Gallbladder disease is a commonly cited complication of oral estrogen use. The WHI studies reported an increased risk for cholecystitis, cholelithiasis, and cholecystectomy among participants taking oral estrogen or estrogen–progestogen therapy. Therefore, transdermal estrogen, which bypasses the liver's first-pass effect, is an alternative to oral therapy for individuals at high risk for cholelithiasis.[6]

Estrogens

Estrogens are naturally occurring hormones or synthetic steroidal or nonsteroidal compounds with estrogenic activity. The primary indication for systemic estrogen-based MHT is the relief of moderate and severe vasomotor and vulvovaginal symptoms. The initial dose should be the lowest effective dose for symptom control.

Adverse Effects Common adverse effects of estrogen include nausea, headache, breast tenderness, and heavy bleeding. More serious adverse effects include increased risk for CHD, stroke, VTE, breast cancer, and gallbladder disease. Transdermal estradiol is associated with a lower incidence of breast tenderness and deep vein thrombosis than oral estrogen.[6,42]

Dosage and Administration (5) Use of MHT at doses lower than those prescribed historically (ie, prior to the WHI study) is effective in reducing bone loss and managing menopausal symptoms (see Table 102-1).[80-83] A dose of 0.625 mg/day in oral conjugated estrogen is equivalent to 1 mg/day of oral 17β-estradiol, which is equivalent to 0.05/day of transdermal estradiol.[84] Low-dose estrogen regimens include 0.3 mg conjugated estrogens, 0.5 mg micronized 17β-estradiol, and 0.014 to 0.0375 mg transdermal 17β-estradiol patch.[6] Topical gels, sprays, and creams are also available in low doses. Lower doses typically have fewer adverse effects and may have better overall benefit-risk profiles than standard doses. The lowest effective dose of estrogen, consistent with individualized patient treatment goals and assessment of safety and effectiveness, should be used.[48] With advancing age, dose of hormone therapy should be reduced or tapered.

Various systemically administered estrogens (typically oral and transdermal) are equally effective for replacement therapy (Table 102-4). Estrogens can be administered orally, percutaneously (transdermal patches and topical products), intravaginally (creams, tablets, rings, or inserts), intramuscularly, and even subcutaneously in the form of implanted pellets. The choice of estrogen delivery (product, route, and method) should be determined in consultation with the patient to ensure acceptability and enhance adherence. In general, the oral and transdermal routes are used most frequently.

Oral Estrogen Oral conjugated equine estrogen has been available for more than 70 years. Oral CEE is prepared from the urine of pregnant mares and is composed of estrone sulfate (50%-60%) and multiple other equine estrogens such as equilin and 17α-dihydroequilin.

Estradiol is the predominant and most active form of endogenous estrogens. A micronized form of estradiol (produced by a technique that yields extremely small particles of the pure hormone) is readily absorbed from the small intestines. When given orally, estradiol is metabolized by the intestinal mucosa and the liver during the first hepatic passage, and only 10% reaches circulation as free estradiol. Metabolism of estrogen is partly mediated by the cytochrome P450 3A4 isoenzyme. Gut and liver metabolism converts a large proportion of estradiol to the less-potent estrone. Thus, measurement of serum estradiol is not useful for monitoring oral estrogen replacement. The principal metabolites of micronized estradiol are estrone and estrone sulfate. Administration of estradiol via the oral route results in estrone concentrations that are five to seven times those of estradiol. Ethinyl estradiol is a highly potent semisynthetic estrogen that has similar activity following administration by the oral or nonoral route.

Orally administered estrogens stimulate the synthesis of hepatic proteins and increase the circulating concentrations of sex hormone-binding globulin, which, in turn, may compromise the bioavailability of androgens and estrogens.

Other Routes of Estrogen Administration Nonoral routes of estrogen administration may offer both advantages and disadvantages compared with the oral route, but long-term data are not available. As the nonoral forms of estrogens bypass the GI tract, they avoid first-pass liver metabolism. These routes of estradiol delivery result in a more physiologic estradiol-to-estrone ratio (estradiol concentrations greater than estrone concentrations), as seen in the normal premenopausal state.

(6) When compared with standard oral estrogen doses, transdermal therapy offers no significant increase in triglycerides, C-reactive protein, sex hormone binding globulin, and blood pressure.[6] Use of transdermal estrogen has also been associated with a lower risk of deep vein thrombosis and possibly stroke and coronary artery disease.[6,21,25] Transdermal estrogen patches share the advantages of other nonoral estrogen routes and have the added advantage of delivering estradiol to the general venous circulation at a continuous rate. The matrix transdermal systems (estrogen in adhesive) generally are well tolerated, and fewer than 5% of individuals experience skin reactions. The incidence of skin irritation diminishes when the application site is rotated. Topical anti-inflammatory products (eg, hydrocortisone cream) can be applied for managing the rashes, and switching to another transdermal patch is often a viable option.

Topical gels, sprays, and emulsions are convenient forms of systemic estrogen therapy, but variability in drug absorption has been noted with some formulations. Intravaginal creams, tablets, inserts, and rings are used for treatment of urogenital (vulvar and vaginal) atrophy. Pharmacologically they are sustained-release delivery systems that can maintain adequate estradiol concentrations. While most products provide local estrogen, one intravaginal-ring product (Femring®) is designed to achieve systemic concentrations of estrogen and is also indicated for treatment of moderate-to-severe vasomotor symptoms. Estradiol pellets (for subcutaneous implantation), containing pure crystalline 17β-estradiol, have been available for more than 60 years. They are inserted subcutaneously into the

TABLE 102-4 FDA-Approved Estrogen Products for Menopausal Hormone Therapy

Medication	Brand Name[a]	Initial Dose/Low Dose	Usual Dose Range	Comments
Systemic Estrogen Products (for the treatment of moderate and severe vasomotor symptoms ± urogenital symptoms)				
Oral estrogens[b]				
Conjugated equine estrogens	Premarin	0.3 or 0.45 mg once daily	0.3-1.25 mg once daily	Dosage form available as 0.3, 0.45, 0.625, 0.9, 1.25 mg
Esterified estrogens (75%-85% estrone + 6%-15% equilin)	Menest	0.3 mg once daily	0.3-1.25 mg once daily	Administer 3 weeks on and 1 week off Dosage form available as 0.3, 0.625, 1.25 mg
Micronized 17β-estradiol	Estrace generics	1 mg once daily	1 or 2 mg once daily	Administer 3 weeks on and 1 week off Dosage form available as 0.5, 1, 2 mg
Transdermal estrogens patches				
17β-Estradiol	Alora	0.025 mg/day (patch applied twice weekly)[c]	0.025-0.1 mg/day (patch applied twice weekly)[c]	Dosage form available as 0.025, 0.05, 0.075, 0.1 mg/day
	Climara	0.025 mg/day (patch applied once weekly)[c]	0.025-0.1 mg/day (patch applied once weekly)[c]	Dosage form available as 0.025, 0.0375, 0.05, 0.06, 0.075, 0.1 mg/day
	Menostar	0.014 mg/day (patch applied once weekly)[c,d]	0.014 mg/day (patch applied once weekly)[c,d]	Dosage form available as 0.014 mg/day
	Minivelle, Vivelle, Vivelle Dot	0.025 mg/day (patch applied twice weekly)[c]	0.025-0.1 mg/day, 0.05 is standard dose (patch applied twice weekly)[c]	Dosage form available as 0.025, 0.0375, 0.05 (standard dose), 0.075, 0.1 mg/day
Other topical forms of estrogen				
17β-Estradiol topical gel	EstroGel 0.06% metered-dose pump	–	1.25 g/day once daily (contains 0.75 mg estradiol)	Apply from wrist to shoulder
	Elestrin 0.06% metered-dose pump	–	1-2 unit doses once daily (1 unit dose: 0.87 g, which contains 0.52-mg estradiol)	Apply to upper arm
	Divigel 0.1% (topical once daily)	0.25 g once daily	0.25-1 g (provides 0.25-1 mg of estradiol)	Apply to upper thigh. Dosage form available as 0.25, 0.5, 0.75, 1 mg
17β-Estradiol transdermal spray	Evamist	1 spray once daily	1-3 sprays once daily (1.53 mg of estradiol per spray)	Apply to inner surface of forearm
Vaginal estrogens				
Estradiol acetate vaginal ring	Femring	12.4 mg every 3 months	12.4-, 24.8-mg ring (delivers 0.05- or 0.1-mg estradiol/day)	
Intravaginal Estrogen Products (for the treatment of urogenital symptoms only/low systemic exposure)				
Conjugated equine estrogens (CEE) vaginal cream	Premarin		0.5-2 g/day (contains 0.625 mg CEE per g)	Administer 21 days on and 7 days off
17β-Estradiol vaginal cream	Estrace	500 mg to 1 g daily for 2 weeks, then 500 mg to 1 g one to three times weekly; or 2-4 g daily for 1 or 2 weeks then gradually reduced to ½ initial dosage for similar period	Maintenance dose of 0.5-1 g, one to three times weekly	Dosage form available as tube containing 1½ oz (45 mL) with calibrated applicator for delivery of 1, 2, 3, or 4 g
17β-Estradiol vaginal ring	Estring	2 mg ring replaced every 90 days	2 mg ring (delivers 0.0075 mg/day) replaced every 90 days	
17β-Estradiol vaginal insert	Imvexxy	1 vaginal insert (4 μg) daily for 2 weeks, then reduce to 1 insert twice weekly	4 or 10 μg twice weekly, every 3-4 days	
Estradiol hemihydrate vaginal tablet	Vagifem Yuvafem Generics	10 μg once weekly for 2 weeks, then twice weekly	10 μg twice weekly	

[a]US brand names.

[b]Orally administered estrogens stimulate synthesis of hepatic proteins and increase circulating concentrations of sex hormone-binding globulin, which in turn may compromise the bioavailability of androgens and estrogens. Individuals with elevated triglyceride concentrations or significant liver function abnormalities are candidates for nonoral estrogen therapy.

[c]Do not apply estrogen patches on or near breasts. Avoid waistline as patch may rub off with tight-fitting clothing.

[d]FDA-approved for prevention of postmenopausal osteoporosis only.

[e]Not available in the United States.

anterior abdominal wall or buttock. Pellets are difficult to remove and may continue to release estradiol for a long time after insertion. Implantation should not be repeated until serum estradiol concentrations have fallen to values similar to those at the midfollicular phase of the menstrual cycle. Although FDA-approved estradiol pellets are not available in the United States, some healthcare providers prescribe and implant compounded bioidentical hormone pellet therapy.[84]

7 Progestogens

Because of the increased risk of endometrial hyperplasia and endometrial cancer with estrogen monotherapy (ie, unopposed estrogen), use of systemic estrogen in individuals with an intact uterus must always be accompanied by a progestogen or tissue-selective estrogen complex (estrogen/bazedoxifene) for endometrial protection.[85] Some data suggest that progestins may also improve vasomotor symptoms,[86,87] but their use for this purpose is not considered first-line or standard therapy.

Progestogens reduce nuclear estradiol receptor concentrations, suppress DNA synthesis, and decrease estrogen bioavailability by increasing the activity of endometrial 17-hydroxysteroid dehydrogenase, an enzyme responsible for converting estradiol to estrone.[88]

The term progestogen is a catch-all term that includes both progesterone products that are structurally identical to the hormone produced by the body and synthetic progestins that have progestogenic effects but are structurally different than the natural hormone.[89] The first generation of progestins included the C-19 androgenic progestin norethindrone (also known as norethisterone), norgestrel, and levonorgestrel. More recent preparations have included the C-21 progestins dydrogesterone (not currently available in the United States) and medroxyprogesterone acetate (MPA), which are less androgenic. Drospirenone, a synthetic progestin analog of the potassium-sparing diuretic spironolactone, has both antiandrogenic and antialdosterone properties. Micronized progesterone is also available and is structurally identical to the natural hormone. The most commonly used oral progestogens are MPA, micronized progesterone, and norethindrone acetate.[90] The latter can also be administered transdermally in the form of a combined estrogen–progestogen patch. Preparations containing MPA have shown to have higher thrombotic risks.[48]

Although data are limited, oral micronized progesterone and dydrogesterone (not currently available in the United States) are considered as the first-line progestogens (safe alternative) because it is effective for endometrial hyperplasia, is metabolically neutral, and does not increase the risk of either breast cancer or CHD in studies to date.[91]

Adverse Effects Common adverse effects of progestogens include irritability, weight gain, bloating, and headache. Changing from a cyclic to a continuous-combined regimen or changing from one progestogen to another may decrease the incidence or severity of untoward effects. Adverse effects of progestogens are difficult to evaluate and can vary with the agent administered. Some individuals experience "premenstrual-like" symptoms, such as mood swings, bloating, fluid retention, and sleep disturbance. Newer methods and routes of progestogen delivery (eg, locally by an intrauterine device that releases levonorgestrel or a progesterone-containing bioadhesive vaginal gel) may be associated with fewer adverse effects.

Dosage and Administration Several progestogen regimens designed to prevent endometrial hyperplasia are available for use in individuals with an intact uterus (Table 102-5). Progestogens can be used continuously (resulting in endometrial atrophy) or cyclically (resulting in monthly withdrawal bleeding). For cyclic use, the progestogen must be taken for a sufficient period of time during each cycle. In general, a minimum of 12 to 14 days of progestogen therapy per month is required for complete protection against estrogen-induced endometrial hyperplasia. For individuals with a history of hysterectomy, use of progestogens is not needed. However, in individuals with endometriosis who have had a hysterectomy, the use of a progestogen along with estrogen may minimize endometriosis exacerbations.

TABLE 102-5 Progestogen Dosing for Endometrial Protection (Cyclic Administration)

Progestogen	Dosage
Medroxyprogesterone acetate	5-10 mg/day for 12-14 days per calendar month (oral dosage form available as 2.5-, 5-, 10-mg tablets)
Micronized progesterone	200 mg/day for 12-14 days per calendar month (oral dosage form available as 100- and 200-mg tablets)
Norethindrone acetate	5 mg/day for 12-14 days per calendar month (oral dosage form available as 2.5- and 5-mg tablets)

Menopausal Hormone Therapy Regimens

Many products have been used for MHT, and most include an estrogen and a progestogen in various regimens, routes, and administration schedules. Continuous combined hormone regimen with synthetic progestin reduce the risk of endometrial cancer, whereas sequential combined hormone regimen with synthetic progestin and continuous combined and sequential combined with natural progestins increase the risk of endometrial cancer depending on the dose and duration of use.[64] Additionally, tissue-selective estrogen complex product (estrogen/bazedoxifene) is available for once-daily dosing. Common combination MHT regimens are described in Table 102-6.

Cyclic (Sequential) Estrogen–Progestogen Treatment Estrogen typically is administered continuously (daily). A progestogen is coadministered with the estrogen for 12 to 14 days of a 28-day cycle.[90] The progestogen causes scheduled withdrawal bleeding in approximately 80% to 90% of users. With this regimen, bleeding usually begins 1 to 2 days after the last progestogen dose. Occasionally, bleeding begins during the latter phase of progestogen administration.

Continuous Combined Estrogen–Progestogen Treatment Continuous combined estrogen–progestogen administration (both estrogen and progestogen are administered daily) results in endometrial atrophy and the absence of vaginal bleeding. Continuous combined MHT is more acceptable than traditional cyclic therapy if individuals prefer to avoid the monthly withdrawal bleeding. However, unpredictable spotting or bleeding may occur initially, which usually resolves within 6 to 12 months. Individuals who recently have undergone menopause have a higher risk for excessive, unpredictable bleeding while receiving continuous therapy; thus, this regimen is best reserved for those who are at least 2 years postmenopausal. This method of treatment can be achieved either by using commercially available oral and transdermal preparations or by administering systemic estrogen along with the use of the levonorgestrel-releasing intrauterine system. This combination offers the best protection against endometrial hyperplasia and cancer.[21] The continuous combined estrogen–progestogen regimen (using conjugated equine estrogens 0.625 mg/day plus medroxyprogesterone acetate 2.5 mg/day) led to a decreased risk of endometrial cancer in the WHI study.[16]

Intermittent Combined Estrogen–Progestogen Treatment The intermittent combined estrogen–progestogen regimen, also called *continuous-pulsed estrogen–progestogen* or

TABLE 102-6 Common Combination Menopausal Hormone Therapy Regimens

Regimen	Brand name	Dosage
Oral Regimens		
Conjugated equine estrogen (CEE) + medroxyprogesterone acetate (MPA)	Prempro (continuous)	0.625 mg CEE/2.5 mg MPA, 0.625 mg CEE/5 mg MPA daily; Low-dose: 0.3 mg CEE/1.5 mg MPA, 0.45 mg CEE/1.5 mg MPA daily
	Premphase (continuous cyclic)	0.625 mg CEE daily only in the first 2 weeks of a 4-week cycle then 0.625 mg daily CEE + 5 mg MPA daily in the last 2 weeks of a 4-week cycle
Conjugated equine estrogen (CEE) + bazedoxifene	Duavee (continuous)	0.45/20 mg daily
Ethinyl estradiol (EE) + norethindrone acetate (NETA)	Generic, Femhrt (continuous) Fayvolv (continuous)	Femhrt: 2.5 μg EE/0.5 mg NETA daily Fyavolv: 2.5 μg EE/0.5 mg NETA daily, 5 μg EE/1 mg NETA daily
Estradiol (E) + drospirenone (DRSP)	Angeliq (continuous)	1 mg E/0.5 mg DRSP daily Low dose: 0.5 mg E/0.25 mg DRSP daily
Estradiol (E) + norgestimate	Prefest (estrogen/intermittent progestogen)	1 mg E daily for first 3 days then 1 mg E/0.09 mg norgestimate daily for next 3 days; this pattern is repeated continuously
Estradiol (E) + norethindrone acetate (NETA)	Activella (continuous) Mimvey (continuous) Amabelz (continuous)	1 mg E/0.5 mg NETA daily Low-dose: 0.5 mg E/0.1 mg NETA daily
Estradiol (E) + progesterone	Bijuva (continuous)	1 mg E/100 mg progesterone daily
Transdermal Regimens		
Estradiol + norethindrone acetate patch	CombiPatch (continuous) CombiPatch (continuous cyclic)	Continuous: 0.05/0.14 mg, 0.05/0.25 mg (apply 1 patch twice weekly) Continuous cyclic: 0.05 mg of an estradiol only patch (apply 1 patch twice weekly) in the first 2 weeks of a 4-week cycle then either dose of the CombiPatch (apply 1 patch twice weekly) in the last 2 weeks of a 4-week cycle
Estradiol (E) + levonorgestrel patch	Climara Pro (continuous)	0.045 mg E/0.015 mg/day (apply 1 patch once weekly)

CEE, conjugated equine estrogen; DRSP, drospirenone; E, estradiol; EE, ethinyl estradiol; NETA, norethindrone acetate; MPA, medroxyprogesterone acetate.

pulsed-progestogen, consists of 3 days of estrogen therapy alone, followed by 3 days of combined estrogen and progestogen, which is then repeated without interruption. This regimen is designed to lower the incidence of uterine bleeding. It is based on the assumption that pulsed-progestogen administration will prevent downregulation of progesterone receptors that can be produced by continuous combined regimens. The lower progestogen dose induces fewer adverse effects and can be better tolerated. The long-term effect of intermittent combined regimens in endometrial protection is undetermined.

Compounded Bioidentical Hormone Therapy

Bioidentical hormone products are those that contain hormones that are chemically identical molecules to those produced by the body. There are FDA-approved products containing bioidentical hormones (eg, 17β-estradiol, progesterone). Compounded bioidentical hormone therapy (CBHT) is terminology used to describe hormone therapy formulations that are custom-prepared (ie, compounded) for individual patients, often involving the use of measuring and monitoring hormone levels in blood and/or other body fluids such as saliva.[25] Hormones that are commonly used in CBHT include estrone, estradiol, estriol, progesterone, testosterone, DHEA, and thyroid hormone. Although claims have been made to suggest that compounded bioidentical hormones are safer and more "natural" alternatives to commercially available preparations, there is a paucity of evidence regarding the efficacy, safety, and pharmaceutical quality of these products. Furthermore, saliva testing is often used to adjust hormone levels, and there is no scientific evidence to support this practice. Bioidentical hormones carry the same risks as traditional hormone therapy products. Several major medical organizations have released statements to dissuade patients and clinicians from CBHT and its use is only recommended only when there is a medical need for an unusual dosing regimen or ingredients or when patients have allergies to FDA-approved therapies.[6,25,92,93]

Other Treatments for Menopause-Related Symptoms

In individuals who have contraindications to MHT use, prefer not to take estrogen and/or progestogen, or cannot tolerate estrogen and/or progestogen administration, a number of other medications may be considered, depending on the goals of therapy.[6,17,19] These include the prescription medications testosterone, SERMs, and tibolone as well as nonhormonal prescription medications (eg, selective serotonin reuptake inhibitors). Tibolone is a gonadomimetic synthetic steroid in the norpregnane family with combined estrogenic, progestogenic, and androgenic activity. It has been in use for several decades in Europe for the treatment of menopausal symptoms and prevention of osteoporosis but is currently not approved in the United States.

Alternatives to estrogen for treatment of hot flashes include selective serotonin reuptake inhibitors (eg, paroxetine, fluoxetine, citalopram, escitalopram), dual serotonin and norepinephrine reuptake inhibitors (eg, venlafaxine, desvenlafaxine), clonidine, gabapentin, and pregabalin (Table 102-7). Progestogens (eg, MPA, megesterol acetate) alone may be an option for some individuals (eg, those with a history of VTE), but weight gain, vaginal bleeding, and other adverse effects often limit their use. Progestogens cannot be considered nonhormonal agents for the treatment of hot flashes for individuals in whom MHT is contraindicated. For this group of patients, selective serotonin reuptake inhibitors such as paroxetine mesylate and serotonin-norepinephrine reuptake inhibitors such as venlafaxine are considered by some to be a first-line

TABLE 102-7 Alternatives to Estrogen for Treatment of Hot Flashes[a]

Medication	Brand Name[b]	Initial Dose	Usual Dose Range	Comments
Venlafaxine	Effexor, Effexor XR	37.5 mg	37.5-75 mg/day	Adverse effects include nausea, headache, somnolence, dizziness, insomnia, nervousness, xerostomia, anorexia, constipation, diaphoresis, weakness, and hypertension
Desvenlafaxine	Pristiq	50 mg	50-100 mg/day	Adverse effects include nausea, headache, somnolence, dizziness, insomnia, xerostomia, anorexia, constipation, diaphoresis, and weakness
Paroxetine, paroxetine CR[c]	Brisdelle,[d] Paxil, Paxil CR, Pexeva	7.5 mg/day (Brisdell formulation),[d] 10 mg/day (paroxetine), or 12.5 mg/day (paroxetine CR)	7.5 mg/day,[d] 10-20 mg/day or 12.5-25 mg/day	Adverse effects include nausea, somnolence, insomnia, headache, dizziness, xerostomia, constipation, diarrhea, weakness, and diaphoresis
Citalopram		10 mg/day	10-20 mg/day	Adverse effects include drowsiness, insomnia, diaphoresis, nausea, xerostomia, dose-dependent QTc prolongation
Escitalopram		10 mg/day, start with 5 mg/day in sensitive or older individuals and titrate up	10-20 mg/day	Adverse effects include headache, insomnia, nausea, increased sweating, fatigue, and somnolence. Decreased libido and anorgasmia
Clonidine patch	Catapres-TTS (transdermal)	0.1 mg/day (0.1 mg/24 hour patch)	0.1-0.3 mg/day (available as 0.1, 0.2, or 0.3 mg/24 hour patch)	Adverse effects include drowsiness, dizziness, hypotension, and dry mouth, especially with higher doses
Pregabalin	Lyrica	50 mg/day	75-150 mg twice/day	Adverse effects include drowsiness, dizziness, dry mouth, edema, blurred vision, weight gain, impaired concentration
Gabapentin	Gralise, Neurontin, generics	300 mg at bedtime	900 mg/day (divided in three daily doses), doses up to 2,400 mg/day (divided in three daily doses) have been studied	Adverse effects include somnolence and dizziness; these symptoms often can be obviated with a gradual increase in dosing

CR, controlled release; XR, extended release.

[a]Treatment of postmenopausal hot flashes is an off-label indication in the United States for all medications listed except for one formulation of paroxetine (paroxetine mesylate).

[b]US brand names.

[c]Other selective serotonin reuptake inhibitors (eg, citalopram, escitalopram, fluoxetine, and sertraline) have also been studied and may be used for the treatment of hot flashes.

[d]The brand Brisdelle contains 7.5 mg of paroxetine and is FDA-approved to treat moderate-to-severe vasomotor symptoms of menopause. This specific product is not FDA-approved for treating psychiatric conditions.

therapy.[17] However, in breast cancer patients, certain selective serotonin reuptake inhibitors (paroxetine and fluoxetine) could interfere with metabolism of endocrine therapies, such as tamoxifen via cytochrome P450 2D6 inhibition (tamoxifen requires activation to its active metabolites by cytochrome P450 2D6).[17,21] Gabapentin has demonstrated beneficial effect for reducing the frequency and severity of vasomotor symptoms. Higher effective doses may limit its use due to adverse events at such doses, including drowsiness, dizziness, and loss of coordination. However, it may be a reasonable option for individuals with disrupted sleep and hot flashes when administered in the evening. Pregabalin has demonstrated benefit at alleviating vasomotor symptoms, but is less well studied.[21] Clonidine has also been shown to be more effective for hot flashes compared to placebo but its adverse effects (eg, sedation, dry mouth, and hypotension) are not always well tolerated. It is also less effective than the previously described nonhormonal treatment options.[21]

Androgens The therapeutic use of testosterone in females is controversial. In the United States, there are currently no FDA-approved testosterone products for use in females. Androgens have important biologic effects in females, acting both directly via androgen receptors in tissues, such as bone, skin fibroblasts, hair follicles, and sebaceous glands, and indirectly via the aromatization of testosterone to estrogen in the ovaries, bone, brain, adipose tissue, and other tissues. There is a natural decline in androgen production with aging, and pathophysiologic states affecting ovarian and adrenal function, such as adrenal insufficiency and hypopituitarism, as well as bilateral oophorectomy, are associated with androgen deficiency in females. Androgens are produced by both the adrenal glands and the ovaries in females and include 5α-dihydrotestosterone, androstenedione, dehydropepiandrosterone (DHEA), dehydropepiandrosterone-sulfate (DHEA-S), and testosterone. A cluster of symptoms that characterize androgen insufficiency in females, manifested as diminished sense of well-being, persistent or unexplained fatigue, and sexual function changes such as decreased libido, decreased sexual receptivity, and decreased pleasure has been reported.[12] A recent meta-analysis of 36 randomized, controlled trials involving 8,480 postmenopausal females concluded that testosterone therapy significantly improved sexual function in those with low sexual desire causing distress, when compared to placebo or estrogen/estrogen-progestogen therapy.[10] In 2019 the Global Consensus Position Statement on the Use of Testosterone Therapy for Females was published and endorsed by 11 professional societies across the world, including the North American Menopause Society, and in 2021, a clinical practice guideline was published.[39,94] The guideline recommends that testosterone therapy can be considered in postmenopausal females with hypoactive sexual desire disorder causing significant distress, after thoroughly discussing the risks and benefits and obtaining informed consent. If an approved female formulation is not available, the guideline recommends using one-tenth of a standard male dose of 1% transdermal testosterone or about 300 μg/day to achieve the normal premenopausal physiological range. However, compounded products are not recommended. Transdermal (patch, gel, cream, or spray) formulations are preferred and oral and intramuscular formulations are not recommended due to the possibility of supraphysiologic testosterone levels and adverse effects. Patients on testosterone therapy should be closely monitored for both efficacy and safety.[39] Effects from excessive testosterone dosage include virilization, acne, hair growth, fluid retention, weight gain, and lipid effects (increase in LDL-cholesterol and decrease in total cholesterol, triglyceride, and HDL-cholesterol). The lipid effects have been reported with oral but not with transdermal testosterone products.[95] Androgenic effects of testosterone therapy are rare when the testosterone level does not exceed the premenopausal range.[39] Further studies are required to determine the long-term (>24 months) safety of testosterone in females including effects on breast cancer and cardiovascular risks.[39] Androgens should not be used during pregnancy or lactation or in individuals with suspected androgen-dependent neoplasia.

Dehydroepiandrosterone (DHEA) DHEA is a precursor hormone in the synthesis of estrone, estradiol, and testosterone and is classified as a dietary supplement in the United States. It has been used off-label for a number of conditions, including fertility and treatment of menopausal symptoms. Intravaginal DHEA (cream, gel, suppositories) was previously only available as compounded formulations but a prescription version (in the form of an insert) has been approved by the FDA for treatment of moderate-to-severe dyspareunia at a dose of 6.5 mg once daily at bedtime. Premarketing clinical trials reported a significant improvement in moderate-to-severe dyspareunia symptoms and decrease in vaginal dryness compared to placebo.[96] Intravaginal administration of prasterone conveys only a local effect on the vaginal tissue; the serum concentrations of estradiol, testosterone, and DHEA were within the normal range for postmenopausal participants after 12 weeks of treatment in one clinical trial.[97] Prasterone's FDA labeling does not carry the same boxed warnings for VTE, endometrial hyperplasia, or other risks that are present in estrogen-containing products. However, the product labeling does warn against the use of prasterone in individuals with a history of, or suspected, breast cancer, given that prasterone is a precursor to estrogen. Prasterone is also contraindicated in individuals with undiagnosed AUB. The most common adverse effects of intravaginal prasterone are vaginal discharge and abnormal Pap smear.[98]

Selective Estrogen Receptor Modulators (SERMs) Selective estrogen receptor modulators are a group of nonsteroidal compounds that are chemically distinct from estradiol. They act as estrogen agonists in some tissues, such as bone, and as estrogen antagonists in other tissues, such as breast and endometrial tissue, through specific, high-affinity binding to the estrogen receptor. Individual SERMs differ in their activity and tissue specificity resulting in varying patterns of estrogen-receptor agonism in some tissues and estrogen-receptor antagonism in others.[99]

The ideal SERM would protect against osteoporosis and decrease the incidence of breast, endometrial, and colorectal cancer and CHD without exacerbating menopausal symptoms or increasing the risk of VTE or gallbladder disease. To date, no SERM meets these ideals. Tamoxifen, the first-generation SERM (a nonsteroidal triphenylethylene derivative), has estrogen antagonist activity on the breast and estrogen-like agonist activity on bone and endometrium. The second-generation SERM raloxifene, a nonsteroidal benzothiophene derivative, is used to reduce the risk of postmenopausal osteoporosis and invasive breast cancer, and also for treatment of postmenopausal osteoporosis. Raloxifene is antiestrogenic at the endometrium and has an increased incidence of hot flashes compared to placebo.[100]

The third-generation SERM, bazedoxifene, in conjunction with conjugated estrogens forms a tissue-selective estrogen complex (TSEC) and is FDA-approved for use in moderate-to-severe vasomotor symptoms and prevention of osteoporosis.[99,101] This agent has a favorable breast, endometrial, and ovarian safety profile, even after prolonged use.[11] While this TSEC has demonstrated high effectiveness for vasomotor symptoms (approximately 75% reduction),[11,102] SERMs alone do not alleviate, and may even exacerbate vasomotor symptoms, and also increase the risk for VTE.

Ospemifene is an orally administered third-generation SERM approved by the FDA for the treatment of moderate-to-severe dyspareunia and moderate-to-severe vaginal dryness from menopausal vulvar and vaginal atrophy due to menopause. Ospemifene's labeling carries a boxed warning about its estrogenic effect on the endometrium as there is an increased risk of endometrial hyperplasia and endometrial cancer in an individual with a uterus who takes unopposed estrogen therapy. Ospemifene labeling also includes a boxed warning about the possible risk of stroke and VTE.[103]

Adverse Effects Depending on the tissue selectivity, several SERMs are associated with hot flashes and less often with leg cramps. The SERMs can increase the risk of VTE and fatal stroke to a degree similar to that of oral estrogen, but the degree of risk is product specific.[6] Common adverse effects (greater than or equal to 5%) of bazedoxifene include muscle spasms, nausea, diarrhea, dyspepsia, upper abdominal pain, oropharyngeal pain, dizziness, and neck pain.[104] Common adverse effects of ospemifene include hot flashes, vaginal discharge, muscle spasm, headache, vaginal hemorrhage, and hyperhidrosis.[103]

Dose and Administration Conjugated estrogens/bazedoxifene is supplied as 0.45/20-mg tablets and is taken once daily. Ospemifene is a 60-mg tablet taken once daily with food. Other available SERMs are also dosed orally once daily.

Complementary and Alternative Medicine Some patients prefer to use natural remedies due to a belief that they are safer. However, randomized, placebo-controlled trials of complementary and alternative therapies have been equivocal and have not established the safety and efficacy of herbal remedies, homeopathic treatments, or acupuncture for the prevention or treatment of hot flashes.

Phytoestrogens Phytoestrogens are plant compounds with estrogen-like biologic activity and relatively weak estrogen receptor-binding properties, resulting in physiologic effects in humans. Epidemiologic studies suggest that consumption of a phytoestrogen-rich diet, which is common in traditional Asian societies, may be associated with a lower risk of endometrial and ovarian cancer.[105]

The biologic potencies of phytoestrogens vary as most of these compounds are nonsteroidal and are less potent than synthetic estrogens. The main classes of phytoestrogens are isoflavones, lignans, coumestans, and prenylflavonoids.[105] The most commonly studied phytoestrogen is the isoflavone class, with genistein and daidzein being the most abundant active components of isoflavones. The concentration of isoflavones per gram of soy protein varies considerably among preparations. Also, a single plant often contains more than one class of phytoestrogen. Common food sources of phytoestrogens include soybeans (isoflavones), oilseeds such as flaxseed (lignans), alfalfa sprouts and pinto beans (coumestans), and hops and beer (prenylflavonoids).[105]

Mild estrogenic effects have been seen in postmenopausal individuals with phytoestrogen consumption. A systematic review indicated that high levels of genistein extracts reduce the number of daily hot flashes compared with placebo without harmful endometrial effects when used for up to 2 years.[106] A limitation of this review is that many of the studies included were of poor quality and short duration. A more recent meta-analysis of randomized, controlled trials concluded that compared to placebo, phytoestrogens reduce the frequency of hot flashes and vaginal dryness but not in night sweats.[107]

Phytoestrogens decrease LDL and triglyceride concentrations with no significant change in HDL concentrations.[108] Furthermore, phytoestrogens have the ability to inhibit LDL oxidation and normalize vascular reactivity in estrogen-deprived primates.[108] Common adverse effects include constipation, bloating, and nausea.[109]

A meta-analysis reported that phytoestrogen use is not associated with increased rates of endometrial cancer, vaginal bleeding, and breast cancer.[109] Large, long-term studies are needed to further document the effects of phytoestrogens on the breast, bone, and endometrium. Furthermore, before phytoestrogens can be considered an alternative to conventional MHT in postmenopausal individuals, additional data are needed to clarify differences among classes of phytoestrogens, including dosing, biologic activity, safety, and efficacy.

Other Complementary and Alternative Options Black cohosh (*Cimicifuga racemosa* or *Actaea racemosa*), a widely used herbal supplement, may not offer substantial benefits for relief of vasomotor symptoms. A systematic review and meta-analysis concluded that black cohosh was not associated with a reduction in hot flashes.[107] This substance does not have strong intrinsic estrogenic properties but may act through the serotonergic system. Although it is generally well tolerated, hepatotoxicity has been reported and it is unclear if this is due to the herb itself or is a result of adulteration of the commercially available products.[110] The long-term effects of black cohosh are unknown. Other herbals and alternative treatments that may be used include dong quai, red clover leaf (contains phytoestrogens), and ginseng. These have not been shown to be effective in the treatment of menopausal symptoms and may carry the risk of adverse events.[6,107,111] Complementary and alternative therapies should not be recommended to treat menopausal symptoms.

Personalized Pharmacotherapy

8 The severity of menopausal symptoms varies widely between individuals. The decision to use MHT must be personalized and based on several parameters, including vasomotor and vulvovaginal symptoms, age, fracture risk, cardiovascular disease risk, breast cancer risk, and thromboembolism risk. MHT is not indicated for prevention of chronic diseases of aging and its initiation should be considered for healthy symptomatic individuals who are within 10 years of the onset of menopause or younger than 60 years and who do not have contraindications to therapy.[6,23] The treatment regimen (estrogen only or combined estrogen–progestogen, dose, route of administration) and duration should be based on the individualized risk versus benefit analysis for each patient.[16]

Long-term use of MHT or initiation in older individuals is associated with greater risks. Once advised of increased risks associated with continuing MHT beyond age 60 years, extending therapy may be acceptable under close medical supervision. For example, in those with severe and persistent menopausal symptoms, use should not be discontinued based solely on age but rather individualized based on assessment of potential risks and benefits.[6]

Estrogen therapy is the most effective treatment for moderate and severe vasomotor symptoms, impaired sleep quality, and vulvovaginal symptoms of menopause (Fig. 102-1). A thorough discussion of the risks and benefits of MHT should be completed with the patient so that they can weigh the risks and benefits versus alternatives and make a rational decision about MHT use. For a healthy recently menopausal individuals with vasomotor symptoms, the benefits of hormonal therapy generally outweigh the risks, including control of vasomotor symptoms, treatment of urogenital atrophy, and prevention of postmenopausal bone loss. Nonetheless, VTE and stroke are concerning short-term risks.

Menopausal hormone therapy should be tailored for optimal formulation, dose, route of delivery, and counseling should be based on age, years since menopause, and hysterectomy status. All types and routes of administration of estrogen are equally effective in relieving vasomotor symptoms and vulvovaginal atrophy.[6] A dose-dependent relationship between estrogen administration and suppression of hot flashes is well established. Some females, especially younger individuals, may require a higher than average dose of estrogen to suppress symptoms, while those with hot flashes at the time of menopause require lower estrogen doses.[112] Initiation of therapy with low doses of estrogen often will minimize adverse effects, such as breast tenderness and unscheduled bleeding. Transdermal estradiol is less likely than oral estrogen to cause nausea and headache. In many cases changing from one estrogen regimen to another can alleviate certain adverse effects.

If MHT is to be initiated, medication therapy should also take into account the potential for interactions, including those involving the cytochrome P450. For example, the CYP450 isoenzyme 3A4, metabolizes estrogen, the SERM ospemifene, and the progestin medroxyprogesterone. Inducers or inhibitors of these enzymes may either decrease or increase, respectively, therapeutic effects or result in adverse effects. Similarly, selection of nonhormonal drug therapy options should take into account the potential for interactions with other prescription and nonprescription medications. Selective serotonin reuptake inhibitors and serotonin norepinephrine reuptake inhibitors can have major interactions with other drugs also affecting CYP450 2D6 and 3A4 (see Chapter 88, "Depressive Disorders"). Patients using vaginal estrogen creams or nonestrogen vaginal moisturizers should be warned that products with oil-based lubricants or vehicles can weaken latex condoms, which can decrease protection against sexually transmitted infections. Pharmacodynamic drug interactions (eg, additive adverse effects) should also be considered.

EVALUATION OF THERAPEUTIC OUTCOMES

The relief of moderate and severe hot flashes is the primary goal of MHT. In order to adequately assess treatment effect, individuals should be encouraged to continue their MHT regimen for at least 1 month. The main reasons for discontinuing MHT are adverse effects such as bleeding, breast tenderness, bloating, and "premenstrual-like symptoms." Reducing the dose or changing the regimen or the route of administration can minimize these effects. Alternatively, if vasomotor symptoms are not controlled adequately with a lower-dose regimen, increasing the estrogen dose may be a reasonable option. Therefore, after the menopausal individual begins MHT, a brief follow-up visit 6 weeks later may be useful to discuss patient concerns and to evaluate the patient for symptom relief, adverse effects, and patterns of withdrawal bleeding. Individuals receiving MHT should be seen by the clinician for annual monitoring (Table 102-8).

The main indication for MHT is relief of menopausal symptoms. Many individuals have no difficulty abruptly stopping MHT; others develop vasomotor symptoms after discontinuation. Although these symptoms may be mild and resolve over a few months, in some the symptoms are severe and intolerable. There is no evidence that gradual discontinuation of MHT reduces the recurrence of hot flashes compared with sudden discontinuation.[6]

CONCLUSION

Menopause is a natural life event—not a disease. Therefore, the decision to use MHT must be individualized based on the severity of

TABLE 102-8 Management of Patients Taking Hormone Therapy Regimens

Initiation of Hormone Therapy

Hormone therapy should be used only as long as vasomotor symptom control is necessary

Six-Week Follow-up Visit

- To discuss patient concerns about hormone therapy
- To evaluate the patient for symptom relief, adverse effects, and patterns of withdrawal bleeding (if continuous sequential hormone therapy is given)

Medication	Common Adverse Effects	Monitoring Parameter	Suggested Change
Estrogen		Persistence of hot flashes	Increase estrogen dose
Estrogen	Breast tenderness		Reduce estrogen dose; switch to a transdermal regimen
Progestogen	Bloating Premenstrual-like symptoms		Switch to another progestogen or bazedoxifene

Annual Follow-up Visit

Annual monitoring: medical history, physical examination (including pelvic examination), blood pressure measurement, and routine endometrial cancer surveillance (as indicated). Additional follow-up is determined based on the patient's initial response to therapy and the need for any modification of the regimen

Breast examinations: annual mammograms (scheduled based on patient's age and risk factors)

Osteoporosis prevention: BMD should be measured in individuals 65 years and older and in those younger than 65 years with risk factors for osteoporosis. Repeat testing should be performed as clinically indicated

In individuals taking sequential hormone therapy	Transvaginal ultrasound, and where indicated an endometrial biopsy should be performed if vaginal bleeding occurs at any time other than the expected time of withdrawal bleeding or when heavier or more prolonged withdrawal bleeding occurs (if endometrial pathology cannot be excluded by endovaginal ultrasonography, further evaluation may be required, such as hysteroscopy)
In individuals taking continuous combined hormone therapy	Endometrial evaluation should be considered when irregular bleeding persists for more than 6 months after initiating therapy

BMD, bone mineral density.

TABLE 102-9 Evidence-Based Hormone Therapy Guidelines for Menopausal Symptom Management

Recommendation	Recommendation Level
In the absence of contraindications, estrogen-based postmenopausal hormone therapy should be used for treatment of moderate-to-severe vasomotor symptoms	Level 1
Systemic or vaginal estrogen therapy may be used for treatment of urogenital symptoms and vaginal atrophy. However, if a patient is only experiencing bothersome GSM, low-dose vaginal estrogen therapy is recommended as first-line therapy before systemic therapy	Level 1
The type of MHT, dose, formulation, route of administration, and duration of use should be carefully considered to meet individual treatment goals for a patient. Periodic reassessment of therapy should consider changes in an individual's health, and ongoing risks and benefits of the current therapy strategy	Level 3
Postmenopausal individuals taking estrogen-based therapy should be informed about potential risks. Benefits likely outweigh risks of initiating MHT for symptomatic individuals younger than 60 years of age or within 10 years of menopause onset	Level 1
Studies demonstrate varying risks for estrogen-only therapy and estrogen and progestin therapy (eg, breast cancer risk)	Level 2
Appropriate counseling and a decision regarding duration of MHT use includes assessment of individual risk (personal and familial) for hormone sensitive cancer, osteoporosis, stroke, venous thromboembolism, and coronary heart disease	Level 3
Endometrial protection is required for individuals with an intact uterus using systemic estrogen therapy. An adequate dose and duration of progestogen or combined estrogen and progestogen or CEE with bazedoxifene is recommended to avoid endometrial hyperplasia	Level 1
Progestogen therapy is not recommended with use of low-dose (local) vaginal estrogen therapy	Level 1
Lower doses or switching to transdermal delivery of hormone therapy may be considered as an individual ages or develops hypertriglyceridemia	Level 3
Compounded bioidentical hormone therapy is not recommended due to safety concerns regarding dosing, lack of studies demonstrating safety and efficacy	Level 1

CEE, conjugated equine estrogen; GSM, Genitourinary Syndrome of Menopause; MHT, menopausal hormone therapy.

North American Menopause Society's Level of Recommendation: Level 1, based on good and consistent scientific evidence; Level 2, based on limited or inconsistent scientific evidence; Level 3, based primarily on consensus and expert opinion.

Data from Reference 6.

menopausal symptoms and the risk for cardiovascular disease, breast cancer, thromboembolism, and osteoporotic fracture (Table 102-9).

The WHI trial reported increased risk of cardiovascular disease, breast cancer, stroke, and thromboembolic disease among participants using continuous combined therapy with CEE plus MPA compared with placebo. In the estrogen-alone arm of the study, CEE had no effect on cardiovascular disease or breast cancer risk compared to placebo, but an increased risk of stroke and thromboembolic disease was noted in those who received estrogen. The WHI trial also demonstrated that quality of life and cognition were no better in the group receiving MHT than in the placebo group, and that MHT increases dementia risk in participants aged 65 years or older. Recent studies suggest dose, duration, and timing (early or late menopause) of therapy may alter the benefit-risk profile and should be considered for individual patients.

In the absence of contraindications, MHT is the most effective treatment for managing postmenopausal symptoms, such as hot flashes, night sweats, and vaginal dryness. For many individuals, the benefits of short-term use of MHT for the relief of menopausal symptoms, far outweighs any risks. For symptoms of genital atrophy alone, the use of local, nonsystemic estrogen, nonhormonal lubricants and moisturizers, or ospemifene should be considered.

Long-term use of MHT cannot be recommended routinely for osteoporosis prevention given the availability of alternative therapies, such as bisphosphonates. For long-term MHT use, the potential harm (cardiovascular disease, breast cancer, and thromboembolism) outweighs the potential benefits. MHT should not be used for prevention of CHD. Individuals with cardiovascular risk factors (eg, hypertension and lipid abnormalities) can benefit from reduction of these risk factors through interventions such as weight loss, lipid-lowering therapy, and physical activity.

ABBREVIATIONS

AUB	abnormal uterine bleeding
AMH	anti-Mullerian hormone
BMD	bone mineral density
CBHT	compounded bioidentical hormone therapy
CEE	conjugated equine estrogens
CIMT	carotid intima-media thickness
CHD	coronary heart disease
FMP	final menstrual period
FSH	follicle-stimulating hormone
GI	gastrointestinal
GnRH	gonadotropin-releasing hormone
GSM	genitourinary syndrome of menopause
HDL	high-density lipoprotein
HR	hazard ratio
LDL	low-density lipoprotein
LH	luteinizing hormone
MHT	menopausal hormone therapy
MPA	medroxyprogesterone acetate
NETA	norethindrone acetate
o-CEE	oral conjugated equine estrogens
SERM	selective estrogen receptor modulator
STRAW	Stages of Reproductive Aging Workshop
TSEC	tissue-selective estrogen complex
VTE	venous thromboembolism
WHI	Women's Health Initiative
WHIMSY	Women's Health Initiative Memory Study of Younger Women

REFERENCES

1. Shifren JL, Gass ML. The North American Menopause Society recommendations for clinical care of midlife women. *Menopause.* 2014;21:1038–1062.
2. Takahashi TA, Johnson KM. Menopause. *Med Clin North Am.* 2015;99:521–534.
3. Harlow SD, Gass M, Hall JE, et al. Executive summary of the Stages of Reproductive Aging Workshop + 10: Addressing the unfinished agenda of staging reproductive aging. *J Clin Endocrinol Metab.* 2012;97:1159–1168.
4. Victoria M, Labrosse J, Krief F, et al. Anti Müllerian hormone: More than a biomarker of female reproductive function. *J Gynecol Obstet Hum Reprod.* 2019;48(1):19–24. 10.1016/j.jogoh.2018.10.015 30352309.
5. Hall JE. Endocrinology of the menopause. *Endocrinol Metab Clin North Am.* 2015;44(3):485–496. 10.1016/j.ecl.2015.05.010 26316238.
6. The NAMS 2017 Hormone Therapy Position Statement Advisory Panel. The 2017 hormone therapy position statement of The North American Menopause Society. *Menopause.* 2017;24:728–753.
7. 2019 surveillance of menopause: Diagnosis and management (NICE guideline NG23). London: National Institute for Health and Care Excellence (UK). https://www.nice.org.uk/guidance/ng23/resources/menopause-diagnosis-and-management-pdf-1837330217413Dec2019, Accessed September 22, 2021.
8. Society of Obstericians and Gynaecologists of Canada Obsterics and Gynaecology, Twelve things physicians and patients should question. Choosing Wisely Canada. https://choosingwiselycanada.org/obstetrics-and-gynaecology/. September 2020. Last accessed September 22, 2021.
9. Gartoulla P, Worsley R, Bell RJ, et al. Moderate to severe vasomotor and sexual symptoms remain problematic for women aged 60 to 65 years. *Menopause.* 2015;22(7):694–701. 10.1097/GME.0000000000000383 25706184.
10. El Khoudary SR, Greendale G, Crawford SL, et al. The menopause transition and women's health at midlife: A progress report from the Study of Women's Health Across the Nation (SWAN). *Menopause.* 2019;26(10):1213–1227. 10.1097/GME.0000000000001424 31568098.
11. Mirkin S, Komm B, Pickar JH. Conjugated estrogen/bazedoxifene tablets for the treatment of moderate-to-severe vasomotor symptoms associated with menopause. *Women's Health.* 2014;10:135–146.
12. Scavello I, Maseroli E, Di Stasi V, et al. Sexual health in menopause. *Medicina (Kaunas).* 2019;55(910.3390/medicina55090559 31480774.
13. The 2020 genitourinary syndrome of menopause position statement of The North American Menopause Society. *Menopause.* 2020;27(9):976–992. 10.1097/GME.0000000000001609 32852449.
14. Maki PM, Kornstein SG, Joffe H, et al. Guidelines for the evaluation and treatment of perimenopausal depression: Summary and recommendations. *Menopause.* 2018;25:1069–1085.
15. Thornton K, Chervenak J, Neal-Perry G. Menopause and sexuality. *Endocrinol Metab Clin North Am.* 2015;44:649–661.
16. Manson JE, Chlebowski RT, Stefanick ML, et al. Menopausal hormone therapy and health outcomes during the intervention and extended poststopping phases of the Women's Health Initiative randomized trials. *JAMA.* 2013;310:1353–1368.
17. North American Menopause Society. Nonhormonal management of menopause-associated vasomotor symptoms: 2015 Position statement of The North American Menopause Society. *Menopause.* 2015;22:1155–1172.
18. Kagan R, Kellogg-Spadt S, Parish SJ. Practical treatment considerations in the management of genitourinary syndrome of menopause. *Drugs Aging.* 2019;36(10):897–908. 10.1007/s40266-019-00700-w 31452067.
19. Baber RJ, Panay N, Fenton A. 2016 IMS Recommendations on women's midlife health and menopause hormone therapy. *Climacteric.* 2016;19(2):109–150. 10.3109/13697137.2015.1129166 26872610.
20. Stuenkel CA, Davis SR, Gompel A, et al. Treatment of symptoms of the menopause: An Endocrine Society Clinical Practice Guideline. *J Clin Endocrinol Metab.* 2015;100:3975–4011.
21. Cobin RH, Goodman NF. American Association of Clinical Endocrinologists and American College of Endocrinology Position Statement on Menopause—2017 Update. *Endocr Pract.* 2017;23:869–880.
22. American College of Obstetrics and Gynecology. ACOG Practice Bulletin No. 141: Management of menopausal symptoms. *Obstet Gynecol.* 2014;123:202–216. (Reaffirmed 2018).
23. North American Menopause Society. The North American Menopause Society statement on continuing use of systemic hormone therapy after age 65. *Menopause.* 2015;22:693.
24. de Villiers TJ, Hall JE, Pinkerton JV, et al. Revised global consensus statement on menopausal hormone therapy. *Climacteric.* 2016;19:313–315.
25. Santoro N, Braunstein GD, Butts CL, Martin KA, McDermott M, Pinkerton JV. Compounded bioidentical hormones in endocrinology practice: An Endocrine Society scientific statement. *J Clin Endocrinol Metab.* 2016;101:1318–1343.
26. Lee SR, Cho MK, Cho YJ, et al. The 2020 Menopausal Hormone Therapy Guidelines. *J Menopausal Med.* 2020;26(2):69–98. 10.6118/jmm.20000 32893509.
27. Management of osteoporosis in postmenopausal women: The 2021 position statement of The North American Menopause Society. *Menopause.* 2021;28(9):973–997. 10.1097/GME.0000000000001831 34448749.
28. Grossman DC, Curry SJ, Owens DK, et al. Hormone therapy for the primary prevention of chronic conditions in postmenopausal women: US Preventive Services Task Force recommendation statement. *JAMA.* 2017;318:2224–2233.
29. Russo E, Caretto M, Giannini A, et al. Management of urinary incontinence in postmenopausal women: An EMAS clinical guide.

Maturitas. 2021;143:223–230. 10.1016/j.maturitas.2020.09.005 33008675.

30. Gottlieb Scott Statement from FDA Commissioner Food Drug Administration. https://www.fda.gov/news-events/press-announcements/statement-fda-commissioner-scott-gottlieb-md-efforts-safeguard-womens-health-deceptive-health-claims. July 2018, Accessed October 25, 2021.
31. Mension E, Alonso I, Tortajada M, et al. Vaginal laser therapy for genitourinary syndrome of menopause: Systematic review. *Maturitas.* 2021;21:S0378–5112. 10.1016/j.maturitas.2021.06.005 34217581.
32. Crandall CJ, Hovey KM, Andrews CA, et al. Breast cancer, endometrial cancer, and cardiovascular events in participants who used vaginal estrogen in the Women's Health Initiative Observational Study. *Menopause.* 2018;25:11–20.
33. Manson JE, Aragaki AK, Rossouw JE, et al. Menopausal hormone therapy and long-term all-cause and cause-specific mortality: The Women's Health Initiative randomized trials. *JAMA.* 2017;318:927–938.
34. Marjoribanks J, Farquhar C, Roberts H, Lethaby A, Lee J. Long-term hormone therapy for perimenopausal and postmenopausal women. *Cochrane Database Syst Rev.* 2017;1:CD004143.
35. Shufelt C, Bairey Merz CN, Pettinger MB, et al. Estrogen-alone therapy and invasive breast cancer incidence by dose, formulation, and route of delivery: Findings from the WHI observational study. *Menopause.* 2018;25:985–991.
36. Chlebowski RT, Anderson GL, Aragaki AK, et al. Association of Menopausal Hormone Therapy With Breast Cancer Incidence and Mortality During Long-term Follow-up of the Women's Health Initiative Randomized Clinical Trials. *JAMA.* 2020;324(4):369–380. 10.1001/jama.2020.9482 32721007.
37. Manson JE, Aragaki AK, Bassuk SS, et al. Menopausal Estrogen-Alone Therapy and Health Outcomes in Women With and Without Bilateral Oophorectomy: A Randomized Trial. *Ann Intern Med.* 2019;171(6):406–414. 10.7326/M19-0274 31499528.
38. Chlebowski RT, Schwartz AG, Wakelee H, et al. Oestrogen plus progestin and lung cancer in postmenopausal women (Women's Health Initiative trial): A post-hoc analysis of a randomised controlled trial. *Lancet.* 2009;374(9697):1243–1251. 10.1016/S0140-6736(09)61526-9 19767090.
39. Parish SJ, Simon JA, Davis SR, et al. International Society for the Study of Women's Sexual Health Clinical Practice Guideline for the Use of Systemic Testosterone for Hypoactive Sexual Desire Disorder in Women. *J Womens Health (Larchmt).* 2021;30(4):474–491. 10.1089/jwh.2021.29037 33797277.
40. Muka T, Oliver-Williams C, Colpani V, et al. Association of vasomotor and other menopausal symptoms with risk of cardiovascular disease: A systematic review and meta-analysis. *PLoS One.* 2016;11:e0157417.
41. Koh KK, Jin DK, Yang SH, et al. Vascular effects of synthetic or natural progestagen combined with conjugated equine estrogen in healthy postmenopausal women. *Circulation.* 2001;103:1961–1966.
42. Schierbeck LL, Rejnmark L, Tofteng CL, et al. Effect of hormone replacement therapy on cardiovascular events in recently postmenopausal women: Randomised trial. *BMJ.* 2012;345:e6409.
43. Bechlioulis A, Naka KK, Kalantaridou SN, et al. Short-term hormone therapy improves sCD40L and endothelial function in early menopausal women: Potential role of estrogen receptor polymorphisms. *Maturitas.* 2012;71:389–395.
44. Hodis HN, Mack WJ, Henderson VW, et al. Vascular effects of early versus late postmenopausal treatment with estradiol. *N Engl J Med.* 2016;374:1221–1231.
45. Sriprasert I, Hodis HN, Karim R, et al. Differential effect of plasma estradiol on subclinical atherosclerosis progression in early vs late postmenopause. *J Clin Endocrinol Metab.* 2019;104(2):293–300. 10.1210/jc.2018-01600 30272234.
46. Keaney JF Jr, Solomon CG. Postmenopausal hormone therapy and atherosclerosis: Time is of the essence. *N Engl J Med.* 2016;374:1279–1280.
47. Shufelt CL, Manson JE. Menopausal hormone therapy and cardiovascular disease: The role of formulation, dose, and route of delivery. *J Clin Endocrinol Metab.* 2021;106(5):1245–1254. 10.1210/clinem/dgab042 33506261.
48. Oliver-Williams C, Glisic M, Shahzad S, et al. The route of administration, timing, duration and dose of postmenopausal hormone therapy and cardiovascular outcomes in women: A systematic review. *Hum Reprod Update.* 2019;25(2):257–271. 10.1093/humupd/dmy039 30508190.
49. Kim JE, Chang JH, Jeong MJ, et al. A systematic review and meta-analysis of effects of menopausal hormone therapy on cardiovascular diseases. *Sci Rep.* 2020;10(1):20631–20631. 10.1038/s41598-020-77534-9 33244065.
50. Arnett DK, Blumenthal RS, Albert MA, et al. 2019 ACC/AHA Guideline on the Primary Prevention of Cardiovascular Disease: A Report of the American College of Cardiology/American Heart Association Task Force on Clinical Practice Guidelines. *J Am Coll Cardiol.* 2019;74(10):e177–e232. 10.1016/j.jacc.2019.03.010 30894318.
51. ACOG committee opinion no. 556: Postmenopausal estrogen therapy: Route of administration and risk of venous thromboembolism. *Obstet Gynecol.* 2013;121(4):887–890. 10.1097/01.AOG.0000428645.90795.d9 23635705.
52. Ramírez I, De la Viuda E, Baquedano L, et al. The thromboembolic risk in Covid-19 women under hormonal treatment group. *Maturitas.* 2020;138:78–79. 10.1016/j.maturitas.2020.05.021.
53. Prentice RL, Aragaki AK, Chlebowski RT, et al. Randomized trial evaluation of the benefits and risks of menopausal hormone therapy among women 50-59 years of age. *Am J Epidemiol.* 2021;190(3):365–375. 10.1093/aje/kwaa210 33025002.
54. Manson JE, Aragaki AK, Bassuk SS, et al. Menopausal estrogen-alone therapy and health outcomes in women with and without bilateral oophorectomy: A randomized trial. *Ann Intern Med.* 2019;171(6):406–414. 10.7326/M19-0274 31499528.
55. Jordan VC. The new biology of estrogen-induced apoptosis applied to treat and prevent breast cancer. *Endocr Relat Cancer.* 2015;22(1):R1–31. 10.1530/ERC-14-0448 25339261.
56. Santen RJ, Heitjan DF, Gompel A, et al. Underlying Breast Cancer Risk and Menopausal Hormone Therapy. *J Clin Endocrinol Metab.* 2020;105(610). 1210/clinem/dgaa073 32052007.
57. Wang T, Bradshaw PT, Moorman PG, et al. Menopausal hormone therapy use and long-term all-cause and cause-specific mortality in the Long Island Breast Cancer Study Project. *Int J Cancer.* 2020;147(12):3404–3415. 10.1002/ijc.33174 32588422.
58. Zhang GQ, Chen JL, Luo Y, et al. Menopausal hormone therapy and women's health: An umbrella review. *PLoS Med.* 2021;18(8):e1003731–e1003731. 10.1371/journal.pmed.1003731 34339416.
59. Type and timing of menopausal hormone therapy and breast cancer risk: Individual participant meta-analysis of the worldwide epidemiological evidence. *Lancet.* 2019;394(10204):1159–1168. 10.1016/S0140-6736(19)31709-X 31474332.
60. Beral V, Peto R, Pirie K, et al. Menopausal hormone therapy and 20-year breast cancer mortality. *Lancet.* 2019;394:1139. 10.1016/S0140-6736(19)32033-1.
61. Breast cancer risk in American women. Available at: https://www.cancer.gov/types/breast/risk-fact-sheet Accessed October 19, 2021. National Cancer Institute Website.
62. Brusselaers N, Tamimi RM, Konings P, et al. Different menopausal hormone regimens and risk of breast cancer. *Ann Oncol.* 2018;29(8):1771–1776. 10.1093/annonc/mdy212 29917061.
63. Vinogradova Y, Coupland C, Hippisley-Cox J. Use of hormone replacement therapy and risk of breast cancer: Nested case-control studies using the QResearch and CPRD databases. *BMJ.* 2020;371:m3873–m3873. 10.1136/bmj.m3873 33115755.
64. Tempfer CB, Hilal Z, Kern P, et al. Menopausal hormone therapy and risk of endometrial cancer: A systematic review. *Cancers (Basel).* 2020;12(810). 3390/cancers12082195 32781573.
65. Londero AP, Parisi N, Tassi A, et al. Hormone replacement therapy in endometrial cancer survivors: A meta-analysis. *J Clin Med.* 2021;10(1410). 3390/jcm10143165 34300331.
66. Rees M, Angioli R, Coleman RL, et al. European Menopause and Andropause Society (EMAS) and International Gynecologic Cancer Society (IGCS) position statement on managing the menopause after gynecological cancer: Focus on menopausal symptoms and osteoporosis. *Maturitas.* 2020;134:56–61. 10.1016/j.maturitas.2020.01.005 32059825.
67. Brieger KK, Peterson S, Lee AW, et al. Menopausal hormone therapy prior to the diagnosis of ovarian cancer is associated with improved survival. *Gynecol Oncol.* 2020;158(3):702–709. 10.1016/j.ygyno.2020.06.481 32641237.
68. Brennan A, Brennan D, Rees M, et al. Management of menopausal symptoms and ovarian function preservation in women with gynecological cancer. *Int J Gynecol Cancer.* 2021;31(3):352–359. 10.1136/ijgc-2020-002032 33127864.
69. Chlebowski RT, Schwartz AG, Wakelee H, et al. Oestrogen plus progestin and lung cancer in postmenopausal women (Women's Health Initiative trial): A post-hoc analysis of a randomised controlled trial. *Lancet.* 2009;374(9697):1243–1251. 10.1016/S0140-6736(09)61526-9 19767090.
70. Hlatky MA, Boothroyd D, Vittinghoff E, Sharp P, Whooley MA. Quality-of-life and depressive symptoms in postmenopausal women after receiving hormone therapy: Results from the Heart and Estrogen/Progestin Replacement Study (HERS) trial. *JAMA.* 2002;287:591–597.

71. Ott A, Breteler MM, van Harskamp F, Stijnen T, Hofman A. Incidence and risk of dementia. The Rotterdam Study. *Am J Epidemiol.* 1998;147:574–580.
72. Shumaker SA, Legault C, Rapp SR, et al. Estrogen plus progestin and the incidence of dementia and mild cognitive impairment in postmenopausal women. The Women's Health Initiative Memory Study: a randomized controlled trial. *JAMA.* 2003;289(20):2651–2662.
73. Espeland MA, Rapp SR, Shumaker SA, et al. Conjugated equine estrogens and global cognitive function in postmenopausal women: Women's Health Initiative Memory Study. *JAMA.* 2004;291:2959–2968.
74. Espeland MA, Shumaker SA, Leng I, et al. Long-term effects on cognitive function of postmenopausal hormone therapy prescribed to women aged 50 to 55 years. *JAMA Intern Med.* 2013;173:1429–1436.
75. Gleason CE, Dowling NM, Wharton W, et al. Effects of hormone therapy on cognition and mood in recently postmenopausal women: Findings from the randomized, controlled KEEPS—Cognitive and Affective Study. *PLoS Med.* 2015;12:e1001833. Discussion e1001833.
76. Espeland MA, Hogan PE, Fineberg SE, et al. Effect of postmenopausal hormone therapy on glucose and insulin concentrations. PEPI Investigators. Postmenopausal Estrogen/Progestin Interventions. *Diabetes Care.* 1998;21:1589–1595.
77. Kanaya AM, Herrington D, Vittinghoff E, et al. Glycemic effects of postmenopausal hormone therapy: The Heart and Estrogen/progestin Replacement Study. A randomized, double-blind, placebo-controlled trial. *Ann Intern Med.* 2003;138:1–9.
78. Margolis KL, Bonds DE, Rodabough RJ, et al. Effect of oestrogen plus progestin on the incidence of diabetes in postmenopausal women: Results from the Women's Health Initiative Hormone Trial. *Diabetologia.* 2004;47:1175–1187.
79. Norman RJ, Flight IH, Rees MC. Oestrogen and progestogen hormone replacement therapy for peri-menopausal and post-menopausal women: Weight and body fat distribution. *Cochrane Database Syst Rev.* 2000;CD001018.
80. Bachmann GA, Schaefers M, Uddin A, Utian WH. Lowest effective transdermal 17beta-estradiol dose for relief of hot flushes in postmenopausal women: A randomized controlled trial. *Obstet Gynecol.* 2007;110:771–779.
81. Haines C, Yu SL, Hiemeyer F, Schaefers M. Micro-dose transdermal estradiol for relief of hot flushes in postmenopausal Asian women: A randomized controlled trial. *Climacteric.* 2009;12:419–426.
82. Lindsay R, Gallagher JC, Kleerekoper M, Pickar JH. Effect of lower doses of conjugated equine estrogens with and without medroxyprogesterone acetate on bone in early postmenopausal women. *JAMA.* 2002;287:2668–2676.
83. Lindsay R, Gallagher JC, Kleerekoper M, Pickar JH. Bone response to treatment with lower doses of conjugated estrogens with and without medroxyprogesterone acetate in early postmenopausal women. *Osteoporos Int.* 2005;16:372–379.
84. Bioidentical hormone pellet therapy for women. Women's Wellness Center. https://womenswellnessnow.com/service/bioidentical-hormone-pellet-therapy-for-women/. Accessed November 7, 2021.
85. Furness S, Roberts H, Marjoribanks J, Lethaby A. Hormone therapy in postmenopausal women and risk of endometrial hyperplasia. *Cochrane Database Syst Rev.* 2012:CD000402.
86. Hitchcock CL, Prior JC. Oral micronized progesterone for vasomotor symptoms: A placebo-controlled randomized trial in healthy postmenopausal women. *Menopause.* 2012;19:886–893.
87. Prior JC, Hitchcock CL. Progesterone for hot flush and night sweat treatment: Effectiveness for severe vasomotor symptoms and lack of withdrawal rebound. *Gynecol Endocrinol.* 2012;28(suppl 2):7–11.
88. Casper RF. Estrogen with interrupted progestin HRT: A review of experimental and clinical studies. *Maturitas.* 2000;34:97–108.
89. Asi N, Mohammed K, Haydour Q, et al. Progesterone vs. synthetic progestins and the risk of breast cancer: A systematic review and meta-analysis. *Syst Rev.* 2016;5(1):121–121. 10.1186/s13643-016-0294-5 27456847.
90. Stute P, Neulen J, Wildt L. The impact of micronized progesterone on the endometrium: A systematic review. *Climacteric.* 2016;19:316–328.
91. Stevenson JC, Rozenberg S, Maffei S, et al. Progestogens as a component of menopausal hormone therapy: The right molecule makes the difference. *Drugs Context.* 2020;910. 7573/dic.2020-10-1 33312219.
92. Committee opinion No. 532: Compounded bioidentical menopausal hormone therapy. *Obstet Gynecol.* 2012;120(2 Pt 1):411–415. 10.1097/AOG.0b013e318268049e 22825109.
93. McBane SE, Borgelt LM, Barnes KN, Westberg SM, Lodise NM, Stassinos M. Use of compounded bioidentical hormone therapy in menopausal women: An opinion statement of the Women's Health Practice and Research Network of the American College of Clinical Pharmacy. *Pharmacotherapy.* 2014;34:410–423.
94. Davis SR, Baber R, Panay N, et al. Global consensus position statement on the use of testosterone therapy for women. *J Clin Endocrinol Metab.* 2019;104:4660–4666. 10.1210/jc.2019-01603.
95. Islam RM, Bell RJ, Green S, et al. Safety and efficacy of testosterone for women: A systematic review and meta-analysis of randomised controlled trial data. *Lancet Diabetes Endocrinol.* 2019;7(10):754–766. 10.1016/S2213-8587(19)30189-5 31353194.
96. Portman DJ, Goldstein SR, Kagan R. Treatment of moderate to severe dyspareunia with intravaginal prasterone therapy: A review. *Climacteric.* 2019;22:65–72.
97. Ke Y, Labrie F, Gonthier R, et al. Serum levels of sex steroids and metabolites following 12 weeks of intravaginal 0.50% DHEA administration. *J Steroid Biochem Mol Biol.* 2015;154:186–196.
98. Package insert. *Intrarosa (prasterone).* Waltham, MA: AMAG Pharmaceuticals, Inc; 2018.
99. Santen RJ, Kagan R, Altomare CJ, Komm B, Mirkin S, Taylor HS. Current and evolving approaches to individualizing estrogen receptor-based therapy for menopausal women. *J Clin Endocrinol Metab.* 2014;99:733–747.
100. Package insert. *Evista (raloxifene).* Indianapolis, IN: Lilly USA; 2018.
101. Palacios S, Mejia Rios A, Bazedoxifene/conjugated estrogens combination for the treatment of the vasomotor symptoms associated with menopause and for prevention of osteoporosis in postmenopausal women. *Drugs Today (Barc).* 2015;51:107–116.
102. Pinkerton JV, Abraham L, Bushmakin AG, et al. Evaluation of the efficacy and safety of bazedoxifene/conjugated estrogens for secondary outcomes including vasomotor symptoms in postmenopausal women by years since menopause in the Selective estrogens, Menopause and Response to Therapy (SMART) trials. *J Womens Health.* 2014;23:18–28.
103. Package insert. *Osphena (ospemifene).* Bryn Mawr, PA, USA: Duchesnay; 2019 January.
104. Package insert. *Duavee (conjugated estrogens/bazedoxifene).* Philadelphia, PA: Pfizer; 2017.
105. Rietjens I, Louisse J, Beekmann K. The potential health effects of dietary phytoestrogens. *Br J Pharmacol.* 2017;174:1263–1280.
106. Lethaby A, Marjoribanks J, Kronenberg F, Roberts H, Eden J, Brown J. Phytoestrogens for menopausal vasomotor symptoms. *Cochrane Database Syst Rev.* 2013:CD001395.
107. Franco OH, Chowdhury R, Troup J, et al. Use of plant-based therapies and menopausal symptoms: A systematic review and meta-analysis. *JAMA.* 2016;315:2554–2563.
108. Lissin LW, Cooke JP. Phytoestrogens and cardiovascular health. *J Am Coll Cardiol.* 2000;35:1403–1410.
109. Tempfer CB, Froese G, Heinze G, Bentz EK, Hefler LA, Huber JC. Side effects of phytoestrogens: A meta-analysis of randomized trials. *Am J Med.* 2009;122:939–946. e9.
110. National Institutes of Health Office of Dietary Supplements. Updated August 30, 2018. Available at: http://ods.od.nih.gov/factsheets/BlackCohosh-HealthProfessional. Accessed October 29, 2021. Dietary supplements fact sheet: Black cohosh.
111. Nedrow A, Miller J, Walker M, Nygren P, Huffman LH, Nelson HD. Complementary and alternative therapies for the management of menopause-related symptoms: A systematic evidence review. *Arch Intern Med.* 2006;166:1453–1465.
112. Ettinger B. Vasomotor symptom relief versus unwanted effects: Role of estrogen dosage. *Am J Med.* 2005;118(suppl 12B):74–78.

103 Erectile Dysfunction

Mary Lee and Roohollah Sharifi

KEY CONCEPTS

1. The incidence of erectile dysfunction is low in men younger than 40 years of age. The incidence increases as men age likely as a result of concurrent medical conditions that impair the vascular, neurologic, psychogenic, and hormonal systems necessary for a normal penile erection.
2. Many commonly used drugs have sympatholytic, anticholinergic, sedative, or antiandrogenic effects that may exacerbate or contribute to the development of erectile dysfunction. Clinicians should be familiar with these agents and be prepared to adjust drug regimens to minimize adverse effects of these drugs on a patient's erectile function.
3. The first step in clinical management of erectile dysfunction is to identify and, if possible, reverse the underlying causes. Risk factors for erectile dysfunction, including hypertension, diabetes mellitus, smoking, and chronic ethanol abuse, should be addressed and minimized.
4. Specific treatments for erectile dysfunction include vacuum erection devices (VEDs), pharmacologic treatments, psychotherapy, and surgery. Of these, phosphodiesterase type 5 inhibitors are the medications of first choice.
5. The ideal treatment of erectile dysfunction should have a fast onset, be effective, be convenient to administer, be cost-effective, have a low incidence of serious adverse effects, and be free of serious drug interactions.
6. Specific treatment is first initiated with the least invasive modality, including VEDs or oral phosphodiesterase type 5 inhibitors, followed by intracavernosal injections or intraurethral inserts, and finally by surgical insertion of a penile prosthesis.
7. Vacuum erection devices can have a slow onset of action (up to 20 minutes) during initial use and are not discreet; therefore, they are most effective for a couple in a stable relationship.
8. Although phosphodiesterase type 5 inhibitors are convenient and effective regardless of the etiology of erectile dysfunction, they fail in 30% to 40% of patients. Also, phosphodiesterase type 5 inhibitors are contraindicated in patients taking any dosage formulation of nitrate.
9. Testosterone supplementation should be reserved for symptomatic patients with primary, secondary, or mixed hypogonadism who have erectile dysfunction. Testosterone supplementation should not be used by patients with erectile dysfunction who have normal serum testosterone levels.
10. Although intracavernosal injections and intraurethral pellets of alprostadil are effective and independent of the etiology of erectile dysfunction, they fail in up to one-third of patients. To self-administer medication by these routes, patients require training to minimize administration-related adverse effects.

BEYOND THE BOOK

Many medications may cause or worsen erectile dysfunction. Based on the physiology of a normal erection, create a table in which you identify various classes of medications that interfere with the hormonal, vascular, neurologic, or psychogenic factors that are essential for a normal penile erection. In a separate column, identify medications that are most likely to interfere with those physiologic factors and are likely to cause erectile dysfunction.

INTRODUCTION

The National Institutes of Health Consensus Development Panel on Impotence[1] defines erectile dysfunction as the persistent or recurrent failure to achieve or maintain a penile erection to allow for satisfactory sexual intercourse. A persistent failure generally refers to erectile dysfunction for a minimum of 3 months. Patients may refer to the condition as impotence. Erectile dysfunction must be distinguished from disorders of libido or ejaculation, and of infertility, all of which are caused by different pathophysiologic mechanisms and are treated with alternative agents (Table 103-1). A patient may have one or more disorders of sexual and reproductive function. For example, an older man with primary hypogonadism could have both decreased libido and erectile dysfunction. Diagnosing the type of sexual disorders in a patient is key to initiating the most appropriate treatment.

Editors' note: In this and other chapters in Pharmacotherapy, *references to biologic gender (as assigned at birth) are used based on prior literature being discussed or anatomical or physiologic differences. We recognize that not all individuals identify with their gender at birth, and to the degree possible when discussing therapeutics, we avoid the use of references to gender. Use of gender in this chapter refers to the*

TABLE 103-1 Types of Sexual Dysfunction in Men

Type of Dysfunction	Definition
Decreased libido	Decreased sexual drive or desire
Increased libido	Inappropriate and excessive sexual drive or desire
Erectile dysfunction (impotence)	Failure to achieve a penile erection suitable for satisfactory sexual intercourse
Delayed ejaculation/ anejaculation	Commonly referred to as "dry sex"; ejaculation is delayed or absent
Retrograde ejaculation	Ejaculate passes retrograde into the bladder, instead of toward the anterior urethra (antegrade) and out of the penis
Infertility	Sperm are insufficient in number, have abnormal morphology, or have inadequate motility, and fail to fertilize the ovum

language used in prior studies, published guidelines, and other recommendations for diagnosis and treatment based on biological gender and does not necessarily reflect an individual's gender identity.

EPIDEMIOLOGY

1 The incidence of erectile dysfunction is low in men younger than 40 years but increases as men ages. The Massachusetts Male Aging Study, a cross-sectional survey of a random sample of 1,290 men in the Boston area, was conducted during the period from 1987 to 1989. The study reported an overall prevalence of 52% for any degree of erectile dysfunction in men aged 40 to 70 years, with an age-related increase in incidence ranging from 12.4 cases per 1,000 men per year in men aged 40 to 49 years, up to 46.4 cases per 1,000 men per year in men aged 60 to 69 years.[2] In men older than 70 years, the prevalence of erectile dysfunction increases and has been reported to be as high as 80%, depending on the population studied.[2] In the Health Professional Follow-up Study of more than 31,000 male health professionals aged 53 to 90 years, the prevalence of erectile dysfunction was 33%.[3] Interestingly, although the prevalence of erectile dysfunction increases with patient age, many patients fail to seek medical treatment. This may be due to a decrease in sexual activity as males age.

Erectile dysfunction is sometimes assumed to be a symptom of the aging process in men. However, more likely it results from concurrent medical conditions of the patient (eg, hypertension, arteriosclerosis, hyperlipidemia, diabetes mellitus, metabolic syndrome, or psychiatric disorders) or from medications that patients may be taking for these diseases.[1,2] For example, up to 50% of patients with diabetes mellitus develop erectile dysfunction, and medications such as diuretics are associated with a high incidence of erectile dysfunction.

PHYSIOLOGY OF A NORMAL PENILE ERECTION

A normal penile erection requires full functioning of several physiologic systems: vascular, nervous, and hormonal. The patient also must be psychologically receptive to sexual stimuli.

Vascular System

The penis comprises two corpora cavernosa on the dorsal side and one corpus spongiosum on the ventral side. The corpus spongiosum surrounds the urethra and forms the glans penis. The corpora are composed of multiple interconnected sinuses, which can fill with blood to produce an erection. The corpora cavernosa are encased by the tunica albuginea, a fibrous tissue membrane, which has limited distensibility. In the flaccid state, arterial flow into and venous outflow from the corpora are balanced. During the erectile phase, arterial blood flow increases, and blood fills the sinusoids within the corpora. Blood traps in the corpora as the outflow of the subtunical veins is compressed against the tunica albuginea. This prolongs the erection (Fig. 103-1).

Arterial flow into the corpora is enhanced by acetylcholine-mediated vasodilation. Acetylcholine indirectly enhances arterial flow to the corpora and increases sinusoidal filling of the corporal tissue. That is, acetylcholine is a co-neurotransmitter, which works along with other nonpeptidergic intracellular neurotransmitters—including cyclic guanosine monophosphate (cGMP), cyclic adenosine monophosphate (cAMP), or vasoactive intestinal polypeptide—to produce vasodilation. In effect, cGMP and cAMP are secondary messengers that direct desired effects in target tissues.

Specifically, acetylcholine produces an erection probably through two different pathways. Through one pathway, in the presence of sexual stimulation to genital tissue, acetylcholine enhances the production of nitric oxide by endothelial cells and nonadrenergic–noncholinergic neurons. Nitric oxide enhances the activity of guanylate cyclase, which increases the conversion of cyclic guanosine triphosphate to cGMP. cGMP activates a cGMP-dependent kinase, which decreases intracellular calcium concentrations in smooth muscle cells of penile arteries and cavernosal sinuses. As a result, smooth muscle relaxation occurs, which enhances arterial blood flow to and blood filling of the corpora.[4] An erection results.

In an alternative pathway, acetylcholine or prostaglandin E enhances the activity of adenyl cyclase, which increases the conversion of cyclic adenosine triphosphate to cAMP, a potent muscle relaxant. Similar to cGMP, cAMP decreases intracellular calcium concentrations to produce smooth muscle relaxation in cells of the arteries and cavernosal sinuses. Arterial blood flow to and blood filling of the corpora are enhanced, and a penile erection results.

Nervous System and Psychogenic Stimuli

Some erections are mediated by a sacral nerve reflex arc (eg, erections can occur while the patient is sleeping). However, in the conscious patient, sensory sexual stimulation mediates erections via the central nervous system (CNS). That is, when a patient sees an attractive partner, hears sweet words, smells a particular scent, or tastes or touches a pleasant object, these situations can result in an erection. In this case, the patient's brain processes this information, and the nervous impulse is carried down the spinal cord to peripheral cholinergic nerves that innervate the vascular supply to the corpora, resulting in an erection.

The medial preoptic area of the hypothalamus is thought to be that portion of the brain responsible for integrating external stimuli. Here, dopamine exerts a proerectogenic effect, whereas alpha$_2$-adrenergic stimulation causes the penis to become and/or remain flaccid. After moving down the spinal cord, stimulatory nerve impulses travel to the penis by efferent peripheral nerves, including inhibitory sympathetic neurons (T_{11}-L_2), proerectogenic parasympathetic neurons (S_2-S_4), and proerectogenic somatic neurons (S_2-S_4).

In short, acetylcholine produces an erection by working along with other co-neurotransmitters, including cGMP and cAMP. Thus, an erection is mediated neurologically, maintained by arterial blood filling of the corpora, and sustained by occlusion of venous outflow from the corpora.

Detumescence, or the progression of an erect penis to a flaccid state, results from the actions of norepinephrine, which contracts vascular smooth muscle to decrease arterial inflow to the corpora and contracts sinusoidal tissue in the corpora. As a result, venous outflow from the corpora increases.

Hormonal System

Testosterone is principally produced by the testes at a daily rate of 4 to 8 mg and a normal physiologic serum concentration is 300 to 1,100 ng/dL (10.4-38.2 nmol/L). Production follows a circadian pattern with the highest blood levels in the morning and lowest levels in the evening. Physiologically active (free) testosterone comprises only 2% of

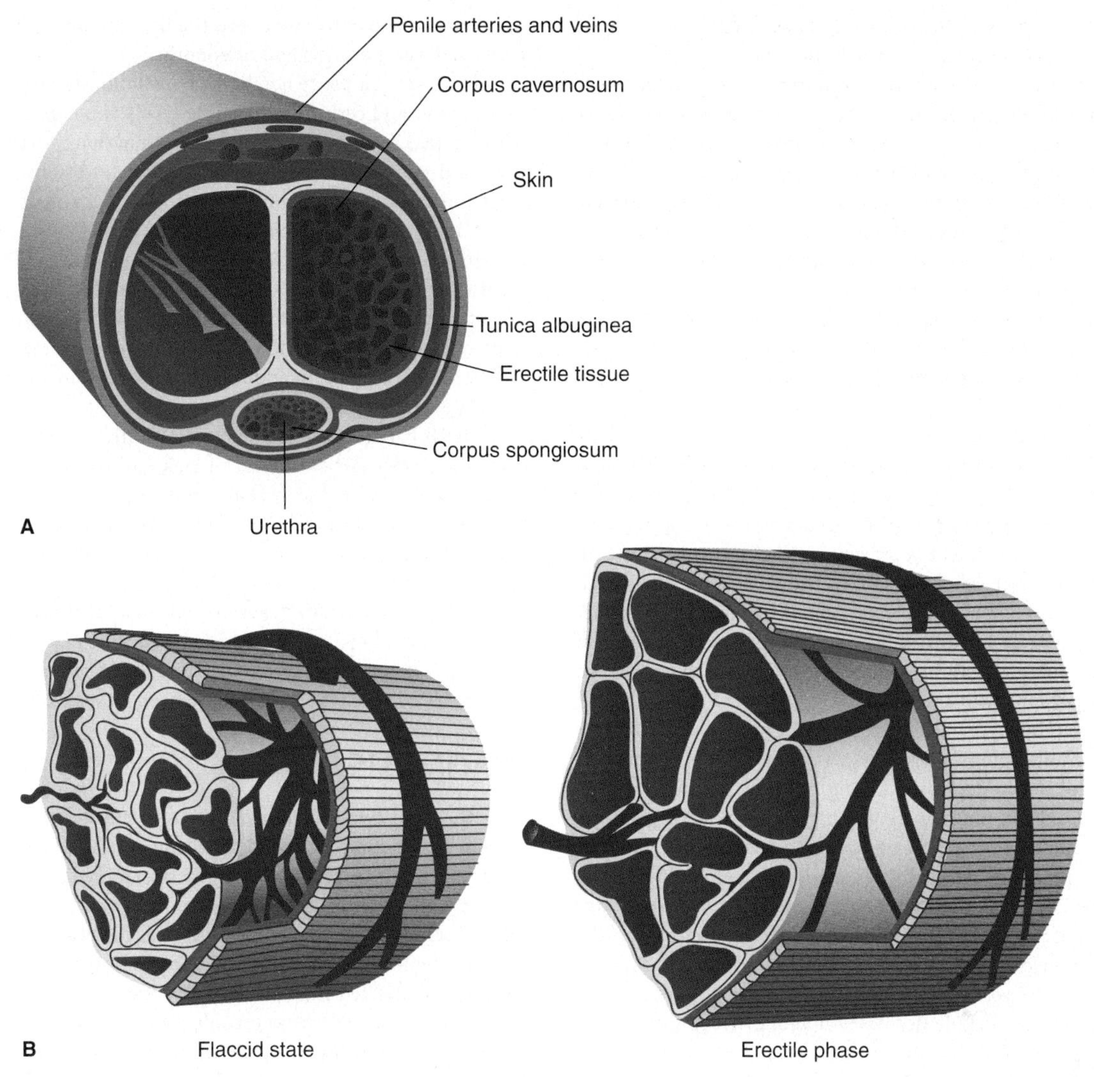

FIGURE 103-1 Microanatomy of and vascular changes in the penis in flaccid and erect states. *(Reprinted, with permission, from Walsh PC, ed. Campbell's Urology, 8th ed. Philadelphia, PA: WB Saunders; 2002:1595, 1697. Copyright © 2002 from Elsevier.)*

circulating blood levels. About 44% of testosterone in the bloodstream is tightly bound to sex hormone-binding globulin and is inactive. Approximately 50% is reversibly bound to albumin and 4% is reversibly bound to corticosteroid-binding globulin; both of these portions of testosterone are in equilibrium with the 2% of testosterone that is not bound. Thus, the bioavailable portion of testosterone is normally 56% and comprises testosterone bound to albumin and corticosteroid-binding globulin, and the unbound or free portion.[5] However, the bioavailable percentage of testosterone can vary considerably with changes in sex hormone-binding globulin. Sex hormone-binding globulin increases with aging, hyperthyroidism, human immunodeficiency virus disease, and hepatic cirrhosis and decreases with obesity, diabetes mellitus, hypothyroidism, nephrotic syndrome, and corticosteroid use.[5]

Testosterone stimulates libido (sexual drive) and increases muscle mass in males. In addition, androgen receptors have been identified in the penile arterial endothelium and are thought to increase cavernosal levels of nitric oxide and cGMP, thereby enhancing vascular processes essential for a penile erection. In addition, androgens may enhance phosphodiesterase type 5 activity and may improve cavernosal nerve function.

ETIOLOGY/PATHOPHYSIOLOGY

Erectile dysfunction can result from any single abnormality or combination of abnormalities of the four systems necessary for a normal penile erection. Vascular, neurologic, or hormonal etiologies of erectile dysfunction are collectively referred to as *organic erectile dysfunction*. Approximately 80% of elderly patients with erectile dysfunction have the organic type. Patients who do not respond to psychogenic stimuli and have no organic cause for dysfunction have *psychogenic erectile dysfunction*.[6]

Diseases that compromise vascular flow to the corpora cavernosum (eg, peripheral vascular disease, arteriosclerosis, and essential hypertension) comprise the most common causes of organic erectile dysfunction.[7] Erectile dysfunction is increasingly recognized as a predictor of cardiovascular disease.[8] This is because penile arteries are small caliber blood vessels when compared to coronary or carotid arteries; the diameters are 1 to 2 mm, 3 to 4 mm, and 5 to 6 mm, respectively. As a result, erectile dysfunction could be one of the first signs of atherosclerosis and may predict future cardiovascular disease.[8]

In addition to decreasing arterial blood flow to the corpora cavernosa, atherosclerosis may cause erectile dysfunction by causing inflammation to or impairing the function of vascular endothelial cells. As a result, nitric oxide release is decreased. Since nitric oxide is essential for the relaxation of cavernosal sinusoidal tissue, tumescence is impaired.[8]

Neurological disorders cause 10% to 20% of all cases of organic erectile dysfunction. Diseases that impair nerve conduction to the central nervous system (eg, Parkinson's disease, epilepsy, stroke, spinal cord injury) or conditions that impair peripheral nerve conduction to the penile vasculature (eg, diabetes mellitus, alcoholic neuropathy) can cause erectile dysfunction.[9]

Patients must be in the proper mental frame of mind to be receptive to sexual stimuli. Patients who suffer from malaise, have reactive depression or performance anxiety, are sedated, or have Alzheimer's disease, hypothyroidism, or mental disorders commonly complain of erectile dysfunction. In most studies, patients with psychogenic erectile dysfunction generally exhibit a higher response rate to various interventions than do patients with organic erectile dysfunction because the former have less severe disease.

Psychogenic causes of erectile dysfunction appear to be more prevalent in men under the age of 40 years of age. Depression, performance anxiety, lack of self-confidence, or partner-related problems are contributory.[10]

Diseases associated with hypogonadism, primary, secondary, or mixed, result in subphysiologic levels of testosterone, which cause diminished sexual drive (decreased libido) and secondary erectile dysfunction. Primary hypogonadism occurs with surgical removal of the testes for the treatment of prostate or testicular cancer or with testicular injury or disease. Secondary hypogonadism may result from hypothalamic or pituitary disorders of luteinizing hormone-releasing hormone or luteinizing hormone, respectively, or elevated prolactin levels, which can be associated with pituitary tumors, or can occur in patients with chronic renal failure.

Late-onset hypogonadism refers to the physiologic changes in testosterone in aging males. The etiology of hypogonadism is mixed. In addition to decreased Leydig cell function in the testes, hypothalamic release of luteinizing-releasing hormone is reduced, the circadian pattern of luteinizing hormone release from the pituitary gland is impaired, and sex hormone-binding globulin production increases.[11] Serum testosterone levels decrease starting at age 40 years by approximately 10% per decade of life. Thus, the prevalence of late-onset hypogonadism ranges from 3.2% and 5.1% in men aged 60 to 69 years and in men aged 70 to 79 years, respectively.[11,12] Symptoms include decreased libido, gynecomastia, small testes, reduced growth of body hair and beard, decreased muscle mass, and increased body fat. Decreased libido is associated with erectile dysfunction and loss of spontaneous morning erections. In addition, patients may complain of a depressed mood and tiredness, which may also contribute to erectile dysfunction. If left untreated, patients develop anemia and osteoporosis.

However, it must be noted that the relationship between erectile dysfunction and serum testosterone levels is complicated. Patients with normal serum testosterone levels may have erectile dysfunction, and patients with subnormal serum testosterone levels may have normal sexual function.[11]

Some patients have multiple factors contributing to the development of erectile dysfunction. Consider the typical older adult with cardiovascular disease, who is a smoker and has hypertension and diabetes mellitus, which are medically treated. The pathophysiology of erectile dysfunction in this patient includes vascular, neurologic, and hormonal origins. In addition, many common antihypertensive medications may cause erectile dysfunction.[13]

Social habits of patients have been linked to erectile dysfunction. The vasoconstrictor effect of cigarette smoking may compromise blood flow to the corpora and decrease cavernosal filling. Excessive ethanol intake may lead to androgen deficiency, peripheral neuropathy, or chronic liver disease, all of which can contribute to erectile dysfunction.

2 Medications may cause erectile dysfunction through similar pathophysiologic mechanisms (Table 103-2). Medications are responsible for approximately 10% to 25% of cases of erectile dysfunction. Two excellent reviews have been published.[14,15]

DIAGNOSIS

With the availability in the late 1990s of effective medications for erectile dysfunction independent of the etiology, diagnostic evaluation of erectile dysfunction became streamlined. Key assessments include a description of the severity of erectile dysfunction, complete medical, psychosocial, and surgical histories, review of concurrent medications, physical examination, assessment of cardiac reserve, and selected clinical laboratory tests.[22]

To assess the severity of erectile dysfunction, the patient should be asked about the quality of sexual intercourse for the past 4 weeks to 6 months. A self-administered standardized questionnaire, such as the International Index of Erectile Function (IIEF), is often used. It is administered before initiation of any treatment and repeated at

TABLE 103-2 Medication Classes That Can Cause Erectile Dysfunction

Drug Class	Proposed Mechanism by Which Drug Causes Erectile Dysfunction	Special Notes
Anticholinergic agents (antihistamines, antiparkinsonian agents, tricyclic antidepressants, phenothiazines)	Anticholinergic activity	• Second-generation nonsedating antihistamines (eg, loratadine, fexofenadine, or cetirizine) are associated with less erectile dysfunction than first-generation agents. • Selective serotonin reuptake inhibitor (SSRI) and multiple receptor reuptake inhibitor antidepressants cause less erectile dysfunction than tricyclic antidepressants. Of the SSRIs, paroxetine, sertraline, fluvoxamine, and fluoxetine cause erectile dysfunction more commonly than venlafaxine, nefazodone, trazodone, bupropion, duloxetine, mirtazapine, escitalopram, or vilazodone.[16] • Phenothiazines with less anticholinergic effect (eg, chlorpromazine) can be substituted in some patients if erectile dysfunction is a problem.
Dopamine antagonists (eg, metoclopramide, phenothiazines)	Inhibit prolactin inhibitory factor, thereby increasing prolactin levels	• Increased prolactin levels inhibit testicular testosterone production; decreased libido results.
Estrogens or drugs with antiandrogenic effects (eg, luteinizing hormone-releasing hormone superagonists, digoxin, spironolactone, ketoconazole, cimetidine)	Suppress testosterone-mediated stimulation of libido	• In the face of decreased libido, a secondary erectile dysfunction develops because of diminished sexual drive.[7]
CNS depressants (eg, barbiturates, narcotics, benzodiazepines, short-term use of large doses of alcohol, anticonvulsants)	Suppress perception of psychogenic stimuli	

(continued)

TABLE 103-2 Medication Classes That Can Cause Erectile Dysfunction (*Continued*)

Drug Class	Proposed Mechanism by Which Drug Causes Erectile Dysfunction	Special Notes
Agents that decrease penile blood flow (eg, diuretics, peripheral β-adrenergic antagonists, or central sympatholytics [methyldopa, clonidine, guanethidine])	Reduce arteriolar flow to corpora	• Any diuretic that produces a significant decrease in intravascular volume can decrease penile arteriolar flow. • Spironolactone has estrogenic effects, and has a high potential to decrease libido and cause erectile dysfunction when used in large doses.[17] • First-generation beta blockers (eg, propranolol) or second-generation agents (eg, atenolol or metoprolol) are associated with more erectile dysfunction than newer generation agents (eg, nebivolol), which possess vasodilatory actions through blockade of alpha adrenoreceptors and release of nitric oxide.[17,18] • Safer antihypertensives include angiotensin-converting enzyme inhibitors, postsynaptic $alpha_1$-adrenergic antagonists (terazosin, doxazosin), calcium channel blockers, and angiotensin II receptor antagonists.[7,19]
Miscellaneous • Finasteride, dutasteride	Erectile dysfunction from 5-alpha reductase inhibitors is thought to result from inhibition of androgen-mediated nitric oxide production by vascular endothelial cells.[20]	• Sexual dysfunction has been reported to persist even after the 5-alpha reductase inhibitor is discontinued.[21]
Lithium carbonate	Unknown mechanism	
Gemfibrozil	Unknown mechanism	
Interferon	Unknown mechanism	
Clofibrate	Unknown mechanism	
Monoamine oxidase inhibitors (eg, phenelzine, isocarboxazid, tranylcypromine)	Unknown mechanism	
Opiates	Unknown mechanism	

SSRI, selective serotonin reuptake inhibitor.

Data from References 6, 14, and 15.

regular intervals during treatment to assess changes. The IIEF is considered a gold standard tool. It includes 15 questions about orgasmic function, libido, erectile function, intercourse satisfaction, and overall satisfaction.[22] Shorter versions of the IIEF are also used in clinical practice. For example, the IIEF-EF includes only the five or six questions that focus on erectile function. The patient responds to each question; each response is scored on a range of 1 to 5. For a six-question IIEF-EF, a score of 26 to 30 is considered normal function, 19 to 25 is mild erectile dysfunction, 13 to 18 is mild-to-moderate erectile dysfunction, 7 to 12 is moderate erectile dysfunction, and 6 or less is severe erectile dysfunction.[23] For a five-question IIEF-EF, a score of 22 to 25 is considered normal function, 17 to 21 is considered mild erectile dysfunction, 12 to 16 is mild-to-moderate erectile dysfunction, and 8 to 11 is moderate erectile dysfunction, and 1 to 7 is severe erectile dysfunction.[23]

Other commonly used questionnaires include the Sexual Health Inventory for Men, Erection Hardness Score, Erectile Dysfunction Inventory for Treatment and Satisfaction, and Treatment Satisfaction Score.[23]

A medical history should be obtained to identify concurrent medical illnesses (eg, hypertension, atherosclerosis, hyperlipidemia, diabetes mellitus, and depression) or surgical procedures (eg, perineal or pelvic) that are risk factors for or are associated with organic or psychogenic erectile dysfunction. Underlying diseases that have not responded to treatment should be addressed before specific treatment for erectile dysfunction is initiated. If the patient smokes cigarettes, drinks excessive amounts of ethanol, or uses recreational drugs, these social habits should be discontinued before specific treatment for erectile dysfunction is started.[24,25]

A complete listing of the patient's prescription and nonprescription medications and dietary supplements should be reviewed by the clinician, who should identify any drugs that could be contributing to erectile dysfunction. If possible, causative agents should be discontinued or the dose should be reduced.

A physical examination of the patient should include a check for hypogonadism (ie, signs of gynecomastia, small testicles, and decreased beard or body hair). The penis should be evaluated for diseases associated with abnormal penile curvature (eg, Peyronie's disease), which are associated with erectile dysfunction. Femoral and lower extremity pulses should be assessed to provide an indication of vascular supply to the genital area. Anal sphincter tone and other genital reflexes should be checked for the integrity of the nerve supply to the penis. A digital rectal examination in patients aged 50 years or older is needed to rule out benign prostatic hyperplasia, which may contribute to erectile dysfunction.

Erectile dysfunction is a potential marker for arteriosclerotic cardiovascular disease. Sexual intercourse and orgasm require a cardiac work equivalent to that needed to vigorously climb two flights of stairs or to walk approximately 1.5 km. In addition, erectogenic drugs may stress the heart.[26] For this reason, a patient's cardiac reserve should be assessed before initiating the treatment for erectile dysfunction. According to the Princeton Consensus Conference guideline, the clinician should take a careful cardiovascular disease history and check for signs and symptoms of cardiovascular disease. Drug treatment for erectile dysfunction is recommended only in patients at low risk of cardiovascular events. Drug treatment should be avoided in patients at high risk of cardiovascular events. For patients at intermediate risk, treadmill testing is indicated; results will stratify patients into low- and high-risk groups, which should be managed accordingly. The risk assessment is described in Table 103-3 and detailed in the Third Princeton Consensus Panel recommendations.[19,26]

Selected laboratory tests should be obtained to identify the presence of underlying diseases that could cause erectile dysfunction.

TABLE 103-3 Recommendations of the Third Princeton Consensus Conference for Cardiovascular Risk Stratification of Patients Being Considered for Phosphodiesterase Inhibitor Therapy

Risk Category	Description of Patient's Condition	Management Approach
Low risk	Has asymptomatic cardiovascular disease with <3 risk factors for cardiovascular disease Has well-controlled hypertension Has mild congestive heart failure (NYHA class I or II) Has mild valvular heart disease Has had a myocardial infarction >8 weeks ago	Patient can be started on phosphodiesterase inhibitor
Intermediate risk	Has ≥3 risk factors for cardiovascular disease Has mild or moderate, stable angina Had a recent myocardial infarction or stroke within the past 2-8 weeks Has moderate congestive heart failure (NYHA class III) History of stroke, transient ischemic attack, or peripheral artery disease	Patient should undergo a complete cardiovascular workup and treadmill stress test to determine tolerance to increased myocardial energy consumption associated with increased sexual activity. Then, reclassify in the low- or high-risk category
High risk	Has unstable or refractory angina, despite treatment Has uncontrolled hypertension Has severe congestive heart failur e (NYHA class IV) Has had a recent myocardial infarction or stroke within the past 2 weeks Has moderate or severe valvular heart disease Has high-risk cardiac arrhythmias Has obstructive hypertrophic cardiomyopathy	Phosphodiesterase inhibitor is contraindicated; sexual intercourse should be deferred

NYHA, New York Heart Association.

Data from References 19 and 26.

CLINICAL PRESENTATION Erectile Dysfunction

General

Men with erectile dysfunction are affected emotionally in different ways, and may present with

- Depression.
- Performance anxiety.
- Marital difficulties and avoidance of sexual intimacy (patients are often brought to a physician by their partners).
- Nonadherence to medications that the patient believes are causing erectile dysfunction.

Symptoms

- Erectile dysfunction or inability to have sexual intercourse, which may or may not be associated with decreased libido and ejaculatory disorders.

Signs

- IIEF questionnaire results are consistent with low satisfaction with the quality of erectile function.
- Medical history may identify concurrent medical illnesses or past surgical procedures that interfere with good vascular flow to the penis, damaged nerve function to the corpora, or mental disorders associated with decreased reception of sexual stimuli.
- Medication history may reveal prescription or nonprescription medications that could cause or contribute to erectile dysfunction.
- Physical examination may reveal signs of hypogonadism (eg, gynecomastia, small testicles, decreased body hair or beard, and decreased muscle mass), which may contribute to erectile dysfunction. The patient may have an abnormally curved penis when erect, decreased pulses in the pelvic region (suggesting impaired vascular flow to the penis), or decreased anal sphincter tone (suggesting impaired nerve function to the corpora). Men older than 50 years should undergo a digital rectal examination to determine whether an enlarged prostate is contributing to the patient's erectile dysfunction.

Assessments

- Conduct IIEF-EF to assess the severity of the patient's erectile dysfunction.[22,23]
- Complete a thorough medical history and check for any psychologic issues (eg, personal relationship issues), social habits (eg, smoking), that might be contributing to erectile dysfunction.[22,24]
- Assess cardiac reserve based on the patient's medical history, signs and symptoms of cardiovascular disease, and treadmill testing, if indicated.

Laboratory Tests

- If the patient has signs of hypogonadism and complains of decreased libido, a serum testosterone concentration may be below the normal range, which would be consistent with a hormonal cause of erectile dysfunction. A low serum testosterone level should always be confirmed with a repeat blood level.
- If the patient has an enlarged prostate noted on digital rectal examination, blood prostate-specific antigen should be measured, especially if the patient is aged 50 or older. If elevated, the patient should be evaluated for a prostate disorder, which could contribute to erectile dysfunction.
- For patients with a history of cardiovascular disease, a fasting glucose and lipid profile is recommended to determine if treatment for risk factors for erectile dysfunction needs to be optimized.

These include a fasting serum blood glucose and lipid profile. Serum testosterone levels should be checked in patients older than 50 years and in younger patients who complain of decreased libido and erectile dysfunction. At least two early morning serum testosterone levels on different days, approximately 4 weeks apart, are needed to confirm the presence of hypogonadism. Within the normal physiologic range for serum total testosterone concentration, sexual drive is usually normal. Because of variability in circulating levels of sex hormone-binding globulin and the lack of precision of available assays, a patient's serum concentration of testosterone should always be interpreted in the context of the patient's symptoms and physical exam findings.[5]

The range of serum total testosterone levels that defines hypogonadism varies among various expert organizations. The Food and Drug Administration (FDA) defines hypogonadism when the serum testosterone concentration is less than 300 ng/dL (10.4 nmol/L) in an adult man, but treatment is indicated only in patients who have symptomatic hypogonadism.

TREATMENT

Desired Outcomes

The goal of treatment is to improve the quantity and quality of penile erections suitable for intercourse and considered satisfactory by the patient and his partner. Simple as this may sound, healthcare providers must ensure that patients and their partners have reasonable expectations before any therapies are initiated. Furthermore, only patients with erectile dysfunction should be treated. Patients who have normal sexual function should not seek—or be encouraged to seek—treatment in an effort to enhance sexual function or enable increased activity. Measures of improvement proposed include a minimum increase of at least 4 points in the IIEF-EF score or achievement of a total score of at least 20.[23] In addition, treatment should be well tolerated and be of reasonable cost.

General Approach to Treatment

3 The Third Princeton Consensus Conference recommendations are a widely accepted multidisciplinary approach to managing erectile dysfunction that maps out a stepwise treatment plan.[26] Since erectile dysfunction, cardiovascular disease, and cardiovascularheir risk factors coexist in many patients, vigorous sexual intercourse can precipitate serious cardiovascular consequences in high-risk patients. Thus, the first step in clinical management of erectile dysfunction is to identify and, if possible, reverse underlying causes. Risk factors for erectile dysfunction, including hypertension, coronary artery disease, dyslipidemia, diabetes mellitus, smoking, or chronic ethanol abuse, should be addressed and minimized.[24,26] Patients should follow a heart-healthy lifestyle, which includes aerobic exercise, weight loss to achieve a normal body mass index, low cholesterol diet, no excessive ethanol intake, and no smoking.[7,17,27-29] In some cases, these types of interventions are sufficient to restore erectile function.[2,6,16,22] However, if erectile dysfunction does not respond to these measures, specific treatment is indicated.

4 5 6 Specific treatments of erectile dysfunction include vacuum erection devices (VEDs), pharmacologic treatments, and surgery. The ideal treatment of this disorder should have a fast onset, be effective, be convenient to administer, be cost-effective, have a low incidence of serious adverse effects, and be free of serious drug interactions (Table 103-4). Generally, when choosing from among treatment approaches, those that are least invasive are selected first; more invasive therapies are reserved for patients who do not respond to first-line agents.

The British Society of Sexual Medicine,[16] 2018 American Urological Association,[22] and the Fourth International Consultation of Sexual Medicine[30] clearly identify oral phosphodiesterase type 5 inhibitors for first-line treatment. VEDs, intracavernosal injection of erectogenic agents, or intraurethral prostaglandin pellets are second-line treatments. Prescribing a particular agent for a patient should be individualized. Surgical intervention should be reserved for patients who fail to respond to first- and second-line treatments. A sample algorithm that guides the selection of treatment is shown in Fig. 103-2.

Nonpharmacologic Therapy

Vacuum Erection Device

A vacuum erection device (VED) is a noninvasive medical device with few contraindications to use. It is available over-the-counter. A patient makes a one-time purchase, and the device can be used repeatedly.

A VED has two parts: a pump, which generates a negative vacuum pressure, and a cylinder, which is closed at one end (Fig. 103-3). The patient applies lubricant to and inserts his penis into the open end of the cylinder, which is then pushed up flush against his lower abdomen to create a vacuum chamber. The lubricant helps maintain a tight seal between the VED and the patient's abdomen. Then, the patient activates the pump to produce a vacuum pressure, which draws arteriolar blood into the corpora cavernosa. To prolong the erection, the patient places constriction bands or tension rings at the base of the erect penis. The bands or rings trap arteriolar blood in the corpora cavernosa and reduce venous outflow from the penis. With the assistance of loading cones to protect the glans, these bands or rings can be rolled over the glans penis onto the erect penile shaft. Alternatively, the bands or rings can be first threaded onto the plastic cylinder before the penis is inserted. Once the penis is erect, the band or ring can be rolled off the cylinder onto the base of the penis. However, some patients prefer to apply the band or ring before the penis is erect.[6,31]

7 The onset of action of the VED is 3 to 20 minutes; a faster onset of 2 to 3 minutes is associated with continued, more experienced use.[31] VEDs are not discreet. That is, a patient's use of a VED is evident to the partner. For this reason, VEDs appear to work best in older patients who are married or who have stable sexual relationships. In this group, VEDs could be considered first-line therapy, and the overall satisfaction rate can be as high as 60% to 80% (range, 27%-94%) in all patients, including those with diabetes mellitus and spinal cord injury.[30,31] VEDs may be used as second-line therapy in patients who do not respond to oral phosphodiesterase type 5 inhibitors,[22] which includes patients who have had a radical prostatectomy or those who do not respond to injectable drug treatments for erectile dysfunction. The combination of a VED with intracavernosal or intraurethral alprostadil[24,32] or a phosphodiesterase type 5 inhibitor is associated with a higher efficacy rate than the use of the VED alone.[16,32,33] As a result, combination therapy sometimes is attempted before penile prosthesis surgery is considered in the patient who fails to respond to a VED alone.

Patients may discontinue using VEDs because they are inconvenient and not discreet. It has been reported that the dropout rate is as high as 56% during the first year of use.[31] Also, 6% to 11% of partners complain that the penis is cool to the touch or is discolored (bluish) in appearance, particularly when constriction bands are used.[22]

Vacuum erection devices are available with battery-operated pumps, which offer convenience, particularly in patients with arthritis of the hands. When choosing a device, patients should select one with a pop-off safety valve that minimizes the likelihood of excessively high vacuum pressure, which can cause penile discomfort, petechiae, or hematoma.[24,31]

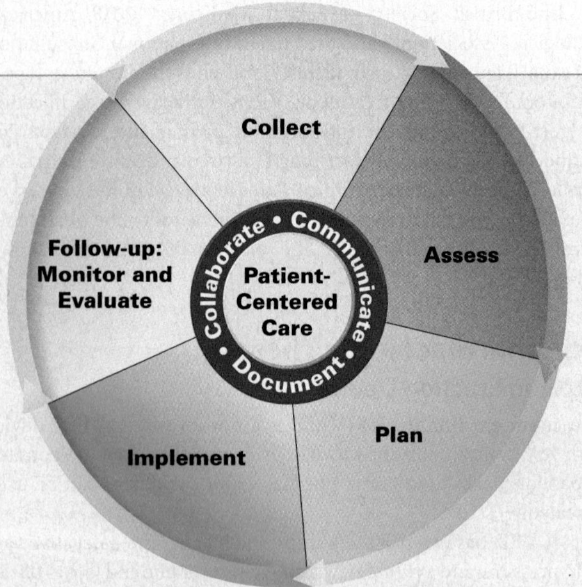

Patient Care Process for the Management of Erectile Dysfunction

The image shows the five fundamental steps included in The Pharmacist's Care Process endorsed by the Joint Commission for Pharmacy Practitioners (2014). The tagline of this process reads collaborate, communicate, and document. The five fundamental steps listed here are collect, assess, plan, implement, and follow-up: monitor and evaluate. All these steps are listed in a circular block diagram.

Collect

- Patient characteristics (eg, age, race)
- Patient history (past medical history, marital/partner status, family history, social—sexual history, situations in which erectile dysfunction occurs, tobacco, recreational drug, or alcohol use, and medication history)
- Current psychologic status (emotional stressors, depression, performance anxiety) (see "Clinical Presentation" box)
- Objective data (see "Diagnosis" section)
    - BP, heart rate (HR), height, weight, and BMI
    - Physical examination to rule out hypogonadism and prostate dysfunction
    - Labs (eg, blood/serum glucose, lipids, testosterone)
    - Cardiovascular risk assessment, if indicated (see the "Diagnosis" section and Table 103-3)
- Administer International Index of Erectile Function screening questionnaire if feasible (see the "Diagnosis" section)
- Current and past medications, including prescription and nonprescription medications, or nonpharmacologic interventions for erectile dysfunction (see Table 103-4)
- If a patient is not responding to a phosphodiesterase type 5 inhibitor, details on how and when a patient is using the medication (see the "Efficacy" subsection under "Phosphodiesterase Type 5 Inhibitor" section)

Assess

- Patient and partner's pattern and frequency of sexual intercourse, their goals for treatment and expectations regarding therapy and its costs
- Patient's physical ability to engage in sexual intercourse
- Presence of conditions that are contraindications to sexual intercourse and to phosphodiesterase type 5 inhibitors (Table 103-3)
- Current use of medications contributing to erectile dysfunction (see Table 103-2)

Plan

- Individualize treatment selection based on the patient's preferences for and perception of the effectiveness of various treatment options, out-of-pocket costs for treatment, and potential adverse effects; patients generally prefer a discreet treatment not obvious to sexual partners and not requiring careful attention to administration timing relative to sexual activity
- Optimize treatment for underlying causes of erectile dysfunction (eg, hypertension, coronary artery disease, dyslipidemia, diabetes mellitus, smoking, chronic ethanol abuse)
- Discontinue medications contributing to erectile dysfunction when possible (Table 103-2)
- Treat hypogonadism when present
- Initiate counseling or psychotherapy for psychogenic causes of erectile dysfunction
- Drug therapy regimen including specific agent(s), dose, route, frequency, and duration; specify the continuation and discontinuation of existing therapies (see Tables 103-4 and 103-5 and Figs. 103-2, 103-3, 103-5, and 103-6); consider the presence of concomitant diseases treatable with agents for erectile dysfunction (eg, daily tadalafil in men who also have benign prostatic hypertrophy)
- Nonpharmacologic or surgical intervention when medications are contraindicated or are not effective (see Figs. 103-2 and 103-3)
- Patient reeducation to salvage patient nonresponders to phosphodiesterase type 5 inhibitor, if appropriate (see "Efficacy" subsection under "Phosphodiesterase Type 5 Inhibitor" section)
- Monitoring parameters including efficacy (eg, BP, cardiovascular events, kidney health), safety (medication-specific adverse effects), and time frame (see Table 103-6)
- Patient education (eg, purpose of treatment, dietary and lifestyle modification, drug therapy)
- Referrals to other providers when appropriate (eg, physician, urologist)

Implement*

- Provide patient education regarding all elements of the treatment plan
- Schedule follow-up for several weeks after therapy initiation

Follow-up: Monitor and Evaluate

- Patient satisfaction with quality and quantity of penile erections
- Presence of adverse effects
- Adjust medication doses or switch to alternative agents as clinically indicated
- Consider alternative devices, drugs, combinations of drugs, or surgical intervention in patients who fail treatment with a single approach

Collaborate with patient, caregivers, and other healthcare professionals.

TABLE 103-4 Dosing Regimens for Selected Drug Treatments for Erectile Dysfunction

Drug	Brand Name*	Initial Dose	Usual Range	Special Population Dose	Other
Phosphodiesterase Inhibitor					
Sildenafil	Viagra	50 mg orally 1 hour before intercourse	25-100 mg 1 hour before intercourse. Limit to one dose per day	In patients aged 65 years and older, start with 25 mg dose. In patients with creatinine clearance less than 30 mL/min (0.5 mL/s) or severe hepatic impairment, limit starting dose to 25 mg. In patients with mild-to-moderate hepatic impairment or those taking strong CYP3A4 inhibitors (eg, itraconazole, ketoconazole, or erythromycin), consider starting with 25 mg. In patients taking protease inhibitors, limit starting dose to 25 mg.	Generic formulations are available. Titrate dose so that erection lasts no more than 1 hour. High-fat foods decrease the rate of absorption by 1 hour. Avoid taking dose with grapefruit juice. Contraindicated with nitrates by any route of administration.
Vardenafil	Levitra[a]	5-10 mg orally 1 hour before intercourse	5-20 mg 1 hour before intercourse. Limit to one dose per day	In patients aged 65 years and older, start with 5-mg Levitra. No dosage adjustment is required in patients with decreased creatinine clearance or mild hepatic impairment. In patients with moderate hepatic impairment, start with 5-mg Levitra. Use not recommended in patients with severe hepatic impairment. In patients taking strong P450 CYP3A4 inhibitors (eg, atazanavir, erythromycin, clarithromycin, ketoconazole, itraconazole), limit starting dose to 2.5 mg in a 24-hour period. In patients on ritonavir, limit dose to 2.5 mg every 72 hours. Not recommended in patients with congenital prolonged QT interval or in patients taking Type 1A or Type 3 antiarrhythmics.	Generic formulations are available. Titrate dose so that erection lasts no more than 1 hour. High-fat foods decrease the rate of absorption by 1 hour. Avoid taking the dose with grapefruit juice. Contraindicated with nitrates by any route of administration.
	Staxyn[b]	10-mg tablet to dissolve on the tongue 1 hour before intercourse	10-mg tablet to dissolve on the tongue 1 hour before intercourse. Limit to one dose per day	Dose of Staxyn requires no adjustment in patients aged 65 years or older, patients with creatinine clearance less than 30 mL/min (0.5 mL/s), or those with mild hepatic impairment. Do not use in patients with moderate or severe hepatic impairment or those taking moderately or highly potent P450 CYP3A4 inhibitors. Do not initiate Staxyn in patients taking *alpha*-adrenergic antagonists.	Generic formulations are available. Staxyn should be taken without any liquid or food. The tablet should be placed on the tongue where it will dissolve. No up-titration of dose is recommended. Do not substitute Staxyn for Levitra, or vice versa.
Tadalafil	Cialis	5-10 mg orally at least 30 minutes before intercourse OR 2.5-5 mg orally once daily	10-20 mg at least 30 minutes before intercourse. Limit to one dose per day 2.5-5 mg once daily. Limit to one dose per day	Dose of tadalafil requires no dosage adjustment in patients aged 65 years or older. In patients with creatinine clearance of 30-50 mL/min (0.5-0.83 mL/s), limit starting dose to 10 mg every 48 hours; if less than 30 mL/min (0.5 mL/s), limit starting dose to 5 mg every 72 hours. In patients with mild-to-moderate hepatic impairment, limit starting dose to 10 mg every 24 hours. Do not use in patients with severe hepatic impairment. In patients taking potent P450 CYP3A4 inhibitors, limit starting dose to 10 mg every 72 hours (if using it on demand) or 2.5 mg daily (if using a continuous daily regimen).	Generic formulations are available. Titrate dose so that erection lasts no more than 1 hour. Food does not affect rate or extent of drug absorption. Avoid taking dose with grapefruit juice. Contraindicated with nitrates by any route of administration. When taken with large amounts of ethanol, tadalafil may cause orthostatic hypotension.
Avanafil	Stendra	100 mg orally 15 minutes before intercourse	50-200 mg orally 15 minutes before intercourse. Limit to one dose per day	Dosage adjustment needed in patients aged 65 years or older. In patients with creatinine clearance of 30-89 mL/min (0.5-1.49 mL/s) or those with mild-to-moderate hepatic impairment, no dosage adjustment is needed. Not recommended if creatinine clearance is less than 30 mL/min (0.5 mL/s), if the patient has severe hepatic disease, or if the patient is taking potent P450 CYP3A4 inhibitors. If the patient is taking moderate P450 CYP3A4 inhibitors (eg, erythromycin, fluconazole), the maximum recommended dose is 50 mg every 24 hours.	Titrate dose so that erection lasts no more than 1 hour. May be taken with or without food. Avoid taking dose with grapefruit juice. Contraindicated with nitrates by any route of administration. When taken with large amounts of ethanol, avanafil may cause orthostatic hypotension.

(*continued*)

TABLE 103-4 Dosing Regimens for Selected Drug Treatments for Erectile Dysfunction (*Continued*)

Drug	Brand Name[a]	Initial Dose	Usual Range	Special Population Dose	Other
Prostaglandin E_1					
Alprostadil intracavernosal injection	Caverject, Edex	2.5-mcg intracavernosally 5-10 minutes before intercourse	10-40 mcg 5-10 minutes before intercourse. Maximum recommended dose is 60 mcg. Limit to not more than one injection per day and not more than three injections per week with a 24-hour interval between doses. Give each dose over 5-10 seconds	In older adults, use the lowest effective dose. No specific dosage adjustment provided in labeling for patients with hepatic or renal impairment.	Titrate dose to achieve an erection that lasts 1 hour. Patient will require training on aseptic intracavernosal injection technique. Avoid intracavernosal injections in patients with sickle cell anemia, multiple myeloma, leukemia, severe coagulopathy, schizophrenia, poor manual dexterity, severe venous incompetence, severe cardiovascular disease, or Peyronie's disease.
Alprostadil intraurethral pellet	Muse	125-250 mcg intraurethrally 5-10 minutes before intercourse	250-1,000 mcg just before intercourse. Limit to not more than two doses per day	In older adults, use the lowest effective dose. No specific dosage adjustment provided in labeling for patients with hepatic or renal impairment.	Patient will require training on proper intraurethral administration techniques. Use applicator provided to administer medications to avoid urethral injury.
Testosterone Supplements[c]					
Methyltestosterone	Methitest	10 mg once daily	10-50 mg once daily	No dosage adjustment provided in labeling for patients with renal or hepatic impairment or older adults.	Not recommended for use due to extensive first-pass hepatic catabolism and because it is associated with hepatotoxicity. May cause fluid retention in patients with renal or hepatic disease.
Testosterone cypionate intramuscular injection	Depo-Testosterone	100-200 mg every 2-4 weeks	200-400 mg every 2-4 weeks (up to 6 weeks)	No dosage adjustment provided in labeling for patients with renal or hepatic impairment or older adults.	During the dosing interval, supraphysiologic serum concentrations of testosterone are produced during a portion of the dosing interval. This has been linked to mood swings and infertility.
Testosterone enanthate intramuscular injection		100-200 mg every 2-4 weeks	200-400 mg every 2-4 weeks (up to 6 weeks)	No dosage adjustment provided in labeling for patients with renal or hepatic impairment or older adults.	During the dosing interval, supraphysiologic serum concentrations of testosterone are produced during a portion of the dosing interval. This has been linked to mood swings and infertility.
Testosterone undecanoate intramuscular injection	Aveed	750 mg as a single dose	750 mg as a single dose on Day 0, Week 4, and then 750 mg every 10 weeks	No dosage adjustment provided in labeling for patients with renal or hepatic impairment or older adults. Contraindicated in patients with serious hepatic or renal disease.	Only available in facilities certified through a Risk Evaluation and Mitigation Strategy Program. Administer by deep intramuscular injection into gluteal muscle. Avoid intravascular injection, which can lead to pulmonary oil embolism.
Testosterone transdermal patch	Androderm	4 mg as a single dose at bedtime	2-6 mg as a single dose at bedtime. Titrate dose 2 weeks after initiating a dose. Multiple patches may be needed to achieve dose needed.	No dosage adjustment is provided in labeling for patients with renal or hepatic impairment or older adults.	When administered at bedtime, serum concentrations of testosterone in the usual circadian pattern are produced. Apply to those body sites recommended in the package labeling: upper arm, back, abdomen, and thigh. Rotate application sites every 7 days. May have to apply multiple patches at one time to achieve appropriate serum testosterone level. Avoid swimming, showering, or washing administration site for 3 hours after patch application.

TABLE 103-4 Dosing Regimens for Selected Drug Treatments for Erectile Dysfunction

Drug	Brand Name[*]	Initial Dose	Usual Range	Special Population Dose	Other
Testosterone gel	AndroGel 1% (25 mg/2.5 g) Testim 1% (25 mg/2.5 g)	5-10 g of gel (equivalent to 50-100 mg testosterone, respectively) as a single dose in the morning	5-10 g of gel (equivalent to 50-100 mg testosterone, respectively) as a single dose in the morning. Titrate dose at 14-day intervals	No dosage adjustment provided in labeling for patients with renal or hepatic impairment or older adults.	Cover application site to avoid inadvertent transfer to others. Avoid swimming, showering, or washing administration site for 2 hours after gel application. Apply to those sites recommended in the product labeling. For Androgel, apply to shoulders, upper arms, or abdomen. For Testim, apply to shoulders or upper arms only. Children and women should avoid contact with unclothed or unwashed application sites. Patients should wash hands with soap and water after administration of transdermal testosterone product. For patients who have difficulty measuring the appropriate dose using tubes of gel, it is also available in premeasured dose packets or from a pump dispenser. REMS assessments must be submitted to the FDA.
	AndroGel 1.62% (20.25 mg/1.25 g)	2 pumps (equivalent to 40.5 mg testosterone) as a single dose in the morning	2-4 pumps (equivalent to 40.5-81 mg) as a single dose in the morning. Titrate dose 14-28 days after starting treatment	No dosage adjustment provided in labeling for patients with renal or hepatic impairment or older adults.	Apply to shoulders and upper arms. Avoid swimming, showering, or washing administration site for 2 hours after application. Same precautions as listed above for 1% gel. REMS assessments must be submitted to the FDA.
Testosterone transdermal spray	Fortesta 2% (10 mg/ actuation)	4 sprays (equivalent to 40-mg testosterone) every morning	4-7 sprays (equivalent to 40-70 mg testosterone) every morning. Titrate dose up at 14- to 35-day intervals	No dosage adjustment provided in labeling for patients with renal or hepatic impairment or older adults.	Must prime pump by pushing on pump three times. Apply to front or inner thighs only. Cover application site to avoid inadvertent transfer to others. Avoid swimming, showering, or washing administration site for 2 hours after spray application. Children and women should avoid contact with unclothed or unwashed application sites. Patients should wash hands with soap and water after administration of transdermal testosterone product. REMS assessments must be submitted to the FDA.
Testosterone transdermal solution	Axiron (30 mg/ actuation)	One pump spray (equivalent to 30-mg testosterone) to left or right axilla daily	One to four pump sprays (equivalent to 30-120 mg testosterone, respectively) to axilla daily. If dose is more than one pump spray, divide total dose between axillae. Titrate dose at 14- to 35-day intervals	No dosage adjustment provided in labeling for patients with renal or hepatic impairment or older adults.	Limit application to axilla. Apply antiperspirant or deodorant before Axiron. If applying multiple spray doses to an axilla, apply one spray, let dry, then apply second dose. Avoid swimming, showering, or washing administration site for 2 hours after application. REMS assessments must be submitted to the FDA.

(continued)

TABLE 103-4 Dosing Regimens for Selected Drug Treatments for Erectile Dysfunction *(Continued)*

Drug	Brand Name*	Initial Dose	Usual Range	Special Population Dose	Other
Testosterone intranasal gel	Natesto (5.5 mg/ actuation)	2 pump actuations in nostrils (equivalent to 1 pump actuation per nostril, total dose of 11 mg) three times a day	2 pump actuations in nostrils (equivalent to 1 pump actuation per nostril, total dose of 11 mg) three times a day. If serum testosterone level is not corrected with this dose, it is recommended to switch to an alternative testosterone supplement	No dosage adjustment provided in labeling for patients with renal or hepatic impairment or older adults.	Administer each dose 6 to 8 hours apart. Prime pump by inverting and depressing pump 10 times. Blow nose before application. After administration, press on nostrils and lightly massage. Do not blow nose or sniff for 1 hour after administration. Do not administer with any other intranasal product, except decongestants. Discontinue if patient has rhinitis. If patient develops severe rhinitis, temporarily switch to an alternative testosterone replacement product until rhinitis resolves. Avoid use in patients with chronic nasal conditions, sinusitis, or after nasal or sinus surgery.
Testosterone subcutaneous implant pellet	Testopel 75 mg/ pellet	150-450 mg (equivalent to 2-6 pellets) as a single dose every 3-6 months	150-450 mg as a single dose every 3-6 months	No dosage adjustment recommended for renal or hepatic impairment or older adults.	Trained health professional is required to administer the dose. Use sterile implanter kit. Administration of the dose requires a forearm incision and local anesthesia to subcutaneously implant dose. Clinical onset is delayed for 3-4 months after initial dose. Generic formulations are available in higher strengths: 100 or 200 mg per pellet.

*Common brand names are included in this table. Medications may be available with other brand names or as generic formulation.

[a]Levitra brand was discontinued in April 2021. Vardenafil is available as generic formulation.

[b]Staxyn brand was discontinued in April 2021. Vardenafil is available as generic formulation.

[c]This listing includes only those testosterone supplements approved for treating hypogonadism associated with aging. Testosterone enanthate auto-injector and oral testosterone undecanoate are not included for this reason.

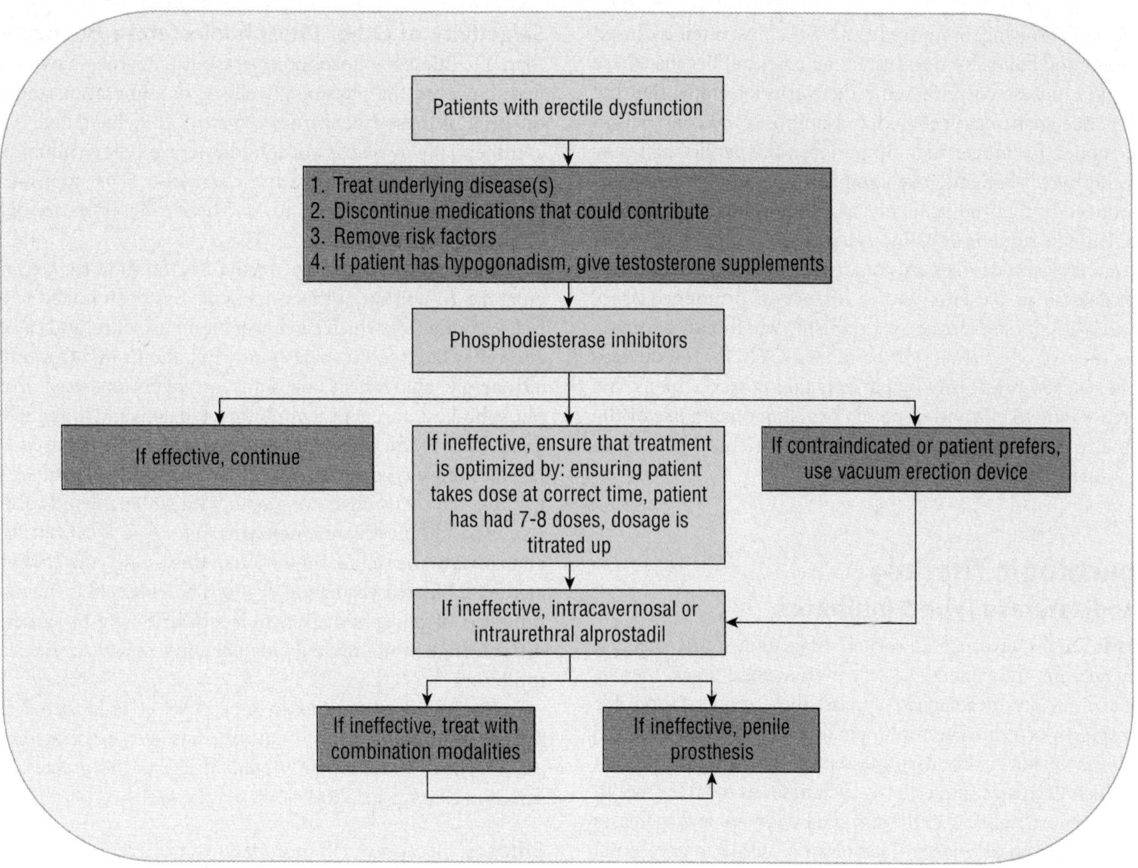

FIGURE 103-2 Algorithm for selecting treatment for erectile dysfunction.

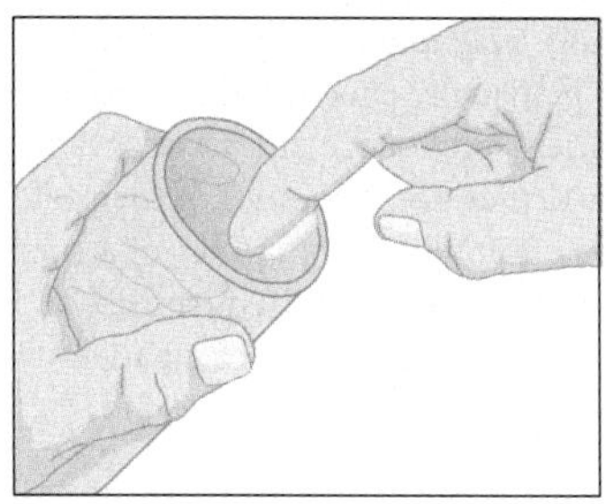

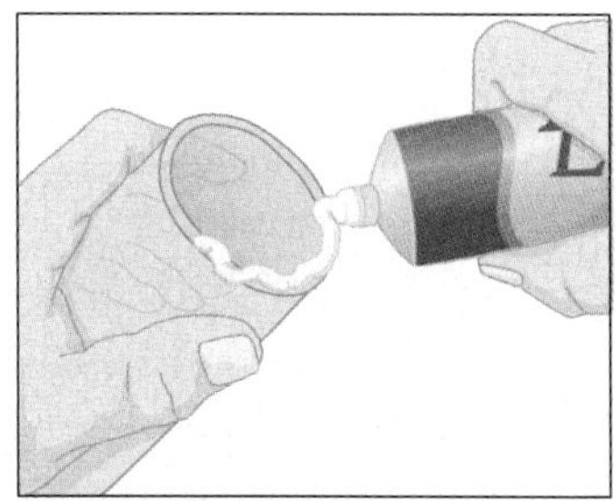

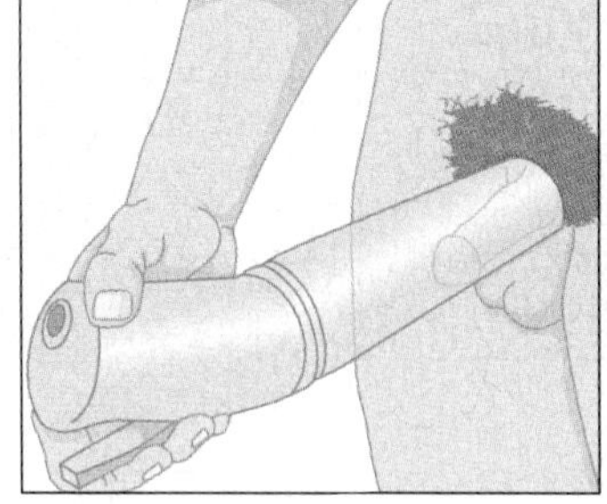

FIGURE 103-3 Technique for using a vacuum erection device. *(Reprinted, with permission, from Osbon Erec Aid Esteem Vacuum Therapy System User Guide. Eden Prairie, MN: TIMM Medical Technologies.)*

Penile pain, bruising, or injury from VEDs most often is caused by the constriction bands used to sustain an erection. Because these rings trap blood in the corpora and reduce arteriolar flow into the penis, the penile shaft may feel cold and numb. If the constriction bands are applied for longer than 30 minutes, the penile shaft may turn blue and hurt.[22] Patients may complain that a hinge-like erection is produced in that the penis pivots on the rubber ring or tension band. Patients sometimes fail to ejaculate.[24]

Vacuum erection devices are contraindicated in patients with sickle cell disease or patients with a history of prolonged erections. These patients are prone to priapism, which can be exacerbated by the use of constriction bands with VEDs. The devices also should be used cautiously by patients taking warfarin, as this agent increases the likelihood of penile bruising during use of the device. Finally, VEDs are contraindicated in patients with severe penile curvature.

Pharmacologic Therapy

Phosphodiesterase Type 5 Inhibitors

Mechanism In the presence of sexual stimulation, nitric oxide is released by neurons and endothelial cells in cavernosal tissue, thereby enhancing the activity of guanylate cyclase, the enzyme responsible for the conversion of guanylate triphosphate to cGMP (Fig. 103-4).[22] cGMP is a vasodilatory secondary messenger that activates protein kinase G, which decreases intracellular calcium levels, relaxes smooth muscle, enhances arterial flow to the corpora cavernosa, and increases blood filling of cavernosal sinuses. Catabolism of cGMP in cavernosal tissue is mediated by phosphodiesterase isoenzyme type 5.

Four competitive, reversible inhibitors of the phosphodiesterase isoenzyme type 5 are marketed for erectile dysfunction in the United States (Table 103-5). Chemically, they are nonhydrolyzable analogs of cGMP and they act by decreasing catabolism and maintaining high concentrations of cGMP in the corpora cavernosa. In effect, this sustains a penile erection. However, these medications are not specific for phosphodiesterase isoenzyme type 5. They also inhibit other phosphodiesterase isoenzymes in other tissues and organs, which produces some of the unwanted side effects of this medication class.[34]

Selectivity of Other Phosphodiesterase Isoenzymes More than 11 different phosphodiesterase isoenzymes have been identified; however, the physiologic effects of stimulation and inhibition of some of these isoenzymes remain to be elucidated.[13,34] The four commercially available phosphodiesterase type 5 inhibitors exhibit variable selectivity for phosphodiesterase 5 as opposed to phosphodiesterase types 1, 6, and 11. These differences are displayed in Table 103-5.

Phosphodiesterase isoenzyme 1 is found in the peripheral vasculature. Inhibition of this isoenzyme has been linked with peripheral vasodilation, which can lower blood pressure, and cause flushing and reflex tachycardia, particularly in patients taking nitrates, alpha-adrenergic antagonists, or some antihypertensives.[37] Among the phosphodiesterase type 5 inhibitors, tadalafil and avanafil have much less selectivity for phosphodiesterase type 1 as compared with phosphodiesterase type 5. As a result, tadalafil and avanafil are less likely to cause hypotension as compared with sildenafil and vardenafil.[36,37]

Phosphodiesterase isoenzyme type 6 is localized to the rods and cones of the retina. Inhibition of this isoenzyme has been associated with blurred vision and cyanopsia. Sildenafil is the most potent inhibitor of phosphodiesterase isoenzyme type 6, vardenafil is an intermediate inhibitor, and tadalafil and avanafil are the least potent inhibitors.[35,37]

Phosphodiesterase isoenzyme type 11 is localized to skeletal muscle. Inhibition of this isoenzyme has been associated with myalgia and back muscle pain. Tadalafil exerts the greatest inhibitory activity against phosphodiesterase type 11.[35,37]

Efficacy Because of their apparent effectiveness, convenient oral route of administration, and comparatively low incidence of serious adverse effects, phosphodiesterase type 5 inhibitors are first-line therapy for erectile dysfunction. They allow for discreet use. Although not based on direct comparison trials, all four commercially available phosphodiesterase type 5 inhibitors are considered to be equally effective and comparable in safety and tolerability.[13,34] Patient preference studies show that some patients may choose a particular agent because of the preferences of the sexual partner or the onset, duration, or cost of a specific medication.[38] For example, for a patient with infrequent sexual intercourse, sildenafil or vardenafil is a good choice; for a patient with frequent sexual intercourse,

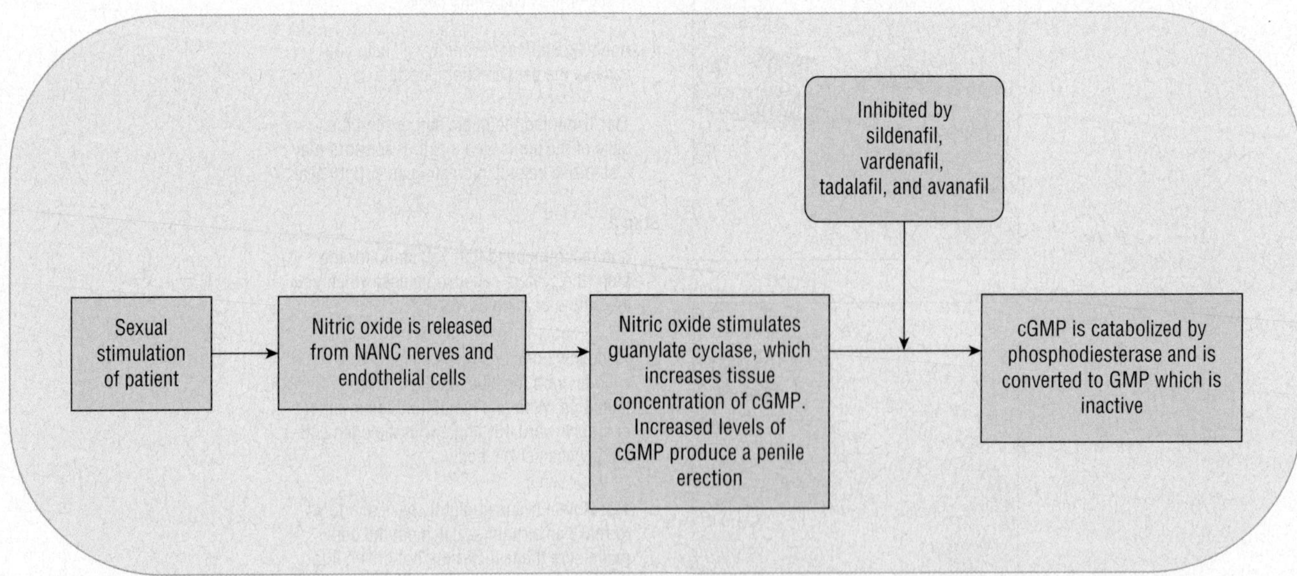

FIGURE 103-4 Mechanism of action of phosphodiesterase type 5 inhibitors. All inhibit catabolism of cGMP, a vasodilatory secondary messenger. (cGMP, cyclic guanosine monophosphate; NANC, nonadrenergic noncholinergic.)

TABLE 103-5 Pharmacodynamics and Pharmacokinetics of Phosphodiesterase Inhibitors

	Sildenafil (Viagra)	Vardenafil (Levitra/Staxyn)	Tadalafil (Cialis)	Avanafil[36,37] (Stendra)
Inhibits PDE-5	Yes	Yes	Yes	Yes
Inhibits PDE-1	Yes	Yes	Minimally	Minimally
Inhibits PDE-6	Yes	Yes	No	Mildly
Inhibits PDE-11	No	No	Yes	No
Onset of action (min)	60	25-60	30	15-30
Time to peak plasma level (hours)	0.5-1	0.7-0.9/1.5	2	0.5-0.8
Oral bioavailability (%)	40	15/21-44	36	15
Fatty meal decreases rate and/or extent of oral absorption?	Yes	Yes/No[a]	No	Yes. Fatty meal decreases rate but not extent of absorption.
Mean plasma half-life (hours)	3.7	4.4-4.8/4-6	18	5
Active metabolite	Yes	Yes/Yes	No	Yes
Is CYP 3A4 principally responsible for metabolism?	Yes	Yes	Yes	Yes
Other CYP enzymes responsible for metabolism	CYP 2C9, CYP 2C19, CYP 2D6, CYP 1A2	CYP 3A5, CYP 2C9	None	CYP 2C9
Percentage of dose excreted in feces	80	91-95/91-95	61	62
Percentage of dose excreted in urine	13	2-6/2-6	36	21
Clinical onset (minutes)	60	30/60	60	25-40
Duration (hours)	2-4, up to 12	4-5/4-6	24-36	6+

[a]When Staxyn is taken with water, the area under the curve decreases by 29%.

Data from References 34 and 35.

tadalafil may be preferred; and for a patient with unscheduled periodic intercourse, a fast-acting agent like vardenafil ODT may be preferred.[39]

Usual starting and maintenance dose regimens are included in Table 103-4.

In the presence of sexual stimulation and in doses of 25 to 100 mg, sildenafil produces satisfactory erections in 56% to 82% of patients, independent of the etiology of erectile dysfunction. Similar results are documented in the product labeling for the other agents in this class (65%-80% for vardenafil, 62%-77% for tadalafil, and 57%-77% for avanafil). The change in IIEF-EF score for a phosphodiesterase inhibitor is approximately 5.6 to 7.4 points.[25] Response rates are in the lower range for patients with diabetes mellitus or after radical prostatectomy, or those with severe vascular disease, probably due to neuropathy, or surgery-related nerve damage.[22] The effectiveness of the drugs appears to be dose-related.

8 Approximately 30% to 40% of patients do not respond to phosphodiesterase type 5 inhibitors.[22] At least half of nonresponders benefit from education on proper use of the drugs.[32] Therefore, follow-up is always recommended after a phosphodiesterase type 5 inhibitor is initiated to see if additional education is needed for the following points: (a) patients must engage in sexual stimulation (foreplay) for the best response[16,22]; (b) sildenafil and vardenafil should be taken on an empty stomach, at least 2 hours before meals, for the fastest response, but tadalafil and avanafil can be taken without regard to meals; (c) patients who do not respond to the first dose should continue with the phosphodiesterase type 5 inhibitor for at least seven to eight doses before failure is declared, as increasing success rates are reported with sequential dose administration[16,32]; (d) some patients require dosage titration up to 100-mg sildenafil, 20-mg vardenafil, 20-mg tadalafil, or 200-mg avanafil for a response[13]; (e) patients should avoid excessive alcohol intake, which can cause drowsiness and hypotension and worsen erectile dysfunction; (f) treatment of concomitant medical illnesses that contribute to erectile dysfunction (eg, diabetes mellitus, hypertension, and hypogonadism) should be optimized (if the patient has depression because of divorce or loss of a sexual partner, or has performance anxiety, psychologic counseling may be helpful).[22]

The phosphodiesterase type 5 inhibitors should not be used by patients with normal erectile function. Also, according to FDA-approved labeling, the drugs should not be used in combination with other forms of therapy for erectile dysfunction because prolonged erections (which may lead to priapism) may result.[22] Phosphodiesterase type 5 inhibitors should be avoided in patients predisposed to developing priapism, including men with sickle cell anemia, leukemia, or multiple myeloma.

Long-term use of phosphodiesterase type 5 inhibitors for up to 10 consecutive years continues to be effective and is not associated with tachyphylaxis.[6] The voluntary discontinuation rate among patients has been reported as high as 50% after 6 to 24 months of treatment, despite a positive treatment response.[13] This phenomenon is likely due to the high out-of-pocket costs of phosphodiesterase type 5 inhibitors, the inconvenient process of obtaining the medication, adverse drug effects, the patient's loss of interest in sexual intercourse, partner-related problems (marital problems/no partner) or the efficacy of the medication being below the patient's expectations because of worsening of the patient's underlying erectile dysfunction disease.[6,40,41]

Despite the initial effectiveness of phosphodiesterase type 5 inhibitors and the measures to salvage patients with reeducation, some patients with severe vascular or neurologic disease will show minimal or no response to maximum doses of a phosphodiesterase type 5 inhibitor. Various strategies have been attempted in this subgroup of patients, including the following:

1. The effectiveness of switching from one phosphodiesterase type 5 inhibitor to another when the patient does not respond to an initial agent is controversial, although it is clear that some patients prefer one agent over another.[24] Controlled clinical trials in larger patient groups are needed before this strategy is used as routine treatment.
2. Switching the patient from an as needed to a daily regimen of tadalafil may be reasonable when the patient has

difficulty coordinating the timing of tadalafil before meals or sexual intercourse.[6,42] However, a daily dose regimen is more expensive than an on-demand regimen.

3. Adding an as-needed shorter-acting phosphodiesterase inhibitor to a low daily dose of tadalafil regimen.[16]
4. High-dose phosphodiesterase type 5 inhibitor treatment (eg, sildenafil 200 mg) has been used anecdotally. However, such doses are also associated with a higher frequency of adverse effects.[43]
5. In older patients (age greater than or equal to 65 years) with late-onset hypogonadism and erectile dysfunction, correcting the former with testosterone supplementation improves the response to a phosphodiesterase type 5 inhibitor.[22,32]
6. Phosphodiesterase type 5 inhibitors have been combined with intracavernosal or intraurethral alprostadil in selected patients. This allows combining agents with 2 different vasodilatory MOA.[22,44]

Pharmacokinetic parameters of the phosphodiesterase inhibitors are listed in Table 103-5.[35]

Sildenafil and the conventional oral formulation of vardenafil have similar pharmacokinetic profiles. Both drugs have a 1-hour onset of action and short duration of action. Oral absorption is significantly delayed by 1 hour when either drug is taken within 2 hours of a fatty meal.[35] An oral disintegrating tablet (ODT) formulation of vardenafil, which dissolves on the tongue, has 1.2- to 1.4-fold higher bioavailability than the conventional oral tablet when taken without water. Unlike the conventional tablet, the ODT formulation should be taken without water, which allows discretion, and is not susceptible to a drug-food interaction. In addition, the ODT dissolves on the tongue and does not require swallowing. Thus, patients with dysphagia, who comprise almost 25% of patients who are 50 years of age or older, could easily use this formulation.[34,39] When compared with the other phosphodiesterase type 5 inhibitors, tadalafil has a slower onset of action of 2 hours and a prolonged duration of action up to 36 hours. Food does not affect the rate of absorption of tadalafil. Tadalafil offers greater spontaneity for patients, as one dose can last through an entire weekend and it allows for multiple acts of sexual intercourse over multiple days with a single dose. Avanafil has an onset of action of 15 minutes; its onset is faster than, but is similar in duration to sildenafil and vardenafil. A high-fat meal will delay the absorption and reduce total amount absorbed by avanafil.[16,24,37]

The onset of action of these agents has undergone reexamination to assess how soon after drug administration patients can expect to have an erection suitable for intercourse. Although up to 50% of patients may develop an erection within 20 to 30 minutes of sildenafil 100 mg, vardenafil 20 mg, tadalafil 20 mg, or avanafil 200 mg, the rest of the patients may require a full hour to achieve an adequate erectile response.[35] Therefore, patients should be instructed to allow adequate time for the drug to work. In addition, sildenafil and vardenafil have been reported to be effective in some patients up to 12 hours after dosing, and tadalafil is effective up to 36 hours after dosing, which is long after plasma concentrations have declined. It has been hypothesized that this may be due to the continued intracellular action of the phosphodiesterase type 5 inhibitor. Further study is needed to determine if avanafil's duration of action is longer than 6 hours.

Concomitant ingestion of ethanol with phosphodiesterase type 5 inhibitors can result in orthostatic hypotension and drowsiness. Therefore, the manufacturer recommends that patients avoid ethanol when taking these medications.

All four phosphodiesterase type 5 inhibitors are hepatically catabolized principally by the cytochrome P450 3A4 microsomal isoenzyme. Other P450 isoenzymes and/or other hepatic enzymes are minor routes of catabolism (see Table 103-5). Sildenafil has an active metabolite, which is excreted primarily in the urine. Tadalafil has a clinically insignificant active metabolite. However, 36% of tadalafil drug is renally eliminated. Thus, both sildenafil and tadalafil doses should be reduced in patients with significant renal impairment. Vardenafil and avanafil have active metabolites that are largely excreted in feces. No specific dosage reduction of these medications is recommended in patients with reduced renal function because of the intermittent nature of the dosing schedule. However, avanafil is not recommended when the creatinine clearance is less than 30 mL/min (0.5 mL/s) (see Table 103-5).

Dosing The usual oral doses of the phosphodiesterase type 5 inhibitors are listed in Table 103-4. Sildenafil, vardenafil (oral swallow tablets), and avanafil should be taken on demand at least 30 to 60 minutes before sexual intercourse. Vardenafil ODT and tadalafil should be taken 15 minutes and 2 hours, respectively, before sexual intercourse. The agents vary as to whether doses must be adjusted for patients aged 65 years and older and those with compromised hepatic or renal function. Patients should be advised to take no more than the amount prescribed and not more than one dose per day.[45] Doses higher than those recommended have been described in the published literature (eg, sildenafil 200 mg).[43] However, such dosing regimens have not consistently produced improved erectile responses.

For patients who do not respond to an adequate course of on-demand phosphodiesterase type 5 inhibitors for erectile dysfunction, daily low dosing of tadalafil may improve endothelial function in cavernosal tissue. That is, regular use of phosphodiesterase type 5 inhibitors may activate endothelial nitric oxide synthase, increase local concentrations of cGMP, which may increase oxygen tension, improve blood flow, and reduce endothelial damage and fibrosis in the corpora cavernosa.[46] Other potential advantages of this daily low dosing regimen include a lower potential for dose-related adverse effects and increased spontaneity of sexual intercourse. However, disadvantages of the daily low-dose regimen are the high cost of treatment; patients with more severe erectile dysfunction, who may require higher doses of a phosphodiesterase type 5 inhibitor, may not respond.[22,28,47] Although clinical trials of daily dosing of tadalafil 10 and 20 mg[48,49] have been published, the only FDA-approved labeling is for daily dosing of tadalafil 2.5 or 5 mg.

Adverse Effects Most adverse effects of the phosphodiesterase type 5 inhibitors are mild or moderate and are self-limited; and tolerance to the adverse effects develops with continued use.[28,47,50,51] The rates of drug discontinuation because of adverse effects are low, ranging from 2.1% to 25%, and are similar for all four agents. In usual doses, the most common adverse effects are headache (11%), facial flushing (12%), dyspepsia (5%), nasal congestion (3.4%), and dizziness (3%), all of which are dose-related and result from vasodilation or smooth muscle relaxation secondary to inhibition of phosphodiesterase isoenzyme type 1 or 5 in cardiac or vascular tissues.[47,50] However, some differences in the adverse reaction profile do exist. Sildenafil and vardenafil use is associated with more vascular and ocular adverse effects due to its inhibition of phosphodiesterase type 1 and 6, and tadalafil is associated with more lower back and limb pain and myalgia due to its greater inhibition of phosphodiesterase type 11.[35,50-52] Avanafil may be the best-tolerated agent because of its highly selective inhibition of phosphodiesterase type 5 and short half-life.[36-38,53]

Sildenafil and vardenafil produce an 8 to 10 mm Hg decrease in systolic and a 5 to 8 mm Hg decrease in diastolic blood pressure starting approximately 1 hour after a dose is taken and lasting for 4 hours. Most patients are asymptomatic as a result of these blood pressure changes, but some patients, particularly those taking multiple antihypertensives or nitrates or those with baseline hypotension, may develop dizziness or palpitations. Avanafil and tadalafil produce decreases in systolic and diastolic blood pressure that are smaller than those associated with sildenafil and vardenafil, although the decrements may be greater when they are used along with other antihypertensives or α-adrenergic antagonists.[47] All phosphodiesterase type 5 inhibitors must be used with caution in patients with cardiovascular disease because of the cardiac risk inherent to vigorous sexual activity. The management approach for such patients, as described in the recommendations of the Princeton Consensus Guideline Conference III,[26] should be applied to all the patients in whom phosphodiesterase type 5 inhibitors are being considered for use (see Table 103-3). If a patient who has cardiovascular disease develops angina during sexual intercourse after having taken a phosphodiesterase type 5 inhibitor, the patient should immediately stop and rest for the next 5 to 10 minutes. If angina does not resolve after 20-30 minutes, or if the patient develops additional anginal symptoms, the patient should be taken to the nearest emergency room.[54]

Sildenafil, vardenafil, and avanafil cause increased sensitivity to light, blurred vision, or transient loss of blue–green color discrimination in 2% to 3% of patients. This adverse effect is dose-related with the incidence increasing to 40% to 50% in patients taking sildenafil 200 mg.[47,55] These effects result from inhibition of phosphodiesterase type 6 in the photoreceptor cells of retinal rods and cones. Visual adverse effects commonly occur 1 to 2 hours after oral dosing when peak serum concentrations are achieved.[55] Avanafil has moderate and tadalafil has minimal to no inhibitory activity against phosphodiesterase type 6, and they are associated with a lower incidence of visual adverse effects (less than 1%) when compared to sildenafil and vardenafil.[47] Nevertheless, according to current product labeling, all phosphodiesterase type 5 inhibitors should be stopped immediately if the patient reports vision loss and should be used cautiously in patients at risk for retinitis pigmentosa, a genetic disease associated with retinal phosphodiesterase deficiency.

Nonarteritic anterior ischemic optic neuropathy (NAION) is a sudden, unilateral, painless blindness, which may be irreversible. Isolated cases of NAION have been associated with phosphodiesterase type 5 inhibitor use.[50] NAION has developed at variable and unpredictable times after starting a phosphodiesterase type 5 inhibitor, ranging from 6 hours to months or years after the first dose. Although a cause–effect relationship has not been established, it has been proposed that the blood pressure-lowering effects of these medications may decrease blood flow to the optic nerve and lead to a sudden unilateral decrease in vision.[56] Because NAION may lead to permanent vision loss, the FDA has required inclusion of warnings on the product labeling of phosphodiesterase type 5 inhibitors. Specifically, before receiving these agents, patients at risk for NAION should be evaluated by an ophthalmologist, risk factors for NAION should be addressed, and the patient should be cautioned against using a phosphodiesterase type 5 inhibitor.[47,50,56]

Patients at risk of NAION include a wide variety of patients: those with glaucoma, macular degeneration, diabetic retinopathy, dyslipidemia, or hypertension, those who have undergone eye surgery or have experienced eye trauma, patients who are aged 50 years or more, or smokers. A patient who experiences sudden vision loss in one eye while taking a phosphodiesterase type 5 inhibitor should be evaluated for NAION before continuing treatment. If NAION is present, the phosphodiesterase type 5 inhibitor should be discontinued as there is a 15% to 25% risk of developing NAION in the other eye in the ensuing 5 to 10 years.[56]

Acute unilateral hearing loss has also been reported after use of a phosphodiesterase type 5 inhibitor. A cause–effect relationship has not been established. In the cases reported, the hearing loss occurred within 1 to 3 days of starting treatment; it was variably accompanied by tinnitus or vertigo, and often resulted in residual hearing loss despite discontinuation of the phosphodiesterase type 5 inhibitor.[47] The product labeling now includes a warning that a phosphodiesterase type 5 inhibitor should be immediately stopped, and the patient should see a physician if sudden hearing loss develops.[50]

Priapism is a rare adverse effect of phosphodiesterase type 5 inhibitors, particularly sildenafil and vardenafil. Priapism has been associated with excessive doses of the phosphodiesterase type 5 inhibitor or when they are used along with other erectogenic drugs.[24]

Sildenafil use has been associated with an increased risk of melanoma. The proposed mechanism is that phosphodiesterase type 5 inhibition activates *BRAF*, a human gene that produces a protein that causes proliferation of melanoma cells. However, a cause–effect relationship has not been established.[57,58]

Recommendations for adverse effect monitoring are included in Table 103-6.

Drug Interactions Approximately 8% of patients taking organic nitrates may develop sudden, severe hypotension if they also take a phosphodiesterase type 5 inhibitor. Decreased blood pressure results from two major factors: (a) organic nitrates on their own produce hypotension and (b) organic nitrates are nitric oxide donors, which can stimulate the activity of guanylate cyclase and increase tissue levels of cGMP.[35,54] For this reason, phosphodiesterase type 5 inhibitor use is contraindicated in patients taking nitrates given by any route at scheduled times or intermittently. Furthermore, nitrates should be withheld for 24 hours after sildenafil, vardenafil, or avanafil administration and for 48 hours after tadalafil administration.[26,35] Furthermore, if a patient who has taken a phosphodiesterase type 5 inhibitor requires medical treatment of angina, non-nitrate-containing agents (eg, calcium channel blocker, β-adrenergic antagonist, and morphine) should be used.

If severe hypotension occurs after exposure to nitrates and a phosphodiesterase type 5 inhibitor, the patient should be placed in a Trendelenburg position and aggressive fluid administration initiated. If severe hypotension continues, parenteral β-adrenergic agonists (eg, dopamine) should be administered cautiously.[26]

Once a phosphodiesterase type 5 inhibitor has been discontinued, a nitrate may be taken 24 hours after the last dose of sildenafil, vardenafil, or avanafil, or 48 hours after the last dose of tadalafil.[54]

Interestingly, dietary sources of nitrates, nitrites, or L-arginine (a precursor for nitrates) do not interact with phosphodiesterase type 5 inhibitors. This is because dietary sources do not increase circulating or tissue levels of nitric oxide in humans.

The phosphodiesterase type 5 inhibitors have a low potential to interact with most antihypertensive medications.[16,17,19] However, small decreases in blood pressure with clinically symptomatic orthostatic hypotension have been described in some patients taking phosphodiesterase type 5 inhibitors and α-adrenergic antagonists. The degree of hypotension that develops is dependent on several factors: (a) stability of patient's blood pressure prior to taking both drugs; (b) dose of the α-adrenergic antagonist used; (c) particular α-adrenergic antagonist used; (d) particular phosphodiesterase type 5 inhibitor used; and (e) timing of administration of both drugs. The drug interaction produces less hypotension when the patient has stable blood pressure prior to taking both drugs; a low dose of alpha-adrenergic antagonist is taken; a uroselective (eg, tamsulosin or silodosin) or extended-release formulation of an α-adrenergic antagonist (eg, alfuzosin, or modified-release doxazosin) is used; tadalafil is preferentially prescribed over sildenafil, vardenafil, or avanafil; and an interval of 4 to 6 hours separates the doses of the α-adrenergic antagonist and phosphodiesterase type 5 inhibitor.[24,39]

Hepatic metabolism of all four phosphodiesterase type 5 inhibitors can be inhibited by strong enzyme inhibitors of CYP 3A4, including fluvoxamine, fluoxetine, nefazodone, verapamil, diltiazem, cimetidine, erythromycin, clarithromycin, itraconazole, ketoconazole, fluconazole itraconazole, atazanavir, indinavir, ritonavir, saquinavir, and grapefruit juice. Potent CYP 3A4 inhibitors may increase plasma levels of phosphodiesterase type 5 inhibitors by threefold or more. Lower starting doses of phosphodiesterase type 5 inhibitor should be used in these patients to minimize dose-related

TABLE 103-6 Drug Monitoring Table

Drug	Adverse Drug Reaction	Monitoring Parameter	Comments
Phosphodiesterase Inhibitor			
Sildenafil	• Headache • Flushing • Dyspepsia • Nasal congestion • Cyanopsia • NAION • Hypotension • Priapism • Hearing loss	• Clinical symptoms of erectile dysfunction • Visual complaints, loss of vision • Hearing loss • Blood pressure • Pulse	• Discontinue sildenafil if the patient has any visual or hearing loss and refer the patient to a physician • If the patient is taking any antihypertensives, stabilize blood pressure before starting sildenafil • If the patient develops priapism, he should proceed to the emergency department • If the patient has a bleeding disorder, use cautiously
Vardenafil	• Headache • Flushing • Dyspepsia • Nasal congestion • Cyanopsia • NAION • Hypotension • QT interval prolongation on EKG • Priapism • Hearing loss	• Clinical symptoms of erectile dysfunction • Visual complaints, loss of vision • Hearing loss • Blood pressure • Pulse • Palpitations or dizziness	• Discontinue vardenafil if the patient has any visual or hearing loss and refer the patient to a physician • If the patient is taking any antihypertensives, stabilize blood pressure before starting vardenafil • If the patient has palpitations or dizziness, check EKG. If QT prolongation is present, refer the patient for appropriate medical care • If the patient develops priapism, he should proceed to the emergency department • If the patient has a bleeding disorder, use cautiously
Tadalafil	• Headache • Flushing • Dyspepsia • Nasal congestion • Cyanopsia • Hearing loss • NAION • Hypotension • Lower back or lower extremity pain or myalgia • Priapism	• Clinical symptoms of erectile dysfunction • Visual complaints, loss of vision • Hearing loss • Blood pressure • Pulse • Palpitations or dizziness • Myalgia	• Discontinue tadalafil if the patient has any visual or hearing loss and refer the patient to a physician • If the patient is taking any antihypertensives, stabilize blood pressure before starting tadalafil • If the patient develops priapism, he should proceed to the emergency department • If the patient has a bleeding disorder, use cautiously • Muscle pain is dose-related
Avanafil	• Headache • Flushing • Dyspepsia • Nasal congestion • Cyanopsia • Hearing loss • NAION • Hypotension • Priapism	• Clinical symptoms of erectile dysfunction • Visual complaints, loss of vision • Blood pressure • Pulse • Palpitations or dizziness • Hearing loss	• Discontinue avanafil if the patient has any visual or hearing loss and refer the patient to a physician • If the patient is taking any antihypertensives, stabilize blood pressure before starting avanafil • If the patient develops priapism, he should proceed to the emergency department • If the patient has a bleeding disorder, use cautiously
Prostaglandin E_1			
Alprostadil, intracavernosal	• Penile pain • Hematoma at injection site • Priapism • Hypotension • Fibrotic nodules along penile shaft • Decreased blood pressure • Dizziness	• Clinical symptoms of erectile dysfunction • Presence of hematoma or fibrotic nodules • Blood pressure • Pulse	• Penile pain responds to acetaminophen • To avoid hematoma, apply pressure to injection site for 5-10 minutes after injection • If the patient develops priapism, he should proceed to the emergency department • Fibrotic nodules are rare but may occur after repeated injections. These may cause curvature of the penis during an erection and this requires assessment by a urologist • Hypotension and dizziness are uncommon and are associated with inadvertent venous injection of the drug
Alprostadil, intraurethral	• Aching pain in penis, testicles, legs, and perineum • Urethral burning, bleeding, or tearing • Priapism • Hypotension • Dizziness • Female partner may experience vaginal pain and burning sensation	• Clinical symptoms of erectile dysfunction • Urethral injury as evidenced by pain, bleeding, or tissue damage • Blood pressure • Pulse	• Burning pain usually resolves spontaneously. If urethral injury is suspected, this requires assessment by a urologist. Pain experienced by the female partner is due to leakage of medication from male urethra into vagina. Pain will usually resolve spontaneously • If the patient develops priapism, he should proceed to the emergency department • Hypotension and dizziness are uncommon, occurring in only 2%-3% of patients, and are associated with systemic absorption of the drugs • Alprostadil is embryotoxic and contact must be avoided if the female sex partner is pregnant. Males should use condoms if female is pregnant

(continued)

TABLE 103-6 Drug Monitoring Table (*Continued*)

Drug	Adverse Drug Reaction	Monitoring Parameter	Comments
Testosterone Supplements			
Methyltestosterone	• Sodium and water retention • Hyperlipidemia • Polycythemia • Gynecomastia • Sleep apnea, worsening • Increased libido • Mood swings • Oligospermia • Hepatotoxicity • Venous thromboembolism • Prostate enlargement	• Clinical symptoms of erectile dysfunction • Physical exam for edema • Blood pressure • Serum lipids, hematocrit, hepatic transaminases, prostate-specific antigen, serum testosterone	• Discontinue if the patient has signs of hepatoxicity. If hematocrit exceeds 55% (0.55), methyltestosterone should be discontinued. Testosterone supplements may worsen lower urinary tract symptoms (LUTS) in patients with BPH. It is contraindicated in patients with untreated prostate cancer or men with breast cancer. May increase the risk of nonfatal myocardial infarction or death. Use precautiously in patients with a significant cardiovascular history. Discontinue if venous thromboembolism is suspected
Testosterone cypionate or enanthate Testosterone undecanoate	• Sodium and water retention • Hyperlipidemia • Polycythemia • Gynecomastia • Sleep apnea, worsening • Increased libido • Oligospermia • Mood swings • Hepatotoxicity • Venous thromboembolism • Prostate enlargement • Injection site pain, pruritis • Pulmonary oil microembolism (POME), testosterone undecanoate only • Anaphylactic reactions • Prostate enlargement • Sodium and water retention • Hyperlipidemia • Polycythemia • Gynecomastia • Sleep apnea, worsening • Increased libido • Oligospermia • Mood swings • Hepatotoxicity	• Clinical symptoms of erectile dysfunction • Physical exam for edema • Blood pressure • Serum lipids, hematocrit, hepatic transaminases, prostate-specific antigen • Clinical symptoms of erectile dysfunction • Physical exam for edema, cough, shortness of breath • Blood pressure • Serum lipids, hematocrit, hepatic transaminases, prostate-specific antigen	• Discontinue if the patient has signs of hepatoxicity. If hematocrit exceeds 55% (0.55), testosterone supplement should be discontinued. Testosterone supplements may worsen LUTS in patients with BPH. It is contraindicated in patients with untreated prostate cancer or men with breast cancer. These formulations produce supraphysiologic serum concentrations of testosterone. Mood swings have been reported with these agents. May increase the risk of nonfatal myocardial infarction or death. Use cautiously in patients with a significant cardiovascular history. Discontinue if venous thromboembolism is suspected • Discontinue if the patient has signs of hepatoxicity. If hematocrit exceeds 55% (0.55), testosterone supplement should be discontinued. Testosterone supplements may worsen LUTS in patients with BPH. It is contraindicated in patients with untreated prostate cancer or men with breast cancer. These formulations produce supraphysiologic serum concentrations of testosterone. Mood swings have been reported with these agents. May increase the risk of nonfatal myocardial infarction or death. Use cautiously in patients with a significant cardiovascular history. Discontinue if venous thromboembolism is suspected • Signs of POME include cough, dyspnea, chest pain, and syncope, usually within 30 minutes of testosterone undecanoate injection. This medication should only be administered by a healthcare provider or in setting which is certified through a Risk Evaluation and Mitigation Strategy program
Testosterone patch	• Sodium and water retention • Hyperlipidemia • Gynecomastia • Sleep apnea, worsening • Increased libido • Contact dermatitis • Application site erythema, pruritus • Prostate enlargement	• Clinical symptoms of erectile dysfunction • Physical exam for edema • Blood pressure • Serum lipids, hematocrit, hepatic transaminases, prostate-specific antigen, serum testosterone	• Testosterone supplements may worsen LUTS in patients with BPH. It is contraindicated in patients with untreated prostate cancer or men with breast cancer. Contact dermatitis has been associated with the alcohol-based agent used to enhance transdermal drug absorption. It responds to topical corticosteroids. Of significance, hepatotoxicity has not been reported with transdermal patches. May increase the risk of nonfatal myocardial infarction or death. Use precautiously in patients with a significant cardiovascular history. Discontinue if venous thromboembolism is suspected. Adverse effects of mood swings and polycythemia are less likely with patch than with injectable formulations
Testosterone transdermal gel/spray/axillary solution	• Sodium and water retention • Hyperlipidemia • Polycythemia • Gynecomastia • Sleep apnea, worsening • Increased libido • Dermatitis • Application site erythema • pruritis, • Prostate enlargement	• Clinical symptoms of erectile dysfunction • Physical exam for edema • Blood pressure • Serum lipids, hematocrit, hepatic transaminases, prostate-specific antigen, serum testosterone	• Do not interchange topical formulations. Testosterone supplements may worsen LUTS in patients with BPH. It is contraindicated in patients with untreated prostate cancer or men with breast cancer. Use is contraindicated in pregnant women or women who are likely to become pregnant, or women who breast feed infants. Women and children who have inadvertent skin exposure to these formulations may become virilized. If hematocrit exceeds 55% (0.55), testosterone supplement should be discontinued. May increase the risk of nonfatal myocardial infarction or death. Use precautiously in patients with a significant cardiovascular history. Discontinue if venous thromboembolism is suspected. With transdermal sprays, REMS assessments must be submitted to the FDA

(*continued*)

TABLE 103-6 Drug Monitoring Table (*Continued*)

Drug	Adverse Drug Reaction	Monitoring Parameter	Comments
Testosterone gel, intranasal	• Rhinorrhea, nose bleeds, nose pain • Sore throat • Sodium and water retention • Hyperlipidemia • Polycythemia • Gynecomastia • Sleep apnea, worsening • Increased libido • Dermatitis • Application site erythema pruritis • Prostate enlargement	• Clinical symptoms of erectile dysfunction • Physical exam for edema • Blood pressure • Serum lipids, hematocrit, hepatic transaminases, prostate-specific antigen, serum testosterone	• Discontinue if severe rhinitis occurs. • Testosterone supplements may worsen LUTS in patients with BPH. It is contraindicated in patients with untreated prostate cancer or men with breast cancer. Use is contraindicated in pregnant women or women who are likely to become pregnant, or women who breast feed infants. Women and children who have inadvertent skin exposure to these formulations may become virilized. If hematocrit exceeds 55% (0.55), testosterone supplement should be discontinued. May increase the risk of nonfatal myocardial infarction or death. Use precautiously in patients with a significant cardiovascular history. Discontinue if venous thromboembolism is suspected. With transdermal sprays, REMS (risk evaluation and mitigation strategies) assessments must be submitted to the US Food and Drug Administration
Testosterone subcutaneous implant	• Sodium and water retention • Hyperlipidemia • Polycythemia • Gynecomastia • Sleep apnea, worsening • Increased libido • Mood swings • Oligospermia • Hepatotoxicity • Prostate enlargement • Pain and infection at the implant site	• Clinical symptoms of erectile dysfunction • Physical exam for edema • Blood pressure • Serum lipids, hematocrit, hepatic transaminases, prostate-specific antigen, serum testosterone	• Subcutaneous pellet implant may be extruded with loss of the dose. Androgen-related adverse effects may persist for a long time after drug administration unless the implant is removed. If hematocrit exceeds 55% (0.55), testosterone implant should be removed. Testosterone supplements may worsen LUTS in patients with BPH. It is contraindicated in patients with untreated prostate cancer or men with breast cancer. May increase the risk of nonfatal myocardial infarction or death. Use cautiously in patients with a significant cardiovascular history. Discontinue if venous thromboembolism is suspected

LUTS, lower urinary tract symptoms.

adverse effects, including cyanopsia, hypotension, flushing, nasal congestion, and priapism (see Table 103-4). Similarly, CYP 3A4 inducers, including rifampin, carbamazepine, phenytoin, and phenobarbital, can decrease plasma levels of phosphodiesterase type 5 inhibitors. Higher starting doses of phosphodiesterase type 5 inhibitors should be used in these patients.

If used with type 1A antiarrhythmics (eg, quinidine or procainamide) or type 3 antiarrhythmics (eg, sotalol, amiodarone), vardenafil can prolong the QT interval. This is a unique drug interaction of vardenafil and not a pharmacologic class effect.

Testosterone Replacement Regimens

Mechanism 9 Testosterone replacement regimens supply exogenous testosterone and restore serum testosterone levels to the normal range of 300 to 1,100 ng/dL (10.4-38.2 nmol/L). In so doing, testosterone replacement regimens correct symptoms of hypogonadism, which include malaise, loss of muscle strength, depressed mood, and decreased libido.[11]

Testosterone can directly stimulate androgen receptors in the CNS and is thought to be responsible for maintaining normal sexual drive. In addition, testosterone may stimulate nitric oxide synthase, thereby increasing cavernosal concentrations of nitric oxide, and enhancing the effects of phosphodiesterase type 5 in cavernosal tissue.[11] Testosterone may also enhance relaxation and blood filling of the corpora cavernosa by downregulating RhoA-ROCK, an enzymatic pathway responsible for calcium transport into penile smooth muscle cells.[59]

Indications Although multiple guidelines on testosterone replacement have been published, four commonly used ones include the recommendations from the Endocrine Society,[12] British Society for Sexual Medicine,[16] American Urological Association,[60] and the European Association of Urology.[61] A recent comparison of published guidelines is also available.[62]

Testosterone replacement regimens are indicated in symptomatic patients with primary, secondary, or mixed hypogonadism, as confirmed with serum concentrations of testosterone. Although the threshold serum total testosterone level that defines hypogonadism varies with specific published guidelines, usually a serum total testosterone less than 230 to 350 ng/dL (8.0-12.2 nmol/L) is used.[11,12,60]

Serum testosterone concentrations typically are measured in the early morning between 7 am and 11 am because the secretion pattern of this hormone follows a circadian pattern, with highest serum concentrations in the morning hours and the lowest level at night (approximately 10 pm). A low measured serum testosterone level is confirmed with a repeat measurement on a separate day, optimally 4 weeks later. Confirmation of a low serum testosterone level is essential because of an approximate 10% intra-individual variation of measured levels and variable performance characteristics of various testosterone assays.[11,12,60,61] Simultaneous serum luteinizing hormone levels help to distinguish patients with primary hypogonadism, who have elevated luteinizing hormone levels, from those with secondary hypogonadism, who have decreased luteinizing hormone levels.[12] In men with equivocal serum total testosterone levels, it is recommended to obtain free testosterone levels.[63]

Testosterone replacement regimens should never be administered to men with normal serum testosterone levels, patients who have asymptomatic hypogonadism, or patients with isolated erectile dysfunction as the only sign of hypogonadism.

Efficacy Testosterone replacement regimens restore muscle strength and sexual drive, promote erythropoiesis, and improve mood, cognition, and bone density in adult patients with hypogonadism.[12,59,60] Testosterone replacement regimens do not directly correct erectile dysfunction; instead, they improve libido, thereby correcting secondary erectile dysfunction. Although testosterone replacement regimens may correct the serum testosterone level within days, observable clinical improvements make take weeks after the start of testosterone replacement. For example, increased libido may be evident at 6 weeks, improvements in erectile dysfunction or increase in muscle mass may take months. For this reason, a minimum effective clinical trial is considered 3 to 6 months.[12,60]

No additional benefit has been demonstrated for large doses of testosterone, which can increase the serum testosterone level from the low end to the upper end of the normal range or to the above-normal range.[60]

Testosterone replacement regimens can be administered parenterally, orally, transdermally, or intransally (see Table 103-4).[63] Intramuscular injections of testosterone enanthate and cypionate are the preferred treatment for symptomatic patients with primary or secondary hypogonadism because they are effective, inexpensive, and not associated with the bioavailability problems or hepatotoxic adverse effects of oral androgens.[60] Patients generally require dosing every 2 to 4 weeks. A longer-acting depot intramuscular formulation of testosterone undecanoate, which can be dosed every 10 weeks, offers greater convenience but is more expensive than testosterone enanthate or cypionate. Testosterone undecanoate has been associated with pulmonary oil embolism and anaphylactic reactions that can necessitate hospitalization.[60] For this reason, testosterone undecanoate is restricted to settings certified through a Risk Evaluation and Mitigation Strategies Program. A subcutaneous implant of testosterone pellets lasts 3 to 6 months, but it requires a surgical incision in the forearm. Extrusion has been reported in up to 8.5% of treated patients and results in loss of drug effect.

Oral formulations are associated with hepatotoxicity and are not recommended.[60] Although convenient for the patient, testosterone patches, gels, and sprays are much more expensive than testosterone enanthate or cypionate.[60] An intranasal testosterone gel formulation avoids inadvertent transfer of testosterone to others, as can occur with some other transdermal gel formulations. However, the intranasal formulation must be taken 3 times a day, which is inconvenient.[63] Therefore, the transdermal and nasal formulations should be reserved for patients who refuse injectable testosterone.

The ideal testosterone replacement regimen would mimic the normal circadian pattern of serum testosterone concentrations such that peak and trough concentrations occur in the early morning and late afternoon, respectively; produce serum concentrations in the normal range; produce serum concentrations of dihydrotestosterone and estradiol, which are metabolites of testosterone, that mimic the normal physiologic pattern; and produce minimal adverse effects. The ideal replacement regimen should be inexpensive and be convenient for the patient to use. Table 103-4 compares commercially available testosterone replacement regimens for these characteristics and shows that an ideal regimen has yet to be identified.[59-62]

The dropout rate with testosterone supplementation is high. Approximately 30% and 85% of patients stop testosterone replacement after 6 and 12 months, respectively. The reasons for this include the cost of the medication, slow onset of response, and inadequate perceived benefit.[12]

Pharmacokinetics Natural testosterone has poor oral bioavailability because of extensive first-pass hepatic metabolism; therefore, large doses must be taken. To improve oral bioavailability, alkylated derivatives were formulated. Of these derivatives, methyltestosterone and fluoxymesterone are more resistant to hepatic catabolism and can be taken in smaller daily doses, which are theoretically safer. However, oral alkylated derivatives of testosterone are not metabolized to dihydrotestosterone or estradiol, are associated with a higher incidence of serious hepatotoxicity, and therefore are not preferred for management of hypogonadism.

Several testosterone esters have been formulated for intramuscular injection, with different durations of action (see Table 103-4). The shorter-acting testosterone propionate, which required dosing three times per week, has been discontinued and replaced with testosterone cypionate or enanthate, which can be dosed every 2, 4, or 6 weeks in most patients. These testosterone formulations produce supraphysiologic serum testosterone levels 2 to 4 days after each dose, which have been linked to mood swings and polycythemia in some patients.[60]

After the first and second doses, which are given 4 weeks apart, intramuscular injections of testosterone undecanoate generally last 10 weeks. An even longer-acting parenteral testosterone is available as a subcutaneous implant for dosing every 3 to 6 months.[60]

Transdermal testosterone replacement regimens can be delivered as once-daily patches or gel. For convenience, the gel is available in premeasured dose packets or in a pump dispenser. Testosterone patches increase serum testosterone levels to the normal range in 2 to 6 hours. Serum testosterone levels return to baseline 24 hours after patch or gel administration. However, unlike oral or injectable supplements, transdermal testosterone patches applied at bedtime or testosterone gel applied each morning produce physiologic patterns of serum testosterone levels throughout the day. Although these formulations are often described as producing more "natural" hormone levels, the clinical importance of this biochemical effect is unknown.[60]

The original Testoderm brand patch was formulated for scrotal application. Scrotal skin is thinner and has a richer vascular supply than does the skin on the arms or thighs. Therefore, application of Testoderm patches produced excellent absorption of the hormone. However, the patch could detach when the scrotum became damp or moist, when the patient exercised, or if the scrotum was excessively hairy. Due to its inconvenient site of application, the scrotal patch is no longer commercially available in the United States.

For improved convenience, Androderm patches are formulated for application to the upper arms, back, abdomen, or thighs. The addition of absorption enhancers and adhesives has been linked to a higher incidence of contact dermatitis with Androderm patches compared with the original Testoderm scrotal patch or to gel formulations.

When compared to patches, testosterone gel 1% formulation (AndroGel) is applied in much larger doses (5 or 10 g each day) to the skin of the shoulders, upper arms, or abdomen. The hormone is absorbed quickly, within 30 minutes, but several hours may be required for complete absorption of the dose. For this reason, the patient should be reminded to wait at least 2 hours after application before showering. To prevent inadvertent transfer of testosterone gel to others, the patient should thoroughly wash his hands with soap and water after administration of a dose, allow the application site to dry undisturbed for several minutes before dressing or covering it, and ensure that there is no contact with clothing contaminated with the gel by children and female members of the household.[60]

A high-strength testosterone gel (1.62%) formulation is also available. It allows administration of a daily dose with a smaller amount of gel. It should be applied to the shoulder or upper arms.

Dosing Table 103-4 lists the usual doses for testosterone replacement regimens. Three to 6 months is considered as an adequate treatment trial with a particular dose.[12] Thus, a dose should not be increased until the patient has used one particular dose for at least this time period. The recommended target serum testosterone level is the mid normal range,[11,60] or 450 to 600 ng/dL (15.6-20.8 nmol/L).[60,62] Repeated serum testosterone levels that exceed the normal range or produce adverse effects will necessitate a dosage reduction or increased interval between drug doses. Table 103-7 provides guidance on the timeline for monitoring serum testosterone levels based on the particular testosterone formulation used. After starting treatment, patients should be reassessed in 1 to 3 months. The patient's libido, mood, and quality of life may improve in 3 to 4 weeks, erectile function may improve in 6 months, but other symptoms of hypogonadism (eg, bone density) may take longer to resolve. If the patient responds to treatment and serum testosterone levels have returned to normal, the patient can be followed up annually. At each visit, the use of a validated self-assessment tool (eg, Androgen Deficiency in Aging Men Questionnaire) can assist the physician in gauging the patient's response to treatment.[64]

TABLE 103-7 Timing of Serum Testosterone Level Monitoring in Patients on Testosterone Replacement Regimens

When to Monitor Serum Testosterone Levels	
Oral testosterone tablets/capsules	2-3 hours after dose for peak level only.
Intramuscular testosterone cypionate or enanthate	Midpoint of dosing interval or measure trough level right before the fourth dose.
Intramuscular testosterone undecanoate	Just before each subsequent injection or measure level halfway between 10-week dosing interval.
Transdermal testosterone gel	Depending on the formulation, just before dose in the morning 2-4 weeks after start of therapy or after a dose adjustment.[65]
Transdermal patch	Before the next dose 2 weeks after start of therapy or after a dose adjustment.
Axillary solution	2-8 hours after application and 2 weeks after starting therapy or after a dosage adjustment.
Intranasal testosterone gel	1 month after starting treatment, measure trough level right before a dose.
Testosterone subcutaneous implant	3-6 months after implantation, obtain trough level just before next dose.

Data from Reference 60.

Once an optimal dose of a patient's testosterone replacement regimen has been established and the patient has received treatment for at least 3 months, the prescriber should consider discontinuing the regimen if the patient's symptoms of hypogonadism show no improvement.[66]

Before initiating any testosterone replacement regimen in patients 40 years and older, patients should be screened for breast cancer, benign prostatic hyperplasia, and prostate cancer. All are testosterone-dependent conditions and theoretically could be worsened by exogenous administration of testosterone. However, no confirmed cases of prostate cancer caused by testosterone supplementation in a hypogonadal patient have been documented.[67] Nevertheless, untreated prostate cancer is a contraindication to androgen supplementation. To screen for prostate disorders, a prostate-specific antigen serum concentration should be obtained, and a digital rectal examination of the prostate performed particularly in men who are 50 years of age or older. These tests are generally repeated at 1-year intervals after treatment is started. Also, since testosterone supplementation has been reported to worsen severe sleep apnea or edema of congestive heart failure, caution should be exercised in using testosterone in patients with these disorders.[12,60]

Other baseline tests that are recommended include hematocrit and liver function tests. These should be repeated 3 and 6 months after the start of a testosterone replacement regimen. If normal, these tests can be repeated annually thereafter. If the hematocrit exceeds 55% (0.55), the testosterone replacement regimen should be withheld to avoid polycythemia and its consequences.

Adverse Effects Testosterone replacement regimens can cause sodium retention, which can lead to weight gain, or exacerbate hypertension, congestive heart failure, and edema (Table 103-6). Although serum lipoprotein perturbations may occur, testosterone replacement regimens have a neutral effect in that they decrease both total cholesterol and high-density lipoprotein cholesterol levels. Two retrospective studies associated testosterone supplementation with an increased risk of myocardial infarction and stroke.[68,69] Although these studies did not show a cause–effect relationship and are considered inconclusive, the FDA included a labeling warning that testosterone supplementation may lead to cardiovascular disease and physicians should discuss this potential risk with patients before initiating treatment. This was prompted by a significant increase in testosterone use in the United States, inadequate monitoring of serum testosterone levels prior to and during testosterone supplementation, and the potential hazards of using testosterone supplementation in elderly patients with cardiovascular risk factors.[70]

Since then, some prospective clinical trials have documented the safe use of testosterone replacement regimens in patients with risk factors for cardiovascular disease and these were included in a recent meta-analysis.[66,71] Nevertheless, in view of the product labeling, prescribers are advised to discuss the potential risks of testosterone replacement regimens with patients before initiating treatment, and to carefully monitor patients for adverse effects.[62] For patients who have had a myocardial infarction, stroke, or worsening of congestive heart failure, a testosterone replacement regimen should be delayed for at least 6 months.[11,61]

Gynecomastia can occur because of conversion of testosterone to estrogen in peripheral tissues. This has been reported most often in patients with liver cirrhosis or those who are obese.

Oral alkylated testosterone replacement regimens have caused hepatotoxicity, ranging from mild elevations of hepatic transaminases to serious liver diseases, including peliosis hepatis (hemorrhagic liver cysts), hepatocellular and intrahepatic cholestasis, and benign or malignant tumors. For this reason, parenteral or transdermal testosterone replacement regimens are preferred.

Transdermal testosterone patches may cause contact dermatitis, which responds well to topical corticosteroids. This adverse effect has been associated with the presence of permeation enhancers, which are added to patch formulations. If the dermatitis from the patch formulation becomes problematic, testosterone gel is associated with a lower incidence of contact dermatitis.

Erythrocytosis occurs most often in patients receiving parenteral testosterone formulations. If the increase in hematocrit is mild, decreasing the dose of testosterone replacement is all that is needed. However, if the hematocrit exceeds 55% (0.55) testosterone injections should be stopped and can be replaced with a transdermal testosterone product.[60]

Although testosterone supplementation in men with late-onset hypogonadism has not been shown to cause prostate cancer, it should not be given to men with known prostate cancer that has not been treated.[60,72]

Alprostadil

Mechanism Alprostadil, also known as prostaglandin E_1, stimulates adenyl cyclase, resulting in increased production of cAMP, a secondary messenger that activates protein kinase A, which decreases intracellular calcium concentrations and causes smooth muscle relaxation of the arterial blood vessels and sinusoidal tissues in the corpora. This results in enhanced blood flow to and blood filling of the corpora.[38,51] Because it does not require nitric oxide to produce its clinical effects, patients with erectile dysfunction due to diseases that are associated with an impaired nitric oxide pathway (eg, diabetes mellitus, post radical prostatectomy, patients in whom phosphodiesterase type 5 inhibitors are contraindicated, and patients who fail phosphodiesterase type 5 treatment) may respond to alprostadil.[38,39]

Alprostadil is commercially available as an intracavernosal injection (Caverject and Edex) and as an intraurethral insert (medicated urethral system for erection [MUSE]).

Indications Both commercially available formulations of alprostadil are FDA-approved as monotherapy for management of erectile dysfunction.

The efficacy of the intracavernosal injection may be related to the excellent bioavailability of the drug when injected directly into the corpora cavernosum. In contrast, intraurethral alprostadil doses generally are several hundred times larger than intracavernosal doses. This is because intraurethral alprostadil must be absorbed from the urethra, through the corpus spongiosum, and into the corpus cavernosum, where it exerts its full proerectogenic effect.

Although several other agents, including papaverine and phentolamine, have been used off-label for intracavernosal therapy, alprostadil is preferred. This is because intracavernosal alprostadil has been approved by the FDA for erectile dysfunction, it does not require extemporaneous compounding, and it has a low potential for causing prolonged erections and priapism.

Both formulations of alprostadil are considered more invasive than VEDs or phosphodiesterase type 5 inhibitors. For this reason, intracavernosal alprostadil is generally prescribed after patients do not respond to or cannot use less invasive interventions. Intracavernosal alprostadil is preferred over intraurethral alprostadil because of its greater effectiveness. Intracavernosal alprostadil may be preferred in patients with diabetes mellitus, who are accustomed to injectable drug therapy and may have peripheral neuropathies, which decrease the patient's perception of pain upon injection. Intraurethral alprostadil is generally reserved as a treatment of last resort for patients who do not respond to other less invasive and more effective forms of therapy, and who refuse surgery.

Intracavernosal Alprostadil

Efficacy The overall efficacy of intracavernosal alprostadil is 70% to 90%.[22] Three characteristics of intracavernosal alprostadil include the following:

1. The effectiveness of alprostadil is dose related. The mean duration of erection is directly related to the dose of alprostadil administered and ranges from 12 to 44 minutes.
2. A higher percentage of patients with psychogenic and neurogenic erectile dysfunction respond to alprostadil at a lower dose compared to patients with vasculogenic erectile dysfunction.
3. Tolerance does not appear to develop with continued use of intracavernosal alprostadil at home.

10 Although 70% to 75% of patients respond to intracavernosal alprostadil, a high proportion of patients elect to discontinue its use over time. Depending on the study and the length of observation, 30% to 50% of patients voluntarily discontinue therapy, usually during the first 6 to 12 months, and this increases to 54% and 67% after 2 to 4 years, respectively.[22,38] After 10 years, less than 5% of patients continue intracavernosal injections. Common reasons for discontinuation include lack of perceived effectiveness; inconvenience of administration; an unnatural, nonspontaneous erection; needle phobia; penile pain, loss of interest; or cost of therapy.

Approximately one-third of patients do not respond to usual doses of intracavernosal alprostadil. In these patients, intracavernosal alprostadil has been used successfully along with VEDs. Such combination therapy can be attempted by patients before transitioning to more invasive surgical procedures.[32] Alternatively, intracavernosal injections of synergistic combinations of vasoactive agents that act by different mechanisms have been used. For example, papaverine is a nonspecific phosphodiesterase inhibitor that increases cavernosal concentrations of cAMP and cGMP, and phentolamine is an α-adrenergic antagonist that blocks detumescence (thereby prolonging an erection). Intracavernosal drug combinations typically produce an erection that lasts longer than an erection produced by any one of the agents in the mixture. In addition, because of the low dosage of each agent in the combination, fewer systemic and local fibrotic adverse effects develop compared with high-dose monotherapy. For example, when used in low-dose combination regimens, papaverine is less likely to induce hypotension and liver dysfunction, and phentolamine is less likely to induce tachycardia and hypotension.[6,22] However, such intracavernosal drug combinations are not commercially available and must be extemporaneously compounded. Several different two- or three-drug formulations have been used, but no one formulation is considered a standard.[22,32] Finally, intracavernosal alprostadil has been used in combination with phosphodiesterase type 5 inhibitors; however, this use is an unlabeled indication.[22,32]

Pharmacokinetics Intracavernosal injection should be administered into only one corpus cavernosum. From this injection site, the drug will reach the other corpus cavernosum through vascular communications between the two corpora. Alprostadil acts rapidly, with an onset of 5 to 15 minutes. The duration is directly related to the dose. Within the usual dosage range of 2.5 to 20 mcg, the duration of erection is not more than 1 hour. Higher doses are expected to exhibit a longer duration of action. Local 15-hydroxy dehydrogenase in the corpora cavernosum quickly converts alprostadil to inactive metabolites. Any alprostadil that escapes into the systemic circulation is deactivated on first pass through the lungs. Hence, the plasma half-life of alprostadil is approximately 5 to 10 minutes, and the potential for systemic and local adverse effects is negligible.[22,30] Dose modification is not necessary in patients with renal or hepatic disease.

Dosing The usual dose of intracavernosal alprostadil is 10 to 20 mcg, with a maximum recommended dose of 60 mcg. Doses greater than 60 mcg have not produced any greater improvement in penile erection but may cause hypotension or prolonged erections lasting more than 1 hour. The dose should be administered 5 to 10 minutes before intercourse. The manufacturer recommends that patients be slowly titrated up to the minimally effective dosage to minimize the likelihood of hypotension. Under a health professional's supervision, patients should be started with a 1.25-mcg dose, which can be increased in increments of 1.25 to 2.50 mcg at 30-minute intervals up to the lowest dose that produces a firm erection for 1 hour and does not produce adverse effects. In clinical practice, this process is rarely done because it is time-consuming.[28] Thus, many physicians start the patient on 10 mcg and move quickly up the dosage range to identify the best dose for the patient. To avoid adverse effects, patients should receive not more than one injection per day and not more than three injections per week with a 24-hour interval between doses (see Table 103-4).

Intracavernosal injections should be performed using a 0.5-in. (1.3 cm), 27- or 30-gauge needle. A tuberculin syringe or a syringe prefilled with diluent as supplied by the manufacturer should be used to ensure precise measurement of doses. Patients with needle phobia, poor vision, or poor manual dexterity can use commercially available autoinjectors to facilitate administration of intracavernosal alprostadil.[30]

Intracavernosal injections require that the patient or the sexual partner practice good aseptic techniques (to avoid infection), have good manual skills and visual ability, and be comfortable with injection techniques. When practicing self-injection, the patient should use one hand to firmly hold the glans penis against his thigh to expose the lateral surface of the shaft. The injection should be made at right angles into one of the lateral surfaces of the proximal third of the penis. The injection should never be made into the dorsal or ventral surface of the penis. This will prevent inadvertent injection of the drug into arteries on the dorsal surface or the urethra on the ventral surface. After the injection, the penis should be massaged to help distribute the drug into the opposite corpus cavernosum. Injection sites should be rotated with each dose. Finally, manual pressure should be applied to the injection site for 5 minutes to reduce the likelihood of hematoma formation (Fig. 103-5).

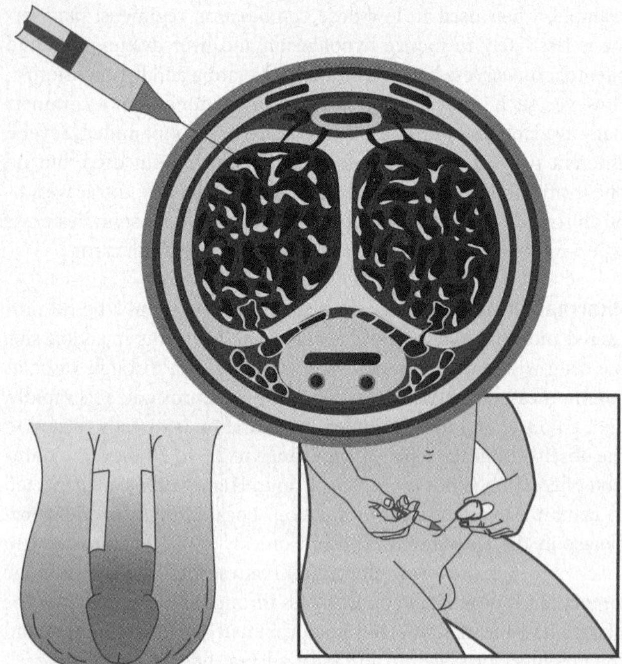

FIGURE 103-5 Technique for administration of intracavernosal injections. *(Source: Caverject [package insert]. New York, NY: Pfizer Inc.; 2006. https://www.pfizer.com/products/product-detail/caverject. Accessed November 1, 2018.)*

Once the optimal dosage of intracavernosal alprostadil is established, the patient should return for routine medical follow-up every 3 to 6 months. Some patients subsequently require dosage adjustment, largely attributed to worsening of the underlying disease that is contributing to the erectile dysfunction.

Adverse Effects Intracavernosal alprostadil is most commonly associated with local adverse effects. Hematoma and bruising at the injection site occur most often during the first year of therapy. These effects are largely the result of poor injection technique. To minimize the risk of injection site hematomas, patients should apply pressure to the injection site for 5 minutes after each dose. Similarly, infection at the injection site has been reported. Meticulous aseptic technique is necessary to prevent this complication.

Cavernosal plaques or areas of fibrosis at injection sites form in approximately 2% to 12% of patients.[51] When they occur, the patient should suspend further injections for 2 to 4 months or until the plaques resolve. These plaques may cause penile curvature, similar to Peyronie's disease, which makes sexual intercourse difficult or impossible. The cause of corporal fibrosis and plaque formation is unknown. This adverse effect may be caused by poor injection technique or by alprostadil itself. Although patients have developed corporal fibrosis, alprostadil may be less likely to cause this adverse effect compared to other intracavernosal drug combinations, such as phentolamine or papaverine. Unlike cavernosal fibrosis associated with large doses and repeated administration of papaverine, penile scarring secondary to alprostadil appears to be unpredictable.

Alprostadil causes penile pain in approximately 10% to 44% of patients. The pain has been described as a burning discomfort or dull pain near the injection site or during the erection, which generally does not persist after the penis becomes flaccid. The pain usually is mild, generally does not require discontinuation of therapy, and often abates even with continued treatment.[22] However, 2% to 5% of patients discontinue taking alprostadil because of severe pain. The pain can be managed by oral analgesics (eg, acetaminophen), if necessary. One investigator has recommended adding procaine to intracavernosal alprostadil, but this may mask the signs of more serious adverse effects of the drug or of penile injury during intercourse, and is not recommended. The mechanism of this adverse reaction is poorly understood. Alprostadil may intrinsically produce pain. In addition, the pain may be a result of the pH of the parenteral solution. Alprostadil is acidic, and the commercially available Caverject formulation is buffered with sodium citrate, a weak base, to reduce pain on injection.[6]

Priapism, a prolonged, painful erection lasting more than 1 hour, occurs in 1% to 15% of treated patients. It occurs most often during the dose titration period and is rare thereafter. Blood sludging in the corpora can lead to tissue hypoxia and irreversible cavernosal fibrosis and scarring. The risk for this complication is greatest for erections that persist beyond 4 to 6 hours. Patients are advised to seek medical attention immediately when drug-induced erections last more than 4 hours, as this may progress to a urologic emergency.[22] Its management includes supportive care, including analgesics for pain and sedatives for anxiety. In addition, needle aspiration of sludged blood in the corpora or intracavernosal injection of α-adrenergic agonists (eg, phenylephrine) has been used. These procedures facilitate venous drainage of the corpora, allowing venous outflow to "catch up" with arterial inflow.[6,30]

The likelihood of prolonged erections with intracavernosal alprostadil is dose related. Therefore, to prevent this adverse effect, the lowest effective dose should be used, and the dose should be titrated to ensure that the duration of the erection is not more than 1 hour.

Intracavernosal alprostadil rarely causes systemic adverse effects, owing to the agent's local catabolism in cavernosal tissue and rapid deactivation in pulmonary tissue (if any of the drug escapes into the systemic circulation). However, large doses greater than 20 mcg are associated with dizziness and hypotension in some patients and is one reason why such large doses are not commonly used.

Intracavernosal injection therapy should be used cautiously by patients at risk for priapism, including patients with sickle cell disease, leukemia, or multiple myeloma. It should be used cautiously by patients who may develop bleeding complications secondary to injections, including patients with thrombocytopenia or those taking anticoagulants. It also should be used cautiously by patients who use poor-quality injection technique, including patients with psychiatric disorders, obese patients (who may not be able to reach or see the penile injection site), patients who are blind, patients with severe arthritis, or patients with abnormal penile anatomy.[22,24]

Intraurethral Alprostadil

Efficacy 10 Intraurethral alprostadil inserts are marketed as MUSE, which contains a medication pellet inside a prefilled urethral applicator. Multiple studies show this product has an overall effectiveness rate of 43% to 65%[22] compared with 70% to 90% for intracavernosal alprostadil. Its decreased effectiveness and inconvenient administration method have resulted in this product being considered a second- or third-line treatment option for patients with erectile dysfunction.[67] However, some patients have responded to intraurethral alprostadil even though they did not respond to intracavernosal alprostadil or sildenafil.[73]

Intraurethral alprostadil has been combined with a VED to improve treatment response.[30,32]

The voluntary dropout rate is high and has been reported to be 57% and 75% after 3 and 15 months, respectively.[22] Intraurethral alprostadil should be avoided in patients with urethral stricture or urethritis, or if the female partner is pregnant.

Pharmacokinetics Following intraurethral instillation, alprostadil is absorbed quickly through the urethra, into the corpus spongiosum, and then into the corpora cavernosum.[24] As much as 80%

of each dose is absorbed by the urethra and corpus spongiosum in less than 10 minutes, with peak absorption occurring in 20 to 25 minutes. An estimated 20% of each dose is delivered to the corpora cavernosum. As with intracavernosal injections of alprostadil, any drug absorbed into the systemic circulation is rapidly metabolized on first pass through the lungs.

The onset after intraurethral insertion is similar to that of intracavernosal injection, 5 to 10 minutes, and the duration is 30 to 60 minutes.

Dosing The usual dosage range of intraurethral alprostadil is 125 to 1,000 mcg, but 500 mcg is typically needed in most patients.[22] It is recommended that the first dose be administered under the supervision of a health professional.[24] The dose should be administered 5 to 10 minutes before sexual intercourse. Not more than two doses per day are recommended. Before administration, the patient should be advised to empty his bladder, voiding completely (see Table 103-4).

Similar to intracavernosal injection treatments, intraurethral insertion of alprostadil requires good manual and visual skills to minimize the risk of urethral injuries. Intraurethral alprostadil is supplied in a prefilled intraurethral applicator. The patient should void first to moisten the urethra. With one hand the patient holds the glans penis, and with the other hand, the patient inserts the intraurethral applicator 0.5 in. (1.3 cm) into the urethra. The drug pellet is then pushed into the urethra. The penis should be massaged to enhance drug dissolution in the urethral fluids and drug absorption (Fig. 103-6).

Adverse Effects The urethra can be injured because of an improper administration technique. Injuries can lead to urethral bleeding or stricture and difficulty voiding. Patients should receive complete education about optimal administration procedures before starting treatment.

Urethral pain has been reported in 24% to 43% of patients. Usually, it is mild and does not require discontinuation of treatment. Approximately 6% of female sexual partners may experience vaginal burning, itching, or pain, which probably is related to transfer of alprostadil from the man's urethra to the woman's vagina during intercourse.[22,30]

Prolonged painful erections (priapism) have been rarely reported. Syncope and dizziness have been reported rarely (only 2%-3% of patients) and likely are related to use of excessively large doses.

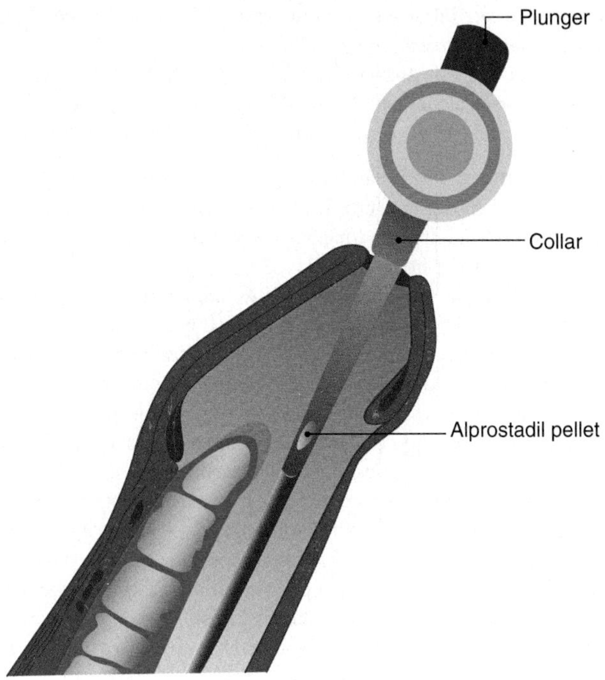

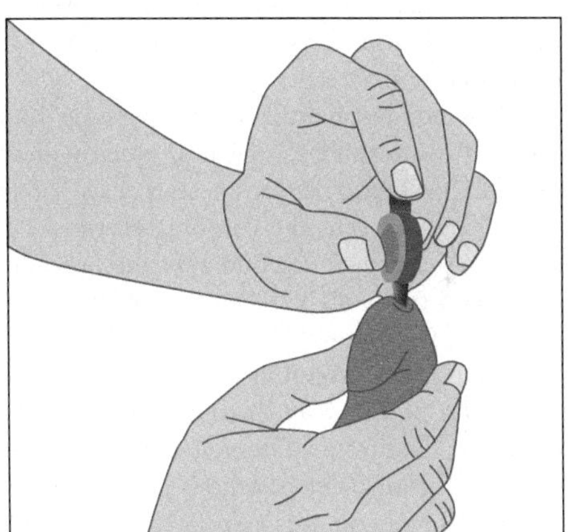

FIGURE 103-6 Technique for administration of intraurethral alprostadil with a medicated urethral system for erection applicator. (*Source: Muse [package insert]. Mountain View, CA: Vivus, Inc.; 2003. https://medlibrary.org/lib/rx/meds/muse. Accessed November 1, 2018.*)

Unapproved Agents

A variety of other commercially available and investigational agents have been used for management of erectile dysfunction. Although it is beyond the scope of this chapter to discuss all of them, some of the more commonly used agents are discussed here.

Yohimbine Yohimbine, a tree-bark derivative also known as *yohimbe*, is widely used as an aphrodisiac. Yohimbine is a central α-2-adrenergic antagonistic that increases catecholamines and improves mood. Some investigators believe that yohimbine has peripheral proerectogenic effects. Yohimbine may reduce peripheral α-adrenergic tone, thereby permitting a predominant cholinergic tone, which could result in a vasodilatory response.[22,51] The usual oral dose is 6 to 15 mg three times per day.

Based on a meta-analysis of published studies that concluded that yohimbine is only mildly efficacious for psychogenic erectile dysfunction, the American Urological Association has cautioned against the use of yohimbine.[22] In addition, yohimbine can cause many systemic adverse effects, including anxiety, insomnia, tachycardia, and hypertension.

Papaverine Papaverine is a nonspecific phosphodiesterase type 5 inhibitor that decreases metabolic catabolism of cAMP in cavernosal tissue. As a result of enhanced tissue levels of cAMP, smooth muscle relaxation occurs. Cavernosal sinusoids fill with blood, and a penile erection results.

Papaverine is not FDA-approved for erectile dysfunction. Intracavernosal papaverine alone is not commonly used for management of erectile dysfunction because the large doses required to achieve a therapeutic effect also produce dose-related adverse effects, such as priapism, corporal fibrosis, hypotension, and hepatotoxicity.[22] Papaverine is more often administered in lower doses combined with phentolamine and/or alprostadil. A variety of formulas have been used, but no one mixture has been proven better than other mixtures. Combination formulations are considered safer and are associated with the potential for fewer serious adverse effects than high doses of any one of these agents.

A portion of each papaverine dose is systemically absorbed, and its prolonged plasma half-life of 1 hour contributes to adverse effects. The usual dose of papaverine is 7.5 to 60 mg when used as a single agent for intracavernosal injection. When used in combination, the dose decreases to 0.5 to 20 mg.

If treated with papaverine, patients with a history of underlying liver disease or alcohol abuse should undergo liver function testing at baseline and every 6 to 12 months during continued treatment.

Phentolamine Phentolamine is a competitive nonselective α-adrenergic blocking agent. It reduces peripheral adrenergic tone and enhances cholinergic tone. As a result, it improves cavernosal filling and is proerectogenic.[22]

Phentolamine has most often been administered as an intracavernosal injection. Monotherapy is avoided because large doses are required for an erection, and at these large doses systemic hypotensive adverse effects would be prevalent. Most often, phentolamine has been used in combination with other vasoactive agents for intracavernosal administration. A ratio of 30-mg papaverine to 0.5 to 1 mg phentolamine is typical, and the usual dose ranges from 0.1 to 1 mL of the mixture. Such a mixture minimizes systemic hypotensive adverse effects.

Hypotension is the most common adverse effect of intracavernosal phentolamine. It is more common and more severe with large doses or in patients with a poor injection technique who have injected into a vein (rather than the cavernosa). Prolonged erections have been reported in patients who used excessive doses of intracavernosal medications in combination.

Surgical Therapy

Penile Prostheses Surgical insertion of a penile prosthesis is the most invasive treatment of erectile dysfunction. It is reserved for patients who do not respond to or who are not candidates for less invasive medical treatments or devices.

Prosthesis insertion requires anesthesia, an operating room, and a skilled urologist. Two prostheses are widely used: malleable and inflatable. Malleable or semirigid prostheses consist of two bendable rods that are inserted into the corpora cavernosa. The patient appears to have a permanent erection after the procedure; the patient is able to bend the penis into position at the time of intercourse.[22,31,74,75]

The inflatable prosthesis has several mechanical parts, including a pump, reservoir, and fillable cylinders. Once it is manually activated, a pump transfers fluid from a reservoir into the cylinders in the corpora cavernosa. The inflatable prosthesis produces a more natural erection, and for this reason, it is associated with a higher patient satisfaction rate than a malleable prosthesis.[72,73] The patient develops an erection only when the device is activated. Inflatable prostheses are available as 2- or 3-piece devices; fewer mechanical parts are associated with fewer malfunctions. With improvements in technology, inflatable devices can be placed during shorter surgical procedures and have a low 10-year mechanical failure rate (5%-15%) as compared with the original inflatable prostheses (Fig. 103-7).[22,74]

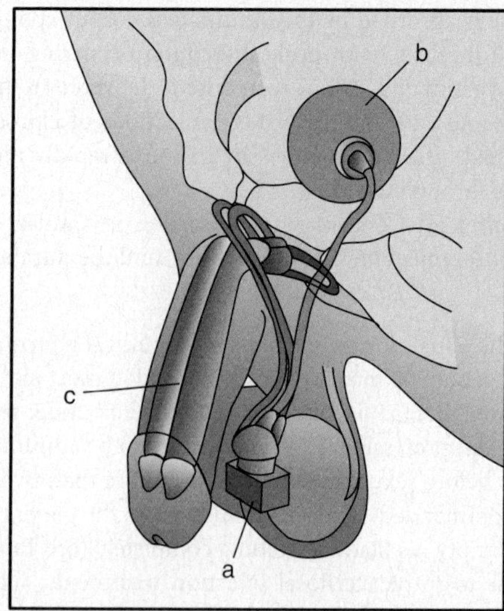

FIGURE 103-7 Example of surgically implanted penile prosthesis. (a, activation mechanism; b, reservoir with fluid for inflating prosthesis; c, inflatable rods in corpora.) *(Reprinted from the National Institutes of Health/National Institute of Diabetes and Digestive and Kidney Diseases.)*

Penile prostheses provide penile rigidity suitable for vaginal intercourse and are associated with a greater than 90% patient satisfaction rate, which is generally higher than that observed with any other drug treatment or VED. The surgical success rate after insertion is 82% to 98%.[74]

Adverse effects of prosthesis insertion can occur early or late after the surgical procedure. The most common early complication is infection. Late complications include mechanical failure of the prosthesis, erosion of the rods through the penis, or late-onset infection. Although some salvage procedures have been devised, in many cases the prosthesis requires removal.[75]

EVALUATION OF THERAPEUTIC OUTCOMES

The primary therapeutic outcomes of specific treatments for erectile dysfunction include (a) improvement in the quantity and quality of penile erections suitable for intercourse and (b) avoidance of adverse drug reactions and drug interactions.

At baseline and after the patient has completed a clinical trial period of several weeks with a specific treatment for erectile dysfunction, the physician should conduct assessments to determine whether the quality and quantity of penile erections have improved. A patient's level of satisfaction is highly individualized, depending on his lifestyle and expectations. Therefore, a patient who has successful intercourse once per week might be completely satisfied, whereas another patient might judge this to be unsatisfactory. Patients with unrealistic expectations in this regard must be identified and counseled by clinicians to avoid adverse effects of excessive use of erectogenic agents.

Failure to improve the quality and quantity of penile erections suitable for intercourse after an appropriate clinical trial period with a specific treatment for erectile dysfunction occurs in a significant percentage of patients. In this case, physicians generally take the following steps to:

1. Ensure that the patient has been prescribed a maximum tolerated medication dose and has an adequate clinical trial of a specific treatment before discarding it as ineffective.
2. Switch to another drug (see Fig. 103-2).
3. Reserve surgical treatment for patients who do not respond to drug treatment.

CONCLUSION

Erectile dysfunction is a common disorder of aging men. Its incidence is higher in patients with underlying medical disorders that compromise the vascular, neurologic, hormonal, or psychogenic systems necessary for a normal penile erection. Medications are common causes of erectile dysfunction. By correcting the underlying etiology, erectile dysfunction can often be reversed without the use of specific treatments. When treatment of erectile dysfunction is needed, the least invasive options should be used first because they produce the lowest incidence of serious adverse effects. Phosphodiesterase type 5 inhibitors are first-line treatment. If this fails or if the patient cannot use a phosphodiesterase type 5 inhibitor, a VED or intracavernosal injection or intraurethral alprostadil can be initiated. If this treatment fails, the patient can attempt a combination of intracavernosal alprostadil and VED, combination intracavernosal therapy, or intraurethral alprostadil. If this treatment fails, the patient may require insertion of a penile prosthesis. Some insurance companies do not reimburse for drug treatments for erectile dysfunction, so cost is an important issue for patients. Clinicians should provide clear and simple advice. Patient confidentiality and privacy, which are extremely important to men with erectile dysfunction, should be maintained at all times.

ABBREVIATIONS

cAMP	cyclic adenosine monophosphate
cGMP	cyclic guanosine monophosphate
CNS	central nervous system
IIEF	International Index of Erectile Function
LUTS	lower urinary tract symptoms
NAION	nonarteritic anterior ischemic optic neuropathy
REMS	risk evaluation and mitigation strategies
VED	vacuum erection device

REFERENCES

1. NIH Consensus Development Panel on Impotence. Impotence. NIH Consensus Development Panel on Impotence. *JAMA.* 1993;270(1):83–90.
2. Johannes CB, Aranjo AB, Feldman HA, et al. Incidence of erectile dysfunction in men 40–69 years old: Longitudinal results from the Massachusetts Male Aging Study. *J Urol.* 2000;163(2):460–463.
3. Bacon CG, Mittleman MA, Kawachi I, et al. Sexual function in men older than 50 years of age: Results from the health professionals follow-up study. *Ann Intern Med.* 2003;139(3):161–168.
4. Andersson KE. Mechanisms of penile erection and basis for pharmacological treatment of erectile dysfunction. *Pharmacol Rev.* 2011;63(4):811–859. doi:10.1124/pr.111.004515
5. Livingston M, Kalansooriya A, Hartland AJ, et al. Serum testosterone levels in male hypogonadism: Why and when to check-a review. *Int J Clin Pract.* 2017(Nov);71(11):e12995. doi:10.1111/ijcp.12995
6. McMahon CG. Current diagnosis and management of erectile dysfunction. *Med J Aust.* 2019(Jun);210(10):469–476. doi:10.5694/mja2.50167
7. Patel JP, Lee EH, Mena-Hurtado CI. Evaluation and management of erectile dysfunction in the hypertensive patient. *Curr Cardiol Rep.* 2017(Aug);19(9):89. doi:10.1007/s11886-017-0889-z
8. Imprialos K, Koutsampasopoulos K, Manolis A, Doumas M. Erectile dysfunction as a cardiovascular risk factor: Time to step up? *Curr Vasc Pharmacol.* 2021;19(3):301–312. doi:10.2174/1570161118666200414102556
9. Moussa M, Papatsoris A, Abou Chakra MA, et al. Erectile dysfunction in common neurological conditions: A narrative review. *Arch Ital Urol Androl.* 2020(Dec 21);92(4). doi:10.4081/aiua.2020.4.371
10. Nguyen HMT, Gabrielson AT, Hellstrom WJG. Erectile dysfunction in young men—A review of the prevalence and risk factors. *Sex Med Rev.* 2017(Oct);5(4):508–520. doi:10.1016/j.sxmr.2017.05.004
11. Nieschlag E. Late-onset hypogonadism: A concept comes of age. *Andrology.* 2020(Nov);8(6):1506–1511. doi:10.1111/andr.12719
12. Bhasin S, Brito JP, Cunningham GR, et al. Testosterone therapy in men with hypogonadism: An Endocrine Society clinical practice guideline. *J Clin Endocrinol Metab.* 2018(May 1);103(5):1715–1744. doi:10.1210/jc2018-00229
13. Voznesensky I, DeLay KJ, Hellstrom WJG. Advances in pharmacotherapy for erectile dysfunction and associated cardiac output. *Expert Opin Pharmacother.* 2016(Dec);17(17):2281–2289. doi:10.1080/146566.2016.1241766
14. Imprialos KP, Stavropoulos K, Doumas M, et al. Sexual dysfunction, cardiovascular risk, and effects of pharmacotherapy. *Curr Vasc Pharmacol.* 2018(Jan);16(2):130–142. doi:10.2174/15701611115666170609101502
15. Razdan S, Greer AB, Alameddine M, et al. Effect of prescription medications on erectile dysfunction. *Postgrad Med J.* 2018(Mar);94(1109):171–178. doi:10.1136/postgradmedj-2017-135233
16. Hackett G, Kirby M, Edwards D, et al. British Society for Sexual Medicine guidelines on adult testosterone deficiency, with statements for UK practice. *J Sex Med.* 2017(Dec);14(12):1504–1523. doi:10.1016/J.JSXM.2017.10.067
17. Hernandez-Cerda J, Bertomeu-Gonzalez V, Zuazola P, Cordero A. Understanding erectile dysfunction in hypertensive patients: The need for good patient management. *Vasc Health Risk Manag.* 2020(Jun 12);16:231–239. doi:10.2147/VHRM.S223331
18. Manolis A, Doumas M, Ferri C, Mancia G. Erectile dysfunction and adherence to antihypertensive therapy: Focus on β-blockers. *Eur J Intern Med.* 2020(Nov);81:1–6. doi:10.1016/j.ejim.2020.07.009
19. Patel JP, Lee EH, Mena-Hurtado CI, Walker CN. Evaluation and management of erectile dysfunction in the hypertensive patient. *Curr Cardiol Rep.* 2017;19:89. doi:10.1008/s11886-017-0889-z
20. Corona G, Tirabassi G, Santi D, et al. Sexual dysfunction in subjects treated with inhibitors of 5α-reductase for benign prostatic hyperplasia: A comprehensive review and meta-analysis. *Andrology.* 2017(Jul);5(4):671–678. doi:10.1111/andro.12353
21. Traish AM. Post-finasteride syndrome: A surmountable challenge for clinicians. *Fertil Steril.* 2020 Jan;113(1):21–50. doi:w.1016/j.fertnstert.2019.11.030
22. Burnett AL, Nehra A, Breau RH, et al. Erectile dysfunction: AUA Guideline. *J Urol.* 2018(Sep);200(3):633–641. doi:10.1016/j.juro.2018.05.004
23. Yafi FA, Huynh LM, Ahlering T, Rosen R. What is a "validated questionnaire"? A critical review of erectile function assessment. *J Sex Med.* 2020(May);17(5):849–860. doi:10.1016/j.jsm.2020.02.005
24. Bennett N Jr. Sexual dysfunction-behavioral, medical, and surgical treatment. *Med Clin N Am.* 2018(Mar);102(2):349–360. doi:10.1016/j.mcna.2017.10.010
25. Capogrosso P, Ventimiglia E, Oreggia D, et al. Medical treatment of erectile dysfunction: Too many medical prescriptions. *Urologia.* 2017(Aug 17;84(3):121–129.
26. Nehra A, Jackson G, Miner M, et al. The Princeton III Consensus recommendations for the management of erectile dysfunction and cardiovascular disease. *Mayo Clin Proc.* 2012(Aug);87(8):766–778. doi:10.1016/j.mayocp.2012.06.015
27. Duca Y, Calogero AE, Cannarella R, et al. Erectile dysfunction, physical activity and physical exercise: Recommendations for clinical practice. *Andrologia.* 2019(Jun);51(5):e13264. doi:10.1111/and.13264.
28. Mitidieri E, Cirino G, d'Emmanuele di Villa Bianca RD, Sorrentino R. Pharmacology and perspectives in erectile dysfunction in man. *Pharmacol Ther.* 2020(Apr);208:107493. doi:10.1016j.pharmthera.2020.107493 0163-7258
29. La J, Roberts NH, Yafi FA. Diet and men's sexual health. *Sex Med Rev.* 2018(Jan);6(1):54–68. doi.org/10.1016/jsxmr.2017.07.004
30. Hatzimouratidis K, Salonia A, Adaikan G, et al. Pharmacotherapy for erectile dysfunction: Recommendations from the Fourth International Consultation for Sexual Medicine (ICSM 2015). *J Sex Med.* 2016(Apr);13(4):465–488. doi:10.1016/j.jsxm.2016.01.016
31. Trost LW, Munarriz R, Wang R, et al. External mechanical devices and vascular surgery for erectile dysfunction. *J Sex Med.* 2016(Nov);13(11):1579–1617. doi:10.1016/j.jsxm.2016.09.008
32. Lee M, Sharifi R. Non-invasive management options for erectile dysfunction when a phosphodiesterase type 5 inhibitor fails. *Drugs Aging.* 2018(Mar);35(3):175–187. doi:10.1007/s40266-018-0528-4
33. Zhang DL, Chen Z, Wang FX, et al. Adding a vacuum erection device to regular use of tadalafil improves penile rehabilitation after posterior urethroplasty. *Asian J Androl.* 2019(Nov-Dec);21(6):582–586. doi:10.4103/aja.aja_50_19
34. Scaglione F, Donde S, Hassan TA, Jannini EA. Phosphodiesterase type 5 inhibitors for the treatment of erectile dysfunction: Pharmacology and clinical impact of the sildenafil citrate orodispersible tablet formulation. *Clin Ther.* 2017(Feb);39(2):370–377. doi:10.1016/j.clinthera.2017.01.001
35. Hong JH, Kwon YS, Kim IY. Pharmacodynamics, pharmacokinetics, and clinical efficacy of phosphodiesterase-5 inhibitors. *Expert Opin Drug Metab Toxicol.* 2017(Feb);13(2):199–192. doi:10.1080/1742555.2017.1244265
36. Boeri L, Capogrosso P, Ventimiglia E, et al. Avanafil-a further step to tailoring patient needs and expectations. *Expert Rev Clin Pharmacol.* 2016(Sep);9(9):1171–1181. doi:10.1080/17512433.2016.1195261
37. Zurawin JL, Stewart CA, Anaissie JE, et al. Avanafil for the treatment of erectile dysfunction. *Expert Rev Clin Pharmacol.* 2016(Sep);9(9):1163–1170. doi:10.1080/17512433.2016.1212655
38. Le TV, Tsambarlis P, Hellstrom WJG. Pharmacodynamics of the agents used for the treatment of erectile dysfunction. *Expert Opin Drug Metab Toxicol.* 2019(Feb 4);15(2):121–131. doi:10.1080/17425255.2019.1560421

39. Zucchi A, Costantini E, Scroppo FI, et al. The first-generation phosphodiesterase 5 inhibitors and their pharmacokinetic issues. *Andrology*. 2019(Nov);7(6):804–817. doi:10.1111/andr.12683
40. Yafi FA, Jenkins L, Albersen M, et al. Erectile dysfunction. *Nat Rev Dis Primers*. 2016(Feb 4);2:16003. doi:10.1038/nrdp.2016.3
41. Corona G, Rastrelli G, Burri A, et al. First-generation phosphodiesterase type 5 inhibitors dropout: A comprehensive review and meta-analysis. *Andrology*. 2016(Nov);4(6):1002–1009. doi:10.1111/andr.12255
42. Peng Z, Yang L, Dong Q, et al. Efficacy and safety of tadalafil once-a-day versus tadalafil on-demand in patients with erectile dysfunction: A systematic review and meta-analyses. *Urol Int*. 2017;99(3):343–352. doi:10.1159/000477496
43. McMahon CG. High dose sildenafil as a salvage therapy for severe erectile dysfunction. *Int J Impot Res*. 2002;14(6):533–538.
44. Moncada I, Martinez-Salamanca J, Ruiz-Castane E, Romero J. Combination therapy for erectile dysfunction involving a PDE5 inhibitor and alprostadil. *Int J Impot Res*. 2018(Oct);30(5):203–208.
45. Irwin GM. Erectile dysfunction. *Prim Care*. 2019(Jun);46(2):249–255. doi:10.1016/j.pop.2019.02.006
46. Osmonov DK, Junemann KP, Bannowsky A. The "Kiel Concept: Of long-term administration of daily low-dose sildenafil initiated in the immediate post-prostatectomy period: Evaluation and comparison with the international literature on penile rehabilitation. *Sex Med Rev*. 2017(Jul);5(3):387–392. doi.org/10.1016/jsxmr.2017.03.002
47. Ventimiglia E, Capogrosso P, Montorsi F, Salonia A. The safety of phosphodiesterase type 5 inhibitors for erectile dysfunction. *Expert Opin Drug Saf*. 2016;15(2):141–152. doi:10.1517/14740338.2016.1131818
48. McMahon C. Efficacy and safety of daily tadalafil in men with erectile dysfunction previously unresponsive to on demand tadalafil. *J Sex Med*. 2004(Nov);1(3):292–300. doi:10.1111/j.1743-6109.04042
49. McMahon C. Comparison, efficacy, and tolerability of on demand tadalafil and daily dosed tadalafil for the treatment of erectile dysfunction. *J Sex Med*. 2005(May);2(3):415–425. doi:10.1111/j.1743-6109.2005.20360.x
50. Yafi FA, Sharlip ID, Becher EF. Update on the safety of phosphodiesterase type 5 inhibitors for the treatment of erectile dysfunction. *Sex Med Rev*. 2018(Apr);6(2):242–252. doi:10.1016/j.sxmr.2017.08.001
51. Gul M, Serefoglu EC. An update on the drug safety of treating erectile dysfunction. *Expert Opin Drug Saf*. 2019(Oct);18(10):965–975. doi:10.1080/1440338.2019.1659244
52. Gong B, Ming M, Xie W, et al. Direct comparison of tadalafil with sildenafil for the treatment of erectile dysfunction: A systematic review and meta-analysis. *Int Urol Nephrol*. 2017(Oct);49(10):1731–1740. doi:10.1007/s11255-017-1644-5
53. Madiera CR, Tonin FS, Fachi MM, et al. Efficacy and safety or oral phosphodiesterase 5 inhibitors for erectile dysfunction: A network meta-analysis and multicriteria decision analysis. *World J Urol*. 2021(Mar);39(3):953–962. doi/org/10.1007/s00345-020-03233-9
54. Kloner RA, Goggin P, Goldstein I, et al. A new perspective on the nitrate-phosphodiesterase type 5 inhibitor interaction. *J Cardiovasc Pharmacol Ther*. 2018(Sept);23(5):375–386. doi:10.1177/1074248418771896
55. Moschos MM, Nitoda E. Pathophysiology of visual disorders induced by phosphodiesterase inhibitors in the treatment of erectile dysfunction. *Drug Des Devel Ther*. 2016(Oct 19);8:3407–3413. doi:102147/DDDT.S118015
56. Pomeranz HD. Erectile dysfunction agents and nonarteritic anterior ischemic optic neuropathy. *Neurol Clin*. 2017(Feb);35(1):17–27. doi:10.1016/j.ncl.2016.08.007
57. Loeb S, Ventigmiglia E, Salonia A, et al. Meta-analysis of the association between phosphodiesterase inhibitors (PDE5Is) and risk of melanoma. *J Natl Cancer Inst*. 2017(Aug);109(8):djx086. doi:10.1093/jnci/djx086
58. Han X, Han Y, Zheng Y, et al. Use of phosphodiesterase type 5 inhibitors and risk of melanoma: A meta-analysis of observational studies. *Onco Targets Ther*. 2018(Feb);11:711–720. doi:10.2147/OTT.s142637
59. Rastrelli G, Guaraldi F, Reismann Y, et al. Testosterone replacement therapy for sexual symptoms. *Sex Med Rev*. 2019(Jul);7(3):464–475. doi:10.1016/j.sxmr.2018.11.005
60. Mulhall JP, Trost LW, Brannigan RE, et al. Evaluation and management of testosterone deficiency: AUA guideline. *J Urol*. 2018(Aug);200(2):423–32. doi:10.1016/j.juro.2018.03.115
61. Dohle GR, Arver S, Bettochi C, et al. EAU guidelines office, 2018. Available at https://uroweb.org/guideline/male-hypogonadism/. Last accessed October 2, 2021.
62. Salter CA, Mulhall JP. Guideline of guidelines: Testosterone therapy for testosterone deficiency. *BJU Int*. 2019(Nov);124(5):722–729. doi:10.1111/bju.14899
63. Anon. Testosterone nasal gel (Natesto) for hypogonadism. *Med Lett Drugs Ther*. 2015 (May 11);57(1468):73–74.
64. Morely JE, Charlton E, Patrick P, et al. Validation of a screening questionnaire for androgen deficiency in aging males. *Metabolism*. 2000(Sept);49(9):1239–1242. doi:10.1053/meta.2000.8625
65. Sansone A, Sansone M, Selleri R, et al. Monitoring testosterone replacement therapy with transdermal gel: When and how? *J Endocrinol Invest*. 2019(Dec);41(12):1491–1496. doi.org/10.1007/s40618-019-01082-x
66. Elkhoury FF, Rambhatla A, Mills JN, Rajfer J. Cardiovascular health, erectile dysfunction, and testosterone replacement: Controversies and correlations. *Urology*. 2017(Dec);110:1–8. doi:10.1016/j.urology.2017.07.030
67. Karakus S, Burnett AL. The medical and surgical treatment of erectile dysfunction: A review and update. *Can J Urol*. 2020(Aug);27(S3):28–35.
68. Vigen R, O'Donnell CI, Baron AE, et al. Association of testosterone therapy with mortality, myocardial infarction and stroke in men with low testosterone levels. *JAMA*. 2013(Nov);310(17):1829–1836. doi:10.1001/jama.2013.280386
69. Finkle WD, Greenland S, Ridgeway GK, et al. Increased risk of nonfatal myocardial infarction following testosterone therapy prescription in men. *PLoS One*. 2014(Jan);9(1):e85805. doi:10.1371/jouornal.pone.00885805.ecollection2014
70. Elsherbiny A, Tricomi M, Bhatt D, Dandapantula HK. State-of-the-art: a review of cardiovascular effects of testosterone replacement therapy in adult males. *Curr Cardiol Rep*. 2017(Apr);19(4):35. doi:10.1007/s11886-017-0838-x
71. Corona G, Rastrelli G, Pasquale G, et al. Testosterone and cardiovascular risk: Meta-analysis of interventional studies. *J Sex Med*. 2018;15(6):820–838. doi:10.1016/j.jsxm.2018.04.641
72. Santella C, Renoux C, Yin H, et al. Testosterone replacement therapy and the risk of prostate cancer in men with late-onset hypogonadism. *Am J Epidemiol*. 2019(Sep);188(9):1666–1673. doi:10.1093/aje/kwz138
73. Engel JD, McVary KT. Transurethral alprostadil as therapy for patients who withdrew from or failed prior intracavernous injection therapy. *Urology*. 1998(May);51(5):687–692. doi:10.1016/s0090-4295(98)0093-4
74. Barnard JT, Cakir OO, Ralpah D, Yafi FA. Technological advances in penile implant surgery. *J Sex Med*. 2021(Jul);18(7):1158–1166. doi:10.1016/j.jsxm.2021.04.011
75. Scherzer NK, Dick B, Gabrielson AT, et al. Penile prosthesis complications: Planning, prevention, and decision making. *Sex Med Rev*. 2019(Apr);7(2):349–359. doi.org/10.1016/j.sxmr.2018.04.002

104

Benign Prostatic Hyperplasia

Mary Lee and Roohollah Sharifi

KEY CONCEPTS

1. Although symptomatic benign prostatic hyperplasia (BPH) is rare in men younger than 50 years, it is common in men aged 60 years and older. Prostate growth is androgen-dependent. Symptoms commonly result from both static and dynamic factors.

2. BPH symptoms may be exacerbated by medications, including antihistamines, phenothiazines, tricyclic antidepressants, and anticholinergic agents. In these cases, discontinuing the causative agent can relieve symptoms.

3. For patients with mild disease who are asymptomatic or have mildly bothersome symptoms and no complications of BPH disease, watchful waiting is indicated. Watchful waiting includes behavior modification, lifestyle modification, discontinuation of medications that contribute to voiding symptoms, and return visits to the physician at 6- or 12-month intervals for assessment of worsening symptoms or signs of bladder outlet obstruction.

4. If symptoms progress to a moderate or severe level, drug therapy or surgery is indicated. α_1-Adrenergic antagonists quickly relieve voiding symptoms, but do not prevent disease progression. 5α-Reductase inhibitors delay symptom progression and reduce the incidence of BPH-related complications in patients with prostates of at least 30 to 40 g, but may not reduce voiding symptoms for 3 to 6 months.

5. All α_1-adrenergic antagonists are equally effective in relieving BPH symptoms. Older second-generation immediate-release formulations of α_1-adrenergic antagonists (eg, terazosin, doxazosin) can cause adverse cardiovascular effects, mainly first-dose syncope, orthostatic hypotension, and dizziness. For patients who cannot tolerate these hypotensive adverse effects, a third-generation, pharmacologically uroselective α_{1A}-adrenergic antagonist (eg, tamsulosin, silodosin) or an extended-release formulation of alfuzosin, a second-generation, functionally uroselective agent, is a good alternative.

6. 5α-Reductase inhibitors are useful primarily for patients with large prostates greater than 40 g who wish to avoid surgery and cannot tolerate the side effects of α_1-adrenergic antagonists. 5α-Reductase inhibitors have a slow onset of action, taking up to 6 months to exert maximal clinical effects, which is a disadvantage of their use, especially as single-drug therapy for BPH. In addition, decreased libido, erectile dysfunction, and ejaculation disorders are common adverse effects, which may be troublesome in sexually active patients.

7. Phosphodiesterase type 5 inhibitors can be used in patients with moderate-to-severe BPH and erectile dysfunction. They improve obstructive and irritative voiding symptoms, but do not significantly increase urinary flow rate or reduce postvoid residual (PVR) urine volume. Hence, a phosphodiesterase type 5 inhibitor is considered less effective than an α-adrenergic antagonist for BPH. A phosphodiesterase type 5 inhibitor may be used alone; however, symptom improvement and an increase in peak urinary flow rate have been demonstrated when it is used along with an α-adrenergic antagonist or a 5α-reductase inhibitor.

8. Anticholinergic agents are indicated in patients with moderate-to-severe lower urinary tract symptoms (LUTS) with a predominance of irritative voiding symptoms. In this case, the drugs are commonly added to an existing regimen of an α_1-adrenergic antagonist or a 5α-reductase inhibitor. Because older patients are at high risk of systemic and central nervous system anticholinergic adverse effects, uroselective anticholinergic agents or those with a low potential to cross the blood brain barrier are preferred over nonuroselective agents. To minimize the risk of acute urinary retention, anticholinergics should be used cautiously in patients when baseline PVR urine volume is greater than 100 to 150 mL. In addition, the anticholinergic medication burden should be assessed by examining the patient's medication profile before starting an anticholinergic agent.

9. β_3-Adrenergic agonists relax the detrusor muscle to increase the bladder's storage capacity and prolong the interval between voidings. These medications are indicated for treatment of overactive bladder symptoms, including urgency and nocturia, which mimic irritative lower urinary tract voiding symptoms. Thus, a β_3-adrenergic agonist is an alternative to an anticholinergic agent in patients with irritative voiding symptoms that do not respond to α_1-adrenergic antagonists or in patients who cannot tolerate anticholinergic adverse effects.

10. Surgery is indicated for severe symptoms of BPH for patients who do not respond to or do not tolerate drug therapy, or for patients with complications of BPH. It is the most effective mode of treatment because it relieves symptoms and increases peak urinary flow rate in the greatest number of men with BPH. However, the two conventional techniques, transurethral resection of the prostate (TURP) and open prostatectomy, are associated with the highest rates of complications, including retrograde ejaculation and erectile dysfunction. Moreover, because medications are first-line treatment for patients with moderate-to-severe symptoms of BPH, patients who are surgical candidates are often older and more frail. Therefore, minimally invasive surgical procedures are often sought by patients and urologists. Such procedures relieve symptoms and are associated with a lower rate of adverse effects and do not require hospitalization, but they have higher reoperation rates than the standard procedures.

BEYOND THE BOOK

Go to a reference text on anatomy and physiology and review the section on the biological male genitourinary tract. Draw a diagram of these organs that shows the anatomical relationship of the kidneys, ureters, urinary bladder, prostate, urethra, and testicles. Then explain how an enlarged prostate could cause obstruction of urinary outflow from the bladder and lead to overflow incontinence, recurrent urinary tract infection, and renal failure.

INTRODUCTION

Benign prostatic hyperplasia (BPH) is the most common benign neoplasm of American men. A nearly ubiquitous condition among elderly men, BPH is of major societal concern, given the large number of men affected, the progressive nature of the condition, and the healthcare costs associated with it. This chapter discusses BPH and its available treatments: watchful waiting, α_1-adrenergic antagonists, 5α-reductase inhibitors, phosphodiesterase inhibitors, anticholinergic agents, β_3-adrenergic agonist, and surgery. The limitations of phytotherapy are described.

Editors' note: In this and other chapters in Pharmacotherapy, *references to biologic gender (as assigned at birth) are used based on prior literature being discussed or anatomical or physiologic differences. We recognize that not all individuals identify with their gender at birth, and to the degree possible when discussing therapeutics, we avoid use of references to gender. In this chapter, gender is used in discussing prior studies, published guidelines, and other recommendations for diagnosis and treatment based on biological gender and does not necessarily reflect an individual's gender identity.*

EPIDEMIOLOGY

According to the results of autopsy studies, approximately 80% of older men develop histologic evidence of BPH. About half of the patients with microscopic changes develop an enlarged prostate gland, and as a result, they may develop symptoms including difficulty emptying urine from the urinary bladder. Approximately half of symptomatic patients eventually require treatment. Thus, the disease can be characterized by three stages: Benign prostatic hyperplasia (BPH), benign prostatic enlargement (BPE), and benign prostatic obstruction (BPO). While BPH itself may not require treatment, some patients with BPE, depending on the size of the prostate, will be at risk of developing complications of BPH. In these patients, 5α-reductase inhibitors can reduce disease complications and delay the need for prostate surgery. In patients with moderate-to-severe BPO, bothersome voiding symptoms require medical or surgical treatment.

1 The peak incidence of clinical BPH occurs between ages 63 and 65 years. Symptomatic disease is uncommon in men younger than 50 years, but some urinary voiding symptoms are present by the time men reach 60 years of age. The Boston Area Normative Aging Study estimated that the cumulative incidence of clinical BPH was 78% for patients at age 80 years.[1] Similarly, the Baltimore Longitudinal Study of Aging projected that approximately 60% of men at least 60 years old develop clinical BPO.[2]

NORMAL PROSTATE PHYSIOLOGY

Located anterior to the rectum, the prostate is a small heart-shaped, chestnut-sized gland located below the urinary bladder. It surrounds the proximal urethra like a doughnut.

Soft, symmetric, and mobile on palpation, a normal prostate gland in an adult man weighs 15 to 20 g. Physical examination of the prostate must be done by digital rectal examination during which the prostate is manually palpated by inserting a finger into the rectum. Thus, the prostate is examined through the rectal wall.

The prostate gland comprises three layers: an innermost transition zone, a middle central zone, and an outermost peripheral zone.

The prostate has two major functions: (a) to secrete fluids that make up a portion (20%-40%) of the ejaculate volume and (b) to provide secretions with antibacterial effect possibly related to its high concentration of zinc.

ETIOLOGY

The etiologies of BPH include: (a) patient age of 40 years or more; (b) the stimulatory effect of androgens; (c) increased α-adrenergic tone in smooth muscle of the prostate and prostatic urethra; and (d) chronic inflammation of the prostate.

Patient Age of 40 Years or More

At birth, the prostate is the size of a pea and weighs approximately 1 g. The prostate remains that size until the boy reaches puberty. At that time, the prostate undergoes its first growth spurt, growing to its normal adult size of 15 to 20 g by the time the man is 25 to 30 years old. The prostate remains this size until the patient reaches the age of 40 years, when a second growth spurt begins and continues for the rest of his lifetime. During this second growth spurt, BPE develops.[3]

Stimulatory Effect of Androgens and Increased α-Adrenergic Tone

The prostate gland comprises three types of tissue: epithelial tissue, stromal tissue, and the capsule. Epithelial tissue, also known as *glandular tissue*, produces prostatic secretions. These secretions are delivered into the urethra during ejaculation and contribute to the total ejaculate volume. Androgens stimulate epithelial tissue growth. Stromal tissue, also known as *smooth muscle tissue*, is embedded predominantly with α_1-adrenergic receptors, predominately of the α_{1A} subtype. Stimulation of these receptors by norepinephrine causes smooth muscle contraction, which results in an extrinsic compression of the urethra, reduction of the urethral lumen, and decreased urinary bladder emptying. The normal prostate is composed of a higher amount of stromal tissue than epithelial tissue, as reflected by a stromal-to-epithelial tissue ratio of 2:1. This ratio is exaggerated to 5:1 for patients with BPH, which explains why α_1-adrenergic antagonists are quickly effective for symptomatic management and why 5α-reductase inhibitors reduce an enlarged prostate gland by only 25%.[3] The capsule, or outer shell of the prostate, is composed of fibrous connective tissue and smooth muscle, which also is embedded with α_1-adrenergic receptors. When stimulated with norepinephrine, the capsule contracts around the prostatic urethra (Fig. 104-1).

Testosterone is the principal testicular androgen in males, whereas androstenedione is the principal adrenal androgen. These two hormones are responsible for penile and scrotal enlargement, increased muscle mass, and maintenance of the normal male libido. These androgens are converted by 5α-reductase in target cells to dihydrotestosterone (DHT), an active metabolite. Two types of 5α-reductase exist. Type I enzyme is localized to sebaceous glands in the frontal scalp, liver, and skin, although a small amount is in the prostate. DHT produced at these target tissues causes acne and increased body and facial hair. Type II enzyme is localized to the prostatic stroma, genital tissue, and hair follicles of the scalp. In the prostate, DHT induces growth and enlargement of the gland.[3]

In prostate cells, DHT has greater affinity for intraprostatic androgen receptors than testosterone, and DHT forms a more stable complex with the androgen receptor. Thus, DHT is considered

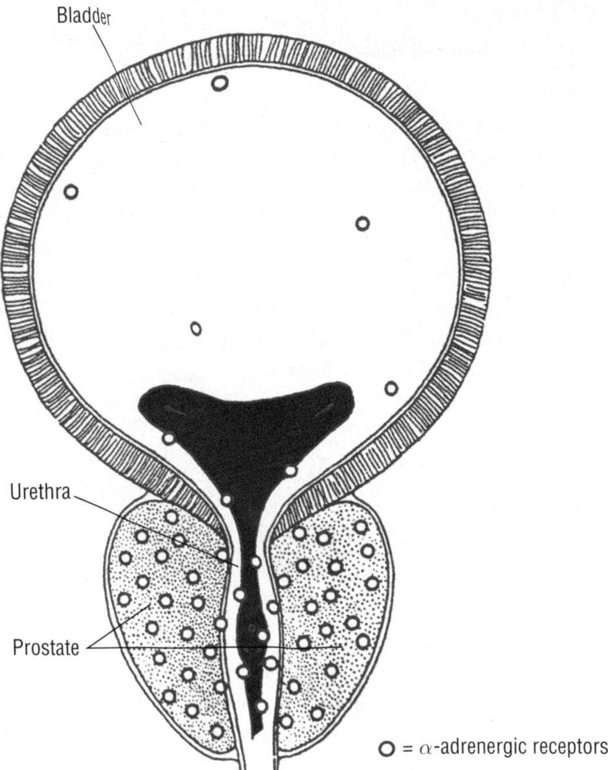

FIGURE 104-1 Representation of the anatomy of α-adrenergic receptor distribution in the prostate, urethra, and bladder. *(Reproduced from Narayan P, Indudhara R. Pharmacotherapy for benign prostatic hyperplasia. Western Journal of Medicine. 1994;161(5):495-506. Copyright © 1994 with permission from BMJ Publishing Group Ltd.)*

a more potent androgen than testosterone in the prostate. Of note, despite the decrease in testicular androgen production in the aging male, intracellular DHT levels in the prostate remain normal, probably due to increased activity of intraprostatic 5α-reductase.[4]

Estrogen, a product of peripheral metabolism of androgens, is believed to stimulate the growth of the stromal portion of the prostate gland. Estrogens are produced when testosterone and androstenedione are converted by aromatase enzymes in peripheral adipose tissues.[4] In addition, estrogens may induce the androgen receptor.[2] As men age, the ratio of serum levels of testosterone to estrogen decreases as a result of a decline in testosterone production by the testes and increased adipose tissue conversion of androgen to estrogen.

Chronic Inflammation of the Prostate

Chronic inflammation stimulates stromal cell growth in the prostate. In addition, inflammation causes cytokine release, which stimulates glandular epithelial tissue proliferation and transition zone enlargement. Proposed triggers for chronic inflammation include dyslipidemia, low serum testosterone, and hyperestrogenism, which have all been associated with metabolic syndrome, a common disorder of aging men and those with BPH.[5-7]

PATHOPHYSIOLOGY

Although the precise pathophysiologic mechanisms causing BPH remain unclear, the role of intraprostatic DHT and type II 5α-reductase in the development of BPH is evidenced by several observations:

1. BPH does not develop in men who are castrated before puberty.
2. Patients with type II 5α-reductase enzyme deficiency do not develop BPH.
3. Castration causes an enlarged prostate to shrink.
4. Administration of testosterone to orchiectomized dogs of advanced age produces BPH.

The pathogenesis of BPH is often described as resulting from both static and dynamic factors. Static factors relate to anatomic enlargement of the prostate gland, which produces a physical block at the bladder neck and thereby obstructs urinary outflow. Enlargement of the gland depends on androgen stimulation of epithelial tissue and estrogen stimulation of stromal tissue in the prostate. Dynamic factors relate to excessive α-adrenergic tone of the stromal component of the prostate gland, bladder neck, and posterior urethra, which results in contraction of the prostate gland around the urethra and narrowing of the urethral lumen.[5,7]

Obstructive voiding symptoms of BPH disease, which include decreased force of the urinary stream and incomplete bladder emptying, may result from static and/or dynamic factors, and this must be recognized when drug therapy is considered. For instance, some patients may present with obstructive voiding symptoms, but have prostates of normal size. In these patients, dynamic factors likely are responsible for the symptoms. However, for patients with enlarged prostate glands, static and dynamic factors likely are working in concert to produce the observed symptoms. Moreover, the likelihood of developing moderate-to-severe obstructive voiding symptoms is directly related to the increasing size of the prostate gland.[5,7]

Dynamic factors may be accentuated if the patient becomes stressed or is in pain. In these situations, increased α-adrenergic tone may precipitate excessive contraction of prostatic stromal tissue. When the stressful event resolves, voiding symptoms often improve.[2]

Irritative voiding symptoms of BPH disease, which include urinary frequency and urgency, result from long-standing bladder outlet obstruction. As BPH progresses, the bladder muscle undergoes hypertrophy so that it can generate a greater contractile force to empty urine past the anatomic obstruction at the bladder neck. Decompensation eventually occurs and the hypertrophied bladder muscle is no longer able to generate adequate contractile force; the bladder becomes ineffective in emptying urine. Acute urinary retention, recurrent urinary tract infections, and renal failure complicate progressive, untreated disease.[8]

MEDICATION-RELATED SYMPTOMS

2 Medications in several pharmacologic categories should be avoided for patients with BPH because they may exacerbate symptoms. Testosterone replacement regimens, used to treat primary or secondary hypogonadism, deliver additional substrate that can be metabolized to DHT by the prostate. Although no cases of BPH have been reported because of exogenous testosterone administration, cautious use is advised for older patients with prostatic enlargement. α-Adrenergic agonists, used as oral or intranasal decongestants (eg, pseudoephedrine, ephedrine, or phenylephrine), can stimulate α-adrenergic receptors in the prostate, resulting in muscle contraction. By decreasing the caliber of the urethral lumen, bladder emptying may be compromised. β-Adrenergic agonists (eg, terbutaline) may cause relaxation of the bladder detrusor muscle, which prevents bladder emptying.[6] Drugs with significant anticholinergic adverse effects (eg, antihistamines, phenothiazines, tricyclic antidepressants, or anticholinergic drugs used as antispasmodics or to treat Parkinson's disease) may decrease contractility of the urinary bladder detrusor muscle. For patients with BPH who have a narrowed urethral lumen, loss of effective detrusor contraction could result in

CLINICAL PRESENTATION Benign Prostatic Hyperplasia

General

- A patient is in no acute distress unless he has moderate-to-severe symptoms or complications of BPH.

Symptoms

- Obstructive symptoms: Slow urinary stream, intermittency, hesitancy, straining to urinate, incomplete emptying, dribbling
- Irritative symptoms: Urgency, frequency, nocturia

Signs

- Digital rectal examination reveals an enlarged prostate (>20 g) with no nodules or indurations; prostate is soft, symmetric, and mobile.

Laboratory Tests

- Increased blood urea nitrogen (BUN) and serum creatinine with long-standing, untreated bladder outlet obstruction, elevated prostate-specific antigen (PSA) level

Other Diagnostic Tests

- Increased American Urological Association (AUA) Symptom Score, decreased urinary flow rate (<10 mL/s), and increased PVR urine volume

acute urinary retention, particularly for patients with significantly enlarged prostate glands and a PVR urine volume greater than 150 mL. Diuretics, particularly in large doses, can produce polyuria, which may present as urinary frequency, similar to that experienced by patients with BPH.[8]

CLINICAL PRESENTATION

Patients with BPH can present with a variety of symptoms and signs of disease. All symptoms of BPH can be divided into two categories: obstructive and irritative.

Obstructive symptoms, also known as *prostatism* or *bladder outlet obstruction*, result when dynamic and/or static factors reduce bladder emptying. The force of the urinary stream becomes diminished, urinary flow rate decreases, and bladder emptying is incomplete and slow. Patients report urinary hesitancy and straining and a weak urine stream. Urine dribbles out of the penis, and the urinary bladder always feels full, even after patients have voided. Some patients state that they need to press on their bladder to force out the urine. In severe cases, patients may go into urinary retention when bladder emptying is not possible. In these cases, suprapubic pain can result from bladder overdistension.

Approximately 50% to 80% of patients have irritative voiding symptoms, which typically occur late in the disease course. Irritative voiding symptoms include urinary frequency and urgency. Patients may report waking up every 1 to 2 hours at night to void (nocturia), which significantly reduces quality of life.

Symptoms of BPH vary over time. Symptoms may improve, remain stable, or worsen spontaneously. Thus, BPH is not necessarily a progressive disease; approximately 85% of patients with BPH have stable symptoms when evaluated 4 years after initial diagnosis.[8] Between one-third and two-thirds of men with mild disease stabilize or improve without treatment over 2.5 to 5 years.[2,9] However, worsening symptoms and complications of BPH develop in patients, particularly those with a prostate gland volume greater than 30 to 40 mL or PSAs of 1.4 ng/mL (mcg/L) or greater.[2,9] A patient with a prostate volume of 30 mL or more is three times more likely to develop acute urinary retention.

Collectively, obstructive and irritative voiding symptoms and their negative impact on a patient's quality of life are referred to as *lower urinary tract symptoms* (LUTS). However, LUTS is not pathognomonic for BPH and may be caused by other diseases, such as neurogenic bladder or urinary tract infection.[2]

Another presentation of BPH is silent prostatism. Patients have LUTS but adapt to the symptoms and do not voluntarily complain about them. Such patients do not present for medical treatment until complications of BPH disease arise or a spouse brings in the symptomatic patient for medical care.

When BPH progresses, it can produce complications that include the following:

1. Acute, painful urinary retention, which can lead to acute renal failure.
2. Persistent or intermittent gross hematuria when tissue growth exceeds its blood supply.
3. Overflow urinary incontinence or unstable bladder.
4. Recurrent urinary tract infection that results from urinary stasis.
5. Bladder diverticula.
6. Bladder stones.
7. Chronic renal failure from long-standing bladder outlet obstruction.

Approximately 17% to 20% of patients with symptomatic BPH require treatment because of disease complications.[7] Men older than 70 years with large prostates of more than 40 g and a PVR urine volume greater than 100 mL are three times more likely to have severe symptoms or suffer from acute urinary retention and to require prostatectomy than patients with smaller prostates. Thus, a serum PSA level of 1.4 ng/mL (mcg/L) or greater has been used as a surrogate marker for an enlarged prostate gland to identify patients at risk for developing complications of BPH disease and has been used to guide selection of the most appropriate treatment modality in some patients.[9]

DIAGNOSTIC EVALUATION

Because the obstructive and irritative voiding symptoms associated with BPH are not unique to the disease and can be presenting symptoms of other genitourinary tract disorders, including prostate or bladder cancer, neurogenic bladder, prostatic calculi, or urinary tract infection, the patient presenting with signs and symptoms of BPH must be thoroughly evaluated.

A careful medical history should be taken to ensure that a complete listing of symptoms is collected to identify concomitant disorders that may be contributing to voiding symptoms. The

TABLE 104-1 Categories of BPH Disease Severity Based on Symptoms and Signs

Disease Severity	AUA Symptom Score[a]	Typical Symptoms and Signs
Mild	≤7	Asymptomatic Peak urinary flow rate ≥10 mL/s PVR urine volume ≤25-50 mL
Moderate	8-19	Peak urinary flow rate <10 mL/s PVR urine volume >25-50 mL Plus obstructive voiding symptoms and irritative voiding symptoms (signs of detrusor instability)
Severe	≥20	All of the above plus 1 or more complications of BPH[a]

[a]Score range, 0-35.

AUA, American Urological Association; BPH, benign prostatic hyperplasia; BUN, blood urea nitrogen; PVR, postvoid residual urine volume.

medical history should be followed by a thorough medication history, including all prescription and nonprescription medications and dietary supplements that the patient is taking. Any drugs that could be causing or exacerbating the patient's symptoms should be identified. If possible, the suspected drugs should be discontinued or the dosing regimen modified to ameliorate the voiding symptoms.

The patient should undergo a physical examination, including a digital rectal examination, although the size of the prostate gland may not correspond to symptoms. Some patients have only a slightly enlarged gland and yet have bothersome or even serious voiding difficulties. Other patients have intravesical enlargement of the prostate gland (ie, the gland grows into the urinary bladder and produces a ball-valve blockage of the bladder neck). This type of prostate enlargement is not palpable on digital examination.

The patient's perception of the severity of BPH symptoms guides selection of a particular treatment modality in a patient. To evaluate the patient's perceptions objectively, validated instruments, such as the AUA Symptom Score (Table 104-1), are commonly used. Using this tool, the patient rates the "bothersomeness" of seven obstructive and irritative voiding symptoms.[9] A patient's perception of bothersomeness is often based on how much these symptoms interfere with daily activities or cause worry or embarrassment in social settings. Each item is rated for severity on a scale from 0 to 5, such that 35 is the maximum score and is consistent with the most severe symptoms. Patients usually are stratified into the three groups shown in the table based on disease severity for the purposes of deciding a treatment approach.

In addition, the patient can complete a voiding diary in which he records the number of voids, the volume of each void, and voiding symptoms each day for several days. This information is used to evaluate symptom severity and tailor recommendations for lifestyle modifications that may ameliorate symptoms.

The only clinical laboratory test that must be performed is a urinalysis. Because many of the voiding symptoms of BPH could be caused by other urologic disorders, a urinalysis can help screen for hematuria, urolithiasis, and infection. To screen for prostate cancer, another common cause of glandular enlargement, a PSA test may be performed for patients aged 40 years or more, with at least a 10-year life expectancy, in whom the potential benefit of diagnosing the disorder will be outweighed by the cost of the test.[9]

Objective measures of bladder emptying include peak and average urinary flow rate (normal is at least 10 mL/s). These measures are determined using an uroflowmeter, which checks the rate of urine flow out of the bladder. This is a quick noninvasive outpatient procedure in which the patient is instructed to drink water until his bladder feels full and then the patient's urinary flow is clocked during voiding. A low urinary flow rate (<10-12 mL/s) implies failure of bladder emptying due to obstruction or a functional disorder of the detrusor muscle. A patient with such a low urinary flow rate has a fourfold greater risk of acute urinary retention than patients with higher urinary flow rates.[5,7]

Another objective measure is PVR urine volume (normal is 0 mL), which is assessed using abdominal ultrasonography. A PVR urine volume of 25 to 50 mL or more implies failure of bladder emptying and a predisposition for urinary tract infections, whereas a PVR of 100 mL or more has been associated with progressive worsening of BPH symptoms if no specific treatment is initiated.[10]

Because of a weak correlation among voiding symptoms, prostate size, and urinary flow rate, most physicians use a combination of measures, including the patient's assessment of symptoms along with objective evaluation of urinary outflow, PVR, and presence of complications of BPH to determine the need for treatment.

Many other tests can be performed if additional information is needed to assess the severity of BPH disease and its complications, to assist in the preoperative assessment of the patient, or to distinguish prostate enlargement due to BPH from that caused by prostate cancer. Tests include a serum BUN and creatinine, voiding cystometrogram, transrectal ultrasound of the prostate, IV pyelogram, renal ultrasound, and prostate biopsy.

TREATMENT

The goals of treatment are to control symptoms, as evidenced by a minimum of a three-point decrease in the AUA symptom index, prevent progression of BPH disease by reducing the risk of developing complications, and delay the need for surgical intervention.

As a disease of symptoms, BPH is treated by relieving bothersome symptoms. However, selection of a single best treatment for a patient must consider the variable costs and adverse effects of treatment options, the inability to predict the course of the disease in an individual patient, and the potential benefit that may occur in a comparatively small number of treated patients.

The 2021 AUA Guidelines on Management of Benign Prostatic Hyperplasia[9] is the principal tool used in the United States and is similar to the 2021 European Guidelines[11] (Fig. 104-2). In a patient with BPH, BPE, or BPO, if symptoms are mild, watchful waiting is recommended. If symptoms are moderate-to-severe with erectile dysfunction, an α-adrenergic antagonist, a phosphodiesterase inhibitor, or both are recommended. If symptoms are moderate-to-severe with a small prostate and low PSA, an α-adrenergic antagonist is recommended. If symptoms are moderate-to-severe with a large prostate and increased PSA, consider a 5α-reductase inhibitor plus an α-adrenergic antagonist. If symptoms are moderate-to-severe with predominant irritative voiding symptoms, consider an α-adrenergic antagonist plus an anticholinergic agent, or an α-adrenergic antagonist plus mirabegron. If symptoms are severe and the patient has complications of BPH or is not responding to medication therapy, surgical intervention is indicated.[9,11]

Although phytotherapy is used by some patients alone or along with conventional medications for BPH, head-to-head comparisons with FDA-approved treatments are lacking; consequently, such herbals cannot be recommended at this time.[9,11]

3 Patients with mild disease are asymptomatic or have mildly bothersome symptoms and have no complications of BPH disease. These patients can be managed with watchful waiting, which entails having the patient return for reassessment at intervals of 6 to 12 months. At each return visit, the patient should complete a standardized, validated survey tool to assess severity of symptoms, and

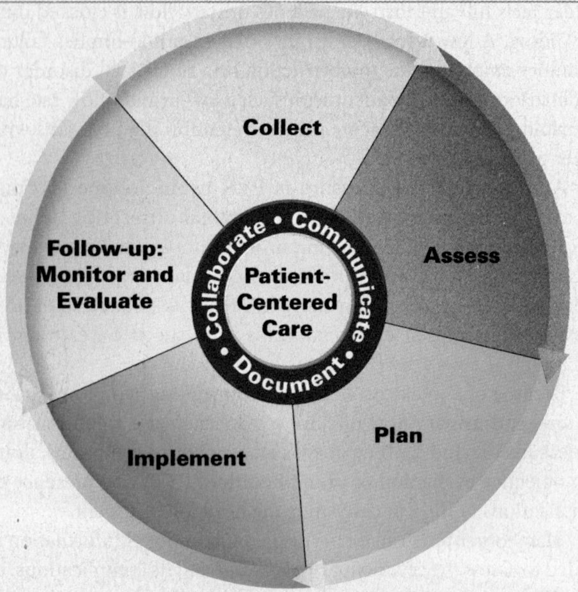

Patient Care Process for Benign Prostatic Hyperplasia

The image shows the five fundamental steps included in The Pharmacist's Care Process endorsed by the Joint Commission for Pharmacy Practitioners (2014). The tagline of this process reads collaborate, communicate, and document. The five fundamental steps listed here are collect, assess, plan, implement, and follow-up: monitor and evaluate. All these steps are listed in a circular block diagram.

Collect

- Patient characteristics (eg, age, race)
- Patient history (past medical history, family history, social—tobacco, recreational drug, or alcohol use)
- Presence of bladder symptoms that are obstructive (slow urinary stream, intermittency, hesitancy, straining to urinate, incomplete emptying, dribbling) and/or irritative (urgency, frequency, nocturia) (see Clinical Presentation box)
- Patient's perception of bothersomeness of voiding symptoms using American Urological Association (AUA) Symptom Score (see Diagnostic Evaluation section)
- Current and past medications, including prescription and nonprescription medications or nonpharmacologic interventions for BPH and medications perceived as causing BPH (see Medication-Related Symptoms section)
- Objective data (see Diagnostic Evaluation section and Clinical Presentation box)
  - BP, heart rate (HR), height, weight, and body mass index (BMI)
  - Digital rectal examination
  - Labs (eg, urinalysis, blood urea nitrogen, serum creatinine, prostate-specific antigen)
  - Urinary flow rates and postvoid residual volume

Assess

- Disease severity (see Table 104-1); patient's views on watchful waiting (in mild cases), medical treatment (in moderate-to-severe cases), and surgery (in severe cases)
- Need for further evaluation based on laboratory and examination findings
- Size of prostate by digital rectal exam or transrectal ultrasound of the prostate
- Presence of BPH, prostate cancer, prostatitis, all of which can cause lower urinary tract symptoms (LUTS)

Plan*

- Dietary and lifestyle modifications to avoid problematic symptoms and situations (see Medication-Related Symptoms section and Clinical Presentation box)
- Interventions as indicated to encourage heart-healthy lifestyle, smoking cessation, weight loss if needed, management of other chronic diseases
- Drug therapy regimen including specific agent(s), dose, route, frequency, and duration; specify the continuation and discontinuation of existing therapies (see Fig. 104-2 and Tables 104-2, 104-3, and 104-4), advantages or disadvantages of single drug versus combination therapy
- Monitoring parameters including efficacy (symptom relief) and safety (medication-specific adverse effects) (see Table 104-5)
- Patient education (eg, purpose of treatment, dietary and lifestyle modification, drug therapy)
- Comparison of during treatment responses by repeating AUA Symptom Score or using a voiding diary (see Diagnostic Evaluation section)
- Referrals to other providers when appropriate (eg, physician, urologist)

Implement*

- Provide patient education regarding all elements of treatment plan
- Use motivational interviewing and coaching strategies to maximize adherence
- Schedule follow-up

Follow-up: Monitor and Evaluate

- Determine BPH goal attainment
- Presence of adverse effects
- Patient adherence to treatment plan using multiple sources of information

Collaborate with patient, caregivers, and other healthcare professionals.

objective signs of disease should be assessed using measurements of urinary flow rate and PVR urine volume. Watchful waiting should be accompanied by patient education about the disease and behavior modification to avoid practices that exacerbate voiding symptoms. Behavior modification includes restricting fluids close to bedtime, minimizing caffeine and alcohol intake, frequent emptying of the bladder during waking hours or before long trips (to avoid overflow incontinence and urgency), smoking cessation, and avoiding drugs that could exacerbate voiding symptoms.[3,8,12,13] At each visit, physicians should assess the patient's risk of developing acute urinary retention by evaluating the patient's prostate size or using PSA as a surrogate marker of prostate enlargement.[14]

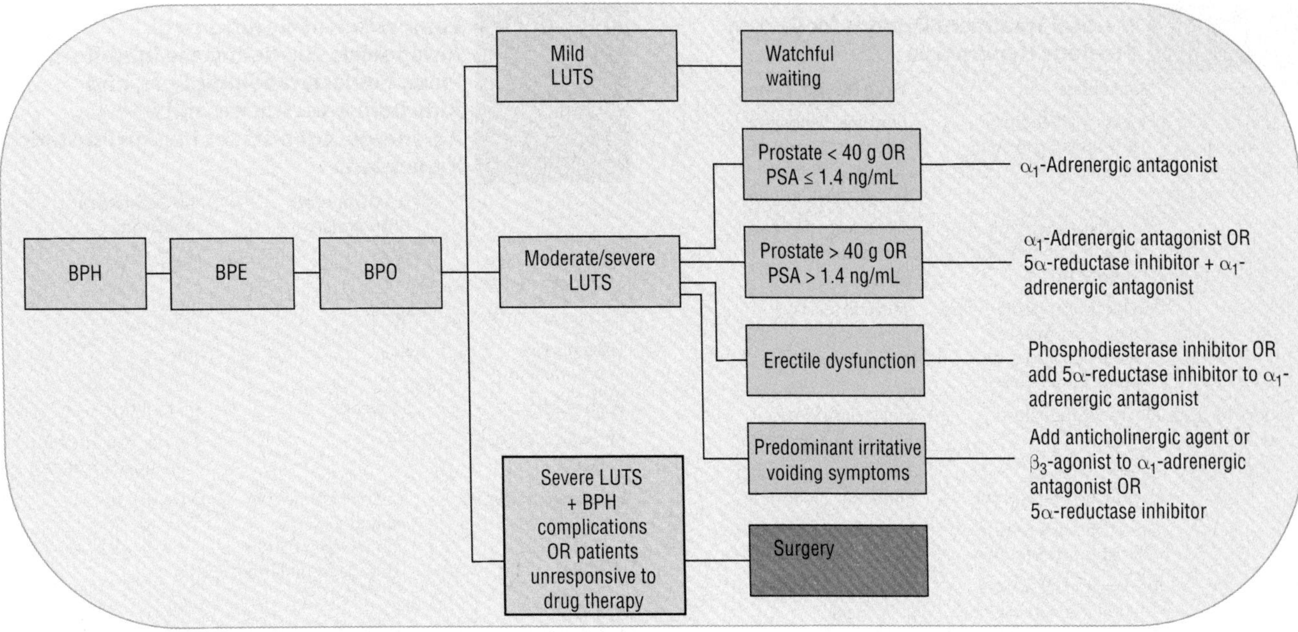

FIGURE 104-2 Management algorithm for benign prostatic hyperplasia (BPH).

4 If symptoms progress to the moderate or severe level, or the patient perceives his symptoms to be bothersome, the patient should be offered specific treatment. In these patients, watchful waiting delays—but does not decrease—the need for prostatectomy. In symptomatic patients, watchful waiting can lead to intractable urinary retention, increased PVR urine volumes, and significant voiding symptoms.[9,11] Recommended medical treatment options include drug therapy with an α_1-adrenergic antagonist or 5α-reductase inhibitor, a combination of an α_1-adrenergic antagonist and a 5α-reductase inhibitor, a phosphodiesterase inhibitor alone or combined with an α_1-adrenergic antagonist or 5α-reductase inhibitor, or the addition of an anticholinergic agent or a β_3-agonist to an α_1-adrenergic antagonist or 5α-reductase inhibitor particularly if the patient has significant irritative voiding symptoms that are not responsive to an α_1-adrenergic antagonist alone or 5α-reductase inhibitor alone.

Patients with serious complications of BPH or patients who do not respond to drug therapy should be offered surgical intervention. Drug therapy is considered an interim measure for such patients because it delays worsening of complications and the need for surgical intervention.[9]

Desired Outcomes

The desired outcomes of treatment include reducing LUTS as evidenced by an improvement of AUA Symptom Score by at least three points, an increase in the peak urinary flow rate, and a normalization of PVR to less than 50 mL. In addition, treatment should prevent the development of disease complications and reduce the need for surgical intervention. Treatment should be well tolerated and be cost-effective.

General Approach to Treatment

In selecting the most appropriate treatment for an individual patient, consideration should be given to the severity and quality of the patient's LUTS, the likelihood of developing complications of BPH (based on size of the prostate gland or the PSA level), the patient's preference for medical versus surgical intervention, the patient's risk for adverse effects of treatment, and the cost of treatment.

Concurrent medical illnesses of the patient should also be considered. For example, if the patient has erectile dysfunction and moderate LUTS, then a phosphodiesterase inhibitor might be preferred over an α_1-adrenergic antagonist. If the patient has overactive bladder syndrome and BPH, irritative voiding symptoms may require the addition of an anticholinergic agent or a β_3-adrenergic agonist. If medical treatment is initiated, the patient's level of renal function should be assessed, as the daily dose of some α-adrenergic antagonists and some anticholinergics require modification to avoid accumulation.

Nonpharmacologic Therapy

BPH is a chronic, nonfatal medical illness. All patients should be encouraged to initiate and maintain a heart-healthy lifestyle, including a low-fat diet, high intake of plenty of fresh fruits and vegetables, regular physical exercise, and no smoking.[15] Patients who have overweight or obesity should be encouraged to lose weight. Those with diabetes mellitus, dyslipidemia, or hypertension should be advised to optimize management of those disorders.[5,8] The patient should avoid excess consumption of caffeine-containing beverages (which may induce diuresis). Patients should void before retiring to bed at night and before long car rides.

Pharmacologic Therapy

Drug therapy for BPH can be categorized into three types: agents that relax prostatic smooth muscle (reducing the dynamic factor), agents that interfere with testosterone's stimulatory effect on prostate gland enlargement (reducing the static factor), and agents that relax bladder detrusor muscle (improving the urine storage capacity of the bladder) (Tables 104-2 and 104-3). Of the agents that relax prostatic smooth muscle, second- and third-generation α_1-adrenergic antagonists have been most widely used. These agents relax the intrinsic urethral sphincter and prostatic smooth muscle, thereby enhancing urinary outflow from the bladder. Phosphodiesterase inhibitors also relax bladder neck and prostatic smooth muscle. α_1-Adrenergic antagonists and phosphodiesterase inhibitors do not reduce prostate size. Of the agents that interfere with testosterone's stimulatory effect on prostate gland size, the only agents approved by the FDA

TABLE 104-2 Medical Treatment Options for Benign Prostatic Hyperplasia

Category	Mechanism	Drug (Brand Name)
Reduces dynamic factor	Blocks α_1-adrenergic receptors in prostatic stromal tissue	Prazosin (Minipress)[a] Alfuzosin (Uroxatral) Terazosin (Hytrin) Doxazosin (Cardura)
	Blocks α_{1A}-adrenergic receptors in prostatic stromal tissue	Tamsulosin (Flomax) Silodosin (Rapaflo)
	Inhibits phosphodiesterase type 5 in prostate, urethra, bladder, and pelvic blood vessels	Tadalafil (Cialis)
Reduces static factor	Blocks 5α-reductase enzyme	Finasteride (Proscar) Dutasteride (Avodart)
	Blocks DHT at its intracellular receptor	Bicalutamide (Casodex)[a] Flutamide (Eulexin)[a]
	Blocks pituitary release of luteinizing hormone	Leuprolide (Lupron)[a] Goserelin (Zoladex)[a]
	Blocks pituitary release of luteinizing hormone and blocks androgen receptor	Megestrol acetate (Megace)[a]
Relaxes detrusor muscle	Blocks muscarinic receptors in detrusor muscle of bladder	Tolterodine (Detrol)[a] Oxybutynin (Ditropan)[a] Trospium (Sanctura)[a] Solifenacin (Vesicare)[a] Darifenacin (Enablex)[a] Fesoterodine (Toviaz)[a]
	Stimulates β_3-adrenergic receptors in detrusor muscle of bladder	Mirabegron (Myrbetriq)[a] Vibegron (Gemtesa)[a]

[a]Not FDA-approved for treatment of benign prostatic hyperplasia.

are 5α-reductase inhibitors (eg, finasteride, dutasteride). Other agents that interfere with androgen stimulation of the prostate have not been popular in the United States because of the many adverse effects associated with their use. The luteinizing hormone-releasing hormone superagonists leuprolide and goserelin decrease libido and can cause erectile dysfunction, gynecomastia, and hot flashes. Antiandrogens (eg, bicalutamide, flutamide) produce nausea, diarrhea, gynecomastia, and hepatotoxicity. Finally, antimuscarinic agents and β_3-adrenergic agonists relax the detrusor muscle, which reduces irritable voiding symptoms, improves urine storage capacity of the bladder, and increases the interval between voidings.[9,11-13]

Selection of a medical treatment for a patient with moderate-to-severe symptoms should be determined on a case-by-case basis after the patient and provider discuss the risks, benefits, and costs of various treatments. With drug therapy for BPH, patients must understand that the benefits continue only as long as the medication is taken.

If possible, drug therapy should be initiated with a single agent, usually an α_1-adrenergic antagonist, which is faster acting and more effective than a 5α-reductase inhibitor. In addition, α_1-adrenergic antagonists are effective in reducing LUTS independent of prostate size and have no effect on PSA. Some are also available as less-expensive generic formulations. A 5α-reductase inhibitor is a good first-choice agent for symptomatic patients with a significantly enlarged prostate (>40 g) and an elevated PSA greater than or equal to 1.4 ng/mL (mcg/L). Such patients are at risk for developing complications of BPH, and typically combination drug therapy with an α_1-adrenergic antagonist and a 5α-reductase inhibitor is prescribed. The pharmacologic rationale for such a combination is that using two drugs with different mechanisms of action can be more effective than either drug alone. Also combination drug therapy quickly

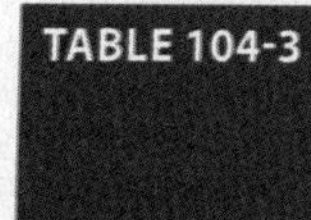

TABLE 104-3 Comparison of α_1-Adrenergic Antagonists, 5α-Reductase Inhibitors, Phosphodiesterase Inhibitors, and Anticholinergic Agents and β_3-Adrenergic Agonists for Benign Prostatic Hyperplasia

	α_1-Adrenergic Antagonists	5α-Reductase Inhibitors
Relaxes prostatic smooth muscle	Yes	No
Decreases prostate size	No	Yes
Halts disease progression	No	Yes
Peak onset	1-6 weeks	3-6 months
Efficacy in relieving BOO	++	++ (for patients with enlarged prostates)
Frequency of dosing	One to two times per day, depending on the agent and dosage formulation	Once per day
Decreases PSA	No	Yes
Sexual dysfunction adverse effects	EJD	Decreased libido, ED, EJD
Cardiovascular adverse effects	Yes	No
	Phosphodiesterase Inhibitors	**Anticholinergic Agents**
Relaxes prostatic smooth muscle	Yes	No
Decreases prostate size	No	No
Halts disease progression	No	No
Peak onset	4 weeks	1-2 weeks
Efficacy in relieving BOO	+	+ (irritative symptoms only)
Frequency of dosing	Once per day	Once per day
Decreases prostate-specific antigen	No	No
Sexual dysfunction adverse effects	No	ED
Cardiovascular adverse effects	Yes (mild hypotension)	Yes (tachycardia)
	β_3-Adrenergic Agonists	
Relaxes prostatic smooth muscle	No	
Decreases prostate size	No	
Halts disease progression	No	
Peak onset	2 weeks, but may take up to 8 weeks	
Efficacy in relieving BOO	+ (irritative symptoms only)	
Frequency of dosing	Once per day	
Decreases prostate-specific antigen	No	
Sexual dysfunction adverse effects	No	
Cardiovascular adverse effects	Yes (hypertension)	

BOO, bladder outlet obstruction; BPH, benign prostatic hyperplasia; ED, erectile dysfunction; EJD, ejaculation disorder; PSA, prostate-specific antigen.

+ Notation is a quantitative assessment.

relieves symptoms, delays disease progression, and reduces the need for surgical intervention. Since it is more expensive and associated with more adverse effects than single-drug therapy, combination drug therapy should be reserved for those patients who will benefit the most from it.

For patients with both erectile dysfunction and BPH, a phosphodiesterase inhibitor alone or in combination with an α_1-adrenergic antagonist may be used. However, it should be noted that a phosphodiesterase inhibitor alone will only relieve LUTS, and will not produce a clinically significant increase in urinary flow rate or a decrease in PVR. Therefore, a phosphodiesterase inhibitor is generally considered less effective than an α_1-adrenergic antagonist.

For patients with a predominance of irritative voiding symptoms, an anticholinergic agent could be added to an existing drug regimen for BPH. To reduce the risk of developing systemic anticholinergic adverse effects, a uroselective anticholinergic agent may be prescribed. To avoid the risk of developing acute urinary retention, an anticholinergic agent should be used cautiously when the patient's PVR is greater than 250 to 300 mL. Mirabegron and vibegron are more expensive than many anticholinergic agents. Therefore, they should be reserved as an add-on treatment for patients with irritative voiding symptoms who cannot tolerate anticholinergic adverse effects.

α_1-Adrenergic Antagonists

Three generations of α-adrenergic antagonists have been used to treat BPH. They all relax smooth muscle in the prostate and bladder neck. Because antagonism of presynaptic α_2-adrenergic receptors produces tachycardia and arrhythmias, first-generation α-adrenergic agents, such as phenoxybenzamine, have been replaced by the second-generation postsynaptic α_1-adrenergic antagonists and third-generation uroselective postsynaptic α_{1A}-adrenergic antagonists.

5 The second- and third-generation α_1-adrenergic antagonists are considered equally effective for treatment of BPH.[9,16] These agents generally improve the AUA Symptom Score by 30% to 40%, decreasing the AUA Symptom Index by three to six points, within 1 to 6 weeks, depending on the need for dose titration; increase urinary flow rate by 2 to 3 mL/s in 60% to 70% of treated patients; and reduce PVR urine volume.[3,12,16] With continued use, durable clinical benefit has been demonstrated for years.[9] Their effectiveness in reducing BPH symptoms and the severity of adverse effects are dose-dependent.[9] They have no effect on prostate volume. α_1-Adrenergic antagonists do not reduce PSA levels, preserving the utility of this prostate cancer marker in this high-risk population.[9]

Older, immediate-release, second-generation α_1-adrenergic antagonists, and tamsulosin are available as inexpensive generic formulations, which may be desirable in selected patients.

Second-Generation α_1-Adrenergic Antagonists

Second-generation agents include prazosin, terazosin, doxazosin, and alfuzosin. These are all nonselective α_1-adrenergic antagonists. At the usual doses used to treat BPH, immediate-release formulations of prazosin, terazosin, and doxazosin antagonize peripheral vascular α_1-adrenergic receptors. As a result, first-dose syncope, orthostatic hypotension, and dizziness are characteristic adverse effects. In older adults, such adverse effects could lead to falls and bone fractures.[3,15,17] To improve tolerance to these adverse effects, therapy should start with a low dose of 1 mg daily and then should be slowly titrated up to a full therapeutic dose over several weeks. Additive blood-pressure-lowering effects commonly occur when these agents are used with antihypertensive agents, which limit the use of these agents for some patients. These agents differ in terms of duration of action and dosage formulation. Prazosin requires twice- to thrice-daily dosing and has significant cardiovascular adverse effects. For these reasons, it is not recommended in the current AUA guidelines for treatment of BPH.[9] Extended-release dosage formulations of doxazosin and alfuzosin offer the convenience of once-daily dosing, treatment initiation with a full therapeutic dose, and decreased dose-related hypotension because they produce lower peak serum concentrations than immediate-release products.

An α_1-adrenergic antagonist is not preferred as single-drug therapy for treatment of both BPH and hypertension in a patient. In the Antihypertensive and Lipid-Lowering Treatment to Prevent Heart Attack Trial (ALLHAT) of 24,000 patients with hypertension, doxazosin produced more congestive heart failure than amlodipine, lisinopril, or chlorthalidone.[18] Thus, both the AUA and the Joint National Committee on Prevention, Detection, Evaluation and Treatment of High Blood Pressure[9,19] recommend that patients with BPH and hypertension be treated with separate and appropriate drug treatment for each medical condition.

When using immediate-release formulations of the second-generation α_1-adrenergic antagonists terazosin and doxazosin, slow titration up to a therapeutic maintenance dose is necessary to minimize orthostatic hypotension and first-dose syncope. Conservatively, dosages should be increased in an orderly stepwise process, at 2- to 7-day intervals, depending on the patient's response to the medication. A faster titration schedule can be used as long as the patient does not develop orthostatic hypotension or dizziness. Two sample titration schedules for terazosin are as follows:

Schedule 1: Slow titration

- Days 4 to 14: 2 mg at bedtime
- Weeks 2 to 6: 5 mg at bedtime
- Weeks 7 and on: 10 mg at bedtime

Schedule 2: Quicker titration

- Days 1 to 3: 1 mg at bedtime
- Days 4 to 14: 2 mg at bedtime
- Weeks 2 to 3: 5 mg at bedtime
- Weeks 4 and on: 10 mg at bedtime

In addition, patients should take their dose at bedtime so that they can sleep through hypotensive side effects that are most likely to occur when peak blood levels are achieved. Patients should continue taking the drug as long as they continue to respond to it. Durable responses for 10 years have been reported for doxazosin.[9]

Alfuzosin is considered functionally and clinically uroselective in that usual doses used to treat BPH are less likely than other second-generation agents to cause cardiovascular adverse effects in animal or human models.[9] This clinical effect has been observed more often with the once-daily, extended-release formulation of alfuzosin, which is the only commercially available formulation in the United States. Its clinical uroselectivity has been postulated to be due to higher concentrations of alfuzosin achieved in the prostate versus serum after usual doses,[20,21] absence of high peak serum levels with the extended-release formulation, and the fixed dosing schedule of the extended-release formulation. Extended-release alfuzosin dosing is FDA-approved for 10 mg daily, with no dose titration increase. This formulation is particularly convenient for patients who have difficulty remembering varying doses needed for uptitration dosing schedules.

Third-Generation α_1-Adrenergic Antagonists

Three subtypes of α_1-adrenergic receptors exist: (a) α_{1A}, which comprise 70% to 75% of the α-adrenergic receptors in the prostate, bladder neck, prostatic urethra, seminal vesicles, spermatic duct, and vas deferens (when stimulated, smooth muscle contraction and the emission phase of ejaculation occurs)[20,21]; (b) α_{1B}, which cause peripheral arterial smooth muscle contraction when stimulated; and (c) α_{1D}, which are found in the detrusor muscle of the bladder, prostate, urethra, and brain, but their function remains to be defined.[22]

Third-generation α_1-adrenergic antagonists preferentially inhibit α_{1A}-adrenergic receptors. Tamsulosin and silodosin are the only third-generation α_{1A}-adrenergic antagonists available in the United States. Blockade of these receptors relaxes smooth muscle of the prostate and bladder neck and improves bladder emptying in patients with BPH, but blockade is likely to cause ejaculatory disorders. In addition, both of these agents have low affinity for vascular α_{1B}-adrenergic receptors, which explains why hypotension is not as frequent with usual daily doses as compared with second-generation agents.[9]

Silodosin has 50-fold greater selectivity for the α_{1A}-adrenergic receptor than the α_{1D}-adrenergic receptor and has 100-fold greater selectivity for the α_{1A}-adrenergic receptor than the α_{1B}-adrenergic receptor.[9,23] Silodosin demonstrates greater pharmacologic uroselectivity than tamsulosin, which has a 10-fold greater selectivity for the α_{1A}-adrenergic receptor than the α_{1D}-adrenergic receptor and has 2.5-fold greater selectivity for the α_{1A}-adrenergic receptor than the α_{1B}-adrenergic receptor.[24] These pharmacologic differences are not associated with a significant difference in efficacy, but there is a higher incidence of ejaculatory disorders as an adverse effect in silodosin-treated patients as opposed to tamsulosin-treated patients.[23-25]

The uroselectivity of α_{1A}-adrenergic receptors has multiple implications. Dose titration is minimal; therefore, patients can start treatment with a therapeutic dose of tamsulosin 0.4 mg daily or silodosin 8 mg daily. Patients can be instructed to take the dose anytime during the day. It should be noted that the product labeling of tamsulosin and silodosin state that they should be taken 30 minutes after the same meal every day. Food decreases their oral bioavailability, reduces the peak serum concentration of the drug, and lowers the risk of hypotensive adverse effects. The onset of peak action is quick, in the range of 1 week. Increasing the daily dose of tamsulosin to 0.8 mg daily produces inconsistent improvements in effectiveness but does increase adverse effects.[26] These agents are well tolerated in patients with well-controlled hypertension; and the addition of tamsulosin to furosemide, enalapril, nifedipine, and atenolol does not result in hypotension.[27]

As compared with tamsulosin, silodosin requires dosage reduction in patients with a creatinine clearance of 30 to 50 mL/min (0.5-0.83 mL/s), is contraindicated in patients with severe hepatic insufficiency or a creatinine clearance less than 30 mL/min (0.5 mL/s), and has the potential to produce more adverse effects because of elevated plasma concentrations if used concurrently with potent CYP 3A4 inhibitors (eg, clarithromycin, itraconazole, ketoconazole, ritonavir) or P-glycoprotein inhibitors (eg, cyclosporine). Silodosin also causes more ejaculatory dysfunction than tamsulosin.[25,28] Finally, silodosin is commercially available from only one source, whereas tamsulosin is available as a generic formulation.

The usual doses of α_1-adrenergic antagonists are summarized in Table 104-4.

Adverse Effects Approximately 10% to 12% of patients discontinue taking second-generation α_1-adrenergic antagonists because of adverse effects, especially those that affect the cardiovascular system (eg, syncope, dizziness, hypotension).[9,11] Patients who tolerate hypotension poorly should avoid immediate-release formulations of second-generation α_1-adrenergic antagonists. This includes patients with poorly controlled angina, serious cardiac arrhythmias, patients with reduced circulating volume, patients with untreated hypertension, and patients taking multiple antihypertensives.[15] Alfuzosin, extended-release doxazosin, or a third-generation α_1-adrenergic antagonist is preferred in these patients.

Tiredness and asthenia, anejaculation and retrograde ejaculation, flu-like symptoms, and nasal congestion are the most common dose-related adverse effects of tamsulosin and silodosin. These adverse effects are extensions of their α_{1A}-adrenergic antagonist activity and are dose-related, but with proper education patients likely will not discontinue treatment. However, if the patient is sexually active and ejaculatory dysfunction is problematic, switching the patient from a third-generation to a second-generation α_1-adrenergic antagonist has been effective.[27,29-32]

Tamsulosin use has been associated with dementia based on analysis of a cohort of patients in the Medicare database from 2006 to 2012.[33] It was hypothesized that dementia was due to blockade of α_{1A}-adrenergic receptors in the brain, as this association was not found with second-generation α_1-adrenergic antagonists.[33] However, conflicting data showing no such association have also been reported.[34]

Floppy iris syndrome has been associated with doxazosin, silodosin, and tamsulosin use, although the number of reported cases is highest with tamsulosin.[35] The mechanism for this adverse reaction is related to blockade of α_{1A}-adrenergic receptors in iris dilator muscles. As a result, during cataract surgery, pupillary constriction occurs despite the use of mydriatic agents and the iris billows out (floppy iris), both of which complicate the procedure or can increase the likelihood of postoperative complications, including posterior capsular rupture, retinal detachment, residual retained lens material, or endophthalmitis. Permanent loss of vision can result.[35,36]

Patients who are taking α_1-adrenergic antagonists and who plan to undergo cataract surgery should inform their ophthalmologist that they are taking this medication so that appropriate measures can be taken during eye surgery, for example, use of iris retractors, pupillary expansion rings, or potent mydriatic agents.[36] No benefit has been demonstrated with holding the α_1-adrenergic antagonist preoperatively.

For patients who are scheduled to have cataract surgery, and who have not yet started an α_1-adrenergic antagonist, they should be advised to delay the start of the α_1-adrenergic antagonist until surgery has been completed.[3,9]

Patients with severe sulfa allergy should avoid tamsulosin.

Drug Interactions Caution is needed when CYP 3A4 inhibitors—for example, cimetidine and diltiazem—are used with α_1-adrenergic antagonists because a drug-drug interaction could lead to decreased metabolism of the latter agents. In contrast, concurrent use of potent CYP 3A4 stimulators such as carbamazepine and phenytoin may increase hepatic catabolism of α_1-adrenergic antagonists.

Phosphodiesterase inhibitors (eg, sildenafil, vardenafil, tadalafil) may produce hypotension if used in large doses along with α_1-adrenergic antagonists. The mechanisms for this interaction are related to the intrinsic vasodilatory effects of phosphodiesterase inhibitors and the higher susceptibility of elderly patients to venous pooling because of autonomic incompetence.[37] The prevalence of hypotension depends on the specific phosphodiesterase inhibitor and α_1-adrenergic antagonist agent, specifically the combination of tadalafil and a third-generation α_{1A}-adrenergic antagonist is least likely to produce a clinically significant drug interaction, as compared with other combinations.[38] Therefore, a patient's blood pressure should be stabilized on the α_1-adrenergic antagonist before starting a phosphodiesterase inhibitor. In addition, patients who are taking phosphodiesterase inhibitors with α_1-adrenergic antagonists should have their blood pressure monitored closely when initiating combined drug use.

5α-Reductase Inhibitors

6 Finasteride competitively inhibits type II 5α-reductase, the predominant isoform of the enzyme in the prostate, which suppresses intraprostatic DHT by 80% to 90%, and decreases serum DHT levels by 70%.[9] Dutasteride is a nonselective inhibitor of type I and II 5α-reductase. It more quickly and completely suppresses intraprostatic DHT production and decreases serum DHT levels by 90%.[39] However, direct comparison clinical trials show no advantages of

TABLE 104-4 Dosing of Drugs Used in Treatment of Benign Prostatic Hyperplasia

Drug	Brand Name	Initial Dose	Usual Dose	Special Population Dose
α-Adrenergic Antagonists				
Prazosin	Minipress	0.5 mg twice a day orally	1-5 mg twice a day orally	To uptitrate the dose, double the dose every 2 weeks.
Terazosin	Hytrin	1 mg at bedtime orally	10-20 mg daily orally	Take extra care if the patient is taking other drugs that lower blood pressure. No dosage adjustment is required for patients with renal or hepatic impairment.
Doxazosin	Cardura	1 mg daily orally	8 mg daily orally	When switching from the immediate- to the extended-release formulation, start with 4 mg of the extended-release formulation no matter what maintenance dose of immediate-release doxazosin the patient is taking. No dosage adjustment is required for patients with renal or hepatic impairment.
	Cardura XL	4 mg daily orally	4-8 mg daily	
Alfuzosin	Uroxatral	10 mg daily orally	10 mg daily orally (no dose titration)	This is an extended-release formulation, and it should not be chewed or crushed. The drug should be taken after meals and used cautiously in patients with creatinine clearance less than 30 mL/min (0.5 mL/s). No dosage adjustment is required for patients with mild hepatic impairment. It is contraindicated in patients with moderate-to-severe hepatic impairment.
Tamsulosin	Flomax	0.4 mg daily orally	0.4-0.8 mg daily orally	This is an extended-release formulation, and it should not be chewed or crushed. The drug should be taken after meals. No dosage adjustment is needed in patients with renal or liver impairment.
Silodosin	Rapaflo	8 mg daily orally	8 mg daily orally (no dose titration)	This drug is contraindicated when creatinine clearance is less than 30 mL/min (0.5 mL/s). If creatinine clearance is 30-50 mL/min (0.5-0.83 mL/s), use 4 mg daily orally, preferably after the same meal each day. No dosage adjustment is required for patients with mild-to-moderate hepatic impairment. Should not be given to patients on potent CYP 3A4 inhibitors or with severe hepatic impairment.
5α-Reductase Inhibitors				
Finasteride	Proscar	5 mg daily orally	5 mg daily orally	No dosage adjustment in patients with renal impairment. Use cautiously in patients with hepatic impairment.
Dutasteride	Avodart	0.5 mg daily orally	0.5 mg daily orally	No dosage adjustment in patients with renal impairment. Use cautiously in patients with hepatic impairment.
Dutasteride + tamsulosin	Jalyn	1 tablet (equivalent to 0.5-mg dutasteride + 0.4-mg tamsulosin) daily orally	1 tablet daily orally	No dosage adjustment needed in patients with renal or moderate hepatic impairment.
Phosphodiesterase Inhibitor				
Tadalafil	Cialis	5 mg daily orally	5 mg daily orally	If creatinine clearance is 30-50 mL/min (0.5-0.83 mL/s), use 2.5 mg daily orally. Do not use if creatinine clearance is less than 30 mL/min (0.5 mL/s). Use cautiously in patients with mild-moderate hepatic impairment. Avoid in patients with severe hepatic impairment.
Anticholinergic Agents				
Darifenacin	Enablex	7.5 mg daily orally	7.5-15 mg daily orally	This is an extended-release formulation and it should not be chewed or crushed. To uptitrate the dose, double the dose after 2 weeks. If the patient is taking a potent CYP3A4 inhibitor (eg, ketoconazole, itraconazole, ritonavir, nelfinavir, and clarithromycin), do not exceed 7.5 mg daily orally. No dosage adjustment is needed for patients with renal impairment. Use a maximum dose of 7.5 mg daily for patients with moderate hepatic impairment. Do not use in patients with severe hepatic impairment.
Fesoterodine	Toviaz	4 mg daily orally	4-8 mg daily orally	This is an extended-release formulation, and it should not be chewed or crushed. If the patient is taking a potent CYP3A4 inhibitor (eg, ketoconazole, itraconazole, ritonavir, nelfinavir, and clarithromycin), do not exceed 4 mg daily orally. If the creatinine clearance is less than 30 mL/min (0.5 mL/s), do not exceed 4 mg daily orally. Use is not recommended in patients with severe hepatic impairment.
Oxybutynin	Ditropan	5 mg two to three times a day orally	5-10 mg two to three times a day orally	Increase daily dose at 5-mg increments at weekly intervals. No specific dosing modifications available for patients with renal or hepatic impairment; use cautiously in these patients.
	Ditropan XL	5 mg daily orally	5-30 mg daily orally	This is an extended-release formulation, and it should not be crushed or chewed. Increase daily dose at 5-mg increments at weekly intervals. No specific dosing modifications available for patients with renal impairment; use cautiously in these patients.
	Oxytrol TDS	1 patch (3.9-mg oxybutynin) twice weekly	1 patch (3.9 mg) twice weekly	This is a transdermal patch. Apply to abdomen, hip, or buttock. Rotate application site. Do not expose patch to sunlight. No specific dosing modifications available for patients with renal or hepatic impairment; however, use cautiously in these patients.
	Gelnique 10% gel	1-g gel (100-mg oxybutynin) daily	1-g gel (100-mg oxybutynin) daily	This is available as premeasured dose packets. Apply to abdomen, thighs, upper arms, or shoulders. Wash hands after application. Do not bathe, shower, or swim for 1 hour after application. Cover application site with clothing until medication dries on skin. Rotate application site daily. No specific dosing modifications available for patients with renal or hepatic impairment; use cautiously in these patients.

(continued)

TABLE 104-4 Dosing of Drugs Used in Treatment of Benign Prostatic Hyperplasia (*Continued*)

Drug	Brand Name	Initial Dose	Usual Dose	Special Population Dose
Solifenacin	VESIcare	5 mg daily orally	5-10 mg daily orally	If the creatinine clearance is less than 30 mL/min (0.5 mL/s) or the patient has moderate hepatic impairment, do not exceed 5 mg daily orally. Do not use if the patient has severe hepatic impairment. If the patient is taking a potent CYP3A4 inhibitor (eg, ketoconazole, itraconazole, ritonavir, nelfinavir, and clarithromycin), do not exceed 5 mg daily orally.
Tolterodine	Detrol	2 mg twice daily orally	1-2 mg twice daily orally	If the patient has significant renal impairment or severe hepatic impairment, limit dose to 1 mg twice a day.
	Detrol LA	4 mg daily orally	2-4 mg daily orally	This is an extended-release formulation, and it should not be chewed or crushed. If the creatinine clearance is 10-30 mL/min (0.17-0.5 mL/s) or the patient has mild-moderate hepatic impairment, do not exceed 2 mg daily orally. If the creatinine clearance is less than 10 mL/min (0.17 mL/s), do not use Detrol LA. If the patient has severe hepatic impairment, use of the extended-release formulation is not recommended.
Trospium	Sanctura	20 mg twice daily orally	20 mg twice daily orally	Avoid alcohol ingestion for 2 hours after a dose. Use cautiously in patients with moderate-severe hepatic impairment. In patients older than 75 years, use the immediate-release formulation and start with 20 mg daily orally. If the creatinine clearance is less than 30 mL/min (0.5 mL/s), use 20-mg immediate-release formulation.
	Sanctura XR	60 mg daily orally	60 mg daily orally	This is an extended-release formulation, and it should not be chewed or crushed. This is not recommended in patients with creatinine clearance less than 30 mL/min (0.5 mL/s). This should be used cautiously in patients with severe hepatic impairment.
β_3-Adrenergic Agonist				
Mirabegron	Myrbetriq	25 mg daily orally	25-50 mg daily orally	This is an extended-release formulation. Do not chew, crush, or divide tablet. In patients with a creatinine clearance of 15-29 mL/min (0.25-0.48 mL/s) or those with moderate hepatic impairment, the maximum daily dose should be 25 mg daily. This drug is not recommended in patients with creatinine clearance less than 15 mL/min (0.25 mL/s) or those with severe hepatic impairment.
Vibegron	Gemtesa	75 mg daily orally	75 mg daily orally (no dose titration)	This tablet may be crushed and administered in applesauce or put into a glass of water for ease of administration. No dosage adjustment for patients with a creatinine clearance of 15 mL/min (0.25 mL/s) or more. Do not use in patients with creatinine clearance less than 15 mL/min (0.25 mL/s). No dosage adjustment for patients with mild-to-moderate hepatic impairment. Do not use in patients with severe hepatic impairment.

these pharmacodynamic differences between these two agents.[39] 5α-Reductase inhibitors are indicated for management of moderate-to-severe BPH disease for patients with enlarged prostate glands of at least 40 g or a PSA greater than 1.4 ng/dL (mcg/L).[9,11,40,41] For such patients, 5α-reductase inhibitors may slow disease progression and decrease the risk of disease complications, thereby decreasing the ultimate need for surgical intervention. When taken continuously for 4 or 6 years, dutasteride or finasteride, respectively, has been shown to decrease the risk of acute urinary retention and prostatectomy.[3,42,43] For patients with severe disease, these agents generally should be used with a 6-month short course of an α_1-adrenergic antagonist; the latter will provide fast symptom relief until the 5α-reductase inhibitor starts to work. 5α-Reductase inhibitors may be preferred for patients with BPH and an enlarged prostate gland who have uncontrolled arrhythmias, have poorly controlled angina, are taking multiple antihypertensive agents, or are unable to tolerate hypotensive adverse effects of α_1-adrenergic antagonists.[13]

5α-Reductase inhibitors also reduce or stop prostate-related bleeding by inhibiting prostatic vascular endothelial growth factor. Thus, the prevalence of gross hematuria in patients with BPH may be reduced with treatment of 5α-reductase inhibitors.[9]

5α-Reductase inhibitors reduce prostate size by 25%, increase peak urinary flow rate by 1.6 to 2.0 mL/s, improve voiding symptoms in approximately 30% of treated patients, and produce few serious adverse effects.[9,11,12]

Compared with α_1-adrenergic antagonists, 5α-reductase inhibitors have several disadvantages. 5α-Reductase inhibitors have a delayed peak onset of clinical effect, which is undesirable for patients with bothersome symptoms. Long-term treatment is needed; an adequate minimum period for a clinical trial is 6 to 12 months. In addition, patients experience less objective improvement of the AUA Symptom Score and urinary flow rate with 5α-reductase inhibitors than with α_1-adrenergic antagonists.[9] 5α-Reductase inhibitors cause more sexual dysfunction than α_1-adrenergic receptor antagonists; therefore, physicians consider 5α-reductase inhibitors to be the second-line agents for treatment of BPH in sexually active males (Tables 104-3 and 104-5).[9,44]

Prostate Cancer and 5α-Reductase Inhibitors In the Prostate Cancer Prevention Trial, patients with BPH who had large prostate glands and a PSA level less than 3 ng/mL (mcg/L) were prescribed finasteride 5 mg daily for up to 7 years. Finasteride reduced the 7-year prevalence of prostate cancer by 25%.[45] However, finasteride was associated with a 27% increase in the number of patients who developed high-grade prostate cancer, which usually is invasive. Although originally thought to be a disadvantage of finasteride use, it is now thought that the higher incidence of prostate cancer was due to biopsy sampling bias. That is, since finasteride reduces the size of the prostate gland, this results in increased sensitivity of sampling biopsies to detect prostate cancer.[46]

Another clinical trial produced similar results. The Reduction by Dutasteride in Prostate Cancer Events (REDUCE) study compared the effect of 4 years of continuous use of dutasteride versus placebo on reducing the incidence of prostate cancer in more than 6,700 men at high risk for developing prostate cancer. At the end of the study, dutasteride-treated patients had a 22.8% decreased relative

TABLE 104-5 Monitoring of Drugs Used in Treatment of Benign Prostatic Hyperplasia

Drug	Adverse Reaction	Monitoring Parameter	Comment
α_1-Adrenergic antagonists	Syncope Lightheadedness Orthostatic hypotension Tachycardia Nasal congestion Ejaculatory dysfunction Priapism Floppy iris syndrome	Blood pressure Heart rate	If prescribing an immediate-release formulation, start the patient on the lowest possible dose and instruct the patient to take the first dose at bedtime. Slowly uptitrate the dose over several weeks. Stabilize the patient's blood pressure on the α_1-adrenergic antagonist before adding any other hypotensive agent. If the patient needs cataract surgery, instruct the patient to inform the ophthalmologist so that appropriate measures can be taken during the procedure to prevent intraoperative complications. If the patient has a painful erection lasting longer than 4 hours, the patient should seek immediate medical attention.
5α-Reductase inhibitors	ED Decreased libido Ejaculatory dysfunction Gynecomastia	PSA	The patient's PSA level should decrease by 50% if he is adherent to therapy.
Phosphodiesterase inhibitor	Headache Dizziness Nasal congestion Dyspepsia Back pain Myalgia Hearing loss Vision loss	Blood pressure Pulse Hearing loss Changes in vision	If the patient experiences hearing or vision loss, discontinue tadalafil.
Anticholinergic agents	Dry mouth Constipation Headache Tachycardia Blurry vision Acute urinary retention Drowsiness Confusion Angioedema Anaphylaxis ED	Mental status Bowel habits Ability to urinate	Adverse effects are dose-related and generally reversible. Patients with signs of severe allergic reaction need immediate medical attention.
β_3-Adrenergic agonist	Hypertension Tachycardia Dry mouth Nausea Constipation Diarrhea Headache Nasopharyngitis Impaired cognition	Blood pressure Bowel habits	Adverse effects are dose-related and generally reversible.

ED, erectile dysfunction; PSA, prostate-specific antigen.

risk of prostate cancer. Of the patients with biopsy-positive prostate cancer, a similar number of patients in each treatment group developed high-grade tumors (Gleason grade 7-10) with no statistical difference between the groups.[47]

Thus, when finasteride is administered long-term to patients with BPH, it could be useful as chemoprophylaxis in patients with a family history of prostate cancer or in men of African descent who have an increased risk of developing prostate cancer. Although a cause-effect relationship has not been established, the possibility of developing a high-grade prostate cancer should be discussed with the patient before initiating a 5α-reductase inhibitor for prevention of prostate cancer.[45,48]

Dosing Table 104-6 compares the pharmacokinetic properties of finasteride and dutasteride. They both exhibit good oral bioavailability, are extensively metabolized by the liver, and are highly protein bound. The principal difference is in the drugs' half-life: 5 to 6 hours for finasteride and 5 weeks for dutasteride. Although dutasteride's long half-life may allow for intermittent dosing as opposed to daily dosing, insufficient clinical data are available to recommend such a dosing schedule.

Maximal reductions in prostate volume or symptom improvement may not be evident for 12 months, but noticeable changes from baseline should occur after 6 months of continuous treatment.

TABLE 104-6 Comparison of Pharmacokinetic Properties of Finasteride and Dutasteride

	Finasteride	Dutasteride
Daily oral dose (mg)	5	0.5
Dosage formulation	Tablet	Capsule
Effect of food on absorption	No effect	No effect
% Oral bioavailability	63	60
Time to peak absorption (hours)	1-2	2-3
Elimination half-life	5-6 hours	5 weeks
% Protein binding	90	99

Patients must continue to take 5α-reductase inhibitors as long as they respond. Durable responses to finasteride and dutasteride have been reported with continued treatment for 6 years[43] and 4 years,[40] respectively. Upon discontinuation of the drug, prostate size and voiding symptoms generally return to baseline.

No clinically relevant drug interactions have been reported with 5α-reductase inhibitors.

Adverse Effects 5α-Reductase inhibitors can produce sexual dysfunction, and this has led to discontinuation of therapy in up to

12% of treated patients in one-pooled analysis.[40] Decreased libido has been reported in 2% to 10% of treated patients.[44] Erectile dysfunction has been reported in 3% to 16% of patients.[40,44] This could be secondary to ejaculation disorders or a drug-induced decrease in DHT and subsequent inhibition of nitric oxide synthase (which is needed to produce nitric oxide, a vasodilatory substance) in cavernosal tissue.[32] Although sexual dysfunction often improves with time as the patient continues to take the medication, decreased libido and erectile dysfunction may persist after discontinuation of the 5α-reductase inhibitors.[49-51] The role of 5α-reductase inhibitors in causing erectile dysfunction is not clear, as older adult men with BPH commonly develop erectile dysfunction as they age or have concurrent medical illnesses or concomitant drug therapies that may predispose to the development of sexual dysfunction.

Ejaculation disorders (dry sex or delayed ejaculation) have been reported in 3% to 8% of treated patients.[49,50] These disorders, which are possible results of decreased prostatic secretion, are reversible with drug discontinuation. In one analysis, dutasteride was associated with a higher frequency of sexual dysfunction than finasteride.[52]

Other minor adverse effects include nausea, abdominal pain, asthenia, dizziness, flatulence, headache, rash, muscle weakness, and gynecomastia.[9,53] Mental depression and an increased risk of self-harm have been associated with the first 1.5 years of treatment with a 5α-reductase inhibitor; however, a cause-effect relationship has not been established.[54,55]

5α-Reductase inhibitors are in FDA pregnancy category X, which means that they are contraindicated in pregnant females. Exposure of the male fetus to finasteride may produce pseudohermaphroditic offspring with ambiguous genitalia, similar to those of patients with a rare genetic deficiency of type II 5α-reductase. Because of this teratogenic effect, women who are pregnant or seeking to become pregnant should not handle 5α-reductase inhibitor tablets and should not have contact with semen from men being treated with 5α-reductase inhibitors. Women health professionals of childbearing age should handle this product with protective gloves if they might be pregnant.

Effects of 5α-Reductase Inhibitors on PSA DHT stimulates prostate epithelial cells to produce PSA. Since 5α-reductase inhibitors inhibit intracellular conversion of testosterone to DHT, these medications can decrease PSA production.

Usual doses of 5α-reductase inhibitors produce a median reduction of serum PSA levels of 50% at months 6 to 12 after the start of treatment. To interpret a PSA level in a patient being treated with a 5α-reductase inhibitor, it is generally recommended that the actual measured level be doubled to get an estimate of the true level.[9] This formula applies particularly when the baseline PSA value is 4 ng/mL (mcg/L) or more.[56] PSA levels must be measured and a digital rectal examination should be performed before treatment begins. After 6 months of therapy, the patient should have a repeat PSA. This PSA level can be used as the new baseline for the patient. Alternatively, when compared to the pretreatment PSA, if the during-treatment level does not decline by 50% but the patient has been adherent to the 5α-reductase inhibitor regimen, he should be evaluated for prostate cancer. Annually thereafter, the patient should have a PSA assay and digital rectal examination if the patient has a 10-year life expectancy. Patients with an increase in PSA level of 0.3 ng/mL (mcg/L) or more above the baseline nadir level should be evaluated for prostate cancer[9] or noncompliance to the prescribed regimen.

Phosphodiesterase Type 5 Inhibitors

7 Several observations led to the use of phosphodiesterase type 5 inhibitors for management of BPH. (1) BPH and erectile dysfunction are often present concurrently in the same patient. (2) The pathophysiology of BPH and erectile dysfunction may be common in so far as both disorders may be associated with increased smooth muscle contraction and pelvic atherosclerosis. (3) Improvement of BPH symptoms has been reported to ameliorate erectile dysfunction; and vice versa. (4) Using a phosphodiesterase type 5 inhibitor with a 5α-reductase inhibitor is reasonable as the former will effectively treat erectile dysfunction, a side effect of the latter.[9,57]

Phosphodiesterase type 5 inhibitors relax smooth muscle in the prostate, urethra, bladder neck, and pelvic blood vessels, probably by increasing cGMP. By so doing, phosphodiesterase type 5 inhibitors interrupt the Rho-protein kinase pathway (which regulates smooth muscle contraction mediated by endothelin and α-adrenergic stimulation), improve perfusion of pelvic organs and oxygenation to tissue,[57] and possibly decrease inflammation.[58]

In multiple clinical trials of patients with moderate LUTS, tadalafil caused a mean two-point improvement in both obstructive and irritative voiding symptoms using the AUA Symptom Index Score or International Prostate Symptom Score (IPSS), with the level of improvement similar to that observed with α_1-adrenergic antagonists.[58,59] However, no or minimal increase in urinary flow rate or reduction in PVR occurred with tadalafil alone. Tadalafil 2.5 mg was inferior to 5 mg, and doses of 10 or 20 mg were not superior to 5 mg.[60] This is the basis of the current product labeling dose of tadalafil 5 mg daily for BPH. The onset of clinical symptom improvement is within 4 weeks.[60] Tadalafil is more effective for BPH in younger men with symptomatic LUTS. It may be that these patients are more likely to be sexually active. Therefore, when treating both BPH and erectile dysfunction, tadalafil improves a patient's perception of the medication's effectiveness.[37]

A few other BPH studies have employed sildenafil 50 or 100 mg daily, vardenafil 10 mg twice a day, or tadalafil 10 or 20 mg daily.[60] Based on a recent meta-analysis, all phosphodiesterase type 5 inhibitors produce comparable improvements of LUTS, but tadalafil is the only one that has been FDA-approved for the treatment of BPH.[60] Tadalafil has the longest plasma half-life and longest duration of action among the phosphodiesterase type 5 inhibitors. This pharmacokinetic characteristic is conducive for the treatment of BPH, which is a chronic illness.

Dosing Recommendations The recommended tadalafil dose is 5 mg daily. Based on the limited clinical benefit, cost, and potential adverse effects of tadalafil, its use should be reserved for patients with both BPH and erectile dysfunction. Patients with known cardiovascular disease should be assessed and stratified according to the Princeton Consensus Panel guidelines[61] to identify those patients who can safely use tadalafil. If used in combination with an α-adrenergic antagonist, precautions should be taken to minimize hypotension, specifically, the patient's blood pressure should be stabilized on the α_1-adrenergic antagonist before adding tadalafil.[37] If used in combination with a 5α-reductase inhibitor, tadalafil may be used instead of an α-adrenergic antagonist, and the combination may be associated with less sexual dysfunction, particularly in younger, sexually active patients.

Adverse Effects The most common adverse effects with tadalafil are headache, flushing, gastroesophageal reflux, sinusitis, visual disturbances, and back pain, which are generally mild and reversible and do not require discontinuation of therapy. Headache and dizziness are related to the vasodilatory effect of tadalfil. If tadalafil is an add-on to an existing α_1-adrenergic antagonist and the patient is at risk of hypotensive adverse effects, it is recommended that: (a) the patient's blood pressure be stabilized on the α_1-adrenergic antagonist before tadalafil is started; (b) once tadalafil is started, separate its administration from the α_1-adrenergic antagonist by 4 hours; and (c) preferentially prescribe tamsulosin, silodosin, or alfuzosin as opposed to other α_1-adrenergic antagonists. Back pain has been linked to tadalafil's inhibition of phosphodiesterase type 11. This usually responds to acetaminophen or a nonsteroidal anti-inflammatory agent.

Drug Interactions Nitrates by any route of administration are contraindicated in patients taking tadalafil.

Anticholinergic Agents

Five types of muscarinic receptors have been identified: (1) M_1 that concentrate in the brain, stomach, and salivary glands; (2) M_2 that comprise 71% to 75% of the muscarinic receptors in the urinary bladder and also are found in the gastrointestinal tract and the atrioventricular node of the heart; (3) M_3 comprise 25% to 29% of the muscarinic receptors in the urinary bladder, and are also distributed in salivary glands, gastrointestinal tract, airways, and eyes; (4) M_4 that are found in the urinary bladder and central nervous system; and (5) M_5 that are found in the brain and eyes. Although M_2 receptors predominate in the urinary bladder, increased M_3 receptor stimulation has been linked with irritative bladder symptoms and overactive bladder syndrome. For this reason, M_3 selective anticholinergic agents (eg, solifenacin and tolterodine) are considered uroselective. However, since M_3 receptors are widely distributed in other organ systems, this explains why darifenacin, a uroselective anticholinergic agent, causes dry mouth, constipation, and mydriasis.[8,9]

8 Treatment with an α_1-adrenergic antagonist, 5α-reductase inhibitor, or surgery may improve urinary flow rate and bladder emptying; however, the patient may still complain of irritative voiding symptoms, which mimic those of overactive bladder syndrome. A variety of anticholinergic agents have been added to an α-adrenergic antagonist regimen to relieve these symptoms.[9,11]

By blocking muscarinic receptors in the detrusor muscle, anticholinergic agents can reduce uninhibited detrusor contractions, a sequela of prolonged bladder outlet obstruction. Thus, irritative voiding symptoms are reduced. The peak clinical effect is observable in several weeks. It is recommended that a patient should be reevaluated 4 to 6 weeks after starting an anticholinergic agent for BPH. These agents do not improve urinary flow rate or consistently improve AUA symptom scores. Because older patients are sensitive to the central nervous system adverse effects and dry mouth, such patients should be started on the lowest effective dose and then slowly titrated up.[9,11] Anticholinergic agents are contraindicated in patients with narrow angle glaucoma, urinary or gastric retention, or severely decreased intestinal motility. The total anticholinergic burden should be considered prior to making the decision to initiate an anticholinergic agent if the patient is already taking other anticholinergic agents (eg, antipsychotic, antidepressant, antihistamine, antiparkinsonian agents). When multiple anticholinergic agents are taken concurrently, anticholinergic adverse effects, including dry mouth, nausea, constipation, blurred vision, and confusion, will more likely occur and be more severe.

For patients who poorly tolerate systemic anticholinergic adverse effects, options include darifenacin, which is a uroselective M_3 receptor antagonist; anticholinergics, which preferentially inhibit M_3 receptors more than other receptors (eg, solifenacin)[62]; transdermal oxybutynin, which bypasses first-pass hepatic metabolism to an active metabolite with anticholinergic adverse effects; or extended-release formulations of anticholinergic agents (eg, tolterodine), which produce lower peak plasma concentrations as compared to immediate-release formulations. For older adults at risk of sedation and confusion from anticholinergic agents, trospium or fesoterodine has a lower propensity to cross the blood-brain barrier and may be a good choice.[63]

In the presence of BPH, anticholinergic agents can cause acute urinary retention in patients with poor detrusor contractility. Therefore, before prescribing an anticholinergic agent, a PVR urine volume should be measured; it should be 100 to 150 mL or less.[9] By so doing, patients at high risk of acute urinary retention would be excluded from treatment.

β_3-Adrenergic Agonists

Approximately 95% of the β-adrenergic receptors in the urinary bladder are of the β_3 subtype. When stimulated, β_3-adrenergic receptors increase production of cyclic adenosine monophosphate (cAMP), which relaxes the detrusor muscle.[9,11]

9 β_3-Adrenergic agonists relax the detrusor muscle during the storage phase of the micturition cycle, thereby reducing irritative voiding symptoms, increasing urinary bladder capacity, and increasing the interval between voidings. They do not inhibit voiding or reduce urinary flow rate, nor do they increase PVR urine volume or cause acute urinary retention.[64] The clinical efficacy of these agents for LUTS is comparable to that of anticholinergic agents, but they are better tolerated. They do not produce anticholinergic adverse effects, nor do they cause acute urinary retention.

β_3-Adrenergenic agonists are indicated for symptomatic management of overactive bladder syndrome, which presents with symptoms that overlap with the irritative component of LUTS. For this reason, they are used as an alternative to anticholinergic agents in patients with LUTS, when irritative symptoms persist despite treatment with an α_1-adrenergic antagonist or 5α-reductase inhibitor.[64] The usual starting dose of mirabegron is 25 mg daily, increasing to 50 mg daily if needed. Increasing the dose to 100 mg is no more effective than 50 mg. A usual daily dose of 25 mg daily is recommended for patients with impaired renal function (creatinine clearance of 15-20 mL/min [0.25-0.33 mL/s]) or moderate hepatic impairment. Mirabegron should not be used in patients with severe hepatic dysfunction or a creatinine clearance less than 15 mL/min (0.25 mL/s).

Vibegron offers several potential advantages over mirabegron. It does not penetrate the blood brain barrier, has no significant blood pressure effects, and may be faster acting than mirabegron. For patients who have difficulty swallowing a tablet, it may be crushed and mixed with applesauce or stirred into a glass of water. Vibegron also does not cause significant interactions with cytochrome 3A4, 2D6, or 2C9.[64]

Adverse effects of mirabegron include mild headache, dry mouth, nausea, diarrhea, constipation, nasopharyngitis, and in rare cases QT-interval prolongation. None of these adverse effects cause discontinuation of treatment. Mirabegron increases systolic blood pressure by 0.5 to 1 mm Hg and heart rate by 1 bpm. Although these increases are generally small, older adults with BPH often have essential hypertension and the concern is that this may be worsened by mirabegron. Therefore, patients with uncontrolled hypertension or a systolic or diastolic blood pressure of 180 mm Hg or 110 mm Hg or higher, respectively, should avoid mirabegron. Regular blood pressure monitoring is advised in patients with poorly controlled blood pressure, significant congestive heart failure, cardiomyopathy, or patients who are 80 years of age or older.[9,11]

Combination Drug Therapy

Many drug combinations have been used for BPH. Typically, patients begin treatment with one medication and additional medications are added when LUTS does not improve or BPH symptoms worsen. To further reduce irritative voiding symptoms in a patient who is already taking an α_1-adrenergic antagonist, an anticholinergic agent, β_3-adrenergic agonist, or a phosphodiesterase type 5 inhibitor may be added.[8] When used alone, a 5α-reductase inhibitor has a slow onset of action. To achieve faster symptom relief, an α_1-adrenergic antagonist, anticholinergic agent,[65] β_3-adrenergic agonist, or a phosphodiesterase inhibitor[63,66] can be added. When any drug combination is used, the benefit of reducing bothersome symptoms must be balanced by the increased risk of adverse effects and drug interactions, higher cost of treatment, lower rates of adherence to treatment, and modest improvement in objective measures of BPH improvement.[63,65] Table 104-7 summarizes commonly prescribed combination regimens.

TABLE 104-7 Commonly Prescribed Combination BPH Regimens, Indications, and Precautions

Combination Regimen	Rationale	Comments
α_1-Adrenergic antagonist + 5α-reductase inhibitor	Moderate/severe LUTS with enlarged prostate gland of 40 g or more (or PSA >1.4 ng/mL [mcg/L])	These patients are at risk of developing complications of long-standing BPH.
α_1-Adrenergic antagonist + anticholinergic agent OR 5α-reductase inhibitor + anticholinergic agent	Moderate/severe LUTS with irritative symptoms not responding to an α_1-adrenergic antagonist alone[12] OR Moderate/severe LUTS with enlarged prostate gland of 40 g or more, and irritative symptoms	Use these combinations cautiously in patients already taking medications with anticholinergic effects/side effects. Avoid in patients with postvoid residual urine volume that is greater than 100 to 150 mL. Preferentially choose an anticholinergic agent with less likelihood to cross the blood brain barrier and cause confusion (eg, solifenacin).[14]
α_1-Adrenergic antagonist + β_3-adrenergic agonist OR 5α-reductase inhibitor + β_3-adrenergic agonist	Moderate/severe LUTS with irritative symptoms not responding to an α_1-adrenergic antagonist alone OR Moderate/severe LUTS with enlarged prostate gland of 40 g or more and irritative symptoms	Preferred regimen for patients with poor tolerance to side effects of anticholinergic agents. Do not use this combination in patients with unstable hypertension.
α_1-Adrenergic antagonist + phosphodiesterase inhibitor	Moderate/severe LUTS with irritative or obstructive symptoms not responding to an α_1-adrenergic antagonist alone[66] OR Moderate/severe LUTS with concomitant erectile dysfunction	This combination may cause hypotension. To minimize, preferentially use alfuzosin, tamsulosin, or silodosin when also prescribing tadalafil.[55]
5α-Reductase inhibitor+ phosphodiesterase inhibitor	Moderate/severe LUTS with enlarged prostate gland of 40 g or more and with irritative or obstructive symptoms not responding to a 5α-reductase inhibitor alone	The phosphodiesterase inhibitor can offset erectile dysfunction of 5α-reductase inhibitor.[9]

BPH, benign prostatic hypertrophy; LUTS, lower urinary tract symptoms.

Of all the combination medication regimens, an α_1-adrenergic antagonist plus a 5α-reductase inhibitor has been extensively studied and is recommended to use at the outset for patients with both moderate-to-severe symptoms and an enlarged prostate gland of at least 40 g and PSA of at least 1.4 ng/mL (mcg/L). Such patients are at high risk for disease progression, as evidenced by symptom worsening and development of disease complications, including acute urinary retention, recurrent urinary tract infection, or the need for surgical intervention.[67]

In the landmark Multiple Treatment of Prostate Symptoms Study (MTOPS), a combination regimen of finasteride and doxazosin for 5 years was shown to prevent symptom progression by 66%, decrease the risk of developing acute urinary retention by 81%, and decrease the need for prostate surgery by 67%. Moreover, urinary symptom improvement and higher urinary flow rates at 15 to 18 months were observed in patients treated with combination therapy, as compared with monotherapy with finasteride alone or doxazosin alone.[67] In another key clinical trial, the Combination of Avodart and Tamsulosin (COMBAT) study, dutasteride versus tamsulosin versus a combination of dutasteride and tamsulosin were evaluated in patients with prostate glands of 40 mL or greater and PSA of 1.5 ng/mL (mcg/L) or higher. The combination regimen was more effective in reducing symptoms 9 months after the start of treatment than dutasteride alone or tamsulosin alone. In addition, after a long-term follow-up of 4 years, the combination of dutasteride and tamsulosin prevented disease progression and reduced the need for prostate surgery.[68]

Although not proven by direct comparison trials, any combination of 5α-reductase inhibitor and α_1-adrenergic antagonist probably is similarly effective for patients with the aforementioned characteristics. The disadvantages of a combination regimen include increased medication cost, decreased adherence to multidrug treatment regimens, and an increased incidence of adverse drug effects (eg, sexual dysfunction).[62]

When this combination is used to prevent BPH progression, patients must continue both medications. Studies have shown if the 5α-reductase inhibitor is discontinued, LUTS recurs, and the prostate size may increase.[62] However, when the combination is used for LUTS in patients who are not at risk of BPH complications, the α_1-adrenergic antagonist may be discontinued after 6 or 9 months of continuous treatment with the 5α-reductase inhibitor.[9,11]

Surgical Interventions

10 The gold standard for treatment of patients with complications of BPH is prostatectomy.[9,11] Surgical intervention is indicated for patients with moderate-to-severe symptoms, who are not responsive to or cannot tolerate adverse effects of drug therapy, who are noncompliant with drug therapy, or who prefer surgical intervention. Surgical intervention is always indicated for patients with complications of BPH, including acute urinary retention not responsive to drug treatment, chronic urinary retention associated with decreased renal function or overflow urinary incontinence, urolithiasis, recurrent urinary tract infection, or recurrent hematuria.[9,11] Surgical removal of the prostatic adenoma offers the highest rate of symptom improvement, but it also has the highest complication rate.

With the availability of 5 medical treatment options for the treatment of BPH, most symptomatic patients are first managed medically. As a result, the number of surgeries for BPH has decreased significantly and the patients who are treated surgically for BPH tend to be older and more likely to have sarcopenia and/or frailty.[69-71] This has stimulated the technology development of a plethora of lasers and miniaturization of tools to expand the number and type of minimally invasive surgical procedures, which can be performed on an outpatient basis with local anesthesia, result in less blood loss, are less expensive than chronic medical treatment for BPH, and are associated with fewer adverse events than conventional prostatectomy procedures, which include transurethral resection of the prostate (TURP) or open prostatectomy.[11,70] However, all minimally invasive surgical procedures are also associated with a smaller improvement in voiding symptoms and a higher reoperation rate and shorter time to recurrence of LUTS than TURP or open prostatectomy.[11,70]

With TURP, an endoscopic resectoscope with a loop electrocautery inserted through the urethra is used to remove the inside core of the prostatic adenoma. This enlarges the opening at the bladder neck and prostatic urethra. Often performed as outpatient surgery, this procedure produces on average a peak urinary flow rate increase by 10 mL/s and improves the AUA Symptom Score by 10 to 18 points in approximately 90% of patients.[9,11] A common complication of TURP is retrograde ejaculation, occurring in up to 75% of patients. Bleeding, urinary incontinence, and erectile dysfunction occur in smaller, but significant numbers of patients (2%-15%).[70] Approximately 2% to 10% and 12% to 15% of patients require second surgeries within 5 and 8 years, respectively.[70]

A conventional open prostatectomy requires a suprapubic or perineal incision to allow the surgeon to remove the entire prostate gland. This procedure is reserved for large prostate glands of 80 to 100 g or more, and is a good choice when the patient has concurrent bladder stones or bladder diverticuli that can be corrected at the same time. Open prostatectomy is being performed laparoscopically or robotically. This procedure requires that the patient to be hospitalized. Once the entire prostate gland is excised along with the internal urethral sphincter, the urinary bladder and remaining urethra must be reconnected. The incision is stabilized by leaving an indwelling urethral catheter in place for 1 or 2 weeks. Adverse effects include bleeding, urinary and soft tissue infection, retrograde ejaculation in 77% of patients, erectile dysfunction in 16% to 33% of patients, and urinary incontinence in 2% of patients. The reoperation rate is 3% to 5% at 10 years.[9,70]

Table 104-8 lists common minimally invasive surgical procedures for BPH. Although the AUA guidelines include recommended indications for each procedure largely based on prostate gland size, additional key considerations include the availability of technology at the facility, skill and expertise of the surgeon, patient preference for one type of procedure over another, whether the patient's health insurance covers the cost of the procedure, and associated adverse effects of the procedure.

Phytotherapy

Although phytotherapy is widely used in Europe for the management of BPH, the published data on herbal agents are largely inconclusive and conflicting. Studies often lack placebo controls, which are essential for assessing treatments for BPH because spontaneous regression of mild symptoms can occur. Furthermore, because these agents are marketed under the Dietary Supplements Health and Education Act, their efficacy, safety, and quality are not regulated by the FDA. For these reasons, herbal products—including saw palmetto berry (*Serenoa repens*), stinging nettle (*Urtica dioica*), South African star grass (*Hypoxis rooperi*), pumpkin seed (*Cucurbita pepo*),

TABLE 104-8 Common Minimally Invasive Surgical Procedures for BPH

Procedure	Methodology	Indication	Comment
Transurethral incision of the prostate (TUIP)	Multiple incisions of the bladder neck widen the bladder neck to increase bladder emptying. Prostate tissue is not removed.	Best in men with small prostates 30 mL or less. Has outcomes similar to TURP.	The reoperation rate for TUIP is slightly higher than with TURP.
Prostatic urethral lift (Urolift)	Adjustable nitinol and stainless steel implants are inserted transurethrally. These implants tack open the obstructing prostate lobes and enhance bladder emptying. Prostate tissue is not removed.[71-73]	Indicated for prostate glands that are 30 to 80 mL. This procedure may be a good option for sexually active men as it appears to preserve erectile and ejaculatory function.[72-74]	Unsuitable for men with obstructing median lobes, prostates greater than 80 mL, or men with urinary retention.
Potassium titanyl phosphate (KTP or Green Light); Laser vaporization of the prostate	The laser is inserted transurethrally. The laser fiber vaporizes and coagulates prostate tissue. No tissue is available for pathologic analysis.	Indicated for prostate glands that are less than 80 mL. Some prostate tissue is removed. Laser vaporization may be preferred over TURP in patients with frailty, those taking anticoagulants, or those at risk of bleeding.[75]	
Robotic waterjet treatment (Aquablation)	Using image guidance and robotics, a cystoscope with ablation probe is inserted transurethrally. A targeted saline jet stream resects the prostate.[75-77] Resection time is less than 10 minutes. The saline is not heated, which reduces thermal injury to tissue.	Indicated for prostate glands that are 30 to 80 mL. May be a good option for sexually active patients, as sexual function appears to be unaffected by the procedure.	
Water vapor thermal therapy (Rezum)	Water vapor is heated using a bedside radiofrequency device. Vapor energy is delivered to and injected into the prostate transurethrally, and it causes cell necrosis. The procedure includes 4 or 5 injections.[78] This modality produces localized necrosis of the prostate without damaging the urethra since the prostatic pseudocapsule is resistant to heated water vapor.[78]	Indicated for prostate glands that are 30 to 80 mL, or in patients with an enlarged median lobe.[70,71,78] May be a good option for sexually active patients, as sexual function appears to be unaffected by the procedure.	It may take up to 3 months for peak clinical effects to be evident. This is because necrosed prostate tissue must be resorbed. Avoid this procedure in patients with implanted urethral sphincters or penile prosthesis.[78]
Thulium (ThuLEP) or Holmium (HoLEP); Laser Enucleation of the Prostate	Transurethrally, a resectoscope peels the prostate away from its capsule. The prostate is morcellated in the bladder and then extracted. The laser is then used for hemostasis.	Indicated for large prostate glands that are greater than 80 mL. Excised prostate tissue is removed and available for pathologic review. Laser prostatectomy is preferred over conventional therapy in patients who are taking anticoagulants or have a risk of bleeding.[79,80]	

Data from Reference 70.

and African plum (*Pygeum africanum*)—are not recommended for treatment of BPH.[14] Excellent reviews on phytotherapy for BPH have been published.[9,81]

EVALUATION OF THERAPEUTIC OUTCOMES

The primary therapeutic outcome of BPH therapy is improvement of voiding symptoms with minimal treatment-related adverse effects. As a disease for which therapy is directed at the voiding symptoms that the patient finds most bothersome, assessment of outcomes depends on the patient's perceptions of the effectiveness of therapy. Use of a validated, standardized instrument, such as the AUA Symptom Score, for assessing patient's voiding symptoms is important in this process.[9,11] A clinically significant improvement is generally associated with a decrease in score of three points or more. The efficacy of any new medication or medication combination for treatment of BPH should be assessed 6 to 12 weeks after its start. Symptomatic improvement of LUTS is expected, although 5α-reductase inhibitors will require at least 6 months to shrink an enlarged prostate.[9,11,16]

For patients being considered for surgical treatment, objective measures of bladder emptying are useful and include the urinary flow rate and PVR urine volume (see Diagnostic Evaluation section).

Because this patient population is at high risk for prostate cancer, PSA should be measured and a digital rectal examination performed annually if a patient has a life expectancy of at least 10 years. For patients taking 5α-reductase inhibitors, a second PSA taken 6 months after the start of treatment should be compared with baseline measurements. If the patient is suspected of having developed renal impairment as a consequence of long-standing bladder outlet obstruction, then BUN and serum creatinine should be evaluated at regular intervals.

CONCLUSION

A ubiquitous disease of aging men, symptomatic BPH requires medical attention to preserve the patient's quality of life and to prevent disease complications, many of which can be life-threatening in this patient population. In men who have no or mildly bothersome symptoms, watchful waiting and behavior modification are the best treatment approach, as BPH remains stable or even regresses in approximately half of these men.

For patients with voiding symptoms that are moderately to severely bothersome, pharmacotherapy is indicated. An α_1-adrenergic antagonist is the agent of first choice. Second-generation agents include terazosin, doxazosin, and alfuzosin, and third-generation agents include tamsulosin and silodosin. Immediate-release formulations of terazosin and doxazosin cause more cardiovascular adverse effects than do extended-release formulations (eg, doxazosin or alfuzosin), or uroselective α_{1A}-adrenergic agents (eg, tamsulosin, silodosin, or alfuzosin). 5α-Reductase inhibitors are preferred drug treatment for patients with enlarged prostates greater than 40 g who poorly tolerate the hypotensive adverse effects of α_1-adrenergic antagonists. However, 5α-reductase inhibitors have a slow onset of action. For patients who do not respond to monotherapy, combination drug therapy could be attempted.

The combination of 5α-reductase inhibitor and α_1-adrenergic antagonist is well established for patients at high risk of developing complications of BPH. In this subset of patients, continuous use of both medications is necessary.

For patients with both moderate-to-severe LUTS and erectile dysfunction, a phosphodiesterase inhibitor alone or combined with an α-adrenergic antagonist may be prescribed. For patients with moderate-to-severe LUTS with a predominance of irritative voiding symptoms, an anticholinergic agent, mirabegron, or a phosphodiesterase inhibitor may be added to an existing drug treatment regimen for BPH. Before starting an anticholinergic agent in a patient with BPH, the patient's PVR should be less than 100 to 150 mL.

For patients who do not respond to or cannot tolerate adverse effects of medical therapy, or who have complications of BPH, surgery is required. Although it has more adverse complications than pharmacotherapy or watchful waiting, TURP is considered the gold standard. Minimally invasive surgical procedures are an attractive alternative for older patients with frailty, as the procedures can be performed on an outpatient basis using local anesthesia. The risk of serious adverse effects are less with a minimally invasive surgical procedure than with TURP.

ABBREVIATIONS

ALLHAT	Antihypertensive and Lipid-Lowering Treatment to Prevent Heart Attack Trial
AUA	American Urological Association
BPE	benign prostatic enlargement
BPO	benign prostatic obstruction
BPH	benign prostatic hyperplasia
BUN	blood urea nitrogen
cAMP	cyclic adenosine monophosphate
cGMP	cyclic guanosine monophosphate
COMBAT	Combination of Avodart and Tamsulosin (Study)
CYP	cytochrome P-450
DHT	dihydrotestosterone
GI	gastrointestinal
IPSS	International Prostate Symptom Score
LUTS	lower urinary tract symptoms
MTOPS	Multiple Treatment of Prostate Symptoms (Study)
PSA	prostate-specific antigen
PVR	postvoid residual (pertains to urine volume)
REDUCE	Reduction by Dutasteride in Prostate Cancer Events
TURP	transurethral resection of the prostate
TUIP	transurethral incision of the prostate

REFERENCES

1. Glynn RJ, Campion EW, Bouchard GR, Silbert JE. The development of benign prostatic hyperplasia among volunteers in the Normative Aging Study. *Am J Epidemiol.* 1985;121(1):78–90.
2. Egan KB. The epidemiology of benign prostatic hyperplasia associated with lower urinary tract symptoms: Prevalence and incident rates. *Urol Clin North Am.* 2016;43(3):289–297.
3. Langan RC. Benign prostatic hyperplasia. *Prim Care.* 2019;46(2):223–232.
4. Rastrelli G, Vignozzi L, Corona G, Maggi M. Testosterone and benign prostatic hyperplasia. *Sex Med Rev.* 2019;7(2):259–271.
5. Skinder D, Zacharia I, Studen J, Covino J. Benign prostatic hyperplasia: A clinical review. *JAAPA.* 2016;29(8):19–23.
6. Nickel JC, Roehrborn CG, Castro-Santamaria R, et al. Chronic prostate inflammation is associated with severity and progression of benign prostatic hyperplasia, lower urinary tract symptoms and risk of acute urinary retention. *J Urol.* 2016; 196(5):1493–1498.
7. Madersbacher S, Sampson N, Culig Z. Pathophysiology of benign prostatic hyperplasia and benign prostatic enlargement: A mini-review. *Gerontology.* 2019;65(5):458–464.
8. Barkin J, Habert J, Wong Am, Lee LYT. The practical update for family physicians in the diagnosis and management of overactive bladder and lower urinary tract symptoms. *Can J Urol.* 2017; 24 (5 supplement 1):1–11.
9. Lerner LB, McVary KT, Barry MJ, et al. Management of benign prostatic hyperplasia/lower urinary tract symptoms: AUA Guideline 2021, part 1, initial work-up and medical management. *J Urol.* 2021 (https://doi.org/0.1097/JU.0000000000002183). Last accessed 8/30/2021.
10. Wasson JH, Reda DJ, Bruskewitz RC, et al. A comparison of transurethral surgery with watchful waiting for moderate symptoms

of benign prostatic hyperplasia. The Veterans Affairs Cooperative Study Group on Transurethral Resection of the Prostate. *N Engl J Med.* 1995;332(2):75–79.

11. Gravas S, Cornu JN, Gacci M, et al. EAU Guidelines on management of non-neurogenic male LUTS. EAU Guidelines EAN presented at the EAU Annual Congress, Milan 2021 (ISBN 9-8-94-92611-13-4. http://uroweb.org/guidelines/compilations-of-all-guidelines). Last accessed 8/31/2021.
12. Rossanese M, Crestani A, Inferrera A, et al. Medical treatment for benign prostatic hyperplasia: Where do we stand. *Urologia.* 2019;86(3):115–121.
13. Berkseth KE, Thirumalai A, Amory JK. Pharmacologic therapy in men's health: Hypogonadism, erectile dysfunction, and benign prostatic hyperplasia. *Med Clin North Am.* 2016;100(4):791–805.
14. Gul ZG, Kaplan SA. BPH: Why do patients fail medical therapy. *Curr Urol Rep.* 2019;20:40 (https://doi.org/10.1007/s11934-019-0899-z).
15. Welk B, McArthur E, Fraser LA, et al. The risk of fall and fracture with the initiation of a prostate-selective α antagonist: A population based cohort study. *BMJ.* 2015;351:h5398 (doi:10.1136/bmj.j5398).
16. Unnikrishnan R, Almassi N, Fareed K. Benign prostatic hyperplasia: Evaluation and medical management in primary care. *Cleve Clin J Med.* 2017;84(1):53–64.
17. Albisinni S, Aoun F, Roumequere T, et al. New treatment strategies for benign prostatic hyperplasia in the frail elderly population: A systematic review. *Minerva Urol Nefrol.* 2017;69(2):119–132.
18. ALLHAT Collaborative Research Group. Major cardiovascular events in hypertensive patients randomized to doxazosin vs chlorthalidone: The Antihypertensive and Lipid-Lowering Treatment to Prevent Heart Attack Trial (ALLHAT). *JAMA.* 2000;283(15):1967–1975.
19. Whelton PK, Carey RM, Aronow WS, et al. 2017 ACC/AHA/AAPA/ABC/ACPM/AGS/APhA/ASH/ASPC/NM/PCNA Guideline for the prevention, detection, evaluation, and management of high blood pressure in adults—a report of the American College of Cardiology/American Heart Association Task Force on Clinical Practice Guidelines. *J Am Coll Cardiol.* 2018;71(19):2199–2269.
20. Mottet N, Bressolle F, Delmas V, et al. Prostatic tissue distribution of alfuzosin in patients with benign prostatic hyperplasia following repeated oral administration. *Eur Urol.* 2003;44(1):101–105.
21. Lepor H. Alpha-blockers for the treatment of benign prostatic hyperplasia. *Urol Clin North Am.* 2016;43(3):311–323.
22. Albisinni S, Biaou I, Marcelis Q, et al. New medical treatments for lower urinary tract symptoms due to benign prostatic hyperplasia and future perspectives. *BMC Urol.* 2016;16(1):58 (doi: 10.1186/s12894-016-0176-0).
23. Villa L, Capogrosso P, Capitanio U, Martini A. Silodosin: An update on efficacy, safety, and clinical indications in urology. *Adv Ther.* 2019;36(1):1–18.
24. Jung JH, Kim J, MacDonald R, et al. Silodosin for the treatment of lower urinary tract symptoms in men with benign prostatic hyperplasia (review). *Cochrane Database Syst Rev.* 2017; Nov 22;11(11): CD012615.
25. Herberts M, Butcher M, Kohler T. The effect of LUTS/BPH and treatments on ejaculatory function. *Curr Urol Rep.* 2016;17(7):48 (doi:10.1007/s11934-016-0604-4).
26. Aharony S, Lam O, Corcos J. Is there a demonstrated advantage to increase tamsulosin dosage in patients with benign prostatic hyperplasia? *Urology.* 2014;84(2):493–494.
27. Bird ST, Delaney JA, Brophy JM, et al. Tamsulosin treatment for benign prostatic hyperplasia and risk of severe hypotension in men aged 40-85 years in the United States: Risk window analyses using between and within patient methodology. *BMJ.* 2013;347:f6320. doi:10.1136/bmj.f6320.
28. Roehrborn CG, Cruz F, Fusco F. α1-Blockers in men with lower urinary tract symptoms suggestive of benign prostatic obstruction: Is silodosin different? *Adv Ther.* 2017;33(12):2110–2121.
29. Belayneh M, Korownyk C. Treatment of lower urinary tract symptoms in benign prostatic hypertrophy with α-blockers. *Can Fam Phys.* 2016;62(9):e523.
30. La Vignera S, Aversa A, Cannarella R, et al. Pharmacological treatment of lower urinary tract symptoms in benign prostatic hyperplasia: Consequences on sexual function and possible endocrine effects. *Expert Opin Pharmacother.* 2021;22(2):179–189.
31. Califano G, Colla Ruvolo CC, Creta M, et al. Focus on silodosin: Pros and cons of uroselectivity. *Res Rep Urol.* 2020;12:669–672.
32. Welliver C, Essa A. Sexual side effects of medical and surgical benign prostatic hyperplasia treatments. *Urol Clin North Am.* 2016;43(3):393–404.
33. Duan Y, Grady JJ, Albertsen PC, Wu ZH. Tamsulosin and the risk of dementia in older men with benign prostatic hyperplasia. *Pharmacoepidemiol Drug Saf.* 2018;27(3):340–348.
34. Tae BS, Jeon BJ, Choi H, et al. α-Blocker and risk of dementia in patients with benign prostatic hyperplasia: A nationwide population based study using the National Health Insurance Database. *J Urol.* 2019;202(2):362–368.
35. Kumar A, Raj A. Intraoperative floppy iris syndrome: An updated review of the literature. *Int Ophthalmol.* 2021 June 29. doi:10.1007/s10792-021-01936-5.
36. Christou Cd, Tsinopoulos I, Ziakas N, Tzamalis A. Intraoperative floppy iris syndrome: Updated perspective. *Clin Ophthalmol.* 2020;14:463–471.
37. Gacci M, Corona G, Salvi M, et al. A systematic review and meta-analysis on the use of phosphodiesterase 5 inhibitors alone or in combination with α-blockers for lower urinary tract symptoms due to benign prostatic hyperplasia. *Eur Urol.* 2012;61(5):994–1003.
38. Goldfischer E, Kowalczyk JJ, Clark WR, et al. Hemodynamic effects of once-daily tadalafil in men with signs and symptoms of benign prostatic hyperplasia on concomitant α1-adrenergic antagonist therapy: Results of a multicenter randomized, double-blind, placebo-controlled trial. *Urology.* 2012;79(4):875–882.
39. Wu C, Kapoor A. Dutasteride for the treatment of benign prostatic hyperplasia. *Expert Opin Pharmacother.* 2013;14(10):1399–1408.
40. Nickel JC, Gilling P, Tammela TL, et al. Comparison of dutasteride and finasteride for treating benign prostatic hyperplasia: The Enlarged Prostate International Comparator Study (EPICS). *BJU Int.* 2011;108(3):388–394.
41. Zatton R, Ficarra V, Novara G. Risk stratification for benign prostatic hyperplasia. *Urologia.* 2017;84(3):153–157.
42. Roehrborn CG, Nickel JC, Andriole GL, et al. Dutasteride improves outcomes of benign prostatic hyperplasia when evaluated for prostate cancer risk reduction: Secondary analysis of the Reduction by Dutasteride of Prostate Cancer Events (REDUCE) trial. *Urology.* 2011;78(3):641–646.
43. Roehrborn CG, Bruskewitz R, Nickel JC, et al. Sustained decrease in incidence of acute urinary retention and surgery with finasteride for 6 years in men with benign prostatic hyperplasia. *J Urol.* 2004;171(3):1194–1198.
44. Welliver C, Butcher M, Potini Y, McVary KT. Impact of alpha blockers, 5-alpha reductase inhibitors and combination therapy on sexual function. *Curr Urol Rep.* 2014;15(10):441. doi:10.1007/s11934-014-0441-2.
45. Thompson IM, Goodman PJ, Tangen CM, et al. The influence of finasteride on the development of prostate cancer. *N Engl J Med.* 2003;349(3):215–224.
46. Thompson IM, Tangen CM, Goodman PJ, et al. Finasteride improves the sensitivity of digital rectal examination for prostate cancer detection. *J Urol.* 2007;177(5):1749–1752.
47. Andriole GL, Bostwick DG, Brawley OW, et al. for the REDUCE Study Group. Effect of dutasteride on the risk of prostate cancer. *N Engl J Med.* 2010;362(13):1192–1202.
48. Theoret MR, Ning YM, Zhang JJ, et al. The risks and benefits of 5α-reductase inhibitors for prostate cancer prevention. *N Engl J Med.* 2011;365(2):97–99.
49. Liu L, Zhao S, Li F, et al. Effect of 5α-reductase inhibitors on sexual function: A meta-analysis and systematic review of randomized controlled trials. *J Sex Med.* 2016;13(9): 1297–1310.
50. Corona C, Tirabassi G, Santi D, et al. Sexual dysfunction in subjects treated with inhibitors of 5α-reductase for benign prostatic hyperplasia: A comprehensive review and meta-analysis. *Andrology.* 2017;5(4):671–678.
51. Traish AM. Post-finasteride syndrome: A surmountable challenge for clinicians. *Fertil Steril.* 2020;113(1):21–50.
52. Kaplan SA, Chung DE, Lee RK, et al. A 5-year retrospective analysis of 5alpha-reductase inhibitors in men with benign prostatic hyperplasia: Finasteride has comparable urinary symptom efficacy and prostate volume reduction, but less sexual side effects and breast complications than dutasteride. *Int J Clin Pract.* 2012;66(11):1052–1055.
53. Meijer M, Thygesen LC, Green A, et al. Finasteride treatment and male breast cancer: A register-based cohort study in four Nordic countries. *Cancer Med.* 2018;7(1):254–260.
54. Welk B, McArthur E, Ordon M, et al. Association of suicidality and depression with 5α-reductase inhibitors. *JAMA Intern Med.* 2017;177(5):683–91.
55. Pietrzk B, Olszanecka-Glinianowicx M, Owczarek A, et al. Depressive symptoms in patients diagnosed with benign prostatic hyperplasia. *Int Urol Nephrol.* 2015;47(3):431–440.

56. Xu D, Ding J, Zhu Y, et al. The new insight of prostate-specific antigen reduction during finasteride therapy in aging men. *Aging Clin Exp Res.* 2016;28(6):1237–1241.
57. Amano T, Earle C, Imao T, et al. Administration of daily 5 mg tadalafil improves endothelial function in patients with benign prostatic hyperplasia. *Aging Male.* 2018;21(1):77–82.
58. Calogero AE, Burgio G, Condorella RA, et al. Treatment of lower urinary tract symptoms/benign prostatic hyperplasia and erectile dysfunction. *Aging Male.* 2018;21(4):272–280.
59. Pattanaik SM, Mavuduru RS, Panda A, et al. Phosphodiesterase inhibitors for lower urinary tract symptoms consistent with benign prostatic hyperplasia. *BJU Int.* 2019;124(1):27–34.
60. Gacci M, Andersson K-E, Chapple C, et al. Latest evidence on the use of phosphodiesterase type 5 inhibitors for the treatment of lower urinary tract symptoms secondary to benign prostatic hyperplasia. *Eur Urol.* 2016;70(1):124–133.
61. Nehra A, Jackson G, Miner M, et al. The Princeton III Consensus Recommendations for the management of erectile dysfunction and cardiovascular disease. *Mayo Clin Proc.* 2012;87(8):766–778.
62. Zhou Z, Cui Y, Wu J, et al. Meta-analysis of the efficacy and safety of combination of tamsulosin plus dutasteride compared with tamsulosin monotherapy in treating benign prostatic hyperplasia. *BMC Urol.* 2019;19:17 (doi.org/10.1186/s12894-019-0446-8).
63. Thomas D, Chughtai B, Kini M, Te A. Emerging drugs for the treatment of benign prostatic hyperplasia. *Expert Opin Emerg Drugs.* 2017;22(3):202–212.
64. Anon. Vebegron (Gemtesa) for overactive bladder. *Med Lett Drugs Ther.* 2021;63(1623): 67–69.
65. Pang R, Zhou XY, Wang X, et al. Anticholinergics combined with alpha-blockers for treating lower urinary tract symptoms related to benign prostatic obstruction. *Cochrane Database System Rev.* 2021, Feb 10;2(2):CD012336.
66. Sebastianelli A, Spatafora P, Morselli S, et al. Tadalafil alone or in combination with tamsulosin for the management for LUTS/BPH and ED. *Curr Urol Rep.* 2020;21(12):56 (doi:10.1007/S11934-020-01009-7)/
67. McConnell JD, Roehrborn CG, Bautista OM, et al. The long-term effect of doxazosin, finasteride, and combination therapy on the clinical progression of benign prostatic hyperplasia. *N Engl J Med.* 2003;349(25):2387–2398.
68. Roehrborn CG, Barkin J, Siami P, et al. Clinical outcomes after combined therapy with dutasteride plus tamsulosin or either monotherapy in men with benign prostatic hyperplasia (BPH) by baseline characteristics: 4-year results from the randomized, double-blind Combination of Avodart and Tamsulosin (CombAT) trial. *BJU Int.* 2011;107(6):946–954.
69. Presicce F, De Nunzio C, Tubaro A. Is early benign prostatic hyperplasia (BPH) treatment worthwhile? *Urologia.* 2017;84(3):142–147.
70. Lerner LB, McVary KT, Barry MJ, et al. Management of lower urinary tract symptoms attributed to benign prostatic hyperplasia. AUA Guideline part II, surgical evaluation and treatment. *J Urol.* 2021; https://doi.org/10.1097/JU.0000000000002184. Last accessed 8/30/2021.
71. Salciccia S, Del Giudice F, Maggi M, et al. Safety and feasibility of outpatient surgery in benign prostatic hyperplasia: A systematic review and meta-analysis. *J Endourol.* 2021;35(4):395–408.
72. Magistro G, Stief C, Woo HH. Mini-review: What is new in Urolift. *Eur Urol Focus.* 2018;4(1):36–39.
73. Das AK, Leong JY, Roehrborn CG. Office-based therapies for benign prostatic hyperplasia: A review and update. *Can J Urol.* 2019;26 (4 suppl 1):2–7.
74. Miller LE, Chughtai B, Dornbier RA, McVary KT. Surgical reintervention rate after prostatic urethral lift: Systematic review and meta-analysis involving over 2,000 patients. *J Urol.* 2020;204(5):1019–2026.
75. Huang SW, Tsai CY, Tseng CS, et al. Comparative efficacy and safety of new surgical treatments for benign prostatic hyperplasia: Systematic review and network meta-analysis. *BMJ.* 2019;367:15919 (doi:10.1136/bmj.15919:10.1136/bmj.15919)
76. Nguyen DD, Barber N, Bidair M, et al. Waterjet ablation therapy for endoscopic resection of prostate tissue trial (WATER) vs WATER II: Comparing Aquablation therapy for benign prostatic hyperplasia in 30-80 and 80-150 mL prostates. *BJU Int.* 2020;125:112–122.
77. National Institute for Health and Care Excellence. NICE Guidance-transurethral water jet ablation for lower urinary tract symptoms caused by benign prostatic hyperplasia. *BJU Int.* 2019;124(3):368–369.
78. Doppalapudi SK, Gupta N. What is new with Rezum water vapor thermal therapy for LUTS/BPH? *Curr Urol Rep.* 2021;22(1):4 (doi.org/10.1107x11934-020-01018-6).; 78. Green Z, Westwood J, Somani BK. What's new in Rezum: a transurethral water vapour therapy for BPH. *Curr Urol Rep.* 2019;20:30 (https://doi.org/10.1007/x11934-019-0903-7).
79. Cornu JN. Bipolar, monopolar, photovaporization of the prostate, or holmium laser enucleation of the prostate-How to choose what's best. *Urol Clin N Am.* 2016;43(3):377–384.
80. Shigemura K, Fujisawa M. Current status of holmium laser enucleation of the prostate. *Int J Urol.* 2018;25(3):206–211.
81. Keehn A, Taylor J, Lowe FC. Phytotherapy for benign prostatic hyperplasia. *Curr Urol Rep.* 2016;17:53. doi:10.1007/s11934-016-0609-z.

105

Urinary Incontinence

Eric S. Rovner, Kristine M. C. Talley, and Sum Lam

KEY CONCEPTS

1. In evaluating urinary incontinence (UI), drug-induced or drug-aggravated etiologies must be ruled out.
2. Accurate diagnosis and classification of UI type are critical to the selection of appropriate pharmacotherapy.
3. Goals of treatment for UI are reduction of symptoms, minimization of adverse effects, and improvement in quality of life.
4. Nonpharmacologic, nonsurgical treatment is the first-line treatment for several types of UI, and should be continued even when drug therapy is initiated.
5. Antimuscarinic agents are second-line treatments for urgency incontinence. Choice of agent should be based on patient characteristics (eg, age, comorbidities, concurrent medications, and ability to adhere to the prescribed regimen).
6. β_3-Adrenergic agonists (mirabegron, vibegron) can be considered in patients who failed to achieve optimal efficacy or cannot tolerate adverse effects of antimuscarinic agents.
7. Duloxetine (approved in Europe only), α-adrenergic receptor agonists, and topical (vaginal) estrogens (alone or together) are the drugs of choice for urethral underactivity (stress urinary incontinence).
8. Assessment of patient outcomes should include efficacy, adverse effects, adherence, and quality of life.
9. Management of UI should target individualized goals and treatment preferences, which may change over time. If therapeutic goals are not achieved with a given agent at optimal dosage for an adequate duration of trial, consider switching to an alternative agent and/or surgery.

BEYOND THE BOOK

Watch one of the two videos titled "Taking Control of Overactive Bladder (OAB)" by the Urology Care Foundation. Reflect on the impact of OAB from the patient's perspective. Available at: https://www.urologyhealth.org/urology-a-z/o/overactive-bladder-(oab)

Next, develop a table with two columns, one titled antimuscarinic agents and one titled β_3-adrenergic agonists. In each column, identify one drug that represents the drug class. Compare the advantages and disadvantages of these two agents when used for the treatment of OAB (efficacy, dosage form, dosing, side effects, drug interactions, drug cost, etc.).

INTRODUCTION

Urinary incontinence (UI) is defined as involuntary loss of urine.[1] It is frequently accompanied by other bothersome lower urinary tract symptoms, such as urgency, increased daytime frequency, and nocturia. It is one of the most common health conditions occurring in adults, and yet it is an underdetected and under-reported problem that can significantly affect quality of life. Patients with UI may have depression as a result of the perceived lack of self-control, loss of independence, and lack of self-esteem, and they often curtail their activities for fear of an "accident." UI may also have serious medical and economic ramifications for untreated or undertreated patients, including perineal dermatitis, worsening of pressure ulcers, urinary tract infections, and falls.

This chapter highlights the epidemiology, etiology, pathophysiology, treatment of stress, urgency, mixed, and overflow UI in men and women.

Editors' note: In this and other chapters in Pharmacotherapy, references to biologic gender (as assigned at birth) are used based on prior literature being discussed or anatomical or physiologic differences. We recognize that not all individuals identify with their gender at birth, and to the degree possible when discussing therapeutics, we avoid use of references to gender. In this chapter on Urinary Incontinence, "men" and "women" are used in discussing prior studies, published guidelines, and other recommendations for diagnosis and treatment based on biological gender and do not necessarily reflect an individual's gender identity.

EPIDEMIOLOGY

UI is highly prevalent, and the impact of this condition is substantial, crossing all racial, ethnic, and geographic boundaries. In addition, lower urinary tract symptoms (eg, urgency, urinary frequency, and nocturia) associated with OAB are also quite debilitating. Evidence from several studies indicates that UI is associated with reduced levels of social and personal activities, increased psychological distress, and overall decreased quality of life.[2] The condition can affect people of all age groups, but the peak incidence of UI, at least in women, occurs around the age of menopause, with a slight decrease in the age group 55 to 60 years, and then a steadily increasing prevalence after the age of 65 years.

Globally, the prevalence of UI ranges between 25% and 45%.[3] Determining the true prevalence of UI is difficult because of problems with definition, reporting bias, and other methodological issues. The condition is stigmatizing as it is associated with considerable embarrassment, as well as real or perceived loss of self-control. Such perceptions may lead to a decrease in reporting, especially self-reporting. Prevalence estimates vary by age, gender, and racial/ethnic group, setting (noninstitutionalized vs institutionalized), and incontinence subtype (stress, urgency, mixed, and overflow UI). Prevalence tends to be highest in women, those of advanced age, and living in long-term care settings.[2] Globally, women have three times the prevalence of urinary incontinence than men. The prevalence of incontinence increases as women age. Ten percent of adult women have incontinence, but this prevalence increases to 40% for women aged 70 years and older.[3] The National Health and Nutrition Examination Survey (NHANES) reported a prevalence rate of 43.8% in noninstitutionalized adults aged 65 years and over, with more than half of women and one-quarter of men reporting urine leakage.[2] Twelve percent of older women had severe or very severe scores on a validated incontinence severity index representing daily urine leakage with more than drops or small splashes, whereas older men had slight or moderate incontinence scores representing less-frequent urine leakage.[2]

Relatively little is known about differences in clinical and epidemiologic characteristics of incontinence across racial or ethnic groups, especially in men. Almost all population-based studies comparing UI prevalence across racial and ethnic groups are from the United States which limits generalizability. The majority of studies report that White women have a higher prevalence of UI overall and stress UI.[4] There is less consistency regarding prevalence of UI subtypes in Black women. In the BACH study, Black women had higher rates of mixed UI,[5] and in the EPI study, Black women had higher rates of urgency UI.[6] Using data from the NHANES program, no racial or ethnic differences were found in UI prevalence in men.[7] However, differences in access to healthcare as well as cultural attitudes and more may contribute to these differences.[8,9] Importantly, there are considerable differences in the causes and treatments of UI between genders.

UI prevalence is highest in nursing home residents, with 36.7% of short-stay residents and 70.3% of long-term residents having bladder control problems.[2] Residents who were aged 85 years and more compared to those aged 65 to 74 years had rates 1.5 times higher for short-term residents and 1.2 higher for long-term residents. UI is associated with several other medical conditions, such as falls,[10] urinary tract infection, skin breakdown, sexual function, and depression.

ETIOLOGY AND PATHOPHYSIOLOGY

Anatomy

The lower urinary tract consists of the bladder, urethra, urinary or urethral sphincter, and surrounding musculofascial structures, including connective tissue, nerves, and blood vessels. The urinary bladder is a hollow organ composed of smooth muscle and connective tissue located deep in the bony pelvis in men and women. The urethra is a hollow tube that acts as a conduit for urine flow out of the bladder. An epithelial cell layer termed the *urothelium*, which is in constant contact with urine, lines the interior surface of both the bladder and the urethra. Previously considered inert and inactive, the urothelium may play an active role in the pathophysiology of many lower urinary tract disorders, including interstitial cystitis/bladder pain syndrome and UI[11] and may be a targeted location for future pharmacologic therapeutic interventions for some types of lower urinary tract dysfunction.[12] The urinary or urethral sphincter is a combination of smooth and striated muscle within and surrounding the proximal portion of the urethra adjacent to the bladder. In the male, the prostate gland lies just beyond the bladder outlet and is intimately associated with the urethral sphincter. Its location accounts for both the favorable effects of pharmacological manipulation on male lower symptoms as well as the risk of UI in males following some types of prostate surgery.

To understand the principles of pharmacotherapy for UI, an understanding of the neuroanatomy and neurophysiology of the bladder and urethra is needed. The primary motor (efferent) input to the detrusor muscle of the bladder is parasympathetic and travels along the pelvic nerves emanating from spinal cord segments S2 to S4. Pharmacologic as well as nonpharmacologic stimulation, modulation, or blockade of afferent and efferent neural pathways between the spinal cord and the lower urinary tract by various mechanisms are important options for treatment for some types of urinary incontinence. Acetylcholine is the primary neurotransmitter at the neuromuscular junction in the human lower urinary tract. Both volitional and involuntary detrusor contractions are mediated by activation of postsynaptic muscarinic receptors by acetylcholine. Of the five known subtypes of muscarinic receptors, the majority of bladder smooth muscle cholinergic receptors are of the M_2 variety. In humans, the ratio of M_2/M_3 receptor numbers is approximately 3:1. However, M_3 receptors are the subtypes responsible for both emptying contractions of normal micturition as well as involuntary bladder contractions that may result in UI.[11] Thus, most pharmacologic antimuscarinic therapy is primarily anti-M_3 based. Administration of such agents results in detrusor smooth muscle relaxation and a reduction of bladder overactivity.

β_3-Adrenergic receptors are found in the lower urinary tract at the level of the detrusor muscle and the urothelium.[11] Although found elsewhere, stimulation of these receptors in the detrusor results in smooth muscle relaxation. Clinically, administration of β_3-agonists is associated with attenuation of bladder contractility and, similar to antimuscarinics, it is used clinically to treat overactive bladder (OAB) and related urgency incontinence. β-Receptors are also located on the urethra but their clinical significance is considered to be negligible.

Clinically relevant α-adrenergic receptors are located at the level of the bladder outlet on the smooth and striated muscle of the urethra.[11] Stimulation of these receptors with α-adrenergic agonists results in increased urethral closure pressure. Such effects are usually not pronounced enough to treat stress urinary incontinence (SUI); however, the use of these agents may result in unwanted adverse effects such as aggravation of bladder outlet obstruction and result in poor bladder emptying (urinary retention), especially in men.

Other potentially relevant motor and sensory pathways, neurotransmitters, and receptors have been identified in the lower urinary tract (eg, transient receptor potential channels, E-series prostaglandin receptors). However, the exact role of such targets, as well as ways of modulating their activity pharmacologically in humans, has yet to be elucidated and further discussion is beyond the scope of this chapter.

Urinary Continence

To prevent incontinence during the bladder filling and storage phase of the micturition cycle, the urethra, or more accurately the urethral sphincter, must maintain adequate closure in order to resist the flow of urine from the bladder at all times until voluntary voiding is initiated. Urethral closure or resistance to flow is maintained to a large degree by the proximal (under involuntary control) and distal (under both voluntary and involuntary control) urinary sphincters. Variable contributions to urethral closure may also come from the urethral mucosa, submucosal spongy tissue, and the overall length of the urethra. During bladder filling and urinary storage, the bladder accommodates increasing volumes of urine flowing in from the upper urinary tract without a significant increase in bladder (intravesical) pressure. The maintenance of a low intravesical pressure despite increasing volumes of urine is a unique property of the bladder and is termed *compliance*. In addition, bladder or detrusor smooth muscle activity is normally suppressed during the filling phase by centrally mediated neural reflexes. Normal bladder emptying occurs with opening of the urethral sphincters concomitant with a volitional bladder contraction. Bladder contraction occurs in a coordinated fashion, resulting in a rise in intravesical pressure. The rise in intravesical pressure is ideally of adequate magnitude and duration to empty the bladder to completion. Opening and funneling of the bladder outlet results in urine flow into the urethra until the bladder is emptied to near completion.

The bladder and urethra normally operate in unison during the bladder filling and storage phase, as well as the bladder emptying phase of the micturition cycle. The smooth and striated muscles of the bladder and urethra are organized during the micturition cycle by a number of reflexes coordinated at the pontine micturition center in the midbrain. Disturbances in the neural regulation of micturition at any level (brain, spinal cord, or pelvic nerves) often lead to characteristic changes in lower urinary tract function that may result in UI.[13,14]

Mechanisms of Urinary Incontinence

Simply stated, UI may occur as a result of abnormalities of only the urethra (including the bladder outlet and urinary sphincter) or only the bladder or as a combination of abnormalities in both. Abnormalities may result in either overactivity or underactivity of the bladder and/or urethra, with resulting development of UI. Although this simple classification scheme excludes extremely rare causes of UI such as congenital ectopic ureters and urinary fistulas, it is useful for gaining a working understanding of the condition and understanding the basis for therapeutic intervention including pharmacotherapy of various lower urinary tract disorders.

Urethral Underactivity (SUI) Stress urinary incontinence is defined as the involuntary loss of urine on effort or physical exertion (including sporting activities) or on sneezing or coughing.[1] The pathophysiology of SUI is related to decreased or inadequate urethral closure forces. In individuals with SUI, the muscular tissues surrounding the urethra that form the urethral sphincter are compromised and thus not able to resist the expulsive forces resulting from transient increases in intra-abdominal pressure during physical activity. Such forces are transmitted to the bladder (an intra-abdominal organ), compressing it to such an extent as to cause the egress of urine through the urethra. SUI is characterized by episodic, usually low-volume urinary leakage but is clearly proportional to the amount of physical exertion or other increases in abdominal pressure such as that related to coughing and sneezing as well as the ambient urethral closure forces.

Risk factors for SUI in woman include pregnancy, childbirth, menopause, cognitive impairment, obesity, and aging.[15] In men, SUI is most commonly the result of prior lower urinary tract surgery and injury to the sphincter mechanism within and external to the urethra. Radical prostatectomy for treatment of adenocarcinoma of the prostate and transurethral resection of the prostate (TURP) is probably the most common proximate causes of SUI in the male. Notably, compared with its prevalence in women, SUI in men is actually quite rare.

SUI may be caused or aggravated by some pharmacologic agents such as α-antagonists and angiotensin-converting enzyme (ACE) inhibitors.[16] α-Antagonists may relax the smooth muscle at the level of the urethral sphincter, resulting in a weakened closure mechanism and the onset of SUI. Alternatively, some α-agonists, such as those used clinically for nasal congestion or weight loss, may improve SUI in some individuals, and may even potentially aggravate some types of voiding problems such as those related to bladder outlet obstruction from an enlarged prostate. An adverse effect of some ACE inhibitors is chronic cough, which can also aggravate existing SUI.

Bladder Overactivity (Urgency Urinary Incontinence [UUI]) Urgency UI is defined as the involuntary loss of urine associated with urgency.[1] This is most often related to detrusor (bladder) overactivity due to involuntary bladder contractions. Bladder overactivity describes the condition in which the detrusor muscle contracts inappropriately during urinary storage that, in the neurologically normal individual, results in a sense of urinary urgency. Overactive bladder is a symptom syndrome characterized by urinary urgency, usually accompanied by increased daytime frequency and/or nocturia, with urinary incontinence (OAB-wet) or without (OAB-dry), in the absence of urinary tract infection or other detectable diseases.[1] The terms *overactive bladder* and *detrusor (bladder) overactivity* are distinct and should not be used interchangeably.

Increased *frequency* is defined as the complaint that micturition occurs more frequently during waking hours than previously deemed normal; numerically, it is often quantified as more than eight times per day. *Urgency* is described as a sudden compelling desire to urinate that is difficult to defer.[1] People with OAB typically have to empty their bladder frequently, and, when they experience a sensation of urgency, they may leak urine if they are unable to reach the toilet quickly. Many patients have associated nocturia (>1 micturition per night) and/or nocturnal incontinence (enuresis). Patients with urgency urinary incontinence (UUI) often, but invariably, experience high-volume urine leakage when it occurs. Although detrusor overactivity may be related to OAB, the former diagnosis requires urodynamic testing while the latter is symptomatically defined.

Most patients with OAB and UUI have no identifiable underlying etiology and thus are classified as "idiopathic." Patients with a combination of a relevant neurologic condition and UI related to involuntary bladder contractions demonstrated on urodynamic testing are classified as having neurogenic detrusor overactivity. Clearly identifiable risk factors for UUI include normal aging, neurologic disease (including stroke, Parkinson's disease, multiple sclerosis, and spinal cord injury), and bladder outlet obstruction resulting in pathological changes to the detrusor muscle (eg, due to benign prostatic hyperplasia [BPH] or prostate cancer).[4]

The pathophysiology of OAB and UUI is not well understood but is likely related to either neurogenic or myogenic factors or a combination of both.[1] A full discussion of these differences is complex and beyond the scope of this chapter. However, in practice, although the cause of UUI is difficult to define, the treatment is identical regardless of etiology and pathophysiology.

Some pharmacologic agents may cause or aggravate UUI. Diuretics will cause the rapid accumulation of urine in the bladder with resulting urinary urgency and frequency that can result in UUI. Alcohol will have similar effects. Anticholinesterase inhibitors may also produce urgency and frequency.

Urethral Overactivity and/or Bladder Underactivity (Overflow Incontinence) Overflow incontinence is urinary leakage resulting from an overfilled and distended bladder that is unable to empty. This type of UI occurs when the bladder is filled to capacity at all times but is unable to empty, causing urine to leak from a distended bladder past a normal or even overactive sphincter. Another term related to overflow incontinence is *chronic urinary retention*.[1]

Overflow incontinence is the result of urethral overactivity, bladder underactivity, or a variable combination of both. Clinically and practically, the most common causes of urethral overactivity in men are anatomic urethral obstruction, including that due to BPH and prostate cancer. In women, urethral overactivity is rare but may result from cystocele formation (with resultant kinking or obstruction of the urethra) or surgical overcorrection following surgery for the repair of SUI (iatrogenic obstruction). In both men and women, overflow UI may be associated with systemic neurologic dysfunction or diseases, such as spinal cord injury or multiple sclerosis.

Bladder underactivity occurs as a result of the detrusor muscle of the bladder becoming suddenly or progressively weakened and eventually losing the ability to voluntarily contract and expel urine

TABLE 105-1 Medications That Influence Lower Urinary Tract Function

Medication	Effect
Diuretics, acetylcholinesterase inhibitors	Polyuria resulting in urinary frequency, urgency
α-Receptor antagonists	Urethral muscle relaxation and stress urinary incontinence
α-Receptor agonists	Urethral muscle contraction (increased urethral closure forces) resulting in urinary retention (more common in men)
Calcium channel blockers	Urinary retention due to reduced bladder contractility
Narcotic analgesics	Urinary retention due to reduced bladder contractility
Sedative hypnotics	Functional incontinence caused by delirium, immobility
Antipsychotic agents	Anticholinergic effects resulting in reduced bladder contractility and urinary retention
Anticholinergics	Urinary retention due to reduced bladder contractility
Antidepressants, tricyclic	Anticholinergic effects resulting in reduced bladder contractility (urinary retention), and α-antagonist effects resulting in reduced urethral smooth muscle contraction (stress incontinence)
Alcohol	Polyuria resulting in urinary frequency, urgency
ACEIs	Cough as a result of ACEIs may aggravate stress urinary incontinence

ACEIs, angiotensin-converting enzyme inhibitors.

during voiding. In the absence of adequate contractility, the bladder is unable to empty completely, and large volumes of residual urine are left after voiding. Both myogenic and neurogenic factors have been implicated in producing the impaired contractility seen in this condition. Clinically, overflow incontinence is most commonly seen in the setting of long-term chronic bladder outlet obstruction in men, such as that due to BPH or prostate cancer, diabetes mellitus, or denervation due to radical pelvic surgery, such as abdominopelvic resection or radical hysterectomy.

1 Many commonly used medications may precipitate or aggravate existing voiding dysfunction and UI (Table 105-1).[17] Agents that increase urethral resistance or closure pressure include α-agonists and tricyclic antidepressants. Over-the-counter cold and cough remedies as well as diet pills may contain agents with α-adrenergic properties and/or antihistaminic properties that can result in voiding dysfunction and urinary retention. Agents that can decrease bladder contractility include anticholinergics, tricyclic antidepressants, calcium channel blockers, narcotic analgesics, and antipsychotics.

Mixed Incontinence and Other Types of Urinary Incontinence Various types of UI may coexist in the same patient. The combination of bladder overactivity resulting in urinary incontinence (urgency UI) and urethral underactivity resulting in urinary incontinence (SUI or stress UI) is termed *mixed incontinence.* The diagnosis is often difficult because of the confusing array of presenting symptoms. Bladder overactivity may also coexist with impaired bladder contractility. This occurs most commonly in the elderly and is termed *detrusor hyperactivity with impaired contractility.*[1]

Functional incontinence (also known as disability-associated urinary incontinence) is not caused by bladder- or urethra-specific factors. It occurs in the presence of a functional inability to reach a toilet or urinal in time because of a physical or mental impairment, such as cognitive or mobility deficits. It is linked to the primary disease process more than any extrinsic or intrinsic deficit of the lower urinary tract. An example of functional incontinence occurs in patients after orthopedic surgery. Following extensive orthopedic reconstructions such as total hip arthroplasty, patients are often immobile secondary to pain or traction. Therefore, patients may be unable to access toileting facilities in a reasonable amount of time and may become incontinent as a result. Treatment of this type of UI may involve simple interventions such as placing a urinal or commode at the bedside that allows for uncomplicated access to toileting. Pharmacologically, functional incontinence can be induced by sedative-hypnotics, narcotic analgesics, and other medications with cognitive adverse effects.

Many localized or systemic illnesses may result in UI because of their effects on the lower urinary tract or the surrounding structures:

1. Dementia/delirium
2. Depression
3. Urinary tract infection (cystitis)
4. Postmenopausal atrophic urethritis or vaginitis
5. Diabetes mellitus
6. Neurologic disease (eg, stroke, Parkinson's disease, multiple sclerosis, spinal cord injury)
7. Pelvic malignancy
8. Constipation
9. Congenital malformations of the urinary tract

Generally, stress UI is considered the most common type of UI and probably accounts for at least a portion of UI in more than half of all incontinent women. Some studies have found that mixed UI (stress UI and urgency UI) is the most common type of UI. However, the proportions of SUI, UUI, and mixed UI vary considerably with age group and gender of patients studied, study methodology, and a variety of other factors.

CLINICAL PRESENTATION

2 UI may present in a number of ways, depending on the underlying pathophysiology. A complete medical and medication history, including an assessment of symptoms and a physical examination, is essential for correctly classifying the type of incontinence and thereby assuring appropriate therapy.

Urine Leakage

UI represents a spectrum of severity in terms of both volume of leakage and degree of bother to the patient. Carefully consider the level of patient discomfort and bother when discussing urine leakage as each individual may or may not desire therapy. A careful and complete history during the patient interview is essential to accurately determine the precise nature of the problem. The onset, nature, timing, and volume of incontinence are recorded as is the use of pads. Use of absorbent products, such as panty liners, pads, or briefs, is an important point of discussion, but the clinician must keep in mind that the use of these products varies among patients. The number and type of pads may not relate to the amount or type of incontinence, as their use is a function of personal preference and hygiene. A high number of absorbent pads may be used everyday by a patient with severe, high-volume UI or, alternatively, by a fastidiously hygienic patient with low-volume leakage who simply changes pads often to prevent wetness or odor. Nevertheless, a large number of pads that are described by the patient as "soaked" is indicative of high-volume urine loss.

Regardless of the volume of urine loss, the desire to seek evaluation for UI in the majority of patients is most commonly elective and therapy is often contingent on the degree of bother to the individual patient. As with the use of absorbent products, patients differ with

CLINICAL PRESENTATION Stress Urinary Incontinence

General

- The patient usually notes UI during activities such as exercise, running, lifting, coughing, and sneezing. Occurs much more commonly in women (generally seen only in men with prior lower urinary tract surgery, neurologic disease, or other injury compromising the sphincter).

Symptoms

- Urine leakage with physical activity (volume is proportional to activity level). No UI with physical inactivity, especially when supine (minimal or no nocturia). May develop urgency and frequency as a compensatory mechanism (or as a separate component of bladder overactivity).

Diagnostic Tests

- Observation of urethral meatus while patient coughs or strains (cough stress test).

TABLE 105-2 Differentiating Bladder Overactivity–Related UI (Urgency Urinary Incontinence) from Urethral Underactivity–Related UI (Stress Urinary Incontinence)

Symptoms	Bladder Overactivity (UUI)	Urethral Underactivity (SUI)
Urgency (strong, sudden desire to void)	Yes	Not common
Frequency with urgency	Yes	Rarely
Leaking during physical activity (eg, coughing, sneezing, lifting)	No	Yes
Amount of urinary leakage with each episode of incontinence	Large if present	Usually small
Ability to reach the toilet in time following an urge to void	No or just barely	Yes
Nocturnal incontinence (presence of wet pads or undergarments in bed)	Yes	Rare
Nocturia (waking to pass urine at night)	Usually	Seldom

SUI, stress urinary incontinence; UUI, urgency urinary incontinence.

regard to the amount of urine loss they will tolerate before considering the condition bothersome enough to seek assistance. However, it is critically important that in some individuals new-onset UI may be the first manifestation of an undiagnosed illness (eg, diabetes, multiple sclerosis), or may occur as a result of treatment or drug therapy of an unrelated condition. It is these individuals who mandate a full evaluation and treatment.

Symptoms

Under the best of circumstances, UI is difficult to categorize based on symptoms alone (Table 105-2). In a study of patients who have SUI based on symptoms and patient history, urodynamics showed that only 72% of patients had SUI as the sole cause of incontinence.[18]

Patients with SUI characteristically complain of urinary leakage with physical activity. Volume of leakage is proportional to the level of activity. They will often leak urine during periods of exercise, coughing, sneezing, lifting, or even when rising from a seated to a standing position. Patients with pure SUI will not have leakage when physically inactive, especially when they are supine. Often they will have little or no UI at night, will not awaken to void during the night (nocturia), will not wet the bed, and often do not even wear absorbent products during the night. Urinary urgency and frequency may be associated with SUI, either as a separate component caused by bladder overactivity (mixed incontinence) or as a compensatory mechanism wherein the patient with SUI learns to toilet frequently to prevent large-volume urine loss during physical activity.

Typical symptoms of UUI and bladder overactivity include frequency, urgency, and high-volume incontinence. Nocturia and nocturnal incontinence are often present. Urine leakage is unpredictable, and the volume loss may be quite large. Patients often wear protection both day and night. Urinary frequency can be affected by a number of factors unrelated to bladder overactivity, including excessive fluid intake (polydipsia) and bladder hypersensitivity states such as interstitial cystitis and urinary tract infection. In some patients, bladder overactivity manifests as UI without awareness in the absence of a sense of urinary urgency or frequency. *Urinary urgency*, a sensation of impending micturition, requires intact sensory input from the lower urinary tract. In patients with spinal cord injury, sensory neuropathies, and other neurologic diseases, a diminished ability to perceive or process sensory input from the lower urinary tract may result in bladder overactivity and UI without urgency or urinary frequency. When bladder contraction occurs without warning and sensation is absent, the condition is referred to as *reflex incontinence*.

Patients with overflow incontinence may present with lower abdominal fullness as well as considerable obstructive urinary symptoms, including hesitancy, straining to void, decreased force of urinary stream, interrupted stream, and a vague sense of incomplete bladder emptying. These patients may also have a significant component of urinary frequency and urgency. In patients with acute urinary retention and overflow incontinence, lower abdominal pain may be present. Although these symptoms are not specific for overflow incontinence, they may warrant further investigation, including an assessment of postvoid residual urine volume.

Signs A presenting complaint of UI mandates a directed physical examination and a brief neurologic assessment. The workup ideally includes an abdominal examination to exclude a distended bladder, neurologic assessment of the perineum and lower extremities, pelvic examination in women (looking especially for evidence of prolapse or hormonal deficiency), and genital and prostate examination in men. Perineal skin maceration, erythema, breakdown, and ulceration may be indicative of chronic, severe UI. Patients with chronic incontinence, especially those who are obese, may also manifest fungal infections of the skin of the perineum and upper thighs.

SUI can usually be objectively demonstrated by having the patient cough or strain during the examination and observing the urethral meatus for a sudden spurt of urine (cough stress test). In women, SUI may be associated with varying degrees of vaginal prolapse, including cystourethrocele (bladder and urethral prolapse).

In both men and women, digital rectal examination provides an opportunity to assess neurological integrity by checking ambient

CLINICAL PRESENTATION Urgency Urinary Incontinence

General

- Can have bladder overactivity and UI without urgency if sensory input from the lower urinary tract is absent.

Symptoms

- Urinary frequency (>8 micturitions per day), urgency with or without UI; nocturia (≥1 micturition per night) and enuresis may be present.

Diagnostic Tests

- Urodynamic studies are the gold standard for diagnosis for the diagnosis of detrusor overactivity when the finding of involuntary bladder contractions on the study reproduces the patient's symptoms. Urinalysis and urine culture should be negative (rule out urinary tract infection as the cause of frequency).

CLINICAL PRESENTATION Overflow Incontinence (Chronic Urinary Retention)

General

- Important but uncommon type of UI in both men and women. Urethral overactivity is usually due to prostatic enlargement (men) or cystocele formation or surgical overcorrection following stress incontinence surgery in women. Bladder underactivity resulting in overflow incontinence can result from many causes including neurogenic disease, diabetes, and postoperatively from pelvic surgery (eg, radical hysterectomy).

Symptoms

- Lower abdominal fullness, hesitancy, straining to void, decreased force of stream, interrupted stream, sense of incomplete bladder emptying. May have urinary frequency and urgency. Abdominal pain if acute urinary retention is present.

Signs

- Increased postvoid residual urine volume.

Diagnostic Tests

- Assessment of postvoid residual urine either by imaging (ultrasound, etc.) or by catheterization. Renal function tests to rule out renal failure due to chronic urinary retention.

rectal tone, perianal sensation, and the integrity of the sacral reflex arc (eg, anal wink) as well as assess the patient's ability to perform a voluntary pelvic floor muscle contraction (ie, Kegel exercise), which may be an important factor in deciding on appropriate therapy. In men, a digital examination of the prostate assesses for the presence of prostate cancer, inflammation, and BPH.

A targeted neurologic examination includes assessment of reflexes, rectal tone, and sensory or motor deficits in the lower extremities, which might be indicative of systemic or localized neurologic disease. Neurologic diseases have the potential to affect bladder and sphincter function and thus may have significant implications in the incontinent patient.

Prior Medical or Surgical Illness UI may present in the setting of concurrent, seemingly unrelated illnesses. New-onset UI may be the initial manifestation of systemic illnesses such as diabetes mellitus, metastatic malignancies, and neurologic diseases such as Parkinson's disease, brain tumors, and multiple sclerosis. Central nervous system (CNS) disease, or injury above the level of the pons, generally results in symptoms of bladder overactivity and UUI. Spinal cord injury or disease may manifest as bladder overactivity and UUI or as overflow incontinence, depending on the spinal level and completeness of the injury or disease.

Medications may have wide-ranging effects on lower urinary tract function (see Table 105-1). A thorough inquiry into the use of new medications in the setting of recent-onset UI may show a relationship. Acute UI manifesting in the immediate postoperative setting may be secondary to a number of factors, including surgical manipulation and immobility, and to a number of medications, especially opioid analgesics and sedative-hypnotics.

Prior surgery may have effects on lower urinary tract function. UI following prostate surgery in men is highly suggestive of injury to the sphincter and resultant SUI. Pelvic surgery for benign and malignant conditions may result in denervation or injury to the lower urinary tract. This includes bowel surgery and gynecologic procedures. For example, new-onset total UI following gynecologic surgery suggests intraoperative urinary tract injury and subsequent development of a postoperative genitourinary fistula. Radiation therapy to the pelvis for malignant disease (eg, prostate cancer or cervical cancer) may result in injury to the bladder or urethra and subsequent UI.

In women, UI may be related to several gynecologic factors including childbirth, hormonal status, and prior gynecologic surgery, although the relationship of some of these factors to UI has come under debate.[19] Pregnancy and childbirth, particularly vaginal delivery, are associated with SUI and pelvic prolapse. Significant SUI in the nulliparous woman is uncommon. UI that becomes progressive at or around menopause suggests a hormonal component that may be responsive to estrogen or hormone replacement therapy.

UI may present in the setting of other significant pelvic floor disorders, signs, and symptoms. Constipation, diarrhea, fecal incontinence, dyspareunia, sexual dysfunction, and pelvic pain may be related to UI. A history of gross hematuria in the setting of UI mandates further urologic investigation, including radiologic imaging of the upper urinary tract and cystoscopy. Acute dysuria with or without hematuria in the setting of UI suggests cystitis. Urinalysis and urine culture should be performed in these patients.

TREATMENT

Desired Outcomes

3 The efficacy goals for the management of UI include restoration of continence, reduction of the number of UI episodes, and prevention of complications (perineal dermatitis, pressure ulcers, falls, etc.). Other desired outcomes are minimization of adverse treatment consequences and cost, improvement in the patient's quality of life, lesser care burden, and reduced risk of nursing home placement.

General Approach to Treatment

Nonsurgical, nonpharmacologic intervention is the first-line treatment for UI. Drug therapy may be considered in patients whose UI is not adequately controlled by nonpharmacologic therapies and in those who have no major contraindications to drug treatment. In general, pharmacotherapy provides a better response when combined with behavioral interventions.[20] Selection of agent should be based on the type of UI, and patient characteristics (eg, age, comorbidities, concurrent drug therapies, ability to maintain medication adherence). Surgery can be considered when the degree of bother or lifestyle compromise is sufficient and other nonsurgical interventions are undesired or ineffective.

Antimuscarinic agents have been the mainstay of pharmacotherapy for OAB and UUI. According to the American Urological Association (AUA) guideline,[21] clinicians should avoid antimuscarinic agents in patients with narrow-angle glaucoma unless approved by the treating ophthalmologist. Antimuscarinic agents should be cautiously used in patients with frailty, impaired gastric emptying, or a history of urinary retention, or in those who are taking other drugs with anticholinergic properties. When one agent offers inadequate symptom control and/or unacceptable adverse drug events, consider a dose modification or switching to another agent. Before initiating antimuscarinic therapy, patients should be informed of adverse effects and strategies to minimize them. Before abandoning effective antimuscarinic therapy, clinicians should manage constipation and dry mouth (bowel regimen, fluid management, dose modification, or alternative antimuscarinics).[21] β_3-Agonists are newer drug alternatives for UUI.

Nonpharmacologic Nonsurgical Treatment

4 Nonpharmacologic, nonsurgical treatment of UI is recommended as the first-line treatment at a primary care level. It is the only option for patients in whom pharmacologic and/or surgical management is inappropriate or undesired. Examples of patients who fulfill these criteria for nonpharmacologic treatment include those with mild-to-moderate symptoms and who do not want to take medication; those with comorbid conditions that place them at high risk for adverse effects from drug therapy; those who are not medically fit for surgery; those who plan future pregnancies (which may adversely affect long-term surgical outcomes); those with overflow incontinence whose condition is not amenable to surgery or drug therapy; and those who are delaying surgery or do not want to undergo surgery.[22]

Nondrug interventions for UI include behavioral interventions, external neuromodulation, anti-incontinence devices, and supportive interventions (Table 105-3).[21] Behavioral interventions are generally the first-line treatment for SUI, UUI, and mixed UI. Interventions include lifestyle modifications, voiding schedule regimens, and pelvic floor muscle rehabilitation based on the patient's treatment preferences. Notably, both stress and urgency urinary incontinence are associated with obesity. Several studies have demonstrated that weight loss benefits patients with UI.[23] Because the key to success with any type of behavioral intervention is motivation of patients or caregivers, these individuals must be active participants in developing a treatment plan. Regular follow-up is needed to help motivate patients and caregivers, provide reassurance and support, and monitor treatment outcomes. Patients should be informed that it takes 8 to 12 weeks for behavioral interventions to be effective.

External neuromodulation may include nonimplantable electrical stimulation (EStim), percutaneous tibial nerve stimulation (PTNS), or extracorporeal magnetic stimulation (MStim). Electrical stimulation is typically prescribed when traditional pelvic floor muscle rehabilitation has failed. Anti-incontinence devices such as bed alarms, catheters, pessaries, penile clamps, and external collection devices are reserved for special situations depending on patients' UI symptoms, cognitive and mobility status, and overall health status. Supportive interventions such as physical therapy may be beneficial for patients with muscle weakness and slow gait to reach the toilet in a timelier manner, and absorbent products will provide greater confidence in dealing with unpredictable urine loss. Penile clamps and external collection devices are available for men and women with significant functional impairment.

Surgical Treatment

Only rarely does surgery play a role in the initial management of UI. In the absence of secondary complications from UI (eg, skin breakdown or infection), the decision to surgically treat symptomatic UI should be based on the premise that the degree of bother or lifestyle compromise to the patient is great enough to warrant an elective operation, and that nonsurgical therapy either is undesired or has been ineffective.

Successful application of surgery depends mostly on defining the underlying abnormalities responsible for UI (bladder vs urethra, underactivity vs overactivity). Once the underlying factors are determined, other considerations include renal function, sexual function, severity of leakage, history of abdominal or pelvic surgery, presence of concurrent abdominal or pelvic pathology requiring surgical correction, and finally the patient's suitability for the procedure and willingness to accept the risks of surgery.

If patients with uncomplicated SUI become dissatisfied with the initial management approaches of pelvic floor exercises, medications, and/or behavioral modification, surgical treatment assumes the primary role. Surgical correction of female SUI (urethral underactivity) is directed toward either (a) repositioning the urethra and/or creating a backboard of support, or otherwise stabilizing the urethra and bladder neck in a well-supported retropubic (intra-abdominal) position that is receptive to changes in intra-abdominal pressure; or (b) improving the sealing mechanism and/or creating compression or otherwise augmenting the urethral resistance provided by the intrinsic sphincteric unit, with (ie, sling) or without (ie, periurethral injectable bulking agents) urethral and bladder neck support.

Bulking agents are injected into the urethra at the level of the urinary sphincter as an office-based procedure and are generally considered quite safe. However, their durability and efficacy are likely inferior to other options.[24]

Midurethral synthetic slings have become the most common approach to the treatment of SUI in women in the United States. These can be inserted as outpatient procedures that have shorter convalescence periods and allow faster return to usual activities compared with many of the older procedures. These procedures are generally felt to be highly durable and efficacious. However, safety concerns have been expressed regarding the implantation of surgical mesh in some patients, the implications of which are yet to be fully clarified.[25]

SUI in men is rare in the absence of prior pelvic surgery, injury, or neurologic disease. When it occurs, SUI in men can be treated in

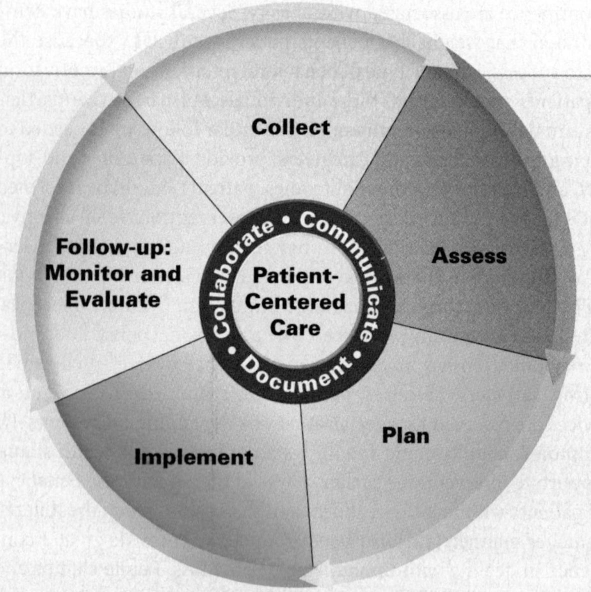

Patient Care Process for Urinary Incontinence

The image shows the five fundamental steps included in The Pharmacist's Care Process endorsed by the Joint Commission for Pharmacy Practitioners (2014). The tagline of this process reads collaborate, communicate, and document. The five fundamental steps listed here are collect, assess, plan, implement, and follow-up: monitor and evaluate. All these steps are listed in a circular block diagram.

Collect

- Patient characteristics (eg, age, sex, pregnancy status, drug allergy profile)
- Patient medical and genitourinary surgical history including coexisting conditions that may influence UI
- Obstetric and menstrual history in women
- Past conservative, medical, and surgical treatment of UI
- Social history (tobacco/ethanol use; caffeine and fluid intake; environmental issues; exercise; availability of family caregiver, if relevant)
- Current medications (see Table 105-1) including over-the-counter (OTC), herbal products, and dietary supplements
- Objective data
  - Lab tests: urinalysis ± urine culture; if infected, treat and reassess if appropriate
  - Cough stress test to demonstrate stress UI (if appropriate)
  - Postvoid residual urine by bladder ultrasound or catheterization (if suspected urinary retention/overflow incontinence)

Assess

- Urinary symptoms including bladder diary (see Table 105-2)
- Presence of bowel symptoms or vaginal prolapse symptoms (in women); estrogen status in women
- Quality of life, treatment preferences, and goals
- Mental status, body mass index, physical dexterity, and mobility
- Abdominal, rectal, prostate (in men), neurological, and pelvic examination (in women)

Plan*

- Nonpharmacological interventions based on UI severity and subtype (see Table 105-3)
- Drug therapy regimen for urgency UI, if indicated (see Table 105-5)
- Monitoring parameters (see Tables 105-6 and 105-7); frequency and timing of follow-up
- Patient education (eg, purpose of treatment, dietary and lifestyle modification, drug-specific information)
- Self-monitoring for resolution of UI symptoms and drug adverse events (if indicated)
- Referrals to other providers when appropriate (eg, urologist, urogynecologist, continence nurse practitioner, physical therapist)

Implement*

- Provide patient education regarding all elements of treatment plan
- Use motivational interviewing and coaching strategies to maximize adherence
- Schedule follow-up (eg, adherence assessment, treatment response)

Follow-up: Monitor and Evaluate

- Monitor for patient response in 1 or 2 weeks after therapy initiation
- Assess efficacy after a minimum of 4 weeks to assess drug efficacy
- Resolution of UI symptoms
- Presence of adverse effects (eg, Table 105-7), or drug interactions
- Patient adherence to treatment plan using multiple sources of information
- Reevaluate efficacy and necessary duration of therapy every 3 to 6 months

Collaborate with patient, caregivers, and other healthcare professionals.

a number of ways.[26] Bulking agents can be injected periurethrally and submucosally into the region of the external urinary sphincter but have fallen out of favor due to poor short- and long-term outcomes. This approach is less effective and far less durable than alternative surgical procedures, although it can be performed in the office setting without the need for general anesthesia. The artificial urinary sphincter is generally considered to be the gold standard for treatment of male SUI.[27] Placement of this manually operated silicone device has been associated with high long-term success and satisfaction rates.[27] Male slings and external urethral compression devices placed through a perineal incision are alternatives to the artificial urinary sphincter in some individuals with mild-to-moderate SUI.[28] However, long-term efficacy and safety data on large numbers of patients is lacking.[29]

TABLE 105-3 Nonpharmacologic Management of Urinary Incontinence

Intervention	Description	Patient Characteristics
Lifestyle Modifications		
Behavioral changes (eg, fluid and caffeine modifications, smoking cessation, weight loss, constipation prevention)	Self-management strategies targeted toward reducing or eliminating risk factors that cause or exacerbate UI	Used as first-line therapies or in combination with pharmacological treatment in patients with stress, urgency, and mixed incontinence
Scheduling Regimens		
Timed voiding	Toileting on a fixed schedule where interval does not change, typically every 2 hours during waking hours	Used for patients with cognitive or physical impairments causing disability-associated incontinence
Habit training	Scheduled toiletings with adjustments of voiding intervals (longer or shorter) based on patient's voiding pattern	Used for institutionalized or homebound patients with cognitive or physical impairments
Prompted voiding	Scheduled toiletings that require prompts to void from a caregiver, typically every 2 hours; patient assisted in toileting only if response is positive; used in conjunction with operant conditioning techniques for rewarding patients for maintaining continence and appropriate toileting	Used for patients who are functionally able to use toilet or toilet substitute, able to feel urge sensation, and able to request toileting assistance appropriately; primarily used in institutional settings or in homebound patients with an available caregiver
Bladder training	Scheduled toiletings with progressive voiding intervals; includes teaching urgency suppression strategies using relaxation and distraction techniques, self-monitoring, and use of reinforcement techniques; sometimes combined with drug therapy	Used for stress, urgency, and mixed incontinence in patients who are cognitively intact, able to toilet, and motivated to comply with training program
Pelvic Floor Muscle Rehabilitation		
Pelvic floor muscle exercises (eg, Kegel exercises)	Regular practice of pelvic floor muscle contractions; may involve use of pelvic floor muscle contraction for prevention of stress leakage and urge inhibition	Used for stress, urgency, and mixed incontinence in patients who can isolate and correctly contract pelvic floor muscles; requires cognitively intact and highly motivated patient
Biofeedback	Use of electronic or mechanical instruments to display visual or auditory information about neuromuscular or bladder activity; used to teach correct pelvic floor muscle contraction or urge inhibition; home trainers available	Used for stress, urgency, and mixed incontinence in patients who have the capability to learn voluntary control through observation and are motivated; used in conjunction with pelvic floor muscle exercises
Vaginal weight training	Active retention of increasing vaginal weights; typically used in combination with pelvic floor muscle exercises at least twice per day	Women with stress incontinence who are cognitively intact, can correctly contract pelvic floor muscles, able to stand, and have sufficient vaginal vault and introitus to retain cone, and are highly motivated; contraindicated in patients with moderate-to-severe pelvic organ prolapse
External Neuromodulation		
Nonimplantable electrical stimulation	Application of electrical current through vaginal, anal, surface, or fine needle electrodes; used to inhibit bladder overactivity and improve awareness, contractility, and efficacy of pelvic floor muscle contraction; handheld stimulators for home use are available	Used for stress, urgency, and mixed incontinence in patients who are highly motivated; contraindicated in patients with diminished sensory perception; urinary retention, history of cardiac arrhythmia, cardiac pacemakers, implantable defibrillators, pregnant or attempting pregnancy; vaginal or anal electrodes are contraindicated in moderate or severe pelvic organ prolapse
Percutaneous tibial nerve stimulation	Application of a pulsed electrical current through a fine needle electrode placed externally near the tibial nerve	Used for treatment of overactive bladder with urinary urgency, frequency, and urgency incontinence; contraindicated in patients with pacemakers or implantable defibrillators, prone to excessive bleeding, or women who are pregnant
Extracorporeal magnetic electrical stimulation	Pulsed magnetic stimulation to pelvic floor musculature causing depolarization of motor neurons, thus inducing pelvic floor muscle contraction; stimulation is provided through a specially designed chair that contains a device for producing a pulsing magnetic field	Used for treatment of stress, urgency, and mixed incontinence; contraindicated in patients with demand cardiac pacemakers or metallic joint replacements; may be useful treatment option when other approaches fail or are not feasible
Alternative Medicine Therapies		
Acupuncture	Involves insertion of disposable sterile fine stainless steel needles into points on the skin that are thought to suppress or stimulate spinal and/or supraspinal reflexes to the bladder and/or urethra	Used for stress, urgency, and mixed incontinence and UI due to spinal cord injury
Anti-Incontinence Devices		
Bed or pant alarms	Sensor devices that respond to wetness; used to awaken or alert individuals via noise or vibrating mechanism	Primarily used for nocturnal enuresis in children; system available for monitoring incontinence in home care and institutional environments

(*continued*)

TABLE 105-3 Nonpharmacologic Management of Urinary Incontinence (*Continued*)

Intervention	Description	Patient Characteristics
Pessaries	Intravaginal devices designed to support the bladder neck, relieve minor-to-moderate pelvic organ prolapse, and change pressure transmission to the urethra	Used for female stress incontinence and mild-to-moderate pelvic organ prolapse; in postmenopausal women, topical estrogen therapy is typically prescribed to prevent ulceration and breakdown of vaginal tissue; requires good manual dexterity to manipulate device
Urethral insert (women only)	Intraurethral device	Used in female stress incontinence with stress incontinence who are cognitively intact and have good manual dexterity
Urethral compression device (men only)	Penile clamp	Used in men patients with stress incontinence who are cognitively intact and have good manual dexterity
External collection devices (men only)	Condom catheter with leg bag	Used in men with urgency, stress, and overflow incontinence and in those with functional impairments
External urine collection devices for women	Female external catheter with suction wicking system that pulls urine through collector tubing into collection canister	Used in women with incontinence related to functional impairments in rehabilitation and hospital settings
Catheters	Disposable, intermittent urethral catheters and indwelling urethral and suprapubic catheters	Used for overflow incontinence; used in patients who are bed-bound or with significant mobility impairments and severe incontinence; those with terminal illness; those with sacral pressure ulcers until healing occurs
Supportive Interventions		
Toileting substitutes and other environmental modifications	Female and male urinals, bedside commodes, elevated toilet seats, grab bars, and frames	Used for patients with mobility impairments that make reaching toilet in timely fashion difficult
Absorbent products	Variety of reusable and disposable liners, pads, male drip collectors, male guard, collector undergarment, fitted brief, and pant systems; some products contain a polymer that absorb and wick urine away from the body	Used for all types of incontinence
Physical therapy	Gait and/or strength training	Used for older patients with mobility impairments that make reaching a toilet in timely fashion difficult

Most patients with UUI are managed nonsurgically with a combination of behavioral modification, pelvic floor exercises, and pharmacologic therapy. However, for patients refractory to such measures, invasive therapy can be beneficial. Posterior tibial nerve stimulation is an office-based percutaneous treatment for UUI or OAB. Therapy consists of weekly 30-minute treatments with a needle placed posteriorly to the medial malleolus of the ankle for 3 months.[30] Efficacy is similar to or slightly better than oral pharmacotherapy. However, long-term efficacy and safety data are lacking.

Surgery for the treatment of UUI generally consists of implantation of a sacral nerve stimulator (neuromodulation) or endoscopic office-based injection of botulinum toxin directly into the detrusor muscle.[31,32] Neuromodulation is a staged surgical procedure in which a neurostimulator lead is placed transforaminally at the level of sacral spinal cord root S3. Its exact mechanism is unknown, but the device may exert its favorable effects on urination and UUI by rebalancing the afferent and efferent nerve impulses to the lower urinary tract and pelvic floor. The injection of botulinum toxin is performed in the office generally with local anesthesia. Following transurethral injection directly into the detrusor muscle using a small needle in a template fashion, the toxin is taken up by the local neurons. The intracellular toxin cleaves SNAP-25, a cystoplasmic protein critical for the attachment of neurotransmitter containing vesicles to the cell membrane at the nerve terminal. As the vesicles containing neurotransmitter are unable to fuse to the cell membrane and release its contents into the synaptic cleft, neural transmission to the postsynaptic muscle fascicle is interrupted. This results in a graded, initially irreversible but transient weakness and paralysis of the affected muscle. The duration of effect of the toxin is about 4 to 8 months, after which repeat injection is necessary to maintain effect. The therapeutic algorithm involving these two choices for treatment of refractory UUI is evolving, and is determined largely by patient preference.[33]

Few surgical treatments for bladder underactivity are effective. After an appropriate evaluation for reversible causes, the most effective management of this condition is intermittent self-catheterization performed by the patient or a caregiver three or four times per day. Sacral nerve stimulation (neuromodulation) has shown some efficacy in this patient population, but success rates for detrusor underactivity (nonobstructive urinary retention) are inferior to that seen for the indication of urgency UI with urinary frequency and urgency.[34] Proper patient selection for this therapy remains poorly defined. Alternative methods of management that are less satisfactory or more invasive include indwelling urethral or suprapubic catheters and urinary diversion.

Urethral overactivity is most commonly caused by anatomic obstruction. Anatomic obstruction in men is most often caused by benign prostatic enlargement. Treatments may include transurethral surgical resection of the prostate (see Chapter 104, "Benign Prostatic Hyperplasia"). Rarely, bladder outlet obstruction is caused by a functional obstruction at the level of the bladder neck or external sphincter. Hypertrophy of the smooth muscle fibers at the level of the bladder neck in men and women may result in obstruction to the flow of urine. In patients who do not respond to pharmacologic therapy with α-adrenergic receptor antagonists, endoscopic incision using the cystoscope (resectoscope) is highly effective in treating this uncommon condition.

Pharmacologic Therapy

Urgency Urinary Incontinence

5 Antimuscarinic agents and β_3-adrenergic agonists are the second-line drug treatments for urgency UI. Table 105-4 summarizes

TABLE 105-4 AUA Guideline for Treatment of Overactive Bladder in Adults

Recommendation	Evidence Strength Grade[a]
First-Line Treatments	
Behavioral therapies (eg, bladder training, bladder control strategies, pelvic floor muscle training, fluid management)	B
Behavioral therapies may be combined with pharmacologic therapies	C
Second-Line Treatments	
Oral antimuscarinics or β_3-adrenergic agonist as second-line therapy	B
If an IR and an ER formulation are available, prefer ER formulations because of lower rates of dry mouth	B
Transdermal oxybutynin (patch or gel) may be offered	C
Combination therapy with an oral antimuscarinic and a β_3-adrenergic agonist is acceptable for patients refractory to monotherapy with either class of drug	C
Third-Line Treatments	
Intradetrusor onabotulinum toxin A (100 units) in carefully selected patients who have been refractory to first- and second-line OAB treatments[b]	B
Peripheral tibial nerve stimulation in a carefully selected patient population	C
Sacral neuromodulation in carefully selected patients with severe refractory OAB symptoms or in those who are not candidates for second-line therapy and are willing to undergo a surgical procedure	C

AUA, American Urological Association; ER, extended-release; IR, immediate-release; OAB, overactive bladder.

[a]When sufficient evidence existed, the body of evidence for a particular treatment was assigned a strength rating of A (high), B (moderate), or C (low). Both B and C indicate that benefits outweigh risks/burdens.

[b]The patient must be able and willing to return for frequent postvoid residual evaluation and able and willing to perform self-catheterization if necessary.

AUA recommendations for treating OAB in adults.[21] Table 105-5 lists the usual dosage for approved agents for OAB or UUI. Table 105-6 suggests common monitoring parameters for these agents.

Antimuscarinic agents (see Table 105-5) antagonize muscarinic receptors and suppress premature detrusor contractions, thereby enhance bladder storage. They have similar contraindications, precautions, and side-effect profiles, with incidence/severity varies with each individual agent.[35] These agents improve quality of life, and are considered equally effective based on clinical efficacy in reducing UI episodes, decreasing micturitions per day, and increasing urine volume voided per micturition.[36] Antimuscarinic agents may worsen cognitive function, especially in older adults. Also, they may antagonize the therapeutic effects of acetylcholine esterase inhibitors indicated for dementia.

Oxybutynin Oxybutynin immediate release (IR) is the oldest and least expensive treatment for UUI. It gives substantial nonurinary antimuscarinic effects, including orthostatic hypotension, sedation, and weight gain (see Table 105-6).[37] These adverse effects may jeopardize medication adherence and prevent dose escalation. Its multiple daily dosing may be too complicated for patients with cognitive impairment or those who are taking multiple medications. Consider dose reduction if side effects become bothersome. Use sugarless gum, hard candy, or a saliva substitute for dry mouth and increase fluid/fiber intake, physical activity, and/or laxative therapy for constipation.

An extended-release (XL) formulation of oxybutynin is an alternative therapy in patients who cannot tolerate IR formulation. It delivers a controlled amount of oxybutynin over a 24-hour period, and has a reduced first-pass metabolism. It gives a lower concentration of active metabolite, *N*-desethyloxybutynin, which is associated with dry mouth as a side effect.[38] In short-term studies, oxybutynin XL was better tolerated than oxybutynin IR, and at least as effective as tolterodine IR or long acting (LA) in managing urinary symptoms.[38] Drug interactions may occur when oxybutynin is used with other anticholinergic drugs, potent CYP3A4 inhibitors (eg, itraconazole, miconazole, erythromycin, and clarithromycin), and acetylcholinesterase inhibitors.[38]

Nonoral formulations of oxybutynin are available for better tolerability. The oxybutynin transdermal system (TDS) is the first OTC treatment for OAB in women aged 18 years or older. It has a similar efficacy as oxybutynin IR or tolterodine LA.[39,40] It bypasses first-pass hepatic and gut metabolism and is more tolerable (anticholinergic side effects <10%).[39] It has been associated with improved quality of life and work productivity. Patients should apply oxybutynin TDS to dry, intact skin on the abdomen, hip, or buttocks every 3 to 4 days (twice weekly). Rotating application site at least weekly helps to minimize local reactions: pruritus (14%-17%) and erythema (6%-9%).[39]

Oxybutynin topical gel causes less dry mouth than oral oxybutynin (6.1% vs 73.1%).[41-43] In older patients with frailty, long-term use warrants proper monitoring for cognitive impairment and anticholinergic effects.[44] Patients should not apply sunscreen within 30 minutes before or after application or shower within 1 hour after application. They should also avoid the transfer of gel to others via vigorous skin contact at the application site; avoid open fires or exposure to smoking until the alcohol-based gel has dried.[41,42]

Tolterodine Tolterodine is a competitive muscarinic receptor antagonist that is as effective as oxybutynin IR, but gives better tolerability and thus medication adherence.[45] Tolterodine is predominantly eliminated by hepatic metabolism, which is partially under the control of genetic polymorphism.[46] The principal metabolic pathway in extensive metabolizers involves oxidation of the parent drug by CYP isoenzyme 2D6 to the active 5-hydroxymethyl metabolite (DD01). In CYP2D6 poor metabolizers (approximately 7% of the US population), the principal metabolic pathway involves CYP3A4. Because tolterodine is principally metabolized by CYP3A4 in this case, monitor for impaired drug limitation when given concomitantly with CYP3A4 inhibitors (eg, fluoxetine, sertraline, fluvoxamine, macrolide antibiotics, azole antifungals, and grapefruit juice). Concurrent use of fluoxetine, a dual inhibitor of CYP2D6 and 3A4 can significantly increase tolterodine level.[46] Caution is also advised with individuals who carry nonfunctional CYP2D6*13 allele.[46,47] The maximum benefit from tolterodine may take up to 8 weeks after therapy initiation or dose escalation.[46] The most common adverse effects of tolterodine are dry mouth, dyspepsia, headache, constipation, and dry eyes. Of note, patients who have known hypersensitivity to fesoterodine fumarate should not receive tolterodine because both agents are metabolized to DD01. Monitor for QT prolongation with concomitant use of Class IA (eg, quinidine, procainamide) or Class III (eg, amiodarone, sotalol) antiarrhythmic medications.[47]

Tolterodine long acting (LA) offers a convenient once-daily dosing and causes less dry mouth than IR formulation.[48] It also improves OAB symptoms in men who were taking α-adrenergic blockers.[49] It may take up to 8 weeks to see maximum benefit after starting therapy or dose escalation.[48]

Fesoterodine Fumarate Fesoterodine fumarate is also indicated for symptoms of urinary frequency, urgency, or urgency incontinence. It is a prodrug that is metabolized to its active metabolite, 5-hydroxymethyl tolterodine (also a metabolite of tolterodine), by

TABLE 105-5 Dosing of Medications Approved for OAB or UUI

Drug	Brand Name	Initial Dose	Usual Range	Special Population Dose	Comments
Anticholinergics/Antimuscarinics					
Oxybutynin IR	Ditropan	2.5 mg twice daily	2.5-5 mg two to four times daily		Titrate in increments of 2.5 mg/day every 1-2 months; available in oral solution
Oxybutynin XL	Ditropan XL	5-10 mg once daily	5-30 mg once daily		Adjust dose in 5-mg increments at weekly interval; swallow whole
Oxybutynin TDS	Oxytrol Oxytrol for Women (OTC)		3.9 mg/day apply one patch twice weekly		Apply every 3-4 days; rotate application site
Oxybutynin gel 10%	Gelnique		One sachet (100 mg) topically daily		Apply to clean and dry, intact skin on abdomen, thighs or upper arms/shoulders; contains alcohol
Oxybutynin gel 3%	Gelnique 3%		Three pumps (84 mg) topically daily		Same as above
Tolterodine IR	Detrol		1-2 mg twice daily	1 mg twice daily if patient is taking CYP3A4 inhibitors, or with renal/hepatic impairment	Avoid in patients with creatinine clearance less than 10 mL/min (0.17 mL/s) or severe hepatic impairment
Tolterodine LA	Detrol LA		2-4 mg once daily	2 mg once daily in those who are taking CYP3A4 inhibitors (ketoconazole, itraconazole, clarithromycin, or ritonavir), with hepatic impairment (Child-Pugh class A or B), or severe renal impairment [creatinine clearance 10 to 30 mL/min (0.17-0.50 mL/s)]	Swallow whole; avoid in patients with creatinine clearance ≤10 mL/min (0.17 mL/s) or severe hepatic impairment
Trospium chloride IR	Sanctura		20 mg twice daily	20 mg once daily in patient age ≥75 years or creatinine clearance ≤30 mL/min (0.5 mL/s)	Take 1 hour before meals or on empty stomach; patient age ≥ 75 years should take at bedtime
Trospium chloride ER	Sanctura XR		60 mg once daily	Avoid in patient age ≥75 years or creatinine clearance ≤30 mL/min (0.5 mL/s)	Take 1 hour before meals or on empty stomach; swallow whole
Solifenacin	VESIcare	5 mg daily	5-10 mg once daily Pediatric: use suspension dosed based on body weight	5 mg daily if patient is taking CYP3A4 inhibitors or with creatinine clearance ≤30 mL/min (0.5 mL/s) or moderate hepatic impairment; avoid in severe hepatic impairment	Swallow whole
Darifenacin ER	Enablex	7.5 mg once daily	7.5-15 mg once daily	7.5 mg daily if patient is taking potent CYP3A4 inhibitors or with moderate hepatic impairment; avoid in severe hepatic impairment	Titrate dose after at least 2 weeks; swallow whole
Fesoterodine ER	Toviaz	4 mg once daily	4-8 mg once daily	4 mg daily if patient is taking potent CYP3A4 inhibitors or with creatinine clearance ≤30 mL/min (0.5 mL/s); avoid in severe hepatic impairment	Prodrug (metabolized to 5-hydroxymethyl tolterodine); swallow whole
β_3-Adrenergic Agonist					
Mirabegron ER	Myrbetriq	25 mg once daily	25-50 mg once daily	25 mg once daily if creatinine clearance 15-29 mL/min (0.25-0.49 mL/s) or moderate hepatic impairment; avoid in patients with ESRD or severe hepatic impairment	Swallow whole
Vibegron	Gemtase	75 mg once daily		Avoid in patients with end-stage kidney disease with or without hemodialysis, or severe hepatic impairment	Swallow whole. Tablets may be crushed and mixed with applesauce

CYP, cytochrome P450 enzyme; ER, extended-release; ESRD, end-stage renal disease; IR, immediate release; LA, long acting; OAB, overactive bladder; OTC, over-the-counter; TDS, transdermal system; UUI, urge urinary incontinence; XL, extended release.

nonspecific plasma esterases.[50] In a short-term study, fesoterodine was better than tolterodine ER 4 mg and placebo on reducing UUI episodes, micturitions, urgency, and improving health-related quality of life. However, fesoterodine caused more dry mouth (28% vs 13%) and constipation (4% vs 3%).

More patients discontinued fesoterodine therapy due to adverse events (5% vs 3%).[51] The most common adverse effects of fesoterodine are dose-related dry mouth (27%), constipation (5.1%), dyspepsia (2%), and dry eyes (1.6%).[50] The most common adverse effects of fesoterodine are dose-related dry mouth (27%), constipation (5.1%), dyspepsia (2%), and dry eyes (1.6%).

Trospium Chloride Trospium chloride, a quaternary ammonium anticholinergic, is a second-generation antimuscarinic agent for urgency UI. Trospium chloride is poorly absorbed after oral administration (<10%), and food reduces bioavailability by 70% to 80%. It

TABLE 105-6 Monitoring of Medications Approved for OAB or UUI

Drug	Adverse Drug Reaction	Monitoring Parameters	Comments
Antimuscarinic			
Oxybutynin IR Oxybutynin XL Oxybutynin TDS Oxybutynin gel 10% Oxybutynin gel 3% Tolterodine IR Tolterodine LA Trospium chloride IR Trospium chloride ER Solifenacin Darifenacin ER Fesoterodine ER	Anticholinergic adverse effects: dry mouth, constipation, headache, dyspepsia, dry eyes, blurred vision, cognitive impairment, tachycardia, sedation, orthostatic hypotension Application site reactions (topical agents): pruritus, erythema	Contraindications and precautions: urinary retention, gastric retention, severely decreased GI motility, angioedema, myasthenia gravis, uncontrolled narrow-angle glaucoma Worsening of renal/hepatic condition or concomitant drug therapy, which may necessitate dosage reduction or drug cessation Mental status change or risk for falls in elderly or frail patients	In general, ER, LA, XL, and topical products are associated with fewer anticholinergic adverse effects, particularly dry mouth Possible transference of drug from topical application Avoid open fire or smoke until alcohol-based gel has dried
β_3-Adrenergic Agonist			
Mirabegron ER	Hypertension, nasopharyngitis, urinary tract infection, headache	Precautions: urinary retention, severe uncontrolled hypertension Worsening of renal/hepatic condition, which may necessitate dosage reduction or drug cessation Increased effect of narrow therapeutic index drugs that are CYP2D6 substrates QT prolongation	Mirabegron is a CYP2D6 inhibitor; may increase digoxin level
Vibegron	Headache, nasopharyngitis, hot flashes, gastrointestinal symptoms, upper respiratory tract infection	Precautions: bladder flow obstruction, hepatic/renal impairment	Minor substrate of CYP3A4, P-glycoprotein/ABCB1; may increase digoxin level

CYP, cytochrome P450 enzyme; ER, extended-release; IR, immediate release; LA, long acting; OAB, overactive bladder; TDS, transdermal system; UUI, urge urinary incontinence; XL, extended release.

is principally cleared by the renal route (60%). Metabolites account for approximately 40% of the excreted dose following oral administration. The major metabolic pathway is hypothesized as ester hydrolysis with subsequent conjugation. CYP is not expected to contribute significantly to the elimination of trospium. The plasma half-life is approximately 20 hours; with renal clearance about 30 L/hr. Active tubular secretion is a major route of elimination for trospium. When creatinine clearance is less than 30 mL/min (0.50 mL/s), drug exposure and drug concentration are significantly increased.[45]

Trospium chloride IR was noninferior to oxybutynin IR, but was associated with less dry mouth.[52] Anticholinergic side effects occur more often in patients aged 75 years and older due to pharmacodynamics changes (ie, increased sensitivity). Trospium may interact with other drugs that are eliminated by active tubular secretion via competition (eg, procainamide, pancuronium, morphine, vancomycin, and tenofovir).[45] Trospium chloride extended-release offers once-daily dosing with established efficacy and safety in patients with OAB.[53] Trospium is eliminated primarily unchanged in the urine; thus it is not recommended in patients with severe renal impairment. It interacts with alcohol (increased drowsiness), antacid (increase or decrease trospium exposure), and metformin (reduced trospium level by 34%).[54] It must be taken on an empty stomach (1 hour before or 2 hours after meals) as food decreases the bioavailability by up to 60%.[53] Common adverse effects with trospium chloride ER are dry mouth (11%), constipation (9%), dizziness (2%), dry eyes (1.6%), flatulence (1.6%), nausea (1.4%), and abdominal pain (1.4%).[54]

Solifenacin Succinate Solifenacin succinate is a second-generation antimuscarinic agent indicated for the treatment of OAB with urgency incontinence, urgency, and urinary frequency.[55] It is also indicated for neurogenic detrusor overactivity in children 2 years or older and adolescents.[56] Solifenacin is associated with less dry mouth than oxybutynin IR (35% vs 83%). It is well absorbed (bioavailability 88%) and taken without regard to food. It is principally eliminated via metabolism (CYP3A4) and renal excretion of metabolites. It has a terminal disposition half-life of 50 to 60 hours.[55]

The recommended dose of solifenacin is 5 mg once daily with or without food. If the drug is well tolerated, the dose can be increased to 10 mg once daily. See Table 105-6 for dose adjustment based on renal/hepatic impairment and drug interactions. The most common adverse reactions of solifenacin are dry mouth (11%-28%), constipation (5%-13%), urinary tract infection (4%-5%), and blurred vision (3%-5%). It interacts with CYP3A4 inhibitors and inducers; close patient monitoring is required. Prolonged corrected QT intervals have been reported with high-dose solifenacin.[55]

Darifenacin Darifenacin is another second-generation antimuscarinic for the management of OAB or UUI. It improves urinary symptoms, and quality of life.[57,58] The bioavailability of extended-release (ER) formulation is low (25%), and is affected by CYP2D6 genotype and treatment dose. Darifenacin is extensively metabolized, with cumulative urinary excretion of the parent compound less than 10%. The 2D6 and 3A4 isoenzymes of CYP are responsible for darifenacin metabolism. Thus, pharmacogenomic profile may impact the clinical response to darifenacin.[59] With a mean terminal disposition half-life of 3 to 5 hours (depending on CYP2D6 metabolizer status), an ER formulation is needed to allow once-daily dosing.[60] Darifenacin ER should be initiated at 7.5 mg once daily, and may be increased to 15 mg once daily after 2 weeks to target clinical response. See Table 105-6 for dose adjustment based on renal/hepatic impairment and drug interactions. It must be swallowed whole without chewing, dividing, or crushing. Common adverse reactions are constipation (21%), dry mouth (19%), headache (7%), dyspepsia (5%), and nausea (4%). Darifenacin may interact with substrates of CYP2D6 (flecainide, thioridazine, and tricyclic antidepressants).[60]

Mirabegron Mirabegron is approved by FDA for the treatment of OAB with symptoms of UUI, urgency, and urinary frequency.

6 Mirabegron is another first-line drug treatment for managing UUI. It increases bladder capacity by relaxing the detrusor smooth muscle during the storage phase of the urinary bladder fill-void cycle through the activation of β_3-adrenergic receptors. Similar

to antimuscarinic agents, it is modestly effective and reduces urinary frequency and incontinence episodes by less than one per day. It is associated with nonsignificant improvements in UUI, urgency episodes, and quality-of-life measures. It has been shown to have similar efficacy as with tolterodine ER.[21,61] It reduces mean number of incontinence episodes per 24 hours, mean number of micturitions per 24 hours, and increased mean volume voided per micturition. The efficacy is usually seen during 4 to 8 weeks of therapy.[62]

Mirabegron reaches its peak plasma concentrations at approximately 3.5 hours and has an oral bioavailability of 29% to 35%. It achieves steady state within 7 days of therapy. It can be taken with or without food. Mirabegron is extensively distributed in the body, with a volume of distribution of approximately 1,670 L. It has protein binding of approximately 71% to both albumin and α_1-acid glycoprotein. Mirabegron is metabolized via multiple pathways involving dealkylation, oxidation, glucuronidation, and amide hydrolysis. It has two inactive metabolites (16% and 11% of total exposure), respectively. Isoenzymes CYP2D6 and 3A4 play a limited role in its elimination. Poor metabolizers of CYP2D6 had an increased mean peak concentration and drug exposure compared to extensive metabolizers of CYP2D6 (16% and 17%, respectively). Other enzymes that are involved in mirabegron metabolism include butylcholinesterase, uridine diphospho-glucuronosyltransferases (UGT), and possibly alcohol dehydrogenase.

Total body clearance of mirabegron is about 57 L/hr, with a terminal elimination half-life of 50 hours. Renal clearance equals approximately 13 L/hr, primarily through active tubular secretion along with glomerular filtration. The urinary elimination of unchanged mirabegron is dose dependent and ranges from 6% to 12% after a daily dose of 25 to 100 mg.[61]

Mirabegron should be initiated at 25 mg once daily, and may titrate upward to 50 mg once daily after 8 weeks, based on individual efficacy and tolerability; limit dose to 25 mg once daily in patients with severe renal impairment or moderate hepatic disease. Mirabegron is available in ER tablets, and should be swallowed whole with water without chewing, dividing, or crushing. It should be avoided in patients with end-stage renal disease, severe hepatic impairment, or severe uncontrolled hypertension (≥180/110 mm Hg). Most commonly reported adverse reactions were hypertension (7%-11%), nasopharyngitis (4%), urinary tract infection (3%-6%), and headache (3%-4%). Patient should be monitored for increased blood pressure and urinary retention, particularly in patients with bladder outlet obstruction or those who are taking anticholinergic drugs.[62] Mirabegron has similar adverse effects (except less dry mouth) when compared with tolterodine ER. Blood pressure and heart rate changes were minimal (<1 mm Hg and <2 beats/min, respectively).[21] Mirabegron is a moderate inhibitor of CYP2D6, and may affect the dosage requirement for some 2D6 substrates (eg, metoprolol and desipramine). Thus, drug-level monitoring for certain medications with a narrow therapeutic range, such as thioridazine, flecainide, and propafenone, is advised.[61] The efficacy and safety of combination therapy with mirabegron (25 or 50 mg) and solifenacin (5 mg) have been evaluated in clinical trials.[63-65] Combination therapy demonstrated improved efficacy without significant increase in side effects as seen in monotherapy.[21]

Vibegron Vibegron is approved by FDA for the treatment of OAB with symptoms of UUI, urgency, and urinary frequency in adults.

Like mirabegron, vibegron is a β_3-adrenergic receptor agonist. It activates β_3-adrenergic receptors in the bladder, resulting in relaxation of the detrusor smooth muscle during the urine storage phase, thus increasing bladder capacity. Vibegron reaches its peak plasma concentrations within 1 to 3.5 hours of administration and has a protein binding of 50%. The usual dose is 75 mg once daily with or without food.

Vibegron is extensively distributed in the body, with a volume of distribution of approximately 6,000 L. It is metabolized via minor metabolism hepatically via CYP3A4. It has a terminal elimination half-life of 30 hours and is excreted unchanged in feces (54%) and urine (19%).[66] Other β_3-adrenergic agonists in development include solabegron, ritobegron, and vibegron.[67-69]

TABLE 105-7 Adverse Event Incidence Rates (%) with Approved Drugs for Bladder Overactivity[a]

Drug	Dry Mouth	Constipation	Dizziness	Vision Disturbance
Oxybutynin IR	71	15	17	10
Oxybutynin XL	61	13	6	14
Oxybutynin TDS	7	3	NR	3
Oxybutynin gel	10	1	3	3
Tolterodine	35	7	5	3
Tolterodine LA	23	6	2	4
Trospium chloride IR	20	10	NR	1
Trospium chloride XR	11	9	NR	2
Solifenacin	20	9	2	5
Darifenacin ER	24	18	2	2
Fesoterodine ER	27	5	NR	3
Mirabegron ER	3	3	3	NR
Vibegron	<1	2	<1	<1

IR, immediate release; LA, long acting; NR, not reported; TDS, transdermal system; XL, extended release; XR/ER, extended release.

[a]All values constitute mean data, predominantly using product information from the manufacturers.

Table 105-7 lists the frequencies for the most common adverse events for all approved treatment oral agents based on manufacturers' product information.

Other Anticholinergics and Antimuscarinics Tricyclic antidepressants are generally no more effective than oxybutynin IR, and give bothersome and potentially serious adverse effects (eg, orthostatic hypotension, cardiac conduction abnormalities, dizziness, and confusion). They are also potentially life-threatening in overdose. Therefore, their use should be limited to individuals who have one or more additional medical indications for these agents (eg, depression or neuropathic pain); patients with mixed UI (because of their effect of decreasing bladder contractility and increasing outlet resistance); and possibly those with nocturnal incontinence associated with altered sleep patterns. Desipramine and nortriptyline have lower incidences of adverse effects; they may be preferred over imipramine and doxepin. However, because of their lower anticholinergic activity, they may not be as effective. Propantheline, flavoxate, dicyclomine, and hyoscyamine are not recommended for urgency UI.

Botulinum Toxin A Enthusiasm is considerable for the application of botulinum toxin A for treatment of voiding dysfunction. Botulinum toxin is a naturally occurring powerful muscle relaxant produced by *Clostridium botulinum*. Injected into smooth or striated muscle, botulinum toxin acts as a neurotoxin by temporarily paralyzing the muscle. The mechanism of action of the paralytic effect is generally ascribed to prevention of the release of the neurotransmitter acetylcholine into the synapse at the neuromuscular junction, although other pathways in neurotransduction may also be affected.

This compound is commercially produced for medical use in a number of conditions such as muscle spasticity, hyperhidrosis, and cosmetic reduction of skin wrinkles. It is indicated for the treatment of detrusor overactivity associated with neurologic condition and OAB.[62,70,71] Intradetrusor onabotulinumtoxin A is recommended by AUA as the third-line treatment in adult patients with refractory

OAB.[21] In the lower urinary tract, it has also been used to treat external urethral sphincter spasticity by direct injection into the external urethral sphincter.

Botulinum toxin is delivered into the detrusor muscle (intravesical injection) using a cystoscope equipped with a needle. The usual dosage is between 100 and 300 units/session. It is injected through the needle directly into the bladder muscle in 10 to 30 injections spaced over 5 to 10 minutes. The procedure is carried out as an outpatient procedure without general anesthesia. The duration of therapeutic effect varies, lasting usually from 4 to 8 months. Repeat injections are necessary to maintain the beneficial effects.[71]

The adverse effects of botulinum toxin A when used in the urinary tract most frequently include dysuria, hematuria, urinary tract infection, and urinary retention. Urinary retention occurs in up to 20% of treated individuals and persists until the paralytic effects have worn off (up to 6-8 months). Therapeutic and adverse effects may not become evident for 3 to 7 days, presumably because this period of time is required for uptake of the toxin following injection.[62,71]

Intravesical (ie, bladder) injection of botulinum toxin A in patients with refractory OAB resulted in increased bladder capacity, increased bladder compliance, and improved quality of life.[62,71] Adverse effects include urinary tract infection and urinary retention.[71] Comparative data with placebo and other interventions, long-term safety and efficacy outcomes, and data regarding the optimal dose of botulinum toxin for idiopathic OAB are needed.

An alternative mechanism of delivery other than intravesical injection would greatly improve the appeal of this agent as needle injection can be painful in some individuals. Results of an open-label trial of intravesical botulinum toxin A in dimethylsulfoxide in 21 women with refractory idiopathic detrusor overactivity demonstrated a significant reduction in the frequency of incontinence episodes without any effect on postvoid residual urine volumes.[72] Further studies are needed in this regard.

Catheterization Combined with Medications Patients with UUI and an elevated postvoid residual urine volume due to retention may require intermittent self-catheterization along with frequent voiding between catheterizations. If intermittent catheterization is not possible, surgical placement of a suprapubic catheter may be necessary. Use of a chronic indwelling catheter should be avoided because of the increased occurrence of urinary tract infections and nephrolithiasis.

Regardless of catheterization status, patients may experience symptom relief with judicious use of oxybutynin (IR, XL, or TDS formulations), tolterodine (IR or LA formulations), trospium chloride, solifenacin, fesoterodine, darifenacin, or mirabegron, as these agents relax the detrusor muscle and enhance bladder storage. Patients with UUI and symptoms of urinary retention may also benefit from an α-adrenergic receptor antagonist that relaxes the internal bladder sphincter (eg, prazosin, terazosin, doxazosin, tamsulosin, silodosin, and alfuzosin). Although theoretically of benefit, bethanechol, a cholinergic agonist, has not been demonstrated effective in improving bladder emptying in well-done trials. In addition, it causes numerous bothersome (eg, muscle and abdominal cramping and diarrhea) and potentially life-threatening adverse effects and should not be used in patients with asthma or heart disease.[22]

Urethral Underactivity

7 Urethral underactivity, or SUI, may be aggravated by agents with α-adrenergic receptor blocking activity, including prazosin, terazosin, doxazosin, tamsulosin, alfuzosin, silodosin, methyldopa, clonidine, guanfacine, and labetalol. The goal of therapy for SUI is to improve the urethral closure mechanism by stimulating α-adrenergic receptors in the smooth muscle of the bladder neck and proximal urethra, enhancing the supportive structures underlying the urethral epithelium, or enhancing the positive effects of serotonin and norepinephrine in the afferent and efferent pathways of the micturition reflex.[73]

Estrogens Local and systemic estrogens have been used extensively for the pharmacologic management of SUI since the 1940s. Estrogens are believed to work via several mechanisms, including enhancement of the proliferation of urethral epithelium, local circulation, and numbers and/or sensitivity of urogenital α-adrenergic receptors. However, a trial has questioned whether estrogens exert a stimulatory effect on vaginal collagen production, at least over the short-term.[74]

A meta-analysis of 34 trials evaluating the use of local or systemic estrogen therapy on UI in postmenopausal women found that systematic administration of estrogen alone or in combination with progesterone resulted in UI worsening.[75] In fact, observational studies have documented that oral or systemic estrogen use is associated with an increased risk of UI compared with that in nonusers.[76] There was some evidence that vaginal estrogen (vaginal cream or pessaries) may improve UI, and reduce urgency and frequency. The long-term effects of this therapy in older women are unknown. A recent meta-analysis of 17 trials of local estrogen compared to placebo or no treatment found beneficial effects on UI and OAB symptoms and some urodynamic parameters.[77] Different forms of vaginal estrogen (ring, pessary) have similar improvements in urinary symptoms (SUI, UUI, frequency, urgency). Studies comparing vaginal estrogen alone or in combination with antimuscarinic drugs (tolterodine or oxybutynin) or pelvic floor muscle exercises found greater improvement in subjective measures of UI in the combination approach. If estrogens are to be used for treatment of UI or OAB in postmenopausal women, only topical products should be administered, potentially combined with other treatment modalities such as pelvic floor muscle exercises or antimuscarinic drugs.

α-Adrenergic Receptor Agonists Numerous open trials have supported the use of a variety of α-adrenergic receptor agonists in SUI, including ephedrine, norfenefrine, phenylpropanolamine, and midodrine. Phenylpropanolamine was withdrawn from the US market in 2000 because of a risk for stroke in women using the agent.[78] Patients may obtain the drug from international sources or via Internet. If so, individuals with the contraindications listed later in the chapter (especially coronary artery disease and/or cardiac arrhythmias) should be warned against self-treatment with this or other α-adrenergic receptor agonists.

Placebo-controlled comparative trials with phenylpropanolamine, norfenefrine, and norephedrine support the modest efficacy of these agents for treatment of mild or moderate SUI.[79] These agents have been found to variably affect maximum urethral closure pressure and functional urethral length. Adverse effects include hypertension, headache, dry mouth, nausea, insomnia, and restlessness. Contraindications to the use of these agents include the presence of hypertension, tachyarrhythmias, coronary artery disease, myocardial infarction, cor pulmonale, hyperthyroidism, renal failure, and narrow-angle glaucoma.

Several studies have evaluated whether the clinical and urodynamic effects of a combination of estrogen and an α-adrenergic receptor agonist exceed those of the individual therapies in SUI.[79] In general, combination therapy has resulted in somewhat superior clinical and urodynamic responses compared with monotherapy, including severity of complaints, amount of urine lost per episode, number of daily voluntary micturitions, number of leakage episodes per day, patient preference, pad use, maximum urethral closure pressure, functional urethral length, and pressure transmission ratio.

Duloxetine Duloxetine, a dual inhibitor of serotonin and norepinephrine reuptake (SNRI), was approved in 2004 for treatment of depression and painful diabetic neuropathy in the United States.[80] It is approved for SUI in Europe only. It is believed to affect central serotoninergic and noradrenergic regions, which are involved in ascending and descending control of urethral smooth muscle and the external urethral sphincter. These mechanisms facilitate the bladder-to-sympathetic reflex pathway, increasing urethral and external urethral sphincter muscle tone during the storage phase.

Duloxetine is metabolized by CYP2D6 and 1A2 enzymes to form multiple metabolites and then eliminated in the urine. Duloxetine may increase the concentrations, drug exposure, and half-lives of CYP2D6 substrates (eg, desipramine). Meanwhile, the drug concentration of duloxetine can be increased by CYP2D6 inhibitors (eg, paroxetine) and CYP1A2 inhibitors (eg, fluvoxamine).[80] Moderate hepatic dysfunction (Child-Pugh class B) significantly increases mean AUC and terminal disposition half-life of duloxetine. Mild or moderate renal impairment (creatinine clearance 30-80 mL/min [0.50-1.33 mL/s]) does not affect drug disposition. In severe renal impairment (hemodialysis patients), mean peak plasma concentration and AUC are both increased 100%, whereas metabolite concentrations are increased up to 900%.[80]

In six large, double-blinded, randomized, placebo-controlled clinical trials that evaluated duloxetine for SUI, duloxetine therapy produced significant reductions in UI episode frequency and number of micturitions per day, improvement in incontinence quality-of-life questionnaire scores and patient self-assessment, and increase in mean micturition interval. Results were independent of baseline UI severity (severity based on incontinent episode frequency). Significant intergroup differences were seen by week 4. However, cure rates were generally not improved by duloxetine. When evaluating the absolute differences between treatments, the actual benefit of duloxetine was generally quite modest. Duloxetine also reduced incontinence episodes and improved quality of life in men with SUI after radical prostatectomy.[81]

A randomized, placebo-controlled clinical trial evaluated the effects of duloxetine (80 mg daily), pelvic floor muscle training (PFMT), and the combination of both modalities on incontinent episode frequency, incontinence-related quality of life, pad use, and patient global impression of change. Sham PFMT was used in the placebo group. Results indicated that duloxetine plus PFMT were probably additive in effect and that combination therapy afforded greater improvement than either monotherapy.[82]

The adverse events associated with duloxetine may make adherence problematic. In the SUI trials, treatment-emergent adverse events occurred in 68% to 93% of duloxetine and 50% to 72% of placebo recipients. Premature study withdrawal rates (due to adverse events) were as high as up to 33%. The most common adverse events reported with duloxetine were nausea (≤46%), headache (≤27%), constipation (≤27%), dry mouth (≤22%), and insomnia (≤14%). Of interest, the drug may be associated with small increases in blood pressure (such as venlafaxine, another SNRI) and withdrawal symptoms (sleep disturbances). Unfortunately, adherence to long-term therapy is quite poor due to a combination of adverse events and lack of efficacy.[83]

Despite these negatives, duloxetine is the first drug approved by a regulatory agency for treating SUI in Europe. Based on studies conducted to date, a dosage regimen of 40 to 80 mg/day (in one or two doses) is reasonable. Gradual dose titration (40 mg daily for 2 weeks, then 80 mg daily) helps reduce the risks of nausea, dizziness, and premature drug discontinuation. If cessation of duloxetine is desired, consider tapering the dosage by 50% for 2 weeks before discontinuation to avoid withdrawal symptoms.

Venlafaxine Venlafaxine is another SNRI. A double-blind, randomized, placebo-controlled clinical trial has demonstrated the benefit of venlafaxine 75 mg once daily for 12 weeks over placebo in terms of incontinence episode frequency, voiding interval, quality of life, and patient global impression of improvement. Nausea occurred in 40% of the venlafaxine group compared with 15% of the placebo group.[84]

Overflow Incontinence

Overflow incontinence secondary to benign or malignant prostatic hyperplasia may be amenable to pharmacotherapy. For management of malignant prostatic disease, see Chapter 154, "Prostate Cancer." The pharmacotherapy of BPH is discussed in Chapter 104.

EVALUATION OF THERAPEUTIC OUTCOMES

8 Assessment of patient outcomes should include efficacy, side effects, adherence, and quality of life. During long-term management of UI, patient-specific clinical signs and symptoms of most distress ("bother") to the individual must be monitored. A daily diary may be useful in this regard. Some of the short-form instruments used in incontinence research for measuring symptom impact and condition-specific quality of life can be used in clinical monitoring. In addition, quantitating the use of ancillary supplies, such as pads, may be useful.

9 The main goal of therapy is to minimize the signs and symptoms most bothersome to the patient, as well as the use of pads and other ancillary supplies or devices. Total elimination of UI signs and symptoms may not be possible, and patients and practitioners need to mutually establish realistic goals of therapy. Because the therapies for UI frequently have nuisance adverse effects (eg, anticholinergic effects such as dry mouth, constipation, and sedation) that may compromise regimen adherence, the presence and severity of adverse effects must be carefully elicited at each visit to the healthcare practitioner. Queries of the patient and caregiver regarding CNS effects are important in elderly or frail patient as these effects can be severe enough to cause loss of independent living skills. Emergence of adverse effects may necessitate drug dosage adjustment or use of alternative strategies (eg, chewing sugarless gum, sucking on hard sugarless candy, or use of saliva substitutes in xerostomia) or even drug discontinuation. Patient should be encouraged to persist with a particular treatment for 4 to 8 weeks before declaring treatment failure. Nonresponders to an antimuscarinic should be offered at least one other antimuscarinic and/or dose modification attempted to obtain a better balance between efficacy and side effects.

ABBREVIATIONS

ACE	angiotensin-converting enzyme
AUA	American Urological Association
AUC	area under the plasma or serum concentration-versus-time curve
BPH	benign prostatic hyperplasia
CNS	central nervous system
CYP	cytochrome P450
DD01	5-hydroxymethyl metabolite
ER	extended-release
EStim	electrical stimulation
FDA	Food and Drug Administration
IR	immediate release
LA	long acting
MStim	magnetic stimulation
OAB	overactive bladder
PFMT	pelvic floor muscle training
PTNS	peripheral tibial nerve stimulation
SNRI	serotonin and norepinephrine reuptake
SUI	stress urinary incontinence
TDS	transdermal system
UI	urinary incontinence
UGT	uridine diphospho-glucuronosyltransferases
UUI	urgency urinary incontinence
XL	extended release

REFERENCES

1. D'Ancona C, Haylen B, Oelke M, et al. Standardisation Steering Committee ICS and the ICS Working Group on Terminology for Male Lower Urinary Tract & Pelvic Floor Symptoms and Dysfunction. The International Continence Society (ICS) report on the terminology for adult male lower urinary tract and pelvic floor symptoms and dysfunction. *Neurourol Urodyn.* 2019;38(2):433–477. doi:10.1002/nau.23897.
2. Gorina Y, Schappert S, Bercovitz A, et al. Prevalence of incontinence among older Americans. National Center for Health Statistics. *Vital Health Stat.* 3(36), 2014.
3. Milsom I, Gyhagen M. The prevalence of urinary incontinence. *Climacteric.* 2019; 22(3):217–222. doi:10.1080/13697137.2018.1543263.
4. Milson I, Altman D, Cartwright R, et al. Epidemiology of urinary incontinence (UI) and other lower urinary tract symptoms (LUTS), pelvic organ prolapse (POP), and anal (AI) incontinence. In: Abrams P, Cardozo L, Wagg A, Wein A, eds. *Incontinence.* 6th ed. Paris: Health Publications Ltd; 2006:17–24.
5. Tennsted SL, Link CL, Steers WD, et al. Prevalence of and risk factors for urine leakage in a racially and ethnically diverse population of adults: the Boston Area Community Health (BACH) Survey. *Am J Epidemiol.* 2008;167:390–399.
6. Fenner DE, Trowbridge ER, Patel DA, et al. Establishing the prevalence of incontinence study: Racial differences in women's patterns of urinary incontinence. *J Urol.* 2008;179:1455–1460.
7. Markland AD, Goode PS, Redden DT, et al. Prevalence of urinary incontinence in men: Results from the National Health and Nutrition Examination Survey. *J Urol.* 2010;184:1022–1027.
8. Bump RC. Racial comparisons and contrasts in urinary incontinence and pelvic organ prolapse. *Obstet Gynecol.* 1993;81:421–425.
9. Burgio KL, Matthews KA, Engel BT. Prevalence, incidence and correlates of urinary incontinence in healthy, middle-aged women. *J Urol.* 1991;146:1255–1259.
10. Moon S, Chung HS, Kim YJ, et al. The impact of urinary incontinence on falls: A systematic review and meta-analysis. *PLoS One.* 2021;19;16(5):e0251711. doi:10.1371/journal.pone.0251711
11. Andersson KE, Chapple C, Cardozo L, et al. Pharmacological treatment of urinary incontinence. In: Abrams P, Cardozo L, Khoury S, Wein A, eds. *Incontinence*, 5th ed. International Consultation on Urological Disease European Association of Urology (ICUD-EAU). 2013:623–672.
12. Kanai A, Wyndaele JJ, Andersson KE, et al. Researching bladder afferents-determining the effects of β(3)-adrenergic receptor agonists and botulinum toxin type-A. *Neurourol Urodyn.* 2011;30(5):684–691.
13. Fowler C. Integrated control of the lower urinary tract—Clinical perspective. *Br J Pharmacol.* 2006;147(suppl 2):s14–s24.
14. Blok BF. Brain control of the lower urinary tract. *Scand J Urol Nephrol Suppl.* 2002;(210):11–15.
15. Abrams P, Andersson KE, Apostolidis A, et al. 6th International Consultation on Incontinence. Recommendations of the International Scientific Committee: Evaluation and treatment of urinary incontinence, pelvic organ prolapse and faecal incontinence. *Neurourol Urodyn.* 2018;37:2271–2272.
16. Ruby CM, Hanlon JT, Boudreau RM, et al. Health, aging and body composition study. The effect of medication use on urinary incontinence in community-dwelling elderly women. *J Am Geriatr Soc.* 2010;58(9):1715–1720.
17. Hall SA, Yang M, Gates MA, et al. Associations of commonly used medications with urinary incontinence in a community based sample. *J Urol.* 2012;188(1):183–189.
18. James M, Jackson S, Shepard A, Abrams P. Pure stress leakage symptomatology: Is it safe to discount detrusor instability? *Br J Obstet Gynaecol.* 1999;106:1255–1258.
19. Fritel X, Ringa V, Quiboeuf E, Fauconnier A. Female urinary incontinence, from pregnancy to menopause: A review of epidemiological and pathophysiological findings. *Acta Obstet Gynecol Scand.* 2012;91(8):901–910.
20. Balk EM, Rofeberg VN, Adam GP, Kimmel HJ, Trikalinos TA, Jeppson PC. Pharmacologic and nonpharmacologic treatments for urinary incontinence in women: A systematic review and network meta-analysis of clinical outcomes. *Ann Intern Med.* 2019;170(7):465–479. doi:10.7326/M18-3227.
21. Lightner DJ, Gomelsky A, Souter L, Vasavada SP. Diagnosis and treatment of overactive bladder (non-neurogenic) in adults: AUA/SUFU guideline. *J Urol.* 2019;202(3):558–563. doi:10.1097/ju.0000000000000309.
22. Dumoulin C, Adewuyi T, Booth J, et al. Adult conservative management. In: Abrams P, Cardozo L, Wagg A, Wein A, eds. *Incontinence*, 6th ed. International Consultation on Urological Disease (ICUD); 2017:1443–1628.
23. Sheridan W, Da Silva AS, Leca BM, et al. Weight loss with bariatric surgery or behaviour modification and the impact on female obesity-related urine incontinence: A comprehensive systematic review and meta-analysis. *Clin Obes.* 2021:e12450. doi:10.1111/cob.12450.
24. Kirchin V, Page T, Keegan PE, Atiemo K, Cody JD, McClinton S. Urethral injection therapy for urinary incontinence in women. *Cochrane Database Syst Rev.* 201215;2:CD003881.
25. Koski ME, Rovner ES. Implications of the FDA statement on transvaginal placement of mesh: The aftermath. *Curr Urol Rep.* 2014;15(2):380.
26. Sandhu JS. Treatment options for male stress urinary incontinence. *Nat Rev Urol.* 2010;7(4):222–228.
27. Wilson LC, Gilling PJ. Post-prostatectomy urinary incontinence: A review of surgical treatment options. *BJU Int.* 2011;107(suppl 3):7–10.
28. Nash S, Aboseif S, Gilling P, et al. Four-year follow-up on 68 patients with a new post-operatively adjustable long-term implant for post-prostatectomy stress incontinence: ProACT™. *Neurourol Urodyn.* 2019;38:248–253.
29. Welk BK, Herschorn S. The male sling for post-prostatectomy urinary incontinence: A review of contemporary sling designs and outcomes. *BJU Int.* 2012;109(3):328–344.
30. Peters KM, Macdiarmid SA, Wooldridge LS, et al. Randomized trial of percutaneous tibial nerve stimulation versus extended-release tolterodine: Results from the overactive bladder innovative therapy trial. *J Urol.* 2009;182(3):1055–1061.
31. Van Kerrebroeck PE, Marcelissen TA. Sacral neuromodulation for lower urinary tract dysfunction. *World J Urol.* 2012;30(4):445–450.
32. Rovner E, Kennelly M, Schulte-Baukloh H, et al. Urodynamic results and clinical outcomes with intradetrusor injections of onabotulinum toxin A in a randomized, placebo-controlled dose-finding study in idiopathic overactive bladder. *Neurourol Urodyn.* 2011;30(4):556–562.
33. Shepherd JP, Lowder JL, Leng WW, Smith KJ. InterStim sacral neuromodulation and botox botulinum—A toxin intradetrusor injections for refractory urge urinary incontinence: A decision analysis comparing outcomes including efficacy and complications. *Female Pelvic Med Reconstr Surg.* 2011;17(4):199–203.
34. van Kerrebroeck PE, van Voskuilen AC, Heesakkers JP, et al. Results of sacral neuromodulation therapy for urinary voiding dysfunction: Outcomes of a prospective, worldwide clinical study. *J Urol.* 2007; 178(5):2029–2034.
35. Shamliyan T, Wyman JF, Ramakrishnan R, Sainfort F, Kane RL. Benefits and harms of pharmacologic treatment for urinary incontinence in women: A systematic review. *Ann Intern Med.* 2012;156(12):861–874, W301–W310.
36. Maman K, Aballea S, Nazir J, et al. Comparative efficacy and safety of medical treatments for the management of overactive bladder: A systematic review and mixed treatment comparison. *Eur Urol.* 2014;65:755–765.
37. Ortho-McNeil-Janssen Pharmaceuticals. Ditropan (Oxybutynin) Package Insert. Raritan, NJ: Ortho-McNeil-Janssen; 2012.
38. Janssen Pharmaceuticals. Ditropan XL (Oxybutynin Chloride) Extended-Release Tablets Package Insert. Titusville, NJ: Janssen Pharmaceuticals; 2015.
39. Activis Pharma. Oxytrol (Oxybutynin Transdermal System) Package Insert. Parsippany, NJ: Activis Pharma; 2015.
40. Cartwright R, Srikrishna S, Cardozo L, Robinson D. Patient-selected goals in overactive bladder: A placebo controlled randomized double-blind trial of transdermal oxybutynin for the treatment of urgency and urge incontinence. *BJU Int.* 2011;107(1):70–76.
41. Activis Pharma. Gelnique 3% (Oxybutynin Chloride 3% Gel) Package Insert. Parsippany, NJ: Activis Pharma; 2015.
42. Activis Pharma. Gelnique (Oxybutynin Chloride 10% Gel) Package Insert. Corona, CA: Activis Pharma; 2015.
43. Sand PK, Davila GW, Lucente VR, et al. Efficacy and safety of oxybutynin chloride topical gel for women with overactive bladder syndrome. *Am J Obstet Gynecol.* 2012;206(2):168.e1–e6.
44. Esin E, Ergen A, Cankurtaran M, et al. Influence of antimuscarinic therapy on cognitive functions and quality of life in geriatric patients treated for overactive bladder. *Aging Ment Health.* 2015;19:217–223.
45. Allergan. Sanctura (Trospium Chloride) Tablets Package Insert. Irvine, CA: Allergan; 2012.
46. Pharmacia & Upjohn. Detrol (Tolterodine) Package Insert. New York, NY: Pharmacia & Upjohn; 2012.
47. Pharmacogenomic effect/ADR for tolterodine. Available at: https://go.drugbank.com/pharmaco/genomics/DBSNPE004890. Accessed November 22, 2021.

48. Pharmacia & Upjohn. Detrol LA (Tolterodine Tartrate Extended Release Capsule). New York, NY: Pharmacia & Upjohn; 2011.
49. Chapple CR, Herschorn S, Abrams P, et al. Efficacy and safety of tolterodine extended-release in men with overactive bladder symptoms treated with an α-blocker: Effect of baseline prostate-specific antigen concentration. *BJU Int.* 2010;106(9):1332–1338.
50. Pfizer Laboratories, Toviaz (Fesoterodine Fumarate Extended-Release Tablets) Package Insert. New York, NY: Pfizer; 2014.
51. Kaplan SA, Schneider T, Foote JE, et al. Superior efficacy of fesoterodine over tolterodine extended release with rapid onset: A prospective, head-to-head, placebo-controlled trial. *BJU Int.* 2011;107(9):1432–1440.
52. Zellner M, Madersbacher H, Palmtag H, et al. Trospium chloride and oxybutynin hydrochloride in a German study of adults with urinary urge incontinence: Results of a 12-week, multicenter, randomized, double-blind, parallel-group, flexible-dose noninferiority trial. *Clin Ther.* 2009;31(11):2519–2539.
53. Sand PK, Rovner ES, Watanabe JH, Oefelein MG. Once-daily trospium chloride 60 mg extended release in subjects with overactive bladder syndrome who use multiple concomitant medications: Post hoc analysis of pooled data from two randomized, placebo-controlled trials. *Drugs Aging.* 2011;28(2):151–160.
54. Allergan, Sanctura XR (Trospium Chloride Extended-Release Capsules) Package Insert. Irvine, CA: Allergan; 2012.
55. Astellas Pharma Technologies. Vesicare (Solifenacin Succinate) Package Insert. Norman, Oklahoma: Stellas Pharma Technologies; 2013.
56. Newgreen D, Bosman B, Hollestein-Havelaar A, et al. Long-term safety and efficacy of solifenacin in children and adolescents with overactive bladder. *J Urol.* 2017;198(4):928–936. doi:10.1016/j.juro.2017.05.038.
57. Dwyer P, Kelleher C, Young J, et al. Long-term benefits of darifenacin treatment for patient quality of life: Results from a 2-year extension study. *Neurourol Urodyn.* 2008;27(6):540–547.
58. Abrams P, Kelleher C, Huels J, et al. Clinical relevance of health-related quality of life outcomes with darifenacin. *BJU Int.* 2008;102(2):208–213.
59. Darifenacin. Available at: https://go.drugbank.com/drugs/DB00496. Accessed November 22, 2021
60. Warner Chilcott. Enablex (Darifenacin Extended Release) Package Insert. Rockaway, NJ: Warner Chilcott; 2013.
61. Astellas Pharma Technologies. Myrbetriq (Mirabegron) Package Insert. Norman, OK: Astellas Pharma Technologies; 2015.
62. Duthie JB, Vincent M, Herbison GP, Wilson DI, Wilson D. Botulinum toxin injections for adults with overactive bladder syndrome. *Cochrane Database Syst Rev.* 2011;(12):CD005493.
63. Abrams P, Kelleher C, Staskin D, et al. Combination treatment with mirabegron and solifenacin in patients with overactive bladder: Exploratory responder analyses of efficacy and evaluation of patient-reported outcomes from a randomized, double-blind, factorial, dose-ranging, Phase II study (SYMPHONY). *World J Urol.* 2017;35:827–838.
64. Gratzke C, van Maanen R, Chapple C, et al. Long-term safety and efficacy of mirabegron and solifenacin in combination compared with monotherapy in patients with overactive bladder: A randomised, multicentre phase 3 study (SYNERGY II). *Eur Urol.* 2018;74:501–509.
65. Drake MJ, Chapple C, Esen AA, et al. BESIDE study investigators. Efficacy and safety of mirabegron add-on therapy to solifenacin in incontinent overactive bladder patients with an inadequate response to initial 4-Week solifenacin monotherapy: A randomised double-blind multicentre phase 3B study (BESIDE). *Eur Urol.* 2016;70:136–145.
66. Urovant Sciences Inc. Vibegron (Gemtesa) Package Insert. Irvine, CA: Urovant Sciences Inc; 2020.
67. Thiagamoorthy G, Cardozo L, Robinson D. Current and future pharmacotherapy for treating overactive bladder. *Expert Opin Pharmacother.* 2016;17:1317–1325.
68. Mitcheson HD, Samanta S, Muldowney K, et al. Vibegron (RVT-901/MK-4618/KRP-114V) administered once daily as monotherapy or concomitantly with tolterodine in patients with an overactive bladder: A multicenter, phase IIb, randomized, double-blind, controlled trial. *Eur Urol.* 2019;75):274–282.
69. Yoshida M, Takeda M, Gotoh M, et al. Efficacy of novel β(3) - adrenoreceptor agonist vibegron on nocturia in patients with overactive bladder: A post-hoc analysis of a randomized, double-blind, placebo-controlled phase 3 study. *Int J Urol.* 2019;26:369–375.
70. Anger JT, Weinberg A, Suttorp MJ, et al. Outcomes of intravesical botulinum toxin for idiopathic overactive bladder symptoms: A systematic review of the literature. *J Urol.* 2010;183(6):2258–2264.
71. Dmochowski R, Chapple C, Nitti VW, et al. Efficacy and safety of onabotulinum toxin A for idiopathic overactive bladder: A double-blind, placebo controlled, randomized, dose ranging trial. *J Urol.* 2010;184(6):2416–2422.
72. Petrou SP, Parker AS, Crook JE, et al. Botulinum A toxin/dimethylsulfoxide bladder instillations for women with refractory idiopathic detrusor overactivity: A phase I/II study. *Mayo Clin Proc.* 2009;84:702–706.
73. Tsakiris P, de la Rosette JJ, Michel MC, et al. Pharmacologic treatment of male stress urinary incontinence: Systematic review of the literature and levels of evidence. *Eur Urol.* 2008;53:53–59.
74. Jackson S, James M, Abrams P. The effect of oestradiol on vaginal collagen metabolism in postmenopausal women with genuine stress incontinence. *BJOG.* 2002;109:339–344.
75. Cody JD, Jacobs ML, Richardson K, et al. Oestrogen therapy for urinary incontinence in post-menopausal women. *Cochrane Database Syst Rev.* 2012. Issue 10, Art. No.: CD001405. doi:10.1002/14651858.CD001405.pub2.
76. Grady D, Brown JS, Vittinghoff E, et al. Postmenopausal hormones and incontinence: The Heart & Estrogen/Progestin Replacement Study. *Obstet Gynecol.* 2001;97:116–120.
77. Weber MA, Kleijn MH, Langendam M, et al. Local oestrogen for pelvic floor disorders: A systematic review. *PLOS One.* 2015 Sep 18; 10(9):e013625.
78. Kernan WN, Viscoli CM, Brass LM, et al. Phenylpropanolamine and the risk of hemorrhagic stroke. *N Engl J Med.* 2000:343:1826–1832.
79. Alhasso A, Glazener CM, Pickard R, N'dow J. Adrenergic drugs for urinary incontinence in adults. *Cochrane Database Syst Rev.* 2005;3: CD001842.
80. Eli Lilly Canada Inc. Cymbalta (duloxetine) Package Insert. Toronto, Ontario. 2016.
81. Cornu JN, Merlet B, Ciofu C, et al. Duloxetine for mild to moderate postprostatectomy incontinence: Preliminary results of a randomised, placebo-controlled trial. *Eur Urol.* 2011;59(1):148–154.
82. Ghoneim GM, VanLeeuwen JS, Elser DM, et al. A randomized controlled trial of duloxetine alone, pelvic floor muscle training alone, combined treatment and no active treatment in women with stress urinary incontinence. *J Urol.* 2005;173:1647–1653.
83. Bump RC, Voss S, Beardsworth A, et al. Long-term efficacy of duloxetine in women with stress urinary incontinence. *Br J Urol Int.* 2008;102:214–218.
84. Erdinc B, Gurates B, Celik H, et al. The efficacy of venlafaxine in the treatment of women with stress urinary incontinence. *Arch Gynecol Obstet.* 2009;279:343–348.

Function and Evaluation of the Immune System

e106

Daniel A. Zlott and Geoffrey M. Thiele

KEY CONCEPTS

1. Cells of the immune system are derived from the pluripotent stem cell. Hematopoiesis is closely regulated to maintain adequate numbers of different cell types. The development of these different cells or cell lineages depends on cell-to-cell interactions and hematopoietic growth factors.
2. Upon activation, dendritic cells (DCs) express higher concentrations of major histocompatibility complex class II molecules, B7-1, B7-2, CD40, ICAM-1, and LFA-3 molecules than other antigen-presenting cells (APCs). They also produce more IL-12. These differences may explain why DCs are the most efficient APC.
3. A T-lymphocyte expresses hundreds of T-cell receptors (TCRs). All the TCRs expressed on the surface of an individual T-lymphocyte have the same antigen specificity.
4. An immature B-lymphocyte expresses thousands of membrane-bound surface immunoglobulin (sIg) as IgM (monomeric) or IgD, all with the same specificity (ie, antigen-binding site). Upon antigen stimulation and T-cell help, the immature B-lymphocyte matures (proliferates, class-switches and becomes a plasma cell) to secrete different isotypes (eg, IgM [pentamer], IgA, immunoglobulin G [IgG], and IgE) with the same specificity as the original membrane-bound sIg.
5. Serum protein electrophoresis determines the total concentration of all circulating proteins, including the immunoglobulins (ie, IgG, IgA, IgM, IgD, and IgE). The concentration of the individual isotypes can be determined with isotype-specific quantification methods. Most clinical laboratories measure only IgG, IgM, and IgA because they are the most prevalent isotypes in the bloodstream. In patients with allergic disorders, measurement of IgE is rarely useful.
6. An understanding of the mechanism of action of immunomodulators allows a clinician to anticipate potential adverse drug reactions. The benefit of manipulating immune responses must be balanced with the potential consequences and long-term sequela (eg, tumor growth, infections, autoimmune reactions) of such manipulation.

BEYOND THE BOOK

Watch the following video to learn more about the different ways clinicians use the immune system to treat cancer. IMMUNOTHERAPY: The Path to a Cancer Cure (For Clinicians), https://www.youtube.com/watch?v=UbFjiWOBErA. As you read the chapter, note which strategies for modulating the immune response for therapeutic purposes were discussed in the video.

INTRODUCTION

The immune system is a complex network of barriers, organs, cellular elements, and molecules that interact to defend the body against invading pathogens. The *immune system* is actually composed of two distinct systems of immunity: innate immunity and adaptive immunity. Innate immunity includes a series of nonspecific barriers (physical and chemical), along with cellular and molecular elements strategically deployed and positioned to prevent or quickly neutralize infection. Adaptive immunity works in concert with the innate immune system. In contrast to innate immunity, adaptive immunity constantly evolves and adapts to invading pathogens. The hallmarks of the adaptive immune response are *diversity*, *memory*, *mobility*, *self-versus-nonself discrimination*, *redundancy*, *replication*, and *specificity*.[1] *Diversity* is the capability of the immune system to respond to many different pathogens or strains of pathogens. Immunological *memory* ensures a quicker and more vigorous response to a subsequent encounter with the same pathogen.

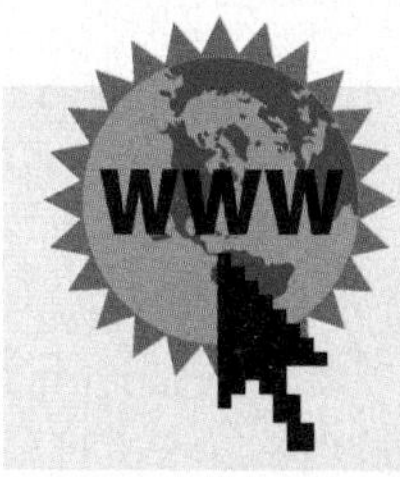

The complete chapter, learning objectives, and other resources can be found at **www.pharmacotherapyonline.com.**

Systemic Lupus Erythematosus

107

Beth H. Resman-Targoff

KEY CONCEPTS

1. Systemic lupus erythematosus (SLE) is considered a disease primarily of young women, but it can occur in anyone. The prevalence and severity vary with sex, race, ethnicity, and socioeconomic factors.
2. Understanding the etiology of SLE and environmental factors that can initiate or exacerbate the disease may make it possible to avoid those triggers.
3. SLE is an autoimmune disease characterized by the presence of autoantibodies, some of which may play a role in the pathogenesis of the disease. An understanding of disease mechanisms can lead to targeted drug therapy.
4. SLE is a multisystem disease that can involve almost any organ and may present in many different ways. Therapy is determined by the manifestations in each patient, which may change and fluctuate in severity over time.
5. Lifestyle changes can modify risk factors for SLE flares and complications.
6. The overall goals of therapy are to prevent disease flares and involvement of other organs, decrease disease activity and prevent damage, achieve and maintain remission, reduce use of corticosteroids, and improve quality of life, while minimizing adverse drug reactions and costs. Most patients with SLE should receive hydroxychloroquine alone or in combination with other therapy appropriate for the disease manifestations.
7. Pregnancy planning is essential for good outcomes. Pregnancy outcomes are best when the disease is controlled before conception. Drugs used to treat SLE may adversely affect fertility and the fetus.
8. Antiphospholipid antibodies are associated with arterial and venous thrombosis and obstetric complications.
9. Many drugs can induce a lupus-like syndrome. The manifestations and laboratory findings may be different between the traditional drug-induced lupus and that seen with tumor necrosis factor-alpha inhibitors.
10. Since SLE can present in many different ways, it is difficult to design standard response criteria. The development of appropriate criteria is essential for the approval of new drugs.

BEYOND THE BOOK

Lupus Canada: review the Living with Lupus Section (https://lupuscanada.org/living-with-lupus/)

Summarize what you learned about SLE from the Personal Stories section (https://lupuscanada.org/living-with-lupus/personal-stories/).

What questions would you have if you developed lupus?

INTRODUCTION

Systemic lupus erythematosus (SLE) is an autoimmune disease associated with autoantibody production. The term "lupus" (Latin for wolf) was first used in medieval Europe to describe erosive lesions that looked like skin that had been bitten by a wolf. In the 1800s, it was recognized that other organs may be affected and we now know that SLE is a multisystem disease. The common finding in SLE is the production of autoantibodies.[1] This is an exciting time in the management of SLE because a better understanding of disease mechanisms has led to the development of new drugs. In addition, new response criteria are evolving to show efficacy of drugs, even with the background of standard therapy. This led to the first approval of a drug for the treatment of SLE in over 50 years with a new indication 9 years later. Two more drugs were approved for SLE management. Despite these advances, control of this disease remains a challenge. It has a myriad of manifestations and many of the drugs used to treat it are not approved for this indication. As a result, the dosing of many of the drugs considered to be standard-of-care therapy must be personalized.

EPIDEMIOLOGY

1 Systemic lupus erythematosus occurs most frequently in women of reproductive age (15-45 years).[2] This is especially characteristic of the disease in non-White women. The epidemiology of SLE depends on the population studied, method used to define cases, and definition of SLE.[3] These can have profound effects on estimates of incidence and prevalence, disease activity and severity, and mortality. In the US Medicare population, the incidence ranges from 3.7 to 49 per 100,000 person-years and the prevalence is 48 to 366.6 per 100,000 persons. The global incidence ranges from 1.5 to 11 per 100,000 person-years with a prevalence of 13 to 7,713.5 per 100,000 individuals, but there are little data from some parts of the world.[3] Rates are nine times higher in women than in men so the overall population statistics can be misleading.[2] It is affected by ethnicity, which includes genetic, geographic, cultural, social, and other aspects within a group. Rates are higher in non-White than in the White population.[4] It is most common in those of African origin, but is also more common in people of Asian, Arab, and Hispanic background, and Native American people (called First Nations in Canada) than in White people.[4,5] Most people are of mixed race, so race by itself can be difficult to analyze. Non-White patients tend to have an earlier onset, more severe disease, and a higher mortality rate, but it can be difficult to separate out the influence of

socioeconomic factors, comorbidities, and access to medical care.[3] The disease tends to be more severe in men and children, and those with onset at a later age (over 50 years) have poor outcomes.[4]

Survival rates have improved with better therapy and earlier diagnosis and initiation of treatment. The standardized mortality ratio for SLE is two to three times higher than in the general population, most related to more cardiovascular and renal disease and infections.[3] Overall SLE survival is 95% at 5 years and 92% at 10 years after diagnosis. This is reduced to about 88% at 10 years with lupus nephritis and even less than that in African American patients with lupus nephritis.[6] The survival rate may be lower in men, but the small number of males in most studies makes this difficult to determine.[4]

ETIOLOGY

2 The exact etiology of SLE is unknown but many factors play a role in the disease. Some are predisposing factors and others are involved in the disease mechanisms. Categories of these elements include genetic influences, epigenetic regulation of gene expression, environmental factors, hormones, and abnormalities in immune cells and cytokines.[7]

The incidence of SLE is increased in affected families. First-degree relatives of patients with SLE are 20 times more likely to develop the disease than those in a general population.[8] Ten percent of patients with SLE have relatives with the disease. The concordance rate is 24% to 69% for identical twins and 2% to 5% for fraternal twins and other full siblings.[9] The genetic predisposition to SLE results from the interplay between several genes. In rare cases, it results primarily from a single abnormal gene.[7] The major histocompatibility complex (MHC) class II alleles HLA-DR2 and HLA-DR3 are known to be linked to SLE. An increasing number of other gene loci have been associated with the disease.[10] Gene expression is regulated by deoxyribonucleic acid (DNA) methylation and histone modifications. These epigenetic changes can cause alterations that may influence SLE. Interestingly, hydralazine and procainamide, two drugs that may induce lupus, inhibit DNA methylation.[11]

In a genetically susceptible individual, environmental triggers can initiate or exacerbate the disease. The type of trigger may influence specific organ involvement. Cigarette smoke has many toxic combustion byproducts that can react with DNA molecules and increase cell apoptosis, NETosis, or necrosis. Chronic smokers with greater than 10 pack-year smoking history are more likely to have elevated titers of anti-double-stranded DNA (anti-dsDNA) and antiphospholipid antibodies.[12,13] Cigarette smoking damages the skin and worsens disease and quality of life.[14] Ultraviolet light can cause DNA damage and keratinocyte apoptosis with the release of cytokines and stimulation of the immune system causing skin injury and possible systemic flares.[14] Viruses may trigger SLE and the Epstein–Barr virus has been implicated.[10] Other implicated triggers include other infections; air pollution; medications; silica and asbestos; heavy metals such as uranium, cadmium, and lead; and polycyclic aromatic hydrocarbons used to make dyes, plastics, and pesticides.[14-16]

The higher prevalence in women suggests that hormones such as estrogens and progesterones play a role in SLE, but the presence of the X chromosome may also contribute. The TLR7 gene on the X chromosome increases susceptibility to autoimmune disease. The incidence of SLE is increased 14-fold in men with Klinefelter (XXY) syndrome and 2.5-fold in women with XXX syndrome, and decreased in women with Turner (XO) syndrome as compared to normal subjects.[17]

PATHOPHYSIOLOGY

3 Systemic lupus erythematosus is a multisystem disease characterized by disorders of the innate and adaptive immune systems (Fig. 107-1). T- and B-lymphocyte activation and signaling are altered in SLE and there is abnormal clearance of apoptotic debris containing nuclear material which can stimulate immune responses.[10] The number of plasma cells is increased in active SLE and these cells produce autoantibodies, which can cause tissue damage. Neutrophil dysfunction can increase the risk of infection.[18] Antibodies directed at dsDNA are seen in about 60% to 70% of patients with SLE and less than 0.5% of patients without the disease.[10] The titers of anti-dsDNA may fluctuate with disease activity and may predict disease flare. Some autoantibodies may play a role in the pathogenesis of clinical features of SLE; these autoantibodies may target Ro/SSA (antigen Ro/Sjögren syndrome A, ribonucleoprotein complex), La/SSB (antigen La/Sjögren syndrome antigen B, RNA-binding protein), C1q (subunit of the C1 complement component), Sm (nuclear particles), *N*-methyl-D-aspartate (NMDA) receptor (amino acid released by neurons), phospholipids, nucleosomes (from apoptotic cellular debris), and histones (protein core of nucleosomes). The autoantibodies can be present for many years before SLE is clinically apparent and they may be associated with specific organ involvement, such as anti-dsDNA, anti-Ro, anti-La, anti-C1q, and anti-Sm with lupus nephritis, and anti-NMDA associated with central nervous system (CNS) lupus.[10]

The exact mechanism of autoantibody tissue destruction is unclear. Immune complexes form when autoantibodies bind to nuclear material and deposit in tissues.[10] They activate the complement cascade, leading to an influx of inflammatory cells and tissue injury.[18] Autoantibodies might also directly react with proteins in tissues. Antibodies to blood cells can cause cytopenias.[10] Antibodies against phospholipids can lead to thrombosis and fetal loss.[19]

T-cell abnormalities contribute to the immune disorders observed in SLE. There are increased T helper cells type 2 and 17 and diminished number and function of T regulatory (Treg) cells. Cytokines, such as tumor necrosis factor-alpha (TNF-α), interferon-gamma, and interleukin-10, produced by activated T-cells can stimulate B-cells.[10]

Cytokines play multiple roles in SLE and contribute to inflammation and tissue damage. Interleukin-10 stimulates B-cell proliferation and autoantibody production in renal cells and may affect skin and joint symptoms.[10] Increased T-cell production of interleukin-17 correlates with disease activity and may contribute to kidney and other tissue damage.[10,18] Interleukin-2 is decreased, which is important for Treg function and restriction of interleukin-17.[18] Plasmacytoid dendritic cells secrete type I interferon, which has a role in the pathogenesis of SLE and may correlate with disease severity. High concentrations of type I interferon are associated with mucocutaneous inflammation and high interferon-γ with nephritis and arthritis.[20] B-lymphocyte stimulator (BLyS), also known as B-cell activating factor of the TNF family (BAFF), increases survival and promotes differentiation of B-cells.[21] Interleukin-6 promotes production of antibodies and may play a role in lupus nephritis.[10] The role of TNF-α in SLE is unclear. It is harmful in some patients and protective in others.[10]

CLINICAL PRESENTATION

4 Systemic lupus erythematosus is an autoimmune disease that can involve almost any organ and may present in different ways. This can make it difficult to establish a diagnosis and an extensive workup may be needed to determine the full extent of involvement and to exclude other possible etiologies for the manifestations. Fatigue is common, but does not help distinguish SLE from other diseases.[22] SLE should be considered for patients with arthritis, mucocutaneous features, noninfectious fever, leukopenia, hemolytic anemia, serositis, and unexplained proteinuria.[22] Arthritis is experienced by 85% of patients with SLE.[13] SLE may present differently in men and women. In a Swedish study, men were found to have more severe disease with

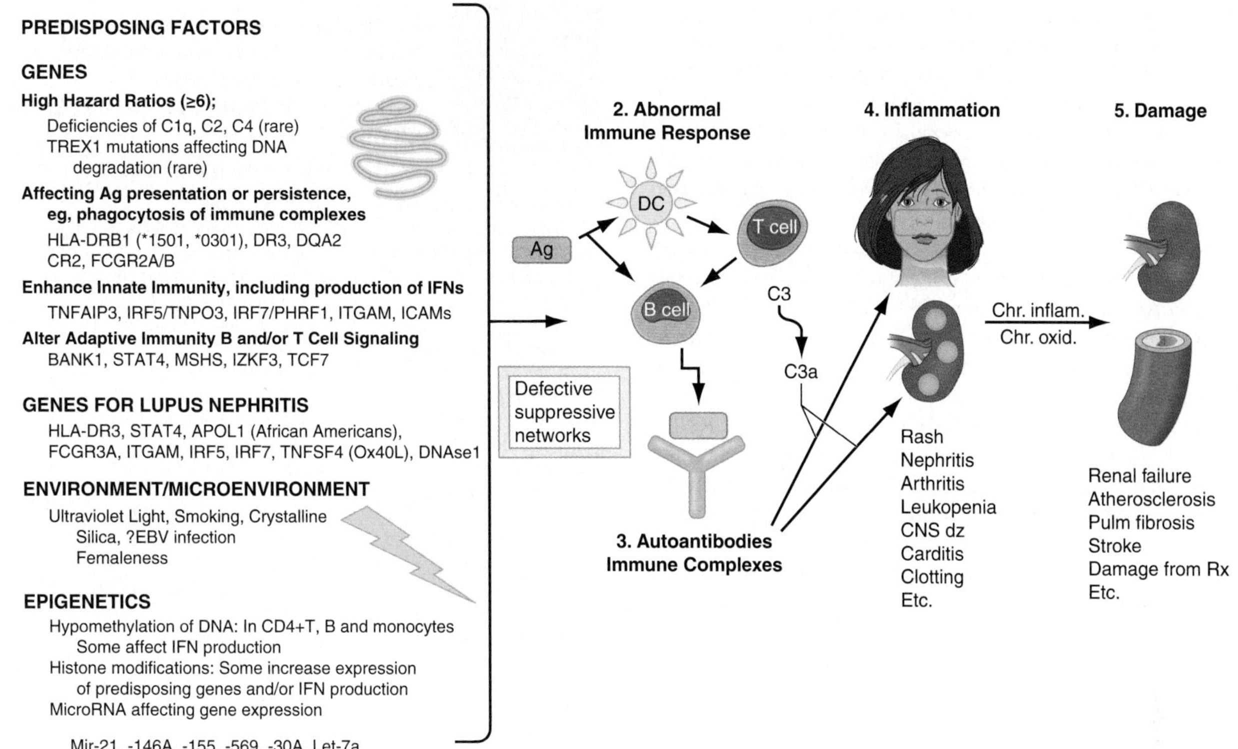

FIGURE 107-1 Pathogenesis of systemic lupus erythematosus (SLE). Pathogenesis is related in large part to the production of increased quantities and immunogenic forms of nucleic acids and other self-antigens, which drive autoimmune-inducing activation of innate immunity, autoantibodies, and T-cells. Interactions between genes, environment, and epigenetic changes drive increased autophagy, Ag presentation, neutrophil NETosis, autoantibody formation with increased plasma cells, and production of pathogenic effector T-cells in Th1, Th17, and Tfh subsets, with ineffective regulatory networks. (Ag, antigen; C1q, complement system; C2, C3, C4, complement components; CNS, central nervous system; DC, dendritic cell; EBV, Epstein-Barr virus; HLA, human leukocyte antigen; IFN, interferon UV, ultraviolet.) *(Reproduced, with permission, from Loscalzo J, Fauci A, Kasper D, Hauser S, Longo D, Jameson J. Harrison's Principles of Internal Medicine 21e; 2022. New York, NY: McGraw Hill; 2019.)*

CLINICAL PRESENTATION Systemic Lupus Erythematosus

Symptoms

- Fatigue, depression, anxiety, photosensitivity, joint pain, headache, weight loss, nausea/abdominal pain

Signs

- Rash, alopecia, fever, oral and nasal ulcers, arthritis, renal dysfunction, seizure, psychosis, pleuritis, pleural effusion, cardiovascular disease, pericarditis/myocarditis, heart murmur, hypertension, anemia, leukopenia, thrombocytopenia, lymphadenopathy, Raynaud's phenomenon, vasculitis

Diagnostic Tests

- Serology: autoantibodies, antiphospholipid antibodies, complement; inflammatory markers: C-reactive protein, erythrocyte sedimentation rate; blood chemistries; complete blood count; urinalysis; lumbar puncture; renal biopsy

increased propensity for renal disorders and serositis. Skin manifestations were more common in women.[23] Race and ethnicity may also affect the specific manifestations and severity.[13]

Disease manifestations fluctuate with 70% of patients experiencing a relapsing-remitting course.[13] The presence of ANA may be used as a screening test for SLE. Most patients with SLE have these antibodies, but they are not specific for the disease.[24]

An international group of SLE researchers developed and validated criteria for classification of SLE in 2012. These are called the Systemic Lupus International Collaborating Clinics (SLICC) classification criteria and were developed to identify patients with the disease for clinical studies. *They are not intended to establish a diagnosis in an individual patient* but may help assess the likelihood that a patient has SLE. The widely used American College of Rheumatology (ACR) criteria were developed in 1982 and revised in 1997. The 1997 version was not validated. The SLICC criteria are more clinically relevant and sensitive than the 1997 ACR criteria. When validated, the SLICC criteria had a sensitivity of 97% and specificity of 84% compared to 83% and 93% for the 1997 ACR criteria.[24,25] The number of criteria was expanded from 11 to 17 and, unlike the 1997 ACR criteria, they are divided into clinical and immunologic parameters. The 1997 ACR criteria required 4 of the 11 elements to be present, serially or simultaneously. To satisfy the SLICC criteria, a patient must still meet at least four of the elements, but now these must include at least one clinical and one immunologic criterion or the patient must have biopsy-proven lupus nephritis with positive ANA or anti-dsDNA antibodies.[25] It may be possible to classify patients earlier in their disease course as having SLE with the SLICC criteria. An updated version of the SLICC criteria added weights to the variables.[26] These have both a sensitivity and specificity of 89%, but were not considered superior to the original SLICC criteria.[26] New classification criteria that focus on early diagnosis were developed through a collaboration of the ACR and the European Alliance of Associations for Rheumatology (formerly European League Against Rheumatism) (EULAR).[24] An abbreviated version of the SLICC criteria, with comparison to the 1997 ACR and the EULAR/ACR criteria, is shown in Table 107-1. The EULAR/ACR criteria require an entry criterion of an ANA positive at a titer of at least 1:80. They include seven clinical and three immunology domains with points assigned only for the most heavily weighted element in each domain. The elements could be present on at least one occasion and must not have an alternative explanation. There must be at least one clinical criterion. A score of at least 10 is required for the classification of SLE. These have a sensitivity of 96% and a specificity of 93%. The criteria worked well in all genders, ethnicities, ages, and disease duration.[22] Some may feel that calculation of weights is more cumbersome. Ultimately, the choice of criteria depends on the study investigators and the population studied.[26]

The SELENA-SLEDAI Flare Index defines an SLE flare as "changes in the SLEDAI score and/or individual manifestations and/or changes in treatment and/or need for hospitalization and/or changes in PGA."[13] The assessor must consider the increase in disease activity to be clinically significant, sufficient to consider a change or an increase in treatment. A need to increase a prednisone dose or hospitalization for SLE is especially pertinent.[13]

Some skin involvement is seen in up to 93% of patients with SLE and is the first sign of systemic disease in up to 25% of patients.[14] Cutaneous lupus is two to three times more common than SLE.[27] This can be disfiguring and affect a patient's health-related quality of life.[28] Four main types of cutaneous lupus erythematosus have been observed. They may occur with or without SLE and one-third of patients have two or more forms of cutaneous lupus.[29] *Acute cutaneous* lupus erythematosus is typically seen in patients with SLE and is characterized by a photosensitive malar rash over the cheeks and nose with sparing of the nasolabial folds. This is commonly called a "butterfly" rash. The malar rash is present in up to 52% of patients with SLE at the time of diagnosis. There can also be a generalized form with erythematous macules and papules in a photodistributed pattern.[27] *Subacute cutaneous* lupus erythematosus is highly photosensitive and is manifested by annular or papulosquamous lesions that usually heal without scarring.[27] It can be accompanied by musculoskeletal complaints such as arthralgias and arthritis, and proteinuria.[30] About 60% to 80% of these patients are ANA positive and 70% have anti-Ro/SSA autoantibodies. It is often seen in young to middle-aged Caucasian women and is more common than other types of cutaneous lupus erythematosus in patients with drug-induced lupus. About half of patients with subacute cutaneous lupus erythematosus meet the criteria for SLE.[27] Many subtypes of *chronic* cutaneous lupus erythematosus have been identified. The most common is discoid lupus, which is confined to the head and neck in most patients, but can also affect mucosal surfaces. It carries a high risk for scarring alopecia.[27] Discoid lupus progresses to SLE in less than 5% of patients.[30] Discoid lupus is more common in African American patients with a 5.4-fold higher risk than in Caucasian patients.[14,31] Some consider *intermittent* cutaneous lupus erythematosus to be a fourth form of cutaneous lupus.[31]

Lupus nephritis is present at the time of SLE diagnosis in about 25% to 50% of adult patients and 60% of patients develop it during the disease course. It is more common in African American, Hispanic, and Asian patients than in White patients and more prevalent in men than in women. It is also more common in those with juvenile-onset SLE than those with adult-onset lupus.[32] The International Society of Nephrology/Renal Pathology Society devised a classification system for lupus nephritis based on histologic findings: Class I: minimal mesangial; Class II: mesangial proliferative; Class III: focal (less than 50% of glomeruli involved); Class IV: diffuse (50% or more of glomeruli involved); Class V: membranous; and Class VI: advanced sclerosing (at least 90% globally sclerosed glomeruli without residual activity). Patients with nephritis may also have hypertension and accelerated atherosclerosis.[32]

TABLE 107-1 2012 Systemic Lupus International Collaborating Clinics Classification Criteria for Systemic Lupus Erythematosus (SLICC) vs. 2019 EULAR/ACR Criteria for SLE

Clinical Criteria-SLICC	Clinical Domains-EULAR/ACR	Weight
1. Nonscarring alopecia	*Mucocutaneous*	
2. Oral OR nasal ulcers	Non-scarring alopecia	2
3. Chronic cutaneous lupus/ discoid rash	Oral ulcers	2
	Subacute cutaneous OR discoid lupus	4
4. Acute/subacute cutaneous lupus /malar rash[a]/photosensitive rash[a]	Acute cutaneous lupus	6
	Musculoskeletal	
5. Arthritis/synovitis or tenderness	Joint involvement	6
	Serosal	
6. Serositis (pleuritis, pericarditis)	Pleural or pericardial effusion	5
7. Renal (urine protein-to-creatinine ratio [or 24-hour urine protein] representing 500-mg protein/24 hr OR red blood cell casts)	Acute pericarditis	6
	Renal	
	Proteinuria >0.5 g/24 h	4
	Renal biopsy Class II or V nephritis	8
	Renal biopsy Class III or IV nephritis	10
8. Neurologic (seizure, psychosis, mononeuritis multiplex, myelitis, peripheral or cranial neuropathy, acute confusional state)	*Neuropsychiatric*	
	Delirium	2
	Psychosis	3
	Seizure	5
	Hematologic	
9. Leukopenia OR lymphopenia[b,c]	Leukopenia[c]	3
	Thrombocytopenia[d]	4
10. Thrombocytopenia[b,d]	Autoimmune hemolysis	4
11. Hemolytic anemia[b]	*Constitutional*	
	Fever (temperature >38.3°)	2
Immunologic Criteria	**Immunology Domains**	**Weight**
1. Antinuclear antibody (ANA)	*ANA at titer $\geq$ 1:80 required*	
	SLE-specific antibodies	
2. Anti-double-stranded DNA (dsDNA)[e]	Anti-dsDNA antibody OR Anti-Smith antibody	6
3. Anti-Sm[e]	*Antiphospholipid antibodies*	
4. Antiphospholipid antibody (lupus anticoagulant, anticardiolipin, anti-β_2-glycoprotein I, false positive rapid plasma reagin test for syphilis)[e]	Anticardiolipin antibodies OR Anti-β2GP1 antibodies OR Lupus anticoagulant	2
	Complement proteins	
	Low C3 OR low C4	3
	Low C3 AND low C4	4
5. Low complement (C3, C4, CH50)		
6. Direct Coombs test (without hemolytic anemia)		

[a]In the ACR Criteria, malar rash and photosensitivity are two separate criteria.

[b]In the ACR Criteria, hemolytic anemia, leukopenia, lymphopenia, and thrombocytopenia count as one criterion.

[c]Leukopenia is defined as <4,000 cells/mm^3 [4 × 10^9/L]; lymphopenia is <1,000 cells/mm^3 [1 × 10^9/L]

[d]Thrombocytopenia is defined as <100,000/mm^3 [100 × 10^9/L]

[e]In the ACR Criteria, anti-dsDNA, anti-Sm, and antiphospholipid antibody count as one criterion.

Data from References 24-26

The central, peripheral, and autonomic nervous systems can be involved in SLE. The prevalence of this involvement is around 56.3% with 93.1% CNS and 6.9% peripheral, but depends on the population studied and methods for detecting the involvement.[33] About 50% of neuropsychiatric events appear within the first 3 to 5 years after the onset of SLE. Events can be categorized as ischemic, involving antiphospholipid antibodies, thrombosis, and immune complexes. These are often focal. Others result from an autoimmune-mediated neuroinflammatory pathway and are more likely diffuse in their manifestations. Only about one-third of neuropsychiatric events can be attributed to SLE.[33] Mild nonspecific neuropsychiatric findings such as headache, mood disorders, anxiety, and mild cognitive dysfunction are very common in SLE and are sometimes excluded in estimating prevalence. Findings more indicative of neuropsychiatric lupus include cerebrovascular disease (ischemic stroke and/or transient ischemic attack) and seizures; severe cognitive dysfunction, acute confusional state, peripheral neuropathy, and psychosis; and less commonly chorea, movement disorders, cranial nerve neuropathies, and aseptic meningitis.[33,34] Risk factors include general SLE disease activity, prior neuropsychiatric events, and presence of antiphospholipid antibodies. It is important to assess contributing factors and to rule out other possible etiologies of these manifestations such as medication use, infection, and metabolic abnormalities. The diagnostic approach will vary depending on the clinical presentation and preliminary findings, but can include a thorough history and physical, lumbar puncture with cerebrospinal fluid analysis (mostly to exclude infection), electroencephalogram, serology, complete blood count, blood chemistries, neuropsychological assessment of cognitive function, nerve conduction studies, and magnetic resonance imaging. An attribution algorithm to determine the likelihood of neuropsychiatric SLE was developed by a study group of the Italian Society of Rheumatology. It scores on timing with respect to SLE onset, nonspecific events, confounding factors, and favoring factors.[34]

Cardiovascular disease is a leading cause of death in patients with SLE.[3] Patients with SLE can not only present with pericarditis, myocarditis, and pulmonary arterial hypertension, but they are also at increased risk for accelerated atherosclerosis.[13,32] This is probably related to the chronic inflammation associated with the disease and adverse drug reactions to the drugs (eg, high-dose corticosteroids) used to treat it. Antiphospholipid antibodies and type I interferons may play a role in the pathogenesis.

Hematologic manifestations are often associated with SLE. Autoimmune cytopenias such as thrombocytopenia, leukopenia, and hemolytic anemia may be observed.[13]

TREATMENT

Desired Outcomes

The goal of therapy should be identified. Ideally, the goal should be remission, but complete remission with the absence of clinical activity and no use of glucocorticoids or immunosuppressive therapy is rare. Achieving low disease activity based on assessment scores with use of antimalarials, prednisone doses no more than 7.5 mg, and well-tolerated immunosuppressive drugs can halt damage and prevent flares.[35] Patients should be involved in treatment decisions, taking into account their preferences, priorities, and pregnancy plans. Therapy should be designed to prevent disease flares and involvement of other organs, decrease disease activity and prevent damage, achieve and maintain remission, reduce use of corticosteroids, and improve quality of life, while minimizing adverse drug reactions and costs. Success in achieving these outcomes depends on disease severity and the type and extent of organ impairment. In general, the prognosis is better if lupus is limited to skin and musculoskeletal findings. The worst prognosis is seen with renal or CNS involvement.[32,33] Hydroxychloroquine is recommended for all patients with SLE and is the cornerstone of therapy.[35] Survival and quality of life have improved with a better understanding of disease mechanisms and new therapeutic options. Mortality is affected by SLE disease activity, cardiovascular risks, and infections.

General Approach

Patients with SLE should be counseled about the importance of lifestyle modifications such as protection from the sun, smoking cessation, exercise, and weight control. The need for immunizations should be assessed with consideration of appropriate timing with respect to immunosuppressive drug use. The effects of disease activity and treatment on pregnancy outcomes should be discussed. Patients should be evaluated and treated for comorbidities such as hypertension, hyperlipidemia, and depression.

Treatment of SLE depends on the patient's symptoms, organ involvement, comorbidities, and other patient-specific factors. Mild symptoms can be managed with nonsteroidal anti-inflammatory drugs (NSAIDs) with or without other analgesics.[36] Antimalarial drugs have numerous beneficial effects in SLE and many experts feel that most patients with the disease should always receive one of these drugs.[35] Corticosteroids are used to treat most forms of SLE and up to 57% to 86% of patients receive continuous/chronic therapy.[37] The need for osteoporosis prevention should be assessed.[38] If the above therapy is ineffective or major organs are involved, immunosuppressive or immunomodulatory drugs are added.[36] The specific treatment is determined by the organs involved and severity of the disease (Fig. 107-2).[39] Belimumab for lupus nephritis, anifrolumab, and voclosporin are approved drugs that have not been incorporated into guidelines other than by class. Patients must be educated about the importance of adherence to treatment. Only 25% to 57% of patients with SLE are adherent to their medications and up to 33% discontinue therapy after 5 years.[40] The expected time for response to lupus medications also needs to be discussed because patients may interpret delayed onset as ineffectiveness.

Nonpharmacologic Therapy

5 Patient perceptions of well-being and quality of life are affected not only by disease activity, but also by social support, coping mechanisms, feelings of helplessness, and abnormal illness-related behaviors.[36] Good social support can improve outcomes, in part by making it easier for patients and their families to navigate the healthcare system and utilize resources.[41] Counseling and support groups may help patients' mental well-being and coping mechanisms, but do not affect SLE disease activity. Aerobic exercise may help decrease patients' risk for cardiovascular events and osteoporosis and may also improve fatigue, depression, anxiety, and sleep disturbances, which are frequently experienced in SLE.[42] Exercise can also help with weight loss. Obesity is associated with worse patient-reported outcomes including quality of life and disease activity.[43]

Since photosensitivity is common in SLE, patients should wear protective clothing and broad-brim hats and use sunscreens with UV-A and UV-B filters to protect themselves from the sun.[30] Since there is systemic absorption of sunscreen ingredients, the FDA recommends use of barrier sunscreens that contain zinc oxide or titanium dioxide as being safer.[44] Sunscreens should be applied in sufficient quantity (about 2 mg/cm^3) 20 to 30 minutes before sun exposure. People with SLE should avoid tanning salons.[30]

Patients should be counseled to stop smoking. Smoking cessation is important, not only because it decreases cardiovascular risk, but because smoking can exacerbate SLE and diminish the effectiveness of antimalarials and belimumab.[12] Smoking damages the skin, resulting in increased cutaneous lupus disease activity and worse quality of life.[14]

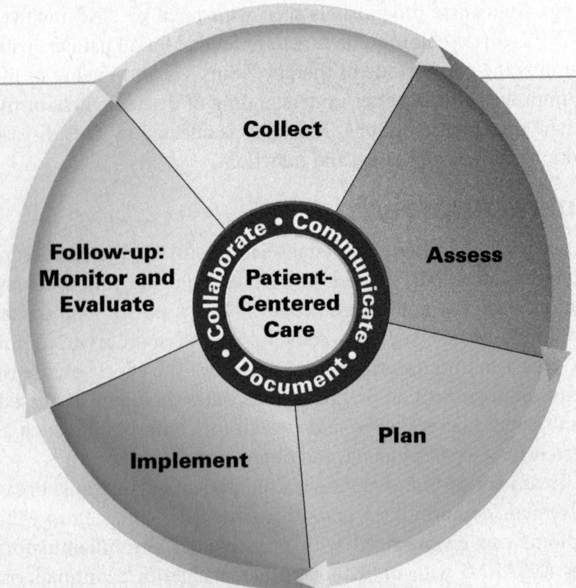

Patient Care Process for Systemic Lupus Erythematosus

The illustration shows that patient-centered care includes collaboration, communication, and documentation. The actions associated with the care are collect, assess, plan, implement, and follow-up by monitoring and evaluating.

Collect

- Patient characteristics (eg, age, race, sex, pregnancy status)
- Patient history (past medical, pregnancies and outcomes, symptoms, family, social—dietary habits, alcohol, and tobacco use)
- Current medications and prior lupus medication use
- Immunization history
- Objective data (see Clinical Presentation box and Table 107-1)
  - BP, heart rate, height, weight, and BMI; other physical examination findings
  - Labs (metabolic panel, Scr, BUN, urinalysis, CBC, ANA, antiphospholipid antibodies, direct Coombs test, other lupus-associated antibodies, complement, inflammatory markers [ESR, CRP])
  - Other diagnostic tests when indicated (eg, ECG, CXR, skin, or kidney biopsy)

Assess

- Presence of cutaneous, renal, neurologic, hematologic, cardiac, or pleural manifestations of lupus
- Evidence of antiphospholipid syndrome (thromboembolic events, miscarriages)
- Current medications that could be associated with drug-induced lupus
- Appropriateness and effectiveness of current lupus regimen (see Figs. 107-2 and 107-3)
- Psychological effects of lupus

Plan*

- Tailored lifestyle modifications (eg, diet, exercise, weight management, protection from sun, smoking cessation, keeping warm if Raynaud's phenomenon occurs)
- Drug therapy regimen including specific medications based on disease manifestations, dose, route, frequency, and duration; specify the continuation and discontinuation of existing therapies (see Figs. 107-2 and 107-3 and Tables 107-2 and 107-3)
- Monitoring parameters including efficacy (eg, skin manifestations, cardiovascular events, thromboembolic events, miscarriages, kidney health, neurologic events), safety (medication-specific adverse drug reactions), and time frame
- Patient education (eg, purpose of treatment, dietary and lifestyle modifications, drug therapy, pregnancy considerations, osteoporosis prevention if taking corticosteroids)
- Self-monitoring of skin and BP—where and how to record results
- Immunizations as needed; consider timing of live vaccines with respect to immunosuppressive drug use and pregnancy
- Referrals to other providers when appropriate (eg, physician, dietician, counselor)

Implement

- Provide patient education regarding all elements of treatment plan
- Use motivational interviewing and coaching strategies to maximize adherence
- Schedule follow-up

Follow-up: Monitor and Evaluate

- Determine goal attainment based on disease manifestations
- Presence of adverse drug reactions
- Occurrence of cardiovascular events, infections, and development/progression of kidney or other organ impairment
- Patient adherence to treatment plan using multiple sources of information

**Collaborate with patient, caregivers, and other healthcare professionals.*

Pharmacologic Therapy

6 Treatment is personalized based on the manifestations of SLE in the patient. It consists of a combination of immunosuppression and symptomatic and supportive therapies. The only drugs approved by the FDA for treatment of SLE are aspirin, prednisone, hydroxychloroquine, belimumab, anifrolumab, and voclosporin. The use of other drugs for SLE, even those considered "standard of care," is considered "off-label" use. For many of these drugs, the optimal doses and duration of therapy for induction and maintenance of response in SLE have not been determined. Ideally, drugs should be safe, effective, and affordable.[45]

Organization or expert task force treatment recommendations have been published for lupus nephritis, neuropsychiatric lupus,

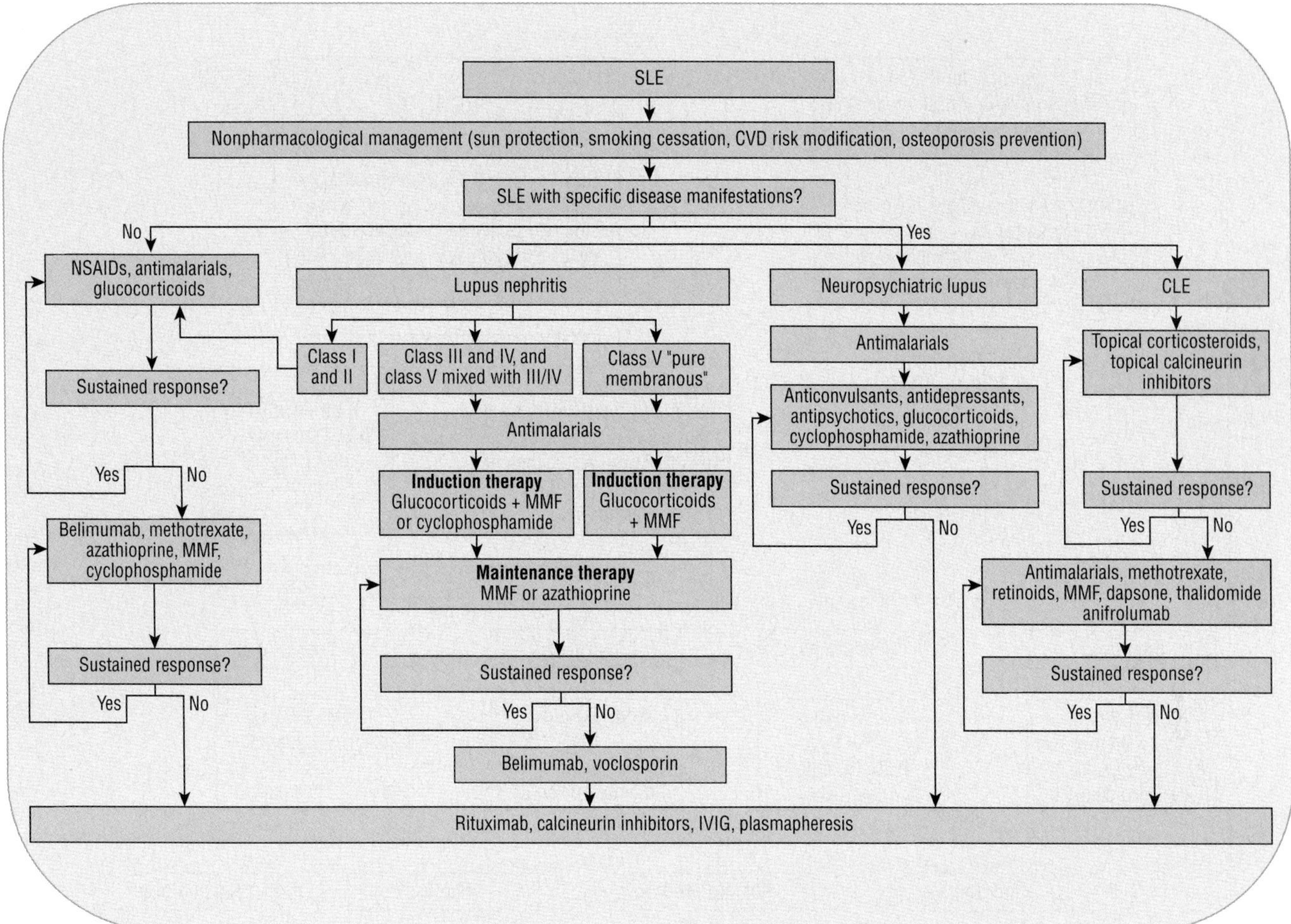

FIGURE 107-2 Algorithm for the treatment of SLE. (CLE, cutaneous lupus erythematosus; CVD, cardiovascular disease; IVIG, intravenous immunoglobulin; MMF, mycophenolate mofetil; SLE, systemic lupus erythematosus.) *(Reprinted, with permission, from Xiong W, Lahita RG. Pragmatic approaches to therapy for systemic lupus erythematosus. Review. Nat Rev Rheumatol. 2014;10(2):97–107.)*

and antiphospholipid antibody carriers.[6,19,46,47] An ACR committee developed guidelines for screening, treatment, and management of lupus nephritis.[6] All patients with nephritis should receive hydroxychloroquine to reduce damage and flares. An angiotensin-converting enzyme inhibitor or angiotensin receptor blocker can reduce proteinuria by about 30% in those with proteinuria of 0.5 g/day or more and delay progression of renal disease. Blood pressure should be maintained at no more than 130/80 mm Hg. Patients with low-density lipoprotein cholesterol greater than 100 mg/dL (2.59 mmol/L) should receive a statin to prevent accelerated atherosclerosis. More specific treatment is based on the type of nephritis. The first two classes, minimal mesangial and mesangial proliferative lupus nephritis, do not usually need immunosuppressive therapy. Focal and diffuse lupus nephritis (Classes III and IV) are treated similarly with aggressive use of glucocorticoids and immunosuppressive therapy. Figure 107-3 shows the induction regimens for these patients and the levels of evidence to support the recommendations. White patients with Western or Southern European backgrounds respond as well to low-dose IV cyclophosphamide ("Euro-Lupus" regimen of 500 mg every 2 weeks for six doses) as to high-dose regimens (500-1,000 mg/m^2 body surface area once a month for six doses) (Level B evidence). African American and Hispanic patients respond less well to IV cyclophosphamide than do White or Asian patients. Those of African or Hispanic origin may respond better to mycophenolate mofetil than to cyclophosphamide.[32] Asian patients require lower doses of mycophenolate mofetil (Level C evidence).[6] Patients with a combination of Class V with III or IV would be treated similar to those with only III or IV. The initial cyclophosphamide or mycophenolate mofetil therapy should be continued for 6 months unless proteinuria or serum creatinine worsens by 50% or more at 3 months (Level A evidence). After 6 months of induction therapy, patients who have improved can be maintained on mycophenolate mofetil or azathioprine, with low doses of corticosteroids if needed. Patients with pure Class V, membranous lupus nephritis, and nephrotic range proteinuria of more than 3 g/day should receive induction therapy with mycophenolate mofetil 2 to 3 g/day with prednisone 0.5 mg/kg/day for 6 months (Level A evidence). Those who improve can be maintained on mycophenolate mofetil 1 to 2 g/day or azathioprine 2 mg/kg/day. Patients who do not respond should be treated with cyclophosphamide 500 to 1,000 mg/m^2/month for 6 months with IV pulse glucocorticoids, followed by prednisone 0.5 to 1 mg/kg/day.[6] Maintenance therapy should be continued for at least 3 to 5 years in complete renal remission and some experts recommend not less than 6 years since the risk of flares decreases after that. Tapering of therapy should start with glucocorticoids, followed by immunosuppressives.[47] Patients with advanced sclerosing lupus nephritis (Class VI) should be considered for renal replacement therapy.[6] EULAR/European Renal Association-European Dialysis and Transplant Association updated their guidelines for management of lupus nephritis in 2019.[47] They recommend a renal biopsy for any patient with SLE and evidence of kidney involvement such as persistent proteinuria of 0.5 g/24 hr or more or a urine protein to creatinine ratio of at least 500 mg/g in morning first void urine (Level 2b, Grade B). The overall recommendations are similar to those of the ACR with some key differences. They recommend the higher initial dose of cyclophosphamide only for patients at high risk for kidney failure. They suggest the addition of a calcineurin inhibitor (especially tacrolimus) to mycophenolate

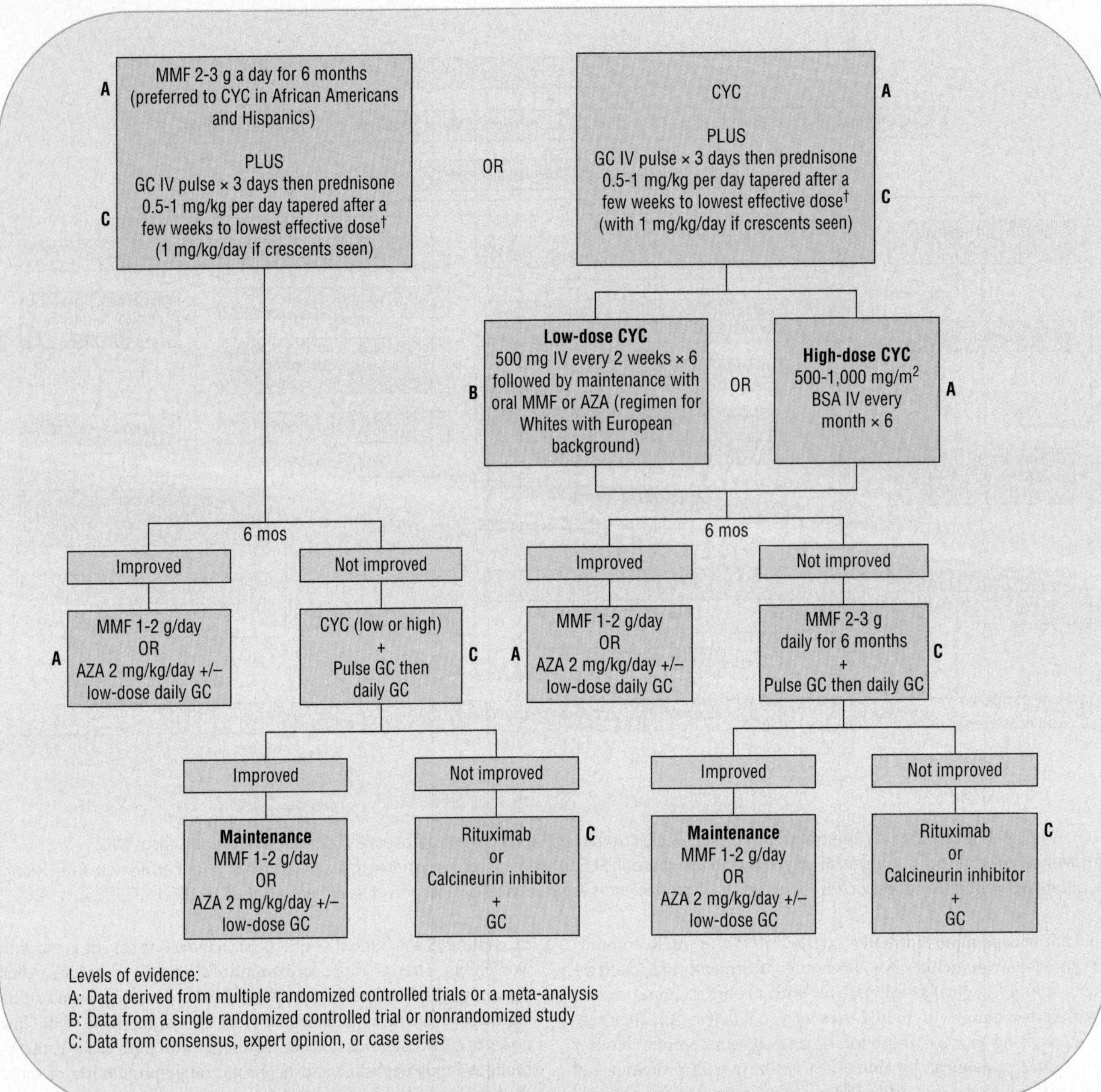

FIGURE 107-3 American College of Rheumatology guidelines for therapy for Class III/IV lupus nephritis. (AZA, azathioprine; BSA, body surface area; GC, glucocorticoids; MMF, mycophenolate mofetil.) *Preference of MMF over cyclophosphamide (CYC) in patients who desire to preserve fertility. †Recommended background therapies discussed in text. *(Reprinted, with permission, from Hahn BH, McMahon MA, Wilkinson A, et al. American College of Rheumatology guidelines for screening, treatment, and management of lupus nephritis. Arthritis Care Res (Hoboken). 2012;64(6):797–808.)*

mofetil as alternative initial therapy, especially for patients with nephrotic range proteinuria or the calcineurin inhibitor as monotherapy for pure Class V nephritis. Another difference is after intravenous pulse doses of methylprednisolone (total dose 500-2,500 mg), oral prednisone should be started at a dose of 0.3 to 0.5 mg/kg/day for up to 4 weeks, then tapered to a dose of 7.5 mg/day or less by 3 to 6 months (Level 2b/C). For pure Class V, the prednisone should be started at 20 mg/day and tapered to 5 mg/day or less by 3 months (Level 2b/C).[47] Since proteinuria at 12 months is a good predictor of risk for end-stage renal disease, a goal of therapy is at least a 50% decrease in proteinuria at 6 months with less than 0.5 to 0.7 g/24 hr by 12 months. It may take longer to reach this goal if the patient initially has nephrotic-range proteinuria.[47] They noted the promising results of trials adding belimumab, voclosporin, rituximab, or obinutuzumab to standard-of-care therapy for lupus nephritis.

A task force of the European League Against Rheumatism (EULAR) developed recommendations for the management of neuropsychiatric lupus. Treatment depends on the manifestations. Symptomatic therapy (eg, anticonvulsants and antidepressants) should be given as needed. More specific treatment depends on whether the problem is determined to be inflammatory or thrombotic or both. If there is inflammation or neurotoxic damage in the presence of generalized SLE activity, glucocorticoids alone or in conjunction with immunosuppressive drugs such as azathioprine or cyclophosphamide should be given (Strong evidence). If the condition does not respond, other treatments such as plasma exchange, IV immunoglobulin, or rituximab can be tried. If the problem is related to moderate-to-high titers of antiphospholipid antibodies and/or thrombosis, anticoagulants and/or inhibitors of platelet aggregation should be used (Sufficient evidence).[46] Recommendations have not significantly changed over the years. Antimalarials may decrease the risk for seizures and brain atrophy through their anti-inflammatory and antithrombotic effects. Results of clinical trials of rituximab, belimumab, anifrolumab, and mycophenolate mofetil have been promising.[33]

Arthralgias and arthritis are common in SLE.[48] Patients often have prolonged morning stiffness and mild-to-moderate joint swelling. Treatment can include low-dose glucocorticoids and antimalarials. If these are inadequate, methotrexate can be added.[48] NSAIDs should be avoided or used with great caution because of their adverse renal effects.[47] For refractory cases, other disease-modifying antirheumatic drugs such as leflunomide, azathioprine, mycophenolate mofetil, or tacrolimus may be tried.[49] Although there is concern about drug-induced lupus with TNF-α inhibitors, successful use of etanercept for resistant lupus arthritis has been reported.[49]

The first step in the management of cutaneous lupus erythematosus is counseling patients to protect themselves from ultraviolet light and stop smoking as described above.[14] Drug treatment is personalized based on the extent and severity of involvement. Recent guidelines from EULAR, the European Dermatology Forum/European Academy of Dermatology and Venereology, and S2k recommend topical therapy as first-line treatment for cutaneous lupus.[35,50] Topical corticosteroids are commonly used, but may not provide adequate clearing of lesions when used alone.[44] The choice of corticosteroid depends on the location of application. Low-potency corticosteroids (eg, fluocinolone acetonide 0.01% and hydrocortisone acetate 1%) should be used on areas with thin skin such as the face and groin, mid-potency (eg, triamcinolone acetonide, and hydrocortisone valerate or butyrate) for trunk and extremities, and high potency (eg, clobetasol propionate and betamethasone dipropionate) for thick-skin areas such as scalp, soles, and palms. Creams or, for more severe disease, ointments, are used on the body, and foams or solutions on the scalp.[44] Intralesional triamcinolone acetonide may be considered, but should not be repeated more often than every 4 to 6 weeks.[50] To avoid the adverse drug reactions of topical corticosteroids, such as skin atrophy, telangiectasias, and steroid-induced dermatitis, the lowest effective potency and duration of therapy should be used. A common recommendation is to use topical corticosteroids for 2 weeks (not more than a few), then only on weekends for maintenance.[44] Alternatively or in addition, topical calcineurin inhibitors such as pimecrolimus or tacrolimus may be used. Other topical products that have been tried are R-salbutamol, Janus kinase inhibitors, clindamycin, and retinoids.[44] Antimalarials have photoprotective effects and are commonly used as first-line systemic therapy in the management of severe or disseminated cutaneous lupus.[50] If hydroxychloroquine alone is ineffective, quinacrine (mepacrine), if available from compounding pharmacies, may be added.[44] For refractory disease, other systemic drugs such as corticosteroids, methotrexate, mycophenolate mofetil, azathioprine, dapsone, thalidomide, lenalidomide, baricitinib, oral retinoids, or biologics (eg, rituximab, belimumab, or anifrolumab) may be added.[44] Patients should be screened for glucose-6-phosphate dehydrogenase (G6PD) deficiency before getting dapsone.[50] Vitamin D should also be considered. It has some immunomodulating effects and patients with cutaneous lupus may be vitamin D deficient because of their sun avoidance.[50] More studies are needed to support the use of these drugs in patients with cutaneous lupus. The choice of agents may be guided by other organ involvement.

Dosing information for selected drugs is given in Table 107-2. Since most of the drugs used to treat SLE are not FDA-approved for

TABLE 107-2 Dosing of Drugs Used to Treat Systemic Lupus Erythematosus

Drug	Brand Name	Initial or Starting Dose	Usual Range or Maintenance Dose	Special Population Doses	Comments (adverse drug reactions, special populations)
NSAIDs/salicylates	Various drugs				Caution in patients with renal insufficiency, cardiovascular disease, gastrointestinal problems
Glucocorticoids	Deltasone (prednisone), Medrol (prednisolone)	0.3-1 mg/kg/day PO	Prefer ≤5-10 mg/day PO		Dose depends on organ involvement and severity; initial dose may be given for 4-6 weeks, then tapered for maintenance; no standard dose
	Solu-Medrol (methylprednisolone)	100-1,000 mg IV daily × 3			Severe disease; later, dose tapered and changed to PO
Hydroxychloroquine	Plaquenil	400 mg PO daily or 200 mg twice daily	200-400 mg PO daily	Dosing adjustment may be needed with renal or hepatic dysfunction	Dose should not exceed 5 mg/kg/day actual weight to minimize retinopathy risk
Belimumab	Benlysta	10 mg/kg IV every 2 weeks × 3 or SLE: 200 mg SC weekly Lupus nephritis: 400 mg SC weekly × 4	10 mg/kg IV every 4 weeks or 200 mg SC weekly	No adjustment for hepatic impairment; no adjustment for renal impairment if CrCl ≥15 mL/min (0.25 mL/s); no studies in pregnant or breastfeeding women	IV infusion over 1 hour; consider premedication to prevent infusion and hypersensitivity reactions; observe for infusion reaction after first two infusions ; if switching from IV to SC for SLE, give first SC dose 1-4 weeks after last IV dose; if for nephritis, switch 1-2 weeks after last IV dose

(continued)

TABLE 107-2 Dosing of Drugs Used to Treat Systemic Lupus Erythematosus (*Continued*)

Drug	Brand Name	Initial or Starting Dose	Usual Range or Maintenance Dose	Special Population Doses	Comments (adverse drug reactions, special populations)
Voclosporin	Lupkynis	23.7 mg PO every 12 hours	23.7 mg PO every 12 hours	Dose adjustment for renal or hepatic impairment	Do not use if baseline BP >165/105 mm Hg or baseline eGFR ≤45 mL/min/1.73 m^2
Anifrolumab-fnia	Saphnelo	300 mg IV every 4 weeks	300 mg IV every 4 weeks		IV infusion over 30 minutes; risk of hypersensitivity and infusion reactions
Cyclophosphamide	Cytoxan	500-1,000 mg/m^2 BSA IV every month × 6 or 500 mg IV every 2 weeks × 6		Dosing adjustment might be needed with renal dysfunction; low and high doses may have equivalent efficacy in White patients with European background	Infertility in women and men, teratogenicity of concern
Mycophenolate mofetil	Cellcept	2-3 g/day PO divided into 2-3 doses for 6 months	0.5-3 g/day PO	Lower doses may be needed in Asian patients (1.5-2 g/day) than non-Asian patients; may be more effective than cyclophosphamide in Black and Hispanic patients	Contraindicated in pregnancy
	Myfortic (enteric coated mycophenolate sodium)	720 mg PO twice daily	360 mg PO twice daily		
Azathioprine	Imuran	2 mg/kg/day PO	1.5-2 mg/kg/day PO	Pregnant patients ≤2 mg/kg/day	Lower dose if thiopurine methyltransferase (TPMT) deficient
Methotrexate	Trexall, Otrexup, Rasuvo, RediTrex, Xatmep	5-15 mg PO or SC weekly	15-25 mg PO or SC weekly		Decrease toxicity by giving with folic acid Avoid use in elderly or if GFR <30 mL/min (0.5 mL/s)
Rituximab	Rituxan	375 mg/m^2 BSA IV weekly × 4 or 500-1,000 mg IV on days 1 and 15		Variable doses have been used	Alternative for patients refractory to other treatments; may be more effective in Black patients

BSA, body surface area; CrCl, creatinine clearance; IV, intravenously; NSAIDs, nonsteroidal anti-inflammatory drugs; PO, orally.

that indication, the doses given are based on other uses for those drugs. Table 107-3 lists adverse drug reactions and drug monitoring parameters. Selected issues concerning the drugs are discussed below.

Nonsteroidal Anti-inflammatory Drugs

Nonsteroidal anti-inflammatory drugs (NSAIDs) are used as first-line treatment for arthritis, musculoskeletal complaints, fever, and serositis.[39] They are not disease-modifying, but are used to relieve symptoms.[51] Low-dose aspirin is used in patients with antiphospholipid antibodies.[19] One concern with NSAIDs is that they can decrease renal function which can complicate evaluation of lupus nephritis. They have the potential to increase cardiac events in patients who already are at elevated risk. Other adverse drug reactions include hepatotoxicity, gastrointestinal (GI) bleeding, and aseptic meningitis.[39]

Corticosteroids

Corticosteroids, as monotherapy or as adjuncts to other treatments, can control flares and maintain low disease activity in SLE. Their effects have a rapid onset, whereas other therapies may take months or over a year to achieve their maximum benefits. The corticosteroids can be used topically or systemically.

Although corticosteroids have been used to manage SLE since the 1950s, optimal doses, duration of therapy, and tapering regimens have not been determined. High doses given in a pulse IV administration regimen are generally free of serious adverse drug reactions and rapidly produce strong immunomodulatory effects. They are used to treat flares and quickly reduce inflammation. Doses should slowly be tapered down to the lowest effective dose.[52] Corticosteroids are the foundation for treatment of most forms of SLE, but high-dose oral corticosteroid use is associated with increased lupus organ damage accrual, infection, and death. Oral maintenance doses should be kept as low as possible with pulse methylprednisolone doses used for disease flares and in combination with other drugs that are steroid-sparing.[52]

Common adverse drug reactions to low (prednisone less than 7.5 mg/day)-to-moderate (7.5-30 mg/day) doses are shown in Table 107-3. Although higher doses may be divided, single morning doses may be associated with fewer adverse drug reactions and less adrenal suppression. Chronic use of any dose is associated with cardiovascular complications, psychological disturbances, glaucoma, cataracts, hyperglycemia, weight gain, avascular necrosis of bone, and osteoporosis.[37] Corticosteroids decrease absorption of vitamin D and increase catabolism of 25(OH) vitamin D and 1,25$(OH)_2$ vitamin D. According to the 2017 ACR guideline for the prevention and treatment of glucocorticoid-induced osteoporosis, all patients taking prednisone at a dose of 2.5 mg daily or more for at least 3 months should optimize calcium and vitamin D intake in addition to lifestyle changes such as balanced diet, maintenance of recommended

TABLE 107-3 Monitoring of Drugs Used to Treat Systemic Lupus Erythematosus

Drug	Adverse Drug Reaction	Monitoring Parameter	Comments
NSAIDs/salicylates	Gastrointestinal bleeding, hepatic toxicity, renal toxicity, hypertension, cardiovascular events, aseptic meningitis	CBC[a], platelets[a], creatinine[a], urinalysis, AST/ALT[a], blood pressure[a]	Antihypertensive effects of calcium channel blockers affected less than other classes
Glucocorticoids, systemic	Osteoporosis, cataracts, glaucoma, hyperglycemia/diabetes, hypertension, dyslipidemia, thinning of the skin, weight gain, fat redistribution, sleep/mood disturbances	Blood pressure[a], serum glucose[a], lipid panel[a], bone densitometry, ophthalmic examinations	Patients should receive osteoporosis preventive therapy; high doses of systemic corticosteroids are associated with infections, myopathy, psychological disturbances, osteonecrosis, and stroke
Glucocorticoids, topical	Skin atrophy, telangiectasias, dermatitis	Skin appearance	Avoid prolonged use, especially of high-potency steroids
Hydroxychloroquine	Retinal toxicity, gastric intolerance, rash, skin hyperpigmentation	Funduscopic and automated visual field examinations, consider spectral domain optical coherence tomography, multifocal electroretinogram, or fundus autofluorescence (frequency depends on risk), CBC, AST/ALT, albumin, chemistry panel, creatinine	Risk for retinal toxicity increased with doses >5 mg/kg/day actual body weight, more than 5 years therapy, renal or macular disease, or concurrent tamoxifen use
Belimumab	Infusion reactions, hypersensitivity, nausea, diarrhea, fever, nasopharyngitis, bronchitis, insomnia, pain in extremity, depression, migraine	Monitor for serious infections, hypersensitivity/infusion reactions, worsening depression, mood changes, or suicidal thoughts	No live vaccines 30 days before or during belimumab therapy; consider premedication with antipyretic and antihistamine
Voclosporin	Infections, lymphomas, other malignancies; QT interval increase, hyperkalemia, neurotoxicity	Monitor for infections, BP, eGFR, potassium, electrocardiogram	Limit sun exposure; reduce dose if given with CYP3A4 inhibitors
Anifrolumab-fnia	Upper respiratory tract infections, nasopharyngitis, herpes zoster, anaphylaxis, angioedema	Monitor for infections	Insufficient data on use during pregnancy or lactation
Cyclophosphamide	Myelosuppression, opportunistic infections, hemorrhagic cystitis, bladder malignancy, infertility	CBC[b], platelets[b], creatinine, AST/ALT, urinalysis[b], urine cytology[a], PAP test[a]	Greater risk for cystitis with oral form than IV; decrease with hydration and mesna
Mycophenolate mofetil	Myelosuppression, nausea, vomiting, diarrhea	CBC[c], platelets[c], creatinine, chemistry panel, AST/ALT, chest x-ray	Gastrointestinal side effects may limit use and compliance; these symptoms may be less with an enteric-coated form
Azathioprine	Myelosuppression, hepatotoxicity	CBC[c,d], platelets[c,d], creatinine[e], AST/ALT[c,f], chemistry panel[e], albumin, TPMT assay, PAP test	Test thiopurine methyltransferase (TPMT) before starting; toxicity greatly increased if deficient
Methotrexate	Hepatic, hematologic, pulmonary toxicity, stomatitis	CBC[c,g], platelets[c,g], creatinine[c,g], AST/ALT[c,g], albumin[c,g], bilirubin, chemistry panel[h], alkaline phosphatase[c], chest x-ray	Check hepatitis B and C serologies before starting if at risk
Rituximab	Infusion reactions, infections, neutropenia, mucocutaneous reactions, fever, fatigue, progressive multifocal leukoencephalopathy	CBC[i], platelets[i], creatinine, vital signs, human antichimeric antibody (HACA) titers	Consider pretreatment with acetaminophen, diphenhydramine, corticosteroid to decrease infusion reactions

[a]52 weeks

[b]4 weeks

[c]12 weeks

[d]Every 1-2 weeks after dose change

Monitoring parameters should be checked at baseline and at interval noted:

[e]26 weeks

[f]Every 2 weeks after dose change

[g]2-4 weeks during 3 months after dose change

[h]8 weeks

[i]8-16 weeks

Data from References 51, 52, 68, and 98.

weight, smoking cessation, and limiting alcohol intake. Additional treatment is based on Fracture Risk Assessment Tool (FRAX) score (Conditional recommendation-limited data).[38] To avoid adrenal insufficiency, patients on chronic corticosteroid therapy should not have treatment stopped abruptly. Some clinicians will increase doses during times of stress such as surgery because of concerns regarding adrenal insufficiency and hypotension, but this can increase the risk of hyperglycemia, postoperative infections, and impaired wound healing. These supraphysiologic doses may not be necessary for minor/intermediate intensity surgeries such as joint arthroplasty in adults taking less than 20 mg/day prednisone.[53] For major surgeries, patients may be given hydrocortisone 50 mg IV intraoperatively and every 8 hours after surgery until the patient's usual oral dose can be resumed.[54] Prolonged use of topical corticosteroids can lead to atrophy of the skin and telangiectasias (small dilated blood vessels).[44]

Antimalarials

The antimalarials, such as chloroquine and hydroxychloroquine, have long been used in rheumatology practice. Hydroxychloroquine has fewer adverse reactions and is the preferred drug. In the past, hydroxychloroquine was primarily used for skin and joint manifestations of SLE, but most experts believe that all patients, including pregnant and lactating women, with SLE should receive hydroxychloroquine. There is high-quality evidence that shows it prevents lupus flares and improves long-term survival; moderate-quality evidence that it protects against bone mass loss, and has protective effects against thrombosis and irreversible organ damage.[55] It has a beneficial effect on lipids and fasting blood glucose, decreases the risk of thrombosis in patients with antiphospholipid antibodies, and decreases infections. It can allow corticosteroid doses to be decreased.[52] When given to patients with some findings consistent with SLE, it can delay the time for them to fully meet criteria for the disease. Patients receiving hydroxychloroquine often have disease flares when the drug is discontinued.[56]

Hydroxychloroquine has anti-inflammatory, immunomodulatory, and antithrombotic effects. It reduces concentrations of inflammatory cytokines such as interleukins 1, 2, 6, 17, and 22, interferon alpha and gamma, and TNF-α. It alters antigen presentation and T-cell proliferative responses. Its key activity may be decreasing activation of toll-like receptors, which are important in innate immunity and autoimmune diseases. It reduces platelet aggregation and thrombosis.[56] Finally, it may reduce cardiovascular risk factors such as hyperlipidemia and diabetes mellitus and improve survival.[52] The LUMINA (LUpus in MInorities, NAture vs nurture) multiethnic study found that hydroxychloroquine has a protective effect on survival. It may delay the development of renal damage and the occurrence of integument damage (severe skin damage including scarring, ulcers, and scarring alopecia).[55,56]

Although some studies showed reduced disease activity and flares with hydroxychloroquine whole blood concentrations over 1,000 ng/mL (μg/L; 2,980 nmol/L), other studies where doses were adjusted to achieve that concentration did not show better disease control. Studies of cutaneous lupus showed good improvement at 750 ng/mL (μg/L; 2230 nmol/L), while others considered 500 ng/mL (μg/L; 1490 nmol/L) to be the minimum therapeutic concentration. Hydroxychloroquine concentration monitoring may be used as a measure of adherence to therapy.[57] The drug is primarily eliminated by the kidneys and has a long tissue half-life of about 40 to 50 days. Low concentrations may therefore be an indicator of consistent nonadherence or abnormal metabolism.[57] It may take 2 to 8 weeks to see the therapeutic effects of hydroxychloroquine and up to 3 to 6 months for maximum clinical efficacy.[57]

Adverse drug reactions with hydroxychloroquine are usually mild. Most common are GI and skin reactions and they usually improve with dose reduction.[56] Prolongation of the QT interval on electrocardiograms is rare at the doses used for SLE.[52] The main concern is retinal toxicity, but the incidence is low and may be less than that seen with chloroquine. The cumulative risk depends on the duration of therapy and is less than 1% in patients receiving the drug at recommended doses for 5 years, less than 2% up to 10 years, and less than 5% after 20 years.[58] Major risk factors are the duration of use over 5 years, daily doses more than 5 mg/kg actual body weight, concurrent use of tamoxifen, or preexisting kidney dysfunction or macular disease. Advanced retinal damage has a characteristic bull's-eye appearance on funduscopic examination and is irreversible, but this should not be seen with appropriate monitoring. Patterns of damage are different in East Asian patients. Early recognition of damage may minimize vision loss. The current ACR/American Academy of Dermatology/American Academy of Ophthalmology 2020 monitoring recommendations are to have baseline screening tests within the first few months, including retinal examination with optical coherence tomography and automated visual fields. After 5 years, patients should begin annual examinations unless the patient is considered to be at high risk, in which case yearly testing would begin earlier. If there are suspicious findings, other tests such as multifocal electroretinogram and fundus autofluorescence should be performed. If toxicity is suspected, the drug should be discontinued or the patient counseled about risks of blindness versus disease flares.[58]

Biologic Agents

Since autoantibody formation is an important feature of SLE, B-cells are a logical target for SLE therapy. B-lymphocyte stimulator (BLyS) is a cytokine that is important for B-cell survival, maturation, and differentiation. Belimumab is a fully human IgG1-λ monoclonal antibody that binds to soluble BLyS, which prevents BLyS from binding to receptors on B-cells and promotes apoptosis of B-lymphocytes. Belimumab is FDA-approved for treatment of autoantibody-positive active SLE in addition to standard therapy. It was the first drug approved by the FDA in over 50 years for management of SLE.[21] Approval of intravenous belimumab was based on two international phase III trials: BLISS-76, conducted primarily in Europe and North America, and BLISS-52, which was carried out in Eastern Europe, South America, and the Asia-Pacific region. These trials had strict entry criteria and used the new SLE Responder Index (SRI) assessment criteria. For both studies, the primary efficacy endpoint was the SRI at 52 weeks. Entry requirements included positive ANA or anti-dsDNA, and active SLE (SELENA-SLEDAI [measure of disease activity] score of 6 or greater) while receiving standard treatment (prednisone, NSAIDs, antimalarials, and/or immunosuppressive drugs [but not IV cyclophosphamide or other biologics]). Patients had to be on stable therapy for at least 30 days. The most common organ systems involved were musculoskeletal and mucocutaneous. Patients with severe active lupus nephritis or CNS lupus were excluded. Patients received belimumab 1 mg/kg, 10 mg/kg, or placebo by IV infusion every 2 weeks for two doses, then every 4 weeks, in addition to their standard therapy. There were restrictions on concomitant medications, and those became stricter as the studies progressed. The response rate was significantly higher in the group receiving belimumab 10 mg/kg as compared to placebo in both studies. Patients receiving belimumab also had greater improvement in health-related quality of life and fatigue. Patients of African descent did not benefit from belimumab.[21] However, later studies such as the EMBRACE trial, reported favorable responses to belimumab in all racial and ethnic groups.[21,59] Open-label trials showed extended benefit to 10 years. The 52-week BLISS-SC trial showed the safety and efficacy of subcutaneously administered belimumab and patients preferred the convenience of self-administration.[21] Belimumab was approved by the FDA for treatment of lupus nephritis based on the 2-year BLISS-LN study. This international double-blind study compared belimumab to placebo added to standard therapy. Significantly more patients in the belimumab group achieved the primary efficacy renal response of urinary protein to creatinine ratio of 0.7 or less, an eGFR no worse than 20% below the pre-flare value or an eGFR of at least 60 mL/min/1.73 m^2, and no rescue therapy use.[60]

Rituximab is a chimeric monoclonal antibody directed at the CD20 antigen on B-cells.[61] Although many case reports and open-label trials have reported beneficial effects of rituximab in SLE, randomized, placebo-controlled trials of rituximab have not demonstrated efficacy in SLE. The largest of these trials was the EXPLORER (Efficacy and Safety of Rituximab in Moderately-to-Severely Active Systemic Lupus Erythematosus) trial, which evaluated patients with extrarenal involvement treated with rituximab and immunosuppressive drugs and the LUNAR (LUpus Nephritis Assessment with Rituximab) trial that examined use of rituximab with mycophenolate mofetil and corticosteroids in patients with lupus nephritis.[61] The negative trial results could be related to the short duration of the trials, overuse of corticosteroids, high background immunosuppressive regimens, or the choice of endpoints.[45] Further improvement was observed in the second year of therapy. Exploratory analyses of specific patient subgroups or different response criteria suggested some benefit. In a small study of rituximab given shortly after diagnosis, followed by mycophenolate mofetil and hydroxychloroquine, about 90% of the patients with lupus nephritis achieved a complete or partial remission without oral corticosteroids.[45] It may serve as an alternative therapy in refractory lupus nephritis, severe hematological lupus, and some CNS manifestations of the disease and is included in some guidelines.[33,45] It may also prove useful for maintenance therapy, as a steroid-sparing agent, or when preservation of fertility is desired.[61]

Other drugs targeting B-cells are being investigated in SLE. Examples of these are other anti-CD20 monoclonal antibodies such as ofatumumab, ocrelizumab, and obinutuzumab.[45] Other biologic agents have been tried in SLE with varying degrees of success, often failing in large phase III clinical trials.[45] In general, biologic drugs should not be combined. However, depletion of B-cells is associated with an increase in BAFF/BLyS and some ongoing trials use rituximab in sequence or together with belimumab to treat SLE.[45]

Anifrolumab is a fully human IgG1κ monoclonal antibody that targets type I interferons through binding the type I interferon receptor subunit 1.[51] It was studied in the MUSE, TULIP-1, and TULIP-2 trials. Patients had moderate-to-severe SLE while taking one or more standard therapies including oral corticosteroids, antimalarials, and immunosuppressives. Those with severe lupus nephritis or neuropsychiatric lupus were excluded. Most of the subjects had active skin and joint disease. After the SRI endpoint was not reached in TULIP-1, the protocol for TULIP-2 was changed to use a new endpoint—BICLA, a composite of BILAG, SLEDAI-2K, and Physician Global Assessment. Anifrolumab decreased flares and disease activity by week 8 to 12 and was steroid-sparing. Severe skin disease improved by CLASI scores. Patients with overexpression of type I interferon-regulated genes (high interferon gene signature) may respond better to anifrolumab.[51]

As discussed later, TNF-α inhibitors may induce lupus. However, good results have been observed with etanercept as long-term treatment of refractory lupus arthritis.[49]

Immunosuppressive Drugs

Cyclophosphamide has long been used to treat severe or refractory organ involvement in SLE such as lupus nephritis, neuropsychiatric lupus, vasculitis, and hematologic disease.[52] Its role in therapy is being redefined because of the availability of newer drugs, as discussed elsewhere in this chapter. Response rate and dosing requirements may vary with patient race.[52]

Cyclophosphamide is an alkylating agent that causes cross-linkage of DNA and inhibits B- and T-cell proliferation and antibody production.[48] The drug can potentially cause hemorrhagic cystitis and bladder cancer due to acrolein, a metabolite of the drug that concentrates in the bladder.[62] The risk is greater with oral administration, higher cumulative doses, and in smokers. Intermittent pulse IV doses, hydration, and frequent voiding may decrease the risk of these adverse drug reactions. With oral administration, patients are advised to take the drug in the morning and to drink fluids for several hours. Adherence is not good with this regimen. With IV administration, IV fluids are begun before administration of the cyclophosphamide and continued for several hours after. Patients are encouraged to maintain oral hydration for 72 hours. Another method to decrease bladder toxicity is to give sodium-2-mercaptoethane sulfonate (mesna), which binds acrolein and prevents its harmful effects on the bladder. Although mesna is sometimes used with high-dose cyclophosphamide, it is only FDA-approved for use with ifosfamide. Mesna used with daily oral cyclophosphamide is expensive and inconvenient based on available dosage forms. The recommended mesna regimen with IV pulse doses of cyclophosphamide is to give IV doses, each equivalent to 20% of the cyclophosphamide dose, 15 to 30 minutes before the cyclophosphamide, then 4 and 8 hours after. Since oral mesna is about 50% bioavailable, the 4- and 8-hour mesna doses after cyclophosphamide may be given orally, each in doses equivalent to 40% of the administered dose of cyclophosphamide.[62] In practice, a variety of mesna regimens are used. The effectiveness of mesna for uroprotection in patients receiving cyclophosphamide for rheumatologic diseases has been questioned.

Mycophenolic acid (MPA) reversibly inhibits the enzyme inosine 5-monophosphate dehydrogenase (IMPDH), which is important for de novo synthesis of purine (guanosine) nucleotides. This inhibits lymphocyte proliferation, chemotaxis, and antibody production. Genetic polymorphisms of the IMPDH proteins may influence the effects of MPA, but routine testing is not recommended at this time.[47] The drug also has other immunomodulating effects such as induction of activated T-cell apoptosis, inhibition of adhesion molecule expression, and fibroblast proliferation.[48]

Mycophenolate mofetil is about 94% absorbed and is hydrolyzed to MPA, its active form. MPA is bound to albumin, so unbound drug concentrations can be affected by changes in albumin. MPA is glucuronidated in the liver to an inactive metabolite, mycophenolic glucuronide. The metabolite is excreted in the urine but also undergoes enterohepatic recycling, with conversion back to the active form. Some studies have reported better lupus nephritis response with higher trough MPA concentrations or 12-hour MPA areas under the curve, but optimal values have not been determined and these did not correlate with toxicity, so measurement is not common practice.[57] Larger trials may support the benefits of individualized dosing based on therapeutic drug monitoring.[32]

Mycophenolate mofetil has been extensively studied in the treatment of lupus nephritis. It is at least as effective as cyclophosphamide for induction therapy and as effective as azathioprine for maintenance treatment.[32] The Aspreva Lupus Management Study (ALMS) was an international study of lupus nephritis. The 6-month induction phase showed mycophenolate mofetil to be equivalent in efficacy in White and Asian patients to monthly IV pulse doses of cyclophosphamide.[32] Black and Hispanic patients responded better to mycophenolate. The response to therapy at 6 months correlated with the baseline complement C4 concentration, time since diagnosis of lupus nephritis, and eGFR. Normalization of complement C3 and/or C4 and reduction in proteinuria of at least 25% at 8 weeks also predicted renal improvement at 6 months.[63] Responders at 6 months entered a 36-month maintenance phase in which mycophenolate mofetil was superior to azathioprine in maintaining renal response and preventing disease relapse. Although adverse drug reactions occurred in more than 97% of patients in both groups, more patients receiving azathioprine withdrew from the study due to adverse drug reactions than those receiving mycophenolate mofetil.[64] The MAINTAIN trial did not find a difference in the rate of renal flare with mycophenolate mofetil compared to azathioprine 5 and 10 years after induction with low-dose IV cyclophosphamide. The difference in these results compared to the ALMS trial may be related to the difference in induction therapy, selection of patients for the maintenance phase, and in populations studied. The MAINTAIN trial studied predominantly (83%) White European patients, whereas the larger ALMS trial included a more racially diverse population (56% non-Caucasian patients). The MAINTAIN trial did find a correlation between achieving a proteinuria value of less than 0.5 g/day at 12 months and good long-term renal outcome.[65]

Mycophenolate mofetil is preferred for maintenance therapy if it is used for induction.[47]

Mycophenolate mofetil may also be useful for nonrenal manifestations of SLE such as cutaneous lupus, hemolytic anemia, thrombocytopenia, vasculitis, and musculoskeletal and neuropsychiatric diseases, and can be steroid-sparing.[52]

The most common adverse drug reactions with mycophenolate mofetil are gastrointestinal complaints and infections.[52] These may be severe enough to require discontinuation of therapy. The adverse drug reactions may be managed with a reduction in dose.[48] Use of an enteric-coated form of mycophenolate sodium may decrease gastrointestinal symptoms. Hematologic effects ranging from cytopenias to red cell aplasia may also be seen. Teratogenicity has been reported with mycophenolate mofetil and it is contraindicated in pregnancy.[66]

Azathioprine is a purine analog that is metabolized to mercaptopurine. It inhibits nucleic acid synthesis and affects cellular and humoral immune functions.[39,67] Mercaptopurine is inactivated by thiopurine methyltransferase (TPMT). Patients should have TPMT testing before receiving azathioprine.[65] If the activity of that enzyme is low, patients may experience more severe toxicity. Myelosuppression and gastrointestinal adverse effects correlate with TPMT polymorphism, but hepatotoxicity may not. Other metabolic pathways are also involved in the elimination of azathioprine.[67] The metabolism of azathioprine and mercaptopurine is inhibited by allopurinol and febuxostat. If the combination of these drugs is to be used, a reduction in azathioprine dose is required.[68] Azathioprine is less effective than cyclophosphamide for induction therapy in lupus nephritis, but it can be an alternative to mycophenolate mofetil for maintenance treatment.[32] Azathioprine may also be used for SLE-related arthritis, serositis, and mucocutaneous manifestations. It has steroid-sparing effects, allowing the use of lower doses of corticosteroids.[39]

Methotrexate is an inhibitor of dihydrofolate reductase, which is needed for DNA synthesis and cell proliferation.[36] Its toxicities are reduced by folic acid administration. It is dosed once weekly in the management of SLE. It is used for musculoskeletal, skin, and serosal disease and as a steroid-sparing drug.[52]

Calcineurin is a serine-threonine phosphatase that stimulates hyperactivation of T-cells, resulting in cytokine release and costimulation of B-cells with release of autoantibodies. Calcineurin also adversely affects podocytes which are important for maintaining the glomerular filtration barrier in the kidneys. Calcineurin inhibitors decrease inflammation and proteinuria.[2] Voclosporin, a calcineurin inhibitor, was the first oral drug approved by the FDA for the treatment of active lupus nephritis. Voclosporin is an analog of cyclosporine with much higher immunosuppressive effect. Voclosporin is used in combination with mycophenolate mofetil and corticosteroids. Approval was based on the randomized double-blind AURORA 1 trial that compared voclosporin to placebo added to mycophenolate mofetil and rapidly tapered oral corticosteroids in patients with active class III to V lupus nephritis. The primary endpoint was complete renal response defined as urinary protein to creatinine ratio of 0.5 mg/mg or less, with an eGFR of at least 60 mL/min/1.73 m^2 (or no decrease from baseline of more than 20%), use of no more than 10 mg prednisone equivalent per day, and no rescue medication at 52 weeks. This response was achieved in 40.8% of those receiving voclosporin compared to 22.5% on placebo.[69] The interim analysis for Aurora 2, a 104-week extension study of AURORA 1, showed that patients receiving voclosporin maintained reductions in proteinuria with no change in mean eGFR at 30 months of treatment.[70]

Other calcineurin inhibitors have also been used to treat lupus nephritis and may be a treatment option for women who are pregnant or breastfeeding.[2] Tacrolimus has a different structure with higher immunosuppressive effects and less nephrotoxicity than cyclosporine. Most of the tacrolimus studies have been conducted in Asian populations. It has been used as monotherapy for induction and maintenance therapy. It has also been used in combination with mycophenolate mofetil for induction therapy for patients with nephrotic range proteinuria.[2] The most recent European recommendations for treatment of lupus nephritis include a calcineurin inhibitor (especially tacrolimus) as alternative monotherapy for class V nephritis (Level 2b/B) or in combination with mycophenolate for patients with nephrotic range proteinuria (Level 1b/B).[47]

Janus-kinase inhibitors such as tofacitinib and baricitinib are being studied for musculoskeletal and cutaneous lupus with some success.[45] Numerous other immunosuppressive drugs have been used in SLE, especially in patients who have contraindications to the agents already discussed or who cannot tolerate them, or those whose disease is refractory to conventional treatment.

Alternative Treatments

Patients receiving conventional treatment for SLE frequently feel they have unmet needs. Often these are psychosocial and may include anxiety or depression. These needs can lead patients to try alternative therapies. Clinicians should have an open dialogue with patients about these therapies so that patients will report them. This allows practitioners to monitor for interactions with other treatments and to guide patients to therapies with greater potential for benefit and less for harm.[71]

Complementary and alternative medicine includes health systems, products, and practices that are outside the realm of conventional medicine. In general, these have not been evaluated in randomized controlled trials involving SLE patients.[71]

Concentrations of dehydroepiandrosterone (DHEA), a weak adrenal androgen, are typically decreased in SLE. DHEA supplementation may offer some limited benefit for patients' assessment of disease activity, steroid effects on bone mineral density, and time to flares in SLE.[71] Effects on oral ulcers and alopecia have also been studied.[72]

Vitamin D concentrations are decreased in SLE, especially in patients with high disease activity and those with darker skin pigmentation (eg, African American patients). A contributing factor to the deficiency is that patients are instructed to protect themselves from sunlight because of the photosensitivity that accompanies SLE.[73] Another factor may be polymorphisms in the gene involved in vitamin D degradation. Vitamin D deficiency is associated with high concentrations of inflammatory cytokines. Deficiencies not only affect bone health, but low vitamin D concentrations may also be associated with greater SLE disease activity, insulin resistance, and fatigue.[74] Low concentrations also correlate with increased cardiovascular risk factors such as hypertension and hyperlipidemia. B- and T-lymphocytes, dendritic cells, macrophages, and neutrophils have vitamin D receptors, which suggests a role for vitamin D in both innate and adaptive immune processes.[74] Baseline 25(OH) vitamin D concentrations should be checked with a current goal of at least 30 ng/mL (75 nmol/L).[50] Some suggest a daily intake of vitamin D3 of 30 to 50 μg (1,000-2,000 IU). This is especially important for patients taking corticosteroids.

Special Populations

Pregnancy and Contraception

7 Pregnancy planning with assessment of risk factors is key for achieving good outcomes for women with SLE and healthy babies. ACR issued recommendations for reproductive health in patients with rheumatic and musculoskeletal diseases.[75] The guideline summarizes information about pregnancy, contraception, assisted reproductive technologies, fertility preservation, hormone replacement therapy, breastfeeding, and use of medications. It distinguishes SLE with and without antiphospholipid antibodies in its recommendations. Timing of pregnancies with respect to disease activity and potential use of teratogenic medications makes

contraception counseling very important. Women should be educated about fertility issues related to age and effects of medications. Cyclophosphamide therapy is associated with ovarian insufficiency, although the low-dose regimen may have minimal impact on ovarian reserve.[52] This is especially of concern in older women who wish to conceive. Estrogen-containing oral contraceptives or hormone replacement therapy are associated with SLE flares and with thrombosis, especially in women with antiphospholipid antibodies or other risk factors. The risk of flares is low in patients with stable disease.[76] Combined estrogen-progestin pill or vaginal ring or progestin-only oral contraceptives or intrauterine devices (IUDs) can be offered to women whose SLE is inactive or stable active and who do not have antiphospholipid antibodies (low-moderate strength of evidence).[75] Short-term use of hormone replacement therapy may be considered for women with severe menopausal symptoms who have stable/inactive disease and do not have antiphospholipid antibodies (moderate evidence). Copper or progestin IUDs and progestin implants are considered to be highly effective and may be better choices for contraception in patients with SLE. Since mycophenolate can reduce the effectiveness of oral contraceptives, IUDs or two other forms of contraception are recommended for patients taking that drug. The IUDs or progestin-only pills are recommended for those with antiphospholipid antibodies. Progestin-only pills are considered effective and are an alternative for those who do not want an IUD. The copper IUD may increase menstrual bleeding and cramping after insertion. However, these symptoms decrease with the progestin IUD, which may be a consideration for patients receiving anticoagulants.

Pregnancy during SLE is considered to be high risk. The risk of maternal mortality, cesarean delivery, preterm labor, lupus nephritis flares, gestational diabetes, preeclampsia, Hemolysis with Elevated Liver tests and Low Platelets (HELLP) and the risk of thrombotic, infectious, and hematologic complications are increased.[36,66,77] Fetal risks include fetal loss, preterm birth, preterm premature rupture of membranes, and intrauterine growth restriction.[66] Preeclampsia occurs in 13% to 35% of women with SLE[66] and is defined as hypertension and proteinuria (greater than 300 mg/24 hr) that develop for the first time after 20 weeks of gestation.[78] This can be difficult to distinguish from lupus nephritis. The risk for preterm preeclampsia is decreased with daily use of low-dose aspirin begun before 16 weeks gestation.[66] Hydroxychloroquine also protects against preeclampsia.[79] Flares during pregnancy may be difficult to identify because they share characteristics of a normal pregnancy.[77] The complications are more likely in patients with active disease, especially lupus nephritis. If the mother has anti-Ro/SSA or anti-La/SSB antibodies, the fetus is at risk for neonatal lupus with rash, hematologic, hepatic, and cardiac abnormalities including heart block. These risks decrease with continued use of hydroxychloroquine.[77] Treatment of pregnant women with antiphospholipid antibodies is discussed below. Pregnancy should be discouraged in patients with severe pulmonary hypertension, advanced renal insufficiency, severe restrictive lung disease, heart failure, or a history of severe preeclampsia. It is also not advised within 6 months of a severe SLE flare, active lupus nephritis, or a stroke. The best pregnancy outcomes are observed in patients who have had inactive disease for at least 6 months prior to the pregnancy. Drugs used to control the SLE should be those, such as hydroxychloroquine, that can be continued throughout the pregnancy and may decrease the risk of flares, disease activity, and heart block in at-risk pregnancies.[77] Any potentially teratogenic drugs (eg, methotrexate, mycophenolate, cyclophosphamide, and thalidomide) should be stopped before attempting pregnancy.[75] The time before conception is 1 to 3 months for methotrexate and thalidomide, more than 6 weeks for mycophenolate, and 3 months for cyclophosphamide. This also allows time to evaluate whether disease activity is still controlled. Leflunomide should be removed through the oral cholestyramine elimination procedure (8 g three times a day for 11 days with confirmation of undetectable serum concentrations) preferably before conception or at least when pregnancy is confirmed.[75,77] Close monitoring and disease management of the mothers and fetuses are essential during pregnancy. The risks of drug use and harmful effects of disease flare need to be considered.[80] If a flare occurs and an immunosuppressive drug is required during the pregnancy, azathioprine may be considered because limited placental transfer occurs and the fetal liver is unable to metabolize it to its active form.[81,82] The dose should not exceed 2 mg/kg/day. Calcineurin inhibitors (cyclosporine, tacrolimus) are alternative choices. Supplements with calcium, vitamin D, and folic acid should be offered.[80,81] If corticosteroids are needed, maintenance doses should be kept as low as possible (preferably 7.5 mg or less) to decrease the risk of gestational diabetes mellitus, hypertension, infections, pre-eclampsia, and premature rupture of membranes.[66,77] Patients on long-term steroid therapy may need stress doses at the time of delivery. Fluorinated corticosteroids (such as dexamethasone or betamethasone) cross the placenta and should be avoided unless they are being used to treat the fetus.[66] Cyclophosphamide should only be used during the second or third trimester of pregnancy if alternatives failed and the mother's life is in danger.[80,81] If treatment of hypertension is needed, methyldopa, beta-blockers (except atenolol), or calcium channel blockers are considered safe, although there are some concerns about fetal bradycardia and intrauterine growth restriction with beta-blockers.[81] Labetalol is the preferred beta-blocker. Angiotensin-converting enzyme inhibitors and angiotensin receptor blockers may cause fetal malformations, oligohydramnios, and fetal renal damage.[81] NSAIDs should be discouraged in the preconception period due to concerns of NSAID-induced unruptured follicle syndrome and in the first trimester due to increased risk of miscarriage.[81] They should not be used in the third trimester of gestation because they increase the risk of premature closure of the ductus arteriosus, oligohydramnios, neonatal renal failure, and pulmonary hypertension. The safety of selective COX-2 inhibitors during pregnancy is not known. The safety of biologics is also not known, but they can be used preconception. The 2020 ACR guideline strongly recommends continuing certolizumab (which lacks an Fc chain) during pregnancy since minimal placental transfer occurs.[75] The guideline conditionally recommends discontinuation of other TNF-α inhibitors (infliximab, etanercept, adalimumab, golimumab) in the third trimester when placental transfer increases. The guideline also conditionally recommends stopping anakinra, belimumab, abatacept, tocilizumab, secukinumab, and ustekinumab once pregnancy is confirmed. Rituximab given during the second half of pregnancy can cause neonatal B-cell depletion and should be avoided unless the woman has severe life- or organ-threatening disease.[75] There is insufficient data on the safety of tofacitinib, baricitinib, and apremilast for any recommendation, but they likely cross the placenta.[75] The ACR guideline also included recommendations regarding men planning to father a child. Since cyclophosphamide can damage sperm, it is strongly recommended that men stop cyclophosphamide 12 weeks prior to attempted conception and consider sperm cryopreservation before starting treatment. It conditionally recommends discontinuation of thalidomide 4 weeks before.

SLE–Antiphospholipid Syndrome Overlap

8 The antiphospholipid antibodies are a group of antibodies including anticardiolipin, anti-β-2-glycoprotein I, and lupus anticoagulant. They can promote clotting and pregnancy morbidity.[83] Complement also plays a key role in antiphospholipid syndrome (APS) pathogenesis.[84] The diagnosis of APS requires at least one clinical and one laboratory feature. The clinical aspects are vascular events such as venous or arterial thrombi and/or obstetric complications. The obstetric complications meeting the criteria are three or more unexplained consecutive miscarriages before the 10th week of gestation, one or more unexplained deaths of fetuses at or beyond the 10th week of gestation, and one or more births of infants before the 34th week of gestation associated with eclampsia or severe preeclampsia

or features of placental insufficiency.[85] Adverse pregnancy outcomes are especially associated with the presence of lupus anticoagulant.[66] Laboratory criteria are the presence of antiphospholipid antibodies on two separate occasions, 12 weeks apart.[85] Antiphospholipid antibodies are found in about 40% of patients with SLE, but less than 40% of those experience thrombotic events.[84] Patients at high risk for thrombotic and obstetric events are those with lupus anticoagulant or a combination of two or three antiphospholipid antibodies or the presence of persistently high antiphospholipid antibody titers.[19] Patients with isolated positive anticardiolipin or anti-β_2-glycoprotein I at low-medium titers, especially if transiently positive, are considered to be at low risk. Patients with thrombosis often have other cardiovascular risk factors (such as hypertension, hyperlipidemia, smoking, or use of estrogen-containing medications) or an underlying autoimmune disease such as SLE.[84] It is recommended that any modifiable factors be controlled. In deciding choice, intensity, and duration of treatment, the clinician should balance benefits with the patient's risk of bleeding. Consideration should also be given to whether thrombotic events are associated with identified transient precipitating factors. A EULAR Task Force developed recommendations for the management of APS in adults that consider individual risk assessments (Table 107-4).[19]

Patients with antiphospholipid antibodies may also have a false-positive test for syphilis (rapid plasma reagin).[18] Other common manifestations of APS are cognitive impairment, thrombocytopenia, stroke or transient ischemic attack, chorea, migraine, glomerulonephritis, avascular necrosis of bones, heart valve lesions, and livedo reticularis.[82]

It is not clear how to treat pregnant women with antiphospholipid antibodies. Low-dose aspirin (75-100 mg) should be considered during pregnancy for those with a high antiphospholipid profile but no history of thrombosis or pregnancy complications (Level 5/D).[19] Those with no history of thrombosis but who have experienced at least three spontaneous miscarriages before 10 weeks gestation and those with fetal loss at 10 weeks or later should be treated with low-dose aspirin and prophylactic doses of heparin (Level 2b/B). Self-administration of low-molecular-weight heparin may be more convenient for patients. Not only does heparin have anticoagulant effects, but it also has anti-inflammatory and immunomodulating properties and can inhibit complement activation.[86] Hydroxychloroquine should also be considered. Those with a history of delivery before 34 weeks gestation associated with eclampsia or severe preeclampsia or placental insufficiency should receive low dose aspirin alone or with prophylactic doses of heparin (Level 2b/B).[19] If women have recurrent obstetric complications despite receiving aspirin and heparin, clinicians should increase the heparin dose to therapeutic (Level 5/D) or consider adding hydroxychloroquine (Level 4/D) or low-dose prednisolone (Level 4/D) in the first trimester. Pregnant patients with APS and a history of thrombosis should receive low-dose aspirin with therapeutic doses of heparin (Level 4/C).[19] Warfarin is teratogenic and should be avoided during pregnancy, especially during the first trimester.[77] If low-molecular-weight heparin is used, it should be switched to unfractionated heparin 4 weeks before the anticipated delivery date. The heparin should be discontinued at the start of labor or 8 hours before a planned cesarean delivery.[87] All women with APS should receive anticoagulation with prophylactic doses of heparin, low-molecular-weight heparin, or warfarin for 6 weeks postpartum. Women without thrombosis risks may benefit from just 7 to 10 days of low-molecular-weight heparin.[83] Both heparin and warfarin are safe during breastfeeding.[84]

Clinicians can achieve better control of APS by adding hydroxychloroquine, statins, and vitamin D to standard therapy.[84] For patients who do not respond to conventional APS treatment or for whom it is contraindicated, alternative therapies include other platelet inhibitors, corticosteroids, rituximab, and the complement inhibitor, eculizumab. The role of direct acting oral anticoagulants is not clear. They should not be used for patients who are triple antibody positive or those with arterial thrombi.[19] They may be considered for patients with a low risk profile and no history of arterial thrombosis with a difficult to control international normalized ratio on warfarin.[35]

The most severe form of APS is called catastrophic and is associated with widespread thrombosis, multiorgan failure, and high mortality.[83] Any precipitating factors should be investigated and managed.[19] Treatment consists of combination therapy with

TABLE 107-4 Recommendations for Thromboprophylaxis in Patients with Systemic Lupus Erythematosus and Antiphospholipid Antibodies

Recommendation	Level of Evidence/Grade of Recommendation
Asymptomatic aPl carriers with no history of thrombosis or pregnancy complications, low-dose aspirin is recommended	2a/B
Patients with no history of thrombosis or pregnancy complications with high-risk aPl profile, low-dose aspirin is recommended	2a/B
Patients with no history of thrombosis or pregnancy complications with low-risk aPl profile, low-dose aspirin can be considered	2b/C
Nonpregnant women with a history of obstetric complications, low-dose aspirin is recommended	2b/B
Patients with APS and first venous thrombosis, warfarin with INR 2-3 is recommended	1b/B
If unprovoked first thrombosis, long-term treatment recommended	2b/B
If provoked first thrombosis, treat as usual	5/D
If provoked first thrombosis with high aPl profile, consider longer treatment	5/D
Patients with APS and recurrent venous thrombosis on warfarin with INR 2-3, consider adding low-dose aspirin or increasing INR target to 3-4 or change to low-molecular-weight heparin	4-5/D
Patients with APS and first arterial thrombosis, warfarin recommended over low-dose aspirin	2b/C
Patients with APS and first arterial thrombosis, warfarin with INR 2-3 or 3-4 recommended	1b/B
Patients with APS and first arterial thrombosis, warfarin with INR 2-3 and low-dose aspirin can be considered	4/C
Patients with APS and recurrent arterial thrombosis on warfarin with INR 2-3, consider adding low-dose aspirin or increasing INR target to 3-4 or change to low-molecular-weight heparin	4-5/D

aPl, antiphospholipid antibodies; APS, antiphospholipid syndrome.

Levels of Evidence: 1a: systematic review of randomized controlled trials (RCTs); 1b: individual RCT; 2a: systematic review of cohort studies; 2b: individual cohort study (and low-quality RCT); 3a: systematic review of case-control studies; 3b: individual case-control study; 4: case series and poor-quality cohort and case–control studies; 5: expert opinion

Grade of Recommendation: A: consistent level 1 studies; B: consistent level 2 or 3 studies, or extrapolations from level 1 studies; C: level 4 studies or extrapolations from level 2 or 3 studies; D: level 5 evidence or troublingly inconsistent or inconclusive studies of any level

Data from Reference 19.

glucocorticoids, heparin, and plasma exchange or intravenous immunoglobulins. If ineffective, rituximab or eculizumab may be considered.

Drug-Induced Lupus

9 Up to 15% of cases of SLE and up to 30% of cases of subacute cutaneous lupus erythematosus can be attributed to drugs.[88] About 15,000 to 30,000 new cases are reported each year in the United States.[11] These are idiosyncratic reactions precipitated by the interplay of genetic predisposition, concurrent illnesses, environmental factors, and other drugs or foods. Various pathophysiologic mechanisms have been proposed for different drugs in inducing lupus. Most drugs are small molecules that can induce an immune response by binding to larger molecules such as proteins, a process called haptenization. Another proposed mechanism is interference with macrophage uptake of apoptotic or necrotic cells, leading to accumulation of self-antigens. A more recently described mechanism is stimulation of neutrophil extracellular traps (NETs; NETosis), a form of neutrophil cell death that also results in self-antigens that stimulate autoreactive T- or B-cells.[89] Other possible mechanisms are dysregulation and hypomethylation of T-cells.[16]

There are no standard diagnostic criteria because the manifestations of drug-induced lupus are so diverse. The diagnosis is based on lupus-like findings in a patient with no history of the disease and the temporal relationship with the drug, including onset at least 1 month after initiation and improvement in symptoms within days to months after the drug is discontinued. The time frame, however, can be variable. The patient will often have laboratory findings such as a positive ANA or anti-histone antibodies, but usually not anti-dsDNA or anti-Sm antibodies.[90]

Many drugs of varied classes have been implicated. The drugs with the highest risk for inducing traditional symptomatic drug-induced lupus are procainamide (20%) and hydralazine (5%-8%), especially with hydralazine doses over 200 mg/day or a cumulative dose of more than 100 g.[90] It is more common in patients who are slow acetylators.[89] The incidence of positive ANAs with these drugs is 80% to 90% and 50%, respectively.[90] Common manifestations include arthralgias, arthritis, and myalgias. Constitutional symptoms such as fever, fatigue, anorexia, and weight loss are common.[11] Other clinical features include rash, pleuritis, pericarditis, and autoimmune hepatitis. Glomerulonephritis, CNS disease, and hematologic abnormalities are rare in drug-induced lupus.[11] The risk and types of reactions vary depending on the offending drug. Laboratory abnormalities associated with drug-induced lupus include positive ANA and antibodies to histones. Other antibodies such as anti-Sm, anti-dsDNA, and antineutrophil cytoplasmic antibodies (ANCA) may be seen with some drugs. A drug with moderate risk for lupus is quinidine. The incidence of quinidine- and procainamide-induced lupus is declining because of decreasing use of the drugs and use of lower doses. Over 100 drugs of many different classes have been implicated and are considered to be of low risk. Other drugs with well-established links to lupus are minocycline, isoniazid, methyldopa, carbamazepine, and chlorpromazine.[11] A variant of the syndrome is drug-induced subacute cutaneous lupus, which has been most associated with terbinafine and TNF-α inhibitors, but also with calcium channel antagonists, thiazide diuretics, angiotensin-converting enzyme inhibitors, chemotherapeutic agents, phenytoin, carbamazepine, and proton pump inhibitors.[16] The mean age for this syndrome is 59 years; more patients are women, and positive ANA, anti-Ro/SSA, and anti-La/SSB are common, but fewer have anti-histone antibodies than those with drug-induced SLE.[16,89] It may occur after weeks to years of therapy.[89] Chronic cutaneous lupus has been reported with fluorouracil, TNF-α inhibitors, antifungals, and rarely intravenous immunoglobulins.[16] Drug-induced lupus can take weeks to months for skin lesions to resolve after the offending drug has been stopped.[11]

A separate category of drug-induced lupus involves TNF-α inhibitors, such as infliximab, etanercept, adalimumab, golimumab, and certolizumab pegol, and is called TNF-α Antagonist Induced Lupus-like Syndrome (TAILS).[11] These drugs, especially chimeric infliximab, are known to induce autoantibodies. Proposed mechanisms for TNF-α inhibitor-induced lupus are that they induce cell apoptosis, increase the risk for bacterial infection, or suppress T-helper 1 immune response and favor T-helper 2 response. It is common for patients receiving these drugs to develop positive ANAs, anti-dsDNA of the IgM subtype, and extractable nuclear antibodies. Antihistone antibodies are less commonly seen than with other drug-induced lupus. As with traditional drug-induced lupus, the risk of clinical lupus is low compared to the numbers that develop autoantibodies.[90] Rashes and hypocomplementemia are more common features with TNF-α inhibitors than traditional drug-induced lupus.[91] Arthralgias, arthritis, fever, and weight loss are also seen. Renal, hematologic, and neurologic disorders are rare.[11] The underlying diseases being treated with these drugs may be a factor in the development of the observed reactions.

The primary treatment for drug-induced lupus is discontinuation of the implicated drug. Some patients require treatment with corticosteroids or other topical or systemic drugs based on the type and severity of the manifestations. If patients do not improve, a diagnosis of idiopathic SLE should be considered.[11]

Immunizations

Patients with SLE are at increased risk for infections because of immune dysfunction caused by their disease and immunosuppressive therapy. It is important to try to protect patients against these infections, but there are areas of concern regarding the safety and efficacy of vaccines in patients with SLE.[92] SLE cases developing or flaring after vaccine administration have been reported, but the actual risk is low when considering how many people receive immunizations.[93] These reactions may be a response to adjuvants added to increase the immunogenicity of vaccines and could be part of the syndrome called "ASIA—Autoimmune/inflammatory Syndrome Induced by Adjuvants."[93] Another concern is that immunosuppressed patients may have an impaired response to vaccines such as influenza and pneumococcal as compared with healthy individuals. Revaccination may be needed in some cases.[92] Whenever possible, to achieve the best response, vaccines should be administered when SLE is stable and prior to initiating immunosuppressive medications. Non-live vaccines are considered safe in immunosuppressed patients. It is recommended that SLE patients receive pneumococcal vaccine because they are particularly susceptible to *Streptococcus pneumoniae* infections. They should also receive annual influenza vaccines. Those considered to be at risk should be immunized against hepatitis A and B.[92] Live-attenuated virus vaccines, such as measles–mumps–rubella, varicella, intranasal influenza, and yellow fever, are generally contraindicated in patients receiving immunosuppressive therapy. They should be avoided with consideration of risks versus benefits in patients taking high doses of immunosuppressive drugs. Doses of corticosteroids equivalent to prednisone 20 mg/day or more given for at least 2 weeks, methotrexate at 0.4 mg/kg/week or more, and azathioprine at 3 mg/kg/day or higher are considered immunosuppressive.[92] Measles–mumps–rubella boosters for patients on low-grade immunosuppression at risk for measles may be an exception. Non-live vaccines should preferably be given 2 weeks before starting immunosuppressive drugs if possible.[94] Live vaccines should be given at least 4 weeks before starting immunosuppressive drugs.[92] The recombinant zoster vaccine can be given during therapy with immunosuppressive drugs but should not be given during pregnancy. The same pregnancy delay should be observed for live vaccines and the human papilloma vaccine. The meningococcal serogroup B vaccine should only be given during pregnancy if benefits outweigh risks.[95] B-cell–depleting therapy such as rituximab suppresses the humoral response to vaccines, so vaccines should be given 6 months after and 4 weeks before the next course of B-cell–depleting therapy.[92] A patient taking a B-cell–depleting therapy who has a high-risk exposure to tetanus should receive passive immunization with tetanus immunoglobulins. Immunosuppressed patients with SLE should receive a third dose of the same mRNA COVID-19 vaccine at least 28 days after the two-dose primary series.[95]

EVALUATION OF THERAPEUTIC OUTCOMES

10 Patients must be assessed for the activity and extent of lupus and monitored for adverse drug reactions. Monitoring for specific drugs is listed in Table 107-3. Many instruments have been developed and modified over the years to assess SLE therapy in trials. It is difficult to assess SLE therapy because milder forms of the disease may fluctuate, regardless of treatment.[96] Examples of measures of disease activity include the Systemic Lupus Erythematosus Disease Activity Index (SLEDAI) and British Isles Lupus Assessment Group (BILAG). The SLEDAI is a measure of global disease activity that scores 24 manifestations as present or not. Modifications include the SELENA (Safety of Estrogens in Lupus Erythematosus National Assessment)-SLEDAI and SLEDAI-2000 (SLEDAI-2K). The SLEDAI-2K modified some of the elements and has been used in recent trials. Another variation is the SLEDAI-2KG that adds a weighted score based on glucocorticoid dose. BILAG measures clinical disease activity in eight organ systems compared to the prior assessment with a score of 0 to 4. The organ domains are given scores of A to E based on severity with A being severe, B moderate, C mild, D no activity, and E no history. An update of this instrument is the BILAG-2004. Individually, these indices were inadequate for showing superiority of new drugs over standard therapy. To overcome this problem, belimumab investigators developed the Systemic Lupus Erythematosus Responder Index (SRI) assessment criteria. The SRI has three components: (a) reduction in disease activity by SELENA-SLEDAI by at least 4 points; (b) no new BILAG A and no more than one new BILAG B score; and (c) less than 0.3 point increase (worsening) in physician global assessment (PGA). The PGA assesses patients' general health status. The BILAG-based Combined Lupus Assessment (BICLA) was used to demonstrate the efficacy of anifrolumab. It is defined as improvement in moderate-severe BILAG-2004 activity, no worsening in global and organ-specific disease activity, and no treatment failure. Other proposed instruments are the S2K RI-50 that measures partial improvement and the Lupus Low Disease Activity State (LLDA).[96] Another important assessment of therapy is health-related quality of life (HRQoL), which may use a patient-reported outcomes tool such as the generic 36-item Health Survey Short Form (SF-36) or one designed for cutaneous lupus.[28]

The Cutaneous Lupus Erythematosus Disease Area and Severity Index (CLASI) may be used for a more comprehensive assessment of disease activity and damage in cutaneous lupus erythematosus and response to therapy.[96]

A British Society for Rheumatology working group developed guidelines for managing SLE in adults. Patients should regularly be evaluated for SLE manifestations, adverse drug reactions, and comorbidities. Those with active disease should be assessed at least every 1 to 3 months with blood pressure, urinalysis, renal function, anti-dsDNA antibodies, complement concentrations, C-reactive protein, complete blood count, and liver function tests with further testing as warranted. Clinical and laboratory assessments should be performed every 6 to 12 months in patients with inactive disease and no organ damage, and more frequently if abnormalities are found.[97]

CONCLUSION

Much progress has been made in understanding the disease processes that lead to the development of SLE. This has led to the development of new drugs that target those disease pathways. Drug approval has been achieved by designing new tools for the assessment of drug efficacy. Therapeutic success is difficult to show when the "placebo" group is receiving standard treatment that usually includes drugs not approved for management of SLE. Practitioners can increase treatment success by educating patients on the importance of adherence to recommended life-style changes and medication regimens.

ABBREVIATIONS

ACR	American College of Rheumatology
ALMS	Aspreva Lupus Management Study
ANA	antinuclear antibody
ANCA	antineutrophil cytoplasmic antibodies
Anti-dsDNA	anti-double-stranded DNA
aPl	antiphospholipid antibodies
APRIL	a proliferation-inducing ligand
APS	antiphospholipid syndrome
BAFF	B-cell activating factor of the TNF family
BICLA	BILAG-based Combined Lupus Assessment
BILAG	British Isles Lupus Assessment Group
BLyS	B-lymphocyte stimulator
CLASI	Cutaneous Lupus Erythematosus Disease Area and Severity Index
CNS	central nervous system
DHEA	dehydroepiandrosterone
DNA	deoxyribonucleic acid
eGFR	estimated glomerular filtration rate
EULAR	European League Against Rheumatism, now European Alliance of Associations for Rheumatology
G6PD	glucose-6-phosphate dehydrogenase
HELLP	hemolysis with elevated liver tests and thrombocytopenia
HRQoL	health-related quality of life
IMPDH	inosine 5-monophosphate dehydrogenase
IL	interleukin
IUD	intrauterine device
La/SSB	antigen La/Sjögren syndrome B antigen
Mesna	sodium-2-mercaptoethane sulfonate
MHC	major histocompatibility complex
MPA	mycophenolic acid
NET	neutrophil extracellular trap
NMDA	*N*-methyl-D-aspartate
NSAID	nonsteroidal anti-inflammatory drug
PGA	physician global assessment
Ro/SSA	antigen Ro/Sjögren syndrome A antigen
RCT	randomized controlled trial
SELENA-SLEDAI	Safety of Estrogens in Lupus Erythematosus: National Assessment-Systemic Lupus Erythematosus Disease Activity Index
SF-36	Medical Outcomes Survey Short Form-36
SLE	systemic lupus erythematosus
SLICC	Systemic Lupus International Collaborating Clinics
SPF	sun protection factor
SRI	SLE Responder Index
TAILS	TNF-α inhibitor-induced lupus syndrome
TNF-α	tumor necrosis factor-alpha
TPMT	thiopurine methyltransferase
Treg	T regulatory cell

REFERENCES

1. Barnett R. Systemic lupus erythematosus. *Lancet.* 2016;387(10029):1711. doi:https://dx.doi.org/10.1016/S0140-6736(16)30266-5
2. Rafael-Vidal C, Altabás I, Pérez N, et al. Calcineurin and systemic lupus erythematosus: The rationale for using calcineurin inhibitors in the treatment of lupus nephritis. *Int J Mol Sci.* 2021;22(3):1263. doi:10.3390/ijms22031263
3. Barber MRW, Drenkard C, Falasinnu T, et al. Global epidemiology of systemic lupus erythematosus. *Nat Rev Rheumatol.* 2021;17(9):515–532. doi:https://dx.doi.org/10.1038/s41584-021-00668-1
4. Pons-Estel GJ, Ugarte-Gil MF, Alarcon GS. Epidemiology of systemic lupus erythematosus. *Expert Rev Clin Immunol.* 2017;13(8):799–814. doi:https://dx.doi.org/10.1080/1744666X.2017.1327352
5. Stojan G, Petri M. Epidemiology of systemic lupus erythematosus. *Curr Opin Rheumatol.* 2018;30(2):144–150. doi:10.1097/BOR.0000000000000480
6. Hahn BH, McMahon MA, Wilkinson A, et al. American College of Rheumatology guidelines for screening, treatment, and management of lupus nephritis. *Arthritis Care Res (Hoboken).* 2012;64(6):797–808. doi:http://dx.doi.org/10.1002/acr.21664
7. Lim SS, Drenkard C. Epidemiology of lupus: An update. *Curr Opin Rheumatol.* 2015;27(5):427–432. doi:10.1097/BOR.0000000000000198
8. Niewold TB. Advances in lupus genetics. *Curr Opin Rheumatol.* 2015;27(5):440–447. doi:https://dx.doi.org/10.1097/BOR.0000000000000205
9. Chen LY, Shi ZR, Tan GZ, et al. Systemic lupus erythematosus with and without a family history: A meta-analysis. *Lupus.* 2018;27(5):716–721. doi:https://dx.doi.org/10.1177/0961203317739133
10. Azevedo PC, Murphy G, Isenberg DA. Pathology of systemic lupus erythematosus: The challenges ahead. *Methods Mol Biol.* 2014;1134:1–16. doi:http://dx.doi.org/10.1007/978-1-4939-0326-9_1
11. Vaglio A, Grayson PC, Fenaroli P, et al. Drug-induced lupus: Traditional and new concepts. *Autoimmun Rev.* 2018;17(9):912–918. doi:https://dx.doi.org/10.1016/j.autrev.2018.03.016
12. Parisis D, Bernier C, Chasset F, et al. Impact of tobacco smoking upon disease risk, activity and therapeutic response in systemic lupus erythematosus: A systematic review and meta-analysis. *Autoimmun Rev.* 2019;18(11):102393. doi:https://dx.doi.org/10.1016/j.autrev.2019.102393
13. Fanouriakis A, Tziolos N, Bertsias G, et al. Update on the diagnosis and management of systemic lupus erythematosus. *Ann Rheum Dis.* 2021;80(1):14–25. doi:https://dx.doi.org/10.1136/annrheumdis-2020-218272
14. Hile GA, Kahlenberg JM. Immunopathogenesis of skin injury in systemic lupus erythematosus. *Curr Opin Rheumatol.* 2021;33(2):173–180. doi:10.1097/bor.0000000000000770
15. Gulati G, Brunner HI. Environmental triggers in systemic lupus erythematosus. *Semin Arthritis Rheum.* 2018;47(5):710–717. doi:https://dx.doi.org/10.1016/j.semarthrit.2017.10.001
16. Borucki R, Werth VP. Cutaneous lupus erythematosus induced by drugs: Novel insights. *Expert Rev Clin Pharmacol.* 2020;13(1):35–42. doi:https://dx.doi.org/10.1080/17512433.2020.1698290
17. Lv J, Feng Y, Qian Y, et al. Klinefelter's syndrome with systemic lupus erythematosus and atrial fibrillation. *Lupus.* 2019;28(12):1477–1479. doi:10.1177/0961203319877256
18. Tsokos GC, Lo MS, Reis PC, et al. New insights into the immunopathogenesis of systemic lupus erythematosus. *Nat Rev Rheumatol.* 2016;12:716. doi:10.1038/nrrheum.2016.186
19. Tektonidou MG, Andreoli L, Limper M, et al. EULAR recommendations for the management of antiphospholipid syndrome in adults. *Ann Rheum Dis.* 2019;78(10):1296–1304. doi:https://dx.doi.org/10.1136/annrheumdis-2019-215213
20. Gensous N, Boizard-Moracchini A, Lazaro E, et al. Update on the cellular pathogenesis of lupus. *Curr Opin Rheumatol.* 2021;33(2):190–196. doi:10.1097/bor.0000000000000775
21. Blair HA, Duggan ST. Belimumab: A review in systemic lupus erythematosus. *Drugs.* 2018;78(3):355–366. doi:https://dx.doi.org/10.1007/s40265-018-0872-z
22. Aringer M, Johnson SR. Systemic lupus erythematosus classification and diagnosis. *Rheum Dis Clin North Am.* 2021;47(3):501–511. doi:10.1016/j.rdc.2021.04.011
23. Ramírez Sepúlveda JI, Bolin K, Mofors J, et al. Sex differences in clinical presentation of systemic lupus erythematosus. *Biol Sex Differ.* 2019;10(1):60. doi:10.1186/s13293-019-0274-2
24. Aringer M, Costenbader K, Daikh D, et al. 2019 European League Against Rheumatism/American College of Rheumatology Classification Criteria for Systemic Lupus Erythematosus. *Arthritis Rheumatol.* 2019;71(9):1400–1412. doi:https://doi.org/10.1002/art.40930
25. Petri M, Orbai AM, Alarcon GS, et al. Derivation and validation of the Systemic Lupus International Collaborating Clinics classification criteria for systemic lupus erythematosus. *Arthritis Rheum.* 2012;64(8):2677–2686. doi:http://dx.doi.org/10.1002/art.34473
26. Petri M, Goldman DW, Alarcon GS, et al. Comparison of the 2019 European Alliance of Associations for Rheumatology/American College of Rheumatology Systemic Lupus Erythematosus Classification Criteria with two sets of earlier systemic lupus erythematosus classification criteria. *Arthritis Care Res (Hoboken).* 2021;73(9):1231–1235. doi:https://dx.doi.org/10.1002/acr.24263
27. Kus KJB, LaChance AH, Vleugels RA. Recognition and management of cutaneous connective tissue diseases. *Med Clin North Am.* 2021;105(4):757–782. doi:https://dx.doi.org/10.1016/j.mcna.2021.04.011
28. Ogunsanya ME, Cho SK, Hudson A, et al. Validation and reliability of a disease-specific quality-of-life measure in patients with cutaneous lupus erythematosus. *Br J Dermatol.* 2019;180(6):1430–1437. doi:https://doi.org/10.1111/bjd.17636
29. Shi Y, Li M, Liu L, et al. Relationship between disease activity, organ damage and health-related quality of life in patients with systemic lupus erythematosus: A systemic review and meta-analysis. *Autoimmun Rev.* 2021;20(1):102691. doi:https://doi.org/10.1016/j.autrev.2020.102691
30. Worm M, Zidane M, Eisert L, et al. S2k guideline: Diagnosis and management of cutaneous lupus erythematosus—Part 1: Classification, diagnosis, prevention, activity scores. *J Dtsch Dermatol Ges.* 2021;19(8):1236–1247. doi:https://doi.org/10.1111/ddg.14492
31. Petty AJ, Floyd L, Henderson C, et al. Cutaneous lupus erythematosus: Progress and challenges. *Curr Allergy Asthma Rep.* 2020;20(5):12. doi:10.1007/s11882-020-00906-8
32. Anders HJ, Saxena R, Zhao MH, et al. Lupus nephritis. *Nat Rev Dis Prim.* 2020;6(1):7. doi:https://dx.doi.org/10.1038/s41572-019-0141-9
33. Govoni M, Hanly JG. The management of neuropsychiatric lupus in the 21st century: Still so many unmet needs? *Rheumatology (Oxford).* 2020;59(Suppl5):v52–v62. doi:10.1093/rheumatology/keaa404
34. Govoni M, Bortoluzzi A, Padovan M, et al. The diagnosis and clinical management of the neuropsychiatric manifestations of lupus. *J Autoimmun.* 2016;74:41–72. doi:https://dx.doi.org/10.1016/j.jaut.2016.06.013
35. Fanouriakis A, Kostopoulou M, Alunno A, et al. 2019 update of the EULAR recommendations for the management of systemic lupus erythematosus. *Ann Rheum Dis.* 2019;78(6):736–745. doi:https://dx.doi.org/10.1136/annrheumdis-2019-215089
36. Lisnevskaia L, Murphy G, Isenberg D. Systemic lupus erythematosus. *Lancet.* 2014;384(9957):1878–1888. doi:http://dx.doi.org/10.1016/S0140-6736(14)60128-8
37. Kasturi S, Sammaritano LR. Corticosteroids in lupus. *Rheum Dis Clin North Am.* 2016;42(1):47–62, viii. doi:https://dx.doi.org/10.1016/j.rdc.2015.08.007
38. Buckley L, Guyatt G, Fink HA, et al. 2017 American College of Rheumatology guideline for the prevention and treatment of glucocorticoid-induced osteoporosis. *Arthritis Care Res (Hoboken).* 2017;69(8):1095–1110. doi:https://dx.doi.org/10.1002/acr.23279
39. Xiong W, Lahita RG. Pragmatic approaches to therapy for systemic lupus erythematosus. Review. *Nat Rev Rheumatol.* 2014;10(2):97–107. doi:http://dx.doi.org/10.1038/nrrheum.2013.157
40. Mehat P, Atiquzzaman M, Esdaile JM, et al. Medication nonadherence in systemic lupus erythematosus: A systematic review. *Arthritis Care Res (Hoboken).* 2017;69(11):1706–1713. doi:https://dx.doi.org/10.1002/acr.23191
41. Mazzoni D, Cicognani E, Prati G. Health-related quality of life in systemic lupus erythematosus: A longitudinal study on the impact of problematic support and self-efficacy. *Lupus.* 2017;26(2):125–131. doi:https://dx.doi.org/10.1177/0961203316646459
42. Rodriguez Huerta MD, Trujillo-Martin MM, Rua-Figueroa I, et al. Healthy lifestyle habits for patients with systemic lupus erythematosus: A systemic review. *Semin Arthritis Rheum.* 2016;45(4):463–470. doi:https://dx.doi.org/10.1016/j.semarthrit.2015.09.003
43. Patterson SL, Schmajuk G, Jafri K, et al. Obesity is independently associated with worse patient-reported outcomes in women with systemic lupus erythematosus. *Arthritis Care Res (Hoboken).* 2019;71(1):126–133. doi:10.1002/acr.23576
44. Shi H, Gudjonsson JE, Kahlenberg JM. Treatment of cutaneous lupus erythematosus: Current approaches and future strategies. *Curr Opin Rheumatol.* 2020;32(3):208–214. doi:https://dx.doi.org/10.1097/BOR.0000000000000704

45. Leandro M, Isenberg DA. Rituximab—The first twenty years. *Lupus.* 2021;30(3):371–377. doi:https://dx.doi.org/10.1177/0961203320982668
46. Bertsias GK, Ioannidis JP, Aringer M, et al. EULAR recommendations for the management of systemic lupus erythematosus with neuropsychiatric manifestations: Report of a task force of the EULAR standing committee for clinical affairs. *Ann Rheum Dis.* 2010;69(12):2074–2082. doi:http://dx.doi.org/10.1136/ard.2010.130476
47. Fanouriakis A, Kostopoulou M, Cheema K, et al. 2019 Update of the Joint European League Against Rheumatism and European Renal Association-European Dialysis and Transplant Association (EULAR/ERA-EDTA) recommendations for the management of lupus nephritis. *Ann Rheum Dis.* 2020;79(6):713–723. doi:https://dx.doi.org/10.1136/annrheumdis-2020-216924
48. Kiriakidou M, Ching CL. Systemic lupus erythematosus. *Ann Intern Med.* 2020;172(11):ITC81–ITC96. doi:https://dx.doi.org/10.7326/AITC202006020
49. Cortés-Hernández J, Egri N, Vilardell-Tarrés M, et al. Etanercept in refractory lupus arthritis: An observational study. *Semin Arthritis Rheum.* 2015;44(6):672–679. doi:http://dx.doi.org/10.1016/j.semarthrit.2015.01.006
50. Worm M, Zidane M, Eisert L, et al. S2k guideline: Diagnosis and management of cutaneous lupus erythematosus—Part 2: Therapy, risk factors and other special topics. *J Dtsch Dermatol Ges.* 2021;19(9):1371–1395. doi:10.1111/ddg.14491
51. Tanaka Y, Tummala R. Anifrolumab, a monoclonal antibody to the type I interferon receptor subunit 1, for the treatment of systemic lupus erythematosus: An overview from clinical trials. *Mod Rheumatol.* 2021;31(1):1–12. doi:https://dx.doi.org/10.1080/14397595.2020.1812201
52. Ruiz-Irastorza G, Bertsias G. Treating systemic lupus erythematosus in the 21st century: New drugs and new perspectives on old drugs. *Rheumatology.* 2020;59(Suppl5):v69–v81. doi:https://dx.doi.org/10.1093/rheumatology/keaa403
53. Goodman SM, Springer B, Guyatt G, et al. 2017 American College of Rheumatology/American Association of Hip and Knee Surgeons guideline for the perioperative management of antirheumatic medication in patients with rheumatic diseases undergoing elective total hip or total knee arthroplasty. *Arthritis Rheumatol.* 2017;69(8):1538–1551. doi:https://doi.org/10.1002/art.40149
54. MacKenzie CR, Goodman SM. Stress dose steroids: Myths and perioperative medicine. *Curr Rheumatol Rep.* 2016;18(7):47. doi:https://dx.doi.org/10.1007/s11926-016-0595-7
55. Ponticelli C, Moroni G. Hydroxychloroquine in systemic lupus erythematosus (SLE). *Expert Opin Drug Saf.* 2017;16(3):411–419. doi:https://dx.doi.org/10.1080/14740338.2017.1269168
56. Costedoat-Chalumeau N, Dunogue B, Morel N, et al. Hydroxychloroquine: A multifaceted treatment in lupus. *Presse Med.* 2014;43(6 Pt 2):e167–e180. doi:http://dx.doi.org/10.1016/j.lpm.2014.03.007
57. Mok CC. Therapeutic monitoring of the immuno-modulating drugs in systemic lupus erythematosus. *Expert Rev Clin Immunol.* 2017;13(1):35–41. doi:https://dx.doi.org/10.1080/1744666X.2016.1212659
58. Rosenbaum JT, Costenbader KH, Desmarais J, et al. American College of Rheumatology, American Academy of Dermatology, Rheumatologic Dermatology Society, and American Academy of Ophthalmology 2020 joint statement on hydroxychloroquine use with respect to retinal toxicity. *Arthritis Rheumatol.* 2021;73(6):908–911. doi:https://dx.doi.org/10.1002/art.41683
59. Ginzler E, Guedes Barbosa LS, D'Cruz D, et al. Phase III/IV, randomized, fifty-two-week study of the efficacy and safety of belimumab in patients of Black African ancestry with systemic lupus erythematosus. *Arthritis Rheumatol.* 2022;74(1):112–123. doi:https://doi.org/10.1002/art.41900
60. Furie R, Rovin BH, Houssiau F, et al. Two-year, randomized, controlled trial of belimumab in lupus nephritis. *N Engl J Med.* 2020;383(12):1117–1128. doi:10.1056/NEJMoa2001180
61. Eko SL, van Vollenhoven RF. Rituximab and lupus: A promising pair? *Curr Rheumatol Rep.* 2014;16(9):444. doi:http://dx.doi.org/10.1007/s11926-014-0444-5
62. Monach PA, Arnold LM, Merkel PA. Incidence and prevention of bladder toxicity from cyclophosphamide in the treatment of rheumatic diseases: A data-driven review. *Arthritis Rheum.* 2010;62(1):9–21. doi:http://dx.doi.org/10.1002/art.25061
63. Dall'Era M, Stone D, Levesque V, et al. Identification of biomarkers that predict response to treatment of lupus nephritis with mycophenolate mofetil or pulse cyclophosphamide. *Arthritis Care Res (Hoboken).* 2011;63(3):351–357. doi:http://dx.doi.org/10.1002/acr.20397
64. Dooley MA, Jayne D, Ginzler EM, et al. Mycophenolate versus azathioprine as maintenance therapy for lupus nephritis. *N Engl J Med.* 2011;365(20):1886–1895. doi:http://dx.doi.org/10.1056/NEJMoa1014460
65. Tamirou F, D'Cruz D, Sangle S, et al. Long-term follow-up of the MAINTAIN Nephritis Trial, comparing azathioprine and mycophenolate mofetil as maintenance therapy of lupus nephritis. *Ann Rheum Dis.* 2016;75(3):526–531. doi:https://dx.doi.org/10.1136/annrheumdis-2014-206897
66. Petri M. Pregnancy and systemic lupus erythematosus. *Best Pract Res Clin Obstet Gynaecol.* 2020;64:24–30. doi:https://dx.doi.org/10.1016/j.bpobgyn.2019.09.002
67. Liu YP, Xu HQ, Li M, et al. Association between thiopurine S-methyltransferase polymorphisms and azathioprine-induced adverse drug reactions in patients with autoimmune diseases: A meta-analysis. *PLoS ONE.* 2015;10(12):e0144234. doi:10.1371/journal.pone.0144234
68. Schmajuk G, Yazdany J. Drug monitoring in systemic lupus erythematosus: A systematic review. *Semin Arthritis Rheum.* 2011;40(6):559–575. doi:http://dx.doi.org/10.1016/j.semarthrit.2010.07.010
69. Heo YA. Voclosporin: First approval. *Drugs.* 2021;81(5):605–610. doi:https://dx.doi.org/10.1007/s40265-021-01488-z
70. Saxena AMC, Coeshall A. Voclosporin for lupus nephritis: Interim analysis of the AURORA 2 extension study [abstract 1425]. *Arthritis Rheumatol.* 2021;73(Suppl 10)
71. Greco CM, Nakajima C, Manzi S. Updated review of complementary and alternative medicine treatments for systemic lupus erythematosus. *Curr Rheumatol Rep.* 2013;15(11):378. doi:http://dx.doi.org/10.1007/s11926-013-0378-3
72. Hannon CW, McCourt C, Lima HC, et al. Interventions for cutaneous disease in systemic lupus erythematosus. *Cochrane Database Syst Rev.* 2021;3:CD007478. doi:https://dx.doi.org/10.1002/14651858.CD007478.pub2
73. Dall'Ara F, Cutolo M, Andreoli L, et al. Vitamin D and systemic lupus erythematosus: A review of immunological and clinical aspects. *Clin Exp Rheumatol.* 2018;36(1):153–162.
74. Shoenfeld Y, Giacomelli R, Azrielant S, et al. Vitamin D and systemic lupus erythematosus—The hype and the hope. *Autoimmun Rev.* 2018;17(1):19–23. doi:https://dx.doi.org/10.1016/j.autrev.2017.11.004
75. Sammaritano LR, Bermas BL, Chakravarty EE, et al. 2020 American College of Rheumatology guideline for the management of reproductive health in rheumatic and musculoskeletal diseases. *Arthritis Rheumatol.* 2020;72(4):529–556. doi:https://dx.doi.org/10.1002/art.41191
76. Sammaritano LR. Contraception and preconception counseling in women with autoimmune disease. *Best Pract Res Clin Obstet Gynaecol.* 2020;64:11–23. doi:https://dx.doi.org/10.1016/j.bpobgyn.2019.09.003
77. Lateef A, Petri M. Systemic lupus erythematosus and pregnancy. *Rheum Dis Clin North Am.* 2017;43(2):215–226. doi:https://dx.doi.org/10.1016/j.rdc.2016.12.009
78. Moroni G, Doria A, Giglio E, et al. Maternal outcome in pregnant women with lupus nephritis. A prospective multicenter study. *J Autoimmun.* 2016;74:194–200. doi:https://dx.doi.org/10.1016/j.jaut.2016.06.012
79. Ruiz-Irastorza G, Martin-Iglesias D, Soto-Peleteiro A. Update on antimalarials and systemic lupus erythematosus. *Curr Opin Rheumatol.* 2020;32(6):572–582. doi:https://dx.doi.org/10.1097/BOR.0000000000000743
80. Andreoli L, Bertsias GK, Agmon-Levin N, et al. EULAR recommendations for women's health and the management of family planning, assisted reproduction, pregnancy and menopause in patients with systemic lupus erythematosus and/or antiphospholipid syndrome. *Ann Rheum Dis.* 2017;76(3):476–485. doi:https://dx.doi.org/10.1136/annrheumdis-2016-209770
81. Taulaigo AV, Moschetti L, Ganhao S, et al. Safety considerations when using drugs in pregnant patients with systemic lupus erythematosus. *Expert Opin Drug Saf.* 2021;20(5):523–536. doi:10.1080/14740338.2021.1893298
82. Belizna C, Meroni PL, Shoenfeld Y, et al. In utero exposure to azathioprine in autoimmune disease. Where do we stand? *Autoimmun Rev.* 2020;19(9):102525. doi:https://doi.org/10.1016/j.autrev.2020.102525
83. Uthman I, Noureldine MHA, Ruiz-Irastorza G, et al. Management of antiphospholipid syndrome. *Ann Rheum Dis.* 2019;78(2):155–161. doi:10.1136/annrheumdis-2018-213846
84. Pons-Estel GJ, Andreoli L, Scanzi F, et al. The antiphospholipid syndrome in patients with systemic lupus erythematosus. *J Autoimmun.* 2017;76:10–20. doi:https://dx.doi.org/10.1016/j.jaut.2016.10.004

85. Gomez-Puerta JA, Cervera R. Diagnosis and classification of the antiphospholipid syndrome. *J Autoimmun.* 2014;48-49:20–25. doi:http://dx.doi.org/10.1016/j.jaut.2014.01.006
86. Alijotas-Reig J. Treatment of refractory obstetric antiphospholipid syndrome: The state of the art and new trends in the therapeutic management. *Lupus.* 2013;22(1):6–17. doi:http://dx.doi.org/10.1177/0961203312465782
87. Baer AN, Witter FR, Petri M. Lupus and pregnancy. *Obstet Gynecol Surv.* 2011;66(10):639–653. doi:http://dx.doi.org/10.1097/OGX.0b013e318239e1ee
88. Haugaard JH, Kofoed K, Gislason G, et al. Association between drug use and subsequent diagnosis of lupus erythematosus. *JAMA Dermatol.* 2020;156(11):1199–1207. doi:https://dx.doi.org/10.1001/jamadermatol.2020.2786
89. He Y, Sawalha AH. Drug-induced lupus erythematosus: An update on drugs and mechanisms. *Curr Opin Rheumatol.* 2018;30(5):490–497. doi:https://dx.doi.org/10.1097/BOR.0000000000000522
90. Araujo-Fernandez S, Ahijon-Lana M, Isenberg DA. Drug-induced lupus: Including anti-tumour necrosis factor and interferon induced. *Lupus.* 2014;23(6):545–553. doi:http://dx.doi.org/10.1177/0961203314523871
91. Lomicova I, Suchy D, Pizinger K, et al. A case of lupus-like syndrome in a patient receiving adalimumab and a brief review of the literature on drug-induced lupus erythematosus. *J Clin Pharm Ther.* 2017;42(3):363–366. doi:https://dx.doi.org/10.1111/jcpt.12506
92. Furer V, Rondaan C, Heijstek MW, et al. 2019 update of EULAR recommendations for vaccination in adult patients with autoimmune inflammatory rheumatic diseases. *Ann Rheum Dis.* 2020;79(1):39–52. doi:10.1136/annrheumdis-2019-215882
93. Garg M, Mufti N, Palmore TN, et al. Recommendations and barriers to vaccination in systemic lupus erythematosus. *Autoimmun Rev.* 2018;17(10):990–1001. doi:https://dx.doi.org/10.1016/j.autrev.2018.04.006
94. Friedman MA, Winthrop K. Vaccinations for rheumatoid arthritis. *Curr Opin Rheumatol.* 2016;28(3):330–336. doi:10.1097/BOR.0000000000000281
95. Centers for Disease Control and Prevention (CDC). Vaccines & immunizations. Accessed January 13, 2022. https://www.cdc.gov/vaccines/
96. Tofighi T, Morand EF, Touma Z. Systemic lupus erythematosus outcome measures for systemic lupus erythematosus clinical trials. *Rheum Dis Clin North Am.* 2021;47(3):415–426. doi:10.1016/j.rdc.2021.04.007
97. Gordon C, Amissah-Arthur MB, Gayed M, et al. The British Society for Rheumatology guideline for the management of systemic lupus erythematosus in adults. *Rheumatology (Oxford).* 2018;57(1):e1–e45. doi:https://dx.doi.org/10.1093/rheumatology/kex286
98. Yazdany J, Panopalis P, Gillis JZ, et al. A quality indicator set for systemic lupus erythematosus. *Arthritis Rheum.* 2009;61:370–377. doi:10.1002/art.24356

e108

Drug Allergy

Mary L. Staicu, Christopher M. Bland, and Bruce M. Jones

KEY CONCEPTS

1. Drug allergy accounts for 6% to 10% of adverse drug reactions to medications. Most of these immune events are mediated by IgE or activated T cells.
2. Three theories—the prohapten/hapten concept, the p-i concept, and the altered repertoire model—have been proposed to explain how drugs stimulate an immune response.
3. Anaphylaxis is an acute, life-threatening allergic reaction involving multiple organ systems that generally begins within 1 hour but almost always within 2 hours after exposure to the inciting allergen. Anaphylaxis requires prompt treatment to restore respiratory and cardiovascular functions. Epinephrine is the drug of first choice and should be administered to counteract bronchoconstriction and peripheral vasodilation. Intravenous fluids should be administered aggressively to restore intravascular volume.
4. Factors that influence the likelihood of drug allergy are the drug's chemical composition, whether the drug contains proteins of nonhuman origin, the route of drug administration, and the individual's sensitivity as determined by genetics or environmental factors. For some drugs, the presence of specific human leukocyte antigen alleles is a risk factor for allergic skin reactions.
5. Ideally, cephalosporins should be avoided in patients with a history of an immediate penicillin allergy, but the risk of an allergic cross-response to a cephalosporin, even in a person with a positive penicillin skin test result, is low. Similarities in the R1 side chain of the agents should be considered when assessing the risk of β-lactam cross-reactivity.
6. Cross-reactivity between sulfonamide antibiotics and nonantibiotics is low. The low cross-reactive rate may be explained by differences in the chemical structures and reactive metabolites of sulfonamide antibiotics and nonantibiotics.
7. In susceptible patients, aspirin and other nonsteroidal anti-inflammatory drugs (NSAIDs) can produce two general types of reactions, urticaria/angioedema and rhinosinusitis/asthma. Most patients with aspirin sensitivity who require aspirin for the prevention of cardiovascular disease can safely undergo and complete a graded challenge or induction of drug tolerance (previously known as desensitization).
8. Fewer than 1% of patients receiving nonionic radiocontrast agents experience some type of adverse reaction. Of the variety of reactions reported, about 90% are nonimmediate and mostly urticarial, with severe immediate reactions occurring as infrequently as 0.02%.
9. The basic principles of management of allergic reactions to drugs or biologic agents include (a) discontinuation of the medication or offending agent when possible; (b) treatment of the adverse clinical signs and symptoms; and (c) substitution, if necessary, of another agent.
10. The penicillin skin test is the reference standard for evaluating the risk of immediate hypersensitivity to penicillin. Skin testing can demonstrate the presence of penicillin-specific immunoglobulin E, if present, and predict immediate reactions. Skin testing is not indicated for non-IgE-mediated reactions.
11. When an allergenic drug is considered medically necessary and no therapeutic alternative or reliable skin testing method exists, three options are available to the clinician: induction of drug tolerance, graded dose challenge, or rechallenge.

BEYOND THE BOOK

Listen to the podcast series entitled "The Itch: An SIDP Podcast Miniseries on Penicillin Allergy" (broadcast on June 26, 2019): https://sidp.org/podcasts/ (or https://sidp.pinecast.co/ and click "Back in time"). These podcasts led by drug allergy experts in the pharmacy field discuss various topics including myth-busting with regards to penicillin allergies (#1), how to successfully implement penicillin skin testing (#2), and finally "lessons learned from the front-line" (#3) to help those interested in developing a comprehensive penicillin allergy assessment and skin test program.

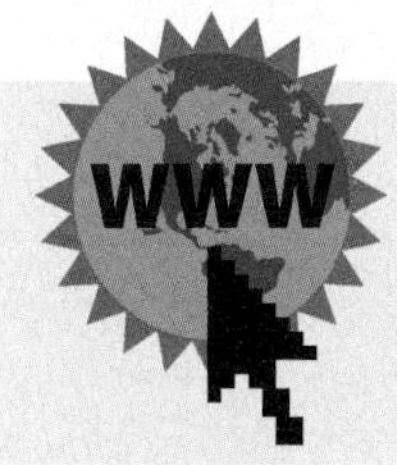

The complete chapter, learning objectives, and other resources can be found at **www.pharmacotherapyonline.com.**

109

Solid-Organ Transplantation

Nicholas W. Lange, David M. Salerno, and Douglas L. Jennings

KEY CONCEPTS

1. Generally, patients receive a combination of two to four immunosuppressive drugs in order to minimize individual drug toxicities as well as block different pathways of the immune response.
2. Antibody preparations that target specific receptors on T cells are classified based on their ability to deplete lymphocyte counts. Most lymphocyte-depleting antibodies are associated with infusion-related reactions, whereas non-depleting agents are generally well tolerated.
3. While the calcineurin inhibitors (CNI) tacrolimus and cyclosporineare the backbone of most immunosuppressive regimens, they are associated with serious adverse effects.
4. Calcineurin inhibitor-induced nephrotoxicity is one of the most common adverse effects observed in solid-organ transplant recipients. Therapeutic drug monitoring is used to optimize the use of calcineurin inhibitors and limit toxicity.
5. Corticosteroids are often a component of immunosuppressive protocols. Their adverse effects have led to steroid-minimizing and steroid-free immunosuppressive regimens. Corticosteroids, however, remain a first-line treatment for allograft rejection.
6. Azathioprine and mycophenolic acid derivatives inhibit T-cell proliferation by altering purine synthesis. Bone marrow suppression is the most significant adverse effect associated with these agents.
7. Sirolimus and everolimus inhibit the mTOR (mammalian target of rapamycin) receptor, which alters T-cell responses to IL-2. The adverse effects associated with these agents include leukopenia, thrombocytopenia, anemia, hyperlipidemia, and impaired wound healing.
8. Immunosuppressive agents are frequently involved in drug-drug and drug-food interactions; thus careful assessments of entire drug regimens are paramount.
9. Long-term allograft and patient survival are limited by chronic rejection, cardiovascular disease, infection, and malignancy.

BEYOND THE BOOK

Visit the International Society for Heart and Lung Transplantation Website <https://ishlt.org>. This Website contains many useful links, including links to many registries that track outcomes in patients who have undergone heart or lung transplantation. Access the International Thoracic Organ Transplant (TTX) Registry Data slides <https://ishltregistries.org/registries/slides.asp>, and review the Adult Heart Transplantation Statistics. Focus on the slides that pertain to immunosuppression regimens and outcomes. This will aid in the ASSESS and PLAN steps in the patient care process.

INTRODUCTION

Solid-organ transplantation provides a potentially life-saving treatment for patients with end-stage kidney, liver, lung, heart, and intestinal diseases. Over 300 US hospitals offer transplant services, and pharmacists are an integral part of the transplant team.[1] In 2016, almost 600 pharmacists were members of the American College of Clinical Pharmacy's Transplant Practice and Research Network, and more than 65% of responding centers have a pharmacist on their transplant teams.[2] The Centers for Medicare and Medicaid Services regulations require that transplant programs have a multidisciplinary team including representatives from medicine, nursing, nutrition, social services, transplant coordination, and a clinician with experience in pharmacology. While the regulations do not specifically state that each center must include a pharmacist, a pharmacist provides the necessary expertise in transplant pharmacotherapy.

Since 1980, over 630,000 transplants have been performed in the United States, with over half being kidney transplants. A recent analysis estimated that since 1987 over 2.27 million life-years have been saved by transplantation, with an average of 4.3 years per patient.[3] Demand for transplantation continues to grow; since 2010, there has been growth in transplant volume across most all organ types (kidney = 37%, liver = 41%, heart = 52%, lung = 52%).[1] This has been made possible through iterative improvements in the way in which sparsely available organs are allocated to patients with end-stage organ disease. Living donors now account for one-third of all kidney transplants, more than any other organ. Living-donor liver transplantation is also becoming increasingly more common. Efforts to expand the cadaveric donor pool have included relaxation of age restrictions, development of better preservation solutions, deployment of machine perfusion pumps, use of "extended-criteria" and non-heart-beating donors, and the transplantation of split liver allografts into different liver transplant recipients. An increase in deaths related to drug overdose has also resulted in an increased number of organs, often times from donors infected with hepatitis C virus (HCV). With the availability of curative treatments for HCV infection, some transplant recipients may be willing to accept

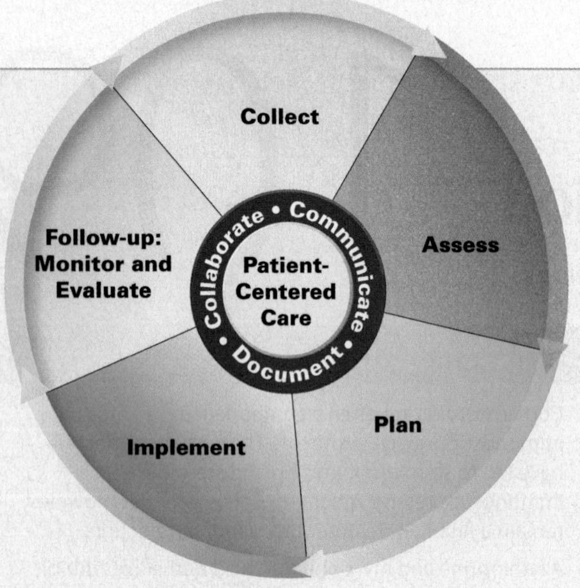

Patient Care Process for Solid-Organ Transplant Recipient*

Collect

- Patient characteristics (eg, age, sex, pregnancy status)
- Patient medical history (personal and family)
- Social history (eg, tobacco/ethanol use/marijuana), dietary habits
- Current medications including OTC agents, herbal products, dietary supplements
- Objective data
  - Blood pressure (BP), heart rate (HR), respiratory rate (RR), temperature (T), height, weight, O_2-saturation
  - Labs including the measure of end-organ function, hemoglobin (Hgb), platelets, serum creatinine (SCr), immunosuppressant concentrations, white blood cell (WBC) count

Assess

- Presence of over immunosuppression: infectious, adverse drug events
- Presence of under immunosuppression: evidence of end-organ compromise/rejection
- Assess risks based on patient-specific risk factors and time post-transplant

Plan**

- Drug therapy regimen including specific immunosuppressive agents, dose, route, frequency, and duration (Fig. 109-2)
- Monitoring parameters including efficacy (eg, signs and symptoms of rejection) and safety (eg, CBC, SCr, constitutional symptoms); frequency and timing of follow-up
- Patient education (eg, purpose of treatment, dietary and lifestyle restriction, drug-specific information, medication administration)
- Signs and symptoms of rejection (urine output, BP, pain, fever) or infection (temperature) (see Table 109-3)
- Self-monitoring for signs/symptoms of adverse effects (see Table 109-6)
- Referrals to other providers when appropriate

Implement

- Provide patient education regarding all elements of the treatment plan
- Use motivational interviewing and coaching strategies to maximize adherence
- Schedule follow-up (eg, CNI concentration, SCr)

Follow-up: Monitor and Evaluate

- Maintenance of graft functions
- Presence of adverse effects (eg, nephrotoxicity, tremor, hyperglycemia, hypertension, nausea, vomiting) (see Tables 109-6 and 109-7)
- Immunosuppressant TDM results (TAC, CSA, SIR, EVR); adjust IS dose as needed
- Patient adherence to treatment plan using multiple sources of information
- Re-evaluate immunosuppression/anti-infective goal of therapy every 3 months

*New solid-organ transplant recipient in the immediate post-op period.
**Collaborate with patient, caregivers, and other healthcare professionals.

a transplant from and HCV-infected donor. Although controversial, creation of a regulated system for compensating individuals financially for the "donation" of a kidney has been suggested.[4]

Despite these efforts, thousands of people on transplantation waiting lists die each year. Current initiatives to improve organ allocation have included allocation primarily on "medical necessity" versus time on the waiting list. Dialysis can be used for an extended period of time to partially replace the function of the kidneys, and more than half of recent heart transplant recipients receive left ventricular assist devices as a bridge to transplantation. Such life-extending therapies are not readily available for liver and lung transplant candidates, however.

Patient and graft survival rates following transplantation have improved dramatically over the past 30 years as a result of advances in pharmacotherapy, surgical techniques, organ preservation, and the postoperative management of patients (Table 109-1). In this chapter, the epidemiology of end-stage kidney, liver, lung, and heart diseases is briefly reviewed, the pathophysiology of organ rejection is presented, the pharmacotherapeutic options for individualized immunosuppressive regimens are explored in great detail, and the unique complications of these regimens along with the therapeutic challenges they present are discussed.

KIDNEY

Etiology of End-Stage Kidney Disease

End-stage kidney disease is defined as a glomerular filtration rate (GFR) of <15 mL/min/1.73 m^2 (0.14 mL/s/m^2) or receipt of renal

TABLE 109-1 Organ-Specific Patient and Graft Survival Rates

	Patient Survival (%)		Graft Survival (%)	
Organ	**1 year**	**5 years**	**1 year**	**5 years**
Kidney				
Living donor	97.9	89.4	97.5	85.6
Deceased donor	94.3	80.4	93.2	74.5
Liver				
Living donor	96.2	77.6	93	77.3
Deceased donor	93.8	71.9	92.1	71.9
Heart				
Cardiomyopathy			91.6	79.4
Coronary artery disease			89.1	71.9
Lung				
Single	85.8	35.8	85.4	45.5
Double	83.3	47.3	87.3	55.7

replacement therapy.[5] The most common causes of end-stage kidney disease (ESKD) leading to transplantation are diabetes, hypertension, glomerulonephritis, and polycystic kidney disease.[6]

Epidemiology

The number of prevalent ESKD patients in 2018 was 785,883, which increased by 3.2% relative to 2017.[7] The adjusted prevalence of ESKD increased to 2,242 cases per 1 million people in 2018 (a new high). The vast majority of patients with ESKD undergo intermittent hemodialysis treatment at a medical facility, though a growing percent of patients undergo home hemodialysis or peritoneal dialysis. The number of patients on the kidney transplant waiting list as of December 31, 2019, was 101,337 which was relatively unchanged compared to those on the waiting list as of December 31, 2014.[6] In 2019, a total of 24,273 kidney transplants were performed. This was an approximate 10% increase relative to the total number of kidney transplants performed in 2018.[6] This was largely driven by deceased donor transplants secondary to increasing acceptance of organs procured from HCV-positive donors. Patients who do not have compatible living donors are placed onto a national waiting list for a deceased donor kidney. Deceased donor kidneys are allocated by the Kidney Allocation System, which considers patient-specific factors such as time on the wait list or time undergoing dialysis, high degree of immune-sensitization, and patient age.[8,9]

At 1-year and 5-year post-transplantation, graft survival was 95.7% and 83.2%, respectively, among patients who underwent deceased donor transplantation between 2012 and 2014. Alternatively, recipients who underwent surgery in the same time period but received a kidney transplant from a living donor experienced 1-year and 5-year graft survival rates of 96.9% and 91.4%, respectively.[6] Median patient survival after kidney transplantation is 12 years.[10]

Physiologic Consequences of Transplantation

The glomerular filtration rate of a successfully transplanted kidney may be near normal almost immediately after transplantation. In some patients, however, the concentration of standard biochemical indicators of kidney function, such as serum creatinine and blood urea nitrogen, may remain elevated for several days or even weeks to months. Standard formulas used to predict drug dosing rely on a stable serum creatinine and thus may be inaccurate or misleading immediately following transplantation. Although the allograft is able to remove uremic toxins from the body, it may take several weeks for other physiologic complications of ESKD—such as anemia, calcium and phosphate imbalance, and altered lipid profiles—to resolve. The renal production of erythropoietin and 1-hydroxylation of vitamin D may return toward normal early in the postoperative period. Because the onset of physiologic effects may be delayed, continuation of the patient's pre-transplantation vitamin D, calcium supplementation, and/or phosphate binders may sometimes be warranted. Patients should be monitored for hypophosphatemia and hypercalcemia for the first few days to weeks after kidney transplantation.

Delayed graft function (DGF) is characterized by the need for dialysis in the first post-operative week.[11] The incidence of DGF in deceased donor kidney transplantation ranges from 10% to 50% and results in a slower return of the kidney's excretory, metabolic, and synthetic functions. DGF is associated with a prolonged hospital stay, higher costs, difficulty managing immunosuppression, slower patient rehabilitation, and lower graft survival.[12] Other early causes of impaired kidney function such as ureteral obstruction, renal artery stenosis, or other technical vascular complications, thrombosis, or rejection should be distinguished from DGF.

General Immunosuppressive Strategy Considerations

Induction

Potent immunosuppressive agents administered parenterally around the time of transplant surgery are referred to as induction therapies. The goal of administering induction immunosuppression is to prevent early cellular- or antibody-mediated.[13] Induction therapies are antibody preparations given most typically along with high doses of corticosteroids. They can be categorized as depleting or non-depleting.[14] Depleting agents include anti-thymocyte globulin preparations (Thymoglobulin, Atgam) and alemtuzumab, whereas the only non-depleting agent is basiliximab. In 2019, 91% of kidney transplant recipients received induction immunosuppression at the time of transplantation.[6] Among kidney transplant recipients at a higher risk for rejection (eg, those undergoing repeat transplantation or those with pre-formed antibodies against their donor) depleting agents should be preferentially administered due to their superiority at preventing acute rejection.[15-17]

Maintenance

Maintenance immunosuppressive therapies are administered to transplant recipients for the duration of the functional life of their transplanted organ, also with the goal of preventing acute rejection. Maintenance immunosuppression regimens are most commonly composed of different agents targeting different pathways or immune system effector cells to ensure adequate immunosuppression as well as increase drug tolerability. The most commonly deployed agents in maintenance immunosuppressive cocktails include the calcineurin inhibitors, anti-metabolites, mammalian target of rapamycin (mTOR) inhibitors, co-stimulation antagonists, and corticosteroids.[18] Between the two available calcineurin inhibitors, tacrolimus is more potent and is generally preferred over cyclosporine due to a decrease in the incidence of acute rejection.[19,20] Similarly, mycophenolate is generally the preferred anti-metabolite relative to azathioprine.[21] These drugs will all be reviewed in detail later in this chapter.

In 2019, the vast majority of kidney transplant recipients were initiated on regimens consisting of tacrolimus (a calcineurin inhibitor; CNI), mycophenolate (an anti-metabolite), +/− a corticosteroid.[6] Belatacept, a co-stimulation antagonist that first gained FDA approval for use in kidney transplantation in 2011, has been incorporated into CNI-sparing or CNI-avoiding immunosuppressive regimens in kidney transplant recipients owing to its more tolerable side effect profile and potential to improve long-term patient and graft outcomes.[22,23]

LIVER

Etiology of End-Stage Liver Disease

Noncholestatic cirrhosis (hepatitis C, alcoholic cirrhosis, hepatitis B, nonalcoholic steatohepatitis, and autoimmune hepatitis) is the primary cause of end-stage liver disease, and more than 70% of liver transplant recipients have been diagnosed with one of these conditions.[24] Other indications for transplantation include acute liver failure, autoimmune hepatitis, primary biliary cholangitis, and primary sclerosing cholangitis. Nonalcoholic steatohepatitis represents a growing indication for liver transplantation, while hepatitis C-related indications are declining.

In general, active substance abuse has been a contraindication to liver transplantation, but given the high mortality for acute alcoholic hepatitis and the current lack of viable treatments, this is an area of growing research worldwide. A number of US centers have expanded transplantation in this patient population.[25] Additionally, active or recent malignancy is a contraindication to any transplantation, with the exception of hepatocellular carcinoma meeting specified criteria for liver transplantation.[26,27]

Epidemiology

According to the CDC National Center for Health Statistics 2018 report, there are 4.5 million adults diagnosed with liver disease in the United States, which resulted in nearly 45,000 deaths attributable to liver disease.[28] In 2019, the total prevalence of patients on the United States liver transplant waitlist was over 25,000. However, only 8,896 patients underwent liver transplantation.[24]

Liver allografts are allocated based on a United Network for Organ Sharing-adapted Model for End-stage Liver Disease (MELD) score.[29,30] This score—which is calculated from the patient's serum creatinine concentration, total serum bilirubin concentration, international normalized ratio, and serum sodium concentration—accurately predicts short-term mortality in patients with cirrhosis. Patients listed for liver transplants are prioritized based on acuity, as measured by MELD score, rather than time on the waitlist.

The median survival after liver transplantation is 11 years and is increasing in recent years. Graft failure occurred in 6.6% of deceased-donor liver transplant recipients at 6 months and 8.9% at 1 year for transplants performed in 2018. Five-year and 10-year patient survival is now 80% and 60%, respectively.[24]

Physiologic Consequences of Transplantation

The physiologic consequences of liver transplantation are complex, involving changes in both its metabolic and synthetic function. Postoperatively, the liver transplant recipient will likely have many fluid, electrolyte, and nutritional abnormalities. Biliary tract dysfunction may alter the absorption of fats and fat-soluble drugs.[31] Poor absorption of the lipid-soluble drug cyclosporine improves after successful liver transplantation and reestablishment of bile flow. Vitamin E deficiency and its neurologic complications are usually reversed after successful liver transplantation. In stable adult liver transplant patients, the concentrations of retinol and tocopherol are similar to those seen in normal healthy subjects, indicating recovery of liver production and excretion of bile salts needed for fat-soluble vitamin absorption. Table 109-2 summarizes the effects of liver transplantation on metabolism and renal elimination that are seen in the immediate postoperative period. Most of these changes resolve as liver function normalizes.

TABLE 109-2 Perioperative Changes in Drug Disposition and Elimination Following Liver Transplantation

	Result	Comment
Serum proteins		
↓ Albumin	↑ Free fraction of drugs usually bound to albumin	Diazepam, salicylic acid binding greater in liver transplant than in chronic liver disease because of endogenous binding inhibitors (up to 45 days post-transplant)
↑ Alpha-1-acid glycoprotein	Lower unbound fraction of drugs	Lidocaine
Metabolism/elimination		
Microsomal enzymes	↑ CYP2E1 activity	Increased drug metabolism (induction)
	↔ CYP2D6	Unaffected
	↓ CYP activity	Decreased drug elimination (inhibition)
Oxidation	Stable	
Conjugation	Normalizes after transplant	
Biliary function	↓ Absorption of lipophilic compounds	
	↑ Cyclosporine metabolites in blood	
Renal elimination	Elimination of gentamicin, vancomycin, cephalosporins less than predicted by serum creatinine	Renal elimination of metabolites limited

General Immunosuppressive Strategy Considerations

Induction

Antibody therapy is seldom used as induction in liver transplantation. In 2019, nearly 80% of liver transplant centers in the United States did not utilize induction therapy (with the exception of corticosteroids) due to the reduced immunogenicity of liver allografts relative to other solid organs.[24] Instead, both basiliximab and antithymocyte globulin have been utilized to allow for a delay in the introduction of CNIs in the setting of residual hepatic encephalopathy or renal dysfunction post-transplant.[32-34]

Maintenance

Maintenance immunosuppressive therapy for liver recipients in most transplant centers includes a CNI with an anti-metabolite agent with or without steroids.[24] More than 60% of transplant centers use three initial agents, though regimens consisting of two or four agents have also been utilized. mTOR inhibitors are infrequently used in maintenance regimens in liver transplant recipients, and use has been muted by an FDA-boxed warning outlining a risk of hepatic artery thrombosis when used within 30 days of transplant.[35] Belatacept is not utilized post-liver transplantation secondary to an increase in mortality following its use.[36]

LUNG

Etiology of End-Stage Lung Disease

End-stage lung disease is generally defined as the inability of the lungs to carry out routine gas exchange.[37] The most common causes of end-stage lung disease leading to transplantation are restrictive lung diseases (eg, idiopathic pulmonary fibrosis, sarcoidosis), cystic fibrosis, chronic obstructive pulmonary disease

(COPD), and pulmonary arterial hypertension.[38] The Pulmonary Transplantation Council of the International Society for Heart and Lung Transplantation (ISHLT) released an updated consensus document in 2014 outlining recommendations for selecting lung transplant candidates, which dictates that transplantation should only be offered to patients who (1) are at high risk (>50%) of death within 2 years if transplantation is not performed, (2) have a high likelihood (>80%) of surviving at least 90 days post-operatively, and (3) have a high likelihood (>80%) of surviving at least 5-year post-transplant assuming there is adequate lung allograft function.[39]

Epidemiology

There is no universally accepted definition for the diagnosis of end-stage lung disease and thus quantifying the incidence is challenging. Rather, conditions that lead to lung disease may have their own respective stages to quantify disease severity, such as with COPD. The Global Initiative for Chronic Obstructive Lung Disease defines stage 4 lung disease as an FEV_1 of <30% expected.[40] The number of patients on the lung transplant waiting list as of December 31, 2019, was 1,423 which was reduced compared to those on the waiting list as of December 31, 2014 (n = 1,683) due to the increasing rate of lung transplants performed annually.[38] In 2019, a total of 2,759 lung transplants were performed which was an increase of 7.6% relative to 2018.[38] Lung transplants are allocated on the basis of the Lung Allocation Score (LAS), which is calculated using patient-specific factors predictive of survival while on the waitlist as well as factors predictive of survival 1-year post-transplant.[41]

Relative to all other solid-organ transplant recipients, those patients who undergo lung transplantation experience the lowest overall survival at all measured time points.[38] In 2016, data analyzed from the ISHLT registry of all lung transplant recipients who underwent transplant between 1990 and 2014 indicated that median patient survival was 5.8 years.[42] Ten-year survival is approximately 33%.

Physiologic Consequences of Transplantation

In the absence of graft dysfunction, gas exchange and parameters of ventilation (tidal volume, minute ventilation, respiratory rate, etc.) after lung transplantation are generally normal relative to those of an otherwise healthy patient without lung disease. Notable differences in pulmonary physiology and function do exist, however. An impaired cough reflex and impaired mucociliary clearance due to at least partial pulmonary denervation increase the risk of infection.[43] Phrenic nerve injury during complex transplant surgery may lead to diaphragmatic paralysis, which complicates post-transplant rehabilitation and is associated with prolonged hospitalization.[44] Right ventricular dysfunction may be observed in the setting of post-operative pulmonary arterial hypertension (see Chapter 46).[45] Among recipients of single lung transplants (as compared to double lung transplantation), infections may develop in the allograft from a native lung source.[46] The upper airways are also a potential source of pulmonary infection, especially among patients with cystic fibrosis, who are often colonized with multi-drug resistant bacteria prior to transplantation.[47] Allograft dysfunction, regardless of the underlying causes, manifests most commonly as shortness of breath due to impaired gas exchange.

General Immunosuppressive Strategy Considerations

Induction

In 2019, 78% of lung transplant recipients received induction immunosuppression at the time of transplantation.[38] Evidence guiding the selection of induction agents in lung transplantation is often of lower quality. Single-center, retrospective evaluations generally indicate a lower incidence of acute rejection but a higher incidence of infections among recipients of depleting agents.[48]

Maintenance

In 2019, the vast majority of lung transplant recipients were initiated on regimens consisting of tacrolimus, mycophenolate, and a corticosteroid.[38] Tacrolimus is the only FDA-approved immunosuppressive agent for use in lung transplants, which can complicate lung transplant recipients' access to their necessary, life-sustaining medications.[49]

A serious, immunologically mediated complication post-lung transplantation is the development of bronchiolitis obliterans syndrome (BOS), also referred to as chronic lung allograft dysfunction (CLAD) or chronic rejection. There are no universally effective treatments for the management of BOS, but various therapeutic approaches have promise in preventing its development. These strategies may include the use of mTOR inhibitors in maintenance immunosuppression as well as the addition of azithromycin, montelukast, and even statins into medication regimens.[50-54]

HEART

Etiology of End-Stage Heart Disease

Advanced heart failure (ie, stage D) can be defined in several ways. Typically these patients have advanced symptoms (eg, New York Heart Association class III or IV) despite maximal medical management. Many patients with advanced heart failure will be frequently admitted to hospital, and most cannot tolerate adequate doses of standard heart failure drug therapies such as ACE inhibitors and beta-blockers.[55] Once in the advanced stage of the disease, patients have an expected 1-year mortality risk of 80% or greater without a heart transplant or a left-ventricular assist device implantation.[56] Idiopathic cardiomyopathy and ischemic heart disease account for heart failure in more than 90% of heart transplantation recipients.[57] Other etiologies include uncontrolled hypertension, valvular disease, genetic cardiomyopathy, chronic alcohol abuse, amyloidosis, cardiac sarcoidosis, congenital heart disease, peripartum cardiomyopathy, and retransplantation for graft atherosclerosis or dysfunction. The role of heart transplant as a therapeutic option for patients with heart failure is discussed in Chapter 36.

Epidemiology

From 2008 to 2019, the number of new listings for heart transplant in the United States increased by 42.5%, from 2,867 to 4,086.[57] The number of candidates awaiting heart transplant increased by 42.6% over 2008 to 2019, from 5,304 to 7,562. The median wait time in 2018 to 2019 was 5.1 months, the lowest in the past decade. The number of heart transplants performed in the United States has steadily risen, albeit slowly, and in 2019 was at 3,597. Adult death rates after heart transplant continued to decline; of those who underwent transplant in 2018, 6.4% died by 6 months and 7.9% died by 1 year.[57] The median survival after heart transplant surgery is 12 to 13 years.[58]

Physiologic Consequences of Transplantation

In the native heart, the sympathetic and parasympathetic nervous systems exert powerful control over heart rate and contractile force. During the surgery, the transplanted heart is denervated and no longer responds to physiologic stimuli and pharmacologic agents in a normal manner.[59] In situations requiring an increased heart rate such as exercise or hypotension, the denervated heart is unable to increase heart rate but instead relies on increasing the stroke volume. Later in the course of exercise or hypotension, heart rate increases in response to circulating catecholamines. While the maximum exercise capacity of heart transplant recipients is below normal, most patients are able to resume normal lifestyles and participate in reasonably vigorous activities.[59]

A number of autoregulatory and physiologic responses present in the normal heart are interrupted or blunted for the first 6 weeks after transplantation. The donor sinus node function may be impaired as the result of the preservation regimen, direct surgical trauma at excision, the presence of long-acting antiarrhythmics (eg, amiodarone) taken prior to transplant by the recipient, and a lack of "conditioning" responsiveness to catecholamines.[60] Consequently, the transplanted heart generally requires chronotropic support with either dobutamine, dopamine, or pacing in the perioperative period to maintain a heart rate greater than 110 beats/minute and satisfactory hemodynamics (ie, blood pressure, urine output, and tissue perfusion).[61]

Right ventricular function is frequently impaired, presumably as a result of preservation regimen injury and elevated pulmonary vascular resistance. Common treatments for right-heart failure include intra- or postoperative administration of pulmonary vasodilators (eg, nitric oxide) and inotropic agents like milrinone and dobutamine.[62]

A "restrictive" hemodynamic pattern may be present initially but usually improves in 6 weeks following transplantation. Donor–recipient size mismatch may contribute to early post-transplantation hemodynamic abnormalities characterized by higher right and left ventricular end-diastolic pressures. Tachyarrhythmia (eg, nonsustained ventricular tachycardia) is usually transient and may result from the use of catecholamines or milrinone.

Myocardial depression frequently occurs as a result of non-immune-related graft injury from cold ischemia and generally requires temporary inotropic support with agents such as dobutamine, milrinone, and epinephrine. Severe forms of myocardial depression/injury can manifest as sustained hypotension and low cardiac output—a syndrome known as primary graft dysfunction (PGD)—which can be severe enough to require temporary mechanical circulatory support.[63]

General Immunosuppressive Strategy Considerations

Induction

The available evidence does not suggest a consistent benefit for induction immunosuppression in terms of improving post-transplant survival or reducing rates of acute rejection after heart transplantation. As such, the use of induction therapy is not uniform, and fewer than 50% of heart transplant recipients receive this therapy at the time of surgery.[64] Considerations favoring the use of induction therapy after heart transplantation include high-risk immunologic features (ie, allosensitization) or the need to delay calcineurin inhibitor initiation in the setting of renal injury. Of the available agents, basiliximab is the most commonly used agent for induction, followed by thymoglobulin.[64]

Maintenance

The standard maintenance immunosuppression regimen immediately after heart transplantation is triple therapy with a calcineurin inhibitor (usually tacrolimus), mycophenolate mofetil, and prednisone. While most patients will remain on tacolimus and mycophenolate long-term, prednisone is frequently tapered off by the end of the first post-transplant year.[64] If patients develop chronic rejection or renal injury from calcineurin inhibitors, mTOR inhibitor can be substituted either for tacolimus or mycophenolate as long-term immunosuppression.[65] To date, newer agents like belatacept have not been studied after heart transplantation.

PATHOPHYSIOLOGY OF REJECTION

Rejection of a transplanted organ can take place at any time following surgery. Rejection can be differentiated based on time from transplantation (eg, early vs late) and/or by the pathophysiologic processes that underlie the rejection. Classically, this would include hyperacute rejection, acute, or chronic rejection, with further immunologic classification as either cellular rejection, antibody-mediated rejection, or some combination thereof.

General Concepts

Rejection is primarily mediated by activation of alloreactive lymphocytes (Fig. 109-1). T-cells and antigen-presenting cells (APC) such as B-cells, macrophages, and dendritic cells coordinate to create a toxic, inflammatory milieu targeting non-self tissue (eg, the transplanted organ).[66]

Chromosome 6 contains an extremely polymorphic region of DNA known as the human leukocyte antigen (HLA) system, which encodes the blueprint for the expression of self-antigen on every nucleated cell in the body.[67] The first event that occurs in the complex sequence of organ rejection is the recognition of foreign, non-self molecules. This is facilitated primarily by APC that recognizes either class I (eg, HLA-A, -B, and -C) or class II (HLA-DR, -DP, and -DQ) antigens that are expressed throughout the allograft. Antigen-specific T-cell activation proceeds, leading to graft injury/destruction. The specifics of this immune cascade of organ rejection are discussed in Chapter e106.

Hyperacute Rejection

Hyperacute rejection occurs when pre-formed donor-specific antibodies are present in the recipient at the time of the transplant. These may be anti-HLA antibodies or anti-ABO antibodies between donor and recipient with incompatible blood group types. Due to the "primed" nature of this immune response, it can be evident within minutes of graft reperfusion. Tissue damage is mediated through antibody-dependent, cell-mediated cytotoxicity, or through activation of the complement cascade. The ischemic damage to the microvasculature rapidly results in tissue necrosis and ultimately graft failure.[68]

Hyperacute rejection has become uncommon in solid-organ transplantation with the advent and subsequent advancement of crossmatching. A positive lymphocytotoxic crossmatch presents a serious risk for graft failure even if hyperacute rejection does not occur.[69] A negative crossmatch does not entirely rule out the possibility of hyperacute rejection because non-HLA antigens on the vascular endothelium can serve as targets of donor-specific antibodies.

Acute Cellular Rejection

Acute rejection is the most common form of allograft rejection, typically occurring in the first few months following transplantation, though it can occur at any time during the life of the allograft. With acute cellular rejection, alloreactive T-lymphocytes appear in the circulation and infiltrate the allograft through the vascular endothelium. Cytotoxic T-cells specifically target and damage functioning cells in the allograft. At the same time, local release of lymphokines attracts and stimulates macrophages to cause tissue damage through a delayed hypersensitivity-like mechanism. These immunologic and inflammatory events lead to nonspecific signs and symptoms that may include pain and tenderness over the graft site, fever, and lethargy. End-organ dysfunction is often evident, especially in patients with higher-grade ACR (Table 109-3). Strategies to reverse acute cellular rejection include the addition of an additional maintenance agent(s), bolus corticosteroids with a taper, and possibly lymphocyte-depleting therapy (Fig. 109-2).

Antibody-Mediated Rejection

Antibody-mediated rejection (AMR), sometimes referred to as vascular or humoral rejection, is characterized by the presence of donor-specific antibodies directed against HLA antigens present on

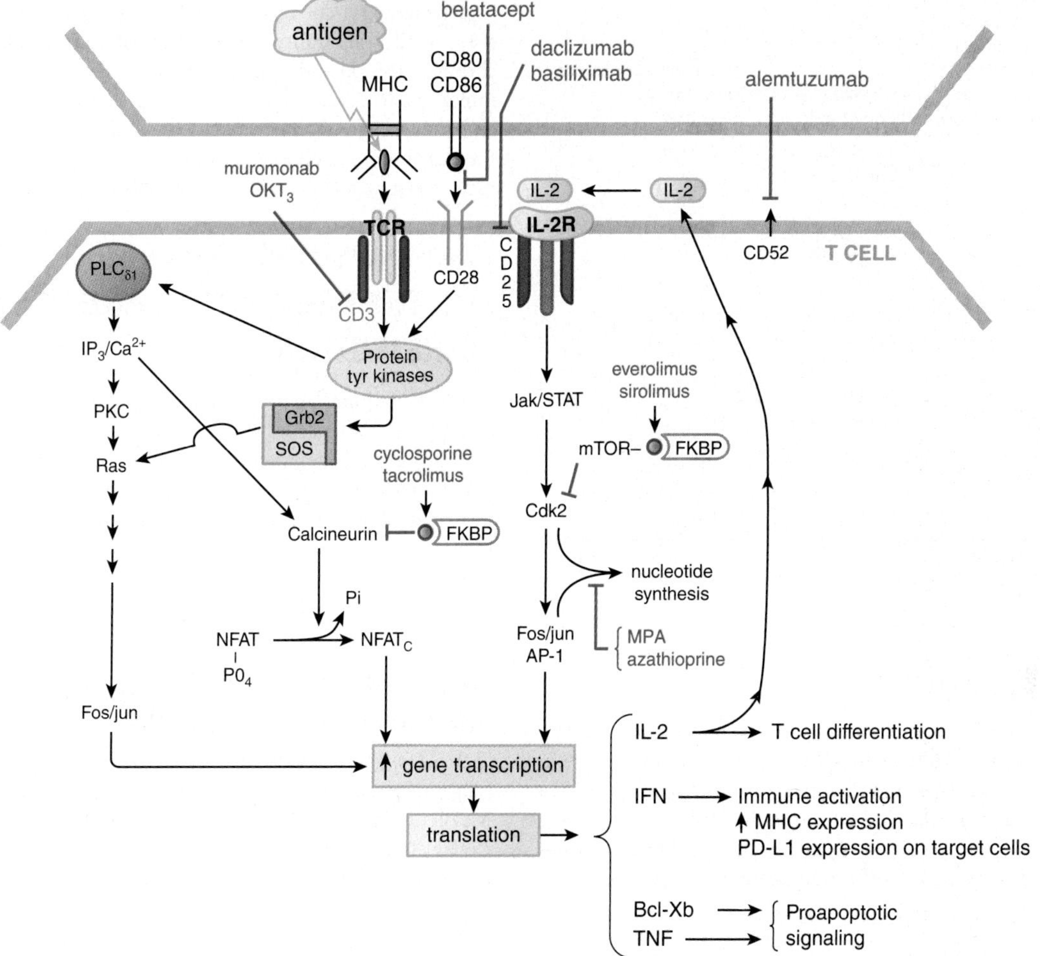

FIGURE 109-1 T-cell activation and sites of action of immunosuppressive agents. The TCR recognizes antigens bound to the MHC. A costimulatory signal is required for T-cell activation: the CD80/CD86-CD28 interaction from the APC to the T cell. Activation leads to IL-2 production (in a positive-feedback loop) and a host of other events, some of which are bracketed in the lower right-hand corner. Numerous agents are available to suppress T-cell activation. Belatacept blocks the CD80/CD86-CD28 interaction. Cyclosporine and tacrolimus bind to immunophilins (cyclophilin and FKBP, respectively), forming a complex that inhibits the phosphatase calcineurin and the calcineurin-catalyzed dephosphorylation that permits translocation of NFAT into the nucleus. NFAT is required for transcription of IL-2 and other growth and differentiation–associated cytokines (lymphokines). Sirolimus (rapamycin) and everolimus work downstream of the IL-2R, binding to FKBP; the FKBP-sirolimus complex binds to and inhibits the mTOR, a kinase involved in cell cycle progression (proliferation). MMF and azathioprine inhibit nucleic acid synthesis, thereby inhibiting T-cell proliferation. The antibody muromonab (OKT3) inhibits TCR function via interaction with its CD3 component. Daclizumab and basiliximab block IL-2 signaling by interacting with the alpha subunit of the IL-2R complex (CD25). Several antibodies can block the systemic effects of released TNF. Alemtuzumab, by binding to CD52, marks the cell for destruction, thereby depleting $CD52^+$ cells. (APC, antigen-presenting cell; FKBP, FK506-binding protein; IFN, interferon; IL-2R, interleukin 2 receptor; MHC, histocompatibility complex; mTOR, mammalian target of rapamycin; NFAT; nuclear factor of activated T lymphocytes; OKT3, muromonab CD3; PD-L1, programmed death ligand 1.) *(Adapted from Immunosuppressants and Tolerogens, Brunton LL, Hilal-Dandan R, Knollmann BC. Goodman & Gilman's: The Pharmacological Basis of Therapeutics, 13e; 2017.)*

the allograft vascular endothelium. The antibodies activate complement, which leads to the formation of the membrane attack complex that directly damages the allograft tissue and further attracts inflammatory cells. The resultant damage is histologically distinct from cellular rejection and involves microvascular injury.[70] Definitive diagnosis of AMR is based on the presence of three clinical features: presence of donor-specific antibodies, immunofluorescence staining of complement deposits in the microvasculature, and evidence of allograft dysfunction.[71,72] Circulating immune complexes often precede humoral rejection. This form of rejection is less common than cellular rejection and often occurs in the first 3 months after transplantation.[71] An increased risk of humoral rejection is associated with female sex, elevated PRA, and a positive crossmatch.[72] Strategies to reverse humoral rejection may include plasmapheresis, often in combination with intravenous immunoglobulin, high-dose intravenous corticosteroids, lymphocyte-depleting agents, proteasome inhibitors, rituximab, and augmented background maintenance immunosuppression.

TABLE 109-3 Acute Cellular Rejection After Transplant

	Percent of Patients with ≥1 Rejection Event Within the First Year Post-transplant	Signs/Symptoms of Rejection	Monitoring Strategies for Detecting Rejection
Kidney	7.1%	Elevated SCr, BUN, reduced UOP	Biopsy
Liver	12.3%	Elevated AST/ALT/Alkaline Phosphatase	Biopsy
Lung	16%	Reduced PFT, hypoxia, shortness of breath	PFT, bronchoscopy, biopsy
Heart	25.1%	Reduced ejection fraction, new dysrhythmia, overt heart failure	Right heart catheterization, echocardiogram, electrocardiogram, biopsy

SCr, serum creatinine; BUN, blood urea nitrogen; UOP, urine output; AST, aspartate transaminase; ALT, alanine transaminase; PFT, pulmonary function tests.

Chronic Rejection

Chronic rejection is a major cause of graft loss. It presents as a slow and indolent form of ACR, in which the humoral immune system and antibodies against the vascular endothelium appear to play a role. Persistent perivascular and interstitial inflammation is a common finding. As a result of the complex interaction of multiple drugs and diseases over time, it is difficult to delineate the true nature of chronic rejection. While chronic rejection of the kidney, liver, or lung allograft is generally not amenable to drug therapy, 3-hydroxy-3-methylglutaryl-coenzyme A (HMGCoA) reductase inhibitors are given to all heart transplant recipients to decrease the incidence of chronic rejection and prolong survival (Table 109-4).[73] The mTOR inhibitors sirolimus and everolimus may also decrease the incidence and slow progression of cardiac allograft vasculopathy; however, these agents are hampered by side effects and cannot be used in the early post-transplant setting (Table 109-4).[73]

IMMUNOSUPPRESSIVE MEDICATIONS FOR THE PREVENTION AND TREATMENT OF REJECTION

Rejection is both prevented and treated with combination drug therapy. A multi-drug approach is rational because immunotherapy agents have potentially synergistic mechanisms of action. Furthermore, the use of a multi-drug immunosuppression regimen may allow the use of lower doses of individual agents, thus reducing the severity of dose-related adverse effects (Fig. 109-2). Immunosuppression protocols tend to be medical center specific, and further tailoring of patient-specific regimens is standard practice.[61,74,75]

Depleting Antibody Therapies

Anti-thymocyte Globulin (ATG)

Two ATG formulations are available in the United States: ATG (Atgam, Pfizer, New York, NY), an equine polyclonal antibody, and RATG (Thymoglobulin, Genzyme, Cambridge, MA), a rabbit polyclonal antibody. The rabbit preparation is less immunogenic and hence has improved tolerability over the equine preparation.

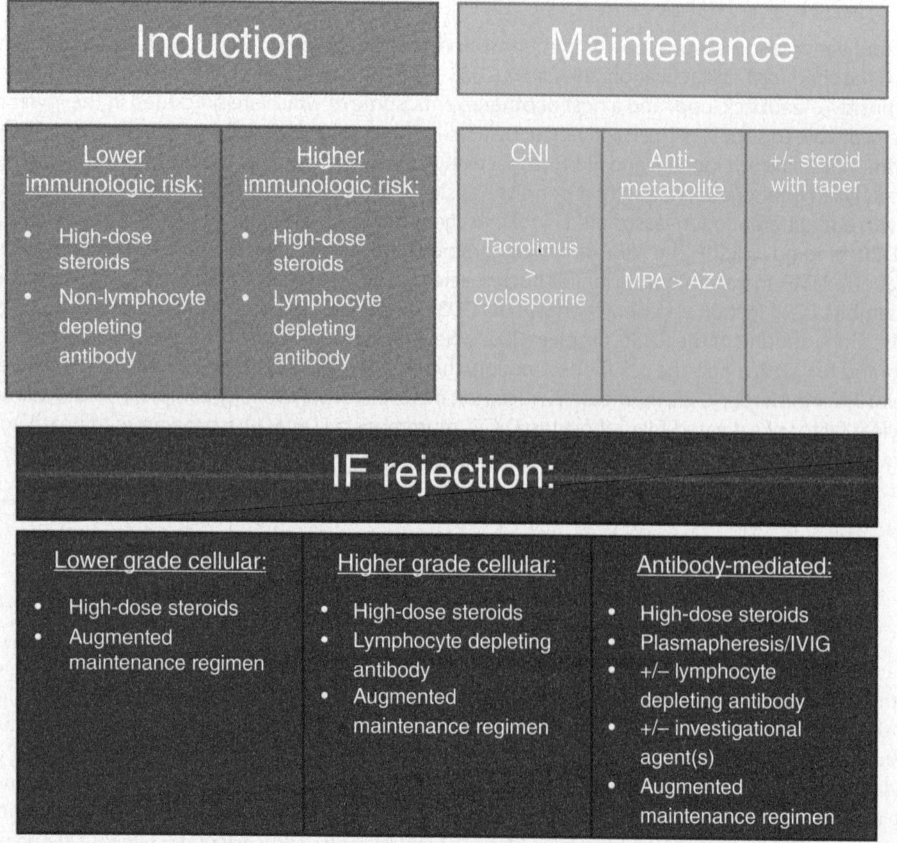

FIGURE 109-2 Representative immunosuppression regimen following solid-organ transplantation. (MPA, mycophenolic acid; AZA, azathioprine; IVIG, intravenous immune globulin.)

TABLE 109-4 Strategies for Preventing Cardiac Allograft Vasculopathy (CAV)

Drug Class	Drugs	Dose	Timing of Initiation
Statins	Pravastatin Simvastatin Atorvastatin Rosuvastatin	20-40 mg daily 5-20 mg daily 10-40 mg daily 5-20 mg daily	Prior to hospital discharge
mTOR inhibitors	Everolimus Sirolimus	0.75 mg twice daily 1-2 mg daily	Not recommended to initiate within 6 months of transplant due to impaired wound healing. However, greatest benefit is realized if started within 1-2 years
Glycemic control	Insulin, other anti-hyperglycemic agents	Titrate to euglycenmia	Immediately post-transplant
Prevent ACR[a]	Tacrolimus Cyclosporine	Titrate to center-specific trough values	Immediately post-transplant
Prevent CMV infection[b]	Valganciclovir	900 mg daily (adjusted for kidney function)	Immediately post-transplant

ACR, acute cellular rejection; CMV, cytomegalovirus.

[a]Episodes of acute cellular rejection increase the subsequent risk of developing CAV.

[b]CMV infection has been linked to accelerated development of CAV. Prophylaxis with valganciclovir is only recommended in recipients at high risk of infection post-transplant.

Pharmacology/Mechanism of Action Because of their polyclonal antibody nature, both ATG and RATG exert their immunosuppressive effect by binding to a wide array of lymphocyte receptors such as CD2, CD3, CD4, CD8, CD25, and CD45. Binding of ATG or RATG to the various receptors results in complement-mediated lysis and subsequent lymphocyte depletion. While T cells are the major lymphocytic target for the compounds, other blood cell components such as B cells and other leukocytes are also affected (see Fig. 109-1).

Pharmacokinetics ATG is poorly distributed into lymphoid tissue and binds primarily to circulating lymphocytes, granulocytes, and platelets. The terminal half-life of ATG is 5.7 days. RATG has a volume of distribution of 0.12 L/kg, and its terminal half-life in kidney transplant recipients is significantly longer than ATG at 30 days.[76] Peak plasma concentrations are reached after 5 to 7 days of ATG or RATG infusions.

Efficacy ATG and RATG are used for the treatment of acute allograft rejection or as induction therapy to prevent acute rejection.[77] When compared head-to-head in kidney transplant recipients, RATG resulted in less frequent and less severe acute rejection episodes, fewer serious adverse events and was superior with respect to the composite endpoint including freedom from death, graft loss, or rejection.[78] RATG received regulatory approval as induction therapy in kidney transplantation.[79] As such, RATG is both preferred over ATG for induction and treatment of rejection in solid-organ transplant recipients.

Use of RATG in liver transplantation as part of a steroid avoidance protocol is associated with similar rates of patient and graft survival and acute rejection compared with dual or triple therapy.[34] In kidney transplant, RATG is associated with improved graft survival at 5 years as compared with equine ATG. Quadruple-drug therapy results in similar rates of patient and graft survival in heart transplant recipients, with a lower rate of acute rejection at 1 year compared with triple-drug therapy. Outcomes associated with RATG in lung transplantation have not consistently demonstrated favorable outcomes related to acute rejection or patient and graft survival.[80,81]

Adverse Effects Most adverse effects reported with ATG and RATG are related to the lack of specificity for lymphocytes. Dose-limiting myelosuppression (leukopenia, anemia, and thrombocytopenia) occurs frequently. Other adverse effects include anaphylaxis, hypotension, hypertension, tachycardia, dyspnea, urticaria, and rash. Serum sickness is seen more frequently with ATG than with RATG. Nephrotoxicity is rare in the absence of serum sickness. Infusion-related febrile reactions are common; therefore, all patients should be pre-medicated with acetaminophen, diphenhydramine, and corticosteroids. Finally, as with any immunosuppressive agent, ATG and RATG are associated with an increased risk of infections—particularly viral infections—and malignancy.

Drug-Drug and Drug-Food Interactions There are no known drug or food interactions with ATG or RATG.

Dosing and Administration ATG doses range from 10 to 30 mg/kg/day as a single dose for 7 to 14 days. A skin test (test dose) is required prior to administration of the initial dose of ATG. RATG is a more potent compound and is administered at doses of 1 to 1.5 mg/kg/day as a single daily dose for 7 to 14 days for acute rejection or for 3 to 10 days for induction of immunosuppression. ATG and RATG should both be administered through a central line or through a high-flow vein with an in-line 0.22-micron filter over at least 4 hours to minimize phlebitis and thrombosis.[76] Heparin and hydrocortisone are commonly added to the infusion to minimize phlebitis and thrombosis.[76]

Alemtuzumab

Alemtuzumab is approved for use in B-cell chronic lymphocytic leukemia.[82] However, its effects on depleting both T and B lymphocytes make it useful in solid-organ transplants. While alemtuzumab is not FDA-approved for solid-organ transplantation, it is widely recognized as a viable therapeutic option for induction or treatment of acute rejection. In 2012, commercial distribution of alemtuzumab ceased for transplantation and leukemia, requiring centers to enroll in a distribution program for ongoing medication access.

Pharmacology/Mechanism of Action Alemtuzumab is a humanized monoclonal antibody against the CD52 surface antigen found on both T and B lymphocytes, as well as macrophages, monocytes, eosinophils, and natural killer cells. When alemtuzumab binds to the CD52 surface antigen, antibody-dependent lysis occurs, which removes both T and B lymphocytes from the blood, bone marrow, and organs, resulting in complete lymphocyte depletion.[82]

Pharmacokinetics The pharmacokinetics of alemtuzumab in solid-organ transplantation patients have not been investigated. In patients with B-cell chronic lymphocytic leukemia, the volume of distribution of alemtuzumab after repeated dosing is 0.18 L/kg. The mean half-life after the first 30 mg dose is 11 hours, but increases to 6 days after 12 weeks of therapy. The extrapolation of these pharmacokinetic data to solid-organ transplantation is difficult because of the differences in dosing strategies used for the FDA indication. One or two doses of alemtuzumab result in complete and prolonged lymphocyte depletion. Following administration, B lymphocyte counts return to normal within 3 to 12 months. T lymphocytes, however, remain depressed for as long as 3 years following administration.[82,83]

Efficacy Alemtuzumab is effective as induction therapy for the prevention of acute rejection in kidney, liver, heart, pancreas, intestinal, and lung transplants.[84] Additionally, alemtuzumab has been used to successfully treat acute rejection following transplantation and is effective for corticosteroid- and antibody-resistant rejection.[72]

Adverse Effects Adverse effects of alemtuzumab are primarily infusion-related, hematologic, and infectious. Because alemtuzumab causes complete lymphocyte depletion and associated cytokine release, infusion-related reactions include rigors, hypotension, fever, shortness of breath, bronchospasms, and chills. The potential for developing these reactions can be reduced by administering pre-medications such as acetaminophen, corticosteroids, and diphenhydramine or by administering smaller doses and escalating the dose gradually. Subcutaneous administration may also reduce the incidence of infusion reactions.[85] Hematologic effects include pancytopenia, neutropenia, thrombocytopenia, and lymphopenia.

Drug-Drug and Drug-Food Interactions No drug or food interactions have been noted with alemtuzumab.

Dosing and Administration Several dosing regimens have been proposed for alemtuzumab in solid-organ transplantation. The most common dosing strategy is 30 mg administered intravenously or subcutaneously as a single dose; some centers administer a second dose 1 to 5 days after transplantation. Other dosing strategies assessed include 0.3 mg/kg/dose, as a single- or multiple-dose regimen, and, finally, two 20-mg doses given on the day of transplantation and the first postoperative day.[82]

Non-Depleting Antibody Therapy

Basiliximab

Basiliximab, a chimeric monoclonal antibody (25% murine) is the only available IL-2 receptor antagonist currently marketed in the United States. It is approved for use in kidney transplantation but is also extensively used in other organ transplants as well.[86]

Pharmacology/Mechanism of Action Basiliximab exerts its immunosuppressive effect by specifically binding with high affinity to the α-chain (CD25) on the surface of activated T lymphocytes (see Fig. 109-1). Binding of basiliximab to the IL-2 receptor prevents IL-2-mediated activation and proliferation of T cells, a critical step in clonal expansion of T cells and the development of allograft rejection. Saturation of the IL-2 receptor occurs rapidly and confers an immunosuppressive effect that lasts for 4 to 6 weeks after administration.[86]

Pharmacokinetics Most of the pharmacokinetic data available for basiliximab was derived following administration to kidney transplant recipients. Caution must be used when extrapolating this information to other transplant recipients. The volume of distribution is approximately 8 L, and it has a half-life of approximately 7 days. Clearance is increased in patients who have received a liver transplant, and it may be necessary in patients with greater than 10 L of ascites to receive an additional dose of basiliximab on postoperative day 8.[87]

Efficacy Basiliximab is approved for use in kidney transplantation in combination with cyclosporine and corticosteroids, although induction therapy has also been evaluated in liver, lung, and heart transplant recipients. Use of basiliximab in liver transplant recipients has been increasing as a means of delaying CNI initiation in the setting of acute kidney injury.[32,33] A meta-analysis of basiliximab efficacy in kidney transplantation concluded that IL-2 receptor antagonists reduced the risk of rejection with no increases in graft loss, infectious complications, malignancy, or death.[86] Similar results were seen in liver transplant patients.[88]

IL-2 receptor antagonists offer a reasonable addition to calcineurin inhibitor—or corticosteroid-sparing protocols. While CNI therapy cannot be completely avoided in most cases, IL-2 receptor antagonists allow for delayed use or reduced doses of CNIs, thus minimizing the risk of nephrotoxicity in the early post-transplantation period.[33]

Adverse Effects Relatively few adverse effects have been observed with basiliximab. In contrast to lymphocyte-depleting agents, basiliximab is not associated with infusion-related reactions. However, since the marketing of basiliximab, an increased number of hypersensitivity reactions have been reported. Development of anti-idiotypic antibodies to the murine portion occurs rarely.[88] There appears to be no increased risk of malignancy.

Drug-Drug and Drug-Food Interactions While cyclosporine and tacrolimus serum concentrations may increase in patients receiving concomitant basiliximab therapy, this interaction is not considered clinically.[86]

Dosing and Administration Basiliximab is usually administered as two 20-mg intravenous doses, intraoperatively and again on postoperative day 4. Basiliximab is compatible with both 0.9% sodium chloride and 5% dextrose and can be administered either centrally or peripherally over 20 to 30 minutes in a volume of 50 mL.

Other Antibody Therapy

Immune Globulin

Immune globulin (more commonly intravenous immune globulin; IVIG) preparations are derived from human plasma and contain a mixture of antibodies that exert immunomodulatory effects. IVIG is often used prophylactically in solid-organ transplant recipients who are at particularly high risk for antibody-mediated rejection due to the presence of pre-formed DSA at the time of transplant surgery. IVIG may also be used for a variety of other post-transplant complications, including in the management of both cellular and antibody-mediated rejection, hypogammaglobulinemia, and many others that are beyond the scope of this text.

Pharmacology/Mechanism of Action IVIG is thought to exert its immunomodulatory properties via a number of mechanisms, including inducing B-cell apoptosis and inhibition of complement.[72]

Pharmacokinetics IVIG has a small volume of distribution (0.05-0.13 L/kg) and upon administration, immune globulin remains primarily in the intravascular compartment. The half-life varies by IVIG preparation but is generally between 14 and 28 days.[89]

Efficacy When administered to sensitized patients awaiting kidney transplantation, IVIG results in reductions in circulating DSA.[90] Pre-transplant IVIG administration (in combination with plasmapheresis) that achieves desensitization may yield a mortality benefit in kidney transplant recipients owing to dialysis liberation.[91] IVIG leads to similar outcomes compared to anti-CD3 monoclonal antibody (OKT3) in patients being treated for steroid-resistant rejection.[92] IVIG is also often used in the setting of chronic antibody-mediated rejection, though supporting evidence for this practice is lacking.[93]

Adverse Effects IVIG infusions can be complicated by reactions that include rash, chills, headaches, shortness of breath, or hypotension. For this reason, pre-medications are routinely administered. IVIG has also been known to rarely cause acute kidney injury (more frequently associated with sucrose-containing formulations due to osmotic diuresis), hemolysis, aseptic meningitis, and thromboembolism.[72]

Drug-Drug and Drug-Food Interactions There are no known drug or food interactions with IVIG.

Dosing and Administration IVIG doses range from 0.1 to 2 g/kg as either a single dose or doses that are administered sequentially, depending on the indication for use. IVIG infusions should generally begin at slower infusion rates to assess patient tolerability before up-titrating. If IVIG is being administered on the same day as plasmapheresis, then it should be administered after because immune globulin is removed by pheresis.

Maintenance Agents

The goal of maintenance immunosuppression is to prevent rejection while minimizing drug-related toxicity. As patients progress through the post-transplant course, the risk of acute rejection decreases and the need for pharmacologic immunosuppression is lessened. With few exceptions, maintenance immunosuppression can never be withdrawn following transplantation and thus one or more agents are required lifelong.

Calcineurin Inhibitors

Cyclosporine and tacrolimus are the two calcineurin inhibitors (CNIs) currently used for most solid-organ transplant recipients. More than 90% of transplant recipients receive tacrolimus as part of their immunosuppressive regimen.[94]

Pharmacology/Mechanism of Action Calcineurin inhibitors block T-cell proliferation by inhibiting the production of IL-2 and other cytokines by T cells (see Fig. 109-1). Cyclosporine and tacrolimus bind to unique cytoplasmic immunophilins: cyclophilin and FK-binding protein-12 (FKBP12), respectively. The drug-immunophilin complex inhibits the action of calcineurin, an enzyme that activates the nuclear factor of activated T cells, which is, in turn, responsible for the transcription of several key cytokines necessary for T-cell activity, including IL-2. IL-2 is a potent T-cell growth factor and ultimately is responsible for activation and clonal expansion.

Pharmacokinetics The calcineurin inhibitors are highly lipophilic compounds, with variable but generally low bioavailability of approximately 30% (range: 5%-60%). Unlike tacrolimus, cyclosporine depends on bile for intestinal absorption, which further increases inter- and intra-patient variability.

Because of the high variability in absorption of cyclosporine a microemulsion formulation was developed. Both forms are available commercially in the United States and are referred to as "cyclosporine, USP," and "cyclosporine, USP [MODIFIED]." The two formulations are not bioequivalent and should not be used interchangeably. The modified formulation is self-emulsifying and forms a microemulsion spontaneously with aqueous fluids in the gastrointestinal tract, making it less dependent on bile for absorption. This translates into a greater rate and extent of absorption and decreased intra-individual variability in pharmacokinetic parameters. The relative bioavailability of the microemulsion formulation is 60%, and peak concentrations are reached within 1.5 to 2 hours after oral administration. Tacrolimus, on the other hand, has a more predictable absorption pattern, reaching peak concentrations within 1 to 3 hours with bioavailability of approximately 20%.[95]

Following oral absorption, both cyclosporine and tacrolimus are highly protein bound. Ninety percent of cyclosporine is bound to lipoproteins in the blood while 99% of tacrolimus is bound primarily to plasma proteins, including albumin and α_1-acid glycoprotein, and red blood cells. Cyclosporine is distributed widely into tissue and body fluids, resulting in a large and variable volume of distribution, ranging from 3 to 5 L/kg. Because of the high concentration of FKBP12 that is found in red blood cells, tacrolimus is distributed primarily in the vasculature, with a volume of distribution of 0.8 to 1.9 L/kg. Both drugs are extensively metabolized by cytochrome P450 3A4 (CYP3A4) in both the gut and the liver, which accounts for their numerous drug interactions that are highlighted in Table 109-5.[83,84,95,96] Cyclosporine and tacrolimus are both excreted primarily in the feces.

TABLE 109-5 The Impact of Concomitant Medications on Immunosuppressive Concentrations

Medications	TAC	CSA	MPA	mTOR Inhibitors
Anti-Infectives				
Clotrimazole	↑	↑		↑
Fluconazole	↑	↑		↑
Ketoconazole	↑	↑		↑
Voriconazole	↑	↑		↑
Itraconazole	↑	↑		↑
Posaconazole	↑	↑		↑
Erythromycin	↑	↑		↑
Clarithromycin	↑	↑		↑
Azithromycin	↑	↑		↑
Levofloxacin	↑	↑		
Metronidazole			↓	
Selective gut decontamination			↓	
Nafcillin	↓	↓	↓	↓
Rifampin	↓	↓	↓	↓
Lopinavir/Ritonavir	↑	↑		
Saquinavir				
Efavirenz	↓	↓		
Glecaprevir/pibrentasvir	↑	↑		↑
Letermovir	↑	↑		↑
Cobicistat	↑	↑		↑
Cardiovascular				
Verapamil	↑	↑		↑
Diltiazem	↑	↑		↑
CNS				
Carbamazepine	↓	↓		↓
Phenytoin	↓	↓		↓
Phenobarbital	↓	↓		↓
Immunosuppressants				
Cyclosporine			↓	↑
Tacrolimus				
Sirolimus		↑		
Everolimus		↑		
Mycophenolic acid		↓		

Efficacy Both cyclosporine and tacrolimus are currently approved for prophylaxis of organ rejection in kidney, liver, and heart transplantation. They are both used as primary immunosuppression in lung transplant recipients despite not being approved for this purpose. The microemulsion formulation of cyclosporine has demonstrated equivalent or superior efficacy in kidney, liver, and heart transplantation recipients relative to the non-modified formulation. Tacrolimus and cyclosporine demonstrate equivalent efficacy as primary immunosuppression in regard to overall patient mortality, but tacrolimus is the preferred CNI owing to its superiority in preventing acute rejection.[97]

Adverse Effects The adverse effects of immunosuppressants are presented in Table 109-6. The nephrotoxic potential of both drugs is equal and is often related to the dose and duration of exposure. Neurotoxicity typically manifests as tremors, headache, and peripheral neuropathy; occasionally, however, seizures have been observed. Tacrolimus may be associated with an increased occurrence of neurologic complications compared with cyclosporine.[97]

TABLE 109-6 Comparison of Common Adverse Effects of Maintenance Immunosuppressants

System/Adverse Effect	AZA	MPA	CNI	Steroids	mTOR	Bela
Neurologic						
Headache			X			
Tremors			X			
Seizures			X			
Mood changes				X		
Cardiovascular						
Hypertension			X	X		
Hyperlipidemia			X	X	X	
Peripheral edema						X
Gastrointestinal						
Nausea	X	X	X	X		
Diarrhea		X	X			X
Vomiting	X					
Bleeding				X		
Hepatotoxicity	X		X			
Renal						
Nephrotoxicity			X		X	
Hyperkalemia			X			
Hypomagnesemia			X			
Urinary tract infection						X
Hematologic						
Anemia						X
Leukocytosis						
Leukopenia	X	X			X	
Neutropenia						X
Thrombocytopenia	X	X			X	
Cosmetic						
Acne				X		
Alopecia			TAC			
Gingival hyperplasia			CSA			
Hirsutism			CSA			
Weight gain				X		
Endocrine						
Hyperglycemia			X	X		
Osteoporosis				X		

AZA, azathioprine; Bela, belatacept; CNI, calcineurin inhibitor; CSA, cyclosporine; MPA, mycophenolic acid; mTOR, mammalian target of rapamycin inhibitor; TAC, tacrolimus.

Cyclosporine has a greater propensity to cause hypertension and hyperlipidemia compared with tacrolimus.[98,99] Conversely, hyperglycemia is more common with tacrolimus than with cyclosporine but is often reversible when doses of tacrolimus are reduced.[98] Cyclosporine is associated with cosmetic effects, such as hirsutism and gingival hyperplasia, which may be managed by converting from cyclosporine to tacrolimus. Tacrolimus, in contrast, may cause alopecia, which is usually self-limiting and reversible.

Calcineurin Inhibitor-Associated Nephrotoxicity Two types of nephrotoxicity can occur with calcineurin inhibitors. Acute nephrotoxicity is seen early and is dose-dependent and reversible, but chronic nephropathy is more problematic. Clinical manifestations of calcineurin inhibitor nephrotoxicity include elevated serum creatinine and blood urea nitrogen concentrations, hyperkalemia, hyperuricemia, proteinuria, and a decreased fractional excretion of sodium. Calcineurin inhibitor nephrotoxicity is the leading cause of impaired kidney function following a non-renal solid-organ transplant, a complication associated with reduced overall patient survival.[100]

The predominant mechanism for calcineurin inhibitor nephrotoxicity is renal vasoconstriction, primarily of the afferent arteriole, resulting in increased renal vascular resistance, decreased renal blood flow by up to 40%, reduced glomerular filtration rate by up to 30%, and increased proximal tubular sodium reabsorption with a reduction in urinary sodium and potassium excretion. A number of other mechanisms have been implicated, including changes in the renin–angiotensin–aldosterone system, prostaglandin synthesis, nitrous oxide production, sympathetic nervous system activation, and calcium handling.[101]

Several approaches have been proposed to reduce calcineurin inhibitor nephrotoxicity, including delaying administration immediately postoperatively in patients at high-risk for nephrotoxicity (using alternative induction protocols including an IL-2 receptor antagonist or antilymphocyte globulin), reducing the calcineurin inhibitor dosage to target lower blood concentrations (if feasible

TABLE 109-7 Differential Diagnosis of Acute Rejection and Cyclosporine or Tacrolimus Nephrotoxicity

	Nephrotoxicity in Renal Transplant Recipients	
	Acute Rejection	CSA or TAC Nephrotoxicity
History	Often <4 weeks postoperatively	Often >6 weeks postoperatively
Clinical presentation	Fever	Afebrile
	Hypertension	Hypertension
	Weight gain	Graft nontender
	Graft swelling/tenderness	Good urine output
	Decreased daily urine volume	
Laboratory biopsy	Rapid rise in SCr	Gradual rise in SCr
	Normal or sub-therapeutic CSA or TAC concentration	Elevated CSA or TAC concentration, especially over long periods of time
	Interstitial lymphocytic infiltrates, peritubular capillaritis, +/- new donor-specific antibodies	Interstitial fibrosis, tubular atrophy, glomerular thrombosis, arterial inflammation

SCr, serum creatinine; CSA, cyclosporine; TAC, tacrolimus.

clinically), and avoiding other nephrotoxins (eg, aminoglycosides, amphotericin B, angiotensin-converting enzyme inhibitors and non-steroidal anti-inflammatory agents) when possible.[101,102] No proven therapies consistently prevent or reverse the nephrotoxic effects of calcineurin inhibitors.

In patients who have received a kidney transplant, it is often difficult to differentiate calcineurin inhibitor nephrotoxicity from kidney allograft rejection. Because the clinical features of acute kidney allograft rejection and calcineurin inhibitor nephrotoxicity overlap considerably, a kidney biopsy is often necessary to differentiate the two (Table 109-7). However, differentiating between chronic kidney allograft rejection and calcineurin inhibitor nephrotoxicity may be more difficult because in addition to clinical signs and symptoms, biopsy findings may also be similar.

Drug-Drug and Drug-Food Interactions Drug interactions occur frequently with the calcineurin inhibitors because they are substrates for CYP3A4 and P-glycoprotein.[83,84,96] The most commonly administered drugs that are known to alter cyclosporine and tacrolimus concentrations are highlighted in Table 109-5. Inhibitors of CYP3A4, such as -azole antifungals, protease inhibitors, diltiazem or erythromycin, can increase drug concentrations, whereas drugs that induce CYP3A4 activity, such as phenytoin or rifampin, can decrease drug concentrations.[96]

Cyclosporine, and to a lesser extent, tacrolimus, are inhibitors of CYP3A4 and P-glycoprotein.[95,103] The inhibitory effects of cyclosporine and tacrolimus on CYP3A4 can be seen with weaker substrates, such as the HMG-CoA reductase inhibitors ("statins"). Concomitant administration of a calcineurin inhibitor with an HMG-CoA reductase inhibitor may result in an increase in the HMG-CoA reductase inhibitor concentrations (particularly those metabolized by CYP3A4), which increases the risk of HMG-CoA reductase inhibitor adverse effects, most notably myopathy.[104] Patients should be monitored for clinical signs of myopathy when receiving HMG-CoA reductase inhibitors in combination with cyclosporine and tacrolimus. The interaction appears to be more pronounced between cyclosporine and HMG-CoA reductase inhibitors due to inhibition of organic anion-transporter proteins (OATP) by cyclosporine.[105]

Consistency in the administration of the calcineurin inhibitors with regard to meals and food intake is important to sustain an effective concentration–time profile. High-fat meals can enhance both plasma clearance and the volume of distribution of cyclosporine by more than 60%.[106] Food reduces the rate and extent of tacrolimus absorption, and a high-fat meal may further delay gastric emptying and reduce the maximum achieved serum concentration (C_{max}) and the area under the concentration–time curve (AUC).[95] Furocoumarins such as quercetin, naringin, and bergamottin—found in grapefruit juice—are potent inhibitors of CYP3A4 and may increase both cyclosporine and tacrolimus concentrations. The AUC and C_{max} of cyclosporine may be increased by more than 55% and 35%, respectively.

Dosing and Administration Initial oral cyclosporine doses range from 6 to 10 mg/kg/day administered in divided doses every 12 hours. Oral tacrolimus doses usually are in the range of 0.1 to 0.3 mg/kg/day in divided doses administered every 12 hours. An extended-release tablet formulation of tacrolimus (Envarsus XR®) has greater bioavailability than the immediate-release formulation and thus a lower recommended daily starting dose (0.14 mg/kg/day).[107] Children often require higher doses to maintain therapeutic drug concentrations, up to 14 to 18 mg/kg/day for cyclosporine and 0.3 mg/kg/day for tacrolimus. Astagraf XL®, another extended-release tacrolimus formulation, and Envarsus XR® are not interchangeable. Astagraf XL® (or Advagraf®) is generally converted from standard tacrolimus formulations on a mg:mg basis, whereas Envarsus® XR has greater bioavailability than the immediate release tacrolimus and thus a 20% reduction in total daily dose is recommended.[95,107,108]

If oral administration is not possible, both CSA and TAC can be administered intravenously. Intravenous cyclosporine should be converted at approximately one-third of the total daily oral dosage since administration by this route avoids first-pass metabolism. The usual intravenous dose of cyclosporine is 0.5 to 2 mg/kg/day, given as a continuous infusion or as a single or twice-daily injection. Intravenous tacrolimus should be converted at approximately one-fourth of the total daily oral dosage, with doses ranging from 0.03 to 0.05 mg/kg/day, and must be administered by continuous infusion.

Therapeutic Drug Monitoring Calcineurin inhibitor trough blood concentrations should be measured routinely to optimize therapy. Both drugs can be measured by radio immunoassay (RIA) or high-performance liquid chromatography (HPLC), which is recognized as the reference procedure.[106] Therapeutic target ranges are assay specific. The specific goal concentration for both drugs is dependent on transplant type, time after transplantation, and concomitant immunosuppression, among other factors. However, target tacrolimus trough concentrations early post-transplantation (ie, 0-3 months) are around 8 to 15 ng/mL (mcg/L; 9.9-18.6 nmol/L) and are reduced over time as clinically tolerated/feasible. Drug concentrations should be measured frequently (daily or three times per week) following initiation of the drug and during the stabilization period after transplantation. With time, blood concentrations can be measured less frequently.

Cyclosporine trough concentrations are poorly predictive of rejection but are the most commonly utilized strategy for therapeutic drug monitoring. In the early post-transplantation period, goal cyclosporine trough concentrations range from 250 to 350 ng/mL (mcg/L; 210-290 nmol/L) and are similarly reduced over time. Alternative strategies, including AUC and peak concentration determination, have been suggested to better correlate with rejection.[106] Limited sampling techniques using two to five blood samples within the first 4 hours after an oral dose have been used to determine AUC and values greater than 4,400 ng/mL/hr correlated with a reduction in rejection.[106,109] Cyclosporine peak concentration (C_{peak}) has also been found to correlate with rejection and toxicity. Some transplantation centers have adopted this strategy to manage cyclosporine concentrations because of the convenience and reduced cost associated with the measurement of a single blood concentration. The suggested therapeutic range for C_{peak} cyclosporine concentrations is 1,500 to 2,000 ng/mL (μg/L; 1,250-1,660 nmol/L) for the first few months after transplant and 700 to 900 ng/mL (μg/L; 580-750 nmol/L) after 6 to 12 months.[106]

Current therapeutic drug monitoring does not ensure complete avoidance of either toxicity or rejection. Intra-patient variability with tacrolimus has been associated with both graft rejection and development of *de novo* donor-specific antibodies. Other measures of CNI exposure such as time in therapeutic range (TTR), commonly employed to measure the adequacy of warfarin monitoring, are positively associated with superior outcomes in lung transplant recipients. Prospective implementation of these findings has not been employed to drive outcomes but may be an opportunity to identify patients at heightened risk for poor outcomes and modify their clinical monitoring.[109-111]

Corticosteroids

Corticosteroids have been used since the beginning of the modern transplantation era. Despite their many adverse events, they continue to be a cornerstone of immunosuppression regimens in many transplant centers.[94] The most commonly used corticosteroids are methylprednisolone and prednisone.

Pharmacology/Mechanism of Action Corticosteroids block cytokine activation by binding to corticosteroid response elements, thereby inhibiting IL-1, IL-2, IL-3, IL-6, γ-interferon, and tumor necrosis factor-α synthesis. Additionally, corticosteroids interfere with cell migration, recognition, and cytotoxic effector mechanisms.[112]

Pharmacokinetics Prednisone is converted to prednisolone, its active moiety, in the liver and has multiple effects on the immune system. Prednisone is rapidly absorbed from the GI tract, achieving peak concentrations in 1 to 3 hours in transplant recipients. Bioavailability is greater than 90%. In kidney transplant recipients, the pharmacokinetic half-life is short, 2 to 4 hours, but the pharmacodynamic effects extend beyond the time that concentrations are measurable, permitting daily administration.[112]

Efficacy The efficacy of corticosteroids is irrefutable based on the decades of clinical experience. Systematic studies comparing corticosteroid-free immunosuppressive agent combinations with conventional therapy are difficult to perform because of the many of potential combinations that now exist. Nevertheless, corticosteroid-free immunosuppressive agent combinations with newer, more specific immunosuppressants hold promise and may be more commonly used in the future.[113]

Adverse Effects Adverse effects of prednisone that occur in more than 10% of patients include increased appetite, insomnia, indigestion, and mood changes. Side effects that occur less often but which are seen with high doses or prolonged therapy include cataracts, hyperglycemia, hirsutism, bruising, acne, sodium and water retention, hypertension, bone growth suppression, and ulcerative esophagitis. The adverse effects of corticosteroids are summarized in Table 109-6.

Drug-Drug and Drug-Food Interactions Barbiturates, phenytoin, and rifampin induce hepatic metabolism of prednisolone and thus may decrease the effectiveness of prednisone. Prednisone decreases the effectiveness of vaccines and toxoids.[112]

Dosing and Administration An intravenous corticosteroid, commonly high-dose methylprednisolone (250-1,000 mg), is given at the time of most solid-organ transplant surgeries and over consecutive days for the treatment of acute rejection. The dose of methylprednisolone is tapered and usually discontinued when oral prednisone is initiated. Prednisone doses are tapered progressively over several weeks to months, as dictated by center-specific protocols. It is preferable to administer corticosteroids in the early morning to mimic the body's diurnal release of cortisol. Prednisone should be taken with food to minimize GI upset. Abrupt corticosteroid discontinuation is not generally recommendable; tapering should be gradual because of the risk for suppression of the hypothalamic–pituitary–adrenal axis. While conversion to alternate-day regimens or complete withdrawal of prednisone in patients with stable post-transplantation courses has been used with success in some transplantation centers, corticosteroids are often continued for the entire life of the functional graft.[112]

Antimetabolites

Antimetabolites have been used since the early days of transplantation because they prevent the proliferation of lymphocytes. Azathioprine, long considered a part of the "gold standard" regimen with cyclosporine and corticosteroids, has largely been supplanted by mycophenolic acid derivatives which are more specific in their effects on lymphocytes and have fewer side effects.

Mycophenolic Acid Derivatives

Two formulations of mycophenolic acid (MPA) are currently available in the United States: mycophenolate mofetil—the morpholinoethyl ester of MPA—and mycophenolate sodium, which is available as an enteric-coated formulation of the sodium salt of MPA.

Pharmacology/Mechanism of Action The immunosuppressive effect of MPA is exerted through non-competitive binding to inosine monophosphate dehydrogenase (IMPDH), the key enzyme responsible for guanosine nucleotide synthesis via the de novo pathway. Inhibition of IMPDH results in decreased nucleotide synthesis and diminished DNA polymerase activity, ultimately reducing lymphocyte proliferation.[114] Although MPA inhibits both types of IMPDH: IMPDH I, expressed by all cells in the body, and IMPDH II, which is expressed only in T and B lymphocytes, it is more specific for IMPDH II.[114] T and B lymphocytes only use the de novo pathway for nucleotide synthesis (see Fig. 109-1), making MPA specific for these cells. Other cells within the body have a salvage pathway by which they can synthesize nucleotides, making them less susceptible to the actions of MPA and thereby reducing, but not eliminating, the potential for the hematologic adverse effects seen with azathioprine. In addition to decreasing lymphocyte proliferation, MPA may also downregulate the activation of lymphocytes.[115]

Pharmacokinetics Because MPA is unstable in an acidic environment, mycophenolate mofetil acts as a prodrug that is readily absorbed from the GI tract, after which it is rapidly and completely converted to MPA by the liver. The enteric coating of mycophenolate sodium protects MPA from the acidic gastric pH and allows MPA to be released directly into the small intestine for absorption. The absolute bioavailability of mycophenolate mofetil and mycophenolate sodium is 94% and 72% of the active moiety, respectively. Peak concentrations of mycophenolate mofetil are reached within 1 to 2 hours following oral administration, while the enteric coating of mycophenolate sodium delays absorption and peak concentrations are not reached until 4 hours after administration.[115]

MPA is extensively bound (97%) to albumin and is eliminated by the kidney and also undergoes glucuronidation in the liver to an inactive glucuronide metabolite (MPAG) that is subsequently excreted in the bile and urine. Enterohepatic cycling of MPAG can lead to deconjugation, thereby recirculating MPA into the bloodstream. This can account for 10% to 60% of total MPA exposure and results in a second peak 6 to 12 hours after oral administration. The half-life of MPA is 18 hours.[115]

Efficacy Mycophenolate mofetil is approved for use in kidney, liver, and heart transplantation and is recommended as a component of maintenance immunosuppression regimens for most all solid-organ transplant recipients.[61,75] Compared to azathioprine, mycophenolate treatment in patients receiving cyclosporine and corticosteroids leads to a significant improvement in patient and graft survival at 1 and 3 years.[115]

Mycophenolic acid derivatives are a key component of calcineurin inhibitor–sparing protocols. MPA monotherapy has been associated with an unacceptable rejection rate. Combination of MPA with sirolimus, on the other hand, resulted in improved kidney function with no change in acute rejection incidence or patient and graft survival.[115]

Adverse Effects Unlike cyclosporine and tacrolimus, MPA is not associated with nephrotoxicity, neurotoxicity, or hypertension. The most common side effects are related to the GI tract, including nausea, vomiting, diarrhea, and abdominal pain (see Table 109-6), which occur with similar frequency during intravenous and oral therapy. Strategies to reduce GI symptoms are not well established. Changing formulation may or may not improve symptoms and it is clear that dose reduction and discontinuation increase the risk of rejections.[115] Mycophenolic acid also has hematologic effects, such as leukopenia and anemia, particularly with higher doses, and may be associated with the rare but serious adverse event of progressive multifocal leukoencephalopathy (PML).[115]

Drug-Drug and Drug-Food Interactions Food has no effect on MPA AUC, but it delays the absorption and decreases MPA C_{max} by 40% and 33% when mycophenolate mofetil and mycophenolate sodium, respectively, are administered. Concomitant administration with aluminum- and magnesium-containing antacids decreases the AUC of MPA, though the significance of this interaction is not likely clinically relevant.[115] Administration of iron may produce similar results, but this has not been tested. Concomitant administration of mycophenolate mofetil with pantoprazole decreases MPA concentrations and systemic exposure in healthy volunteers. The same effect is not observed with mycophenolate sodium. Reduced MPA exposure does not impact graft outcomes in all patients.

Acyclovir, commonly used in kidney transplant recipients for the treatment and prevention of viral infections, competes with MPAG for renal tubular secretion. AUCs of both entities are increased during concomitant acyclovir and MPA administration. No pharmacokinetic interaction with other antiviral agents has been demonstrated; but, there is potential for additive pharmacodynamic effects such as bone marrow suppression.

Decreased MPA trough concentrations are observed when MPA is administered with cyclosporine compared with those achieved when MPA is given with tacrolimus or sirolimus.[115] This interaction is most likely a result of cyclosporine inhibition of multidrug-resistance-associated protein 2 (MRP2), which inhibits the enterohepatic recycling of MPAG, resulting in decreased MPA concentrations.[115] Cyclosporine decreases MPA concentrations by approximately 40% to 50% compared to tacrolimus.[83] To achieve equivalent MPA and MPAG serum concentrations, it may be necessary to administer higher doses of MPA with cyclosporine compared to tacrolimus. Antibiotics may also interfere with enterohepatic recycling of MPAG by decreasing bacterial-mediated de-glucuronidation in the colon.[115] MPA concentrations may also be reduced in the setting of concomitant corticosteroid administration, owing to the induction of glucuronidation caused by steroids.[116]

Dosing and Administration Mycophenolate mofetil is currently available in both oral and intravenous formulations. Although intravenous administration of equal doses closely mimics oral administration, the two cannot be considered bioequivalent. Mycophenolate sodium is only available as an oral formulation. To optimize immunosuppression and minimize adverse effects, MPA is most commonly administered in two divided doses given every 12 hours. The total daily dose for kidney and liver transplants is typically 2 g/day for mycophenolate mofetil and 1.44 g/day for mycophenolate sodium. The total daily dose in heart transplant recipients is commonly 3 g/day, with a target trough concentration of greater than 1.5 μg/mL (mg/L; 4.7 μmol/L).[61] The recommended pediatric dose is 600 mg/m^2 for mycophenolate mofetil and 400 mg/m^2 for mycophenolate sodium, in two divided doses.

While therapeutic drug monitoring of MPA may be of value it remains controversial.[117-119] Plasma appears to be the most appropriate medium in which to measure MPA for therapeutic drug monitoring, due to the relationship between target plasma MPA concentrations and improved clinical outcomes in patients receiving concomitant CNIs and corticosteroids. For example, patients with trough MPA concentrations between 1.0 and 3.5 μg/mL (mg/L; 3.1-10.9 μmol/L) experience fewer complications. Unbound concentrations as opposed to total MPA concentrations may be the most relevant to measure, especially in patients with liver disease, hypoalbuminemia, and severe infection.[115] Trough concentrations may not be accurate in predicting total drug exposure during a 12-hour interval and thus AUC monitoring has been proposed as the most appropriate measure of MPA drug exposure to guide therapy.[115] Better outcomes are associated with MPA AUC concentrations of greater than 42.8 μg/mL (mg/L; 134 μmol/L) per hour (by HPLC), although a reference range of 30 to 60 μg/mL (mg/L; 94-188 μmol/L) has been proposed.[119] The correlation between MPA AUC values and adverse effects is low. The best means to evaluate MPA concentrations, the acceptable targets for each method, and the appropriate strategy to monitor MPA concentrations remain unclear.[119]

Azathioprine

Azathioprine, a prodrug for 6-mercaptopurine (6-MP), has been used as an immunosuppressant in combination with corticosteroids since the earliest days of the modern transplantation era. Its use has dramatically declined with the availability of newer immunosuppressants, but it remains an option for patients intolerant of other medications.[61,75]

Pharmacology/Mechanism of Action Azathioprine is an inactive compound that is converted rapidly to 6-MP in the blood and is subsequently metabolized by three different enzymes. Xanthine oxidase, found in the liver and GI tract, converts 6-MP to the inactive final end product, 6-thiouric acid. Thiopurine *S*-methyltransferase (TPMT), found in hematopoietic tissues and red blood cells, methylates 6-MP to an inactive metabolite, 6-methylmercaptopurine. Finally, hypoxanthine-guanine phosphoribosyltransferase is the first step responsible for converting 6-MP to 6-thioguanine nucleotides (6-TGNs), the active metabolites, which are incorporated into nucleic acids, ultimately disrupting both the salvage and de novo pathways of DNA, RNA, and protein synthesis. This process is toxic to the cell and renders the cell unable to proliferate (see Fig. 109-1). Eventually, 6-TGNs are catabolized by xanthine oxidase and thiopurine *S*-methyltransferase to inactive products.[118]

Pharmacokinetics Oral bioavailability of azathioprine is approximately 40%. Metabolism of 6-MP is primarily by xanthine oxidase to inactive metabolites, which are excreted by the kidneys. The half-life of azathioprine is short, approximately 12 minutes. The half-life of 6-MP is longer, ranging from 0.7 to 3 hours. However, it is the activity of the 6-TGNs that determines the pharmacodynamic half-life of the drug which has been estimated to be 9 days.[120]

Adverse Effects Dose-limiting adverse effects of azathioprine are often hematologic (see Table 109-6). Leukopenia, anemia, and thrombocytopenia can occur within the first few weeks of therapy and can be managed by dose reduction or discontinuation of azathioprine. Other common adverse effects include nausea and vomiting, which can be minimized by taking azathioprine with food. Alopecia, hepatotoxicity, and pancreatitis are less common adverse effects of azathioprine and are reversible on dose reduction or discontinuation. Activity of TPMT can affect the occurrence of adverse effects with azathioprine. Approximately 10% of the population has intermediate TPMT activity and 0.3% has low activity of the enzyme. In both scenarios, the incidence of leukopenia and hepatotoxicity is increased.

Drug-Drug and Drug-Food Interactions The xanthine oxidase inhibitors allopurinol and febuxostat increase azathioprine and 6-MP concentrations by as much as fourfold.[120] The metabolic pathways shift to favor the production of 6-TGNs, which ultimately results in increased bone marrow suppression and pancytopenia. Doses of azathioprine should be reduced by at least 50% to 75% when allopurinol is added to a patient's drug regimen.

Dosing and Administration Usual initial doses of azathioprine range from 1 to 3 mg/kg/day orally. An intravenous formulation exists but is variably available and thus infrequently used in clinical practice.

Mammalian Target of Rapamycin (mTOR) Inhibitors

Two mTOR inhibitors have been approved in the United States for use in transplantation. Sirolimus, also known as rapamycin, is an immunosuppressive macrolide antibiotic that is structurally similar to tacrolimus, and is effective in reducing the risk of acute rejection. Everolimus, a synthetic derivative of sirolimus that was approved in the United States in 2009, was developed to improve upon the pharmacokinetics of sirolimus.

Pharmacology/Mechanism of Action Sirolimus and everolimus both bind to FKBP12, forming a complex that binds to mTOR, which inhibits the body's response to cytokines (see Fig. 109-1). IL-2 stimulates mTOR to activate kinases that ultimately advance the cell cycle from G1 to the S phase. Thus, these drugs reduce T-cell proliferation by inhibiting the cellular response to IL-2 and progression of the cell cycle.[121,122]

Pharmacokinetics Bioavailability after oral administration is low for both, only 14% to 20%, with peak concentrations being reached within 1 to 2 hours.[121,122] Both have large volumes of distribution, 5.6 to 16.7 L/kg for sirolimus and between 128 and 529 L for everolimus. Both are metabolized primarily by CYP3A4 in the gut and the liver. Likewise, both are also substrates for P-glycoprotein. The half-life for sirolimus is 60 hours but can be as long as 110 hours in patients with liver dysfunction, while that of everolimus is much shorter (18-35 hours).[121,122]

Efficacy Sirolimus is approved for the prevention of rejection in kidney transplant recipients when given in combination with corticosteroids and cyclosporine, or after withdrawal of cyclosporine in patients with low-to-moderate immunologic risk. Sirolimus is also effective in combination with tacrolimus or mycophenolate in kidney transplants, with patient survival rates greater than 99% and graft survival rates greater than 96%.[112] Combination therapy with sirolimus and mycophenolate can be used to avoid the use of calcineurin inhibitors and decrease the risk of nephrotoxicity. Everolimus is approved for use in both kidney and liver transplantation. In kidney transplant recipients, it was evaluated in combination with basiliximab, cyclosporine, and corticosteroids, whereas in liver transplant recipients, it was initiated at least 30 days after transplantation in combination with reduced-dose tacrolimus and corticosteroids. Everolimus has also been used with tacrolimus with similar results as sirolimus.[123] Everolimus appears to have less of an effect on wound healing and thus may potentially be used earlier after transplantation.

Early cyclosporine withdrawal has been studied in patients receiving sirolimus-based immunosuppressive protocols. Ideal candidates are patients who have not had a recent or severe rejection episode and have adequate kidney function 3 months after transplant. Rejection occurred in 5.6% of patients after discontinuation of cyclosporine and no difference in graft survival was noted. Long-term follow-up (2 years) showed improved kidney function and blood pressure without an increase in acute rejection or graft loss in patients who discontinued cyclosporine.[112] Similar results have been demonstrated with everolimus.[123]

mTOR inhibitors have demonstrated efficacy to reduce CNI use and nephrotoxicity in liver, heart, and lung transplant patients.[122] mTOR inhibitors have also been investigated in liver transplant patients as a means to reduce the recurrence of hepatitis C and hepatocellular carcinoma.[122] They may also reduce the incidence of chronic rejection after heart transplantation.[65,73]

Adverse Effects Both everolimus and sirolimus are associated with dose-related myelosuppression. Thrombocytopenia is usually seen within the first 2 weeks of sirolimus therapy but generally improves with continued treatment; leukopenia and anemia are also typically transient.[121,122] Sirolimus trough serum concentrations greater than 15 ng/mL (μg/L; 16 nmol/L) have been correlated with thrombocytopenia and leukopenia.[121] Hypercholesterolemia and hypertriglyceridemia are also common in patients receiving everolimus or sirolimus. The proposed mechanism of this adverse effect is overproduction of lipoproteins or inhibition of lipoprotein lipase. Peak cholesterol and triglyceride concentrations are often seen within 3 months of sirolimus initiation but usually decrease after 1 year of therapy and can be managed by reducing the dose, discontinuing sirolimus, or initiating therapy with an HMG-CoA reductase inhibitor or fibric acid derivative. Dyslipidemia associated with sirolimus may not be a major risk factor for early cardiovascular complications following kidney transplantation.[121] Delayed wound healing and dehiscence could be a result of inhibition of smooth muscle proliferation and intimal thickening.[121] For this reason, mTOR inhibitors are infrequently administered to transplant recipients in the immediate post-operative period. Mouth ulcers are observed in as many as 60% of patients treated with sirolimus and appear to be dose-related.[121] Reversible interstitial pneumonitis has been described in kidney, liver, and heart-lung transplantation recipients.[112] Despite their similarities, everolimus and sirolimus do have some differences likely related to differences in distribution. Sirolimus appears to enhance CSA neurotoxicity and both CSA and TAC nephrotoxicity, whereas everolimus did not.[122] Other adverse effects of sirolimus include increased liver enzymes, hypertension, rash, acne, diarrhea, and arthralgia (see Table 109-6).

Drug-Drug and Drug-Food Interactions The major metabolic pathway for everolimus and sirolimus is CYP3A4; thus, the drug interactions mediated by induction or inhibition of the CYP3A4 enzyme system are similar to those seen with cyclosporine and tacrolimus (see Table 109-5). Administration of the microemulsion formulation of cyclosporine with sirolimus increases the AUC and trough sirolimus serum concentrations: this has not been observed with the standard formulation of cyclosporine. Conversely, cyclosporine concentrations and AUC are increased when it is given concomitantly with sirolimus. The mechanism is proposed to be competitive binding to CYP3A4 and P-glycoprotein.[121,122] Concomitant administration of tacrolimus does not affect sirolimus concentrations.[121] Although everolimus AUC was increased by the administration of a single dose of the microemulsion cyclosporine formulation, no specific recommendations for dose timing are given. It should be expected, however, that any changes in CSA dose may also necessitate a modification of everolimus dose and increased attention to therapeutic drug monitoring.[121]

As with cyclosporine and tacrolimus, grapefruit juice increases sirolimus concentrations. Administration of sirolimus with a high-fat meal is associated with a delayed rate of absorption, decreased C_{max}, and increased AUC, indicating an increased drug exposure, whereas the half-life remains unchanged.[121] Conversely, administration of everolimus with a high-fat meal was associated with decreases in both C_{max} and AUC.[122]

Dosing and Administration The fixed sirolimus dosing regimen, approved for concomitant use with cyclosporine, includes a loading dose of 6 to 15 mg followed by 2 or 5 mg daily, respectively. However, loading doses are no longer recommended in clinical practice due to an increase in side effects. Therapeutic monitoring of sirolimus is routinely performed using whole-blood concentrations measured by HPLC, which is specific for the parent compound. For everolimus, a starting dose of 0.75 mg twice daily is indicated in regimens that contain cyclosporine, corticosteroids, and basiliximab induction. Target serum concentrations are 3 to 8 ng/mL (mcg/L; 3.1-8.4 nmol/L).

Co-Stimulatory Signal Inhibitor

Belatacept, derived from abatacept, is the only drug currently approved for use in solid-organ transplantation in this class of immunosuppressive agents. Belatacept may ultimately replace calcineurin inhibitors in the majority of immunosuppressive regimens given the lack of toxicities frequently seen with CNIs, especially nephrotoxicity.[23] Belatacept is only approved for kidney transplantation.

Pharmacology/Mechanism of Action Belatacept is a selective co-stimulation blocker that binds co-stimulatory ligands (CD80 and CD86) on antigen-presenting cells, preventing interaction with CD28 on T cells (see Fig. 109-1). The interaction of CD80 and CD86 with CD28 is required for the initiation of "signal 2," the co-stimulatory signal that leads to the activation and proliferation of T-cells. Thus, blockade of CD80 and CD86 prevents T-cell activation.[124]

Pharmacokinetics Belatacept, which is only available as an intravenous formulation, has a volume of distribution of 0.11 L/kg, a half-life of approximately 11 days and is not affected by impaired kidney or liver function.

Efficacy Belatacept and cyclosporine exhibit similar efficacy in terms of both patient and graft survival in first time kidney transplant recipients. Cyclosporine users experienced more chronic allograft nephropathy at month 12, while the belatacept users experienced more frequent and more severe ACR. Despite this, the measured GFR was 13 to 15 mL/min (0.22-0.25 mL/s) higher in the belatacept group compared to the cyclosporine group, a trend that persisted for 7 years.[125] Additionally, belatacept-treated patients had better blood pressure control and lower lipid concentrations as well as less diabetes than CNI-treated patients. This finding may underlie the mortality difference observed at 7 years of follow-up.[23] Compared to tacrolimus, ACR is more common among kidney transplant recipients receiving belatacept, whereas the incidence of metabolic and neurologic toxicities is less common.[126] Conversion from CNI-based regimens to belatacept in kidney transplant recipients with stable kidney function leads to improved GFR from baseline.[127,128] However, acute rejection occurs more frequently in patients who switch to belatacept, compared with patients who remain on CNI.[23]

Use of belatacept in liver transplant patients has been associated with increased graft loss and death.[36,124] There is limited post-marketing experience with belatacept in heart and lung transplant recipients, though this is an area of ongoing interest.[127,129]

Adverse Effects Belatacept is generally well tolerated. Adverse effects among belatacept recipients include anemia, neutropenia, diarrhea, urinary tract infections, headache, and peripheral edema.[23] Patients who are Epstein-Barr virus (EBV) naïve experienced a higher incidence of post-transplant lymphoproliferative disease (PTLD). PTLD typically occurs within the first 18 months of treatment and the majority occur in the central nervous system. There was no increase in incidence of PTLD in patients who are EBV-seropositive. As a result, belatacept carries a boxed warning for PTLD and is contraindicated in patients who are EBV-seronegative. Belatacept has been associated with progressive multifocal leukoencephalopathy (PML).[23]

Drug-Drug and Drug-Food Interactions There are no known drug or food interactions with belatacept.

Dosing and Administration Potential belatacept recipients must be screened for EBV-serostatus prior to initiation of therapy. Only patients who are EBV-seropositive should receive belatacept due to the increased risk of PTLD in EBV-seronegative patients. As a primary immunosuppressant for first time kidney transplants, belatacept is administered as 10 mg/kg intravenously over 30 minutes on days 0, 5, 14, 28, and at the end of weeks 8 and 12. Thereafter, the dose is reduced to the maintenance dose of 5 mg/kg administered IV over 30 minutes every 4 weeks beginning at week 16.

When converting to belatacept from a CNI-based regimen, the proposed dosing schedule is 5 mg/kg IV administered every 2 weeks for 5 doses on days 0, 14, 28, 42, and 56, then every 4 weeks thereafter. The CNI dose should be decreased by 50% after the second dose of belatacept and then discontinued after the fourth dose.[23]

Investigational Agents

Rituximab

Rituximab is a chimeric monoclonal antibody against the CD20 receptor found on selected populations of B cells. While it is FDA-approved for non-Hodgkin lymphoma and rheumatoid arthritis, it has also been used for the treatment and prevention of antibody-mediated rejection and post-transplant lymphoproliferative disorders.[130] In highly sensitized patients, rituximab administration prior to transplant suppresses alloantibody levels.[131] However, when used in kidney transplant recipients with active AMR, administration of rituximab has failed to consistently demonstrate efficacy.[132] In PTLD, rituximab is most effective in patients with CD20-positive malignancies.[130]

Bortezomib

Bortezomib, a proteosomal inhibitor that is FDA-approved for the treatment of multiple myeloma, has been used in the treatment of AMR. Among patients with AMR who received four doses of bortezomib 1.3 mg/m^2 on days 1, 4, 7, and 11 with plasmapheresis, bortezomib was effective in lowering DSA by 50%.[72] Another series showed a benefit of bortezomib over rituximab.[72] However, bortezomib is associated with a high incidence of side effects (up to 33% required hospitalization) that may include diarrhea/dehydration, nausea, edema, thrombocytopenia, infections, and peripheral neuropathy.[72]

EVALUATION OF THERAPEUTIC OUTCOMES

The success of transplantation can be measured in terms of length of graft and patient survival as well as improvements in quality of life. Several donor and recipient factors that have an impact on graft and patient survival have been identified. The greatest risks to short-term graft survival are technical/surgical complications and acute rejection. Routine surveillance of appropriate biochemical markers and serum drug concentrations is essential to minimize the potential for acute rejection. These parameters should be assessed daily to weekly for the first 1 to 3 months after transplantation.

TABLE 109-8 Laboratory Monitoring After Transplantation

	1-2 Weeks	1 Month	2-4 Months	4-12 Months	>12 Months
SCr/BUN	Daily	1-2 times per week	Every 1-2 weeks	Monthly	Every 1-2 months
Chemistries[a]	Daily	1-2 times per week	Every 1-2 weeks	Monthly	Every 1-2 months
Liver function tests[b]					
Kidney or heart recipient	Once	Once	Monthly	Every 1-3 months	Every 1-3 months
Liver recipient	Daily	1-3 times per week	Every 1-2 weeks	Monthly	Every 1-2 months
Immunosuppressant concentrations	Daily	1-2 times per week	Every 1-2 weeks	Monthly	Every 1-2 months
Complete blood count[c]	Daily	1-2 times per week	Every 1–2 weeks	Monthly	Every 1-2 months
Lipid panel[d]	Once	Every 3 months	Every 3 months	Every 3 months	Every 3 months
HbA_{1c}	Once	Every 3 months	Every 3 months	Every 3 months	Every 3 months

BUN, blood urea nitrogen; HbA_{1c}, hemoglobin A1c; SCr, serum creatinine.

[a]Chemistries include sodium, potassium, chloride, CO_2 content, magnesium, calcium, phosphorus, and blood glucose.

[b]Liver function tests include total bilirubin, aspartate transaminase (AST), alanine transaminase (ALT), gamma glutamyl transpeptidase (GGTP), and alkaline phosphatase.

[c]Complete blood count includes white blood cells (WBC), red blood cells (RBC), platelets, and +/- differential.

[d]Lipid panel includes total cholesterol, low-density lipoprotein (LDL), high-density lipoprotein (HDL), and triglyceride.

Monitoring for recipients of all solid-organ transplants should include complete blood counts, serum electrolyte concentrations, serum creatinine and blood urea nitrogen concentrations, and the appropriate serum drug concentrations. Liver function tests should also be evaluated using the same schedule in liver transplantation recipients. Routine biopsies are necessary to monitor for acute rejection in lung and heart transplantation recipients. As the time after transplantation increases, the frequency of monitoring decreases. Once 3 months have elapsed after transplantation, monitoring of these parameters can be reduced to biweekly or monthly for most patients. Table 109-8 depicts a typical post-transplantation laboratory monitoring plan. Long-term graft survival of all solid-organ transplants is limited by chronic rejection, a complication with few effective therapies which often necessitates re-transplantation.

IMMUNOSUPPRESSION-RELATED COMPLICATIONS

A fine counterbalance exists between under and over-immunosuppression. Beyond the first year post-transplant, death with a functioning graft is mostly attributed to cardiovascular disease, infection, and malignancy.[133] CNIs and corticosteroids, mainstays of maintenance immunosuppression, both contribute to cardiovascular disease-related risk factors including new-onset hypertension, diabetes, hyperlipidemia, and chronic kidney disease. All immunosuppressive agents inherently increase the risk of infection and impair cancer-related surveillance, which may lead to either de novo cancer post-transplant or cancer recurrence.[134] Routine surveillance including assessment and treatment of cardiovascular risk factors, along with vaccinations and age-appropriate cancer screening, are vital to ensure long-term patient survival. The following sections will review immunosuppression-related complications including cardiovascular disease, infections, and malignancy.

Cardiovascular Disease

Cardiovascular disease is a leading cause of morbidity and mortality in transplant patients.[135] Hypertension, hyperlipidemia, and diabetes are common complications in transplanted recipients and are independent risk factors for cardiovascular disease.

Hypertension

Corticosteroids, tacrolimus, cyclosporine, and impaired kidney graft function may all contribute to post-transplantation hypertension. Calcineurin inhibitor-associated hypertension may be due to increased endothelin production as well as stimulation of the sympathetic and renin-angiotensin systems.[136] In addition to the propensity to cause peripheral vasoconstriction, CNIs promote sodium retention, resulting in extracellular fluid volume expansion. Tacrolimus appears to have less potential to induce hypertension following transplantation than cyclosporine.[99,136,137]

Dihydropyridine calcium channel blockers have traditionally been the first-line agents to treat hypertension after transplantation.[136] They may ameliorate the nephrotoxic effects of CNIs and improve renal hemodynamics.[138] ACEIs and angiotensin II receptor blockers have traditionally been avoided in kidney transplantation recipients, especially in the perioperative period, because of the potential for hyperkalemia and negative influence on glomerular filtration rate. When ACEIs or angiotensin II receptor blockers are used in patients after transplant, serum creatinine and potassium concentrations should be monitored closely. If the increase in serum creatinine is greater than 30% within 1 to 2 weeks after initiating ACEIs or angiotensin II receptor blockers, then other alternatives should be considered (see Chapter 65).

Multiple antihypertensive agents are usually necessary to achieve the goal of blood pressure in transplant recipients; consequently, the addition of a β-blocker, diuretic, or centrally acting antihypertensive may also be necessary. Calcineurin inhibitor-induced hypertension is often salt-sensitive, making it responsive to diuretics. Central-acting agents (eg, clonidine) are used often as adjunctive therapy in transplantation recipients who are unable to achieve blood pressure control with first-line pharmacotherapy agents. There are no universal goals for blood pressure in transplant recipients. Most guidelines indicate a goal between 130-140/80-90 depending on other compelling co-morbid disease states.[136]

Hyperlipidemia

Hyperlipidemia may be exacerbated by corticosteroids, calcineurin inhibitors, and mTOR inhibitors.[74,75] Corticosteroids promote insulin resistance and a decrease in lipoprotein lipase activity, as well as excessive triglyceride production. CNIs may decrease the activity of the low-density lipoprotein (LDL) receptor or lipoprotein lipase, altering LDL catabolism.[74] Tacrolimus appears to have less potential than cyclosporine to induce hyperlipidemia.[99] Controversy remains whether the management of hyperlipidemia in transplant recipients should be more aggressive than current guidelines for the general population (see Chapter 32).[75,139] Aggressive lipid lowering may not only arrest the progress or prevent the complications of atherosclerosis but may also promote graft survival in kidney and heart transplant recipients. Current recommendations suggest monitoring lipid panels 2 to 3 months after transplantation and annually thereafter.[61,75]

HMG-CoA reductase inhibitors should be used with caution in transplantation recipients because of the risk of rhabdomyolysis when these agents are combined with CNIs.[104] However, beyond their impact on hyperlipidemia, HMG-CoA reductase inhibitors also have immunomodulatory effects on MHC expression and T-cell activation, and they reduce cardiac allograft rejection and extend life in heart transplant recipients.[104]

Concurrent use of simvastatin and cyclosporine is contraindicated due to the increased risk of rhabdomyolysis.[139] The concurrent use of medications known to increase the risk of myopathy (such as gemfibrozil) should be avoided.[104] Baseline and follow-up creatinine phosphokinase measurements (every 6 months) have proven useful in identifying patients with subclinical rhabdomyolysis. HMG-CoA reductase inhibitors not metabolized by CYP3A4 may be preferred owing to their diminished risk of CNI-associated drug-drug interactions. Close monitoring of liver function is recommended in all transplant recipients.[75,139]

For transplant patients who have hypertriglyceridemia refractory to dietary intervention, fish oil and fibric acid derivatives are generally well-tolerated, effective alternatives (see Chapter 32). Fibric acid derivatives are most effective in lowering serum triglyceride concentrations. The novel PCSK9 inhibitors have been used in heart transplant recipients who are intolerant to HMG-CoA reductase inhibitors or those who require further LDL lowering therapy, but evidence to support this practice in other solid-organ transplant recipients is lacking.[140]

Post-Transplantation Diabetes Mellitus

Corticosteroids and CNIs can impair glucose control in patients with pre-existing diabetes and may cause post-transplantation diabetes mellitus (PTDM) in 5% to 30% of solid-organ transplant recipients.[70,75,98] Corticosteroids induce insulin resistance and impair peripheral glucose uptake, whereas CNIs appear to inhibit insulin production.[74] Tacrolimus seems to be more diabetogenic than cyclosporine.[99] Other possible risk factors that have been identified for PTDM include African American race or Hispanic ethnicity, age greater than 40 years at time of transplant, family history, and obesity, as well as CMV and hepatitis C virus infection.[74]

Up to 40% of patients with PTDM will require insulin therapy.[74] In patients with post-transplant diabetes who can be adequately managed with only oral hypoglycemics, agents such as dipeptidyl peptidase 4 (DPP-4) inhibitors, thiazolidinediones (TZDs), and sulfonylureas may be reasonable choices. Agents that do not undergo extensive renal elimination may be preferred to reduce the incidence of hypoglycemia and toxicity in the setting of drug accumulation due to end-organ dysfunction. Metformin should be used with caution because of the risk of lactic acidosis in those with impaired kidney function but is generally well-tolerated and may be associated with improved long-term outcomes.[141] Short-term use of SGLT2 inhibitors has been endorsed in transplant patients.[142]

Frequent blood glucose monitoring is imperative in the early postoperative phase to improve glucose control and to identify those with PTDM. Changes in kidney function secondary to CNI-associated nephrotoxicity, acute rejection, or other causes in kidney transplant recipients may affect elimination of many hypoglycemic agents, including insulin, and may result in hyper- or hypoglycemia. Dose changes of immunosuppressant drugs also affects glycemic control. Tapering of immunosuppressive medications may result in reduced insulin requirements, whereas corticosteroid pulses for the treatment of rejection may result in increased insulin requirements.

Infection

Increased risk of infection is a natural consequence of pharmacologic immunosuppression. Many infections in solid-organ transplant recipients, including cytomegalovirus and fungal infections, are reviewed in Chapter 145.

Polyomavirus-associated nephropathy (PVAN) is an important cause of impaired kidney function in kidney transplant recipients.[143] Primary infection with BK virus occurs in childhood as an asymptomatic infection in 50% to 90% of the general population. The precise mechanism of transmission is not clear but is suspected to be via the oral or respiratory routes. The virus may remain latent primarily in the genitourinary tract until reactivation as the result of compromised immune function. Reactivation can be detected by measuring the presence of BK virus in the urine or plasma, a finding that is seen in approximately 30% to 40% of kidney transplant recipients, although it does not progress to nephropathy in the majority of patients. However, BK viremia (if it develops) has been noted to progress to allograft nephropathy in 50% of patients.[143] The development of BK virus nephropathy results in graft loss in about 46% of affected patients.[143]

All kidney transplant recipients should be screened for urinary BK virus replication monthly for the first 3 to 6 months after transplant, and every 3 months thereafter for the first year.[75,143] Screening for BK virus in serum should also occur any time the serum creatinine is elevated without a known cause and after treatment of acute rejection. Treatment of BK virus should be initiated when plasma concentrations persist above 10,000 copies/mL (10×10^6/L).[75,143] The first line of treatment is to reduce immunosuppressive medications, targeting tacrolimus trough concentrations of <6 ng/mL (mcg/L; 7.4 nmol/L), cyclosporine <150 ng/mL (mcg/L; 125 nmol/L), sirolimus troughs <6 ng/mL (mcg/L; 6.6 nmol/L) or total daily mycophenolate mofetil doses of <1,000 mg.

Malignancy

Although advances in immunosuppression have decreased the incidence of acute rejection and increased patient survival, they have also increased the solid-organ transplant recipients' lifetime exposure to immunosuppression. While the precise mechanism is unclear, post-transplantation malignancy seems to be related to the overall level of immunosuppression, as evidenced by a difference in the rates of malignancy associated with quadruple versus triple versus dual immunosuppressant regimens. The risk of *de novo* malignancy in transplantation recipients is increased threefold to fivefold relative to the general population, and the risk of lung and colon cancers may be as much as doubled in kidney transplant recipients.[115,144] A number of cancers that are uncommon in the general population occur with much higher prevalence in transplantation recipients: post-transplantation lymphomas and lymphoproliferative disorders (PTLD), Kaposi sarcoma, renal carcinoma, in situ carcinomas of the uterine cervix, hepatobiliary tumors, and anogenital carcinoma are a few examples.[144]

Skin cancers are the most common malignancy. Factors that may predispose transplant recipients to skin cancers include sun exposure, the use of immunosuppressive medications, and concomitant use of medications that increase the risk of phototoxicity.[145] The mTOR inhibitors have a theoretical benefit in reducing the development of malignancy by way of antiproliferative effects. In fact, a decreased incidence of malignancy may be observed in patients receiving mTOR inhibitors versus CNIs, and conversion to mTOR inhibitors may result in regression of Kaposi sarcoma.[144]

PTLD encompasses a broad spectrum of disorders, ranging from benign polyclonal hyperplasia to malignant monoclonal lymphomas. Factors that predispose patients to PTLD include Epstein-Barr virus seronegativity at transplantation and intense immunosuppression, particularly with lymphocyte-depleting agents. Non-renal transplantation recipients are more likely to develop PTLD secondary to the intensive immunosuppression used to reverse rejection. Treatment of life-threatening PTLD generally includes severe reduction or cessation of immunosuppression. Other options include systemic chemotherapy or rituximab.[144]

Post-transplantation malignancies appear at an average of 5 years after transplantation and their incidence increases with the increasing length of follow-up. As many as 72% of solid-organ transplant recipients surviving greater than 20 years may be affected. Malignancy accounts for 11.8% of deaths after cardiac transplantation and is the single most common cause of death in the 6th to the 10th post-transplant years.[144]

CLINICAL BOTTOM LINE

Transplantation is a lifesaving therapy for several types of end-organ failure. Advances in the understanding of transplant immunology have produced an unprecedented number of choices in terms of immunosuppression. The increasing number of effective immunosuppressive therapies offers clinicians diverse ways to prevent allograft rejection.

However, the vast array of currently available immunosuppressive agents make it increasingly difficult to evaluate their long-term efficacy. Clinicians must be keenly aware of the adverse effects of immunosuppressive medications and their management in order to optimize the care of the transplanted patient.

ABBREVIATIONS

ACEI	angiotensin-converting enzyme inhibitor
ACR	acute cellular rejection
AMR	antibody-mediated rejection
APC	antigen-presenting cell
ATG	antithymocyte globulin
ATN	acute tubular necrosis
AUC	area under the concentration curve
C_2	concentration 2 hours after dose
C_{peak}	peak concentration
CI	calcineurin inhibitors
CMV	cytomegalovirus
CYP	cytochrome P450 liver enzyme system
DAA	direct acting antivirals
DGF	delayed graft function
EBV	Epstein-Barr virus
ESKD	end-stage kidney disease
FKBP	FK506-binding protein
GI	gastrointestinal
HBIg	hepatitis B immunoglobulin
HLA	human leukocyte antigen
HMGCoA	hydroxy-3-methylglutaryl-coenzyme A
HPLC	high-performance liquid chromatography
IFN	interferon
IFTA	interstitial fibrosis and tubular atrophy
IL-2R	interleukin 2 receptor
IMPDH	inosine monophosphate dehydrogenase
LAS	lung allocation score
LDL	low-density lipoprotein
MELD	model for end-stage liver disease
MHC	major histocompatibility complex
6-MP	6-mercaptopurine
MPA	mycophenolic acid
MPAG	mycophenolic acid glucuronide
MRP2	multidrug-resistance-associated protein 2
mTOR	mammalian target of rapamycin
NFAT	nuclear factor of activated T lymphocytes
NODAT	new-onset diabetes after transplantation
OATP	organic anion-transporter proteins
OKT3	muromonab-CD3
PD-L1	programmed death ligand 1
PML	progressive multifocal leukoencephalopathy
PRA	panel of reactive antibodies
PSI	proliferation signal inhibitor
PTLD	post-transplantation lymphoproliferative disorder
PVAN	polyomavirus associated nephropathy
RIA	radioimmunoassay
REMS	risk evaluation and mitigation strategy
TPMT	thiopurine S-methyltransferase

REFERENCES

1. OPTN/SRTR 2019 Annual Data Report: Introduction. *Am J Transplant.* 02 2021;21(Suppl 2):11-20. 10.1111/ajt.16493
2. Alloway RR, Dupuis R, Gabardi S, et al. Evolution of the role of the transplant pharmacist on the multidisciplinary transplant team. *Am J Transplant.* Aug 2011;11(8):1576–83. 10.1111/j.1600-6143.2011.03601.x
3. Rana A, Gruessner A, Agopian VG, et al. Survival benefit of solid-organ transplant in the United States. *JAMA Surg.* Mar 1 2015;150(3):252–9. 10.1001/jamasurg.2014.2038
4. Working Group on Incentives for Living D, Matas AJ, Satel S, et al. Incentives for organ donation: Proposed standards for an internationally acceptable system. *Am J Transplant.* Feb 2012;12(2): 306–312. doi:10.1111/j.1600-6143.2011.03881.x
5. Levey AS, Eckardt KU, Tsukamoto Y, et al. Definition and classification of chronic kidney disease: a position statement from Kidney Disease: Improving Global Outcomes (KDIGO). *Kidney Int.* Jun 2005;67(6):2089–100. doi:10.1111/j.1523-1755.2005.00365.x
6. Hart A, Lentine KL, Smith JM, et al. OPTN/SRTR 2019 Annual Data Report: Kidney. *Am J Transplant.* 02 2021;21(Suppl 2):21–137. doi:10.1111/ajt.16502
7. Johansen KL, Chertow GM, Foley RN, et al. US Renal Data System 2020 Annual Data Report: Epidemiology of Kidney Disease in the United States. *Am J Kidney Dis.* 04 2021;77(4 Suppl 1):A7–A8. 10.1053/j.ajkd.2021.01.002
8. U.S. Department of Health and Human Services, Health Resources and Services Administration, Organ Procurement and Transplantation Network. How Organ Allocation Works. U.S. Department of Health and Human Services. Accessed April 7, 2019. https://optn.transplant.hrsa.gov/learn/about-transplantation/how-organ-allocation-works/
9. U.S. Department of Health and Human Services, Health Resources and Services Administration, Organ Procurement and Transplantation Network. Kidney Donor Profile Index (KDPI) Guide for Clinicians. U.S. Department of Health and Human Services. Accessed April 7, 2019. https://optn.transplant.hrsa.gov/resources/guidance/kidney-donor-profile-index-kdpi-guide-for-clinicians/
10. Rana A, Godfrey EL. Outcomes in solid-organ transplantation: Success and stagnation. *Tex Heart Inst J.* 02 2019;46(1):75–76. 10.14503/THIJ-18-6749
11. Lim MA, Bloom RD. Medical therapies to reduce delayed graft function and improve long-term graft survival: Are we making progress? *Clin J Am Soc Nephrol.* 01 2020;15(1):13–15. 10.2215/CJN.13961119
12. Ojo AO, Wolfe RA, Held PJ, Port FK, Schmouder RL. Delayed graft function: Risk factors and implications for renal allograft survival. *Transplantation.* Apr 1997;63(7):968–974. 10.1097/00007890-199704150-00011
13. Wiseman AC. Induction therapy in renal transplantation: Why? What agent? What dose? We may never know. *Clin J Am Soc Nephrol.* Jun 2015;10(6):923–925. 10.2215/CJN.03800415
14. Kirk AD. Induction immunosuppression. *Transplantation.* Sep 2006;82(5):593–602. 10.1097/01.tp.0000234905.56926.7f
15. Hanaway MJ, Woodle ES, Mulgaonkar S, et al. Alemtuzumab induction in renal transplantation. *N Engl J Med.* May 2011;364(20):1909–1919. 10.1056/NEJMoa1009546
16. Brennan DC, Daller JA, Lake KD, Cibrik D, Del Castillo D, Group TIS. Rabbit antithymocyte globulin versus basiliximab in renal transplantation. *N Engl J Med.* Nov 2006;355(19):1967–77. 10.1056/NEJMoa060068

17. Noël C, Abramowicz D, Durand D, et al. Daclizumab versus antithymocyte globulin in high-immunological-risk renal transplant recipients. *J Am Soc Nephrol.* Jun 2009;20(6):1385–92. 10.1681/ASN.2008101037
18. Wiseman AC. Immunosuppressive medications. *Clin J Am Soc Nephrol.* Feb 2016;11(2):332–43. 10.2215/CJN.08570814
19. Group USMFLS. A comparison of tacrolimus (FK 506) and cyclosporine for immunosuppression in liver transplantation. *N Engl J Med.* 10 1994;331(17):1110–1115. 10.1056/NEJM199410273311702
20. Levy G, Villamil F, Samuel D, et al. Results of lis2t, a multicenter, randomized study comparing cyclosporine microemulsion with C2 monitoring and tacrolimus with C0 monitoring in de novo liver transplantation. *Transplantation.* Jun 2004;77(11):1632–1638. 10.1097/01.tp.0000129095.51031.42
21. Wiesner R, Rabkin J, Klintmalm G, et al. A randomized double-blind comparative study of mycophenolate mofetil and azathioprine in combination with cyclosporine and corticosteroids in primary liver transplant recipients. *Liver Transpl.* May 2001;7(5):442–450. 10.1053/jlts.2001.23356
22. Perez CP, Patel N, Mardis CR, Meadows HB, Taber DJ, Pilch NA. Belatacept in solid organ transplant: Review of current literature across transplant types. *Transplantation.* 09 2018;102(9):1440–1452. 10.1097/TP.0000000000002291
23. Vincenti F, Rostaing L, Grinyo J, et al. Belatacept and long-term outcomes in kidney transplantation. *N Engl J Med.* Jan 2016;374(4):333–343. 10.1056/NEJMoa1506027
24. Kwong AJ, Kim WR, Lake JR, et al. OPTN/SRTR 2019 annual data report: Liver. *Am J Transplant.* 02 2021;21(Suppl 2):208–315. 10.1111/ajt.16494
25. Weeks SR, Sun Z, McCaul ME, et al. Liver transplantation for severe alcoholic hepatitis, updated lessons from the world's largest series. *J Am Coll Surg.* Apr 2018;226(4):549–557. 10.1016/j.jamcollsurg.2017.12.044
26. Mazzaferro V, Regalia E, Doci R, et al. Liver transplantation for the treatment of small hepatocellular carcinomas in patients with cirrhosis. *N Engl J Med.* Mar 1996;334(11):693–699. 10.1056/NEJM199603143341104
27. Wald C, Russo MW, Heimbach JK, Hussain HK, Pomfret EA, Bruix J. New OPTN/UNOS policy for liver transplant allocation: Standardization of liver imaging, diagnosis, classification, and reporting of hepatocellular carcinoma. *Radiology.* Feb 2013;266(2):376–382. 10.1148/radiol.12121698
28. MA V, DL B, A J. Tables of Summary Health Statistics for U.S. Adults: 2018 National Health Interview Survey. National Center for Health Statistics. Accessed July 26, 2021. http://www.cdc.gov/nchs/nhis/SHS/tables.htm
29. Quante M, Benckert C, Thelen A, Jonas S. Experience since MELD implementation: How does the new system deliver? *Int J Hepatol.* 2012;2012:264015. 10.1155/2012/264015
30. Kim WR, Biggins SW, Kremers WK, et al. Hyponatremia and mortality among patients on the liver-transplant waiting list. *N Engl J Med.* Sep 2008;359(10):1018–1026. 10.1056/NEJMoa0801209
31. Venkataramanan R, Habucky K, Burckart GJ, Ptachcinski RJ. Clinical pharmacokinetics in organ transplant patients. *Clin Pharmacokinet.* Mar 1989;16(3):134–161. 10.2165/00003088-198916030-00002
32. Verna EC, Farrand ED, Elnaggar AS, et al. Basiliximab induction and delayed calcineurin inhibitor initiation in liver transplant recipients with renal insufficiency. *Transplantation.* Jun 2011;91(11):1254–1260. 10.1097/TP.0b013e318218f0f5
33. Lange NW, Salerno DM, Sammons CM, Jesudian AB, Verna EC, Brown RS. Delayed calcineurin inhibitor introduction and renal outcomes in liver transplant recipients receiving basiliximab induction. *Clin Transplant.* 2018;32(12):e13415. 10.1111/ctr.13415
34. Yoo MC, Vanatta JM, Modanlou KA, et al. Steroid-free Liver transplantation using rabbit antithymocyte globulin induction in 500 consecutive patients. *Transplantation.* Jun 2015;99(6):1231–1235. 10.1097/TP.0000000000000477
35. Massoud O, Wiesner RH. The use of sirolimus should be restricted in liver transplantation. *J Hepatol.* Jan 2012;56(1):288–290. 10.1016/j.jhep.2011.06.012
36. Klintmalm GB, Feng S, Lake JR, et al. Belatacept-based immunosuppression in de novo liver transplant recipients: 1-year experience from a phase II randomized study. *Am J Transplant.* Aug 2014;14(8):1817–1827. 10.1111/ajt.12810
37. Hemmila MR, Napolitano LM. Severe respiratory failure: Advanced treatment options. *Crit Care Med.* Sep 2006;34(9 Suppl):S278–S290. 10.1097/01.CCM.0000233788.96388.D8
38. Valapour M, Lehr CJ, Skeans MA, et al. OPTN/SRTR 2019 annual data report: Lung. *Am J Transplant.* 02 2021;21(Suppl 2):441–520. 10.1111/ajt.16495
39. Weill D, Benden C, Corris PA, et al. A consensus document for the selection of lung transplant candidates: 2014—An update from the Pulmonary Transplantation Council of the International Society for Heart and Lung Transplantation. *J Heart Lung Transplant.* Jan 2015;34(1):1–15. 10.1016/j.healun.2014.06.014
40. Ekberg-Aronsson M, Pehrsson K, Nilsson JA, Nilsson PM, Löfdahl CG. Mortality in GOLD stages of COPD and its dependence on symptoms of chronic bronchitis. *Respir Res.* Aug 2005;6:98. 10.1186/1465-9921-6-98
41. Egan TM, Edwards LB. Effect of the lung allocation score on lung transplantation in the United States. *J Heart Lung Transplant.* Apr 2016;35(4):433–439. 10.1016/j.healun.2016.01.010
42. Yusen RD, Edwards LB, Dipchand AI, et al. The Registry of the International Society for Heart and Lung Transplantation: Thirty-third adult lung and heart-lung transplant report-2016; Focus theme: Primary diagnostic indications for transplant. *J Heart Lung Transplant.* 10 2016;35(10):1170–1184. 10.1016/j.healun.2016.09.001
43. Studer SM, Levy RD, McNeil K, Orens JB. Lung transplant outcomes: A review of survival, graft function, physiology, health-related quality of life and cost-effectiveness. *Eur Respir J.* Oct 2004;24(4):674–685. 10.1183/09031936.04.00065004
44. Maziak DE, Maurer JR, Kesten S. Diaphragmatic paralysis: A complication of lung transplantation. *Ann Thorac Surg.* Jan 1996;61(1):170–173. 10.1016/0003-4975(95)00823-3
45. Hoeper MM, Benza RL, Corris P, et al. Intensive care, right ventricular support and lung transplantation in patients with pulmonary hypertension. *Eur Respir J.* 01 2019;53(1). 10.1183/13993003.01906-2018
46. Horvath J, Dummer S, Loyd J, Walker B, Merrill WH, Frist WH. Infection in the transplanted and native lung after single lung transplantation. *Chest.* Sep 1993;104(3):681–685. 10.1378/chest.104.3.681
47. Renders N, Verbrugh H, Van Belkum A. Dynamics of bacterial colonisation in the respiratory tract of patients with cystic fibrosis. *Infect Genet Evol.* Jul 2001;1(1):29–39. 10.1016/s1567-1348(01)00004-1
48. Scheffert JL, Raza K. Immunosuppression in lung transplantation. *J Thorac Dis.* Aug 2014;6(8):1039–1053. 10.3978/j.issn.2072-1439.2014.04.23
49. Klintmalm GB, Kaplan B, Kirk AD. FDA jeopardizes the lives of lung transplant recipients and in the process severely increases the cost to develop new immunosuppression. *Am J Transplant.* 04 2019;19(4):971–972. 10.1111/ajt.15215
50. Johnson BA, Iacono AT, Zeevi A, McCurry KR, Duncan SR. Statin use is associated with improved function and survival of lung allografts. *Am J Respir Crit Care Med.* May 2003;167(9):1271–1278. 10.1164/rccm.200205-410OC
52. Strueber M, Warnecke G, Fuge J, et al. Everolimus versus mycophenolate mofetil de novo after lung transplantation: A prospective, randomized, open-label trial. *Am J Transplant.* 11 2016;16(11):3171–3180. 10.1111/ajt.13835
51. Sacher VY, Fertel D, Srivastava K, et al. Effects of prophylactic use of sirolimus on bronchiolitis obliterans syndrome development in lung transplant recipients. *Ann Thorac Surg.* Jan 2014;97(1):268–274. 10.1016/j.athoracsur.2013.07.072
53. Ruttens D, Verleden SE, Vandermeulen E, et al. Prophylactic azithromycin therapy after lung transplantation: Post hoc analysis of a randomized controlled trial. *Am J Transplant.* Jan 2016;16(1):254–261. 10.1111/ajt.13417
54. Ruttens D, Verleden SE, Demeyer H, et al. Montelukast for bronchiolitis obliterans syndrome after lung transplantation: A randomized controlled trial. *PLoS One.* 2018;13(4):e0193564. 10.1371/journal.pone.0193564
55. Crespo-Leiro MG, Metra M, Lund LH, et al. Advanced heart failure: A position statement of the Heart Failure Association of the European Society of Cardiology. *Eur J Heart Fail.* 2018;20(11):1505–1535. 10.1002/ejhf.1236
56. Mehra MR, Domanski MJ. Should left ventricular assist device should be standard of care for patients with refractory heart failure who are not transplantation candidates?: left ventricular assist devices should be considered standard of care for patients with refractory heart failure who are not transplantation candidates. *Circulation.* Dec 2012;126(25):3081–3087. 10.1161/CIRCULATIONAHA.111.079301
57. Colvin M, Smith JM, Ahn Y, et al. OPTN/SRTR 2019 annual data report: Heart. *Am J Transplant.* 02 2021;21(Suppl 2):356–440. 10.1111/ajt.16492
58. Moayedi Y, Fan CPS, Cherikh WS, et al. Survival outcomes after heart transplantation: Does recipient sex matter? *Circ Heart Fail.* 10 2019;12(10):e006218. 10.1161/CIRCHEARTFAILURE.119.006218

59. Deng MC. Cardiac transplantation. *Heart.* Feb 2002;87(2):177–184.
60. Wright M, Takeda K, Mauro C, et al. Dose-dependent association between amiodarone and severe primary graft dysfunction in orthotopic heart transplantation. *J Heart Lung Transplant.* Nov 2017;36(11):1226–1233. 10.1016/j.healun.2017.05.025
61. Costanzo MR, Dipchand A, Starling R, et al. The International Society of Heart and Lung Transplantation Guidelines for the care of heart transplant recipients. *J Heart Lung Transplant.* Aug 2010;29(8):914–56. 10.1016/j.healun.2010.05.034
62. Sabato LA, Salerno DM, Moretz JD, Jennings DL. Inhaled pulmonary vasodilator therapy for management of right ventricular dysfunction after left ventricular assist device placement and cardiac transplantation. *Pharmacotherapy.* Aug 2017;37(8):944–955. 10.1002/phar.1959
63. Truby LK, DeRoo S, Spellman J, et al. Management of primary graft failure after heart transplantation: Preoperative risks, perioperative events, and postoperative decisions. *Clin Transplant.* 2019;33(6):e13557. 10.1111/ctr.13557
64. Khush KK, Cherikh WS, Chambers DC, et al. The International Thoracic Organ Transplant Registry of the International Society for Heart and Lung Transplantation: Thirty-sixth adult heart transplantation report—2019; focus theme: Donor and recipient size match. *J Heart Lung Transplant.* 10 2019;38(10):1056–1066. 10.1016/j.healun.2019.08.004
65. Jennings DL, Lange N, Shullo M, et al. Outcomes associated with mammalian target of rapamycin (mTOR) inhibitors in heart transplant recipients: A meta-analysis. *Int J Cardiol.* Aug 2018;265:71–76. 10.1016/j.ijcard.2018.03.111
66. Cozzi E, Colpo A, De Silvestro G. The mechanisms of rejection in solid organ transplantation. *Transfus Apher Sci.* Aug 2017;56(4):498–505. 10.1016/j.transci.2017.07.005
67. Kruskall MS. The major histocompatibility complex: The value of extended haplotypes in the analysis of associated immune diseases and disorders. *Yale J Biol Med.* 1990 Sep-Oct 1990;63(5):477–486.
68. Williams GM, Hume DM, Hudson RP, Morris PJ, Kano K, Milgrom F. "Hyperacute" renal-homograft rejection in man. *N Engl J Med.* Sep 1968;279(12):611–618. 10.1056/NEJM196809192791201
69. Patel R, Terasaki PI. Significance of the positive crossmatch test in kidney transplantation. *N Engl J Med.* Apr 1969;280(14):735–739. 10.1056/NEJM196904032801401
70. Haas M. Pathologic features of antibody-mediated rejection in renal allografts: An expanding spectrum. *Curr Opin Nephrol Hypertens.* May 2012;21(3):264–271. 10.1097/MNH.0b013e3283520efa
71. Fehr T, Gaspert A. Antibody-mediated kidney allograft rejection: Therapeutic options and their experimental rationale. *Transpl Int.* Jun 2012;25(6):623–632. 10.1111/j.1432-2277.2012.01453.x
72. Kim M, Martin ST, Townsend KR, Gabardi S. Antibody-mediated rejection in kidney transplantation: A review of pathophysiology, diagnosis, and treatment options. *Pharmacotherapy.* Jul 2014;34(7):733–744. 10.1002/phar.1426
73. Chih S, Chong AY, Mielniczuk LM, Bhatt DL, Beanlands RS. Allograft vasculopathy: The Achilles' heel of heart transplantation. *J Am Coll Cardiol.* Jul 5 2016;68(1):80–91. 10.1016/j.jacc.2016.04.033
74. Lucey MR, Terrault N, Ojo L, et al. Long-term management of the successful adult liver transplant: 2012 Practice guideline by the American Association for the Study of Liver Diseases and the American Society of Transplantation. *Liver Transpl.* Jan 2013;19(1):3–26. 10.1002/lt.23566
75. Kasiske BL, Zeier MG, Craig JC, et al. Kidney disease: Improving Global Outcomes Transplant Work Group. KDIGO clinical practice guideline for the care of kidney transplant recipients. *Am J Transplant.* Nov 2009;9(Suppl 3):S1–S155. 10.1111/j.1600-6143.2009.02834.x
76. Petite SE, Bollinger JE, Eghtesad B. Antithymocyte globulin induction therapy in liver transplant: Old drug, new uses. *Ann Pharmacother.* Jul 2016;50(7):592–8. 10.1177/1060028016647974
77. Pilch NA, Bowman LJ, Taber DJ. Immunosuppression trends in solid organ transplantation: The future of individualization, monitoring, and management. *Pharmacotherapy.* 01 2021;41(1):119–131. 10.1002/phar.2481
78. Brennan DC, Flavin K, Lowell JA, et al. A randomized, double-blinded comparison of Thymoglobulin versus Atgam for induction immunosuppressive therapy in adult renal transplant recipients. *Transplantation.* Apr 1999;67(7):1011–1018. 10.1097/00007890-199904150-00013
79. Alloway RR, Woodle ES, Abramowicz D, et al. Rabbit anti-thymocyte globulin for the prevention of acute rejection in kidney transplantation. *Am J Transplant.* 08 2019;19(8):2252–2261. 10.1111/ajt.15342
80. Mullen JC, Oreopoulos A, Lien DC, et al. A randomized, controlled trial of daclizumab vs anti-thymocyte globulin induction for lung transplantation. *J Heart Lung Transplant.* May 2007;26(5):504–510. 10.1016/j.healun.2007.01.032
81. Hartwig MG, Snyder LD, Appel JZ, et al. Rabbit anti-thymocyte globulin induction therapy does not prolong survival after lung transplantation. *J Heart Lung Transplant.* May 2008;27(5):547–553. 10.1016/j.healun.2008.01.022
82. Morgan RD, O'Callaghan JM, Knight SR, Morris PJ. Alemtuzumab induction therapy in kidney transplantation: A systematic review and meta-analysis. *Transplantation.* Jun 27 2012;93(12):1179–1188. 10.1097/TP.0b013e318257ad41
83. Kuypers DR. Immunotherapy in elderly transplant recipients: A guide to clinically significant drug interactions. *Drugs Aging.* 2009;26(9):715–737. 10.2165/11316480-000000000-00000
84. Jasiak NM, Park JM. Immunosuppression in solid-organ transplantation: Essentials and practical tips. *Crit Care Nurs Q.* Jul-Sep 2016;39(3):227–240. 10.1097/CNQ.0000000000000117
85. Patel K, Parmar S, Shah S, et al. Comparison of subcutaneous versus intravenous alemtuzumab for graft-versus-host disease prophylaxis with fludarabine/melphalan-based conditioning in matched unrelated donor allogeneic stem cell transplantation. *Biol Blood Marrow Transplant.* Mar 2016;22(3):456–461. 10.1016/j.bbmt.2015.10.022
86. Simulect® (basiliximab) [product information]. East Hanover, NJ: Novartis Pharmaceutical Corporation. 2018.
87. Kovarik JM, Nashan B, Neuhaus P, et al. A population pharmacokinetic screen to identify demographic-clinical covariates of basiliximab in liver transplantation. *Clin Pharmacol Ther.* Apr 2001;69(4):201–209. 10.1067/mcp.2001.114887
88. Cillo U, Bechstein WO, Berlakovich G, et al. Identifying risk profiles in liver transplant candidates and implications for induction immunosuppression. *Transplant Rev (Orlando).* Jul 2018;32(3):142–150. 10.1016/j.trre.2018.04.001
89. Koleba T, Ensom MH. Pharmacokinetics of intravenous immunoglobulin: A systematic review. *Pharmacotherapy.* Jun 2006;26(6):813–827. 10.1592/phco.26.6.813
90. Jordan SC, Tyan D, Stablein D, et al. Evaluation of intravenous immunoglobulin as an agent to lower allosensitization and improve transplantation in highly sensitized adult patients with end-stage renal disease: Report of the NIH IG02 trial. *J Am Soc Nephrol.* Dec 2004;15(12):3256–3262. 10.1097/01.ASN.0000145878.92906.9F
91. Montgomery RA, Lonze BE, King KE, et al. Desensitization in HLA-incompatible kidney recipients and survival. *N Engl J Med.* Jul 2011;365(4):318–326. 10.1056/NEJMoa1012376
92. Casadei DH, del C Rial M, Opelz G, et al. A randomized and prospective study comparing treatment with high-dose intravenous immunoglobulin with monoclonal antibodies for rescue of kidney grafts with steroid-resistant rejection. *Transplantation.* Jan 2001;71(1):53–58. 10.1097/00007890-200101150-00009
93. Moreso F, Crespo M, Ruiz JC, et al. Treatment of chronic antibody mediated rejection with intravenous immunoglobulins and rituximab: A multicenter, prospective, randomized, double-blind clinical trial. *Am J Transplant.* 04 2018;18(4):927–935. 10.1111/ajt.14520
94. U.S. Department of Health and Human Services, Health Resources and Services Administration, OPTN/SRTR Annual Data Report. U.S. Department of Health and Human Services. Accessed April 7, 2019. https://srtr.transplant.hrsa.gov/annual_reports/Default.aspx
95. Knops N, Levtchenko E, van den Heuvel B, Kuypers D. From gut to kidney: Transporting and metabolizing calcineurin-inhibitors in solid organ transplantation. *Int J Pharm.* Aug 16, 2013;452(1-2):14–35. 10.1016/j.ijpharm.2013.05.033
96. Trofe-Clark J, Lemonovich TL. AST Infectious Diseases Community of Practice. Interactions between anti-infective agents and immunosuppressants in solid organ transplantation. *Am J Transplant.* Mar 2013;13(Suppl 4):318–326. 10.1111/ajt.12123
97. Webster AC, Woodroffe RC, Taylor RS, Chapman JR, Craig JC. Tacrolimus versus ciclosporin as primary immunosuppression for kidney transplant recipients: Meta-analysis and meta-regression of randomised trial data. *BMJ.* Oct 2005;331(7520):810. 10.1136/bmj.38569.471007.AE
98. Shivaswamy V, Boerner B, Larsen J. Post-transplant diabetes mellitus: Causes, treatment, and impact on outcomes. *Endocr Rev.* Feb 2016;37(1):37–61. 10.1210/er.2015-1084
99. Lee RA, Gabardi S. Current trends in immunosuppressive therapies for renal transplant recipients. *Am J Health Syst Pharm.* Nov 15, 2012;69(22):1961–1975. 10.2146/ajhp110624

100. Ojo AO, Held PJ, Port FK, et al. Chronic renal failure after transplantation of a nonrenal organ. *N Engl J Med.* Sep 2003;349(10):931–940. 10.1056/NEJMoa021744
101. Salvadori M, Bertoni E. Is it time to give up with calcineurin inhibitors in kidney transplantation? *World J Transplant.* Jun 24, 2013;3(2):7–25. 10.5500/wjt.v3.i2.7
102. Wagner SJ, Brennan DC. Induction therapy in renal transplant recipients: How convincing is the current evidence? *Drugs.* Mar 26, 2012;72(5):671–683. 10.2165/11631300-000000000-00000
103. Amundsen R, Asberg A, Ohm IK, Christensen H. Cyclosporine A- and tacrolimus-mediated inhibition of CYP3A4 and CYP3A5 in vitro. *Drug Metab Dispos.* Apr 2012;40(4):655–661. 10.1124/dmd.111.043018
104. Olyaei A, Greer E, Delos Santos R, Rueda J. The efficacy and safety of the 3-hydroxy-3-methylglutaryl-CoA reductase inhibitors in chronic kidney disease, dialysis, and transplant patients. *Clin J Am Soc Nephrol.* Mar 2011;6(3):664–678. 10.2215/CJN.09091010
105. Heeney SA, Tjugum SL, Corkish ME, Hollis IB. Safety and tolerability of high-intensity statin therapy in heart transplant patients receiving immunosuppression with tacrolimus. *Clin Transplant.* Jan 2019;33(1):e13454. 10.1111/ctr.13454
106. Schiff J, Cole E, Cantarovich M. Therapeutic monitoring of calcineurin inhibitors for the nephrologist. *Clin J Am Soc Nephrol.* Mar 2007;2(2):374–384. 10.2215/CJN.03791106
107. Envarsus XR® (tacrolimus extended-release tablets) [product information]. Cary, NC: Veloxis Pharmaceuticals, Inc. 2018.
108. Kuypers DR. Immunosuppressive drug monitoring: What to use in clinical practice today to improve renal graft outcome. *Transpl Int.* Feb 2005;18(2):140–150. 10.1111/j.1432-2277.2004.00041.x
109. Ensor CR, Iasella CJ, Harrigan KM, et al. Increasing tacrolimus time-in-therapeutic range is associated with superior one-year outcomes in lung transplant recipients. *Am J Transplant.* Jun 2018;18(6): 1527–1533. 10.1111/ajt.14723
110. Del Bello A, Congy-Jolivet N, Danjoux M, et al. High tacrolimus intra-patient variability is associated with graft rejection, and de novo donor-specific antibodies occurrence after liver transplantation. *World J Gastroenterol.* Apr 28, 2018;24(16):1795–1802. 10.3748/wjg.v24.i16.1795
111. Taber DJ, Gebregziabher MG, Srinivas TR, Chavin KD, Baliga PK, Egede LE. African-American race modifies the influence of tacrolimus concentrations on acute rejection and toxicity in kidney transplant recipients. *Pharmacotherapy.* Jun 2015;35(6):569–77. 10.1002/phar.1591
112. Bergmann TK, Barraclough KA, Lee KJ, Staatz CE. Clinical pharmacokinetics and pharmacodynamics of prednisolone and prednisone in solid organ transplantation. *Clin Pharmacokinet.* Nov 2012;51(11):711–741. 10.1007/s40262-012-0007-8
113. Pascual J, Royuela A, Galeano C, Crespo M, Zamora J. Very early steroid withdrawal or complete avoidance for kidney transplant recipients: A systematic review. *Nephrol Dial Transplant.* Feb 2012;27(2):825–832. 10.1093/ndt/gfr374
114. de Jonge H, Naesens M, Kuypers DR. New insights into the pharmacokinetics and pharmacodynamics of the calcineurin inhibitors and mycophenolic acid: Possible consequences for therapeutic drug monitoring in solid organ transplantation. *Ther Drug Monit.* Aug 2009;31(4):416–435. 10.1097/FTD.0b013e3181aa36cd
115. Staatz CE, Tett SE. Pharmacology and toxicology of mycophenolate in organ transplant recipients: An update. *Arch Toxicol.* Jul 2014;88(7):1351–1389. 10.1007/s00204-014-1247-1
116. Cattaneo D, Perico N, Gaspari F, Gotti E, Remuzzi G. Glucocorticoids interfere with mycophenolate mofetil bioavailability in kidney transplantation. *Kidney Int.* Sep 2002;62(3):1060–1067. 10.1046/j.1523-1755.2002.00531.x
117. Knorr JP, Sjeime M, Braitman LE, Jawa P, Zaki R, Ortiz J. Concomitant proton pump inhibitors with mycophenolate mofetil and the risk of rejection in kidney transplant recipients. *Transplantation.* Mar 15 2014;97(5):518–524. 10.1097/01.tp.0000436100.65983.10
118. van Gelder T, van Schaik RH, Hesselink DA. Pharmacogenetics and immunosuppressive drugs in solid organ transplantation. *Nat Rev Nephrol.* Dec 2014;10(12):725–731. 10.1038/nrneph.2014.172
119. Kuypers DR, Le Meur Y, Cantarovich M, et al. Consensus report on therapeutic drug monitoring of mycophenolic acid in solid organ transplantation. *Clin J Am Soc Nephrol.* Feb 2010;5(2):341–358. 10.2215/CJN.07111009
120. Imuran® (azathioprine) [product information]. San Diego, CA: Prometheus Laboratories Inc. 2011.
121. Shihab F, Christians U, Smith L, Wellen JR, Kaplan B. Focus on mTOR inhibitors and tacrolimus in renal transplantation: Pharmacokinetics, exposure-response relationships, and clinical outcomes. *Transpl Immunol.* Jun 2014;31(1):22–32. 10.1016/j.trim.2014.05.002
122. Klawitter J, Nashan B, Christians U. Everolimus and sirolimus in transplantation-related but different. *Expert Opin Drug Saf.* Jul 2015;14(7):1055–1070. 10.1517/14740338.2015.1040388
123. Dantal J. Everolimus: Preventing organ rejection in adult kidney transplant recipients. *Expert Opin Pharmacother.* Apr 2012;13(5): 767–778. 10.1517/14656566.2012.662955
124. Nulojix® (belatacept) [product information]. Princeton, NJ: Bristol-Myers Squibb Company. 2014.
125. Vincenti F, Charpentier B, Vanrenterghem Y, et al. A phase III study of belatacept-based immunosuppression regimens versus cyclosporine in renal transplant recipients (BENEFIT study). *Am J Transplant.* Mar 2010;10(3):535–546. doi:10.1111/j.1600-6143.2009.03005.x
126. Woodle ES, Kaufman DB, Shields AR, et al. Belatacept-based immunosuppression with simultaneous calcineurin inhibitor avoidance and early corticosteroid withdrawal: A prospective, randomized multicenter trial. *Am J Transplant.* 04 2020;20(4):1039–1055. 10.1111/ajt.15688
127. Iasella CJ, Winstead RJ, Moore CA, et al. Maintenance belatacept-based immunosuppression in lung transplantation recipients who failed calcineurin inhibitors. *Transplantation.* Jan 2018;102(1):171–177. 10.1097/TP.0000000000001873
128. Kumar D, LeCorchick S, Gupta G. Belatacept as an alternative to calcineurin inhibitors in patients with solid organ transplants. *Front Med (Lausanne).* 2017;4:60. 10.3389/fmed.2017.00060
129. Launay M, Guitard J, Dorent R, et al. Belatacept-based immunosuppression: A calcineurin inhibitor-sparing regimen in heart transplant recipients. *Am J Transplant.* 02 2020;20(2):553–563. 10.1111/ajt.15584
130. Ramanath V, Nistala R, Chaudhary K. Update on the role of rituximab in kidney diseases and transplant. *Expert Opin Biol Ther.* Feb 2012;12(2):223–233. 10.1517/14712598.2012.646984
131. Kobashigawa JA, Patel JK, Kittleson MM, et al. The long-term outcome of treated sensitized patients who undergo heart transplantation. *Clin Transplant.* 2011 Jan-Feb 2011;25(1):E61–E67. 10.1111/j.1399-0012.2010.01334.x
132. Sautenet B, Blancho G, Büchler M, et al. One-year results of the effects of rituximab on acute antibody-mediated rejection in renal transplantation: RITUX ERAH, a multicenter double-blind randomized placebo-controlled trial. *Transplantation.* Feb 2016;100(2):391–399. 10.1097/TP.0000000000000958
133. Awan AA, Niu J, Pan JS, et al. Trends in the causes of death among kidney transplant recipients in the United States (1996-2014). *Am J Nephrol.* 2018;48(6):472–481. doi:10.1159/000495081
134. Gutierrez-Dalmau A, Campistol JM. Immunosuppressive therapy and malignancy in organ transplant recipients: A systematic review. *Drugs.* 2007;67(8):1167–1198. 10.2165/00003495-200767080-00006
135. Webber A, Hirose R, Vincenti F. Novel strategies in immunosuppression: Issues in perspective. *Transplantation.* May 27 2011;91(10):1057–1064. 10.1097/TP.0b013e3182145306
136. Weir MR, Burgess ED, Cooper JE, et al. Assessment and management of hypertension in transplant patients. *J Am Soc Nephrol.* Jun 2015;26(6):1248–1260. 10.1681/ASN.2014080834
137. James PA, Oparil S, Carter BL, et al. 2014 Evidence-based guideline for the management of high blood pressure in adults: Report from the panel members appointed to the Eighth Joint National Committee (JNC 8). *JAMA.* Feb 5 2014;311(5):507–520. doi:10.1001/jama.2013.284427
138. Grześk G, Wiciński M, Malinowski B, et al. Calcium blockers inhibit cyclosporine A-induced hyperreactivity of vascular smooth muscle cells. *Mol Med Rep.* Jun 2012;5(6):1469–1474. 10.3892/mmr.2012.847
139. Florentin M, Elisaf MS. Simvastatin interactions with other drugs. *Expert Opin Drug Saf.* May 2012;11(3):439–444. 10.1517/14740338.2012.670633
140. Jennings DL, Jackson R, Farr M. PCSK9 inhibitor use in heart transplant recipients: A case series and review of the literature. *Transplantation.* 01 2020;104(1):e38–e39. 10.1097/TP.0000000000002944
141. Vest LS, Koraishy FM, Zhang Z, et al. Metformin use in the first year after kidney transplant, correlates, and associated outcomes in diabetic transplant recipients: A retrospective analysis of integrated registry and pharmacy claims data. *Clin Transplant.* 08 2018;32(8):e13302. 10.1111/ctr.13302

142. Halden TAS, Kvitne KE, Midtvedt K, et al. Efficacy and safety of empagliflozin in renal transplant recipients with posttransplant diabetes mellitus. *Diabetes Care.* 06 2019;42(6):1067–1074. 10.2337/dc19-0093
143. Hirsch HH, Randhawa P, Practice ASTIDCo. BK virus in solid organ transplant recipients. *Am J Transplant.* Dec 2009;9(Suppl 4):S136–S146. doi:10.1111/j.1600-6143.2009.02904.x
144. Bottomley MJ, Harden PN. Update on the long-term complications of renal transplantation. *Br Med Bull.* 2013;106:117–134. 10.1093/bmb/ldt012
145. O'Reilly Zwald F, Brown M. Skin cancer in solid organ transplant recipients: Advances in therapy and management: Part I. Epidemiology of skin cancer in solid organ transplant recipients. *J Am Acad Dermatol.* Aug 2011;65(2):253–261. 10.1016/j.jaad.2010.11.062

110

Osteoarthritis

Lucinda M. Buys and Sara A. Wiedenfeld

KEY CONCEPTS

1. Osteoarthritis (OA) is a common disease. OA prevalence increases with age and number of other chronic conditions, with women more commonly affected than men.
2. Contributors to OA are systemic (age, genetics, hormonal status, obesity, occupational or recreational activity) and/or local (injury, overloading of joints, muscle weakness, or joint deformity).
3. OA is primarily a disease of cartilage that reflects a failure of the chondrocyte to maintain proper balance between cartilage formation and destruction. This leads to loss of cartilage in the joint, local inflammation, pathologic changes in underlying bone, and further damage to cartilage triggered by the affected bone.
4. The most common symptom associated with OA is pain, which leads to decreased function and motion. Pain relief is the primary objective of medication therapy.
5. Manifestations of OA are local, affecting one or a few joints; the knees are most commonly affected, as well as the hips and hands.
6. Nonpharmacologic therapy is the foundation of the treatment plan for all patients with OA. Nonpharmacologic therapy should be initiated before or concurrently with pharmacologic therapy.
7. Based upon efficacy, safety, and cost considerations, scheduled acetaminophen, up to 4 g/day, should be tried initially for pain relief in knee and hip OA. If this fails, nonsteroidal anti-inflammatory drugs (NSAIDs; topical or oral) are recommended, if there are no contraindications.
8. Topical NSAIDs, in lieu of oral NSAIDs, are recommended for patients older than 75 years of age to decrease the risks of systemic toxicity.
9. Strategies to reduce NSAID-induced gastrointestinal (GI) toxicity include the use of nonacetylated salicylates, COX-2 selective inhibitors, or the addition of misoprostol or a proton pump inhibitor.
10. Other agents useful in treating knee OA include intra-articular injections of corticosteroids, duloxetine, or tramadol.

BEYOND THE BOOK

This activity is designed to build skills in developing a safe-and-effective patient-specific PLAN as part of the patient care process.

Create a table of drug treatment options for a patient with knee, hip, and hand osteoarthritis and a history of a myocardial infarction.

INTRODUCTION

Osteoarthritis (OA) is the most common joint disease and one of the leading causes of disability in the United States.[1] Knee OA alone is as important a contributor to disability as cardiovascular (CV) disease and more important than other comorbidities. OA is a common co-occurrence with other chronic health conditions that adversely affect quality of life.[1]

The progressive destruction of articular cartilage has long been appreciated in OA, but OA involves the entire diarthrodial joint, including articular cartilage, synovium, capsule, and subchondral bone, with surrounding ligaments and muscles also playing important roles. Changes in structure and function of these tissues produce clinical OA, characterized by joint pain and tenderness, with decreased range of motion, weakness, joint instability, and disability.

This chapter will review the epidemiology, etiology, pathophysiology, and clinical presentation of OA. It then will focus on nonpharmacologic and pharmacologic treatments for OA. Because millions of persons take medications for OA, the overall risks posed by these medications require careful consideration, particularly by clinicians who treat or advise patients on drug therapy for OA. This chapter examines the risks and benefits of OA treatments, with emphasis on those individuals who have the highest risk for adverse events, to help clinicians maximize benefits and minimize risks to their patients with OA.

EPIDEMIOLOGY

1 During 2013 to 2015, an estimated 54.4 million adults in the United States reported doctor-diagnosed arthritis (osteoarthritis, rheumatoid arthritis, gout, lupus, or fibromyalgia), with 23.7 million reporting arthritis-attributable activity limitation (AAAL).[1] The prevalence of AAAL among adults with arthritis increased by almost 20% over time (2002-2015).[1] Arthritis is projected to affect 78.4 million adults by 2040.[2] OA imposes a tremendous cost burden with combined arthritis-attributable medical expenditures and earnings losses totaling approximately $303 billion dollars in 2013.[3] The US Medical Expenditure Panel Survey found that arthritis-attributable

medical expenditures were $139.8 billion, representing 11% of the total medical expenditures in 2013.[3] Among all adults in the US population, adults with arthritis had the highest overall average cost per person ($9,233), followed by adults with at least one nonarthritis chronic condition ($6,272) and those with no chronic conditions ($1,369).[3] Total hospital costs associated with the specific diagnosis of osteoarthritis were $16.5 billion attributed to 1 million hospital stays in 2013.[4] Arthritis-attributable lost earnings were $163.7 billion with almost half of lost earnings due to lower adjusted per-person earnings for those with arthritis.[3]

Prevalence by Age, Sex, and Race

Prevalence estimates for OA vary depending on the age group of interest, gender, ethnic group, and the specific joint involved. Estimates also depend on the specific means by which OA is assessed and documented. Clinical OA is based on physical exam and patient history, whereas radiographic OA is determined by x-ray or other imaging, and symptomatic OA is based on patient history and physical exam plus x-ray. OA is more prevalent with increasing age. In the United States, the prevalence of self-reported doctor-diagnosed arthritis in the 2013 to 2015 National Health Interview Survey (NHIS) is 22.7% for all persons over age 18, but 49.6% for persons age 65 and older.[1] Prevalence for AAAL among persons with doctor-diagnosed arthritis is 43.5% for all persons over age 18 and 44% for persons age 65 and older.[1] Radiologically confirmed hip OA shows clear trends through all age groups, affecting 1.6% of those between ages 30 and 39, up to a prevalence of 14% in those over 85 years of age.[5] Radiographic hand OA is found in 5% of those aged 40, but in 65% of those older than 80 years of age.[6]

Prevalence of physician-diagnosed arthritis is 26.3% in White populations, and ranges from 11.1% for Asian populations to 21.8% for Black populations.[1] African American men are approximately 35% more likely to have radiographic knee OA and twice as likely to have more severe knee OA than White men.[7] No significant differences were found between the prevalence of knee OA in Black women and White women, but Black women were 50% more likely than White women to have more severe involvement.[7] Among adults with arthritis, the prevalence of severe joint pain is significantly higher in women (29.7%), non-Hispanic Blacks (45.6%), those with less than a high school education (40.2%), and those unable to work (51.9%).[8] Women are also more likely to have inflammatory OA of the proximal and distal interphalangeal joints of the hands, giving rise to the formation of Bouchard and Heberden nodes, respectively (Fig. 110-1).

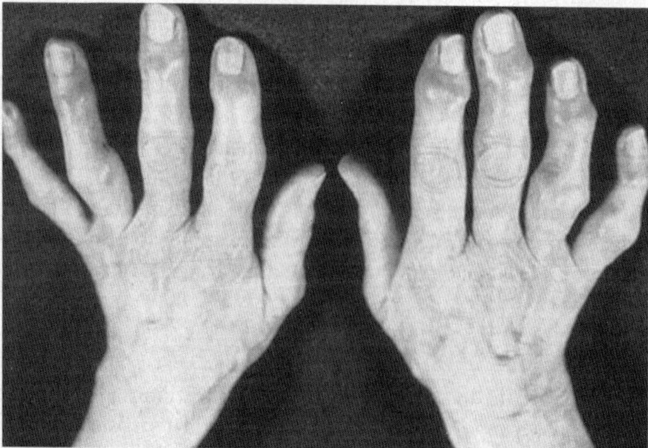

FIGURE 110-1 Heberden nodes (distal interphalangeal joint) noted on all fingers and Bouchard nodes (proximal interphalangeal joint) noted on most fingers. *(Reproduced, with permission, from Johnson BE. Arthritis: Osteoarthritis, gout, and rheumatoid arthritis. In: South-Paul JE, Matheny SC, Lewis EL, eds. CURRENT Diagnosis and Treatment in Family Medicine. 4th ed. New York, NY: McGraw Hill; 2015.)*

Incidence

As the incidence of a disease describes the number of newly diagnosed cases each year, OA poses a challenging situation for determining disease incidence. These reasons include: (1) not all patients with OA seek medical treatment; (2) OA is common within the population; (3) many effective treatments are available over the counter, promoting self-treatment; (4) not all radiographically diagnosed OA is symptomatic and patients may not be formally diagnosed with OA; and (5) many patients have multiple affected joints, making it difficult to track the overall occurrence of OA in these individuals.

ETIOLOGY

2 The etiology of OA is multifactorial and complex, with development of OA depending on interplay between person-level risk factors and joint-level risk factors.[9] Many patients have more than one risk factor for the development of OA. The most common risk factors for the development of OA include age, obesity, sex, occupation, participation in certain sports, history of joint injury or surgery, and genetic predisposition.

Obesity

Obesity is the most important preventable risk factor for OA. This linkage is strongest for knee OA, although hip OA and even hand and wrist OA may be linked with obesity. The etiology of this association of OA in non-weight-bearing joints is thought to be the adverse metabolic and inflammatory effects produced by obesity.[10] As the epidemic of obesity spreads in the United States and in other developed countries, so will the burdens imposed by OA. For every five unit increase in BMI, the risk of knee OA increases 35%.[9] Obesity often precedes OA and contributes to its development, rather than occurring as a result of inactivity from joint pain. In an 11-year study of approximately 30,000 Norwegian men and women, obesity significantly increased the risk of developing OA.[11] Men who were obese at baseline had a 2.8-fold increase in developing knee OA compared to the nonobese men, whereas women who were obese at baseline had a 4.4-fold increased risk in developing knee OA compared to the nonobese women. Also, there was an increased risk for severe knee OA in obese subjects.[11]

Occupation, Sports, and Trauma

OA risk is increased for people in occupations involving excessive mechanical stress. Work that involves prolonged standing, kneeling, squatting, lifting, or moving of heavy objects increases risk of OA. Such occupations include construction, mining, healthcare assistance, factory work, carpentry, and farming.[9] Repetitive motion also contributes to hand OA, with the dominant hand usually affected. Risk for OA depends on the type and intensity of physical activity and whether injury incurred in the activity. Increased risk of OA is associated with participation in activities such as wrestling, soccer, weight lifting, football, and hockey, although recreational participants do not have the increased risk seen in the professional athlete.[12] Studies that have included running, including long distances, have produced decidedly mixed results.[12] In the study of 30,000 Norwegians, exercise intensity was not associated with any increased risk in the obese subjects compared to those of normal weight.[11]

Traumatic knee injury, either during sports or in accidents, significantly increases the risk of knee OA over a 10-year period.[12] These injuries include anterior cruciate ligament tears, meniscal tears, and direct cartilage injuries.[9] Meniscal damage increases the risk of knee OA because of the loss of proper load bearing and shock absorption, and increased focal load on cartilage and on subchondral bone. Quadriceps muscle weakness is also recognized to increase the risk for knee OA, as these muscles are important in maintaining joint stability.[10] As proper alignment of the joint structures is critical to proper function of the joint, knee malalignment increases risk of developing OA. In the person who already has OA, knee malalignment is strongly associated with faster progression of OA.[10]

Genetic Factors

OA is a complex disease with a strong genetic component. The genetic contribution to OA has been supported by many studies and it is estimated that 30% of the risk of OA is genetically determined.[13] There is not a single genetic variant responsible for OA, but likely thousands of loci associated with the complex nature of the disease. Identification of these genetic loci may promote development of agents to prevent OA or to slow or halt its progression. Heberden nodes are 10 times more prevalent in women than in men, for example, with a twofold higher risk if the woman's mother had them. Genetic links have been shown with OA of the first metatarsophalangeal joint and with generalized OA. Twin studies indicate that OA can be attributed substantially to genetic factors.[14]

One approach OA researchers have used is the candidate gene approach which is hypothesis based and focuses on genes with known function which could be plausibly linked with the OA. This approach requires a priori knowledge of disease etiology and only very small regions of the genome can be studied at a time. Studies of 199 candidate genes found that only two variants (COL11A1 and VEGF genes) reached significance.[13] These results confirm that using existing joint biology knowledge to identify genetic variants is unlikely to facilitate the understanding of the genetic risks of OA.

Genome-wide association studies (GWAS) use a hypothesis-free methodology that involves scanning hundreds of thousands or millions of genetic markers, in the form of single-nucleotide polymorphisms (SNPs). Using GWAS studies, at least 21 independent susceptibility loci to OA have been found.[13] A meta-analysis of GWAS with 6,709 knee OA cases and 44,439 controls revealed that the Chrom7Q22 locus was highly significantly associated with knee OA. The locus also included six genes which code for proteins that are known to be expressed in joint tissues.[15]

It is quite likely that the genetic risk of developing OA, like many other diseases, is determined by a combination of genetic differences. This underscores the point that understanding of the genetics and pathology of OA is in its early stages.

PATHOPHYSIOLOGY

OA falls into two major etiologic classes. *Primary (idiopathic) OA*, the more common type, has no identifiable cause. *Secondary OA* is that associated with a known cause such as inflammation, trauma, metabolic or endocrine disorders, and congenital factors.[16]

The old view of OA as a "wear-and-tear" or degenerative disease, largely focused on joint cartilage, has long been superseded by an appreciation of the dynamic nature of OA and that it represents a failure of the joint and surrounding tissues.[10] Some changes in the OA joint may reflect compensatory processes to maintain function in the face of ongoing joint destruction. Not only biomechanical forces but also inflammatory, biochemical, and immunologic factors are involved. An appreciation of the biology and function of normal cartilage can aid in understanding osteoarthritic cartilage and is summarized below.

Normal Cartilage

Function, Structure, and Composition of Cartilage

Articular cartilage possesses viscoelastic properties that provide lubrication with motion, shock absorbency during rapid movements, and load support. In synovial joints, articular cartilage is found between the synovial cavity on one side and a narrow layer of calcified tissue overlying subchondral bone on the other side (Fig. 110-2).[16,17] The layer of cartilage is narrow, with human medial femoral articular cartilage being approximately 2 to 3 mm thick.

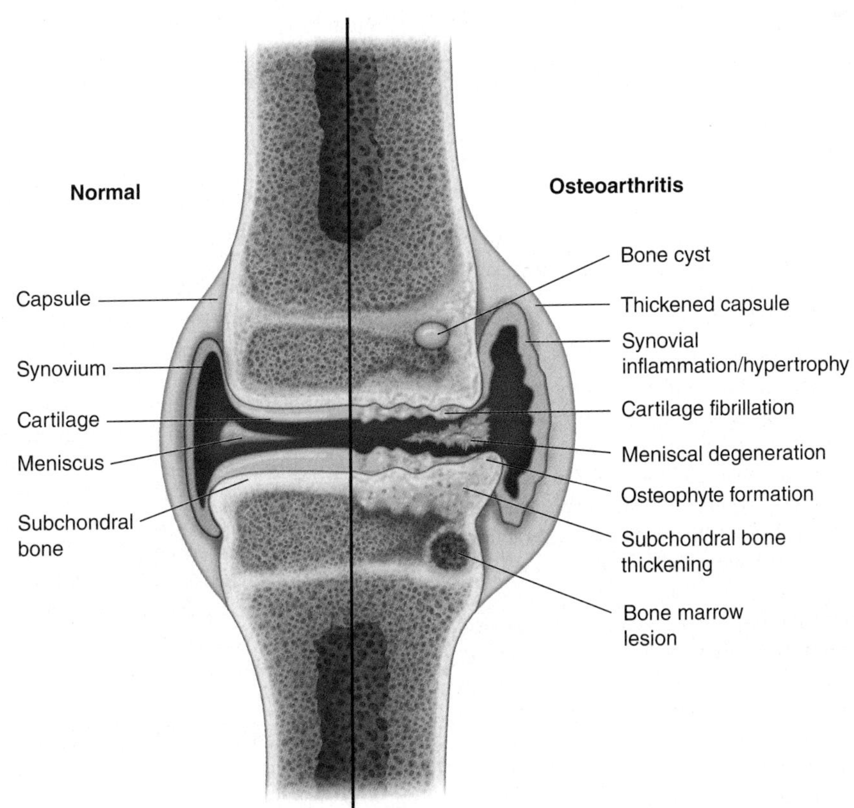

FIGURE 110-2 Characteristics of osteoarthritis in the diarthrodial joint. *(Reprinted, with permission, from Loeser RF. Age-related changes in the musculoskeletal system and the development of osteoarthritis. Clin Geriatr Med. 2010;26(3):371-386.)*

Despite this, healthy articular cartilage in weight-bearing joints withstands millions of cycles of loading and unloading each year. Cartilage is easily compressed, losing up to 40% of its original height when a load is applied. Compression increases the area of contact and disperses force more evenly to underlying bone, tendons, ligaments, and muscles. In addition, cartilage is almost frictionless, and together with its compressibility, this enables smooth movement in the joint, distributes load across joint tissues to prevent damage, and stabilizes the joint.

Strength, a low coefficient of friction, and compressibility of cartilage derive from its unique structure. Cartilage is a complex, hydrophilic, extracellular matrix (ECM). It is approximately 70% water, 10% collagen, 8% proteoglycans, chondrocytes, other proteins, and long hyaluronic acid molecules.[18] The two major structural components in articular cartilage are type II collagen and aggrecans.[16] Type II collagen has a tightly woven triple helical structure, which provides the tensile strength of cartilage. Aggrecan is a proteoglycan linked with hyaluronic acid, providing the long aggrecan molecules a high negative charge. These are squeezed together by surrounding fibrils of type II collagen. The strong electrostatic repulsion of proteoglycans held in close proximity gives cartilage the ability to withstand further compression. Within the cartilage ECM, chondrocytes, the only cells in cartilage, are responsible for laying down all the components of cartilage.

Normal cartilage turnover helps repair and restore cartilage in response to demands of joint loading and during physical activity. In adults, cartilage chondrocyte metabolism is slow and is regulated by growth factors, including bone morphogenetic protein 2, insulin-like growth factor-1, and transforming growth factor, and by catabolism and proteolysis stimulated by matrix metalloproteinases (MMPs), tumor necrosis factor-α (TNF-α), interleukin-1, and other cytokines. Tissue inhibitors of metalloproteinase (TIMP) also contribute to the balance by restraining the catabolic actions of MMPs. If cartilage is injured, chondrocytes react by removing the damaged areas and increasing synthesis of matrix constituents to repair and restore cartilage.[17]

Other components supporting healthy joints are the joint protective mechanisms, such as muscles bridging the joint, sensory receptors in feedback loops to regulate muscle and tendon function, supporting ligaments, and subchondral bone that has shock-absorbent properties.

Finally, note that adult articular cartilage is avascular, with chondrocytes nourished by synovial fluid. With movement and cyclic loading and unloading of joints, nutrients flow into the cartilage, whereas immobilization reduces nutrient supply. This is one of the reasons that normal physical activity is beneficial for joint health.

Osteoarthritic Cartilage

3 Important contributors to the development of OA are local mechanical influences, genetic factors, inflammation, and aberrant chondrocyte function leading to loss of articular cartilage.[16,19] At a molecular level, OA pathophysiology involves the interplay of dozens, if not hundreds, of extracellular and intracellular molecules with roles including chondrocyte regulation, phenotypic changes, proteolytic degradation of cartilage components, and interactions between articular cartilage, underlying subchondral bone, and the joint synovium.[10,19]

OA most commonly begins with damage to articular cartilage, through trauma or other injury, excess joint loading from obesity or other reasons, or instability or injury of the joint that causes abnormal loading. In response to cartilage damage, chondrocyte activity increases in an attempt to remove and repair the damage. Depending on the degree of damage, the balance between breakdown and resynthesis of cartilage can be lost, and a vicious cycle of increasing breakdown can lead to further cartilage loss and apoptosis of chondrocytes.[10,19] Studies have revealed several aspects of the complex nature of OA.

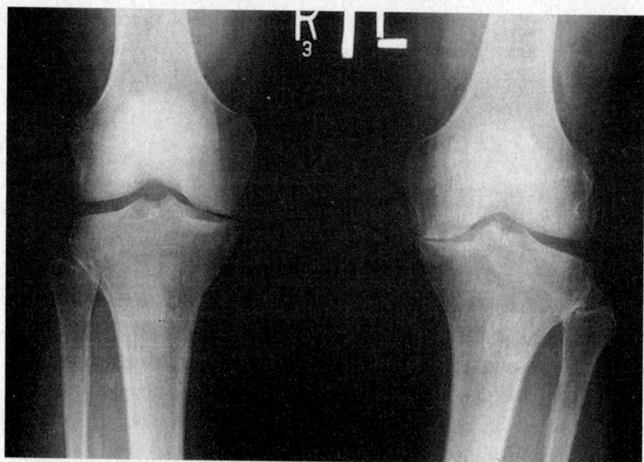

FIGURE 110-3 Plain x-ray films of the knee demonstrating joint space narrowing. *(Reproduced, with permission, from Johnson BE. Arthritis: Osteoarthritis, gout and rheumatoid arthritis. In: South-Paul JE, Matheny SC, Lewis EL, eds. CURRENT Diagnosis & Treatment in Family Medicine. 4th ed. New York, NY: McGraw Hill; 2015.)*

There is increased appreciation of the role of tissues beyond cartilage, within the joint and surrounding subchondral bone.[19] Subchondral bone undergoes pathologic changes that may precede, coincide with, or follow damage to the articular cartilage. In OA, subchondral bone releases vasoactive peptides and MMPs, and damage to subchondral bone may trigger further damage to articular cartilage.[18] Neovascularization and subsequent increased permeability of the adjacent cartilage contribute further to cartilage loss.

Joint space narrowing results from loss of cartilage, which can lead to a painful, deformed joint (Fig. 110-3). Remaining cartilage softens and develops fibrillations (vertical clefts into the cartilage), followed by splitting off of more cartilage and exposure of underlying bone.[18] During this time, adjacent subchondral bone undergoes further pathologic changes, cartilage is eroded completely, leaving denuded subchondral bone, which becomes dense, smooth, and glistening (eburnation). A more brittle, stiffer bone results, with decreased weight-bearing ability and development of sclerosis and microfractures. New bone formations or osteophytes also appear at joint margins, distant from cartilage destruction and are thought to arise from local and humoral factors. There is direct evidence that osteophytes can help stabilize osteoarthritic joints.[16]

In the joint capsule and synovium, inflammatory changes and pathologic changes can occur.[19] Contributors to inflammation may include crystals or cartilage shards in synovial fluid. Other possible factors are interleukin-1, prostaglandin E_2, TNF-α, and nitric oxide that are found in synovial fluid. With inflammatory changes in the synovium, effusions and synovial thickening occur.

4 The pain of OA is not related to the destruction of cartilage but arises from the activation of nociceptive nerve endings within the joint by mechanical and chemical irritants.[10,16] OA pain may result from distension of the synovial capsule by increased joint fluid, microfracture, periosteal irritation, or damage to ligaments, synovium, or the meniscus. Consequently, x-ray changes in OA correlate poorly with pain severity.

CLINICAL PRESENTATION

Diagnosis

5 The diagnosis of OA is made through history, physical examination, characteristic radiographic findings, and laboratory testing.[20] The major diagnostic goals are (1) to discriminate between primary

CLINICAL PRESENTATION Osteoarthritis

Age

- Usually occurs in older adults (≥65 years of age)

Gender

- Age <45 years more common in men
- Age >45 years more common in women

Symptoms

- Pain
- Deep, aching character
- Pain on motion
- Stiffness in affected joints
- Resolves with motion, recurs with rest ("gelling phenomenon")
- Usually duration <30 minutes
- Often related to weather
- Limited joint motion
- May result in limitations of activities of daily living
- Instability of weight-bearing joints

Signs, history, and physical examination

- Monoarticular or oligoarticular, asymmetrical involvement
- Hands
  - Distal interphalangeal joints
    - Herberden nodes (osteophytes or bony enlargements) (Fig. 110-1)
  - Proximal interphalangeal joints
    - Bouchard's nodes (osteophytes)
  - First metacarpal joint
    - Osteophytes give characteristic square appearance to hands
- Knee
  - Pain related to climbing stairs
  - Transient joint effusion
  - Genu varum ("bow-legged")
- Hips
  - Groin pain during weight-bearing exercises
  - Stiffness, especially after activity
  - Limited joint movement
- Spine
  - Lumbar involvement is most common at L3 and L4
  - Paresthesia
  - Loss of reflexes
- Feet
  - Typically involves the first metatarsophalangeal joint
- Shoulder, elbow, acromioclavicular, sternoclavicular, temporomandibular joints may also be affected
- Observation on joint examination
  - Bony proliferation or occasional synovitis
  - Local tenderness
  - Crepitus
  - Limited motion with passive/active movement
  - Deformity
- Radiologic evaluation
  - Early mild OA
    - Radiographic changes are often absent
  - Progressive OA
    - Joint space narrowing (Fig. 110-3)
    - Subchondral bone sclerosis
    - Marginal osteophytes
- Late OA
  - Abnormal alignment of joints
  - Effusions

and secondary OA and (2) to clarify the joints involved, severity of joint involvement, and response to prior therapies, providing a basis for a treatment plan. The American College of Rheumatology has published traditional diagnostic criteria and "decision trees" for OA diagnosis.[20] As with all guidelines, the authors stress these are for assisting the clinician rather than replacing clinical judgment. For example, traditional criteria are as follows: (1) For hip OA, a patient must have pain in the hip and at least two of the following three: an erythrocyte sedimentation rate <20 mm/hr (5.6 μm/s), femoral or acetabular osteophytes on radiography, or joint space narrowing on radiography. This provides a sensitivity of 89% and a specificity of 91%. For a clinical diagnosis of knee OA, a patient must have pain at the knee and osteophytes on radiography plus one of the following: age older than 50 years, morning stiffness no more than 30 minutes, crepitus on motion, bony enlargement, bony tenderness, or no palpable warmth. This provides a sensitivity of 95% and a specificity of 69%. The addition of laboratory or radiographic data further improves accuracy of diagnosis. Criteria for hand OA have also been published.[21]

Prognosis

The prognosis for patients with primary OA is variable and depends on the joint involved. If a weight-bearing joint or the spine is involved, considerable morbidity and disability are possible. In the case of secondary OA, the prognosis depends on the underlying cause. Treatment of OA may relieve pain or improve function but does not reverse preexisting damage to the joint.

TREATMENT

Desired Outcome

Management of the patient with OA begins with a diagnosis based on a careful history, physical examination, radiographic findings, and an assessment of the extent of joint involvement. Treatment should be tailored to each individual. Goals are (1) to educate the patient, family members, and caregivers; (2) to relieve pain and stiffness; (3) to maintain or improve joint mobility; (4) to limit functional impairment; and (5) to maintain or improve quality of life.[24,25] About half of the US population has one chronic health condition, with 25% having two or more conditions.[26] With nearly 25% of the US adults with at least one chronic health condition having arthritis, it is essential that comprehensive patient-centered medication management is provided to these patients to maximize treatment goals for OA and other chronic conditions, while minimizing medication-related adverse outcomes.

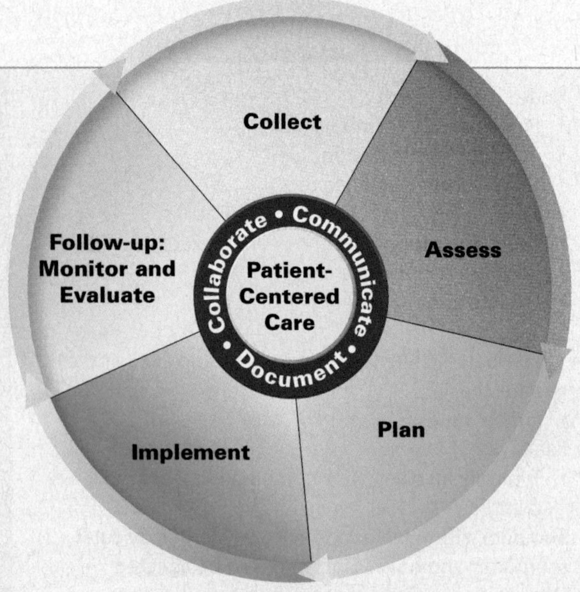

Patient Care Process for the Management of Osteoarthritis

The image shows the five fundamental steps included in The Pharmacist's Care Process endorsed by the Joint Commission for Pharmacy Practitioners (2014). The tagline of this process reads collaborate, communicate, and document. The five fundamental steps listed here are collect, assess, plan, implement, and follow-up: monitor and evaluate. All these steps are listed in a circular block diagram.

Collect

- Patient characteristics (eg, age, weight, height, race, sex, pregnant)
- Patient history (past medical, family, social—trauma, diet, exercise, alcohol use)
- Symptom information: type and location of pain, duration, effect of motion and rest, range of motion and limitations on activities, joint instability
- Current and past medications, including nonprescription agents and dietary supplements, and medications' relief of symptoms
- Objective data
  - Physical examination, appearance of joints
  - Radiologic evaluation—changes in joints, subchondral bone sclerosis, effusions
  - Body mass index (presence of overweight or obesity)

Assess

- Distribution and severity of joint involvement
- Impact of symptoms on patients' movements, health-related quality of life, amount of disability

Plan

- Patient education about disease, prognosis, treatment options, application and use of topical products
- Nonpharmacologic therapy (see Table 110-1)—weight loss (if overweight or obese), exercise, surgery (for severe pain or functional disability)
- Drug therapy regimen including specific analgesics, dose, route, frequency, and duration; specify the continuation and discontinuation of existing therapies (see Figs. 110-4 and 110-5 and Tables 110-2 and 110-3)
- Monitoring parameters including efficacy (eg, symptom relief) and safety (medication-specific adverse effects) (see Table 110-3)
- Self-monitoring of symptoms, exercise, and weight—where and how to record results
- Referrals to other providers when appropriate (eg, physician, orthopedic surgeon, physical therapist, dietician)

Implement*

- Provide patient education regarding all elements of treatment plan
- Use motivational interviewing and coaching strategies to maximize adherence
- Schedule follow-up

Follow-up: Monitor and Evaluate

- Assess symptom relief, effectiveness of weight loss and exercise programs
- Presence of adverse effects (see Table 110-3), including CV and renal effects of NSAIDs and hepatic effects of acetaminophen
- Closely monitor proper use of opioids, including dependence, addiction, tolerance, hyperalgesia, and diversion (see text); joint replacement may be preferred to chronic opioids
- Patient adherence to treatment plan using multiple sources of information

Collaborate with patient, caregivers, and other healthcare professionals.

General Approach to Treatment

Treatment for each OA patient depends on the distribution and severity of joint involvement, comorbid disease states, concomitant medications, and allergies. Management for all individuals with OA should begin with both oral and written patient education, a customized activity and exercise program, and weight loss, if the patient is overweight or obese.[24,25] A multidisciplinary intervention for knee OA initiated by pharmacists has been shown to improve adherence to OA guideline recommendations, decrease pain scores, and improve functional assessment scores.[27] These types of multidisciplinary disease state management programs that implement strategies to provide comprehensive care should be offered to all OA patients to maximize outcomes.

The primary objective of medication is to alleviate pain.[24,25] Scheduled acetaminophen, up to 4 g/day, should be tried initially (knee, hip), if contraindications are not present. Application of topical NSAIDs over specific joints (knee, hands) and topical capsaicin (hands) are recommended as initial therapy. Nonsteroidal anti-inflammatory drugs (NSAIDs) or possibly a cyclooxygenase-2 (COX-2)–selective inhibitor (celecoxib) can be prescribed after

TABLE 110-1 Nonpharmacologic Interventions in the Treatment of OA

Intervention	Strength of Recommendation
Exercise	Strong
Weight loss (if overweight)	Strong
Patient education	Strong
Use of assistive device (ie, cane)	Moderate
Use of shoe insoles	Moderate
Application of heat	Moderate
Use of fitted knee braces	Minimal
Lateral patellar taping	Minimal
Passive exercise alone	Minimal

Data from References 22 and 23.

Robustness of recommendation: Strong—fully supported by evidence-based guidelines; Moderate—supported by evidence-based guidelines; Minimal—little support by evidence-based guidelines.

careful risk assessment if additional pain control is needed. Intra-articular corticosteroid injections (knee or hip) can relieve pain and are offered concomitantly with oral analgesics or after failed trials of first-line medications, depending on the practitioner's preference. With centrally acting serotonin reuptake inhibition and analgesic properties, tramadol can also be considered if acetaminophen or topical treatment is ineffective or not tolerated.

Consideration may also be given to duloxetine or, rarely, hyaluronic acid injections when additional pain control is needed for knee OA. When symptoms are persistent or there is significant loss of function, joint replacement can be appropriate if the patient is a surgical candidate.

There is general agreement that glucosamine and/or chondroitin and topical medications lack uniform efficacy in the treatment of hip and knee OA pain and are not preferred treatment options.

Nonpharmacologic Therapy

6 Nonpharmacologic therapy is an integral part of the treatment plan for all patients with OA.[24,25,28] Nonpharmacologic therapy is the only available treatment that has been shown to delay the progression of OA.[2,29] Delaying the progression of OA through active participation in nonpharmacologic therapy is critical to prevent future functional impairment. Patient-specific characteristics such as (1) number and location of affected joints, (2) degree of functional impairment, (3) body mass index, (4) motivation, and (5) overall health status determine which nonpharmacologic therapies should be offered. Nonpharmacologic therapy should be ongoing treatment for all patients, even those who require pharmacologic therapy for pain control (Table 110-1).[2,28,29]

Patient Education

The first step in OA treatment is patient education about the disease process, the extent of OA, the prognosis, and treatment options. Education is paramount, in that OA is often seen as a wear-and-tear disease, an inevitable consequence of aging for which nothing helps. Even worse, patients may resort to the use of alternative but unproven medications or treatments. Organizations such as the Arthritis Foundation provide a wealth of educational information for patients regarding OA, OA medications, and local clinics and agencies offering physical and economic assistance. Exercise, weight loss, and nutritional information are also available. Most educational information is readily available online for patient use. Several mobile applications are available to provide education, track symptoms and exercise, and encourage better self-management of OA.

The benefits of patient education have been documented in a variety of programs.[22,28] These programs are provided across a wide spectrum of delivery methods: from trained volunteers using telephone calls to group sessions for patient support to one-on-one educational sessions with physical therapists or nurse educators. While nearly all of these delivery methods are effective, cost of delivery is highly variable. Long-term cost-effectiveness is important for sustainability of these patient education programs.

Weight Loss

The association between OA and obesity has been well established. Studies also indicate a strong association between increasing BMI and surgical replacement of the hip and knee joints.[30] Weight loss of amounts as small as 4% body weight can lessen OA pain in the knee.[31] Greater amounts of weight loss, especially when associated with regular exercise improve joint function and substantially lessen pain.[2,29] Modest weight loss (5%) has been shown to provide some relief in obese patients with OA but the goal should be an initial decrease in body weight of at least 10% to provide significant reductions in pain.[30] The Intensive Diet and Exercise for Arthritis trial (IDEA) found that after 18 months, overweight and obese adults with knee OA who participated in the diet and exercise treatment group had less inflammation, less pain, better function, and better quality of life.[32] Weight loss requires a motivated patient, but all patients with OA who also have obesity and overweight should be encouraged and supported in their efforts to optimize their body size. Effective behavior change strategies should be employed to promote weight loss in patients with OA.[29]

Exercise

Exercise programs can improve joint function and can decrease disability, pain, and analgesic use by OA patients.[2,33] Low-impact aerobic exercise including both land- and water-based methods are preferred.[34] Exercises can be taught and then observed before the patient exercises at home. The frequency, types of exercise, and setting of exercise are still uncertain, but patients who exercise have decreased pain and increased physical function.[35] The patient should be instructed to decrease the number of repetitions if severe pain develops with exercise.

Some regular exercise should be encouraged for all patients with OA.[25] With weak or deconditioned muscles, the load is transmitted excessively to the joints; weight-bearing activities can exacerbate symptoms. Many patients fear that exercise will promote further joint damage and avoid exercise as a means to protect the joint. However, avoidance of regular exercise by those with hip or knee OA leads to further deconditioning and/or weight gain. Further weight gain and deconditioning leads to more pain and impaired joint function, promoting a downward spiral of disability. Exercise therapy in addition to patient education has been shown to decrease or postpone the need for hip replacement surgery in patients with hip OA.[36]

Referral to the physical and/or occupational therapist is especially helpful for developing a customized exercise plan for patients with functional disabilities. The therapist can assess muscle strength and joint stability and recommend exercises and assistive and orthotic devices, such as canes, walkers, braces, heel cups, splints, or insoles for use during exercise or daily activities. Heat or cold treatments help to maintain and restore joint range of motion and to reduce pain and muscle spasms. Warm baths or warm water soaks may decrease pain and stiffness. Heating pads should be used with caution, especially in the elderly. Patients should be warned not to fall asleep on the heat source or to lie on it for more than brief periods to avoid burns.

Surgery

Surgery can be recommended for OA patients with functional disability and/or severe pain unresponsive to medical therapy.[37] Total

TABLE 110-2 Dosing of Medications for Osteoarthritis

Drug	Brand Name	Starting Dose	Usual Range	Special Population Dose	Other
Oral analgesics					
Acetaminophen	Tylenol	325-500 mg three times a day	325-650 mg every 4-6 hours or 1 g three to four times/day	Chronic alcohol intake, hepatic disease	Contained in many combination analgesics
Tramadol Tramadol ER	Ultram Ultram ER	25 mg in the morning 100 mg daily	Titrate dose in 25-mg increments to reach a maintenance dose of 50-100 mg three times a day Titrate to 200-300 mg daily	Creatinine clearance <30 mL/min (0.5 mL/s)—maximum dose is 200 mg daily Do not use if creatinine clearance <30 mL/min (0.5 mL/s)	May need to taper dose upon discontinuation to prevent withdrawal symptoms
Hydrocodone/acetaminophen	Lortab, Vicodin, Norco	5 mg/325 mg three times daily	2.5-10 mg/325-650 mg three to five times daily	Titrate dose slowly in older adults (age >65 years)	Maximum dose limited by total daily dose of acetaminophen
Oxycodone/acetaminophen	Percocet	5 mg/325 mg three times daily	2.5-10 mg/325-650 mg three to five times daily	Titrate dose slowly in older adults (age >65 years)	Maximum dose limited by total daily dose of acetaminophen
Topical analgesics					
Capsaicin 0.025% or 0.15%	Capzasin-HP		Apply to affected joint three to four times per day		—
Diclofenac 1% gel	Voltaren		Apply 2 or 4 g per site as prescribed, four times daily		
Diclofenac 1.3% patch	Flector		Apply one patch twice daily to the site to be treated, as directed		
Diclofenac 2% solution	Pennsaid		Apply 40 mg (two pump actuations) twice daily		
Intra-articular corticosteroids					
Triamcinolone	Kenalog	5-15 mg/joint	10-40 mg/large-joint (knee, hip, shoulder)	If multiple joints injected, maximum total dose is usually 80 mg	Often administered concomitantly with a local anesthetic
Methylprednisolone acetate	Depo-Medrol	10-20 mg/joint	20-80 mg/large-joint (knee, hip, shoulder)	10-40 mg for medium joints (elbows, wrists)	
Nonsteroidal anti-inflammatory drugs (NSAIDs)					
Aspirin, plain, buffered, or enteric-coated	Bayer, Ecotrin, Bufferin	325 mg three times a day	325-650 mg four times a day		Doses of 3,600 mg/day are needed for anti-inflammatory activity
Celecoxib	Celebrex	100 mg daily	100 mg twice daily or 200 mg daily		
Diclofenac XR Diclofenac IR	Voltaren-XR Cataflam	100 mg daily 50 mg twice a day	100-200 mg daily 50-75 mg twice a day		
Diflunisal	Dolobid	250 mg twice a day	500-750 mg twice a day		
Etodolac	Lodine	300 mg twice a day	400-500 mg twice a day		
Fenoprofen	Nalfon	400 mg three times a day	400-600 mg three to four times a day		
Flurbiprofen	Ansaid	100 mg twice a day	200-300 mg/day two to four divided doses		
Ibuprofen	Motrin, Advil	200 mg three times a day	1,200-3,200 mg/day in three to four divided doses		Available OTC and Rx
Indomethacin Indomethacin SR	Indocin Indocin SR	25 mg twice a day 75 mg SR once daily	Titrate dose by 25-50 mg/day until pain controlled or maximum dose of 50 mg three times a day Can titrate to 75 mg SR twice daily if needed		
Ketoprofen	Orudis	50 mg three times a day	50-75 mg three to four times a day		
Meclofenamate	Meclomen	50 mg three times a day	50-100 mg three to four times a day		
Mefenamic acid	Ponstel	250 mg three times a day	250 mg four times a day		FDA approval for 1 week of therapy

(continued)

TABLE 110-2 Dosing of Medications for Osteoarthritis (*Continued*)

Drug	Brand Name	Starting Dose	Usual Range	Special Population Dose	Other
Meloxicam	Mobic	7.5 mg daily	15 mg daily		
Nabumetone	Relafen	500 mg daily	500-1,000 mg one to two times a day		
Naproxen	Naprosyn	250 mg twice a day	500 mg twice a day		
Naproxen sodium Naproxen sodium DR	Anaprox, Aleve Naprelan	220 mg twice a day	220–550 mg twice a day 375-750 mg twice a day		Available OTC and Rx
Oxaprozin	Daypro	600 mg daily	600-1,200 mg daily		
Piroxicam	Feldene	10 mg daily	20 mg daily		
Salsalate	Disalcid	500 mg twice a day	500-1,000 mg two to three times a day		

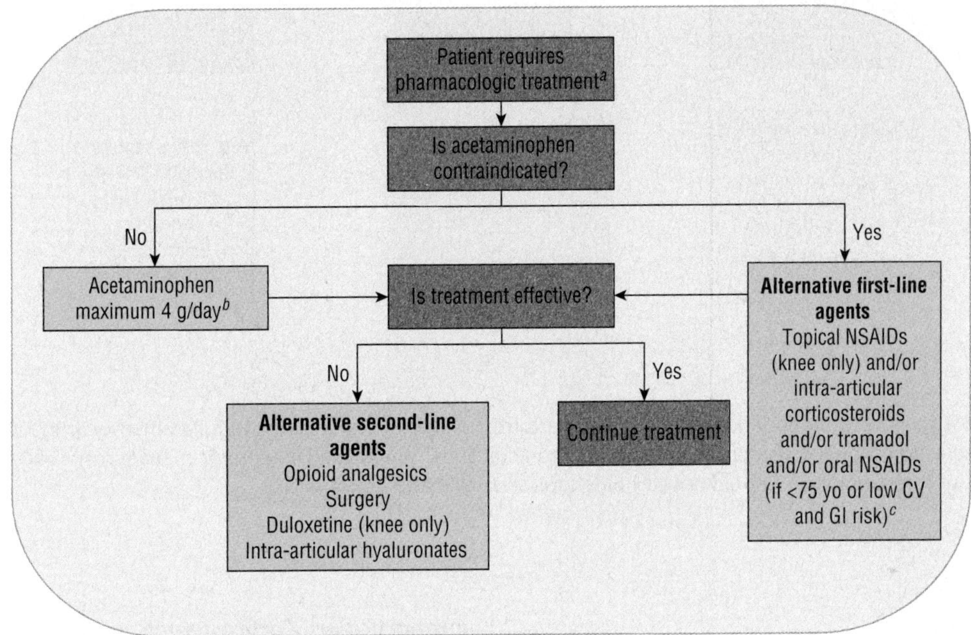

FIGURE 110-4 Treatment recommendations for knee and hip osteoarthritis. (CV, cardiovascular; GI, gastrointestinal; NSAID, nonsteroidal anti-inflammatory drug.)
[a]Selection of a medication should consider patient-specific characteristics. [b]The patient must be counseled regarding all acetaminophen-containing products. [c]When used for chronic management of OA, consider addition of a proton-pump inhibitor.

joint replacement surgeries are quite common and expected to increase. Over 1 million total hip and knee replacement procedures are performed each year in the United States. Seven million individuals are living with an artificial knee or hip, including 620,000 people who have both.[23] Although total knee arthroplasty can decrease pain and improve function for many patients, about 20% experience little or no improvement in pain, disability, and/or quality of life.[38] Patients who are obese are less likely to have improvement in symptoms from knee arthroplasty. Patients also experience less pain and decreased length of hospitalization after surgery if they participate in a supervised exercise program for the first two months that begins on the day of surgery.[39]

Total joint arthroplasty is responsible for a large portion of the direct medical costs associated with OA in the United States. The cost-effectiveness of total knee arthroplasty has been evaluated for a Medicare-age population.[40] Calculations were based on Medicare claims data and costs and outcomes data. Cost projections were calculated for lifetime costs as well as quality-adjusted life expectancy (QALE) for different risk populations and across low-volume to high-volume hospitals. Although total knee arthroplasty was found to be cost-effective across hospital settings and patient risk categories, the procedure was found to be most cost-effective when performed in high-volume centers. The cost-effectiveness of knee arthroplasty was evaluated against nonsurgical management. Knee arthroplasty was cost-effective at both low and high levels of improvement in pain and function in patients with severe knee OA.[41] Direct medical costs associated with joint replacement will continue to increase at a rate higher than predicted rates due to increasing willingness of patients to undergo joint replacement surgery.[3]

Pharmacologic Therapy

Drug therapy in OA is targeted at relief of pain. OA is commonly seen in older individuals who have other medical conditions, and OA treatment is often long term. As such, a conservative and patient-centered approach to drug treatment is warranted (see Figs. 110-4 and 110-5).[24,25,28] Even when pharmacologic therapy is initiated, appropriate nondrug therapies should be continued and reinforced. Specific drug therapy recommendations depend on which joint(s) are affected, response to previous trials of medication, and patient comorbidities.

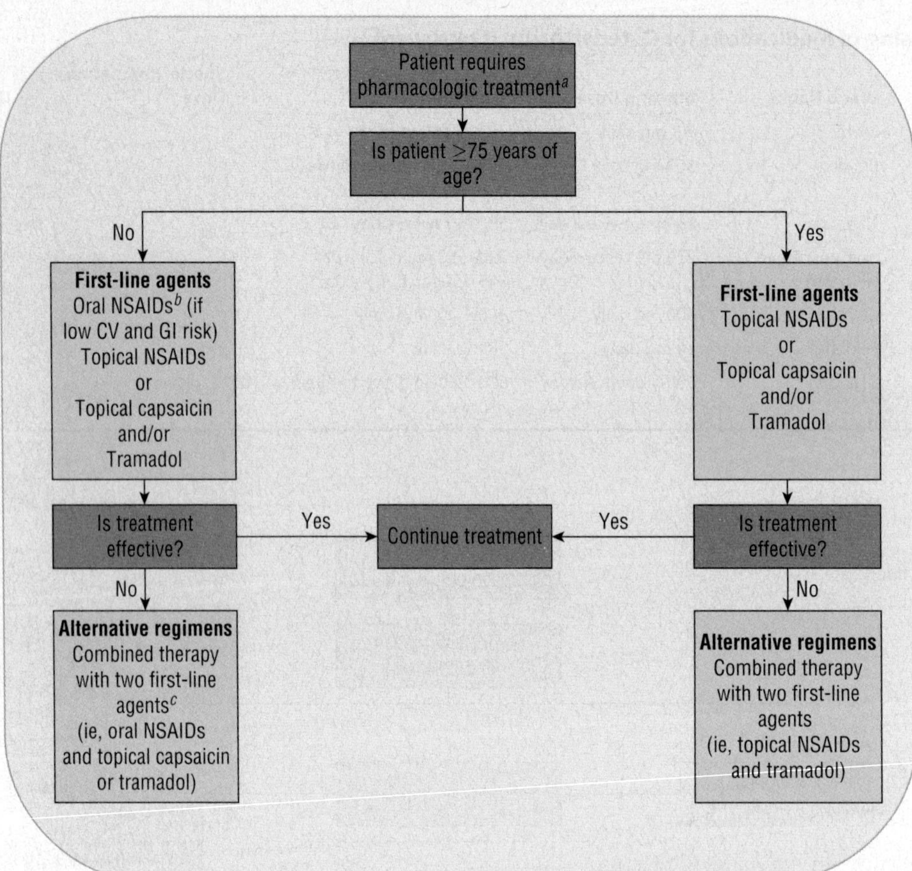

FIGURE 110-5 Treatment recommendations for hand osteoarthritis. (NSAID, nonsteroidal anti-inflammatory drug.) [a]Selection of a medication should consider patient-specific characteristics. [b]When used for chronic management of OA, consider addition of a proton-pump inhibitor. [c]Should not combine topical NSAIDs and oral NSAIDs.

Knee and Hip OA

First-Line Treatments

Acetaminophen 7 The American College of Rheumatology, as well as others, recommend acetaminophen as a first-line treatment for knee and hip OA.[24,25,42] Acetaminophen has been extensively studied in the treatment of knee and hip OA and is more effective than placebo in controlling OA pain.[43] Compared with oral NSAIDs, acetaminophen may be modestly less effective, but have lower risk of serious GI and CV adverse events and as a consequence is preferred to oral NSAIDs as first-line treatment.[28,42]

Oral NSAIDs The American College of Rheumatology and other key groups recommend nonspecific or COX-2 selective NSAIDs, depending on patient risk factors, as a first-line option for knee and hip OA if the patient fails acetaminophen.[25,26,41] Nonselective and COX-2 selective NSAIDs pose higher risks for GI, renal, and CV adverse events compared to acetaminophen. COX-2 inhibitors carry less risk for both minor and serious GI adverse events in comparison to nonselective NSAIDs (with the exception of diclofenac).[42]

Topical NSAIDs—Knee Only 8 The American College of Rheumatology and other authorities recommend topical NSAIDs as a first-line option for knee OA if the patient fails acetaminophen and is preferred to oral NSAIDs for those older than age 75 years.[24,25,42] Topical NSAIDs provide pain relief for OA similar to that obtained with oral NSAIDs but with fewer GI adverse events. Topical NSAIDs offer a favorable safety profile and aren't associated with systemic adverse effects. The most common adverse effect of topical NSAIDs is a localized skin reaction.[44]

Intra-articular Corticosteroids Intra-articular corticosteroid injections are recommended as alternative first-line treatment for both knee and hip OA when pain control with acetaminophen or NSAIDs is suboptimal.[24,25] Injections can also be administered with concomitant oral analgesic therapy as needed for additional pain control. Intra-articular corticosteroids are generally safe and well tolerated, but should not be administered more frequently than once every 3 months due to risks of systemic adverse effects.

Tramadol Tramadol is recommended as an alternative first-line treatment of knee and hip pain due to OA in patients who have failed treatment with scheduled full-dose acetaminophen and topical NSAIDs, who are not appropriate candidates for oral NSAIDs, and who are not able to receive intra-articular corticosteroids.[25] Tramadol can also be safely added to partially effective acetaminophen or oral NSAID therapy. Less data are available to support the use of tramadol as monotherapy for OA pain.

Second-Line Treatments

Opioid Analgesics The American College of Rheumatology recommends opioid analgesics as the primary second-line medication for both knee and hip OA.[25] Opioids may be considered in patients who have not had an adequate response to both nonpharmacologic and first-line pharmacologic therapies. Patients who are at high surgical risk, precluding joint arthroplasty, are also candidates for opioid therapy. When compared to nonopioid medications in a 12-month randomized trial, opioids were not found to be superior in improving pain-related function.[45] Adverse effects, including serious events, limit the routine use of opioids in the treatment of OA pain.

TABLE 110-3 Monitoring of Medications Used in Osteoarthritis Treatment

Drug	Adverse Drug Reactions	Monitoring Parameters	Comments
Oral analgesics			
Acetaminophen	Hepatotoxicity	Total daily dose limits	Use caution with multiple acetaminophen-containing products—total 4 g limit (or less in patients with hepatic dysfunction)
Tramadol	Nausea, vomiting, somnolence	No routine labs recommended	Drug-drug interaction with other serotonergic medications
Opioids	Sedation, constipation, nausea, dry mouth, hormonal changes	No routine labs recommended	Risks of addiction, dependence, and drug diversion
NSAIDs	Dyspepsia, CV events, GI bleeding, renal impairment	BUN/Creatinine, Hgb/Hct, blood pressure	Risks higher in those older than 75 years of age
Topical analgesics			
Capsaicin	Skin irritation and burning	Inspection of areas of application	Wash hands thoroughly after application
NSAIDs	Skin itching, rash, irritated dyspepsia, CV events, GI bleeding, renal impairment	Inspection of areas of application. As needed: BUN/Creatinine, Hgb/Hct, blood pressure	Wash hands thoroughly after application. Avoid oral NSAID or aspirin other than cardioprotective dose. Ensure patient applies gel, solution, or patch correctly
Injectable drugs			
Intra-articular corticosteroids	Hypertension, hyperglycemia	Glucose, blood pressure	HPA axis suppression if used too frequently
Intra-articular hyaluronates	Local joint swelling, stiffness, pain	No routine labs recommended	Less effective than intra-articular corticosteroids; expensive

Duloxetine—Knee Only Duloxetine can be used as adjunctive treatment in patients with knee OA who have had a partial response to first-line analgesics.[24,25] It may be a preferred second-line medication in patients with both neuropathic and musculoskeletal OA pain. Duloxetine has demonstrated efficacy primarily as add-on therapy when there has been less than optimal response to acetaminophen or oral NSAIDs.[46,47] Reduction in pain occurs at about 4 weeks after initiation.[48] Adverse events associated with duloxetine in the treatment of knee OA are most commonly GI, with nausea, vomiting, and constipation being the most common. The recommended dose is 60 mg once daily. However, some patients may benefit from higher doses, up to a maximum dose of 120 mg daily.[48] Adverse events have been reported in OA trials that most commonly used doses of 60 mg/day. A higher dose is associated with an increased risk of adverse reactions.

Intra-articular Hyaluronic Acid The American College of Rheumatology, NICE, and others do not routinely recommend the use of intra-articular hyaluronic acid injections for knee OA pain.[24,25,28] HA injections do not provide clinically meaningful improvement in pain and/or function scores, although some studies may report statistical differences in scores. These agents may be associated with serious adverse events such as increased pain, joint swelling, and stiffness. Limited efficacy and risks of serious events limit the routine use of these agents.

Hand OA

First-Line Treatments

NSAIDs The American College of Rheumatology and NICE recommend topical NSAIDs as a first-line option for hand OA.[28] Application of diclofenac gel compared to placebo topical product for hand OA provided significant relief.[21] No difference was found between the efficacy of oral and topical NSAIDs. Local adverse effects were seen more with topical versus oral NSAIDs but GI adverse effects were more common with oral NSAIDs.[49,50] Efficacy with topical NSAIDs was reported quickly, within 1 to 2 weeks.[21]

Oral NSAIDs are recommended as an alternative first-line treatment for hand OA by the American College of Rheumatology and as second-line therapy in the NICE guidelines.[25,28] For the person who cannot tolerate local skin reactions or who received inadequate relief from topical NSAIDs, oral NSAIDs can offer relief, but the patient then faces increased risk for GI, renal, and CV adverse events.

Topical Capsaicin Capsaicin cream is recommended as an alternative first-line treatment for hand OA.[25] Clinical trial data supporting the use of capsaicin for the treatment of hand OA is limited to small studies, but demonstrates about 50% reduction in pain scores.[21] Adverse effects associated with capsaicin are primarily skin irritation and burning; therefore, it is a reasonable therapeutic alternative for patients who are not able to take oral NSAIDs.

Tramadol Tramadol is recommended by the American College of Rheumatology as an alternative first-line treatment for OA of the hand.[25] No studies in hand OA with tramadol have been performed.[21] In clinical practice, tramadol is a therapeutic option for patients who do not respond to topical therapy and are not candidates for oral NSAID treatment due to high GI, CV, or renal risks. Tramadol may also be used in combination with partially effective acetaminophen, topical therapy, or oral NSAIDs.

Drug Class Information

Highlights of drug information is presented here. This section is not intended to be all inclusive but aims to provide pertinent drug information to facilitate the safe-and-effective use of these medications in patients with OA.

First-Line Treatments

Acetaminophen

Pharmacology and Mechanism of Action Acetaminophen is understood to act within the central nervous system (CNS) by inhibiting synthesis of prostaglandins, agents that enhance pain sensations. Acetaminophen prevents prostaglandin synthesis by blocking the action of central cyclooxygenase (COX). Acetaminophen is well absorbed after oral administration, with bioavailability of 60% to 98%. It achieves peak concentrations within 1 to 2 hours. It is inactivated in the liver by conjugation with sulfate or glucuronide, and its metabolites are renally excreted.

Adverse Effects Although acetaminophen is one of the safest analgesics for younger individuals without comorbidities, it carries greater risk in frail older adults.[51] Serious hepatotoxicity, including fatalities, have been well documented with acetaminophen overdose (see Chapter e8, "Clinical Toxicology," for treatment of acetaminophen overdose).[52] Unintentional overdoses of acetaminophen are due to a variety of circumstances including narrow therapeutic window at the maximum dose (4 g/day), interpatient differences in sensitivity to liver injury from acetaminophen, a wide array of nonprescription and prescription products that contain acetaminophen, which may be hard for patients to identify on the label, and consumers' lack of knowledge about the association of acetaminophen and serious liver injury.

Acetaminophen-related hepatotoxicity is dose-dependent. Even at therapeutic doses, acetaminophen may cause transient liver enzyme elevations and potentially hepatotoxicity.[53,54] The most common risk factor for liver failure in patients who take acetaminophen is chronic alcohol intake.[55] The FDA has recommended that chronic alcohol users (three or more drinks daily) avoid acetaminophen intake as it increases the risk of liver damage or GI bleeding. Other individuals are not at increased risk of GI bleeding.

Drug-Drug Interactions and Drug-Food Interactions Drug interactions with acetaminophen can occur; for example, isoniazid can increase the risk of hepatotoxicity. Chronic ingestion of maximal doses of acetaminophen may intensify the anticoagulant effect for patients taking warfarin; such individuals may need closer monitoring. Although food decreases the maximum serum concentration of acetaminophen by approximately half, the overall efficacy is unchanged.

Dosing and Administration When used for chronic OA, acetaminophen should be administered in a scheduled manner. It may be taken with or without food. Acetaminophen can be taken at 325 to 650 mg every 4 to 6 hours, but the total dose must not exceed 4 g daily (see "Adverse Effects" section above). FDA labeling requirements warn patients about potential liver toxicity if they inadvertently ingest more than the recommended dose when using multiple products containing acetaminophen. Additionally, prescription analgesics containing acetaminophen are limited to 325 mg/tablet to further decrease the opportunity for inadvertent overdose. Acetaminophen should be avoided in the setting of chronic alcohol intake or in those with underlying liver disease.

Oral Nonsteroidal Anti-inflammatory Drugs

Pharmacology and Mechanism of Action NSAIDs reduce pain, inflammation, and fever by preventing synthesis of tissue prostaglandins and related prostanoids, which play a role in triggering these symptoms. All NSAIDs bind (reversibly) to the cyclooxygenase 2 (COX-2) enzyme, blocking its action and thus prostanoid production. Blockade of prostaglandin synthesis by inhibiting COX enzymes (mainly COX-2) is thought to account for NSAIDs ability to relieve pain and inflammation (Fig. 110-6).[56] Nonselective NSAIDs were developed prior to extensive knowledge of COX enzymes, but in fact they block both COX-2 and COX-1. COX-1 has required "housekeeping" functions such as gastroprotection. COX-2 inhibitors selectively block COX-2 but not COX-1 activity.

The various NSAIDs exhibit several pharmacokinetic similarities, including high oral availability, high protein binding, and absorption as active drugs (except for sulindac and nabumetone, which require hepatic conversion for activity). There is a broad range of serum half-lives for different NSAIDs, which influence dosing frequency, and potentially, compliance with therapy.[57] Elimination of NSAIDs largely depends on hepatic inactivation, with a small fraction of active drug being renally excreted. NSAIDs penetrate joint fluid, reaching approximately 60% of blood levels.

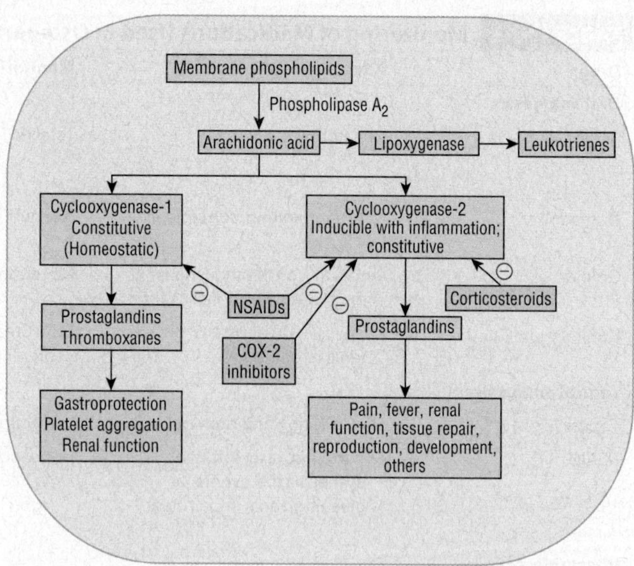

FIGURE 110-6 Pathway of synthesis for prostaglandins and leukotrienes. COX-1 and COX-2 are cyclooxygenase-1 and cyclooxygenase-2 enzymes, respectively. The minus (–) sign indicates inhibitory influence. Prostaglandins include PGE_2 and PGI_2; the latter is also known as prostacyclin.

Adverse Effects

Gastrointestinal Effects of Nonselective NSAIDs The most common adverse effects of NSAIDs involve the GI tract. NSAIDs can cause minor symptoms such as nausea and dyspepsia as well as more serious effects such as ulcers and bleeding.[58-60] All NSAIDs increase ulcer risk, but the serious GI complications associated with NSAIDs include perforations, gastric outlet obstruction, and bleeding. These important GI complications occur in 1.5% to 4% of patients per year. NSAIDs are so widely used that these small percentages translate into substantial morbidity and mortality. Moreover, the risk increases substantially for patients with risk factors including a longer duration of NSAID usage, higher dosage, age older than 60 years, past history of peptic ulcer disease of any cause, history of alcohol use, concomitant use of glucocorticoids, and/or anticoagulants.[56] A patient treated with NSAIDs has a three to five times higher risk of developing GI complications than a patient not treated with these medications.[61]

9 Options are available to reduce the GI risk of traditional NSAIDs. (1) Take the lowest dose possible and take only when needed. (2) Take the prostaglandin analog, misoprostol four times daily that reduces the rate of ulcers and serious GI complications. Many patients cannot tolerate the GI adverse events of misoprostol, especially diarrhea. (3) Take a proton pump inhibitor (PPI) or a full-dose H2 blocker daily. The PPI and the H2 blocker do reduce minor GI complaints and reduce the risk of ulcers but are not rigorously proven to decrease the serious complications, possibly because of lack of power to detect rare events.[61]

Another choice that is available to reduce risk of GI events with an NSAID is to take a COX-2 selective inhibitor ("coxib").[58,60] Celecoxib is the only coxib available in the United States. Because this drug does not block the "housekeeping" gene, it may not have the same GI risks, but it is not without GI risk.[55] A meta-analysis showed that COX-2 selective inhibitors were associated with significantly fewer gastroduodenal ulcers and clinically important ulcer complications. Celecoxib has been shown to be as safe to the upper GI tract as a nonselective NSAID plus a PPI.[62] Another concern is the risk associated with NSAID use in patients taking aspirin for cardioprotection. The GI risk is lower in patients taking a coxib medication and low-dose aspirin than a nonselective NSAID. However, in patients with high GI risk the combination may still be harmful and gastroprotection is appropriate.[62]

Dosing and Administration Administration of NSAIDs must be tailored to the individual patient with OA. Selection of an NSAID depends on the prescriber's experience, medication cost, patient preference, allergies, toxicities, and adherence issues. Individual patient response differs among NSAIDs, so if an inadequate response is obtained with one NSAID, another NSAID may yet provide benefit.[25,28]

Cardiovascular Risk of COX-2 Inhibitors and Traditional NSAIDs Both nonselective and selective NSAIDs are associated with an increased risk for hypertension, stroke, myocardial infarction (MI), and death. NSAIDs should be avoided in patients with known active ischemic heart disease, cerebrovascular disease, and moderate-to-severe heart failure.[56] The mechanism for the CV effects of NSAIDs is not entirely clear.[61] NSAIDs are associated with hypertension, increased preload, volume expansion, and reduced sodium excretion.[63] A large meta-analysis showed some differences among NSAIDs in terms of vascular risk. The risks of diclofenac and ibuprofen were similar to that of coxibs but naproxen was not associated with an increased risk of major vascular events. Overall, coxibs were found to increase vascular risk by approximately one-third.[64] Several randomized controlled trials have compared NSAIDs to evaluate CV safety and found celecoxib to be noninferior to other NSAIDs in terms of CV events. However, the celecoxib dose in these trials was lower than the doses previously reported to be associated with increased CV risk. In these trials, more patients also discontinued celecoxib due to lack of efficacy compared to other NSAIDs.[64,65]

In February 2014, an advisory committee to the FDA met to discuss the data relating the CV risk and NSAIDs. After their review it was decided to strengthen the warning label for nonaspirin NSAIDs, warning patients on the risk of heart attack and stroke. The updated labeling warns that CV events can happen at any point during NSAID therapy and the risk may increase with longer treatment and higher doses. The FDA concluded that there was insufficient evidence that the risk of any NSAID was higher or lower than another. An increased risk for CV events is present even in patients with no underlying CV disease. The data reviewed also showed patients taking an NSAID following a first MI were more likely to die in the first year following the MI.[66] Strategies to reduce CV risk with NSAIDs are not well documented. Naproxen may present less CV risk than coxibs and diclofenac at higher doses and therefore seems prudent to consider this when choosing a specific NSAID.[61,62,66]

Other Toxicities Associated with NSAIDs NSAIDs may cause kidney diseases, including acute renal insufficiency, sodium retention, acute interstitial nephritis, renal papillary necrosis, and accelerated chronic kidney disease. In a trial evaluating NSAID safety, serious renal events occurred at a significantly lower rate in the celecoxib group compared to the ibuprofen group but when celecoxib was compared to naproxen the difference in renal events was not significant.[67] Sodium retention has been reported to occur in up to 25% of NSAID-treated patients. This effect may be clinically important to cause exacerbations of congestive heart failure.[63] Clinical features of these NSAID-induced renal syndromes include increased serum creatinine and blood urea nitrogen, hyperkalemia, elevated blood pressure, peripheral edema, and weight gain. Patients at high risk are those with conditions associated with decreased renal blood flow or taking certain medications. Examples are those with chronic renal insufficiency, congestive heart failure, severe hepatic disease, and nephrotic syndrome, those of advanced age, or those taking diuretics, angiotensin-converting enzyme inhibitors, cyclosporine, or aminoglycosides (Fig. 110-7).

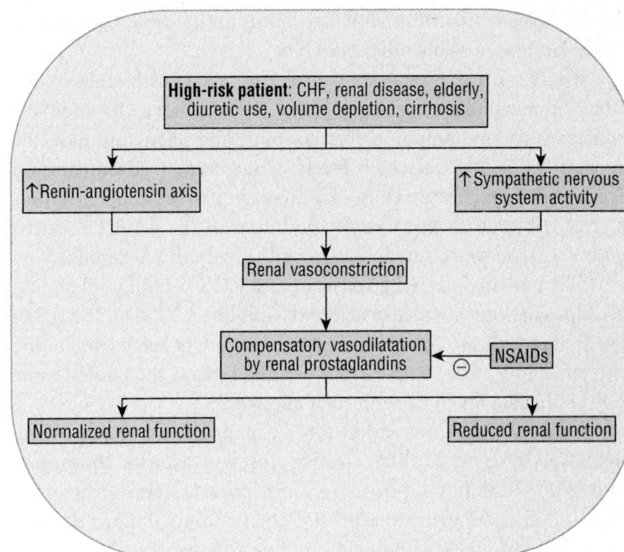

FIGURE 110-7 Mechanisms implicated in NSAID-induced renal injury. The minus (–) sign indicates inhibitory influence. (CHF, congestive heart failure; NSAIDs, nonsteroidal anti-inflammatory drugs.)

Close monitoring is advisable for high-risk patients taking an NSAID, with monitoring of serum creatinine at baseline and within 3 to 7 days of drug initiation. For those with impaired renal function, the National Kidney Foundation recommends acetaminophen over NSAIDs, although acetaminophen may pose risks, as discussed above.

Coxibs and NSAIDs uncommonly cause drug-induced hepatitis; the two NSAIDs most frequently implicated are diclofenac and sulindac. Patient monitoring should include periodic liver enzymes (aspartate aminotransferase and alanine aminotransferase), with cessation of therapy if these values exceed two to three times the upper limit of normal. Hepatotoxicity associated with NSAIDs is responsible for about 10% of medication-induced liver injury.[68]

Other toxic effects of NSAIDs include hypersensitivity reactions, rash, and CNS complaints of drowsiness, dizziness, headaches, depression, confusion, and tinnitus.[57] NSAIDs should be avoided for patients with asthma who are aspirin-intolerant.

All nonspecific NSAIDs inhibit COX-1–dependent thromboxane production in platelets and thus increase bleeding risk. Unlike aspirin, celecoxib and nonspecific NSAIDs inhibit thromboxane formation reversibly, with normalization of platelet function 1 to 3 days after the drug is stopped. Warfarin and celecoxib are metabolized by the cytochrome P450 isoenzyme CYP2C9; thus, patients receiving warfarin and COX-2 inhibitors should be followed closely.

Finally, if misoprostol is taken for GI protection, great care is indicated. Because of its abortifacient properties, misoprostol is contraindicated in pregnancy and in women of childbearing age who are not maintaining adequate contraception. It must be dispensed in its original container, which carries a warning for these individuals. Misoprostol is also available in a combination product with diclofenac, which bears the same restrictions as misoprostol alone.

Drug-Drug Interactions Avoidance of concomitant use, or anticipation and careful monitoring, can often prevent serious events when potentially interacting drugs are being considered. The most potentially serious interactions include the use of NSAIDs with lithium, warfarin, other agents that increase bleeding risk, oral hypoglycemics, methotrexate, antihypertensives, angiotensin-converting enzyme inhibitors, β-blockers, and diuretics.[57] In addition, there are probable drug interactions with tacrolimus for ibuprofen, naproxen, diclofenac, and possibly other NSAIDs.

Specific drug interactions are also seen with celecoxib.[69] Celecoxib metabolism is primarily via CYP2C9.[69] Cytochrome P450 inducers such as rifampin, carbamazepine, and phenytoin have the potential to reduce celecoxib levels. Concomitant administration of celecoxib with fluconazole can increase plasma concentrations of celecoxib, due to fluconazole inhibition of the CYP2C9 isoenzyme. Because warfarin and celecoxib are both metabolized by CYP2C9, patients receiving warfarin and COX-2 inhibitors should be followed closely. Because celecoxib inhibits CYP2D6, it has the potential to increase concentrations of a variety of agents, including antidepressants. Celecoxib is a sulfonamide and is thus noted to be contraindicated for those with sulfa allergies.[69]

Another drug interaction has been noted for those taking some NSAIDs and cardioprotective doses of aspirin. Ibuprofen, used at doses of 400 mg or more, may block aspirin's antiplatelet effect if it is taken prior to aspirin. Patients taking ibuprofen have been advised to take a single dose of ibuprofen at least 30 minutes after taking aspirin, or to take their aspirin at least 8 hours after taking ibuprofen. It is possible that other nonselective NSAIDs, such as naproxen, also may cause such interactions. The ACR recommends that patients taking aspirin who need an oral NSAID for OA choose an NSAID other than ibuprofen or COX-2 selective inhibitors.[25] Acetaminophen does not interfere with the antiplatelet effect of aspirin.

Topical NSAIDs

Pharmacology and Mechanism of Action The mechanism of action of topical NSAIDs is considered to be through inhibition of the COX-2 enzyme in tissues near the site of application. Studies show significant placebo effects which could result from rubbing the product into the skin, which may have a counterirritant effect. Topical NSAIDs are significantly more efficacious compared to placebo vehicle in reducing pain due to musculoskeletal conditions, including osteoarthritis. Most trials have shown topical diclofenac to be as effective as oral NSAIDs, including both oral diclofenac and other comparators.[42,50,70] Diclofenac 1% gel as well as the newer diclofenac solution and diclofenac patches are approved in the United States for osteoarthritis.

Adverse Effects Compared to oral NSAIDs, topical NSAIDs are associated with many fewer GI adverse events and fewer adverse events overall, except for local application site reactions. In comparison to placebo or oral NSAIDs, topical NSAID use is associated with more local adverse events, most often mild skin reactions such as itching or rash, but with few serious adverse effects. Meta-analyses and reviews have found similar tolerability between topical NSAIDs and placebo. Topical NSAIDs have not shown a significant link between their use and increased risk of CV events.[44] From 1% to 15% of topical NSAIDs enter the systemic circulation, but usually less than 5% contribute to its greater safety profile.[70,71]

Drug-Drug Interactions Interactions listed for topical diclofenac are the same as those listed above for oral NSAIDs. The most potentially serious interactions include the use of NSAIDs with lithium, warfarin, and other agents that increase bleeding risk, oral hypoglycemics, methotrexate, antihypertensives, angiotensin-converting enzyme inhibitors, β-blockers, and diuretics. Other topical agents have not been studied with the product and there could be changes in tolerability and absorption of diclofenac. For all of these interactions, as there is only a small percentage of diclofenac absorbed, the risks are likely significantly less than that with oral drug, but the patient and provider should monitor appropriately for these interactions with any of these drugs the patient is taking. Patients should avoid oral NSAIDs while using topical products to minimize additive adverse effects. Care should be taken to avoid contact with the eyes or open wounds and to wash hands after application (except when treating hand OA).

Dosing and Administration Diclofenac 1% gel (Voltaren®) can be used for hand or knee OA or other joints amenable to topical application (eg, not the hip or shoulder) and is available as an OTC product. It is applied four times daily using the dose measuring cards provided by the manufacturer. Four grams of gel is recommended for application to the affected area in the lower limb (eg, foot, ankle, knee) four times daily. For use on the upper extremities (eg, hand, wrist, elbow), the dose is 2 g four times daily. Diclofenac solution (Pennsaid®), only approved for knee OA, is available as a 2% solution. The 2% diclofenac solution is available in a meter-dose pump. It is applied as two actuations or 40 mg twice daily to the affected knee(s). The entire dose should be pumped into the palm of the hand then applied evenly to the knee. The diclofenac patch (180-mg diclofenac epolamine) is applied twice daily. If the patch doesn't stick well, the patient can tape edges with first-aid tape. Patient counseling is important to carefully explain how to apply the topical products. Other counseling points include hand washing after use, avoidance of touching the eyes, nose, or mouth directly after use, and how long to wait before dressing, putting on gloves, showering, and so forth.

Pharmacoeconomic Impact of NSAIDs The highest costs associated with the pharmacotherapy of OA are hospitalization for treatment of NSAID-related complications, particularly serious GI adverse events. Historically, gastroprotective therapy or the use of COX-2–selective inhibitors for low-risk patients has not been cost-effective because of the number needed to treat to prevent serious events is large, but most PPIs are generic, multisource products, making concomitant treatment with PPIs effective.[72] Pharmacoeconomic considerations for OA involve the selection of therapy for the initial treatment of patients with OA. Use of the nonprescription analgesic acetaminophen as initial therapy has greatly reduced medication costs in comparison with the use of NSAIDs, many of which are by prescription only. Oral NSAID costs vary considerably, depending on the medication, daily dose, and regimen selected. As oral NSAIDs as a class are therapeutically similar, the use of a less-expensive agent such as nonprescription ibuprofen or naproxen or a multisource generic product may minimize the cost. More expensive NSAIDs can be prescribed if neither of these offers benefit after a 2-week trial at sufficient doses. Prescription-only topical NSAIDs are significantly more costly than oral agents. Over-the-counter diclofenac products are likely to have a similar cost compared to many generic prescription oral NSAIDs. Costs related to the serious complications associated with oral NSAID therapy are likely to outweigh the costs associated with topical diclofenac in any form, making prescription status products cost-effective.

Intra-articular Corticosteroids

Pharmacology and Mechanism of Action 10 The anti-inflammatory properties of corticosteroids as a class are the primary mechanism of pain relief in the treatment of OA. These properties decrease the formation and release of prostaglandins, kinins, liposomal enzymes, and histamine. These actions decrease erythema, swelling, heat, and tenderness of the inflamed joints.[25,73] Aspiration of the effusion and injection of glucocorticoid are carried out aseptically, with examination of the aspirate recommended to exclude crystalline arthritis or infection. Several randomized, placebo-controlled, double-blind studies have shown that intra-articular corticosteroids are superior to placebo in alleviating knee pain and stiffness caused by OA but with a relatively short duration.[73] The most commonly used corticosteroids for intra-articular use are triamcinolone acetonide and methylprednisolone acetate. The branched esters of triamcinolone and methylprednisolone are preferred by practitioners because of the reduced solubility that allows the agents to remain in the joint space longer.[74,75]

Adverse Events Adverse events associated with intra-articular injection of corticosteroids can be local or systemic in nature. Systemic adverse events are the same as with any other systemic corticosteroid and can include hyperglycemia, edema, elevated blood pressure, flushing, dyspepsia, and hypercortisolism. There is an acute 2- to 3-day rise in blood glucose in patients with diabetes following a single corticosteroid injection. The risk of systemic side effects can be lessened by limiting the dose of the corticosteroid since doses greater than 40 mg for triamcinolone or methylprednisolone have not been shown to provide any additional benefit.[74] Local adverse effects can include infection in the affected joint, osteonecrosis, tendon rupture, and skin atrophy at the injection site. Systemic corticosteroid therapy is not recommended in OA, given the lack of proven benefit and the well-known adverse effects with long-term use.

Dosing and Administration Average doses for injection of large joints in adults are 40 mg of triamcinolone and methylprednisolone acetate. Local anesthetics such as lidocaine or bupivacaine are commonly combined with corticosteroids to provide rapid pain relief.[74] This therapy is generally limited to three or four injections per year due to the potential systemic effects of corticosteroids and because the need for more frequent injections indicates little response to the therapy.

After injection, the patient should minimize activity and stress on the joint for several days. Initial pain relief may be seen within 24 to 72 hours after injection, with peak pain relief about 7 to 10 days after injection and lasting up to 4 to 8 weeks.

Capsaicin

Pharmacology and Mechanism of Action Capsaicin, isolated from hot peppers, releases and ultimately depletes substance P from afferent nociceptive nerve fibers. Substance P has been implicated in the transmission of pain in arthritis, and capsaicin cream has demonstrated to have moderate efficacy compared to placebo in clinical trials.[51] Due to the larger surface area and distance from the site of application to the joint, it is not expected that application of capsaicin would provide efficacy in the treatment of hip OA.

Adverse Effects Adverse events associated with capsaicin are primarily local, including burning, stinging, and/or erythema that usually subsides with repeated application. Systemic effects are rare.[51] The FDA has issued a public drug safety communication notifying consumers that rare cases of severe burns have been reported.[76] Some patients may experience coughing associated with application.

Dosing and Administration To be effective, capsaicin must be used regularly, and it may take up to 2 weeks to take effect. Use is recommended four times a day.[51] Patients should be counseled not to get the cream in their eyes or mouth. Patients should also notify their healthcare provider immediately if they experience pain, swelling, or blistering skin at the site of application.

Capsaicin is a nonprescription product available as a cream, gel, solution lotion, or patch in concentrations ranging from 0.025% to 0.15%.

Tramadol

Pharmacology and Mechanism of Action Tramadol, an analgesic with affinity for the μ-opioid receptor, as well as weak inhibition of the reuptake of norepinephrine and serotonin neurotransmitter, has shown moderate pain improvement for patients with OA when compared with placebo.[77,78] Tramadol is also modestly effective as add-on therapy for patients taking concomitant acetaminophen, NSAIDs, or COX-2–selective inhibitors. Tramadol may be helpful for patients who cannot take NSAIDs or COX-2–selective inhibitors.

Adverse Events Opioid-like adverse effects such as nausea, vomiting, dizziness, constipation, headache, and somnolence are common with tramadol. These occur in 45% to 84% of treated patients.[79] Although the frequency of adverse effects is high, the severity of these effects is less than for NSAIDs, as tramadol use is not associated with life-threatening GI bleeding, CV events, or renal failure. The most notable serious adverse event associated with tramadol use is seizures. Withdrawal symptoms can occur if tramadol is stopped abruptly. Older adults are significantly more likely to experience adverse events.[79] Tramadol was initially not classified as a controlled substance but was rescheduled as a class IV controlled substance due to its potential for dependence, addiction, and diversion.

Drug-Drug Interaction Medications that lower the seizure threshold should be used with caution in patients taking tramadol. These include tricyclic antidepressants, first-generation antipsychotic medications, and cyclobenzaprine, as well as others. There is also an increased risk of serotonin syndrome (see Chapter 88, "Depressive Disorders," for description) when tramadol is used concomitantly with other serotonergic medications, including duloxetine.

Dosing and Administration Tramadol should be initiated at a lower dose (100 mg/day) and may be titrated as needed for pain control to a dose of 200 mg/day, with a maximum dose of 400 mg/day. Tramadol is available in a combination tablet with acetaminophen and as an extended-release tablet or capsule.

Second-Line Treatments

Opioid Analgesics Opioid analgesics may be useful for patients who experience limited pain relief with acetaminophen, oral NSAIDs, intra-articular injections, or topical therapy or who cannot tolerate the side effect profile of these agents.[55] For patients with underlying conditions that limit the use of first-line analgesics, opioid analgesics can effectively relieve acute OA pain. A common clinical scenario includes the patient who cannot take oral NSAIDs because of renal failure or CV disease. Patients in whom all other treatment options have failed and who are at high surgical risk, precluding joint arthroplasty, are also candidates for opioid therapy. It is important to carefully use opioids to promote safety. The CDC recommends only prescribing opioids if the benefits from pain control and function outweigh the risk. The best practices for prescribing opioid include using the lowest effective dose and the smallest quantity needed; providing patients with information on how to use, store, and dispose of opioid medications; and avoiding combinations of opioids and sedating medications unless there is a specific indication to do so. Opioid use should be assessed at least every 3 months, evaluating patient progression toward functional treatment goals, risks of harm, and adverse effects.[80]

Adverse effects are common in opioid-treated patients with OA. More than 75% of patients in clinical trials experience at least one typical opioid-related (ie, nausea, somnolence, constipation, dry mouth, and dizziness) adverse effect. Although this is not an unexpected finding, it serves as a reminder to use opioids cautiously in elderly patients who may be more susceptible to adverse effects.

Opioid dependence, addiction, tolerance, hyperalgesia, and issues surrounding drug diversion are more serious adverse effects associated with long-term treatment. Prescription opioid misuse/abuse/addiction is a major public health concern with the CDC reporting around 46 deaths every day from prescription opioid overdose.[81] Patients should be educated on the risks of taking opioids, including addiction, overdose, and death.

If pain is poorly controlled and limits activities of daily living, and the patient has sufficiently good cardiopulmonary health to undergo major surgery, joint replacement may be preferable to continued reliance on opioids.

Duloxetine Duloxetine is a centrally acting dual-reuptake inhibitor of both serotonin and norepinephrine, although norepinephrine reuptake inhibition does not occur until doses reach 60 mg/day. While the most common pain target in OA is peripheral nociceptive pain, there is some evidence that chronic nociceptive pain leads to central pain sensitization thereby lowering the pain threshold.[47] Duloxetine provides pain relief through the blocking of central pain transmitters, including serotonin and norepinephrine.

Adverse effects commonly associated with duloxetine therapy include nausea, dry mouth, constipation, and anorexia. Expected neurologic adverse effects include fatigue, somnolence, and dizziness. Rare, but serious adverse events associated with duloxetine include Stevens-Johnson syndrome and liver failure. Patients should be notified to contact their healthcare provider immediately if they develop a rash while taking duloxetine.

Particular care should be taken to avoid the use of duloxetine with other serotonergic medications including tramadol. As tramadol is a first-line treatment recommendation for OA, the likelihood of encountering this combination is high. Concomitant use of duloxetine with other medications that increase serotonin concentrations increases the risk of serotonin syndrome.

Hyaluronic Acid Injections Hyaluronate is a naturally occurring component of cartilage and synovial fluid. Exogenous intra-articular hyaluronate is available as a treatment for the symptoms of knee OA. The goal of intra-articular HA is to provide and maintain intra-articular lubrication. HA may also have anti-inflammatory, analgesic, and chondroprotective effects on the articular cartilage and joint synovium.[82] Evidence has not shown intra-articular HA to have a clinically significant benefit involving pain relief and functional improvement and therefore does not support the routine use of HA.[83] Most HA products are injected once weekly for either 3 or 5 weeks, depending on the specific agent administered. Patients are generally advised to repeat the injection schedule by six months if they are satisfied with the previous course.[73] Strenuous or prolonged weight-bearing activities should be avoided for 48 hours after treatment. Routinely, most of the improvement is expected from 5 to 13 weeks after injection with some effect still occurring at 24 weeks.[82] Injections are generally well tolerated, although acute joint swelling, effusion, and stiffness can occur. Local skin reactions, including rash, ecchymosis, and pruritus, have also been reported. Local adverse effects are more frequent in products from animal origin. Rarely, systemic adverse events including hypersensitivity reactions have occurred. Joint infections are rare but have been reported.

At this time, the effect of HA injections on knee OA is modest at best.[82] These agents are expensive because the treatment includes both drug costs and administration costs. Patient expectations and cost effectiveness must be considered before choosing HA injection.[73]

Glucosamine and Chondroitin Interest in chondroitin and glucosamine was spurred initially by anecdotal reports of benefit in animals and humans and by the ability of these substances to stimulate proteoglycan synthesis from articular cartilage in vitro. Over the past decade, enthusiasm for these agents has waned as additional efficacy data has become available to the point that the American College of Rheumatology conditionally recommends against the use of glucosamine and chondroitin.[25] Glucosamine, alone or in combination, has not been shown to provide uniform improvements in pain control or functional status in patients with OA of the knee or hip.[84]

Numerous trials have examined the safety and efficacy of glucosamine and chondroitin; however, the duration of these studies has been relatively short. The efficacy of glucosamine and chondroitin was evaluated after 2 years and was found not to be statistically superior to placebo.[85] The combination of glucosamine and chondroitin was well tolerated. There has previously been some concern that glucosamine may worsen diabetes or asthma; however, with 2-year follow-up this was not substantiated.[85] When the combination of glucosamine and chondroitin was compared to celecoxib in patients with knee OA, it was noninferior in the reduction of pain at 6 months. The combination was well tolerated and the authors suggest glucosamine and chondroitin as a potential safe alternative for patients with CV or GI conditions.[86]

Because glucosamine and chondroitin are marketed in the United States as dietary supplements, neither the products nor their purity is adequately regulated by the FDA. The potential consequences related to the lack of regulatory oversight for these products can affect both efficacy and safety. Products containing less than labeled doses can compromise efficacy, while those containing ingredients not included on the labeling can compromise safety. A variety of brand name and generic products are available in various doses and formulations.

EVALUATION OF THERAPEUTIC OUTCOMES

For persons with OA, treatment decisions and pharmacotherapy monitoring are patient specific. The patient's situation and individual needs should be considered when devising a treatment plan. Is the patient bothered primarily by pain, by limitations in activity, or with concerns about side effects from medications? Does the patient understand what OA is and why certain treatments are useful?

When the patient is first being assessed for the possibility of OA, the diagnosis is often straightforward, including history and physical exam, plain films of the affected joint(s), and lab tests. The older patient with unilateral knee pain, limited range of motion, no palpable warmth, crepitus, and without prolonged morning stiffness and other suspicious findings is highly likely to have knee OA. It is still reasonable to obtain x-rays that may help follow disease over time (although joint space narrowing often does not correlate with the extent of pain or difficulty walking). Basic labs to help decide what pharmacologic therapy is possible (eg, no NSAIDs with poor renal function), assessment of pain using a visual analog scale, range of motion for affected joints. Additional tests of OA severity may include measurement of grip strength, 50 ft (~15 m) walking time, patient and physician global assessment of OA severity, and assessment of ability to perform activities of daily living. Once the patient is assessed and diagnosed, patient and family education is essential. Nondrug therapy may include a referral for physical and/or occupational therapy services, where the therapists can help to maintain and improve range of motion. Referral for nutritional counseling and weight loss may also be necessary if the patient is overweight or obese. These interventions may decrease pain and facilitate improved activity for OA patients.

Although all patients must be provided with nonpharmacologic therapies, results from these interventions usually require weeks to months. In the meantime, the patient needs pain relief. First-line therapy continues to be acetaminophen. Adverse events with acetaminophen are uncommon, although it is important that the patient understand the maximum daily dose limits and all possible sources of acetaminophen-containing products. Although some do well on acetaminophen, many do not achieve sufficient pain relief. A step up to oral NSAIDs or second-line therapy might be necessary but poses significant risks beyond acetaminophen. A switch to NSAIDs requires careful consideration of the patient's age and comorbidities, renal function, history of GI problems, hypertension, and CV health. Periodic monitoring would include open-ended questions followed by direct questions relating to the commonest adverse effects associated with the respective medication. For an oral NSAID, symptoms of abdominal pain, heartburn, nausea, or change in stool color provide valuable clues to the presence of GI complications, although serious GI complications can occur without warning. Patients should be monitored for the development of hypertension, weight gain, edema, skin rash, and CNS adverse effects such as headaches and drowsiness. Baseline serum creatinine, complete blood count, and serum transaminases are repeated at 6- to 12-month intervals to identify GI, renal, and hepatic toxicities.

Topical NSAIDs have demonstrated efficacy in OA of the hand and knee and are as effective as oral NSAIDs. Although they carry the same CV, renal, and GI warnings, their area under the concentration–time curve (AUC) for a typical dose is only a few percent of the AUC from an equivalent dose of oral NSAID. Topical NSAIDs' most common side effects are local, with irritated skin, rash, or itching, usually mild, and with many fewer adverse effects of CV, GI, or renal nature. These agents are a welcome addition to the limited treatment modalities for the common, costly, painful, and often disabling disease of OA. It is important that the patient apply the topical products appropriately to achieve maximum benefit and avoid adverse events.

For patients receiving intra-articular corticosteroids, pain relief should begin with 2 to 3 days and last 4 to 8 weeks. Patients should be advised about possible injection site reactions, as well as possible systemic effects, especially for those with hypertension or diabetes, as there is a potential for increased blood pressure or blood glucose. For patients receiving opioids or tramadol, relief from pain should occur rapidly. Frail or elderly patients should be monitored carefully and cautioned about sedation, dysphoria, nausea, risk of falls, and constipation. Special additional monitoring should include strategies to assess development of opioid tolerance, addiction, misuse, and diversion.

CONCLUSION

OA is a common, slowly progressive disorder that affects diarthrodial joints and is characterized by progressive deterioration of articular cartilage, subchondral sclerosis, and osteophyte production. Clinical manifestations include gradual onset of joint pain, stiffness, and limitation of motion. The primary treatment goals are to reduce pain, maintain function, and prevent further destruction. An individualized approach based on education, rest, exercise, weight loss as needed, and analgesic medication can succeed in meeting these goals. Recommended drug treatment starts with acetaminophen ≤4 g/day and topical analgesics as needed. If acetaminophen is ineffective, oral NSAIDs may be used in appropriately selected patients, often providing satisfactory relief of pain and stiffness. Individuals at increased risk for toxicity from NSAIDs, especially for GI, CV, or renal events, deserve special attention. Celecoxib may have safety advantages in some OA patients, but its safety relative to other NSAIDs and its role in OA remains poorly defined. Adjunctive therapy with tramadol, intra-articular corticosteroids, and duloxetine may be helpful in patients with poorly controlled pain. Experimental therapy aimed at preventing the progression of OA requires further clinical investigation before entering widespread clinical use.

ABBREVIATIONS

AAAL	arthritis-attributable activities limitations
AUC	area under the concentration–time curve
BMI	body mass index
CNS	central nervous system
COX	cyclooxygenase
CV	cardiovascular
ECM	extracellular matrix
FDA	Food and Drug Administration
GI	gastrointestinal
GWAS	genome-wide linkage studies
HA	hyaluronic acid
IDEA	Intensive Diet and Exercise for Arthritis
IR	immediate release
MI	myocardial infarction
MMP	matrix metalloproteinase
NICE	National Institute for Health and Clinical Excellence
NSAID	nonsteroidal anti-inflammatory drug
OA	osteoarthritis
OARSI	Osteoarthritis Research International
PPI	proton pump inhibitor
QALE	quality-adjusted life expectancy
SNPs	single-nucleotide polymorphisms
SR	sustained release
TIMP	tissue inhibitors of metalloproteinase
TNF-α	tumor necrosis factor-α

REFERENCES

1. Barbour KE, Helmick CG, Boring M, Brady TJ. Vital signs: Prevalence of doctor-diagnosed arthritis and arthritis-attributable activity limitation—United States, 2013–2015. *MMWR Morb Mortal Wkly Rep.* 2017;66(9):246–253.
2. Hootman JM, Murphy LB, Omura JD, et al. Health care provider counseling for physical activity or exercise among adults with arthritis—United States, 2002 and 2014. *MMWR Morb Mortal Wkly Rep.* 2018;66(5152):1398–1401.
3. Murphy LB, Cisternas MG, Pasta DJ, Helmick CG, Yelin EH. Medical expenditures and earnings losses among US adults with arthritis in 2013. *Arthritis Care Res (Hoboken).* 2018;70(6):869–876.
4. Torio C (AHRQ), Moore B (Truven Health Analytics). National inpatient hospital costs: The most expensive conditions by payer, 2013. HCUP statistical brief #204.
5. Dagenais S, Garbedian S, Wai EK. Systematic review of the prevalence of radiographic primary hip osteoarthritis. *Clin Orthop Relat Res.* 2009;467(3):623–637.
6. Feydy A, Pluot E, Guerini H, Drape JL. Osteoarthritis of the wrist and hand, and spine. *Radiol Clin North Am.* 2009;47(4):723–759.
7. Jordan JM. An ongoing assessment of osteoarthritis in African Americans and Caucasians in North Carolina: The Johnston county osteoarthritis project. *Trans Am Clin Climatol Assoc.* 2015;126:77–86.
8. Barbour KE, Boring M, Helmick CG, Murphy LB, Qin J. Prevalence of severe joint pain among adults with doctor-diagnosed arthritis—United States, 2002–2014. *MMWR Morb Mortal Wkly Rep.* 2016;65(39):1052–1056.
9. Johnson VL, Hunter DJ. The epidemiology of osteoarthritis. *Best Pract Res Clin Rheumatol.* 2014;28(1):5–15.
10. Glyn-Jones S, Palmer AJ, Agricola R, et al. Osteoarthritis. *Lancet.* 2015;386(9991):376–387.
11. Mork PJ, Holtermann A, Nilsen TI. Effect of body mass index and physical exercise on risk of knee and hip osteoarthritis: Longitudinal data from the norwegian HUNT study. *J Epidemiol Community Health.* 2012;66(8):678–683.
12. Vina ER, Kwoh CK. Epidemiology of osteoarthritis: Literature update. *Curr Opin Rheumatol.* 2018;30(2):160–167.
13. Warner SC, Valdes AM. Genetic association studies in osteoarthritis: Is it fairytale? *Curr Opin Rheumatol.* 2017;29(1):103–109.
14. Munk HL, Svendsen AJ, Hjelmborg J, Sorensen GL, Kyvik KO, Junker P. Heritability assessment of cartilage metabolism. A twin study on circulating procollagen IIA N-terminal propeptide (PIIANP). *Osteoarthritis Cartilage.* 2014;22(8):1142–1147.
15. Evangelou E, Valdes AM, Kerkhof HJ, et al. Meta-analysis of genome-wide association studies confirms a susceptibility locus for knee osteoarthritis on chromosome 7q22. *Ann Rheum Dis.* 2011;70(2):349–355.
16. Felson DT, Neogi T Osteoarthritis. In: Jameson JL, Fauci AS, Kasper DL, Hauser SL, Longo DL, Loscalzo J, eds. *Harrison's Principles of Internal Medicine.* 20th ed. New York, NY: McGraw-Hill Education; 2017. accessmedicine.mhmedical.com/content.aspx?aid=1155953712.
17. Loeser RF. Age-related changes in the musculoskeletal system and the development of osteoarthritis. *Clin Geriatr Med.* 2010;26(3):371–386.
18. Kumar V, Abbas AK, Aster J. Bones, joints, and soft tissue tumors. *Robbins Basic Pathology.* 10th ed. New York: Elsevier, Inc.; 2018.
19. Loeser RF, Goldring SR, Scanzello CR, Goldring MB. Osteoarthritis: A disease of the joint as an organ. *Arthritis Rheum.* 2012;64(6):1697–1707.
20. American College of Rheumatology. Available at http://www.rheumatology.org/publications/.
21. Kloppenburg M. Hand osteoarthritis-nonpharmacological and pharmacological treatments. *Nat Rev Rheumatol.* 2014;10(4):242–251.
22. Zhang W, Doherty M, Leeb BF, et al. EULAR evidence based recommendations for the management of hand osteoarthritis: Report of a task force of the EULAR standing committee for international clinical studies including therapeutics (ESCISIT). *Ann Rheum Dis.* 2007;66(3):377–388.

23. Maradit Kremers H, Larson DR, Crowson CS, et al. Prevalence of total hip and knee replacement in the United States. *J Bone Joint Surg Am.* 2015;97(17):1386–1397.
24. Bennell KL, Hunter DJ, Hinman RS. Management of osteoarthritis of the knee. *BMJ.* 2012;345:e4934.
25. Hochberg MC, Altman RD, April KT, et al. American College of Rheumatology 2012 recommendations for the use of nonpharmacologic and pharmacologic therapies in osteoarthritis of the hand, hip, and knee. *Arthritis Care Res (Hoboken).* 2012;64(4):465–474. 10.1002/acr.21596 22563589.
26. Qin J, Theis KA, Barbour KE, et al. Impact of arthritis and multiple chronic conditions on selected life domains—United States, 2013. *MMWR Morb Mortal Wkly Rep.* 2015;64(21):578–582.
27. Marra C, Cibere J, Grubisic M, et al. Pharmacist initiated intervention trial in osteoarthritis (PhIT-OA): A multidisciplinary intervention for knee osteoarthritis. *Arthritis Care Res (Hoboken).* 2012;64(12):1837–1845.
28. National Institute for Health and Care Excellence. Available at https://www.nice.org.uk/guidance/cg177. Updated 2014. Accessed August 25, 2015. Osteoarthritis care and management in adults.
29. Guglielmo D, Hootman JM, Murphy LB, et al. Health care provider counseling for weight loss among adults with arthritis and overweight or obesity—United States, 2002–2014. *MMWR Morb Mortal Wkly Rep.* 2018;67(17):485–490.
30. Bliddal H, Leeds AR, Christensen R. Osteoarthritis, obesity and weight loss: Evidence, hypotheses and horizons—a scoping review. *Obes Rev.* 2014;15(7):578–586.
31. Vincent HK, DeJong G, Mascarenas D, Vincent KR. The effect of body mass index and hip abductor brace use on inpatient rehabilitation outcomes after total hip arthroplasty. *Am J Phys Med Rehabil.* 2009;88(3):201–209.
32. Messier SP, Mihalko SL, Legault C, et al. Effects of intensive diet and exercise on knee joint loads, inflammation, and clinical outcomes among overweight and obese adults with knee osteoarthritis: The IDEA randomized clinical trial. *JAMA.* 2013;310(12):1263–1273.
33. Qin J, Barbour KE, Nevitt MC, et al. Objectively measured physical activity and risk of knee osteoarthritis. *Med Sci Sports Exerc.* 2018;50(2):277–283.
34. Nelson AE, Allen KD, Golightly YM, Goode AP, Jordan JM. A systematic review of recommendations and guidelines for the management of osteoarthritis: The chronic osteoarthritis management initiative of the U.S. bone and joint initiative. *Semin Arthritis Rheum.* 2014;43(6):701–712.
35. Regnaux JP, Lefevre-Colau MM, Trinquart L, et al. High-intensity versus low-intensity physical activity or exercise in people with hip or knee osteoarthritis. *Cochrane Database Syst Rev.* 201510):CD010203. doi: 10.1002/14651858.CD010203.pub2.
36. Svege I, Nordsletten L, Fernandes L, Risberg MA. Exercise therapy may postpone total hip replacement surgery in patients with hip osteoarthritis: A long-term follow-up of a randomised trial. *Ann Rheum Dis.* 2015;74(1):164–169.
37. Gossec L, Paternotte S, Maillefert JF, et al. The role of pain and functional impairment in the decision to recommend total joint replacement in hip and knee osteoarthritis: An international cross-sectional study of 1909 patients. Report of the OARSI-OMERACT task force on total joint replacement. *Osteoarthritis Cartilage.* 2011;19(2):147–154.
38. Skou ST, Roos EM, Laursen MB, et al. Total knee replacement plus physical and medical therapy or treatment with physical and medical therapy alone: A randomised controlled trial in patients with knee osteoarthritis (the MEDIC-study). *BMC Musculoskelet Disord.* 2012;13:67.
39. Weber KL, Jevsevar DS, McGrory BJ. AAOS clinical practice guideline: Surgical management of osteoarthritis of the knee: Evidence-based guideline. *J Am Acad Orthop Surg.* 2016;24(8):e94–e96.
40. Losina E, Walensky RP, Kessler CL, et al. Cost-effectiveness of total knee arthroplasty in the united states: Patient risk and hospital volume. *Arch Intern Med.* 2009;169(12):1113–1121. discussion 1121–2.
41. Waimann CA, Fernandez-Mazarambroz RJ, Cantor SB, et al. Cost-effectiveness of total knee replacement: A prospective cohort study. *Arthritis Care Res (Hoboken).* 2014;66(4):592–599.
42. Chou R, McDonagh MS, Nakamoto E, Griffin J. Analgesics for osteoarthritis: An update of the 2006 comparative effectiveness review. comparative effectiveness review no. 38. (prepared by the oregon evidence-based practice center under contract HHSA 290 2007 10057 I). *Agency for Healthcare Research and Quality.* 2011;No. 11(12)-EHC076-EF.
43. Bannuru RR, Schmid CH, Kent DM, Vaysbrot EE, Wong JB, McAlindon TE. Comparative effectiveness of pharmacologic interventions for knee osteoarthritis: A systematic review and network meta-analysis. *Ann Intern Med.* 2015;162(1):46–54.
44. Barkin RL. Topical nonsteroidal anti-inflammatory drugs: The importance of drug, delivery, and therapeutic outcome. *Am J Ther.* 2015;22(5):388–407.
45. Krebs EE, Gravely A, Nugent S, et al. Effect of opioid vs nonopioid medications on pain-related function in patients with chronic back pain or hip or knee osteoarthritis pain: The SPACE randomized clinical trial. *JAMA.* 2018;319(9):872–882.
46. Frakes EP, Risser RC, Ball TD, Hochberg MC, Wohlreich MM. Duloxetine added to oral nonsteroidal anti-inflammatory drugs for treatment of knee pain due to osteoarthritis: Results of a randomized, double-blind, placebo-controlled trial. *Curr Med Res Opin.* 2011;27(12):2361–2372.
47. Hochberg MC, Wohlreich M, Gaynor P, Hanna S, Risser R. Clinically relevant outcomes based on analysis of pooled data from 2 trials of duloxetine in patients with knee osteoarthritis. *J Rheumatol.* 2012;39(2):352–358.
48. Brown JP, Boulay LJ. Clinical experience with duloxetine in the management of chronic musculoskeletal pain. A focus on osteoarthritis of the knee. *Ther Adv Musculoskelet Dis.* 2013;5(6):291–304.
49. Altman RD. Pharmacological therapies for osteoarthritis of the hand: A review of the evidence. *Drugs Aging.* 2010;27(9):729–745.
50. Altman RD, Barthel HR. Topical therapies for osteoarthritis. *Drugs.* 2011;71(10):1259–1279.
51. Taylor N. Nonsurgical management of osteoarthritis knee pain in the older adult. *Clin Geriatr Med.* 2017;33(1):41–51.
52. Department of Health and Human Services. *Federal Register.* 2009; 81.
53. Watkins PB, Kaplowitz N, Slattery JT, et al. Aminotransferase elevations in healthy adults receiving 4 grams of acetaminophen daily: A randomized controlled trial. *JAMA.* 2006;296(1):87–93.
54. Larson AM, Polson J, Fontana RJ, et al. Acetaminophen-induced acute liver failure: Results of a United States multicenter, prospective study. *Hepatology.* 2005;42(6):1364–1372.
55. O'Neil CK, Hanlon JT, Marcum ZA. Adverse effects of analgesics commonly used by older adults with osteoarthritis: Focus on non-opioid and opioid analgesics. *Am J Geriatr Pharmacother.* 2012;10(6):331–342.
56. Meara AS, Simon LS. Advice from professional societies: Appropriate use of NSAIDs. *Pain Med.* 2013;14(suppl 1):S3–S10.
57. McEvoy GK. *AHFS Drug Information.* Bethesda, MD: American Society of Health-System Pharmacists, Inc.; 2012ISBN 978-1-58528-247-0.
58. Lanas A. Nonsteroidal anti-inflammatory drugs and cyclooxygenase inhibition in the gastrointestinal tract: A trip from peptic ulcer to colon cancer. *Am J Med Sci.* 2009;338(2):96–106.
59. Moore N, Scheiman JM. Gastrointestinal safety and tolerability of oral non-aspirin over-the-counter analgesics. *Postgrad Med.* 2018;130(2):188–199.
60. Rostom A, Moayyedi P, Hunt R; Canadian Association of Gastroenterology Consensus Group. Canadian consensus guidelines on long-term nonsteroidal anti-inflammatory drug therapy and the need for gastroprotection: Benefits versus risks. *Aliment Pharmacol Ther.* 2009;29(5):481–496.
61. Patricio JP, Barbosa JP, Ramos RM, Antunes NF, de Melo PC. Relative cardiovascular and gastrointestinal safety of non-selective non-steroidal anti-inflammatory drugs versus cyclo-oxygenase-2 inhibitors: Implications for clinical practice. *Clin Drug Investig.* 2013;33(3):167–183.
62. Scarpignato C, Lanas A, Blandizzi C, et al. Safe prescribing of non-steroidal anti-inflammatory drugs in patients with osteoarthritis—An expert consensus addressing benefits as well as gastrointestinal and cardiovascular risks. *BMC Med.* 2015;13:55. doi: 10.1186/s12916-015-0285-8.
63. Crofford LJ. Use of NSAIDs in treating patients with arthritis. *Arthritis Res Ther.* 2013;15(suppl 3):S2.
64. Coxib and traditional NSAID Trialists' (CNT) Collaboration; Bhala N, Emberson J, Merhi A, et al. Vascular and upper gastrointestinal effects of non-steroidal anti-inflammatory drugs: Meta-analyses of individual participant data from randomised trials. *Lancet.* 2013;382(9894):769–779.
65. Antman EM. Evaluating the cardiovascular safety of nonsteroidal anti-inflammatory drugs. *Circulation.* 2017;135(21):2062–2072.
66. Bello AE, Holt RJ. Cardiovascular risk with non-steroidal anti-inflammatory drugs: Clinical implications. *Drug Saf.* 2014;37(11):897–902.

67. Nissen SE. Cardiovascular safety of celecoxib, naproxen, or ibuprofen for arthritis. *N Engl J Med.* 2017;376(14):1390.
68. Meunier L, Larrey D. Recent advances in hepatotoxicity of non steroidal anti-inflammatory drugs. *Ann Hepatol.* 2018;17(2):187–191.
69. Celebrex® [package insert]. Available at: http://labeling.pfizer.com/ShowLabeling.aspx?id=793. Accessed June 2016. Pfizer, Inc. NY; May 2016.
70. Derry S, Moore RA, Rabbie R. Topical NSAIDs for chronic musculoskeletal pain in adults. *Cochrane Database Syst Rev.* 2012;9:CD007400.
71. Conaghan PG, Dickson J, Grant RL, Guideline Development Group. Care and management of osteoarthritis in adults: Summary of NICE guidance. *BMJ.* 2008;336(7642):502–503.
72. Latimer N, Lord J, Grant RL, et al. Cost effectiveness of COX 2 selective inhibitors and traditional NSAIDs alone or in combination with a proton pump inhibitor for people with osteoarthritis. *BMJ.* 2009;339:b2538.
73. Ayhan E, Kesmezacar H, Akgun I. Intraarticular injections (corticosteroid, hyaluronic acid, platelet rich plasma) for the knee osteoarthritis. *World J Orthop.* 2014;5(3):351–361.
74. Law TY, Nguyen C, Frank RM, Rosas S, McCormick F. Current concepts on the use of corticosteroid injections for knee osteoarthritis. *Phys Sportsmed.* 2015;43(3):269–273.
75. Pyne D, Ioannou Y, Mootoo R, Bhanji A. Intra-articular steroids in knee osteoarthritis: A comparative study of triamcinolone hexacetonide and methylprednisolone acetate. *Clin Rheumatol.* 2004;23(2):116–120.
76. FDA Drug Safety Communication, September 13, 2012. Available at http://fda.gov./Drugs/DrugSafety/ucm318858.htm. Accessed September 10, 2015.
77. Cepeda MS, Camargo F, Zea C, Valencia L. Tramadol for osteoarthritis: A systematic review and metaanalysis. *J Rheumatol.* 2007;34(3):543–555.
78. Howes F, Buchbinder R, Winzenberg TB. Opioids for osteoarthritis? weighing benefits and risks: A cochrane musculoskeletal group review. *J Fam Pract.* 2011;60(4):206–212.
79. Langley PC, Patkar AD, Boswell KA, Benson CJ, Schein JR. Adverse event profile of tramadol in recent clinical studies of chronic osteoarthritis pain. *Curr Med Res Opin.* 2010;26(1):239–251.
80. Dowell D, Haegerich TM, Chou R. CDC guideline for prescribing opioids for chronic pain—United States, 2016. *JAMA.* 2016;315(15):1624–1645.
81. Centers for Disease Control and Prevention (CDC). 2018 annual surveillance report of drug-related risks and outcomes—United States; surveillance special report. Centers for Disease Control and Prevention, U.S. Department of Health and Human Services. Accessed August 8, 2018 from https://www.cdc.gov.drugoverdose/pdf/pubs/2018cdc-drug-surveillance-report.pdf.
82. Hunter DJ. Viscosupplementation for osteoarthritis of the knee. *N Engl J Med.* 2015;372(11):1040–1047.
83. Jevsevar D, Donnelly P, Brown GA, Cummins DS. Viscosupplementation for osteoarthritis of the knee: A systematic review of the evidence. *J Bone Joint Surg Am.* 2015;97(24):2047–2060.
84. Wandel S, Juni P, Tendal B, et al. Effects of glucosamine, chondroitin, or placebo in patients with osteoarthritis of hip or knee: Network meta-analysis. *BMJ.* 2010;341:c4675.
85. Sawitzke AD, Shi H, Finco MF, et al. The effect of glucosamine and/or chondroitin sulfate on the progression of knee osteoarthritis: A report from the glucosamine/chondroitin arthritis intervention trial. *Arthritis Rheum.* 2008;58(10):3183–3191.
86. Hochberg MC, Martel-Pelletier J, Monfort J. Combined chondroitin sulfate and glucosamine for painful knee osteoarthritis: A multicentre, randomised, double-blind, non-inferiority trial versus celecoxib. *Ann Rheum Dis.* 2015;75(1):37–44.

111

Rheumatoid Arthritis

Stephanie Gruber, Bianca Harris, and Susan Hylland

KEY CONCEPTS

1. The etiology of rheumatoid arthritis is unknown but is thought to result from a combination of genetic and environmental factors.
2. Rheumatoid arthritis is a systemic autoimmune condition in which inappropriate activation of innate and adaptive immune responses cause inflammation leading to bone, cartilage, and synovium erosion.
3. The primary goal of treatment includes targeting disease remission/low disease activity ultimately aiming at enhancing quality of life.
4. Care should be provided by a rheumatology-trained clinician.
5. Optimizing mental health and completing physical therapy are both crucial nonpharmacologic therapies in addition to providing comprehensive disease and treatment education.
6. Drug treatment should be started as soon as a diagnosis is established.
7. Choice of therapy depends on the level of disease activity, comorbid health conditions, patient preference, and often insurance coverage.
8. Nonsteroidal anti-inflammatory drugs, analgesics, and corticosteroids are used as adjunctive therapy to disease-modifying antirheumatic drug therapy.
9. Response to therapy is evaluated by patient subjective reports, physical examination, laboratory markers, and imaging.

BEYOND THE BOOK

Direct-to-consumer advertising refers to the marketing of products to patients rather than healthcare professionals. This is a common marketing strategy, particularly for pharmaceutical products. Watch the following advertisements for tofacitinib and adalimumab:

- https://www.ispot.tv/ad/O1Z1/xeljanz-mornings-raking
- https://www.ispot.tv/ad/wrWz/humira-food-drive

Reflect on the promotional materials by considering the following questions:

- What is the general feeling generated by the commercials?
- What actions or activities do the commercials focus on?
- What additional concerns might one have after hearing about the possible side effects of this biologic product?

Watching the adalimumab commercial would lead patients to the product Website to do their own research: https://www.humira.com. Explore the Website and reflect on the following questions:

- How user-friendly is the Website? What resources are available for patients?
- What specifically is HUMIRA Complete?
- Where is the injection education video located on the Website?
- Would you direct patients to watch this video?
- What resources would you use from this Website, if any, for your patient education in clinic?

One of the counseling points for adalimumab is to contact your provider prior to having any surgeries or receiving any vaccinations. Make a chart of which immunizations a patient can and cannot receive while using this injectable medication.

INTRODUCTION

Autoimmune conditions cause the body to produce an inappropriate immune response against its own healthy tissue. Rheumatoid arthritis (RA) is a common, chronic, progressive autoimmune condition that primarily affects the joint and synovium but can also have detrimental effects on organ systems throughout the body. It can have substantial and devastating effects on one's ability to function and complete basic activities of daily living. The exact etiology of RA is unknown, but treatment options are numerous. Comprehensive treatment plans are developed under the guidance of a rheumatology specialist and through a process of shared decision making with the patient.

EPIDEMIOLOGY

RA is one of the more common autoimmune conditions. The annual incidence is about 40 individuals per 100,000. Worldwide disease prevalence is approximately 1% with some variance for race and geographic location.[1] This prevalence corresponds most closely with North American and Northern European countries; however, native American-Indian populations have the highest prevalence noted (approximately 5%-6%). Southern European, Eastern Asian, and African countries have a lower prevalence.[1] Women are twice as likely to develop the disease compared with men.[2]

RA generally presents in the fifth decade of life with increasing prevalence up to the eighth decade of life.[3] RA can affect children age 16 years or younger; in these patients, the condition is referred to as juvenile RA. This chapter focuses only on the clinical management of adult RA. Compared with the general population, individuals with RA have higher rates of disability claims and workplace limitations and lower rates of employment.[4] Loss of productivity has been associated with lower annual earnings.[2,4]

The mortality rate in patients with RA is higher than that of the general population. Cardiovascular (CV) disease is the leading cause of death in RA and presents the greatest concern. Patients with RA have a higher risk of major adverse CV events, and RA disease activity is a predictor of increased CV risk. The risk of death is also increased by infections, malignancy, depression, and pulmonary disease. The expected life expectancy of patients with RA is 3 to 10 years less than the general population.[5-7]

Despite advancements in therapy, mortality trends have not changed drastically, though one could argue additional time is required to detect changes in survival data. Other common comorbid autoimmune diseases include insulin-dependent diabetes mellitus and autoimmune thyroid disease.[6,7]

ETIOLOGY

1 The specific cause of RA is unknown. The disease results from a mix of genetic susceptibility and nongenetic factors combined with a triggering event. Genetic polymorphisms seem to play a large role based on descriptive epidemiologic studies. There is a thought that multiple genes are involved, specifically those of the human leukocyte antigen (HLA) system.[8] Genetics also seems to play a role based on familial studies. In studies of the development of RA in twins, monozygotic twins had a higher concordance than dizygotic twins.[9] Patients with a first-degree relative with RA are at a higher risk of having RA themselves when nongenetic factors are standardized.[10]

There is some variability regarding the role of hormonal regulation and the likelihood of RA development, particularly with estrogen. Evidence is conflicting as to whether pregnancy status affects the risk of RA. Pregnancy is often associated with disease remission in the last trimester, but flares commonly occur in the acute postpartum period.[8] There is also controversial evidence showing female oral contraceptives may protect against or postpone disease development. Testosterone may have a protective effect, as men with low testosterone levels are more likely to have RA.

Nongenetic or environmental factors possibly associated with RA include cigarette use, coffee consumption, and obesity.[8] Cigarette smoking has been tied to increased disease activity, increased biomarkers, and poor prognoses.[6] Ties are weaker for disease development with heavy coffee consumption and obesity.[11,12] Dietary choices have been reported by patients to both positively and negatively impact disease severity or progression.[13] Occupational hazards, such as exposure to silica, may also play a role in susceptibility to disease.[14]

Additional factors, aside from those mentioned above, are needed to trigger the disease itself. An infectious process is hypothesized to be the primary trigger. The Epstein–Barr virus and retroviruses are most commonly associated with the disease.[8] Infections of *Mycoplasma* spp. and *Porphyromonas gingivalis* have been suspected as bacterial triggers, but no true link has been found to show their causality.[15] Further studies are required to help uncover the exact etiology of RA.

PATHOPHYSIOLOGY

2 The role of the immune system is to detect foreign matter, build a response, and neutralize the threat. In RA, the immune system cannot discriminate between self and nonself. This results in cell proliferation, inflammation, and destruction of tissues and fluids throughout one's own body.

The immune cascade and inflammatory pathway dysregulation associated with RA is multifactorial (Fig. 111-1). Overstimulation of the innate immune system is thought to be one of the earliest histologic changes in RA. T cells display an activated surface phenotype with high allele expression of HLA and CD 27, increasing their affinity for lymphokines. Activated T cells stimulate B cells, causing production of autoantibodies. These autoantibodies form large complexes that deposit throughout the body. Antibodies to immunoglobulin G (IgG) have a strong correlation to the pathogenesis and poor prognosis of RA and are known as rheumatoid factor (RF). B cells also produce proinflammatory cytokines, including tumor necrosis factor (TNF) and the interleukin (IL) system, which are responsible for inducing expression of adhesion molecules on the endothelium, further enhancing T-cell proliferation and differentiation, encouraging cell migration, and regulating matrix modeling.[16-18]

Other mechanisms of pathogenesis include overexpression of tumor suppressor gene *p53*, which prevents normal DNA repair and interferes with appropriate cell apoptosis (programmed cell death), and increased presence of anticitrullinated protein antibodies (ACPA). ACPA positivity is associated with a poorer prognosis in patients with RA.[19,20]

A variety of histological changes occur within the synovium, given the above pathological processes. Synovial tissue typically attaches to the skeletal tissues and the bone-cartilage joint cavity and provides a protective shield for the synovial interstitium and a nutrient-rich environment for cartilage. Migration of lymphocytes, macrophages, and mononuclear cells into the synovium and

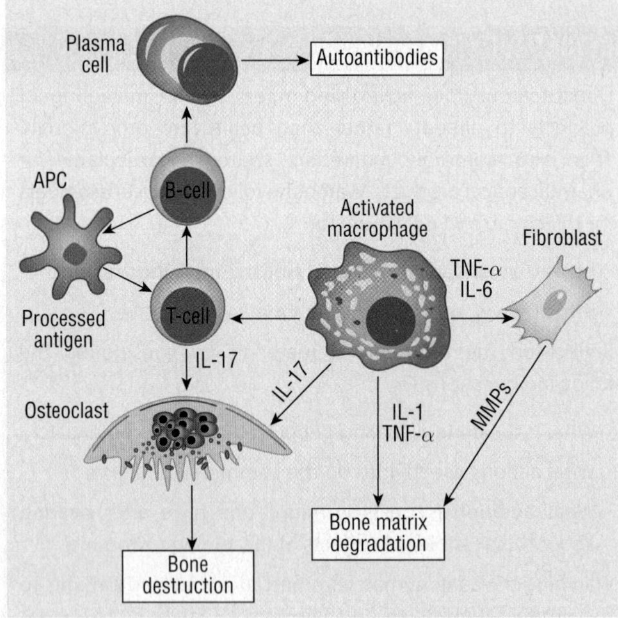

FIGURE 111-1 Pathogenesis of the inflammatory response. Antigen-presenting cells process and present antigens to T cells, which may stimulate B cells to produce antibodies and osteoclasts to destroy and remove bone. Macrophages stimulated by the immune response can stimulate T cells and osteoclasts to promote inflammation. They also can stimulate fibroblasts, which produce matrix metalloproteinases to degrade the bone matrix and produce proinflammatory cytokines. Activated T cells and macrophages release factors that promote tissue destruction, increase blood flow, and result in cellular invasion of synovial tissue and joint fluid. (APC, antigen-presenting cell; IL, interleukin; MMP, matrix metalloproteinase; TNF-α, tumor necrosis factor α.)

synovial cavity are some of the earliest histologic changes in RA. With the increased mass to the synovium comes hypertrophy and subsequently angiogenesis, which is needed to bring the necessary oxygen and nutrients to the environment. Angiogenesis is initiated by the proinflammatory cytokines and driven by factors such as IL-8, prostaglandins, vascular endothelial growth factor, and macrophage angiogenic factor. As the vessels develop, cytokines also stimulate further migration of both innate and adaptive immune systems into the synovium, causing inflammation. The inflamed, fibrotic synovium found in RA is known as a pannus. The pannus invades cartilage and bone around it, thereby promoting further destruction and dysregulation.[21-24]

Cytokines in the cartilage drive the generation of reactive nitrogen and oxygen species while increasing chondrocyte catabolism, inhibiting chondrocyte anabolism, and increasing extracellular matrix destruction. Proinflammatory cytokines travel to the bone, provide the source for receptor activator of NFkB ligand (RANKL), and enhance the differentiation and activity of osteoclasts leading to bone matrix destruction.[25-28]

Circulating immune complexes and T cells have been found in the extra-articular involvement of RA. Chronic inflammation in vascular endothelial and visceral, cutaneous, and pleural tissues leads to complications including vasculitis, fibrosis, anemia, and renal amyloidosis.[21,29]

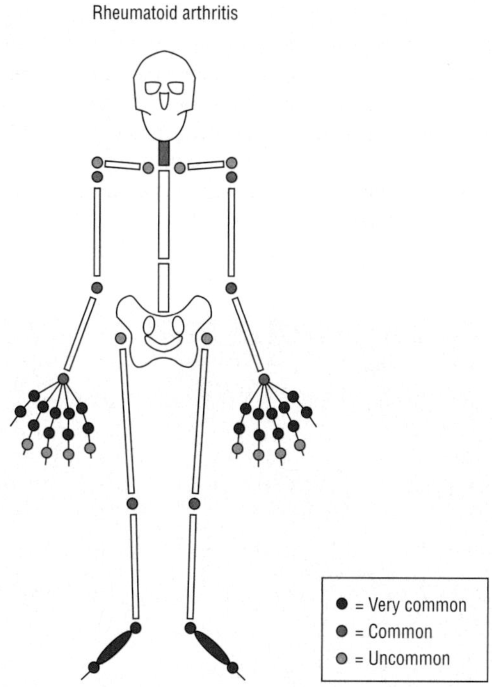

FIGURE 111-2 Patterns of joint involvement in rheumatoid arthritis.

CLINICAL PRESENTATION

Joint Involvement

Patients with RA often present with involvement of synovial-lined peripheral joints, typically in a symmetrical fashion (Fig. 111-2). The joints of the hands, feet, wrists, and ankles are most commonly involved. Elbows, knees, shoulders, hips, cervical spine, and temporomandibular joints may also be affected.

Classic features of RA are the presence of swelling and prolonged morning stiffness, often for more than 30 minutes. Joint swelling is caused by proliferation of synovium or effusion within the joint capsule. On physical examination, joint swelling may be visible or detected by palpation of soft spongy tissue along joint lines. A swollen joint may appear erythematous, and the overlying skin may feel warmer than surrounding tissue. In contrast, the swelling associated with osteoarthritis is due to bony enlargement and not typically associated with signs of inflammation.

RA of the hands more specifically involves the metacarpophalangeal, proximal interphalangeal, and wrist joints, while sparing

CLINICAL PRESENTATION Rheumatoid Arthritis

Joint Involvement

- Hands, wrists, ankles, and feet are most commonly affected, often bilaterally
- Presence of warmth and swelling with or without pain
- Prolonged morning stiffness, often for longer than 30 minutes in duration
- Decreased functionality
- Symptoms present for 6 weeks or more
- Subluxations and deformities possible with advanced disease

Extra-articular Involvement

- Generalized fatigue, weakness, and decreased mood are nonspecific implications of disease
- Rheumatoid nodules can be found on extensor or pleural lining surfaces
- Interstitial lung disease or pleural disease
- Vasculitis
- Keratoconjunctivitis sicca, scleritis, or Sjögren's syndrome
- Pericarditis, cardiac conduction abnormalities, or myocarditis
- Felty syndrome or anemia

Laboratory Findings

- Rheumatoid factor is detected in 70% to 80% of patients with RA with higher titers, which reflects increased sensitivity and more progressive disease
- Anticyclic citrullinated antibodies are more specific for disease, particularly early stage, and generally indicate more aggressive disease
- Erythrocyte sedimentation rate and C-reactive proteins may indicate the presence of a nonspecific inflammatory process
- Synovial fluid analysis through joint aspiration typically demonstrates a high white blood cell count in the absence of crystals or infection

Radiography

- In early stages of RA, it may show soft tissue swelling and joint space narrowing
- In late-stage disease, it may show joint subluxations, deviations, and secondary arthritis

distal interphalangeal joints (Fig. 111-3). Pain and swelling commonly affect joint range of motion and grip strength. Wrist swelling may lead to focal nerve compression, causing symptoms of carpal tunnel syndrome. Untreated, long-term joint inflammation may lead to bony erosions, subluxations, and deformities (Figs. 111-4 and 111-5). These changes may alter the mechanics of hand function, reducing grip strength and making it difficult to perform usual daily activities.

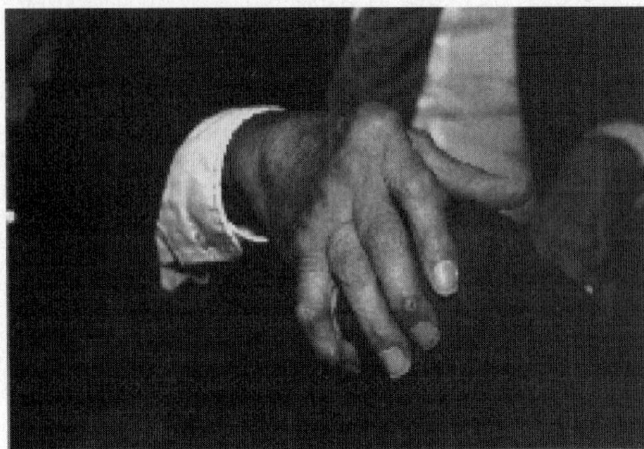

FIGURE 111-3 Typical hand deformities of rheumatoid arthritis showing ulnar deviation of the fingers and swelling of the metacarpophalangeal and proximal interphalangeal joints. *(Reproduced, with permission, from Brunicardi FC, Anderson DK, Billiar TR, et al. Schwartz's Principles of Surgery. 8th ed. New York: McGraw Hill; 2005.)*

When patients with RA have involvement of the joints of the feet, walking may be difficult because of metatarsophalangeal, midfoot, and ankle joint inflammation. Untreated long-term inflammation may lead to subluxations of the metatarsal heads causing bunion formation, hammer toe deformities, or overlapping digits (Figs. 111-4 and 111-5). Affected joints are then subject to ulceration of the skin overlying joint deformities secondary to pressure caused by footwear.

Other parts of the body are also affected by pathophysiologic changes in RA. Pain and decreased range of motion in the elbow and shoulder joints may be the result of joint inflammation or inflammation of the tendons and bursae around the joints. Chronic synovial inflammation of the knee may lead to effusions, pain, and loss of range of motion. Synovitis of the knee may cause the formation of a fluid collection behind the knee called a popliteal (Baker) cyst. Eventually, chronic knee joint inflammation may lead to cartilage loss and muscle atrophy, which can result in laxity of the ligamentous structures that support the knee and ultimately instability. The hip joint, a large axial joint, is less commonly involved in RA, but may manifest with joint effusion and long-term accelerated cartilage loss.

Spinal involvement in RA, when present, occurs in the upper cervical vertebrae. Inflammation of the synovial-lined portions of the first and second cervical vertebrae (C1-C2) can lead to neck pain and stiffness. Long-term RA activity at this joint may lead to instability and subluxation, putting patients at risk for spinal cord compression, although this complication is rare.

The temporomandibular joint of the jaw is also a synovial lined joint and, when affected, patients with RA may experience malocclusion and difficulty chewing.

Extra-articular Involvement

Although joint involvement is the hallmark finding in RA, it is important to recognize that this is ultimately a multisystem inflammatory

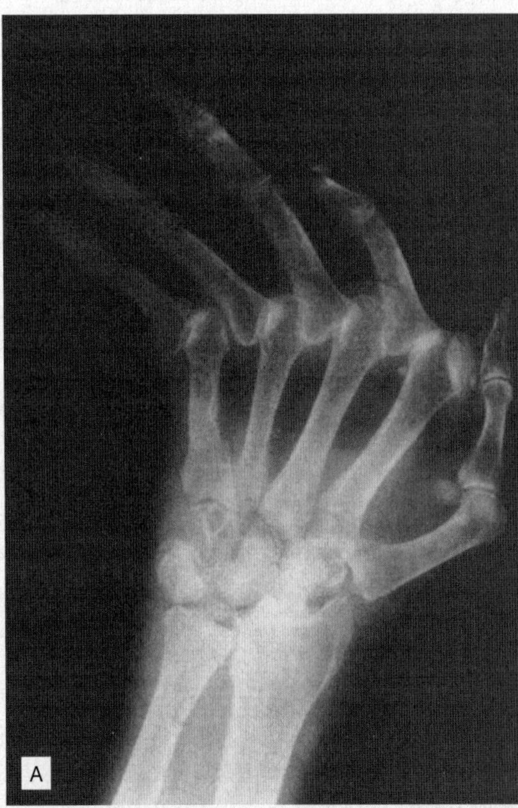

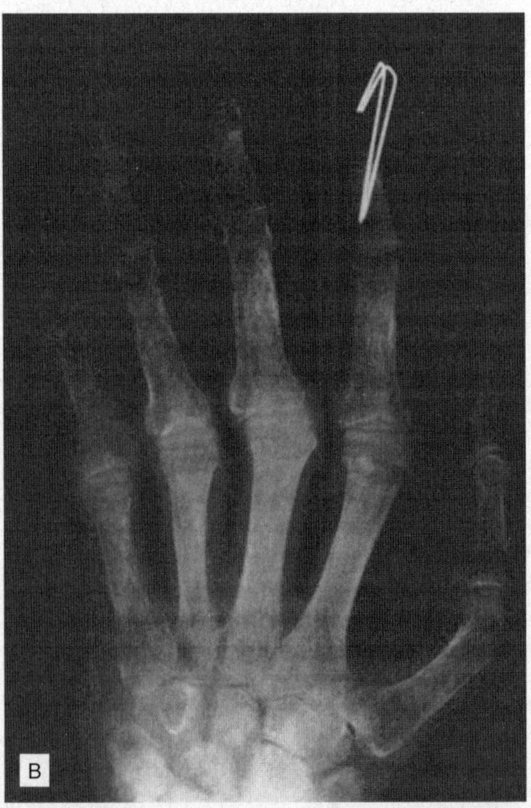

FIGURE 111-4 Radiographs of hands of patient with rheumatoid arthritis showing erosions and subluxations of the metacarpophalangeal joints with ankylosis of the carpal bones of both wrists. *(Reproduced with permission from Papadopoulos DV, Bednar MS, Davidson A, Schmidt CC. Hand surgery. In: McMahon PJ, Skinner HB. eds. Current Diagnosis & Treatment in Orthopedics, 6th Edition. McGraw Hill; 2021.)*

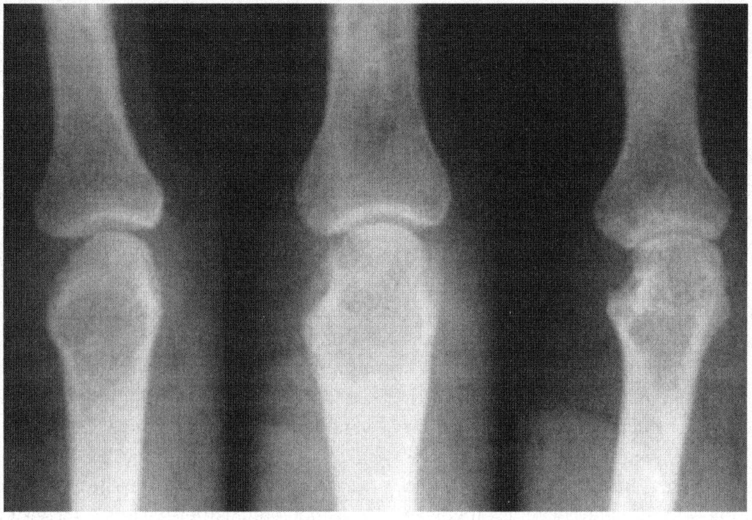

FIGURE 111-5 Radiograph showing soft tissue swelling, joint space narrowing, and erosions in the metacarpophalangeal joints. *(Reprinted, with permission, from Jonsson A, Borg A, Hannesson, et al. Film-screen vs digital radiography in rheumatoid arthritis of the hand: An ROC analysis. Acta Radiologica. 1994;35(4):312.)*

disease. Patients with high-titer RF or ACPA have a higher likelihood of extra-articular manifestations.

Rheumatoid Nodules

Rheumatoid nodules occur in 20% to 35% of patients with RA at some point during their disease course.[30] Rheumatoid nodules are subcutaneous collections of palisading macrophages surrounded by lymphocytes and fibroblasts, which can vary in size from several millimeters to several centimeters. They are most commonly found on the extensor surfaces of the elbows, forearms, and hands but also may be seen on the feet and at other pressure points. They also may develop in the lung or pleural lining of the lung. Rheumatoid nodules usually are asymptomatic and do not require any special intervention. They do not necessarily improve with treatments targeting RA activity and can accelerate in growth during treatment with methotrexate.[31]

Pulmonary Complications

Interstitial lung disease (ILD) is the most common pulmonary manifestation of rheumatoid disease. Frequently ILD is not overtly clinically apparent, but it can be seen on high-resolution CT imaging in up to 33% of patients with RA without symptoms of cough or dyspnea.[32] The most frequent patterns of ILD seen in RA are the usual interstitial pneumonia and nonspecific interstitial pneumonia. Smoking increases the risk of this complication.[33]

Pleural disease is common in RA, and while most commonly asymptomatic, it may result in pleural effusion.[34] Rheumatoid nodules may also develop in lung tissue and may be difficult to distinguish from infection or malignancy on chest imaging. Interstitial pneumonitis is a rare but potentially life-threatening complication of RA. Treatments directed at treating articular manifestations of rheumatoid arthritis frequently do not control pulmonary manifestations.

Vasculitis

Rheumatoid vasculitis is a rare complication of RA seen in patients with long-standing seropositive disease. Invasion of arterial walls by inflammatory cells results in narrowing of the vessel lumen, producing tissue ischemia and infarct. Skin is the most common tissue involved, and infarcts of distal fingers or toes are usually of little consequence. Vasculitis may also involve skin in the lower extremities, producing ulcers that may first appear to be stasis ulcers but are painful due to the ischemic arterial component.

When more severe or visceral rheumatoid vasculitis is present, patients commonly show constitutional symptoms such as weight loss, fever, or failure to thrive. Infarction of vessels supplying blood to nerves can cause motor deficits, such as a foot drop. Renal involvement of vasculitis may lead to a necrotizing glomerulonephritis. Rarely, involvement of medium-sized vessels can result in life-threatening complications with visceral involvement similar to that seen in polyarteritis nodosa.

Rheumatoid vasculitis requires aggressive immunosuppressive therapy to prevent serious complications. Fortunately, the incidence of rheumatoid vasculitis has dramatically decreased with the advent of the routine use of disease-modifying antirheumatic drugs (DMARDs) and biologic therapies with the intent of treating patients with RA to target remission.[35]

Ocular Manifestations

Ocular manifestations of RA include keratoconjunctivitis sicca and inflammation of the sclera, episclera, cornea, and uveal tract. Inflammation and subsequent atrophy of the lacrimal glands may result in decreased tear formation, causing dry and itchy eyes, a condition usually termed *keratoconjunctivitis sicca*. When this condition is observed in association with RA, it is referred to as "secondary Sjögren's syndrome."

Inflammation of the superficial layers of the sclera is called *episcleritis* and is a generally self-limiting manifestation. *Scleritis* is a more serious vascular inflammation of the cornea, episclera, and uvea, as it is painful and threatens vision. Scleritis in RA is typically a sign of uncontrolled systemic inflammation and warrants prompt and aggressive immunosuppression to preserve vision.

Cardiac Involvement

RA is believed to be an independent risk factor for coronary artery disease and is associated with an increased risk of cardiovascular mortality. A meta-analysis published in 2008 concluded that the risk of cardiovascular mortality was 59% higher in patients with RA than in the general population.[36]

The risk for cardiovascular disease is higher in those with more active inflammation and is reduced with treatment, particularly with methotrexate.[37] Pericarditis may occur, although the development of clinically evident pericarditis with tamponade is a rare complication. Cardiac conduction abnormalities and aortic valve incompetence, caused by aortic root dilation, may occur. Myocarditis is a rare complication of RA.

Hematologic Involvement

A small subset of patients with more severe, long-standing, seropositive RA will go on to develop splenomegaly and neutropenia; this is known as *Felty syndrome*. Neutropenia leads to an increased susceptibility to recurrent bacterial infection. Treatment with immunosuppressive therapy, typically methotrexate, with the goal of reversing immune system dysfunction, will usually improve granulocyte counts.

Large granular lymphocyte leukemia (LGL) is an indolent leukemia characterized by a clonal proliferation of large granular lymphocytes. Often patients with LGL require no therapy, unless neutropenia is severe leading to recurrent infections. LGL is treated with immunosuppression. The majority of experience has involved the use of methotrexate, cyclophosphamide, or cyclosporine.[38]

Other Complications

Lymphadenopathy may occur in patients with RA, and when present, it warrants a workup for infection or malignancy. Amyloidosis is a rare complication of longstanding RA and may lead to renal and gastrointestinal complications. Osteoporosis in patients with RA is almost two times higher than in patients without RA.[39]

Laboratory Findings

The complete blood count can be altered by RA or its treatment. A mild-to-moderate normocytic anemia is commonly due to anemia of chronic disease. It is important to differentiate anemia of chronic disease from anemia associated with complications of therapy, such as gastritis induced by nonsteroidal anti-inflammatory drugs (NSAIDs) or bone marrow suppression from immunosuppressive therapy. Thrombocytosis is a common finding with active RA since platelets are generally considered an acute phase reactant and tend to rise and fall in correlation with inflammation in many patients. Thrombocytopenia may also result as a side effect of immunosuppressive therapy. Neutropenia is associated with Felty syndrome and LGL, but it also may be a side effect of immunosuppressive drugs. Leukocytosis is seen commonly as a result of corticosteroid treatment.

The erythrocyte sedimentation rate (ESR) and C-reactive proteins (CRP) are nonspecific markers of inflammation that are usually elevated in patients with active RA. They may be used as an aid in following RA activity.

A positive RF is detected in 70% to 80% of patients with RA. In general, higher titers of RF increase the sensitivity and indicate a potentially more severe disease course. A positive RF (two times the upper limit of normal) in a patient with consistent clinical features of inflammatory arthritis is fairly specific for rheumatoid arthritis. However, a positive RF, especially with a low titer in a patient without clinical evidence of inflammatory arthritis, has low specificity for RA. Many patients with hepatitis C have a positive rheumatoid factor, as do many patients with Sjögren's syndrome, sarcoidosis, and certain infections.

Anticyclic citrullinated antibodies have a slightly lower sensitivity to the RF, being found in 57% (range, 12%-93%) of patients with RA, but ACPAs are more specific (96%) and may be detectable early in the disease.[40] The presence of ACPA, in general, predicts a more aggressive course of disease and increased risk of joint erosions. In contrast to RF, ACPAs are not typically present in patients with hepatitis C. Many rheumatologists order both tests in evaluating new patients.

Antinuclear antibodies (ANAs) are detected in 25% of patients with RA as a result of their disease. The presence of a positive ANA in a workup of polyarthritis may initially lead to a diagnostic challenge, since they are more commonly seen in systemic lupus erythematosus, systemic sclerosis, and mixed connective tissue disease, all of which can have arthritis as a presenting feature. However, patients with RA who have a positive ANA would not be expected to be positive for more specific antibodies for connective tissue disorders, including anti-ds DNA antibodies, anti-Smith antibodies, anti-SCL 70 antibodies, or anti-RNP antibodies.

Synovial fluid analysis may be performed during the initial diagnosis or follow-up in patients with RA to rule out crystalline disease or infection in swollen joints (especially joints that are swollen out of proportion to the rest of the clinical examination). Synovial fluid analysis of involved joints typically reveals white blood cell counts of 1,500 to 25,000/mm^3 (1.5×10^9 to 25×10^9/L) but may be higher in those with active RA.[41]

Plain radiographs in RA are often normal at the time of disease presentation. The earliest plain radiographic findings typically include soft tissue swelling and periarticular osteoporosis on hand and foot x-rays. As RA progresses, joint space narrowing occurs as a result of cartilage degradation, and marginal erosions (at the margins of the joint capsules) may occur, typically in the ulnar styloid, metacarpophalangeal and proximal interphalangeal joints of the hands (Fig. 111-5), and the metatarsophalangeal joints of the feet. In advanced stages of RA, radiographs may show deformities including joint subluxations, ulnar deviation of the metacarpophalangeal joints, and secondary osteoarthritis. Many DMARD and biologic therapies halt the progression of erosive changes in RA. Serial joint radiographs may be used in addition to clinical findings as a way of evaluating disease progression and adequacy of therapy.

DIAGNOSTIC CRITERIA

In 2010, the American College of Rheumatology (ACR) and European League Against Rheumatism (EULAR) updated their classification criteria for RA.[42] The revised criteria allow for identification of patients at an earlier stage of disease, such as synovitis of one small joint in the absence of an alternative diagnosis. Early identification of patients with RA may allow for earlier treatment geared toward preventing structural damage to joints.

The criteria use a scoring system which assigns points based upon the number and types (small and large) of joints involved. The presence of RF or ACPA and elevated acute phase reactants (CRP and ESR) result in additional points. A duration of symptoms of 6 weeks or more provides an additional point. A total score of 6 or more out of a possible total score of 10 is considered diagnostic for RA (Table 111-1).[42] Not all patients with RA will score 6 or greater initially but may evolve to higher scores over time.

TABLE 111-1 ACR/EULAR Rheumatoid Arthritis Classification Criteria

Criteria	Score
Low-positive RF or ACPA	2
High-positive RF or ACPA	3
High ESR or CRP	1
Duration of symptoms ≥6 weeks	1
Joint Involvement (at least one joint not explained by another disease)	
2-10 large joints	1
1-3 small joints (± large joint)	2
4-10 small joints (± large joint)	3
>10 joints (at least one small joint)	5

ACR/EULAR, American College of Rheumatology/European League Against Rheumatism; ACPA, anticitrullinated protein antibodies; CRP, C-reactive protein; ESR, eosinophil sedimentation rate; RF, rheumatoid factor.

Patients with inflammatory arthritis who have negative RF and ACPA may be diagnosed with RA if they fulfill further criteria otherwise characteristic of RA. In addition, a number of other inflammatory arthritic conditions are managed similarly to seropositive rheumatoid arthritis; these include psoriatic arthritis, reactive arthritis, ankylosing spondylitis, and arthritis associated with inflammatory bowel disease.

TREATMENT

Desired Outcomes

The ACR as well as the EULAR guidelines recommend a treat-to-target approach when treating patients with RA rather than a non-targeted treatment approach. If remission cannot be achieved, low disease activity is an acceptable alternative target. This treatment approach is supported by superior clinical outcomes compared with usual care. In general, RA treatment is directed toward reducing inflammation and symptoms, including joint pain and stiffness. Most of the therapies used to treat RA slow the disease progression and thus the progression of irreversible joint damage, which can help decrease disability and improve quality of life.[43]

General Approach to Treatment

3 4 Available pharmacologic therapies do not reverse joint damage that has already occurred. Therefore, early aggressive treatment of RA is imperative. Early treatment of RA results in improved outcomes. Patients with a shorter disease duration are more likely to respond to treatment.[44,45] Nonpharmacologic therapies also play a role in the management of RA and encourage patients to take an active role in managing their disease.[46] Therefore, the approach to the treatment of RA should include both pharmacologic and

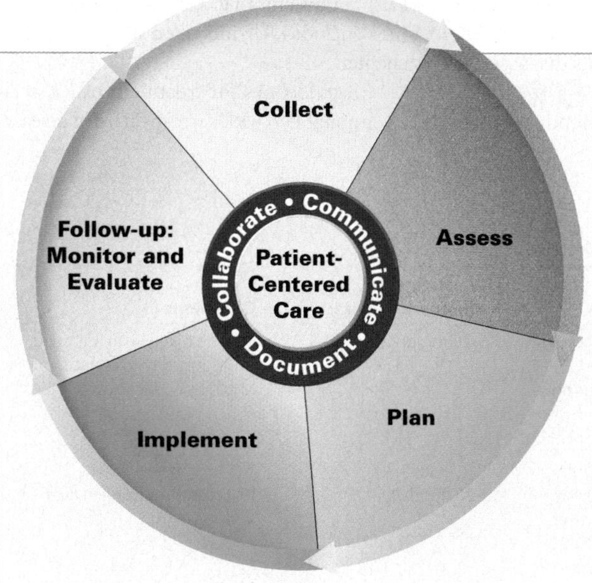

Patient Care Process for Rheumatoid Arthritis

The image shows the five fundamental steps included in The Pharmacist's Care Process endorsed by the Joint Commission for Pharmacy Practitioners (2014). The tagline of this process reads collaborate, communicate, and document. The five fundamental steps listed here are collect, assess, plan, implement, and follow-up: monitor and evaluate. All these steps are listed in a circular block diagram.

Collect

- Patient characteristics (eg, age, sex, pregnancy status, insurance)
- Social history (eg, tobacco/alcohol use, activity)
- Patient medical history (eg, health conditions, immunizations, recent infections)
- Family medical history (eg, autoimmune conditions)
- Current medications
- Past RA medication trials
- Subjective symptom report
- Objective data such as blood pressure, labs (eg, ESR, CRP, CBC), imaging (eg, DEXA, x-ray films, ultrasound), physical examination (eg, number of tender/swollen joints)

Assess

- Patient subjective report (eg, pain score, duration of morning joint stiffness, adherence to therapy, injection technique/medication storage, side effects to drug therapy, disability, fatigue)
- Change in number of tender/swollen joints, labs, or imaging
- Cardiovascular risk factors
- Infection risk and upcoming procedures
- Patient treatment preference (utilize motivational interviewing as appropriate)

Plan*

- Drug therapy (see Table 111-2)
- Referrals when appropriate (eg, tobacco treatment clinic, podiatry, mental health, social work, physical and/or occupational therapy)
- Patient education (eg, dosing, side effects, infection risk management, symptom self-monitoring)
- Order follow-up labs based on therapy chosen (see Table 111-4)

Implement*

- Provide patient education regarding rationale for and follow-up of treatment plan
- Provide patient with written medication changes, time frame for follow-up, and clinic/emergency contact information
- Coordinate and schedule follow-up

Follow-up: Monitor and Evaluate

- Subjective symptom changes and impact on daily activities
- Presence of adverse effects and infections
- Laboratory results as indicated for therapy
- Patient adherence to treatment plan
- Time frame dependent on treatment plan (generally every 1-3 months)

Collaborate with a rheumatologist.

nonpharmacologic methodologies. Ultimately, care should be coordinated by a healthcare provider trained in rheumatology.

Nonpharmacologic Treatment

5 Nonpharmacologic approaches for the treatment of RA include referrals to occupational and physical therapy, mental health, social work, reviewing pain coping skills, and providing patient education. Both mental and physical health are important in patients with RA, as central neuroendocrine and dopaminergic pathways may be involved in both RA disease activity and physical and mental health. Patients with RA are also more likely to be affected by mood disorders and may benefit from referrals to specialty providers as appropriate.[47]

Patient education should involve disease state education as well as medication education related to potential adverse effects and how to appropriately administer injectable agents. Physical therapy is beneficial for reducing pain and inflammation while preserving joint function. The benefits of exercise and physical activity, including aerobic activity and muscle-strengthening exercises, have been demonstrated to improve RA-related disease outcomes. Assistive devices and orthoses such as braces and supports are useful to improve pain and function. Occupational therapy can be effective and provide several benefits such as exercises, appropriate footwear, and splinting.[46] Weight loss can help decrease the stress on joints. Surgical options, including joint replacements, are reserved for patients with more severe disease where there may have significant cartilage loss.

Pharmacologic Therapy

Currently available therapies used to treat RA and also slow the progression of the disease include conventional and biologic DMARDs and the small-molecule agents tofacitinib, baricitinib, and upadacitinib. Conventional DMARDs include methotrexate, leflunomide, sulfasalazine, and hydroxychloroquine. Biologic DMARDs fall into two categories: tissue necrosis factor (TNF) inhibitor biologics (adalimumab, etanercept, certolizumab, golimumab, and infliximab) and non-TNF biologics (abatacept, tocilizumab, rituximab, anakinra, and sarilumab). Tofacitinib, baricitinib, and upadacitinib are oral synthetic DMARDs that are also Janus Kinase (JAK) inhibitors. Many of the therapies used to treat RA are also indicated and used in the treatment of other conditions such as psoriatic arthritis and ankylosing spondylitis, conditions that are outside the scope of this chapter. Table 111-2 includes RA-indicated dosages for the agents discussed in this chapter.

6 7 The current ACR guidelines for treatment of RA recommend initiation of conventional DMARDs irrespective of disease

TABLE 111-2 Usual Doses for Disease-Modifying Antirheumatic Drugs

Drugs	Brand Names	Routes of Administration	Starting Doses	Usual Ranges or Maintenance Doses	Comments
Methotrexate	Rasuvo Trexall Otrexup (SubQ)	Oral, SubQ, IM	Oral: 7.5 mg once weekly or 2.5 mg every 12 hours for 3 doses once weekly SubQ/IM: 7.5 mg once weekly	7.5-20 mg once weekly	May be given with folic acid 1-5 mg/day to reduce adverse reactions
Leflunomide	Arava	Oral	Loading dose: 100 mg daily for 3 days, then 20 mg daily or 10-20 mg daily without loading dose	10-20 mg daily	Not recommended in liver disease (ALT >3 times ULN)
Hydroxychloroquine	Plaquenil	Oral	200 mg twice daily or 400 mg daily	200 mg twice daily or 400 mg daily	Take with food or milk; use with caution in renal or hepatic impairment
Sulfasalazine	Azulfidine	Oral	500 mg once or twice daily	1,000 mg twice daily (maximum dose is 3,000 mg/day if inadequate response after 12 weeks of 2,000 mg/day)	Not recommended in renal or hepatic impairment
Etanercept	Enbrel	SubQ	50 mg once weekly or 25 mg twice weekly	Same as starting dose	
Infliximab	Remicade	IV	3 mg/kg at 0, 2, 6 weeks, and then every 8 weeks	3-10 mg/kg every 4-8 weeks	Given in combination with methotrexate therapy; pretreat with methylprednisolone, acetaminophen, and antihistamine
Adalimumab	Humira	SubQ	40 mg every 2 weeks	40 mg every 2 weeks (may increase to 40 mg once weekly if not taking methotrexate)	
Certolizumab	Cimzia	SubQ	400 mg at 0, 2, 4 weeks	200 mg every other week or 400 mg every 4 weeks	
Golimumab	Simponi	SubQ	50 mg once monthly	Same as starting dose	
Rituximab	Rituxan	IV	1,000 mg in 2 doses given 2 weeks apart	Initial dose may be repeated every 16-24 weeks based on response	Pretreat with methylprednisolone, acetaminophen, and antihistamine

(continued)

TABLE 111-2 Usual Doses for Disease-Modifying Antirheumatic Drugs (*Continued*)

Drugs	Brand Names	Routes of Administration	Starting Doses	Usual Ranges or Maintenance Doses	Comments
Abatacept	Orencia	IV, SubQ	IV: <60 kg: 500 mg, 60-100 kg: 750 mg, >100 kg: 1,000 mg at 0, 2, and 4 weeks or initial IV dose followed by 125 mg subcutaneously within 24 hours SubQ: 125 mg weekly	IV: dose based on weight every 4 weeks SubQ: 125 mg weekly	
Tocilizumab	Actemra	IV, SubQ	IV: 4 mg/kg every 4 weeks SubQ: <100 kg: 162 mg every other week, >100 kg 162 mg weekly	IV: 4-8 mg/kg every 4 weeks (maximum 800 mg per infusion) Subcutaneously: <100 kg: 162 mg every other week, followed by an increase to weekly injections if needed, >100 kg: 162 mg weekly	Can increase the metabolism of CYP3A4 substrates
Tofacitinib	Xeljanz	Oral	IR: 5 mg twice daily ER: 11 mg daily	Same as starting dose	5 mg once daily in moderate-to-severe renal insufficiency, moderate hepatic impairment, or concomitant CYP3A4 or CYP2C19 inhibitors
Upadacitinib	Rinvoq	Oral	ER: 15 mg daily	Same as starting dose	Use is not recommended in severe hepatic impairment.
Baricitinib	Olumiant	Oral	2 mg daily	Same as starting dose	eGFR 30-60 mL/min/1.73 m^2: 1 mg daily; use is not recommended with eGFR <30 mL/min/1.73 m^2; use is not recommended in severe hepatic impairment; dosage adjustment for concomitant strong organic anion transporter 3: 1 mg daily.
Anakinra	Kineret	SubQ	100 mg once daily	Same as starting dose	
Sarilumab	Kevzara	SubQ	200 mg every 2 weeks	Same as starting dose	

ALT, alanine transaminase; CYP, cytochrome P; ER, extended release; IR, immediate release; ULN, upper limit of normal; IM, intramuscular; SubQ, subcutaneous; IV, intravenous.

activity in treatment-naïve patients (Fig. 111-6) once a diagnosis is established. The preferred conventional DMARD is methotrexate unless a contraindication to its use exists.[48,49] In practice, choice of therapy may ultimately be dependent on level of disease activity, comorbid health conditions, patient preference, and often insurance coverage.

The ACR guidelines recommend treatment with DMARD monotherapy for patients with early RA—defined as duration of disease/symptoms of less than 6 months—and low disease activity. Double or triple DMARD therapy is recommended if disease activity is moderate or high. A biologic agent can be used as monotherapy or with conventional DMARD(s) in patients with moderate or high disease activity. Tofacitinib would be an alternate option if disease activity remains moderate or high with combination conventional DMARDs. If disease activity remains moderate or high despite DMARD or biologic agents, a low-dose glucocorticoid can be added for the shortest duration of time necessary. Low-dose glucocorticoid is defined as prednisone 10 mg/day or less or an equivalent amount of another glucocorticoid. If patients achieve remission, DMARDs and biologic agents can be tapered; however, patients should remain on DMARD therapy at some level.

In patients with established RA—defined as duration of disease/symptoms for 6 months or more—treatment with DMARD monotherapy is recommended despite disease activity in DMARD-naïve patients. Combination conventional DMARDs or a biologic DMARD or tofacitinib can be used if disease activity remains moderate or high after an adequate trial with DMARD monotherapy. In patients who are on TNF inhibitor monotherapy with moderate or high disease activity, one or two DMARDs can be added to the TNF inhibitor. A non-TNF biologic can be used in place of a TNF inhibitor if disease activity remains moderate or high on a TNF inhibitor. This is recommended over tofacitinib. Therapy can be switched to another non-TNF biologic if a single non-TNF biologic is unable to adequately control disease activity. If courses of two TNF inhibitors have not adequately controlled disease activity, a non-TNF biologic can be initiated. Tofacitinib can be initiated if disease activity persists despite multiple TNF inhibitors in patients for whom non-TNF biologics are not an option. Glucocorticoids can be added if disease flares occur or are inadequately controlled despite DMARD, TNF inhibitor, or non-TNF biologic therapy.[41] It is worth mentioning that the newer JAK inhibitors, baricitinib and upadacitinib, were not yet approved at the time of these ACR guidelines and, therefore, only tofacitinib is listed specifically.

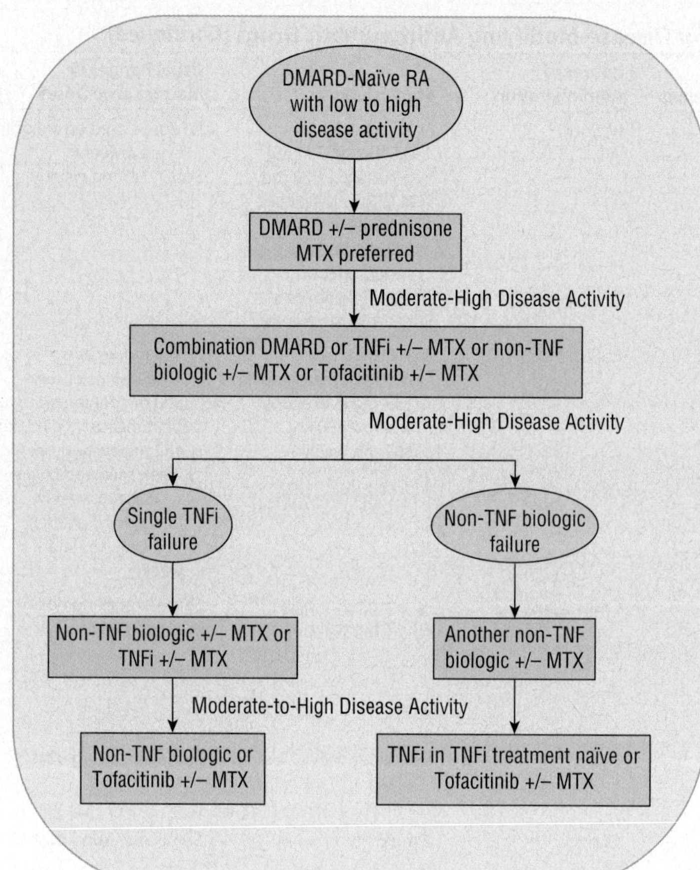

FIGURE 111-6 Treatment algorithm for rheumatoid arthritis based on the American College of Rheumatology guidelines. (DMARD, disease-modifying antirheumatic drug; MTX, methotrexate; TNF, tumor necrosis factor.) *(Data from Reference 50.)*

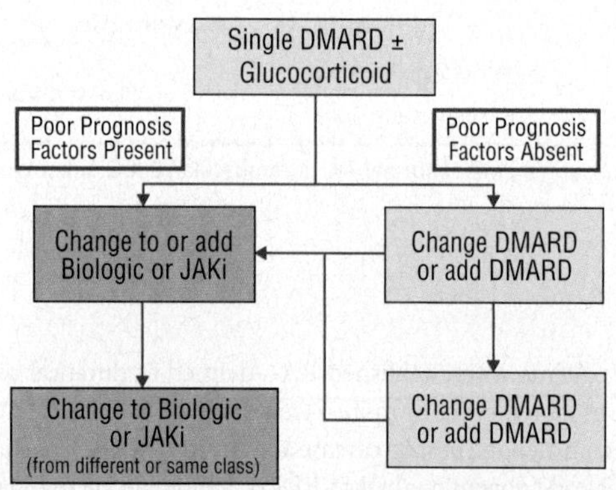

FIGURE 111-7 Simplified treatment algorithm for rheumatoid arthritis based on the EULAR 2019 update. (DMARD, disease-modifying antirheumatic drug; JAKi, Janus kinase inhibitor.)

In contrast to the ACR guidelines, the 2019 EULAR guidelines delineates treatment recommendations based on past therapy, clinical response, and presence of poor prognostic factors (Fig. 111-7). Poor prognostic factors are defined as high disease activity, early joint damage, positive RF or ACPA, and failure of >2 conventional DMARDs. Dosages and therapies should be reassessed no later than 3 months after the initiation or change. The algorithm also provides dose reduction recommendations for persistent disease remission of at least 6 months in duration, especially if having tapered glucocorticoid therapy. It is not recommended that all pharmacologic treatment be completely discontinued.[50]

8 DMARDs can take weeks to months to take effect in patients with RA. NSAIDs and/or glucocorticoids, as well as other analgesics such as acetaminophen, can provide symptomatic relief and have a more rapid onset of action than DMARDs; they are often used as "bridge" therapy. NSAIDs do not impact disease progression, and corticosteroids have several side effects associated with their use, making both less desirable choices for long-term use.

Conventional Disease-Modifying Antirheumatic Drugs

Methotrexate Methotrexate is the DMARD of choice for most patients unless its use is contraindicated. Methotrexate has been used in the treatment of RA for several decades and has a sustained clinical response over time and a glucocorticoid-sparing effect.[51] It can be taken as monotherapy or in combination with other DMARDs.

Methotrexate is a structural analogue of folic acid that inhibits dihydrofolate reductase. Dihydrofolate reductase is the enzyme responsible for reducing dihydrofolic acid to folinic acid, the active intracellular metabolite. Through this action, methotrexate inhibits DNA synthesis and repair and cellular replication.[52]

Methotrexate is taken once weekly and is typically given in either tablet form or as a subcutaneous injection. It is also available as an intramuscular injection. The absorption of oral methotrexate is highly variable. At low doses (≤30 mg/m^2), oral bioavailability is about 60%, and this decreases at higher doses. Methotrexate is about 50% protein bound and is excreted by the kidney, about 80% to 90% unchanged.[52] Injectable methotrexate has a higher bioavailability compared with oral methotrexate and thus provides superior clinical efficacy. Injectable methotrexate is typically better tolerated and has less potential to cause gastrointestinal side effects as well.[53] The doses used for the treatment of RA typically range from 7.5 to 20 mg weekly. Doses exceeding 20 mg weekly can increase the risk for toxicities.[52] At doses higher than 15 mg weekly, oral methotrexate may not have significant added clinical benefit; changing to subcutaneous methotrexate may increase bioavailability and clinical benefit.[8] Clinical benefit can be seen 3 to 6 weeks after starting methotrexate therapy.[52]

Methotrexate is teratogenic and is therefore contraindicated in pregnancy and breastfeeding. Additional contraindications include alcoholism, alcoholic liver disease or other chronic liver disease, immunodeficiency, and preexisting hematologic disorders, such as leukopenia and thrombocytopenia. Methotrexate excretion is reduced in renal impairment and may require dose reduction or discontinuation in some cases. Excretion is also reduced in ascites or pleural effusions.[52]

Recommended laboratory monitoring prior to starting methotrexate includes a complete blood count (CBC) with differential, alanine transaminase (ALT), aspartate transaminase (AST), and renal function. These should be monitored every 2 to 4 weeks for 3 months after initiation or following a dose increase, then every 8 to 12 weeks during 3 to 6 months of therapy, and every 12 weeks after 6 months of therapy.[5] A chest x-ray film can be considered before starting methotrexate in patients with underlying lung disease. Hepatitis B, hepatitis C, and tuberculosis screenings should be obtained at baseline in high-risk patients.[54]

Adverse effects of methotrexate include infection, pulmonary complications (eg, interstitial pneumonitis and chronic obstructive pulmonary disease [COPD]), gastrointestinal problems (eg, perforation and diarrhea), hematologic changes (eg, thrombocytopenia and leukopenia), and hepatic toxicities (eg, elevated liver enzymes and cirrhosis). Because methotrexate is a structural analogue of folic acid, it can cause folic acid deficiency; methotrexate should be given with folic acid 1 to 5 mg daily to reduce the incidence of toxicities associated with methotrexate.[52]

Leflunomide Leflunomide, an oral DMARD that inhibits pyrimidine synthesis, can be used as monotherapy or in combination with other DMARDs to treat RA. Leflunomide reduces signs and symptoms of RA, inhibits structural damage, and improves physical function. It is significantly protein bound (>99.3%). The typical maintenance dose used to treat RA is 20 mg daily; the dose can be decreased to 10 mg daily if patients are unable to tolerate higher doses. A loading dose can be given of 100 mg for 3 days to achieve steady state more rapidly, but this may increase the risk for toxicities.

Leflunomide has a half-life of about 2 weeks and may require washout with cholestyramine if rapid elimination is required due to toxicity or incidental pregnancy. Leflunomide is excreted by the kidneys as well as through direct biliary excretion.[9] Baseline monitoring should include a tuberculosis screening, CBC with differential, ALT, AST, and renal function. These should be monitored every 2 to 4 weeks for 3 months after initiation or following a dose increase, then every 8 to 12 weeks during 3 to 6 months of therapy, and every 12 weeks after 6 months of therapy.

Adverse reactions associated with leflunomide include diarrhea, elevated liver enzymes, alopecia, elevated blood pressure, and rash. If ALT is three times the upper limit of normal (ULN), leflunomide should be discontinued. Leflunomide should not be used in pregnant or nursing mothers or in patients with severe hepatic impairment.[55]

Sulfasalazine Sulfasalazine is a prodrug with two metabolites, 5-aminosalicylic acid (5-ASA) and sulfapyridine. The exact mechanism of action of sulfasalazine for the treatment of RA is unknown; [illegible] it has immunomodulating and anti-inflammatory proper- [illegible] be used as monotherapy or in combination with other DMARDs to treat RA. The typical starting dose of sulfasalazine is 500 mg daily or 1 g daily in two divided doses; this can be increased weekly to 2 g daily in two divided doses to minimize the risk of adverse events. Clinical benefit can be seen in 4 weeks, but some individuals may need to be on sulfasalazine for 12 weeks before clinical benefit is achieved. If clinical benefit is not sufficient after 12 weeks of therapy, the dose can be further titrated to 3 g/day in evenly divided doses.

Sulfasalazine is primarily eliminated by the kidney and should be used with caution in renal impairment. Sulfasalazine is contraindicated in sulfonamide or salicylate allergy.[56] Baseline monitoring should include a CBC with differential, ALT, AST, and renal function.[56] These should be monitored every 2 to 4 weeks for 3 months after initiation or following a dose increase, then every 8 to 12 weeks during 3 to 6 months of therapy, and every 12 weeks after 6 months of therapy. Glucose-6-phosphate dehydrogenase deficiency can cause hemolytic anemia; therefore, screening for this prior to initiation should be considered.[57]

Sulfasalazine use is limited by its potential to cause gastrointestinal adverse effects, including diarrhea, nausea, vomiting, and anorexia. Less common adverse effects associated with sulfasalazine include rash, urticaria, blood cell abnormalities (including leukopenia, anemia, and thrombocytopenia), severe hypersensitivity reactions (including Stevens-Johnson syndrome), photosensitivity, elevated liver enzymes, and alopecia. Sulfasalazine can also cause urine and skin discoloration. Sulfasalazine crosses the placenta and is present in breast milk but can be used in pregnant and nursing mothers with caution.[56]

Hydroxychloroquine Hydroxychloroquine is typically used in combination with other DMARDs in patients with RA, but it can be used as monotherapy in mild cases. The mechanism of action in the treatment of RA is not fully understood, but a proposed mechanism for its anti-inflammatory properties is its interference with antigen processing in macrophages and other antigen-presenting cells.[57] Hydroxychloroquine's oral absorption is incomplete and inconsistent, varying from 25% to 100%. It is about 40% protein bound and excreted predominately in the urine.[58]

The typical dose of hydroxychloroquine is 400 mg daily either as one dose or as two divided doses. Clinical benefit is delayed and may take several weeks. The main advantage of hydroxychloroquine use is that it does not require frequent, routine laboratory monitoring because it is not generally associated with infection risk or hepatic, renal, or blood cell abnormalities. The most common adverse effects with hydroxychloroquine are gastrointestinal side effects, including nausea, vomiting, and diarrhea; these can sometimes be mitigated by taking the medication with food or splitting the dose into two doses.[46]

Irreversible retinal damage can occur with hydroxychloroquine use. For patients with risk factors for developing retinal damage, such as low body weight and renal and hepatic impairment, ophthalmologic exams should be conducted annually throughout the treatment with this drug. If patients do not have risk factors for developing retinal damage, an ophthalmologic examination should be completed within 5 years of starting hydroxychloroquine and then repeated annually.[46,59]

Hydroxychloroquine can be continued during pregnancy as there is no increased risk of birth defects or ocular toxicities. Hydroxychloroquine is excreted into the breast milk, and caution should be exercised in nursing mothers.[60]

Biologic Disease-Modifying Antirheumatic Drugs

Biologics agents are genetically engineered protein molecules that have varying mechanisms by which they decrease inflammation. They can be separated into two groups: TNF inhibitor biologics including adalimumab, etanercept, certolizumab, golimumab, and infliximab; and non-TNF biologics including abatacept, tocilizumab, rituximab, anakinra, and sarilumab.

Biologic DMARDs are associated with an increased risk of infection due to their immunosuppressant effects. A tuberculin skin test or interferon gamma release assay (IGRA) blood test should be obtained before starting a biologic to detect and treat latent or active tuberculosis. Patients should also be screened for hepatitis B before starting biologic therapy because of the risk for reactivation.

Biologic agents can be used in combination with conventional DMARDs, but multiple biologics should not be used concomitantly due to additive immunosuppressive effects. In general, if patients are switched from one biologic to another, the new agent should be initiated when the patient is due for a dose of the previous biologic to avoid potential adverse effects. Because of the immunosuppressive effects of these agents, patients should notify their providers if they are being treated for an infection or plan to undergo major surgery while on a biologic or before starting a biologic. A patient's therapy may need to be held until appropriate postsurgical healing and/or resolution of infection can be confirmed.

TNF Inhibitor Biologics

TNF inhibitors block the proinflammatory cytokine TNF-α. Elevated levels of TNF-α are found in the synovial fluid of individuals with RA as well as other rheumatologic conditions. Adalimumab, etanercept, golimumab, certolizumab, and infliximab can take several weeks for clinical benefit to be noted and up to 3 months to achieve full clinical benefit.[61] The place in therapy for these agents is typically when disease activity remains moderate or high despite conventional DMARD therapy.

A major limitation to the use of TNF inhibitors is cost, as they are more expensive than conventional DMARDs. To optimize the use of TNF inhibitors, medication education should include site of administration, expected time to benefit, safe storage, proper disposal, and possible side effects.

Although these agents have similar side effect profile and contraindications, the TNF inhibitors all have differing structures, pharmacokinetics, and dosing schemes. The selection of an agent depends on cost and patient preference for route and frequency of administration. TNF inhibitors should not be used in patients with moderate-to-severe heart failure (New York Heart Association [NYHA] class III/IV), as new-onset and worsening heart failure has been reported with TNF inhibitors. These agents increase the risk of serious infection and malignancies such as lymphoma and skin cancers.

New-onset or exacerbation of demyelinating disorders such as multiple sclerosis has been observed with TNF-α inhibitors. Therapy should be discontinued in patients who develop symptoms of demyelinating disorders, and caution should be exercised in using these agents in this patient population. Before starting TNF inhibitors, patients should be screened for tuberculosis and hepatitis B. During therapy, a CBC with differential should be monitored periodically as TNF inhibitors can cause blood cell disorders including pancytopenia. Other monitoring includes signs/symptoms of malignancy and serious infections.[61]

Certolizumab Certolizumab is a pegylated humanized antibody Fab fragment of TNF-α monoclonal antibody. Because it is not a complete antibody and lacks the Fc region, it does not induce complement activation, antibody-dependent cell-mediated cytotoxicity, or apoptosis. Pegylation allows for delayed elimination and extended half-life. It is available as a prefilled syringe for subcutaneous injection. A loading dose of 400 mg at week 0, 2, and 4 can be given followed by a maintenance dose of 200 mg every other week or 400 mg every 4 weeks.

The most common adverse effects associated with certolizumab are upper respiratory tract infection, rash, and urinary tract infection. The safety and efficacy of certolizumab were evaluated in multiple studies that found that adult patients with moderate-to-severe RA treated with certolizumab had improved clinical response compared with placebo. Structural damage and RA progression was inhibited by certolizumab as compared with placebo plus methotrexate. Patients had improved function when treated with certolizumab compared with placebo.[62]

Adalimumab Adalimumab binds to TNF-α and blocks its interaction with the p55 and p75 cell surface TNF receptors. It is available as a prefilled syringe or pen for subcutaneous injection. Typical dosing for RA is 40 mg every 2 weeks when used with methotrexate. The dose can be increased to 40 mg weekly if it is not being used with methotrexate. Local injection site reactions are the most common adverse event and usually manifest as redness, itching, pain, and swelling.

Adalimumab has been studied as monotherapy, with methotrexate, or as combination therapy with other DMARDs in patients with RA. It improves clinical response, delays the progression of structural damage, and improves function.[61]

Etanercept Etanercept is a recombinant DNA-derived protein composed of TNF receptor linked to the Fc fragment of human IgG1. It is available as a prefilled syringe or pen for subcutaneous injection. Typical dosing for RA is 50 mg once weekly.[63]

The most common adverse effects associated with etanercept use include infections and injection site reactions. Patients treated with etanercept monotherapy and etanercept with methotrexate have improved clinical response. Clinical response was noted within 1 to 2 weeks of starting etanercept, but some patients required 3 months of therapy to demonstrate clinical response. Etanercept plus methotrexate decreased structural damage and progression of RA compared with monotherapy with etanercept or methotrexate. Function was also improved in patients treated with etanercept as compared with placebo.[63]

Golimumab Golimumab is a human monoclonal antibody that binds to human TNF-α. It is available as a prefilled syringe or pen for subcutaneous injection and is typically dosed at 50 mg once monthly. It is also available as an intravenous product that dosed 2 mg/kg at weeks 0 and 4, and then every 8 weeks thereafter.

The most common adverse effects associated with golimumab use are upper respiratory tract infections and nasopharyngitis. Compared with methotrexate monotherapy, golimumab plus methotrexate improves clinical response in patients with RA. Golimumab also improves function in patients as compared with placebo.[64]

Infliximab Infliximab is a chimeric monoclonal antibody that binds to human TNF-α. Infliximab is administered as an IV infusion and typical dosing is 3 mg/kg at weeks 0, 2, and 6, followed by every 8 weeks.

The most common adverse effects associated with infliximab use are infections, infusion-related reactions, headache, and abdominal pain.[41] About 15% of patients develop antibodies to infliximab. Patients who develop these antibodies typically have a higher likelihood of developing an infusion reaction, have increased clearance of infliximab, and therefore decreased efficacy. An electrochemiluminescence immunoassay (ECLIA) can be used to measure infliximab antibodies if this is suspected. When infusion reactions occur with infliximab, they typically begin within 2 hours of infusion. Concomitant use with immunosuppressants such as methotrexate can lessen the likelihood of developing antibodies to infliximab. Premedication with an antihistamine, acetaminophen, and/or a glucocorticoid can help decrease the likelihood of patients developing infusion-related reactions. Patients on infliximab plus methotrexate have an improved clinical response as compared with patients on methotrexate alone. Structural damage and progression of RA [illegible] also delayed.[65]

Non-TNF Biologics

Abatacept Abatacept is a selective co-stimulation modulator that inhibits T-cell activation by binding to CD80 and CD86. This binding blocks the interaction between T cells CD28, thus inhibiting the activation of T cells. Activated T cells are found in the synovial fluid of patients with rheumatologic conditions such as RA and are thought to play a role in the disease. Abatacept is indicated for moderate-to-severe RA and can be used as monotherapy or in conjunction with conventional DMARDs.[66]

Abatacept is typically initiated if disease activity persists in patients after conventional DMARD monotherapy and can be an alternative to TNF inhibitors with or without methotrexate. It can also be initiated in patients who have failed or have had an inadequate response to TNF inhibitors. Abatacept plus methotrexate has similar efficacy and incidence of adverse events as compared with adalimumab plus methotrexate in biologic-naïve patients who had an incomplete response to methotrexate.[67]

Abatacept is available in a prefilled syringe or autoinjector for subcutaneous injection and is given at a dose of 125 mg once weekly. It is also available as a 30-minute IV infusion that is dosed according to body weight (<60 kg: 500 mg; 60-100 kg: 750 mg; >100 kg: 1,000 mg); it is given at 0, 2, and 4 weeks and every 4 weeks thereafter.[66]

The most common side effects associated with abatacept include headache, upper respiratory tract infection, nasopharyngitis, and nausea. Abatacept should be used with caution in patients with COPD; exacerbations have been observed in patients with both COPD and RA on abatacept. Like other biologics, abatacept has also been associated with serious infections and malignancy. Infusion reactions are rare but can include anaphylaxis, hypotension, dyspnea, and urticaria and can occur within 24 hours of intravenous administration.[66]

Tocilizumab Tocilizumab is a monoclonal antibody that inhibits the binding of the proinflammatory cytokine IL-6 to its receptor. Tocilizumab can be used in patients with moderate-to-severe RA who have had an incomplete response to one or more conventional DMARDs and/or TNF inhibitor and can be used as monotherapy or in combination with DMARDs.[68] A study that included patients with severe RA who could not use methotrexate found that tocilizumab monotherapy was more effective in the symptom management of RA compared to adalimumab monotherapy.[69]

Tocilizumab is available as a prefilled syringe for subcutaneous injection with dosing dependent on weight (<100 kg: 162 mg every other week, followed by an increase to weekly injections if needed based on clinical response; >100 kg: 162 mg weekly). It is also available as a 1-hour intravenous infusion at a dose of 4 mg/kg every 4 weeks; the dose can be increased to 8 mg/kg every 4 weeks if needed based on clinical response.[68]

The most common side effects associated with tocilizumab include upper respiratory tract infections, nasopharyngitis, headache, hypertension, increased liver enzymes, and injection site reactions. Infusion reactions can also occur, typically within 24 hours of infusion; these are manifest as headache, rash, pruritus, and urticaria. Tocilizumab can also cause gastrointestinal perforation, neutropenia, and thrombocytopenia as well as serious infections and malignancy. Baseline monitoring recommended should include neutrophils, platelets, lipid panel, AST, and ALT. Neutrophils, platelets, and liver enzymes should also be monitored 4 to 8 weeks after starting therapy and every 3 months thereafter. A lipid panel should be repeated after 4 to 8 weeks of treatment and every 6 months during treatment.[68]

Tocilizumab should not be initiated in patients with an absolute neutrophil count (ANC) of less than 2,000/mm^3 (2 × 10^9/L) or platelet count less than 100,000/mm^3 (100 × 10^9/L); treatment should be discontinued if ANC is less than 500/mm^3 (0.5 × 10^9/L) or platelet count is less than 50,000/mm^3 (50 × 10^9/L). Treatment should not be initiated if liver enzymes are greater than 1.5 times ULN and should be discontinued if liver enzymes are greater than five times ULN. Tocilizumab has the potential to increase the metabolism of drugs that are CYP450 substrates, particularly CYP3A4.[68]

Rituximab Rituximab is a monoclonal antibody that binds the CD20 antigen found on the surface of B cells. Rituximab can be given as monotherapy or in combination with methotrexate and can be initiated in patients with moderate-to-severe RA who have had an incomplete response to one or more TNF inhibitors.[70] Patients who failed one TNF inhibitor had greater reductions in disease activity scores when treated with rituximab than with a second TNF inhibitor.[71]

Rituximab is available as an intravenous infusion and can be given as two 1,000-mg infusions separated by 2 weeks. The recovery of B cells can take several months; therefore, rituximab can be given every 24 weeks. Some patients may not need to receive another dose as often as every 24 weeks; the decision to re-dose should be based on the return of RA symptoms. Rituximab should not be given more frequently than every 16 weeks.[70]

Methylprednisolone 100 mg administered intravenously is recommended 30 minutes before each infusion as well as acetaminophen and an antihistamine to reduce the development and severity of infusion reactions. Side effects that could occur with rituximab treatment include upper respiratory tract infection, nasopharyngitis, urinary tract infection, serious infections, bronchitis, infusion reactions, bowel obstruction/perforation, blood cell disorders, and cardiovascular events.[70] A CBC with differential should be obtained before treatment, with each infusion, and every 2 to 4 months.

Anakinra Anakinra inhibits IL-1, which is involved in inflammatory responses. It can be used in patients with moderate-to-severe RA who have failed one or more DMARDs; however, the ACR did not include this drug in its 2015 RA treatment recommendations due to its infrequent use for the treatment of RA and lack of new data to support its use since 2012. It is a once-daily subcutaneous injection dosed at 100 mg.[72]

Sarilumab Sarilumab is an IL-6 receptor antagonist that is indicated in the treatment of patients with moderate-to-severe RA who have had an incomplete response to one or more DMARDs. The ACR did not include this drug in their RA treatment recommendations because it had been approved when the 2015 recommendations were issued. Sarilumab can be used as monotherapy or with conventional DMARDs. It is a subcutaneous injection of 200 mg administered every 2 weeks.[73]

The most common adverse effects with sarilumab include neutropenia, increased liver enzymes, injection site reactions, and upper respiratory and urinary tract infections. It can also be associated with gastrointestinal perforation and serious infections. Monitoring of this medication should include a baseline tuberculosis screening, CBC with differential, and liver enzymes at baseline, 4 to 8 weeks later, and every 3 months thereafter, and a lipid panel at baseline, 4 to 8 weeks after starting therapy, and then every 6 months. Sarilumab should not be initiated in patients with ANC less than 2,000/mm^3 (2 × 10^9/L), platelets less than 150,000/mm^3 (150 × 10^9/L), or liver enzymes greater than 1.5 times ULN.[73]

The MOBILITY study included patients treated with sarilumab plus methotrexate compared with methotrexate plus placebo; sarilumab plus methotrexate produced a decrease in symptoms, improvement in function, and less progression of RA compared with placebo plus methotrexate.[74] In the TARGET study, sarilumab plus a DMARD reduced the symptoms of RA and improved function compared with placebo plus DMARD.[75]

Target-Specific DMARDs

Janus Kinase (JAK) Inhibitors Tofacitinib and upadacitinib are oral (JAK) inhibitors approved for the treatment of moderate-to-severe rheumatoid arthritis with an inadequate response or intolerance to methotrexate. Baricitinib is a JAK inhibitor approved for the treatment of moderate-to-severe RA with an inadequate response to one or more TNFi therapies. Janus kinases function intracellularly in cell signaling for cytokine-activated receptors. JAK inhibitors bind to and modulate the catalytic activity of JAKs, thus blocking the messaging pathway of multiple pro-inflammatory cytokines and thereby exerting anti-inflammatory effects.[76,77]

JAK inhibitors can be used as monotherapy or in combination with conventional DMARDs and should not be used in combination with biologic DMARDs or other JAK inhibitors. These medications have black box warnings for serious infections including fungal, bacterial, and viral infections; malignancies, including lymphoma; and thrombosis, pulmonary embolism (PE), and deep vein thrombosis (DVT).[76,78,79]

Tofacitinib Tofacitinib is available as a 5-mg immediate-release tablet and an 11-mg extended-release tablet. The recommended dosing is either 5 mg twice daily or 11 mg daily unless a dose reduction is recommended due to hepatic or renal impairment or if used concomitantly with CYP3A4 or CYP2C19 inhibitors.[76,78]

A common measure in studies of RA is *ACR 20* improvement, which is defined as at least a 20% improvement in seven ACR core measures of disease activity, including tender and swollen joints as well as patients' assessment of disease activity and physical function. It has been widely used to measure disease activity and response to therapy in clinical trials. Patients receiving tofacitinib with methotrexate had similar ACR 20 response after 6 months compared with adalimumab with methotrexate and a higher ACR 20 response compared to placebo with methotrexate.[80,81]

Adverse effects that can occur with tofacitinib include upper respiratory tract infection, cardiovascular effects, gastrointestinal perforation, serious infections, ILD, malignancy, nasopharyngitis, diarrhea, and headache. Because tofacitinib can be associated with bone marrow suppression, it should not be initiated when lymphocytes are less than 500 cells/mm^3 (0.5 × 10^9/L) or when ANC is less than 1,000 cells/mm^3 (1 × 10^9/L). Use should be avoided when hemoglobin is less than 9 g/dL (90 g/L; 5.59 mmol/L), and therapy should be interrupted if hemoglobin is less than 8 g/dL (80 g/L; 4.97 mmol/L) or decreases more than 2 g/dL (20 g/L; 1.24 mmol/L). Lymphocyte count should be monitored at baseline and every 3 months thereafter. ANA, platelet counts, and hemoglobin should be monitored at baseline, after 4 to 8 weeks of therapy, and every 3 months thereafter. Tofacitinib can also cause hyperlipidemia; lipids should be monitored 4 to 8 weeks after starting therapy and periodically thereafter. Hepatotoxicity can occur with treatment, and liver function test monitoring is recommended. Use in severe hepatic impairment is not recommended.[76]

An ongoing, open-label study evaluating the safety of tofacitinib 5 mg twice daily and 10 mg twice daily showed that patients with RA, who are 50 years or older with at least one cardiovascular risk factor, had a higher rate of all-cause mortality on tofacitinib 10 mg twice daily versus 5 mg twice daily on TNF inhibitors. These preliminary findings prompted a black box warning of mortality for tofacitinib. Of note, tofacitinib 10 mg twice daily is only FDA-approved for the treatment of ulcerative colitis.[82]

Upadacitinib Upadacitinib is available as a 15-mg extended-release 24-hour oral tablet dosed once daily. No renal dose adjustment is recommended; however, upadacitinib has not been studied in end-stage renal disease (eGFR <15 mL/min/1.73 m^2). It can be utilized in mild-to-moderate hepatic impairment, but use is not recommended in severe hepatic dysfunction. Caution should be exercised when using upadacitinib in patients on strong CYP3A4 inhibitors, and use with strong CYP3A4 inducers is not recommended. Upadacitinib should not be started in patients with absolute lymphocyte count (ALC) less than 500 cells/mm^3 (0.5 × 10^9/L), absolute neutrophil count (ANC) less than 1,000 cells/mm^3 (1 × 10^9/L), or hemoglobin less than 8 g/dL (80 g/L; 4.97 mmol/L).[79]

A phase III, double-blind, randomized controlled trial evaluating the efficacy and safety of upadacitinib compared to placebo or adalimumab in patients with RA and a history of inadequate response to methotrexate showed that upadacitinib was superior to placebo and adalimumab in improving signs, symptoms, and physical function in RA patients. Patients on upadacitinib had significantly less radiographic progression of RA compared to placebo. The safety profile of upadacitinib was similar to adalimumab, except for higher rates of herpes zoster and creatine phosphokinase (CPK) elevations in patients on upadacitinib.[83]

Adverse effects that may occur with upadacitinib include upper respiratory tract infections, neutropenia, lymphocytopenia, nausea, hepatotoxicity, CPK elevations, DVT, PE, increased cholesterol, and gastrointestinal perforation. Therapy should be interrupted if neutropenia, lymphopenia, or anemia occurs past the above ALC and ANC thresholds during treatment.

Recommended monitoring for upadacitinib includes lymphocyte count, ANC, hemoglobin, and liver function tests at baseline and periodically throughout treatment, lipids 12 weeks after initiation and periodically throughout treatment, hepatitis screenings prior to initiation and periodically thereafter, tuberculosis screening at baseline, signs and symptoms of infection during and after therapy, periodic skin examinations, and signs or symptoms of thrombosis throughout treatment.[79]

Baricitinib Baricitinib is available as a 1-mg and 2-mg tablet and is typically dosed at 2 mg daily with eGFR greater than 60 mL/min/1.73 m^2. A dose reduction to 1 mg daily is recommended with eGFR 30 to 60 mL/min/1.73 m^2 and use is contraindicated with eGFR less than 30 mL/min/1.73 m^2. Use in severe hepatic impairment has not been studied and is therefore not recommended. A dose reduction to 1 mg daily is also recommended when used concomitantly with strong organic anion transporter 3 inhibitors, such as probenecid. Baricitinib should not be started in patients with ALC less than 500 cells/mm^3 (0.5 × 10^9/L), ANC less than 1,000 cells/mm^3 (1 × 10^9/L), or hemoglobin less than 8 g/dL (80 g/L; 4.97 mmol/L).[78]

A phase III, double-blind study comparing baricitinib to placebo in patients with RA and inadequate response or intolerance to one or more conventional DMARDs showed that patients on baricitinib had statistically significant improvements in signs and symptoms of RA, including morning stiffness and joint pain, and achieved an ACR20 response compared to placebo. Baricitinib also slowed radiographic progression of RA-related joint damage.[84]

Adverse effects that may occur with baricitinib use include upper respiratory tract infections, herpes zoster infection, hepatotoxicity, hematologic toxicities including anemia, gastrointestinal perforations, thrombosis, lymphocytopenia, neutropenia, increase in SCr and CPK. Therapy should be interrupted if neutropenia, lymphopenia, or anemia occurs past the above ALC and ANC thresholds during treatment.[84]

Recommended monitoring for baricitinib includes lymphocyte, ANC, platelet counts, hemoglobin, and LFTs at baseline and periodically throughout treatment, lipids 12 weeks after therapy and periodically throughout treatment, hepatitis B screening prior to starting therapy, signs and symptoms of infection, abdominal symptoms, and skin examinations periodically.[78]

Other Disease-Modifying Antirheumatic Drugs

Therapies such as azathioprine, cyclosporine, minocycline, and gold salts were previously used to treat RA. With the development of other DMARDs and biologics, they are now used infrequently and have no recent data to support their use.

Nonsteroidal Anti-Inflammatory Drugs NSAIDs inhibit prostaglandin synthesis and can provide anti-inflammatory as well as analgesic effects. However, they do not slow disease progression and should not be used as monotherapy. NSAIDs can provide symptomatic relief from pain and stiffness and can be effective as adjuncts to DMARD therapy in patients with RA. They have a more rapid onset of action than DMARDs and may be beneficial to "bridge" patients while DMARDs take effect.

Although these agents are available without prescription, they still possess potentially serious risks to use. In the United States, NSAIDs carry a Boxed Warning because they increase the risk of serious cardiovascular thrombotic events, including myocardial infarction and stroke.[85] Their use is also associated with serious gastrointestinal bleeding and ulcerations. For more details on NSAIDs, see Chapter 110, "Osteoarthritis."

Glucocorticoids Glucocorticoids have been used in the treatment of RA for their anti-inflammatory and immune-modulating effects.[84] Although these agents slow the progression of RA, glucocorticoids should not be used as monotherapy in the treatment of RA, particularly due to the potential for serious, long-term adverse effects. Therefore, they should be used at the lowest effective dose for the shortest period of time. According to the ACR, short-term glucocorticoid is defined as less than 3 months of therapy and low-dose glucocorticoid is defined as prednisone 10 mg/day or less or its equivalent.

Glucocorticoids can be administered orally or intramuscularly. They act systemically to decrease inflammation and pain. Intra-articular injections administered directly into joints can provide a local decrease in inflammation and pain relief. The intra-articular route is associated with fewer systemic adverse effects because of the limited systemic action. Intra-articular injections should not be repeated more often than every 3 months because of the potential for accelerated loss of cartilage in the joint. Oral glucocorticoids are absorbed almost completely in the gastrointestinal tract, metabolized in the liver, and eliminated in the urine. Typically, oral glucocorticoids, such as prednisone, are taken once daily. Intramuscular glucocorticoids such as triamcinolone acetonide and methylprednisolone acetate can be administered instead of oral steroids based on patient preference or in patients who may not adhere to daily oral therapy. This can also be used in place of an intra-articular injection when multiple joints are involved. To avoid withdrawal associated with hypothalamus–pituitary–adrenal (HPA) axis suppression, glucocorticoids should not be stopped abruptly but should be tapered, especially when used for long term or at high doses. Intramuscular glucocorticoids provide patients with a physiologic taper.

Similar to NSAIDs, glucocorticoids can be used to "bridge" patients while DMARDs take effect. They can also be used as adjuncts to DMARDs at the lowest dose possible in patients with refractory disease. High-dose, short-term bursts can be used as needed for acute flares of RA symptoms, followed by tapering to the lowest effective dose to control symptoms or until discontinued over several days.[86]

Use of long-term glucocorticoids is limited by adverse effects, which include fluid retention, hyperglycemia, hypertension, behavioral and mood changes, increased appetite, weight gain, electrolyte imbalances, impaired healing, hirsutism, Cushing syndrome, HPA axis suppression, osteonecrosis of femoral and humeral heads, osteoporosis and fractures, myopathy, glaucoma, and cataracts.[87,88] The lowest effective dose for the shortest period of time should be used to minimize the potential for these adverse effects. Patients with RA are at a higher risk of developing osteoporosis, and the use of long-term glucocorticoids doubles this risk. In a study of prednisone 7.5 mg daily, patients lost an average of 9.5% of bone in the spine over 20 weeks of treatment.[88] For more information on glucocorticoid-induced bone loss, see Chapter 112, "Osteoporosis."

Special Populations

Pregnancy and Lactation

Data on the safety of a majority of the medications used to treat RA during pregnancy and breastfeeding are limited, and a majority of medications with available safety data in this population have been associated with adverse effects. The potential risks of becoming pregnant should be discussed with women of childbearing age who are being treated for RA, and contraception counseling should be discussed for those not planning on becoming pregnant. Approximately 20% to 40% of patients with RA achieve remission during the third trimester of pregnancy and remission is more common in women with RF-negative RA.[89]

Because of risks associated with paternal exposure to DMARDs, family planning for male patients should also be taken into account when developing treatment plans.[89]

In women who want to become pregnant, therapies that are contraindicated in pregnancy such as methotrexate and leflunomide should be discontinued. Medications that are unsafe during pregnancy or have inadequate data to determine safety, such as abatacept, tocilizumab, rituximab, tofacitinib, and anakinra, should also be discontinued. Disease activity should then be monitored. For symptom control, NSAIDs, acetaminophen, and glucocorticoids can be considered. DMARDs that can be used during pregnancy include hydroxychloroquine and sulfasalazine.[89] Newer medications including upadacitinib, baricitinib, and sarilumab do not have sufficient data available to determine safety during pregnancy.[73,78,79]

There is no increase in congenital malformations with use of TNF inhibitors and therefore they may be considered for use during the first part of pregnancy.[89,90] Specifically, etanercept and certolizumab may be continued throughout pregnancy.[90]

For women who are breastfeeding, methotrexate and leflunomide are contraindicated. NSAIDs, acetaminophen, hydroxychloroquine, sulfasalazine, and glucocorticoids are preferred. TNF inhibitors, anakinra, abatacept, rituximab, tocilizumab, tofacitinib, sarilumab, baricitinib, and upadacitinib do not have sufficient evidence to recommend safe use during breastfeeding.[79,89] Since TNF inhibitors are large protein molecules, little to no drug is likely to be found in breastmilk.[90]

For male patients with RA, methotrexate should be held for 3 months before conception, and sulfasalazine may need to be held if the patient is having difficulty with fertility. There is limited data on adverse outcomes with leflunomide. TNF inhibitors can disrupt spermatogenesis, but use could be considered. Adverse outcomes have been reported with rituximab and abatacept.[89]

Serious Infections

In patients with a history of serious infections, combination DMARDs are recommended over TNF inhibitors. Abatacept can be considered over TNF inhibitors; in a study of patients hospitalized for an infection while on TNF inhibitors, abatacept was associated with the lowest risk of a subsequent infection compared with other biologics.[43]

In patients who screen positive for tuberculosis via either a tuberculin skin test or IGRA, a chest x-ray film should be obtained to determine if the patient has latent or active tuberculosis infection. If the chest x-ray film is positive, a sputum for acid-fast bacillus (AFB) can be collected to rule out active tuberculosis. If this is negative, then the patient likely has latent tuberculosis and a biologic DMARD or tofacitinib can be started or resumed after completing at least 1 month of treatment for latent tuberculosis. If the test is positive, then the patient likely has active tuberculosis and a biologic DMARD or tofacitinib can be started or resumed after the patient has completed treatment for active tuberculosis.[43]

Hepatitis

In patients with hepatitis B infection who are receiving treatment for hepatitis B, treatment of RA should be the same as in patients without a history of hepatitis. In patients with prior exposure to hepatitis B, RA treatment should be the same as unexposed patients, with monitoring of viral load every 6 to 12 months. In patients with history of untreated hepatitis B, treatment of hepatitis B should be considered prior to initiating immunosuppressive therapies.

Patients who are being treated for hepatitis C should not be treated differently than patients without hepatitis C. TNF inhibitors can be used in patients with hepatitis C when they are being treated for this viral infection. In patients with untreated hepatitis C, DMARDs are recommended over TNF inhibitors. Methotrexate and leflunomide should be avoided due to potential effects on the liver; instead, hydroxychloroquine or sulfasalazine should be considered.[43]

Malignancy

In patients with previous melanoma and nonmelanoma skin cancer, DMARDs are preferred over biologic agents and tofacitinib. DMARDs are less immunosuppressive than biologics, decreasing the risk of skin cancer with DMARDs compared with other RA therapies. However, in patients with low-grade skin cancer with history of prior treatment, biologics could be considered with close monitoring of the skin by a dermatologist.

In patients with previously treated lymphoproliferative disorders, rituximab use is recommended over TNF inhibitors because of the known increased risk of lymphoma with TNF inhibitors. Also, rituximab is an FDA-approved treatment for some lymphoproliferative disorders. Combination DMARDs, abatacept, or tocilizumab can be considered over TNF inhibitors. Patients with a history of previously treated solid organ malignancy should be treated as patients without this history.[43]

Heart Failure

TNF inhibitors should be avoided in patients with NYHA II, III, or IV heart failure because of the potential for TNF inhibitors to worsen heart failure or cause new-onset heart failure. If patients develop signs of worsening heart failure on TNF inhibitors, this therapy should be discontinued. Combination DMARDs, non-TNF biologics, or tofacitinib would be recommended as alternative therapies.[43]

Comorbidity Management

Cardiovascular Risk Reduction

RA poses as a risk factor for CV disease; this is likely the result of multiple factors present in patients with RA, including chronic inflammation. Therefore, part of RA management is to also manage cardiovascular disease risk. To lower CV disease risk, RA disease activity should be as low as possible. Lifestyle recommendations should be discussed with patients including smoking cessation, regular exercise, and healthy diet.

Other factors that contribute to CV disease—such as hypertension, hyperlipidemia, and diabetes—should be screened for and treated appropriately. NSAIDs should be used with caution, especially in patients with established CVD. Glucocorticoid use should be minimized and tapered to the lowest possible dose due to their potential ill effects on blood glucose and blood pressure.[91]

Osteoporosis

RA is associated with an increased incidence of osteoporosis, falls, and fractures. Glucocorticoid use can increase the potential for these risks. Published recommendations for osteoporosis screening in patients with RA vary greatly. The American Association of Clinical Endocrinologists recommends screening all postmenopausal women with an increased risk of secondary osteoporosis, including those with RA. Canadian recommendations include osteoporosis screening for all patients older than 50 years of age who have RA.[92]

In patients with RA who have low bone mineral density, treatment should be considered based on estimated 10-year probability of a major osteoporotic fracture or hip fracture risk.[92] Vitamin D supplementation and calcium intake should also be assessed and optimized.

According to the ACR, patients on long-term glucocorticoids who are 40 years of age or older should have bone mineral density testing at least within 6 months of initiating glucocorticoids, and fracture risk should be estimated using FRAX. In patients younger than 40 years of age, bone mineral density testing should be considered at least within 6 months of initiating glucocorticoids if the patient has a history of an osteoporotic fracture or has significant risk factors for developing osteoporosis.[93]

Immunizations

Live vaccines should not be given during treatment with biologics but instead should be given before starting therapy when possible and avoided for at least 3 months after immunosuppressants are discontinued.[6] This is because of the inability of the immunocompromised patient to mount an appropriate immune response to the vaccine. Live vaccines can be given to patients on methotrexate (the doses used in RA typically do not produce enough immunosuppression to cause concern), leflunomide, sulfasalazine, and hydroxychloroquine. Inactivated vaccines can be administered while patients are on conventional DMARDs, TNF and non-TNF biologics, and JAK inhibitors; however, efficacy of the vaccine may be reduced if the patient is on methotrexate or biologic agents.[43]

Several influenza vaccines are available, including inactivated influenza vaccine (IIV), recombinant influenza vaccine (RIV), and the intranasal live-attenuated influenza vaccine (LAIV). Patients with RA should receive the influenza vaccine yearly before initiating and during therapy. The IIV and RIV can be administered to all patients on conventional DMARDs, TNF inhibitors, non-TNF biologics, and JAK inhibitors and who do not have other contraindications to the vaccine. The high-dose inactivated influenza vaccine that is licensed for individuals 65 years of age or older can be given to RA patients regardless of concomitant RA drug therapy.

The available hepatitis B vaccines—either a three-dose series over 6 months (Recombivax HB, Engerix-B), a newer recombinant product (Heplisav-B) that is given in two doses 1 month apart, or a three-dose series in combination with hepatitis A protection (Twinrix)—are licensed for use in adults. These can be given before initiating or while on therapy for RA, but patients on immunosuppressive agents may have a reduced response to the vaccine. The series can be completed as directed in product labeling without regard for RA therapy. The Centers for Disease Control and Prevention (CDC) immunization schedule states that Heplisav-B can be used as a substitute for a dose of a three-dose series hepatitis B vaccine; however, two doses of Heplisav-B still need to be given at least 4 weeks between doses in order for the series to be complete.

Tetanus, diphtheria, acellular pertussis (Tdap) is an inactivated vaccine that should be given to adults who have not received a dose of Tdap as an adult or child. A dose of Td or Tdap is then recommended every 10 years.

The two inactivated pneumococcal vaccines, the pneumococcal polysaccharide vaccine (PPSV, Pneumovax 23) and the pneumococcal conjugated vaccine (PCV, Prevnar 13), should be administered to patients with acquired immunodeficiencies, including patients with RA who are receiving biologic therapy. PCV13 is administered to such patients who are 19 to 64 years of age followed by PPSV23 at least a year later. Another dose of PPSV23 should be given 5 years later. At age 65 or older, an additional dose of PPSV23 should be given at least 5 years after the most recent dose of PPSV23.[94,95]

The Advisory Committee on Immunization Practices (ACIP) no longer recommends routine PCV13 use for all adults >65 years old. Instead, shared clinical decision making for PCV13 use is recommended for adults age 65 years and older who do not have an immunocompromising condition. Due to the nature of RA and its immunocompromising therapies, the updated recommendation does not change immunization practices with respect to this health condition.[96]

A recombinant, adjuvant zoster vaccine to prevent herpes zoster was approved in 2017 (Shingrix) and is recommended for adults aged 50 years and older. It is administered as two doses at 0 and 2 to 6 months. The safety of this vaccine in patients with certain comorbid conditions, including RA, still needs to be determined.[97,98] An older zoster vaccine, Zostavax, is a live vaccine that is contraindicated in patients with RA who are on immunosuppressive therapies; Shingrix is now the preferred vaccine over Zostavax, according to the CDC.[9]

EVALUATION OF THERAPEUTIC OUTCOMES

9 An assessment of disease activity should be conducted at baseline and at each follow-up visit for patients with RA to evaluate disease control and therapeutic response. The evaluation of therapeutic outcomes should be based largely on the patient's subjective improvement of RA symptoms with respect to joint pain, swelling and tenderness, morning stiffness, and fatigue, as well as on a patient's ability to perform activities of daily living. A physical examination should also be conducted at each visit to evaluate the number of swollen and/or tender joints to obtain objective data. This can also help clinicians evaluate loss of joint mobility and deformity. As detailed in Table 111-3, several useful tools can guide clinicians in the objective measurement of disease activity.

Laboratory monitoring of acute phase reactants such as CRP and ESR can be useful in assessing inflammation. Plain radiographs of the hands, wrists, and forefeet should be obtained at baseline as well as every 2 years in patients with low disease activity or in remission. Little-to-no evidence of RA disease progression should be evident on this imaging if drug therapy is effective. Imaging may be needed more frequently in patients with moderate or high disease activity. If patients have radiographic changes on imaging that indicate RA disease progression—such as periarticular osteopenia, bone erosions, or joint space narrowing—drug therapy should be modified.[98]

It is also important to monitor and assess for adverse effects of the medications used to treat RA as detailed in Table 111-4.

TABLE 111-3 Assessment Tools to Measure Rheumatoid Arthritis Disease Activity

Assessment Tool	Scale	High Disease Activity	Moderate Disease Activity	Low Disease Activity	Remission
Clinical Disease Activity Index (CDAI)	0 to 76	>22	>10 to 22	>2.8 to 10	≤2.8
Disease Activity Score (DAS28)	0 to 9.4	>5.1	≥3.2 to ≤5.1	≥2.6 to <3.2	<2.6
Patient Activity Scale (PAS) or PASII	0 to 10	≥8.0	>3.7 to <8.0	>2.5 to 3.7	0 to 2.5
Routine Assessment of Patient Index Data 3 (RAPID-3)	0 to 10	>4.0 to 10	>2 to 4	>1.0 to 2.0	0 to 1.0
Simplified Disease Activity Index (SDAI)	0 to 86	>26	>11 to ≤26	>3.3 to ≤11.0	≤3.3

TABLE 111-4 Adverse Drug Reactions and Monitoring Recommended for Disease-Modifying Antirheumatic Drugs

Drugs	Adverse Drug Reactions	Initial Monitoring	Maintenance Monitoring
NSAIDs	GI ulceration, bleeding, and perforation, renal damage	SCr, CBC every 2-4 weeks after starting therapy	Same as initial plus stool guaiac every 6-12 months
Corticosteroids	Fluid retention, hyperglycemia, hypertension, behavioral and mood changes, increased appetite, weight gain, electrolyte imbalances, impaired healing, hirsutism, Cushing syndrome, HPA axis suppression, osteonecrosis of femoral and humeral heads, osteoporosis and fractures, myopathy, glaucoma, cataracts	Glucose, CBC periodically, blood pressure every 3-6 months	Same as initial
Hydroxychloroquine	Retinal damage, rash, diarrhea	Ophthalmologic exam (fundus examination plus visual fields and spectral-domain optical coherence tomography if maculopathy present) within 5 years of starting therapy	Ophthalmologic exam annually if risk factors for retinal damage present or annually beginning after 5 years of use if no risk factors
Methotrexate	Infection, hepatic fibrosis, cirrhosis, interstitial pneumonitis, stomatitis, rash, GI perforation, diarrhea, thrombocytopenia, leukopenia	SCr, CBC with differential, AST, ALT, hepatitis B and C screening, tuberculosis screening	SCr, CBC with differential, AST, ALT, every 2-4 weeks for 3 months after starting or following a dose increase, then every 8-12 weeks during 3-6 months of therapy, and every 12 weeks after 6 months of therapy, signs of infection
Leflunomide	Hepatitis, diarrhea/nausea, alopecia, elevated blood pressure	CBC with differential, SCr, ALT, AST, blood pressure	CBC with differential, SCr, ALT, AST every 2-4 weeks for 3 months after starting or following a dose increase, then every 8-12 weeks during 3-6 months of therapy, and every 12 weeks after 6 months of therapy; blood pressure periodically
Sulfasalazine	Rash, nausea, vomiting, diarrhea, photosensitivity, alopecia	CBC with differential, SCr, ALT, AST	CBC with differential, SCr, ALT, AST every 2-4 weeks for 3 months after starting or following a dose increase, then every 8-12 weeks during 3-6 months of therapy, and every 12 weeks after 6 months of therapy

(continued)

TABLE 111-4 Adverse Drug Reactions and Monitoring Recommended for Disease-Modifying Antirheumatic Drugs (*Continued*)

Drugs	Adverse Drug Reactions	Initial Monitoring	Maintenance Monitoring
Tocilizumab	Local injection-site reactions, infection, malignancy, GI perforation, neutropenia, thrombocytopenia	Tuberculosis screening, hepatitis B screening, CBC with differential, AST, ALT, FLP	AST, ALT, CBC with differential every 4-8 weeks after starting then every 3 months; FLP after 4-8 weeks of starting then every 6 months, signs/symptoms of infection and malignancy
Upadacitinib	Infection, malignancy, GI perforations, upper respiratory tract infections, neutropenia, lymphocytopenia, nausea, hepatotoxicity, CPK elevation, thrombosis, increased cholesterol	Tuberculosis screening, hepatitis screening, CBC with differential, LFTs, FLP	CBC with differential, FLP, LFTs, hepatitis screening periodically
Baricitinib	Infection, malignancy, upper respiratory tract infections, herpes zoster infection, hepatotoxicity, hematologic toxicities including anemia, gastrointestinal perforations, thrombosis, lymphocytopenia, neutropenia, increase in SCr and CPK	CBC with differential, LFTs, FLP, tuberculosis, and hepatitis screening	CBC with differential, LFTs, FLP periodically
Anakinra	Local injection-site reactions, infection, malignancy	CBC with differential, tuberculosis screening, SCr, hepatitis B screening	CBC with differential every 3 months up to 1 year, SCr periodically, signs/symptoms of infection and malignancy
Etanercept, adalimumab, golimumab, certolizumab	Local injection-site reactions, infection, malignancy	Tuberculosis screening, hepatitis B screening, CBC with differential	Periodic skin examination, signs/symptoms of infection and malignancy, CBC with differential periodically
Infliximab	Immune reactions, infection, malignancy	Tuberculosis screening, hepatitis B screening, CBC with differential, LFTs	CBC with differential, LFTs, signs/symptoms of infection and malignancy
Rituximab	Immune reactions, infection, malignancy	Tuberculosis screening, hepatitis B screening, CBC with differential	CBC with differential prior to each treatment course and at 2- to 4-month intervals, signs/symptoms of infection
Abatacept	Immune reactions, infection, malignancy	Tuberculosis screening, hepatitis B screening	Signs/symptoms of infection and malignancy
Tofacitinib	Infection, malignancy, GI perforations, upper respiratory tract infections, headache, diarrhea, nasopharyngitis	Tuberculosis screening, hepatitis B screening, CBC with differential, Hgb, LFTs, FLP, HR, and blood pressure	CBC with differential and Hgb after 4-8 weeks and every 3 months, FLP after 4-8 weeks and periodically, LFTs periodically, periodic skin examinations, HR and blood pressure, signs/symptoms of infection and malignancy
Sarilumab	Local injection-site reactions, infection, malignancy	Tuberculosis screening, hepatitis B screening, CBC with differential, LFTs, lipid panel	CBC with differential and LFTs 4-8 weeks after starting and then every 3 months, FLP 4-8 weeks after starting and every 6 months during therapy, signs/symptoms of infection and malignancy

ALT, alanine transaminase; AST, aspartate transaminase; CBC, complete blood count; CPK, creatine phosphokinase; FLP, fasting lipid panel; GI, gastrointestinal; HPA, hypothalamic–pituitary–adrenal; LFTs, liver function tests; SCr, serum creatinine.

CONCLUSION

Rheumatoid arthritis is an autoimmune condition that impacts approximately 1% of the population. It is a systemic, progressive disease that can lead to disability and decreased quality of life. The course of therapy is variable but includes both nonpharmacologic and pharmacologic therapies. A patient-centered, comprehensive treatment plan should be initiated as soon as a diagnosis is established to target disease remission or low disease activity. Though a treatment plan should be created with a trained rheumatologist, other clinicians should be utilized for their expertise, such as social work, mental health, and physical/occupational therapy. Chosen pharmacologic treatment is dependent on level of disease activity, past medication trials, comorbidities, and patient-preference. Though the etiology of RA is unclear, we can expect further research to be conducted to determine its cause to help design additional targeted therapies, including expansion of the role of biosimilars.

ABBREVIATIONS

ACIP	Advisory Committee on Immunization Practices
ACPA	anticitrullinated protein antibodies
ACR	American College of Rheumatology
ALC	absolute lymphocyte count
ALT	alanine aminotransferase
AST	aspartate aminotransferase
ANA	antinuclear antibody
ANC	absolute neutrophil count
ANTI-CCP	anti-citrullinated C protein
BID	twice daily
CBC	complete blood count
CPK	creatine phosphokinase
CRP	C-reactive protein
CT	computed tomography
CYP450	cytochrome P450

DEXA	dual-energy x-ray absorptiometry
DMARDs	disease-modifying antirheumatic drugs
eGFR	estimated glomerular filtration rate
ESR	erythrocyte sedimentation rate
EULAR	European League Against Rheumatism
EX	extended release
FDA	Food and Drug Administration
GI	gastrointestinal
HLA	human leukocyte antigen
Hgb	hemoglobin
HPA	hypothalamic–pituitary–adrenal
IgG	immunoglobulin G
IL	interleukin
IM	intramuscular
IR	immediate release
IV	intravenous
ILD	interstitial lung disease
JAK	Janus kinase
LFTs	liver function tests (includes AST/ALT, T bilirubin, Alkaline Phosphatase)
LGL	large granular lymphocyte leukemia
MO	month
MTX	methotrexate
NSAIDs	nonsteroidal anti-inflammatory drugs
NYHA	New York Heart Association
PBM	pharmacy benefit managers
RA	rheumatoid arthritis
RANKL	receptor activator of NFkB ligand
RF	rheumatoid factor
SCr	serum creatinine
SubQ	subcutaneous
TNF	tumor necrosis factor
ULN	upper limit of normal
US	ultrasound

REFERENCES

1. Cross M, Smith E, Hoy D, et al. The global burden of rheumatoid arthritis: Estimates from the global burden of disease 2010 study. *Ann Rheum Dis* 2014;73(7):1316–1322.
2. Sullivan P, Ghushchyan V, Huang X, Globe D. Influence of rheumatoid arthritis on employment, function, and productivity in a nationally representative sample in the United States. *J Rheumatol.* 2010;37(3):544–549.
3. Silman AJ, Hochberg MC. Descriptive epidemiology of rheumatoid arthritis. In: Hochberg MC, Silman AJ, Smolen JS, Weinblatt ME, Weisman MH, eds. *Rheumatoid Arthritis.* Philadelphia, PA: Mosby Elsevier; 2009;15–22.
4. Martikainen JA, Kautiainen H, Rantalaiho V, Puolakka K. Long-term work productivity costs due to absenteeism and permanent work disability in patients with early rheumatoid arthritis: A Nationwide Register Study of 7831 Patients. *J Rheumatol.* 2016;34(26):2101–2015.
5. Gibofsky A. Overview of epidemiology, pathophysiology, and diagnosis of rheumatoid arthritis. *Am J Manag Care.* 2012;18:S295–S302.
6. Myasoedova E, Davis J III, Crowson C, Gabriel S. Epidemiology of rheumatoid arthritis: Rheumatoid arthritis and mortality. *Curr Rheumatol Rep.* 2010;12:379–385.
7. Carmona L, Cross M, Williams B, et al. Rheumatoid arthritis. *Best Pract Res Clin Rheumatol.* 2010;24:733–745.
8. Silman AJ, Pearson JE. Epidemiology and genetics of rheumatoid arthritis. *Arthritis Res Ther.* 2002;4(3):S265.
9. Silman AJ, MacGregor AJ, Thomson W, et al. Twin concordance rates for rheumatoid arthritis: Results from a nationwide study. *Br J Rheumatol.* 1993;32(10):903.
10. Hemminki K, Li X, Sundquist J, Sundquist K. Familial associations of rheumatoid arthritis with autoimmune diseases and related conditions. *Arthritis Rheum.* 2009;60(3):661.
11. Bridges SL Jr, White DW, Worthing AB, et al. The science behind biosimilars: Entering a new era of biologic therapy. *Arthritis Rheumatol.* 2018;70(3):334–344.
12. Pedersen M, Jacobsen S, Garred P, et al. Strong combined gene-environment effects in anti-cyclic citrullinated peptide-positive rheumatoid arthritis: A nationwide case-control study in Denmark. *Arthritis Rheum.* 2007;56(5):1446.
13. Tedeschi SK, Frits M, Cui J, et al. Diet and rheumatoid arthritis symptoms: Survey results from a rheumatoid arthritis registry. *Arthritis Care Res (Hoboken).* 2017;69(12):1920–1925.
14. Khuder SA, Peshimam AZ, Agraharam S. Environmental risk factors for rheumatoid arthritis. *Rev Environ Health.* 2002;17(4):307.
15. Wegner N, Lundberg K, Kinloch A, et al. Autoimmunity to specific citrullinated proteins gives the first clues to the etiology of rheumatoid arthritis. *Immunol Rev.* 2010;233(1):34.
16. Jiang H, Chess L. Regulation of immune response by T cells. *N Engl J Med.* 2006;354:1166–1176.
17. Youinou P, Taher TE, Pers J-O, et al. B lymphocyte cytokines and rheumatoid autoimmune disease. *Arthritis Rheum.* 2009;60:1873–1880.
18. Uesugi M, Hayashi T, Jasin HE. Covalent cross-linking of immune complexes by oxygen radicals and nitrite. *J Immunol.* 1998;161:1422.
19. Firestein GS, Echeverri F, Yeo M, et al. Somatic mutations in the p53 tumor suppressor gene in rheumatoid arthritis synovium. *Proc Natl Acad Sci USA.* 1997;94:10895.
20. Huizinga TW, Amos CI, van der Helm-van Mil AH, et al. Refining the complex rheumatoid arthritis phenotype based on specificity of the HLA-DRB1 shared epitope for antibodies to citrullinated proteins. *Arthritis Rheum.* 2005;52:3433.
21. John Hopkins Arthritis Center. RA Pathophysiology. Available at: https://www.hopkinsarthritis.org/arthritis-info/rheumatoid-arthritis/ra-pathophysiology-2/. Last accessed, September 14, 2018.
22. Deane KD, O'Donnell CI, Hueber W, et al. The number of elevated cytokines and chemokines in preclinical seropositive rheumatoid arthritis predicts time to diagnosis in an age-dependent manner. *Arthritis Rheum.* 2010;62:3161.
23. Hill JA, Southwood S, Sette A, et al. Cutting edge: The conversion of arginine to citrulline allows for a high-affinity peptide interaction with the rheumatoid arthritis-associated HLA-DRB1*0401 MHC class II molecule. *J Immunol.* 2003;171:538.
24. Hitchon CA, El-Gabalawy HS. The synovium in rheumatoid arthritis. *Open Rheumatol J.* 2011;5(1:M3):107–114.
25. Brennan FM, McInnes IB. Evidence that cytokines play a role in rheumatoid arthritis. *J Clin Invest.* 2008;118:3537–3545.
26. Choy EH, Panayi GS. Cytokine pathways and joint inflammation in rheumatoid arthritis. *N Engl J Med.* 2001;344(12):907–916.
27. Catrina AI, af Klint E, Ernestam S, et al. Anti-tumor necrosis factor therapy increases synovial osteoprotegerin expression in rheumatoid arthritis. *Arthritis Rheum.* 2006;54:76.
28. Gravallese EM. Bone destruction in arthritis. *Ann Rheum Dis.* 2002;61(S2):ii84–ii86.
29. Jasin HE, Taurog JD. Mechanisms of disruption of the articular cartilage surface in inflammation. Neutrophil elastase increases availability of collagen type II epitopes for binding with antibody on the surface of articular cartilage. *J Clin Invest.* 1991;87:1531.
30. Turesson C, Jacobsson LT. Epidemiology of extra-articular manifestations in rheumatoid arthritis. *Scand J Rheumatol.* 2004;33(2):65.
31. Patatanian E, Thompson DF. A review of methotrexate-induced accelerated nodulosis. *Pharmacotherapy.* 2002;22(9):1157.
32. Gochuico BR, Avila NA, Chow CK, et al. Progressive preclinical interstitial lung disease in rheumatoid arthritis. *Arch Intern Med.* 2008;168(2):159.
33. Lake F, Proudman S. Rheumatoid arthritis and lung disease: From mechanisms to a practical approach. *Semin Respir Crit Care Med.* 2014;35(2):222–238.
34. Balbir-Gurman A, Yigla M, Nahir AM, Braun-Moscovici Y. Rheumatoid pleural effusion. *Semin Arthritis Rheum.* 2006;35(6):368.
35. Bartels C, Bell C, Rosenthal A, Shinki K, Bridges A. Decline in rheumatoid vasculitis prevalence among US veterans: A retrospective cross-sectional study. *Arthritis Rheum.* 2009;60(9):2553.
36. Aviña-Zubieta JA, Choi HK, Sadatsafavi M, Etminan M, Esdaile JM, Lacaille D. Risk of cardiovascular mortality in patients with rheumatoid arthritis: A meta-analysis of observational studies. *Arthritis Rheum.* 2008;59(12):1690.
37. Wallberg-Jonsson S, Johansson H, Ohman ML, Rantapaa-Dahlqvist S. Extent of inflammation predicts cardiovascular disease and overall mortality in seropositive rheumatoid arthritis. A retrospective cohort study from disease onset. *J Rheumatol.* 1999;26(12):2562–2571.

38. Lamy T, Loughran TP Jr. How I treat LGL leukemia. *Blood.* 2011;117(10):2764.
39. Hauser B, Riches PL, Wilson JF, Horne AE, Ralston SH. Prevalence and clinical prediction of osteoporosis in a contemporary cohort of patients with rheumatoid arthritis. *Rheumatology (Oxford).* 2014;53(10):1759.
40. Whiting PF, Smidt N, Sterne JA, et al. Systematic review: Accuracy of anti-citrullinated Peptide antibodies for diagnosing rheumatoid arthritis. *Ann Intern Med.* 2010;152(7):456.
41. Dougados M. Synovial fluid cell analysis. *Baillieres Clin Rheumatol.* 1996;10(3):519.
42. Aletaha D, Neogi T, Silman AJ, et al. Arthritis 2010 Rheumatoid arthritis classification criteria: An American College of Rheumatology/European League Against Rheumatism collaborative initiative. *Rheum.* 2010;62(9):2569.
43. Solomon DH, Bitton A, Katz JN, et al. Treat to Target in rheumatoid arthritis: Fact, fiction or hypothesis? *Arthritis Rheumatol.* 2014;66(4):775–782.
44. Demoruelle MK, Deane KD. Treatment strategies in early rheumatoid arthritis and prevention of rheumatoid Arthritis. *Curr Rheumatol Rep.* 2012;14(5):472–480.
45. Anderson JJ, Wells G, Verhoeven AC, et al. Factors predicting response to treatment in rheumatoid arthritis: The importance of disease duration. *Arthritis Rheum.* 2000;43:22–29.
46. Vliet Vlieland TP, Van Den Ende CH. Nonpharmacological treatment of rheumatoid arthritis. *Curr Opin Rheumatol.* 2011; 23(3):259–264.
47. Sturgeon JA, Finan PH, Zautra AJ. Affective disturbance in rheumatoid arthritis: Psychological and disease-related pathways. *Nat Rev Rheumatol.* 2016;12(9):532.
48. Smolen JS, Landewé RBM, Bijlsma JWJ, et al. EULAR recommendations for the management of rheumatoid arthritis with synthetic and biological disease-modifying antirheumatic drugs: 2019 update. *Ann Rheum Dis.* 2020;79(6):685–699. 31969328.
49. Weinblatt ME. Efficacy of methotrexate in rheumatoid arthritis. *Br J Rheumatol.* 1995;34(Suppl 2):43–48.
50. Methotrexate [package insert]. Huntsville, AL: DAVA Pharmaceuticals, Inc; https://www.accessdata.fda.gov/drugsatfda_docs/label/2016/008085s066lbl.pdf.
51. Bianchi G, Caporali R, Todoerti M, et al. Methotrexate and rheumatoid arthritis: Current evidence regarding subcutaneous versus oral routes of administration. *Adv Ther.* 2016;33:369–378.
52. Kremer JM, Alarcon GS, Lightfoot RW Jr, et al. Methotrexate for rheumatoid arthritis. Suggested guidelines for monitoring liver toxicity. American College of Rheumatology. *Arthritis Rheum.* 1994;37(3):316–328.
53. Arava [package insert]. Bridgewater, NJ: Sanofi-Aventis U.S. LLC; 2011, https://www.accessdata.fda.gov/drugsatfda_docs/label/2011/020905s022lbl.pdf.
54. Azulfidine [package insert]. New York, NY: Pfizer; 2012, https://www.accessdata.fda.gov/drugsatfda_docs/label/2012/007073s125lbl.pdf.
55. Fox RI. Mechanism of action of hydroxychloroquine as an antirheumatic drug. *Semin Arthritis Rhem.* 1993;23(2 Suppl 1):82–91.
56. Tett SE, Day RO, Cutler DJ. Concentration-effect relationship of hydroxychloroquine in rheumatoid arthritis: A cross sectional study. *J Rheumatol.* 1993;20(11):1874–1879.
57. Marmor MF, Kellner U, Lai TY, et al. American Academy of Ophthalmology. Recommendations on screening for chloroquine and hydroxychloroquine retinopathy (2016 revision). *Ophthalmology.* 2016;123(6):1386–1394.
58. Plaquenil [package insert]. St. Michael, Barbados: Concordia Pharmaceuticals; January 2017. Available at: https://www.accessdata.fda.gov/drugsatfda_docs/label/2017/009768s037s045s047lbl.pdf.
59. Humira [package insert]. North Chicago, IL: Abbvie: August 2018. Available at: https://www.rxabbvie.com/pdf/humira.pdf.
60. Cimzia [package insert]. Smyrna, GA: UCB; May 2018, https://www.cimzia.com/sites/default/files/docs/CIMZIA_full_prescribing_information.pdf.
61. Enbrel [package insert]. Thousand Oaks, CA: Immunex Corporation; December 2012. Available at: https://www.accessdata.fda.gov/drugsatfda_docs/label/2012/103795s5503lbl.pdf.
62. Simponi [package insert]. Horsham, PA: Janssen Biotech; August 2011, https://www.accessdata.fda.gov/drugsatfda_docs/label/2011/125289s0064lbl.pdf.
63. Remicade [package insert]. Horsham, PA: Janssen Biotech; November 2013. Available at: https://www.accessdata.fda.gov/drugsatfda_docs/label/2013/103772s5359lbl.pdf.
64. Orencia [package insert]. Princeton, NJ: Bristol-Meyers Squibb; March 2017. Available at: https://packageinserts.bms.com/pi/pi_orencia.pdf.
65. Weinblatt ME, Schiff M, Valente R, et al. Head-to-head comparison of subcutaneous abatacept versus adalimumab for rheumatoid arthritis: Findings of a phase IIIb, multinational, prospective, randomized study. *Arthritis Rheum.* 2013;65(1):28–38.
66. Actemra [package insert]. South San Francisco, CA: Genentech; May 2018. Available at: https://www.gene.com/download/pdf/actemra_prescribing.pdf.
67. Gabay C, Emery P, van Vollenhoven R, et al. Tocilizumab monotherapy versus adalimumab monotherapy for treatment of rheumatoid arthritis (ADACTA): A randomised, double-blind, controlled phase 4 trial. *Lancet.* 2013;381(9877):1541–1550.
68. Rituxan [package insert]. South San Francisco, CA: Genentech; June 2018. Available at: https://www.gene.com/download/pdf/rituxan_prescribing.pdf.
69. Chatzidionysiou K, van Vollenhoven RF. Rituximab versus anti-TNF in patients who previously failed one TNF inhibitor in an observational cohort. *Stand J Rheumatol.* 2013;42(3):190–195.
70. Kineret [package insert]. Stockholm, Sweden: Swedish Orphan Biovitrum AB; December 2012. Available at: https://www.accessdata.fda.gov/drugsatfda_docs/label/2012/103950s5136lbl.pdf.
71. Kevzara [package insert]. Bridgewater, NJ: Sanofi-Aventis U.S.; May 2017. Available at: https://www.accessdata.fda.gov/drugsatfda_docs/label/2017/761037s000lbl.pdf.
72. Genovese MC, Fleischmann R, Kivitz AJ, et al. Sarilumab plus methotrexate in patients with active rheumatoid arthritis and inadequate response to methotrexate: Results of a phase III study. *Arthritis Rheumatol.* 2015;67(6):1424–1437.
73. Strand V, Really M, Chen CI, et al. Sarilumab improves patient-reported outcomes in rheumatoid arthritis patients with inadequate response/intolerance to tumor necrosis factor inhibitors. *RMD Open.* 2017;3:e000416.
74. Xeljanz [package insert]. New York, NY: Pfizer; May 2018. Available at: http://labeling.pfizer.com/ShowLabeling.aspx?id=959.
75. Dowty ME, Lin TH, Jesson MI, et al. Janus kinase inhibitors for the treatment of rheumatoid arthritis demonstrate similar profiles of in vitro cytokine receptor inhibition. *Pharmacol Res Perspect.* 2019;7(6):e00537–e00537.
76. Olumiant [package insert]. Indianapolis, IN: Eli Lilly; May 2018. Available at: https://www.accessdata.fda.gov/drugsatfda_docs/label/2018/207924s000lbl.pdf.
77. Rinvoq [package insert]. North Chicago, IL: AbbVie Inc; August 2019. Available at: https://www.accessdata.fda.gov/drugsatfda_docs/label/2019/211675s000lbl.pdf.
78. van Vollenhoven RF, Fleischmann R, Cohen S, et al. Tofacitinib or adalimumab versus placebo in rheumatoid arthritis. *N Engl J Med.* 2012;367(6):508–519.
79. Felson DT, LaValley MP. The ACR20 and defining a threshold for response in rheumatic disease: Too much of a good thing. *Arthritis Res Ther.* 2017;16(1):101.
80. Xeljanz XR (tofacitinib): Drug safety communication—due to an increased risk of blood clots and death with higher dose. Available at: https://www.fda.gov/safety/medical-product-safety-information/xeljanz-xeljanz-xr-tofacitinib-drug-safety-communication-due-increased-risk-blood-clots-and-death.
81. Fleischmann R, Pangan AL, Song IH, et al. Upadacitinib versus placebo or adalimumab in patients with rheumatoid arthritis and an inadequate response to methotrexate: Results of a Phase III, double-blind, randomized controlled trial. *Arthritis Rheumatol.* 2019;71(11):1788–1800.
82. Dougados M, van der Heijde D, Chen YC, et al. Baricitinib in patients with inadequate response or intolerance to conventional synthetic DMARDs: Results from the RA-BUILD study. *Ann Rheum Dis.* 2017;76(1):88–95.
83. Kineret [package insert]. Stockholm, Sweden: Swedish Orphan Biovitrum AB; December 2012. Available at: https://www.accessdata.fda.gov/drugsatfda_docs/label/2012/103950s5136lbl.pdf.
84. Kavanaugh A, Wells AF. Benefits and risks of low-dose glucocorticoid treatment in the patient with rheumatoid arthritis. *Rheumatology (Oxford).* 2014;53(10):1742–1751.
85. Rayos [package insert]. Deerfield, IL: Horizon Pharma USA; July 2012. Available at: https://www.accessdata.fda.gov/drugsatfda_docs/label/2012/202020s000lbl.pdf.
86. Da Silva JAP, Jacobs JWG, Kirwan JR, et al. Safety of low dose glucocorticoid treatment in rheumatoid arthritis: Published evidence and prospective trial date. *Ann Rheum Dis.* 2006;65(3):285–293.
87. Krause ML, Makes A. Management of rheumatoid arthritis during pregnancy: Challenges and solutions. *Open Access Rheumatol.* 2016;8:23–26.

88. Skorpen CG, Hoeltzenbein M, Tincani A, et al. The EULAR points to consider for use of antirheumatic drugs before pregnancy, and during pregnancy and lactation. *Ann Rheum Dis.* 2016;75:795–810.
89. Agca R, Heslinga SC, Rollefstad S, et al. EULAR recommendations for cardiovascular disease risk management in patients with rheumatoid arthritis and other forms of inflammatory joint disorders: 2015/2016 Update. *Ann Rheum Dis.* 2016;0:1–12.
90. Jeremiah MP, Unwin BK, Greenawald MH, et al. Diagnosis and management of osteoporosis. *Am Fam Physician.* 2015;92(4):261–268.
91. Buckley L, Guyana G, Fink HA, et al. 2017 American College of Rheumatology guideline for the prevention and treatment of glucocorticoid-induced osteoporosis. *Arthritis Rheumatol.* 2017;69(8):1521–1537.
92. Centers for Disease Control and Prevention. Recommended immunization schedule for adults aged 19 years or older, United States, 2018. Available at: https://www.cdc.gov/vaccines/schedules/downloads/adult/adult-combined-schedule.pdf. Last assessed, September 10, 2018.
93. Centers for Disease Control and Prevention. Pneumococcal vaccine timing for adults. Available at: https://www.cdc.gov/vaccines/vpd/pneumo/downloads/pneumo-vaccine-timing.pdf. Last assessed, September 10, 2018.
94. Matanock A, Lee G, Gierke R, et al. Use of 13-valent pneumococcal conjugate vaccine and 23-valent pneumococcal polysaccharide vaccine among adults aged ≥65 years: Updated recommendations of the Advisory Committee on Immunization Practices. *MMWR Morb Mortal Wkly Rep.* 2019;68(46):1069–1075.
95. Shingrix [package insert]. Research Triangle Park, NC: GlaxoSmithKline Biologicals; October 2017. Available at: https://gsksource.com/pharma/content/dam/GlaxoSmithKline/US/en/Prescribing_Information/Shingrix/pdf/SHINGRIX.PDF.
96. Khanna D, Ranganath VK, Fitzgerald J, et al. Increased radiographic damage scores at the onset of seropositive rheumatoid arthritis in older patients are associated with osteoarthritis of the hands, but not with more rapid progression of damage. *Arthritis Rheum.* 2005;52(8):2284.
97. Fraenkel L, Bathon JM, England BR, et al. 2021 American College of Rheumatology guideline for the treatment of rheumatoid arthritis. *Arthritis Care Res (Hoboken).* 2021;73(7):924–939.
98. Smolen JS, Landewé RBM, Bijlsma JWJ, et al. EULAR recommendations for the management of rheumatoid arthritis with synthetic and biological disease-modifying antirheumatic drugs: 2019 update. *Ann Rheum Dis.* 2020;79(6):685–699.

112

Osteoporosis

Mary Beth O'Connell, Jill S. Borchert, Erin M. Slazak, and Joseph P. Fava

KEY CONCEPTS

1. Osteoporosis is a public health epidemic that affects all ages, genders, races, and ethnicities. Lifestyle behaviors, diseases, and medications should be reviewed to identify the risk factors for developing osteoporosis and osteoporotic fractures. Healthcare professionals should identify and resolve reversible risks. Secondary causes of bone loss should be explored, especially for patients with early-onset or severe osteoporosis.
2. Bone physiology and pathophysiology are complex involving coupled bone resorption and formation in bone remodeling processes. These processes result from many different cell lines, transmitters, pathways, and biofeedback systems. As these processes become more delineated, additional targets are identified for medications.
3. All patients taking medications known to increase bone loss, falls, and fractures should practice a bone-healthy lifestyle, be evaluated for a switch to a safer alternative medication, and/or be considered for osteoporosis therapy. The most common causes of medication-induced osteoporosis are long-term oral glucocorticoids and certain chemotherapeutic agents.
4. Ten-year probabilities for a major osteoporotic and hip fracture can be estimated for women (postmenopausal to 90 years old) and men (50-90 years old) with the fracture risk assessment tool (FRAX) tool. This tool is a questionnaire that can be used in any setting, including pharmacies, health fairs, and clinics. Central bone mass densitometry can determine bone mass, predict fracture risk, and influence patient and provider treatment decisions.
5. Throughout life, everyone should practice a bone-healthy lifestyle, which emphasizes regular exercise, nutritious diet, tobacco avoidance, minimal alcohol use, and fall prevention to prevent and treat osteoporosis.
6. Treatment should be considered for postmenopausal women and men older than 50 years who have a low-trauma hip or vertebral fracture, T-score of −2.5 or less at the femoral neck, total hip, or spine, or low bone mass (T-score between −1.0 and −2.5) and a FRAX 10-year probability of major osteoporotic fracture of 20% or more or hip fracture of 3% or more. Patients with secondary causes might receive therapy at younger ages or higher T-scores.
7. The recommended dietary calcium intake for American adults is 1,000 to 1,200 mg of elemental calcium daily with diet as the preferred source. Supplements are added when diet is insufficient.
8. The recommended daily dietary vitamin D intake for American adults is 600 units and for older adults 800 units. Some organizations and guidelines recommend higher doses of at least 800 to 1,000 units daily. Vitamin D intake is achieved through sun exposure, fortified foods, and supplements. Vitamin D insufficiency and deficiency, defined as 25-hydroxyvitamin D (25[OH] vitamin D) concentrations of less than 30 ng/mL (mcg/L; 75 nmol/L) and less than 20 ng/mL (mcg/L; 50 nmol/L) respectively, are common in Americans. Higher vitamin D daily intakes and/or replenishment doses are then required.
9. Alendronate, risedronate, zoledronic acid, and denosumab decrease vertebral, hip, and nonvertebral fractures and are first-line osteoporosis treatments for those with high fracture risk. Therapy continues for about 5 years in mild osteoporosis and 5 to 10 years in moderate-to-severe osteoporosis. Other antiresorptive (ibandronate, raloxifene), anabolic (abaloparatide, teriparatide), and combination anabolic and antiresorptive (romosozumab) medications are alternatives. These medications decrease osteoporotic fracture risk but not hip fractures. In patients with very high fracture risk, sequential therapy with abaloparatide, romosozumab, or teriparatide followed by an antiresorptive agent is recommended.
10. Adherence to osteoporosis medications is suboptimal. Poor adherence is associated with less fracture prevention. Healthcare professionals should assess medication administration technique and adherence at each visit, provide education, and resolve medication-related problems.

BEYOND THE BOOK

Create a team of three classmates. Each team member selects one of the below patients to workup. This activity is useful to enhance your understanding of the COLLECT, ASSESS, and PLAN steps in the patient care process, the osteoporosis treatment algorithm, and individualization of patient care.

In your patient workup:

- Identify osteoporosis risks and secondary causes.
- Calculate a FRAX score (https://www.sheffield.ac.uk/FRAX/).

- Estimate calcium intake (https://www.osteoporosis.foundation/educational-hub/topic/calcium-calculator).
- Determine the calcium and vitamin D Institute of Medicine recommended daily intakes and deficits.
- Develop a prevention or treatment plan.
- Present your patient's risk factors, assessments, and treatment plan to each other.
- Compare and contrast these three women's cases and treatment plans.

Patient 1: A 57-year-old White, nonsmoking woman living in the United States. Patient's weight is 77 kg and height is 5 ft 6 in (168 cm). She has had no previous fractures and has no family history of fracture. Her T-scores are femoral neck −2.2 and spine −2.0. She has hypertension, hyperlipidemia, and GERD. The patient's current medications are omeprazole (Prilosec), atorvastatin (Lipitor), and amlodipine (Norvasc). The patient reports no vitamins or supplements. The patient drinks 1 glass of milk daily and eats 1 serving of yogurt daily. She does not drink alcohol.

Patient 2: A 67-year-old Hispanic woman living in the United States. Patient's weight is 77 kg and height is 5 ft 6 in (168 cm). She has had no previous fractures but her mother had a hip fracture. Her T-scores are femoral neck −2.4 and spine −2.0. She has hypertension, diabetes type 2, and hyperlipidemia. The patient's current medications are canagliflozin (Invokana), atorvastatin (Lipitor), and enalapril (Vasotec). The patient reports taking Centrum(R) Silver(R) Women's 50+ every day. Social history: the patient drinks 1 glass of milk daily and eats 1 serving of yogurt daily. She smokes tobacco products but does not drink alcohol.

Patient 3: A 77-year-old Asian woman living in the United States. Patient's weight is 77 kg and height is 5 ft 6 in (168 cm). She has had no previous fractures and no family history of fracture. Her T-scores are femoral neck −2.6 and spine −2.9. She has diabetes type 2, rheumatoid arthritis, hypertension, and lactose intolerance. The patient's current medications are metformin (Glucophage), lisinopril (Prinivil), adalimumab (Humira), and celecoxib (Celebrex) as needed. Prior to adalimumab, she had used prednisone 5 to 10 mg daily for over 5 years. The patient uses no vitamins or supplements. The patient drinks 1 glass of fortified soy milk daily and eats 1 serving of tofu daily. She does not drink alcohol or smoke.

INTRODUCTION

1 Osteoporosis is a bone disorder characterized by low bone density, impaired bone architecture, and compromised bone strength that predisposes a person to increased fracture risk. Osteoporosis is a major public health threat, with about 50% of people 50 years of age and older expected to develop this disease.[1] In the United States, 10.2 million Americans are estimated to have osteoporosis.[2] An additional 43.4 million Americans are estimated to have low bone density and are at risk for osteoporosis. Attention to bone health is required throughout life. Osteoporosis and osteoporotic fractures are multifactorial conditions, beginning at birth with genetics and continuing throughout life due to health behaviors that influence bone growth and maintenance, skeletal factors that lead to compromised bone strength, and nonskeletal factors that lead to falls (Fig. 112-1). Healthcare professionals should educate people about bone-healthy lifestyles and empower them to practice these health behaviors. Osteoporosis is underdiagnosed and undertreated. Bone health screenings, osteoporosis prevention programs, accurate diagnoses, and optimal medication management are needed to prevent and treat osteoporosis and prevent fractures.

Editors' note: In this and other chapters in Pharmacotherapy, *references to biologic sex (as assigned at birth) are used based on prior literature being discussed or anatomical or physiologic differences. We recognize that not all individuals later identify with their sex at birth, and to the degree possible when discussing therapeutics, we avoid use of references to gender. In this chapter on Osteoporosis, "men" and "women" are used in discussing prior studies, published guidelines, and other recommendations for diagnosis and treatment based on biological sex and do not necessarily reflect an individual's gender identity.*

EPIDEMIOLOGY

1 Low bone density, osteoporosis, and osteoporotic fractures are common in all people, with race and ethnic differences in osteoporosis detection, treatment and outcomes likely due to health disparities.[3,4] The prevalence of osteoporosis in women is 16.5%.[4] Low bone density was estimated to occur in 45% of non-Hispanic White, 43% of Mexican American, and 30% of non-Hispanic Black women aged 50 years and older.[3,5] Osteoporosis affects 13.4% of Mexican American, 10.2% of non-Hispanic White, and 4.9% of non-Hispanic Black women aged 50 years and older. Disease prevalence greatly increases with age; from 7% in women aged 50 to 59 years to 35% in women aged 80 years and older.[4] White American (17%) and Hispanic American (14%) women have the highest fragility fracture rate followed by Black American (6%) women.

Although more prevalent in women, men can also have low bone density and osteoporosis. Based on FRAX estimates, approximately 16% of men aged 50 years and older have low bone density rising to 46% in men aged 80 years and older.[6] Osteoporosis rises from 3% in men aged 50 to 59 years to 11% in men aged 80 years and older.[5] Osteoporosis prevalence also varies by race and ethnicity in men: 6% in Mexican American, 4% in non-Hispanic White American, and 1% in non-Hispanic Black American men.[3,5]

Fragility wrist and vertebral fractures are common throughout adulthood, with hip fractures more common in older adults. Although osteoporosis is common in adults with fractures, 12% of fracture patients have normal BMD and 52% have low bone density, supporting fractures can occur in all.[7]

Gender differences in osteoporotic fractures exist with 70% occurring in women and 30% in men.[2] As a woman ages, her risk of any fracture increases from 10% at age 50 years to 22% at 80 years old; with hip fractures increasing from 0.3% to 9% over the same time frame.[8] For men over the same time frame, fracture risk increases from 7% to 8% and hip fracture increases from 0.2% to 3%. Fracture outcomes are worse for people of color.[3]

Osteoporosis creates an economic health burden. In 2011, 1.7 million hospitalizations occurred for fragility fractures with 3 million osteoporotic fractures expected in 2025.[9] By 2025, osteoporosis treatment costs are estimated to be about $25 billion.[2] Because of associated morbidity, hip fracture is the most costly complication of osteoporosis, accounting for almost 72% of fracture costs. Osteoporosis costs exceed costs for breast cancer, heart attack, or stroke.

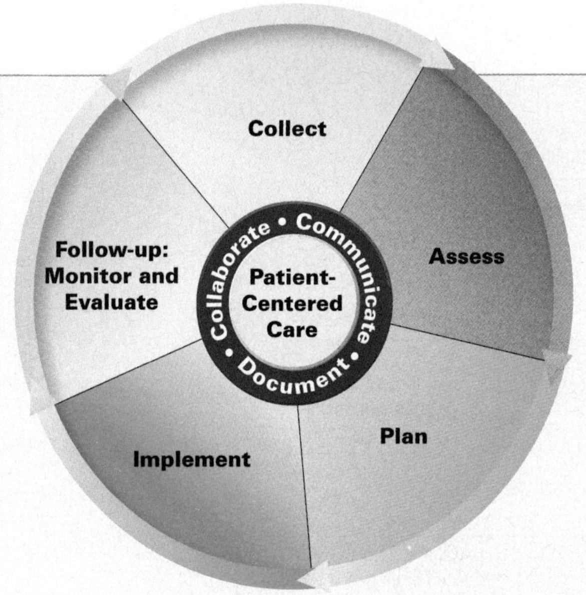

Patient Care Process for Osteoporosis

The image shows the five fundamental steps included in The Pharmacist's Care Process endorsed by the Joint Commission for Pharmacy Practitioners (2014). The tagline of this process reads collaborate, communicate, and document. The five fundamental steps listed here are collect, assess, plan, implement, and follow-up: monitor and evaluate. All these steps are listed in a circular block diagram.

Collect

- Patient characteristics (eg, age, sex, race, ethnicity, postmenopausal status)
- Medical history (personal and family; eg, maximum height, falls, fractures, dental issues, gastroesophageal reflux/heartburn, and for women age at menarche and menopause)
- Social history (eg, tobacco and alcohol use, physical activity, and dietary habits, including calcium-containing food and beverage intake)
- Current medications including calcium and vitamin D, dietary supplements, multivitamins, and herbal product use
- Past medications (eg, hormone therapy and medications causing osteoporosis; see Table 112-3)
- Objective data
  - Height, weight
  - Laboratory results (see Table 112-4) and secondary causes
  - Central dual-energy x-ray absorptiometry (DXA) at the spine and hip
  - Fracture evidence (eg, vertebral fracture assessment [VFA], radiographs)

Assess

- Adequacy of dietary calcium and calcium/vitamin D supplement intakes
- Bone mineral density (BMD): Categorize lowest T-score as normal, low bone mass, or osteoporosis
- FRAX 10-year risk of major osteoporotic fractures and hip fracture
- Laboratory data and presence of secondary causes (see Tables 112-2 and 112-3)
- Patient preferences including injectable medications and concern about adverse effects
- Potential barriers to adherence (eg, administration route, frequency, cost, health literacy)

Plan

- Medication regimen including specific agent, dose, route, frequency, and duration (see Fig. 112-3, Tables 112-7 and 112-8), and calcium and vitamin D supplements as necessary
- Monitoring parameters including efficacy (eg, BMD, fracture, 25(OH)-vitamin D concentration) and safety (eg, common and serious adverse effects, serum creatinine, calcium). Include frequency and timing of follow-up

Implement*

- Provide patient education regarding treatment plan (eg, purpose of treatment, dietary calcium sources, medication-specific administration/injection technique in patient's primary language, adverse effects) (see Tables 112-7 and 112-8)
- Consider risk communication tool to explain medication benefit and rare adverse effects
- Schedule laboratory tests as needed and DXA (generally 2-5 years after initiation)
- Schedule referrals when appropriate (eg, physical therapist for fall prevention, dietitian)
- For zoledronic acid, coordinate with infusion center for administration
- For nongeneric therapies, coordinate prior authorization process as necessary

Follow-up: Monitor and Evaluate*

- Patient adherence to treatment plan and administration instructions
- Presence of adverse effects (see Table 112-8)
- BMD, fractures, falls, and laboratory parameters
- Changes in habits (eg, dietary calcium, exercise, alcohol, and tobacco use)
- Re-evaluate duration of therapy after 1 year (romosozumab), 2 years (abaloparatide, teriparatide), 3 years (intravenous bisphosphonate), 5 years (oral bisphosphonate), or as suggested by response to therapy and adverse effects

Collaborate with patient, caregivers, and other healthcare professionals.

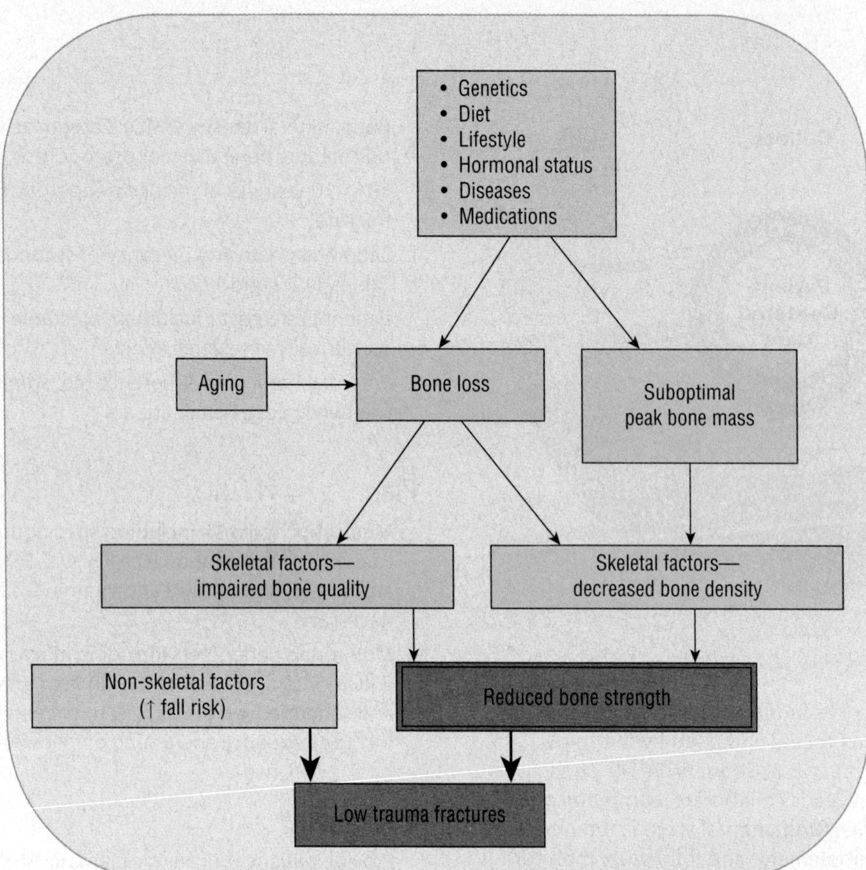

FIGURE 112-1 Etiology of osteoporosis and osteoporotic fractures.

ETIOLOGY

1 Figure 112-1 depicts a model describing osteoporosis and fracture etiology. The major risk factors (see Table 112-1) influencing bone loss are hormonal status, genetics, exercise, aging, nutrition, lifestyle, concomitant diseases, and medications. Nonhormonal risk factors are similar between women and men.

Low Bone Density

BMD is a major predictor of fracture risk. Every standard deviation decrease in BMD in women represents a 10% decrease in bone mass and a 1.6- to 2.6-fold increase in fracture risk.[2] In contrast, increasing peak bone mass in younger years by 10% was estimated to create 13 more years without a fracture in older women.[16] Low BMD can occur as a result of failure to reach a normal peak bone mass, bone loss, or both. Genetics accounts for 50% to 85% of peak bone mass variability.[4,14] Bone loss occurs when bone resorption exceeds bone formation, which also can result from high bone turnover when the number or depth of bone resorption sites greatly exceeds the rate and ability of osteoblasts to form new bone. Women and men begin to lose a small amount of bone mass starting in the third to fourth decade of life, about 0.5% to 1% per year.[12,14] During perimenopause and menopause, bone loss occurs predominantly due to increases in bone resorption. By age 80 years, 30% of a woman's bone mass is lost.[4] Older adults steadily lose bone mass as a consequence of an accelerated rate of bone remodeling combined with reduced bone formation.

Impaired Bone Quality

Bone strength is highly affected by the quality of the bone's composition and its structure and is a better predictor of fracture than BMD.[9] Changes in bone mass do not fully reflect changes in bone thinning and decreased connectivity, both related to strength. BMD explains only 70% of femur and 44% of spine bone strength. Even women with normal bone mass (3.4%) and low bone mass (5.3%) fracture, rates slightly lower than women with osteoporotic bone mass (6.8%). Accelerated bone turnover can increase the amount of immature bone that is not adequately mineralized. Sex differences exist with thinning of trabeculae, with aging in men causing less bone quality damage and impaired bone strength than in women.[12] With aging, fracture risk increases for a given T-score, partly related to bone quality changes; for example, at a T-score of −2.5, a 50-year-old postmenopausal woman has about a 4% probability of a hip fracture, whereas a 70-year-old woman has about a 9% probability.[23]

Falls

Each year, 15% to 45% of community-dwelling older adults and up to 60% of nursing home residents fall, with more women falling than men.[4,24] Hip fractures only occurred in 1% to 2% of falls; however, 90% of hip fractures resulted from a fall.[8,25] Falls lead to accidental death in about 70% of older adults.[24] Inpatient and outpatient fall care is expensive.[24] The risk factors for falls overlap with the risk factors for osteoporosis and osteoporotic fractures.[2,24] Environmental factors also contribute to falls (eg, electric cords, throw rugs, and poor lighting).

PATHOPHYSIOLOGY

Normal Bone Physiology

2 The skeleton has two types of bone. Cortical bone makes up the majority of the skeleton (80%) and is found mostly in the long bones

TABLE 112-1 Risk Factors for Osteoporosis and Osteoporotic Fractures

Low bone mineral density (BMD)[a]
Female sex[a]
Advanced age[a]
Race/ethnicity[a]
History of a previous fragility (low-trauma) fracture including radiographic vertebral fracture as an adult[a] (especially clinical vertebral fracture or hip fracture)
Osteoporotic fracture in a first-degree relative (especially parental hip fracture[a])
Low body weight or body mass index[a]
Premature menopause[b]
Secondary osteoporosis[a,b]
Rheumatoid arthritis[a]
Past or present systemic oral glucocorticoid therapy (prednisolone 5 mg daily or more for >3 months)[a,c]
Current smoking[a,c]
Alcohol intake of 2 or more drinks/day[a,c]
Low calcium intake
Low physical activity or immobilization
Vitamin D insufficiency and deficiency
Recent falls
Cognitive impairment
Impaired vision

[a]Factors included in World Health Organization fracture risk assessment tool (FRAX).

[b]Secondary causes included in the FRAX tool are type 1 diabetes, osteogenesis imperfecta as an adult, long-standing untreated hyperthyroidism, hypogonadism, premature menopause, chronic malnutrition, malabsorption, and chronic liver disease.

[c]Risk is higher with greater exposure.

Data from References 2, 4, and 10-13.

(eg, forearm and hip).[14] Trabecular bone is found mostly in the vertebrae and ends of long bones. This bone type is metabolically more active compared with cortical bone due to a much higher bone turnover rate because of its large surface area and honeycomb-like shape.

Bone is made of collagen and mineral components.[9,14] The collagen component gives bone its flexibility and energy-absorbing capability. The mineral component (mostly calcium and phosphorus), which accounts for 50% to 70% of bone mass, gives bone its stiffness and strength. The correct balance of these substances is needed for bone to adequately accommodate stress and strain and resist fractures. Imbalances can impair bone quality and lead to reduced bone strength.

Bone strength reflects the integration of bone mass, bone strength and quality (composition and microarchitecture).[9,16] Bone mass increases rapidly throughout childhood and adolescence. Peak bone mass is attained by age 18 to 25 years. Peak bone mass is highly dependent on genetic factors, which accounts for 60% to 80% of the variability. The remaining 20% to 40% is influenced by modifiable factors such as nutritional intake (eg, calcium, vitamin D, and protein), exercise, adverse lifestyle practices (eg, smoking), hormonal status, and certain diseases and medications (see Tables 112-2 and 112-3). Optimizing peak bone mass is important for preventing osteoporosis. The higher the peak bone mass, the more bone a person can lose before being at an increased fracture risk. As the microarchitecture of bone deteriorates, the bone strength greatly decreases.

Bone remodeling is a dynamic process that occurs continuously throughout life (see Fig. 112-2A-C).[14,17] One to two million tiny sections of bone are in the process of remodeling at any given time.

TABLE 112-2 Select Medical Conditions Associated with Osteoporosis in Children and Adults

Endocrine/Hormonal
Primary or secondary ovarian failure
Testosterone deficiency
Hyperthyroidism
Cushing's syndrome (hypercortisolism)
Growth hormone deficiency (in children)
Hyperparathyroidism
Diabetes, type 1 and type 2
Gastrointestinal
Nutritional disorders (eg, anorexia nervosa)
Malabsorptive states (eg, Crohn's disease, celiac disease, cystic fibrosis, gastrectomy, and bariatric surgery)
Chronic liver disease (eg, primary biliary cirrhosis)
Disorders of Calcium Balance
Hypercalciuria
Calcium and or vitamin D deficiency
Inflammatory Disorders
Rheumatoid arthritis
Chronic Illness
Chronic kidney disease
Malignancies (eg, multiple myeloma, lymphoma, and leukemia)
Human immunodeficiency virus infection/acquired immunodeficiency syndrome
Organ transplant
Disuse/Immobility
Immobilization
Muscular dystrophy
Multiple sclerosis
Stroke/cerebrovascular accident
Genetic
Osteogenesis imperfecta
Cystic fibrosis
Hemochromatosis
Hypophosphatasia

Data from References 2, 4, and 10-16.

Within these sections, the bone remodeling activities of bone resorption and bone formation are coupled and balanced. Bone remodeling is triggered to repair microdamage to the skeleton and serves to support calcium homeostasis by maintaining a normal serum calcium, releasing calcium from the bone into the blood stream as needed. Within an active bone remodeling unit, osteoclasts (bone resorbing cells) work to resorb bone during the resorptive phase, then this process reverses and osteoblasts (bone-forming cells) work to form bone during the formation phase. Osteoblasts then become incorporated into the bone matrix as osteocytes or cover the surface as lining cells, both with bone-communication activities. The unit then becomes inactive and enters a quiescent phase. If remodeling becomes unbalanced and bone resorption surpasses bone formation or if the phases become uncoupled and bone resorption occurs without adequate formation, a decrease in BMD results. Osteocytes and lining cells play key roles in the process and can trigger a new remodeling cycle.

Three schemas show the overview and molecular level details of the bone remodeling cycle. Schema (A) on the top gives the overview of remodeling process with the six steps involved in bone remodeling: Step 1 = initiation, Step 2 and

TABLE 112-3 Select Medications Associated with Increased Bone Loss and/or Fracture Risk

Medications	Comments
Antiseizure therapy (phenytoin, carbamazepine, phenobarbital, and valproic acid)	↓ BMD and ↑ fracture risk; increased vitamin D metabolism leading to low 25(OH) vitamin D concentrations
Aromatase inhibitors (eg, letrozole and anastrozole)	↓ BMD and ↑ fracture risk; reduced estrogen concentrations
Calcineurin inhibitors (eg, cyclosporine and tacrolimus)	↓ BMD and ↑ fracture risk; increase osteoclast activity
Glucocorticoids (long-term oral therapy)	↓ BMD and ↑ fracture risk; increased bone resorption and decreased bone formation, and decreased calcium absorption and reabsorption; dose and duration dependent; see "Special Populations" section
Gonadotropin-releasing hormone agonists (eg, leuprolide and goserelin) or analogs (ganirelix)	↓ BMD and ↑ fracture risk; decreased sex hormone production
Heparin (unfractionated, UFH) or low molecular weight heparin (LMWH)	↓ BMD and ↑ fracture risk (UFH >>> LMWH) with long-term use (eg, >6 months); decreased osteoblast replication and increased osteoclast function
Loop diuretics (eg, furosemide)	↑ fracture risk; increased calcium renal elimination
Medroxyprogesterone acetate depot administration	↓ BMD, fracture risk unknown; possible BMD recovery with discontinuation; decreased estrogen concentrations
Nucleoside/nucleotide reverse transcriptase inhibitors (NRTIs) (tenofovir disoproxil fumarate > other NRTIs)	↓ BMD, fracture risk unknown; greater risk when combined with pharmacological boosters
Proton pump inhibitor therapy (long-term therapy)	↓ BMD and ↑ fracture risk; possible calcium malabsorption secondary to acid suppression for calcium carbonate salts
Selective serotonin reuptake inhibitors	↓ BMD and ↑ fracture risk; decreased osteoblast activity
Sodium glucose cotransporter 2 (SGLT2) inhibitors (canagliflozin; class effect uncertain)	↓ BMD and ↑ fracture risk; alteration in calcium and phosphate homeostasis; increased bone resorption
Thiazolidinediones (pioglitazone and rosiglitazone)	↓ BMD and ↑ fracture risk; decreased osteoblast function
Thyroid—excessive supplementation	↓ BMD and ↑ fracture risk associated with suppressed serum TSH; possible increase in bone resorption
Vitamin A—excessive chronic intake (>10,000 units of retinol form)	↓ BMD and ↑ fracture risk; decreased osteoblast activity and increased osteoclast activity

BMD, bone mineral density; TSH, thyroid-stimulating hormone.

Data from References 2, 14, and 17-22.

3 = resorption, Step 4 =reversal, Step 5 = formation, and Step 6 = quiescence. The schema (B) in the middle gives the molecular level detail of major pathways during bone resorption (mainly steps 2 and 3). The schema (C) at the bottom gives the molecular level detail of major pathways during bone formation (mainly steps 4 and 5). Hence, steps 2 to 5 are also points of osteoporosis medication targets. A mature osteoclast is formed from hematopoietic stem cell under the action of receptor activator of nuclear factor kappa β ligand (RANKL), interleukins 1 and 6 (IL-1, IL-6), macrophage colony stimulating factor (m-CSF), parathyroid hormone (PTH), parathyroid-releasing protein (PTHrP), 1,25(OH) vitamin D, tissue growth factor-β (TGF-β), prostaglandin E2 (PGE_2), insulin-like growth factor (IGF), sclerostin, integrins, platelet-derived growth factor, bone morphometric proteins (BMP), fibroblast growth factor (FGF), and tumor necrosis factor-α (TNF-α).

The signaling of the bone remodeling cycle through the steps from resorption through quiescence is highly complex.[14,17] Many cytokines, growth factors, and hormones influence each step. The complete physiology of bone remodeling is not fully known but appears to begin with signals from lining cells or osteocytes that are triggered by stress, microfractures, biofeedback systems responsive to cytokines and growth factors and potentially certain diseases and medications (see Fig. 112-2B, step 1). A major stimulus for hematopoietic stem cell differentiation to become mature osteoclasts is the receptor activator of nuclear factor kappa β ligand (RANKL), which is a cytokine emitted from osteoblasts or osteocytes in step 2. IL-1, IL-6, m-CSF, PTH through RUNX2/cbfa1, PTHrP, 1,25(OH) vitamin D, TGF-β, PGE_2 IGF, sclerostin, and TNF-α stimulate RANKL release, whereas estrogen and calcitonin inhibit RANKL release. RUNX2/cbfa1 also inhibit osteoprotegerin. The RANKL then binds to the receptor activator of nuclear factor kappa β (RANK) on the surface of osteoclast precursors initiating differentiation. The RANKL also stimulates mature osteoclast activation and bone adherence via $\alpha_v\beta_3$ integrins to resorb bone (step 3). This step is influenced by TGF-β, IGF 1 and 2, platelet-derived growth factor, BMP, and FGF. After bone attachment, the osteoclasts secrete hydrogen and chloride ions and proteinases, such as cathepsin K, collagenase, gelatinase, tartrate-resistant acid phosphate isoenzyme 5 (TRACP5b), and matrix metalloproteases (MMP) to dissolve the mineralized bone. Hydrogen ion production is under nonreceptor tyrosine kinase (Src) control, which needs to be bound to other compounds such as E3 ubiquitin ligase (Cbl), focal adhesion kinase (FAK), and phosphatidylinositol 3-kinase (PI3K).

After bone is resorbed and a cavity is created, osteoclasts produce cytokines and growth factors to elicit osteoblast differentiation from mesenchymal stem cells, maturation, and activity (step 4).[14,17] Osteoblast differentiation can be inhibited by PPARγ, which directs mesenchymal cell maturation to adipocytes instead of osteoblasts. However, leptin produced by adipocytes can stimulate bone formation. Mature osteoblasts and osteocytes produce osteoprotegerin (OPG) that binds to RANKL, thereby stopping bone resorption. Leucine-rich repeat-containing G protein (LGR4) also binds RANKL and stops resorption.

The process of bone formation is complicated (see Fig. 112-2C).[14,17] First, wingless tail ligands (Wnt) bind to low-density lipoprotein receptor–related protein 5 or 6 (LRP5/6) and a frizzled coreceptor. Wnt binding is influenced by PTH and PTHrP, which fit into the same receptor PTH1R, IGF-1, and irisin, which is increased during exercise. Next, LRP5/6 binds to disheveled cytoplasmic protein (DSH), which then binds to axin. Axin now cannot bind to glycogen synthase kinase-3β (GSK-3β), thereby preventing degradation of β-catenin by casein kinase 1α (Csk1α) (step 5). Irisin also increases β-catenin. Accumulated β-catenin then enters the nucleus and binds to T-cell-specific transcription factor 4/lymphoid enhancer factor 1 (TCF/LEF). This complex signals target genes to create proteins to fill the resorption cavity with osteoid. Growth hormone and IGF-1 also increase bone collagen production. Next mineralization of bone with calcium, magnesium, and phosphorus follows to give the new matrix strength.

Once the cavity is mineralized, bone formation can be stopped through multiple signaling processes.[14,17] Secreted frizzled-related proteins (sFRP) or Wnt inhibitory factor 1 (WIF1) can bind to Wnt, preventing it from binding to LRP 5/6. Both sclerostin and Dickkopf-1 (Dkk-1 or Kremen) are secreted from

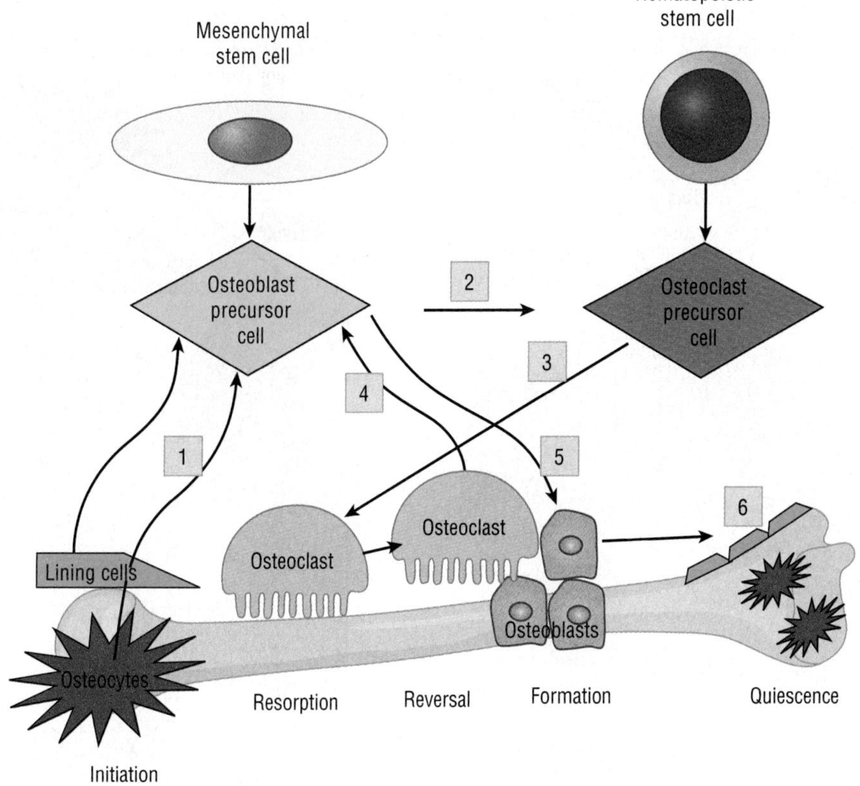

A

B

FIGURE 112-2 (*Continued*)

osteocytes and bind to LRP5/6, which also prevents Wnt from binding with LRP 5/6. Axin can then bind to adenomatous polyposis coli (APC), Csk1α, and GSK-3β, which then can cause β-catenin degradation, osteoblast apoptosis, and the end of osteoblastic activity (step 6). The mature osteoblasts can become lining cells or osteocytes.

Quiescence is the phase when bone is at rest until another remodeling cycle is initiated.[14,17] Later, osteocytes can trigger initiation of a new remodeling cycle through secretion of sclerostin or RANKL to stimulate osteoclasts and bone resorption.

Hormones can influence the remodeling steps. Estrogen has many positive effects on the bone remodeling process in people of

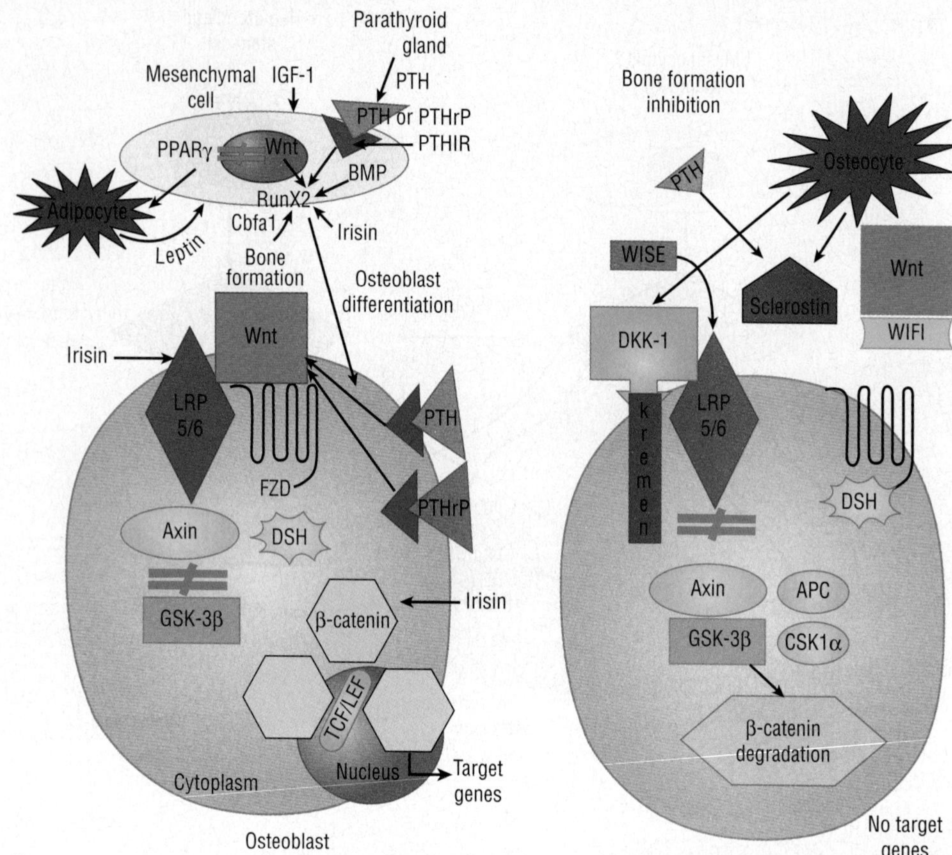

FIGURE 112-2 Bone remodeling cycle. *(A)* Overview of remodeling process, Step 1 = initiation, Steps 2 and 3 = resorption, Step 4 = reversal, Step 5 = formation, and Step 6 = quiescence. *(B)* Molecular level detail of major pathways during bone resorption steps 2 and 3, which also showcase osteoporosis medication targets. *(C)* Molecular level detail of major pathways during bone formation steps 4 and 5, which also showcase osteoporosis medication targets.[14,17] (APC, adenomatous polyposis coli; BMP, bone morphogenetic protein; Ca^{++}, elemental calcium; cbfa1, core-binding factor alpha 1; Cbl, E3 ubiquitin ligase; Cl^-, chloride ion; Csk1α, casein kinase 1α Dkk-1, Dickkoff1; DSH, disheveled cytoplasmic protein; FAK, focal adhesion kinase; GSK-3β, glycogen synthase kinase-3β; H^+, hydrogen ion; IGF-1, insulin-like growth factor 1; LGR4, leucine-rich repeat-containing G protein; LRP5/6, lipoprotein-receptor–related protein 5 or 6; m-CSF, macrophage-colony-stimulating factors; Mg^{++}, magnesium; MMP, matrix metalloproteinases; NF-kβ, nuclear factor kappa beta; NCP, noncollagenous proteins; OPG, osteoprotegerin; Phos, phosphorous; PI3K, phosphatidylinositol 3-kinase; PPARγ, peroxisome proliferator-activated receptor; PTH, parathyroid hormone; PTH1R, PTH and PTHrP receptor; PTHrP, parathyroid hormone-related protein; RANK, receptor activator of nuclear factor-kβ; RANKL, receptor activator of nuclear factor-kβ ligand; RunX2, runt-related transcription factor; Scr, nonreceptor tyrosine kinase; sFRP, secreted frizzled-related proteins; TCF/LEF, T cell specific transcription factor 4/lymphoid enhancer factor 1; TRACP 5b, tartrate-resistant acid phosphate isoenzyme 5; TRAF-6, tumor necrosis factor receptor associated factor 6; WIFI, Wnt inhibitory factor 1; WISE, Wnt modulator insurface ectoderm; Wnt, wingless tail ligands.)

both genders. Most of estrogen's actions help to maintain a normal bone resorption rate.[26] Estrogen suppresses the proliferation and differentiation of osteoclasts and increases osteoclast apoptosis. Estrogen decreases the production of several cytokines that are potent stimulators of osteoclasts, including IL-6, IL-7, IL-17, TNF-α, and m-CSF, and increases IL-4, IL-10, TGF-β, and TGF-α, which increases osteoclast apoptosis. Estrogen also decreases RANKL and increases OPG to reduce osteoclastogenesis.

Most of testosterone's bone effects relate to its metabolism to estradiol and the above estrogen bone effects; however, testosterone does have some direct and indirect effects on osteoblasts.[13,27] Testosterone increases osteoblast proliferation and differentiation directly via the androgen receptor, and indirectly by increasing TGF-β, IGF-2, and decreasing IL-6 stimulation of osteoclasts. Testosterone also increases muscle strength, which can decrease falls leading to fractures. Leydig cells secrete insulin-like factor 3 (INSL3) that stimulates relaxin family peptide receptor 2 (RXFP2) thereby increasing osteoblast and osteocyte functions.[13] A 25-hydroxylase is also secreted that increases vitamin D metabolism to 25(OH) vitamin D.

Bone physiology has many genomic and genetic influences. Isolating one or a few genes for correction will unlikely resolve the problems in an aging population for whom osteoporosis is a common problem.[16] Genetic mutations do result in bone disorders such as osteoporosis, osteogenesis imperfecta, and juvenile idiopathic osteoporosis. Heredity is important since family history, especially of a hip fracture in a parent, is a strong risk factor for osteoporosis development and fracture.

At least 56 loci have been identified that influence BMD and 14 loci for fracture risk, ranging from impacts on bone resorption (RANKL, OPG) to formation (Wnt, LRP5, and sclerostin).[28,29] Calcium, vitamin D, and estrogen receptors are also under genetic influence. Studies are conflicting as to whether an association exists between response to currently available antifracture medications and genetic profiles. Genetic modulation is in its infancy for osteoporosis prevention and treatment, but epigenomics and gene editing might lead to the creation of new medications and/or the ability to tailor medication choices to an individual's genetic profile.[29]

Calcium Homeostasis, Vitamin D, and Parathyroid Hormone

2 Calcium homeostasis is maintained by vitamin D and PTH, which influence calcium gastrointestinal (GI) absorption and renal reabsorption. Calcium absorption under normal conditions is approximately 30% and is improved with vitamin D sufficiency.[30,31] Calcium absorption is lower in the winter due to decreased exposure to required ultraviolet light that converts cholesterol in the skin to vitamin D. Absorption is reported to be higher in obesity, which is associated with greater vitamin D storage. Calcium absorption is predominantly an active rate-limited process in the duodenum and jejunum, which is controlled by many hormones, such as 1,25-dihydroxyvitamin D (1,25[OH] vitamin D), estrogen, and transient receptor potential cation channel subfamily V member 6 (TRPV6). A calcium transporter (calmodulin or calbindin) is required to bring calcium from the gut into the tissue wall and then across the enterocyte. Calcium is extruded into the circulation via calcium (Ca^{++}) adenosine triphosphatase (ATPase) and the sodium-calcium exchanger. Throughout the intestine, paracellular passive calcium diffusion occurs. This diffusion accounts for less than 15% of absorbed calcium, is not rate limited, and possibility is sensitive to 1,25(OH) vitamin D. Solvent drag plays a minor role in calcium absorption.

When the calcium-sensing receptor on parathyroid cells detects low serum calcium, PTH production increases. PTH then directly (minimal effect) and indirectly (predominant effect via increasing calcitriol production) causes calcium reabsorption by the kidney.[30,32] Calcium reabsorption increases as 25(OH) vitamin D concentrations increase, plateauing around 10 to 15 ng/mL (mcg/L; 25-37 nmol/L). Loop diuretics decrease, and thiazide diuretics increase calcium resorption in the kidney.

Sometimes, the increased fractional calcium absorption is insufficient to maintain normal serum calcium, requiring bone resorption for correction.[30,31] Consistent and high concentrations of PTH and calcitriol increase RANKL and decrease OPG, resulting in increased osteoclast activity, which releases calcium from bone to restore calcium homeostasis. Of note, low PTH concentrations for a short time (eg, teriparatide) increase bone formation.

Active 1,25(OH) vitamin D concentrations depend on skin conversion, dietary and supplemental intake, and PTH control.[30,32] The sun's ultraviolet B rays convert 7-dehydrocholesterol in the skin to cholecalciferol (vitamin D_3), which is the most abundant vitamin D source. A few foods contain ergocalciferol (vitamin D_2). Supplements and multivitamins contain cholecalciferol or ergocalciferol. Subsequent conversion of cholecalciferol and ergocalciferol to 25-hydroxyvitamin D (25[OH] vitamin D; calcidiol) occurs in the liver, and then, PTH stimulates conversion of 25(OH) vitamin D via 25(OH) vitamin D-1α-hydroxylase (CYP27B1) to its final active form, 1,25-dihydroxyvitamin D (calcitriol; 1,25[OH] vitamin D), in the kidney. Calcitriol binds to the intestinal vitamin D receptor (VDR) and then increases the action of calcium-binding proteins calmodulin and calbindin. As a result, the intestinal absorption of calcium and phosphorus is increased. The feedback system is completed with CYP27B1 activity inhibited by adequate calcium and phosphorus, and FGF23 inhibiting PTH synthesis.

Postmenopausal Osteoporosis

2 Estrogen deficiency causes significant bone density loss and compromises bone architecture.[4,26,66] Estrogen deficiency increases proliferation, differentiation, and activation of new osteoclasts and prolongs survival of mature osteoclasts. Interleukins 7 and 17, TNF-α, and interferon γ increase and TGF-β decreases resulting in more RANKL and less OPG. Loss of estrogen also increases calcium excretion and decreases calcium gut absorption through decreases in TRPV6 activity and 1,25(OH) vitamin D binding proteins. Estrogen deficiency can also be seen in other settings such as anorexia nervosa and lactation, and from medications, such as prolonged depot medroxyprogesterone acetate implants, aromatase inhibitors, and gonadotropin releasing hormone agonists.

Accelerated bone loss of both mass and strength begins during perimenopause (1-5 years premenopause) and continues up to 10 years after menopause due to increased bone resorption that exceeds bone formation.[2] During this time, increased bone loss can be as high as 2% per year, with total BMD loss due to menopause about 10% to 12%.[4] About 30% of peak bone mass is lost by the age of 80 years. Bone strength decreases by about 2.5% per year.[9] The number of remodeling sites increases, and resorption pits are deeper and inadequately filled by normal osteoblastic function. During menopause, trabecular bone is most susceptible, leading predominantly to vertebral and wrist fractures. Initially, women with early menopause (ie, before the age of 40 years) due to natural or induced causes have lower BMD than matched premenopausal women. After the age of 70 years, risk for fractures and low bone density becomes the same between the groups.

Male Osteoporosis

2 Men lose about 0.8% of bone mass per year after the age of 60 years and 20% experience hypogonadism in their older adult years.[12] Men are at a lower risk for developing osteoporosis and osteoporotic fractures because of larger bone size, greater peak bone mass and connectivity, increase in bone width with aging, fewer falls, and shorter life expectancy. With aging, sex hormone binding globulin increases, which results in less free testosterone and thereby less testosterone available for conversion to estrogen. Estrogen inhibits bone resorption in men; however, androgen deficiency increases RANKL release and bone resorption. Mortality rate after a fracture is greater for men (19.5%) than women (12.5%).

Male osteoporosis results from aging or secondary causes (see Tables 112-2 and 112-3).[12,13,27] The most common risk factors for men are smoking, alcohol abuse, low body weight, weight loss, age, long-term glucocorticoid use, androgen deprivation therapy, and low testosterone concentrations. Medical conditions and medications that cause hypogonadism can increase bone loss. Although many causes and serious fracture outcomes, osteoporosis is underdiagnosed in men.

Age-Related Osteoporosis

2 Age-related bone mass and strength loss begin after peak bone mass is reached.[16] About 0.5%-1% of BMD is loss each year after the age of 30 years in men and until menopause for women.[4] Bone loss accelerates to 2% for 1 to 3 years before and 5 to 10 years post menopause before returning to normal aging bone loss.[4] After the age of 60 years, bone loss for both sexes is 1% to 1.5% per year.[8] Age-related osteoporosis occurs in older adults because of accelerated bone turnover rate and reduced osteoblast bone formation.[23,90] These bone changes occur from hormone deficiencies; calcium and vitamin D deficiencies due to changes in intake, absorption, and metabolism; decreased production or function of cytokines or other bone biochemicals; decreased molecular signaling; increase in redox status and free radical formation; increase in adipocytes; decreased body water; telomere shortening; and less exercise. Fracture risk for a given BMD value increases with aging.[8] For example, at a T-score of −2.5, a 50-year-old postmenopausal woman has about a 4% probability of a hip fracture, whereas a 70-year-old woman has about a 9% probability.[23] Hip fracture risk rises dramatically in older adults because of the cumulative loss of cortical and trabecular bone and an increased risk for falls.

Sarcopenia increases with aging with risk factors similar to osteoporosis.[14] The decrease in muscle strength and function results in weakness and balance instability leading to a greater likelihood of falls and fractures. Falls accounted for 87% of fractures in older adults.

Illness-Induced Secondary Causes of Osteoporosis

1 2 A secondary medical cause of osteoporosis is common (see Table 112-2). Symptoms, laboratory test results, certain diseases and medications, and/or a decreased Z-score from a DXA can suggest a secondary cause, warranting a more comprehensive workup.

Medication-Induced Secondary Causes of Osteoporosis

1 3 Medication-related reductions in BMD and associated fractures are a common secondary cause of osteoporosis. Table 112-3 lists select medications associated with bone loss and/or fracture risk as well as the proposed mechanisms of bone loss.[18-22] Alternative medications should be used when possible, with consideration given to patients' individual risk and baseline BMD status. When these medications cannot be avoided, periodic re-assessment of benefits and risks should be performed, as reversal of bone loss might be possible upon discontinuation of some of these medications. Two of the most common causes of medication-induced osteoporosis, glucocorticoids, and certain cancer chemotherapies are discussed later in this chapter.

CLINICAL PRESENTATION

Table 112-4 outlines the clinical presentation of osteoporosis. Osteoporosis is a silent disease, frequently not detected until a fracture is experienced or noticed on x-ray. Many vertebral fractures are asymptomatic, with patients sometimes attributing mild back pain to other factors, such as advanced age or work. Some new vertebral fractures present with moderate-to-severe back pain that can radiate down the leg. The pain usually subsides after 2 to 4 weeks; however, residual chronic back pain can persist. Multiple vertebral fractures decrease height and sometimes curve the spine (kyphosis or lordosis). Patients with a nonvertebral fracture frequently present with severe pain, swelling, and reduced function and mobility at the fracture site.

Consequences of Osteoporosis

Osteoporosis can lead to fragility/low-trauma fractures defined as fracture that occurs as a result of a fall from standing height or less or with minimal to no trauma.[2] Fractures of the vertebrae, hip, forearm, and humerus are considered major osteoporotic fractures, whereas other fractures are generally not considered osteoporosis-related. Osteoporotic fractures can lead to increased morbidity and mortality and decreased quality of life. Pain and physical deformity are common, and these changes can lead to other health consequences.[4] For example, severe kyphosis can lead to respiratory problems as a result of compression of the thoracic region and GI complications such as poor nutrition from intra-abdominal compression. Depression is common because of fear of falling/fracture, pain, loss of self-esteem from physical deformity, and loss of independence and mobility after fracture.

Hip fractures are associated with the greatest increase in morbidity and mortality. After a hip fracture, 40% of patients have mobility limitations, 50% no longer can live independently or require long-term care (25%), and about 12% to 20% die within the year from complications of the hip fracture or other comorbid disease processes.[2,8] Men have a higher 1-year mortality rate after hip fracture than women.[12] People of color have greater morbidity and mortality after a fracture than non-Hispanic White people.[3]

TABLE 112-4 Clinical Presentation of Osteoporosis

General
- Many patients are unaware they have osteoporosis until testing or fracture.
- Fractures can occur after bending, lifting, or falling, or independent of any activity.

Symptoms
- Frequently asymptomatic
- Pain
- Immobility
- Depression, fear, and low self-esteem from physical limitations and deformities

Signs
- Shortened stature (>1.5 in. [4 cm] loss from maximum height; >0.8 in. [2 cm] loss in 1 year), kyphosis, or lordosis
- Fragility (low-trauma) vertebral, hip, wrist, or forearm fracture

Laboratory tests
- Routine tests: comprehensive metabolic profile (creatinine, calcium, phosphorous, electrolytes, alkaline phosphatase, and albumin), 25(OH) vitamin D, thyroid-stimulating hormone, complete blood count, total testosterone (for men), and 24-hour urine calcium and creatinine concentrations
- Bone turnover markers (eg, serum NTX, serum CTX, and serum PINP) are sometimes used, especially to determine if high bone turnover exists
- Additional testing if the patient's history, physical examination, or initial laboratory and or diagnostic tests suggest a specific secondary cause (eg, intact parathyroid hormone, free testosterone, serum parathyroid, and celiac panel)

Other diagnostic tests
- Spine and hip bone density measurement using central dual-energy x-ray absorptiometry (DXA)
- Vertebral fracture assessment (VFA) with DXA technology
- Radiograph ordered for other reasons that shows low bone density
- Radiograph to confirm fracture
- Balance and mobility tests

CTX, C-terminal crosslinking telopeptide of type 1 collagen; NTX, N-terminal crosslinking telopeptide of type 1 collagen; PINP, procollagen type 1 N-terminal propeptide.

Data from References 2, 4, 6, 10, 21, 33, and 34.

Wrist fractures occur more commonly in younger postmenopausal women and are frequently a result of a fall on an outstretched hand. Although they cause less disability than other fracture sites, negative outcomes include prolonged pain and weakness, and difficulty with activities such as meal preparation, using a keyboard, and lifting at work.

Once a low-trauma fracture has occurred, the risk for subsequent fractures goes up exponentially.[8] Vertebral fractures, even if asymptomatic, are a major predictor of a future fracture with up to a five- to seven-fold increase in future vertebral fractures and an increased risk at other sites.[4] Patients with a hip fracture have a 2% to 10% chance of a second hip fracture.[4]

Patient Assessment

Laboratory tests and other assessments are described in Table 112-4. Height should be measured annually using a wall-mounted stadiometer. Low bone density (sometimes called osteopenia) reported on routine radiographs is a sign of significant bone loss and requires further evaluation for osteoporosis. Additional tests will be required that are specific to potential secondary causes (Tables 112-2 and 112-3). In addition to physical examination and laboratory tests, patients can be assessed with risk factor assessment tools, osteoporosis quality of life questionnaires, peripheral and central DXA, ultrasonography, and bone turnover markers (BTM).

Risk Factor Assessment

The aim of an initial osteoporosis risk assessment screening is to identify those patients who are at risk for osteoporosis and osteoporotic fractures (see Table 112-1) and/or would benefit from further evaluation or pharmacologic intervention. The most commonly used assessment is the fracture risk assessment (FRAX) tool[2]; the Garvan tool[35] is another option.

4 The FRAX tool was created to be used for screening and diagnosis.[2] It can be used without DXA results; however, estimates improve when T-scores are available. This tool uses 11 risk factors: age, race/ethnicity, sex, previous fracture, parent history of hip fracture, body mass index, glucocorticoid use (current use or past use for three or more months of the equivalent of at least 5 mg of prednisolone daily), current smoking, alcohol use of three or more drinks per day, rheumatoid arthritis, and select secondary causes of osteoporosis (see Table 112-1); with optional entry for femoral neck BMD (g/cm^2 or T-score). The FRAX tool calculates an individual's percent probability of any major osteoporotic fracture and hip fracture in the next 10 years. Each country establishes cut-off points for fracture risk treatment decisions. For the United States, they are 20% or higher for major osteoporotic fracture and 3% or higher for hip fracture. Most guidelines use these universal cutoffs, but others are beginning to recommend age-adjusted FRAX cutoffs to prevent undertreatment of younger people and overtreatment of older people or create a middle zone in which BMD would be needed to determine treatment.[34] For example, for a 55-year-old person, a 10% 10-year risk of major osteoporotic fracture would be used, and for an 80-year-old person, 30% would be used. For postmenopausal women younger than 65 years, a 10-year major osteoporotic fracture risk of greater than 8.4% would result in a referral for a central DXA.[2,36] Some important risk factors for fracture, for example, falls, multiple fractures, recent fracture, or other common secondary causes, are not accommodated in the FRAX model.

The Garvan calculator uses four risk factors (age, sex, low-trauma fracture, and falls) with the option to also use BMD.[2,6,35] It calculates 5- and 10-year risk estimates of any osteoporotic/fragility fracture and hip fracture. This tool corrects some disadvantages of the FRAX tool since it includes falls and number of previous fractures, but it does not use as many other risk factors.

Screening Using Peripheral Bone Mineral Density Devices

Peripheral bone density devices that use DXA (pDXA) or quantitative ultrasonography (QUS) are helpful as screening tools to determine which patients require further evaluation with central DXA or for decision making if central DXA testing is not available.[2,36,37] Peripheral DXA of the forearm, heel, or finger uses a low amount of radiation and requires personnel with special training. Quantitative ultrasonography at the heel and other peripheral sites uses sound waves without radiation, and specially trained personnel are not needed. The heel is the only skeletal site at which QUS has been validated.[37] The QUS has better fracture predictive value than pDXA and has demonstrated the ability to predict fractures in postmenopausal women and in men 65 years of age or older. The specific peripheral T-score threshold for referral is not universally defined and varies by device. These tests should not be used for diagnosis or for monitoring response to therapy.[37]

Peripheral devices are considerably less expensive than central DXA, easy to use, portable, fast (less than 5 minutes), and can predict general fracture risk. They are popular for screening patients at health fairs and community pharmacies. Patients already identified as being at high risk for osteoporosis based on risk factors, fragility fracture, or secondary causes for osteoporosis should be referred for central DXA testing.

Central Dual-Energy X-Ray Absorptiometry

4 BMD measurements at the hip or spine can be used to assess fracture risk, establish the diagnosis and severity of osteoporosis, and confirm osteoporosis following a low-trauma fracture.[2,34] Multiple techniques are available for measurement of BMD and include DXA, quantitative computed tomography (QCT), digital x-ray radiogrammetry, and radiographic absorptiometry. Central DXA is the most widely used technique and preferred for making therapeutic decisions.[37] It has high precision, short scan times, low-radiation dose (comparable to the average daily dose from natural background), and stable calibration. Measurements of lumbar spine, femoral neck, and total hip BMD are recommended with the lowest BMD value used for diagnosis. The forearm (distal third of the radius) can be used as an alternative if the preferred areas cannot be scanned.[2,4,34,37] Trabecular bone score (TBS) is a newer technology available on some densitometers that can provide measurements of bone quality and microarchitecture. Low TBS is independently associated with increased fractures and can be used in combination with BMD and FRAX scores to better identify those at increased fracture risk.

Several consensus guidelines and position statements are consistent in recommending central BMD testing for all women aged 65 years or older, men aged 70 years or older, postmenopausal women younger than 65 years and men 50 to 69 years old with risk factors for fracture, and patients with an identified secondary cause for bone loss.[2,4,12,37] The US Preventive Services Task Force (USPSTF) provides similar recommendations for screening in women 65 years or older and in women under the age of 65 years with additional risk factors as determined by a clinical risk assessment tool, such as FRAX.[36] This group, however, has concluded that current data are insufficient to make recommendations for screening in men. Patients with a fragility fracture do not need a DXA for an osteoporosis diagnosis, but the results are helpful for determining the severity of osteoporosis and as a baseline for monitoring response to therapy.[2] The DXA results can also help patients make decisions about the need for lifestyle changes and prescription osteoporosis medications. In the absence of a suspected or known secondary cause for osteoporosis or a history of a low-trauma fracture, central BMD testing is not recommended for children,[15] women,[38] or men younger than 50 years.[13]

A central DXA BMD report provides the actual bone density value (in g/cm^2), T-score, and Z-score.[37] The T-score is used for diagnosis and is a comparison of the patient's BMD to the mean BMD of a healthy, young (20-29 year olds), and sex-matched White reference population. It is not adjusted for age, race, or ethnicity. The T-score is the number of standard deviations from the mean of the reference population.[37] The Z-score is similar but compares the patient's BMD to the mean BMD for a healthy sex- and age-matched population. The patient's race and ethnicity should be used for the Z-score if available. The Z-score is sometimes helpful in determining whether a secondary cause for osteoporosis is present and is used for diagnosis (value ≤ -2.0) in children, premenopausal women, and men younger than 50 years. The actual bone density value is most useful for serial monitoring of therapy response. Follow-up BMD is recommended every 1 to 3 years by some guidelines,[2,4] although other guidelines recommend every 5 years in postmenopausal women.[1,34] The DXA results after medication initiation need to be above the machine's least significant change to be clinically relevant. For patients with normal bone density or those in the upper range of low bone mass, time between follow-up scans can be lengthened. Most insurance carriers, including Medicare, cover BMD testing every 2 years.

Using the spine DXA image, a VFA can be performed to assess for vertebral fractures that might otherwise go undetected.[2,4,37] Each vertebra is visually evaluated for fracture and fractures are assessed for severity. This result becomes important for treatment decisions in patients with low bone mass. Because many vertebral fractures are asymptomatic, VFA is recommended for those at high risk of an undiagnosed vertebral fracture. This includes patients with a T-score less than -1.0 when one or more of the following criteria are also present: women aged at least 70 years or men aged at least 80 years; a historical height loss of more than 1.5 in. (4 cm); a self-reported but undocumented prior vertebral fracture; or patients on glucocorticoid therapy (≥5 mg prednisone or equivalent daily for 3 months or more).

Laboratory Tests

Routine laboratory testing (see Table 112-4) is used for initial bone health assessment.[2,4,10,12,15] To evaluate secondary causes, additional testing is conducted, which will be specific to the suspected secondary cause.

Bone Turnover Markers

BTM are commonly used in clinical trials and sometimes in clinical practice.[2,4] They can be used to assess bone pathophysiology, predict fracture risk, monitor response to osteoporosis medications, evaluate medication adherence, and determine the need for restarting bisphosphonates after a drug holiday. Although many BTMs exist, serum carboxyterminal propeptide of type-I collagen (PINP) and bone-specific alkaline phosphatase (BSAP) are the preferred bone formation markers, and serum C-terminal telopeptide type-1 collagen (CTX) is the preferred bone resorption marker. Response to osteoporosis therapy can be measured with BTMs as early as 2 to 3 months; however, monitoring is usually done 3 to 6 months after osteoporosis medication initiation. Goal values would be at or below median premenopausal concentrations for antiresorptive medications and significant increase for formation medications.[2] Circadian variability, seasonal variations, food intake, recent exercise, some diseases and conditions, and assay variability can affect results and decrease utility in clinical practice. Fasting morning samples should be obtained with repeat tests done at the same facility with the same assay to decrease interassay variability. Of note, fractures increase BTMs for a short time frame. These tests can be expensive with coverage varying by health insurance plan. As an alternative, bone-specific alkaline phosphatase can be used, which is usually covered.

Diagnosis of Osteoporosis

6 The diagnosis of osteoporosis is based on a low-trauma fracture or femoral neck, total hip and/or spine DXA using World Health Organization (WHO) T-score thresholds.[2] Low bone mass (preferred term) or osteopenia is a T-score between –1 and –2.5, and osteoporosis is a T-score at or below –2.5. Although these definitions are based on data from postmenopausal white women, they are also applied to perimenopausal women, men aged 50 years and older, and adults from different races and ethnicities. The diagnosis of osteoporosis in children,[15] premenopausal women,[11] and men under 50 years of age[13] should be based on a Z-score at or less than –2.0 in combination with other risk factors or fracture. Without a history of clinically significant fracture, children, premenopausal women, and men are given a diagnosis of bone mass below the expected range for age.

PREVENTION AND TREATMENT

Desired Outcomes

The primary goal of osteoporosis care should be prevention. Optimizing skeletal development and peak bone mass accrual in childhood, adolescence, and early adulthood will ultimately reduce the future incidence of osteoporosis. Once low bone mass or osteoporosis develops, the objective is to improve or stabilize bone mass and strength, and prevent fractures. In patients who have already suffered osteoporotic fractures, reducing pain and deformity, improving functional capacity, improving quality of life, and reducing future falls and fractures are the main goals.

General Approach to Prevention and Treatment

5 6 A bone-healthy lifestyle should begin at birth and continue throughout life. The foundation of osteoporosis prevention and treatment is a bone-healthy lifestyle. Supplements and medications are used when lifestyle habits are insufficient or suboptimal, osteoporosis has developed, and/or a low-trauma fracture occurs. Guidelines and position statements recommend considering prescription therapy in any postmenopausal woman or man aged 50 years and older presenting with one of the following scenarios: a hip or vertebral fracture; T-score of −2.5 or lower at the femoral neck, total hip, or spine; or low bone mass (T-score between −1.0 and −2.5 at the femoral neck, total hip, or spine) with a FRAX 10-year probability of hip fracture of 3% or more or any major osteoporosis-related fracture of 20% or more. Figure 112-3 provides an osteoporosis management algorithm for postmenopausal women and men aged 50 years and older that incorporates both nonpharmacologic and pharmacologic approaches.

Nonpharmacologic Therapy

5 Nonpharmacologic therapy, referred to as a bone-healthy lifestyle, includes proper nutrition, moderation of alcohol intake, smoking cessation, exercise, and fall prevention. A bone-healthy lifestyle that is employed early in life will help to optimize peak bone mass, and if continued throughout life, it will minimize bone loss over time. A bone-healthy lifestyle not only maintains or increases BMD but it also helps decrease falls and fragility fractures.

Diet

5 Overall, a diet well balanced in nutrients and minerals with limited salt, alcohol, and caffeine use are important for bone health. Adequate amounts of calcium and vitamin D have documented impacts on bone health. Protein is required for bone, thus the recommended dietary allowances (RDAs) of 0.8 g/kg body weight per day is recommended for adults increasing to 1 to 1.2 g/kg body weight in older adults and to 1.5 g/kg body weight for some chronic illnesses.[8] Magnesium, boron, and vitamin K have a physiologic role in bone development and maintenance but either no or insufficient data exist to establish them independently as supplemental agents for prevention and treatment of osteoporosis. Some of these agents are included in calcium combination products and are found in multivitamins. Strontium ranelate has documented positive bone effects and is marketed in Europe for prevention of osteoporosis.

Eating disorders are associated with increased bone loss and fractures.[11,15] Being thin or having anorexia nervosa are well known to decrease bone mass. In the past, obesity was thought protective due to increased estrogen production and stimulation of bone remodeling due to weight bearing; however, emerging literature suggests adipocytes have negative impacts on bone health.

Calcium

5 7 Adequate calcium intake is necessary for calcium homeostasis throughout life, bone development during growth, and bone maintenance thereafter. The Institute of Medicine (IOM) recommended calcium intakes are based on age and gender (Table 112-5).[2,34,39] These values represent the average daily amount needed to meet requirements for 97% to 98% of healthy people. Higher intakes might be needed when concomitant diseases and medications known to negatively affect calcium and vitamin D homeostasis exist. Ingesting calcium-containing and/or calcium-fortified foods and beverages is the preferred method to achieve daily calcium requirements. Dairy products generally have the highest amount of calcium per serving and are available in low-fat options. Some food sources result in good calcium absorption but have low elemental calcium content (eg, broccoli). Carbohydrates increase calcium absorption, whereas phylates (eg, beans, seeds, wheat bran) and oxalates (eg, spinach and rhubarb) decrease absorption.[6,35]

People should be encouraged to evaluate their food and beverage intake to determine if they are receiving adequate amounts of calcium. To calculate the amount of calcium in a serving of food,

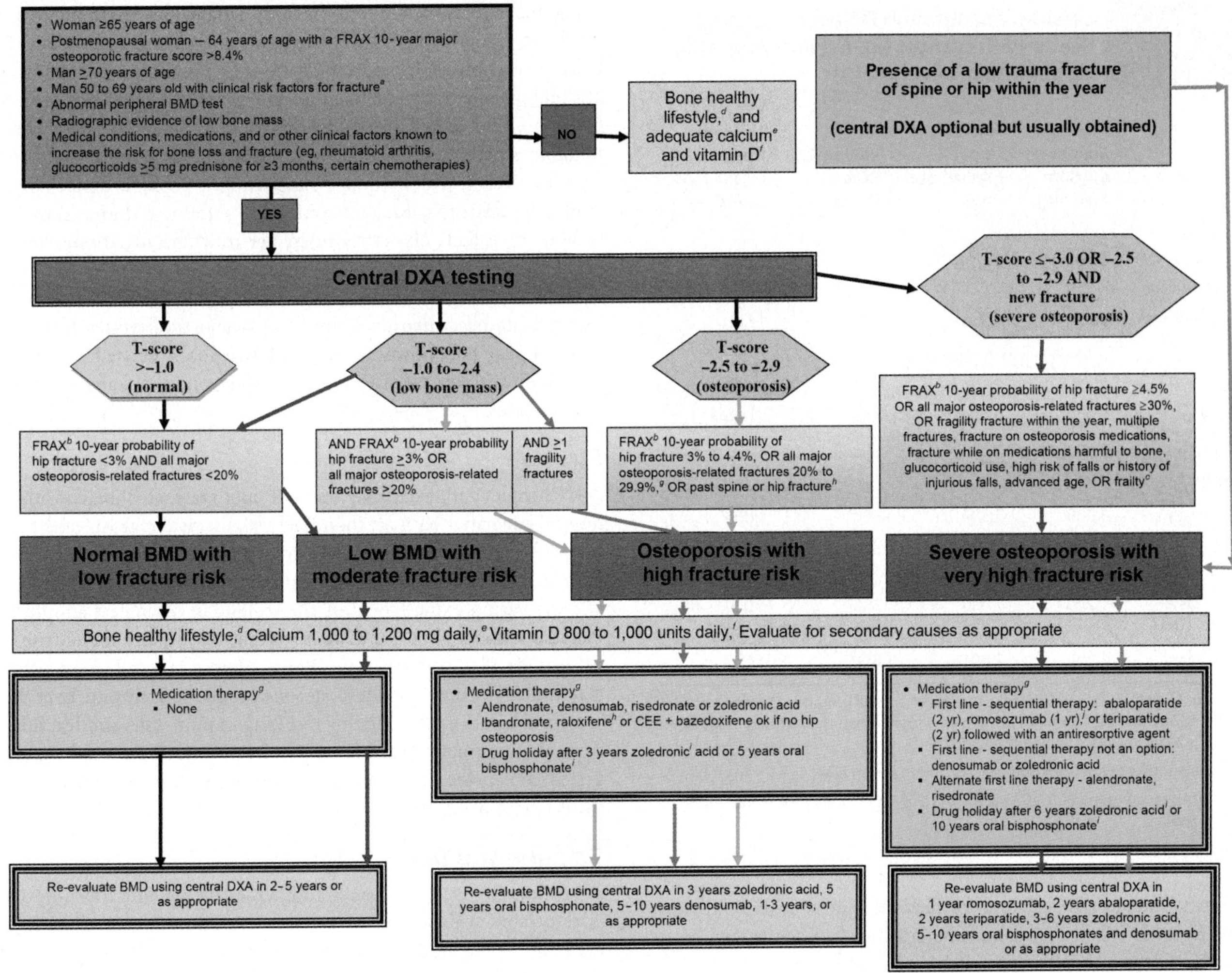

FIG. 112-3 [a]aMajor clinical risk factors for fracture: advanced age, current smoker, low body weight or body mass index, personal history of fracture as an adult (after age 50 years), history of osteoporosis/low trauma fracture in a first-degree relative, excessive alcohol intake.

[b]Some providers use age adjusted FRAX thresholds versus set thresholds for all age groups.

[c]Fragility fracture is high risk for ES guidelines, and very high risk for AACE/ACE guideline.

[d]Bone-healthy lifestyle includes well-balanced diet with adequate calcium, vitamin D, and protein intakes; smoking cessation; limited alcohol intake; weight-bearing/resistance exercises; and fall prevention.

[e]Dietary calcium preferred. If diet is inadequate, supplement as necessary.

[f]Higher vitamin D doses might be needed to achieve 25(OH) vitamin D concentrations >30 ng/mL.

[g]Some increased BMD effects will be seen for women using menopausal hormonal therapy and for men using testosterone for hypogonadism. For women and men on hormonal therapy and at high risk or very high risk for osteoporotic fractures, an osteoporosis medication will also be prescribed, creating a case for combination therapy.

[h]Raloxifene option for postmenopausal women < 60 years old with low hip fracture, stroke, and venous thromboembolic risk and high breast cancer risk.

[i]Restart therapy when BMD goes below T-score ≤−2.5 or a fracture; alternative is to use raloxifene or denosumab, or in some cases a bone formation medication during the drug holiday.

jDo not use romosozumab in patients with at high risk for or past myocardial infarction and/or stroke.

(BMD, bone mineral density; CEE, conjugated equine estrogens, DXA, dual-energy x-ray absorptiometry, FRAX = World Health Organization fracture risk assessment tool)

Data from references 1,3,7,42, and 43

consumers can add a zero to the percent of the daily value listed on food labels. For example, a serving of milk (8 oz. [~240 mL]) has 30% of the daily value of calcium. This translates to 300-mg calcium per serving. Websites can be used to identify foods and beverages high in calcium.[31]

Although many foods and beverages are high in calcium, the average daily dietary calcium intake is insufficient in many children and adults.[31] In addition, lactose intolerance limits dietary calcium intake. The incidence in Asian Americans (15%-100%), Native Americans (79%), African Americans (75%), and Hispanic Americans (51%) are higher than in White Americans (21%).[41] Patients with lactose-intolerance have several options to increase dietary calcium intake, including products containing lactase (Lactaid®), lactose-reduced milk, lactose-free milk, calcium-fortified milk alternatives (eg, soy and almond milk), certain aged cheeses, or yogurt with active cultures along with other nondairy calcium-fortified products (eg, orange juice, breakfast cereals, and energy bars). Vegan diets sometimes have insufficient calcium intake, but

TABLE 112-5 Calcium and Vitamin D Recommended Dietary Allowances (RDAs) and Tolerable Upper Intake Levels (ULs)

Group and Ages	Elemental Calcium RDA (mg)	Calcium Tolerable Upper Intake Level (mg)	Vitamin D RDA (units)[a]	Vitamin D Tolerable Upper Intake Level (units)
Infants				
Birth to 6 months	200[b]	1,000	400[b]	1,000
7-12 months	260[b]	1,500	400[b]	1,500
Children				
1-3 years	700	2,500	600	2,500
4-8 years	1,000	2,500	600	3,000
9-18 years	1,300	3,000	600	4,000
Adults				
19-50 years	1,000	2,500	600[b,c]	4,000
51-70 years (men)	1,000	2,000	600[b,c]	4,000
51-70 years (women)	1,200	2,000	600[b,c]	4,000
>70 years	1,200	2,000	800[b,c]	4,000

[a]Some guidelines recommend intake to achieve a 25(OH) vitamin D concentration of >30 ng/mL (mcg/L; 75 nmol/L),[1,3,8] which is higher than the Institute of Medicine goal of >20 ng/mL (mcg/L; 50 nmol/L).[40]

[b]Adequate intake (evidence insufficient to determine an RDA).

[c]Guidelines recommend 800-1,000 units[1] or 1,000-2,000 units[3,8] for adults with osteoporosis.

Data from References 2, 34, and 39.

products such as tofu, calcium-fortified milk alternatives, and juices can be used. When diet cannot be enhanced to achieve adequate intakes, calcium supplements will be required.

Vitamin D

5 8 Table 112-5 also lists the IOM recommended adequate intakes for Vitamin D.[2,34,39] The three main sources of vitamin D are sunlight (conversion of 7-dehydrocholesterol to vitamin D3), diet, and supplements. Vitamin D3 comes from oily fish, eggs, and fortified dairy products. Vitamin D2 comes from fungi and eggs (chickens given vitamin D2 in their diet). Websites can be used to identify the few foods high in vitamin D.[42] To calculate the amount of vitamin D in a serving of food, consumers can multiply the percent daily value of vitamin D listed on the food label by 4 (eg, 20% vitamin D = 80 units).

The overall prevalence of hypovitaminosis D (<20 ng/mL [mcg/L; 50 nmol/L]) in American adults has been estimated at 29%; with higher prevalence ratios observed in those who are older than 60 years, from a minority, have lower education levels, obese, physically inactive, and/or current smokers.[43] Low vitamin D concentrations can result from insufficient intake, dietary fat malabsorption, decreased sun exposure, decreased skin production, and/or decreased liver and renal metabolism. Endogenous synthesis of vitamin D can be decreased by factors that affect exposure to or decrease skin penetration of ultraviolet B light rays. Sunscreen use, full body coverage with clothing (eg, women wearing veils and full-length dresses), and darkly pigmented skin can all decrease vitamin D production. Seasonal variations in vitamin D concentrations are also seen with nadirs in late winter and peaks in late summer. Because few foods are naturally high or fortified with vitamin D, most people, especially older adults, require supplementation to achieve IOM recommended adequate intakes.

Isoflavones

5 Phytoestrogens (isoflavones, lignans, and coumestans) are plant-derived compounds that possess weak estrogenic agonist and antagonist effects throughout the body. Isoflavones are found in soy products, lignans in seeds, berries, and grains, and coumestans in peas, beans, broccoli, and alfalfa sprouts. Genistein and daidzein are biologically active isoflavones found in soybeans. Isoflavones, genistein, and daidzein are also available as single-agent or combination supplements. Isoflavones produce estrogenic activity and increase IGF-1. The evidence supporting a positive bone benefit from phytoestrogen intake is conflicting with most studies showing little or no effect. The effect is greater on trabecular bone. Doses and products studied are quite varied with potentially more BMD activity with higher doses. Spine but not hip BMD is increased in some studies when compared to placebo. Isoflavones from soy foods appear safe; however, more information is needed, especially in women with breast cancer and for isoflavone supplements versus food sources.[44]

Alcohol

3 Chronic and excessive but not moderate alcohol consumption is associated with an increased risk for osteoporosis and fractures.[2,45] Alcohol increases bone resorption by increasing RANKL and decreases bone formation by inhibiting Wnt signaling pathway and increasing oxidative stress that results in osteoblast apoptosis. Patients with alcohol-use disorder might also have poor nutrition, decreased calcium absorption, altered vitamin D metabolism, estrogen inhibition, decreased testosterone production, chronic liver disease, and balance impairments resulting in more falls and fractures. Typical recommendations for alcohol consumption should be suggested, which are not to exceed 2 drinks per day for women and 3 drinks per day for men.

Caffeine and Tea

5 Although results are conflicting, excessive caffeine consumption is associated with increased calcium excretion, increased rates of bone loss, and a modestly increased risk for fracture.[45] Greater negative effects are seen in women. Ideally, caffeine consumption should be limited to two servings or less per day. For those with greater intakes, the increased calcium excretion might be compensated by additional calcium intake. Chronic tea drinking might have a positive benefit on bone mass, but no fracture outcomes exist.

Smoking

5 Cigarette smoking is an independent risk factor for osteoporosis and is associated with increased relative risk for fracture at all sites.[46] The effect is dose- and duration-dependent, but even passive smoking shows adverse effects on BMD. The negative bone effects are associated with reduced intestinal calcium absorption, lower 25(OH) vitamin D concentrations possibly due to increased hepatic metabolism, an increase in bone resorption from a decrease in production and increase in metabolism of estradiol leading to an increase in RANKL and decrease in OPG, decrease in osteoblasts and bone formation secondary to increase in cortisol and dehydroepiandrosterone sulfate, and impairment of osteoid production and mineralization.[16,46] The detrimental effects of smoking on physical function and balance can contribute to an increased risk of falls. Per guidelines, counseling patients of all ages on smoking cessation can help to optimize peak bone mass, minimize bone loss, and ultimately reduce fracture risk[2]; however, few studies have explored these outcomes.[46]

Exercise

5 Physical activity or exercise is an important nonpharmacologic approach to preventing osteoporotic fractures. Exercise increases bone mechanical strain, especially in weaker bone, thus stimulating osteocytes leading to bone resorption and then new stronger bone formation.[9] Weight-bearing exercise inhibits myostatin, which increases muscle and bone mass and decreases fat mass, and sclerostin and Dickoff-1, which prevents them from stopping bone

formation.[17] Irisin is increased by exercise leading to increased bone formation by stimulating runX2, LRP 5/6, and β-catenin. Exercise can decrease the risk of falls and fractures by stabilizing bone density and improving muscle strength, coordination, balance, and mobility.[2,14,16,47] Physical activity is especially important early in life since peak bone mass is gained at that time and lack of exercise during growth can lead to suboptimal loading/straining, decreased stimulation of bone deposition, and reduced peak bone mass.[9] Although bone mass might not increase, bone strength will increase in older adults. All people of any age who are medically fit should be encouraged to perform a moderate-intensity weight-bearing activity (eg, running), plyometric (eg, jumping, hopping, bounding), and resistance activity (eg, weight machines, free weights, or elastic bands). Walking, swimming, cycling, and yoga have less impact on osteogenics but are still important. People at risk of osteoporosis should participate in exercise, including weight-bearing activities, at least three to four times weekly for 30 to 40 minutes per session. Adult recommendations for exercise from the American Heart Association can be suggested, which are 150 minutes of moderate-intensity aerobic exercise weekly or 75 minutes of vigorous-intensity exercise per week, and moderate- to high-intensity muscle strengthening at least twice a week.[48]

Fall Prevention

5 Risk of falling increases with advanced age predominantly as a result of balance, gait, and mobility problems, poor vision, reduced muscle strength, impaired cognition, multiple medical conditions (eg, arrhythmias, postural hypotension, Alzheimer's disease, and Parkinson disease), and polypharmacy (especially psychoactive, cardiovascular, diabetes, seizure, and pain medications).[2,24] The ability to adapt to falls also decreases with aging. Older adults are more likely to sustain a hip or pelvic fracture because they tend to fall backward or sideways instead of forward.

Because of the link between falls and fractures, all older adults should be asked at least annually if they have fallen. The US Centers for Disease Control and Prevention have created an assessment tool.[49] If an older adult scores 4 or more, a comprehensive falls assessment should be conducted. Many other assessment tools exist to evaluate falls.

Generally, intervention programs that are multifactorial have greater effects on decreasing falls, fractures, other injuries, and nursing home and hospital admissions than single interventions.[2,24,40,47,50] Medication profiles should be reviewed for any unnecessary medications that can affect cognition and balance, and potentially increase fall risk. Consideration should be given to deprescribing or substitution with safer medications. Although Vitamin D supplementation has been advocated to reduce falls and fractures in some guidelines, the most recent USPSTF recommendation states the evidence is inadequate to prescribe this therapy for fall and fracture prevention. Maintenance of a regular individualized exercise program, such as tai chi, resistance training, and strengthening, should be recommended to improve body strength, balance, and agility. Other recommendations include resolving heart rate/rhythm irregularities, low blood pressure, and vision and foot problems, and using proper footwear. A home environment safety assessment is helpful to identify environmental solutions to decrease falls.[24,40,51] External hip protectors are specialized undergarments designed to pad the area surrounding the hip, decreasing the force of impact from a sideways fall.[8] Conflicting results and poor adherence limit their use. Many patient education materials exist with the US Centers for Disease Control and Prevention older adult falls prevention program being an excellent resource for patients and providers.[40]

Vertebroplasty and Kyphoplasty

During vertebroplasty and kyphoplasty cement is injected into fractured vertebra(e) for patients with debilitating pain from vertebral compression fractures. Although used to stabilize damaged vertebrae, reduce pain, and decrease opioid intake, this therapy is decreasing based on results showing effects that are similar to sham interventions, being short-term, and having no major pain benefit, and or are associated with vertebral fracturing around the cement, cement leakage into the spinal column, and nerve damage (rare).[52] The AACE/ACE guideline lists vertebral augmentation as an uncertain therapy due to limited data, potential for adverse treatment outcomes, and lack of long-term effects.[2]

Pharmacologic Therapy

9 Because nonpharmacologic interventions alone are frequently insufficient to prevent or treat osteoporosis, medication therapy is often necessary. Osteoporosis medication effects on fracture risk and BMD (Table 112-6), dosing (Table 112-7), and adverse effects and monitoring (Table 112-8) are described. Medication use should be combined with a bone-healthy lifestyle. People of color were less likely to receive osteoporosis prescription medications[3]; thus, health disparities need to be resolved to provide osteoporosis prevention to all women and men.

The North American Menopause Society guidelines for postmenopausal women, Endocrine Society guideline for postmenopausal women, the American Association of Clinical Endocrinologists and American College of Endocrinology guideline for postmenopausal women, the American College of Physicians guideline for women and men, and the Bone Health and Osteoporosis Foundation guideline for women and men provide guidance on osteoporosis prevention and treatment strategies.[1,2,4,39]

Medication Treatments of First Choice

9 Alendronate, risedronate, zoledronic acid, and denosumab reduce both hip and vertebral fracture risks.[2] Abaloparatide, calcitonin, ibandronate, raloxifene, romosozumab, and teriparatide reduce vertebral but not hip fracture risks. Estrogen and testosterone therapies are not used for osteoporosis treatment, but when prescribed for other conditions will have a positive bone effect.[27] In theory, sequential therapy starting with bone formation medications and followed by antiresorption medications is recommended, especially in patients with osteoporosis and very high risk for fracture. Formation medication cost and injectable dosage forms limit sequential therapy as initial therapy. The algorithm (see Fig. 112-3) helps determine for whom medication therapy should be used. In general, prescription therapy combined with adequate intakes of calcium and vitamin D should be considered for any postmenopausal woman or man aged 50 years and older presenting with a fragility fracture, osteoporosis, or low bone mass combined with a FRAX 10-year probability of hip fracture of 3% or more or any major osteoporosis-related fracture of 20% or more. Type of fracture risk (spine, hip, or both) will also determine medication of choice. Calcitonin is a last-line therapy. The use of osteoporosis prescription medications in children,[10,15,57,58] premenopausal women,[11] and men younger than 50 years[12,13] occurs in special cases and is generally related to secondary medical and medication causes or genetic disorders.

Antiresorptive Therapies

Antiresorptive therapies include calcium, vitamin D, bisphosphonates, denosumab, estrogen agonists/antagonists (EAA), tissue selective estrogen complexes (TSEC), calcitonin, estrogen, and testosterone.

Calcium Supplementation 7 Calcium imbalance can result from inadequate dietary intake, decreased fractional calcium absorption, enhanced calcium excretion, and diseases and medications altering these processes. Adequate calcium intake (see Table 112-5) is considered a foundation for osteoporosis prevention and treatment in the guidelines and should be combined with

TABLE 112-6 Fracture and Bone Mineral Density Effects of Osteoporosis Medications from Pivotal Fracture Trials[a] in Postmenopausal Women

Medication	Vertebral Fracture	Nonvertebral Fracture	Hip Fracture	% Change in Spine BMD[b]	% Change in Hip BMD[b,c]
Abaloparatide	86%↓	43%↓	↔	10.4%↑	4.3%↑
Bazedoxifene	35%-42%↓	↔[d]	↔	2.1-3.0%↑	0.5%↑
Bazedoxifene with conjugated equine estrogens	ND	ND	ND	0.24%-1.6%↑	0.2%-1.5%↑
Bisphosphonates	41%-70%↓	20%-38%↓[e]	28%-50%↓[f]	3.1%-6.0%↑	1.8%-4.0%↑
Calcitonin	33%↓	↔	↔	3%↑	↔
Denosumab	68%↓	20%↓	40%↓	9.2%↑	6.0%↑
Estrogen with or without a progestogen	33%-40%↓	13%-27%↓	30%-50%↓	3.5%-7%↑[f]	1.7%-5%↑[g]
Raloxifene	30%-68%↓[h]	↔	↔	2.6%↑	2.1%↑
Romosozumab	73%↓	ND/19%↓[i]	ND/38%↓[i]	11.3%-13.7%↑[g]	4.1%-6.9%↑
Teriparatide	65%↓	53%↓	↔	8.6%-9.7%↑	3.5%↑

[a]Fracture reductions are relative risk reductions, no head to head fracture studies except for raloxifene and bazedoxifene. Data should only be used for relative between class comparisons. Clinical trials have different patient samples and study designs. Most pivotal fracture trials were of 3-year duration except for abaloparatide (2 years), romosozumab (1 year) and teriparatide (18 months) studies.

[b]Relative to placebo; may vary based on duration of therapy and timing relative to menopause.

[c]Total hip (alendronate, ibandronate, zoledronic acid, bazedoxifene, denosumab, estrogen, abaloparatide, teriparatide, romosozumab) or femoral neck (calcitonin, estrogen, risedronate, and raloxifene).

[d]50% decreases in nonvertebral fractures in subgroup of high-risk postmenopausal women (very low BMD and/or previous fractures).

[e]Risedronate and zoledronic acid only; nonvertebral fracture reductions with ibandronate were not significant.

[f]Alendronate, risedronate, and zoledronic acid only; hip fracture data not reported with ibandronate.

[g]Data obtained from nonpivotal fracture trials.

[h]Includes data from a pivotal bazedoxifene trial with raloxifene as one of the comparators.

[i]Second year results after 1 year of romosozumab followed by alendronate or denosumab for 1 year.

[j]Includes data from teriparatide versus romosozumab study.

%, percent; BMD, bone mineral density; ↓, decrease; ↑, increase; ↔, no significant change; ND, no data.

Data from References 1, 2, 4, 39, and 53-56.

TABLE 112-7 Dosing of Medications for Osteoporosis

Medication	Brand Name	Dose	Comments
Antiresorptive Medications—Nutritional Supplements			
Calcium	Various	Adequate daily intake: *IOM:* 200-1,200 mg/day, varies per age; see Table 112-5); supplement dose is the difference between required adequate intake and dietary intake. Immediate-release doses should be <500-600 mg.	Recommend food sources first to achieve goal intake. Available in different salts including carbonate and citrate, absorption of other salts not fully quantified. Different formulations including chewable, liquid, gummy, softgel, drink, and wafer; different combination products. Review package to determine number of units per serving size and desired amount of elemental calcium. Give calcium carbonate with meals to improve absorption.
Vitamin D D3 (cholecalciferol) D2 (ergocalciferol)	**Over the counter** • Tablets, 400, 1,000, and 2,000 units • Capsules, 400, 1,000, 2,000, 5,000, and 10,000 units • Gummies, 300, 500, and 1,000 units • Drops, 300, 400, 1,000, and 2,000 units/mL or drop • Solution, 400 and 5,000 units/mL • Spray, 1,000 and 5,000 units/spray • Creams and lotions, 500 and 1,000 units per ¼ teaspoonful **Prescription** • Capsule, 50,000 units • Solution, 8,000 units/mL	Adequate daily intake: IOM: 400-800 units/day to achieve adequate intake (see Table 112-5); guidelines: 800-2,000 units orally daily; if low 25(OH) vitamin D concentrations, malabsorption, or altered metabolism higher doses (>2,000 units daily) might be required. Vitamin D deficiency: 5,000 units or higher daily preferred over 50,000 units orally once to twice weekly for 8-12 weeks; repeat as needed. Higher doses until therapeutic concentrations reached.	Vegetarians and vegans need to read label to determine if the vitamin D source is plant-based. Slight advantage of D3 over D2 for increasing serum 25(OH) vitamin D concentrations. For drops, make sure measurement is correct for desired dose. Ability of sprays, lotions, and creams to resolve deficiencies or maintain adequate intakes is unknown.

(Continued)

TABLE 112-7 Dosing of Medications for Osteoporosis (*Continued*)

Medication	Brand Name	Dose	Comments
Antiresorptive Prescription Medications			
Bisphosphonates			
Alendronate	Fosamax Fosamax Plus D Binosto (effervescent tablet)	Treatment: 10 mg orally daily or 70 mg orally weekly Prevention: 5 mg orally daily or 35 mg orally weekly	Generic available, effervescent tablet is brand only. 70-mg dose is available as a tablet, effervescent tablet, solution, or combination tablet with 2,800 or 5,600 units of vitamin D3. Administered in the morning on an empty stomach with 6-8 ounces (180-240 mL) of plain water. Do not eat and remain upright for at least 30 minutes following administration. Do not coadminister with any other medications or supplements, including calcium and vitamin D. Caution if CrCl <35 mL/min (0.58 mL/s).
Ibandronate	Boniva	Treatment: 150 mg orally monthly, 3-mg intravenous quarterly Prevention: 150 mg orally monthly	Generics available. Administration instructions same as alendronate, except must delay eating and remain upright for at least 60 minutes. Caution if CrCl <30 mL/min (0.50 mL/s).
Risedronate	Actonel Atelvia (delayed-release)	Treatment and prevention: 5 mg orally daily, 35 mg orally weekly, 150 mg orally monthly	Generics available. 35-mg dose is also available as a delayed-release product. Administration instructions same as for alendronate, except delayed-release product is taken immediately following breakfast with at least 120 mL (ounces) of plain water. Caution if CrCl <30 mL/min (0.50 mL/s).
Zoledronic acid	Reclast	Treatment: 5-mg intravenous infusion yearly Prevention: 5-mg intravenous infusion every 2 years	Generic available. Can premedicate with acetaminophen to decrease infusion reactions. Contraindicated if CrCl <35 mL/min (0.58 mL/s). Also marketed under the brand name Zometa (4 mg) with different dosing for oncology-related indications.
RANK Ligand Inhibitor			
Denosumab	Prolia	Treatment: 60-mg subcutaneously every 6 months	Administered by a healthcare practitioner. Correct hypocalcemia before administration. Also marketed under the brand name Xgeva (70 mg/mL) with different dosing for treatment of hypercalcemia of malignancy, multiple myeloma, bone metastases from solid tumors, and giant cell tumor of bone.
Estrogen Agonist/Antagonist and Tissue Selective Estrogen Complex			
Raloxifene	Evista	60 mg daily	Generic available.
Bazedoxifene with conjugated equine estrogens (CEE)	Duavee	20 mg plus 0.45 mg CEE daily	For postmenopausal women with a uterus; no progestogen needed. Bazedoxifene monotherapy available in some countries.
Calcitonin			
Calcitonin (salmon)	Fortical	200 units (1 spray) intranasally daily, alternating nares every other day.	Nasal formulation only available as a generic. Refrigerate nasal spray until opened for daily use, then room temperature. Prime with first use. Also available as a subcutaneous injection.
Formation Medications			
Recombinant Human Parathyroid Hormone (PTH 1-34 units)			
Teriparatide	Forteo Bonsity	20-mcg subcutaneously daily	First dose sitting or lying. Refrigerate before and after each use. Use new needle with each dose. Inject in thigh or abdomen. Discard after 28 days or if cloudy. Forteo and Bonsity not interchangeable.

(*Continued*)

TABLE 112-7 Dosing of Medications for Osteoporosis (*Continued*)

Medication	Brand Name	Dose	Comments
Human Parathyroid Hormone–Related Peptide (PTHrP [1-34]) Analog			
Abaloparatide	Tymlos	80-mcg subcutaneously daily for up to 2 years	First dose sitting or lying. Refrigerate before use then keep at room temperature. Use new needle with each dose. Inject in abdomen. Discard after 30 days.
Formation and Antiresorptive Medication			
Sclerostin Inhibitor			
Romosozumab	Evenity	210-mg subcutaneously monthly for 1 year; administered as two single use 105-mg/1.17-mL prefilled syringes	Correct hypocalcemia before administration. Refrigerate. Leave at room temperature for at least 30 minutes before use. Provider administration, exploring patient self-administration. Inject in abdomen, thigh, or upper arm; preferably each injection at a different site.

IOM, Institute of Medicine; NSAID, nonsteroidal anti-inflammatory drug.

TABLE 112-8 Medication Adverse Reactions and Monitoring

Medication	Adverse Reactions	Monitoring Parameters	Comments
Antiresorptive Medications—Nutritional Supplements			
Calcium	Constipation, gas, upset stomach, kidney stones	Dietary calcium intake, constipation	Education about a bowel healthy lifestyle (eg, adequate water, fiber, and exercise).
Vitamin D	Hypercalcemia, hypercalciuria, weakness, headache, somnolence, nausea Rare: cardiac rhythm disturbance	Serum 25(OH) vitamin D concentration, symptoms	Adverse effects usually not experienced until 25(OH) vitamin D concentration more than 100-150 ng/mL (mcg/L; 250-375 nmol/L), which are generally not achieved with recommended therapeutic doses.
Antiresorptive Prescription Medications			
Bisphosphonates			
Bisphosphonates	Dyspepsia (oral), transient or chronic musculoskeletal pain, nausea, transient flu-like illness (injectable) Rare: GI perforation, ulceration, and/or bleeding (oral); osteonecrosis of the jaw; atypical femoral shaft fracture, severe musculoskeletal pain	Bone density, fractures, GI symptoms, muscle aches Serum calcium for zoledronic acid	Adherence is suboptimal, thus it should be assessed frequently. Assess correct use of product with refills. Risk outweighs benefit in pregnancy, use prior to or during pregnancy might cause fetal medication exposure.
RANK Ligand Inhibitor			
Denosumab	Back pain, arthralgia, eczema, dermatitis, and infection Rare: osteonecrosis of the jaw, atypical femoral shaft fracture	Bone density, fractures, serum calcium	REMS: Medication guide and monitoring plan due to risks of hypocalcemia, osteonecrosis of the jaw, atypical femoral shaft fractures, serious infections, and dermatologic adverse reactions. Contraindicated in pregnancy.
Estrogen Agonist/Antagonist and Tissue Selective Estrogen Complex			
Raloxifene	Hot flushes, leg pain, spasms, or cramps, peripheral edema, venous thromboembolism (warm swollen leg, chest pain, shortness of breath, coughing up blood, and change in vision)	Bone density, fractures, hot flushes, leg cramps, and blood clots	Contraindicated in pregnancy. Warning for fatal stroke; rare events predominantly seen in women at high-risk for stroke.
Bazedoxifene with conjugated equine estrogens	Similar to raloxifene and estrogens	Bone density, fractures, leg cramps, blood clots	Contraindicated in pregnancy.
Calcitonin			
Calcitonin (salmon)	Rhinitis, epistaxis	Bone density, fractures, nasal irritation	Limited information regarding use in pregnancy.
Formation Prescription Medications			
Recombinant Human Parathyroid Hormone (PTH 1-34 units) Analog			
Teriparatide	Orthostasis with first few injections, pain at injection site, nausea, headache, dizziness, leg cramps, increase in uric acid, transient hypercalcemia, hypercalciuria	Bone density, fractures, trough serum calcium concentration 1 month after therapy initiation, urinary calcium if prior hypercalciuria or active urolithiasis	If serum calcium is high (>10.6 mg/dL [2.65 mmol/L]), calcium intake should be decreased. Warning about osteosarcoma in rats and therefore contraindicated in patients at high risk for this adverse event. In pregnancy, adverse events noted in animal studies. Not for use in pregnancy.

(*Continued*)

TABLE 112-8 Medication Adverse Reactions and Monitoring (*Continued*)

Medication	Adverse Reactions	Monitoring Parameters	Comments
Human Parathyroid Hormone–Related Peptide [PTHrP (1-34)] Analog			
Abaloparatide	Orthostasis with first few injections, pain at injection site, headache, dizziness, leg cramps, increase in uric acid, hypercalcemia, hypercalciuria	Bone density, fractures, serum calcium concentration, urinary calcium if prior hypercalciuria or active urolithiasis	Warning about osteosarcoma in rats and therefore contraindicated in patients at high risk for this adverse event. Not for use in pregnancy.
Formation and Antiresorptive Prescription Medication			
Sclerostin Inhibitor			
Romosozumab	Arthralgias, headache, muscle spasms, hypocalcemia, mild injection site pain, myocardial infarction, stroke, cardiovascular death. Antibody production with some neutralizing, an effect on efficacy or toxicity not reported. Rare: osteonecrosis of the jaw, atypical femoral fractures	Bone density, fractures, joint pain, injection site, serum calcium prior to and during therapy	Box warning about myocardial infarction, stroke, and cardiovascular death. Not for use in pregnancy.

REMS, risk evaluation and mitigation strategies.

Data from Reference 1; product prescribing labeling.

vitamin D, especially when osteoporosis medications are taken.[2,34,39] If dietary intake cannot be increased to achieve adequate intake, calcium supplements can be used.

Efficacy Calcium generally maintains BMD, although small BMD increases (0.6%-1.8%) have been documented.[2,59] These BMD effects are less than those observed with other osteoporosis medications. A USPSTF report states insufficient data exist to support using calcium and vitamin D supplementation to reduce fracture incidence.

Adverse Events Calcium's most common adverse reaction, constipation, can first be treated with increased water intake, dietary fiber, and exercise. If still unresolved, smaller and more frequent calcium administration or a lower total daily dose can be tried. Calcium carbonate can create gas and cause upset stomach. Calcium citrate, a formulation with fewer GI side effects, is often recommended if calcium carbonate is not tolerated.

Calcium supplementation when combined with vitamin D can increase the risk of kidney stone formation. However, in some cases, calcium binds to oxalate in the gut, which decreases urinary oxalate excretion thereby decreasing kidney stones. Increased fluid intake and decreased salt intake might be warranted to prevent kidney stones. Calcium supplements resulting in total calcium intakes above the upper limit of intake can slightly increase coronary artery calcification and cardiovascular disease events.[1,31,60]

Interactions Since calcium carbonate requires acid for disintegration, medications such as proton pump inhibitors and histamine type-2 receptor antagonists can decrease absorption from the carbonate product.[31] Fiber laxatives can also decrease the absorption of calcium if given concomitantly. Calcium can decrease the oral absorption of some medications including iron, tetracyclines, quinolones, bisphosphonates, and thyroid supplements.

Dosing and Administration Many patients, especially those aged 60 years or older, do not ingest sufficient dietary calcium and therefore require supplements. To ensure adequate calcium absorption, 25(OH) vitamin D concentrations should be at least 10 to 15 ng/mL (mcg/L; 25-37 nmol/L). Because fractional calcium absorption is dose-limited, maximum single doses of 500 to 600 mg or less of elemental calcium are recommended.[2] Despite this, slow-release and/or absorbable calcium formulations (eg, Citracal Slow Release 1,200) are available in doses of 1,200 mg and advertised to be taken once daily. These high-dose products are sometimes two 600-mg tablets that can be taken at different times. Supplemental doses this high are usually not needed unless a severe dietary deficiency of calcium exists. Calcium carbonate is the salt of choice as it contains the highest amount of elemental calcium (40%) and is typically the least expensive. Calcium carbonate should be taken with meals, which increases gastric acidity resulting in product disintegration and dissolution. Calcium citrate (21% elemental calcium) has acid-independent absorption and does not need to be administered with meals. Although tricalcium phosphate contains 38% elemental calcium, calcium-phosphate complexes could limit overall calcium absorption. This product might be helpful in patients with hypophosphatemia that cannot be resolved with increased dietary intake.

Disintegration and dissolution rates vary significantly between products and lots. Products labeled United States Pharmacopeia "USP Verified" should be recommended. This indicates that the products have undergone the voluntary USP verification program, which ensures that the product contains the ingredients shown on the label at the stated strength/potency, and has been produced using safe, clean, and controlled manufacturing processes as specified by the USP and the US Food and Drug Administration (FDA). Products from unrefined oyster shell or coral calcium should not be recommended because of concerns for high concentrations of lead and other heavy metals. Some calcium products come in alternative dosage forms (eg, chewable tablets, dissolvable tablets, and liquid), which can be beneficial for select patients with issues such as swallowing large tablets. For all products, encourage patients to read the labeling carefully as the serving size is often more than just one tablet. In addition, product labeling sometimes recommends taking doses providing 1,000 to 1,200 mg/day, which often provides more calcium than needed to meet IOM requirements and could exceed tolerable upper limits when dietary calcium intake is adequate.

Some commercial calcium supplements contain other nutrients associated with bone physiology such as magnesium, vitamin K, "natural estrogens," or isoflavones. Minimal BMD and no fracture data exist for these combination products. These products are also typically more expensive. Additionally, combining too many vitamins and supplements might exceed upper-tolerable nutrient limits and increase toxicities.

Vitamin D Supplementation 8 The IOM recommends adequate intakes of vitamin D from diet and/or supplementation for all ages (see Table 112-5). Current osteoporosis guidelines recommend slightly higher vitamin D maintenance doses (800-2,000 units daily).[2,34,38]

The desired therapeutic range for vitamin D is controversial. The IOM defines 20 ng/mL (50 nmol/L; 1 ng/mL = 2.5 nmol/L) as the cut point for normal 25(OH) vitamin D, below which a patient would be considered deficient. Current guidelines recommend treating patients with osteoporosis to a concentration of at least 20 ng/mL (mcg/L; 50 nmol/L) or 30 to 50 ng/mL (mcg/L; 75-125 nmol/L) 25(OH) vitamin D. Concentrations higher than 50 to 60 ng/mL (mcg/L; 125-150 nmol/L) can be associated with adverse effects.[2,38]

The major effects of vitamin D are achieved with 25(OH) vitamin D concentrations between 6 and 20 ng/mL (mcg/L; 15-50 nmol/L), including increasing calcium absorption (16 ng/mL [mcg/L; 40 nmol/L]) and decreasing BMD loss (up to 20 ng/mL [mcg/L; 50 nmol/L]).[61] Daily vitamin D doses of 500 to 700 units generally are sufficient to achieve vitamin D concentrations more than 20 ng/mL (mcg/L; 50 nmol/L), leading some experts to suggest the higher daily doses recommended in guidelines are not warranted. Other experts state not everyone achieves a 25(OH) vitamin D concentration greater than 30 ng/mL (mcg/L; 75 nmol/L), and therefore recommend 800 to 2,000 units daily, especially in adults at high risk or with osteoporosis. Furthermore, since most products are inexpensive and safe, the higher recommended doses are appropriate.[2,34,39] These higher recommendations are within the upper limit for vitamin D in adults, which is 4,000 units daily.

Serum 25(OH) vitamin D is the best indicator of total body vitamin D status.[42] Interassay variability exists; thus, the same laboratory should be used for repeat testing. Measurement of 25(OH) vitamin D concentration can be considered in anyone with high risk for low vitamin D, low bone density, history of a low-trauma fracture, frequent falls, unexplained muscle weakness, and/or bone pain.

Efficacy Supplemental vitamin D given at doses of 700 to 800 units per day significantly reduces the incidence of both hip and nonvertebral fractures.[2] Small increases in BMD, improvement in muscle strength, and improvement in balance have also been observed. Several studies have analyzed the effect of supplemental vitamin D on falls; however, the USPSTF recommends against the use of supplemental vitamin D specifically for fall prevention.[24]

Interactions Some medications can induce vitamin D metabolism including rifampin, phenytoin, barbiturates, valproic acid, and carbamazepine. Vitamin D absorption can be decreased by cholestyramine, colestipol, orlistat, and mineral oil. Vitamin D can enhance the absorption of aluminum; therefore aluminum-containing products should be avoided to prevent aluminum toxicity.

Dosing and Administration Dosing of supplemental vitamin D should be based on IOM adequate intakes (see Table 112-5) or to achieve a 25(OH) vitamin D concentration of ≥30 ng/mL (mcg/L; 75 nmol/L), especially in those with osteoporosis.[2] Almost 30% of older adults have hypovitaminosis D (≤20 ng/mL [mcg/L; 50 nmol/L]), with higher prevalence in Black (72%) and Hispanic (43%) patients.[43,62] Replenishment doses will first be required in these patients before recommended maintenance doses.

Vitamin D can be taken as a single-agent or combination product. Supplements and multivitamins contain vitamin D3 or D2. Synthesized vitamin D3 can be made from irradiated sheep's wool and vitamin D2 from irradiated mushrooms. Guidelines suggest either product for prevention and treatment of vitamin D deficiency. Current guidelines recommend dosing with 5,000 units once daily for 8-12 weeks to achieve a target 25(OH) vitamin D concentration of ≥30 ng/mL (mcg/L; 75 nmol/L), followed by a maintenance dose of 1,000 to 2,000 units daily.[2,63] The preferred dosage form is vitamin D_3 (cholecalciferol).[2] Higher-dose prescription vitamin D regimens have less support[8] but are sometimes used,[63] especially when adherence and cost are concerns. An example regimen is 50,000 units given once weekly for 8 to 12 weeks, or until the 25(OH) vitamin D concentration reaches 30 ng/mL (mcg/L; 75 nmol/L), followed by 1,000 to 2,000 units daily to maintain this concentration. More than one multivitamin or large doses of cod liver oil daily are no longer advocated because of the risk of hypervitaminosis A, which can increase bone loss. Because the half-life of vitamin D is about 1 month, approximately 3 months of therapy are required before a new steady state is achieved and a repeat 25(OH)-vitamin D concentration should be obtained to assess efficacy of therapy.

Individuals with deficient concentrations of vitamin D are at risk for osteomalacia, a condition that can be mistaken for osteoporosis, which is characterized by decreased mineralization or "softening" of bone matrix. In patients who are pregnant, obese, or with disorders (eg, celiac disease, cystic fibrosis, Crohn's disease, chronic kidney disease) or medications (eg, anticonvulsants, glucocorticoids, antifungals, and antiretroviral medications used in treatment of acquired immunodeficiency syndrome) affecting vitamin D absorption and/or metabolism, higher doses and more frequent monitoring might be required.

Bisphosphonates 9 Alendronate, risedronate, and intravenous zoledronic acid are approved by the FDA for postmenopausal, male, and glucocorticoid-induced osteoporosis. Intravenous and oral ibandronate and some specialized oral formulations of other bisphosphonates are indicated only for postmenopausal osteoporosis.

Pharmacology Bisphosphonates mimic pyrophosphate, an endogenous bone resorption inhibitor.[2,64] Bisphosphonate antiresorptive activity results from binding to hydroxyapatite in bone with preference for areas with active bone remodeling. This leads to decreased osteoclast maturation, number, recruitment, bone adhesion, and life span.

Pharmacokinetics

Oral bisphosphonate bioavailability is less than 1% and is greatly decreased with concomitant food and beverages.[64,65] Within 24 hours of administration, bisphosphonates undergo rapid skeletal uptake and any medication not incorporated into bone is renally excreted. Elimination decreases linearly with declining renal function. Incorporation into bone gives bisphosphonates long biologic half-lives of up to 10 years. Bisphosphonates differ in the strength of binding to bone (zoledronic acid greater than alendronate which is greater than ibandronate which is greater than risedronate) with zoledronic acid having the greatest bone absorption and longest bone retention.

Efficacy Bisphosphonates consistently provide fracture risk reduction and BMD increases (see Table 112-6) with noted difference in sites of fracture reduction between agents.[53] Fracture clinical trial data are from daily oral bisphosphonate or annual intravenous therapy, not weekly, monthly, or quarterly regimens.[65] Bisphosphonate comparative fracture prevention trials do not exist. Hip-fracture reduction has not been demonstrated with daily oral ibandronate; however, the study might have been underpowered.[2] Because of the lack of hip-fracture reduction data, ibandronate is not a first-line therapy (see Fig. 112-3). Annual intravenous zoledronic acid has documented secondary fracture prevention and a decrease in mortality when given after a first hip fracture.[53] Administration of intravenous zoledronic acid at an extended 18-month interval in women 65 years of age or older with osteopenia also decreased both vertebral and nonvertebral fractures over 6 years.

Bone turnover reaches an equilibrium with a lower rate of bone turnover evident within 3 to 6 months of bisphosphonate starting therapy, which results in BMD increases and a reduced fracture risk seen within the first 6 to 12 months.[53,65] For all bisphosphonates, increases in BMD are typically greater at the spine than at the hip.[53] Small increases in BMD continue for 4 to 5 years before plateauing. After discontinuation, the increased BMD is sustained for a prolonged period of time that varies based on different binding affinities of the individual bisphosphonates.[2] Because of the sustained effects, drug holidays can be considered for bisphosphonates.

The BMD increases with alendronate, risedronate, zoledronic acid, and oral ibandronate in men are similar to those in postmenopausal women.[6] Because of a lack of fracture data from pivotal trials in men, bisphosphonates are only FDA indicated to increase BMD, not to reduce fracture risk in men. However, no evidence suggests that efficacy profiles are expected to be different in men.

Adverse Effects Oral bisphosphonates are well tolerated if patients are selected for therapy appropriately and the patient takes them correctly (see Table 112-8). Patients with creatinine clearances (CrCl) less than 30 to 35 mL/min (0.50-0.58 mL/s), who have serious GI conditions (abnormalities of the esophagus that delay emptying, such as stricture or achalasia), or who are pregnant should not take bisphosphonates. Some evidence suggest bisphosphonates can be used in select patients with age-related decline in renal function without added adverse effects.

GI complaints, including heartburn and dyspepsia, are one of the most common reasons cited by patients for discontinuing therapy.[2,65] While these mild GI effects are common, bisphosphonates are also associated with rare severe GI events, such as esophageal erosion, ulcer, or GI bleeding. If GI adverse events occur, switching to a different bisphosphonate or less frequent administration schedule might resolve the problem. Patients should be encouraged to discuss GI complaints with a healthcare provider. Intravenous zoledronic acid or ibandronate can be used for patients with GI contraindications or intolerances to oral bisphosphonates. Other common bisphosphonate adverse effects include injection reactions and musculoskeletal pain. If severe musculoskeletal pain occurs, the medication can be discontinued temporarily or permanently. Acute phase reactions (eg, fever, flu-like symptoms, myalgias, and arthralgias) are typically associated with intravenous administration, but rarely reported with oral bisphosphonates. This reaction usually diminishes with subsequent administration.

Rare adverse effects include osteonecrosis of the jaw (ONJ) and subtrochanteric femoral (atypical) fractures.[2] ONJ occurs more commonly in patients with cancer, receiving higher-dose intravenous bisphosphonate therapy. In osteoporosis, the incidence of ONJ is 0.001% to 0.01%. Maxillary or mandibular bone surgery and poor oral hygiene are dental-specific risk factors for development of ONJ. When possible, major dental work should be completed before bisphosphonate initiation. For patients already on therapy, some practitioners withhold bisphosphonate therapy during and after major dental procedures, but no data exist to support any benefit of such practice. Atypical femoral shaft fractures are rare but can occur without trauma. Some evidence suggests the risk could increase with longer duration of bisphosphonate use (greater than 5 years). Since some patients with atypical fracture experience prodromal thigh or hip pain, any such pain should be evaluated.

Interactions Because of poor bioavailability, oral bisphosphonates should not be administered at the same time as other medications. The administration instructions described below should be followed.

Dosing and Administration Because bioavailability is poor for bisphosphonates and to minimize GI side effects, each oral tablet should be taken with at least 6 ounces (~180 mL) of plain water (not coffee, juice, mineral water, or milk) at least 30 minutes (60 minutes for ibandronate) before consuming any food, supplements (including calcium and vitamin D), or medications (see Table 112-7). The patient should also remain upright (ie, either sitting or standing) for at least 30 minutes after alendronate and risedronate and 1 hour after ibandronate administration. For patients with swallowing difficulties (eg, stroke and tube feeding), an effervescent tablet form of alendronate, which is dissolved in 4 ounces (~120 mL) of room temperature water, could be used. This formulation has the same food restrictions as traditional oral tablets. In contrast, delayed-release risedronate is available, and it is administered immediately following breakfast with at least 4 ounces (~120 mL) of plain water. A patient who misses a weekly dose can take it the next day. If more than 1 day has lapsed, that dose is skipped. If a patient misses a monthly dose, it can be taken up to 7 days before the next administration.

Before intravenous bisphosphonates are used, the patient's serum calcium concentration must be normal. Serum creatinine should be monitored before each dose of zoledronic acid. The intravenous products need to be administered by a healthcare provider. The quarterly ibandronate injection is given intravenously over 15 to 30 seconds or can be diluted and given with a syringe pump. Zoledronic acid should be infused once yearly over at least 15 minutes with a pump. Acetaminophen can be given to decrease acute phase reactions.

Although these medications are effective, adherence is poor and results in decreased effectiveness.[2,66] Adherence is improved with once-weekly bisphosphonate administration over daily therapy; however, it is unclear if once-monthly therapy improves adherence more. While dosing frequency is a common barrier to adherence, adverse effects and concerns about adverse effects remain important predictors of adherence and persistence. Using decision aids in discussions about medication therapy choices and periodic follow-up with a healthcare professional could improve adherence and persistence to therapy. These decision aids visually display the pros of bisphosphonate therapy (ie, fracture avoidance) to the cons (ie, adverse effects) based on an individualized fracture risk.[67] To help overcome barriers associated with oral dosing frequency, intravenous ibandronate and zoledronic acid could be used as alternatives.

Duration The ideal duration of bisphosphonate therapy is not known.[2] Bisphosphonates are deposited into the bone and continue to suppress bone turnover after discontinuation. Some adverse effects, such as atypical fracture, are associated with duration of therapy. To balance risk and benefit, some clinicians recommend a "bisphosphonate/drug holiday," defined as disruption of therapy during which medication effects exist with a plan for medication reinstitution. Two randomized, double-blind studies with a bisphosphonate/drug holiday after therapy with alendronate for 5 years or zoledronic acid for 3 years showed a continued fracture benefit after discontinuation of therapy. Because a beneficial response was predicted by hip T-score, experts recommend that a bisphosphonate holiday could be considered in postmenopausal women after 5 years of oral bisphosphonates or 3 years of intravenous bisphosphonates if no significant fracture history, hip BMD T-score is above −2.5, and fracture risk is not high. In women initially with very high fracture-risk who remain high-risk, continuing oral bisphosphonates for 10 years or intravenous bisphosphonates for 6 years should be considered. These recommendations are based on limited data and questions remain regarding what therapy to reinitiate and the applicability of this approach for men and patients with glucocorticoid-induced osteoporosis. Patients should be monitored during the drug holiday and restarting therapy considered if fractures occur or if there are significant BMD losses.

Denosumab (9) Denosumab is approved by FDA for the treatment of osteoporosis in postmenopausal women and men at high risk for fracture. It is also approved for glucocorticoid-induced osteoporosis and to increase bone mass in men receiving androgen deprivation therapy for nonmetastatic prostate cancer and in women receiving adjuvant aromatase inhibitor therapy for breast cancer who are at high risk for fracture.

Pharmacology Denosumab is a fully human monoclonal antibody that binds to RANKL, blocking its ability to bind to its RANK receptor on the surface of osteoclast precursor cells and mature osteoclasts.[68] Denosumab inhibits osteoclastogenesis and increases osteoclast apoptosis.

Pharmacokinetics Following subcutaneous injection, rapid suppression of bone turnover occurs within 12 hours.[68,69] Denosumab achieves peak concentration in approximately 10 days. The half-life is approximately 25 days, and the concentration slowly declines over a period of 4 to 5 months. The medication does not accumulate with repeated dosing at 6-month intervals. No dosage adjustment is necessary in renal impairment; however, hypocalcemia is more common in severe renal impairment. No studies have been conducted in hepatic impairment.

Efficacy Over 3 years, denosumab significantly decreased vertebral fractures, nonvertebral fractures, and hip fractures in postmenopausal women with low bone density (see Table 112-6).[53] Continued increases in BMD are demonstrated with long-term treatment over 10 years. For postmenopausal women previously treated with oral bisphosphonates, switching to denosumab for 1 year provided greater increases in BMD at the spine and hip over switching to zoledronic acid; however, fracture outcomes are unknown.[2] Denosumab is not incorporated into bone and drug holidays are not recommended. Upon medication discontinuation, a rapid increase in bone turnover above baseline is noted with a corresponding loss of protection against vertebral fractures and case reports of multiple vertebral fracture. Therefore, for those with high fracture risk, denosumab therapy should be continued or alternative antiresorptive therapy (ie, bisphosphonate) should be initiated if denosumab is discontinued.

Adverse Events In trials up to 10 years in duration, denosumab was generally well tolerated (see Table 112-8).[2] Dermatologic reactions not specific to the injection site and serious infections were noted in initial clinical trials, although an increased incidence has not been noted in long-term, follow-up trials nor with denosumab used in higher doses (Xgeva) for oncologic indications.[2]

As with bisphosphonates, rare, serious adverse effects from bone turnover suppression have been reported with denosumab including ONJ and atypical femoral fracture.[68] Major dental work should be completed before use when possible. Hypocalcemia can occur and any existing hypocalcemia should be corrected prior to use. Severe hypocalcemia is more common in patients with underlying kidney dysfunction. The manufacturer recommends monitoring of serum calcium, magnesium, and phosphorus within 14 days of administration in those with a CrCl less than 30 mL/min (0.50 mL/s).

Interactions No interactions have been identified with denosumab.

Dosing and Administration Denosumab is administered subcutaneously in the upper arm, upper thigh, or abdomen by a healthcare professional including pharmacists in some states. The product is available as a refrigerated prefilled syringe that can be stored at room temperature up to 14 days before administration (see Table 112-7).

Duration After 5 to 10 years of therapy, patients should be reevaluated for medication continuation, discontinuation, or switching to a different medication.

Mixed Estrogen Agonists/Antagonists and Tissue Selective Estrogen Complexes (9) Raloxifene is a second-generation mixed estrogen agonist/antagonist (EAA; previously known as a selective estrogen receptor modulator, or SERM) approved by the FDA for prevention and treatment of postmenopausal osteoporosis and for reducing the risk of invasive breast cancer in postmenopausal women with and without osteoporosis. Raloxifene might be considered as a treatment option for women with no to minimal postmenopausal symptoms at low risk for hip fracture and with an increased breast cancer risk. Bazedoxifene is a third-generation EAA combined with conjugated equine estrogens (CEE) making it a TSEC that is approved by FDA for prevention of postmenopausal osteoporosis and vasomotor menopausal symptoms.[55,56] Bazedoxifene with CEE can be considered for younger postmenopausal women with a uterus, menopausal symptoms, and at risk for osteoporosis.[2,4,55,56]

Pharmacology EAAs bind with α- and β-estrogen receptors and coactivators or corepressors to cause varying agonist or antagonist effects at different tissue sites.[55,56] Raloxifene is an agonist at bone receptors and antagonist at breast receptors and has minimal effect on the uterus. Bazedoxifene is an agonist at bone, and antagonist at the uterus and breast; however, reduction in breast cancer risk has not yet been demonstrated in large-scale clinical trials.

Pharmacokinetics Food has a nonsignificant effect on absorption, which is about 2% for raloxifene and 6% for bazedoxifene due to extensive presystemic glucuronidation.[56,70,71] Raloxifene is 95% protein bound. The half-life of both raloxifene and bazedoxifene is 28 hours. EAAs are predominantly metabolized via glucuronidation and eliminated in the feces.

Efficacy Raloxifene and bazedoxifene decrease vertebral but not hip fractures. In a post hoc analysis of the Multiple Outcomes with Raloxifene Evaluation trial, raloxifene decreased nonvertebral fractures in postmenopausal women with the most severe vertebral fractures at baseline. Bazedoxifene also decreased nonvertebral fractures in a subgroup of women with a higher fracture risk at baseline.[55,56] The fracture prevention effects of bazedoxifene combined with CEE are not known. EAAs increase spine and hip BMD, but to a lesser extent than bisphosphonates (see Table 112-6). Raloxifene's vertebral fracture prevention is greater in women without previous fracture.[4] Upon discontinuation, the medication effect of EAAs is lost, with bone loss returning to age- or disease-related bone loss rates. EAAs have a positive impact on the lipid profile but have not demonstrated a benefit on cardiovascular disease.[4,55]

Adverse Events Hot flushes are common with raloxifene but decreased with bazedoxifene with CEE (see Table 112-8).[55,56,70,71] Raloxifene rarely causes endometrial thickening and bleeding; bazedoxifene decreases these adverse events making progestogen therapy unnecessary when it is combined with CEE. Leg cramps and muscle spasms are also common with both medications. Thromboembolic events are uncommon (less than 1.5%), but can be fatal. In large trials, no change in overall death, cardiovascular death, or overall stroke incidence was seen with raloxifene; however, a slight increase in fatal stroke (0.7/1,000 women – year difference) was documented, which resulted in a boxed warning for raloxifene.[55] Fatal stroke with raloxifene occurred most frequently in women with an increased risk of stroke at baseline. Bazedoxifene with CEE also has all the adverse effects listed for estrogens as a class including increased thromboembolic events.

Interactions Because of raloxifene's highly protein bound nature (95%), when given concomitantly with other highly protein bound medications, like warfarin, a potential for binding interactions exists and, therefore, monitoring of both medications is suggested. Cholestyramine can decrease raloxifene absorption. Rifampin, phenytoin, carbamazepine, and phenobarbital can decrease bazedoxifene concentrations by inducing intestinal and liver uridine diphosphate glucuronosyltransferase (UGT) metabolism. Estrogen metabolism is altered with CYP3A4 and CYP1A2 inducers and inhibitors.

Dosing and Administration EAAs/TSECs are administered orally once daily (see Table 112-7).[70,71] They are contraindicated for women with an active or past history of venous thromboembolic disease, pregnancy, or childbearing potential. Therapy should be stopped if a patient anticipates extended immobility. Women at high risk for a stroke or coronary events and those with known coronary artery disease, peripheral vascular disease, atrial fibrillation, or a prior history of cerebrovascular events might not be good candidates for EAAs/TSECs. These medications should be used with caution in patients with severe liver impairment or moderate-to-severe renal impairment due to a lack of data. Bazedoxifene with CEE has all the contraindications and precautions for estrogens as a class.

Calcitonin (9) Calcitonin is FDA-indicated for osteoporosis treatment for women who are at least 5 years past menopause.[72] Intranasal calcitonin therapy (200 units daily) decreases vertebral fractures alone with no fracture reduction demonstrated with higher and lower doses (see Table 112-6).[2] Once calcitonin is discontinued, the benefits are lost over the next 1 to 2 years. A meta-analysis revealed a higher incidence of cancer in patients taking calcitonin. While the FDA found that evidence was insufficient for a causal relationship, calcitonin is considered a last-line therapy since there are more effective treatment options. Intranasal calcitonin might provide some short-term pain relief to some patients with acute vertebral fractures.

Dosing and Administration Some patients do not like to administer medications intranasally (see Table 112-7). In clinical trials of calcitonin, a high dropout rate exists. If the nasal product is used for vertebral fracture pain, calcitonin should be prescribed for short-term (4 weeks) treatment and should not be used in place of other more effective and less-expensive analgesics nor should it preclude the use of more appropriate osteoporosis therapy.

Hormone Therapies

Estrogen In women, estrogens with or without a progestogen significantly decrease fracture risk and bone loss (see Table 112-6).[2,4,34,36] Estrogen therapy is approved by FDA for prevention of postmenopausal osteoporosis but not for treatment. For women going through early menopause, estrogen therapy can be considered when protection against bone loss is needed in addition to reduction of vasomotor symptoms.[4,73] Other anti-osteoporosis therapies are reserved for treatment closer to the average age of natural menopause. Estrogens should not be prescribed solely for the prevention or treatment of osteoporosis if other anti-osteoporosis therapies can be used.[1,2,38] Oral and transdermal estrogens at equivalent doses and continuous or cyclic hormone therapy regimens have similar BMD effects. Effect on BMD is dose-dependent, with some benefit seen with lower estrogen doses. Fracture risk reduction has not been demonstrated with the lower doses. When estrogen therapy is discontinued, bone loss accelerates and fracture protection is lost. A complete discussion of adverse events, drug interactions, dosing, and administration for estrogen can be found in Chapter 102, "Hormone Therapy in Women."

Testosterone No fracture data are available, but some data demonstrate BMD improvements with testosterone use.[74] Testosterone is used to treat hypogonadism in men, but an osteoporosis medication should be added when risk for osteoporotic fracture is high.[12,74] A complete discussion of adverse events, drug interactions, dosing, and administration for testosterone products for men can be found in Chapter 103, "Erectile Dysfunction."

Formation Medications

Parathyroid Hormone Analogs

9 Abaloparatide is an analog of PTHrP and teriparatide is an analog of PTH.[2,54] These agents are FDA-indicated for the treatment of postmenopausal women with osteoporosis at high risk for fracture defined as multiple risk factors for fracture, a history of osteoporotic fracture, or failed or intolerant to other therapies. Teriparatide is additionally approved by FDA for osteoporosis in men who are at high risk for fracture or intolerant to other osteoporosis medications and glucocorticoid-induced osteoporosis. Patients who have a very high fracture risk, history of osteoporotic fracture, low bone density (eg, T-score less than −3.5), or have failed or are intolerant of previous bisphosphonate therapy could be candidates for PTH analog therapy.

Pharmacology Teriparatide is a recombinant human product representing the first 34 amino acids in human PTH.[54] Unlike continuous PTH effects from primary hyperparathyroidism that can decrease BMD, when administered intermittently (ie, subcutaneously once daily) teriparatide increases bone formation with a minor increase in bone resorption for a net anabolic effect. Abaloparatide is a synthetic analog of PTHrP sharing the first 22 amino acids but with differing amino acids at positions 23 to 34. While both agents bind to the PTH type I receptor, abaloparatide binds with higher affinity to the RG confirmation, which results in an increased anabolic effect. Further, abaloparatide demonstrates less of an effect on activating bone resorption and remodeling than teriparatide. With both medications bone mass is improved.

Pharmacokinetics Bioavailability for teriparatide and abaloparatide are 95% and 36%, respectively. The peptides are cleared through hepatic and extrahepatic pathways, with a half-life of 1 hour and 1.7 hours, respectively. Increases in the area under the curve are noted with decreasing renal function but there are no dosage adjustments noted in renal insufficiency. No studies have been performed in hepatic impairment. Alternative delivery formulations are being investigated.[54]

Efficacy Two years of teriparatide or abaloparatide reduce vertebral and nonvertebral fracture risk in postmenopausal women (see Table 112-6).[53] Compared with alendronate, teriparatide has demonstrated reductions in vertebral fracture rates in patients taking glucocorticoids; however, no reductions in nonverterbral fractures were evident.[54] Lumbar spine BMD increases are greater than with antiresorptive agents. Observational data for teriparatide suggest a similar fracture benefit in men; no data are available regarding abaloparatide use in men. Discontinuation of parathyroid hormone analog therapy results in a decrease in BMD, which can be alleviated with subsequent antiresorptive therapy.[2]

Adverse Events Transient hypercalcemia can occur and is less common with abaloparatide than with teriparatide (3.4% vs 6.4%, respectively) (see Table 112-8).[54] Because of an increased incidence of osteosarcoma in rats, both medications contain a box warning against use in patients at increased baseline risk for osteosarcoma (eg, Paget's bone disease, unexplained elevations of alkaline phosphatase, pediatric patients, young adults with open epiphyses, or patients with prior radiation therapy involving the skeleton). This adverse effect has not been seen in humans.

Interactions An increased calcium concentration could be a concern in patients on digoxin therapy.

Dosing and Administration Teriparatide and abaloparatide are commercially available as a prefilled pen delivery device (see Table 112-7). A daily subcutaneous injection is delivered to the abdominal area with site rotation. Teriparatide can also be given in the thigh. The administration of the first dose should take place with the patient either sitting or lying down in case orthostatic hypotension occurs. Both medications should be stored in the refrigerator before first use. After first use, abaloparatide can be kept at room temperature for up to 30 days. In contrast, teriparatide must be returned for storage in the refrigerator after each use and special precautions must be taken for travel. The teriparatide pen should be discarded after 28 days. Due to the theoretical risk for osteosarcoma, these medications are generally limited to 2 years of use cumulatively in a patient's lifetime with additional use of teriparatide considered on a risk-benefit basis. In select patients, a second trial with teriparatide can be tried. Suboptimal adherence is documented to decrease efficacy.

Besides the conditions listed above, parathyroid hormone analogs should not be used in patients with hypercalcemia, metabolic bone diseases other than osteoporosis, metastatic or skeletal cancers, previous radiation therapy, or premenopausal women of childbearing potential.

Formation and Antiresorptive Medication

Romosozumab

9 Romosozumab is approved by FDA for postmenopausal women at high risk for fracture defined as multiple risk factors for fracture, a history of osteoporotic fracture, or failed or intolerant to other

therapies. This medication might be the anabolic osteoporosis medication of choice for patients with previous radiation therapy,[2] and those at risk for osteosarcoma and hypercalcemia.[75]

Pharmacology Romosozumab is a humanized monoclonal antibody that binds to sclerostin to prevent inhibition of bone formation and decrease bone resorption, an activity that separates this medication from other anabolic medications.[54,75] By binding sclerostin, Wnt signaling can continue to increase gene transcription, which results in increased osteoblast synthesis, differentiation, and bone matrix building. This medication inhibits bone resorption by decreasing RANKL and m-CSF, and increasing OPG.

Pharmacokinetics About 50% to 70% of a dose is absorbed. Peak serum concentrations after subcutaneous administration are reached within 3 to 4.5 days, with no accumulation with subsequent doses. Romosozumab has a half-life of 6 to 7 days.

Efficacy After 1 year of romosozumab, vertebral fractures are statistically decreased by 73%, with a nonsignificant decrease in nonvertebral fractures by 25% in postmenopausal women (see Table 112-6).[2,39,54,75] Fracture prevention was higher if the study participants in Latin America were removed from the multi-country study analysis because this cohort had lower fracture rates even in the placebo arm. Fracture risk was also decreased by 48% for vertebral fractures, 19% for nonvertebral fractures, and 38% for hip fractures after 1 year of romosozumab followed by 1 year of alendronate. Lumbar spine and hip BMD statistically increased after 1 year of romosozumab treatment. To prevent BMD loss after discontinuation, therapy with denosumab or alendronate for 1 year after romosozumab resulted in BMD continuing to increase at hip and bone sites. Vertebral, femoral neck, and hip BMD and hip bone strength increased after romosozumab therapy in postmenopausal women who had received at least 3 years of prior bisphosphonate therapy.[73] These BMD increases were not as large as reported in bisphosphonate naïve women but were greater than teriparatide therapy BMD effects after bisphosphonate therapy. Comparing published results in postmenopausal women, romosozumab might be better to prevent hip fractures compared to abaloparatide and teriparatide while these last agents might be better for vertebral fracture prevention.[75] Romosozumab increased BMD in men by 12.1% at the lumbar spine, 2.5% total hip, and 2.2% femoral neck, all significantly different than placebo after 1 year of therapy.[54] Fracture data were not captured in men.

Adverse Effects Headache and arthralgia were the most common adverse effects, followed by hypercalcemia (<1%) (see Table 112-8).[2,39,54] Mild injection site irritation occurred in 6% to 8% of patients. Romosozumab antibodies developed in 10% to 20% patients, sometimes being transient. The antibodies generally are not neutralizing antibodies nor did they alter efficacy. Serious cardiovascular events have been reported in a few trials, but the incidence is low (<2.5%) and not much higher nor significantly different from the alendronate treatment arm (1.9%) in postmenopausal women at 1 year. The serious cardiovascular events increased to 6.5% and 6.1%, respectively, after both arms were switched to alendronate for year 2. In men, the cardiovascular event rates were 4.9% in men receiving romosozumab versus 2.5% receiving placebo. Myocardial infarction, stroke, and cardiovascular death are listed as a boxed warning. Romosozumab should not be used within 1 year of a myocardial infarction or stroke and benefit risk evaluation should be conducted in patients at risk for these conditions or with these conditions in their past medical history. Rare cases of ONJ and atypical femoral fractures have been reported. Because Wnt signaling is also related to malignancies, the medication-induced increased activity could be a concern. However, this adverse effect was not seen in the premarketing clinical trials.

Interactions None

Dosing and Administration The medication comes as two prefilled syringes requiring refrigeration until administered by a healthcare provider. Each syringe is injected into two different sites during the same visit (see Table 112-7). Patient self-administration is being explored.

Sequential and Combination Therapy

9 In sequential therapy, an anabolic agent is given first to increase bone remodeling units and bone mass, followed by an antiresorptive agent to continue with bone formation. Although this sequential therapy is recommended in the guidelines, in practice this regimen is generally reserved for patients with severe osteoporosis because of the cost of anabolic agents. Starting with an antiresorptive first and then switching to teriparatide results in lower BMD compared to starting with the bone formation medication first. Thus starting teriparatide after antiresorption therapy is not preferred.[2] However, this therapy will be used, especially for patients who have fractured or continue to lose bone mass while on antiresorptive therapy. Romosozumab can be used after previous treatment with parathyroid hormone analogs.[2] Small increases in BMD can be seen when switching from an oral bisphosphonate to denosumab. Switching to denosumab thus can be used during a bisphosphonate drug holiday or for bisphosphonate treatment failures (ie, BMD decreases or fracture).

Because of no documented fracture benefit, increased cost, concern for dual suppression of bone turnover, and potential for more adverse effects, combination therapy is rarely used.[2,53,54] Combination therapy of two antiresorptive agents or two anabolic agents did not increase bone mass compared to monotherapy even though they have different pharmacologic properties. Combination of teriparatide with oral bisphosphonates generally resulted in less BMD gains than monotherapy, and thus is not used. Combination teriparatide and denosumab resulted in greater hip BMD effects, but long-term results were generally similar to sequential therapy. Estrogen therapy combined with a bisphosphonate did not increase bone mass more than monotherapy. Antiresorptive therapy can be initiated after estrogen discontinuation to help negate the accelerated bone loss that occurs once estrogen is stopped. For postmenopausal women with menopause symptoms and an osteoporosis diagnosis, an osteoporosis medication should be prescribed along with menopausal hormone therapy. When raloxifene is used for breast cancer prevention, sometimes another antiresorptive agent will be prescribed, especially if hip fracture risk is high.

SPECIAL POPULATIONS

Osteoporosis is a particular threat in some subgroups because of age, genetic abnormalities, diseases, and medications.

Children and Adolescents

6 Osteoporosis in children and adolescents is uncommon but can lead to significant pain, deformity, and chronic disability. Pediatric osteoporosis is due to genetic disorders such as osteogenesis imperfecta and idiopathic juvenile osteoporosis, or secondary causes including chronic inflammatory diseases, growth hormone deficiency, celiac disease, diabetes, anorexia nervosa, and glucocorticoid use (see Tables 112-2 and 112-3 for other causes). Female athlete triad and anorexia nervosa, which are common in this age group, can lead to osteoporosis and fractures.

The diagnosis and treatment of osteoporosis in children and adolescents are challenging. Low bone mass is defined as a Z-score of −2.0 or less (adjusted for gender, age, and race/ethnicity) or T-score <−2.5 when adult height has been achieved using central DXA of the spine or total body minus head.[10,15] Ability to lie still during the DXA and radiation doses of some tests create concerns for this age group. Routine DXA monitoring is not required[10]; however, some criteria for this test have been suggested.[15] An osteoporosis diagnosis requires a DXA Z-score of −2.0 or less and 2 long-bone fractures by age of 10 or 3 long-bone fractures by the age of 19.[10]

DXA monitoring is done every 1 to 2 years for bone health and annually for children on bisphosphonate therapy.[10] Spine x-rays can also be monitored every 6 months to 2 years. Genetic testing might be required to identify an underlying cause.[15]

The first step in management is correcting any underlying primary or secondary causes and instituting a bone-healthy lifestyle especially adequate calcium, vitamin D, and exercise.[10,15,58] This step includes weight gain for anorexia nervosa and decreased exercise intensity for those with the female athlete triad.

Pharmacologic treatment has been used for children and adolescents with low bone mass and fragility fractures. Unlike adults, many children can reshape vertebral fractures and reclaim more BMD with treatment.[58] Growth hormone can be helpful in children with a documented deficiency but has no effect if no underlying deficit.[57] The optimal osteoporosis medication, dose, and duration of therapy are unknown and can vary by age and cause of osteoporosis. More safety data are needed.[15,58]

Bisphosphonates can be used off-label in children/adolescents but should be discontinued when the Z-score goes above −2.0.[10] Children and adolescents on glucocorticoids frequently need bisphosphonate therapy for longer periods.[10,15,58] For children less than 40 kg, the alendronate dose is 5 mg/day or 35 mg/week and risedronate is 15 mg/week.[10] Zoledronic acid is dosed 0.0125 to 0.05 mg/kg (maximum dose 4 mg) every 6 to 12 months. A major concern with bisphosphonates is their effect on longitudinal bone growth and modeling. Fracture healing, skeletal growth/maturation, and the appearance of growth plates do not appear to be impaired by bisphosphonates. Because bisphosphonates are released from bone for many years and cross the placenta, teratogenic effects are also a concern. Bisphosphonates should not be used if pregnancy is planned within the year. Pediatric experience with denosumab is limited but positive.[57]

Teriparatide has a box warning to avoid use in children due to a concern for osteosarcoma. Newer agents have not been evaluated in pediatric patients.

Premenopausal Women

6 Clinically significant bone loss and fractures in healthy premenopausal women are rare.[73] Risk factors are similar between premenopausal and postmenopausal osteoporosis. While bone loss occurs during pregnancy and lactation, it is usually gained back 6 to 12 months after pregnancy or breastfeeding is complete. Secondary causes are involved in 50% to 90% of premenopausal women with osteoporosis (see Tables 112-2 and 112-3) for the bone loss.[11] Common secondary causes in this group are amenorrhea, anorexia nervosa, glucocorticoid use, and celiac disease. Premenopausal women with prior fracture have a higher risk of postmenopausal osteoporotic fractures.[11,73,76]

Routine bone density screening should not be performed in healthy premenopausal women. Premenopausal women with known osteoporosis risk factors and low-trauma fractures can undergo central DXA examinations.[73] In this case, the Z-score is used, with Z-scores of −2.0 or less defined as bone mass below the expected range for age.[11,37,73,76] The categorization of osteopenia or osteoporosis based on T-score alone should be avoided in premenopausal women unless there is a history of low-trauma fracture or a secondary cause of osteoporosis.

Pharmacologic therapy for osteoporosis should be used with caution in premenopausal women as antifracture efficacy and safety have not been adequately demonstrated.[11,73] All premenopausal women should practice a bone-healthy lifestyle, including adequate calcium and vitamin D intake. Secondary causes of bone loss should be resolved. For example, gaining weight and resumed menses are more effective in correcting bone loss secondary to anorexia nervosa than oral contraceptives.[73,76] If the contributing factor cannot be eliminated, for example, chemotherapy or glucocorticoids, pharmacological therapy can be considered. Women with an unidentified cause for osteoporosis and no history of fracture should be treated with a bone-healthy lifestyle and watchful waiting.

Osteoporosis medication safety during pregnancy and breastfeeding have not been adequately studied. While some data suggest that use prior to conception and during the first trimester of pregnancy is safe, bisphosphonates are generally not used in women of childbearing age due to concern for fetal harm resulting from the long half-lives of these agents.[73,76] Bisphosphonate use should be avoided within 12 months of conception and use of contraceptive agents should be encouraged to reduce the likelihood of becoming pregnant during therapy. Human data on the safety of denosumab and bone-forming agents such as teriparatide in pregnancy are lacking; however, some animal data suggest congenital defects following exposure. Therefore, these agents should be avoided during pregnancy.[11]

Older Adults

Although osteoporosis, osteoporotic fractures, and postfracture morbidity and mortality increase with age, osteoporosis is underdiagnosed and undertreated in older adults. One-third of older adults older than 65 years old and about 50% of older adults older than 80 years old fall annually; with 20% to 30% of these falls resulting in moderate to severe injury.[2] More than 50% of women older than 75 years old have osteoporosis. Fewer than 25% of older adults had a DXA completed or received osteoporosis medications after a fracture. After a hip fracture, more than 50% of older adult women will require assistance including long-term nursing home residence (25%).[2,4] Only 33% of nursing home residents with an osteoporosis diagnosis or past fracture received an osteoporosis medication, even though 89% of them were considered at high risk for a fracture.[77] Hypogonadism is present in about 29% of older men.[12] Sarcopenia resulting in decreased muscle mass and function is prevalent in older adults[8] and is associated with increased falls and fractures.[78]

Guidelines recommend central DXA for adults aged 65 years and older; however, all older adults are not evaluated for osteoporosis. Reference standards for osteoporosis assessment tools are generally not available for the oldest older adults (eg, maximum age for FRAX is 90 years). In clinical practice, estimates for a 90-year-old person are applied to those adults older than 90 years. FRAX slightly overestimates, whereas ultrasound underestimates osteoporosis in nursing home residents. In an older adult with falls, the Garvan calculator might be preferred since it includes falls, whereas FRAX does not.[2]

Older adults should practice a bone-healthy lifestyle, ingest adequate calcium and vitamin D, and implement measures to prevent falls (see above sections).[2,8,12,14,79] While some guidelines recommend adequate amounts of calcium and vitamin D, the USPSTF feels evidence is insufficient to support fall and fracture prevention with supplementation. Lactose intolerance and hypercholesterolemia increase with aging and can lead to lower calcium intake from dairy products, which can increase the need for calcium supplements. Limited sun exposure due to frailty and institutional residence can increase the need for vitamin D supplementation for bone and muscle health. Protein intakes of 1 g/kg/day (up to 1.5 g/kg/day for some chronic illnesses) are suggested, and these also help with decreasing sarcopenia. Exercise might be difficult in older adults due to osteoarthritis or limited by underlying cardiac and respiratory diseases. However, walking and lifting light weights can still stimulate bone remodeling. Encouraging older adults to do a home safety evaluation for falls can assist with fracture prevention. Multidisciplinary fall prevention programs with multiple interventions generally have greater impact on fall prevention than single discipline or single intervention.[47] Exercise is a major component of these interventions. Many fall prevention materials are available without cost on the Internet.

Some data exist to support osteoporosis medication benefits in older adults; however, data are limited for the oldest older adults.[8,14,75] In a Medicare study, antiosteoporotic medications after a fracture lowered subsequent fracture risk by 21%. When deciding whether to use prescription medications in older adults, the following factors need to be taken into consideration: remaining life span, ability to take and afford medications, cognitive function, swallowing ability, GI disorders, polypharmacy, desire to avoid additional medications, and regimen complexity. Challenges with oral bisphosphonate administration requirements exist for older adults who are bed bound, have difficulties swallowing, have fluid restrictions for cardiovascular or kidney diseases, forget to drink adequate amounts of fluid, or cannot stay upright for the given time. Diuretics, nephrotoxic medications, and dehydration can increase acute and chronic renal failure when zoledronic acid is administered too quickly.[2]

The cost of antiosteoporosis medications can quickly cause an older adult with the Medicare Part D (medications) to enter the coverage gap, or "donut hole," which is the period when out-of-pocket medication expenses can be higher. Having to pay for antiosteoporosis medications might create adherence problems. Sometimes not initiating or stopping osteoporosis medications might be warranted for older adults with conditions such as severe Alzheimer disease or during palliative or hospice care. Comprehensive medication reviews and deprescribing can decrease all-cause mortality and potentially inappropriate medication use but does not increase nor decrease falls.[50]

Chronic Kidney Disease

Low BMD and fractures occur in patients with chronic kidney disease (CKD, glomerular filtration rate (GFR) less than 60 mL/min/1.73 m^2 [0.58 mL/s/m^2]), using chronic dialysis, and/or after kidney transplant.[80] Some medications for CKD and transplant can further compromise bone health. Fractures occur earlier and have greater 1-year mortality rates (64%). Osteoporosis and decreased renal function due to aging are different from other chronic kidney disease-mineral and bone disorders (CKD-MBD) such as renal osteodystrophy (see Chapter 69 "Calcium and Phosphorus Homeostasis" and Chapter 62 "Chronic Kidney Disease"), which can be related to high bone turnover, adynamic bone, or a combination of both. A DXA with VFA when appropriate can be used to assess bone loss and FRAX can be used to determine fracture risk; however, neither assessment distinguishes between renal and nonrenal causes of bone loss.[81] The DXA result can underestimate fracture risk since changes in bone quality from CKD are not captured. Similarly, FRAX can underestimate risk since renal failure is not included as a risk factor. When the diagnosis of the underlying bone disease pathophysiology could influence treatment, a bone biopsy can be conducted but is no longer a Kidney Disease Improving Global Outcomes (KDIGO) requirement.[80] Laboratory tests such as serum calcium, 25(OH) vitamin D, intact PTH, and serum phosphorus can help with identifying underlying CKD-MBD. Non-kidney-retained BTM such as bone-specific alkaline phosphatase (BSAP), PINP and tartrate-resistant acid phosphatase 5b (TRAP 5b) can be used to monitor therapy and guide reinstitution of therapy after a bisphosphonate drug holiday.[81] Other markers are being investigated.[80]

The first treatment step is to manage underlying disease conditions, including calcium and vitamin D abnormalities, hyperphosphatemia, and hyperparathyroidism (discussed in Renal Disorders chapters of this textbook).[80] Limited data exist on osteoporosis medications for patients with CKD, dialysis, and/or post kidney transplant.[2,80,81] Calcium intake is preferred by diet with supplements used only to achieve RDAs when diet is insufficient. A 25(OH) vitamin D level is obtained to assess bone health with vitamin D treatment prescribed as needed to maintain therapeutic concentrations, which are the same as non-CKD patient recommendations. Sometimes 1,25-$(OH)_2$-vitamin D might also be used for underlying CKD-induced deficiencies, creating a need for adding prescription calcitriol therapy to over-the-counter vitamin D therapy.

Osteoporosis medication studies in patients with CKD are lacking and often with insufficient sample sizes or were post hoc analyses.[2,80,81] Denosumab is not renally eliminated and thus can be used. When denosumab is used in CKD-MBD or dialysis, serum calcium levels need to be monitored since these patients can develop hypocalcemia, especially if also receiving calcium-sensing receptor agonists. According to product labeling, oral bisphosphonates are not recommended and zoledronic acid is contraindicated if CrCl is less than 30 or 35 mL/min (0.50 or 0.58 mL/s). However, guidelines suggest bisphosphonates can be used, particularly when decreased renal function is the result of aging alone. Insufficient data exist to support lower doses for shorter durations, which have been suggested to account for decreased renal bisphosphonate elimination. Dialysis does eliminate bisphosphonates, but if the dose is given after dialysis, a lower dose or longer interval is suggested.[80] Bisphosphonates should not be given at the same time as phosphate binders or other medications. Patients with CKD should be reassessed in 3 years or after a fracture for bisphosphonate continuation decisions. Raloxifene is not suggested for patients with severe renal impairment. Teriparatide can help patients with adynamic bone and those with low PTH and BMD but not for patients with high bone turnover. A role for abaloparatide and romosozumab could exist since these medications are not renally eliminated, do not accumulate in bone, and can overcome some CKD-MBDs; however, little evidence is available to guide use. Since many patients with decreased renal function have cardiovascular disease, use of romosozumab might be limited. Fracture risk increases with osteoporosis medication discontinuation, so a post-discontination plan is needed. Kidney and/or bone specialists usually provide care to patients with significant kidney disease and osteoporosis.

Drug-Induced Osteoporosis

Glucocorticoid-Induced Osteoporosis 3 Glucocorticoid use is the most common cause of medication-induced osteoporosis. Up to 40% of patients taking chronic oral glucocorticoids will experience a clinical fracture or show evidence of vertebral fracture on x-ray.[82,83] In patients who take 2.5 to 7.5 mg/day of prednisone or the equivalent, the relative risk of vertebral fracture doubles and the relative risk of hip fracture increases by 50%.[84] All glucocorticoid doses and formulations have been associated with increased bone loss and fractures; however, risk is much greater with prednisone doses of 5 mg or more daily or equivalent and with oral therapy versus inhaler and intranasal therapy.[84,85] Although a well-documented risk, many patients receiving glucocorticoids are not evaluated or treated for glucocorticoid-induced osteoporosis (GIO); therefore, greater vigilance by all healthcare professionals is needed.[82,84]

Bone losses with glucocorticoids are rapid with up to 12% loss over the first year. The greatest decrease occurs in the first 3 to 6 months of therapy. Afterward, bone loss is about 2% to 3% per year.[84] The risk of fracture increases within 3 months of initiating glucocorticoid therapy and peaks at 1 year. Trabecular bone is affected more than cortical bone; therefore, vertebral fractures are more common. The pathophysiology of glucocorticoid-induced bone loss is multifactorial.[83] Glucocorticoids decrease bone formation through decreased proliferation and differentiation and enhanced apoptosis of osteoblasts. They can interfere with the bone's natural repair mechanism through increased apoptosis of osteocytes. Glucocorticoids increase RANKL and decrease OPG, leading to an increase in the number of osteoclasts and increased bone resorption. They can reduce estrogen and testosterone concentrations. A negative calcium balance is created from decreased calcium absorption and increased urinary calcium excretion via alterations in calcium transporters. The underlying disease requiring glucocorticoids (see Table 112-2) also can negatively affect bone metabolism.

FRAX and central DXA are recommended by current guidelines for evaluation, though neither adequately accounts for the rapid increase in fracture risk following glucocorticoid initiation.[82,83] Since FRAX does not account for specific dose, duration or accumulation of glucocorticoids, scores must be adjusted based on prednisone dose or equivalent.[82] For those taking more than 7.5 mg or equivalent per day, FRAX risk of major osteoporotic fracture should be increased by 15% (ie, multiplied by 1.15) and FRAX risk of hip fracture by 20% (ie, multiplied by 1.2). Based on glucocorticoid-adjusted FRAX estimates of the 10-year risk of major osteoporotic fracture and hip fracture, the patients are risk stratified into low, moderate, and high risk for fracture. Criteria for classification into a risk category is detailed in Table 112-9. An initial BMD assessment is recommended prior to or within 6 months of glucocorticoid initiation for adults 40 years of age or older and for adults under the age of 40 with a history of fragility fracture or other risk factors. Repeat BMD testing is recommended every 2 to 3 years during osteoporosis therapy for those taking high-glucocorticoid doses (30 mg of prednisone or more per day or a cumulative dose greater than 5 g in the past year), a fracture 18 months or more after starting osteoporosis therapy, medication adherence or absorption concerns, or other risk factors for osteoporosis. VFA is also suggested for patients receiving 5 mg or more prednisone or equivalent daily for 3 months or more.[37]

TABLE 112-9 Classification of Fracture Risk in Patients Treated with Glucocorticoids

Fracture Risk	Adults ≥40 Years Old	Adults <40 Years Old
Low	FRAX[a] 10-year risk of major osteoporotic fracture <10% FRAX[a] 10-year risk of hip fracture ≤1%	None of the risk factors listed below for moderate- or high-fracture risk
Moderate	FRAX[a] 10-year risk of major osteoporotic fracture 10%-19% FRAX[a] 10-year risk of hip fracture >1% and <3%	Hip or spine BMD Z-score <−3.0, or rapid bone loss (≥10% at the hip or spine over 1 year) and continuing glucocorticoid therapy with ≥7.5 mg/day for ≥6 months
High	History of osteoporotic fracture, or hip or spine BMD T-score ≤−2.5 in men ≥50 years old and postmenopausal women, or FRAX[a] 10-year risk of major osteoporotic fracture ≥20%, or FRAX[a] 10-year risk of hip fracture ≥3%	Prior osteoporotic fracture

[a]If glucocorticoid treatment is >7.5-mg prednisone or equivalent per day, the FRAX risk score should be multiplied by 1.15 for major osteoporotic fracture and by 1.2 for hip fracture and then used to determine overall fracture risk.

Date from Reference 82.

All patients using glucocorticoids should practice a bone-healthy lifestyle and minimize glucocorticoid exposure when possible.[82-84] All patients starting or receiving glucocorticoid therapy (any dose or duration) should consume 1,000 to 1,200 mg elemental calcium and 600 to 800 units of vitamin D daily or more to achieve therapeutic 25(OH) vitamin D concentrations. Minimizing fall risk is important. Osteoporosis prevention counseling should occur for all patients using this medication for three months or more regardless of dose. Glucocorticoids should be used at the lowest dose and for the shortest duration possible. Upon discontinuation of glucocorticoid therapy, fracture risk decreases and BMD increases, though they might not increase to baseline levels.[84]

Alendronate, risedronate, zoledronic acid, denosumab, and teriparatide are approved by FDA for GIO.[84] The current guidelines from the American College of Rheumatology divide recommendations for prescription osteoporosis medication use in GIO by fracture risk and age (see Tables 112-9 and 112-10).[82] Therapy recommendations are based on comparative efficacy, potential for toxicity, and cost.

Oral bisphosphonates are recommended first-line, though intravenous bisphosphonates can be used in patients who are not adherent or unable to take the oral preparations. Teriparatide is recommended for patients who cannot use a bisphosphonate, and denosumab is recommended if neither a bisphosphonate nor teriparatide can be used. Denosumab is not recommended first-line for GIO due to limited safety data in this population. Consideration should be given to potential risk of infection in patients taking immunosuppressive agents or biologic therapies. Raloxifene does not have an FDA indication for GIO, but does have some clinical data documenting improved BMD at the lumbar spine in patients taking glucocorticoids.[84] It is recommended only in postmenopausal women if no other osteoporosis medications can be used. Standard osteoporosis therapy doses are used. The recommendations are similar for women of childbearing potential who do not plan to become pregnant and are using effective contraception or are not sexually active.[82]

Patients receiving glucocorticoids are considered high risk, and, therefore, a bisphosphonate drug holiday is generally not considered

TABLE 112-10 Therapy to Prevent or Treat Glucocorticoid-Induced Osteoporosis in Adults Beginning Long-Term Glucocorticoid Treatment (≥2.5-mg Prednisone or Equivalent Per Day for ≥3 Months)

Patient Population	Low-Fracture Risk	Moderate-Fracture Risk	High-Fracture Risk
All	Optimize calcium and vitamin D intake; bone-healthy lifestyle	Optimize calcium and vitamin D intake; bone-healthy lifestyle	Optimize calcium and vitamin D intake; bone healthy lifestyle
Adults age ≥40 years	No prescription osteoporosis therapy	Oral bisphosphonate alternatives: IV bisphosphonate, teriparatide, denosumab, or raloxifene[b]	Oral bisphosphonate alternatives: IV bisphosphonate, teriparatide, denosumab, or raloxifene[b]
Adults age <40 years	No prescription osteoporosis therapy	Oral bisphosphonate alternatives: IV bisphosphonate, teriparatide, or denosumab	Oral bisphosphonate alternatives: IV bisphosphonate, teriparatide, or denosumab
Women of childbearing potential[c,d]	No prescription osteoporosis therapy	Oral bisphosphonate alternative: teriparatide	Oral bisphosphonate alternatives: teriparatide, IV bisphosphonate, or denosumab

IV, intravenous.

[a]Listed in order of preference; abaloparatide and romosozumab were not yet approved during guideline development.

[b]Recommended only for postmenopausal women when other alternative therapies cannot be used.

[c]Women of childbearing potential who do not intend to become pregnant during the osteoporosis treatment period and are using effective birth control or are not sexually active.

[d]Fetal risks from osteoporosis medications during pregnancy.

Data from Reference 82.

after 5 years. Bisphosphonate treatment for 7 to 10 years is recommended if patients continue glucocorticoid use. Since glucocorticoids can cause hypogonadism, sometimes hormone therapy will be prescribed. The hormonal therapy for correcting hypogonadism symptoms most likely will have some positive bone effects as well.

Cancer Treatment–Induced Bone Loss

3 Cancers, some associated treatments and metastatic bone disease can cause bone loss and osteoporosis.[59,63] Medications used to treat hormone-responsive cancers—such as aromatase inhibitors and androgen deprivation therapy, and some cytotoxic chemotherapies—are associated with a reduction in BMD. Chemotherapy-induced ovarian failure can enhance bone loss. Glucocorticoids used as chemotherapy, chemotherapy premedication, and/or treatment for chemotherapy-induced nausea and vomiting also increase bone loss in patients with cancer.

Central DXA screening is advocated for patients at high risk for osteoporosis, which would include certain chemotherapies and cancers.[59] Patients with at least 1 risk factor should be offered BMD testing with central DXA. In patients on medications that cause bone loss or whose BMD is near the threshold of treatment with FRAX, BMD testing should be offered every 2 years or more frequently considering the results of the BMD and anticipated bone loss, but not more than annually. FRAX can be used to estimate the risk for osteoporotic fracture; however, it has not been validated in patients with cancer. When using FRAX, secondary osteoporosis can be checked "yes" when premature menopause and/or hypogonadism caused by chemotherapy and cancer are present, though fracture risk is likely still underestimated in this group.[86]

Certain osteoporosis medications are used to prevent bone loss or treat osteoporosis due to chemotherapy, cancer, and metastases. Bisphosphonates and denosumab decrease chemotherapy-induced bone loss and in some trials, reduce fractures.[59] Most research has been conducted in women with breast cancer and men with prostate cancer. Raloxifene decreases the risk of invasive breast cancer in high-risk women.[2,34] Due to risk of osteosarcoma, teriparatide and abaloparatide are specifically contraindicated in patients with bone metastases or prior radiation to the skeleton. Zoledronic acid and denosumab are used for cancer-related hypercalcemia and skeletal-related events.[63] They are marketed with different product names for these indications since dosages are much higher than for osteoporosis. For additional information see Chapter 150, "Supportive Care in Cancer."

EVALUATION OF THERAPEUTIC OUTCOMES

Monitoring of Patient-Centered Care Plan

10 Assessment of adherence and tolerability of medication should be performed during each encounter patients have with the healthcare system. Having patients repeat back instructions for medication administration will help identify administration problems and enable timely correction. Assessment of fracture, back pain, and height loss can help identify worsening osteoporosis.

The role of routine monitoring of BMD via central DXA is controversial and recommendations vary since change in BMD is only one component of fracture risk.[2,87] Nonetheless, decreases in BMD while on treatment are associated with increases in fracture risk compared to stable or increased BMD. Since BMD continues to decrease with aging, no change from baseline can be an acceptable response. However, BMD is considered a failure if BMD significantly decreases while on treatment. This treatment failure could indicate nonadherence, a lack of response, or the presence of secondary causes contributing to continued bone loss.[2] To minimize test variability, BMD testing should be performed on the same DXA machine. A statistical change needs to be greater than the least significant change for that specific piece of equipment based on local data with the team of technicians.

The AACE/ACE guidelines recommend central DXA every 1 to 2 years after medication initiation until BMD is stable at which time the interval for reassessment could be lengthened.[2] The Endocrine Society guidelines recommend waiting 3 years for zoledronic acid, 5 years for other bisphosphonates, and 5 to 10 years for denosumab.[39] Financial support for testing at intervals less than 2 years might not be provided by insurance plans. In patients with conditions associated with higher rates of bone loss (eg, glucocorticoid use and certain chemotherapy agents), more frequent monitoring might be warranted.

Like central DXA, BTM can be used to identify nonadherence and lack of response to therapy.[2] The markers are measured 3 to 6 months after therapy initiation and compared to baseline values.[2,88] Significant changes need to be greater than the least significant change for that test.[2] Because no consensus on result interpretation and high-test variability exists, these tests are not routinely ordered.

Osteoporosis Services

10 Despite the availability of effective therapies, many patients (approximately 70%) are not being evaluated or do not receive appropriate osteoporosis therapy.[2] In fact, the proportion of patients receiving osteoporosis medication following a hip fracture has decreased. People of color receive even fewer DXA screenings and less medication therapy, and have poorer results after a fracture.[3] To combat this trend, many institutions are implementing an Own the Bone program or a fracture liaison service, which is generally an interprofessional, multifaceted program to increase treated patient numbers, enhance adherence, and improve osteoporosis treatment outcomes. All providers and programs should work to decrease health disparities in osteoporosis prevention and treatment.[3] Communicating risk is important for people to understand their risk for and consequences of fractures, especially in relation to other medical conditions.[2] Community pharmacists and other healthcare professionals can provide osteoporosis screenings using the FRAX tool to estimate fracture risk in the community, especially at health fairs. Osteoporosis prevention and treatment services have been clinically successful in community pharmacies and in ambulatory care settings. At 1 year, only 26% to 56% of patients still use their osteoporosis medications. Thus, all healthcare professionals should identify and resolve barriers to optimal medication initiation and adherence. The main reasons for nonadherence are medication cost, fear of adverse effects, resistance to medication use, and perceived lack of medication need. Routine follow-up with healthcare professionals and enhanced risk-benefit communication tools could improve treatment and adherence rates. Databases can be used to identify patients after a low-trauma fracture who have not had a DXA screening or osteoporosis medication started. Patient medication assistance programs can be used to decrease cost.

To improve patient care, the US Centers for Medicare and Medicaid Services have created this quality measure—the percent of women 50 to 85 years old with a recent fracture that is screened or treated within 6 months.[1,44,89] Financial incentives tied to these measures could help bridge the gap in quality of care.

CONCLUSION

Osteoporosis prevention begins at birth and continues throughout life by practicing a bone-healthy lifestyle (adequate calcium and vitamin D intake, exercise, no smoking, minimal alcohol use, and fall prevention). Generally, osteoporosis occurs in postmenopausal women and older men; however, the disease can occur in all ages because of secondary causes such as genetics, diseases, and medications. FRAX tool can be used for screening and to assist in identifying patients at high risk for fracture requiring treatment. Central DXA can be used for osteoporosis screening, diagnosis, and monitoring.

Alendronate, risedronate, zoledronic acid, and denosumab are first-line therapies for those with high fracture risk since these medications decrease hip, nonvertebral, and vertebral fractures. Abaloparatide, romosozumab, and teriparatide are the only medications that can build bone; however, cost, subcutaneous administration, and lack of hip fracture prevention limit their use. Although medications decrease fracture risk, prescribing of osteoporosis medications and patient adherence to them is suboptimal. All healthcare professionals need to be actively involved with people of all ages to provide osteoporosis education and counseling, prevent osteoporosis development across the lifespan, treat osteoporosis, and improve medication adherence to prevent osteoporotic fractures.

ABBREVIATIONS

25(OH) vitamin D	25-hydroxyvitamin D/calcidiol
APC	adenomatous polyposis coli
ATPase	adenosine triphosphatase
BMD	bone mineral density
BMP	bone morphometric proteins
BSAP	bone-specific alkaline phosphatase
BTM	bone turnover markers
Ca^{++}	Calcium
Cbfa1	core-binding factor alpha 1
Cbl	E3 ubiquitin ligase
CEE	conjugated equine estrogens
Csk1α	casein kinase 1α
CKD-MBD	chronic kidney disease-mineral and bone disorder
CrCl	creatinine clearance
CTX	c-terminal type 1 collagen telopeptide
Dkk-1	Dickkoff-1
DPD	deoxypyridinoline
DSH	disheveled cytoplasmic protein
DXA	dual-energy x-ray absorptiometry
EAA	estrogen agonist antagonist
FAK	focal adhesion kinase
FDA	US Food and Drug Administration
FGF	fibroblast growth factor
FRAX	World Health Organization fracture risk assessment tool
GFR	glomerular filtration rate
GI	gastrointestinal
GIO	glucocorticoid-induced osteoporosis
GSK-3β	glycogen synthase kinase-3β
ICTP	c-terminal telopeptide
IGF	insulin-like growth factor
IOM	Institute of Medicine
LGR4	leucine-rich repeat-containing G protein
LRP5/6	lipoprotein-receptor related protein
m-CSF	macrophage-colony stimulating factor
MMP	matrix metalloproteases
NF-Kβ	nuclear factor kappa β
NHANES	National Health and Nutrition Examination Survey
NTX	n-terminal type 1 collagen telopeptide
OCN	osteocalcin
ONJ	osteonecrosis of the jaw
OPG	osteoprotegerin
P13K	phosphatidyl inositol 3-kinase
pDXA	peripheral dual-energy x-ray absorptiometry
PICP	procollagen type 1 carboxy(C)-terminal propeptide
PINP	procollagen type 1 amino(N)-terminal propeptide
PPARγ	peroxisome proliferator-activated receptor gamma
PTH	parathyroid hormone
PTHrP	parathyroid hormone-related protein
QCT	quantitative computed tomography
QUS	quantitative ultrasound
RANK	receptor activator of nuclear factor-kappa β
RANKL	receptor activator of nuclear factor-kappa β ligand
RDA	recommended dietary allowances
runX2	runt-related transcription factor
Scr	nonreceptor tyrosine kinase
sFRP	secreted frizzled related proteins
TBS	trabecular bone score
TCF/LEF	T-cell-specific transcription factor 4/lymphoid enhancer factor 1
TGF-β	tissue growth factor-β
TNF-α	tumor necrosis factor-α
TRACP5b	tartrate-resistant acid phosphatase isoenzyme 5
TRPV6	transient receptor potential cation channel subfamily V member 6
TSEC	tissue selective estrogen complex
UL	upper limits
USP	United States Pharmacopeia
USPSTF	United States Preventive Services Task Force
VDR	vitamin D receptor
VFA	vertebral fracture assessment
WIFI	Wnt inhibitory factor 1
WISE	Wnt modulator insurface estoderm
WHO	World Health Organization
Wnt	wingless tail ligands

REFERENCES

1. Qaseem A, Forciea MA, McLean RM, et al. Treatment of low bone density or osteoporosis to prevent fractures in men and women: A clinical practice guideline update from the American College of Physicians. *Ann Intern Med.* 2017;11:818–839. 10.7326/M15-1361.
2. Camacho PM, Petak SM, Binkley N, et al. American Association of Clinical Endocrinologists/American College of Endocrinology clinical practice guidelines for the diagnosis and treatment of postmenopausal osteoporosis-2020 update. *Endocr Pract.* 2020;Suppl 1:1–46. doi:10.4158/gl-2020-0524suppl
3. Noel SE, Santos MP, Wright NC. Racial and ethnic disparities in bone health and outcomes in the United States. *J Bone Miner Res.* October2021;36(10):1881–1905. 10.1002/jbmr.4417.
4. Management of osteoporosis in postmenopausal women: The 2021 position statement of the North American Menopause Society. *Menopause.* 2021;9:973–997. doi:10.1097/gme.0000000000001831
5. Wright NC, Looker AC, Saag KG, et al. The recent prevalence of osteoporosis and low bone mass in the United States based on bone mineral density at the femoral neck or lumbar spine. *J Bone Miner Res.* 2014;11:2520–2526. doi:10.1002/jbmr.2269
6. Adler RA. Update on osteoporosis in men. *Best Pract Res Clin Endocrinol Metab.* 2018;5:759–772. doi:10.1016/j.beem.2018.05.007
7. Carlson BC, Robinson WA, Wanderman NR, et al. The American Orthopaedic Association's Own the Bone® database: A national quality improvement project for the treatment of bone health in fragility fracture patients. *Osteoporos Int.* 2018;9:2101–2109. 10.1007/s00198-018-4585-7.
8. Bouvard B, Annweiler C, Legrand E. Osteoporosis in older adults. *Joint Bone Spine.* 2021;3:105135. doi:10.1016/j.jbspin.2021.105135
9. Troy KL, Mancuso ME, Butler TA, et al. Exercise early and often: Effects of physical activity and exercise on women's bone health. *Int J Environ Res Public Health.* 2018;5. doi:10.3390/ijerph15050878
10. Galindo-Zavala R, Bou-Torrent R, Magallares-López B, et al. Expert panel consensus recommendations for diagnosis and treatment of secondary osteoporosis in children. *Pediatr Rheumatol Online J.* 2020;1:20. doi:10.1186/s12969-020-0411-9
11. Pepe J, Body JJ, Hadji P, et al. Osteoporosis in premenopausal women: A clinical narrative review by the ECTS and the IOF. *J Clin Endocrinol Metab.* 2020;105:dgaa306. doi:10.1210/clinem/dgaa306
12. Rinonapoli G, Ruggiero C, Meccariello L, et al. Osteoporosis in men: A review of an underestimated bone condition. *Int J Mol Sci.* 2021;4. doi:10.3390/ijms22042105

13. Porcelli T, Maffezzoni F, Pezzaioli LC, et al. Management of endocrine disease: Male osteoporosis: Diagnosis and management—should the treatment and the target be the same as for female osteoporosis? *Eur J Endocrinol.* 2020;3:R75–r93. doi:10.1530/eje-20-0034
14. Barnsley J, Buckland G, Chan PE, et al. Pathophysiology and treatment of osteoporosis: Challenges for clinical practice in older people. *Aging Clin Exp Res.* 2021;4:759–773. doi:10.1007/s40520-021-01817-y
15. Mäkitie O, Zillikens MC. Early-onset osteoporosis. *Calcif Tissue Int.* 2021. doi:10.1007/s00223-021-00885-6
16. Zhu X, Zheng H. Factors influencing peak bone mass gain. *Front Med.* 2021;1:53–69. doi:10.1007/s11684-020-0748-y
17. Saad FA. Novel insights into the complex architecture of osteoporosis molecular genetics. *Ann NY Acad Sci.* 2020;1:37–52. doi:10.1111/nyas.14231
18. Watts NB. Adverse bone effects of medications used to treat non-skeletal disorders. *Osteoporos Int.* 2017;10:2741–2746. doi:10.1007/s00198-017-4171-4
19. Jackson K, Moseley KF. Diabetes and bone fragility: SGLT2 inhibitor use in the context of renal and cardiovascular benefits. *Curr Osteoporos Rep.* 2020;5:439–448. 10.1007/s11914-020-00609-z.
20. Panday K, Gona A, Humphrey MB. Medication-induced osteoporosis: Screening and treatment strategies. *Ther Adv Musculoskelet Dis.* 2014;5:185–202. doi:10.1177/1759720X14546350
21. Mirza F, Canalis E. Management of endocrine disease: Secondary osteoporosis: Pathophysiology and management. *Eur J Endocrinol.* 2015;3:R131–151. doi:10.1530/EJE-15-0118
22. Clinical Info HIV.gov. Guidelines for the use of antiviral agents in adults and adolescents living with HIV. Available at https://clinicalinfo.hiv.gov/en/guidelines/adult-and-adolescent-arv/whats-new-guidelines. Accessed September 7, 2021.
23. Burr DB. Changes in bone matrix properties with aging. *Bone.* 2019;85–93. doi:10.1016/j.bone.2018.10.010
24. Casey CM, Caulley J, Phelan EA. The intersection of falls and dementia in primary care: Evaluation and management considerations. *Med Clin N Am.* 2020;5:791–806. doi:10.1016/j.mcna.2020.06.003
25. Blain H, Miot S, Bernard PL. How can we prevent falls? In: Falaschi P, Marsh D eds. *Orthogeriatrics: The Management of Older Patients with Fragility Fractures.* Cham (CH): Springer 2021:273–290.
26. Uehara IA, Soldi LR, Silva MJB. Current perspectives of osteoclastogenesis through estrogen modulated immune cell cytokines. *Life Sci.* 2020;117921. doi:10.1016/j.lfs.2020.117921
27. Shigehara K, Izumi K, Kadono Y, et al. Testosterone and bone health in men: A narrative review. *J Clin Med.* 2021;3. doi:10.3390/jcm10030530
28. Marini F, Brandi ML. Pharmacogenetics of osteoporosis. *Best Pract Res Clin Endocrinol Metab.* 2014;6:783–793. doi:10.1016/j.beem.2014.07.004
29. Kim KT, Lee YS, Han I. The role of epigenomics in osteoporosis and osteoporotic vertebral fracture. *Int J Mol Sci.* 2020;24. doi:10.3390/ijms21249455
30. Bringhurst FR DM, Kronenberg HM. Bone and mineral metabolism in health and disease. In: Jameson JL FA, Kasper DL, et al. eds. *Harrison's Principles of Internal Medicine.* New York: McGraw-Hill Companies, Inc.: 2018:1–23.
31. U.S. Department of Health and Human Services. Calcium fact sheet for health professionals, Available at https://ods.od.nih.gov/factsheets/Calcium-HealthProfessional/. Accessed September 7, 2021.
32. Barrett KE, Barman SM. Hormonal control of calcium & phosphate metabolism & the physiology of bone. *Ganong's Review of Medical Physiology.* 2019; 26 ed. McGraw Hill.https://accesspharmacy.mhmedical.com/content.aspx?bookid=2525§ionid=204295758.
33. LeBoff MS, Greenspan SL, Insogna KL, et al. The clinician's guide to prevention and treatment of osteoporosis. *Osteoporos Int.* Published online April 28, 2022. https://doi.org/10.1007/s00198-021-05900-y.
34. Kanis JA, Cooper C, Rizzoli R, et al. European guidance for the diagnosis and management of osteoporosis in postmenopausal women. *Osteoporos Int.* 2019;1:3–44. doi:10.1007/s00198-018-4704-5
35. Garvan Institute. Fracture risk calculator. Available at https://www.garvan.org.au/promotions/bone-fracture-risk/calculator/. Accessed September 7, 2021.
36. Curry SJ, Krist AH. United States Preventive Services Task Force. Screening for osteoporosis to prevent fractures: US Preventive Services Task Force recommendation statement. *JAMA.* 2018;24:2521–2531. 10.1001/jama.2018.7498.
37. International Society for Clinical Densitometry. Adult official positions of ISCD: Indications for bone mineral density (BMD) testing. Available at https://iscd.app.box.com/s/5r713cfzvf4gr28q7zdccg2i7169fv86. Accessed September 7, 2021.
38. Eastell R, Rosen CJ, Black DM, et al. Pharmacological management of osteoporosis in postmenopausal women: An Endocrine Society clinical practice guideline. *J Clin Endocrinol Metab.* 2019;5:1595–1622. doi:10.1210/jc.2019-00221
39. Shoback D, Rosen CJ, Black DM, et al. Pharmacological management of osteoporosis in postmenopausal women: An endocrine society guideline update. *J Clin Endocrinol Metab.* 2020;3:587–594. doi:10.1210/clinem/dgaa048
40. US Centers for Disease Control and Prevention. Older adult fall prevention. Available at https://www.cdc.gov/falls/. Accessed September 7, 2021.
41. Jansson-Knodell CL, Krajicek EJ, Savaiano DA, et al. Lactose intolerance: A concise review to skim the surface. *Mayo Clinic Proc.* 2020;7:1499–1505. doi:10.1016/j.mayocp.2020.04.036
42. National Institutes of Health Office of Dietary Supplements. Vitamin D fact sheet for health professionals. Available at https://ods.od.nih.gov/factsheets/VitaminD-HealthProfessional/#en1. Accessed September 7, 2021.
43. Liu X, Baylin A, Levy PD. Vitamin D deficiency and insufficiency among US adults: Prevalence, predictors and clinical implications. *Br J Nutr.* 2018;8:928–936. doi:10.1017/S0007114518000491
44. Gómez-Zorita S, González-Arceo M, Fernández-Quintela A, et al. Scientific evidence supporting the beneficial effects of isoflavones on human health. *Nutrients.* 2020;12. doi:10.3390/nu12123853
45. Sheng B, Li X, Nussler AK, et al. The relationship between healthy lifestyles and bone health: A narrative review. *Medicine.* 2021;8:e24684. doi:10.1097/md.0000000000024684
46. Tarantino U, Cariati I, Greggi C, et al. Skeletal system biology and smoke damage: From basic science to medical clinic. *Int J Mol Sci.* 2021;12. doi:10.3390/ijms22126629
47. Dautzenberg L, Beglinger S, Tsokani S, et al. Interventions for preventing falls and fall-related fractures in community-dwelling older adults: A systematic review and network meta-analysis. *J Am Geriatr Soc.* 2021. doi:10.1111/jgs.17375
48. American Heart Association. Association recommendations for physical activity in adults and kids. Available at https://www.heart.org/en/healthy-living/fitness/fitness-basics/aha-recs-for-physical-activity-in-adults. Accessed September 7, 2021.
49. Centers for Disease Control and Prevention. Resource algorithm for fall risk, assessment, and intervention. Available at https://www.cdc.gov/steadi/pdf/STEADI-Algorithm-508.pdf. Accessed September 7, 2021.
50. Bloomfield HE, Greer N, Linsky AM, et al. Deprescribing for community-dwelling older adults: A systematic review and meta-analysis. *J Gen Int Med.* 2020;11:3323–3332. doi:10.1007/s11606-020-06089-2
51. Minnesota Safety Council. Fall prevention home safety checklist what you can do to prevent falls. Available at https://www.minnesotasafetycouncil.org/SeniorSafe/fallcheck.pdf. Accessed September 7, 2021.
52. Wei H, Dong C, Zhu Y, et al. Analysis of two minimally invasive procedures for osteoporotic vertebral compression fractures with intravertebral cleft: A systematic review and meta-analysis. *J Orthopaed Surg Res.* 2020;1:401. doi:10.1186/s13018-020-01938-6
53. Lorentzon M. Treating osteoporosis to prevent fractures: Current concepts and future developments. *J Intern Med.* 2019. doi:10.1111/joim.12873
54. McClung MR. Role of bone-forming agents in the management of osteoporosis. *Aging Clin Exp Res.* 2021;4:775–791. doi:10.1007/s40520-020-01708-8
55. Pinkerton JV, Thomas S. Use of SERMs for treatment in postmenopausal women. *J Steroid Biochem Mol Biol.* 2014;142:142–154. 10.1016/j.jsbmb.2013.12.011.
56. Yavropoulou MP, Makras P, Anastasilakis AD. Bazedoxifene for the treatment of osteoporosis. *Exp Opin Pharmacother.* 2019;10:1201–1210. doi:10.1080/14656566.2019.1615882
57. Sakka SD, Cheung MS. Management of primary and secondary osteoporosis in children. *Ther Adv Musculoskelet Dis.* 2020;1759720x20969262. doi:10.1177/1759720x20969262
58. Ward LM. Part 2: When should bisphosphonates be used in children with chronic illness osteoporosis? *Curr Osteoporos Rep.* 2021;3:289–297. doi:10.1007/s11914-021-00672-0
59. Shapiro CL, Van Poznak C, Lacchetti C, et al. Management of osteoporosis in survivors of adult cancers with nonmetastatic disease: ASCO clinical practice guideline. *J Clin Oncol.* 2019;31:2916–2946. doi:10.1200/jco.19.01696
60. Kahwati LC, Weber RP, Pan H, et al. Vitamin D, calcium, or combined supplementation for the primary prevention of fractures in community-dwelling adults: Evidence report and systematic review for the US Preventive Services Task Force. *JAMA.* 2018;15:1600–1612. doi:10.1001/jama.2017.21640

61. Reid IR. Vitamin D effect on bone mineral density and fractures. *Endocrinol Metab Clin N Am.* 2017;4:935–945. doi:10.1016/j.ecl.2017.07.005
62. Ames BN, Grant WB, Willett WC. Does the high prevalence of vitamin D deficiency in African Americans contribute to health disparities? *Nutrients* 2021;13(2):499. 10.3390/nu13020499.
63. Coleman R, Hadji P, Body JJ, et al. Bone health in cancer: ESMO clinical practice guidelines. *Ann Oncol.* 2020;12:1650–1663. doi:10.1016/j.annonc.2020.07.019
64. Cremers S, Drake MT, Ebetino FH, et al. Pharmacology of bisphosphonates. *Br J Clin Pharmacol.* 2019. doi:10.1111/bcp.13867
65. Maraka S, Kennel KA. Bisphosphonates for the prevention and treatment of osteoporosis. *BMJ.* 2015;h3783. doi:10.1136/bmj.h3783
66. Rizzoli R. Postmenopausal osteoporosis: Assessment and management. *Best Pract Res Clin Endocrinol Metab.* 2018;5:739–757. doi:10.1016/j.beem.2018.09.005
67. Mayo Clinic. Bone health choice decision aid. Available at https://osteoporosisdecisionaid.mayoclinic.org/. Accessed September 7, 2021.
68. Anastasilakis AD, Polyzos SA, Makras P. Therapy of endocrine disease: Denosumab vs bisphosphonates for the treatment of postmenopausal osteoporosis. *Eur J Endocrinol.* 2018;1:R31–R45. doi:10.1530/EJE-18-0056
69. Zaheer S, LeBoff M, Lewiecki EM. Denosumab for the treatment of osteoporosis. *Expert Opin Drug Metab Toxicol.* 2015;3:461–470. doi:10.1517/17425255.2015.1000860
70. Evista. Prescribing information. Eli Lilly and Company; 2021. Accessed September 7, 2021. https://dailymed.nlm.nih.gov/dailymed/drugInfo.cfm?setid=fcaaa6dc-74e8-4fb8-800c-5574bf0f8de9.
71. Duavee. Prescribing information. US Pharmaceuticals; 2021. Accessed September 7, 2021. https://dailymed.nlm.nih.gov/dailymed/drugInfo.cfm?setid=e16705d8-4472-4f83-96ac-69fa2be066cb.
72. US Food and Drug Administration. Questions and answers: Changes to the indicated population for miacalcin (calcitonin-salmon). Avalable at https://www.fda.gov/Drugs/DrugSafety/PostmarketDrugSafetyInformationforPatientsandProviders/ucm388641.htm. Accessed September 7, 2021
73. Langdahl BL. Osteoporosis in premenopausal women. *Curr Opin Rheumatol.* 2017;4:410–415. doi:10.1097/BOR.0000000000000400
74. Bhasin S, Brito JP, Cunningham GR, et al. Testosterone therapy in men with hypogonadism: An Endocrine Society clinical practice guideline. *J Clin Endocrinol Metab.* 2018;5:1715–1744. 10.1210/jc.2018-00229.
75. Cosman F, Dempster DW. Anabolic agents for postmenopausal osteoporosis: How do you choose? *Curr Osteoporos Rep.* 2021;2:189–205. doi:10.1007/s11914-021-00663-1
76. Cohen A. Premenopausal osteoporosis. *Endocrinol Metabol Clin N Am.* 2017;1:117–133. doi:10.1016/j.ecl.2016.09.007
77. Zarowitz BJ, Cheng LI, Allen C, et al. Osteoporosis prevalence and characteristics of treated and untreated nursing home residents with osteoporosis. *J Am Med Dir Assoc.* 2015;4:341–348. doi:10.1016/j.jamda.2015.01.073
78. Woo J. Sarcopenia. *Clin Geriatr Med.* 2017;3:305–314. doi:10.1016/j.cger.2017.02.003
79. United States Preventive Services Task Force. Interventions to prevent falls in community-dwelling older adults: US Preventive Services Task Force recommendation statement. *JAMA.* 2018;16:1696–1704. 10.1001/jama.2018.3097.
80. Hampson G, Elder GJ, Cohen-Solal M, et al. A review and perspective on the assessment, management and prevention of fragility fractures in patients with osteoporosis and chronic kidney disease. *Endocrine.* 2021;3:509–529. doi:10.1007/s12020-021-02735-9
81. Evenepoel P, Cunningham J, Ferrari S, et al. European consensus statement on the diagnosis and management of osteoporosis in chronic kidney disease stages g4-g5d. *Nephrol Dial Transplantat.* 2021;1:42–59. 10.1093/ndt/gfaa192.
82. Buckley L, Guyatt G, Fink HA, et al. 2017 American College of Rheumatology guideline for the prevention and treatment of glucocorticoid-induced osteoporosis. *Arthritis Care Res.* 2017;8:1095–1110. doi:10.1002/acr.23279
83. Chiodini I, Merlotti D, Falchetti A, et al. Treatment options for glucocorticoid-induced osteoporosis. *Expert Opin Pharmacother.* 2020;6:721–732. doi:10.1080/14656566.2020.1721467
84. Buckley L, Humphrey MB. Glucocorticoid-induced osteoporosis. *N Engl J Med.* 2018;26:2547–2556. doi:10.1056/NEJMcp1800214
85. Whittier X, Saag KG. Glucocorticoid-induced osteoporosis. *Rheum Dis Clin North Am.* 2016;1:177–189, x. doi:10.1016/j.rdc.2015.08.005
86. Gielen E, Bergmann P, Bruyere O, et al. Osteoporosis in frail patients: A consensus paper of the Belgian Bone Club. *Calcif Tissue Int.* 2017;2:111–131. doi:10.1007/s00223-017-0266-3
87. Compston JE, McClung MR, Leslie WD. Osteoporosis. *Lancet.* 2019;10169:364–376. doi:10.1016/S0140-6736(18)32112-3
88. Jain S. Role of bone turnover markers in osteoporosis therapy. *Endocrinol Metab Clin North Am.* 2021;2:223–237. doi:10.1016/j.ecl.2021.03.007
89. Centers for Medicare and Medicaid Services. CMS Measures Inventory Tool. Osteoporosis management in women who had a fracture. Available at https://cmit.cms.gov/CMIT_public/ViewMeasure?MeasureId=4082. Access September 7, 2021.
90. Pignolo RJ, Law SF, Chandra A. Bone aging, cellular senescence, and osteoporosis. *JBMR Plus.* 2021;4:e10488. doi:10.1002/jbm4.10488

113 Gout and Hyperuricemia

Michelle A. Fravel and Michael E. Ernst

KEY CONCEPTS

1. Treatment of hyperuricemia in the absence of a history of gout (ie, asymptomatic hyperuricemia) is not recommended.
2. An acute gout flare can be treated effectively with short courses of nonsteroidal anti-inflammatory drugs (NSAIDs), corticosteroids, or low-dose colchicine.
3. Initiation of a xanthine oxidase inhibitor may be considered in patients with one of the following indications for urate-lowering therapy (ULT): (a) one or more subcutaneous tophi, (b) evidence of joint damage by radiography, (c) two or more gout flares per year, (d) more than one previous gout flare but infrequent flares (less than two per year), (e) first gout flare in the presence of CKD stage 3 or greater, serum uric acid >9 mg/dL (535 µmol/L), or urolithiasis.
4. The goal serum urate concentration when using ULT is less than 6 mg/dL [357 µmol/L].
5. Allopurinol is the preferred ULT given its preferable safety and efficacy profile.
6. Uricosuric drugs have limited efficacy in patients with impaired kidney function [CKD stage 3 or greater].
7. Pegloticase should be reserved for patients in whom treatment with a xanthine oxidase inhibitor, uricosuric, and other interventions have failed to achieve the serum uric acid target, and who continue to have frequent gout flares (two or more per year) or non-resolving subcutaneous tophi.
8. Low-dose colchicine, NSAID, or oral corticosteroid therapy should be administered to minimize the risk of acute gout attacks during the first 3 to 6 months of initiating ULT; therapy can be extended beyond this time period if gout flares persist.
9. Uric acid nephrolithiasis should be treated with adequate hydration (2 L/day) and 30 to 80 mEq/day (mmol/day) of potassium bicarbonate or potassium citrate.
10. Patients with hyperuricemia or a history of gouty arthritis should be evaluated for commonly associated comorbidities (eg, hypertension, diabetes, CKD, cardiovascular disease), and implement lifestyle modifications and aggressive management of risk factors (eg, weight loss, reduction of alcohol intake, control of blood pressure, glucose, and lipids).

BEYOND THE BOOK

Watch the video entitled "Gout and pseudogout" from Khan Academy (Available at: https://www.youtube.com/watch?app=desktop&v=1O3F-b8FfDY&list=PL5JaZVPnPe4YY4F2P50R14mjAy3gr2giX&index=11). This 10-minute video provides a brief overview of the pathophysiology of gout versus pseudogout. The video is useful to enhance student's understanding of differences in pathophysiology and how they impact the treatment approach for each disorder, as well as the COLLECT and ASSESS steps in the patient care process.

INTRODUCTION

The term gout describes an inflammatory response to precipitation of monosodium urate (MSU) crystals in both articular and non-articular tissues.[1] The underlying metabolic disorder of gout is an elevated serum uric acid level (hyperuricemia), which is defined physiochemically as a serum that is supersaturated with monosodium urate and begins to exceed the limit of solubility (concentrations above 6.8 mg/dL [404 µmol/L]). Although hyperuricemia is fundamental to the development of gout, the mere presence of hyperuricemia itself is often an asymptomatic condition.[2,3]

EPIDEMIOLOGY

The prevalence of gout varies widely across the world, with many factors potentially contributing to the variance, including genetics, dietary habits, and socioeconomic factors.[4] Although the prevalence of gout continues to be highest in high-income countries, the overall global burden of gout has increased over the past 50 years, likely due to the aging population and increasing rates of obesity.[4,5] According to the National Health and Nutrition Examination Survey (NHANES), NHANES 2007-2016, the prevalence of gout among adults in the United States is 3.9%, corresponding to an estimated 9.2 million people.[5] Although this represents a 1.2% increase in prevalence compared with NHANES survey data from 1988 to 1994, the rate has remained stable between 2007 and 2016.[6]

Elevated serum urate concentrations are the single most important risk factor for the development of gout, and the relationship between the risk of an attack of acute gouty arthritis and serum urate concentration is linearly correlated. The 5-year cumulative risk of gout for patients with serum urate concentrations less than 7 mg/dL (416 µmol/L) is 0.6%, compared with a risk of 30.5% in those with urate concentrations exceeding 10 mg/dL (595 µmol/L).[2] Sustained elevation of serum urate is virtually essential for the development of gout; however, hyperuricemia does not always lead to gout, and many patients with hyperuricemia remain asymptomatic. For example, even in patients with severe hyperuricemia (>10 mg/dL [595 µmol/L]), fewer than 50% develop gout over a 15-year period.[3]

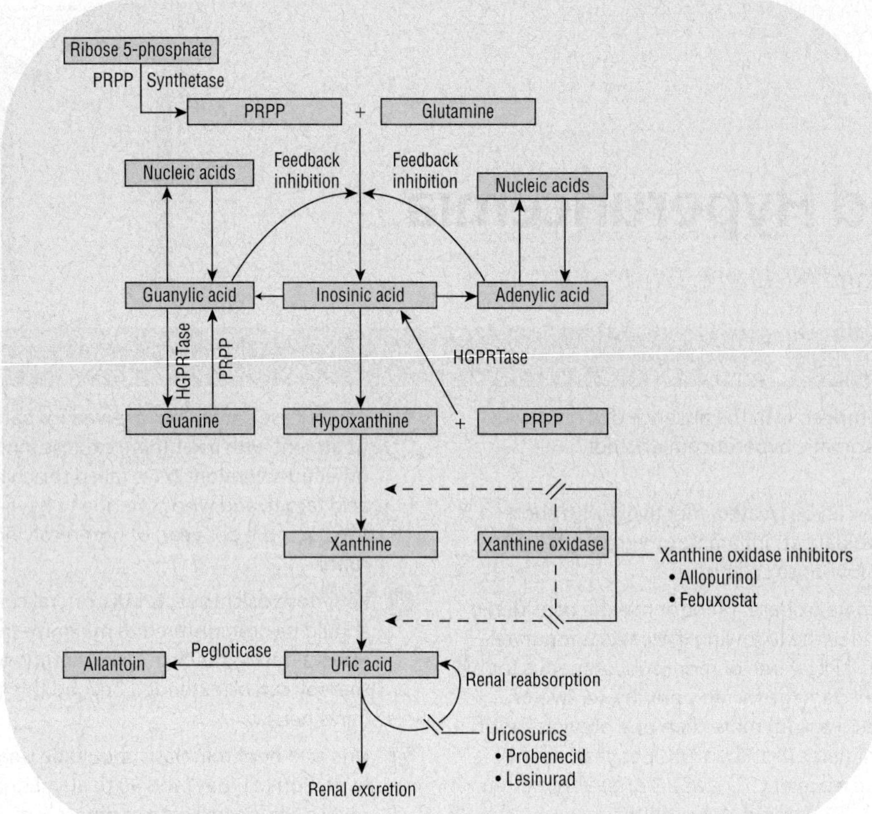

FIGURE 113-1 Uric acid pathway and targets of drug action. (HGPRT, hypoxanthine-guanine phosphoribosyltransferase; PRPP, phosphoribosyl pyrophosphate.)

Gout and hyperuricemia are more common in older adults, with the highest prevalence (8.7%) observed in those 80 years of age and older, compared with just 0.7% in those between the ages of 20 and 39 years.[5] Obesity is associated with a twofold increased risk for gout.[7] Dietary and lifestyle factors linked to obesity have also been independently associated with gout. These include consumption of alcohol, sugary beverages, and red meat, along with a sedentary lifestyle.[8]

Gout affects men about 2 to 3 times more often than women in the United States; however, the impact of sex on the risk of gout and hyperuricemia varies among different ethnicities, with a risk ratio as high as 8:1 for men compared to women in Korea.[5,9] Serum uric acid concentrations in women approach those of men once menopause has occurred due to loss of estrogen-influenced uricosuria; thus, in older age groups the gap between male and female patients narrows, and approximately half of newly diagnosed cases of gout are observed in women.[10,11] Gout in men younger than 30 years of age, or in premenopausal women, may indicate an inherited enzyme defect or the presence of kidney disease.

ETIOLOGY AND PATHOPHYSIOLOGY

In humans, the production of uric acid is the terminal step in the degradation of purines (Fig. 113-1). Uric acid serves no known physiologic purpose and is a waste product. Normal uric acid concentrations are near the limits of urate solubility, because of the delicate balance that exists between the amount of urate produced and excreted.[1] Humans have higher uric acid concentrations than other mammals because they do not express the enzyme uricase, which converts uric acid into the more soluble allantoin.[1]

Gout occurs exclusively in humans in whom a miscible pool of uric acid exists. Under normal conditions, the amount of accumulated uric acid is about 1,200 mg in men and about 600 mg in women. The size of the urate pool is increased severalfold in individuals with gout. This excess accumulation may result from either overproduction or underexcretion of uric acid. Several conditions are associated with either decreased kidney clearance or an overproduction of uric acid, leading to hyperuricemia. Table 113-1 lists some of these conditions.

TABLE 113-1 Conditions Associated with Hyperuricemia

Primary gout	Obesity
Diabetic ketoacidosis	Sarcoidosis
Myeloproliferative disorders	Congestive heart failure
Lactic acidosis	Impaired kidney function
Lymphoproliferative disorders	Down syndrome
Starvation	Lead toxicity
Chronic hemolytic anemia	Hyperparathyroidism
Toxemia of pregnancy	Acute alcoholism
Pernicious anemia	Hypoparathyroidism
Glycogen storage disease type 1	Acromegaly
Psoriasis	Hypothyroidism
Hypoxanthine-guanine phosphoribosyltransferase deficiency	Phosphoribosylpyrophosphate synthetase overactivity
Polycythemia vera	Berylliosis
Kidney transplantation	

Overproduction of Uric Acid

The purines from which uric acid is produced originate from three sources: dietary purine, conversion of tissue nucleic acid into purine nucleotides, and de novo synthesis of purine bases. The purines derived from these three sources enter a common metabolic pathway leading to the production of either nucleic acid or uric acid. Under normal circumstances, uric acid may accumulate excessively if production exceeds excretion. The average human produces about 600 to 800 mg of uric acid each day. Dietary purines play an unimportant role in the generation of hyperuricemia in the absence of some derangement in purine metabolism or elimination. However, diet modifications are an important first step for patients who develop symptomatic hyperuricemia.

Several enzyme systems regulate purine metabolism. Abnormalities in these regulatory systems can result in overproduction of uric acid. Uric acid may also be overproduced as a consequence of increased breakdown of tissue nucleic acids and excessive rates of cell turnover, as observed with myeloproliferative and lymphoproliferative disorders, polycythemia vera, psoriasis, and some types of anemias. Cytotoxic medications used to treat these disorders can result in overproduction of uric acid secondary to lysis and breakdown of cellular matter.

Two enzyme abnormalities resulting in an overproduction of uric acid have been well described (Fig. 113-1). The first is an increase in the activity of phosphoribosyl pyrophosphate (PRPP) synthetase, which leads to an increased concentration of PRPP. PRPP is a key determinant of purine synthesis and uric acid production. The second is a deficiency of hypoxanthine-guanine phosphoribosyltransferase (HGPRT). HGPRT is responsible for the conversion of guanine to guanylic acid and hypoxanthine to inosinic acid. These two conversions require PRPP as the co-substrate and are important reactions involved in the synthesis of nucleic acids. A deficiency in the HGPRT enzyme leads to increased metabolism of guanine and hypoxanthine to uric acid and to more PRPP to interact with glutamine in the first step of the purine pathway.[1] Complete absence of HGPRT results in the childhood Lesch–Nyhan syndrome, characterized by choreoathetosis, spasticity, intellectual disability, and markedly excessive production of uric acid. A partial deficiency of the enzyme may be responsible for marked hyperuricemia in otherwise normal, healthy individuals.

Underexcretion of Uric Acid

Normally, uric acid does not accumulate as long as production is balanced with elimination. About two-thirds of the daily uric acid production is excreted in the urine and the remainder is eliminated through the gastrointestinal (GI) tract after enzymatic degradation by colonic bacteria.

TABLE 113-2 Drugs Capable of Inducing Hyperuricemia and Gout

Diuretics	Ethanol	Ethambutol
Nicotinic acid	Pyrazinamide	Cytotoxic drugs
Salicylates (<2 g/day)	Testosterone	Cyclosporine

A decline in the urinary excretion of uric acid to a concentration below the rate of production leads to hyperuricemia and an increased miscible pool of sodium urate. Almost all the urate in plasma is freely filtered across the glomerulus. The concentration of uric acid appearing in the urine is determined by multiple renal tubular transport processes in addition to the filtered load. Evidence favors a four-component model including glomerular filtration, tubular reabsorption, tubular secretion, and post-secretory reabsorption.

Approximately 90% of filtered uric acid is reabsorbed in the proximal tubule, probably by both active and passive transport mechanisms. There is a close linkage between proximal tubular sodium reabsorption and uric acid reabsorption, so conditions that enhance sodium reabsorption (eg, dehydration) also lead to increased uric acid reabsorption. The exact site of tubular secretion of uric acid has not been determined; this too involves an active transport process. Post-secretory reabsorption occurs somewhere distal to the secretory site. Table 113-2 lists the drugs that decrease renal clearance of uric acid through modification of filtered load or one of the tubular transport processes.[12] By enhancing renal urate reabsorption, insulin resistance is also associated with gout.

CLINICAL PRESENTATION

1 Gout is diagnosed clinically by the presence of symptoms, rather than laboratory tests of uric acid. In fact, asymptomatic hyperuricemia discovered incidentally generally requires no therapy because many individuals with hyperuricemia will never experience an attack of gout.[2,3] These patients should still be encouraged to implement lifestyle measures to reduce serum urate concentrations.

Acute Gouty Arthritis

A classic acute attack of gouty arthritis is characterized by rapid and localized onset of excruciating pain, swelling, and inflammation. The attack is typically monoarticular at first, most often affecting the

CLINICAL PRESENTATION Acute Gouty Arthritis

General

- Gout classically presents as an acute inflammatory monoarthritis. The first metatarsophalangeal joint is often involved ("podagra"), but any joint of the lower extremity can be affected and occasionally gout will present as a monoarthritis of the wrist or finger. The spectrum of gout also includes nephrolithiasis, gouty nephropathy, and aggregated deposits of sodium urate (tophi) in cartilage, tendons, synovial membranes, and elsewhere.

Signs and Symptoms

- Fever, intense pain, erythema, warmth, swelling, and inflammation of involved joints.

Laboratory Tests

- Elevated serum uric acid concentrations; leukocytosis.

Other Diagnostic Tests

- Observation of MSU crystals in synovial fluid or a tophus.
- For patients with long-standing gout, radiographs may show asymmetric swelling within a joint on or subcortical cysts without erosions.

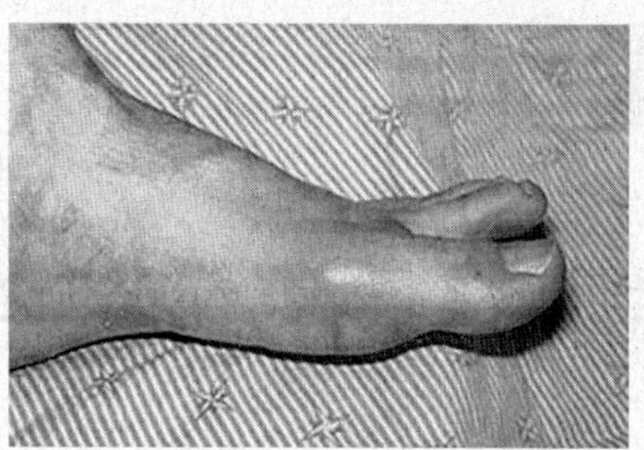

FIGURE 113-2 Acute gout attack of the first metatarsophalangeal joint. *(Reproduced with permission from Imboden J, Hellmann DB, Stone JH. Current Rheumatology Diagnosis &Treatment. 2nd ed. New York: McGraw Hill, 2004:316.)*

TABLE 113-3 Clinical Manifestations of Gout

Acute gout	Monoarticular arthritis Frequently attacks the first metatarsophalangeal joint ("podagra"), although other joints of the lower extremities are also frequently involved Affected joint is swollen, erythematous, and tender
Interval gout	Asymptomatic period between attacks
Tophaceous gout	Deposits of monosodium urate crystals in soft tissues Complications include soft tissue damage, deformity, joint destruction, and nerve compression syndromes such as carpal tunnel syndrome
Atypical gout	Polyarthritis affecting any joint, upper or lower extremity May be confused with rheumatoid arthritis or osteoarthritis
Gouty nephropathy	Nephrolithiasis Acute and chronic kidney disease

first metatarsophalangeal joint (great toe) and then, in order of frequency, the insteps, ankles, heels, knees, wrists, fingers, and elbows. In one-half of initial attacks, the first metatarsophalangeal joint is affected, a condition commonly referred to as podagra (Fig. 113-2). Up to 90% of patients with gout will experience podagra at some point in the course of their disease.[2]

Atypical presentations of gout also occur. For older adults, gout can present as a chronic polyarticular arthritis that can be confused with rheumatoid arthritis or osteoarthritis. Table 113-3 summarizes the different clinical manifestations of gout.

The predilection of acute gout for peripheral joints of the lower extremity is probably related to the low temperature of these joints combined with high intra-articular urate concentration. Synovial effusions are likely to occur transiently in weight-bearing joints during the course of a day with routine activity. At night, water is reabsorbed from the joint space, leaving behind a supersaturated solution of monosodium urate (MSU), which can precipitate attacks of acute arthritis. Attacks generally begin at night with the patient awakened from sleep by excruciating pain.

The development of crystal-induced inflammation involves several chemical mediators causing vasodilation, increased vascular permeability, complement activation, and chemotactic activity for polymorphonuclear leukocytes.[1] Phagocytosis of urate crystals by the leukocytes results in rapid lysis of cells and a discharge of lysosomal and proteolytic enzymes into the cytoplasm. The ensuing inflammatory reaction is associated with intense joint pain, erythema, warmth, and swelling. Fever is common, as is leukocytosis. Untreated attacks may last from 3 to 14 days before spontaneous recovery.

TABLE 113-4 Differential Diagnosis of Gout

1. Pseudogout (calcium pyrophosphate crystal-related arthritis)
2. Rheumatoid disease
3. Psoriatic arthritis
4. Osteoarthritis
5. Septic arthritis/bursitis
6. Cellulitis
7. Osteomyelitis
8. Unrelated hyperuricemia (as in psoriasis, hypertension) when joint pain is not caused by gout

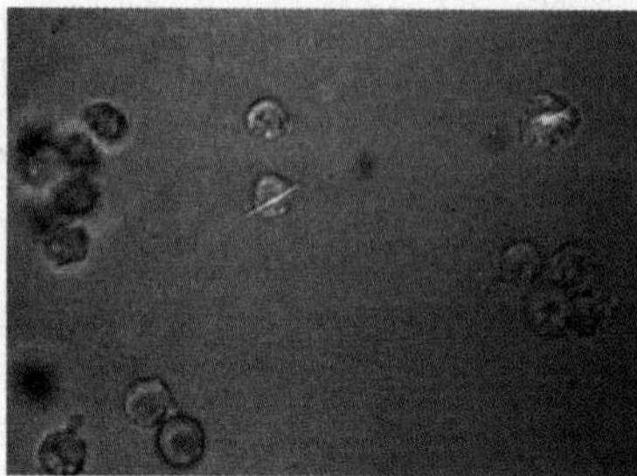

FIGURE 113-3 Urate crystal ingested by a polymorphonuclear leukocyte in synovial fluid. *(Reproduced with permission from Imboden J, Hellmann DB, Stone JH. Current Rheumatology Diagnosis &Treatment. 2nd ed. New York: McGraw Hill, 2004:317.)*

Although acute attacks of gouty arthritis may occur without apparent provocation, several conditions may precipitate an attack. These include stress, trauma, alcohol ingestion, infection, surgery, rapid lowering of serum uric acid by ingestion of uric acid-lowering agents, and ingestion of certain drugs known to elevate serum uric acid concentrations (Table 113-2). The natural course of an acute flare, if left untreated, varies among patients and may resolve after several hours or may take up to 2 weeks. Furthermore, acute flares of gouty arthritis may initially occur infrequently. Over time the duration of untreated attacks may become longer and the interval between attacks may shorten if appropriate measures to correct hyperuricemia are not undertaken. Later in the disease, tophaceous deposits of MSU in the skin or subcutaneous tissues may be found. These tophi are often found on the hands, wrists, elbows, or knees. It takes 10 or more years for tophi to develop.

Diagnostic Evaluation

Table 113-4 lists the differential diagnosis of gout.[10] A definitive diagnosis of gout requires aspiration of synovial fluid from the affected joint and identification of intracellular crystals of monosodium urate monohydrate in synovial fluid leukocytes.[1] Identification of MSU crystals are highly dependent on the experience of the observer. Crystals are needle-shaped, and when examined under polarizing light microscopy, they are strongly negatively birefringent (Fig. 113-3). Crystals can be observed in synovial fluid during asymptomatic periods.[13] If an affected joint is tapped, the resulting synovial fluid may have white cells and appear purulent. Such findings should always raise the question of infection. If any clinical features of infection are present, such as high fever, elevated white blood cell count, multiple joints affected, or an identified source of infection, proper diagnosis and treatment are critical. Patients with gout can have septic arthritis. Diabetes, alcohol abuse, and advanced age increase the likelihood of septic arthritis.

In lieu of obtaining a synovial fluid sample from an affected joint to inspect for urate crystals, a clinical diagnosis may be supported by the following characteristics: monoarticular involvement of a foot or ankle joint, previous similar episode, rapid onset of severe pain and swelling (peak pain intensity in <24 hours), erythema, male sex, presence of cardiovascular disease, and hyperuricemia. However, this approach has limitations, including a failure to recognize atypical gout presentations and the fact that serum uric acid concentrations can be normal or even low during an acute gout attack.[10,14] Radiographs may show evidence of MSU crystal deposits; however, ultrasound may be more helpful in the identification of tophi or a double contour sign at cartilage surfaces, which is specific for articular urate deposits.[15] The presence of chondrocalcinosis on radiographs may indicate pseudogout (see additional discussion on pseudogout below). Table 113-5 summarizes the European League Against Rheumatism (EULAR) evidence-based diagnostic principles for gout.[15]

The American College of Rheumatology (ACR) and EULAR have also jointly developed recommendations for the classification of gout to assist in identifying subjects potentially eligible for enrollment into clinical trials of gout treatments.[16] Although it is specifically stated that the recommendations should not be used clinically to diagnose gout, the classification system may be a useful reference when evaluating a patient presenting with symptoms suggestive of gout. The recommendations utilize a point-based system that incorporates clinical, laboratory, and imaging information, which can be used when a patient presents with at least one episode of swelling, pain, or tenderness in a peripheral joint or bursa but has no evidence of MSU crystals. An online calculator is available at http://goutclassificationcalculator.auckland.ac.nz/.

Other crystal-induced arthropathies that may resemble gout on clinical presentation are caused by calcium hydroxyapatite crystals and calcium pyrophosphate dihydrate crystals (calcium pyrophosphate deposition disease [CPDD] or "pseudogout"), which are associated with calcific periarthritis, tendinitis, and arthritis.[17-19] Pseudogout is relatively common, occurring in up to 7% of all adults in Europe and the United States. Furthermore, its prevalence increases with age, doubling with every decade over 60 years.[17] Identification of calcium pyrophosphate crystals in the synovial fluid of an affected joint in combination with positive radiology findings (eg, chondrocalcinosis, hook-like osteophytes, and axial skeletal involvement) are key methods used for diagnosis of pseudogout. Importantly, calcium pyrophosphate crystals differ from uric acid crystals in that they are positively birefringent when exposed to light microscopy. Furthermore, the clinical picture may provide clues as pseudogout rarely presents with podagra and more commonly affects the knee or wrist. Although initial management of an acute flare of pseudogout is similar to the approach used for treatment of gout, management of chronic pseudogout may require use of hydroxychloroquine, methotrexate, and, ultimately, joint replacement. Recommended therapies used to prevent gout by lowering uric acid will not impact the progression of pseudogout. For these reasons, differentiating between pseudogout and gout, although challenging, is important to insure successful clinical outcomes.

TABLE 113-5 EULAR Recommendations for Diagnosis of Gout

Recommendations	Level of Evidence	Grade of Evidence
1. Searching for crystals in synovial fluid or tophus aspirates is recommended in every person with suspected gout, because demonstration of MSU crystals allows a definitive diagnosis of gout.	2b	B
2. Gout should be considered in the diagnosis of any acute arthritis in an adult. When synovial fluid analysis is not feasible, a clinical diagnosis of gout is supported by the following suggestive features: monoarticular involvement of a foot (especially the first MTP) or ankle joint; previous similar acute arthritis episodes; rapid onset of severe pain and swelling (at its worst in <24 hours); erythema; male gender; and associated cardiovascular diseases and hyperuricemia. These features are highly suggestive, but not specific, for gout.	2b	B
3. Synovial fluid aspiration and examination for crystals in any patient with undiagnosed inflammatory arthritis is recommended.	3	C
4. The diagnosis of gout should not be made on the presence of hyperuricemia alone.	2a	B
5. When a clinical diagnosis of gout is uncertain and crystal identification is not possible, patients should be investigated with imaging (see #6 below) to search for MSU crystal deposition and features of any alternative diagnosis.	1b	A
6. Plain radiographs are indicated to search for imaging evidence of MSU crystal deposition but have limited value for the diagnosis of gout flare. Ultrasound scanning can be more helpful in establishing a diagnosis in patients with suspected gout flare or chronic gouty arthritis by detection of tophi not evident on clinical examination, or a double contour sign at cartilage surfaces, which is highly specific for urate deposits in joints.	1b	A
7. Risk factors for chronic hyperuricemia should be searched for in every person with gout; these include chronic kidney disease; obesity, medications (including diuretics, low-dose aspirin, cyclosporine, tacrolimus); excess consumption of alcohol (particularly beer and spirits), non-diet sodas, red meat, and shellfish.	1a	A
8. Systematic assessment for the presence of associated comorbidities in people with gout is recommended, including obesity, kidney disease, hypertension, ischemic heart disease, heart failure, diabetes, and dyslipidemia.	1a	A

EULAR, The European League Against Rheumatism; MSU, monosodium urate.

Data from Reference 20.

Level of Evidence: 1A = meta-analysis of cohort studies, 1B = meta-analysis of case-control studies, 2A = cohort studies, 2B = case-control studies, 3 = non-comparative descriptive studies, 4 = expert option.

Grade of Evidence: A = category 1 evidence, B = category 2 evidence or extrapolated recommendations from category 1 evidence, C = category 3 evidence or extrapolated recommendations from category 2 evidence, D = category 4 evidence or extrapolated recommendations from category 3 evidence.

Uric Acid Nephrolithiasis

Clinicians should be suspicious of hyperuricemic states in patients who present with kidney stones, as nephrolithiasis occurs in approximately 14% of patients with gout.[20] The frequency of urolithiasis depends on serum uric acid concentrations, acidity of the urine, and urinary uric acid concentration. Typically, patients with uric acid nephrolithiasis have a urinary pH of less than 6 and frequently less than 5.5. When acidic urine is saturated with uric acid, spontaneous precipitation of stones may occur.

Other factors that predispose individuals to uric acid nephrolithiasis include excessive urinary excretion of uric acid and highly concentrated urine. In addition to pure uric acid stones, hyperuricosuric individuals are at increased risk for mixed uric acid–calcium oxalate stones and pure calcium oxalate stones.

Gouty Nephropathy

There are two types of gouty nephropathy: acute uric acid nephropathy and chronic urate nephropathy.[21] In acute uric acid nephropathy, acute kidney injury occurs as a result of blockage of urine flow secondary to massive precipitation of uric acid crystals in the collecting ducts and ureters. This syndrome is a known complication for patients with myeloproliferative or lymphoproliferative disorders and is a result of massive malignant cell turnover, particularly after initiation of chemotherapy.

Chronic urate nephropathy is caused by the long-term deposition of urate crystals in the renal parenchyma. Microtophi may form, with a surrounding giant-cell inflammatory reaction. A decrease in the kidneys' ability to concentrate urine and the presence of proteinuria may be the earliest pathophysiologic disturbances. Hypertension and nephrosclerosis are common associated findings. Although kidney failure occurs in a higher percentage of gouty patients than expected, it is not clear if hyperuricemia per se has a harmful effect on the kidneys. The chronic kidney disease seen in individuals with gout may result largely from the coexistence of hypertension, diabetes mellitus, and atherosclerosis.

Tophaceous Gout

Tophi (urate deposits) are uncommon in the general population of patients with gout, but are a late complication of untreated hyperuricemia. The most common sites of tophaceous deposits for patients with recurrent acute gouty arthritis are the base of the fingers, olecranon bursae, ulnar aspect of the forearm, Achilles tendon, knees, wrists, and hands (Fig. 113-4).[21] Eventually, even the hips, shoulders, and spine may be affected. In addition to causing obvious deformities, tophi may damage surrounding soft tissue, cause joint destruction and pain, and can even lead to nerve compression syndromes including carpal tunnel syndrome.

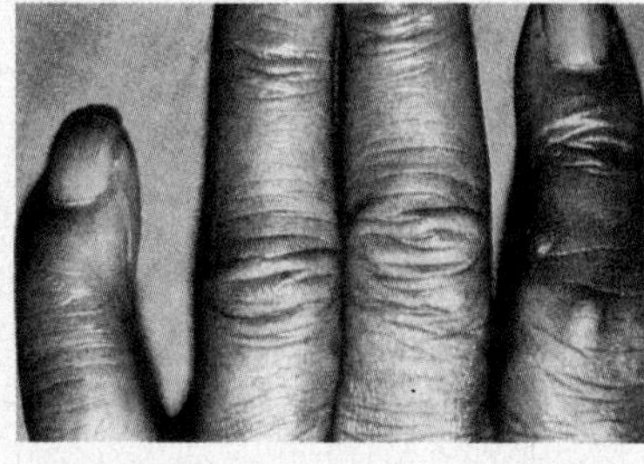

FIGURE 113-4 Tophaceous gout with subcutaneous nodule almost breaking through the skin. *(Reproduced with permission from South-Paul JE, Matheny SC, Lewis EL. Current Diagnosis and Treatment in Family Medicine. New York: McGraw Hill, 2004:275.)*

TREATMENT

Desired Outcomes

The goals in the treatment of gout are to terminate the acute attack, prevent recurrent attacks of gouty arthritis, and prevent complications associated with chronic deposition of urate crystals in joints and tissues. These can be accomplished through a combination of pharmacologic and nonpharmacologic methods, including focused patient education efforts. Several organizations, including ACR, EULAR, and the American College of Physicians, have developed guidelines for the management of gout.

The first-ever ACR evidence- and consensus-based guidelines for the management of gout were published in 2012 and were most updated in 2020.[22-24] These guidelines provide specific recommendations for treatment of acute gout attacks, management of hyperuricemia in gout, and anti-inflammatory prophylaxis of acute gout during initiation of ULT. Tables 113-6 and 113-7 summarize dosing and monitoring information for available pharmacotherapy used in management and prevention of gout.

General Approach to Treatment

Treatment of gout can be separated into three categories: (1) treatment of the pain and inflammation associated with an acute gout attack, (2) use of ULT to prevent recurrence of future gout attacks, and (3) use of anti-inflammatory prophylaxis to prevent acute gout attacks during initiation of urate-lowering therapy, which can occur paradoxically as a result of the rapid decline in serum urate after initiation of these therapies. Each of these categories will be covered in further detail throughout the remainder of the treatment section of this chapter.

Acute Gouty Arthritis

Nonpharmacologic Therapy

Nonpharmacologic therapies have an important role in modifying the underlying hyperuricemia and reducing the risk of an acute gout attack before one occurs. However, nonpharmacologic therapies for treatment of an acute gout attack are limited and are recommended strictly as adjuvants.

Local ice application to the affected joint is the most effective adjuvant.[24] Localized ice application results in significantly greater pain reduction in those receiving the therapy compared with those not treated with ice.[25] Complementary and alternative medicines, including vitamin C, flaxseed, cherry, and celery root, are not recommended for treatment of acute gout due to unproven benefit.[23,24]

Pharmacologic Therapy

2 For most patients, acute attacks of gouty arthritis may be treated successfully with NSAIDs, corticosteroids, or colchicine. The ACR guidelines recognize these three monotherapies equally as first-line treatments of acute gout.[23,24,26,27] Treatment should commence as soon as possible after the onset of an attack. In more severe cases involving inadequate response to first-line therapy, combination first-line therapy or off-label use of IL-1 inhibitor therapy may be considered (Fig. 113-5).[23,26]

Nonsteroidal Anti-Inflammatory Drugs NSAIDs are a mainstay of therapy for acute attacks of gouty arthritis because of their excellent efficacy and minimal toxicity with short-term use. Indomethacin has been historically favored as the NSAID of choice for acute gout flares, but there is little evidence to support one NSAID as being more efficacious than another. Three agents (indomethacin, naproxen, and sulindac) have US Food and Drug Administration (FDA)-approved labeling for the treatment of gout, although several

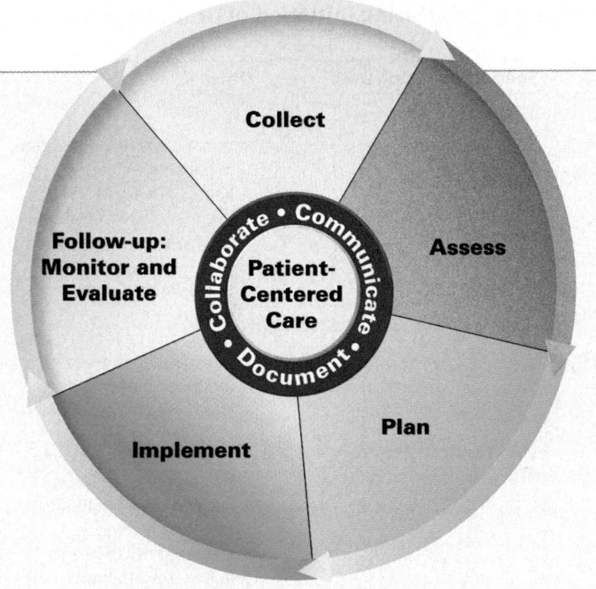

Patient Care Process for Gout

Collect

- Patient characteristics (eg, age, sex, ethnicity)
- Patient medical history (see Table 113-1)
- Dietary habits that may lead to increased uric acid concentrations, including alcohol consumption, intake of high purine foods, and products containing high-fructose corn syrup
- Current medications that may contribute to hyperuricemia (see Table 113-2)
- Subjective report of acute gout symptoms
- Objective data
  - o Blood pressure (BP), height, weight
  - o Labs including uric acid, serum creatinine (SCr)
  - o Synovial fluid aspirate

Assess

- Presence of acute gout (see Tables 113-3 and 113-5)
- Presence of hyperuricemia (>6.8 mg/dL [404 μmol/L])
- Indication for urate-lowering therapy (see Table 113-6)
- Optimal therapy given the patient-specific characteristics (see Table 113-9)
- Presence of other cardiovascular risk factors (eg, hypertension, diabetes)

Plan*

- Drug therapy regimen, including a specific agent for the treatment of acute gout: dose, route, frequency, and duration (see Table 113-6)
- Monitoring parameters for efficacy (eg, resolution of pain) and safety (eg, signs and symptoms of adverse effects associated with selected therapy), frequency and timing of follow-up
- Drug therapy regimen including specific agent for treatment of hyperuricemia if indicated: dose, route, frequency, and duration (see Table 113-6)
- Patient education (eg, the purpose of treatment vs prevention, dietary and lifestyle modification, drug-specific information, medication counseling; see Table 113-6)
- Self-monitoring for resolution of gout symptoms and occurrence of medication side effects
- Referrals to other providers when appropriate (eg, rheumatologist, dietitian)

Implement*

- Provide patient education regarding all elements of the treatment plan
- Use motivational interviewing and coaching strategies to maximize adherence
- Schedule follow-up (eg, assessment of uric acid, SCr, adherence)

Follow-up: Monitor and Evaluate

- Resolution of gout symptoms (eg, pain)
- Presence of adverse effects (eg, diarrhea [colchicine], agitation [corticosteroids], rash or allopurinol hypersensitivity syndrome [allopurinol])
- Uric acid concentrations [allopurinol, febuxostat] (adjust dose as needed to achieve uric acid <6.0 mg/dL [357 μmol/L])
- Patient adherence to treatment plan using multiple sources of information

**Collaborate with patients, caregivers, and other healthcare professionals.*

others are likely to be effective.[23] The most important determinant of therapeutic success is not which NSAID is chosen, but rather, how soon it is initiated. Early initiation of treatment is more likely to be effective than if delayed; therefore, ensuring patients have a plan to access therapy on their own when needed (referred to as the "medication-in-pocket" strategy) is an important cornerstone of an optimized gout management strategy.[24] Following resolution of the attack, tapering of NSAID therapy may be considered, especially in patients with comorbidities such as impaired hepatic or kidney function where prolonged therapy would be undesirable.[23] Resolution of an acute attack for most patients generally occurs within 5 to 8 days after initiating therapy.

All NSAIDs have the potential to cause similar adverse effects. The most common areas affected include the gastrointestinal (GI) system (gastritis, bleeding, perforation), kidneys (renal papillary necrosis, reduced glomerular filtration rate), cardiovascular system (sodium and fluid retention, increased blood pressure), and central nervous system (CNS) (impaired cognitive function, headache, dizziness). Caution should be exercised when using NSAIDs in individuals with a history of peptic ulcer disease, congestive heart failure, uncontrolled hypertension, impaired kidney function, coronary artery disease, or who are concurrently receiving anticoagulants or antiplatelets. Patients with active peptic ulcer disease, decompensated congestive heart failure, chronic kidney disease, or a history of hypersensitivity to aspirin or other NSAIDs should not be prescribed an NSAID.

Selective cyclooxygenase-2 (COX-2) inhibitors present a potentially less risky alternative to nonselective NSAIDs in patients with

TABLE 113-6 Pharmacotherapy of Acute Gout, Anti-Inflammatory Prophylaxis During Initiation of Urate-Lowering Therapy and Hyperuricemia in Gout[a]

Drug	Brand Name	Initial Dose	Usual Range	Special Population Dose	Other
Acute Gout					
NSAIDs					In general, not recommended in patients with advanced kidney disease as NSAID use may decrease kidney function; use with caution in patients with mild to moderate kidney impairment Use caution in patients taking anticoagulants given increased bleeding risk when used in combination with NSAIDs Use caution in patients with heart failure as NSAIDs can contribute to fluid retention leading to increased risk of heart failure exacerbation
Etodolac	Lodine, various	300 mg twice daily	300-500 mg twice daily		
Fenoprofen	Nalfon, various	400 mg three times daily	400-600 mg three to four times daily		
Ibuprofen	Advil, various	400 mg three times daily	400-800 mg three to four times daily		
Indomethacin	Indocin	50 mg three times daily	50 mg three times daily initially until pain is tolerable then rapidly reduce to complete cessaion		
Ketoprofen	Orudis, various	75 mg three times daily or 50 mg four times daily	50-75 mg three to four times daily	Severe kidney impairment (GFR <25 mL/min [0.42 mL/s]): 100 mg maximum daily dose Mildly impaired kidney function: 150 mg maximum daily dose Impaired liver function with serum albumin <3.5 g/dL (35 g/L): 100 mg maximum daily dose	
Naproxen	Naprosyn, various	750 mg followed by 250 mg every 8 hours until the attack has subsided		Not recommended in severe kidney impairment (creatinine clearance <30 mL/min [0.5 mL/s])	
Piroxicam	Feldene	20 mg once daily or divided twice daily			
Sulindac	Clinoril	200 mg twice a day	150-200 mg twice daily for 7-10 days		
Meloxicam	Mobic	5 mg daily	7.5-15 mg daily	Not recommended if creatinine clearance <15 mL/min (0.25 mL/s)	
Celecoxib	Celebrex	800 mg followed by 400 mg on day one then 400 mg twice daily for 1 week			Option for patients with GI contraindications to nonselective NSAIDs; unclear risk-to-benefit ratio now due to cardiovascular concerns
Colchicine	Colcrys	1.2 mg initially, followed by 0.6 mg 1 hour later, with ongoing anti-inflammatory therapy until the flare resolves		See Table 113-8	Dose adjustment recommended when used with selected CYP3A4 and P-glycoprotein inhibitors
Corticosteroids					
Oral		0.5 mg/kg prednisone equivalent daily for 5-10 days followed by discontinuation or 0.5 mg/kg daily for 2-5 days followed by tapering for 7-10 days	30-60 mg prednisone equivalent once daily for 3-5 days, then taper in 5-mg decrements spread over 10-14 days until discontinuation		The use of an oral methylprednisolone dose pack may be considered
Intramuscular		Triamcinolone acetonide 60 mg IM once; methylprednisolone 100 mg IM once	Triamcinolone acetonide 60 mg IM once; methylprednisolone 100-150 mg IM daily for 1-2 days		Administration of intramuscular triamcinolone is to be followed by oral prednisone or prednisolone

(Continued)

TABLE 113-6 Pharmacotherapy of Acute Gout, Anti-Inflammatory Prophylaxis During Initiation of Urate-Lowering Therapy and Hyperuricemia in Gout[a] (*Continued*)

Drug	Brand Name	Initial Dose	Usual Range	Special Population Dose	Other
Intra-articular	Kenalog	Triamcinolone acetonide 10 mg (large joints), 5 mg (small joints)	Triamcinolone acetonide 10-40 mg (large joints), 5-20 mg (small joints)		Intra-articular administration is acceptable when only one to two joints involved and should be used in combination with NSAIDs, colchicine, or oral corticosteroids
Corticotropin	H.P. Acthar Gel	20-40 units IM or SC	Dose may be repeated as clinically indicated; a dose of 40-80 units every 24-72 hours is used for other inflammatory conditions		Contraindicated for IV administration
Interleukin-1 inhibitors					Reserve use for refractory cases
Anakinra	Kineret	100 mg SC daily for 5 days			
Canakinumab	Ilaris	Single dose 150 mg SC			
Anti-Inflammatory Prophylaxis During Initiation of Urate-Lowering Therapy					
NSAIDs			Lowest effective dosage		
Colchicine	Colcrys	0.6 mg daily	0.6 mg once or twice daily	See Table 113-8	
Prednisone or prednisolone		≤10 mg daily			
Interleukin-1 inhibitors					Reserve use for refractory cases Studied for 16-week duration
Rilonacept	Arcalyst	320 mg loading dose followed by 160 mg weekly (SC)			
Canakinumab	Ilaris	Single SC dose (50 mg-300 mg) or four times weekly SC dosing (50 mg—50 mg—25 mg—25 mg)			
Hyperuricemia in Gout					
Xanthine oxidase inhibitors					
Allopurinol	Lopurin, Zyloprim	100 mg daily	100-800 mg daily to achieve serum urate concentration <6 mg/dL (357 μmol/L)	Start at dose of 50 mg daily for patients with a glomerular filtration rate <30 mL/min/1.73 m² (0.29 mL/s/m²)	
Febuxostat	Uloric	40 mg daily	40-80 mg/daily	No dosage adjustment necessary for patients with mild-moderate kidney impairment (creatinine clearance 30-89 mL/min [0.5-1.49 mL/s]) Insufficient data in patients with creatinine clearance <30 mL/min (0.5 mL/s)	
Uricosurics					
Probenecid	Probalan	250 mg twice daily for 1 week	500-2,000 mg/day (target serum urate concentration <6 mg/dL [357 mol/L])	Not recommended if creatinine clearance <50 mL/min (0.83 mL/s)	

(*Continued*)

TABLE 113-6 Pharmacotherapy of Acute Gout, Anti-Inflammatory Prophylaxis During Initiation of Urate-Lowering Therapy and Hyperuricemia in Gout[a] (*Continued*)

Drug	Brand Name	Initial Dose	Usual Range	Special Population Dose	Other
Lesinurad	Zurampic	200 mg once daily in combination with a xanthine oxidase inhibitor		Not recommended if creatinine clearance <45 mL/min (0.75 mL/s) Not studied in patients with severe hepatic disease Contraindicated in tumor lysis syndrome and Lesch-Nyhan syndrome	Should be used in combination with a xanthine oxidase inhibitor due to increased risk of acute kidney injury with lesinurad monotherapy Use is not recommended in patients taking allopurinol doses <300 mg daily (normal kidney function) or <200 mg daily (creatinine clearance <60 mL/min [1 mL/s]) Not currently marketed in the United States
Combination Therapy					
Lesinurad/ Allopurinol	Duzallo	Lesinurad 200 mg/ allopurinol 300 mg: one tablet daily		Lesinurad 200 mg/allopurinol 200 mg: one tablet daily recommended if creatinine clearance is 45-60 mL/min (0.75-1 mL/s) Not recommended if creatinine clearance <45 mL/min (0.75 mL/s)	See above for lesinurad and allopurinol comments Not currently marketed in the United States
Other					
Pegloticase	Krystexxa	8 mg IV every 2 weeks			Optimal treatment duration has not been established Reserved for patients with refractory gout who have failed other therapies and continue to have frequent gout flares (≥2 flares/year) OR who have non-resolving subcutaneous tophi

[a]Agents available in the United States.

CYP, cytochrome P; GFR, glomerular filtration rate; IM, intramuscular; IV, intravenous; NSAID, nonsteroidal anti-inflammatory drug; SC, subcutaneous.

TABLE 113-7 Drug Monitoring

Drug	Adverse Drug Reaction	Monitoring Parameter	Comments
NSAIDs	Impaired kidney function (acute and chronic) gastritis (worse with concurrent aspirin), fluid retention, blood pressure elevation	Therapeutic Resolution of pain Avoidance of gout attacks when used for prophylaxis Toxic Blood pressure Kidney function Edema Dark stools	Avoid in patients with peptic ulcer disease, active bleeding Use caution in heart failure, dehydration, impaired kidney function Consider coadministration with a proton-pump inhibitor when used long term for patients at risk for GI bleeding
Systemic corticosteroids	GI upset, increased appetite, nervousness/restlessness, transient glucose intolerance, fluid retention, blood pressure elevation	Therapeutic Resolution of pain Avoidance of gout attacks when used for prophylaxis Toxic Glucose levels in patients with diabetes	Limit duration of therapy in patients with diabetes
Intra-articular corticosteroids	Injection pain, rebound arthritis	Therapeutic Resolution of pain Toxic Signs of rebound arthritis (pain relief followed by reemergence of pain)	Avoid if joint sepsis cannot be ruled out
Corticotropin	Increased appetite, nervousness/restlessness, transient glucose intolerance, fluid retention, blood pressure elevation	Therapeutic Resolution of pain	Requires intact pituitary–adrenal axis Less effective for patients receiving long-term oral corticosteroid therapy

(*Continued*)

TABLE 113-7 Drug Monitoring (*Continued*)

Drug	Adverse Drug Reaction	Monitoring Parameter	Comments
Colchicine	Dose-dependent GI adverse effects (diarrhea, nausea, vomiting), rare myelosuppression, and reversible neuromyopathy	Therapeutic Resolution of pain Avoidance of gout attacks when used for prophylaxis Toxic GI symptoms Complete blood count	
Interleukin-1 inhibitors	Injection site reaction, neutropenia, immune hypersensitivity reaction, infectious disease, malignancy	Therapeutic Resolution of pain Avoidance of gout attacks when used for prophylaxis Toxic Neutrophil count (prior to initiation, monthly for the first 3 months of therapy then after 6, 9, and 12 months of therapy) Temperature (periodically to detect infection)	Safety for use in acute gout and gout prophylaxis during initiation of urate-lowering therapy has not yet been established; not FDA-approved for use in gout
Allopurinol	Rash, potential for fatal hypersensitivity syndrome	Therapeutic Serum urate level Reduced frequency of gout attacks Toxic Rash Kidney function	Testing for the HLA-B*5801 allele prior to starting allopurinol is recommended for patients of Southeast Asian (eg, Han Chinese, Korean, Thai) and African descent
Febuxostat	Liver enzyme elevation, nausea, arthralgias, and rash	Therapeutic Serum urate level Reduced frequency of gout attacks Toxic Liver function tests Kidney function	Use not recommended in patients with cardiovascular disease
Probenecid	Urolithiasis	Therapeutic Serum urate level Reduced frequency of gout attacks Toxic Kidney function	Avoid in patients with CKD (stage 3 or greater)
Pegloticase	Acute gout attack during treatment initiation, anaphylaxis, GI symptoms (constipation, nausea, vomiting), chest pain, nasopharyngitis	Therapeutic Serum urate levels Reduced frequency of gout attacks Toxic Signs/symptoms of anaphylaxis following infusion	Reserved for patients with severe gout refractory to conventional therapies
Lesinurad	Acute gout attack during treatment initiation, headache, GERD, major adverse cardiovascular events have been observed although a causal relationship has not been established	Therapeutic Serum urate levels Reduced frequency of gout attacks Toxic Kidney function	Reserved for patients with hyperuricemia associated with gout who do not achieve target serum uric acid levels with conventional therapies Can be used in both urate overproduction and urate underexcretion Must be used in combination with a xanthine oxidase inhibitor due to increased risk of acute kidney injury with monotherapy Not currently marketed in the United States

FDA, Food and Drug Administration; GERD, gastroesophageal reflux disease; GI, gastrointestinal; NSAID, nonsteroidal anti-inflammatory drug; CKD, chronic kidney disease.

GI issues.[28] Specific COX-2 inhibitors, etoricoxib and lumiracoxib, have demonstrated efficacy in the treatment of acute gout; however, these agents are not available in the United States. The effectiveness of high-dose celecoxib (1,200 mg on day 1 followed by 400 mg twice daily thereafter) in the treatment of acute gout has been established, but concerns regarding the cardiovascular risk of COX-2 inhibitors must be considered when using these agents (see Chapter 110, Osteoarthritis, for further discussion of COX-2 inhibitors).[29]

Corticosteroids Corticosteroids have historically been reserved for treatment of acute gout flares when contraindications to other therapies exist, largely due to lack of evidence from controlled clinical trials. However, evidence indicates that corticosteroids are equivalent to NSAIDs in the treatment of acute gout flares.[30,31] They can be used either systemically or by intra-articular injection. With systemic therapy, a hypothetical risk exists for a rebound attack upon steroid withdrawal; therefore, gradual tapering is often employed when discontinuing. Examples of appropriate tapers include 0.5 mg/kg daily for 5 to 10 days followed by abrupt discontinuation, 0.5 mg/kg daily for 2 to 5 days followed by tapering for 7 to 10 days, or using a methylprednisolone dose pack—a 6-day regimen that starts with 24 mg on day 1 and decreases by 4 mg each day.[23]

Intra-articular administration of triamcinolone acetonide in a dose of 20 to 40 mg may be useful in treating acute gout limited to one or two joints. Injection should be done under an aseptic technique in a joint determined not to be infected. A single intramuscular injection of a long-acting corticosteroid, such as methylprednisolone, followed by a short course of oral corticosteroid therapy is another recognized therapeutic approach to the treatment of acute gout.[23] Alternatively, intramuscular corticosteroid monotherapy could be considered in patients with multiple affected joints who are unable to take oral therapy.

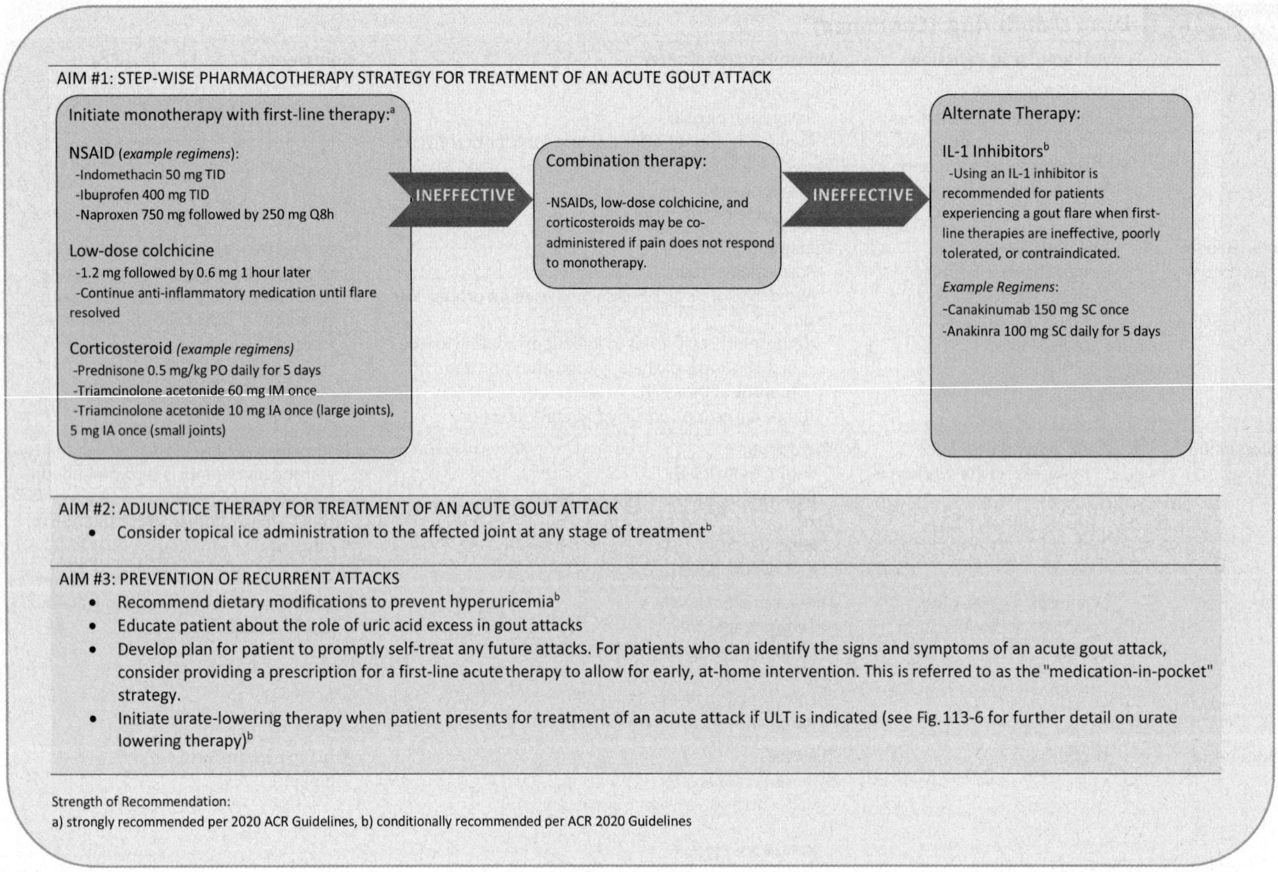

AIM #1: STEP-WISE PHARMACOTHERAPY STRATEGY FOR TREATMENT OF AN ACUTE GOUT ATTACK

Initiate monotherapy with first-line therapy:[a]

NSAID (*example regimens*):
- Indomethacin 50 mg TID
- Ibuprofen 400 mg TID
- Naproxen 750 mg followed by 250 mg Q8h

Low-dose colchicine
- 1.2 mg followed by 0.6 mg 1 hour later
- Continue anti-inflammatory medication until flare resolved

Corticosteroid (*example regimens*)
- Prednisone 0.5 mg/kg PO daily for 5 days
- Triamcinolone acetonide 60 mg IM once
- Triamcinolone acetonide 10 mg IA once (large joints), 5 mg IA once (small joints)

INEFFECTIVE →

Combination therapy:

- NSAIDs, low-dose colchicine, and corticosteroids may be co-administered if pain does not respond to monotherapy.

INEFFECTIVE →

Alternate Therapy:

IL-1 Inhibitors[b]
- Using an IL-1 inhibitor is recommended for patients experiencing a gout flare when first-line therapies are ineffective, poorly tolerated, or contraindicated.

Example Regimens:
- Canakinumab 150 mg SC once
- Anakinra 100 mg SC daily for 5 days

AIM #2: ADJUNCTICE THERAPY FOR TREATMENT OF AN ACUTE GOUT ATTACK
- Consider topical ice administration to the affected joint at any stage of treatment[b]

AIM #3: PREVENTION OF RECURRENT ATTACKS
- Recommend dietary modifications to prevent hyperuricemia[b]
- Educate patient about the role of uric acid excess in gout attacks
- Develop plan for patient to promptly self-treat any future attacks. For patients who can identify the signs and symptoms of an acute gout attack, consider providing a prescription for a first-line acute therapy to allow for early, at-home intervention. This is referred to as the "medication-in-pocket" strategy.
- Initiate urate-lowering therapy when patient presents for treatment of an acute attack if ULT is indicated (see Fig. 113-6 for further detail on urate lowering therapy)[b]

Strength of Recommendation:
a) strongly recommended per 2020 ACR Guidelines, b) conditionally recommended per ACR 2020 Guidelines

FIGURE 113-5 Comprehensive management of an acute gout attack. (IM, intramuscular; IA, intra-articular; SC, subcutaneous.) *(Data from FitzGerald JD, Dalbeth N, Mikuls TB, 2020 American College of Rheumatology Guideline for the Management of Gout. Arthritis Care Res. 72:744–760.)*

The adverse effects of corticosteroids are generally dose and duration dependent. Short-term use for treatment of acute attacks is generally well tolerated. Corticosteroids should be used with caution for patients with diabetes as they can increase blood sugar. In addition, patients with a history of GI problems, bleeding disorders, cardiovascular disease, and psychiatric disorders should be monitored closely for exacerbation of these conditions. Long-term corticosteroid use should be avoided because of the increased risk for osteoporosis, hypothalamic–pituitary axis suppression, cataracts, and muscle deconditioning.

Corticotropin, or adrenocorticotropic hormone (ACTH), which stimulates the adrenal cortex to produce cortisol and corticosterone, can be administered to treat acute gout. A dose of 25 to 40 international units given subcutaneously and repeated as needed has been recommended in the past for treatment of acute gout.[23] Studies with ACTH are limited, but it provides similar efficacy to systemic anti-inflammatory doses of corticosteroids.[32] Unfortunately, access to ACTH has been impacted following changes in the manufacturer of ACTH in 2007. This change in ownership resulted in a dramatic increase in the price of the medication such that it is no longer a viable treatment option.[33] The ACR guidelines support use of other first-line agents over ACTH primarily due to reduced cost effectiveness with ACTH.[24]

Colchicine Colchicine is an antimitotic drug that is highly effective at relieving acute attacks of gout.[34] When begun within the first 24 hours of an acute attack, colchicine produces a response in two-thirds of patients within hours of administration.[35] Although it is highly effective, oral colchicine can cause dose-dependent GI adverse effects, including nausea, vomiting, and diarrhea. Other important non-GI adverse effects include neutropenia and axonal neuromyopathy, which may be worsened for patients taking other myopathic drugs such as β-hydroxy-β-methylglutaryl-coenzyme A (HMG-CoA) reductase inhibitors (statins) or for those with impaired kidney function.

Colchicine was used for many years to treat acute gouty arthritis, but as an unapproved drug without having undergone formal FDA review for safety and efficacy. In 2009, the FDA-approved a 0.6-mg tablet of colchicine (under the brand name Colcrys®) for oral use, which was followed by an order for all unapproved colchicine products to stop manufacturing within 90 days. Following enforcement of market exclusivity for the branded colchicine product, use of colchicine to treat acute gouty arthritis declined immediately thereafter due to the significant cost.[36] Colchicine is now once again available generically; however, increased cost remains a potential barrier given the unique patent agreements established which may reduce competition among generic producers until 2029.[37]

One benefit of the 2009 FDA approval of Colcrys® was new information on dosing. A substantially lower dose of colchicine (1.2 mg initially, followed by a single 0.6 mg dose 1 hour later) is as effective as traditionally used higher doses (continued hourly dosing until symptoms subside or GI symptoms become intolerable).[38] In addition to the low-dose regimen, the ACR guidelines also suggest that following the low-dose colchicine regimen, anti-inflammatory medication may be continued until the flare resolves.[24] This off-label dosing recommendation is based upon pharmacokinetic data that suggest that colchicine concentrations begin to decline 12 hours after administration.[38]

Postmarketing safety information suggests an increased risk of adverse events for patients receiving colchicine administered concurrently with P-glycoprotein or cytochrome P450 3A4 inhibitors (eg, clarithromycin or cyclosporine) (Table 113-8).[39] These interactions are thought to result in an increased colchicine concentration. Colchicine should also be used carefully for patients with impaired kidney and hepatic function. Colchicine dosing recommendations in these special situations are listed in Table 113-8.

Management of Hyperuricemia in Gout

Nonpharmacologic Therapy

Following treatment and resolution of an acute gout attack, the focus should shift to the prevention of future episodes. Recurrent gout attacks can be prevented by maintaining low uric acid concentrations. Although both nonpharmacologic and pharmacologic efforts to maintain low uric acid concentrations are critical in the management of gout, nonadherence with ULT is common.[40] A likely explanation for this lack in patient adherence is the silent nature of intercritical gout (the period of time between two gout attacks). Patient education, therefore, is a critical first step in the management of hyperuricemia.[24] Education should address the recurrent nature of the disease and reinforce the objective of each lifestyle/dietary modification and medication therapy recommended.

Weight loss through caloric restriction and exercise should be promoted in all patients with gout and hyperuricemia who are overweight/obese, as this may enhance renal excretion of urate.[24] Specifically, the urate-lowering effect of the DASH diet (Dietary Approaches to Stop Hypertension) has been examined. This diet includes vegetables, fruits, whole grains, reduced-fat dairy, lean meats, beans, and nuts along with avoidance of foods high in saturated fats and sweetened beverages/foods. Studies have demonstrated a reduction of ~1.0 mg/dL (~60 μmol/L) in serum uric acid levels in patients with hyperuricemia who adhere to the diet.[41,42] Restriction of alcohol intake can also aid in the management of gout, as increased alcohol consumption has been associated with an increased risk of gout attacks.[43,44] Acute ingestions of alcohol cause lactic acidemia, which reduces renal urate excretion, and long-term

TABLE 113-8 Colchicine Dosing in Special Situations/Colchicine Drug Interactions

	Treatment of Acute Gout Flares	Prophylaxis of Gout Flares
Impaired Kidney Function[a]		
Mild/moderate (creatinine clearance = 30-80 mL/min [0.5-1.33 mL/s])	Dose adjustment not required	Dose adjustment not required
Severe (creatinine clearance <30 mL/min [0.5 mL/s])	Dose adjustment not required; treatment course should be repeated no more than once every 2 weeks	0.3 mg daily (starting dose)
Dialysis	Single 0.6 mg dose; treatment course should not be repeated more than once every 2 weeks	0.3 mg twice weekly (starting dose)
Hepatic Impairment[b]		
Mild/moderate	Dose adjustment not required	Dose adjustment not required
Severe	Dose adjustment not required; treatment course should be repeated no more than once every 2 weeks	Dose reduction should be considered
Colchicine Drug Interactions		
Strong CYP3A4 inhibitors • Atazanavir • Clarithromycin • Darunavir/ritonavir • Indinavir • Itraconazole • Ketoconazole • Lopinavir/ritonavir • Nefazodone • Nelfinavir • Ritonavir • Saquinavir • Telithromycin • Tipranavir/ritonavir	Single 0.6 mg dose followed by 0.3 mg 1 hour later; dose to be repeated no earlier than 3 days	0.3 mg once every other day to 0.3 mg once daily
Moderate CYP3A4 inhibitors • Amprenavir • Aprepitant • Diltiazem • Erythromycin • Fluconazole • Fosamprenavir • Grapefruit juice and related citrus products • Verapamil	Single 1.2 mg dose; dose to be repeated no earlier than 3 days	0.3 g-0.6 mg daily (0.6 mg dose may be given as 0.3 mg twice daily)
P-glycoprotein inhibitors • Cyclosporine • Ranolazine	Single 0.6 mg dose; dose to be repeated no earlier than 3 days	0.3 mg once every other day to 0.3 mg once daily

[a]Treatment of gout flares with colchicine is not recommended in patients with impaired kidney function who are receiving colchicine for prophylaxis.

[b]Treatment of gout flares with colchicine is not recommended in patients with hepatic impairment who are receiving colchicine for prophylaxis.

alcohol intake promotes production of purines as a by-product of the conversion of acetate to acetyl coenzyme A in the metabolism of alcohol.[45] The ACR guidelines conditionally recommend limiting alcohol use in all gout patients.[24] The guidelines also conditionally recommend limiting consumption of high-fructose corn syrup and purine-rich foods (organ meats and some seafood), which have also been linked to uric acid elevation.

Consumption of cherry-containing products, such as cherries and tart cherry extract, has received considerable attention and a wide variety of non-FDA-regulated supplements purporting benefits for gout are available. Uric acid lowering associated with cherry consumption has been demonstrated, although a physiologic mechanism for this effect has not been described.[46] For example, cherry intake over a 2-day period was associated with a 35% lower risk of gout attacks compared with no intake.[47] Randomized controlled trials are needed to better establish the role of cherry products before they can be recommended for management of hyperuricemia. Furthermore, the caloric and sugar content of each cherry-containing product should be considered. Since many patients with hyperuricemia can benefit from weight loss, use of these caloric-dense products is not optimal.

Another strategy to lower uric acid before initiating urate-lowering pharmacotherapy is to evaluate the patient's medication list for potentially unnecessary drugs that may elevate uric acid concentrations. Additionally, when clinically appropriate, medications that increase serum uric acid levels may be switched to equally effective medications without this effect (Table 113-2). Although the presence of gout is not an absolute contraindication to the use of thiazide diuretics in hypertensive patients, the ACR guidelines conditionally recommend that hydrochlorothiazide, specifically, be switched to an alternative antihypertensive medication when feasible.[24] This is particularly important if the patient has had frequent gout attacks or continues to have an elevated serum uric acid concentration despite appropriate therapy for gout. Importantly, the ACR guidelines specifically highlight the importance of continuing low-dose aspirin when used for an appropriate indication in patients with gout, despite its uric acid elevating properties.[24]

Pharmacologic Therapy

After the first attack of acute gouty arthritis, a decision to institute prophylactic urate-lowering pharmacotherapy may be considered. This decision should carefully balance risk and benefit.

(3) The ACR guidelines recognize the occurrence of frequent gout flares (two or more attacks per year) as an indication for pharmacologic ULT. Other indications include the presence of one or more tophus and radiographic evidence of damage attributable to gout. A conditional recommendation for ULT initiation exists for patients who have experienced more than one gout attack, but who have infrequent flares (fewer than two per year), as well as for patients experiencing their first flare who have CKD (stage 3 or greater), serum uric acid level greater than 9 mg/dL (535 μmol/L), or urolithiasis.[24] ACR guidelines conditionally recommend that pharmacologic ULT can be safely started during an acute gout attack, citing evidence that initiation of ULT during an acute attack did not prolong duration or worsen severity of the attack compared to delayed initiation.[24,48-50]

Reduction in serum urate concentrations can be accomplished pharmacologically by decreasing the synthesis of uric acid (xanthine oxidase inhibitors) or by increasing the renal excretion of uric acid (uricosurics).

The ACR guidelines provide a step-wise approach to the treatment of hyperuricemia in patients with gout (Fig. 113-6).[24]

A xanthine oxidase inhibitor, allopurinol, is recommended as first-line therapy, with an alternate xanthine oxidase inhibitor, febuxostat, as second-line therapy for those with a contraindication or intolerance to allopurinol or who do not achieve target serum urate. In refractory cases, combination therapy including a xanthine oxidase inhibitor plus an agent with uricosuric properties may be considered. Finally, in severe cases, in which the patient is not achieving the target serum uric acid level and is continuing to experience frequent gout flares or non-resolving tophi despite preferred treatments, pegloticase is recommended.

(4) The target serum uric acid concentration identified by ACR guidelines is less than 6 mg/dL (357 μmol/L).[24]

Given that the factors associated with uric acid elevation are typically persistent throughout life, urate-lowering therapy is usually prescribed for long-term use. Furthermore, long-term ULT administration has been demonstrated to be more effective in controlling gouty attacks compared to intermittent administration.[51] For these reasons, ACR guidelines recommend indefinite ULT in patients in whom therapy is indicated.[24]

Xanthine Oxidase Inhibitors (5) Xanthine oxidase inhibitors reduce uric acid by impairing the ability of xanthine oxidase to convert hypoxanthine to xanthine and xanthine to uric acid (Fig. 113-1). Because they are efficacious for prophylaxis in both underexcreters and overproducers of uric acid, xanthine oxidase inhibitors are the most widely prescribed agents for the long-term prevention of recurrent attacks of gout. There are two commercially available xanthine oxidase inhibitors, allopurinol and febuxostat.

Allopurinol is an effective urate-lowering agent,[52] but not all patients are able to take it due to adverse effects, and long-term adherence with allopurinol is low.[40] Mild adverse effects such as skin rash, leukopenia, GI problems, headache, and urticaria can occur with allopurinol administration. A more severe adverse reaction known as "allopurinol hypersensitivity syndrome," which includes severe rash (toxic epidermal necrolysis, erythema multiforme, or exfoliative dermatitis), hepatitis, interstitial nephritis, and eosinophilia, reportedly occurs in approximately 1:1,000 patients and is associated with a 20% to 25% mortality rate.[22] The annual incidence rate of allopurinol hypersensitivity is up to 4.68 per 1,000 patients. Risk factors associated with the development of allopurinol hypersensitivity include female sex, age above 60 years, initial starting dose of allopurinol exceeding 100 mg/day, kidney disease, cardiovascular disease, and use of allopurinol for treatment of asymptomatic hyperuricemia.[53] Additionally, the presence of the *HLA-B*5801* allele is associated with increased risk for allopurinol hypersensitivity syndrome (see Pharmacotherapy Considerations later in the chapter).

As evidence has linked higher starting doses of allopurinol with an increased incidence of allopurinol hypersensitivity syndrome, conservative initial dosing is important.[54] ACR guidelines recommend that allopurinol be started at a dose no greater than 100 mg daily in patients with normal kidney function and limited to 50 mg daily in patients with chronic kidney disease (stage 3 or worse).[22,24,26] Despite the cautious approach of initiating at lower doses in patients with CKD, titrating allopurinol to the maximum approved dose has been proven to be safe and effective in this population.[24,55,56] Ideally, the dose of allopurinol should be gradually titrated based on serial serum uric acid measurements until the serum urate target is met, up to a maximum dose of 800 mg/day.[24] During titration, patients should be educated about the signs and symptoms of a serious reaction, including pruritus and rash.

Similar to allopurinol, febuxostat lowers serum urate concentrations in a dose-dependent manner.[57] The recommended starting dose is 40 mg daily and this can be titrated to the maximum FDA-approved dose of 80 mg daily. Although febuxostat and allopurinol may have similar efficacy in serum uric acid lowering and reduction in gout flares,[58,59] an increase in all-cause mortality and cardiovascular mortality has been shown with febuxostat compared to allopurinol.[58] These findings are reflected

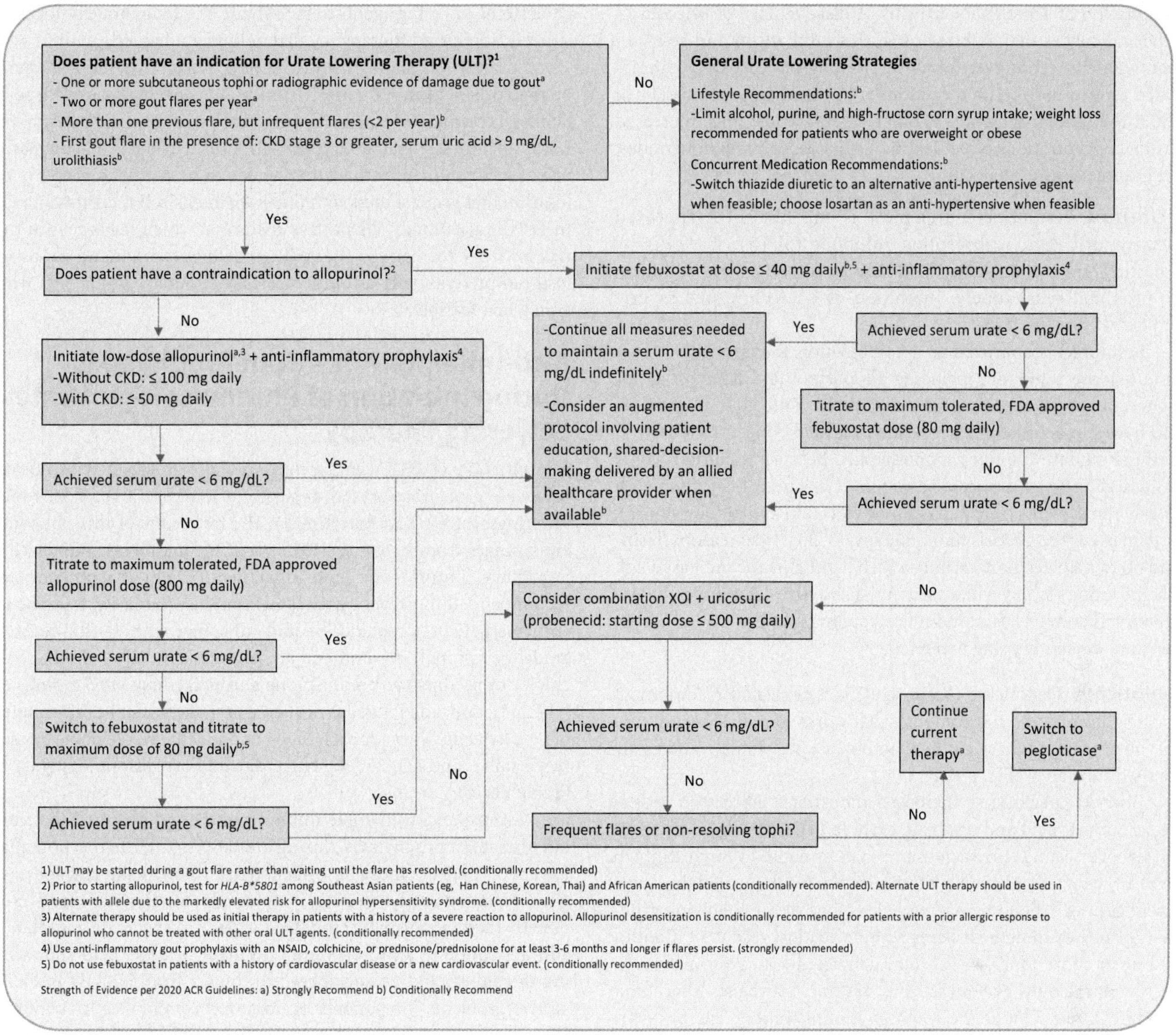

FIGURE 113-6 Algorithm for management of hyperuricemia. (CKD, chronic kidney disease; XOI, xanthine-oxidase inhibitor.) Serum urate levels expressed as 6 mg/dL is equivalent to 357 μmol/L. *(Data from FitzGerald JD, Dalbeth N, Mikuls TB, 2020 American College of Rheumatology Guideline for the Management of Gout. Arthritis Care Res. 72:744–760.)*

in an FDA black box warning stating that febuxostat should be reserved for patients unable to take allopurinol.[60] Consistent with this warning, the ACR guidelines recommend febuxostat as an alternative urate-lowering therapy in patients unable to tolerate or unresponsive to allopurinol. Additionally, the guidelines suggest switching to an alternative oral urate-lowering medication in patients taking febuxostat who have a history or cardiovascular disease or a new CVD-related event.[24]

Uricosuric Drugs 6 Uricosuric drugs increase the renal clearance of uric acid by inhibiting post-secretory renal proximal tubular reabsorption of uric acid. One uricosuric, probenecid, is available for use in the United States. An alternative uricosuric, benzbromarone, is available in Europe but not in the United States. A third uricosuric, lesinurad, is FDA-approved in the United States but is not currently marketed.[10] Uricosurics offer an alternative and complementary mechanism to xanthine oxidase inhibitors to enhance serum uric acid lowering. Although this class of medications can contribute to meaningful urate lowering and is well tolerated overall, uricosuric therapy is associated with less efficacy in patients with impaired kidney function and, therefore, is not generally recommended in patients with moderate-to-severe CKD (stage 3 or greater).[24,61]

Probenecid Probenecid is given initially at a dose of 250 mg twice daily for 1 to 2 weeks and then 500 mg twice daily for 2 weeks. Thereafter, the daily dose is increased by 500 mg increments every 1 to 2 weeks until satisfactory control is achieved or a maximum dose of 2 g is reached. Uricosuric therapies, through their action to increase the elimination of uric acid (Fig. 113-1), cause marked uricosuria and may cause stone formation. Probenecid, specifically, has been associated with a 9% to 11% risk of urolithiasis.[22] For this reason, patients with a history of urolithiasis should not use uricosuric drugs.[24,61] The maintenance of adequate fluid intake when using uricosuric therapy is important to diminish the possibility of uric acid stone formation.[61]

In addition to urolithiasis, adverse effects associated with uricosuric therapy include GI irritation, rash/hypersensitivity, and precipitation of acute gouty arthritis. A disadvantage of uricosurics is that salicylates may interfere with this mechanism and result in treatment failure; however, low doses (325 mg/day or less) of enteric-coated aspirin may be used cautiously. In addition, probenecid can inhibit the tubular secretion of other organic acids; thus, increased plasma concentrations of penicillins, cephalosporins, sulfonamides, and indomethacin can occur.

Lesinurad Lesinurad (Zurampic®) is the first FDA-approved selective uric acid reabsorption inhibitor (SURI). It works by inhibiting urate transporter 1 (URAT1), a transporter found in the proximal renal tubule. Inhibition of URAT1 results in uric acid excretion (Fig. 113-1).

Lesinurad is approved as a combination therapy with a xanthine oxidase inhibitor (including allopurinol and febuxostat) for the treatment of hyperuricemia associated with gout in patients who have not achieved target serum uric acid concentrations with xanthine oxidase inhibitor monotherapy. Because lesinurad works by increasing renal uric acid secretion, it has been associated with adverse renal events (serum creatinine elevation and kidney stones), particularly when used as monotherapy.[62,63] For these reasons, lesinurad carries a black box warning which highlights the increased risk of acute kidney injury when used in the absence of xanthine oxidase inhibitor therapy.[63] Lesinurad retains approval in the United States, but is not currently being marketed.

Pegloticase Pegloticase (Krystexxa®) is a pegylated recombinant uricase administered intravenously that works to reduce serum uric acid by converting uric acid to allantoin, a water-soluble and easily excreted substance (Fig. 113-1).

Biweekly pegloticase therapy demonstrates efficacy in reducing serum uric acid and resolving tophi in patients with severe gout and hyperuricemia (uric acid more than or equal to 8 mg/dL [476 μmol/L]) who fail or have a contraindication to allopurinol therapy.[64] Severe gout is defined by having at least one of the following criteria: (a) three or more gout flares within the most recent 18 months, (b) one or more tophi, or (c) joint damage due to gout. Although clearly efficacious, pegloticase has several drawbacks that limit widespread use. One is the route of administration. The biweekly IV infusions of pegloticase must be given over no less than 2 hours, a potential inconvenience to many patients. Furthermore, given potential infusion-related allergic reactions, patients must be treated with antihistamines and corticosteroids before therapy. Cost is another major consideration. Pegloticase is estimated to cost several thousand dollars per month, not including administration costs associated with an IV infusion.[65] This represents a significantly greater cost burden compared with other ULT.[65]

The ideal duration of pegloticase therapy is unknown. Other ULTs such as allopurinol or febuxostat are typically used indefinitely in patients with gout and hyperuricemia. Immunogenicity issues associated with pegloticase therapy may limit the duration with which it may be used effectively. Patients may develop pegloticase antibodies that result in a loss of efficacy after several months.[64]

7 Given these many limitations and the narrow patient population in which the drug has been studied, ACR guidelines recommend reserving use of pegloticase for patients with refractory gout for whom all other urate-lowering therapies have failed to reach target serum uric acid and who continue to have frequent gout flares (two or more per year), or who have non-resolving tophi.

Miscellaneous Urate-Lowering Agents Fenofibrate has been demonstrated to reduce uric acid levels as an ancillary benefit by increasing the clearance of hypoxanthine and xanthine, leading to a sustained reduction in serum urate concentrations. Reductions of 20% to 30% in urate concentrations have been observed with fenofibrate use.[66,67] Despite demonstrated urate-lowering effects, ACR guidelines recommend against adding or switching cholesterol-lowering agents to fenofibrate,[24] as fenofibrate is not considered a preferred therapy in current lipid guidelines.

Losartan, an angiotensin II receptor antagonist, has also demonstrated benefit in reducing serum urate concentrations independent of its primary mechanism, angiotensin receptor antagonism.[68,69] Losartan inhibits renal tubular reabsorption of uric acid and increases urinary excretion, and this effect seems to be a unique property of losartan that is not shared with other angiotensin II receptor antagonists.[70] In addition, it alkalinizes the urine, which helps reduce the risk for stone formation. The ACR guidelines recommend choosing losartan preferentially as antihypertensive therapy in patients with gout when feasible.[24]

Anti-Inflammatory Gout Prophylaxis During Initiation of Pharmacologic Urate-Lowering Therapy

8 Initiation of ULT can prompt an acute attack of gout due to remodeling of urate crystal deposits in joints as a result of rapid lowering of urate concentrations.[23] The frequency of this phenomenon ranges from as few as 25% up to 75% of patients.[71] Given this possibility, prophylactic anti-inflammatory pharmacotherapy is recommended to prevent gout attacks and, secondarily, to assist in ensuring patient acceptance of, and adherence with, ULT. The ACR guidelines strongly recommend anti-prophylaxis with NSAIDs, colchicine or prednisone/prednisolone during the first 3 to 6 months of ULT initiation, and longer as needed if gout flares persist.[24] Examples of prophylactic doses for each medication include: colchicine 0.6 mg twice daily, naproxen 250 mg twice/day, and prednisone 10 mg daily (Table 113-6).

Given the considerable duration of therapy required for anti-inflammatory prophylaxis during initiation of ULT, the potential for adverse effects must be considered. Although the risk for gastric ulceration and bleeding is relatively small with short-term NSAID therapy normally employed when treating acute gout flares, administration of a proton-pump inhibitor or other acid-suppressing therapy should be considered to protect from NSAID-induced gastric problems for patients on long-term prophylactic therapy.[23] Prolonged corticosteroid therapy may be linked to many adverse effects not experienced with short-term therapy used for acute treatment (ie, hyperglycemia, Cushing syndrome, fluid retention, hypertension, osteoporosis, glaucoma, depression/euphoria). Therefore, when used for longer-term anti-inflammatory prophylaxis, these risk must be considered.

Cost is another major consideration when selecting prophylactic pharmacotherapy given the need for an extended duration of therapy (3 to 6 months of therapy compared to approximately 1 week for acute gout treatment). Although generic colchicine again became commercially available in 2015, the lack of competition among manufacturers of generic colchicine may allow the cost per tablet to remain high well into the future.[37,72] The cost of colchicine, if not covered by insurance, remains a potential challenge to therapy for certain patients making NSAIDs and corticosteroids more affordable options for patients.

Investigational Drugs

Prior to the approvals of febuxostat in 2009 and pegloticase in 2010, several decades passed without the release of any new pharmacotherapeutic agents for the treatment of gout. Given the increased prevalence of gout and the presence of both treatment intolerance and treatment refractory cases, discovery of novel therapies continues to be a focus of ongoing research.[73]

Interleukin-1 Inhibitors

During acute gout attacks, urate crystals elicit an inflammatory response that triggers the production of interleukin-1 (IL-1).[10] This finding has led to the investigational use of IL-1 inhibitors in the treatment and prevention of acute gout.

Two IL-1 inhibitors, anakinra and canakinumab, have demonstrated efficacy in the treatment of acute gout.[74-76] Neither is approved for the treatment of acute gout by the FDA, and their use remains off-label. As such, the ACR guidelines suggest that use of IL-1 inhibitors should be reserved for treatment for patients experiencing an acute gout attack for whom first-line treatments are ineffective, poorly tolerated, or contraindicated.[24]

Limited evidence also suggests efficacy of IL-1 inhibitors in the prevention of acute gout during the first 16 weeks of ULT initiation (subcutaneous rilonacept 320-mg loading dose followed by 160 mg weekly and subcutaneous canakinumab single dose [50-300 mg] or four times weekly dosing [50 mg—50 mg—25 mg—25 mg]).[76-78] Given the limited evidence and lack of FDA approval for this indication, the ACR guidelines do not provide a recommendation for the use of IL-1 inhibitors for anti-inflammatory prophylaxis during initiation of ULT.

Other Investigational Agents

Several investigational agents intended to be used for the management of gout are at various stages of development. Uricosurics in development include verinurad and arhalofenate.[73] Arhalofenate also suppresses the production of IL-1β which may potentially lead to a reduction in gout flares, in addition to urate lowering.[79] Other novel mechanisms of action include purine nucleoside phosphorylase (PNP) inhibition (ulodesine) and glucose transporter 9 (GLUT9) inhibition (tranilast).[76,78] Other agents include a xanthine oxidase inhibitor, topioxostat, and a uricase, pergsiticase. Continued research will ultimately define the role of these agents in the management of gout and hyperuricemia.

Nephrolithiasis

9 The medical management of uric acid nephrolithiasis includes hydration sufficient to maintain a urine volume of at least 2 to 3 L/day, alkalinization of urine, avoidance of purine-rich foods, moderation of protein intake, and reduction of urinary uric acid excretion.

Maintenance of a 24-hour urine volume of at least 2 L with an adequate intake of fluids is desirable for all patients with gout, but especially for those who form stones. Alkalinizing agents should be used with the objective of making the urine less acidic. Urine pH should be maintained at 6 to 6.5.[80] In this pH range, up to 85% of uric acid will be in the form of the soluble urate ion.

Reduction of urine acidity is usually accomplished by the administration of potassium bicarbonate or potassium citrate 30 to 80 mEq/day (mmol/day).[80] Administration of alkali via sodium salts is a less desirable option for two reasons. First, the sodium-induced volume expansion will increase sodium excretion and can secondarily cause hypercalcemia because calcium passively follows the reabsorption of sodium in the proximal tubule and loop of Henle. In the presence of uric acid, the resultant hypercalcemia can lead to calcium oxalate stone formation. Second, older patients with uric acid kidney stones may also have hypertension, heart failure, or impaired kidney function. Because of these conditions, they should not be overloaded with alkalinizing sodium salts or unlimited fluid intake, as these can worsen these conditions.[80]

Carbonic anhydrase inhibitors (eg, acetazolamide and topiramate) produce rapid and effective urinary alkalinization; however, they are not recommended because they cause metabolic acidosis and hypocitraturia which may result in increased urinary saturation of calcium salts and calcium stone formation.[80]

The mainstay of drug therapy for recurrent uric acid nephrolithiasis is xanthine oxidase inhibitors. They are effective in reducing both serum and urinary uric acid concentrations, thus preventing the formation of calculi.

Uric Acid Lowering in the Absence of Gout

Asymptomatic Hyperuricemia

Questions are often raised regarding the use of drug therapy to treat hyperuricemia in patients who have never experienced a gout attack (ie, asymptomatic hyperuricemia). The purported benefits include prevention of acute gouty arthritis, tophi formation, nephrolithiasis, and chronic urate nephropathy. Furthermore, gout is associated with many comorbidities (eg, CKD, hypertension, obesity, heart failure, diabetes, myocardial infarction, stroke) and increasing levels of hyperuricemia have been associated with increased prevalence of these comorbidities.[81] Drug treatment of asymptomatic hyperuricemia to mitigate development of these conditions is not recommended, as it has not been demonstrated that uric acid lowering therapy prevents disease in such individuals.[10,82,83] Nevertheless, an incidental finding of hyperuricemia should prompt further evaluation of other cardiovascular risk factors.

Pharmacotherapy Considerations

While the ACR guidelines provide clear recommendations regarding use of pharmacotherapy in the management of gout and hyperuricemia, application of these recommendations requires personalization to fit the needs of a specific patient. When making therapeutic choices for an individual, it is critical to evaluate the adverse effect profile of a particular pharmacotherapeutic agent while considering a patient's baseline risk for those unwanted effects. This involves an analysis of patient demographics and comorbidities.

Allopurinol hypersensitivity syndrome is perhaps the most concerning adverse effect of all potential side effects associated with gout therapies, given the high mortality rate associated with this reaction. As such, it would be ideal if patients at high risk for developing this syndrome could be screened for and, consequently, guided to alternative therapy. The *HLA-B*5801* allele has been associated with a significant increase risk for allopurinol hypersensitivity syndrome. Patients of Korean, Han Chinese, Thai, and African descent have been identified as having a high prevalence of this allele and, therefore, at increased risk for allopurinol hypersensitivity syndrome. For this reason, the ACR guidelines recommend that *HLA-B*5801* testing be pursued before allopurinol initiation in these specific populations.[24] For those found to be positive, alternative therapy should be used.[84]

Certain comorbidities may warrant dose adjustment of some gout therapies or, in certain instances, complete avoidance of certain medications. For example, patients with impaired kidney function should generally avoid NSAID therapy and should receive colchicine at reduced doses. Patients with GI disease should also avoid NSAID therapy and may not be able to tolerate colchicine therapy; in these patients, corticosteroid therapy may be a better option. Patients with uncontrolled diabetes may experience hyperglycemia with use of corticosteroids and, therefore, should avoid these agents and preferably use NSAIDs or colchicine instead. In addition to comorbidities, polypharmacy and cost considerations may affect treatment decisions in an individual patient. The comprehensive management of gout provides ample opportunity for pharmacists to apply medication expertise, and care models incorporating pharmacists in the management of gout have demonstrated improved outcomes compared to standard practice.[85] Refer to Table 113-9 for an overview of important factors to consider when personalizing pharmacotherapy for an individual patient with gout.

Evaluation of Therapeutic Outcomes

Follow-up of patients with gout depends on the frequency of attacks and on the medications used to treat symptoms. For a patient who is experiencing a first attack of gout, long-term therapy is generally not indicated; however, patients having a first attack should be educated about the likelihood of recurrence and what to do if another attack

TABLE 113-9 Pharmacotherapy Considerations in Gout

Conditions and Situations	Limitations to Pharmacotherapy	Alternative Therapies
Impaired Kidney Function	NSAIDs may lead to exacerbation of kidney impairment	Consider reduced-dose colchicine or corticosteroids for short-term treatment of acute gout Consider reduced-dose colchicine for prophylaxis during initiation of urate-lowering therapy
	Uricosuric therapy is ineffective in patients with impaired kidney function	Consider allopurinol or febuxostat
	Lesiurad is not indicated in patients with impaired kidney function	Consider allopurinol or febuxostat for first-line urate-lowering therapy; consider pegloticase for refractory cases
GI disease	Colchicine may cause GI upset and diarrhea	Consider corticosteroids for treatment of acute gout If monoarticular, consider joint injection
	NSAIDs may cause GI bleeding or ulceration	Consider gastroprotection with coadministration of proton-pump inhibitor when NSAID therapy is used Consider colchicine or corticosteroids for treatment of acute gout Consider low-dose colchicine for prophylaxis during initiation of urate-lowering therapy
Congestive heart failure	NSAIDs may cause a congestive heart failure exacerbation	Consider colchicine for treatment of acute gout Consider colchicine for prophylaxis during initiation of urate-lowering therapy
	Concurrent use of diuretic may increase serum urate	If diuretic remains necessary, consider initiating urate-lowering therapy Consider losartan as a therapy for congestive heart failure given its uricosuric properties
Hypertension	Diuretics may increase uric acid	Consider losartan as alternative or additional antihypertensive therapy given its uricosuric properties Consider non-diuretic anti-hypertensive agents as alternative therapy Consider addition of urate-lowering therapy if diuretic remains necessary
	NSAIDs may worsen blood pressure control	Consider colchicine or corticosteroids for treatment of acute gout Consider colchicine for prophylaxis during initiation of urate-lowering therapy
Polypharmacy	CYP3A4 inhibitors and P-glycoprotein inhibitors interact with colchicine leading to elevated colchicine levels	Reduce the dose of colchicine used for the treatment and prophylaxis of acute gout Consider NSAIDs or corticosteroids for treatment of acute gout Consider NSAIDs for prophylaxis during initiation of urate-lowering therapy
	Added pharmacotherapy may be undesirable in a patient with a large medication burden	Consider losartan as urate-lowering therapy in patients with comorbid hypertension Consider fenofibrate as urate-lowering therapy in patients with hypertriglyceridemia
Financial limitations	Febuxostat and colchicine are considerably more costly compared with other gout treatments	Consider allopurinol as urate-lowering therapy Consider NSAIDs or corticosteroids for treatment of acute gout Consider NSAIDs for prophylaxis of gout during initiation of urate-lowering therapy

CYP, cytochrome P450; GI, gastrointestinal; NSAID, nonsteroidal anti-inflammatory drug.

occurs. Approximately 60% of patients have a second attack within the first year, and 78% have a second attack within 2 years. Only 7% of patients do not have a recurrence within a 10-year period.[39]

Baseline blood work for patients receiving ULT chronically should include kidney function (serum creatinine), liver enzymes (aspartate aminotransferase, alanine aminotransferase), complete blood count, and electrolytes. There is generally no need to recheck these laboratory parameters for patients undergoing acute therapy with an NSAID or colchicine of limited duration. However, for patients requiring long-term therapy or prophylaxis, they should be rechecked every 6 to 12 months or as clinically indicated. For patients suspected of having an acute attack of gouty arthritis, it is reasonable to check a serum uric acid concentration, particularly if it is not the first attack and a decision is to be made regarding initiation of prophylactic therapy. However, clinicians should be mindful that acute gouty arthritis can occur in the presence of normal serum uric acid concentrations.[1] During titration of ULT, serial uric acid measurements should be obtained; once the urate target is achieved, uric acid should be monitored periodically (every 6-12 months).[10] This monitoring regimen is recommended not only to insure appropriate dosing of ULT, but also to serve as an assessment of patient adherence given the known adherence issues with ULTs. 10 Because of the high rates of comorbidities associated with gout, including diabetes mellitus, CKD, hypertension, obesity, coronary heart disease, heart failure, and stroke, an elevated uric acid concentration or an acute attack of gout should prompt evaluation for these related comorbidities and implementation of appropriate risk reduction measures.[81] Additionally, clinicians should look for possible underlying causes of hyperuricemia that may be actionable, such as medications (eg, diuretics, niacin, calcineurin inhibitors), obesity, malignancy, and alcohol abuse. Nonpharmacologic options include encouraging patients to exercise, lose weight, and reduce their consumption of alcohol and syrup-sweetened sodas. Periodic follow-up is necessary to address progress on these goals.

CONCLUSION

Hyperuricemia can be asymptomatic without complications, or it may lead to acute attacks of gouty arthritis, chronic gout, and uric acid nephrolithiasis. Treatment of asymptomatic hyperuricemia is not recommended, although lifestyle modifications (eg, weight loss, reduction of alcohol intake, control of blood pressure) should be encouraged to help reduce serum urate and improve overall health.

Acute gouty arthritis responds well to short courses of NSAIDs, colchicine, or corticosteroids to treat the underlying inflammatory response. The management of uric acid nephrolithiasis includes hydration and alkalinization of the urine. Prevention of recurrent gouty arthritis or recurrent nephrolithiasis, as well as the treatment of chronic gout, requires hypouricemic therapy with either a xanthine oxidase inhibitor, uricosuric, or a combination of both therapies. Allopurinol is the ULT with the strongest safety and efficacy profile, making it the first-line choice for prevention of gout attacks in patients needing prophylactic therapy who do not have contraindications. Finally, anti-inflammatory prophylaxis with colchicine, NSAID, or an oral corticosteroid is indicated during the initiation of ULT to prevent the development of acute gout due to the rapid mobilization or urate.

ABBREVIATIONS

ACR	American College of Rheumatology
ACP	American College of Physicians
ACTH	adrenocorticotropic hormone
CKD	chronic kidney disease
CNS	central nervous system
COX-2	cyclooxygenase-2
EULAR	European League Against Rheumatism
FDA	Food and Drug Administration
GI	gastrointestinal
GLUT9	glucose transporter 9
HGPRT	hypoxanthine-guanine phosphoribosyltransferase
IL-1	interleukin-1
MSU	monosodium urate
NSAID	nonsteroidal anti-inflammatory drug
PNP	purine nucleoside phosphorylase
PRPP	phosphoribosyl pyrophosphate (synthetase)
SURI	selective uric acid reabsorption inhibitor
ULT	urate-lowering therapy
URAT1	urate transporter 1
USP	United States Pharmacopeia

REFERENCES

1. Keenan R TM, Pillinger M. Etiology and Pathogenesis of Hyperuricemia and Gout. In: Firestein GS BR, Gabriel SE, Koretzky GA, McInnes IB, O'Dell JR, eds. *Firestein & Kelly's Textbook of Rheumatology*. 11 ed. Philadelphia, PA: Elsevier Inc.; 2021.
2. Campion EW, Glynn RJ, DeLabry LO. Asymptomatic hyperuricemia. Risks and consequences in the Normative Aging Study. *Am J Med.* 1987;82:421–426. DOI:10.1016/0002-9343(87)90441-4
3. Dalbeth N, Phipps-Green A, Frampton C, et al. Relationship between serum urate concentration and clinically evident incident gout: an individual participant data analysis. *Ann Rheum Dis.* 2018;77:1048–1052. DOI:10.1136/annrheumdis-2017-212288
4. Kuo CF, Grainge MJ, Zhang W, et al. Global epidemiology of gout: prevalence, incidence and risk factors. *Nat Rev Rheumatol.* 2015;11:649–662. DOI:10.1038/nrrheum.2015.91
5. Chen-Xu M, Yokose C, Rai SK, et al. Contemporary Prevalence of Gout and Hyperuricemia in the United States and Decadal Trends: The National Health and Nutrition Examination Survey, 2007-2016. *Arthritis Rheumatol.* 2019;71:991–999. DOI:10.1002/art.40807
6. Zhu Y, Pandya BJ, Choi HK. Prevalence of gout and hyperuricemia in the US general population: the National Health and Nutrition Examination Survey 2007-2008. *Arthritis Rheum.* 2011;63:3136–3141. DOI:10.1002/art.30520
7. Juraschek SP, Miller ER 3rd, Gelber AC. Body mass index, obesity, and prevalent gout in the United States in 1988-1994 and 2007-2010. *Arthritis Care Res (Hoboken).* 2013;65:127–132. DOI:10.1002/acr.21791
8. Choi HK. A prescription for lifestyle change in patients with hyperuricemia and gout. *Curr Opin Rheumatol.* 2010;22:165–172. DOI:10.1097/BOR.0b013e328335ef38
9. Kim JW, Kwak SG, Lee H, et al. Prevalence and incidence of gout in Korea: data from the national health claims database 2007-2015. *Rheumatol Int.* 2017;37:1499–1506. DOI:10.1007/s00296-017-3768-4
10. Dalbeth N, Gosling AL, Gaffo A, et al. Gout. *Lancet.* 2021;397:1843–1855. DOI:10.1016/s0140-6736(21)00569-9
11. Neogi T. Clinical practice. Gout. *N Engl J Med.* 2011;364:443–452. DOI:10.1056/NEJMcp1001124
12. Ben Salem C, Slim R, Fathallah N, et al. Drug-induced hyperuricaemia and gout. *Rheumatology (Oxford).* 2017;56:679–688. DOI:10.1093/rheumatology/kew293
13. Agudelo CA, Weinberger A, Schumacher HR, et al. Definitive diagnosis of gout by identification of urate crystals in asymptomatic metatarsophalangeal joints. *Arthritis Rheum.* 1979;22:559–560. DOI:10.1002/art.1780220521
14. Zhao T, Lv X, Cao L, et al. Renal excretion is a cause of decreased serum uric acid during acute gout. *Int J Rheum Dis.* 2018;21:1723–1727. DOI:10.1111/1756-185x.13348
15. Richette P, Doherty M, Pascual E, et al. 2018 Updated European League Against Rheumatism evidence-based recommendations for the diagnosis of gout. *Annals of the Rheumatic Diseases.* 2020;79:31–38. DOI:10.1136/annrheumdis-2019-215315
16. Neogi T, Jansen TL, Dalbeth N, et al. 2015 Gout classification criteria: an American College of Rheumatology/European League Against Rheumatism collaborative initiative. *Ann Rheum Dis.* 2015;74:1789–1798. DOI:10.1136/annrheumdis-2015-208237
17. Rosenthal AK, Ryan LM. Calcium Pyrophosphate Deposition Disease. *N Engl J Med.* 2016;374:2575–2584. DOI:10.1056/NEJMra1511117
18. Schumacher HR. Crystal-induced arthritis: an overview. *Am J Med.* 1996;100:46s–52s. DOI:10.1016/s0002-9343(97)89546-0
19. Macmullan P, McCarthy G. Treatment and management of pseudogout: insights for the clinician. *Ther Adv Musculoskelet Dis.* 2012;4:121–131. DOI:10.1177/1759720X11432559
20. Hoff LS, Goldenstein-Schainberg C, Fuller R. Nephrolithiasis in gout: prevalence and characteristics of Brazilian patients. *Adv Rheumatol.* 2019;60:2. DOI:10.1186/s42358-019-0106-4
21. Edwards N, Choi H, Terkeltaub R. Gout. In: Klippel J, Stone S, Crofford L, Other X, eds. *Primer on the Rheumatic Diseases.* 13 ed. New York, NY: Springer Science+Business Media; 2008.
22. Khanna D, Fitzgerald JD, Khanna PP, et al. 2012 American College of Rheumatology guidelines for management of gout. Part 1: systematic nonpharmacologic and pharmacologic therapeutic approaches to hyperuricemia. *Arthritis Care Res (Hoboken).* 2012;64:1431–1446. DOI:10.1002/acr.21772
23. Khanna D, Khanna PP, Fitzgerald JD, et al. 2012 American College of Rheumatology guidelines for management of gout. Part 2: therapy and antiinflammatory prophylaxis of acute gouty arthritis. *Arthritis Care Res (Hoboken).* 2012;64:1447–1461. DOI:10.1002/acr.21773
24. FitzGerald JD, Dalbeth N, Mikuls T, et al. 2020 American College of Rheumatology Guideline for the Management of Gout. *Arthritis Rheumatol.* 2020;72:879–895. DOI:10.1002/art.41247
25. Schlesinger N, Detry MA, Holland BK, et al. Local ice therapy during bouts of acute gouty arthritis. *J Rheumatol.* 2002;29:331–334.
26. Richette P, Doherty M, Pascual E, et al. 2016 Updated EULAR evidence-based recommendations for the management of gout. *Ann Rheum Dis.* 2017;76:29–42. DOI:10.1136/annrheumdis-2016-209707
27. Qaseem A, Harris RP, Forciea MA. Management of Acute and Recurrent Gout: A Clinical Practice Guideline From the American College of Physicians. *Ann Intern Med.* 2017;166:58–68. DOI:10.7326/m16-0570

28. van Durme CM, Wechalekar MD, Buchbinder R, et al. Non-steroidal anti-inflammatory drugs for acute gout. *Cochrane Database Syst Rev.* 2014:Cd010120. DOI:10.1002/14651858.CD010120.pub2
29. Schumacher HR, Berger MF, Li-Yu J, et al. Efficacy and tolerability of celecoxib in the treatment of acute gouty arthritis: a randomized controlled trial. *J Rheumatol.* 2012;39:1859–1866. DOI:10.3899/jrheum.110916
30. Rainer TH, Cheng CH, Janssens HJ, et al. Oral Prednisolone in the Treatment of Acute Gout: A Pragmatic, Multicenter, Double-Blind, Randomized Trial. *Ann Intern Med.* 2016;164:464–471. DOI:10.7326/m14-2070
31. Xu L, Liu S, Guan M, et al. Comparison of Prednisolone, Etoricoxib, and Indomethacin in Treatment of Acute Gouty Arthritis: An Open-Label, Randomized, Controlled Trial. *Med Sci Monit.* 2016;22:810–817. DOI:10.12659/msm.895749
32. Siegel LB, Alloway JA, Nashel DJ. Comparison of adrenocorticotropic hormone and triamcinolone acetonide in the treatment of acute gouty arthritis. *J Rheumatol.* 1994;21:1325–1327.
33. Sánchez Fernández I, Amengual-Gual M, Gaínza-Lein M, et al. Cost-effectiveness of adrenocorticotropic hormone versus oral steroids for infantile spasms. *Epilepsia.* 2021;62:347–357. DOI:10.1111/epi.16799
34. van Echteld I, Wechalekar MD, Schlesinger N, et al. Colchicine for acute gout. *Cochrane Database of Systematic Reviews.* 2014. DOI:10.1002/14651858.CD006190.pub2
35. Ahern MJ, Reid C, Gordon TP, et al. Does colchicine work? The results of the first controlled study in acute gout. *Aust N Z J Med.* 1987;17: 301–304. DOI:10.1111/j.1445-5994.1987.tb01232.x
36. Kesselheim AS, Franklin JM, Kim SC, et al. Reductions in use of colchicine after FDA enforcement of market exclusivity in a commercially insured population. *J Gen Intern Med.* 2015;30: 1633–1638. DOI:10.1007/s11606-015-3285-7
37. McCormick N, Wallace ZS, Yokose C, et al. Prolonged increases in public-payer spending and prices after unapproved drug initiative approval of colchicine. *JAMA Intern Med.* 2021;181:284–287. DOI:10.1001/jamainternmed.2020.5017
38. Terkeltaub RA, Furst DE, Bennett K, et al. High versus low dosing of oral colchicine for early acute gout flare: Twenty-four-hour outcome of the first multicenter, randomized, double-blind, placebo-controlled, parallel-group, dose-comparison colchicine study. *Arthritis Rheum.* 2010;62:1060–1068. DOI:10.1002/art.27327
39. Gutman AB. The past four decades of progress in the knowledge of gout, with an assessment of the present status. *Arthritis Rheum.* 1973;16:431–445. DOI:10.1002/art.1780160402
40. Scheepers L, van Onna M, Stehouwer CDA, et al. Medication adherence among patients with gout: a systematic review and meta-analysis. *Semin Arthritis Rheum.* 2018;47:689–702. DOI:10.1016/j.semarthrit.2017.09.007
41. Juraschek SP, Gelber AC, Choi HK, et al. Effects of the Dietary Approaches to Stop Hypertension (DASH) diet and sodium intake on serum uric acid. *Arthritis Rheumatol.* 2016;68:3002–3009. DOI:10.1002/art.39813
42. Tang O, Miller ER 3rd, Gelber AC, et al. DASH diet and change in serum uric acid over time. *Clin Rheumatol.* 2017;36:1413–1417. DOI:10.1007/s10067-017-3613-x
43. Zhang Y, Woods R, Chaisson CE, et al. Alcohol consumption as a trigger of recurrent gout attacks. *Am J Med.* 2006;119:800.e813–808. DOI:10.1016/j.amjmed.2006.01.020
44. Neogi T, Chen C, Niu J, et al. Alcohol quantity and type on risk of recurrent gout attacks: an internet-based case-crossover study. *Am J Med.* 2014;127:311–318. DOI:10.1016/j.amjmed.2013.12.019
45. Schlesinger N. Management of acute and chronic gouty arthritis: present state-of-the-art. *Drugs.* 2004;64:2399–2416. DOI:10.2165/00003495-200464210-00003
46. Haidari F Jr., Mohammad Shahi M, Keshavarz SA, et al. Inhibitory effects of Tart Cherry (Prunus cerasus) juice on xanthine oxidoreductase activity and its hypouricemic and antioxidant effects on rats. *Malays J Nutr.* 2009;15:53–64.
47. Zhang Y, Neogi T, Chen C, et al. Cherry consumption and decreased risk of recurrent gout attacks. *Arthritis Rheum.* 2012;64:4004–4011. DOI:10.1002/art.34677
48. Hill EM, Sky K, Sit M, et al. Does starting allopurinol prolong acute treated gout? A randomized clinical trial. *J Clin Rheumatol.* 2015;21:120–125. DOI:10.1097/rhu.0000000000000235
49. Taylor TH, Mecchella JN, Larson RJ, et al. Initiation of allopurinol at first medical contact for acute attacks of gout: a randomized clinical trial. *Am J Med.* 2012;125:1126–1134.e1127. DOI:10.1016/j.amjmed.2012.05.025
50. Feng X, Li Y, Gao W. Significance of the initiation time of urate-lowering therapy in gout patients: a retrospective research. *Joint Bone Spine.* 2015;82:428–431. DOI:10.1016/j.jbspin.2015.02.021
51. Perez-Ruiz F, Herrero-Beites AM, Carmona L. A two-stage approach to the treatment of hyperuricemia in gout: the "dirty dish" hypothesis. *Arthritis Rheum.* 2011;63:4002–4006. DOI:10.1002/art.30649
52. Seth R, Kydd ASR, Buchbinder R, et al. Allopurinol for chronic gout. *Cochrane Database of Systematic Reviews.* 2014. DOI:10.1002/14651858.CD006077.pub3
53. Yang CY, Chen CH, Deng ST, et al. Allopurinol Use and Risk of Fatal Hypersensitivity Reactions: A Nationwide Population-Based Study in Taiwan. *JAMA Intern Med.* 2015;175:1550–1557. DOI:10.1001/jamainternmed.2015.3536
54. Stamp LK, Taylor WJ, Jones PB, et al. Starting dose is a risk factor for allopurinol hypersensitivity syndrome: a proposed safe starting dose of allopurinol. *Arthritis Rheum.* 2012;64:2529–2536. DOI:10.1002/art.34488
55. Stamp LK, Chapman PT, Barclay M, et al. Allopurinol dose escalation to achieve serum urate below 6 mg/dL: an open-label extension study. *Ann Rheum Dis.* 2017;76:2065–2070. DOI:10.1136/annrheumdis-2017-211873
56. Stamp LK, Chapman PT, Barclay ML, et al. A randomised controlled trial of the efficacy and safety of allopurinol dose escalation to achieve target serum urate in people with gout. *Ann Rheum Dis.* 2017;76:1522–1528. DOI:10.1136/annrheumdis-2016-210872
57. Becker MA, Schumacher HR Jr., Wortmann RL, et al. Febuxostat compared with allopurinol in patients with hyperuricemia and gout. *N Engl J Med.* 2005;353:2450–2461. DOI:10.1056/NEJMoa050373
58. White WB, Saag KG, Becker MA, et al. Cardiovascular safety of febuxostat or allopurinol in patients with gout. *N Engl J Med.* 2018;378:1200–1210. DOI:10.1056/NEJMoa1710895
59. Mackenzie IS, Ford I, Nuki G, et al. Long-term cardiovascular safety of febuxostat compared with allopurinol in patients with gout (FAST): a multicentre, prospective, randomised, open-label, non-inferiority trial. *Lancet.* 2020;396:1745–1757. DOI:10.1016/s0140-6736(20)32234-0
60. ULORIC. Febuxostat. Deerfield, IL: Takeda Pharmaceuticals, 2021.
61. Vargas-Santos AB, Neogi T. Management of gout and hyperuricemia in CKD. *Am J Kidney Dis.* 2017;70:422–439. DOI:10.1053/j.ajkd.2017.01.055
62. Perez-Ruiz F, Sundy JS, Miner JN, et al. Lesinurad in combination with allopurinol: results of a phase 2, randomised, double-blind study in patients with gout with an inadequate response to allopurinol. *Ann Rheum Dis.* 2016;75:1074–1080. DOI:10.1136/annrheumdis-2015-207919
63. Tausche AK, Alten R, Dalbeth N, et al. Lesinurad monotherapy in gout patients intolerant to a xanthine oxidase inhibitor: a 6 month phase 3 clinical trial and extension study. *Rheumatology (Oxford).* 2017;56:2170–2178. DOI:10.1093/rheumatology/kex350
64. Sundy JS, Baraf HS, Yood RA, et al. Efficacy and tolerability of pegloticase for the treatment of chronic gout in patients refractory to conventional treatment: two randomized controlled trials. *JAMA.* 2011;306:711–720. DOI:10.1001/jama.2011.1169
65. Shannon JA, Cole SW. Pegloticase: a novel agent for treatment-refractory gout. *Ann Pharmacother.* 2012;46:368–376. DOI:10.1345/aph.1Q593
66. Feher MD, Hepburn AL, Hogarth MB, et al. Fenofibrate enhances urate reduction in men treated with allopurinol for hyperuricaemia and gout. *Rheumatology (Oxford).* 2003;42:321–325. DOI:10.1093/rheumatology/keg103
67. Waldman B, Ansquer JC, Sullivan DR, et al. Effect of fenofibrate on uric acid and gout in type 2 diabetes: a post-hoc analysis of the randomised, controlled FIELD study. *Lancet Diabetes Endocrinol.* 2018;6:310–318. DOI:10.1016/s2213-8587(18)30029-9
68. Würzner G, Gerster JC, Chiolero A, et al. Comparative effects of losartan and irbesartan on serum uric acid in hypertensive patients with hyperuricaemia and gout. *J Hypertens.* 2001;19:1855–1860. DOI:10.1097/00004872-200110000-00021
69. Miao Y, Ottenbros SA, Laverman GD, et al. Effect of a reduction in uric acid on renal outcomes during losartan treatment: a post hoc analysis of the reduction of endpoints in non-insulin-dependent diabetes mellitus with the Angiotensin II Antagonist Losartan Trial. *Hypertension.* 2011;58:2–7. DOI:10.1161/hypertensionaha.111.171488
70. Shahinfar S, Simpson RL, Carides AD, et al. Safety of losartan in hypertensive patients with thiazide-induced hyperuricemia. *Kidney Int.* 1999;56:1879–1885. DOI:10.1046/j.1523-1755.1999.00739.x
71. Borstad GC, Bryant LR, Abel MP, et al. Colchicine for prophylaxis of acute flares when initiating allopurinol for chronic gouty arthritis. *J Rheumatol.* 2004;31:2429–2432.

72. RetailMeNot RxSaver. Colchicine. Available at: https://rxsaver.retailmenot.com/prescriptions/prices?distance=20&filter=allopurinol&zipCode=52240. Accessed 3/12/2019.
73. Pascart T, Richette P. Investigational drugs for hyperuricemia, an update on recent developments. *Expert Opin Investig Drugs.* 2018;27:437–444. DOI:10.1080/13543784.2018.1471133
74. Janssen CA, Oude Voshaar MAH, Vonkeman HE, et al. Anakinra for the treatment of acute gout flares: a randomized, double-blind, placebo-controlled, active-comparator, non-inferiority trial. *Rheumatology (Oxford).* 2019. DOI:10.1093/rheumatology/key402
75. Schlesinger N, Alten RE, Bardin T, et al. Canakinumab for acute gouty arthritis in patients with limited treatment options: results from two randomised, multicentre, active-controlled, double-blind trials and their initial extensions. *Ann Rheum Dis.* 2012;71:1839–1848. DOI:10.1136/annrheumdis-2011-200908
76. Schlesinger N, Mysler E, Lin HY, et al. Canakinumab reduces the risk of acute gouty arthritis flares during initiation of allopurinol treatment: results of a double-blind, randomised study. *Ann Rheum Dis.* 2011;70:1264–1271. DOI:10.1136/ard.2010.144063
77. Schumacher HR Jr., Sundy JS, Terkeltaub R, et al. Rilonacept (interleukin-1 trap) in the prevention of acute gout flares during initiation of urate-lowering therapy: results of a phase II randomized, double-blind, placebo-controlled trial. *Arthritis Rheum.* 2012;64:876–884. DOI:10.1002/art.33412
78. Sundy JS, Schumacher HR, Kivitz A, et al. Rilonacept for gout flare prevention in patients receiving uric acid-lowering therapy: results of RESURGE, a phase III, international safety study. *J Rheumatol.* 2014;41:1703–1711. DOI:10.3899/jrheum.131226
79. Shahid H, Singh JA. Investigational drugs for hyperuricemia. *Expert Opin Investig Drugs.* 2015;24:1013–1030. DOI:10.1517/13543784.2015.1051617
80. Wiederkehr MR, Moe OW. Uric acid nephrolithiasis: a systemic metabolic disorder. *Clin Rev Bone Miner Metab.* 2011;9:207–217. DOI:10.1007/s12018-011-9106-6
81. Zhu Y, Pandya BJ, Choi HK. Comorbidities of gout and hyperuricemia in the US general population: NHANES 2007-2008. *Am J Med.* 2012;125:679–687.e671. DOI:10.1016/j.amjmed.2011.09.033
82. Gaffo AL, Calhoun DA, Rahn EJ, et al. Effect of Serum Urate Lowering With Allopurinol on Blood Pressure in Young Adults: A Randomized, Controlled, Crossover Trial. *Arthritis Rheumatol.* 2021;73:1514–1522. DOI:10.1002/art.41749
83. Badve SV, Pascoe EM, Tiku A, et al. Effects of allopurinol on the progression of chronic kidney disease. *N Engl J Med.* 2020;382:2504–2513. DOI:10.1056/NEJMoa1915833
84. Jutkowitz E, Dubreuil M, Lu N, et al. The cost-effectiveness of HLA-B*5801 screening to guide initial urate-lowering therapy for gout in the United States. *Semin Arthritis Rheum.* 2017;46:594–600. DOI:10.1016/j.semarthrit.2016.10.009
85. Latif Z, Abhishek A. Are doctors the best people to manage gout? Is there a role for nurses and pharmacists? *Curr Rheumatol Rep.* 2018;20:14. DOI:10.1007/s11926-018-0722-8

114 Glaucoma

Richard Fiscella, Ohoud Owaidhah, and Deepak P. Edward

KEY CONCEPTS

1. Primary open-angle glaucoma (POAG) or ocular hypertension is more prevalent outside Asia than primary angle-closure glaucoma (PACG).
2. In any form of glaucoma, reduction of intraocular pressure (IOP) is essential.
3. IOP is an important risk factor for glaucoma, but the most important considerations are progression of glaucomatous changes in the back of the eye (optic disk and nerve fiber layer) and visual field changes when diagnosing and monitoring for POAG or ocular hypertension.
4. Optic nerve changes often occur before visual field changes are exhibited.
5. Reduction in IOP prevents progression or even onset of glaucoma.
6. Newer medications simplify treatment regimens for patients. Prostaglandin analogs are considered the most potent topical medications for reducing IOP and flattening diurnal variations in IOP.
7. Local adverse events are common with topical glaucoma medications, but patient education and reinforcing adherence are essential to prevent glaucoma progression.

BEYOND THE BOOK

Watch the video from Dr. Henry Jampel, a leading glaucoma specialist, entitled "Using Eye Drops to Treat Glaucoma" from The Wilmer Eye Institute (https://www.youtube.com/watch?v=IR7nH1kXsBY). Proper administration of eye drops is critical prior to discussing glaucoma medication with a patient. The video presents common mistakes associated with eye drop administration, the proper technique for administering eye drops, and frequently asked questions about using eye drops in glaucoma. It is a useful tool for the students to help ensure that the proper use of eye drops in glaucoma in the ASSESS and IMPLEMENT steps for the Patient Care Process.

INTRODUCTION

Glaucomas are a group of ocular disorders that lead to an optic neuropathy characterized by changes in the optic nerve head (optic disk) that is associated with loss of visual sensitivity and field. Increased intraocular pressure (IOP) is thought to play an important role in the pathogenesis of glaucoma, but it is not a diagnostic criterion for glaucoma. Consistently elevated IOP without signs or symptoms of glaucoma is called ocular hypertension (OHT).

Two major types of glaucoma have been identified: open angle and closed angle. Primary open-angle glaucoma (POAG) accounts for the great majority of cases in North America, while primary angle-closure glaucoma (PACG) is more prevalent in Asia. Either type can be a primary inherited disorder, congenital, or secondary to disease, trauma, or drugs and can lead to serious complications. Both primary and secondary glaucomas may be caused by a combination of open-angle and closed-angle mechanisms (Table 114-1 and Fig. 114-1). Patients with consistently high IOP or patients with clinical findings suspicious of early glaucomatous changes are called "glaucoma suspects."[1,2]

BASIC CONCEPTS

Aqueous Humor Dynamics and IOP

An understanding of IOP and aqueous humor dynamics will assist the reader in understanding the drug therapy of glaucoma.[1-6]

Aqueous humor is a clear fluid and ultrafiltrate of the serum that fills and helps to form the anterior and posterior chambers of the eye.[7] It is formed in the ciliary body and its epithelium through both filtration and secretion. Because ultrafiltration depends on pressure gradients, blood pressure and IOP changes influence aqueous humor formation. Osmotic gradients produced by active secretion of sodium and bicarbonate and possibly by other solutes such as ascorbate from the ciliary body epithelial cells into the aqueous humor result in the movement of water from the pool of ciliary

TABLE 114-1 General Classification of Glaucoma

I. Primary glaucoma
  a. Open angle
  b. Angle closure
    1. With pupillary block
    2. Without pupillary block
II. Secondary glaucoma
  a. Open angle
    1. Pretrabecular
    2. Trabecular
    3. Posttrabecular
  b. Angle closure
    1. Without pupillary block
    2. With pupillary block
III. Congenital glaucoma
IV. Others

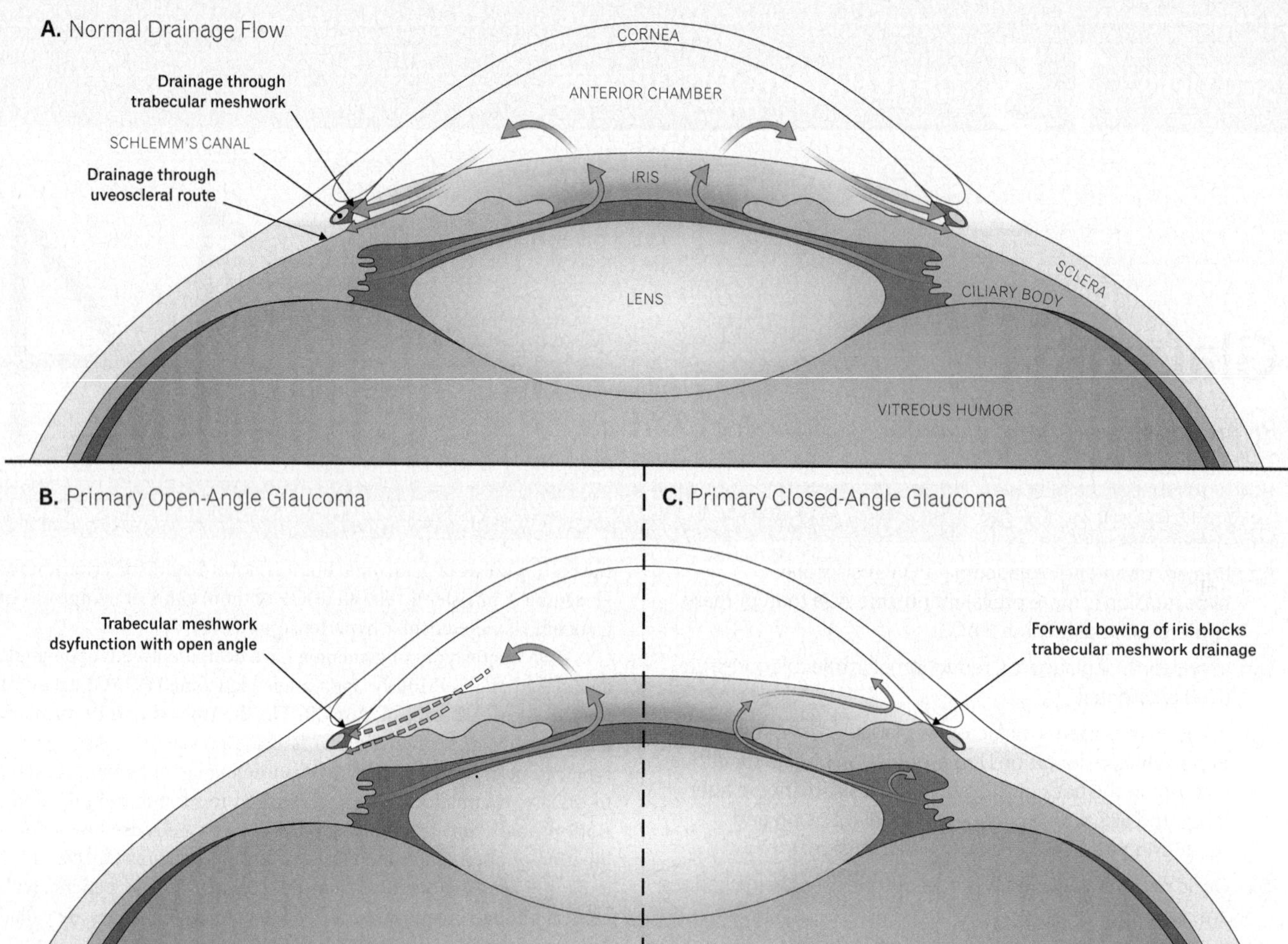

FIGURE 114-1 Aqueous humor drainage pathways in normal eyes and eyes with glaucoma. The cross-section demonstrates aqueous humor drainage in the normal healthy eye, and in primary open-angle glaucoma (POAG) and primary angle closure glaucoma (PACG). The three diagrams indicate the following aqueous humor pathways: (*A*) healthy eye, (*B*) POAG, and (*C*) PACG. Aqueous humor exits the anterior chamber by two routes: The trabecular meshwork (conventional) with approximately 80%-85% of outflow through to Schlemm's canal and the rest of the aqueous humor filtering through the uveoscleral (unconventional) outflow pathway (ciliary body and the suprachoroidal space). POAG is often associated with increased resistance to aqueous humor drainage at the trabecular meshwork. In PACG the drainage pathway is often obstructed by the iris. *(Figure by Lauren Kalinoski, MS, CMI. Courtesy University of Illinois at Chicago Department of Ophthalmology, Chicago, Illinois).*

stromal ultrafiltrate into the posterior chamber, forming aqueous humor. Carbonic anhydrase (primarily isoenzyme type II), α- and β-adrenergic receptors, and sodium- and potassium-activated adenosine triphosphatases are found on the ciliary epithelium and appear to be involved in this secretion of the solutes sodium and bicarbonate.

Receptor systems controlling aqueous inflow have not been elucidated fully. Pharmacologic studies suggest that β-adrenergic agents increase inflow, whereas α_2-adrenergic blocking, β-adrenergic blocking dopamine-blocking, carbonic anhydrase-inhibiting, melatonin-1 agonist, and adenylate cyclase-stimulating agents decrease aqueous inflow. Aqueous humor produced by the ciliary body is secreted into the posterior chamber at a rate of approximately 2 to 3 μL/min. The pressure in the posterior chamber produced by the constant inflow pushes the aqueous humor between the iris and lens and through the pupil into the anterior chamber of the eye (see Fig. 114-1).[1-6]

Aqueous humor in the anterior chamber leaves the eye by two routes: (a) filtration through the trabecular meshwork (conventional outflow) to the Schlemm's canal (80%-85%) and (b) through the ciliary body and the suprachoroidal space (uveoscleral outflow or unconventional outflow) (see Fig. 114-1). Cholinergic agents such as pilocarpine appear to increase outflow by physically opening the meshwork pores secondary to ciliary muscle contraction. The nitric oxide group on latanoprost bunod is believed to cause trabecular relaxation and increased trabecular meshwork outflow. ROCK inhibitors are believed to increase aqueous humor outflow through the trabecular meshwork. Prostaglandins are thought to result in remodeling of extracellular matrix in the meshwork, thereby increasing mainly uveoscleral outflow. The uveoscleral outflow of aqueous humor is increased by prostaglandin analogs, and α_2-adrenergic agonists. Constant inflow of aqueous humor from the ciliary body and resistance to outflow result in an IOP great enough to produce an outflow rate equal to the inflow rate (see Fig. 114-1). Novel adenosine receptor agonists, cannabinoids, serotonin agents, and dopamine agonists also increase aqueous humor outflow and reduce IOP.[1-4,6]

The median IOP measured in large populations is 15.5 ± 2.5 mm Hg (2.1 ± 0.3 kPa); however, the distribution of pressures around the mean is skewed to the right (toward higher readings). IOP is not constant and changes with pulse, blood pressure, forced expiration or coughing, neck compression, and posture. Gender, general health, and lifestyle (eg, smoking) are some factors that may have a long-term effect on the IOP.[5,7-11] The amount of caffeine in one cup of caffeinated coffee (182 mg) increases IOP by about 1 mm Hg (0.1 kPa) after 90 minutes; this increase in IOP is not clinically relevant. Patients who have thinner corneas, have had laser refractive eye surgery (LASIK), or have had cataract surgery demonstrate falsely low IOP readings. IOP is measured by tonometry: indentation tonometry, applanation tonometry, or a noncontact method using an air pulse. Newer methods of tonometry include the Pascal tonometer, Icare™ rebound tonometer, and a contact lens-based investigational device that can remotely monitor 24-hour IOP changes from baseline.[7] These methods may result in slightly different pressure readings. IOPs consistently greater than 21 mm Hg (2.8 kPa) are found in 5% to 8% of the general population. The incidence increases with age, such that "abnormal" (ie, >22 mm Hg [2.9 kPa]) IOP is found in 15% of those 70 to 75 years of age. Intermittently very high IOP (>40 mm Hg [5.3 kPa]) is found in patients with PACG.

IOP demonstrates considerable circadian variation (often referred to as *diurnal* IOP or the IOP during the daily 24-hour cycle) primarily because of changes in the rate of aqueous humor formation. This circadian variation results in a minimum IOP at approximately 6 pm and a maximum IOP at awakening, although some studies suggest that both healthy and glaucoma patients may have their highest IOP at night after falling asleep.[1-6,8-14] Low systemic blood pressure in conjunction with high IOPs (decreased ocular perfusion pressure) at night can result in optic nerve head damage. Generally, the circadian IOP variation is less than 3 to 4 mm Hg (0.4-0.5 kPa); however, it may be greater for patients with glaucoma. This circadian variation and the variable relationship of IOP with visual loss make measurement of IOP a poor screening test for glaucoma. Controlling circadian increases in IOP is thought to be important in the prevention of disease progression. Prostaglandin analogs and carbonic anhydrase inhibitors (CAIs) reduce nocturnal IOP, whereas beta blockers and alpha-2 adrenergic agents have minimal effects.[1-6,8-15]

Although increased IOP within any range is associated with a higher risk of glaucomatous damage, it is both an insensitive and nonspecific diagnostic and monitoring tool. Of individuals with IOP between 21 and 30 mm Hg (2.8-4.0 kPa), only 0.5% to 1% per year will develop optic disk changes and visual field loss (ie, glaucoma) over 5 to 15 years. However, more subtle retinal damage, such as alteration of color vision or decreased contrast sensitivity, occurs in a higher percentage of patients with IOPs greater than 21 mm Hg (2.8 kPa), and the incidence of visual field defects increases to as high as 28% in individuals with IOPs above 30 mm Hg (4.0 kPa). For a given IOP finding, the risk of developing glaucoma increases with older age, family history of glaucoma, lower ocular perfusion pressure, lower blood pressure, thinner central cornea, optic disc hemorrhage, larger cup-to-disk ratio, and specific visual fields findings. For patients with preexisting optic nerve damage, the worse the existing damage, the more sensitive the eye is to a given IOP. As many as 20% to 30% of patients with glaucomatous visual field loss have an IOP of less than 21 mm Hg (2.8 kPa) (called *normal-tension glaucoma*, referring to the normal IOP). Thus, the absolute IOP is a less-precise predictor of optic nerve damage. More direct measurements of therapeutic outcome, such as optic disk examination and visual field evaluation, also must be used as monitors of disease progression. Taking the above factors into consideration, glaucoma medications that provide maximal reduction of IOP over 24 hours and have minimal influence on blood pressure may be advantageous in treating glaucoma patients.[1-5,8-17]

Optic Disk and Visual Fields

The optic disk is the portion of the optic nerve ophthalmoscopically visible as it leaves the eye. It consists of approximately 1 million retinal ganglion nerve cell axons, blood vessels, and supporting connective tissue structures (lamina cribrosa). The small depression within the disk is termed the *cup*. A normal physiologic cup does not extend beyond the optic nerve rim and has a varying diameter of less than one-third to one-half that of the disk (cup-to-disk ratio: 0.33-0.5). Table 114-2 lists the common alterations of the optic disk found in glaucoma. These disk changes result from optic nerve axonal degeneration and remodeling of the supporting structures. As the nerve axons die, the cup becomes larger in relation to the whole disk. A loss of retinal nerve fiber layer might be visualized in glaucoma patients with detectable visual field loss (see Fig. 114-2). This pattern of changes is consistent with visual field losses and loss of visual sensitivity seen in glaucoma.[1-6,8-15] Damage to the optic nerve can be documented by optic disk photographs, and disease stability or progression may be monitored by examining sequential photographs. Newer methods of assessing damage to the retinal nerve fiber layer and optic disk have been described. These include scanning laser polarimetry (GDX), confocal laser ophthalmoscopy (Heidelberg retinal tomography, or HRT), and optical coherence tomography (OCT). These methods offer the ability to assess the damage to the optic nerve quantitatively.

Determination of the visual field allows the assessment of optic nerve damage and is an important monitoring parameter in the treatment. However, visual field changes typically lag behind optic disk changes, and a loss of 25% to 35% of retinal ganglion cells is usually required before detectable visual field defects are noted. The peripheral visual field is measured using a visual field instrument called a *perimeter*. Characteristic visual field loss occurs in glaucoma (Fig. 114-2; see also Table 114-2), but loss of central visual acuity usually does not occur until late in the disease. Other indicators, such as color vision changes and contrast sensitivity, may allow earlier and more sensitive detection of glaucomatous changes.[1-4]

TABLE 114-2 Optic Disk and Visual Field Findings in Patients with Glaucoma

Optic disk
Cup-to-disk ratio >0.5
Progressive increase in cup size
Cup-to-disk ratio asymmetry >0.2
Vertical elongation of the cup
Excavation of the cup
Increased exposure of lamina cribrosa
Pallor of the cup
Splinter hemorrhages
Cupping to edge of disk
Notching of the cup (usually superior or inferior)
Nerve fiber defects
Visual field findings
General peripheral field constriction
Isolated scotomas (blind spots)
Nasal visual field depression ("nasal step")
Enlargement of blind spot
Large arc-like scotomas
Reduced contrast sensitivity
Reduced peripheral acuity
Altered color vision

Genetics

Glaucoma is often inherited as a complex multifactorial disease, but it can also be inherited as a Mendelian autosomal-dominant or autosomal-recessive trait form. The common age-related adult-onset glaucoma, like POAG, although containing heritability of some significance, is more complex and is influenced by environmental factors. Genetic studies have more clearly defined the underlying molecular events responsible for the Mendelian forms of the disease. However, the chromosome locations identified may play some factor in the more complex forms. Several major gene loci associated

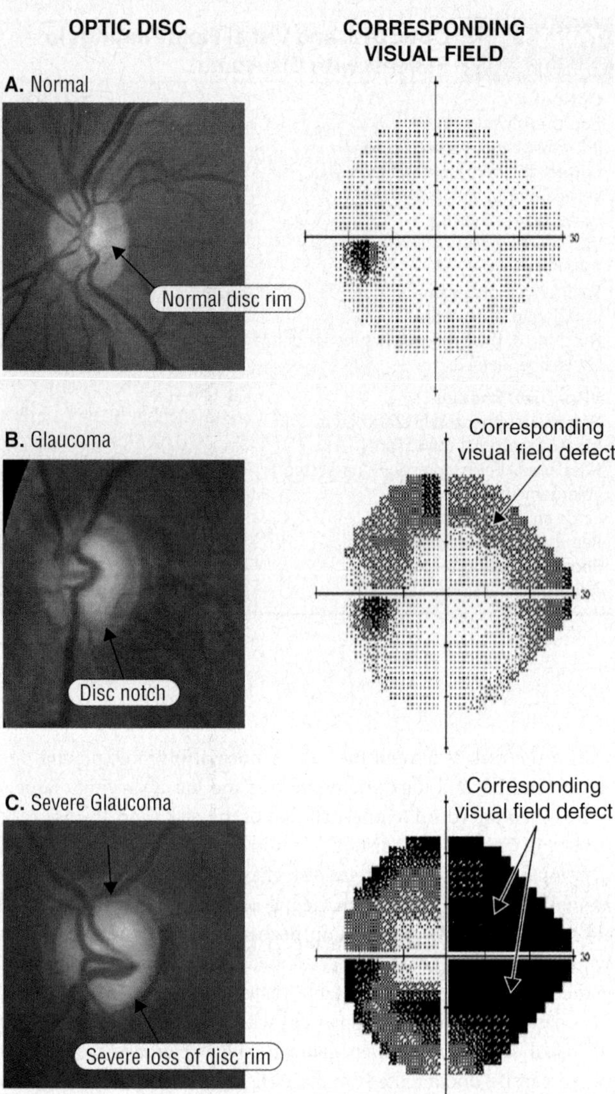

FIGURE 114-2 Normal, moderate glaucoma, and severe glaucoma disc damage and their corresponding visual fields. (*A*) The photograph shows the normal optic disc, and the corresponding visual field test shows a normal visual field. The physiologic "blind spot" (dark area on the visual field) corresponds to the location of the optic nerve. (*B*) The eye with moderate glaucoma shows an enlarged cup and thinning of the inferior neuro-retinal rim with the arrowhead pointing to the optic disc notch. Note the arrow pointing to the corresponding superior visual field defect. The physiologic "blind spot" corresponds to the location of the optic nerve. (*C*) In severe glaucoma, there is severe loss of the optic disc rim and enlargement of the cup (see arrows). The corresponding visual field shows a significant loss of visual field in both superior and inferior hemifields. *(Courtesy University of Illinois at Chicago Department of Ophthalmology, Chicago, Illinois, and King Khaled Eye Specialist Hospital, Riyadh, Saudi Arabia.)*

with POAG have been identified. The molecular mechanism of how mutations in any of these genes result in increased IOP with loss of visual field has not been determined. The future of genetic studies in glaucoma will include the discovery of new glaucoma genes, determination of clinical phenotypes associated with these genes and mutations, understanding how environmental factors interact, and developing a database that can be used for further testing.

Genome-wide association studies have identified new loci that are associated with clinically relevant optic disc parameters, including the optic disc area and vertical cup-to-disc ratio. Genes associated with chronic angle-closure glaucoma have also been identified. Improved understanding of the genetic origins of POAG may lead to new diagnostic tools and therapies that target the underlying causes of the disease.[1-4,14,18]

Epidemiology of Ocular Hypertension, Glaucoma Suspects, and Open-Angle Glaucoma

1 Overall, OHT occurs in 4.5% of non-Hispanic Whites in the United States. The frequency increases to 7.7% of those older than 79 years.[19-22] The number of glaucoma suspects (ie, consistently high IOP or suspicious eye findings) is thought to be 3 to 6 million individuals in the United States. Approximately 2% of glaucoma suspects who are left untreated will progress to glaucoma each year.[7]

Open-angle glaucoma (OAG) is the second leading cause of blindness, affecting up to 4 million individuals in the United States and up to 70 million individuals worldwide. More than 135,000 persons in the United States and about 6 to 7 million in the world have glaucoma-related bilateral blindness. The prevalence rate varies with age, race, diagnostic criteria, and other factors. In the United States, OAG occurs in 1.5% of the population older than 30 years, 1.3% of Whites, and 3.5% of Blacks. Data have also suggested that the prevalence of OAG and ocular hypertension is also high among Latinos of Mexican ancestry, with approximately 4.74% and 3.56% of people affected, respectively.[23]

The incidence of OAG increases with increasing age. The incidence of the disease for patients aged 80 years is 3% in Whites and 5% to 8% in Blacks. In addition to increased IOP, age, and ethnicity, the risk of glaucoma increases with family history, thinner central corneal thickness, lower ocular perfusion pressure, Type II diabetes, myopia, and certain genetic mutations.[7,14,18-21]

Etiology of Open-Angle Glaucoma

2 The specific cause of glaucomatous optic neuropathy is presently unknown. Previously, increased IOP was considered to be the sole cause of the damage; however, it is now recognized that IOP is only one of the many factors associated with the development and progression of glaucoma. Increased susceptibility of the optic nerve to ischemia (a reduced or dysregulated blood flow), excitotoxicity, autoimmune reactions, and other abnormal physiologic processes are likely additional contributory factors. Damage of the optic nerve ganglion occurs at the point at which ganglion and blood vessels pass through the perforated supportive collagen lamina cribosa of the optic disc. The outcome of these processes is believed to be apoptosis of the retinal ganglion cells, which results in axonal degeneration and finally permanent loss of vision. Neuronal loss also extends beyond the optic nerve to the lateral geniculate nucleus and visual cortex. POAG may represent a number of distinct diseases or conditions that simply manifest the same symptoms. Susceptibility to visual loss at a given IOP varies considerably; some patients do not demonstrate damage at high IOPs, whereas other patients have progressive visual field loss despite an IOP in the normal range (normal-tension glaucoma).[1-5,7]

Although IOP poorly predicts which patients will have visual field loss, the risk of visual field loss clearly increases with increasing IOP within any range. Lowering IOP, no matter what the pretreatment IOP, reduces the risk of glaucomatous progression or may even prevent the onset to early glaucoma in patients with ocular hypertension.[1-4,7,8,10,11]

The mechanism by which a certain level of IOP increases the susceptibility of a given eye to nerve damage remains controversial. Multiple mechanisms are likely to be operative in a spectrum of combinations to produce the death of retinal ganglion cells and their axons in glaucoma. Pressure-sensitive astrocytes and other cells in the optic disk supportive matrix may produce changes and remodeling of the disk, resulting in axonal death. Vasogenic theories suggest that optic nerve damage results from insufficient blood flow to the retina secondary to the increased perfusion pressure required in the eye, dysregulated perfusion, or vessel wall abnormalities and results in degeneration of axonal fibers of the retina. Another theory suggests that the IOP may disrupt axoplasmal flow at the optic disk.[7]

Focus on the mechanisms of the retinal ganglion cell apoptosis and the role of excessive glutamate and nitric oxide found in glaucoma patients has broadened the focus of drug therapy research to include evaluation of agents that act as neuroprotectants. Such agents may be particularly useful for patients with normal-pressure glaucoma, in whom pressure-independent factors may play a relatively larger role in disease progression. These agents would target risk factors and underlying pathophysiologic mechanisms of disease other than IOP.[7,10,24]

Pathophysiology of Open-Angle Glaucoma

3 As stated previously, optic nerve damage in POAG can occur at a wide range of IOPs, and the rate of progression is highly variable. Patients may exhibit pressures in the 20 to 30 mm Hg (2.7-4.0 kPa) range for years before any disease progression is noticed in the optic disk or visual fields. That is why POAG is often referred to as the "sneak thief of sight."

Clinical Presentation of Open-Angle Glaucoma

POAG is a bilateral, often asymmetric, genetically determined disorder constituting 60% to 70% of all glaucomas and 90% to 95% of primary glaucomas in the United States (see the "Clinical Presentation" box). An increased IOP is not required for diagnosis of POAG. Symptoms do not present until substantial visual field constriction occurs. Central visual acuity typically is maintained, even in the late stages of the disease. Even though POAG is a bilateral disease, it may have greater IOP and progression and severity in one eye. As such, each eye is treated individually.[7]

4 Detection and diagnosis involve evaluation of the optic disk and retinal nerve fiber layer, assessment of the visual fields, and measurement of IOP. The presence of characteristic disk changes and visual field loss with or without increased IOP confirms the diagnosis of glaucoma. Typical disk changes and field loss occurring at an IOP of less than 21 mm Hg (2.8 kPa) account for 20% to 30% of patients and are referred to as *normal-tension glaucoma*. Elevated IOP (>21 mm Hg [2.8 kPa]) without disk changes or visual field loss is observed in 5% to 7% of individuals (*glaucoma suspects*) and is referred to as *ocular hypertension*. New technologies such as OCT, retinal nerve fiber analyzers, or confocal scanning laser tomography of the optic nerve head may allow early identification of signs of glaucomatous retinal changes in ocular hypertensives, thus allowing for earlier initiation of therapy.[7]

Secondary OAG has many causes, including exfoliation syndrome, pigmentary glaucoma, systemic diseases, trauma, surgery, ocular inflammatory diseases, and medications. A system for classifying secondary glaucomas into pretrabecular, trabecular, and posttrabecular forms has been proposed. This classification allows drug therapy to be chosen on the basis of the pathogenic mechanism involved. In pretrabecular forms, a normal meshwork is covered and does not permit aqueous humor outflow. Trabecular forms of secondary glaucoma result from either an alteration of meshwork or an accumulation of material in the intertrabecular spaces. The posttrabecular forms result primarily from disorders causing increased episcleral venous blood pressure.

CLINICAL PRESENTATION

Prognosis of Open-Angle Glaucoma

5 In most cases of POAG, the overall prognosis is excellent when it is discovered early and treated adequately. Even patients with advanced visual field loss can have continued visual field loss reduced if the IOP is maintained at low enough pressures (often <10-12 mm Hg [1.3-1.6 kPa]). Medications will control IOP successfully in 60% to 80% of patients over a 5-year period. Progression of visual field loss still occurs in 8% to 20% of patients despite reaching standard therapy IOP goals. However, for untreated patients and for those who fail to achieve target IOP reduction, up to 80% have continued visual field loss. Estimates of progression to bilateral blindness in treated patients range from 4% to 22%. Compared to placebo, each 1 mm Hg (0.1 kPa) in IOP reduction reduces the risk of disease progression by at least 10% and up to 19%.[7,24] After 2 years, visual field loss occurred in 25.6% of placebo patients compared to 15.2% of those treated with latanoprost.[25] Thus, the keys to medical treatment of POAG are an effective, well-tolerated drug regimen, close monitoring of therapy, and adherence.[26,27]

Epidemiology of PACG

The incidence of PACG varies by the ethnic group, with a higher incidence in individuals of Inuit, Chinese, and Asian-Indian descent. Incidence rates of 1% to 4% have been reported in these populations.[7] Because of the high frequency of PACG in populous Asia, PACG accounts for approximately one-third of glaucoma worldwide. PACG accounts for a disproportionately high proportion of blindness (estimated at up to 50%) worldwide.[28-30]

Etiology Primary Angle-Closure Glaucoma (Acute ACG and CACG)

In North America, PACG accounts for a minority of cases of primary glaucoma. When severe acute angle-closure glaucoma (ACG) occurs, it may need to be treated as an emergency to avoid visual loss. PACG results from mechanical blockage of the (usually normal) trabecular meshwork by the peripheral iris. Partial or complete blockage of the meshwork occurs intermittently, potentially resulting in extreme fluctuations between normal IOP with no symptoms and very high IOP with symptoms of acute PACG. Between attacks of PACG, the IOP is usually normal unless the patient has concomitant POAG or nonreversible blockage of the meshwork with synechiae ("creeping" angle closure) that develops over time in the narrow-angle eye. PACG occurs in patients with inherited shallow anterior chambers (often seen in small eyes), which produce a narrow angle between the cornea and iris or tight contact between the iris and lens (pupillary block) (see Fig. 114-1C). The presence of a narrow angle is determined mainly by visualization of the angle by gonioscopy. Other tests for PACG involve provocation of an angle-closure–induced IOP increase. These tests, which attempt to produce angle closure through mydriasis (darkroom test or mydriasis test) or gravity (prone test), are rarely performed in the clinical setting.

Two major types of classic, reversible PACG have been described: PACG with pupillary block and PACG without pupillary block. PACG with pupillary block results when the iris is in firm contact with the lens. This produces a relative block of aqueous flow through the pupil to the anterior chamber (pupillary block), resulting in a bowing forward of the iris, which blocks the trabecular meshwork. PACG with pupillary block occurs most commonly when the pupil is in mid-dilation. In this position, the combination of pupillary block and relaxed iris allows the greatest bowing of the iris; however, angle closure may occur during miosis or mydriasis.

PACG can occur without significant pupillary block for patients with an abnormality called a *plateau iris*. The ciliary processes in these cases are situated anteriorly, which indent the iris forward and cause closure of the trabecular meshwork, especially during mydriasis. The mydriasis produced by anticholinergic drugs or any other drug results in precipitation of both types of PACG glaucoma, whereas drug-induced miosis may produce pupillary block.[7,30]

CLINICAL PRESENTATION Glaucoma

General

- Glaucoma can be detected in otherwise asymptomatic patients, or patients can present with characteristic symptoms, especially vision loss. POAG is a chronic, slowly progressive disease found primarily in patients older than 50 years, whereas PACG is more typically associated with symptomatic acute episodes or may be slowly progressive like POAG

Symptoms

- POAG: None until substantial visual field loss occurs
- PACG: Nonsymptomatic or prodromal symptoms (blurred or hazy vision with halos around lights that is caused by a hazy, edematous cornea, and occasionally headache) may be present. Acute episodes produce symptoms associated with a cloudy, edematous cornea, ocular pain, or discomfort, nausea, vomiting, abdominal pain, and diaphoresis

Signs

- POAG: Disk changes and visual field loss (see Table 114-2); IOP can be normal or elevated (>21 mm Hg [2.8 kPa])
  - Mild: Optic disk abnormalities with normal visual field with standard perimetry
  - Moderate: Optic disk changes plus visual field abnormalities in one hemifield that are not within 5 degrees of central visual fixation
  - Severe: Optic disk changes with visual field loss in both hemifields and loss within 5 degrees of central fixation and abnormalities in at least one hemifield
- Acute Angle-Closure Glaucoma (ACG): Acute, hyperemic conjunctiva, cloudy cornea, shallow anterior chamber, and occasionally an edematous and hyperemic optic disk; IOP is generally elevated markedly (40-90 mm Hg [5.3-12.0 kPa]) when symptoms are present
- Chronic (CACG): Disk changes and visual field loss (see Table 114-2); IOP can be normal or elevated (>21 mm Hg [2.8 kPa])

Laboratory Tests

- None

Other Diagnostic Tests

- Emerging tests include optical coherence tomography, retinal nerve fiber analyzers, and confocal scanning laser tomography of the optic nerve. Pachymetry is crucial to detect a thin cornea that has been proved to be associated with visual field progression in open-angle glaucomas

Pathophysiology of PACG

The mechanism of IOP elevation in PACG is clearer than that of POAG. In PACG, a physical blockage of trabecular meshwork is present. In many cases, single or multiple episodes of high IOP that in some patients may exceed 40 mm Hg (5.3 kPa) and result in optic nerve damage. Very high IOP (>60 mm Hg [8.0 kPa]) may result in permanent loss of visual field within a matter of hours to days.

One type of CAG, known as "creeping" angle closure, occurs in patients with narrow angles in which the iris adheres to the trabecular meshwork and may result in continuously increased IOP in ranges more similar to those of POAG, and the clinical behavior is similar to POAG, with individuals differing in the degree and rapidity of visual loss from any given elevated IOP.[30]

Clinical Presentation of Angle-Closure Glaucoma

Most patients with untreated PACG typically experience intermittent nonsymptomatic or prodromal symptoms brought on by precipitating events (see the "Clinical Presentation" box). Increased IOP during such prodromal episodes is not great enough or long enough to produce the other symptoms of a full-blown attack. Such prodromal attacks last 1 to 2 hours, at which time pupillary block is broken by further mydriasis or miosis, or when miosis or mydriasis occurs in patients with plateau iris. The rate at which IOP increases may be a determinant of when full-blown symptoms occur. Visual fields demonstrate generalized constriction or typical glaucomatous defects as seen in POAG. In approximately 25% of patients, severe attacks may occur, and if prolonged, total loss of vision may occur if the IOP is high enough. Tonometry reveals IOPs as high as 40 to 90 mm Hg (5.3-12.0 kPa). Patients who have developed adhesions between the iris and meshwork (anterior synechiae) may have chronic IOP elevation with intermittent spikes of high IOP when angle closure occurs.[7,30]

Drug-Induced Glaucoma

A number of medications are associated with increased IOP or carry labeling that cautions against use of the medication in glaucoma patients. The potential for a medication to produce or worsen glaucoma depends on the type of glaucoma and whether the patient is treated adequately.[7,31-35] Patients with treated, controlled POAG are at minimal risk of induction of an increase in IOP by systemic medications with anticholinergic properties or vasodilators; however, for patients with untreated glaucoma or uncontrolled POAG, the potential of these medications to increase IOP should be considered. Topical anticholinergic agents used to produce mydriasis may result in an increase in IOP. Potent anticholinergic agents such as atropine or homatropine are most likely to increase IOP. Weaker anticholinergics, such as tropicamide, that produce less cycloplegia are less likely to increase IOP and are favored, along with phenylephrine, when mydriasis is desired for POAG patients. Inhaled, nasal, topical, or systemic glucocorticoids may increase IOP for both normal individuals and patients with POAG.

Patients with POAG appear to be particularly susceptible to glucocorticoid-induced increases in IOP. Glucocorticoids reduce the facility of aqueous humor outflow through the trabecular meshwork. The decreased facility of outflow appears to result from the accumulation of extracellular material blocking the trabecular channels. The potential of a glucocorticoid to increase IOP is related to its anti-inflammatory potency and intraocular penetration. Thus, patients should be treated with the lowest potency and dose and for the shortest time possible when steroids are indicated.

For patients predisposed to CAG (ie, narrow anterior chambers), angle closure may be produced by any drug that causes

TABLE 114-3 Drugs That May Induce or Potentiate Increased Intraocular Pressure

Open-angle glaucoma
Ophthalmic corticosteroids (high risk)
Systemic corticosteroids
Nasal/inhaled corticosteroids
Fenoldopam
Ophthalmic anticholinergics
Succinylcholine
Vasodilators (low risk)
Cimetidine (low risk)
Closed-angle glaucoma
Topical anticholinergics
Topical sympathomimetics
Systemic anticholinergics
Heterocyclic antidepressants
Low-potency phenothiazines
Antihistamines
Ipratropium
Benzodiazepines (low risk)
Theophylline (low risk)
Vasodilators (low risk)
Systemic sympathomimetics (low risk)
CNS stimulants (low risk)
Serotonin-selective reuptake inhibitors
Imipramine
Venlafaxine
Topiramate
Tetracyclines (low risk)
Carbonic anhydrase inhibitors (low risk)
Monoamine oxidase inhibitors (low risk)
Topical cholinergics (low risk)

mydriasis (eg, anticholinergics). A wide range of sulfa compounds causes idiosyncratic reactions that result in lens swelling and anterior choroidal effusions with anterior movement of the iris and lens, resulting in angle closure. The topical use of anticholinergics or sympathomimetic agents most likely will result in angle closure. Systemic and inhaled anticholinergic and sympathomimetic agents also must be used with caution in such patients. As discussed previously, potent miotic agents such as echothiophate may produce angle closure by increasing pupillary block. Table 114-3 lists the drugs associated with potentiation of glaucoma.

TREATMENT

Treatment for Glaucoma Suspect and Ocular Hypertension

Treatment of the patients with possible glaucoma (ocular hypertension; ie, patients with IOP >22 mm Hg [2.9 kPa]) is less controversial with the recent results of the Ocular Hypertensive Treatment Study (OHTS) than it was in the past.[10] The OHTS helped to identify risk factors for treatment. Patients with IOPs higher than 25 mm Hg (3.3 kPa), vertical cup-to-disk ratio of more than 0.5, and central corneal thickness of less than 555 μm are at greater risk for developing glaucoma. Risk factors such as family history of glaucoma, Black, Latino/Hispanic ethnicity, severe myopia, and patients with only one eye must also be taken into consideration when deciding which individuals need treatment.

Patients without risk factors typically are not treated and are monitored for the development of glaucomatous changes. The use of risk calculators has been suggested as a means of determining who are at greatest risk in developing glaucoma. It is hoped that with future improvement in such calculators, one would be able to tailor treatment to those at greatest risk for developing glaucoma.

Patients with significant risk factors usually are treated with a well-tolerated topical agent such as a prostaglandin analog or β-blocking agent. Other options include a α_2-agonist (brimonidine), a topical carbonic anhydrase inhibitor (CAI), or netarsudil, depending on individual patient characteristics. Therapy may be initiated in one eye to assess tolerance and efficacy compared to the contralateral eye; however, because each eye may respond differently to a medication as well as possible contralateral effects, IOP response may be compared to baseline in individual eyes.

The goal of therapy is to lower the IOP to a level associated with a decreased risk of optic nerve damage, usually at least a 20%, if not a 25% to 30% decrease from the baseline IOP. Greater decreases may be required in high-risk patients or those with higher initial IOPs. Drug therapy should be monitored by measurement of IOP, examination of the optic disk, assessment of the visual fields, and evaluation of the patient for drug adverse effects and compliance with therapy. Patients who are unresponsive to or intolerant of a drug should be switched to an alternative agent rather than given an additional drug. Partial responders may be treated with combinations of well-tolerated topical medications (prostaglandins, beta-blockers, brimonidine, or a CAI). The use of multiple combinations of topical agents or when first-line agents fail to reduce IOP depends on the risk-to-benefit assessment of each patient. Some clinicians prefer to discontinue all medications for patients who fail to respond adequately to simple topical therapy, closely monitor for the development of disk changes or visual field loss, and treat again when such changes occur. The cost and inconvenience of frequent adverse effects of multiple-combination therapies, pilocarpine, cholinesterase inhibitors, and oral CAIs generally result in an unfavorable risk-to-benefit ratio for glaucoma suspect patients.[3,4,7,32-34,36,37]

Treatment for Open-Angle Glaucoma

All patients with elevated IOP and characteristic optic disk changes and/or visual field defects not caused by other factors (ie, glaucoma by definition) should be treated. Recent findings that one in five patients with "normal" IOP and glaucomatous retinal nerve findings (ie, normal-tension glaucoma) do not have progression of visual field loss if left untreated have prompted recommendations to monitor normal-tension glaucoma patients without immediate threat of loss of central vision and to treat only when progression is documented. Some controversy exists as to whether the initial therapy of glaucoma should be surgical trabeculectomy (filtering procedure), argon or selective laser trabeculectomy, or medical therapy.[7,32-34,36-43] Drug therapy remains the most common initial treatment modality. Drug therapy of patients with documented glaucomatous change with either elevated or normal IOP is initiated in a stepwise manner (Fig. 114-3), starting with a single, well-tolerated topical agent. The goal of therapy is to prevent further visual loss. A "target" IOP is chosen based on a patient baseline IOP and the amount of existing visual field loss. Typically, an initial target IOP reduction of 25% to 30% is desired. Greater reductions may be desired for patients with very high baseline IOPs or advanced visual field loss. Patients with normal baseline IOPs (normal-tension glaucoma) may have target IOPs of less than 10 to 12 mm Hg (1.3-1.6 kPa).[7]

Pharmacotherapeutic Approach

6 Medications most commonly used to treat glaucoma are the prostaglandin analogs, nonselective β-blockers, brimonidine (a α_2-agonist), the topical CAIs, and the fixed combination products of timolol/dorzolamide, timolol/brimonidine, brimonidine/brinzolamide, or timolol/prostaglandins (non-United States). Effective and acceptable safety profiles include latanoprostene bunod and netarsudil.[7,32-34,36,37]

The prostaglandin analogs are often recommended as first-line therapy. They offer once-daily dosing, better IOP reduction, better 24-hour IOP control, good tolerance, and availability of lower-cost

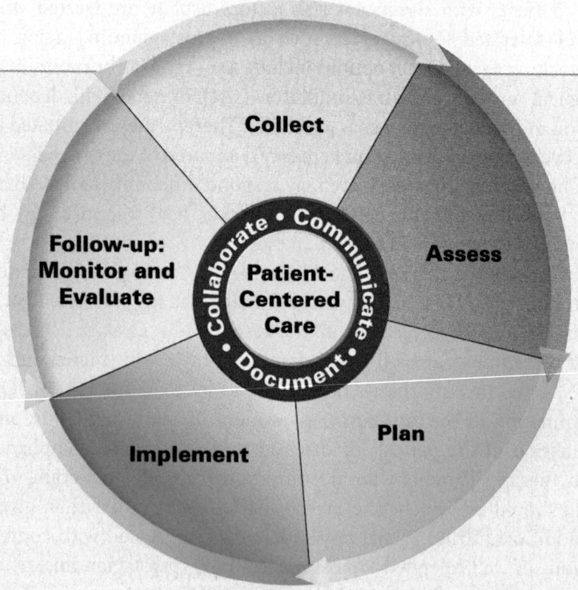

Patient Care Process for the Management of Glaucoma

The image shows the five fundamental steps included in the Pharmacist's Care Process endorsed by the Joint Commission for Pharmacy Practioners (2014). The tagline of this process reads collaborate, communicate, and document. The five fundamental steps listed here are collect, assess, plan, implement, and follow-up: monitor and evaluate. All these steps are listed in a circular block diagram.

Collect

- Patient characteristics (eg, age, race, sex, and pregnant)
- Patient history (past medical, family history of glaucoma, social, and date and results of past eye examinations)
- Changes in vision (see Fig. 114-2)
- Current medications, including nonprescription agents and topically applied products, including eye drops (see Table 114-3 for agents that affect intraocular pressure [IOP])
- Objective data (see the "Clinical Presentation" box)
  - IOP measurements
  - Disc changes and abnormalities—bilateral, symmetrical?
  - Visual field changes and losses

Assess

- If PACG is suspected, manage or refer as ophthalmologic emergency
- Presence of conditions that can produce secondary cases of open-angle glaucoma (eg, exfoliation syndrome, pigmentary glaucoma, systemic diseases, trauma, surgery, ocular inflammatory diseases, and medications [see Table 114-3])
- Current medications that may contribute to or worsen glaucoma (see Table 114-3)
- Past history of adverse effects to agents used in the treatment of glaucoma
- Identify target IOP goal based on past history and current situation

Plan*

- Drug therapy regimen designed to achieve target IOP, including specific agent(s), dose, route, frequency, and duration; specify the continuation and discontinuation of existing therapies (see Fig. 114-3 and Table 114-4)
- Monitor IOP for target reductions (usually at least 20% reduction from baseline IOP, if not a reduction of 25% to 30%, at 4 to 6 weeks after therapy begins, and for adverse effects [eg, local intolerance or reactions, altered iris pigmentation within 2 years of treatment initiation, hypertrichosis, hyperpigmentation of lids or lashes]
- Referrals to other providers when appropriate (eg, ophthalmologist)

Implement*

- Provide patient education regarding all elements of treatment plan
- Provide extensive education about administration of eye drops, separation of doses, and reinforcement of importance of adherence to preservation of vision
- Use motivational interviewing and coaching strategies to maximize adherence
- Schedule follow-up, usually 4 to 6 weeks after therapy starts and every 3 to 4 months once target IOPs are achieved

Follow-up: Monitor and Evaluate

- Measure IOP
- Optic disc and visual fields
- Adverse effects to medications
- Adherence to treatment and drug administration technique

**Collaborate with patient, caregivers, and other healthcare professional.*

generics (see Fig. 114-3). The topical β-blockers have a long history of successful use, providing a combination of clinical efficacy and general tolerability. Brimonidine and topical CAIs are also well tolerated and effective agents, but often considered second-line agents (to prostaglandins and beta blockers).[7] The role of newer agents such as latanoprostene bunod and netarsudil are not established but will likely be used (individually or in combination) in patients not inadequately responding to or intolerant of other agents. Therapy optimally is started as a single agent; it can be started in one eye (except for patients with very high IOP or advanced visual field loss) to evaluate drug efficacy and tolerance, although response may differ between contralateral eyes. Monitoring of therapy should be individualized. Initial check for IOP response to therapy is typically done 4 to 6 weeks after the medication is started. Once IOPs reach acceptable levels, the IOP is monitored every 3 to 4 months or longer if there is prolonged control (over 6-12 months) without progression. More frequent monitoring is necessary if IOP target is not achieved, disease progression is noted, and after any change in drug therapy.[7]

Visual fields and disk changes are typically monitored every 6 to 12 months or earlier if the glaucoma is unstable or there is suspicion of disease worsening. Patients should always be questioned regarding adherence to and tolerance of prescribed therapy. Initial IOP response does not predict long-term IOP control, as tachyphylaxis to IOP reduction and or disease progression may occur.

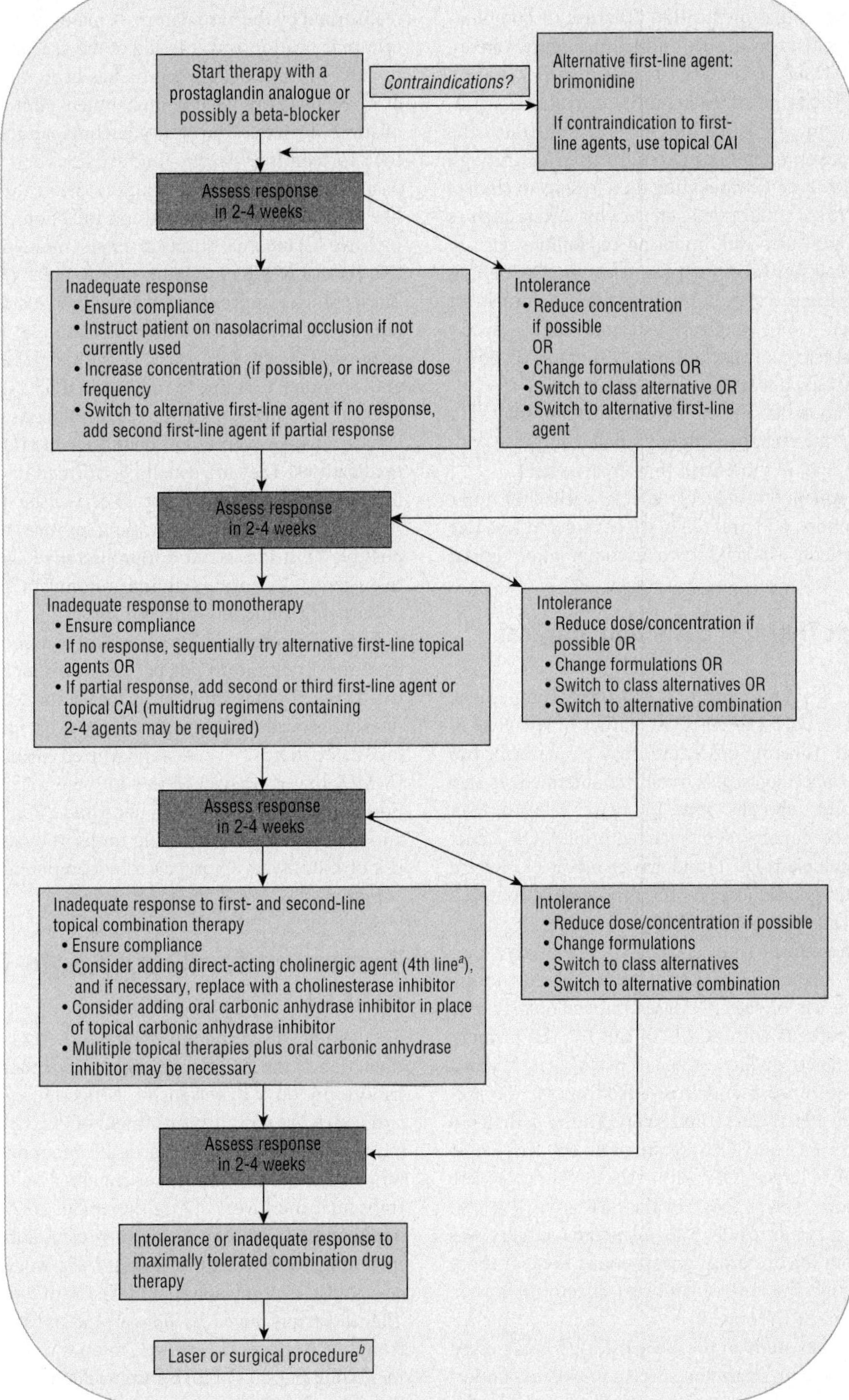

FIGURE 114-3 Algorithm for the pharmacotherapy of open-angle glaucoma. [a]Fourth-line agents are not commonly used any longer or are commercially unavailable. [b]Most clinicians believe the laser procedure should be performed earlier (eg, after three-drug maximum, poorly adherent patient). (CAI, carbonic anhydrase inhibitor.)

The value of an agent with which the patient has shown a drop in IOP following an initial response can be measured by discontinuing the medication completely and determining if an increase in IOP occurs. Patients responding to but intolerant of initial therapy may be switched to another drug. For patients failing to respond to an initial drug, a switch to an alternative agent should be considered. If only a partial response occurs, addition of another topical drug to be used in combination is a possibility. A number of drugs or drug combinations may need to be tried before an effective and well-tolerated regimen is identified. Prostaglandin agonists, beta blockers, brimonidine, CAI, and pilocarpine may be used in various combinations. Generally adding a second drug results in a less than additive reduction in IOP. Using more than one drop per dose does not improve response, and it increases the likelihood of adverse effects and the cost of therapy. When using more than one medication, separation of drop instillation of each agent by at least 5 minutes is suggested to provide optimal ocular absorption. Combination products reduce the number of daily doses, possibly improving adherence and preventing washout effect seen when a second medication is administered too soon after the initial medication. The use of combination products also reduces exposure to ophthalmic preservatives. Ocular surface disease (OSD) secondary to glaucoma therapy will often manifest as superficial punctate keratitis, tear-film instability, or allergy.[44] In-vivo and animal studies have demonstrated the toxic effects of preservatives, often benzalkonium chloride through various mechanisms. However, extrapolating these results to clinical use is difficult because these studies must control for effects such as blinking, tear dilution and turn over, buffering capabilities, etc., of the human eye. While many crossover clinical trials show benefit to preservative-free therapies, there are a multitude that demonstrate no improvement. Patients with medication-related OSD may try treatment with artificial tears, anti-inflammatory therapy, or possibly preservative-free therapy if feasible.

The IOP response to ocular hypotensive medication may vary with corneal thickness. The response might be better in those with normal or thin corneas than in those with thicker structures.

Because of the frequency of adverse effects, carbachol, topical cholinesterase inhibitors, and oral CAIs are considered last-line agents to be used for patients who fail less-toxic combination topical therapy.

Nonpharmacologic Therapy: Laser and Surgical Procedures

When drug therapy fails, is not tolerated, or is excessively complicated, surgical procedures such as laser trabeculoplasty (argon or selective) or a surgical trabeculectomy (filtering procedure) may be performed to improve outflow. Laser trabeculoplasty is usually an intermediate step between drug therapy and trabeculectomy. The newer selective laser trabeculoplasty (SLT) procedure has demonstrated similar IOP reduction as argon laser trabeculoplasty (ALT) and may be repeatable. Recent studies have demonstrated good efficacy for this procedure in comparison with medical treatment options for POAG.

A multicenter randomized clinical trial (LiGHT Study) conducted at six hospitals in the United Kingdom compared the use of eye drops versus the use of selective laser trabeculoplasty as a first-line treatment in patients with POAG or OHT.[45] The primary outcome was health-related quality of life (HRQoL) at 3 years. Secondary outcomes were cost and cost-effectiveness, disease-specific HRQoL, clinical effectiveness, and safety. Of the patients in the SLT group, 74.2% (95% CI 69.3-78.6) required no eye drops at 36 months to maintain IOP at target. IOPs within the target range were achieved in slightly more eyes of those in the SLT group (93.0%) than among those using eye drops (91.3%). Glaucoma surgery was needed for 11 patients in the eye drops group versus none of those who received SLT initially. The HRQoL and cost-effectiveness were also more favorable in the SLT group.[45,46]

A real-world outcomes study in the United Kingdom assessed baseline factors associated with treatment success in patients undergoing their first recorded SLT. The main outcome measures were change from baseline in IOPs and glaucoma medication use with failure defined as any further glaucoma procedure post-SLT or IOP of greater than 21 mm Hg (2.8 kPa), IOP reduction of less than 20%, or an increase in glaucoma medications from baseline. The majority failed SLT within 1 year, and efficacy was better in patients with higher baseline IOP but did not differ by glaucoma severity or concurrent use of IOP-lowering medication.[46] As these studies show, many factors must be considered for patients with glaucoma when choosing a laser treatment option.

Procedures with higher complication rates, such as those involving placement of draining tubes or destruction of the ciliary body (cyclodestruction), may be required when other methods fail (see Figs. 114-1 and 114-2).[7]

Surgical methods for reduction of IOP involve the creation of a channel through which aqueous humor can flow from the anterior chamber to the subconjunctival space (filtering bleb), where it is reabsorbed by the vasculature. A major reason for failure of the procedure is healing and scarring of the site. The use of aqueous shunts or valves to manage glaucoma has been increasing, and the results of a recent study have demonstrated improved safety and efficacy of these devices. However, glaucoma surgery is still plagued with the shortcomings despite modifications and improvements over the past century, including potentially vision-threatening complications like hypotony, wound leaks, and infections.[40,41,47] MIGS (Minimally Invasive Glaucoma Surgery) offers micro incisions and implants that reduce IOP by targeting various areas of the outflow pathway.[47] These can be approached from either inside the eye (ab-interno) (eg, iStent, Hydrus, Trabectome, XEN 45, suprachoroidal shunts) or outside the eye (ab-externo) (eg, canaloplasty, Gold micro shunt, and Stegman Canal Expander).[47] MIGS can be considered as an alternative to medical therapy in an effort to address adherence challenges, adverse events, and quality-of-life (QOL) issues with topical medications. They are usually performed in combination with cataract surgery (eg, iStent, Hydrus) or as a solo procedure (XEN 45).

Modification of the healing process to maintain patency is possible with the use of antiproliferative agents. The antiproliferative agents, 5-fluorouracil and mitomycin C, are used for patients undergoing glaucoma-filtering surgery to improve success rates by reducing fibroblast proliferation and consequent scarring. Although used most commonly for patients with increased risk for suboptimal surgical outcome (after cataract surgery and a previous failed filtering procedure), the use of these agents also improves success in low-risk patients.[40,41,47] A standardized formulation of mitomycin C (MMC) that is prepacked in a kit with a fixed dose and concentration was approved by the US Food and Drug Administration in 2012 and is commercially available under the name "Mitosol." Off-label use of mitomycin C prepared by compounding pharmacies is also common.

Treatment for Acute Angle-Closure Crisis (AACC)

The goal of initial therapy for acute AACC with high IOP is rapid reduction of the IOP to preserve vision and to avoid surgical or laser iridectomy on a hypertensive, congested eye. Iridectomy (laser or surgical) is the definitive treatment of PACG; it produces a hole in the iris that permits aqueous humor flow to move directly from the posterior chamber to the anterior chamber, opening up the block at the trabecular meshwork. Drug therapy of an AACC typically involves administration of one or more topical antiglaucoma medications including miotics (eg, pilocarpine), secretory inhibitors (β-blockers, α_2-agonist, or topical/systemic CAIs), or a prostaglandin agonist.[6,30] The miosis produced by pilocarpine pulls the peripheral iris away from the meshwork. However, miotics may worsen angle closure by increasing pupillary block and producing anterior movement of the lens because of drug-induced accommodation. The aqueous secretory inhibitors and pilocarpine may not be effective due to ischemia of the ciliary body and pupillary sphincter, respectively. Now, the urge to use excessive amounts of topical agents must be resisted. A hyperosmotic agent such as mannitol or glycerin may be needed to temporarily reduce IOP and restore response to the topical agents.

An osmotic agent also is commonly administered because these drugs produce the most rapid decrease in IOP. Oral glycerin 1 to 2 g/kg can be used if an oral agent is tolerated; if not, IV mannitol 1 to 2 g/kg should be used. Osmotic agents reduce IOP by withdrawing water from the eye secondary to the osmotic gradient between the blood and the eye. These drugs are among the first-line agents in the short-term treatment of an AACC or other forms of acute very high IOP elevations. Topical corticosteroids often are used to reduce the ocular inflammation and reduce the development of synechiae in PACG eyes. Patients failing therapy altogether will require an emergency iridectomy. Once the IOP is controlled, iridectomy is performed on the affected eye as well as the contralateral eye (if narrow angles are present). As reported in the EAGLE study, for patients who are older than 50 years and with other specific inclusion criteria, an alternative approach involves crystalline lens extraction since it plays a role in PACG pathology.[48]

Laser peripheral iridotomy can prevent acute angle closure glaucoma in patients at risk. However, its role on preventing the conversion of an angle-closure suspect to PACG is modest.[31,49] Long-term drug therapy is not used unless IOP remains high because of the presence of synechiae blocking the trabecular meshwork or concurrent POAG. In such cases, the pharmacotherapeutic approach is essentially identical to that for the POAG patient, or laser or surgical procedures are performed.[30]

PHARMACOLOGIC AGENTS USED IN GLAUCOMA

Prostaglandin Analogs

The prostaglandin analogs, including latanoprost, travoprost, bimatoprost, and tafluprost, reduce IOP by increasing the uveoscleral and, to a lesser extent, trabecular outflow of aqueous humor. Some differences in receptor sites and mechanisms of action may exist between the two prostaglandins (latanoprost, travoprost, and tafluprost) and the prostamide (bimatoprost). However, both classes appear to produce collagen changes in the matrix of the ciliary body and trabecular meshwork. Bimatoprost may be slightly more effective in lowering IOP, getting a larger percentage of patients to lower IOPs, and for patients unresponsive to latanoprost. If the patient does not respond to one prostaglandin agonist, a switch to another may be beneficial.[39,42,50] Generic forms of some prostaglandin analogs are now available, reducing the cost to patients for these agents. Tafluprost is available as a preservative-free solution, which may be useful in patients intolerant of common ophthalmic preservatives or those with corneal surface disorders.

Reduction in IOP with once-daily doses of prostaglandin analogs (a 25%-35% reduction) is often greater than that seen with timolol 0.5% twice daily. In addition, nocturnal control of IOP is improved compared with timolol.[7,42,50] The drugs are administered at nighttime, although they are probably as effective if given in the morning.

Prostaglandin analogs are well tolerated and produce fewer systemic adverse effects than timolol. Local ocular tolerance generally is good, but ocular reactions such as punctate corneal erosions and conjunctival hyperemia do occur. Local intolerance occurs in 10% to 25% of patients with these agents.[7,33,36,37,51]

With prostaglandin analogs, altered iris pigmentation occurs in 15% to 30% of patients, particularly those with mixed-color irises (blue-brown, green-brown, blue-gray-brown, or yellow-brown eyes), which become browner in color over 3 to 12 months. The change in iris pigmentation will often appear within 2 years, and long-term consequences of this pigment change appear to be mostly cosmetic but irreversible upon discontinuation. Hypertrichosis is common and reverses upon discontinuation of the drug. Hyperpigmentation around the lids and lashes has also been reported and appears to reverse upon discontinuation. Loss of periorbital fat has been reported, which may lead to apparent enophthalmos and sunken eye, especially when used unilaterally.

Topical prostaglandin analogs may produce rates of corneal thinning that are slightly higher than ongoing age-related changes. This effect is unlikely to be clinically relevant.[24,33,36,37,51,52]

These agents have occasionally been associated with uveitis, and caution is recommended for patients with ocular inflammatory conditions. Cases of cystoid macular edema and worsening of herpetic keratitis have been reported.

Prostaglandin analogs can be used in combination with other antiglaucoma agents for additional IOP control because of their unique mechanism of action. Given their excellent efficacy and side-effect profile, prostaglandin analogs provide effective monotherapy or adjunctive therapy for patients who are not responding to or tolerating other agents. Long-term studies demonstrate that these agents are safe, efficacious, and well tolerated in glaucoma therapy.[24,33,36,37,51,52] Various fixed combination prostaglandin products, often with timolol, are available in Canada and overseas.

Latanoprostene bunod is a newer agent approved for use in patients with OAG and OHT.[50,51,53] This agent is a prodrug of latanoprost and is also metabolized to a nitric-oxide–donating moiety, thus providing dual mechanisms for increasing aqueous outflow. This agent produces IOP reduction similar to or greater than that with timolol. Adverse effects are similar to that seen with pure prostaglandin analogs.

The first intraocular biodegradable, implant of bimatoprost (Durysta), is another newer product indicated for patients with OAG and OHT. It is administered intracamerally (into the anterior chamber of the affected eye). The bimatoprost implant has potential to improve adherence and reduce treatment burden in glaucoma. In a randomized, 20-month, evaluator-masked, phase 3 clinical study, efficacy (IOP lowering) and safety of bimatoprost 10- and 15-mcg implants were evaluated. Bimatoprost implants 10 mcg (n = 198) or 15 mcg (n = 198) on day 1 were noninferior to timolol in IOP lowering after administration at baseline and weeks 16 and 32 of the trial. Corneal and inflammatory treatment-emergent adverse events of interest (eg, corneal endothelial cell loss, iritis) were higher with bimatoprost implants than timolol and highest with the 15-μg dose implants. One year after the third administration of bimatoprost implants, IOP was controlled in most study participants. The risk-benefit assessment favored the commercial approval for the 10-mcg implant, and the US Food and Drug Administration approved that dose for a single administration in each eye for the life of the patient. Ongoing studies are evaluating other administration regimens.[26,47] The bimatoprost implant has potential for improving adherence and reducing treatment burden in glaucoma.

β-Blocking Drugs

The topical β-blocking agents are one of the most commonly used antiglaucoma medications (Table 114-4). β-Blockers lower IOP by 20% to 30% with a minimum of local ocular adverse effects. Beta blockers have minimal effects on nocturnal IOP. These are commonly one of the agents of first choice—along with prostaglandin analogs—in treating POAG if no contraindications exist.[7,33,36,37,51]

The β-blocking agents produce ocular hypotensive effects by decreasing the production of aqueous humor by the ciliary body without producing substantial effects on aqueous humor outflow facility. The mechanism by which β-blockers decrease aqueous humor inflow remains controversial, but it is most frequently attributed to β_2-adrenergic receptor blockade in the ciliary body.

Five ophthalmic β-blockers are presently available: timolol, levobunolol, metipranolol, carteolol, and betaxolol. Timolol, levobunolol, and metipranolol are nonspecific β-blocking agents, whereas betaxolol is a relatively β_1-selective agent. Carteolol is a nonspecific blocker with intrinsic sympathomimetic activity. Despite differences in potency, selectivity, lipophilicity, and intrinsic sympathomimetic activity, the five agents reduce IOP to a similar degree, although betaxolol has been reported to produce somewhat less lowering of IOP than timolol and levobunolol. Levobunolol, which possesses alpha-adrenergic effects, may be more effective than timolol and betaxolol in reducing postcataract surgery IOP increases and may be more effective in controlling IOP than other agents when given as aqueous solutions on a once-daily schedule (up to 70% of patients). Timolol in the form of a gel-forming solution (Timoptic-XE) provides equivalent IOP control with once-daily administration when

TABLE 114-4 Topical Drugs Used in the Treatment of Open-Angle Glaucoma

Drug	Pharmacologic Properties	Common Brand Names/Generic	Dosage Form	Strength (%)	Usual Dose[a]	Mechanism of Action
β-Adrenergic blocking agents						
Betaxolol	Relative β_1 selective	Generic	Solution	0.5	One drop twice a day	All reduce aqueous production of ciliary body
		Betoptic-S	Suspension	0.25	One drop twice a day	
Carteolol	Nonselective, intrinsic sympathomimetic activity	Generic	Solution	1	One drop twice a day	
Levobunolol	Nonselective	Betagan/Generic	Solution	0.25, 0.5	One drop twice a day	
Metipranolol	Nonselective	OptiPranolol	Solution	0.3	One drop twice a day	
Timolol	Nonselective	Timoptic, Betimol, Istalol/Generic	Solution	0.25, 0.5	One drop every day—one to two times a day	
		Timoptic-XE/ Generic	Gelling solution	0.25, 0.5	One drop every day[a]	
Adrenergic agonists						
α_2-Adrenergic agonists						
Apraclonidine	Specific α_2-agonists	Iopidine	Solution	0.5, 1	One drop two to three times a day	Both reduce aqueous humor production; brimonidine known to also increase uveoscleral outflow; only brimonidine has primary indication
Brimonidine		Alphagan P 0.1/ Generic 0.2, 0.15	Solution	0.2, 0.15, 0.1	One drop two to three times a day	
Cholinergic agonists direct acting						
Carbachol	Direct and indirect acting	Carboptic, Isopto Carbachol	Solution	1.5, 3	One drop two to three times a day[a]	All increase aqueous humor outflow through trabecular meshwork
Pilocarpine	Direct acting	Isopto Carpine, Pilocar/Generic	Solution	1, 2, 4	One drop two to three times a day[a]	
					One drop four times a day	
Cholinesterase inhibitors						
Echothiophate	Indirect acting cholinesterase inhibitor	Phospholine Iodide	Solution	0.125	Once or twice a day	
Carbonic anhydrase inhibitors						
Topical						
Brinzolamide	Carbonic anhydrase type II inhibition	Azopt	Suspension	1	Two to three times a day	All reduce aqueous humor production of ciliary body
Dorzolamide		Trusopt/Generic	Solution	2	Two to three times a day	
Systemic						
Acetazolamide		Generic	Tablet	125 mg, 250 mg	125-250 mg two to four times a day	
		Injection	500 mg/vial	250-500 mg		
		Diamox Sequels	Capsule	500 mg	500 mg twice a day	
Methazolamide		Generic	Tablet	25 mg, 50 mg	25-50 mg two to three times a day	
Prostaglandin analogs						
Latanoprost	Prostanoid agonist	Xalatan/Generic	Solution	0.005	One drop every night	Increases aqueous uveoscleral outflow and to a lesser extent trabecular outflow

(continued)

TABLE 114-4 Topical Drugs Used in the Treatment of Open-Angle Glaucoma (*Continued*)

Drug	Pharmacologic Properties	Common Brand Names/Generic	Dosage Form	Strength (%)	Usual Dose[a]	Mechanism of Action
Latanoprostene Bunod	Prostanoid agonist	Vyzulta	Solution	0.024	One drop every night	
Bimatoprost	Prostamide agonist	Lumigan 0.01/ Generic 0.03	Solution	0.01, 0.03	One drop every night	
		Durysta 10 mcg	Intracameral biodegradable implant	One implant per eye for the life of the patient		
Travoprost	Prostanoid agonist	Travatan Z/ GenericTravoprost	Solution	0.004	One drop every night	
Tafluprost	Prostanoid agonist	Zioptan/Saflutan	Preservative free solution	0.0015	One drop every night	
Rho Kinase Inhibitors						
Netarsudil	Rho Kinase Inhibitor	Rhopressa	Solution	0.02	One drop every night	
Combinations						
Timolol–dorzolamide		Cosopt Generic	Solution	Timolol 0.5/ Dorzolamide 2	One drop twice daily	
Timolol–brimonidine		Combigan	Solution	Timolol 0.5/ Brimonidine 0.2	One drop twice daily	
Brinzolamide–brimonidine		Simbrinza	Suspension	Brinzolamide 1/ Brimonidine 0.2	One drop three times daily	
Netarsudil-latanoprost		Rocklatan	Solution	Netarsudil 0.02/ Latanoprost 0.005	One drop every night	

[a]Use of nasolacrimal occlusion will increase the number of patients. Successfully treated with longer dosage intervals.

compared with the same concentration of the aqueous solution administered twice daily. The choice of a specific β-blocking agent generally is based on differences in adverse effect potential, individual patient response, and cost. Treatment with topical β-blockers may result in tachyphylaxis (short-term escape and long-term drift) in 20% to 25% of patients. The mean IOP reduction from baseline may be smaller for patients receiving topical β-blockers with concurrent systemic β-blockers.[33,36,37]

Local adverse effects with β-blockers usually are tolerable, although stinging on application occurs commonly, particularly with betaxolol solution (less with betaxolol suspension) and metipranolol. Other local effects include dry eyes, corneal anesthesia, blepharitis, blurred vision, and, rarely, conjunctivitis, uveitis, and keratitis. Some local reactions may be a result of preservatives used in the commercially available products. Switching from one agent to another or switching the type of formulation may improve tolerance in patients experiencing local adverse effects.

Systemic effects are the most important adverse effects of β-blockers. Drug absorbed systematically may produce decreased heart rate, reduced blood pressure, negative inotropic effects, conduction defects, bronchospasm, CNS effects, and alteration of serum lipids and may block the symptoms of hypoglycemia. The β_1-specific agents' betaxolol and possibly carteolol (as a consequence of intrinsic sympathomimetic activity) are less likely to produce the systemic adverse effects caused by β-adrenergic blockade, such as the cardiac effects and bronchospasm, but a real risk still exists. The use of timolol as a gel-forming liquid or betaxolol as a suspension allows for administration of fewer drugs per day and, therefore, reduces the chance for systemic adverse effects compared with the aqueous solutions.

Because of their systemic adverse effects, all ophthalmic β-blockers should be used with caution for patients with pulmonary diseases, sinus bradycardia, second- or third-degree heart block, congestive heart failure, atherosclerosis, diabetes, and myasthenia gravis, as well as for patients receiving oral β-blocker therapy. The use of the nasolacrimal occlusion (ELC; see Patient Education below for description) technique during administration reduces the risk or severity of systemic adverse effects, as well as optimizes response. Overall, β-adrenergic blocking agents are well tolerated by most patients, and most potential problems can be avoided by appropriate patient evaluation, drug choice, and monitoring of drug therapy. For patients failing or having an inadequate response to single-drug therapy with a β-blocking agent, the addition of a topical CAI, prostaglandin analog, or the α_2-adrenergic receptor agonist brimonidine usually will result in additional IOP reduction.[7,33,36,37,51]

α_2-Adrenergic Agonists

Brimonidine and the less lipid-soluble and less receptor-selective apraclonidine are α_2-adrenergic agonists structurally similar to clonidine. Apraclonidine is indicated and brimonidine is effective for prevention or control of postoperative or postlaser treatment increases in IOP. Brimonidine has a primary indication in open-angle glaucoma and is considered a second-line agent (often after a prostaglandin or beta blocker) or adjunctive agent. Apraclonidine is generally used only in short term after ocular surgery due to high incidence of loss of control of IOP (tachyphylaxis) and a more severe and prevalent ocular allergy rate.

Alpha-2 agonists reduce IOP by decreasing the rate of aqueous humor production (some increase in uveoscleral outflow also occurs with brimonidine). The drugs reduce IOP by 18% to 27% at peak (2-5 hours) and by 10% at 8 to 12 hours. Comparative trials demonstrate a reduction in IOP similar to that obtained with 0.5% timolol. The use of brimonidine 0.2% every 8 to 12 hours provides maximum IOP-lowering effects in long-term use. The use of ELC (see Patient Education below) may improve response and allow the longer dosing frequency (ie, every 12 hours). These agents have minimal effects on nocturnal IOP. Combinations of α_2-agonists with β-blockers, prostaglandin analogs, or CAIs produce additional IOP reduction.

An allergic-type reaction characterized by lid edema, eye discomfort, foreign-object sensation, itching, and hyperemia occurs in approximately 30% of patients with apraclonidine. Brimonidine produces this adverse effect in up to 8% of patients. This reaction commonly necessitates drug discontinuation. Systemic adverse effects with brimonidine include dizziness, fatigue, somnolence, dry mouth, and possibly a slight reduction in blood pressure and pulse. α_2-Agonists should be used with caution for patients with cardiovascular diseases, renal compromise, cerebrovascular disease, and diabetes, as well as in those taking antihypertensives and other cardiovascular drugs, monoamine oxidase inhibitors, and tricyclic antidepressants.

Brimonidine is also contraindicated in infants because of apneic spells and hypotensive reactions. In terms of overall efficacy and tolerability, brimonidine approximates that achieved with β-blockers.[7,33,36,37,51]

Brimonidine Purite 0.15% or 0.1% is a formulation of brimonidine in a lower concentration than the original product that contains a less corneal-toxic preservative than the commonly employed benzalkonium chloride. The newer formulations are as effective as the original because the more neutral pH of brimonidine Purite (0.15% pH 7.2; 0.1% pH 7.7) allows for higher concentrations of brimonidine in the aqueous humor with a similar reduction in IOP and a reduced incidence of ocular allergy.

A randomized clinical trial of topical brimonidine 0.2% twice daily preserved visual field better than treatment with topical timolol maleate 0.5% in patients with OAG and statistically normal IOP.[23] The IOP-lowering efficacy was similar between the two medications, suggesting that this finding was consistent with a non-IOP-related mechanism, possibly a neuroprotective action. However, validation of a neuroprotective role for brimonidine requires further research to confirm these results.[23,54] The combination product timolol 0.5% and brimonidine 0.2% (Combigan) may provide additional IOP lowering than either agent alone.

Carbonic Anhydrase Inhibitors

Topical Agents

CAIs reduce IOP by decreasing ciliary body aqueous humor secretion. CAIs appear to inhibit aqueous production by blocking active secretion of sodium and bicarbonate ions from the ciliary body to the aqueous humor.[7,33,51] The topical CAIs dorzolamide and brinzolamide are well tolerated and are considered second line (after prostaglandins and beta blockers) for monotherapy or adjunctive therapy of POAG and ocular hypertension. These drugs reduce IOP by 15% to 26%.

Topical CAIs generally are well tolerated. Local adverse effects include transient burning and stinging, ocular discomfort and transient blurred vision, tearing, and, rarely, conjunctivitis, lid reactions, and photophobia. A superficial punctate keratitis occurs in 10% to 15% of patients. Brinzolamide produces more blurry vision but is less stinging than dorzolamide. Systemic adverse effects are unusual despite the accumulation of drug in red blood cells. Because of their favorable adverse-effect profile, topical CAIs provide a useful alternative agent for monotherapy or adjunctive therapy for patients with inadequate response to or who are unable to use other agents. The drugs may add additional IOP reduction for patients using other single or multiple topical agents. The usual dose of a topical CAI is one drop every 8 to 12 hours. Administration every 12 hours produces somewhat less IOP reduction than administration every 8 hours. The use of ELC should optimize response to CAI given at any interval.[7,33] The combination product timolol 0.5% and dorzolamide 2% (Cosopt) is dosed twice daily and produces equivalent IOP lowering to each product dosed separately. Both dorzolamide and timolol/dorzolamide (Cosopt) are now available as generic formulations. The combination product brimonidine 0.2% and brinzolamide 1% (Simbrinza) is available dosed three times daily.

Systemic CAI Agents

Systemic CAIs are indicated for patients failing to respond to or tolerate maximum topical therapy. Systemic and topical CAIs should not be used in combination because no data exist concerning improved IOP reduction, and the risk for systemic adverse effects is increased. Oral CAIs reduce aqueous humor inflow by 40% to 60% and IOP by 25% to 40%. The available systemic CAIs (see Table 114-4) produce equivalent IOP reduction but differ for potency, adverse effects, dosage forms, and duration of action. Despite their excellent effects on elevated IOP of any etiology, the systemic CAIs frequently produce intolerable adverse effects. As a result, CAIs are considered third-line agents in the treatment of POAG and often used for short-term administration to lower IOP.

On average, only 30% to 60% of patients are able to tolerate oral CAI therapy for prolonged periods. Intolerance to CAI therapy results most commonly from a symptom complex attributable to systemic acidosis and including malaise, fatigue, anorexia, nausea, weight loss, altered taste, depression, and decreased libido. Other adverse effects include renal calculi, increased uric acid, blood dyscrasias, diuresis, and myopia. Elderly patients do not tolerate CAIs as well as younger patients. The available CAIs produce the same spectrum of adverse effects; however, the drugs differ in the frequency and severity of the adverse effects listed.

CAIs should be used with some caution in patients with sulfa allergies (all CAIs, topical or systemic, contain sulfonamide moieties, although cross-sensitivity is thought to be very low), sickle cell disease, respiratory acidosis, pulmonary disorders, renal calculi, electrolyte imbalance, hepatic disease, renal disease, diabetes mellitus, or Addison's disease. Concurrent use of a CAI and a diuretic may rapidly produce hypokalemia. High-dose salicylate therapy may increase the acidosis produced by CAIs, whereas the acidosis produced by CAIs may increase the toxicity of salicylates.[7,33,36,37,51]

Rho Kinase Inhibitors

Netarsudil is the first approved agent in a new class of antiglaucoma medications, Rho kinase inhibitors.[51,53] Netarsudil reduces IOP by increasing trabecular meshwork outflow. Once-daily (in the evening) administration of a 0.02% solution reduces both daytime and nighttime IOP. Efficacy appears to be similar to that of beta blockers. Netarsudil may be used in combination with other antiglaucoma agents. The most common local side effects are conjunctival hyperemia, conjunctival hemorrhage, and corneal verticillate. Systemic effects are rare. Patients with OAG or OHT who are taking as many as four ocular hypotensive medications showed modest IOP reduction when netarsudil was added to their regimen.[13]

A combination of netarsudil/latanoprost ophthalmic solution 0.02%/0.005% (Rocklatan) was approved in the United States. Rocklatan provided superior IOP reduction compared to either netarsudil or latanoprost products alone. However, discontinuation rates at 12 months occurred in 20.6%, 23.0%, and 1.7% of patients receiving netarsudil/latanoprost, netarsudil, and latanoprost, respectively.[28]

Parasympathomimetic Agents

The parasympathomimetic (cholinergic) agents reduce IOP by increasing aqueous humor trabecular outflow. The increase in outflow is a thought to be a result of physically pulling open the trabecular meshwork secondary to ciliary muscle contraction, thereby reducing resistance to outflow. These agents may actually reduce uveoscleral outflow. Their use as primary or even adjunctive agents in the treatment of glaucoma has decreased significantly because of local ocular adverse effects and/or frequent dosing requirements.

Pilocarpine, the parasympathomimetic agent of choice in POAG, is available as an ophthalmic solution (see Table 114-4). Pilocarpine produces similar (20%-30%) reductions in IOP as those seen with β-blocking agents. Pilocarpine in POAG is initiated as 1% solution, one drop three to four times daily. The use of ELC improves response and reduces the need for an every 6-hour dosing frequency. The use of one drop of 2% pilocarpine every 6 to 12 hours and ELC provides optimal response in many patients. Both drug concentration and frequency may be increased if IOP reduction is inadequate. Patients with darkly pigmented eyes frequently require higher concentrations of pilocarpine than do patients with lightly pigmented eyes. Concentrations of pilocarpine above 4% rarely improve IOP control in patients.

Ocular adverse effects of pilocarpine include miosis, which decreases night vision and vision in patients with central cataracts. Visual field constriction may be seen secondary to miosis and should be considered when evaluating visual field changes in a glaucoma patient. Pilocarpine ciliary muscle contraction produces accommodative spasm, particularly in young patients still able to accommodate (prepresbyopic). Pilocarpine may also produce frontal headache, brow ache, periorbital pain, eyelid twitching, and conjunctival irritation or injection early in therapy, which tends to decrease in severity over 3 to 5 weeks of continued therapy.

Cholinergics produce a breakdown of the blood–aqueous humor barrier and may result in a worsening of an ocular inflammatory reaction or condition. Systemic cholinergic adverse effects of pilocarpine such as diaphoresis, nausea, vomiting, diarrhea, cramping, urinary frequency, bronchospasm, and heart block can be seen. Other adverse effects associated with direct-acting miotics include retinal tears or detachment, allergic reaction, permanent miosis, cataracts, precipitation of CAG, and, rarely, miotic cysts of the pupillary margin.

Carbachol is a potent direct-acting miotic agent; its duration of action is longer than that of pilocarpine (8-10 hours) because of resistance to hydrolysis by cholinesterases. This drug also may act as a weak inhibitor of cholinesterase. Patients with an inadequate response to or intolerance of pilocarpine as a result of ocular irritation or allergy frequently do well on carbachol. The ocular and systemic adverse effects of carbachol are similar to but more frequent, constant, and severe than those of pilocarpine.[33] Clinical use of carbachol is limited.

Echothiophate is a cholinesterase inhibitor and is used in the treatment of POAG. It is a long-acting, relatively irreversible agent (limited commercial availability; see Table 114-4). This agent is a potent inhibitor of pseudocholinesterase, but also inhibits true cholinesterase. Because of the serious ocular and systemic toxic effects of echothiophate, it is reserved primarily for patients who are either not responding to or are intolerant of other therapy. Because of its cataractogenic properties, most ophthalmologists use this agent only for patients without lenses (aphakia) and for patients with artificial lenses (pseudophakia). The ocular and periocular parasympathomimetic adverse effects are more common and more severe than with pilocarpine or carbachol.

In addition to the parasympathomimetic effects, echothiophate may produce severe fibrinous iritis (particularly with the irreversible inhibitors), synechiae, iris cysts, conjunctival thickening, occlusion of the nasolacrimal ducts, and cataracts. The inhibition of systemic pseudocholinesterase by echothiophate decreases the rate of succinylcholine hydrolysis, resulting in prolonged muscle paralysis. Echothiophate should be discontinued at least 2 weeks before procedures in which succinylcholine is used.

The role of echothiophate in glaucoma is limited by its frequency and potential toxicity. For phakic patients, cholinesterase inhibitors should be administered only if intolerance or failure results with other antiglaucoma medications. Echothiophate provides additional IOP-lowering effects when used with β-blockers, CAIs, and sympathomimetic (adrenergic) agents. Only one concentration of this agent (0.125%) is currently available. A once-daily administration frequency should be used for most patients unless very high IOP is present.

The use of ELC likely improves response, reduces systemic adverse effects, and should be performed by all patients administering echothiophate. The drug should be used with caution for patients with asthma, retinal detachments, narrow angles, bradycardia, hypotension, heart failure, Down's syndrome, epilepsy, Parkinsonism, peptic ulcer, and ocular inflammation, as well as in those receiving cholinesterase inhibitor therapy for myasthenia gravis or exposure to carbamate or organophosphate insecticides and pesticides.

Future Drug Therapies

It is hoped that new agents, improved formulations, and novel approaches to the reduction of IOP and other methods of prevention of glaucomatous visual field loss will provide more effective and better-tolerated therapies. Most areas of glaucoma development continue to focus on drugs that reduce IOP by either reducing aqueous production or increasing outflow. The efficacy and safety of omidenepag isopropyl (OMDI) 0.002%, a selective, nonprostaglandin, prostanoid EP2 receptor agonist, were evaluated in comparison with latanoprost 0.005% in participants with POAG or OHT. OMDI 0.002% was noninferior to latanoprost 0.005% in reducing IOP and was well tolerated.[7]

Classes of drugs in development include adenosine-1 receptor agonists, cannabinoids, serotonin agonists, dopamine agonists, nitric oxide/carbon dioxide modulators, and hydroxysteroid dehydrogenase inhibitors. Agents that are neuroprotective and act through mechanisms other than IOP reduction are also in development and are likely to be part of glaucoma therapy in the future.[24,52-54]

Development of new long-acting topical formulations (such as nanoparticulates), implants, ocular inserts, and drug-eluting punctal plugs may provide improved patient convenience and medication adherence in the future.[28]

EVALUATION OF THERAPEUTIC OUTCOMES

The ultimate goal of drug therapy for the patient with glaucoma is to preserve visual function through reduction of IOP to a level at which no further optic nerve damage occurs. Because of the poor relationship between IOP and optic nerve damage, no specific target IOP exists. Indeed, drugs used to treat glaucoma may act in part to halt visual field loss through mechanisms separate from or in addition to IOP reduction, such as improvements in retinal or choroidal blood flow. Often a 25% to 30% reduction is desired, but greater reductions (40%-50%) may be desired for patients with initially high IOPs. For patients with glaucoma, an IOP of less than 21 mm Hg (2.8 kPa) generally is desired, with progressively lower target pressures needed for greater levels of glaucomatous damage. Even lower IOPs (possibly even below 10 mm Hg [1.3 kPa]) are required for patients with very advanced disease, those showing continued damage at higher IOPs, and those with normal-tension glaucoma and pretreatment pressures in the low-to-middle teens. The IOP considered acceptable for a patient is often a balance of desired IOP and acceptable treatment-related toxicity and of patient quality of life.

PATIENT EDUCATION

7 An important consideration for patients failing to respond to drug therapy is adherence. Poor adherence or nonadherence occurs in 25% to 60% of glaucoma patients.

A large percentage of patients also fail to use topical ophthalmic drugs correctly. Patients should be taught the following procedure:

1. Wash and dry the hands; shake the bottle if it contains a suspension.
2. With a forefinger, pull down the outer portion of the lower eyelid to form a "pocket" to receive the drop.
3. Grasp the dropper bottle between the thumb and fingers with the hand braced against the cheek or nose and the head held upward.
4. Place the dropper over the eye while looking at the tip of the bottle; then look up and place a single drop in the eye.
5. The lids should be closed (but not squeezed or rubbed) for 5 minutes after instillation. This increases the ocular availability of the drug and reduces systemic absorption.
6. Recap bottle and store as instructed.

Note that many patients are physically unable to administer their own eye drops without assistance. ELC also should be used to improve ocular bioavailability and reduce systemic absorption.[7] The patient induces ELC for 5 minutes by gently closing the eyes. ELC decreases nasolacrimal drainage of drug, thereby decreasing the amount of drug available for systemic absorption by the nasopharyngeal mucosa. The use of ELC may improve drug response significantly, reduce adverse effects, and allow less-frequent dosing intervals and the use of lower drug concentrations.

The use of more than one drop per dose increases costs, does not improve response significantly, and may increase adverse effects. When two drugs are to be administered, instillations should be separated by at least 5 minutes (preferably 10 minutes) to prevent the drug administered first from being washed out. The patient should be taught not to touch the dropper bottle tip with eye, hands, or any surface.

Adherence to glaucoma therapy usually is inadequate, and it always should be considered as a possible cause of drug therapy failure. Assessment of adherence by healthcare providers generally is poor; so all patients should be encouraged continually to administer prescribed therapy diligently as instructed. To improve adherence, the patient, family, and care providers should be fully informed of the expectations of therapy and the need to continue therapy despite a lack of symptoms. Possible adverse effects of the medication and ways to reduce them should be discussed. Adherence will be improved by good communication, simplified and well-tolerated dosing regimens, reminder devices, education, close monitoring, and individualized care planning.[7,43]

ABBREVIATIONS

CAG	closed-angle glaucoma
CAI	carbonic anhydrase inhibitor
IOP	intraocular pressure
ELC	eyelid closure
OAG	open-angle glaucoma
OHT	ocular hypertension
OHTS	Ocular Hypertensive Treatment Study
POAG	primary open-angle glaucoma

REFERENCES

1. Jonas JB, Aung T, Bourne RR, Bron AM, Ritch R. Glaucoma. *Lancet.* 2017:390:2183–2193.
2. Weinreb RN, Aung T, Madeiros FA. The pathophysiology and treatment of glaucoma. *JAMA.* 2014;311:1901–1911.
3. Kwon YH, Fingert JH, Kuehn MH, Alward WLM. Primary open-angle glaucoma. *N Engl J Med.* 2009;360:1113–1124.
4. Wax MB, Camras CB, Fiscella RG, et al. Emerging perspectives in glaucoma: Optimizing 24-hour control of intraocular pressure. *Am J Ophthalmol.* 2002;133:S1–S10.
5. American Academy of Ophthalmology PPP Glaucoma Committee. *Preferred Practice Pattern Guidelines. Primary Open-Angle Glaucoma PPP 2020.* www.aao.org/preferred-practice-pattern/primary-open-angle-glaucoma-ppp Nov 2020.
6. Leske MC, Heijl A, Hussein M, et al. Factors for glaucoma progression and the effect of treatment: The early manifest glaucoma trial. *Arch Ophthalmol.* 2003;121:48–56.
7. American Academy of Ophthalmology PPP Glaucoma Committee. Primary open-angle glaucoma suspect PPP 2020. www.aao.org/preferred-practice-pattern/primary-open-angle-glaucoma-suspect-ppp Nov2020.
8. Collaborative Normal-Tension Glaucoma Study Group. Comparison of glaucomatous progression between untreated patients with normal-tension glaucoma and patients with therapeutically reduced intraocular pressures. *Am J Ophthalmol.* 1998;126:487–497.
9. Brandt JD, Beiser JA, Gordon MO, et al. Ocular Hypertension Treatment Study (OHTS) Group. Central corneal thickness and measured IOP response to topical ocular hypotensive medication in the Ocular Hypertension Treatment Study. *Am J Ophthalmol.* 2004;138:717–722.
10. Kass MA, Heuer DK, Higginbotham EJ, et al. The ocular hypertension treatment study: A randomized trial determines that topical ocular hypotensive medication delays or prevents the onset of primary open-angle glaucoma. *Arch Ophthalmol.* 2002;120:701–713. discussion 829, 830.
11. Chauhan BC, Mikelberg FS, Balaszi AG, et al. Canadian glaucoma study 2. Risk factors for the progression of open-angle glaucoma. *Arch Ophthalmol.* 2008;126:1030–1036.
12. Van Veldhuisen PC, Schwartz AL, Gaasterland DE, et al. The advanced glaucoma intervention study (AGIS): 7. The relationship between control of intraocular pressure and visual field deterioration. *Am J Ophthalmol.* 2000;130:429–440.
13. Prager Alisa J, Tang Minjia, Pleet Alexander L., et al. Effectiveness and Tolerability of netarsudil in combination with other ocular hypotensive agents. *Ophthalmol. Glaucoma.* 2021.10.1016/j.ogla.2021.03.014.
14. Mansouri Kaweh, Medeiros Felipe A, Tafreshi Ali, et al. Continuous 24-hour monitoring of intraocular pressure patterns with a contact lens sensor. *Arch. Ophthalmol.* 2012;130:1534. 10.1001/archophthalmol.2012.2280.
15. Goel M, Picciani G, Lee RK, Bhattacharya SK. Aqueous humor dynamics: A review. *Open Ophthalmol J.* 2010;4:52–59.
16. Hoy SM. Netarsudil ophthalmic solution 0.02%: First global approval. *Drugs.* 2018;78:389–396.
17. Mansouri K, Medeiros FA, Tafreshi A, Weinreb RN. Continuous 24-hour monitoring of intraocular pressure patterns with a contact lens sensor: Safety, tolerability, and reproducibility in patients with glaucoma. *Arch Ophthalmol.* 2012;13:1–6. doi:10.1001/archophthalmol.2012.2280.
18. Miller MA, Fingert JF, Bettis DI. Genetics and genetic testing for glaucoma. *Curr Opin Ophthalmol.* 2017, 28:133–138.
19. Wiggs JL. Genetic etiologies of glaucoma. *Arch Ophthalmol.* 2007;125:30–37.
20. Gordon MO, Torri V, Miglior S, et al. Ocular Hypertension Treatment Study Group; European Glaucoma Prevention Study Group. Validated prediction model for the development of primary open-angle glaucoma in individuals with ocular hypertension. *Ophthalmology.* 2007;114:10–19.
21. Quigley HA, Broman AT. The number of people with glaucoma worldwide in 2010 and 2020. *Br J Ophthalmol.* 2006;90:262–267.
22. Brandt JD, Gordon MO, Beiser JA, et al. Ocular Hypertension Treatment Study Group. Changes in central corneal thickness over time: The ocular Hypertension Treatment Study. *Ophthalmology.* 2008;115:1550–1556.
23. Krupin T, Liebmann JM, Greenfield DS, et al. A randomized trial of brimonidine versus timolol in preserving visual function: Results from the low-pressure Glaucoma Treatment Study. *Am J Ophthalmol.* 2011;151:671–681.
24. Kolko M. Present and new treatment strategies in the management of glaucoma. *The Open Ophthalmol J.* 2015:9(suppl 1:M5):89–100.
25. Garway-Heath DF, Crabb DP, Bunce C, et al. Latanoprost for open angle glaucoma (UKGTS): A randomized, multicenter, placebo controlled trial. *Lancet.* 2015;385:1295–1304.
26. Nucci C, Russo R, Martucci A, et al. New strategies for neuroprotection in glaucoma, a disease that affects the central nervous system. *Eur J Pharmacol.* 2016;787:119–126.
27. Li T, Lindsley K, Rouse B, et al. Comparative effectiveness of first line medications for primary open-angle glaucoma. A systematic review and network meta-analysis. *Ophthalmology.* 2016;123:129–140.
28. Ostler Erik, Rhee Douglas, Burney Edward, et al. Advances in medical therapy for glaucoma. *Curr. Opin. Ophthalmol.* 2020;32:129–133. 10.1097/icu.0000000000000740.

29. Medeiros Felipe A, Walters Thomas R, Kolko Miriam, et al. Phase 3, Randomized, 20-Month Study of Bimatoprost Implant in Open-Angle Glaucoma and Ocular Hypertension (ARTEMIS 1). *Ophthalmology.* 2020;127:1627–1641. 10.1016/j.ophtha.2020.06.018.
30. Wright C, Tawfik MA, Waisbourd M, Katz LJ. Primary angle-closure glaucoma: An update. *Acta Ophthalmologica.* 2016;94(3):217–225.
31. He Mingguang, Jiang Yuzhen, Huang Shengsong, et al. Laser peripheral iridotomy for the prevention of angle closure: A single-centre, randomised controlled trial. *Lancet.* 2019;393:1609–1618. 10.1016/s0140-6736(18)32607-2.
32. Zheng W, Dryja TP, Wei Z, et al. Systemic medication associations with presumed advanced or uncontrolled primary open-angle glaucoma. *Ophthalmology.* 2018;125(7):984–993.
33. Murphy RM, Bakir B, O'Brien C, et al. Drug-induced bilateral secondary angle-closure glaucoma: A literature synthesis. *J Glaucoma.* 2016;25:99–105.
34. American Academy of Ophthalmology Glaucoma Panel. Preferred Practice Pattern Guidelines. Primary Angle Closure. https://www.aao.org/preferred-practice-pattern/primary-angle-closure-disease-ppp. 2020.
35. Tripathi RC, Tripathi BJ, Haggerty C. Drug-induced glaucomas. *Drug Saf.* 2003;26:749–767.
36. Kanner E, Tsai JC. Glaucoma medications. Use and safety in the elderly population. *Drugs Aging.* 2006;23:321–332.
37. Han JA, Frishman WH, Sun SW, et al. Cardiovascular and respiratory considerations with pharmacotherapy of glaucoma and ocular hypertension. *Cardiol Rev.* 2008;16:95–108.
38. Katz LJ, Steinmann WC, Kabir A, et al. Selective laser trabeculoplasty versus medical therapy as initial treatment of glaucoma: A prospective, randomized trial. *J Glaucoma.* 2012;21:460–468.
39. Law SK. Switching within glaucoma medication class. *Curr Opin Ophthalmol.* 2009;111:1439–1448.
40. Habash AA, Aljasim LA, Owaidhah O, Edward DP. A review of the efficacy of mitomycin C in glaucoma filtration surgery. *Clin Ophthalmol.* 2015;9:1945–1951.
41. Singh K, Mehta K, Shaikh NM, et al. Trabeculectomy with intraoperative mitomycin C versus 5-fluorouracil. *Ophthalmology.* 2000;107:2305–2309.
42. van der Valk R, Webers CA, Schouten JSAG, et al. Intraocular pressure-lowering effects of all commonly used glaucoma drugs. A meta-analysis of randomized clinical trials. *Ophthalmology.* 2005;112:1177–1185.
43. Gray TA, Orton LC, Henson D, et al. Interventions for improving adherence to ocular hypotensive therapy. *Cochrane Database Syst Rev.* 2009;2:CD006132. doi:10.1002/14651858.CD006132.pub2.
44. Anwar Z, Wellik SR, Galor A. Glaucoma therapy and ocular surface disease: Current literature and recommendations. *Curr Opin Ophthalmol.* 2013;24:136–143.
45. Gazzard Gus, Konstantakopoulou Evgenia, Garway-Heath David, et al. Selective laser trabeculoplasty versus eye drops for first-line treatment of ocular hypertension and glaucoma (LiGHT): A multicentre randomised controlled trial. *Lancet.* 2019;393:1505–1516. 10.1016/s0140-6736(18)32213-x.
46. Khawaja Anthony P, Campbell Joanna H, Kirby Nicholas, et al. Real-world outcomes of selective laser trabeculoplasty in the United Kingdom. *Ophthalmology.* 2020;127:748–757. 10.1016/j.ophtha.2019.11.017.
47. Pillunat LE, Erb C, Junemann AGM, Kimmich F. Micro-invasive glaucoma surgery (MIGS): A review of surgical procedures using stents. *Clin Ophthalmol.* 2017;11:1583–1600.
48. Mott M, Aref A, Azura-Blanco A, Gedde S. Clear lens extraction: First-line treatment for primary angle-closure glaucoma? *EyeNet Magazine.* https://www.aao.org/eyenet/article/clear-lens-extraction-for-pacg Nov2017.
49. Baskaran Mani, Kumar Rajesh S, Friedman David S, et al. The Singapore Asymptomatic Narrow Angles Laser Iridotomy Study (ANA-LIS): 5 year results of a Randomized Controlled Trial. *Ophthalmology.* 202110.1016/j.ophtha.2021.08.017.
50. Hoy SM. Latanoprosene bunod. Ophthalmic solution 0.024%: A review in open angle glaucoma and ocular hypertension. *Drugs.* 2018;78:773–780.
51. Schmidl D, Schmetterer L, Gashofer G, Pops-Cherecheanu A. Pharmacotherapy of glaucoma. *J Ocul Pharmcol Thera.* 2015;31:63–77.
52. Bucolo C, Salomone S, Drago F, Reibaldi M, Longo A, Uva MG. Pharmacological management of ocular hypertension: Current approaches and future perspective. *Curr Opin Pharmacol.* 2013;13:50–55.
53. Dikopf MS, Vajaranant TS, Edward DP. Topical treatment of glaucoma: Established and emerging pharmacology. *Exp Opin Pharmacol.* 2017;18:885–898.
54. Aihara M, Lu F, Kawata H, et al. Omidenepag isopropyl versus latanoprost in primary open-angle glaucoma and ocular hypertension. *Am J Ophthalmol.* 2020;220:53–63. 10.1016/j.ajo.2020.06.003.

115

Age-Related Macular Degeneration

Alisa K. Escano and Casey S. Washington

KEY CONCEPTS

1. The hallmark sign of age-related macular degeneration (AMD) is the development of drusen in the macula. Drusen are yellow deposits of lipids between the retinal pigment epithelial and Bruch's membrane that can develop with age.
2. AMD is identified as the leading cause of blindness in the industrialized world and a top cause of blindness worldwide.
3. The two most important risk factors for AMD are age and smoking.
4. The goal of treatment is to slow progression of AMD and prevent severe visual impairment or blindness.
5. Smoking cessation is the main modifiable risk factor that will slow progression of AMD. Pharmacists and other health professionals can play a vital role in helping people stop smoking.
6. Antioxidant vitamins and minerals may prevent cellular damage in the retina caused by the formation of free radicals through light absorption. Use may benefit patients the most with medium- or large-sized drusen and/or geographic atrophy in at least one eye.
7. For most patients with wet AMD and choroidal neovascularization, the use of intravitreal vascular endothelial growth factor (VEGF) inhibitors and other inhibitor-like drugs have led to improvement in visual acuity.
8. The appeal of the ranibizumab treat and extend (TREX) approach is the reduction of office visits and medication cost.
9. VEGF inhibitors and antioxidant vitamins and minerals are the only pharmacologic therapies available that have been shown to improve and stabilize visual acuity in patients with intermediate to advanced AMD.

BEYOND THE BOOK

Watch the first three age-related macular degeneration videos from the National Eye Institute at https://youtube.com/playlist?list=PLNol8zIT_P1Bjl8o7HNMCybk1tA3s0SIN. These short videos totaling 3 minutes provide a brief overview to age-related macular degeneration and animation of the pathophysiology. These videos are useful to enhance student understanding regarding the COLLECT and ASSESS steps in the patient care process.

INTRODUCTION

Age-related macular degeneration (AMD) is a neurodegenerative disease that produces irreversible loss of central vision due to damage to the macula, the center region of the retina. AMD is a leading cause of blindness due to age-related changes in the macula and, specifically, the photoreceptor–retinal pigment epithelial (RPE) complex.[2]

A general familiarity with the anatomy of the eye including the macula and photoreceptor–RPE complex will aid in understanding the disease and treatment mechanisms (Figs. 115-1 and 115-2).[3,4] The macula in the middle of the retina is responsible for all central vision, a significant part of color vision, and the fine detail images. The photoreceptor cells of the macula identify light and then transfer the information to the brain to produce an image. Central vision is needed to read, write, drive, watch television, and other typical activities of daily living. AMD reduces central vision, visual acuity, and blue-yellow color sensitivity leading to significant disability (Fig. 115-3).[5]

(1) The hallmark sign of AMD is the development of drusen in the macula. Drusen are yellow deposits of lipids between the RPE and Bruch's membrane that can develop with age (Fig. 115-4). Bruch's membrane is an extracellular layer separating the RPE from choroidal capillaries in the eye. Small drusen without additional abnormalities have a lower risk of progression to severe disease than large drusen.

Two distinct types of AMD have been identified: geographic atrophy (GA) "dry" and choroidal neovascularization (CNV), exudative "wet" (Fig. 115-5). Disease progression is unpredictable as visual disturbances do not correlate with drusen formation. Patients can monitor visual changes with an Amsler grid by using one eye at a time and looking for any distortions in the grid (Fig. 115-6).

The American Academy of Ophthalmology defines AMD by the presence of one of the following criteria[1]:

- Presence of at least intermediate-size drusen (63 μm or larger in diameter)
- RPE abnormalities (hypopigmentation or hyperpigmentation)
- Reticular pseudodrusen
- Presence of any of the following features: RPE GA, CNV, polypoidal choroidal vasculopathy, retinal angiomatous proliferation

EPIDEMIOLOGY

(2) With longer life expectancy, the incidence of vision impairment from macular diseases increased 62% from 1990 to 2010.[6] AMD is identified as the leading cause of vision impairment in the industrialized world and a top cause of blindness worldwide, in addition to diabetic retinopathy, glaucoma, cataracts, and under-correction

of refraction error.[7-9] Drusen development and AMD diagnosis can occur at any age, although usually after the age of 50 years. The prevalence of AMD is 8.69% for adults 45 to 85 years of age.[10] Rates of AMD increase nonlinearly with age affecting 6% to 10% of people aged 65 years or older and more than 20% to 25% of who have reached the age of 75 years.[11,12]

Dry AMD is the most common type diagnosed in 80% to 90% of patients and 10% to 20% may progress to wet AMD.[7,11] The more severe wet AMD is associated with progressive vision loss and makes up only 10% to 20% of AMD diagnoses yet is responsible for 90% of the vision loss of AMD.[8]

In the United States, 2.8 million individuals have advanced or intermediate forms of AMD, with expectations to reach 5.44 million by 2050.[10,11] Cases of early AMD in the United States totaled 9.1 million in 2010 with expectations to increase to 17.8 million by 2050.[10]

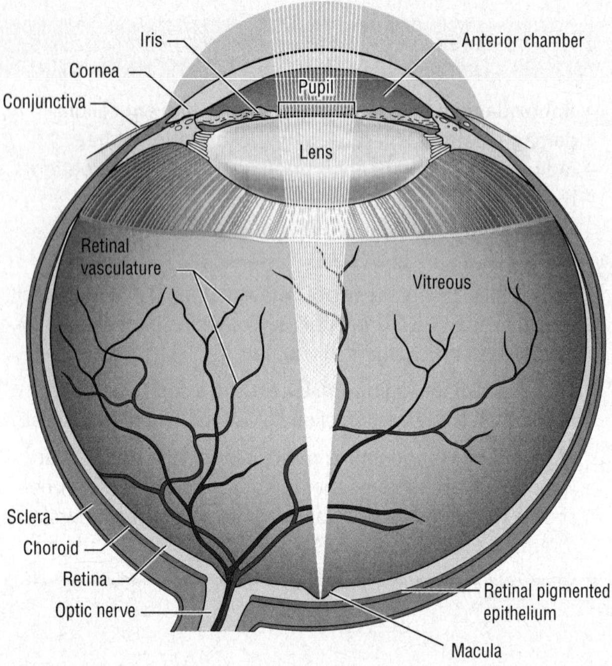

FIGURE 115-1 Anatomy of the eye. The macula, in the center of the retina, is responsible for central vision, color vision, and fine details.

Risk Factors

3 The two most important risk factors for AMD are older age and smoking. Additional risk factors for AMD include ethnicity and genetics, both of which are nonmodifiable. In addition to smoking, modifiable risk factors include hypertension, body-mass index (BMI), and cardiovascular disease (Table 115-1).[8]

The risk of development of AMD increases exponentially with age, with risk at the age of 75 years 2 to 3 times that at 65 years. A 2014 worldwide meta-analysis found a higher prevalence of AMD in European compared to Asian, Hispanic, and African populations.[6,8] The Salisbury Eye Evaluation evaluated the prevalence of AMD of White and Black Americans and found higher prevalence of large drusen, focal hyperpigmentation, and GA in white participants, suggesting there may be a mechanism of protection against fundus abnormalities in the central zone for Black participants.[9]

Genetics

Several genetic factors are associated with increasing risk, progression, and protection from AMD.[8] The complement factor H (CFH)–related gene on chromosome 1 binds to factor C3b and is involved in regulation of the innate immune system. This regulation is defective with a homozygous Y402H polymorphism of *CFH*, causing alteration at the C3b site leading to an up-regulation of inflammation, affecting vascular endothelial growth factor (VEGF) expression, and increasing the risk of AMD by 7.4-fold.[13]

Other genetic variants associated with increased risk of AMD include the ARMS2/HtrA serine peptidase 1 (*HtrA1*) genes, hepatic lipase (*LIPC*) gene, and the rs3775291 variant in the toll-like receptor 3 (*TLR3*) gene.[8,13] Despite publications suggesting genetic testing

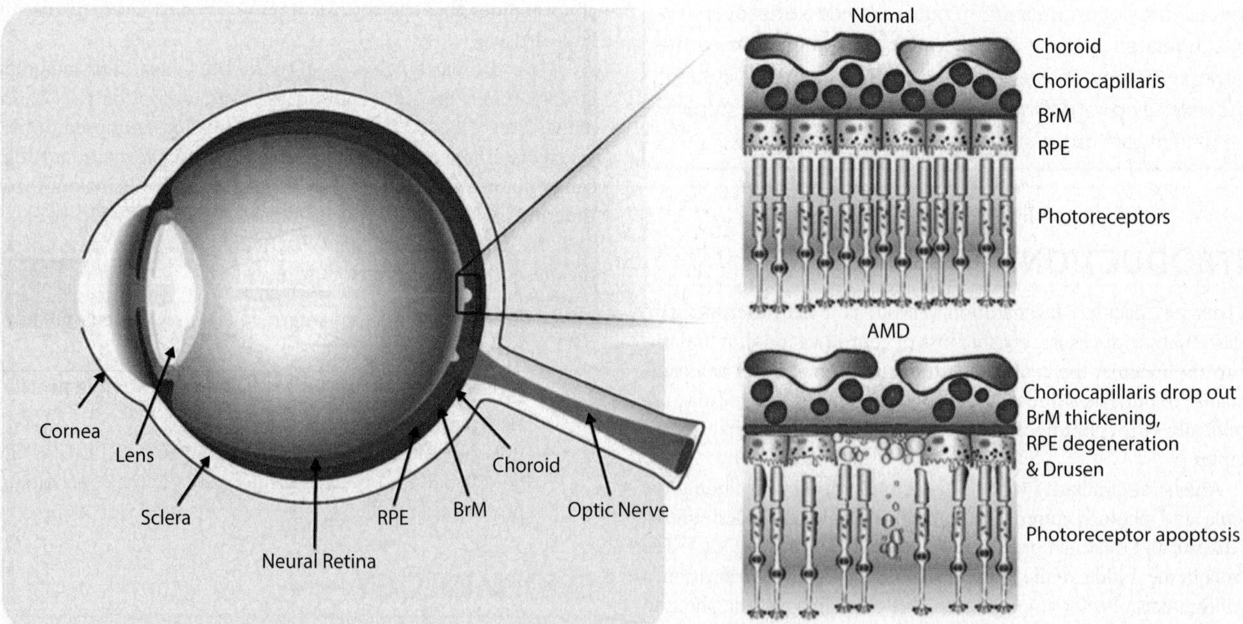

FIGURE 115-2 Detailed anatomy of the photoreceptor–RPE complex. The photoreceptor–RPE complex in the normal state and in a state with AMD that shows the breakdown of the RPE with drusen formation and apoptosis of photoreceptors contributing to the loss of vision with AMD. *(Reproduced, with permission, from Chichagova V, Hallam D, Collin J, Zerti D, Dorgau B, Felemban M, Lako M, Steel DH. Cellular regeneration strategies for macular degeneration: past, present and future. Eye (Lond). 2018 May;32(5):946-971.)*

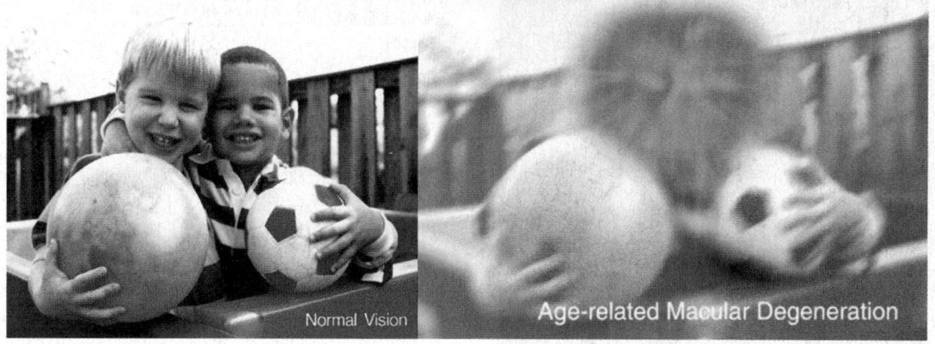

FIGURE 115-3 Effects of the loss of central vision with AMD. *(From National Eye Institute, National Institutes of Health, Washington, DC.)*

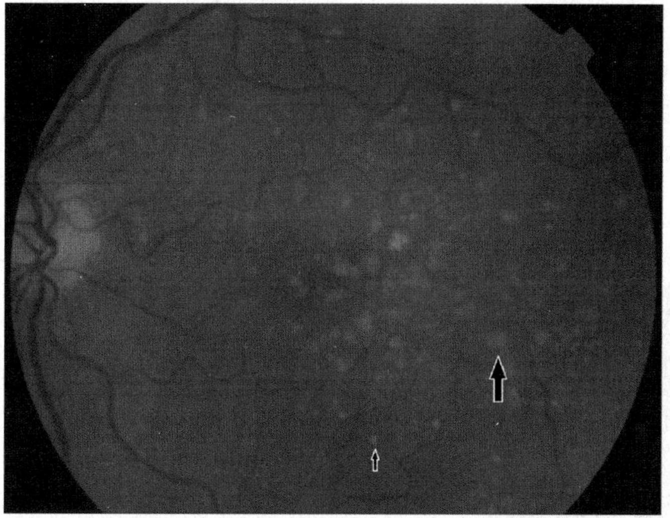

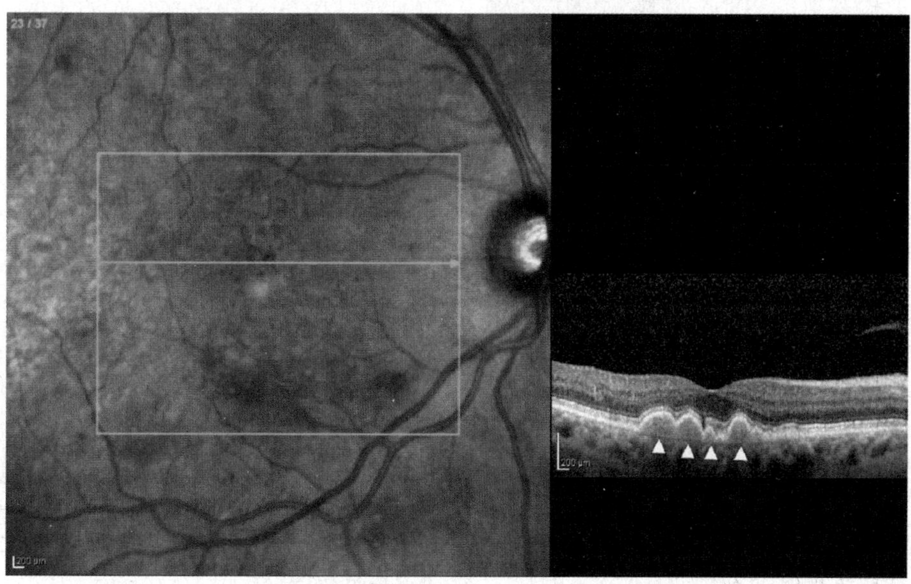

FIGURE 115-4 Age-related macular degeneration (AMD). (*A*) Discrete (**small arrow**) and large confluent (**large arrow**) drusen. (*B*) Optical coherence tomography scan of large confluent drusen (**arrowheads**). *(Reproduced, with permission, from Riordan-Eva P, Augsburger JJ, eds. Vaughan & Asbury's General Ophthalmology. 19th ed. New York: McGraw Hill; 2018.)*

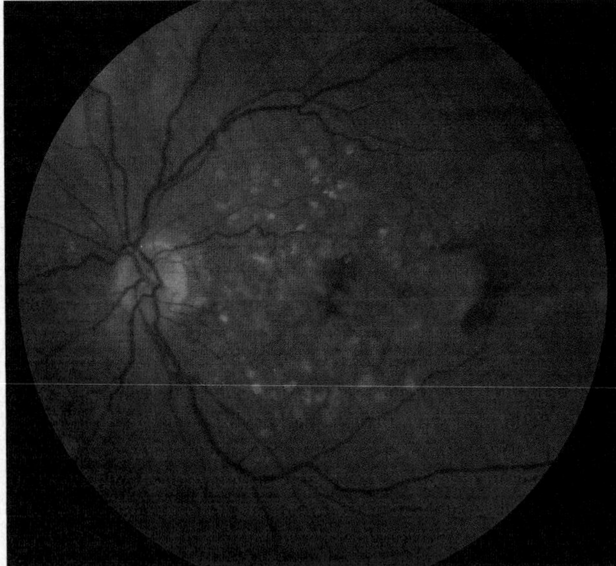

FIGURE 115-5 Age-related macular degeneration consisting of scattered yellow drusen in the macula (dry form) and a crescent of fresh hemorrhage temporal to the fovea from a subretinal neovascular membrane (wet form). *(Reproduced, with permission, from Jameson JL, Fauci AS, Kasper DL, Hauser SL, Longo DL, Loscalzo J, eds. Harrison's Principles of Internal Medicine. 20th ed. New York, NY: McGraw Hill; 2019.)*

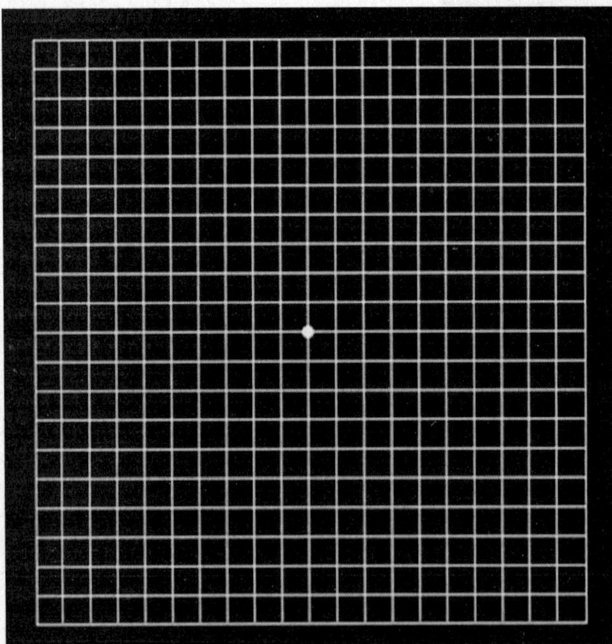

FIGURE 115-6 Amsler grid for monitoring vision by tracking any distortions in the grid lines while focusing on the center dot. *(Reproduced, with permission, from Riordan-Eva P, Augsburger JJ, eds. Vaughan & Asbury's General Ophthalmology. 19th ed. New York: McGraw Hill; 2018.)*

may be helpful, genetic tests are not recommended in patient care at this time because of inconclusive data.[14,15]

Smoking

Because it is a modifiable risk factor, smoking is important for health professionals to address; it is associated with an increased risk of AMD.[8] Studies have consistently found an increased risk across different populations of early, wet, and dry AMD with current smoking and former smoking within the last 20 years.[8]

TABLE 115-1 Risk Factors for AMD

Factor		Increased Risk	Protective
Age (years)	<55		✓
	55-75	✓	
	>75	✓	
Ethnicity	European	✓	
Race[a]	Wite	✓	
	Black		✓
Genetics	Y402H	✓	
	ARMS2/HtrA1	✓	
	LIPC	✓	
	rs3775291	✓	
Gender[b]	Female	✓	
Smoking	Active	✓	
	History	✓	
Diet	Omega-3 fatty acids		✓
	High fat	✓	
	Lutein		✓
	Fruit and vegetables		✓
	Nitrates		✓
Physical activity			✓
Medications	Statins		✓

[a]Take into consideration race is a socially created categorization and not determinable by genetic testing.

[b]Gender nonbinary inclusive studies have not been performed; consult www.transhealth.ucsf.edu/guidelines.[33]

Smoking cessation is a staple in the care plan for patients at risk for and with a prior diagnosis of AMD due to the ability to slow progression. The Australian government added warnings to cigarette packs regarding the risk of blindness related to data from AMD.[16] In 2014, the United States Department of Health & Human Services published a report of the damage smoking can do to health; however, the warnings on cigarettes in the United States are opposed by the tobacco industry.[17,18]

Diet

Diets higher in saturated, transunsaturated, polyunsaturated, and monounsaturated fatty acids (FAs) are associated with higher prevalence and progression of AMD compared to diets with lower intake of fat.[8] Interestingly, FA in nuts and fish was protective. Omega-3 FA intake can decrease the risk of AMD by up to 30%.[8]

Antioxidant intake has also proven important in AMD.[19] Lutein, zeaxanthin, zinc, and vitamins C and E had varying results when evaluating supplements and dietary intake. Combining types of antioxidants, through a varied diet, tends to have better results.[20-22] A recent population-based cohort study found that patients who followed a diet consisting of 200 g of vegetables per day, fruit twice daily, and fish twice a week had a significantly reduced risk of AMD.[20] Dietary nitrate intake of 142 g/day, from vegetable and nonvegetable sources, was also found to reduce incidence of early AMD.[23]

Additional Risk Factors

AMD can loosely be linked to atherosclerosis and cardiovascular disease.[8,24] Risk factors of these disease states overlap, including hypertension, which is associated with a higher incidence of wet AMD. Obesity and inactivity are also associated with increased risk of early and late AMD.[25] 3-Hydroxy-3-methyl-glutaryl-coenzyme

A (HMG-CoA) reductase inhibitors (statins) are associated with a potential modest reduction in risk of early AMD and a protective effect against wet AMD; the drugs show no benefit or harm with respect to risk of dry AMD.[26] Aspirin was thought to increase the chance of developing wet AMD, but results have been conflicting and the minimal increase in the risk of wet AMD is less than the benefit in using aspirin for cardiovascular disease in older adults.[8,27]

Ultraviolet radiation exposure, especially in people with light-colored eyes, has also shown an increase in the risk of AMD.[28] Thyroid dysfunction and thyroxine use have both shown an association with increased AMD diagnosis.[29] Medications have also been associated with AMD including nitroglycerin, beta-blockers, chloroquine derivatives, and phenothiazines.[30] Environmental safety is a prudent component to evaluate due to unsafe chemicals and the need for a focus on sustainability in healthcare.[31] Pesticide exposure was correlated to AMD diagnosis in the Agriculture Health Study reporting that exposure to insecticides and herbicides is a modifiable risk factor for AMD.[32]

ETIOLOGY

AMD is a neurodegenerative disease with ocular inflammation and autoimmunity in combination with additional causes of RPE dysfunction and atrophy including the effects of aging, external environmental factors, and genetic factors.[8] Abnormal processing of complement, lipid, angiogenic, inflammatory, and extracellular matrix pathways contribute to the detrimental changes, but the pathogenesis of AMD is not fully understood. Oxidative stress and complement activation can increase RPE secretion of VEGF-A, which is associated with angiogenesis.

Wet AMD has CNV, which are new blood vessels created in the choroidal region of the eye. There are different types of wet AMD determined by how the CNV occurs and how it affects the RPE.[8] In type 1, formerly referred to as "occult," CNV is categorized by lesions with leakage of blood or plasma proteins from immature choroidal blood vessels that remain below the RPE.[8] The extra volume may cause pigment epithelial detachment. Type 1 can progress to type 2. In type 2, often referred to as classic, lesions push through and are visible above the RPE. Type 3 has retinal angiomatous proliferation meaning the choroidal and retinal vessels link together. Retinal macrophages are increased and are a hallmark sign of CNV.[34]

Dry AMD has been labeled a metabolic storage disease, due to the excessive buildup of lipofuscin, a nondegradable debris that accumulates in the RPE with age or other toxic accumulations between the RPE and Bruch's membrane.[35] The deposits on the semipermeable Bruch's membrane interfere with efflux, increasing stress and inflammation on the RPE (Fig. 115-3). This stress, in addition to cigarette smoking and aging, increases lipofuscin that interferes with lipid metabolism. The extra volume shifts the original layers of the RPE complex resulting in GA.

Alzheimer's disease, Parkinson's disease, amyotrophic lateral sclerosis, and Huntington's disease are other common neurodegenerative diseases of aging potentially related to AMD.

A reduction in quality of life (QOL) is common with AMD.[36] Clinical depression is reported in one-third of patients, twice the rate of peers without AMD, and this risk increases as vision deteriorates.[8,37] A significant decline in participation in valued activities such as hobbies can occur, which has been found to increase the risk of depression. Additionally, a meta-analysis reported an association of AMD, specifically late AMD, with an increased risk of all-cause and cardiovascular mortality.[38]

PATHOPHYSIOLOGY

The presence and type of drusen on the retina upon examination can predict the progression of AMD. Drusen are yellow-white deposits made up of protein and lipids that appear on a layer of the retina known as the Bruch's membrane, a thin, semipermeable membrane that operates as a basement membrane for the retinal epithelium and mediates the metabolic exchange between the retina and the choroid (Fig. 115-3). While the exact cause of drusen is unknown, several hypotheses suggest that drusen are composed of lipids and cellular debris accumulation from the rods and cones of the retina that are not fully eliminated. While drusen are not a cause of or diagnostic of AMD, the presence of drusen on examination can increase a person's risk of developing AMD. Patients younger than 50 years should consider hereditary factors for macular disease if signs and symptoms similar to AMD are present.[8]

Drusen can be classified as hard or soft (Fig. 115-4). Drusen that are small, round, well-defined spots located far away from one another on the retina are called "hard" drusen. Hard drusen are not a large cause for concern for vision loss or AMD as they may never progress to AMD or may be slow to progress. Most people over the age of 50 years have hard drusen present on their retina, and these are considered a natural consequence of aging. Soft drusen increase the risk for AMD (specifically wet AMD); these are larger drusen, are not well-defined with blurred edges, and are often clustered closer together on the retina. The presence of large, soft drusen is associated with vision loss and an increased risk for progression to AMD. Soft drusen can also lead to RPE detachment through the disruption of the retinal layers.

Dry AMD

Atrophic or dry AMD is a painless disease of the macula resulting in a gradual loss of vision. The most common form of AMD, dry AMD can progress slowly and is less threatening to central vision loss compared to wet AMD. Dry AMD is characterized by subretinal hard and soft drusen deposits, the thinning of the macula, RPE atrophy, and hyperpigmentation of the retina. The cause of dry AMD is unknown, but studies indicate that it may be related to inflammation, genetics, and environmental factors such as smoking and diet.[24,25]

Dry AMD is usually diagnosed in patients older than 50 years. As the eye ages, the macula begins to thin and break down. Early detection, self-care, and reduction of risk factors through better diet, smoking cessation, and vitamin supplementation can help to slow progression of the disease.

Dry AMD that progresses to the advanced stage—when there is progressive and irreversible loss of RPE, choriocapillaris, and photoreceptors leading to a loss of central vision—is called GA.[39] Severe GA can also progress to wet AMD.

Dry AMD usually affects both eyes, but in some patients, only one eye is affected. Patients with dry AMD in one eye may not have noticeable symptoms because the healthier eye will overcompensate for the eye affected by AMD. The patient's peripheral vision is not affected by dry AMD, so the vision loss may not be obvious in the early stages of the disease.

Symptoms of dry AMD are as follows[39]:

- Difficulty reading or driving (eg, increasing blurriness of written words)
- Visual distortion (eg, straight lines appearing bent)
- Blurred images (eg, difficulty recognizing faces)
- Difficulty seeing in low or dim light; bright light may be needed to see better
- Decreasing central vision
- Colors may not appear as bright as they once were

Wet AMD

CNV, or exudative AMD, is typically referred to as wet AMD and is advanced AMD.[8,40] Wet AMD is characterized by the loss of central vision caused by CNV, which is the abnormal growth of new blood vessels from the choroid into the macula and retina. These abnormal blood vessels can leak blood or fluid into the retina and can form pockets of fluid between the choroid and the RPE; these can be seen as bumps in the macula and cause a disruption in central vision. The patient will see dark spots (floaters) in their central vision because of the pockets of fluid and wavy lines instead of straight lines because their macula is no longer smooth. The presence of drusen that are large and soft and RPE hyperpigmentation increases the risk of the development of wet AMD.

VEGF plays an important role in the pathogenesis of wet AMD. VEGF is a specific and potent regulator of angiogenesis and is responsible for the abnormal growth of blood vessels. One isoform, VEGF-A, is most strongly associated with angiogenesis in ocular diseases and is therefore a target for VEGF inhibitors for the treatment of wet AMD.[8,41]

Like dry AMD, wet AMD may affect one or both eyes. Once the patient has progressed to wet AMD, vision loss may be rapid if treatment is not initiated promptly to address the leaky blood vessels. Symptoms of wet AMD are similar to dry AMD and also include the presence of dark spots in the patient's central vision; peripheral vision is not affected. Patients at high risk of wet AMD should have regular eye examinations to assess functional change.

Classification of AMD

AMD can be classified using different systems. Most practitioners use the Age-Related Eye Disease Study (AREDS) classification or the more recently developed Beckman Classification system (Table 115-2), which is based on the presence and size of drusen and pigmentary changes.[8,42]

TABLE 115-2 Classification of Age-Related Macular Degeneration

Clinical Classification	Characteristics
Normal aging changes	Small drusen ≤63 μm No pigmentary abnormalities
Early AMD	Medium-sized drusen >63 μm and ≤125 μm No pigmentary abnormalities
Intermediate AMD	Large drusen >125 μm and/or any pigmentary abnormalities
Late AMD	Neovascular AMD and/or GA
AREDS Classification	
No AMD (Category)	No or few small drusen
Early AMD (Category 2)	Multiple small drusen Few intermediate drusen Mild abnormalities in the retinal pigment epithelium
Intermediate AMD (Category 3)	Any of the following: • Numerous intermediate drusen • At least one large drusen • GA
Advanced AMD (Category 4)	One or more of the following: • GA of the retinal pigment epithelium involving the foveal center • Neovascular maculopathy that includes the following: • CNV • Serous and/or hemorrhagic detachment of the neurosensory retina or retinal pigment epithelium • Retinal hard exudates • Subretinal and subretinal pigment epithelium fibrovascular proliferation • Disciform scar (subretinal fibrosis)

AREDS, Age-Related Eye Disease Study; AMD, age-related macular degeneration.

Early AMD

AREDS defines early AMD based on the presence of a few small (<63 μm) to medium (63-124 μm) drusen. The patient may or may not have pigment epithelial abnormalities in the macula. Patients diagnosed with early AMD have a low risk of progressing to advanced AMD after 5 years of stable disease.[42]

Intermediate AMD

Intermediate AMD has been defined by the AREDS as having one or more large drusen (≥125 μm in diameter) or evidence of extensive medium drusen (63-124 μm) or in one or both eyes. Patients with intermediate AMD have a much greater chance of progression to advanced AMD if left untreated. If, at baseline diagnosis, drusen are present only in one eye, there is approximately an 18% chance that the disease will progress to advanced AMD after 5 years. If medium to large drusen are present in both eyes, the risk of progression to advanced AMD increases to 26% after 5 years.[42] Upon diagnosis, patients should begin a discussion with their physician about the risks and benefits of delayed progression or stabilized visual acuity with the available treatment options.

Reticular pseudodrusen, also called subretinal drusenoid deposits, may appear in patients with intermediate AMD. These are difficult to identify upon examination, and diagnosis may require the use of fundus autofluorescence, infrared reflectance, and/or spectral domain optical coherence tomography (SD-OCT). The presence of pseudodrusen is associated with the progression of intermediate AMD.[8,43-46]

Advanced AMD

AREDS defines advanced AMD as neovascular AMD or GA present in the macula. In patients with advanced AMD, at least one eye is affected, with a complete loss of visual acuity. According to AREDS, the risk of progression of visual acuity loss in the unaffected eye is 35% to 50% at 5 years.[47] Patients with GA may have a slower loss of visual acuity compared with patients with neovascular AMD.[8]

CLINICAL PRESENTATION

AMD can present without symptoms, or patients may have complaints of central vision loss, including scotoma (a dark patch in the middle of their vision), or distorted vision. Patients are typically older than 50 years. In dry AMD, patients may complain of the need for a bright light or a magnifying glass while reading or trouble seeing while driving. Wet AMD presents as metamorphopsia, the distortion of straight lines. Acute vision loss requires urgent evaluation and care.

TREATMENT

4 The goal of treatment is to slow progression of AMD and prevent severe visual impairment or blindness. It should be noted that while pharmacotherapeutic options do exist, there is not enough supportive evidence to advocate for one treatment option over another to prevent progression to advanced AMD. For patients with intermediate AMD, studies support the use of antioxidant vitamins and minerals to slow progression to advanced AMD. In patients with wet AMD, the use of anti-VEGF agents, photodynamic therapy (PDT), and even surgery has been studied in an attempt to slow progression to vision loss. Assessment of the patient by the physician and informed discussion with the patient evaluating the risks and benefits of treatment are necessary before treatment begins.

CLINICAL PRESENTATION Age-Related Macular Degeneration

Signs

- Distortion when viewing the Amsler grid (Fig. 115-6)
- Dilated eye examination with a slit-lamp instrument to observe and measure
  - Dry: drusen, GA present as hypopigmentation or hyperpigmentation
  - Wet: subretinal fluid or hemorrhage, which requires other diagnostic tests

Laboratory Tests

- None

Diagnosis Tests

- Subretinal evaluation using fluorescein dye retinal angiography, optical coherence tomography, or fundus autofluorescence

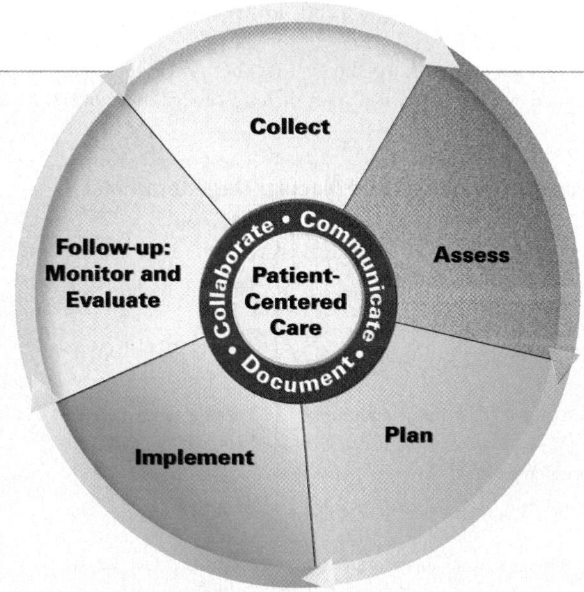

Patient Care Process for Management of Age-Related Macular Degeneration

The image shows the five fundamental steps included in The Pharmacist's Care Process endorsed by the Joint Commission for Pharmacy Practitioners (2014). The tagline of this process reads collaborate, communicate, and document. The five fundamental steps listed here are collect, assess, plan, implement, and follow-up: monitor and evaluate. All these steps are listed in a circular block diagram.

Collect

- Patient characteristics (age, sex, distance from treatment center, burden of follow-up visits, satisfaction, financial burden of treatment)
- Patient history (past medical, family history of AMD, social, smoking; date, frequency, and results of past eye examinations)
- Changes in vision (see Fig. 114-3 in the Glaucoma chapter and Fig. 115-5)
- Current medications
- Objective data (see the "Clinical Presentation" box)
- Visual field changes and losses
- Macula changes

Assess

- QOL
- Vision status (general, near, distance, peripheral)
- Mental health
- Smoking status
- Current treatment
- Functional status including driving, dependency, and role difficulties and activities of daily living (ADLs)

Plan

- Drug therapy regimen designed to prevent progression of the disease and preserve visual acuity, including specific agent(s), dose, route, frequency, and duration; specify the continuation and discontinuation of existing therapies (see Table 115-4)
- Referral to an ophthalmologist as needed

Implement*

- Provide patient education regarding all elements of the treatment plan
- Provide education on diet and functional/lifestyle changes, adherence to medications, and use of the Amsler grid
- Use motivational interviewing and coaching strategies to maximize adherence
- Schedule follow-up, usually 4 to 8 weeks, or as needed for specific medications

Follow-up: Monitor and Evaluate

- Monitor vision with Amsler grid (Fig. 115-6)
- Visual fields and diagnostic tests
- Adverse effects to medications
- Adherence to treatment
- Functional status
- Disease/treatment burden; financial burden

**Collaborate with patient, caregivers, and other healthcare professionals.*

Smoking Cessation

5 For all patients with dry AMD, smoking cessation is crucial to include as the first-line nonpharmacotherapeutic treatment option. Smoking cessation is the primary modifiable risk factor that can slow progression of AMD.

Health professionals, particularly pharmacists, can play a vital role in providing patient counseling and assistance with choosing the appropriate over-the-counter (OTC) nicotine replacement therapy (NRT) options for patients. A Cochrane review evaluated evidence supporting the effectiveness of community pharmacists and their role in helping patients achieve smoking cessation. Well-trained, community pharmacists who provide behavioral counseling and education on choosing the appropriate NRT were able to help patients achieve smoking cessation goals. In the community setting, behavioral counseling and education for at least 1 month yielded positive smoking cessation rates.[39,48] Because most smoking cessation products in the United States are widely available OTC, community pharmacists have an opportunity to make a significant impact by helping a patient choose the appropriate NRT agent and dose while also providing the necessary counseling to support the patient (see Chapter 86, "Substance-Related Disorders: Alcohol, Nicotine, and Caffeine").

Antioxidant Vitamins and Minerals

6 Several studies looked at the benefit of antioxidant vitamins and minerals in slowing the progression of AMD.[42] These trials are based on the hypothesis that antioxidant vitamins and minerals may prevent cellular damage in the retina caused by the formation of free radicals through light absorption. Use may benefit patients the most with medium or large drusen and/or GA in at least one eye.

Patient-specific factors must be considered before recommending available antioxidant vitamins and minerals to patients with dry AMD (Table 115-3). AREDS evaluated the effects of high doses of vitamins E, C, and beta-carotene plus zinc (once-daily doses of vitamin E 400 IU, vitamin C 500 mg, beta carotene 15 mg, zinc 80 mg as zinc oxide, and copper 2 mg as cupric oxide) in patients with AMD with an average follow-up of 6.3 years. Compared with placebo, the supplements decreased the progression to visual acuity loss significantly in patients with intermediate and advanced disease in both the wet and dry forms of AMD. Patients with mild or borderline AMD did not demonstrate a benefit. The use of zinc alone in patients with AMD has significantly lowered the risk of progression to advanced AMD.[42]

Previous studies have shown that the use of beta-carotene is associated with an increased risk of lung cancer in smokers, thus

TABLE 115-3 Selected[a] Commercially Available Vitamin Products Useful in Age-Related Macular Degeneration

Brand Names	Active Ingredients	Dosage Forms	Directions
AREDS Formulation			
Preservision AREDS	Vitamin E 400 IU, vitamin C 452 mg, beta carotene 28,640 IU, zinc 69.6 mg as zinc oxide, and copper 1.6 mg as cupric oxide	Softgel, tablet	**Softgels**: 1 softgel twice daily **Tablets**: 2 tablets twice daily
AREDS 2 Formulation			
Preservision AREDS 2	Vitamin E 400 IU, vitamin C 500 mg, zinc 80 mg as zinc oxide, and copper 2 mg as cupric oxide, lutein 10 mg, zeaxanthin 2 mg	Softgel, chewable	1 softgel twice daily
Miscellaneous formulations containing components of the AREDS and AREDS 2 ingredients			
Pro-Optic	Vitamin E 200 IU, vitamin C 500 mg, zinc 25 mg, copper 2 mg, lutein 10 mg, zeaxanthin 2 mg	Capsule	1 capsule daily
Equate Vision Formula with Lutein, Zexanthin & Omega-3 50+	Vitamin E 30 IU, vitamin C 150 mg, zinc 9 mg, copper 1 mg, omega-3 250 mg, lutein 5 mg, zexanthin 1 mg	Tablet, softgel	1 tablet/softgel daily with food
Equate Vision Formula with Lutein	Vitamin A 1,000 IU, vitamin C 200 mg, vitamin E 60 IU, zinc 40 mg, selenium 55 mcg, copper 2 mg, lutein 2 mg	Tablet	1 tablet daily
Visivite AREDS 2 Eye Vitamin	Vitamin C 500 mg, vitamin E 400 IU, zinc 40 mg as zinc oxide, copper 1 mg as copper oxide, lutein 10 mg, zeaxanthin 2 mg	Capsule	1 capsule twice daily with meals
ActiveEyes AREDS 2	Vitamin E 266 mg, vitamin C 500 mg, zinc 80 mg as zinc oxide, copper 2 mg as copper gluconate, lutein 10 mg, zeaxanthin 2 mg (per 2 capsules)	Capsule	1 capsule twice daily
EyePromise AREDS 2	Vitamin C 500 mg, vitamin D3 2,000 IU, vitamin E 400 IU, fish oil EE 250 mg, mixed tocopherols 20 mg, alpha lipoic acid 10 mg, zeaxanthin 10 mg, lutein 10 mg	Softgel	1 softgel twice daily
Viteyes Classic AREDS 2	Vitamin C 500 mg, vitamin E 400 IU, zinc 25 mg as zinc oxide, copper 1.2 mg as cupric oxide, lutein 10 mg, zeaxanthin 2 mg	Capsule	1 capsule twice daily with meals
Dr. Krawitz Eye Vitamins Macular Support	Vitamin E 100IU, vitamin C 500 mg, zinc 40 mg, copper 1 mg, lutein 15 mg, zeaxanthin 3 mg, calcium 115 mg, vitamin B6 20 mg, selenium 200 mcg, bilberry 50 mg, alpha lipoic acid 20 mg, grape seed extract 20 mg, L-gluthione 10 mg	Soy free, GMO free, gluten free, sugar free vegetarian capsule	2 capsules daily
MaxiVision Ocular Formula	Vitamin C 500 mg, vitamin D3 600 IU, vitamin E 400 IU, zinc 25 mg, copper 1.6 mg, lutein 20 mg, zeaxanthin 4 mg	Capsule	2 capsules per day during a meal
Systane I-Caps AREDS	Vitamin E 400 IU, vitamin C 425 mg, beta carotene 28,640 IU, zinc 69.6 mg, copper 1.6 mg	Softgel, coated tablet	1 tablet/softgel twice daily
Systane I-Caps AREDS 2	Vitamin E 400 IU, vitamin C 500 mg, zinc 25 mg, copper 2 mg, lutein 10 mg, zeaxanthin 2 mg	Softgel, chewable tablet	1 softgel/tablet twice daily
Ocuvite Eye Vitamin & Mineral Supplement 50+	Vitamin E 20 mg, vitamin C 150 mg, zinc 9 mg, copper 1 mg, lutein 5 mg, zeaxanthin 1 mg, omega-3 fatty acids 250 mg	Softgel	1 softgel twice daily

[a]Not an all-inclusive list.

limiting its use in this population to nonsmokers only.[49] In the AREDS 2 study, beta-carotene was replaced with lutein 10 mg and zeaxanthin 2 mg; other components of the AREDS formulation of antioxidant vitamins and minerals remained the same. The replacement combination reduced the progression of AMD and therefore would be a reasonable substitute for beta-carotene in patients with AMD who smoke.[50]

The antioxidant property of saffron and its effect on visual acuity in AMD was studied in a small number of patients older than 50 years with mild-to-moderate AMD. Study participants received saffron 20 mg/day for 3 months and were followed for 6 months. Participants who received saffron and the antioxidant vitamin cocktail studied in the AREDS study demonstrated a modest improvement in visual function compared with placebo. Continued study of saffron in a larger sample of this patient population is needed to fully support its use in improving visual acuity in AMD.[51]

Specific Treatments for Wet AMD

Decisions about specific therapies for wet AMD must take into account the risks and benefits of the various therapies and the likelihood of visual recovery. Patients with smaller, more recent drusen are more likely to benefit from therapy. Therapies discussed below—VEGF inhibitors, PDT, and surgical therapy—are specific for wet AMD.

VEGF Inhibitors and Inhibitor-Like Drugs

7 For most patients with wet AMD and CNV, the use of intravitreal VEGF inhibitors and other inhibitor-like drugs has improved visual acuity and decreased blindness in about 50% of treated patients.[41] VEGF is a potent endothelial cell-specific mitogen and vascular permeability factor that is produced by many cells in the body including tumor cells, macrophages, and platelets.[8] As discussed earlier, VEGF-regulated CNV is a major cause of vision loss caused by the growth of new abnormal blood vessels through the Bruch membrane into the subretinal space. VEGF inhibitors play a pivotal role in preventing neovascularization in patients with wet AMD by preventing the growth of new blood vessels into the retina. Inhibition of VEGF in AMD can limit the progression of AMD and stabilize or reverse vision loss. Early initiation of VEGF inhibitors can have a significant effect on vision outcomes. Delay in therapy after early AMD symptoms have appeared has been associated with poor vision outcomes post-VEGF inhibitor initiation.[8]

Three recombinant humanized monoclonal antibodies—bevacizumab, ranibizumab, and brolucizumab-dbll—exert their mechanism of action as VEGF inhibitors. By acting as VEGF inhibitors in AMD, these monoclonal antibodies inhibit neovascularization within the retina by preventing the growth and leakage of new blood vessels into the retina, thus slowing the loss of vision.

Bevacizumab is a humanized monoclonal antibody approved by the US Food and Drug Administration (FDA) for ovarian, non-small-cell lung, glioblastoma, and colorectal cancers and is used off label intravitreally for wet AMD. It exerts its effect on all isoforms of VEGF. Compared with ranibizumab, bevacizumab is much less expensive.[52] Structurally, ranibizumab and bevacizumab are different but related monoclonal antibodies.

Ranibizumab is a fragmented monoclonal antibody that was genetically engineered to have an increased binding affinity for all biologically active forms of VEGF, allowing for increased VEGF inhibition. This is achieved by a modification of the amino acid sequence in ranibizumab.

Studies comparing the efficacy of bevacizumab to ranibizumab given monthly or as needed have found that both drugs improve visual acuity, with no significant differences seen in efficacy.[53,54] Both drugs also demonstrated similar safety data, with no differences seen in mortality, hospitalizations, or atherothrombotic events.

8 Ranibizumab has been studied for efficacy in increasing and maintaining visual acuity using a treat and extend (TREX) approach to dosing compared to the traditional monthly dosing (Table 115-4).

TABLE 115-4 Medications Used in the Treatment of Age-Related Macular Degeneration

Medication	Brand Names	Usual Doses	Notes
Antioxidant Vitamins: described in Table 115-3			
Monoclonal Antibody VEGF Inhibitors: inhibit neovascularization within the retina by preventing the growth and leakage of new blood vessels into the retina			
Bevacizumab	Avastin	Intravitreal: 1.25 mg monthly for 3 months, then may be given monthly or as needed based on monthly ophthalmic assessment	
Ranibizumab	Lucentis	Intravitreal: 0.5 mg once a month (approximately every 28 days) TREX dosing Frequency may be reduced (eg, 4-5 injections over 9 months) after the first 3 injections or may be reduced after the first 4 injections to once every 3 months if monthly injections are not feasible	A regimen averaging 4-5 doses over 9 months is expected to maintain visual acuity and an every 3-month dosing regimen has reportedly resulted in a ~5 letter (1 line) loss of visual acuity over 9 months, as compared to monthly dosing which may result in an additional ~1-2 letter gain
Ranibizumab-nuna	Byooviz	Intravitreal: 0.5 mg once a month (approximately every 28 days) TREX dosing Frequency may be reduced (eg, 4-5 injections over 9 months) after the first 3 injections or may be reduced after the first 4 injections to once every 3 months if monthly injections are not feasible	A regimen averaging 4-5 doses over 9 months is expected to maintain visual acuity and an every 3-month dosing regimen has reportedly resulted in a ~5 letter (1 line) loss of visual acuity over 9 months, as compared to monthly dosing which may result in an additional ~1-2 letter gain
Brolucizumab-dbll	Beovu	Intravitreal: 6 mg once per month (approximately every 25-31 days) for 3 months, followed by 6 mg once every 8 to 12 weeks	
Nonmonoclonal antibody VEGF inhibitors			
Aflibercept	Eylea	Intravitreal: 2 mg once every 4 weeks for the first 12 weeks, followed by 2 mg once every 8 weeks	Some patients may require every 4-week dosing after the first 12 weeks
Pegaptanib[a]	Macugen	Intravitreal: 0.3 mg once every 6 weeks	Does not improve visual acuity in patients with new-onset wet AMD

[a]Pegaptanib is not currently available in the United States.

The appeal of the ranibizumab TREX approach is the reduction of office visits and cost of the medication. Visual acuity was maintained with the TREX approach in patients with wet AMD following the initial monthly injections for 3 months, and costs associated with monthly office visits for treatment and ophthalmic examinations were decreased.[55] The TREX method in patients using ranibizumab is thus preferred over monthly injections.[54,55] Premedication prior to injection is not generally necessary with bevacizumab or ranibizumab.

Brolucizumab-dbll is a humanized single-chain antibody fragment that inhibits the VEGFR-1 and VEGFR-2 receptors by binding to three major VEGF-A isoforms. It is the latest VEGF inhibitor to be approved by FDA. Two studies that established efficacy of brolucizumab-dbll compared the monoclonal antibody to aflibercept for 48 weeks. Both of the studies found brolucizumab-dbll noninferior to the control group with regard to improvement in visual acuity. Doses studied for brolucizumab-dbll were 3 mg and 6 mg given every 12 weeks following an 8-week loading dose phase. If the patient improved or remained stable, doses were continued at 12-week intervals for a total of 48 weeks; if the disease worsened, dosing intervals were reduced to every 8 weeks. The control group was administered aflibercept 2 mg every 8 weeks for the 48-week study period.[56]

In addition to being noninferior to aflibercept, brolucizumab-dbll 6 mg doses were able to maintain the dosing interval at 12 weeks in more than 50% of the study participants throughout the 48-week study period. Additionally, a statistically significant difference was observed in the decrease in visual acuity in patients treated with brolucizumab-dbll 6 mg compared to aflibercept 2 mg after week 16 of the treatment. Overall, the studies concluded that the brolucizumab-dbll treatment is noninferior to aflibercept with improving visual acuity as measured by the mean best-corrected visual acuity change from baseline.[56]

VEGF Inhibitor Biosimilars

Ranibizumab-nuna, the first biosimilar of ranibizumab, was approved by the FDA with indications of dry AMD, macular edema, and myopic CNV. Another biosimilar currently under investigation for approval is bevacizumab-vikg (ONS-5010). The indications being studied for bevacizumab-vikg are dry AMD, DME, and branch retinal vein occlusion.[57]

The VEGF inhibitor drugs aflibercept and pegaptanib are also administered intravitreally in wet AMD. These drugs are pharmacologically classified as VEGF inhibitors and are not monoclonal antibodies such as bevacizumab or ranibizumab. Aflibercept and pegaptanib are primarily used in patients who have an insufficient response in visual acuity improvement to ranibizumab and bevacizumab.

The first VEGF inhibitor approved by the FDA for use in wet AMD was pegaptanib. Pegaptanib was approved by the FDA in 2004. Randomized controlled trials at the time of approval demonstrated efficacy with the 0.3-mg dose injected into the vitreous every 6 weeks, but pegaptanib does not improve visual acuity in patients with new-onset wet AMD compared with other VEGF inhibitors.[8] For these reasons, it is rarely used in clinical practice and has been discontinued in the United States.

Aflibercept is a pan-VEGF-A and placental growth factor blocker that exerts its action in wet AMD by competing for binding with VEGF-A.[8] It was approved by the FDA in 2011.

Aflibercept is dosed by intravitreal injections of three monthly loading doses, followed by 2 mg injected intravitreally every 4 to 8 weeks. While some patients may require every 4-week injections, there was no additional efficacy noted in the clinical trials in doses administered every 4 weeks compared with every 8 weeks. Therefore, in patients receiving aflibercept 2 mg every 8 weeks, the benefit is improvement of visual acuity without the burden and risk of monthly intravitreal injections or monitoring.

Efficacy and safety tolerability are similar between the two VEGF inhibitors, with the advantage being that aflibercept had the potential for a reduced administration schedule at every 2 months and a reduced monthly cost compared with aflibercept. Overall, it is unknown if there is a standard optimal dosing schedule for VEGF inhibitors.

Adherence with these medications is imperative to maintain the visual acuity gains achieved.[58] If therapy is not continued, the gains can be lost. Counseling patients on the importance of adherence, risks of nonadherence, and options if cost is prohibitive are needed for the continued benefit of VEGF therapy.

Agents in the Pipeline

Faracimab is a new agent in development with a combined mechanism of action.[59] In addition to being a VEGF inhibitor targeting VEGF-A, faracimab also inhibits angiopoietin isoform 2 (Ang-2), which is a growth factor in the Ang-Tie pathway, a main pathway involved in angiogenesis.[60] Inhibition of Ang-2 can improve vascular permeability. Several multicenter phase 2 trials have demonstrated the efficacy of faracimab, providing a therapeutic option that may be administered less frequently than monthly ranizumab therapy and maybe more efficacious at improving visual acuity.[61-63]

An ocular implant device designed to provide continuous delivery of ranizumab has recently been approved for use in patients with dry AMD and who has received at least 2 doses of a VEGF inhibitor intravitrealy with an improved response to therapy. Once implanted, the device will deliver a continuous dose of ranizumab. One other advantage to this device is that it only requires refilling every 6 months in a physician's office in a manner similar to receiving a traditional intravitreal injection of ranizumab.[64]

Photodynamic Therapy for Wet AMD

PDT is initiated in patients with wet AMD who fail to demonstrate an improvement in visual acuity with the use of VEGF inhibitors alone. PDT for AMD is performed by the intravenous injection of a photosensitizing dye, verteporfin, followed by activation of the dye using a photo laser applied through the use of a specialized contact lens. A physician then shines a laser into the patient's eye, focused on a localized area. The laser activates the dye, causing the formation of a thromboembolism within the abnormal blood vessels below the macula. The thromboembolism seals off the abnormal blood vessels, preventing further leakage of the fluid into the retina that is causing difficulty in vision.

PDT may be used with or without VEGF inhibitors in patients whose visual acuity has worsened while on treatment with VEGF inhibitors alone.[8] When used at least once in combination with the VEGF inhibitors ranibizumab or bevacizumab, it can help improve and maintain visual acuity with continued VEGF inhibitor administration. Several randomized controlled trials with verteporfin and ranibizumab indicate that the combination therapy of VEGF inhibitors with PDT was more effective in improving and maintaining visual acuity and required fewer PDT treatments than with PDT alone, yet more studies are needed.[8,65]

A meta-analysis of randomized clinical trials comparing the combination therapy of bevacizumab and PDT to bevacizumab monotherapy concluded that patients treated with combination PDT + bevacizumab required significantly less injections of bevacizumab with similar effects on visual acuity improvement and ocular side effects compared to bevacizumab monotherapy.[66] Results have been conflicting with aflibercept plus PDT usage and changes in visual acuity. A randomized trial was unable to demonstrate benefit in combination over monotherapy alone due to insufficient patients meeting criteria for dual therapy.

Side effects of PDT are light sensitivity for several days following the procedure and pain in the eye. Patient counseling should include instructions on avoiding exposure to direct sunlight, wearing dark sunglasses and protective clothing when outside, and using OTC analgesics such as acetaminophen for pain. Patients may experience blurry vision that is temporary and will subside. However, worsening vision or increasing eye pain should be reported to a physician.

Surgical Therapy

Management of AMD using surgical techniques is varied and requires further investigation. Surgical therapy is usually reserved in patients with substantial macular hemorrhages that lack a response to VEGF inhibitor therapy.

The most effective surgery for these patients has been the removal of submacular hemorrhages following the administration of tissue plasminogen activator (tPa) into the retina.[67] Visual acuity improves following surgery; however, it declines over time without the continued use of a VEGF inhibitor to decrease CNV.

Thermal laser photocoagulation is a surgical procedure that involves the use of a thermal laser seal to stop the leakage of fluid from abnormal blood vessel growth under the macula. The heat from the laser seals the abnormal, leaky blood vessels, preventing further fluid leakage and subsequent loss of visual acuity. The negative aspect of this procedure is that it can also destroy surrounding healthy retinal tissue as it seals the leaky blood vessels. Because of this risk, thermal laser photocoagulation is not used to seal vessels located directly under the center of the macula. Thermal laser photocoagulation does not restore vision loss in advanced AMD and should be used as early as possible in therapy to help prevent progression of the disease. Because of these limitations, thermal laser photocoagulation is rarely used in clinical practice.

Antioxidant Vitamins, Beta Carotene, and Zinc

As discussed earlier, antioxidant vitamins and minerals may be useful in delaying progression to advanced AMD in patients with the presence of drusen. The choice of vitamin formulation should be considered based on the patient's history of smoking. Smokers with AMD should be counseled to use only the vitamin formulation that contains lutein and zeaxanthin, whereas nonsmokers can use the formulations containing either beta-carotene or lutein and zeaxanthin. Attention should be paid to amount of vitamin E the patient is consuming daily to avoid vitamin E overdose with the use of other multivitamin supplements.

Daily doses should consist of vitamin C 500 mg, vitamin E 400 IU, lutein 10 mg, zeaxanthin 2 mg, zinc oxide 80 mg, and copper (cupric oxide) 2 mg. Beta-carotene 15 mg may be used in lieu of lutein and zeaxanthin in nonsmokers.

Statin Therapy

The use of statins to prevent the onset of AMD and progression of early AMD to late AMD has been evaluated in several randomized placebo-controlled studies. Epidemiologic data suggest a link between patients with atherosclerotic disease and AMD, and the use of statins may exert a protective effect in patients with AMD.[26,68] The rationale is that drusen are composed of lipid deposits that accumulate within the retinal layers. The effects of statins on drusen are hypothesized to be through a number of different mechanisms. Through the serum lipid lowering, statins may alter the formation of lipid deposits on the Bruch's membrane.[17] Statins may also exert a protective effect against atherosclerosis and AMD by preserving the vascular supply to the outer retina.[18] There may also be an intraocular anti-inflammatory effect through the inhibition of VEGF. In AMD, elevated levels of VEGF may play a role in the development of CNV. Finally, statins may interfere with secretion of metalloproteinases, which when released play a role in the rupture of lipid plaques and neovascular development.[19]

Several studies have examined the effect of statins on preventing or reducing progression of AMD to vision loss. Studies evaluating simvastatin indicated there may be a benefit in patients with early AMD; however, sample sizes were small in one study and in the largest study, 30% of patients were lost to follow-up.[17,20] In both studies, no benefit was observed in patients with advanced AMD to support statin therapy. In a small pilot study of patients with advanced AMD, intensive therapy with atorvastatin 80 mg daily indicated a possible regression in drusen size and vision improvement, but a larger study should be conducted to confirm these effects.[21]

Overall, statin therapy is not recommended for the treatment of patients with AMD alone, as results from larger studies would be needed to support use.[8] Statins may be used in AMD patients with other indications such as a diagnoses of atherosclerosis, coronary artery disease, or hyperlipidemia.

Prevention of AMD

Antioxidant vitamins and minerals have not been proven to prevent the onset of AMD in patients with risk factors such as drusen.[69] One trial indicated that there may be some benefit in the use of B vitamins in preventing the onset of AMD. The study compared folic acid 2.5 mg/day, pyridoxine 50 mg/day, and cyanocobalamin 1 mg/day to placebo in women with an increased risk of cardiovascular disease without AMD. After 7 years of follow-up, more women in the placebo group had evidence of AMD compared to the treatment group. Additional studies with larger patient populations are needed to confirm these results. However, it is promising that the use of B vitamins may be beneficial in reducing the risk of AMD in women with cardiovascular disease.[70]

Diets rich in the omega-3 fatty acids, eicosapentaenoic acid (EPA), and docosahexaenoic acid (DHA) found in fish and plant-based omega-3 FA, such as alpha-linolenic acid (ALA), may play a role in decreasing the progression to advanced AMD in patients with intermediate AMD, as seen in several subsets of studies.[8] However, there is insufficient evidence to say that dietary modification can prevent AMD formation.[8,71]

As previously discussed, smoking cessation is imperative (Table 115-1).

EVALUATION OF THERAPEUTIC OUTCOMES

The overall goal of therapy for macular degeneration is to prevent vision loss through slowing down progression of the disease and preserving visual acuity.

9 VEGF inhibitors and antioxidant vitamins and minerals are the only pharmacologic therapies available that have been shown to improve and stabilize visual acuity in patients with intermediate to advanced AMD. It is important to counsel the patient when discussing the treatment options that they are not curative and may only serve to improve visual acuity from baseline. Current pharmacologic therapy options will require repeated long-term administration to maintain visual acuity.

No pharmacologic therapy has been shown to prevent AMD in patients with high-risk factors for development. Studies are conflicting regarding the implementation of a diet high in omega-3 fatty acids such as EPA and DHA found in fish and plant-based omega 3 fatty acid supplements, such as ALA for prevention of AMD. More studies are needed to fully support this indication.

CONCLUSION

Age-related macular degeneration remains one of the leading causes of blindness globally. Its impact on the QOL of the aging adult can be tremendous. Early detection of this disease is the key to preserving visual acuity and allows early initiation of pharmacologic therapy to help stabilize and slow vision loss.

ABBREVIATIONS

ALA	alpha-linolenic acid
AMD	age-related macular degeneration
AREDS	Age-Related Eye Disease Study
CFH	complement factor H
CNV	choroidal neovascularization
DHA	docosahexaenoic acid
EPA	eicosapentaenoic acid
FA	fatty acid
FDA	Food and Drug Administration
GA	geographic atrophy
HtrA1	ARMS2/HtrA serine peptidase 1
LIPC	hepatic lipase
NRT	nicotine replacement therapy
OTC	over the counter
PDT	photodynamic therapy
QOL	quality of life
RPE	retinal pigment epithelium
TLR3	toll-like receptor 3
TREX	treat and extend
US	United States
VEGF	vascular endothelial growth factor

REFERENCES

1. Shah N, Dakin SC, Dobinson S, Tufail A, Egan CA, Anderson RS. Visual acuity loss in patients with age-related macular degeneration measured using a novel high-pass letter chart. *Br J Ophthalmol.* 2016;100(10):1346–1352. Available at: https://www.ncbi.nlm.nih.gov/pubmed/26846435.
2. Hunt LA, Nijjar B, Stead A. Chapter 14: Sensory function, function related to the skin and pain: Health conditions. In: Bonder B, Bello-Haas VD, eds. *Functional Performance in Older Adults*. Philadelphia, PA: F. A. Davis Company; 2018.
3. Mathew R, Sivaprasad S, Augsburger JJ, Corrêa ZM. Retina. In: Riordan-Eva P, Augsburger JJ, eds. *Vaughan & Asbury's General Ophthalmology*. 19th ed. New York, NY: McGraw-Hill. Available at: http://accessmedicine.mhmedical.com.proxy.library.vcu.edu/content.aspx?bookid=2186§ionid=165517649.
4. Horton J. Disorders of the eye. In: Jameson J, Fauci AS, Kasper DL, Hauser SL, Longo DL, Loscalzo J, eds. *Harrison's Principles of Internal Medicine*. 20th ed. New York, NY: McGraw-Hill. Available at: http://accessmedicine.mhmedical.com.proxy.library.vcu.edu/content.aspx?bookid=2129§ionid=192011900.
5. Chang DF. Ophthalmologic examination. In: Riordan-Eva PAJ, ed. *Vaughan & Asbury's General Ophthalmology*. 19th ed. New York, NY: McGraw-Hill. Available at: http://accessmedicine.mhmedical.com.proxy.library.vcu.edu/content.aspx?bookid=2186§ionid=165516032.
6. Wong WL, Su X, Li X, et al. Global prevalence of age-related macular degeneration and disease burden projection for 2020 and 2040: A systematic review and meta-analysis. *Lancet Glob Health.* 2014;2(2):106. Accessed December 30, 2021. doi:10.1016/S2214-109X(13)70145-1.
7. Chou R, Dana T, Bougatsos C, Grusing S, Blazina I. Screening for impaired visual acuity in older adults: Updated evidence report and systematic review for the US preventive services task force. *JAMA.* 2016;315(9):915–933. Accessed December 30, 2021. doi:10.1001/jama.2016.0783.
8. American Academy of Ophthalmology Retina/Vitreous Panel. *Age-Related Macular Degeneration Preferred Practice Pattern®*. San Francisco, CA: American Academy of Ophthalmology; 2019. Updated November 2021. Available at: https://www.aao.org/Assets/ca4e92da-1e00-470b-aa28-56ed2bac2efb/637714766764570000/age-related-macular-degeneration-ppp-2021-update-pdf.
9. Bressler SB, Muñoz B, Solomon SD, West SK. Racial differences in the prevalence of age-related macular degeneration: The salisbury eye evaluation (SEE) project. *Arch Ophthalmol.* 2008;126(2):241–245. Accessed December 30, 2021. doi:10.1001/archophthalmol.2007.53.
10. Jonas JB, Bourne RRA, White RA, et al. Visual impairment and blindness due to macular diseases globally: A systematic review and meta-analysis. *Am J Ophthalmol.* 2014;158(4):808–815. Accessed December 30, 2021. doi:10.1016/j.ajo.2014.06.012.
11. Al-Zamil WM, Yassin SA. Recent developments in age-related macular degeneration: A review. *Clin Interv Aging.* 2017;12:1313. Accessed December 30, 2021. doi:10.2147/CIA.S143508.
12. Kahn HA, Leibowitz HM, Ganley JP, et al. The framingham eye study. I. Outline and major prevalence findings. *Am J Epidemiol.* 1977;106(1):17–32. Accessed December 30, 2021.
13. Kumaramanickavel G. Age-related macular degeneration: Genetics and biology. *Asia Pac J Ophthalmol (Phila).* 2016;5(4):229–235. Available at: https://www.ncbi.nlm.nih.gov/pubmed/27488064.
14. Chew EY, Klein ML, Clemons TE, Agrón E, Abecasis GR. Genetic testing in persons with age-related macular degeneration and the use of the AREDS supplements: To test or not to test? *Ophthalmology.* 2015;122(1):212–215. Available at: https://www.clinicalkey.es/playcontent/1-s2.0-S0161642014010124.
15. Wittes J, Musch DC. Should we test for genotype in deciding on age-related eye disease study supplementation? *Ophthalmology.* 2015;122(1):3–5. Available at: https://www.clinicalkey.es/playcontent/1-s2.0-S0161642014010392.
16. Adams A, Gelles EB. *Letters.* New York, NY: Library of America; 2016;275:1386–1387. Available at: https://www.ncbi.nlm.nih.gov/pmc/articles/PMC1772857/.
17. US Department of Health & Human Services. The health consequences of Smoking—50 years of progress: A report of the surgeon general, 2014 | SurgeonGeneral.gov. Available at: https://www.surgeongeneral.gov/library/reports/50-years-of-progress/index.html. Updated 2014. Accessed December 30, 2021.
18. Products CfT. Labeling—cigarette graphic health warnings. Web site. Available at: https://www.fda.gov/tobaccoproducts/labeling/labeling/ucm257774.htm. Accessed December 30, 2021.
19. Ranard KM, Jeon S, Mohn ES, Griffiths JC, Johnson EJ, Erdman JW. Dietary guidance for lutein: Consideration for intake recommendations is scientifically supported. *Eur J Nutr.* 2017;56(suppl 3):37–42. Accessed December 30, 2021. doi:10.1007/s00394-017-1580-2.
20. de Koning-Backus APM, Buitendijk GHS, Kiefte-de Jong JC, et al. Intake of vegetables, fruit, and fish is beneficial for age-related macular degeneration. *Am J Ophthalmol.* 2018. Accessed December 30, 2021. doi:10.1016/j.ajo.2018.09.036.
21. Chew EY, Clemons TE, Sangiovanni JP. Lutein + zeaxanthin and omega-3 fatty acids for age-related macular degeneration: The age-related eye disease study 2 (AREDS2) randomized clinical trial. *JAMA.* 2013;309(19): Available at: http://parlinfo.aph.gov.au/parlInfo/search/display/display.w3p;query=library/jrnart/2465549.
22. Zampatti S, Ricci F, Cusumano A, Marsella LT, Novelli G, Giardina E. Review of nutrient actions on age-related macular degeneration. *Nutr Res.* 2014;34(2):95–105. Available at: https://www.clinicalkey.es/playcontent/1-s2.0-S0271531713002674.
23. Gopinath B, Liew G, Kifley A, et al. Association of dietary nitrate intake with the 15-year incidence of age-related macular degeneration. *J Acad Nutr Diet.* 2018. Available at: https://jandonline.org/article/S2212-2672(18)30276-4/fulltext.
24. Wu J, Uchino M, Sastry SM, Schaumberg DA. Age-related macular degeneration and the incidence of cardiovascular disease: A systematic review and meta-analysis. *PLoS ONE.* 2014;9(3):e89600. Available at: https://www.openaire.eu/search/publication?articleId=dedup_wf_001::591efe6bcfc631a2f27e50df59cf19dc.
25. McGuinness MB, Le J, Mitchell P, et al. Physical activity and age-related macular degeneration: A systematic literature review and meta-analysis. *Am J Ophthalmol.* 2017;180:29–38. Available at: https://www.clinicalkey.es/playcontent/1-s2.0-S0002939417302180.
26. Ma L, Wang Y, Du J, Wang M, Zhang R, Fu Y. The association between statin use and risk of age-related macular degeneration. *Sci Rep.* 2015;5:18280. Accessed December 30, 2021. doi:10.1038/srep18280.
27. Ye J, Xu YF, He JJ, Lou LX. Association between aspirin use and age-related macular degeneration: A meta-analysis. *Invest Ophthalmol Vis Sci.* 2014;55(4):2687–2696. doi:10.1167/iovs.13-13206.
28. Klein BEK, Howard KP, Iyengar SK, et al. Sunlight exposure, pigmentation, and incident age-related macular degeneration. *Invest Ophthalmol Vis Sci.* 2014;55(9):5855–5861. Accessed December 30, 2021.
29. Gopinath B, Liew G, Kifley A, Mitchell P. Thyroid dysfunction and ten-year incidence of age-related macular degeneration. *Invest Ophthalmol Vis Sci.* 2016;57(13):5273–5277. Accessed December 30, 2021. doi:10.1167/iovs.16-19735.
30. Klein R, Myers CE, Klein BE. Vasodilators, blood pressure-lowering medications, and age-related macular degeneration: The Beaver Dam Eye Study [published correction appears in *Ophthalmology.* 2016

Apr;123(4):923]. *Ophthalmology*. 2014;121(8):1604–1611. doi:10.1016/j.ophtha.2014.03.005.
31. Modenese A, Gobba F. Macular degeneration and occupational risk factors: A systematic review. *Int Arch Occup Environ Health*. 2019;92(1):1–11. doi:10.1007/s00420-018-1355-y.
32. Montgomery MP, Postel E, Umbach DM, et al. Pesticide use and age-related macular degeneration in the agricultural health study. *Environ Health Perspect*. 2017;125(7):077013. Accessed December 30, 2021. doi:10.1289/EHP793.
33. Center of Excellence for Transgender Health, Department of Family and Community Medicine, University of California San Francisco, ed. *Guidelines for the primary and gender-affirming care of transgender and gender nonbinary people*. 2nd ed.; 2016. Deutsch M.B., ed. Available at: www.transhealth.ucsf.edu/guidelines.
34. Jager MJ. Macrophages and macular degeneration. *J Ophthalmic Vis Res*. 2014;9(1):1–2. Available at: https://www.ncbi.nlm.nih.gov/pmc/articles/PMC4074466/.
35. Zając-Pytrus HM, Pilecka A, Turno-Kręcicka A, Adamiec-Mroczek J, Misiuk-Hojło M. The dry form of age-related macular degeneration (AMD): The current concepts of pathogenesis and prospects for treatment.. *Adv Clin Exp Med*. 2015;24(6):1099–1104. doi:10.17219/acem/27093.
36. Chatziralli I, Mitropoulos P, Parikakis E, Niakas D, Labiris G. Risk factors for poor quality of life among patients with age-related macular degeneration. *Semin Ophthalmol*. 2017;32(6):772–780. Available at: https://doi-org.proxy.library.vcu.edu/10.1080/08820538.2016.1181192.
37. Dillon L, Gandhi S, Tang D, et al. Perspectives of people with late age-related macular degeneration on mental health and mental wellbeing programmes: A qualitative study. *Ophthalmic Physiol Opt*. 2021;41(2):255–265. doi:10.1111/opo.12779.
38. Xin X, Sun Y, Li S, Xu H, Zhang D. Age-related macular degeneration and the risk of all-cause and cardiovascular mortality: A meta-analysis of cohort studies. *Retina*. 2018;38(3):497–507. doi:10.1097/IAE.0000000000001741.
39. Sadda SR, Chakravarthy U, Birch DG, Staurenghi G, Henry EC, Brittain C. Clinical endpoints for the study of geographic atrophy secondary to age-related macular degeneration. *Retina (Philadelphia, Pa.)*. 2016;36(10):1806–1822. Available at: https://www.ncbi.nlm.nih.gov/pubmed/27652913.
40. Spaide RF, Jaffe GJ, Sarraf D, et al. Consensus Nomenclature for Reporting Neovascular Age-Related Macular Degeneration Data: Consensus on Neovascular Age-Related Macular Degeneration Nomenclature Study Group [published correction appears in Ophthalmology. 2020 Oct;127(10):1434-1435]. *Ophthalmology*. 2020;127(5):616–636. doi:10.1016/j.ophtha.2019.11.004.
41. Sloan FA, Hanrahan BW. The effects of technological advances on outcomes for elderly persons with exudative age-related macular degeneration. *JAMA Ophthalmology*. 2014;132(4):456–463. http://dx.doi.org/10.1001/jamaophthalmol.2013.7647. doi:10.1001/jamaophthalmol.2013.7647.
42. Age-Related Eye Disease Study Research Group. A randomized, placebo-controlled, clinical trial of high-dose supplementation with vitamins C and E, beta carotene, and zinc for age-related macular degeneration and vision loss: AREDS report no. 8. *Arch Ophthalmol*. 2001;119(10):1417–1436. Accessed December 30, 2021.
43. Curcio CA, Messinger JD, Sloan KR, McGwin G, Medeiros NE, Spaide RF. Subretinal drusenoid deposits in non-neovascular age-related macular degeneration: Morphology, prevalence, topography, and biogenesis model. *Retina (Philadelphia, Pa.)*. 2013;33(2):265–276. Available at: https://www.ncbi.nlm.nih.gov/pubmed/23266879.
44. Sarks J, Arnold J, Ho I, Sarks S, Killingsworth M. Evolution of reticular pseudodrusen. *Br J Ophthalmol*. 2011;95(7):979–985. Available at: https://www.ncbi.nlm.nih.gov/pubmed/21109695.
45. Zweifel SA, Imamura Y, Spaide TC, Fujiwara T, Spaide RF. Prevalence and significance of subretinal drusenoid deposits (reticular pseudodrusen) in age-related macular degeneration. *Ophthalmology*. 2010;117(9):1775–1781. Available at: https://www.clinicalkey.es/playcontent/1-s2.0-S0161642010000552.
46. Ueda-Arakawa N, Ooto S, Tsujikawa A, Yamashiro K, Oishi A, Yoshimura N. Sensitivity and specificity of detecting reticular pseudodrusen in multimodal imaging in Japanese patients. *Retina (Philadelphia, Pa.)*. 2013;33(3):490–497. Available at: https://www.ncbi.nlm.nih.gov/pubmed/23403515.
47. Ferris FL, Davis MD, Clemons TE, et al. A simplified severity scale for age-related macular degeneration: AREDS report no. 18. *Arch Ophthalmol*. 2005;123(11):1570–1574. Available at: http://dx.doi.org/10.1001/archopht.123.11.1570.
48. Sinclair HK, Bond CM, Stead LF. Community pharmacy personnel interventions for smoking cessation. *Cochrane Database Syst Rev*. 2004;1:CD003698. Available at: https://www.ncbi.nlm.nih.gov/pubmed/14974031.
49. Druesne-Pecollo N, Latino-Martel P, Norat T, et al. Beta-carotene supplementation and cancer risk: A systematic review and meta-analysis of randomized controlled trials. *Int J Cancer*. 2010;127(1):172–184. Available at: https://onlinelibrary.wiley.com/doi/abs/10.1002/ijc.25008.
50. Chew EY, Clemons T, et al. AREDS2 Research Group. The age-related eye disease study 2 (AREDS2): Study design and baseline characteristics (AREDS2 report number 1). *Ophthalmology*. 2012;119(11):2282–2289.
51. Broadhead GK, Grigg JR, McCluskey P, Hong T, Schlub TE, Chang AA. Saffron therapy for the treatment of mild/moderate age-related macular degeneration: A randomised clinical trial. *Graefe's archive for clinical and experimental ophthalmology = Albrecht von Graefes Archiv fur klinische und experimentelle Ophthalmologie*. 2018;1–10. Available at: https://www.ncbi.nlm.nih.gov/pubmed/30343354.
52. Brown GC, Brown MM, Rapuano S, Boyer D. Cost-utility analysis of VEGF inhibitors for treating neovascular age-related macular degeneration. *Am J Ophthalmol*. 2020;218:225–241. doi:10.1016/j.ajo.2020.05.029.
53. Berg K, Pedersen TR, Sandvik L, Bragadóttir R. Comparison of ranibizumab and bevacizumab for neovascular age-related macular degeneration according to LUCAS treat-and-extend protocol. *Ophthalmology*. 2015;122(1):146–152. Available at: doi:10.1016/j.ophtha.2014.07.041. https://www.clinicalkey.es/playcontent/1-s2.0-S016164201400685X.
54. Wykoff CC, Croft DE, Brown DM, et al. Prospective trial of treat-and-extend versus monthly dosing for neovascular age-related macular degeneration: TREX-AMD 1-year results. *Ophthalmology*. 2015;122(12):2514. Available at: https://www.ncbi.nlm.nih.gov/pubmed/26391465.
55. Silva R, Berta A, Larsen M, Macfadden W, Feller C, Monés J. Treat-and-extend versus monthly regimen in neovascular age-related macular degeneration. *Ophthalmology*. 2018;125(1):57–65. Available at: https://www.sciencedirect.com/science/article/pii/S0161642017310254.
56. Dugel PU, Koh A, Ogura Y, et al. HAWK and HARRIER: Phase 3, Multicenter, Randomized, Double-Masked Trials of Brolucizumab for Neovascular Age-Related Macular Degeneration. *Ophthalmology*. 2020;127(1):72–84. doi:10.1016/j.ophtha.2019.04.017.
57. Outlook Therapeutics. ONS-5010/LYTENAVATM OVERVIEW. https://outlooktherapeutics.com/lytenava-overview/. Published 2019. Accessed December 7, 2021.
58. Ehlken C, Helms M, Böhringer D, Agostini HT, Stahl A. Association of treatment adherence with real-life VA outcomes in AMD, DME, and BRVO patients. *Clin Ophthalmol*. 2018;12:13–20.
59. Nicolò M, Ferro Desideri L, Vagge A, Traverso CE. Faricimab: An investigational agent targeting the Tie-2/angiopoietin pathway and VEGF-A for the treatment of retinal diseases. *Expert Opin Investig Drugs*. 2021;30(3):193–200. doi:10.1080/13543784.2021.1879791.
60. Akwii RG, Sajib MS, Zahra FT, Mikelis CM. Role of angiopoietin-2 in vascular physiology and pathophysiology. *Cells*. 2019;8(5):471. https://doi.org/10.3390/cells8050471.
61. Sahni J, Dugel PU, Patel SS, et al. Safety and efficacy of different doses and regimens of faricimab vs ranibizumab in neovascular age-related macular degeneration: The AVENUE Phase 2 randomized clinical trial. *JAMA Ophthalmol*. 2020;138(9):955–963. doi:10.1001/jamaophthalmol.2020.2685.
62. Khanani AM, Patel SS, Ferrone PJ, et al. Efficacy of Every four monthly and quarterly dosing of faricimab vs ranibizumab in neovascular age-related macular degeneration: The STAIRWAY Phase 2 randomized clinical trial. *JAMA Ophthalmol*. 2020;138(9):964–972. doi:10.1001/jamaophthalmol.2020.2699.
63. Sahni J, Patel SS, Dugel PU, Khanani AM, Jhaveri CD, Wykoff CC, Hershberger VS, Pauly-Evers M, Sadikhov S, Szczesny P, Schwab D, Nogoceke E, Osborne A, Weikert R, Fauser S. Simultaneous inhibition of angiopoietin-2 and vascular endothelial growth factor-A with faricimab in diabetic macular edema: BOULEVARD phase 2 randomized trial. *Ophthalmology*. 2019;126(8):1155–1170. doi:10.1016/j.ophtha.2019.03.023. Epub 2019 Mar 21. PMID: 30905643.
64. SUSVIMO [package insert]. South San Francisco, CA: Genentech, Inc: 2021. Accessed December 30, 2021. Available at: https://www.susvimo-hcp.com/.
65. Su Y, Wu J, Gu Y. Photodynamic therapy in combination with ranibizumab versus ranibizumab monotherapy for wet age-related macular degeneration: A systematic review and meta-analysis. *Photodiagnosis Photodyn Ther*. 2018;22:263–273. doi:10.1016/j.pdpdt.2018.05.002.

66. Wei Q, Liu J, Liu Q, et al. Combination of bevacizumab and photodynamic therapy vs. bevacizumab monotherapy for the treatment of wet age-related macular degeneration: A meta-analysis of randomized controlled trials. *Exp Ther Med.* 2018;16(2):1187–1194. doi:10.3892/etm.2018.6305.
67. Chang W, Garg SJ, Maturi R, et al. Management of thick submacular hemorrhage with subretinal tissue plasminogen activator and pneumatic displacement for age-related macular degeneration. *Am J Ophthalmol.* 2014;157(6):1250–1257. Available at: https://www.clinicalkey.es/playcontent/1-s2.0-S0002939414000701.
68. Vavvas DG, Daniels AB, Kapsala ZG, et al. Regression of some high-risk features of age-related macular degeneration (AMD) in patients receiving intensive statin treatment. *EBioMedicine.* 2016;5:198–203. Available at: https://www.sciencedirect.com/science/article/pii/S2352396416300299.
69. Evans JR, Lawrenson JG. Antioxidant vitamin and mineral supplements for preventing age-related macular degeneration. *Cochrane Database Syst Rev.* 2017;7:CD000253. Available at: https://www.ncbi.nlm.nih.gov/pubmed/28756617.
70. Christen WG, Glynn RJ, Chew EY, Albert CM, Manson JE. Folic acid, vitamin B6, and vitamin B12 in combination and age-related macular degeneration in a randomized trial of women. *Arch Intern Med.* 2009;169(4):335–341.
71. Lawrenson JG, Evans JR. Omega 3 fatty acids for preventing or slowing the progression of age-related macular degeneration. *The Cochrane Database of Syst Rev.* 2015;(4):CD010015. Available at: https://www.ncbi.nlm.nih.gov/pubmed/25856365.

Drug-Induced Ophthalmic Disorders

e116

Rena A. Gosser

KEY CONCEPTS

1. The eye is highly susceptible to drug toxicity due to its extensive vasculature.
2. When ophthalmic disorders occur, all medications and biologic agents, irrespective of the route of administration, are potential causes.
3. It is difficult to fully quantify the incidence of drug-induced ophthalmic disorders due to the variety of causative factors and side-effect reporting behaviors of clinicians.
4. The most common drug-induced ophthalmic disorders include dry eye, cataract, intraoperative floppy iris syndrome, optic neuropathy, and retinopathy.
5. The severity of drug-induced ophthalmic disorders varies and depends on dose, pharmacokinetics, genetic predisposition, age, extremes of body weight, and/or duration of exposure.
6. Health professionals and patients should discuss potential drug-induced ophthalmic disorders to ensure awareness, prompt identification, management, and treatment.

BEYOND THE BOOK

Watch the following videos available from the US National Library of Medicine MedlinePlus for a brief overview of the anatomy and function of the eye. These videos provide the necessary foundation and will assist in understanding the mechanisms of drug-induced ophthalmic disorders.

Seeing: https://medlineplus.gov/ency/anatomyvideos/000109.htm (3:22)

Blinking: https://medlineplus.gov/ency/anatomyvideos/000010.htm (1:01)

INTRODUCTION

1 The eye is an important, complex organ of the nervous system. It is composed of specialized tissues and complex structures that collectively contribute to the body's ability to visually process the environment (Fig. e116-1).[1–3] The sequence for normal, functioning eyes begins with the eyelid, which opens to allow exposure to light, bathes the eye with tear film, and helps remove waste. The eye receives light through the cornea, a clear tissue at the front of the eye. The light then proceeds through the aqueous humor and enters the pupil. The light continues through the pupil, which regulates the amount of light entering the eye to the lens. The lens changes thickness and shape to bend the received light and send it through the vitreous humor to the retina at the back of the eye.[1–3] The retina then transforms the light into electrical impulses, which travel through the optic nerve to the brain. The brain then translates these impulses into the image that is seen. The function of each structure of the eye is summarized in Table e116-1.[2,3]

1 2 Disruption at any structure or step in the process can lead to dysfunction of the eye. This can result from many factors. Exposure to toxic substances, including medications, is one such cause of dysfunction. The combination of a rich blood supply and extensive vasculature allows for ocular exposure to systemically administered medication. The blood-aqueous and blood-retinal barriers are capable of keeping most compounds away from the eye; however, some medications are able to bypass the junctions within cells and reach the eye.[4] The eye is the second most common organ to display drug toxicities, with the liver considered most common.[5]

3 It is difficult to accurately quantify the incidence of drug-induced ophthalmic disorders overall.[4,6] All medications have the potential to induce side effects, irrespective of the mode of administration. Side effects may range from mild to severe and can affect any area of the eye. Many but not all drug-induced ophthalmic disorders are well documented in the literature; lack of clinician or patient reports is a limiting factor. Despite any potential gaps in the literature, it is important to establish causality between an ophthalmic side effect and medication use. A popular tool used by clinicians to establish the likelihood of causality is the adverse drug reaction probability scale, commonly known as the Naranjo scale.[7] The Naranjo scale is composed of scored questions the clinician should use to assess an adverse drug reaction. Categories of definite, probable, possible, and doubtful are assigned based on the score.[7]

This chapter will discuss drug-induced ophthalmic disorders seen with commonly prescribed medications in clinical practice. A review of drug-induced glaucoma will not be covered in this chapter, as it is discussed in Chapter 114, "Glaucoma."

DRUG-INDUCED OPHTHALMIC REACTIONS

Dry Eye Disease

4 Dry eye disease (DED), also known as dry eye syndrome or keratoconjunctivitis sicca, is a common ophthalmic disorder that affects the quality of life for millions of people around the world.[6,8]

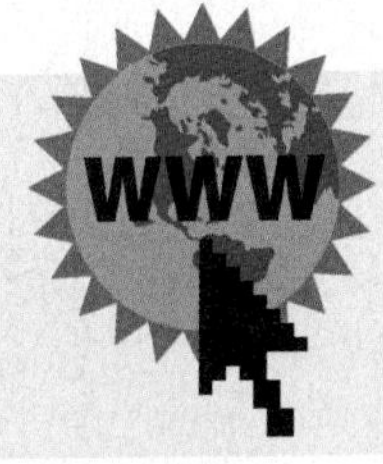

The complete chapter, learning objectives, and other resources can be found at **www.pharmacotherapyonline.com.**

117 Acne Vulgaris

Debra Sibbald and Cathryn Sibbald

KEY CONCEPTS

1. Acne is a highly prevalent disorder affecting adolescents and adults, with a large psychosocial impact.
2. The etiology of this complex disease originates from multiple causative and contributory factors, including genetics and environment. The diagnosis is based on the patient's history and clinical presentation.
3. Acne is a disease of the pilosebaceous unit. Elements of pathogenesis involve defects in epidermal keratinization, androgen secretion, sebaceous function, bacterial growth, inflammation, and immunity.
4. Acne vulgaris is a chronic disorder which cannot be "cured." Goals of treatment and prevention include control and alleviation of symptoms by reducing the number and severity of lesions, slowing progression, limiting disease duration and recurrence, prevention of long-term disfigurement associated with scarring and hyperpigmentation, and avoidance of psychologic suffering. Targeting goals may increase patient adherence to therapy.
5. The most critical target for treatment is the microcomedone. Minimizing or reversing follicular occlusion will arrest the pathogenic acne cascade and involve combining treatment measures to target all pathogenic elements.
6. Nondrug measures are aimed at long-term prevention and treatment. Patients should eliminate aggravating factors, maintain a balanced, low-glycemic load diet, and control stress. Cleanse twice daily with mild soap or soapless cleanser and use only oil-free cosmetics. Comedone extraction in approximately 10% of patients produces immediate cosmetic improvement. Shave infrequently as possible, using a sharp blade or electric razor.
7. First-, second-, and third-line therapies should be appropriate for the severity and staging of the clinical presentation and directed toward control and prevention.
8. Treatment regimens should be tapered over time, adjusting to response. Combine the smallest number of agents at the lowest possible dosages to ensure efficacy, safety, avoidance of resistance, and patient adherence.
9. Once control is achieved, maintenance regimens should be simplified to continue with some suppressive therapy. Therapy must be continued beyond 8 weeks: efficacy is assessed through comedonal and inflammatory lesion count, control or progression of severity, and management of associated anxiety or depression. Safety end points include monitoring for treatment adverse effects.
10. Motivate the patient to continue long-term therapy through empathic and informative counseling.

BEYOND THE BOOK

Watch the video entitled "Acne" by Dr Sheilagh Maguiness, pediatric dermatologist, available on the Society for Pediatric Dermatology Website (https://tinyurl.com/saa9t4s). This 5-minute video provides a brief overview regarding information patients need to know about acne vulgaris. The video is useful to enhance student understanding regarding what information to provide to patients regarding causes of acne, triggers, cleansing, over-the-counter and prescription options, directions for use, and precautions. It gives a brief summary of take-home points useful to direct counseling.

INTRODUCTION

In this chapter, we review the latest developments in understanding acne vulgaris and its treatment. The contents provide an analysis of the physiology of the pilosebaceous unit; the epidemiology, etiology, and pathophysiology of acne; relevant treatment with nondrug measures; and comparisons of pharmacologic agents, including drugs of choice recommended in best-practice guidelines. Options include a variety of alternatives such as retinoids, antimicrobial agents, hormones, and light therapy. Formulation principles are discussed in relation to drug delivery. Patient assessment, general approaches to individualized therapy plans, and monitoring evaluation strategies are presented.

EPIDEMIOLOGY

1 Acne vulgaris is a chronic disease and the most common one treated by dermatologists. There is a high degree of variability in prevalence, age of onset, distribution, severity, and age of resolution.

The lifetime prevalence of acne approaches 90%, with the highest incidence in adolescents; it affects 9.4% of the general population, with trends reflecting higher rates in urban areas compared to rural villages, although these rates are subject to selection and detection bias due to differential access to providers.[1]

The onset of acne vulgaris during puberty occurs at a younger chronologic age in girls than boys (12% age 25-58 vs 3% in males of the same age) and periodic premenstrual flares may continue until menopause. It is triggered in children by the initiation of androgen production by the adrenal glands and gonads, and it usually subsides after the end of growth. However, to some degree, most patients continue to have symptoms into their mid-twenties, and there is evidence that the duration of acne may last into middle age for most women, recorded in 54% of women and 40% of men older than 25 years of age.[2] In puberty, acne is often more severe in boys in about 15% of cases, which is 10-fold greater than in girls. Women often have more severe forms during adulthood. When untreated, acne usually lasts for several years until it spontaneously remits. After the disease has ended, scars and dyspigmentation are not uncommon permanent negative outcomes.

Genetic factors have been recognized; there is a high concordance among identical twins, and there is also a tendency toward severe acne in patients with a positive family history of acne.

There are believed to be no gender differences in acne prevalence. A systematic review included five studies, with a pooled odds ratio of 1.07 (95% CI 0.42-2.7, males with reference to females), suggesting only a slightly higher odds in males.[3]

An international group of epidemiologists, community medicine specialists, and anthropologists have questioned whether acne might be predominantly a disease of Western civilization.[4] They assert that since acne vulgaris is nearly universal in westernized societies (afflicting 79%-95% of the adolescent population), one causative factor might be the Western glycemic diet. While this hypothesis is based on the observation that primitive societies subsisting on traditional (low glycemic) diets have no acne, the theory awaits validation and acceptance by the dermatologic community.

ETIOLOGY

2 Acne is a multifactorial disease. Genetic, racial, hormonal, dietary, and environmental factors have been implicated in its development. Its psychologic impact can be severe.

Four major etiologic factors are involved in the development of acne: increased sebum production, due to hormonal influences; alteration in the keratinization process and hyperproliferation of ductal epidermis; bacterial colonization of the duct with *Propionibacterium acnes*; and production of inflammation with release of inflammatory mediators in acne sites. These are reviewed in the "Pathophysiology" section later in this chapter.

The role of heredity in acne has not been clearly defined; however, there is a significant tendency toward more serious involvement if one or both parents had severe acne during their youth.

Environmental factors play a major role in determining the severity and extent of acne and may influence the choice of topical treatments. Heat and humidity may induce comedones; pressure or friction caused by protective devices such as helmets, shoulder pads, or pillows, and excessive scrubbing or washing can exacerbate existing acne by causing microcomedones to rupture. Pressure may cause acne lesions to form in patients who do not have acne vulgaris: this variant is called *mechanical acne*. Friction, wool, or other rough textured fabrics and occlusive clothing may also be mechanical irritants. Hair styles that are low on the forehead or neck may cause excessive sweating and occlusion, exacerbating acne. In most cases acne is worse in winter and improves during the summer, suggesting a salutary effect of sunlight. However, in some cases, exposure to sunlight worsens the disease.[5] Studies examining the relationship between tobacco smoking and acne show inconsistent results; however, dermatologists have begun to counsel people to quit tobacco smoking as a potential auxiliary treatment for acne.

The importance of psychologic factors in this prolonged and capricious condition has been repeatedly stressed. Two-thirds of affected teenagers wish that they could speak with their physician and healthcare provider about acne, but only one-third do. Emotions, such as intense anger and stress, can exacerbate acne, causing flares or increasing mechanical manipulation: picking, excoriating, or pinching lesions sometimes subconsciously or in sleep. This is probably the result of increased glucocorticoid secretion by the adrenal glands, which appears to potentiate the effects of androgens.[6]

Dietary influences Current investigations explore associations between dietary influences and acne. Under study are dietary influences as factors in acne development as well as potential treatment modalities. This follows the dismissal of overinterpreted 40-year-old, poorly designed studies that disavowed potential effects of dietary ingestions on acne.[7-9] Three primary influences on development include dairy and growth factors in milk; whey protein in milk; and hyperglycemic-load diets.

A series of studies have linked consumption of dairy products with acne.[10,11] Acne has been positively associated with the reported quantity of milk ingested, particularly skim milk.[12] The Nurses Health Retrospective Study examining diet during high school in 47,355 women found an association between acne and milk intake, suggesting natural hormonal components of milk and/or other bioactive molecules in milk could exacerbate acne.[13]

Lactoferrin is a whey milk protein with anti-inflammatory activity. Lactoferrin-enriched fermented milk ameliorated acne vulgaris, selectively decreasing triacylglycerols in skin surface lipids.[13] Lactoferrin administered as a dietary supplement twice daily in mild-to-moderate acne vulgaris led to an overall improvement in acne lesion counts in adolescents and young adults.[14]

A meta-analysis of observational studies examined association of dairy intake and acne in children, adolescents, and young adults. Any dairy product—including milk, yogurt, and cheese—was associated with an increased odds ratio for acne in individuals aged 7 to 30 years; however, studies were heterogeneous in design, making comparisons difficult.[15]

Other studies suggest a role for insulin-like growth factor (IGF), increased by ingestion of high glycemic loads.[16,17] The strongest evidence supports a high-glycemic-load (HGL) diet as a significant factor in acne. In a randomized controlled trial, patients who eliminated high glycemic index foods showed a significant reduction in acne. Those who consumed a low-glycemic-load diet compared with a conventional HGL diet had improvements of facial acne after 12 weeks. Accompanying changes in physical and endocrinologic parameters suggest that decreases in total energy intake, body weight, and indices of androgenicity and insulin resistance may also be associated with observed improvements in acne.[18] Another study reported an improvement in acne and insulin sensitivity in low-glycemic-load diets compared with controls, suggesting nutrition-related lifestyle factors play a role in acne etiology.[19] Independent effects of weight loss versus dietary intervention need to be isolated. In an Australian study, participants who consumed low-glycemic-load diets had no reported cases of acne.[12]

Other studies showed correlations between increases in the ratio of saturated to monoun-saturated fatty acids, acne lesion counts, and increased sebum outflow, suggesting a possible role of desaturase enzymes in sebaceous lipogenesis and the clinical manifestation of acne. These require further investigation.[20]

Univariate and multivariate analyses were used to examine results of a 2015 French survey of individuals (age 15-24 years) reporting or not reporting acne with associated epidemiologic variables. Daily consumption of chocolate and sweets (odds ratio 2.38) and regular use of cannabis (odds ratio 2.88) was independently and highly associated with acne. Smoking tobacco (>10 cigarettes daily) was highly protective. Respective roles of sugar, lipids, and milk were not investigated.[21]

The role of dietary factors in the development or progression of acne vulgaris cannot be dismissed. The practical recommendations would be to avoid excess sugar and skim milk. Further studies are ongoing, including reviewing antioxidants from nutritional and topical sources and probiotics as potential acne-fighting agents.[12]

PATHOPHYSIOLOGY

3 The pathogenesis of acne includes hyperseborrhea, abnormal follicular keratinization, and *Propionibacterium acnes* proliferation in the pilosebaceous unit. Recent research has shed some new light on the involvement of the sebaceous gland, as well as on the pro-inflammatory activity of the cutaneous microbiome. Acne progresses through the following four major stages:

1. Increased sebum production by the sebaceous gland
2. *P. acnes* follicular colonization (and bacterial lipolysis of sebum triglycerides to free fatty acids)
3. Release of inflammatory mediators
4. Increased follicular keratinization

Improved understanding of acne development on a molecular level suggests that acne is a disease that involves both innate and adaptive immune systems and inflammatory events. Receptors that regulate sebaceous lipid metabolism work in concert with receptors regulating epidermal growth and differentiation. Acne can be considered as a model of immune-mediated chronic inflammatory skin disease: an innate immune response that is not able to control *P. acnes* followed by a Th1-mediated adaptive immune response that becomes self-maintaining independently from *P. acnes* itself.[22]

Acne usually begins in the prepubertal period, when the adrenal glands mature, and progresses as androgen production and sebaceous gland activity increase with gonad development. During puberty, alteration of the sebaceous lipid profile, called dysseborrhea, together with stress, irritation, cosmetics, and potential dietary factors lead to inflammation and formation of different types of acne lesions.[23]

As shown in Fig. 117-1, acne results from the development of an obstructed sebaceous follicle, called a *microcomedone*. Sebaceous glands increase their size and activity in response to circulating androgens. Most patients with acne do not overproduce androgens (with some exceptions); instead, they have sebaceous glands that are hyperresponsive to androgens.[24] Patients with acne have a significantly greater number of lobules per gland compared with unaffected individuals.

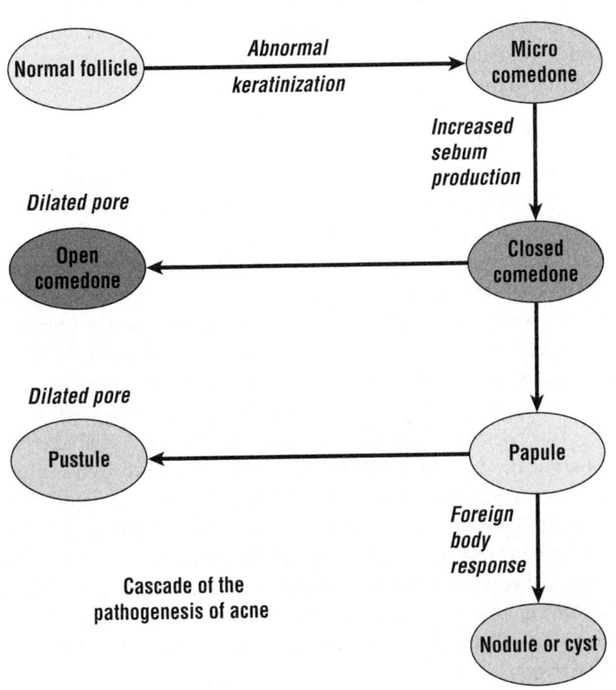

FIGURE 117-1 Cascade of the pathogenesis of acne. *(Reprinted, with permission, from Mills OH, Kligman AM. Comedogenicity of sunscreens: Experimental observations in rabbits. Arch Dermatol. 1982;18(6):417-419.)*

Sebum production is induced by different receptors expressed by the sebaceous gland. Involved are the histamine receptor (activated by histamines); the hormonal DHT receptor (activated by androgens); the neuromodulator receptor (mainly substance P); and corticotrophin-releasing hormone (CRH) receptor (mainly activated by stress); molecular research has identified three other receptors that are expressed by the sebocyte and control sebum production. Each of these newly identified receptors is activated by a dietary substance.[23]

The peroxisome proliferator-activated receptors are stimulated by free fatty acids and cholesterol, which act in concert with retinoid X receptors to regulate epidermal growth and differentiation as well as lipid metabolism.

The insulin-like growth factor (IGF)-1 receptor is stimulated by sugar to increase lipid formation, mediated by sterol response element binding proteins. The leptin receptor is stimulated by fat. Leptin is responsible for creating lipid droplets within the sebocyte and induces pro-inflammatory enzyme and cytokine (interleukin [IL]-6 and IL-8) secretion as well.[23]

The sebaceous gland also acts as an endocrine organ in response to changes in androgens and other hormones. Oxidized squalene can stimulate hyperproliferative behavior of keratinocytes, and lipoperoxides produce leukotriene B4, a powerful chemoattractant.[24] The composition of sebum is changed, with a reduction in linoleic acid. The growth of keratinocytes changes. The infrainfundibulum increases its keratinization of cells with hypercornification and development of the microcomedone, the primary lesion of both noninflammatory and inflammatory acne.[22] Cells adhere to each other in an expanding mass, which forms a dense keratinous plug. Androgen hormones could be a stimulus to pilosebaceous duct hypercornification. Sebum, produced in increasing amounts by the active gland, becomes trapped behind the keratin plug and solidifies, contributing to open or closed comedone formation.

Interleukin-1-α upregulation contributes to the development of comedones independently of colonization with *P. acnes*. A relative linoleic acid deficiency has also been described.[24]

A prominent role is played by the follicular colonization by *P. acnes*. *P. acnes* displays several activities which promote the development of acne lesions, including the promotion of follicular hyperkeratinization; the induction of sebogenesis; and the stimulation of an inflammatory response by the secretion of proinflammatory molecules and by the activation of innate immunity, followed by a *P. acnes*–specific adaptive immune response. In addition, *P. acnes*–independent inflammation mediated by androgens or by a neurogenic activation, followed by the secretion in the skin of proinflammatory neuropeptides, can occur in acne lesions.[22]

The pooling of sebum in the follicle provides ideal substrate conditions for proliferation of the anaerobic bacterium *P. acnes*, generating a T-cell response, which results in inflammation.[25] *P. acnes* produces a lipase that hydrolyzes sebum triglycerides into free fatty acids. These free fatty acids may trigger the changes that lead to an increase in keratinization and microcomedone formation.[26,27] This closed comedone, or whitehead, is the first clinically visible lesion of acne. It takes approximately 5 months to develop. The closed comedone is almost completely obstructed to drainage and has a tendency to rupture.[28-30]

As the plug extends to the upper canal and dilates its opening, an open comedone, or blackhead, is formed. Its dark color is not due to dirt but to either oxidized lipid and melanin or to the impacted mass of horny cells. The cylindrically shaped, open comedone is very stable and may persist for a long time as soluble substances and liquid sebum escape more easily. Acne that is characterized by open and closed comedones is termed *noninflammatory acne*.

Acne produces chemotactic factors and promotes the synthesis of tumor factor-α and interleukin-1β. Cytokine induction by *P. acnes* occurs. Both recruitment of polymorphs into the follicle during the inflammatory process and release of *P. acnes*–generated chemokines lead to pus formation. The pus eventually bursts on the surface with resolution of the inflammation or into the dermis. *P. acnes* also produces enzymes that increase the permeability of the follicular wall, causing it to rupture, releasing keratin, hair, and lipids and irritating free fatty acids into the dermis. Several different types of inflammatory lesions may form, including pustules, nodules, and cysts and may lead to scarring.

Postinflammatory hyperpigmentation (PIH) and scarring are two sequelae of acne. A time delay of up to 3 years between acne onset and adequate treatment correlates to degree of scarring and emphasizes the need for early therapy.[7,8]

CLINICAL PRESENTATION

To correctly diagnose acne vulgaris, the clinician considers patient assessment, which includes distinguishing all the presenting signs and symptoms of the clinical presentation, reviewing diagnostic and assessment considerations (see Clinical Presentation box), as well as considering psychosocial issues, differential diagnosis, and the possibility of drug-induced acne.

Psychosocial Issues

Acne causes profound negative psychological and social effects on the quality of life (QOL) of patients. Assessment of acne's impact on QOL is an important consideration in clinical decision-making. The negative impact of facial acne is one of the primary motivators for patients to seek and to adhere to treatment.[34] The European Dermatology Forum S3-Guideline for the Treatment of Acne recommended adopting a QOL measure as an integral part of acne management.[35] Specific QOL indicators represent patients' perceptions of and reactions to their health. Assessing QOL impairment in patients with acne may aid in management by evaluating psychologic impact, which may not correlate with clinical severity; aid in detection of depression or need for psychologic care; and improve therapeutic outcomes.

Acne adversely affects all aspects of QOL. In addition to documentation regarding acne-specific QOL impairment, acne impact on general health and psychologic status has been assessed for relationship between sociodemographic variables, disease severity, and mental status on QOL of acne sufferers. In a report of 195 cases, acne impact on health status was worse compared to other chronic diseases. Authors concluded acne is not a minor disease in comparison with other chronic conditions. Age of onset is capable to influence general health quality (GHQ status), which in turn affects QOL.[36] Patients with acne experience functioning and emotional effects from their skin disease comparable with those experienced by patients with psoriasis, and patients with severe acne reported levels of social, psychological, and emotional problems as great as those reported by patients with chronic disabling asthma, epilepsy, diabetes, back pain, or arthritis.[35]

The European Academy of Dermatology and Venereology Task Force on QOL and Patient Oriented Outcomes and the Task Force on Acne, Rosacea and Hidradenitis Suppurativa have documented the QOL instruments that have been used in acne patients, with information on validation, purposes of their usage, description of common limitations and mistakes in their usage, and overall recommendations.[35]

There are many global scales that have been used to evaluate acne. Some include the World Health Organization Quality of Life (WHOQOL), Skindex,[37] the Dermatology QOL Index,[38] and the Children's Dermatology Life Quality Index (CDLQI). Examples of acne-specific scales include the Acne-specific QOL questionnaire,[39] the Acne QOL Scale,[40] the Acne Disability Index (ADI), and the Cardiff Acne Disability Index (CADI).[35] The Acne QOL Scale was developed to measure the impact of facial acne across four domains (acne symptoms, role-emotional, self-perception, and role-social) of health-related QOL. Health-state utilities (such as time trade-off [TTO]) are quantitative measures of patient preferences of health outcomes ranging from 0 (death) to 1 (perfect health) and can be used in clinical trials as outcome measures of treatment effects. TTO utilities for acne in the range of 0.94 to 0.96 can be compared with those of other diseases (eg, 0.92 for epilepsy, 0.94 for myopia), and help to identify the impact of acne on self-perception and psychologic functioning.[41]

Differential Diagnosis

Acne vulgaris is rarely misdiagnosed. The conditions most commonly mistaken for acne vulgaris include rosacea, perioral dermatitis, gram-negative folliculitis, and drug-induced acne.[42]

Acne rosacea (adult acne) is a chronic, progressive relapsing condition occurring after age of 30 years in fair-complexioned persons. The diagnosis is clinical and based on history and physical findings. There are four subtypes: erythematotelangiectatic changes (erythema, flushing, telangiectasia [spider veins], stinging and burning); progressing to papular-pustular changes (inflammatory lesions, with edema, papules, and pustules on central facial areas such as nose, cheeks, chin, and forehead); phymatous changes (thickened skin and prominent pores on nose, ears, chin, and eyelids); and ocular changes (foreign body sensation, dryness, burning, eyelid erythema).

Rosacea has key differences from acne vulgaris. Onset is not linked to androgens or endocrine changes; and comedones are not usually present. Aggravating factors include endogenous triggers: ingestion of alcohol, spicy foods, or hot drinks (especially those containing caffeine), smoking; and exogenous triggers: overexposure to sunlight; exposure to temperature extremes, heat and humidity, friction, irritating cosmetics, and steroids. Treatment may include antibiotics, particularly doxycycline (low, anti-inflammatory dose) or erythromycin, topical metronidazole, pimecrolimus or azelaic acid as well as agents to reduce erythema (alpha adrenergics).[43]

Perioral dermatitis occurs primarily in young women and adolescents and is characterized by erythema, scaling, and papulopustular lesions commonly clustered around the nasolabial folds, mouth, and chin. The cause is unknown.[44]

Gram-negative folliculitis (*Proteus, Pseudomonas, Klebsiella*) may complicate acne, with a sudden change to pustules or large inflammatory cysts occurring after long-term treatment of acne with oral antibiotics. Folliculitis may be caused by staphylococci. There is a sudden onset of superficial pustules around the nose, chin, and cheeks. Patients with suspected folliculitis should be referred.[45]

Several conditions include acne vulgaris as a characteristic component, and understanding the mechanisms involved in these syndromes provides insight into the pathogenesis of acne. These include polycystic ovary syndrome (elevated androgen levels); PAPA syndrome (pyogenic arthritis, pyoderma gangrenosum, acne; early onset arthritis with increased inflammatory activity), and SAPHO syndrome (synovitis, acne, pustulosis, hyperostosis, osteitis syndrome; sterile inflammatory arthro-osteitis, with *P. acnes* as a possible trigger).[25]

Drug-Induced Acne

In addition to the conditions induced by drugs that are presented in Chapter e121, "Drug-Induced Dermatologic Disorders," acneiform eruptions can also be caused by medications. Drug-induced acne is monomorphic, either comedonal with some inflammation

CLINICAL PRESENTATION Acne Vulgaris

Lesion Type: Acne Vulgaris Can Be Noninflammatory or Inflammatory

- Noninflammatory acne is characterized by open and closed comedones that develop from the subclinical microcomedo
- The closed comedo is visible as a 1 to 2 mm whitehead most easily seen when the skin is stretched. It is often inconspicuous with no visible follicular opening
  - Is the first clinical sign of acne
  - Has a tendency to rupture
- The open comedo or blackhead is large, approximately 2 to 5 mm, and dark-topped with contents extruding
  - is relatively stable
- Inflammatory acne is traditionally characterized as having papulopustular and/or nodular lesions, which may arise from the microcomedo or from noninflammatory clinically apparent lesions
- A pustule is formed from a superficial aggregation of neutrophils
  - Appears as a raised white lesion filled with pus, usually less than 5 mm in diameter
  - Superficial pustules usually resolve within a few days without scarring
- A nodule is produced through deeper, dermal, inflammatory infiltration
  - Is the most severe variant of acne
  - Appears as warm, tender, firm lesions, with a diameter of 5 mm or greater
  - May be suppurative or hemorrhagic within the dermis, may involve adjacent follicles and sometimes extend down to fat
- Cysts are suppurative nodules named because they resemble inflamed epidermal cysts
  - Cystic acne may show double comedones, resulting from prior inflammation and fistulous links between neighboring sebaceous units
- Progression of inflammatory lesions
  - Pustules and cysts often rupture spontaneously and drain a purulent or bloody but odorless discharge[31]
  - Inflammatory lesions may itch as they erupt and can be tender or painful. Nodules may develop exudative sinus tracts resulting in tissue destruction
  - Often resolution of these lesions leaves erythematous or pigmented macules that can persist for months or longer, especially in dark-skinned individuals
- Nodules and deep lesions may result in scarring

Regions of Involvement

- Acne lesions can occur anywhere on the body apart from the palms and soles
  - Are usually located on the face, back, neck, shoulders, and chest
  - May extend to buttocks or extremities
- One or more anatomic areas may be involved in any given patient
- The pattern of involvement, once present, tends to remain constant
- Comedones frequently have a midfacial distribution in childhood and, when evident early, are indicative of a poor prognosis
- Skin, scalp, and hair are frequently oily

Severity Grading Taxonomies

US Food and Drug Administration (FDA) Investigator Global Assessment 2005[31]

Type 1	Almost clear: rare noninflammatory lesions with no more than 1 small IL
Type 2	Mild, some noninflammatory lesions, no more than a few inflammatory lesions (papules/pustules only, no nodules)
Type 3	Moderate: many noninflammatory lesions, some inflammatory lesions, no more than one nodule
Type 4	Severe: up to many noninflammatory and inflammatory lesions, but no more than a few nodular lesions

European Union Guidelines Clinical Classification[32,33]

I	Comedonal acne
II	Mild-to-moderate papulopustular (MMPP) acne
III	Severe papulopustular acne, moderate nodular acne (*this level combines FDA types 3 and 4, above*)
IV	Severe nodular acne, conglobate acne (*this is an additional level beyond the FDA types above*)

Diagnostic and Assessment Considerations

Palliating factors	Sunlight
Provoking factors	Premenstrual flares, humid environments, excessive sweating; exposure to chemicals; occlusive clothing; friction; oily cosmetics; manual manipulation; stress; diet (high glycemic load, dairy)
Associated symptoms	Itch, pain, fever
Medical conditions	May contribute to or coexist with acne, including endocrine factors (eg, irregular menses, hirsutism, alopecia), pregnancy, atopy
Allergies	May cause acne symptoms, or present a contraindication to therapy
Medication history	Products may cause or interact with acne signs and symptoms
Social habits	Diet or smoking
Family history	Genetic predisposition to acne
Psychosocial issues	Assess global and disease-specific quality of life (QOL) indicators or health-state utilities

or papular–pustular. Drugs most commonly implicated in inducing comedonal/inflammatory acne include those with hormonal effects (steroids, OCP), halogens (iodide, bromide), vitamins (B_2, B_6, B_{12}), tuberculostatic drugs (isoniazid, ethambutol), lithium salts, antiepileptics (phenytoin), cyclosporine, and azathioprine. Drugs that most commonly induce papular–pustular reactions include anti-inflammatory medications (NSAIDs), sulfamethoxazole–trimethoprim, cephalosporins, and diltiazem.

Systemic corticosteroids can cause a pustular inflammatory form of acne, especially on the trunk. Onset is abrupt at 2 to 6 weeks after initiation of therapy. Acne has also been associated with most of the potent topical steroids, but not with hydrocortisone, which lacks the ability to inhibit protein synthesis. Discontinuation of the steroid results in an initial worsening of appearance due to removal of the anti-inflammatory action of the steroid itself. Caution patients about this reaction, which can be subdued through judicious use of topical hydrocortisone.[44-47]

Antiepileptics and tuberculostatics are the most commonly implicated in drug-induced acne, followed by lithium. Other heavy metals inducing acne include cobalt (in vitamin B_{12}).[48] Halogens, especially an excess of iodide in seafood, salt, and health foods, can exacerbate acne. In addition, halogens can provoke de novo acne lesions in individuals who have increased external exposure often due to occupational contact, or pool or hot tub disinfection; this variant is called *chloracne*.

In addition, certain minor ingredients in cosmetics have been implicated in cosmetic acne, including isopropyl myristate, cocoa butter, and fatty acids.

TREATMENT

The first step in determining a safe and efficacious treatment regimen for acne vulgaris is to establish desired outcomes for the patient, regarding both short- and long-term goals.

Desired Outcomes (Goals of Treatment)

4 Acne vulgaris is treated as a chronic disease, as it demonstrates typical chronicity characteristics: manifests as either acute outbreaks or slow onset; patterns of recurrence or relapse; a prolonged course; and psychologic and social impact. There are two governing principles: the chronic nature warrants early and aggressive treatment, and maintenance therapy is often needed for optimal outcomes.

Acne requires long-term control. This must be stressed with the patient to encourage adherence to lengthy treatment regimens, which address management of current symptoms and signs and preventive measures.

Basic goals of treatment include alleviation of symptoms by reducing the number and severity of lesions (objective and subjective grading) and improving appearance, slowing progression, limiting duration and recurrence, prevention of long-term disfigurement associated with scarring and hyperpigmentation, and avoidance of psychologic suffering.

A significant percentage change in lesion counts is desirable: most patients empirically validate a margin of 10% to 15% reduction in facial lesion counts as appropriate. Patient global self-assessment of acne improvement is a primary outcome.

General Approach to Treatment

5 The most critical treatment target is the microcomedone. Eliminating follicular occlusion will arrest the whole acne cascade. Nondrug and pharmacologic treatment and preventive measures should be directed toward cleansing, reducing triggers, and combination therapy targeting all four pathogenic mechanisms. Combination therapy is often more effective than single therapy and may decrease side effects and minimize resistance or tolerance to individual treatments.

The approach to acne management is largely determined by:

1. Severity index
2. Lesion type: predominantly noninflammatory or inflammatory
3. Treatment preferences including patient choices
4. Cost implications
5. Skin type and/or ethnic group
6. Patient age
7. Adherence
8. Response to previous therapy
9. Presence of scarring
10. Psychologic effects
11. Family history of persistent acne

Topical therapy is the standard of care for mild-to-moderate acne. Those with moderate-to-severe acne will require systemic therapy.

Topical treatments work only where applied. To reduce new lesion development, they must be applied to the entire affected area rather than individual spots. Most cause initial skin irritation, which may result in nonadherence or discontinuation. Irritation can be minimized by starting with lower strengths and gradually increasing frequency or dose. Where irritation persists, changing formulation from alcoholic solutions to washes, gels, or more moisturizing creams or lotions might help.

6 7 First-line, second-line, and third-line therapies should be selected and altered as appropriate for the severity and staging of the clinical presentation. Treatment is directed at control, not cure. Regimens should be tapered over time, adjusting to response. Combine the smallest number of agents at the lowest possible dosages to ensure efficacy, safety, avoidance of resistance, and patient adherence. Once control is achieved, simplify the regimen but continue with some suppressive therapy. As it takes 8 weeks for a microcomedone to mature, therapy must be continued beyond this duration to assess efficacy. With the exception of topical antibiotics, most topical preparations may be used for years as needed.

Lesions typically recur for years. Microcomedones significantly decrease during therapy but rebound almost immediately after therapy is discontinued. The strategy for treating acne includes an induction phase followed by a maintenance phase, further supported by adjunctive treatments and/or cosmetic routines. Routine maintenance therapy involves regular use of appropriate agents to ensure remission and reduce potential for recurrence of visible lesions.

For successful long-term treatment, maintenance therapy must be tolerable, appropriate for the patient's lifestyle and convenience, continuing months to years, depending on age. Education about pathophysiology of acne and the psychosocial benefits of clearer skin are compelling reasons for patient adherence to consistent therapy to sustain remission.

Nonpharmacologic Therapy

8 9 Encourage patients with acne to discontinue or avoid aggravating factors, including occlusion from mechanical factors or cosmetics, maintain a balanced, low-glycemic-load diet, and control stress. By being empathic and informative during counseling, the health professional may motivate the patient to continue long-term therapy.[1,4,43] One of the first approaches to nondrug management of acne is attention to cleansing techniques. Shaving recommendations, comedone extraction, dietary considerations, issues relating to ultraviolet light, and prevention of cosmetic acne should be reviewed with patients.

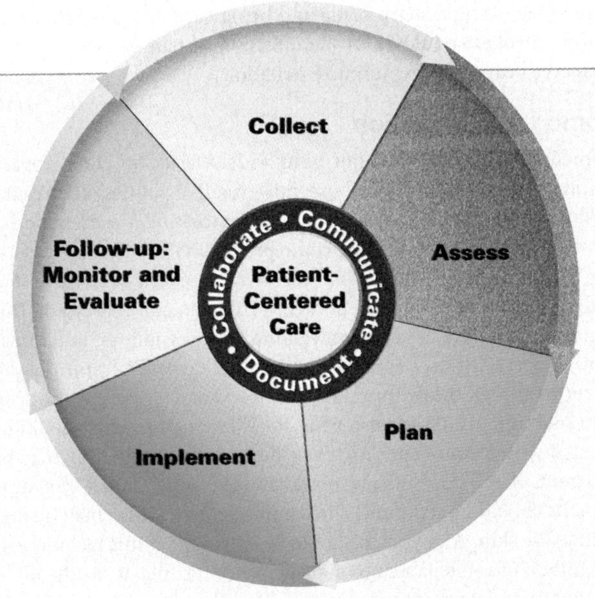

Patient Care Process for Acne Vulgaris

The image shows the five fundamental steps included in The Pharmacist's Care Process endorsed by the Joint Commission for Pharmacy Practitioners (2014). The tagline of this process reads collaborate, communicate, and document. The five fundamental steps listed here are collect, assess, plan, implement, and follow-up: monitor and evaluate. All these steps are listed in a circular block diagram.

Collect

- Patient characteristics (eg, age, race, sex, weight [body mass index], pregnant)
- Patient medical history (personal and family history, especially of acne or scarring, adrenal abnormalities)
- Social history (eg, psychosocial issues) and dietary habits including intake of glycemic foods, dairy, and sugary drinks (see Clinical Presentation/Diagnostic and Assessment Considerations; also section "Etiology")
- Current medications including OTC drug and nondrug measures, prescription drugs (eg, contraceptives) sunscreens, herbal products, dietary supplements, and prior acne medication use
- Current cosmetic use, including makeup, coverups, and cleansers
- Current use of devices (eg, comedone extractors)
- Inhaled systemic or contact allergies to drugs, cosmetics, foods, vehicle ingredients or excipients
- Objective data
  - o Fitzpatrick phototype
  - o Labs if relevant to monitoring for hepatic or renal function

Assess

- Presence of provoking factors or contributing factors (see Clinical Presentation/Diagnostic and Assessment Considerations) (eg, hormonal or adrenal anomalies: presence of vellus hair on females; in children: early age of onset [age 1-7 years], body odor, hair in axillary and pubic areas; and adrenal: rapid growth in children)
- Severity: number, type, and region of lesions; presence of scarring
- Hyperpigmentation of healed lesions (postinflammatory hyperpigmentation)
- Ability/willingness to adhere to long-term therapy
- Emotional status (eg, presence of anxiety, depression)

Plan*

- Goals: clear existing and prevent new lesions; reduce scarring, hyperpigmentation, and psychological impact
- Discontinuation of provoking habits, botanicals, or drug or nondrug measures
- Cleansing routine
- Drug therapy regimen including dietary, nonpharmacologic, and pharmacologic approaches
- Monitoring parameters including efficacy (eg, improvement or resolution of lesions and time frame) and safety (eg, sign and symptoms worsening, irritation, or allergy); frequency and timing of follow-up
- Patient education (eg, purpose of treatment, dietary and lifestyle modification, drug-specific information, medication administration, or application technique)
- Self-monitoring for resolution of acne symptoms, occurrence of scarring, when to seek emergency medical attention
- Referrals to other providers when appropriate (eg, behavioral health, dietitian)

Implement*

- Provide patient education regarding all elements of treatment plan
- Use motivational interviewing and coaching strategies to maximize adherence
- Schedule follow-up, adherence assessment

Follow-up: Monitor and Evaluate

- Improvement or resolution of acne symptoms (eg, noninflammatory or inflammatory lesions)
- Prevention of complications (eg, scarring, infection)
- Slow progression
- Presence of adverse effects
- Patient adherence to treatment plan using multiple sources of information
- Reevaluate duration of therapy every 3 months

**Collaborate with patient, caregivers, and other healthcare professionals.*

Cleansing

A systematic review of clinical evidence for washing and cleansers reported that they are common interventions. Cleansers are indicated in all patients with acne. However, the clinical evidence for their efficacy is not well understood.[49]

Twice-daily face washing may be superior to either once-daily or more frequent washing. Washing too frequently in an attempt to remove surface oils has no added benefit and is not likely helpful, as surface lipids do not affect acne. Contributory lipids are deep in the follicle and are not removed through washing. Antiseptic cleansers, while producing a clean, refreshed feeling, remove only surface dirt, oil, and aerobic bacteria. They do not affect *P. acnes*. Patients should wash no more than twice daily with a mild, nonfragranced opaque or glycerin soap or a soapless cleanser.

Bar soaps are subclassified into true soaps, comprising an alkali and a fatty acid, syndet bars, which use synthetic surfactants, and combars, which include features of both. A study has suggested syndet bars may be superior to true soaps as an acne vulgaris cleansing agent.[50]

Soapless cleansers are an alternative to soaps.[51] Soaps are the most widely used cleansing products, but do not lend themselves to efficient delivery of active drug. Two main disadvantages exist. As soaps are rinsed off, the deposit of active agent is limited, and the high pH required in soaps may degrade some active ingredients and be less tolerable on sensitive skin. Soaps produce a drying effect on the skin due to detergent action. As medicated cleansers require increased contact time, this drying action is pronounced, especially with peeling agents.

Gentle liquid cleansers often contain surfactant systems to remove dirt, sebum, bacteria, and corneocytes from the skin surface. Oil is dispersed from the skin into the surfactant system; however, the active ingredient is sometimes trapped and removed upon rinsing. The balance between cleanliness and drying or irritation should also be considered. Most patients prefer products with foaming action, and these must contain additional secondary surfactants to enhance the foam and condition the skin.

There is no evidence that any particular washing regimen is superior. Evidence-based studies on the use of cleanser or medicated cleansers are lacking or poorly designed with small numbers of patients.[52] It is also difficult to compare studies of different nonprescription formulations even when the same active ingredient is used, as differences in the composition of vehicle may affect cutaneous penetration and vehicles themselves may affect acne. Avoid cream-based cleansers. Scrubbing should be minimized to prevent follicular rupture.

Because the acid pH of skin has an antimicrobial effect, it has been proposed that lowering lesional surface pH (with products such as Herpifix, marketed in Europe) may be correlated to the number of acne lesions. Studies are planned.

Synthetic polyester cleansing sponges abrade the skin surface, removing superficial debris. Considering the structure of comedones, they are unlikely to unseat these lesions. Sponges are available in soft or coarse textures, with or without soap. Circular or rubbing motions will increase irritation. Instruct patients to use single, gentle, continuous strokes on each side of the face, from the midline out toward the ears.

Cationic-bond strips are activated by water. As the strip dries, the cation bonds with the anionic dirt and oil in the pores and removes it when the strip is peeled off.

Shaving

Boys and men with acne should try electric and safety razors to determine which is more comfortable for shaving. When using a safety razor, the beard should be softened with soap and warm water or shaving gel. Shaving should be done as lightly and infrequently as possible, using a sharp blade and being careful to avoid nicking lesions. Strokes should be in the direction of hair growth, shaving each area only once, to minimize irritation.

Comedone Extraction

Comedone extraction has not been widely tested in clinical trials despite long-standing clinical use; however, it is painless and results in immediate cosmetic improvement. Pretreatment with a peeler for 4 to 6 weeks often facilitates the procedure.[47] Following cleansing with hot water, a comedone extractor is placed over the lesion and gentle pressure applied until the contents are expressed. This removes unsightly lesions, preventing progression to inflammation. A correctly sized extractor allows the central keratin plug to extrude through the opening. The small end of a plastic eye dropper, with bulb removed, may also be used. These instruments should be cleaned with alcohol after each use. Some initial reddening may be apparent. If the contents are not expressed with modest pressure, patients should not continue since improper extraction may further irritate the skin. A physician should be consulted if this technique is too difficult for the patient to manage. Since the follicle is difficult to remove completely, comedones may recur between 25 and 50 days following expression. Fewer than 10% of comedone extractions are a complete success, but the process is useful when done properly.[31]

Comedo removal may be helpful in the management of comedones resistant to other therapies. While the procedure cannot affect the clinical course of the disease, it can improve the patient's appearance, which may encourage adherence with the treatment program.

Ultraviolet Light

Although ultraviolet light was recommended in the past for desquamation, the practice is no longer advisable because of the well-established carcinogenic and photoaging effects of ultraviolet exposure. Moreover, inflamed skin is more susceptible to the damaging effects of ultraviolet light. Patients taking tretinoin may show heightened sensitivity.[52]

Before exposure to sunlight, patients with acne should apply sunscreens (sun protection factor [SPF] 15) in alcohol- or oil-free bases and avoid using the acnegenic benzophenones. Sunscreen should be applied as the first product.

Prevention of Cosmetic Acne

Persistent low-grade acne is frequently caused by heavy cosmetic use in women after their mid-twenties. Adolescent acne in younger women may be exacerbated with makeup overuse. The problem is perpetuated when resultant blemishes are concealed with more cosmetics.

Patients should be advised to discontinue oil-containing cosmetics and avoid cosmetic multistep regimens applying various cream-based cleansers and cover-ups. These are commercially advertised and often available with promotional bonuses through Internet shopping. Three-step basic systems usually combine medicated and nonmedicated ingredients. The product names used in marketing these preparations may not make apparent the inclusion of therapeutic agents. Initial steps usually involve cleansers, in lotions or creams, which may contain a multitude of unnecessary ingredients, including medicated peelers, oils, fragrances, and preservatives. Active ingredients including salicylic acid, sulfur, or benzoyl peroxide are often included in subtherapeutic or low doses. The second step is generally a water- or alcohol-based "toner" or "refresher," which might contain medicated mild comedolytic agents such as α-hydroxy acids (eg, glycolic acid), or even a humectant such as glycerin. The final product, often called intensive or repairing solutions, usually contains the lowest strength of peelers such as benzoyl peroxide, sulfur, or salicylic acid; plus potentially sensitizing fragrances and preservatives; or oil-soluble sunscreens not identified on the label. Bases may have significant oil content. There may be additional products such as masks or spot treatments that supplement the base routine of three steps. Multiple-step cosmetic programs are often costly and should be avoided in favor of simple cleansers and more effective single-ingredient peelers at optimal concentrations.

The term *noncomedogenic* may refer to either water-based vehicles or products that are free of substances known to induce comedones. They are not necessarily oil-free. Water-based cosmetics may contain significant amounts of oil in the form of undiluted vegetable oils, lanolin, fatty acid esters (butyl stearate, isopropyl myristate), fatty acids (stearic acid), fatty acid alcohols, cocoa butter, coconut oil, red veterinary petrolatum, and sunscreens containing benzophenones. Water-based products are more likely to contribute to pore blockage than oil-free products.

Oil-free makeups are well tolerated and lipstick, eye shadow, eyeliner, eyebrow pencils, and loose face powders are relatively innocuous. Heavier, oil-based preparations, particularly moisturizers and hairsprays, clog pores and accelerate comedone formation.[53]

Patients should restrict cosmetic use including makeup, moisturizers, or sunscreens to products labeled oil-free rather than water-based. Cover-up cosmetics for acne are available in several skin tones and in lotion and cream forms. They often contain peeling agents, antibacterial agents, or hydroquinone. Most contain sulfur. They may be applied as cosmetics two or three times daily, over the entire face or to individual lesions. Because the spread time of oil-free makeup is decreased, best results are achieved if applied to one-quarter of the face at a time. Topical medication should be applied after gentle cleansing and a foundation lotion may be used sparingly as a concealer.[54-56]

Because the action of most therapeutic acne agents is to dry the skin, the use of nonspecific moisturizers is counterproductive. Active agents, such as α-hydroxy acids (glycolic, lactic, pyruvic, and citric acids), may be present in a cosmetic formulation, since they reduce corneocyte adhesion.[57] Patients with acne should be restricted to oil-free α-hydroxy acid products unless necessary because of treatment with strong drying agents or isotretinoin.

Cosmetics, if correctly prescribed, may improve the performance of the therapy, whereas incorrect procedures and/or inadequate cosmetics may worsen acne. Clinicians should make informed decisions about the role of various cosmetics and to identify the appropriate indications and precautions. The choice of the most effective product should take into consideration the ongoing pharmacologic therapy and acne type/severity as well.[58]

Vehicles

Topical medication is a staple in treating mild-to-moderate acne because it is an efficient way to deliver medication to the site of action and involves decreased risk of exposure to ingredients. Since local irritation from the vehicle can lead to poor adherence and outcomes, it is essential to choose a vehicle which is effective and well tolerated. Topical agents are absorbed primarily through passive diffusion via appendageal transcellular or intracellular pathways. As the active drug travels, it may undergo chemical changes in the skin or by the vehicle.[59]

The formulation of an acne vehicle must consider the technical characteristics of maintaining and delivering the drug in an active state together with the need for an elegant product that is well tolerated and the patient will enjoy using, so that it is more likely to be applied as required and deliver the full benefit. Physically and chemically, the vehicle will be used with one or more of the following goals: reduce excess oil, control bacteria associated with acne, reduce the effects of hyperkeratinization, and unclog pores. Performance, safety, and stability should be maximized while addressing technical and commercial factors.

Immiscible liquids might be delivered in oil-in-water or water-in-oil emulsions. In addition to having undesirable oil content, these vehicles also contain humectants, thickeners, preservatives, and fragrance, all of which may be problematic.

Solutions are simpler formulations. They are often used as the soaking liquid for fibrous cloth wipe products. The shelf life depends upon whether multiple wipe packages are resealable, and whether the solvent volatility will affect storage and active agent availability or cause crystallization. Solutions are used mainly with topical antibiotics, which are often dissolved in specific types of alcohol. Although some antibiotics are only soluble in ethyl alcohol, isopropyl alcohol is generally better able to remove oil from the skin surface and is preferred for nonmedicated vehicles. Solutions and washes can be more easily applied to large areas such as the back.[60] Nongreasy solutions, gels, lotions, and creams should be selected as bases for topical acne preparations. Lotions and creams will contain some oil-phase ingredients. Discourage moisturizers and oil-based products. Lotions are slightly less drying than gels, and creams are more emollient. Gels are very useful as they are mixtures of water or alcohol and totally oil free. Many gels contain ethanol or isopropyl alcohol. Propylene glycol is sometimes present in small amounts to add viscosity and lessen the drying effects of strong peeling agents. Gels are drying but may cause a burning irritation in some patients and may prevent certain kinds of cosmetics from adhering to the skin.[53] Propylene glycol gels are easy to apply and dry without a visible or sticky film. Nonalcoholic gels may be so effective and less drying than alcoholic solutions. Alcoholic or acetone gels are usually more drying and provide better penetration of the active ingredient.

Consider the patient's skin type and preferences in the choice of vehicle for topical agents. Patients with oily skin often prefer vehicles with higher proportions of alcohol (solutions and gels), while those with dry or sensitive skin prefer nonirritating lotions and creams. Hydrating and emollient products are often recommended to patients using drying treatment therapies, such as isotretinoin, to control adverse effects and improve adherence to treatment. Lotions can be used with any skin type and can be easily spread over hair-bearing skin, but they will cause burning or dryness if they contain propylene glycol. Compatibility of vehicles and agents with cosmetics should also be considered.

The focus of innovation has been optimal formulations of problematic drugs. A fixed topical alcohol-free aqueous gel combination of clindamycin phosphate 1.2% and tretinoin 0.025% given once daily simplifies administration and encourages adherence. Creamy wash and gel hydrophase options for benzoyl peroxide reduce the irritation of this drug.[61]

The importance of vehicle effects in topical therapy has been demonstrated in placebo effect literature.[61] The percent contribution of vehicle (placebo) toward efficacy of reduction of lesions counts of eight commonly prescribed topical preparations at the end of 10 to 12 weeks of daily administration has been reported as a mean value of 55% (range 35%-82%).

How to Use Topical Preparations

Topical preparations should not be applied to individual lesions but to the whole area affected by acne to prevent new lesions from developing. Care should be advised in applying around the eyelid, mouth, and neck (to avoid chafing). Lotions should be applied with a cotton swab once or twice a day after washing or at bedtime if they leave a visible residue. Skincare products may cause skin dryness and redness particularly at the early stages of the treatment. Should this occur, the product should be applied more infrequently, the treatment should be stopped for a while or another topical product tried. To reduce irritation a topical vehicle with high water content may be applied over the medicinal product after a few minutes; the irritation usually subsides as the skin becomes accustomed to the topical skincare product.

Psychologic Approaches, Hypnosis, and Biofeedback

The psychologic effects of acne may be profound. The American Academy of Dermatology expert workgroup unanimously concluded that effective acne treatment can improve the emotional outlook of patients.[62] There is weak evidence of the possible benefit of biofeedback-assisted relaxation and cognitive imagery.[63,64]

Dressings

A pilot double-blind, randomized study of 20 patients has shown some benefit of treatment with a hydrocolloid acne dressing when compared with tape dressings for improving mild-to-moderate inflammatory acne vulgaris. Results showed greater reduction over 3 to 7 days in the overall severity of acne and inflammation, along with greater improvement in redness, oiliness, dark pigmentation, and sebum casual level. Less ultraviolet B light reaches the skin surface with the hydrocolloid dressing in place.[65,66]

Pharmacologic Therapy

Successful pharmacologic therapy must address one of the four mechanisms involved in the pathogenesis of acne. Numerous agents are available that prove one or more of these actions and are therefore effective. However, the choice of active pharmacologic therapy depends on severity.

Mechanisms of drug action relating to acne pathogenesis are illustrated in Fig. 117-2.

Drug Treatments of First Choice

There is concordance among key opinion leaders in different settings regarding recommendations for drugs of choice for management of acne—the Global Alliance 2018 and the 2016 European Guidelines.[24,32,67]

Managing Acne

For comedonal, noninflammatory acne Active agents of first choice include those that correct the defect in keratinization by producing exfoliation most efficaciously. Topical retinoids, in particular, adapalene, or a fixed combination with a retinoid (eg, adapalene plus benzoyl peroxide) can be recommended as drugs of choice.[24,32] Benzoyl peroxide or azelaic acid or salicylic acid can be considered, as alternatives (lower strength recommendation).[24,32] Limitations can apply that may necessitate the use of a treatment with a lower strength of recommendation as a first-line therapy (eg, financial resources and reimbursement limitations, legal restrictions, availability, drug licensing). Because the comedone is the initial lesion even in inflammatory acne, these agents are used to correct the defect in keratinization in all cases of acne.

For mild-to-moderate papulopustular inflammatory acne It is important to reduce the population of *P. acnes* in the follicle and the generation of its extracellular products and inflammatory effects. Either the fixed-dose combination (adapalene and benzoyl peroxide) or benzoyl peroxide or topical retinoid or azelaic acid is strongly recommended as first choice therapy (high strength recommendation).[24,32,67] In case of more widespread disease, for the treatment of **moderate papulopustular inflammatory acne**, the fixed-dose combination is preferred, with or without hormonal therapy and/or antibiotic, particularly if the trunk is involved.[67]

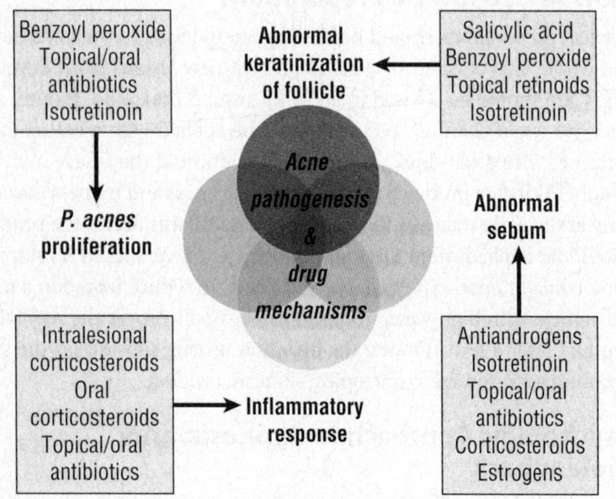

FIGURE 117-2 Acne pathogenesis and drug mechanisms.

Low-strength recommendations are offered as considerations for treatment if there are limitations that apply in selecting a first-choice agent. The choices would be blue light monotherapy, alternate combination therapy (such as fixed-dose combination of erythromycin and tretinoin, fixed-dose combination of isotretinoin and erythromycin) or oral zinc. In case of more widespread disease, a combination of a systemic antibiotic with either benzoyl peroxide or with adapalene in fixed combination with benzoyl peroxide can be considered.[24,32]

For moderately severe or severe papulopustular or moderate nodular acne The fixed-dose combination with an oral antibiotic is preferred. Alternatively, oral isotretinoin or oral hormonal therapy can also be added.[68] If there are limitations to use these agents, considerations could be given to oral antiandrogens in combination with oral antibiotics or topical treatments, or systemic antibiotics in combination with benzoyl peroxide (low strength recommendation).

Managing Very Severe Acne

For nodular or conglobate acne In males, monotherapy with oral isotretinoin is strongly recommended as the drug of first choice (high strength recommendation).[24,32] As alternative agents, a retinoid fixed combination or oral antibiotics can be recommended. For females, oral isotretinoin plus antiandrogenic hormonal therapy is preferred. Alternatively a fixed combination retinoid with oral antibiotics (consider high dose) and/or oral antiandrogenic hormonal therapy can be recommended.[68]

For maintenance therapy for acne The most frequently recommended agents are topical retinoids or retinoid and benzoyl peroxide fixed dose combinations.[67] The most extensively studied maintenance treatment (four controlled trials) has been adapalene regimens.[24,32] Other published options include tazarotene or tretinoin. In general, maintenance therapy is begun after a 12-week induction and continues for 3 to 4 months. Continuing improvement using this schema is achieved, with relapse occurring when patients stop treatment, suggesting a longer duration of maintenance therapy is likely to be beneficial. Topical azelaic acid is an alternative to topical retinoids for acne maintenance therapy, with advantageous efficacy and safety profiles for long-term therapy. To minimize antibiotic resistance, long-term therapy with antibiotics is not recommended as an alternative to topical retinoids. If an antimicrobial effect is desired, the addition of benzoyl peroxide to topical retinoid therapy is preferred.

Published Guidelines

In general, recommendations should be based on critical appraisal and interpretation of the literature combined with clinical experience. There is considerable heterogeneity in the acne literature. The large number of products and product combinations, and the scarcity of comparative studies, has led to disparate opinions and few recommendations are evidence based. Various evidence-based guidelines, available from multiple American, Canadian, European, Scandinavian, and South African sources from 2005 to 2018, do not provide concordance or clarity on all issues.

The 2016 European Guidelines for the Treatment of Acne focus primarily on major treatments, but do not review general management issues such as psychologic determinants, scarring, and diet.[24,69] Where relevant, specific information from multiple sources will be integrated into the therapy section that follows.

An expert committee of the American Academy of Dermatology redefined guidelines for acne therapy in 2016 (Table 117-1).[68] These guidelines address the management of adolescent and adult patients presenting with acne but not the consequences of disease, including the scarring, postinflammatory erythema, or postinflammatory hyperpigmentation. In 2009, the Global Alliance to Improve Outcomes in Acne updated their 2003 recommendations to review new information about pathophysiology and treatment and included current published data on relevant issues.[70] In 2018, the Global Alliance published a further update providing relevant clinical guidance to healthcare practitioners managing patients with acne, with an emphasis on areas where the evidence base may be sparse or needs interpretation for daily practice. They provided 10 consensus recommendations, based on the 2016 American Academy and European Guidelines.[67]

The Alliance recommendations statements were as follows[67]:

1. Retinoids have an essential role in treatment of acne. For most patients with inflammatory acne, comedonal acne, or both, a topical retinoid plus benzoyl peroxide is first-line therapy.24,68,69
2. The role of antibiotics in acne therapy has changed. Neither topical nor systemic antibiotics should be used as monotherapy for acne treatment.69,71
3. Oral isotretinoin should be first-line therapy for very severe (cystic and conglobate) acne.69
4. Oral isotretinoin therapy should proceed until full clearance of acne. Additional studies are needed to define a total cumulative dose that maintains remission.
5. Acne flare with oral isotretinoin can be minimized by initiating therapy at a low dose.
6. Most patients with acne should receive maintenance therapy with a topical retinoid.
7. Azelaic acid cream 20% or gel 15% is a useful acne treatment in pregnant women and patients with acne and PIH.
8. At present, devices that use laser, intense pulsed light, or photodynamic therapy should not be considered first-line treatment for inflammatory acne.
9. A minority of women 25 years of age have acne lesions localized only to the lower face. Topical retinoids with or without benzoyl peroxide are important components in therapy of adult acne.
10. Early and effective treatment is important to minimize potential risk for acne scarring.

TABLE 117-1 Evidence Chart for Recommendations for Managing Acne Vulgaris

Recommendation	Strength of Recommendation	Level of Evidence
Grading/classification system	B	II, III
Microbiologic testing	B	II, III
Endocrinologic testing	B	I, II
Topical therapies		
Benzoyl peroxide	A	I, II
Topical antibiotics (eg, clindamycin, minocycline, and erythromycin)	A	I, II
Combination of topical antibiotics and benzoyl peroxide	A	I
Topical retinoids (eg, tretinoin, adapalene, tazarotene, and trifarotene)	A	I, II
Combination of topical retinoids and benzoyl peroxide/topical antibiotic	A	I, II
Azelaic acid	A	I
Dapsone	A	I, II
Salicylic acid	B	II
Systemic antibiotics		
Tetracyclines (eg, doxycycline, minocycline, and sarecycline)	A	I, II
Macrolides (eg, azithromycin and erythromycin)	A	I
Trimethoprim (with or without sulfamethoxazole)	B	II
Limiting treatment duration and concomitant/maintenance topical therapy	A	I, II
Hormonal agents		
Combined oral contraceptives	A	I
Spironolactone	B	II, III
Oral corticosteroids	B	II
Isotretinoin		
Conventional dosing	A	I, II
Low-dose treatment for moderate acne	A	I, II
Monitoring	B	II
iPLEDGE and contraception	A	II
Miscellaneous therapies and physical modalities		
Chemical peels	B	II, III
Intralesional steroids	C	III
Complementary and alternative therapies (eg, tea tree oil, herbal, and biofeedback)	B	II
Role of diet in acne effect of glycemic index	B	II
Dairy consumption	B	II

Data from Reference 68.

General Information Regarding Efficacy and Safety

The guidelines and recommendations of the American Academy of Dermatology considered the efficacy and safety of various treatments, such as topical agents, systemic antibacterial agents, hormonal agents, isotretinoin, miscellaneous therapies, complementary and alternative therapies, and dietary restriction, based on levels of evidence and best clinical practice.[68] More specific information about the efficacy and safety of each of these specific modalities is outlined below in sections on each individual agent.

Alternative Drug Treatments

Complementary and Alternative Medications People with acne often turn to complementary and alternative medicine (CAM), such as herbal medicine, acupuncture, and dietary modifications, because of their concerns about the adverse effects of conventional medicines. Although these products might be well tolerated, very limited data exist regarding their safety and efficacy.

There is increasing interest in the use of CAM as adjuvant or single therapies: in America, 7% people report using a complementary medicine, and 2% report seeing a complementary medicine practitioner.[72] Traditional Chinese medicine has been widely used to treat acne for many years, based on a diagnosis from a traditional Chinese medicine perspective according to the different syndromes of acne.

The Cochrane collaboration undertook a systematic review, reported in 2015, to assess the effectiveness and safety of any CAM in the management of acne vulgaris. This included 35 studies, with a total of 3,227 participants in parallel-group randomized controlled trials (or the first phase data of randomized cross-over trials) of any kind of CAM, compared with no treatment, placebo, or other active therapies, in people with a diagnosis of acne vulgaris. The primary outcome was improvement of clinical signs assessed through skin lesion counts. Some evidence from single studies showed low-glycemic-load diet, tea tree oil, and pollen bee venom (PBV) may have an effect reducing total skin lesion counts and acne severity scores. However, small sample sizes and poor methodological quality limited the strength of the evidence. Evidence from other existing randomized controlled trials does not support the use of herbal medicine, acupuncture, or wet-cupping therapy for the treatment of acne vulgaris. The evidence for a secondary outcome (number of participants with remission) for herbal medicine versus antibiotic was uncertain. Two trials reported QOL showed the benefit of herbal medicine compared with western drugs. From the review of 31 studies, the Cochrane review cautioned there is a lack of evidence to support the use of other CAMs, such as aloe vera, copaiba essential oil, dried fruit of *Berberis vulgaris*, or seaweed oligosaccharides for the treatment of this condition. Most studies were done in a traditional Chinese medicine context; therefore, results might be less generalizable to western medicine. The review highlights potential adverse effects from herbal medicine (dizziness, dry mouth, nausea, diarrhea, or stomach upset); acupuncture (pain, itchiness, or redness); and tea tree oil gel (pruritus, dryness, burning sensations, and skin flaking).[73]

A 2018 review focused on the use of essential oils and aromatherapy in acne, examining existing evidence from small pilot studies.[74] It reaffirmed there is only weak clinical evidence that tea tree oil 5% may be used as an alternative acne therapy. Several agents may be helpful as complementary therapy due to biologic plausibility, including lactobacillus-fermented *Chamaecyparis obtuse*, copaiba, sandalwood oil, rosemary extract, jeju essential oil, and Korean citrus, but concluded there is little supportive clinical evidence.

The use of botanical preparations that are nonstandardized should be discouraged in favor of traditional quality-controlled preparations that have evidence of efficacy. The lack of appropriate data, absence of quality assessment, and inconsistencies in search methodology suggest that CAM cannot be recommended for acne therapy now.

Glycolic Acid Another agent considered alternative therapy for acne vulgaris is glycolic acid. The efficacy and tolerability of a 0.1% retinaldehyde/6% glycolic acid combination (Diacneal) has been evaluated for mild-to-moderate acne vulgaris.[75] Physician and patient ratings of acne symptom severity and tolerance performed at baseline and months 1, 2, and 3 showed mean numbers of papules, pustules, and comedones were significantly reduced from month 1 on, demonstrating that glycolic acid is effective and well tolerated in mild-to-moderate acne vulgaris.

Both glycolic acid–based, salicylic acid or salicylic acid derivative–based (eg, lipohydroxyacid), and amino fruit acid–peeling preparations have been used in the treatment of acne. There is very little evidence from clinical trials published in peer-reviewed literature supporting the efficacy of peeling regimens.[62] Topical corneolytics, including retinaldehyde/glycolic acid or lactic acid, induce a comedolytic effect and may also facilitate skin absorption of topical drugs.[58] Further research on the use of peeling in the treatment of acne needs to be conducted to establish best practices for this modality.

Hydroquinone To control pigmentation, hydroquinone, which reversibly damages melanocytes, has been used as a hypopigmenting agent in concentrations of 2% to 4%, in preparations of clear or tinted gels, which are more drying, and as vanishing or opaque, flesh-tinted creams, with or without α-hydroxy acids or sunscreens. Hydroquinone causes fading of epidermal but not dermal pigmentation. Onset of response is usually 3 to 4 weeks, and the depigmentation lasts for 2 to 6 months but is reversible. While effective in the removal of melanin, hydroquinone has been clinically found to be a possible carcinogen and causes a blue-black discoloration known as ochronosis.[76]

After considering new data and information on the safety of hydroquinone, the FDA issued a proposed ruling in 2006 about hydroquinone products. The FDA proposed reversing earlier rules that hydroquinone is generally recognized as safe and effective. The FDA has not yet issued a final ruling on the status of nonprescription hydroquinone, and many physicians consider a ban unnecessary, given the lack of convincing evidence of carcinogenic risk to humans and the rarity of ochronosis occurrence.

Treatment of Scarring Drug and nondrug measures for scar resolution are important in acne vulgaris because many patients are scarred despite adequate treatment and scarring carries an emotional toll. Interventions for atrophic scars might be aided through early identification of patients at risk using a risk assessment tool for scar development. One such tool incorporates four factors: worst ever severity of acne, duration of acne, family history of atrophic acne scars, and lesion manipulation behaviors.[77]

Effective procedures for treatment of scarring focus on resurfacing techniques. For patients with mild scarring, nonprescription α-hydroxy acids may be used, while severe scarring may be corrected with other treatment modalities that require consultation with a dermatologist. Dermabrasion, local or subcuticular excision, collagen implants, chemical peels (eg, 70% glycolic acid, trichloroacetic acid), and laser therapy have been used to improve scarring. Atrophic scars can be treated with laser resurfacing. Usually the scar is not completely removed, but a more cosmetically acceptable result is achieved. Keloids and hypertrophic scars can be treated with intralesional triamcinolone, cryotherapy, topical steroids, and silicone sheeting. Surgical options for scars include excision, augmentation with collagen or fat, chemical peels, subcision, and injection of autologous fibroblasts.

Special Populations

About 20% of young infants (2-3 months of age) develop papules, pustules, and less commonly closed or open comedones, primarily on the cheeks, due to placental transfer of maternal androgens (neonatal acne). The acne subsides within a few months with regular maturation. Boys are affected more often than girls because of a transient increase in testosterone secretion during the third and fourth month of intrauterine life. *Malassezia* spp. may be involved in pathogenesis.[31] Resolution occurs without therapy.[78] Infants with neonatal acne may have more severe teenage acne.[31]

The treatment of acne in children is similar to treatment for adults. Because topical therapies may be more irritating in children, initiation with low concentrations is preferred. Systemic treatments should be reserved for more extensive cases. Erythromycin is preferred over tetracyclines for children younger than 9 years of age because tetracyclines can affect growing cartilage and teeth.

Although treatment with isotretinoin has numerous potential minor adverse effects in patients of all ages, an uncommon complication in young patients is premature epiphyseal closure. This generally occurs when isotretinoin is administered in high doses, thus limiting long-term therapy.

There is a growing population of women seeking acne therapy and a clinical perception that acne in women requires systemic treatment. Analyses of clinical trials have shown that topical therapy can be efficacious in this group. Most patients have an acne presentation similar to adolescent acne, with mixed inflammatory and noninflammatory lesions on multiple facial areas (not limited to the mandibular area). Topical therapy with a retinoid and antimicrobial can be a good option. Data support the use of retinoids, including adapalene/benzoyl peroxide in both 0.1% and 0.3% concentrations, tretinoin 0.04%, and a retinaldehyde 0.1%/glycolic acid/6% cream. Among antimicrobial agents, both dapsone and clindamycin/benzoyl peroxide have efficacy if a topical retinoid is added. Azelaic acid 15% gel has also shown good results in a small study. Hormonal therapy, including oral contraceptives (OCs), can play an important role in management of acne in women and is typically used in combination with topical acne therapy.[67]

Selecting appropriate treatment in pregnant women can be challenging because many acne therapies are teratogenic; all topical and especially oral retinoids should be avoided. Oral therapies, such as tetracyclines and antiandrogens, are also contraindicated in pregnancy. Topical and oral treatment with erythromycin may be considered.

Acne in skin of color is an increasing problem, presenting unique challenges. Postinflammatory hyperpigmentation (PIH), a hypermelanotic reaction to skin inflammation, is a common occurrence in patients with acne, particularly in those with darker skin and those who excoriate their lesions, affecting all genders and ages. It has a prolonged duration and can be more bothersome than active acne lesions. Prevention (including sun protection) and early treatment of underlying acne-associated inflammation effectively is a primary approach to PIH management. Chemical peels, lasers, and other light therapies may also be used for PIH; however, these methods can also cause pigmentation problems so should be used with care. Topical retinoids also improve pigmentation by inhibiting melanosome transfer to keratinocytes and increasing epidermal turnover, lessening pigmentation. It is important for the patient to be aware that many PIH lesions resolve spontaneously, but slowly.[67]

A variety of topical agents have studies that specifically included patients with skin of color, confirming their safe use in this population. These include all the currently available topical retinoids, benzoyl peroxide, azelaic acid, clindamycin, dapsone, and clascoterone. A key goal of therapy in this population is to minimize postinflammatory hyperpigmentation from irritating topical agents, with an emphasis on use of hydrating cleansers and non-comedogenic moisturizers.[79]

Another important counseling point is to emphasize sun protective measures to minimize the darkening effects of UV irradiation on postinflammatory hyperpigmentation. Recommendations include use of a broad-spectrum sunscreen, protective clothing, and inclusion of vitamin D–rich foods or supplementation.[76]

Drug Class Information

This section reviews the pharmacology and mechanisms as related to pathophysiology for pharmacologic options recommended in the guidelines for mild, moderate, and severe acne. It will also review evidence of efficacy and safety as well as kinetics, interactions, dosing, and administration when relevant.

Topical Therapies Topical therapy agents are available over the counter or by prescription. The choice of therapy can be influenced by age of the patient, site of involvement, extent and severity of disease, and patient preference. Topical therapies may be used as monotherapy, in combination with other topical agents, or in combination with oral agents in both initial control and maintenance. Strength of recommendations for treatment of acne with topical therapies is shown in Table 117-2.

Exfoliants (Peeling Agents) Exfoliants induce continuous mild drying and peeling by primary irritation, damaging the superficial layers of the skin, and inciting inflammation. This stimulates mitosis, thickening the epidermis, and increasing horny cells, scaling, and erythema. A decrease in sweating results in a dry, less oily surface and may superficially resolve pustular lesions.

In the past, a rabbit model was used to study the efficacy of topical exfoliants in retarding tar-induced comedone formation and accelerating their loss (comedolysis). In this animal model, retinoic acid (tretinoin) was most active, compared with benzoyl peroxide and salicylic acid, which were respectively less active. Data from peer-reviewed literature regarding the efficacy of sulfur, resorcinol, sodium sulfacetamide, aluminum chloride, and zinc are limited. Traditional nonprescription exfoliants, including phenol, resorcinol, beta-naphthol, sulfur, Vleminckx solution, and sodium thiosulfate, are weak or ineffective. These agents are not comedolytic given that they affect the superficial epidermis rather than the hair canal. They have been supplanted by superior effective agents. Linoleic acid–rich phosphatidylcholine combined with 4% nicotinamide is suggested as an emulsion treatment that may be effective in normalization of follicular hyperkeratinization, and also provide anti-inflammatory effects.[80,81]

Resorcinol Although sulfur and resorcinol have been used for many years in the treatment of acne, evidence from peer-reviewed literature supporting their efficacy is lacking.[67] The phenol derivative resorcinol is less keratolytic than salicylic acid. It is noted to be both bactericidal and fungicidal. Products containing resorcinol 1% to 2% have been used for acne, often in combination with other peeling agents such as sulfur or salicylic acid. The FDA considers resorcinol 2% and resorcinol monoacetate 3%, in combination with sulfur 3% to 8%, to be safe and effective and that the combination may enhance the activity of sulfur. However, the FDA is not convinced that resorcinol and resorcinol acetate are safe and effective when used as single ingredients, and has placed such products in category II (not generally recognized as safe and effective, or misbranded).[81]

Resorcinol is an irritant and sensitizer and should not be applied to large areas of the skin or on broken skin. It produces a reversible, dark brown scale on some dark-skinned individuals.

Protective packaging is important as resorcinol is reactive to light and oxygen. It has good solubility in both water and alcohol and is heat stabile. Thus, it is incorporated into a variety of products, including emulsions.[82]

Salicylic Acid Salicylic acid, a β-hydroxy acid, is a comedolytic agent that is available over the counter in 0.5% to 2% strengths. Clinical trials demonstrating the efficacy or safety of salicylic acid in acne are limited, although it has been used for many years.[67] It is a natural ingredient in many plants such as willow tree or willow bark, and it penetrates the pilosebaceous unit. The comedolytic action depends on concentration: concentrations in commercial preparations (<2%-3%) are generally low. Concentrations less than 2% may in fact increase keratinization, while those between 3% and 6% are keratolytic, softening the horny layer and producing shedding of scales. Its mechanism remains unresolved, attributed to either reduced cohesion of corneocytes or shedding of epidermal cells, rather than breakdown of keratin.

Salicylic acid has no effect on the mitotic activity of normal epidermis and does not influence disordered cornification.[83] It may provide mild antibacterial value, as it is active against *P. acnes*. It offers slight anti-inflammatory activity at concentrations ranging from 0.5% to 5%. Its efficacy against comedones helps to prevent development of inflamed lesions, thus providing a delayed efficacy.[84]

Salicylic acid is effective. As a peeling agent, its relative strength compared with others in this class varies according to the model used in measurement. It is slightly *less* potent than equal-strength benzoyl peroxide when measured with the rabbit ear animal model, and slightly *more* potent when measured with a biologic microcomedone model.[84] Its anti-inflammatory properties may help dry inflammatory lesions.[82] Its comedolytic properties are considered less potent than topical retinoids. It is often used when patients cannot tolerate a topical retinoid because of skin irritation.[85]

Its keratolytic effect may enhance the absorption of other agents. Salicylic acid is a mild irritant and may cause some degree of local skin peeling and discomfort (burning or reddening). It is not a sensitizer. Although the FDA recognizes salicylic acid as safe

TABLE 117-2 Monitoring of Medications Used in Acne Treatment and Maintenance Therapy

Medications	Adverse Drug Effects	Monitoring Parameters	Comments
Exfoliants			
Resorcinol	Irritant and sensitizer	Degree and/or changes in signs or symptoms of irritancy (redness, discomfort, peeling, skin breakdown, or dermatitis)	Should not be applied to large areas of the skin or on broken skin
Sulfur	Avoid eye contact—slight ophthalmic and skin irritation	Degree and/or changes in signs or symptoms of irritancy (redness, discomfort, peeling, skin breakdown, or dermatitis). Discontinue use if excessive irritation results	
Salicylic acid	Mild irritant—burning and reddening, local skin peeling	Degree and/or changes in signs or symptoms of irritancy (redness, discomfort, peeling, skin breakdown, or dermatitis)	Begin with a low concentration and increase as tolerance develops Not a sensitizer
Retinoids			
Isotretinoin	Side effects: mucocutaneous (most common), musculoskeletal, and ophthalmic systems Common: dryness of mucus membranes (lips, mouth, eyes, nose) dry skin, itching, hair loss, thirst, back pain, myalgia, headaches, and central nervous system effects Increased cholesterol Teratogenic Sun sensitivity Depression and suicide—controversial	Test for pregnancy twice before starting Contraceptive measures must be started 1 month prior, continued during the 2 months of treatment and for at least 1 month after stopping treatment (but normally 4 months) Laboratory monitoring during therapy should include triglycerides, cholesterol, transaminases, and complete blood counts (before, during, and after treatment) Degree and/or changes in signs or symptoms of irritancy to skin (redness, discomfort, peeling, skin breakdown, or dermatitis) Degree and/or changes in signs or symptoms of irritancy to mucous membranes (mouth, nose, eyes) Instances of headache or central nervous system symptoms Note prior psychiatric symptoms, monitor patients at each visit for early recognition of changes in mood or psychological well-being (before, during, and after treatment)	Drying agents must be discontinued Sun-avoidance strategies and sunscreen use recommended Vitamin A supplementation Use moisturizers (lip balm, nasal moisturizers, eye lubricants, temporary removal of contacts) Most adverse effects, such as cheilitis, and dry nose, eyes and mouth, are temporary and resolve after the drug is discontinued Advise patients about a possible risk of depression and suicidal behavior
Tretinoin/retinoic acid	Common: erythema, dryness, burning, photosensitization Rare: true contact allergy Use cautiously in pregnancy (Irritation: tazarotene > retinoic acid > adapalene)	Degree and/or changes in signs or symptoms of irritancy to skin (redness, discomfort, peeling, skin breakdown, or dermatitis) Skin changes in areas of sun exposure—dermatitis or hives	Additive effects with concomitant topical drying medications, such as products with high concentrations of alcohol, astringents, or abrasive soaps Gels and creams are less irritating than solutions Sun-avoidance strategies and sunscreen use recommended
Adapalene	Side effects include erythema, xerosis, burning and desquamation Less irritation than other retinoids Photoirritation or sensitization	Degree and/or changes in signs or symptoms of irritancy to skin (redness, discomfort, peeling, skin breakdown, or dermatitis) Skin changes in areas of sun exposure—dermatitis or hives	Less photosensitivity than other agents Sun-avoidance strategies and sunscreen use recommended
Tazarotene	Side effects include irritation, erythema, xerosis, burning, and desquamation	Skin changes in areas of sun exposure—dermatitis or hives	Contraindicated in pregnancy due to the large surface area Short contact therapy, 1-5 minutes every other night, gradually increasing to overnight advocated for dosing in patients with sensitive skin Oily complexions may tolerate twice daily, short contact time
Topical Antimicrobial Agents			
Benzoyl peroxide	Dryness and peeling appear after a few days, erythema, burning, pruritus Rare reports of contact allergic dermatitis May bleach hair and clothing Body odor, odor on clothes and bedsheets Irritation is concentration dependent—most frequent with 10% gel Irritation from gels used as vehicles—water-based < alcohol = acetone	Once tolerance is achieved, the strength may be increased to 5% or the base changed to the acetone or alcohol gels, or to paste Degree and/or changes in signs or symptoms of irritancy to skin (redness, discomfort, peeling, skin breakdown, or dermatitis) Hives	Increased skin irritation or drying effect with other medications, soaps, and cosmetics with strong drying effect Chemically incompatible with retinoic acid Cross-reactions with other sensitizers, such as Peruvian balsam, cinnamon, and other benzoic acid derivatives (topical anesthetics)
Clindamycin	Erythema, peeling, itching, dryness, and burning	Signs or symptoms of irritancy to skin (redness, discomfort, peeling, skin breakdown, or dermatitis)	

(continued)

TABLE 117-2 Monitoring of Medications Used in Acne Treatment and Maintenance Therapy (*Continued*)

Medications	Adverse Drug Effects	Monitoring Parameters	Comments
Oral Antibiotics			
Erythromycin	Gastrointestinal upset (nausea, vomiting, diarrhea) Vaginal candidiasis	If gastrointestinal adverse effects occur, monitor hydration Vaginal discharge	Drug interactions: Inhibits CYP1A2 and CYP3A4: carbamazepine, cyclosporine, theophylline, and warfarin Safe in pregnant women and children
Tetracyclines	Gastrointestinal intolerance: (tetracycline > erythromycin > doxycycline = minocycline) Vaginal candidiasis Photosensitivity is dose-dependent (doxycycline > tetracycline)	Vaginal discharge Skin changes in areas of sun exposure—dermatitis or hives	Contraindicated in pregnant women or in children younger than 9 years of age Absorption decreased by food, chelated by antacids and milk To be taken on an empty stomach
Minocycline	Drug-induced lupus Pigment changes in skin, mucous membranes, and teeth Hepatitis Urticaria Dose-related dizziness (resolves with dose titration) Autoimmune hepatitis and hypersensitivity syndrome	Vaginal discharge Skin changes in areas of sun exposure—dermatitis or hives Changes or discoloration of skin, teeth, or mucous membranes Monitor degree of dizziness as dose is titrated Signs of hypersensitivity syndrome: fever, dermatitis, blistering reactions; systemic symptoms such as malaise, changes in blood pressure, or renal function	Contraindicated in pregnant women or in children younger than 9 years of age Decreased gastrointestinal absorption with Fe, Ca, Mg, Al Sun-avoidance strategies and sunscreen use recommended
Doxycycline	Gastrointestinal upset Photosensitizer (especially at higher doses)	If gastrointestinal side effects occur, monitor hydration Skin changes in areas of sun exposure—dermatitis or hives	Contraindicated in pregnant women or in children younger than 9 years of age Sun-avoidance strategies and sunscreen use recommended
Antisebum			
Combination oral contraceptives	Breakthrough bleeding, headache Serious: venous thromboembolism, hepatotoxicity	Spotting or bleeding	Oral antibiotics may decrease contraceptive efficacy—(significance controversial)
Spironolactone	Common: hyperkalemia, menstrual irregularity, gynecomastia, breast tenderness	Menstrual signs Breast changes	
Anti-inflammatory			
Azelaic acid	Primary: pruritus, burning, stinging, and tingling Other: erythema, dryness, rash, peeling, irritation, dermatitis, and contact dermatitis in less than 1% of patients	Skin changes in areas of sun exposure—dermatitis or hives	Adverse reactions are generally transient and mild in nature
Dapsone	Short- and long-term safety and efficacy demonstrated Peeling, dryness, and erythema	Skin changes in areas of sun exposure—dermatitis or hives	Does not induce phototoxicity or photoallergy in human dermal safety studies Medications such as rifampin, anticonvulsants, trimethoprim/sulfamethoxazole, and St John's wort may increase formation of dapsone hydroxylamine (toxicity)

Al, aluminum; Ca, calcium; CYP, cytochrome P450; Fe, iron; Mg, magnesium.

and effective, the compound offers no advantages over more modern topical agents such as benzoyl peroxide.[81,83,85]

Salicylic acid products are often used as first-line therapy for mild acne because of their widespread availability without a prescription in a variety of formulations. Both wash-off and leave-on preparations are well tolerated. Lower concentrations are sometimes combined with sulfur to produce an additive keratolytic effect. Concentrations up to 5% to 10% can be used for acne, beginning with a low concentration and increasing as tolerance to the irritation develops. However, the maximum strength allowed in nonprescription acne products is 2%. In high concentrations of 20% to 30% in hydroethanolic vehicles, salicylic acid, either alone or in combination, can be used as a peeling agent for comedonal acne and hyperpigmentation. It extrudes closed and open comedones several days after peel, but it must be applied under strict control to offer this adjunctive benefit when treating acne vulgaris.[86]

Sulfur Sulfur medications often lessen the severity of acne, presumably because of keratolytic and antibacterial action. Sulfur helps to resolve comedones by an exfoliant action. Its popularity is due to its ability to quickly resolve pustules and papules, mask and conceal lesions (as a thick foundation lotion), and produce irritation leading to skin peeling and mild antibacterial action. Sulfur is used in the precipitated or colloidal form in concentrations of 2% to 10%, because it is practically insoluble in water and must be well dispersed. Its stability depends on effective maintenance of the dispersion.[82] Sulfur compounds (eg, sulfides, thioglycolates, sulfites, thiols, cysteines, and thioacetates) are also available and somewhat weaker.

Sulfur can cause slight ophthalmic and dermatologic irritation, and patients should be cautioned to avoid eye contact. Use should be discontinued if excessive irritation results. Although it is often combined with salicylic acid or resorcinol to increase its effect, its use is limited by its offensive odor and the availability of more effective agents.[87]

Topical Retinoids Topical retinoids are prescription vitamin A derivatives with well-documented, randomized, double-blind, placebo-controlled trials supporting their use for acne treatment.[68] Multiple agents are available in a variety of strengths and formulations: tretinoin, adapalene, tazarotene, and trifarotene. Each retinoid binds to a different set of retinoic acid receptors conferring slight differences in activity, tolerability, and efficacy: tretinoin to alpha, beta, and gamma; tazarotene and adapalene, selectively, to beta and gamma; and trifarotene to gamma. Binding to specific nuclear receptors reduces inflammation, and inhibits sebocyte proliferation and differentiation, which reduces sebum production.

Retinoids are the most powerful available peeling agents since normal epithelial cell differentiation is a vitamin A–dependent process. There is no consensus about the relative efficacy of currently available topical retinoids and oral isotretinoin. They are the core of topical therapy because of their ability to target key stages in the development of the disease: they are comedolytic, resolve the precursor microcomedone lesion, and are anti-inflammatory.

Retinoids act to reduce obstruction within the follicle and therefore are useful in the management of both comedonal and inflammatory acne. As a group, they are highly active peelers as they reverse abnormal keratinocyte desquamation.[88] They improve acne vulgaris by inhibiting microcomedone formation, diminishing the number of mature comedones and subsequently, inflammatory lesions. They also normalize follicular epithelium maturation and desquamation. Topical retinoids, unlike isotretinoin, do not decrease production of sebum, but primarily decrease inflammation, normalize keratinocyte differentiation, and increase keratinocyte proliferation and migration.[88]

Retinoids also facilitate acne lesion clearance through secondary effects of loosening and decreasing corneocytes. This increases skin permeability, facilitates absorption of other agents, such as antimicrobials or benzoyl peroxide, and increases penetration of oral antibiotics into the follicular canal. As a result, the overall duration of antibiotic treatment decreases, and the possibility of resistance lessens. Therefore, combination products with oral or topical antimicrobials are available for increased efficacy, faster onset of effects, decreased total antibiotic use and risk of resistance, and shorter duration of treatment.[88] Retinoids may also improve and prevent postinflammatory hyperpigmentation often seen in people with darker complexions who have acne.

Retinoic acid (vitamin A acid or tretinoin) is a powerful exfoliant that slows the desquamation process, reducing numbers of both microcomedones and comedones.[26] Gels and creams are less irritating than solutions.

Stable and fast acting, adapalene has significant anti-inflammatory and comedolytic properties.[88-92] It causes epidermal and follicular epithelium hyperplasia, increased desquamation, keratinocyte differentiation, and loosening of corneocyte connections. Its anti-inflammatory effect is due to the inhibition of oxidative metabolism of arachidonic acid and inhibition of chemotactic reponses.[92] It is better at reducing inflammatory lesions and total lesion count[91] and causes less local irritation because of its mechanisms and receptor specificity than tretinoin or tazarotene.[90-96] Release from lotions and hydroalcoholic gels is more effective than from creams and aqueous gels and a microsphere gel formulation may be less irritating.[88,93] It is a good first-line therapy for colder climates or in patients with sensitive skin.[76]

Adapalene is generally regarded as effective but less irritating than other topical retinoids.[54,70] It is available in fixed-dose combinations in specialized gel vehicles with benzoyl peroxide to increase the efficacy in comparison with monotherapies. This strategy allows for the synergy of adapalene effects on normalizing desquamation with reduction of inflammation due to benzoyl peroxide action against *P. acnes*. Adapalene gel 0.1% is approved in the United States as a nonprescription product for once-daily application by patients aged 12 years and older.

Tazarotene has superior efficacy to parent retinoids, reducing both noninflammatory and ILs. While its exact mechanism is unknown, it is thought to activate retinoid receptors and thereby affect keratinocyte differentiation, and inhibit proinflammatory transcription factors to decrease cell proliferation and inflammation.[47] It penetrates skin but accumulates in the upper dermis. It is as effective as adapalene in reducing noninflammatory and IL counts when applied half as frequently. Compared with tretinoin, it is as effective for comedonal and more effective for inflammatory lesions when applied once daily. Tazarotene foam 0.1% can be used as an alternative vehicle to the gel with less systemic absorption and is a safe and effective formulation.[87,97,98] Tazarotene is not degraded by sunlight.[26]

Trifarotene is a topical selective agonist of RAR-γ, a receptor expressed in skin and not in internal organs. It was evaluated in two vehicle-controlled, 12-week, randomized double-blind studies of more than 2,000 patients aged 9 years and older, with 20% to 30% decrease in both noninflammatory and inflammatory lesions on the face and trunk. In an open-label extension of continued use, more than 70% of patients achieved an Investigator Global Assessment score of 0 or 1 by 52 weeks. It is approved in the United States as a once-daily application to the trunk and face in patients 9 years and older.[99]

Isotretinoin is a systemic retinoid that is reviewed separately below.

Retinoids tend to produce remissions that are maintained for extended periods of time, provided the accompanying irritation does not impede patient adherence. Side effects, including dryness, peeling, erythema, and irritation, can be mitigated by reduced frequency of application. Given any single agent, higher concentrations may be more efficacious, but with greater side effects. The vehicle of any particular retinoid may also decrease tolerability.[91,92] Most retinoids are unstable and insoluble in water.

Topical retinoids should be used cautiously in pregnancy and tazarotene is contraindicated. Tretinoin and adapalene are in FDA category C, while tazarotene, based on large-surface-area use in psoriasis (see Chapter 118, "Psoriasis"), is in FDA category X.[31] Trifarotene should be avoided in pregnancy. Cases of birth defects in the babies of females using trifarotene have been reported, as has adverse effects in pregnant rabbits given trifarotene orally during the period of organogenesis. The drug is also present in the breast milk of rats being fed the medications, and the manufacturer therefore recommends caution, with application only to small areas that would be unlikely to result in systemic absorption and avoidance of application to the nipples.

Skin type and age may influence tolerability in addition to the choice of vehicle. Oily skin may be more resistant, and darker skin is more prone to postinflammatory hyperpigmentation due to retinoid dermatitis. To decrease irritation, start with the lowest concentration and increase as tolerated. Application of retinoids should be at night, a half hour after cleansing, starting with every other night for 1 to 2 weeks to adjust to irritation. Short contact time starting with 2 minutes and adding 30 seconds per dose can be advised for patients with sensitive skin or in the winter, discontinuing and resuming after a 3-day rest if undue irritation results. Doses can be increased after 4 to 6 weeks if there is no irritation. Gels and creams are less irritating than solutions.

Some formulations of tretinoin are not photostable and should be applied in the evening. Tretinoin also may be oxidized and inactivated by the coadministration of benzoyl peroxide. It is recommended that the two agents be applied at different times. Tretinoin microsphere formulation, adapalene, and tazarotene do not have similar restrictions. Topical retinoids have been associated with an increased risk of photosensitivity; concurrent daily sunscreen can be used to reduce the risk of sunburn.

Adapalene and tazarotene are photo-irritants (not photosensitizers), and sun avoidance and sunscreen use are imperative.[88]

These agents enhance any other topical acne regimen and allow for maintenance of clearance after discontinuation of oral therapy. Since retinoids are ideal for comedonal acne, when used in combination with other agents, they can address all acne variants. Adapalene is available in combination with benzoyl peroxide, and tretinoin is available combined with clindamycin phosphate 1.2%/tretinoin 0.025% gel, approved for those age 12 years or older.[67]

The therapy of acne in children younger than 12 years of age with products approved by the FDA has expanded. Fixed combination benzoyl peroxide 2.5%/adapalene 1% gel and trifarotene are approved for patients 9 years of age or older, and tretinoin 0.05% micronized tretinoin gel for patients 10 years of age or older. All other retinoids are approved by the FDA for patients 12 years of age or older. Current data show that retinoids in younger patients are effective and are not associated with increased irritation or risk.[67]

Overall, topical retinoids are the cornerstone of acne treatment and provide safe, effective, and economical means of treating all but the most severe cases of acne vulgaris. They should be the first step in moderate acne, alone or in combination with antibiotics and benzoyl peroxide, reverting to retinoids alone for maintenance once adequate results are achieved. Their lack of effect in inducing bacterial resistance enables long-term maintenance of remission.

Antibacterial Agents Choices for antibacterial therapy include benzoyl peroxide, prescription topical and systemic antibiotics, and combination products. These drugs kill *P. acnes* and inhibit the production of proinflammatory mediators by organisms that are not killed.[26]

Benzoyl Peroxide Benzoyl peroxide is a bactericidal agent that has proven effective in the treatment of acne. It kills *P. acnes* through the release of free oxygen radicals and is also mildly comedolytic. No resistance to this agent has been reported, and the addition of benzoyl peroxide to regimens of antibiotic therapy enhances results and may reduce resistance development.

Benzoyl peroxide is a derivative of coal tar and was first used for acne vulgaris in the mid-1960s, becoming popular once stable formulations aimed at its heat-lability were developed in the mid-1970s.[95] These preparations are the single most useful group of topical nonprescription drugs. Used alone or in combination, benzoyl peroxide is the standard of care for mild-to-moderate papular-pustular acne. It is an agent of first choice when combined with adapalene for most patients with mild-to-moderate inflammatory acne vulgaris and a second choice alternative for patients with noninflammatory comedonal acne.[24,32,67] A systematic review of 22 trials using benzoyl peroxide for acne vulgaris provided evidence that it reduces acne-lesion count, although high-quality evidence is not robust enough for firm conclusions.[100]

Benzoyl peroxide is well absorbed through the stratum corneum and concentrates in the pilosebaceous unit.[101] It has three principal actions useful in both noninflammatory and inflammatory acne. It produces powerful anaerobic antibacterial activity due to slow release of oxygen, thereby acting against gram-positive and gram-negative bacteria, yeasts, and fungi. This nonspecific antibacterial mechanism does not induce resistance with long-term use.[101] It has a rapid (within 2 hours) bactericidal effect that lasts at least 48 hours. As a result, it may decrease the number of inflamed lesions within 5 days. As an indirect effect, it induces suppression of sebum production; it does not reduce skin surface lipids, but is effective in reducing free fatty acids, which are comedogenic agents and triggers of inflammation.[101] Topical benzoyl peroxide 5% lowers free fatty acids 50% to 60% after daily application for 14 days and decreases aerobic bacteria by 84% and anaerobic bacteria (primarily *P. acnes*) by 98%.

Benzoyl peroxide is also comedolytic. While earlier rabbit model studies showed a benzoyl peroxide effect greater than that of salicylic acid, these animal comedones were not physiologic but induced by tar. More recent studies using native microcomedones show an anticomedogenic effect that is only comparatively slight, compared with tretinoin or salicylic acid.[102-104]

Finally, a supplementary benefit of benzoyl peroxide is an indirect anti-inflammatory action, which is due either to its antibacterial or oxidizing effects. This has been reported in several studies and thus can be used to support treatment of predominantly inflamed lesions.[101] The drug's antiacne effect is augmented by increased blood flow, dermal irritation, local anesthetic properties, and promotion of healing.[105-108] Because the primary effect of benzoyl peroxide is antibacterial, it is most effective for inflammatory acne. Many patients with noninflammatory comedonal acne will respond to its peeling action.

Benzoyl peroxide is available in a variety of preparations without a prescription such as topical washes, foams, creams, or gels, and can be used as leave-on or wash-off agents. There is no clear superiority of different preparations in terms of effectiveness. Newer delivery systems to enhance efficacy and tolerability are also being investigated. Strengths available for acne therapy range from 2.5% to 10%. Total skin contact time and formulation can affect efficacy. Lower concentrations (eg, 2.5%-5%), water-based, and wash-off agents may be better tolerated in patients with more sensitive skin.

Cleansers containing benzoyl peroxide are available as nonprescription liquid washes and solid bars of various strengths. The desquamative and antibacterial effectiveness in a soap or wash is minimized by limited contact time and removal with proper rinsing. Alcohol and acetone gels facilitate bioavailability and may be more effective, while water-based vehicles are less irritating and better tolerated. Paste vehicles are stiffer and more drying than ointments or creams, which facilitate absorption and allow the active ingredients to stay localized.

Concentrations of 2.5%, 5%, and 10% in a water-based gel have been compared with the vehicle alone. The 2.5% formulation is equivalent to the 5% and 10% formulation in reducing the number of inflammatory lesions. The lower strength may not be as effective a peeler compared to higher strengths, which is due to an irritancy reaction. Thus, irritant side effects with the 2.5% gel are less frequent than with the 10% gel but are equivalent to the 5% gel. The lowest concentration of benzoyl peroxide should be used for treating patients with easily irritated skin and may lessen irritation when used in combination topical therapy with comedolytic agents.

Therapy is limited by staining and bleaching of hair, bedsheets, and clothing, concentration-dependent irritation, and uncommonly contact allergy. It produces a mild primary irritant dermatitis that subsides with continued use and is more likely to occur in those with fair complexions, a tendency to irritancy, or propensity to sunburn. This irritation is dependent on the concentration and the vehicle, being higher with alcoholic gels compared with emulsion bases.[102] There are rare reports of contact allergic dermatitis. Cross-reactions with other sensitizers, notably Peruvian balsam and cinnamon, are well established. It may cross-sensitize to other benzoic acid derivatives such as topical anesthetics. Concomitant use of an abrasive cleanser may initiate or enhance sensitization.[109]

Another side effect is body odor from breakdown of the benzoyl peroxide that remains on clothing and bedsheets.

Benzoyl peroxide has been combined with prescription agents to improve efficacy, reduce dosing strengths, decrease irritation, and reduce resistance of antibiotics.[110-113]

Benzoyl peroxide is combined with topical retinoids for an antimicrobial effect or used in conjunction with an antimicrobial. It reduces the likelihood of antibiotic resistance. For long-term maintenance therapy, it is recommended as a highly efficient bactericidal agent to be added to a topical retinoid.[24,32]

The adjunctive use of clindamycin/benzoyl peroxide gel with tazarotene cream promotes greater efficacy and may also enhance tolerability. Increased tolerability might be attributed to emollients in the clindamycin/benzoyl peroxide gel formulation.[114] A patented gel formulation of benzoyl peroxide 5%/clindamycin phosphate 1% (clindamycin) containing dimethicone and glycerin was studied both as a monotherapy and in combination with topical retinoid use. Certain additives, such as silicates and specific humectants, reduced irritation by maintaining barrier integrity.[115]

When using single-agent preparations of benzoyl peroxide, the weakest concentration (2.5%) in a water-based formulation is preferred for anyone with a history of skin irritation.[115] There are many suggested routines to initiate therapy. One is to gently cleanse the skin and apply the preparation for 15 minutes the first evening, avoiding the eyes and mucous membranes. A mild stinging and reddening will appear. Each evening the time should be doubled until the product is left on for 4 hours and subsequently all night. Dryness and peeling will appear after a few days. Once tolerance is achieved, the strength may be increased to 5% or the base changed to the acetone or alcohol gels, or to paste. Alternatively, benzoyl peroxide can be applied for 2 hours for four nights, 4 hours for four nights, and then left on all night. It is important to wash the product off in the morning. Other drying agents should be discontinued. Patients with very sensitive skin or demonstrated sensitivity to benzoyl peroxide should not use the product, and it should be discontinued if irritation becomes severe upon use. Contact with eyes, lips, or mouth should be avoided.

A sunscreen is recommended if benzoyl peroxide is used. To avoid interactions, apply the sunscreen during the day and the benzoyl peroxide at night.

Topical Antibacterials Topical antibiotics for acne accumulate in the follicle, where they can have antibacterial effects (the primary mechanism for efficacy in acne) and anti-inflammatory actions. These agents are best used in combination with benzoyl peroxide (wash-off or leave-on), which increases efficacy and decreases the development of resistant bacterial strains. Monotherapy with topical antibiotics in the management of acne is not recommended because of the development of antibiotic resistance.[116,117] Macrolides, including topical erythromycin and topical clindamycin, are effective and well-tolerated, well-established acne treatments.

Clindamycin is available as a single agent for topical acne therapy. Topical erythromycin has reduced efficacy in comparison with clindamycin because of resistance of cutaneous staphylococci and *P. acnes*.[68] More than 50% of *P. acnes* strains are resistant to topical macrolides. Resistant strains are usually resistant to all macrolides.[118]

Current recommendations discourage topical antibiotic monotherapy in favor of combination therapy with benzoyl peroxide and topical retinoids. Addition of benzoyl peroxide or topical retinoids to the macrolide antibiotic regimen is more effective than monotherapy and mitigates against survival of resistant *P. acnes* populations.

Clindamycin is the preferred macrolide because of potent action, lack of absorption, and its systemic use is limited because it can cause pseudomembranous colitis when given orally or by injection. It is available as a single ingredient topical preparation and can also be combined with benzoyl peroxide. A topical fixed-dose clindamycin phosphate 12% and benzoyl peroxide 30% combination gel once daily was more effective and twice daily at least as effective as clindamycin alone twice daily, with an early onset of action and an acceptable safety and tolerability profile.[119] Erythromycin is available alone and in combination with retinoic acid or benzoyl peroxide. Stable, fixed-combination agents are available with erythromycin 3%/benzoyl peroxide 5%, clindamycin 1%/benzoyl peroxide 5%, and clindamycin 1%/benzoyl peroxide 3.75%. Combination agents may enhance adherence with treatment regimens. Some topical antibiotic–benzoyl peroxide combinations require refrigeration.[62] Tolerance with these agents is excellent; clindamycin alone is pregnancy category B.[68]

Other topical antibiotics that are being studied include fluoroquinolones, such as nadifloxacin and minocycline, but these are not approved for use in patients with acne by FDA. Minocycline 4% foam is approved by FDA for topical treatment of patients aged 9 years and older with inflammatory lesions of nonnodular moderate-to-severe acne vulgaris. Its use has been evaluated in 3 large randomized, double-blind, vehicle-controlled study in patients with moderate-to-severe acne. Once-daily application for 12 weeks was associated with a decrease in inflammatory lesion count of approximately 13% to 17% compared with 10% to 17% with vehicle alone. It is generally well tolerated, with the most common adverse effects including headache (3%), mild erythema (14.2%), inflammatory/postinflammatory hyperpigmentation (12.4%), and xerosis (6.8%).[120]

Minocycline is formulated in a yellow base, which can stain fabrics but does not permanently stain skin, and there are no reports to date of drug-induced pigmentation associated with topical application. There are additionally no reports to date of bacterial resistance with topical minocycline. It is broken down by benzoyl peroxide; they should be applied 8 hours apart when used concurrently.

Oral Antibacterials Overview: a systematic evidence-based review of scientific evidence of the efficacy of oral antibiotics for acne was published in 2017. Due to heterogeneity in trials, there is insufficient evidence to support one type, dose, or duration of oral antibiotic over another in terms of efficacy and summarized key points.[121]

- The use of oral antibiotics is reserved for patients with moderate-to-severe inflammatory acne.
- Tetracyclines are considered first-line therapy, while macrolides and trimethoprim/sulfamethoxazole are acceptable alternative agents.
- It is recommended that oral antibiotics be prescribed with concurrent topical therapy for improved efficacy and to combat antibiotic resistance.
- The choice of antibiotic should be determined based on the side effect profile, resistance, cost, and consensus guidelines.
- Oral antibiotics used in the treatment of acne may have unintended effects on nontarget bacteria, and the clinical implications of this warrant further exploration.

Systemic antibiotics are a standard of care in the management of moderate and severe acne and treatment-resistant forms of inflammatory acne. There is evidence to support the use of tetracycline, doxycycline, minocycline, erythromycin, trimethoprim-sulfamethoxazole, trimethoprim, and azithromycin. Studies do not exist for the use of ampicillin, amoxicillin, or cephalexin. However, any antibiotic that can reduce the *P. acnes* population in vivo and interfere with the organism's ability to generate inflammatory agents should be effective.[62] Although erythromycin is effective, use should be limited to those who cannot use one of the tetracyclines (ie, pregnant women or children under 8 years of age because of the potential for damage to the skeleton or teeth). Ciprofloxacin, trimethoprim-sulfamethoxazole, and trimethoprim alone are also effective in instances where other antibiotics cannot be used or for patients who do not respond to conventional treatment.[81,122]

The tetracycline antibiotic family has multiple modes of action, well-understood antibacterial effects, and anti-inflammatory effects that target an additional aspect of pathogenesis.[116,122,123] Through calcium chelation, they inhibit neutrophil and monocyte chemotaxis. Concentrations below the antibiotic threshold still inhibit inflammation and improve both acne vulgaris and acne rosacea.

Tetracycline is no longer the drug of choice in this family; disadvantages include diet-related effects on absorption and the drug's lower anti-inflammatory and antibacterial activity.

The incidence of significant adverse effects with oral antibiotic use is low. However, adverse effect profiles may be helpful for each systemic antibiotic used in the treatment of acne. Vaginal candidiasis may complicate the use of all oral antibiotics.[62] Doxycycline is very commonly a photosensitizer especially at higher doses.

Minocycline has been associated with pigment deposition in the skin, mucous membranes, and teeth, particularly among patients receiving long-term therapy and/or higher doses of the medication. In some instances this is irreversible. Pigmentation occurs most often in acne scars, anterior shins, and mucous membranes. Minocycline may cause dose-related dizziness, which resolves with dose titration; urticaria; hypersensitivity syndrome, autoimmune hepatitis, a systemic lupus erythematosus-like syndrome; and serum sickness-like reactions.[62,116]

The Cochrane collaboration has conducted a review into the efficacy and safety of minocycline, examining 39 randomized controlled trials. These studies show that minocycline is an effective treatment for moderate-to-severe inflammatory acne but present no evidence to support the first-line use of minocycline in acne treatment. The drug is more lipophilic, may act more quickly, and can be taken once daily. However, people treated with minocycline are at a significantly greater risk of developing an autoimmune syndrome than those given tetracycline or no treatment.[124]

Sarecycline (Seysara) is a new, oral, narrow-spectrum tetracycline-derived antibiotic with anti-inflammatory properties. It is specifically indicated for the treatment of inflammatory lesions of non-nodular moderate-to-severe acne vulgaris in patients 9 years of age or older. The mechanism of action in treating acne vulgaris is not known. Sarecycline should be taken with or without food once daily at a weight-based tiered dosage (60 mg if 33-54 kg, 100 mg if 55-84 kg, and 150 mg if 85-136 kg). To reduce the risk of esophageal irritation and ulceration, sarecycline should be administered with adequate amounts of fluid.

The FDA approval of sarecycline in October 2018 was based on two identically designed, large, multicenter, randomized, double-blind, placebo-controlled, phase III studies that assessed use in a total of 2,002 participants 9 years of age or older with moderate-to-severe facial acne vulgaris. Data demonstrated that once-daily sarecycline 1.5 mg/kg significantly improved acne severity based on Investigator's Global Assessment (IGA) success and significantly reduced inflammatory lesion count versus placebo at week 12. Study 1: IGA success, 21.9% versus 10.5%, and mean absolute reduction in number of inflammatory lesions, 15.3 versus 10.2. Study 2: IGA success, 22.6% versus 15.3%, and mean absolute reduction in inflammatory lesions, 15.5 versus 11.1.[125-127]

Bacterial resistance to antibiotics is an increasing problem in acne therapy, particularly because treatments are used over a long period of time.[116] The development of strains with unidentified mutations suggests new evolving mechanisms of resistance. Combined resistance to clindamycin and erythromycin is much more common than resistance to tetracycline. Use of topical antibiotics can lead to resistance largely confined to the skin of treated sites, whereas oral antibiotics can lead to resistance in commensal flora at all body sites. Resistance is more common in patients with moderate-to-severe acne and in countries with high outpatient antibiotic sales. Resistance is disseminated primarily by person-to-person contact, and thus the spread occurs frequently.

There have been an increasing number of reports of systemic infections caused by resistant *P. acnes* in nonacne patients after surgery. A transmission of factors conferring resistance to bacteria other than *P. acnes* has been described.

The most likely consequence of resistance is decreased clinical efficacy of antibiotic-based treatment regimens compared with that in patients with fully susceptible flora.

Studies on *P. acnes* resistance have highlighted the need for treatment guidelines to restrict the use of antibiotics to limit the emergence of resistant strains. Patients with less severe forms of acne should not be treated with oral antibiotics, and where possible such therapy should be limited to the shortest feasible duration (eg, 6-8 weeks). Local patterns of resistance should be considered. The use of systemic antibiotics should be limited (both indication and duration) and topical antibiotic monotherapy should be avoided.

Guidelines advocate early use of combination therapy with retinoids. Often, when oral antibiotics are combined with topical agents, the antibiotic may be discontinued after 6 months of therapy. Nearly 70% of patients with acne require antibiotics for 12 weeks or less if aggressive retinoid therapy is introduced during that time.[116]

Another potential strategy is to eliminate the use of antibiotics and combine other topical agents. Neither retinoids nor benzoyl peroxide creates selective pressure for resistance and is one combination option. Although this approach has been evaluated for efficacy and safety, there is limited evidence of its effect on microbial resistance. In one open label study of adapalene and benzoyl peroxide, baseline counts of antibiotic resistant strains of *P. acnes* were reduced by week 4.[116]

Stricter cross-infection control measures are recommended when assessing acne. Any topical or systemic antibiotic therapy should be combined when possible with broad-spectrum antibacterial agents such as benzoyl peroxide. In addition, isotretinoin use should be initiated earlier in indicated patients, rather than prolonging antibiotic courses.[24,69]

Other Topical Agents A tyrosine kinase inhibitor, azelaic acid has been used in patients with sensitive skin or of Fitzpatrick skin types IV or greater because of the lightening effect of the product on dyspigmentation.[67]

Azelaic acid possesses activity against all four pathogenic factors that produce acne. It has anti-inflammatory and antibacterial activities. Azelaic acid also normalizes keratinization, which accounts for its anticomedogenic effect. It is a competitive inhibitor of mitochondrial oxidoreductases and of 5-α-reductase, inhibiting the conversion of testosterone to 5-dehydrotestosterone. It also possesses bacteriostatic activity to both aerobic and anaerobic bacteria including *P. acnes*. Azelaic acid is an antikeratinizing agent, displaying antiproliferative cytostatic effects on keratinocytes and modulating the early and terminal phases of epidermal differentiation.[103] It may produce hypopigmentation. Inhibition of thioredoxin reductase by azelaic acid provides a rationale for its depigmenting property.

Azelaic acid 20% cream is used in the treatment of mild-to-moderate inflammatory acne, has an excellent safety profile with minimal adverse effects, and is well tolerated in comparison with other acne treatments. The most common adverse effects are pruritus, burning, stinging, and tingling; these are reported in 1% to 5% of patients. These are generally transient and mild in nature. Other adverse reactions, such as erythema, dryness, rash, peeling, irritation, dermatitis, and contact dermatitis, were reported in fewer than 1% of patients.

Azelaic acid has been effective in clinical trials studied with topical 2% erythromycin, topical 5% benzoyl peroxide gel, and topical 0.05% tretinoin cream in the treatment of mild-to-moderate inflammatory acne. However, the agent has limited efficacy, compared with other antiacne therapies.[62] It is an alternative to first choice therapy for comedonal and all types inflammatory acne, particularly in combination. It is an alternative to topical retinoids for maintenance therapy as its efficacy and safety profile are advantageous for long-term therapy.[24,32,67]

Azelaic acid should be applied twice a day, in the morning and evening. A majority of patients with inflammatory lesions may experience an improvement in their acne within 4 weeks of beginning treatment. However, treatment may be continued over several months, if necessary.

Azelaic acid is in a pregnancy category B and should only be used in pregnant women if medically necessary. Patients with dark complexions should be monitored for early signs of hypopigmentation.

Dapsone, a synthetic sulfone, is available topically as 5% and 7.5% gels for acne, and may be used in sulfonamide-allergic patients. Dapsone's utility is attributable to its anti-inflammatory and antimicrobial properties that improve both inflammatory and noninflammatory acne, with more prominent effects occurring in inflammatory lesions. In clinical trials, topical dapsone showed modest-to-moderate efficacy, primarily in the reduction of inflammatory lesions. Short- and long-term safety and efficacy have been demonstrated.[128]

In a study of 101 adult women with mild-to-moderate inflammatory facial acne and sensitive skin for 12 weeks, topical 5% dapsone gel was effective and minimally irritating. Response to dapsone appears to be influenced by gender, with female patients experiencing a significantly greater reduction in acne lesion counts and a significantly higher clinical success rate following 12 weeks of treatment.[129]

Topical 5% dapsone gel is recommended to be used twice daily for acne. Conversely, dapsone 7.5% gel is indicated once daily. It received FDA approval for use in patients aged 12 years and older based on a pair of 12-week, double-blind, placebo-controlled, randomized trials that included more than 4,300 participants with acne. In these studies, a Global Acne Assessment Score of 0 or 1 with at least a two-grade improvement was achieved in 30% of patients assigned to dapsone 7.5% gel, compared with 21% of vehicle-treated controls. It was extremely well tolerated, with application site dryness and itching rates similar to placebo.[130]

Topical dapsone is especially beneficial for patients exhibiting sensitivities or intolerance to conventional antiacne agents.[131]

Combination therapy with dapsone and topical retinoids may be indicated if comedonal components are present. Topical dapsone 5%, alone or in combination, with adapalene 0.1% or benzoyl peroxide 4% has been safe and efficacious but may be more irritating than other topical agents.[131,132]

Intralesional Steroids Intralesional corticosteroid injections are effective for individual inflammatory acne nodules. The effect of intralesional injection with corticosteroids (eg, triamcinolone acetonide) is a well-established and recognized treatment for large inflammatory lesions. Cystic acne improved in patients receiving intralesional steroids.[62] Rapid improvement and decreased pain are noted.

Systemic absorption of steroids may occur with intralesional injections. Adrenal suppression was observed in one study. The injection of intralesional steroids may be associated with local atrophy. Lowering the concentration and/or volume of steroid may minimize these complications.

Hormonal Agents Two topical antiandrogen treatments are now available: clascoterone and topical spironolactone. Systemic antiandrogen agents include oral contraceptives and systemic spironolactone.

Clascoterone is an androgen receptor inhibitor with a greater ability to inhibit inflammatory cytokine synthesis from sebocytes compared to spironolactone. It has been approved in a 1% cream formulation for topical treatment of acne vulgaris in patients 12 years and older based on two randomized, double-blind, vehicle-controlled trials of 1,421 participants 12 years and older with moderate-to-severe facial acne vulgaris. Overall, 62% of participants were female, and 91% were White, with a mean age of 19.7 years. After 12 weeks of twice-daily application, clascoterone cream 1%, produced a significant reduction in absolute noninflammatory lesions from baseline to −19.4 (both trials) versus −13.0 and −10.8 with vehicle, respectively, as well as a reduction in inflammatory lesions from baseline to −19.3 and −20.0 versus −15.5 and −12.6 with vehicle, respectively. The most common side effects were erythema, pruritus, edema, stinging, and burning.[133]

In contrast to systemic spironolactone, topical clascoterone can be used in both males and females. There are no human data on use in pregnancy, but subcutaneous exposure to doses 8 to 39 times maximal recommended human doses resulted in increased malformations in rats and postimplantation loss and resorptions in rabbits. There are no data on safety in lactation or detection of drug or metabolite in human milk.[134]

Oral Contraceptives Estrogen-containing oral contraceptives can be useful in the treatment of acne in some women. Those approved by the FDA for the management of acne contain norgestimate with ethinyl estradiol and norethindrone acetate with ethinyl estradiol. There is good evidence and consensus opinion that other estrogen-containing oral contraceptives are also equally effective.[62]

The mechanism of action of combination oral contraceptives (COCs) in the treatment of acne is based on their antiandrogenic properties. These hormones decrease androgen production at the level of the ovary and also increase sex hormone-binding globulin, binding free circulating testosterone and rendering it unavailable to bind and activate the androgen receptor. In addition, COCs reduce 5-α-reductase activity and block the androgen receptor.[68]

The risks of COCs must be weighed against the risks of the condition that they are treating or preventing. If COCs are used exclusively for acne, their risks must be compared to the risks of acne. It is important to remember that FDA approval of all COCs for acne specifies that they are approved for the treatment of acne in women who also desire contraception. COCs carry cardiovascular risks, and breast cancer risks in some women, and low estrogen may affect bone mass. However, decreased risks of colorectal, ovarian, and endometrial cancers have been shown.

Oral contraceptives may improve acne for many women with clinical and laboratory findings of hyperandrogenism and in women without these findings.[68]

The Cochrane collaboration conducted a review in 2012 to determine the effectiveness of COCs for the treatment of facial acne compared with placebo or other active therapies. Thirty-one trials with a total of 12,579 women were reviewed.[134]

Combination oral contraceptive use reduced inflammatory and noninflammatory facial lesion counts, severity grades, and self-assessed acne in nine placebo comparison trials, according to the review.

Most studies assessed women over six treatment cycles, which might not be adequate for a chronic condition like acne. In two trials, patients were more likely to discontinue because of adverse events, suggesting even if COCs improve acne, women might not be willing to accept long-term use for acne because of other side effects.

The review concluded that COCs should be considered for women with acne who also want an oral contraceptive.

A meta-analysis review of 32 randomized controlled trials comparing use of antibiotics to oral contraceptive agents for acne concluded that although antibiotics may be superior at 3 months, oral contraceptive agents are equivalent to antibiotics at 6 months in reducing acne lesions and may be a better first-line alternative to systemic antibiotics for long-term acne management in women.[135]

Spironolactone Spironolactone is an antiandrogenic compound that decreases testosterone production and competitively inhibits binding of testosterone and dihydrotestosterone to androgen receptors in the skin. Spironolactone may cause hyperkalemia, primarily with higher doses or in patients with cardiac or renal compromise. Routine use occasionally causes menstrual irregularity. A 5% spironolactone gel, studied in patients with increased sebum secretion, resulted in a decrease in the total acne lesions with no significant efficacy under the acne severity index.[136,137]

A single center review of 80 female patients with acne treated with systemic spironolactone (median age 19 years; range 14-20) reported complete response in 22.5% of patients, and complete or partial response greater than 50% in 58.8% of subjects. The median dose was 100 mg, and median time to initial and maximal responses were 3 and 5 months, respectively. Responders were more likely to have jawline distribution of acne (70.3% vs 56.3%) and cyclic flares (75% vs 56.3%), although this was not significant. Only three patients experienced side effects (rash, breast tenderness, diarrhea, and headache) and discontinued treatment. There were no reports of symptoms of hypotension, although blood pressure and potassium were not routinely checked in the cohort.[138]

Although not currently FDA approved for the treatment of acne, the 2016 AAD work group supports the use of spironolactone in the management of acne in select women.[68]

Oral Corticosteroids Oral corticosteroids have two potential modes of activity in the treatment of acne. One study demonstrated that low-dose corticosteroids suppress adrenal activity in patients who have proven adrenal hyperactivity.[139] Low-dose prednisone in doses ranging from 5 to 15 mg daily, administered alone or with high estrogen containing COCs, has efficacy in the treatment of acne and seborrhea. Expert opinion is that short courses of higher dose oral corticosteroids may be beneficial in patients with highly inflammatory disease. Long-term adverse effects of corticosteroids prohibit use as a primary therapy for acne.[68]

Oral Isotretinoin Isotretinoin has been revolutionary for acne treatment. The risk of potential adverse effects must be weighed against its ability to prevent lifelong and permanent physical and psychologic scarring.[140]

Oral isotretinoin is an isomer of retinoic acid that has been used for many years and is approved by the FDA for the treatment of severe recalcitrant acne vulgaris. Its use results in decreased sebum production, acne lesions, and acne scarring, along with a decrease in symptoms of anxiety and depression. The 2016 AAD guidelines recommend use of oral isotretinoin in patients with moderate acne that is treatment-resistant or that produces physical scarring or significant psychosocial distress.

Oral isotretinoin is a natural metabolite of vitamin A. Its mechanism is elusive, as it does not bind to retinoid receptors. It reduces sebogenesis and may also inhibit sebaceous gland activity, growth of *P. acnes*, and inflammation, and improve follicular epithelial differentiation.[141] Systemic isotretinoin exerts a primary effect on comedogenesis, causing a decrease in size and reduction in formation of new comedones.[26] Isotretinoin is the only drug treatment for acne that produces prolonged remission.

The teratogenic effects of oral retinoid therapy are well documented, and it should be prescribed only by those physicians knowledgeable in its appropriate administration and monitoring. Individuals capable of becoming pregnant who are of child-bearing potential must enroll in the approved pregnancy prevention and management program (ie, iPLEDGE) to be treated with isotretinoin. Two different forms of contraception must be started 1 month before and continue at least 1 month (but normally 4 months) after therapy and pregnancy monitoring undertaken before, during, and after therapy.[140]

The efficacy of conventional isotretinoin treatment (0.5-1.0 mg/kg/day for 16-32 weeks, reaching a cumulative dose of 120-150 mg/kg) for acne has been well established. The approved dosage of isotretinoin is 0.5 to 2.0 mg/kg/day.

Initial flaring can be minimized by initiation of lower doses (ie, 0.5 mg/kg/day or less). Many reports document efficacy of low-dose and intermittent isotretinoin treatment. Lower doses can be used for longer time periods, with a total cumulative dose of 120 to 150 mg/kg or the dose can be lowered to 20 mg on alternate days after an initial 2 months of therapy with higher dosage.[142-144] Reports suggest that low-dose regimens are superior to other regimens (conventional or intermittent) in terms of patient satisfaction, tolerability, and efficacy in patients with moderate acne. In patients with severely inflamed acne, an even greater initial dose reduction may be required or pretreatment with oral corticosteroids considered.

Some patients experience a relapse of acne after the first course of treatment with isotretinoin. A retrospective review compared 82 patients who completed two courses of isotretinoin to 160 patients with only one course. Patients receiving a second course had shorter time from clear date to end of the treatment (32.0 ± 43.3 days compared with 65.4 ± 65 days).[145] Despite the small number of patients and retrospective nature of these data, waiting for 2 months without new lesions has been adopted by some practitioners to minimize risk of relapse after achieving target cumulative dosing.

The 2016 AAD guidelines support initiation of isotretinoin at 0.5 mg/kg/day when appropriate, subsequently increasing to a full dose of 1 mg/kg/day after the first month as tolerated, with a goal cumulative dose between 120 and 150 mg/kg. One recent study of 116 patients found that a cumulative dose of 220 mg/kg or more may result in lower relapse rates, but confirmation will require study in larger populations.[68]

Isotretinoin is highly lipophilic and best absorbed when taken with food. One novel formulation is less dependent on the presence of fat in the gut for absorption.[146] When prescribed, drying agents must be discontinued and replaced with moisturizers.

Because isotretinoin is a vitamin A derivative, it interacts with many of the biologic systems of the body, and consequently has a significant pattern of adverse effects. The pattern is similar to that seen in hypervitaminosis A. Side effects include those of the mucocutaneous (most common), musculoskeletal, and ophthalmic systems, as well as headaches and central nervous system effects. Most adverse effects, including cheilitis and dry nose, eyes, and mouth, are transient and resolve with drug discontinuation.[140] Laboratory monitoring during therapy should include triglycerides, cholesterol, transaminases, and complete blood counts.

Mood disorders, depression, suicidal ideation, and suicides have been reported sporadically in patients taking this drug. A causal relationship has not been established. These symptoms are quite common in adolescents and young adults, the age range of patients who are likely to receive isotretinoin.

Issues regarding responsible and informed use Published data and expert opinion differ with respect to the use of isotretinoin as first-line or reserve therapy, optimal dosing, and risk of depression.[140]

Although some persist in reserving isotretinoin use only for severe acne, nodular or conglobate acne that has not responded to appropriate antibiotics and topical therapy, delaying use of isotretinoin, the most effective choice, poses an ethical problem.[147] Opinions vary on whether or not to restrict use to patients under 12 years and whether to avoid lasers, peelers, or wax epilation for at least 6 months after discontinuation of therapy.[148]

The causal relationship between the use of isotretinoin and risk of depression continues to be scrutinized with no consensus. The issue is complex as depression and suicidal ideation occur with severe acne in the absence of isotretinoin.

There are instances in which withdrawal of isotretinoin has resulted in improved mood, and reintroduction of isotretinoin has resulted in the return of mood changes. Treatment of severe acne with isotretinoin is often associated with mood improvement.[62] There is epidemiologic evidence that the incidence of these events is lower in patients treated with isotretinoin than in an age-matched general population. There is also evidence that the risk of depressed mood is no greater during isotretinoin therapy than during therapy of an age-matched acne group treated with conservative therapy.[62]

A 2016 review on isotretinoin controversies, facts, and recommendations concluded despite common misperceptions, there is weak evidence for increased incidence of depression, suicidality, or inflammatory bowel disease with isotretinoin use, and data indicate that transient increases in transaminases and lipid levels do not typically necessitate discontinuation of therapy.[149]

In 2017, a systematic review and meta-analysis of the literature, with 31 studies, concluded isotretinoin treatment for acne did not appear to be associated with an increased risk for depression and that the treatment of acne appears to ameliorate depressive symptoms.[150] Current literature regarding the association with depression and suicide was reexamined in 2018. It reconfirmed that while those with a personal or family history of mental disorder might be at risk, further studies are needed and no conclusions can be drawn.[151] The current literature is insufficient to support a meaningful causative association, but important study limitations exist. In the absence of definitive evidence, an idiosyncratic effect cannot be excluded. This disputed association remains an important area for future research. Given the prevalence of depression, anxiety, and suicidal ideation/suicide in the general population, and especially the adolescent population who may be candidates for isotretinoin therapy, the prescribing physician should continue to monitor for these symptoms at each visit for early recognition, advise patients about a possible risk of depression and suicidal behavior, and make therapeutic decisions within the context of each individual patient.[68]

Light Therapy

Light therapies are believed to work by killing *P. acnes* and by damaging and shrinking sebaceous glands, reducing sebum output and have few[152] or temporary[153,154] adverse effects. Light therapies may be used once or twice weekly as a course of 6 to 10 treatments, with each irradiation lasting 10 to 20 minutes.[154] *P. acnes* produce endogenous porphyrins that absorb light to form highly reactive singlet oxygen, which destroys the bacteria.[154] There is still debate about the effectiveness of different wavelengths.[154] Since porphyrins have peak absorption at blue light wavelengths, blue light is often used to treat acne. Red light is also absorbed by porphyrins and can penetrate deeper into the skin,[155] where it may directly affect inflammatory mediators. Other light therapies attempt to selectively target and damage sebaceous glands directly, reducing their size and thus sebum output.[156] These include infrared lasers, low-energy pulsed dye lasers, and radiofrequency devices.[154]

Photodynamic therapy (PDT) uses specific light-activating creams, which are absorbed into the skin and amplify the response to light therapy but tend to produce more severe adverse effects. There are concerns that PDT may interfere with the skin's natural immune mechanisms[157,158] and cause long-term skin damage.

Light therapies, previously expensive and accessed privately via dermatologists or clinics, are increasingly popular. Home-use blue light therapy is now available. Patients find it easier to comply with light treatments because of their short duration.

Very few trials compare light therapy with conventional acne treatments. The European evidence-based guidelines concluded published evidence is scarce and standardized treatment protocols and widespread experience are lacking. Due to conflicting or insufficient evidence, these guidelines did not make a recommendation for or against treatment of comedonal, MMPP, or severe papulopustular/nodular acne with monotherapy visible light, visible or infrared wavelength lasers, or intense pulsed light or PDT. Blue light has a low strength recommendation as a consideration for MMPP.[24,69] An ongoing Cochrane review protocol continues to investigate the current state of evidence for use of light therapy in acne.[159]

Pharmacologic Cleansing Options

Medicated Soaps and Washes Medicated soaps, washes, and foams may contain topical antiseptics such as triclosan; peeling agents such as salicylic acid, sulfur; antimicrobials such as benzoyl peroxide, clindamycin, or azelaic acid, alone or in combination in low concentrations. They may be nonprescription or prescription status.[160] Most washes should remain on the skin from 15 seconds to 5 minutes followed by thorough rinsing. This limits the amount of time the active ingredient is in contact with the skin. Other cleansers are applied after washing and left on the skin without rinsing.

Quaternary ammonium compounds are cationic detergents that are inactivated quickly in the presence of organic material such as sebum. The duration of action of these products is short.

Antiseptic cleansers that have been studied include hexachlorophene, chlorhexidine, and povidone-iodine. Use of hexachlorophene has since been banned in nonprescription products by the UFDA because of neurotoxicity concerns. Bacteriostatic soaps containing hexachlorophene, carbanilides, and salicylanilides (halogenated hydroxyphenols) may alter normal flora or be acnegenic. Few ordinary soaps induce acne. However, acne patients are particularly susceptible to comedogenic contactants, and if these soaps are applied several times daily for long periods, they may become troublesome.

Soaps containing coal tar, which can induce folliculitis, are not indicated for acne.

In a very small group of patients in an 8-week, double-blind, randomized clinical trial, a combination cleanser containing triclosan, azelaic acid, and salicylic acid produced a greater histopathologic decrease in inflammatory response compared with a nonmedicated cleanser, but there was no significant difference in noninflammatory lesions in either group.[161] A rebound tendency was noted for the nonmedicated cleanser with respect to inflammatory lesions at 4 weeks. Authors concluded that nonmedicated cleansers were an easier and cheaper way of managing patients with mild acne.

Chlorhexidine inhibits in vitro growth of *P. acnes*.[162] A 4% chlorhexidine gluconate preparation in a detergent base is as effective as benzoyl peroxide washes in patients with mild acne, and both preparations reduced the number of inflammatory and noninflammatory lesions after 8 and 12 weeks, compared with vehicle alone.[161] However, further evidence is lacking, and irritation is a side effect.[49]

Glycolic 1%, an alpha-hydroxy acid (AHA), has been used as a cleanser. AHAs cause desquamation by decreasing basal corneocyte cohesion and limiting follicular occlusion. AHA-containing formulations may be considered in the treatment of acne in light of mechanistic similarities with better validated antikeratinization agents such as retinoids.[49]

Alcohol-detergent medicated pads, impregnated with salicylic acid 0.5%, have reduced inflammatory lesions and open comedones in mild-to-moderate acne. This type of medication is less abrasive, not rinsed off, and convenient.[163]

Alcohol-detergent wipes, swabs, or "pledgets" impregnated with antibiotics, such as clindamycin or lincomycin, are available. The antibiotic is deposited in low concentrations on the surface of the skin and may not penetrate to the depths of the pilosebaceous duct. Although patients may like the convenience and perception of using an active agent, they should not be recommended over simple cleansing.

Abrasives consist of finely divided particles of fused aluminum or plastic together with cleansing and wetting agents. Abrasives peel and remove surface debris and may assist resorption of papules and pustules. Despite vigorous rubbing, removal of comedones is not accomplished. Particles containing active agents, such as sodium tetraborate decahydrate, dissolve on use, and their abrasiveness is therefore limited.[163] The effectiveness of an abrasive cleanser with and without polyethylene granules showed no difference in results in patients with mild-to-moderate acne. These products are not

TABLE 117-3 Monitoring Therapy for Acne: Parameters and Frequency

Person Responsible and Frequencies for Monitoring:

Patient: daily while on drug therapy; Pharmacist: every 4-8 weeks of therapy or next pharmacy visit

Parameter	Time Frame/Degree of Change	Actions
Short-Term Effectiveness End Points (Acne Resolution/Control)		
Lesion count	Decrease by 10%-25% within 4-8 weeks, with control, or more than a 50% decrease within 2-4 months	If end points are not achieved, refer to a physician for further therapy
Comedones	Resolve by 3-4 months	
Inflammatory lesions	Resolve within a few weeks	
Anxiety, depression	Achieve control or improvement within 2-4 months	
Long-Term Effectiveness End Points (Acne Resolution/Control)		
Progression of severity	No progression of severity	If end points are not achieved, refer to a physician for further therapy
Recurrent episodes	Lengthening of acne-free periods throughout therapy	
Scarring or pigmentation	No further scarring or pigmentation throughout therapy	
Safety End Points (Treatment Side Effects)		
Dermatitis, increased dryness, gastrointestinal upset, photosensitivity	No adverse effects	Refer to a physician for alternate therapy, dose reduction, discontinuation or additive palliative treatment, or preventative measures for adverse effects

TABLE 117-4 Monitoring Care Plans for Acne Types I Through IV

Acne Type	Description	Suggested Options	Follow-up Action If Patient Responds	Follow-up Action If Patient Does Not Respond in 3 Months	Adjustment in Therapy If Patient Does Not Respond Adequately to Previous Action
Type I	Mainly comedones with an occasional small inflamed papule or pustule; no scarring present	Topical retinoid or a fixed combination with a retinoid is the drug of choice; can also consider benzoyl peroxide or azelaic acid or salicylic acid	Continue until lesions are completely cleared and then stop or taper therapy	Treat as Type II acne	
Type II	Comedones and more numerous papules and pustules (mainly facial); mild scarring	Fixed-dose combination (adapalene and benzoyl peroxide) or benzoyl peroxide or topical retinoid or azelaic acid; if more severe, fixed-dose combination is preferred, with or without hormonal therapy and/or antibiotic, particularly if the trunk is involved	Continue until lesions are completely cleared and then stop or taper therapy	Treat as Type III acne	
Type III	Numerous comedones, papules and pustules, spreading to the back, chest, and shoulders, with an occasional cyst or nodule; moderate scarring	Fixed-dose combination with an oral antibiotic is preferred; oral isotretinoin or oral hormonal therapy can also be added	Oral antibiotics typically are prescribed for daily use over 4-6 months, with subsequent tapering and discontinuation as acne improves. Other agents can also be stopped or tapered now	Add oral contraceptive or antiandrogen (women only)	Oral isotretinoin (except in women who are or who may become pregnant); consider safety end points (potential adverse effects) before initiating therapy
Type IV	Numerous large cysts on the face, neck, and upper trunk; severe scarring	For males, monotherapy with oral isotretinoin or a retinoid fixed combination or oral antibiotics; for females, oral isotretinoin plus antiandrogenic hormonal therapy is preferred, or a fixed combination retinoid with oral antibiotics (consider high dose) and/or oral antiandrogenic hormonal therapy	Oral antibiotics typically are prescribed for daily use over 4-6 months, with subsequent tapering and discontinuation as acne improves Other agents can also be stopped or tapered now	If no response after 3-6 months, oral isotretinoin (except in women who are or who may become pregnant). Consider safety end points (potential adverse effects) before initiating therapy	

indicated in most cases but may be used in a patient who responds empirically.[164]

EVALUATION OF THERAPEUTIC OUTCOMES

10 Provide a monitoring framework for patients with acne. Parameters should be monitored by the patient and recorded in a diary. Therapy should be appropriately tapered in response to improvement or resolution. The healthcare professional should be responsible for ensuring that the treatment plan remains on schedule and is effective with no adverse effects. The patient should be contacted within 2 to 3 weeks to determine progress.

Acne is poorly understood by adolescents. These patients often lack knowledge of the cause of the disorder and aggravating factors, indications for self-care versus prescription treatment, expected onset of effect, sequence of the healing process, duration of treatment, appropriate application of topical agents, maximal achievable effects, expected adverse effects, safety concerns, and the benefit to QOL. Clinicians should review patient understanding of each of these important factors to ensure patient adherence. There is often a need to supplement counseling sessions with written materials to which the patient can refer at home.

Good adherence is the key to treatment success. Other strategies to increase adherence include use of once-daily regimens, online follow-up visits, and remote digital imaging for ongoing lesion assessment.[165,166] A randomized controlled trial compared the effectiveness of automated online counseling to standard web-based education on improving acne knowledge. While both models had a significant increase in knowledge from baseline, after 12 weeks, mean improvement in knowledge was higher in the automated counseling group than in the standard Website group. The automated counseling Website group rated their educational material more useful and more enjoyable to view than did the standard Website group. Internet-based patient education appears to be an effective method of improving acne knowledge among adolescents.[167]

Monitoring of the Pharmaceutical Care Plan

Tables 117-2 to 117-4 provide a guide for monitoring patients with acne. Table 117-2 outlines individual drugs, their most common adverse effects, parameters to monitor, and issues to note. Table 117-3 outlines general effectiveness and safety end points, monitoring parameters, and degree of change and time frames for short- and long-term outcomes. Table 117-4 is a guide for monitoring acne patients with consideration to the severity grading of acne types I through IV.

CONCLUSION

Considerable gaps remain in the understanding of acne, despite all that is known about the pathogenesis of acne and the mechanisms of effective drugs for controlling its symptoms, progression, and complications at structural, biochemical, and physiologic levels. It is still not possible to precisely define the cause of one of the most common skin diseases, nor is it possible to identify a cure for a condition that affects a very large proportion of the global population.

ABBREVIATIONS

BGA	best guideline acne
CAM	complementary and alternative medicine
COC	combination oral contraceptive
CRH	corticotropin-releasing hormone
FDA	Food and Drug Administration
GHQ	general health quality
HGL	high glycemic load
IGF	insulin-like growth factor
MMPP	mild-to-moderate papulopustular
P. acnes	*Propionibacterium acnes*
PAPA	pyogenic arthritis, pyoderma gangrenosum, acne
PBV	pollen bee venom
PDT	photodynamic therapy
QOL	quality of life
SAPHO	synovitis, acne, pustulosis, hyperostosis, osteitis syndrome
SPF	sun protection factor
TTO	time trade-off

REFERENCES

1. Tan JKL, Bhate K. A global perspective on the epidemiology of acne. *British Journal of Dermatology*. 2015;172:3–12. doi:10.1111/bjd.13462.
2. Smithard A, Glazebrook C, Williams HC. Acne prevalence, knowledge about acne and psychological morbidity in mid-adolescence: A community-based study. *Br J Dermatol.* 2001;41:577–580.
3. Heng AHS, Chew FT. Systematic review of the epidemiology of acne vulgaris. *Scientific Reports*. 2020;10. doi:10.1038/s41598-020-62715-3.
4. Kubba R, Bajaj AK, Thappa DM, et al. Acne in India: Guidelines for management—IAA Consensus Document: Epidemiology of acne. *Indian J Dermatol Venereol Leprol.* 2009;75(suppl 1):S3.
5. Shalita AR. Acne vulgaris: Pathogenesis and treatment. *Cosmet Toiletries*. 1983;98:57–60.
6. Malus M, LaChance PA, Lamy L, Macaulay A, Vanasse M. Priorities in adolescent health care: The teenagers' viewpoint. *J Fam Pract.* 1987;25:159–162.
7. Rosenberg EW. Acne diet reconsidered. *Arch Dermatol.* 1981;117(4):193–195.
8. Fulton JE, Plewig G, Kligman AM. Effect of chocolate on acne vulgaris. *JAMA*. 1969;210(11):2071–2074.
9. Anderson PC. Foods as the cause of acne. *Am Fam Physician*. 1971;3(3): n102–n103.
10. Adebamowo CA, Spiegelman D, Danby FW, Frazier AL, Willett WC, Holmes MD. High school dietary dairy intake and teenage acne. *J Am Acad Dermatol.* 2005;52(2):207–214.
11. Danby FW. Acne and milk, the diet myth, and beyond. *J Am Acad Dermatol.* 2005;52(2):360–362.
12. Bowers J. Diet and acne. *Dermatology World*. 2011:31–34.
13. Kim J, Ko Y, Park YK, et al. Dietary effect of lactoferrin-enriched fermented milk on skin surface lipid and clinical improvement of acne vulgaris. *Nutrition*. 2010;26(9):902–909.
14. Mueller EA, Trapp S, Frentzel A, et al. Efficacy and tolerability of oral lactoferrin supplementation in mild to moderate acne vulgaris: An exploratory study. *Curr Med Res Opin*. 2011;27(4):793–797.
15. Juhl CR, Bergholdt HKM, Miller IM, Jemec GBE, Kanters JK, Ellervik C. Dairy intake and acne vulgaris: A systematic review and meta-analysis of 78,529 children, adolescents, and young adults. *Nutrients*. 2018;10(8):1049. doi:10.3390/nu10081049.
16. Thiboutot D. Acne: Hormonal concepts and therapy. *Clin Dermatol.* 2004;22:419–428.
17. Cappel M, Mauger D, Thiboutet D. Correlation between serum levels of insulin-like growth factor 1, dehydroepiandrosterone sulfate, and dihydrotestosterone and acne lesion counts in adult women. *Arch Dermatol.* 2005;141(3):333–338.
18. Smith RN, Mann NJ, Braue A, et al. The effect of a high protein, low-glycemic load diet versus a conventional high-glycemic load diet on biochemical parameters associated with acne vulgaris: A randomized, investigator-masked controlled trial. *J Am Acad Dermatol.* 2007;57(2):247–256.
19. Smith RN, Mann NJ, Braue A, Mäkeläinen H, Varigos GA. A low-glycemic-load diet improves symptoms in acne vulgaris patients: A randomized controlled trial. *Am J Clin Nutr.* 2007;86(1):107–115. doi:10.1093/ajcn/86.1.107.
20. Smith RN, Braue A, Varigos GA, Mann NJ. The effect of a low glycemic load diet on acne vulgaris and the fatty acid composition of skin surface triglycerides. *J Dermatol Sci.* 2008;50(1):41–52.

21. Wolkenstein P, Misery L, Amici JM, et al. Smoking and dietary factors associated with moderate-to-severe acne in French adolescents and young adults: Results of a survey using a representative sample. *Dermatology*. 2015;230(1):34–39.
22. Antiga E, Verdelli A, Bonciani D, et al. Acne: A new model of immune-mediated chronic inflammatory skin disease. *Giornale Italiano di Dermatologia e Venereologia*. 2015;150(2):247–254.
23. Dréno B. What is new in the pathophysiology of acne, an overview. *J Eur Acad Dermatol Venereol*. 2017;31(S5):8–12. https://doi.org/10.1111/jdv.14374.
24. Gollnick HP, Bettoli V, Lambert J, et al. A consensus-based practical and daily guide for the treatment of acne patients. *J Eur Acad Dermatol Venereol*. 2016;30(9):1480–1490. doi:10.1111/jdv.13675.
25. Chu A. Acne vulgaris. In: Lebwohl MG, Heyman WR, Berth-Jones J, Couslon I, eds. *Treatment of Skin Diseases*. 2nd ed. Philadelphia, PA: Mosby Elsevier; 2006:6–12.
26. Dreno B, Poli F. Epidemiology of acne. *Dermatology*. 2003;206:7–10.
27. Tucker SB, Rogers S, Winkleman RK. Inflammation in acne vulgaris: Leukocyte attraction and cytotoxicity by comedonal material. *J Invest Dermatol*. 1985;74:21–25.
28. Winston MH, Shalita AR. Acne vulgaris. *Pediatr Clin North Am*. 1991;38(4):889–903.
29. Plewig G, Kligman AM. The dynamics of primary comedo formation. In: Plewig G, Kligman AM, eds. *Acne: Morphogenesis and Treatment*. New York: Springer-Verlag; 1975:58–107.
30. Puissegur-Lupo M. Acne vulgaris, treatments and their rationale. *Postgrad Med*. 1985;78(7):76–88.
31. Batra RS. Acne. In: Arndt KA, Tsu JTS, eds. *Manual of Dermatologic Therapeutics*. 7th ed. Philadelphia, PA: Lippincott, Williams and Wilkins; 2007:3–18.
32. Nast A, Rosumeck S, Erdmann R, Alsharif U, Dressler C, Werner RN. Methods report on the development of the European evidence-based (S3) guideline for the treatment of acne: Update 2016. *J Eur Acad Dermatol Venereol*. 2016;30(8):e1–e28. doi:10.1111/jdv.13783.
33. U.S. Department of Health and Human Services/Food and Drug Administration Center for Drug Evaluation and Research Guidance for Industry. Acne vulgaris: Developing drugs for treatment. http://www.fda.gov/dowloads/Drugs/GuidanceComplianceRegulatoryInformation/GuidancesCM071292.pdf. 2005.
34. Harrison-Atlas R, Bernhard JD, O'Connor RC, Weinraub LF. What to do when typical teenage acne strikes. *JCOM*. 1996;3:9.
35. Chernyshov PV, Zouboulis CC, Tomas-Aragones L, et al. Quality of life measurement in acne. Position paper of the European Academy of Dermatology and Venereology Task Forces on Quality of Life and Patient Oriented Outcomes and Acne, Rosacea and Hidradenitis Suppurativa. *J Eur Acad Dermatol Venereol*. 2018;32(2):194–208. doi:10.1111/jdv.14585.
36. Pagliarello C, Di Pietro C, Tabolli S. A comprehensive health impact assessment and determinants of quality of life, health and psychological status in acne patients. *Giornale Italiano di Dermatologia e Venereologia*. 2015;150(3):303–308.
37. Chren MM, Lasek RJ, Quinn LM, et al. Skindex, a quality-of-life measure for patients with skin disease. Reliability, validity and responsiveness. *J Invest Dermatol*. 1996;107(5):707–713.
38. Finlay AY, Khan GK. Dermatology Quality of Life Index (DLQI): A simple practical measure for routine clinical use. *Clin Exp Dermatol*. 1994;19(3):210–216.
39. Girman CJ, Hartmaier S, Thiboutot D, et al. Evaluating health-related quality of life in patients with facial acne: Development of a self-administered questionnaire for clinical trials. *Qual Life Res*. 1996;5(5):481–490.
40. Gupta MA, Johnson AM, Gupta AK. The development of an acne quality of life scale: Reliability, validity and relationship to subjective acne severity in mild to moderate acne vulgaris. *Acta Derm Venereol*. 1998;78(6):451–456.
41. Wang KC, Zane LT. Recent advances in acne vulgaris research: Insights and clinical implications. In: James WD, ed. *Advances in Dermatology*. Philadelphia, PA: Elsevier; 2008:197–209.
42. Johnson BA, Nunley JR. Topical therapy for acne vulgaris: How do you choose the best drug for each patient? *Postgrad Med J*. 2000; 107(3):69–80.
43. Steinhoff M, Schauber J, Leyden JJ. New insights into rosacea pathophysiology: A review of recent findings. *J Am Acad Dermatol*. 2013;69:S15–S26.
44. Habif TP. Acne, rosacea, and related disorders. In: Klein EA, Menczer BS, eds. *Clinical Dermatology*. Toronto: Mosby; 1990:756.
45. Kelly AP. Acne and related disorders. In: Sams WM, Lynch PJ, eds. *Principles and Practice of Dermatology*. New York: Churchill Livingstone; 1990:1014.
46. MacDonald Hull S, Sunliffe WJ. The use of a corticosteroid cream for immediate reduction in the clinical signs of acne vulgaris. *Acta Derm Venereol*. 1989;69(5):452–453.
47. Brodell RT, O'Brien MR. Topical corticosteroid-induced acne: Three treatment strategies to break the "addiction cycle." *Postgrad Med*. 1999;106(6):225–229.
48. Hitch JM. Acneform eruption induced by drugs and chemicals. *JAMA*. 1969;200:879.
49. Stringer T, Nagler A, Orlow SJ, Oza VS. Clinical evidence for washing and cleansers in acne vulgaris: A systematic review. *J Dermatol Treatment*. 2018;29(7):688–693. doi:10.1080/09546634.2018.1442552.
50. Choi YS, Suh HS, Yoon MY, et al. A study of the efficacy of cleansers for acne vulgaris. *J Dermatol Treat*. 2010;21(3):201–205.
51. Boothroyd S. Topical therapy and formulation principles. In: Webster GF, Rawlings AV, eds. *Acne and Its Therapy*. New York: Informa Healthcare USA; 2007:253–274.
52. Food and Drug Administration. Non-prescription drugs. 2009. Available at: http://www.fda.gov/OHRMS/DOCKETS/98fr/78n-0065-npr0003.pdf.
53. Russell JJ. Topical therapy for acne. *Am Fam Physician*. 2000;61(2):357–365.
54. Epinette WW, Gresit MC. Osols II. The role of cosmetics in postadolescent acne. *Cutis*. 1982;29(5):500–514.
55. Plewig G, Kligman AM. Acne cosmetica. In: Plewig G, Kligman AM, eds. *Acne: Morphogenesis and Treatment*. New York: Springer-Verlag; 1975;226–229.
56. Mills OH, Kligman AM. Comedogenicity of sunscreens. Experimental observations in rabbits. *Arch Dermatol*. 1982;18(6):417–419.
57. Cappel M, Mauger D, Thiboutet D. Correlation between serum levels of insulin-like growth factor 1, dehydroepiandrosterone sulfate, and dihydrotestosterone and acne lesion counts in adult women. *Arch Dermatol*. 2005;141:333–338.
58. Dall'oglio F, Tedeschi A, Fabbrocini G. Cosmetics for acne: Indications and recommendations for an evidence-based approach. *Giornale Italiano di Dermatologia e Venereologia*. 2015;150(1):1–11.
59. Hoffman LK, Bhatia N, Zeichner J, Kircik LH. Topical vehicle formulations in the treatment of acne. *J Drugs Dermatol*. 2018;17(6 suppl):s6–s10.
60. Thiboutot DM. New treatments and therapeutic strategies for acne. *Arch Fam Med*. 2000;9:179–187. 10.1001/archfami.9.2.179.
61. Chiou WL. Low intrinsic drug activity and dominant vehicle (Placebo) effect in the topical treatment of acne vulgaris. *Int J Clin Pharmacol Therapeut*. 2012;50(6):434–437.
62. Strauss JS, Kowchk DP, Leyden JJ, et al. Guidelines of care for acne vulgaris management. *J Am Acad Dermatol*. 2007;56:651–663.
63. Ellerbroek WC. Hypotheses toward a unified field theory of human behavior with clinical application to acne vulgaris. *Perspect Biol Med*. 1973;16:240–262.
64. Hughes H, Brown BW, Lawlis GF, Fulton JE Jr. Treatment of acne vulgaris by biofeedback relaxation and cognitive imagery. *J Psychosom Res*. 1983;27:185–191.
65. Chao CM, Lai WY, Wu BY, Chang HC, Huang WS, Chen YF. A pilot study on efficacy treatment of acne vulgaris using a new method: Results of a randomized double-blind trial with Acne Dressing. *J Cosmet Sci*. 2006;57(2):95–105.
66. Rhei LD, Zatz JL, Motwani MR. Targeted delivery of actives from topical treatment products to the pilosebaceous unit. In: Webster GF, Rawlings AV, eds. *Acne and Its Therapy*. New York: Informa Healthcare USA; 2007:223–252.
67. Thiboutot DM, Dréno B, Abanmi A, et al. Practical management of acne for clinicians: An international consensus from the Global Alliance to Improve Outcomes in Acne. *J Am Acad Dermatol*. 2018;78(2 suppl 1):s1–s23.e. doi:10.1016/j.jaad.2017.09.078.
68. Zaenglein AL, Pathy AL, Schlosser BJ, et al. Guidelines of care for the management of acne vulgaris. *J Am Acad Dermatol*. 2016;74(5):945–973. doi:10.1016/j.jaad.2015.12.037.
69. Nast A, Dréno B, Bettoli V, et al. European evidence-based (S3) guideline for the treatment of acne: Update 2016—short version. *J Eur Acad Dermatol Venereol*. 2016;30(8):1261–1268. doi:10.1111/jdv.13776.
70. Thiboutot D, Gollnick H, Bettoli V, et al. New insights into the management of acne: An update from the Global Alliance to Improve Outcomes in Acne Group. *J Am Acad Dermatolog*. 2009;60:S1–S50.
71. Dréno B, Thiboutot DM, Gollnick H, et al. Antibiotic stewardship in dermatology: Limiting antibiotic use in acne. *Eur J Dermatol*. 2014;24(3):330–334. doi:10.1684/ejd.2014.2309.
72. Eisenberg DM, Davis RB, Ettner SL, et al. Trends in alternative medicine use in the United States, 1990–1997: Results of a follow-up national survey. *JAMA*. 1998;280(18):1569–1575.

73. Cae H, Liu JP, Smith CA, et al. Complementary therapies for acne vulgaris (Review). The Cochrane collaboration, issue 1. New York: Wiley; 2015. Available at: http://www.thecochranelibrary.com.
74. Winkelman WJ. Aromatherapy, botanicals, and essential oils in acne. *Clin Dermatol.* 2018;36(3):299–305. doi:10.1016/j.clindermatol.2018.03.004.
75. Poli F, Ribet V, Lauze C, Adhoute H, Morinet P. Efficacy and safety of 0.1% retinaldehyde/6% glycolic acid (Diacneal) for mild to moderate acne vulgaris. A multicentre, double-blind, randomized, vehicle-controlled trial. *Dermatol.* 2005;210(suppl 1):14–21.
76. Food and Drug Administration. Non-prescription drugs. 2009. Available at: http://www.fda.gov/OHRMS/DOCKETS/98fr/78n-0065-npr0003.pdf.
77. Tan J, Thiboutot D, Gollnick H, et al. Development of an atrophic acne scar risk assessment tool. *J Eur Acad Dermatol Venereol.* 2017;31(9):1547–1554. doi:10.1111/jdv.14325.
78. Katsambas AD, Katoulis AC, Stavropoulos P. Acne neonatorum: A study of 22 cases. *Int J Dermatol.* 1999;38(2):128–130.
79. Andriessen A, Rodas DA, Gameros P, et al. Over the counter products for acne treatment and maintenance in Latin America: A review of current clinical practice. *J Drugs Dermatol.* 2021;20:244–250. 10.36849/jdd.5779.
80. Brown S. Therapeutic potpourri. *Dermatol Clin.* 1989;7(1):71–74.
81. Sykes NL, Webster GF. Acne: A review of optimum treatment. *Drugs.* 1994;48(1):59–70.
82. Zouboulis CC. Moderne aknetherapie. *Akt Dermatol.* 2003;29:49–57.
83. Zander E, Weisman S. Treatment of acne vulgaris with salicylic acid pads. *Clin Ther.* 1992;14:247–253.
84. Gross G. Benzoyl peroxide and salicylic acid therapy. In: Webster GF, Rawlings AV, eds. *Acne and Its Therapy*. New York: Informa Healthcare USA; 2007:117–136.
85. Shalita AR. Treatment of mild and moderate acne vulgaris with salicylic acid in an alcohol-detergent vehicle. *Cutis.* 1981;28:556–561.
86. Kligman D, Kligman AM. Salicylic acid as a peeling agent for the treatment of acne. *Cosmetic Dermatol.* 1997;10:44–47.
87. Lin AN, Reimer RJ, Carter DM. Sulfur revisited. *J Am Acad Dermatol.* 1988;18:553–558.
88. Kroshinsky D, Shalita AR. Topical retinoids. In: Webster GF, Rawlings AV, eds. *Acne and Its Therapy*. New York: Informa Healthcare USA; 2007:103–112.
89. Galvin SA, Gilbert R, Baker M, Guibal F, Tuley MR. Comparative tolerance of adapalene 0.1% gel and six different tretinoin formulations. *Br J Dermatol.* 1998;139(suppl 52):34–40.
90. Mills OH Jr, Berger RS. Irritation potential of a new topical tretinoin formulation and a commercially-available tretinoin formulation as measured by patch testing in human subjects. *J Am Acad Dermatol.* 1998;38:S11–S16.
91. Jeremy AHT, Holland DB, Roberts SG, et al. Inflammatory events are involved in acne lesion initiation. *J Invest Dermatol.* 2003;139:897–900.
92. Shroot B, Michel S. Pharmacology and chemistry of adapalene. *J Am Acad Dermatol.* 1997;36(6):S96–S103.
93. Brogden R, Goa K. Adapalene: A review of its pharmacological properties and clinical potential in the management of mild to moderate acne. *Drugs.* 1997;53(3):511–519.
94. Weiss JS, Shavin JS. Adapalene for the treatment of acne vulgaris. *J Am Acad Dermatol.* 1998;39(2):50–54.
95. Verschoore M, Langner A, Wolska M, Jablonska S, Czernielewski J, Schaefer H. Vehicle controlled study of CD 271 lotion in the topical treatment of acne vulgaris. *J Invest Dermatol.* 1993;100:221.
96. Kakita L. Tazarotene versus tretinoin or adapalene in the treatment of acne vulgaris. *J Am Acad Dermatol.* 2000;43(2 pt 3):851–854.
97. Feldman SR, Werner CP, Alio Saenz AB. The efficacy and tolerability of tazarotene foam, 0.1%, in the treatment of acne vulgaris in 2 multicenter, randomized, vehicle-controlled, double-blind studies. *J Drugs Dermatol: JDD.* 2013;12(4):438–446.
98. Jarratt M, Werner CP, Alió Saenz AB Tazarotene foam versus tazarotene gel: a randomized relative bioavailability study in acne vulgaris. *Clin Drug Investig.* 2013;33(4):283–9. 10.1007/s40261-013-0065-1 23456673.
99. Cosio T, Di Prete M, Gaziano R, et al. Trifarotene: A current review and perspectives in dermatology. *Biomedicines.* 2021;9:237. 10.3390/biomedicines9030237.
100. Mohd Nor NH, Aziz Z. A systematic review of benzoyl peroxide for acne vulgaris. *J Dermatolog Treat.* 2013;24(5):397–386.
101. Gross G. Benzoyl peroxide and salicylic acid therapy. In: Webster GF, Rawlings AV, eds. *Acne and Its Therapy*. New York: Informa Healthcare USA; 2007:117–136.
102. Zander E, Weisman S. Treatment of acne vulgaris with salicylic acid pads. *Clin Ther.* 1992;14:247–253.
103. Zouboulis CC. Moderne aknetherapie. *Akt Dermatol.* 2003;29:49–57.
104. Gollnick H, Schramm M. Topical drug treatments in acne. *Dermatol.* 1998;196:119–125.
105. Cotterill JA. Benzoyl peroxide. *Acta Derm Venereol.* 1980;89(suppl):57–63.
106. Cunliffe WJ, Holland KT. The effect of benzoyl peroxide on acne. *Acta Derm Venereol.* 1981;61(3):267–269.
107. Lassus A. Local treatment of acne. A clinical study and evaluation of the effect of different concentrations of benzoyl peroxide gel. *Curr Med Res Opin.* 1981;7(6):370–373.
108. Cunliffe WJ, Dodman B, Eady R. Benzoyl peroxide in acne. *Practitioner.* 1978;220(3):470–482.
109. Maddin S. Benzoyl peroxide. *Can J Dermatol.* 1989;1(4):92.
110. Bowman S, Gold M, Nasir A, Vamvakias G. Comparison of clindamycin/benzoyl peroxide, tretinoin plus clindamycin, and the combination of clindamycin/benzoyl peroxide and tretinoin plus clindamycin in the treatment of acne vulgaris: A randomized, blinded study. *J Drug Dermatol.* 2005;4(5):611–618.
111. Korkut C, Piskin S. Benzoyl peroxide, adapalene, and their combination in the treatment of acne vulgaris. *J Dermatol.* 2005;2(3):169–173.
112. Bikowski JB. Clinical experience results with clindamycin 1% benzoyl peroxide 5% gel (Duac) as monotherapy and in combination. *J Drug Dermatol.* 2005;4(2):164–171.
113. Burkhart CG, Burkhart CN. Treatment of acne vulgaris without antibiotics: Tertiary amine-benzoyl peroxide combination vs. benzoyl peroxide alone (Proactiv Solution). *Int J Dermatol.* 2007;46(1):89–93.
114. Tanghetti E, Abramovits W, Solomon B, Loven K, Shalita A. Tazarotene versus tazarotene plus clindamycin/benzoyl peroxide in the treatment of acne vulgaris: A multicenter, double-blind, randomized parallel-group trial. *J Drugs Dermatol.* 2006;5(3):256–261.
115. Del Rosso JQ, Tanghetti E. The clinical impact of vehicle technology using a patented formulation of 5%/clindamycin 1% gel: Comparative assessments of skin tolerability and evaluation of combination use with a topical retinoid. *J Drug Dermatol.* 2006;5(2):160–164.
116. Webster G. Antimicrobial therapy in acne. In: Webster GF, Rawlings AV, eds. *Acne and Its Therapy*. New York: Informa Healthcare USA; 2007:97–102.
117. Austin BA, Fleischer AB Jr. The extinction of topical erythromycin therapy for acne vulgaris and concern for the future of topical clindamycin. *J Dermatolog Treat.* 2017;28(2):145–148. doi:10.1080/09546634.2016.1214234.
118. Walsh TR, Efthimiou J, Dréno B. Systematic review of antibiotic resistance in acne: An increasing topical and oral threat. *Lancet Infect Dis.* 2016;16(3):e23–e33. doi:10.1016/S1473-3099(15)00527-7.
119. Kawashima M, Hashimoto H, Alio Saenz AB, et al. Clindamycin phosphate 12%-benzoyl peroxide 30% fixed-dose combination gel has an effective and acceptable safety and tolerability profile for the treatment of acne vulgaris in Japanese patients: A phase III, multicentre, randomised, single-blinded, active-controlled, parallel-group study. *Br J Dermatol.* 2015;172(2):494–503.
120. Onge Erin St., Mobley WC. Minocycline topical foam: A new drug for the treatment of acne. *Ann Pharmacother.* 2020;55:105–110. 10.1177/1060028020939926.
121. Bienenfeld A, Nagler AR, Orlow SJ. Oral antibacterial therapy for acne vulgaris: An evidence-based review. *Am J Clin Dermatol.* 2017;18(4):469490. doi:10.1007/s40257-017-0267-z.
122. Bottomly WW, Cunliffe WJ. Oral trimethoprim as a third line antibiotic in the management of acne vulgaris. *Dermatol.* 1993;187:193–196.
123. Dalzeil K, Dykes PJ, Marks R. The effect of tetracycline and erythromycin in a model of acne-type inflammation. *Br J Exp Pathol.* 1987;68:6770.
124. Garner SE, Eady A, Bennett C, et al. Minocycline for acne vulgaris: Efficacy and safety (review). The Cochrane Collaboration, Issue 9. New York: Wiley; 2012. Available at: http://www.thecochranelibrary.com.
125. Deeks ED. Sarecycline: First global approval. *Drugs.* 2019;79(3):325–329. doi:10.1007/s40265-019-1053-4.
126. Zhanel G, Critchley I, Lin L-Y, Alvandi N. Microbiological profile of sarecycline, a novel targeted spectrum tetracycline for the treatment of acne vulgaris. *Antimicrob Agents Chemother.* 63(1):pii:e01297-18. doi:10.1128/AAC.01297-18.
127. Moore A, Green LJ, Bruce S, et al. Once-daily oral sarecycline 1.5 mg/kg/day is effective for moderate to severe acne vulgaris: Results from

two identically designed, phase 3, randomized, double-blind clinical trials. *J Drugs Dermatol.* 2018;17(9):987–996.

128. Draelos ZD, Carter E, Maloney JM, et al. Two randomized studies demonstrate the efficacy and safety of dapsone gel, 5% for the treatment of acne vulgaris. *J Am Acad Dermatol.* 2007;56(3):439. e1–e10.
129. Lynde CW, Andriessen A. Cohort study on the treatment with dapsone 5% gel of mild to moderate inflammatory acne of the face in women. *SKINmed.* 2014;12(1):15–21.
130. Tanghetti E, Harper JC, Oefelein MG. The efficacy and tolerability of dapsone 5% gel in female vs male patients with facial acne vulgaris: Gender as a clinically relevant outcome variable. *J Drugs Dermatol: JDD.* 2012;11(12):1417–1421.
131. Fleischer ABJr, Shalita A, Eichenfield LF, et al. Dapsone gel 5% in combination with adapalene gel 0.1%, benzoyl peroxide gel 4% or moisturizer for the treatment of acne vulgaris: A 12-week, randomized, double-blind study. *J Drugs Dermatol.* 2010;9(1):33–40.
132. Gamble R, Dunn J, Dawson A, et al. Topical antimicrobial treatment of acne vulgaris: An evidence-based review. *Am J Clin Dermatolgol.* 2012;13(3):141–152.
133. Hebert A, Thiboutot D, Stein GL, et al. Efficacy and safety of topical clascoterone cream, 1%, for treatment in patients with facial acne. *JAMA Dermatology.* 2020;156:621. doi:10.1001/jamadermatol.2020.0465.
134. Arowojolu AO, Gall MR, Lopez LM, et al. Combined oral contraceptive pills for treatment of acne. The Cochrane Collaboration, Issue 7. New York: Wiley; 2012. Available at: http://www.thecochranelibrary.com.
135. Koo EB, Petersen TD, Kimball AB. Meta-analysis comparing efficacy of antibiotics versus oral contraceptives in acne vulgaris. *J Am Acad Dermatol.* 2014;71(3):4509.
136. Afzli BM, Yaghoobi E, Yaghoobi R, et al. Comparison of the efficacy of 5% topical spironolactone gel and placebo in the treatment of mild and moderate acne vulgaris: A randomized controlled trial. *J Dermatol Treat.* 2012;23(1):21–25.
137. Plovanich M, Weng QY, Mostaghimi A. Low usefulness of potassium monitoring among healthy young women taking spironolactone for acne. *JAMA Dermatol.* 2015;151:941–944. 10.1001/jamadermatol.2015.34.
138. Roberts EE, Nowsheen S, Davis DMR, et al. Use of spironolactone to treat acne in adolescent females. *Pediatric Dermatology.* 2020;38:7276. doi:10.1111/pde.14391.
139. Nader S, Rodriguez-Rigau LJ, Smith KD, Steinberger E. Acne and hyperandrogenism: Impact of lowering androgen levels with glucocorticoid treatment. *J Am Acad Dermatol.* 1984;11:256–259.
140. Lowenstein EB, Lowenstein EJ. Isotretinoin systemic therapy and the shadow cast upon dermatology's downtrodden hero. *Clin Dermatol.* 2011;29:652–661.
141. Rawlings AV. The molecular biology of retinoids and their receptors. In: Webster GF, Rawlings AV, eds. *Acne and Its Therapy.* New York: Informa Healthcare USA; 2007:45–53.
142. Agarwal US, Besarwal RK, Bhola K. Oral isotretinoin in different dose regimens for acne vulgaris: A randomized comparative trial. *Indian J Dermatol Venereol Leprol.* 2011;77(6):688–694.
143. Lee JW, Yoo KH, Park KY, et al. Effectiveness of conventional, low-dose and intermittent oral isotretinoin in the treatment of acne: A randomized, controlled comparative study. *Br J Dermatol.* 2011;164(6):1369–1375.
144. Berk DR. Effectiveness of conventional, low-dose and intermittent oral isotretinoin in the treatment of acne: A randomized, controlled comparative study—comment. *Br J Dermatol.* 2011;165(1):205.
145. Tran Patrick T, Berman Hannah S, Leavitt E, et al. Analysis of factors associated with relapse in patients on their second course of isotretinoin for acne vulgaris. *J Am Acad Dermatol.* 2021;84:856–859. 10.1016/j.jaad.2020.10.030.
146. Webster GF, Leyden JJ, Gross JA. Results of a Phase III, double-blind, randomized, parallel-group, non-inferiority study evaluating the safety and efficacy of isotretinoin-Lidose in patients with severe recalcitrant nodular acne. *J Drugs Dermatol: JDD.* 2014;13(6):665–670.
147. European Directive for systemic isotretinoin prescription. EMEA—Committee for Proprietary Medicinal Products (CPMP). 2012. Available at: http://www.ema.europa.eu/docs/en_GB/document_library/Referrals_document/Isotretinoin_29?WC500010882.pdf.
148. Layton AM, Dreno B, Gollnick HPM, et al. A review of the European Directive for prescribing systemic isotretinoin for acne vulgaris. *J Eur Acad Dermatol Venereol.* 2006;20:773–776.
149. Bauer LB, Ornelas JN, Elston DM, Alikhan A. Isotretinoin: Controversies, facts, and recommendations. *Expert Rev Clin Pharmacol.* 2016;9(11):1435–1442. doi:10.1080/17512433.2016.1213629.
150. Huang YC, Cheng YC. Isotretinoin treatment for acne and risk of depression: A systematic review and meta-analysis. *J Am Acad Dermatol.* 2017;76(6):1068–1076.e9. doi:10.1016/j.jaad.2016.12.028.
151. Oliveira JM, Sobreira G, Velosa J, Telles Correia D, Filipe P. Association of isotretinoin with depression and suicide: A review of current literature. *J Cutan Med Surg.* 2018;22(1):58–64. doi:10.1177/1203475417719052.
152. Elman M, Slatkine M, Harth Y. The effective treatment of acne vulgaris by a high-intensity, narrow band 405–420 nm light source. *J Cosmet Laser Ther.* 2003;5:111–117.
153. Friedman PM, Jih MH, Kimyai-Asadi A, Goldberg LH. Treatment of inflammatory facial acne vulgaris with the 1450-nm diode laser: A pilot study. *Dermatol Surg.* 2004;30:147–151.
154. Mariwalla K, Rohrer TE. Use of lasers and light-based therapies for treatment of acne vulgaris. *Lasers Surg Med.* 2005;37(5):333–342.
155. Ross EV. Optical treatments for acne. *Dermatol Ther.* 2005;18(3):253–266.
156. Lloyd JR, Mirkov M. Selective photothermolysis of the sebaceous glands for acne treatment. *Lasers Surg Med.* 2002;31(2):115–120.
157. Böhm M, Luger TA. The pilosebaceous unit is part of the skin immune system. *Dermatol.* 1998;196(1):75–79.
158. Seaton E, Mouser PE, Charakida A, Alam S, Seldon PM, Chu AC. Investigation of the mechanism of action of nonablative pulsed-dye laser therapy in photorejuvenation and inflammatory acne vulgaris. *Br J Dermatol.* 2006;155(4):748–755.
159. Car J, Car M, Hamilton F, et al. Light therapies for acne (protocol). The Cochrane Collaboration, Issue 4. New York: Wiley; 2009. Available at: http://www.thecochranelibrary.com.
160. Choi YS, Suh HS, Yoon MY, et al. A study of the efficacy of cleansers for acne vulgaris. *J Dermatol Treat.* 2010;21(3):201–205.
161. Shalita AR. Treatment of mild and moderate acne vulgaris with salicylic acid in an alcohol-detergent vehicle. *Cutis.* 1982;28(11): 556–568.
162. Stoughton RB, Leyden JJ. Efficacy of 4 percent chlorhexidine gluconate skin cleanser in the treatment of acne vulgaris. *Cutis.* 1987;39(6):551–553.
163. Arndt KA. Acne. In: Arndt KA, ed. *Manual of Dermatologic Therapeutics.* 4th ed. Toronto: Little Brown; 1989:3–13.
164. Fulgha CC, Caltalano PM, Childers RC, et al. Abrasive cleansing in the management of acne vulgaris. *Arch Dermatol.* 1982;118(9):658–659.
165. Watson AJ, Bergman H, Williams CM, et al. A randomized trial to evaluate the efficacy of online follow-up visits in the management of acne. *Arch Dermatol.* 2010;146(4):406–411.
166. Bergman H, Tsai KY, Seo SJ, et al. Remote assessment of acne: The use of acne grading tools to evaluate digital skin images. *Telemed J E Health.* 2009;15(5):426–430.
167. Tuong W, Wang AS, Armstrong AW. Comparing the effectiveness of automated online counseling to standard web-based education on improving acne knowledge: A randomized controlled trial. *Am J Clin Dermatol.* 2015;16(1):55–60.

118

Psoriasis

Rebecca M. Law and Wayne P. Gulliver

KEY CONCEPTS

1. Patients with psoriasis have a lifelong illness that may be visible and emotionally distressing. There is a strong need for empathy and a caring attitude in interactions with these patients.
2. Psoriasis is a progressive T-lymphocyte–mediated systemic inflammatory disease that results from a complex interplay between multiple genetic factors and environmental influences. Genetic predisposition and precipitating "trigger" factors play a role in the "march of psoriasis." This march of innate and adaptive immune responses results in clinical expressions (eg, keratinocyte proliferation) and is linked to systemic psoriatic comorbidities.
3. Diagnosis of psoriasis is usually based on recognition of the characteristic psoriatic lesion and not based on laboratory tests.
4. Treatment goals for patients with psoriasis use "treat to target" strategies to reduce disease morbidity and improve quality of life. They serve to minimize signs such as plaques and scales, alleviate symptoms such as pruritus, reduce the frequency of flare-ups, improve the patient's quality of life ensure appropriate treatment of associated comorbid conditions, such as metabolic syndrome, psoriatic arthritis, or clinical depression, and minimize treatment-related morbidity.
5. Management of patients with psoriasis generally involves both nonpharmacologic and pharmacologic therapies.
6. Nonpharmacologic alternatives such as stress reduction and the liberal use of moisturizers may be beneficial and should always be considered and initiated when appropriate.
7. Pharmacologic alternatives for psoriasis include topical agents, phototherapy, and systemic agents (both traditional/nonbiologic and biologic agents).
8. Pharmacologic therapy is generally guided by the severity of disease and its impact on the patient's quality of life, advancing from topical agents to phototherapy to systemic agents as needed.
9. Rotational therapy (ie, rotating systemic drug interventions) is a means to minimize drug-associated toxicities. However, continuous treatment has replaced rotational or sequential therapy and is now the standard of care for many dermatologists. Rotational and sequential therapy are used in pediatrics. Sequential therapy may be needed for biologics.
10. Some biologic agents have proven efficacy for psoriasis; however, there are differences among these agents, including mechanism of action, duration of remission, and adverse-effect profile. Biologics are often used for moderate-to-severe psoriasis and may be first-line therapy especially if comorbidities exist.

BEYOND THE BOOK

What does psoriasis look like? Search online for images of the skin manifestations of the various types of psoriasis (as described in Table 118-1). In particular, for plaque psoriasis (the most common phenotype), search for images of scalp, trunk/limb, hands, and nail involvement (oil spots). This activity is useful to enhance students understanding of the ASSESS step in the patient care process.

INTRODUCTION

Psoriasis is a chronic disease that waxes and wanes. It is never cured, and it is now known to be associated with multiple comorbidities including heart disease, diabetes, and metabolic syndrome. The signs and symptoms of psoriasis may subside totally (go into remission) and then flare up again (exacerbation). Triggers include stress, seasonal changes, and some drugs. Disease severity may vary from mild to disabling. Psoriasis imposes a burden of disease that extends beyond the physical dermatologic manifestations.

(1) Patients with psoriasis often have a lifelong illness that may be visible and emotionally distressing. There is a strong need for empathy and a caring attitude in interactions with these patients. Thus, management of this condition is necessarily long term and multifaceted, and management modalities may change according to the severity of the illness at the time.

EPIDEMIOLOGY

Psoriasis is the most common immune-mediated inflammatory disease worldwide. In the United States, psoriasis affects about 8 million people, or approximately 3% of the population.[1] The prevalence in countries varies between 0.09% and 11.4%, with differing reasons for the wide range.[2] Climate, sun exposure, and ethnicity are thought to affect prevalence, but correlation between latitude and prevalence is weak.[3]

According to the largest population-based survey—the Multinational Assessment of Psoriasis and Psoriatic Arthritis (MAPP)—the prevalence of psoriasis ranges from 1.4% in Spain to 3.3% in Canada, with the United States at 2.2% and the overall prevalence of psoriasis at 1.9%.[4] Lower frequencies of between 0.4% and 0.7% are seen for people of African and Asian descent.[3] Of interest is the fact that psoriasis is seldom seen in North and South American aboriginal Indians. It affects males and females equally.[5] Psoriasis can present at any age.[4] The majority of patients (approximately 75%)

have onset before the age of 40 years,[5] but psoriasis has been observed at birth and as late as the ninth decade of life.[5]

Prevalence increases are roughly linear over the life course (about 0.12% at age 1 year to 1.2% at age 18).[3] Many studies report two peak ages of onset: at 20 to 30 years and again at 50 to 60 years of age.[4,5]

ETIOLOGY

2 Psoriasis is a T-lymphocyte–mediated systemic inflammatory disease that results from a complex interplay between multiple genetic factors and environmental influences. Genetic predisposition coupled with some precipitating factor triggers an abnormal immune response, resulting in the initial psoriatic skin lesions. This has been called the "march of psoriasis"[6,7] to reflect the innate and adaptive immune responses that are present. This march leads to expressions of psoriasis with keratinocyte proliferation being central to the clinical presentation of psoriasis and is likely responsible for various comorbidities as a consequence of the chronic inflammation associated with psoriasis.[3,6] For example, there is an association between psoriasis and cardiovascular disease, which is an ongoing, two-way interplay.[6,7] The concept is that systemic inflammation enhances insulin resistance, causing endothelial dysfunction, leading to atherosclerosis and coronary events.[8]

Genetics

Dermatologists have recognized the familial tendencies of psoriasis for many years. Approximately 30% of patients have a first-degree relative with psoriasis, and the risk of psoriasis increases with the number of affected relatives.[4] Monozygotic twins have a concordance rate in the 80% range. Rates of family history in a psoriasis family range between 36% and 91%.[9,10] A study using the founder population of Newfoundland and Labrador noted that more than 80% of the patients had a positive family history.

The bimodal distribution of this disease (prevalence peaking at 20-30 years and again at 50-60 years) may represent two distinct forms of psoriasis, with early-onset psoriasis much more likely to possess a genetic marker highly associated with psoriasis.[4]

There are psoriasis susceptibility genes and variants that reside on various chromosomes. The psoriasis susceptibility locus 1 (*PSORS1*) on chromosome 6p is a key gene locus, accounting for up to 50% of disease heritability.[3] In 2009, studies of the Newfoundland and Labrador population confirmed that major histocompatibility complex antigen HLA-Cw6 and tumor necrosis factor (TNF)-α as major psoriasis susceptibility genes, along with interleukin (IL)-23 loci that had previously been reported.[5,11] The findings have been confirmed in multiple populations worldwide.[12]

Roughly 40 additional loci are thought to be associated with psoriasis.[3] Corresponding genes to these loci are involved in pathogenesis pathways in the immune system (adaptive and innate). There is a general role for T cells and a specific role for TH17 lymphocytes in psoriasis pathogenesis and as indicators of psoriasis risk.[3]

Predisposing Factors and Precipitating Factors

Injury to the skin, infection, drugs, smoking, alcohol consumption, obesity, and psychogenic stress have been implicated in the development of psoriasis. Examples of these precipitating factors include a horsefly bite causing skin trauma and resulting in new-onset psoriasis (known as the *Koebner phenomenon*),[13] a viral or streptococcal infection, or the use of β-adrenergic blockers.[14] Factors exacerbating preexisting psoriasis include drugs[14] (eg, lithium, nonsteroidal anti-inflammatory drugs [NSAIDs], antimalarials such as chloroquine, β-adrenergic blockers, fluoxetine, and withdrawal of corticosteroids), and psoriatic patients commonly have exacerbations during times of stress.[3,14,15] Smoking cigarettes has been shown in two international studies to be a risk factor for psoriasis.[16] Lifestyle intervention to mitigate risk factors has been recommended.[17]

PATHOPHYSIOLOGY

Psoriasis is a common chronic inflammatory disease that involves both adaptive and innate immunity.[3] It is an immune-mediated disease in which the skin inflammatory changes are dependent on immune cells and their cytokines.[4] The interaction between dermal dendritic cells, activated T cells of the TH-1, TH-17 lineage in concert with a multitude of cytokines and growth factors are responsible for the epidermal hyperplasia and dermal inflammation that is seen in the skin of patients with psoriasis. Cross-talk between the innate and adaptive immune system mediated by cytokines including TNF-α, interferon-gamma, and interleukin-1 is a major research focus.[3]

Comorbidities

It is well documented that psoriasis patients have significantly associated comorbidities.[3,4,6,7,16] Approximately 75% of patients will have at least one comorbid condition, and many will have multiple comorbidities.[4] Psoriatic arthritis (PsA) is one of the most common and well-known extracutaneous manifestations of the disease.[4,16] Other associated comorbidities include metabolic syndrome, other immune-mediated disorders such as Crohn's disease, multiple sclerosis, and some psychological illnesses (anxiety, depression, and alcoholism).[18] Also, malignancies such as cutaneous T-cell lymphoma are associated with psoriasis, and melanoma and nonmelanoma skin cancer are associated with psoriasis treatments.

The National Psoriasis Foundation published a clinical consensus on psoriasis comorbidities with recommendations for screening and addressing issues such as cardiovascular risk, metabolic syndrome, and obesity.[19] The importance of screening for comorbidities in psoriasis patients cannot be overemphasized: nearly half of the psoriatic patients older than 65 years have at least three comorbidities (with two-thirds of this patient population having two or more comorbidities).[20] The presence of specific comorbidity in a patient with psoriasis may influence the choice of pharmacotherapy.

PsA usually develops after the onset of psoriasis,[5] typically 10 years later,[18] with a range of 5 to 12 years.[4] However, 10% to 15% of patients report that the PsA appeared first.[5] The prevalence of PsA in psoriatic patients is about 30%[3,18] but varies by disease severity.[18] In one US study, the prevalences were 14% for patients with mild psoriasis, 18% for those with moderate psoriasis, and 56% for patients with severe psoriasis.[21] PsA most commonly presents as polyarticular peripheral arthritis but can vary widely with peripheral and/or axial, monoarticular, or polyarticular patterns.[4] The severity of PsA also varies widely and does not necessarily correlate with the severity of skin findings.[4] TNF-α and HLA-Cw6 are linked to both PsA and psoriasis.[22] Although immunomodulating treatments for psoriasis (such as methotrexate or TNF-α inhibitors) are useful for PsA, NSAIDs effective for joint symptoms of PsA may exacerbate psoriasis.

Metabolic syndrome is a cluster of risk factors including abdominal obesity, atherogenic dyslipidemia, hypertension, insulin resistance or glucose intolerance, prothrombotic state, and a proinflammatory state.[19] Patients with psoriasis are at increased risk of developing metabolic syndrome.[3,19] The syndrome is a strong predictor of cardiovascular diseases, stroke, and diabetes.[19,23,24] Patients with this syndrome are three times as likely to have a myocardial infarction (MI) or stroke, twice as likely to die from the MI or stroke, and five times as likely to develop type 2 diabetes.[19] A 2010 retrospective analysis of pooled data from three clinical trials (M02-528, CHAMPION, and REVEAL) showed that patients with psoriasis have a 28% and 12% increased 10-year risks of coronary heart disease (CHD) and stroke, respectively.[24]

Psychiatric/psychologic comorbidities include depression, suicidal ideation and suicide, anxiety, and poor self-esteem.[16] A recent meta-analysis reported that more than 25% of psoriasis patients had depressive symptoms and more than 10% were clinically depressed.[16,25] In comparison to control subjects, psoriasis patients had significantly more depression symptoms with an odds ratio (OR) of 1.57% (95% CI 1.40–1.76) for clinical depression (using the International Classification of Diseases codes) and had an OR of 4.24 (95% CI 1.53–11.76) for antidepressant use.[16,25]

Patients with psoriasis also have a decreased life expectancy and increased rates of mortality. Psoriasis is an independent risk factor for atherosclerosis, especially for younger patients with severe disease.[19] A 2006 study found that a relative risk (RR) of death for a 30-year-old person with severe psoriasis was 3.10, after controlling for traditional cardiovascular risk factors (eg, age, gender, hypertension, dyslipidemia, diabetes mellitus, smoking, body mass index [BMI], C-reactive protein [CRP], and family history of cardiovascular disease).[19,26] Three epidemiological meta-analyses identified increased cardiovascular mortality risk (relative risk: 1.39, 1.37, 1.2) and stroke (relative risk 1.56, 1.59, and 1.21) for psoriatic patients.[3] Only patients with severe psoriasis are associated with a higher cardiovascular disease risk.[16] Moderate-to-severe psoriasis may be associated with an increased risk of chronic kidney disease.[16]

Systemic treatment of psoriasis with anti-inflammatory agents—in particular, methotrexate and some biologic therapies—may have protective effects against cardiovascular death, MI, and stroke/cerebrovascular disease.[27,28] However, the use of systemic retinoids does not.[28]

Types of Psoriasis

Plaque psoriasis, also known as *psoriasis vulgaris*, is the most common type of psoriasis (Table 118-1) and is seen in about 90% of psoriasis patients. Plaque psoriasis presents as shown in the Clinical Presentation box.

CLINICAL PRESENTATION: PSORIASIS

Signs and Symptoms of Plaque Psoriasis	Description (from Reference 16)
Lesions (plaques)	Erythematous
	Red-violet in color
	At least 0.5 cm in diameter
	Well demarcated—clearly distinguished from normal skin
	Typically covered by silver, flaking scales—scale removal is accompanied by fine points of bleeding (the "Auspitz sign")
	Lesions may develop at sites of trauma or injury (the "Koebner phenomenon")
Skin involvement	Either as single lesions at predisposed areas (eg, knees, elbows)
	Or
	Generalized over a wide BSA
	Mild psoriasis: ≤5% BSA involvement
	Moderate psoriasis: PASI ≥8 (higher in trials of biologics)
	Severe psoriasis: The rule of tens: PASI ≥10 or DLQI ≥10 or BSA ≥10% (in some phototherapy trials, BSA ≥20% used as lower limit)
	Categories in the European consensus: Mild psoriasis: BSA ≤10 and PASI ≤10 and DLQI ≤10. Moderate-to-severe psoriasis: (BSA >10 or PASI >10) and DLQI >10
Pruritus	More than 50% of patients with psoriasis have associated pruritus
	May be severe in some patients and may require treatment to minimize excoriations from constant scratching
Other associated concerns	This condition may also be physically debilitating or socially isolating with significant quality-of-life issues for the patient
	Potential comorbidities: PsA, depression, hypertension, obesity, diabetes mellitus, Crohn's disease, anxiety, alcoholism

BSA, body surface area; DLQI, Dermatology Life Quality Index; PASI, psoriasis area and severity index; PsA, psoriatic arthritis.

TABLE 118-1 Phenotypic Classifications of Psoriasis

Plaque (psoriasis vulgaris)
Flexural and/or intertriginous (inverse psoriasis)
Seborrheic
Scalp
Acrodermatitis of Hallopeau
Palm and/or soles
Generalized pustular psoriasis
Guttate
Erythrodermic

Up to 30% of patients with psoriasis have associated PsA[3] but this varies by disease severity.[18] Although nail involvement (psoriatic onychodystrophy) can occur with any type of psoriasis, it is seen in up to 90% of patients with PsA.[16] Fingernails are involved in about 50% of all patients with psoriasis and toenails are involved in 35% of patients.[16]

DIAGNOSTIC CONSIDERATIONS

3 The diagnosis of psoriasis is based on recognition of the characteristic psoriatic lesion and not on laboratory tests. Diagnostic testing is rarely performed as a biopsy may be suggested but is not diagnostic of psoriasis.

Psoriasis is traditionally classified into mild, moderate, or severe disease. In 2011, a European consensus (19 countries) formalized the definition of disease severity and treatment goals and defined plaque psoriasis severity as two main categories: mild versus moderate-to-severe. This became the basis for defining treatment goals in the 2015 European guidelines.[29,30] Both classification systems are in use today. In 2017 the Medical Board of the National Psoriasis Foundation (NPF) used a consensus-building (Delphi) process to establish treatment goals/targets in psoriasis (discussed later).[31] In clinical practice, assessment of the severity of disease includes both an objective evaluation of the extent and symptoms as well as a subjective evaluation of the impact of disease on the patient's quality of life.[16] Assessment typically includes measures of symptom and involvement such as body surface area (BSA), Psoriasis Area and Severity Index (PASI), or Physician's Global Assessment (static PGA), as well as quality-of-life measures such as the Dermatology Life Quality Index (DLQI) or the Short Form (SF-36) Health Survey.[4,16]

Classification of psoriasis as mild, moderate, moderate-severe, or severe disease is generally based on skin lesions and BSA or PASI measurements (see Clinical Presentation box). Practically, to give a rough estimate of BSA involvement, palm size is approximately 1% BSA, head and neck involvement is approximately 10% BSA, both upper limbs approximately 20% BSA, trunk involvement (front and back) approximately 30% BSA, and both lower limbs approximately 40% BSA. The DLQI and other indicators of the disease's impact on a patient's quality of life may also play a role. In 2020, an international group using a Delphi consensus process suggested that in lieu of severity, patients with psoriasis should be classified as either candidates for topical therapy or candidates for systemic therapy32; however, this classification differs from the 2021 AAD/NPF treatment guidelines that are discussed later in this chapter.

TREATMENT

Treatment of psoriasis is based on managing the underlying pathophysiology. Agents that modulate the abnormal immune response, such as topical corticosteroids (TCS) and biologic agents, are important treatment strategies for psoriasis. Topical therapies that affect cell turnover, such as retinoids, are also effective for psoriasis. In addition, nonpharmacologic therapies are effective adjuncts and should be considered for all patients with psoriasis. A treatment regimen should always be individualized, taking into consideration severity of disease, patient responses, and tolerability to various interventions. Furthermore, if comorbidities exist, they must be taken into treatment considerations and managed early. Optimal psoriasis care needs to maintain a focus on the patient's overall health-related quality of life.

Desired Outcomes

4 Goals of treatment[15]:

- Minimizing or eliminating the visible signs of psoriasis, such as plaques and scales
- Alleviating pruritus and minimizing excoriations
- Reducing the frequency of flare-ups

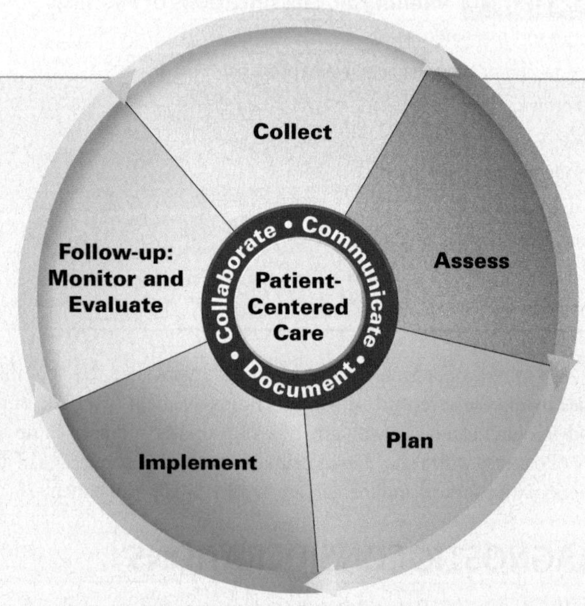

Patient Care Process for Management of Psoriasis

Collect

- Patient characteristics (eg, age, sex, pregnancy status)
- Patient medical history (personal and family)
- Patient description of history of psoriasis, subjective complaints of itch, and other symptoms
- Signs associated with severity of psoriasis (eg, areas of involvement)
- Signs associated with severity of itch (eg, excoriations, sleep disturbances)
- Signs of other comorbid illnesses (PsA, depression, anxiety, poor self-esteem, Crohn's disease, and metabolic syndrome–associated diseases, eg, dyslipidemia, hypertension, and obesity)
- Signs of secondary skin infections
- Symptoms of stress or distress (personal and family/caregiver)

Assess

- Type of psoriasis (plaque psoriasis being most common)
- Severity of psoriasis—classified into mild, moderate, or severe disease. Mild psoriasis: ≤5% BSA involvement. Moderate psoriasis: PASI ≥8 (higher in trials of biologics). Severe psoriasis: the rule of tens: PASI ≥10 or DLQI ≥10 or BSA ≥10% (in some phototherapy trials, BSA ≥20% used as lower limit). Categories in the European consensus: Mild psoriasis: BSA ≤10 and PASI ≤10 and DLQI ≤10. Moderate-to-severe psoriasis: (BSA >10 or PASI >10) and DLQI >10. Both classifications are in use in North America.
- Severity of itch
- Ability/willingness to pay for medical treatment options
- Emotional concerns for patient and caregiver (if any) and the level of disease-associated stress

Plan

- Determine an appropriate treatment approach, that is, topical or phototherapy or systemic therapy or a combination of treatments
- Determine specific therapeutic agents/treatments of choice
- Recommend the most appropriate therapies (nonpharmacologic and pharmacologic) for this patient's psoriasis
- Manage the itch with appropriate nonpharmacologic and pharmacologic therapies

Implement*

- Provide patient education regarding all elements of treatment plan
- Use motivational interviewing and coaching strategies to maximize adherence
- Provide information about prevention of future flare-ups

Follow-up: Monitor and Evaluate

- Contact patient/caregiver in 1 to 3 weeks (or as recommended based on the specific drug therapy) to follow-up about the efficacy of recommended therapies and any issues with the treatment regimen
- Ensure that appropriate monitoring parameters for efficacy and potential adverse effects have been put in place (eg, follow-up lab tests as needed)
- Reinforce preventive measures including continuation of maintenance therapy
- Ensure that patient/caregiver has been connected to other health resources as needed for follow-up (eg, a psychologist for stress reduction therapy)

Collaborate with patient, caregivers, and other healthcare professionals.

- Ensuring appropriate treatment of associated comorbid conditions such as PsA, hypertension, dyslipidemia, diabetes, or clinical depression, and ensuring follow-up care for other conditions by appropriate healthcare providers
- Screening for and managing lifestyle factors which may trigger exacerbations (eg, stress, smoking, obesity)[32]
- Minimizing nonspecific triggers such as mild trauma (scratching, piercings, tattoos), sunburn, chemical irritants, environmental/workplace factors[3]
- Optimizing the patient's overall health-related quality of life
- Providing guidance or counseling as needed (eg, stress-reduction techniques, smoking cessation programs)
- Avoiding or minimizing adverse effects from treatments used (topical, phototherapy, and/or systemic)
- Providing cost-effective therapy

Evaluation of Therapeutic Outcomes

Successful management of psoriasis should include not only clearance of skin lesions, which may take weeks to months depending on the severity of disease, but also control of associated conditions such as itching, and, importantly, comorbidities, including dyslipidemia, hypertension, PsA, and clinical depression as discussed earlier. The ultimate goal is to provide enough control of this chronic disease and its comorbidities (if present) so that the patient's quality of life is optimized.

The 2011 European consensus defined induction and maintenance phases and provided separate treatment goals for induction and maintenance.[29,30] The induction phase is defined as the first 16 weeks of treatment for drugs with a rapid induction to remission (such as adalimumab or infliximab), extending the phase to 24 weeks of treatment for less rapidly effective drugs (such as methotrexate or etanercept).[30] To be considered successful therapy, a treatment regimen should result in a reduction of PASI greater than or equal to 75%, or PASI of 50% to 75% coupled with a DLQI less than 5.[30] Otherwise, treatment modifications should be considered. Treatment goals should be assessed at 10 to 16 weeks and then every 8 weeks thereafter.[30]

In 2017, the NPF-led US consensus recommended earlier treatment response targets: An acceptable treatment response at 3 months after starting new therapies (ie, induction phase) is either BSA 3% or less, or BSA improvement of 75% or more from baseline; the target response at 3 months after starting new therapies is BSA 1% or less.[31] During the maintenance phase, evaluation should occur every 6 months with the target response being BSA 1% or less at every 6 months of maintenance evaluation.[31]

It is important to treat beyond clearing visible skin lesions. Psoriasis is a dermatological inflammatory disorder where the goal is to manage both skin lesions and associated diseases."[32] Comorbidities and trigger factors must be managed as early as possible.

General Approach to Treatment

5 Management of patients with psoriasis generally involves both nonpharmacologic and pharmacologic therapies. Nonpharmacologic management strategies are important and should be used for all patients with psoriasis, regardless of the severity of disease. Pharmacologic therapies are always tailored to the individual patient with psoriasis, and different treatment strategies would be used depending on psoriatic disease severity, presence or absence of comorbid illnesses, and any special considerations such as hepatic or renal dysfunction.

Nonpharmacologic Management Strategies

6 Nonpharmacologic alternatives may be beneficial and should always be considered and initiated when appropriate.[15] These include stress-reduction strategies, moisturizers, oatmeal baths, and skin protection using sunscreens.[33]

In particular, stress reduction has been shown to improve both the extent and severity of psoriasis, and includes methods such as guided imagery and stress-management clinics. Liberal use of nonmedicated moisturizers, applied ad lib, helps to maintain skin moisture, reduces skin shedding, controls associated scaling, and may reduce pruritus. Oatmeal baths further reduce pruritus and with regular use may minimize the need for systemic antipruritic drugs.

Sunscreens, preferably with a sun protection factor (SPF) of 30 or more, should be regularly used because sunburns can trigger an exacerbation of psoriasis. Irritation to the skin should be minimized—harsh soaps or detergents should not be used. Cleansing should be done with tepid water and preferably with lipid-free and fragrance-free cleansers.[15,33]

For patients with comorbidities such as dyslipidemia, obesity, or cardiovascular disease, cessation of nicotine and alcohol consumption, diet management, and increasing physical activity can be important interventions.[6,32]

Pharmacologic Therapies

7 Pharmacologic alternatives for psoriasis are topical agents, phototherapy, and systemic agents, including biologic agents (formerly referred to as biologic response modifiers or BRMs).

Drug Treatments of First Choice

8 9 For limited or mild-to-moderate disease, topical treatments are the mainstay of care.[34] Phototherapy and photochemotherapy are used in moderate-to-severe cases.[35] For patients presenting with extensive or moderate-to-severe disease, systemic therapies with or without the use of topical treatments are the usual standard of care.[36,37] Newer systemic treatments such as biologic agents may be the treatments of choice, especially for patients with comorbidities such as PsA or if traditional systemic treatments (such as methotrexate or cyclosporine) are contraindicated.[37] See the "Systemic Therapy with Biologic Agents" section about guidelines for transitioning from traditional nonbiologic systemic agents to biologics.

Once the disease is under control, therapy is reduced in intensity to the least potent, least toxic agent(s) that maintain(s) control. Rotational therapy (ie, rotating systemic drug interventions) may minimize drug-associated toxicities; however, continuous treatment has replaced rotational or sequential therapy and is now the standard of care for many dermatologists. Sequential therapy may be needed for biologics.

Different treatment algorithms are used, depending on the severity of the plaque psoriasis (Figs. 118-1 and 118-2). The European consensus categorizes psoriasis as mild or moderate-to-severe with mild disease treated topically and moderate-to-severe disease treated systemically. The Canadian Psoriasis Guidelines Addendum Committee[16]

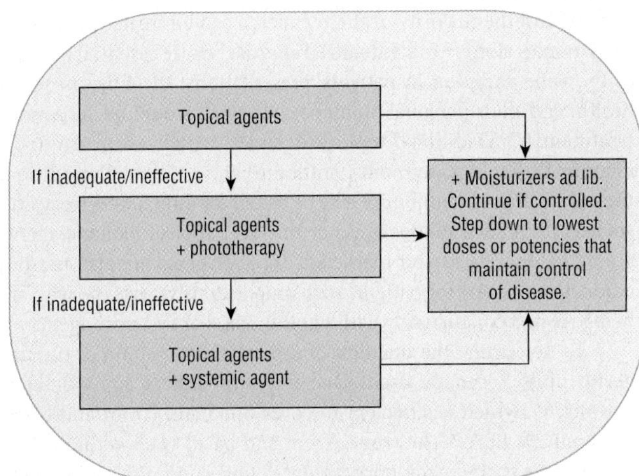

FIGURE 118-1 Treatment algorithm for mild-to-moderate psoriasis.

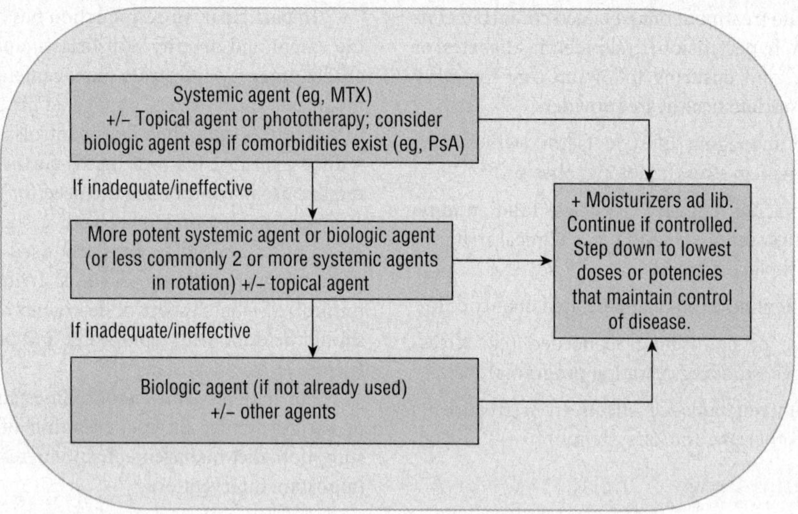

FIGURE 118-2 Treatment algorithm for moderate-to-severe psoriasis. (See section "Systemic Therapy with Biologic Agents" for details: choosing a biologic and guidelines for transitioning from traditional systemic therapies to biologics.)

and the British Association of Dermatologists have recommendations for first and alternate choices for biologics (if used)—see the "Systemic Therapy with Biologic Agents" section for details.

Published Guidelines or Treatment Protocols There are treatment guidelines for both Canada (the Canadian Dermatology Association [CDA])[16] and the United States (American Academy of Dermatology [AAD]).[38-41] In addition, the National Psoriasis Foundation (NPF) has guidelines for use of cyclosporine and methotrexate[42,43] and jointly with AAD for use of topical and alternative medicines in management of psoriasis.[40] In 2011, a 19-country European conference provided a consensus document focusing on disease severity and treatment goals, which ultimately resulted in updated European treatment guidelines in 2015.[29] In 2016, the CDA provided a guideline addendum which updated each chapter of the 2009 guidelines, and in particular, provided more information on use of biologics for treatment of psoriasis.[16] This was followed by new biologics guidelines from the British Association of Dermatologists (BAD) in 2017,[44] and updated joint AAD-NPF biologics guidelines in 2019.[45] AAD-NPF also provided psoriasis guidelines with special attention paid to comorbidities in 2019.[46] As mentioned earlier, the NPF provided guidance about psoriasis treatment targets in 2017 via a consensus study (Delphi method).[31] These guidelines represent the current standards of care.

Topical Therapies

Approximately 80% of patients with psoriasis have mild-to-moderate disease, and the majority of these patients can be treated with topical therapies alone.[40] Individualized approaches are essential because of the wide variation in patients' presentations, their psychosocial health, and their personal opinions as to what would be acceptable treatment.[14,16] Traditional topical therapies include corticosteroids, vitamin D_3 analogs, retinoids, anthralin, and coal tar. In addition, topical calcineurin inhibitors may be useful for difficult-to-treat sites such as the intertriginous areas or the face. Topical biologic agents are being developed and marketed. Topical agents are also used as adjunctive therapy for patients with more extensive disease, who are being treated concurrently with phototherapy or systemic agents.

To determine the quantity of topical agents required, the fingertip unit[47,48] can be used. One fingertip unit is approximately 500 mg,[40,47] which is sufficient to cover one hand (front and back) or about 2% BSA.[48] The trunk (front and back) is about 30% BSA; to cover the entire trunk once, about 15 fingertip units, or 7,500 mg (7.5 g), would be required.

In the United States, the current (2021) treatment guidelines recommend TCS of varying strengths as first-line treatment for limited psoriasis,[40,49] used either as monotherapy or in conjunction with nonsteroidal topical agents; and potency can be enhanced with different vehicles, and as needed by occlusion.[49] Case-based discussions illustrating the guidelines were published in 2010.[49]

In a 2012 systematic review of topical and phototherapies for psoriasis by dermatologists in France, nine recommendations based on evidence and expert opinion are offered. However, quality literature was limited, and the recommendations relating to optimal steroid use and optimal first-line treatment for psoriasis did not reach 80% consensus.[47]

Corticosteroids TCS have been the mainstay of therapy for the majority of patients with psoriasis for over half a century. They are generally well tolerated, although adverse effects can occur, including systemic ones on occasion. Table 118-2 provides a summary of TCS formulations—including ointments, creams, gels, foams, lotions, sprays, shampoos, tape, and solutions—and potencies.

The most important distinction between corticosteroids is their potency differences. Various potency classification systems are available and Table 118-2 is a compilation with 7 potency classes similar to the 2021 AAD-NPF classification.[40] A comparison of potency classification systems was recently published.[54] Superpotent (class I) TCS provides rapid onset of efficacy but has the greatest risk of adverse effects. Their use should be limited in scope (body area) and duration (2-4 weeks). Clobetasol-17-propionate and betamethasone dipropionate were effective in clearing or markedly improving psoriasis in 75% to 80% of patients in about 3 weeks.[55] Lowest potency TCS should be used on the face and skin folds.

Salt forms of corticosteroids affect potency. For example, betamethasone dipropionate is superpotent to high potency (formulation dependent), whereas betamethasone valerate is medium to lower-mid potency (formulation dependent).

The choice of vehicle affects corticosteroid potency: Ointments, being the most occlusive, enhance drug penetration and provide the most potent formulations. However, patients may prefer a less greasy formulation, such as a cream or lotion for daytime use, although they may be willing to apply the more effective ointment-based corticosteroid during the night.[40] Providing additional occlusion will increase drug penetration of a topical preparation, resulting in enhanced potency. For example, flurandrenolide cream and lotion are potency class 5, but flurandrenolide tape was found to have higher efficacy than diflorasone diacetate ointment (potency class 1).[40,56]

TABLE 118-2 Topical Corticosteroid Potency Chart

Potency Rating	Corticosteroid—Topical Preparations
Class 1: Superpotent	Betamethasone dipropionate 0.05% ointment (Diprolene and Diprosone ointment)
	Clobetasol propionate 0.05% lotion/spray/shampoo/foam (Clobex lotion/spray/shampoo, OLUX and OLUX-E foam)
	Clobetasol propionate 0.05% cream, gel, solution (scalp), ointment (Cormax, Temovate, Dermovate)
	Diflorasone diacetate 0.05% ointment (Florone, Psorcon, ApexiCon)
	Halobetasol propionate 0.05% cream, lotion, ointment (Ultravate)
	Flurandrenolide tape 4 μg/cm² (Cordran)
Class 2: Potent	Amcinonide 0.1% ointment (Cyclocort, Amcort)
	Betamethasone dipropionate 0.05% cream/gel (Diprolene cream, gel, and Diprosone cream)
	Desoximetasone 0.25% cream, gel, ointment (Topicort)
	Diflorasone diacetate 0.05% ointment (ApexiCon, Florone, Psorcon)
	Fluocinonide 0.05% cream, gel, ointment (Lidex)
	Halcinonide 0.1% cream (Halog)
Class 3: Upper mid-strength	Amcinonide 0.1% cream (Cyclocort)
	Betamethasone valerate 0.1% ointment (Betnovate/Valisone)
	Diflorasone diacetate 0.05% cream (Psorcon, Florone, ApexiCon)
	Fluticasone propionate 0.005% ointment (Cutivate)
	Mometasone furoate 0.1% ointment (Elocon)
	Triamcinolone acetonide 0.5% cream and ointment (Aristocort)
Class 4: Mid-strength	Betamethasone valerate 0.12% foam (Luxiq)
	Betamethasone dipropionate 0.05% spray (Sernivo)
	Clocortolone pivalate 0.1% cream (Cloderm)
	Desoximetasone 0.05% cream and gel (Topicort LP)
	Fluocinolone acetonide 0.025% ointment (Synalar)
	Fluocinolone acetonide 0.2% cream (Synalar-HP)
	Hydrocortisone valerate 0.2% ointment (Westcort)
	Mometasone furoate 0.1% cream, lotion, solution (Elocon)
	Triamcinolone acetonide 0.1% ointment (Kenalog)
Class 5: Lower mid-strength	Betamethasone dipropionate 0.05% lotion (Diprosone)
	Betamethasone valerate 0.1% cream and lotion (Betnovate/Valisone)
	Desonide 0.05% lotion, ointment, gel (DesOwen, Tridesilon)
	Fluocinolone acetonide 0.01% shampoo (Capex)
	Fluocinolone acetonide 0.01%, 0.025%, 0.03% cream (Synalar)
	Flurandrenolide 0.05% cream and lotion (Cordran)
	Fluticasone propionate 0.05% cream and lotion (Cutivate)
	Hydrocortisone butyrate 0.1% ointment, lotion, cream (Locoid, Locoid Lipocream)
	Hydrocortisone probutate 0.1% cream (Pandel)
	Hydrocortisone valerate 0.2% cream (Westcort)
	Prednicarbate 0.1% cream and ointment (Dermatop)
	Triamcinolone acetonide 0.1% cream, ointment and lotion (Kenalog)
Class 6: Mild (low potency)	Alclometasone dipropionate 0.05% cream and ointment (Aclovate)
	Betamethasone valerate 0.05% cream and ointment (Valisone)
	Desonide 0.05% cream, ointment, gel (DesOwen, Desonate, Tridesilon)
	Desonide 0.05% foam (Verdeso)
	Fluocinonide acetonide 0.01% cream and solution (Synalar)
	Fluocinonide acetonide 0.01% FS oil (Derma-Smoothe)
Class 7: Least Potent	Hydrocortisone 0.5%, 1%, 2%, 2.5% cream, lotion, spray, and ointment (various brands)

Data from References 54-57.

Despite their widespread use, there have been few large-scale, randomized placebo-controlled corticosteroid trials and even fewer head-to-head comparisons with other therapies. The most comprehensive review to date is the analysis of topical psoriasis therapies done in 2002 but recent studies aren't included so this review was already somewhat out of date when published.[16,57] This systematic review found that all TCS treatments considered were efficacious and significantly better than placebo; and that the highest potency corticosteroids were the most efficacious, followed by vitamin D_3 analogs.[16] The French group in 2012 found variable efficacy in their systematic review, noting that recommendations about topical steroid use should be mostly based on expert opinion, and that maintenance intermittent treatment may prolong remission.[58] In addition, TCS used in combination with other agents—topical, systemic, or biologic—may be mutually beneficial. For example, the concomitant use of a second agent may provide a steroid-sparing effect; or the TCS may enhance the efficacy of the second agent. Specifics are discussed in various sections below.

Corticosteroids have anti-inflammatory, antiproliferative, immunosuppressive, and vasoconstrictive effects.[34,40] These are mediated through a variety of mechanisms. Mechanisms of action include binding to intracellular corticosteroid receptors and regulation of gene transcription (in particular, those which code for proinflammatory cytokines).[34,40]

Appropriate use of TCS should include an assessment of disease severity and disease location as well as knowledge of the patient's preference and age. Lower potency TCS should be used for infants and lesions on the face, intertriginous areas, and areas with thin skin. For other areas of the body in adults, mid- to high-potency agents are generally recommended as initial therapy.[40] The highest potency TCS are generally reserved for patients with thick plaques or recalcitrant disease, such as plaques on palms and soles. The use of potency class 1 corticosteroids should be limited to a duration of 2 to 4 weeks,[40] recognizing that the risk of cutaneous and systemic side effects increases with continued use.

Cutaneous adverse effects include skin atrophy, acne, contact dermatitis, hypertrichosis, folliculitis, hypopigmentation, perioral dermatitis, striae, telangiectases, and traumatic purpura.[16,40] Systemic adverse effects have been reported not only with superpotent corticosteroids but also with extended or widespread use of mid-potency agents.[40] Systemic adverse effects include hypothalamic–pituitary–adrenal (HPA) axis suppression and less commonly Cushing's syndrome, osteonecrosis of the femoral head, cataracts, and glaucoma.[40]

Tachyphylaxis can occur with prolonged use, although its clinical significance is difficult to verify.[16] It is recommended that the frequency of use be gradually reduced once clinical response is seen, although there are no established tapering regimens.[40] The French group recommended twice-weekly maintenance therapy.[47] Other approaches include transitioning to weaker potency agents or combination with other nonsteroidal topical therapies.[40] Pulse dosing has also been used to minimize tachyphylaxis and adverse effects.[59]

Vitamin D_3 Analogs Topical vitamin D_3 analogs include calcipotriol (calcipotriene), calcitriol (the active metabolite of vitamin D), and tacalcitol. Calcipotriol and calcitriol are currently available in the United States and Canada and tacalcitol is available in the United Kingdom. Calcitriol is only available in ointment form; however, calcipotriol is available in ointment, cream, foam, solution, and gel suspension formulations.[34] Other analogs currently under study include maxacalcitol and becocalcidiol. Their mechanisms of action include binding to vitamin D receptors, which results in inhibition of keratinocyte proliferation and enhancement of keratinocyte differentiation.[16] They also have immunosuppressive properties such as inhibiting proinflammatory cytokine production (eg, IL-2 and IFN-gamma) leading to inhibition of T-lymphocyte activity.[16]

Topical calcitriol can be used as first-line monotherapy or in combination regimens for patients with mild plaque psoriasis.[16] The efficacy of calcitriol has been established in large, randomized, double-blind clinical trials.[16] The efficacy of calcipotriol for patients with mild psoriasis is also well established in randomized double-blind placebo-controlled trials. In head-to-head comparison studies with other topical agents, calcipotriol was found to be more effective than anthralin (dithranol)[60] and comparable or slightly more effective than potency class 3 (upper mid-strength) TCS ointments such as betamethasone valerate 0.1% ointment.[16,61,62] In an analysis of topical psoriasis therapies done in 2002,[57] calcipotriol was found to be as effective as all but the most potent TCS.[16,57] Combination therapy with a TCS is particularly effective[63] and is also discussed later in the chapter.

Vitamin D_3 analogs are generally well tolerated and have a good safety profile in comparison with other topical therapies.[63] They have been considered the safest long-term topical treatments.[3] Cutaneous adverse effects most commonly include a mild irritant contact dermatitis; others include burning, pruritus, edema, peeling, dryness, and erythema.[16,40] These adverse effects may be mitigated with continued use.[40] Systemic adverse effects, including hypercalcemia and parathyroid hormone suppression, are rare unless patients are using more than the recommended maximum of 5-mg calcipotriol (100 g of calcipotriol 50 μg/g cream or ointment) per week[16,40] or if there is underlying renal disease or impaired calcium metabolism.[40] When applied sparingly over a BSA <30%, the risk of hypercalcemia is remote.[47]

Calcipotriol is inactivated by ultraviolet A (UVA) light, thus it should be applied after rather than before UVA light exposure.[40] Calcipotriol can be inactivated by acidic substances and thus should not be used with salicylic acid in treating psoriasis.[34] It may also be partially degraded by hydrocortisone valerate.[34] However, calcipotriol is stable with other TCS[63] and stable combinations available in the United States include: calcipotriol and betamethasone dipropionate ointment and suspension (Taclonex) and calcipotriol and betamethasone dipropionate foam (Enstilar).[34] The combination of calcipotriol with betamethasone dipropionate in either ointment or foam results in enhanced efficacy when compared with either agent used alone.[34]

Retinoids Tazarotene is a topical retinoid that acts through the following mechanisms: normalizing abnormal keratinocyte differentiation, diminishing keratinocyte hyperproliferation, and clearing the inflammatory infiltrate in the psoriatic plaque.[16,40] It is effective in clearing psoriatic plaque lesions and achieving remission.

In a placebo-controlled trial of tazarotene 0.1% and 0.05% gels for patients with plaque psoriasis, tazarotene provided a 50% or greater improvement in 63% (0.1% gel) and 50% (0.05% gel) of patients, respectively, after 12 weeks of use.[64] The therapeutic benefit is maintained for 12 weeks after cessation of therapy.[64] Later clinical trials with tazarotene 0.1% and 0.05% creams versus a placebo vehicle provided similar findings.[65] The 2012 systematic review similarly found that about 50% of patients experienced a 50% or more improvement with no difference in formulations.[47] In comparison to other agents, tazarotene 0.1% gel has similar efficacy to calcipotriol 0.005% ointment (in a small study) but is less effective than clobetasol propionate 0.05% cream.[16] It may be combined with TCS to enhance efficacy and reduce irritation.[34] Fixed combinations are marketed, for example, halobetasol propionate and tazarotene lotion 0.01%/0.045% (Duobrii) received FDA approval in April 2019.

Adverse effects of tazarotene include a high incidence of irritation at the site of application, a dose-dependent effect.[16] This results in burning, itching, and erythema, which can occur in lesional and perilesional skin.[40] Irritation may be reduced by using the cream formulation, lower concentration, alternate-day application, or short-contact (30-60 minutes) treatment.[40] Ad lib use of moisturizers is also beneficial. Tazarotene is also potentially photosensitizing, due to thinning of the epidermis that can occur with continued use.[40]

Tazarotene is contraindicated in pregnancy and should not be used in women of childbearing age unless effective contraception is being used. (All retinoids are potentially teratogenic including topically applied agents. See under section "Retinoids" for further details.)

Anthralin Anthralin is not as commonly used as other topical therapies currently available for psoriasis; however, there are situations where its use is appropriate and efficacious. It has a direct antiproliferative effect on epidermal keratinocytes,[16,34] normalizing keratinocyte differentiation.[40] Although the exact mechanism of action is unknown, it may have a direct effect on mitochondria[40,66] and reduce the mitotic activity of epidermal cells.[34] It also prevents T-lymphocyte activation.[40] Small placebo-controlled studies demonstrated efficacy for anthralin used continuously or as short contact (1 minute of treatment).[40]

Short-contact anthralin therapy (SCAT) is usually the preferred regimen, where the anthralin ointment is applied only to the thick plaque lesions for 2 hours or less and then wiped off.[15,40] To minimize irritation, it can be applied for 5 to 10 minutes daily initially then titrating up the application time to 20 to 30 minutes or more as tolerated.[34] Because lesions are generally well demarcated, zinc oxide ointment or a nonmedicated stiff paste should be applied to the surrounding normal skin to protect it from irritation and burning. Anthralin should be used with caution, if at all, on the face and intertriginous areas because of the risk of severe skin irritation.[40]

Concentrations for SCAT range from 1% to 4% or as tolerated; concentrations for continuous anthralin therapy vary from 0.05% to 0.4%. Aside from significant and often severe skin irritation, other adverse effects include folliculitis and allergic contact dermatitis, but these are uncommon.

Anthralin powder causes skin irritation. People who handle the dry anthralin powder should avoid skin contact (eg, by wearing gloves while compounding).[15]

Coal Tar Coal tar was one of the earliest agents used to treat psoriasis. It is keratolytic and may have antiproliferative and anti-inflammatory effects.[15,34] Coal tar formulations include crude coal tar and tar distillates (liquor carbonis detergens—LCD) in ointments, creams, and shampoos. Because of limited efficacy coupled with patient acceptance and compliance issues, coal tar preparations are less commonly used today, especially in North American and European[47] countries.

A 2007 comparative study in Thailand reported that betamethasone valerate was significantly more effective than coal tar.[16,67] Although coal tar may have similar efficacy as calcipotriol,[16] it has a slower onset of action.[16] In addition, coal tar has an unpleasant odor and will stain clothing; thus, it may be cosmetically unappealing to patients. LCD 15% solution was shown to be cosmetically acceptable, well tolerated, and effective when compared with calcipotriol 0.005% cream.[16,68]

Adverse effects include folliculitis, acne, local irritation, and phototoxicity.[16] It is carcinogenic in animals, but for human, no convincing data have emerged regarding carcinogenicity with topical use.[40]

Coal tar concentrations as used in psoriasis treatments (0.5%-5%) are considered safe by the FDA.[69] However, occupational exposure to coal tar, especially in high concentrations such as coal tar used in industrial paving, was reported to increase the risk of lung cancer, scrotal cancer, and skin cancer.[40] The risk of teratogenicity when used in pregnancy is likely to be small, if it exists.[40,69]

Salicylic Acid Salicylic acid has keratolytic properties and has been used in various formulations including shampoos or bath oils for patients with scalp psoriasis. In combination with TCS, it enhances steroid penetration, thus increasing efficacy.[34] It should not be used in combination with ultraviolet B (UVB) light phototherapy because of a filtering effect that may reduce UVB efficacy.[34] It should not be used with calcipotriol as it inactivates calcipotriol upon contact.[34] Systemic absorption and toxicity can occur, especially when applied to more than 20% BSA[34] or when used for patients with renal impairment.

Avoid the use of salicylic acid in children. However, it may be used for limited and localized plaque psoriasis in pregnancy.[40]

Calcineurin Inhibitors Topical calcineurin inhibitors such as pimecrolimus 1% cream (Elidel) are marketed for the treatment of inflammatory skin diseases such as atopic dermatitis.[70-72] They are not FDA-approved for psoriasis but are used off-label. Pimecrolimus was found effective for plaque psoriasis when used under occlusion[71] and also effective for patients with moderate-to-severe inverse psoriasis (intertriginous areas are affected).[72] Because this cream is less irritating than calcipotriol and also avoids steroid adverse effects such as skin atrophy, it may be a useful alternative for patients with lesions in intertriginous areas or on the face.[34] Janus Kinase (JAK) Inhibitors Janus Kinase (JAK) Inhibitors Tofacitinib (topical and systemic) and ruxolitinib (topical) are nonbiologic JAK inhibitors. Tofacitinib is currently used off-label for plaque psoriasis (topical and oral) but is indicated for psoriatic arthritis (oral use), rheumatoid arthritis, ankylosing spondylitis, and ulcerative colitis. If used systemically, the dosage must be adjusted for moderate-to-severe renal impairment and moderate hepatic impairment, Tofacitinib is not recommended in severe hepatic impairment. Ruxolitinib is currently indicated for atopic dermatitis.

Combination Topical Therapies Combining agents from different drug classes may be particularly useful in enhancing efficacy or minimizing toxicity.[40] Refer to the "Combination Therapies" section for further information.

Phototherapies and Photochemotherapy

Phototherapy has been used for treating psoriasis for years and is still an important treatment modality today. It has been known for centuries that some skin diseases improve with sun exposure, and clinical studies with phototherapies have been reported since the late 19th century.[38] Phototherapy consists of using nonionizing electromagnetic radiation, either UVA or UVB, as light therapy to treat psoriatic lesions.[73]

UVB is given alone as either broadband or narrowband UVB (NB-UVB), currently with NB-UVB being the preferred method. UVB is also given as photochemotherapy with topical agents such as crude coal tar (Goeckerman regimen)[73] or anthralin (Ingram regimen) for enhanced efficacy.[38]

UVA is generally given with a photosensitizer, such as oral psoralens, to enhance efficacy—this regimen is known as PUVA (photochemotherapy with oral methoxypsoralen and ultraviolet A light).[73]

With respect to comparative efficacy, NB-UVB is more efficacious than broadband UVB, but may be slightly less effective than PUVA.[38,74] PUVA is effective in the majority of patients, with the potential for long remissions.[38] A meta-analysis showed that more patients are still clear at 6 months with PUVA versus with NB-UVB.[74] However, because of greater availability of UVB treatment centers, more evidence available now of the efficacy of UVB treatments for psoriasis (in particular, NB-UVB), and especially the increasing concerns about PUVA toxicities (including skin cancers), phototherapy for psoriasis currently uses UVB or NB-UVB where available. Failure of NB-UVB may justify PUVA therapy.[73]

UVB interferes with protein and nucleic acid synthesis, leading to decreased proliferation of epidermal keratinocytes.[38] UVA has similar effects on epidermal keratinocytes. However, because of deeper penetration into the dermis, it also has effects on dermal dendritic cells, fibroblasts, endothelial cells, mast cells, and skin-infiltrating inflammatory cells including granulocytes and T lymphocytes.[38]

Adverse effects of phototherapy include erythema, pruritus, xerosis, hyperpigmentation, and blistering, especially with higher dosages. It should be used with caution for patients with photosensitivity concerns, and drug interactions include photosensitizing medications such as tetracyclines. Patients must be provided with eye protection during UVB, NB-UVB, or PUVA treatments, and for 24 hours[73] or the remainder of the day[38] after PUVA treatments. In addition, patients receiving PUVA therapy may experience gastrointestinal symptoms such as nausea or vomiting, which may be minimized by taking the oral psoralens with food or milk.[38] For patients also receiving oral retinoids plus PUVA (RE-PUVA), the UVA dose should be reduced by one-third.[38] Long-term PUVA use can lead to photoaging and the development of PUVA lentigines. Psoralens bind to proteins in the lens of the eye; thus, there is a potential for increased cataract formation.

Furthermore, although UVB has a theoretical risk of photocarcinogenesis, the risk is significantly higher with PUVA and is dose related.[38,73] A meta-analysis reported a 14-fold increase in the incidence of squamous cell carcinoma (SCC) in patients receiving high-dose PUVA when compared with low-dose PUVA, with SCC of the male genitalia particularly elevated.[38,75] PUVA may also increase the risk of basal cell carcinoma and possibly melanoma,[38] which may occur 15 years after the first treatment.[73] Thus, the use of phototherapy or photochemotherapy is contraindicated in patients with a history of melanoma or multiple nonmelanoma skin cancers.

Targeted phototherapy using excimer lasers that selectively target psoriatic lesions without affecting normal skin is an option being studied and early results are promising, although blistering and burning of treated lesions are more common, and long-term safety has not been established.[38]

Systemic Therapies

Systemic therapies are the mainstay of treatment for patients with moderate-to-severe psoriasis, with topical therapies remaining as useful adjuncts. However, as discussed below under combination therapies, topical calcipotriol and betamethasone dipropionate ointment may provide sufficient disease control for some patients.[16,76] Conversely, a subset of patients with limited disease may have debilitating symptoms and the use of systemic therapies would be warranted.[39] This may include disease involving "sensitive areas" with significant impact on quality of life (QoL).[54] Systemic therapies include the following traditional agents: acitretin, cyclosporine, methotrexate, mycophenolate mofetil (MMF), and hydroxyurea; as well as the biologic agents, specifically adalimumab, alefacept, etanercept, infliximab, ustekinumab, secukinumab, and newer agents certolizumab, ixekixumab, brodalumab, guselkumab, tildrakizumab, risankizumab, and others at various stages of development.

Acitretin In the 1980s, etretinate became the first oral retinoid, or vitamin A acid derivative, available for the treatment of psoriasis. It has since been replaced by acitretin, its active metabolite.

Retinoids may be less effective than methotrexate or cyclosporine when used as monotherapy, although the initial response may be more rapid than methotrexate for patients with severe inflammatory forms of psoriasis. Acitretin is more commonly used in combination with topical calcipotriol or phototherapy.[16,39] Its efficacy is dose dependent.[39] Although low-dose acitretin (25 mg/day) is safer and better tolerated than higher-dose (50 mg/day) therapy,[16] low-dose acitretin is not recommended as monotherapy for psoriasis.

Common adverse effects of acitretin include hypertriglyceridemia and mucocutaneous adverse effects such as dryness of the eyes, nasal and oral mucosa, chapped lips, cheilitis, epistaxis, xerosis, brittle nails, and burning or sticky skin.[16,39] Less commonly, "retinoid dermatitis" may occur. Ophthalmologic changes include photosensitivity, decreased color vision, and impaired night vision.[29] GI side effects including hepatitis and jaundice are rare with liver enzyme elevations usually being transient.[29] Periungual pyogenic granulomas are sometimes seen after long-term use of acitretin.[39] Rarely, skeletal abnormalities—such as disseminated idiopathic skeletal hyperostosis (DISH) syndrome—may occur.[16]

All retinoids are teratogenic and are absolutely contraindicated in pregnancy, including topical retinoids. Acitretin should not be used for women of childbearing age unless they are able and willing to use effective birth control not only for the duration of acitretin therapy but also for at least 2 years after discontinuing the agent.[16,29,39] Blood donation (men and women) is not permitted during and for at least a year after treatment.[29] Ethanol should be avoided during therapy and for 2 months after drug discontinuation because it causes the transesterification of acitretin to etretinate, which has a much longer elimination half-life.

Cyclosporine Cyclosporine is a systemic calcineurin inhibitor. The more bioavailable microemulsion formulation, Neoral, was approved by the FDA in 1997 for the treatment of psoriasis and rheumatoid arthritis.[42]

Cyclosporine is efficacious for both inducing remissions and as maintenance therapy for patients with moderate-to-severe plaque psoriasis. It is also effective in treating pustular, erythrodermic, and nail psoriasis.[42] The 2009 Canadian Guidelines recommended that cyclosporine be normally reserved for intermittent use in periods up to 12 weeks for most patients with psoriasis, for treatment failures, in crisis management, and as a bridge to other therapies such as biologics.[16] Other recommendations are for periods of 1 year or up to 2 years.[42] Risk of toxicity increases with treatment duration: intermittent short-course therapy (<12 weeks) is preferable since this significantly reduces the risk of nephrotoxicity as compared to continuous therapy.[16,29,42]

In comparative randomized controlled trials (RCTs), cyclosporine was significantly more effective than etretinate[77] and similar or slightly better in efficacy than methotrexate.[16,42,78] After inducing remission, maintenance therapy using low doses (1.25-3.0 mg/kg/day) may prevent relapse.[42] The dose should always be titrated to the lowest effective dose for maintenance. In one placebo-controlled study, the relapse rate was 42% for patients on 3.0 mg/kg/day versus 84% for patients on placebo.[79] For patients discontinuing cyclosporine, a gradual taper of 1 mg/kg/day each week may prolong the time before relapse, as compared with abrupt discontinuation.[39,42] Abrupt discontinuation resulted in a dramatic rebound of psoriasis in a few cases.[16] Because more than half of patients discontinuing cyclosporine will relapse within 4 months, patients should be provided with appropriate alternative treatments shortly before or after discontinuing cyclosporine therapy.[42]

Adverse effects of cyclosporine include cumulative renal toxicity, hypertension, and hypertriglyceridemia. The latter two are particularly significant for patients with prior elevation of diastolic blood pressure or triglycerides.[16] Hypertriglyceridemia can occur in up to 15% of patients with psoriasis who are treated with cyclosporine, although this effect is generally reversible upon cessation of therapy.[39] The cyclosporine-induced blood pressure elevation is dose-related, based on a Cochrane systematic review.[80]

The risk of SCC and other nonmelanoma skin cancers increases with duration of treatment[16] and with prior PUVA treatments.[39] Thus, although continuous therapy for up to 2 years may be efficacious,[42] it should be used only in a subset of patients[16] in whom renal function is monitored with annual determinations of glomerular filtration rate (GFR) and monthly measurements of blood pressure and creatinine clearance, with more frequent measurements during the initial 6 weeks of treatment.[16]

Baseline blood pressure, serum creatinine, serum urea nitrogen, triglycerides, complete blood count, uric acid, potassium, and magnesium should be obtained before initiating therapy, every 2 weeks for the first 12 weeks of therapy, and monitored monthly thereafter during therapy.[16,42] If the serum creatinine increases to 25% above the patient's baseline on two occasions (2 weeks apart), the cyclosporine dosage needs to be decreased by 25% to 50%, and serum creatinine rechecked as often as every other week for 1 month. If the serum creatinine does not return to within 10% of the patient's baseline value, a further dose decrease of 25% to 50% should be considered. If the value continues to be greater than 10% above the patient's baseline value, consider discontinuing cyclosporine therapy.[42] (*Note*: A 25% above-baseline cutoff for dosage reduction is the manufacturer's recommendation; the NPF consensus guidelines continue to recommend a 30% cutoff.)[42] Age-appropriate malignancy screening should also be done, and patients should be seen for dental examinations at least yearly because of the risk of gingival hyperplasia.[42]

As a cytochrome P450 isoenzyme 3A4 (CYP3A4) substrate, cyclosporine has significant drug interactions. Serum concentration monitoring is not routinely needed for patients with psoriasis because doses used are lower than in transplant recipients, although monitoring may be advisable for patients taking interacting drugs.

Drugs that can increase cyclosporine concentrations include calcium channel blockers (verapamil, diltiazem, and nicardipine), amiodarone, thiazide diuretics, macrolide antibiotics, allopurinol, oral contraceptives, ezetimibe, selective serotonin reuptake inhibitors (fluoxetine, sertraline), fluoroquinolones (ciprofloxacin, norfloxacin), antifungals (ketoconazole, itraconazole, fluconazole, voriconazole), and cimetidine.[42] Grapefruit juice will also increase cyclosporine concentrations.

Drugs that can reduce cyclosporine concentrations include anticonvulsants (carbamazepine, oxcarbazepine, phenobarbital, phenytoin, valproic acid), rifampin, efavirenz, and St. John's wort.[42]

Conversely, cyclosporine may also affect the drug levels of some drugs. Concurrent use of potentially interacting drugs should be avoided when possible.

Methotrexate For decades, methotrexate has been the mainstay of systemic therapy for patients with moderate-to-severe psoriasis. It has direct anti-inflammatory benefits due to its effects on T-cell gene expression and also has cytostatic effects.[16] It is more efficacious than acitretin and similar or slightly less efficacious than cyclosporine.[16,43]

Although it also has a significant adverse-effect profile, methotrexate is generally considered a safer alternative than cyclosporine unless there are preexisting contraindications such as liver disease. In some head-to-head clinical studies, more patients dropped out of the cyclosporine treatment arms due to adverse effects.[39,43] While biologic agents are undoubtedly more efficacious, they are much more costly, and some insurance companies require an inadequate response or intolerance to methotrexate (the gold standard) as a prerequisite for approving their use.[43] In a recent placebo-controlled comparative study with adalimumab (CHAMPION), the efficacy of methotrexate was 36% versus 80% for adalimumab and 19% for placebo.[81] Adalimumab also provided a more rapid response; however, the duration of remission is unclear.

Initial doses of 7.5 to 15 mg once weekly may be increased to 20 to 25 mg/week if the response is inadequate at 8 to 12 weeks, with appropriate adverse effect monitoring. Low-dose methotrexate (7.5 to 10 mg/week) in combination with a biologic agent is also recommended.[29] Methotrexate can be used continuously for years or decades with sustained benefits.[16] Methotrexate inhibits folate biosynthesis; and the use of folate supplementation during prolonged methotrexate therapy as seen in dermatology remains controversial. Although some experts recommend folate supplementation for all patients receiving methotrexate for psoriasis, others add folate only when patient issues occur, such as gastrointestinal adverse effects or early bone marrow toxicity (as manifested by an increased mean corpuscular volume) that can be caused by megaloblastic anemia.[39,43] Lack of folate supplementation has also been listed as a risk factor for hepatotoxicity from methotrexate use.[43] One small placebo-controlled study suggested that folate supplementation may result in a slight decrease in efficacy of treatment,[82] but the study methodology has been questioned.[39,43]

The most significant adverse effect is cumulative liver toxicity, and the total lifetime dose of methotrexate must be monitored. Traditionally, patients received a pretreatment liver biopsy and subsequent biopsies when a cumulative dose of 1.5 g is reached. Liver biopsy is the gold standard for assessing histological changes and provides an invasive marker of liver fibrosis. It is recognized that pretreatment liver biopsies may not be practical or appropriate in all cases.[16,43] It has also been recommended that a baseline liver biopsy be delayed for 2 to 6 months so that medication efficacy and tolerability can first be established[43] (ie, intention to continue with methotrexate use). Risk factors for hepatotoxicity from methotrexate include the following: a history of or current alcohol consumption, persistent abnormal liver chemistry studies, history of liver disease including chronic hepatitis B or C, family history of inheritable liver disease, history of significant exposure to hepatotoxic drugs or chemicals, diabetes mellitus, obesity, and hyperlipidemia.[39,43] For patients without preexisting risk factors for hepatotoxicity, it is recognized that they would likely have a low risk of fibrosis and would not require a baseline liver biopsy; furthermore, consideration can be made to continue methotrexate treatment for these patients without biopsies at all, to perform a liver biopsy after 3.5 to 4.0 g total cumulative dose, or to switch therapy to an alternate drug at that point.[39,43]

Currently, liver biopsies are reserved for select high-risk patients. Noninvasive blood serology (FIB-4, Fibrosure, Fibrometer or Hepascore) and LFT monitoring should be performed at baseline prior to starting methotrexate to assess the risk for hepatotoxicity. The additional use of type III serum procollagen as additional monitoring would be ideal, but this is not readily available in the US.[39] The procollagen type III N-terminal peptide (P3NP or PIIINP) serum level is the 2015 European recommendation for MTX monitoring - prior to starting MTX and every 3 months thereafter.[29] As a precaution, a systematic review and meta-analysis of the diagnostic accuracy of noninvasive markers of liver fibrosis in patients with psoriasis taking methotrexate concluded that the clinical utility of LFTs, P3NP, and liver ultrasound is poor, and that if these tests are used in isolation, a significant proportion of patients with liver fibrosis may remain unidentified.[83]

Other adverse effects include significant nausea, pulmonary toxicity, pancytopenia, acute myelosuppression, megaloblastic anemia, and a small but significant increase in lymphoma.[16] Although rare, pancytopenia can occur anytime with the use of low-dose weekly methotrexate and even after single doses of methotrexate.[39] Informing patients about the early symptoms of pancytopenia (dry cough, nausea, fever, dyspnea, cyanosis, stomatitis/oral symptoms, and bleeding) may aid early detection.[29] Methotrexate is an abortifacient and is teratogenic and is absolutely contraindicated in pregnancy. After methotrexate therapy is discontinued, it is recommended that men continue effective birth control for 3 months (since one cycle of spermatogenesis is 74 days), and women should be on effective birth control for at least one ovulatory cycle.[16,39]

Significant drug interactions include serum albumin binding interactions with salicylates, phenytoin, sulfonamides/trimethoprim, ciprofloxacin, and thiazide diuretics, potentially increasing toxicity. Drugs that can reduce methotrexate renal elimination (such as acidic drugs, including salicylates or vitamin C) will also increase serum methotrexate levels and hence increase toxicity. In addition, drugs with hepatotoxic potential may pose an additive risk with methotrexate use.[39]

Janus Kinase (JAK) Inhibitors: Tofacitinib *Tofacitinib* is a potent and selective inhibitor of the JAK family of kinases. It inhibits JAK1, JAK2, JAK3, and to a lesser extent TyK2.[84] Inhibition of JAK1 and JAK3 blocks signaling through common receptors for cytokines including IL2, IL4, IL7, IL9, IL15, and IL21.[84] JAK1 inhibition also attenuates signaling by other proinflammatory cytokines (ie, IL6 and Type I interferons).[84]

Tofacitinib is both a topical agent (see above) and an oral agent with a recommended dosage of 5 mg twice daily (or 11 mg of the tofacitinib XR once daily) taken with or without food; the XR tablets must be swallowed whole and cannot be split, crushed, or chewed.[84] There are potential drug interactions with CYP450 substrates—potent CYP3A4 inhibitors (eg, ketoconazole) or modest CYP3A4 plus potent CYP2C19 inhibitions (eg, fluconazole) may increase tofacitinib exposure and potent CYP3A4 inducers (eg, rifampin) may reduce tofacitinib exposure.[84]

Systemic Therapy with Biologic Agents

10 Biologic agents have exploded onto the treatment scenario for many immune conditions, including psoriasis. More and more biologic agents have proven efficacy for psoriasis and have been or approved for use, with many more being used off-label or in various stages of development. Currently available biologic agents include *tumor necrosis factor-α (TNF-α) inhibitors* (etanercept, infliximab, adalimumab, certolizumab), ustekinumab, *IL-17 inhibitors* (secukinumab, ixekixumab, brodalumab), *IL-23 inhibitors* (guselkumab, tildrakizumab, risankizumab), and others. They are recommended for consideration as first-line therapies alongside conventional systemic agents for moderate-to-severe disease. There are differences among these agents, including mechanism of action, duration of remission, and adverse-effect profile. In addition to biologic agents, there are biosimilars to established biologic agents (eg, Amjevita is a biosimilar to adalimumab [Humira]).

General Concerns and Precautions What precautions are needed when using biologics for treating psoriasis? In general, because of their immunomodulatory effects, there is an increased risk of infection with most of these agents, including serious infections such as sepsis, new-onset or reactivation of tuberculosis, and opportunistic infections such as histoplasmosis, cryptococcosis, aspergillosis, candidiasis, and pneumocystis. The use of live or live-attenuated vaccines during therapy is generally contraindicated. Because biologics are relatively new on the market, the risks of rare but serious adverse effects or those with a longer latency period may still be unrecognized or unreported. Further, clinical trial experience is limited for some biologics, and adequate postmarketing or long-term data are not available. Likewise, safety data on vulnerable populations such as children or women planning a pregnancy are usually absent.[85] There may be more safety data with earlier biologics which had approval for use in rheumatoid arthritis; however, it is the newer classes of biologics which are showing most promise. A 2018 publication concisely addresses the adverse reactions known to-date of biologics used in dermatology—both as indicated and off-label use.[86] In 2020, a Canadian panel of experts (psoriasis, pediatric dermatology, consensus process) considered efficacy and safety of biologics and provided recommendations for use of three biologics in children with moderate-to-severe plaque psoriasis, including a treatment algorithm.[86]

A more recently recognized concern about using biologics is that their efficacy may not be sustainable for much more than three years, that is, there is a loss of effect over time. For example, the British Association of Dermatologists (BAD) Biologic Interventions Register (BAD-BIR) has registered a 53% overall probability of drug survival by year 3, that is, about 50% failure.[85] BAD-BIR currently has more than 10,000 registrations including children.[85] Current data also suggest that failure of one biologic may negatively impact the efficacy of the next, as seen in psoriasis studies.[85] From experience with biologics for rheumatoid diseases, it appears that, after three biologic agents are used, other agents are less likely to be efficacious—there may be a similar phenomenon with their use in psoriasis.

Place in Therapy and Transitioning from Other Therapies Biologics are often considered for patients with moderate-to-severe psoriasis when other systemic agents are inadequate or relatively contraindicated, or if comorbidities such as active PsA exists. Biologic agents are sometimes recommended for first-line therapy, alongside conventional systemic agents, for patients with moderate-to-severe psoriasis; however, in practice, drug access due to cost considerations may be a limiting factor. The availability of biosimilars may mitigate this to some extent. British Association of Dermatologists (BAD) recommends biologics in methotrexate and cyclosporine failure/intolerance/contraindication; when psoriasis has significant impact on physical, psychological, or social functioning and (a) the psoriasis is extensive (BSA >10 or PASI >=10) or (b) the psoriasis is severe at localized sites and associated with significant functional impairment and/or high levels of distress (eg, nail disease or involvement of high-impact and difficult-to-treat sites such as the face, scalp, palms, soles, flexures, and genitals).[44]

Are there guidelines for transitioning from traditional systemic therapies to biologics? BAD provides some transitioning strategies in their 2017 guidelines[44]: (1) In stable disease, aim to allow 1 month to elapse between the last dose of any current standard systemic immunosuppressive therapy (except MTX) and the planned date of biologic initiation; (2) start a biologic with no drug washout period in patients taking MTX, or on other therapies where a drug washout period would lead to unstable disease; (3) when standard systemic immunosuppressant therapy cannot be stopped (eg, if a disease flare would be severe or hazardous), rationalize the use of therapy and stop as soon as possible (eg, when a minimum response has been achieved).[44]

Biologics may be appropriate/preferred as first-line therapy if comorbidities exist. For example, biologics such as infliximab or adalimumab would be an appropriate treatment option for patients with both plaque psoriasis and active PsA. Biologics currently available for the treatment of psoriasis and/or PsA include adalimumab, brodalumab, certolizumab, etanercept, guselkumab, infliximab, ixekixumab, risankizumab, secukinumab, tildrakizumab, ustekinumab, and others at various stages of development.[37]

Tumor Necrosis Factor-α Inhibitors: Adalimumab, Certolizumab, Etanercept, and Infliximab The regulation of TNF-α production is associated with various inflammatory conditions, including rheumatoid arthritis, inflammatory bowel disease, ankylosing spondylitis, PsA, and psoriasis.[16,37,41,44,45] Elevated TNF-α levels are seen in both the affected skin and serum of patients with psoriasis; and these elevated levels have a significant correlation with psoriasis severity.[41] The biologic agents adalimumab, certolizumab, etanercept, and infliximab are TNF-α inhibitors; this class of agents is effective for psoriasis and PsA.[16,37,41,44,45,87,88]

There are safety concerns common to TNF-α inhibitors, mainly from observations made through their use in rheumatoid arthritis and inflammatory bowel disease and more recently in psoriasis.[87-89] One concern is an increased risk of bacterial, mycobacterial, invasive fungal (disseminated or extrapulmonary histoplasmosis, aspergillosis, coccidioidomycosis), viral, parasitic, or other opportunistic infections—most commonly upper respiratory tract infections, and less commonly serious infections including sepsis, new-onset or reactivation tuberculosis, and opportunistic infections.[16,41,87-90] There have been reports of serious pulmonary and disseminated histoplasmosis, coccidioidomycosis, and blastomycosis infections, sometimes with fatal outcomes when these infections were not consistently recognized and promptly treated in the patients taking TNF-α inhibitors.[90]

A second concern is the development or worsening of autoimmune diseases such as peripheral and central demyelinating disorders including multiple sclerosis and drug-induced lupus-like syndromes.[16,41,89] Although there is no definitive causal relationship, it is recommended that anti-TNF agents be avoided in patients with established demyelinating diseases (eg, multiple sclerosis), and treatment discontinued in patients with suspected demyelination during therapy.[89] A third concern is the potential increased risk of malignancies such as lymphoma,[16,89,90] melanoma, and nonmelanoma skin cancer.[41] A fourth concern is the potential for other cutaneous adverse effects including vasculitis, granulomatous reactions, cutaneous infections, psoriasiform eruptions, and infusion or injection site reactions.[88] Flares of pustular psoriasis have been reported primarily for patients undergoing treatment for nondermatologic conditions such as rheumatoid arthritis.[16] A fifth concern is the risk of hematologic toxicity including neutropenia (more commonly reported)[89,90] and rare reports of other hematologic events including pancytopenia and aplastic anemia.[90]

There is also a sixth concern about chronic heart failure (CHF): worsening congestive heart failure (CHF) and new-onset CHF have been reported during the use of these agents. TNF-α inhibitors are contraindicated in patients with preexisting moderate-to-severe CHF (NYHA class III/IV),[29,41,90] and those with milder CHF should have their TNF-α inhibitors withdrawn at the onset of new symptoms or worsening of preexisting CHF.[41]

Although the above are safety concerns common to adalimumab, certolizumab, etanercept, and infliximab, their safety profiles are not identical. For example, the risk for tuberculosis (TB) is lowest with etanercept and may be highest with infliximab.[16] Nonetheless, they are contraindicated in patients with active TB.[29] Patients should be evaluated for active or latent TB prior to therapy and considered for a yearly PPD.[16,41] CBC and LFTs are also recommended prior to and periodically during therapy.[29] In addition, pretreatment C-reactive protein (CRP), hepatitis serology (HBV, HCV), and HIV testing have been recommended.[29] They are safe to use in pregnancy.[41] However, some manufacturers have cautioned that, since these agents cross the placenta, infants exposed in utero may be at higher risk of infections and live vaccines would therefore be contraindicated for several months after birth.[90]

Adalimumab is a human monoclonal antibody that provides rapid and efficacious control of psoriasis.[16,41] Adalimumab is indicated for adults with psoriasis, particularly when psoriatic arthropathy is a consideration.[44] Clinical trials in patients with moderate-to-severe psoriasis have shown dramatic results. A 2006 12-week RCT with open-label extension to 52 weeks showed significant improvement within 1 week of therapy, with complete or nearly complete clearance in some patients, and clinical benefits were maintained for at least 1 year with continuous therapy for most patients.[16,91] There is evidence that some patients may achieve/maintain PASI 90 through at least 160 weeks of treatment.[16]

A pivotal 2008 52-week RCT (REVEAL) with an initial 16-week double-blind placebo-controlled (DBPC; period A) phase followed by a 17-week open-label phase (period B) followed by a 19-week DBPC phase (period C) showed a 71% PASI 75 response for adalimumab-treated patients versus 7% for placebo-treated patients at week 16. All patients received open-label adalimumab from weeks 17 through 32. At week 33, patients achieving PASI 75 were rerandomized to adalimumab or placebo; patients achieving PASI 50 but <75 were continued on open-label adalimumab; and therapy for patients with PASI <50 was discontinued. At week 52, 5% of patients rerandomized to adalimumab lost adequate response versus 28% of patients rerandomized to placebo. Adalimumab was continued at 40 mg every other week. The study showed that adalimumab can produce rapid and dramatic results which can be sustained on continued use, in patients with moderate-to-severe psoriasis.[92]

An additional 3-year open-label extension study for patients in REVEAL showed that in patients with sustained initial PASI 75 responses, adalimumab efficacy was maintained for more than 3 years of continuous therapy, and maintenance was best at PASI 100. Some patients with PASI <75 in REVEAL also achieved long-term PASI 75 responses.[87]

For comparative studies, as discussed in the "Methotrexate" section, a head-to-head study showed that adalimumab was significantly more efficacious than methotrexate.[81] For patients who have an inadequate response to other psoriasis treatments (including etanercept), adalimumab is a good alternative.[16]

Adalimumab is given as 80 mg subcutaneously in the first week, then 40 mg the following week, and thereafter 40 mg every other week continuously.[16,29,41,90] More frequent dosing has been explored.[16] For PsA, adalimumab is given as 40 mg subcutaneously every other week, with concomitant use with other medications (analgesics, DMARDs, glucocorticoids, methotrexate, and NSAIDs) allowed, according to product labeling.

Adverse effects in adalimumab clinical trials including the 3-year extension were similar to those already described for this class of biologics.[90]

Etanercept was one of the earliest biologics available on the market for use in inflammatory diseases. It has demonstrated efficacy for rheumatoid arthritis. It was approved for use in PsA in the United States in June 2002 and approved in 2004 for use in moderate-to-severe psoriasis. It is also approved for treatment of juvenile rheumatoid arthritis and ankylosing spondylitis. Thus, as opposed to some of the other biologics approved for psoriasis, etanercept has been extensively used in rheumatology for both adults and children.

The dosing of etanercept in psoriasis differs from its other indications, reflective of the dosing regimens found to be effective for psoriasis in clinical trials. Etanercept is used continuously, given as 50 mg subcutaneously twice weekly for the first 12 weeks, followed by 25 mg twice weekly[16] or 50 mg once weekly.[29,41] Significant improvement was seen in about 50% of patients in clinical trials by week 12 and more than 50% of participants by week 24; with continuing therapy, weaker responders continued to improve for up to 1 year.[16,41,93] Continuing therapy using 50 mg twice weekly regimens is being explored and may provide greater benefit.[16] Etanercept was efficacious in children and adolescents (aged 4-17 years) with plaque psoriasis dosed at 0.8 mg/kg (maximum 50 mg) once weekly.[94] The dosing of etanercept for active PsA is 50 mg by subcutaneous injection once weekly. In patients with moderate-to-severe psoriasis with active PsA, etanercept 50 mg twice weekly for 12 weeks followed by 50 mg once weekly for an additional 12 weeks can be considered, according to product labeling.

Infliximab also received approval for rheumatologic diseases before psoriasis and was on the market before adalimumab. Infliximab is more efficacious than etanercept. A 2011 open-label study showed that psoriatic patients with an inadequate response to etanercept had rapid and sustained improvement when switched to infliximab.[95] Unlike etanercept or adalimumab, infliximab is a chimeric antibody with both murine and human components; thus, antibodies to the drug can develop, resulting in infusion reactions[41,45] and loss of clinical efficacy.[45] The standard dosing regimen is the same for plaque psoriasis and PsA: three IV infusions of 5 mg/kg given over a 6-week induction period, followed by regular infusions every 8 weeks.[41] This 8-week gap between infusions is longer than with other agents, thus increasing the risk of infusion reactions and loss of efficacy due to antibody development in comparison to other biologics.[45]

Clinical response is seen rapidly. In a pivotal phase III RCT, 76% and 70% of patients achieved PASI 75 by week 10 (after 3 doses of infliximab at 5 mg/kg and 3 mg/kg respectively), and PASI 90 was achieved by 45% and 37%, respectively[45,96]; however, the response dropped to about 50% by week 50.[96,97] Combining infliximab with other therapies may enhance response. Methotrexate can reduce the immunogenicity of infliximab, which minimizes the risk of antibody development to infliximab and a consequent loss of clinical response.[45] Enhanced clinical response has been seen in psoriasis and PsA.[45] Thus, the joint AAD-NPF guidelines recommend that the addition of methotrexate to infliximab should be considered strongly for all patients.[45] They caution that the long-term safety of this combination is currently unknown.[45] Infliximab has been combined with TCS and a vitamin D analog to augment efficacy but rigorous evidence supporting this combination is currently lacking.[45]

In addition to antibody development and infusion reactions, serious adverse events, including fatal cases of hepatosplenic T-cell lymphomas, have been reported rarely with infliximab use.[41] Cutaneous adverse effects include nonmelanoma skin cancers; however, these were mostly seen in patients with prior exposure to UV therapy, including NB-UVB and PUVA.[89] Other rare instances of cholecystitis and autoimmune hepatitis, which may be a class effect for TNF-α inhibitors, have also been reported.[16]

Certolizumab pegol is a humanized antigen-binding fragment of a monoclonal antibody that is further conjugated with a polyethylene glycol moiety. This binds to TNF-α, blocking its interaction with TNF receptors.[45] A phase II RCT showed PASI 75 achieved in 75% and 83% of patients by week 10, on doses of 200 mg or 400 mg every other week, respectively, versus 7% for the placebo group.[45,98] Recommended certolizumab dosing is 400 mg (as 2 × 200-mg subcutaneous injections) every 2 weeks, with a dose-reduced regimen for patients under 90 kg (198 lb): 400 mg (as 2 × 200-mg subcutaneous injections) initially and at weeks 2 and 4, followed by 200 mg every other week.[45,99] Recommended initial certolizumab dosing in active PsA is 400 mg (as 2 × 200-mg subcutaneous injections) once and then repeat at weeks 2 and 4. Maintenance dosing for active PsA is 200 mg subcutaneously every other week or 400 mg every 4 weeks, according to product labeling.

IL-12/IL-23 Inhibitors: Ustekinumab *Ustekinumab* is an IL-12/23 monoclonal antibody approved for the treatment of moderate-to-severe plaque psoriasis and/or active PsA alone or in combination with methotrexatein adults 18 years or older.[16,26] It has a higher drug survival rate than TNF-α inhibitors, that is, longer duration of efficacy with continued treatment.[45] There is evidence that some patients may maintain PASI 90 through at least 244 weeks of treatment.[16] One study found that patients who had not used a biologic before (ie, biologic-naïve) or were using methotrexate concomitantly had longer survival.[45,100] Ustekinumab was significantly more efficacious than etanercept but less efficacious than the IL-17 inhibitors secukinumab or ixekizumab in clinical trials.[41] Ustekinumab has demonstrated long-term efficacy and safety for up to 5 years.[16] In addition, it is effective for difficult-to-treat areas, including hand and foot (either palmoplantar plaque or pustular), nail, and scalp psoriasis.[41]

Ustekinumab selectively targets IL-12 and IL-23, two cytokines that play a role in the pathogenesis of psoriasis.[29,45] It binds to their shared p40 protein subunit, thus preventing interaction with their cell surface IL-12Rβ1 receptor.[101] This shared binding may allow ustekinumab to exert its clinical effects in both psoriasis and PsA through interruption of the TH1 and TH17 cytokine pathways, central to both disease conditions.[101]

Ustekinumab can provide a rapid response that is seen within 2 weeks of initiating treatment.[45,102,103] Two large randomized placebo-controlled trials (PHOENIX 1[97] and PHOENIX 2[98]) demonstrated clinical efficacy of ustekinumab, with approximately 70% of patients achieving 75% skin clearance after two doses and maintaining the response for 1 year with continued treatment. The improvements were dramatic. Ustekinumab is effective in treating difficult-to-treat areas, such as hand and foot (palmoplantar plaque or pustular), nail, and scalp psoriasis.[45] In active PsA, ustekinumab demonstrated a greater proportion of ACR20 response at week 24 when compared to placebo in adult patients, according to product labeling. There was also a greater proportion of patients on ustekinumab with no or less radiographic progression at week 24 when compared with placebo.

The impact of ustekinumab on patients' health-related QoL was evaluated in the PHOENIX 2 trial.[104] Patients showed a significant improvement not only in skin-related QoL, but also in symptoms of anxiety and depression (as assessed by the Hospital Anxiety and Depression Scale).[103] The subset of patients with PsA in PHOENIX 1 and PHOENIX 2 also showed significant improvement in QoL, anxiety, and depression.[105]

Weight-based dosing rather than fixed-dose was found to be clinically significant for efficacy in PHOENIX 1 and PHOENIX 2—heavier patients required a higher dose.[106] Serum ustekinumab concentrations were also affected by weight.[106] Clinical response is related to serum ustekinumab levels achieved.[101] Manufacturer-recommended dosing is 45 mg for patients weighing 100 kg (220 lb) or less, and 90 mg for those of higher weights. Ustekinumab is administered subcutaneously at weeks 0 and 4, then every 12 weeks thereafter as maintenance therapy.[16,101] This dosing regimen is the same for active PsA alone or in combination with methotrexate. In cases where a loss of response is detected in the patient, the dose can be increased from 45 mg every 12 weeks to 90 mg every 8 weeks to improve response.[16]

Cumulative 3-year safety data from PHOENIX 1 and 2 have been published[107,108] and there is 5-year safety data.[89] Common adverse effects include upper respiratory infections, headache, fatigue, pruritus, back pain, injection site reactions, and arthralgia, with the most common events being headache and nasopharyngitis.[107] Ustekinumab does not exacerbate atopic diseases.[107] Serious adverse effects include those seen with other biologics, including serious tubercular, fungal, viral infections, and cancers. No evidence of a dose-response to infection rates was seen.[108] Serious infections and malignancy rates did not increase with long-term ustekinumab treatment for up to 3 years.[107,108] In addition, a reversible posterior leukoencephalopathy syndrome (RPLS) has been reported.[88,89] Regarding major adverse cardiovascular events (MACE), 5-year follow-up of clinical trials did not show an increased risk with ustekinumab.[89,109] Recommended monitoring parameters (pretreatment and every 3–6 months thereafter) include complete blood count, liver enzymes, serum creatinine, and renal status. In addition, pretreatment CRP and testing for hepatitis B and C and human immunodeficiency virus have been recommended.[29] Contraindications include clinically important active infection (including untreated latent TB) and hypersensitivity to the drug or excipients.

IL-17 Inhibitors: Secukinumab, Ixekizumab, Brodalumab, and Bimekizumab IL-17 is a proinflammatory cytokine. It is a key cytokine in the pathogenesis of psoriasis—binding to receptors on keratinocytes leads to increased inflammation and recruitment of inflammatory cell types, resulting in the characteristic psoriatic plaques.[37]

IL-17 inhibitors are useful in blocking this process. These agents have comparable efficacies, and some adverse effects are similar, such as an increased risk of infection—in particular mucocutaneous *Candida* infection.[45] Patients with a history of or active inflammatory bowel disease (IBD) may experience worsening or reactivation, and IL-17 inhibitors should be avoided in these patients.[45] Neutralizing antibodies to specific IL-17 inhibitors have been reported, and their presence may be associated with lower serum concentrations of the biologic and reduced efficacy.[45]

Secukinumab is a fully human IgG1κ monoclonal antibody that selectively binds and inhibits IL-17A, thus inhibiting the release of chemokines and other proinflammatory mediators. It was approved in the United States and Canada in 2015 for the treatment of moderate-to-severe plaque psoriasis in adult patients who are candidates for systemic therapy or phototherapy.[45,110] The approval was based on the results of four RCTs (including ERASURE and FIXTURE)[111] that included more than 2,000 patients. Secukinumab was shown to induce a rapid response with clinically significant greater PASI rates by week 12, and continued treatment was associated with sustained high responses through week 52.[111]

The CLEAR study compared secukinumab to ustekinumab in participants with plaque psoriasis and found greater efficacy at week 16 with secukinumab.[112] Secukinumab showed greater efficacy at 300 mg than at 150 mg in several RCTs and is equally safe.[45] Thus, the recommended dosing regimen for plaque psoriasis is 300 mg (as two subcutaneous injections of 150 mg) at weeks 0, 1, 2, and 3, followed by 300 mg as a maintenance dose starting at week 4.[45,110] However, a 150-mg dose may be acceptable for some patients.[45,111] The 300-mg dose may be more effective in treating head, neck, nail, palmoplantar, erythrodermic, and generalized pustular psoriasis.[45,113–116] A loading dose may be considered for active PsA. If a loading dose is given, subsequent dosing includes 150 mg subcutaneously every week up to week 4 and then every 4 weeks thereafter. If a loading dose is not given, 150 mg subcutaneously every 4 weeks is recommended, with consideration of increasing the dose to 300 mg every 4 weeks if the disease persists, according to product labeling. Adverse effects from clinical trials commonly included nasopharyngitis, headache, upper respiratory tract infection, diarrhea, and uncommonly included neutropenia and detection of anti-secukinumab antibodies.[45,110,111]

Ixekizumab is a humanized IgG4 monoclonal antibody that neutralizes IL-17A.[45] Binding to IL-17A prevents it from binding to its target IL-17 receptor, thus reducing/attenuating the expression of cytokines including interferon-gamma, IL-17, IL-22, and Il-23.[37] It is indicated for moderate-to-severe psoriasis; pivotal clinical trials include UNCOVER-1, UNCOVER-2, UNCOVER-3, and IXORA-S.[37,45] UNCOVER-3 was a phase 3 RCT that showed that ixekizumab was superior to etanercept after a 12-week induction phase.[34,117] The percentages of patients achieving PASI 75, PASI 90, and PASI 100 were 84%, 65%, and 35% with ixekizumab versus 53%, 26%, and 7% with etanercept, respectively.[45,117] Placebo responses were 7%, 3.1%, and 0%, respectively.[117] IXORA-S was a phase 3 RCT comparing efficacy of ixekizumab with ustekinumab at the label doses. At week 12, patients achieving PASI 90 were 73% with ixekizumab versus 42% with ustekinumab.[45,118] Ixekizumab is also efficacious for palmoplantar (nonpustular), nail, scalp, erythrodermic, inverse, and generalized pustular psoriasis.[45]

Recommended dosing for ixekizumab in patients with plaque psoriasis is an initial dose of 160 mg (self-administered subcutaneously) followed by 80 mg every 2 weeks until week 12, followed by a maintenance phase of 80 mg every 4 weeks thereafter.[37,45] Dosing for active PsA is 160 mg (as two 80 mg injections) subcutaneously at week 0, then 80 mg every 4 weeks. If the patient has plaque psoriasis with active PsA, dosing for plaque psoriasis as described above is recommended. Adverse events from clinical trials include nasopharyngitis, URTI, injection site reactions, with the most serious being cellulitis (0.4%); MACE was rare (one patient with a stroke).[37] Neutralizing anti-ixekizumab antibodies develop over time and are associated with reduced drug concentrations and loss of efficacy.[45]

Brodalumab is a fully human IgG2 anti-IL-17RA monoclonal antibody that binds to the IL-17 receptor A and blocks the biologic activities of cytokines including IL-17A, IL-17F, IL-17A/F, IL-17A/F heterodimer, IL-17C, and IL-17E (also known as IL-25).[37,45] Pivotal clinical trials include IMAGINE-1, IMAGINE-2, and IMAGINE-3. In both IMAGINE-2 and IMAGINE-3, brodalumab at 210-mg doses had higher PASI 90 and PASI 100 response rates than ustekinumab.[37,45] Brodalumab is also efficacious in erythrodermic, nail, scalp, generalized pustular psoriasis, and PsA.[45] Recommended dosing is 210 mg subcutaneously self-injected on weeks 0, 1, and 2 then 210 mg every 2 weeks.[45]

The most frequent adverse effects in clinical trials of brodalumab were arthralgia, headache, fatigue, diarrhea, oropharyngeal pain, nausea, and infections were seen in 25% of patients (mostly URTI, nasopharyngitis, UTI, bronchitis, influenza, and nonserious skin and mucosal *Candida* infections).[37] The most serious potential risk is suicidal ideation or behavior which occurred in 34 of 4,464 patients treated with brodalumab (ie, a rate of 0.37 per 100 participant-years).[37] Thus, brodalumab has a black box warning, and it is contraindicated in patients with suicidal ideation, recent suicidal behavior, or history of suicidal ideation. In addition, brodalumab is only available through a risk evaluation and mitigation strategy (REMS) program,[37,45] the SILIQ REMS.[45]

IL-23 Inhibitors: Guselkumab, Tildrakizumab, Risankizumab Acting through a transcription pathway, IL-23 induces a population of T-helper cells (designated as TH17 cells) with a unique inflammatory gene signature that is important in the pathogenesis of psoriasis and other autoimmune diseases.[119] IL-23 inhibitors block/bind to the p19 subunit of IL-23.[45] Neutralizing antibodies to specific IL-17 inhibitors have been reported and their presence may be associated with lower serum concentrations of the biologic and reduced efficacy.[45] In patients on these agents who are not responding adequately, dose escalation may be needed or other modalities (eg, TCS, vitamin D analogs, methotrexate, or UVB) added.[45]

Guselkumab is a fully human IgG1 lambda monoclonal antibody that blocks the p19 subunit of IL-23.[45] A phase 3 RCT (VOYAGE 2) comparing guselkumab with adalimumab and placebo found greater efficacy at week 16 (PASI 90 was 70% vs 47% for adalimumab and 2.4% for placebo).[120] Furthermore, 66% of adalimumab nonresponders switched to guselkumab reached PASI 90 at week 48.[45,120] The recommended guselkumab dose for active PsA and plaque psoriasis is 100 mg subcutaneously at weeks 0 and 4, and every 8 weeks thereafter.[45] The agent has also been shown to be effective for scalp, nail, and plaque-type palmoplantar psoriasis.[45]

Tildrakizumab is a humanized IgG1 monoclonal antibody designed to selectively block IL-23 by binding to the p19 subunit.[45] A phase 3 RCT (reSURFACE 2) comparing two doses of tildrakizumab (200 mg and 100 mg) to etanercept and placebo found greater efficacy at week 12 with either dose of tildrakizumab than with etanercept (66% of patients on tildrakizumab 200 mg achieving PASI 75 and 61% for tildrakizumab 100 mg, compared with 48% for etanercept and 6% with placebo).[121] PASI 90 was achieved by 37% (200-mg dose), 39% (100-mg dose), 21% (etanercept), and 1% (placebo) of participants.[45,121] The recommended dose is 100 mg subcutaneously administered *only by a healthcare provider* at weeks 0 and 4, and every 12 weeks thereafter.[45]

Risankizumab is a humanized IgG1 monoclonal antibody that selectively inhibits IL-23 by binding to the p19 subunit; it is more efficacious than ustekinumab.[45,122,123] The agent received FDA and Health Canada approvals in April 2019 for treatment of moderate-to-severe plaque psoriasis. The approval decisions were supported by positive results from four phase 3 RCTs: ultIMMa-1, ultIMMa-2, IMMhance, and IMMvent.[122,123] From clinical trials, at week 12, PASI 90 for risankizumab was about 75% (90 mg and 180 mg doses pooled) versus about 40% to 45% for ustekinumab (weight-based dosing).[45,122] Recommended dosing is risankizumab 75 mg subcutaneously for 2 doses (totaling 150 mg) at weeks 0 and 4, followed by 150 mg as two injections every 12 weeks thereafter.

Switching Between Biologic Agents Switching between biologic agents to possibly improve efficacy, safety, and/or tolerability is a useful consideration. Biologics that develop neutralizing antibodies may have reduced efficacy over time (secondary failure),[45] and sustainability for more than 3 years is currently a treatment target for a biologic agent—and 3 years is not that long a time for a chronic disease such as psoriasis.

Switching to another biologic even within its own class of biologics may restore efficacy. However, not all switches result in improvement, and there are no recommendations for specific switches in the US guidelines, nor recommendations for the duration interval between discontinuing one biologic and starting another.[45]

BAD provided some general recommendations in its 2020 guidelines: Consider using a 1-month washout period, or the length of the treatment cycle (whichever is longer), between the last dose of the current biologic therapy and the planned date of a new biologic initiation.[44] BAD also recommended taking into consideration the pharmacology of the agents, the patient's clinical circumstances, and the patient's views on the risks and benefits of transitioning option(s).[44]

Combination Therapies

Combination therapies may be beneficial in the management of plaque psoriasis: generally to either enhance efficacy or minimize toxicity. As shown in Figs. 118-1 and 118-2, combinations can include two topical agents, a topical agent plus phototherapy, a systemic agent plus topical therapy, a systemic agent plus phototherapy, two systemic agents used in rotation, or a biologic agent with either a systemic agent or a topical agent.

The combination of a TCS and a topical vitamin D_3 analog is particularly useful. This was shown in several studies to be efficacious and safe, with less skin irritation than monotherapy with either agent, and the combination product containing calcipotriol and betamethasone dipropionate ointment has demonstrated efficacy in RCTs for patients with relatively severe psoriasis.[16,40] The combination may also be steroid sparing.[40]

The combination of retinoids with phototherapy has also been shown to increase efficacy. Because retinoids may be photosensitizing and increase the risk of burning after ultraviolet (UV) light exposure, doses of phototherapy should be reduced to minimize adverse effects. An RCT with tazarotene and broadband UVB not only showed significant enhancement of UVB efficacy but also reduced the number of UVB treatment sessions needed for response.[38,40,124] The combination of acitretin and broadband UVB reduced the number of needed treatments, compared with UVB alone.[16,125] Acitretin with NB-UVB (RE-UVB) was highly effective for patients with difficult-to-control psoriasis.[40,126] The combination of acitretin and PUVA (RE-PUVA) also showed greater efficacy than monotherapy with either agent.[38,127] RE-PUVA can be used to achieve clearance with up to a twofold reduction in total UV exposure.[16] Phototherapy has also been used with other topical agents, such as UVB with coal tar (Goeckerman regimen)[73] to increase treatment response because coal tar is also photosensitizing.

Cyclosporine and calcipotriol/betamethasone dipropionate in combination is superior to cyclosporine alone.[29] Cyclosporine may also be successfully used with SCAT; however, it should not be used with PUVA due to reduced efficacy and the potential increased risk of cutaneous malignancies.[42]

The combination of MTX and UVB is synergistic.[39,43] MTX in combination with biologics is beneficial. MTX has been effectively used in conjunction with etanercept, infliximab, adalimumab, ustekinumab, and others. MTX in combination with adalimumab or infliximab is widely used in rheumatology, and low-dose MTX (eg, 7.5-10 mg once per week) is likely sufficient to reduce the formation of anti-biologic-antibodies and increase the respective trough levels of adalimumab or infliximab.[29] Infliximab given concurrently with MTX or azathioprine may result in a lower incidence of infusion reactions to infliximab.[41]

Biologics used in combination with nonbiologic therapies are being explored and recommended, sometimes with just a theoretical rationale (ie, without RCT backup yet). In particular, the concept of increasing biologic survival with the addition of an immunosuppressive agent that reduces the development of neutralizing biologic antibodies is gaining acceptance as experience and clinical evidence accumulate with their use. Newer biologics whose use is associated with neutralizing antibodies are often used together with an immunosuppressive agent such as MTX.[45]

Other Drug Treatments

Selective Phosphodiesterase-4 (PDE4) Inhibitors: Crisaborole, Apremilast A relatively new approach to management of inflammatory skin conditions such as psoriasis and atopic dermatitis (AD) is targeted inhibition of phosphodiesterase 4 (PDE4).[128] PDE4 inhibition causes an increase in intracellular cyclic AMP (cAMP), which leads to multiple effects, including reduced production of proinflammatory mediators.[128]

Apremilast is an oral tablet approved in the United States and Canada for patients with active PsA or moderate-to-severe psoriasis. It has shown efficacy and safety in 2 Phase III RCT (ESTEEM 1 and ESTEEM 2) for patients with psoriasis.[129] Recommended dosing is 10 mg on day 1, 10 mg twice daily on day 2, 10 mg in the morning and 20 mg in the evening on day 3, 20 mg twice daily on day 4, 20 mg in the morning, and 30 mg in the evening on day 5, then 30 mg twice daily thereafter. Dosing if renally impaired (CrCl <30 mL/min [0.5 mL/s]) is 10 mg in the morning on days 1 to 3; titrate using morning doses only (skip evening doses) to 20 mg on days 4 and 5, with the maintenance dose of 30 mg once daily in the morning thereafter.

Apremilast may be taken without regard to food; however, it should not be crushed, chewed, or split. There are drug interactions: the levels/effects of apremilast may be decreased by bosentan, CYP3A4 inducers (moderate and strong); dabrafenib, deferasirox, ivosidenib, lorlatinib, pitolisant, sarilumab, siltuximab, tocilizumab, and St. John's wort.[130]

Crisaborole is a topical PDE4 inhibitor approved for atopic dermatitis.

Mycophenolate Mofetil Mycophenolate mofetil (MMF) is a systemic agent occasionally used for patients with resistant cases of moderate-to-severe psoriasis.[16] This is not an approved indication in either Canada or the United States (off-label use).

A few reports and small studies are available describing the efficacy of MMF when used as monotherapy or adjuvant therapy.[131] In addition, one small study evaluated the switch for eight patients with severe psoriasis from cyclosporine to MMF after a washout period of 2 to 4 weeks. On cyclosporine, seven of these patients had deteriorating renal function and hypertension, and one experienced loss of efficacy.[132] After the switch to MMF, there was a significant loss of psoriasis control in five of the eight patients, but also a significant improvement in renal function for six patients.[131,132]

Conversely, another small study evaluated the sequential use of MMF followed by cyclosporine in eight patients with moderate-to-severe psoriasis.[133] There was significant improvement with MMF in all patients, and all patients further improved when switched to cyclosporine.[133]

MMF has some uncommon but significant adverse effects, including increased incidence of opportunistic infections such as cytomegalovirus, cryptococcosis, candidiasis, and *Pneumocystis jirovecii*.[3,131] Cases of progressive multifocal leukoencephalopathy have also been reported.[131] There may be an associated risk of malignancy.[134]

Hydroxyurea Hydroxyurea is an antimetabolite usually used for cancer treatments, but it has also been used in the systemic treatment of psoriasis for more than 30 years.[16,39] It is still occasionally tried for patients with recalcitrant severe psoriasis, although biologics may be a better option for these patients.

Hydroxyurea has been compared with MTX for patients with moderate-to-severe psoriasis.[135] Weekly regimens showed greater efficacy for MTX with a faster clearance rate, although hydroxyurea was also efficacious. The authors concluded that weekly doses of hydroxyurea may be an alternative to MTX for patients experiencing intolerable MTX side effects or who have reached the recommended cumulative MTX dose.[135]

Adverse effects of hydroxyurea include significant bone marrow suppression, lesional erythema, localized tenderness, and reversible hyperpigmentation.[16,135]

Complementary and Alternative Medicines

The use of complementary and alternative medicine (CAM) among patients with psoriasis is common, with a prevalence of 43% to 69% in various studies.[136] Most of these patients use herbs, special diets, or dietary supplements in conjunction with their usual antipsoriatic medications and not as replacements. Most patients do not discuss CAM use with their physicians.[136]

A 2009 systematic review of RCTs found that, although there is a large body of literature on CAM use in psoriasis, the quality of most studies was relatively low.[136] CAM agents and interventions with documented clinical efficacy in psoriasis include *Mahonia aquifolium*, fish oil, climatotherapy (Dead Sea salts), and stress reduction techniques.

Mahonia aquafolium (Oregon grape, Mountain grape, or barberry but *not* European barberry) is an evergreen native to southern British Columbia, western Oregon, and northern Idaho. The rhizome and root contain berberine as the primary active constituent. Berberine is an alkaloid that inhibits keratinocyte growth and reduces keratinocyte proliferation, and it also has antibacterial and antifungal activities. In at least two clinical trials, *Mahonia aquifolium* was efficacious in reducing disease severity: in one randomized placebo-controlled study, a *Mahonia aquifolium* 10% preparation applied topically twice daily resulted in a significant improvement in the PASI score and the Quality of Life Index (QLI), compared with placebo.[137] Adverse effects in clinical trials included rash, burning sensation, redness, and itching.

Fish oil contains two important long-chain polyunsaturated fatty acids—eicosapentaenoic acid (EPA) and docosahexaenoic acid (DHA). EPA and DHA are omega-3 fatty acids. They act as substrates competing with arachidonic acid for cyclooxygenase and lipoxygenase, thus reducing the production of proinflammatory molecules in psoriatic plaques.[136] Several randomized placebo-controlled and/or comparative trials for patients with psoriasis have demonstrated efficacy of fish oils. One study comparing EPA plus etretinate to etretinate monotherapy found significantly greater efficacy with the combination of EPA plus etretinate.[138]

Climatotherapy refers to the practice of traveling to the Dead Sea and sunbathing and/or bathing in the sea—the beneficial effects are likely from the high salinity of the sea and UV rays.[136] Several studies have demonstrated efficacy, including two studies using saline spa baths. One study used highly concentrated (25%-27%) saline spa baths plus UVB compared with UVB alone, and the other used low concentrated (4.5%-12%) saline spa bath plus UVB again compared with UVB alone. In both studies, the clinical response was significantly better with the saline spa bath plus UVB combination.[136,139,140]

Stress-reduction techniques have inconsistently shown some benefit. One randomized study demonstrated that both meditation or meditation and imagery were efficacious as adjunctive treatments for patients with scalp psoriasis.[141] A second randomized study for patients with psoriasis receiving either UVB or PUVA therapy showed that the addition of a mindfulness-based stress-reduction audiotape played during light treatments reduced response times for patients receiving UVB but not PUVA therapy.[142] This confirmed the belief that psychological stress plays a role in psoriasis. More recently, in a case-control study of risk factors during the year before the onset of psoriasis, stressful life events were found to be significant.[143,144]

Personalized Pharmacotherapy

Despite the availability of good quality evidence and clinical practice guidelines, patients with psoriasis are still often undertreated or inappropriately managed.[30] A 2007 study in the United States involving 1,657 patients from National Psoriasis Foundation surveys found that 40% of patients with psoriasis were receiving no current treatment; of those, 27% had psoriasis involving >10% BSA.[145] In addition, those receiving care may be undertreated.[145] Early access to care and adherence may also be issues.

Patient-specific therapies that take into consideration comorbid illnesses, adherence, and pharmacoeconomic issues in addition to the patient's psoriatic manifestations and responses to treatments are important, and will ultimately improve the quality of care. Treatment goals need to be patient-specific and defined for both short-term and long-term management time frames.[30] Without optimizing patient care, the concern is that patients with poorly managed psoriasis may follow a "diminished" life course compared with the course they might have taken if they did not have psoriasis, as the disease has significant psychological, social, and economic impacts in addition to its physical manifestations.[146]

To this end, a current focus is defining frameworks,[146] specific treatment goals,[29,30] and targets[31] for implementation of practice guidelines, as described earlier in this chapter. The reader is encouraged to review the noted references for further information.

Special Populations

Psoriasis in Children Psoriasis affects approximately 1% of children, with the most common onset during adolescence. One third of patients with psoriasis had onset of symptoms during the pediatric years.[147] Pediatric psoriasis is more often attributable to direct precipitating factors such as skin trauma, infections, drugs, or stress.[16,148] Compared with adults, plaque lesions in children are often smaller, thinner, and less scaly, which can make diagnosis more difficult. Face and flexures are more commonly involved than for adults. Psoriatic diaper rash can occur up to age 2. PsA is rare.[16]

Psoriasis in children is associated with cardiovascular risk factors and metabolic syndrome.[16] Cardiovascular risk factors include being overweight, obesity, hyperlipidemia, hypertension, high blood glucose, and diabetes.[16] Obesity and excessive waist circumference (central adiposity) are higher in children with severe psoriasis, and in general, are higher in childhood psoriasis than in adults.[16,149] Adolescent girls who are overweight are at increased risk of later developing moderate-to-severe psoriasis, suggesting that obesity precedes the onset of psoriasis.[16,150]

Thus, nonpharmacologic management strategies in children also include minimizing cardiovascular risk factors and the development of the metabolic syndrome. The importance of maintaining a healthy lifestyle with good eating habits, exercise, and weight balance is crucial information to communicate to the child/adolescent and caregivers.

Topical treatment is the standard-of-care for children with psoriasis.[16,151] Vitamin D_3 analogues (calcipotriene, calcipotriol, and calcitriol) have a corticosteroid-sparing function; this is an important advantage for pediatric patients. Calcipotriol with or without TCS has been recommended as treatment of first choice[16,151] because it produces minimal adverse effects.[16] Since children's skin is thinner and better hydrated than that of adults, they are at higher risk of drug absorption leading to systemic adverse effects. If a TCS is needed, the lowest potency TCS that provides control should be used, and it should be tapered as the lesions improve.

Combination products with calcipotriol and betamethasone dipropionate are effective and have FDA approval for use in children 12 years and older. Calcipotriol/betamethasone dipropionate ointment applied once daily for up to 4 weeks at a time has been recommended by AAD-NPF as a safe and effective treatment for children 12 years and older with mild-to-moderate plaque psoriasis, and the suspension has been recommended for once-daily use up to 8 weeks for mild-to-moderate scalp psoriasis. Due to the expense of combination products, individual products are often prescribed for simultaneous use in various regimens (e.g. once daily for the first 2 weeks, then reduced to weekends for topical corticosteroids and weekdays for the vitamin D analogue). To minimize corticosteroid use, combination therapy can be transitioned to topical vitamin D monotherapy when the condition improves.[147]

If long-term calcipotriol is used, monitoring of ionized calcium is recommended because of the risk of hypercalcemia.[16] Topical calcineurin inhibitors have been recommended as first-line therapy for psoriasis of the face, genitalia, and body folds. Rotational therapy with topical vitamin D analogues, topical calcineurin inhibitors, emollients, tar-based therapies, and topical corticosteroids should be considered in children as steroid-sparing regimens.[147,151] For treatment-resistant or moderate-to-severe psoriasis, anthralin has been suggested, before considering short-term UVB in adolescents.[16,151] NB-UVB is recommended as a treatment option for moderate-to-severe pediatric plaque and guttate psoriasis.[147] For treatment-resistant or moderate-to-severe psoriasis, anthralin is suggested, followed by short-term UVB in adolescents.[16,151]NB-UVB is recommended as a treatment option for moderate-to-severe pediatric plaque and guttate psoriasis.[147]

Systemic therapies (traditional nonbiologic and biologic) are appropriate for children with moderate-to-severe and recalcitrant psoriasis[16,86,147,151] or in the presence of comorbidities such as psoriatic arthritis.[147] In general, the goal with all systemic therapies in children is to control or clear the disease, provide maintenance disease stability for several months, then taper to the lowest effective dose and ultimately transition off systemic therapies if possible. If not possible, long-term maintenance at the lowest effective dose using the least toxic therapy is the preferred approach. MTX can provide near to complete clearance and has been recommended as the systemic treatment of choice in the Canadian guidelines[16] and recommended as effective systemic therapy in the AAD-NPF guidelines. MTX can be safely used to control severe childhood psoriatic episodes and then withdrawn as lesions improve.[16] Folate supplementation is recommded. Regular monitoring for liver and blood toxicity is required.[16] Other nonbiologic systemic agents such as cyclosporine and acitretin may also be used in children.[86,147]

Biologic agents recommended in the 2020 AAD-NPF guidelines for use in children include etanercept, adalimumab, infliximab, and ustekinumab.[147] Etanercept has been recommended as a third-line option in the 2016 Canadian guidelines.[16] A 2020 Canadian consensus summarizing the most recent evidence on the use of biologics for moderate-to-severe plaque psoriasis in pediatrics provides an algorithm that includes the biologics etanercept, adalimumab.[86] A randomized controlled trial in 211 children and adolescents (4-17 years) with moderate-to-severe plaque psoriasis showed that etanercept significantly reduced disease severity; however, four serious adverse events occurred (ovarian cyst requiring removal, gastroenteritis, gastroenteritis-associated dehydration, and left basilar pneumonia).[148] Etanercept has been studied in children with polyarticular juvenile rheumatoid arthritis without new safety concerns emerging.[16] Ustekinumab and adalimumab's safety profiles are also continuing to be evaluated.[16]

Biologics can be safely combined with topical corticosteroids, with or without a topical vitamin D analogue, to augment effectiveness for the treatment of moderate-to-severe plaque psoriasis in children.[147]

Phototherapy should be used with caution, especially for younger children, because of long-term carcinogenic risks and phototoxicities. For older children and adolescents with severe, extensive, or treatment-resistant disease, UVB (in particular, NB-UVB) may be a treatment option.[16]

Psoriasis in Pregnancy Hormonal changes in pregnancy can improve symptoms for patients with plaque psoriasis. In one study, 55% of patients showed improvements during pregnancy.[16,153] For patients with more than 10% BSA involvement who reported improvement, lesions decreased by more than 80% during pregnancy.[153] This appeared to correlate with high estrogen but not progesterone levels.[153] Thus, some pregnant women may require minimal treatment for their psoriasis.

Some antipsoriatic drugs have significant teratogenic risks, making them contraindicated in pregnancy. Thus, women of childbearing potential must use effective birth control during therapy, and may need to continue effective contraception after discontinuing therapy for a period of time, as discussed in detail throughout this chapter. In addition, some drugs may carry known teratogenic risks in animal studies or have limited available data for use in pregnancy in humans.

UVB has been considered the safest treatment for extensive psoriasis during pregnancy. It is recommended for patients with widespread disease not controlled by topical agents. One problem with this therapy is an increased potential for reactivation of herpes simplex, which may be transmitted to the infant at delivery.[16]

For more detailed information about antipsoriatic drugs in pregnancy, a systematic, drug-by-drug review of case reports and case-control studies is available.[154] The 2009 Canadian Guidelines provides a drug-by-drug summary of recommendations for topical agents, phototherapy, and systemic agents in pregnancy.[16] The 2015 European S3 Guidelines provides a discussion about most appropriate treatments for women with a wish for pregnancy in the near future, and which treatments to avoid.[29]

Psoriasis in Older Adults Age-related changes in organ function/drug clearance and greater drug sensitivity increase the risk of adverse drug events for elderly patients with psoriasis.

MTX is hepatotoxic and should be used with caution in older adults. Cyclosporine has nephrotoxic potential and may also increase blood pressure. Both drugs have significant drug interactions, and polypharmacy, common in older patients, makes management of interactions challenging.

In addition, older patients may have preexisting comorbidities, such as hyperlipidemia and metabolic syndrome, and this may further limit drug selection. Adalimumab is equally efficacious in patients aged 65 years or older who may have higher incidences of hypertension, hyperlipidemia, depression, obesity, and diabetes.[155] Adverse-effect profiles were similar between subgroups (various weights and comorbidities) with no significant differences in serious adverse events.[155] Ustekinumab requires no dosage adjustments for renal or hepatic impairments and geriatric dosing is the same as for adults younger than 65 years, with the dose based on weight. Secukinumab also requires no dosage change in older adults and those with renal/hepatic impairment.

Topical psoriasis treatments are often prescribed for older adults as first-line therapy[16]; however, even with topicals, adverse effects—including systemic ones—can occur with greater frequency in these patients.[16]

Psoriasis in Patients with a History of Solid Tumors As discussed throughout this chapter, many antipsoriatic therapies carry significant cancer risks. PUVA, systemic therapies such as cyclosporine, and some biologics are associated with increased risks of oncologic disorders.

A systematic review of the risk of malignancy associated with therapies for moderate-to-severe psoriasis confirmed the following[134]: PUVA is associated with an increased risk of cutaneous SCC and malignant melanoma; UVB is a much safer therapeutic modality than PUVA; cyclosporine increases risks of lymphoma, internal malignancies, and skin cancers; methotrexate may be associated with increased melanoma and Epstein-Barr virus–associated lymphomas; MMF may be associated with lymphoproliferative disorders; and the malignancy risk may be increased for biologic agents, especially the TNF-α inhibitors.[134]

The 2009 Canadian guidelines recommend that TNF-α inhibitors be used with caution for patients with a history of malignancy or existing malignancies, and the T-cell modulator alefacept (now voluntarily withdrawn from the US and Canadian markets) is contraindicated for these patients.[16] There are currently registry safety databases (PSOLAR,[156] BADBIR,[157] PsoBest[158,159]) for biologics; over time, these will provide biologic-specific and updated safety information.[159] Known risks in general include the development of neoplasms such as nonmelanoma skin cancer.[89]

Coronavirus Disease 2019 Risk in Patients Receiving Biologics for Psoriasis During the coronavirus disease 2019 (COVID-19) pandemic caused by severe acute respiratory syndrome coronavirus 2 (SARS-CoV-2), there was concern around increased risk of infection in patients receiving ongoing biologic therapy for psoriasis.

A study exploring the incidence of COVID-19 in 1,830 patients with psoriasis who were receiving various biologics (etanercept, ustekinumab, ixekizumab, secukinumab, and guselkumab) found a COVID-19 incidence rate (IR) of 9.7 (95% CI 3.9-20.1) per 10,000 person-months in patients with psoriasis versus an IR of 11.5 (95% CI 11.4-11.7) per 10,000 person-months in the general population. This study was conducted in northeast Italy (the Veneto region comprising Verona, Padua, and Vicenza) with data collected between February 20, 2020, and June 1, 2020, during the height of an initial wave of the COVID-19 pandemic in this region. Only six cases of COVID-19 occurred among 1,830 patients with psoriasis compared with 19,154 cases among 4,905,854 people in the general population. Of the six COVID-19–positive patients with psoriasis, four were hospitalized with interstitial pneumonia with no deaths. These results were contrary to the expectation that the incidence and severity of COVID-19 would be higher in patients with psoriasis as they had a higher prevalence of known comorbidities (hypertension, cardiovascular diseases, diabetes) than those in the general population.[160]

Pharmacoeconomic Considerations

10 The wide gap in costs of agents for psoriasis makes economics and availability of insurance or other coverage important considerations in formulating a therapeutic plan.

The biologics are often considered for patients with moderate-to-severe psoriasis when less-expensive traditional systemic agents are inadequate or relatively contraindicated. Biologics have also been recommended as first-line therapy, alongside conventional systemic agents, for patients with moderate-to-severe psoriasis; however, in practice, drug access secondary to cost considerations can limit use. These agents may be needed early, though, for some patients with comorbidities, such as PsA.

A pharmacoeconomic analysis of biologics in the treatment of psoriasis suggests that the cost-to-benefit ratio for biologics may be favorable.[161] This analysis was performed in 2009 when available biologics were fewer and more expensive than today. More recent analyses indicate wide variations when clinical outcomes are factored into costs of recently marketed agents.[162]

CONCLUSION

Psoriasis is a lifelong illness with no known cure. Significant comorbidities may coexist. Treatment should be patient-specific, with consideration given to disease severity, patient risk factors, age, and comorbidities. Newer treatment modalities, including numerous biologics, are now parts of the armamentarium available in the management of this disease.

ABBREVIATIONS

BAD	British Association of Dermatologists
BADBIR	British Association of Dermatologists Biologic Interventions Register
BMI	body mass index
BRM	biologic response modifier (This term has been replaced by "biologic agents.")

BSA	body surface area
CAM	complementary and alternative medicine
CDA	Canadian Dermatology Association
CHD	coronary heart disease
CHF	chronic heart failure
COVID-19	Coronavirus Disease 2019
CRP	C-reactive protein
CYP3A4	cytochrome P450 isoenzyme 3A4
DBPC	double-blind placebo-controlled
DHA	docosahexaenoic acid
DISH	disseminated (or diffuse) idiopathic skeletal hyperostosis
DLQI	Dermatology Life Quality Index
EPA	eicosapentaenoic acid
FDA	Food and Drug Administration
GFR	glomerular filtration rate
HLA-C	major histocompatibility complex antigen
HPA	hypothalamic–pituitary–adrenal
IL	interleukin
MACE	major adverse cardiovascular events
MMF	mycophenolate mofetil
MI	myocardial infarction
NPF	National Psoriasis Foundation
NSAIDs	nonsteroidal anti-inflammatory drugs
NB-UVB	narrowband ultraviolet B (311-nm ultraviolet B light)
OR	odds ratio
PASI	Psoriasis Area and Severity Index
PGA	Physician's Global Assessment
PsA	psoriatic arthritis
PUVA	psoralens with ultraviolet A light
QoL	quality of life
QLI	Quality of Life Index
RCT	randomized controlled trial
RE-PUVA	retinoid plus PUVA (as combination therapy)
RE-UVB	retinoid plus NBUVB (as combination therapy)
RPLS	reversible posterior leukoencephalopathy syndrome
RR	relative risk
SARS-COV2	severe acute respiratory syndrome coronavirus
SCAT	short-contact anthralin therapy
SCC	squamous cell carcinoma
SF-36	Short Form Health Survey
SPF	sun protection factor
TB	tuberculosis
TNF-α	tumor necrosis factor-α
UV	ultraviolet
UVA	ultraviolet A (315-400 nm ultraviolet A light)
UVB	ultraviolet B, or broadband UVB (28-315 nm ultraviolet B light)

REFERENCES

1. Armstrong AW, Mehta MD, Schupp Clayton W., et al. Psoriasis prevalence in adults in the United States. *JAMA Dermatology* 2021;157:940–946. 10.1001/jamadermatol.2021.2007.
2. World Health Organization. Global report on psoriasis. https://apps.who.int/iris/bitstream/handle/10665/204417/9789241565189_eng.pdf.psoriasis?sequence=1. 2016, Accessed Feb. 28, 2022.
3. Boehncke WH, Schon MP. Psoriasis. *Lancet.* 2015; 386:983–994.
4. Kimmel GW, Lebwohl M. Psoriasis: Overview and diagnosis. In: Bhutani T, Liao W, Nakamura M, eds. *Evidence-Based Psoriasis, Diagnosis and Treatment*. Cham, Switzerland: Springer International Publishing AG; 2018;1–16. A textbook in the series Updates in Clinical Dermatology, with series editors Berth-Jones J, Gob CL, and Maibach HI. http://www.springer.com/series/13203.
5. Gulliver WP, Pirzada SM. Psoriasis: More than skin deep. In: Saeland S, ed. *Recent Advances in Skin Immunology*. Kevala, India: Research Signpost; 2008:167–179.
6. Reich K. The concept of psoriasis as a systemic inflammation: Implications for disease management. *J Eur Acad Dermatol Venereol.* 2012;26(suppl 2):3–11.
7. Boehncke WH, Boehncke S, Tobin AM, Kirby B. The 'psoriatic march': A concept of how severe psoriasis may drive cardiovascular comorbidity. *Exp Dermatol.* 2011;147:1031–1039.
8. Grozdev I, Korman N, Tsankov N. Psoriasis as a systemic disease. *Clinics Dermatol.* 2014;32:343–350.
9. Farber E, Bright R, Nall M. Psoriasis: A questionnaire survey of 2144 patients. *Arch Dermatol.* 1974;98:248–259.
10. Farber EM, Nall ML, Watson W. Natural history of psoriasis in 61 twin pairs. *Arch Dermatol.* 1974;109:207–211.
11. Nall L, Gulliver WP, Charmley P, et al. Search for the psoriasis susceptibility gene: The Newfoundland Study. *Cutis.* 1999;64:323–329.
12. Nair RP, Duffin KC, Helms C, et al. Genome-wide scan reveals association of psoriasis with IL-23 and NF-κB pathways. *Nat Genet.* 2009;41:199–204.
13. Raychaudhuri SP, Jiang W-Y, Raychaudhuri SK. Revisiting the Koebner phenomenon. *Am J Pathol.* 2008;172:961–971.
14. Basavaraj KH, Ashok NM, Rashmi R, Praveen TK. The role of drugs in the induction and/or exacerbation of psoriasis. *Int J Dermatol.* 2010;49:1351–1361.
15. Law RM. Chapter 64: Psoriasis. In: Chisholm-Burns M, ed. *Pharmacotherapy Principles and Practice.* 3rd ed. New York: McGraw-Hill; 2013:1127–1141.
16. Papp KA, Gulliver W, Lynde CW, Poulin Y. Canadian Guidelines for the Management of Plaque Psoriasis. 1st Edition, June 2009. Available at: (Steering Committee). Also see: Canadian Psoriasis Guidelines Addendum Committee. Addendum to the Canadian Guidelines for the Management of Plaque Psoriasis, May 2016. *J Cutan Med Surg.* 2016;20(5):375-431. Available at: https://dermatology.ca/dermatologists/guidelines/psoriasis. Also see: Canadian Psoriasis Guidelines Addendum Committee. Addendum to the Canadian Guidelines for the Management of Plaque Psoriasis, May 2016. *J Cutan Med Surg.* 2016;20(5):375-431. Available at: https://www.ncbi.nlm.nih.gov/pmc/articles/PMC5014087/. Accessed Feb. 28, 2022.
17. Boehncke S, Boehncke WH. 'Upgrading' psoriasis responsibly. *Exp. Dermatol.* 2014;23:710–711.
18. Guenther L, Gulliver W. Psoriasis comorbidities. *J Cutan Med Surg.* 2009;13(suppl 2>):S77–S87.
19. Kimball AB, Gladman D, Gelfand JM, et al. National Psoriasis Foundation clinical consensus on psoriasis comorbidities and recommendations for screening. *J Am Acad Dermatol.* 2008;58:1031–1042.
20. Gulliver WP. Importance of screening for comorbidities in psoriasis patients. *Expert Rev Dermatol.* 2008;3:133–135.
21. Gelfand JM, Gladman Dd, Mease PJ, et al. Epidemiology of psoriatic arthritis in the population of the United States. *J Am Acad Dermatol.* 2005;53:573–577.
22. Rahman P, O'Reilly DD. Psoriatic arthritis genetic susceptibility and pharmacogenetics. *Pharmacogenomics.* 2008;9:195–205.
23. Wilson PW, D'Agostino RB, Parise H, et al. Metabolic syndrome as a precursor of cardiovascular disease and type 2 diabetes mellitus. *Circulation.* 2005;112:3066–3072.
24. Kimball AB, Guerin A, Latremouille-Viau D, et al. Coronary heart disease and stroke risk in patients with psoriasis: Retrospective analysis. *Am J Med.* 2010;123:350–357.
25. Dowlatshani EA, Wakkee M, Arends LR, et al. The prevalence and odds of depressive symptoms and clinical depression in psoriasis patients: A systematic review and meta-analysis. *J Invest Dermatol.* 2014;136(6):1542–1551.
26. Gelfand JM, Neimann AL, Shin DB, et al. Risk of myocardial infarction in patients with psoriasis. *JAMA.* 2006;296:1735–1741.
27. Ahlehoff O, Skov L, Gislason G, et al. Cardiovascular disease event rates in patients with severe psoriasis treated with systemic anti-inflammatory drugs: A Danish real-world cohort study. *J Intern Med.* 2013;273(2):197–204.
28. Lan CC, Ko YC, Yu HS, et al. Methotrexate reduces the occurrence of cerebrovascular events among Taiwanese psoriatic patients: A nationwide population-based study. *Acta Derm Venereol.* 2012;92(4):349–352.
29. European S3-Guidelines on the systemic treatment of psoriasis vulgaris. Updated 2015. EDF in cooperation with EADV and IPC. *J Eur Acad Dermatol Venereol.* 2015;29(12):e1–22. Available at: https://www.edf.one/dam/jcr:d0c615a6-0631-4bf7-9f87-c8f95c21ab9b/European%20

S3-Guidelines%20on%20the%20systemic%20treatment%20of%20 psoriasis%20(2).pdf.
30. Mrowietz U. Implementing treatment goals for successful long-term management of psoriasis. *J Eur Acad Dermatol Venereol.* 2012;26(suppl 2):12–20.
31. Armstrong AW, Siegel MP, Bagel J, et al. From the Medical Board of the National Psoriasis Foundation: Treatment targets for plaque psoriasis. *J Am Acad Dermatol.* 2017;76(2):290–298.
32. Strober B, Ryan C, van de Kerkhof P, et al. Recategorization of psoriasis severity: Delphi consensus from the International Psoriasis Council. *J Am Acad Dermatol.* 2020;82:117–122.
33. Law RMT, Gulliver WP. Chapter 110: Psoriasis. In: Schwinghammer TL, Koehler JM, eds. *Pharmacotherapy Casebook and Instructor's Guide: A Patient-Focused Approach.* 12th ed. New York: McGraw-Hill; 2023.
34. Jeon C, Sekhon S, Bhutani T, Koo J. Topical treatments. In: Bhutani T, Liao W, Nakamura M, eds. *Evidence-Based Psoriasis, Diagnosis and Treatment. (A textbook in the series Updates in Clinical Dermatology, with series editors Berth-Jones J, Gob CL, and Maibach HI, at http://www.springer.com/series/13203).* Cham, Switzerland: Springer International Publishing AG; 2018;17–29.
35. Griffith JL, Zarbo AJ, Lim HW. Phototherapy and photochemotherapy. In: Bhutani T, Liao W, Nakamura M, eds. *Evidence-Based Psoriasis, Diagnosis and Treatment. (A textbook in the series Updates in Clinical Dermatology, with series editors Berth-Jones J, Gob CL, and Maibach HI, at http://www.springer.com/series/13203).* Cham, Switzerland: Springer International Publishing AG; 2018;31–53.
36. Beck KM, Yang EJ, Afifian L, et al. Oral agents for psoriasis. In: Bhutani T, Liao W, Nakamura M, eds., et al. *Evidence-Based Psoriasis, Diagnosis and Treatment. (A textbook in the series Updates in Clinical Dermatology, with series editors Berth-Jones J, Gob CL, and Maibach HI, at http://www.springer.com/series/13203).* Cham, Switzerland: Springer International Publishing AG; 2018;55–71.
37. Sekhon S, Jeon C, Liao W. Biologics. In: Bhutani T, Liao W, Nakamura M, eds. *Evidence-Based Psoriasis, Diagnosis and Treatment. (A textbook in the series Updates in Clinical Dermatology, with series editors Berth-Jones J, Gob CL, and Maibach HI, at http://www.springer.com/series/13203).* Cham, Switzerland: Springer International Publishing AG; 2018;73–92.
38. Elmets CA, Lim HW, Stoff B, et al. Joint American Academy of Dermatology–National Psoriasis Foundation guidelines of care for the management and treatment of psoriasis with phototherapy. *J Am Acad Dermatol.* 2019;81:775–804.
39. Menter A, Gelfand JM, Connor C, et al. Joint American Academy of Dermatology–National Psoriasis Foundation guidelines of care for the management of psoriasis with systemic nonbiologic therapies. *J Am Acad Dermatol.* 2020;82:1445–1486.
40. Elmets CA, Korman NJ, Prater EF, et al. Joint AAD–NPF guidelines of care for the management and treatment of psoriasis with topical therapy and alternative medicine modalities for psoriasis severity measures. *J Am Acad Dermatol.* 2021;84:432–470.
41. Menter A, Gottlieb A, Feldman SR, et al. Guidelines of care for the management of psoriasis and psoriatic arthritis—section 1. Overview of psoriasis and guidelines of care for the treatment of psoriasis with biologics. *J Am Acad Dermatol.* 2008;58:826–850.
42. Rosmarin DM, Lebwohl M, Elewski BE, et al. Cyclosporine and psoriasis: 2008 National psoriasis Foundation Consensus Conference. *J Am Acad Dermatol.* 2010;62:838–853.
43. Kalb RE, Strober B, Weinstein G, Lebwohl M. Methotrexate and psoriasis: 2009 National Psoriasis Foundation Consensus Conference. *J Am Acad Dermatol.* 2009;60:824–837.
44. Smith CH, Yiu ZZN, Bale T, et al. British Association of Dermatologists guidelines for biologic therapy for psoriasis 2020: A rapid update. *Br J Dermatol.* 2020;183(3):628–637. 10.1111/bjd.19039.
45. Menter A, Strober BE, Kaplan DH, et al. Joint AAD-NPF guidelines of care for the management and treatment of psoriasis with biologics. *J Am Acad Dermatol.* 2019;80(4):1029–1072.
46. Elmets CA, Leonardi CL, Davis DMR, et al. Joint AAD-NPF guidelines of care for the management and treatment of psoriasis with awareness and attention to comorbidities. *J Am Acad Dermatol.* 2019;80(4):1073–1113.
47. Paul C, Gallini A, Archier E, et al. Evidence-based recommendations on topical treatment and phototherapy of psoriasis: Systematic review and expert opinion of a panel of dermatologists. *J Eur Acad Dermatol Venereol.* 2012;26(suppl 3):1–10.
48. Long CC, Finlay AY. The finger-tip unit—A new practical measure. *Clin Exp Dermatol.* 1991;16:444–447.
49. Menter A, Korman NJ, Elmets CA, et al. Guidelines of care for the management of psoriasis and psoriatic arthritis. Section 6. Guidelines of care for the treatment of psoriasis and psoriatic arthritis: Case-based presentations and evidence-based conclusions. *J Am Acad Dermatol.* 2011;65:137–174.
50. Data from The National Psoriasis Foundation—Mild Psoriasis: Steroid potency chart. http://www.psoriasis.org/netcommunity/sublearn03_mild_potency.
51. Rosso JD, Friedlander SF Corticosteroids: Options in the era of steroid-sparing therapy. *J Am Acad Dermatol.* 2005;53:S50–S58.
52. Leung DYM, Nicklas RA, Li JT, et al. Disease management of atopic dermatitis: An updated practice parameter. *Ann Allergy Asthma Immunol.* 2004;93:S1–S17.
53. Jeon C, Sekhon S, Bhutani T, Koo J Topical Treatments. In: Bhutani T, Liao W, Nakamura M eds. *Evidence-Based Psoriasis, Diagnosis and Treatment.* Table 2.1 Switzerland: Springer International Publishing AG; 2018 (A textbook in the series Updates in Clinical Dermatology, with series editors Berth-Jones J, Gob CL, and Maibach HI, at http://www.springer.com/series/13203).
54. Bowie AC, Tadrous M, Egeberg A, et al. Agreement and correlation between different topical corticosteroid potency classification systems. *JAMA Dermatol.* 2022;158(7):796–800.
55. Katz HI, Hien NT, Prawer SE, et al. Superpotent topical steroid treatment of psoriasis vulgaris: Clinical efficacy and adrenal function. *J Am Acad Dermatol.* 1987;16(4):804–811.
56. Krueger GG, O'Reilly MA, Weidner M, et al. Comparative efficacy of once-daily flurandrenolide tape versus twice-daily diflorasone diacetate ointment in the treatment of psoriasis. *J Am Acad Dermatol.* 1998;38:186–190.
57. Mason J, Mason AR, Cork MJ. Topical preparations for the treatment of psoriasis: A systemic review. *Br J Dermatol.* 2002;146:351–364.
58. Castela E, Archier E, Devaux S, et al. Topical corticosteroids in plaque psoriasis: A systematic review of efficacy and treatment modalities. *J Euro Acad Dermatol Venereol.* 2012;26(suppl 3):36–46.
59. Katz HI, Prawer SE, Medansky RS, et al. Intermittent corticosteroid maintenance treatment of psoriasis: A double-blind multicenter trial of augmented betamethasone dipropionate ointment in a pulse dose treatment regimen. *Dermatol.* 1991;183:269–274.
60. Wall ARJ, Poyner TF, Menday AP. A comparison of treatment with dithranol and calcipotriol on the clinical severity and quality of life in patients with psoriasis. *Br J Dermatol.* 1998;139:1005–1011.
61. Cunliffe WJ, Berth-Jones J, Claudy A, et al. Comparative study of calcipotriol (MC 903) ointment and betamethasone 17-valerate ointment in patients with psoriasis vulgaris. *J Am Acad Dermatol.* 1992;26:736–743.
62. Kragballe K, Gjertsen BT, De Hoop D, et al. Double-blind, right/left comparison of calcipotriol and betamethasone valerate in treatment of psoriasis vulgaris. *Lancet.* 1991;337:193–196.
63. Devaux S, Castela A, Archier E, et al. Topical vitamin D analogues alone or in association with topical steroids for psoriasis: A systematic review. *J Euro Acad Dermatol Venereol.* 2012;26(suppl 3):52–60.
64. Weinstein GD, Krueger GG, Lowe NJ, et al. Tazarotene gel, a new retinoid, for topical therapy of psoriasis: Vehicle-controlled study of safety, efficacy, and duration of therapeutic effect. *J Am Acad Dermatol.* 1997;37:85–92.
65. Weinstein GD, Koo JY, Krueger GG, et al. Tazarotene cream in the treatment of psoriasis: Two multicenter, double-blind, randomized, vehicle-controlled studies of the safety and efficacy of tazarotene cream 0.05% and 0.1% applied once daily for 12 weeks. *J Am Acad Dermatol.* 2003;48:760–767.
66. McGill A, Frank A, Emmett N, et al. The anti-psoriatic drug anthralin accumulates in keratinocyte mitochondria, dissipates mitochondrial membrane potential, and induces apoptosis through a pathway dependent on respiratory competent mitochondria. *FASEB J.* 2005;19:1012–1014.
67. Thawornchaisit P, Harncharoen K. A comparative study of tar and betamethasone valerate in chronic plaque psoriasis: A study in Thailand. *J Med Assoc Thai.* 2007;90:1997–2002.
68. Alora-Palli MB, Perkins AC, Van Cott A, et al. Efficacy and tolerability of a cosmetically acceptable coal tar solution in the treatment of moderate plaque psoriasis: A controlled comparison with calcipotriene (calcipotriol) ream. *Am J Cli Dermatol.* 2010;11(4):275–283.
69. Cosmetic Ingredient Review Expert Panel. Final safety assessment of coal tar as used in cosmetics. *Int J Toxicol.* 2008;27(suppl 2):1–24.
70. Stuetz A, Grassberger M, Meingassner JG. Pimecrolimus (Elidel, SDZ ASM 981)—Preclinical pharmacologic profile and skin selectivity. *Semin Cutan Med Surg.* 2001;20:233–241.
71. Mrowietz U, Graeber M, Brautigam M, et al. The novel azomycin derivative SDZ ASM 981 is effective for psoriasis when used topically under occlusion. *Br J Dermatol.* 1998;139:992–996.
72. Gribetz C, Ling M, Lebwohl M, et al. Pimecrolimus cream 1% in the treatment of intertriginous psoriasis: A double-blind, randomized study. *J Am Acad Dermatol.* 2004;51:731–738.

73. Matz H. Phototherapy for psoriasis: What to choose and how to use: Facts and controversies. *Clin Dermatol.* 2010;28:73–80.
74. Archier E, Devaux S, Castela E, et al. Efficacy of Psoralen UV-A therapy vs. narrowband UV-B therapy in chronic plaque psoriasis: A systematic literature review. *J Euro Acad Dermatol Venereol.* 2012;26(suppl 3):11–21.
75. Stern RS. Genital tumors among men with psoriasis exposed to psoralens and ultraviolet A radiation (PUVA) and ultraviolet B radiation: The photochemotherapy follow-up study. *N Engl J Med.* 1990;322:1093–1097.
76. Anstey AV, Kragballe K. Retrospective assessment of PASI 50 and PASI 75 attainment with a calcipotriol/betamethasone dipropionate ointment. *Int J Dermatol.* 2006;45:970–975.
77. Mahrie G, Schulze HJ, Farber L, et al. Low-dose short-term cyclosporine versus etretinate in psoriasis: Improvement of skin, nail, and joint involvement. *J Am Acad Dermatol.* 1995;32:78–88.
78. Heydendael VM, Spuls POL, Opmeer BC, et al. Methotrexate versus cyclosporine in moderate-to-severe chronic plaque psoriasis. *N Engl J Med.* 2003;349:658–665.
79. Shupack J, Abel E, Bauer E, et al. Cyclosporine as maintenance therapy in patients with severe psoriasis. *J Am Acad Dermatol.* 1997;36:423–432.
80. Robert N, Wong GWK, Wright JM. Effect of cyclosporine on blood pressure. *Cochrane Database Syst Rev.* 2010;(1):CD007893.
81. Saurat JH, Stingl G, Dubertret L, et al. Efficacy and safety results from the randomized controlled comparative study of adalimumab vs. methotrexate vs. placebo in patients with psoriasis (CHAMPION). *Br J Dermatol.* 2008;158:558–566.
82. Salim A, Tan E, Ilchyshyn A, et al. Folic acid supplementation during treatment of psoriasis with methotrexate: A randomized, double-blind, placebo-controlled trial. *Br J Dermatol.* 2006;154:1169–1174.
83. Maybury CM, Samarasekera E, Douiri A, et al. Diagnostic accuracy of noninvasive markers of liver fibrosis in patients with psoriasis taking methotrexate: A systematic review and meta-analysis. *Br J Dermatol.* 2014;170(6):1237–1247. doi:10.1111/bjd.12905.
84. Tofacitinib (Xeljanz) product monograph. https://labeling.pfizer.com/ShowLabeling.aspx?id=959. Accessed Feb. 28, 2022.
85. Puig L, Gulliver W. eds. Volume 53: Adverse Reactions to Biologics. Part of the series Current Problems in Dermatology. Series editors Itin P, Jemec GBE. Karger AG, Basel (Switzerland), 2018. ISBN 978-3-318-06100-0.
86. Lansang P, Bergman JN, Fiorillo L, et al. Management of pediatric plaque psoriasis using biologics. *J Am Acad Dermatol.* 2020;82(1):213–221.
87. Gordon K, Papp K, Poulin Y, et al. Long-term efficacy and safety of adalimumab in patients with moderate to severe psoriasis treated continuously over 3 years: Results from an open-label extension study for patients from REVEAL. *J Am Acad Dermatol.* 2012;66:241–251.
88. Moustou A-E, Matekovits A, Dessinioti C, et al. Cutaneous side effects of anti-tumor necrosis factor biologic therapy: A clinical review. *J Am Acad Dermatol.* 2009;61:486–504.
89. Lockwood SJ, Prens LM, Kimball AB. Adverse reactions to biologics in psoriasis. In: Puig L, Gulliver W. eds. *Adverse Reactions to Biologics.* Part of the series Current Problems in Dermatology. Series editors Itin P, Jemec GBE. Karger AG, Basel (Switzerland), 2018. Vol 53:1-14. ISBN 978-3-318-06100-0.
90. Adalimumab (Humura) product monograph Date of Revision: Apr. 21, 2021. http://www.abbvie.ca/content/dam/abbviecorp/ca/en/docs/HUMIRA_PM_EN.pdf. Accessed Feb. 28, 2022.
91. Gordon KB, Langley RG, Leonard C, et al. Clinical response to adalimumab treatment in patients with moderate to severe psoriasis: Double-blind, randomized controlled trial and open-label extension study. *J Am Acad Dermatol.* 2006;55:598–606.
92. Menter A, Tyring SK, Gordon K, et al. Adalimumab therapy for moderate to severe psoriasis: A randomized, controlled phase III trial. *J Am Acad Dermatol.* 2008;58:106–115.
93. Leonardi CL, Powers JL, Matheson RT, et al. Etanercept as monotherapy in patients with psoriasis. *N Engl J Med.* 2003;349:2014–2022.
94. Paller AS, Siegfried EC, Langley RG, et al. Etanercept treatment for children and adolescents with plaque psoriasis. *N Engl J Med.* 2008;358:241–251.
95. Gottlieb AB, Kalb RE, Blauvelt A, et al. The efficacy and safety of infliximab in patients with plaque psoriasis who had an inadequate response to etanercept: Results of a prospective, multicenter, open-label study. *J Am Acad Dermatol.* 2011;67:642–650.
96. Menter A, Feldman SR, Weinstein GD, et al. A randomized comparison of continuous vs intermittent infliximab maintenance regimens over 1 year in the treatment of moderate-to-severe plaque psoriasis. *J Am Acad Dermatol.* 2007;56:e1–e15.
97. Reich K, Nestle FO, Papp K, et al. Infliximab induction and maintenance therapy for moderate-to-severe psoriasis: A phase III, multicenter, double-blind trial. *Lancet.* 2005;366:1367–1374.
98. Reich K, Ortonne JP, Gottlieb AB, et al. Successful treatment of moderate to severe plaque psoriasis with the PEGylated Fab' certolizumab pegol: Results of a phase II randomized, placebo-controlled trial with a re-treatment extension. *Br J Dermatol.* 2012;167(1):180–190.
99. Goffe B, Papp K, Gratton D, et al. An integrated analysis of thirteen trials summarizing the long-term safety of alefacept in psoriasis patients who have received up to nine courses of therapy. *Clin Ther.* 2005;27:1912–1921.
100. Shalom G, Cohen AD, Ziv M, et al. Biologic drug survival in Israeli psoriasis patients. *J Am Acad Dermatol.* 2017;76(4):662–666. e661.
101. Stelara (ustekinumab injection). Stelara (ustekinumab injection). Stelara (ustekinumab injection). Stelara (ustekinumab injection). https://www.janssenlabels.com/package-insert/product-monograph/prescribing-information/STELARA-pi.pdf. Accessed Feb. 28, 2022.
102. Leonardi C, Kimball AB, Papp K, et al. Efficacy and safety of ustekinumab, a human interleukin-12/23 monoclonal antibody, in patients with psoriasis: 76-Week results from a randomized, double-blind, placebo-controlled trial (PHOENIX 1). *Lancet.* 2008;371:1665–1674.
103. Papp KA, Langley RG, Lebwohl M, et al. Efficacy and safety of ustekinumab, a human interleukin-12/23 monoclonal antibody, in patients with psoriasis: 52-Week results from a randomized, double-blind, placebo-controlled trial (PHOENIX 2). *Lancet.* 2008;371:1675–1684.
104. Langley RG, Feldman SR, Han C, et al. Ustekinumab significantly improves symptoms of anxiety, depression, and skin-related quality of life in patients with moderate-to-severe psoriasis: Results from a randomized, double-blind, placebo-controlled phase III trial. *J Am Acad Dermatol.* 2010;63:457–465.
105. Sofen H, Wasel N, Yeilding N, et al. Ustekinumab improves overall skin response and health-related quality of life, in a subset of moderate to severe psoriasis patients with psoriatic arthritis: Analysis of PHOENIX 1 and 2. *J Am Acad Dermatol.* 2011 Feb;64(2 suppl 1):AB156.
106. Lebwohl M, Yeilding N, Szapary P, et al. Impact of weight on the efficacy and safety of ustekinumab in patients with moderate to severe psoriasis: Rationale for dosing recommendations. *J Am Acad Dermatol.* 2010;63:571–579.
107. Lebwohl M, Leonardi C, Griffiths CEM, et al. Long-term safety experience of ustekinumab in patients with moderate-to-severe psoriasis (part I of II): Results from analyses of general safety parameters from pooled phase 2 and 3 clinical trials. *J Am Acad Dermatol.* 2012;66:731–741.
108. Gordon KB, Papp KA, Langley RG, et al. Long-term safety experience of ustekinumab in patients with moderate to severe psoriasis (part II of II): Results from analyses of infections and malignancy from pooled phase II and III clinical trials. *J Am Acad Dermatol.* 2012;66:742–751.
109. Bissonnette R, Kerdel F, Naldi L, Papp K, et al. Evaluation of risk of major adverse cardiovascular events with biologic therapy in patients with psoriasis. *J Drugs Dermatol.* 2017;16(10):1002–1013.
110. Secukinumab (Cosentyx) product monograph. https://www.novartis.us/sites/www.novartis.us/files/cosentyx.pdf. Accessed Feb. 28, 2022.
111. Langley RG, Elewski BE, Lebwohl M, et al. Secukinumab in plaque psoriasis: Results of two Phase 3 trials. *N Engl J Med.* 2014;371(4):326–338. Available at: http://www.nejm.org/doi/pdf/10.1056/NEJMoa1314258.
112. Blauvelt A, Reich K, Tsai TF, et al. Secukinumab is superior to ustekinumab in clearing skin of subjects with moderate-to-severe plaque psoriasis up to 1 year: Results from the CLEAR study. *J Am Acad Dermatol.* 2017;76(1):60–69. e69.
113. Kircik L, Fowler J, Weiss J, et al. Efficacy of secukinumab for moderate-to-severe head and neck psoriasis over 52 weeks: Pooled analysis of four phase 3 studies. *Dermatol Ther (Heidelv).* 2016;6(4):627–738.
114. Polesie S, Lidjolm AG. Secukinumab in the treatment of generalized pustular psoriasis: A Case report. *Acta Derm Venereol.* 2017;97(1):124–125.
115. Weng HJ, Wang TS, Tsai TF. Clinical experience of secukinumab in the treatment of erythrodermic psoriasis: A case series. *Br J Dermatol.* 2018;178(6):1439–1440.
116. Mugheddu C, Atzori L, Lappi A, et al. Successful secukinumab treatment of generalized pustular psoriasis and erythrodermic psoriasis. *J Eur Acad Dermatol Venereol.* 2017;31(9):e420–e421.
117. Griffiths CE, Reich K, Lebwohl M, et al. Comparison of ixekizumab with etanercept or placebo in moderate-to-severe psoriasis (UNCOVER-2 and UNCOVER-3): Results from two phase 3 randomized trials. *Lancet.* 2015;386(9993):541–551.

118. Reich K, Pinter A, Lacour JP, et al. Comparison of ixekizumab with ustekinumab in moderate-to-severe psoriasis: 24-Week results from IXORA-S, a phase III study. *Br J Dermatol.* 2017;177(4):1014–1023.
119. Gaffen SL, Jain R, Garg AV, Cua DJ. IL-23-IL-17 immune axi: Discovery mechanistic understanding, and clinical testing. *Nat Rev Immunol.* 2014;14(9):585–600.
120. Reich K, Armstrong AW, Foley P, et al. Efficacy and safety of guselkumab, an anti-interleukin-23 monoclonal antibody, compared with adalimumab for the treatment of patients with moderate to severe psoriasis with randomized withdrawal and retreatment: Results from the phase III, double-blind, placebo- and active comparator-controlled VOYAGE 2 trial. *J Am Acad Dermatol.* 2017;76(3):418–431.
121. Reich K, Papp KA, Blauvelt A, et al. Tildrakizumab versus placebo or etanercept for chronic plaque psoriasis (reSURFACE 1 and reSURFACE 2): Results from two randomised controlled, phase 3 trials. *Lancet.* 2017;390(100091):276–288.
122. Gordon KB, Strober B, Lebwohl M, et al. Efficacy and safety of risankizumab in moderate-to-severe plaque psoriasis (UltiMMa-1 and UltiMMa-2): Results from two double-blind, randomized, placebo-controlled and ustekinumab-controlled phase 3 trials. *Lancet.* 2018 Aug 25;392(10148):650–661.
123. Al-Janabi A, Jabbar-Lopez ZK, Griffiths CEM, Yiu ZZN. Risankizumab vs. ustekinumab for plaque psoriasis: A critical appraisal. *Br J Dermatol.* 2019;180(6):1348–1351.
124. Koo JY, Lowe NJ, Lew-Kaya DA, et al. Tazarotene plus UVB phototherapy in the treatment of psoriasis. *J Am Acad Dermatol.* 2000;43:821–828.
125. Lowe NJ, Prystowsky JH, Bourget T, et al. Acitretin plus UVB therapy for psoriasis: Comparisons with placebo plus UVB and acitretin alone. *J Am Acad Dermatol.* 1991;24:591–594.
126. Spuls PI, Rozenblit M, Lebwohl M. Retrospective study of the efficacy of narrow band UVB and acitretin. *J Dermatol Treat.* 2003;14(suppl):17–20.
127. Tanew A, Guggenbichler A, Honigsmann H, et al. Photochemotherapy for severe psoriasis without or in combination with acitretin: A randomized, double-blind comparison study. *J Am Acad Dermatol.* 1991;25:682–684.
128. Kitzen JM, Pergolizzi JV, Taylor R, Raffa RB. Crisaborole and apremilast: PDE4 inhibitors with similar mechanism of action, different indications for management of inflammatory skin conditions. *Pharmacology & Pharmacy.* 2018;9:357–381.
129. Crowley J, Thaci D, Joly P, et al. Long-term safety and tolerability of apremilast in patients with psoriasis: Pooled safety analysis for ≥156 weeks from 2 Phase 3, randomized, controlled trials (ESTEEM 1 and 2). *J Am Acad Dermaol.* 2017;77:310–317.
130. Lexicomp 2022, Wolters Kluwer Clinical Drug Information, Inc. Lexi-Drugs: Apremilast.
131. Orvis AK, Wesson SK, Breza TS, et al. Mycophenolate mofetil in dermatology. *J Am Acad Dermatol.* 2009;60:183–199.
132. Davidson SC, Morris-Jones R, Powles AV, et al. Change of treatment from cyclosporin to mycophenolate mofetil in severe psoriasis. *Br J Dermatol.* 2000;143:405–407.
133. Pedraz J, Dauden E, Delgado-Jimenez Y, et al. Sequential study on the treatment of moderate-to-severe chronic plaque psoriasis with mycophenolate mofetil and cyclosporin. *J Eur Acad Dermatol Venereol.* 2006;20:702–706.
134. Patel RV, Clark LN, Lebwohl M, et al. Treatments for psoriasis and the risk of malignancy. *J Am Acad Dermatol.* 2009;60:1001–1017.
135. Ranjan N, Sharma NL, Shanker V, et al. Methotrexate versus hydroxycarbamide (hydroxyurea) as a weekly dose to treat moderate-to-severe chronic plaque psoriasis: A comparative study. *J Dermatol Treat.* 2007;18:295–300.
136. Smith N, Weymann A, Tausk FA, et al. Complementary and alternative medicine for psoriasis: A qualitative review of the clinical trial literature. *J Am Acad Dermatol.* 2009;61:841–856.
137. Bernstein S, Donsky H, Gulliver W, et al. Treatment of mild to moderate psoriasis with Relieva, a Mahonia aquifolium extract—A double-blind, placebo-controlled study. *Am J Ther.* 2006;13:121–126.
138. Danno K, Sugie N. Combination therapy with low-dose etretinate and eicosapentaenoic acid for psoriasis vulgaris. *J Dermatol.* 1998;25:703–705.
139. Brochow T, Schiener R, Franke A, et al. A pragmatic randomized controlled trial on the effectiveness of highly concentrated saline spa water baths followed by UVB compared to UVB only in moderate to severe psoriasis. *J Altern Complement Med.* 2007;13:725–732.
140. Brochow T, Schiener R, Franke A, et al. A pragmatic randomized controlled trial on the effectiveness of low concentrated saline spa water baths followed by ultraviolet B (UVB) compared to UVB only in moderate to severe psoriasis. *J Eur Acad Dermatol Venereol.* 2007;21:1027–1037.
141. Gaston L, Crombez J, Lassonde M, et al. Psychological stress and psoriasis: Experimental and prospective correlational studies. *Acta Derm Venereol.* 1991;156:37–43.
142. Kabat-Zinn J, Wheeler E, Light T, et al. Influence of a mindfulness meditation-based stress reduction intervention on rates of skin clearing in patients with moderate to severe psoriasis undergoing phototherapy (UVB) and photochemotherapy (PUVA). *Psychosom Med.* 1998;60:625–632.
143. Treloar V. Integrative dermatology for psoriasis: Facts and controversies. *Clin Dermatol.* 2010;28:93–99.
144. Naldi L, Chatenoud L, Linder D, et al. Cigarette smoking, body mass index, and stressful life events as risk factors for psoriasis: Results from an Italian case-control study. *J Invest Dermatol.* 2005;125:61–67.
145. Horn EJ, Fox KM, Patel V, et al. Are patients with psoriasis undertreated? Results of National Psoriasis Foundation survey. *J Am Acad Dermatol.* 2007;57:957–962.
146. Augustin M, Alvaro-Gracia JM, Bagot M, et al. A framework for improving the quality of care for people with psoriasis. *J Euro Acad Dermatol Venereol.* 2012;26(suppl 4):1–16.
147. Menter A, Cordoro KM, Davis DMR, et al. Joint American Academy of Dermatology-National Psoriasis Foundation guidelines of care for the management and treatment of psoriasis in pediatric patients. *J Am Acad Dermatol.* 2020;82(1):161–201.
148. Benoit S, Hamm H. Childhood psoriasis. *Clin Dermatol.* 2007;25:555–562.
149. Paller AS, Mercy K, Kwasny MJ, et al. Association of pediatric psoriasis severity with excess and central adiposity: An international cross-sectional study. *JAMA Dermatol.* 2013;149(2):166–176.
150. Bryld LE, Sorensen TI, Andersen KK, et al. High body mass index in adolescent girls precedes psoriasis hospitalization. *Acta Derm Venereol.* 2010;90(5):488–493.
151. De Jager MEA, de Jong EMG, van de Kerkhof PCM, et al. Efficacy and safety of treatments for childhood psoriasis: A systematic literature review. *J Am Acad Dermatol.* 2010;62:1013–1030.
152. Paller AS, Siegfried EC, Langley RG, et al. Etanercept treatment for children and adolescents with plaque psoriasis. *N Engl J Med.* 2008;358:241–251.
153. Murase JE, Chan KK, Garite TJ, et al. Hormonal effect on psoriasis in pregnancy and postpartum. *Arch Dermatol.* 2005;141:601–606.
154. Lam J, Polifka JE, Dohil MA. Safety of dermatologic drugs used in pregnant patients with psoriasis and other inflammatory skin diseases. *J Am Acad Dermatol.* 2008;59:295–315.
155. Menter A, Gordon KB, Leonardi CL, et al. Efficacy and safety of adalimumab across subgroups of patients with moderate to severe psoriasis. *J Am Acad Dermatol.* 2010;63:448–456.
156. Papp KA, Strober B, Augustin M, et al. PSOLAR: Design, utility, and preliminary results of a prospective, international disease-based registry of patients with psoriasis who are receiving, or are candidates for, conventional systemic treatments or biologic agents. *J Drugs Dermatol.* 2012;11:1210–1217.
157. Islandar IY, Ashcroft DM, Warren RB, et al. Patterns of biologic therapy use in the management of psoriasis: Cohort study from the British Association of Dermatologists Biologic Interventions Register (BADBIR). *Br J Dermatol.* 2017;176:1297–1307.
158. Augustin M, Spehr C, Radtke MA, et al. German psoriasis registry PsoBest: Objectives, methodology and baseline data. *J Ktsch Dermatol Ges.* 2014;12:48–57.
159. Reich K, Mrowietz U, Radtke MA, et al. Drug safety of systemic treatments for psoriasis: Results from the German Psoriasis Registry PsoBest. *Arch Dermatol Res.* 2015;307:875–883.
160. Piaserico S, Gisondi P, Cazzaniga S, et al. Lack of evidence for an increased risk of severe COVID-19 in psoriasis patients on biologics: A cohort study from Northeast Italy. *Am J Clin Dermatol.* 2020;21:749–751.
161. Poulin Y, Langley R, Teiseira HD, et al. Biologics in the treatment of psoriasis: Clinical and economic overview. *J Cutan Med Surg.* 2009;13(suppl 2):S49–S57.
162. Blauvelt A, Burge R, Malatestinic W, et al. Cost per cumulative clinical benefit of biologic therapies for patients with plaque psoriasis: A systematic review. J Managed Care Specialty Pharmacy 2021;27:84–94. 10.18553/jmcp.2021.27.1.084.

119

Atopic Dermatitis

Rebecca M. Law and Wayne P. Gulliver

KEY CONCEPTS

1. Atopic dermatitis is a chronic skin disorder involving inflammation associated with intense pruritus (itching), a hallmark symptom. Management of atopic dermatitis must always include appropriate management of the associated pruritus.
2. Atopic dermatitis is associated with other atopic diseases such as asthma and allergic rhinitis in the same patient or family. The three conditions are known as the *atopic triad*.
3. The prevalence of atopic dermatitis has increased two- to threefold in many developed and developing countries during the past three decades. Age and country or regional differences, with some countries, show no change or even a decrease. Rural areas have lower prevalence rates.
4. There are genetic and environmental factors in the pathogenesis and pathophysiologic manifestations of atopic dermatitis. The inheritance pattern is not straightforward. More than one gene may be involved in the disease, with the filaggrin gene (*FLG*) being a key player. Other genes coding for specific cytokines are also involved.
5. Atopic dermatitis usually presents in infants and young children. The clinical presentation differs somewhat depending on the age of the patient.
6. Disease severity can be determined by using SCORAD (Severity Scoring of Atopic Dermatitis). This composite index assesses both signs and symptoms to classify overall disease severity as mild, moderate, or severe, which is useful in determining appropriate treatment approach.
7. Secondary bacterial skin infections are common in patients with atopic dermatitis and must be promptly treated.
8. Management of atopic dermatitis must always include appropriate nonpharmacologic management of any controllable environmental factors, such as avoidance of identified triggers. These may include aeroallergens (eg, mold, grass, pollen), foods (eg, peanuts, eggs, tomatoes), chemicals (eg, detergents, soaps), clothing material (eg, wool, polyester), temperature (eg, excessive heat), and humidity (eg, low humidity).
9. Nonpharmacologic management of atopic dermatitis entails managing the symptoms associated with pruritus and encouraging appropriate skin care habits such as proper bathing techniques and the copious use of moisturizers, which is a standard of care.
10. Topical corticosteroids (TCS) are the drugs of first choice for atopic dermatitis.
11. Topical calcineurin inhibitors (TCI), that is, tacrolimus and pimecrolimus, are alternate treatment options for adults and children over the age of 2 years.
12. Phototherapy is a second-line treatment when TCS and TCI fail.
13. Biologic agents and JAK inhibitors may be an option for severe atopic dermatitis in adults and adolescents (not approved in children).
14. This chronic illness has substantial socioeconomic impact. The burden of disease is significant, and the societal cost is magnified by undertreatment.

BEYOND THE BOOK

Some of the treatment modalities for atopic dermatitis are also used in psoriasis. Review the discussion about topical corticosteroids (including the corticosteroid potency chart) in Chapter 118, "Psoriasis," in this textbook.

INTRODUCTION

1 Atopic dermatitis (AD) is a chronic, pruritic inflammatory skin disease. It is often referred to as *eczema*, which is a general term for several types of skin inflammation. AD is the most common type of eczema (Table 119-1).[1] Pruritus is the hallmark symptom and presentation and is responsible for much of the disease burden borne by patients and their families.[2]

2 This form of dermatitis is commonly associated with a personal or family history of other atopic disorders, such as allergic rhinitis and asthma[2] (collectively known as the *atopic triad*). AD has been considered the start of the "atopic march"[2]; however, the association with other atopic conditions is multifactorial and complex since this progression does not happen in all cases.[2] The disease can have periods of exacerbation, or flare-ups, followed by periods of remission. These flare-ups may be disruptive to the patient's quality of life and may affect the entire family. Disease flare-ups may be difficult to manage and may be complicated by secondary infections. About one-half (estimate up to 65%) of cases in children first manifest before the age of 1 year[1-4]; these cases are termed *early onset atopic dermatitis*.[3,5] Onset of AD is most common between 3 and 6 months of age.[2] Approximately 85% to 90% of patients develop symptoms before the age of 5 years.[2]

About 10% to 30% of children with AD will have the same skin condition continuing into their adulthood.[2] Early and severe onset,

TABLE 119-1 Types of Eczema (Dermatitis)

- **Allergic contact eczema (dermatitis):** A red, itchy, weepy reaction where the skin has come into contact with a substance that the immune system recognizes as foreign, such as poison ivy or certain preservatives in creams and lotions.
- **Atopic dermatitis:** A chronic skin disease characterized by itchy, inflamed skin.
- **Contact eczema (dermatitis):** A localized reaction that includes redness, itching, and burning where the skin has come into contact with an allergen (an allergy-causing substance) or with an irritant such as an acid, cleaning agent, or other chemical.
- **Dyshidrotic eczema:** Irritation of the skin on the palms of hands and soles of the feet characterized by clear, deep blisters that itch and burn.
- **Neurodermatitis:** Scaly patches of the skin on the head, lower legs, wrists, or forearms caused by a localized itch (such as an insect bite) that become intensely irritated when scratched.
- **Nummular eczema:** Coin-shaped patches of irritated skin—most common on the arms, back, buttocks, and lower legs—that may be crusted, scaling, and extremely itchy.
- **Seborrheic eczema:** Yellowish, oily, scaly patches of skin on the scalp, face, and occasionally other parts of the body.
- **Stasis dermatitis:** A skin irritation on the lower legs, generally related to circulatory problems.

Data from Reference 1.

family history of AD, and early allergen sensitizations are risk factors for a prolonged course.[3] Furthermore, patients who have apparently outgrown their disease may continue to have sensitive hyperreactive skin and might have recurrences after long symptom-free periods.[3] However, onset after the age of 30 years is much less common and is often caused by exposure to harsh or wet conditions[1] such as repeated skin trauma or exposure to harsh chemicals.

EPIDEMIOLOGY

3 The prevalence of AD is generally said to have increased two- to threefold in developed and developing countries during the past three decades.[5] In developed countries, an estimated 15% to 30% of children and 2% to 10% of adults are affected.[3,5,6] The prevalence has increased worldwide, as earlier prevalence rates were estimated at 10% to 15% in children.[4] In developed countries, the lifetime prevalence seems to have plateaued at 10% to 20%, whereas in many developing countries, the lifetime prevalence may be lower but continues to increase.[3]

3 The largest international study of the prevalence of AD found both age and country differences in prevalence rates.[7] This was the International Study of Asthma and Allergies in Childhood (ISAAC), which was conducted in three phases.[8] The strength of this study was the use of a uniformly validated methodology that allowed a direct comparison of results from pediatric populations worldwide.[9] ISAAC Phase One included 700,000 children from 156 centers in 56 countries between 1992 and 1998. ISAAC Phase Two studied allergic causes from 30 centers in 22 countries. ISAAC Phase Three repeated a multicountry cross-sectional survey (1999–2004) and included 187,943 children aged 6 to 7 years from 64 centers in 35 countries and 302,159 adolescents aged 13 to 14 years from 105 centers in 55 countries. For children aged 6 to 7 years, most countries showed an increase of two standard deviations (SDs) in mean annual prevalence over a 5- to 10-year period. In contrast, for adolescents aged 13 to 14 years, the trends differ from country to country. Large increases in prevalence were seen in developing countries (eg, Mexico, Chile, Kenya, and Algeria, and seven countries in Southeast Asia). But in other countries with formerly high prevalences, the mean annual prevalence in eczema symptoms has either leveled off or decreased. Most of the largest decreases (SD ≥2) in prevalence were reported from developed countries in northwest Europe (eg, the United Kingdom, Ireland, Sweden, Germany) and New Zealand.[7] The ISAAC study has suggested that a maximum prevalence plateau of approximately 20% has emerged.[7,8]

There were no differences according to the sex of the study participant, or with gross national income at a country level.[7] This is consistent with other reports that AD affects males and females at approximately the same rate.[1] There is a lower prevalence of AD in rural areas when compared with urban areas,[2] suggesting a link to the *hygiene hypothesis*,[10,11] which postulates that the absence of early childhood exposure to infectious agents increases susceptibility to allergic diseases.[10-12] In contrast, children attending daycare centers before 3 months of age have less atopy and asthma in later childhood,[11,12] and areas with diffuse and chronic helminth infestations have a low prevalence of allergic diseases.[12] In addition, a European birth cohort study involving 1,133 newborns showed that children born to farm families had a lower prevalence of sensitization to seasonal inhaled allergens such as grass pollen.[11,13] Maternal exposure during pregnancy (ie, prenatal exposure) to animal sheds correlated with the lower prevalence rate in the farm children. However, there were no differences in prevalence related to inhaled perennial allergens. Parasitic infections decreased the risk of allergen sensitization.[11] A systematic review reported that exposures to endotoxin, farm animals, and dogs may protect against AD.[14]

Reported risk factors associated with higher prevalence include urban environment, higher socioeconomic status, higher level of family education, a family history of AD, female gender (after age 6 years), and smaller family size.[8] However, more recent studies are conflicting. There are no consistent findings that higher socioeconomic status or male/female gender affect the risk of AD.[2] Urban living does increase the risk of AD, but studies attempting to identify causative environmental agents have been inconclusive.[2] Strongly associated risk factors include a family history of AD, and functional mutations in the *FLG* gene.[2]

ETIOLOGY

4 AD is a complex genetic disease that arises from gene-gene and gene-environment interactions. There are two major groups of genes involved. First, there are the genes encoding for epidermal or other epithelial structural proteins. Second, there are genes encoding for the major elements of the immune system.[5] However, the diagnosis of AD remains clinical, as there is no reliable biomarker to distinguish AD from other inflammatory conditions.[15]

The inheritance pattern is not straightforward. More than one gene is likely involved in the disease. There is an increased risk for a child to have AD if there is a family history of other atopic diseases, such as hay fever or asthma. The risk of AD is two- to threefold higher in children with one atopic parent and three- to fivefold higher if both parents are atopic.[2] Studies of identical twins show that a person whose identical twin has AD is seven times more likely to have AD than someone in the general population.[1] And a person whose fraternal twin has AD is three times more likely to have AD than someone in the general population.[1] Another estimate is 80% concordance in monozygous twins and 20% in heterozygous twins.[10]

Thus, genetic predispositions to developing AD exist. There is a genetic predisposition in patients with atopy to demonstrate T-helper (Th_2) predominance—hence increased Th_2 cell activity.[3] At least 32 susceptibility loci have been identified through gene-mapping studies, but they explain less than 20% of the estimated heritability.[3] The strongest known genetic risk factor for AD is null mutations in filaggrin (FLG).[3] The filaggrin gene (*FLG*) on chromosome 1q21.3 encodes for a key structural protein in epidermal differentiation.[3] FLG mutations also cause the semidominant skin-scaling disorder ichthyosis vulgaris, characterized by abnormal skin dryness and palmer hyperlinearity, which are features often found in

AD.[3] More specifically, there are several possible genes on the chromosomes 3q21, 1q21, 16q, 17q25, 20p, and 3p26. Of these chromosomes, 1q21 has the highest linkage region. This region has a family of epithelium-related genes called the epidermal differentiation complex.[5] One of these genes is the *FLG*, on chromosome 1q21.3, which encodes for profilaggrin that degrades to filaggrin proteins.[2] Filaggrin proteins play key roles in epidermal differentiation, including terminal differentiation of the epidermis and formation of the skin barrier (including the stratum corneum).[2,16] Filaggrin breakdown products are natural moisturizers and contribute to epidermal hydration and barrier function.[2] Mutations or deficiency of *FLG* result in an abnormality in permeability barrier function.[16] Patients with AD who carry FLG mutations have more persistent disease, a higher incidence of skin infections with herpes virus (eczema herpeticum) and a greater risk for multiple allergies.[16] However, FLG mutation is neither necessary nor sufficient to cause AD. Up to 60% of carriers will not develop AD, and many patients with AD do not carry an FLG mutation.[3]

Epidermal barrier dysfunction is a prerequisite for the penetration of high-molecular-weight allergens in pollens, house dust mite products, microbes, and food.[5] In mice studies, this barrier abnormality lowers irritability thresholds, and enhanced cutaneous allergen penetration.[16] In humans, two common FLG variants (*R501X* and *2282del4*) with an estimated combined allele frequency of about 6% have been identified in individuals of European descent.[17] Eighteen other less common variants have also been identified in Europeans, with an additional 17 mutations restricted to individuals of Asian descent.[17] Each of these variants leads to nonsense mutations that either prevent or severely diminish the production of filaggrin in the epidermis.[17] Mutations of FLG occur mainly in patients with early onset AD and may be associated with the development of asthma in patients with AD.[5,17] However, FLG mutations are identified in only 30% of European patients with AD, implying that other genetic mutations affecting other epidermal structures may be important (eg, changes in the cornified envelope proteins involucrin and loricrin, or lipid composition).[5]

4 There are other genes encoding for the immune system that may be associated with AD, especially those on chromosome 5q31-33.[5] These genes code for cytokines that regulate IgE synthesis. Cytokines are produced by helper T cells (TH_0, TH_1, TH_2, TH_3).[11] T-helper type 1 (TH_1) cells produce cytokines that suppress immunoglobulin E (IgE) production (eg, interferon-γ and interleukin-12 [IL-12]).[5] T-helper type 2 (TH_2) cells produce cytokines that increase IgE production (eg, IL-5 and IL-13).[5,18] In patients with AD, there is an imbalance between TH_1 and TH_2 immune responses. These patients are genetically predisposed to TH_2 predominance, seen as increased TH_2 cell activity.[2,5,9,18] Increased TH_2 activity causes the release of IL-3, IL-4, IL-5, IL-10, and IL-13, resulting in blood eosinophilia, increased total serum IgE, and increased growth and development of mast cells.[2,5,11,18] This is seen in the initial and acute phase of AD.[9] In addition, these cytokines affect the maturation of B cells and cause a genomic rearrangement in these cells that favors isotype class switching from immunoglobulin M (IgM) to IgE.[5] As discussed below, epidermal Langerhans cells (LCs) and dendritic cells (DCs) with high-affinity IgE receptors uptake allergens and mediate the inflammatory response.[11]

In summary, FLG deficiency alone can provoke a barrier abnormality in the epidermis and predispose to the development of AD by enhancing allergen absorption through the skin.[19] Furthermore, there is complex relationships, including genetic and nongenetic risk factors, that modify an individual's susceptibility to allergic disease.[20] Complex genetic factors contribute to the increased susceptibility to AD (FLG mutations and gene-gene interactions). These, along with environmental factors such as food allergens[21] (gene-environment interactions), result in the pathophysiologic changes and clinical presentations associated with AD.

PATHOPHYSIOLOGY

4 The initial mechanisms that trigger inflammatory changes in the skin in patients with AD are unknown. Neuropeptides, irritation, or pruritus-induced scratching may be causing the release of proinflammatory cytokines from keratinocytes. Alternatively, allergens in the epidermal barrier or in food[21] may cause T-cell mediated but IgE-independent reactions. Allergen-specific IgE is not a prerequisite.[5] Characteristic features in pathophysiology are skin barrier dysfunction and immune deviation toward TH_2 with subsequent increased IgE.[10] The disease is further complicated by microbial colonization with pathologic organisms resulting in increased susceptibility for skin infections.[10]

As discussed above, skin barrier dysfunction plays a critical role in the development of AD,[10,11,16,22] with loss of function mutations in *filaggrin* being a major risk factor.[16,22] Other factors may include a deficiency of skin barrier proteins, increased peptidase activity, lack of certain protease inhibitors, and lipid abnormalities.[22] There must be epidermal barrier dysfunction for high-molecular-weight allergens in pollens, house dust mite particles, microbes, and foods to penetrate the skin barrier. Atopic skin has reduced antimicrobial peptides (AMPs). AMPs are normally produced by keratinocytes, sebocytes, and mast cells, and they form a chemical shield on the surface of the skin. Reduced AMPs result in a diminished antimicrobial barrier, which correlates with increased susceptibility to infections and superinfections seen in these patients.[23]

Upon penetration of the epidermal barrier, allergens are met by DCs. DCs are antigen-presenting cells populating the skin, respiratory tract, and mucosa of the GI tract (ie, at the front line of pathogen entry).[24] DCs then enhance TH_2 polarization, resulting in increased production of IgE. Keratinocytes in the skin of patients with AD also produce high levels of an IL-7–like protein, which again drives DCs to enhance TH_2 polarization. Epidermal DCs in patients with AD bear IgE and express its high-affinity receptor (FcεRI).[25-27] Total serum IgE is often elevated in patients with AD,[1,2] especially during an exacerbation.

However, on initial presentation, patients with early onset AD generally do not have increased total serum IgE levels (ie, there is no detectable IgE-mediated allergic sensitization). IgE-mediated allergic sensitization may occur several weeks or months after the initial AD lesions, although in some children—mostly girls—this sensitization never occurs.[5] Furthermore, elevated total serum IgE is not specific to AD and can be associated even with nonatopic conditions.[2]

Other potential biomarkers discovered include serum CD30, macrophage-derived chemoattractant (MDC), interleukins (IL)-12, -16, -18, and -31, and thymus and activation-regulated chemokine (TARC); however, to date none of them have shown reliable sensitivity nor specificity for clinical use.[2]

Predisposing Factors

4 Several factors can predispose patients to development of AD. These include climate, infection, genetics, environmental aeroallergens, urban versus rural living, breastfeeding and time of weaning, obesity, pollution/tobacco smoke, and food/diet. A Western diet with high amounts of sugar and polyunsaturated fatty acids, a small family size, a high education level in the household, living in urban settings, and living in regions with low exposure to UV radiation and low humidity are all factors that may increase the risk of AD.[3]

Hot and extremely cold climates are both poorly tolerated by patients with AD. Dry weather, common in the winter, causes increased skin dryness. Hot weather causes increased sweating, resulting in pruritus.

Patients with AD are commonly colonized by *Staphylococcus aureus* bacteria. Clinical infections with *S. aureus* frequently cause flare-ups of AD.

As discussed previously, genetics plays a role in AD. Family history of AD is a strong risk factor.

4 Exposure to environmental aeroallergens is another risk factor. Dust mites, pollens, molds, cigarette smoke, and dander from animal hair or skin may worsen the symptoms of AD.[13]

The role of food as antigens in the pathogenesis of AD is still not fully understood.[3,21] Preliminary results (mostly animal studies) indicate that defects in the skin and gut barrier function may facilitate sensitization to food allergens.[21] Small amounts of environmental foods (low-dose exposure from foods on tabletops, hands, dust) may penetrate the skin barrier and be taken up by LCs, leading to TH_2 responses and IgE production.[28] However, early high-dose oral food consumption induces oral tolerance. The timing and balance of cutaneous and oral exposure determines whether a child will have allergy or tolerance.[28] Increased serum IgE antibodies to a particular food is evidence of sensitization to a food and is consistent with—although not proof of—a food allergy.[1,29] Eczema may frequently be a manifestation of food allergy,[28] and patients with AD have a higher prevalence of food allergy than those in the general population.[1] Conversely, there is a belief that food allergy may be caused by AD, and in most patients with coexisting AD and food allergy, AD precedes the food allergy. (The assumption is that AD is a causal risk factor for asthma and systemic allergen sensitization in the context of FLG mutations.[16]) Regardless, the two conditions coexist, and the likelihood of an infant or child with AD also having food allergy or other allergies must be kept in mind.[29]

There is a known epidermal barrier dysfunction in AD, allowing for increased low-level skin permeability to allergenic foods. Certain foods may trigger acute reactions including urticaria and anaphylaxis. The most commonly reported allergenic foods are hen's eggs, cow's milk, peanuts, wheat, soy, tree nuts, shellfish, and fish.[1,30] Individual food allergies, such as peanut allergy, have increased in prevalence in the past decade[28,29]; new food allergies may also be increasing in prevalence, particularly kiwi allergy[28,31] and sesame seed allergy.[28,32] Allergies to seafood, peanuts, and tree nuts are more likely to persist into adulthood, while allergies to cow's milk, hen's eggs, wheat, and soy generally resolve by late-childhood.[21] Consistent with the oral tolerance concept, early results from recent studies using sublingual and oral immunotherapy to specific food allergens (eg, cow's milk or peanut) indicate that it may be possible to induce oral tolerance, and that it may be possible to desensitize children to some allergenic foods.[33] Nine to 12 months of immunotherapy were needed to observe the beneficial effect and "the present evidence does not warrant routine recommendation" by the AAD.[34] Injectable allergen-specific immunotherapy is also being studied.[34] National Institute of Allergy and Infectious Diseases (NIAID) suggests limited food allergy testing (ie, cow's milk, eggs, wheat, soy, peanut) if a child <5 years old has moderate-to-severe AD and persistent disease despite optimal therapy.[29,34] For more information about management of food allergies the reader is directed to the 2010 NIAID-sponsored expert panel's report, available at www.niaid.nih.gov.[29]

CLINICAL PRESENTATION

Diagnosis of AD is generally based on clinical presentation (Table 119-2).[1] There is no objective diagnostic test or reliable biomarker for the clinical confirmation of AD.[1-3] On occasion, skin biopsy specimens or other tests (eg, total and/or allergen-specific serum IgE, potassium hydroxide preparation, patch testing, and/or genetic testing) may be used to rule out other or associated skin conditions.[2] *Filaggrin* gene mutations may be associated with persistent and more severe AD as well as early onset cases.[22]

Atopic dermatitis follows a relapsing course.[34,35] Studies reviewing the natural course of the disease usually describe the disease pattern as persistent, intermittent, or in remission.[8] A 2004 study found that 43% were in complete remission after the age of 2 years, with 19% having persistent disease and 38% an intermittent pattern.[8]

TABLE 119-2 Skin Features Associated with Atopic Dermatitis

- **Atopic pleat (Dennie–Morgan fold):** An extra fold of skin that develops under the eye.
- **Headlight sign:** Sparing of the skin on top of the nose.
- **Herthoge's sign:** Thinning or absence of the lateral portions of the eyebrows.
- **Cheilitis:** Inflammation of the skin on and around the lips.
- **Hyperlinear palms:** Increased number of skin creases on the palms.
- **Hyperpigmented eyelids:** Eyelids that have become darker in color from inflammation or hay fever.
- **Ichthyosis:** Dry, rectangular scales on the skin.
- **Keratosis pilaris:** Small, rough bumps, generally on the face, upper arms, and thighs.
- **Lichenification:** Thick, leathery skin resulting from constant scratching and rubbing.
- **Papules:** Small raised bumps that may open when scratched and become crusty and infected.
- **Urticaria:** Hives (red, raised bumps) that may occur after exposure to an allergen, at the beginning of flares, or after exercise or a hot bath.

5 The clinical presentation of AD differs depending on the age of the patient. In infancy, the earliest onset of AD usually occurs between 3 and 6 months of age, with 60% of patients developing symptoms within the first year of life, and 85% to 90% having developed symptoms before the age of 5 years.[1,2] The initial presentation in infancy is an erythematous, papular skin eruption that may first appear on the cheeks and chin as a patchy facial eruption which may progress to red, scaling, oozing skin.[1] The eruption shows a centrifugal distribution affecting the malar region of the cheeks, forehead, scalp, chin, and behind the ears while sparing the central areas (ie, the nose and paranasal creases). Sparing of the skin on top of the nose is a characteristic feature (known as the "headlight sign"), and there is thinning or absence of the lateral portions of the eyebrows (known as the Herthoge's sign).[3] Lesions occur in the flexor surfaces, such as antecubital and popliteal fossae. Over the next few weeks and as the infant becomes more mobile and begins crawling, the lesions spread to the extensors of the lower legs, and eventually the entire body may be involved, with sparing of the groin, axillary region, and the nose.[1,2,35] These lesions are associated with uncontrollable itchiness, and the infant will become irritable and may try to rub his or her face to relieve the itch. Scratching may occur quite early, and infants with AD may scratch themselves continuously, even during sleep.[2] Sleep disruption occurs in up to 60% of children with AD, increasing to 80% or more during exacerbations.[2] Excessive rubbing or scratching may result in excoriation and predispose the patient to secondary infections.

In childhood, the skin is often dry, flaky, rough, cracked, and may bleed because of scratching. With repeated scratching and rubbing, the skin becomes lichenified. Lichenification, usually localized to the flexural folds of the extremities, is characteristic of childhood AD in older children and in adults.[35] Lichenification signifies repeated rubbing of the skin and is seen mostly over the folds, bony protuberances, and forehead.[35] Excoriations and crusting are also commonly seen, along with secondary infections. Sometimes increased folds are seen underneath the eyes (so-called Dennie–Morgan folds).[35] Lesions are still most commonly seen in the flexor surfaces of the body, particularly the flexural creases of the antecubital and popliteal fossae.[35]

Sleep disturbances also occur. One study reported that there are both brief and longer awakenings associated with scratching episodes that affect sleep efficiency in school-age children with AD.[36]

In adulthood, lesions are more diffuse with underlying erythema. The face is commonly involved and may be dry and scaly. Lichenification may again be seen. A brown macular ring around

TABLE 119-3 Clinical Features in the Diagnosis of Atopic Dermatitis

Essential Features (Must Be Present):

- Pruritus
- Eczema (acute, subacute, chronic)
  - Typical morphology and age-specific patterns
    Facial, neck, external involvement (infants, children)
    Flexural lesions (any age group)
    Sparing of groin and axillary regions
  - Chronic or relapsing history

Important Features (Seen in Most Cases, Supports the Diagnosis of AD):

- Early age of onset
- Atopy
  - Personal/family history
  - IgE reactivity
- Xerosis

Data from Reference 2.

TABLE 119-4 Major and Minor Signs and Symptoms of Atopic Dermatitis

Major Indicators

- Pruritus (intense itching)
- Characteristic rash in locations typical of the disease
- Chronic or repeatedly occurring symptoms
- Personal or family history of atopic disorders (eczema, hay fever, asthma)

Selected Minor Indicators

- Early age of onset
- Dry skin that may also have patchy scales or rough bumps
- Increased serum IgE
- Numerous skin creases on the palms
- Hand or foot involvement
- Inflammation around the lips
- Nipple eczema
- Susceptibility to skin infection
- Positive allergy skin tests

Data from Reference 1.

the neck, representing a localized deposit of amyloid, is typical but not always present.[35]

In people of color, skin lesions may present in a different manner, often with a perifollicular distribution.

Although no objective diagnostic test confirms the presence of AD,[1,2] some signs, symptoms, and other factors are commonly used in its diagnosis. These include pruritus, early age of onset, eczematous skin lesions that vary with age, chronic and relapsing courses, dry and flaky skin, IgE reactivity, family or personal history of asthma or hay fever, or other atopic diseases (Tables 119-3 and 119-4).[2,35] Allergy skin testing has little utility in AD, although negative results may help rule out certain substances as triggers; however, positive results may be unrelated to disease activity, and false positives are common.[1]

1 Pruritus is a quintessential feature of AD, and a diagnosis cannot be made if there is no history of itching.[1-4,35] Scratching and rubbing itchy atopic skin further irritates the skin, increases inflammation, and exacerbates itchiness.[3] Atopic skin can itch during sleep. This nighttime itching is a problem for many infants and children with the disease, since there is no conscious control of scratching during sleep.[1,2] Pruritus is the symptom that most affects the health-related quality of life for most patients with AD. In studies, more than 50% of patients rated their pruritus as bothersome or extremely bothersome and reported that they often or always experienced intolerable symptoms.[35]

Pruritus can be triggered by a variety of factors. The most common triggers of itch have been reported as heat and perspiration (96%), wool (91%), emotional stress (81%), certain (usually vasodilatory) foods (49%), alcohol (44%), upper respiratory infections (36%), and house dust mites (>35%).[35,36]

Once pruritus occurs, the surrounding normally nonpruritic skin area (whether inflamed or noninflamed) may be sensitive and react to light stimuli and begin itching (a process known as *allokinesis*). Allokinesis is typical of AD.[35,36] As a result of allokinesis, patients with AD may experience pruritic attacks when their skin is touched accidentally by mechanical factors such as clothing, especially wool products.[36]

Elevated serum IgE may be seen, consistent with the genetically predetermined dominance of TH_2 cytokines causing increased IgE. In addition, increased serum IgE antibodies to a particular food, consistent with a food allergy, is common in patients with AD. Serum-based tests for allergen-specific IgE (formerly a radioallergosorbent test referred to as RAST) are used to screen for allergy to a specific substance or substances.[34] (Most labs use large autoanalyzers that rely on fluorescent or chemiluminesent labels rather than radiolabels to identify reactions, so RAST does not describe the technique used.) In some cases, allergen-specific IgE tests may be used to monitor immunotherapy or to see if a child has outgrown a specific allergy. The negative predictive value is high (>95%) but the specificity and positive predictive value are low (40%-60%).[34] Negative results help to rule out a food allergy, whereas positive (elevated) allergen-specific IgE test results only signify sensitization and require clinical correlation and confirmation.[34] The level of IgE may not correlate with the severity of an allergic reaction or with the severity of AD.

With respect to IgE reactivity, several candidate genes that encode cytokines involved in the regulation of IgE synthesis have been identified, notably on chromosome 5q31-33.[2] Increased Th_2 activity leads to release of IL-3, IL-4, IL-5, IL-10, and IL-13, which causes eosinophilia, increases IgE, and increases the growth and development of mast cells.[35] In addition to eosinophils and mast cells, basophils and newly identified innate immune cells called group 2 innate lymphoid cells (ILC2s) have been shown to underlie the pathogenesis of AD.[35] The above cytokines also affect B-cell maturation, causing a genomic rearrangement that favors isotype class switching from IgM to IgE.[2] Th_{17} cells have been found to be elevated, with its role not yet clearly defined.[35]

A clinically useful set of criteria for the diagnosis of AD is as follows: atopy, pruritus, eczema, and altered vascular reactivity.

Disease Severity

6 Disease severity can be classified as mild, moderate, or severe. Assessing the severity of AD includes subjective symptoms and objective signs—in particular, the subjective evaluations relating to pruritus and sleep disturbance are particularly important. Composite scores assessing both signs and symptoms must be used to assess overall disease severity.[36] SCORAD (Scoring of Atopic Dermatitis) is a composite score developed by the European Task Force of Atopic Dermatitis (ETFAD), where a SCORAD score >50 defines severe AD, and one <25 considered mild AD.[36] There is also a Patient-Oriented SCORAD (PO-SCORAD) which is also useful since it can be administered independent of the physician; and the PO-SCORAD correlates well with SCORAD.[36] In addition, there is an objective assessment tool for visible lesions called EASI (Eczema Area and Severity Score) which is often used together with a subjective symptom assessment tool called POEM (Patient-Oriented Eczema Measures); this pair of tests is especially useful in the clinical trial setting.[36] Both SCORAD and PO-SCORAD are available as apps from the Eczema Foundation at https://www.fondation-dermatite-atopique.org/en/healthcare-professionals-space (Fig. 119-1).

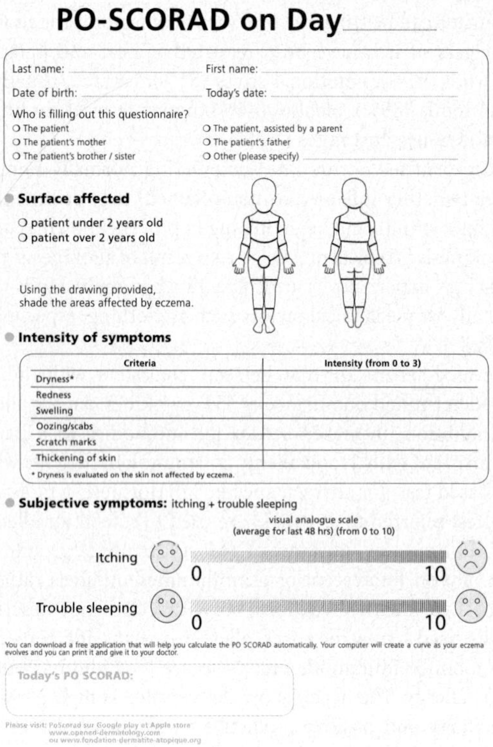

PO-SCORAD on Day______

Last name: ______ First name: ______

Date of birth: ______ Today's date: ______

Who is filling out this questionnaire?
- ○ The patient
- ○ The patient, assisted by a parent
- ○ The patient's mother
- ○ The patient's father
- ○ The patient's brother / sister
- ○ Other (please specify) ______

Surface affected

- ○ patient under 2 years old
- ○ patient over 2 years old

Using the drawing provided, shade the areas affected by eczema.

Intensity of symptoms

Criteria	Intensity (from 0 to 3)
Dryness*	
Redness	
Swelling	
Oozing/scabs	
Scratch marks	
Thickening of skin	

* Dryness is evaluated on the skin not affected by eczema.

Subjective symptoms: itching + trouble sleeping

visual analogue scale
(average for last 48 hrs) (from 0 to 10)

Itching 0 — 10

Trouble sleeping 0 — 10

You can download a free application that will help you calculate the PO SCORAD automatically. Your computer will create a curve as your eczema evolves and you can print it and give it to your doctor.

Today's PO SCORAD:

Please visit: PoScorad sur Google play et Apple store
www.opened-dermatology.com
ou www.fondation-dermatite-atopique.org

FIGURE 119-1 Example of use of SCORAD tool for atopic dermatitis disease severity assessment. A composite score of 40.8 would be consistent with moderate disease. *(SCORAD and PO-SCORAD copyright © Pr JF Stalder, Eczema Foundation, 2020. Reprinted with permission.)*

Complications

7 Patients with AD are prone to skin infections. Atopic skin is drier and the stratum corneum has weakened protective abilities; combined with the abnormal skin barrier function and immune defense, there is an increased risk of secondary bacterial skin infections with staphylococci or streptococci, and viral infections such as herpes simplex or even fungal infections.[1,2] Constant scratching to relieve pruritus may cause excoriations, further compromising the integrity of the skin barrier. *S. aureus* is a common cause of secondary bacterial infections in AD.[3,10] Binding of *S. aureus* is enhanced by skin inflammation as seen in AD. Many patients with AD are colonized with *S. aureus* and may have exacerbations after skin infections of this organism.[10] Secondary bacterial infections may present as yellowish crusty lesions and should be promptly treated. Oral (systemic) antibiotics are generally more effective than topical treatment.[1]

Patients with AD are also more prone to disseminated infections with herpes simplex or vaccinia virus. Severe viral infections such as eczema herpeticum or eczema vaccinatum might be linked to the severity of atopy. Eczema herpeticum is a severe widespread skin infection with herpes simplex virus (HSV) that occurs in up to 3% of patients, in particular those with severe disease.[3] *Molluscum contagiosum* virus infection may be seen in children and adolescents with AD.[3] Smallpox vaccination is contraindicated in patients with AD.

TREATMENT

Desired Outcomes

In treating patients with AD, clinicians generally have the following clinical goals in mind:

1. Provide symptomatic relief—control the itching.
2. Control the AD.
3. Identify and, when possible, eliminate triggers and environmental aeroallergens.
4. Identify and minimize predisposing factors for exacerbations including any stressors.
5. Prevent future exacerbations.
6. Provide any social and psychological support needed for the patient, family, and caregivers.
7. Minimize or prevent adverse events from medications and other treatment modalities.
8. Treat to cure any secondary skin infections, if present.

Successful management of AD should include not only clearance of skin lesions, which may take days to weeks depending on the severity of disease—and this determines the type of treatment regimen—but also controls of the itch, minimizing or eliminating triggers, monitoring the patient to minimize or prevent adverse events from medications or other treatment modalities, and providing adequate social and psychological support for the patient, family, and caregivers.

The ultimate goal is to provide enough control of this chronic disease so that future exacerbations are prevented, thus ensuring that the patient's quality of life is minimally affected by AD. Because the course of the disease evolves over time, management strategies may change. Mild disease can be managed by reactive therapy, moderate-to-severe disease will require proactive therapy to maintain disease control.[36]

8 Both nonpharmacologic and pharmacologic therapies are important in managing the signs and symptoms of AD. Nonpharmacologic strategies include identifying and minimizing or eliminating preventable risk factors, such as known triggers and allergens, as well as appropriate skin care.[30,36]

Treatment guidelines and protocols for AD are available. These are listed in Table 119-5. At the time this chapter was prepared for publication, the American Academy of Dermatology (AAD) was updating its 2014 guidelines in a series of publications.[37] The reader is encouraged to access the online version of this chapter for updates.

Nonpharmacologic Therapy

8 9 Nonpharmacologic approaches to the treatment of infants and children with AD include the following[30,36,38]:

1. Apply moisturizers frequently throughout the day. Moisturizers are a standard of care for AD and there is strong evidence that their use can reduce disease severity and the need for pharmacologic intervention.[30,36,38] Long-term moisturizer therapy improves AD associated xerosis.[36] Even stand-alone use of moisturizers for 1 week improves mild-to-moderate AD flares.[39] Daily use of moisturizers from birth may reduce the development of AD in a high-risk population.[36,40]
2. Give lukewarm baths. There is insufficient evidence for patients with AD to recommend the addition of oils, emollients, or most other additives to bath water, or the use of acidic spring water.[38]
3. Apply moisturizer immediately after bathing. There is no standard for the frequency or duration of bathing appropriate for those with AD.[38]
4. Use nonsoap cleansers (which are neutral to low pH, hypoallergenic, fragrance free). Limited use.[38]
5. Use wet-wrap therapy (with or without TCS) during flare-ups for patients with moderate-to-severe AD. "Wet wrap" is applying damp tubular elasticized bandages and occlusive dressing to the limbs—this promotes skin hydration

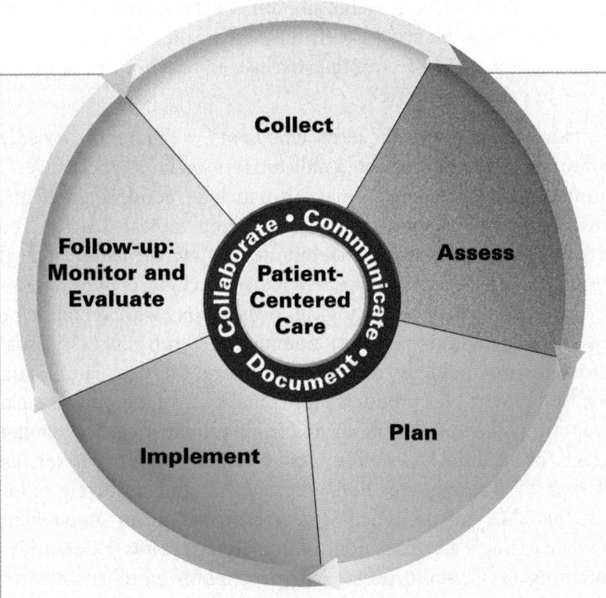

Patient Care Process for Atopic Dermatitis

An illustration shows that patient-centered care includes collaboration, communication, and documentation. The actions associated with the care are collect, assess, plan, implement, and follow-up by monitoring and evaluating.

Collect

- Patient characteristics (eg, age, sex, pregnancy status)
- Patient medical history (personal and family)
- Patient/caregiver description of history of atopic dermatitis, subjective complaints of itch and other symptoms
- Signs associated with severity of itch (eg, excoriations, sleep disturbances)
- Signs associated with severity of atopic dermatitis (eg, areas of involvement)
- Signs of secondary skin infections
- Signs of caregiver stress or distress

Assess

- Severity of atopic dermatitis—classify into mild, moderate, or severe disease (eg, using SCORAD)
- Severity of itch
- Ability/willingness to pay for medical treatment options
- Emotional/psychological concerns (for patient and caregiver, if any)

Plan*

- Determine an appropriate treatment approach, that is, proactive versus reactive therapy
- Recommend the most appropriate therapies (nonpharmacologic and pharmacologic) for atopic dermatitis and itch
- Recommend the most appropriate treatment (treat to cure) and ongoing preventative strategies for secondary skin infection, if present
- Recommend management strategies for caregiver stress or distress, if needed

Implement

- Provide patient education regarding all elements of treatment plan
- Use motivational interviewing and coaching strategies to maximize adherence
- Provide information about prevention of future flare-ups

Follow-up: Monitor and Evaluate

- Contact patient/caregiver in 1 to 2 weeks to follow up about the efficacy of recommended therapies and any issues with the treatment regimen
- Ensure that appropriate monitoring parameters for efficacy and potential adverse effects have been put in place (eg, follow-up lab tests as needed)
- Reinforce preventive measures including continuation of proactive therapy, if implemented
- Ensure that patient/caregiver has been connected to other health resources as needed for follow-up (eg, a dermatologist, psychologist)

**Collaborate with patient, caregivers, and other healthcare professionals.*

and absorption of emollients and TCS,[11] reducing disease severity and water loss.[11,38]

6. Keep child's fingernails filed short.
7. Select clothing made of soft cotton fabrics.
8. Consider using sedating antihistamines to reduce scratching at night.
9. Keep the child cool; avoid situations in which overheating occurs.
10. Learn to recognize skin infections and seek treatment promptly.
11. Attempt to distract the child with activities to keep him or her from scratching.
12. Identify and remove irritants and allergens.

Hydration is crucial, and adequate skin hydration is a fundamental part of managing AD.[30,36,38] Transepidermal water loss is greater in atopic skin than in normal skin. Thus, any measures to improve skin moisturization, such as liberal use of moisturizers, would be beneficial. Moisturizers are a standard of care and may be steroid sparing.[10,36,38] They are useful for both prevention and maintenance therapy.[10,38,41,42] They can be categorized based on their specific effects on the skin:

1. *Occlusives*: These agents provide an oily layer on the skin surface to slow transepidermal water loss, increasing the moisture content of the stratum corneum. These are the best moisturizers for patients with AD.
2. *Humectants*: In the stratum corneum, these agents increase the water-holding capacity. However, they are not useful

TABLE 119-5 Useful Sources of Information About Treatment of Atopic Dermatitis

Published Guidelines or Treatment Protocols

- Davis DMR Drucker AM, Alikhan A et al. AAD guidelines: awareness of comorbidities associated with atopic dermatitis in adults. *J Am Acad Derm* 2022. Published pre-print Jan 24, 2022 https://doi.org/10.1016/j.jaad.2022.01.009
- Wollenberg A, Barbarot S, Bieber T, et al. Consensus-based European guidelines for treatment of atopic eczema (atopic dermatitis) in adults and children: part I & part II. *J Eur Acad Dermatol Venereol* 2018;32(5):657–682 & 850-878.
- Wong ITY, Tsuyuki RT, Cresswell-Melville A, et al. Guidelines for the management of atopic dermatitis (eczema) for pharmacists. *Can Pharm J (Ott)* 2017;150(5):285-297.
- Gooderham M, Lynde CW, Papp K, et al. Review of systemic treatment options for adult atopic dermatitis. *J Cutan Med Surg* 2017;21(1):31-39.
- Eichenfield LF, Tom WL, Chamlin SL, et al. Guidelines of care for the management of atopic dermatitis. Section 1. Diagnosis and assessment of atopic dermatitis. *J Am Acad Dermatol* 2014;70:338-351.
- Eichenfield LF, Tom WL, Berger TG, et al. Guidelines of care for the management of atopic dermatitis. Section 2. Management and treatment of atopic dermatitis with topical therapies. *J Am Acad Dermatol* 2014;71:116-132.
- Sidbury R, Davis DM, Cohen DE, et al. Guidelines of care for the management of atopic dermatitis. Section 3. Management and treatment with phototherapy and systemic agents. *J Am Acad Dermatol* 2014;71:327-349.
- Sidbury R, Tom WL, Bergman JN, et al. Guidelines of care for the management of atopic dermatitis. Section 4. Prevention of disease flares and use of adjunctive therapies and approaches. *J Am Acad Dermatol* 2014; published online September 25, 2014. http://dx.doi.org/10.1016/j.jaad.2014.08.038.
- Eichenfield LF, Boguniewicz M, Simpson E, et al. Translating atopic dermatitis management guidelines into practice for primary care providers. *Pediatrics* 2015;136(3). http://www.pediatrics.org/cgi/doi/10.1542/peds.2014-3678.
- Rubel D, Thirumoorthy T, Soebaryo W, et al. Consensus guidelines for the management of atopic dermatitis: An Asia-Pacific perspective. *J Dermatol* 2013;40:160-171.
- Baron SE, Cohen SN, Archer CB. British Association of Dermatologists and Royal College of General Practitioners. Guidance on the diagnosis and clinical management of atopic eczema. *Clin Exp Dermatol* 2012;37(suppl 1):7-12.
- Izadi N, Leung DYM. Clinical approach to the patient with refractory atopic dermatitis. *Ann Allergy Asthma Immunol* 2018;120:23-33.
- Simpson EL. Atopic dermatitis: A review of topical treatment options. *Curr Med Res Opin* 2010;26(3):633-640.
- Carbone A, Siu A, Patel R. Pediatric atopic dermatitis: A review of the medical management. *Ann Pharmacother* 2010;44:1448-1458.
- National Institute of Arthritis and Musculoskeletal and Skin Diseases. Handout on Health: Atopic Dermatitis. US Department of Health and Human Services. NIH Publication No. 09-4272. May 2013, www.niams.nih.gov/Health_Info/Atopic_Dermatitis/default.asp.
- Lynde C, Barber K, Claveau J, et al. Canadian practical guide for the treatment and management of atopic dermatitis. *J Cutan Med Surg* 2005;8 (suppl 5):1-9. http://www.springerlink.com/content/r5432000056r2748/fulltext.html.

Useful Websites

- National Institute of Arthritis and Musculoskeletal and Skin Diseases (NIAMS), US National Institutes of Health: http://www.niams.nih.gov/Health_Info/Atopic_Dermatitis/default.asp
- American Academy of Allergy Asthma & Immunology (AAAAI): http://www.aaaai.org/conditions-and-treatments/allergies/Skin-Allergy.
- American Academy of Dermatology: https://www.aad.org/education/clinical-guidelines, http://www.jaad.org/article/S0190-9622(13)01095-5/fulltext.
- DermNet NZ: http://dermnetnz.org/dermatitis/atopic.html.

in patients with AD because they have a stinging effect on open skin. Humectants act by drawing moisture from their surroundings to attract water to the skin surface. In humid environments, this works well; however, in dry and low humidity environments, humectants can draw water from deeper parts of the skin, thus further drying out the skin. Thus, they are not recommended for patients with AD.

3. *Emollients*: These agents smooth out the surface of the skin by filling the spaces with droplets of oil. As moisturizers, these are less effective than occlusives, but they can be useful in patients with AD.

However, note that the term "emollients" is often more broadly used to mean *all* nonmedicated moisturizers, including occlusives.[36] Nonmedicated "emollients" may also include active ingredients, softening the delineation of emollients from topical drugs.[36] The 2018 European consensus guideline defines *emollients* as "topical formulations with vehicle-type substances lacking active ingredients" and *emollients plus* as "topical formulations with vehicle-type substances and additional active, nonmedicated substances."[36] Usual ingredients in emollients can include mineral oil, petrolatum, and urea.[36] Emollient-plus products may contain active ingredients such as saponins, flavonoids, riboflavins from protein-free oat plantlet extracts, or bacterial lysates from *Aquaphilus dolomiae* or *Vitreoscilla filiformis*.[36,43] These lysates both improve AD and positively influence the skin microbiome.[36,44] A cream based on *Aquaphilus dolomiae* extracts alleviates nonhistaminergic pruritus.[45] Ceramide-containing OTC moisturizers and prescription emollient devices (PEDs) with distinct ratios of lipids mimic endogenous compositions. However, to date these have not shown superiority in AD.[38]

The humidity in the home should be kept at or above 50% and the room temperature kept on the cool side.[46]

Appropriate skin care is crucial in preventing flare-ups.[1] A daily skin care routine should include the following[46]:

1. Using scent-free moisturizers liberally as needed each day. Large quantities can be used.
2. Bathing in lukewarm water (never hot) for 5 to 10 minutes, once or twice daily.[30,36,38] Adding a capful of emulsifying oil[10] may help the body retain moisture; baths are better than showers. Bathing daily for 10 to 20 minutes may be desirable as long as a thick moisturizer is applied afterward. A 20-minute soak followed by immediate application of topical anti-inflammatory agents (eg, TCS) without towel drying is known as the "soak and smear" technique and is useful when the topical anti-inflammatory agent alone is inadequate.[38] Bathing twice daily during disease flares may also be a useful method for enhancing skin penetration of topical therapies and for debridement of crusting and staphylococcal colonization. The skin should be lightly towel dried (pat to dry, avoid rubbing or brisk drying).[1,46]
3. Scent-free moisturizer should then be applied while the skin is still moist or slightly damp (eg, within 3 minutes of towel drying).[46] Some fragrance-free moisturizers include Aveeno Baby Soothing Relief Moisture Cream, CeraVe lotion, Cetaphil, Neutrogena Hand Cream, and Vanicream products. Lotions may be used on the scalp and other hairy areas and for mild dryness on the face, trunk, and limbs; creams are more occlusive than lotions; ointments are the most occlusive and can be used for drier, thicker, or more scaly areas.[46]
4. Using nonsoap skin cleansers[1] may cause less skin irritation. Lipid- and fragrance-free skin cleansers may be particularly advantageous (eg, CeraVe facial cleansers [Foaming, Hydrating], CeraVe Eczema Body Wash, Cetaphil Gentle Skin Cleanser, Free and Clear Liquid Cleanser, Spectro Derm Cleanser, and Trisan Antibacterial Skin Cleanser). Aquanil, Dove, Neutrogena, and pHisoderm sensitive skin products have also been recommended as low-irritant products, and some are lipid free.
5. Avoiding alcohol-containing topical products including lotions, swabs, and wipes, as they may be drying.
6. Clothing should be double-rinsed. Mild detergents should be used to wash clothing, with no bleach or fabric softener.

Pharmacologic Therapy

Current treatment recommendations are based on disease severity, with reactive therapy appropriate for mild disease, and proactive therapy for moderate or severe AD—severe disease most appropriately managed initially with systemic therapy in a hospital setting (see Fig. 119-2).

Reactive therapy is the traditional treatment modality where anti-inflammatory agents are used only during disease flares with moisturizers used alone between flare-ups. Proactive therapy includes a predefined, long-term, anti-inflammatory treatment applied intermittently (usually twice weekly) together with moisturizers and a predefined appointment schedule for clinical examinations which begins *after* all lesions have been successfully treated. The duration of proactive therapy is usually adapted to disease severity and persistence.[36]

Topical Corticosteroids

10 *Topical corticosteroids* (TCS) are the standard of care to which other treatments are compared.[10,11,30,36,38,42] They remain the drug treatment of choice for AD. However, despite their extensive use, supporting data are limited regarding optimal corticosteroid concentrations, duration and frequency of therapy, and quantity of application.[10,38] The use of long-term intermittent application of TCS was beneficial and safe in two randomized controlled trials (RCTs); however, independent studies of other formulations are needed.

(a) Treatment recommendation for atopic eczema: adult

- For every phase, *additional* therapeutic options should be considered
- Add antiseptics/antibiotics in cases of superinfection
- Consider compliance and diagnosis, if therapy has insufficient effect
- Refer to guideline text for restrictions, especially for treatment marked with[1]
- Licensed indications are marked with[2], off-label treatment options are marked with[3]

Severe: SCORAD >50 / or persistent eczema	Hospitalization; systemic immunosuppression: cyclosporine A[2], short course of oral glucocorticosteroids[2], dupilumab[1,2], methotrexate[3], azathioprin[3], mycophenolate mofetil[3]; PUVA[1]; alitretinoin[1,3]
Moderate: SCORAD 25-50 / or recurrent eczema	Proactive therapy with topical tacrolimus[2] or class II or class III topical glucocorticosteroids[3], wet wrap therapy, UV therapy (UVB 311 nm, medium dose UVA1), psychosomatic counseling, climate therapy
Mild: SCORAD <25 / or transient eczema	Reactive therapy with topical glucocorticosteroids class II[2] or depending on local cofactors: topical calcineurin Inhibitors[2], antiseptics incl. silver[2], silver coated textiles[1]
Baseline: Basic therapy	Educational programmes, emollients, bath oils, avoidance of clinically relevant allergens (encasings, if diagnosed by allergy tests)

(b) Treatment recommendation for atopic eczema: children

- For every phase, *additional* therapeutic options should be considered
- Add antiseptics/antibiotics in cases of superinfection
- Consider compliance and diagnosis, if therapy has insufficient effect
- Refer to guideline text for restrictions, especially for treatment marked with[1]
- Licensed indications are marked with[2], off-label treatment options are marked with[3]

Severe: SCORAD >50 / or persistent eczema	Hospitalization, systemic immunosuppression: cyclosporine A[3], methotrexate[3], azathioprin[3], mycophenolate mofetil[1,3]
Moderate: SCORAD 25-50 / or recurrent eczema	Proactive therapy with topical tacrolimus[2] or class II or III topical glucocorticosteroids[3], wet wrap therapy, UV therapy (UVB 311 nm)[1], psychosomatic counseling, climate therapy
Mild: SCORAD <25 / or transient eczema	Reactive therapy with topical glucocorticosteroids class II[2] or depending on local cofactors: topical calcineurin inhibitors[2], antiseptics incl. silver, silver coated textiles
Baseline: Basic therapy	Educational programmes, emollients, bath oils, avoidance of clinically relevant allergens (encasings, if diagnosed by allergy tests)

FIGURE 119-2 Stepwise treatment for atopic dermatitis in adults and children. *(Reprinted, with permission, from Wollenberg A, Barbarot S, Bieber T, et al. Consensus-based European guidelines for treatment of atopic eczema (atopic dermatitis) in adults and children: Part I & part II. J Eur Acad Dermatol Venereol. 2018;32(5):657–682.)*

To maximize the anti-inflammatory benefit and minimize adverse effects, the choice of TCS should be matched with the severity and site of disease. Low-potency TCS, such as hydrocortisone 1%, are suitable for the face, and medium-potency TCS, such as betamethasone valerate 0.1%, may be used for the body. For longer-duration maintenance therapy, low-potency TCS are recommended.[38] Mid-strength and high-potency TCS should be used for short-term management of exacerbations.[38] There is no established optimum regimen for controlling flare-ups—starting with a short burst of high-potency TCS to rapidly control active disease followed by a rapid taper in potency is equally acceptable as using the lowest-potency agent thought to be needed then adjusting upward in potency if treatment fails.[38] Although twice-daily application is the usual clinical practice, there is some evidence of efficacy with once-daily use of some potent TCS.[38] Daily TCS applications are recommended until the inflammatory lesions are significantly improved—which may take up to several weeks at a time. Once control is achieved, either (a) stop the TCS and use moisturizers alone until the next flare-up, or (b) apply a TCS once or twice weekly to areas of the patient's body where frequent/repeated flare-ups occur—this method has reduced rates of relapse for those patients who experience frequent flare-ups at the same body sites[38] and should be used as proactive therapy in patients with moderate-to-severe AD.[36] There are different potencies for corticosteroids which should be used to guide therapy. (For a corticosteroid potency comparison chart, see Table 118-2 in Chapter 118, or visit the National Psoriasis Foundation Website at http://www.psoriasis.org/netcommunity/sublearn03_mild_potency.) Children should be treated with less-potent corticosteroids than adults.[36] Ultrahigh- and high-potency TCS, such as betamethasone dipropionate 0.05% or clobetasone propionate 0.05%, are typically reserved for short-term treatment of lichenified areas in adults.[41] After the lesions have cleared or significantly improved, a lower-potency agent (the least potent TCS that is effective)[38] should be used for maintenance when appropriate.[41] Potent fluorinated TCS should be avoided not only on the face, but also the genitalia and the intertriginous areas, and in young infants.[36]

It is also important to remember that altering the local environment through hydration and/or occlusion (eg, wet-wrap therapy)[11] as well as changing the vehicle[47] may alter the absorption and effectiveness of the TCS.[10] Some vehicles are better suited for certain body areas,[47] such as a lotion for the scalp and hairy areas. Foams may be more cosmetically pleasing to some patients, as they easily disappear into the skin. The surface area of the skin involved and the skin thickness also play a role. In addition, tachyphylaxis is a clinical concern, but there is little experimental documentation.

TCS are efficacious for the itch in addition to improving lesions, and itch is the key symptom for evaluation of response to treatment.[36] Tapering should not be initiated before the itch has largely improved.[36] Dose tapering has been suggested to avoid withdrawal rebound—with various tapering strategies such as to a less potent TCS or by reducing the frequency of application to intermittent treatment (eg, twice weekly).[36] Dose tapering also minimizes side effects.

Adverse effects of TCS may be systemic in nature, and they are directly related to the steroid potency, duration of use, and other factors as discussed above. Local adverse effects include striae distendae (stretch marks) and skin atrophy, perioral dermatitis, acne, rosacea, telangiectasias (rubeosis steroidica), purpura, focal hypertrichosis, a "dirty neck" (cutis punctata linearis colli), spontaneous scars (pseudocicatrices stellaires), and allergic contact dermatitis (often related to the vehicle but may be due to the corticosteroid).[36,38,48] Inappropriate, long-term use of potent TCS on the face can cause a facial rosacea-like disease with persistent erythema, burning and stinging sometimes called the "red face syndrome" or "corticosteroid addiction syndrome."[36] In infants, inappropriate use of high-potency TCS can cause granuloma gluteal infantum or iatrogenic Cushing's disease.[36] The potential for systemic adverse effects is related to the potency of the TCS, the site of application, the occlusiveness of the preparation, the percentage of body surface area covered, and the duration of use. Potential systemic side effects include hypothalamic-pituitary-adrenal (HPA) axis suppression, infections, hyperglycemia, cataracts, glaucoma, and growth retardation (in children).[1,36,38,46,48] However, growth retardation may also be related to the chronicity of the illness rather than to TCS use or dietary factors. Although less likely, systemic adverse effects can occur with low-potency TCS. For example, a phase II study of a mild-potency corticosteroid (desonide 0.05% foam) in children and adolescents 3 months to 17 years showed that 4% (3 out of 75) of patients experienced mild reversible HPA-axis suppression after a 4-week treatment period.[49]

When TCS therapy has failed for efficacy or safety reasons, numerous agents and interventions can be used as alternative or add-on therapy in patients with AD. Some of these interventions are steroid sparing.

Topical Calcineurin Inhibitors

11 Topical immunomodulators, such as the topical calcineurin inhibitors (TCIs): tacrolimus ointment (Protopic) and pimecrolimus cream (Elidel), have been shown to reduce the extent, severity, and symptoms of AD in adults and children.[10,36,38,41,42] TCIs inhibit the activation of key cells involved in AD, including T cells and mast cells, blocking the production of proinflammatory cytokines and mediators.[38] Tacrolimus also decreases the number and costimulatory ability of epidermal DCs.[38] Pimecrolimus has more favorable lipophilic characteristics and, in animal studies, appears to preferentially distribute to the skin as opposed to the systemic circulation.[50] Both tacrolimus ointment and pimecrolimus cream are approved for AD in adults and children older than 2 years.[10,36,38,41,42] Although clinical trials conducted in younger infants (eg, 2-23 months old) showed significant efficacy without appreciable adverse effects, use in children younger than 2 years is not Food and Drug Administration (FDA)-approved.[51] Tacrolimus 0.03% ointment is approved for moderate-to-severe AD for children aged 2 years and older, with the 0.1% ointment limited to ages 16 years and older; pimecrolimus 1% cream is approved for mild-to-moderate AD for ages 2 years and older.[51] There is limited data comparing TCS with tacrolimus or pimecrolimus. However, it is known that simultaneous combination of TCS with TCI at the same site does not seem to provide greater benefit.[36] Using a TCI at sensitive skin sites such as face and skin folds while using TCS at other sites may be a useful strategy. Unlike TCS, long-term use of TCI does not cause skin atrophy[38]; however, an initial acute site reaction is fairly common.[36]

Proactive therapy (intermittent) using TCI is cost-effective for patients with moderate and severe AD.[36,52,53] However, cost-effectiveness of first-line treatment with TCI has not yet been conclusively demonstrated.[36]

The FDA has a black-box warning for both tacrolimus ointment and pimecrolimus cream about their potential cancer risk, but no causal relationship has been proven between use of a TCI and the development of lymphoma or nonmelanoma skin cancer in humans.[44] However, there is a theoretical potential of local skin carcinogenesis as discussed below. Thus, both tacrolimus and pimecrolimus are recommended for use as second-line treatments for short-term and noncontinuous chronic use in AD,[10,36,38,41,42] when the continued use of TCS is ineffective or inadvisable.[36,38] They may be appropriate in patients with corticosteroid-related adverse effects, patients with large body-surface areas of disease, patients unresponsive to TCS, or other reasons where treatment with TCS is inadvisable. Children and adults with a weakened or compromised immune system should not be treated with these agents.[38] Unlike TCS, TCI can be used on all body locations for prolonged periods,[36] although episodic use is recommended. They may be used as twice-weekly long-term therapy for maintenance.[11,36,52,53] They may be used as steroid-sparing agents (sequentially or concomitantly with TCS).[36,38]

The most common adverse effect of TCI is transient discomfort (burning sensation) at the application site.[36,38] Some patients may experience a transient worsening of skin conditions; and these transient side effects are more often seen with tacrolimus than pimecrolimus, and if applying to acutely inflamed skin.[36] Generalized viral infections (eg, eczema herpeticum, eczema molluscatum) have been reported.[36] There is a theoretical potential for local skin carcinogenesis as seen in animal studies, or for systemic effects if high blood levels are reached (eg, increased susceptibility to infections due to immunosuppressive effects).[51] Because of the theoretical possible risk of cutaneous malignancy in humans,[36,38] and the known long-term use of systemic cyclosporine being associated with increased photocarcinogenicity in solid organ transplant patients, sun protection is recommended.[11,36,46] However, it may be that the use of TCI has no association with increased risk of nonmelanoma skin cancer, other malignancies, or photocarcinogenicity.[54,55] Nonetheless, patients should be encouraged to apply a high sun protection factor (SPF) broad-spectrum sunblock daily to all exposed skin (ie, SPF 30 or higher); and this counseling should especially be emphasized for those patients with the highest risk of developing skin cancer, including patients with red hair and/or Fitzpatrick skin types I and II, and patients receiving phototherapy or using tanning beds.[46]

TCI are effective in relieving the associated pruritus. Both tacrolimus and pimecrolimus significantly relieve pruritus even after the first few days of treatment, in both children and adults (studies report relief after just 3 days).[10]

Coal Tar

Although tar preparations had been widely used for AD and have been recommended as alternative topical therapy, few RCTs support their efficacy.[38] Their anti-inflammatory properties are not well characterized, and part of the improvement may be the result of a placebo effect, which can be significant in AD.

Coal tar products are also staining and malodorous, although newer products may be more cosmetically acceptable. They are not recommended on acutely inflamed skin, since this may result in additional skin irritation.

The use of coal tar in pregnancy has not been studied. Few data are available about tar excretion into breast milk; in addition, safety in children has not been established.[56] Adverse effects include tar folliculitis, acneiform eruptions, irritant dermatitis, burning, stinging, photosensitivity, and a risk of tar intoxication if used extensively in a young child.[56] Although animal studies showed that tar components can be converted to carcinogenic and mutagenic entities, there is inconclusive epidemiologic evidence supporting the claim that human use of topical tar preparations in dermatology leads to skin cancer.[56]

Selective Phosphodiesterase-4 Inhibitors

Crisaborole and apremilast are small-molecule phosphodiesterase (PDE)-4 inhibitors. Cyclic nucleotide PDEs break down cAMP and cGMP into inactive metabolites and there is increased PDE activity in AD, creating a proinflammatory state that may result in stimulation of Th_2 cells to release inflammatory mediators.[57,58] PDE-4 inhibitors inhibit the increased PDE activity; and crisaborole ointment is FDA-approved for treatment of mild-to-moderate AD in adults and children 2 years of age or older.[36] (Apremilast is approved for psoriasis and psoriatic arthritis [see Chapter 118, "Psoriasis," in this textbook].)[57] However, a pilot study of apremilast in patients with moderate-to-severe AD demonstrated moderate improvement of skin lesions, pruritus, and quality of life,[58] and it has also shown success for moderate-to-severe AD in children.[59]

Other Topical Therapies

Patients with moderate-to-severe AD who have frequent bacterial infections may benefit from dilute bleach baths with intranasal mupirocin—one study showed enhanced clinical improvement.[38] Janus kinase (JAK) inhibitors have shown evidence of efficacy for atopic dermatitis when administered either topically and orally. Topical JAK inhibitors include ruxolitinib and tofacitinib.[36]

Phototherapy

12 Phototherapy is effective for AD and is recommended[10,11,36,60] as second-line treatment when the disease is not controlled by TCS and/or TCI.[36,60] Although rarely used in prepubertal children, it is not contraindicated.[36] Both natural (heliotherapy) and artificial sources of UV radiation are effective.[36] UV light sources on the skin have immunosuppressive, immunomodulating, anti-inflammatory, and antipruritic effects.[36] A known mechanism of action is immunomodulation through apoptosis of inflammatory cells, inhibition of LCs, and alteration of cytokine production.[36] There are other potential benefits. Phototherapy may be steroid sparing, allowing for the use of lower-potency TCS, or even eliminating the need for maintenance by TCS in some cases. Phototherapy can be used for acute or maintenance therapy in children and adults with AD.[60] Phototherapy may also help prevent secondary bacterial skin infections, commonly seen in patients with AD. UVB radiation reduces *S. aureus* skin colonization.[36,61] However, in a few patients, phototherapy may worsen the AD; it is not recommended in patients whose disease flares up when exposed to sunlight. Relapse following cessation of therapy frequently occurs.[10]

Phototherapy may consist of either ultraviolet light therapy alone, or ultraviolet light therapy alongside drug or topical ointment (commonly called photochemotherapy). Psoralens plus ultraviolet A light (PUVA) is one type of photochemotherapy. The photosensitizer (psoralens) is administered either topically or in a bath immediately prior to ultraviolet A (UVA) light therapy. Topical ointments (such as crude coal tar) may also be used concomitantly with ultraviolet light therapy (eg, Crude coal tar + ultraviolet B [UVB] light) to increase efficacy.

Ultraviolet lamps include UVA (315-400 nm), UVA1 (340-400 nm), broadband UVB (BB-UVB) (280-315 nm), and narrowband UVB (NB-UVB) (311 nm). Phototherapies used for AD have included PUVA, high- or medium-dose UVA1, BB-UVB, and NB-UVB.[10,60] No definitive recommendation can be made to differentiate between the various phototherapies.[60] NB-UVB is more effective than BB-UVB therapy and is generally the most commonly recommended light treatment and it has a better side-effect profile than UVA or PUVA.[10,60] BB-UVB may not effectively treat the scalp and skinfold areas. Medium-dose UVA1 is effective for patients with an acute exacerbation of severe AD; however, the effect may be relatively short-lived and symptoms may recur within 3 months of stopping therapy.[60] Medium-dose UVA1 is considered similar in efficacy as NB-UVB; and high-dose UVA1 is preferred in severe cases when available.[10] There is weaker evidence supporting the use of PUVA in AD[47] and it is not first-choice.[10]

Patients need to wear eye protection during ultraviolet (UV) light therapy to prevent damage to the retina. Short-term adverse effects include erythema, skin pain, skin burning or sunburn, pruritus, and pigmentation.[60] Long-term adverse effects include premature aging of the skin (photoaging), lentigines, photosensitive eruptions, folliculitis, photo-onycholysis, HSV reactivation, facial hypertrichosis, and skin cancer.[60] For example, PUVA has been associated with squamous cell carcinoma and possibly melanoma, which may occur years after PUVA therapy has ceased. UVA therapy may also cause cataract formation.[60]

To minimize a possible initial flare-up, co-medication of TCS and moisturizers has been suggested at the beginning of phototherapy.[36]

Other light therapies include short-wave visible light (>380 nm) ("blue light")—in uncontrolled pilot studies, photopheresis, and devices such as 308-nm monochromatic excimer lasers and pulsed-dye lasers—experimental.[36]

Systemic Therapies

Systemic therapies for the treatment of AD are generally not well studied. Small case series or open studies are available for some agents, but few well-conducted RCTs exist. Agents described in published papers have included systemic corticosteroids, cyclosporine, interferon-γ, azathioprine, methotrexate, mycophenolate mofetil, intravenous immunoglobulin (IVIG), and biologic agents.[10,60] Systemic therapies are indicated in AD care only for the subset of adult and pediatric patients in whom optimized topical regimens and/or phototherapy do not adequately control the disease, or where the quality of life is substantially affected.[60]

Systemic corticosteroids, although sometimes used for rapid disease suppression, are generally not recommended due to an unfavorable risk-benefit profile.[11,36,41,60] A 2017 systematic review of systemic treatment options for adults with AD gave no recommendations for use of systemic corticosteroids due to limited available evidence.[15] The 2018 European consensus guidelines recommended the following regarding oral corticosteroids for patients with AD: (1) restricted use, largely limited to adult patients; (2) short-term use (up to 1 week) in acute flare-ups only in exceptional cases; (3) daily dose not to exceed 0.5 mg/kg bodyweight; (4) use even more cautiously in children than in adults; (5) no long-term use.[36] Short courses of oral corticosteroids may lead to atopic flares/rebound.[11,60]

Cyclosporine is effective for AD and is considered the first-line treatment option when systemic therapy for AD is warranted, that is, for severe, recalcitrant AD,[10,11,15,36,60] but its usefulness is also limited by significant side effects, including hypertension and nephrotoxicity. Combination with UV therapy is not recommended, and effective UV protection should be used.[36] There is also the potential for significant drug-drug and drug-food (eg, grapefruit juice) interactions. It should be reserved for short-term use in adults (and more cautiously in children) with severe refractory disease.[11,60] Maximal benefit is usually seen after 2 to 6 weeks of use and relapse may occur quickly after cessation of therapy.[10,11,60] Treatment durations recommended are 6 to 9 months[11] and up to 1 year—this is off-label use in the United States and Canada.[60] European guidelines are for 2 years then to switch to another treatment if possible, but shorter intervals of 3 to 6 months are usually recommended; and cyclosporine is approved for AD in many European countries.[36] In a meta-analysis of eight RCTs, cyclosporine was more efficacious than placebo, with reduced body surface area, erythema, sleep loss, and glucocorticoid use. However, all scores were back to pretreatment levels 8 weeks after ending cyclosporine therapy.[10] An earlier study (2000) comparing intermittent to continuous cyclosporine therapy in children 12 to 16 years of age showed efficacy in some children on intermittent therapy (thus with a lower cumulative cyclosporine dose and minimizing toxicity); however, continuous cyclosporine therapy provided enhanced sustained improvement.[36,62]

Recombinant interferon-γ may be effective in a subset of patients with AD.[10] It may be an alternative for refractory AD (adults and children).[60] Two randomized placebo-controlled trials in patients with severe AD demonstrated significant improvement in symptoms.[63,64] Short-term adverse effects, such as headache, myalgias, and chills, occurred in substantial proportions of study patients. Transient liver transaminase elevations and granulocytopenia have also occurred. There is no recommended optimal dose.[60]

Azathioprine,[60,65] *methotrexate,*[60,66] *mycophenolate mofetil,*[60] and IVIG have shown efficacy in small case series or open-label studies primarily in adults with recalcitrant AD. There are two RCTs with azathioprine as monotherapy which showed efficacy, improving both QOL and AD.[60,65] Additional RCTs are needed. Oral methotrexate, with a long history of pediatric use for various inflammatory conditions, is effective in a case series of children (aged 2-16 years) with severe AD[66] and has also shown efficacy in adults.[60]

13 *Biologic agents* are beginning to be approved for AD in some countries. The safety and efficacy of various biologic agents in patients with AD have been studied, mostly in case reports, small case series, or open-label studies with a limited number of patients; however, larger randomized, placebo-controlled trials are now available.[36] Dupilumab, a fully human monoclonal antibody that blocks the common α-chain of the receptor for interleukin-4 and intereukin-13, was approved by the FDA in April 2017 for treating moderate-to-severe adult AD.[36] Dupilumab is a down-regulator of the JAK-STAT pathway. Clinical outcomes (SCORAD, EASI, IGA, BSA) as well as patient-reported outcomes (DLQI, pruritus rating scales) were improved in various phase I to III clinical trials in adults with AD.[67] Clinical trials in children are ongoing at the time of writing (NCT02407756) as well as open-label studies evaluating long-term safety and efficacy of repeat doses in children, adolescents, and adults with previous participation in dupilumab clinical trials (NCT02612454, NCT01949311).[15] Dupilumab's safety profile is superior to conventional immunosuppressives such as cyclosporine or methotrexate; its most relevant side effects being conjunctivitis and injection site reactions.[67] Safety in pregnancy is unknown at the time of writing. A recent review of systemic treatment options for adults with AD discussed trials with other biologics including infliximab, mepolizumab, omalizumab, rituximab, and ustekinumab.[15] Some of these trials showed little to no improvement; however, a case series of ustekinumab use showed promising results and was well tolerated.[15] Nemolizumab is another biologic with some promise in a recent clinical trial especially in reducing pruritus.[36] The TNF-α inhibitors infliximab and etanercept is effective in a few patients but not others, and adverse events have included infusion reactions with flushing and dyspnea, urticaria, and recurrent skin infections of methicillin-resistant *S. aureus*. Similarly, omalizumab, rituximab, and alefacept have been shown in a few case reports and small case series to be somewhat effective. A case report series of omalizumab plus IVIG showed significant clinical improvement.[68] However, an RCT with omalizumab showed no clinical improvement in AD despite reducing IgE levels.[60] Therapy of AD with traditional biologics (eg, rituximab, omalizumab, or ustekinumab) is not recommended.[36]

Upadacitinib and abrocitinib are oral selective JAK-1 inhibitors approved by the FDA for treatment of moderate-to-severe atopic dermatitis. Upadacitinib was compared to dupilumab in a 24-week, head-to-head, phase 3b multicenter RCT in adults with moderate-to-severe AD with results showing superior efficacy of upadacitinib vs dupilumab in Eczema Area and Severity Index (EASI75) ($p = 0.006$) and all secondary endpoints such as worst pruritis NRS.[69] There were other clinical trials with upadacitinib involving adults and children older than 12 years, and it has received FDA approval for use at 15 and 30 mg once daily as monotherapy for those age groups. Abrocitinib has received FDA approval based on the results of five clinical trials for use in adults only, at 100 and 200 mg doses, with the 200 mg dose reserved for patients unresponsive to the 100 mg dose. Both products carry a warning of increased risk of serious infections, mortality, malignancy, major adverse cardiovascular events, and thrombosis.

Alitretinoin is a retinoid with anti-inflammatory and antiproliferative effects licensed in some European countries for treatment of hand eczema.[36] It may improve both extrapalmar and hand lesions in AD patients and may be used for atopic hand eczema in adult patients of non-childbearing potential unresponsive to TCS therapy.[36]

Oral antihistamines are used widely; however, there is mixed evidence of efficacy in AD control.[36,60] There is some evidence that oral sedating antihistamines used at night may benefit patients with AD with poor sleep due to pruritus.[11,60]

Complementary and Alternative Therapies

Traditional Chinese herbal therapy has been studied in placebo-controlled trials and provide temporary benefit for patients with severe AD. However, the effectiveness may wear off despite continued treatment, and long-term toxicity is unknown.[10,70] A recent meta-analysis of seven RCTs attempted to evaluate the efficacy and safety of oral Chinese medicines for AD and concluded that traditional Chinese herbal medicines significantly improved symptom severity and was well tolerated; however, the studies were of poor quality and did not allow for valid conclusions to be drawn about tolerability and routine use.[71] Additional studies are needed.

Probiotics and *prebiotics* may prove to be beneficial for prevention and treatment of AD. Probiotics are live microorganisms (bacteria or fungi) that confer a health benefit on the host when administered in adequate amounts.[72] Prebiotics are nondigestable compounds that lead to favorable changes in the gut microbiome.[72] The term "synbiotics" refers to products that contain both probiotics and prebiotics.[72]

Although earlier studies of *probiotics* had mixed results, more recent clinical trials showed evidence of benefit in both prevention and treatment of AD.[72-75] The most common species of probiotics used include *Lactobacillus rhamnosus GG, Lactobacillus casei, Lactobacillus plantarum, Lactobacillus johnsonii, Bifidobacterium lactis*, and *Saccaromues boulardii*.[72] A meta-analysis of 25 clinical trials concluded that probiotics significantly reduced the risk of atopic sensitization when given prenatally.[72,73] A double-blind RCT showed that probiotics reduced the SCORAD index and serum cytokines in AD patients.[72,74] A randomized trial of oral *Bifidobacterium bifidum* in 40 infants newly diagnosed with AD noted a significant reduction in the SCORAD index posttreatment in the infants receiving the probiotic versus no change in those who did not.[75]

Prebiotics are nondigestible oligosaccharides including fructooligosaccharides, galactooligosaccharides, lactulose, and inulin. These can stimulate the growth of selective beneficial gut bacteria, in particular lactobacilli and bifidobacteria.[72] In the colon, prebiotics are fermented into short chain fatty acids (SCFAs) including butyrate, acetate, and propionate. The SCFAs may alter the gut microbiome. For example, transgalactooligosaccharides increase the number of bifidobacteria and modify the colonic fermentation metabolism of the gut flora.[76] Prebiotics have shown benefits for various disease conditions including hypercholesterolemia, *Clostridium difficile*–associated diarrhea, and allergic conditions such as AD.[72] Two recent meta-analyses have shown a 32% reduced incidence of pediatric AD[77] and that the combination of galactooligosaccharide and fructooligosaccharide reduced AD incidence.[78]

Immunotherapy using allergen-specific desensitization techniques in controlled settings for patients with AD may also be beneficial, and much research is ongoing including RCTs. A recent review and meta-analysis of immunotherapy in patients with AD showed significant efficacy.[11,79] More research is also needed to adequately assess the role of homeopathy, hypnotherapy, acupuncture, massage therapy, and biofeedback therapy in the treatment of AD.

Patient Considerations

14 AD may have significant implications not only for the patients themselves, but also their families and caregivers. The burden of AD needs to be addressed. There is strong evidence that AD in adults is associated with select allergic, atopic, immune-mediated, mental health, and bone health comorbidities and skin infections.[37] In addition, patients with refractory AD may need further follow-up to rule out other diagnoses, confirm adequate/appropriate first-line therapy use, rule out/minimize exacerbating factors, and implement second-line therapies.[80]

In 2006, an international study of 2,002 patients and caregivers from eight countries addressed the effect of AD on the lives of patients and society.[81] This European study found that, on average, patients experienced nine flares per year, with those having severe disease experiencing more flares and taking significantly longer to clear. The flares were associated with disturbed sleep, and 86% of patients avoided at least one type of everyday activity. Schoolwork performance and productivity were negatively affected. Patients missed an average of 2.5 days of school or work per year, and an analysis of adult patient performance at work and occupational absence showed that the social cost of lost productivity could amount to more than 2 billion Euros per year across the European Union. There were also emotional consequences; half of the patients experienced depression or unhappiness about their condition, and one-third reported that AD had eroded their self-confidence. In addition, concern about adverse effects from TCS treatments resulted in poor adherence to therapy. On average, patients endured the symptoms of AD without initiating specific treatment 47% of the time they had an exacerbation. Approximately one-half of the respondents were concerned about using TCS, and 58% restricted them to particular sites, 39% used them less frequently or for shorter time periods than prescribed, and 66% used them as a last resort. The study concluded that AD is "an undertreated disease that has a significant, yet mostly avoidable, negative effect on patients, their caregivers, and society."[81]

The above conclusion is echoed in more recent reports. In 2018 and 2019, studies relating to the burden of disease from the United States, Canada, and internationally were published. In a 2018 US cross-sectional study, 1,519 adult patients with AD reported a multidimensional burden of disease that is higher with greater disease severity and inadequate disease control.[82] Patients with moderate/severe AD (830/1519) reported more severe itching and pain, greater adverse effects on sleep, higher prevalence of anxiety and depression, and greater health-related QoL impairment. About 103/1,519 patients had inadequate disease control despite treatment with systemic immunomodulators or phototherapy, and they reported higher burdens of itch and sleeping symptoms versus those with controlled disease.[82] Sleep symptoms included trouble sleeping (significant on PO-SCORAD), longer sleep latency, more frequent sleep disturbances, and greater need for OTC sleep medications.[82] Results from two 2018 Canadian online national cross-sectional surveys included the burden of moderate-to-severe AD on pediatric patients.[83] For the adult patients: 87% (187/216) reported that their daily life was negatively affected by their disease, with experiences ranging from dysfunctional sleep (79%, ie, 148/187), anxiety (64%, ie, 120/187), avoidance of social activities (48%, ie, 90/187), avoidance of physical activity (47%, ie, 88/187), and avoidance of intimacy (40%, ie, 75/187). In addition, 32% reported difficulty accessing treatments and 41% felt that their treatment needs were unmet. Only 9% reported that their disease was well controlled, and 78% reported they had lived for over 1 year with inadequate treatment for their disease. For the pediatric patients: 78% (253/361) had sleep disturbances, 51% avoided social activities, 30% had anxiety issues, 20% missed school due to their AD—and of these, 23% have missed 10 days or more within the past year.[83] Regardless of treatment modalities, most survey respondents felt that their child's AD is not well controlled—85% have used three or more treatment modalities for their child's AD, and 80% of respondents find the recommended care regimen for their child's AD challenging.[83]

In 2019, data from a 2016 National Health and Wellness Survey conducted in France, Germany, Italy, Spain, and the United Kingdom was published with comparisons between controls without AD matched to patients with self-reported AD (both $n = 1{,}860$).[84] Self-reported comorbidities were significantly more prevalent in patients with AD compared to those without AD and these included anxiety, depression, and sleep disturbances. There was reduced health-related QoL as well as a significant impact on work productivity (ie, presenteeism and overall work impairment) and the ability to undertake activities. There was also greater healthcare utilization.[84]

Even though there is likely selection bias due to the self-reporting nature of these surveys, the results from these (and others) should alert healthcare professionals to the continuing unmet health, psychosocial, and educational needs associated with AD.

Patient communication may be a key step—treating them as partners in their own (or their child's) care, with regular contact, advice, and support. Healthcare professionals play an integral role in providing patient and caregiver education and support about this disease and specific treatment plans. The importance of adequate and appropriate education for the patient, family, and caregivers about AD and its management cannot be overemphasized. Patients should be involved in their own care whenever possible. Timely access to dermatology consultation may be another key factor—in the above Canadian survey only 27% (123/451) of respondents are managed by a dermatologist—wait times for appointments were 3 months or longer (46%) and in 25% of cases were 6 months or longer.[81] Limited access to care is a societal issue.

EVALUATION OF THERAPEUTIC OUTCOMES

- Contact patient/caregiver in 1 to 2 weeks to follow-up about the efficacy of recommended therapies and any issues with the treatment regimen. Continuing regular follow-up is recommended to monitor for adherence and address other issues and patient concerns (eg, QoL issues as discussed above).
- Ensure that appropriate monitoring parameters for efficacy and potential adverse effects have been put in place (eg, follow-up lab tests as needed).
- Reinforce preventive measures including continuation of proactive therapy, if implemented.
- Ensure that patient/caregiver has been connected to other health resources as needed for follow-up (eg, a dermatologist, psychologist, and social worker).

CONCLUSION

AD is a chronic skin condition that generally presents at an early age. It affects the patient, family, caregivers, and our society and is optimally managed by multidisciplinary care. Nonpharmacologic management strategies are important in treatment; these include appropriate skin care, hydration, avoidance of triggers, and psychosocial support and management. Community pharmacists are in a prime position to support patients, physicians, and other health professionals because patients with AD (and caregivers of children with AD) may initially seek nonprescription treatments.[30] The pharmacologic treatment strategy may be proactive or reactive depending on disease severity. Treatment alternatives continue to emphasize TCS as the standard of care; others being TCIs and other topical agents, wet wrap therapy, and UV therapy. For severe/recalcitrant disease, systemic therapies including cyclosporine and biologics may be warranted. A 2018 review provides a step-wise clinical approach to the patient with refractory AD which include ruling out other diagnoses, confirming first-line therapies, and ruling out exacerbating factors before using second-line therapies; further, a multidisciplinary approach to address behavioral factors (poor adherence, improper technique, habitual scratching, depression, sleep disturbance, stress) is described (eg, habit reversal training for the itch-scratch cycle).[80] Patient and caregiver education and support about AD and treatment strategies is critical to optimize treatment outcomes. Successful outcomes result when patients and caregivers are partners with healthcare professionals in the management of this chronic disease.

ACKNOWLEDGMENT

The authors gratefully acknowledge the contributions of Dr. P.G. Kwa to previous editions of this chapter.[1]

ABBREVIATIONS

AD	atopic dermatitis
AMP	antimicrobial peptide
BB-UVB	broadband ultraviolet B light (280-315 nm)
DC	dendritic cell
ETFAD	European Task Force of Atopic Dermatitis
FDA	Food and Drug Administration
FLG	filaggrin gene
GI	gastrointestinal
HPA	hypothalamic-pituitary-adrenal
IgE	immunoglobulin E
IgM	immunoglobulin M
IL	interleukin
ISAAC	International Study of Asthma and Allergies in Childhood
IVIG	intravenous immunoglobulin
JAK	Janus kinase
MDC	macrophage-derive chemoattractant
NB-UVB	narrowband ultraviolet B light (311 nm)
NIAID	National Institute of Allergy and Infectious Diseases
PDE	phosphodiesterase
PUVA	psoralens plus ultraviolet A light
RAST	radioallergosorbent test
RCT	randomized controlled trial
SCFAs	short-chain fatty acids
SCORAD	Scoring of Atopic Dermatitis
SD	standard deviation
SPF	sun protection factor
TARC	thymus and activation-regulated chemokine
TCIs	topical calcineurin inhibitors
TCS	topical corticosteroids
TH_1	T-helper cell type 1
TH_2	T-helper cell type 2
UV	ultraviolet
UVA	ultraviolet A
UVB	ultraviolet B

REFERENCES

1. National Institute of Arthritis and Musculoskeletal and Skin Diseases. Atopic Dermatitis. US Department of Health and Human Services. 2018. Available at: https://www.niams.nih.gov/health-topics/atopic-dermatitis. Accessed February 5, 2022.
2. Eichenfield LE, Tom WL, Chamlin SI, et al. Guidelines of care for the management of atopic dermatitis. Section 1. Diagnosis and assessment of atopic dermatitis. *J Am Acad Dermatol.* 2014;70:338–351.
3. Weidinger S, Novak N. Atopic dermatitis. *Lancet.* 2016 (March 12);387(10023):1109–1122.
4. Hanifin JM. Epidemiology of atopic dermatitis. *Immunol Allergy Clin North Am.* 2002;22:1–24.
5. Bieber T. Mechanisms of disease: Atopic dermatitis. *N Engl J Med.* 2008;358:1483–494.
6. Williams H, Flohr C. How epidemiology has challenged 3 prevailing concepts about atopic dermatitis. *J Allergy Clin Immunol.* 2006;118:209–213.
7. Williams H, Stewart A, von Mutius E, Cookson W, et al. Is eczema really on the increase worldwide? *J Allergy Clin Immunol.* 2008;121:947–954.
8. DaVeiga SP. Epidemiology of atopic dermatitis: A review. *Allergy Asthma Proc.* 2012;23:227–234.
9. Nutten S. Atopic dermatitis: Global epidemiology and risk factors. *Ann Nutr Metab.* 2015;66(suppl 1):8–16.

10. Wollenberg A, Barbarot S, Bieber T, et al. Consensus-based European guidelines for treatment of atopic eczema (atopic dermatitis) in adults and children: Part I & part II. *J Eur Acad Dermatol Venereol.* 2018;32(5):657–682.
11. Plotz SG, Wiesender M, Todorova A, Ring J. What is new in atopic dermatitis/eczema? *Expert Opin Emerging Drugs.* 2014;19(4):441–458.
12. Akdis CA. New insights into mechanisms of immunoregulation in 2007. *J Allergy Clin Immunol.* 2008;122:700–709.
13. Ege MJ, Herzum I, Buchele G, et al. Prenatal exposure to a farm environment modifies atopic sensitization at birth. *J Allergy Clin Immunol.* 2008;122:407–412.
14. Flohr C, Yeo L. Atopic dermatitis and the hygiene hypothesis revisited. *Curr Probl Dermatol.* 2011;41:1–34.
15. Gooderham M, Lynde CW, Papp K, et al. Review of systemic treatment options for adult atopic dermatitis. *J Cutan Med Surg.* 2017;21(1):31–39.
16. Irvine AD, McLean WH, Leung DY. Filaggrin mutations associated with skin and allergic diseases. *N Eng J Med.* 2011;365(4):1315–1327.
17. Rodriguez E, Baurecht H, Herberich E, et al. Meta-analysis of filaggrin polymorphisms in eczema and asthma: Robust rick factors in atopic disease. *J Allergy Clin Immunol.* 2009;123:1361–1370.
18. Honey B, Steinhoff M, Ruzicka T, Leung DYM. Cytokines and chemokines orchestrate atopic skin inflammation. *J Allergy Clin Immunol.* 2006;118:178–189.
19. Leung DYM. Our evolving understanding of the functional role of filaggrin in atopic dermatitis. *J Allergy Clin Immunol.* 2009;124:494–495.
20. Steinke JW, Rich SS, Borish L. Genetics of allergic disease. *J Allergy Clin Immunol.* 2008;121(suppl):S384–S387.
21. Heratizadeh A, Wichmann K, Werfel T. Food allergy and atopic dermatitis: How are they connected? *Curr Allergy Asthma Rep.* 2011;11:284–291.
22. Sicherer SC, Leung DYM. Advances in allergic skin disease, anaphylaxis and hypersensitivity reactions to foods, drugs, and insects in 2008. *J Allergy Clin Immunol.* 2009;123:319–327.
23. Schauber J, Gallo RL. Antimicrobial peptides and the skin immune defense system. *J Allergy Clin Immunol.* 2008;122:261–266.
24. Novak N, Bieber T. Dendritic cells as regulators of immunity and tolerance. *J Allergy Clin Immunol.* 2008;121(suppl):S370–S374.
25. Biebe T, de la Salle H, Wollenberg A, et al. Human epidermal Langerhans cells express the high affinity receptor for immunoglobulin E (Fc epsilon RI). *J Exp Med.* 1992;175:1285–1290.
26. Wang B, Rieger A, Kilgus O, et al. Epidermal Langerhans cells from normal human skin bind monomeric IgE via Fc epsilon RI. *J Exp Med.* 1992;175:1353–1365.
27. Novak N, Bieber T. The role of dendritic cell subtypes in the pathophysiology of atopic dermatitis. *J Am Acad Dermatol.* 2005;53(suppl 2):S171–S176.
28. Lack G. Epidemiologic risks for food allergy. *J Allergy Clin Immunol.* 2008;121:1331–1336.
29. Boyce JA, Assa'ad AH, Burks AW, et al. Guidelines for the diagnosis and management of food allergy in the United States. Report of the NIAID-sponsored expert panel. *J Allergy Clin Immunol.* 2010;126(6 suppl):S1–S58. Available at: https://www.niaid.nih.gov/diseases-conditions/food-allergy. Accessed February 5, 2022.
30. Wong ITY, Tsuyuki RT, Cresswell-Melville A, et al. Guidelines for the management of atopic dermatitis (eczema) for pharmacists. *Can Pharm J.* 2017;150(5):285–297.
31. Lucas JSA, Lewis SA, Jourihane JO'B. Kiwi fruit allergy: A review. *Pediatr Allergy Immunol.* 2003;14:420–428.
32. Cohen A, Goldberg M, Levy B, et al. Sesame food allergy and sensitization in children: The natural history and long-term follow-up. *Pediatr Allergy Immunol.* 2007;18:217–223.
33. Burks AW, Laubach S, Jones SM. Oral tolerance, food allergy, and immunotherapy: Implications for future treatment. *J Allergy Clin Immunol.* 2008;121:1344–1350.
34. Sidbury R, Tom WL, Bergman JN, et al. Guidelines of care for the management of atopic dermatitis. Section 4. Prevention of disease flares and use of adjunctive therapies and approaches. *J Am Acad Dermatol.* December 2014;71(6):1218–1233. 10.1016/j.jaad.2014.08.038.
35. Kim BS. Atopic Dermatitis. Medscape eMedicine updated Oct 30, 2018. Available at: http://emedicine.medscape.com/article/1049085-overview. Accessed November 19, 2018.
36. Wollenberg A, Barbarot S, Bieber T, et al. Consensus-based European guidelines for treatment of atopic eczema (atopic dermatitis) in adults and children: Part I. *J Eur Acad Dermatol Venereol.* 2018;32:657–682.
37. Davis Dawn MR, Drucker Aaron M, Alikhan Ali, et al. AAD Guidelines: Awareness of comorbidities associated with atopic dermatitis in adults. *J Am Acad Dermatol.* 2022. 10.1016/j.jaad.2022.01.009.
38. Eichenfield LF, Tom WL, Berger TG, et al. Guidelines of care for the management of atopic dermatitis. Section 2. Management and treatment of atopic dermatitis with topical therapies. *J Am Acad Dermatol.* 2014;71:116–132.
39. Angelova-Fischer I, Neufang G, Jung K, et al. A randomized, investigator-blinded efficacy assessment study of stand-alone emollient use in mild to moderately severe atopic dermatitis flares. *J Eur Acad Dermatol Venereol.* 2014;(suppl 3):9–15.
40. Horimukai K, Morita K, Narita M, et al. Application of moisturizer to neonates prevents development of atopic dermatitis. *J Allergy Clin Immunol.* 2014;134:824–830. e6.
41. Rubel D, Thirumoorthy T, Soebaryo W, et al. Consensus guidelines for the management of atopic dermatitis: An Asia-Pacific perspective. *J Dermatol.* 2013;40:160–171.
42. Baron SE, Cohen SN, Archer CB. British Association of Dermatologists and Royal College of General Practitioners. Guidance on the diagnosis and clinical management of atopic eczema. *Clin Exp Dermatol.* 2012;37(suppl 1):7–12.
43. Aries MF, Hernandez-Pigeon H, Vaissiere C, et al. Anti-inflammatory and immunomodulatory effects of *Aquaphilus dolomiae* extract on in vitro models. *Clin Cosmet Investig Dermatol.* 2016;9:421–434.
44. Bianchi P, Theunis J, Casas C, et al. Effects of a new emollient-based treatment on skin microflora balance and barrier function in children with mild atopic dermatitis. *Pediatr Dermatol.* 2016;33:175–171.
45. Fostini AC, Georgescu V, Decoster CI, Girolomini G. A cream based on *Aquaphilus dolomiae* extracts alleviates non-histaminergic pruritus in humans. *Eur J Dermatol.* 2017;27:317–318.
46. Law RM, Kwa PG, Maibach HI, et al. Atopic dermatitis: The itch that erupts when scratched. In: Schwinghammer TL, ed., et al. *Pharmacotherapy Casebook: A Patient-Focused Approach.* 11th ed. New York: McGraw-Hill; 2020.
47. Rosso JD, Friedlander SF. Corticosteroids: Options in the era of steroid-sparing therapy. *J Am Acad Dermatol.* 2005;53:S50–S58.
48. Hengge UR, Ruzicka T, Schwartz RA, et al. Adverse effects of topical glucocorticosteroids. *J Am Acad Dermatol.* 2006;54:1–15.
49. Hebert AA; Desonide Foam Phase III Clinical Study Group. Desonide foam 0.05%: Safety in children as young as 3 months. *J Am Acad Dermatol.* 2008;59:334–340.
50. Stuetz A, Grassberger M, Meingassner JG. Pimecrolimus (Elidel, SDZ ASM 981)—Preclinical pharmacologic profile and skin selectivity. *Semin Cutan Med Surg.* 2001;20:233–241.
51. Berger TG, Duvic M, Van Voorhees AS, Frieden IJ. The use of topical calcineurin inhibitors in dermatology: Safety concerns. *J Am Acad Dermatol.* 2006;54:818–823.
52. Healy E, Bentley A, Fidler C, Chambers C. Cost-effectiveness of tacrolimus ointment in adults and children with moderate and severe atopic dermatitis: Twice-weekly maintenance treatment vs. standard twice-daily reactive treatment of exacerbations from a third party payer (U.K. National Health Service) perspective. *Br J Dermatol.* 2011;164:387–395.
53. Thaci D, Chambers C, Sidu M, et al. Twice-weekly treatment with tacrolimus 0.03% ointment in children with atopic dermatitis: Clinical efficacy and economic impact over 12 months. *J Eur Acad Dermatol Venereol.* 2010;24:1040–1046.
54. Margolis DJ, Abuabara K, Hoffstad OJ, et al. Association between malignancy and topical use of pimecrolimus. *JAMA Dermatol.* 2015;151:594–599.
55. Deleuran M, Vewtergaard C, Volund A, et al. Topical calcineurin inhibitors, topical glucocorticoids and cancer in children: A nationwide study. *Acta Derm Venereol.* 2016;96:834–835.
56. Pughdal KV, Schwartz RA. Topical tar: Back to the future. *J Am Acad Dermatol.* 2009;61:294–302.
57. Kitzen JM, Pergolizzi JV, Taylor R, et al. Crisaborole and apremilast: PDE4 inhibitors with similar mechanism of action, different indications for management of inflammatory skin conditions. *Pharmacology & Pharmacy.* 2018;9:357–381.
58. Samrao A, Berry TM, Goreshi R, Simpson EL. A pilot study of an oral phosphodiesterase inhibitor (apremilast) for atopic dermatitis in adults. *Arch Dermatol.* 2012;148:890–1108.
59. Saporito RC, Cohen DJ. Apremilast use for moderate-to-severe atopic dermatitis in pediatric patients. *Case Rep Dermatol.* 2016;8:179–184.
60. Sidbury R, Davis DM, Cohen DE, et al. Guidelines of care for the management of atopic dermatitis. Section 3. Management and treatment with phototherapy and systemic agents. *J Am Acad Dermatol.* 2014;71:327–349.
61. Dotterud LK, Wilsgaard T, Vorland LH, et al. The effect of UVB radiation on skin microbiota in patients with atopic dermatitis and health controls. *Int J Circumpolar Health.* 2008;67:254–260.

62. Harper JI, Ahmed I, Barclay G, et al. Cyclosporin for severe childhood atopic dermatitis: Short course versus continuous therapy. *Br J Dermatol.* 2000;142:52–58.
63. Hanifin JM, Schneider LC, Leung DY, et al. Recombinant interferon gamma therapy for atopic dermatitis. *J Am Acad Dermatol.* 1993;28:189–197.
64. Jang IG, Yang JK, Lee HJ, et al. Clinical improvement and immunohistochemical findings in severe atopic dermatitis treated with interferon gamma. *J Am Acad Dermatol.* 2000;42:1033–1040.
65. Meggitt SJ, Gray JC, Reynolds NJ. Azathioprine doses by thiopurine methyltransferase activity for moderate-to-severe atopic eczema: A double-blind, randomized controlled trial. *Lancet.* 2006;367:839–846.
66. Rouse C, Siegfried E. Methotrexate for atopic dermatitis in children. *J Am Acad Dermatol.* 2008;58(2 suppl 2):AB7, abstract P608.
67. Seegraber M, Srour J, Walter A, et al. Dupilumab for treatment of atopic dermatitis. *Expert Rev Clin Pharmacol.* 2018;11(5):467–474.
68. Toledo F, Silvestre JF, Munoz C. Combined therapy with low-dose omalizumab and intravenous immunoglobulin for severe atopic dermatitis. Report of four cases. *J Eur Acad Dermatol Venereol.* 2012;26:1325–1327.
69. Blauvelt Andrew, Teixeira Henrique D, Simpson Eric L, et al. Efficacy and safety of upadacitinib vs dupilumab in adults with moderate-to-severe atopic dermatitis. *JAMA Dermatology.* 2021;157:1047–1055. 10.1001/jamadermatol.2021.3023.
70. Koo J, Arain S. Traditional Chinese medicine for the treatment of dermatologic disorders. *Arch Dermatol.* 1998;134:1388–1393.
71. Tan HY, Zhang AL, Chen DC, et al. Chinese herbal medicine for atopic dermatitis: A systematic review. *J Am Acad Dermatol.* 2013;69:295–230.
72. Patel R, DuPont HL. New approaches for bacteriotherapy: Prebiotics, new-generation probiotics, and synbiotics. *Clin Infect Dis.* 2015;60(suppl 2):S108–S121.
73. Elazab N, Mendy A, Gasana J, et al. Probiotic administration in early life, atopy, and asthma: A meta-analysis of clinical trials. *Pediatrics.* 2013;132:e666–e676.
74. Yesilova Y, Calka O, Akdeniz N, et al. Effect of probiotic on the treatment of children with atopic dermatitis. *Ann Dermatol.* 2012;24:189–193.
75. Lin RJ, Qiu LH, Guan RZ, et al. Protective effect of probiotics in the treatment of infantile eczema. *Experimental and Therapeutic Medicine.* 2015;9:1593–1596.
76. Bouhnik Y, Flourie B, D'Agay-Abensour L, et al. Administration of transgalato-oligosaccharides increases fecal bifidobacteria and modifies colonic fermentation metabolism in healthy humans. *J Nutr.* 1997;127:444–448.
77. Baquerizo Nole KL, Yim E, Keri JE. Probiotics and prebiotics in dermatology. *J Am Acad Dermatol.* 2014;71:814–821.
78. Osborn DA, Sinn J. Prebiotics in infants for prevention of allergy. *Cochrane Database Syst Rev.* 2013;3.
79. Bae JM, Choi YY, Park CO, et al. Efficacy of allergen-specific immunotherapy for atopic dermatitis: A systematic review and meta-analysis of randomized controlled trials. *J Allergy Clin Immunol.* 2013;132:110–117.
80. Izadi N, Leung DYM. Clinical approach to the patient with refractory atopic dermatitis. *Ann Allergy Asthma Immunol.* 2018;120(1):23–33.e1. doi:10.1016/j.anai.2017.09.061.
81. Zuberbier T, Orlow SJ, Paller AS, et al. Patient perspectives on the management of atopic dermatitis. *J Allergy Clin Immunol.* 2006;118:226–232.
82. Simpson EL, Guttman-Yassky E, Margolis DJ, et al. Association of inadequately controlled disease and disease severity with patient-reported disease burden in adults with atopic dermatitis. *JAMA Dermatol.* 2018;154(8):903–912. doi:10.1001/jamadermatol.2018.1572.
83. Bridgman AC, Eshtiaghi P, Cresswell-Melville A, Ramien M, Drucker AM. The burden of moderate to severe atopic dermatitis in Canadian children: A cross-sectional survey. *J Cutan Med Surg.* 2018;22(4):443–444. doi:10.1177/1203475418761859.
84. Eckert L, Gupta S, Gadkari A, Mahajan P, Gelfand JM. Burden of illness in adults with atopic dermatitis: Analysis of National Health and Wellness Survey data from France, Germany, Italy, Spain, and the United Kingdom. *J Am Acad Dermatol.* 2019;81(1):187–195. doi:10.1016/j.jaad.2019.03.037.

Alopecia

Rebecca M. Law, Le Hanh Dung Do, and Howard I. Maibach

120

KEY CONCEPTS

1. The hair cycle consists of three phases: anagen, catagen, and telogen. These are not synchronized across all hair follicles. Different factors regulate each phase of the hair cycle.
2. Pattern hair loss (or androgenetic alopecia) is an inherited condition in which androgens play a key role.
3. Inflammation plays an important role in alopecia. Inflammatory infiltrates are evident in androgenetic alopecia and alopecia areata. Alopecia areata is the most frequent cause of inflammation-induced alopecia. Chronic inflammation may lead to the destruction of the hair follicle, resulting in irreversible hair loss.
4. Scarring hair loss (or cicatricial alopecia) leading to irreversible hair loss can be caused by chronic inflammation or secondary to burns, cancer, trauma, radiation, or other diseases such as lichen planopilaris and chronic cutaneous lupus erythematosus.
5. Thinning of hair or hair loss is usually the only clinical sign of alopecia. Other symptoms (eg, itching, pain, burning, or prickly discomfort) would suggest other underlying disease conditions. Dermatologic diseases can cause hair loss, which varies from mild, nonscarring, and reversible to scarring and irreversible.
6. Alopecia can be distressing, affecting the quality of life and causing psychological problems. Psychosocial support and counseling must not be overlooked.
7. Treatment and management strategies of alopecia should be as cause-specific as possible. Identified causes (eg, iron deficiency, tinea capitis) should be treated and/or eliminated as soon as practically feasible.
8. Treatment for androgenetic alopecia includes topical minoxidil, oral 5α-reductase inhibitors (finasteride, dutasteride) for men, hormonal therapy for women, and miscellaneous therapies including nutritional supplements and laser light therapy with variable efficacy.
9. Treatment for alopecia areata includes intralesional corticosteroids, topical corticosteroids, high-dose oral corticosteroids, topical minoxidil, topical immunotherapy, topical and systemic biologic agents (in particular JAK inhibitors), azathioprine and other immunosuppressive agents, and other miscellaneous therapies.
10. Treatment of alopecia in patients of color should include cultural sensitivity for hair stigma (patient hair differs from perceived societal norm) and hair discordance (racial discordance between health professionals and patients seeking care for alopecia).

BEYOND THE BOOK

Read this continuing medical education article: "Hair Loss: Common Causes and Treatment," by T. Grant Phillips, W. P. Slomiany, and R. Allison.[1]

INTRODUCTION

Having a full head of hair is of some importance to most adults and children. Alopecia, defined in the Oxford Dictionary as "the partial or complete absence of hair from areas of the body where it normally grows," is a condition with a myriad of causes. This chapter reviews normal hair growth and physiology and discusses some of the known causes and types of alopecia.

ANATOMY AND PHYSIOLOGY OF THE HAIR FOLLICLE

Hair covers most of the human body and grows both outside and inside of the skin. The external part is keratinized nonliving hair shaft, and the living follicles are located below the skin surface. The visible dead shaft mostly remains constant, while the living follicles continuously regenerate.[2,3]

The hair follicle is part of the human skin. It begins in the dermis with the hair bulb and the hair shaft, which extend through the epidermis and out into the external environment. The dermis provides support for the hair bulb, hair shaft, and other skin structures and appendages. The hair follicle and the sebaceous gland form a pilosebaceous unit with a common duct opening into the environment (Fig. 120-1). (For discussions of other components in skin, refer to Chapter e121, "Drug-Induced Dermatologic Disorders.")

The hair shaft comprises three layers from outside to inside: the cuticle, the cortex, and the medulla. The cuticle consists of hard, colorless cells that overlap. This outermost layer is responsible for elasticity and resiliency; it determines the general condition of the hair. The cortex contains melanin and thus determines hair color. It also contains keratin and determines whether the hair is straight or curly. The innermost layer is the medulla, which plays an important role in supporting the structure of hair.

Below the skin surface, the hair follicle is divided into upper and lower segments by the insertion site of the arrector pili muscle. The upper segment comprises the infundibulum and the isthmus (Fig. 120-2). The infundibulum is a funnel-shaped cavity that serves as a reservoir of the sebaceous gland. It is filled with sebum, and

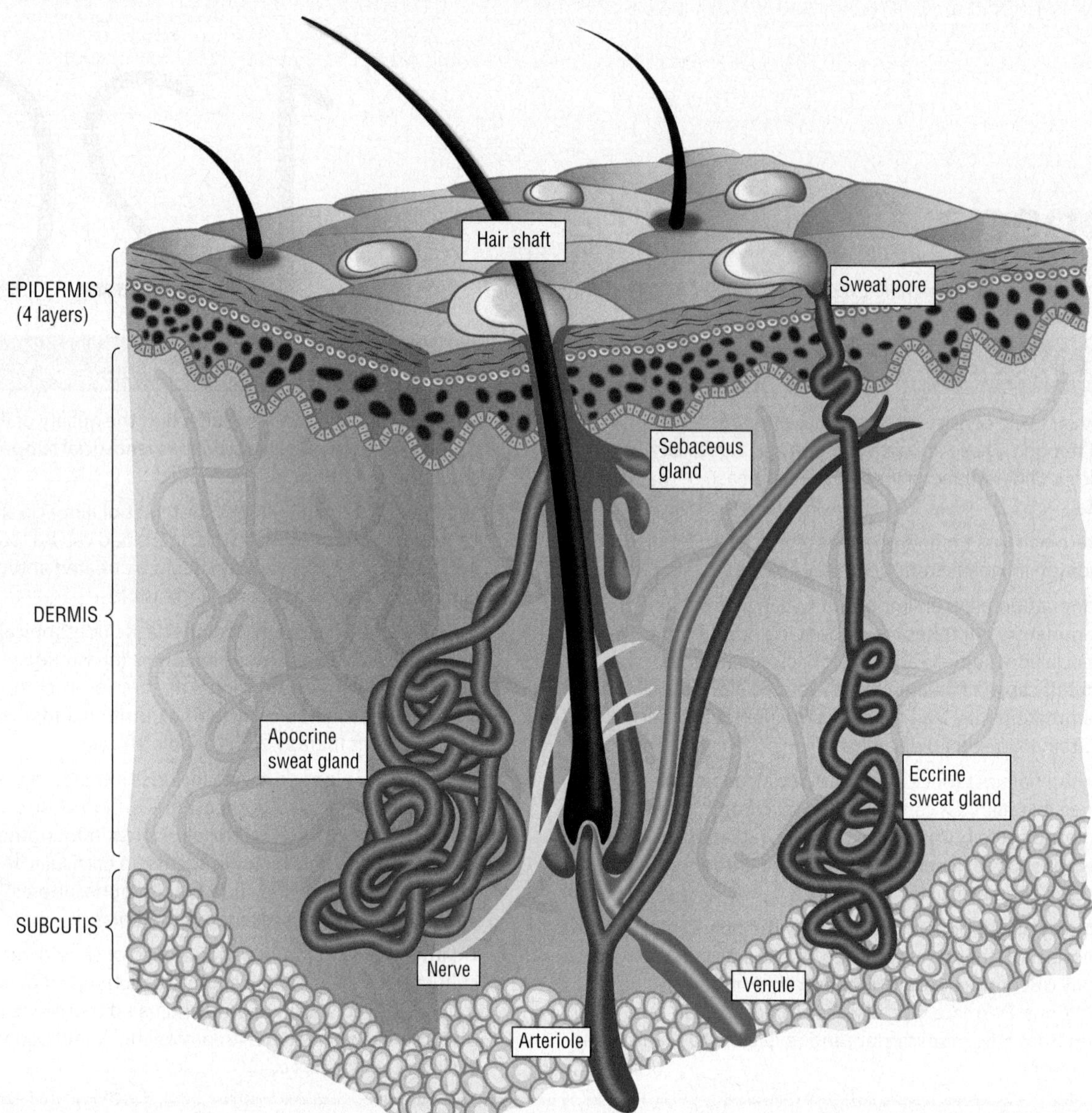

FIGURE 120-1 The hair follicle and its relationship to other structures and appendages of the human skin. Refer to Chapter e121, "Drug-Induced Dermatologic Disorders," for discussions about other components in skin. *(Original artwork courtesy of Rebecca Law, ©2018 by R Law, all rights reserved.)*

covered by an impermeable stratum corneum. The isthmus lies below the infundibulum, and it connects the duct of the sebaceous gland to the arrector pili muscle. The lower segment of the hair follicle contains the stem and the hair bulb. Adamson's fringe is the boundary between anucleate cells in the stem and nucleated cells in the bulb. The hair bulb contains nerve fibers, a capillary network, and loose connective tissue called the dermal papilla. Nerves and arterioles that supply the follicles are arranged as a plexus, arising from the subcutaneous fat to the dermis. The dermal papilla is a pear-shaped structure that consists of active cells and growth factors, which can induce hair growth and pigmentation.

The Hair Cycle

1 The hair cycle consists of three phases; these are not synchronized among all hair follicles. The phases are the anagen, catagen, and telogen phases, followed by an intermediary "returning to anagen" phase (Fig. 120-3).[4]

Most of the hairs are in the *anagen phase* (also known as the growth phase). At the beginning of this phase, hair stem cells multiply, grow downward into the dermis, and differentiate into the hair shaft,[5] where the melanocytes start producing pigment. While the anagen phase of short hairs (eg, eyelashes, eyebrows, hairs on arms, and legs) lasts around 1 month, those of longer scalp hairs can last up to 6 years. Scalp hairs of an adult grow at a rate of about 1 mm per 3 days.

The anagen phase is regulated by factors as listed in column 1 of Table 120-1. Since hairs in this phase are growing, regulation is mostly by growth factors.

Overall, about 1% to 3% of hairs are in the *catagen phase* (also known as the transition phase). It begins when the anagen phase ends. The hair follicle starts to undergo apoptosis and reduces in size. The keratinocytes decrease proliferation, melanocytes decrease the production of pigments, and the hair shaft is no longer lengthened. The dermal papilla is transformed into a cluster of inactive cells along with the shrinking hair follicle. This phase lasts about 2 to 3 weeks.

The catagen phase is regulated by factors as listed in column 2 of Table 120-1.[7] Note that Interleukin 1b (IL-1b) and tumor necrosis

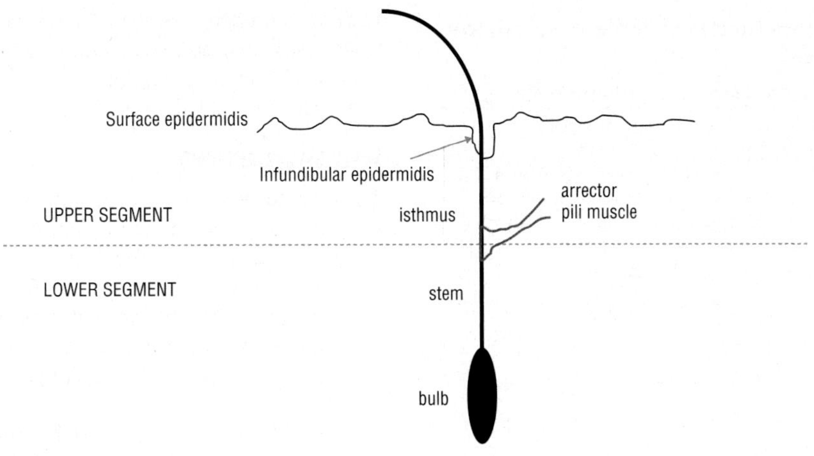

FIGURE 120-2 The hair follicle.

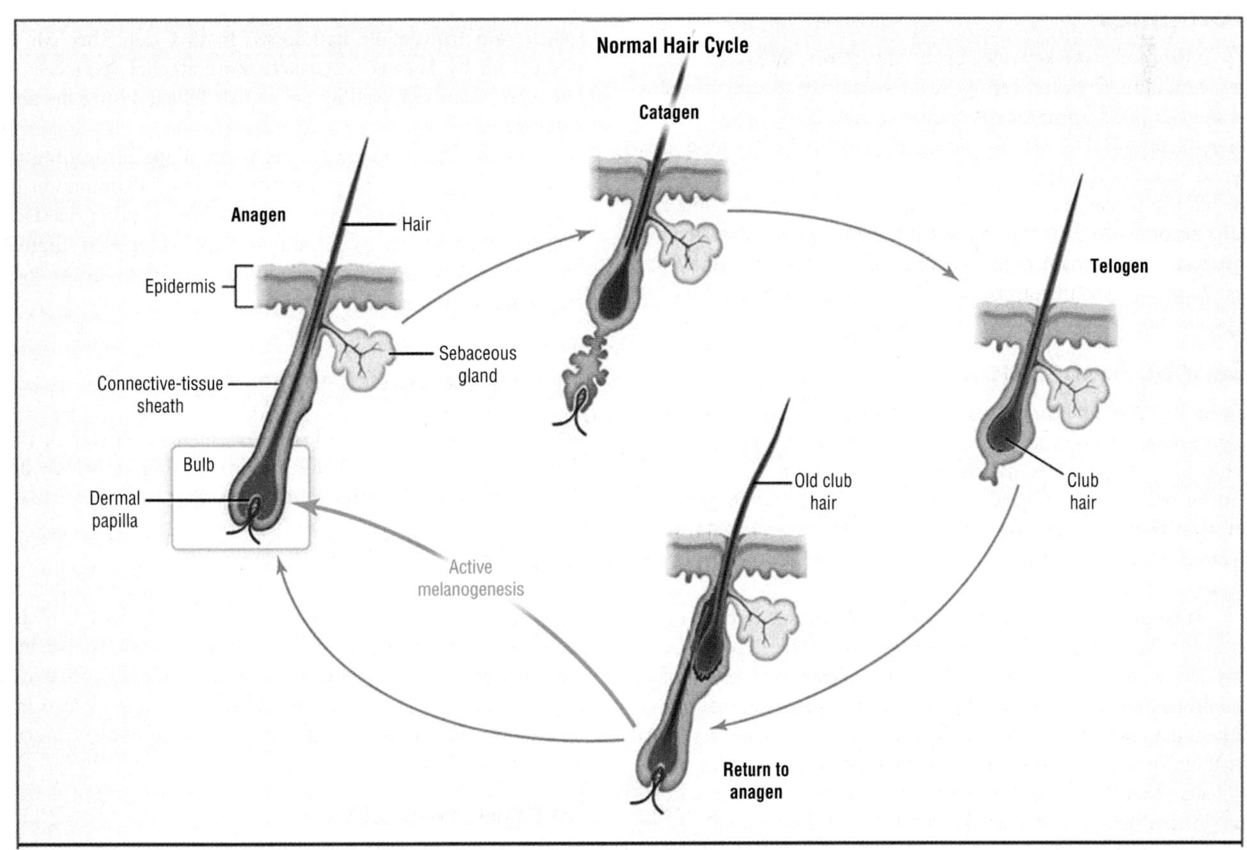

FIGURE 120-3 The normal hair cycle. *(Reprinted with permission from Gilhar A, Etzioni A, Paus R. Alopecia areata. N Engl J Med. 2012;366(16):1515–1525.)*

factor α (TNF-α) aid the inhibition of growth factors, leading to a decrease in proliferation of hair follicles.

The *telogen phase* begins after the catagen phase ends and lasts for 1 to 3 months, with 10% to 15% of hairs. The hair and the dermal papilla go into a resting phase and melanocytes go into apoptosis.

This phase is regulated by various hormones (thyroid hormones, androgens, prolactin, ACTH, and others) as listed in column 3 of Table 120-1. In the end, the hair falls out (*exogen phase*) at a usual rate of 50 to 100 scalp hairs per day.

The follicle rests for a few weeks and then proceeds to the growth phase with the multipotent stem cells from the bulge area. Generally, hair grows until the fourth decade of life. After that age period, the majority of hair follicles are in the catagen and telogen phases, which leads to thinning of the hair, and baldness.

TABLE 120-1 Regulatory Factors of Three Phases in the Hair Cycle

Anagen Phase	Catagen Phase	Telogen Phase
Bone morphogenetic protein (BMP) Sonic hedgehog WNT proteins and receptors Insulin-like growth factor-1 (IGF-1) Fibroblast growth factor-7 (FGF-7) Hepatic growth factor (HGF) Vascular endothelial growth factor (VEGF)	FGF-5 Transforming growth factor β1 (TGF-β1) Interleukin 1b (IL-1b) Neurotrophins NT-3, NT-4 Bone morphogenetic protein BMP2/4 Tumor necrosis factor α (TNF-α)	Androgens Prolactin Adrenocorticotropic hormone (ACTH) Retinoids and thyroid hormones Estrogen FGF-5 BMP-4[6]

PATHOPHYSIOLOGY

Hormones

2 Androgens play a key role in pattern hair loss, which is an inherited condition characterized by scalp sensitivity to dihydrotestosterone (DHT). Testosterone is converted into DHT by the enzyme 5α-reductase. DHT binds to androgen receptors in the same manner as testosterone, but with much greater affinity. DHT shortens the telogen phase, leading to more rapid hair loss. With aging, new hairs become insufficient to replace the shed ones and contribute to alopecia. This mechanism is observed both in male and female pattern hair loss. Treatment protocols for alopecia using inhibitors of 5α-reductase are proven to be effective.[8]

Genetic Association

2 In the 1990s and early 2000s, observations that there is a resemblance between alopecia in fathers and sons led to suggestions that genes from some autosomal chromosomes were the cause of male pattern baldness. Postulated genes included the insulin gene, the 5α-reductase genes, and the hairless gene.[9] However, further investigations[10-12] found only a weak association between those genes and male pattern alopecia.

Maternal inheritance of male pattern alopecia with their investigation of variants of androgen receptor locus on the X chromosome was demonstrated.[13] This implied that the phenotypic resemblance should be higher between affected males and their maternal grandfathers than between affected males and their fathers. However, the attributable risk from this case–control study was only 0.46, which indicated that the remaining risk fraction was due to other autosomal loci, which may explain the similarity of the alopecia pattern between fathers and sons.

Genetic predisposition has been shown for alopecia areata (AA) through a genome-wide association study that identified eight susceptibility loci and 139 single-nucleotide polymorphisms associated with the activation and proliferation of T-cells, IL-2 receptors, natural killer cell receptors, genes expressed in the hair follicle, and other factors.[14] A follow-up study established IL-13 and KIAA0350/CLEC16A as susceptibility loci for AA.[15] Research is ongoing.

Hair Cycle Dynamics

The hair cycle itself was one of the key factors in alopecia.[16] As mentioned above, maximal hair length is achieved in the *anagen phase.* If this phase is too short, patients may present with shortened hair. In some cases, the *anagen* duration may significantly decline, which may lead to empty follicular pores.[17] A shortened *anagen phase* leads to a premature progression to the *telogen phase*, which contributes to a decrease in hair diameter (clinically seen as fine hair) and hair loss. Patients also present with longer duration of the *telogen phase* and latency to the next hair cycle. This lag worsens the effect of alopecia.

Inflammation

3 Inflammation plays an important role in alopecia. Lymphohistiocytic infiltrate in the perifollicular area was shown, with collagen deposition four times higher in patients with male pattern alopecia than in normal controls.[18] Morphometric and ultrastructural analyses of the transitional zones in patients with male pattern alopecia were performed and found a significant increase in the number of mast cells and lymphocytes around the follicular epithelium.[19]

A study in 2012 also showed greater eosinophilic infiltration around lower hair follicles and mononuclear cell count in diffuse AA.[20] A 2012 review described AA as an autoimmune inflammatory disorder in which hair follicles are attacked by a mixed inflammatory cell infiltrate containing T-cells, natural killer cells, mast cells, and dendritic cells.[4]

Scarring

3 Chronic inflammation may lead to the destruction of the hair follicle and irreversible hair loss.[21] In this case, the hair follicle is replaced by fibrous tissue and the epithelial stem cells in the bulge are destroyed, leading to the hair follicle losing the ability to regenerate.[22]

4 Scarring alopecia (or cicatricial alopecia) leading to irreversible hair loss can be caused by chronic inflammation or secondary to burns, cancer, trauma, radiation, or other diseases such as lichen planopilaris and chronic cutaneous lupus erythematosus. This type of scarring alopecia is discussed further in the "Scarring Hair Loss" section.

CLINICAL PRESENTATION

5 Thinning of hair or hair loss is usually the only sign of alopecia. Other symptoms such as itching, pain, burning, or prickly discomfort may suggest other underlying conditions.

Anagen Hair Loss

Anagen hair loss or anagen effluvium usually has a sudden onset.[23] Patients present with the chief complaint of short hair and the inability to grow longer hair. The hair can be thin, sparse, but usually not fragile. Empty follicles can also be seen. Most cases of anagen effluvium are reversible and hair can regrow in 6 months. Common causes and presentations of anagen effluvium are listed in Table 120-2.

Telogen Hair Loss

Telogen hair loss or telogen effluvium starts with thinning of hair, especially at the temples. It is a noninflammatory alopecia, usually of sudden onset.[2] Patients can lose 300 to 500 hairs a day, which is 2 to 3 times more than usual hair loss in a healthy individual. Hairs appear to be short, thin, and lacking melanin.

Telogen effluvium is usually seen 3 months after a medical condition that stops hair growth, such as childbirth, surgery, hormonal imbalance, or medications. The *telogen phase* normally lasts for about 3 months; if the condition is caused by drugs, hair can regrow after 4 months of drug withdrawal. The various systemic medical conditions affect the scalp, resulting in nonscarring alopecia. Medical causes include iron deficiency, thyroid hormone deficiency, systemic lupus erythematosus, syphilis, bacterial infections, and viral infection (herpes zoster). Medical and other causes are listed in Table 120-3.

TABLE 120-2 Characteristics of Hair Loss in Anagen Effluvium

Causes	Presentations
Autoimmune disease—severe diffuse alopecia areata[20]	Diffuse and rapid hair shedding with exclamation point hairs, usually starts with a round patch, then spreads in a multilocular pattern.
Chemotherapy-induced alopecia[24]	Patients who recently received anticancer chemotherapeutic agents, radiation treatment, and other medications. Not all anticancer agents/treatments cause hair loss.
	Usually, recovery occurs within 6 months of treatment completion/drug discontinuation.
Inherited/congenital condition—loose anagen syndrome[25]	Predominantly seen in young girls between 2 and 6 years, but sometimes in boys. Diffuse or patchy alopecia often seen in the occiput.

TABLE 120-3 Causes of Telogen Effluvium

Pregnancy
Psychological stress
Fever, infection, hemorrhage, surgery
Weight loss
Autoimmune diseases (most common is systemic lupus erythematosus), thyroid hormone deficiency
Localized telogen effluvium following hair transplantation[26]
Vitamin or mineral deficiency—iron deficiency is a common cause of hair loss in women
Medications: contraceptives, anticoagulants, anticonvulsants, isotretinoin, warfarin

TABLE 120-4 Male and Female Pattern Hair Loss

Male Pattern Hair Loss	Female Pattern Hair Loss
Gradual loss of the frontal hairline early in the process.	The frontal hairline is often preserved. Gradual thinning leading to widening of the part line.
Gradual thinning in the vertex and temporal areas.	Thinning hair on the mid-frontal area of the scalp. Diffuse pattern. Hair loss is generally less severe than that which occurs in males.

TABLE 120-5 Dermatological Diseases That Can Cause Hair Loss

Diseases	Presentations
Tinea capitis[28]	Gray patch (scaling with patchy hair loss), black dot, and diffuseal opecia. But on occasions, severely inflammatory and raised lesions can occur.
Psoriatic alopecia[29]	Often nonscarring and regrows after a few months. Complete destruction of the follicle leads to the inability to regrow.
Seborrheic dermatitis of the scalp[30]	From mild desquamation to honey-colored crusts attached to scalp and hair leading to alopecia. May reach into forehead as scaly erythematous border known as "corona seborrheica."
Allergic contact dermatitis of the scalp[31]	Mild hair loss 2-4 months after the episode of scalp dermatitis.
Pityriasis rubra pilaris[32]	Eczematous changes of the skin, ichthyosiform scale on lower extremities, coarse laminated palmoplantar keratoderma, and alopecia.
Erythroderma (a generalized disease)	Generalized erythema and exfoliation, patients sometimes present with malaise, fever or hypothermia, pruritus, diffuse alopecia, keratoderma, nail dystrophy, ectropion, pitting edema, lymphade nopathy, tachycardia, and high-output cardiac failure.[33]

Androgenetic Alopecia

Distinct patterns of hair loss are seen in boys/men and girls/women (Table 120-4).

2 Male pattern hair loss, or androgenetic alopecia (AGA), is the most common type of hair loss; it most often occurs in adult males.[23] AGA is caused by the effects of DHT in specific areas of the scalp such as the vertex and the temporal scalp. Patients usually have a vivid memory of a transitional time from having thick, long pigmented hairs to thinner, shorter hairs with less pigment.

A few women present with male pattern hair loss (AGA) caused by excessive levels of androgens, which leads to thinning hair on the mid-frontal area, but the condition is usually milder than in men. Polycystic ovarian syndrome (PCOS) and congenital adrenal hyperplasia are the common causes of male pattern hair loss in women.

Female pattern hair loss (FPHL or female AGA) usually presents with preservation of the frontal hairline with widening of the part line and reduced hair volume. These women are mostly losing their hair with age and hormone tests are normal. The Ludwig Classification is often used to describe FPHL, with Type I being minimal thinning that can be camouflaged with hair styling techniques and Type III being diffuse thinning with a see-through appearance on the top of the scalp.[27]

Dermatological Disease

3 4 5 Dermatological conditions on the scalp may result in scarring or nonscarring patchy hair thinning and alopecia. Table 120-5 provides some common diseases and their presentations.

Scarring Hair Loss

3 4 Scarring hair loss, or cicatricial alopecia, can be primary or secondary to indirect causes, such as burns, cancer, trauma, or radiation. Table 120-6 provides common causes of scarring hair loss and their presentations.

Alopecia Areata

3 Alopecia areata (AA) is the most frequent cause of inflammation-induced hair loss, affecting perhaps 4.5 million people in the United States.[4] AA affects both children and adults, with prevalence rates peaking between the ages of 20 and 40 years; up to 66% of AA patients are younger than 30 years and only 20% are older than 40 years.[4] Although AA generally occurs equally in males and females,[4,34] one study involving subjects 21 to 30 years found male dominance.[35]

AA is a nonscarring, autoimmune inflammatory disease that manifests in the hair follicles and can affect the nails in up to two-thirds of patients.[36] Due to the autoimmune nature of the disease, hair-follicle specific autoantibodies may be detected and other autoimmune conditions may be associated. There is a familial tendency with an especially high concordance rate in monozygotic twins, and genetic polymorphisms have been identified in multiple regions of the human genome.[34]

AA presents as an acute, patchy alopecia (with a well-circumscribed solitary or multiple patches) that is most commonly seen on the scalp but can be elsewhere in the body.[36,37] Patches up to 2 cm (~0.8 in.) in diameter can suddenly appear overnight then extend

TABLE 120-6 Characteristics of Scarring Hair Loss

Causes	Presentations
Lichen planopilaris	<10% scalp involvement (localized) Generalized Rapidly progressing Itchy, multifocal, or central patches with follicular hyperke ratosis and perifollicular erythema; nonscalp areas may be affected
Chronic cutaneous lupus erythematosus	Single or multifocal patches with pronounced activity in the center of the patch, ulceration, follicular plugging, atrophy, and depigmentation
Frontal fibrosing alopecia	Band-like distribution around the frontal hairline; may be present in eyebrows
Central centrifugal cicatricial alopecia	Resembles lichen planopilaris; burning, scaling, and itchiness may occur
Brocq pseudopelade	Small and/or large, irregular patches of hair loss on the scalp with no detectable symptoms or inflammation; end-stage burnout
Folliculitis decalvans	Single patch of complete alopecia that expands circumferentially, slowly over years; typically found on hair-bearing periphery of scalp; pustules, honey-colored crusting, tufting; nonscalp involvement is rare
Dissecting cellulitis of the scalp	Multiple fluctuant nodules found across the scalp, often interconnected by sinus tracts; may be associated with acne conglobata: discharge is common and should be cultured

TABLE 120-7 Classifications of Alopecia Areata

Types	Descriptions
Patchy AA	The most common type; localized hair loss; patchy; most commonly on scalp, sometimes involving beard area
AA totalis	Total hair loss on the scalp
AA universalis	Complete hair loss in all hair-bearing areas
Acute diffuse and total alopecia	Short clinical course ranging from a little hair loss to total baldness; favorable prognosis; rapid disease resolution, sometimes without treatment
Diffuse AA	Diffuse hair loss; can mimic telogen effluvium
Ophiasis	Hair loss only on the sides of the scalp (occipital areas) and the nape
Sisapho	A rare condition in which hair loss spares the sides of the scalp (occipital areas) and the nape and usually affects the central scalphis
Reticular patches	Several patches of AA coalescing to form a reticular pattern

Data from References 4 and 34.

TABLE 120-8 Common Causes of Hair Loss in Children

Tinea capitis
Alopecia areata
Telogen effluvium
Traction alopecia
Diffuse hair loss with abnormal texture
Trichotillomania
Hair abnormalities with atopic eczema
Folliculitis decalvans

circumferentially at a rate of about 1 cm/week (0.4 in./week); the hair loss consists of hair breakage close to or just below the skin surface. As a result, black dots can be seen on dermoscopy, with characteristic "exclamation mark" hairs—that is, hairs where the distal hair shaft is broader than the proximal end—around the margins of the patch of hair loss.[4] Table 120-7 lists the types of AA.

AA involves abnormality in the hair cycle (shortened and disordered) due to the activity of inflammatory mediators released by a mixed inflammatory cell infiltrate (Fig. 120-4).[4]

Alopecia in Children

Hair loss in the pediatric population is more common than expected—about 7.5% of pediatric patients in dermatology practices.[38] Although sharing many features with alopecia in adults, children may present with unique associations that require further examination.

A 5-year study in Jordan[38] showed that the three most common causes of alopecia in children are tinea capitis (40.5%), AA (17.6%), and telogen effluvium (17%). Tinea capitis is often straightforward with additional findings, such as itchy erythema and scaly border. However, in some communities, parents use unknown topical/herbal creams, some of which contain corticosteroids, and these can mask the presentation of tinea capitis. Therefore, potassium hydroxide (KOH) testing plays an important role in etiologic diagnosis.

Autoimmune diseases were found in 13.5% of the pediatric AA cases, including diabetes, hypothyroidism, and vitiligo. In pediatric AA, the male:female ratio is 3:2,[38] compared to 1:2.3 in adults.[39]

Telogen effluvium in children is commonly caused by a prior low-grade fever.[38] All of these cases presented with a healthy scalp, normal hair texture, and regular bulb of telogen hair. This condition was seen more in female children, usually within 4 to 6 months before coming to the clinic.

Approximately 20% of the examined cases had some elements of traction alopecia,[38] with female predominance and occurring at the hairline. Moreover, some cases showed follicular pustules and perifollicular inflammation. This type of hair loss may be more common than the 20% seen, as traction alopecia is easily noticed by parents and reversed by wearing a loosened hair style, perhaps making it underrepresented in the clinic.

Trichotillomania is an impulse-control disorder where patients consciously or unconsciously pull, twist, or twirl their hair. It is a relatively common disorder in children. The mean age of onset is at about age 13 years, and it affects an estimated 4% of the population. Patients usually present with frontoparietal patches of alopecia that progress posteriorly and bare patches are typical. Trichoscopy shows broken hair shafts of various lengths typically with frayed "split ends." The condition is associated with problems of self-esteem and social avoidance. Complications include infection, skin damage, and scarring.[1,40]

The above and other causes of hair loss in children are listed in Table 120-8.

COMPLICATIONS

6 Like other medical conditions, alopecia can be distressing, affecting the quality of life and causing psychological problems.[41] Loss of normal scalp hair increases the risk of sunburn and injury. Moreover, studies have shown that hair loss can be associated with depression, low self-esteem, and feelings of unattractiveness. Some studies show that men with hair loss are perceived, based solely on appearance, to be not as attractive and successful as men without hair loss. This is further discussed below in the "Hair Stigma" section.

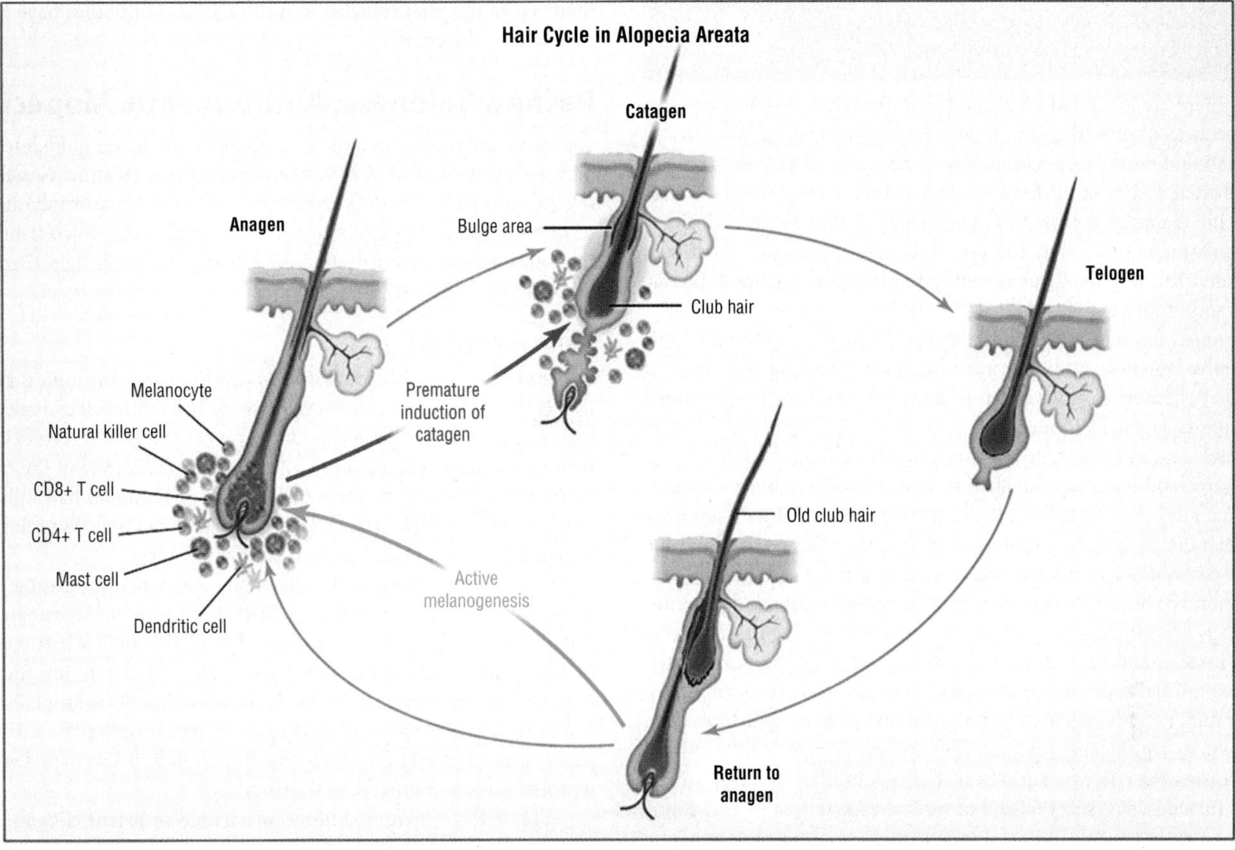

FIGURE 120-4 The hair cycle in alopecia areata. *(Reprinted with permission from Gilhar A, Etzioni A, Paus R. Alopecia areata. N Engl J Med. 2012;366(16):1515–1525.)*

DIAGNOSIS

Diagnosis of alopecia usually can be made clinically: by a meticulous patient history plus skin and hair examination. In cases of less certainty, further workup may be warranted.

Regarding patient history, the essential points to obtain include time of onset, course of hair loss, past medical history (autoimmune disease, medications, procedures, or surgery), and family history of alopecia. In children, physical and mental development should also be obtained. Then, an extensive physical evaluation can be performed to assess whether the patient has hypotrichosis or alopecia, the type of alopecia, hair shaft anomalies, hair quality, and other conditions of the scalp, including erythema, edema, pustules, scaling, atrophy, or scarring.

For hair examination, the hair tug and pull test is clinically popular since it is quick and easy to use, and it can also be done at multiple locations on the scalp for a more thorough assessment. This test distinguishes between loss from follicles and loss due to hair shaft fragility. First, the patient's hairs are separated into a 4- to 6-mm diameter bundle (approximately 50-60 hairs). The tug portion of the test involves gentle holding of hairs between the thumb and index finger near their root, then tugging with the other hand on the same strand at its distal part. The tug test is positive if more than 10% of the hairs fracture, suggesting hair shaft fragility. The pull test involves holding a hair close to the root between the thumb and index finger, then use a slight force to pull the hair out, causing mild discomfort but not pain. In general, telogen hairs are more likely to be extracted than anagen hairs. Furthermore, microscopic observation of the hair root can help distinguish anagen hairs (long sheath shaped) and telogen hairs (club shaped).[42]

In the case of suspected fungal infection, the wood lamp examination is an efficient test. For the test to be accurate, the hairs should be free of all hair applications such as deodorants or moisturizers. After the surroundings are darkened, the wood lamp is turned on and held about 5 to 10 in. (~12-25 cm) away from the skin. Some common fluorescent colors are listed in Table 120-9.

TABLE 120-9 Common Colors Shown on Wood Lamp Examination

Conditions/Organisms	Fluorescent color
Pityriasis versicolor by *Malassezia*	Yellowish or orange
Malassezia folliculitis	Bluish-white
Tinea capitis by *Microsporum* species	Blue-green
Tinea capitis by *Trichophyton schoenleinii*	Dull blue

Bacterial or viral infection usually can be further diagnosed with swabs for stain or culture.

In suspected cases of iron deficiency, complete blood count, ferritin, total iron-binding capacity, and transferrin saturation should be tested. If a female patient presents with alopecia along with virilization, clinicians should order dehydroepiandrosterone (DHEA) sulfate and testosterone analysis. Other systemic conditions such as lupus or hypothyroidism/hyperthyroidism can be assessed using their specific laboratory findings.

Alopecia in general does not need a biopsy for diagnosis, but this is sometimes performed for research purposes. Hairs can be biopsied transversely and may show miniaturization, especially in cases of AGA or telogen effluvium.

Genetic Testing in Androgenetic Alopecia

As mentioned in the pathophysiology section, many genetic factors may contribute to alopecia. However, more research is still needed before clinicians can reach a consensus in the screening test for AGA. Therefore, no genetic testing is officially recommended.

TREATMENT

7 There are a myriad of distinct and diverse causes and types of alopecia as discussed above; thus, treatment or management strategies should be as cause-specific as possible. Identified causes should be treated and/or eliminated as soon as practically feasible. Cause-specific management/treatment strategies include several considerations—infections, chemotherapy, iron deficiency, other nutritional deficiencies, physiological or emotional trauma, trichotillomania, and autoimmune diseases.

Infectious causes should be treated with the appropriate anti-infective agent(s) and treatment regimen (whether systemic or topical therapy as appropriate). Tinea capitis, which commonly manifests as patchy alopecia and usually caused by a *Trichophyton* species, requires a systemic antifungal with oral terbinafine or itraconazole and not a topical agent (it does not penetrate hair follicles sufficiently). See Chapter 143, "Superficial Fungal Infections," for further discussion of the treatment of mycotic infections of the scalp.

Chemotherapy-induced alopecia is generally a reversible and temporary condition. However, for the patient undergoing chemotherapy, having their hair fall out—seeing clumps of hair on pillows and brushes and bald areas on their head—may be emotionally distressing. Cold caps and scalp cooling systems reduce the amount of chemotherapeutic agents reaching the hair follicles and have been shown to significantly reduce the amount of hair loss[43] without increasing the risk of scalp skin metastases.[44] Other nondrug strategies include wigs, scarves/hats or other head coverings, and counseling/psychological support. Limited studies of topical or systemic drug therapies for prevention and treatment (using alopecia treatments discussed below) have not been that promising especially in preventing hair loss,[24] and the risk for affecting chemotherapy efficacy or toxicity must be kept in mind, even with nutraceuticals.[24] Reassuring the patients that hair regrowth will happen may be comforting and letting them know that occasionally the hair grows back differently (eg, may be fuller or curlier) can provide a positive outlook.

Iron deficiency is a known and reversible cause of alopecia. In this case, appropriate treatment is iron replacement therapy followed by iron supplementation once iron stores are replenished. Iron-deficiency anemia is further discussed in Chapter 122, "Anemias."

Other *nutritional deficiencies* including specific trace element deficiencies should be corrected if found, as these may possibly play a role in alopecia. For example, there may be an association between copper deficiency and AGA; decreased copper level in the frontal zones of scalp hair and serum were found in both men and women with AGA when compared with their respective matched controls and the differences were statistically significant.[45] There may also be an association between defective copper metabolism and trichorrhexis nodosa, although there are many other possible causes, including hypothyroidism and Menkes disease.[1]

Any physiologic or emotional *trauma or stressors* that preceded the alopecia could be the inciting cause. If the traumatic events or stressors are still present and ongoing, management strategies to ameliorate them would be helpful (eg, mindfulness techniques, relaxation clinics, counseling, or psychotherapy).

Trichotillomania may be treated via nonpharmacologic and/or pharmacotherapy—the optimal treatment is unknown, and psychiatric referral may be indicated. Cognitive behavior therapy and selective serotonin reuptake inhibitors (SSRIs) may be effective, and using both together may be more effective than either treatment used alone. Olanzapine and clomipramine may also be effective.[46]

Alopecia that is thought to be associated with *autoimmune diseases* as discussed above (eg, SLE, hypothyroidism) sometimes improves with treatment of the specific autoimmune disorder. Antibodies (eg, thyroid-antimicrosomal antibodies) may be involved in the pilar follicles, as antifollicular antibodies have been reported in alopecia.[47]

Pattern Baldness: Androgenetic Alopecia

8 There are recent reviews[1,48,49] and evidence-based guidelines[50,51] on the treatment of AGA in women and in men. Treatments include topical minoxidil, oral 5α-reductase inhibitors (finasteride, dutasteride) for men, hormonal therapies for women, and miscellaneous therapies including nutritional supplements and laser light therapy, with variable efficacy.

Male Baldness

Topical Therapy: Minoxidil *Minoxidil* (2% or 5%) topical solution is the most common treatment for male baldness. It can prevent the progression of baldness and improve hair density and thickness, with hair regrowth being more robust at the vertex than in the frontal area of the head.[52] Its exact mechanism of action on hair follicles remains unclear. However, the main benefits seen may be prolongation of the anagen phase and hair shaft diameter.[51]

The 5% concentration has been recommended for greater efficacy; a randomized controlled trial (RCT) comparing 5% versus 2% minoxidil in men aged 18 to 49 years found 45% higher hair counts in those given 5% versus those given 2%.[53] There is insufficient evidence to recommend the 5% foam over the 5% solution.[50] The response to treatment should be assessed at 6 months.[50] If successful, treatment needs to continue indefinitely as hair loss recurs when treatment is interrupted or discontinued.[1,50]

Side effects of minoxidil lotion include transient telogen hair shedding—an indication that minoxidil is stimulating telogen follicles to re-enter anagen[50]—this usually normalizes within a few weeks to months and therapy should be continued and not stopped.[50] Hypertrichosis is more common with the 5% concentration and may reflect incorrect application. To minimize drug contamination of the pillow and inadvertent contact with the face during sleep, patients should be advised to use the medication at least 2 hours before going to bed.[50] Irritant and contact dermatitis sometimes occur. Minoxidil is an antihypertensive agent when used systemically, and uncommon to rare side effects of topical administration are related to its systemic effects on blood pressure: dizziness, headache, hypotension, tachycardia, or chest pain.

Systemic Therapy: Finasteride, Dutasteride The 5α-reductase enzyme converts testosterone to DHT, the main androgen causing AGA. There are two types of 5α-reductases in humans: type I is primarily found in liver, skin, and scalp; and type II is found in the prostate, genitourinary tract, and hair follicle.[50] 5α-Reductase inhibitors were originally marketed for treatment of benign prostatic hyperplasia (BPH), and their efficacy for AGA was an incidental finding based on a "side effect" of BPH treatment.

Finasteride is a selective type II 5α-reductase inhibitor that reduces scalp production of DHT. Multiple RCTs have shown significant increases in total hair counts and/or other hair growth benefits in men at 6 months,[54,55] 12 months,[56,57] and 24 months.[58] A dose-ranging study found benefits at all doses greater than 0.2 mg/day but no greater difference between 5 mg/day versus 1 mg/day.[54] Thus, the recommended dose for male pattern baldness is finasteride 1 mg/day (the dose for BPH is 5 mg/day). A 4-year study (2-year observation, 2-year finasteride) found that hair follicles that can still produce a thick hair fiber responded to finasteride 1 mg/day by reducing the hair cycle lag phase by 40% (thus initiating active growth more rapidly) and increasing the duration of the anagen phase by 23%.[58] However, miniaturized hair follicles (ie, those that were producing thinner hair, defined as <40 μm thick) did not respond to finasteride.[58] This may be useful in future for patient selection and may be an explanation for nonresponders. In 2019, a follow-up study by the same investigators assessing finasteride pharmacodynamics in responders found

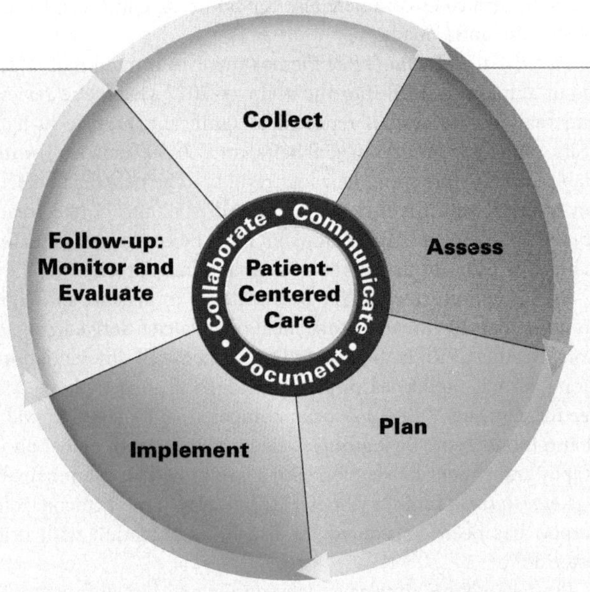

Patient Care Process for Androgenetic Alopecia

The image shows the five fundamental steps included in The Pharmacist's Care Process endorsed by the Joint Commission for Pharmacy Practitioners (2014). The tagline of this process reads collaborate, communicate, and document. The five fundamental steps listed here are collect, assess, plan, implement, and follow-up: monitor and evaluate. All these steps are listed in a circular block diagram.

Collect

- Patient characteristics (eg, age, sex, pregnancy status if female)
- Patient medical history (personal and family)
- Patient description of history of the alopecia
- Signs associated with severity of androgenetic alopecia (eg, areas of involvement)
- Signs or symptoms of other conditions (ie, differential diagnosis—could this be a condition other than androgenetic alopecia? Symptoms such as itching, pain, burning, or prickly discomfort may suggest underlying conditions. If the alopecia is seen in a female, is polycystic ovarian syndrome [PCOS] or congenital adrenal hyperplasia present?)

Assess

- Severity of androgenetic alopecia—can quantify using hair counts, hair density measurements, and assessing the areas of involvement
- Relevant lab work, if needed (eg, check parameters that would rule out PCOS. Refer to the Acne case in the Casebook for discussion of relevant labs for PCOS.)
- Ability/willingness to pay for treatment options
- Emotional/psychological concerns

Plan

- Determine an appropriate treatment approach or various optional approaches (ie, topical vs systemic pharmacotherapy vs natural health products/nutritional supplements vs other approaches [mesotherapy, low-level laser light therapy, hair restoration surgery, cosmetic coverings]). Determine if psychosocial support is needed.
- Discuss with the patient various options to determine the most appropriate therapies (nonpharmacologic and pharmacologic) for the patient. Discuss options for psychosocial support if needed.

Implement*

- Provide patient education regarding all elements of treatment plan. Patient counseling points for various agents follow.
  - If topical therapy with minoxidil lotion is used: (1) Transient hair shedding may initially occur (indicating that minoxidil is stimulating hair follicles to re-enter a growth phase called anagen). This usually normalizes within a few weeks to months of starting therapy and treatment should be continued and not stopped. (2) To minimize drug contamination of the pillow and then inadvertent transfer to the face during sleep, use minoxidil lotion at least 2 hours before going to bed.
  - If systemic therapy with finasteride or dutasteride is used: (1) The medication must be swallowed whole and not chewed or crushed. (2) The medication may harm a growing fetus; pregnant women should not ingest or touch broken tablets. This also includes women seeking to become pregnant (including pharmacists, other health professionals, and caregivers). (3) The medication may cause sexual dysfunction. (4) Bloodwork may be needed (liver function tests) to monitor for potential side effects. (5) There are potential interactions with other medications—please check with your physician or pharmacist.
- Use motivational interviewing and coaching strategies to maximize adherence when needed.
- Provide information about prevention/minimization of further hair loss (eg, appropriate hair care). Provide information about psychosocial support options, if needed.

Follow-up: Monitor and Evaluate

- Contact patient in 3 and 6 months to follow-up about the efficacy of recommended therapies and any issues with the treatment regimen.
- Ensure that appropriate monitoring parameters for efficacy and potential adverse effects have been put in place. Ensure follow-up lab tests if needed are in place (eg, liver function tests when finasteride or dutasteride is used).
- Reinforce preventive measures including appropriate hair care.

**Collaborate with patient, caregivers, and other healthcare professionals.*

finasteride-dependency and a rebound effect when finasteride was discontinued: after 12 months off-treatment, viable drug-responsive hair follicles began to rapidly miniaturize; and by 30 months off-treatment, 94% had miniaturized, which worsened the alopecia.[59] The authors concluded that drug dependency and a rebound phenomenon are new findings for finasteride use in alopecia.[59]

Side effects of finasteride include orthostatic hypotension, dizziness, decreased libido, impotence, and ejaculatory disorder. Two recent systematic reviews identified growing concerns about sexual dysfunctions[8,60] and patient counseling should be provided prior to starting treatment.[8] Finasteride is extensively metabolized; monitoring parameters include liver function tests (LFTs) prior to starting therapy and repeated every 6 months.[61] Finasteride is teratogenic (risk category X), and crushed or broken tablets should not be touched by pregnant women or women seeking to become pregnant (including pharmacists, other health professionals, and caregivers), as exposure to the active ingredient can occur.

Dutasteride is a double inhibitor of both type I and type II 5α-reductase. It is only approved for BPH in men (and not for AGA) in the United States and Canada, although it is approved in other countries (eg, Korea) for AGA. RCTs have shown that dutasteride 0.5 mg/day has efficacy in 6 months without significant side effects[62] and that in comparison with finasteride 1 mg/day or placebo, it is significantly more efficacious.[55] Total hair counts (2.54 and 1.13 cm diameter [1 and 0.44 in. diameter]) and hair width but not terminal hair counts (2.54 cm diameter [1 in. diameter]) were significantly greater at 24 weeks with dutasteride compared with finasteride or placebo.[55] Incidences of sexual dysfunction and breast disorders were similar between dutasteride and finasteride but lower in the placebo group.

Also similar to finasteride, dutasteride is teratogenic (risk category X), and skin contact with the active ingredient (if tablet is broken or crushed) should be avoided. Tablets should be swallowed whole and not chewed or crushed. There is a potential association with high-grade prostate cancer, but the risk is low. Dutasteride is also extensively metabolized; its already-long half-life (5 weeks) increases with age. Its concentration/pharmacodynamic effects may be increased during concomitant therapy with strong CYP3A4 inhibitors.

The most concerning side effect for 5α-reductase inhibitors (finasteride, dutasteride) appears to be sexual dysfunction. A 2019 systematic review and meta-analysis of adverse sexual effects of finasteride or dutasteride as treatment for male AGA evaluated 15 RCTs (4,495 participants).[60] This study found an overall 1.57-fold risk of any adverse sexual effects associated with the use of either finasteride 1 mg/day or dutasteride 0.5 mg/day; when analyzed separately, finasteride had a 1.66-fold risk and dutasteride had an increased risk that was not statistically significant (RR 1.37, 95% CI 0.81-2.32).[60] But there were many fewer dutasteride RCTs, which may account for the wide confidence interval.

Miscellaneous Therapies Many other cosmetic, pharmaceutical, nutraceutical, and food products are marketed as alternative therapies for alopecia. But most of these have little to no clinical evidence of efficacy, especially robust RCTs. However, health practitioners should be somewhat knowledgeable about alternative therapies, as patients may be using them and/or have questions—for instance, if they have heard of or are considering these options.[50]

Mesotherapy is the microinjection of medications, vitamins, or other substances into the mesoderm (the middle layer of skin). Medications have included dutasteride, minoxidil, or other active ingredients. An RCT comparing mesotherapy to topical 5% minoxidil found little difference in the two types of treatments, the only difference being a variation of hair shaft diameter at 1 month that was not present at 4 months (the end of the study).[63] The mesohair solution contained 56 ingredients, including 24 amino acids, 13 vitamins, 4 coenzymes, 4 nucleic acids, 5 minerals, and 2 reducing agents, and the active ingredients decapeptide 4, acetyl decapeptide, and copper tripeptide.[63] A study of mesotherapy using 1 mL of dutasteride 0.01% demonstrated significant improvement after 9 months, but only 6 patients (5 males, 1 female) participated in the trial.[64]

Low-level laser (light) therapy (LLLT) can stimulate hair growth by scalp vasodilatation, but the exact mechanism is unclear.[65] LLLT devices are available commercially for home or clinic use in the United States and Canada.[66]

Platelet-rich plasma (PRP) therapy involves intradermal injections of autologous PRP into the scalp. A 2017 systematic review found that 7 of 14 studies reported a significant increase in hair density, ranging from 12.3 to 45.9 hairs/cm^2 (80-300 hairs/in.^{2}) with variable hair thickness and hair loss results.[67] The beneficial effects seem to begin with the first treatment and peak after 3 to 5 treatments, then attenuates and treatments must be continued to maintain benefits. Side effects include local irritation and pain.[66,67]

PRP is concentrated autologous platelets in plasma, and contains more than 20 growth factors, including platelet-derived growth factors. In AGA, PRP is thought to induce stem cell differentiation, prolong dermal papilla cell survival, prolong the anagen phase, and other mechanisms.[68] PRP has been compared to topical minoxidil and at 6 months, the PRP group scored higher in both global photography and patient satisfaction with a hair growth questionnaire.[69]

Ketoconazole inhibits the DHT pathway, and ketoconazole shampoo has been considered for use in combination with oral finasteride.[70]

Prostaglandin F2 analogues latanoprost and bimatoprost topical therapy are being studied for use in AGA. Early results seem promising.[70]

Topical valproic acid 8.3% spray was found to increase hair count in a recent RCT.[71] Alopecia is a fairly common adverse effect of systemic valproic acid.

Hair restoration surgery involves hair transplantation, scalp reduction surgery, or a combination of both.

Natural health products—including biotin, melatonin, saw palmetto, black cohosh, dong quai, false unicorn, chaste berry, and red clover—have been used in treatment of alopecia. Some of these may have anti-androgenic or estrogen-promoting activities.[65] However, there is scant evidence of efficacy as hair growth promoters in men, as shown in these summaries:

1. A small 2017 RCT of a combination traditional Chinese medicine (TCM) containing six herbal ingredients (*Ginseng Radix, Astragali Radix, Angelicae Sinensis Radix, Ligustri Fructus, Rehmannia glutinosa*, and *Eclipta prostrata* Linn.) versus placebo showed that 9 of 17 patients receiving TCM had increased hair growth versus 2 of 17 in the placebo group, a statistically significant difference. However, of the 9 responders in the TCM group, 1 minimally improved, 5 moderately improved, and only 3 showed significant improvement.[72]
2. Biotin is popularly used for AGA; although it is known that genetic biotinidase deficiency results in hair loss and biotin was found to reverse valproic acid–induced alopecia in a few patients, robust evidence is lacking.[73]
3. In contrast, a well-designed 2017 RCT of a commercially available product called Lambdapil (1,000 mg L-Cysteine, 100 mg *Serenoa repens*, 7.14 mg *Equisetum arvense L*, 0.5 mg silicon, 10 mg zinc, 16 mg vitamin B3, 6 mg vitamin B5, 1.4 mg vitamin B6, 50 μg D-biotin, 40 mg taurine), which enrolled both men and women in a 6 month placebo-controlled RCT using high-level methodology, found that Lambdapil increased the anagen/telogen ratio in men, with a 3.7% increase in anagen hair and an increase in hair volume. Quality of life was also improved.[74] (Results of the use of this product in women are discussed in the next section.)

Female Hair Loss

The majority of female hair loss is FPHL or female pattern AGA; however, women with PCOS also can develop male pattern baldness. A 2016 Cochrane review of interventions for FPHL reported moderate- to low-quality evidence of efficacy for minoxidil, low-quality evidence of efficacy for finasteride, and moderate- to low-quality evidence of efficacy for.[49] Hormonal therapy, nutraceuticals, and mesotherapy were not included in the review, although there are promising RCTs of these approaches. Other possibilities such as prostaglandin analogs are too early in development for review. Recently published management strategies include other hormone-modulating treatments (dutasteride, spironolactone, cyproterone acetate, flutamide), ketoconazole shampoo, platelet-rich plasma, microneedling, as well as updated comments on prostaglandin analogues (latanoprost, bimatoprost), light therapy, topical hormonal treatments, and hair transplant.[75]

Topical *minoxidil* 2% has been approved for use in females with AGA, but not the 5% concentration. Many RCTs using 2% minoxidil in women have shown efficacy, and pooled data from six studies (5 using 2%, 1 using 1%) confirmed the observation, with 157 of 593 patients demonstrating a moderate-to-marked increase in hair growth when compared with placebo (RR 1.93, 95% CI 1.51-2.47).[49] In 8 pooled studies (1,242 participants), there was a significant increase in total hair count (13.2/cm^2 [85/in.^{2}]) compared with placebo.[49] Four studies (1,006 participants) comparing minoxidil 2% versus 5% did not show a difference, although the quality of the evidence was moderate to low.[49] If successful, it should be continued indefinitely.[75] Women should be informed about transient telogen hair loss within the first few months of treatment and possible hypertrichosis as a side effect of treatment.[75] Minoxidil, including topical use, is contraindicated in pregnancy and lactation.

Oral *minoxidil* at low doses of 0.25 to 2.5 mg/day may be an option if unresponsive or intolerant to topical minoxidil treatment.[75] However, significant drops in blood pressure may occur, especially if other anti-hypertensive medications are used concomitantly.

Topical and oral prostaglandin analog treatments may be promising. Latanoprost, travoprost, and bimatoprost are prostaglandin analogs that are used for glaucoma, which caused eyelashes to grow as a side effect; they promote hair growth by prolonging the anagen phase. Blocking the prostaglandin D2 receptor (GPR44) may help to increase hair growth.[75] Setipiprant (KITH-105) is an oral GPR44 receptor inhibitor. Studies are ongoing but still too early to provide general guidance.

5α-Reductase inhibitors are not approved for use in females. One RCT showed efficacy with *finasteride* 1 mg/day in women with AGA while two others did not.[49] Higher doses (2.5-5 mg/day) have shown efficacy consistently[75-78] and are used in practice.[75] Patient selection and dose used may be key—at 1 mg/day four women with hyperandrogenism showed improvement with finasteride[79] but not postmenopausal women without hyperandrogenism.[48,80] However, at a dose of 5 mg/day, 86 mostly postmenopausal Asian women without hyperandrogenism showed significant increases in mean hair density and mean hair thickness after 12 months of treatment.[77] Studies in premenopausal women have shown conflicting results.[80] *Dutasteride* is a more potent 5α-reductase inhibitor that can lower serum DHT levels by more than 90%[80] and effectiveness has been reported in a 46-year-old woman.[81] Precautions and concerns with handling broken tablets are even more of an issue if used by a woman, as the drug is contraindicated in pregnancy and in women of childbearing age.

Hormonal therapy with antiandrogens with or without estrogens has shown some efficacy. In particular, *cyproterone acetate* was compared with topical minoxidil; results showed greater efficacy for minoxidil in women without hyperandrogenism and greater efficacy for cyproterone acetate in women with multiple symptoms of hyperandrogenism.[82] Cyproterone acetate may be more effective in a birth control formulation (eg, Diane or Diane-35, which is available in Canada and Europe but not in the United States). Suggested regimens for use in premenstrual women are either 100 mg/day on days 5 to 15 alongside ethinyl estradiol 50 μg on days 5 to 25, or 50 mg/day on days 1 to 10 with ethinyl estradiol 35 μg on days 1 to 21.[75] For postmenopausal women, a suggested regimen is cyproterone acetate 50 mg/day.[75]

Spironolactone has antiandrogenic activities and has been considered the most commonly used, off-label antiandrogen for the treatment of FPHL and hirsutism[48]; however, published studies are limited. An open intervention study found spironolactone to be equally effective when compared with cyproterone acetate.[83]

Flutamide has potent antiandrogenic effects and has shown efficacy for FPHL in clinical trials. In a 4-year prospective cohort study in which flutamide was used in annually reduced doses of 250 mg/day, 125 mg/day, and 62.5 mg/day, flutamide was used either alone or with an oral contraceptive reduced alopecia scores. The maximum drug effect occurred after 2 years and was maintained for the duration of the 4-year study.[84] The regimen of annually reduced doses was a dose-ranging attempt to minimize side effects; the study showed that the dose of 62.5 mg/day maintained efficacy with complete hepatic tolerability and high adherence. At the dose of 250 mg/day, the dropout rate was 4% due to drug-related hepatic changes.[84] Monitor serum transaminases at baseline, monthly for the first 4 months and periodically thereafter.[75,85]

Natural health products and nutritional supplements may be beneficial. RCTs showing efficacy are as follows[81]:

1. A 2015 RCT of a nutritional supplement combination (460-mg fish oil [exact amounts of EPA and DHA unspecified], 460-mg black currant seed oil, antioxidants [1-mg lycopene, 30-mg vitamin C, 5-mg vitamin E])[86,87] versus placebo in 120 women found that 62% of the supplement group had increased hair density compared with 28% in the placebo group. Anagen hair increased significantly and telogen hair decreased significantly in the supplement group.[86,87]
2. The well-designed 2017 RCT of Lambdapil as discussed in an earlier section enrolled both women with acute Telogen effluvium (aTE) and men with AGA in a 6-month, placebo-controlled design using high-level methodology. Results in women showed an increase in hair volume (slight to moderate) and an improved quality of life.[74]
3. A topical botanical lotion that acts by increasing Bcl-2, perifollicular Langerhans and mast cells, and perifollicular collagen was found in a 2018 single-blinded RCT to increase hair density, improve Dermatology Life Quality Index, and increase the anagen:telogen ratio at 24 weeks.[88]

LLLT increased the total hair count in women with FPHL in several studies.[49,89] A 2019 meta-analysis of 8 papers comprising a total of 11 RCTs found that LLLT device used (comb vs helmet) and the duration of treatment (short vs long) did not appear to matter. Thus, LLLT appears promising and is a potentially effective treatment for AGA.[89] Majority of studies to date have shown an overall improvement in hair regrowth, thickness, and patient satisfaction.[75] To this end, the FDA has approved various LLLT devices for use in AGA and these are available commercially. LLLT is usually well tolerated, with side effects that include scalp dryness, itching, tenderness, and a warm sensation.[75]

Platelet-Rich Plasma may be a promising option for female AGA[75,90]; however, current European Guidelines for AGA in women and men concluded that there is insufficient evidence to support its use.[75,91]

Mesotherapy containing nutritional supplements has been compared with topical minoxidil 5% lotion. No significant differences were found with regard to hair density or hair loss, but the mesotherapy group had a greater increase in the number of hair follicles.[92]

Hair transplantation is a viable option if other medical therapies are unsuccessful.[75] Cosmetic methods such as wigs, scarves, and hats are other alternatives.

Ketoconazole shampoo has been recommended for female AGA if seborrheic dermatitis or sebopsoriasis is present.[75]

Androgenetic Alopecia in Children

Familial predisposition may be present. Nonetheless, if AGA is seen in a prepubertal child, an endocrine evaluation is strongly recommended.[93] AGA in an adolescent is not uncommon and topical minoxidil may be effectively used.[42,94] One case report of AGA seen in a 15-year-old girl was successfully treated with topical minoxidil and oral contraceptives.[95]

Alopecia Areata

Alopecia areata (AA) can be emotionally devastating to a person and can cause a significant impact on the patient's quality of life and self-esteem.[4] It can cause stigmatization[34] (see the "Hair Stigma and Hair Discordance" section). It may lead to clinical depression, anxiety, and/or social phobia. Management and treatment of the psychological impact of AA must not be overlooked.

9 Curative therapy for AA does not yet exist; however, there is a high rate of spontaneous remission even with no pharmacotherapy.[4] Alopecia totalis and alopecia universalis are more resistant to treatment. Due to the autoimmune and inflammatory nature of AA, effective pharmacotherapy primarily involves immunosuppressive agents used systemically, intralesionally, and/or topically. Treatments that may be effective include high-dose oral corticosteroids, intralesional corticosteroids, topical corticosteroids, topical minoxidil, topical immunotherapy, systemic and topical biologic agents (in particular the Janus kinase inhibitors discussed later in this section), azathioprine and other immunosuppressive agents, and a few miscellaneous agents. Robust RCTs are lacking or limited for some of these therapies; some treatments may not be suitable for children with AA.

Intralesional corticosteroids are the treatment of choice in adults.[34] The best-tested immunosuppressive treatment is intradermal (intralesional) triamcinolone acetonide (5-10 mg/mL) every 2 weeks[4] or every 4 to 6 weeks.[34] Monthly intervals would be more convenient for the patient. An effective method is to inject 0.1 mL of solution into multiple sites at 1 cm (0.4 in.) apart, into the deep dermis, with a maximum volume of 20 mL injected at each clinic visit.[34] This treatment stimulates regrowth in more than 60% of patients.[4] If there is no improvement at 6 months or if significant atrophy is noted, treatment should be discontinued.

Hydrocortisone acetate (25 mg/mL) is an alternative. Side effects include pain at injection sites, localized skin atrophy, and hypopigmentation. Dermal atrophy usually recovers over 3 to 6 months.[34] Relapses are common with treatment discontinuation.[4]

Topical corticosteroids (TCS) are commonly used, especially in children (since scalp injections are painful) and in those adults with less than 50% scalp involvement.[4] High-potency TCS such as clobetasol propionate used under occlusion is more effective since this may further increase potency. (As an aside, although keloid is an entirely different disease entity, a recent RCT found that clobetasol propionate 0.05% cream under silicone occlusion dressing was equally efficacious and had fewer adverse effects compared with intralesional triamcinolone.[96]) Treatment for AA may need to be continued for 3 months before regrowth is seen.[34] Monitor for topical and potentially systemic side effects since potent TCS are being used.[97] Folliculitis is a common side effect. Refer to Chapter 118, "Psoriasis/Psoriatic Arthrtis," for a corticosteroid potency comparison chart and for a detailed discussion of TCS side effects. A recent article about rational and ethical use of TCS also provides a summary.[97]

Systemic corticosteroids are efficacious in patients with AA. However, their side effects profile limits their use to short treatment periods of 2 to 3 months. Pulse dosing (eg, once weekly) is used to minimize systemic side effects. Regimens include prednisolone 0.5 mg/kg/day (usually of 40-50 mg/day) daily for 3 months,[34] prednisolone 200 mg once weekly for 3 months,[4] or dexamethasone 0.1 mg/kg/day (mean dose about 8 mg) on 2 consecutive days once weekly for at least 4 months and then slowly tapered or discontinued (with some patients on treatment for 2 years).[98] This dexamethasone regimen was used in 31 patients with alopecia totalis or alopecia universalis, and complete response was seen in 22 patients (71%) and partial response in 3 patients (10%). The mean time to response was 1.55 months, and the mean duration of therapy was 12.9 months (range 4-24 months). Adverse effects were seen in 10 of 31 patients (32%), including weight gain in 9 patients and Cushing syndrome, striae, and irritability in 1 patient each.

Relapses are seen after treatment is discontinued and sometimes during treatment.[98] Pulse therapy with high-dose systemic steroids has been used in other studies and may be an option for severe, extensive, or recalcitrant AA.

Biologic agents have exploded on the treatment scene for many dermatologic inflammatory disorders such as psoriasis, atopic dermatitis (AD), and AA, including the subtypes alopecia totalis (AT) and alopecia universalis (AU). Some biologic agents may be used topically for AA, and some have been successfully used in children and adolescents.

Janus kinase (JAK) inhibitors (tofacitinib, ruxolitinib, baricitinib) are a promising new class of biologic treatment for AA.[99,100] A JAK-STAT (signal transducer and activator of transcription) signaling pathway is important in the hair growth cycle, with key genes being highly expressed in the catagen and telogen phases but suppressed in the anagen phase.[99] JAK inhibitors inhibit the JAK-STAT pathway, resulting in various immunologic changes that result in prolonging the anagen phase, angiogenesis, stimulating/activating the proliferation of hair stem cells, and other changes, which all manifest in hair regrowth, as shown in these studies[99]:

1. Studies and case reports of oral and topical *tofacitinib* demonstrate efficacy in adults and children with AA, including AA subtypes AT and AU.[100] Patients with AA may have greater response than patients with AA subtypes. Systemic treatments may be more effective than the topical route. Using the Severity of Alopecia Tool (SALT), a cohort study of oral tofacitinib 5 to 10 mg twice daily in 90 adults with AA and subtypes, found that 58% improved their SALT score by 50% or more over 4 to 18 months of treatment. Patients with AA showed a greater degree of change in SALT than those with alopecia totalis or universalis (82% vs 59%).[100] A retrospective review of 13 adolescents with AA treated with tofacitinib 5 mg twice daily found a 90% median improvement in SALT score (1%-100%), and there are many other recent studies.[100] A retrospective review of children under 12 years with AA, AT, or AU treated with tofacitinib identified three children aged 5 years or younger who failed previous treatment before tofacitinib and who responded to tofacitinib 2.5 mg daily for 4 days then 5 mg daily for 3 days each week (one child with >90% hair regrowth after 12 months of treatment and the other two children with >50% improvement by 6 months and 21 months, respectively).[101] Results with topical JAK inhibitors are poorer than with oral agents. Topical tofacitinib or ruxolitinib were applied to eyebrow regions/upper eyelids/scalp in 6 pediatric patients aged 3 to 17 years with AA, and responses were only seen in 3 patients.[102] Additional clinical studies are under way.
2. Fewer reports and studies have examined the use of *ruxolitinib;* however, there are reports of efficacy in hair regrowth in a few patients with AT who had failed therapy with tofacitinib.[103] Encouraging results and additional studies are under way.
3. There is one case report of oral *baricitinib* being effective in AA as an incidental finding, and other JAK inhibitors are on

the horizon, including filgotinib and decernotinib, which are being tested for rheumatoid arthritis.

Dupilumab is a new class of biologic agents (an IL-4 receptor-α-antagonist) marketed for AD. It was found to trigger hair regrowth in two case reports of AD patients using dupilumab for AD: one case was a patient with long-standing AT[104] and the other case was a patient with long-standing AU.[105]

Methotrexate is a systemic immunosuppressive agent which may be an option for AA with extensive hair loss where other treatments have been ineffective. If efficacious, regrowth may be seen in 3 months with full regrowth in 6 to 12 months. Methotrexate is more efficacious when used with prednisone or prednisolone (various regimens). A regimen starting with IV methylprednisolone (500 mg/d × 3 days, then monthly × 3 cycles) prior to starting oral methotrexate has also shown efficacy in several studies.[106] Various dosing regimens of methotrexate have been used, most with starting doses of 2.5-10 mg/week and increasing to 15-25 mg/week.[106] In adults and children with severe AA, response to methotrexate was better in adults than in children, confirming that combination treatment with a corticosteroid results in higher complete response rates than methotrexate used alone.[106] Tapering often resulted in recurrence.[106]

Azathioprine has also been successfully used to treat AU including recalcitrant cases in adults (nonresponders to oral corticosteroids and topical immunotherapy with diphencyprone). A case study of 14 adult patients showed a complete response in 6 of 14 patients (43%). No identifiable prognostic factors were found, and adverse effects included elevated liver enzymes (1 patient), pancreatitis (1 patient), bone marrow suppression (1 patient), and diarrhea (2 patients); treatment had to be discontinued in 4 patients.[107]

Other agents have been tried for treating AA over the years with varying levels of success, including topical anthralin,[108,109] topical diphenylcyclopropenone,[109] topical calcineurin inhibitors, and oral cyclosporine. None of these is commonly used today because of inconsistent efficacy and/or side effects.

Loss of Eyelashes and Eyebrows

Bimatoprost (Latisse) 0.03% drops is FDA approved for treatment of hypotrichosis of the eyelashes, discovered due to increased eyelash growth observed through usual use for elevated intraocular pressure in glaucoma. One drop is applied along the skin of the upper eyelid at the base of eyelashes once daily at bedtime. Beneficial effects may take months to be seen.[110,111] Bimatoprost 0.03% solution has also shown efficacy in hypotrichosis of the eyebrows.[112]

HAIR CARE IN THE PATIENT WITH ALOPECIA

Patients suffering from alopecia may attempt to manipulate their hair to hide their hair loss and to make their head of hair appear fuller; however, most methods may actually further damage the hair and are not recommended. Chemical processing such as hair weaving or hair straightening can further damage the hair and cause hair breakage.

All hair dyes can damage the hair with the exception of temporary hair dyes. Temporary hair dyes have particle sizes that are too large to penetrate through the cuticle, which minimizes hair damage and accounts for their temporary nature (they are removed by a single shampooing).

Heat denatures the keratin protein structure of the hair shaft and turns the water in the hair shaft into steam. This can physically remove the cuticular scale as the steam escapes from the hair shaft. Without the structural protection afforded by the cuticular scale, the hair breaks easily. Heat-damaged hair is known as bubble hair and cannot be repaired. Frequent hair combing or brushing may also damage the hair by encouraging cuticle removal.[113]

Hair should be combed or brushed only when dry, and excessive combing or brushing should be avoided. Brushing the hair 100 strokes a day and massaging the scalp vigorously with the brush are not appropriate for the patient with alopecia.[113]

Hair conditioners coat the hair shaft and smooth the cuticle, and they should be routinely used. Instant conditioners that are applied after shampooing and rinsed out coat the hair shaft with a thin dimethicone or quaternary ammonium compound to temporarily "glue down" loosened cuticular scales. Supplementing these with a leave-in conditioner can provide a thicker coating to further protect the hair until the next shampoo. Hair conditioners reduce combing friction, improve hair shine, increase hair softness, minimize static electricity, and reduce frizziness.[113]

HAIR STIGMA AND HAIR DISCORDANCE

"Beauty standards of hair are a form of bias."[114] Men, women, adolescents, and children are often distressed when there is hair loss, or when their hair is perceived as "different" from the societal norm—such as in minoritized people of color. Adolescents and children in particular may be subject to bullying by their peers, sometimes just for having a head of hair that looks different.[115] In 2019, an anti-bullying song/video was released and a cosmetic manufacturer partnered in an anti-bullying campaign.[114,115]

Imagine the potential stigmatization/bullying situation if the person had patchy AA or AA totalis? This is involuntary hair loss which is quite different from people who have chosen to shave their heads such as monks. Stigmatization affects adults as well. Healthcare professionals should be cognizant of the psychosocial impact on their patient's quality of life. A 2015 review of the burden of disease for patients with AA reported rates for depression (8.8%) and generalized anxiety disorder (18.2%), both significantly higher than in the general population (about 1%-2%).[41] This review also found that the rate of psychiatric comorbidity was influenced by the age of onset of AA, with an increased risk of depression in patients aged <20 years and increased risks of anxiety and obsessive-compulsive disorder in patients aged 40 to 59 years.[41]

Similarly, in patients with AGA or other forms of alopecia, the psychosocial impact must not be overlooked. Even with temporary anagen hair loss (such as chemotherapy-induced alopecia), the onset is usually sudden and may be absolutely traumatizing to the patient.

In addition, hair discordance may be present between a healthcare professional and an alopecia patient of color seeking care. There may be patient discomfort and/or a negative perception of the ability of the healthcare professional to meet their care needs. A survey of Black women with alopecia reported that some physicians did not touch their hair, and some were unfamiliar with their usual hair care routine.[116] Another recent study noted that alopecia is one of the most common conditions for patients of African descent being seen by a dermatologist.[117]

Thus, healthcare professionals should be cognizant that hair stigma and hair discordance may be potential issues. Being aware of common cultural hair care practices and being empathetic in interactions with the patient with alopecia are important components of care.

An approach to examining tightly coiled hair for patients with hair loss in race-discordant patient-physician interactions is available, describing appropriate actions, tips for hair examination, and sample language appropriate for the interaction.[118]

CONCLUSION

Alopecia is the visible result of many diverse causes, some of which may be temporary and easily reversible and others refractory to therapy. Identifying the cause is key. Management/treatment of alopecia should be as cause-specific as possible. In addition, psychosocial support should always be considered.

ABBREVIATIONS

ACTH	adrenocorticotropic hormone
AA	alopecia areata
AD	atopic dermatitis
AGA	androgenetic alopecia
AT	alopecia totalis (or alopecia areata totalis)
aTE	acute telogen effluvium
AU	alopecia universalis (or alopecia areata universalis)
BMPs	bone morphogenetic proteins
BPH	benign prostatic hyperplasia
CI	confidence interval
DHEA	dehydroepiandrosterone
DHT	dihydrotestosterone
F	female
FGF	fibroblast growth factor
FPHL	female pattern hair loss
HGF	hepatic growth factor
IGF	insulin-like growth factor
IL	interleukin
JAK-STAT	Janus Kinase-signal transducer and activator of transcription
KOH	potassium hydroxide
LFTs	liver function tests
LLLL	low-level laser light
M	male
NT	neurotrophins
PCOS	polycystic ovarian syndrome
PRP	platelet-rich plasma
QoL	quality of life
RCT	randomized controlled trial
RR	risk ratio
SALT	severity of Alopecia Tool
SLE	systemic lupus erythematosus
SSRI	selective serotonin reuptake inhibitor
TCM	traditional Chinese medicine
TCS	topical corticosteroids
TGF	transforming growth factor
TNF	tumor necrosis factor
WNT	aportmanteau created from the name Wingless and the name Int-1
VEGF	vascular endothelial growth factor

REFERENCES

1. Phillips TG, Slomiany WP, Allison R. Hair loss: Common causes and treatment. *Am Fam Physician*. 2017;96(6):371–378.
2. Buffoli B, Rinaldi F, Labanca M, et al. The human hair: From anatomy to physiology. *Int J Dermatol.* 2014;53(3):331–341. doi:0.1111/ijd.12362.
3. Mandt N, Troilius A, Drosner M. Epilation today: Physiology of the hair follicle and clinical photo-epilation. *J Investig Dermatol Symp Proc.* 2005;10(3):271–274.
4. Gilhar A, Etzioni A, Paus R. Alopecia areata. *N Engl J Med.* 2012;366(16):1515–1525. doi:10.1056/NEJMra1103442.
5. Yang CC, Cotsarelis G. Review of hair follicle dermal cells. *J Dermatol Sci.* 2010;57(1):2–11. doi:10.1016/j.jdermsci.2009.11.005.
6. Erdoğan B. (2017, May 03). Anatomy and physiology of hair. Retrieved May 22, 2019, from https://www.intechopen.com/books/hair-and-scalp-disorders/anatomy-and-physiology-of-hair.
7. Schneider MR, Schmidt-Ullrich R, Paus R. The hair follicle as a dynamic miniorgan. *Curr Biol.* 2009;19(3):R132–R142. doi:10.1016/j.cub.2008.12.005.
8. Mysore V, Shashikumar BM. Guidelines on the use of finasteride in androgenetic alopecia. *Indian J Dermatol Venereol Leprol.* 2016;82(2):128–134. doi:10.4103/0378-6323.177432.
9. Juárez-Rendón KJ, Rivera Sánchez G, Reyes-López MÁ, et al. Alopecia Areata. Current situation and perspectives. *Arch Argent Pediatr.* 2017;115(6):e404–e411. doi:10.5546/aap.2017.eng.e404.
10. Ellis JA, Stebbing M, Harrap SB. Insulin gene polymorphism and premature male pattern baldness in the general population. *Clin Sci (Lond).* 1999;96(6):659–662.
11. Ellis JA, Stebbing M, Harrap SB. Genetic analysis of male pattern baldness and the 5alpha-reductase genes. *J Invest Dermatol.* 1998;110(6):849–853.
12. Hillmer AM, Kruse R, Macciardi F, et al. The hairless gene in androgenetic alopecia: Results of a systematic mutation screening and a family-based association approach. *Br J Dermatol.* 2002;146(4):601–608.
13. Hillmer AM, Hanneken S, Ritzmann S, et al. Genetic variation in the human androgen receptor gene is the major determinant of common early-onset androgenetic alopecia. *Am J Hum Genet.* 2005;77(1):140–148. doi:10.1086/431425.
14. Petukhova L, Duvic M, Hordinsky M, et al. Genome-wide association study in alopecia areata implicates both innate and adaptive immunity. *Nature.* 2010;466(7302):113–117. doi:10.1038/nature09114.
15. Jagielska D, Redler S, Brockschmidt FF, et al. Follow-up study of the first genome-wide association scan in alopecia areata: IL13 and KIAA0350 as susceptibility loci supported with genome-wide significance. *J Invest Dermatol.* 2012;132(9):2192–2197. doi:10.1038/jid.2012.129.
16. Courtois M, Loussouarn G, Hourseau C, Grollier JF. Hair cycle and alopecia. *Skin Pharmacol.* 1994;7(1-2):84–89.
17. Guarrera M, Rebora A. Anagen hairs may fail to replace telogen hairs in early androgenic female alopecia. *Dermatology.* 1996;192(1):28–31.
18. Kibar M, Aktan S, Bilgin M. Scalp dermatoscopic findings in androgenetic alopecia and their relations with disease severity. *Ann Dermatol.* 2014;26(4):478–484. doi:10.5021/ad.2014.26.4.478.
19. Cranwell W, Sinclair R, et al. Male androgenetic alopecia. [Updated 2016 Feb 29]. In: Feingold KR, Anawalt B, Boyce A, et al., eds. *Endotext [Internet].* South Dartmouth (MA): MDText.com, Inc; 2000. Available at: https://www.ncbi.nlm.nih.gov/books/NBK278957/
20. Zhao Y, Zhang B, Caulloo S, Chen X, Li Y, Zhang X. Diffuse alopecia areata is associated with intense inflammatory infiltration and CD8+ T cells in hair loss regions and an increase in serum IgE level. *Indian J Dermatol Venereol Leprol.* 2012;78(6):709–714.
21. Filbrandt R, Rufaut N, Jones L, Sinclair R. Primary cicatricial alopecia: Diagnosis and treatment. *CMAJ.* 2013;185(18):1579–1585. doi:10.1503/cmaj.111570.
22. Harries MJ, Sinclair RD, Macdonald-Hull S, Whiting DA, Griffiths CE, Paus R. Management of primary cicatricial alopecias: Options for treatment. *Br J Dermatol.* 2008;159(1):1–22. doi:10.1111/j.1365-2133.2008.08591.x.
23. Piraccini BM, Alessandrini A. Androgenetic alopecia. *G Ital Dermatol Venereol.* 2014;149(1):15–24.
24. Rubio-Gonzalez B, Juhász M, Fortman J, Mesinkovska NA. Pathogenesis and treatment options for chemotherapy-induced alopecia: A systematic review. *Int J Dermatol.* 2018;57(12):1417–1424. doi:10.1111/ijd.13906.
25. Dhurat RP, Deshpande DJ. Loose anagen hair syndrome. *Int J Trichology.* 2010;2(2):96–100. doi:10.4103/0974-7753.77513.
26. Loh SH, Lew BL, Sim WY. Localized telogen effluvium following hair transplantation. *Ann Dermatol.* 2018;30(2):214–217. doi:10.5021/ad.2018.30.2.214.
27. Harvard Health Publishing. Harvard Medical School. Treating female pattern hair loss. https://www.health.harvard.edu/staying-healthy/treating-female-pattern-hair-loss. November 14, 2018; August 24, 2019.
28. Hay RJ. Tinea capitis: Current status. *Mycopathologia.* 2017;182(1-2):87–93. doi:10.1007/s11046-016-0058-8.
29. Almeida MC, Romiti R, Doche I, Valente NY, Donati A. Psoriatic scarring alopecia. *An Bras Dermatol.* 2013;88(6 suppl 1):29–31. doi:10.1590/abd1806-4841.20132241.
30. Borda LJ, Wikramanayake TC. Seborrheic dermatitis and dandruff: A comprehensive review. *J Clin Investig Dermatol.* 2015;3(2). doi:10.13188/2373-1044.1000019.
31. Tosti A, Piraccini BM, van Neste DJ. Telogen effluvium after allergic contact dermatitis of the scalp. *Arch Dermatol.* 2001;137(2):187–190.
32. Brown F, Badri T. Pityriasis Rubra Pilaris. [Updated 2019 February 22]. In: *StatPearls [Internet].* Treasure Island (FL): StatPearls Publishing; 2019. Available at: https://www.ncbi.nlm.nih.gov/books/NBK482436/.
33. Rothe MJ, Bialy TL, Grant-Kels JM. Erythroderma. *Dermatol Clin.* 2000 Jul;18(3):405–415.
34. Perera E, Yip L, Sinclair R. Alopecia areata. In: Ioannides D, Tosti A, eds. *Alopecias—Practical Evaluation and Management. Curr Probl Dermatol.* Basel: Karger, 2015;47:67–75. doi:10.1159/000369406.

35. Kyriakis KP, Paltatzidou K, Kosma E, Sofouri E, Tadros A, Rachioti E. Alopecia areata prevalence by gender and age. *J Eur Acad Dermatol Venereol.* 2009;23(5):572–573. doi:10.1111/j.1468-3083.2008.02956.x.
36. Amin SS, Sachdeva S. (n.d.). Alopecia areata: An update. Retrieved May 22, 2019, from http://jpad.com.pk/index.php/jpad/article/view/346.
37. Seetharam KA. Alopecia areata: An update. *Indian J Dermatol Venereol Leprol.* 2013;79(5):563–575. doi:10.4103/0378-6323.116725.
38. Al-Refu K. Hair loss in children: Common and uncommon causes; clinical and epidemiological study in Jordan. *Int J Trichology.* 2013;5(4):185–189. doi:10.4103/0974-7753.130393.
39. Lundin M, Chawa S, Sachdev A, Bhanusali D, Seiffert-Sinha K, Sinha AA. Gender differences in alopecia areata. *J Drugs Dermatol.* 2014;13(4):409–413.
40. Lacarrubba F, Micali G, Tosti A. Scalp dermoscopy or trichoscopy. *Curr Probl Dermatol.* 2015;47:21–32. doi:10.1159/000369402.
41. Villasante Fricke AC, Miteva M. Epidemiology and burden of alopecia areata: A systematic review. *Clin Cosmet Investig Dermatol.* 2015;8:397–403. doi:10.2147/CCID.S53985.
42. Xu L, Liu KX, Senna MM. A practical approach to the diagnosis and management of hair loss in children and adolescents. *Front Med (Lausanne).* 2017;4:112. doi:10.3389/fmed.2017.00112.
43. Torborg L. Mayo Clinic Q & A: Cold cap therapy can reduce hair loss caused by chemotherapy. January 30, 2018. Mayo Clinic. Available at: https://newsnetwork.mayoclinic.org/discussion/mayo-clinic-q-and-a-cold-cap-therapy-can-reduce-hair-loss-caused-by-chemotherapy/. Accessed May 19, 2019.
44. Cold caps and scalp cooling systems. March 11, 2019. BreastCancer.org. Available at: https://www.breastcancer.org/tips/hair_skin_nails/cold-caps. Accessed May 19, 2019.
45. Skalnaya MG. Chapter 17: Copper deficiency a new reason of androgenetic alopecia? Pharmacology and Nutritional Intervention in the Treatment of Disease. Available at: http://dx.doi.org/10.5772/58416. Accessed April 30, 2019.
46. Ninan PT, Rothbaum BO, Marsteller FA, et al. A placebo-controlled trial of cognitive-behavioural therapy and clomipramine in trichotillomania. *J Clin Psychiatry.* 2000;61(1):47–50.
47. Likhitkar M, Shakur AA, Bansal KK, Pande M. Alopecia—Reason and possible treatments. *MOJ Drug Design Development & Therapy.* 2018;2(5):198–208.
48. Fabbrocini G, Cantelli M, Masarà A, Annunziata MC, Marasca C, Cacciapuoti S. Female pattern hair loss: A clinical, pathophysiologic, and therapeutic review. *Int J Womens Dermatol.* 2018;4(4):203–211. doi:10.1016/j.ijwd.2018.05.001.
49. van Zuuren EJ, Fedorowicz Z, Schoones J. Interventions for female pattern hair loss. *Cochrane Database Syst Rev.* 2016;2016(5):CD007628. doi:10.1002/14651858.CD007628.pub4.
50. Blumeyer A, Tosti A, Messenger A, et al.; European Dermatology Forum (EDF). Evidence-based (S3) guideline for the treatment of androgenetic alopecia in women and in men. *J Dtsch Dermatol Ges.* 2011;9(suppl 6):S1–S57. doi:10.1111/j.1610-0379.2011.07802.x.
51. Lee WS, Lee HJ, Choi GS, et al. Guidelines for management of androgenetic alopecia based on BASP classification—The Asian Consensus Committee guideline. *J Eur Acad Dermatol Venereol.* 2013;27(8):1026–1034. doi:10.1111/jdv.12034.
52. Torres F. Androgenetic, diffuse and senescent alopecia in men: Practical evaluation and management. In: Ioannides D, Tosti A, eds. *Alopecia—Practical Evaluation and Management. Curr Probl Dermatol.* Basel: Karger; 2015;47:33–44. doi:10.1159/000369403.
53. Olsen EA, Dunlap FE, Funicella T, et al. A randomized clinical trial of 5% topical minoxidil versus 2% topical minoxidil and placebo in the treatment of androgenetic alopecia in men. *J Am Acad Dermatol.* 2002;47(3):377–385.
54. Roberts JL, Fiedler V, Imperato-McGinley J, et al. Clinical dose ranging studies with finasteride, a type 2 5alpha-reductase inhibitor, in men with male pattern hair loss. *J Am Acad Dermatol.* 1999;41(4):555–563.
55. Gubelin Harcha W, Barboza Martínez J, Tsai TF, et al. A randomized, active- and placebo-controlled study of the efficacy and safety of different doses of dutasteride versus placebo and finasteride in the treatment of male subjects with androgenetic alopecia. *J Am Acad Dermatol.* 2014;70(3):489–498 e3. doi:10.1016/j.jaad.2013.10.049.
56. Stough DB, Rao NA, Kaufman KD, Mitchell C. Finasteride improves male pattern hair loss in a randomized study in identical twins. *Eur J Dermatol.* 2002;12(1):32–37.
57. Van Neste D, Fuh V, Sanchez-Pedreno P, et al. Finasteride increases anagen hair in men with androgenetic alopecia. *Br J Dermatol.* 2000;143(4):804–810.
58. Van Neste D. Natural scalp hair regression in preclinical stages of male androgenetic alopecia and its reversal by finasteride. *Skin Pharmacol Physiol.* 2006;19(3):168–176.
59. Neste DV. (2019, May 12). Maintenance of optimised hair growth from viable terminal scalp hair follicles at baseline with oral finasteride in male pattern hair loss and first evidence of a "drug dependency" and a post-finasteride "rebound effect". Retrieved May 22, 2019. Available at: https://onlinelibrary.wiley.com/doi/abs/10.1111/srt.12707.
60. Lee S, Lee YB, Choe SJ, Lee WS. Adverse sexual effects of treatment with finasteride or dutasteride for male androgenetic alopecia: A systematic review and meta-analysis. *Acta Derm Venereol.* 2019;99(1):12–17. doi:10.2340/00015555-3035.
61. Torres F. Androgenetic, and senescent alopecia in men: Practical evaluation and management. In: Ioannides D, Tosti A, eds. *Alopecia—Practical Evaluation and Management. Curr Probl Dermatol.* Basel: Karger; 2015:47:33–44. doi:10.1159/000369403.
62. Eun HC, Kwon OS, Yeon JH, et al. Efficacy, safety, and tolerability of dutasteride 0.5 mg once daily in male patients with male pattern hair loss: A randomized, double-blind, placebo-controlled, phase III study. *J Am Acad Dermatol.* 2010;63(2):252–258. doi:10.1016/j.jaad.2009.09.018.
63. Gajjar PC, Mehta HH, Barvaliya M, Sonagra B. Comparative study between mesotherapy and topical 5% minoxidil by dermoscopic evaluation for androgenic alopecia in male: A randomized controlled trial. *Int J Trichology.* 2019;11(2):58–67. doi:10.4103/ijt.ijt_89_18.
64. Saceda-Corralo D, Rodrigues-Barata AR, Vañó-Galván S, Jaén-Olasolo P. Mesotherapy with dutasteride in the treatment of androgenetic alopecia. *Int J Trichology.* 2017;9(3):143–145. doi:10.4103/ijt.ijt_73_16.
65. McElwee KJ, Shapiro JS. Promising therapies for treating and/or preventing androgenic alopecia. *Skin Therapy Lett.* 2012;17(6):1–4.
66. Jones MC. (2018, August 17). Treatment Options for Androgenetic Alopecia. Retrieved May 22, 2019. Available at: https://www.uspharmacist.com/article/treatment-options-for-androgenetic-alopecia.
67. Picard F, Hersant B, Niddam J, Meningaud JP. Injections of platelet-rich plasma for androgenic alopecia: A systematic review. *J Stomatol Oral Maxillofac Surg.* 2017;118(5):291–297. doi:10.1016/j.jormas.2017.06.011.
68. Cervelli V, Garcovich S, Bielli A, et al. The effect of autologous activated platelet rich plasma (AA-PRP) injection on pattern hair loss: Clinical and histomorphometric evaluation. *Biomed Res Int.* 2014;2014. doi:10.1155/2014/760709.
69. Verma K, Tegta GR, Verma G, Gupta M, Negi A, Sharma R. A study to compare the efficacy of platelet-rich plasma and minoxidil therapy for the treatment of androgenetic alopecia. *Int J Trichology.* 2019;11(2):68–79. doi:10.4103/ijt.ijt_64_18.
70. Kelly Y, Blanco A, Tosti A. Androgenetic alopecia: An update of treatment options. *Drugs.* 2016;76(14):1349–1364. doi:10.1007/s40265-016-0629-5.
71. Jo SJ, Shin H, Park YW, et al. Topical valproic acid increases the hair count in male patients with androgenetic alopecia: A randomized, comparative, clinical feasibility study using phototrichogram analysis. *J Dermatol.* 2014;41(4):285–291.
72. Lee CY, Wei CC, Yu MC, et al. Hair growth effect of traditional Chinese medicine BeauTop on androgenetic alopecia patients: A randomized double-blind placebo-controlled clinical trial. *Exp Ther Med.* 2017;13(1):194–202. doi:10.3892/etm.2016.3935.
73. Sonthalia S, Daulatabad D, Tosti A. (2016, January 23). Hair Restoration in Androgenetic Alopecia: Looking Beyond Minoxidil, Finasteride and Hair Transplantation. Retrieved May 22, 2019. Available at: https://www.omicsonline.org/open-access/hair-restoration-in-androgenetic-alopecia-looking-beyond-minoxidil-finasteride-and-hair-transplantation-jctt1000105.php?aid=68395.
74. Narda M, Aladren S, Cestone E, Nobile V. (2017, November 30). Efficacy and Safety of a Food Supplement Containing L-cystine, Serenoa repens Extract and Biotin for Hair Loss in Healthy Males and Females. A Prospective, Randomized, Double-blinded, Controlled Clinical Trial. Available at: https://www.omicsonline.org/open-access/efficacy-and-safety-of-a-food-supplement-containing-lcystine-serenoa-repens-extract-and-biotin-for-hair-loss-in-healthy-males-and-2471-9323-1000127-96167.html.
75. Starace M, Orlando G, Alessandrini A, Piraccini BM. Female androgenic alopecia: An update on diagnosis and management. *Am J Clin Dermatol.* 2020;21(1):69–84.
76. Won YY, Lew BL, Sim WY. Clinical efficacy of oral administration of finasteride at a dose of 2.5 mg/day in women with female pattern hair loss. *Dermatol Ther.* 2018;31(2):e12588.

77. Yeon JH, Jung JY, Choi JW, et al. 5 mg/day finasteride treatment for normoandrogenic Asian women with female pattern hair loss. *J Eur Acad Dermatol Venereol.* 2011;25:211–214.
78. Oliveira-Soares R, E Silva JM, Correia MP, Andre MC. Finasteride 5 mg/day treatment of patterned hair loss in normo-androgenetic postmenopausal women. *Int J Trichol.* 2013;5:22–25.
79. Shum KW, Cullen DR, Messenger AG. Hair loss in women with hyperandrogenism: Four cases responding to finasteride. *J Am Acad Dermatol.* 2002;47(5):733–739.
80. Ioannides D, Lazaridou E. Female pattern hair loss. *Curr Probl Dermatol.* 2015:47:45–54. doi:10.1159/000369404.
81. Olszewska M, Rudnicka L. Effective treatment of female androgenic alopecia with dutasteride. *J Drugs Dermatol.* 2005;4(5):637–640.
82. Vexiau P, Chaspoux C, Boudou P, et al. Effects of minoxidil 2% vs. cyproterone acetate treatment on female androgenetic alopecia: A controlled, 12-month randomized trial. *Br J Dermatol.* 2002;146(6):992–999.
83. Sinclair R, Wewerinke M, Jolley D. Treatment of female pattern hair loss with oral antiandrogens. *Br J Dermatol.* 2005;152(3):466–473.
84. Paradisi R, Porcu E, Fabbri R, Seracchioli R, Battaglia C, Venturoli S. Prospective cohort study on the effects and tolerability of flutamide in patients with female pattern hair loss. *Ann Pharmacother.* 2011;45(4):469–475. doi:10.1345/aph.1P600.
85. Azarchi S, Bienenfeld A, Lo Sicco K et al. Androgens in women: Hormone modulating therapies for skin disease (part II). *J Am Acad Dermatol.* 2019;80(6):1509–1521. doi:10.1016/j.jaad.2018.08.061.
86. Le Floc'h C, Cheniti A, Connétable S, Piccardi N, Vincenzi C, Tosti A. Effect of a nutritional supplement on hair loss in women. *J Cosmet Dermatol.* 2015;14(1):76–82. doi:10.1111/jocd.12127.
87. Torkos S, Gazella K. (2015, April). Essential Fatty Acids and Antioxidants Benefit Women With Female Pattern Hair Loss. Retrieved May 22, 2019. Available at: https://www.naturalmedicinejournal.com/journal/2015-04/essential-fatty-acids-and-antioxidants-benefit-women-female-pattern-hair-loss.
88. Katoulis AC, Liakou AI, Alevizou A, et al. Efficacy and safety of a topical botanical in female androgenetic alopecia: A randomized, single-blinded, vehicle-controlled study. *Skin Appendage Disord.* 2018;4(3):160–165. doi:10.1159/000480024.
89. Liu KH, Liu D, Chen YT, Chin SY. Comparative effectiveness of low-level laser therapy for adult androgenic alopecia: A system review and meta-analysis of randomized controlled trials. *Lasers Med Sci.* 2019;34(6):1063–1069.
90. Starace M, Alessandrini A, D'Acunto C, et al. Platelet-rich plasma on female androgenetic alopecia: Tested on 10 patients. *J Cosmet Dermatol.* 2019;18(1):59–64.
91. Kanti V, Messenger A, Dobos G, et al. Evidence-based (S3) guideline for the treatment of androgenetic alopecia in women and men. *Eur Acad Dermatol.* 2018;32(1):11–22.
92. Hunter N, Sayed K, Hay RA, Allam R, Hussein N. Comparing the efficacy of mesotherapy to topical minoxidil in the treatment of female pattern hair loss using ultrasound biomicroscopy: A randomized controlled trial. *Acta Dermatovenerol Croat.* 2019;27(1):1–7.
93. Tosti A, Iorizzo M, Piraccini BM. Androgenetic alopecia in children: Report of 20 cases. *Br J Dermatol.* 2005;152(3):556–559.
94. Price VH. Androgenetic alopecia in adolescents. *Cutis.* 2003;71(2):115–121.
95. Rodrigues M, Antunes I, Magalhães S, et al. Androgenic alopecia: An entity to consider in adolescence. *Case Reports.* 2017; 2017:bcr-2017-220679.
96. Nor NM, Ismail R, Jamil A, Shah SA, Imran FH. A randomized, single-blind trial of clobetasol propionate 0.05% cream under silicone dressing occlusion versus intra-lesional triamcinolone for treatment of keloid. *Clin Drug Investig.* 2017;37(3):295–301. doi:10.1007/s40261-016-0484-x.
97. Rathi SK, D'Souza P. Rational and ethical use of topical corticosteroids based on safety and efficacy. *Indian J Dermatol.* 2012;57(4):251–259. doi:10.4103/0019-5154.97655.
98. Vañó-Galván S, Hermosa-Gelbard Á, Sánchez-Neila N, et al. Pulse corticosteroid therapy with oral dexamethasone for the treatment of adult alopecia totalis and universalis. *J Am Acad Dermatol.* 2016;74(5):1005–1007.
99. Triyangkulsri K, Suchonwanit P. Role of janus kinase inhibitors in the treatment of alopecia areata. *Drug Des Devel Ther.* 2018;12:2323–2335. doi:10.2147/DDDT.S172638.
100. Liu LY, Craiglow BG, Dai F, King BA. Tofacitinib for the treatment of severe alopecia areata and variants: A study of 90 patients. *J Am Acad Dermatol.* 2017;76(1):22–28. doi:10.1016/j.jaad.2016.09.007.
101. Dai YX, Chen CC. Tofacitinib therapy for children with severe alopecia areata. *J Am Acad Dermatol.* 2019;80(4):1164–1166. doi:10.1016/j.jaad.2018.12.041.
102. Bayart CB, DeNiro KL, Brichta L, Craiglow BG, Sidbury R. Topical Janus kinase inhibitors for the treatment of pediatric alopecia areata. *J Am Acad Dermatol.* 2017;77(1):167–170. doi:10.1016/j.jaad.2017.03.024.
103. Liu LY, King BA. Ruxolitinib for the treatment of severe alopecia areata. *J Am Acad Dermatol.* 2019;80(2):566–568. doi:10.1016/j.jaad.2018.08.040.
104. Penzi LR, Yasuda M, Manatis-Lornell A, Hagigeorges D, Senna MM. Hair regrowth in a patient with long-standing alopecia totalis and atopic dermatitis treated with dupilumab. *JAMA Dermatol.* 2018;154(11):1358–1360. doi:10.1001/jamadermatol.2018.2976.
105. Smogorzewski J, Sierro T, Compoginis G, Kim G. Remission of alopecia universalis in a patient with atopic dermatitis treated with dupilumab. *JAAD Case Rep.* 2019;5(2):116–117. doi:10.1016/j.jdcr.2018.11.007.
106. Phan K, Ramachandran V, Sebaratnam DF. Methotrexate for alopecia areata: A systematic review and meta-analysis. *J Am Acad Dermatol.* 2019;80(1):120–127.e2.
107. Vañó-Galván S, Hermosa-Gelbard Á, Sánchez-Neila N, et al. Treatment of recalcitrant adult alopecia areata universalis with oral azathioprine. *J Am Acad Dermatol.* 2016;74(5):1007–1008. doi:10.1016/j.
108. Fiedler-Weiss VC, Buys CM. Evaluation of anthralin in the treatment of alopecia areata. *Arch Dermatol.* 1987;123(11):1491–1493.
109. Spano F, Donovan JC. Alopecia areata: Part 2: Treatment. *Can Fam Physician.* 2015;61(9):757–761.
110. Jha AK, Sarkar R, Udavan UK et al. Bimatoprost in dermatology. *Ind Dermatol Online J.* 2018;9(3):224–228.
111. Barron-Hernandez YL, Tosti A. Bimatoprost for the treatment of eyelash, eyebrow, and scalp alopecia. *Expert Opin Invest Drugs.* 2017;26(4):515–522. doi:10.1080/13543784.2017.1303480.
112. Riahi RR, Cohen PH. Topical treatment of eyebrow hypotrichosis with bimatoprost 0.03% solution: Case report and literature review. *Cureus.* 2018;10(5):e2666. doi:10.7759/cureus.2666.
113. Draelos ZD. Hair care and dyeing. *Curr Probl Dermatol.* 2015;47:121–127. doi:10.1159/000368412.
114. Dove US (a skin care product company). YouTube. Beauty standards of hair are a form of bias. Available at: https://www.youtube.com/watch?v=agptI1_1C40. August 25, 2019.
115. Rowland K. YouTube. Crown. Available at: https://www.youtube.com/watch?v=LUkqY-pR5EU. August 25, 2019.
116. Gorbatenko-Roth K, Prose N, Kundu RV, Patterson S. Assessment of Black patients' perception of their dermatology care. *JAMA Dermatol.* 2019;155(10):1129–1134. doi:10.1001/jamadermatol.2019.2063.
117. Gaulding JV, Gutierrez D, Bhatia BK et al. Epidemiology of skin diseases in a diverse patient population. *J Drugs Dermatol.* 2018;17(10):1032–1036.
118. Grayson C, Heath C. An approach to examining tightly coiled hair among patients with hair loss in race-discordant patient-physician interactions. *JAMA Dermatol.* 2021;157(5):505–506.

Dermatologic Drug Reactions, Contact Dermatitis, and Common Skin Conditions

e121

Rebecca M. Law, David T. S. Law, and Howard I. Maibach

KEY CONCEPTS

1. Patients presenting with a skin condition should be interviewed thoroughly regarding signs and symptoms, urgency, other subjective complaints, and medication history. The skin eruption should be carefully assessed to help distinguish between a disease condition and a drug-induced skin reaction.
2. Drug-induced skin reactions may be caused by systemic or topical medications and can be irritant (if topical route) or allergic (topical or systemic route) in nature.
3. Allergic drug reactions can be classified into exanthematous, urticarial, blistering, and pustular eruptions. Exanthematous reactions include maculopapular rashes and drug hypersensitivity syndrome. Urticarial reactions include urticaria, angioedema, and serum sickness-like reactions. Blistering reactions include fixed drug eruptions, Stevens-Johnson syndrome, and toxic epidermal necrolysis (SJS/TEN). Pustular eruptions include acneiform drug reactions and acute generalized exanthematous pustulosis. Other drug-induced skin reactions include hyperpigmentation and photosensitivity. Genotyping may help identify patients at higher risk of a severe reaction.
4. Not all skin reactions are drug induced. In clinical practice, a diagnosis of drug-induced skin reaction is often a diagnosis of exclusion (ie, the diagnosis is reached after other possible diagnoses have been ruled out).
5. Contact dermatitis is a common skin disorder caused either by an irritant contactant or an allergic/sensitizing contactant, resulting in irritant contact dermatitis (ICD) or allergic contact dermatitis (ACD).
6. An ICD is confined to the area of chemical contact, whereas an ACD may extend beyond the areas of contact. However, it may sometimes be difficult to differentiate an ICD from an ACD.
7. Patch testing is a criterion standard for the diagnosis of ACD—the crucial investigative and diagnostic method used together with a detailed clinical history and physical examination/workup.
8. The first goals of therapy in the management of contact dermatitis involve identification, withdrawal, and avoidance of the offending agent. A thorough history, including occupational history, must be carefully reviewed for potential contactants.
9. Other goals of therapy for contact dermatitis include providing symptomatic relief, implementing preventive measures, and providing coping strategies and other information for patients and caregivers.
10. Photoaging is premature skin aging most commonly due to sun exposure.
11. Skin cancers include squamous cell carcinoma, basal cell carcinoma, and malignant melanoma.
12. Skin manifestations of COVID-19 infection go beyond the chilblains-like lesions commonly called "COVID-toes," and may also present as morbilliform/maculopapular, papulosquamous, vesicular, urticarial, or erythema multiform-like lesions. In addition, purpuric pressure ulcers or vascular lesions (petechiae, purpura, and livedo) may present in patients with COVID-19.

BEYOND THE BOOK

Review Chapter e17 "Skin Care and Minor Dermatologic Conditions" in this textbook for background on skin structure and function, transdermal drug absorption, and definitions of macules, papules, nodules, and nevi. In particular, the section on "Sun Damage—Issues and Prevention" is a precursor to the sections on "Photoaging" and "Skin Cancers and Precancerous Conditions" in this chapter.

INTRODUCTION

As the fictional character, Lois Lane said, "... the light always returns to show us things familiar ... and things entirely new, or long overlooked. It shows us new possibilities, and challenges us to pursue them ... you can see it. All you have to do is look ..." (Justice League movie, 2017).[1]

This chapter builds on concepts from Chapter e17, Skin Care and Minor Dermatologic Conditions, the first concept in dermatology is learning how to look at the skin. The reader is strongly encouraged to review that chapter prior to reading this one.

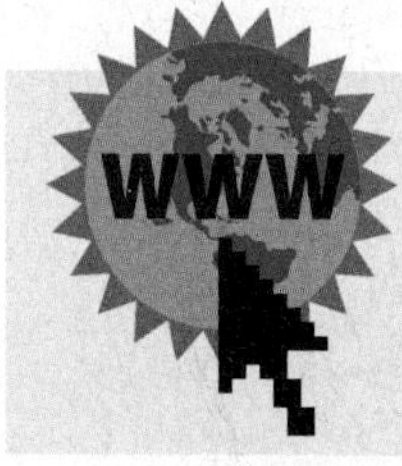

The complete chapter, learning objectives, and other resources can be found at **www.pharmacotherapyonline.com.**

122 Anemias

Kristen M. Cook and Devon M. Greer

KEY CONCEPTS

1. Anemia is a group of diseases characterized by a decrease in either hemoglobin (Hb) or the volume of red blood cells (RBCs), which results in decreased oxygen-carrying capacity of the blood. Anemia is defined by the World Health Organization (WHO) as Hb less than 13 g/dL (130 g/L; 8.07 mmol/L) in men and less than 12 g/dL (120 g/L; 7.45 mmol/L) in women.
2. Acute onset anemias are most likely to present with tachycardia, lightheadedness, and dyspnea. Chronic anemia often presents with weakness, fatigue, headache, vertigo, and pallor.
3. Iron-deficiency anemia (IDA) is characterized by decreased ferritin levels (most sensitive marker) and serum iron, and decreased transferrin saturation. Hb and hematocrit decrease later. RBC morphology includes hypochromia and microcytosis. Most patients are adequately treated with oral iron therapy, although parenteral iron therapy is necessary in some patients.
4. Vitamin B_{12} deficiency, a macrocytic anemia, can be due to inadequate intake, malabsorption syndromes, and inadequate utilization. Anemia caused by lack of intrinsic factor, resulting in decreased vitamin B_{12} absorption, is called *pernicious anemia*. Neurologic symptoms can be present and can become irreversible if the vitamin B_{12} deficiency is not treated promptly. Oral or parenteral therapy can be used for replacement.
5. Folic acid deficiency, a macrocytic anemia, results from inadequate intake, decreased absorption, and increased folate requirements. Treatment consists of oral administration of folic acid, even for patients with absorption problems. Adequate folic acid intake is essential in women of childbearing age to decrease the risk of neural tube defects in their children.
6. Anemia of inflammation (AI) is a newer term used to describe both anemia of chronic disease and anemia of critical illness. AI is a diagnosis of exclusion. It results from chronic inflammation, infection, or malignancy and can occur as early as 1 to 2 months after the onset of the disease. The serum iron level is usually decreased, but in contrast to IDA, the serum ferritin concentration is normal or increased. Treatment is aimed at correcting the underlying pathology. Anemia of critical illness occurs within days of acute illness.
7. Anemia is a common problem in older adults, although not an inevitable complication of aging. Low Hb concentrations are not "normal" in older adults. Anemia is associated with an increased risk of hospitalization and mortality, reduced quality of life, and decreased physical functioning in older adults.
8. IDA is a leading cause of infant morbidity and mortality worldwide. Age- and sex-adjusted norms must be used to interpret laboratory results for pediatric patients. Primary prevention of IDA is the goal because physical and mental developmental delays can be irreversible.

BEYOND THE BOOK

Watch the Khan Academy video on the pathophysiology of anemia:

https://tinyurl.com/5n8eb5dx

Write a paragraph that explains the pathophysiology of anemia to a patient. You can only use patient friendly language.

INTRODUCTION

Anemia affects almost one-third of the world's population, with developing countries carrying the highest burden.[1] Anemia is defined by the WHO as hemoglobin (Hb) less than 13 g/dL (130 g/L; 8.07 mmol/L) in men or less than 12 g/dL (120 g/L; 7.45 mmol/L) in women.[2] In the United States, about 3 million people have anemia.[3] Millions of people are unaware they have anemia, making it one of the most underdiagnosed conditions in the United States. Iron deficiency is the leading cause of anemia worldwide, accounting for as many as 50% of cases.[2] Although nutritional deficiencies occur less often in the United States, they can occur in at risk populations (discussed in more detail later). Anemia is not an innocent bystander because it can affect both length and quality of life. Retrospective observational studies of hemodialysis patients and heart failure patients suggest that anemia is an independent risk factor for mortality.[4] In addition, anemia significantly influences morbidity in patients with end-stage renal disease, chronic kidney disease, and heart failure.[5] Anemia is associated with psychomotor and cognitive abnormalities in children. Similarly, anemia is associated with cognitive dysfunction in patients with renal failure or cancer, and among community-dwelling elders.[6] Anemia during pregnancy is

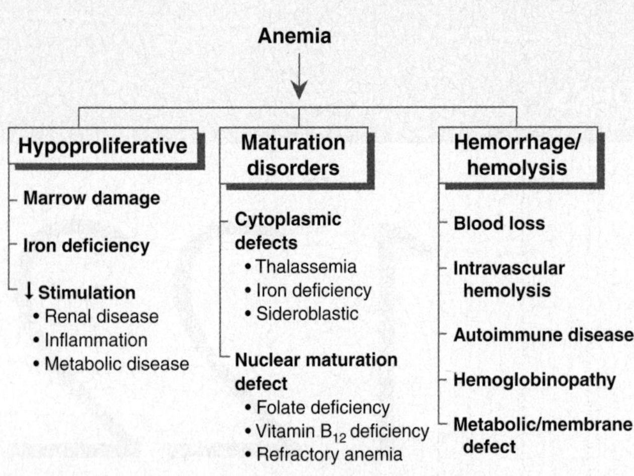

FIGURE 122-1 Functional classification of anemia.

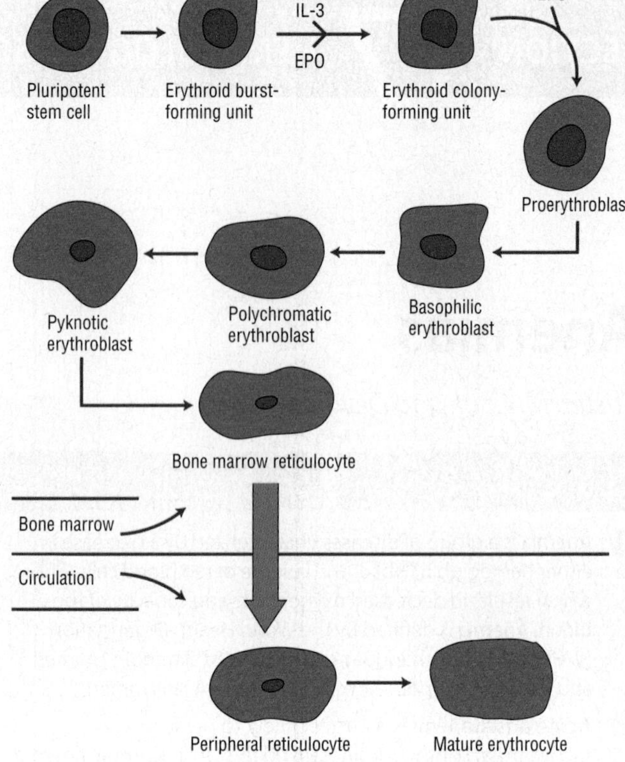

FIGURE 122-2 Erythrocyte maturation sequence.

associated with increased risk for low birth weights, preterm delivery, and perinatal mortality.[7] Maternal IDA may be associated with postpartum depression in mothers and poor performance by offspring on mental and psychomotor tests. In older adults, anemia is associated with a greater risk for falls and dementia.[8] Global goals of treatment in anemic patients are to alleviate signs and symptoms, correct the underlying etiology, and prevent recurrence of anemia.

1 Anemia is a group of diseases characterized by a decrease in Hb or circulating red blood cells (RBCs), resulting in reduced oxygen-carrying capacity of the blood. Anemia can result from inadequate RBC production, increased RBC destruction, or blood loss. It can be a manifestation of systemic disorders, such as infection, chronic renal disease, or malignancy. Anemia is often a sign of underlying pathology, and rapid diagnosis of the cause may be essential.

Figure 122-1 shows the functional classification of anemia. This chapter focuses on some of the most common causes of anemia—IDA, vitamin B_{12} or folic acid deficiency, and anemia of inflammation (AI) (eg, anemia of chronic disease [ACD]). Some of the other common causes of anemia are discussed in other chapters (cancer, renal disease). Drugs can also cause hematologic disorders, including anemia.

Characteristic changes in the RBC size based on erythrocyte indices can be the first step in the morphologic classification and understanding of the anemia. Anemia can be classified by RBC size such as macrocytic, normocytic, or microcytic. Both vitamin B_{12} deficiency and folic acid deficiency are macrocytic anemias. An example of a microcytic anemia is iron deficiency, whereas a normocytic anemia may be associated with recent blood loss or chronic disease. More than one etiology of anemia can occur concurrently. Mixed anemias occur more commonly in older adults.

Microcytic anemias result from a quantitative deficiency in Hb synthesis, usually due to iron deficiency or impaired iron utilization. As a result, erythrocytes containing insufficient Hb are formed. Microcytosis and hypochromia are the morphologic abnormalities that provide evidence of impaired Hb synthesis.

Macrocytic anemias can be divided into megaloblastic and nonmegaloblastic anemias. The type of macrocytic anemia can be distinguished microscopically by peripheral blood smear examination. Megaloblasts are distinctive cells that express a biochemical abnormality of impaired DNA synthesis, resulting in unbalanced cell growth. Megaloblastic anemias may affect all hematopoietic cell lines. The most common causes of megaloblastic anemia discussed in this chapter are vitamin B_{12} and folate deficiency. Nonmegaloblastic macrocytic anemias may arise from liver disease, hypothyroidism, hemolytic processes, and alcoholism.

MATURATION AND DEVELOPMENT OF RED BLOOD CELLS

In adults, RBCs are formed in the marrow of the vertebrae, ribs, sternum, clavicle, pelvic (iliac) crest, and proximal epiphyses of the long bones. In children, most bone marrow space is hematopoietically active to meet increased RBC requirements.

In normal RBC formation, a pluripotent stem cell yields an erythroid burst-forming unit. Erythropoietin (EPO) and cytokines such as interleukin-3 and granulocyte-macrophage colony-stimulating factor stimulate this cell to form an erythroid colony-forming unit in the marrow (Fig. 122-2). During this process, the nucleus becomes smaller with each division, finally disappearing in the normal erythrocyte. Hb and iron are incorporated into the gradually maturing RBC, which eventually is released from the marrow into the circulating blood as a reticulocyte. The maturation process usually takes about 1 week. The reticulocyte loses its nucleus and becomes an erythrocyte within several days. The circulating erythrocyte is a non-nucleated, nondividing cell. More than 90% of the protein content of the erythrocyte consists of the oxygen-carrying molecule Hb. Erythrocytes have a normal survival time of about 120 days.[9]

Stimulation of Erythropoiesis

The hormone EPO, 90% of which is produced by the kidneys, initiates and stimulates RBC production. Erythropoiesis is regulated by a feedback loop (Fig. 122-3). The primary mechanism of action of EPO is to prevent apoptosis, or programmed cell death, of erythroid precursor cells and allow their proliferation and subsequent maturation. A decrease in tissue oxygen concentration signals the kidneys to increase the production and release of EPO into the plasma, which increases production and maturation of RBCs. Under normal circumstances, the RBC mass is kept at an almost constant level by EPO matching new erythrocyte production to the natural rate of loss

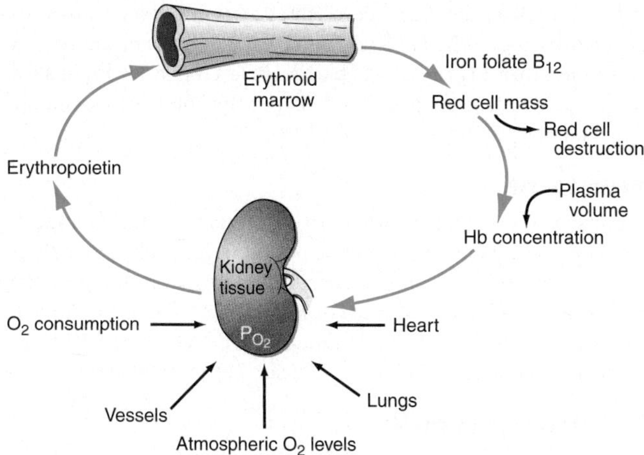

FIGURE 122-3 Physiologic regulation of red cell production by tissue oxygen tension. *(Reproduced, with permission, from Adamson JW, Longo DL. Anemia and polycythemia. In: Longo DL, Fauci AS, Kasper DL, et al., eds. Harrison's Principles of Internal Medicine. 18th ed. New York: McGraw Hill; 2012.)*

of RBCs. Early appearance of large quantities of reticulocytes in the peripheral circulation (reticulocytosis) is an indication of increased RBC production.[9]

Incorporation of Iron into Heme

Iron is an essential part of Hb. The specific plasma transport protein transferrin delivers iron to the bone marrow for incorporation into the Hb molecule. Transferrin enters cells by binding to transferrin receptors, which circulate and then attach to cells needing iron. Fewer transferrin receptors are present on the surface of cells that do not need iron, thus preventing iron-replete cells from receiving excess iron.[10]

Circulating transferrin normally is about 30% saturated with iron. Transferrin delivers extra iron to other body storage sites, such as the liver, marrow, and spleen, for later use. This iron is stored within macrophages as ferritin or hemosiderin. Ferritin consists of a Fe^{3+} hydroxyphosphate core surrounded by a protein shell called *apoferritin*. Hemosiderin can be described as compacted ferritin molecules with an even greater iron-to-protein shell ratio. Physiologically it is a more stable, but less available, form of storage iron. Since total body iron storage is generally reflected by ferritin levels, low serum ferritin levels provide strong evidence of IDA.[9]

Normal Destruction of Red Blood Cells

Phagocytic breakdown destroys older blood cells, primarily in the spleen but also in the marrow (Fig. 122-4). The Hb in RBCs destroyed by intravascular hemolysis becomes attached to haptoglobin and is carried back to the marrow for processing in the normal manner.[11]

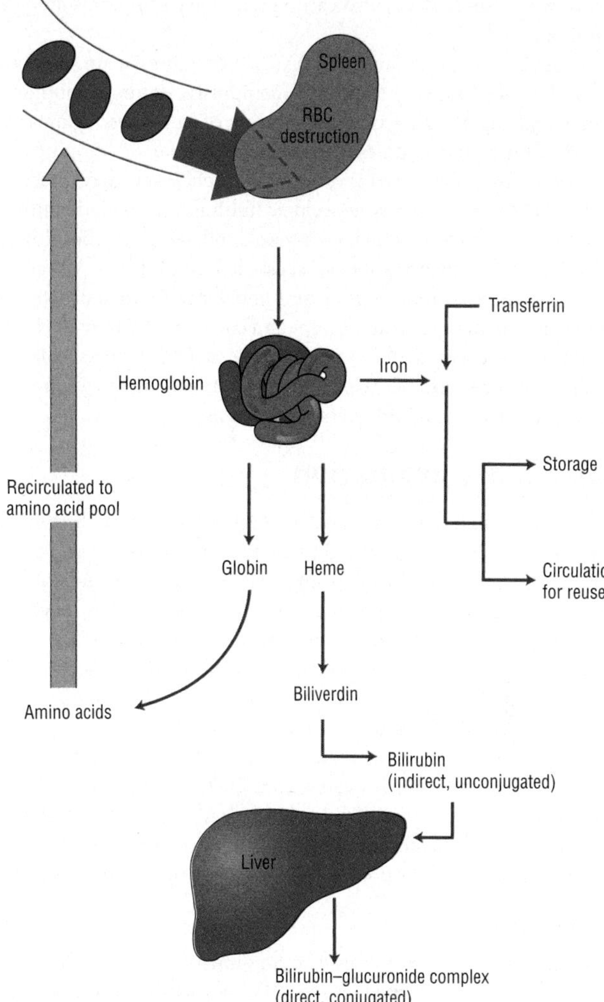

FIGURE 122-4 Destruction of red blood cells.

DIAGNOSIS OF ANEMIA

General Presentation

History, physical examination, and laboratory testing are used to evaluate the patient with anemia. The workup determines if the patient is bleeding and investigates potential causes of the anemia, such as increased RBC destruction, bone marrow suppression, and iron deficiency. Diet can be important in identifying the causes of anemia. Additionally, information about concurrent nonhematologic disease states and a drug history are essential when evaluating the cause of the anemia (Chapter e125, "Drug-Induced Hematologic Disorders"). History of blood transfusions and exposure to toxic chemicals also should be obtained.

Presenting signs and symptoms of anemia depend on its rate of development and the patient's age and cardiovascular status. The severity of symptoms does not always correlate with the degree of anemia. Healthy patients may acclimate to low Hb concentrations if the anemia develops slowly. Mild anemia often is associated with no clinical symptoms and may be found incidentally upon obtaining a complete blood count (CBC) for other reasons. The signs and symptoms in older adults with anemia may be incorrectly attributed to their age or concomitant disease states. Older adults may not tolerate lower levels of Hb in the same way that younger persons do. Similarly, patients with cardiac or pulmonary disease may be less tolerant of mild anemia. Premature infants with anemia may be asymptomatic or have tachycardia, poor weight gain, increased supplemental oxygen needs, or episodes of apnea or bradycardia.

2 Anemia of rapid onset is most likely to present with cardiopulmonary symptoms such as palpitations, angina, lightheadedness, and shortness of breath due to decreased oxygen delivery to tissues or hypovolemia in those with acute bleeding. The patient also may have tachycardia and hypotension.

If onset is more chronic, presenting symptoms may include fatigue, weakness, headache, orthopnea, dyspnea on exertion, vertigo, faintness, sensitivity to cold, and pallor. These traditional signs of anemia have limited sensitivity and specificity and may be misinterpreted. With chronic bleeding, equilibration within the extravascular space occurs, so cardiopulmonary symptoms are less common.

Possible manifestations of IDA include glossal pain, smooth tongue, reduced salivary flow, pica (compulsive eating of nonfood items), and pagophagia (compulsive eating of ice). These symptoms are not likely to appear unless the anemia is severe.

Neurologic findings in vitamin B_{12} deficiency may precede hematologic changes. Early neurologic findings may include numbness and paraesthesias, which are typically bilateral and affect lower limbs more frequently. Ataxia, spasticity, diminished vibratory sense, decreased proprioception, and imbalance may occur later as demyelination of the dorsal columns and corticospinal tract develop. Vision changes may result from optic nerve involvement. Psychiatric findings include irritability, personality changes, memory impairment, depression, and infrequently, psychosis.

Laboratory Evaluation

The initial evaluation of anemia involves a CBC (including RBC indices), reticulocyte index, and possibly an examination of a stool sample for occult blood if bleeding is suspected. The results of the initial evaluation determine the need for other studies, such as examination of a peripheral blood smear. Based on laboratory test results, anemia can be categorized into three functional defects: RBC production failure (hypoproliferative), cell maturation ineffectiveness, or increased RBC destruction or loss (see Fig. 122-1).

Figure 122-5 shows a broad, general algorithm for the diagnosis of anemia based on laboratory data. There are many exceptions and additions to this algorithm, but it can serve as a guide to the typical presentation of common types and causes of anemia. The algorithm is less useful in the presence of more than one cause of anemia.

Hemoglobin

Values given for Hb represent the amount of Hb per volume of whole blood. The higher values seen in males are due to stimulation of RBC production by androgenic steroids, while the lower values in females reflect the decrease in Hb as a result of blood loss during menstruation. The Hb level can be used as a rough estimate of the oxygen-carrying capacity of blood. Hb levels may be diminished because of a decreased quantity of Hb per RBC or a decrease in the actual number of RBCs.

Hematocrit

Expressed as a percentage, hematocrit (Hct) is the actual volume of RBCs in a unit volume of whole blood. It is generally about three times the Hb value (when Hb is expressed in g/dL). An alteration in this ratio may occur with abnormal cell size or shape and often indicates pathology. A low Hct indicates a reduction in either the number or the size of RBCs or an increase in plasma volume.

Red Blood Cell Count

The RBC count is an indirect estimate of the Hb content of the blood; it is an actual count of RBCs per unit of blood.

Red Blood Cell Indices

Wintrobe indices describe the size and Hb content of the RBCs and are calculated from the Hb, Hct, and RBC count. RBC indices, such as mean corpuscular volume (MCV) and mean corpuscular hemoglobin (MCH), are single mean values that do not express the variation that can occur in cells.

Mean Corpuscular Volume MCV represents the average volume of RBCs. It may reflect changes in MCH. Cells are considered macrocytic if they are larger than normal, microcytic if they are smaller than normal, and normocytic if their size falls within normal limits. Folic acid– and vitamin B_{12}–deficiency anemias yield macrocytic cells, whereas iron deficiency is an example of a microcytic anemia. When IDA (decreased MCV) is accompanied by folate deficiency (increased MCV), the overall MCV may be normal. Failure to understand that the MCV represents an average RBC size can cause the clinician to potentially overlook some causes of the anemia.

CLINICAL PRESENTATION Anemia

General

- Patients may be asymptomatic or have vague complaints
- Patients with vitamin B_{12} deficiency may develop neurologic complications
- In AI, signs and symptoms of the underlying disorder often overshadow those of the anemia

Symptoms

- Decreased exercise tolerance
- Fatigue
- Dizziness
- Irritability
- Weakness
- Palpitations
- Vertigo
- Shortness of breath
- Chest pain
- Neurologic symptoms in vitamin B_{12} deficiency

Signs

- Tachycardia
- Pale appearance (most prominent in conjunctivae)
- Decreased mental acuity
- Increased intensity of some cardiac valvular murmurs
- Diminished vibratory sense or gait abnormality in vitamin B_{12} deficiency

Laboratory Tests

- Hemoglobin, hematocrit, and RBC indices may remain normal early in the disease and then decrease as the anemia progresses
- Serum iron is low in IDA and AI
- Ferritin levels are low in IDA and normal or elevated in AI
- Total iron-binding capacity is high in IDA and is low or normal in AI
- Mean cell volume is elevated in vitamin B_{12} deficiency and folate deficiency
- Vitamin B_{12} and folate levels are low in their respective types of anemia
- Homocysteine is elevated in vitamin B_{12} deficiency and folate deficiency
- Methylmalonic acid is elevated in vitamin B_{12} deficiency

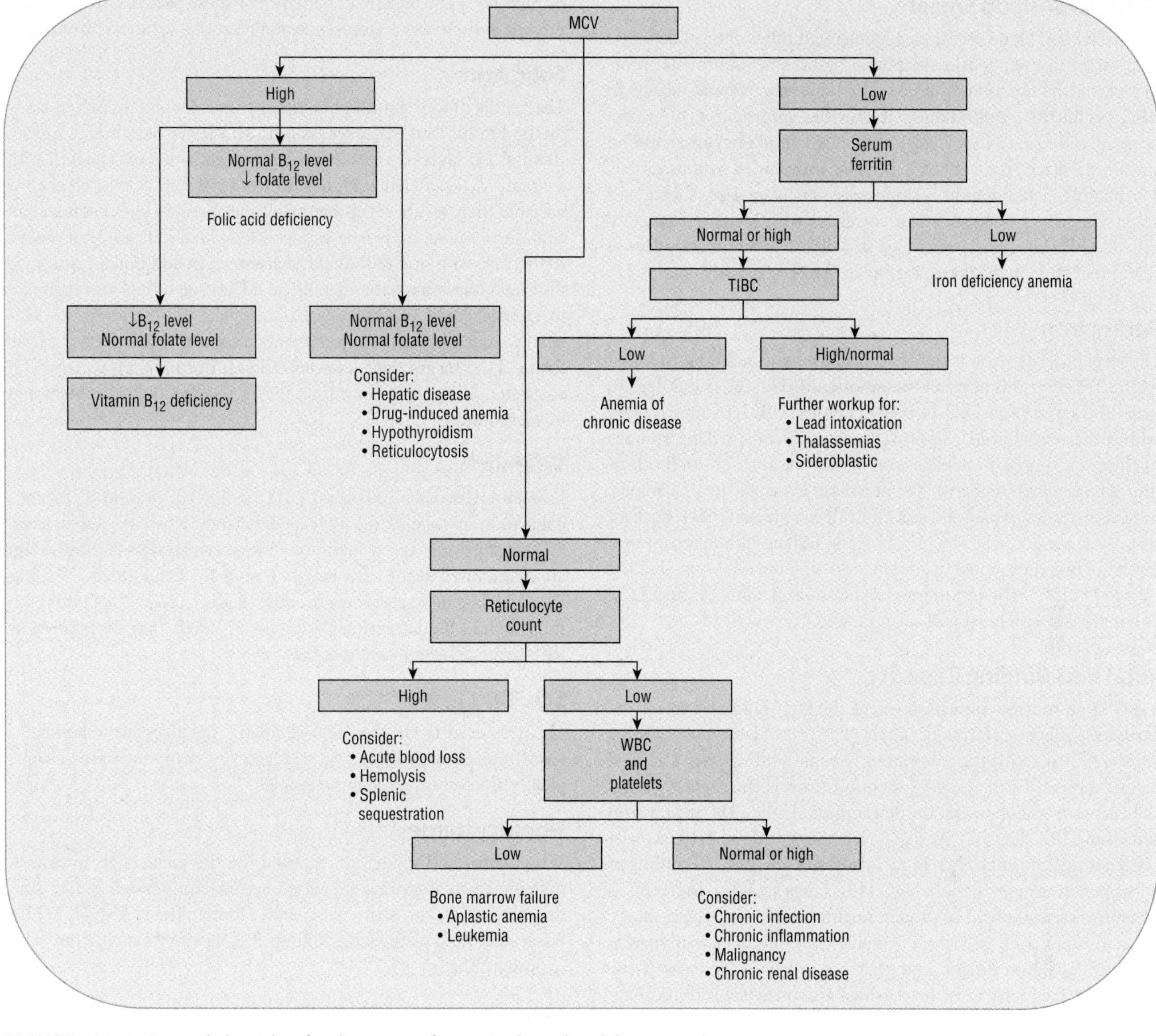

FIGURE 122-5 General algorithm for diagnosis of anemias based on laboratory data.

Mean Corpuscular Hemoglobin MCH is the amount of Hb in a RBC, and usually increases or decreases with the MCV. Two morphologic changes, microcytosis and hypochromia, can reduce MCH. A microcytic cell contains less Hb because it is a smaller cell, while a hypochromic cell has a low MCH because of the decreased concentration of Hb present in the cell. Cells can be both microcytic and hypochromic, as seen with IDA. The MCH alone cannot distinguish between microcytosis and hypochromia. The most common cause of an elevated MCH is macrocytosis (eg, vitamin B_{12} or folate deficiency).

Mean Corpuscular Hemoglobin Concentration The concentration of Hb per volume of cells is the mean cell Hb concentration (MCHC). Because MCHC is independent of cell size, it is more useful than MCH in distinguishing between microcytosis and hypochromia. A low MCHC indicates hypochromia; a microcyte with a normal Hb concentration will have a low MCH but a normal MCHC. A decreased MCHC is seen most often in IDA.

Total Reticulocyte Count

The total reticulocyte count is an indirect assessment of new RBC production. It reflects how quickly immature RBCs (reticulocytes) are produced by bone marrow and released into the blood. Reticulocytes circulate in the blood about 2 days before maturing into RBCs. About 1% of RBCs are normally replaced daily, representing a reticulocyte count of 1%. The reticulocyte count in normocytic anemia can differentiate hypoproliferative marrow from a compensatory marrow response to anemia (see Fig. 122-5). A lack of reticulocytosis in anemia indicates impaired RBC production. Examples include iron deficiency, B_{12} deficiency, ACD, malnutrition, renal insufficiency, and malignancy. A high reticulocyte count may be seen in acute blood loss or hemolysis.

Red Blood Cell Distribution Width

The higher the red blood cell distribution width (RDW), the more variable is the size of the RBCs. The RDW increases in early IDA because of the release of large, immature, nucleated RBCs to compensate for the anemia, but this change is not specific for IDA. The RDW can also be helpful in the diagnosis of a mixed anemia. A patient can have a normal MCV yet have a wide RDW. This finding indicates the presence of microcytes and macrocytes, which would yield a "normal" average RBC size. The use of RDW to distinguish IDA from ACD is not recommended.

Peripheral Blood Smear

The peripheral blood smear can supplement other clinical data and help establish a diagnosis. Peripheral blood smears provide information on the functional status of the bone marrow and defects in RBC production. Additionally, it provides information on variations in cell size (anisocytosis) and shape (poikilocytosis). Blood smears are placed on a microscope slide and stained as appropriate. Morphologic examination includes assessment of size, shape, and color. The extent of anisocytosis correlates with increased range of cell sizes. Poikilocytosis can suggest a defect in the maturation of RBC precursors in the bone marrow or the presence of hemolysis.

Serum Iron

The level of serum iron is the concentration of iron bound to transferrin. Transferrin is normally about one-third bound (saturated) to iron. The serum iron level of many patients with IDA may remain within the lower limits of normal because a considerable amount of time is required to deplete iron stores. Serum iron levels show diurnal variation (higher in the morning, lower in the afternoon), but this variation is probably not clinically significant.[12] Since serum iron levels are decreased by infection and inflammation, serum iron levels are best interpreted in conjunction with the total iron-binding capacity (TIBC). The serum iron level decreases with IDA and ACD and increases with hemolytic anemias and iron overload.

Total Iron-Binding Capacity

TIBC is an indirect measurement of the iron-binding capacity of serum transferrin. Normally, about 30% of available iron binding sites are filled. With this laboratory test, all binding sites are filled to measure TIBC; the excess (unbound) iron is then removed and the serum iron concentration determined. Unlike the serum iron level, the TIBC does not fluctuate over hours or days. TIBC usually is higher than normal when body iron stores are low. The finding of a low serum iron level and a high TIBC suggests IDA. The TIBC is actually a measurement of protein serum transferrin, which can be affected by a variety of factors. Patients with infection, malignancy, inflammation, liver disease, and uremia may have a decreased TIBC and a decreased serum iron level, which are consistent with the diagnosis of ACD.

Percentage Transferrin Saturation

The ratio of serum iron level to TIBC indicates transferrin saturation. It reflects the extent to which iron-binding sites are occupied on transferrin and indicates the amount of iron readily available for erythropoiesis. It is expressed as a percentage, as described in the following formula:

$$\text{Transferrin saturation} = \frac{\text{serum iron}}{\text{TIBC}} \times 100$$

Transferrin normally is 20% to 50% saturated with iron. In IDA, transferrin saturation of 15% or lower is commonly seen.[11] Transferrin saturation is a less sensitive and specific marker of iron deficiency than ferritin levels.

Serum Ferritin

The serum concentration of ferritin (storage iron) is proportional to total iron stores and therefore is the best indicator of iron deficiency or iron overload. Ferritin levels indicate the amount of iron stored in the liver, spleen, and bone marrow cells. Low serum ferritin levels are virtually diagnostic of IDA. In contrast, serum iron levels may decrease in both IDA and ACD. Since serum ferritin is an acute phase reactant, chronic infection or inflammation can increase its concentration independent of iron status, masking depleted tissue stores. This limits the utility of the serum ferritin if the level is normal or high for a chronically ill patient. For these patients, iron, even if present in these tissue stores, may not be available for erythropoiesis.

Folic Acid

The results of folic acid measurements vary depending on the assay method used. Decreased serum folic acid levels (less than 4 ng/mL [9 nmol/L]) indicate a folate deficiency anemia that may coexist with a vitamin B_{12}–deficiency anemia. Erythrocyte folic acid levels are less variable than serum levels because they are slow to decrease in an acute process such as drug-induced folic acid deficiency and slow to increase with oral folic acid replacement. In addition, erythrocyte folic acid levels have the theoretical advantage of less susceptibility to rapid changes in diet and alcohol intake. Limitations with sensitivity and specificity do exist with measurements of erythrocyte folate. If the serum folate concentration is normal for a patient with suspected folate deficiency, then the erythrocyte folate level should be measured.[13]

Vitamin B_{12}

Low levels (less than 200 pg/mL [148 pmol/L]) of vitamin B_{12} (cyanocobalamin or cobalamin) indicate deficiency. However, a deficiency may exist prior to the recognition of low serum levels. Serum values are maintained at the expense of vitamin B_{12} tissue stores. Vitamin B_{12} and folate deficiency may overlap, thus serum levels of both vitamins should be determined. Vitamin B_{12} levels may be falsely low with folate deficiency and pregnancy.[11]

Schilling Test

This test used to be the "gold standard" for assessing vitamin B_{12} absorption. Due to its cost, unavailable test components, and complexity, the test is no longer available.[14]

Homocysteine

Vitamin B_{12} and folate are required for the conversion of homocysteine to methionine. Increased serum homocysteine may suggest vitamin B_{12} or folate deficiency. Homocysteine levels can also be elevated in patients with vitamin B_6 deficiency, renal failure, and hypothyroidism.[15]

Methylmalonic Acid

A vitamin B_{12} coenzyme is needed to convert methylmalonyl coenzyme A to succinyl coenzyme A. Patients with vitamin B_{12} deficiency have increased concentrations of serum methylmalonic acid (MMA), which is a more specific marker for vitamin B_{12} deficiency than homocysteine. MMA levels are not elevated in folate deficiency because folate does not participate in MMA metabolism. Levels of both MMA and homocysteine usually are elevated prior to the development of hematologic abnormalities and reductions in serum vitamin B_{12} levels.[11]

IRON-DEFICIENCY ANEMIA

Epidemiology

Iron deficiency is the most common nutritional deficiency in developing and developed countries. Data from the National Health and Nutrition Examination Survey (NHANES) indicate the prevalence of iron deficiency in the United States in toddlers (1-2 years) and women of childbearing age is 7% and 12%, respectively.[16] Iron deficiency may precede the appearance of anemia because of the wide normal ranges for Hb and Hct.

Iron Balance

The normal iron content of the body is about 3 to 4 g. Iron is a component of Hb, myoglobin, and cytochromes. About 2 g of the iron exists in the form of Hb, and about 130 mg exists as iron-containing proteins such as myoglobin. About 3 mg of iron is bound to transferrin in plasma, and 1,000 mg of iron exists as storage iron in the form of ferritin or hemosiderin. The rest of the iron is stored in other tissues such as cytochromes.[12] Due to the toxicity of inorganic iron, the body has an intricate system for iron absorption, transport, storage, assimilation, and elimination. Hepcidin is a regulator of intestinal iron absorption, iron recycling, and iron mobilization from hepatic stores. It is a peptide hormone made in the liver, distributed in plasma, and excreted in urine. Hepcidin inhibits efflux of iron through ferroportin. Hepcidin synthesis is increased by iron loading and inflammation and decreased by iron deficiency and erythropoietic activity. Hepcidin is induced during infections and inflammation, which allows iron to sequester in macrophages, hepatocytes, and enterocytes.[158] As a result, hepcidin is likely an important mediator of AI. Hepcidin is usually suppressed in IDA.[17] Hepcidin testing is not routinely available.[18]

Most people lose about 1 mg of iron daily. Menstruating women can lose up to 0.6% to 2.5% more per day. Pregnancy requires additional iron and a blood donation can result in as much as 250 mg of iron loss;[19] these individuals are at higher risk for deficiency.

The daily recommended dietary allowance for iron is 8 mg in adult males and postmenopausal females and 18 mg in menstruating females. Children require more iron because of growth-related increases in blood volume, and pregnant women have an increased iron demand brought about by fetal development. In the absence of hemochromatosis, iron overload does not occur because only the amount of iron lost per day is absorbed. The amount of iron absorbed from food depends on body stores, the rate of RBC production, the type of iron provided in the diet, and the presence of any substances that may enhance or inhibit iron absorption.

Heme iron is found in meat, fish, and poultry, and is about three times more absorbable than the nonheme iron found in vegetables, fruits, dried beans, nuts, grain products, and dietary supplements. Gastric acid and other dietary components such as ascorbic acid increase the absorption of nonheme iron. Dietary components that form insoluble complexes with iron (phytates, tannates, and phosphates) decrease absorption. Phytates, a natural component of grains, brans, and some vegetables, can form poorly absorbed complexes and partially explain the increased prevalence of IDA in poorer countries, where grains and vegetables compose a disproportionate amount of the normal diet. Polyphenols bind iron and decrease nonheme iron absorption when large amounts of tea or coffee are consumed with a meal. Although the mechanism is unknown, calcium inhibits absorption of both heme and nonheme iron. Finally, because gastric acid improves iron absorption, patients who have had a gastrectomy or achlorhydria have decreased iron absorption.[20,21]

Etiology

Iron deficiency results from prolonged negative iron balance, which can occur due to increased iron demand or hematopoiesis, increased loss, or decreased intake/absorption. The onset of iron deficiency depends on an individual's initial iron stores and the imbalance between iron absorption and loss. Multiple etiologic factors usually are involved. Certain groups at higher risk for iron deficiency include children younger than 2 years, adolescent girls, pregnant/lactating females, and those older than 65 years. Blood loss should initially be considered a cause of IDA in adults.[22] Blood loss may occur as a result of many disorders, including trauma, hemorrhoids, peptic ulcers, gastritis, GI malignancies, arteriovenous malformations, diverticular disease, copious menstrual flow, nosebleeds, and postpartum bleeding. In less industrialized nations, the risk of IDA is largely related to dietary factors.

Pregnant women should be screened for anemia at their first prenatal visit, but the United States Preventive Services Task Force (USPSTF) no longer recommends routine screening for IDA in all asymptomatic pregnant women.[23] If a pregnant patient is anemic on screening, they should be evaluated for all types of anemia, with iron deficiency being the most common. The Centers for Disease Control and Prevention (CDC) recommends initiation of low-dose iron supplements or prenatal vitamins with 30 mg/day of iron at each woman's first prenatal visit to compensate for the increased iron demands during pregnancy.[24]

Medication history, specifically regarding recent or past use of iron, alcohol, corticosteroids, anticoagulants, aspirin, and nonsteroidal anti-inflammatory drugs (NSAIDs), is a vital part of the history to assess bleeding risk. Other possible causes of hypochromic microcytic anemia include AI, thalassemia, sideroblastic anemia, and heavy metal (mostly lead) poisoning (see Fig. 122-4).

Pathophysiology

Iron is vital to the function of all cells. Manifestations of iron deficiency occur in three stages. In the initial stage, iron stores are reduced without reduced serum iron levels and can be assessed with serum ferritin measurement. The stores allow iron to be utilized when there is an increased need for Hb synthesis. Once stores are depleted, there still is adequate iron from daily RBC turnover for Hb synthesis. Further iron losses would make the patient vulnerable to anemia development. In the second stage, iron deficiency occurs when iron stores are depleted, and Hb is above the lower limit of normal for the population, but may be reduced for a given patient. Findings include reduced transferrin saturation and increased TIBC. The third stage occurs when the Hb falls to less than normal values.

Laboratory Findings

3 Abnormal laboratory findings for patients with IDA generally include low serum iron and ferritin levels and high TIBC. In the early stages of IDA, RBC size is not changed. Low ferritin concentration is the earliest and most sensitive indicator of iron deficiency. However, ferritin may not correlate with iron stores in the bone marrow because renal or hepatic disease, malignancies, infection, or inflammatory processes may increase ferritin values.[12] Hb, Hct, and RBC indices usually remain normal in early stages. In the later stages of IDA, Hb, and Hct fall below normal values, and a microcytic hypochromic anemia develops. Even slightly abnormal Hb and Hct levels may indicate significant depletion of iron stores and should not be ignored. In terms of RBC indices, MCV is reduced earlier in IDA than Hb concentration.

Transferrin saturation (ie, serum iron level divided by the TIBC) is helpful for assessing IDA. Low values may indicate IDA, although low serum transferrin saturation values also may be present in inflammatory disorders. The TIBC may help to differentiate the diagnosis in these patients. Elevated TIBC levels suggest IDA, while low values represent inflammatory disease.

TREATMENT

Desired Outcomes

The outcomes for all types of anemia include reversal of hematologic parameters to normal, return of normal function and quality of life, and prevention or reversal of long-term complications, such as neurologic complications of vitamin B_{12} deficiency.

Dietary Supplementation and Oral Iron Preparations

The severity and cause of IDA determine the approach to treatment. Treatment is focused on replenishing iron stores. Because iron deficiency can be an early sign of other illnesses, treatment of the underlying disease may aid in the correction of iron deficiency.

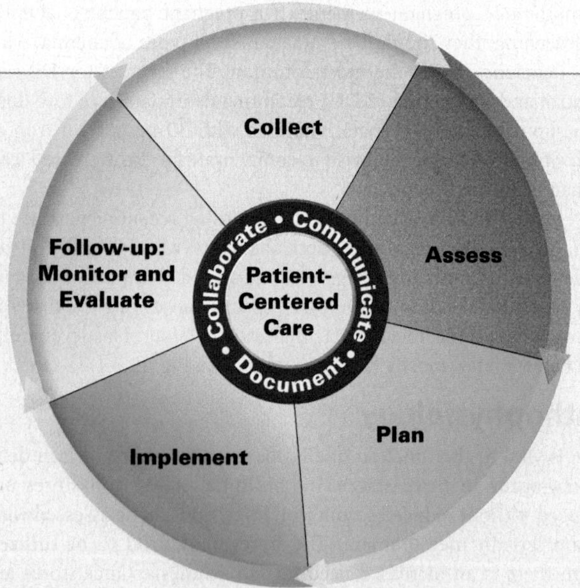

Patient Care Process for Anemia

The image shows the five fundamental steps included in The Pharmacist's Care Process endorsed by the Joint Commission for Pharmacy Practitioners (2014). The tagline of this process reads collaborate, communicate, and document. The five fundamental steps listed here are collect, assess, plan, implement, and follow-up: monitor and evaluate. All these steps are listed in a circular block diagram.

Collect

- Patient characteristics (eg, age, race, sex, pregnancy)
- Patient history (eg, past medical history, dietary habits, physical activity, alcohol intake, smoking status, chemical exposure)
- Symptoms of anemia (eg, fatigue, weakness, chest pain, dizziness, pallor, see "Clinical Presentation: Anemia" box)
- Current medications (including over-the-counter and supplements)
- Objective data (see "Clinical Presentation: Anemia" box)
  - o Blood pressure (BP), heart rate (HR)
  - o Labs (CBC, iron studies, vitamin B_{12}, folate, homocysteine, MMA, etc.)

Assess

- Underlying disease states (blood loss, heart failure, chronic renal disease, HIV, malignancy; see Table 122-1)
- Dietary habits and potential social factors contributing to nutritional deficiencies
- Acuity of symptoms and need for transfusion or hospitalization
- Current medications that may contribute to or worsen anemia or blood loss
- Lab results to determine underlying etiology of anemia for proper treatment selection or attainment of treatment goals
- Ability to self-inject medications (eg, cyanocobalamin)

Plan*

- Dietary interventions for nutritional deficiencies
- Initiate appropriate drug therapy treatment based on etiology (correct formulation, strength, dosing, frequency, and address pertinent drug interactions [see Table 122-3 for iron product selection/drug interactions])
- Monitoring for efficacy and safety (labs and symptom improvement, corrected etiology if possible, adverse drug reactions)
- Patient education (expectations/purpose of treatment, adverse effects, diet modifications, etc.)
- Improved treatment of underlying pathologies if contributing to anemia of chronic disease

Implement*

- Educate patient on treatment interventions and treatment expectations
- Reinforce adherence to treatment plan for short- and long-term success
- Schedule patient for follow-up at appropriate intervals

Follow-up: Monitor and Evaluate

- Lab values within 4 weeks after treatment initiation
- Tolerability of medications
- Symptom improvement (eg, fatigue, pallor, weakness, dizziness, neuropathy)
- If minimal improvement or worsening, determine whether etiology of anemia was correct

**Collaborate with patient, caregivers, and other healthcare professionals.*

Treatment of IDA usually consists of administration of oral or parenteral iron preparations. Examples of foods that are high in iron include animal liver, fortified cereals/oatmeal, beef, eggs, spinach, lentils, tofu, and beans. Iron is best absorbed from meat, fish, and poultry. These foods as well as certain iron-fortified cereals can help treat IDA if diet is a major factor in deficiency. Milk and tea reduce absorption of iron and should be consumed in moderation. In many cases of IDA, oral administration of iron therapy with soluble Fe^{2+} iron salts is an appropriate first step.

Fe^{2+} sulfate, succinate, lactate, fumarate, glutamate, and gluconate have similar oral absorption. Ferric citrate was approved by the Food and Drug Administration (FDA) in 2017 to treat IDA in adults with chronic kidney disease who are not on dialysis (see Chapter 63). Iron is best absorbed in the reduced Fe^{2+} form, with maximal absorption occurring in the duodenum, primarily due to the acidic medium of the stomach. Slow-release, sustained-release, or enteric coated iron preparations may not undergo sufficient dissolution until they reach the small intestine. In the alkaline environment of the small intestine, iron tends to form insoluble complexes, which significantly reduces absorption. The dose of iron replacement therapy depends on the patient's ability to tolerate the administered iron. Tolerance of iron salts improves with a small initial dose and gradual escalation to the full dose. For patients with IDA, the generally recommended dose is about 150 to 200 mg of elemental iron daily, usually in two

TABLE 122-1 Oral Iron Products

Iron Salt	Percent Elemental Iron	Common Formulations and Elemental Iron Provided
Ferrous sulfate	20	60-65 mg/324-325 mg tablet 44 mg/5 mL elixir 15 mg/1 mL solution
Ferrous gluconate	12	38 mg/325 mg tablet 28-29 mg/240-246 mg tablet
Ferrous fumarate	33	66 mg/200 mg tablet 106 mg/324-325 mg tablet
Ferric maltol	100	30 mg/30 mg

TABLE 122-2 Iron Salt-Drug Interactions

Drugs That Decrease Iron Absorption	Drugs Affected by Iron
Al', Mg', and Ca^{2+}-containing antacids Tetracycline and doxycycline $Histamine_2$ antagonists Proton-pump inhibitors Cholestyramine	Levodopa ↓ (chelates with iron) Methyldopa ↓ (decreases efficacy of methyldopa) Levothyroxine ↓ (decreased efficacy of levothyroxine) Penicillamine ↓ (chelates with iron) Fluoroquinolones ↓ (forms ferric ion quinolone complex) Tetracycline and doxycycline ↓ (when administered within 2 hours of iron salt)

or three divided doses to maximize tolerability. If patients cannot tolerate this daily dose of elemental iron, smaller amounts of elemental iron (eg, single 325-mg tablet of Fe^{2+} sulfate) usually are sufficient to replace iron stores, although at a slower rate. Table 122-1 lists the percentage of elemental iron of commonly available iron salts. Iron preferably is administered at least 1 hour before meals because food can interfere with iron absorption. Many patients must take iron with food because they experience GI upset when iron is administered on an empty stomach.

Lower amounts of iron can be given and produce similar results with better tolerability. Hepicidin, a protein that regulates iron absorption, may play a role in oral iron dosing. A large dose of iron in the morning may elevate hepicidin levels and prevent further iron absorption of subsequent doses for at least the rest of the day, potentially up to 48 hours later.[25] Furthermore, once daily dosing of iron may result in a lower amount of iron being absorbed versus every other day dosing.[26] These studies have led some to propose that oral iron could be dosed every other day, particularly if the patient has difficulty tolerating a larger daily dose of oral iron. However, no long-term studies have been conducted to support this dosing strategy.

Adverse drug reactions to therapeutic doses of iron are primarily GI in nature and consist of dark discoloration of feces, constipation or diarrhea, nausea, and vomiting. GI effects usually are common, dose-related, and are similar among iron salts when equivalent amounts of elemental iron are administered. Administration of smaller amounts of iron with each dose or administration with meals may minimize these adverse effects. Histamine-2 blockers or proton-pump inhibitors reduce gastric acidity and may impair iron absorption. Table 122-2 lists important drug interactions with iron.

Failure to respond to iron treatment regimens necessitates reevaluation of the patient's condition. Common causes of treatment failure include poor patient adherence, inability to absorb iron, incorrect diagnosis, continued bleeding, or a concurrent inflammatory condition that impairs a full response. Even when iron deficiency is present, response may be impaired when a coexisting cause for anemia exists. Rarely a patient has diminished ability to absorb iron, most often due to previous gastrectomy, such as gastric bypass surgery, or celiac disease. Regardless of the form of oral therapy used, treatment should continue for 3 to 6 months after the anemia is resolved to allow for repletion of iron stores and to prevent relapse. Patients should be instructed to store oral iron out of reach of children and pets as small amounts can result in a fatal overdose. Treatment for acute iron poisoning is discussed in Chapter e8, "Clinical Toxicology."

Parenteral Iron Therapy

Indications for parenteral iron therapy include intolerance to oral, malabsorption, and nonadherence. Patients with significant blood loss who refuse transfusions and cannot take oral iron therapy also may require parenteral iron therapy. Parenteral iron therapy should also be considered, possibly first line, in patients with inflammatory bowel disease and those with gastric bypass/gastric resection due to poor oral absorption.[27] Parenteral iron therapy is also used for patients with chronic kidney disease (see Chapter 63), especially those undergoing hemodialysis, and for some cancer patients receiving chemotherapy on erythropoiesis-stimulating agents (ESAs; Chapter 150). Seven different parenteral iron preparations available in the United States are low molecular weight iron dextran, ferric gluconate, iron sucrose, ferumoxytol, ferric derisomaltose, ferric pyrophosphate citrate, and ferric carboxymaltose (Table 63-4). They differ in their molecular size, pharmacokinetics, bioavailability, and adverse effect profiles. Although toxicity profiles of these agents differ, clinical studies indicate that each is efficacious. High molecular weight iron dextran parenteral preparations have been previously associated with more anaphylactic reactions. The high molecular weight product is no longer available. The low molecular weight has a lower risk of these reactions, but it requires a test dose prior to full dose administration. Fatal reactions have also occurred in patients who tolerated the test dose with the high molecular weight product. The safety profile of parenteral iron is largely assessed by spontaneous reports to the FDA and observational studies. All parenteral iron preparations carry a risk for anaphylactic reactions but the risk is lower than that for high molecular weight iron dextran.[28,29] The FDA recommends that resuscitation equipment and trained staff be available during administration of all iron dextran preparations. A concern with parenteral iron is that iron may be released too quickly and overload the ability of transferrin to bind it, leading to free iron reactions that can interfere with neutrophil function.

Iron dextran, a complex of Fe^{3+} hydroxide and the carbohydrate dextran, contains 50 mg of iron/mL and can be given via the intramuscular or IV route. Different brands of iron dextran are available and differ in their molecular weight. They are not interchangeable. The intramuscular route is no longer used routinely and requires Z-tract injection technique.[30] Methods of IV administration include multiple injections or an infusion of a diluted preparation. This latter method often is referred to as total dose infusion.

Total replacement doses of IV iron dextran can be given as a single dose, but this method of administration is not FDA-approved. A test dose is still required. Patients who receive total dose infusions are at higher risk for adverse drug reactions, such as arthralgias, myalgias, flushing, malaise, and fever. Patients with preexisting immune-mediated diseases, such as active rheumatoid arthritis or systemic lupus erythematosus, are at high risk for adverse drug reactions because of their hyperreactive immune response.[31]

Ferric gluconate is a complex of iron bound to one gluconate and four sucrose molecules in a repeating pattern. Ferric gluconate is available in an aqueous solution. No direct transfer of iron from the Fe^{3+} gluconate to transferrin occurs. The complex is taken up quickly by the mononuclear phagocytic system and has a half-life of about 1 hour in the bloodstream. Ferric gluconate produces fewer anaphylactic reactions than iron dextran does. Adverse drug reactions of sodium ferric gluconate include cramps, nausea, vomiting, flushing, hypotension, intense upper gastric pain, rash, and pruritus.[32]

Iron sucrose is a polynuclear iron (III) hydroxide in sucrose complex. Following IV administration of iron sucrose, the iron is released directly from the circulating iron sucrose to transferrin and is taken up by the mononuclear phagocytic system and metabolized. The half-life is about 6 hours, with a volume of distribution similar to that of iron dextran.[33] Adverse drug reactions include leg cramps and hypotension.

Ferumoxytol is FDA-approved to treat iron deficiency in adults with chronic kidney disease and adults with IDA who have not responded to oral iron. No test dose is required but anaphylaxis can occur and patients should be observed for at least 30 minutes after each dose. A warning was added in 2015 due to case reports of fatal and nonfatal anaphylactic reactions to the product. It should not be used in patients who previously had an allergic reaction to other iron preparations. Ferumoxytol can also interfere with magnetic resonance imaging (MRI) scans and the radiologist should be notified if the patient has received this medication within 3 months of the scan.[34]

Ferric carboxymaltose received approval for treatment of IDA in those who have failed oral iron therapy or who have intolerance to oral therapy. The approval of this product was delayed due to hypophosphatemia seen in clinical trials. No additional warnings were required and no clinical issues related to hypophosphatemia have been reported. This product can also be given in a two-dose regimen or a single-dose regimen. It is also approved for chronic kidney disease patients not on hemodialysis.[35]

Ferric derisomaltose is approved for patients with IDA who have intolerance to oral iron or an unsatisfactory response to oral iron, as well as patients with chronic kidney disease who do not depend on hemodialysis. This product can be given as a single- or multi-dose regimen.

Increased risk for infection is a concern with parenteral iron preparations because iron is a growth factor for some bacteria, but a meta-analysis reported that IV iron does not increase the risk for infection.[36] Parenteral iron products are discussed in more detail in Chapter 63.

MEGALOBLASTIC ANEMIAS

Macrocytic anemias are divided into megaloblastic and nonmegaloblastic anemias. Macrocytosis, as seen in megaloblastic anemias, is caused by abnormal DNA metabolism resulting from vitamin B_{12} or folate deficiency. It can also be caused by administration of various drugs, such as hydroxyurea, zidovudine, cytarabine, methotrexate, azathioprine, 6-mercaptopurine, and cladribine. In vitamin B_{12}– or folate-deficiency anemia, megaloblastosis results from interference with folic acid- and vitamin B_{12}–interdependent nucleic acid synthesis in the immature erythrocyte (Fig. 122-6).

Although vitamin B_{12} and folate deficiency are common causes of macrocytosis, other possible causes must be considered if these deficiencies are not found. These can include aplastic anemia, myelodysplastic syndromes, alcohol abuse, and multiple myeloma. Macrocytosis is the most typical morphologic abnormality associated with excessive alcohol consumption. Even with adequate folate and vitamin B_{12} levels and the absence of liver disease, patients with high alcohol intake may present with an alcohol-induced macrocytosis. Cessation of alcohol ingestion resolves the macrocytosis within a couple of months.

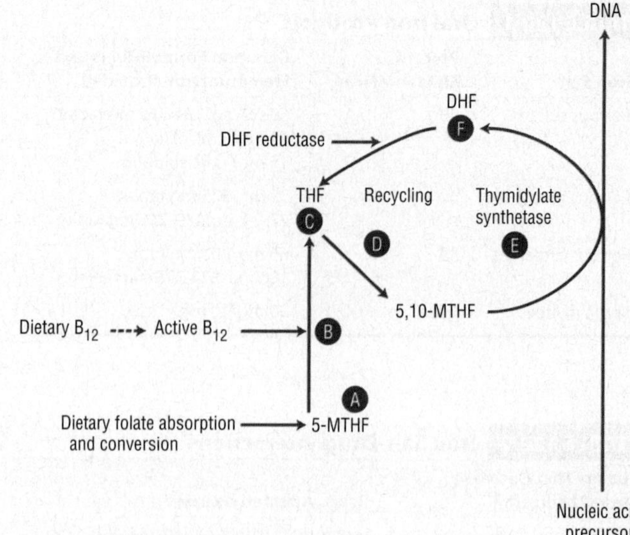

FIGURE 122-6 Drug-induced megaloblastosis.

Vitamin B_{12}–Deficiency Anemia

The exact prevalence of vitamin B_{12}–deficiency anemia in the United States is unknown. Risk increases with age.[37] One study conducted in the United States and the United Kingdom found that the prevalence of vitamin B_{12} deficiency increased from about 6% in adults younger than 60 years to 20% in those older than 60 years.[38] Gastric acid–suppressing agents may inhibit cobalamin release from food, and their use is associated with an increased risk. Older adults in the United States have a high prevalence (up to 15%) of elevated MMA levels and associated low or low-normal vitamin B_{12} levels, likely due to atrophic gastritis and malabsorption of food-bound vitamin B_{12}.[37]

Etiology

4 The three major causes of vitamin B_{12} deficiency are inadequate intake, malabsorption syndromes, and inadequate utilization. Inadequate dietary consumption of vitamin B_{12} is rare. It usually occurs only in patients who are strict vegans without supplementation, chronic alcoholics, and older adults who consume a "tea and toast" diet because of financial limitations or poor dentition. Decreased vitamin B_{12} absorption can occur with loss of intrinsic factor by autoimmune mechanisms (such as pernicious anemia, in which gastric parietal cells are selectively damaged), chronic atrophic gastritis, or stomach surgery. One of the most frequent causes of low serum B_{12} levels results from the inability of vitamin B_{12} to be cleaved and released from proteins in food because of inadequate gastric acid production. Treatment of *Helicobacter pylori* may improve vitamin B_{12} status because this bacterial infection is a cause of chronic gastritis.[39] Vitamin B_{12} deficiency may occasionally result from overgrowth of bacteria in the bowel that uses vitamin B_{12} or from injury or removal (from Crohn's disease or small bowel surgery, respectively) of ileal receptor sites where vitamin B_{12} and the intrinsic factor complex are absorbed. Blind loop syndrome, Whipple disease, Zollinger–Ellison syndrome, tapeworm infestations, intestinal resections, tropical sprue, surgical resection of the ileus, pancreatic insufficiency, inflammatory bowel disease, advanced liver disease, tuberculosis, and Crohn's disease may contribute to the development of vitamin B_{12} deficiency.[37] Metformin may reversibly decrease B_{12} absorption, likely due to its effects on the intestinal mucosa in the ileum and calcium homeostasis. Low B_{12} related to metformin can occur within months of starting the medication, but it is more likely after 5 years and some clinicians will monitor B_{12} in patients receiving long-term metformin therapy or those with a poor oral intake

of vitamin B_{12}.[40] Proton pump inhibitors and histamine-2 receptor antagonists may also contribute to vitamin B_{12} deficiency because an acidic environment is needed for vitamin B_{12} to be absorbed in the GI tract from food.[41] Long-term use of these agents for 2 or more years increases the risk of deficiency.[41]

Pathophysiology

Vitamin B_{12} works closely with folate in the synthesis of building blocks for DNA and RNA, is essential in maintaining the integrity of the neurologic system, and plays a role in fatty acid biosynthesis and energy production. It is a water-soluble vitamin obtained exogenously by ingestion of meat, fish, poultry, dairy products, and fortified cereals. The body stores several years of vitamin B_{12}, of which about 50% is in the liver. The recommended daily allowance is 2 μg in adults and 2.6 μg in pregnant or breast-feeding women. The average Western diet provides 5 to 15 μg of vitamin B_{12} daily, of which 1 to 5 μg is absorbed.[37] Vitamin B_{12} deficiency can take several years to develop following vitamin deprivation.

Once dietary cobalamin enters the stomach, pepsin and hydrochloric acid release the cobalamin from animal proteins. The cobalamin then binds with intrinsic factor that serves as a cell-directed carrier protein similar to transferrin for iron. This complex attaches to mucosal cell receptors in the distal ileum, the intrinsic factor is discarded, and the cobalamin is bound to transport proteins (transcobalamin I, II, and III). Passive diffusion is an alternate pathway for vitamin B_{12} absorption independent of intrinsic factor or an intact terminal ileum and accounts for about 1% of vitamin B_{12} absorption.[37]

Vitamin B_{12} deficiency can cause neurologic and hematologic complications. They usually start with bilateral paraesthesia in the extremities; deficits in proprioception and vibration can also be present. If not treated, this can progress to ataxia, dementia-like symptoms, psychosis, and vision loss. In children, prolonged deficiency can lead to poor brain development.[14,42] Patients with unexplained neuropathies should be evaluated for vitamin B_{12} deficiency.

Laboratory Findings

In macrocytic anemias, MCV is elevated, but some patients deficient in vitamin B_{12} may have a normal MCV. If there is a coexisting cause of microcytosis, the MCV may not be elevated.[36] A peripheral blood smear shows macrocytosis accompanied by hypersegmented polymorphonuclear leukocytes (one of the earliest and most specific indications of this disease), oval macrocytes, anisocytosis, and poikilocytosis. Serum lactate dehydrogenase and indirect bilirubin levels may be elevated as a result of hemolysis or ineffective erythropoiesis.[14] Other laboratory findings include a low reticulocyte count, low serum vitamin B_{12} level (less than 200 pg/mL [148 pmol/L]), and low Hct.

In the early stages of vitamin B_{12} deficiency, classic signs and symptoms of megaloblastic anemia may not be evident, and serum levels of vitamin B_{12} may be within normal limits or borderline low (200-300 pg/mL [148-221 pmol/L]). Therefore, measurement of MMA and homocysteine may be useful because these parameters are typically the first to change. Because MMA and homocysteine are involved in enzymatic reactions that depend on vitamin B_{12}, vitamin B_{12} deficiency leads to accumulation of these metabolites. Elevations in MMA are more specific for vitamin B_{12} deficiency. Homocysteine is also elevated in several other situations including folate deficiency, chronic renal disease, alcoholism, smoking, and use of steroid or cyclosporine therapy.[42]

Blood levels of vitamin B_{12} should be drawn for all patients with suspected vitamin B_{12} deficiency. Vitamin B_{12} values less than 200 pg/mL (148 pmol/L) are diagnostic for B_{12} deficiency. Subclinical vitamin B_{12} deficiency is sometimes found with vitamin B_{12} levels of 200 to 300 pg/mL (148-221 pmol/L).[43] Some patients with clinical B_{12} deficiency manifesting as neurological disease have normal hematological parameters.

The Schilling test was once performed to determine whether replacement of vitamin B_{12} should occur via an oral or parenteral route due to pernicious anemia, but evidence now shows that oral replacement is as efficacious as parenteral supplementation because of the vitamin B_{12} absorption pathway independent of intrinsic factor.[37,44]

TREATMENT

Early treatment is important because neurologic damage may be irreversible if the deficiency is not detected and corrected within months. In addition to replacement therapy, any underlying etiology that is treatable, such as bacterial overgrowth, should be corrected. Indications for starting oral or parenteral therapy include megaloblastic anemia or other hematologic abnormalities and neurologic disease from deficiency.[42] Those with borderline low levels of B_{12} but no hematologic abnormalities should be followed at yearly intervals; monitoring MMA and homocysteine may also be useful.[42] Patients should be counseled on the types of foods high in vitamin B_{12} content such as fortified cereals, fish, animal liver, milk, clams, and yogurt. Oral vitamin B_{12} replacement is indicated for those without neurologic complications or significant symptoms and can be used effectively to treat pernicious anemia because of passive absorption, independent of intrinsic factor.[15] Cyanocobalamin is used primarily in the United States while hydroxycobolamin may be used in other countries. The typical dose for oral therapy is cyanocobalamin 1,000 μg once daily. Higher doses of (1,000-2,000 μg) of vitamin B_{12} may be given to patients with malabsorption and is as effective as intramuscular administration in achieving hematologic and neurologic responses.[37,44] If vitamin B_{12} levels are marginally low and either MMA or both MMA and homocysteine levels are elevated, oral administration of 1,000 μg of vitamin B_{12} daily should be strongly considered.[45] Timed-release preparations of oral cobalamin should be avoided.[46] Nonprescription 1,000 μg cobalamin tablets are available, among several other strengths at a low cost. Oral replacement may be as effective as parenteral administration in achieving hematologic and neurologic responses.[37,38] However, parenteral therapy is usually given if patients have neurologic or severe anemia symptoms to protect against further progression. A commonly used initial parenteral vitamin B_{12} regimen consists of daily intramuscular or deep subcutaneous injections of 1,000 μg of cyanocobalamin for 1 week to saturate vitamin B_{12} stores in the body and resolve clinical manifestations of the deficiency. After that, it can be given weekly for 1 month and monthly thereafter for maintenance. The series of daily parenteral injections may be omitted if administration is difficult or inconvenient. In this case, the parenteral injection is then given weekly, sometimes for longer than 1 month. Patients can be instructed to give these injections at home to avoid the cost of an office visit and convenience. After symptoms have resolved and hematologic indices and vitamin B_{12} levels have normalized, patients can be converted from parenteral therapy to oral maintenance therapy.[47] When patients are converted from the parenteral to the oral form of cobalamin, oral cobalamin daily can be initiated on the due date of the next injection. Vitamin B_{12} should be continued for life in patients with pernicious anemia.

In addition to the oral and parenteral forms, vitamin B_{12} is available as a nasal spray for patients in remission following intramuscular vitamin B_{12} therapy who have no neurologic involvement. The nasal spray is administered once weekly. Intranasal administration should be avoided for patients with nasal diseases or those receiving medications intranasally in the same nostril. Patients should not administer the spray 1 hour before or after ingestion of hot foods or beverages, which can impair cobalamin absorption. The efficacy of the nasal spray formulation has not been well studied and may have variable absorption. It should be used for maintenance therapy only after hematologic parameters have normalized.

Potential adverse drug reactions with vitamin B_{12} replacement therapy are rare. Uncommon adverse drug reactions are headache, weakness, and hypokalemia.

Folic Acid Deficiency Anemia

Epidemiology

Folic acid deficiency is one of the most common vitamin deficiencies occurring in the United States, largely because of its association with excessive alcohol intake and pregnancy. Fortification of grain products in the 1990s increased folate intake across the United States. According to data from the National Health and Nutrition Examination Survey (NHANES), most people in the United States intake adequate dietary amounts of folate and only 0.5% of children aged 1 to 18 years have folate deficiency.[48]

Etiology

5 Major causes of folic acid deficiency include inadequate intake, decreased absorption, and increased folate requirements. Poor eating habits make this deficiency more common in older adults, teenagers whose diets consist of "junk food," and individuals with alcoholism, food insecurity, chronic illness, or dementia. Folic acid absorption may decrease for patients who have malabsorption syndromes or received certain drugs. In patients with alcoholism with poor dietary habits, alcohol interferes with folic acid absorption and utilization at the cellular level and decreases hepatic stores of folic acid.

Increased folate requirements may occur when the rate of cellular division is increased, as seen in pregnant women; patients with hemolytic anemia, malignancy, chronic inflammatory disorders such as Crohn's disease, rheumatoid arthritis, or psoriasis; patients undergoing long-term dialysis; burn patients; and adolescents and infants during their growth spurts. This hyperutilization eventually can lead to anemia, particularly when the daily intake of folate is borderline, resulting in inadequate replacement of folate stores.

Several drugs have been reported to cause a folic acid deficiency. Some drugs (eg, azathioprine, 6-mercaptopurine, 5-fluorouracil, hydroxyurea, and zidovudine) directly inhibit DNA synthesis. Other drugs are folate antagonists and inhibit dihydrofolate reductase; the most toxic is methotrexate (other examples include pentamidine, trimethoprim, and triamterene). A number of drugs (eg, phenytoin, carbamazepine, valproate, primidone) antagonize folate via poorly understood mechanisms but are thought to reduce vitamin absorption by the intestine (see Chapter e125). Since folic acid doses as low as 1 mg/day may affect serum phenytoin levels, routine folic acid supplementation is not generally recommended.[42] Alcohol can also interfere with folic acid absorption, likely through its effects on the intestinal mucosa.[41]

Pathophysiology

Folic acid is a water-soluble vitamin readily destroyed by cooking or processing. It is necessary for the production of DNA and RNA. It acts as a methyl donor to form methylcobalamin, which is used in the remethylation of homocysteine to methionine. Because humans are unable to synthesize sufficient folate to meet total daily requirements, they depend on dietary sources. Major dietary sources of folate include fresh, green leafy vegetables, citrus fruits, yeast, mushrooms, dairy products, and animal organs such as liver and kidney. Once absorbed, dietary folate must be converted to the active form tetrahydrofolate through a cobalamin-dependent reaction. In 1997, the United States mandated that grain products be fortified with folic acid to increase the dietary intake of folate. This amount of supplementation was chosen to decrease the incidence of neural tube defects without masking occult vitamin B_{12} deficiency.

As a result of grain product fortification, neural tube defect frequency has decreased by 25% to 30%.[49] Although body demands for folate are high because of high rates of RBC synthesis and turnover, the minimum daily requirement is 50 to 100 μg. In the general population, the recommended daily allowance for folate is 400 μg in nonpregnant females, 600 μg in pregnant females, and 500 μg in lactating females.[45] Because the body stores about 15 to 30 mg of folate, primarily in the liver, cessation of dietary folate intake can result in deficiency in months.[50]

Laboratory Findings

It is critically important to rule out vitamin B_{12} deficiency when folate deficiency is suspected to prevent neurologic complications developing from vitamin B_{12} deficiency. Laboratory changes associated with folate deficiency are similar to those seen in vitamin B_{12} deficiency, except serum vitamin B_{12} and MMA levels are normal. Serum folate levels less than 2 ng/mL (4.5 nmol/L) are considered low, although normal ranges may vary between institutions. The RBC folate level (less than 150 ng/mL [340 nmol/L]) also declines, and levels remain constant throughout the life span of the erythrocyte.[11] The RBC folate levels may not provide additional information beyond the serum folate level. If serum or erythrocyte folate levels are borderline, serum homocysteine usually is increased with a folic acid deficiency. If serum MMA levels also are elevated, vitamin B_{12} deficiency must be ruled out given that folate does not participate in MMA metabolism.

TREATMENT

Therapy for folic acid deficiency consists of administration of exogenous folic acid to normalize hematologic labs, replace body stores, and resolve signs and symptoms. In most cases, 1 mg daily is sufficient to replace stores; doses of 1 to 5 mg daily may be necessary in cases of deficiency due to malabsorption. Parenteral folic acid is available but rarely necessary. Synthetic folic acid is almost completely absorbed by the GI tract and is converted to tetrahydrofolate without cobalamin. Therapy should continue for about 4 months if the underlying cause of the deficiency can be identified and corrected to allow for clearance of all folate-deficient RBCs from the circulation. Examples of foods high in folic acid include beef liver, fortified cereals, lentils, green leafy vegetables, orange juice, and rice. They should be encouraged in the diet. Long-term folate administration may be necessary in patients with chronic conditions associated with increased folate requirements. Low-dose folate therapy (500 μg daily) can be administered when anticonvulsant drugs produce a megaloblastic anemia so that discontinuation of anticonvulsant therapy may not be necessary. Adverse drug reactions have not been reported with folic acid doses used for replacement therapy. It is considered nontoxic at high doses and is rapidly excreted in the urine.

Although megaloblastic anemia during pregnancy is rare, the most common cause is folate deficiency. Periconceptional folic acid supplementation is recommended to decrease the occurrence and recurrence of neural tube defects (eg, anencephaly and spinal bifida). Folic acid supplementation at a dose of 400 μg daily is recommended for all women. Women who have previously given birth to offspring with neural tube defects or those with a family history of neural tube defects should ingest 1 to 4 mg daily of folic acid.[49,51,52] Higher levels of folic acid supplementation should not be attained via ingestion of excess multivitamins because of the risk of fat-soluble vitamin toxicity.[52] Prenatal vitamins usually have a higher amount of folic acid as compared with general multivitamins to ensure adequate supplementation is attained. It is essential that women in their childbearing years maintain adequate folic acid intake.

ANEMIA OF INFLAMMATION

Epidemiology

6 AI is a term used to describe both ACD and anemia of critical illness. This term was developed to reflect the inflammatory process resulting in disturbances in iron homeostatis underlying both types of anemia. The onset of anemia of critical illness is rapid, generally over days, and often occurs in a hospital setting due to tissue damage and acute inflammatory changes. ACD has a similar mechanism, but develops over months to years from an underlying chronic condition. Globally, AI is one of the most common forms of anemia, particularly among older adults, although its prevalence is not known due to the complex and multifaceted nature of the disease. ACD is associated with common disease states that may mimic the symptoms of anemia, which causes the diagnosis of ACD to be sometimes overlooked in the outpatient setting. Anemia of critical illness is a common complication in critically ill patients and is found almost universally in this patient population.[53]

Etiology

AI is an anemia traditionally associated with infectious or inflammatory processes, tissue injury, and conditions associated with the release of proinflammatory cytokines. The etiology of AI can be multifactorial and the diagnosis is usually one of exclusion. A comprehensive history of the illness is important to help rule out other potential causes of anemia. Although it may be difficult to delineate between IDA and AI, it is important to exclude IDA as the true or competing etiology. Various conditions associated with ACD may predispose patients to blood loss (malignancy, GI blood loss from treatments with aspirin, NSAIDs, or corticosteroids). ACD is often observed in patients with diseases containing an inflammatory component lasting longer than 1 to 2 months, although it can occur in conditions with a more rapid onset of several weeks, such as pneumonia. Anemia associated with human immunodeficiency virus (HIV), autoimmune conditions, cancer, and heart failure are common forms of AI. The degree of anemia in ACD generally reflects the severity of the underlying disease.

Factors that contribute to anemia in critically ill patients include sepsis, frequent blood sampling, surgical blood loss, immune-mediated functional iron deficiency, decreased production of endogenous EPO, reduced RBC life span, and active bleeding, especially in the GI tract. A combination of these factors often exists, creating a rapid anemic state over days. Additional comorbid factors include coagulopathies and nutritional deficits such as poor oral intake and altered absorption of vitamins and minerals, including iron, vitamin B_{12}, and folate.[54] Deleterious effects of anemia include an increased risk of cardiac-related morbidity and mortality, especially for patients with known cardiovascular disease. Persistent tissue hypoxia can result in cerebral ischemia, myocardial ischemia, multiple organ deterioration, lactic acidosis, and death. The consequences of anemia in critically ill patients may be enhanced because of the increased metabolic demands of critical illness. Weaning anemic patients from mechanical ventilation may be more difficult, as low Hg has been identified as a potential risk factor for poor outcomes.[55,56] This is likely due to Hg's critical role in oxygen delivery; low Hg has been associated with increased work of breathing and cardiac output.[57-59]

Pathophysiology

AI is a hypoproliferative response to stimulation of the cellular immune system by various underlying disease processes. The pathogenesis of AI is multifactorial and is characterized by a blunted EPO response to anemia, an impaired proliferation of erythroid progenitor cells, and a disturbance of iron homeostasis. Increased iron uptake and retention occur within cells. The RBCs have a shortened life span, and the bone marrow's capacity to respond to EPO is inadequate to maintain normal Hb concentration. The cause of this defect is uncertain but related to impaired release of iron from bone marrow cells. Iron availability to erythroid progenitor cells is therefore limited. Various cytokines, such as interleukin-1, interferon-γ, interleukin-6, and tumor necrosis factor released during illness, may inhibit the production or action of EPO or the production of RBCs.[60] These cytokines also upregulate hepcidin, a small peptide that regulates iron availability. Increased hepcidin inhibits iron absorption from the gastrointestinal tract and prevents release from macrophages which are elevated during inflammation. Inflammation also increases the uptake of iron by macrophages reducing free iron for erythropoiesis.[60,61]

TABLE 122-3 Laboratory Value Differences Between Anemia of Inflammation and Iron-Deficiency Anemia

	Anemia of Inflammation	Iron-Deficiency Anemia
Iron	↓	↓
Transferrin	↓ or NL	↑
Transferrin saturation	↓	↓
Ferritin	↑ or NL	↓
Soluble transferrin receptor	NL	↑

NL, normal limits.

Laboratory Findings

ACD tends to be a mild (Hb greater than 9.5 g/dL [95 g/L; 5.90 mmol/L]) or moderate (Hb greater than 8 g/dL [80 g/L; 4.97 mmol/L]) anemia.[60] No definitive test can confirm the diagnosis of AI. The clinician should maintain a high index of suspicion for any patient with a chronic inflammatory or neoplastic disease. AI may coexist with IDA and folic acid deficiency because many patients with these conditions have poor dietary intake. Examination of the bone marrow, although not routinely performed, reveals an abundance of iron, suggesting that the release mechanism for iron is the central defect. Patients with AI usually have a decreased serum iron level, but unlike patients with IDA, their TIBC is decreased and their serum ferritin level is normal or increased. Ferritin is an acute phase reactant and is often elevated during inflammation, helping to delineate AI from IDA. Transferrin saturation is typically decreased. AI usually is normocytic and normochromic with mildly depressed Hb. Patients with concurrent AI and IDA usually have microcytes and a more severe anemia. Table 122-3 shows lab values seen in AI and IDA. Erythrocyte survival may be reduced for patients with AI, but a compensatory erythropoietic response does not occur. A low reticulocyte count indicates underproduction of RBCs.[60] As discussed in the IDA section, hepcidin levels are not routinely used for diagnosis but would likely be elevated in a patient with ACD.[62]

TREATMENT

Treatment of AI depends on the underlying etiology. Resolution of the underlying condition may prompt recovery from anemia. Guidelines exist for management of anemia in patients with cancer or chronic kidney disease. Although the goals of therapy should include treating the underlying disorder and correcting reversible causes of anemia, accomplishment of these goals may not be feasible nor completely reverse hematologic and physiologic abnormalities. If AI is mild and does not affect the patient's quality of life or progression of other disease states, additional therapy may not be needed.

Iron supplementation is effective only if iron deficiency is present and should not be utilized for AI in its absence. During inflammation, oral or parenteral iron therapy may not be as effective. Absorption is impaired because of downregulation of ferroportin and iron diversion mediated by cytokines.[60] Because iron is a required nutrient for proliferating microorganisms, supplementation may also theoretically increase the risk of infections. Therefore, iron therapy should be reserved for patients with an established iron deficiency.[60]

ESAs have been used to stimulate erythropoiesis for patients with symptomatic AI since a relative EPO deficiency exists in comparison to the degree of anemia. Similar to endogenous EPO, response to exogenous ESA may be blunted in AI. Two agents are available: recombinant epoetin alfa and recombinant darbepoetin alfa. Although both agents share the same mechanism of action, darbepoetin alfa has a longer half-life and can be administered less frequently. ESAs are FDA-approved for AI due to chronic kidney disease and HIV infection, as well as anemia due to malignancy, but are sometimes used off label for AI due to other underlying causes. The initial dosages of epoetin alfa and darbepoetin alfa are 50 to 100 Units/kg three times per week and 0.45 μg/kg once weekly, respectively. Response to ESAs varies depending on dose and cause of the anemia. Higher doses may be required to overcome hyporesponsiveness. Since ESAs are more effective when the marrow has an adequate supply of iron, cobalamin, and folic acid, these agents should be used in combination with iron therapy.

Iron deficiency can occur in patients treated with ESAs, so close monitoring of iron levels is necessary. Some patients develop "functional" iron deficiency, in which the iron stores are normal but the supply of iron to the erythroid marrow is less than necessary to support the demand for RBC production. Therefore, many practitioners routinely supplement ESA therapy with oral or IV iron therapy to maintain a serum ferritin ≥100 ng/mL (mcg/L; 225 pmol/L) or serum transferrin saturation (TSAT) ≥20%. Potential toxicities of exogenous ESA administration include increases in blood pressure, nausea, headache, fever, bone pain, and fatigue. Less-common adverse drug reactions include seizures, thrombotic events, and allergic reactions such as rashes and local reactions at the injection site. Tumor progression with these agents can also occur and is discussed in Chapter 150. Further discussion of dosing guidelines and potential adverse outcomes of ESA treatment in populations for which treatment is FDA-approved are discussed in Chapters 63 and 150. If ESAs are used, the practitioner must monitor to ensure the patient's Hb does not exceed 12 g/dL (120 g/L; 7.45 mmol/L) with treatment or that Hb does not rise greater than 1 g/dL (10 g/L; 0.62 mmol/L) every 2 weeks since both of these events have been associated with increased mortality and cardiovascular events.[63] Continued monitoring of Hb should be considered every 2 to 4 weeks thereafter. If no rise in Hb is seen after 8 weeks of optimal therapy, the patient should be considered EAS nonresponsive and therapy may be discontinued.

Transfusions of packed red blood cells are effective but should be limited to situations in which oxygen transport is inadequate due to concomitant medical problems and symptomatic patients with insufficient time to respond to other methods. RBC transfusions should be strongly considered for severe AI with complications involving bleeding. Liberal use of transfusions to correct anemia in critical illness can result in adverse patient outcomes.[53] Transfusion risks may include transmission of blood-borne infections, development of autoantibodies, transfusion reactions, and iron overload. Transfusions begin to be considered in most situations for those with severe anemia (Hb less than 7-8 g/dL [70-80 g/L; 4.34-4.97 mmol/L]).[64]

Critically ill patients require the necessary substrates of iron, folic acid, and vitamin B_{12} for RBC production. Parenteral iron is generally preferred in this population because patients often are undergoing enteral therapy or because of concerns regarding inadequate iron absorption. The disadvantage of parenteral therapy is the theoretical risk of infection, hypersensitivity reactions, including anaphylaxis, and hypotension during infusion.

ESAs have been used to treat the anemia of critical illness, but they are not FDA-approved for this indication. In critically ill patients, the use of ESAs did not significantly reduce mortality or length of ICU stay.[65] The few randomized controlled trials which evaluated ESAs in this patient population did not consistently show a decrease in transfusion requirements in ESA-treated patients.[66] Additionally, their use is often limited by the rapid progression of anemia in this setting and the increased risk of thrombotic events with their use. Further investigation is necessary to determine the effectiveness of ESAs in critically ill patients.

Many critically ill patients receive RBC transfusions despite the inherent risks associated with transfusions. Stored RBCs may not function as well as endogenous blood. Although RBC transfusions may increase oxygen delivery to tissues, cellular oxygen may not increase.[67] Transfusion practices in ICUs vary, and clinicians use different Hb concentrations as thresholds for administering transfusions. The decision to use transfusions must consider the risks, including transmission of infections; volume overload, especially for patients with renal or heart failure; iron overload; and immune-mediated reactions such as febrile reactions, hemolysis, and anaphylaxis. The clinician also must consider administrative, logistic, and economic factors, including the shortage of blood supplies.

The recognition of hepcidin in the regulation of iron homeostasis and its role in ACD has led to interest in new agents targeted at hepcidin. Mechanisms for these novel agents include inhibition of hepcidin production, circulating hepcidin, or hepcidin-inducing cytokines, including interleukin-6.

Prolyl hydroxylases have become potential targets for AI because they regulate hypoxia-inducible factors, which increase endogenous EPO formation and iron delivery. Prolyl hydroxylase inhibitors are in clinical trials to treat anemia in patients on hemodialysis.

ANEMIA IN OLDER ADULTS

Epidemiology

7 Anemia is one of the most common clinical problems observed in older adults, with about 20% of people aged 85 years and older affected.[68] Older patients with the highest incidence of anemia are those who are hospitalized, followed by residents of nursing homes and other institutions, with an estimated rate of 31% to 40%.[69] Although anemia is common in older adults, it should not be regarded as an inevitable outcome of aging. The body's set point of Hb does not fall with age. An underlying cause can be identified in about two-thirds of older patients. Undiagnosed and untreated anemia has been associated with adverse outcomes, including all-cause hospitalization, hospitalization secondary to cardiovascular disease, and all-cause mortality.[70] Anemia is an independent predictor of death and major clinical adverse events in older adults with stable symptomatic coronary artery disease.[71] Anemia can exacerbate neurologic and cognitive conditions and can adversely influence quality of life and physical performance in older adults.[72] Anemia may be an indication of serious diseases such as cancer.

Pathophysiology

Aging is associated with a progressive reduction in hematopoietic reserve, which increases the risk of anemia in times of hematopoietic stress.[73] Dysregulation of proinflammatory cytokines, most notably interleukin-6, may inhibit EPO production or interact with EPO receptors.[74] Although Hb levels may remain normal, the diminished marrow reserve leaves older adults more susceptible to other causes of anemia. Renal insufficiency, which also is common in older adults, may reduce the ability of the kidneys to produce EPO. Older patients often have a normal creatinine level but a diminished glomerular filtration rate. Myelodysplastic syndromes are another common cause of anemia in older adults, but most anemia cases in older adults are multifactorial.

Etiology

In the acute care setting, the most common causes of anemia in older adults are chronic disease (35%), unexplained (17%), and iron deficiency (15%), whereas in community-based outpatient clinics, the most common causes are unexplained (36%), infection (23%), and chronic disease (17%).[75] Another common problem in older adults is vitamin B_{12} deficiency. The most common causes of clinically overt vitamin B_{12} deficiency are food or cobalamin malabsorption (more than 60% of cases) and pernicious anemia (15%-20% of cases).[76]

One often overlooked major factor that may contribute to anemia in the older population is nutritional status. Cognitive and functional impairments in the older population may create barriers for patients to obtain and prepare a nutritious diet. Nutritional deficiencies that are not severe enough to affect the hematopoietic system in the younger population may contribute to anemia in older adults. Edentulous or older adults who may be too ill to prepare their meals are at risk for nutritional folate deficiency. Risk factors for inadequate folate intake in older adults include low caloric intake, inadequate consumption of fortified cereals, and failure to take a vitamin/mineral supplement. However, unlike vitamin B_{12} levels, folate levels often increase rather than decline with age. High folic acid intake can occur if older adults regularly take a supplement and consume fortified cereals.[77,78]

Bleeding with resultant iron deficiency in older adults may be due to carcinoma, peptic ulcer, atrophic gastritis, drug-induced gastritis, postmenopausal vaginal bleeding, or bleeding hemorrhoids. Older women have a much lower incidence of IDA compared with younger, menstruating women. Until proven otherwise, iron deficiency in older adults should be considered a sign of chronic blood loss. Steps should be taken to rule out bleeding, especially from the GI or female reproductive tract. AI is more common in older adults, as diseases that contribute to AI such as cancer, infection, and rheumatoid arthritis are more prevalent in this population.

Laboratory Findings

For practical purposes, it is best to use usual adult reference values and WHO criteria for laboratory tests in older adults. Anemia in older adults usually is normocytic and mild, with Hb values ranging between 10 and 12 g/dL (100-120 g/L; 6.21-7.45 mmol/L) in most anemic patients.[68] Evaluation of an older patient should be similar to strategies described previously for younger adults, perhaps with more emphasis on identifying occult blood loss and vitamin B_{12} deficiency. Vitamin B_{12} deficiency may be present even when plasma levels of vitamin B_{12} are within the normal range, but elevated MMA levels will reveal the deficiency. A refractory macrocytic anemia in older adults should raise suspicion of a myelodysplastic syndrome.

TREATMENT

Treatment of anemia in older adults is the same as that described for each type of anemia previously discussed in this chapter. With IDA, it is essential to treat the underlying cause, if known (ie, bleeding), and administer iron supplementation. Lower doses of iron supplementation are often recommended in older adults (eg, 325 mg of ferrous sulfate once daily or every other day) to decrease the incidence of GI adverse effects, which can lead to additional morbidity and poor adherence. Vitamin B_{12} can be repleted orally or parenterally. The dose for oral therapy is 1,000 to 2,000 μg daily depending on anemia severity and has been shown to be as effective as intramuscular injections. As with oral iron therapy, reticulocytosis often occurs within a week of Vitamin B_{12} therapy. Folate deficiency is treated with folic acid supplementation at 1 mg daily. The goal of treatment of AI is resolution of the underlying cause, although curing the underlying chronic illness in older adults can be difficult. Routine treatment with ESAs is not standard of care for AI in older adults.

ANEMIA IN PEDIATRIC POPULATIONS

Epidemiology

8 Globally, anemia is a significant cause of morbidity and mortality in pediatrics with an incidence as high as 47% in pre-school aged children and the highest concentration of patients found in Africa and Southeast Asia.[79] In the United States, the WHO reported the incidence of anemia in the pediatric population as 6% in 2011.[80] IDA accounts for the most cases of anemia in children and the prevalence of iron deficiency is reported to be as high as 20% in low-income families, likely due to diet.[81] IDA is a leading cause of infant mortality around the world.[82] Data from NHANES III indicated that 9% of children ages 12 to 36 months in the United States had iron deficiency and 3% had IDA.[83,84] Lack of a normal Hb at birth directly affects nonstorage iron and increases the risk of IDA in the first 3 to 6 months of life. An anemia of prematurity most commonly occurs 3 to 12 weeks after birth in infants younger than 32 weeks gestation and can spontaneously resolve by 3 to 6 months. Additional causes of anemia in pediatrics include "physiologic anemia" in newborns, G6PD deficiency, and thalassemia.

Etiology

The age of the child can yield some clues regarding the etiology of the anemia. From birth to 3 months, a "physiologic anemia" is the most common cause of anemia due to a decrease in erythropoiesis post-birth. At 3 to 6 months, hemoglobinopathy is more frequently encountered, as IDA is rare prior to 6 months of age. Iron deficiency becomes the most frequent etiology of anemia in toddler through adolescent years. The optimal amount of nutritional iron and folate required varies among individuals based on life-cycle stages. Two peak periods place children at risk of developing IDA. The first peak occurs during late infancy and early childhood, when children undergo rapid body growth, have low levels of dietary iron, and exhaust stores accumulated during gestation. The second peak occurs during adolescence, which is associated with rapid growth, poor diets, and onset of menses in girls. Some studies suggest that overweight children are at significantly higher risk for IDA. Proposed factors include genetic influences; physical inactivity, leading to decreased myoglobin breakdown and lower amounts of released iron into the blood; and inadequate diet with limited intake of iron-rich foods.[85]

Conditions in the newborn period that can lead to IDA include prematurity, low iron intake, and insufficient maternal iron consumption, particularly during the third trimester of pregnancy when 60% to 80% of fetal iron storage occurs. However, there is insufficient data to suggest that treatment of IDA in pregnant women will prevent IDA in newborns. Premature infants are at increased risk for IDA because of their smaller total blood volume, increased blood loss through phlebotomy, and poor GI absorption. Factors leading to unbalanced iron metabolism in infants include insufficient iron intake, early introduction of cow's milk, intolerance of cow's milk, medications, and malabsorption. Dietary deficiency of iron in the first 6 to 12 months of life is less common today because of the increased use of iron supplementation during breast-feeding and use of iron-fortified formulas. Iron deficiency becomes more common when children change to regular diets.

When screening for iron deficiency in young children, a careful dietary history can help identify children at risk. High iron needs and the tendency to eat fewer iron-containing foods contribute to the etiology of iron deficiency during adolescence.

Other causes of microcytic anemia include thalassemia, lead poisoning, and sideroblastic anemia. Normocytic anemias in children include infection with human parvovirus B19 and glucose-6-phosphate dehydrogenase (G6PD) deficiency. In the setting of G6PD deficiency, a thorough review of potential drug and toxin exposure around the onset of anemia will be helpful to determine an offending agent. Macrocytic anemias are caused by deficiencies in vitamin B_{12} and folate, chronic liver disease, hypothyroidism, and myelodysplastic disorders. Folic acid deficiency usually is due to inadequate dietary intake, but human milk and cow's milk provide adequate sources. Vitamin B_{12} deficiency due to nutritional reasons is rare but may occur due to congenital pernicious anemia.

Pathophysiology

In contrast to anemias in adults, which tend to be manifestations of a broader underlying pathology, anemias in the pediatric population are more often due to a primary hematologic abnormality. In newborn infants, "physiologic anemia" is often due to reduced EPO production.[86] Erythropoiesis also decreases during this time as a result of increased tissue oxygenation.

Hemoglobinopathy is often suspected in infants with anemia between the ages of 3 to 6 months because IDA is rare during this period. Potential causes include sickle cell anemia, thalassemia, and G6PD deficiency. Thalassemia is an inherited condition in which the Hgb structure is compromised leading to anemia of various degrees based on the subtype of thalassemia. This condition is most frequently seen in patients of Mediterranean and Southeast Asian heritage.[81] G6PD deficiency is an X-linked disorder most frequently seen in patients of Asian, Mediterranean, and African descent.[87] The lack of this enzyme reduces the RBC's protection against oxidative injury by limiting the glutathione available. Glutathione in RBCs rapidly inactivates oxidants preventing cellular injury. G6PD is an important enzyme in the formation of glutathione and a deficiency in this enzyme ultimately leads to hemolysis and anemia after exposure to an oxidant, such as dapsone, primaquine, or fava beans.

IDA should be suspected in microcytic anemia of children after 6 months of age. The amount of iron present at birth depends on gestational length and weight. Iron stores from birth are mostly depleted by 6 months of age. The addition of iron supplements and iron-enriched foods is important to maintain iron levels and prevent the development of IDA.

Laboratory Findings

When evaluating laboratory values for pediatric patients, the clinician must use age- and sex-adjusted norms. It is important to know that many blood samples are capillary samples, such as heel or finger sticks, which may have slightly different results than venous samples. The USPSTF has concluded that evidence is insufficient to recommend for or against routine screening for IDA in asymptomatic low-risk children aged 6 to 12 months. Hb is a sensitive test for iron deficiency, but it has low specificity in childhood anemias. If an abnormality is found, a CBC should be ordered to evaluate MCV and determine whether the anemia is microcytic, normocytic, or macrocytic. A peripheral blood smear and reticulocyte count also may be helpful. The peripheral blood smear can indicate the etiology based on RBC morphology, and the reticulocyte count helps differentiate between decreased RBC production and increased RBC destruction or loss. Other laboratory tests include serum iron, ferritin, TIBC, and transferrin saturation. Laboratory markers of hemolysis, including increased bilirubin, lactate dehydrogenase, and decreased haptoglobin, can identify hemolytic anemias, including G6PD deficiency and thalassemia. A G6PD deficiency screening test may be indicated if hemolysis is present. Mild hereditary anemias may produce a mild hypochromic microcytic anemia that can be confused with IDAs. The RDW may be high with iron deficiency and is more likely to be normal with thalassemia. Laboratory features of anemia of prematurity include normocytic normochromic cells, low reticulocyte count, low serum EPO concentrations, and decreased RBC precursors in bone marrow. Laboratory diagnosis of vitamin B_{12} and folate deficiency in children is similar to that of adults.

TREATMENT

Primary prevention of IDA in infants, children, and adolescents is the most appropriate goal because delays in mental and motor development are potentially irreversible. In 2015, the USPSTF published revised recommendations to screen and supplement iron deficiency in the United States, focusing on children and pregnant women. They concluded that the current evidence is insufficient to evaluate the benefits and harms of routine screening in asymptomatic children ages 6 to 24 months and routine use of iron supplementation in pregnant women to improve fetal outcomes.[88] Screening should be restricted to high risk children, including those with poor growth and insufficient iron intake. Routine iron supplementation for exclusively breastfed infants at 1 mg/kg/day is recommended by the American Academy of Pediatrics (AAP) beginning at 4 months until appropriate iron-containing foods are introduced. Fair evidence was found that iron supplementation (eg, iron-fortified formula or iron supplements) improves neurodevelopmental outcomes in children at risk for IDA. Due to the widespread use of iron-enriched formula, additional supplementation is rarely necessary in formula-fed infants.[80]

Interventions likely to prevent anemia include diverse foods with bioavailable forms of iron, food fortification for infants and children, and individual supplementation. Routine screening for iron deficiency in nonpregnant adolescents is recommended only for those with risk factors, which include vegetarian diets, malnutrition, low body weight, chronic illness, or history of heavy menstrual blood loss.

For infants aged 9 to 12 months with a mild microcytic anemia, the most cost-effective treatment is a therapeutic trial of iron. Fe^{2+} sulfate at a dose of 3 to 6 mg/kg/day of elemental iron divided once or twice daily between meals for 4 weeks is recommended. In children who respond, iron should be continued for 2 more months to replace storage iron pools, along with dietary intervention and patient education.[89] Liquid iron preparations can occasionally stain teeth. Kids should be advised to brush teeth or rinse out their mouth after administration. Parenteral iron therapy has a limited role and is rarely necessary.

For the macrocytic anemias in children, folate can be administered at a dose of 1 mg daily. However, vitamin B_{12} deficiency due to congenital pernicious anemia requires lifelong vitamin B_{12} supplementation. Dose and frequency should be titrated according to clinical response and laboratory values. No data regarding the use of oral vitamin B_{12} supplementation in children is available.

Treatment of normocytic anemias is based on underlying cause.

EVALUATION OF THERAPEUTIC OUTCOMES

For IDA, a positive response to a trial of oral iron therapy is characterized by modest reticulocytosis in days, with an increase in Hb starting after about 2 weeks with continued rapid rise in Hb. As the Hb level approaches normal, the rate of increase slows progressively.

Hb should reach a normal level after about 2 months of therapy and often sooner.[12] If the patient does not develop reticulocytosis, reevaluation of the diagnosis or iron replacement therapy is necessary. Iron therapy should continue for a period sufficient for complete restoration of iron stores. Serum ferritin concentrations should return to the normal range prior to discontinuation of iron. The time interval required to accomplish this goal varies, although at least 6 to 12 months of therapy usually is warranted.

When large amounts of parenteral iron are administered, by either total dose infusion or multiple intramuscular or IV doses, the patient's iron status should be closely monitored. Patients receiving regular IV iron should be monitored for clinical or laboratory evidence of iron toxicity or overload. Iron overload may be indicated by abnormal hepatic function tests, serum ferritin greater than 800 ng/mL (800 μg/L [1,800 pmol/L]), or transferrin saturation greater than 50%. Serum ferritin and transferrin saturation should be measured in the first week after larger IV iron doses. Hb and Hct should be measured weekly, and serum iron and ferritin levels should be measured at least monthly.

Most patients with vitamin B_{12}–deficiency anemia respond rapidly to vitamin B_{12} therapy. The typical patient will experience improved strength and well-being within a few days of treatment initiation. Reticulocytosis is evident in 3 to 5 days. Hb begins to rise after the first week and should normalize in 1 to 2 months.[90] CBC and serum cobalamin levels usually are drawn 1 to 2 months after initiation of therapy and 3 to 6 months thereafter for surveillance monitoring. Homocysteine and MMA levels can be repeated 2 to 3 months after initiation of replacement therapy to evaluate for normalization of levels, although levels begin to decrease in 1 to 2 weeks. Neuropsychiatric signs and symptoms can be reversible if treated early. If permanent neurologic damage has resulted, progression should cease with replacement therapy. Slow response to therapy or failure to observe normalization of laboratory results may suggest the presence of an additional abnormality such as iron deficiency, thalassemia trait, infection, malignancy, nonadherence, or misdiagnosis.

In folic acid deficiency anemia, symptomatic improvement, as evidenced by increased alertness and appetite, often occurs early during treatment. Reticulocytosis begins in the first week. Hct begins to rise within 2 weeks and should reach normal levels within 2 months. MCV initially increases because of an increase in reticulocytes but gradually decreases to normal.

One of the earliest responses with ESA use is an increased blood reticulocyte count, which usually occurs in the first few days. Baseline iron status should be checked before and during treatment, as many patients receiving ESAs require supplemental iron therapy. The optimal form and schedule of iron supplementation are not known. Hb levels should be monitored twice a week until stabilized. Hb should also be monitored twice weekly for 2 to 6 weeks after a dose adjustment.[54] A fall in Hb during ESA therapy may indicate a need for iron supplementation or signal occult blood loss. Baseline and periodic monitoring of iron, TIBC, transferrin saturation, or ferritin levels may be useful in optimizing iron repletion and limiting the need for ESAs. Patients who do not respond to 8 weeks of optimal dosage should not continue taking ESAs. Target Hb levels should be 11 to 12 g/dL (110-120 g/L; 6.83-7.45 mmol/L). Cost is an issue with ESA therapy. Therefore, drug cost must be weighed against the effects on transfusions and hospitalizations.

In older adults, responses and treatment monitoring are similar as that described for the general adult population. If the reticulocyte count rises but the anemia does not improve, inadequate absorption of iron or continued blood loss should be suspected. As with any form of anemia, symptomatic improvement should be evident shortly after starting therapy and Hb/Hct should begin to rise within a few weeks of initiating therapy. A key component of symptom assessment among older adults is the functional domain. Patients should be asked about changes in self-care abilities, mobility, and stamina.

Therapeutic outcomes are assessed in children by monitoring Hb, Hct, and RBC indices 4 to 8 weeks after initiation of iron therapy. For premature infants, Hb or Hct should be monitored weekly.

CONCLUSION

Anemia affects many patients across the lifespan, impacting morbidity and mortality. The causes of anemia can vary and includes genetic disorders, nutritional deficiencies, chronic disease, and acute illness. Identification of the correct cause of anemia through lab assessment is key to selecting the appropriate treatment and monitoring plan. While anemia can sometimes be a symptom or complication of another disease or deficiency, it is important for clinicians to understand the disease and how to treat it.

ABBREVIATIONS

ACD	anemia of chronic disease
AI	anemia of inflammation
CBC	complete blood count
CDC	Centers for Disease Control and Prevention
EPO	erythropoietin
ESA	erythropoiesis-stimulating agent
Fe^{2+}	ferrous iron
Fe^{3+}	ferric iron
G6PD	glucose-6-phosphate dehydrogenase
Hb	hemoglobin
Hct	hematocrit
HIV	human immunodeficiency virus
IDA	iron-deficiency anemia
MCH	mean corpuscular hemoglobin
MCHC	mean corpuscular hemoglobin concentration
MCV	mean corpuscular volume
MMA	methylmalonic acid
NHANES	National Health and Nutrition Examination Survey
NSAID	nonsteroidal anti-inflammatory drugs
RBC	red blood cell
RDW	red blood cell distribution width
TIBC	total iron-binding capacity
USPSTF	United States Preventive Services Task Force
WHO	World Health Organization

REFERENCES

1. Kassebaum NJ; GBD 2013 Anaemia Collaborators. The global burden of anemia. *Hematol Oncol Clin North Am.* 2016;30(2):247–308. doi:10.1016/j.hoc.2015.11.002
2. Nutritional anaemias: Tools for effective prevention and control. Geneva: World Health Organization; 2017.
3. Patient Education Anemia. American Society of Hematology. https://www.hematology.org/education/patients/anemia. Last accessed, January 25, 2022.
4. Nissenson A. Anemia not just an innocent bystander. *Arch Intern Med.* 2003;163:1400–1404.
5. Mozaffarian D. Anemia predicts mortality in severe heart failure: The prospective randomized amlodipine survival evaluation (PRAISE). *J Am Coll Cardiol.* 2003;1933–1939.
6. Chaves PHM, Carlson MC, Ferrucci L, et al. Association between mild anemia and executive function impairment in community-dwelling older women: The Women's Health and Aging Study II. *J Am Geriatr Soc.* 2006;54:1429–1435.
7. Anemia in pregnancy. ACOG Practice Bulletin No. 95. American College of Obst and Gynecologists. *Obstet Gynecol.* 2008;112:201–207.
8. Gaskell H, Derry S, Andrew Moore R, McQuay HJ. Prevalence of anaemia in older persons: Systematic review. *BMC Geriatr.* 2008;8:1. doi:10.1186/1471-2318-8-1.

9. Prchal JT, Thiagarajan P. Erythropoiesis. In: Kaushansky K, Lichtman MA, Beutler E, et al, eds. *Williams Hematology.* 8th ed. New York: McGraw-Hill; 2010:453–458.
10. Wians FH, Urban JE, Keffer JH, Kroft SH. Discriminating between iron deficiency anemia and anemia of chronic disease using traditional indices of iron status vs. transferrin receptor concentration. *Am J Clin Pathol.* 2001;115:112–118.
11. Beutler E. Destruction of erythrocytes. In: Kaushansky K, Lichtman MA, Beutler E, et al, eds. *Williams Hematology.* 8th ed. New York: McGraw-Hill; 2010:449–454.
12. Beutler E. Disorders of iron metabolism. In: Kaushansky K, Lichtman MA, Beutler E, et al, eds. *Williams Hematology.* 8th ed. New York: McGraw-Hill; 2010:565–606.
13. Galloway M, Rushworth L. Red cell or serum folate? Results from the National Pathology Alliance benchmarking review. *J Clin Pathol.* 2003;56:924–926.
14. Green R. Folate, cobalamin, and megaloblastic anemias. In: Kaushansky K, Lichtman MA, Beutler E, et al, eds. *Williams Hematology.* 8th ed. New York: McGraw-Hill; 2010:533–564.
15. Dharmarajan TS, Norkus EP. Approaches to vitamin B_{12} deficiency. Early treatment may prevent devastating complications. *Postgrad Med.* 2001;110:99–105.
16. Cusick SE, Mei Z, Freedman DS, et al. Unexplained decline in the prevalence of anemia among US children and women between 1988-1994 and 1999-2002. *Am J Clin Nutr.* 2008;88:1611–1617.
17. Goodnough LT, Nemeth E, Gan T. Detection, evaluation, and management of iron restricted erythropoiesis. *Blood.* 2010;116:4754–4761.
18. Camaschella C. Iron-deficiency anemia. *N Engl J Med.* 2015;372:1832–1843.
19. Killip S, Bennett J, Chambers M. Iron deficiency anemia. *Am Fam Physician.* 2007;75:671–678.
20. Hershko C, Ianculovich M, Souroujon M. A hematologist's view of unexplained iron deficiency anemia in males: Impact of *Helicobacter pylori* eradication. *Blood Cells Mol Dis.* 2007;38:45–53.
21. Ems T, St Lucia K, Huecker MR. Biochemistry, Iron Absorption. [Updated 2021 Apr 26]. In: StatPearls [Internet]. Treasure Island (FL): StatPearls Publishing; 2022 Jan-. Available from: https://www.ncbi.nlm.nih.gov/books/NBK448204/
22. Ganz T. Hepcidin—A regulator of intestinal iron absorption and iron recycling by macrophages. *Best Pract Res Clin Haematol.* 2005;18:171–182.
23. McDonagh M, Cantor A, Bougatsos C, et al. Routine iron supplementation and screening for iron deficiency anemia in pregnant women: A systematic review to update the US Preventive Services Task Force recommendation. Agency for Healthcare Research and Quality (US); US Preventive Services Task Force Evidence Syntheses, Rockville, 2015.
24. Anemia in Pregnancy: ACOG Practice Bulletin, Number 233. *Obstet Gynecol.* 2021;138(2):e55–e64. doi:10.1097/AOG.0000000000004477.
25. Moretti D, Goede JS, et al. Oral iron supplements increase hepcidin and decrease iron absorption from daily or twice-daily doses in iron-depleted young women. *Blood.* 2015;126:1981–1989. doi:10.1182/blood-2015-05-642223.26289639.
26. Stoffel NU, Cercamondi CI, Brittenham G, et al. Iron absorption from oral iron supplements given on consecutive versus alternate days and as single morning doses versus twice-daily split dosing in iron-depleted women: Two open-label, randomised controlled trials. *Lancet Haematol.* 2017;4(11):e524–e533. doi:10.1016/S2352-3026(17)30182-5.29032957.
27. Gasche C, Berstad A, Befrits R, et al. Guidelines on the diagnosis and management of iron deficiency and anemia in inflammatory bowel diseases. *Inflamm Bowel Dis.* 2007;13:1545–1553.
28. Faich G, Strobos J. Sodium Fe^{3+} gluconate complex in sucrose: Safer IV iron therapy than iron dextrans. *Am J Kidney Dis.* 1999;33:464–470.
29. Chandler G, Harchowal J, Macdougall IC. Intravenous iron sucrose: Establishing a safe dose. *Am J Kidney Dis.* 2001;38:988–991.
30. Silverstein SB, Gilreath JA, Rodgers GM. Intravenous iron therapy: A summary of treatment options and review of guidelines. *J Pharm Practice.* 2008;21:431–443.
31. Munoz M, Garcia-Erce JA, Remacha AF. Disorders of iron metabolism: Part II: Iron deficiency and iron overload. *J Clin Pathol.* 2011;64:287–296.
32. Ferrlecit [package insert]. Morristown, NJ: Watson Pharma; 2015.
33. Venofer [package insert]. Shirley, NY: American Regent; 2015.
34. Feraheme [package insert]. Lexington, MA: AMAG Pharmaceuticals; 2015.
35. Injectafer [package insert]. Shirley, NY: American Regent; 2013.
36. Avni T, Bieber A, Grossman A, et al. The safety of intravenous iron preparations: Systematic review and meta-analysis. *Mayo Clin Proc.* 2015;90:12–23.
37. Oh RC, Brown DL. Vitamin B_{12} deficiency. *Am Fam Physician.* 2003;67:979–986, 993–994.
38. Hunt A, Harrington D, Robinson S. Vitamin B12 deficiency. *BMJ.* 2014;349:g5226.
39. Kaptan K, Beyan C, Ural AU, et al. *Helicobacter pylori*—Is it a novel causative agent in vitamin B_{12} deficiency? *Arch Intern Med.* 2000;160:1349–1353.
40. Mazokopakis EE, Starakis IK. Recommendations for diagnosis and management of metformin-induced vitamin B12 (Cbl) deficiency. *Diabetes Res Clin Pract.* 2012 Sep;97(3):359–67. doi:10.1016/j.diabres.2012.06.001. Epub 2012 Jul 7. PMID: 22770998.
41. Hesdorffer CS, Longo DL. Drug-induced megaloblastic anemia. *NEJM.* 2015;373:164–958.
42. Hoffbrand AV. Megaloblastic anemias. In: Longo DL, Fauci AS, Kasper DL, Hauser SL, Jameson JL, Loscalzo J, eds. *Harrison's Principles of Internal Medicine.* 18th ed. New York: McGraw-Hill; 2012:chap 105.
43. Green R. Indicators for assessing folate and vitamin B-12 status and for monitoring the efficacy of intervention strategies. *Am J Clin Nutr.* 2011;94(Suppl):666S–672S.
44. Vidal-Alaball J, Butler CC, Cannings-John R, et al. Oral vitamin B_{12} versus intramuscular vitamin B_{12} for vitamin B_{12} deficiency. *Cochrane Database Syst Rev.* 2005;3:CD004655.
45. Cravens DD, Nashelsky J, Oh RC. How do we evaluate a marginally low B_{12} level? *J Fam Pract.* 2007;56:62–63.
46. Solomon LR. Oral vitamin B_{12} therapy: A cautionary note. *Blood.* 2004;103:2863.
47. Lane LA, Rojas-Fernandez C. Treatment of vitamin B_{12}-deficiency anemia: Oral versus parenteral therapy. *Ann Pharmacother.* 2002;36:1268–1272.
48. U.S. Department of Agriculture, Agricultural Research Service. What We Eat in America, 2013-2014. 2017.
49. Pitkin RM. Folate and neural tube defects. *Am J Clin Nutr.* 2007;85:285S–288S.
50. Yang Q, Cogswell ME, Hamner HC, et al. Folic acid source, usual intake, and folate and vitamin B-12 status in US adults: National Health and Nutrition Examination Survey (NHANES) 2003-2006. *Am J Clin Nutr.* 2010;91:64–72.
51. Yerby MS. Clinical care of pregnant women with epilepsy: Neural tube defects and folic acid supplementation. *Epilepsia.* 2003;44(Suppl 3):33–40.
52. American College of Obstetricians and Gynecologists (ACOG). Neural Tube Defects. ACOG Practice Bulletin No. 44. Washington, DC: American College of Obstetricians and Gynecologists; 2003.
53. Corwin HL, Gettinger A, Pearl RG, et al. The CRIT Study: Anemia and blood transfusion in the critically ill—Current clinical practice in the United States. *Crit Care Med.* 2004;32:39–52.
54. Rodriguez RM, Corwin HL, Gettinger A, et al. Nutritional deficiencies and blunted erythropoietin response as cause of anemia of critical illness. *J Crit Care.* 2001;16:36–41.
55. Silver MR. Anemia in the long-term ventilator-dependent patient with respiratory failure. *Chest.* 2005;128(Suppl):568S–575S.
56. Lai YC, Ruan SY, Huang CT, Kuo PH, Yu CJ. Hemoglobin levels and weaning outcome of mechanical ventilation in difficult-to-wean patients: A retrospective cohort study. *PLoS One.* 2013;8:e73743. 10.1371/journal.pone.0073743.24015310.
57. Schönhofer B, Wenzel M, Geibel M, Köhler D. Blood transfusion and lung function in chronically anemic patients with severe chronic obstructive pulmonary disease. *Crit Care Med.* 1998;26:1824–1828.
58. Leach RM, Treacher DF. The pulmonary physician in critical care * 2: Oxygen delivery and consumption in the critically ill. *Thorax.* 2002;57:170–177.
59. Ouellette DR. The impact of anemia in patients with respiratory failure. *Chest.* 2005;128(5 Suppl 2):576S–582S. doi:10.1378/chest.128.5_suppl_2.576S.16306056.
60. Weiss GW, Goodnough LT. Anemia of chronic disease. *N Engl J Med.* 2005;352:1011–1023.
61. Adamson J. The anemia of inflammation/malignancy: Mechanisms and management. *Hematol Am Soc Hematol Educ Program.* 2008;159–165.
62. Poggiali E, Migone De Amicis M, Motta I. Anemia of chronic disease: A unique defect of iron recycling for many different chronic diseases. *Eur J Intern Med.* 2014;25:12–17.
63. Procrit [package insert]. Thousand Oaks, CA: Amgen, 2009.
64. Carson JL, Guyatt G, Heddle NM, et al. Clinical Practice Guidelines From the AABB: Red Blood Cell Transfusion Thresholds and Storage. *JAMA.* 2016 Nov 15;316(19):2025–2035. doi:10.1001/jama.2016.9185. PMID: 27732721.

65. Zarychanski R, Turgeon AF, McIntyre L, Fergusson DA. Erythropoietin-receptor agonists in critically ill patients: A meta-analysis of randomized controlled trials. *CMAJ.* 2007;177:725–734. doi:10.1503/cmaj.071055.17823140.
66. Rudis M, Jacobi J, Hassan E, et al. Managing anemia in the critically ill patient. *Pharmacotherapy*. 2004;24:229–247.
67. Hébert PC, Wells G, Martin C, et al. Do blood transfusions improve outcomes related to mechanical ventilation? *Chest.* 2001;119:1850–1857.
68. Guralnik JM, Eisenstaedt RS, Ferrucci L, et al. Prevalence of anemia in person 65 years and older in the United States: Evidence for a high rate of unexplained anemia. *Blood.* 2004;104:2263–2268.
69. Carmel R. Anemia and aging: An overview of clinical, diagnostic, and biological issues. *Blood Rev.* 2001;15:9–18.
70. Culleton BF, Manns BJ, Zhang J, et al. Impact of anemia on hospitalization and mortality in older adults. *Blood.* 2006;107:3841–3846.
71. Muzzarelli S, Pfisterer M, TIME Investigators. Anemia as independent predictor of major events in elderly patients with chronic angina. *Am Heart J.* 2006;152:991–996.
72. Woodman R, Ferrucci L, Guralnik J. Anemia in older adults. *Curr Opin Hematol.* 2005;12:123–128.
73. Balducci L, Hardy CL, Lyman GH. Hematopoietic growth factors in the older cancer patient. *Curr Opin Hematol.* 2001;8:170–187.
74. Eisenstaedt R, Penninx BW, Woodman RC. Anemia in the elderly: Current understanding and emerging concepts. *Blood Rev.* 2006;20:213–226.
75. Balducci L. Epidemiology of anemia in the elderly: Information on diagnostic evaluation. *J Am Geriatr Soc.* 2003;51(Suppl):S2–S9.
76. Andres E, Loukili N, Noel E, et al. Vitamin B_{12} (cobalamin) deficiency in elderly patients. *CMAJ.* 2004;171:251–259.
77. Mulligan JE, Greene GW, Caldwell M. Sources of folate and serum folate levels in older adults. *J Am Diet Assoc.* 2007;107:495–499.
78. Ford ES, Bowman BA. Serum and red blood cell folate concentrations, race, and education: Findings from the third National Health and Nutrition Examination Survey. *Am J Clin Nutr.* 1999;69:476–481.
79. McLean E, Cogswell M, Egli I, Wojdyla D, de Benoist B. Worldwide prevalence of anaemia, WHO Vitamin and Mineral Nutrition Information System, 1993-2005. *Public Health Nutr.* 2009;12:444–454. doi:10.1017/S1368980008002401.18498676.
80. Wang M. Iron deficiency and other types of anemia in infants and children. *Am Fam Physician.* 2016;93:270–278. 26926814.
81. Khan L. Anemia in childhood. *Pediatr Ann.* 2018;47(2):e42–e47. doi:10.3928/19382359-20180129-01.29446792.
82. Milman N. Iron prophylaxis in pregnancy—General or individual and in which dose? *Ann Hematol.* 2006;85:821–828.
83. Recommendations to prevent and control iron deficiency in the United States. *Morb Mortal Wkly Rep.* 1998;47:1–36.
84. Moy RJ. Prevalence, consequences and prevention of childhood nutritional iron. *Clin Lab Haematol.* 2006;28:291–298.
85. Nead KG, Halterman JS, Kaczorowski JM, et al. Overweight children and adolescents: A risk group for iron deficiency. *Pediatrics.* 2004;114:104–108.
86. Palis J, Segel GB. Hematology of the fetus and newborn. In: Prchal JT, Kaushansky K, Lichtman MA, Kipps TJ, Seligsohn U, eds. *Williams Hematology*. 8th ed. New York: McGraw-Hill; 2010.
87. Nkhoma ET, Poole C, Vannappagari V, Hall SA, Beutler E. The global prevalence of glucose-6-phosphate dehydrogenase deficiency: A systematic review and meta-analysis. *Blood Cells Mol Dis.* 2009;42(3):267–278. doi:10.1016/j.bcmd.2008.12.005.19233695.
88. Siu AL. Screening for iron deficiency anemia and iron supplementation in pregnant women to improve maternal health and birth outcomes: U.S. Preventive Services Task Force Recommendation Statement. *Ann Intern Med.* 2015;163(7):529–536. doi:10.7326/M15-1707.26344176.
89. Kazal LA. Prevention of iron deficiency in infants and toddlers. *Am Fam Physician.* 2002;66:1217–1224.
90. Snow CF. Laboratory diagnosis of vitamin B_{12} and folate deficiency. *Arch Intern Med.* 1999;159:1289–1298.

123

Coagulation Disorders

Heidi Trinkman, Timothy L. McCavit, and Lauren Duran

KEY CONCEPTS

1. Hemophilia is an inherited bleeding disorder resulting from a congenital deficiency in factor VIII or IX.
2. The goal of therapy for hemophilia is to prevent bleeding episodes and their resulting long-term complications and to arrest bleeding if it occurs.
3. Recombinant factor concentrates usually are the first-line treatment of hemophilia because they have the lowest risk of infection.
4. Inhibitor formation is the most significant treatment complication in hemophilia and is associated with significant morbidity and decreased quality of life.
5. Recombinant factor VIIa is effective for the treatment of acute bleeds in patients with hemophilia A or B who have developed inhibitors.
6. The goal of therapy for von Willebrand disease (vWD) is to increase von Willebrand factor (vWF) and factor VIII levels to prevent bleeding during surgery or arrest bleeding when it occurs.
7. vWF concentrates are the agents of choice for treatment of type 3 vWD and some type 2 vWD, and for serious bleeding in type 1 vWD.
8. Desmopressin acetate often is effective for the treatment of type 1 vWD. It also may be effective for the treatment of some forms of type 2 vWD in addition to mild-to-moderate hemophilia A.

BEYOND THE BOOK

Create a Venn diagram to compare hemophilia A and B. Within the diagram, be sure to include pertinent disease state information such as clinical manifestations, incidence, and recommended treatment. List specific short- and long-acting products used in each type, as well as treatment modalities that may be common to both.

INTRODUCTION

The coagulation system is intricately balanced and designed to stop bleeding at the site of vascular injury through complex interactions between the vascular endothelium, platelets, procoagulant proteins, anticoagulant proteins, and fibrinolytic proteins. Hemostasis stops bleeding at the site of vascular injury through the formation of an impermeable platelet and fibrin plug. Three key mechanisms facilitate hemostasis including vascular constriction, primary platelet plug formation (primary hemostasis), and clot propagation through fibrin formation (secondary hemostasis). Derangements in this system can lead to either bleeding or thrombosis. Bleeding disorders are the result of a coagulation factor defect, a quantitative or qualitative platelet defect, or enhanced fibrinolytic activity.

COAGULATION FACTORS

Secondary hemostasis facilitates propagation and stabilization of the initial platelet plug formed in primary hemostasis through the formation of fibrin on the activated platelet surface. This step is initiated via the tissue factor pathway and is vital for adequate hemostasis. Coagulation factors circulate as inactive precursors (zymogens). Activation of these coagulation proteins leads to a cascading series of proteolytic reactions. At each step, a clotting factor undergoes limited proteolysis and becomes an active protease (designated by a lowercase "a," as in Xa).

The coagulation factors can be divided into three groups based on biochemical properties: vitamin K–dependent factors (II, VII, IX, and X), contact activation factors (XI and XII, prekallikrein, and high-molecular-weight kininogen), and thrombin-sensitive factors (V, VIII, XIII, and fibrinogen). Biologic half-life and blood product source varies by coagulation factor.

CLINICAL MANIFESTATIONS AND DIAGNOSIS

The diagnosis of coagulation disorders is established from a detailed clinical history, physical examination, and laboratory test results. The clinical history should ascertain if there is a family history of bleeding or known bleeding disorders. Laboratory testing can distinguish bleeding disorders caused by defects in the coagulation pathways, fibrinolytic pathways, or alterations in the number or function of platelets. Table 123-1 describes common coagulation tests.

HEMOPHILIA

1 Hemophilia is a bleeding disorder that results from a congenital deficiency in a plasma coagulation protein. Hemophilia A (classic hemophilia) is caused by a deficiency of factor VIII and hemophilia B (Christmas disease) is caused by a deficiency of factor IX. Hemophilia affects about 400,000 males worldwide.[1] The incidence

TABLE 123-1 Laboratory Procedures

Procedure	Identifies	Possible Cause of Abnormal Value	Clinical Manifestations
Prothrombin time (PT)	Factors I, II, V, VII, X	Newborn Vitamin K deficiency Inherited factor deficiencies[a] Warfarin therapy Liver disease Lupus anticoagulant (rare) Afibrinogenemia Dysfibrinogenemia	Bleeding following surgery, trauma, etc. Easy bruising
Activated partial thromboplastin time (aPTT)	Factors I, II, V, VIII, IX, X	Inherited factor deficiencies[a] Lupus anticoagulant Heparin therapy Liver disease Afibrinogenemia Dysfibrinogenemia	Joint and muscle bleeding Bleeding after surgery, trauma, etc.
	High-molecular-weight kininogen (HMWK), prekallikrein		No bleeding manifestations
	Factor XII		Increased incidence of thrombotic disease possible with severe factor XII deficiency
	Factor XI		Variable bleeding tendency Bleeding following surgery, trauma, etc.
Thrombin time (TT)	Fibrinogen Inhibitors of fibrin aggregation	Afibrinogenemia Dysfibrinogenemia Heparin therapy	Lifelong hemorrhagic disease Variable clinical symptoms from asymptomatic to either a bleeding diathesis or prothrombotic
Platelet count	Thrombocytopenia	Quantitative platelet disorder, type 2B von Willebrand disease, immune thrombocytopenia, other cause of thrombocytopenia	Mucocutaneous bleeding
Platelet function analyzer	Platelet function	Qualitative platelet defects, von Willebrand disease, antiplatelet therapy Also prolonged in anemia and thrombocytopenia[b]	Mucocutaneous bleeding
Platelet aggregation	Gold standard to assess platelet function	Qualitative platelet defects, antiplatelet medications	Mucocutaneous bleeding
Euglobulin clot lysis time (ECLT)	Fibrinolytic defect	A decreased ECLT indicates hyperfibrinolysis, which indicates an abnormality in the fibrinolytic pathway including plasminogen activator inhibitor 1 deficiency, α_2-plasminogen inhibitor deficiency Hypofibrinogenemia	Bleeding after trauma or surgical procedures especially in oral and urogenital areas

[a]Bleeding manifestations depend on factor levels.

[b]Insensitive to mild platelet defects and has fallen out of favor as a screening test

of hemophilia A is about 1 in 5,000 male births and hemophilia B occurs in 1 in 30,000 male births.[2] Hemophilia A constitutes 80% to 85% of all patients with hemophilia with the other 15% to 20% being hemophilia B.[1] The incidence of hemophilia is not affected by race.

About one-third of patients with hemophilia have a negative family history, presumably representing a spontaneous mutation.[1] Both hemophilia A and hemophilia B are recessive X-linked diseases, which means that the defective gene is located on the X chromosome. The disease primarily affects only males while females are carriers. Since affected males have the abnormal allele on their X chromosome and no matching allele on their Y chromosome, their sons would be normal (assuming the mother is not a carrier) and their daughters would be obligatory carriers. Female carriers have one normal allele and, therefore, do not usually have a bleeding tendency, although female carriers have lower factor VIII levels than females who are not carriers.[3] Sons of a female carrier and a normal male have a 50% chance of having hemophilia and daughters have a 50% chance of being carriers. Thus, there is a "skipped generation" mode of inheritance in which the female carriers do not express the disease but can pass it on to the next male generation. Hemophilia has been observed in a small number of females. It can occur if both factor VIII and IX genes are defective or if a female patient has only one X chromosome as in Turner syndrome.[4]

In 1984, researchers isolated and cloned the human factor VIII gene. It is a large gene, consisting of 186 kilobases (kb).[5] More than 2,000 unique mutations in the factor VIII gene, including point mutations, deletions, and insertions, have been reported.[6] Deletions and nonsense mutations are often associated with the more severe forms of factor VIII deficiency because functional factor VIII is not produced. In 1993, researchers identified an inversion in the factor VIII gene at intron 22 that accounts for almost 30% to 45% of severe hemophilia A gene abnormalities.[1] That discovery has greatly simplified carrier detection and prenatal diagnosis in families with this gene mutation.

The factor IX gene, cloned and sequenced in 1982, consists of only 34 kb and is significantly smaller than the factor VIII gene.[5] Unlike the factor VIII gene in patients with severe hemophilia A, the factor IX gene in patients with hemophilia B has no predominant mutation. Direct gene mutation analysis is simpler in hemophilia B because of the smaller gene size, and to date more than 1,000 different mutations have been reported.[7] Most of these mutations are single base-pair substitutions. About 3% of factor IX gene mutations are deletions or complex rearrangements, and the presence of these mutations is associated with a severe phenotype.[1]

Hemophilia B Leyden is a rare variant in which factor IX levels initially are low but rise at puberty. The mechanism of this disorder is controversial. Some propose that the binding of the androgen receptor and other transcription factors are responsible. Other molecular mechanisms for age-related gene regulation have been discovered and implicated in factor IX Leyden.[8] Identification of this genotype is clinically important because it confers a better prognosis.

Clinical Presentation and Diagnosis

The characteristic bleeding manifestations of hemophilia include palpable ecchymosis, bleeding into joint spaces (hemarthroses), muscle hemorrhages, and excessive bleeding after surgery or trauma. The severity of clinical bleeding generally correlates with the degree of deficiency of either factor VIII or factor IX. Factor VIII and factor IX activity levels are measured in units per milliliter, with 1 unit/mL representing 100% of the factor found in 1 mL of normal plasma.[2] Normal plasma levels range from 0.5 to 1.5 units/mL (50%-150%). Patients with less than 0.01 units/mL (1%) of either factor are classified as having severe hemophilia, those with between 0.01 and 0.05 units/mL (1%-5%) are moderate, and those with between 0.05 and 0.4 units/mL (5%-40%) have mild hemophilia.

Patients with severe disease experience frequent spontaneous hemorrhages, while those with moderate disease have excessive bleeding following mild trauma and rarely experience spontaneous hemarthroses. Patients with mild hemophilia may have few symptoms that their condition can be undetected for many years and they usually have excessive bleeding only after significant trauma or surgery. Disease severity does not always correlate with disease manifestations. Those with severe disease (<1% [0.01 units/mL] factor activity) may occasionally not display a severe phenotype, while some with milder forms of the disease may have more severe bleeding. Prolonged bleeding after circumcision is a common presenting sign. Most patients will have some manifestation of the disease sometime after their first year of life when they begin to walk and increase their risk of bleeding due to falling.[1]

The diagnosis of hemophilia should be considered in any male with unusual bleeding. A family history of bleeding is helpful in the diagnosis but is absent in up to 50% of patients with about one-third representing spontaneous mutations and the remaining secondary to unrecognized family history.[5] Brothers of patients with hemophilia should be screened; sisters should consider undergoing carrier testing. Laboratory testing in patients with hemophilia will usually reveal an isolated prolonged partial thromboplastin time and they will have a decreased factor VIII or factor IX level.

Patients with severe hemophilia A should be tested for the common factor VIII gene inversions. In patients with severe hemophilia A who lack an inversion mutation or in patients with moderate or mild hemophilia A, the gene can be sequenced to determine the exact mutation if needed. The exact mutation can determine carrier status but is not done routinely because it is very costly and does not change therapy. Techniques to determine the genetic mutation in patients with hemophilia B are similar, but no predominant mutation like the factor VIII inversion has been found. The smaller size of the factor IX gene facilitates direct DNA mutational analysis.[7]

Hemophilia can be diagnosed prenatally, if desired, by chorionic villus sampling in gestational weeks 9 to 14 or by amniocentesis after 15 to 17 weeks of gestation.[1,9] These are invasive procedures with a 0.5% to 1% chance for pregnancy loss so it is not routinely done.[9] A new noninvasive method uses cell-free fetal DNA in maternal circulation to determine the sex of the fetus; more invasive testing is required for a male fetus.[9] This method was used to successfully identify hemophilia mutations but is still experimental and requires further validation.[10]

Treatment: Hemophilia

2 The comprehensive care of hemophilia requires an interprofessional team approach. The patient is best managed in specialized centers with trained personnel and appropriate laboratory, radiologic, and pharmaceutical services.[1] The healthcare team should include hematologists, orthopedic surgeons, nurses, physical therapists, dentists, genetic counselors, psychologists, pharmacists, case managers, and social workers who have experience in caring for patients with bleeding disorders. The goal for comprehensive hemophilia care is to prevent bleeding episodes and their long-term sequelae so that patients with hemophilia can live full, active, and productive lives.

Patients with hemophilia should receive routine immunizations, including immunization against hepatitis B. Hepatitis A vaccine is also recommended for patients with hemophilia because of the risk (albeit small) of transmitting the causative agent through factor concentrates. The administration of vaccines is preferred subcutaneously in patients with severe disease.[1,11] If intramuscular administration is required, the use of a small-gauge needle with cold compresses and pressure to the site can prevent excessive bleeding.

A few special considerations apply to the perinatal care of male infants of hemophilia carriers. Intracranial or extracranial hemorrhage occurs in 1% to 2% of newborns with hemophilia.[7] Vacuum extraction and forceps delivery increase the risk of cranial bleeding. Elective cesarean section does not prevent intracranial bleeding. The optimal mode of delivery or the use of prophylactic factor replacement in male infants of hemophilia carriers is controversial.[1] Circumcision should be postponed until a diagnosis of hemophilia is excluded. Factor levels can be assayed from cord blood samples or

CLINICAL PRESENTATION Hemophilia

Signs and Symptoms

- Ecchymoses (palpable/raised)
- Hemarthroses (especially knee, ankle, and elbow)
- Joint pain
- Joint swelling and erythema
- Decreased range of motion
- Muscle hemorrhage
- Swelling at the site of muscle bleeding
- Pain with motion of affected muscle
- Signs of nerve compression
- Significant anemia from an iliopsoas or thigh bleed
- Oral bleeding with dental extractions or trauma
- Hematuria
- Intracranial hemorrhage (spontaneous or following trauma)
- Excessive bleeding with surgery

Laboratory Testing

- Prolonged aPTT
- Decreased factor VIII or factor IX level
- Normal prothrombin time
- Normal platelet count
- Normal von Willebrand factor antigen and activity
- Normal bleeding time

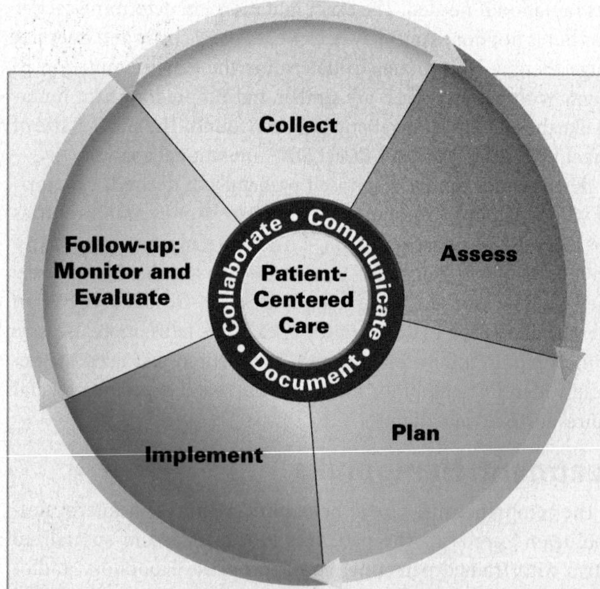

Patient Care Process for Coagulation Disorders

The image shows the five fundamental steps included in The Pharmacist's Care Process endorsed by the Joint Commission for Pharmacy Practitioners (2014). The tagline of this process reads collaborate, communicate, and document. The five fundamental steps listed here are collect, assess, plan, implement, and follow-up: monitor and evaluate. All these steps are listed in a circular block diagram.

Collect

- Patient characteristics (age, sex, etc.)
- Patient medical history (including family history and bleeding history)
- Social history (level of activity, extracurricular activities)
- Medication list, especially aspirin, nonsteroidal anti-inflammatory drugs [NSAIDs], other antiplatelet medications and anticoagulants
- Labs—clotting factors

Assess

- Presence of active bleeding (see "Clinical Manifestations and Diagnosis" section and Table 123-1)
- Presence of common clinical manifestations in bleeding disorders (easy bruising, bleeding after surgery, mucocutaneous bleeding, prolonged menses, etc., and Table 123-1).
- Factor level and the need for prophylactic management

Plan*

- Determine drug therapy regimen (dose, route, frequency, and duration) (see Table 123-3 and "Treatment: Hemophilia" section)
- Monitoring parameters (signs/symptoms of bleeding, frequency of bleeding episodes)
- Patient education/counseling (control of bleeding episodes, administration of drug therapy, when to seek medical attention)
- Continued care at a Hemophilia Treatment Center (or comparable clinic with a comprehensive care team)

Implement

- Provide education and reinforcement of the treatment plan
- Improve adherence through motivational interviewing and open discussions about patient care and the treatment plan
- Schedule regular clinic appointments to assess adherence, bleeding episodes, and to tailor patient therapy

Follow-up: Monitor and Evaluate

- Control and resolution of bleeding signs and symptoms
- Number of bleeding episodes (improvement since beginning care, need for adjustment in the treatment plan)
- Factor level activity (tailor factor doses to patient-specific levels)
- Adherence to the treatment plan (prophylactic and as-needed therapy, seeking medical attention)

Collaborate with patients, caregivers, and other healthcare professionals.

from peripheral venipuncture. Arterial puncture should be avoided because of the risk of hematoma formation. If an infant has hemophilia, many clinicians recommend a screening head ultrasound to rule out an intracranial hemorrhage prior to discharge from the nursery.[1,12]

Prophylaxis

The prevention of bleeding episodes and their resulting long-term complications is the mainstay of treatment for hemophilia. This can be accomplished through the regular administration of factor products or non-factor products to maintain hemostasis and prevent bleeding. It should begin early in life (before the age of 3 years old) to prevent musculoskeletal complications associated with joint or muscle bleeds. The goal of prophylaxis is to maintain a minimum factor activity or hemostasis level which would allow the patient to live a healthy and active life. Prophylaxis for patients with severe hemophilia is considered to be the standard of care recommended by the World Health Organization and the World Federation of Hemophilia (WFH).[1] Prophylaxis is sometimes required in patients with moderate hemophilia but is rarely used in patients with mild hemophilia.

Age at initiation of prophylaxis is a strong predictor of long-term clinical outcomes. Primary prophylaxis is started at a young age (usually before age 2 years), prior to the onset of joint bleeding.[13] Secondary prophylaxis begins after significant joint bleeding has already occurred.[13] In 2001, the Medical and Scientific Advisory Council of the National Hemophilia Foundation of the United States recommended primary prophylaxis beginning at age 1 to 2 years for children with severe hemophilia.

Prophylaxis with Factor Replacement Prophylactic factor replacement therapy is the regular intravenous administration of the deficient factor to maintain adequate activity levels to prevent

TABLE 123-2 Factor Concentrates

Plasma Derived	Recombinant	Extended Half-Life
• **Factor VIII** • Hemofil M • Koate DVI • Monoclate P • **Factor VIII + vWF** • Alphanate • Humate P • Wilate • **Factor IX** • AlphaNine • Mononine • **PCC** • Bebulin • Kcentra • Profilnine • **aPCC** • FEIBA	• **Factor VIII** • Advate • Afstyla • Helixate • Kogenate • Kovaltry • Obizur (PS) • Recombinate • Nuwiq • NovoEight (BDD) • Xyntha (BDD) • **Factor IX** • BeneFIX • Ixinity • Rixubis • **Factor VII** • NovoSeven • **vWF** • Vonvendi	• **Factor VIII** • Adynovate (PEG) • Jivi (PEG) • Eloctate (Fc-IgG) • **Factor IX** • Alprolix (Fc-IgG) • Idelvion (FP) • Rebinyn (PEG)

BDD, B-domain deleted; Fc-IgG, fusion protein IgG; FP, fusion protein–albumin; PCC, prothrombin complex concentrate; PEG, pegylated; PS, porcine sequenced; vWF, von Willebrand Factor.

bleeding. This effectively converts severe hemophilia into a milder form of the disease. The rationale for this approach is that patients with moderate hemophilia rarely experience spontaneous hemarthroses, and they have a much lower risk of chronic arthropathy. Many clinical trials proved the efficacy of a prophylactic approach in pediatric patients both in previously treated and untreated patients. The common finding is that prophylaxis prevented joint damage and decreased the frequency of joint and other hemorrhages.[13,14]

The dosing for prophylactic regimens varies considerably and no one regimen has been proven to be superior. Early on, patients with hemophilia A would be dosed on an every other day or three times a week regimen of standard half-life (SHL) factor VIII. For hemophilia B, the usual dosing of standard half-life factor IX would be twice weekly because of the intrinsically longer half-life.[1] The recent introduction of extended half-life factor products has made prophylaxis a more feasible approach (see Table 123-2). Patients with hemophilia A can now be dosed with an extended half-life product at 3- to 5-day intervals depending on their individual response.[14,15] Similarly, patients with hemophilia B can be dosed with an extended half-life product once weekly or every 10 to 14 days.[15] The extended half-life factor products allow for a much more ambitious dosing approach achieving higher activity levels in the mild and non-hemophilic range for substantial periods of time.[1]

Prophylactic factor replacement therapy comes with its own set of challenges. In addition to the paucity of standardized regimens, a significant challenge is the high cost of this approach. The cost to treat a patient with hemophilia A in the United States is about $300,000 per year.[16] Other issues to consider are the inconvenience to families and possible difficulties with adherence. Central venous lines may be necessary for frequent administration of factor concentrates, particularly in children younger than 2 years, who are at the age when primary prophylaxis is considered. Potential complications of central venous access include surgical risks, infection, and catheter-related deep-vein thrombosis.[1]

Prophylaxis with Nonfactor Products While prophylaxis with factor products has been the mainstay of hemophilia treatment, the landscape is changing with the development of new therapeutic approaches and products for hemostasis. Non-factor replacement products for prophylaxis differ from the factor products in that they obtain hemostasis through unique mechanisms. This is an area of growing research. The only commercially available product for this purpose is emicizumab for hemophilia A. Emicizumab is a recombinant, humanized, bispecific monoclonal antibody that bridges activated factor IX and factor X, performing the function of the missing activated factor VIII in maintaining hemostasis in patients with hemophilia A. Due to its unique structure, the risk of developing neutralizing antibodies to the drug is low and it is not affected by the patient's preexisting inhibitors (neutralizing antibodies) to factor VIII if present. Due to a prolonged half-life of 4 weeks, it can be administered in a single subcutaneous injection once weekly and in some cases every 2 to 4 weeks. The safety and efficacy of emicizumab has been demonstrated in children and adults with hemophilia A for prophylaxis therapy in the HAVEN 1-4 trials.[17,18]

In patients with inhibitors, emicizumab is much more effective than previously utilized prophylaxis modalities such as recombinant activated factor VII or activated prothrombin complex concentrates (aPCC). In non-inhibitor patients, emicizumab reduces the annual bleeding rate, or ABR even lower than some reported trials in patients receiving factor replacement prophylaxis. The subcutaneous administration of emicizumab is allowing prophylaxis to start even earlier in children 6 to 12 months of age without the need for indwelling central lines. It avoids the peaks and troughs associated with prophylactic factor replacement therapy and is much more convenient for patients and families potentially increasing adherence and thereby improved outcomes.[1]

With the success of emicizumab and the promise of future non-factor products on the way, the concepts and definitions of prophylaxis for hemophilia patients are shifting to be more inclusive of a wide variety of mechanisms of action and modalities of administration. The WFH is proposing a new definition based on outcomes rather than doses of products used or age of initiation. They propose the following as a modern definition of prophylaxis: the regular administration of a hemostatic agent/agents with the goal of preventing bleeding in people with hemophilia while allowing them to lead active lives and to achieve a quality of life comparable to a non-hemophilic individual.[1]

Hemophilia A

Therapy for hemophilia has undergone dramatic advances over the past few decades. Fifty years ago, the administration of fresh-frozen plasma was the only available treatment. The introduction of cryoprecipitate in the early 1960s allowed more specific therapy for hemophilia A.[19] Intermediate-purity factor VIII and IX plasma-derived concentrates became available in the 1970s.[19] Plasma-derived factor concentrates are made from the donations of thousands of people. Contamination of plasma pools with hepatitis B, hepatitis C, and the human immunodeficiency virus (HIV) during the late 1970s and early 1980s resulted in transmission to a large portion of patients with hemophilia. Since the mid-1980s, plasma-derived concentrates have been manufactured with a variety of virus-inactivating techniques, including dry heat, pasteurization, and treatment with chemicals (eg, solvent detergent mixtures).[5] Since 1986, no transmission of HIV through factor concentrates to patients with hemophilia in the United States has been reported.[5] Protein purification techniques, introduced in the 1990s, led to the production of high-purity plasma-derived concentrates with increased amounts of factor VIII or factor IX relative to the product's total protein content. Recombinant factor VIII and then factor IX also became available in the 1990s.[19] Significant improvements have been made with recombinant products in limiting the risk of infectious transmission from albumin used to stabilize some of the products. Like plasma-derived products, these products use viral inactivation steps. With each subsequent generation of recombinant factor VIII products, the use of human proteins has been reduced.[19]

Significant advancements have taken place in the development of long-acting factor VIII and IX products some of which are

Food and Drug Administration approved and commercially available. Methods for prolonging the half-life of these products include pegylation and Fc fusion.[20] Pegylation is thought to increase half-life by protecting the factor from receptor-mediated uptake and enzymatic catabolism. It reduces renal clearance and levels of neutralizing antibodies due to steric hindrance.[19] Protein fusion has also been a successful approach to prolonging the half-life of factor products. This method fuses factor VIII or IX to another human protein with a long circulatory half-life such as albumin or immunoglobulin G (IgG). These fused proteins then bind to the neonatal Fc receptor, or FcRn, present in the acidified endosomes of the endothelial cells. This binding protects the factor fusion product from targeted lysosomal degradation and facilitates recycling of the neonatal Fc receptor ligands at the endothelial surface resulting in a prolonged systemic half-life of the factor.[21,22]

Table 123-2 summarizes many of the factor VIII products available in the United States. Most patients are treated with high-purity products, which generally have the lowest risk of transmitting infectious disease and are therefore recommended as first-line agents.[1] Recombinant products, when available, are generally used rather than plasma-derived products.

Recombinant Factor VIII 3 Recombinant factor VIII is produced with recombinant DNA technology and is derived from cultured Chinese hamster ovary cells or baby hamster kidney cells transfected with the human factor VIII gene.[5] Since these products are not derived from blood donations, the risk of transmitting infections through administration of recombinant factor VIII is low and recombinant products are generally favored over plasma-derived products. A small risk of viral infection of the cell lines used to produce the clotting factor still remains. Furthermore, human or animal proteins are used in the production process of some recombinant products.[19] Therefore, these products have a theoretical risk of transmitting infection, although hepatitis and HIV infection have never been reported with their use.[5] First-generation recombinant factor VIII products contain human albumin as a stabilizing protein.[5] Second-generation recombinant factor VIII products add sugar instead of human albumin as a stabilizer, but human albumin is used in the culture process. Several products are manufactured specifically with the B domain of the factor VIII gene deleted, yielding a smaller protein product.[5,23] This B domain does not appear to be necessary for coagulation function and may serve as a binding site for neutralizing antibodies. Third-generation recombinant factor VIII products do not contain human protein either in the culture or in the stabilization processes.[19]

Plasma-Derived Factor VIII Products The recombinant factor VIII products are comparable in effectiveness to plasma-derived products.[5] Several different plasma-derived factor VIII products are available (Table 123-2). These products are derived from the pooled plasma of thousands of donors and therefore have the potential to transmit infection. Donor screening, testing of plasma pools for evidence of infection, viral reduction through purification steps, and viral inactivation procedures (eg, dry heat, pasteurization, and solvent detergent treatment) have resulted in a safer product. No cases of HIV transmission from factor concentrates have been reported since 1986.[5] However, isolated cases of hepatitis C infection with the use of plasma-derived products have been reported.[5] Additionally, outbreaks of hepatitis A viral infections associated with plasma-derived products have been reported, likely because solvent detergent treatment does not inactivate this nonenveloped virus. Finally, possible infection with unidentified viruses not inactivated by the currently used methods remains a concern. In addition, Prion disease may be present in plasma-derived factor products.[24]

Factor VIII concentrates can be classified according to their level of purity, which refers to the specific activity of factor VIII in the product. Cryoprecipitate is a low-purity product that also contains vWF, fibrinogen, and factor XIII. The American Association of Blood Banks standards call for a minimum of 80 international units of factor VIII per cryoprecipitate pack.[5] This product is no longer considered a primary treatment of factor VIII deficiency in countries where factor VIII concentrates are available because cryoprecipitate does not undergo a viral inactivation process. Intermediate-purity products have a specific factor VIII activity of 5 units/mg of protein and high-purity products have up to 2,000 units/mg of protein.[5] Ultrahigh-purity plasma-derived products are prepared with monoclonal antibody purification steps and have a specific activity of 3,000 units/mg of protein prior to addition of albumin as a stabilizer.

Factor VIII: Dosing Appropriate dosing of factor VIII concentrate depends on the half-life of the infused factor, the patient's body weight, and the location and severity of the bleed. The presence or absence of an inhibitory antibody to factor VIII and the titer of this antibody also influence treatment. Recovery studies, which measure the immediate postinfusion factor level, and survival studies, which assess the half-life of the factor, can establish patient-specific pharmacokinetics. The location and magnitude of the bleeding episode determine the percent correction to target as well as the duration of treatment. Serious or life-threatening bleeding requires peak factor levels of greater than 0.75 to 1 units/mL (75%-100%); less severe bleeding may be treated with a goal of 0.3 to 0.5 units/mL (30%-50%) peak plasma levels. Table 123-3 provides general guidelines for the management of bleeding in different locations.

Factor VIII is a large molecule that remains in the intravascular space. Therefore, the plasma volume (about 50 mL/kg) can be used to estimate the volume of distribution. In general, each unit of factor VIII concentrate infused per kilogram of actual body weight results in a 2% rise in plasma factor VIII levels.[1] The following equation can be used to calculate an initial dose of factor VIII:

$$\text{Factor VIII (units)} = (\text{Desired level} - \text{Baseline level}) \times 0.5 \times (\text{Weight [in kilograms]})$$

The baseline level usually is omitted from the equation when it is negligible compared to the desired level. The half-life of factor VIII ranges from 8 to 15 hours. It is generally necessary to administer 50% of the initial dose about every 12 hours to sustain the desired level of factor VIII. A single treatment may be adequate for minor bleeding, such as oral bleeding or slight muscle hemorrhages. However, because of the potential for long-term joint damage with hemarthroses, 2 or 3 days of treatment is often recommended for these bleeds. Serious bleeding episodes may require maintenance of 70% to 100% (0.7-1.0 units/mL) factor activity for 1 week or longer. As previously mentioned, factor VIII dosing depends on several variables, and each case must be considered individually. Individualized pharmacokinetics may help guide treatment, particularly for serious bleeding episodes.

Alternatively, factor VIII can be administered as a continuous infusion when prolonged treatment is required (eg, in the perioperative period or for serious bleeding episodes). Infusion rates ranging from 2 to 4 units/kg/hr usually are given in fixed-dose continuous infusion protocols, with the aim of maintaining a steady-state level of 60% to 100% (0.6-1.0 units/mL).[25] Administration of factor concentrate via continuous infusion may reduce factor requirements by 20% to 50% because unnecessarily high peaks of factor VIII that occur with bolus injections are avoided. A gradual decrease in factor VIII clearance during the first 5 to 6 days of treatment contributes to the lower factor concentrate requirements. Daily monitoring of factor level can help determine the appropriate rate of infusion.

Administration of factor VIII concentrate via continuous infusion is safe and effective, and it may be more convenient than bolus therapy for hospitalized patients.[26] Concerns about the stability of the formulations appear to be unwarranted, as most high-purity factor VIII concentrates remain stable for at least 7 days

TABLE 123-3 Guidelines for Factor Replacement Therapy for Hemorrhage in Hemophilia A and B

Site of Hemorrhage	Desired Hemostatic Factor Level (% of Normal)	Comments
Joint	50%-70%, 2-3 days	Rest/immobilization/physical therapy rehabilitation following bleed; several doses may be necessary to prevent or treat target joint
Muscle	30%-50% for most sites 70%-100% for thigh, iliopsoas, or nerve compression	Risk of significant blood loss with a thigh or iliopsoas bleed; bed rest for iliopsoas or thigh bleeding
Oral mucosa	30%-50%	May try antifibrinolytic or topical thrombin prior to factor replacement for minor bleeding; higher factor levels are needed for tongue swelling or risk of airway compromise; antifibrinolytic therapy should be used following factor replacement
Gastrointestinal	Initially 100%, then 40%-60%	Endoscopy is highly recommended; antifibrinolytic therapy may be useful; continue until healing occurs
Hematuria	30%-50% if no trauma 70%-100% if traumatic	If no pain or trauma, consider bed rest and fluids for 24 hours; factor should be given if hematuria persists; evaluate if hematuria persists; if trauma to abdomen or back, perform imaging and give aggressive factor replacement
Central nervous system	Initially 100%, then 50%-100% for 10-21 days	Lumbar puncture requires prophylactic factor coverage
Trauma or surgery	Initially 100%, then 50%-100% until wound healing complete	The perioperative and postoperative management plan must be in place preoperatively; evaluation for inhibitors is crucial prior to elective surgery

after reconstitution.[26] However, exposure of factor VIII to light for 10 hours after reconstitution can decrease activity by 30% (0.3 units/mL).[26] Therefore, it would be prudent to shield the container with foil wrap or an appropriate bag.

Other Pharmacological Therapy Treatment with desmopressin acetate often is adequate for minor bleeding episodes in patients with mild hemophilia A. A synthetic analog of the antidiuretic hormone vasopressin, desmopressin causes the release of vWF and factor VIII from endogenous endothelial storage sites. It is most effective in patients with higher baseline factor VIII levels (0.1-0.15 units/mL [10%-15%]).[25] The recommended dose of desmopressin is 0.3 mcg/kg diluted in 50 mL of normal saline and infused IV over 15 to 30 minutes.[25] Patients with mild or moderate hemophilia A should undergo a desmopressin trial to determine their response to this medication. At least a twofold rise in factor VIII to a minimal level of 0.3 units/mL (30%) within 60 minutes is considered an adequate response.[1,25] Infusion of desmopressin can be repeated daily for up to 2 to 3 days. Tachyphylaxis, an attenuated response with repeated dosing, may develop after that time due to the depletion of factor stores. The factor increase after the second dose of desmopressin is about 30% lower than after the initial dose.[27] Factor concentrate therapy may be necessary if the patient requires additional treatment. Factor levels should be monitored to ensure that an adequate response has been achieved. Treatment with desmopressin will not result in hemostasis in patients who have severe hemophilia and those who are only marginally responsive. Desmopressin should not be used as primary therapy for life-threatening bleeding episodes such as intracranial hemorrhage or for major surgical procedures.[1]

Desmopressin can be administered intranasally via a concentrated nasal spray.[25] It elicits a slower and less marked response, with a peak effect in 60 to 90 minutes after administration, which is somewhat longer than with IV administration.[25,27] The dosage is one spray (150 mcg) in one nostril for patients who weigh less than 50 kg and two sprays (one in each nostril, 300 mcg total) for those who weigh more than 50 kg.[25] The nasal spray may serve as an alternative to the IV formulation, especially in patients with mild bleeding episodes. Few adverse drug reactions are associated with desmopressin. The most commonly observed adverse drug reaction is facial flushing.[27] Less frequently reported adverse drug reactions include mild headaches, increased heart rate, and decreased blood pressure. Desmopressin can cause water retention because of its antidiuretic effects, which may lead to severe hyponatremia. This may be a particular problem in children younger than 2 years and, therefore, should be used with caution in this age group.[25] Fluid restriction for 24 hours after the desmopressin dose and monitoring of urine output are recommended with desmopressin administration.[25]

Antifibrinolytic therapy inhibits clot lysis and therefore is a useful adjunctive therapy for the treatment of hemophilia, primarily with mucocutaneous bleeding. Antifibrinolytic agents are particularly beneficial for the treatment of oral bleeding because of a high concentration of fibrinolytic enzymes in saliva. Antifibrinolytic therapy can also be helpful as adjuvant therapy in GI bleeding, epistaxis, and menorrhagia. Antifibrinolytic therapy should be used with caution in patients with urinary bleeding, due to the risk of obstruction and subsequent renal toxicity. The two available antifibrinolytics include aminocaproic acid and tranexamic acid. Aminocaproic acid is given at a dosage of 100 mg/kg (maximum 6 g) every 6 hours and can be administered orally or IV.[5] The dosage of tranexamic acid is 25 mg/kg (maximum 1.5 g) orally every 6 to 8 hours.[5]

Hemophilia B

Therapeutic options for hemophilia B have improved greatly over the past several years, first with the development of monoclonal antibody-purified plasma-derived products and then with the licensure of recombinant factor IX. Products available in the United States for treatment of hemophilia B are listed in Table 123-2.

Recombinant Factor IX Recombinant factor IX was not available until 1998, which is 6 years after the first recombinant factor VIII product.[19] The first commercially available recombinant factor IX is produced in Chinese hamster ovary cells transfected with the factor IX gene. Since blood and plasma products are not used to produce recombinant factor IX or to stabilize the final product, recombinant factor IX has an excellent viral safety profile.[5] Clinical trials have proved the safety and efficacy of the product in the treatment of acute bleeding episodes and in the management of bleeding associated with surgical procedures.[5] Although the half-life of recombinant factor IX is similar to that of the plasma-derived products, recovery is about 30% lower.[25] As a result, doses of recombinant factor IX concentrate must be higher than those of plasma-derived products to achieve equivalent plasma levels. Because individual pharmacokinetics may vary, recovery and survival studies should be performed to determine optimal treatment.[5] Recombinant factor IX is considered the treatment of choice for hemophilia B.[1]

Plasma-Derived Factor IX Products High-purity factor IX plasma concentrates have been available in the United States since the early 1990s.[5,19] These products are derived from plasma through biochemical purification and monoclonal immunoaffinity techniques. Other viral inactivation measures, such as solvent detergent or chemical treatment, are also used. High-purity factor IX concentrates have excellent efficacy in the treatment of bleeding episodes and in the control of bleeding associated with surgical procedures.[25] Their viral safety profile has been reported to be excellent and the risk of thromboembolic complications is low.

Before the high-purity products were approved for use, hemophilia B patients were treated with factor IX concentrates that also contained other vitamin K–dependent proteins (factors II, VII, and X), known as prothrombin complex concentrates (PCCs). These products contain small amounts of activated factors generated during processing, and their use has been associated with thrombotic complications, including deep-vein thrombosis, pulmonary embolism, myocardial infarction, and disseminated intravascular coagulation.[5,25] The risk of these complications is highest in patients receiving high or repeated doses of PCCs, in those with hepatic disease (the liver produces antithrombotic factors and removes the activated factors from circulation), in neonates, and in patients who have experienced crush injuries or who are undergoing major surgery.[5] Concomitant use of PCCs and antifibrinolytics should be avoided because of the risk for thrombosis. Because of the lower purity of PCCs and their thrombogenic potential, these products are not first-line treatment for hemophilia B.

Factor IX: Dosing Factor IX is a relatively small protein. Unlike factor VIII, it is not limited to the intravascular space; it also passes into the extravascular compartment.[5] Therefore, it has a volume of distribution that is about twice that of factor VIII. For plasma-derived factor IX concentrates, each unit of factor IX infused per kilogram of actual body weight results in about a 1% (0.01 units/mL) rise in the plasma level of factor IX (range, 0.67%-1.28% [0.0067-0.0128 units/mL]).[5] The following equation can be used to calculate the initial dose:

$$\text{Plasma} - \text{derived factor IX (units)} = (\text{Desired level} - \text{Baseline level}) \times (\text{Weight [in kilograms]})$$

As with the factor VIII dose calculation, the baseline level term can be omitted from the formula if it is negligible compared to the desired level. Because recovery of recombinant factor IX is lower than that of the plasma-derived products, the following adjustment is made:

Pediatric dosing:

$$\text{Recombinant factor IX (units)} = (\text{Desired level} - \text{Baseline level}) \times 1.4 \times (\text{Weight [in kilograms]})$$

Adult dosing:

$$\text{Recombinant factor IX (units)} = (\text{Desired level} - \text{Baseline level}) \times 1.2 \times (\text{Weight [in kilograms]})$$

A recovery study to determine optimal dosing is recommended for patients who receive recombinant factor IX because of the wide interpatient variability in pharmacokinetics. Because the half-life of factor IX is about 24 hours, dosing can be less frequent than with factor VIII. Table 123-3 provides general guidelines for dosing factor IX based on the site and severity of the bleeding episode.[25]

Treatment of Inhibitors

4 Neutralizing antibodies to factors VIII and IX, known as *inhibitors*, develop in a subset of patients with hemophilia. The development of an inhibitor is the most serious complication of factor replacement therapy and is associated with considerable morbidity and a decreased quality of life. The incidence of new factor VIII inhibitors in patients with severe factor VIII deficiency is about 30%.[28] Inhibitors are less common in patients with mild or moderate hemophilia occurring in about 5% to 10% of patients.[1] The risk of developing inhibitors in patients with hemophilia B is much lower, occurring in only 3% of patients.[5]

An inhibitor is a polyclonal high-affinity IgG directed against the factor VIII or IX protein. Inhibitors interfere with infused factor concentrate, rendering them ineffective. The presence of an inhibitor is suspected when a decreased clinical response to factor replacement is observed or it may be discovered incidentally on routine laboratory screening. Inhibitors are measured with the Bethesda assay, and titers are reported in Bethesda units (BUs). One BU is the amount of inhibitor needed to inactivate half of the factor VIII or factor IX in a mixture of inhibitor-containing plasma and pooled normal plasma.[5] Patients with inhibitors to factor VIII or factor IX are divided into two groups: low responders, who have low levels of inhibitors (5 BU/mL), and high responders who have higher inhibitor levels (>5 BU/mL) and develop an increase in antibody titer after exposure (anamnestic response).[5,29]

Most inhibitors develop in childhood, after relatively few exposure days (median 9-12 days).[30] Patients with severe hemophilia are much more likely to develop inhibitors than those with milder forms of the disease.[29] It is possible that the low levels of factor produced in patients with mild or moderate hemophilia induce immune tolerance in these individuals. In contrast, factor levels are undetectable in patients with severe hemophilia, so infused factor VIII is regarded as a foreign protein, which may provoke an antibody response. The rate of inhibitor formation varies even among patients with identical mutations, which suggests that host factors modify the risk. The development of an inhibitor is the result of a complex interaction between a patient's immune system and genetic and environmental risk factors.

The type of factor product administered to patients may influence the risk of developing inhibitors. An international, multicenter, randomized, open-label clinical trial named Survey of Inhibitors in Plasma-Product Exposed Toddlers, or SIPPET, was designed to evaluate the incidence of inhibitor development in previously untreated or minimally treated patients with hemophilia A exposed to plasma-derived factor products compared to recombinant products.[31] The results of this pivotal trial showed that patients receiving recombinant factor VIII products had a significantly higher incidence of developing inhibitors compared to those receiving plasma-derived products.

Therapy for patients with inhibitors involves the treatment of acute bleeding episodes and treatment directed at eradicating the inhibitor. The inhibitor titer, the site and magnitude of bleeding, and the patient's past response to bypassing therapy determine the approach to the treatment of acute bleeding. For patients with a low inhibitor titer, the administration of high doses of the specific factor often can control bleeding episodes. Two to three times the usual replacement dose and more frequent dosing intervals are often necessary to overcome the antibody. Factor-level monitoring and clinical assessments help to evaluate the adequacy of treatment. Additional supportive measures, such as immobilization and administration of antifibrinolytic agents, should be used, where appropriate.[1]

Treatment of acute bleeds in patients with high-titer inhibitors can be complicated and require the use of alternative agents. In the presence of a high-titer inhibitor, it is impossible to administer enough factor VIII or factor IX to neutralize the antibody and achieve a hemostatic plasma level. Therefore, the treatment of bleeding episodes consists of agents that bypass the factor to which the antibody is directed. These bypassing agents include PCCs, aPCCs, and recombinant factor VIIa. PCCs contain the vitamin

K–dependent factors II, VII, IX, and X. Small quantities of activated factors are present in these products. Activated PCCs contain greater quantities of the activated factors, primarily factor X and prothrombin. The only available aPCC product in the United States is FEIBA® (Factor Eight Inhibitor Bypassing Agent). The recommended dosage is 50 to 100 units/kg administered every 8 to 12 hours, depending on the severity of the bleeding episode and the maximum dose should not exceed 200 units/kg/day.[15] Activated PCCs appear to be more effective than PCCs and are preferred in patients with inhibitors. As previously mentioned, serious thrombotic complications, including pulmonary emboli, deep-vein thrombosis, and myocardial infarction, have been associated with the use of PCCs and aPCCs.[15] Other minor adverse drug reactions include dizziness, nausea, hives, flushing, and headaches. Patients with factor IX inhibitors occasionally develop severe allergic reactions in response to infusion of factor IX-containing products, so these patients should be monitored closely.[29]

5 Recombinant factor VIIa is effective for the treatment of acute bleeds in patients with hemophilia A or B who have developed inhibitors. Recombinant factor VIIa is a bypassing agent that is thought to be hemostatically active only at the site of tissue injury where the tissue factor is present. Recombinant factor VIIa is not a plasma-derived product, so both viral transmission and anamnestic responses to factor VIII or factor IX are unlikely. The initial recommended dose for bleeding episodes is 90 mcg/kg.[15] However, depending on a patient's response, higher doses up to 300 mcg/kg can be used. A drawback is the product's short half-life, which necessitates initial dosing every 2 hours. Continuous infusion of recombinant factor VIIa, which may be more convenient and cost-effective, has been reported.[32] Patients treated with bypassing agents must be monitored clinically because no laboratory test directly measures the effectiveness of treatment.

Both recombinant factor VIIa and aPCCs are effective in the treatment of bleeding for patients with inhibitors. In determining which bypassing product to use in an individual patient, the clinician must consider multiple factors. In a patient with a newly diagnosed inhibitor, it is prudent to use recombinant factor VIIa because aPCCs contain a small amount of factor VIII or IX and increase the inhibitor titer. It is also important to consider an individual's response to specific bypassing agents because of the significant variability in response between individuals. In some patients, bleeding can be unresponsive to monotherapy and may require alternating products.[33] Due to the risk of developing thrombosis or disseminated intravascular coagulation from alternating bypassing agents, this therapy should be used with caution and only in an inpatient setting.[15]

In the past, plasma-derived porcine factor VIII was an alternative therapeutic option for patients who have hemophilia A and inhibitors. It was removed from the market secondary to contamination with porcine parvovirus. The rationale for its use is that porcine factor VIII is enough like human factor VIII to participate in the coagulation cascade, yet most factor VIII inhibitors have absent or only weak neutralizing activity against nonhuman factor VIII making this an effective agent to treat an acute bleed. Unfortunately, cross-reactivity with porcine factor VIII does occur, and a high titer of antibody against porcine factor VIII can develop and hypersensitivity to porcine proteins can occur. A recombinant porcine factor VIII has been approved, but only for the treatment of acute bleeds in patients with acquired hemophilia A.[15,34]

The hemostatic therapies for patients with an inhibitor have limited effectiveness leading to significant morbidity and a decreased quality of life. The ideal therapy for patients with an inhibitor is total eradication so that optimal hemostatic treatment with either factor VIII or IX is possible. At this time, the only proven method for inhibitor eradication is immune tolerance induction (ITI), which involves the regular infusion of factor VIII to induce antigen-specific tolerance. This approach is not recommended for patients with hemophilia B who have developed inhibitors due to the risk of hypersensitivity reactions and anaphylaxis associated with factor IX administration in this group.

Multiple immune tolerance registries were established to help determine patient- and treatment-related factors associated with immune tolerance outcome.[35] Across these registries, a patient's peak historical factor VIII inhibitor titer (<200 BU) and the inhibitor titer at the time of ITI induction (<10 BU) were associated with successful immune tolerance. The overall ITI success rate from these registries ranges from 51% to 79%; the variability is likely related to a lack of standardization in study methodologies, treatment protocols, and eradication definitions.[35,36]

The relationship between factor VIII dose and ITI success rate is not clear. A variety of different dosing regimens, ranging from 25 units/kg every other day to more than 200 units/kg every day, have been used. The International Immune Tolerance Registry demonstrated improved ITI success with high doses (200 IU/kg), while the North American and Spanish Immune Tolerance Registries showed improved success with lower dosing strategies.[36] The International Immune Tolerance Study is a multicenter randomized clinical trial that compared high-dose (200 units/kg/day) to low-dose (50 units/kg three times/week) regimens in patients with severe hemophilia A and high titer inhibitors (>5 BU).[35] This study was stopped early due to an increased risk of bleeding events in the low-dose arm. At the stopping point, the proportion of ITI success was not significantly different between the two arms, but the time to achieve ITI success was shorter in the high-dose arm. Because the study was stopped early, it lacked statistical power to demonstrate therapeutic equivalence below the 30% boundary of equivalence. A high-dose strategy achieves tolerance at a faster rate, which explains the lower bleeding rate.

Some studies report better success rates for ITI in patients receiving plasma-derived factor products containing vWF, which may be related to the role of vWF in factor VIII function, stabilization, and immunogenicity.[37] vWF binding to the C2 domain of factor VIII, a common site for inhibitor formation, may result in epitope masking and decreased inhibitor activity. The use of vWF-containing products may also extend the plasma half-life of factor VIII during ITI; thus, increasing antigen presentation and possibly contributing to its overall success.[37]

Although not commonly used in ITI protocols, immune modulation can improve tolerance success. Agents such as cyclophosphamide and intravenous immune globulin have been used to reduce inhibitor titers and make ITI more successful.[1] Another immune modulating agent, rituximab, an anti-CD20 monoclonal antibody that inhibits B-cells and interferes with IgG production, has been used with some success. In a phase II trial of rituximab in patients with high titer inhibitors, only 3 out of 16 subjects (18.8%) had a major response (decline in the inhibitor to <5 BU without an increase in the inhibitor titer after rechallenge to factor VIII).[38] When used as a single agent in previously treated patients with inhibitors, rituximab had a modest effect, but further studies are needed to determine the activity of rituximab combined with ITI. Figure 123-1 summarizes the therapeutic options in the management of acute bleeding in patients with hemophilia A and inhibitors.

Gene Therapy

Hemophilia is an excellent candidate for gene therapy because tight control of gene expression is not required. Even low levels of factor expression can reduce bleeding episodes in patients with severe hemophilia, which is similar to the rationale for prophylactic factor replacement. The goal of gene therapy is to achieve a sustainable factor activity level of over 5% (0.05 units/mL), which is sufficient to convert patients with severe disease to a much milder phenotype.[39,40] If a treatment strategy could produce consistent factor activity levels

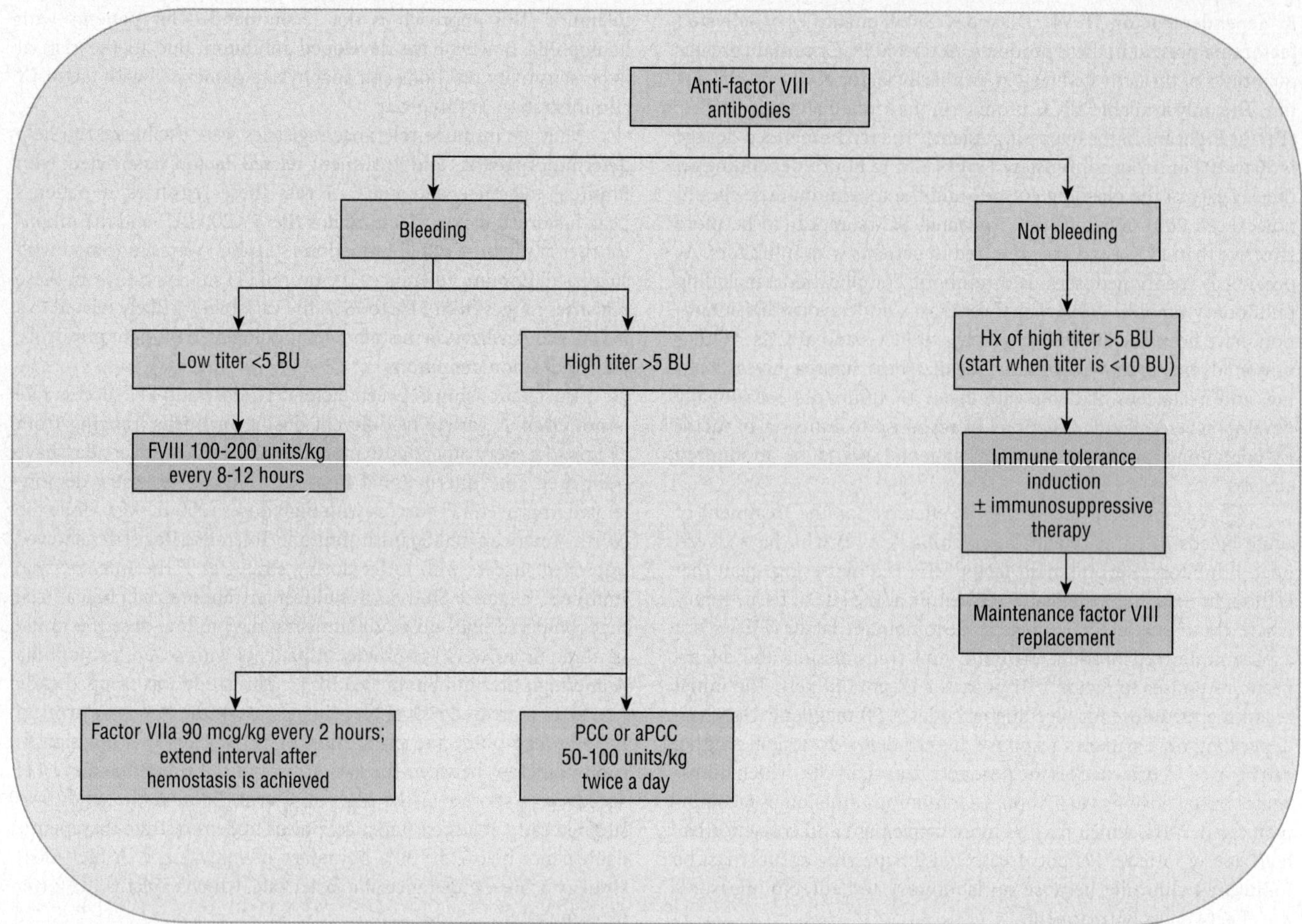

FIGURE 123-1 Treatment algorithm for the management of patients with hemophilia A and factor VIII antibodies. (aPCC, activated prothrombin complex concentrate; BU, Bethesda unit; PCC, prothrombin complex concentrate.)

of around 50% (0.5 units/mL), it would be considered curative.[40] Potential benefits to gene therapy include patient convenience, viral safety, and decreased cost. Possible drawbacks to gene therapy include a risk of inhibitor formation, tumorigenesis related to possible integration of the viral vector, possible germline transmission of the viral vector, and concerns about long-term gene expression.

Gene therapy for the treatment of hemophilia remains in the early clinical stages. Advances are most apparent in hemophilia B, which has been attributed to the smaller size (about 1.4 kb) of its complementary DNA (cDNA).[40] A landmark clinical trial reported the results of a single peripheral venous infusion of an adenovirus associated factor IX transgene vector under the control of a liver-restricted promoter in six patients with severe hemophilia B.[41] All of the study subjects showed long-term (over 2 years) expression of the factor IX transgene with therapeutic levels of factor IX (plateau factor IX levels from 1% to 6% [0.01-0.06 units/mL]).[41]

Gene therapy for factor VIII deficiency has been challenging due to the considerably larger size of its cDNA (about 9 kb).[40] The development of B-domain deleted factor VIII has been beneficial in allowing a smaller amount of cDNA to be able to be packaged into a single vector. A multi-year follow-up of the original clinical trial of Adeno-associated virus (AAV) serotype 5 human factor VIII (hFVIII) SQ (valoctocogene roxaparvovec) was published reporting safety and efficacy data for up to 3 years in the original 15 patients enrolled in this dose escalating study. Patients were enrolled into four escalating dose cohorts. All patients experienced at least one adverse drug reaction; however, all of these were considered mild and transient. No participants dropped out of the study. After 3 years of follow-up one patient had factor VIII levels in the non-hemophilic range, 11 patients had levels in the mild hemophilic range, one patient in the moderate hemophilic range, and two patients (dose level one and dose level two) still have factor VIII levels in the severe hemophilic range. So far this 3-year follow-up does show that the decline in factor levels over time does decrease. No cellular immune response was consistently detected against factor VIII or the AAV serotype 5 capsid in any patient. No factor VIII inhibitors or other antibodies directed to components of factor VIII have been detected in any of the patients.[40]

Other areas of gene therapy are being explored for the treatment of hemophilia. Platelets derived from hematopoietic stem cells may be able to deliver factor VIII or IX directly into the circulation. Lentiviral vectors are being explored for gene therapy due to their much larger packaging capacities compared to the adeno-associated viral vector AAV. The area of gene editing is also being explored for patients with hemophilia using zinc finger nucleases or clustered regularly interspaced short palindromic repeats (CRISPR) approaches.[41]

Pain Management

Pain, both acute and chronic, can be a common occurrence in patients with hemophilia. The most likely cause of acute pain is bleeding, and treatment should include factor replacement to stop the bleeding, and PRICE (Protect, Rest, Ice, Compression, and Elevation).[1,42] Acetaminophen can be used for mild pain, although narcotic analgesia may be required for more severe pain. NSAIDs impair platelet function and may complicate bleeding. For this reason, nonspecific NSAIDs are not routinely recommended during acute bleeding episodes. Cyclooxygenase-2 inhibitors have less antiplatelet activity and are an option for acute and chronic pain management.[1,42]

Chronic pain in patients with hemophilia is typically secondary to hemophilic arthropathy. Hemophilic arthropathy is the direct result of recurrent hemarthrosis. Persistent blood in the joint leads to inflammation, synovial hypertrophy and inflammation, cartilage destruction, and finally bony erosion. Cyclooxygenase-2 inhibitors can also help manage chronic pain. Surgical interventions may help to alleviate chronic pain. Synovectomy (removal of the hypertrophied synovium) can reduce chronic pain from recurrent bleeding. Patients with more advanced joint disease could benefit from joint replacement.

Surgery

In patients with severe hemophilia, the dose of replacement factor required in the perioperative period will depend on the surgery, the inhibitor status, and the patient's previous response to factor products. Ideally, the patient's factor activity level should be maintained in the range of 50% to 100% (0.5-1.0 units/mL) depending on clinical status and type of procedure. Intermittent dosing or continuous infusion factor replacement may accomplish this goal.[1,32,43] Before surgery, factor concentrate is usually infused to obtain a plasma level of 1 unit/mL (100%). Replacement therapy is continued to maintain plasma levels greater than 0.5 units/mL (50%) for 5 to 7 days or longer, depending on the type of surgery and the patient's clinical response. Preoperative evaluation for elective procedures should include measurement of an inhibitor titer no longer than 2 weeks prior to procedure and assessment of the recovery and half-life of infused factor in the patient.[1] For those patients with inhibitors undergoing surgical procedures, there is evidence to support the use of both activated factor VII and aPCCs.[1,32]

Evaluation of Therapeutic Outcomes

The main goal in the treatment of hemophilia is to control and prevent bleeding episodes and their long-term sequelae such as chronic arthropathies. Pharmacologic and nonpharmacologic interventions should be aimed at achieving this goal. Treatment response can be monitored through clinical parameters such as cessation of bleeding and resolution of symptoms. Monitoring plasma factor levels also may be helpful, particularly for severe bleeding episodes. Home therapy for administration of factor concentrates is common among patients with hemophilia because this approach can lead to earlier treatment and more independence for the patient. Diaries in which the patient documents symptoms, the dose of factor replacement, adjuvant therapies used, and treatment response can help the caregiver to evaluate the success of home therapy. Monitoring the number and type of bleeding episodes and trough plasma factor levels can evaluate the adequacy of prophylactic regimens. Pharmacokinetically driven dosing for prophylactic factor could optimize therapy, reduce bleeding, and decrease overall factor consumption for the patient.[44] Physical examination with evaluation of joint range of motion and radiographic imaging of target joints can evaluate the long-term success of preventing and treating arthropathies.[44]

Clinicians should check for the development of inhibitors, especially in patients with severe disease and exposure to factor concentrates, at least yearly and with any suspicion of poor treatment response. The development of inhibitors challenges the management and control of bleeding episodes. A full understanding of the clinical situation and the titer of the inhibitor are mandatory to address all treatment options for each patient. Because no laboratory test measures the effectiveness of bypassing therapy in patients with inhibitors, close clinical monitoring for worsening or resolution of symptoms is essential for optimizing the outcome.[1]

VON WILLEBRAND DISEASE

von Willebrand disease (vWD) is the most common congenital bleeding disorder in the United States and in the world, with a prevalence of 0.1% to 1%.[45] vWD refers to a family of disorders caused by a quantitative and/or qualitative defect of vWF, a glycoprotein that plays a role in both platelet aggregation and coagulation (Table 123-4). vWF mediates platelet adhesion to injured blood vessel sites and promotes platelet aggregation. It binds factor VIII and protects it from degradation by plasma proteases, thus prolonging its half-life. Unlike hemophilia, vWD has an autosomal inheritance pattern, resulting in an equal frequency of disease in males and females. Diagnosis of vWD may be more prevalent in females due to female-specific hemostatic challenges, such as child birth and menstruation.

Transcription and translation produce a large primary product that subsequently undergoes complex modifications, resulting in vWF multimers of various sizes. vWF is synthesized in endothelial cells, where it is either stored in Weibel–Palade bodies or secreted constitutively. It is also synthesized in megakaryocytes and stored in α-granules, from which it is released following platelet activation.[46,47]

vWF is important for both primary and secondary hemostasis. In response to vascular injury, it promotes platelet adhesion by interacting with the glycoprotein Ib receptor on platelets.[47] It can facilitate platelet aggregation by binding to the platelet glycoprotein IIb/IIIa receptor, although fibrinogen is the main ligand for this receptor.[48] The highest-molecular-weight vWF multimers are the most important in platelet adhesion because their large surface area contains numerous binding sites for various ligands and receptors. vWF is also the carrier molecule for circulating factor VIII, protecting it from premature degradation and removal.[46,47] A deficiency of vWF reduces the half-life of factor VIII and decreases plasma factor VIII levels. Therefore, vWF plays a dual role in hemostasis, affecting both platelet function and coagulation.

Classification of von Willebrand Disease

vWD consists of a heterogeneous group of disorders that can be classified into three major subtypes. The National Institutes of Health has developed a classification scheme that characterizes vWD according to both the quantity of the von Willebrand clotting factors and their functionality (Fig. 123-2). Types 1 and 3 are associated with quantitative defects in vWF; type 2 mutations refer to functional abnormalities in vWF (qualitative defects).[45,47,48] It is important to determine disease subtype because it influences treatment.

TABLE 123-4 von Willebrand Disease—Blood Tests

von Willebrand factor (vWF)
Large multimeric glycoprotein that is necessary for normal platelet adhesion, normal bleeding time, and stabilization of factor VIII
von Willebrand factor antigen (vWF:Ag)
Antigenic determinant(s) on vWF measured by immunoassays; usually low in types 1 and 2; virtually absent in type 3
Ristocetin cofactor activity (RCo)
Functional assay of vWF activity based on platelet aggregation with ristocetin. Reduced by the same degree as vWF:Ag in types 1 and 3, but to a greater extent in type 2 disease (except 2B)
Glycoprotein Ib with gain-of-function mutation (vWF:GPIbM)
Functional assay of vWF binding to a fragment of recombinant glycoprotein Ib; usually low in types 1 and 2; virtually absent in type 3
Glycoprotein Ib with ristocetin-dependent binding (vWF:GPIbR)
Functional assay utilizing ristocetin, recombinant glycoprotein Ib fragments, and microparticles, rather than whole platelets; usually low in types 1 and 2; virtually absent in type 3

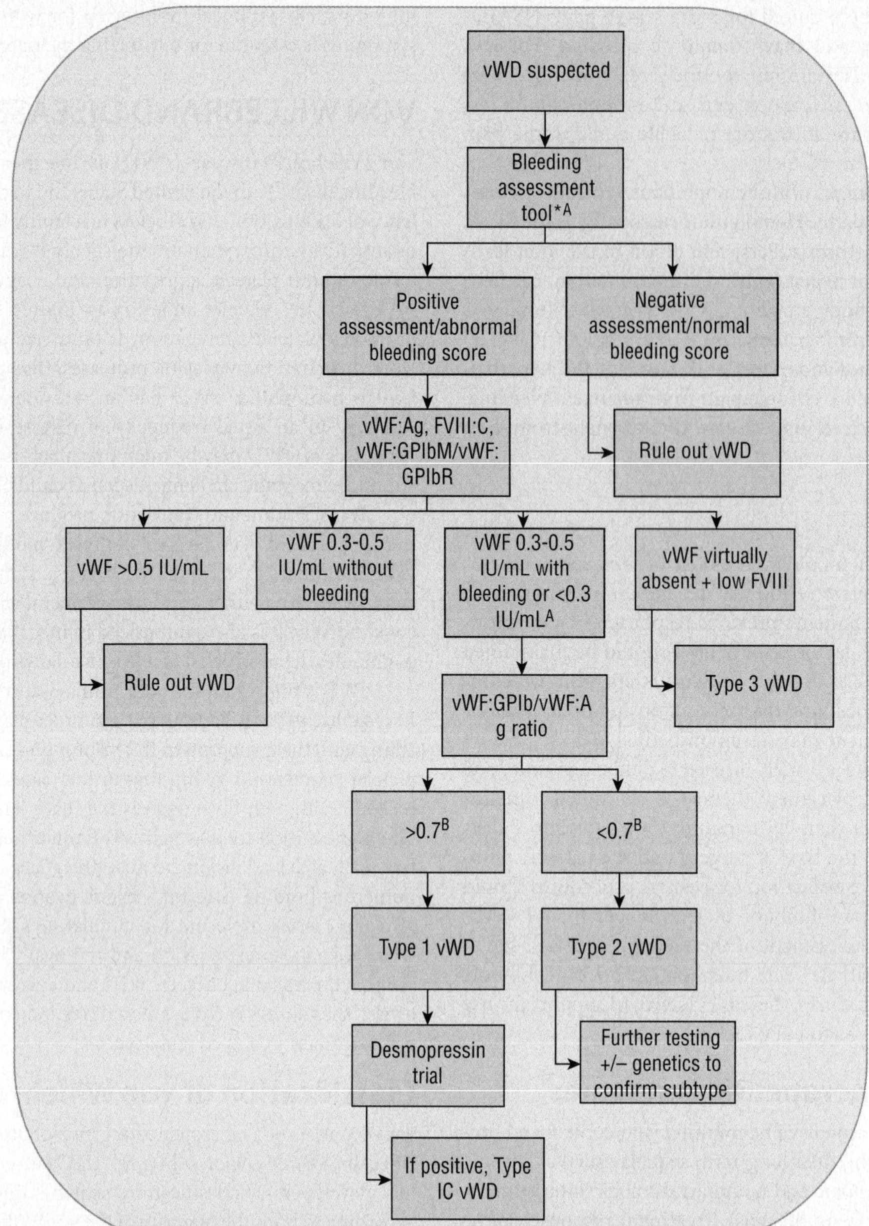

FIGURE 123-2 Classification and Diagnosis of vWD. *Patients with an intermediate or strong probability of vWD should not rely on bleeding assessment tools to guide blood specific testing.
Guideline recommendations:
A = Strong recommendation. Most individuals should follow the recommended course of action. Decision-making tools are not likely to be needed to help patients make decisions which align with their beliefs.
B = Conditional recommendation. Different choices will be appropriate for different patents. Decision aids may be helpful to ensure clinical management aligns with values, preferences, and acceptable risks. *(Adapted from James PD, Connell NT, Ameer B, et al. ASH ISTH NHF WFH 2021 guidelines on the diagnosis of vonWillebrand disease. Blood Adv. 2021;5(1):280–300.)*

Type 1 vWD is the most common type, accounting for 70% to 85% of cases.[48,49] It is characterized by a mild-to-moderate quantitative reduction in the level of vWF (although its multimeric structure is normal) and a similar reduction in the level of factor VIII. It usually is inherited in an autosomal dominant fashion with variable penetrance and expression.[47] Bleeding symptoms often are very mild to moderate.[47] Patients with vWD can experience mucocutaneous bleeding, such as nosebleeds, bruising, gastrointestinal, or menstrual bleeding. Subjects may be at risk of bleeding following surgery, traumatic injury, or childbirth.[47] Type 1C vWD is characterized by increased clearance of vWF and may be identified by a desmopressin trial (preferred), or measuring the ratio of vWF propeptide to antigen.[45]

Type 2 vWD, diagnosed in 20% to 30% of affected patients, is characterized by a qualitative abnormality of vWF.[50] Bleeding manifestations may be more severe than with type 1 disease. Inheritance most often is autosomal dominant but may be recessive.[47] Type 2 vWD can be subdivided into four variants. Type 2A is the most frequent subtype and is characterized by a reduced vWF–platelet interaction and an absence of high- and intermediate-molecular-weight factor multimers. Type 2B is a less common variant characterized by an abnormal vWF that has an increased affinity for the platelet glycoprotein Ib receptor. This subtype is associated with thrombocytopenia, which is usually mild. In addition, high-molecular-weight forms of vWF are usually absent. A platelet-type pseudo-vWD has been characterized in which vWF is normal but a defect in the platelet glycoprotein Ib receptor causes an increased affinity for normal vWF.[47] As a result, platelet-type pseudo-vWD is phenotypically similar to type 2B disease but should be distinguished from it because the treatment is different. Type 2M arises from a qualitative defect in vWF that impairs its binding to platelets; it is similar to type 2A, except there is no measurable reduction in the high-molecular-weight multimers.[47] Finally, type 2N vWD (Normandy) is a rare form of the disease in which vWF has a markedly reduced affinity for factor VIII. This subtype leads to a moderate-to-severe reduction of factor VIII plasma levels with normal vWF levels.[47]

Type 3 vWD refers to a severe quantitative variant of the disease in which vWF is nearly undetectable and factor VIII levels are very low (<20 IU/dL [0.2 IU/mL]). Genetic defects in the vWF gene are null alleles in 80% of patients with type 3 disease, supporting the severe lack of vWF in this subtype.[50] Type 3 vWD is rare and accounts for less than 5% of all cases.[50] The clinical phenotype is severe, reflecting major deficits in primary hemostasis and coagulation.

Acquired von Willebrand Syndrome is a rare bleeding disorder that is similar to the congenital form of the disease. It is primarily associated with autoimmune disorders, such as systemic lupus erythematosus, lymphoproliferative disorders, myeloproliferative disorders, cardiovascular diseases, and certain neoplastic diseases, such as Wilms' tumor and lymphoma.[49] Certain medications have been associated with acquired vWD, most notably valproic acid, griseofulvin, and ciprofloxacin.[51,52] Bleeding manifestations vary from mild to severe, and the condition often resolves with treatment of the underlying disease. Various mechanisms have been proposed, including autoantibodies to vWF resulting in rapid removal from the plasma, adsorption to tumor cells or activated platelets, increased proteolysis, or mechanical destruction.[49]

Clinical Presentation and Diagnosis

Two evidence-based guidelines regarding vWD were updated in early 2021; one focusing on diagnosis and the other on treatment (discussed later). The American Society of Hematology (ASH), the International Society on Thrombosis and Haemostasis (ISTH), the National Hemophilia Foundation (NHF), and the WFH formed a multidisciplinary panel to investigate and prioritize clinical questions and outcomes, assess current evidence, and make recommendations.[45]

When a patient has a lifelong history of mucocutaneous bleeding and a family history of abnormal bleeding, vWD should be suspected. A bleeding assessment tool (BAT) should be utilized as a screening measure to determine if a patient warrants specific blood testing for vWD. Many BATs exist, and there is not one recommended over another in the current guidelines.[45] Abbreviated examples of questions which may be included in a BAT are listed in Table 123-5. For patients with a low probability of vWD, such as those seen in a primary care setting, a BAT is recommended for initial screening. A positive bleeding assessment should determine specific blood testing over nonstandardized clinical assessment.[45] For patients with an intermediate probability of vWD, for example, those referred to hematology, current guidelines recommend against relying on a BAT to determine specific blood testing for diagnosis.[45] Several different laboratory tests are helpful in the diagnosis of this hemostatic abnormality.

Specific laboratory tests for the diagnosis of vWD include measurement of vWF antigen (vWF:Ag) level, factor VIII assay, determination of vWF ristocetin cofactor (vWF:RCo) activity, and vWF multimer analysis (see Table 123-4). Unfortunately, these levels vary considerably and often indeterminate or unreliable results can lead to confusion in the diagnosis. For example, the cutoff normal values for vWF:Ag, vWF:RCo, and other specialized tests vary between laboratories. This coupled with the natural variation of plasma concentrations of vWF can complicate interpretation of these results.[47] Plasma concentrations of vWF increase with age, stress, cigarette smoking, exercise, pregnancy starting in the second trimester, infection, and with the use of certain medications such as

TABLE 123-5 Questions to Ask Patients—Bleeding Assessment Tools

Have you ever experienced epistaxis?
- If so, was it spontaneous?
- What interventions were required?
- When and how often did you experience these symptoms?

Have you ever experienced easy/frequent bruising, ecchymosis, or other cutaneous bleeding?
- If so, how often has this occurred?
- What medical interventions were required?
- Where was the location and size of the bleed?

Have you ever experienced prolonged bleeding from minor wounds?
- If so, did you require medical management? Please describe the intervention(s).

Have you ever experienced hematuria and/or gastrointestinal bleeding?
- If so, specify the type of bleeding (hematuria, melena, hematochezia, etc.).

Have you experienced bleeding in the oral cavity (gum bleeding, spontaneous or minor manipulation)?
- How often does this occur and when did it begin?
- Have you required medical management? If so, please describe.

Have you experienced menorrhagia?
- What medical intervention has been required?
- At what age did this symptom begin?

Have you experienced post-partum hemorrhage?
- How long after birth did this symptom occur?

CLINICAL PRESENTATION Von Willebrand Disease

Signs and Symptoms

- Clinical manifestations are variable; some patients are asymptomatic
- Mucocutaneous bleeding: epistaxis, gingival bleeding with minor manipulation, menorrhagia
- Easy bruising
- Abnormal bleeding after surgery, childbirth, or dental procedures
- Severe cases: musculoskeletal bleeding

corticosteroids, high-dose estrogen oral contraceptives, and desmopressin. Repeated test measurements may be necessary due to this physiologic variability.[47]

Electroimmunoassay, immunoradiometric assay, or enzyme-linked immunosorbent assay, or ELISA, can be used to quantify vWF:Ag.[47] vWF:Ag levels are known to vary with different ABO blood types. Individuals with type O blood exhibit up to a 25% decrease in vWF levels when compared to those with type A due to increased plasma protein clearance.[47] The vWF:Ag level is usually low in types 1 and 2 vWD and virtually absent in type 3 disease. Factor VIII levels are normal or mildly decreased in patients with type 1 or 2 disease and very low (<10% [0.1 units/mL]) in those with type 3 disease.[47]

Ristocetin, an antibiotic that causes platelet aggregation in the presence of functional vWF, is used to measure vWF activity. The Ristocetin cofactor activity usually is reduced in parallel to vWF:Ag levels in types 1 and 3 disease and decreased to a greater extent than vWF:Ag in type 2 disease (except type 2B).[47] Low-dose ristocetin-induced platelet agglutination is useful for further distinguishing type 2B disease, as a low concentration of ristocetin induces excessive aggregation in type 2B disease.[47] When this measure is used, there is the potential for false results due to defects in vWF's ability to bind ristocetin due to genetic variants in the vWF gene.[48,54]

Newer, platelet-dependent assays are now recommended over the vWF:RCo activity test due to their lower coefficients of variation and higher reproducibility. Because glycoprotein Ib binding activity is reduced in most types of vWD, this measurement can guide diagnosis. The first assay functions independently of ristocetin and instead introduces gain-of-function mutations to GPIbα (glycoprotein Ib alpha), therefore allowing it to bind vWF in vitro, spontaneously. The vWF:GPIbM assay provides greater precision with lower limits of detection compared to previous tests but is available.[48,55] Another assay still utilizes ristocetin, but also incorporates recombinant glycoprotein Ib fragments adhered to microparticles, rather than whole platelets. This assay may be susceptible to similar genetic variants as the vWF:RCo assay; however, greater sensitivity and less variation have been observed.[54]

vWF, secreted as high-molecular-weight multimers, is cleaved in plasma to increasingly small protein fragments. The distribution of these multimer sizes can help determine the type of vWD. All multimer sizes are present in type 1 disease, whereas reduced levels of intermediate- and high-molecular-weight multimers are characteristic of type 2 disease. Patients with type 3 disease lack all sizes of vWF multimers. Molecular genetic testing for vWD is now a feasible option in some instances. Genetic testing may clarify diagnostic uncertainty that may remain after coagulation testing and clinical evaluation, and may be especially useful in diagnosing type 2B and 2N vWD.[45,47] Figure 123-2 illustrates the diagnostic algorithm recommended by the guidelines for types 1 and 2 vWD. Type 3 vWD is not addressed in the most recent guidelines, as diagnosis is relatively straight forward for these patients. vWF is virtually absent in type 3 disease (<3 IU/dL [0.03 IU/mL]), with an associated low FVIII level.

Treatment: von Willebrand Disease

6 The specific type of vWD and the location and severity of bleeding determine the approach to treatment. The guidelines from ASH, ISTH, NHF, and WFH cover recommendations ranging from prophylaxis in severe disease to heavy menstrual bleeding.[53] The comprehensive care of patients with vWD requires an interprofessional team approach. The desired outcome is to prevent bleeding episodes and their short-term and long-term consequences so that patients with vWD can live active and productive lives. Local measures, including prolonged pressure, ice, and topical thrombin, often can control superficial bleeding. Systemic treatment is used for bleeding that cannot be controlled in this manner and for the prevention of bleeding with surgery. The goal of systemic therapy is to correct platelet adhesion and coagulation defects by stimulating the release of endogenous vWF or by administering products that contain vWF and factor VIII or vWF alone.[53] General guidelines for the treatment of vWD are shown in Table 123-6.

Replacement Therapy

7 The treatment of choice for patients with severe vWD, including types 2B, 2M, and 3 vWD and for patients with type 1 or 2A vWD who are unresponsive to desmopressin, is replacement therapy with vWF concentrate.[53] Several virus-inactivated, intermediate- or high-purity plasma-derived factor VIII concentrates contain sufficient amounts of functional vWF for treatment in this patient population (see Table 123-2). Ultrahigh-purity (monoclonal antibody-derived) plasma-derived products contain only negligible amounts of vWF and recombinant factor VIII products contain no vWF and are inadequate for treatment of vWD. The evolution of replacement therapy over the past several decades has improved the therapy options available to patients, particularly with severe disease.[56]

Recombinant vWF alone was approved by the US Food and Drug Administration (FDA) in 2015 for on-demand treatment and

TABLE 123-6 Management Recommendations—ASH–ISTH–NHF–WFH Guidelines

Clinical Question	Recommendation	Strength of Recommendation
Prophylaxis	In vWD with severe and frequent bleeds, long-term prophylaxis is suggested, rather than no prophylaxis.	Conditional
Desmopressin trial and administration	If desmopressin in an option (primarily Type 1) and vWF <0.30 IU/mL, trial of desmopressin is suggested. The panel suggests against treating with desmopressin in the absence of a trial first.	Conditional
Antithrombotic therapy	In patients with vWD and cardiovascular disorders requiring anticoagulants or antiplatelet agents, use of these agents is suggested over no therapy.	Conditional
Major surgery	Target vWF and FVIII activity levels ≥0.50 IU/mL for at least 3 days after surgery.	Conditional
Minor surgery/invasive procedures	Target vFW activity levels ≥0.50 IU/mL using desmopressin or factor concentrate along with tranexamic acid.	Conditional
Gynecology—heavy menstrual bleeding	Hormonal therapy or tranexamic acid is suggested over desmopressin.	Conditional

Abbreviated recommendations from the 2021 Guidelines on treatment of vWD. Additional recommendations can be found in the source document. Strength of Recommendations: *Strong:* Most individuals should follow the recommended course of action. Decision-making tools are not likely to be needed to help patients make decisions which align with their beliefs. *Conditional:* Different choices will be appropriate for different patents. Decision aids may be helpful to ensure clinical management aligns with values, preferences, and acceptable risks. *(Data from Reference 53.)*

control of bleeding episodes as well as perioperative management of bleeding in patients with vWD. Unlike plasma-derived vWF, recombinant products have no exposure to the ADAMTS13 (a disintegrin and metalloprotease with thrombospondin type 1 motif, member 13) which cleave large multimers.[57] Ultralarge and high-molecular-weight multimers are necessary for optimal platelet plug formation, making recombinant products ideal.[56,57]

Cryoprecipitate was one of the earliest forms of replacement therapy for vWD. It contains about 80 to 100 units of vWF per unit (5-10 times more vWF and factor VIII than fresh-frozen plasma), and it was the mainstay of therapy for vWD. However, because cryoprecipitate is not always virally inactivated, it should not be used as first-line treatment and is no longer recommended in the United States or Europe.[56]

Other Pharmacological Therapy

8 Desmopressin stimulates the endothelial cell release of vWF and factor VIII. It is temporarily effective for patients with vWD who have adequate endogenous stores of functional vWF, which includes most patients with type 1 disease and some patients with type 2A disease. Conversely, desmopressin is not appropriate for patients with type 3 disease, who lack stores of vWF. Desmopressin usually is not recommended for the treatment of type 2B disease because the release of additional abnormal vWF may exacerbate thrombocytopenia, but it has been reported to be beneficial in some patients with type 2B disease.[58] If desmopressin is used for the treatment of type 2B disease, close monitoring is necessary.

The dose of desmopressin used for treatment of vWD is identical to that used for treatment of mild factor VIII deficiency, 0.3 mcg/kg given IV over 15 to 30 minutes.[15] Patients with vWD generally have a better response to desmopressin than those with hemophilia, with an average three- to fivefold increase in vWF and factor VIII levels.[48] These levels remain elevated for about 6 to 8 hours. The response to desmopressin in a given patient usually is consistent, and a desmopressin trial should determine if the medication likely will be effective for the individual. Desmopressin is preferable to use of plasma-derived products for patients who have an adequate response because desmopressin does not carry a risk of viral transmission. An added benefit is the substantially lower cost of desmopressin compared to the plasma-derived and recombinant products. (For a discussion of the adverse drug reactions of desmopressin, see "Hemophilia: Other Pharmacologic Therapy" section.)

Desmopressin can be administered every 12 to 24 hours, but the response diminishes with repeated treatment. After three to four doses, desmopressin often is no longer effective and alternative replacement therapy may be necessary if prolonged treatment is required. Laboratory monitoring, including vWF:Ag measurements, factor VIII assays, vWF:activity assessments, and clinical examinations, will determine the adequacy of treatment.[58] Intranasal administration of desmopressin, at the same dosage as that used for mild factor VIII deficiency, can be useful for the treatment of mild bleeding episodes. One or two doses administered at the start of menses may help control menorrhagia. Oral contraceptives may also be very effective in controlling this symptom (see Table 123-6). Antifibrinolytic agents, such as aminocaproic acid and tranexamic acid, may be of special value in bleeds associated with tissues rich in plasminogen activators, such as the mouth, especially with tooth extractions.[58] These agents can also be used in the management of epistaxis, GI bleeding, and menorrhagia. However, these agents should be avoided in urinary tract bleeding because of the risk of thrombosis and obstruction.

In acquired vWD, low levels of plasma vWF are the result of accelerated removal of protein from plasma through the action of different pathogenic mechanisms. Acquired vWD may be associated with monoclonal gammopathy, lymphoproliferative or myeloproliferative syndromes, or autoimmune disorders. Cardiovascular disease, such as aortic stenosis and congenital cardiac defects, are increasing in the literature as causes of acquired vWD. Intravenous immune globulin remains a therapeutic option in acquired vWD, along with vWF concentrate and/or desmopressin.[51]

Gene Therapy

Patients with the most severe bleeding phenotypes of vWD (type 3 and some severe cases of types 1 and 2) may be the most likely candidates for gene therapy, which offers the potential of a long-term, if not lifelong, correction of vWF deficiency. Preclinical trials are being conducted to test the feasibility of gene transfer in the management of vWD.[59]

Evaluation of Therapeutic Outcomes

Since the main goal in the treatment of vWD is to prevent or control bleeding and the consequences of such bleeding, bleeding episodes can be monitored via clinical and laboratory parameters. Monitoring the number and types of bleeding episodes and measurement of plasma concentrations of vWF and factor VIII make it possible to evaluate the effectiveness of specific prophylactic and treatment regimens. As with hemophilia patients, assessment of patients' activities of daily living gives clinicians a better appreciation of the success of the treatment plan.

OTHER CONGENITAL FACTOR DEFICIENCIES

Rare bleeding disorders constitute 3% to 5% of all inherited coagulation factor deficiencies.[60] These rare bleeding disorders include congenital deficiencies in fibrinogen, in factors II, V, VII, X, XI, and XIII, and in combinations of factor deficiencies. Contact factor abnormalities, including deficiencies in factor XII, high-molecular-weight kininogen, and prekallikrein, prolong the aPTT but do not lead to any bleeding diathesis. Identification of these disorders is important so that inappropriate treatment is not given. The only contact factor deficiency associated with bleeding symptoms is factor XI deficiency. Also known as hemophilia C, this deficiency is particularly common in people of Ashkenazi Jewish descent.[61] Bleeding manifestations are variable. Bleeding usually does not occur spontaneously, but excessive bleeding may occur after trauma or surgery. Most other deficiencies are inherited as autosomal recessive disorders and are rare. Some patients with abnormal molecules, such as a dysfibrinogenemia, may have an increased tendency to develop thromboembolic disease. Most of these deficiencies are treated with fresh-frozen plasma. Newer specific concentrates are becoming available. For example, a factor XIII plasma-derived concentrate is available, and recombinant factor VIIa is approved for use in patients with congenital VII deficiency. Cryoprecipitate, which is rich in fibrinogen, or fibrinogen concentrates (RiaSTAP®), can be used to treat patients with fibrinogen deficiency or dysfunctional fibrinogen (dysfibrinogenemia).

COMPLICATIONS OF REPLACEMENT THERAPY

As discussed previously, the transmission of blood borne infectious diseases is a concern when blood and blood-derived products are used. Most patients with hemophilia who received plasma-derived products were infected with hepatitis viruses and HIV during the 1980s prompting the development of viral inactivation methods for use during the manufacturing of factor concentrates.[15] All available plasma-derived factor concentrates come from screened donors and undergo viral inactivation procedures in an effort to reduce the risk of viral transmission. Heat treatment, which includes dry and wet heat, is one method of viral inactivation. Wet heat is applied while the concentrate is in suspension or in solution (pasteurization) and is more effective than dry heat. Other methods of viral inactivation include chemical (solvent detergent) and affinity chromatography with monoclonal antibodies. Solvent detergent treatment inactivates lipid-coated viruses, such as HIV and hepatitis B and C, but it is not effective against parvovirus B19, transfusion transmitted virus, hepatitis A, or prions.[5] Parvovirus B19 is found in both plasma-derived and recombinant factor VIII concentrates (due to the use of albumin as a stabilizer in some recombinant products).[5,19] Parvovirus B19 may be particularly important for patients with hemophilia and HIV infection because it can cause chronic anemia in patients with immune deficiency.

Other complications associated with factor administration include allergic reactions, fever, chills, urticaria, and nausea. PCCs and aPCCs also have the potential to cause thromboembolic complications, including deep-vein thrombosis, pulmonary embolism, myocardial infarction, and disseminated intravascular coagulation, likely related to the presence of activated factors.[15] Antifibrinolytic agents should not be given to patients receiving PCCs or aPCCs to avoid thrombotic complications.

Porcine factor VIII, used in the treatment of patients with inhibitors to factor VIII, is not known to transmit human viruses. However, allergic-type reactions (eg, fever, chills, skin rashes, nausea, and headaches) have been reported.[15] Patients who experience these reactions can be treated with steroids and/or diphenhydramine. Thrombocytopenia is another potential complication of porcine factor VIII use.[15]

CONCLUSION

Coagulation disorders, such as hemophilia and vWD, affect a small subset of the overall population, but their treatment can be costly and complicated, requiring knowledgeable health professionals and an interprofessional team approach for optimal outcomes to be achieved. Exciting progress is being made in the development of new strategies for treating these types of disorders. The development of new factor products with improved pharmacokinetic properties, non-factor replacement therapy, as well as the advances in gene therapy may soon redefine the therapeutic landscape for these patients and improve their overall experience.

ABBREVIATIONS

AAV	adeno-associated virus
ADAMTS13	a disintegrin and metalloprotease with thrombospondin type 1 motif, member 13
aPCC	activated prothrombin complex concentrate
aPTT	activated partial thromboplastin time
ASH	American Society of Hematology
BAT	bleeding assessment tool
BU	Bethesda unit
cDNA	circulating DNA
HIV	human immunodeficiency virus
IgG	immunoglobulin G
ISTH	International Society on Thrombosis and Haemostasis
ITI	immune tolerance induction
NHF	National Hemophilia Foundation
NSAID	nonsteroidal anti-inflammatory drug
PCC	prothrombin complex concentrate
PRICE	Protect, Rest, Ice, Compression, and Elevation
SIPPET	Survey of Inhibitors in Plasma-Product Exposed Toddlers
vWD	von Willebrand disease
vWF	von Willebrand factor
vWF:Ag	von Willebrand factor antigen
vWF:RCo	von Willebrand factor ristocetin cofactor
vWF:GPIbM	von Willebrand factor glycoprotein Ib mutational assay
WFH	World Federation of Hemophilia

REFERENCES

1. Srivastava A, Brewer AK, Mauser-Bunschoten EP, et al. Guidelines for the management of hemophilia. *Haemophilia.* 2013;19:e1–e47.
2. Wynn TT, Gumuscu B. Potential role of a new PEGylated recombinant factor VIII for hemophilia. *J Blood Med.* 2016;7:121–128.
3. World Federation of Hemophilia. Carriers and Women with Hemophilia. 2012. Available at: http://www1.wfh.org/publication/files/pdf-1471.pdf.
4. Shahriari M, Bazrafshan A, Moghadam M, Karimi M. Severe hemophilia in a girl infant with mosaic Turner syndrome and persistent hyperplastic primary vitreous. *Blood Coagul Fibrinolysis.* 2016;27:352–353.
5. Lee C, Berntorp E, Hoots W, eds. *Textbook of Hemophilia.* 3rd ed. Chichester, West Sussex, UK: Wiley-Blackwell; 2014.
6. Structural Immunology Group, University of College London. Factor VIII (F8). 2021. Available at: http://www.factorviii-db.org.
7. Structural Immunology Group, University of College London. Factor IX Gene (F9). 2021. Available at: https://www.factorix.org/.
8. Funnell APW, Crossley M. Hemophilia B Leyden and once mysterious cis-regulatory mutations. *Trends in Genetics.* 2014;30:18–23.
9. Davies GA, Poon MC, Rydz N, Goodyear D. Attitudes toward prenatal diagnosis and pregnancy management in carriers of hemophilia: A qualitative analysis exploring the views of carriers in Southern Alberta. *Blood.* 2016;128:4742.
10. Xu XP, Gan HY, Li FX, et al. A method to quantify cell-free fetal DNA fraction in maternal plasma using next generation sequencing: Its application in non-invasive prenatal chromosomal aneuploidy detection. *PLoS ONE.* 2016;11:1–13.
11. Carpenter SL, Soucie JM, Presley MV, et al. Hepatitis B vaccination is effective by subcutaneous route in children with bleeding disorders: A universal data collection database analysis. *Haemophilia.* 2015;21:e39–e43.
12. Streif W, Knöfler R. Perinatal management of haemophilia. *Hämostaseologie.* 2020;40:226–232. doi: 10.1055/a-1141-1252.
13. Acharya SS. Advances in hemophilia and the role of current and emerging prophylaxis. *Am J Manag Care.* 2016;22:S116–S125.
14. Berntorp E, Andersson NG. Prophylaxis for haemophilia in the era of extended half-life factor VIII/factor IX products. *Semin Thromb Hemost.* 2016;42:518–525.
15. Lexicomp Online®, Pediatric & Neonatal Lexi-Drugs®, Hudson, Ohio: Lexi-Comp, Inc.; 2018.
16. Chen SL. Economic costs of hemophilia and the impact of prophylactic treatment on patient management. *Am J Manag Care.* 2016;22(5 suppl):s126–s133.
17. Oldenburg J, Mahlangu JN, Kim B, et al. Emicizumab prophylaxis in hemophilia A with inhibitors. *N Engl J Med.* 2017;377:809–818.
18. Mahlangu J, Oldenburg J, Paz-Priel I, et al. Emicizumab prophylaxis in patients who have hemophilia A without inhibitors. *N Engl J Med.* 2018;379:811–822.
19. Aledort LM. The evolution of comprehensive haemophilia care in the United States: Perspectives from the frontline. *Haemophilia.* 2016;22:676–683.
20. Berntorp E, Shapiro AD. Modern haemophilia care. *Lancet.* 2012;379:1447–1456.
21. Negrier C, Karim FA, Lepatan LM, et al. Efficacy and safety of long-acting recombinant fusion protein linking factor IX with albumin in haemophilia B patients undergoing surgery. *Haemophilia.* 2016;22:e259–e266.
22. Nolan B, Mahlangu J, Perry D, et al. Long-term safety and efficacy of recombinant factor VIII Fc fusion protein (rFVIIIFc) in subjects with hemophilia A. *Haemophilia.* 2015;22:72–80.
23. Dube E, Bonnefoy A, Merien C, et al. A prospective surveillance study of inhibitor development in haemophilia A patients following a population switch to a third-generation B-domain-deleted recombinant factor VIII. *Haemophilia.* 2018;24:236–244.
24. Urwin P, Thanigaikumar K, Ironside JW, et al. Sporadic Creutzfeldt-Jakob disease in 2 plasma product recipients, United Kingdom. *Emerging Inf Diseases.* 2017;23:893–897.

25. Micromedex® Healthcare Series. Greenwood Village, CO: Thomson Reuters (Healthcare). Updated September 21, 2021.
26. Prelog T, Dolnicar MB, Kitanovaski L. Low-dose continuous infusion of factor VIII in patients with haemophilia A. *Blood Transfus.* 2016;14:474–480.
27. Loomans JI, Kruip MJHA, Carcao M, et al. Desmopressin in moderate hemophilia A patients: A treatment worth considering. *Haematologica.* 2018;103:550–557.
28. Shima M, Lillicrap D, Kruse-Jarres R. Alternative therapies for the management of inhibitors. *Haemophilia.* 2016;22:36–41.
29. Ljung RCR. How I manage patients with inherited haemophilia A and B and factor inhibitors. *Br J Haematol.* 2018;180:501–510.
30. Konkle BA. Impacting inhibitor development in hemophilia A. *Blood.* 2017;130:1689–1690.
31. Peyvandi F, Manucci PM, Garagiola I, et al. A randomized trial of factor VIII and neutralizing antibodies in hemophilia A. *N Engl J Med.* 2016;374:2054–2064.
32. Santagostino E, Escobar M, Ozelo M, et al. Recombinant activated factor VII in the treatment of bleeds and for the prevention of surgery-related bleeding in congenital haemophilia with inhibitors. *Blood Rev.* 2015;29(suppl 1):S9–S18.
33. Antunes SV, Tangada S, Stasyshyn O, et al. Randomized comparison of prophylaxis and on-demand regimens with FEIBA NF in the treatment of haemophilia A and B with inhibitors. *Haemophilia.* 2014;20:65–72.
34. Mannucci PM, Franchini M. Porcine recombinant factor VIII: An additional weapon to handle anti-factor VIII antibodies. *Blood Transfus.* 2017;15:365–368.
35. Valentino LA, Kempton CL, Kruse-Jarres R, et al. US guidelines for immune tolerance induction in patients with haemophilia a and inhibitors. *Haemophilia.* 2015;21:559–567.
36. Collins P, Chalmers E, Alamelu J, et al. First-line immune tolerance induction for children with severe haemophilia A: A protocol from the UK Haemophilia Centre Doctors' Organisation Inhibitor and Paediatric Working Parties. *Haemophilia.* 2017;23:654–659.
37. Batsuli G, Meeks SL, Herzog RW, et al. Innovating immune tolerance induction for haemophilia. *Haemophilia.* 2016;22(S5):31–35.
38. Jiang L, Liu Y, Zhang L, et al. Rituximab for treating inhibitors in people with inherited severe hemophilia. *Cochrane Database Syst Rev.* 2017;7:1465–1858.
39. Giangrande P. The future of hemophilia treatment: Longer-acting factor concentrates versus gene therapy. *Semin Thromb Hemost.* 2016;42:513–517.
40. Pasi KJ, Rangarajan S, Mitchell N, et al. Multiyear follow-up of AAV5-hFVIII-SQ gene therapy for hemophilia A. *NEJM.* 2020;382:29–40. doi: 10.1056/nejmoa1908490.
41. van den Berg HM. A cure for hemophilia within reach. *N Engl J Med.* 2017;377:2592–2593.
42. Auerswald G, Dolan G, Duffy A, et al. Pain and pain management in haemophilia. *Blood Coagul Fibrinolysis.* 2016;27:1–10.
43. Mensah PK, Gooding R. Surgery in patients with inherited bleeding disorders. *Anaesthesia.* 2015;70(suppl 1):112–120.
44. Pasca S, Milan M, Sarolo L, Zanon E. PK-driven prophylaxis versus standard prophylaxis: When tailored treatment may be a real and achievable cost-saving approach in children with severe hemophilia A. *Thrombosis Research.* 2017;157:58–63.
45. James PD, Connell NT, Ameer B, et al. ASH ISTH NHF WFH 2021 guidelines on the diagnosis of von Willebrand disease. *Blood Adv.* 2021;5(1):280–300. doi: 10.1182/bloodadvances.2020003265.
46. Swami A, Kaur V. von Willebrand disease: A concise review and update for the practicing physician. *Clin Appl Thromb Hemost.* 2017;23:900–910.
47. Ng C, Motto DG, Di Paola J. Diagnostic approach to von Willebrand disease. *Blood.* 2015;125:2029–2037.
48. Sharma R, Flood VH. Advances in the diagnosis and treatment of von Willebrand disease. *Blood.* 2017;130:2386–2391.
49. Mital A. Acquired von Willebrand syndrome. *Adv Clin Exp Med.* 2016;25(6):1337–1344. doi: 10.17219/acem/64942.
50. Leebeek FWG, Eikenboom JCJ. von Willebrand disease. *N Engl J Med.* 2016;375:2067–2080.
51. Franchini M, Mannucci PM. Acquired von Willebrand syndrome: Focused for hematologists. *Haematologica.* 2020;105(8):2032–2037. doi: 10.3324/haematol.2020.255117.
52. Kumar R, Vidaurre J, Gedela S. Valproic acid-induced coagulopathy. *Pediatr Neurol.* 2019;98:25–30. doi: 10.1016/j.pediatrneurol.2019.04.019.
53. Connell NT, Flood VH, Brignardello-Petersen R, et al. ASH ISTH NHF WFH 2021 guidelines on the management of von Willebrand disease. *Blood Adv.* 2021;5(1):301–325. doi: 10.1182/bloodadvances.2020003264.
54. Boender J, Eikenboom J, van der Bom JG, et al. Clinically relevant differences between assays for von Willebrand factor activity. *J Thromb Haemost.* 2018;16:2413–2424. doi: 10.1111/jth.14319.
55. Patzke J, Favaloro EJ. Laboratory testing for von Willebrand Factor activity by Glycoprotein Ib Binding Assays (VWF:GPIb). *Methods Mol Biol.* 2017;1646:453–460. doi: 10.1007/978-1-4939-7196-1_33.
56. Peyvandi F, Kouides P, Turecek PL, et al. Evolution of replacement therapy for von Willebrand disease: From plasma fraction to recombinant von Willebrand factor. *Blood Rev.* 2019;38:100572–100572. doi: 10.1016/j.blre.2019.04.001.
57. Gill JC, Castaman G, Windyga J, et al. Hemostatic efficacy, safety, and pharmacokinetics of a recombinant von Willebrand factor in severe von Willebrand disease. *Blood.* 2015;126:2038–2046.
58. Laffan MA, Lester W, O'Donnell JS, et al. The diagnosis and management of von Willebrand disease: A United Kingdom Haemophilia Centre Doctors Organization guideline approved by the British Committee for Standards in Haematology. *Br J Haematol.* 2014;167:453–465.
59. Portier I, Vanhoorelbeke K, Verhenne S, et al. High and long-term von Willebrand factor expression after *Sleeping Beauty* transposon-mediated gene therapy in a mouse model of severe von Willebrand disease. *J Thromb Haemost.* 2018;16:592–604.
60. James P, Salomon O, Mikovic D, et al. Rare bleeding disorders—Bleeding assessment tools, laboratory aspects and phenotype and therapy of FXI deficiency. *Haemophilia.* 2014;20:71–75.
61. Franchini M, Marano G, Pupella S, et al. Rare congenital bleeding disorders. *Ann Transl Med.* 2018;6:331.

124

Sickle Cell Disease

Jin Han, Santosh L. Saraf, and Victor R. Gordeuk

KEY CONCEPTS

1. Sickle cell disease is an inherited disorder caused by a defect in the gene for β-globin, a component of hemoglobin. It is considered to be a qualitative hemoglobinopathy. Patients can have one defective gene (sickle cell trait) or two defective genes (sickle cell disease).
2. Although sickle cell disease usually occurs in persons of African ancestry, other ethnic groups can be affected. Multiple mutation variants are responsible for differences in clinical manifestations.
3. Sickle cell disease involves multiple organ systems. Usual clinical signs and symptoms include anemia, pain, splenomegaly, and pulmonary symptoms. Sickle cell disease is diagnosed through routine newborn screening programs available in all 50 states. Early diagnosis allows early preventive and comprehensive care.
4. Patients with sickle cell disease are at risk for infection. Prophylaxis against pneumococcal infection reduces death during childhood.
5. Hydroxyurea decreases the risk of painful episodes, but patients treated with hydroxyurea require careful monitoring.
6. Neurologic complications caused by vasoocclusion and hemolysis can lead to stroke. Screening with transcranial Doppler ultrasound to identify children at risk accompanied by chronic transfusion therapy programs can decrease the risk of overt and silent stroke in children with sickle cell disease.
7. Patients with fever greater than 38.5°C (101.3°F) should be evaluated, and appropriate antibiotics administered immediately, including coverage for encapsulated organisms, especially pneumococcal organisms.
8. Pain episodes can often be managed at home. Hospitalized patients require parenteral analgesics. Analgesic options include opioids, nonsteroidal anti-inflammatory agents, and acetaminophen. The patient characteristics and the severity of the pain should determine the choice of agent and regimen.
9. Patients with sickle cell disease should be followed regularly for healthcare maintenance issues and monitored for changes in organ function.

BEYOND THE BOOK ACTIVITY

https://tinyurl.com/tel4648

Watch the short video entitled "Sickle Cell Anemia" in the DNA Learning Center. This short 1-minute video provides 3D animation of the gene mutation resulting in sickle cell disease.

https://tinyurl.com/vb4g9ye

Then listen to the podcast in EM Basic by Dr Jared Walker on evaluation and management of sickle cell disease in the emergency room.

INTRODUCTION

1 Sickle cell syndromes, which can be divided into sickle cell trait (SCT) and sickle cell disease (SCD), are a group of hereditary conditions characterized by the presence of sickle cell hemoglobin (HbS) in red blood cells (RBCs). SCT is the heterozygous inheritance of one normal β-globin gene producing hemoglobin A (HbA) and one sickle gene, producing HbS (HbAS). Individuals with SCT are usually asymptomatic. SCD can be of homozygous or compounded heterozygous inheritance. Homozygous HbS (HbSS) has historically been referred to as sickle cell anemia (SCA), which now also includes HbSβ^0-thal due to similarities in clinical severity. The heterozygous inheritance of HbS with another qualitative or quantitative β-globin mutation results in sickle cell hemoglobin C (HbSC), sickle cell β-thalassemia (HbSβ^+-thal and HbSβ^0-thal), and some other rare phenotypes.[1-4]

Over the years, progress has been made in our understanding of the relationship between clinical severity and genotype, as well as the pathological cascades leading to complications and morbidities associated with SCD. Ongoing research focuses on disease modification, organ damage prevention, and curative treatment. Advances in the care of patients with SCD have increased life expectancy to adulthood. Therefore, the transition from pediatric to adult medical care has become a focus to further improve survival and quality of life.[1-7]

SCD is a chronic illness with financial and emotional challenges for patients and their caregivers and high economic impact on society. Frequent hospitalizations can interrupt schooling and result in employment difficulties.[8,9] Acute complications of the disease can be unpredictable, rapidly progressive, and life-threatening. Later in life, chronic organ damage and cognitive or emotional impairment can develop.[3,7,10,11] Because of the complexity of the illness, comprehensive care must be available to all patients and that all providers have a good understanding of disease progression and management.[1,10,11]

EPIDEMIOLOGY

2 SCD affects millions of people worldwide. The condition is most common in people with African heritage.[2,3] The most common SCD genotype is HbSS (60%-65%), followed by HbSC (25%-30%), HbSβ^+-thal, and HbSβ^0-thal (5%-10%). Other variants account for less than 1% of patients.[1,2,5] The prevalence of SCD is highest in sub-Saharan Africa. The sickle mutation can also be found in the Arabian Peninsula, the Indian subcontinent, and the Mediterranean region.[1,3-5] An estimated 300,000 children are born each year with SCD-HbSS and another 50,000 to 100,000 births per year for other forms of SCD.[8] In the United States, about 100,000 Americans have SCD with a prevalence of 1 in 2,500 newborns of all ethnicities, 1 in 365 Black births, and 1 in 36,000 Hispanic births.[1,5]

The prevalence of SCD in a region is determined by the frequency of SCT. An estimated 300 million people are carriers worldwide.[12] The distribution of SCT reflects the survival advantage in regions where malaria is endemic as the gene mutation offers partial protection against serious malarial infection. Since RBCs carrying the abnormal sickle hemoglobin (Hb) prevent the normal growth and development of *Plasmodium falciparum* within RBCs, individuals with SCT are more likely to survive an acute malarial illness.[13] The overall incidence of SCT reported in the United States is 15.5 per 1,000 newborns, with a rate of 7.3% in Black, 0.6% in Hispanics, and 0.3% in White.[14,15]

ETIOLOGY

Normal hemoglobin (HbA) is composed of two α-chains and two β-chains ($\alpha_2 \beta_2$). The biochemical defect that leads to the development of HbS involves the substitution of valine for glutamic acid as the sixth amino acid in the β-polypeptide chain. Another abnormal hemoglobin, hemoglobin C (HbC), is produced by the substitution of lysine for glutamic acid as the sixth amino acid in the β-chain. Structurally, the α-chains of HbS, HbA, and HbC are identical. Therefore, it is the chemical differences in the β-chain that account for sickling and its related sequelae.[1-4]

Homozygous HbSS, the most common form of SCD, occurs when an individual inherits both maternal and paternal β-globin alleles that code for HbS. Figures 124-1 to 124-4 show the probability of inheritance with each pregnancy for the offspring of parents with HbA, SCT, and HbSS. β-Thalassemia is a quantitative hemoglobinopathy resulting from a genetic defect in β-globin production that may vary from no β-globin production (β^0) to some β-globin production (β^+). β-Thalassemia can be co-inherited with HbS.

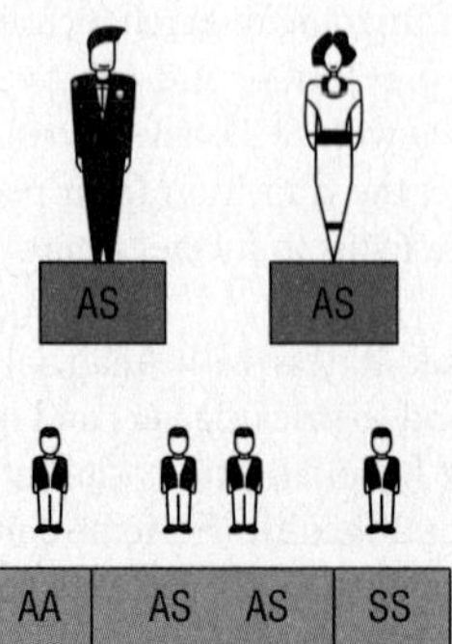

FIGURE 124-1 Sickle cell gene inheritance scheme for both parents with SCT. Possibilities with each pregnancy: 25% normal (AA); 50% SCT (AS); 25% SCA (SS). (A, normal hemoglobin; S, sickle cell hemoglobin.)

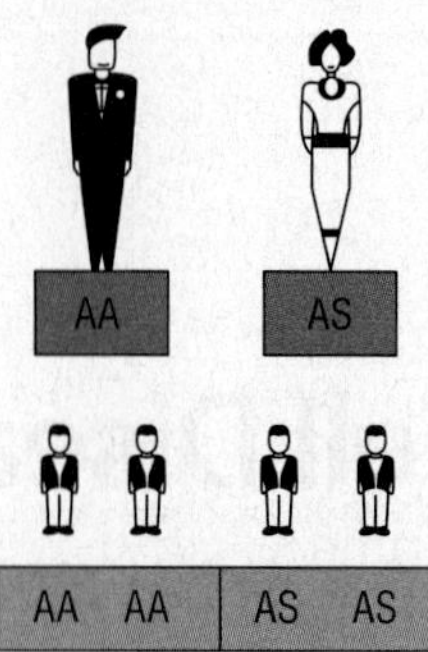

FIGURE 124-2 Sickle cell gene inheritance scheme for one parent with SCT and one parent with no sickle cell gene. Possibilities with each pregnancy: 50% normal (AA); 50% SCT (AS). (A, normal hemoglobin; S, sickle cell hemoglobin.)

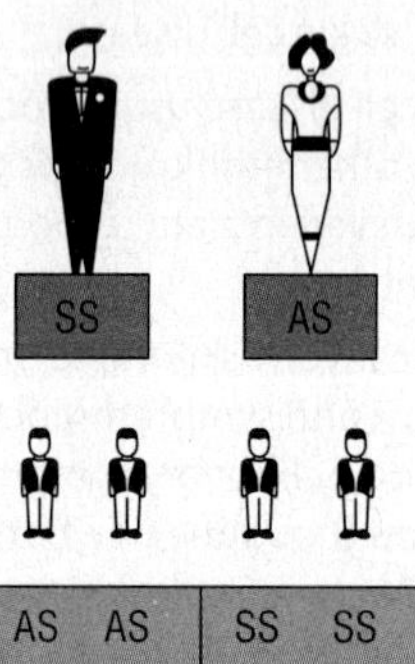

FIGURE 124-3 Sickle cell gene inheritance scheme for one parent with SCT and one parent with SSA (SS). Possibilities with each pregnancy: 50% SCA (SS); 50% SCT (AS). (A, normal hemoglobin; S, sickle cell hemoglobin.)

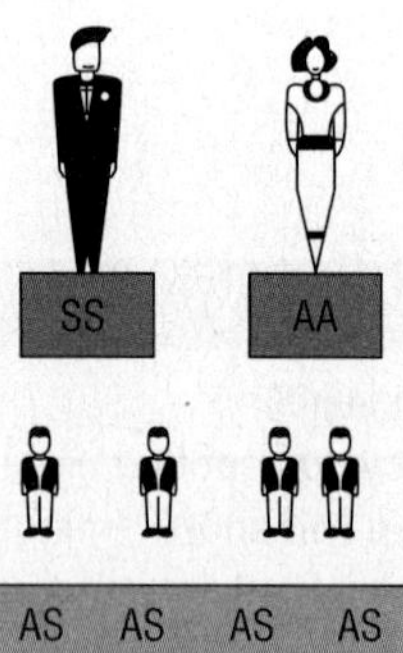

FIGURE 124-4 Sickle cell inheritance scheme for one parent without sickle cell gene and one parent with SCA. Possibilities with each pregnancy: 100% SCT (AS). (A, normal hemoglobin; S, sickle cell hemoglobin.)

Individuals with HbSS and HbSβ^0-thal have a more severe course than those with HbSC and HbSβ^+-thal and are now both referred to as SCA.[2,4,10]

SCD is most commonly found among people with ancestors from sub-Saharan Africa, India, Saudi Arabia, and Mediterranean countries. Genetic analysis shows that the haplotype containing the sickle mutation found in Arabic patients differs from the haplotype in those of African descent. These haplotype variants associated with different geographic regions may be responsible for variations in the clinical manifestations and response to therapy.[1-3,7] The three most common haplotypes in the United States are the Bantu haplotype, characterized by severe disease; the Senegal haplotype, characterized by mild disease; and the Benin haplotype, characterized by a course intermediate to that of the other two haplotypes. Although there are a number of other haplotypes seen around the world, the major types outside of the United States are found in Saudi Arabia and Cameroon, both with milder courses of illness.[1-3,7,10,16] Other genetic modifiers such as coincident α-thalassemia and the levels of fetal hemoglobin concentration also affect the clinical severity of SCD.[1]

PATHOPHYSIOLOGY

Normal adult RBCs contain predominantly HbA (96%-98%). Other forms of Hb are HbA_2 (2%-3%) and fetal Hb (<1%). Normal RBCs have a biconcave shape and are able to deform to squeeze through capillaries. Fetal hemoglobin (HbF) is a tetramer of two α-globin chains and two γ-globin chains ($\alpha_2\gamma_2$) that is present predominantly in fetal RBCs.[2,3,7,13] Prior to birth, HbF is the predominant Hb type. At around 32-week gestation, a switch from the production of γ chains to β-chains occurs and consequently an increase in HbA production occurs. Increased HbF production occurs under severe erythroid stress, such as anemia, after hematopoietic stem cell transplantation (HSCT) or chemotherapy, or in the hereditary condition, hereditary persistence of fetal hemoglobin (HPFH), where a mutation in the β-globin gene cluster results in continued HbF production after birth. HPFH is a benign, asymptomatic condition.[2,3,17] HbF does not participate in the formation of the HbS polymer, so its presence in the HbSS RBC in sufficient quantity can prevent the sickling phenomenon described below.

In the pathogenesis of SCD, the following are responsible for the various clinical manifestations: impaired circulation, destruction of RBCs with release of RBC content to the plasma, stasis of blood flow, and ongoing inflammatory responses. These changes result directly from two major disturbances involving RBCs: abnormal Hb polymerization and membrane damage (Fig. 124-5).

The solubilities of HbS and HbA are the same under conditions of normal oxygenation, but the solubility of deoxygenated HbS is reduced because of the valine substitution. Deoxy-HbS leads to intermolecular binding and formation of thin bundles of fibers, which initially are unstable. However, the increased binding of deoxy-HbS eventually results in cross-linked fibers and stable polymers. This process is influenced by mean corpuscular Hb concentration, temperature, intracellular pH, and the circulating amount of HbS. Polymerization allows deoxygenated Hb molecules to exist as a semisolid gel that protrudes into the cell membrane, leading to distortion of RBCs (sickle shaped) and loss of deformability. The presence of sickled RBCs increases blood viscosity and encourages sludging in the capillaries and postcapillary venules. Such obstructive events lead to local tissue hypoxia, which tends to accentuate the pathologic process.[4,18,19]

When reoxygenated, polymers within the RBCs disassemble and the RBCs eventually return to normal shape. This process contributes to vasoocclusion because the HbS-containing RBCs are able to enter the microvasculature when oxygenated, but sickle as Hb releases oxygen to the tissues. The cycle of sickling and unsickling results in damage to the cell membrane, loss of membrane flexibility, and rearrangement of surface phospholipids. Membrane damage also alters ion transport, resulting in potassium and water loss, which can lead to a dehydrated state enhancing the formation of sickled forms. After continual repetitions of the process, the RBCs develop into rigid irreversibly sickled cells (ISCs). Unlike the reversible sickled cells, which have normal morphology when oxygenated, ISCs are elongated cells that remain sickled when oxygenated. The more rigid membranes of these ISCs retard flow, particularly through the microcirculation. In addition, sickled RBCs tend to adhere to vascular endothelial cells, which further increases polymerization and obstruction.[1,6,18,19]

Intermolecular binding and polymer formation are reduced by HbF and to a lesser degree by HbA_2. RBCs that contain HbF sickle less readily than cells without. ISCs, not surprisingly, have a low HbF level. Increased levels of HbF, as in the case of the Saudi Arabian

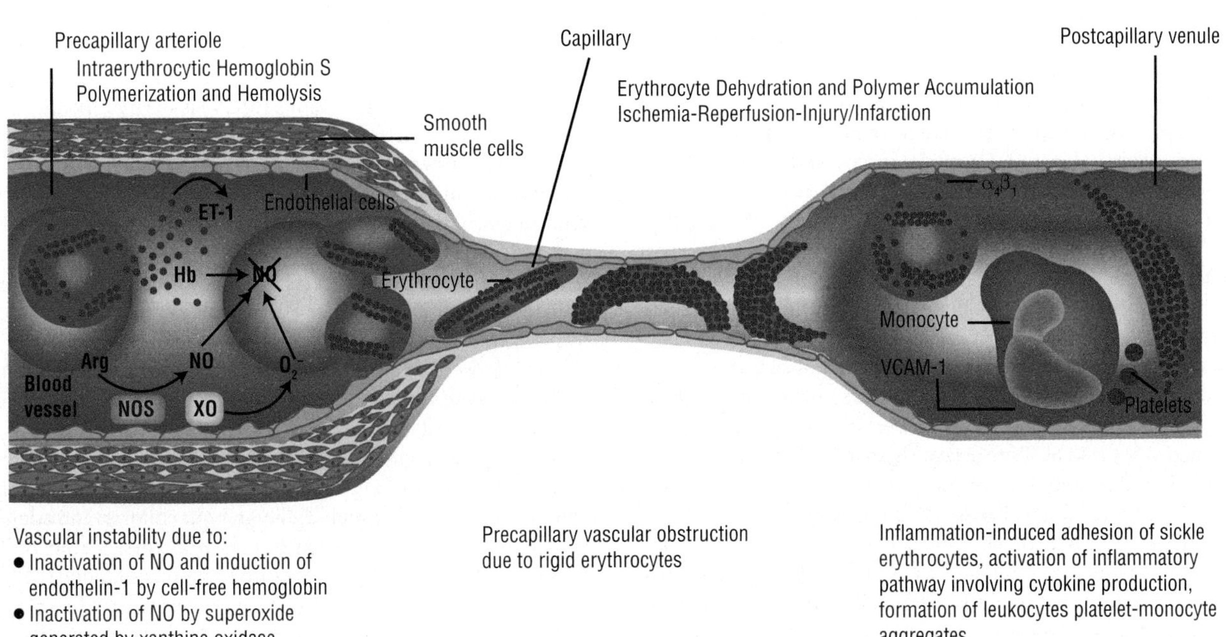

FIGURE 124-5 Pathophysiology of sickle cell disease. (Arg, arginine; ET-1, endothelin-1; NO, nitric oxide; NOS, nitrous oxide synthase; VCAM-1, vascular cell adhesion molecule 1; XO, xanthine oxidase.) *(Reproduced, with permission, from Kato GJ, Gladwin MT. Sickle cell disease. In: Hall JB, Schmidt GA, Wood LDH. Principles of Critical Care. 3rd ed. New York: McGraw Hill, 2005:1658.)*

haplotype, result in a more benign form of SCD. The amount of HbF and HbA_2 in relation to HbS influences the clinical manifestations and accounts for some of the variability in severity among SCD genotypes.[2,3,5]

Intravascular destruction of sickle cells occurs at an accelerated rate. The stress of repetitive sickle–unsickle cycles leads to damage to the cell membrane that promotes recognition and removal of the damaged RBCs by macrophages. Rigid ISCs are easily trapped, resulting in short circulatory survival and chronic hemolysis. The typical sickle cell survives for about 10 to 20 days, while the life span of a normal RBC is 120 days.[7,10] Anemia triggers the release of immature RBCs (reticulocytes) from the bone marrow prematurely. Surface adhesion proteins of reticulocytes adhere to the endothelium in postcapillary venules, further decreasing the movement of mature HbS-containing RBCs through the microvessels.[1-3]

SCD is a complex disease of inflammation as evidenced by leukocytosis, particularly an increase in monocytes and neutrophil counts. Coagulation abnormalities in SCD are the result of continuous activation of the hemostatic system or disorganization of the membrane layer. Sickled cells interact with leukocytes, endothelial cells, and platelets to form an occlusive clot. Hemolysis releases free Hb resulting in generation of reactive oxygen species, nitric oxide (NO) depletion, and vascular inflammation. Chronic NO depletion contributes to vasoconstriction, activation of platelets and adhesion molecules such as vascular cell adhesion molecule 1 and production of the potent vasoconstrictor peptide endothelin-1.[2,3,6,13,20]

Obstruction of blood flow in the spleen by sickle cells can result in functional asplenia, defined as the loss of splenic function with an intact spleen, and eventually splenic atrophy. These patients can have deficient opsonization. Impaired splenic function increases susceptibility to infection by encapsulated organisms, particularly pneumococcal bacteria.[1,5,13]

TABLE 124-1 Clinical Features of Sickle Cell Trait and Common Types of Sickle Cell Disease

Type	Clinical Features
Sickle cell trait (SCT)	Rare painless hematuria; heavy exercise under extreme conditions can provoke gross hematuria and complications (normal Hb)
Sickle cell anemia (SCA- HbSS)	Pain episodes, microvascular disruption of organs (spleen, liver, bone marrow, kidney, brain, and lung), gallstones, priapism, leg ulcers; anemia (Hb 6-9 g/dL [60-90 g/L; 3.72-5.59 mmol/L])
Sickle cell hemoglobin C (HbSC)	Painless hematuria and rare aseptic necrosis of bone; pain episodes are less common and occur later in life; other complications are ocular disease and pregnancy-related problems; mild anemia (Hb 9-14g/dL [90-140 g/L; 5.59-8.69 mmol/L])
Sickle cell β^+-thalassemia (HbSβ^+-thal)	Rare pain; milder severity than HbSS because of the production of some HbA; Hb 9-12 g/dL (90-120 g/L; 5.59-7.45 mmol/L) with microcytosis
Sickle cell β^0-thalassemia (HbSβ^0-thal)	No HbA production; severity similar to SCA; Hb 7-9 g/dL (70-90 g/L; 4.34-5.59 mmol/L) with microcytosis

Data from References 1-4, and 22-24.

CLINICAL PRESENTATION

3 Since 2006, universal newborn screening for SCD is performed in all 50 states. The sensitivity and specificity of screening methods such as isoelectric focusing, high-performance liquid chromatography, and Hb electrophoresis approach 100%. For infants with a positive screening result, a second test should be performed before 2 months of age to confirm the diagnosis. More than 98% newborns in the United States are screened for SCD. Some infants with SCD may not be identified because of extreme prematurity, prior blood transfusion, inability to contact family, and/or immigration from countries where universal screening is not performed.[4,8,21] SCD involves multiple organ systems, and its clinical manifestations vary greatly among genotypes (Table 124-1).[2,21,22]

Persons with SCT are usually asymptomatic. However, under certain extreme situations where Hb oxygenation is altered, RBC sickling can occur in SCT. Sickling of RBCs in the renal medulla, an area with low-oxygen tension, can result in the inability to concentrate urine. Individuals with such impairment can be at risk of dehydration. Microscopic hematuria has been observed, and gross hematuria can occur after heavy exercise. Other reported complications associated with SCT are delayed hemorrhage after eye trauma, venous thromboembolism (VTE), particularly pulmonary embolism, and chronic kidney disease.[12,23] Individuals with SCT should be cautious when participating in exercise under extreme conditions, such as athletic or military training. The US Sudden Death in Athletes Registry reported that 0.9% of 2,462 deaths occurred in athletes with SCT. The events in those 23 athletes with SCT were sudden cardiovascular collapse followed by several minutes of gradually worsening symptoms including dyspnea, fatigue, and weakness during or after vigorous physical activity.[24] Preventive strategies such as gradual conditioning, adequate rest, and hydration are recommended to minimize the risk of sudden death in personnel undergoing athletic or military training.[12,24]

The cardinal features of SCD are hemolytic anemia and vasoocclusion. In individuals with HbSS, anemia usually develops from 4 to 6 months after birth. The delay is due to the presence of HbF in fetal RBCs. HbF production is gradually replaced by HbS, leading to the clinical manifestations of the disease, such as pain and swelling of the hands and feet, commonly referred to as *hand-and-foot syndrome* or *dactylitis* in infants.[4,5,10]

The common clinical signs and symptoms associated with HbSS include chronic anemia and pallor, fever, arthralgia, scleral icterus, abdominal pain, weakness, anorexia, fatigue, hematuria, and enlargement of the liver, spleen, and heart. Laboratory findings include low hemoglobin level around 6 to 9 g/dL (60-90 g/L; 3.72-5.59 mmol/L), elevated reticulocytes of 10% to 25%, elevated lactate dehydrogenase, and elevated platelet and white blood cell (WBC) counts. Mean corpuscular volume (MCV) is normal. The peripheral blood smear demonstrates sickled RBC forms.[4,22]

Individuals with HbSC disease usually present with less severe symptoms than HbSS. The condition is characterized primarily by mild anemia (Hb levels of 9-14 g/dL [90-140 g/L; 5.59-8.69 mmol/L] and reticulocytes of 5%-10%), persistence of splenomegaly into adult life, and excessive target cells in the peripheral blood smear. In individuals with heterozygous HbSβ-thalassemia syndrome, severity of disease depends on the thalassemia mutation involved.[4,22]

Many factors can influence disease severity and mortality in children and adults with SCD. Markers for disease severity in children include dactylitis before 1 year of age, average Hb less than 7 g/dL (70 g/L; 4.34 mmol/L) in the second year of life, and leukocytosis in the absence of infection. Reticulocytosis has been associated with increased death and morbidity in both children and adults.[25,26] Early acute chest syndrome (ACS) during the first 3 years of life is a predictor for recurrent episodes throughout childhood. Children with concomitant SCD and asthma have an increased risk of ACS and pain episodes and increased mortality. Factors associated with decreased survival in adults with SCD include frequency of sickle cell pain, elevated WBC, cerebrovascular events, renal failure, proteinuria, and pulmonary hypertension.[25-28] With improved survival for SCD, chronic manifestations of the disease contribute to the

CLINICAL PRESENTATION Sickle Cell Disease

General

- Most patients in the United States with SCD are diagnosed during newborn screening
- Patients usually have a history of anemia and vasoocclusive pain crisis

Symptoms

- Acute or chronic pain, painful swelling of hands and feet, weakness, anorexia, and fatigue

Signs

- Chronic anemia and pallor, scleral icterus, hematuria, and enlargement of spleen

Laboratory Tests

- Hemoglobin electrophoresis shows over 90% hemoglobin S without the presence of hemoglobin A for the HbSS or HbSβ^0 genotype, about 50% hemoglobin S and C respectively for the HbSC genotype. Low hemoglobin level, elevated reticulocytes, elevated lactate dehydrogenase, and elevated platelet and WBC count. The peripheral blood smear demonstrates sickled RBC forms.

increased morbidity later in life. Additionally, genetic modifiers also affect the severity of SCD. For example, BCL11A is associated with the HbF concentration, and coincident α thalassemia reduces hemolysis.[1]

COMPLICATIONS

Acute Complications

Fever and Infection

Functional asplenia and failure to make antibodies against encapsulated organisms contribute to the high risk of overwhelming sepsis in individuals with SCD. Penicillin prophylaxis and vaccination have significantly reduced the overall risk of *Streptococcus pneumonia* bacteremia, but nonvaccine serotypes of *Streptococcus pneumonia* have been reported.[4,6,13,29] Children with SCD remain at a greater risk of invasive pneumococcal infections when compared to those with other underlying diseases or healthy children.[29,30] Other encapsulated organisms are *Haemophilus influenzae, Neisseria meningitidis,* and *Salmonella,* with the latter known to cause osteomyelitis and pneumonia in SCD. *Mycoplasma pneumoniae* and *Chlamydia pneumoniae* should be considered in older children with infiltrates on chest radiograph. Viral infections such as respiratory syncytial virus, influenza, and parvovirus B19, can result in severe morbidity.[4,31] In children with SCD admitted for bacteremia, coagulase-negative *Staphylococcus* was associated with central venous access; this infection should be considered for those with a permanent indwelling venous catheter. In adults, overt pneumococcal bacteremia is less common. Pathogens such as *Staphylococcus aureus* and gram-negative organisms are associated with immunosuppression, indwelling catheter, and bone and joint infections.[5,32]

All patients with SCD with fever greater than 38.5°C (101.3°F) must be evaluated for infection or sepsis and considered for empiric antibiotic therapy; those with temperature 39.5°C (103.1°F) and appearing ill should be hospitalized. Lumbar puncture may be needed, especially in young and toxic-appearing children.[3,4,22,32]

Children with SCD may experience an aplastic crisis, which is characterized by a decrease in the reticulocyte count, the rapid development of severe anemia, and hypoplastic bone marrow (Table 124-2). An aplastic crisis is most often associated with a viral infection, particularly parvovirus B19.[3,4]

Neurologic

Neurologic abnormalities and cognitive deficits are well documented in patients with SCD. Vasoocclusive processes can lead to cerebrovascular occlusion that manifests as signs and symptoms of overt stroke (Table 124-2). The risk of stroke is highest for HbSS and lowest for HbSβ^+-thal. The incidence of cerebral infarction in HbSS is 11% by age 20 years and 24% by age 45 years with a recurrence rate as high as 70% in 3 years. The highest risk occurs during the first decades, in particular ages 2 to 5 years. The risk is lowest before age 2 secondary to the protective effect of HbF. Ischemic strokes occur in 54% of cerebrovascular accidents with the highest risk before age 10 years and after 30 years of age, whereas hemorrhagic strokes are more common when patients are in their twenties and are associated with poor outcome.[1,4,19,36,38]

In addition to neurologic examination, evaluation of acute events includes computed tomography scan and magnetic resonance imaging (MRI) of the brain. Asymptomatic or silent infarcts are detected by screening MRI. Transcranial Doppler ultrasound (TCD) is important in primary stroke prevention to identify children between 2 and 16 years with abnormal cerebral artery velocities, which are associated with a 40% risk of overt stroke in the subsequent 3 years. Other imaging studies are magnetic resonance angiogram to evaluate for cerebral vasculopathy in patients with persistently abnormal TCD, overt stroke or silent stroke; and magnetic resonance venography to evaluate for cerebral vein thrombosis. In addition, electroencephalography can be helpful in patients with a history of seizure.[4,5,22,36]

About 10% to 30% of individuals who have HbSS with no prior history of stroke have changes on MRI of the brain consistent with infarction or ischemia. Silent cerebral infarcts can be associated with an increased risk of stroke, decreased neurocognitive function, behavioral changes, and poor academic performance.[39] Neurological complications predispose aging adult patients to dementia. Finally, lower intelligence, visual-motor impairments, and neuropsychological dysfunction have been reported in patients not affected by acute or silent strokes and are associated with severity of anemia.[4,5,22,39]

Acute Chest Syndrome

ACS, defined as a new pulmonary infiltrate associated with fever and/or respiratory symptoms, is the second most common cause of hospitalization and a leading cause of death among individuals with SCD (Table 124-2).[1,33,34] The primary causes of ACS are pulmonary vascular occlusion and infection. Vascular occlusion can be caused by fat emboli released from bone marrow, VTE, or direct adhesion of RBCs to the pulmonary vasculature resulting in a vicious cycle of inflammation, hypoxia, and injury to the lung. The most common infectious pathogens causing ACS are *M. pneumonia,*

TABLE 124-2 Acute Sickle Cell Complications

Acute chest syndrome[a]
Clinical features: Peak incidence between ages 2 and 4 years. Clinically resembles pneumonia. Viral causes are more common in children than adults. Hypoxia is associated with outcome.
Signs and symptoms: New radiographic pulmonary infiltrate with one or more of the following: cough, dyspnea, tachypnea, chest pain, fever, wheezing, and new-onset hypoxia (greater than 2% decrease from baseline).
Evaluation: Chest x-ray, CBC, Type and Screen, frequent O_2 monitoring, sputum culture, serology for respiratory organisms.
Acute splenic sequestration[b]
Clinical features: Acute exacerbation of anemia due to sequestration of large blood volume by the spleen. More commonly seen in patients with functioning spleens (eg, infants with HbSS and older children and rarely adults with HbSC disease); onset often is associated with viral or bacterial infections; recurrences are common and can be fatal.
Signs and symptoms: Sudden onset of fatigue, dyspnea, and distended abdomen; rapid decrease in Hb and Hct with elevated reticulocyte count, abdominal pain, splenomegaly, vomiting, hypotension, and shock.
Evaluation: Close monitoring of vital signs, spleen size, and oxygen saturation, CBC, reticulocyte count, type and screen and blood cultures.
Aplastic crisis[c]
Clinical features: Acute decrease in Hb with decreased reticulocyte count (usually <1%); transient suppression of RBC production in response to bacterial or viral infection, most common being parvovirus B19.
Signs and symptoms: Headache, fatigue, dyspnea, pallor, and tachycardia; can also present with fever, upper respiratory or gastrointestinal infection symptoms.
Evaluation: CBC, reticulocyte count, type and screen, cultures (blood, urine, and throat), evaluation of viral infection (eg, parvovirus titers).
Overt stroke[d]
Clinical features: Sudden onset but often proceeded by a transient ischemic attack. Commonly seen in patients with HbSS and HbSβ^0-thal genotypes.
Signs and symptoms: Headache, paralysis or weakness, aphasia, visual disturbances, facial droop and convulsions.
Evaluation: Imaging, CBC, reticulocyte count, HbS quantification, type and screen, prothrombin time, activated partial thromboplastin time, and basic chemistry.
Vasoocclusive pain episodes[e]
Clinical features: Acute painful infarction without changes in Hb; almost all patients with SCA will have episodes of acute pain. Recurrent acute pain results in bone, joint, and organ damage and chronic pain. Vasoocclusive episodes most commonly involve the bones, liver, spleen, brain, lungs, and penis. Acute pain in long bones can be accompanied by signs of inflammation, making it difficult to differentiate from osteomyelitis. Abdominal involvement can resemble a surgical abdomen. Precipitating factors include infection, extreme weather conditions, swimming, excessive physical activity, dehydration, and stress.
Signs and symptoms: Deep throbbing pain; local tenderness, erythema, and swelling can be seen. Fever and leukocytosis are common. Dactylitis usually occurs in young infants. Jaundice and increased transaminases can be present if the liver is involved.
Evaluation: Frequent physical examination, CBC, reticulocyte count, and urinalysis. Based on symptomatology, the following may be needed: needle aspiration to rule out osteomyelitis, abdominal studies (radiograph, computed tomography scan, etc.), liver function tests, bilirubin, blood culture, and chest radiograph.

[a]Data from References 1, 4, 33, and 34.
[b]Data from References 1, 4, 13, 22, and 35.
[c]Data from References 2–4, 22, and 32.
[d]Data from References 1, 2, 4, 22, and 36.
[e]Data from References 1, 3, 4, 22, and 37.
Hct, hematocrit.

respiratory syncytial virus, *C. pneumoniae*, *Staphylococcus aureus*, and *Streptococcus pneumoniae*.[1,4,33,34]

Risk factors for ACS and recurrence include young age, lower HbF, higher leukocytes, history of asthma or bronchial hyper-responsiveness, smoke exposure, and recent history of stroke (overt or silent) or vasoocclusion. Genotype and haplotype also influence risk. Patients with HbSS and HbSβ^0-thal have a higher risk than those with HbSC and HbSβ^+-thal and the risk is higher with African haplotypes than that of Saudi Arabia.[1,4,33,34]

ACS is more common in children but more severe in adults. Hypoxia is a predictor of severity and outcome. In severe cases, computed tomography scan, perfusion scintigraphy, transthoracic echocardiography, and bronchoscopy may be helpful to identify the etiology. Pulmonary changes often involve the lower lobes of the lungs and may cause pleural effusions. Bilateral infiltrates or multiple lobe involvement is associated with poor prognosis.[4,33,34] Pulmonary manifestations must be recognized early and managed aggressively as ACS can rapidly progress to pulmonary failure and death.[33,34]

Priapism

Stasis and sickling of RBCs within the sinusoids of the corpora cavernosa is the primary mechanism of priapism, a sustained painful erection of the penis. The pathophysiology of priapism at the molecular level includes abnormal NO signaling as the result of chronic NO depletion. Stuttering priapism is repeated intermittent attacks up to several hours before remission; ischemic priapism is a persistent painful erection greater than 4 hours and should be considered an emergency. Thirty percent to 45% of boys/men with SCD will present with at least one episode of priapism during their lifetime. The first episodes often occur during childhood. Impotence has been reported after repeated episodes and is directly related to the duration prior to treatment.[1,22,40]

Sickle Cell Pain

Acute episodes of pain are the most common reason for seeking treatment in SCD (Table 124-2). The usual cause of sickle cell pain is microvascular occlusion in the bone marrow. Although fever, infections, dehydration, hypoxia, acidosis, and sudden temperature alterations can precipitate pain, episodes are often unpredictable with no known triggers.[1,4,22] Dactylitis (hand-and-foot syndrome) is a subtype of sickle cell pain occurring in infancy and early childhood that usually does not result in permanent damage.[1,22] Each painful episode is associated with residual damage from inflammation that worsens with recurrence leading to more serious complications such as ACS.[37]

Sickle cell pain may be localized or migratory and is continuous and throbbing. The most common locations are the back, chest, and extremities but pain can occur in any location such as the abdomen or the head and lead to confusion with other acute complications such as stroke.[1,22] Risk factors associated with painful episodes include older age, iron overload, higher Hb, and lower HbF.[2,4,37]

Splenic Sequestration

Splenic sequestration is the sudden massive enlargement of the spleen resulting from the sequestration of sickled RBCs in the splenic parenchyma (Table 124-2). Hct and Hb concentrations fall dramatically with associated reticulocytosis and no evidence of marrow failure or accelerated hemolysis. The trapping of the sickled RBCs by the spleen leads to a decrease in circulating blood volume, which can result in hypotension and shock. The condition is most often seen in infants and children because their spleens are intact; it can cause sudden death in young children due to hypovolemia. Splenic enlargement may also be acutely painful due to rapid capsular expansion. Over time, repeated splenic infarctions lead to autosplenectomy and the spleen can no longer become engorged. Sequestration usually occurs between 1 and 4 years of age for children with HbSS and HbSβ^0-thal and not at older ages because autoinfarction usually is completed by then. For HbSC and HbSβ^+-thal, autoinfarction is delayed and sequestration can occur even during adulthood.[1,4,13,22,35]

Venous Thromboembolism

Patients with SCD are susceptible to VTE due to a hypercoagulable state, endothelial dysfunction, and impaired blood flow. In addition to inflammation and hemostatic abnormalities associated with the disease, other risk factors for thrombosis include central venous access, decreased mobility, and frequent hospitalizations. An increased risk of VTE, deep vein thrombosis, and pulmonary embolism has been reported to be independent of hospitalization frequency.[7,11,13,41] Prevalence rates of 7.4% by age 30 and 11.3% by age 40 were reported.[7] In addition, a recurrence rate of about 25% has been reported.[11] D-dimer testing cannot be used to detect deep vein thrombosis because elevated D-dimers are found in more than 90% of patients with SCD as a result of hemolysis.[13] Awareness of VTE is essential when evaluating patients presenting with ACS or vasoocclusive episodes. Management of VTE is based on the anticoagulation guidelines for the general public and the role of prophylaxis in patients with SCD is unclear.[7]

Chronic Complications

Pulmonary

Over 90% of children survive into adulthood, increasing the contribution of pulmonary manifestations to the morbidity and mortality of SCD. Physical exam and history should be performed to identify signs and symptoms of respiratory conditions such as asthma, restrictive lung disease, and chronic obstructive pulmonary disease. Pulmonary function testing is recommended in symptomatic patients but not as a routine screening tool. Lower predicted FEV1% was associated with earlier death in SCD.[2]

Pulmonary hypertension, defined as a resting mean pulmonary arterial pressure of 25 mm Hg or greater by right heart catheterization, is associated with increased morbidity and mortality in SCD. Symptoms of pulmonary hypertension include shortness of breath during normal activities, fatigue, syncope, and peripheral edema. A less invasive test, tricuspid regurgitant jet velocity by Doppler echocardiography, is frequently performed initially to estimate systolic pulmonary arterial pressure, but this test is not diagnostic of pulmonary hypertension. Serum N-terminal pro-brain natriuretic peptide (NT-pro-BNP) measurement is an alternative test that can be used to estimate the risk of pulmonary hypertension in patients with normal renal function when Doppler echocardiography is not an option. The American Thoracic Society recommends assessment of mortality risk with noninvasive (indirect) or invasive direct measurement to guide management of pulmonary hypertension (Table 124-3).[22,42,43]

Airway inflammation and hyper-responsiveness are common in SCD. Therefore, careful screening for respiratory symptoms in adults and children with SCD is essential. Asthma and wheezing (with or without a diagnosis of asthma) in individuals with SCD have been associated with ACS and vasoocclusive pain episodes and increased mortality. Symptoms of asthma exacerbation can overlap with ACS making it difficult to differentiate the two.[1,4,13,27] For the management of asthma, the National Asthma Education and Prevention Program asthma management guideline should be utilized and inhaled corticosteroids are first line for persistent symptoms.[27]

Skeletal and Skin Diseases

Musculoskeletal complications from vasoocclusion are common in SCD and have a significant impact on quality of life. Osteonecrosis, particularly of the femoral or humeral heads, causes chronic pain, permanent damage, and disability.[11,44] Low bone mineral density can occur early with a prevalence of over 70% reported in adults with SCD. Osteopenia and osteoporosis associated with low bone formation have been reported in individuals with SCD.[4,45] Vitamin D deficiency is common in SCD, especially in children, and is associated with increased bone fragility and vasoocclusive pain episodes.[3-5] Children with SCD also have an increased incidence of osteomyelitis; the organism most often responsible is *Salmonella*.[4,45] Septic arthritis occurs in up to 5% of children but is rare in adults.[44] In addition to necrosis of joints, chronic leg ulcers, most commonly seen in the medial and lateral malleolus (ankles), can become a difficult and painful problem for adults. Ulcers are often seen after trauma or infection and are usually slow to heal.[5,22]

Ocular Manifestations

Ocular problems seen in patients with SCD include orbital and retinal manifestation. The incidence of proliferative sickle retinopathy and vitreous hemorrhage is up to 50%. Vasoocclusion in the eye can occur as early as 20 months of age. Clinically detectable retinal diseases usually occur during adolescence and early adulthood. Orbital involvement is uncommon but has a high potential for severe vision loss. Despite less systemic manifestations, individuals with HbSC develop serious retinal complications more often and earlier than those with HbSS. Lack of visual symptoms does not indicate the absence of ocular manifestations. Annual retinal examination starting at age 10 years is recommended for patients with SCD to prevent blindness from retinopathy and other complications.[22,46]

TABLE 124-3 Risk Stratification and Management Recommendation for Pulmonary Hypertension

	Recommendations	Strength	Evidence Quality
Increased risk for mortality[a]	Hydroxyurea	Strong	Moderate
Increased risk for mortality, unresponsive or not candidates for hydroxyurea	Chronic transfusion therapy	Weak	Low
RHC-confirmed PH, venous thromboembolism, no risk factors for hemorrhage	Indefinite anticoagulant therapy	Weak	Low
Elevated TRV alone	No PAH therapy[b]	Strong	Moderate
Elevated NT-pro-BNP alone	No PAH therapy[b]	Strong	Moderate
RHC-confirmed marked elevation of pulmonary vascular resistance, normal pulmonary artery wedge pressure, presence of related symptoms	• A trial of prostacyclin agonist or endothelin receptor antagonist • Phosphodiesterase-5 inhibitor should not be used as first-line therapy	Weak Moderate	Very low Moderate

[a]Increased risk for mortality: (1) Tricuspid regurgitant jet velocity (TRV) greater than or equal to 2.5 m/s, (2) an N-terminal pro-brain natriuretic peptide (NT-pro-BNP) level greater than or equal to 16 pg/mL (ng/L; 1.9 pmol/L), or (3) right heart catheterization (RHC)-confirmed pulmonary hypertension (PH).

[b]PAH therapy: (1) prostacyclin agonist (epoprostenol, treprostinil, iloprost), (2) soluble guanylate cyclase stimulator (riociguat), (3) endothelin receptor antagonist (bosentan, macitentan, ambrisentan), and (4) phosphodiesterase-5 inhibitor (sildenafil, vardenafil, tadalafil).

Data from References 42 and 43.

Hepatobiliary Diseases

Cholelithiasis is a common complication of SCD resulting from chronic hemolysis and increased bilirubin production, leading to biliary sludge and/or stone formation. The risk of gallstones increases with age: 12% for age 2 to 4 years, 43% by age 15 to 18 years, and 70% to 75% in adults. Cholecystitis, exemplified by pain in the right upper quadrant, can be confused with an acute sickle pain episode in the abdomen. Mild baseline hepatomegaly and elevation of liver function tests can occur in individuals with SCD. Cirrhosis occurred in 18% of young adults with SCD. Causes for the development of chronic hepatic disease include repeated occlusion in the liver, iron overload, and hepatitis.[22,47]

Cardiac Diseases

Cardiovascular complications associated with anemia, including cardiac enlargement and various murmurs, can occur in patients with SCD. Patients experience varying degrees of exertional dyspnea, tachycardia, and palpitation because of the decreased oxygen-carrying capacity of the blood. Left ventricular diastolic dysfunction has been reported in 18% of adults with SCD and is associated with increased mortality, especially in patients with pulmonary hypertension. Left ventricular stiffness and left ventricular hypertrophy have been reported, and can progress to diastolic dysfunction later in life. Acute myocardial infarction in adults with SCD may be under-recognized due to the high incidence of sickle cell acute chest pain.[1,10,48]

Renal Diseases

Renal dysfunction in SCD begins during infancy, as evidenced by glomerular hyperfiltration. Other manifestations include the inability to concentrate urine, hematuria, tubular acidosis, papillary necrosis, glomerulonephritis, microalbuminuria, and proteinuria. Enuresis, as a result of increased urine production, occurs in 42% of children ages 6 to 8 and 9% in young adults ages 18 to 20. Microalbuminuria, present in 42% of adults with the HbSS disease, is typically the first sign of chronic kidney disease, which has been associated with increased mortality.[6,7,22,49,50] In adults with SCD, cystatin C may better correlate with eGFR compared to serum creatinine.[7]

TREATMENT

Desired Outcomes

The goal of treatment is to reduce hospitalizations, complications, and mortality as well as improve quality of life. Management involves the use of general measures to meet the unique demands with the goal of preventing or treating complications of the disease. When an acute complication occurs, the type and severity of the episode determine the appropriate therapeutic plan.

With the availability of public health programs and comprehensive care, most children in developed countries survive through childhood and the burden of reducing mortality has shifted to focus on adults with SCD.[1,7,10] The life expectancy for individuals with SCD is lower than the general population by at least 20 years and a particularly vulnerable period appears to be during the transition to adult medical care.[4,7] Outcome evaluation for management of SCD should include assessment of health-related quality of life in both adults and children.

All patients with SCD should receive regularly scheduled comprehensive medical evaluations. Because of the complexity of the disease, an interprofessional team is needed to provide high-quality medical care, education, counseling, and psychosocial support. Appropriate comprehensive care can have a positive impact on both longevity and quality of life. This care includes the use of evidence-based treatment combining general symptomatic supportive care, preventative medical therapies, and specific disease modifying therapies aimed at altering hematologic capacity and function.

Routine Health Maintenance

SCD is a complex chronic disease involving multiple organs. In addition to the preventive care recommended for the general population, individuals with SCD also need health maintenance and screenings that focus on minimizing complications (Table 124-4).

Growth and development in children with SCD should be monitored as delayed growth and sexual maturation are common.[4,10,39] Depression, anxiety, and other behavior issues are more common in children and adults with SCD than in the general population and have a significant impact on quality of life. Psychosocial supports are essential elements of care for individuals with SCD as well as their caretakers.[9,55] Pregnancy introduces an increased risk for the mother with SCD and for the fetus. Reproductive counseling and education should be incorporated into the care of individuals with SCD.[22,56]

Immunizations

Administration of routine immunizations is crucial preventive care in managing SCD. Children 6 months and older and adults with SCD should receive influenza vaccine annually. The COVID-19 vaccine should also be recommended to individuals with SCD. The most updated immunization and catch-up schedules are provided by the Centers for Disease Control and Prevention (http://www.cdc.gov/vaccines/schedules).

Impaired splenic function increases susceptibility to infection by encapsulated organisms, particularly *Streptococcus pneumoniae*. Prior to the routine use of penicillin prophylaxis and the development of pneumococcal vaccines, invasive pneumococcal disease was 20- to 100-fold more common in children with SCD than in healthy children. Reduced mortality has been associated with the introduction of pneumococcal vaccines.[1,4]

Two different pneumococcal vaccines are available. The 13-valent pneumococcal conjugate vaccine (PCV13) induces good antibody responses in infants and children less than 2 years of age. Immunization with the PCV13 is recommended for all children, regardless of SCD status, younger than 24 months of age. Infants should receive the first dose after 6 weeks of age. Two additional doses should be given at 2-month intervals, followed by a fourth dose at age 12 to 15 months. The 23-valent pneumococcal polysaccharide vaccine (PPSV23) is recommended for all children with functional or acquired asplenia but must be given after 2 years of age because of poor antibody response. To cover different serotypes, PPSV23 should be given starting at 2 years of age, and be administered 2 months after the last dose of the PCV13. A booster dose of PPSV23 is recommended 5 years after the first dose. Both pneumococcal vaccines are recommended for adults with certain medical conditions, including SCD (Table 124-4).[51]

The risk of meningococcal disease is also higher in SCD and vaccination is recommended for individuals with functional or acquired asplenia. Two types of meningococcal vaccines are available: (1) quadrivalent (serogroups A, C, Y, and W-135) meningococcal conjugate vaccines (MenACWY-CRM and MenACWY-D) and (2) meningococcal group B vaccine (MenB-FHbp and Menb-4C). Infants with functional asplenia should receive four-dose series with MenACWY-CRM at 2, 4, 6, and 12 months. Children over 2 years and adults with functional or acquired asplenia should receive a primary immunization series with two doses of the quadrivalent vaccine given 8 weeks apart. MenACWY-D should be given at age 2 years or older and at least 4 weeks after completion of all PCV13. A booster is recommended every 5 years for individuals with SCD.[22,52,54] Group B meningococcal vaccination is given to children with functional asplenia 10 years of age or older as a two-dose (MenB-FHbp or Menb-4C) or three-dose (MenB-FHbp) immunization series and these two vaccines are not interchangeable (Table 124-4).[52,54]

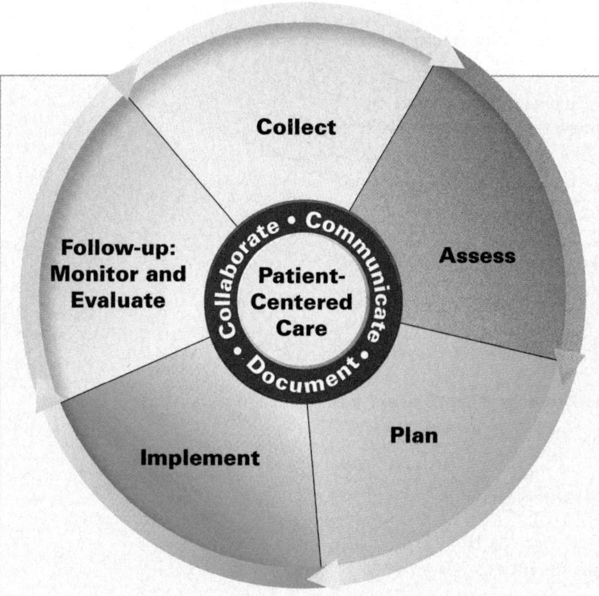

Patient Care Process for Vasoocclusive Episodes

The image shows the five fundamental steps included in The Pharmacist's Care Process endorsed by the Joint Commission for Pharmacy Practitioners (2014). The tagline of this process reads collaborate, communicate, and document. The five fundamental steps listed here are collect, assess, plan, implement, and follow-up: monitor and evaluate. All these steps are listed in a circular block diagram.

Collect

- Patient characteristics (eg, age, sex, sickle cell disease genotypes)
- Patient medical history (include organ function and psychosocial issues)
- Immunization history
- Social history (eg, tobacco use)
- Pain diary
- Medication use
- Blood transfusion history
- Objective data
  - Vital signs: blood pressure, heart rate, respiratory rate, height, weight, O_2 saturation
  - Labs: complete blood count (CBC), reticulocytes, basic chemistry, lactate dehydrogenase, ferritin, urine analysis, hemoglobin fractionation
  - Additional labs or imaging per presenting symptoms (see Table 124-2)

Assess

- Hemodynamic stability
- Pain scale
- Adherence to home medication
- Sign or symptom associated with sickle cell acute complications (see Table 124-2)

Plan*

- Fluid
- Pain management (see Table 124-6)
- Initiate antibiotics if febrile
- Oxygen

Implement

- Provide education on current pain regimen
- Develop individualized plan for pain management
- Evaluate for initiation of hydroxyurea, L-glutamine, voxelotor, crizanlizumab
- Schedule follow-up

Follow-up: Monitor and Evaluation

- Ongoing evaluation of pain level
- Monitor for adverse drug reactions of pain medication and initiate supportive care if needed

**Collaborate with patients, caregivers, and other healthcare professionals.*

Pharmacologic Therapy

Penicillin

4 Penicillin prophylaxis until at least 5 years of age is recommended in children with SCD HbSS or HbSβ⁰-thal, even if they have received PCV13 or PPSV23 immunization, as prophylaxis against invasive pneumococcal infections. An effective regimen that reduces the risk of pneumococcal infections by 84% is penicillin V potassium at a dosage of 125 mg orally twice daily until the age of 3 years, followed by 250 mg twice daily until the age of 5 years. Individuals who are allergic to penicillin can be given erythromycin 20 mg/kg/day. Penicillin prophylaxis is not routinely given in older children, based on a study demonstrating no benefit over placebo beyond the age of 5 years. However, continuation of oral pneumococcal prophylaxis should be considered on a case-by-case basis and is recommended for anyone with a history of invasive pneumococcal infection or surgical splenectomy.[22,32]

Hydroxyurea

HbF reduces polymer formation of HbS due to its high oxygen affinity and its inability to polymerize with HbS. Higher HbF levels are associated with decreased RBC sickling and RBC adhesion and observational studies show a relationship between higher HbF concentration and lower severity of SCD. Individuals with SCD and low HbF levels experience more frequent pain and higher mortality. HbF levels of 20% or greater are associated with a lower risk of acute sickle cell complications. Based on these observations, HbF induction has become a treatment modality for patients with SCD.

Hydroxyurea, a chemotherapeutic agent, stimulates HbF production and increases the number of HbF-containing reticulocytes and intracellular HbF. The drug inhibits DNA synthesis by blocking the conversion of ribonucleoside to deoxyribonucleotides. The exact mechanism of HbF production is unknown, but its myelosuppressive effect stimulates stress erythropoiesis, triggers rapid erythroid regeneration, and shifts erythrocyte Hb production to HbF. In addition, hydroxyurea increases NO levels, reduces neutrophils and monocytes, has antioxidant properties, alters the RBC membrane, increases RBC deformability by increasing intracellular water content, and decreases RBC adhesion to the endothelium.

Hydroxyurea is FDA-approved for patients 2 years of age and older with recurrent moderate-to-severe painful crises to reduce

TABLE 124-4 Health Maintenance

Invasive Pneumococcal Infection Prevention
1. Oral penicillin until age 5 for children with HbSS/Sβ°-thal
   a. Discontinue penicillin prophylaxis at age 5 unless have had splenectomy or invasive pneumococcal infection
2. Consider no penicillin prophylaxis for children with HbSC disease and HbSβ⁺-thal unless they have had a splenectomy

Immunization
1. All individuals should receive immunization according to the Advisory Committee on Immunization Practices
2. Pneumococcal Vaccine
   a. All infants should receive complete series of PCV13
   b. All children should receive PPSV23 at age 2 years and second dose at age 5 years
   c. Children age 2-5 years with incomplete PCV13 vaccination
      i. Unvaccinated or less than three doses PCV13: Two doses of PCV13 with second dose 8 weeks apart
      ii. Received three doses of PCV13 but none after 12-month of age: One dose of PCV13
      iii. Give two doses of PPSV23 after the PCV13 series completed. First dose at least 8 weeks after PCV13 and second dose at least 5 years later
   d. Children age 6-18 years not received PCV13 should receive one dose of PCV13.
   e. Children age 6-18 years not received PPSV23 should receive two doses of PPSV23. First dose at least 8 weeks after PCV13 and second dose at least 5 years later
   f. Adults age 19-64 years not previously received PCV13 or PPSV23:
      i. One dose PCV13
      ii. Two doses PPSV23. First dose at least 8 weeks after PCV13 and second dose at least 5 years later
   g. Adults age 19-64 years previously received PPSV23
      i. One dose PCV13 at least 1 year after last PPSV23
      ii. One dose of PPSV23 at least 5 years after first dose and no sooner than 8 weeks after PCV13
3. Haemophilus Influenza (Hib) Vaccine
   a. Children age greater than 5 years who have not previously received Hib vaccine should receive one dose
4. Meningococcal Vaccine (indicated for persons have functional or anatomic asplenia)[a]
   a. Four-dose primary series to be administered with MenACWY-CRM (2, 4, 6, and 12 months)
   b. Booster dose to be administered with MenACWY-CRM or MenACWY-D
      i. Primary series completed prior to age 7: Booster dose 3 years after primary series and repeat every 5 years thereafter
      ii. Primary series completed age 7 or older: Booster dose 5 years after primary series and repeat every 5 years thereafter
   c. Unvaccinated children 7-23 months: Two doses of MenACWY-CRM with second dose at least 12 weeks after the first dose AND after first birthday
   d. Unvaccinated children age 2 years or older and adults: Two doses of MenACWY-CRM or MenACWY-D 8-12 weeks apart
      i. MenACWY-D to be given at least 4 weeks after completion of all PCV13 doses
   e. Adults previously vaccinated should receive MenACWY-CRM or MenACWY-D every 5 years
   f. Serogroup B Meningococcal (MenB): Age 10 or older
      i. MenB-FHbp (Trumenba®): Three-dose series (at 0, 1-2, and 6 months); or two-dose series (at 0 and 6 months)
      ii. MenB-4C (Bexsero®): Two-dose series at least 1 month apart
5. Influenza vaccine annually for age 6 months and older

Renal
1. Screen for proteinuria by age 10 and annually if negative
2. Initiate ACE inhibitor for adults with microalbuminuria or proteinuria without apparent cause

Pulmonary Hypertension (PH)
1. Noninvasive tests (Doppler echocardiography or alternatively, serum NT-pro-BNP measurement) can be used to assess mortality risk
2. Echocardiogram to screen for PH and associated cardiac problems by age 8 for those with frequent cardiorespiratory symptoms
3. The optimal frequency for Doppler echocardiography is unknown but every 1-3 years seems to be reasonable
4. Children with evidence of PH by echocardiogram should be further evaluated: Pulmonary function test, polysomnography, oxygenation assessment, and thromboembolic disease
5. Cardiac catheterization should be performed before initiation of PAH-specific therapy

Ophthalmological Evaluation
1. Dilated eye examination begins at age 10 and rescreen at 1-2 year intervals

Stroke Prevention
1. Children with SCA: Transcranial Doppler (TCD) annually beginning at age 2 until at least age 16
2. Chronic transfusion therapy for stroke prevention in children with elevated (>200 cm/s) TCD results

[a]Brand name for meningococcal vaccine: MenACWY-CRM (Menveo®) and MenACWY-D (Menactra®)

Data from References 22, 32, 35, 42, and 51-54.

PCV13, 13-valent conjugate pneumococcal vaccine; PPSV23, 23-valent pneumococcal polysaccharide vaccine; ACE Inhibitor, angiotensin converting enzyme inhibitor; PAH, pulmonary artery hypertension; PH, pulmonary hypertension.

the frequency of painful crises and the need for blood transfusions. The Multicenter Study of Hydroxyurea in Sickle Cell Anemia (MSH Trial) was the first double-blind, placebo-controlled randomized controlled trial of hydroxyurea in adults with SCD. In that study, hydroxyurea significantly reduced the frequency of painful episodes, risk of ACS, need for blood transfusions, and number of hospitalizations in adults with SCD. A follow-up study showed a 40% reduction in mortality with hydroxyurea over a 9-year period and this trend continued when the original 299 patients from the MSH study were followed for 17.5 years.[10,26,57,58]

Studies in pediatric patients reported similar results to the MSH Trial with no adverse effects on growth and development. Some patients treated with hydroxyurea had possible recovery or preservation of splenic and brain function, including cognitive performance. The Transcranial Doppler with Transfusions Converting to Hydroxyurea study (TWiTCH) closed early after interim analysis showed that hydroxyurea was not inferior to chronic blood transfusions to prevent primary stroke. However, the Stroke with Transfusions Changing to Hydroxyurea (SWiTCH) trial also closed early when the interim analysis showed that hydroxyurea was inferior to chronic transfusions to prevent recurrent stroke. Therefore, chronic transfusion with iron chelation to treat transfusion-related iron overload is the preferred therapy to prevent stroke.[10,26,57,58] Initiating hydroxyurea early, prior to the development of complications may be beneficial. The Pediatric Hydroxyurea Phase III Clinical Trial (BABY HUG) randomized young children ages 9 to

18 months to hydroxyurea or placebo. Although investigators found no significant difference in the primary endpoints (splenic and renal function), children treated with hydroxyurea had fewer episodes of pain and dactylitis with no significant toxicities.[6,57,59] Hydroxyurea reduced the risk of painful events, ACS, renal enlargement, hospitalizations, and transfusions. In addition, improved urine concentration ability as demonstrated by higher urine osmolality was reported.[57,58] In a retrospective study of hydroxyurea therapy in children aged 3 to 18 years with SCD, a significant reduction in mortality, fewer hospitalizations and emergency visits, and shorter hospital stays were reported.[60]

The most common adverse drug reaction of hydroxyurea is bone marrow suppression, resulting in neutropenia, thrombocytopenia, anemia, and decreased reticulocyte count. These hematologic adverse drug reactions usually recover within 2 weeks of therapy discontinuation. Other adverse drug reactions include dry skin and hyperpigmentation of skin or nails.[4,22,57,59] Long-term adverse effects of hydroxyurea therapy in patients with SCD are not fully known, although no serious adverse effects were reported in the long-term (17.5 years) follow-up study of the MSH trial. There is no delays in growth or puberty, increased risk of infections, or genotoxicity for children.[61] Myelodysplasia, acute leukemia, and chronic opportunistic infection associated with T-lymphocyte abnormalities have been reported in other patient populations treated with higher doses of hydroxyurea. Reproductive toxicity is also a concern. High-dose hydroxyurea is teratogenic in animals, but normal pregnancies have been reported in women with SCD who received hydroxyurea during pregnancy.[57]

Although hydroxyurea was only FDA-approved for patients age 2 years and older with SCD in 2017, the agent has been used in pediatric patients for years.[1,3,4,22] Clinical indications for hydroxyurea include frequent painful episodes, severe symptomatic anemia, a history of ACS, or other severe vasoocclusive complications (Table 124-5). The starting dose for adults is 15 mg/kg/day rounded to the nearest 500 mg as a single daily dose. A lower dose of 5 to 10 mg/kg/day is used for patients with chronic kidney disease. The recommended initial dose for children is 20 mg/kg. Dosage can be increased by 5 mg/kg up to a maximum of 35 mg/kg in 8-week intervals if the patient does not demonstrate adverse drug reactions and blood counts are stable (Fig. 124-6). Hydroxyurea dosage should be individualized based on response and toxicity. In general, 3 to 6 months of therapy are required before improvement is observed. Medication adherence can be an issue. Since the MCV generally increases as the level of HbF increases, monitoring MCV is an inexpensive and convenient method to monitor response and adherence.[1,3,4,22,57]

5 Patients receiving hydroxyurea should be closely monitored for toxicity. Blood counts should be checked every 2 weeks during dose titration and every 4 to 8 weeks thereafter. Treatment should be interrupted if hematologic indices fall below the following values: absolute neutrophil count, 2,000 cells/mm^3 (2×10^9/L); platelet count, 80,000 cells/mm^3 (80×10^9/L); hemoglobin, 5 g/dL (50 g/L; 3.1 mmol/L); or reticulocytes, 80,000 cells/mm^3 (80×10^9/L) if the Hb concentration is less than 9 g/dL (90 g/L; 5.59 mmol/L). Other laboratory abnormalities warranting temporary discontinuation of therapy are a 50% increase in serum creatinine and a 100% increase in transaminases. After recovery has occurred, treatment should be resumed at a dose that is 5 mg/kg/day lower than the dose associated with toxicity. If no toxicity occurs after 12 weeks with the lower dose, the dose can be increased by 2.5 to 5 mg/kg/day. If the increased dose produces hematologic toxicity, the patient should be maintained at the last tolerated dose with no further escalation except for normal growth or weight gain.[22,57,58]

L-Glutamine

Sickled RBCs are susceptible to oxidative damage leading to hemolysis and vasoocclusion. Glutamine, an essential amino acid, is a precursor for nicotinamide adenine dinucleotide (NAD$^+$) synthesis. There is an increased uptake of glutamine by sickle RBCs, mainly to produce NAD$^+$. Children with SCD have lower glutamine levels; an increase of NAD$^+$ can potentially restore the redox balance in oxidative stressed cells.

In a phase III double-blind, placebo-controlled trial, L-glutamine significantly reduced the median number of pain episodes and the number of hospitalizations over the study period of 48 weeks. L-glutamine was well tolerated overall but nausea, noncardiac chest pain, fatigue, and musculoskeletal pain were more commonly reported in the L-glutamine group.[62]

L-glutamine was FDA-approved in July 2017, becoming the first product approved for pediatric patients with SCD and the first new treatment for adults in almost 20 years. It is indicated for patients with SCD age 5 and older to reduce the acute complications of SCD. The product is available in 5-g packets and should be mixed with 8 ounces of liquid (~240 mL) or 4 to 6 ounces (~110-170 g) of food. The recommended dose is based on weight: 5 g twice a day for less than 30 kg; 10 g twice a day for 30 to 65 kg and 15 g twice a day for greater than 65 kg. The most common gastrointestinal adverse drug reactions are constipation, abdominal pain, and nausea.[63]

TABLE 124-5 Recommendations on Hydroxyurea Therapy

	Recommendation	Strength	Evidence Quality
Adults with HbSS or HbSβ^0-thalassemia			
• Three or more sickle cell–associated moderate-to-severe pain crises per year	Treat with hydroxyurea	Strong	High
• Sickle cell–associated pain that interferes with daily activities and quality of life		Strong	Moderate
• History of severe and/or recurrent ACS		Strong	Moderate
• Severe symptomatic chronic anemia that interferes with daily activities or quality of life		Strong	Moderate
Infants 9 months of age and older, children, and adolescents with HbSS or HbSβ^0-thalassemia regardless of clinical severity	Offer hydroxyurea	Strong	High (age 9-42 months); Moderate (>42 months)
Sickle nephropathy with persisting proteinuria despite therapy	Consider hydroxyurea	Weak	Low
Chronic hypoxia	Treat with hydroxyurea	Strong	Low
HbSC or HbSβ$^+$-thalassemia with recurrent sickle cell–associated pain that interferes with daily activities or quality of life	Consider hydroxyurea	Moderate	Low
History of stroke and unable to implement chronic transfusion	Initiate hydroxyurea	Moderate	Low

Data from References 57 and 58.

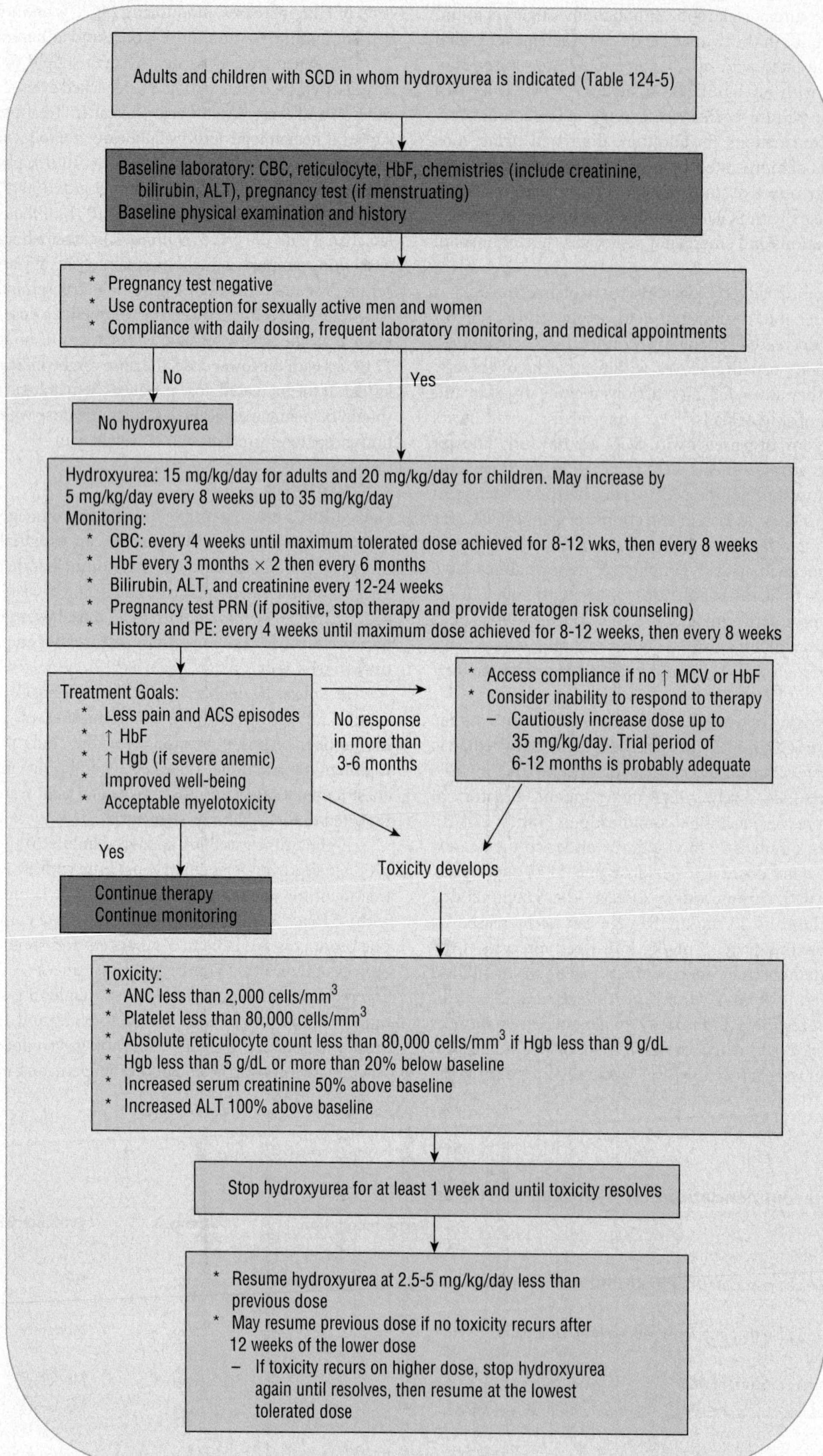

FIGURE 124-6 Hydroxyurea use in sickle cell disease. Blood test results expressed in SI units that are consistent with toxicity are $<2 \times 10^9$/L for ANC; $<80 \times 10^9$/L for platelets; $<80 \times 10^9$/L for absolute reticulocyte count if Hb <90 g/L (5.59 mmol/L); and Hb <50 g/L (3.10 mmol/L). (ALT, alanine aminotransferase; ANC, absolute neutrophil count; PE, physical examination; PRN, as needed.) (*Data from References 1, 3, 4, and 22.*)

Crizanlizumab

Adherence of erythrocytes and leukocytes to the endothelium causes vascular obstruction in SCD and increased severity of the disease. The expression of adhesion molecules, including P-selectin, on the surface of endothelial cells and platelets, contributes to this process. Blockage of P-selectin reduces the adhesion of sickle erythrocytes and leukocytes, and improves microvascular blood flow. Thus, P-selectin plays an important role in vasoocclusion and microcirculatory abnormalities in SCD.[8,9]

Crizanlizumab is a monoclonal antibody against P-selectin. In a phase II double-blind, randomized, placebo-controlled trial (the SUSTAIN trial), high-dose crizanlizumab (5 mg/kg) significantly reduced the annual rate of vasoocclusive crises from 2.98 per year in the placebo group to 1.63 per year (45% reduction) and increased the median time to the first vasoocclusive crisis. The risk of serious adverse drug reactions was similar between crizanlizumab and placebo groups, with arthralgia, diarrhea, pruritus, vomiting, and chest pain more common in the crizanlizumab group.[10]

Crizanlizumab was granted FDA approval in November 2019; it is indicated for patients ≥16 years old with SCD. It is available as an intravenous (IV) solution (100 mg/10 mL). The dosing regimen is 5 mg/kg once every 2 weeks for the first two doses, followed by 5 mg/kg once every 4 weeks.

Voxelotor

The sickling and unsickling process of erythrocytes due to HbS polymerization damages the cell membrane and results in hemolysis. It contributes to SCD-related complications, including anemia, pulmonary hypertension, leg ulcers, priapism, and chronic kidney disease, and can be mitigated by inhibiting HbS polymerization.[11]

In a phase III double-blind, randomized, placebo-controlled trial (the HOPE trial), 274 patients with SCD were randomly assigned to the placebo, the 900 mg or the 1,500 mg voxelotor group. The percentage of patients with an Hb increase of more than 1 g/dL (10 g/L; 0.62 mmol/L) after 24-week treatment was significantly higher in the 1,500 mg voxelotor group than in the placebo group. The voxelotor group also experienced improvement in the hemolytic markers. The risk of adverse drug reactions was comparable in all three groups, with headache and diarrhea reported in ≥20% of the 1,500 mg voxelotor group.[12] Similar results were observed after 72-week treatment.[13]

In November 2019, FDA approved voxelotor for the treatment of SCD in patients ≥12 years of age. It is available in oral tablet of 500 mg, and the recommended dose is 1,500 mg taken once daily, with a dose adjustment to 1,000 mg once daily in severe hepatic impairment (Child Pugh class C). As a CYP3A4 substrate, concomitant use of voxelotor with strong CYP3A4 inducers or inhibitors should be avoided, or dose adjusted if not avoidable.

Chronic Transfusion Therapy

RBC transfusions play an important role in the management of SCD. In acute illness, transfusions can be life-saving. Chronic transfusion programs can prevent complications of SCD. The primary indication for chronic transfusion is primary and secondary stroke prevention and amelioration of organ damage.[4,64] Blood transfusions can be administered as a simple transfusion, a manual exchange or an automated exchange called erythrocytapheresis. Exchange transfusion frequently requires permanent venous access and is associated with higher cost but has the advantage of increasing normal (donor) HbA, limiting volume, minimizing hyperviscosity, and limiting transfusional iron overload.[22]

6 Chronic transfusions should be considered in children with SCD and adults with previous stroke or children with abnormal TCD measurements.[22] Prophylactic transfusions reduced the incidence of first stroke from 16% to 2% over a 2-year period in children 2 to 16 years of age who were at an increased risk for stroke based on abnormal annual TCD screening.[64] In children with an overt stroke, chronic transfusions reduced stroke recurrence from about 50% to about 10% over 3 years. Chronic transfusions may also be useful in patients with severe or recurrent ACS, debilitating pain, chronic organ failure, intractable leg ulcers, severe chronic anemia with cardiac failure, and complicated pregnancies, although support for the efficacy of chronic transfusion in these situations is limited.[65]

The goal of transfusions is to achieve and maintain an HbS concentration of less than 30% of total hemoglobin in the primary and secondary prevention of neurologic complications. Transfusions are usually given every 3 to 4 weeks, but the frequency of transfusion is adjusted to maintain the desired HbS levels. The risk of recurrent stroke decreases after 2 years of transfusion therapy and, in the absence of recurrent stroke, many clinicians will liberalize the HbS goal to less than 50%.[4,64] The optimal duration of primary prophylactic transfusion therapy in children with abnormal TCD is not clear. Based on the results of the TWiTCH trial, some patients can safely transition to hydroxyurea therapy after normalization of TCD and no evidence of cerebral vasculopathy with at least a 6-month overlap in transfusions and hydroxyurea therapy. Discontinuation of transfusions has been associated with a 50% stroke recurrence rate within 12 months in children with a previous stroke and abnormal blood flow velocity on TCD. For secondary stroke prevention, transfusions should be continued indefinitely.[4,57,64] Hydroxyurea could be started prior to discontinuation of transfusion for secondary stroke prevention with at least a 6-month overlap with transfusions. However, the phase III trial of switching hydroxyurea for transfusion in secondary stroke prevention, the SWiTCH trial, was closed early due to an increased risk of recurrent strokes in the hydroxyurea arm when compared to the transfusions arm.[38] The National Institutes of Health recommends hydroxyurea for prevention of recurrent stroke only if implementation of a transfusion program is not possible.[22]

Although the benefits of transfusion therapy are clear in some clinical situations, its role in other situations such as priapism or an acute pain episode remains controversial.[22] The risks of transfusion therapy must be weighed against possible benefits. The risks associated with transfusion therapy include alloimmunization (sensitization to the blood received), hyperviscosity, transfusion-transmitted viral infections, volume overload, iron overload, and nonhemolytic transfusion reactions. The use of leukocyte-reduced RBC transfusions in chronically transfused patients can reduce the risk of nonhemolytic transfusion reactions.[4,64,65] All patients should be immunized with hepatitis A and B vaccines. Other viruses that can be transmitted through blood products are parvovirus B19, hepatitis C, cytomegalovirus, and HIV.[32,64]

Alloimmunization or alloantibody formation results from antigen differences on the red cell surface between the primarily Caucasian donor pool and recipients with SCD and can cause delayed hemolytic transfusion reactions (DHTRs). Alloimmunization occurs in 19% to 37% of SCD patients who receive RBC transfusions and can make it difficult to find cross-matched blood. To prevent alloimmunization, patients receiving chronic transfusions should receive the best cross-matched blood including extended typing of other RBC antigens especially C, E, and Kell or full RBC phenotyping.[22,64,65]

The development of alloimmunization can be life threatening for individuals with SCD. DHTRs usually occur within 7 to 10 days after transfusion of blood to which the recipient is immunized, but it can occur as early as 2 days or as late as 20 days after transfusion. During a DHTR, patients develop worsening pain, especially abdominal pain, severe anemia due to hemolysis of the transfused unit and reticulocytopenia, further aggravating the anemia. Subsequent transfusions can further worsen the clinical situation because of the presence of multiple antibodies making cross-matching difficult. Life-threatening events can be treated with steroids and intravenous immunoglobulin. Recombinant erythropoietin has been used in patients with reticulocytopenia.[22,64,65] Recovery, as evidenced by reticulocytosis with a gradual increase in the Hb level, may occur only after further transfusions are withheld. Although some patients tolerate further transfusions after recovery, especially if the donor unit is negative for the offending alloantibody, others cannot avoid recurrent transfusions and may experience another hemolytic transfusion reaction. Rituximab has been used to prevent recurrent DHTR. It is generally preferable to prevent the development of DHTR by performing RBC phenotyping and, at a minimum, transfusing individuals with blood that is C, E, and Kell negative.[4,22,65]

Transfusional iron overload is an important complication of RBC transfusions and patients should be instructed to not take iron supplements.[64,65] Abnormal liver biopsy results showing mild-to-moderate inflammation, fibrosis, or cirrhosis have been reported. Iron overload assessments, including serum ferritin and liver function tests, should be performed semiannually. Iron overload can be confirmed by liver biopsy or less invasively by MRI.[22,65] Three chelating agents are available. Deferoxamine has been used as a chelating agent for decades but must be administered by subcutaneous or intravenous infusion. The oral chelation agents, deferasirox and deferiprone, are as effective as deferoxamine with acceptable safety profiles in long-term studies up to 5 years.[66-68] Deferasirox is available in two forms. Exjade® is a dissolving tablet given once daily on an empty stomach starting at 20 mg/kg/day. Jadenu® is given as a film-coated tablet or sprinkle granule once daily on an empty stomach or with a light meal starting at a lower dose of 14 mg/kg/day. The common adverse drug reactions for deferasirox are transient skin rash and gastrointestinal symptoms such as nausea, vomiting, diarrhea, and abdominal pain. However, some patients may prefer film-coated tablets as it is more palatable and can be taken with food. Deferiprone has good oral bioavailability but a short half-life. The usual starting dose for deferiprone is 75 mg/kg/day, given in three divided doses. Similar to deferasirox, the common adverse drug reactions for deferiprone are rashes and gastrointestinal symptoms but the most concerning adverse drug reactions are neutropenia and agranulocytosis. For patients who require more aggressive management, deferoxamine in combination with either oral agent has been reported.[66-69]

Allogeneic Hematopoietic Stem Cell Transplantation

Allogeneic HSCT is a curative therapy for patients with SCD. The overall and disease-free survival rate for children and young adults with human leukocyte antigen (HLA)-matched sibling donors has been reported at 95% to 98% and 87% to 92%, respectively.[70,71] The reported incidences of acute and chronic graft-versus-host disease (GVHD) ranged from 5% to 17% and 0% to 3%, respectively. Other complications included seizures, marrow rejection, and sepsis. Improved growth, stabilization or improvement of CNS abnormalities, and recovery of splenic dysfunction were observed in post-transplant patients with SCD, but gonadal failure and delayed sexual development in girls requiring hormonal replacement have been reported.[72]

The optimal candidates for matched sibling donor transplant are SCD patients with severe disease (HbSS and HbSβ^0) prior to the onset of SCD symptoms, but the procedure should also be considered in patients with a history of stroke, elevated TCD velocity, recurrent ACS, recurrent pain, red cell alloimmunization on chronic transfusion protocol, pulmonary hypertension, and sickle nephropathy.[73,74] Unfortunately, many children who are eligible for HSCT do not have an HLA-matched sibling donor and unrelated HLA-matched transplants are associated with higher transplant-related mortality. However, matched unrelated allogeneic HSCT is considered for SCD patients who are younger than 16 years of age and have severe complications from SCD. Because allogeneic HSCT performed in young children before organ damage and alloimmunization occur is associated with increased success, counseling and screening for HLA-matched sibling donors during the first year of life is recommended. The risks associated with allogeneic HSCT must be carefully considered, as the transplant-related mortality rate is about 5% to 10%, and graft rejection is about 10%. Other risks associated with allogeneic HSCT include secondary malignancies. Neurologic events, such as intracranial hemorrhage and seizures during transplant, were seen more frequently in patients with a history of stroke.[73,74] Tacrolimus and cyclosporine should be used with caution and the blood pressure aggressively controlled due to the increased risk of posterior reversible encephalopathy syndrome, estimated to be 22%, with calcineurin inhibitors in SCD patients undergoing allogeneic HSCT.[75]

Umbilical cord blood is another potential donor source of hematopoietic stem cells with some advantages over marrow donors, including a lower incidence of severe GVHD and a larger donor pool from which to select donors, but such advantages are offset by longer time to engraftment and a higher rate of graft rejection.[72-74] Several protocols are under investigation with haploidentical donors, such as parents, for patients with recurrent stroke on chronic transfusions or severe SCD symptoms with no HLA-matched sibling donors. Recent studies with haploidentical donors have reported stable engraftment and low rates of acute and chronic GVHD, leading to similar outcomes compared to HSCT with HLA-matched donors.[76]

HSCT with myeloablative conditioning has traditionally been limited to children and young adults with SCD due to an increased risk of GVHD or transplant-related mortality with older age.[77] HSCT with HLA-matched donors and nonmyeloablative conditioning regimens resulted in mixed donor-recipient chimerism, reversal of acute SCD complications, and low rates of transplant-related toxicity or GVHD.[70-72,74] Conditioning with alemtuzumab, total body irradiation, and post-transplant sirolimus in adults with SCD up to the age of 65 years old resulted in stable engraftment in 87% of recipients with no observed chronic GVHD.[78]

TREATMENT OF COMPLICATIONS

Parents and older children should be educated on the signs and symptoms of complications and conditions that require urgent evaluation. During acute illness, patients should be evaluated promptly because deterioration can occur rapidly. Fluid balance should be maintained as either dehydration or fluid overload can worsen complications associated with SCD. Oxygen saturation by pulse oximetry should be maintained at least 92% or at baseline. New or increasing supplemental oxygen requirements should be investigated.

Acute Sickle Cell Pain

Hydration and analgesia are the mainstays of treatment for vasoocclusive (painful) episodes (Table 124-6). Patients with mild pain crises can be treated as outpatients with rest, increased fluid intake, warm compresses, and oral analgesics. Hospitalization is necessary for moderate-to-severe pain or when oral analgesics fail to relieve pain. A pain episode may be precipitated by several risk factors including infection. In the setting of pain and fever, an infectious etiology should be considered and appropriate empiric therapy should be initiated. In patients with severe symptomatic anemia, transfusions may be indicated. Fluid replacement given intravenously or orally to correct or prevent hydration at 1 to 1.5 times the maintenance requirement is recommended. Close monitoring of fluid status is essential as aggressive hydration, particularly with sodium-containing fluids, can lead to volume overload, ACS, and heart failure.[4,10,13,22]

The frequency and severity of acute pain episodes associated with SCD are variable. Pain should be assessed and analgesic therapy should be tailored for each patient and each individual episode.

TABLE 124-6 Management of Acute Pain of Sickle Cell Disease

Principles

1. Treat underlying precipitating factors
2. Avoid delays in analgesia administration
   a. Initiate analgesic within 30 minutes of triage or 60 minutes of registration
3. Use pain scale to assess severity
4. Choice and dose of initial analgesic should be based on the home regimen, previous pain pattern, history of response, current status, and other medical conditions. The following initial dosages may be considered if an individualized plan unavailable:
   a. Morphine (IV): 0.1-0.15 mg/kg/dose for less than 50 kg; 5-10 mg/dose for greater than 50 kg
   b. Hydromorphone (IV): 0.015-0.02 mg/kg for less than 50 kg; 1.5 mg/dose for greater than 50 kg
   c. Ketorolac 0.5 mg/kg IV up to 30 mg/dose
5. Schedule pain medication; avoid as-needed dosing
6. Provide rescue dose for breakthrough pain
7. If adequate pain relief can be achieved with one or two doses of morphine, consider outpatient management with a weak opioid; otherwise hospitalization is needed for parenteral analgesics
8. Frequently assess to evaluate pain severity and adverse drug reactions; titrate dose as needed
9. Treat adverse effects of opioids as part of pain management
10. Consider nonpharmacologic intervention (eg, relaxation techniques, guided imagery, deep breathing)
11. Transition to oral analgesics as the patient improves; choose an oral agent based on previous history, anticipated duration, and ability to swallow tablets; if sustained-release products are used, a product with a rapid onset is also needed for breakthrough pain

Analgesic regimens

Mild-to-moderate pain: nonopioid ± weak opioid

Moderate-to-severe pain: weak opioid or low dose of a strong opioid ± nonopioid

Severe pain: strong opioid + nonopioid

Other adjunct therapy

Hydration, heating pads, relaxation, and distraction

Nonopioid analgesic including transdermal lidocaine and NSAIDs

Laxatives for constipation

Antihistamine for itching

Antiemetics for nausea or vomiting

Data from References 4, 10, 11, 79–81, and 82.

Several verbal and nonverbal pain assessment tools are available to measure pain intensity, but these tools have not been validated for sickle cell pain. Pain scales validated for use in children, such as the Wong-Baker FACES scale, should be used in pediatric patients with SCD pain. The healthcare provider should choose one tool appropriate for age and use it to assess pain. However, numeric scales alone should not be the only assessment of pain severity. Other useful information to guide the choice of analgesics includes previous effective agents and their dosages, response to therapy and previous clinical course, and duration of pain episodes.[10,83,84] Individualized patient-specific protocols and standardized pathways improve the quality of pain management.[79,81,85]

8 Aggressive therapy that relieves pain and enables the patient to attain maximum functional ability should be initiated in patients with acute pain. Mild-to-moderate pain should be treated with nonsteroidal anti-inflammatory drugs (NSAIDs) or acetaminophen, unless there are contraindications to their use. Ketorolac may be useful for patients requiring intravenous therapy. Because of the increased risk of gastrointestinal bleeding, the duration of therapy should be limited to 5 days or less. NSAID use has been associated with acute nonreversible kidney failure in a patient with SCD and should be done with caution and monitoring of renal function.[82] When acetaminophen is used, it is important to monitor the total dose of acetaminophen administered because of the risk of hepatic toxicity. Patients may also be receiving the agent for fever or another acetaminophen-containing product for pain. If mild-to-moderate pain persists, an opioid can be added.[10,22,79,80,83]

Severe pain should be treated aggressively until the pain is tolerable. Commonly used opioids include morphine, hydromorphone, fentanyl, and methadone. The weak opioids, codeine, and hydrocodone are used to manage mild-to-moderate pain usually in the outpatient setting. Some patients have clinically demonstrated inadequate relief to analgesic dosing with codeine. Some individuals who failed oral therapy with codeine were found to have a polymorphism in the *CYP2D6* gene resulting in a poor metabolizer phenotype. The CYP2D6 enzyme mediates the metabolism of codeine to morphine.[83,86] These results can lead to early discontinuation of codeine analgesics if no response is seen after their first dose and use of alternative oral analgesics for the treatment of pain at home. Meperidine has no advantages as an analgesic and many disadvantages. Meperidine toxicity is caused by accumulation of the metabolite normeperidine, which can cause adverse drug reactions in the central nervous system, ranging from dysphoria to seizures. Effective combination therapy, such as an NSAID and an opioid, can enhance analgesic efficacy while decreasing adverse drug reactions.

Both prior history and current assessment should be considered in the management of acute sickle cell pain. For patients whose typical pain improves in a short time, preparations with a short duration of action are appropriate. For patients whose pain requires many days to resolve, sustained-release preparations combined with a short-acting product for breakthrough pain are more appropriate. If the patient has been on long-term opioid therapy at home, tolerance can develop. In these cases, acute pain should be treated with an opioid of different potency or a larger dose of the same medication. Low dose ketamine has been evaluated as an adjunct therapy for individuals with severe pain despite high dose opioid therapy. The consensus guidelines on the use of intravenous ketamine for acute pain management recommends that ketamine may be considered for opioid-dependent or -tolerant patients with acute or chronic sickle cell pain. The dosing range is not well defined but the guideline recommends the bolus dose not to exceed 0.35 mg/kg and the infusion rate not to exceed 1 mg/kg/hr.[87]

Intravenous opioids provide a rapid onset of action and therefore are preferred for severe pain. Intramuscular injections should be avoided. Children may actually deny pain due to fear of injections. Analgesics should be titrated to pain relief. In patients with continuous pain, the analgesic should be given as a scheduled dose or continuous infusion. Continuous infusion has the advantage of less fluctuation of blood levels between dosing intervals. As needed dosing is only indicated for breakthrough pain. Patient-controlled analgesia (PCA) is commonly prescribed for severe pain episodes. When used properly, PCA allows patients to have control over pain therapy and minimizes the lag time between perception of pain and administration of analgesics. PCA use reduces the cumulative dosage required for pain control. Another route of administration to produce rapid pain relief is intranasal administration of an opioid such as fentanyl. The transdermal fentanyl patch has also been used successfully, but its role in sickle cell acute pain crisis is unclear because of its slow onset of pain relief (12-16 hours) and fixed dosage form, which makes it difficult to titrate the dose.[4,10,11,13,80,83]

Chronic Sickle Cell Pain

As the number of adults living with SCD increases due to improved survival, the prevalence of disease morbidities including chronic pain also increases. As outpatients, 55% of adults reported pain in more than half of the days and 29% of adults reported pain on 95% of the days. The 2014 Export Panel Report described pain as chronic when it lasts more than 3 months. Diagnostic criteria for chronic SCD pain syndrome are available.[88]

Treatment of chronic pain in SCD requires an interprofessional team approach. Most physicians with expertise in treating SCD follow established guidelines for chronic pain. Much of the research has focused on the prevention of pain and the management of acute pain episodes. Central sensitization, neurogenic inflammation, and peripheral neural sensitization have been hypothesized to play a role in the development of chronic SCD pain.[34,40] The evidence supports other medications such as selective serotonin reuptake inhibitors, serotonin–norepinephrine reuptake inhibitors, and anticonvulsants commonly used to treat chronic pain in patients with SCD. In a pilot study, pregabalin reduced pain and improved quality of life scores.[89] Nonpharmacological interventions such as acupuncture, massage, cognitive behavioral therapy, and relaxation therapy have also been used as adjunct therapy.

Episodic Transfusions for Acute Complications

Indications for acute blood transfusion include: (1) acute exacerbation of baseline anemia, such as aplastic crisis if the anemia is severe, hepatic or splenic sequestration, or severe hemolysis; (2) ACS, stroke, intrahepatic cholestasis, or acute multisystem organ failure; and (3) preparation for procedures that require the use of general anesthesia.[22] Acute transfusion is not indicated for priapism, uncomplicated pain or asymptomatic anemia. Simple transfusion or partial exchange transfusion can be used, though red cell exchange has superior outcomes when compared to simple transfusion in overt stroke. If simple transfusion is used, volume overload leading to congestive heart failure can occur if anemia is corrected too rapidly in patients with severe anemia. Acute increases in hemoglobin level to greater than 10 g/dL (100 g/L; 6.21 mmol/L) can cause hyperviscosity and should be avoided.[3,22]

Infection and Fever

Fever in a patient with SCD should be considered a medical emergency with rapid administration of intravenous antibiotics due to the risk of overwhelming sepsis. Patients with SCD should be evaluated as soon as possible for any fever greater than 38.5°C (101.3°F). Criteria for hospitalization include an infant younger than 1 year, history of previous bacteremia or sepsis, temperature greater than 39.5°C (103.1°F), WBC greater than 30,000 cells/mm^3 (30×10^9/L) or less than 5,000 cells/mm^3 (5×10^9/L), platelets less than 100,000 cells/mm^3 (100×10^9/L), or evidence of other acute complications or toxic appearance. Outpatient management can be considered in older nontoxic children with reliable family caregivers. Antibiotic choice should provide adequate coverage for encapsulated organisms.[4,22,32,90]

7 Ceftriaxone should be used for outpatient management because it provides coverage for 24 hours unless the patient has received ceftriaxone in the previous 8 weeks and then ampicillin should be given due to ceftriaxone-induced hemolysis.[91] For patients with cephalosporin allergy, clindamycin can be used. Vancomycin should be considered for acutely ill children or if *Staphylococcus* is suspected. Vancomycin trough levels should be closely monitored to ensure therapeutic levels are attained while minimizing the 4.5-fold greater risk for acute kidney injury with this antibiotic.[92,93] A macrolide antibiotic should be added if *M. pneumoniae* is suspected such as in ACS. Penicillin prophylaxis should be discontinued while the patient is receiving broad-spectrum antibiotics. Acetaminophen or ibuprofen can be used for fever control. Increased fluid requirement may be present because of poor oral intake and/or increased insensible losses contributing to dehydration.[13,32]

Cerebrovascular Accidents

Patients with acute neurologic events must be hospitalized and monitored closely. Physical and neurologic examination should be performed every 2 hours. Acute treatment for children should include exchange transfusion to maintain Hb at about 10 g/dL (100 g/L; 6.21 mmol/L) and HbS less than 30%, anticonvulsants for patients with a seizure history, and therapy for increased intracranial pressure if needed. Chronic transfusion therapy should be initiated for children with ischemic stroke as discussed earlier. In adults presenting with ischemic stroke related to atherosclerotic disease and not occlusion by sickled red cells, thrombolytic therapy should be administered if it is less than 3 hours since the onset of symptoms.[13,22,36,94]

Acute Chest Syndrome

All patients with SCD admitted for a vasoocclusive crisis should use incentive spirometry frequently (eg, at least every 2 hours while awake) to reduce atelectasis development. In addition, proper management of pain is important. The goal is to provide relief while avoiding analgesic-induced hypoventilation. Appropriate fluid therapy is important as overhydration can cause pulmonary edema. For patients who develop ACS, early use of broad-spectrum antibiotics, including a macrolide or quinolone in adults, is recommended. Infection is a common cause of ACS and can involve gram-positive, gram-negative, or atypical bacteria as well as viral infection. Oxygen therapy is indicated for all patients who are hypoxic. In a patient with a history of reactive airway disease, asthma or wheezing on examination, a trial of bronchodilators is appropriate. Transfusions are indicated for severe ACS with worsening hypoxia and increased work of breathing.[13,33,34]

Steroids can decrease inflammation and endothelial cell adhesion. Their use can decrease the duration of hospitalization and need for transfusions and other supportive care but can also increase the readmission rate for other SCD-related complications. Another potential therapy is NO, which relaxes and dilates blood vessels. Its hematologic effects include inhibition of platelet aggregation and reduction in the polymerization tendency of HbS. Marked improvement of pulmonary status and cardiac output were reported in some patients with ACS.[33,34]

Priapism

Stuttering priapism, episodes that last a few minutes to 2 hours, may resolve spontaneously with exercise, warm bath, and oral analgesics. Prolonged episodes lasting more than 2 to 3 hours require prompt medical attention. The initial goals of treatment are to provide appropriate analgesic therapy, reduce anxiety, produce detumescence, and preserve testicular function and fertility. Treatment given within 4 to 6 hours can usually reduce erection. Aggressive hydration and adequate pain control should be initiated. Heat (hot water bottles, hot packs, or sitz baths) can provide comfort without precipitating a pain crisis. Although transfusions have been given to these patients, they are not recommended because they are not efficacious and may be associated with severe neurologic sequelae if the Hb concentration is raised too precipitously.[40,95]

Clinicians have used both vasoconstrictors and vasodilators in the treatment of priapism. Vasoconstrictors, such as diluted phenylephrine (10 mcg/mL) or epinephrine (1 mcg/mL), are thought to work by forcing blood out of the corpus cavernosum into the venous return. In one uncontrolled, open-label study, aspiration followed by intra-penile irrigation of epinephrine was well tolerated and effective in 37 of 39 episodes. The procedure should be performed by a urologist with experience in the treatment of priapism.[13,40,95]

Vasodilators, such as terbutaline and hydralazine, relax the smooth muscle of the vasculature. This relaxation allows oxygenated arterial blood to enter the corpus cavernosum, which displaces or washes out the damaged sickle cells. Terbutaline has been used to treat priapism, but it has not been formally studied in patients with SCD.[40,95] Antiandrogens, bicalutamide and finasteride, have been used in SCD for treatment of recurrent or refractory priapism without major adverse drug reactions.[95] Surgical interventions used in severe refractory priapism have included a variety of shunt procedures. These surgical procedures have been successful in some cases, but they have a high failure rate and potentially serious complications, which include impotence, skin sloughing, cellulitis, and urethral fistulas.[40,95]

Modalities to prevent priapism are limited and not well studied. Pseudoephedrine (30 or 60 mg/day given orally at bedtime) and leuprolide, a gonadotropin-releasing hormone, have been used. In one case report, a single oral sildenafil dose at onset of priapism aborted episodes. However, long-term studies of sildenafil show an increase in the frequency of pain episodes.[40,95] The results of a randomized, double-blind, placebo-controlled trial to evaluate efficacy and safety of sildenafil at a dose of 50 mg/day to prevent recurrent episodes was inconclusive partly due to a small sample size.[96] Hydroxyurea promotes NO release but its effect on priapism has not been established.[97] Some clinicians transfuse patients to maintain an HbS level less than 30% to prevent recurrent priapism. Duration of such regimens should be limited to 6 to 12 months. Long-term chronic transfusions to prevent priapism are not recommended.[22,95]

Aplastic Crisis

Treatment of aplastic crisis is primarily supportive. Most patients recover spontaneously within 5 to 10 days. The only treatment may be blood transfusion if the anemia is severe or symptomatic. The reticulocyte count is used to detect the suppression of RBC production and the need for transfusion. The most common cause, parvovirus B19, is contagious and infected patients should be placed in isolation. In addition, contact with pregnant healthcare providers should be avoided because parvovirus infection during the midtrimester of pregnancy can result in hydrops fetalis and stillbirth.[4,13,32]

Splenic Sequestration

Splenic sequestration is a major cause of mortality in young children with SCD. The sequestration of RBCs in the spleen can result in a rapid drop of hemoglobin, leading to hypovolemia, shock, and death. Immediate treatment with fluid resuscitation and blood transfusions is indicated to correct hypovolemia. Broad-spectrum antibiotic therapy, which includes coverage for *Streptococcus pneumoniae* and *H. influenzae*, can also be beneficial if the patient is febrile as infection can precipitate sequestration.[1,4,22]

Recurrent episodes occur in about half of patients and are associated with increased mortality. Options for the management of recurrence include observation and splenectomy.[22] Increased risk of invasive infection after splenectomy is a concern in young children, but most experts agree individuals with HbSS develop splenic dysfunction as early as 6 months of age and have acquired asplenia by 5 years of age and by 10 to 12 years for those with HbSC. Splenectomy is probably indicated, even after a single sequestration crisis, if that sequestration was life-threatening. Splenectomy should be considered after repetitive episodes, even if they are less serious. For children younger than 2 years of age, some experts recommend chronic blood transfusions to prevent sequestration and delay splenectomy until the age of 2 years, when the risk of post splenectomy septicemia is lower and pneumococcal vaccination has been completed. Splenectomy should also be considered for patients with chronic hypersplenism.[4,13,22,35]

EVALUATION OF THERAPEUTIC OUTCOMES

9 For infants younger than 1 year, medical evaluations every 2 to 4 months are recommended. Beyond 2 years of age, evaluation can be extended to every 6 to 12 months with modifications depending on the severity of the illness. Routine laboratory evaluation includes complete blood cell counts and reticulocyte counts every 3 to 6 months up to 2 years of age, then every 6 to 12 months; HbF level should be screened annually until 2 years of age. The laboratory evaluation should be performed every 2 to 3 months if the patient is receiving hydroxyurea therapy. Renal, hepatobiliary, and pulmonary function should be evaluated annually. TCD screening is recommended to start at age 2 years and to be performed annually for children with HbSS and HbSβ^0. Ophthalmologic examination to screen for retinopathy is recommended at around age 10 to 12 years for those with HbSC and 14 years for HbSS. In patients with recurrent ACS, pulmonary function tests should be done to establish baseline values and identify declines in lung function as well as an evaluation to screen for lower airway hyper-responsiveness.

Immunizations and prophylactic antibiotics must be given. When infections do occur, appropriate antibiotic therapy should be initiated, and the patient should be monitored for laboratory and clinical improvement. The effectiveness of hydroxyurea can be measured as a decrease in the number, severity, and duration of sickle cell pain episodes. HbF concentrations or MCV values can be used as a biomarker of the patient's response to therapy. When painful episodes do occur, the effectiveness of analgesics can be measured by subjective assessments made by the patient and healthcare practitioners. The success of poststroke blood transfusions can be measured by clinical progression or the occurrence of subsequent strokes.

CONCLUSION

SCD is an inherited disorder in the β-globin gene and involves multiple organ systems. Common complications include vasoocclusive pain crisis, ACS infection, stroke, pulmonary hypertension, etc. Several pharmacologic therapies are available. Hydroxyurea, L-glutamine, and crizanlizumab decrease the frequency of pain crises. Voxelotor increases the Hb level. Transfusion therapy and allogeneic HSCT are also used to manage SCD. Changes in organ function and other healthcare maintenance issues need to be monitored regularly.

ABBREVIATIONS

ACS	acute chest syndrome
DHTR	delayed hemolytic transfusion reactions
GVHD	graft-versus-host disease
HbA	hemoglobin A
HbAS	one normal (hemoglobin A) and one sickle cell hemoglobin (hemoglobin S) gene
HbC	hemoglobin C
HbF	fetal hemoglobin
HbS	sickle cell hemoglobin
HbSβ$^+$-thal	hemoglobin sickle cell β$^+$-thalassemia
HbSβ^0-thal	hemoglobin sickle cell β^0-thalassemia
HbSC	one sickle cell hemoglobin (hemoglobin S) gene and one hemoglobin C gene
HbSS	homozygous sickle cell hemoglobin (hemoglobin S)
HLA	human leukocyte antigen
HPFH	hereditary persistence of fetal hemoglobin
HSCT	hematopoietic stem cell transplantation
ISC	irreversibly sickled cell
MCV	mean corpuscular volume
MRI	magnetic resonance imaging
MSH	Multicenter Study of Hydroxyurea in Sickle Cell Anemia
NO	nitric oxide
NSAID	nonsteroidal anti-inflammatory drug
NT-pro-BNP	N-terminal pro-brain natriuretic peptide
PAH	pulmonary artery hypertension
PCA	patient-controlled analgesia
PCV13	13-valent pneumococcal conjugate vaccine
PPSV23	23-valent pneumococcal polysaccharide vaccine
RBC	red blood cell
SCA	sickle cell anemia

SCD	sickle cell disease
SCT	sickle cell trait
TCD	transcranial Doppler ultrasound
VTE	venous thromboembolism
WBC	white blood cell

REFERENCES

1. Alrayyes S, Baghdan D, Haddad RY, et al. Sickle cell disease: An overview of the disease and its systemic effects. *Dis Mon.* 2018;64:283–289.
2. Piel FB, Steinberg MH, Rees DC. Sickle cell disease. *N Engl J Med.* 2017;376:1561–1573.
3. Ware RE, de Montalembert M, Tshilolo L, Abboud MR. Sickle cell disease. *Lancet.* 2017;390:311–323.
4. Quinn CT. Sickle cell disease in childhood: From newborn screening through transition to adult medical care. *Pediatr Clin North Am.* 2013;60:1363–1381.
5. Brousse V, Makani J, Rees DC. Management of sickle cell disease in the community. *BMJ.* 2014;348:1765–1773.
6. Meier ER. Treatment options for sickle cell disease. *Pediatr Clin North Am.* 2018;65:427–443.
7. Thein MS, Igbineweka NE, Thein SL. Sickle cell disease in the older adult. *Pathology.* 2017;49:1–9.
8. Chakravorty S, Williams TN. Sickle cell disease: A neglected chronic disease of increasing global health importance. *Arch Dis Child.* 2015;100:48–53.
9. Madani BM, Raddadi R, Jaouni S, et al. Quality of life among caregivers of sickle cell disease patients: A cross sectional study. *Health Qual Life Outcomes.* 2018;16:176–184.
10. Kanter J, Kruse-Jarres R. Management of sickle cell disease from childhood through adulthood. *Blood Rev.* 2013;27:279–287.
11. Lanzkron S, Haywood C Jr. The five key things you need to know to manage adult patients with sickle cell disease. *Hematology Am Soc Hematol Educ Program.* 2015;2015:420–425.
12. Key NS, Connes P, Derebail VK. Negative health implications of sickle cell trait in high income countries: From the football field to the laboratory. *Br J Haematol.* 2015;170:5–14.
13. Lovett PB, Sule HP, Lopez BL. Sickle cell disease in the emergency department. *Hematol Oncol Clin North Am.* 2017;31:1061–1079.
14. Dueker ND, Della-Morte D, Rundek T, et al. Sickle cell trait and renal function in Hispanics in the United States: The Northern Manhattan Study. *Ethn Dis.* 2017;27:11–14.
15. Ojodu J, Hulihan MM, Pope SN, Grant AM. Incidence of sickle cell trait—United States, 2010. *MMWR Morb Mortal Wkly Rep.* 2014;63:1155–1158.
16. Saraf SL, Molokie RE, Nouraie M, et al. Differences in the clinical and genotypic presentation of sickle cell disease around the world. *Paediatr Respir Rev.* 2014;15:4–12.
17. Serjeant GR, Serjeant BE, Hambleton IR, et al. A plea for the newborn diagnosis of Hb S-hereditary persistence of fetal hemoglobin. *Hemoglobin.* 2017;41:216–217.
18. Kuypers FA. Hemoglobin S polymerization and red cell membrane changes. *Hematol Oncol Clin North Am.* 2014;28:155–179.
19. Telen MJ. Beyond hydroxyurea: New and old drugs in the pipeline for sickle cell disease. *Blood.* 2016;127:810–819.
20. Conran N, Belcher JD. Inflammation in sickle cell disease. *Clin Hemorheol Microcirc.* 2018;68:263–299.
21. Therrell BL Jr, Lloyd-Puryear MA, Eckman JR, Mann MY. Newborn screening for sickle cell diseases in the United States: A review of data spanning 2 decades. *Semin Perinatol.* 2015;39:238–251.
22. National Institutes of Health, National Heart Lung and Blood Institute. Evidence-Based Management of Sickle Cell Disease: Expert Panel Report. Available at http://www.nhlbi.nih.gov/health-pro/guidelines/sickle-cell-disease-guidelines/. Accessed October 15, 2018.
23. Naik RP, Derebail VK, Grams ME, et al. Association of sickle cell trait with chronic kidney disease and albuminuria in African Americans. *JAMA.* 2014;312:2115–2125.
24. Maron BJ, Zipes DP, Kovacs RJ, et al. Eligibility and disqualification recommendations for competitive athletes with cardiovascular abnormalities: Preamble, principles, and general considerations: A scientific statement from the American Heart Association and American College of Cardiology. *Circulation.* 2015;132:e256–e261.
25. Maitra P, Caughey M, Robinson L, et al. Risk factors for mortality in adult patients with sickle cell disease: A meta-analysis of studies in North America and Europe. *Haematologica.* 2017;102:626–636.
26. Meier ER, Fasano RM, Levett PR. A systematic review of the literature for severity predictors in children with sickle cell anemia. *Blood Cells Mol Dis.* 2017;65:86–94.
27. De A, Manwani D, Rastogi D. Airway inflammation in sickle cell disease: A translational perspective. *Pediatr Pulmonol.* 2018;53:400–411.
28. Elmariah H, Garrett ME, De Castro LM, et al. Factors associated with survival in a contemporary adult sickle cell disease cohort. *Am J Hematol.* 2014;89:530–535.
29. Martin OO, Moquist KL, Hennessy JM, Nelson SC. Invasive pneumococcal disease in children with sickle cell disease in the pneumococcal conjugate vaccine era. *Pediatr Blood Cancer.* 2018;65:e26713.
30. Payne AB, Link-Gelles R, Azonobi I, et al. Invasive pneumococcal disease among children with and without sickle cell disease in the United States, 1998 to 2009. *Pediatr Infect Dis J.* 2013;32:1308–1312.
31. Sadreameli SC, Reller ME, Bundy DG, et al. Respiratory syncytial virus and seasonal influenza cause similar illnesses in children with sickle cell disease. *Pediatr Blood Cancer.* 2014;61:875–878.
32. Sobota A, Sabharwal V, Fonebi G, Steinberg M. How we prevent and manage infection in sickle cell disease. *Br J Haematol.* 2015;170:757–767.
33. Farooq S, Abu Omar M, Salzman GA. Acute chest syndrome in sickle cell disease. *Hosp Pract.* 2018;46:144–151.
34. Howard J, Hart N, Roberts-Harewood M, et al. Guideline on the management of acute chest syndrome in sickle cell disease. *Br J Haematol.* 2015;169:492–505.
35. Brousse V, Elie C, Benkerrou M, et al. Acute splenic sequestration crisis in sickle cell disease: Cohort study of 190 paediatric patients. *Br J Haematol.* 2012;156:643–648.
36. Kassim AA, Galadanci NA, Pruthi S, DeBaun MR. How I treat and manage strokes in sickle cell disease. *Blood.* 2015;125:3401–3410.
37. Darbari DS, Ballas SK, Clauw DJ. Thinking beyond sickling to better understand pain in sickle cell disease. *Eur J Haematol.* 2014;93:89–95.
38. Brousse V, Kossorotoff M, de Montalembert M. How I manage cerebral vasculopathy in children with sickle cell disease. *Br J Haematol.* 2015;170:615–625.
39. Glass P, Brennan T, Wang J, et al. Neurodevelopmental deficits among infants and toddlers with sickle cell disease. *J Dev Behav Pediatr.* 2013;34:399–405.
40. Anele UA, Le BV, Resar LM, Burnett AL. How I treat priapism. *Blood.* 2015;125:3551–3558.
41. Brunson A, Lei A, Rosenberg AS, White RH, et al. Increased incidence of venous thromboembolism in sickle cell disease patients: Risk factors, recurrence and impact on mortality. *Br J Haematol.* 2017;178:319–326.
42. Abman SH, Hansmann G, Archer SL, et al. Pediatric Pulmonary Hypertension: Guidelines from the American Heart Association and American Thoracic Society. *Circulation.* 2015;132:2037–2099.
43. Klings ES, Machado RF, Barst RJ, et al. An official American Thoracic Society clinical practice guideline: Diagnosis, risk stratification, and management of pulmonary hypertension of sickle cell disease. *Am J Respir Crit Care Med.* 2014;189:727–740.
44. Vanderhave KL, Perkins CA, Scannell B, Brighton BK. Orthopaedic manifestations of sickle cell disease. *J Am Acad Orthop Surg.* 2018;26:94–101.
45. Osunkwo I. An update on the recent literature on sickle cell bone disease. *Curr Opin Endocrinol Diabetes Obes.* 2013;20:539–546.
46. Do BK, Rodger DC. Sickle cell disease and the eye. *Curr Opin Ophthalmol.* 2017;28:623–628.
47. Shah R, Taborda C, Chawla S. Acute and chronic hepatobiliary manifestations of sickle cell disease: A review. *World J Gastrointest Pathophysiol.* 2017;8:108–116.
48. Gladwin MT. Cardiovascular complications and risk of death in sickle-cell disease. *Lancet.* 2016;387:2565–2574.
49. Nath KA, Hebbel RP. Sickle cell disease: Renal manifestations and mechanisms. *Nat Rev Nephrol.* 2015;11:161–171.
50. Sharpe CC, Thein SL. How I treat renal complications in sickle cell disease. *Blood.* 2014;123:3720–3726.
51. Bennett N. Use of 13-valent pneumococcal conjugate vaccine and 23-valent pneumococcal polysaccharide vaccine for adults with immunocompromising conditions: Recommendations of the Advisory Committee on Immunization Practices (ACIP). *MMWR Morb Mortal Wkly Rep.* 2012;61:816–819.
52. Patton ME, Stephens D, Moore K, MacNeil JR. Updated Recommendations for Use of MenB-FHbp Serogroup B Meningococcal Vaccine: Advisory Committee on Immunization Practices, 2016. *MMWR Morb Mortal Wkly Rep.* 2017;66:509–513.

53. Cohn AC, MacNeil JR, Clark TA, et al. Use of 13-valent pneumococcal conjugate vaccine and 23-valent pneumococcal polysaccharide vaccine among children aged 6-18 years with immunocompromising conditions: Recommendations of the Advisory Committee on Immunization Practices (ACIP). *MMWR Morb Mortal Wkly Rep.* 2013;62:521–524.
54. Cohn AC, MacNeil JR, Clark TA, et al. Prevention and control of meningococcal disease: Recommendations of the Advisory Committee on Immunization Practices (ACIP). *MMWR Recomm Rep.* 2013;62(RR-2):1–28.
55. Sehlo MG, Kamfar HZ. Depression and quality of life in children with sickle cell disease: The effect of social support. *BMC Psychiatry.* 2015;15:78–85.
56. Smith-Whitley K. Reproductive issues in sickle cell disease. *Hematology Am Soc Hematol Educ Program.* 2014;2014:418–424.
57. Qureshi A, Kaya B, Pancham S, et al. Guidelines for the use of hydroxycarbamide in children and adults with sickle cell disease: A British Society for Haematology Guideline. *Br J Haematol.* 2018;181:460–475.
58. Wong TE, Brandow AM, Lim W, Lottenberg R. Update on the use of hydroxyurea therapy in sickle cell disease. *Blood.* 2014;124:3850–3857.
59. Thornburg CD, Files BA, Luo Z, et al. Impact of hydroxyurea on clinical events in the BABY HUG trial. *Blood.* 2012;120:4304–4310.
60. Lobo CL, Pinto JF, Nascimento EM, Moura PG, Cardoso GP, Hankins JS. The effect of hydroxcarbamide therapy on survival of children with sickle cell disease. *Br J Haematol.* 2013;161:852–860.
61. Rana S, Houston PE, Wang WC, et al. Hydroxyurea and growth in young children with sickle cell disease. *Pediatrics.* 2014;134:465–472.
62. Niihara Y, Miller ST, Kanter J, et al. A phase 3 trial of l-glutamine in sickle cell disease. *N Engl J Med.* 2018;379:226–235.
63. Endari™ [package insert]. Torrance, CA: Emmaus Medical; 2017.
64. Chou ST. Transfusion therapy for sickle cell disease: A balancing act. *Hematology Am Soc Hematol Educ Program.* 2013;2013:439–446.
65. Smith-Whitley K, Thompson AA. Indications and complications of transfusions in sickle cell disease. *Pediatr Blood Cancer.* 2012;59:358–364.
66. Calvaruso G, Vitrano A, Di Maggio R, et al. Deferiprone versus deferoxamine in sickle cell disease: Results from a 5-year long-term Italian multi-center randomized clinical trial. *Blood Cells Mol Dis.* 2014;53:265–271.
67. Chaudhary P, Pullarkat V. Deferasirox: Appraisal of safety and efficacy in long-term therapy. *J Blood Med.* 2013;4:101–110.
68. Vichinsky E, Torres M, Minniti CP, et al. Efficacy and safety of deferasirox compared with deferoxamine in sickle cell disease: Two-year results including pharmacokinetics and concomitant hydroxyurea. *Am J Hematol.* 2013;88:1068–1073.
69. Ware HM, Kwiatkowski JL. Evaluation and treatment of transfusional iron overload in children. *Pediatr Clin North Am.* 2013;60:1393–1406.
70. Fitzhugh CD, Abraham AA, Tisdale JF, Hsieh MM. Hematopoietic stem cell transplantation for patients with sickle cell disease: Progress and future directions. *Hematol Oncol Clin North Am.* 2014;28:1171–1185.
71. Walters MC, De Castro LM, Sullivan KM, et al. Indications and results of HLA-identical sibling hematopoietic cell transplantation for sickle cell disease. *Biol Blood Marrow Transplant.* 2016;22:207–211.
72. Thompson LM, Ceja ME, Yang SP. Stem cell transplantation for treatment of sickle cell disease: Bone marrow versus cord blood transplants. *Am J Health Syst Pharm.* 2012;69:1295–1302.
73. Angelucci E, Matthes-Martin S, Baronciani D, et al. Hematopoietic stem cell transplantation in thalassemia major and sickle cell disease: Indications and management recommendations from an international expert panel. *Haematologica.* 2014;99:811–820.
74. King A, Shenoy S. Evidence-based focused review of the status of hematopoietic stem cell transplantation as treatment of sickle cell disease and thalassemia. *Blood.* 2014;123:3089–3094.
75. Gaziev J, Marziali S, Paciaroni K, et al. Posterior reversible encephalopathy syndrome after hematopoietic cell transplantation in children with hemoglobinopathies. *Biol Blood Marrow Transplant.* 2017;23(9):1531–1540. doi:10.1016/j.bbmt.2017.05.033 28602890.
76. de la Fuente J, Dhedin N, Koyama T, et al. Haploidentical bone marrow transplantation with post-transplantation cyclophosphamide plus thiotepa improves donor engraftment in patients with sickle cell anemia: Results of an international learning collaborative. *Biol Blood Marrow Transplant.* 2019;25(6):1197–1209. doi:10.1016/j.bbmt.2018.11.027 30500440.
77. Gluckman E, Cappelli B, Bernaudin F, et al. Sickle cell disease: An international survey of results of HLA-identical sibling hematopoietic stem cell transplantation. *Blood.* 2017;129(11):1548–1556. doi:10.1182/blood-2016-10-745711 27965196.
78. Alzahrani M, Damlaj M, Jeffries N, et al. Non-myeloablative human leukocyte antigen-matched related donor transplantation in sickle cell disease: Outcomes from three independent centres. *Br J Haematol.* 2021;192(4):761–768. doi:10.1111/bjh.17311.
79. Krishnamurti L, Smith-Packard B, Gupta A, Campbell M, et al. Impact of individualized pain plan on the emergency management of children with sickle cell disease. *Pediatr Blood Cancer.* 2014;61:1747–1753.
80. Telfer P, Bahal N, Lo A, Challands J. Management of the acute painful crisis in sickle cell disease: A re-evaluation of the use of opioids in adult patients. *Br J Haematol.* 2014;166:157–164.
81. Tanabe P, Silva S, Bosworth HB, et al. A randomized controlled trial comparing two vaso-occlusive episode (VOE) protocols in sickle cell disease (SCD). *Am J Hematol.* 2018;93:159–168.
82. Han J, Saraf SL, Lash JP, Gordeuk VR. Use of anti-inflammatory analgesics in sickle-cell disease. *J Clin Pharm Ther.* 2017;42:656–660.
83. Brandow AM, DeBaun MR. Key components of pain management for children and adults with sickle cell disease. *Hematol Oncol Clin North Am.* 2018;32:535–550.
84. Naegeli AN, Heath L, Zhou C, et al. Psychometric properties of a modified version of the faces pain scale-revised (Modified FPS-R) to evaluate worst pain in children and adolescents with sickle cell anemia. *J Pediatr Hematol Oncol.* 2018;40:499–503.
85. Kavanagh PL, Sprinz PG, Wolfgang TL, et al. Improving the management of vaso-occlusive episodes in the pediatric emergency department. *Pediatrics.* 2015;136:e1016–1025.
86. Yee MM, Josephson C, Hill CE, et al. Cytochrome P450 2D6 polymorphisms and predicted opioid metabolism in African American children with sickle cell disease. *J Pediatr Hematol Oncol.* 2013;35:e301–e305.
87. Schwenk ES, Viscusi ER, Buvanendran A, et al. Consensus guidelines on the use of intravenous ketamine infusions for acute pain management from the American Society of Regional Anesthesia and Pain Medicine, the American Academy of Pain Medicine, and the American Society of Anesthesiologists. *Reg Anesth Pain Med.* 2018;43:456–466.
88. Dampier C, Palermo TM, Darbari DS, et al. AAPT diagnostic criteria for chronic sickle cell disease pain. *J Pain.* 2017;18:490–498.
89. Schlaeger JM, Molokie RE, Yao Y, et al. Management of sickle cell pain using pregabalin: A pilot study. *Pain Manag Nurs.* 2017;18:391–400.
90. Ellison AM, Smith Whitley K, Kittick M, et al. A standardized clinical pathway to decrease hospital admissions among febrile children with sickle cell disease. *J Pediatr Hematol Oncol.* 2018;40:111–115.
91. Neuman G, Boodhan S, Wurman I, et al. Ceftriaxone-induced immune hemolytic anemia. *Ann Pharmacother.* 2014;48:1594–1604.
92. Han J, Zhang X, Oderinde J, et al. Increased vancomycin dosing requirements in sickle cell disease due to hyperfiltration-dependent and independent pathways. *Haematologica.* 2017 Aug;102(8):e282–e284. doi:10.3324/haematol.2017.169128.
93. Saraf SL, Viner M, Rischall A, et al. HMOX1 and acute kidney injury in sickle cell anemia. *Blood.* 2018 Oct 11;132(15):1621–1625. doi:10.1182/blood-2018-05-853929.
94. Adams RJ, Cox M, Ozark SD, et al. Coexistent sickle cell disease has no impact on the safety or outcome of lytic therapy in acute ischemic stroke: Findings from Get With The Guidelines-Stroke. *Stroke.* 2017;48:686–691.
95. Olujohungbe A, Burnett AL. How I manage priapism due to sickle cell disease. *Br J Haematol.* 2013;160:754–765.
96. Burnett AL, Anele UA, Trueheart IN, et al. Randomized controlled trial of sildenafil for preventing recurrent ischemic priapism in sickle cell disease. *Am J Med.* 2014;127:664–668.
97. Anele UA, Mack AK, Resar LMS, Burnett AL. Hydroxyurea therapy for priapism prevention and erectile function recovery in sickle cell disease: A case report and review of the literature. *Int Urol Nephrol.* 2014;46:1733–1736.

Drug-Induced Hematologic Disorders

e125

Elisa M. Greene and Tracy M. Hagemann

KEY CONCEPTS

1. The most common drug-induced hematologic disorders are aplastic anemia, agranulocytosis, megaloblastic anemia, hemolytic anemia, and thrombocytopenia.
2. Drug-induced hematologic disorders are rare adverse drug reactions (ADRs) associated with drug therapy.
3. The incidence of rare ADRs is usually established by postmarketing surveillance and reporting.
4. Rechallenging a patient with an agent suspected of inducing a blood disorder is not generally recommended.
5. Drug-induced hematologic disorders can occur by two mechanisms: direct drug or metabolite toxicity or an immune reaction.
6. The primary treatment of drug-induced hematologic disorders is the removal of the drug in question and symptomatic support of the patient.

BEYOND THE BOOK

Watch the video entitled "Part 1: Anemia: Pathophysiology and Diagnostic Approach" (https://accessmedicine.mhmedical.com/MultimediaPlayer.aspx?MultimediaID=16442308) in AccessMedicine by Scott Stern, MD. This can be found by clicking on Multimedia, Lectures, Diagnostic Reasoning, then Part 1: Anemia (https://accessmedicine.mhmedical.com/MultimediaPlayer.aspx?MultimediaID=16442308). This 21-minute video provides an overview of the foundational knowledge of anemia, the approach to evaluate a patient with anemia, common causes of anemias, and differential diagnosis for different types of anemias. This video increases student understanding regarding the COLLECT and ASSESS steps in the patient care process.

INTRODUCTION

1 Hematologic disorders have long been a potential risk of modern pharmacotherapy. Granulocytopenia (agranulocytosis) was reported in association with one of medicine's early therapeutic agents, sulfanilamide, in 1938.[1] Some agents cause predictable hematologic disease (eg, antineoplastics), but others induce idiosyncratic reactions not directly related to the drugs' pharmacology. The most common drug-induced hematologic disorders are aplastic anemia, agranulocytosis, megaloblastic anemia, hemolytic anemia, and thrombocytopenia.

2 The incidence of idiosyncratic drug-induced hematologic disorders varies depending on the condition and the associated drug. Few epidemiologic studies have evaluated the actual incidence of these adverse reactions, but these reactions are rare. Women are generally more susceptible than men to the hematologic effects of drugs. The incidence varies based on geography, which suggests that genetic differences may be important determinants of susceptibility. Drug-induced thrombocytopenia is the most common drug-induced hematologic disorder, with reports suggesting that between 0.1% and 5% of patients who receive heparin develop heparin-induced thrombocytopenia (HIT).[2,3] The Berlin Case-Control Surveillance Study was conducted from 2000 to 2009 to assess the incidence and risks of drug-induced hematologic disorders and found that almost 30% of all cases of blood dyscrasias were "possibly" attributable to drug therapy.[4]

Although drug-induced hematologic disorders are less common than other types of adverse reactions, they are associated with significant morbidity and mortality. Aplastic anemia is the leading cause of death followed by thrombocytopenia, agranulocytosis, and hemolytic anemia.[5] Similar to most other adverse drug reactions (ADRs), drug-induced hematologic disorders are more common in older individuals than in the young; the risk of death is also greater with increasing age.

3 The MedWatch program supported by the Food and Drug Administration (FDA)[6] is the most common avenue for postmarketing surveillance to establish the incidence of ADRs. The FDA's Adverse Event Reporting System (FAERS) is the database that contains the reports submitted to the FDA and supports the post-marketing safety and surveillance program for both drug and therapeutic biologic products. It has a dashboard that allows the public to search for human adverse events that have been reported by the pharmaceutical industry, healthcare providers, and consumers. Many facilities have similar drug-reporting programs to follow ADR trends and to determine whether an association between a drug and an ADR is causal or coincidental. These programs enable practitioners to confirm that an adverse event is the result of drug therapy rather than one of many other potential causes; general guidelines are readily available.[7,8]

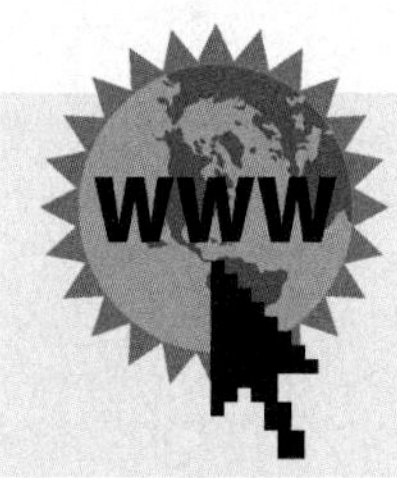

The complete chapter, learning objectives, and other resources can be found at **www.pharmacotherapyonline.com.**

Laboratory Tests to Direct Antimicrobial Pharmacotherapy

e126

Jordan R. Smith, Brian J. Werth, and Katie E. Barber

KEY CONCEPTS

1. Understanding the difference between normal host microbiota and typical pathogens will help determine whether a patient is truly infected or merely colonized.

2. Direct examination of tissue and body fluids by Gram stain provides rapid information about the causative pathogen.

3. Isolation of the offending organism by culture or rapid diagnostic testing assists in the diagnosis of infection and allows for more definitive directed treatment.

4. Development of molecular testing systems (or rapid diagnostic testing) has improved our ability to diagnose infections and determine the antimicrobial susceptibilities for numerous pathogens, including fastidious or slow-growing mycobacteria and viruses.

5. *In vitro* antimicrobial susceptibility testing has limitations and often cannot truly mimic the conditions found at the site of an infection. This can cause discordance between *in vitro* susceptibility results and *in vivo* response to antimicrobial therapy.

6. Laboratory evaluation of antimicrobial activity is an important component of the pharmacotherapeutic management of infectious diseases.

7. When used appropriately, rapid automated susceptibility test systems appear to improve therapeutic outcomes of patients with infection, especially when they are linked with other clinical information systems.

8. Understanding the fundamentals of antimicrobial pharmacodynamic properties will help the clinician make drug selection and dosing decisions in situations where robust clinical data are lacking.

9. Routine monitoring of serum concentrations is currently used for a select few antimicrobials, eg, aminoglycosides and vancomycin, in an attempt to minimize toxicity and maximize efficacy.

10. Appropriate timing for the collection of serum samples when measuring antimicrobial serum concentrations is crucial to ensure that valid pharmacokinetic data are generated.

11. Monitoring of aminoglycoside serum concentrations and the use of extended-interval dosing can help maximize the probability of therapeutic success and minimize the probability of aminoglycoside-related toxicity for certain infections.

12. Vancomycin and aminoglycoside serum concentration monitoring should be routinely done to ensure adequate serum concentrations, minimize toxicity, and avoid the potential for resistance.

13. Antimicrobial pharmacodynamics has become a crucial consideration for the selection of both empirical and pathogen-directed therapy in the current era of antimicrobial resistance.

14. Optimization of antimicrobial pharmacodynamic parameters such as the ratio of the peak serum concentration to minimum inhibitory concentration (MIC) or the time that the antibiotic serum concentration remains above the MIC or the ratio of the area under the concentration-time curve to the MIC can improve infection treatment outcomes.

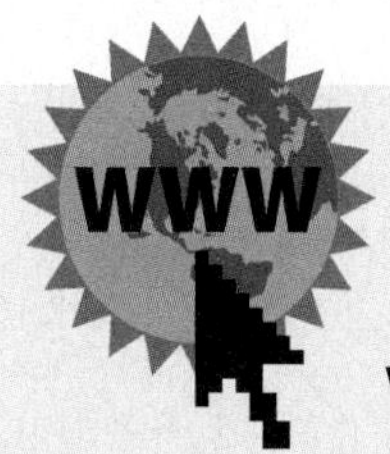

The complete chapter, learning objectives, and other resources can be found at **www.pharmacotherapyonline.com.**

Antimicrobial Regimen Selection

127

Katie B. Olney and David S. Burgess

KEY CONCEPTS

1. Every attempt should be made to obtain specimens for culture and sensitivity testing prior to initiating antibiotics.
2. Empirical antibiotic therapy should be based on knowledge of likely pathogens for the site of infection, information from patient history (eg, recent hospitalizations, work-related exposure, travel, and pets), and local susceptibility.
3. Patients with delayed dermatologic reactions (ie, rash) to penicillin generally can receive cephalosporins. Patients with type I hypersensitivity reactions (ie, anaphylaxis) to penicillins should not receive cephalosporins. Alternatives to the β-lactam antimicrobials include aztreonam, quinolones, sulfonamide antibiotics, or vancomycin based on type of coverage indicated.
4. Renal function should be considered for every patient who is to receive antibiotics. Hepatic function should be considered for drugs eliminated through the hepatobiliary system, such as clindamycin, erythromycin, and metronidazole.
5. All concomitant drugs and nutritional supplements should be reviewed when an antibiotic is added to a patient's therapy to ensure drug-drug interactions will be avoided.
6. Combination antibiotic therapy may be indicated for polymicrobial infections (eg, intra-abdominal and gynecologic infections), to produce synergistic killing, or to prevent the emergence of resistance.
7. All patients receiving antibiotics should be monitored for resolution of infectious signs and symptoms (eg, decreasing temperature and white blood cell count) and adverse drug events.
8. Antibiotics with the narrowest effective spectrum of activity are preferred. Antibiotic route of administration should be evaluated daily, and conversion from IV to oral therapy should be attempted as signs of infection improve for patients with functioning GI tracts (general exceptions are endocarditis and CNS infections).
9. Patients not responding to an appropriate antibiotic treatment in 2 to 3 days should be reevaluated to ensure (a) the correct diagnosis, (b) that therapeutic drug concentrations are being achieved, (c) that the patient is not immunosuppressed, (d) that appropriate source control has been achieved (ie, abscess and foreign body), or (e) that resistance has not developed.
10. The main goals of antimicrobial stewardship programs (ASPs) are to optimize antimicrobial selection, dosing, duration, and route of administration while minimizing adverse drug events and the emergence of antimicrobial resistance.

BEYOND THE BOOK

KS is a 65-year-old woman with a past medical history significant for uterine cancer and total abdominal hysterectomy, for which they received radiation and chemotherapy. They present to the emergency department with complaints of nausea, vomiting, and flank pain. Their vital signs and laboratory values are as follows:

Laboratory Values
C-reactive protein: 224 mg/dL (2,240 mg/L)
WBC: 22,600 cells/mm^3 (22.6 × 10^9/L)
Bands: 10%

Vitals
Blood pressure: 95/58
Temperature: 39.4°C (103 °F)
Heart rate: 136 beats/min

1. Which of the following statements regarding microbiologic studies is false?
   A. Obtaining cultures prior to administration of antimicrobial therapy may improve culture yield.
   B. Ideally two sets of blood cultures should be obtained peripherally from two different sites 1 hour apart.
   C. Coagulase-negative staphylococci recovered from blood cultures always warrant antimicrobial treatment.
   D. Urine cultures should be evaluated in conjunction with results of the urinalysis to confirm infection.
2. Which of the following is an important consideration when selecting empiric antimicrobial therapy for this patient?
   A. Prior antimicrobial use
   B. Site of infection and the organisms most likely present
   C. Prior knowledge of colonization or infections
   D. All of the above
3. Which of the following criteria must be met prior to transitioning a patient to oral antibiotic therapy?
   A. Re-culture twice daily to ensure adequate microbiological cure
   B. Lack of fever for 8 to 24 hours
   C. Resolution of electrolyte abnormalities
   D. Decrease in C-reactive protein

INTRODUCTION

Antimicrobials are among the most widely used classes of drugs.[1] In the United States, expenditures for antimicrobial agents exceed $8 billion annually. Approximately 20% to 50% of inpatient antibiotic use, 40% to 75% of nursing home antibiotic use, and 30% of outpatient antibiotic use is considered unnecessary or inappropriate.[2] The use of antibiotics is the main driver in creating selective pressure for the emergence of antimicrobial resistant pathogens; nevertheless, antibiotic overuse remains common. Selecting appropriate antimicrobial agent(s) to treat an infection has proven to be a challenging task.[3] Although the choice of a single agent or a combination of agents should be individualized for each patient, certain general principles of therapy should guide the selection of specific drugs (Table 127-1).

The initial selection of antimicrobial therapy is nearly always empirical, which is prior to documentation and identification of the offending organism. Infectious diseases generally are acute, and a delay in antimicrobial therapy can result in serious morbidity or even mortality. Thus, empirical antimicrobial therapy selection should be based on information gathered from the patient's history and physical examination and results of Gram stains or of rapidly performed tests on specimens from the infected site. This information, combined with knowledge of the most likely offending organism(s) and an institution's local susceptibility patterns, should result in a rational selection of antibiotics to treat the patient. This chapter introduces a systematic approach to the selection of antimicrobial therapeutic regimens.

CONFIRMING THE PRESENCE OF INFECTION

An infectious disease diagnosis is determined by assessing the presence of signs and symptoms of an infection, determining the site of infection, and establishing a microbiological diagnosis, when possible.

Fever

Aberrations of temperature reaching >38°C (100.4°F) or <36°C (96.8°F) are indicative of systemic inflammation, and may often be seen in patients presenting with infectious disease processes. Body temperature is controlled by the hypothalamus. In addition, the circadian rhythm, a built-in temperature cycle, is also operational. The daily temperature rhythm can vary for each individual. In a healthy person, the internal thermostat is set between the morning low temperature and the afternoon peak as controlled by the circadian rhythm. During fever, the hypothalamus is reset at a higher temperature level.

Fever is defined as a controlled elevation of body temperature above the normal range. The average normal body temperature range taken orally is 36.7°C to 37°C (98°F–98.6°F). Body temperatures obtained rectally generally are 0.6°C (1°F) higher and axillary temperatures are 0.6°C (1°F) lower than oral temperatures, respectively. Skin temperatures are also less than the oral temperature but can vary depending on the specific measurement method. Fever can be a manifestation of disease states other than infection. Collagen vascular (autoimmune) disorders and several malignancies can have fever as a manifestation. Fever of unknown or undetermined origin is a diagnostic dilemma and is reviewed extensively elsewhere.[4]

Many drugs have been identified as causes of fever. *Drug-induced fever* is defined as persistent fever in the absence of infection or other underlying condition. The fever must coincide temporally with the administration of the offending agent and disappear promptly on its withdrawal, after which the temperature remains normal. Possible mechanisms of drug-induced fever are either a hypersensitivity reaction or development of antigen–antibody complexes that result in the stimulation of macrophages and the release of interleukin 1 (IL-1). While fever is not a common drug effect (accounting for no more than 5% of all drug reactions), it should be suspected when obvious reasons for fever are not present. Almost any medication can produce fever, but β-lactam antibiotics, anticonvulsants, allopurinol, hydralazine, nitrofurantoin, sulfonamides, phenothiazines, and methyldopa are responsible more often than others.

Noninfectious etiologies of fever can be referred to as "false-positives." Although these certainly can confuse the clinician, even more troublesome are false-negatives: the absence of fever in a patient with signs and symptoms consistent with an infectious disease. Careful questioning of the patient or family is vital to assess the ingestion of any medication that can mask fever (eg, aspirin, acetaminophen, nonsteroidal anti-inflammatory agents, and corticosteroids). The use of antipyretics should be discouraged during the treatment of infection unless absolutely necessary because they can mask a poor therapeutic response. Moreover, elevated body temperature, unless very high (greater than 40.5°C [105°F]), is not harmful and may be beneficial.

White Blood Cell Count

Most infections result in elevated white blood cell (WBC) counts (leukocytosis) because of the increased production and mobilization of granulocytes (neutrophils, basophils, and eosinophils), lymphocytes, or both to destroy invading microbes. The generally accepted range of normal values for WBC counts is between 4,000 and 10,000 cells/mm^3 (4×10^9 and 10×10^9/L). Values above or below this range hold important prognostic and diagnostic value.

Bacterial infections are associated with elevated granulocyte counts, often with immature forms (band neutrophils) seen in peripheral blood smears. Mature neutrophils are also referred to as *segmented neutrophils* or *polymorphonuclear* (PMN) *leukocytes*. The presence of immature forms (left shift) is an indication of an increased bone marrow response to the infection. With infection, peripheral WBC counts can be very high, but they are rarely higher than 30,000 to 40,000 cells/mm^3 (30×10^9/L to 40×10^9/L). Because leukocytosis indicates the normal host response to infection, low leukocyte counts after the onset of infection indicate an abnormal response and generally are associated with a poor prognosis.

The most common granulocyte defect is neutropenia, a decrease in absolute numbers of circulating neutrophils. A thorough description of the consequences of neutropenia is given in Chapter 145, "Infections in Immunocompromised Patients." Lymphocytosis, even with normal or slightly elevated total WBC counts, generally is associated with tuberculosis and viral or fungal infections. Increases

TABLE 127-1 Systematic Approach for Selection of Antimicrobials

Confirm the presence of infection
Careful history and physical examination
Signs and symptoms
Predisposing factors
Identification of the pathogen (see Chapter e126, "Laboratory Tests to Direct Antimicrobial Pharmacotherapy")
Collection of infected material
Stains
Serologies
Culture and sensitivity
Selection of presumptive therapy considering every infected site
Host factors
Drug factors
Monitor therapeutic response
Clinical assessment
Laboratory tests
Assessment of therapeutic failure

in monocytes can be associated with tuberculosis or lymphoma, and increases in eosinophils can be associated with allergic reactions to drugs or infections caused by metazoa. Many types of infections can be accompanied by a completely normal WBC count and differential.

Local Signs

The classic signs of pain and inflammation can manifest as swelling, erythema, tenderness, and purulent drainage. Unfortunately, these are only visible if the infection is superficial or in a bone or joint. The manifestations of inflammation in deep-seated infections (eg, meningitis, pneumonia, endocarditis, and urinary tract infection) must be ascertained by examining tissues or fluids. For example, the presence of neutrophils in spinal fluid, lung secretions (sputum), or urine is highly suggestive of a bacterial infection.

Symptoms referable to an organ system must be sought out carefully because not only do they help in establishing the presence of infection, but they also aid in narrowing the list of potential pathogens. For example, a febrile patient with complaints of flank pain and dysuria may be presenting with pyelonephritis. In this situation, enteric gram-negative bacilli, especially *Escherichia coli*, are the predominant pathogens. If a febrile patient has no symptoms suggestive of an organ system but only constitutional complaints, the list of possible infectious diseases is lengthy.[4] A febrile individual with cough and sputum production may have a pulmonary infection. What is not so evident, however, is the etiologic organism in this situation, because pneumonia can be bacterial, viral, or fungal in etiology.[5] In this situation, attention to the patient's history and background disease states is important. Even more important is a careful examination of the infected material (in this case sputum) to ascertain the identity of the pathogen.

IDENTIFICATION OF THE PATHOGEN

Microbiological Studies

1 Identification and antimicrobial susceptibility of a pathogen are the most important factors in determining the choice of antimicrobial therapy. Generally, infected body materials must be sampled, if at all possible or practical, before or concurrently with institution of any antimicrobial therapy for two reasons. First, a Gram stain of the material might reveal bacteria, or an acid-fast stain might detect mycobacteria or actinomycetes. Second, the premature use of antimicrobials can suppress the growth of pathogens that might result in false-negative cultures results or alterations in the cellular and chemical composition of infected fluids. This is particularly true in patients with vertebral osteomyelitis, urinary tract infections, subacute endocarditis, meningitis, and septic arthritis.[11]

Blood cultures should be performed in the acutely ill febrile patient. Blood culture collection should coincide with sharp elevations in temperature, suggesting the possibility of microorganisms or microbial antigens in the bloodstream. Ideally, blood should be obtained from peripheral sites as two sets (one set consists of an aerobic bottle and one set an anaerobic bottle) from two different sites approximately 1 hour apart to optimize culture yield. In selected infections, bacteremia is qualitatively continuous (eg, endocarditis), so cultures can be obtained at any time.[10]

In addition to the infected materials produced by the patient (eg, blood, sputum, urine, stool, and wound or sinus drainage), other less accessible fluids or tissues must be obtained if they are suspected to be the infected site (eg, spinal fluid in meningitis and joint fluid in arthritis). Abscesses and cellulitic areas also should be aspirated.

When a pathogenic microorganism is identified, the next step for the majority of clinical microbiological laboratories is antimicrobial susceptibility testing (AST) that measures the ability of a select organism to grow in the presence of an antimicrobial agent. These methods are described in detail in Chapter e126. Once a microorganism is identified and its susceptibilities are known, antimicrobial therapy should be tailored to the specific pathogen.

Over the last decade, there has been an explosion in the development of rapid diagnostic methods that provide simultaneous organism identification and resistance marker detection. These methods include nonamplified probe technologies (peptide nucleic-acid-fluorescence in situ hybridization), proteomics, and nucleic acid amplification methods combined with microarray technologies. These tests can significantly reduce time to organism identification, thereby reducing time to effective antimicrobial therapy. Rapid diagnostic tests reduce overall antimicrobial use, length of hospital stay, and mortality among patients with infectious diseases.[12-16]

Interpreting Results

After a positive Gram stain, culture results, or both are obtained, the clinician must be cautious in determining whether the organism recovered is a true pathogen, a contaminant, or a part of the normal flora (see Chapter e126). The latter consideration is especially problematic with cultures obtained from the skin, oropharynx, nose, ears, eyes, throat, and perineum. These surfaces are heavily colonized with a wide variety of bacteria, some of which can be pathogenic in certain settings. For example, coagulase-negative staphylococci are found in cultures of all the aforementioned sites, yet are seldom regarded as pathogens unless recovered from multiple blood cultures, venous access catheters, or prosthetic devices.

Cultures of specimens from purportedly infected sites that are obtained by sampling from or through one of these contaminated areas might contain significant numbers of the normal flora. For example, asymptomatic bacteriuria, or bacterial colonization of the genitourinary tract in the absence of symptoms, is common even in healthy individuals. The treatment of asymptomatic bacteriuria is an important contributor to inappropriate antimicrobial use and promotion of resistance.[17] Careful consideration of a patient's presenting symptoms, risk factors, and history are essential to discern true infection from colonization.

Particularly problematic are expectorated sputum specimens that must be evaluated carefully by determination of the presence of squamous epithelial cells and leukocytes.[4] A predominance of epithelial cells in sputum specimens reduces the likelihood that recovered bacteria are pathogenic, especially when multiple types of organisms are seen on Gram stain. In contrast, the discovery of leukocytes in large numbers with one predominant type of organism is a more reliable indicator of a valid collection and quality sample. In general, however, sputum evaluation has poor sensitivity and specificity as a diagnostic test.[5]

Gram-staining techniques, culture methods, and serologic identification, as well as susceptibility testing, are discussed in detail in Chapter e126. Emphasis must be placed on the proper collection and handling of specimens and careful assessment of Gram stain or other test results in guiding the clinician toward appropriate selection of initial antimicrobial therapy.[18]

SELECTION OF PRESUMPTIVE THERAPY

2 In many instances, empiric therapy must be instituted before microbiological results are available. To select rational antimicrobial therapy for a given clinical situation, a variety of factors must be considered. These include the severity and acuity of the disease, local epidemiology and antibiogram, patient history, host factors, factors related to the drugs used, and the necessity for using multiple agents. In addition, there are generally accepted drugs of choice for the treatment of most pathogens (see Appendix 123-1).

Antibiogram

Drugs of choice are compiled from a variety of sources and are intended as guidelines rather than as specific rules for antimicrobial use. These choices are influenced by local antimicrobial susceptibility data rather than information published by other institutions or national compilations. Each institution should publish an annual summary of antibiotic susceptibilities (antibiogram) for organisms cultured from patients. Antibiograms contain both the number of nonduplicate isolates for common species and the percentage susceptible to the antibiotics tested. To further guide empirical antibiotic therapy, some hospitals publish unit-specific antibiograms in unique patient care areas, such as intensive care units or burn units.

Susceptibility of bacteria can differ substantially among hospitals within a community. For example, the prevalence of hospital-acquired methicillin-resistant *Staphylococcus aureus* (HA-MRSA) in some centers is quite high, whereas in other centers the problem might be nonexistent. This particular situation will influence the selection of therapy for possible *S. aureus* infection, where the clinician must choose either a β-lactam or vancomycin. The problem of differing susceptibilities is not limited only to gram-positive bacteria but also is evident in gram-negative organisms, and all drug classes are affected.

Patient History

Empirical therapy is directed at organisms that are known to cause the infection in question. These organisms are discussed for different sites of infection in Chapters 124–143. To define the most likely infecting organisms, a careful history and physical examination must be performed. The place where the infection was acquired should be determined, for example, the home (community acquired), nursing home environment, or hospital acquired (nosocomial). Nursing home patients can be exposed to potentially more resistant organisms because they are often surrounded by ill patients who are receiving antibiotics. Important considerations when selecting empiric antimicrobial therapy include: (1) prior knowledge of colonization or infections, (2) previous antimicrobial exposure, (3) the site of infection and the most likely pathogens, and (4) local antibiogram and resistance patterns for important pathogens. Other questions to ask infected patients regarding the history of present illness include: (1) Are any other people sick at home, especially children? (2) Are any unusual pets kept in the home? (3) Where are you employed (ie, are you exposed to contaminated meat or infectious biohazards)? and (4) Has there been any recent travel (ie, to endemic areas of fungal infections or developing countries)?

Host Factors

Several host factors should be considered when evaluating a patient for antimicrobial therapy. The most important factors are drug allergies, age, pregnancy, genetic or metabolic abnormalities, renal and hepatic function, site of infection, concomitant drug therapy, and underlying disease states.

Allergy

3 Anaphylactic allergy to an antimicrobial agent generally precludes its use. Careful assessment of allergy histories must be performed because many patients confuse common adverse drug effects (ie, GI disturbance) with true allergic reactions.[19-21] Among the most commonly cited antimicrobial allergies are those to penicillin, penicillin-related compounds, or both. In the absence of complete penicillin skin testing capabilities, a rule of thumb for giving cephalosporins to patients allergic to penicillin is to avoid giving them to patients who give a good history for immediate or accelerated reactions (eg, anaphylaxis, laryngospasm) and to give them under close supervision in patients with a history of delayed reactions, such as a rash.[19] If a gram-negative infection is suspected or documented, therapy with a monobactam may be appropriate because cross-reactivity with other β-lactams is nonexistent, with the exception of isolated cross-reactivity in ceftazidime-allergic patients.

Age

The patient's age is an important factor both in identifying the likely etiologic organism and in assessing pharmacokinetic alterations that may impact the patient's ability to eliminate the drug(s) to be used. The best example of an age determinant of organisms is in bacterial meningitis, where the pathogens differ as the patient grows from the neonatal period through infancy and childhood into adulthood.[6,7]

The impact of age on pharmacokinetics is exemplified in the neonatal population. Neonates have several pharmacokinetic alterations that may lead to variations in drug absorption, distribution, and metabolism. At birth, infants have reduced phase I (eg, cytochrome P450 enzymatic) and phase II (eg, glucuronidation and acetylation) metabolism that develops rapidly throughout the first year of life. Phase II metabolism occurs primarily through sulfation from birth through the first few months of life and is eventually replaced by glucuronidation and acetylation. In addition, neonates have more body water content that results in a larger volume of distribution and variations in gastric emptying time leading to alterations in drug absorption. Each of these alterations result in the need for adjustments in antibiotic dosing regimens.[22] Additional special drug considerations for pediatric patients include availability of dosage formulations (eg, concentration of liquid dosage forms and availability of tablet strengths) and compliance-enhancing features (eg, palatability).

The major physiologic change in persons older than 65 years of age is a decline in the number of functioning nephrons that, in turn, results in decreased renal function.[23] This is usually manifested by an increased incidence of side effects caused by antimicrobials that are eliminated renally.

Pregnancy

During pregnancy, not only is the fetus at risk for drug teratogenicity, but the pharmacokinetic disposition of certain drugs can be altered.[24-27] Penicillins, cephalosporins, and aminoglycosides are cleared from the peripheral circulation more rapidly during pregnancy. This is probably a result of marked increases in intravascular volume, glomerular filtration rate, and hepatic and metabolic activities. The net result is that maternal serum antimicrobial concentrations can be as much as 50% lower during this period than in the nonpregnant state. Increased dosages of certain compounds might be necessary to achieve therapeutic levels during late pregnancy.[26]

Metabolic or Genetic Variation

Inherited or acquired metabolic abnormalities will influence the therapy of infectious diseases in a variety of ways. For example, patients with impaired peripheral vascular flow may not absorb drugs given by intramuscular injection. In addition, certain metabolic states can predispose patients to enhanced drug toxicity. For instance, patients who are phenotypically slow acetylators of isoniazid are at greater risk for peripheral neuropathy.[28] Patients with severe deficiency of glucose-6-phosphate dehydrogenase can develop significant hemolysis when exposed to such drugs as sulfonamides, nitrofurantoin, nalidixic acid, antimalarials, and dapsone. Although mild deficiencies are found in African Americans, the more severe forms of the disease generally are confined to persons of eastern Mediterranean origin. Another example is the antiretroviral drug abacavir, which is associated with a severe hypersensitivity reaction, consisting of fever, rash, abdominal pain, and respiratory distress. This risk has been associated with the presence of a human leukocyte antigen allele HLA-B*5701. Routine screening for the presence of this allele before initiating treatment with abacavir is a recommendation in the current HIV treatment guidelines. Furthermore, the hepatic cytochrome P450 system is a major pathway for a large number of antimicrobials. While differential host expressions of these enzymes occur, insufficient clinical data are available to recommend routine screening for antimicrobial therapy.

Organ Dysfunction

4 Patients with diminished renal or hepatic function may have pharmacokinetic alterations resulting in altered antibiotic exposure. These alterations often necessitate dose individualization and therapeutic drug monitoring, especially in critically ill populations. Because many of the commonly used antimicrobials are primarily cleared by the kidneys, it is imperative to adjust the dosing regimen as clinically appropriate.[29,30] However, there are many etiologies for altered serum creatinine concentrations aside from renal dysfunction (eg, sepsis, immobility-related cachexia) and inappropriate assessment of these concentrations may lead to inaccurate estimations of glomerular filtration rate (GFR) and creatinine clearance (CrCl).[31] Renal dose adjustment of antibiotics should be delayed for the first 48 hours of illness in patients admitted with acute kidney injury (AKI) being treated for infectious diseases.[32] Clinicians should always consider patient-specific factors, severity of illness, and pathogens of concern when making dose adjustments based on measured serum creatinine concentrations. Nephrotoxic medications (eg, aminoglycosides) are generally avoided in patients with severe liver disease.[33]

Concomitant Drugs

5 Any concomitant therapy that the patient is receiving can influence the drug selection, dose, and monitoring. For instance, administration of isoniazid to a patient who is also receiving phenytoin can result in phenytoin toxicity secondary to inhibition of phenytoin metabolism by isoniazid. Furthermore, drugs that possess similar adverse effect profiles can increase the risk for effects (ie, two drugs that cause nephrotoxicity or neutropenia). A detailed review of drug interactions is beyond the scope of this chapter, but an excellent textbook on this subject is available.[34] Lists of potentially severe drug-drug interactions are provided in Table 127-2.

Concomitant Disease States

Concomitant disease states can influence the selection of therapy. Certain diseases will predispose patients to a particular infectious disease or will alter the type of infecting organism. For example, patients with diabetes mellitus and resulting peripheral vascular disease often develop infections of the lower extremity soft tissue. Moreover, the alterations in peripheral blood flow associated with

TABLE 127-2 Major Drug–Drug Interactions with Antimicrobials

Antimicrobial	Interacting Agent(s)	Mechanism of Action/Effect	Clinical Management
Aminoglycosides	Neuromuscular blocking agents	Additive toxicity of neuromuscular-blocking agents	Monitor therapy
	Nephrotoxins (N) or ototoxins (O) (eg, amphotericin B [N], cisplatin [N/O], cyclosporine [N], furosemide [O], NSAIDs [N], radiocontrast [N], vancomycin [N])	Additive toxicity	Monitor renal function, obtain regular audiograms for patients receiving prolonged or repeated courses of aminoglycosides
	β-lactams	Aminoglycoside degradation	Separate administration and flush line thoroughly between doses of aminoglycoside and β-lactam therapy
Amphotericin B	Nephrotoxins (eg, aminoglycosides, cyclosporine, foscarnet)	Additive nephrotoxicity	Monitor renal function
Azoles	See Chapter 144		
Foscarnet	Pentamidine IV	Increased risk of severe nephrotoxicity and hypocalcemia	Monitor renal function and serum calcium
Isoniazid	Carbamazepine, phenytoin	Decreased metabolism of carbamazepine and phenytoin, resulting in increased serum concentrations	Monitor for signs and symptoms of phenytoin and carbamazepine and phenytoin toxicity (eg, nausea, vomiting, nystagmus, ataxia)
Macrolides/azalides	Digoxin	Decreased digoxin bioavailability and metabolism	Monitor digoxin SDC
	Theophylline	Decreased metabolism of theophylline	Monitor theophylline SDC
Metronidazole	Ethanol (drugs containing ethanol)	Disulfiram-like reaction	Avoid
Fluoroquinolones	Other QTc-prolonging agents (eg, antiemetics, macrolides, azoles, antidepressants, etc.)	Prolonged QTc interval	Monitor ECG at baseline and periodically while on concomitant QTc-prolonging therapy
	Multivalent cations	Decreased absorption of fluoroquinolone	Separate administration by at least 2 hours
Rifampin	Azoles, cyclosporine, methadone, propranolol, oral contraceptives, tacrolimus, warfarin	Increased of metabolism of interacting agent via rifampin induction of CYP-450 metabolism resulting in decreased serum concentrations	Avoid
Sulfonamides	Sulfonylureas, phenytoin, warfarin	Decreased metabolism of interacting agent resulting in increased serum concentrations	Monitor blood glucose, SDC of interacting agent, and PT
Doxycycline	Multivalent cations	Decreased absorption of tetracycline	Separate administration by at least 2 hours

the disease and perhaps altered immunity make such infections more difficult to treat than in nondiabetics. Patients with chronic lung disease or cystic fibrosis develop frequent pulmonary infections that can be caused by somewhat different microorganisms than are found in otherwise normal hosts.

Patients with immunosuppressive diseases, such as malignancies or acquired immunologic deficiencies, are highly predisposed to infections, and the types of causative or pathogenic organisms can be vastly different from what would be expected (see Chapter 145, "Infections in Immunocompromised Patients"). For instance, patients undergoing chemotherapy for acute forms of leukemia often are profoundly granulocytopenic and are predisposed to infections caused by bacteria and fungi.[35] Patients with acquired immunodeficiency syndrome (AIDS) are more likely to become infected with less common opportunistic pathogens (see Chapter 148, "Human Immunodeficiency Virus"). Many factors predisposing to infection are related to disruption of the host's integumentary barriers. For example, trauma, burns, and iatrogenic wounds induced in surgery can lead to a substantial risk of infection depending on the severity and location of the injury or disruption. For a complete discussion of the various risks involved in surgical procedures, see Chapter 146, "Antimicrobial Prophylaxis in Surgery."

DRUG FACTORS

Pharmacokinetic and Pharmacodynamic Considerations

Integration of both pharmacokinetic and pharmacodynamic properties of an agent is important when choosing antimicrobial therapy to ensure efficacy and to prevent resistance.[36] Early researchers relied solely on pharmacokinetic properties such as the area under the (drug concentration) curve (AUC), maximum observed concentration (peak), and drug half-life to optimize therapy. Pharmacodynamics is the study of the relationship between drug concentration and the effects on the microorganism. There is an important relationship between both pharmacokinetic and microbiologic parameters that has resulted in measurements such as AUC:minimal inhibitory concentration (MIC) ratio, peak:MIC ratio, and time (*T*) the concentration is above MIC ($T>$MIC).[37-41]

Aminoglycosides exhibit concentration-dependent bactericidal effects. An example of the integration of pharmacokinetics and microbiologic activity is the use of high-dose, once-daily aminoglycosides. For these regimens, the drug is given as a single large daily dose to maximize the peak:MIC ratio. Aminoglycosides also possess a post-antibiotic effect (persistent suppression of organism growth after concentrations decrease below the MIC) that contribute to the success of high-dose, once-daily administration. Fluoroquinolones exhibit concentration-dependent killing activity, but optimal killing is characterized by the AUC:MIC ratio.

β-Lactams display time-dependent bactericidal effects. Killing activity is enhanced only marginally if drug concentration exceeds the MIC. Therefore, the important pharmacodynamic relationship for these antimicrobials is the duration that drug concentrations exceed the MIC ($T >$ MIC). Effective dosing regimens require serum drug concentrations to exceed the MIC for at least 40% to 60% of the dosing interval. *In vitro, in vivo* animal, and human clinical trials have demonstrated improved pharmacodynamic attainment and clinical efficacy with continuous or prolonged infusions of β-lactams.[37] A detailed discussion on antimicrobial pharmacokinetics–pharmacodynamics is beyond the scope of this chapter. However, excellent sources of information on this topic are available.[36,42,43]

Tissue Penetration

The importance of tissue penetration varies with site of infection. Some of the difficulties in interpreting data include a lack of correlation with clinical outcomes and poor understanding of whether the antimicrobial agents are present in a biologically active form. An example of the former problem is the recognized efficacy of drugs with low biliary fluid concentrations in the treatment of cholecystitis, cholangitis, or both and the absence of the enhanced efficacy of drugs whose primary route of elimination is biliary excretion of active drug. An example of the latter difficulty is with penetration to deep infections, such as abscesses, where various factors such as acid pH, WBC products, and various enzymes can inactivate even high concentrations of certain drugs. The CNS is one body site where antimicrobial penetration is relatively well defined, and correlations with clinical outcomes are established.[6,11,44] Cerebrospinal fluid (CSF) concentrations of antimicrobial agents necessary to cure bacterial meningitis have been defined, and drugs that do not reach significant concentrations in the CSF should be either avoided or instilled directly, if feasible. Caution must be exercised when selecting an antimicrobial agent for clinical use on the basis of tissue or fluid penetration. Body fluids where drug concentration data are clinically relevant include CSF, urine, ocular, synovial fluid, and peritoneal fluid. More attention should be paid to clinical efficacy, antimicrobial spectrum, and toxicity than to comparative data on penetration into a given body site.

The proper route of administration for an antimicrobial depends on the site of infection. Parenteral therapy is warranted when patients are being treated for febrile neutropenia or deep-seated infections such as meningitis, endocarditis, and osteomyelitis. Severe pneumonia often is treated initially with IV antibiotics and switched to oral therapy as clinical improvement is evident.[5,22,45] Patients treated in the ambulatory setting for bacterial upper respiratory tract infections (eg, pharyngitis, bronchitis, sinusitis, and otitis media), lower respiratory tract infections, skin and soft-tissue infections, uncomplicated urinary tract infections, and selected sexually transmitted diseases can usually receive oral therapy.

Drug Toxicity

It is incumbent on health professionals to avoid toxic drugs whenever possible. Antibiotics associated with CNS toxicities, usually when not dose-adjusted for renal function, include penicillins, cephalosporins, quinolones, and imipenem. Hematologic toxicities generally are manifested with prolonged use of β-lactam antimicrobials, vancomycin, or sulfamethoxazole/trimethoprim. Reversible nephrotoxicity classically is associated with aminoglycosides and vancomycin. Irreversible ototoxicity can occur with aminoglycosides. In the outpatient setting, patients must be counseled regarding photosensitivity with azithromycin, quinolones, tetracyclines, pyrazinamide, and sulfamethoxazole/trimethoprim. Lastly, all antibiotics have been implicated in causing diarrhea and colitis secondary to *Clostridium difficile* (see Chapter 136, "Gastrointestinal Infections and Enterotoxigenic Poisonings").[46] List of potential antibiotic adverse drug reactions is provided in Table 127-3.

Aside from consideration of drug toxicity, some antimicrobial use requires more intensive risk–benefit analysis. An example of this is the decision to use isoniazid for treatment of latent tuberculosis. Because the hepatotoxicity of isoniazid increases in frequency with age, older persons (greater than 45 years of age) who have latent tuberculosis must have additional risk factors for tuberculosis to balance the potential toxic effects. These include immunosuppression, or immunocompromising conditions, including HIV. Older patients without additional risk factors are more likely to suffer toxicity from isoniazid than derive benefit from its use.

COMBINATION ANTIMICROBIAL THERAPY

6 In selecting a drug regimen for a given patient, consideration must be given to the necessity of using more than one drug empirically. Inappropriate or inadequate antimicrobial therapy has been

TABLE 127-3 Antimicrobial Adverse Drug Reactions

Antimicrobial Class	Adverse Drug Reaction	Monitoring Parameters	Comments
Penicillins	Rash, N/V/D, hypersensitivity reactions including anaphylaxis, LFT elevations, interstitial nephritis, cytopenias, hemorrhagic cystitis, *C. difficile* colitis	Hypersensitivity reactions (eg, bronchospasm, anaphylaxis) CBC with differential Renal function Hepatic function	Immediate IgE-mediated anaphylaxis incidence is <0.05%.
Cephalosporins	Rash, N/V/D, hypersensitivity reactions including anaphylaxis, LFT elevations, interstitial nephritis, cytopenias, Coomb's positive hemolytic anemia, *C. difficile* colitis	Hypersensitivity reactions (eg, bronchospasm, anaphylaxis) CBC with differential Renal function Hepatic function	
Carbapenems	Rash, N/V/D, hypersensitivity reactions including anaphylaxis, LFT elevations, interstitial nephritis, cytopenias, eosinophilia, *C. difficile* colitis	Hypersensitivity reactions (eg, bronchospasm, anaphylaxis) CBC with differential Renal function Hepatic function	Clinically significant cross-sensitivity reactions in penicillin-allergic patients reported to be as low as 1%. Incidence of seizures more frequent in patients who are elderly, have history of seizure disorders, or who have renal dysfunction.
Monobactams	Rash, diarrhea, nausea, LFT elevations, *C. difficile* colitis, thrombocytopenia	CBC with differential Renal function Hepatic function	May be used in patients with anaphylactic penicillin allergy. *Note:* Isolated cross-reactivity has been described in ceftazidime-allergic patients due to a shared R-side chain.
Aminoglycosides	Tubular necrosis and renal failure (reversible), vestibular and cochlear toxicity, anemia, hypersensitivity	Renal function (daily) SDC Obtain regular audiology exams in patients with prolonged or cumulative exposure to aminoglycosides	Nephrotoxicity is more common in patients with the following risk factors: elderly, history of renal dysfunction, concomitant administration of nephrotoxic drugs, and prolonged duration of therapy. Ototoxicity can be irreversible.
Glycopeptides	Red person syndrome, phlebitis, renal dysfunction, neutropenia, leukopenia, eosinophilia, thrombocytopenia, drug fever	Renal function SDC CBC with differential if on prolonged therapy	Red person syndrome is associated with rapid infusion and nonspecific histamine release; prolonging vancomycin infusion and pre-medicating with antihistamines often mitigates occurrence.
Lipopeptides	Elevations in serum creatinine phosphokinase (CPK) levels, rhabdomyolysis, eosinophilic pneumonia.	Renal function CPK at baseline and weekly (or more frequently in patients with prior or concomitant statin, renal dysfunction, or patients with baseline elevations in CPK)	Daptomycin doses should be held in the setting of: (1) CPK elevation >5× the upper limit of normal (ULN) in patients who have symptoms of rhabdomyolysis or (2) CPK elevation >10× the ULN in patients who are asymptomatic. Daptomycin may be restarted if CPK level returns to baseline.
Oxazolidinones	Myelosuppression (thrombocytopenia, leukopenia, and anemia), peripheral neuropathy, optic neuropathy, lactic acidosis, diarrhea, nausea, serotonin syndrome	Monitor for signs and symptoms of serotonin syndrome in patients receiving concomitant serotonergic agents CBC with differential For prolonged therapy, monitor visual acuity	Myelosuppression is reversible and associated with treatment duration > 2 weeks.
Tetracyclines	GI upset, N/V/D, hepatotoxicity, esophageal ulcerations, photosensitivity, azotemia, visual disturbances, vertigo, hyperpigmentation, hemolytic anemia, pseudotumor cerebri, pancreatitis, *C. difficile* colitis	CBC with differential Renal function Hepatic function	Vestibular symptoms more frequent in women than in men. Avoid use during pregnancy. The American Academy of Pediatrics (AAP) provides guidance on utilization of doxycycline in pediatrics: doxycycline may be used ***without regard to patient age*** for treatment durations ≤21 days.
Chloramphenicol	Myelosuppression, aplastic anemia, "gray baby syndrome," optic neuritis, peripheral neuropathy, digital paresthesias, GI upset, *C. difficile* colitis, hypersensitivity reactions	CBC with differential (baseline and daily) Renal function Hepatic function SDC (particularly in children and in patients with hepatic or renal insufficiency)	Bone marrow suppression associated with doses >4 g/day. Use has fallen out of favor due to significant toxicities.
Rifamycines	Red discoloration of urine, tears, contact lens, sweat, hepatotoxicity, GI upset, flu-like syndrome, hypersensitivity, thrombocytopenia, leukopenia, drug fever, interstitial nephritis	CBC with differential (baseline and daily) Renal function Hepatic function (LFTs, bilirubin)	Increased potential for hepatitis with concomitant hepatotoxic drugs (ie, TB drugs).
Macrolides/azalide	GI intolerance, diarrhea, prolonged QTc, cholestatic hepatitis, reversible ototoxicity, torsade de pointes, rash, hypothermia, exacerbation of myasthenia gravis	Hepatic function in high-risk patients ECG (baseline and periodically if on multiple QTc-prolonging agents or if prolonged QTc at baseline)	

(*continued*)

TABLE 127-3 Antimicrobial Adverse Drug Reactions (*Continued*)

Antimicrobial Class	Adverse Drug Reaction	Monitoring Parameters	Comments
Clindamycin	Diarrhea, *C. difficile* colitis, nausea, vomiting, generalized rash, hypersensitivity	Signs/symptoms of *C. difficile* Hepatic function (if prolonged therapy)	
Fluoroquinolones	GI intolerance, headache, malaise, insomnia, dizziness, photosensitivity, QTc prolongation, tendon rupture, peripheral neuropathy, crystalluria, seizure, interstitial nephritis, Stevens-Johnson syndrome, allergic pneumonitis, *C. difficile* colitis	Renal function Signs and symptoms of encephalopathic changes (eg, confusion, hallucinations, and tremor)	Tendon rupture more frequently seen in the elderly and kidney, heart, and lung transplant recipients, and with concurrent use of corticosteroids.
Polymyxins	Nephrotoxicity, neurotoxicity (paresthesia, vertigo, ataxia, blur red vision, slurred speech), neuromuscular blockade, bronchospasms (when administered via inhalation)	CBC with differential (baseline and daily) Renal function (baseline and daily) Signs of neurotoxicity (eg, peripheral paresthesias, blurred vision, apnea, muscle weakness)	Nephrotoxicity is dose-dependent.
Sulfonamides and trimethoprim	GI intolerance, rash, hyperkalemia, bone marrow suppression (eg, anemia with folate deficiency, thrombocytopenia, and leukopenia), serum sickness, hepatitis, photosensitivity, crystalluria with azotemia, urolithiasis, methemoglobinemia, Stevens-Johnson syndrome, toxic epidermal necrolysis, pancreatitis, interstitial nephritis	Hypersensitivity reactions (eg, bronchospasm, anaphylaxis) and rash CBC with differential Renal function Hepatic function Serum potassium	HIV-infected patients are at increased risk for developing adverse drug reactions. Methemoglobinemia due to severe G6PD deficiency.
Metronidazole	N/V/D, headache, metallic taste, dark urine, peripheral neuropathy, disulfiram reactions with alcohol, insomnia, stomatitis, dysarthria	CBC with differential (baseline and periodically during prolonged therapy) Hepatic function Signs of neurotoxicity	Peripheral neuropathy is reversible and associated with prolonged treatment.

CBC, complete blood count; CPK, creatine phosphokinase; LFT, liver function test; SDC, serum drug concentrations; TB, tuberculosis.

associated with increased morbidity and mortality.[47] Combinations of antimicrobials generally are used to broaden the spectrum of coverage for empirical therapy, achieve synergistic activity against the infecting organism, and mitigate the emergence of resistance.[48,49]

Broadening the Spectrum of Coverage

Increasing the coverage of antimicrobial therapy generally is necessary in two scenarios. The first scenario is in mixed infections where multiple organisms are likely to be present. This is the case in intra-abdominal and female pelvic infections, in which a variety of aerobic and anaerobic bacteria can produce disease.[50] Traditionally, a combination of a drug active against aerobic gram-negative bacilli (such as an aminoglycoside) and a drug active against anaerobic bacteria (such as metronidazole) is selected. Options for monotherapy which possess good activity against both of these types of organisms, include the β-lactam/β-lactamase inhibitor combinations and carbapenems. The second scenario is for critically ill patients with presumed healthcare-associated infections in which an increased spectrum of activity is desirable.[45] Healthcare-associated infections are frequently caused by multidrug resistant pathogens; combination therapy is often used in this setting to ensure that at least one of the antimicrobials will be active against the pathogen(s).

Synergism

The achievement of synergistic antimicrobial activity is advantageous for some serious bacterial infections. Laboratory tests to identify synergy between antibiotic combinations are described in Chapter e126. Traditionally, combinations of aminoglycosides and β-lactams have been used because these drugs together generally act synergistically against a wide variety of bacteria. However, the data supporting superior efficacy of synergistic over nonsynergistic combinations are weak. At best, synergistic combinations produce better results in infections caused by *Enterococcus* species.[42-44]

The most obvious example of the use of synergy is the treatment of enterococcal endocarditis. The causative organism is usually only inhibited by penicillins, but it is killed rapidly by the addition of gentamicin or ceftriaxone to a penicillin. The need for bactericidal activity in the treatment of endocarditis underscores the need for these synergistic combinations.[9,10]

Preventing Resistance

The use of antimicrobial combinations to prevent the emergence of resistance is applied widely but not often realized. The only circumstance where this has been clearly effective is in the treatment of tuberculosis. The prevalence of resistance to a first-line drug such as isoniazid or rifampin in a population of organisms may be as high as 1 in 10^6 to 10^8. Because the bacterial load in a patient with active tuberculosis often exceeds this, two drugs are given to reduce the likelihood of encountering resistance to less than 1 in 10. There is ample evidence from *in vitro* data and experimental bacterial infections that combinations of drugs with different mechanisms are effective in the prevention of the emergence of resistance.

Disadvantages of Combination Therapy

Although there are potentially beneficial effects from combining drugs, there also are potential disadvantages, including increased cost, greater risk of drug toxicity, and superinfection with even more resistant bacteria.[9,51] The combination of two or more antibiotics can result in antagonistic effects. For example, the effect of antagonism may be evident when one drug induces β-lactamase production and another drug is β-lactamase unstable.

MONITORING THERAPEUTIC RESPONSE

7 After antimicrobial therapy has been instituted, the patient must be monitored carefully for a therapeutic response. Culture and

sensitivity reports from specimens sent to the microbiology laboratory must be reviewed and the therapy changed accordingly. Use of agents with the narrowest spectrum of activity against identified pathogens is recommended. If anaerobes are suspected, even if they are not identified, anti-anaerobic therapy should be continued.

Patient monitoring should include many of the same parameters used to diagnose the infection. The WBC count and temperature should start to normalize. Physical complaints from the patient also should diminish (ie, decreased pain, shortness of breath, cough, or sputum production). Appetite should improve. However, radiologic improvement can lag behind clinical improvement.

Determinations of serum (or other fluid) levels of antimicrobials can be useful in ensuring outcome, preventing toxicity, or both. Vancomycin, aminoglycosides, and voriconazole are examples of antimicrobials that require routine monitoring of serum concentrations. Achievement of adequate aminoglycoside concentrations within the first few days of therapy of gram-negative infection has been correlated with better therapeutic outcome.[52]

Changes in the volume of distribution can have a significant impact on the efficacy and safety of therapy. An unexpectedly low volume of distribution (such as in the dehydrated patient) will result in higher, potentially toxic drug concentrations, whereas a larger-than-expected volume of distribution (such as in patients with edema or ascites) will result in low, potentially subtherapeutic concentrations. The most effective methods use measured serum concentrations of the drugs rather than estimations from renal function tests to assess true drug clearance from the body.

8 As patients improve clinically, the route of administration should be reevaluated. Transitioning therapy from parenteral to oral (step-downtherapy) has become an accepted practice for many infections.[5,22] Criteria that should be present to justify a switch to oral therapy include (a) overall clinical improvement, (b) lack of fever for 8 to 24 hours, (c) decreased WBC count, and (d) a functioning GI tract. Drugs that exhibit excellent oral bioavailability when compared with IV formulations include fluoroquinolones, clindamycin, doxycycline, metronidazole, linezolid, and trimethoprim–sulfamethoxazole.

FAILURE OF ANTIMICROBIAL THERAPY

9 A variety of factors may be responsible for an apparent lack of response to therapy. Patients who fail to respond over 2 to 3 days require a thorough reevaluation. It is possible that the disease is not infectious or is not bacterial in origin, or there is an undetected pathogen in a polymicrobial infection. Other factors include those directly related to drug selection, the host, or the pathogen. Laboratory error in identification, susceptibility testing, or both (presence of inoculum effect or resistant subpopulations) is a rare cause of antimicrobial failure.

Failures Caused by Drug Selection

Factors related directly to the drug selection include an inappropriate drug selection, dosage, or route of administration. Malabsorption of a drug product because of GI disease (such as a short-bowel syndrome) or a drug interaction (such as complexation of fluoroquinolones with multivalent cations resulting in reduced absorption) can lead to potentially subtherapeutic serum concentrations. Accelerated drug elimination is also possible. This can occur in patients with cystic fibrosis or during pregnancy, when more rapid clearance or larger volumes of distribution can result in low serum concentrations, particularly for aminoglycosides. A common cause of failure of therapy is poor penetration into the site of infection. This is especially true for sites such as the CNS, eye, and prostate gland. Drug failure also can result from drugs that are highly protein bound or that are chemically inactivated at the site of infection.

Failures Caused by Host Factors

Host defenses must be considered when evaluating a patient who is not responding to antimicrobial therapy. Patients who are immunosuppressed (eg, granulocytopenia from chemotherapy or AIDS) may respond poorly to therapy because their defenses are inadequate to eradicate the infection despite seemingly adequate drug regimens. A good example is the poor response of infection in granulocytopenic patients that is seen when their WBC counts remain low during therapy. This contrasts with a much better response when granulocyte counts increase during therapy. Other host factors are related to the need for surgical drainage of abscesses or removal of foreign bodies, necrotic tissue, or both. If these situations are not corrected, they result in persistent infection and, occasionally, bacteremia despite adequate antimicrobial therapy.

Failures Caused by Microorganisms

There are two types of resistance: intrinsic and acquired. Intrinsic is when the antimicrobial agent never had activity against the bacterial species. For example, gram-negative bacteria are naturally resistant to vancomycin because the drug cannot penetrate the outer membrane of gram-negative bacteria. Acquired resistance is when the antimicrobial agent was originally active against the bacterial species but the genetic makeup of the bacteria has changed so the drug can no longer be effective.[53] The strategies used by bacteria to develop acquired resistance are primarily classified into three general mechanisms of resistance: (a) alteration in the target site, (b) changes in membrane permeability (eg, upregulation of efflux pumps, porin channel alterations), and (c) enzymatic inactivation. Bacteria can use one or more of these mechanisms against a specific antibiotic or antibiotic class. Furthermore, a single mechanism of resistance can result in resistance to multiple related or unrelated classes of antibiotics.

Enzymatic inactivation through production of β-lactamases can be either plasmid or chromosomally mediated. In addition, the expression of β-lactamases can be induced or constitutive. There are now multiple types and classes of β-lactamases identified, which is beyond the scope of this chapter. However, there are several outstanding publications discussing all of the different types of β-lactamases.[4,54-56] The increase in resistance among bacteria is believed to be a result of continued overuse of antimicrobials in the community, as well as in hospitals, and the increasing prevalence of immunosuppressed patients receiving long-term suppressive antimicrobials for the prevention of infections. These resistance patterns are regionally variable, and susceptibility patterns in the community (or hospital) should be monitored closely to promote judicious antimicrobial selection.[57]

Enterococci have been isolated with multiple resistance patterns and may be resistant to β-lactams (by virtue of β-lactamase production, altered penicillin-binding proteins, or both), vancomycin (via alterations in peptidoglycan synthesis), and aminoglycosides (via enzymatic degradation). *Streptococcus pneumoniae* tends to be highly susceptible to penicillin, vancomycin, levofloxacin, moxifloxacin, and third-generation parenteral cephalosporins. However, resistance to penicillin, certain cephalosporins (including oral third-generation cephalosporins), and macrolides has become increasingly more common. Newer antimicrobial agents such as linezolid and ceftaroline have demonstrated increased activity against penicillin and cephalosporin-resistant *S. pneumoniae.*

Treatment of an infection caused by AmpC β-lactamase producing organisms (eg, *Enterobacter* sp., *Citrobacter* sp., *Serratia marcescens*, indole-positive Proteae, *Acinetobacter* sp., or *Pseudomonas aeruginosa*) with any penicillin, cephalosporin (with the exception of cefepime), or aztreonam is strongly discouraged. Although such therapy may produce an initial clinical response by eradicating some susceptible bacteria in the population, patients will likely experience

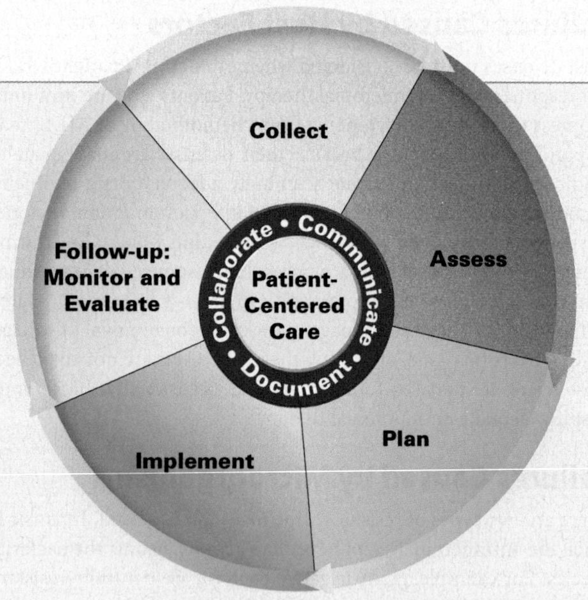

Patient Care Process for Infectious Diseases

The image shows the five fundamental steps included in The Pharmacist's Care Process endorsed by the Joint Commission for Pharmacy Practitioners (2014). The tagline of this process reads collaborate, communicate, and document. The five fundamental steps listed here are collect, assess, plan, implement, and follow-up: monitor and evaluate. All these steps are listed in a circular block diagram.

Collect

- Patient presenting features (eg, age, allergies, predisposing factors)
- Patient medication history (including timing and duration of previous antibiotic use)
- Patient medical history (including past infection and culture data)
- Patient social history (eg, ethanol or illicit drug use)
- Objective data
  - Blood pressure (BP), heart rate (HR), respiratory rate (RR), temperature, height, weight
  - Labs including complete blood count (CBC) with differential and serum creatinine (SCr)
  - Cultures with susceptibilities from appropriate sites for which infectious process is a concern
  - Objective confirmation of presence of infection

Assess

- Hemodynamic stability (eg, systolic BP <90 mm Hg, HR >90 bpm, O_2 saturation <90% [0.9], Respiratory rate > 20 or $PaCO_2$ <32 mm Hg [4.3 kPa])
- Allergy history (including: agent(s), type of reaction, timing of reaction onset, agent(s) (if utilized) to abort reaction, etc.)
- Antimicrobial history (eg, timing, duration, and agent selection)
- Culture history (eg, prior positive cultures and susceptibilities)
- Presence of risk factors for multi-drug resistant infections (eg, recent broad-spectrum antimicrobial exposure, immunocompromising factors)
- Presence of medications with drug-drug interactions; see Table 127-2

Plan*

- Drug therapy regimen including specific antibiotic(s), dose, route, frequency, and duration
- Monitoring parameters including efficacy (eg, fever curve, complete blood count with differential) and safety (eg, nephrotoxicity, hypersensitivity reactions, CPK elevation); see Table 127-3
- Patient education (eg, purpose of therapy, medication administration, drug-drug interactions, and adverse effects); see Tables 127-2 and 127-3
- Monitoring for resolving signs and symptoms of infection and finalized culture results/susceptibilities
- Therapeutic drug monitoring based on pharmacokinetic/pharmacodynamic properties of agent (eg, AUC:MIC, Peak:MIC, trough concentrations) as appropriate
- Schedule follow-up as necessary

Implement*

- Provide patient education regarding all elements of treatment plan
- Schedule follow-up for laboratory monitoring and physical assessment as appropriate

Follow-up: Monitor and Evaluate

- Resolution of signs and symptoms of infection (eg, fever, erythema, leukocytosis, etc.)
- Presence of adverse effects (eg, nephrotoxicity, hypersensitivity reactions, CPK elevation); see Table 127-3
- Therapeutic drug monitoring based on pharmacokinetic/pharmacodynamic properties of agent (eg, AUC:MIC, Peak:MIC, trough concentrations)

**Collaborate with patient, caregivers, and other healthcare professionals.*

treatment failure within a few days as the highly resistant AmpC-producing subpopulations have a selective advantage and are uninhibited by these agents. AmpC β-lactamase producing organisms usually retain susceptibility to cefepime and carbapenems but are resistant to all other β-lactams. Non-β-lactam therapy, including trimethoprim/sulfamethoxazole, aminoglycosides, and fluoroquinolones are additional agents that may be utilized once susceptibilities are known. Host defenses are extremely important in this scenario and debilitated patients with pulmonary infections, abscesses, or osteomyelitis are at high risk for drug failure. In these situations, a combination regimen to prevent the emergence of resistance or the use of carbapenem may be warranted for empirical therapy.

ANTIMICROBIAL STEWARDSHIP

10 The importance of the selection and continuation of appropriate antimicrobial therapy in acute care hospitals are part of a wide movement that is referred to as "antimicrobial stewardship." Antimicrobial stewardship programs are aimed at optimizing antimicrobial selection, dosing, route, and duration of therapy to maximize clinical cure or prevention of infection while limiting the unintended consequences, such as the emergence of resistance, adverse drug events, and cost. Many institutions have developed an antibiotic stewardship program. The team is generally a multidisciplinary group including representation from microbiology, infection control, administration, information technology, pharmacy including infectious disease-trained clinical pharmacists, and physicians from several disciplines, including infectious disease. Components of antimicrobial stewardship activities include formulary restriction, prospective audit and feedback of antimicrobial prescriptions to clinicians, education, use of clinical order sets and guidelines, de-escalation of therapy, and intravenous to oral antimicrobial conversion.[58,59]

Antibiotic Formulary

One of the main roles of an antimicrobial stewardship team is to decide which antibiotics to include on their formularies. The decision to have a formulary remains controversial; however, restricting choices does encourage familiarity with a core of antibiotics for residents and attending physicians. Open formularies allow the empirical use of any commercially available antibiotics, with recommended guidelines for changes when culture and sensitivity results are finalized. The implementation of the guidelines and restrictions requires the cooperation of the entire medical staff. Education is vital to the success of the antibiotic formulary.

Attention must be paid to the literature on antimicrobials to assist in the selection of therapy. Evidence-based practice guidelines from the Infectious Diseases Society of America can aid clinicians to direct appropriate therapy for specific infectious disease syndromes. In addition, the results from prospective, controlled, randomized clinical trials should be evaluated whenever possible when considering appropriate antimicrobial therapy. Results from prelicensing open trials offer only limited information that can be useful in this regard because patients in these trials generally are not seriously ill and are not infected with multiple resistant bacteria. Other confounding factors found in most clinical situations are excluded by virtue of the study design. Therefore, comparative data in more seriously ill patients are essential for the appropriate application of new agents.

Post-marketing trials are also important because results can demonstrate superiority of one regimen over another, as it relates to efficacy, safety, or cost-effectiveness. Appropriate antimicrobial therapy can change as new organisms are discovered, susceptibility patterns change, new drugs become available, and new clinical trial results are published. Classical thinking in the treatment of infectious diseases will continue to change and evolve to maintain antimicrobial efficacy. Optimal use of modern antimicrobials is just beginning to be defined.

ABBREVIATIONS

AIDS	acquired immunodeficiency syndrome
AST	antimicrobial susceptibility testing
AUC	area under the curve
CSF	cerebrospinal fluid
ESBL	extended-spectrum β-lactamase
HA-MRSA	hospital-acquired methicillin-resistant *Staphylococcus aureus*
IL-1	interleukin 1
MIC	minimal inhibitory concentration
PBP	penicillin-binding protein
PMN	polymorphonuclear
WBC	white blood cell

REFERENCES

1. Suda KJ, Hicks LA, Roberts RM, et al. Antibiotic expenditures by medication, class, and healthcare setting in the United States, 2010-2015. *Clin Infect Dis.* 2018;66(2):185–190. 10.1093/cid/cix773.
2. Centers for Disease Control and Prevention (CDC) Improve Antibiotic Use Initiative 2020 [updated 2020-11-05]. Available from: https://www.cdc.gov/sixeighteen/hai/index.htm#anchor_1603387115.
3. Tamma PD, Aitken SL, Bonomo RA, et al. Infectious Diseases Society of America Guidance on the treatment of extended-spectrum β-lactamase producing enterobacterales (ESBL-E), carbapenem-resistant enterobacterales (CRE), and pseudomonas aeruginosa with difficult-to-treat resistance (DTR-P. aeruginosa). *Clin Infect Dis.* 2021;72(7):e169–e183. 10.1093/cid/ciaa1478.
4. Bennett J, Dolin R, Blaser M. *Mandell, Douglas, and Bennett's Principles and Practice of Infectious Diseases.* 9th ed. Philadelphia, PA: Elsevier Health Sciences; 2020.
5. Metlay JP, Waterer GW, Long AC, et al. Diagnosis and Treatment of Adults with Community-acquired Pneumonia. An Official Clinical Practice Guideline of the American Thoracic Society and Infectious Diseases Society of America. *Am J Respir Crit Care Med.* 2019;200(7):e45–e67. doi: 10.1164/rccm.201908-1581ST.
6. van Ettekoven CN, van de Beek D, Brouwer MC. Update on community-acquired bacterial meningitis: Guidance and challenges. *Clin Microbiol Infect.* 2017;23(9):601–606. 10.1016/j.cmi.2017.04.019.
7. McGill F, Heyderman RS, Panagiotou S, et al. Acute bacterial meningitis in adults. *Lancet.* 2016;388(10063):3036–3047. 10.1016/s0140-6736(16)30654-7.
8. Berbari EF, Kanj SS, Kowalski TJ, et al. 2015 Infectious Diseases Society of America (IDSA) Clinical Practice Guidelines for the Diagnosis and Treatment of Native Vertebral Osteomyelitis in Adults. *Clin Infect Dis.* 2015;61(6):e26–e46. doi: 10.1093/cid/civ482.
9. Liu C, Bayer A, Cosgrove SE, et al. Clinical practice guidelines by the infectious diseases society of america for the treatment of methicillin-resistant *Staphylococcus aureus* infections in adults and children. *Clin Infect Dis.* 2011;52(3):e18–e55. 10.1093/cid/ciq146.
10. Baddour LM, Wilson WR, Bayer AS, et al. Infective endocarditis in adults: Diagnosis, antimicrobial therapy, and management of complications: A scientific statement for healthcare professionals from the American Heart Association. *Circulation.* 2015;132(15):1435–1486. 10.1161/cir.0000000000000296.
11. Tunkel AR, Hasbun R, Bhimraj A, et al. 2017 Infectious Diseases Society of America's Clinical Practice Guidelines for Healthcare-Associated Ventriculitis and Meningitis. *Clin Infect Dis.* 2017;64(6):e34–e65. doi: 10.1093/cid/ciw861.
12. Timbrook TT, Morton JB, McConeghy KW, et al. The effect of molecular rapid diagnostic testing on clinical outcomes in bloodstream infections: A systematic review and meta-analysis. *Clin Infect Dis.* 2017;64(1):15–23. 10.1093/cid/ciw649.
13. Messacar K, Hurst AL, Child J, et al. Clinical impact and provider acceptability of real-time antimicrobial stewardship decision support for rapid diagnostics in children with positive blood culture results. *J Pediatric Infect Dis Soc.* 2017;6(3):267–274. 10.1093/jpids/piw047.
14. Pardo J, Klinker KP, Borgert SJ, et al. Clinical and economic impact of antimicrobial stewardship interventions with the FilmArray blood culture identification panel. *Diagn Microbiol Infect Dis.* 2016;84(2):159–64. doi: 10.1016/j.diagmicrobio.2015.10.023.
15. MacVane SH, Nolte FS. Benefits of adding a rapid PCR-based blood culture identification panel to an established antimicrobial stewardship program. *J Clin Microbiol.* 2016;54(10):2455–2463. 10.1128/jcm.00996-16.
16. Mahrous AJ, Thabit AK, Elarabi S, et al. Clinical impact of pharmacist-directed antimicrobial stewardship guidance following blood culture rapid diagnostic testing. *J Hosp Infect.* 2020;106(3):436–446. doi: 10.1016/j.jhin.2020.09.010.
17. Nicolle LE, Gupta K, Bradley SF, et al. Clinical practice guideline for the management of asymptomatic bacteriuria: 2019 Update by the Infectious Diseases Society of America. *Clin Infect Dis.* 2019;68(10):1611–1615. doi: 10.1093/cid/ciz021.
18. McPherson R, Pincus M. *Henry's Clinical Diagnosis and Management by Laboratory Methods.* 23rd ed. Philadelphia, PA: Elsevier Health Sciences; 2017.

19. Shenoy ES, Macy E, Rowe T, et al. Evaluation and management of penicillin allergy: A review. *Jama*. 2019;321(2):188–199. doi: 10.1001/jama.2018.19283.
20. Vorobeichik L, Weber EA, Tarshis J. Misconceptions surrounding penicillin allergy: Implications for anesthesiologists. *Anesth Analg*. 2018;127(3):642–649. doi: 10.1213/ane.0000000000003419.
21. Sacco KA, Bates A, Brigham TJ, et al. Clinical outcomes following inpatient penicillin allergy testing: A systematic review and meta-analysis. *Allergy*. 2017;72(9):1288–1296. 10.1111/all.13168.
22. Bradley JS, Byington CL, Shah SS, et al. The management of community-acquired pneumonia in infants and children older than 3 months of age: Clinical practice guidelines by the Pediatric Infectious Diseases Society and the Infectious Diseases Society of America. *Clin Infect Dis*. 2011;53(7):e25–76. 10.1093/cid/cir531.
23. Hommos MS, Glassock RJ, Rule AD. Structural and functional changes in human kidneys with healthy aging. *J Am Soc Nephrol*. 2017;28(10):2838–2844. doi: 10.1681/asn.2017040421.
24. Muanda FT, Sheehy O, Bérard A. Use of antibiotics during pregnancy and the risk of major congenital malformations: A population based cohort study. *Br J Clin Pharmacol*. 2017;83(11):2557–2571. 10.1111/bcp.13364.
25. Tasnif Y, Morado J, Hebert MF. Pregnancy-related pharmacokinetic changes. *Clin Pharmacol Ther*. 2016;100(1):53–62. doi: 10.1002/cpt.382.
26. Briggs GGF, Roger K, Towers, Craig V, Forinash, Alicia B. *Drugs in Pregnancy and Lactation: A Reference Guide to Fetal and Neonatal Risk*. 11th Edition. Philadelphia, PA: Lippincott Williams & Wilkins (LWW); 2017.
27. Bookstaver PB, Bland CM, Griffin B, et al. A review of antibiotic use in pregnancy. *Pharmacotherapy*. 2015;35(11):1052–1062. 10.1002/phar.1649.
28. Devaleenal Daniel B, Ramachandran G, Swaminathan S. The challenges of pharmacokinetic variability of first-line anti-TB drugs. *Expert Rev Clin Pharmacol*. 2017;10(1):47–58. doi: 10.1080/17512433.2017.1246179.
29. Lea-Henry TN, Carland JE, Stocker SL, et al. Clinical pharmacokinetics in kidney disease: Fundamental principles. *Clin J Am Soc Nephrol*. 2018;13(7):1085–95. doi: 10.2215/cjn.00340118.
30. Lewis SJ, Mueller BA. Antibiotic dosing in patients with acute kidney injury: "Enough but not too much". *J Intensive Care Med*. 2016;31(3):164–176. 10.1177/0885066614555490.
31. Ulldemolins M, Roberts JA, Lipman J, et al. Antibiotic dosing in multiple organ dysfunction syndrome. *Chest*. 2011;139(5):1210–1220. 10.1378/chest.10-2371.
32. Crass RL, Rodvold KA, Mueller BA, et al. Renal dosing of antibiotics: Are we jumping the gun? *Clin Infect Dis*. 2019;68(9):1596–1602. 10.1093/cid/ciy790.
33. European Association for the Study of the Liver. EASL Clinical Practice Guidelines for the management of patients with decompensated cirrhosis. *J Hepatol*. 2018;69(2):406–460. 10.1016/j.jhep.2018.03.024.
34. Rodvold KA, Piscitelli SC, Rodvold K, et al. *Drug Interactions in Infectious Diseases*. 3rd ed. New York: Totowa, NJ: Humana Press: Imprint: Humana; 2011.
35. Freifeld AG, Bow EJ, Sepkowitz KA, et al. Clinical practice guideline for the use of antimicrobial agents in neutropenic patients with cancer: 2010 update by the infectious diseases society of america. *Clin Infect Dis*. 2011;52(4):e56–e93. doi: 10.1093/cid/cir073.
36. Drusano GL. Pharmacokinetics and pharmacodynamics of antimicrobials. *Clin Infect Dis*. 2007;45 (Suppl 1):S89–S95. doi: 10.1086/518137.
37. Guilhaumou R, Benaboud S, Bennis Y, et al. Optimization of the treatment with beta-lactam antibiotics in critically ill patients-guidelines from the French Society of Pharmacology and Therapeutics (Société Française de Pharmacologie et Thérapeutique-SFPT) and the French Society of Anaesthesia and Intensive Care Medicine (Société Française d'Anesthésie et Réanimation-SFAR). *Crit Care*. 2019;23(1):104. doi: 10.1186/s13054-019-2378-9.
38. Sumi CD, Heffernan AJ, Lipman J, et al. What antibiotic exposures are required to suppress the emergence of resistance for Gram-negative bacteria? A systematic review. *Clin Pharmacokinet*. 2019;58(11):1407–1443. doi: 10.1007/s40262-019-00791-z.
39. Rybak MJ, Le J, Lodise TP, et al. Therapeutic monitoring of vancomycin for serious methicillin-resistant Staphylococcus aureus infections: A revised consensus guideline and review by the American Society of Health-System Pharmacists, the Infectious Diseases Society of America, the Pediatric Infectious Diseases Society, and the Society of Infectious Diseases Pharmacists. *Am J Health Syst Pharm*. 2020;77(11):835–864. 10.1093/ajhp/zxaa036.
40. Thabit AK, Hobbs ALV, Guzman OE, et al. The pharmacodynamics of prolonged infusion β-lactams for the treatment of pseudomonas aeruginosa infections: A systematic review. *Clin Ther*. 2019;41(11):2397–2415. doi: 10.1016/j.clinthera.2019.09.010.
41. Labreche MJ, Graber CJ, Nguyen HM. Recent updates on the role of pharmacokinetics-pharmacodynamics in antimicrobial susceptibility testing as applied to clinical practice. *Clin Infect Dis*. 2015;61(9):1446–1452. 10.1093/cid/civ498.
42. Ritchie David J. Antimicrobial pharmacodynamics in theory and clinical practice: Antimicrobial pharmacodynamics in theory and clinical practice, second edition. *Clinical Infectious Diseases*. 2008;46(12):1942. doi: 10.1086/588473.
43. Ambrose PG, Bhavnani SM, Rubino CM, et al. Pharmacokinetics-pharmacodynamics of antimicrobial therapy: It's not just for mice anymore. *Clin Infect Dis*. 2007;44(1):79–86. doi: 10.1086/510079.
44. Kumta N, Roberts JA, Lipman J, et al. A systematic review of studies reporting antibiotic pharmacokinetic data in the cerebrospinal fluid of critically ill patients with uninflamed meninges. *Antimicrob Agents Chemother*. 2020;65. 110.1128/aac.01998-20.
45. Kalil AC, Metersky ML, Klompas M, et al. Management of adults with hospital-acquired and ventilator-associated pneumonia: 2016 Clinical Practice Guidelines by the Infectious Diseases Society of America and the American Thoracic Society. *Clin Infect Dis*. 2016;63(5):e61–e111. 10.1093/cid/ciw353.
46. McDonald LC, Gerding DN, Johnson S, et al. Clinical Practice Guidelines for Clostridium difficile Infection in Adults and Children: 2017 Update by the Infectious Diseases Society of America (IDSA) and Society for Healthcare Epidemiology of America (SHEA). *Clin Infect Dis*. 2018;66(7):987–994. 10.1093/cid/ciy149.
47. Pogue JM, Kaye KS, Cohen DA, et al. Appropriate antimicrobial therapy in the era of multidrug-resistant human pathogens. *Clin Microbiol Infect*. 2015;21(4):302–312. 10.1016/j.cmi.2014.12.025.
48. Tamma PD, Cosgrove SE, Maragakis LL. Combination therapy for treatment of infections with gram-negative bacteria. *Clin Microbiol Rev*. 2012;25(3):450–470. 10.1128/cmr.05041-11.
49. Kengkla K, Kongpakwattana K, Saokaew S, et al. Comparative efficacy and safety of treatment options for MDR and XDR Acinetobacter baumannii infections: A systematic review and network meta-analysis. *J Antimicrob Chemother*. 2018;73(1):22–32. 10.1093/jac/dkx368.
50. Mazuski JE, Tessier JM, May AK, et al. The Surgical Infection Society revised guidelines on the management of intra-abdominal infection. *Surg Infect (Larchmt)*. 2017;18(1):1–76. 10.1089/sur.2016.261.
51. Paul M, Lador A, Grozinsky-Glasberg S, et al. Beta lactam antibiotic monotherapy versus beta lactam-aminoglycoside antibiotic combination therapy for sepsis. *Cochrane Database of Systematic Reviews*. 2014(1). doi: 10.1002/14651858.CD003344.pub3.
52. Roger C, Louart B, Elotmani L, et al. An international survey on aminoglycoside practices in critically ill patients: The AMINO III study. *Annals of Intensive Care*. 2021;11. 110.1186/s13613-021-00834-4.
53. Partridge SR, Kwong SM, Firth N, et al. Mobile genetic elements associated with antimicrobial resistance. *Clin Microbiol Rev*. 2018;31. 4 10.1128/cmr.00088-17.
54. Ruppé É, Woerther PL, Barbier F. Mechanisms of antimicrobial resistance in Gram-negative bacilli. *Ann Intensive Care*. 2015;5(1):61. doi: 10.1186/s13613-015-0061-0.
55. Bush K. The ABCD's of β-lactamase nomenclature. *J Infect Chemother*. 2013;19(4):549–59. doi: 10.1007/s10156-013-0640-7.
56. Bush K, Jacoby GA. Updated functional classification of beta-lactamases. *Antimicrob Agents Chemother*. 2010;54(3):969–976. doi: 10.1128/aac.01009-09.
57. Strich JR, Heil EL, Masur H. Considerations for empiric antimicrobial therapy in sepsis and septic shock in an era of antimicrobial resistance. *J Infect Dis*. 2020;222(Suppl 2):S119–S131. 10.1093/infdis/jiaa221.
58. Barlam TF, Cosgrove SE, Abbo LM, et al. Implementing an antibiotic stewardship program: Guidelines by the Infectious Diseases Society of America and the Society for Healthcare Epidemiology of America. *Clin Infect Dis*. 2016;62(10):e51–e77. 10.1093/cid/ciw118.
59. (CDC) CfDCaP. CDC. *Core Elements of Hospital Antibiotic Stewardship Programs*. Atlanta, GA: US Department of Health and Human Services, CDC; 2019.

APPENDIX 127-1: DRUG(S) OF CHOICE, *ALTERNATIVE(S)*

GRAM-POSITIVE COCCI

Organism	Drug(s) of Choice	*Alternatives*
Enterococcus faecalis Serious infections	Ampicillin, penicillin G (± gentamicin or ceftriaxone)	*Vancomycin daptomycin,[a] linezolid*
Enterococcus faecalis Urinary tract infection	Ampicillin, amoxicillin	*Fosfomycin, nitrofurantoin*
Enterococcus faecium *Recommend consultation with ID specialist*	Vancomycin, linezolid, daptomycin[a]	*Eravacycline, omadacycline*
Methicillin-susceptible *Staphylococcus aureus* (MSSA)	Nafcillin, oxacillin, cefazolin	*Daptomycin,[a] trimethoprim/sulfamethoxazole, clindamycin,[b] BL/BLI*
Methicillin-resistant *Staphylococcus aureus* (MRSA) Serious infections	Vancomycin, daptomycin[a]	*Linezolid, ceftaroline*
Methicillin-resistant *Staphylococcus aureus* (MRSA) SSTIs, CAP	Doxycycline, trimethoprim/sulfamethoxazole	*Clindamycin, linezolid, oritivancin, tedizolid, telavancin, dalbavancin*
Group A *Streptococcus* (*S. pyogenes*)	Penicillin G (± clindamycin *or* linezolid)[c]	*Erythromycin, azithromycin, clarithromycin*
Group B *Streptococcus* (*S. agalactiae*)	Penicillin G, ampicillin, amoxicillin	*Cephalexin, clindamycin,[b] vancomycin, azithromycin*
Group C, F, G *Streptococcus*	Penicillin G, penicillin V, ampicillin	*Daptomycin,[a] clindamycin, cefazolin*
Viridans group *Streptococcus*	Penicillin G	*Ceftriaxone, cefotaxime, vancomycin doxycycline*
Penicillin-susceptible *Streptococcus pneumoniae*	Penicillin G, ampicillin, amoxicillin	*Ceftriaxone, doxycycline*
Penicillin-resistant *Streptococcus pneumoniae*	Ceftriaxone, vancomycin	*Levofloxacin, moxifloxacin, vancomycin, linezolid, ceftaroline*

GRAM-NEGATIVE COCCI

Organism	Drug(s) of Choice	*Alternatives*
Moraxella catarrhalis	Ampicillin/sulbactam, amoxicillin/clavulanate	*Trimethoprim/sulfamethoxazole, doxycycline, azithromycin, ceftriaxone*
Neisseria gonorrhoeae	Ceftriaxone	*Gentamicin + azithromycin*
Neisseria meningitides	Penicillin G, ceftriaxone	*Moxifloxacin, ampicillin*

GRAM-POSITIVE BACILLI

Organism	Drug(s) of Choice	*Alternatives*
Clostridium perfringes	Penicillin G (± clindamycin)	*Metronidazole, ceftriaxone, ampicillin, piperacillin/tazobactam, meropenem, imipenem/cilastatin*
Clostridioides difficile (formerly *Clostridium difficile*)	PO vancomycin, fidaxomicin	*Metronidazole*

GRAM-NEGATIVE BACILLI

Organism	Drug(s) of Choice	*Alternatives*
Acinetobacter spp.	Cefepime, meropenem, imipenem/cilastatin, ampicillin/sulbactam	*amikacin, fluoroquinolone, minocycline, piperacillin/tazobactam, tigecycline, trimethoprim/sulfamethoxazole*
Bacteroides spp.	Metronidazole	*BL/BLI[f], meropenem, imipenem, cefoxitin*
Enterobacter spp.	Cefepime, meropenem, imipenem/cilastatin	*Trimethoprim/sulfamethoxazole, amikacin, piperacillin/tazobactam, fluoroquinolone[e], tigecycline*
Escherichia coli	Ceftriaxone	*Cefepime, BL/BLI, fluoroquinolone[e], trimethoprim/sulfamethoxazole, cephalexin, nitrofurantoin (cystitis), carbapenem[g]*
Haemophilus influenzae	Ampicillin/sulbactam, ceftriaxone *If* β-lactamase-negative, *may use ampicillin*	*Trimethoprim/sulfamethoxazole, azithromycin, fluoroquinolone[e], carbapenem[g]*
Klebsiella pneumoniae	Ceftriaxone, BL/BLI	*Cefepime, carbapenem[g], fluoroquinolone[e]*
Legionella spp.[d]	Levofloxacin, moxifloxacin, azithromycin	*Erythromycin, ciprofloxacin*
Pasteurella multocida	Ampicillin/sulbactam	*Penicillin G, doxycycline, trimethoprim/sulfamethoxazole*
Proteus mirabilis	Ceftriaxone	*Penicillin G, BL/BLI[f], cefepime*

(continued)

GRAM-NEGATIVE BACILLI		
Organism	**Drug(s) of Choice**	***Alternatives***
Indole-positive *Proteus* (ie, *Providencia spp., Morganella morganii*)	Cefepime, meropenem, imipenem/cilastatin	*Trimethoprim/sulfamethoxazole, amikacin, piperacillin/tazobactam, fluoroquinolone*[e]*, minocycline, tigecycline*
Pseudomonas aeruginosa	Cefepime, meropenem, amikacin, tobramycin, imipenem/cilastatin, piperacillin/tazobactam	*Ceftazidime, ciprofloxacin, levofloxacin, aztreonam*
Salmonella typhi	Ceftriaxone	*Ciprofloxacin, levofloxacin, sulfamethoxazole/ trimethoprim, carbapenem*[g]
Serratia marcescens	Cefepime, meropenem, imipenem/cilastatin	*Trimethoprim/sulfamethoxazole, amikacin, piperacillin/tazobactam, fluoroquinolone*[e]
Stenotrophomonas maltophilia	Trimethoprim/sulfamethoxazole	*Minocycline, levofloxacin*[h]

MISCELLANEOUS MICROORGANISMS		
Organism	**Drug(s) of Choice**	***Alternatives***
Chlamydia pneumoniae	Azithromycin, clarithromycin, doxycycline	*Levofloxacin, moxifloxacin*
Mycoplasma pneumoniae	Azithromycin, clarithromycin, doxycycline	*Levofloxacin, moxifloxacin*
Treponema pallidum	Penicillin G	*Ceftriaxone*

MULTI-DRUG RESISTANT (MDR) GRAM-NEGATIVE ORGANISMS		
Organism	**Drug(s) of Choice**	***Alternatives***
Any ESBL-positive *Enterobacterales* Infections outside the urinary tract	Carbapenem[g]	*Trimethoprim/sulfamethoxazole*[i]*, fluoroquinolone*[e]
Any ESBL-positive *Enterobacterales* Pyelonephritis	Trimethoprim/sulfamethoxazole	*Carbapenem*[g]*, levofloxacin, ciprofloxacin*
Any ESBL-positive *Enterobacterales* Cystitis	Nitrofurantoin	*Trimethoprim/sulfamethoxazole, levofloxacin, ciprofloxacin*
Any *Enterobacterales* positive for KPC carbapenemase	Meropenem/vaborbactam, ceftazidime/ avibactam, imipenem/cilastatin/relebactam	*Cefiderocol*
Any *Enterobacterales* positive for ametallo-β-lactamase (ie, VIM, NDM, or IMP)	Ceftazidime/avibactam + aztreonam	*Cefiderocol*
Any *Enterobacterales* positive for OXA-48 carbapenemase	Ceftazidime/avibactam	*Cefidericol*
***Pseudomonas aeruginosa* resistant to all routinely tested β-lactams**	Ceftolozane/tazobactam	*Ceftazidime/avibactam, imipenem/cilastatin/ relebactam, cefiderocol*

"Recommendations in chart are assuming in vitro susceptibility"

ESBL: extended-spectrum β-lactamase; GAS: Group A *Streptococcus;* CAP: community acquired pneumonia; SSTIs: skin and soft tissue infections; BL/BLI: β-Lactam/ β-lactamase inhibitor.

[a]Daptomycin does not achieve appreciable CNS concentrations and therefore would not be recommended for treatment of meningitis.

[b]Clindamycin is not an appropriate alternative for treatment of bloodstream or CNS infections.

[c]Both clindamycin and linezolid provide anti-toxin activity against GAS and selection of agent dependent upon patient-specific factors.

[d]May consider the addition of rifampin for serious *Legionella* infections.

[e]Fluoroquinolones: ciprofloxacin, levofloxacin, moxifloxacin.

[f]β-Lactam/β-lactamase inhibitor combination: ampicillin–sulbactam, piperacillin–tazobactam, ticarcillin–clavulanate, amoxicillin–clavulanate.

[g]Carbapenem: meropenem, imipenem/cilastatin, ertapenem.

[h]Levofloxacin should not be used as monotherapy for treatment of *Stenotrophomonas maltophilia*.

[i]Oral step-down therapy to trimethoprim/sulfamethoxazole, levofloxacin, or ciprofloxacin may be considered after (1) susceptibility to the oral agent is demonstrated, (2) patients are afebrile and hemodynamically stable, (3) appropriate source control is achieved, and (4) there are no issues with intestinal absorption.

Central Nervous System Infections

128

Delaney E. Hart, Christina Koutsari, Michael A. Wankum, and Ramy H. Elshaboury

KEY CONCEPTS

1. The four most common causative pathogens of acute community-acquired bacterial meningitis in the United States are *Streptococcus pneumoniae*, group B *Streptococcus*, *Neisseria meningitidis*, and *Haemophilus influenzae* type b, although routine vaccinations are having a dramatic effect on the incidence and distribution of these pathogens.
2. In cases of bacterial meningitis, initial findings can include (a) presenting signs and symptoms: fever, headache, nuchal rigidity (the classic triad), Brudzinski's or Kernig's sign, and altered mental status; and (b) abnormal cerebrospinal fluid (CSF) chemistries: elevated white blood cell (WBC) count (>1,000 cells/mm^3 [1.0 × 10^9/L]), elevated protein (>50 mg/dL [500 mg/L]), and decreased glucose levels (<45 mg/dL [2.5 mmol/L]).
3. Main microbiologic tests that should be obtained include Gram stain and culture of the CSF and blood. In patients with negative CSF Gram stain and culture, molecular testing such as polymerase chain reaction (PCR) has additive value in the pathogen(s) identification.
4. Three primary goals of treatment in meningitis include (a) eradication of infection, (b) amelioration of signs and symptoms, and (c) prevention of the development of neurologic sequelae, such as seizures, deafness, coma, and death.
5. When selecting antibiotics, the clinician must consider the antibiotic concentration at the site of infection and the spectrum of antibacterial activity. Empirical choices should be based on age, predisposing conditions, vaccination history, comorbidities, and local susceptibility patterns.
(a) Either ceftriaxone or cefotaxime with vancomycin is a reasonable initial choice for empirical coverage of community-acquired meningitis in adult patients.
(b) Meningitis due to *Listeria monocytogenes* is more common in infants and elderly. Therefore, ampicillin—with or without gentamicin—should be empirically added to antimicrobial regimens in these age groups.
6. Empirical coverage with an appropriate antibiotic should be started as soon as possible when clinical suspicion of meningitis exists. If there is a delay in obtaining a lumbar puncture (even 30-60 minutes), or if the patient is to undergo neuroimaging, the first dose of antibiotic(s) should not be withheld.
7. Antibiotic dosages for the treatment of meningitis should be optimized to ensure adequate CNS therapeutic concentrations.
8. The duration of antibiotic treatment for acute bacterial meningitis has not been standardized. However, it is generally based on the causative organism and the individual case, and may range from 7 to 21 days.
9. Close contacts and relatives of the index case should be assessed for appropriate chemoprophylaxis and vaccinations, particularly for *N. meningitidis* and *H. influenzae* meningitis.
10. Steroid treatment includes dexamethasone of 0.15 mg/kg per dose given four times daily for 2 to 4 days in infants and children with proven or strongly suspected *H. influenzae* type b meningitis. Steroids should be started 10 to 20 minutes prior to, or at least concomitant with, the first dose of antibiotics.

BEYOND THE BOOK

Find the Infectious Diseases Society of America (IDSA) guidelines for the diagnosis and treatment of neurocysticercosis infection. Assume that a male patient who is 90 kg and has normal kidney function requires treatment. Create a treatment regimen with drug, dose (both in mg/kg and in mg), dosing interval, and monitoring parameters for each recommended agent. When are antiparasitic agents used and when are they not given? The purpose of this activity is to enhance your ability to find evidence-based guidelines and apply them to clinical practice.

INTRODUCTION

Central nervous system (CNS) infections are caused by a variety of pathogens, including bacteria, viruses, fungi, and parasites. CNS infections result from hematogenous spread from a primary infection site, seeding from a parameningeal focus, reactivation from a latent site, trauma, neurosurgery, or CNS congenital defects. Newer diagnostic techniques have enabled more rapid and definitive diagnosis, thus reducing the number of unknown "aseptic meningitis" diagnoses and improving targeted therapy. Bacteria resistant to multiple antibiotics present new challenges in the management of CNS infections. This chapter presents the epidemiology, etiology, pathophysiology, therapy, and prophylaxis of common CNS infections.

EPIDEMIOLOGY

The incidence of acute, community-acquired bacterial meningitis is approximately 0.7 to 0.9 per 100,000 persons annually in developed countries, including the United States and Western Europe.[1] In the United States, this corresponded to approximately 4,100 annual cases of acute community-acquired bacterial meningitis, excluding epidemics, between 2003 and 2007 resulting in approximately 500 deaths.[2] In stark contrast, incidence rates of meningitis in the region of sub-Saharan Africa average 10 to 40 cases per 100,000 people per year.[1] This region, also known as the "meningitis belt," is characterized by seasonal and explosive epidemics putting at least 350 million individuals at risk for meningitis annually.[3]

The estimated incidence of brain abscesses is 0.3 to 1.3 per 100,000 people per year but can be considerably higher in high-risk groups, such as patients with HIV/AIDS.[4] The global reported incidence of encephalitis varies according to the population studied, and due to differences in definitions and research methodology. The reported incidence in western settings ranges from 0.7 to 13.8 per 100,000 for all ages: 0.7 to 12.6 per 100,000 adults and 10.5 to 13.8 per 100,000 children. The incidence peaks in the young and the elderly.[5,6] In the United States, there are approximately 20,000 encephalitis-related hospitalizations and 1,400 deaths per year.[7,8]

ETIOLOGY

1 *Streptococcus pneumoniae* remains the leading cause of acute community-acquired bacterial meningitis in the United States with an incidence rate of 0.3 per 100,000 people in 2010.[9] *Neisseria meningitidis* and *Haemophilus influenzae* type b (Hib) have also been important causes of acute bacterial meningitis but their incidence has decreased substantially in the past several decades, mainly due to introduction of effective vaccinations. *S. pneumoniae* remains the leading cause of bacterial meningitis, followed by Hib, *N. meningitidis*, and other bacterial, viral, and fungal causes.[10]

Hib was the most commonly identified cause of bacterial meningitis until the introduction of the Hib conjugate vaccine in 1987 (at 18 months of age) and 1991 (at 2 months of age) in the United States. Hib vaccination had a profound population-wide effect on incidence of Hib meningitis, and in 2016 Hib was the least common cause of meningitis.[10] Targeted meningococcal vaccinations for high-risk infants, adolescents, and adults have similarly impacted the epidemiology and risk of meningococcal meningitis following the availability of meningococcal vaccines in the United States.[11]

Organisms causing healthcare-associated ventriculitis and meningitis differ markedly from those causing community-acquired bacterial meningitis. The most likely pathogens associated with CSF shunt and drain infections are coagulase-negative staphylococci, *Staphylococcus aureus, Propionibacterium (now Cutibacterium) acnes*, and gram-negative bacilli (including *Escherichia coli*, Enterobacter species, Citrobacter species, Serratia species, and *Pseudomonas aeruginosa*).[12]

Infectious encephalitis is caused by many viruses, bacteria, parasites, and fungi.[5,13,14] Noninfectious processes can also cause encephalitis and, as a result, the etiology remains unknown in 20% or more of encephalitis cases. Viral encephalitis in the United States is often caused by enteroviruses, herpes viruses, and arboviruses.[7,15,16]

ANATOMY AND PHYSIOLOGY OF THE CENTRAL NERVOUS SYSTEM

Meninges

The skull and vertebrae protect the CNS from blunt or penetrating trauma (Fig. 128-1). The brain is suspended in these structures by CSF and is surrounded by the meninges. The meninges are made up of three separate membranes: dura mater, arachnoid, and pia mater.[17] Dura mater, or pachymeninges, lies directly beneath and is adherent to the skull. The other two membranes are referred to collectively as leptomeninges. Pia mater lies directly over brain tissue. Arachnoid, the middle layer, lies between the dura mater and the pia mater. The subarachnoid space, located between the arachnoid and the pia mater, is the conduit for CSF. Meningitis refers to

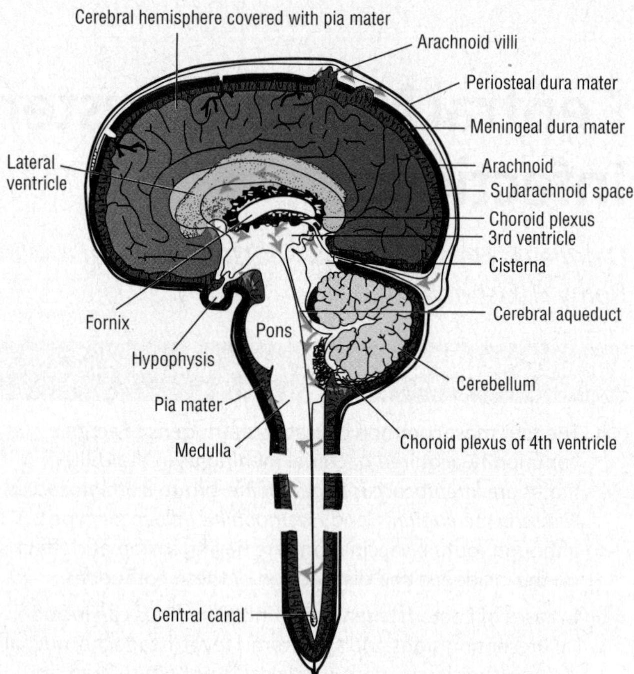

FIGURE 128-1 Diagram of the central nervous system.

inflammation of the subarachnoid space or spinal fluid, whereas encephalitis is an inflammation of the brain tissue itself. Since infectious microorganisms frequently are an underlying cause of these inflammatory processes, the terms "meningitis," "encephalitis," and "meningoencephalitis" are frequently used to denote an infectious process.[18]

Cerebrospinal Fluid

Approximately 85% of the CSF is produced within the third, fourth, and lateral ventricles by the choroid plexus (Fig. 128-1). CSF volume in the CNS is related to patient age: infants have approximately 40 to 60 mL of CSF, older children have 60 to 100 mL, while adults have 115 to 160 mL. Normally, CSF is produced at the rate of approximately 500 mL/day and flows unidirectionally downward through the spinal cord. The CSF is removed by the arachnoid villi and vertebral venous plexus located in the spinal cord and does not recommunicate with the point of production.[18]

2 The CSF normally is clear, with a protein content of less than 50 mg/dL (500 mg/L), a glucose concentration of approximately 50% to 60% of the simultaneous peripheral serum glucose concentration, and a pH of approximately 7.4. Also, it typically contains fewer than 5 WBCs per mm^3 (5×10^6/L), all of which should be lymphocytes (Table 128-1).[3,19] As meninges become inflamed, CSF abnormalities can be used diagnostically as markers of CNS infections.

Blood–Brain Barrier/Blood–CSF Barrier

Natural barriers to the exchange of drugs and endogenous compounds among the blood, brain, and CSF are the blood–brain barrier (BBB) and the blood–CSF barrier (BCSFB) (Fig. 128-2). The BBB consists of tightly joined capillary endothelial cells. Drug entry into brain tissue is accomplished by direct passage through the capillary endothelial cells and further penetration of the glial cells that envelop the capillary structure.[18] Passage of drugs into the CSF is controlled by the BCSFB. This barrier is created by ependymal cells of the choroid plexus, which function as an active-transport system similar to the renal tubular epithelial cells. The inflammatory process

TABLE 128-1 Mean Values of the Components of Normal and Abnormal Cerebrospinal Fluid

Type	Normal	Bacterial	Viral	Fungal	Tuberculosis
WBC (cells/mm³ or 10^6/L)	<5 (<30 in newborns)	1,000-5,000	50-1,000	20-500	25-500
Differential[a]	Monocytes	Neutrophils	Lymphocytes	Lymphocytes	Lymphocytes
Protein (mg/dL)	<50 (500 mg/L)	Elevated	Mild elevation	Elevated	Elevated
Glucose (mg/dL)	45-80 (2.5-4.4 mmol/L)	Low	Normal	Low	Low
CSF/blood glucose ratio	50%-60%	Decreased	Normal	Decreased	Decreased

[a]Data from References *3 and 19.*

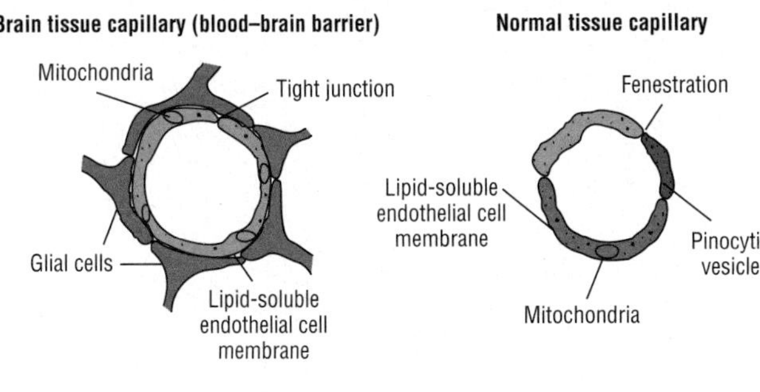

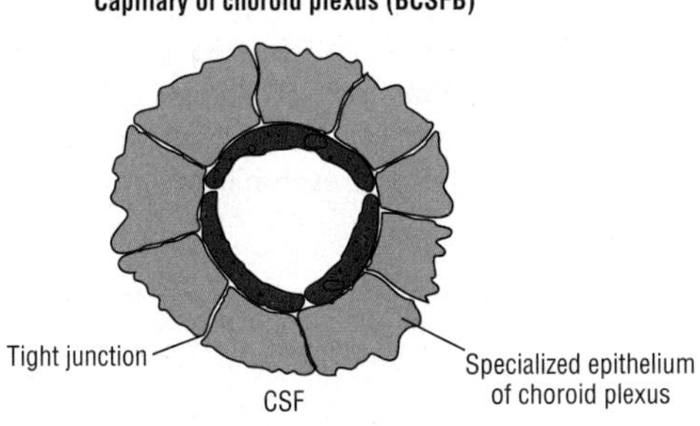

FIGURE 128-2 Schematic representation of a blood–cerebrospinal fluid barrier capillary, brain tissue capillary, and normal tissue capillary.

associated with meningitis can also inhibit the active-transport system of the choroid plexus.

PATHOPHYSIOLOGY OF THE CNS INFECTION

The development of bacterial meningitis involves four main processes: (1) mucosal colonization and bacterial invasion of the host and CNS; (2) bacterial replication in the subarachnoid space; (3) pathophysiologic alterations resulting in progressive inflammation; and (4) increased intracranial pressure (ICP) and cerebral edema leading to neuronal damage.[3,20] Many bacteria that cause meningitis initially colonize the mucous membranes of the upper respiratory tract. Immunoglobulins (Ig), such as secretory IgA, are found in high concentrations within nasopharyngeal secretions and work to inhibit bacterial colonization. However, this mucus barrier is deteriorated by IgA proteases secreted by bacteria, which allows bacteria to adhere to the host cell surface receptors.

Bacterial pathogens tightly attach to nasopharyngeal epithelial cells and are then phagocytized into the host's bloodstream. Invasion into the bloodstream occurs either transcellularly (passing through the cells) or paracellularly (between cells). After accessing the patient's bloodstream, bacteria must overcome the host's defense mechanisms. Commonly, CNS bacterial pathogens produce an extensive polysaccharide capsule resistant to neutrophil phagocytosis and complement opsonization. Capsular polysaccharides activate the alternate complement pathway, which promotes phagocytosis and clearance of infecting pathogens. Patients unable to activate the alternative complement pathway, such as those with asplenia or sickle cell anemia, are predisposed to bacterial infections caused by encapsulated microorganisms and, therefore, are at increased risk for meningitis. Most cases of acute bacterial meningitis likely occur following bacteremia, but the high incidence of pneumococcal meningitis in patients with sinusitis and otitis media suggests that direct spread to the CNS can also occur.[3]

Although the exact site and mechanism of bacterial invasion into the CNS is unknown, invasion into the subarachnoid space may occur by continuous exposure of the CNS to large bacterial inoculum. Micro-organisms utilize three main mechanisms to directly transit the blood–brain barrier: transcellular route, paracellular route, and lytic mechanism.[21] Host defense mechanisms within the subarachnoid space are inadequate to combat bacterial pathogens. Therefore, bacteria replicate freely within the CSF. Although in most cases of bacterial meningitis the neurological syndrome is caused by the pathogen having invaded into the CNS, some bacteria such as the Shiga toxin-producing *Escherichia coli* (*E. coli*) attack from outside the CNS using toxins.[22]

The effects of meningitis, namely inflammation within the subarachnoid space and the ensuing neurologic damage, are not necessarily a direct result of the pathogens themselves. The neurologic sequelae occur due to the activation of the host's inflammatory pathways, a process induced by the pathogen or its products. Bacterial cell lysis and subsequent death can result in the release of cell-wall components, such as lipopolysaccharide (LPS), lipid A (endotoxin), lipoteichoic acid, teichoic acid, and peptidoglycan, depending on whether the pathogen is gram-positive or gram-negative (Fig. 128-3). These cell-wall components cause capillary endothelial cells and CNS macrophages to release cytokines (interleukin-1 [IL-1] and tumor necrosis factor [TNF]) and other inflammatory mediators (IL-6, IL-8, platelet-activating factor [PAF], nitric oxide, arachidonic acid metabolites [eg, prostaglandin and prostacycline], and macrophage-derived proteins). Proteolytic products and toxic oxygen radicals are released from the capillary endothelium, causing an alteration in the permeability of the BBB. Platelet-activating factor activates the coagulation cascade, and arachidonic acid metabolites stimulate vasodilation. These events propagate other sequential events that can lead to cerebral edema, ICP, CSF pleocytosis, decreased cerebral blood flow, cerebral ischemia, and possibly death.

CLINICAL PRESENTATION AND DIAGNOSIS

Clinical presentation of CNS infections varies with host age, immune status, duration of illness, and the specific pathogen causing the infection.

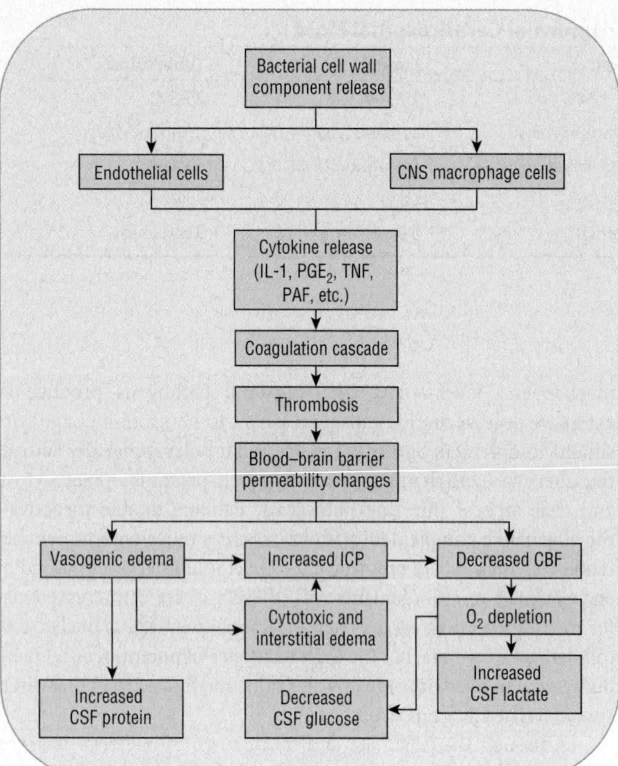

FIGURE 128-3 Hypothetical schema of pathophysiologic events that occur during bacterial meningitis. (CBF, cerebral blood flow; CSF, cerebrospinal fluid; ICP, intracranial pressure; IL-1, interleukin-1; PAF, platelet-activating factor; PGE_2, prostaglandin E_2; TNF, tumor necrosis factor.)

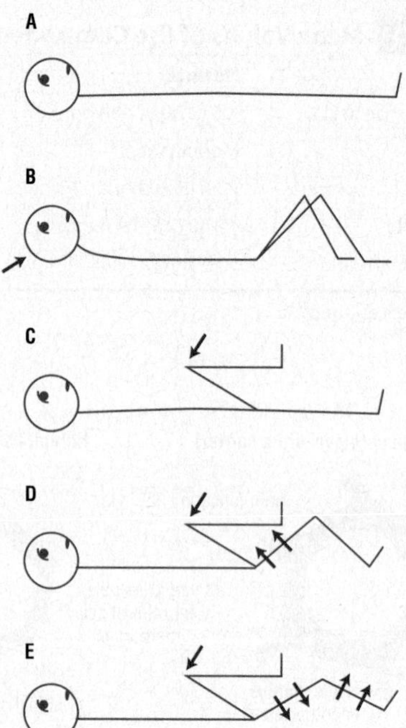

FIGURE 128-4 (A and B) Brudzinski's neck signs. (B) Hip and knee flexion occurs as a result of flexion of the neck. (C to E) Brudzinski's leg signs. (C) Patient's leg is flexed by examiner (*arrow*). (D) The contralateral leg begins to flex—identical contralateral sign (*arrows*). (E) The contralateral leg now begins to extend spontaneously, resembling a little kick (*arrows*).

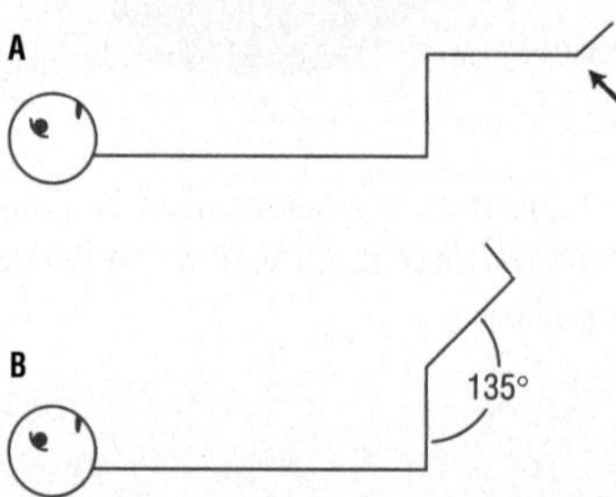

FIGURE 128-5 Kernig's sign. (A) Knees are raised to form a 90-degree angle relative to the trunk, and the examiner attempts to extend the knees. (B) Once the knee angle reaches approximately 135° contracture or extensor spasm occurs.

Signs and Symptoms

2 Classic signs and symptoms of acute bacterial meningitis include fever, nuchal rigidity, altered mental status (the classic triad), chills, nausea, vomiting, photophobia, and severe headache. Kernig's and Brudzinski's signs may also be present but are poorly sensitive and frequently absent in children (Figs. 128-4 and 128-5). Additionally, clinical signs and symptoms in young children may include bulging fontanelle, apneas, purpuric rash, irritability, refusal to eat, and convulsions. The classic triad occurs in <50% of adult patients with acute bacterial meningitis.[23] However, up to 95% of patients exhibit at least two of the following symptoms: fever, nuchal rigidity, headache, and altered mental status. Purpuric and petechial skin lesions may indicate meningococcal involvement, although lesions may also be present with *H. influenzae* meningitis.[24]

As opposed to acute bacterial meningitis, symptoms of chronic meningitis, defined as 4 weeks of symptoms of meningitis or meningoencephalitis, can be present over weeks and months. Examples include *Mycobacterium tuberculosis* and fungal meningitis (eg, due to Cryptococcus, Histoplasma, or Aspergillus species). Early symptoms of chronic meningitis may include headache, nausea, and decreased memory or comprehension, while later symptoms may include double vision, cranial nerve palsies, unsteady gait, emesis, and confusion.[19]

The clinical manifestations of brain abscess depend on the size and location of the space-occupying lesion. Common symptoms include headache, focal neurologic deficits, motor speech disorder, ataxia, fever, nystagmus, seizures, and vomiting. The clinical course can be indolent or fulminant depending on the virulence of the pathogen.

The classical clinical features of infective encephalitis in adults include fever, abnormal mental status (often with severe headache), nausea, and vomiting. Seizures can also be the initial presenting feature of patients with infectious encephalitic processes affecting the cortex.[5,14] Lastly, ill children cannot often adequately describe symptoms such as headache, whereas infants commonly have nonspecific symptoms similar to those for other acute illnesses including feeding and respiratory difficulties.[13]

Diagnostic Tests

3 CSF examination is essential for establishing diagnosis of bacterial meningitis, identifying the pathogen, and performing susceptibility testing. CSF polymorphonuclear pleocytosis, an elevated CSF protein of >50 mg/dL (500 mg/L), and a CSF glucose concentration of <50% of the simultaneously obtained peripheral value suggest bacterial meningitis (Table 128-1).[3,19] However, the values for CSF

glucose, protein, and WBC found with bacterial meningitis overlap significantly with those with viral, tuberculous, and fungal meningitis (Table 128-1). Therefore, CSF WBC count and CSF glucose and protein concentrations cannot always distinguish the different etiologies of meningitis. CSF culture is the gold standard for diagnosis of bacterial meningitis and is positive in 80% to 90% of patients with community-acquired bacterial meningitis if the CSF sample is obtained before the start of antibiotics.[24] In addition, Gram stain is a rapid, inexpensive, and accurate method to assess the presence of bacteria in CSF. However, the sensitivity of the Gram stain depends on the causative microorganism, so that its aggregate diagnostic yield is 90% in pneumococcal, 70% to 90% in meningococcal, 50% in *H. influenzae*, and only 25% to 35% in *L. monocytogenes* meningitis.[25]

In patients presenting with new-onset seizures, signs of space-occupying lesions, or moderate-to-severe impairment of consciousness, cranial imaging via magnetic resonance imaging (MRI), or cranial computed tomography (CT) should precede a lumbar puncture. MRI is generally preferred, as it more clearly identifies areas of cerebral edemas and has higher specificity and sensitivity than CT.[26] Neuroimaging or CSF cultures should not delay initiation of appropriate antibiotic therapy as doing so can result in a poor outcome in this disease.

3 In patients with suspected CNS bacterial infection, blood cultures are strongly recommended and should be collected before the first dose of antibiotics. Blood cultures identify the causative organism in 50% to 80% of cases, although the yield decreases by 20% if the patient has received antibiotics.[24] CSF viral cultures are insensitive for the diagnosis of viral encephalitis/meningitis. Patients with suspected encephalitis should have a CSF PCR test for HSV1, HSV2, VZV, and enteroviruses, as this will identify ~90% of cases due to known viral pathogens.[27]

Models have been developed in an attempt to predict the likelihood of acute community-acquired bacterial versus viral meningitis. Expert opinions and guidelines have systematically evaluated these models and identified concerns that limit their use in clinical practice.[24,27] Limitations include <100% sensitivity (risk of false-negative results), application limited to age-specific cohorts in which the models were developed, and ability to only differentiate between acute bacterial versus viral meningitis when in clinical practice other causes are also considered.

CSF lactate may be useful in differentiating between bacterial and other types of meningitis.[12,27] In a meta-analysis of 1,881 adult and pediatric patients, CSF lactate had a sensitivity of 93% and a specificity of 96% in differentiating bacterial from aseptic meningitis, when the specimen was collected before antibiotics. However, administration of antibiotics reduced sensitivity to 49%, suggesting that the usefulness of CSF lactate is compromised in patients who have already received antimicrobial therapy.[28] CSF and/or serum procalcitonin (PCT) may be useful markers for bacterial cause in community-acquired and healthcare-associated meningitis.[29,30] However, more studies are needed to confirm the impact of PCT monitoring on clinical outcomes, establish cut-off values, and evaluate cost-effectiveness.

3 Polymerase chain reaction (PCR) techniques can rapidly diagnose CNS infections and may be particularly useful in patients who have received antimicrobial therapy before lumbar puncture, have negative cultures, or when the organism is fastidious or fails to grow in conventional culture.[5,12,27] In addition to individual PCR tests, a multiplex PCR panel can simultaneously and rapidly (within ~1 hour) detect six bacterial, seven viral, and two yeast targets directly from CSF specimens; however, more studies are needed to establish performance in clinical practice.[31] Antimicrobial stewardship programs when combined with rapid diagnostic bloodstream tests have been shown to optimize antimicrobial use, though more data is needed in antimicrobial stewardship initiatives with CNS PCR tests.[32] Routine cultures are necessary for the detection of pathogens not covered by the multiplex PCR panel and for antibiotic susceptibility testing. 16s rRNA molecular testing and next generation sequencing are also emerging as diagnostic tools for CNS infections.[33,34] Ribosomal 16s is part of the 30s ribosomal subunit in bacteria. By identifying species-level 16s sequences, this testing can detect a causative pathogen for patients whose cultures are negative. Due to low positivity, high cost, and slow turnaround time, ribosomal 16s testing should be applied on a case by case basis.[35]

Latex agglutination has little incremental value and is not a recommended routine diagnostic modality for rapid determination of bacterial etiology of meningitis.[12,26,27] More studies are needed to determine whether immunochromatographic antigen testing has incremental value in the diagnosis of bacterial meningitis.

Diagnosis of tuberculous meningitis employs acid-fast stain, culture, and PCR of the CSF. The standard diagnostic tests for fungal meningitis include culture, direct microscopic examination of stained and unstained specimens of CSF, antigen detection of cryptococcal or histoplasma, and antibody assay of serum and/or CSF.

TREATMENT

Desired Outcome

4 Goals for the treatment of CNS infections should include prompt and effective eradication of infection, amelioration of signs and symptoms, and reduction of morbidity and mortality. Key elements include initiation of appropriate anti-infective and supportive care, and prevention of disease through timely introduction of vaccination and chemoprophylaxis. Understanding appropriate selection of anti-infective agents and the issues surrounding their CNS penetration will assist in meeting the goals of treatment.

General Approach to Treatment, Nonpharmacologic and Supportive Therapy

5 Until a pathogen is identified, prompt empiric antibiotic coverage is needed. Based on the patient's profile (ie, allergies, age, and concurrent medical conditions), extent of antibiotic CNS penetration, spectrum of activity, and local susceptibility patterns, appropriate recommendations should be made. Therapy should last at least 48 to 72 hours or until an infectious process has been ruled out (Tables 128-2 and 128-3).[26,27,36]

6 Acute bacterial meningitis is a neurologic emergency. An empiric antimicrobial therapy should be initiated as soon as possible after a diagnosis is suspected.[26] The first dose of antibiotics should not be withheld, even when lumbar puncture is delayed or neuroimaging is being performed. It is strongly recommended that the time period from suspected diagnosis to initiation of antibiotic treatment should not exceed 1 hour.[27]

Supportive care, particularly early in the course of treatment, is important. Administration of fluids, electrolytes, antipyretics, and analgesics may be indicated for patients presenting with a possible CNS infection. Additionally, venous thromboembolism prophylaxis, antiepileptic therapy, and ICP monitoring may be needed. Patients may require the administration of osmotic diuretics such as mannitol 25% or hypertonic saline to maintain an ICP of less than 15 mm Hg (2 kPa) and a cerebral perfusion pressure of 60 mm Hg (8 kPa) or more. Other supportive care measures may include respiratory and circulatory supports, gastrointestinal (GI) care, and maintaining normal body temperature.

Although supportive treatment may be indicated in certain patients with acute bacterial meningitis, the routine use of adjuvant mannitol, acetaminophen, antiepileptic agents, or hypertonic saline is not recommended according to the European guidelines.[27]

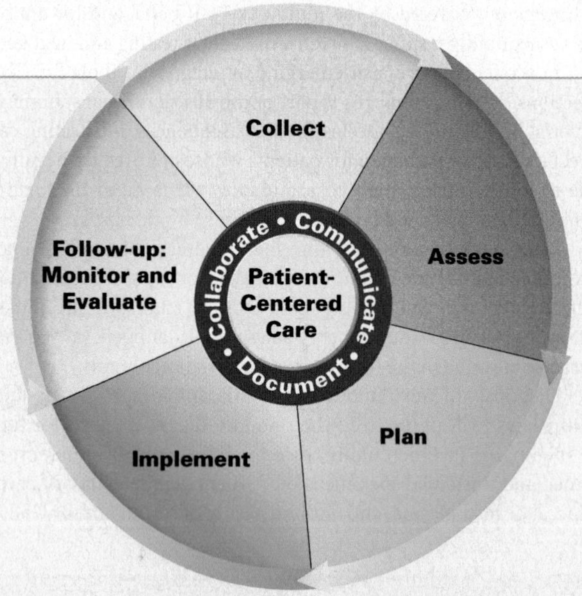

Patient Care Process for CNS Infections

The image shows the five fundamental steps included in The Pharmacist's Care Process endorsed by the Joint Commission for Pharmacy Practitioners (2014). The tagline of this process reads collaborate, communicate, and document. The five fundamental steps listed here are collect, assess, plan, implement, and follow-up: monitor and evaluate. All these steps are listed in a circular block diagram.

Collect

- Patient characteristics (eg, age, sex, weight, height, pregnancy/breastfeeding status, allergies)
- Patient medical history (personal and family)
- Social history (eg, alcohol/illicit drug use, recent travel, home residence, exposure to animals) and dietary habits including intake of unpasteurized dairy products
- Current medication use including anti-infective and immunomodulating agents
- Vaccination history (eg, PCV13, PPSV23, Hib, MenACWY, MenB, influenza, COVID-19)
- Objective data
  - Vitals (eg, temperature, blood pressure, pulse, respiratory rate), and laboratories (white blood cell count, lactate, procalcitonin, serum creatinine, blood urea nitrogen)
  - Blood/CSF examination, cultures, Gram stain, PCR, 16s rRNA, smear, AFB, serology radiologic imaging (MRI, CT)

Assess

- Presence of risk factors (eg, vaccination history, immunocompromised status, asplenia, recent dental procedure, endocarditis, consumption of unpasteurized dairy products, central venous catheter, CSF shunt)
- Signs and symptoms (eg, temperature >100.4 °F [38 °C], nuchal rigidity, headache, Kernig's and Bruzinski's signs [Figs. 128-4 and 128-5], CSF characteristics [Table 128-1], radiographic evidence, pathogen identification)
- Local susceptibilities of suspected/proven pathogen(s)
- Source control of focal infection (eg, minimally invasive aspiration of brain abscess)
- Barriers for successful completion of therapeutic regimen
- Candidates for chemoprophylaxis

Plan*

- Evidence-based empiric drug therapy regimen including anti-infective agent(s) with good CNS penetration (Table 128-3), dose, route, frequency, and duration (see Tables 128-2 and 128-5, the sections "Healthcare-Associated Ventriculitis and Meningitis," "Bacterial Brain Abscess," "Viral Encephalitis," and "CNS Infections in Special Populations").
- Definitive anti-infective therapy if specific pathogen identified (Tables 128-4 and 128-5, sections as above)
- Corticosteroid use when indicated
- Monitoring parameters including efficacy (eg, fever, mental status, meningismus, white blood cell count, radiologic resolution of focal infection, drug monitoring) and safety (eg, renal function, drug-drug interactions); frequency and timing of follow-up
- Patient education (eg, purpose of treatment, invasive procedures, drug-specific information)
- Referrals to other providers when appropriate (eg, infectious diseases, neurologist, interventional radiologist)

Implement*

- Provide patient education regarding all elements of treatment plan
- Ensure effective transitions of care
- Schedule follow-up if treatment continues as outpatient (eg, SCr, adherence assessment, radiographic imaging)

Follow-up: Monitor and Evaluate

- Resolution of CNS infection symptoms (eg, fever, nuchal rigidity, headache, altered mental status)
- Presence of adverse effects (eg, acute renal injury, electrolyte abnormalities, QT interval prolongation)
- Patient adherence to treatment plan using multiple sources of information
- Duration of therapy based on evidence-based guidelines, clinical and radiologic progress

Collaborate with patient, caregivers, and other healthcare professionals.

Furthermore, therapeutic hypothermia and glycerol are contraindicated because they have been associated with a higher mortality rate.[37,38] However, a Cochrane meta-analysis including 1,272 patients (mostly children under 16 years) demonstrated no effect of glycerol on mortality.[39]

7 Several factors influence the transfer of antibiotic from capillary blood into the CNS. Notably, antibiotic penetration is increased through inflamed meninges due to damage to tight junctions between capillary endothelial cells and reduction of the activity of energy-dependent efflux pumps in the choroid plexus responsible

TABLE 128-2 Bacterial Meningitis: Most Likely Etiologies and Empiric Therapy by Age Group

Age	Most Likely Organisms	Empirical Therapy[a]
<1 month	*S. agalactiae* Gram-negative enterics[b] *L. monocytogenes*	Ampicillin + cefotaxime *or* ampicillin + aminoglycoside
1-23 months	*S. pneumoniae* *N. meningitidis* *H. influenzae* *S. agalactiae*	Vancomycin[c] + third-generation cephalosporin (cefotaxime *or* ceftriaxone)
2-50 years	*N. meningitidis* *S. pneumoniae*	Vancomycin[c] + third-generation cephalosporin (cefotaxime *or* ceftriaxone)
>50 years	*S. pneumoniae* *N. meningitidis* Gram-negative enterics[b] *L. monocytogenes*	Vancomycin[c] + ampicillin + third-generation cephalosporin (cefotaxime *or* ceftriaxone)

[a]Data from References *26 and 27*.

[b]*E. coli, Klebsiella* spp., *Enterobacter* spp. common.

[c]Vancomycin use should be based on local incidence of penicillin-resistant *S. pneumoniae* and until cefotaxime or ceftriaxone minimum inhibitory concentration results are available.

Strength of recommendation: (A) Good evidence to support a recommendation for use; should always be offered. (B) Moderate evidence to support a recommendation for use; should generally be offered.[26]

Quality of evidence: (i) Evidence from one or more properly randomized, controlled trial. (ii) Evidence from one or more well-designed clinical trial, without randomization; from cohort or case-controlled analytic studies (preferably from one or more center) or from multiple time-series. (iii) Evidence from opinions of respected authorities, based on clinical experience, descriptive studies, or reports of expert committees.[26]

TABLE 128-3 Penetration of Anti-infective Agents into the CSF[a]

Therapeutic Levels in CSF With or Without Inflammation	
Acyclovir	Levofloxacin
Chloramphenicol	Linezolid
Ciprofloxacin	Metronidazole
Fluconazole	Moxifloxacin
Flucytosine	Pyrazinamide
Foscarnet	Rifampin
Fosfomycin	Sulfonamides
Ganciclovir	Trimethoprim
Isoniazid	Voriconazole
Therapeutic Levels in CSF With Inflammation of Meninges	
Ampicillin ± sulbactam	Imipenem
Aztreonam	Meropenem
Cefepime	Nafcillin
Cefotaxime	Ofloxacin
Ceftazidime	Penicillin G
Ceftriaxone	Piperacillin/tazobactam[b]
Cefuroxime	Pyrimethamine
Colistin	Quinupristin/dalfopristin
Daptomycin	Ticarcillin ± clavulanic acid[b]
Ethambutol	Vancomycin
Nontherapeutic Levels in CSF With or Without Inflammation	
Aminoglycosides	Cephalosporins (second generation)[d]
Amphotericin B	Doxycycline[e]
β-Lactamase inhibitors[c]	Itraconazole[f]
Cephalosporins (first generation)	

[a]Data from Reference *36*.

[b]May not achieve therapeutic levels against organisms with higher MIC, as in *P. aeruginosa*. Tazobactam does not penetrate BBB.

[c]Includes clavulanic acid, sulbactam, and tazobactam.

[d]Cefuroxime is an exception.

[e]Documented effectiveness for *B. burgdorferi*.

[f]Achieves therapeutic concentrations for *Cryptococcus neoformans* therapy.

for movement of penicillins and, to a lesser extent, fluoroquinolones and aminoglycosides (Table 128-3). Antibiotics having low molecular weights are passed more easily through biologic barriers than compounds of higher molecular weight. Furthermore, only non-ionized antibiotics at physiologic or pathologic pH are capable of diffusion. Highly lipid-soluble compounds penetrate more readily than water-soluble compounds. Antibiotics not extensively bound to plasma proteins provide a larger free fraction of drug capable of passing into the CSF. However, passage of large, polar antibiotics into the CSF may be assisted by a carrier transport system. Antibiotic dosages in the treatment of CNS infections must be optimized to ensure adequate penetration to the site of infection.

Challenges of CSF penetration were traditionally overcome by direct instillation of antibiotics intrathecally or intraventricularly. Advantages of direct instillation, however, must be weighed against the risks of invasive CNS procedures and adverse effects. Intraventricular delivery may be necessary in patients who have shunt infections that are difficult to eradicate or who cannot undergo surgical management.[26] Antimicrobial agents often utilized for bacterial meningitis treatment have adequate CSF penetration, which has limited the need for direct CNS instillation for this type of infection. The Infectious Diseases Society of America (IDSA) guidelines for healthcare-associated meningitis and ventriculitis recommend considering the use of intraventricular antibiotics only in patients who fail or respond poorly to systemic treatment.[12]

8 Although the length of treatment for acute bacterial meningitis is generally based on the causative organism, there is no universally accepted standard (Table 128-4).[12,26,27] Meningitis caused by *S. pneumoniae* has been treated successfully with 10 to 14 days of antibiotic therapy, while cases caused by *N. meningitidis* or *H. influenzae* usually can be treated with a 7-day course. In contrast, a longer duration (21 days or more) has been recommended for patients with *L. monocytogenes*, gram-negative or pseudomonal meningitis. Nonetheless, antibiotic treatments for bacterial meningitis should be individualized, and some patients may require prolonged courses.

ACUTE BACTERIAL MENINGITIS

Causative Organisms

Streptococcus pneumoniae (Pneumococcus or Diplococcus)

9 *S. pneumoniae* continues to be the leading cause of community-acquired bacterial meningitis in patients 2 months of age or older. It accounts for approximately 40% to 50% of bacterial meningitis cases in the United States, with an overall case fatality rate of ~8% to 22%.[2,9,40] Despite declining rates of pneumococcal meningitis since the introduction of PCV7 and PCV13 vaccinations in 2000 and 2010, respectively, case fatality rate has not significantly changed from the pre-PCV7 era.[2,41] Pneumonia, bloodstream infection, endocarditis, CSF leak secondary to head trauma, splenectomy, alcoholism, sickle cell disease, and bone marrow transplantation may predispose the patient to the development of pneumococcal meningitis. Coma, hearing impairment, and seizures are common neurologic complications due to *S. pneumoniae* meningitis.

TABLE 128-4 Antimicrobial Agents of First Choice and Alternative Choice in the Treatment of Meningitis Caused by Gram-Positive and Gram-Negative Microorganisms

Organism	Antibiotics of First Choice	Alternative Antibiotics	Recommended Duration of Therapy
Gram-Positive Organisms			
Streptococcus pneumoniae[a]			10-14 days
Penicillin susceptible MIC ≤0.06 mcg/mL (mg/L)	Penicillin G or Ampicillin (A-III)	Cefotaxime (A-III), Ceftriaxone (A-III), Cefepime (B-II), or Meropenem (B-II)	
Penicillin resistant MIC >0.06 mcg/mL (mg/L)	Vancomycin[b,c] + Cefotaxime or Ceftriaxone (A-III)	Moxifloxacin (B-II)	
Ceftriaxone resistant MIC >0.5 mcg/mL (mg/L)	Vancomycin[b,c] + Cefotaxime or Ceftriaxone (A-III)	Moxifloxacin (B-II)	
Staphylococcus aureus			14-21 days
Methicillin susceptible	Nafcillin or Oxacillin (A-III)	Vancomycin (A-III) or Meropenem (B-III)	
Methicillin resistant	Vancomycin[b,c] (A-III)	Trimethoprim-sulfamethoxazole or Linezolid (B-III)	
Group B *Streptococcus*	Penicillin G or Ampicillin (A-III) ± Gentamicin[b,c]	Ceftriaxone or Cefotaxime (B-III)	14-21 days
S. epidermidis	Vancomycin[b,c] (A-III)	Linezolid (B-III)	14-21 days[d]
L. monocytogenes	Penicillin G or Ampicillin ± Gentamicin[b,c,e] (A-III)	Trimethoprim-sulfamethoxazole (A-III), Meropenem (B-III)	≥21 days
Gram-Negative Organisms			
Neisseria meningitis			7-10 days
Penicillin susceptible	Penicillin G or Ampicillin (A-III)	Cefotaxime or Ceftriaxone (A-III)	
Penicillin resistant	Cefotaxime or Ceftriaxone (A-III)	Meropenem or Moxifloxacin (A-I)	
Haemophilus influenzae			7-10 days
β-lactamase negative	Ampicillin (A-III)	Cefotaxime (A-III), Ceftriaxone (A-III), Cefepime (A-III), or Moxifloxacin (A-III)	
β-lactamase positive	Cefotaxime or Ceftriaxone (A-I)	Cefepime (A-I) or Moxifloxacin (A-III)	
Enterobacteriaceae[f]	Cefotaxime or Ceftriaxone (A-II)	Cefepime (A-III), Moxifloxacin (A-III), Meropenem (A-III), or Aztreonam (A-III)	21 days
Pseudomonas aeruginosa	Cefepime or Ceftazidime (A-II) ± Tobramycin[b,c] (A-III)	Ciprofloxacin (A-III), Meropenem (A-III), Piperacillin plus Tobramycin[a,b] (A-III), Colistin sulfomethate[g] (B-III), Aztreonam (A-III)	21 days

[a]Data from References *12, 26, and 27*.

[b]Direct CNS administration may be considered if failed conventional treatment.

[c]Monitor serum drug levels.

[d]Based on clinical experience; no clear recommendations.

[e]European guidelines recommend adding gentamicin for the first 7 days of treatment.

[f]Includes *E. coli* and *Klebsiella* spp.

[g]Should be reserved for multidrug-resistant pseudomonal or Acinetobacter infections for which all other therapeutic options have been exhausted.

See Table 128-2 footnotes for rating scale of evidence.

5 Based on resistance patterns, penicillin should not be used as empiric therapy if *S. pneumoniae* is suspected. Furthermore, appropriate Clinical Laboratory Standards Institute (CLSI)-approved testing of all CSF isolates for penicillin resistance is recommended. Ceftriaxone and cefotaxime have served as alternatives to penicillin in the treatment of penicillin-nonsusceptible pneumococci. Of note, higher minimum inhibitory concentration (MIC) with cephalosporins and higher cephalosporin resistance rates were noted in penicillin-resistant isolates, with the exception of ceftaroline.[42] Therapeutic approaches to cephalosporin-resistant pneumococci include the addition of vancomycin or, to a lesser extent, rifampin. The combination of vancomycin and ceftriaxone can be used as empirical treatment until antimicrobial susceptibility data are available.[25-27]

Given the limited therapeutic options for penicillin- and cephalosporin-resistant pneumococcal meningitis, newer agents have been evaluated. Meropenem is approved for the treatment of bacterial meningitis in children aged 3 months and older and has shown similar clinical and microbiologic efficacies to cefotaxime or ceftriaxone. Meropenem is recommended as an alternative to a third-generation cephalosporin in penicillin-nonsusceptible isolates. Some caution is warranted with the use of imipenem for CNS infections, given the risk of drug-induced seizures, especially when doses are not properly adjusted for declining renal function. Of note, seizures may be caused by meningitis itself or imipenem, and the cause is often difficult to differentiate. Levofloxacin and moxifloxacin represent additional therapeutic options with favorable activity against multidrug-resistant pneumococci and good penetration into the CSF.[12,43]

Intravenous linezolid, daptomycin, and ceftaroline have also emerged as viable therapeutic options for treating multidrug-resistant gram-positive infections. Linezolid in combination with ceftriaxone has been used to treat limited cases of pneumococcal meningitis with outcomes similar to standard treatment.[44] Further research is required to delineate the clinical utility of therapeutic options such as daptomycin and ceftaroline and determine their place in therapy.[45,46]

Pneumococcal vaccines help reduce the risk of invasive pneumococcal disease (IPD). Virtually all serotypes of *S. pneumoniae* exhibiting intermediate or complete resistance to penicillin are included in the 23-serotype pneumococcal polysaccharide vaccine (PPSV23). Use of the heptavalent pneumococcal conjugate vaccine (PCV7), introduced in 2000, significantly reduced the incidence of invasive pneumococcal infections, including sepsis and meningitis. However, in the decade following its introduction, rate of invasive disease caused by non-PCV7 strains increased considerably, especially serotype 19A, leading to the development of a newer vaccine with expanded coverage. In 2010, the FDA approved PCV13 to replace PCV7. In the first 3 years after the introduction of PCV13 in the United States, investigators estimated over 30,000 cases of IPD and 3,000 deaths were potentially averted.[47] Between 1998 and 2018, rates of IPD in the United States among children and adults have steadily decreased since PCV7 and PCV13 introductions.[48]

For current recommendations on vaccinations against pneumococcal disease and high-risk groups, refer to Chapter 147, "Vaccines, Toxoids, and Other Immunobiologics" in this book and the current guidelines by the Advisory Committee on Immunization Practices (ACIP).

Neisseria meningitidis (Meningococcus)

1 *N. meningitidis* is a leading cause of bacterial meningitis among children and young adults in the United States and around the world.[2,49] Incidence of meningococcal disease in the United States has been declining from 1.2 cases per 100,000 population in the 1990s to 0.1 cases per 100,000 population in 2018. Incidence peaks in infants <1-year-old (0.93 cases per 100,000 population) with a second peak in adolescents and young adults 16 to 23 years of age (0.23 cases per 100,000 population).[50] Five of the thirteen serogroups of *N. meningitidis* (A, B, C, Y, and W) are primarily responsible for invasive meningococcal disease. The proportion of cases caused by each serogroup varies by age group. Serogroup B causes ~65% of meningococcal disease among children <5 years old.[49]

N. meningitidis is spread by direct person-to-person close contact, including respiratory droplets and pharyngeal secretions. Close contacts of patients contracting meningococcal meningitis are at an increased risk of developing meningitis. Secondary cases of meningitis usually develop within the first week following exposure but may take up to 60 days after contact with the index case.[11] Clusters of disease are associated with crowding as in schools, dormitories, and military barracks. Other significant risk factors for meningococcal disease include complement deficiency, anatomic or functional asplenia, HIV infection, and passive or active smoking.[11]

The presence of petechiae may be the primary clue that the underlying pathogen is *N. meningitidis*.[25] Patients may also have an obvious or subclinical picture of disseminated intravascular coagulation (DIC). Deafness unilaterally or bilaterally may develop early or late in the disease course.

5 Third-generation cephalosporins (ie, cefotaxime and ceftriaxone) are the recommended empiric treatment for meningococcal meningitis (Table 128-4).[26,27] When final culture results are available, penicillin G or ampicillin is recommended for penicillin-susceptible isolates. Meropenem and fluoroquinolones are also suitable alternatives for the treatment of penicillin nonsusceptible meningococci. The recommended duration of therapy is typically 7 days if there is good clinical response.[26] Antimicrobial chemoprophylaxis of close contacts should be started as soon as possible (ideally <24 hours after identification of the index patient). There was an 84% reduction in the risk of invasive meningeal disease for 30 days after the index case when household contacts were given chemoprophylaxis. Ciprofloxacin and rifampin are the two most used chemoprophylactic agents, although antibiotic resistance can develop when meningococcal isolates are exposed to rifampin.[51] For further discussion on who should receive prophylaxis, interested readers can refer to current recommendations by the Centers for Disease Control and Prevention (CDC).[11]

Two types of meningococcal vaccines are available in the United States: two quadrivalent polysaccharide protein conjugate vaccine directed against serogroups A, C, W, and Y and two MenB vaccines directed against serogroup B meningococcal vaccine. The quadrivalent meningococcal conjugate vaccine is recommended for all people 11 to 12 years old with a booster dose at 16 years of age. Among adolescents ages 13 to 17 years old in the United States, 88.9% received ≥1 dose of the MenACWY vaccine in 2019.[52] Additionally, the outer membrane vesicle meningococcal B vaccine (MeNZB) is being assessed for vaccine effectiveness against gonorrhea in young adults, due to the 80% to 90% genetic homology in primary sequences between *N. gonorrhoeae* and *N. meningitidis*.[53] For full details on vaccine availability and vaccination recommendations in various age groups and for those with significant risk factors, refer to Chapter 147, "Vaccines, Toxoids, and Other Immunobiologics" in this book and the current recommendations from the ACIP.

Haemophilus influenzae Type b

1 Widespread vaccination of infants and children has resulted in a dramatic decline in the global incidence of Hib meningitis from 31 to 5 per 100,000 children aged <5 years in 2000 and 2015, respectively.[54] Similarly, the global Hib meningitis case fatality ratio fell from 44% in 2000 to 23% in 2015. Interested readers can refer to Chapter 147, "Vaccines, Toxoids, and Other Immunobiologics" in this book for information on recommended Hib vaccine dosing and administration schedules. In neonates, infection is acquired intrapartum by aspiration of amniotic fluid or by contact with genital tract secretions containing the organism. In older children and adults, Hib meningitis should suggest the presence of other underlying conditions, including otitis media, epiglottitis, sinusitis, pneumonia, diabetes mellitus, sickle cell, asplenia, alcoholism, and immunodeficiency.

5 Third-generation cephalosporins (cefotaxime and ceftriaxone) are the drugs of choice for empiric therapy for Hib meningitis as they are active against β-lactamase–producing and non-β-lactamase–producing strains. Cefepime and fluoroquinolones are suitable alternatives regardless of β-lactamase activity. Ampicillin can be used if the isolate is susceptible. Beta-lactamase-negative, ampicillin-resistant strains of *H. influenzae* have been described and some experts recommend caution in using ampicillin when the penicillin minimum inhibitory concentration is 1 to 2 mcg/mL.[55] Recommended duration of treatment is 7 days (adults) or 7 to 10 days (children).[26,27]

Dexamethasone is beneficial for treatment of infants and children with Hib meningitis to diminish the risk of hearing loss, if given before or concurrently with the first dose of antimicrobial agent(s).[26,27,56] All invasive (including meningitis) cases should be reported to the local public health department.

9 Chemoprophylaxis is indicated to reduce the risk of secondary invasive Hib disease in close contacts by eliminating nasopharyngeal and oropharyngeal carriages of *H. influenzae*. For prophylaxis, rifampin should be administered orally (once a day for 4 days; 20 mg/kg/dose; maximum, 600 mg). The dose for infants younger than 1 month is not established; some experts recommend lowering the dose to 10 mg/kg.[56,57]

Streptococcus agalactiae (Streptococcus Group B)

Streptococcus group B (GBS) is a leading cause of meningitis in neonates and young infants, with a case fatality rate of 7.3% in pediatric patients and 20.8% in adult patients.[2] Neurologic sequelae include sight or hearing loss and cerebral palsy. Neonates acquire this infection through vertical transmission while passing through the vaginal canal during birth. GBS is an inhabitant of the human GI and genitourinary tracts. Maternal GBS colonization worldwide was shown to be 18% with regional variation from 11% to 35%.[58]

Early onset GBS infection occurs within the first 24 hours of life (range 0-6 days), whereas late-onset disease typically occurs from 7 to 89 days of age.[59] Universal prenatal screening and intrapartum antimicrobial prophylaxis of GBS-colonized pregnant women have significantly decreased the rate of early onset invasive disease.[60] However, late-onset disease cannot be prevented by intrapartum antimicrobial prophylaxis. Recommended agents for intrapartum prophylaxis are penicillin G or ampicillin, cefazolin (if penicillin allergy with low risk of anaphylaxis), clindamycin (if penicillin allergy with high risk of anaphylaxis and GBS isolate is known to be susceptible to clindamycin), or vancomycin (if penicillin allergy with high risk of anaphylaxis and GBS isolate not susceptible, or unknown susceptibility, to clindamycin). Intrapartum antibiotic prophylaxis should be started promptly to achieve the optimal antibiotic treatment window of at least 4 hours before birth.[61]

Maternal immunization represents a non-antibiotic strategy to prevent both early- and late-onset GBS infection and has been a focus of the WHO.[62] There are currently no licensed GBS vaccines, although some promising conjugate vaccine candidates have been tested for safety and immunogenicity in phase I and II trials.

(5) Ampicillin plus an aminoglycoside is the treatment of choice for a newborn infant with presumptive early onset GBS meningitis. Empiric treatment for late-onset meningitis differs by postnatal age at the time of evaluation. When group B streptococci are identified in culture, penicillin G is the drug of choice, with ampicillin as an acceptable alternative therapy.[59] For infants with uncomplicated meningitis, 14 days of treatment is satisfactory, but longer periods of treatment may be necessary for patients with prolonged or complicated courses; ventriculitis should be treated for at least 4 weeks. Ampicillin or penicillin G is the recommended agent for confirmed GBS meningitis in adults. Addition of an aminoglycoside could also be considered.[26] Alternative agents are third-generation cephalosporins and vancomycin. For adults with meningitis, the recommended duration of antibiotics is 14 to 21 days.

Listeria monocytogenes

L. monocytogenes is a facultative anaerobic, gram-positive, diphtheroid-like organism that multiplies intracellularly. Meningitis due to *L. monocytogenes* primarily affects neonates, alcoholic or immunocompromised individuals (including pregnant women), and the elderly. Invasive infections in healthy young individuals remain rare. *L. monocytogenes* is implicated in approximately 10% of meningitis cases in patients older than 65 years of age and carries a case fatality rate of approximately 18% in the United States.[2]

Transmission usually involves colonization of the patient's gastrointestinal tract with the organism, which then penetrates the gut lumen to seed the bloodstream. Soft cheeses and raw produce are common causes of listeriosis outbreaks. Coleslaw, unpasteurized milk, ready-to-eat foods, and raw beef and poultry have also been identified as sources of this foodborne pathogen. Invasive disease includes bacteremia, meningitis, meningoencephalitis, or cerebritis. Infection of the CNS may be diffuse or localized.

(5) (8) Treatment of *L. monocytogenes* meningitis should consist of penicillin G or ampicillin. The addition of aminoglycoside is also recommended in proven infection for both children and adults. Trimethoprim-sulfamethoxazole and meropenem are recommended alternative agents, whereas there is less clinical experience with linezolid and fluoroquinolones. Despite *in vitro* activity against *L. monocytogenes*, intravenous vancomycin has been associated with high failure rates in patients with *L. monocytogenes* meningitis. Also, third-generation cephalosporins lack *in vitro* activity against *L. monocytogenes*. Patients should be treated for a minimum of 21 days.[26,27]

A national prospective study from France of 252 cases of neurolisteriosis showed significantly greater mortality in patients who received adjunctive dexamethasone within the first 24 hours.[63] This deleterious effect suggests that adjunctive dexamethasone should be avoided in the treatment of neurolisteriosis.

Dexamethasone as an Adjunctive Treatment for Acute Bacterial Meningitis

In addition to antibiotics, dexamethasone is a commonly used adjunctive therapy in the treatment of acute bacterial meningitis to immunomodulate the inflammatory response. Corticosteroids inhibit the production of TNF and IL-1, both potent proinflammatory cytokines.

A systematic review of 25 randomized controlled trials involving 4,121 participants showed that corticosteroid use in bacterial meningitis was associated with lower rates of hearing loss and short-term neurological sequelae in adults and children, but there was no mortality benefit in high-income countries. No beneficial effects were observed in low-income countries. Additionally, subgroup analyses demonstrated a 16% reduction in overall mortality in pneumococcal meningitis and a 66% reduction in severe hearing loss in children with *H. influenzae* meningitis.[64]

(1) Routine use of dexamethasone in meningitis is not without controversy. A potential concern is that adjunctive dexamethasone therapy may reduce the penetration of antibiotics into the CSF by inhibiting or reducing meningeal inflammation. Appropriate concentrations of vancomycin in CSF may be obtained even when adjunctive dexamethasone is used, but the small number of subjects studied limits the generalization of these findings.[65] Recommendations by practice guidelines call for the use of adjunctive dexamethasone in infants and children (6 weeks of age and older) with *H. influenzae* meningitis.[26] The recommended intravenous dose is 0.15 mg/kg every 6 hours for 2 to 4 days, initiated 10 to 20 minutes prior to or concomitant with the first dose of antibiotics. In infants and children with pneumococcal meningitis, adjunctive dexamethasone may be considered after weighing the potential benefits and possible risks.[26,56] If pneumococcal meningitis is suspected or proven, adults should receive dexamethasone 0.15 mg/kg (up to 10 mg) every 6 hours for 2 to 4 days with the first dose administered 10 to 20 minutes prior to first dose of antibiotics. It is often difficult to ascertain the responsible pathogen on presentation. Therefore, some clinicians and the European guidelines recommend initiating dexamethasone in all patients (adults and children) presenting with suspected or proven community-acquired bacterial meningitis and consider discontinuation only if pathogens other than *H. influenzae* or *S. pneumoniae* are identified. Another difference between the US and European guidelines is that according to the European guidelines, dexamethasone can still be administered up to 4 hours after initiation of antibiotics.[27] Adjunctive dexamethasone in neurolisteriosis has been associated with reduced survival. Therefore, adjunctive dexamethasone should be discontinued if the meningitis is found to be caused by *L. monocytogenes*.[63]

HEALTHCARE-ASSOCIATED VENTRICULITIS AND MENINGITIS

Healthcare-associated meningitis and ventriculitis, formerly referred to as nosocomial meningitis, is a subclass of bacterial meningitis that largely occurs in neurosurgical patients.[12] The disease process in these patients can be more indolent compared to those with community-acquired bacterial meningitis. The most likely pathogens associated with CSF shunt and drain infections are coagulase-negative staphylococci (especially *Staphylococcus epidermidis*), *S. aureus*, *Propionibacterium* (now *Cutibacterium*) *acnes*, and gram-negative bacilli; including *E. coli*, Enterobacter species, Citrobacter species, Serratia species, and *Pseudomonas aeruginosa*. In the presence of prosthetic devices, some of the microorganisms form biofilms which compromise antibiotic penetration.

Diagnosis of healthcare-associated meningitis and ventriculitis can be challenging and should focus on CSF fluid analysis and culture. However, patients may have only modest abnormalities in CSF cell counts. Additionally, CSF Gram stain may be unreliable—particularly in the setting of systemic antibiotic exposure. If possible, antibiotic therapy should be delayed until CSF can be recovered for culture. A negative CSF culture following antimicrobial therapy is not sufficient to exclude healthcare-associated meningitis or ventriculitis.[66] Use of extended hold cultures is encouraged to increase recovery of slow-growing pathogens such as *C. acnes*. If a CSF drain or shunt is removed due to possible infection, then these components should be cultured as well. Blood cultures may be considered in those with ventriculopleural or ventriculoperitoneal shunts but are recommended in those with ventriculoatrial shunts.[12] 1-3-β-D-glucan may be useful in diagnosing fungal meningitis and ventriculitis because of the low sensitivity of CSF culture for fungal pathogens.[67]

Empiric use of broad-spectrum antibiotic therapy is critical for the treatment of healthcare-associated meningitis and ventriculitis because of the variety of organisms implicated in these cases. Empiric treatment should include intravenous vancomycin coupled with an anti-pseudomonal β-lactam such as meropenem, cefepime, or ceftazidime. All agents should be dosed to maximize CNS penetration.[12] Piperacillin-tazobactam is not recommended given the suboptimal CNS penetration of tazobactam. Continuous infusion vancomycin may optimize vancomycin exposure in the CSF but clinical data remain scant.[68]

Once culture results are available, antibiotic therapy can be tailored. Staphylococcus spp. are important causative pathogens in healthcare-associated meningitis and ventriculitis, particularly among patients with intracranial or spinal hardware. For methicillin-susceptible *S. aureus* (MSSA), the treatment of choice is nafcillin or oxacillin. For methicillin-resistant *S. aureus* (MRSA), vancomycin is preferred. Rifampin may be considered for staphylococcal infections if the isolate is susceptible. Rifampin is indicated when there is hardware present for optimal biofilm penetration. If β-lactam or vancomycin therapy is not possible then clinicians may consider linezolid or trimethoprim-sulfamethoxazole. Daptomycin may also be considered although given its limited CNS penetration aggressive dosing is probably necessary (eg, 10-12 mg/kg/day).[12,69]

5 The treatment of meningitis due to *P. aeruginosa* remains a challenge because antibiotics showing good antibacterial activity, such as antipseudomonal penicillins and aminoglycosides, penetrate the CSF moderately or poorly (Table 128-3). Initially, cases of *P. aeruginosa* meningitis should be treated with an extended-spectrum β-lactam such as ceftazidime or cefepime, or alternatively aztreonam, ciprofloxacin, or meropenem depending on local susceptibility patterns. The addition of an aminoglycoside, usually tobramycin, to one of the aforementioned agents can also be considered. Since aminoglycosides penetrate the CSF poorly, their inclusion is to predominantly aid in the treatment of extracerebral infections.

Multidrug-resistant *P. aeruginosa*, Acinetobacter, and carbapenem-resistant Enterobacterales infections are of concern to clinicians because of the limited therapeutic options available. This concern has led to the reemergence of the use of older antibiotics, such as colistin and polymyxin B. Colistin can be used, both intravenously and intrathecally, in the treatment of multidrug-resistant *P. aeruginosa* or Acinetobacter CNS infections. The use of colistin should be reserved for only the most severe cases.

New cephalosporin-β-lactamase inhibitor combination agents (ceftolozane-tazobactam and ceftazidime-avibactam) have yet to be formally studied in patients with CNS infections, but may represent alternative therapies for multidrug resistant gram-negative organisms. For instance, ceftazidime/avibactam resulted in several successful treatments of meningitis caused by a KPC-producing *Klebsiella pneumoniae*.[70,71] Ceftaroline, a novel cephalosporin with affinity for PBP2a has shown promise in a case series of *S. pneumoniae* and *S. aureus* meningitis as well as three other case reports of MRSA meningitis/ventriculopleural shunt infections.[45,72-74] The pharmacokinetic properties of ceftaroline suggest it is probably reliable for CNS infections, particularly if using every 8-hour dosing.

Other gram-negative organisms causing meningitis, excluding *P. aeruginosa* and Acinetobacter spp., most likely can be treated with a third- or fourth-generation cephalosporin, such as cefotaxime, ceftriaxone, ceftazidime, or cefepime. Ceftazidime, however, may not be the best choice of empiric monotherapy for situations where the offending organism is unknown initially due to lack of reliable gram-positive activity. Cefotaxime should be used in place of ceftriaxone in the neonatal period because of the potential of ceftriaxone to displace bilirubin from its albumin-binding sites. Trimethoprim-sulfamethoxazole may offer utility for ventriculitis and meningitis caused by Enterobacterales, given that its penetration into the CSF does not depend on meningeal inflammation. Fluoroquinolones, such as ciprofloxacin, exhibit good penetration into the CSF and are recommended as alternative agents for the treatment of susceptible gram-negative bacilli, including *P. aeruginosa*, when susceptible.

For patients with documented or suspected fungal meningitis or ventriculitis, empiric lipid formulation of liposomal amphotericin B in combination with flucytosine is recommended.[12,75] Once susceptibility is confirmed, fluconazole may be used for Candida spp. recovered from CSF. Echinocandins are large molecules that penetrate poorly into the CNS and are not recommended for fungal meningitis or ventriculitis. For suspected or confirmed Aspergillus spp., the treatment of choice is voriconazole targeting a serum trough level of 2 to 5 mg/L (6 to 14 μmol/L).[12,76]

8 Some patients with meningitis or ventriculitis respond poorly to systemic antibiotic therapy. For these patients intraventricular therapy should be considered. Numerous antimicrobials can be given intraventricularly, including amikacin, amphotericin B deoxycholate, colistimethate sodium, daptomycin, gentamicin, polymyxin B, quinupristin/dalfopristin, tobramycin, and vancomycin. There is no consensus on the optimal dose of intraventricular antimicrobial that should be used; however, some general recommendations are available.[12] If used, intraventricular antibiotic therapy requires vigilance in preparation and administration. Preservative-free product and diluents should be used unless no preservative-free products exist. For patients receiving antimicrobial therapy through a ventricular drain, the drain should be clamped for 15 to 60 minutes to allow antimicrobial equilibration throughout the CSF.

CSF cultures may remain positive for several days or more with a regimen that eventually will be curative. Therapeutic efficacy can be monitored through bacterial colony counts every 2 or 3 days, which should decrease progressively over the period of therapy. Duration of therapy for healthcare-associated meningitis and ventriculitis is based on clinical response and the offending pathogen. For instance, for *P. acnes* and coagulase-negative Staphylococcal spp., IDSA guidelines recommend 10 to 14 days. For *S. aureus* and gram-negative pathogens 14 days or longer is recommended. For those with persistently positive CSF cultures therapy should continue for 10 to 14 days following the last positive culture.[12]

Finally, another important opportunity for antibiotic optimization exists for patients with external ventricular drains (EVDs). Patients with EVD are often given systemic antibiotic therapy (eg, cefazolin) for infection prophylaxis for the duration of EVD placement to prevent ventriculostomy-related infections. However, the Neurocritical Care Society recommended against this practice citing the potential for harm (eg, *Clostridioides difficile* and antimicrobial-resistant pathogens) from the lack of efficacy attributable to antibiotic prophylaxis.[77] Instead the authors recommend administering one dose of antimicrobials prior to EVD insertion, avoiding routine CSF sampling, and using antibiotic-impregnated EVD catheters.

Current guidelines also recommend against extended antibiotic prophylaxis following EVD insertion.[12]

BACTERIAL BRAIN ABSCESS

Brain abscess is a life-threatening focal infection of the brain that begins as a localized area of cerebritis and develops into a collection of pus surrounded by a well-vascularized capsule.[78] In immunocompetent patients, bacteria account for >95% of brain abscesses. Bacteria enter the brain either through contiguous spread (eg, following infection in the oropharynx, middle ear, paranasal sinuses, or neurosurgical procedures and cranial trauma), or hematogenous spread due to distant infections (eg, infective endocarditis, congenital heart disease, dental infection, or pulmonary abscess). Abscess occurs most commonly in the frontal lobe, but can occur in any location.[79] Mortality rates have declined significantly in the past 50 years, with 70% of survivors expected to have no to minimal neurologic sequelae, although data on long-term functional and neuropsychological evaluation are lacking.[80]

2 The clinical presentation varies depending on the number, size, and location of the abscess, and diagnosis can be challenging due to this variable presentation. Headache, mental status changes, focal neurologic deficits, and fever are the most common symptoms of brain abscess. Brain imaging is the cornerstone for the diagnosis of brain abscess, with MRI being the preferred modality over contrast-enhanced CT due to better resolution and differentiation of abscesses from tumors. Blood samples should be collected prior to initiation of antibacterial treatment for anaerobic and aerobic cultures, molecular biology, serology, and other diagnostic tests.

The etiology of brain abscess depends on the initial site of infection and the immune state of the host. Abscesses arising from spread of infection from oropharynx, middle ear, and paranasal sinuses are commonly caused by *S. aureus*, streptococci, and oral anaerobes (eg, Actinomyces spp., Bacteroides spp., Fusobacterium spp., or Peptostreptococcus spp.). Dental infections are associated with abscesses caused by Streptococcus spp. and *Bacteroides fragilis*. Staphylococci and Enterobacterales are commonly involved in postoperative abscesses or those following head trauma. *Toxoplasma gondii, Mycobacterium tuberculosis*, Listeria spp., and Nocardia spp. can also cause brain abscesses and are more commonly seen in immunocompromised patients.[79]

5 All lesions equal to or greater than 2.5 cm in diameter should be stereotactically aspirated or surgically excised and specimens should be sent to the microbiology and pathology laboratory.[78,80] Because brain abscesses are commonly polymicrobial, empiric antimicrobial therapy should include antibiotics with activity against gram-positive, gram-negative, and anaerobic organisms. The antimicrobial agents should penetrate into the abscess cavity and remain active in acidic environments. Most commonly the regimen includes a third- or fourth-generation cephalosporin plus metronidazole. Vancomycin should be added when infection caused by MRSA is suspected. Ceftazidime or cefepime can be used if *P. aeruginosa* is suspected. A carbapenem (such as meropenem) could replace the cephalosporin and metronidazole. In immunocompromised patients, the empiric regimen may be supplemented with voriconazole, and trimethoprim-sulfamethoxazole or sulfadiazine to cover fungi and Nocardia while awaiting definitive results. De-escalation of therapy should occur once a causative organism is identified. Repeated neuroimaging should be performed to monitor for abscess resolution or progression.

Prophylactic anticonvulsant therapy and corticosteroids are not routinely recommended.[80] Corticosteroids are not routinely used in brain abscess, and are typically reserved for use in patients with edema causing increased intracranial pressure, brain shift, or increased risk of cerebral herniation. Intravenous antibiotics have traditionally been administered for 6 to 8 weeks, although shorter or longer durations may be used depending on the clinical and radiologic progress. Given the risk of neurotoxicity with prolonged courses of metronidazole, it may be discontinued once anaerobic pathogens have been ruled out. Oral options can consist of ciprofloxacin, metronidazole, trimethoprim-sulfamethoxazole, and amoxicillin but there is no consensus when transition to oral agents can be safely done.

VIRAL ENCEPHALITIS

Encephalitis refers to inflammation of the brain parenchyma in association with clinical evidence of neurologic dysfunction. "Meningoencephalitis" is a term commonly used to describe meningeal inflammation along with encephalitis. Infectious encephalitis should be distinguished from those patients with encephalopathy (eg, due to metabolic disturbances, intoxications, hypoxia, or systemic infections) or noninfectious encephalitis (eg, postimmunization encephalitis or encephalomyelitis), as they have similar clinical presentations.[14] While a confirmed or probable pathogen is identified in less than 50% of cases, viral etiologies are the most commonly diagnosed.[7,15] Collectively, about 20,000 encephalitis-associated hospitalizations are expected per year in the United States, with a case fatality rate of more than 5%. Of those 20,000 hospitalizations, approximately 20% are due to viral pathogens.

The epidemiology of viral encephalitis in the United States has changed dramatically since the mid-1960s due to the introduction of large-scale polio, rubella, varicella-zoster virus, and mumps immunization programs. The most common causes of viral encephalitis/meningoencephalitis in the United States is enteroviruses, followed by herpes viruses and arboviruses.[7,15,16]

Less common causes include adenoviruses, influenza, rotavirus, corona virus, cytomegalovirus (CMV), varicella-zoster virus, Epstein-Barr virus, West Nile Virus (WNV), and lymphocytic choriomeningitis. In recent years, Powassan, Chikungunya, and Zika viruses have emerged as increasing causes of encephalitis in North America. These arboviruses are transmitted via ticks (Powassan) or mosquitoes (Chikungunya and Zika) and have a diverse spectrum of disease. Of these, Powassan virus has seen the largest increase in incidence; prior to 1999 there was an average of 0.7 cases per year in the United States and Canada. In 2003, the CDC included Powassan virus as a reportable disease, resulting in 181 cases reported between 2010 and 2019, with 43 cases reported in 2019 alone.[81]

Zika virus sparked global attention in 2016 after the first cases of brain developmental disorders in newborns were linked to Zika virus infection of their mothers during pregnancy. Epidemiologic and experimental studies have now provided strong support for causality between Zika virus infection during pregnancy and congenital structural abnormalities of the brain.[82] Since 2019 there have been no confirmed reports of Zika disease transmitted by mosquitoes in the United States.[83] Several vaccine candidates for the prevention of Zika disease are in development, although none are approved for use at this time.

Viral encephalitis is acquired primarily by hematogenous spread or, alternatively, by neuronal spread of the causative pathogen. After entry into the host, viral replication occurs, resulting in dissemination through the reticuloendothelial system or vasculature. Infection of the capillary endothelial cells and choroid plexus may provide a conduit for CNS infections. Viruses such as polio, HSV, and Varicella-zoster virus may also gain access to the CNS by axonal retrograde transmission from peripheral nerve endings. Once a virus gains access to the CNS, the course of infection depends on the virulence of the particular virus and the host immune response. Subsequent neuronal injury is caused by direct cell damage due to viral replication, but inflammatory and immune-mediated responses also contribute to neurological damage.

2 In contrast with purulent meningitis, host response to viral encephalitis is mediated primarily through cytotoxic T-lymphocytes. Increases in concentrations of IL-1, IL-6, and interferon (INF) α, β, and

γ may occur. The clinical syndrome associated with viral encephalitis generally is independent of viral etiology and may vary depending on the patient's age. Common signs in adults include headache, mild fever, nuchal rigidity, malaise, drowsiness, nausea, vomiting, and photophobia. Only fever and irritability may be evident in the infant, and acute bacterial meningitis must be ruled out as a cause of fever when no other localized findings are observed in a child. Duration of symptoms generally is 1 to 2 weeks, and specific manifestations outside the meninges can also occur depending on the viral etiology.

Laboratory examination of the CSF usually reveals a pleocytosis with 100 to 1,000 WBC/mm^3 ($0.1 \times 10^9 - 1 \times 10^9$/L), which are primarily lymphocytic. However, 20% to 75% of patients with viral encephalitis may have a predominance of polymorphonuclear cells on initial examination of the CSF. On repeat lumbar puncture, 90% of patients presenting initially with a predominance of neutrophils experience a shift to a predominance of mononuclear cells. Other laboratory findings include normal to mildly elevated protein concentrations and normal or mildly reduced glucose concentrations (see Table 128-1).

3 As mentioned earlier, pathogens responsible for viral encephalitis are often unidentified. When clinical signs warrant pathogen identification, appropriate laboratory diagnostic techniques, including PCR and serologic testing, should be undertaken. Molecular methods are preferred to conventional laboratory tests, such as viral cultures and brain biopsy, in the diagnosis of viral encephalitis owing to improved sensitivity and specificity, higher yield, and rapid results.[14,84]

Supportive and symptomatic treatments, including seizure control, hemodynamic management, venous thromboembolism prevention, ICP management, and secondary bacterial infection prevention, are of great importance in patients with viral encephalitis due to limited treatment options. Corticosteroid therapy is generally not recommended in most viral encephalitis cases; however, treatment should be considered for patients with cerebral edema and increased ICP.[14]

Although there are numerous pathogenic causes of viral encephalitis, much of the clinical presentation, diagnosis, and treatment are similar. The most commonly isolated viral etiologies are described here. HSV type 1 (HSV1) and type 2 (HSV2) are considered the most common treatable causes of viral encephalitis. Between 2011 and 2014, HSV encephalitis accounted for 8.3% of viral encephalitis-associated hospitalizations.[7,16] HSV1 is associated with encephalitis in adults, whereas HSV2 is associated predominantly with encephalitis in newborns. Sexually active adults may acquire HSV meningitis during or after an attack of genital or rectal HSV, whereas neonates acquire the virus during passage through the vaginal canal of mothers with active HSV infection. HSV PCR on CSF specimens should be performed for all patients with presumed encephalitis. Repeat testing should be considered for patients with an initial negative test after 3 to 7 days.[14] Establishing the correct diagnosis early is paramount due to mortality rates approaching 70% without treatment and, unlike other viral etiologies, effective therapy is available. As a result, empiric therapy of suspected HSV encephalitis is recommended, while results are pending. Delaying antiviral therapy has been consistently associated with increased mortality. Additionally, a clinical decision to treat may need to be made regardless of test results.

Acyclovir is the drug of choice for HSV encephalitis. In adults with normal renal function, acyclovir is usually administered as 10 mg/kg intravenously every 8 hours for 2 to 3 weeks.[14,84] Higher doses of acyclovir (up to 20 mg/kg intravenously every 8 hours) have been used in neonates and are associated with lower mortality rates.[85] HSV resistance to acyclovir has been reported with increasing incidence, particularly in immunocompromised patients with prior or chronic exposures to acyclovir, ranging from 3.5% to 10%.[86] The alternative treatment for acyclovir-resistant HSV is foscarnet. The dose for patients with normal renal function is 40 to 60 mg/kg every 8 to 12 hours for 3 weeks, with the higher dose typically reserved for HIV-infected individuals.[14,84] Ensuring adequate hydration is imperative to decrease risk of acyclovir- and foscarnet-induced nephrotoxicity. In addition, patients receiving foscarnet should be monitored for seizures related to alterations in plasma electrolyte levels. Adult patients who completed standard initial HSV encephalitis treatment followed by long-term antiviral treatment (an additional 3-month course) of oral valacyclovir did not show improvements in neuropsychological testing 12 months later compared to placebo.[87]

Although mosquito bites account for nearly all human cases of WNV, transmissions via blood products, organ transplantation, transplacental transfer, and breast milk have been documented.[16,88] Similar to other arboviruses, the incubation period for WNV ranges from 2 to 14 days, although periods of up to 21 days have been observed in immunocompromised patients. Infection with WNV is asymptomatic in most adults or causes a mild flu-like syndrome characterized by fever, malaise, myalgia, and lymphadenopathy. Among 41,762 reported cases of WNV in the United States between 1999 and 2014, the overall mortality rate was approximately 4% (9% in patients with neuroinvasive disease). In 2020, the CDC reported a total of 557 cases of WNV and 38 deaths. CSF examination of WNV encephalitis typically shows pleocytosis and a slightly elevated CSF protein concentration. Several diagnostic methods have been developed for WNV, including a PCR assay and enzyme-linked immunosorbent assay (ELISA) tests. Treatment is typically supportive, including treatment for seizures and increased ICP, and in the majority of cases, the disease is self-limiting.[88]

CMV has emerged as a major cause of morbidity and mortality in immunocompromised patients, including HIV-infected individuals and transplant recipients on immunosuppressant therapy. CNS infections with CMV are often difficult to treat, with higher failure rates and poor outcomes. Combination therapy with ganciclovir and foscarnet is recommended for induction treatment due to the potential for poor outcomes with monotherapy.[14] In adult patients, ganciclovir 5 mg/kg every 12 hours and foscarnet 60 mg/kg every 8 hours (or 90 mg/kg every 12 hours) for 3 weeks or until symptom resolution are recommended during the induction phase, followed by maintenance phase with either induction agent. Some clinicians may use oral valgancyclovir for maintenance treatment of CMV CNS disease, although the use of this agent is not well established. Other interventions that may improve survival outcomes include the initiation of highly active antiretroviral therapy in untreated HIV-infected patients and reduction of immunosuppression intensity in transplant recipients. Although there is no vaccine for the prevention of CMV disease, there are multiple vaccine candidates in the process for FDA approval.

HIV encephalitis is a common CNS complication associated with AIDS. Frequently, patients may complain of headache, photophobia, or stiff neck at the time of presumed seroconversion. As the disease progresses, neurologic symptoms are frequently reported secondary to other opportunistic infections. Diagnosis of viral encephalitis is difficult because mental status and neurologic examinations are not sensitive enough to detect early changes. Direct evidence of HIV encephalitis can be obtained through CSF culture, p24 antigen testing, and qualitative or quantitative PCR for HIV RNA. Diagnostic workup of coinfections, such as HSV, *Toxoplasma gondii, Mycobacterium tuberculosis*, Aspergillus spp., and Cryptococcus spp., should also be performed. See Chapter 148 "Human Immunodeficiency Virus" for a complete discussion of infectious complications in HIV-positive individuals.

CNS INFECTIONS IN SPECIAL POPULATIONS

This section discusses additional pathogens that can cause CNS infections. For discussion on CNS infections caused by Cryptococcus,

Histoplasma, and Aspergillus species, the interested reader can refer to Chapter 144, "Invasive Fungal Infections." CNS infection due to *Treponema Pallidum* (neurosyphilis) is discussed in Chapter 140, "Sexually Transmitted Diseases."

Bacillus Species

Bacillus anthracis, the causative agent of anthrax, is a nonmotile spore-forming, gram-positive, rod-shaped bacterium. The disease is common in wild and domestic animals. Biodefense experts place *Bacillus anthracis* at or near the top of the list for potential threat agents. It enters the host in the form of spores at the epidermis (cutaneous anthrax), the gastrointestinal epithelium (gastrointestinal anthrax), or the lung mucosa (inhalation anthrax). Anthrax meningitis has been reported with all three clinical forms of anthrax and likely results from hematogenous spread across the blood–brain barrier, generally presenting as hemorrhagic meningitis. Anthrax meningitis is characterized by a fulminant, rapidly progressive clinical course and is nearly always fatal even with treatment. For diagnosis, blood and CSF exam for Gram stain, culture PCR, and toxin assays are recommended.[89]

For the general adult population, empiric treatment for suspected anthrax meningitis should include ≥3 antimicrobial drugs with activity against *B. anthracis*.[89] At least one antimicrobial agent should have bactericidal activity, ≥1 should be a protein synthesis inhibitor for suppression of exotoxin production, and all should have good CNS penetration. A higher percent survival has been observed for patients with anthrax meningitis receiving 3 antimicrobials than those receiving only 2 antimicrobial agents.[90]

5 Empiric regimens that include high doses of intravenous fluoroquinolones (ciprofloxacin preferably, levofloxacin or moxifloxacin) along with a carbapenem (meropenem preferably, doripenem or imipenem/cilastatin) and a protein synthesis inhibitor (e.g., linezolid preferred or clindamycin) are recommended for ≥2 to 3 weeks until clinical criteria for stability are met. Once penicillin susceptibility is confirmed, the carbapenem can be de-escalated to intravenous penicillin G or ampicillin.[89] In addition, adjunctive corticosteroids should be considered.

Bacillus cereus is an unusual cause of CNS infections in immunocompromised patients. Occasional outbreaks may occur in the nosocomial setting. One such outbreak was discovered in a cluster of five patients with AML. All patients were started on vancomycin at time of neurological symptom onset, which is a treatment of choice with frequent resistance to beta-lactams and less frequent documented resistance to carbapenems.[91]

Borrelia burgdorferi (Lyme Disease)

Lyme disease (LD) is caused by the spirochete *Borrelia burgdorferi* and is the most common tick-borne infection in North America and Europe.[92] Lyme neuroborreliosis (LNB) is an infectious disorder of the nervous system caused by *B. burgdorferi* and has been reported in up to 15% of patients with untreated LD. CNS involvement may include meningitis, myelitis, cerebral vasculitis, or encephalitis. Clinical manifestations include fever, headache, fatigue, photosensitivity, confusion, hemiparesis, cerebellar ataxia, painful radiculitis, cranial palsy, and Parkinson-like symptoms among others. Poliomyelitis-like syndromes and acute stroke-like symptoms caused by cerebral vasculitis have been documented but are considered rare. Unlike the European LD, the North American LD is also characterized by a skin rash called erythema migrans.[92,93] There is no international consensus for the diagnosis of Lyme neuroborreliosis (LNB). Diagnosis is based on the presence of neurological symptoms without other obvious reasons, CSF analysis (lymphocytic pleocytosis, moderately elevated protein, normal glucose), intrathecal *B. burgdorferi* antibody production, blood and CSF serologic testing (ELISA plus Western blot), and MRI demonstrating areas of inflammation.[92-94] PCR testing for detection of *B. burgdorferi* in CSF has a sensitivity of <30% with an unknown specificity; therefore, it is not routinely recommended. Parenteral treatment with ceftriaxone once daily is recommended as first-line treatment of LNB.

5 Patients with cranial neuropathy without clinical signs of meningitis may be treated with oral amoxicillin, doxycycline, or cefuroxime axetil. European guidelines also recommend oral doxycycline as a first-line option for patients with symptoms confined to the meninges, cranial nerves, nerve roots, or peripheral nerves based on its CSF penetration, ability to achieve CSF concentrations above the MIC, and several studies showing similar short- and long-term efficacy to various parenteral regimens.[93] Alternative parenteral options to ceftriaxone include cefotaxime or penicillin G. For patients intolerant to β-lactams, oral or intravenous doxycycline is suggested.

Mycobacterium tuberculosis

5 *M. tuberculosis* is the primary cause of tuberculous meningitis and remains the most life-threatening form of extrapulmonary tuberculosis. The incidence of tuberculosis, in general, has decreased to 3 cases per 100,000 individuals in the United States in 2016.[95] The guidelines jointly sponsored by the CDC, IDSA, and the American Thoracic Society recommend an initial regimen of four drugs for empirical treatment of drug-susceptible *M. tuberculosis* in adults. The recommended regimen consists of isoniazid, rifampin, pyrazinamide, and ethambutol for the first 2 months, followed by isoniazid plus rifampin for an additional 7 to 10 months, although the optimal duration has not been defined. Furthermore, initial adjunctive corticosteroid therapy tapered over 6 to 8 weeks is recommended, which provides mortality benefit. The recommended therapy for HIV-positive individuals is similar as that for immunocompetent patients.[95,96] In HIV-infected patients with tuberculous meningitis, antiretroviral therapy should not be initiated in the first 8 weeks of antituberculosis therapy to reduce the risk of immune reconstitution syndrome (IRIS). Therapy should be individualized based on susceptibility patterns and evidence-based guidelines including those by the WHO.[97]

Nocardia

Nocardia is an aerobic, gram-positive bacterium. *Nocardia* species represent a ubiquitous group of environmental bacteria that commonly cause opportunistic infections in immunocompromised individuals. Nevertheless, up to 20% of patients with nocardiosis are apparently healthy, although the presence of nocardiosis might reveal a previously unidentified primary immunodeficiency in immunocompetent patients.[98] Pulmonary nocardiosis is the most common clinical presentation and CNS nocardiosis represents the second most frequently involved organ. The usual presentation of CNS infection is single or multiple brain abscesses. CNS symptoms appear gradually and are nonspecific including headache, nausea, vomiting, seizures, and mental status changes. MRI of the brain is the recommended imaging modality. Specific therapeutic recommendations on the basis of prospective controlled trials for nocardiosis are lacking. In addition, *Nocardia* has inconsistent antimicrobial susceptibility patterns *in vitro*.[99] Thus, the management of nocardiosis must be individualized and isolates should undergo antimicrobial testing for treatment decisions. Surgical management may be necessary in many cases.[100]

5 According to the 2019 guidelines from the American Society of Transplantation for the treatment of nocardia infections in transplant patients, imipenem/cilastatin coadministered with amikacin alone or in a three-drug regimen with trimethoprim-sulfamethoxazole can be used as empiric therapy for cerebral disease or life-threatening disease. In critically ill patients with significant renal dysfunction where it may be desirable to avoid trimethoprim-sulfamethoxazole and aminoglycosides, treatment with linezolid is an option until susceptibility results are available. Alternative

therapies include cefotaxime, ceftriaxone, and minocycline, although some Nocardia species are resistant to these agents, and therefore, use should be guided by susceptibility testing. Nocardiosis appears to be a rare infection in children. Antibiotics reported useful in children are similar to those used in adults. Combined treatment is required until there is evidence of clinical improvement and antimicrobial susceptibility is confirmed. Parenteral therapy is recommended for 3 to 6 weeks followed by appropriate oral therapy for a total of 12 months. After completion of antibiotic therapy, secondary prophylaxis with trimethoprim-sulfamethoxazole can be considered at doses of one double strength tablet daily for adults. However, breakthrough nocardial infections may still occur.[100] Therefore, use of trimethoprim-sulfamethoxazole prophylaxis should not prevent clinicians from considering nocardial infections in differential diagnosis. Patients should be monitored for 1 year after completion of therapy for relapse.

Primary Amoebic Meningoencephalitis (PAM)

Naegleria fowleri is a thermophilic, unicellular parasite that lives in stagnant fresh or brackish waters and causes a rare form of nearly fatal CNS infection known as Primary Amoebic Meningoencephalitis (PAM). Humans acquire PAM when water is insufflated through the nostrils usually while swimming in warm freshwater lakes and rivers. The time from exposure to *N. fowleri* to the onset of symptoms

TABLE 128-5 Dosing of Anti-infective Agents by Age Group

Agent	Infants and Children	Adults	Monitoring/Comments
Antibacterial			
Ampicillin	75 mg/kg every 6 h	2 g every 4 h	
Aztreonam	40mg/kg every 6-8 h	2 g every 6-8 h	Alternative for severe penicillin allergy
Cefepime	50 mg/kg every 8 h	2 g every 8 h	Consider prolonged infusion
Cefotaxime	75 mg/kg every 6-8 h	2 g every 4-6 h	Preferred in neonates
Ceftazidime	50 mg/kg every 8 h	2 g every 8 h	
Ceftriaxone	100 mg/kg daily	2 g every 12 h	Avoid in neonates
Ciprofloxacin	10 mg/kg every 8 h	400 mg every 8-12 h	Consider higher doses for *P. aeruginosa*
Colistin	5 mg/kg/day (package insert dosing)	5 mg/kg/day (package insert dosing)	Consider intraventricular doses Only for MDR organisms Monitor renal function
Gentamicin	2.5 mg/kg every 8 h	2 mg/kg every 8 h or 5-7 mg/kg daily	TDM is recommended
Levofloxacin	—	750 mg daily	May prolong QTc
Linezolid	10 mg/kg every 8-12 h	600 mg every 12 h	May cause thrombocytopenia and peripheral neuropathy
Meropenem	40 mg/kg every 8 h	2 g every 8 h	Consider prolonged infusion
Moxifloxacin	—	400 mg daily	May prolong QTc
Oxacillin/Nafcillin	50 mg/kg every 6 h	2 g every 4 h	Nafcillin preferred if renal dysfunction
Penicillin G	0.05 million Units/kg every 4 h	4 million Units every 4 h	
Polymyxin B	—	1.25-1.5 mg/kg every 12 h	Only for MDR organisms No data in pediatric patients
Tobramycin	2.5 mg/kg every 8 h	2.5 mg/kg every 8 h or 5-7 mg/kg daily	TDM is recommended Monitor renal function
Trimethoprim-sulfamethoxazole	5 mg/kg every 6-12 h	5 mg/kg every 6-12 h	Dose based on trimethoprim
Vancomycin	15 mg/kg every 6 h	15-20 mg/kg every 8-12 h	TDM is recommended Monitor renal function
Antifungals			
Conventional Amphotericin B	1 mg/kg daily	0.7-1 mg/kg daily	Monitor renal function Maintain adequate hydration
Lipid amphotericin B	3-5 mg/kg once daily	3-5 mg/kg daily	Monitor renal function Maintain adequate hydration
Flucytosine	25 mg/kg every 6 h	25 mg/kg every 6 h	Consider TDM to avoid bone marrow suppression
Fluconazole	6-12 mg/kg daily	400-800 mg daily	Monitor liver function
Voriconazole	9mg/kg every 12 h × 2 doses then 8 mg/kg every 12 h	6 mg/kg every 12 h × 2 doses then 4 mg/kg every 12 h	Consider TDM Many drug-drug interactions Monitor liver function
Antivirals			
Acyclovir	10-20 mg/kg every 8 h	10-20 mg/kg every 8 h	Monitor renal function Maintain adequate hydration
Ganciclovir	—	5 mg/kg every 12 h	Monitor renal function
Foscarnet	—	60 mg/kg every 8 h or 90 mg/kg every 12 h	Monitor renal function Maintain adequate hydration

TDM, therapeutic drug monitoring. Data from References *12, 14, 26, and 27.*

is 1 to 9 days. The pathogen migrates to the brain along the olfactory nerve. Signs and symptoms of PAM include severe frontal headache, fever, nausea, vomiting, seizures, altered mental status, hallucinations, and coma.

Even with early recognition of PAM, progression is rapid and the clinical prognosis is poor. PAM is a rare disease that is almost always fatal. In the United States, there have been 148 PAM infections from 1962 through 2019 with only four survivors. PAM disproportionately affects males and children. Several drug combinations have been used for treatment of PAM.[101] Based on treatment regimens used in survivors, the CDC recommend combination therapy with miltefosine (an oral drug used to treat breast cancer and leishmaniasis), azithromycin, rifampin, fluconazole, and conventional amphotericin B (intravenous and intrathecal) and dexamethasone.

Toxoplasma gondii

5 Toxoplasmic encephalitis (TE) is caused by the protozoan *T. gondii*. Approximately 11% of the US population 6 years and older have been infected with *T. gondii*. In other parts of the world, up to 95% of populations are infected. The primary routes of transmission are foodborne, animal-to-human (cats serving as the definitive host), and mother-to-child (congenital).[96,102] TE is typically caused by the reactivation of disease in immunocompromised patients, especially those with AIDS, or intrauterine infection in newborns. Clinical manifestations can range from asymptomatic in healthy, nonpregnant patient to headache, seizures, confusion, hemiparesis, cranial nerve abnormalities, or fever in immunocompromised patients. In congenital toxoplasmosis, patients may also present with hydrocephalus, intracerebral calcification, microcephaly, convulsions, or chorioretinitis.[14,96] Definitive diagnosis of TE requires a clinical sample via a brain biopsy; therefore, TE is presumptively diagnosed on the basis of clinical symptoms, positive serology for antitoxoplasma IgG antibodies, and identification of space-occupying lesions on CT, MRI, or other radiologic imaging. In patients with AIDS, MRI typically shows multiple ring-enhancing lesions.

T. gondii can also be detected by PCR in CSF. However, the sensitivity is low (50%) and the result is usually negative once treatment has started.[96,102] First-line treatment for TE in adults consists of pyrimethamine plus sulfadiazine plus leucovorin. Leucovorin is added to the treatment regimen to reduce the likelihood of hematologic toxicity associated with pyrimethamine. In patients who are unable to tolerate sulfadiazine, due to allergies or impaired renal function, clindamycin may be used as an alternative. Other alternative treatment options are available, including trimethoprim-sulfamethoxazole, but have not been extensively studied. Treatment recommendations are the same in pediatric patients; however, several of the alternative regimens have not been studied in children.[96,102] After completion of initial 6-week therapy, chronic maintenance therapy should be initiated and continued based on risk factors and immune status.

EVALUATION OF THERAPEUTIC OUTCOMES

Because of the potential for rapid deterioration associated with CNS infections, the presence of fever, headache, meningismus (eg, nuchal rigidity, Brudzinski's, or Kernig's sign), and signs of cerebral dysfunction should be evaluated every 4 hours for the initial 3 days and then daily thereafter. The Glasgow Coma Scale should be used in severely ill patients. Trends in improvement and resolution rather than single evaluations in time are more important in monitoring the signs and symptoms of meningitis. Continued therapy should be based on the assessment of clinical improvement, culture, and susceptibility testing results. Once a pathogen is identified, anti-infective therapy should be tailored to the specific pathogen (Tables 128-4 and 128-5). Throughout the course of treatment, efficacy parameters such as signs and symptoms, microbiologic findings, and CSF examination should be followed to evaluate the success of meeting the desired outcomes. If adjunctive dexamethasone is used, careful monitoring of signs and symptoms of gastrointestinal bleeding and hyperglycemia should be employed. Moreover, the use of dexamethasone may interfere with the interpretation of clinical response to treatment, such as resolution of fever.

ABBREVIATIONS

ACIP Advisory Committee on Immunization Practices
AFB acid fast bacillus
AIDS acquired immunodeficiency syndrome
BBB blood–brain barrier
BCSFB blood–cerebrospinal fluid barrier
CBF cerebral blood flow
CDC United States Centers for Disease Control and Prevention
CFH complement factor H
CFU colony forming unit
CLSI Clinical and Laboratory Standards Institute
CMV cytomegalovirus
CNS central nervous system
CSF cerebrospinal fluid
CT computed tomography
DIC disseminated intravascular coagulation
EFNS European Federation of Neurological Societies
EIA enzyme immunoassay
ELISA enzyme-linked immunosorbent assay
EVD external ventricular drains
FDA US Food and Drug Administration
GBS group B *Streptococcus*
Hib *Haemophilus influenzae* type b
HIV human immunodeficiency virus
HSV herpes simplex virus
ICP intracranial pressure
IDSA Infectious Diseases Society of America
Ig immunoglobulin
IL interleukin
IPD invasive pneumococcal disease
INF interferon
IRIS immune reconstitution syndrome
LNB Lyme neuroborreliosis
LPS lipopolysaccharide
MenACWY serogroup A, C, W, Y meningococcal vaccine
MenB serogroup B meningococcal vaccine
MIC minimum inhibitory concentration
MSSA methicillin-susceptible *Staphylococcus aureus*
MRI magnetic resonance imaging
MRSA methicillin-resistant *Staphylococcus aureus*
PAF platelet-activating factor
PAM primary amoebic meningoencephalitis
PBP2a penicillin binding protein 2a
PCR polymerase chain reaction
PCT procalcitonin
PCV7 heptavalent pneumococcal conjugate vaccine
PCV13 13-valent pneumococcal conjugate vaccine
PGE2 prostaglandin E2
PMN polymorphonuclear neutrophil
PPSV23 23-valent pneumococcal polysaccharide vaccine
rRNA ribosomal ribonucleic acid
SNP single-nucleotide polymorphism
TDM therapeutic drug monitoring

TE	toxoplasmic encephalitis
TNF	tumor necrosis factor
WBC	white blood cell
WNV	West Nile virus

REFERENCES

1. Brouwer MC, van de Beek D. Epidemiology of community-acquired bacterial meningitis. *Curr Opin Infect Dis.* 2018;31:78–84.
2. Thigpen MC, Whitney CG, Messonnier NE, et al. Bacterial meningitis in the United States, 1998–2007. *N Engl J Med.* 2011;364:2016–2025.
3. McGill F, Heyderman RS, Panagiotou S, Tunkel AR, Solomon T. Acute bacterial meningitis in adults. *Lancet* 2016;388:3036–3047.
4. Brouwer MC, Coutinho JM, van de Beek D. Clinical characteristics and outcome of brain abscess: systematic review and meta-analysis. *Neurology* 2014;82:806–813.
5. Solomon T, Michael BD, Smith PE, et al. Management of suspected viral encephalitis in adults–Association of British Neurologists and British Infection Association National Guidelines. *J Infect.* 2012;64:347–373.
6. Granerod J, Cousens S, Davies NW, Crowcroft NS, Thomas SL. New estimates of incidence of encephalitis in England. *Emerg Infect Dis.* 2013;19.
7. Vora NM, Holman RC, Mehal JM, Steiner CA, Blanton J, Sejvar J. Burden of encephalitis-associated hospitalizations in the United States, 1998–2010. *Neurology* 2014;82:443–451.
8. Tack DM, Holman RC, Folkema AM, Mehal JM, Blanton JD, Sejvar JJ. Trends in encephalitis-associated deaths in the United States, 1999–2008. *Neuroepidemiology* 2014;43:1–8.
9. Castelblanco RL, Lee M, Hasbun R. Epidemiology of bacterial meningitis in the United States from 1997 to 2010: a population-based observational study. *Lancet Infect Dis.* 2014;14:813–819.
10. Collaborators GBDM. Global, regional, and national burden of meningitis, 1990–2016: a systematic analysis for the Global Burden of Disease Study 2016. *Lancet Neurol.* 2018;17:1061–1082.
11. Cohn AC, MacNeil JR, Clark TA, et al. Prevention and control of meningococcal disease: recommendations of the Advisory Committee on Immunization Practices (ACIP). *MMWR Recomm Rep.* 2013;62:1–28.
12. Tunkel AR, Hasbun R, Bhimraj A, et al. 2017 Infectious Diseases Society of America's Clinical Practice Guidelines for Healthcare-Associated Ventriculitis and Meningitis. *Clin Infect Dis.* 2017;64:e34–e65.
13. Kneen R, Michael BD, Menson E, et al. Management of suspected viral encephalitis in children—Association of British Neurologists and British Paediatric Allergy, Immunology and Infection Group national guidelines. *J Infect.* 2012;64:449–477.
14. Tunkel AR, Glaser CA, Bloch KC, et al. The management of encephalitis: clinical practice guidelines by the Infectious Diseases Society of America. *Clin Infect Dis.* 2008;47:303–327.
15. Bloch KC, Glaser CA. Encephalitis surveillance through the Emerging Infections Program, 1997–2010. *Emerg Infect Dis.* 2015;21:1562–1567.
16. Hasbun R, Rosenthal N, Balada-Llasat JM, et al. Epidemiology of meningitis and encephalitis in the United States, 2011–2014. *Clin Infect Dis.* 2017;65:359–363.
17. Archibald LK, Quisling RG. Central nervous system infections. In: Layon A.J. ed. *Textbook of Neurointensive Care.* London: Springer-Verlag; 2013:427–517.
18. Bleck T, Greenlee J. *Anatomic Considerations in Central Nervous System Infections.* 5th ed. New York: Churchill Livingstone; 2000.
19. Bennett JE DR, Blaser MA. *Mandell, Douglas, and Bennett's Principles and Practice of Infectious Diseases.* Philadelphia, PA: Elsevier Saunders; 2015.
20. Kim KS. Emerging molecular targets in the treatment of bacterial meningitis. *Expert Opin Ther Targets* 2003;7:141–152.
21. Klein RS, Hunter CA. Protective and pathological immunity during central nervous system infections. *Immunity* 2017;46:891–909.
22. Magnus T, Rother J, Simova O, et al. The neurological syndrome in adults during the 2011 northern German *E. coli* serotype O104:H4 outbreak. *Brain* 2012;135:1850–1859.
23. Levin SN, Lyons JL. Infections of the nervous system. *Am J Med.* 2018;131:25–32.
24. Brouwer MC, Thwaites GE, Tunkel AR, van de Beek D. Dilemmas in the diagnosis of acute community-acquired bacterial meningitis. *Lancet* 2012;380:1684–1692.
25. Brouwer MC, Tunkel AR, van de Beek D. Epidemiology, diagnosis, and antimicrobial treatment of acute bacterial meningitis. *Clin Microbiol Rev.* 2010;23:467–492.
26. Tunkel AR, Hartman BJ, Kaplan SL, et al. Practice guidelines for the management of bacterial meningitis. *Clin Infect Dis.* 2004;39:1267–1284.
27. van de Beek D, Cabellos C, Dzupova O, et al. ESCMID guideline: diagnosis and treatment of acute bacterial meningitis. *Clin Microbiol Infect.* 2016;22(Suppl 3):S37–S62.
28. Sakushima K, Hayashino Y, Kawaguchi T, Jackson JL, Fukuhara S. Diagnostic accuracy of cerebrospinal fluid lactate for differentiating bacterial meningitis from aseptic meningitis: a meta-analysis. *J Infect.* 2011;62:255–262.
29. Velissaris D, Pintea M, Pantzaris N, et al. The role of procalcitonin in the diagnosis of meningitis: a literature review. *J Clin Med.* 2018;7.
30. Vikse J, Henry BM, Roy J, Ramakrishnan PK, Tomaszewski KA, Walocha JA. The role of serum procalcitonin in the diagnosis of bacterial meningitis in adults: a systematic review and meta-analysis. *Int J Infect Dis.* 2015;38:68–76.
31. Leber AL, Everhart K, Balada-Llasat JM, et al. Multicenter Evaluation of BioFire FilmArray Meningitis/Encephalitis Panel for Detection of Bacteria, Viruses, and Yeast in Cerebrospinal Fluid Specimens. *J Clin Microbiol.* 2016;54:2251–2261.
32. Beganovic M, McCreary EK, Mahoney MV, Dionne B, Green DA, Timbrook TT. Interplay between Rapid Diagnostic Tests and Antimicrobial Stewardship Programs among Patients with Bloodstream and Other Severe Infections. *J Appl Lab Med.* 2019;3:601–616.
33. Srinivasan L, Pisapia JM, Shah SS, Halpern CH, Harris MC. Can broad-range 16S ribosomal ribonucleic acid gene polymerase chain reactions improve the diagnosis of bacterial meningitis? A systematic review and meta-analysis. *Ann Emerg Med.* 2012;60:609–20e2.
34. Wilson MR, O'Donovan BD, Gelfand JM, et al. Chronic meningitis investigated via metagenomic next-generation sequencing. *JAMA Neurol.* 2018;75:947–955.
35. Aggarwal D, Kanitkar T, Narouz M, et al. Clinical utility and cost-effectiveness of bacterial 16S rRNA and targeted PCR based diagnostic testing in a UK microbiology laboratory network. *Sci Rep.* 2020;10:7965. https://doi.org/10.1038/s41598-020-64739-1.
36. Nau R, Seele J, Djukic M, Eiffert H. Pharmacokinetics and pharmacodynamics of antibiotics in central nervous system infections. *Curr Opin Infect Dis.* 2018;31:57–68.
37. Mourvillier B, Tubach F, van de Beek D, et al. Induced hypothermia in severe bacterial meningitis: a randomized clinical trial. *JAMA* 2013;310:2174–2183.
38. Ajdukiewicz KM, Cartwright KE, Scarborough M, et al. Glycerol adjuvant therapy in adults with bacterial meningitis in a high HIV seroprevalence setting in Malawi: a double-blind, randomised controlled trial. *Lancet Infect Dis.* 2011;11:293–300.
39. Wall EC, Ajdukiewicz KM, Bergman H, Heyderman RS, Garner P. Osmotic therapies added to antibiotics for acute bacterial meningitis. *Cochrane Database Syst Rev.* 2018;2:CD008806.
40. Wahl B, O'Brien KL, Greenbaum A, et al. Burden of Streptococcus pneumoniae and Haemophilus influenzae type b disease in children in the era of conjugate vaccines: global, regional, and national estimates for 2000-15. *Lancet Glob Health* 2018;6:e744–e757.
41. Jacobs DM, Yung F, Hart E, Nguyen MNH, Shaver A. Trends in pneumococcal meningitis hospitalizations following the introduction of the 13-valent pneumococcal conjugate vaccine in the United States. *Vaccine* 2017;35:6160–6165.
42. Pfaller MA, Mendes RE, Duncan LR, Flamm RK, Sader HS. In vitro activities of Ceftaroline and Comparators against Streptococcus pneumoniae isolates from U.S. Hospitals: results from seven years of the AWARE Surveillance Program (2010 to 2016). *Antimicrob Agents Chemother.* 2018;62.
43. Hameed N, Tunkel AR. Treatment of drug-resistant pneumococcal meningitis. *Curr Infect Dis Rep.* 2010;12:274–281.
44. Tsuji Y, Hiraki Y, Matsumoto K, et al. Pharmacokinetics and protein binding of linezolid in cerebrospinal fluid and serum in a case of post-neurosurgical bacterial meningitis. *Scand J Infect Dis.* 2011;43:982–985.
45. Sakoulas G, Nonejuie P, Kullar R, Pogliano J, Rybak MJ, Nizet V. Examining the use of ceftaroline in the treatment of Streptococcus pneumoniae meningitis with reference to human cathelicidin LL-37. *Antimicrob Agents Chemother.* 2015;59:2428–2431.
46. Vivas M, Force E, Garrigos C, et al. Experimental study of the efficacy of daptomycin for the treatment of cephalosporin-resistant pneumococcal meningitis. *J Antimicrob Chemother.* 2014;69:3020–3026.
47. Moore MR, Link-Gelles R, Schaffner W, et al. Effect of use of 13-valent pneumococcal conjugate vaccine in children on invasive pneumococcal disease in children and adults in the United States: analysis of multisite, population-based surveillance. *Lancet Infect Dis.* 2015;15:301–309.

48. Pilishvili T, Gierke R, Farley MM, et al. 1470. Epidemiology of Invasive Pneumococcal Disease (IPD) following 18 years of Pneumococcal Conjugate Vaccine (PCV) use in the United States. *Open Forum Infectious Diseases* 2020;7:S736–S737.
49. Harrison LH, Trotter CL, Ramsay ME. Global epidemiology of meningococcal disease. *Vaccine* 2009;27(Suppl 2):B51–B63.
50. Centers for Disease Control and Prevention. Enhanced Meningococcal Disease Surveillance Report 2018. Available at: https://www.cdc.gov/meningococcal/surveillance/index.html#enhanced-reports. Accessed May 2021.
51. Telisinghe L, Waite TD, Gobin M, et al. Chemoprophylaxis and vaccination in preventing subsequent cases of meningococcal disease in household contacts of a case of meningococcal disease: a systematic review. *Epidemiol Infect.* 2015;143:2259–2268.
52. Centers for Disease Control and Prevention. Meningococcal conjugate (MenACWY) vaccination coverage among adolescents 13–17 years by State HR, and the United States, National Immunization Survey-Teen (NIS-Teen), 2019. Available at: https://www.cdc.gov/vaccines/imz-managers/coverage/teenvaxview/data-reports/menacwy/dashboard/2019.html. Accessed April 2021.
53. Petousis-Harris H, Paynter J, Morgan J, et al. Effectiveness of a group B outer membrane vesicle meningococcal vaccine against gonorrhoea in New Zealand: a retrospective case-control study. *Lancet* 2017;390:1603–1610.
54. Slack MPE. Long term impact of conjugate vaccines on *Haemophilus influenzae* meningitis: narrative review. *Microorganisms* 2021;9.
55. American Academy of Pediatrics. Haemophilus influenzae Infections. In: Kimberlin DW, Brady MT, Jackson MA, Long SS, eds. *Red Book: 2018 Report of the Committee on Infectious Diseases.* American Academy of Pediatrics; 2018; 367–375.
56. Kimberlin DW BM, Jackson MA, Long SS. *Red Book®: 2018 Report of the Committee on Infectious Diseases.* 31st ed. Elk Grove Village, IL: American Academy of Pediatrics; 2018.
57. Briere EC, Rubin L, Moro PL, et al. Prevention and control of Haemophilus influenzae type b disease: recommendations of the advisory committee on immunization practices (ACIP). *MMWR Recomm Rep.* 2014;63:1–14.
58. Russell NJ, Seale AC, O'Driscoll M, et al. Maternal colonization with Group B Streptococcus and Serotype distribution worldwide: systematic review and meta-analyses. *Clin Infect Dis.* 2017;65:S100–S11.
59. Puopolo KM, Lynfield R, Cummings JJ, Committee On F, Newborn, Committee On Infectious D. Management of infants at risk for Group B Streptococcal disease. *Pediatrics* 2019;144.
60. Nanduri SA, Petit S, Smelser C, et al. Epidemiology of invasive early-onset and late-onset Group B Streptococcal disease in the United States, 2006 to 2015: multistate laboratory and population-based surveillance. *JAMA Pediatr.* 2019;173:224–233.
61. Prevention of Group B Streptococcal Early-Onset Disease in Newborns: ACOG Committee Opinion, Number 797. *Obstet Gynecol.* 2020;135:e51–e72.
62. Vekemans J, Moorthy V, Friede M, et al. Maternal immunization against Group B streptococcus: World Health Organization research and development technological roadmap and preferred product characteristics. *Vaccine* 2019;37:7391–7393.
63. Charlier C, Perrodeau E, Leclercq A, et al. Clinical features and prognostic factors of listeriosis: the MONALISA national prospective cohort study. *Lancet Infect Dis.* 2017;17:510–519.
64. Brouwer MC, McIntyre P, Prasad K, van de Beek D. Corticosteroids for acute bacterial meningitis. *Cochrane Database Syst Rev.* 2015CD004405.
65. Ricard JD, Wolff M, Lacherade JC, et al. Levels of vancomycin in cerebrospinal fluid of adult patients receiving adjunctive corticosteroids to treat pneumococcal meningitis: a prospective multicenter observational study. *Clin Infect Dis.* 2007;44:250–255.
66. Rogers T, Sok K, Erickson T, et al. Impact of antibiotic therapy in the microbiological yield of healthcare-associated ventriculitis and meningitis. *Open Forum Infect Dis.* 2019;6:ofz050.
67. Lyons JL, Thakur KT, Lee R, et al. Utility of measuring (1,3)-beta-d-glucan in cerebrospinal fluid for diagnosis of fungal central nervous system infection. *J Clin Microbiol.* 2015;53:319–322.
68. Albanese J, Leone M, Bruguerolle B, Ayem ML, Lacarelle B, Martin C. Cerebrospinal fluid penetration and pharmacokinetics of vancomycin administered by continuous infusion to mechanically ventilated patients in an intensive care unit. *Antimicrob Agents Chemother.* 2000;44:1356–1358.
69. Kullar R, Chin JN, Edwards DJ, Parker D, Coplin WM, Rybak MJ. Pharmacokinetics of single-dose daptomycin in patients with suspected or confirmed neurological infections. *Antimicrob Agents Chemother.* 2011;55:3505–3509.
70. Xipell M, Bodro M, Marco F, Losno RA, Cardozo C, Soriano A. Clinical experience with ceftazidime/avibactam in patients with severe infections, including meningitis and lung abscesses, caused by extensively drug-resistant Pseudomonas aeruginosa. *Int J Antimicrob Agents* 2017;49:266–268.
71. Yasmin M, Hanrahan J, Marshall S, et al. Using therapeutic drug monitoring to treat KPC-producing Klebsiella pneumoniae central nervous system infection with Ceftazidime/Avibactam. *Open Forum Infect Dis.* 2020;7:ofaa349.
72. Balouch MA, Bajwa RJ, Hassoun A. Successful use of ceftaroline for the treatment of MRSA meningitis secondary to an infectious complication of lumbar spine surgery. *J Antimicrob Chemother.* 2015;70:624–625.
73. Kuriakose SS, Rabbat M, Gallagher JC. Ceftaroline CSF concentrations in a patient with ventriculoperitoneal shunt-related meningitis. *J Antimicrob Chemother.* 2015;70:953–954.
74. Cies JJ, Moore WS, 2nd, Enache A, Chopra A. Ceftaroline cerebrospinal fluid penetration in the treatment of a ventriculopleural shunt infection: a case report. *J Pediatr Pharmacol Ther.* 2020;25:336–339.
75. Pappas PG, Kauffman CA, Andes DR, et al. Clinical Practice Guideline for the Management of Candidiasis: 2016 Update by the Infectious Diseases Society of America. *Clin Infect Dis.* 2016;62:e1–e50.
76. Patterson TF, Thompson GR, 3rd, Denning DW, et al. Executive Summary: Practice Guidelines for the Diagnosis and Management of Aspergillosis: 2016 Update by the Infectious Diseases Society of America. *Clin Infect Dis.* 2016;63:433–442.
77. Fried HI, Nathan BR, Rowe AS, et al. The insertion and management of external ventricular drains: an evidence-based consensus statement: a statement for healthcare professionals from the Neurocritical Care Society. *Neurocrit Care* 2016;24:61–81.
78. Sonneville R, Ruimy R, Benzonana N, et al. An update on bacterial brain abscess in immunocompetent patients. *Clin Microbiol Infect.* 2017;23:614–620.
79. Patel K, Clifford DB. Bacterial brain abscess. *Neurohospitalist* 2014;4:196–204.
80. Brouwer MC, van de Beek D. Epidemiology, diagnosis, and treatment of brain abscesses. *Curr Opin Infect Dis.* 2017;30:129–134.
81. Doughty CT, Yawetz S, Lyons J. Emerging causes of Arbovirus Encephalitis in North America: Powassan, Chikungunya, and Zika viruses. *Curr Neurol Neurosci Rep.* 2017;17:12.
82. Garcez PP, Loiola EC, Madeiro da Costa R, et al. Zika virus impairs growth in human neurospheres and brain organoids. *Science* 2016;352:816–818.
83. Centers for Disease Control and Prevention. Zika Virus Statistics and Maps. Available at: https://www.cdc.gov/zika/reporting/index.html. Accessed May 2021.
84. Steiner I, Budka H, Chaudhuri A, et al. Viral meningoencephalitis: a review of diagnostic methods and guidelines for management. *Eur J Neurol.* 2010;17:999–e57.
85. Whitley R. Neonatal herpes simplex virus infection. *Curr Opin Infect Dis.* 2004;17:243–246.
86. Piret J, Boivin G. Resistance of herpes simplex viruses to nucleoside analogues: mechanisms, prevalence, and management. *Antimicrob Agents Chemother.* 2011;55:459–472.
87. Gnann JW, Jr, Skoldenberg B, Hart J, et al. Herpes simplex encephalitis: Lack of clinical benefit of long-term valacyclovir therapy. *Clin Infect Dis.* 2015;61:683–691.
88. Petersen LR, Brault AC, Nasci RS. West Nile virus: review of the literature. *JAMA* 2013;310:308–315.
89. Hendricks KA, Wright ME, Shadomy SV, et al. Centers for Disease Control and prevention expert panel meetings on prevention and treatment of anthrax in adults. *Emerg Infect Dis.* 2014;20.
90. Pillai SK, Huang E, Guarnizo JT, et al. Antimicrobial treatment for systemic anthrax: analysis of cases from 1945 to 2014 identified through a systematic literature review . *Health Secur* 2015;13:355–364.
91. Rhee C, Klompas M, Tamburini FB, et al. Epidemiologic investigation of a cluster of neuroinvasive *Bacillus cereus* infections in 5 patients with acute myelogenous leukemia. *Open Forum Infect Dis.* 2015;2:ofv096.
92. Wormser GP, Dattwyler RJ, Shapiro ED, et al. The clinical assessment, treatment, and prevention of lyme disease, human granulocytic anaplasmosis, and babesiosis: clinical practice guidelines by the Infectious Diseases Society of America. *Clin Infect Dis.* 2006;43:1089–1134.
93. Mygland A, Ljostad U, Fingerle V, et al. EFNS guidelines on the diagnosis and management of European Lyme neuroborreliosis. *Eur J Neurol.* 2010;17:8–16, e1-e4.
94. Garcia-Monco JC, Benach JL. Lyme neuroborreliosis: clinical outcomes, controversy, pathogenesis, and polymicrobial infections. *Ann Neurol.* 2019;85:21–31.

95. Nahid P, Dorman SE, Alipanah N, et al. Executive Summary: Official American Thoracic Society/Centers for Disease Control and Prevention/Infectious Diseases Society of America Clinical Practice Guidelines: treatment of drug-susceptible tuberculosis. *Clin Infect Dis.* 2016;63:853–867.
96. Panel on Opportunistic Infections in Adults and Adolescents with HIV. Guidelines for the prevention and treatment of opportunistic infections in adults and adolescents with HIV: recommendations from the Centers for Disease Control and Prevention, the National Institutes of Health, and the HIV Medicine Association of the Infectious Diseases Society of America. Available at: http://aidsinfo.nih.gov/contentfiles/lvguidelines/adult_oi.pdf. Accessed April 2021.
97. Falzon D, Schunemann HJ, Harausz E, et al. World Health Organization treatment guidelines for drug-resistant tuberculosis, 2016 update. *Eur Respir J.* 2017;49.
98. Lafont E, Conan PL, Rodriguez-Nava V, Lebeaux D. Invasive nocardiosis: disease presentation, diagnosis and treatment – Old questions, new answers? *Infect Drug Resist.* 2020;13:4601–4613.
99. Restrepo A, Clark NM, Infectious Diseases Community of Practice of the American Society of T. Nocardia infections in solid organ transplantation: Guidelines from the Infectious Diseases Community of Practice of the American Society of Transplantation. *Clin Transplant.* 2019;33:e13509.
100. Corsini Campioli C, Castillo Almeida NE, O'Horo JC, et al. Clinical presentation, management, and outcomes of patients with brain abscess due to *Nocardia* species. *Open Forum Infect Dis.* 2021;8:ofab067.
101. Taravaud A, Fechtali-Moute Z, Loiseau PM, Pomel S. Drugs used for the treatment of cerebral and disseminated infections caused by free-living amoebae. *Clin Transl Sci.* 2021.
102. Panel on Opportunistic Infections in HIV-Exposed and HIV-Infected Children. Guidelines for the Prevention and Treatment of Opportunistic Infections in HIV-Exposed and HIV-Infected Children. Department of Health and Human Services. Available at: http://aidsinfo.nih.gov/contentfiles/lvguidelines/oi_guidelines_pediatrics.pdf. Accessed April 2021.

Lower Respiratory Tract Infections

129

Evan J. Zasowski and Martha G. Blackford

KEY CONCEPTS

1. Respiratory infections remain a major cause of morbidity from acute illness in the United States and represent the most common reasons why patients seek medical attention.
2. The majority of pulmonary infections follow colonization of the upper respiratory tract with potential pathogens, whereas microbes less commonly gain access to the lungs via the bloodstream from an extrapulmonary source or by inhalation of infected aerosol particles. The competency of a patient's immune status is an important factor influencing the susceptibility to infection, etiologic cause, and disease severity.
3. An appropriate treatment regimen for a patient with uncomplicated lower respiratory tract infection can be established by evaluating the patient history, physical examination, chest radiograph, and properly collected sputum for culture interpreted in light of current knowledge of the most common lung pathogens and their antibiotic susceptibility patterns within the community.
4. Acute bronchitis is most commonly caused by respiratory viruses and is almost always self-limiting. Therapy targets associated symptoms such as lethargy, malaise, or fever and may include fluids for rehydration. Routine use of antibiotics should be avoided and medication to suppress cough is rarely indicated.
5. Chronic bronchitis is caused by several interacting factors, including inhalation of noxious agents (most prominent are cigarette smoke and exposure to occupational dusts, fumes, and environmental pollution) and host factors including genetic factors and bacterial (and possibly viral) infections. The hallmark of this disease is a chronic cough, accompanied by excessive production, and expectoration of sputum with a persistent presence of microorganisms in the patient's sputum.
6. Treatment of acute exacerbations of chronic bronchitis includes attempts to mobilize and enhance sputum expectoration (chest physiotherapy, humidification of inspired air), oxygen if needed, aerosolized bronchodilators in select patients with demonstrated benefit, and possibly antibiotics.
7. Respiratory syncytial virus is the most common cause of acute bronchiolitis, an infection that mostly affects infants during their first year of life. In the well infant, bronchiolitis usually is a self-limiting viral illness.
8. The most prominent pathogen causing community-acquired bacterial pneumonia in otherwise healthy adults is *Streptococcus pneumoniae*, whereas the most common pathogens causing hospital-acquired pneumonia are *Staphylococcus aureus* and gram-negative aerobic bacilli.
9. Empiric antimicrobial therapy for pneumonia should consist of antibiotic regimens targeting presumed causative pathogens based on clinical presentation and patient-specific characteristics, local epidemiology, and resistance patterns.
10. Microbiologic tests for pneumonia etiology should be performed when clinically indicated and used along with patient clinical response to tailor antibiotic therapy using evidence-based pathogen-directed therapy when possible.

BEYOND THE BOOK

Create a study chart of the following antibiotics with potential utility in lower respiratory tract infections: ceftazidime-avibactam; ceftolozane-tazobactam; meropenem-vaborbactam; cefiderocol, imipenem-relabactam, plazomicin, eravacycline. On the chart include spectrum of activity, pharmacokinetics (ADME), dosing (including need for adjustment in special populations), adverse effects, Food and Drug Administration (FDA)-approved indication(s), level of evidence supporting use in lower respiratory tract infections (none, in vitro/in vivo, case report/series, observational study, randomized controlled trial), and potential place in therapy of lower respiratory tract infections.

INTRODUCTION

1 Respiratory tract infections remain a major cause of morbidity from acute illness in the United States and most likely represent the single most common reason patients seek medical attention. This chapter focuses on bacterial and viral infections involving the lower respiratory tract, which includes the tracheobronchial tree and lung parenchyma.

2 The respiratory tract has an elaborate system of host defenses, including humoral immunity, cellular immunity, and anatomic mechanisms.[1] When functioning properly, respiratory tract host defenses are markedly effective in protecting against pathogen invasion and removing potentially infectious agents from the lungs. For the most part, infections in the lower respiratory tract occur

only when these defense mechanisms are impaired, as in cases of dysgammaglobulinemia or compromised ciliary function, such as that caused by the chronic inflammation accompanying cigarette smoking. In addition, local defenses may be overwhelmed when a particularly virulent microorganism or excessive inoculum invades lung parenchyma. Most pulmonary infections follow colonization of the upper respiratory tract with potential pathogens, which, after achieving sufficiently high concentrations, gain access to the lung via aspiration of oropharyngeal secretions. Less commonly, microbes enter the lung via the blood from an extrapulmonary source or by inhalation of infected aerosolized particles. The specific type of pulmonary infection caused by an invading microorganism is determined by a variety of host factors, including age, anatomic features of the airway, and specific characteristics of the infecting agent.

The most common infections involving the lower respiratory tract are bronchitis, bronchiolitis, and pneumonia. Bronchitis and bronchiolitis are inflammatory conditions of the large and small airways, respectively, of the tracheobronchial tree. The inflammatory process does not extend to the alveoli. Bronchitis frequently is classified as acute or chronic; acute bronchitis occurs in individuals of all ages, whereas chronic bronchitis primarily affects adults. Bronchiolitis is a disease of infancy.

Lower respiratory tract infections in children and adults most commonly result from either viral or bacterial invasion of lung parenchyma. The diagnosis of viral infections rests primarily on the recognition of a characteristic constellation of clinical signs and symptoms. Because treatment of viral respiratory infections is largely supportive, only occasionally does the diagnosis require laboratory confirmation; this is achieved through serologic tests or identification of the organism by culture or antigen detection in respiratory secretions.[2] Laboratory techniques using polymerase chain reaction (PCR), microarrays, and multiplex ligation-dependent probe amplification, to name a few, have emerged to identify specific pathogens rapidly and accurately.[3]

In contrast, because bacterial pneumonia usually necessitates expedient, effective, and specific antibiotic therapy, its management depends, in large part, on an understanding of the risk factors for acquiring pneumonia, predominant pathogens within the community, and, if necessary, isolation of the etiologic agent by culture from lung tissue or secretions.[4-6] The pharynx is colonized with many organisms that can cause pneumonia; therefore, culture of expectorated sputum can be misleading unless the specimen is examined to ensure that it has originated from the lower respiratory tract. The Gram stain provides the easiest method for distinguishing lower from upper respiratory tract secretions; moreover, through determination of the shape and color of the bacteria, the Gram stain frequently narrows the microbiologic differential diagnosis sufficiently to allow accurate initial therapy. Scanned under low-power microscopy, Gram-stained expectorated upper respiratory tract secretions contain many irregularly shaped epithelial cells with little evidence of inflammation and may not reflect the pathogen. In contrast, a lower-tract specimen from a patient with bacterial pneumonia usually contains multiple neutrophils per high-powered field and a single or predominant bacterial species. More aggressive procedures can be performed to more accurately identify responsible pathogens including respiratory secretion samples obtained via bronchoscopy or bronchoalveolar lavage (BAL). Culture of specimens confirmed to originate from the lower tract by Gram stain or collection via BAL provides valuable diagnostic information for the majority of patients with bacterial pneumonia. In addition, pneumonia promotes the release of inflammatory mediators and acute-phase proteins, such as C-reactive protein, which can be significantly elevated in serum in the presence of respiratory tract infections.[7] Unfortunately except for pathogen identification by culture, elevations in C-reactive protein, changes in sputum color or peripheral white blood count, etc., are not specific for determining viral, bacterial, or fungal etiology. Newer genomic testing may aid tremendously in determining the identity of responsible pathogen(s) and then selection of optimal antimicrobial therapy.

3 An appropriate treatment regimen for the patient with an uncomplicated lower respiratory tract infection usually can be established by history, physical examination, chest radiograph, and properly collected sputum cultures interpreted in light of the most common lung pathogens and their antibiotic susceptibility patterns within the community.[2,5] More sophisticated or invasive diagnostic methods (eg, computed tomography, bronchoscopy, and lung biopsy) are reserved for severely ill patients who are unable to expectorate sputum or who are not responding to empirical therapy or for pulmonary infections occurring in immunocompromised patients.[2]

BRONCHITIS

Acute Bronchitis

Epidemiology and Etiology

Acute bronchitis occurs year-round, but more commonly during the winter months. Cough accounts for more than 6 million ambulatory visits annually, underscoring its major financial impact on the healthcare system.[8] Acute bronchitis is characterized by inflammation of the epithelium of the large airways resulting from infection or exposure to irritating environmental triggers (eg, air pollution and cigarette smoke). Acute (viral) infection and/or smoking are the most common precipitants of attacks, which usually manifest initially as a persistent cough.

4 Respiratory viruses are the predominant infectious agents associated with acute bronchitis, accounting for 85% to 95% of occurrences. The most common infecting agents include influenza A and B, respiratory syncytial virus (RSV), and parainfluenza virus, whereas the common cold viruses (rhinovirus and coronavirus) and adenovirus are encountered less frequently. Although far less common, bacterial pathogens are involved in a minority of cases and involve pathogens often associated with community-acquired pneumonia (CAP) including *Mycoplasma pneumoniae, Streptococcus pneumonia, Haemophilus influenzae, Moraxella catarrhalis*, and less commonly *Chlamydophila pneumoniae* and *Bordetella pertussis*, the agent responsible for whooping cough. Although a primary bacterial etiology for acute bronchitis appears rare, secondary bacterial infection may be involved, particularly in patients with underlying disease(s).[8]

Pathogenesis

4 Since acute bronchitis is primarily a self-limiting illness and rarely a cause of death, few data describing the pathology are available. In general, infection of the trachea and bronchi yields inflammation-induced hyperemic and edematous mucous membranes with an increase in bronchial secretions. Destruction of respiratory epithelium can range from mild to extensive and may affect bronchial mucociliary function. In addition, the increase in desquamated epithelial cells and bronchial secretions, which can become thick and tenacious, further impairs mucociliary activity. The probability of permanent damage to the airways as a result of acute bronchitis remains unclear but appears unlikely. However, epidemiologic evaluations support the belief that recurrent acute respiratory infections may be associated with increased airway hyperreactivity and possibly the pathogenesis of asthma, chronic obstructive pulmonary disease (COPD), or possibly the asthma-COPD syndrome.[9,10]

Clinical Presentation

Acute bronchitis usually begins as an upper respiratory infection with nonspecific complaints.[8,11] Cough is the hallmark of acute bronchitis and occurs early. The onset of cough may be insidious or abrupt, and the symptoms persist despite resolution of nasal or nasopharyngeal complaints; cough may persist for up to 3 or more weeks. Frequently, the cough initially is nonproductive, but then progresses, yielding mucopurulent sputum. In older children and adults, the sputum is raised and expectorated; in the young child, sputum often is swallowed and can result in gagging and vomiting. Substantial discomfort may result from the coughing. Dyspnea, cyanosis, or signs of airway obstruction are observed rarely unless the patient has underlying pulmonary disease, such as emphysema or COPD. Fever, when present, rarely exceeds 39°C (102.2°F) and appears most commonly with adenovirus, influenza virus, and *M. pneumoniae* infections. The diagnosis typically is made on the basis of a characteristic history and physical examination and should be differentiated from asthma or bronchiolitis as these latter diseases are usually associated with wheezing, shortness of breath, and hypoxemia. Bacterial cultures of expectorated sputum are of limited use because of the inability to avoid normal nasopharyngeal flora by the sampling technique. Similarly, viral cultures are unnecessary. In the absence of important risk factors, including COPD, congestive heart failure, or immune compromise, throat/sputum cultures have no role in the routine care of patients with acute bronchitis. For the vast majority of affected patients, an etiologic diagnosis is unnecessary and will not change the prescribing of routine supportive care for the management of these patients.

TREATMENT

Desired Outcome

In the absence of a complicating bacterial superinfection, acute bronchitis almost always is self-limiting. The goals of therapy are to provide comfort to the patient and, in the unusually severe case, to treat associated dehydration and respiratory compromise.[8]

General Approach to Treatment

4 Treatment of acute bronchitis is symptomatic and supportive in nature. Reassurance and antipyretics frequently are all that are needed. Bedrest for comfort may be instituted as desired. Patients should be encouraged to drink fluids to prevent dehydration and possibly to decrease the viscosity of respiratory secretions. Mist therapy (use of a vaporizer) may promote the thinning and loosening of respiratory secretions.

Pharmacologic Therapy

Mild analgesic–antipyretic therapy often is helpful in relieving the associated lethargy, malaise, and fever. Aspirin or acetaminophen (650 mg/dose in adults [maximum less than 4 g/day] or 10-15 mg/kg/dose in children [maximum 60-75 mg/kg/day or 5 doses/day]) administered every 4 to 6 hours or ibuprofen (200-800 mg/dose in adults [maximum 3.2 g/day] or 10 mg/kg/dose in children [maximum 40 mg/kg/day]) should be administered every 6 to 8 hours. Aspirin should be avoided in children less than 19 years of age with a fever-causing illness and acetaminophen or ibuprofen used as the preferred agents because of a possible, but unclear and unproven association between aspirin use and the possible development of Reye's syndrome.

Patients may present with mild-to-moderate wheezing. In otherwise healthy patients, no meaningful benefits have been described with the routine use of oral or aerosolized β_2-receptor agonists[11,12] and/or oral or aerosolized corticosteroids. Corticosteroids should be avoided in patients with acute bronchitis. There is no evidence to support the routine use of β_2-receptor agonists in either pediatric or adult patients with acute bronchitis; however, adults with airflow obstruction may have a trend toward improvement in cough.[13] Some clinicians, despite no data, may initiate a brief trial (eg, about 5-7 days) of β_2-receptor agonists and even oral or inhaled corticosteroid for patients with a persistent (more than 14-20 days), troublesome cough. This is rarely, if ever, necessary in patients with uncomplicated acute bronchitis and should be avoided. Cough may persist for 3+ weeks and airway hyperresponsiveness for 5 to 6 weeks in as many as 50% of affected patients. In contrast, COPD patients experiencing an acute exacerbation can benefit from a short course of corticosteroid.

Patients suffering from acute bronchitis frequently medicate themselves with nonprescription cough and cold remedies containing various combinations of antihistamines, sympathomimetics, and antitussives despite the lack of definitive evidence supporting their effectiveness.[8,11] The tendency of these agents to dehydrate bronchial secretions could aggravate and prolong the recovery process. Although not recommended for routine use, persistent, mild cough, which may be bothersome, can be treated with dextromethorphan; more severe coughs may require intermittent codeine or other similar agents.[14] In severe cases, the cough may be persistent enough to disrupt sleep, and use of a mild sedative-hypnotic, concomitantly with a cough suppressant (eg, codeine), may be desirable. However, antitussives should be used cautiously when the cough is productive, and codeine is no longer recommended for use in pediatric patients. The primary or supplemental use of expectorants is questionable because their clinical effectiveness has not been well established.[8]

Routine use of antibiotics for treatment of acute bronchitis should be strongly discouraged due to limited benefit.[8,11,15] In previously healthy patients who exhibit persistent fever or respiratory symptoms for more than 5 to 7 days or for predisposed patients (eg, elderly/frail, COPD, and immune compromised), the possibility of a concurrent bacterial infection should be suspected. When possible, antibiotic therapy should be directed toward anticipated respiratory pathogen(s) (eg, *S. pneumoniae* and *H. influenzae*). *M. pneumoniae*, if suspected by history or if confirmed by culture serology or PCR, can be treated with azithromycin. Alternatively, a fluoroquinolone antibiotic with activity against these suspected pathogens (eg, levofloxacin or moxifloxacin) can be used empirically, but due to the increasing rate of pathogen resistance to current antimicrobial drugs, the use of antibiotics in patients with acute bronchitis should be reserved for only those patients not responding adequately to supportive care and deemed at risk of associated complications. During known epidemics involving the influenza A virus, amantadine or rimantadine may have been effective in minimizing associated symptoms if administered early in the course of the disease; however, treatment with these adamantanes is no longer recommended by the Centers for Disease Control and Prevention (CDC) due to increasing influenza resistance and associated adverse effects (see Chapter 131, "Influenza"). The neuraminidase inhibitors (eg, zanamivir and oseltamivir) and the endonuclease inhibitor baloxavir are active against both influenza A and B viral infections and may reduce the severity and duration of the influenza episode if administered promptly during the onset of the viral infection and are the preferred treatment (see Chapter 131).[12,16] Unfortunately, the incidence of influenza virus resistance to available antiviral drugs is increasing, necessitating reconsideration of how we administer antiviral drugs for prophylaxis and treatment.[12] The concept of antiviral drug combinations has emerged as a successful approach to effectively treat systemic viral infections.[17]

Chronic Bronchitis

Epidemiology and Etiology

Chronic bronchitis, most often a component of COPD, is a clinical diagnosis for a nonspecific, heterogenic disease that primarily affects adults. An in-depth presentation of the spectrum and management of COPD is given in Chapter 45, "Chronic Obstructive Pulmonary Disease"; this section focuses solely on chronic bronchitis. In developed countries, the prevalence of chronic bronchitis is slightly higher in men than in women. Depending on the definition used for chronic bronchitis, 3.4% to 22% of adults have chronic bronchitis and 14% to 74% of COPD patients suffer from chronic bronchitis.[18]

5 Chronic bronchitis is defined as the presence of a chronic cough productive of sputum lasting more than 3 consecutive months of the year for 2 consecutive years without an underlying etiology of bronchiectasis or tuberculosis. The disease is a result of several contributing factors; the most prominent factor is cigarette smoking; however, in nonsmokers who develop chronic bronchitis (4%-22%), other factors may be exposure to occupational dusts, fumes, and environmental pollution, and host factors (eg, genetic factors and bacterial [and possibly viral] infections).[18] The contribution of each of these factors and of others (either alone or in combination) to chronic bronchitis is unknown.[19] Cigarette smoke is a well-known airway irritant and is a predominant factor in the etiology of chronic bronchitis. Although previously assumed the most common etiologic cause of chronic bronchitis, more strict prohibition of public smoking and the resultant decrease in chronic tobacco smokers, particularly in developed countries, underscores the importance of other factors as causes of this chronic disease. Airway irritants including occupational dust, chemicals, or air pollution, either alone or more likely in combination, are also responsible for the pathogenesis of chronic bronchitis and may explain the development in nonsmokers.[18] Furthermore, genomic studies have begun to expand our understanding of the molecular pathways that may have clinical relevance in this heterogeneous disease. Lastly, the influence of recurrent respiratory tract infections during childhood or young adult life on the later development of chronic bronchitis remains obscure, but recurrent respiratory infections may predispose individuals to the development of chronic bronchitis. Whether these recurrent respiratory tract infections are a result of unrecognized anatomic abnormalities of the airways or impaired pulmonary defense mechanisms is unclear.

Chronic bronchitis and emphysema are the two main components of COPD/chronic obstructive lung disease.[20-22] The Global Initiative for Chronic Obstructive Lung Disease (GOLD) guidelines document does not distinguish these two diagnoses (eg, emphysema or chronic bronchitis) in the definition of COPD, but it does define COPD as a disease characterized by airflow obstruction that is not fully reversible and progressive. The GOLD guidelines provide a COPD classification scoring system according to severity that can be helpful in staging patients for intensity of therapy, acute/chronic therapy, and prognosis. Unfortunately, differences in definitions between authoritative organizations may cause confusion in the assignment of patients in clinical trials and thus in assessment and application of study results to clinical care.

Pathogenesis

Chronic inhalation of an irritating noxious substance compromises the normal secretory and mucociliary function of bronchial mucosa.[18] Bronchial biopsy specimens in bronchitic patients underscore the importance of T-cell-derived proinflammatory cytokines (eg, interleukins IL-4, IL-5, IL-13, and interferon gamma) in the pathogenesis and propagation of the observed inflammatory changes. In chronic bronchitis, the bronchial wall is thickened, and the number of mucus-secreting goblet cells on the surface epithelium of both larger and smaller bronchi is increased markedly. In contrast, goblet cells generally are absent from the smaller bronchi of normal individuals. In addition to the increased number of goblet cells, hypertrophy of the mucous glands and dilation of the mucous gland ducts are observed. As a result of these changes, chronic bronchitis has substantially more mucus in the peripheral airways, further impairing normal lung defenses. This increased quantity (overproduction and hypersecretion) of tenacious secretions within the bronchial tree frequently causes mucous plugging of the smaller airways. Accompanying these changes is squamous cell metaplasia of the surface epithelium, edema, and increased vascularity of the basement membrane of larger airways and variable chronic inflammatory cell infiltration. In addition, the amounts of several proteases derived from inflammatory cells are increased and due to COPD-induced defective antiproteases lead to continued destruction of connective tissue. Continued progression of this pathology can result in residual scarring of small bronchi and peribronchial fibrosis augmenting airway obstruction and weakening of bronchial walls.[18]

Clinical Presentation

5 The hallmark of chronic bronchitis is a cough that may range from a mild to a severe and incessant coughing productive of purulent sputum. Coughing may be precipitated by multiple stimuli, including simple, normal conversation. Expectoration of the largest quantity of sputum usually occurs on arising in the morning, although many patients expectorate sputum throughout the day. The expectorated sputum usually is tenacious and can vary in color from white to yellow-green. Patients with chronic bronchitis often expectorate as much as 100 mL/day more than normal. As a result, many patients complain of a frequent bad taste in their mouth and of halitosis. Sputum color provides no prognostic indication of infection or cause of an infectious disease exacerbation, that is, viral versus bacterial cause. Although sputum color of more green and yellow can be a predictor of potentially pathogenic bacteria, this is unreliable clinically.[23] The diagnosis of an acute exacerbation requires consideration of a number of different factors all occurring within a discrete timeframe (eg, increased/worsening respiratory symptoms including dyspnea, sputum volume and/or clearance, and cough). The tracking of the number of acute exacerbations and their consequences (decline in forced expiratory volume in 1 second [FEV1]), persistent/worsening of symptoms annually, is extremely important for prognostication and defining ongoing treatment strategies. Each acute exacerbation of chronic bronchitis results in continual declines in lung function.

The diagnosis of chronic bronchitis is based primarily on clinical assessment and history. Any patient who reports coughing sputum on most days for at least 3 consecutive months each year for 2 consecutive years presumptively has chronic bronchitis.[18] The diagnosis of chronic bronchitis is made only when the possibilities of bronchiectasis, cardiac failure, cystic fibrosis, and lung carcinoma, among others, have been effectively excluded. To be more specific in the diagnosis, some investigators have added the criteria of lost wages for 3 or more weeks. In addition, many clinicians attempt to subdivide their patients based on severity of disease to guide therapeutic interventions. Two primary classification proposals are most often used in an attempt to determine the severity of the underlying disease as well as the occurrence/impending occurrence of an acute exacerbation of chronic bronchitis; for disease severity and acute exacerbations the prognostic tools advocated by GOLD are very helpful including classification based on spirometry ("mild" postbronchodilator FEV1 greater than or equal to 80% predicted to "very severe" postbronchodilator FEV1 less than 30% predicted: see Chapter e43, "Evaluation of Pulmonary Function"); the COPD assessment test (eight-item measure of health status), the Clinical COPD Questionnaire (a measure of clinical control), and the Modified Medical Research Council Questionnaire to predict future mortality. The other simple classification system is that proposed by Anthonisen and colleagues in 1987 that is still used to categorize patients in many therapeutic clinical trials.[24] The use of patient symptom diaries can also be helpful in compliant patients. The importance of accurate classification for grouping patients of similar disease involvement cannot be overemphasized with respect to assessing publications outlining treatment strategies for these patients. These classifications attempt to capture specific phenotypes of chronic bronchitis patients. The typical clinical presentation of chronic bronchitis is listed in Table 129-1. Comparison of the trends in changes in a patient's physical activity, symptoms, and clinical/physical findings from the patient's "routine" is extremely helpful in determining the presence and severity of an acute exacerbation.

In more advanced stages of chronic bronchitis, physical findings associated with cor pulmonale, including cardiac enlargement, hepatomegaly, and edema of the lower extremities, are observed. In general, people with chronic bronchitis tend to maintain at least normal body weight and commonly are obese. Radiographic studies are of limited value in either the diagnosis or follow-up of a patient. The microscopic and laboratory assessments of sputum are used in the overall evaluation of patients with chronic bronchitis. Gram staining of the sputum often reveals a mixture of both gram-positive and gram-negative bacteria, reflecting normal oropharyngeal flora and chronic tracheal colonization (in order of frequency) by non-typable *H. influenzae*, *S. pneumoniae*, and *M. catarrhalis*. Table 129-2 lists the most common bacterial isolates identified from sputum culture for patients experiencing an acute exacerbation of chronic bronchitis. For patients with more severe airflow disease (eg, FEV_1 less than 40% predicted), enteric gram-negative bacilli, *Escherichia coli*, *Klebsiella* species, *Enterobacter* species, and *Pseudomonas aeruginosa* may be significant pathogens during acute exacerbations.

TABLE 129-1 Clinical Presentation of Chronic Bronchitis

Signs and symptoms

Excessive sputum expectoration
Cough
Cyanosis (advanced disease)

Physical examination

Chest auscultation usually reveals inspiratory and expiratory rales, rhonchi, and mild wheezing with an expiratory phase that is frequently prolonged
Hyperresonance on percussion with obliteration of the area of cardiac dullness
Normal vesicular breathing sounds are diminished
Clubbing of digits (advanced disease)
Obesity

Chest radiograph

Increase in anteroposterior diameter of the thoracic cage (barrel chest)
Depressed diaphragm with limited mobility

Laboratory tests

Erythrocytosis (advanced disease), that is, increased hematocrit

Pulmonary function tests

Decreased vital capacity
Prolonged expiratory flow

TABLE 129-2 Common Bacterial Pathogens Isolated from Sputum of Patients with Acute Exacerbation of Chronic Bronchitis

Pathogen	Percent of Cultures
H. influenzae[a,b]	45
M. catarrhalis[a]	30
S. pneumoniae[c]	20
E. coli, *Enterobacter* species, *Klebsiella* species, *P. aeruginosa*	5

[a]Often β-lactamase positive.

[b]Vast majority are nontypable strains.

[c]More than 25% of strains may have intermediate or high resistance to penicillin.

TREATMENT

Desired Outcome

The goals of therapy for chronic bronchitis are twofold: to reduce the severity of chronic symptoms and to ameliorate acute exacerbations and achieve prolonged exacerbation-free intervals.

General Approach to Treatment

The approach to treatment of chronic bronchitis is multifactorial.[18] First and foremost, attempts must be made to reduce the patient's exposure to known bronchial irritants (eg, smoking and workplace pollution). A complete occupational and environmental history for determination of exposure to noxious, irritating gases as well as preference toward cigarette smoking must be assessed. Often easier to discuss than accomplish, reasonable attempts should be made with the patient to reduce or eliminate the number of cigarettes smoked daily and to reduce exposure to secondhand smoke. An organized, coordinated, smoking cessation program, including counseling, possibly hypnotherapy, and the adjunctive use of nicotine substitutes (eg, nicotine gum or patch) or other pharmacotherapy (eg, bupropion and varenicline), may promote the reduction or complete withdrawal from cigarette smoking. Often just as difficult is modification of exposure to irritating substances within the home and workplace.

The importance of pulmonary rehabilitation has been realized in improving the quality of life for patients with chronic respiratory diseases.[25] Pulmonary rehabilitation is broadly defined as an interdisciplinary program individualized for patients with chronic respiratory impairment designed to optimize each patient's physical and social performance and autonomy. A personalized exercise-training program including resistance and aerobic exercise is central to these programs. Pulmonary rehabilitation programs relieve dyspnea and fatigue, improve a patient's emotional function, and enhance their sense of control over their disease and life. These improvements are often moderately large and clinically relevant.[25] The challenge for the future is to determine what components of a comprehensive pulmonary rehabilitation program provide the greatest benefit.

6 Measures to provide chest physiotherapy (eg, pulmonary "toilet") can be instituted.[26] Clearly the cost-effectiveness of chest physiotherapy needs to be better described but their short-term effects have been demonstrated and may be of symptomatic value to many patients experiencing an acute exacerbation of the chronic bronchitis. During acute pulmonary exacerbations of the disease, the patient's ability to mobilize and expectorate sputum may be reduced dramatically. In these instances, attempts at postural drainage techniques, with instruction and or active participation from a respiratory therapist, may assist in promoting clearance of pulmonary secretions. In addition, humidification of inspired air may promote the hydration (liquefaction) of tenacious secretions, allowing for removal that is more productive. Use of aerosolized mucolytic aerosols, such as *N*-acetylcysteine (NAC) and DNAse, is of questionable therapeutic value, particularly considering their propensity to induce bronchospasm (NAC) and their excessive cost. NAC cleaves the disulfide bonds of mucus, decreasing its elastic property that is important for upward mobility and then expectoration. Aerosol mucolytic therapy was associated with a small reduction in acute exacerbations in subjects with chronic bronchitis or COPD and did not cause any harm, improve quality of life, or slow the decline of lung function.[27] The clinical benefit may be greater for chronic bronchitis/COPD patients who have frequent or prolonged exacerbations and are unable to utilize inhaled corticosteroids or long-acting β_2-agonists.[27] Although limited data are available, chronic use of oral or aerosolized bronchodilators may be of benefit by increasing mucociliary and cough clearance. For patients with moderate to severe COPD, combination therapy with a long-acting β_2-agonist

and inhaled corticosteroid led to decreased exacerbations and rescue medication use, while it also improved quality of life, lung function, and symptom scores compared with long-acting β_2-agonist monotherapy.

Pharmacologic Therapy

Patients should be up to date with vaccinations, particularly pneumococcal and an annual influenza vaccine. For patients who consistently demonstrate clinical limitation in airflow, a therapeutic challenge of a short-acting β_2-agonist bronchodilator (eg, as albuterol aerosol) could be considered; however, there is insufficient evidence to recommend the routine use of pharmaceutical agents for cough relief.[18] Pulmonary function tests should be performed before and after β_2-agonist aerosol administration for more objective determination of a patient's propensity to benefit from supplemental aerosol therapy. Regular use of a long-acting β-receptor agonist aerosol (eg, salmeterol and formoterol) in responsive patients is more effective and probably more convenient than short-acting β_2-receptor agonists.[28] The aerosol route for β_2-receptor agonist and/or corticosteroid administration is favored over systemic formulations for improved patient acceptance and compliance and to minimize the number and magnitude of associated adverse effects. Chronic inhalation of a combination long-acting β-receptor agonist (LABA) and a corticosteroid (eg, salmeterol-fluticasone and formoterol-mometasone) improved pulmonary function and quality of life.[29] Long-term use of aerosolized corticosteroid is associated with increased side effects including hoarseness, sore throat, thrush, pneumonia, and osteoporosis; however, caution should be exercised in withdrawing inhaled glucocorticoid administration in patients with severe COPD receiving triple inhalation therapy. A stepwise approach to withdrawing inhaled corticosteroids may minimize the risk for acute exacerbations but a decrease in lung function can still occur after discontinuation.[30]

Inhaled anticholinergic drugs, including ipratropium and tiotropium, have an important role in the chronic management of patients with chronic bronchitis and COPD.[31] Inhaled long-acting muscarinic antagonists (LAMAs) alone or more frequently, when administered in combination with a LABA, improve lung function and symptom control and reduce the number of acute exacerbations. Triple combination inhalation therapy (eg, LABA + LAMA + an inhaled corticosteroid) is being evaluated in patients with more severe COPD with promising findings and its role remains to be defined.[32] Although once prescribed extensively for patients with chronic bronchitis, chronic theophylline therapy is used with decreasing frequency in favor of aerosolized β_2-receptor agonists, LABA, LAMA, etc. Nevertheless, long-acting theophylline remains an effective "add on" therapy for many patients, particularly those with more severe chronic bronchitis/COPD due to the drug's beneficial effects of bronchodilation, improved ciliary function and increased beat frequency, possibly increased mucus hydration, and low cost.[18]

Phosphodiesterase 4 inhibitors (PDE-4), compared with the nonselective phosphodiesterase inhibitor theophylline, only affect phosphodiesterase in the airway smooth muscle, immune cells (eosinophils, monocytes, and neutrophils), and proinflammatory cells. Roflumilast is a highly specific (second generation) PDE-4 inhibitor that is most often reserved for use in patients with moderate to severe COPD. Considering that many of the published studies assessing the viability of second-generation PDE-4 inhibitors in patients with COPD involved patients with chronic cough and increased sputum production, it is inferred that these drugs would be of value in patients with chronic bronchitis as well. The GOLD guidelines suggest roflumilast reduces exacerbations in COPD patients with chronic bronchitis treated with oral glucocorticosteroids. Roflumilast only provides a net benefit to patients at high risk of severe exacerbations.[32,33] A lower 30-day readmission rate in patients hospitalized for COPD with roflumilast therapy was reported.[34] PDE-4 inhibitors improved lung function over placebo and reduced the likelihood of exacerbations; they had little impact on a patient's symptoms or quality of life. Nevertheless, the major limitation to the use of PDE-4 inhibitors is their side effect profiles. Patients receiving roflumilast often experience nausea, vomiting, headache, weight loss, insomnia, and an increased risk of psychiatric events.[35] The exact role of roflumilast in chronic lung disease is evolving but many guidelines suggest its use as add-on therapy for subgroups of patients.[32,35]

Use of antimicrobials for treatment of chronic bronchitis has been controversial, but is becoming more accepted in specific circumstances. Numerous comparative evaluations, including placebo-controlled studies of antibiotic administration for acute and chronic treatment of chronic bronchitis, have suggested clinical benefit. The antibiotics selected most frequently possess variable in vitro activity against the common sputum isolates *H. influenzae*, *S. pneumoniae*, *M. catarrhalis*, and *M. pneumoniae*. Conflicting published results appear independent of the antibiotic used or the regimen compared. A wide disparity that existed in the published results from older studies served as the basis for the enormous controversy about the use of antibiotics for the treatment of acute exacerbations of chronic bronchitis. Overall, good clinical results have been observed with the use of standard short-course antibiotic regimens (eg, macrolides, azalides, oral cephalosporins, and the combination drug amoxicillin-clavulanate, trimethoprim-sulfamethoxazole, and tetracyclines).[36,37] The goal is to select the most effective antibiotic drug for the patient based on their history of previous exacerbations and response to drug therapy. The introduction of genome expression profiling of sputum and other biologic fluids can facilitate specific pathogen diagnosis and focused therapy.[38]

A useful paradigm for the assessment and treatment of acute exacerbations of chronic bronchitis and antibiotic decision making is shown in Fig. 129-1.[39] Many clinicians use the so-called Anthonisen criteria to determine if antibiotic therapy is indicated.[24] With the Anthonisen criteria, if a patient exhibits two of the following three criteria during an acute exacerbation of chronic bronchitis (AECB), the patient will most likely benefit from antibiotic therapy and, thus, should receive a treatment course: (a) increase in shortness of breath; (b) increase in sputum volume; and (c) production of purulent sputum. There are greater healthcare costs for patients who are noncompliant with their antibiotic regimen for their AECB.

The increasing resistance of the common bacterial pathogens to first-line agents further complicates antibiotic selection. As many as 30% to 40% of *H. influenzae* isolates and 95% to 100% of *M. catarrhalis* isolates produce β-lactamases. Moreover, up to 40% of *S. pneumoniae* isolates demonstrate intermediate susceptibility (minimum inhibitory concentration [MIC] 0.125-1 mg/L) or resistance (MIC $\geq$ 2 mg/L) to oral penicillin, with approximately 20% of isolates being highly resistant (MIC > 2 mg/L). Concern regarding *S. pneumoniae* resistance is increasing, and resistance is now greater than or equal to 30% for macrolides. Despite these changes in bacterial susceptibility, the recommendation is to initiate therapy with first-line antimicrobial agents in less severely affected patients (see Fig. 129-1). For patients with more moderate to severe disease, many clinicians will begin antibiotic therapy with the second-line agents, such as amoxicillin-clavulanate, a macrolide (such as azithromycin or clarithromycin, although they are being used less frequently), or a fluoroquinolone, such as levofloxacin and moxifloxacin (see Fig. 129-1).

Regardless of the antibiotic selected, predetermined outcome measures should be monitored closely for each patient to determine the success or failure of the therapeutic intervention. Oral antibiotics with broader antibacterial spectra (eg, amoxicillin-clavulanate and fluoroquinolones) that possess potent in vitro activity against sputum isolates are increasingly becoming first-line antibiotics as initial therapy for treatment of acute exacerbations of chronic bronchitis.

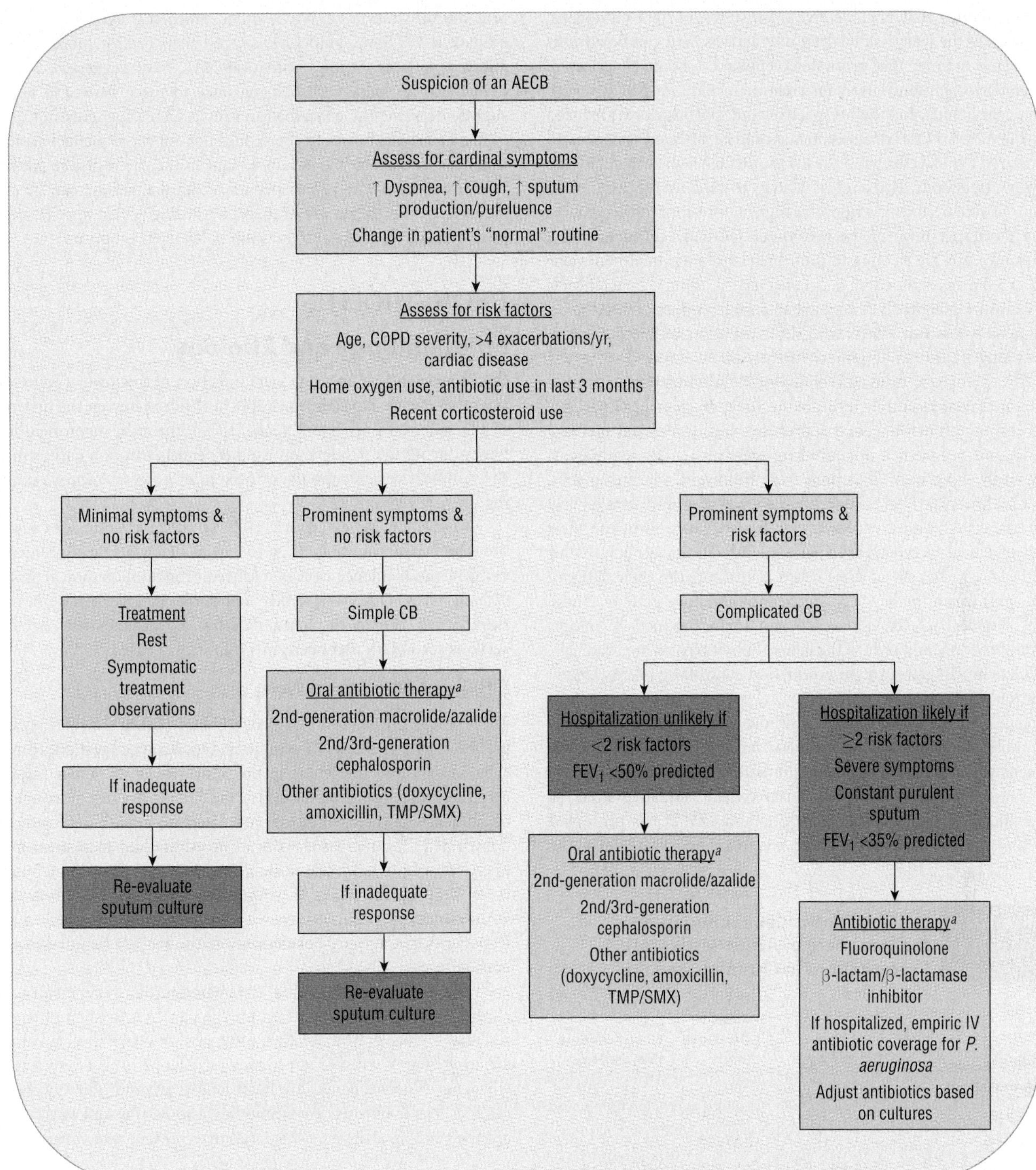

FIGURE 129-1 Clinical algorithm for the diagnosis and treatment of chronic bronchitis patients with an acute exacerbation incorporating the principles of the clinical classification system. (AECB, acute exacerbation of chronic bronchitis; CB, chronic bronchitis; COPD, chronic obstructive pulmonary disease; TMP/SMX, trimethoprim/sulfamethoxazole.)[a]See Table 129-3 for commonly used antibiotics and doses. *(Reprinted, with permission, from Hayes DJ, Meyer K. Acute exacerbations of chronic bronchitis in elderly patients: Pathogenesis, diagnosis, and management. Drugs Aging 2007;24:555–572.)*

An important clinical outcome variable directing drug selection and criteria for beginning antibiotics in individual patients is the infection-free period when they are off antibiotics. The length of the infection-free time period and the change in the number of physician office visits and hospital admissions with a particular antibiotic regimen are extremely important to identify, whenever possible, for each patient. The antibiotic regimen that results in the longest infection-free period defines the "regimen of choice" for specific patients for future acute exacerbations of their disease. Long-term prophylactic antibiotic use may provide a slight benefit in decreasing exacerbation rates, but does not appear to decrease mortality, and markedly increase the emergence and colonization of antibiotic-resistant pathogens. For this reason, most guidelines do not support this indication. However, chronic macrolide/azalide use reduces the incidence of acute exacerbations in COPD patients in a clinically significant manner (macrolide and anti-inflammatory activity addressed later).[39,40]

Antibiotics that are effective against responsible pathogens, demonstrate the least risk of drug interactions, and can be administered in a manner that promotes compliance should be selected. Antibiotics, commonly used for treatment of these patients with chronic bronchitis, and their respective adult starting doses are listed in Table 129-3. Doses of antibiotics should be adjusted as needed to the desired clinical effect and the lowest incidence of acceptable side effects. A frequently used clinical strategy to enhance the duration of symptom-free periods incorporates higher-dose antibiotic regimens using the upper limit of the recommended daily antibiotic dose. More clinicians are electing to limit their antibiotic treatment regimen to 5 days as compelling data continue to support equal efficacy, less exposure potentially reducing bacterial resistance development, and possibly less side effects with short-duration antibiotic therapy versus longer treatment regimens (greater than 7 days).

Except for long-term macrolide/azalide administration, chronic antibiotic therapy is rarely indicated in the management of patients with chronic bronchitis. Such approaches lead to marked increase in cost and occurrence of multidrug-resistant (MDR) pathogens. Conversely, long-term macrolide (erythromycin, clarithromycin, and roxithromycin) or azalide (azithromycin) administration has been associated with a clinically significant reduction in the incidence of acute exacerbations in patients with chronic bronchitis and COPD.[39-41] The benefit of these drugs is attributed to their antibacterial, anti-inflammatory, and immunomodulatory activity. These drugs reduce bacterial adherence and toxin production, inhibit biofilm function, and reduce the generation of oxygen-free radicals, modulate mucin gene protein production controlling mucus hypersecretion, and improve mucociliary clearance. These drugs also decrease neutrophil chemotaxis, promote downregulation of adhesion molecule expression, and inhibit transcription factors leading to decreased production of pro-inflammatory cytokines.[41]

The importance of multifactorial cellular oxidative stress in the pathogenesis of chronic bronchitis and COPD has prompted the study of the efficacy of antioxidants and particularly the oral administration of NAC, other mucolytic agents, and antioxidants.[27,42,43] Some guidelines suggest their use for more severely affected patients. Studies with oral NAC have suggested a dose-dependent response with 600 mg once to twice daily and it may slightly decrease the exacerbation rate in COPD patients not using inhaled steroids; however, there does not appear any effect on lung function. The exact role of antioxidant in the care of these patients remains to be defined—no specific recommendations can be provided until more data are available regarding which specific compound (as well as dose and duration of therapy) is optimal.

TABLE 129-3 Oral Antibiotics Commonly Used for the Treatment of Acute Respiratory Exacerbations in Chronic Bronchitis

Antibiotic	Brand Name	Usual Adult Oral Dose (mg)	Dose Schedule (Doses/Day)
Preferred Drugs			
Ampicillin	–	250-500	3-4
Amoxicillin	–	500-875	2-3
Amoxicillin-clavulanate	Augmentin®	500-875	2-3
Ciprofloxacin	Cipro®	500-750	2
Levofloxacin	Levaquin®	500-750	1
Moxifloxacin	Avelox®	400	1
Doxycycline	Monodox®	100	2
Minocycline	Minocin®	100	2
Tetracycline HCl	–	500	4
Trimethoprim-sulfamethoxazole	Bactrim DS®/ Septra DS®	1 DS	2
Supplemental Drugs			
Azithromycin	Zithromax®	250-500	1
Erythromycin	Ery-Tab®/ Erythrocin®	500	4
Clarithromycin	Biaxin®	250-500	2
Cephalexin	Keflex®	500	4

DS, double-strength tablet (160-mg trimethoprim/800-mg sulfamethoxazole).

BRONCHIOLITIS

Epidemiology and Etiology

7 Bronchiolitis is an acute viral infection of the lower respiratory tract that affects approximately 50% of children during the first year of life and 100% by age 2 years. The occurrence of bronchiolitis peaks during the winter months and persists through early spring. Bronchiolitis remains the major reason for hospital admission during the first year of life.[44]

Respiratory syncytial virus (RSV) is the most common cause of bronchiolitis, accounting for up to 75% of all cases. During epidemic periods, the incidence of RSV-induced bronchiolitis may approach 90% of cases. Other frequently detectable viruses include human rhinovirus, coronavirus, parainfluenza, and adenovirus. Bacteria serve as secondary pathogens in a minority of cases.[44]

Clinical Presentation

The clinical presentation of bronchiolitis (Table 129-4) is often preceded by 1 to 4 days of symptoms (eg, nasal congestion, rhinorrhea, cough, and low-grade fever) indicative of an upper respiratory tract infection. Due to limited oral intake because of coughing combined with fever, vomiting, and diarrhea, infants frequently are dehydrated. The increased work of breathing and tachypnea most likely contribute to increased fluid loss. In most cases, bronchiolitis is self-limiting and typically symptoms improve within 7 to 10 days with resolution within 28 days without the need for hospitalization. In patients who require hospitalization, the average length of stay is approximately 3 days.[45]

The diagnosis of bronchiolitis is based primarily on history and clinical findings. It is important for the clinician to attempt to differentiate between bronchiolitis and a host of other clinical entities affecting infants, which may produce a similar picture of dyspnea and wheezing. Asthma, congestive heart failure, anatomic airway abnormalities, cystic fibrosis, foreign bodies, and gastroesophageal reflux are the primary disease entities that may present with wheezing in

TABLE 129-4 Clinical Presentation of Bronchiolitis

Signs and symptoms

- Prodrome with irritability, restlessness, and mild fever
- Cough and coryza
- Vomiting, diarrhea, noisy breathing, and increased respiratory rate as symptoms progress
- Labored breathing with retractions of the chest wall, nasal flaring, and grunting

Physical examination

- Tachycardia and respiratory rate of 40-80 per minute in hospitalized infants
- Wheezing and inspiratory rales
- Mild conjunctivitis in one-third of patients
- Otitis media in 5%-10% of patients

Laboratory tests

- Peripheral white blood cell count normal or slightly elevated
- Abnormal arterial blood gases (hypoxemia and, rarely, hypercarbia)

children. Isolation of a viral pathogen in the respiratory secretions of a wheezing child establishes a presumptive diagnosis of infectious bronchiolitis. However, identification of specific viral pathogens often is hindered by the limited availability of special virology laboratories. In addition, in the elderly and in immunocompromised patients, antigen detection lacks adequate sensitivity, and patients frequently seek medical care after the acute stage of the infection, thus compromising the ability of the available tests to diagnose RSV. However, the proliferation of commercial enzyme-linked immunosorbent assays and fluorescent antibody staining techniques of nasopharyngeal secretions has increased the ability to identify viral antigens within several hours. Identification of RSV by PCR should be available from most clinical laboratories, but its relevance to the clinical management of bronchiolitis remains obscure and therefore routine testing is not recommended.[45,46]

Multiple clinical laboratory determinations have been used to assist in the management of cases of bronchiolitis. Radiographic evaluation of the chest in children with bronchiolitis yields variable findings and rarely alters therapeutic decisions. Thus, the routine use of chest radiography is not recommended; however, in hospitalized patients who fail to demonstrate expected improvement, they may help to distinguish bronchiolitis from other entities characterized by wheezing so that appropriate treatment may be initiated. In children requiring hospitalization, abnormalities in blood gas tensions are frequent and appear to relate to disease severity. Hypoxemia is common and increases the respiratory drive, whereas hypercarbia is seen in only the most severe cases. Despite the presence of moderate degrees of hypoxemia, clinical cyanosis is unusual.[44]

TREATMENT

Desired Outcome

In the well infant, bronchiolitis usually is a self-limiting illness, and reassurance, antipyretics, and adequate fluid intake usually are all that are necessary while waiting for resolution of the underlying viral infection. In-hospital support is necessary for the child suffering from respiratory failure or marked dehydration; underlying cardiac and pulmonary diseases potentiate these conditions.[45]

General Approach to Treatment

7 Almost all otherwise healthy babies with bronchiolitis can be followed as outpatients. Such infants are treated for fever, provided generous amounts of oral fluids, and observed closely for evidence of respiratory deterioration.[44] In severely affected children, the mainstays of therapy for bronchiolitis are oxygen therapy and IV fluids. In a subset of patients, aerosolized bronchodilators may have a role. For selected infants, particularly those with underlying pulmonary disease, cardiac disease, or both, therapy with the antiviral agent ribavirin can be considered.[47]

Pharmacologic Therapy

7 Aerosolized β_2-adrenergic therapy appears to offer little benefit for most patients and may even be detrimental.[46-48] Given their overall ineffectiveness, neither aerosolized β_2-adrenergic nor nebulized epinephrine therapies are recommended by the American Academy of Pediatrics (AAP) for the treatment of bronchiolitis.[48,49] Multiple studies have supported the AAP recommendations due to insufficient evidence for the effectiveness of bronchodilators in bronchiolitis, although there may be subgroups of patients who might benefit.[48-50]

Similarly, controlled trials of corticosteroids in bronchiolitic infants have not shown therapeutic effects or significant harmful effects, though viral shedding may be prolonged.[45,48] As a result, the routine use of systemically administered corticosteroids is not recommended by the AAP and is therefore discouraged.[46,48] Combination therapy with oral dexamethasone and nebulized epinephrine may act synergistically to reduce hospital admissions and shorten the time to discharge and the duration of symptoms, but the overall clinical benefits is questionable based on study results.[49] Although placing children with bronchiolitis in mist tents has been common practice, no data have documented the effectiveness of this practice.

The AAP guidelines support the use of nebulized hypertonic saline (eg, 3% saline) for the treatment of bronchiolitis in hospitalized infants and children while other international guidelines do not recommend its use.[46,48] As such, although nebulized hypertonic saline has proven to be safe and effective for the symptomatic improvement in patients with bronchiolitis after 1 day of use, there continues to be debate on if it reduces the length of hospital stay.[51]

Ribavirin may offer benefit to a subset of infants with bronchiolitis. Ribavirin, a synthetic nucleoside, possesses in vitro antiviral properties against a variety of RNA and DNA viruses, including influenza A, influenza B, parainfluenza, and adenovirus; it is approved only in aerosolized form against RSV. Use of the aerosol drug formulation requires special equipment (small-particle aerosol generator) and specially trained personnel for administration via oxygen hood or mist tent. Special care must be taken to avoid drug particle deposition and the resulting clogging of respiratory tubing and valves in mechanical ventilators. Among hospital admissions for RSV infection, ribavirin therapy failed to decrease length of hospital stay, number of days in the intensive care unit, or number of days receiving mechanical ventilation. Consequently, the AAP does not recommend the routine use of ribavirin in children with bronchiolitis and most experts recommend reserving use of ribavirin for severely ill patients.[48]

For infants with underlying pulmonary or cardiovascular disease, prophylaxis against RSV may be warranted. When administered monthly during the RSV season, both RSV immune globulin and palivizumab (a monoclonal antibody for RSV) may decrease the number of RSV episodes and the need for hospitalization. Between the two, palivizumab is preferred, given its ease of administration, lack of administration-related adverse effects, and noninterference with select immunizations. Despite continuing research, there is no vaccine marketed for RSV.

PNEUMONIA

Epidemiology

Pneumonia remains one of the most common causes of severe sepsis and the leading infectious cause of death in children and adults in the United States, with a mortality rate as high as 50% depending on the severity of illness.[5,52] Pneumonia occurs throughout the year, with the relative incidence of disease resulting from different etiologic entities varying with the seasons. It occurs in persons of all ages, although the clinical manifestations are most severe in the very young, the elderly, and the chronically ill.

Pathogenesis and Etiology

Inspiration of ambient air constantly exposes the lungs to environmental and infectious particulate matter. Respiratory pathogens enter the lower respiratory tract by one of three routes: (1) direct inhalation of infectious droplets; (2) aspiration of oropharyngeal contents; or (3) hematogenous spread from another infection site. Respiratory host defenses comprise innate and adaptive immunity pathways. These defense mechanisms are preserved in healthy individuals and respiratory pathogens are effectively removed before infection occurs. Conversely, immunocompromised individuals (such as those with cystic fibrosis or prolonged neutropenia) lack robust defense mechanisms and are at higher risk of severe

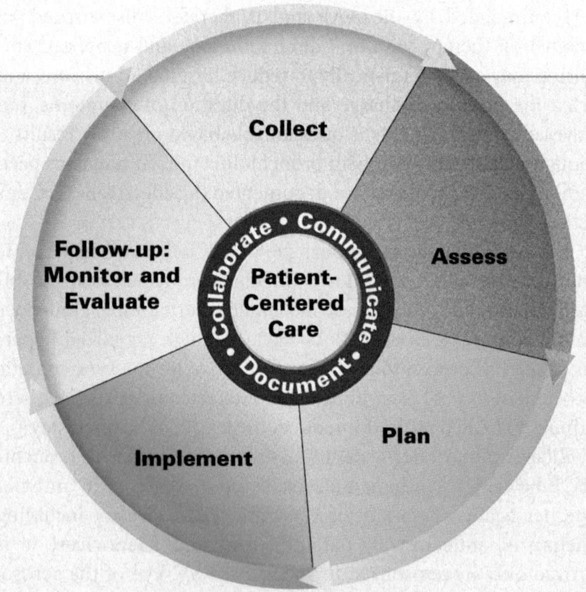

Patient Care Process for Pneumonia

The image shows the five fundamental steps included in The Pharmacist's Care Process endorsed by the Joint Commission for Pharmacy Practitioners (2014). The tagline of this process reads collaborate, communicate, and document. The five fundamental steps listed here are collect, assess, plan, implement, and follow-up: monitor and evaluate. All these steps are listed in a circular block diagram.

Collect

- Patient characteristics (eg, age, sex, pregnancy, drug allergies)
- Patient medical history including comorbid conditions, previous infections, previous hospitalization, and current or recent residence in a nursing facility
- Social history (including tobacco/ethanol/drug use)
- Current and past medications, particularly antimicrobials, immune suppressants, and chemotherapy
- Subjective data
  - Patient-reported risk factors for pneumonia (Table 129-5)
  - Patient-reported pneumonia signs/symptoms (Table 129-6)
  - Timing/location of symptom onset (ie, community vs hospital; time since onset)
- Objective data
  - Temperature, blood pressure (BP), heart rate (HR), respiratory rate (RR), height, weight, O_2-saturation, ventilator settings if applicable
  - Pertinent respiratory physical exam findings (Table 129-6)
  - Diagnostic procedures (such as chest imaging)
  - Labs including CBC and differential, basic metabolic panel, blood gases, and lactate (if sepsis suspected)
  - Current and previous microbiology results including antimicrobial susceptibility when available

Assess

- Likelihood of pneumonia based on history of present illness, physical exam, imaging, and laboratory and microbiologic data
- Severity of illness and mortality risk based on hemodynamics, respiratory status, presence of organ failure, severity score(s) if CAP
- Most likely pathogens and potential for antimicrobial resistance based on age, comorbidities, clinical presentation and diagnostics, pneumonia type (ie, CAP vs HAP vs VAP vs aspiration—Table 129-5), local epidemiology and antimicrobial resistance patterns, previous infections and antibiotic exposure

Plan

- Empiric antimicrobial regimen based on likely pathogen(s) and mortality risk
  - Include drug(s), route of administration, dose, frequency, and duration (Tables 129-8 to 129-10)
- Appropriate monitoring parameters for efficacy, toxicity, and potential modification of therapy (ie, cultures or other tests for etiology when indicated)
  - Include timing (cultures preferably obtained before antimicrobials administered) and frequency
- Provider education including rationale and evidence for recommendation
- Patient education including counseling points/monitoring for efficacy and safety

Implement*

- Clearly and professionally communicate recommendations to prescribers, healthcare team, and/or patient
- Determine consensus treatment plan as an interdisciplinary team
- Follow-up to ensure accurate/appropriate implementation of consensus treatment plan (antimicrobial therapy, diagnostics, and monitoring)

Follow-up: Monitor and Evaluate

- Efficacy monitoring including improvement/resolution of signs/symptoms, physiologic and laboratory data with focus on indicators of infection (temperature, WBC, etc.), respiratory status (RR, oxygenation, ventilator settings), and organ failure/sepsis
- Safety monitoring (including SCr and urine output for nephrotoxicity, etc.)
- Microbiologic cultures and diagnostic tests for etiology
- Assess whether therapy can be narrowed, should be broadened, or requires change based on above monitoring considerations
- When possible, change empiric therapy to pathogen-directed therapy (Table 129-11)
- Design and implement new plan and continual monitoring as needed/appropriate

**Collaborate with patient, caregivers, and other healthcare professionals.*

TABLE 129-5 Pneumonia Classifications and Risk Factors

Type of Pneumonia	Definition	Risk Factors
Community-acquired pneumonia	Pneumonia developing outside the hospital or <48 hours after hospital admission	• Age >65 years • Diabetes mellitus • Asplenia • Chronic cardiovascular, pulmonary, renal, and/or liver disease • Smoking and/or alcohol abuse
Hospital-acquired pneumonia	Pneumonia developing >48 hours after hospital admission	• Witnessed aspiration • COPD, ARDS, or coma • Administration of antacids, H_2-antagonists, or proton pump inhibitor • Supine position • Enteral nutrition, nasogastric tube • Reintubation, tracheostomy, or patient transport • Head trauma, ICP monitoring • Age >60 years • MDR risk (eg, MRSA, MDR *Pseudomonas*) if IV antibiotic use within 90 days
Ventilator-associated pneumonia	Pneumonia developing >48 hours after endotracheal intubation	• Same as hospital acquired • MDR risk with IV antibiotics in past 90 days, septic shock, ARDS preceding VAP, acute renal replacement therapy preceding VAP, or 5+ days of hospitalization preceding VAP

ARDS, acute respiratory distress syndrome; CAP, community-acquired pneumonia; COPD, chronic obstructive pulmonary disease; HAP, hospital-acquired pneumonia; ICP, intracranial pressure; MDR, multidrug-resistant; MRSA, methicillin-resistant *S. aureus*; VAP, ventilator-associated pneumonia.

respiratory infections. Lung infections can also suppress the antibacterial activity of the lung by impairing alveolar macrophage function and mucociliary clearance, thus setting the stage for secondary bacterial pneumonia. Mucociliary transport is also depressed by ethanol and narcotics and by obstruction of bronchi by mucus, tumor, or extrinsic compression. All these factors can severely impair pulmonary clearance of aspirated bacteria. Any alteration of the normal lung microbiome by infection and/or disease can evolve to pneumonia requiring antimicrobial treatment.[53]

Pneumonia is caused by a variety of viral and bacterial pathogens. The causative organism(s) is highly dependent on how and/or where the pneumonia was contacted.[4-6,54] For epidemiologic and treatment purposes, pneumonia is often categorized as either community-acquired or hospital-acquired (Table 129-5).[6] Patients with pneumonia onset outside of the hospital or within 48 hours of hospital admission are considered to have community-acquired pneumonia (CAP). Those with pneumonia onset in the hospital after at least 48 hours of hospitalization are considered to have hospital-acquired pneumonia (HAP). Patients with pneumonia onset following 48 hours of endotracheal intubation are considered to have ventilator-associated pneumonia (VAP).

Community-Acquired Pneumonia

8 The causative pathogen in CAP in adult patients is most commonly viral, with human rhinovirus and influenza most common.[55] The most prominent bacterial pathogen causing CAP in otherwise healthy adults is *S. pneumoniae* accounting for up to 35% of all acute cases. It is particularly prevalent and severe for patients with splenic dysfunction, diabetes mellitus, chronic cardiopulmonary or renal disease, or HIV infection. Other common pathogens include *H. influenzae* (2.5%-45%) and the atypical pathogens *M. pneumoniae*, *Legionella* species, and *C. pneumoniae* (about 20%).[55-57] Although generally less common, *S. aureus* is also an important CAP pathogen in children and adults and is often seen in patients with cystic fibrosis and those recovering from an antecedent viral respiratory infection such as influenza. CAP caused by enteric gram-negative bacteria, including *E. coli* and *K. pneumoniae*, is also uncommon but these pathogens are sometimes identified; most frequently among patients with chronic illness, especially alcoholism and diabetes mellitus.[4] Healthcare-associated pneumonia was a classification that had been previously used to distinguish nonhospitalized patients at risk for MDR pathogens from those likely infected with traditional CAP pathogens; however, it is no longer recommended to risk stratify patients using this designation.[4,6]

Even more so than in adult patients, viral pathogens predominate in CAP among pediatric patients with a prevalence of up to 80% in those less than 2 years of age. Respiratory syncytial virus and human rhinovirus comprise the majority of these infections.[58] Other common viruses in children include parainfluenza, adenovirus, human metapneumovirus, and bocavirus.[5,58] Group B *Streptococcus*, although rare in adults, is the most common cause of bacterial pneumonia among neonates and typically causes a clinical and radiographic picture nearly indistinguishable from hyaline membrane disease.[59] The bacterial causes of CAP outside the neonatal period are generally similar to adults, with *S. pneumoniae* being the major bacterial pathogen in childhood pneumonia.[58] *M. pneumoniae* is also common, particularly among older children. *H. influenzae* type b, once a major childhood pathogen, has become an infrequent cause of pneumonia since the introduction of active vaccination against this organism in the late 1980s.

Hospital-Acquired Pneumonia

8 HAP occurs most commonly in critically ill patients and is usually caused by bacteria.[6] Factors predisposing patients to the development of HAP include high severity of illness, longer duration of hospitalization, supine positioning, witnessed aspiration, coma, acute respiratory distress syndrome, patient transport, and prior antibiotic exposure (Table 129-5). The strongest predisposing factor, however, is mechanical ventilation (intubation). The length of stay for hospital admissions is increased by a mean of 7 to 9 days for patients who develop HAP.[6]

HAP is predominantly caused by gram-negative aerobic bacilli or *S. aureus* and is much more likely to be caused by an MDR isolate.[6] Collectively, the non-lactose fermenting gram-negative bacilli *P. aeruginosa* and *Acinetobacter* spp. are the most common cause of HAP (about 25%-45%).[6] Enteric gram-negative bacilli such as *K. pneumoniae* and *E. coli* are also common (13%-20%).[6] *S. aureus* is also common (12%-21%) with approximately half of these isolates methicillin-resistant.[6] Patients with longer lengths of hospital admission or IV antibiotic use within the previous 90 days preceding HAP development are more likely to have MDR organisms.[6]

HAP can be subclassified as ventilator-associated pneumonia (VAP), which is pneumonia occurring after 48 or more hours of endotracheal intubation.[6] The risk for developing pneumonia in the hospital increases by 6 to 21 times after a patient is intubated because the natural airway defenses against the migration of upper respiratory tract organisms into the lower tract are bypassed.[6] This situation is exacerbated by the wide use of acid-suppressing drugs (eg, H_2-receptor blocking agents and proton pump inhibitors) in the intensive care unit, which increases the pH of gastric secretions and may promote the proliferation of microorganisms in the upper GI tract. Subclinical microaspirations are events that occur routinely in intubated patients and result in the inoculation of bacteria-contaminated gastric contents into the lung and a higher incidence of nosocomial pneumonia.[60] Although generally similar in etiology to HAP, VAP is more likely to be caused by *S. aureus* (20%-30%) and multidrug resistance is more common.[6,61,62]

Aspiration pneumonia is classically treated as a separate entity from CAP or HAP. It was predominantly caused by anaerobic bacteria that commonly colonize the oropharynx. The epidemiologic evidence suggests a decreasing importance of anaerobic bacteria in aspiration pneumonia. Aspiration pneumonia has a bacteriology similar to CAP or HAP, and anaerobic pathogens are less common and typically seen in patients with specific risk factors such as severe periodontal disease or those with specific clinical findings such as necrotizing pneumonia or lung abscess.[54]

Tuberculosis

The acid-fast bacillus *Mycobacterium tuberculosis* causes tuberculosis and is spread person to person by inhalation of droplets. After years of steady decline, the number of cases of pneumonia caused by *M. tuberculosis* in the United States began to increase in the mid- to late 1980s. The new epidemic was a consequence of an increased incidence among prison inmates, IV drug abusers, immigrants, and, most prominently, HIV-infected patients. It is most prominent in urban neighborhoods afflicted with crowded living conditions and poor access to healthcare; thus, groups prone to tuberculosis include the homeless and patients in chronic care facilities and homes for the elderly. Unlike previous eras in which tuberculosis was seen most frequently in elderly men, infection currently is identified in increasing numbers of young adults. MDR strains of *M. tuberculosis* have become more common, and treatment regimens for these patients should involve consultation with a specialist. (See Chapter 135, "Tuberculosis" for a detailed discussion of tuberculosis pathophysiology, diagnosis, and treatment.)

Clinical Presentation and Diagnosis

The common signs, symptoms, physical exam findings, and diagnostic features of patients with pneumonia are listed in Table 129-6. They are both constitutional (fever, chills, malaise) and respiratory (cough, increased sputum production, dyspnea). These signs and symptoms coupled with physical exam findings suggestive of a pulmonary infiltrate, with or without abnormal whiteblood cell (WBC) count or oxygen saturation, can form the basis of a presumed clinical diagnosis of pneumonia. The diagnosis of pneumonia is preferably further strengthened by radiographic evidence such as pulmonary infiltrate(s) on chest x-ray or another chest imaging. Clinical practice guidelines recommend a chest radiograph for all adult patients with suspected pneumonia but only in select pediatric patients with severe CAP (eg, inpatient, signs of hypoxia/respiratory distress).[4-6]

TABLE 129-6 Clinical Presentation of Pneumonia

Signs and symptoms

- Abrupt onset of fever, chills, dyspnea, and productive cough
- Rust-colored sputum or hemoptysis
- Pleuritic chest pain
- Dyspnea

Physical examination

- Tachypnea and tachycardia
- Dullness to percussion
- Increased tactile fremitus, whisper pectoriloquy, and egophony
- Chest wall retractions and grunting respirations
- Diminished breath sounds over affected area
- Inspiratory crackles during lung expansion

Chest radiograph

- Dense lobar or segmental infiltrate

Laboratory tests

- Leukocytosis with predominance of polymorphonuclear cells
- Low oxygen saturation on arterial blood gas or pulse oximetry

Clinical and radiographic data can begin to shape the differential diagnosis of suspected pneumonia pathogens. Pneumonia caused by the atypical pathogens, such as *M. pneumoniae* and *C. pneumoniae,* often has a more gradual onset and overall lower severity compared with other bacterial causes.[64,65] The exception to this is *Legionella pneumophila*, which is an atypical pathogen that often causes severe illness making it a common pathogen in patients with CAP who require ICU admission.[64,118] Patients with atypical pneumonia also commonly have extrapulmonary, constitutional symptoms.[64,65] Atypical pneumonias often demonstrate patchy infiltrates on chest x-ray that are more extensive than clinical symptoms suggest, hence the term "walking pneumonia."[66] Chest radiographs in patients with viral etiology are often diffuse, interstitial compared with the classic lobar or lobular consolidated infiltrates of bacterial pneumonia. Staphylococcal pneumonias often demonstrate cavitary or necrotizing lesions on imaging. Although these general clinical and diagnostic characteristics can be useful, there is considerable overlap in clinical presentation between pneumonia etiologies. These data alone are not sufficiently reliable to differentiate between bacterial, atypical bacterial, and viral etiology.[67] Similarly, the use of biomarkers, such as procalcitonin, is not recommended to differentiate between bacterial and viral pneumonia.[4,6]

10 Following a pneumonia diagnosis based on clinical and radiographic evidence, further diagnostic testing to confirm the diagnosis and determine the etiology may be warranted. Blood cultures and noninvasive sputum cultures (ie, expectorated sputum, sputum induction, or nasotracheal suctioning) are recommended for all adult patients with suspected HAP or VAP.[6] Blood cultures often provide value in determining the causative pathogen, particularly in VAP where approximately 15% of patients have concomitant bacteremia.[68,69] Emphasis is placed on determining an etiology in HAP and VAP due to the high prevalence of MDR organisms and associated risk of ineffective empiric therapy. This allows adjustment of initial empiric therapy into optimal, pathogen-specific therapy.

Confirmation of etiology is less common in CAP, where a microbiologically confirmed etiology is identified in only 7% of cases in clinical practice.[70] As such, empiric treatment of CAP is often continued for the entire duration of therapy without ever determining the causative pathogen. Cultures are only routinely recommended in patients with more severe CAP where knowledge of the causative pathogen and whether the empiric antibiotic regimen is active are most important. In patients treated in the outpatient setting, sputum cultures are not routinely recommended. The exceptions to this are pediatric patients who have experienced failure of initial antibiotics and adult patients treated with empiric antibiotics that cover MRSA and/or *P. aeruginosa*.[4,5] Blood and sputum cultures are recommended in hospitalized adult patients with severe CAP. This includes, but is not limited to, patients with septic shock requiring vasopressors and/or those with respiratory failure requiring mechanical ventilation (Table 129-7). Blood and sputum cultures

TABLE 129-7 Severe CAP Criteria

Major Criteria – 1 or more defines severe CAP

Septic shock with need for vasopressors
Respiratory failure requiring mechanical ventilation

Minor Criteria – 3 or more defines severe CAP

Respiratory rate >30 breaths/min
PaO_2/FIO_2 ratio <250
Multilobar infiltrates
Confusion/disorientation
Uremia (blood urea nitrogen level >20 mg/dL [7.1 mmol/L])
Leukopenia (white blood cell count <4,000 cells/mm³ [4 × 10⁹/L])
Thrombocytopenia (platelet count <100,000/mm³ [100 × 10⁹/L])
Hypothermia (core temperature <36°C)
Hypotension requiring aggressive fluid resuscitation

are also recommended in hospitalized adult patients receiving empiric therapy covering MRSA and/or *P. aeruginosa* or among considered at risk for these pathogens.[4] Sputum Gram stain and culture are recommended for hospitalized children who can produce a sputum sample along with blood cultures in those with moderate/severe CAP.[5] Urinary antigen tests are also available for *S. pneumoniae* and *L. pneumophila*, and are recommended in adults with severe CAP.[4] These tests are more rapid than traditional microbiologic methods and can detect pathogen antigen days (*S. pneumoniae*) to weeks (*L. pneumophila*) after initiation of antibiotic therapy.[71] These tests have a high specificity (90%-99%) but lower sensitivity (50%-80%). This translates to few false-positives and more false-negatives, making it a useful test to "rule in" these pathogens in adult patients.[63,72,73] Rapid diagnostic tests for viruses, including influenza, are also recommended in children with suspected CAP. Influenza nucleic acid amplification testing is also recommended in adult patients when influenza is circulating in the community. A positive result in combination with an absence of clinical factors strongly suggestive of bacterial infection can be used to reduce unnecessary antibiotic use.[5] It would also be prudent to perform nucleic acid amplification testing for SARS-CoV-2 when it is circulating in the community.

Treatment Goals

Eradication of the offending organism through selection of the appropriate antibiotic(s) and subsequent complete clinical cure is the primary goal of therapy of pneumonia. Secondary goals include minimization of the unintended consequences of therapy, including toxicities and selection for secondary infections such a *Clostridioides difficile* or antibiotic-resistant pathogens, and minimizing costs through outpatient and oral therapy when the patient's severity of illness and clinical considerations permit.

General Approach to Treatment

9 Achievement of the goals of therapy for pneumonia treatment requires the provider to follow the principles of good antimicrobial stewardship while ensuring adequate treatment of the potential infection. Comprehensive principles of optimal antimicrobial therapy and infectious diseases stewardship are discussed in detail in Chapter 127, "Antimicrobial Regimen Selection." In general, antimicrobial stewardship involves provision of the right antimicrobial(s) (or lack thereof when infection is not present); at the right time, at the right dose, for the right duration. This is often a balance between providing therapy broad enough to cover likely pathogens but not overly broad resulting in potentially unnecessary drug toxicity, secondary infection, or antibiotic resistance. This also involves continual monitoring of patient clinical status and diagnostic data to support the decision to either continue empiric therapy, narrow or alter therapy, or discontinue therapy if infection is ruled out. This section discusses the selection of antimicrobial regimens in patients with a suspected or confirmed diagnosis of pneumonia.

Following diagnosis of the pneumonia, one of the first treatment decisions is what level of medical care is necessary (ie, outpatient vs inpatient vs inpatient ICU). This decision is ultimately made by a physician and should be based on the patient's severity of illness and subsequent risk of mortality. However, it is important for pharmacists to be able to perform and understand this severity assessment because it should be used to recommend the appropriate diagnostic monitoring and empiric antimicrobial therapy. Multiple severity scores designed to estimate mortality risk in CAP are available for severity assessment.[74,75] The preferred severity score for determining whether hospital admission is appropriate is the Pneumonia Severity Index (PSI), also known as Pneumonia Outcomes Research Team (PORT) score.[4,76] The PSI score utilizes age, comorbidities, physical exam findings, diagnostic test results, and laboratory test results to compute a patient's mortality risk. The PSI score identifies patients with low mortality risk allowing them to be safely treated in the outpatient setting.[4] The extensive laboratory and physiologic data required to calculate the PSI score is often not readily available upon patient presentation or in the outpatient setting.[76] The CURB-65 or CRB-65 scores may be used in these cases.[74,75] These short, simple point systems can easily be applied at the point of care using readily available clinical data. For CURB-65, patients receive 1 point for each criterion present: **C**onfusion, **U**remia (BUN >20 mg/dL [7.1 mmol/L]), **R**espiratory rate ≥30 breaths/min, **B**lood pressure (systolic <90 mm Hg, diastolic ≤60 mm Hg), age ≥65 years. CRB-65 is a simplified version of CURB-65 that does not require knowledge of serum BUN concentration. Patients with CURB-65 or CRB-65 scores <2 are generally candidates for outpatient treatment.[4] Patients with a score of 2 or more are typically admitted to the general ward or ICU.[4] The severe CAP criteria listed in Table 129-7 are recommended to determine whether ICU care is necessary. Patients with one major criteria should be admitted to ICU. Minor criteria should be used in conjunction with clinical judgment when neither of the major criteria is present. Although guidelines do not state a specific number of minor criteria necessitating ICU admission, data indicate patients with three or more minor criteria are often admitted to the ICU in practice.[4]

Empiric Antimicrobial Treatment Treatment of bacterial pneumonia, like the treatment of most infectious diseases, initially involves the empirical use of a relatively broad-spectrum antibiotic therapy that is effective against probable pathogens after appropriate cultures and specimens for laboratory evaluation have been obtained as indicated.[56,77] Therapy should be narrowed to cover specific pathogens after the results of cultures are known in cases where cultures are obtained. Multiple factors can aid in identifying the potential pathogens involved, including when and where the pneumonia was contracted, local pathogen epidemiology and susceptibility patterns, and individual patient factors. These individual patient factors include patient age, previous and current medication history, underlying disease(s), major organ function, and present clinical status. These factors must be evaluated to select an appropriate and effective empirical antibiotic regimen as well as the most appropriate route for drug administration (oral vs parenteral). (For a more detailed discussion on the principles of antibiotic selection, see Chapter 127.)

Because many antibiotics are effective in the treatment of bacterial pneumonia, and superiority of one antibiotic over another is often unclear or difficult to define, there are a variety of recommended empiric antimicrobial regimens for suspected bacterial pneumonia. For a list of potential empiric antimicrobial regimens, based on available clinical practice guidelines, primary literature, and antimicrobial susceptibility and PK/PD, refer to Table 129-8 for adults and Table 129-9 for children. A complete list of antimicrobial agents for specific pathogens is beyond the scope of this chapter and is presented in Chapter 127. Table 129-10 lists dosages for selected antibiotics used for the treatment of bacterial pneumonia.

Community-Acquired Pneumonia

9 Tables 129-8 and 129-9 provide evidence-based guidelines for the treatment of CAP in adults[4] and children,[5] respectively. The bacterial causes are relatively constant, even across geographic areas and patient populations. Unfortunately, pathogen resistance to standard antimicrobials is increasing (penicillin-resistant *S. pneumoniae*, macrolide-resistant *S. pneumoniae*, etc.) and can vary geographically, necessitating careful attention by the clinician to local and regional bacterial susceptibility patterns.[78] Indiscriminate use of antimicrobials for treatment of pneumonia has contributed to the problem of antimicrobial resistance, underscoring the need for defining the optimal antibiotic regimen for each patient. Thus, initial therapy should be based on presumed antibacterial susceptibility.

9 Evidence-based empiric therapy for CAP in adults differs between outpatients, hospitalized patients, and hospitalized patients

TABLE 129-8 Evidence-Based Empirical Antimicrobial Therapy for Pneumonia in Adults[a]

Clinical Setting and/or Patient Characteristics	Usual Pathogens	Empirical Therapy
Outpatient/Community-Acquired		
No at-risk comorbidity (diabetes, heart/lung/liver/renal disease, alcoholism, malignancy, asplenia)	*S. pneumoniae*, *M. pneumoniae*, *H. influenzae*, *C. pneumoniae*, *M. catarrhalis*	Amoxicillin (preferred) OR Doxycycline (2nd preferred) OR Macrolide[b] (non-preferred)
At-risk comorbidity (diabetes, heart/lung/liver/renal disease, alcoholism, malignancy, asplenia) OR immunosuppressive condition/drugs	*S. pneumoniae* (including drug-resistant), *M. pneumoniae*, *H. influenzae*, *C. pneumoniae*, *M. catarrhalis*	Antipneumococcal fluoroquinolone[c] OR β-lactam[d] + EITHER macrolide[b] OR doxycycline
Inpatient/Community-Acquired		
Non-severe CAP	*S. pneumoniae*, *H. influenzae*, *M. pneumoniae*, *C. pneumoniae*, *Legionella* sp.	β-lactam[e] + EITHER macrolide[b] OR doxycycline OR Antipneumococcal fluoroquinolone[c]
	If prior respiratory MRSA (1 year) If prior respiratory *P. aeruginosa* (1 year)	ADD vancomycin OR linezolid AND obtain cultures, de-escalate in 48 hr if MRSA negative and clinically improving
	If prior hospitalization AND IV antibiotic (90 days) locally validated risk factor	ADD[f] cefepime, piperacillin-tazobactam, ceftazidime, imipenem, meropenem, OR aztreonam AND obtain cultures, de-escalate in 48 hr if *P. aeruginosa* negative and clinically improving Obtain cultures, escalate if needed based on results
Severe CAP	*S. pneumoniae*, *H. influenzae*, *M. pneumoniae*, *C. pneumoniae*, *Legionella* sp.	β-Lactam[e] + EITHER macrolide[b] OR antipneumococcal fluoroquinolone[c]
	If prior respiratory MRSA (1 year)	ADD vancomycin OR linezolid AND obtain cultures, de-escalate in 48 hr if MRSA negative and clinically improving
	If prior respiratory *P. aeruginosa* (1 year)	ADD[f] cefepime, piperacillin-tazobactam, ceftazidime, imipenem, meropenem, OR aztreonam AND obtain cultures, de-escalate in 48 hr if *P. aeruginosa* negative and clinically improving
	If prior hospitalization AND IV antibiotic (90 days)	ADD vancomycin OR Linezolid AND ADD[e] cefepime, ceftazidime, imipenem, meropenem, piperacillin-tazobactam, OR aztreonam AND obtain cultures, de-escalate if MRSA/*P. aeruginosa*-negative and clinically improving
Hospital-Acquired Pneumonia		
Low mortality risk[g] AND No MDR HAP[h] risk factors AND Local MRSA prevalence <20%	Non-fermenting gram-negative bacilli[i], enteric gram-negative bacilli, MSSA	Piperacillin-tazobactam, cefepime, levofloxacin, imipenem, OR meropenem
Low mortality[g] risk AND No MDR HAP[h] risk factors AND Local MRSA ≥20% OR unknown	Non-fermenting gram-negative bacilli[i], enteric gram-negative bacilli, MRSA	Piperacillin-tazobactam, cefepime, levofloxacin, ciprofloxacin, imipenem, meropenem, OR aztreonam + vancomycin OR linezolid
High mortality risk[g] OR MDR risk factor(s)[h]	Non-fermenting gram-negative bacilli[i], enteric gram-negative bacilli, MRSA	Double cover *P. aeruginosa* with two of the following, avoiding two from the same class: piperacillin-tazobactam, cefepime, levofloxacin, ciprofloxacin, imipenem, meropenem, aztreonam, gentamicin, tobramycin, amikacin + vancomycin OR linezolid
Ventilator-Associated Pneumonia		
No MDR VAP risk factors[i] AND Local MRSA and gram-negative bacilli-resistance both <10%[j]	Non-fermenting gram-negative bacilli, enteric gram-negative bacilli, MSSA	Piperacillin-tazobactam, cefepime, levofloxacin, imipenem OR meropenem
No MDR VAP risk factors[i] AND Local MRSA ≥10% or unknown AND gram-negative bacilli-resistance <10%[j]	Non-fermenting gram-negative bacilli, enteric gram-negative bacilli, MRSA	Piperacillin-tazobactam, cefepime, levofloxacin, ciprofloxacin, imipenem, meropenem, OR aztreonam + vancomycin OR linezolid
MDR VAP risk factor(s)[i] OR local MRSA and gram-negative bacilli-resistance >10%[j] or unknown	MDR non-fermenting gram-negative bacilli, MDR enteric gram-negative bacilli, MRSA	Double cover *P. aeruginosa* with two of the following, avoiding two from the same class: piperacillin-tazobactam, cefepime, levofloxacin, ciprofloxacin, imipenem, meropenem, aztreonam, gentamicin, tobramycin, amikacin, colistin, polymyxin B + vancomycin OR linezolid
Aspiration Pneumonia		
Community-acquired	*S. pneumoniae*, *M. pneumoniae*, *H. influenzae*, *C. pneumoniae*	Treat as above for CAP
Hospital-acquired	*S. aureus*, *P. aeruginosa* enteric gram-negative bacilli	Treat as above for HAP
	If anaerobes suspected	Treat as above for CAP/HAP using antibiotic with anaerobic coverage OR add clindamycin OR metronidazole

[a]See the section Selection of Antimicrobial Agents.
[b]Macrolide: erythromycin, clarithromycin, and azithromycin.
[c]Antipneumococcal fluoroquinolone: levofloxacin and moxifloxacin.
[d]Infectious Diseases Society of America recommended outpatient β-lactams: high-dose amoxicillin or amoxicillin/clavulanate preferred, cefpodoxime, cefuroxime, ceftriaxone (intramuscular) alternatives.
[e]Infectious Diseases Society of America recommended inpatient β-lactams: ceftriaxone (intravenous), cefotaxime, ampicillin, ampicillin-sulbactam, ceftaroline.
[f]If β-lactam-based CAP regimen selected, substitute antipseudomonal β-lactam for standard CAP β-lactam, unless ceftazidime or aztreonam chosen.
[g]Indicators of high HAP mortality risk: need for ventilator support due to pneumonia; septic shock.
[h]MDR HAP risk factors: receipt of IV antibiotics in previous 90 days; structural lung disease (bronchiectasis or cystic fibrosis).
[i]MDR VAP risk factors: receipt of IV antibiotics in previous 90 days; septic shock; acute respiratory distress syndrome preceding VAP; ≥5 days hospitalization preceding VAP; acute renal replacement therapy preceding VAP.
[j]Resistance to antibiotic being considered for empiric gram-negative monotherapy. MDR, multidrug resistant; MRSA, methicillin-resistant *Staphylococcus aureus*; MSSA, methicillin-sensitive *Staphylococcus aureus*.

TABLE 129-9 Empirical Antimicrobial Therapy for Pneumonia in Pediatric Patients[a]

Clinical Setting and/or Patient Characteristics	Usual Pathogen(s)	Empirical Therapy
Outpatient/Community-Acquired		
<1 month	Group B *Streptococcus*, *H. influenzae* (nontypable), *E. coli*, *S. aureus*, *Listeria* CMV, RSV, adenovirus	Ampicillin-sulbactam, cephalosporin,[b] carbapenem[c] Ribavirin for RSV[d]
1-3 months	*C. pneumoniae*, possibly *Ureaplasma*, CMV, *Pneumocystis carinii* (afebrile pneumonia syndrome) *S. pneumoniae*, *S. aureus*	Macrolide/azalide,[e] trimethoprim–sulfamethoxazole Semisynthetic penicillin[f] OR cephalosporin[g]
Preschool-aged children	Viral (rhinovirus, RSV, influenza A and B, parainfluenzae, adenovirus, human metapneumovirus, coronavirus)	Antimicrobial therapy not routinely required
Previously healthy, fully immunized infants and preschool children with suspected mild-to-moderate bacterial CAP	*S. pneumonia* *M. pneumoniae*, other atypical	Amoxicillin, cephalosporin[b,g] Macrolide/azalide or fluoroquinolone
Previously healthy, fully immunized school-aged children and adolescents with mild-to-moderate CAP	*S. pneumonia* *M. pneumoniae*, other atypical	Amoxicillin, cephalosporin,[b,g] or fluoroquinolone Macrolide/azalide, fluoroquinolone, or tetracycline
Moderate-to-severe CAP during influenza virus outbreak	Influenza A and B, other viruses	Oseltamivir or zanamivir
Inpatient/Community-Acquired		
Fully immunized infants and school-aged children	*S. pneumonia* CA-MRSA *M. pneumoniae*, *C. pneumoniae*	Ampicillin, penicillin G, cephalosporin[b] β-Lactam + vancomycin/clindamycin β-Lactam + macrolide/fluoroquinolone/doxycycline
Not fully immunized infants and children; regions with invasive penicillin-resistant pneumococcal strains; patients with life-threatening infections	*S. pneumoniae*, PCN-resistant MRSA *M. pneumoniae*, other atypical pathogens	Cephalosporin[b] Add vancomycin/clindamycin Macrolide/azalide[e] + β-lactam/doxycycline/fluoroquinolone

[a]See the section Selection of Antimicrobial Agents.

[b]Third-generation cephalosporin: ceftriaxone and cefotaxime. Note that cephalosporins are not active against *Listeria*.

[c]Carbapenem: imipenem–cilastatin and meropenem.

[d]See text for details regarding possible ribavirin treatment for RSV infection.

[e]Macrolide/azalide: erythromycin and clarithromycin/azithromycin.

[f]Semisynthetic penicillin: nafcillin and oxacillin.

[g]Second-generation cephalosporin: cefuroxime and cefprozil.

CAP, community-acquired pneumonia; CMV, cytomegalovirus; MRSA, methicillin resistant *Staphylococcus aureus*; RSV, respiratory syncytial virus.

Data from Reference 5.

TABLE 129-10 Antibiotic Doses for Treatment of Bacterial Pneumonia

		Antibiotic Dose[a]	
Antibiotic Class	**Antibiotic**	**Pediatric**	**Usual Adult Dose**
Penicillin	Ampicillin ± sulbactam	150-200 mg/kg/day IV	2 g IV every 4-6 h (6 hr if ampicillin/sulbactam)
	Amoxicillin ± clavulanate[b]	45-100 mg/kg/day orally	875-2,000 mg orally twice daily
	Piperacillin-tazobactam	200-300 mg/kg/day IV	3.375-4.5 g IV every 6-8 hr
	Penicillin	100,000-250,000 units/kg/day IV	12-24 million units/day in divided doses IV every 4-6 hr
Extended-spectrum cephalosporins	Ceftriaxone	50-75 mg/kg/day IV	1-2 g IV daily
	Cefotaxime	150 mg/kg/day IV	1-2 g IV every 8 hr
	Ceftazidime	90-150 mg/kg/day IV	1-2 g IV every 8 hr
	Cefepime	100-150 mg/kg/day IV	1-2 g IV every 6-8 hr
	Ceftolozane-tazobactam	–	3 g IV every 8 hr
	Ceftazidime-avibactam	–	2.5 g IV every 8 hr
	Cefiderocol		2 g IV every 8 hr
Monobactam	Aztreonam	90-120 mg/kg/day IV	1-2 g IV every 8 hr
Macrolide/azalide	Clarithromycin	15 mg/kg/day orally	0.5-1 g orally once or twice daily
	Erythromycin	30-50 mg/kg/day IV or orally	500 mg IV or orally every 6 to 8 hr
	Azithromycin	10 mg/kg × 1 day (× 2 days if parenteral), and then 5 mg/kg days 2-5 IV or orally	500 mg × 1 day (× 2 days if parenteral), and then 250 mg days 2-5 IV or orally
Fluoroquinolones[c]	Moxifloxacin	–	400 mg IV or orally daily
	Levofloxacin	8-20 mg/kg/day IV or orally	750 mg IV or orally daily
	Ciprofloxacin	30 mg/kg/day IV or orally	400 mg IV every 8 hr/750 mg orally twice daily
Tetracycline[d]	Doxycycline	2-5 mg/kg/day IV or orally	100 mg IV or orally twice daily
	Tetracycline HCl	25-50 mg/kg/day orally	–

(continued)

TABLE 129-10 Antibiotic Doses for Treatment of Bacterial Pneumonia (*Continued*)

		Antibiotic Dose[a]	
Antibiotic Class	**Antibiotic**	**Pediatric**	**Usual Adult Dose**
Aminoglycosides	Gentamicin	7.5-10 mg/kg/day IV	7.5 mg/kg IV daily
	Tobramycin	7.5-10 mg/kg/day IV	7.5 mg/kg IV daily
	Amikacin	15-20 mg/kg/day IV	15-20 mg/kg IV daily
	Plazomicin		15 mg/kg IV daily
Carbapenems	Imipenem	60-100 mg/kg/day IV	500-1,000 mg IV every 6 to 8 hr
	Meropenem	30-60 mg/kg/day IV	500-2,000 mg IV every 6 to 8 hr
	Meropenem-vaborbactam	—	2 g/2 g IV every 8 hr
	Imipenem-relabactam	—	1.25 g every 6 hr
Polymyxins	Colistin	2.5-5 mg/kg/day IV	IV: 300 mg × 1, then 150 mg daily/Neb: 150 mg every 8 hr
	Polymyxin B	15,000-30,000 units/kg/day IV	IV: 2-2.5 mg/kg × 1, then 1.25-1.5 mg/kg every 12 hr
Other	Vancomycin	45-60 mg/kg/day IV	15-20 mg/kg IV every 8-12 hr
	Linezolid	20-30 mg/kg/day IV or orally	600 mg IV or orally every 12 hr
	Clindamycin	30-40 mg/kg/day IV or orally	600 mg IV or orally every 8 hr or 450 mg orally every 6 hr

[a]Doses can be increased for more severe disease and may require modification for patients with organ dysfunction.

[b]Higher-dose amoxicillin and amoxicillin/clavulanate (eg, 90 mg/kg/day) are used for penicillin-resistant *S. pneumoniae*.

[c]Fluoroquinolones have been avoided for pediatric patients because of the potential for cartilage damage; however, they have been used for MDR bacterial infection safely and effectively in infants and children (see text).

[d]Tetracyclines are rarely used in pediatric patients, particularly in those younger than 8 years because of tetracycline-induced permanent tooth discoloration.

admitted to an intensive care unit (see Tables 129-8 and 129-9).[4,5] In adult outpatients, choice of therapy depends on the individual patient's risk for drug-resistant *S. pneumoniae*. Amoxicillin is the preferred treatment for patients at low risk (ie, no at-risk comorbidities). Patients who cannot receive amoxicillin should be treated with doxycycline. Macrolides (such as azithromycin) should only be used when both amoxicillin and doxycycline are contraindicated and local macrolide-resistant *S. pneumoniae* prevalence is low.[4] In patients with specific comorbidities putting them at risk for treatment failure or drug-resistant *S. pneumoniae*, either anti-pneumococcal fluoroquinolone monotherapy (such as levofloxacin or moxifloxacin) or combination therapy consisting of a β-lactam (Table 129-8) plus either a macrolide or doxycycline is indicated to ensure coverage of resistant strains.[4] Empiric therapy of CAP for inpatients differs from that of outpatients in two ways: first, it is usually IV rather than oral route of administration; and second, coverage against drug-resistant *S. pneumoniae* is given to all patients. This reflects the desire to rapidly achieve adequate systemic antimicrobial exposures and increase the likelihood of providing in vitro active therapy in patients with a higher severity of illness where the importance of early appropriate therapy is increased. In patients with severe CAP, therapy should always consist of a combination regimen with a β-lactam backbone (Table 129-8), as these regimens are associated with reduced mortality in patients with bacteremic pneumococcal pneumonia.[79-81]

Coverage of less frequent CAP pathogens, such as MRSA and *P. aeruginosa*, may be considered in patients with specific risk factors for these pathogens.[4] Patients with a positive respiratory culture for MRSA and/or *P. aeruginosa* in the past year should receive empiric coverage for that respective pathogen.[4] Respiratory cultures and/or nasal MRSA PCR tests should be obtained in these patients before antibiotic therapy is administered. The empiric MRSA and/or *P. aeruginosa* coverage should be discontinued in 48 hours if these test results are negative for these pathogens and the patient is clinically improving. Patients who have been hospitalized in the past 90 days who also received IV antibiotics are at increased risk for both MRSA and *P. aeruginosa*. Patients meeting this criteria who have non-severe cap should have cultures and nasal MRSA PCR tests performed. Antibiotics covering MRSA and/or *P. aeruginosa* should be added only if these pathogens are identified. Patients who have been hospitalized in the past 90 days who also received IV antibiotics admitted with severe CAP should receive both empiric MRSA and *P. aeruginosa* coverage and have cultures performed. The MRSA and *P. aeruginosa* coverage should be discontinued after 48 hours if culture results are negative and the patient is clinically improving.[4]

Additional treatment considerations for adult patients with CAP include whether to provide coverage for influenza or SARS-CoV-2 and whether adjunctive corticosteroids are necessary. Nucleic acid amplification testing for influenza should be obtained when influenza and/or SARS-CoV-2 is circulating in the community.[4] Treatment with a neuraminidase inhibitor (such as oseltamivir or peramivir) should be administered only if influenza testing is positive. Adjunctive corticosteroids should only be given to patients with septic shock that is refractory to fluid resuscitation and vasopressor support.[4]

Similar to adult patients, empiric antibiotic regimens for CAP in pediatric patients differ between the outpatient and inpatient setting. However, in pediatric patients, choice of empiric therapy is more dependent on patient age group and immunization status rather than comorbidity. For outpatients, choice of therapy is predominantly based on age group and suspected etiology (ie, typical vs atypical bacteria; viral). Among inpatients, those fully immunized against *S. pneumoniae* and *H. influenzae* type B may be treated with a penicillin antibiotic with or without macrolide for typical coverage as indicated based on clinical suspicion for atypical pneumonia.[5] Empiric regimens in unimmunized patients or in areas with a high prevalence of penicillin-resistant *S. pneumoniae* should consist of third-generation cephalosporin (such as ceftriaxone).[5] Similar to CAP in adults, MRSA is sometimes the causative pathogen. Addition of MRSA coverage (with vancomycin or linezolid) should be considered when clinical suspicion is high (post-viral pneumonia, necrotizing/cavitary radiographic findings).[5]

Hospital-Acquired and Ventilator-Associated Pneumonia

9 Because HAP and VAP have a distinctive epidemiology compared with CAP, empiric antimicrobial regimens for HAP and VAP differ greatly from those for CAP (Table 129-8). Despite this, selection of therapy is based on many of the same principles. As with CAP, knowledge of the local pathogen and antibiotic resistance distribution is important. Antibiotic resistance patterns can vary greatly between institutions in the same city and even within the same institution between hospital units. Because of this, use of institution-specific antibiograms is highly recommended. These antibiograms should ideally also contain separate susceptibility

data specific to the ICU population.[6] Along with local susceptibility, patient-specific factors should weigh heavily in the choice of empiric therapy. Individual risk factors for infection with MRSA and MDR gram-negative bacilli are particularly important in HAP and VAP, as is severity of illness and mortality risk.

The vast majority of HAP cases are caused by gram-negative bacilli, predominantly *P. aeruginosa* and the Enterobacteriaceae, or *S. aureus*.[6] As such, all empiric HAP regimens should consist of at least one antibiotic with coverage against these pathogens, usually an antipseudomonal, antistaphylococcal β-lactam (such as piperacillin/tazobactam or cefepime) or an antipseudomonal, antistaphylococcal fluoroquinolone (such as levofloxacin).[6] While aminoglycosides are useful in treating gram-negative pneumonia in combination with another gram-negative-active antibiotic, they should not be used as monotherapy in pneumonia given the lack of data supporting their use in this manner. Patients contracting the pneumonia in a hospital or hospital unit with an MRSA prevalence of 20% or greater should also receive MRSA coverage with either vancomycin or linezolid.[6] Patients with MDR HAP risk factors, such as receipt of IV antibiotics in the past 90 days or structural lung disease, should also receive MRSA coverage in addition to a second antipseudomonal agent to cover for MDR gram-negative bacilli. An empiric antibiotic regimen containing dual pseudomonal and MRSA coverage is also indicated in patients at high risk of mortality, such as those requiring mechanical ventilation as a result of their pneumonia and those in septic shock.[6] This approach is taken to maximize the likelihood of early effective therapy in those patients where the consequences of delayed appropriate therapy in the event the pathogen is resistant to the empiric regimen are greatest.

Empiric antibiotic regimens for patients with VAP are similar to patients with HAP. In patients with no MDR VAP risk factors, who contracted VAP in a unit with a low prevalence of both MRSA (less than 10%-20%) and of gram-negative bacilli resistance (<10% to an antibiotic being considered for use), monotherapy with an antipseudomonal antibiotic with staphylococcal coverage may be used.[6] Higher MRSA prevalence would indicate the addition of vancomycin or linezolid. Likewise, more than 10% resistance to all antibiotics being considered for gram-negative monotherapy would indicate the need for double antipseudomonal coverage (Table 129-8).[6] Patients at risk for MDR VAP, including those receiving IV antibiotics in previous 90 days, those in septic shock, those with VAP onset after 5 or more days of hospitalization, and those with acute respiratory distress syndrome or receiving renal replacement therapy preceding VAP onset should also receive double pseudomonal and MRSA coverage.[6]

Pathogen-Directed Antimicrobial Therapy

10 Tailoring antimicrobial therapy based on diagnostic test results and patient clinical status is an important aspect of the pharmacotherapy of pneumonia. Utilizing a pathogen-directed antimicrobial regimen can optimize patient outcome using evidence-based antimicrobials for a particular pathogen. It can also mitigate potential negative impacts of ongoing broad-spectrum antimicrobial use, including adverse drug reactions, *C. difficile* infection, and development of further MDR infection.[82-84] When tailoring antimicrobial therapy, it is important to consider both diagnostic test results (chest imaging, Gram stain, respiratory cultures), and patient clinical factors (hemodynamics, temperature, respiratory status, white blood cell counts/differential). In patients who are clinically stable with signs of improving infection, narrowing of therapy should be considered, especially if culture results have identified a likely pathogen with associated susceptibility pattern.[6] Recommendations for directed therapy of common pneumonia pathogens can be found in Table 129-11.

TABLE 129-11 Directed Antimicrobial Therapy for Common Pneumonia Pathogens in Adult Patients

Pathogen	Preferred Antibiotic Therapy	Alternative Antibiotic Therapy
Penicillin-susceptible *S. pneumoniae* (MIC ≤2 mg/L)	Ampicillin, amoxicillin, penicillin G	Ceftriaxone, cefotaxime, macrolide, levofloxacin, moxifloxacin, doxycycline, clindamycin, vancomycin
Penicillin-resistant *S. pneumoniae* (MIC >2 mg/L)	Ceftriaxone, cefotaxime, levofloxacin, moxifloxacin	High-dose amoxicillin (3 g/day), linezolid, clindamycin, vancomycin
Non-β-lactamase-producing *H. influenzae*	Ampicillin (IV), amoxicillin	Fluoroquinolone, doxycycline, azithromycin, clarithromycin
β-Lactamase-producing *H. influenzae*	Ceftriaxone, cefotaxime, ampicillin-sulbactam, amoxicillin-clavulanate	Fluoroquinolone, doxycycline, azithromycin, clarithromycin
Mycoplasma pneumoniae	Macrolide, doxycycline	Fluoroquinolone
Chlamydophila pneumoniae	Macrolide, doxycycline	Fluoroquinolone
Legionella pneumophila	Fluoroquinolone or azithromycin	Doxycycline
MSSA	Cefazolin, antistaphylococcal penicillin	Clindamycin, vancomycin
MRSA	Vancomycin, linezolid	Telavancin, ceftaroline, quinupristin/dalfopristin, clindamycin, sulfamethoxazole/trimethoprim
P. aeruginosa	Antipseudomonal β-lactam[a] or fluoroquinolone[b] based on antimicrobial susceptibility testing results. Can consider adding aminoglycoside if patient in septic shock or at high mortality risk	IV colistin or polymyxin B + inhaled colistin for isolates resistant to all preferred therapies
Acinetobacter spp.	Carbapenem OR ampicillin-sulbactam based on antimicrobial susceptibility testing results	IV colistin or polymyxin B + inhaled colistin for isolates resistant to all preferred therapies
Extended-spectrum β-lactamase-producing gram-negative bacilli	Carbapenem	Piperacillin-tazobactam or cefepime potential options depending on susceptibility/adequate dosing
Carbapenem-resistant organisms	New β-lactam/β-lactamase inhibitors[c] based on antimicrobial susceptibility testing OR IV colistin or polymyxin B + inhaled colistin	

[a]Antipseudomonal β-lactam: piperacillin/tazobactam, cefepime, ceftazidime, meropenem, imipenem/cilastatin, doripenem, aztreonam.

[b]Antipseudomonal fluoroquinolone: ciprofloxacin and levofloxacin.

[c]New β-lactam/β-lactamase inhibitors: ceftazidime/avibactam, meropenem/vaborbactam, ceftolozane/tazobactam.

MIC, minimum inhibitory concentration; MRSA, methicillin-resistant *Staphylococcus aureus*; MSSA, methicillin-sensitive *Staphylococcus aureus*; *PCN*, penicillin.

Directed Therapy of Important Gram-Positive Pathogens

10 Directed therapy for *S. pneumoniae,* the most common bacterial cause of CAP, primarily depends on penicillin susceptibility. For isolates considered susceptible to intravenous penicillin by the CLSI (MIC ≤2 mg/L), a narrow-spectrum penicillin such as penicillin, ampicillin, or amoxicillin is preferred.[4] Alternatively, a cephalosporin antibiotic may be used, or in the case of a severe β-lactam allergy, either a macrolide or antipneumococcal fluoroquinolone (Table 129-11).[4] For penicillin-resistant strains, a third-generation cephalosporin or fluoroquinolone is preferred (Table 129-11). High-dose amoxicillin (3 g/day) may be used for penicillin-intermediate strains (MIC = 4 mg/L).[4] High-dose amoxicillin has efficacy in these situations because resistance of *S. pneumoniae* to penicillins is conferred through a change in penicillin-binding protein resulting in decreased affinity of the antibiotic for the binding site. In the case of penicillins and *S. pneumoniae,* this can be overcome by more aggressive dosing that maximizes achievement of adequate time drug concentration is in excess of the MIC ($t >$ MIC) despite the elevated MIC.[85]

Treatment of *S. aureus* pneumonia is dependent on whether the strain exhibits methicillin resistance. Treatment with an antistaphylococcal penicillin, such as oxacillin, nafcillin, or dicloxacillin, is preferred by the CAP guidelines for methicillin-susceptible strains.[4] Cefazolin is an alternative for methicillin-susceptible strains with fewer clinical data in pneumonia. However, it is an equivalent alternative to an antistaphylococcal penicillin on the basis of data from *S. aureus* bacteremia suggesting equivalence or even superiority.[86] Clindamycin or vancomycin may also be used, although these agents are not preferred for treatment of MSSA infections.[87] The treatment of choice for MRSA pneumonia is either vancomycin or linezolid, which are considered equivalent by infectious Diseases Society of America (IDSA) guidelines.[88-90] Vancomycin is often preferred over linezolid in clinical practice to preserve linezolid susceptibility for infections for which linezolid is one of the few remaining treatment options, such as infections caused by vancomycin-resistant enterococci (VRE). Telavancin, while FDA-approved for HAP/VAP caused by *S. aureus,* is often reserved for alternate therapy due to concerns of nephrotoxicity and potentially increased mortality in the subgroup of patients with a creatinine clearance less than 30 mL/min (0.5 mL/s). Additional alternatives for MRSA pneumonia include quinupristin-dalfopristin, ceftaroline, sulfamethoxazole-trimethoprim, and clindamycin. However, clinical evidence for these alternative options remains limited.[91-93]

Directed Therapy of Important Gram-Negative Pathogens

10 For *H. influenzae,* the most common gram-negative cause of CAP, the choice of directed therapy is dependent on whether the strain is β-lactamase producing. Non-β-lactamase-producing strains may be treated with ampicillin (IV) or amoxicillin (oral).[4] A third-generation cephalosporin (such as ceftriaxone) is the treatment of choice for β-lactamase-producing strains. Alternative therapy for *H. influenzae* includes fluoroquinolone, doxycycline, azithromycin, or clarithromycin.[4] Azithromycin is generally preferred to clarithromycin. A larger proportion of *H. influenzae* strains are susceptible to azithromycin relative to clarithromycin and azithromycin has a more favorable drug interaction profile.[94,95]

P. aeruginosa is a notoriously antibiotic-resistant pathogen that utilizes a variety of mechanisms of resistance, resulting in variable susceptibility patterns. Because of this, directed therapy against *P. aeruginosa* pneumonia is highly dependent on antimicrobial susceptibility results. When susceptible, all antipseudomonal agents recommended for empiric therapy are considered equivalent with respect to clinical outcomes in pneumonia.[6] The exception to this is the aminoglycosides, which are not recommended as monotherapy against *P. aeruginosa* pneumonia. Despite equivalence of most antibiotics in this setting, piperacillin-tazobactam, cefepime, and ceftazidime are generally preferred when susceptible. This is to preserve susceptibility of carbapenems, newer β-lactam/β-lactamase inhibitors, and fluoroquinolones for use in more resistant infections. Another consideration in the directed therapy of *P. aeruginosa* is the utility of combination therapy. Patients receiving monotherapy and combination therapy generally have similar outcomes.[6] However, combination therapy may be associated with reduced mortality in patients with septic shock.[96] Directed combination therapy against *P. aeruginosa* only is recommended in patients in septic shock or at high risk of mortality at the time antimicrobial susceptibility testing results become available.[6]

Enterobacterales, particularly *K. pneumoniae* and *E. coli,* are common causes of both HAP and VAP. Although generally susceptible to the gram-negative active agents recommended for empiric therapy of HAP and VAP, Enterobacteriaceae-producing extended-spectrum β-lactamases (ESBL) capable of hydrolyzing many of the β-lactams commonly used for empiric therapy have become increasingly common.[97-99] Because this diverse family of β-lactamases each has variable affinity for different β-lactams, susceptibility to each β-lactam agent can vary depending on the enzyme (ie, CTX-M, TEM, SHV).[100] Further complicating this is the inoculum effect, whereby β-lactams seemingly susceptible in vitro are hydrolyzed in vivo in the presence of a high-inoculum of ESBL-producing organism.[101] This variable susceptibility has resulted in debate regarding the treatment of choice for these infections. Although the limited evidence from observational studies did not demonstrate superiority of carbapenems over piperacillin/tazobactam or cefepime when the organism is susceptible to these agents, carbapenems are often considered the treatment of choice for serious ESBL infections such as pneumonia.[6] Piperacillin/tazobactam was not as effective meropenem for ceftriaxone-resistant *E. coli* or *K. pneumoniae* bloodstream infections.[102] Based on this, carbapenems will likely continue to be considered the treatment of choice for serious ESBL infections. If piperacillin/tazobactam or cefepime are utilized, it is important to ensure that the isolate is considered fully susceptible by the Clinical and Laboratory Standards Institute (CLSI) and that aggressive dosing strategies to ensure optimal $t >$ MIC are employed.

While initially thought of as reliable, last-line antibiotics for resistant gram-negative infections, resistance to carbapenems due to a variety of mechanisms has emerged. Until recently, few antibiotics retained activity against these organisms, resulting in a resurgence in the use of older, more toxic agents such as the polymyxins (colistin, polymyxin B). Availability of three new β-lactam/β-lactamase inhibitor combinations, ceftolozane-tazobactam, ceftazidime-avibactam, and meropenem-vaborbactam has provided hope for these infections. Ceftazidime/avibactam and meropenem/vaborbactam have in vitro activity against most carbapenem-resistant Enterobacteriaceae (CRE) acquiring resistance via carbapenemase enzymes.[103,104] Although ceftolozane-tazobactam does not have activity against carbapenemase-producing strains, it is active against many carbapenem-resistant *P. aeruginosa* strains where the primary mechanism of carbapenem resistance is change in cell permeability and/or efflux pumps.[105] Clinical data suggest that these new antimicrobials may be superior and less toxic relative to colistin- and/or aminoglycoside-containing regimens.[106-108,119] Coupled with favorable in vitro susceptibility data it seems reasonable to prefer these novel agents to more toxic polymyxin-containing regimens when the isolate is susceptible. Additional new antibiotic therapies with in vitro activity against many MDR pathogens that commonly cause lower respiratory tract infections and varying levels of clinical evidence include cefiderocol, plazomicin, imipenem-cilastatin-relebactam, and eravacycline. For infections that remain resistant to all other available antibiotics, treatment with inhaled polymyxins or aminoglycosides are recommended.[6] Inhaled antibiotics should be given with systemic antibiotics to which the pathogen is susceptible (ie, if only susceptible to colistin, give both inhaled and IV colistin).

Directed Therapy of Important Atypical Pathogens

10 Treatment of pneumonia caused by atypical bacteria, including

C. pneumoniae, *M. pneumoniae*, and *L. pneumophila*, generally consists of either a fluoroquinolone, macrolide, or doxycycline. For *C. pneumoniae* and *M. pneumoniae*, macrolides or doxycycline are preferred agents.[4] Fluoroquinolones or azithromycin is preferred over doxycycline for *Legionella* pneumonia due to the relative paucity of data involving doxycycline for this infection.[4]

Antimicrobial Pharmacokinetic/Pharmacodynamic Considerations

Antimicrobial pharmacokinetics/pharmacodynamics (PK/PD) is an important aspect of optimal antimicrobial therapy for pneumonia. Antibiotic concentrations in respiratory secretions in excess of the pathogen MIC are necessary for successful treatment of pulmonary infections.[109] Thus, ability of an antimicrobial to penetrate into pulmonary secretions is important and must be factored into antimicrobial selection and dosing for pneumonia. The ability of a drug to penetrate respiratory secretions depends on multiple physicochemical factors, including molecular size, lipid solubility, and degree of ionization at serum and biologic fluid pH and the extent of protein binding. Studies evaluating antibiotic concentrations in the pulmonary epithelial lining fluid (ELF) indicate that β-lactams, glycopeptide, and aminoglycosides tend to have ELF to plasma antibiotic concentration ratios less than 1. In contrast, macrolides, fluoroquinolones, and linezolid tend to have ELF to plasma antibiotic concentration ratios much greater than 1. Thus, the latter agents penetrate and concentrate into the ELF to a greater extent.[109]

Although β-lactams, glycopeptides, and aminoglycosides have less extensive ELF penetration, carefully constructed dosing schemes based on PK/PD principles allow these agents to be effective in treating lower respiratory tract infections. Although evidence is conflicting, dosing guided by PK/PD principles may reduce mortality and improve clinical outcome in patients with pneumonia.[6] The use of strategies maximizing antibiotic PK/PD to select antibiotic dosing for HAP and VAP is recommended by the IDSA guidelines.[6] This includes weight-based initial dosing of vancomycin and aminoglycosides followed by measurement of serum antibiotic concentrations to adjust doses through antibiotic therapeutic drug monitoring (TDM) and use of extended or continuous infusion of β-lactams. Dosing and TDM of vancomycin for pneumonia should target achievement of a vancomycin area under the concentration-time curve (AUC) 400-600 mg*hr/L early in the course of therapy.[110,111] This will maximize achievement of AUC/MIC ratios >400 for *S. aureus* isolates with an MIC ≤1 mg/L. Clinical practice guidelines recommend this should preferably be achieved via AUC monitoring.[112] Alternatively, this may be achieved by targeting vancomycin trough concentrations of 15-20 mg/L (10.4-13.8 μmol/L) as surrogate for AUC >400 mg*h/L, although this approach leads to supratherapeutic AUC in a large proportion of patients and a resulting increased risk of vancomycin-associated nephrotoxicity.[13,120] The preferred aminoglycoside dosing strategy for pneumonia, when patient renal function permits, is high-dose once-daily administration. This approach maximizes the AUC:MIC and peak:MIC ratios for efficacy while allowing undetectable serum trough concentrations for a period of time to minimize nephrotoxicity.[113,114] Aminoglycoside peak:MIC ratios ≥10 are typically targeted clinically for pneumonia. We refer the reader to Chapter e126, "Laboratory Tests to Direct Antimicrobial Pharmacotherapy" and Chapter 127 for more in-depth discussion of antibiotic PK/PD concepts.

PATIENT MONITORING, THERAPY MODIFICATION, AND DURATION OF THERAPY

After therapy has been instituted, appropriate clinical parameters should be monitored to ensure the efficacy and safety of the therapeutic regimen. For patients with bacterial infections of the lower respiratory tract, the time to resolution of initial presenting symptoms and the lack of appearance of new associated symptomatology are important to determine.[115] For patients with pneumonia of mild-to-moderate clinical severity, the time to resolution of cough, decreasing sputum production, and fever, as well as other constitutional symptoms of malaise, nausea, vomiting, and lethargy, should be noted. If the patient requires supplemental oxygen therapy, the amount and need should be assessed regularly. A gradual and persistent improvement in the resolution of these symptoms and therapies should be observed. Initial resolution of infection should be observed within the first 2 days of therapy and progression to complete resolution within 5 to 7 days (usually no more than 10 days). Because cultures for causative organism are rarely obtained except for more severe CAP cases, empiric therapy is typically continued for the duration of therapy provided the patient is responding adequately. When cultures are obtained, tailoring therapy to be pathogen-directed as described above is recommended. The majority of hospitalized patients with CAP should be switched from IV to oral therapy when hemodynamically stable, improving clinically as described above, have normal gastrointestinal tract function, and be able to ingest oral medications.[4] The minimum duration of therapy for CAP is 5 days, although CAP is commonly treated for 7 to 10 days.[4] When discontinuing therapy, patients should be afebrile for 48 to 72 hours and have no more than one CAP-related sign of clinical instability (ie, tachycardia, tachypnea, hypotension, hypoxia, altered mental status). Discontinuation of therapy using these criteria starting at day 5 of therapy decreases the duration of antibiotic therapy without reducing cure rates or increasing readmission in non-ICU CAP patients.[116]

For patients with HAP, substantial underlying diseases, or both, additional parameters can be followed, including the magnitude and character of the peripheral blood WBC count, chest radiograph, and blood gas determinations. Similar to patients with less severe disease, some resolution of symptoms should be observed within 2 days of instituting antibiotic therapy. If no resolution of symptoms is observed within 2 days of starting seemingly appropriate antibiotic therapy or if the patient's clinical status is deteriorating, the appropriateness of initial antibiotic therapy should be critically reassessed. The patient should be evaluated carefully for deterioration of underlying concurrent disease(s). Additionally, the clinician should consider the possibility of changing the initial antibiotic therapy to expand antimicrobial coverage not included in the original regimen if the patient's clinical status is worsening or failing to improve after 48 to 72 hours of therapy. The results of initial and follow-up diagnostic tests, such as respiratory cultures, should also be used alongside clinical response to streamline therapy. De-escalation of antibiotic therapy to be more narrow spectrum in patients with HAP/VAP is strongly recommended. This approach may not affect clinical outcomes while reducing excess antibiotic use.[6] The recommended duration of therapy for HAP/VAP is 7 days, as the clinical benefit of longer durations of therapy (≥10 days) is not clear based on available clinical evidence.[6] Serum procalcitonin concentrations in combination with clinical response criteria can be used in the decision to discontinue antibiotic therapy.[6]

Prevention of Pneumonia

Prevention of some cases of pneumonia is possible through the use of vaccines and medications against selected infectious agents. Polyvalent polysaccharide vaccines are available for two of the leading causes of bacterial pneumonia, *S. pneumoniae* and *H. influenzae* type b. Children should be vaccinated against *S. pneumoniae*, *H. influenzae* type b, pertussis, and influenza while caregivers for infants less than 6 months should also be vaccinated against influenza and pertussis. Immune prophylaxis for RSV is only recommended for high-risk infants during RSV season. To minimize the risk of developing VAP, healthcare providers should seek to minimize colonization of the aerodigestive tract, prevent aspiration (head raised 45 degrees), and limit the length of mechanical ventilation of patients.[60] (See Chapter 131 for a full discussion of influenza postexposure prophylaxis and Chapter 147, "Vaccines, Toxoids, and Other Immunobiologics" for vaccines.)[117]

ABBREVIATIONS

AAP	American Academy of Pediatrics
ADME	absorption, distribution, metabolism, and excretion
AECB	acute exacerbation of chronic bronchitis
AUC	area under the concentration-time curve
BAL	bronchoalveolar lavage
CAP	community-acquired pneumonia
CLSI	Clinical and Laboratory Standards Institute
COPD	chronic obstructive pulmonary disease
CRE	carbapenem-resistant Enterobacteriaceae
ELF	epithelial lining fluid
FEV_1	forced expiratory volume in the first second of expiration
GOLD	Global Initiative for Chronic Obstructive Lung Disease
HAP	hospital-acquired pneumonia
HIV	human immunodeficiency virus
LABA	long-acting β-receptor agonist
LAMA	long-acting muscarinic antagonist
MDR	multidrug-resistant
MIC	minimum inhibitory concentration
MRSA	methicillin-resistant *Staphylococcus aureus*
NAC	*N*-acetyl cysteine
PCR	polymerase chain reaction
PDE4	phosphodiesterase 4
PK-PD	pharmacokinetics/pharmacodynamics
RSV	respiratory syncytial virus
SARS	severe acute respiratory syndrome
SARS-CoV	severe acute respiratory syndrome coronavirus
TDM	therapeutic drug monitoring
VAP	ventilator-associated pneumonia
VRE	vancomycin-resistant enterococci
WBC	white blood cell

REFERENCES

1. Eddens T, Kolls JK. Host defenses against bacterial lower respiratory tract infection. *Curr Opin Immunol.* 2012;24(4):424–430.
2. Jaroszewski DE, Webb BJ, Leslie KO. Diagnosis and management of lung infections. *Thorac Surg Clin.* 2012;22(3):301–324.
3. Yan Y, Zhang S, Tang YW. Molecular assays for the detection and characterization of respiratory viruses. *Semin Respir Crit Care Med.* 2011;32(4):512–526.
4. Mandell LA, Wunderink RG, Anzueto A, et al. Infectious Diseases Society of America/American Thoracic Society consensus guidelines on the management of community-acquired pneumonia in adults. *Clin Infect Dis.* 2007;44(suppl 2):S27–S72.
5. Bradley JS, Byington CL, Shah SS, et al. The management of community-acquired pneumonia in infants and children older than 3 months of age: clinical practice guidelines by the Pediatric Infectious Diseases Society and the Infectious Diseases Society of America. *Clin Infect Dis.* 2011;53(7):e25–e76.
6. Kalil AC, Metersky ML, Klompas M, et al. Management of adults with hospital-acquired and ventilator-associated pneumonia: 2016 Clinical Practice Guidelines by the Infectious Diseases Society of America and the American Thoracic Society. *Clin Infect Dis.* 2016;63(5):e61–e111.
7. Lippi G, Meschi T, Cervellin G. Inflammatory biomarkers for the diagnosis, monitoring and follow-up of community-acquired pneumonia: clinical evidence and perspectives. *Eur J Intern Med.* 2011;22(5):460–465.
8. Kinkade S, Long NA. Acute bronchitis. *Am Fam Physician.* 2016;94(7):560–565.
9. Nielsen M, Barnes CB, Ulrik CS. Clinical characteristics of the asthma-COPD overlap syndrome—a systematic review. *Int J Chron Obstruct Pulmon Dis.* 2015;10:1443–1454.
10. Gibson PG, McDonald VM. Asthma-COPD overlap 2015: now we are six. *Thorax.* 2015;70(7):683–691.
11. Smith MP, Lown M, Singh S, et al. Acute cough due to acute bronchitis in immunocompetent adult outpatients. *Chest.* 2020;157:1256–1265. 10.1016/j.chest.2020.01.044.
12. Jefferson T, Jones MA, Doshi P, et al. Neuraminidase inhibitors for preventing and treating influenza in healthy adults and children. *Cochrane Database Syst Rev.* 2014;(4):Cd008965.
13. Becker LA, Hom J, Villasis-Keever M, van der Wouden JC. Beta2-agonists for acute cough or a clinical diagnosis of acute bronchitis. *Cochrane Database Syst Rev.* 2015(9):Cd001726.
14. Martin MJ, Harrison TW. Causes of chronic productive cough: an approach to management. *Respir Med.* 2015;109(9):1105–1113.
15. Smith SM, Fahey T, Smucny J, Becker LA. Antibiotics for acute bronchitis. *Cochrane Database Syst Rev.* 2017;6:Cd000245.
16. Ison MG, Portsmouth S, Yoshida Y, et al. Early treatment with baloxavir marboxil in high-risk adolescent and adult outpatients with uncomplicated influenza (CAPSTONE-2): a randomised, placebo-controlled, phase 3 trial. *Lancet Infect Dis.* 2020;20:1204–1214. 10.1016/s1473-3099(20)30004-9.
17. Dunning J, Baillie JK, Cao B, Hayden FG. Antiviral combinations for severe influenza. *Lancet Infect Dis.* 2014;14(12):1259–1270.
18. Malesker MA, Callahan-Lyon P, Madison MJ, et al. Chronic cough due to stable chronic bronchitis. *Chest.* 2020;158:705–718. 10.1016/j.chest.2020.02.015.
19. Cai Y, Schikowski T, Adam M, et al. Cross-sectional associations between air pollution and chronic bronchitis: an ESCAPE meta-analysis across five cohorts. *Thorax.* 2014;69(11):1005–1014.
20. Celli BR, Decramer M, Wedzicha JA, et al. An official American Thoracic Society/European Respiratory Society statement: research questions in chronic obstructive pulmonary disease. *Am J Respir Crit Care Med.* 2015;191(7):e4–e27.
21. Criner GJ, Bourbeau J, Diekemper RL, et al. Prevention of acute exacerbations of COPD: American College of Chest Physicians and Canadian Thoracic Society guideline. *Chest.* 2015;147(4):894–942.
22. Overington JD, Huang YC, Abramson MJ, et al. Implementing clinical guidelines for chronic obstructive pulmonary disease: barriers and solutions. *J Thorac Dis.* 2014;6(11):1586–1596.
23. Miravitlles M, Kruesmann F, Haverstock D, Perroncel R, Choudhri SH, Arvis P. Sputum colour and bacteria in chronic bronchitis exacerbations: a pooled analysis. *Eur Respir J.* 2012;39(6):1354–1360.
24. Anthonisen NR, Manfreda J, Warren CP, Hershfield ES, Harding GK, Nelson NA. Antibiotic therapy in exacerbations of chronic obstructive pulmonary disease. *Ann Intern Med.* 1987;106(2):196–204.
25. Puhan MA, Gimeno-Santos E, Cates CJ, et al. Pulmonary rehabilitation following exacerbations of chronic obstructive pulmonary disease. *Cochrane Database Syst Rev.* 2016;12(12):CD005305. 10.1002/14651858.cd005305.pub4.
26. McIlwaine MP, Lee Son NM, Richmond ML. Physiotherapy and cystic fibrosis: what is the evidence base? *Curr Opin Pulm Med.* 2014;20(6):613–617.
27. Poole P, Chong J, Cates CJ. Mucolytic agents versus placebo for chronic bronchitis or chronic obstructive pulmonary disease. *Cochrane Database Syst Rev.* 2015;(7):Cd001287.
28. Santus P, Radovanovic D, Paggiaro P, et al. Why use long acting bronchodilators in chronic obstructive lung diseases? An extensive review on formoterol and salmeterol. *Eur J Intern Med.* 2015;26(6):379–384.
29. Kew KM, Dias S, Cates CJ. Long-acting inhaled therapy (beta-agonists, anticholinergics and steroids) for COPD: a network meta-analysis. *Cochrane Database Syst Rev.* 2014;(3):Cd010844.
30. Magnussen H, Disse B, Rodriguez-Roisin R, et al. Withdrawal of inhaled glucocorticoids and exacerbations of COPD. *N Engl J Med.* 2014;371(14):1285–1294.
31. Singh D. New combination bronchodilators for chronic obstructive pulmonary disease: current evidence and future perspectives. *Br J Clin Pharmacol.* 2015;79(5):695–708.
32. Global Initiative for Chronic Obstructive Lung Disease. Global strategy for the diagnosis, management, and prevention of chronic obstructive pulmonary disease. 2021. Available at: www.goldcopd.org. Accessed October 19, 2021.
33. Yu Tsung, Fain Kevin, Boyd Cynthia M, et al. Benefits and harms of roflumilast in moderate to severe COPD. *Thorax.* 2013;69:616–622. 10.1136/thoraxjnl-2013-204155.

34. Fu AZ, Sun SX, Huang X, Amin AN. Lower 30-day readmission rates with roflumilast treatment among patients hospitalized for chronic obstructive pulmonary disease. *Int J Chron Obstruct Pulmon Dis.* 2015;10:909–915.
35. Janjua S, Fortescue R, Poole P. Phosphodiesterase-4 inhibitors for chronic obstructive pulmonary disease. *Cochrane Database Syst Rev.* 2020;5(5):CD002309. 10.1002/14651858.cd002309.pub6.
36. Laopaiboon M, Panpanich R, Swa Mya K. Azithromycin for acute lower respiratory tract infections. *Cochrane Database Syst Rev.* 2015;(3):Cd001954.
37. Lee RA, Centor RM, Humphrey LL, et al. Appropriate use of short-course antibiotics in common infections: best practice advice from the American College of Physicians. *Ann Intern Med.* 2021;174(6):822–827. 10.7326/m20-7355.
38. Euba B, Moleres J, Segura V, et al. Genome expression profiling-based identification and administration efficacy of host-directed antimicrobial drugs against respiratory infection by nontypeable *Haemophilus influenzae. Antimicrob Agents Chemother.* 2015;59(12):7581–7592.
39. Hayes DJ, Meyer K. Acute exacerbations of chronic bronchitis in elderly patients: pathogenesis, diagnosis, and management. *Drugs Aging.* 2007;(24):555–572.
40. Herath SC, Poole P. Prophylactic antibiotic therapy in chronic obstructive pulmonary disease. *JAMA.* 2014;311(21):2225–2226.
41. Spagnolo P, Fabbri LM, Bush A. Long-term macrolide treatment for chronic respiratory disease. *Eur Respir J.* 2013;42(1):239–251.
42. Tse HN, Tseng CZ. Update on the pathological processes, molecular biology, and clinical utility of N-acetylcysteine in chronic obstructive pulmonary disease. *Int J Chron Obstruct Pulmon Dis.* 2014;9:825–836.
43. Fischer BM, Voynow JA, Ghio AJ. COPD: balancing oxidants and antioxidants. *Int J Chron Obstruct Pulmon Dis.* 2015;10:261–276.
44. Meissner HC. Viral bronchiolitis in children. *N Engl J Med.* 2016;374(1):62–72.
45. Pelletier JH, Au AK, Fuhrman D, et al. Trends in bronchiolitis ICU admissions and ventilation practices: 2010–2019. *Pediatrics.* 2021;147(6):e2020039115. 10.1542/peds.2020-039115.
46. Cavaye D, Roberts DP, Saravanos GL, et al. Evaluation of national guidelines for bronchiolitis: AGREEments and controversies. *J Paediatr Child Health.* 2018.
47. Barr R, Green CA, Sande CJ, et al. Respiratory syncytial virus: diagnosis, prevention and management. *Ther Adv Infect Dis.* 2019;6:2049936119865798. 10.1177/2049936119865798.
48. Ralston SL, Lieberthal AS, Meissner HC, et al. Clinical practice guideline: the diagnosis, management, and prevention of bronchiolitis. *Pediatrics.* 2014;134(5):e1474–e1502.
49. Kua KP, Lee SWH. Systematic review and meta-analysis of the efficacy and safety of combined epinephrine and corticosteroid therapy for acute bronchiolitis in infants. *Front Pharmacol.* 2017;8:396.
50. Shanahan KH, Monuteaux MC, Nagler J, et al. Early use of bronchodilators and outcomes in bronchiolitis. *Pediatrics.* 2021;148:e2020040394. 10.1542/peds.2020-040394.
51. Auger KA, Parker MW, Huang B. New method, same answer: we do not know if hypertonic saline helps bronchiolitis. *Pediatrics.* 2018;142(3):e20181868. doi: 10.1542/peds.2018-1868.
52. Nseir S, Mathieu D. Antibiotic treatment for severe community-acquired pneumonia: beyond antimicrobial susceptibility. *Crit Care Med.* 2012;40(8):2500–2502.
53. Segal LN, Rom WN, Weiden MD. Lung microbiome for clinicians. New discoveries about bugs in healthy and diseased lungs. *Ann Am Thorac Soc.* 2014;11(1):108–116.
54. DiBardino DM, Wunderink RG. Aspiration pneumonia: a review of modern trends. *J Crit Care.* 2015;30(1):40–48.
55. Jain S, Self WH, Wunderink RG, et al. Community-acquired pneumonia requiring hospitalization among U.S. adults. *N Engl J Med.* 2015;373(5):415–427.
56. Musher DM, Thorner AR. Community-acquired pneumonia. *N Engl J Med.* 2014;371(17):1619–1628.
57. Prina E, Ranzani OT, Torres A. Community-acquired pneumonia. *Lancet.* 2015;386(9998):1097.
58. Jain S, Williams DJ, Arnold SR, et al. Community-acquired pneumonia requiring hospitalization among U.S. children. *N Engl J Med.* 2015;372(9):835–845.
59. Pettersson K. Perinatal infection with group B streptococci. *Semin Fetal Neonatal Med.* 2007;12(3):193–197.
60. Hunter JD. Ventilator-associated pneumonia. *BMJ.* 2012;344:e3325.
61. Weiner LM, Webb AK, Limbago B, et al. Antimicrobial-resistant pathogens associated with healthcare-associated infections: summary of data reported to the National Healthcare Safety Network at the Centers for Disease Control and Prevention, 2011-2014. *Infect Control Hosp Epidemiol.* 2016;1–14.
62. Jones RN. Microbial etiologies of hospital-acquired bacterial pneumonia and ventilator-associated bacterial pneumonia. *Clin Infect Dis.* 2010;51(suppl 1):S81–S87.
63. Murdoch DR, Laing RT, Mills GD, et al. Evaluation of a rapid immunochromatographic test for detection of *Streptococcus pneumoniae* antigen in urine samples from adults with community-acquired pneumonia. *J Clin Microbiol.* 2001;39(10):3495–3498.
64. Cunha BA, Burillo A, Bouza E. Legionnaires' disease. *Lancet.* 2016;387(10016):376–385.
65. Phin N, Parry-Ford F, Harrison T, et al. Epidemiology and clinical management of Legionnaires' disease. *Lancet Infect Dis.* 2014;14(10):1011–1021.
66. Saraya T, Kurai D, Nakagaki K, et al. Novel aspects on the pathogenesis of *Mycoplasma pneumoniae* pneumonia and therapeutic implications. *Front Microbiol.* 2014;5:410.
67. Huijskens EG, Koopmans M, Palmen FM, van Erkel AJ, Mulder PG, Rossen JW. The value of signs and symptoms in differentiating between bacterial, viral and mixed aetiology in patients with community-acquired pneumonia. *J Med Microbiol.* 2014;63(pt 3):441–452.
68. Agbaht K, Diaz E, Munoz E, et al. Bacteremia in patients with ventilator-associated pneumonia is associated with increased mortality: a study comparing bacteremic vs. nonbacteremic ventilator-associated pneumonia. *Crit Care Med.* 2007;35(9):2064–2070.
69. Kunac A, Sifri ZC, Mohr AM, Horng H, Lavery RF, Livingston DH. Bacteremia and ventilator-associated pneumonia: a marker for contemporaneous extra-pulmonic infection. *Surg Infect (Larchmt).* 2014;15(2):77–83.
70. Bartlett JG. Diagnostic tests for agents of community-acquired pneumonia. *Clin Infect Dis.* 2011;52(suppl 4):S296–S304.
71. Couturier MR, Graf EH, Griffin AT. Urine antigen tests for the diagnosis of respiratory infections: legionellosis, histoplasmosis, pneumococcal pneumonia. *Clin Lab Med.* 2014;34(2):219–236.
72. Dominguez J, Gali N, Blanco S, et al. Detection of *Streptococcus pneumoniae* antigen by a rapid immunochromatographic assay in urine samples. *Chest.* 2001;119(1):243–249.
73. Helbig JH, Uldum SA, Luck PC, Harrison TG. Detection of *Legionella pneumophila* antigen in urine samples by the BinaxNOW immunochromatographic assay and comparison with both Binax Legionella Urinary Enzyme Immunoassay (EIA) and Biotest Legionella Urin Antigen EIA. *J Med Microbiol.* 2001;50(6):509–516.
74. Lim WS, van der Eerden MM, Laing R, et al. Defining community acquired pneumonia severity on presentation to hospital: an international derivation and validation study. *Thorax.* 2003;58(5):377–382.
75. Bauer TT, Ewig S, Marre R, Suttorp N, Welte T. CRB-65 predicts death from community-acquired pneumonia. *J Intern Med.* 2006;260(1):93–101.
76. Fine MJ, Auble TE, Yealy DM, et al. A prediction rule to identify low-risk patients with community-acquired pneumonia. *N Engl J Med.* 1997;336(4):243–250.
77. Ottosen J, Evans H. Pneumonia: challenges in the definition, diagnosis, and management of disease. *Surg Clin North Am.* 2014;94(6):1305–1317.
78. Feldman C, Anderson R. Antibiotic resistance of pathogens causing community-acquired pneumonia. *Semin Respir Crit Care Med.* 2012;33(3):232–243.
79. Martinez JA, Horcajada JP, Almela M, et al. Addition of a macrolide to a beta-lactam-based empirical antibiotic regimen is associated with lower in-hospital mortality for patients with bacteremic pneumococcal pneumonia. *Clin Infect Dis.* 2003;36(4):389–395.
80. Waterer GW, Somes GW, Wunderink RG. Monotherapy may be suboptimal for severe bacteremic pneumococcal pneumonia. *Arch Intern Med.* 2001;161(15):1837–1842.
81. Weiss K, Low DE, Cortes L, et al. Clinical characteristics at initial presentation and impact of dual therapy on the outcome of bacteremic *Streptococcus pneumoniae* pneumonia in adults. *Can Respir J.* 2004;11(8):589–593.
82. Davis ML, Sparrow HG, Ikwuagwu JO, Musick WL, Garey KW, Perez KK. Multicentre derivation and validation of a simple predictive index for healthcare-associated *Clostridium difficile* infection. *Clin Microbiol Infect.* 2018;24(11):1190–1194.
83. Johnson MT, Reichley R, Hoppe-Bauer J, Dunne WM, Micek S, Kollef M. Impact of previous antibiotic therapy on outcome of gram-negative severe sepsis. *Crit Care Med.* 2011;39(8):1859–1865.
84. Shehab N, Patel PR, Srinivasan A, Budnitz DS. Emergency department visits for antibiotic-associated adverse events. *Clin Infect Dis.* 2008;47(6):735–743.
85. Tomasz A. Antibiotic resistance in *Streptococcus pneumoniae. Clin Infect Dis.* 1997;24(suppl 1):S85–S88.

86. Bidell MR, Patel N, O'Donnell JN. Optimal treatment of MSSA bacteraemias: a meta-analysis of cefazolin versus antistaphylococcal penicillins. *J Antimicrob Chemother.* 2018;73(10):2643–2651.
87. McDanel JS, Perencevich EN, Diekema DJ, et al. Comparative effectiveness of beta-lactams versus vancomycin for treatment of methicillin-susceptible *Staphylococcus aureus* bloodstream infections among 122 hospitals. *Clin Infect Dis.* 2015;61(3):361–367.
88. Stevens DL, Herr D, Lampiris H, Hunt JL, Batts DH, Hafkin B. Linezolid versus vancomycin for the treatment of methicillin-resistant *Staphylococcus aureus* infections. *Clin Infect Dis.* 2002;34(11):1481–1490.
89. Wunderink RG, Mendelson MH, Somero MS, et al. Early microbiological response to linezolid vs vancomycin in ventilator-associated pneumonia due to methicillin-resistant *Staphylococcus aureus. Chest.* 2008;134(6):1200–1207.
90. Wunderink RG, Niederman MS, Kollef MH, et al. Linezolid in methicillin-resistant *Staphylococcus aureus* nosocomial pneumonia: a randomized, controlled study. *Clin Infect Dis.* 2012;54(5):621–629.
91. Kaye KS, Udeani G, Cole P, Friedland HD. Ceftaroline fosamil for the treatment of hospital-acquired pneumonia and ventilator-associated pneumonia. *Hosp Pract (1995).* 2015;43(3):144–149.
92. Markowitz N, Quinn EL, Saravolatz LD. Trimethoprim-sulfamethoxazole compared with vancomycin for the treatment of *Staphylococcus aureus* infection. *Ann Intern Med.* 1992;117(5):390–398.
93. Eliakim-Raz N, Hellerman M, Yahav D, et al. Trimethoprim/sulfamethoxazole versus vancomycin in the treatment of healthcare/ventilator-associated MRSA pneumonia: a case-control study. *J Antimicrob Chemother.* 2017;72(3):882–887.
94. Gordon KA, Biedenbach DJ, Jones RN. Comparison of *Streptococcus pneumoniae* and *Haemophilus influenzae* susceptibilities from community-acquired respiratory tract infections and hospitalized patients with pneumonia: five-year results for the SENTRY Antimicrobial Surveillance Program. *Diagn Microbiol Infect Dis.* 2003;46(4):285–289.
95. Hawser S, Morrissey I, Lemos B, Keedy K, Fernandes P. Surveillance of the activity of solithromycin (CEM-101) against bacteria from respiratory tract infections. *Int J Antimicrob Agents.* 2017;50(1):17–22.
96. Kumar A, Zarychanski R, Light B, et al. Early combination antibiotic therapy yields improved survival compared with monotherapy in septic shock: a propensity-matched analysis. *Crit Care Med.* 2010;38(9):1773–1785.
97. Castanheira M, Farrell SE, Krause KM, Jones RN, Sader HS. Contemporary diversity of beta-lactamases among Enterobacteriaceae in the nine U.S. census regions and ceftazidime-avibactam activity tested against isolates producing the most prevalent beta-lactamase groups. *Antimicrob Agents Chemother.* 2014;58(2):833–838.
98. Coque TM, Baquero F, Canton R. Increasing prevalence of ESBL-producing Enterobacteriaceae in Europe. *Euro Surveill.* 2008;13(47):pii=19044.
99. Lukac PJ, Bonomo RA, Logan LK. Extended-spectrum beta-lactamase-producing Enterobacteriaceae in children: old foe, emerging threat. *Clin Infect Dis.* 2015;60(9):1389–1397.
100. Bush K, Jacoby GAw. Updated functional classification of beta-lactamases. *Antimicrob Agents Chemother.* 2010;54(3):969–976.
101. Wu N, Chen BY, Tian SF, Chu YZ. The inoculum effect of antibiotics against CTX-M-extended-spectrum beta-lactamase-producing *Escherichia coli. Ann Clin Microbiol Antimicrob.* 2014;13:45.
102. Harris PNA, Tambyah PA, Lye DC, et al. Effect of piperacillin-tazobactam vs meropenem on 30-day mortality for patients with *E. coli* or *Klebsiella pneumoniae* bloodstream infection and ceftriaxone resistance: a randomized clinical trial. *JAMA.* 2018;320(10):984–994.
103. Zasowski EJ, Rybak JM, Rybak MJ. The beta-lactams strike back: ceftazidime-avibactam. *Pharmacotherapy.* 2015;35(8):755–770.
104. Petty LA, Henig O, Patel TS, Pogue JM, Kaye KS. Overview of meropenem-vaborbactam and newer antimicrobial agents for the treatment of carbapenem-resistant Enterobacteriaceae. *Infect Drug Resist.* 2018;11:1461–1472.
105. Zhanel GG, Chung P, Adam H, et al. Ceftolozane/tazobactam: a novel cephalosporin/beta-lactamase inhibitor combination with activity against multidrug-resistant gram-negative bacilli. *Drugs.* 2014;74(1):31–51.
106. Shields RK, Nguyen MH, Chen L, et al. Ceftazidime-avibactam is superior to other treatment regimens against carbapenem-resistant *Klebsiella pneumoniae* bacteremia. *Antimicrob Agents Chemother.* 2017;61(8):AAC.00883-1.
107. van Duin D, Lok JJ, Earley M, et al. Colistin versus ceftazidime-avibactam in the treatment of infections due to carbapenem-resistant Enterobacteriaceae. *Clin Infect Dis.* 2018;66(2):163–171.
108. Wunderink RG, Giamarellos-Bourboulis EJ, Rahav G, et al. Effect and safety of meropenem-vaborbactam versus best-available therapy in patients with carbapenem-resistant Enterobacteriaceae infections: The TANGO II Randomized Clinical Trial. *Infect Dis Ther.* 2018;7(4):439–455.
109. Rodvold KA, George JM, Yoo L. Penetration of anti-infective agents into pulmonary epithelial lining fluid: focus on antibacterial agents. *Clin Pharmacokinet.* 2011;50(10):637–664.
110. Rybak MJ, Lomaestro BM, Rotschafer JC, et al. Vancomycin therapeutic guidelines: a summary of consensus recommendations from the infectious diseases Society of America, the American Society of Health-System Pharmacists, and the Society of Infectious Diseases Pharmacists. *Clin Infect Dis.* 2009;49(3):325–327.
111. Zasowski EJ, Lodise TP. The importance of individualized vancomycin dosing to ensure optimal exposure early in therapy. *J Clin Pharmacol.* 2018. doi: 10.1002/jcph.1281.
112. Rybak MJ, Le J, Lodise TP, et al. Therapeutic monitoring of vancomycin for serious methicillin-resistant Staphylococcus aureus infections: A revised consensus guideline and review by the American Society of Health-System Pharmacists, the Infectious Diseases Society of America, the Pediatric Infectious Diseases Society, and the Society of Infectious Diseases Pharmacists. *Am J Health Syst Pharm.* 2020;77:835–864. 10.1093/ajhp/zxaa036.
113. Drusano GL, Ambrose PG, Bhavnani SM, Bertino JS, Nafziger AN, Louie A. Back to the future: using aminoglycosides again and how to dose them optimally. *Clin Infect Dis.* 2007;45(6):753–760.
114. Nicolau DP, Freeman CD, Belliveau PP, Nightingale CH, Ross JW, Quintiliani R. Experience with a once-daily aminoglycoside program administered to 2,184 adult patients. *Antimicrob Agents Chemother.* 1995;39(3):650–655.
115. Zasowski E, Butterfield JM, McNutt LA, et al. Relationship between time to clinical response and outcomes among Pneumonia Outcomes Research Team (PORT) Risk Class III and IV hospitalized patients with community-acquired pneumonia who received ceftriaxone and azithromycin. *Antimicrob Agents Chemother.* 2014;58(7):3804–3813.
116. Uranga A, Espana PP, Bilbao A, et al. Duration of antibiotic treatment in community-acquired pneumonia: a multicenter randomized clinical trial. *JAMA Intern Med.* 2016;176(9):1257–1265.
117. Tablan OC, Anderson LJ, Besser R, Bridges C, Hajjeh R. Guidelines for preventing health-care–associated pneumonia, 2003: recommendations of CDC and the Healthcare Infection Control Practices Advisory Committee. *MMWR Recomm Rep.* 2004;53(Rr-3):1–36.
118. Pereira JM, Paiva JA, Rello J. Assessing severity of patients with community-acquired pneumonia. *Semin Respir Crit Care Med.* 2012;33(3):272–283.
119. Pogue JM, Kaye KS, Veve MP, et al. Ceftolozane/tazobactam vs polymyxin or aminoglycoside-based regimens for the treatment of drug-resistant *Pseudomonas aeruginosa. Clin Infect Dis.* 2019;71:304–310. 10.1093/cid/ciz816.
120. Finch NA, Zasowski EJ, Murray KP, et al. A quasi-experiment to study the impact of vancomycin area under the concentration-time curve-guided dosing on vancomycin-associated nephrotoxicity. *Antimicrob Agents Chemother.* 2017;61(12):e01293-17. 10.1128/aac.01293-17.

Upper Respiratory Tract Infections

130

Grace C. Lee, Bradi L. Frei, and Christopher R. Frei

KEY CONCEPTS

1. Many upper respiratory tract infections are due to viral etiologies and will resolve spontaneously without pharmacologic therapy.
2. The most common bacterial causes are *Streptococcus pneumoniae* (acute otitis media and acute rhinosinusitis) and group A β-hemolytic *Streptococcus* (acute pharyngitis).
3. Vaccination against influenza and pneumococcus may decrease the risk of acute otitis media.
4. Distinguishing between viral and bacterial causes for upper respiratory tract infections may be difficult, and antimicrobials are often prescribed inappropriately leading to antimicrobial resistance.
5. When antimicrobials are indicated, amoxicillin or amoxicillin-clavulanate is first-line for acute otitis media, amoxicillin-clavulanate for acute rhinosinusitis, and amoxicillin or penicillin for acute pharyngitis.
6. For acute otitis media, high-dose amoxicillin (80-90 mg/kg/day in two divided doses) is recommended.

BEYOND THE BOOK

Watch the videos entitled "What is an upper respiratory infection (URI)?", "What is sinusitis?", and "Pharyngitis" in Khan Academy. These videos provide an overview of common URI. Compare and contrast infectious etiologies, diagnoses, and clinical presentation of these conditions.

INTRODUCTION

Upper respiratory tract infection is the most common reason for visits to primary care providers. There are over 25 million office visits per year for acute upper respiratory tract infections.[1] Otitis media, rhinosinusitis, and pharyngitis are the three most common upper respiratory tract infections. Although most upper respiratory tract infections typically manifest as mild illnesses, their high incidence and transmissibility places these infections as a leading cause of missed work or school days. The majority of these illnesses are caused by viruses; however, distinguishing patients with viral versus bacterial infection poses challenges as signs and symptoms are generally similar. Upper respiratory tract infections remain the leading condition for antibiotic prescribing, often inappropriately, and thereby serve as catalysts for the emergence and spread of antibiotic resistance. The prudent use of antibiotics for upper respiratory tract infections is critically important.

ACUTE OTITIS MEDIA

Acute otitis media comes from the Latin *oto-* for "ear," *itis* for "inflammation," and *medi-* for "middle"; otitis media, then, is an inflammation of the middle ear. There are three subtypes of otitis media: acute otitis media, otitis media with effusion, and chronic otitis media. Acute otitis media is the subtype with the greatest role for antibiotics and will be discussed in detail.

Epidemiology

Acute otitis media is primarily an infection during childhood and is the most common pediatric infection for prescribing an antibiotic in the United States. There are more than 709 million cases of otitis media worldwide each year; half of these cases occur in children under 5 years of age.[2] Most cases of acute otitis media occur in young children ages 6 to 24 months. Fortunately, the incidence of acute otitis media has declined over the past two decades, and a downward trend in acute otitis media healthcare visits have been observed in children younger than 5 years of age from 2001 to 2011. The introduction of routine pneumococcal vaccinations in infants may have been a major contributor to this decline, coinciding with the introduction of the seven-valent pneumococcal conjugate vaccine (PCV-7) in 2000, that was updated with PCV-13 starting in 2010.[3]

Etiology

(1) Acute otitis media frequently occurs following an initial viral upper respiratory illness (eg, common cold) that often predisposes the patient to a bacterial otitis media. When comprehensive and sensitive microbiologic methods have been used in patients with a diagnosis of acute otitis media, bacteria have been found in more than 80% of cases.[4]

(2) Common bacterial pathogens include *Streptococcus pneumoniae*, nontypeable *Haemophilus influenzae*, and *Moraxella catarrhalis*.[5] *S. pneumoniae* and *H. influenzae* together cause up to 60% of all pediatric cases. *Staphylococcus aureus* including methicillin-resistant *S. aureus* is uncommon in children, although it is an emerging pathogen in adult.

S. pneumoniae is an important cause of acute otitis media. Among children, there has been a dramatic shift in the microbial etiology after the introduction and widespread use of the pneumococcal conjugate vaccines. Specifically, the proportion of *S. pneumoniae* cases has declined over time, and the proportion of *H. influenzae* cases has risen.[4–6]

S. pneumoniae, H. influenzae, and *M. catarrhalis* can all possess resistance to β-lactams. *S. pneumoniae* develops resistance through alteration of penicillin-binding proteins, whereas *H. influenzae* and *M. catarrhalis* produce β-lactamases.

Pathophysiology

Acute otitis media usually follows a viral upper respiratory tract infection that impairs the mucociliary apparatus and causes

CLINICAL PRESENTATION Acute Otitis Media

General

- Cases of acute otitis media often follow viral upper respiratory tract infections or an exacerbation of seasonal allergic rhinitis. Nonverbal children with ear pain might hold, rub, or tug their ear. Infants might cry, be irritable, or have difficulty sleeping.

Signs and Symptoms

- Bulging of the tympanic membrane
- Reduced tympanic membrane mobility (pneumatoscopy)
- Otorrhea
- Otalgia (considered to be moderate or severe if pain lasts at least 48 hours)
- Diminished hearing
- Fever (considered to be severe if temperature is 39°C [102.2°F] or higher)
- Other signs reported include vertigo, nystagmus, and tinnitus

Data from Reference 3.

Eustachian tube dysfunction in the middle ear. The middle ear is the space behind the tympanic membrane, or eardrum. A noninfected ear has a thin, clear tympanic membrane. In otitis media, this space becomes blocked with fluid, resulting in a bulging and erythematous tympanic membrane. Acute otitis media results when bacteria from the nasopharynx enter the inflammatory fluid in the middle ear and are not cleared properly by the mucociliary system. The bacteria proliferate and cause infection. Children tend to be more susceptible to otitis media than adults because the anatomy of their Eustachian tube is shorter and more horizontal, facilitating bacterial entry into the middle ear.[7]

Clinical Presentation

Patients or caregivers frequently characterize acute otitis media as having an acute onset of otalgia (ear pain). For parents of young children, irritability and tugging on the ear are often the first clues that a child has acute otitis media. In adults, an upper respiratory tract infection or seasonal allergic rhinitis episode often predisposes the onset of acute otitis media. In adults it is usually unilateral with ear pain and muffled hearing. If the tympanic membrane is ruptured, a sudden relief of pain followed by purulent otorrhea may be reported.

The diagnosis of acute otitis media includes demonstration of fluid in the middle ear. The American Academy of Pediatrics (AAP) guidelines have stringent diagnostic criteria to ensure accurate diagnosis. Children should be diagnosed with acute otitis media if they have middle ear effusion *and* either (1) moderate-to-severe bulging of the tympanic membrane *or* new onset otorrhea not due to acute otitis externa, or (2) mild bulging of the tympanic membrane *and* onset of ear pain within the last 48 hours or intense erythema of the tympanic membrane. Middle ear effusion should be identified based on pneumatic otoscopy and/or tympanometry.[4]

The diagnoses of acute otitis media and otitis media with effusion are easily confused, and careful attention to history, signs, and symptoms is important. Otitis media with effusion is characterized by fluid in the middle ear without signs and symptoms of acute ear infection, such as pain and a bulging eardrum.[8]

TREATMENT

Desired Outcomes

6 Treatment goals include pain management and prudent antibiotic use.

3 Pneumococcal conjugate vaccine (PCV) and annual influenza vaccination should be assessed in all children according to the Advisory Committee on Immunization Practices (ACIP) schedule from the United States Centers for Disease Control and Prevention.[3] Also, because acute otitis media cases often follow influenza cases, influenza vaccination should be considered as a possible means to prevent acute otitis media.

General Approach to Treatment

The first step in treatment is to differentiate acute otitis media from otitis media with effusion or chronic otitis media, as the latter two types do not necessitate antibiotic therapy. Risk factors and disease severity of acute otitis media are assessed when considering initiation of antibiotic therapy. Amoxicillin is the mainstay of therapy and can overcome penicillin resistance, in many cases, with higher doses. The therapeutic strategy should be changed if complications develop or if symptoms fail to resolve within 3 days.

Pharmacologic Therapy

National clinical practice guidelines for diagnosis and management of acute otitis media (updated in 2013) are focused on children 6 months to 12 years of age with uncomplicated cases and without underlying conditions that may alter the natural course of the disease.[4] The decision to administer antibiotics or initially observe the patient ("watchful waiting") depends on patient age, symptom severity, laterality, and joint decision-making.

- Antibiotic therapy should be initiated for:
- Children 6 months and older with acute otitis media showing severe symptoms (ie, toxic-appearing, persistent ear pain lasting more than 48 hours, or temperature of 39°C [102.2°F] or higher)
- Children 6 months and older with acute otitis media with otorrhea
- Children 6 to 23 months of age, with bilateral acute otitis media
- Observation without initial antibiotic treatment can be considered for:
- Children 6 months and older with nonsevere unilateral acute otitis media without otorrhea
- Children 24 months and older with bilateral acute otitis media without otorrhea

Initial observation (watchful waiting) should be based on joint decision-making with parents/caregivers, and must include a plan to initiate antibiotics if the child's symptoms worsen or decline within 48 to 72 hours of symptom onset.[4] The central principle is to administer antibiotics quickly when the diagnosis is certain, but to withhold antibiotics, at least initially, when the diagnosis is uncertain.

4 Antibiotic therapy for upper respiratory diseases must be balanced with possible increases in adverse drug events and

increased antibiotic pressure to cause bacterial resistance. Systematic reviews and randomized controlled trials suggest a moderate benefit of antibiotics for the treatment of acute otitis media, including a marked decline in suppurative complications, and improved outcomes in both early- and late-phases.[9,10] On the other hand, rates of adverse effects, such as diarrhea and diaper rash are higher for children who receive antibiotics for acute otitis media.

There are no national guideline recommendations for the treatment of acute otitis media among adults. Data regarding the etiologies and safety of withholding antibiotics are limited for adults. Because acute otitis media is unusual among adults without underlying risk factors where complications might be significant, the general recommendation is to treat adults with empiric antibiotic therapy.[5] Choice of antibiotic regimens should be based on (1) coverage of the common bacterial pathogens (see Etiology), and (2) allergy, tolerance, previous exposure to antibiotics, costs, and resistance levels. Table 130-1 lists antibiotic recommendations for acute otitis media.

5 Amoxicillin is the first-line therapy for most children.[4] Exceptions include: children who have received amoxicillin in the last 30 days, have concurrent purulent conjunctivitis, or have a history of recurrent infection unresponsive to amoxicillin. These patients should receive amoxicillin-clavulanate instead of amoxicillin. Patients with otitis conjunctivitis syndrome are more likely to be infected with nontypeable *H. influenzae*, hence the need for a β-lactamase inhibitor (such as clavulanate).[4] Clinicians should reassess the plan if the child's symptoms worsen or decline within 48 to 72 hours of symptom onset.[4]

High-dose amoxicillin (80-90 mg/kg/day in two divided doses) is recommended for most pediatric patients with acute otitis media. Amoxicillin has the best pharmacodynamic profile against drug-resistant *S. pneumoniae* of all available oral antibiotics. In addition, amoxicillin has a long record of safety, possesses a narrow spectrum of activity, is inexpensive, and is more palatable than other options. Higher middle ear fluid concentrations of amoxicillin, as a result of higher dosing, overcome most drug-resistant *S. pneumoniae*.[3] Its excellent efficacy against *S. pneumoniae* outweighs the issue of β-lactamase-producing *H. influenzae* and *M. catarrhalis*, against which amoxicillin may not be effective. This is because both *H. influenzae* and *M. catarrhalis* are more likely than *S. pneumoniae* to lead to a spontaneous resolution of the infection.

A patient who has received amoxicillin in the last 30 days, has concurrent purulent conjunctivitis, or has a history of recurrent infection unresponsive to amoxicillin should receive high-dose amoxicillin-clavulanate (90 mg/kg/day of amoxicillin, with 6.4 mg/kg/day of clavulanate, in two divided doses) instead of amoxicillin. Amoxicillin-clavulanate has activity against β-lactamase-producing *H. influenzae* and *M. catarrhalis* as well as drug-resistant *S. pneumoniae*.[4]

In most adults, the first-line treatment is amoxicillin-clavulanate 875 mg with clavulanate 125 mg orally twice daily. A higher dose of the amoxicillin component (2,000 mg) with clavulanate is recommended for patients with clinical or epidemiologic risk for severe infections or infections due to penicillin nonsusceptible *S. pneumoniae* (those who live in regions with >10% penicillin nonsusceptible *S. pneumoniae*, 65 years and older, immunocompromised, recent hospitalizations, or have used antibiotics in the past month).[5]

Other antibiotic choices include cefdinir, cefuroxime, cefpodoxime, and intramuscular or intravenous ceftriaxone.[4] Second-generation cephalosporins, though β-lactamase stable, are expensive, have an increased incidence of side effects, and may increase selective pressure for resistant bacteria. Furthermore, most cephalosporins do not achieve adequate middle ear fluid concentrations against drug-resistant *S. pneumoniae* for the desired duration of the dosing interval. Amoxicillin and intramuscular ceftriaxone and amoxicillin are the only antibiotics that achieve middle ear fluid concentrations above the minimal inhibitory concentration (MIC) for greater than 40% of the dosing interval. Although single doses of ceftriaxone have been used, daily doses for 3 days are recommended to optimize clinical outcomes.[4] Ceftriaxone is more expensive than amoxicillin, and the intramuscular injections are painful.

Patients with a penicillin allergy can be treated with several alternative antibiotics, including a cephalosporin in patients without history of severe or type 1 penicillin allergy. Use of

TABLE 130-1 Antibiotics and Doses for Acute Otitis Media

Antibiotic	Brand Name	Dose	Comments[a]
Initial Diagnosis			
Amoxicillin	Amoxil®	80-90 mg/kg/day orally divided twice daily	First-line
Amoxicillin-clavulanate	Augmentin®	90 mg/kg/day orally of amoxicillin plus 6.4 mg/kg/day orally of clavulanate, divided twice daily	First-line if certain criteria are present[b]
Cefdinir, Cefuroxime, Cefpodoxime	Omnicef®, Ceftin®, Vantin®	Cefdinir (14 mg/kg/day orally in 1-2 doses), Cefuroxime (30 mg/kg/day orally divided in two daily, Cefpodoxime (10 mg/kg/day orally divided in two daily doses)	Second-line or nonsevere penicillin allergy
Ceftriaxone	Rocephin®	50 mg/kg/day IM or IV once daily for 3 days	Second-line or nonsevere penicillin allergy
Failure at 48-72 Hours			
Amoxicillin-clavulanate[b]	Augmentin®	90 mg/kg/day orally of amoxicillin plus 6.4 mg/kg/day orally of clavulanate, divided twice daily	First-line
Ceftriaxone	Rocephin®	50 mg/kg/day IM or IV once daily for 3 days	First-line or nonsevere penicillin allergy

IM, intramuscular; IV, intravenous

[a]Amoxicillin-clavulanate 90:6.4 or 14:1 ratio is available in the United States; 7:1 ratio is available in Canada (use amoxicillin 45 mg/kg for one dose, amoxicillin 45 mg/kg with clavulanate 6.4 mg/kg for second dose).

[b]If a patient has received amoxicillin in the last 30 days, has concurrent purulent conjunctivitis, or has a history of recurrent infection unresponsive to amoxicillin.

Data from Reference 4.

trimethoprim-sulfamethoxazole and erythromycin-sulfisoxazole is discouraged because of high rates of resistance. Notably, clindamycin lacks efficacy against *H. influenzae*. Cefdinir or azithromycin (Zithromax) should be the first-line antibiotic in those with penicillin allergy based on risk of cephalosporin allergy.

There is ongoing debate regarding the optimal duration of therapy for acute otitis media. Duration is based on age and severity of symptoms. Traditional recommendations call for 10 days of antibiotic therapy; however, some experts have speculated that patients can be treated for as little as 5 to 7 days. Short-course treatment is not recommended in children younger than 2 years of age.[11] In children at least 6 years of age who have uncomplicated acute otitis media, a 5- to 7-day treatment course may be used.[4]

Recurrent acute otitis media is defined as at least three episodes in 6 months or four episodes in 1 year, with one episode in the preceding 6 months. Recurrent episodes are of concern because children younger than 3 years of age are at high risk for hearing loss and language and learning disabilities. Clinicians should avoid prophylactic antibiotics against recurrent episodes, but they may offer tympanostomy tubes (T tubes).[4]

Adjunctive Therapy

Children with acute otitis media should be assessed and treated for pain. Those with pain should be recommended analgesics to reduce pain regardless of the decision to administer antibiotics.[4] This is largely because antibiotics do not reduce pain in the first 24 hours. Furthermore, some children may experience some pain up to 3 to 7 days even after antibiotics are started. Choice of pain treatment depends on possible benefits and risks to the individual patient. Acetaminophen and ibuprofen are mainstays of treatment, are effective analgesics for mild-to-moderate pain, and are readily available. Eardrops with a local anesthetic may offer additional, but brief, benefit over acetaminophen in patients at least 5 years of age.[4] Finally, several studies have documented the large risk reductions in pediatric pneumococcal acute otitis media.[12,13] Thus, routine assessment of vaccination schedules is essential for prevention.

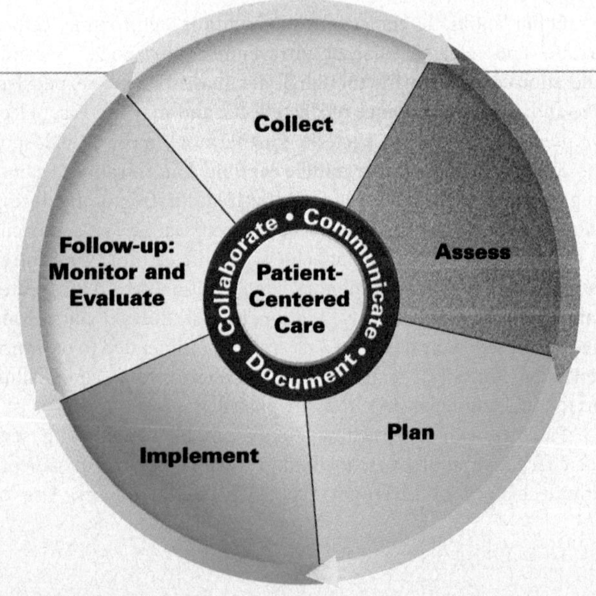

Patient Care Process for Acute Otitis Media

Collect

- Patient characteristics (eg, age, weight)
- Patient history (eg, past infections, current and past antibiotic/antiviral use noting previous failures, medication allergies)
- Determine whether patient has concurrent purulent conjunctivitis
- Objective data:
  - Temperature
  - Signs and symptoms (see Clinical Presentation)
  - Presence of congestion, fullness, purulent discharge, or pain in the ear
  - Presence of redness, fullness, bulging, or limited/absent mobility of the tympanic membrane

Assess

- Infection status, including presence of signs and symptoms
- Determine which symptoms may need additional therapy (eg, ongoing ear pain)
- Use information collected, patient factors (eg, patient age, symptom severity, laterality), and joint decision-making with parents/caregivers to determine whether antibiotics are needed
- If antibiotics are appropriate, determine proper choice of antibiotic, dose, duration, and dosage form
  - Determine if the patient meets criteria for high-dose amoxicillin-clavulanate
  - Determine whether a short-course of therapy (5-7 days) may be appropriate

Plan

- Select drug therapy regimen including specific antibiotic, dose, route, frequency, and duration; specify the continuation and discontinuation of existing therapies (see Table 130-1)
- Monitor efficacy (eg, temperature, pain), safety (eg, medication-specific adverse effects), and time frame
- Educate patient and/or caregiver (eg, purpose of treatment, drug therapy) emphasizing adherence to treatment regimen

Implement*

- Provide patient education regarding the infection and all elements of treatment plan
- Use motivational interviewing and coaching strategies to maximize adherence
- Schedule follow-up, when indicated
- Recommend measures to reduce ear pain, if present

Follow-up: Monitor and Evaluate

- Improvement/resolution of signs and symptoms; reassess the plan if the child's symptoms worsen or decline within 48 to 72 hours of symptom onset
- Presence of adverse effects, particularly allergic reactions and diarrhea
- Patient adherence to treatment plan using multiple sources of information
- Recommend pneumococcal conjugate vaccine and annual influenza vaccination

**Collaborate with patient, caregiver(s), and other healthcare professionals.*

Evaluation of Therapeutic Outcomes

Patients with acute otitis media should be reassessed after 48 to 72 hours. By this time, there should be clinical improvement in the signs and symptoms of infection, including pain, fever, and erythema/bulging of the tympanic membrane. If the patient has not responded and antibiotics were withheld initially, they should be instituted now.[14] If the patient initially received an antibiotic, then the antibiotic should be changed (Table 130-1). A switch in regimen is recommended if there is no clinical improvement by the third day of therapy, given the possibility of infection with a β-lactamase-producing strain of *H. influenzae* or *M. catarrhalis* or with a strain of penicillin-resistant *S. pneumoniae.* Most children will become asymptomatic within 7 days. Tympanocentesis for culture of middle ear fluid can be considered for treatment failure or persistent acute otitis media. It has a therapeutic effect of relieving pain and pressure and can be used to collect fluid to identify the causative agent.

Early reevaluation of the eardrum when signs and symptoms are improving can be misleading because effusions persist. Over a period of 1 week, changes in the eardrum normalize, and the pus becomes serous fluid. Air-fluid levels are apparent behind the eardrum, at which point the stage is now referred to as *otitis media with effusion*. This does not represent ongoing infection, nor are additional antibiotics required.[4]

Immediate reevaluation is appropriate if hearing loss results from persistent middle ear effusions following infection. Complications of otitis media are infrequent but include mastoiditis, bacteremia, meningitis, and auditory sequelae with the potential for speech and language impairment.[4]

ACUTE BACTERIAL RHINOSINUSITIS

Sinusitis is an inflammation and/or infection of the paranasal sinuses, or membrane-lined air spaces, around the nose.[15] The term *rhinosinusitis* is preferred because sinusitis typically also involves the nasal mucosa.[15] Even though the majority of rhinosinusitis infections are viral in origin, antibiotics are frequently prescribed. It is important to differentiate between viral and bacterial rhinosinusitis to avoid unnecessary antibiotic use.

The most current clinical practice guidelines for acute bacterial rhinosinusitis were published in 2012 by the Infectious Diseases Society of America (IDSA) and 2015 by the American Academy of Otolaryngology—Head and Neck Surgery Foundation (AAO-HNSF).[15,16]

Epidemiology

1 Nearly 30 million cases of rhinosinusitis are diagnosed annually in the United States.[17] Adults with rhinosinusitis miss an average of 1 to 2 workdays/year with these infections and experience significant activity, work, and social limitations.[16] Most episodes of acute sinusitis are caused by viral upper respiratory tract infection; however, the lack of clinical criteria to accurately differentiate bacterial from viral infections leads to inappropriate use of antibiotics and remains the fifth leading diagnosis for which antibiotics are prescribed.[14,18]

Etiology

2 Acute bacterial rhinosinusitis is caused, most often, by the same bacteria implicated in acute otitis media: *S. pneumoniae* and nontypeable *H. influenzae.* These organisms are responsible for approximately 50% to 70% of bacterial causes of acute bacterial rhinosinusitis in both adults and children.[15] *M. catarrhalis* is also sometimes implicated in children (approximately 8%-16%) and less commonly in adults.[15] *Streptococcus spp., S. aureus*, gram-negative bacilli, atypical bacteria, and anaerobes are associated less frequently with acute bacterial rhinosinusitis.[15] Healthcare-associated cases can be attributable to pathogens prevalent in the healthcare environment including *S. aureus*, methicillin-resistant *S. aureus* (MRSA), *P. aeruginosa*, *K. pneumoniae*, and other gram negatives; and often are polymicrobial.

Pathophysiology

Acute bacterial rhinosinusitis is often preceded by a viral respiratory tract infection that causes mucosal inflammation. This can lead to obstruction of the sinus ostia—the pathways that drain the sinuses. Mucosal secretions become trapped, local defenses are impaired, and bacteria from adjacent surfaces begin to proliferate. The maxillary and ethmoid sinuses are most frequently involved. The pathogenesis of chronic rhinosinusitis has not been well studied. Whether it is caused by more persistent pathogens or a subtle defect in the host's immune function, some patients develop chronic symptoms after their acute infection. Rarely, life-threatening complications of sinusitis can include meningitis, epidural, or cerebral abscess.

CLINICAL PRESENTATION Acute Bacterial Rhinosinusitis

General

The diagnosis of acute bacterial sinusitis involves assessing signs and symptoms, distinguishing bacterial from viral infection with temporal patterns of the illness. Patients manifest with focused sinonasal symptoms compared to those with viral URIs. Acute sinusitis manifests with up to 4 weeks of purulent nasal drainage.

Signs and Symptoms

- Purulent anterior nasal discharge, purulent or discolored posterior nasal discharge, nasal congestion or obstruction, facial congestion or fullness, facial pain or pressure, fever, headache, ear pain/pressure/fullness, halitosis, dental pain, cough, and fatigue
- Clinical presentations (any of 3) that are most consistent with acute bacterial versus viral rhinosinusitis:
  - i) Onset with *persistent* signs or symptoms compatible, lasting for ≥10 days without any evidence of clinical improvement
  - ii) Onset with *severe* signs or symptoms of high fever (≥39°C [102.2°F]) and purulent nasal discharge or facial pain lasting for at least 3 to 4 consecutive days at the beginning of illness
  - iii) Onset with *worsening* signs or symptoms characterized by new-onset fever, headache, or increase in nasal discharge following a typical viral URI that lasted 5 to 6 days and were initially improving ("double sickening")

Data from Reference 15.

TREATMENT

Desired Outcomes

The goals of treatment for acute bacterial rhinosinusitis are to reduce signs and symptoms, achieve and maintain patency of the ostia, limit antibiotic treatment to those who may benefit, eradicate the bacterial infection with appropriate antibiotic therapy, minimize the duration of illness, prevent complications, and prevent progression from acute disease to chronic disease.

General Approach to Treatment

4 The first step is to differentiate viral and bacterial rhinosinusitis. This is based on disease duration, initial severity of illness, and worsening symptomatology. Viral rhinosinusitis typically improves in 7 to 10 days. In contrast, acute bacterial rhinosinusitis symptoms persist for 10 days or greater without improvement or with worsening symptoms after 10 days, or can manifest worsening after initial improvement ("double-sickness" pattern).[16] Acute bacterial rhinosinusitis may also be suspected if the patient has severe symptoms at the beginning of his/her illness. Management involves antibiotic therapy or watchful waiting based on shared decision making. Amoxicillin-clavulanate is the first-line antibiotic therapy for patients with acute bacterial rhinosinusitis.[15]

Urgent early referral to a specialist is essential for patients exhibiting complicated acute bacterial rhinosinusitis. Indications for referral include high, persistent fevers, periorbital edema or inflammation, mental status changes, visual disturbances, severe headache, immunosuppressive illness, healthcare-associated infections,

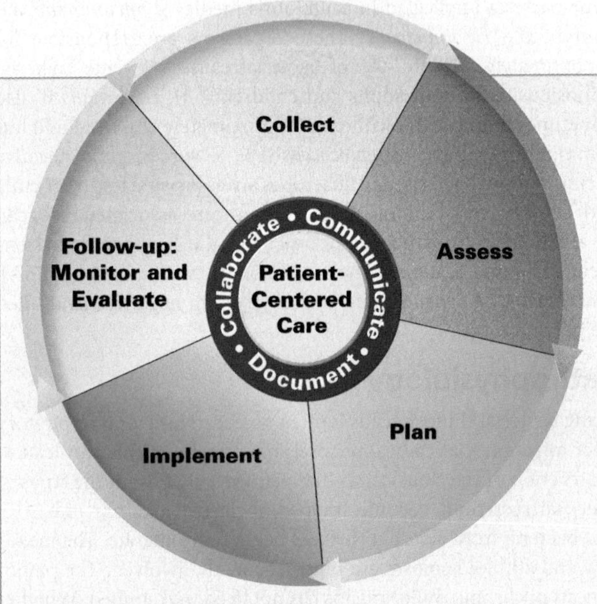

Patient Care Process for Acute Bacterial Rhinosinusitis

Collect

- Patient characteristics (eg, age, weight, comorbidities)
- Patient history (eg, past infections, current and past antibiotic/antiviral use noting previous failures, medication allergies, history of allergic rhinitis)
- Recent healthcare exposures or procedures
- Temporal patterns of symptoms
- Determine whether patient is in daycare, is a daycare worker, or has a child in daycare
- Objective data:
  - Temperature
  - Signs and symptoms (see Clinical Presentation)
  - Presence of congestion, fullness, or pain in the nose, face, or ear
  - Presence of purulent or discolored nasal discharge
  - Other diagnostic tests, when indicated (eg, computerized tomography scan (CT), sinus puncture)

Assess

- Infection status, including presence and severity of signs and symptoms
- Determine which symptoms may need additional therapy (eg, ongoing nose pain)
- Decide if referral is needed (eg, mental status changes, visual disturbances, immunosuppressive illness, nosocomial infections, anatomic defects, unilateral findings)
- Use information collected, patient factors (eg, patient age, symptom severity), and joint decision making with parents/caregivers to determine whether antibiotics are needed
- If antibiotics are appropriate, determine proper choice of antibiotic, dose, duration, and dosage form
  - Determine if the patient meets criteria for high-dose amoxicillin-clavulanate

Plan*

- Select drug therapy regimen including specific antibiotic, dose, route, frequency, and duration; specify the continuation and discontinuation of existing therapies (see Tables 126-2 and 126-3)
- Monitor efficacy (eg, temperature, pain), safety (eg, medication-specific adverse effects), and time frame
- Educate patient and/or caregiver (eg, purpose of treatment, drug therapy) emphasizing adherence to treatment regimen

Implement

- Provide patient education regarding the infection and all elements of treatment plan
- Use motivational interviewing and coaching strategies to maximize adherence
- Schedule follow-up, when indicated
- Recommend symptomatic measures to reduce nose pain and inflammation

Follow-up: Monitor and Evaluate

- Improvement/resolution of signs and symptoms; reassess the plan if the patient's symptoms worsen or decline within 48 to 72 hours of symptom onset
- Presence of adverse effects, particularly allergic reactions and diarrhea
- Patient adherence to treatment plan using multiple sources of information

Collaborate with patient, caregiver(s), and other healthcare professionals.

anatomic defects causing obstruction, unusually severe symptoms, multiple recurrent episodes (three to four times per year), unilateral findings, significant coexisting illnesses, risk factors for unusual or resistant pathogens, and history of antibiotic failure. The specialist may perform computed tomography to assess the severity and extent of disease and identify the underlying causes.

Pharmacologic Therapy

The IDSA published clinical practice guidelines in 2012 that are the primary source for many of the statements in this chapter.[15] Additional guidance and recommendations come from a 2015 update of the 2007 guidelines from AAO-HNSF.[16] There are two major differences in the IDSA and AAO-HNSF guidelines. The AAO-HNSF guidelines endorse watchful waiting, without antibiotics, unless symptoms fail to improve within 7 days.[16] When antibiotics are given, the AAO-HNSF endorses amoxicillin as first-line treatment, instead of amoxicillin-clavulanate.[16] In contrast, the IDSA guidelines support initiating empiric therapy as soon as the clinical diagnosis of acute bacterial rhinosinusitis is established and amoxicillin-clavulanate rather than amoxicillin alone as first-line treatment.[15]

5 Amoxicillin-clavulanate is considered the first-line treatment for acute bacterial rhinosinusitis in children and adults according to IDSA guidelines (Tables 130-2 and 130-3).[15] In contrast, prior guidelines, and the AAO-HNSF guidelines,[16] list amoxicillin as the first-line treatment option due to its safety,

TABLE 130-2 Antibiotics and Doses for Acute Bacterial Rhinosinusitis in Children

Antibiotic	Brand Name	Dose	Comments
Initial Empirical Therapy			
Amoxicillin-clavulanate	Augmentin®	45 mg/kg/day orally twice daily	First line
Amoxicillin-clavulanate	Augmentin®	90 mg/kg/day orally twice daily	Second line
β-Lactam Allergy			
Clindamycin plus cefixime or cefpodoxime	Cleocin®, Suprax®, Vantin®	Clindamycin (30-40 mg/kg/day orally three times daily) cefixime (8 mg/kg/day orally twice daily) or efpodoxime (10 mg/kg/day orally twice daily)	Non-type 1 allergy
Levofloxacin	Levaquin®	10-20 mg/kg/day orally every 12-24 hours	Type 1 allergy
Risk for Antibiotic Resistance or Failed Initial Therapy			
Amoxicillin-clavulanate	Augmentin®	90 mg/kg/day orally twice daily	
Clindamycin plus cefixime or cefpodoxime	Cleocin®, Suprax®, Vantin®	Clindamycin (30-40 mg/kg/day orally three times daily) plus Cefixime (8 mg/kg/day orally twice daily) or Cefpodoxime (10 mg/kg/day orally twice daily)	
Levofloxacin	Levaquin®	10-20 mg/kg/day orally every 12-24 hours	
Severe Infection Requiring Hospitalization			
Ampicillin-sulbactam	Unasyn®	200-400 mg/kg/day IV every 6 hours	
Ceftriaxone	Rocephin®	50 mg/kg/day IV every 12 hours	
Cefotaxime	Claforan®	100-200 mg/kg/day IV every 6 hours	
Levofloxacin	Levaquin®	10-20 mg/kg/day IV every 12-24 hours	

Data from Reference 15.

TABLE 130-3 Antibiotics and Doses for Acute Bacterial Rhinosinusitis in Adults

Antibiotic	Brand Name	Dose	Comments
Initial Empirical Therapy			
Amoxicillin-clavulanate	Augmentin®	500 mg/125 mg orally three times daily, or 875 mg/125 mg orally twice daily	First-line
Amoxicillin-clavulanate	Augmentin®	2,000 mg/125 mg orally twice daily	Second- line
Doxycycline		100 mg orally twice daily or 200 mg orally once daily	Second- line
β-Lactam Allergy			
Doxycycline		100 mg orally twice daily or 200 mg orally once daily	
Levofloxacin	Levaquin®	500 mg orally once daily	
Moxifloxacin	Avelox®	400 mg orally once daily	
Risk for Antibiotic Resistance or Failed Initial Therapy			
Amoxicillin-clavulanate	Augmentin®	2,000 mg/125 mg orally twice daily	
Levofloxacin	Levaquin®	500 mg orally once daily	
Moxifloxacin	Avelox®	400 mg orally once daily	
Severe Infection Requiring Hospitalization			
Ampicillin-sulbactam	Unasyn®	1.5-3 g IV every 6 hours	
Levofloxacin	Levaquin®	500 mg orally once daily	
Moxifloxacin	Avelox®	400 mg orally once daily	
Ceftriaxone	Rocephin®	1-2 g IV every 12-24 hours	
Cefotaxime	Claforan®	2 g IV every 4-6 hours	

Data from Reference 15.

narrow spectrum of activity, good tolerability, and favorable cost. The IDSA guidelines support the choice of amoxicillin-clavulanate based on (a) the emergence of *H. influenzae* as a more common cause of upper respiratory tract infections in children than in the past,[5] and (b) the high prevalence of β-lactam-producing respiratory pathogens in acute bacterial rhinosinusitis (particularly *H. influenzae* and *M. catarrhalis*). The advantage of using amoxicillin-clavulanate, as compared with amoxicillin, is a greater spectrum of coverage. The disadvantages are increased cost, greater risk of adverse effects including diarrhea, and an added risk of hypersensitivity to the clavulanate component.[15]

Symptomatic Management

Symptomatic management for acute rhinosinusitis aims to relieve symptoms due to nasal drainage and obstruction such as pain with use of analgesics. The following are recommended as adjunct to therapy in patients with acute bacterial rhinosinusitis[15]:

- Intranasal saline irrigation with either physiologic or hypertonic saline
- Intranasal corticosteroids as adjunct to antibiotics in the empiric treatment of acute bacterial rhinosinusitis, primarily in patients with a history of allergic rhinitis

Topical or oral decongestants or antihistamines are generally not recommended as adjunctive treatment for acute bacterial rhinosinusitis. These agents can dry mucosa and disturb clearance of mucosal secretions.

High-dose amoxicillin-clavulanate (eg, 2,000 mg twice daily or 90 mg/kg/day twice daily) is recommended in the following situations: (a) geographic regions with high endemic rates (10% or greater) of invasive penicillin-nonsusceptible *S. pneumoniae*, (b) severe infection, (c) attendance at daycare, (d) age less than 2 or greater than 65 years, (e) recent hospitalization, (f) antibiotic use within the last month, and (g) immunocompromised persons.[15] Severe infections are those with "evidence of systemic toxicity with fever of 39°C (102.2°F) or higher, and threat of suppurative complications."[15]

For those with a history of β-lactam allergy, levofloxacin monotherapy is recommended for children or combination therapy with clindamycin plus cefixime or cefpodoxime.[15] Adults with a penicillin allergy may receive doxycycline (not suitable for children), levofloxacin, or moxifloxacin monotherapy.[15] The ISDA guidelines also provide several options for patients at risk for antibiotic resistance, who failed initial therapy, or who have a severe infection requiring hospitalization (Tables 130-2 and 130-3).[15] Notably, cephalosporins are no longer recommended as monotherapy due to variable rates of resistance against *S. pneumoniae*.[15] Combination therapy with a third-generation oral cephalosporin plus clindamycin may be used in regions with high endemic rates of penicillin nonsusceptible *S. pneumoniae*. Macrolides are not recommended because of high rates of *S. pneumoniae* resistance (~30%).[15] Trimethoprim-sulfamethoxazole has not been recommended for some time due to resistance among *S. pneumoniae* and *H. influenzae* (~30-40%).[15]

The duration of therapy for the treatment of uncomplicated acute bacterial rhinosinusitis is 5 to 7 days for most adults. A longer duration of 10 to 14 days is still recommended for children.[15]

Evaluation of Therapeutic Outcomes

If symptoms persist or worsen after 48 to 72 hours of appropriate antibiotic therapy, then the patient should be reevaluated and alternative antibiotics should be considered.[15] Patients who do not respond to first- or second-line therapies should be referred to a specialist and evaluated more aggressively, potentially with direct sinus aspiration or contrast-enhanced computed tomography.[15]

ACUTE PHARYNGITIS

1 2 Pharyngitis is an acute infection of the oropharynx or nasopharynx.[19] The most common presenting symptom is sore throat. It is responsible for 6% of visits by children to their primary care provider annually.[20] Although viral causes are most common, group A β-hemolytic *Streptococcus* (GAS, also known as *S. pyogenes*) is the primary bacterial cause[19]; pharyngitis due to GAS is commonly known as "strep throat," accounting for 20% to 30% of cases among children and 5% to 15% among adults.

Epidemiology

Acute pharyngitis accounts for approximately 15 million healthcare visits per year, resulting in an economic burden of up to $539 million for children alone.[19]

Although all age groups are susceptible, the frequency is much greater in the pediatric population. Children 5 to 15 years of age are most susceptible; parents of school-aged children and those who work with children are also at increased risk.

Seasonal outbreaks occur, and the incidence of GAS is highest in winter and early spring.[19] The incubation period is 2 to 5 days, and the illness often occurs in clusters.[19] Spread occurs via direct contact (usually from hands) with droplets of saliva or nasal secretions, and transmission is thus worse in institutions, schools, families, and crowded areas.[19] Untreated patients with streptococcal pharyngitis are infectious during the acute illness and for another week thereafter. Effective antibiotic therapy reduces the infectious period to about 24 hours.

Acute rheumatic fever is rarely seen in developed countries. In the United States, acute rheumatic fever secondary to GAS infection was a cause of concern in the 1950s and was the major reason for penicillin therapy, but the annual incidence of this disease today is extremely rare (one case or more per 1 million population). Outbreaks have been reported in the United States as recently as the late 1980s and early 1990s. In developing countries, acute rheumatic fever and rheumatic heart disease is widespread affecting an estimated 20 million people worldwide making this a leading cause of cardiac death during the first five decades of life. This risk can be reduced by timely therapy.

Etiology

1 Viruses cause the majority of acute pharyngitis cases. Specific etiologies include rhinovirus (20%), coronavirus (5%), adenovirus (5%), herpes simplex virus (4%), influenza virus (2%), parainfluenza virus (2%), and Epstein–Barr virus (1%) and less frequently coxsackievirus A, cytomegalovirus, and acute human immunodeficiency virus (HIV) infection.[19]

4 GAS is the most common cause of pharyngitis (10%-30% of persons of all ages with pharyngitis) and is the only commonly occurring form of acute pharyngitis for which antibiotic therapy is indicated.[19] In the pediatric population, GAS causes 15% to 30% of pharyngitis cases. In adults, GAS is responsible for 5% to 15% of all symptomatic episodes of pharyngitis.[19] Pharyngitis in a child younger than 3 years of age is rarely caused by GAS.[19]

Other less common causes of acute pharyngitis are groups C and G *Streptococcus, Corynebacterium diphtheriae, Neisseria gonorrhoeae, Mycoplasma pneumoniae, Arcanobacterium haemolyticum, Yersinia enterocolitica*, and *Chlamydia pneumoniae*.[19] Treatment options for these organisms are not addressed in this chapter.

Pathophysiology

Streptococcal pharyngitis results from GAS proliferating in the pharynx, although exact mechanisms are not well defined. Asymptomatic pharyngeal carriers of the organism may have an alteration in host immunity (eg, a breach in the pharyngeal mucosa) and the bacteria of the oropharynx may migrate to cause an infection. Pathogenic

CLINICAL PRESENTATION Group A Streptococcal Pharyngitis

General

- A sore throat of sudden onset that is mostly self-limited.
- Fever and constitutional symptoms resolving in about 3 to 5 days.
- Clinical signs and symptoms are similar for viral causes and nonstreptococcal bacterial causes.

Signs and Symptoms of GAS Pharyngitis

- Sore throat
- Pain on swallowing
- Fever
- Headache, nausea, vomiting, and abdominal pain (especially in children)
- Erythema/inflammation of the tonsils and pharynx with or without patchy exudates
- Enlarged, tender lymph nodes
- Red swollen uvula, petechiae or purple spots on the soft palate, and a scarlatiniform rash

Signs Suggestive of Viral Origin for Pharyngitis

- Conjunctivitis
- Coryza
- Cough

Laboratory Tests

- Throat swab and culture
- Rapid antigen-detection test (RADT)

Data from Reference 19.

factors associated with the organism itself, pyrogenic toxins, hemolysins, streptokinase, and proteinase, may also play a role.

The primary goal of diagnosis is accurate differentiation of GAS from pharyngitis due to other agents (eg, viral). There is broad overlap between the signs and symptoms of pharyngitis from GAS versus viral or nonstreptococcal agents, and thus rarely can be differentiated based on clinical grounds alone even among the most experienced clinicians.

Guidelines from IDSA and the American Heart Association recommend swabbing the throat and testing for GAS in patients with signs and symptoms of streptococcal pharyngitis.[19] Only those with a positive test for GAS require antibiotic treatment.[19] Diagnostic studies are not indicated for children <3 years old because the incidence of streptococcal pharyngitis is uncommon in this age. Laboratory tests should not be performed in patients with clinical features that strongly suggest a viral etiology. This is because a positive test does not necessarily indicate disease. A positive test may simply indicate that the patient is a carrier for GAS and is not actively infected. Approximately 20% of children are carriers of GAS; the prevalence is lower among adults.[19]

Testing for GAS can be performed using a throat swab that can be sent for culture or used for the RADT. Cultures are the gold standard, but they require 24 to 48 hours for results. The RADT is more practical in that it provides results quickly, it can be performed at the bedside, and it is less expensive than culture. If RADT is positive, it does not require a follow-up throat culture.[19] If RADT yields negative test results, it is generally recommended to follow up with a throat culture to confirm the results for children and adolescents, but not necessary in adults.[19] Delaying therapy while awaiting culture results does not affect the risk of complications (though some argue that symptomatic benefit is postponed, and contagion remains), and patients must be educated as to the value of waiting, given the low false-negative rate of RADT.[19] The accurate diagnosis of streptococcal pharyngitis followed by appropriate antimicrobial therapy is important for the prevention of suppurative and nonsuppurative complications including acute rheumatic fever, acute glomerulonephritis, reactive arthritis, peritonsillar abscess, retropharyngeal abscess, cervical lymphadenitis, mastoiditis, otitis media, rhinosinusitis, and necrotizing fasciitis. In addition, accurate diagnosis would allow to improve outcomes, decrease transmission, and minimizing potential inappropriate antimicrobial therapy.

TREATMENT

Desired Outcomes

The goals of treatment for pharyngitis are to improve clinical signs and symptoms, minimize adverse drug reactions and overuse of antibiotics, prevent transmission to close contacts, and prevent acute rheumatic fever and suppurative complications, such as peritonsillar abscess, cervical lymphadenitis, and mastoiditis.[19]

General Approach to Treatment

Once the diagnosis of GAS pharyngitis has been made, the clinician must decide appropriate supportive care, when to initiate antibiotic therapy, the appropriate antibiotic, and the duration of therapy. The selection of appropriate antibiotic therapy will involve careful consideration of cost, safety, efficacy, potential for regimen adherence, and bacterial resistance rates. Clinicians should be aware of local resistance patterns, which may differ from the national patterns.

4 Inappropriate antibiotic use for acute pharyngitis has been a major contributor to the development antimicrobial resistance.[19] Approximately 60% of patients who visit their provider with a complaint of "sore throat are prescribed an antibiotic."[21, 22] This rate is well above the incidence of GAS pharyngitis. Antibiotic therapy should be reserved for those patients with clinical and epidemiologic features of GAS pharyngitis, preferably with a positive laboratory test. Empirical therapy is not recommended; however, if used while results are pending, it is important to discontinue empirical antibiotics once laboratory results come back as negative.

Pharmacologic Therapy

The clinical practice guidelines published by the IDSA in 2012 are the primary source for many of the recommendations in this section.[19] Tables 130-4 and 130-5 outline dosing for acute GAS pharyngitis and chronic carriers of GAS.

5 In the United States there have been no reported cases of penicillin-resistant GAS.[19] Because penicillin and amoxicillin have a narrow spectrum of activity and are readily available, safe, and inexpensive, they are considered to be the treatments of choice.[19]

Amoxicillin often used in place of penicillin V for children with GAS pharyngitis because the suspension is more palatable.[19]

TABLE 130-4 Antibiotics and Doses for Group A β-Hemolytic Streptococcal Pharyngitis

Antibiotic	Brand Name	Dose	Route / Duration	Rating
Preferred Antibiotics				
Penicillin V	Pen-V®	Children: 250 mg twice daily or three times daily. Adolescents and Adults: 250 mg four times daily or 500 mg twice daily	Orally 10 days	IB
Penicillin G benzathine	Bicillin L-A®	<27 kg: 0.6 million units; ≥ 27 kg : 1.2 million units	IM One dose	IB
Amoxicillin[a]	Amoxil®	50 mg/kg once daily (maximum 1 g); 25 mg/kg (maximum 500 mg) twice daily	Orally 10 days	IB
Penicillin Allergy				
Cephalexin	Keflex®	20 mg/kg/dose (maximum 500 mg)	Orally 10 days	IB
Cefadroxil	Duricef®	30 mg/kg once daily (maximum 1 g)	Orally 10 days	
Clindamycin	Cleocin®	7 mg/kg/dose three times daily (maximum 300 mg/dose)	Orally 10 days	IIaB
Azithromycin[b]	Zithromax®	12 mg/kg once daily (maximum 500 mg) for one day, then 6 mg/kg orally once daily (maximum 250 mg) for four days	Orallly 5 days	IIaB
Clarithromycin[b]	Biaxin®	7.5 mg/kg per (maximum 250 mg) twice daily	Orally 10 days	IIaB

These guidelines provide a systematic weighting of the strength of the recommendation (Class I, conditions for which there is evidence and/or general agreement that a given procedure or treatment is beneficial, useful, and effective; Class II, conditions for which there is conflicting evidence and/or a divergence of opinion about the usefulness/efficacy of a procedure or treatment; Class IIa, weight of evidence/opinion is in favor of usefulness/efficacy; Class IIb, usefulness/efficacy is less well established by evidence/opinion; Class III, conditions for which there is evidence and/or general agreement that a procedure/treatment is not useful/effective and in some cases may be harmful) and quality of evidence (A, data derived from multiple randomized clinical trials or meta-analyses; B, data derived from a single-randomized trial or nonrandomized studies; C, only consensus opinion of experts, case studies, or standard of care).

[a]Standard formulation, not extended release.

[b]Resistance of group A β-hemolytic *Streptococcus* (GAS) to these agents may vary and local susceptibilities should be considered with these agents.

Data from Reference 19.

TABLE 130-5 Antibiotics and Doses for Eradication of Group A β-Hemolytic Streptococcal Pharyngitis in Chronic Carriers

Antibiotic	Brand Name	Dose
Clindamycin	Cleocin®	20-30 mg/kg/day orally in three divided doses (maximum 300 mg/dose) for 10 days
Amoxicillin-clavulanate	Augmentin®	40 mg/kg/day orally in three divided doses (maximum 2,000 mg/day of amoxicillin) for 10 days
Penicillin V and rifampin	Pen-V®, Rifadin®	Penicillin V: 50 mg/kg/day orally in four divided doses for 10 days (maximum 2,000 mg/day); Rrifampin: 20 mg/kg/day orally in one dose for the last 4 days of treatment (maximum 600 mg/day)
Penicillin G benzathine and rifampin	Bicillin L-A®, Rifadin®	Penicillin G benzathine: <27 kg—0.6 million units once IM, ≥ 27 kg 1.2 million units once intramuscularly; *and* Rifampin: 20 mg/kg/day orally in two divided doses during last 4 days of treatment with penicillin (maximum 600 mg/day)

Data from Reference 19.

Gastrointestinal (GI) adverse effects and rash are more common with amoxicillin. A once-daily, extended-release formulation of amoxicillin has been approved for treatment of GAS pharyngitis in adults and children aged 12 years and older.[19] In addition, a number of antibiotics have been effective against GAS pharyngitis (Table 130-4). Most oral regimens are administered for 10 days.

In patients with nonanaphylactic penicillin allergy, a first-generation cephalosporin such as cephalexin is recommended for 10 days. For patients with type I immunoglobulin E (IgE)–mediated penicillin allergies, azithromycin, clarithromycin, or clindamycin is recommended for a duration of 10 days except 5 days with azithromycin. Clindamycin resistance among GAS is ~1% and 5% to 8% for macrolides in the United States, but is higher in some other areas of the world.[19]

A few antimicrobials are not recommended for GAS pharyngitis including tetracyclines due to high prevalence of resistance as well as sulfonamides and trimethoprim-sulfamethoxazole due to poor eradication rates for GAS.[19] Older fluoroquinolones such as ciprofloxacin have poor activity against GAS while newer fluoroquinolones have activity against GAS, but are expensive and have an unnecessarily broad spectrum of activity for this treatment for GAS pharyngitis.[19] Treatment early in the course leads to more rapid clinical response in symptoms, decreases contagiousness to others, and can prevent suppurative and nonsuppurative complications. The immediate therapy can be postponed up to 9 days without major nonsuppurative sequela.[19] Clinical guidelines recommend withholding antibiotics unless the patient has a positive laboratory result.[19]

The severity of pharyngitis symptoms and communicability of the disease is less after 24 hours of antibiotic therapy. The duration of therapy for GAS pharyngitis is 10 days, except for benzathine penicillin and azithromycin, to maximize bacterial eradication.[19] A systematic review of short- versus long-course therapies concluded that oral penicillin for 10 days (long course) remains first-line therapy.[23] Although some studies have suggested shorter courses of treatment for pharyngitis, confounding factors from these studies, such as the lack of strict entry criteria or differentiation between new and failed infections, limit the widespread application of short-antibiotic courses now.[19]

Approximately 33% of household contacts of a person with acute GAS pharyngitis harbor GAS in their upper respiratory tracts.[19] Routine testing and/or treating of asymptomatic household contacts of an index patient is not recommended.[19] GAS carriers do not need antimicrobial therapy due to low risk of spreading GAS pharyngitis or developing suppurative or nonsuppurative complications.[18] If tested, it is not necessary to treat asymptomatic carriers. It is difficult to ascertain the cause of symptomatic pharyngitis in carriers of GAS if they do develop symptoms. Clinicians need to differentiate whether the patient is experiencing a repeat GAS infection or a chronic carrier of GAS because laboratory tests will be positive in these patients.[19]

When acute GAS pharyngitis occurs in a carrier, a treatment course of appropriate antibiotics is recommended.[19] Table 130-5 outlines antimicrobials for the eradication of GAS in chronic carriers experiencing symptomatic episodes. In the treatment of recurring episodes of culture-positive GAS pharyngitis, there are several alternative antibiotics which are preferred over penicillin or amoxicillin with GAS carriers. Amoxicillin-clavulanate, clindamycin, penicillin/rifampin combination, and benzathine penicillin G/rifampin combination may be considered for recurrent episodes of pharyngitis to maximize bacterial eradication in potential carriers and to counter copathogens that produce β-lactamases.[19]

Factors that should be considered when personalizing therapy for a patient include allergy status, prior antibiotic use, and adherence. Those with a history of antibiotic use for acne may be at higher risk for resistant strains of GAS. Short-course antibiotics or penicillin G benzathine may be considered in patients with a history of nonadherence. Supportive care should be offered to all patients with acute pharyngitis including antipyretic medications, analgesics, and nonprescription lozenges and sprays containing menthol and topical anesthetics for temporary relief of pain.[19] There are limited data for use of corticosteroids to reduce the symptoms of GAS pharyngitis, and given the risk of adverse effects, their use is not recommended.[19] Because pain is often the primary reason for visiting a physician, emphasis on analgesics such as acetaminophen and nonsteroidal anti-inflammatory drugs to aid in pain relief is strongly recommended.

Evaluation of Therapeutic Outcomes

Most pharyngitis cases are self-limited; however, antibiotics hasten resolution when given early for proven cases of GAS pharyngitis.[19] Generally, fever and other symptoms resolve within 3 to 4 days of onset without antibiotics; however, symptoms will improve 0.5 to 2.5 days earlier with antibiotic therapy.[19] Follow-up testing is generally not necessary for index cases or asymptomatic contacts[19]; however, throat cultures 2 to 7 days after completion of antibiotics are warranted for patients who remain symptomatic or when symptoms recur despite completion of treatment.[19]

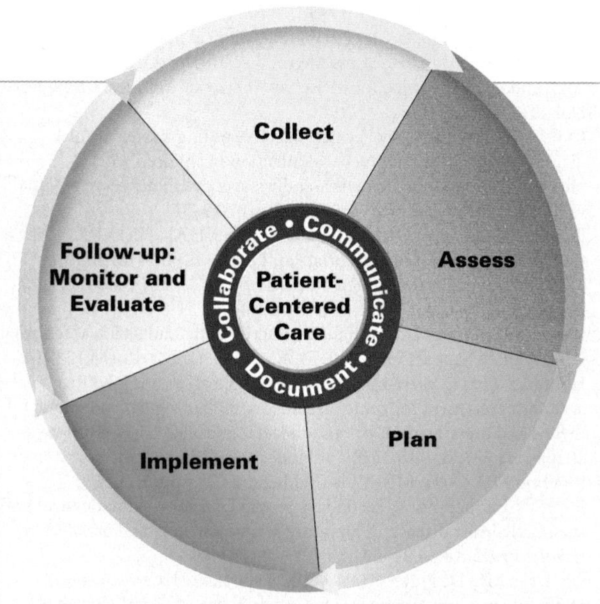

Patient Care Process for Acute Pharyngitis

Collect

- Patient characteristics (eg, age, weight)
- Patient history (eg, past infections including rheumatic fever and rheumatic heart disease, current and past antibiotic/antiviral use noting previous failures, medication allergies)
- Determine whether patient is a school-age child, parent/caregiver of a school-age child, or works with school-age children
- Objective data:
  - Temperature
  - Signs and symptoms (see Clinical Presentation)
  - Other diagnostic tests, when indicated (eg, RADT, throat culture, microbiologic testing)

Assess

- Infection status, including presence of signs and symptoms
- Determine which symptoms may need additional therapy (eg, ongoing throat pain)
- Use information collected, patient factors (eg, patient age, symptom severity), and joint decision making with parents/caregivers to determine whether antibiotics are needed
- If antibiotics are appropriate, determine proper choice of antibiotic, dose, duration, and dosage form

Plan*

- Select drug therapy regimen including specific antibiotic, dose, route, frequency, and duration; specify the continuation and discontinuation of existing therapies (see Tables 130-4 and 130-5)
- Monitor efficacy (eg, temperature, pain), safety (eg, medication-specific adverse effects), and time frame
- Educate patient and/or caregiver (eg, purpose of treatment, drug therapy) emphasizing adherence to treatment regimen
- Recommend self-monitoring of body temperature

Implement*

- Provide patient education regarding the infection and all elements of treatment plan
- Use motivational interviewing and coaching strategies to maximize adherence
- Schedule follow-up, when indicated
- Recommend measures to reduce throat pain, if present

Follow-up: Monitor and Evaluate

- Presence of adverse effects, particularly allergic reactions
- Patient adherence to treatment plan using multiple sources of information
- Inquire if there have been infections among household contacts

**Collaborate with patient, caregiver(s), and other healthcare professionals.*

ABBREVIATIONS

AAO-HNSF	American Academy of Otolaryngology—Head and Neck Surgery Foundation
AAP	American Academy of Pediatrics
ACIP	Advisory Committee on Immunization Practices
MRSA	methicillin-resistant *Staphylococcus aureus*
IM	intramuscular
IV	intravascular
GAS	group A β-hemolytic streptococci
GI	gastrointestinal
IDSA	Infectious Diseases Society of America
IgE	immunoglobulin E
MIC	minimal inhibitory concentration
PCV7	seven-valent pneumococcal conjugate vaccine
RADT	rapid antigen-detection test
T tube	tympanostomy tube
URI	upper respiratory infection

REFERENCES

1. U.S. Department of Health and Human Services, Centers for Disease Control and Prevention, National Center for Health Statistics, National Ambulatory Medical Care Survey: 2015 State and National Summary Tables.
2. Schilder A, Chonmaitree T, Cripps A, et al. Otitis media. *Nat Rev Dis Primers.* 2016;2:160–163. https://doi.org/10.1038/nrdp.2016.63.
3. Marom T, Tan A, Wilkinson GS, Pierson KS, Freeman JL, Chonmaitree T. Trends in otitis media-related health care use in the United States, 2001-2011. *JAMA Pediatr.* 2014;168:68–75.
4. Lieberthal AS, Carroll AE, Chonmaitree T, et al. The diagnosis and management of acute otitis media. *Pediatrics.* 2013;131:e964999.
5. Gaddey HL, Wright MT, Nelson TN. Otitis media: Rapid evidence review. *Am Fam Physician.* 2019;1006:350–356.
6. Jabarin B, Pitaro J, Lazarovitch T, et al. Decrease in pneumococcal otitis media cultures with concomitant increased antibiotic susceptibility in the pneumococcal conjugate vaccines era. *Otol Neurotol.* 2017;38:853–859.
7. Tawfik KO, Ishman SL, Altaye M, Meinzen-Derr J, Choo DI. Pediatric acute otitis media in the era of pneumococcal vaccination. *Otolaryngol Head Neck Surg.* 2017;156:938–945. doi: 10.1177/0194599817699599.
8. Rosenfeld RM, Shin JJ, Schwartz SR, et al. Clinical practice guideline: Otitis media with effusion (update). *Otolaryngol Head Neck Surg.* 2016;154:S1–S41.
9. Tapiainen T, Kujala T, Renko M, et al. Effect of antimicrobial treatment of acute otitis media on the daily disappearance of middle ear effusion: A placebo-controlled trial. *JAMA Pediatr.* 2014;168:635–641.
10. Venekamp RP, Sanders SL, Glasziou PP, Del Mar CB, Rovers MM. Antibiotics for acute otitis media in children. *Cochrane Database Syst Rev.* 2015;6:CD000219.
11. Hoberman A, Paradise JL, Rockette HE, et al. Shortened antimicrobial treatment for acute otitis media in young children. *N Engl J Med.* 2016;375:2446–2456.
12. Tawfik KO, Ishman SL, Altaye M, Meinzen-Derr J, Choo DI. Pediatric acute otitis media in the era of pneumococcal vaccination. *Otolaryngol Head Neck Surg.* 2017;156:938–945. doi: 10.1177/0194599817699599.
13. de Sévaux JL, Venekamp RP, Lutje V, Hak E, Schilder AG, Sanders EA, Damoiseaux RA. Pneumococcal conjugate vaccines for preventing acute otitis media in children. *Cochrane Database Syst Rev.* 2020;11:CD001480. doi: 10.1002/14651858.CD001480.pub6.
14. Harris AM, Hicks LA, Qaseem A. High Value Care Task Force of the American College of Physicians and for the Centers for Disease Control and Prevention. Appropriate antibiotic use for acute respiratory tract infection in adults: Advice for high-value care from the American College of Physicians and the Centers for Disease Control and Prevention. *Ann Intern Med.* 2016;164(6):425–434. doi: 10.7326/M15-1840.
15. Chow AW, Benninger MS, Brook I, et al. IDSA clinical practice guideline for acute bacterial rhinosinusitis in children and adults. *Clin Infect Dis.* 2012;54:e72–e112.
16. Rosenfeld RM, Piccirillo JF, Chandrasekhar SS, et al. Clinical practice guideline (update): Adult sinusitis. *Otolaryngol Head Neck Surg.* 2015;152:S1–S39.
17. Blackwell DL, Villarroel MA, Clarke TC. *Tables of summary health statistics for U.S. adults: 2013 National Health Interview Survey.* Atlanta: Centers for Disease Control and Prevention; 2015. http://www.cdc.gov/nchs/nhis/SHS/tables.htm.
18. Rosenfield RM. Acute sinusitis in adults. *N Engl J Med.* 2016;375:962–70. doi: 10.1056/NEJMcp1601749.
19. Shulman ST, Bisno AL, Clegg HW, et al. Clinical practice guideline for the diagnosis and management of group A streptococcal pharyngitis: 2012 update by the Infectious Diseases Society of America. *Clin Infect Dis.* 2012;55:1279–1282.
20. Cohen JF, Cohen R, Levy C, et al. Selective testing strategies for diagnosing group A streptococcal infection in children with pharyngitis: A systematic review and prospective multicentre external validation study. *Can Med Assoc J.* 2015;187:23–32.
21. Dooling KL, Shapiro DJ, Van Beneden C, Hersh AL, Hicks LA. Overprescribing and inappropriate antibiotic selection for children with pharyngitis in the United States, 1997-2010. *JAMA Pediatr.* 2014;168:1073–1074.
22. Barnett ML, Linder JA. Antibiotic prescribing to adults with sore throat in the United States, 1997-2010. *JAMA Intern Med.* 2014;174:138–140.
23. Holm AE, Llor C, Bjerrum L, Cordoba G. Short- vs. long-course antibiotic treatment for acute Streptococcal Pharyngitis: Systematic review and meta-analysis of randomized controlled trials. *Antibiotics.* 2020;9(11):733. doi: 10.3390/antibiotics9110733.
24. Remond MG, Coyle ME, Mills JE, Maguire GP. Approaches to improving adherence to secondary prophylaxis for rheumatic fever and rheumatic heart disease: A literature review with a global perspective. *Cardiol Rev.* 2016;24:94–98.
25. van Driel ML, De Sutter AI, Keber N, Habraken H, Christiaens T. Different antibiotic treatments for group A streptococcal pharyngitis. *Cochrane Database Syst Rev.* 2013CD004406.

131

Influenza

Jessica C. Njoku

KEY CONCEPTS

1. Influenza is a viral illness associated with high mortality and high hospitalization rates among persons older than 65 years. Aging of the population is contributing to an increased disease burden in the United States.
2. Seasonal influenza epidemics are the result of viral antigenic drift, which is why the influenza vaccine is changed on a yearly basis. Antigenic drift forms the foundation of the recommendation for annual influenza vaccination.
3. The acquisition of a new hemagglutinin and/or neuraminidase by the influenza virus is called *antigenic shift*, which results in a novel influenza virus that has the potential to cause a pandemic.
4. The primary route of influenza transmission is person-to-person via inhalation of respiratory droplets, and transmission can occur for as long as the infected person is shedding virus from the respiratory tract.
5. Clinical diagnosis of influenza is difficult. Classic signs and symptoms include abrupt onset of fever, muscle pain, headache, malaise, nonproductive cough, sore throat, and rhinitis. These signs and symptoms usually resolve within 1 week of presentation.
6. In the United States, the primary mechanism of influenza prevention is annual vaccination. Vaccination not only prevents influenza illness and influenza-related hospitalizations and deaths but may also decrease healthcare resource use and the overall cost to society.
7. The inactivated influenza vaccine (IIV) and the live-attenuated influenza vaccine (LAIV) are commercially available for prevention of seasonal influenza. Both vaccines contain influenza A subtypes H3N2 and H1N1, and influenza B virus, which are initially grown in hens' eggs.
8. Antiviral drugs for prophylaxis of influenza should be considered adjuncts to vaccine and are not replacements for annual vaccination.
9. If used, antiviral drugs should be started within 48 hours of symptom onset to maximize effectiveness.
10. Neuraminidase inhibitors (oseltamivir, zanamivir, and peramivir) and cap-dependent endonuclease inhibitor (baloxavir) have activity against both influenza A and influenza B viruses. Although the adamantanes inherently have activity against influenza A H1N1 viruses, they are no longer used clinically due to overwhelming viral resistance.

BEYOND THE BOOK

Complete the influenza vaccine table

Approved Influenza Vaccines for Different Age Groups—United States

Vaccine	Trade Name	Manufacturer	Dose/ Presentation	Thimerosal Mercury Content (μg Hg/0.5-mL dose)	Age Group	Number of Doses
aIIV4						
IIV4 High Dose						
IIV4						
IIV4						
ccIIV4						
RIV4						
LAIV4						

INTRODUCTION

Influenza causes significant morbidity and mortality, particularly among young children and the elderly. The Centers for Disease Control and Prevention (CDC) estimates that influenza has resulted in 9 to 45 million illnesses, 140,000 to 810,000 hospitalizations, and 12,000 to 61,000 deaths annually since 2010.[1,2] Globally, influenza causes nearly 650,000 deaths each year, with the highest burden among children younger than 5 years and adults 75 years and older.[3] More people die of influenza than of any other vaccine-preventable illness. Significant societal consequences associated with influenza include visits to physicians' offices and emergency departments and days lost from school and/or work. The societal costs associated with influenza are more than $10 billion in healthcare costs and $16.3 billion in indirect costs.[4]

Vaccination is the primary mechanism of influenza prevention in the United States. The antiviral armamentarium for treatment and prophylaxis of influenza is limited, which further emphasizes the importance of prevention with vaccination and appropriate use of infection control measures during outbreaks. Research toward the development of novel antivirals and vaccines is needed for effective control of seasonal epidemics and for pandemic preparedness.

ETIOLOGY AND EPIDEMIOLOGY

1 Influenza infection can occur at any time during the year with the highest rates of influenza-associated illness during the winter months. The highest rate of infection occurs in children, but severe illness, hospitalization, and death occur most commonly among those older than 65 years, young children (younger than 2 years), and those with underlying medical conditions, including pregnancy and cardiopulmonary disorders, which increase their risk of complications from influenza. The seasonal influenza epidemics has resulted in an estimated 9.3 to 49 million influenza-related illnesses, 4.3 to 16.6 million healthcare visits, and between 12,000 and 79,000 deaths annually since 2010.[4] During 2019 to 2020 influenza season alone, influenza resulted in 39 to 56 million illnesses; 18 to 26 million medical visits; 410,000 to 740,000 hospitalizations, and 24,000 to 62,000 deaths.[5] Influenza-associated illness was three times higher among children aged 0 to 4 years compared with those aged 5 to 17 years.[6] Similarly, influenza-associated illness rates among persons 65 years or older were nine times higher than those aged 18 to 49 years, and two times higher among those aged 50 to 64 years.[6] Furthermore, influenza-related hospitalization was highest among individuals age 65 years or older; 327 per 100,000 population.

Influenza activity was unusually low throughout the 2020 to 2021 influenza season both in the United States and globally, despite high levels of testing.[7] Between September 28, 2020, and May 22, 2021, in the United States, 0.2% of respiratory specimens tested by US clinical laboratories were positive for an influenza virus compared with 26.2% and 30.3% at the last three seasons. The low level of influenza activity at 0.8 per 100,000 population during this past season contributed to dramatically fewer influenza illnesses, hospitalizations, and deaths compared with previous seasons. Only one pediatric influenza death was reported during the 2020 to 2021 season compared to 37 (during 2011-2012) and 199 (during 2019-2020). COVID-19 mitigation measures, such as wearing face masks, staying home, hand washing, school closures, reduced travel, increased ventilation of indoor spaces, and physical distancing, have contributed to the decline in 2020 to 2021 influenza incidence, hospitalizations, and deaths.[7] Influenza vaccination may also contributed to reduced illness during the 2020 to 2021 season; however, vaccine intake was not different compared to previous seasons.[8,9]

Vaccination coverage with ≥1 dose of flu vaccine was 58% among children aged 6 months to 17 years, while vaccination coverage among adults ≥18 years was 55%.[8-10] Vaccine coverage was highest among individuals aged 65 years or older (80%). Overall vaccine effectiveness was low at 39% (39% among individuals 65 years or older and 34% for children younger than 9 years).[11] Influenza vaccine effectiveness in 2020 to 2021 was not estimated due to low influenza virus circulation during the 2020 to 2021 influenza season. Deaths associated with influenza often result from secondary bacterial pneumonia, primary viral pneumonia, and/or exacerbation of underlying comorbidities.[12]

Influenza Viruses A, B, and C

Influenza virus types A, B, and C are members of the Orthomyxoviridae family and affect many species, including humans, pigs, horses, and birds. Influenza A and B viruses are the two types that cause disease in humans. Influenza A viruses are responsible for the regular, seasonal epidemics of the flu, whereas influenza B viruses are typically associated with sporadic outbreaks, particularly among residents of long-term care facilities. Influenza A viruses are further categorized into different subtypes based on changes in two surface antigens—hemagglutinin and neuraminidase (NA). Influenza B viruses are not categorized into subtypes.

Hemagglutinin allows the influenza virus to enter host cells by attaching to sialic acid receptors and is the major antigen to which antibodies are directed on exposure.[13] NA allows the release of new viral particles from host cells by catalyzing the cleavage of linkages to sialic acid.[14]

Sixteen hemagglutinin subtypes (H1-H16) and nine NA subtypes (N1-N9) of influenza A have been isolated from birds. However, the only influenza A subtypes that have circulated among humans since the 1918 pandemic (see Antigenic Drift and Antigenic Shift) are H1 to H3 and N1 and N2.[13] The primary subtypes of influenza A that have been circulating among humans for the past three decades are H3N2 and H1N1.

Antigenic Drift and Antigenic Shift

2 Immunity to influenza virus occurs as a result of the development of antibody directed at the surface antigens, particularly hemagglutinin. However, immunity to one influenza subtype does not offer protection against other subtypes or types of influenza. Moreover, immunity to one antigenic variant of a subtype of influenza may not confer protection against other antigenic variants. Antigenic variants are created by point mutations in the surface antigens of a particular subtype, resulting in small changes in the hemagglutinin and/or NA molecules, which is called *antigenic drift*. Antigenic drift is the basis for seasonal epidemics of influenza, the reason for changes in the annual influenza vaccine, and the rationale behind the recommendation for annual vaccination.

3 Antigenic shift occurs when the influenza virus acquires a new hemagglutinin and/or NA via genetic reassortment rather than point mutations.[13] Most likely, the genetic reassortment occurs when an animal that supports the growth of multiple subtypes of influenza, such as a pig, is concurrently infected with two subtypes of the influenza virus. Conversely, antigenic shift may occur directly from avian strains that have gained competency in the human host. Antigenic shift results in the emergence of a novel influenza virus and carries the potential of causing a pandemic. However, novelty alone is insufficient to cause an influenza pandemic; the virus must be able to replicate in humans, spread person-to-person, and affect a susceptible population.[13] Immunity to one subtype of influenza does not confer protection against other subtypes or types.

Spanish Influenza of 1918

The influenza pandemic of 1918 was the most significant infectious disease outbreak known to humans, causing approximately 40 to 50 million deaths in a year, with more than 500,000 deaths occurring in the United States.[14] The pandemic originated in China, but occurred almost concurrently in Europe, Asia, and North America.[14]

The 1918 pandemic was caused by a particularly virulent influenza A H1N1 virus, which was entirely of avian origin.[14] In contrast to the other pandemics of the 20th century, the 1918 pandemic resulted in an unusual mortality pattern. The mortality peaked for those younger than 4 years, those between the ages of 25 and 35 years, and those older than 65 years, which resulted in a W-shaped mortality curve, as opposed to the U- or J-shaped curve typically associated with influenza.[11] Over half of the deaths occurred in persons aged 20 to 40 years. The death toll associated with this pandemic culminated in an almost 10-year drop in the life expectancy of the population at the time.[14]

Asian Influenza of 1957

The Asian flu pandemic began when a new H2 subtype of influenza A surfaced in Hunan province in China in 1957.[13] The virus formed from coinfection with an avian H2N2 virus and a human H1N1 virus in a common host, possibly a pig or a human. The H2N2 virus quickly spread to Japan, South America, the United States, New Zealand, and Europe, resulting in 1 to 2 million deaths worldwide, with 70,000 deaths occurring in the United States.[15] Unlike the Spanish influenza of 1918, the mortality curve for the Asian influenza pandemic was U- or J-shaped, with infants and elderly being most affected.

Hong Kong Influenza of 1968

The H2N2 virus of the Asian influenza circulated in the human population until 1968, when a new H3 subtype emerged in China and Hong Kong following genetic reassortment with the H2N2 virus.[13] The H3N2 virus quickly spread to the United States and later to Europe. This pandemic caused more than 30,000 deaths in the United States and 0.5 to 2 million deaths worldwide. The lower morbidity and mortality associated with the Hong Kong influenza may be explained by previous exposure of the population to the N2 subtype, and the availability of antibiotics for the management of secondary bacterial pneumonia. Similar to the Asian influenza of 1957, the mortality curve for the Hong Kong influenza pandemic was U- or J-shaped, primarily affecting infants and elderly.

Avian Influenza

Influenza viruses are in circulation in southern China during all months of the year.[13] Given this fact and the close proximity of dense populations of people, pigs, and wild and domestic birds, this area proves ideal for the emergence of new influenza viruses via genetic reassortment (antigenic shift) such as avian influenza. Avian influenza infections have been reported with A(H5N1), A(H5N6), A(H7N9), A(H9N2), A(H6N1), and A(H7N4) in China.[16]

The first report of human infection with the avian H5N1 virus occurred in 1997 in Hong Kong.[16] The virus reemerged in 2003 as an antigenically and genetically different virus that has spread widely through wild and domestic bird populations in Asia, Africa, and Europe as well as infecting humans in several countries.[17] From 2003 to 2021, 863 cases and 456 deaths caused by H5N1 infection have been reported. The overall case fatality was 53%.

The novel avian influenza H7N9 virus infection was first reported in humans in 2013, in China.[18] Since then, 1,568 laboratory-confirmed cases of human infection have been reported, including 615 deaths.[17] The majority of avian H7N9 human infection cases have been among those with recent exposure to live poultry or potentially contaminated environments, especially markets where live birds are sold.[18] The overall case fatality was 39%.

In December 2014, the first case of novel avian influenza H5N6 human infection was reported in China,[17] and to date, 25 laboratory-confirmed human cases of avian influenza A(H5N6) virus infection, including six deaths, were reported to the World Health Organization (WHO) from China.[16,17]

The spread of avian influenza viruses from person to person is rare and has been limited, inefficient, and unsustained.[15-18] The precise mode of transmission is unknown, but most cases have occurred as a result of contact with poultry, contaminated environment, and prolonged personal contact.[16] Cases of transmission via aerosolization have not been reported.[16,17] Clinical presentation includes high fever and influenza-like illness, and watery diarrhea without blood may occur up to 1 week prior to respiratory symptoms.[15] Almost all patients have clinically apparent pneumonia. Progression to death, most commonly as a consequence of respiratory failure, occurs at a mean of 9 to 10 days after the onset of illness.[19] The NA inhibitors (oseltamivir, peramivir, and zanamivir) and cap-dependent endonuclease inhibitor (baloxavir marboxil) have activity against influenza A and B viruses (including H1N1), although higher doses of NA inhibitors may be needed for efficacy.[19-21] Two inactivated monovalent influenza vaccines, nonadjuvanted[22] and adjuvanted[23] influenza H5N1 vaccine and an H7N9[24] virus vaccine, are available for vaccination of persons 6 months and older. They are only available to government agencies and for stockpiles.[16] The recommended dose of the nonadjuvanted vaccine is two 1-mL injections given intramuscularly 28 days apart (range, 21-35 days) if 18 to 64 years old,[22] while the nonadjuvanted vaccine dose is two 0.5-mL injections given 21 days apart if adjuvanted vaccine if 18 to 64 years old, or two 0.25-mL injection given 21 days apart if 6 months to 17 years.[23] Individuals at high risk, for example, those who work with poultry and H5N1 poultry outbreak responders, are encouraged to receive annual seasonal influenza vaccine to minimize the risk of coinfection with human and avian influenza A viruses. The potential for avian viruses H5N1 and H7N9 to cause a pandemic is of concern as it could spread more quickly than pandemics of the past because of the mobility of people in today's world.

A severe pandemic, like that of 1918, could cause more than 10 million hospitalizations and more than 2 million deaths, whereas a moderate pandemic, like those of 1957 and 1968, could result in more than 1 million hospitalizations and more than 650,000 deaths in the United States alone.[25-27]

Swine Influenza of 2009

An outbreak of a novel influenza A H1N1 (formerly swine-origin influenza virus [SOIV]) was initially detected in Mexico in March 2009 and subsequently in the United States in April 2009 in California and Texas.[28] The virus then spread throughout North America, Europe, Asia, and subsequently worldwide, prompting the WHO on June 11, 2009, to declare phase 6, indicating widespread human infection, for the influenza pandemic.[29] Since 1998, triple reassortant swine influenza A (H1) viruses, containing genes from swine, avian, and human lineages, have circulated among swine in the United States.[15,28]

The virus, now formally known as influenza A(H1N1) pdm09, has become the predominant influenza A H1N1 in circulation, effectively replacing traditional seasonal influenza A (H1N1).

Several characteristics of the novel influenza A H1N1 outbreak differ from those of a typical seasonal influenza outbreak. Symptomatology associated with the novel influenza includes fever (94%), cough (92%), sore throat (66%), diarrhea (25%), and vomiting (25%).[28,30] An estimated 43 to 89 million cases of 2009 H1N1 occurred between April 2009 and April 2010 with a median of 274,000 hospitalizations. Globally, up to 575,000 H1N1-related deaths were reported; however, this may represent an underestimation of true disease burden.[27,29] The majority of the cases occurred in otherwise healthy children and adults younger than 65 years of age including pregnant women, with the highest incidence reported among those aged 18 to 64 years.[29] Contrary to seasonal influenza, where about 60% of hospitalizations and 90% of deaths occur in people older than or equal to 65 years, approximately 90% and 87% of 2009 H1N1-related hospitalizations and deaths, respectively, occurred in people younger than 65 years. However, like seasonal influenza, people with underlying health conditions had greater risk of hospitalizations and death. Among those who were deceased due to novel H1N1 infection, the median age was ~40 years and 59% of deaths (respiratory and cardiovascular) occurred in Southeast Asia and Africa.[29] The wide spread of 2009 novel influenza was attributed to extensive global trade and travel, such that the virus was detected in 122 countries in 6 weeks as opposed to 6 months with previous pandemics.[27]

Variant Influenza A (H3N2v) 2012

H3N2v is a nonhuman influenza virus that normally circulates in pigs and that has infected humans.[31] In 2011, the US Centers for Disease Control and Prevention (CDC) reported the first case of an influenza infection due to influenza A H3N2 variant virus (H3N2v).[31] Since then, 430 cases have been documented from 17 states resulting in 34 hospitalizations and low mortality.[32] The H3N2v is considered a variant virus because it is different from influenza A viruses circulating among humans. The H3N2v virus contains genes from avian, swine, and human viruses and the M gene from the 2009 H1N1 pandemic virus (A[H1N1]pdm09).[31,32] The virus spreads more readily from pigs to people than other variant viruses, but has limited person-to-person transmission. The main risk factor for infection with the virus based on evaluation of available cases is exposure to pigs, mostly at agricultural fairs.[32] Since the virus is related to human flu viruses from the 1990s, most adults have some immunity against it.[31] Hence, most cases to date have occurred in children, who have little immunity against this virus.[29,32]

The symptoms and severity of H3N2v have mostly been mild and similar to those of seasonal influenza (fever, cough, sore throat, body aches, etc.), but like seasonal influenza, serious illness with H3N2v infection is possible.[29] Vaccination remains key to preventing H3N2v infection. Additionally, the CDC has encouraged people at high risk of influenza complications to stay away from swine barns at fairs.[32] People who are at high risk of serious complications from influenza, including H3N2v virus infection, are children younger than 5 years, people aged 65 years or older, pregnant women, body mass index of 40 or higher, age less than 19 years of age on long-term aspirin- or salicylate-containing drugs, chronic care facility residents, and people with certain chronic medical conditions (asthma, cystic fibrosis, chronic obstructive pulmonary disease, diabetes, heart disease, stroke, sickle cell, kidney and liver disorders, inherited metabolic disorders, immunocompromised, and neurologic or neurodevelopmental conditions).[33] The treatment of H3N2v virus infection is similar to that of seasonal influenza. NA inhibitors and cap-dependent endonuclease inhibitors are the mainstay of treatment. The adamantanes should not be used due to high resistance.

PATHOGENESIS

4 The route of influenza transmission is person-to-person via inhalation of respiratory droplets, which can occur when an infected person coughs or sneezes.[30,34] Transmission may also occur if a person touches an object contaminated with respiratory secretions and then touches his or her mucus membranes. The incubation period for influenza ranges between 1 and 7 days, with an average of 2 days.[34] Transmission can occur for as long as the infected person is shedding virus from the respiratory tract. Adults are considered infectious within 1 day before until 7 days after onset of illness. Children, especially younger children, might potentially be infectious for longer periods (more than 10 days).[35,36] Viral shedding can persist for weeks to months in severely immunocompromised people.

The pathogenesis of influenza in humans is not well understood. The severity of the infection is determined by the balance between viral replication and the host immune response. Severe illness is likely a result of both a lack of ability of host defense mechanisms to inhibit viral replication and an overproduction of cytokines leading to tissue damage in the host.[16,30]

Influenza Diagnostics Tests

Influenza molecular assays

Rapid influenza molecular assays (RIMAs) detect influenza viral RNA in upper respiratory tract specimens utilizing different nucleic acid amplification technologies (NAATs). They have high sensitivity (90%-95%) and high specificity (55%-99%), depending on the virus type, compared with RT-PCR assays.[38] FDA-cleared RIMAs are available for point of care (POC) use that produce results in approximately 15 to 30 minutes.

RT-PCR (real time or multiplex) is a nucleic acid amplification test that can identify the presence of influenza viral RNA or nucleic acids in respiratory specimens with high sensitivity and specificity. It is the most sensitive, specific, and versatile diagnostic test for influenza.[37] Results are available in approximately 45 minutes to several hours (1-6 hours) depending upon the assay, and are frequently used as a confirmatory test.

Rapid influenza diagnostic tests (RIDTs)

RIDTs use enzyme immunoassay (EIA) technology to provide results within 10 to 15 minutes and may have utility in community- and hospital-based outpatient settings because of their rapid processing times. RIDTs allow for differentiation of influenza viruses A and B but none of the RIDTs provide any information about influenza A virus subtypes. Sensitivities for RIDTs range are low often yielding false-negative results, while specificities are high compared with RT-PCR or viral culture.[37,38] For this reason, RIDTs are not recommended for use in hospitalized patients with suspected influenza, and RIMAs are preferred in outpatient settings since CLIA-waived tests are available for POC use.

Immunofluorescence assays (IFAs)

IFAs are antigen detection assays that generally require use of a fluorescent microscope to produce results in approximately 2 to 4 hours with moderate sensitivity and high specificity. One rapid IFA is an RIDT and utilizes an analyzer device to produce results in approximately 15 minutes.[37]

Viral culture

Culture allows for extensive antigenic and genetic characterization of influenza viruses. However, viral culture results do not yield timely results to inform clinical management. Shell-vial tissue culture results may take 1 to 3 days, while traditional tissue-cell viral culture results may take 3 to 10 days.

Serologic testing

Routine serological testing for influenza requires paired acute and convalescent sera, does not provide timely results to help with clinical decision making, is only available at a limited number of public health or research laboratories and is not generally recommended, except for research and public health investigations.

Specimen Collection

Upper respiratory tract specimens should be collected from outpatients for influenza testing as soon after illness onset as possible, preferably within 4 days of symptom onset to increase detection of influenza viruses. Nasopharyngeal specimens are preferred over other upper respiratory tract specimens. If nasopharyngeal specimens are not available, nasal and throat swab specimens should be collected and combined together for influenza testing over single specimens from either site (particularly over throat swabs). Collect endotracheal aspirate or bronchoalveolar lavage fluid specimens from hospitalized patients with respiratory failure receiving mechanical ventilation, including patients with negative influenza testing results on upper respiratory tract specimens, for influenza testing.

PREVENTION

The best means to decrease the morbidity and mortality associated with influenza is to prevent infection through vaccination.[34,35] Appropriate infection control measures, such as hand hygiene, basic respiratory etiquette (eg, cover your cough, throw tissues away), and contact avoidance, are important in preventing the spread of influenza. Additionally, chemoprophylaxis is useful in certain situations.

CLINICAL PRESENTATION Diagnosis of Influenza

General

- The clinical diagnosis of influenza can be difficult because the presentation is similar to a number of other respiratory illnesses. The sensitivity of clinical diagnosis ranges from 40% for children to 70% for adults and largely depends on the relative prevalence of influenza and other respiratory viruses circulating in a community.[34-36]
- The clinical course and outcome are affected by age, immunocompetence, viral characteristics, smoking, comorbidities, pregnancy, and the degree of preexisting immunity.[36]
- Complications of influenza may include exacerbation of underlying comorbidities, primary viral pneumonia, secondary bacterial pneumonia or other respiratory illnesses (eg, sinusitis, bronchitis, otitis), encephalopathy, transverse myelitis, myositis, myocarditis, pericarditis, and Reye's syndrome.[33,36]

Signs and Symptoms

- 5 Classic signs and symptoms of influenza include rapid onset of fever, myalgia, headache, malaise, nonproductive cough, sore throat, and rhinitis.[21,30,36]
- Nausea, vomiting, and otitis media are also commonly reported in children.[35]
- Signs and symptoms typically resolve in approximately 3 to 7 days, although cough and malaise may persist for more than 2 weeks.
- Primary viral pneumonia, occurring predominantly in pregnant women and those with underlying cardiovascular disease, usually begins with fever and dry cough, which changes to a productive cough of bloody sputum. This rapidly progresses to dyspnea, hypoxemia, and cyanosis with radiologic evidence of bilateral interstitial infiltrates.[36]
- Secondary bacterial pneumonia is usually seen in individuals with underlying pulmonary disorders and presents during the early stages of defervescence from the influenza infection. These patients usually present with fever, productive cough, and radiologic evidence of consolidation.[36]

Laboratory Tests

- Complete blood count and chemistry panels should be obtained to assess the overall status of the patient.
- The gold standard for diagnosis of influenza is reverse-transcription polymerase chain reaction (RT-PCR) or viral culture, which can provide information on the specific strain and subtype. Viral culture has a high sensitivity but can take as long as a week to develop, limiting the clinical relevance of the results.[36,37]

Other Diagnostic Tests

- Cultures of potential sites of infection should be obtained if coinfection, superinfection, or secondary infection is suspected.
- Chest radiograph should be obtained if pneumonia is suspected.

Vaccination

6 The primary means of influenza prevention used in the United States is annual vaccination. Vaccination can help prevent hospitalization and death among those at high risk, decrease influenza-like illness, decrease visits to physicians' offices and emergency rooms, decrease otitis media in children, and prevent school and/or work absenteeism. Annual vaccination is recommended for all persons aged 6 months or older and caregivers (eg, parents, teachers, babysitters, nannies) of children younger than 6 months. Vaccination is also recommended for those who live with and/or care for people who are at high risk, including household contacts and healthcare workers.

The ideal time for all influenza vaccination is during October or November to allow for the development and maintenance of immunity during the peak of the influenza season.[34,35] Table 131-1 lists the vaccination coverage rates and goals for various patient populations. Provider recommendation and offer of vaccination was associated with significantly higher vaccine uptake among adults 18 years and older (67%), compared to providers who only recommended but did not offer (48%), and those who neither recommended nor offered (32%).[39] If vaccination rates improved to the Healthy People goal of 70% for all age groups, another 4.6 million illnesses, 2.2 million medical visits, and 65,844 hospitalizations could have been prevented during the 2020 to 2021 influenza season.[10] Vaccine efficacy is highest when influenza virus in circulation is well matched with strains in the vaccine. Mismatched seasons have occurred, and were associated with reduced influenza vaccine uptake and severe influenza infection. TIV (vaccine efficacy 52% vs matched 65%) and LAIV (vaccine efficacy 54% vs matched 83%) provide cross protection against nonmatching circulating strains.[40]

TABLE 131-1 Influenza Vaccination Rates and Goals by Patient Population

Patient Population	Vaccination Coverage (%) 2020-2021	Vaccination Coverage National Goal (2030) (%)
Children aged 6 months to 17 years	58	70
Persons aged 18 years or older	55	70
Nursing home residents	72 (2019-2020)	90
Pregnant women	61	80
Healthcare workers	90 (2018-2019)	90

Data from References 8-10.

7 The two vaccine types available for prevention of seasonal influenza are the inactivated influenza vaccine (IIV) and the live attenuated influenza vaccine (LAIV).[34] IIV is available as trivalent (IIV3) and quadrivalent (IIV4) formulations, while LAIV is a quadrivalent formulation. Both vaccines contain two influenza A subtypes (H3N2 and H1N1) and two influenza B viruses; the specific strains included in the vaccine each year change based

on antigenic drift. The viruses used for both vaccines are initially grown in embryonated hens' eggs, which explains the precautionary measures for vaccination of persons with a severe allergic reaction to eggs.[34] Two other vaccines are produced using non-egg based technologies, recombinant quadrivalent vaccine [RIV4 (Flublok® Quadrivalent)] and cell-culture quadrivalent vaccine [ccIIV4 (Flucelvax Quadrivalent®)], and are safe if the patient has egg allergy. The Advisory Committee on Immunization Practices (ACIP) has made the following recommendations regarding the vaccinations of persons with reports of egg allergy: (1) for persons with a history of severe allergic reaction (eg, anaphylaxis) to any egg-based IIV or LAIV of any valency, the provider can consider administering ccIIV4 or RIV4; (2) for persons with a history of severe allergic reaction (eg, anaphylaxis) to any ccIIV of any valency, the provider can consider administering RIV4; and (3) for persons with a history of severe allergic reaction (eg, anaphylaxis) to any RIV of any valency, the provider can consider administering ccIIV4. Providers can also consider consulting with an allergist to help determine which vaccine component is responsible for the allergic reaction.[34] The CDC encourages individuals to use the Vaccine Adverse Event Reporting System to aide in collecting and analyzing adverse events following influenza vaccinations.[31]

Trivalent and Quadrivalent Influenza Vaccine

7 Intramuscular IIV is FDA-approved for use in people aged 6 months and older regardless of their immune status. For adults and older children, the deltoid is the preferred injection site. Infants and younger children should be vaccinated in the anterolateral thigh. Several commercial products are available and are approved for different age groups (Table 131-2). IIV is made with killed viruses, meaning it cannot cause signs and symptoms of influenza-like illness (Table 131-3). Age and immune status can affect the efficacy of IIV as can the similarity of the vaccine to the viruses in circulation. Fluzone quadrivalent may be given to children aged 6 to 35 months as either 0.25 mL per dose or 0.5 mL per dose. No preference is expressed for one or the other dose volume for this age group. Persons aged ≥3 years should receive 0.5-mL dose volume.[34] Flucelvax® quadrivalent vaccine use has been expanded to include those aged 6 months and older, and is reformulated without egg protein.[34]

In children aged between 6 and 24 months, a 2-year randomized study of intramuscular IIV3 exhibited 89% seroconversion and efficacy of 66% in year 1 and 7% in year 2 versus culture-confirmed influenza.[41] In children aged between 2 and 15 years, the efficacy of IIV3 was 91% and 77% against culture-confirmed influenza A H1N1 and H3N2, respectively. IIVs reduced the risk of influenza and influenza-like illness (ILI) in children.[42] To prevent one case of influenza, five children would need to be vaccinated, and to prevent one case of ILI, 12 children would need to be vaccinated. Therefore, vaccinating children could prevent influenza-related mortality and may also lead to fewer parents taking time off work. Two doses of IIVs are important for children under the age of 9 years, supporting the rationale for the recommendation of a booster dose of IIV at least 4 weeks after the initial dose in children between 6 months and less than 9 years of age if no previous vaccination (see Table 131-2).[34]

IIV is also effective in adult populations under and older than the age of 65 years. Intramuscular IIVs demonstrated a reduction in influenza, ILI, hospitalization, and work absenteeism in healthy adults aged 16 to 65 years.[43] Seventy-one adults would need to be vaccinated to prevent one influenza case, and 29 adults need to be vaccinated to prevent one ILI. In pregnant women, IIVs efficacy was 50% (number needed to vaccinate, NNV 55), and 49% in infants up to 24 weeks (NNV 56).

Adults older than the age of 65 years benefit from influenza vaccination, including prevention of complications, decreased risk of influenza-related hospitalization, and death.[44] However, people in this population may not generate a strong antibody response to the vaccine and may remain susceptible to infection. In patients older than the age of 60 years who do not reside in a long-term care facility, IIV efficacy was 58% against influenza illness.[45] Although the efficacy against influenza illness for those living in long-term care facilities is between 30% and 40%, the vaccine is 50% to 60% effective in preventing influenza-related hospitalization or pneumonia and 80% effective in preventing influenza-related death.[45]

Fluzone HD trivalent induced higher immune response compared with standard IIV3 and offered better protection than SD-IIV3 for persons aged 65 years or older. Fluzone HD prevented 24% more cases of influenza caused by any circulating influenza strain and 51% more cases of influenza caused by strains similar to those contained in the vaccine compared to standard trivalent vaccine. Compared to IIV3, Fluzone HD trivalent would avert 195,958 cases of influenza, 22,567 influenza-related hospitalizations, 5,423 influenza-related deaths, and generate 29,023 more Quality Adjusted Life Years among US seniors.[46] Fluzone HD quadrivalent or Fluad quadrivalent vaccine are preferred vaccines for use in adult patients 65 years and older.[35]

The most frequent adverse effect associated with IIV is soreness at the injection site that lasts for less than 48 hours. IIV may cause fever and malaise in those who have not previously been exposed to the viral antigens in the vaccine.[34] Allergic-type reactions (hives, systemic anaphylaxis) rarely occur after influenza vaccination and are likely a result of a reaction to residual egg protein in the vaccine.

The 1976 swine influenza vaccine was linked to a rise in the incidence of Guillain-Barré syndrome (GBS), and this has propagated the belief that IIV may cause GBS.[47] However, there is insufficient evidence to establish causality. Although several studies have failed to establish a relationship between influenza vaccination and increased frequency of GBS, some studies have demonstrated a small but significant increase in GBS following influenza vaccination.[47] Therefore, vaccination should be avoided in persons who are not at high risk for influenza complications and who have experienced GBS within 6 weeks of receiving a previous influenza vaccine.[34] The potential benefits of influenza vaccination in terms of prevention of severe illness, hospitalization, and mortality significantly outweigh the risks of GBS, and vaccination is recommended for all groups previously discussed.

The multidose vials and a few of the single-dose preparations of intramuscular IIV contain trace to small amounts of a preservative, thimerosal, which is a mercury-containing compound (see Table 131-2). Some individuals are concerned about thimerosal exposure, particularly among children, because of the unfounded belief that thimerosal exposure is linked to the development of autism. No scientifically persuasive evidence exists to suggest harm from thimerosal exposure from a vaccine. Conversely, accumulating evidence reports the lack of harm from such exposure.[48,49] Thus, similar to GBS, the potential benefits of influenza vaccination in terms of prevention of severe illness, hospitalization, and mortality significantly outweigh the theoretical risk associated with thimerosal exposure, and vaccination is recommended for all groups previously discussed. However, to maximize the public health benefit and placate concerned individuals, thimerosal-free vaccine is available (see Table 131-2).

Live-Attenuated Influenza Vaccine

7 LAIV is made with live, attenuated viruses and is approved for intranasal administration in healthy people between 2 and 49 years of age (see Table 131-3). Advantages of LAIV include its ease of administration, intranasal rather than intramuscular administration, and the

TABLE 131-2 Approved Influenza Vaccines for Different Age Groups—United States, 2021-2022 Season

Vaccine	Trade Name	Manufacturer	Dose/Presentation	Thimerosal Mercury Content (μg Hg/0.5 mL dose)	Age Group	Number of Doses
			Quadrivalent IIV (IIV4)			
IIV4	Afluria Quadrivalent	Seqirus	0.25-mL prefilled syringe 0.5-mL prefilled syringe 5-mL multidose vial	0 0 24.5	≥6-35 months ≥3 years ≥6 months (needle/syringe) or 18-64 years via jet injector	1 or 2[a] 1 or 2[a] 1 or 2[a]
IIV4	Fluarix Quadrivalent	GlaxoSmithKline	0.5-mL prefilled syringe	0	≥6 months	1 or 2[a]
IIV4	FluLaval Quadrivalent	GlaxoSmithKline	0.5-mL prefilled syringe 5-mL multidose vial	0 <25	≥6 months ≥6 months	1 or 2[a]
IIV4	Fluzone Quadrivalent[b]	Sanofi Pasteur	0.25-mL prefilled syringe 0.5-mL prefilled syringe 0.5-mL single-dose vial 5-mL multi-dose vial	0 0 0 25	≥6-35 months ≥6 months ≥6 months ≥6 months	1 or 2[a] 1 or 2[a] 1 or 2[a] 1 or 2[a]
			Quadrivalent IIV high dose (IIV4-HD)			
aIIV4 high dose	Fluad Quadrivalent	Seqirus	0.5-mL prefilled syringe	0	≥65 years	1
IIV4 high dose	Fluzone HD Quadrivalent	Sanofi Pasteur	0.7-mL prefilled syringe	0	≥65 years	1
			Cell culture-based quadrivalent IIV (ccIIV4)			
ccIIV4	Flucelvax Quadrivalent	Seqirus	0.5-mL prefilled syringe 5-mL multidose vial	0 25	≥6 months ≥6 months	1 or 2[a] 1 or 2[a]
			Recombinant quadrivalent IIV (RIV4)			
RIV4	Flublok Quadrivalent	Sanofi Pasteur	0.5-mL prefilled syringe	0	≥18 years	1
			LAIV quadrivalent (LAIV4)			
LAIV	FluMist Quadrivalent	AstraZeneca	0.2-mL sprayer	0	2-49 years	1 or 2[c]

[a]Two doses administered at least 4 weeks apart are recommended for children aged 6 months to less than 9 years who are receiving influenza vaccine for the first time or received one dose in the first year of vaccination during the previous influenza season.

[b]Fluzone quadrivalent may be given to children aged 6 to 35 months as either 0.25 mL per dose or 0.5 mL per dose. No preference is expressed for one or the other dose volume for this age group. Persons aged ≥3 years should receive 0.5-mL dose volume.

[c]Two doses administered 4 weeks apart are recommended for children aged 2 years to less than 9 years who are receiving influenza vaccine for the first time.

IIV, inactivated influenza vaccine; aIIV4, adjuvanted inactivated influenza vaccine, quadrivalent, high dose; IIV4, inactivated influenza quadrivalent vaccine; IIV4-HD, inactivated influenza quadrivalent vaccine – high dose; ccIIV4, cell culture-based quadrivalent influenza vaccine; RIV4, recombinant quadrivalent influenza vaccine; LAIV, live-attenuated influenza vaccine.

Note: IIVs and RIV4 may be administered concomitantly or sequentially with other inactivated vaccines or live vaccines. LAIV4 may be given simultaneously with other live or inactivated vaccines. However, after administration of a live vaccine (such as LAIV4), at least 4 weeks should elapse before another live vaccine is administered.

Influenza antiviral medications might reduce the effectiveness of LAIV4 if given within 48 hours before to 14 days after administration of LAIV4. Persons who receive influenza antiviral medications within this period of LAIV4 vaccination can be revaccinated with another appropriate influenza vaccine (eg, IIV or RIV4).

Data from References 34 and 35.

TABLE 131-3 Comparison of Inactivated Influenza Vaccine (IIV) and Live-Attenuated Influenza Vaccine (LAIV)

Characteristic	IIV (IIV3/IIV4)	LAIV
Age groups approved for use	≥6 months	2-49 years
Immune status requirements	Immunocompetent or immunocompromised	Immunocompetent
Viral properties	Inactivated (killed) influenza A (H3N2), A (H1N1), and B viruses	Live-attenuated influenza A (H3N2), A (H1N1), and B viruses
Route of administration	Intramuscular	Intranasal
Immune system response	High serum IgG antibody response	Lower IgG response and high serum IgA mucosal response

Data from References 34 and 35.

potential induction of broad mucosal and systemic immune response.[34] The mucosal response occurs at the site of viral entry and may prevent infection before viral replication occurs. LAIV is more expensive than IIV and is approved for use in a more limited population. Originally licensed as a trivalent vaccine, in 2012, the FDA approved FluMist® Quadrivalent vaccine (LAIV4) for influenza prevention in people aged 2 to 49 years.[34] FluMist® Quadrivalent vaccine which has replaced the trivalent vaccine contains four strains of the influenza viruses, two influenza A strains and two influenza B strains. The inclusion of a second B strain in the vaccine increases the likelihood of adequate protection against circulating influenza B strains.

Studies of FluMist® trivalent, in addition to three new clinical trials with the quadrivalent vaccine in 4,000 children (2-17 years) and adults (18-49 years) in the United States, provide supporting evidence on the efficacy and safety of FluMist® Quadrivalent.[50] Immune responses were similar between FluMist® Quadrivalent and FluMist® trivalent. LAIV4 recipients aged 2 to 5 years had 52.5% and 54.4% fewer cases of influenza illness against matched and mismatched strains, respectively, as compared with IIV3 recipients.[50]

Although LAIV4 is FDA-approved for adults younger than the age of 49 years, LAIV is effective in healthy adults aged between 18 and 64 years.[34] LAIV4 should not be used during pregnancy. Vaccination reduced the number of severe febrile illnesses by 18.8% and febrile upper respiratory tract illnesses by 23.6%.[50] Additionally, vaccination led to fewer days of illness, fewer days lost from work, fewer visits to healthcare providers, and decreased use of prescription antibiotics and nonprescription medications.[50]

Adverse reactions of LAIV are similar among those receiving FluMist® Quadrivalent and FluMist® trivalent. The adverse effects typically associated with LAIV administration include runny nose, congestion, sore throat, and headache. Because LAIV contains live, attenuated viruses, viral shedding may occur for several days following vaccination with LAIV, although this should not be equated with person-to-person transmission.[34] Additionally, because LAIV contains live, attenuated viruses, which carry a theoretical infection risk, LAIV should not be given to immunosuppressed patients or given by healthcare workers who are severely immunocompromised. Moreover, for the reasons discussed in IIV above, LAIV should not be administered to persons with a history of GBS or hypersensitivity to eggs. Vaccine effectiveness of LAIV was 45% against influenza A and B, with 25% protection against influenza A (H1N1) pdm09 compared with unvaccinated children.[34] LAIV is not recommended in several populations, including people older than 50 years and pregnant females, largely because the vaccine has not been studied extensively in these populations. However, many clinicians believe the use of LAIV in these populations is acceptable.[34,50]

Postexposure Prophylaxis

8 Antiviral drugs available for prophylaxis of influenza should be considered adjuncts but are not replacements for annual vaccination. Adamantanes are no longer recommended for prophylaxis or treatment in the United States because of widespread resistance among influenza viruses.[35,51] Neuraminidase (NA) inhibitor antiviral medications are approximately 70% to 90% effective in preventing influenza against susceptible influenza viruses and are useful adjuncts to influenza vaccination.[52] Peramivir is not approved for chemoprophylaxis; however, oseltamivir and zanamivir are effective prophylactic agents against influenza for preventing laboratory-confirmed influenza when used for seasonal prophylaxis (67% and 85% effective for zanamivir and oseltamivir, respectively) and preventing influenza illness among persons exposed to a household contact who was diagnosed with influenza (79%-81% and 68%-89% effective for zanamivir and oseltamivir, respectively). Additionally, oseltamivir was 92% effective against influenza, and also reduced associated complications when used as seasonal prophylaxis among immunized, institutionalized, elderly patients.[35,52] Zanamivir and oseltamivir are 79% to 81% and 68% to 89% effective, respectively, in preventing influenza illness among persons exposed to a household contact who was diagnosed with influenza.[34,51] In 2020, the FDA approved baloxavir for post-exposure prophylaxis of influenza in persons aged 12 years and older.[52] Baloxavir, when administered within 24 hours of the onset of symptoms in persons 12 years of age and older, reduced the risk of household transmission of influenza by 86% compared with placebo.[53] Prophylaxis was begun within 2 days after exposure. Oseltamivir is FDA-approved for chemoprophylaxis in individuals aged 1 year and older. However, the CDC, the American Academy of Pediatrics (AAP), and the Pediatric Infectious Diseases Society (PIDS) provide an expanded recommendation for chemoprophylaxis in those aged 3 months and older.[35,51] All of these agents remain active against all influenza viruses, including influenza A H3N2v. Table 131-4 lists dosing recommendations.

In those patients who did not receive the influenza vaccination and are receiving an antiviral drug for prevention of disease during the influenza season, the medication should optimally be taken for the entire duration of influenza activity in the community. The use of prophylaxis requires clinical judgment and depends on a variety of factors, but prophylaxis for seasonal influenza should be considered during influenza season for the following groups of patients after exposure to an infectious source[35,36,51]:

1. Persons at high risk of serious illness and/or complications who are exposed to an infectious person and cannot be vaccinated.
2. Persons at high risk of serious illness and/or complications who are vaccinated but exposed to an infectious person during the first 2 weeks following vaccination. The development of sufficient antibody titers after vaccination takes approximately 2 weeks.
3. Persons with severe immune deficiency or who may have an inadequate response to vaccination (eg, advanced human immunodeficiency virus [HIV] disease, persons receiving immunosuppressive medications), after exposure to an infectious person.
4. Long-term care facility residents, regardless of vaccination status, when an outbreak has occurred in the institution.

LAIV should not be administered until 48 hours after influenza antiviral therapy has stopped, and influenza antiviral drugs should not be administered for 2 weeks after the administration of LAIV because the antiviral drugs inhibit influenza virus replication.[34,36] No contraindication exists for concomitant use of IIV and influenza antiviral drugs. If chemoprophylaxis is given, it should be administered as soon as possible after exposure, ideally no later than 48 hours after exposure.[36] Postexposure prophylaxis should not be given if >48 hours has elapsed since exposure, and full-dose empiric antiviral treatment should be initiated as soon as symptoms occur, if treatment is indicated. Duration of chemoprophylaxis in a non-outbreak setting is 7 days after the most recent exposure to a close contact with influenza.[36,51]

Pregnant Females and Immunocompromised Hosts

Pregnant females and immunocompromised hosts are special populations at increased risk of influenza complications and are also populations in whom careful consideration must be given in regard to prevention strategies.

Pregnant females, regardless of trimester, should receive annual influenza vaccination with IIV but not with LAIV.[34,36] No studies have demonstrated an increased incidence of adverse effects in mothers or their infants related or potentially related to IIV, but no such data exist for LAIV.[34] Receipt of an influenza vaccination reduced hospitalizations of pregnant females by about 40%.[55] Influenza vaccination of pregnant females reduced hospitalization of their infants by 92% during the first 6 months of life.[54] IIV is also safe for breastfeeding mothers. No data exist for LAIV and breastfeeding mothers, but caution is warranted because of the potential for viral shedding.[34]

Immunocompromised hosts should receive annual influenza vaccination with IIV but not with LAIV. IIV was 100% effective against laboratory-confirmed influenza in HIV-positive patients with no significant effect on viral load or CD4 cell count.[56] HIV-infected persons may benefit from vaccination with high-dose IIV3 due to greater immunogenicity compared to standard-dose vaccine (H1N1, seroprotection rate; 96% vs 87%).[56] In solid-organ transplant recipients high-dose IIV3 (compared with standard dose IIV) resulted in higher immunogenicity.[57] A two-dose vaccination strategy spaced 5 weeks apart in solid-organ transplant recipients elicited greater immune response compared to single dose.[58] Although this suggests a potential benefit from a two-dose regimen, such a regimen is not recommended for solid-organ transplant recipients. Standard annual influenza vaccination and early antiviral therapy were shown to reduce influenza-related morbidity in transplant recipients (solid

TABLE 131-4 Recommended Daily Dosage of Influenza Antiviral Medications for Treatment and Prophylaxis—United States

Drug	Adult Treatment	Adult Prophylaxis[a]	Pediatric Treatment	Pediatric Prophylaxis[a]
		CAP-dependent endonuclease inhibitor		
Baloxavir[b,c]	12 yrs and older: 40 to <80 kg: One 40 mg dose >80 kg: One 80 mg dose	None	FDA approved and recommended for use in children aged 12 yrs or older weighing at least 40 kg. See adult dosage	None
		Neurominidase inhibitors		
Oseltamivir[d,e,f]	75-mg capsule twice daily × 5 days	75-mg capsule daily × 10 days	Term infants 0-8 months: 3 mg/kg/dose twice daily 9-11 months[g]: 3.5 mg/kg/dose twice daily or 3 mg/kg/dose twice daily ≥1 year: ≤15 kg: 30 mg twice daily >15-23 kg: 45 mg twice daily >23-40 kg: 60 mg twice daily >40 kg: 75 mg twice daily Duration: All for 5 days	Not recommended if <3 months 3 to <12 months: 3 mg/kg/dose daily 9-11 months: 3.5 mg/kg/dose daily ≥1 year: ≤15 kg: 30 mg daily >15-23 kg: 45 mg daily >23-40 kg: 60 mg daily >40 kg: 75 mg daily Duration: All for 10 days
Zanamivir	10 mg (2 of 5 mg inhalations) twice daily × 5 days	10 mg (2 of 5 mg inhalations) daily × 10 days	10 mg (2 of 5 mg inhalations) twice daily × 5 days for ≥7 years old	10 mg (2 of 5 mg inhalations) daily for ≥5 years old × 10 days
Peramivir[c,e]	13 yrs and older: One 600 mg dose via intravenous infusion for 15-30 minutes	None	2 to 12 yrs of age: One 12 mg/kg dose, up to 600 mg maximum, via intravenous infusion for a minimum of 15-30 minutes	None

[a]If influenza vaccine is administered, prophylaxis can generally be stopped 14 days after vaccination for noninstitutionalized persons. When prophylaxis is being administered following an exposure, prophylaxis should be continued for 10 days after the last exposure. In persons at high risk for complications from influenza for whom vaccination is contraindicated or expected to be ineffective, chemoprophylaxis should be continued for the duration that influenza viruses are circulating in the community during influenza season.

[b]Time to peak = 4 hours. Food and cations (calcium, aluminum, magnesium, iron) can decrease peak concentration by 48%. Long half-life (79.1 hours) and is metabolized by UDP-glucuronosyltransferase (UGT1A3) and CYP3A4.

[c]For the treatment of uncomplicated influenza with oral baloxavir or intravenous peramivir, a single dose is recommended. Longer daily dosing (oral oseltamivir or intravenous peramivir) can be considered for patients who remain severely ill after 5 days of treatment.

[d]Oseltamivir dosing for preterm infants using their postmenstrual age (ie, gestational age + chronological age): <38 weeks: 1.0 mg/kg/dose twice daily; 38–40 weeks: 1.5 mg/kg/dose twice daily; >40 weeks: 3.0 mg/kg/dose twice daily.[32]

[e]In patients with renal insufficiency, the dose should be adjusted on the basis of creatinine clearance. See https://www.cdc.gov/flu/professionals/antivirals/summary-clinicians.htm.[33,52]

[f]Some experts recommend 150 mg twice daily for severe illness in pregnant women. Optimal dosing for prophylaxis in pregnant women is unknown.[33]

[g]The American Academy of Pediatrics recommends 3.5 mg/kg per dose twice daily; CDC and US Food and Drug Administration (FDA)–approved dosing is 3 mg/kg per dose twice daily for children aged 9 to 11 months.[32,54]

Note: Although amantadine and rimantadine have been used historically for the treatment and prophylaxis of influenza A viruses, due to high resistance, the CDC no longer recommends the use of these agents for the treatment and/or prophylaxis of influenza.

Data from References 35 and 52.

and hematopoietic).[59] Immune responses in patients receiving chemotherapy for either solid or hematologic tumors are lower (fourfold rise, 17%-52%) than in those who had completed chemotherapy (50%-83%) and healthy patients (67%-100%).[60] However, there was lower mortality- and infection-related outcomes with influenza vaccination of immunocompromised adults with cancer.[61]

Large clinical trials evaluating the use of influenza antivirals for prophylaxis are lacking in immunocompromised hosts. Viral shedding occurs for prolonged periods in this population and may promote the development of antiviral resistance, which has been documented with oseltamivir in immunocompromised patients.[35,36]

TREATMENT

When prevention efforts fail or are not used, clinicians must turn to the agents available for treatment of influenza. Antiviral treatment options are limited, particularly in the face of resistance to the adamantanes and oseltamivir. The four primary goals of therapy of influenza are to control symptoms, prevent complications, decrease work and/or school absenteeism, and prevent the spread of infection.

General Approach to Treatment

9 In the era of pandemic preparedness and increasing resistance, early and definitive diagnosis of influenza is crucial. Antiviral drugs are most effective if started within 48 hours of the onset of illness. Moreover, the sooner the antiviral drugs are started after the onset of illness, the more effective they are. Antiviral drugs shorten the duration of illness and provide symptom control. Adjunct agents, such as acetaminophen for fever or an antihistamine for rhinitis, may be used concomitantly with the antiviral drugs.

Nonpharmacologic Therapy

Patients suffering from influenza should get adequate sleep and maintain a low level of activity. They should stay home from work and/or school to rest and prevent the spread of infection. Appropriate fluid intake should be maintained. Cough/throat lozenges, warm tea, or soup may help with symptom control (cough, sore throat).

Pharmacologic Therapy

The Cap-dependent endonuclease inhibitor, baloxavir and NA inhibitors, oseltamivir, zanamivir, and peramivir are the only antiviral drugs available for the treatment and prophylaxis of influenza.[51] Peramivir is the only intravenous formulation commercially

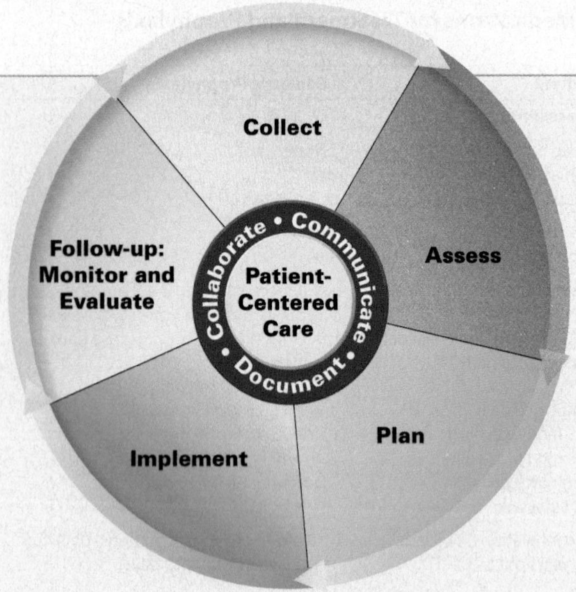

Patient Care Process for Influenza Infection Treatment

The image shows the five fundamental steps included in The Pharmacist's Care Process endorsed by the Joint Commission for Pharmacy Practitioners (2014). The tagline of this process reads collaborate, communicate, and document. The five fundamental steps listed here are collect, assess, plan, implement, and follow-up: monitor and evaluate. All these steps are listed in a circular block diagram.

Collect

- Patient characteristics: age, occupation, travel, lifestyle, immune status, present and past medical history, allergies
- Medication history (include prescription, nonprescription, and other substances); vaccination history; pregnancy status
- Microbiologic results from rapid respiratory viral panel and secondary bacterial infection. Bacterial susceptibility tests when available (see Clinical Presentation: Diagnosis of Influenza)
- Laboratory results, major organ function (particularly, kidney and liver), lactate

Assess

- Assess for medication contraindications and drug interactions
- Determine severity of illness based on vital signs, acute organ dysfunction, and source control (or lack thereof) (see Clinical Presentation: Diagnosis of Influenza)
- Determine at-risk patients for secondary bacterial infection of the respiratory tract, patient's microbiologic history, previous antibiotic exposure, and response to current therapy (see Clinical Presentation: Diagnosis of Influenza)
- Determine if other conditions are present such as chronic lung disease likely to affect outcomes of infection
- Estimate creatinine clearance for drug dosing

Plan*

- Strongly recommend future influenza vaccine if no contraindication is present (Tables 131-2 and 131-3)
- Initiate treatment neuraminidase therapy—oral or inhaled or IV based on severity of illness (Table 131-4)
- Determine influenza treatment goals of therapy with monitoring parameters for each goal (see Goals of Therapy)
- Determine appropriate antibiotic therapy for secondary bacterial infection and monitoring plan
- Establish antimicrobial monitoring goals for efficacy (eg, resolution of infection, clearance of bacteria from blood cultures) and drug toxicity
- Check for drug interactions and dose adjustments based on end-organ function

Implement

- Initiate a neuraminidase inhibitor and continue for ~7 days after identification of illness onset in the last patient (prophylaxis for community outbreak) or 5 days (treatment) or establish a tentative stop date for severely ill patients
- If secondary bacterial infection is suspected, initiate empiric antimicrobial regimen, and deescalate antimicrobial therapy to more narrow-spectrum agents as appropriate based on response and microbiologic data
- Assess patient as needed for response to antiviral medications, and other treatments
- Use measures to minimize adverse events to medications and assess for occurrence of adverse events

Follow-up: Monitor and Evaluate

- Refer patient for other health, wellness, or follow-up services to their identified primary care provider or another provider (provide patient with documentation of referral)
- Determine if patient shows improvement in the signs and symptoms of infection within 48 hours after neuraminidase inhibitor is initiated
- Monitor for emergence of resistant virus
- Monitor for occurrence of secondary bacterial pneumonia

Collaborate with patient, caregiver(s), and other healthcare professionals.

available. The adamantanes (amantadine and rimantadine) are no longer recommended due to high resistance among influenza viruses. A limited discussion of adamantanes can be found in the following section, but the focus will be on oseltamivir, zanamivir, and peramivir.

Adamantanes

The adamantanes (amantadine and rimantadine) block the M2 ion channel, which is specific to influenza A viruses, and inhibit viral uncoating. Historically, the adamantanes were used for the treatment of seasonal influenza A H1N1, as they do not have activity against influenza A H3N2 or influenza B viruses. The novel influenza A H1N1 that emerged during the 2009 to 2010 influenza season, which has now replaced seasonal influenza A H1N1 as the predominant seasonal virus, was resistant to the adamantanes. Since 2009 more than 99% of influenza A H3N2 and H1N1pdm09 were resistant to adamantanes.[51] As a result, the CDC only recommends the use of NA inhibitors for the treatment and prophylaxis of influenza A, until susceptibility of adamantanes is reestablished among influenza A viruses. Resistance to adamantanes is often conferred by a single-point mutation, and this is problematic because it results in cross-resistance to the entire class.[36]

Cap-Dependent Endonuclease Inhibitor

Oral baloxavir marboxil is a Cap-dependent polymerase acidic endonuclease inhibitor that interferes with viral RNA transcription and blocks virus replication.[52] It is approved for use within 48 hours of illness onset, in people aged 12 years and older, for the treatment of acute, uncomplicated influenza in patients who are at high risk for developing serious influenza-related complications, for example, those with chronic conditions like asthma, heart disease, and diabetes. Avoid co-administration of baloxavir with dairy products, calcium-fortified beverages, polyvalent cation-containing laxatives or antacids, or oral supplements (eg, calcium, iron, magnesium, selenium, or zinc).[52] When administered within 48 hours of symptom onset, baloxavir decreased duration of illness by 2.5 days. The safety and efficacy of baloxavir in patients less than 12 years of age or weighing less than 40 kg have not been established. Baloxavir is not recommended for use in pregnant women or breastfeeding mothers. Commonly reported events for baloxavir were diarrhea, bronchitis, nausea, nasopharyngitis, and increased liver enzymes.[52] The recommended doses are listed in Table 131-4.

Neuraminidase Inhibitors

9 10 Oseltamivir, zanamivir, and peramivir are NA inhibitors that have activity against both influenza A and influenza B viruses.[51] Without NA, release of the virus from infected cells is impaired, and, thus, viral replication is decreased. Although no randomized, placebo-controlled trials of antiviral treatment have been conducted in hospitalized influenza patients to establish the efficacy of NA inhibitors, a number of observational studies have reported clinical benefits of NA inhibitors in hospitalized patients, including reduction in duration of hospitalization and risk of death, including ICU patients.[62,63] When administered within 48 hours of the onset of illness, NA inhibitors may reduce the duration of illness by approximately 1 day versus placebo. Neuroaminidase inhibitors shortened symptom duration in adults by 0.5 to 1 day, and improved survival in hospitalized patients.[63] In children, NA inhibitor use resulted in shorter duration of illness and 34% lower risk of otitis media.[64] Treatment of children with laboratory-confirmed influenza with oseltamivir significantly reduced the duration of illness by 17.6 hours.[64] This has a significant effect on not only the quality of life for the patient but also the societal costs associated with influenza. The benefits of treatment are highly dependent on the timing of the initiation of treatment, with the ideal initiation period being within 12 hours of illness onset, up to 48 hours after onset of illness.[35,36,51] Debate still exists regarding the benefit of antiviral administration more than 48 hours after onset. Observational studies have reported a lower risk for severe outcomes with oral oseltamivir started as late as 4 and 5 days after onset of illness in critically ill patients with suspected or confirmed influenza.[65-67] Based upon the available observational data in hospitalized patients with influenza, including ICU patients, initiation of NA inhibitor treatment is recommended as soon as possible for hospitalized patients with suspected or confirmed influenza.

Oseltamivir treatment in adults and adolescents with documented influenza illness resulted in a 27% reduction in overall antibiotic use, a 55% reduction in lower respiratory tract complications (bronchitis, pneumonia), and a 59% reduction in hospitalizations.[68] Zanamivir treatment in adults and adolescents with influenza-like illness resulted in a 28% reduction in antibiotic use and a 40% reduction in lower respiratory tract complications.[69] The data in these studies largely come from healthy individuals rather than those at highest risk for complications associated with influenza. The impact of appropriate treatment in high-risk populations may be even greater than that documented to date.

Oseltamivir is FDA-approved for treatment in those aged 14 days and older, zanamivir for treatment in those older than 7 years, and peramivir for those aged 2 years and older.[51] The CDC, the American Academy of Pediatrics (AAP), and the Pediatric Infectious Diseases Society (PIDS) provide an expanded recommendation for oseltamivir for treatment of infants younger than 14 days.[35,51] The recommended doses vary by agent and age (see Table 131-4). The recommended duration of treatment for both oseltamivir and zanamivir is 5 days, and one dose for 1 day for peramivir.

The FDA-approved single-dose peramivir injection (Rapivab®) for intravenous use for the treatment of acute uncomplicated influenza in people aged 2 years and older.[36,51] Peramivir is as effective as oseltamivir, without severe adverse events.[70,71] It is an effective option in patients who are unable to tolerate or absorb oral or enterically administered oseltamivir due to gastric stasis, malabsorption, or gastrointestinal bleeding. Enteric oseltamivir and intravenous peramivir had similar clinical benefits in hospitalized influenza patients.[70] The benefit of peramivir beyond 1 day has not been demonstrated. Intravenous peramivir at a dosage of 600 mg once daily (10 mg/kg once daily in children) for 5 days plus standard of care did not demonstrate a clinical benefit compared with placebo plus standard of care in hospitalized patients younger than 6 years.[72]

Neuropsychiatric complications consisting of delirium, seizures, hallucinations, and self-injury in pediatric patients (mostly from Japan) have been reported following treatment with oseltamivir, and peramivir. Since influenza itself can be associated with neuropsychiatric manifestations, a causal relationship between oseltamivir or peramivir and neuropsychiatric effects has not been delineated. However, the labels for oseltamivir and peramivir have been updated to include neuropsychiatric events as a precaution, and their occurrence with use of these agents should not be ignored.

Influenza resistance to the NA inhibitors has been documented but cross-resistance between the NA inhibitors has not.[21,51] Antiviral resistance remains relatively low. During the 2018 to 2019 influenza season, 99% of the tested A(H1N1) pdm09 viruses were susceptible to oseltamivir and peramivir, and 100% of the 2009 H1N1 viruses tested were susceptible to zanamivir; 100% of influenza A (H3N2) tested were susceptible to both oseltamivir and zanamivir; and 100% of influenza B viruses tested were susceptible to both oseltamivir and zanamivir.[21,51] Antiviral susceptibility testing of circulating viruses confirmed that seasonal influenza A H3N2 and variant influenza H3N2 maintain susceptibility to oseltamivir, peramivir, and zanamivir.[21] The burden of surveillance rests on clinicians to identify local patterns of influenza circulation to guide antiviral therapy.

Special Populations

There is inadequate data for the use of anti-influenza medications in special populations, such as immunocompromised hosts. Furthermore, there is limited data for use of influenza antivirals during pregnancy. The adamantanes are embryotoxic and teratogenic in rats, and limited case reports of adverse fetal outcomes following amantadine use in humans have been published. Oseltamivir and zanamivir have been used but lack solid safety clinical data in pregnant females. Pregnancy should not be considered a contraindication to oseltamivir or zanamivir use. Oseltamivir is preferred for the treatment of pregnant females because of its systemic activity; however, the drug of choice for chemoprophylaxis is not yet defined. Zanamivir may be preferred because of its limited systemic absorption, but respiratory complications need to be considered, especially in females with underlying respiratory diseases. Both the adamantanes and the NA inhibitors are excreted in breast milk and should be avoided by mothers who are breastfeeding their infants. More studies are needed in these populations who are at high risk for serious disease and complications from influenza.

PANDEMIC PREPAREDNESS

This chapter is not meant to provide an exhaustive review of the biology of influenza or pandemic preparedness. This topic is rapidly changing and interested readers are referred to the following Websites: www.flu.gov, www.who.int/influenza/human_animal_interface/en/, and www.cdc.gov/h1n1flu.

A vital component of pandemic preparedness is forethought—plans must be established for how to effectively triage large numbers of ill patients, prioritize and/or ration vaccine and antivirals, and communicate with the public through mass media during a period of severe labor shortage (a result of stress and illness among healthcare workers) and supply shortfall (a result of societal and economic disruption).

EVALUATION OF THERAPEUTIC OUTCOMES

Patients should be monitored daily for resolution of signs and symptoms associated with influenza, such as fever, myalgia, headache, malaise, nonproductive cough, sore throat, and rhinitis. These signs and symptoms will typically resolve within approximately 1 week. If the patient continues to exhibit signs and symptoms of illness beyond 10 days or a worsening of symptoms after 7 days, a physician visit is warranted as this may be an indication of a secondary bacterial infection. Ideally, antiviral therapy should not be started until influenza is confirmed via the laboratory. However, therapy should be initiated within 48 hours of illness onset, emphasizing the need for rapid diagnosis. Repeat diagnostic tests to demonstrate clearance of the virus are not necessary.

ABBREVIATIONS

AAP	American Academy of Pediatrics
ACIP	Advisory Committee on Immunization Practices
CDC	US Centers for Disease Control and Prevention
DFA	direct fluorescence antibody
EIA	enzyme immunoassay
FDA	Food and Drug Administration
GBS	Guillain-Barré syndrome
GMTs	geometric mean titers
HIV	human immunodeficiency virus
IFA	indirect fluorescence antibody
IIV	inactivated influenza vaccine
IIV3	trivalent influenza vaccine
IIV4	quadrivalent influenza vaccine
LAIV	live-attenuated influenza vaccine
M	matrix
NA	neuraminidase
PIDS	Pediatric Infectious Diseases Society
POC	point of care
PRs	protection rates
RIDTs	Rapid Influenza Diagnostic Tests
RIMAs	rapid influenza molecular assays
RT-PCR	reverse-transcription polymerase chain reaction
SOIV	swine origin influenza virus
VE	vaccine efficacy
WHO	World Health Organization

REFERENCES

1. Rolfes MA, Foppa IM, Garg S, et al. Annual estimates of the burden of seasonal influenza in the United States: A tool for strengthening influenza surveillance and preparedness. *Influenza Other Respir Viruses.* 2018;12(1):132–137.
2. Centers for Disease Control and Prevention. Disease Burden of Influenza. Available at https://www.cdc.gov/flu/about/burden/index.html. August 20, 2021.
3. Iuliano AD, Roguski KM, Chang HH, et al. Global Seasonal Influenza-associated Mortality Collaborator Network. Estimates of global seasonal influenza-associated respiratory mortality: A modelling study. *Lancet.* 2018;391(10127):1285–1300.
4. Yan S, Weycker D, Sokolowski S. US healthcare costs attributable to type A and type B influenza. *Hum Vaccin Immunother.* 2017;13(9):2041–2047.
5. Centers for Disease Control and Prevention. 2019–2020 U.S. Flu Season: Preliminary Burden Estimates. Available at https://www.cdc.gov/flu/about/burden/preliminary-in-season-estimates.htm. Accessed August 20, 2021.
6. Centers for Disease Control and Prevention. Laboratory-Confirmed Influenza Hospitalizations. Available at https://gis.cdc.gov/GRASP/Fluview/FluHospRates.html. Accessed August 20, 2021.
7. 2020–2021 Flu Season Summary. Available at https://www.cdc.gov/flu/season/faq-flu-season-2020-2021.htm. Accessed August 20, 2021.
8. Centers for Disease Control and Prevention. Estimates of Flu Vaccination Coverage, United States, 2020–21 Influenza Season. Available at https://www.cdc.gov/flu/fluvaxview/interactive.htm. Accessed August 20, 2021.
9. Weekly National Flu Vaccination Dashboard https://www.cdc.gov/flu/fluvaxview/dashboard/vaccination-dashboard.html. Accessed August 20, 2021.
10. HHS Vaccines National Strategic Plan for the United States 2021–2025 https://www.hhs.gov/sites/default/files/HHS-Vaccines-Report.pdf. Accessed August 20, 2021.
11. Centers for Disease Control and Prevention. Preliminary Estimates of 2019–20 Seasonal Influenza Vaccine Effectiveness against Medically Attended Influenza from three U.S. Networks. Available at https://www.cdc.gov/flu/vaccines-work/2019-2020.html. Accessed August 20, 2021.
12. Reed C, Chaves SS, Perez A, et al. Complications among adults hospitalized with influenza: A comparison of seasonal influenza and the 2009 H1N1 pandemic. *Clin Infect Dis.* 2014;59(2):166–174.
13. Lagacé-Wiens PR, Rubinstein E, Gumel A. Influenza epidemiology—Past, present, and future. *Crit Care Med.* 2010;38(4 Suppl):e1–9.
14. Morens DM, Taubenberger JK, Harvey HA, et al. The 1918 influenza pandemic: Lessons for 2009 and the future. *Crit Care Med.* 2010;38(4 Suppl):e10–20.
15. Trombetta C, Piccirella S, Perini D, et al. Emerging influenza strains in the last two decades: A threat of a new pandemic? *Vaccines (Basel).* 2015;3(1):172–185.
16. Centers for Disease Control and Prevention. Avian Influenza: Influenza Type A Viruses. Available at https://www.cdc.gov/flu/avianflu/influenza-a-virus-subtypes.htm. Accessed September 10, 2021.
17. World Health Organization. Avian Influenza Weekly Update Number 810. Available at https://www.who.int/westernpacific/emergencies/surveillance/avian-influenza.
18. Anonymous. Avian influenza A(H7N9) virus. Available at http://www.who.int/influenza/human_animal_interface/influenza_h7n9/en/. Accessed July 10, 2021.
19. Nguyen HH. Brown T. Influenza Clinical Presentation. Medscape News. Available at https://emedicine.medscape.com/article/219557-clinical. April 23, 2019; Accessed September 12, 2019.
20. FluView. Weekly U.S. Influenza Surveillance Report 2020–2021 Influenza Season. Available at https://www.cdc.gov/flu/weekly/index.htm. Accessed August 12, 2021.
21. Centers for Disease Control and Prevention. Influenza Antiviral Drug Resistance. Available at https://www.cdc.gov/flu/treatment/antiviralresistance.htm. Accessed August 10, 2021.
22. Anonymous. Influenza virus vaccine, H5N1 [prescribing information]. Swiftwater, PA: Sanofi Pasteur; April 2007.

23. Anonymous. Influenza A (H5N1) virus monovalent vaccine, adjuvanted. Research Triangle Park, NC: GlaxoSmithKline; September 2016.
24. World Health Organization. Summary of status of development and availability of avian influenza A(H7N9) candidate vaccine viruses and potency testing reagents. Available at https://www.who.int/influenza/vaccines/virus/candidates_reagents/summary_a_h7n9_cvv_nh1920_20190220.pdf?ua=1. Accessed October 10, 2019.
25. World Tourism Organization. *International Tourism Highlights*. 2020 ed. Madrid: UNWTO; 2021. doi:https://doi.org/10.18111/9789284422456.
26. U.S. Department of Commerce International Trade Administration/Industry and Analysis National Travel and Tourism Office (NTTO). U.S. Resident Travel to International Destinations Increased Six Percent in 2019. Available at https://travel.trade.gov/tinews/archive/tinews2019/20190402.asp. Accessed August 12, 2021.
27. Saunders-Hastings PR, Krewski D. Reviewing the history of pandemic influenza: Understanding patterns of emergence and transmission. *Pathogens*. 2016;5(4):pii: E66.
28. Centers for Disease Control and Prevention. Update: Novel influenza A (H1N1) virus infections—Worldwide, May 6, 2009. *MMWR Morb Mortal Wkly Rep*. 2009;58:453–458.
29. Dawood FS, Iuliano AD, Reed C, et al. Estimated global mortality associated with the first 12 months of 2009 pandemic influenza A H1N1 virus circulation: A modeling study. *Lancet Infect Dis*. 2012;12:687–695.
30. Uyeki TM. Influenza. *Ann Intern Med*. 2017;167(5):ITC33–ITC48.
31. Blanton L, Wentworth DE, Alabi N, et al. Update: Influenza Activity—United States and Worldwide, May 21–September 23, 2017. *MMWR Morb Mortal Wkly Rep*. 2017;66:1043–1051.
32. Centers for Disease Control and Prevention. Influenza A (H3N2) Variant Virus Outbreaks. Available at http://www.cdc.gov/flu/swineflu/h3n2v-case-count.htm. Accessed July 12, 2021
33. Centers for Disease Control and Prevention. People at High Risk For Flu Complications. Available at https://www.cdc.gov/flu/highrisk/index.htm. Accessed August 12, 2021.
34. Grohskopf LA, Alyanak E, Ferdinands JM, Broder KR, Blanton LH, Talbot HK, Fry AM. Prevention and control of seasonal influenza with vaccines: Recommendations of the Advisory Committee on Immunization Practices, United States, 2021–22 Influenza Season. *MMWR Recomm Rep*. 2021;70(5):1–28.
35. Recommendations for Prevention and Control of Influenza in Children, 2020–2021. Committee on Infectious Diseases. Committee on Infectious Diseases. *Pediatrics*. 2020;146(4):e2020024588.
36. Uyeki TM, Bernstein HH, Bradley JS, et al. Clinical Practice Guidelines by the Infectious Diseases Society of America: 2018 Update on Diagnosis, Treatment, Chemoprophylaxis, and Institutional Outbreak Management of Seasonal Influenza. *Clin Infect Dis*. 2019;68(6):895–902.
37. Centers for Disease Control and Prevention. Influenza testing and clinical algorithms. Available at https://www.cdc.gov/flu/professionals/diagnosis/index.htm. Accessed May 12, 2021.
38. Vos LM, Bruning AHL, Reitsma JB, et al. Rapid molecular tests for influenza, respiratory syncytial virus, and other respiratory viruses: A systematic review of diagnostic accuracy and clinical impact studies. *Clin Infect Dis*. 2019;69(7):1243–1253.
39. Lu PJ, Srivastav A, Amaya A, et al. Association of provider recommendation and offer and influenza vaccination among adults aged ≥18 years—United States. *Vaccine*. 2018;36(6):890–898.
40. Tricco AC, Chit A, Soobiah C, et al. Comparing influenza vaccine efficacy against mismatched and matched strains: A systematic review and meta-analysis. *BMC Med*. 2013;11:153.
41. Hoberman A, Greenberg DP, Paradise JL, et al. Effectiveness of inactivated influenza vaccine in preventing acute otitis media in young children: A randomized controlled trial. *JAMA*. 2003;290(12):1608–1616.
42. Jefferson T, Rivetti A, Di Pietrantonj C, Demicheli V. Vaccines for preventing influenza in healthy children. *Cochrane Database Syst Rev*. 2018;2:CD004879.
43. Demicheli V, Jefferson T, Ferroni E, et al. Vaccines for preventing influenza in healthy adults. *Cochrane Database Syst Rev*. 2018;2:CD001269.
44. DiazGranados CA, Dunning AJ, Kimmel M, et al. Efficacy of high-dose versus standard-dose influenza vaccine in older adults. *N Engl J Med*. 2014;371:635–645.
45. Demicheli V, Jefferson T, Di Pietrantonj C, et al. Vaccines for preventing influenza in the elderly. *Cochrane Database Syst Rev*. 2018;2:CD004876.
46. Chit A, Roiz J, Briquet B, Greenberg DP. Expected cost effectiveness of high-dose trivalent influenza vaccine in US seniors. *Vaccine*. 2015;33(5):734–741.
47. Vellozzi C, Iqbal S, Broder K. Guillain-Barré syndrome, influenza, and influenza vaccination: The epidemiologic evidence. *Clin Infect Dis*. 2014;58(8):1149–1155.
48. Price CS, Thompson WW, Goodson B, et al. Prenatal and infant exposure to thimerosal from vaccines and immunoglobulins and risk of autism. *Pediatrics*. 2010;126:656–664.
49. Taylor LE, Swerdfeger AL, Eslick GD. Vaccines are not associated with autism: An evidence-based meta-analysis of case-control and cohort studies. *Vaccine*. 2014 Jun 17;32(29):3623–3629. doi:10.1016/j.vaccine.2014.04.085.
50. FluMist Quadrivalent Vaccine [prescribing information]. Gaithersburg, MD: MedImmune, LLC; 2019.
51. Centers for Diseases Control and Prevention. Influenza Antiviral Medications: Summary for Clinicians 2021–2022. https://www.cdc.gov/flu/professionals/antivirals/index.htm.
52. XOFLUZA [Prescribing Information]. South San Francisco, CA: Genentech USA, Inc.; 2018.
53. Ikematsu H, Hayden GF, Kawaguchi K, et al. Baloxavir marboxil for prophylaxis against influenza in household contacts. *N Engl J Med*. 2020 Jul 23;383:309.
54. Benowitz I, Esposito DB, Gracey KD, et al. Influenza vaccine given to pregnant women reduces hospitalization due to influenza in their infants. *Clin Infect Dis*. 2010;51(12):1355–1361.
55. Thompson MG, Kwong JC, Regan AK, et al. Influenza vaccine effectiveness in preventing influenza- associated hospitalizations during pregnancy: A Multi-country Retrospective Test Negative Design Study, 2010–2016. *Clin Infect Dis*. 2019;68(9):1444–1453.
56. McKittrick N, Frank I, Jacobson JM, et al. Improved immunogenicity with high-dose seasonal influenza vaccine in HIV-infected persons: A single-center, parallel, randomized trial. *Ann Intern Med*. 2013;158(1):19–26.
57. Natori Y, Shiotsuka M, Slomovic J, et al. A double blind randomized trial of high dose vs. standard dose influenza vaccine in adult solid organ transplant recipients. *Clin Infect Dis*. 2018;66(11):1698–1704.
58. Cordero E, Roca-Oporto C, Bulnes-Ramos A, et al. TRANSGRIPE 1–2 Study Group. Two doses of inactivated influenza vaccine improve immune response in solid organ transplant recipients: Results of TRANSGRIPE 1-2, a randomized controlled clinical trial. *Clin Infect Dis*. 2017;64(7):829–838.
59. Kumar D, Ferreira VH, Blumberg E, et al. A five-year prospective multi-center evaluation of influenza infection in transplant recipients. *Clin Infect Dis*. 2018;67(9):1322–1329.
60. Shehata MA, Karim NA. Influenza vaccination in cancer patients undergoing systemic therapy. *Clin Med Insights Oncol*. 2014;8:57–64.
61. Bitterman R, Eliakim-Raz N, Vinograd I, et al. Influenza vaccines in immunosuppressed adults with cancer. *Cochrane Database Syst Rev*. 2018 Feb 1;2:CD008983.
62. Dominguez A, Romero-Tamarit A, Soldevila N, et al. Effectiveness of antiviral treatment in preventing death in severe hospitalised influenza cases over six seasons. *Epidemiol Infect*. 2018;146(7):799–808.
63. Doll MK, Winters N, Boikos C, et al. Safety and effectiveness of neuraminidase inhibitors for influenza treatment, prophylaxis, and outbreak control: A systematic review of systematic reviews and/or meta-analyses. *J Antimicrob Chemother*. 2017;72(11):2990–3007.
64. Malosh RE, Martin ET, Heikkinen T, et al. Efficacy and safety of oseltamivir in children: Systematic review and individual patient data meta-analysis of randomized controlled trials. *Clin Infect Dis*. 2018;66(10):1492–1500.
65. Muthuri SG, Venkatesan S, Myles PR, et al. Effectiveness of neuraminidase inhibitors in reducing mortality in patients admitted to hospital with influenza A H1N1pdm09 virus infection: A meta-analysis of individual participant data. *Lancet Respir Med*. 2014;2(5):395–404.
66. Katzen J, Kohn R, Houk JL, Ison MG. Early oseltamivir after hospital admission is associated with shortened hospitalization: A five-year analysis of oseltamivir timing and clinical outcomes. *Clin Infect Dis*. 2019;69(1):52–58.
67. Louie JK, Yang S, Acosta M, et al. Treatment with neuraminidase inhibitors for critically ill patients with influenza A (H1N1)pdm09. *Clin Infect Dis*. 2012;55(9):1198–1204.
68. Kaiser L, Wat C, Mills T, et al. Impact of oseltamivir treatment on influenza-related lower respiratory tract complications and hospitalizations. *Arch Intern Med*. 2003;163(14):1667–1672.
69. Kaiser L, Keene ON, Hammond JM, et al. Impact of zanamivir on antibiotic use for respiratory events following acute influenza in adolescents and adults. *Arch Intern Med*. 2000;160(21):3234–3240.
70. Nakamura S, Miyazaki T, Izumikawa K, et al. Efficacy and safety of intravenous peramivir compared with oseltamivir in high-risk patients

infected with influenza A and B viruses: A multicenter randomized controlled study. *Open Forum Infect Dis.* 2017;4(3):ofx129.

71. Lee J, Park JH, Jwa H, Kim YH. Comparison of efficacy of intravenous Peramivir and Oral Oseltamivir for the treatment of influenza: Systematic review and meta-analysis. *Yonsei Med J.* 2017;58(4):778–785.

72. de Jong MD, Ison MG, Monto AS, et al. Evaluation of intravenous peramivir for treatment of influenza in hospitalized patients. *Clin Infect Dis.* 2014;59(12):172–185.

Coronavirus Disease (COVID-19)

e132

Jason M. Pogue, Erin K. McCreary, and Julie Ann Justo

All information in this chapter is current as of August 1, 2022. The COVID-19 pandemic is a rapidly evolving situation with frequently changing information. While this text should serve as a foundational reference, the National Institutes of Health (NIH) and Infectious Diseases Society of America (IDSA) COVID-19 Treatment Guidelines and the Centers for Disease Control and Prevention (CDC) COVID-19 Vaccination site should be referenced electronically for the most current treatment and prevention recommendations.

KEY CONCEPTS

1. Coronavirus disease 2019 (COVID-19), caused by the SARS-CoV-2 virus, is associated with significant morbidity and mortality particularly among patients 65 years of age and older, those with multiple chronic comorbidities, and/or patients of select racial and ethnic backgrounds.
2. The primary route of transmission of SARS-CoV-2 is direct person-to-person respiratory transmission via infected particles (ie, droplets, aerosols). Risk of transmission is greatest for individuals in close contact for a significant period of time, especially while indoors. Transmission can occur from symptomatic, presymptomatic, or asymptomatic individuals.
3. COVID-19 disease progression occurs in three phases of increasing severity: (i) early infection, (ii) pulmonary phase, and (iii) hyperinflammation. The majority of patients recover in the early infection phase; yet a small proportion may progress to the pulmonary and hyperinflammation phases.
4. Signs and symptoms typically emerge 3 to 5 days from onset of infection but may occur sooner or take up to 14 days to manifest. Common symptoms include rhinorrhea, headache, sore throat, sneezing, cough, and fever/chills. Evolving variants manifest differently both with regards to timing and type of symptom onset. Oxygenation status and patient location (hospitalized vs nonhospitalized) are defining characteristics that determine eligibility for specific pharmacotherapy.
5. Symptomatic COVID-19 is diagnosed by a positive nucleic acid amplification test (NAAT) or antigen test for SARS-CoV-2. Asymptomatic infection is a positive test in the absence of symptoms. Probable COVID-19 can be diagnosed by a compatible syndrome in either the absence of viral testing or a negative test. False negative tests are most common early in infection and with use of antigen tests.
6. Four vaccines are available in the United States: two using an mRNA technology platform (Pfizer, Moderna), one using an adenovirus vector platform (Johnson & Johnson), and one using an adjuvanted recombinant spike protein platform (Novovax). All eligible patients should receive a vaccination series as soon as possible to prevent COVID-19.
7. One combination monoclonal antibody product, tixagevimab and cilgavimab, is available for pre-exposure prophylaxis against SARS-CoV-2 for immunocompromised patients who may not mount an adequate immune response to COVID-19 vaccination or for whom vaccination with any available vaccine is not recommended due to history of severe allergy to any vaccine component.
8. Therapeutic management of mild-to-moderate COVID-19 in high-risk, nonhospitalized adult patients should include symptomatic management and either ritonavir-boosted nirmatrelvir, 3 days of remdesivir, or monoclonal antibody therapy. If none of these therapies are available, molnupiravir may be considered.
9. Therapeutic management of severe COVID-19 in hospitalized patients requiring supplemental oxygen should include dexamethasone, remdesivir, and therapeutic anticoagulation unless contraindicated.
10. Therapeutic management of severe to critical illness from COVID-19 in hospitalized patients with rapidly increasing oxygen needs and systemic inflammation should include dexamethasone plus either baricitinib or tocilizumab. These patients should receive only prophylactic dose heparin (unless contraindicated). Remdesivir should not be used in patients requiring mechanical ventilation.

BEYOND THE BOOK

Most U.S. states have a Department of Public Health webpage dedicated to providing COVID-19 information. Conduct a search to find your state's page and familiarize yourself with the categories of information contained within.

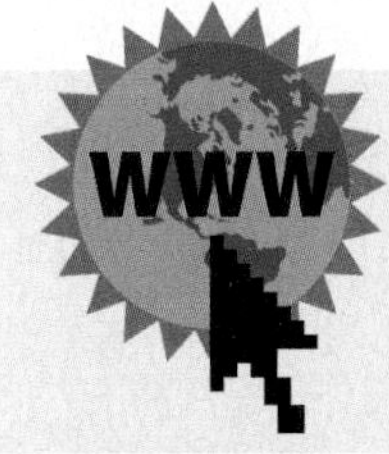

The complete chapter, learning objectives, and other resources can be found at **www.pharmacotherapyonline.com.**

Skin and Soft Tissue Infections

Douglas N. Fish

133

KEY CONCEPTS

1. Folliculitis, furuncles (boils), and carbuncles begin around hair follicles and are caused most often by *Staphylococcus aureus*. Folliculitis and small furuncles are generally treated with warm, moist heat to promote drainage; larger furuncles and carbuncles require incision and drainage. Purulent, moderately severe infections (eg, with fever or other systemic signs of infection) have a higher suspicion for community-associated methicillin-resistant *S. aureus* (MRSA) and empiric treatment should include trimethoprim–sulfamethoxazole or a tetracycline such as doxycycline.
2. Erysipelas, a superficial skin infection with extensive lymphatic involvement, is caused by *Streptococcus pyogenes*. The treatment of choice is penicillin, administered orally or parenterally, depending on the severity of the infection.
3. Impetigo is a superficial skin infection that occurs most commonly in children. It is characterized by fluid-filled vesicles that rapidly develop into pus-filled blisters that rupture to form golden-yellow crusts. Effective therapy includes penicillinase-resistant penicillins (dicloxacillin), first-generation cephalosporins (cephalexin), and topical mupirocin or retapamulin. *S. aureus* is the primary cause of impetigo, with MRSA becoming more common in recent years.
4. Lymphangitis, an infection of the subcutaneous lymphatic channels, is usually caused by *S. pyogenes*. Acute lymphangitis is characterized by the rapid development of fine, red, linear streaks extending from the initial infection site toward the regional lymph nodes, which are usually enlarged and tender. Penicillin is the drug of choice.
5. Cellulitis is an infection of the epidermis, dermis, and superficial fascia most commonly caused by *S. pyogenes* and *S. aureus*. Lesions generally are hot, painful, and erythematous, with nonelevated, poorly defined margins. Oral trimethoprim–sulfamethoxazole, doxycycline, or minocycline is used for initial treatment of suspected MRSA in patients with purulent, moderately severe cellulitis (ie, lesion with purulent drainage or exudate, or nondrainable abscess plus systemic signs of infection). Treatment of nonpurulent cellulitis generally consists of penicillin VK, a penicillinase-resistant penicillin (dicloxacillin), first-generation cephalosporin (cephalexin), or clindamycin for 5 days; coverage for MRSA may be added in certain patients. More severe infections in hospitalized and/or immunocompromised patients should receive empiric therapy with parenteral agents active against streptococci (nonpurulent infections) or both streptococci and MRSA (purulent infections).
6. Necrotizing fasciitis is an uncommon but life-threatening infection of subcutaneous tissue that results in progressive destruction of superficial fascia and subcutaneous fat. Early and aggressive surgical debridement is an essential part of therapy for treatment of necrotizing fasciitis. Mixed infections are treated with broad-spectrum regimens that cover streptococci, gram-negative aerobes, and anaerobes. Infections caused by *S. pyogenes* or *Clostridium* species should be treated with the combination of penicillin and clindamycin.
7. Diabetic foot infections are managed with a comprehensive treatment approach that includes both proper wound care and antimicrobial therapy. Potential pathogens include staphylococci, streptococci, aerobic gram-negative bacilli, and obligate anaerobes. Antimicrobial regimens for diabetic foot infections are based on severity of the infection, expected treatment setting, and risk factors for infection with more resistant pathogens such as MRSA and *Pseudomonas aeruginosa*. Outpatient therapy with oral antimicrobials should be used whenever possible for less severe infections, while more severe infections initially require IV therapy.
8. Prevention is the single most important aspect in the management of pressure injuries. After an injury develops, successful local care includes a comprehensive approach consisting of relief of pressure, proper cleaning (debridement), disinfection, and appropriate antimicrobial therapy if an infection is present. Good wound care is crucial to successful management.
9. All bite wounds (animal or human) should be thoroughly irrigated with large volumes of sterile normal saline, and the injured area should be immobilized and elevated. Depending on the severity of the bite wound, amoxicillin–clavulanic acid or ampicillin–sulbactam is often used for treatment of animal bites because of their coverage of *Pasteurella* species, streptococci, *S. aureus*, and anaerobes typically present in the oral flora of dogs and cats.
10. Antimicrobial prophylaxis (early preemptive therapy) of animal bites is not routinely recommended; however, patients at high risk of infection (eg, immunocompromised, moderate-to-severe bite injuries especially to the hands and face, penetration of the periosteum or joint capsule) should be given prophylactic antimicrobial therapy for 3 to 5 days. Infected bite wounds should be treated for 7 to 14 days with oral or IV antibiotics having activity against *Eikenella corrodens*, streptococci, *S. aureus*, and β-lactamase–producing anaerobes.

BEYOND THE BOOK

Refer to "Chapter 126: Skin and Soft Tissue Infection: A Pain in the Butt Level II" in Pharmacotherapy Casebook: A Patient-Focused Approach, 11e (may be obtained online through AccessPharmacy). After studying the patient presentation, briefly answer Questions 1 through 5 and the Follow-Up Case Questions 1 through 9 regarding patient Jimmie Chipwood's skin and soft tissue infection (SSTI). The purpose of this exercise is to gain experience in applying knowledge regarding SSTI to assess infections in individual patients and develop an appropriate therapeutic plan based on clinical presentation, type and severity of infection, past treatment history, potential causative pathogens, and patient characteristics.

INTRODUCTION

Skin and soft-tissue infections (SSTIs) may involve any or all layers of the skin (epidermis, dermis, subcutaneous fat), fascia, and muscle. They may also spread far from the initial site of infection and lead to more severe complications, such as endocarditis, gram-negative sepsis, or streptococcal glomerulonephritis. Sometimes the treatment of SSTIs may necessitate both medical and surgical management. This chapter presents details of the pathogenesis and management of some of the most common infections involving the skin and soft tissues, ranging in severity from superficial to life-threatening.

EPIDEMIOLOGY

Bacterial infections of the skin can be classified as primary or secondary (Table 133-1).[1-4] Primary bacterial infections usually involve areas of previously healthy skin and are caused by a single pathogen. In contrast, secondary infections occur in areas of previously damaged skin and are frequently polymicrobic. SSTIs are also classified as complicated or uncomplicated. Complicated infections are those that involve deeper skin structures (eg, fascia, muscle layers), require significant surgical intervention, and/or occur in patients with compromised immune function (eg, diabetes mellitus, human immunodeficiency virus [HIV] infection).[3-5] Other categories that are crucial for successful treatment are the differentiation of necrotizing versus non-necrotizing, as well as purulent versus nonpurulent, SSTIs.[3-6] Acute bacterial skin and skin structure infections (ABSSSIs) are a subset of SSTI and specifically denote those more severe bacterial infections of the skin with a lesion size area of at least 75 cm^2 and for which antibiotic therapy is generally considered to be required for successful resolution.[7] The subset of ABSSSI specifically includes cellulitis, erysipelas, wound infection, and major cutaneous abscess.[7]

SSTIs are among the most common infections seen in community and hospital settings.[9,10] However, most infections are mild and are treated in an outpatient setting, making it difficult to accurately quantify community-acquired SSTIs. SSTIs occur in approximately 14 million persons each year, being more common among those 50 years of age and older.[8,9,10] Emergency room visits for SSTIs continue to increase each year, attributed primarily to an increase in community-associated methicillin-resistant *Staphylococcus aureus* (CA-MRSA) cellulitis and abscesses.[3-5,11] Both inpatient admissions and outpatient office visits due to SSTIs increased by approximately 65% over a 9-year period in the early 2000s; during this same period the prevalence of MRSA among SSTIs increased from 29% to 64% in one emergency department.[10,12] In 2011 SSTIs were responsible for over 750,000 hospitalizations and represented approximately 2% of all admissions.[10] Additionally, the frequency of infections caused by drug-resistant gram-positive cocci (particuarly

TABLE 133-1 Bacterial Classification of Important Skin and Soft-Tissue Infections

Primary Infections	
Erysipelas	Group A streptococci (*Streptococcus pyogenes*)
Impetigo	*Staphylococcus aureus* (including methicillin-resistant strains), group A streptococci
Lymphangitis	Group A streptococci; occasionally *S. aureus*
Cellulitis	Group A streptococci, *S. aureus* (potentially including methicillin-resistant strains); occasionally other gram-positive cocci, gram-negative bacilli, and/or anaerobes
Necrotizing fasciitis	
Type I	Anaerobes (*Bacteroides* spp., *Peptostreptococcus* spp.) and facultative bacteria (streptococci, Enterobacterales)
Type II	Group A streptococci
Type III	*Clostridioides perfringens*
Secondary Infections	
Diabetic foot infections	*S. aureus*, streptococci, Enterobacteriaceae, *Bacteroides* spp., *Peptostreptococcus* spp., *Pseudomonas aeruginosa*
Pressure sores	*S. aureus* including methicillin-resistant strains, streptococci, Enterobacterales, *Bacteroides* spp., *Peptostreptococcus* spp., *P. aeruginosa*
Bite wounds	
Animal	*Pasteurella* spp., *S. aureus*, streptococci, *Bacteroides* spp.
Human	*Eikenella corrodens*, *S. aureus*, streptococci, *Corynebacterium* spp., *Bacteroides* spp., *Peptostreptococcus* spp.
Burn wounds	*P. aeruginosa*, Enterobacterales, *S. aureus*, streptococci

Data from References 1, 2, and 8.

S. aureus) has been increasing.[3-6,10,11] While the high incidence of healthcare-associated MRSA (HA-MRSA) has been a major concern for many years, the emergence of CA-MRSA is even more problematic.[3-6,13-20] CA-MRSA are characteristically isolated from patients lacking typical risk factors (eg, prior hospitalization, long-term care facility residence) and are often susceptible to antibiotics such as trimethoprim–sulfamethoxazole, doxycycline, and clindamycin.[13-20] They also differ genetically from HA-MRSA with methicillin resistance carried on the type IV or V staphylococcal chromosomal cassette *mec* (SCC*mec*) element of the *mecA* gene.[1,13,18] CA-MRSA strains often harbor genes for Panton-Valentine leukocidin (PVL), a cytotoxin causing leukocyte destruction and tissue necrosis. In contrast, HA-MRSA strains usually lack genes for PVL and are associated with SCC*mec* alleles I to III.[1,13,15,18] While the incidence of HA-MRSA has declined in recent years,[21] the incidence of CA-MRSA has dramatically increased; nearly half (46%) of all culture-positive SSTIs are caused by MRSA and nearly 50% of all CA-MRSA are isolated from SSTIs.[3-6,9,10,20] Clinicians should suspect CA-MRSA in geographic areas with a high prevalence of these strains, or in recurrent or persistent infections that are not responding to appropriate β-lactam therapy. In addition to the emergence of CA-MRSA, there is also concern about the use of clindamycin for CA-MRSA infections due to the risk of inducible clindamycin resistance in strains that are erythromycin-resistant, but clindamycin-susceptible.[8,15,18,21,23] A double-disk test (D-zone test) is recommended to identify erythromycin-resistant strains with inducible clindamycin resistance if treatment with clindamycin is desired.[4,6,13,15,18,24] A positive D-zone test, indicating the presence of inducible resistance conferred by the *erm* gene, suggests the possibility of the emergence of clindamycin resistance during therapy.[13,15,18,24]

TABLE 133-2 Predominant Microorganisms of Normal Skin

Bacteria

Gram-positive
- Coagulase-negative staphylococci
- Micrococci (*Micrococcus luteus*)
- *Corynebacterium* species (diphtheroids)
- *Propionibacterium* species

Gram-negative
- *Acinetobacter* species

Fungi
- *Malassezia* species
- *Candida* species

Data from References 1, 2, and 8.

ETIOLOGY

The majority of SSTIs are caused by gram-positive organisms present on the skin surface.[2,6,22] Gram-positive bacteria (coagulase-negative staphylococci, diphtheroids) are the predominant flora of healthy skin, with gram-negative organisms being relatively uncommon (Table 133-2).[1,2,8,22] *S. aureus*, as well as a variety of gram-negative bacteria, including *Acinetobacter* species, can be found in moist intertriginous areas (eg, axilla, groin, and toe webs) of the body.[1,2,22,23] Approximately 30% to 35% of healthy individuals are reported to be colonized with *S. aureus* on the skin or in the anterior nares.[1,8,22] Colonization, whether transient or permanent, provides a nidus for infection should the integrity of the epidermis be compromised.[1-3,5,6,8,22]

S. aureus and *S. pyogenes* account for the majority of community-acquired SSTIs.[1,12,15,22] Data from large surveillance studies showed *S. aureus* to be the most common cause of SSTIs in hospitalized patients, with often 30% to 50% of these being caused by MRSA.[8,10,12,13,17,20] Other common healthcare-associated pathogens included *Pseudomonas aeruginosa* (11%), enterococci (9%), and *Escherichia coli* (7%).[6,8,10,13]

PATHOPHYSIOLOGY

The skin serves as a barrier between humans and their environment, therefore functioning as a primary defense mechanism against infections. The skin and subcutaneous tissues normally are extremely resistant to infection but may become susceptible under certain conditions. Although the human skin supports an abundant and diverse microbiome of bacteria and fungi,[1,2,22] several host factors act together to confer protection against skin infections. Continuous renewal of the epidermal layer results in the shedding of keratocytes, as well as skin bacteria.[2,22] In addition, sebaceous secretions are hydrolyzed to form free fatty acids that strongly inhibit the growth of many bacteria and fungi. A normal commensal skin microbiome itself serves a protective function by not allowing space or environmental conditions favorable to colonization with more pathogenic strains.[1,2,22] Conditions that may predispose a patient to the development of skin infections include (a) high concentrations of bacteria (more than 10^5 microorganisms), (b) excessive moisture of the skin, (c) inadequate blood supply, (d) availability of bacterial nutrients, and (e) damage to the corneal layer allowing for bacterial penetration.[2,3,5,8,22,23,25]

The best defense against SSTI is intact skin.[2,22,25] The majority of SSTIs result from the disruption of normal host defenses by processes such as skin puncture, abrasion, or underlying diseases (eg, diabetes).[1-3,5,8,22,25] The nature and severity of the infection depend on both the type of microorganism present and the site of inoculation.

FOLLICULITIS, FURUNCLES, AND CARBUNCLES

1 Folliculitis is inflammation of the hair follicle and is caused by physical injury, chemical irritation, or infection. Infection occurring at the base of the eyelid is referred to as a stye. While folliculitis is a superficial infection with pus present only in the epidermis,[4,15,23] furuncles and carbuncles occur when a follicular infection around the hair shaft extends to involve deeper areas (subcutaneous tissue) of the skin.[4,15,23] A furuncle, commonly known as a *boil*, is a walled-off mass of purulent material arising from a hair follicle.[4,15,23] The lesions are called *carbuncles* when adjacent furuncles coalesce to form a single inflamed area.[4,15,23] This aggregate of infected hair follicles forms deep masses that generally open and drain through multiple sinus tracts.[15,23] *S. aureus* is the most common cause of folliculitis, furuncles, and carbuncles.[4,15,23] Outbreaks of furunculosis caused by *S. aureus* and CA-MRSA have been reported in settings involving close contact (eg, families, prisons), especially when skin injury was common (such as with athletes).[11] In addition, some individuals experience repeated episodes of furunculosis.[23] A major predisposing factor for recurrent infection is the presence of *S. aureus* in the anterior nares.[15,23]

CLINICAL PRESENTATION Folliculitis, Furuncles, and Carbuncles

Folliculitis
- Clustering, pruritic papules localized to hair follicles.
- Generally develop in areas subject to friction and perspiration.
- Papules are generally 5 mm or less in diameter and erythematous.
- Papules evolve into pustules that generally spontaneously rupture in several days.
- Systemic signs (fever, malaise) are uncommon.

Furuncles
- Inflammatory, draining nodule involving a hair follicle.
- Develop in areas subject to friction and perspiration.
- Lesions are discrete, whether occurring as singular or multiple nodules.
- Lesion starts as a firm, tender, red nodule that becomes painful and fluctuant.
- Lesions often drain spontaneously.
- Lesions caused by CA-MRSA often have necrotic centers
- Systemic signs are uncommon.

Carbuncles
- Formed when adjacent furuncles coalesce to form a single inflamed area.
- Form broad, swollen, erythematous, deep, and painful follicular masses.
- Commonly develop on the back of the neck.
- Commonly associated with systemic signs (fever, chills, malaise).
- Bacteremia with secondary spread to other tissues is common.

TREATMENT: FOLLICULITIS, FURUNCLES, AND CARBUNCLES

Desired Outcomes

The goals of treatment include relieving discomfort, preventing further spread of the infection, and preventing recurrence. Controlling recurrent furunculosis is key due to the difficulty in treating chronic furunculosis. Treatments should be effective and inexpensive and have minimal adverse effects.

Pharmacologic Therapy

Table 133-3 summarizes evidence-based treatment recommendations from clinical guidelines for SSTIs.[3,4,8,15,26-28] Treatment of folliculitis generally requires only local measures, such as warm moist

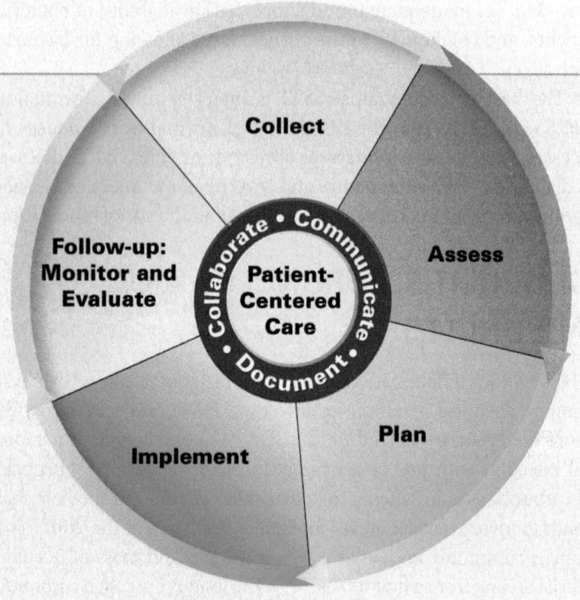

Patient Care Process for the Treatment of Skin and Soft-Tissue Infections (SSTIs)

The image shows the five fundamental steps included in The Pharmacist's Care Process endorsed by the Joint Commission for Pharmacy Practitioners (2014). The tagline of this process reads collaborate, communicate, and document. The five fundamental steps listed here are collect, assess, plan, implement, and follow-up: monitor and evaluate. All these steps are listed in a circular block diagram.

Collect

- Patient characteristics (eg, age, sex, pregnant)
- Patient medical history
- Social history (eg, drug/ethanol use), animal exposures (if bite injury)
- Current and prior medications (eg, antimicrobials, immunosuppressive agents.
- Objective data
  - Weight, temperature, blood pressure (BP), heart rate (HR), respiratory rate (RR), altered mental status (AMS), urine output (UO)
  - Laboratory findings including white blood cells (WBC) with differential, serum creatinine (SCr), liver function tests (LFT), blood glucose (especially for diabetic foot infection)
  - Culture and antimicrobial susceptibility data
  - Physical examination of skin lesions including location, size, appearance, presence of abscesses or ulcers, presence of purulence or drainage
  - Imaging studies (if suspicion for osteomyelitis, necrotizing fasciitis)

Assess

- Specific type of infection (see Clinical Presentation boxes for various SSTIs)
- Classification of infection severity, especially for cellulitis, diabetic foot infection, and pressure sores (see Tables 133-8 and 133-10)
- Risk for infection with specific pathogens (see Tables 133-1 and 133-9)
- Ability/willingness to be treated as outpatient, including potential adherence barriers
- Hemodynamic/clinical stability (eg, SBP <90 mm Hg, HR >100 bpm, RR >22, AMS, decreased UO)
- Contraindications to specific antibiotic therapy (eg, age, allergies, drug-drug/disease interactions)

Plan*

- Antibiotic regimen including specific antimicrobial(s), dose, route, frequency, and duration (see Figs. 133-1 to 133-3; Tables 133-3 to 133-5 and 133-9)
- Monitoring parameters including efficacy (eg, improvement and/or healing of infectious lesions and other symptoms [depending on specific SSTI]), and safety (eg, antibiotic side effects, *Clostridioides difficile*); frequency and timing of follow-up
- Monitoring parameters for specific antibiotics administered to hospitalized patients (see Table 133-6)
- Patient education (eg, purpose of treatment, lifestyle modification, drug- and infection-specific information, medication administration)
- Self-monitoring for resolution of SSTI signs and symptoms, signs of worsening or unresponsive SSTI, when to seek additional medical attention
- Referrals to other providers when appropriate (eg, surgeon, diabetes educator, wound care specialist)

Implement*

- Provide patient and caregiver education regarding all elements of treatment plan
- Use motivational interviewing and coaching strategies to maximize adherence to outpatient antibiotics
- Schedule follow-up as needed for more severe infections (eg, cellulitis, diabetic foot infection, pressure sores, bite wounds)

(continued)

Follow-up: Monitor and Evaluate*

- Resolution of infectious symptoms (depending on specific type of SSTI)
- Presence of adverse effects specific to the antibiotic regimen
- Patient adherence to treatment plan using multiple sources of information
- Presence of drug-drug interactions potentially requiring changes in drug regimens or monitoring plans
- Therapeutic drug levels for specific agents used in hospitalized patients (see Table 133-6)

Collaborate with patient, caregivers, and other healthcare professionals.

compresses or topical therapy (eg, clindamycin, erythromycin, mupirocin, retapamulin, or benzoyl peroxide).[8,23] Topical agents are typically applied two to four times daily for 7 days. Small furuncles generally can be treated with moist heat, which promotes localization and drainage of pus.[4,8,23] Large and/or multiple furuncles and carbuncles require incision and drainage.[4,5,8,13,15,23,27] Systemic antibiotics are usually not necessary unless accompanied by fever or extensive cellulitis.[4,5,15,23] Treatment of more severe infections (eg, accompanied by systemic signs of infection) should include oral trimethoprim–sulfamethoxazole or a tetracycline (doxycycline or minocycline) for 5 to 10 days due to a higher suspicion for MRSA (see Table 133-4 for adult and pediatric doses).[4,5,13,15,23,27] For individuals with nasal colonization, application of mupirocin ointment twice daily in the anterior nares for the first 5 days of each month decreases recurrent furunculosis by almost half.[13,15] Daily chlorhexidine washes and daily washing of personal items such as towels, bedding, and clothes may also be recommended.[15]

Evaluation of Therapeutic Outcomes

Many follicular infections resolve spontaneously without medical or surgical intervention. Lesions should be incised if they do not respond to a few days of moist heat and nonprescription topical agents. Following drainage, most lesions begin to heal within several days without antimicrobial therapy. Any patient who is unresponsive to several days of systemic antibiotic therapy or suffers recurrent infection should have a culture and sensitivity test performed to guide continued antibiotic selection.

ERYSIPELAS

2 Erysipelas is a distinct form of cellulitis involving the more superficial layers of the skin and cutaneous lymphatics.[3,30,31] The intense red color and burning pain associated with erysipelas led to the common name of "St. Anthony's fire." The infection is almost always caused by β-hemolytic streptococci, with the organisms penetrating via small breaks in the skin. Group A streptococci (*S. pyogenes*) are responsible for most infections.[8,15,31] Infections are more common in infants, young children, older adults, and patients with nephrotic syndrome or who are immunocompromised.[4,8,30,31] Erysipelas also commonly occurs in areas of preexisting lymphatic obstruction or edema.[8,13,30,31] Diagnosis is made on the basis of the characteristic lesion.

TREATMENT: ERYSIPELAS

Desired Outcomes

The goal of treatment of erysipelas is rapid eradication of the infection, thereby providing relief of symptoms (pain, tenderness, fever).[30] Preventing recurrent infection is also important as recurrence is a common complication, occurring in approximately 20% of patients.[30] Treatments should be effective and inexpensive, and have minimal adverse effects.

Pharmacologic Therapy

Mild-to-moderate cases of erysipelas are treated with intramuscular procaine penicillin G or oral penicillin VK for 7 to 10 days (see Table 133-4).[8,15,30] Recommended doses and monitoring parameters for selected antibiotics are given in Tables 133-5 and 133-6. Penicillin-allergic patients can be treated with clindamycin. For more serious infections, the patient should be hospitalized and administered IV aqueous penicillin G.[8,15] Marked improvement is seen within 48 hours, and the patient may be switched to oral penicillin to complete the course of therapy.

CLINICAL PRESENTATION Erysipelas

General

- Lower extremities are the most common sites.

Symptoms

- Flu-like symptoms (fever, chills, malaise) common prior to the appearance of the lesion.
- Infected area described as very painful or as a burning pain.

Signs

- Lesion is intensely erythematous and edematous, often with lymphatic streaking.
- Lesion has raised border, which is sharply demarcated from uninfected skin.
- Temperature is often mildly elevated.

Laboratory Tests

- Causative organism usually cannot be cultured from the skin surface.
- Needle aspiration or punch biopsies occasionally identify organism.
- Cultures considered for more severe cases (eg, atypical clinical findings such as fluid-filled blisters).

Other Diagnostic Tests

- Complete blood cell count is often performed, leukocytosis is common.
- C-reactive protein is also generally elevated.

TABLE 133-3 Evidence-Based Recommendations for Treatment of Skin and Soft-Tissue Infections

Recommendations	Recommendation Grade[a]
Folliculitis, Furuncles, Carbuncles	
Gram stain and culture of pus from carbuncles and abscesses are recommended, but treatment without cultures is reasonable in most patients	Strong, moderate
Carbuncles, abscesses, and large furuncles of mild severity should be treated with incision and drainage	Strong, high
Administration of antibiotics with activity against *Staphylococcus aureus* as an adjunct to incision and drainage should be based on the presence or absence of systemic signs of infection	Strong, low
Antibiotics with activity against MRSA are recommended for patients with carbuncles or abscesses of higher severity who have failed initial antibiotic therapy, have severe systemic signs of infection, or are immunocompromised	Strong, low
Erysipelas	
Most infections are caused by *Streptococcus pyogenes*. Penicillin (oral or IV depending on clinical severity) is the drug of choice	A-I
If *S. aureus* is suspected, a penicillinase-resistant penicillin or first-generation cephalosporin should be used	A-I
Impetigo	
Gram stain and culture of pus or exudates should be obtained to help identify causative pathogens	Strong, moderate
Bullous and nonbullous impetigo should be treated with either mupirocin or retapamulin for 5 days	Strong, high
Impetigo should be treated with oral antibiotics active against *S. aureus* unless cultures show streptococci alone. Dicloxacillin or cephalexin is recommended for 7 days. Doxycycline, clindamycin, or sulfamethoxazole–trimethoprim should be used when MRSA is suspected or confirmed	Strong, moderate
Cellulitis	
Cultures of blood or cutaneous aspirates, biopsies, or swabs are not routinely recommended	Strong, moderate
Blood cultures are recommended, and cultures of cutaneous aspirates, biopsies, or swabs should be considered, in patients receiving chemotherapy for malignancies, neutropenia, severe cell-mediated immunodeficiency, immersion injuries, or animal bites	Strong, moderate (blood)
Typical cases of mild nonpurulent cellulitis should be treated with antibiotics active against streptococci	Strong, moderate
Systemic antibiotics are recommended for moderate nonpurulent cellulitis with systemic signs of infection. Use of antibiotics active against methicillin-susceptible *S. aureus* could be considered	Weak, low
Patients with severe nonpurulent cellulitis associated with penetrating trauma, MRSA infection in another location, MRSA nasal colonization, injection drug use, or systemic signs of infection should be treated with vancomycin or other antibiotics active against both MRSA and streptococci	Strong, moderate
Broad-spectrum antibiotic therapy with vancomycin plus piperacillin–tazobactam, imipenem, or meropenem may be considered for empiric treatment of severe nonpurulent cellulitis in severely immunocompromised patients	Weak, moderate (need for broad-spectrum therapy), strong, moderate (recommended broad-spectrum antibiotic regimen if used)
A treatment duration of 5 days is recommended for cellulitis, but may be extended if lack of clinical response within that time	Strong, high
Elevation of the affected area and treatment of predisposing factors are recommended for cellulitis	Strong, moderate
Systemic corticosteroids for 7 days can be considered for adjunctive treatment of cellulitis in nondiabetic patients	Weak, moderate
Patients with mild nonpurulent cellulitis who do not have systemic signs of infection, altered mental status, or hemodynamic instability should be treated as outpatients	Strong, moderate
Hospitalization is recommended for patients with moderate-to-severe nonpurulent cellulitis who have failed outpatient therapy, have poor adherence to therapy, are immunocompromised, or in whom there is a concern for deeper or necrotizing infection	Strong, moderate
Empiric antibiotics for outpatients with purulent cellulitis should provide activity against community-associated MRSA; coverage of β-hemolytic streptococci is likely not required. Mild-to-moderate infections can generally be treated with oral agents (dicloxacillin, cephalexin, clindamycin) unless resistance is high in the community	A-II
Recommended antibiotics for empiric coverage of MRSA in outpatients include orally administered trimethoprim–sulfamethoxazole, doxycycline, minocycline, clindamycin, and linezolid	A-II for all listed options
If coverage of both β-hemolytic streptococci and community-associated MRSA is desired, empiric antibiotic regimens for outpatient therapy include orally administered clindamycin alone; linezolid alone; or trimethoprim–sulfamethoxazole, doxycycline, or minocycline in combination with amoxicillin	A-II for all listed options
Hospitalized patients with complicated or purulent cellulitis should receive IV antibiotics with activity against MRSA pending culture data. Antibiotic options include vancomycin, linezolid, daptomycin, telavancin, and clindamycin	A-I for all except clindamycin; clindamycin A-III
In patients with suspected or definitive serious MRSA infections, an individualized target of the AUC/MIC ratio of 400 to 600 (assuming a vancomycin MIC of 1 mg/L) should be advocated to achieve clinical efficacy while improving patient safety	B-III
Necrotizing Fasciitis	
Patients with severe nonpurulent cellulitis characterized by aggressive infection and associated with signs of systemic toxicity, necrotizing fasciitis, or gas gangrene should have prompt surgical consultation	Strong, low
Early and aggressive surgical debridement of all necrotic tissue is essential	A-III
Necrotizing fasciitis should be empirically treated with broad-spectrum antibiotics such as vancomycin or linezolid plus piperacillin–tazobactam or a carbapenem, or vancomycin or linezolid plus ceftriaxone and metronidazole	Strong, low
Necrotizing fasciitis caused by *S. pyogenes* should be treated with the combination of clindamycin and penicillin	Strong, low

(continued)

TABLE 133-3 Evidence-Based Recommendations for Treatment of Skin and Soft-Tissue Infections (*Continued*)

Recommendations	Recommendation Grade[a]
In the treatment of necrotizing fasciitis caused by methicillin-resistant *S. aureus* infections, trough serum vancomycin concentrations of 15-20 mg/L (10-14 μmol/L) are recommended	B-II
Clostridial gas gangrene (myonecrosis) should be treated with clindamycin and penicillin	A II
Diabetic Foot Infections	
Clinically uninfected wounds should not be treated with antibiotics	A-III
Empiric antibiotic regimens should be selected based on severity of infection and likely pathogens	A-III
Antibiotic therapy should target only aerobic gram-positive cocci in patients with mild-to-moderate infection who have not received antibiotics within the previous month	C-III
Broad-spectrum empiric antibiotic therapy should be initiated in most patients with severe infections, until culture and susceptibility data are available	A-III
Empiric antibiotics directed against *Pseudomonas aeruginosa* are usually unnecessary except in patients with specific risk factors for infection with this pathogen: patient has been soaking feet, patient has failed previous antibiotic therapy with nonpseudomonal agents, or clinically severe infection	A-III
Empiric antibiotics directed against MRSA should be considered in patients with specific risk factors, including prior history of infection or colonization with MRSA, high local prevalence of MRSA (eg, ≥50% for mild infections, ≥30% for severe infection), or clinically severe infection	C-III
Oral agents with high bioavailability may be used in the treatment of most mild, and many moderate, infections	A-II
Parenteral therapy is initially preferred for all severe, and some moderate, infections. After initial response, step-down therapy to oral agents can be considered	C-III
Definitive therapy should be based on results of appropriately collected cultures and sensitivities, as well as clinical response to empiric antimicrobial agents	A-III
Appropriate wound care, in addition to appropriate antimicrobial therapy, is often necessary for healing of infected wounds	A-III
Antibiotic therapy should only be continued until resolution of signs/symptoms of infection, but not necessarily until the wound is fully healed. The duration of therapy should initially be 1-2 weeks for mild infections and 2-3 weeks for moderate-to-severe infection	C-III
Pressure Ulcers	
Optimize the host response by evaluating nutritional status and addressing deficits; stabilizing glycemic control; improving arterial blood flow; and/or reducing immunosuppressant therapy if possible	A-III
Consider the use of topical antiseptics for pressure ulcers that are not expected to heal and are critically colonized/topically infected	B-III
Consider use of silver sulfadiazine in heavily contaminated or infected pressure ulcers until definitive debridement is accomplished	B-III
Consider the use of medical-grade honey in heavily contaminated or infected pressure ulcers until definitive debridement is accomplished	C-III
Limit the use of topical antibiotics on infected pressure ulcers, except in special situations where the benefit to the patient outweighs the risk of antibiotic side effects and resistance	B-III
Use systemic antibiotics for individuals with clinical evidence of systemic infection, such as positive blood cultures, cellulitis, fasciitis, osteomyelitis, systemic inflammatory response syndrome (SIRS), or sepsis	B-III
Animal Bites	
Preemptive early antibiotics should be administered for 3-5 days in patients with any of the following: immunocompromised; asplenic; advanced liver disease; preexisting or resultant edema of the bitten area; moderate-to-severe bite-related injuries, especially to the hands or face; or bite injuries that have penetrated the periosteum or joint capsule	Strong, low
Amoxicillin–clavulanic acid or other antibiotics active against both aerobic and anaerobic bacteria should be used for treatment of infected animal bites	Strong, moderate
Serious infections requiring IV antimicrobial therapy can be treated with a β-lactam/β-lactamase inhibitor combination or second-generation cephalosporin with activity against anaerobes (eg, cefoxitin)	B-II
Penicillinase-resistant penicillins, first-generation cephalosporins, macrolides, and clindamycin should not be used for treatment of infected wounds because of their poor activity against *Pasteurella multocida*	D-III
Human Bites	
Antimicrobial therapy should provide coverage against *Eikenella corrodens*, *S. aureus*, and β-lactamase–producing anaerobes	B-III

[a]Cited evidence-based guidelines utilize different systems for grading the strengths of recommendation and quality of the associated evidence. Qualitative (descriptive) recommendations are from Reference 15; letter- and roman numeral–based recommendations are from the other cited guidelines. Readers are advised to consult the original documents for full explanations of the grading systems and definitions used in individual guidelines.

Strength of recommendation: A, good evidence for use; B, moderate evidence for use; C, poor evidence for use, optional; D, moderate evidence to support not using; E, good evidence to support not using. *Quality of evidence*: I, evidence from ≥1 properly randomized controlled trials; II, evidence from ≥1 well-designed clinical trials without randomization, case–control analytic studies, multiple time series, or dramatic results from uncontrolled experiments; III, evidence from expert opinion, clinical experience, descriptive studies, or reports of expert committees.

Qualitative (descriptive) recommendations: *Strong, high*: strong recommendation, high-quality evidence from well-performed randomized controlled trials (RCTs) or exceptionally strong evidence from unbiased observational studies; *Strong, moderate*: strong recommendation, moderate quality evidence from RCTs with important limitations or exceptionally strong evidence from unbiased observational studies; *Strong, low*: strong recommendation, low-quality evidence for at least 1 critical outcome from observational studies, RCTs with serious flaws, or indirect evidence; *Weak, moderate*: weak recommendation, moderate quality evidence from RCTs with important limitations or exceptionally strong evidence from unbiased observational studies; *Weak, low*: weak recommendation, low-quality evidence for at least one critical outcome from observational studies, RCTs with serious flaws, or indirect evidence.

Data from References 3, 4, 8, 15, and 26-29.

TABLE 133-4 Recommended Oral Drugs for Outpatient Treatment of Mild-to-Moderate Skin and Soft-Tissue Infections

Infection	Adults	Children
Folliculitis	None; warm saline compresses usually sufficient	
Furuncles and carbuncles	Trimethoprim–sulfamethoxazole[a,b] Doxycycline[a,b] Minocycline[a,b]	Trimethoprim–sulfamethoxazole[a,b] Clindamycin[a,b]
Erysipelas	Procaine penicillin G Penicillin VK Clindamycin[a] Erythromycin[a]	Penicillin VK Clindamycin[a] Erythromycin[a]
Impetigo	Mupirocin ointment[a] Retapamulin ointment[a] Dicloxacillin Cephalexin Trimethoprim–sulfamethoxazole[a,b] Clindamycin[a,b] Doxycycline[a,b]	Mupirocin ointment[a] Retapamulin ointment[a] Dicloxacillin Cephalexin Trimethoprim–sulfamethoxazole[a,b] Clindamycin[a,b]
Lymphangitis	Initial IV therapy, followed by penicillin VK Clindamycin[a]	Initial IV therapy, followed by penicillin VK Clindamycin[a]
Cellulitis	Penicillin VK[c] Cephalexin[c] Dicloxacillin[c] Clindamycin[b,c] Trimethoprim–sulfamethoxazole[b,d] Doxycycline[b,d] Minocycline[b,d] Linezolid[b]	Penicillin VK[c] Cephalexin[c] Dicloxacillin[c] Clindamycin[b,c] Trimethoprim–sulfamethoxazole[b,d] Linezolid[b]
Diabetic foot infections	Dicloxacillin Clindamycin Cephalexin Amoxicillin–clavulanate Levofloxacin ± metronidazole or clindamycin[a,e] Ciprofloxacin ± metronidazole or clindamycin[a,e] Moxifloxacin	
Bite wounds (animal or human)	Amoxicillin–clavulanate Doxycycline[a] Moxifloxacin[a] Trimethoprim–sulfamethoxazole + metronidazole or clindamycin[a] Levofloxacin or ciprofloxacin + metronidazole or clindamycin[a] Cefuroxime axetil + metronidazole or clindamycin Dicloxacillin + penicillin VK	Amoxicillin–clavulanate Trimethoprim–sulfamethoxazole + metronidazole or clindamycin[a] Cefuroxime axetil + metronidazole or clindamycin Dicloxacillin + penicillin VK

[a]May be used in patients with penicillin allergy.

[b]Recommended if CA-MRSA is suspected.

[c]For nonpurulent cellulitis when CA-MRSA is not suspected, or purulent cellulitis when CA-MRSA not documented (not penicillin VK).

[d]May be combined with amoxicillin if additional coverage for streptococci is desired.

[e]Fluoroquinolone alone may be suitable for mild infections, while addition of drugs with antianaerobic activity may be recommended for more severe infections.

TABLE 133-5 Drug Dosing[a]

Drug	Brand Name	Usual Dosing Range	Special Population Dose	Other
Oral Agents				
Amoxicillin–clavulanate	Augmentin®	875/125 mg orally every 12 hours	Pediatric: 40 mg/kg (of the amoxicillin component) orally in two divided doses	
Cefaclor	Ceclor®	500 mg orally every 8 hours	Pediatric: 20-40 mg/kg/day (not to exceed 1 g) orally in three divided doses	
Cefadroxil	Duricef®	250-500 mg orally every 12 hours	Pediatric: 30 mg/kg orally in two divided doses	
Cefuroxime axetil	Ceftin®	250-500 mg orally every 12 hours	Pediatric: 20-30 mg/kg orally in two divided doses	
Cephalexin	Keflex®	250-500 mg orally every 6 hours	Pediatric: 25-50 mg/kg orally in four divided doses	
Ciprofloxacin	Cipro®	500-750 mg orally every 12 hours		
Clindamycin	Cleocin®	300-600 mg orally every 6-8 hours	Pediatric: 10-30 mg/kg/day orally in three to four divided doses[3]	May be used for oral treatment of MRSA infection
Delafloxacin	Baxdela®	450 mg orally every 12 hours		May be used for oral treatment of MRSA infection
Dicloxacillin	Dynapen®	250-500 mg orally every 6 hours	Pediatric: 25-50 mg/kg orally in four divided doses	

(continued)

TABLE 133-5 Drug Dosing[a] (Continued)

Drug	Brand Name	Usual Dosing Range	Special Population Dose	Other
Doxycycline	Vibramycin®	100-200 mg orally every 12 hours		May be used for oral treatment of MRSA infection
Erythromycin	E-Mycin® Erythrocin®	250-500 mg orally every 6 hours	Pediatric: 30-50 mg/kg orally in four divided doses[a]	
Levofloxacin	Levaquin®	500-750 mg orally once daily		
Linezolid	Zyvox®	600 mg orally every 12 hours	Pediatric: 20-30 mg/kg/day orally in two to three divided doses	For oral treatment of MRSA infection
Metronidazole	Flagyl®	250-500 mg orally every 8 hours	Pediatric: 30 mg/kg orally in three to four divided doses	
Moxifloxacin	Avelox®	400 mg orally once daily		
Mupirocin ointment	Bactroban®	Apply to affected areas every 8 hours	Pediatric: apply to affected areas every 8 hours	
Penicillin VK	Veetids® Pen-V®	250-500 mg orally every 6 hours	Pediatric: 25,000-90,000 units/kg orally in four divided doses	
Retapamulin ointment	Altabax®	Apply to affected area every 12 hours	Pediatric: apply to affected area every 12 hours	
Tedizolid	Sivextro®	200 mg orally once daily		For oral treatment of MRSA infection
Trimethoprim–sulfamethoxazole	Bactrim® Septra® Cotrimoxazole®	160/800 mg orally every 12 hours	Pediatric: 4-6 mg/kg (of the trimethoprim component) orally every 12 hours	Up to double the usual dose may be considered for oral treatment of MRSA infection
Parenteral Agents				
Ampicillin	Omnipen® Polycillin® Principen®	1-2 g IV every 6 hours	Pediatric: 200-300 mg/kg/day IV in four to six divided doses	
Aztreonam	Azactam®	1 g IV every 6 hours	Pediatric: 100-150 mg/kg/day IV in four divided doses	
Cefazolin	Ancef® Kefzol®	1 g IV every 6-8 hours	Pediatric: 75 mg/kg/day IV in three divided doses	
Cefepime	Maxipime®	1-2 g IV every 12 hours	Pediatric: 100 mg/kg/day IV in two divided doses	
Cefotaxime	Claforan®	1-2 g IV every 6 hours	150-200 mg/kg/day in three to four divided doses	
Cefoxitin	Mefoxin®	1-2 g IV every 6 hours	Pediatric: 30-40 mg/kg/day IV in four divided doses	
Ceftazidime	Fortaz®	1-2 g IV every 8 hours	Pediatric: 150 mg/kg/day IV in three divided doses	
Ceftaroline	Teflaro®	600 mg IV every 12 hours		For MRSA infection
Ceftriaxone	Rocephin®	1 g IV once daily		
Cefuroxime	Zinacef®	0.75-1.5 g IV every 8 hours	Pediatric: 150 mg/kg/day IV in three divided doses	
Ciprofloxacin	Cipro®	400 mg IV every 8-12 hours		
Clindamycin	Cleocin®	300-600 mg IV every 6-8 hours; 600-900 mg IV every 6-8 hours for necrotizing fasciitis	Pediatric: 30-50 mg/kg/day IV in three to four divided doses	
Dalbavancin	Dalvance®	1,000 mg IV once on Day 1 of therapy, followed by 500 mg IV once on Day 8 of therapy; OR 1,500 mg IV once with no additional doses	Pediatric: 22.5 mg/kg (less than 6 years of age) or 18 mg/kg/day (6-18 years of age) IV in one dose	For MRSA infection
Daptomycin	Cubicin®	4 mg/kg IV once daily		For MRSA infection
Delafloxacin	Baxdela®	300 mg IV every 12 hours		For MRSA infection
Doripenem	Doribax®	500 mg IV every 8 hours		
Ertapenem	Invanz®	1 g IV once daily	Pediatric: 30 mg/kg/day IV in one to two divided doses	
Gentamicin	Garamycin®	Traditional: 2 mg/kg loading dose, followed by 1.5 mg/kg IV every 8 hours and guided by measured serum concentrations. Alternative: 5-7 mg/kg IV once daily	Pediatric: 5-7 mg/kg/day IV in three divided doses; doses guided by serum concentrations	

(continued)

TABLE 133-5 Drug Dosing[a] (Continued)

Drug	Brand Name	Usual Dosing Range	Special Population Dose	Other
Imipenem–cilastatin	Primaxin®	250-500 mg IV every 6-8 hours	Pediatric: 40-80 mg/kg/day IV in four divided doses	
Levofloxacin	Levaquin®	500-750 mg IV once daily		
Linezolid	Zyvox®	600 mg IV every 12 hours	Pediatric: 20-30 mg/kg/day IV in two to three divided doses	For MRSA infection
Meropenem	Merrem®	1 g IV every 8 hours	Pediatric: 60 mg/kg/day IV in three divided doses	
Metronidazole	Flagyl®	500 mg IV every 8 hours	Pediatric: 30-50 mg/kg/day IV in three divided doses	
Moxifloxacin	Avelox®	400 mg IV once daily		
Nafcillin	Nafcil®	1-2 g IV every 4-6 hours	Pediatric: 100-200 mg/kg/day IV in four to six equally divided doses	
Oritavancin	Orbactiv® Kimyrsa®	1,200 mg IV once with no additional doses (Orbactive® administered over 3 hours and Kimyrsa® over 1 hour)		For MRSA infection
Penicillin G	Pfizerpen® Bicillin® Wycillin®	1-2 million units IV every 4-6 hours	Pediatric: 100,000-200,000 units/kg/day IV in four divided doses[a]	
Piperacillin–tazobactam	Zosyn®	3.375-4.5 g IV every 6 hours	Pediatric: 250-350 mg/kg/day IV in three to four divided doses	
Procaine penicillin G	Bicillin C-R®	0.6-1.2 million units IM every 12 hours	Pediatric: 25,000-50,000 units/kg (maximum 1.2 million units) IM once daily	
Tedizolid	Sivextro®	200 mg IV once daily		For MRSA infection
Telavancin	Vibativ®	10 mg/kg IV once daily		For MRSA infection
Tigecycline	Tigacil®	100 mg IV once, and then 50 mg IV every 12 hours		
Tobramycin	Nebcin®	Traditional: 2 mg/kg loading dose, followed by 1.5 mg/kg IV every 8 hours and guided by measured serum concentrations. Alternative: 5-7 mg/kg IV once daily	Pediatric: 5-7 mg/kg/day IV in three divided doses; doses guided by serum concentrations	
Vancomycin	Vancocin®	30-40 mg/kg/day IV in two divided doses; dosing guided by serum concentrations to achieve 24-hour AUC/MIC ratios of 400-600 for serious MRSA infections	Pediatric: 60-80 mg/kg/day IV in three to four divided doses; doses guided by serum concentrations	For MRSA infection

IM, intramuscularly; MRSA, methicillin-resistant *S. aureus*.

[a]Dosing guidelines in patients with normal renal function.

TABLE 133-6 Drug Monitoring

Drug	Adverse Reaction	Monitoring Parameters	Comments
Aminoglycosides (tobramycin, gentamicin)	Nephrotoxicity	Serum creatinine, urine output, serum concentrations	Extended-interval ("once-daily") dosing potentially associated with less renal toxicity, similar efficacy to traditional dosing. Goal trough concentration <1 μg/mL (mg/L; 2 μmol/L) during extended-interval dosing
Daptomycin	Myopathy	Serum creatine phosphokinase	Most creatinine phosphokinase elevations will be asymptomatic; risk of myopathy may be increased with concomitant use of HMG-coA reductase inhibitors
Imipenem–cilastatin	CNS toxicities, seizures	Serum creatinine, mental status, CNS function	Increased incidence with higher dose, failure to adjust dose/interval for reduced renal function. Increased risk compared with meropenem or doripenem
Linezolid	Myelosuppression, thrombocytopenia, optic/peripheral neuropathy, serotonin syndrome	CBC, vision changes, serum lactate, heart rate, blood pressure, temperature, myoclonus	Myelosuppression and neuropathy more common with prolonged use. Weak MAO inhibitor, serotonin syndrome possible with other serotonergic drugs such as SSRIs and SNRIs
Nafcillin	Interstitial nephritis	Serum creatinine, urine output	Reversible, requires switch to alternative β-lactam
Vancomycin	Nephrotoxicity, infusion reactions	Serum creatinine, urine output, blood pressure, heart rate, serum concentrations	Dose adjustment required for renal dysfunction. Pretreatment and slow infusion may decrease incidence of infusion reaction. Drug concentrations monitored to achieve goal AUC/MIC ratio of 400-600 for serious infections, including necrotizing fasciitis

CBC, complete blood count; MAO, monoamine oxidase; SNRI, serotonin–norepinephrine reuptake inhibitor; SSRI, selective serotonin reuptake inhibitor.

CLINICAL PRESENTATION Impetigo

General

- Exposed skin, especially the face, is the most common site.

Symptoms

- Pruritus is common.
- Systemic signs and symptoms of infection are minimal.
- Weakness, fever, and diarrhea occasionally seen with bullous form.

Signs

Nonbullous:

- Lesions start as small, fluid-filled vesicles.
- Vesicles rapidly develop into pustules that rupture readily.
- Purulent discharge dries to form characteristic golden-yellow crusts.

Bullous:

- Lesions start as vesicles that rapidly progress into bullae containing clear yellow fluid.
- Bullae soon rupture, forming thin, light brown crusts.
- Regional lymph nodes may be enlarged.

Laboratory Tests

- Cultures should be collected for pathogen identification in more severe cases.
- Crusted tops of lesions should be raised to obtain purulent material at the base for culture.
- Open, draining pustules should not be cultured as they may be colonized with skin flora.

Other Diagnostic Tests

- Complete blood cell count often performed, leukocytosis is common.

Evaluation of Therapeutic Outcomes

Erysipelas generally responds quickly to appropriate antimicrobial therapy. Temperature and white blood cell count should return to normal within 48 to 72 hours. Erythema, edema, and pain also should resolve gradually.

IMPETIGO

3 Impetigo is a superficial skin infection that is seen most commonly in children.[5,23,30,32,33] The infection is generally classified as bullous or nonbullous based on clinical presentation.[5,30,32,33] Impetigo is most common during hot, humid weather, which facilitates microbial colonization of the skin.[4,8,30,32] Minor trauma, such as scratches or insect bites, allows entry of organisms into the superficial layers of skin, and infection ensues.[8,23,30,32] Impetigo is highly communicable and readily spreads through close contact, especially among siblings and children in daycare centers and schools.[8,30,32]

Although historically caused by *S. pyogenes*, *S. aureus* has emerged as a principal cause of impetigo (either alone or in combination with *S. pyogenes*).[23,30,32,33] The bullous form is caused by strains of *S. aureus* capable of producing exfoliative toxins.[23,32,33] The bullous form most frequently affects neonates and children less than 5 years of age,[33,34] and accounts for approximately 30% of all cases of impetigo.[8,32] Similar to other SSTIs, impetigo has been reported to be increasingly due to MRSA.[23,32,33]

TREATMENT: IMPETIGO

Desired Outcomes

The goals of treatment include relieving discomfort, improving the cosmetic appearance of lesions, preventing further spread of the infection, and preventing recurrence. Preventing transmission to others is also important.[32] Treatments should be effective and inexpensive and have minimal adverse effects.[30,32]

Pharmacologic Therapy

Although impetigo may resolve spontaneously, antimicrobial treatment is indicated to relieve symptoms, prevent formation of new lesions, and prevent complications such as cellulitis. A review of interventions for impetigo by the Cochrane Collaboration found that topical mupirocin and oral antibiotics (except penicillin and erythromycin) were equally effective for the treatment of impetigo[34]; topical mupirocin ointment or retapamulin ointment for 5 days are now recommended as first-line treatment of mild cases of impetigo not involving multiple lesions or the face.[15,23,30,32,33] Penicillinase-resistant penicillins (such as dicloxacillin) are preferred for oral treatment because of the increased incidence of infections caused by *S. aureus*.[15,23,32,33] First-generation cephalosporins (eg, cephalexin) are also commonly used.[15,23,30,32,33] Penicillin, administered as a single intramuscular dose of benzathine penicillin G or as oral penicillin VK, is effective for infections known to be caused by *S. pyogenes* but should not be used for empiric therapy of unknown etiology.[23] Penicillin-allergic patients, or those known to be infected with MRSA, can be treated with clindamycin, doxycycline, or trimethoprim–sulfamethoxazole. The duration of therapy is 7 days.[15,30,33] With proper treatment, healing of skin lesions is rapid and occurs without residual scarring. Removal of crusts by soaking in soap and warm water also may be helpful in providing symptomatic relief.[8,30,32]

Evaluation of Therapeutic Outcomes

Clinical response should be seen within 5 to 7 days of initiating antimicrobial therapy for impetigo. Treatment failures could be a result of noncompliance or antimicrobial resistance. A follow-up culture of exudates should be collected for culture and sensitivity, with treatment modified accordingly.

LYMPHANGITIS

4 Acute lymphangitis is an inflammation involving the subcutaneous lymphatic channels. Lymphangitis usually occurs secondary to puncture wounds, infected blisters, or other skin lesions. Most infections are caused by *S. pyogenes*.[35]

CLINICAL PRESENTATION Lymphangitis

General

- Lymphadenitis (acute or chronic inflammation of the lymph nodes) may occur when microorganisms reach the lymph nodes.

Symptoms

- Systemic signs and symptoms (ie, fever, chills, malaise, and headache) often develop rapidly before any sign of infection is evident at the initial site of inoculation, or after the initial lesion has subsided.
- Systemic signs and symptoms often are more profound than would be expected based on examination of the cutaneous lesion.

Signs

- Peripheral lesion associated with proximal red linear streaks directed toward the regional lymph nodes is diagnostic of acute lymphangitis.
- Lymph nodes are enlarged and tender.
- Peripheral edema of the involved extremity is present.
- Thrombophlebitis and acute lymphangitis in the lower extremities may be confused because both are associated with red linear streaking and tender areas; however, in thrombophlebitis, no portal of entry is identifiable.

Laboratory Tests

- Cultures of the affected lesions yield negative results.
- Pathogens identified by Gram stain of the initial lesion if done early in the course of the disease.

Other Diagnostic Tests

- Complete blood cell count is often performed as leukocytosis is common.

TREATMENT: LYMPHANGITIS

Desired Outcomes

The goal of treatment of lymphangitis is rapid eradication of the infection, thereby providing relief of symptoms (pain, tenderness, fever). Prevention of systemic complications is also an important goal as thrombophlebitis and abscess formation are possible. Treatments should be effective and inexpensive and have minimal adverse effects.

Pharmacologic Therapy

Penicillin is the antibiotic of choice. Because these infections are potentially serious and rapidly progressive, initial treatment should be with IV penicillin G 1 to 2 million units every 4 to 6 hours. Parenteral treatment should be continued for 48 to 72 hours, followed by oral penicillin VK for a total of 10 days.[35] Nondrug therapy includes immobilization and elevation of the affected extremity and warm-water soaks every 2 to 4 hours.[35] For penicillin-allergic patients, clindamycin may be used.

Evaluation of Therapeutic Outcomes

Lymphangitis usually responds rapidly to appropriate therapy; signs and symptoms often are decreased markedly or absent within 24 hours of starting antibiotics.

CELLULITIS

5 Cellulitis is an acute infectious process that initially affects the epidermis and dermis and may spread subsequently within the superficial fascia.[3,5,12] Cellulitis is considered a serious disease because of the propensity of the infection to spread through lymphatic tissue and to the bloodstream. *S. pyogenes* and *S. aureus* are the most frequent bacterial causes.[3-6,13,21,30] However, many bacteria have been implicated in various types of cellulitis (Table 133-1). Approximately 4 million patients were hospitalized for cellulitis between 1998 and 2006, representing 10% of all infection-related admissions.[3,10,36] Additionally, hospitalizations and costs related to cellulitis and abscess doubled between 1998 and 2013; the number of visits to ambulatory care clinics and emergency rooms doubled from 4.6 million in 1997 to 9.6 million in 2005.[3,5] The rising incidence of infections caused by methicillin-resistant *S. aureus* (MRSA) is a major concern in both the community and hospital settings and is thought to be the major factor contributing to the dramatic increases in both outpatient visits and hospitalizations.[3,5,14,18,37]

Injection drug users are predisposed to several infectious complications, including abscess formation and cellulitis at the site of injection.[3,5,15] These SSTIs are often polymicrobic and originate from skin and/or oropharyngeal flora, as well as from contaminated needles, syringes, and diluents.[3,5,15] *S. aureus*, including MRSA, is the most common pathogen isolated from injection drug users.[3-5,37] Anaerobic bacteria, especially oropharyngeal anaerobes, are also found commonly, particularly in polymicrobic infections.[3,5,15] Outbreaks caused by *Clostridium* species have also been reported in injection drug users.[15]

Acute cellulitis with mixed aerobic and anaerobic pathogens may occur in persons with diabetes, following traumatic injuries, at sites of surgical incisions to the abdomen or perineum, or where host defenses have been otherwise compromised (eg, vascular insufficiency).[3-5,23] In older patients, cellulitis of the lower extremities also may be complicated by thrombophlebitis. Other complications of cellulitis include local abscess, myositis, osteomyelitis, septic arthritis, bacteremia, endocarditis, and sepsis.[3,5,15,23,30] Such complications of cellulitis may occur in approximately 1% of outpatients but as many as 17% of hospitalized patients.[9]

TREATMENT: CELLULITIS

Desired Outcomes

The goals of therapy of acute bacterial cellulitis are rapid eradication of the infection and prevention of further complications. Effective treatment of cellulitis includes avoidance of unnecessary antimicrobials that contribute to increased resistance, and minimizing toxicities and cost of therapy.

CLINICAL PRESENTATION Cellulitis

General

- A history of an antecedent wound from minor trauma, abrasion, ulcer, or surgery is often present.

Symptoms

- Patients often experience fever, chills, or malaise and complain that the affected area feels hot and painful.
- Systemic findings such as hypotension, dehydration, and altered mental status are common.

Signs

- Characterized by erythema and edema of the skin.
- Lesions are nonelevated and have poorly defined margins.
- Affected areas are warm to touch.
- Inflammation is present with little or no necrosis or suppuration of soft tissue.
- Lesions may be associated with purulent drainage, exudates, and/or abscesses.
- Tender lymphadenopathy associated with lymphatic involvement is common.

Laboratory Tests

- Cultures of fluid should be collected when purulent drainage, exudates, or abscesses are present.
- Gram stain of fluid obtained by injection and aspiration of 0.5 mL of saline (using a small 22-gauge needle) into the advancing edge of the lesion may aid the microbiologic diagnosis but often yields negative results.
- Diagnosis usually is made on clinical grounds rather than by culture.

Other Diagnostic Tests

- Complete blood cell count is often performed as leukocytosis is common.
- Blood cultures often useful because bacteremia may be present in up to 30% of cases.

Drug and Nondrug Management of Cellulitis

Local care of cellulitis includes elevation and immobilization of the involved area to decrease swelling.[3,5,15,23,30] Initial application of cool sterile saline dressings may decrease pain and swelling, and can be followed 1 to 3 days later with moist heat to aid in localization of the cellulitis. Surgical intervention (incision and drainage) is rarely indicated in the treatment of uncomplicated cellulitis, but may play an important role in management of more severe or complicated cases. Antimicrobial therapy is directed against the type of bacteria either documented or suspected to be present based on the clinical presentation and risk factors. Particular attention must be paid to patients with risk factors for more atypical or resistant bacterial pathogens when selecting antibiotics for treatment of cellulitis. Such organisms include particularly MRSA, but also aerobic gram-negative bacteria and anaerobes.

Because staphylococcal and streptococcal cellulitis are indistinguishable clinically,[3-5,30] and because of concern regarding appropriate recognition and treatment of MRSA infections, guidelines from the Infectious Diseases Society of America (IDSA) provide detailed recommendations for empiric antibiotic therapy of cellulitis.[15,27] Antibiotic selection for treatment of cellulitis is chiefly determined by clinical findings such as appearance of the infected lesion and presence of more severe systemic illness. Cellulitis may be broadly classified as either purulent or nonpurulent for purposes of determining likely pathogens and appropriate empiric antibiotic therapy. Purulent cellulitis is defined as infection associated with purulent drainage or exudate in the absence of a simple drainable abscess; the presence of abscesses is also often associated with purulent cellulitis but by definition is the only clinical feature.[4,15,27] Incision and drainage of any abscesses and good wound care are the primary therapies for mild purulent infections when no systemic findings of infection are present. Systemic antibiotic therapy is often unnecessary in such cases.[3-5,27] Antibiotic therapy is recommended along with incision and drainage in patients with more complicated abscesses and/or moderately severe purulent cellulitis including the following: those with systemic signs of infection; multiple sites of infection; rapidly progressive infection in the presence of associated cellulitis; complicating factors such as extremes of age, comorbidities, or immunosuppression; abscesses in areas that are difficult to drain, such as hands, face, and genitalia; or lack of response to previous drainage alone.[3-5,15,23,27] Patients with complicated abscesses and/or moderately severe purulent cellulitis are usually treated as outpatients using orally administered antibiotics with activity against MRSA; infection due to streptococci is less likely in this situation and specific coverage is not required.[3-5,27] Oral agents recommended for moderate purulent cellulitis include trimethoprim–sulfamethoxazole and doxycycline (Fig. 133-1).[3-5,15] Oral linezolid is also recommended in such cases but is more expensive and apparently no more efficacious than other treatment options.[3-5,27,37,38] Tedizolid, an oxazolidinone, is also indicated for the treatment of complicated SSTI. Compared to linezolid, tedizolid may have advantages related to a more convenient dosing schedule and fewer adverse effects and drug interactions. However, tedizolid is likely no more effective than linezolid for SSTI and its role relative to linezolid is still unclear.[15,37,38,39]

Severe purulent cellulitis is defined as purulent infections occurring in patients who have failed incision and drainage plus oral antibiotic therapy, patients with systemic signs of infection (defined as temperature greater than 38°C, heart rate greater than 90 beats/min, respiratory rate greater than 24 breaths/min, or white blood cell count greater than 12,000 [12×10^9/L] or less than 400 cells/μL [0.4×10^9/L]), or immunocompromised patients. Appropriate clinical specimens for culture and susceptibility testing should be collected whenever possible in such patients.[3-5,15,22,27] Patients with severe purulent cellulitis should be hospitalized for empiric treatment with parenteral antibiotics having activity against MRSA. Vancomycin, daptomycin, linezolid or tedizolid, televancin, and ceftaroline are all acceptable treatment options with comparable efficacy in adults (Fig. 133-1).[8,3-6,12,13,15,27,37,38] In children, vancomycin, linezolid, or clindamycin are the preferred treatment options.[3,15,33]

Linezolid, tedizolid, daptomycin, ceftaroline, and telavancin all exhibit excellent activity against resistant gram-positive pathogens.[6,12,37,38,39,40] However, significantly higher cost compared with vancomycin, as well as lack of clearly demonstrated advantages in efficacy, makes them most appropriate for the treatment of

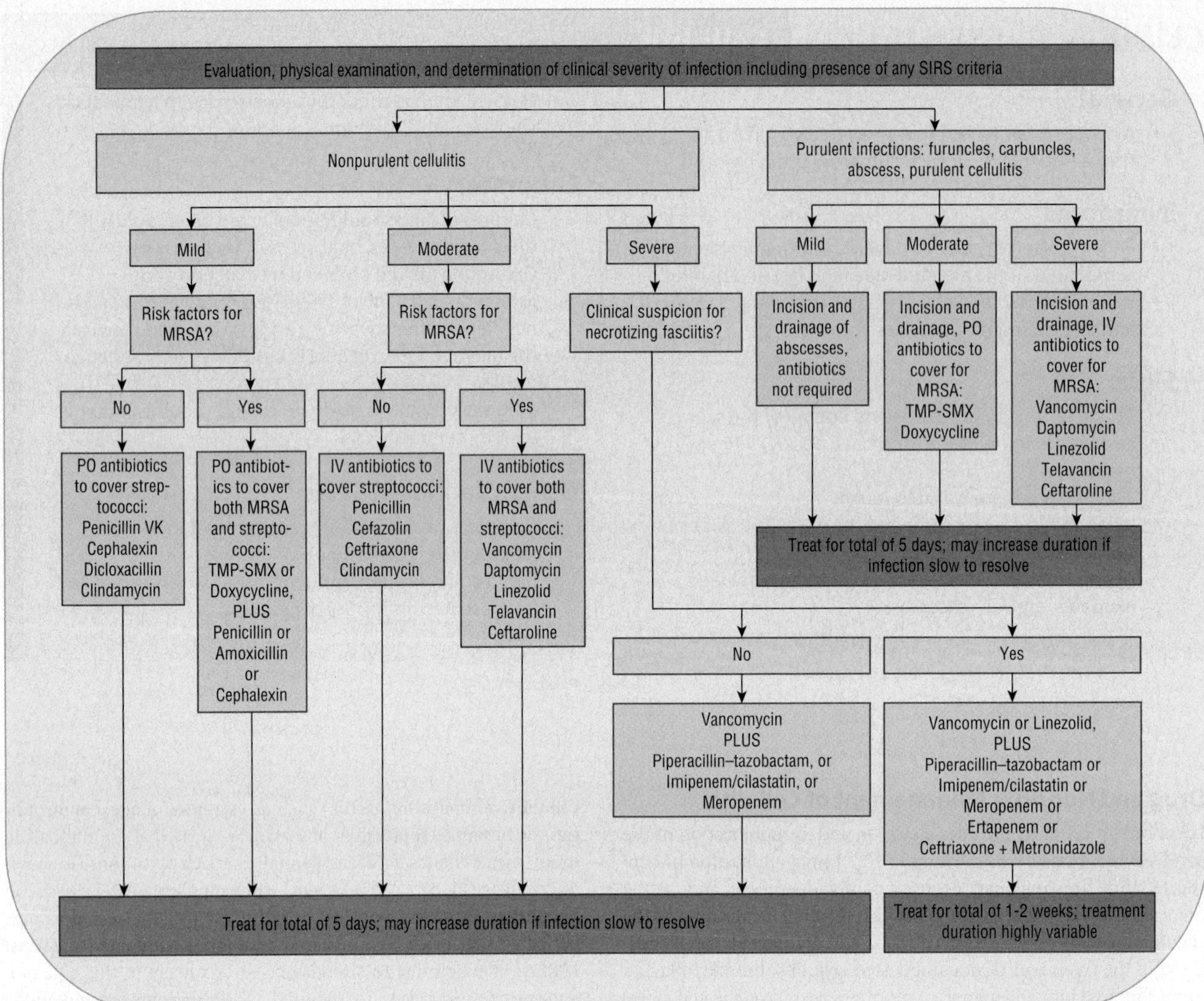

FIGURE 133-1 Recommended treatment algorithm for initial empiric management of selected purulent and nonpurulent skin and soft-tissue infections. (GNR, aerobic gram-negative rods; GPC, aerobic gram-positive cocci; IV, intravenous; MRSA, methicillin-resistant *Staphylococcus aureus*; PO, oral; SIRS, systemic inflammatory response syndrome; TMP-SMX, trimethoprim–sulfamethoxazole.)

complicated or refractory infections, or those documented as caused by multidrug-resistant pathogens, rather than as initial therapy. The availability of orally administered linezolid and tedizolid may provide cost-effective "step-down" options as alternatives to prolonged treatment with parenteral agents for many patients with more complicated infections and/or those patients who require initial hospitalization.[4,6,12,13,37-39]

The appropriate roles of dalbavancin and oritavancin, two newer glycopeptide drugs indicated for the treatment of complicated SSTI and with good activity against MRSA, are not well-defined for the routine management of SSTIs. Dalbavancin exhibits a terminal elimination half-life of approximately 14 days and is administered as a single large dose or two smaller doses given one week apart. Oritavancin has a half-life of approximately 10 days and is administered as a single one-time dose. The ability to provide an entire course of therapy with only one or two doses is attractive in terms of convenience, improved adherence compared to oral therapy, facilitation of early discharge of hospitalized patients, and potential for avoidance of inpatient hospitalization costs through administration in the emergency department, infusion centers, or physician offices. However, drug acquisition costs are higher than other treatment options and there are concerns related to potential lack of patient follow-up for monitoring of severe infections. Although these agents are not routinely used as first-line therapy, they may be considered for individual patients on a case-by-case basis in order to optimize their use.[3-6,12,13,15,23,37,38]

Delafloxacin is a fluoroquinolone with activity against staphylococci including MRSA, streptococci, and gram-negative bacteria including *P. aeruginosa*. Although IV followed by oral delafloxacin is equivalent to vancomycin plus aztreonam in the treatment of ABSSSI, its role is not well-defined and delafloxacin is not routinely recommended for treatment of cellulitis. The ability to transition patients from IV to oral therapy and its broad spectrum of activity may make delafloxacin a potential treatment option for carefully selected patients, particularly those with severe polymicrobial infections.

Carbapenems (ie, imipenem, meropenem, ertapenem, and doripenem) and the penicillin–β-lactamase inhibitor combination antibiotics (ampicillin–sulbactam, piperacillin–tazobactam) are equivalent to standard therapies in adults.[3,8,15] However, the greater cost of these agents without increased efficacy compared with other reliable regimens, particularly given the increasing problem of MRSA, makes them less desirable for empiric therapy except in serious polymicrobic infections.[3,15] Newer β-lactam–β-lactamase inhibitor combination agents such as ceftolozane–tazobactam, ceftazidime–avibactam, and meropenem–vaborbactam have few clinical data in the treatment of SSTIs and should not be used for empiric treatment of severe infections.

Nonpurulent cellulitis is defined as cellulitis without purulent drainage or exudate and no associated abscess. The role of MRSA in these types of infection is not clear, so empiric therapy of nonpurulent cellulitis is directed primarily against Group A β-hemolytic streptococci.[3-5,23] Recommended empiric therapy of mild nonpurulent cellulitis (ie, no focus of purulence or systemic signs of infection) consists of an orally administered β-lactam such as penicillin VK, cephalexin, or dicloxacillin (Fig. 133-1).[3-5,15,21,27] Oral cephalosporins, such as cefadroxil, cefaclor, cefprozil, cefpodoxime proxetil, and cefdinir, are also effective in the treatment of cellulitis but are more expensive.[15,21,23] Oral clindamycin may be used in penicillin-allergic patients.[15,21,23,27] Alternatively, a cephalosporin may be used cautiously for patients without a history of immediate or anaphylactic reactions to penicillin. Patients with moderately severe nonpurulent cellulitis (ie, systemic evidence of infection) or poor adherence to oral therapy should be hospitalized and treated with parenteral antibiotics directed against Group A streptococci. Recommended agents include penicillin VK, ceftriaxone, cefazolin, and clindamycin.[3-5,15,21,33] Hospitalization and treatment with parenteral antibiotics are also recommended for patients with severe nonpurulent cellulitis as indicated by the presence of systemic findings of infection (as previously defined for purulent cellulitis), failure of previous oral antibiotic therapy, immunocompromised states, or presence of clinical signs of deeper infection such as bullae, skin sloughing, hypotension, or organ dysfunction.[3,4,15,21,23] Empiric antibiotics for severe nonpurulent cellulitis should provide a broad spectrum of activity against MRSA and streptococci, as well as gram-negative and anaerobic bacteria. Recommended regimens include vancomycin plus piperacillin–tazobactam, and vancomycin plus imipenem–cilastatin or meropenem.[3,5,15,21,23]

Empiric treatment of MRSA should be considered for patients with either moderate or severe nonpurulent cellulitis that is associated with penetrating trauma, evidence of MRSA infection at another site or nasal colonization with MRSA, injection drug use, or in patients meeting SIRS criteria (fever, tachycardia, tachypnea, or leukocytosis or leukopenia as previously defined).[3,13,15,21,27] Recommended drugs for the coverage of MRSA in this setting are the same as those for purulent cellulitis. Clindamycin has reasonably good activity against β-hemolytic streptococci, but the activities of trimethoprim–sulfamethoxazole and the tetracyclines against this organism are not well-defined.[3,15,23,27] Therefore, if empiric coverage of both MRSA and β-hemolytic streptococci is desired for patients with nonpurulent cellulitis, they should receive clindamycin alone or amoxicillin in combination with trimethoprim–sulfamethoxazole, doxycycline, or minocycline.[3,13,15,23,27] Hospitalized patients with nonpurulent cellulitis who are not initially treated for MRSA should have their antibiotic changed to an agent with activity against MRSA if there is unsatisfactory clinical response.[3,16,23,27] Although often used for treatment of uncomplicated outpatient cellulitis, fluoroquinolones (eg, levofloxacin, moxifloxacin) are not recommended for routine use due to their unnecessarily broad spectrum of activity, concerns for resistance and toxicities, and higher cost compared with other preferred options.

Patients in whom specific pathogens have been identified by culture should have empiric antibiotics narrowed according to susceptibility test results. If documented to be a mild cellulitis secondary to streptococci, oral penicillin VK or intramuscular procaine penicillin G may be administered. Since *S. aureus* susceptibilities are more variable, treatment of documented staphylococcal infections will depend on test results for specific isolates. The usual duration of therapy for outpatient treatment of cellulitis, either purulent or nonpurulent, is 5 days; a longer duration should be considered if the infection has not sufficiently improved within that time.[3,8,15,23,30] A 7 to 14 day course of antibiotics has been recommended for cellulitis in hospitalized patients, but shorter courses (5-7 days) are often as effective as longer courses and should be used whenever possible.[16] In all cases, duration of therapy should be individualized based on patient response.[3,4,15,27]

For cellulitis caused by gram-negative bacilli or a mixture of microorganisms, immediate antimicrobial therapy, as determined by Gram stain, is essential. Surgical debridement of necrotic tissue and drainage may also be appropriate. Gram-negative cellulitis may be treated appropriately with an aminoglycoside (ie, gentamicin or tobramycin), or a first- or second-generation cephalosporin (eg, cephalexin, cefaclor, or cefuroxime). Ceftriaxone, ceftazidime, and fluoroquinolones are also effective in the treatment of cellulitis caused by both gram-negative and gram-positive bacteria.[3,4,8,15] If gram-positive aerobic bacteria are also present on Gram stain, an additional agent such as penicillin G or a penicillinase-resistant penicillin may need to be added to provide coverage against streptococci or staphylococci, respectively, as appropriate.[3,4,27] Addition of an agent active against MRSA (eg, vancomycin) may need to be considered for severe, complicated infections in hospitalized patients.[3,4,6,8,27] Ceftaroline is potentially advantageous in this setting since it has activity against MRSA and streptococci as well as gram-negative aerobic bacteria.

Because some polymicrobic infections may involve anaerobic bacteria, antibiotic therapy may need to be broadened to include agents with good activity against these organisms. Many different treatment regimens are possible depending on the bacteriology of the lesion (Fig. 133-1). Orally administered antibiotics, as monotherapy or in combination regimens, may be appropriately used in the treatment of mild-to-moderate infections in outpatients. Monotherapy or combination regimens of IV antibiotics may be necessary for more severe infections in hospitalized patients. Therapy should be 5 to 7 days in duration, with longer durations potentially needed in patients who do not respond to therapy in that time.[8,3,4,15]

Because gram-negative and mixed aerobic–anaerobic cellulitis can progress quickly to serious tissue damage, therapeutic intervention should be immediate.[8,3,15] If treated early, a rapid response can be seen. Unfortunately, because these infections often occur in patients with compromised immune defenses, they may still progress, even with therapeutic intervention. If the infectious process is secondary to a systemic cause (eg, diabetes), the treatment course often is prolonged and may be associated with high morbidity and mortality.[3,4,8,23]

Infections in injection drug users are treated similar to those in other types of patients.[8,15] Blood cultures must be obtained in these cases because 25% to 35% of patients may be bacteremic.[8,15,22] Also, patients should be assessed for the presence of abscesses; incision, drainage, and culture of these lesions are of extreme importance.[15] Initial antimicrobial therapy while awaiting culture results of abscesses should include broad coverage for gram-negative and anaerobic organisms, in addition to MRSA and streptococci.[8,15,22]

Evaluation of Therapeutic Outcomes

If treated promptly with appropriate antibiotics, the majority of patients with cellulitis are cured rapidly. Culture and sensitivity results should be evaluated carefully for both the adequacy of culture material and the presence of resistant organisms. Additional high-quality samples for culture may be needed for microbiologic analysis. Failure to respond to therapy may also be indicative of an underlying local or systemic problem or a misdiagnosis.

NECROTIZING SOFT-TISSUE INFECTIONS

Necrotizing soft-tissue infections consist of a group of extremely severe infections, associated with high morbidity and mortality, that require early and aggressive surgical debridement in addition to appropriate antibiotics and intensive supportive care.[4-6,23,41-45] Different terms have been used to classify necrotizing infections based on factors such as predisposing conditions, onset of symptoms, pain, skin appearance, etiologic agent, gas production, muscle involvement, and systemic toxicity.[3,4,23,42] However, while many types of necrotizing soft-tissue infections have been designated as unique infectious processes, they all share similar pathophysiologies, clinical features, and treatment approaches.[41-45] The major clinical entities of necrotizing infections are *necrotizing fasciitis* and *clostridial myonecrosis* (gas gangrene).[4,23,41-45]

6 Necrotizing fasciitis is a rare but severe infection of the subcutaneous tissue that may be caused by aerobic and/or anaerobic bacteria and results in progressive destruction of the superficial fascia and subcutaneous fat.[4,23,41-45] Type I necrotizing fasciitis is the most common and accounts for approximately 80% of necrotizing soft-tissue infections.[4,23,41-45] It generally occurs after trauma or surgery and involves a mixture of anaerobes (*Bacteroides*, *Peptostreptococcus*) and facultative bacteria (streptococci and Enterobacterales) that act synergistically to cause destruction of fat and fascia.[4,23,41,42] Type I necrotizing fasciitis is also reported more commonly among injection drug users.[41-44] In type I infections, the skin may be spared, and the speed at which the infection spreads (3-5 days) is somewhat slower than that in type II.[23,42] Necrotizing fasciitis affecting the male genitalia is termed *Fournier's gangrene*.[4,41,42] Type II necrotizing fasciitis is caused by virulent strains of *S. pyogenes* and is commonly referred to as *streptococcal gangrene*.[4,23,41-45] This type of infection has often been called "flesh-eating bacteria" by the lay press. Type II infections may occur in young, previously healthy individuals as well as older individuals with underlying diseases.[4,23,41-45] It differs from type I infections in its clinical presentation. Type II infections have rapidly extending necrosis (ie, 24-72 hours) of subcutaneous tissues and skin, gangrene, severe local pain, and systemic toxicity.[41-45] They are also highly associated with an early onset of shock and organ failure and are present in approximately half the cases of streptococcal toxic shock-like syndrome.[41-45] Of note, MRSA is increasingly reported in type II infections, either as a single organism or in combination with streptococci.[4,23,41-43]

Clostridial myonecrosis (type III necrotizing fasciitis) is a necrotizing infection that involves the skeletal muscle.[4,23,41-45] Type III infections account for less than 5% of necrotizing infections.[42] Gas production and muscle necrosis (myonecrosis) are prominent features of this infection, which readily explains why this infection is commonly referred to as *gas gangrene*.[4,23,41-43] The infection advances rapidly, often over a matter of a few hours.[41-45] Most infections occur after surgery or trauma, with *Clostridium perfringens* identified as the most common etiologic agent.[4,23,41-45]

TREATMENT: NECROTIZING SOFT-TISSUE INFECTIONS

Desired Outcomes

The goals of therapy of acute bacterial cellulitis are rapid eradication of the infection, prevention of further complications, and reduction in mortality. Effective treatment of necrotizing soft-tissue infections

CLINICAL PRESENTATION Necrotizing Soft-Tissue Infections

General

- Most frequently involve the abdomen, perineum, and lower extremities.
- Predisposing factors such as diabetes mellitus, local trauma or infection, or recent surgery often present.
- Rapid diagnosis is critical due to the aggressive nature and high associated mortality (20%-50%).

Symptoms

- Systemic symptoms generally are marked (eg, fever, chills, and leukocytosis) and may include shock and organ failure, especially in patients with type II infections.
- Pain in the affected area and systemic toxicity are characteristically more pronounced than with cellulitis.

Signs

- May be difficult to differentiate between necrotizing fasciitis and cellulitis early in infection.
- Affected area is initially hot, swollen, and erythematous without sharply demarcated margins.
- Affected area is often shiny, exquisitely tender, and very painful.
- Diffuse swelling of the area is followed by the appearance of bullae filled with clear fluid.
- Rapidly progressive infection with the frequent development of a maroon or violaceous color of the skin after several days.
- Infection may rapidly evolve into a cutaneous gangrene, sometimes with myonecrosis.

Laboratory Tests

- Tissue samples should be obtained for histologic examination, and culture and susceptibility testing.
- Clostridial myonecrosis shows little inflammation on histologic examination.

Other Diagnostic Tests

- Surgical exploration is the best and most rapid means of diagnosing necrotizing infections; computed tomography and magnetic resonance imaging may also be helpful.
- Blood samples should be collected for complete blood cell count and chemistry profile, as well as for bacterial culture.
- Laboratory tests that may aid in the diagnosis of necrotizing infections (LRINEC score) include C-reactive protein, white blood cell count, hemoglobin, sodium, creatinine, and glucose.

includes avoidance of unnecessary antimicrobials that contribute to increased resistance, and minimizing toxicities and cost of therapy.

Management of Necrotizing Infections

Immediate and aggressive surgical debridement of all necrotic tissues is essential in all patients with suspected or confirmed necrotizing fasciitis.[4,15,23,41-45] Initial surgical debridement performed greater than 14 hours after the diagnosis of necrotizing infection was independently associated with increased patient mortality, including a 34-fold increased risk of death in patients with septic shock.[41-45] Patients often require repeated surgical intervention following initial debridement to ensure that all necrotic tissue has been removed.[41-45] Type I necrotizing fasciitis must be empirically treated with broad-spectrum antibiotics that include coverage against streptococci, Enterobacterales, and anaerobes. Piperacillin–tazobactam plus vancomycin is specifically recommended as appropriate empiric therapy of necrotizing fasciitis, although a number of antibiotic regimens are also appropriate to successfully treat necrotizing soft-tissue infections (see Fig. 133-1).[4,15] These antibiotic regimens are generally similar to regimens used for polymicrobic cellulitis.[4,8,23,41-45] Antibiotic therapy can be modified after Gram stain and culture reports are available.

If a diagnosis of either type II (streptococcal) or type III (clostridial) necrotizing fasciitis is established, broad-spectrum empiric therapy should be replaced with the combination of penicillin plus clindamycin.[4,15,23,41-45] Although *S. pyogenes* remains susceptible to penicillin, the combination with clindamycin is more effective.[41,43] Several factors have been postulated to explain the greater efficacy of clindamycin, including a mechanism of action (inhibition of protein synthesis) that may cause decreased production of bacterial exotoxins.[4,23,41-45] In addition, clindamycin has immunomodulatory properties that may account for higher efficacy.[41-45] Clindamycin is also effective against some strains of MRSA.[4,23,42] Linezolid has also been suggested for necrotizing fasciitis due to mechanistic properties that are similar to those of clindamycin, but clinical data are fewer in comparison.[4,23,41,42] Hyperbaric oxygen is potentially beneficial for clostridial myonecrosis, but its use is not currently recommended due to lack of clear evidence of improved patient outcomes.[4,15,23,41-45] Likewise, the use of intravenous immunoglobulin (IVIG) has not yet been proven beneficial in the treatment of necrotizing streptococcal infections and its use is not routinely recommended.[4,15,23,41-45]

Evaluation of Therapeutic Outcomes

Because of the high mortality associated with necrotizing infections, rapid and complete debridement of all devitalized and necrotic tissue is essential. Surgical debridement, coupled with appropriate antimicrobial therapy and supportive measures for management of shock and organ failure, should stabilize the patient. Vital signs and laboratory tests should be monitored carefully for signs of resolution of the infection. Change in antimicrobial therapy or additional surgical debridement may be needed in patients who do not show signs of improvement.

DIABETIC FOOT INFECTIONS

Three major types of foot infections are seen in patients with diabetes: deep abscesses, cellulitis of the dorsum, and mal perforans ulcers.[46,47] Most deep abscesses involve the central plantar space (arch) and are caused by minor penetrating trauma or by an extension of infection of a nail or web space of the toes. Infections of the dorsal area generally arise from infections in the toes that are related to routine care of the nails, nail beds, and calluses of the toes. Mal perforans ulcer is a chronic ulcer of the sole of the foot. The ulcer develops on thickened, hardened calluses over the first or fifth metatarsal. Mal perforans ulcers are associated with neuropathic changes, which are responsible for the misalignment of the weight-bearing bones of the foot.[46,47] Osteomyelitis is one of the most serious complications of diabetic foot infection (DFI) and may occur in 30% to 40% of infections.[26,46,47]

Epidemiology

DFI is among the most common complications of diabetes, accounting for as many as 20% of all hospitalizations in patients with diabetes at an annual cost of $200 to $350 million.[26,46,48] Approximately 25% of patients with diabetes develop a foot ulcer during their lifetime; up to 60% of these ulcers involve significant soft-tissue infection and osteomyelitis is present in up to 40%.[26,46-48] Approximately 71,000 lower-extremity amputations, often sequelae of uncontrolled infection, are performed each year on patients with diabetes; this represents up to 80% of all nontraumatic amputations in the United States.[26,46,48] Approximately 40% of patients with diabetes will have recurrence of an ulcer within 12 months, and 20% of patients will undergo additional surgery or amputation of a second limb within 12 months of an initial amputation.[26,46-48]

Etiology

Mild cases of DFI are often monomicrobial. However, more severe infections are typically polymicrobic; up to 60% of hospitalized patients have polymicrobial infections (Table 133-7).[26,46,47,49,50-53] Wide ranges in the frequency of various bacteria in DFI reflect differences in culture techniques as well as variation among different types and severity of infections. Staphylococci and streptococci are the most common pathogens, although gram-negative bacilli and/or anaerobes occur in up to 50% of cases.[49-53] Although *P. aeruginosa* is an important pathogen in DFI, it is usually reported in less than 10% of wounds and is most commonly associated with more severe infections.[26,50] Obligate anaerobes are also more commonly associated with severe infections in patients with chronic foot ischemia.[26,49,50] MRSA is increasingly important in DFI and has been reported in 10% to 30% of infected wounds.[26,50,51,53-55] The presence of MRSA in

TABLE 133-7 Bacterial Isolates from Foot Infections in Diabetic Patients

Organisms	Percentage of Isolates
Aerobes	63-100
Gram-positive	24-100
Staphylococcus aureus (all)	10-80
S. aureus (MRSA)	1-37
Streptococcus spp.	3-37
Enterococcus spp.	2-25
Coagulase-negative staphylococci	6-10
Other gram-positive aerobes	0-19
Gram-negative	16-73
Proteus spp.	3-7
Enterobacter spp.	1-9
Escherichia coli	3-10
Klebsiella spp.	1-6
Pseudomonas aeruginosa	1-48
Other gram-negative bacilli	3-13
Anaerobes	1-40
Peptostreptococcus spp.	4-28
Bacteroides fragilis group	2-9
Other *Bacteroides* spp.	3-6
Clostridium spp.	0-2
Other anaerobes	7-19

Data from References 26, 46, 47, 49, 50-54, and 56.

DFI has been associated with increased risk of treatment failure and worse patient outcomes, but these findings have not been consistent among studies and the clinical relevance of MRSA in this setting is still unclear.[26,47,54]

Identifying causative pathogens from cultures of DFI is often difficult. The chronic nature of DFI means that these wounds are often heavily colonized by organisms not playing a role in the infection. Superficial swab cultures are not as reliable as culture specimens obtained from deep tissues or bone via biopsy, tissue scraping (curettage), or needle aspiration of drainage or abscess fluid.[22,47,51,53] Therefore, cultures and sensitivity tests should be done with specimens obtained from a deep culture of the wound base whenever possible. Before the wound is cultured, it should be scrubbed vigorously with saline-moistened sterile gauze to remove any overlying necrotic debris and further debrided as necessary.[22,26,51] Bone cultures should also be performed when there is diagnostic uncertainty regarding the presence of osteomyelitis or when therapeutic decisions are dependent on knowing the exact etiology of infection.[22,26,47,51,53]

Pathophysiology

Three key factors are involved in the development of diabetic foot ulcers: neuropathy, angiopathy and ischemia, and immunologic defects. Any of these disorders can occur in isolation; however, they frequently occur together.[48]

Neuropathic changes to the autonomic nervous system as a consequence of diabetes may affect the motor nerve supply of small intrinsic muscles of the foot, resulting in muscular imbalance, abnormal stresses on tissues and bone, and repetitive injuries.[46,48] Diminished sensory perception causes an absence of pain and unawareness of minor injuries and ulceration. The sympathetic nerve supply may be damaged, resulting in the absence of sweating that may lead to dry cracked skin and secondary infection.[26,46,48]

Atherosclerosis is more common, appears at a younger age, and progresses more rapidly in the persons with diabetes compared with those without. Individuals with diabetes may have problems with both small vessels (microangiopathy) and large vessels (macroangiopathy) that can result in varying degrees of ischemia, ultimately leading to skin breakdown and infection. Peripheral artery disease is present in up to 50% of persons with diabetes and is strongly associated with impaired wound healing.[49]

Persons with diabetes typically have normal humoral immunity, normal levels of immunoglobulins, and normal antibody responses. Patients with diabetes, however, have impaired phagocytosis and intracellular microbicidal function as compared with nondiabetics; this may be related to angiopathy and low tissue levels of oxygen.[26,46,48] These defects in cell-mediated immunity make patients with diabetes more susceptible to certain types of infection and impair the patients' ability to heal wounds adequately.[46-48]

TREATMENT: DIABETIC FOOT INFECTIONS

Desired Outcomes

7 The goals of therapy in the management of DFI include the following: (a) successfully treat infected wounds by using effective nondrug and antibiotic therapy; (b) prevent additional infectious complications; (c) preserve as much normal limb function as possible; (d) avoid unnecessary use of antimicrobials that contribute to increased resistance; and (e) minimize toxicities and cost while increasing patient quality of life.

Management

Up to 90% of infections can be treated successfully with a comprehensive treatment approach that includes both wound care and antimicrobial therapy.[26,47,51] After carefully assessing the extent of the lesion and obtaining necessary cultures, necrotic tissue must be thoroughly debrided, with wound drainage and amputation as required. Wounds must be kept clean and dressings changed frequently (two to three times daily). Because of the relationship between hyperglycemia and immune system defects, glycemic control must be maximized to ensure optimal wound healing. In addition, the patient's activities should be restricted initially to bed rest for leg elevation and control of edema, if present. Adequate pressure relief from a foot wound (ie, off-loading) is crucial to the healing process.[26,48,51] Finally, appropriate antimicrobials must be initiated.[26,47,48,51] However, the optimal antimicrobial therapy for DFI has yet to be defined. Broad-spectrum empiric therapy that provides coverage of all possible pathogens is not recommended unless the infection is life- or limb-threatening, assuming that

CLINICAL PRESENTATION Diabetic Foot Infections

General

- Infections are much more extensive than they initially appear.

Symptoms

- Patients with peripheral neuropathy often do not experience pain; simple complaints of swelling or edema are common.

Signs

- Clinical signs of infection may not be present secondary to angiopathy and neuropathy.
- Lesions vary in size and clinical features (eg, erythema, edema, warmth, presence of pus, draining sinuses, pain, and tenderness).
- Foul-smelling odor suggests the presence of anaerobic organisms.
- Temperature may be mildly elevated or normal.

Laboratory Tests

- Specimens for culture and sensitivities should be collected.
- Deep-tissue samples obtained during surgical debridement are most useful for culture and susceptibility testing.
- Wounds must be cultured for both aerobic and anaerobic organisms.

Other Diagnostic Tests

- Possible presence of osteomyelitis must also be assessed via radiograph, bone scan, or both, as appropriate.

TABLE 133-8 Classifications and Treatment Strategies for Diabetic Foot Infections of Varying Severity

Clinical Signs/Symptoms of Infection	Infection Severity	Treatment Setting
None	Uninfected	Outpatient management; nonantibiotic wound management only
Local infection present (≥2 of the following): local swelling or induration, erythema, local tenderness or pain, local warmth, purulent discharge		Outpatient or inpatient management according to severity (mild, moderate, or severe) as assessed by additional criteria
Local infection involving only skin and subcutaneous tissue, without involvement of deeper tissues or SIRS criteria present; if erythema is present, must be >0.5 and ≤2 cm around ulcer	Mild	Outpatient management; topical or oral antibiotics
Local infection with erythema >2 cm around ulcer, or involving structures deeper than skin and subcutaneous tissue (eg, abscess, osteomyelitis, septic arthritis, fasciitis); no SIRS criteria present	Moderate	Outpatient (or initial inpatient) management; oral (or initial parenteral) antibiotics
Local infection with ≥2 SIRS criteria: • Temperature >38°C (100.4°F) or <36°C (96.8°F) • HR >90 • RR >20 • WBC >12,000/mm^3 (12 × 10^9/L) or <4,000/mm^3 (4 × 10^9/L), or >10% (0.10) bands	Severe	Inpatient, followed by outpatient, management; initial parenteral antibiotics, followed by switch to oral when possible

Data from Reference 26.

adequate wound care is also being performed.[46-49,51,54] This is particularly true regarding MRSA, *P. aeruginosa*, and anaerobes; the perceived need for empiric coverage of these organisms often leads to use of excessively broad-spectrum drug regimens. Several studies have shown good antimicrobial treatment efficacy despite the fact that the regimens did not have consistently good activity against these particular organisms and no specific regimen has shown clear superiority over another.[46-52,54-56]

Proper selection of empiric antibiotics for DFI begins with thorough patient assessment and classification of the severity of the infection. Specific drug regimens, route of administration, and duration of therapy are all then largely dependent on the severity of infection. Although a number of classification systems are available, the most recent DFI treatment guidelines use those summarized in Table 133-8.[26,46,51] Wounds with no local signs of infection often do not require antibiotic therapy, and the majority of mild, uncomplicated infections can be managed successfully on an outpatient basis with highly bioavailable oral antimicrobials and good wound care (Tables 133-8 and 133-9).[46-49,53] Antibiotics for treatment of mild infections should be largely limited to those with activity against skin flora such as streptococci and methicillin-susceptible *S. aureus* (MSSA), except in those patients with risk factors for infection with other types of pathogens (Fig. 133-2).[46-48,51] Patients with specific risk factors for MRSA (Table 133-9) should empirically receive trimethoprim–sulfamethoxazole or doxycycline orally, while those who have received antibiotics within the past month should also receive empiric antibiotics that provide activity against gram-negative bacilli. Oral antimicrobials should be used cautiously in DFI complicated by osteomyelitis, extensive ulceration, areas of necrosis, or a combination of these. The use of topical antimicrobials, including medical-grade honey, has been advocated for the treatment of DFI in an attempt to minimize the cost of therapy and systemic antibiotic exposure leading to adverse effects and resistance. Although the most recent guidelines allow for consideration of topical therapy in mild infection in selected patients, use of topical agents is quite controversial, inconsistent in proven benefits, and not routinely recommended.[26,47,51,57]

Appropriate initial therapy for patients with moderate-to-severe infection is also dependent on the presence of specific risk factors that increase the likelihood of infection with more resistant pathogens such as *P. aeruginosa* and MRSA (Table 133-9).[26,46,48,51] Many moderate infections can be successfully treated with orally administered antibiotics that provide activity against MSSA, streptococci, and gram-negative aerobic bacilli; coverage of obligate anaerobes may also be considered in patients with chronic or previously treated wounds (Fig. 133-3).[26,46,48,51] The addition of orally administered agents with activity against MRSA is recommended in patients with moderate or severe infection and specific risk factors for MRSA; such patients may also be considered for hospitalization and initial treatment with parenteral antibiotics in order to ensure adequate antibiotics for potentially more complex infections.[26,46,48,50,51] Patients with more extensive or chronically unhealed wounds, even though assessed as moderate in severity, may also be more appropriately treated initially with parenteral antibiotics in the hospital setting.[47-52]

All patients with severe DFI should be hospitalized initially and treated with broad-spectrum IV antibiotics (Table 133-9 and Fig. 133-3).[46-52] Severe infection is considered a risk factor for *P. aeruginosa*, so most patients with severe DFI will be initially started on antipseudomonal antibiotics.[48-51] Many patients will also be initially started on antibiotics that provide activity against MRSA due to risk-versus-benefit considerations, but assessment of risk factors in individual patients is important in order to minimize the use of excessively broad-spectrum antibiotics when possible.

Guidelines for management of DFI include options for both monotherapy and combination regimens (Table 133-9).[26] Monotherapy, along with appropriate medical or surgical management, or both, is often effective in treating DFI, including those in which osteomyelitis is present.[46-52,56] Monotherapy is particularly attractive because of the potential advantages of convenience, cost, and avoidance of toxicities. Microbiologic and clinical cure rates ranging from 60% to 90% may be expected from any of these agents.[46-52,56] Selection of a specific regimen is determined by patient-specific factors including allergies, renal function, history of previous antibiotic use, and cost. In penicillin-allergic patients, metronidazole or clindamycin plus a fluoroquinolone, aztreonam, or possibly a third- or fourth-generation cephalosporin is appropriate.[46-52,56] Vancomycin is also used frequently in severe infections because of its good activity against gram-positive pathogens, with linezolid, daptomycin, and tigecycline specifically recommended as alternatives to vancomycin.[46-52] Tigecycline may be particularly useful in this setting because of its activity against gram-negative aerobes and anaerobic bacteria, thus allowing it to be used as monotherapy for the treatment of mixed infections in patients where coverage of *P. aeruginosa* is not of great concern. Ceftaroline fosamil also has in vitro activity suitable for DFI but has not been studied

TABLE 133-9 Suggested Antibiotic Regimens for Empiric Treatment of Diabetic Foot Infections

Severity of Infection	Probable Pathogens	Drug(s)[a]	Duration of Therapy
Mild	*Staphylococcus aureus* (MSSA) *Streptococcus* spp.	Amoxicillin–clavulanate	1-2 weeks; may increase up to 4 weeks if infection is slow to resolve
	S. aureus (MRSA) • Patients with history of MRSA infection or colonization in past year • Prevalence of MRSA ≥50% in local geographic area • Recent hospitalization	Cephalexin Dicloxacillin Clindamycin Levofloxacin Moxifloxacin[b]	
Moderate-to-severe (initially oral or IV antibiotics for moderately severe infections, IV antibiotics for severe infections)	MSSA *Streptococcus* spp. Enterobacterales Obligate anaerobes	Ampicillin–Sulbactam Cefoxitin Ceftriaxone Imipenem/cilastatin Ertapenem Levofloxacin Moxifloxacin Tigecycline Levofloxacin or ciprofloxacin + clindamycin	Moderately severe infection: 1-3 weeks; severe infection: 2-4 weeks
	MRSA • Patients with history of MRSA infection or colonization in past year • Prevalence of MRSA ≥30% in local geographic area • Recent hospitalization • Infection severe enough that not empirically covering MRSA poses unacceptable risk of treatment failure	Add to one of the above regimens: • Vancomycin • Linezolid • Daptomycin	
	Pseudomonas aeruginosa • Patient has been soaking feet • Patient has previously failed therapy with nonpseudomonal antibiotic regimen • Severe infection	Piperacillin/tazobactam	
	Mixed infections potentially including all of the above	Cefepime, ceftazidime, or aztreonam + metronidazole or clindamycin + vancomycin[c] *or* piperacillin–tazobactam or imipenem–cilastatin or meropenem[b] + vancomycin[c]	

[a]Agents not shown in any particular order of preference.

[b]Not specifically recommended in IDSA guidelines but may be appropriate treatment option.

[c]Linezolid or daptomycin may be used in place of vancomycin.

MRSA, methicillin-resistant *S. aureus*; MSSA, methicillin-susceptible *S. aureus*.

Data from Reference 26.

for this indication. Because many patients already have some degree of diabetic nephropathy that may place them at higher risk of nephrotoxicity, strong recommendations have been made against the use of aminoglycoside antibiotics unless no alternative agents are available.[26,47] When an aminoglycoside is used, care must be taken to avoid further compromising renal function. All antibiotic regimens should be adjusted as necessary for renal dysfunction. There is no defined role for newer broad-spectrum agents such ceftolozane–tazobactam, ceftazidime–avibactam, meropenem–vaborbactam, eravacycline, and delafloxacin; their use in DFI is not recommended.

Duration of therapy for DFI depends on the severity of the infection, ranging from 1 to 2 weeks for mild infections up to 2 to 4 weeks or more for severe infections.[46-52] In the cases of underlying osteomyelitis, treatment should continue for 6 to 12 weeks.[46-52] After healing of the infection has occurred, a well-designed program for the prevention of further infections should be instituted. The use of adjunctive agents such as colony-stimulating factors, growth factors, and hyperbaric oxygen for either prevention or treatment of DFIs is controversial and not widely recommended.[26]

Evaluation of Therapeutic Outcomes

Therapy should be reevaluated carefully after 48 to 72 hours to assess favorable response. Change in therapy (or route of administration, if oral) should be considered if clinical improvement is not observed at this time. For optimal results, drug therapy should be appropriately modified according to information from deep-tissue culture and the clinical condition of the patient. Infections in patients with diabetes often require extended courses of therapy because of impaired host immunity and poor wound healing.

PRESSURE INJURIES

The terms *decubitus ulcer*, *bed sore*, *pressure sore*, and *pressure injury* are often used interchangeably, althought pressure injury is now the preferred term.[29,58-60] The decubitus ulcer and the bed sore are types of pressure injuries. The term *decubitus ulcer* is derived from the Latin word *decumbere*, meaning "lying down." Pressure injuries, however, can develop regardless of a patient's position.

Numerous systems for classification of pressure injuries have been described. The 2016 recommendations of the National Pressure Ulcer Advisory Panel (NPUAP) are shown in Table 133-10. The NPUAP classification system is most commonly used and illustrates various stages of progression through which a pressure injury may pass.[60]

Complications of pressure injuries are common and may be life-threatening. Infection is one of the most serious and most frequently encountered complications of pressure injuries.[58,59] Although most pressure injury wounds are heavily colonized, the majority of these

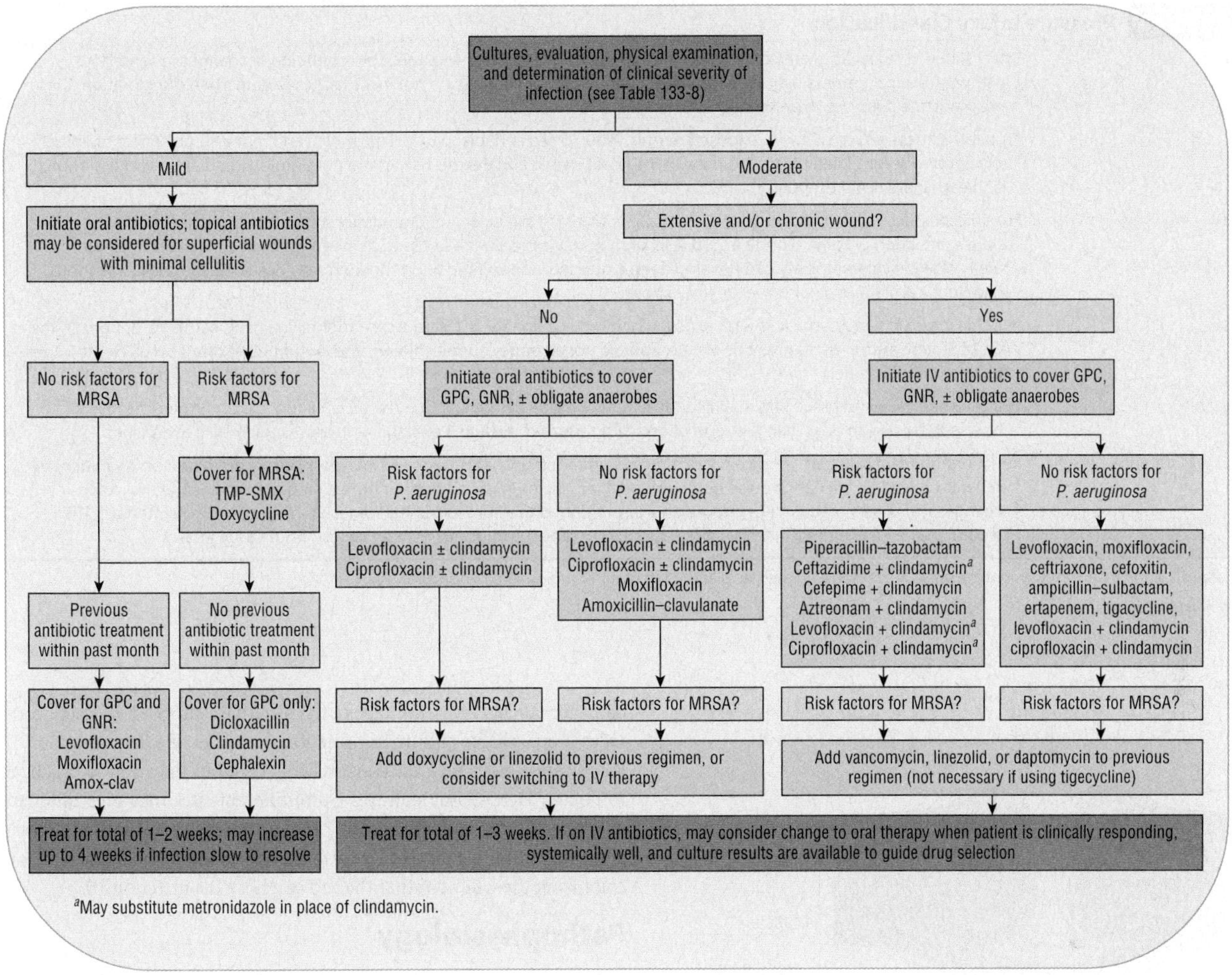

Cultures, evaluation, physical examination, and determination of clinical severity of infection (see Table 133-8)

Mild

Initiate oral antibiotics; topical antibiotics may be considered for superficial wounds with minimal cellulitis

No risk factors for MRSA

Risk factors for MRSA

Cover for MRSA: TMP-SMX Doxycycline

Previous antibiotic treatment within past month

No previous antibiotic treatment within past month

Cover for GPC and GNR: Levofloxacin Moxifloxacin Amox-clav

Cover for GPC only: Dicloxacillin Clindamycin Cephalexin

Treat for total of 1–2 weeks; may increase up to 4 weeks if infection slow to resolve

Moderate

Extensive and/or chronic wound?

No

Initiate oral antibiotics to cover GPC, GNR, ± obligate anaerobes

Risk factors for *P. aeruginosa*

Levofloxacin ± clindamycin
Ciprofloxacin ± clindamycin

No risk factors for *P. aeruginosa*

Levofloxacin ± clindamycin
Ciprofloxacin ± clindamycin
Moxifloxacin
Amoxicillin–clavulanate

Risk factors for MRSA?

Risk factors for MRSA?

Add doxycycline or linezolid to previous regimen, or consider switching to IV therapy

Yes

Initiate IV antibiotics to cover GPC, GNR, ± obligate anaerobes

Risk factors for *P. aeruginosa*

Piperacillin–tazobactam
Ceftazidime + clindamycin[a]
Cefepime + clindamycin
Aztreonam + clindamycin
Levofloxacin + clindamycin[a]
Ciprofloxacin + clindamycin[a]

No risk factors for *P. aeruginosa*

Levofloxacin, moxifloxacin, ceftriaxone, cefoxitin, ampicillin–sulbactam, ertapenem, tigacycline, levofloxacin + clindamycin ciprofloxacin + clindamycin

Risk factors for MRSA?

Risk factors for MRSA?

Add vancomycin, linezolid, or daptomycin to previous regimen (not necessary if using tigecycline)

Treat for total of 1–3 weeks. If on IV antibiotics, may consider change to oral therapy when patient is clinically responding, systemically well, and culture results are available to guide drug selection

[a]May substitute metronidazole in place of clindamycin.

FIGURE 133-2 Recommended treatment algorithm for initial empiric management of mild-to-moderate diabetic foot infections. (GNR, aerobic gram-negative rods; GPC, aerobic gram-positive cocci; MRSA, methicillin-resistant *Staphylococcus aureus*; TMP-SMX, trimethoprim–sulfamethoxazole.)

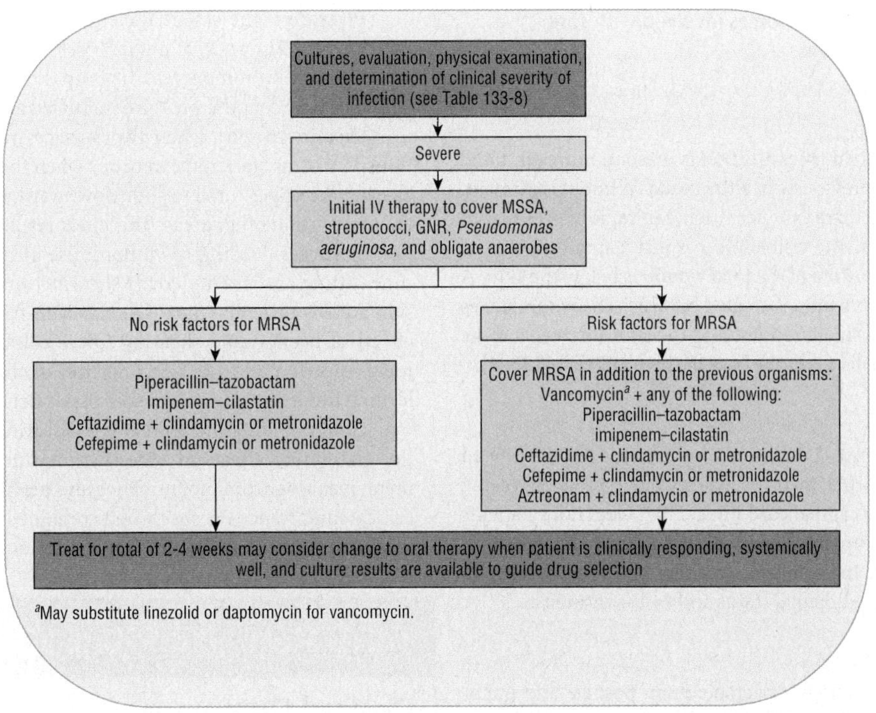

FIGURE 133-3 Recommended treatment algorithm for initial empiric management of severe diabetic foot infections. (GNR, aerobic gram-negative rods; MRSA, methicillin-resistant *Staphylococcus aureus*; MSSA, methicillin-susceptible *S. aureus*.)

TABLE 133-10 Pressure Injury Classification

Stage 1	Intact skin with a localized area of nonblanchable erythema. Presence of blanchable erythema or changes in sensation, temperature, or firmness may precede visual changes. Color changes do not include purple or maroon discoloration; these may indicate deep tissue pressure injury.
Stage 2	Partial-thickness loss of skin with exposed dermis. Wound bed is viable, pink or red, moist, and may also present as an intact or ruptured serum-filled blister. Adipose tissue is not visible and deeper tissues are not visible. Granulation tissue, slough, and eschar are not present.
Stage 3[a]	Full-thickness loss of skin, in which adipose tissue is visible in the ulcer and granulation tissue and epibole (rolled wound edges) are often present. Slough and/or eschar may be visible. Depth of tissue damage varies by anatomical location; areas of significant adiposity can develop deep wounds. Undermining and tunneling may occur. Fascia, muscle, tendon, ligament, cartilage, and/or bone are not exposed.
Stage 4[a]	Full-thickness skin and tissue loss with exposed or directly palpable fascia, muscle, tendon, ligament, cartilage, or bone in the ulcer. Slough and/or eschar may be visible. Epibole (rolled edges), undermining, and/or tunneling often occur. Depth varies by anatomical location.
Unstageable[a]	Full-thickness skin and tissue loss in which the extent of tissue damage within the ulcer cannot be confirmed because it is obscured by slough or eschar. If slough or eschar is removed, a stage 3 or stage 4 pressure injury will be revealed.
Deep-tissue pressure injury	Intact or nonintact skin with localized area of persistent nonblanchable deep red, maroon, purple discoloration or epidermal separation revealing a dark wound bed or blood filled blister. Pain and temperature change often precede skin color changes. This injury results from intense and/or prolonged pressure and shear forces at the bone-muscle interface. The wound may evolve rapidly to reveal the actual extent of tissue injury, or may resolve without tissue loss.

[a]Stage 3, stage 4, and unstageable lesions are unlikely to resolve on their own and often require surgical intervention.

Data from Reference 60.

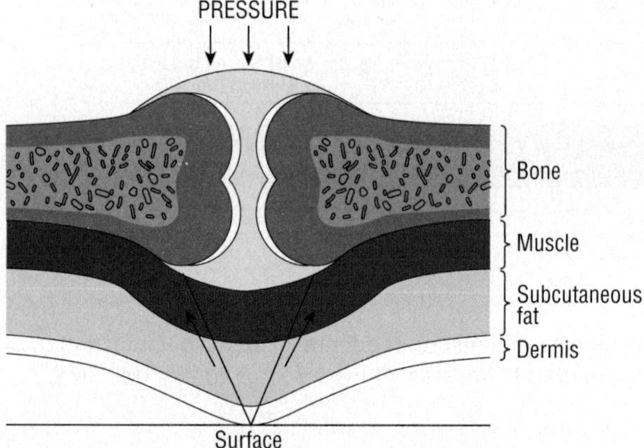

FIGURE 133-4 Distribution of forces involved with sore formation in a conical fashion.

eventually heal.[58,59,61] When true infection is present, however, there is bacterial invasion of previously healthy tissue. Without treatment, an initial small, localized area of ulceration can rapidly progress to large ulcers within days. The visible ulcer is just a small portion of the actual wound[29]; up to 70% of the total wound is below the skin. A pressure-gradient phenomenon is created by which the wound takes on a conical nature; the smallest point is at the skin surface, and the largest portion of the defect is at the base of the ulcer (Fig. 133-4).

Epidemiology

Pressure injuries are most common among chronically debilitated persons, older adults (70% involve persons older than 70 years), and persons with serious spinal cord injury.[29,58,59] Generally, patients who are at risk for pressure injuries are older adults or chronically ill young patients who are immobilized, in either bed or a wheelchair, and who may have altered mental status and/or incontinence.[58,59]

Etiology

Similar to DFIs, a large variety of aerobic gram-positive and gram-negative organisms, as well as anaerobes, frequently are isolated from wound cultures.[24,62] Most pressure injury–related ulcers are heavily colonized with microorganisms, making assessment for infection a clinical challenge.[24,62] Curettage of the ulcer base after debridement provides more reliable culture information than does needle aspiration.[61,62] Biopsy specimens give the most reliable data but may not be practical to obtain. Deep-tissue cultures from different sites may give different results. Cultures collected from pressure ulcers reveal polymicrobial growth. A culture collected by swab is likely to identify surface bacteria colonizing the wound rather than to diagnose the infection.[29,62]

Pathophysiology

Many factors apparently predispose patients to the formation of pressure injuries: paralysis, paresis, immobilization, malnutrition, anemia, infection, and advanced age. Factors thought to be most critical to their formation are pressure, shearing forces, friction, and moisture[29,58,59]; however, there is still a debate as to the exact pathophysiology of pressure injury development.[58,59]

Pressure is the essential element in the formation of pressure injuries.[24,58,59] The areas of highest pressure are generated most often over the bony prominences.[24,58,59] Both the degree of pressure and the length of time that the pressure is applied are important.[58,59]

Shearing occurs when two surfaces move in opposite directions.[24,58,59] This situation can occur when the head of a bed is raised, causing the upper torso to slide downward, transmitting pressure to the sacrum and other areas. This effect results in occlusion or distortion of vessels, leading to compromise of the dermis. At the same time, sitting and gravity create shearing forces; the posterior sacral skin area can become fixed secondary to friction with the bed. The effects of friction and shearing forces combine, resulting in transmission of force to the deep portion of the superficial fascia and leading to further damage of soft-tissue structures.[24,58,59]

Compounding the problems of shearing and friction forces are the macerating effects of excessive moisture in the local environment, resulting from incontinence and perspiration. This factor is of critical importance because when combined with the other forces, it increases the risk of pressure sore formation fivefold.[29,58,59]

TREATMENT: PRESSURE SORES

Desired Outcomes

The primary goal for pressure injuries is prevention. Once pressure injury has developed, the goals of therapy are prevention of

CLINICAL PRESENTATION Pressure Injuries

General

- Most pressure injuries are in the pelvic region and lower extremities; see Fig. 133-5.
- Most common sites: sacral and coccygeal areas, ischial tuberosities, and greater trochanter.

Symptoms

- Patients commonly have other medical problems that may mask signs and symptoms of infection.
- Pain may be present with or without infection; continuous pain may indicate infection.

Signs

- A dark red color on the surface of a pressure injury–related ulcer may indicate local infection.
- Surrounding erythema, swelling, and heat are commonly present with infection.
- Purulent discharge, foul odor, and systemic signs (eg, fever and leukocytosis) of infection may be present.

Laboratory Tests

- Cultures should be collected from either a biopsy or fluid obtained by needle aspiration.

Other Diagnostic Tests

- Complete blood cell count often performed for assessment of potential infection.
- Consider magnetic resonance imaging if suspicious of underlying osteomyelitis.

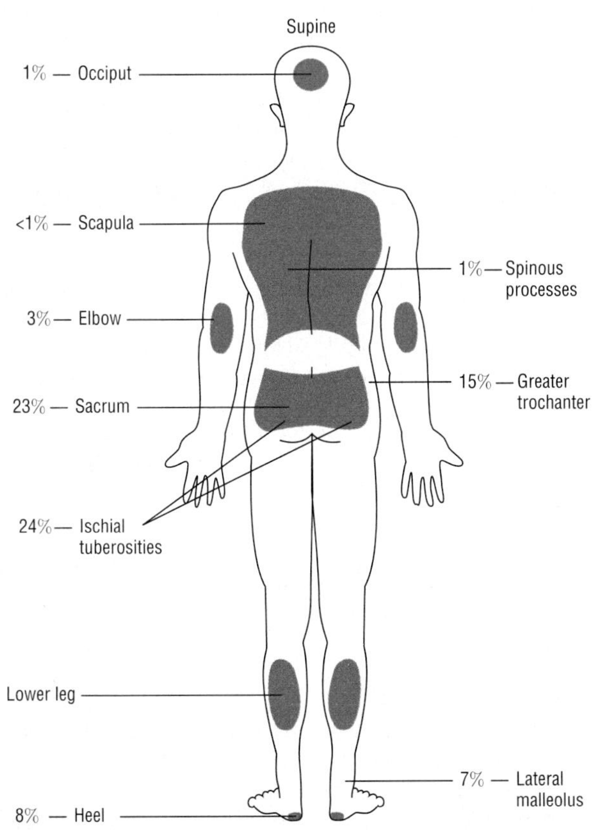

FIGURE 133-5 Supine view of areas where pressure sore injuries tend to occur.

complications (ie, infections), preventing injuries from growing larger, and preventing the development of injuries in other locations.[58,59] Eradication of infection should include good wound care and topical therapies, and avoidance of broad-spectrum antimicrobials unless guided by results from appropriately collected cultures or in patients with bacteremia, sepsis, cellulitis, or osteomyelitis.

Drug and Nondrug Management

8 Prevention is the single most important aspect in the management of pressure injuries. Skin surveillance and frequent repositioning (ie, pressure reduction) are key in preventing pressure injuries.[29,58,59] Prevention is far easier and less costly than the intensive care necessary for the healing and eventual closure of pressure injuries. Of primary importance, then, is the ability to identify patients who are at high risk so that preventive measures may be instituted. Relief of pressure through proper positioning, and periodic repositioning, is probably the single most important factor in preventing pressure injury formation. Relief for a period of only 5 minutes once every 2 hours gives protection against pressure injury formation.[29,58,59,61] Repositioning seated patients every 15 to 60 minutes is also recommended.[29,58,59] Pressure relief devices such as mattresses or overlays filled with air, water, gel, or foam are helpful in preventing pressure injuries.[29] Cushions and ankle or heel protectors should also be encouraged.[29,59] Skin care and prevention of soilage are also important, with the intent being to keep the surface relatively free of moisture. Patients with problems of incontinence should be cleaned frequently, and efforts should be made to keep the involved areas dry.[29,58,59]

The medical approach to the treatment of pressure injuries depends on the stage of the disease. Medical management is indicated for lesions that are of moderate size and relatively shallow depth (stage 1 or 2 lesions) and are not located over a bony prominence. Depending on their location and severity, from 30% to 80% of these injuries will heal without an operation. Surgical intervention is almost always necessary for ulcers that extend through superficial layers or into bone (stage 3, stage 4, and unstageable lesions).[24,56]

The goal of therapy is to clean and decontaminate the ulcer in order to permit formation of healthy granulation tissue that promotes wound healing or prepare the wound for an operative procedure. The main factors to be considered for successful topical therapy (local care) are (a) relief of pressure, (b) debridement of necrotic tissue as needed, (c) wound cleansing, (d) dressing selection, and (e) prevention, diagnosis, and treatment of infection.[29,58,59,61]

Relief of pressure is important once pressure injury has developed. The same repositioning methods and pressure-reducing devices used for preventive care also apply to treatment.[29,58,59,61]

The goals of debridement and cleansing measures are removal of devitalized tissue and reduction of bacterial contamination, which can slow granulation time and impede healing.[29,58,59,61] Debridement can be accomplished by surgical, mechanical, or chemical means.[24,58,59,61] Surgical debridement rapidly removes necrotic material from the wound and is recommended for urgent situations (eg, cellulitis and sepsis).[29,58,59,61] Mechanical debridement involves wet-to-dry dressing changes in which saline-soaked gauze is applied to the wound; after drying, the gauze is removed and with it any adherent necrotic tissue. Other effective mechanical therapies include hydrotherapy (use of the whirlpool [Hubbard tank] to remove necrotic tissue and debris), wound irrigation, and dextranomers (beads placed in the wound to absorb exudate and bacteria).[24,58,59] Chemical debridement includes enzymatic and autolytic agents. Enzymatic debridement involves application of topical debriding agents to remove devitalized tissue. This method is recommended for patients who cannot tolerate surgery or are in a long-term care or home setting.[29,58,59,61] Autolytic debridement involves the use of synthetic dressings that allow devitalized tissue to self-digest via enzymes present in wound fluids. Autolytic debridement is contraindicated in the treatment of infected pressure injuries.[29,58,59,61]

Pressure injury wounds should be cleaned with normal saline.[24,29,59,61] No cleansing solution or technique has demonstrated greater efficacy on healing.[63] Cleansing agents that are cytotoxic, such as povidone–iodine, iodophor, sodium hypochlorite solution, hydrogen peroxide, and acetic acid, should be avoided.[29,58,59,61] Many of these agents destroy granulation tissue and impair healing. Many different types of dressings are available for pressure injuries.[24] Wound dressing materials should keep the wound moist, allow free exchange of air, act as a physical barrier to bacteria, and prevent physical damage.[24,29,59] Controlled studies of the various types of wound dressings have shown no significant differences in healing outcomes.[58,63] Occlusive dressings (hydrocolloid, such as DuoDERM™ or Tegaderm™) and transparent dressings (eg, 3M Tegaderm™) are not recommended for infected wounds.[24,29,59] If occlusive dressings are used, any infection should be controlled or the dressing frequency increased.

Topical antibiotics (silver sulfadiazine, triple antibiotic) or medical grade honey may be considered for a clean ulcer that is not healing or is producing a moderate amount of exudate despite appropriate care.[29,58,59] When used, topical antibiotics should be limited to a 2-week trial or until additional definitive debridement can be performed, whichever comes first.[29,58,59] Systemic treatment of pressure-related ulcers is generally reserved for infections associated with bacteremia, sepsis, cellulitis, fasciitis, or osteomyelitis.[29,58,61] Empiric therapy for infected pressure sores or associated infectious complications should cover MRSA, anaerobes, enterococci, and more resistant gram-negative bacteria such as *Pseudomonas* (see Table 133-5).[58,59] Thereafter, antibiotics should be guided by results from appropriately collected cultures.

Other nonpharmacologic approaches to shorten the healing time have included the use of hyperbaric oxygenation, hydrotherapy, high-frequency/high-intensity sound waves, and electrotherapy.[29,61] Electrical stimulation is the only adjunctive therapy that is proven effective.[29,61] Various comorbid conditions (diabetes mellitus, smoking, peripheral vascular disease, malnutrition) may impair wound healing. Eliminating or optimizing these factors is recommended, although studies have not demonstrated benefit.[24,59]

Evaluation of Therapeutic Outcomes

With appropriate wound care and antimicrobial therapy, infected pressure injuries can heal. A reduction in erythema, warmth, pain, and other signs and symptoms should be seen in 48 to 72 hours.

ANIMAL AND HUMAN BITE WOUNDS

Approximately half the population in the United States will be bitten by either an animal or another human sometime during their lifetimes.[64-66] Animal bites (typically from dogs or cats) are common causes of injury, particularly to children, and are associated with significant risk of infection without prompt attention and appropriate management. Likewise, human bite wounds are often deceptively severe and frequently require aggressive management to reduce the risk of infectious complications. If left untreated, severe soft-tissue infection and osteomyelitis may occur, possibly requiring extensive debridement or amputation.

Epidemiology

Dog bites account for approximately 75% to 90% of all animal bite wounds requiring medical attention.[65] The Centers for Disease Control and Prevention reports that approximately 330,000 individuals seek emergency room attention for dog bites annually; rates of dog bite–related injuries are highest in children aged 5 to 9 years.[66] Most dog bites are to the extremities,[65] but the majority of bites to children less than 5 years of age are to the face and neck.[66] Cat bites are the second most common cause of bite wounds in the United States, accounting for up to 20% of all animal bites.[64] Cat bites occur most commonly on the upper extremities and face, with most injuries reported in women and older adults.[64,67] Human bites are the third most frequent type of bites requiring medical attention.

Infection rates after dog and cat bites are estimated at 20% overall. However, infection may occur in up to 30% to 80% of serious cat bites, a rate more than double that seen with dog bites.[64,67] Also, bite wounds to the hands become infected in 30% to 40% of cases.[64] Patients at greatest risk of acquiring animal bite–related infection have had a puncture wound (usually to the hand), have not sought medical attention within 8 hours of the injury, and are older than 50 years of age.[64,65,67]

Infected human bites can occur as bites from the teeth or from blows to the mouth (clenched-fist injuries). Bites by others can occur to any part of the body, but most often involve the hands. Infectious complications occur in 10% to 50% of patients with human bites.[67]

Etiology

Infections in bite wounds are caused predominantly by mouth flora from the animal or human biter, and from the victim's own skin flora (Table 133-11).[64,65,67-71] Most infections are polymicrobial, with a median of three to nine bacterial isolates per culture.[67-71] *Pasteurella* is the most frequent isolate from both dog and cat bites. *Pasteurella multocida* is part of the normal oral flora of up to 90% of cats; dog bites more commonly involve *P. canis* (approximately 26% of infections).[64,65,67,69] Tularemia (*Pasteurella tularensis*) and cat scratch disease (*Bartonella henselae*) have also been transmitted by cat bites, while rabies is associated with dog bites, particularly in developing countries.[64,65,69,70,72] Human bite wounds are notable for potential involvement of *Eikenella corrodens* in approximately 30% of infections.

Pathophysiology

Animal bites have great potential for infection owing to the pressure that can be exerted during the bite and the vast number of potential pathogens that make up the normal oral flora.[64,65,67-70] Cats' teeth are slender and extremely sharp. Their teeth easily penetrate into bones and joints, resulting in a higher incidence of septic arthritis and osteomyelitis.[67-70] Although a dog's teeth may not be as sharp, they can exert a pressure of 200 to 450 lb/in.^{2} (~1,400-3,100 kPa) and therefore result in a serious crush injury with much devitalized tissue.[64,65,67-70] In addition, the polymicrobic (aerobic and anaerobic) nature of animal bites provides a synergistic relationship, thus making an infection harder to eradicate.[68]

Human bites are more serious and more prone to infection than animal bites, particularly clenched-fist injuries.[68] While the force of a punch may break a bone or sever a tendon or nerve, it most often causes a breach in the capsule of the metacarpophalangeal joint, leading to direct inoculation of bacteria into the joint or bone.[68,70] When the hand is relaxed, the tendons carry bacteria into deeper spaces of the hand, resulting in more extensive infection.[68,70]

TABLE 133-11 Bacterial Isolates from Infections in Animal and Human Bite Wounds

	Percentage of Isolates	
Organisms	**Dog and cat**	**Human**
Aerobes	74-90	44
Pasteurella spp.	50-75	—
Streptococcus spp.	46-50	52-84
S. anginosus	—	52
S. mitis	22	12
S. pyogenes	12	14
S. mutans	12	2
Staphylococcus spp.	35-46	54
S. aureus	20	30
S. epidermidis	18	22
Neisseria spp.	32-35	4
Moraxella spp.	10-35	2
Corynebacterium spp.	12-28	12
Enterococcus spp.	10-12	6
Bacillus spp.	8-11	—
Eikenella corrodens	2	30
Enterobacteriaceae	6-12	8-15
Anaerobes	50-70	40-90
Fusobacterium spp.	32-33	32-34
Porphyromonas spp.	28-30	2
Bacteroides spp.	18-28	4
Prevotella spp.	19-28	22-36
Propionibacterium spp.	18-20	4
Peptostreptococcus spp.	8-16	22
Veillonella spp.	2	24
Mixed aerobic and anaerobic	50-75	40-66

Data from References 67-70.

TREATMENT: BITE WOUNDS

Desired Outcomes

The goals of therapy of bite wounds, whether caused by animals or humans, are twofold: to provide effective prophylaxis against infection, when appropriate, and to achieve rapid eradication of established infection and prevent further complications. Effective treatment of bite wounds includes avoidance of unnecessary antimicrobials that contribute to increased resistance, and minimizing toxicities and cost of therapy.

Management of Bite Wounds

9 Bite wounds should be irrigated thoroughly with a copious volume of sterile water or saline, and the wound washed vigorously with soap or povidone–iodine in order to reduce the bacterial count in the wound.[64,65,67,70] Surgical debridement and immobilization of the affected area are often required in dog and human bites associated with more extensive tissue injury. Clinical failures due to edema have occurred despite appropriate antibiotic therapy.[64] Therefore, it is important to stress to patients that the affected area should be elevated for several days or until edema has resolved. In the case of animal bites, an immunization history of the animal should be obtained. It is also important for the patient's tetanus immune status to be determined. Because transmission of viruses (HIV, herpes, hepatitis B and C) is a possibility with human bites, information about the biter is important. Although the possibility of acquiring HIV through saliva alone is believed to be unlikely, the presence of virus-containing blood in the saliva makes disease transmission possible.[73] Bite victims exposed to blood-tainted saliva may be offered antiretroviral chemoprophylaxis, but each case should be individually assessed based on the potential for significant exposure and potential risks and benefits of antiretroviral therapy.[73]

Patients with clenched-fist injuries should be seen by a specialist in hand care to evaluate for penetration into the synovium, joint capsule, and bone.[15,68] Primary closure for human bites generally is not recommended. Tetanus toxoid and antitoxin may be indicated.

10 All patients with human bite injuries should receive prophylactic antibiotic therapy ("early preemptive therapy") for 3 to 5 days due to high infection risk (Table 133-4).[70,71] Prophylactic antimicrobial agents should be given as soon as possible to all patients, regardless of the appearance of the wound, unless it can be documented that the wound does not involve hands, feet, or joints and penetrates no deeper than the epidermis.[15,70]

The role of prophylactic antimicrobial therapy for early, noninfected animal bite wounds remains controversial.[15,64,65,67,68,70] Recommendations from the IDSA suggest that prophylactic or early preemptive therapy seems to provide only marginal benefit for most patients in the absence of specific factors that increase the risk of infection.[15] The decision to administer prophylactic antibiotics is therefore based on an assessment of wound severity and host immune competence. Specifically, prophylaxis is more strongly recommended in patients with the following factors associated with increased risk for infection: immunocompromised; asplenic; advanced liver disease; preexisting or resultant edema of the affected area; moderate-to-severe bite-related injuries, especially to the hands or face; deep puncture wounds that cannot be adequately irrigated; or bite injuries that have penetrated the periosteum or joint capsule.[15,65] A 3- to 5-day course of prophylactic antibiotics is recommended when such therapy is considered to be appropriate.[15,65,67,68,70]

Empiric antibiotics for the treatment of established infection of bite wounds should be directed at a variety of aerobic and anaerobic flora (Table 133-4). Amoxicillin–clavulanic acid is most commonly recommended for oral outpatient therapy due to excellent activity against all likely pathogens, including *Pasteurella* and *Eikenella*.[15,64,65,67,68,70] Alternative oral agents include moxifloxacin or doxycycline alone; or trimethoprim–sulfamethoxazole, levofloxacin, ciprofloxacin, or a second- or third-generation cephalosporin in combination with metronidazole or clindamycin to provide activity against oropharyngeal anaerobes.[15,64,65,67,68,70] Although the combination of penicillin VK plus dicloxacillin has been recommended traditionally for the treatment of bite wounds, its use has become less common in favor of other alternatives. Failure to provide adequate initial treatment of bite wounds results in treatment failures and increased need for hospitalization for parenteral antibiotics.[15,64,65,67,68-70]

Hospitalization for minor wounds is unnecessary if surgical repair of vital structures is not needed. Patients with clenched-fist or other serious bite injuries and severe resultant infection may be considered for IV antibiotics. Treatment options for patients requiring IV therapy include β-lactam–β-lactamase inhibitor combinations (ampicillin–sulbactam, piperacillin–tazobactam), second-generation cephalosporins with antianaerobic activity (eg, cefoxitin), and ertapenem.[15,70] The combination of doxycycline or fluoroquinolone with metronidazole or clindamycin may be used in patients with severe β-lactam allergies. The length of antimicrobial therapy depends on the severity of the injury/infection. However, therapy should generally be continued for 7 to 14 days.[15,64,74]

Tetanus does not occur commonly after dog bites; however, it is possible. If the immunization history of a patient with anything

CLINICAL PRESENTATION Bite Wounds

General

Animal bites:

- Only general wound care is required for most patients with dog bites who present early (<12 hours) after injury; infection is more likely in patients presenting late (≥12 hours) after injury.

Human bites:

- Most patients with clenched-fist injuries present for medical care after infection is already established.

Symptoms

- Patients often seek medical care for infection-related complaints (ie, pain, purulent discharge, swelling) at the site of the injury.
- Wounds often have a purulent discharge, and decreased range of motion may be present.

Signs

- Erythema, swelling, and clear or purulent discharge at site of infected wound.

Animal bites:

- If *P. multocida* is present, a rapidly progressing cellulitis is observed within 24 to 48 hours of initial injury.
- Fever is often absent.
- Adenopathy or lymphangitis is uncommon.

Human bites:

- Lymphadenopathy is common.
- In clenched-fist injuries, edema may limit the ability of tendons to glide in their sheaths, thereby limiting a joint's range of motion.

Laboratory Tests

- Samples for bacterial cultures (aerobic and anaerobic) should be obtained from infected wounds.
- Wounds seen <8 hours or more than 24 hours after injury that show no signs of infection may not need to be cultured.
- White blood cell counts should be monitored for resolution of infection if initially elevated.

Other Diagnostic Tests

- Radiographic evaluation should be performed if damage to a bone or joint is suspected.

other than a clean, minor wound is unknown, or if the last known vaccination was longer than 10 years ago, tetanus–diphtheria (TD) toxoids should be administered.[74] Both TD toxoids and tetanus immune globulin should be administered to patients who have never been immunized.[70,75]

Because the rabies virus can be transmitted via saliva, rabies may be a potential complication of a bite. When the symptoms of rabies develop after a bite, the prognosis for survival is poor. Roughly 3% of rabies cases documented in animals were in dogs (the most frequent vectors are skunks, raccoons, and bats).[72,76] In the United States, recommendations for postexposure prophylaxis after a dog bite depend on the health of the dog. If the animal is healthy and able to be observed for a 10-day period, active prophylaxis is only required if the dog develops signs of rabies.[67,72] If the dog is known or suspected to be rabid, postexposure procedures should be initiated; current treatment guidelines should be consulted for appropriate management recommendations.[72,76] Outside of the United States, locally applicable guidelines such as those from the World Health Organization should be consulted.[77]

Evaluation of Therapeutic Outcomes

Evaluation of treatment for either animal or human bites should follow the same general guidelines. Bite victims treated on an outpatient basis with oral antimicrobials should be followed up within 24 hours by either phone or office visit.[15] Hospitalization or change to IV therapy should be considered if the infection has progressed. For hospitalized patients with no improvement in signs and symptoms following 24 hours of appropriate therapy, surgical debridement may be needed. Physical therapy may be needed to improve complications such as residual joint stiffness and loss of function, particularly after human bites involving clenched-fist injuries.

ABBREVIATIONS

ABSSSI	acute bacterial skin and skin structure infection
AMS	altered mental status
CA-MRSA	community-associated methicillin-resistant *S. aureus*
DFI	diabetic foot infection
HA-MRSA	healthcare-associated methicillin-resistant *Staphylococcus aureus*
HIV	human immunodeficiency virus
IDSA	Infectious Diseases Society of America
MRSA	methicillin-resistant *Staphylococcus aureus*
MSSA	methicillin-susceptible *Staphylococcus aureus*
NPUAP	National Pressure Ulcer Advisory Panel
PVL	Panton-Valentine leukocidin
SCC*mec*	staphylococcal chromosomal cassette *mec*
SSTI	skin and soft-tissue infection
TD	tetanus–diphtheria

REFERENCES

1. Egert M, Simmering R. The microbiota of the human skin. *Adv Experiment Med Biol.* 2016;902:61–81. doi:10.1007/978-3-319-31248-4_5.
2. Poulakou G, Lagou S, Tsiodras S. What's new in the epidemiology of skin and soft tissue infections in 2018? *Curr Opin Infect Dis.* 2019;32:77–86. doi:10.1097/QCO.0000000000000527.
3. Bystritsky RJ. Cellulitis. *Infect Dis Clin N Am.* 35(2021):49–60. doi:10.1016/j.idc.2020.10.002.
4. Esposito S, Bassetti M, Concia E, et al. Diagnosis and management of skin and soft tissue infections (SSTI). A literature review and consensus statement: An update. *J Chemother.* 2017;29:197–214. doi:10.1080/1120009X.2017.1311398.

5. Rrapi R, Chand S, Kroshinsky D. Cellulitis. A review of pathophysiology, diagnosis, and management. *Med Clin N Am.* 105(2021):723–735. doi:10.1016/j.mcna.2021.04.009.
6. Cardona AF, Wilson SE. Skin and soft tissue infections: A critical review and the role of telavancin in their treatment. *Clin Infect Dis.* 2015;61(Suppl 2):S69–S78. doi:10.1093/cid/civ528.
7. U.S. Food and Drug Administration, Department of Health and Human Services. Guidance for industry. Acute bacterial skin and skin structure infections: Developing drugs for treatment. Available at https://www.fda.gov/regulatory-information/search-fda-guidance-documents/acute-bacterial-skin-and-skin-structure-infections-developing-drugs-treatment. Last accessed, September 28, 2021.
8. Pasternak MS, Swartz MN. Cellulitis, necrotizing fasciitis, and subcutaneous tissue infections. In: Bennett JE, Dolin R, Blaser MJ, eds. *Mandell, Douglas, and Bennett's Principles and Practice of Infectious Diseases*. 9th ed. Philadelphia, PA: Elsevier, Inc.; 2020:1282–1306.e4.
9. Miller LG, Eisenberg DF, Liu H, et al. Incidence of skin and soft tissue infections in ambulatory and inpatient settings, 2005–2010. *BMC Infect Dis.* 2015;15:362. doi:10.1186/s12879-015-1071-0.
10. Kaye KS, Petty LA, Shorr AF, et al. Current epidemiology, etiology, and burden of acute skin infections in the United States. *Clin Infect Dis.* 2019;68(S3):S193–S199. doi:10.1093/cid/ciz002.
11. Poulakou G, Giannitsioti E, Tsiodras S. What is new in the management of skin and soft tissue infections in 2016? *Curr Opin Infect Dis.* 2017;30:158–171. doi:10.1097/QCO.0000000000000360.
12. Pollack CV Jr, Amin A, Ford WT Jr, et al. Acute bacterial skin and skin structure infections (ABSSSI): Practice guidelines for management and care transitions in the emergency department and hospital. *J Emerg Med.* 2015;48:508–519. doi:10.1016/j.jemermed.2014.12.001.
13. Guillamet CV, Kollef MH. How to stratify patients at risk for resistant bugs in skin and soft tissue infections? *Curr Opin Infect Dis.* 2016;29:116–123. doi:10.1097/QCO.0000000000000244.
14. Planet PJ. Life after USA300: The rise and fall of a superbug. *J Infect Dis.* 2017;215(S1):S71–S77. doi:10.1093/infdis/jiw444.
15. Stevens DL, Bisno AL, Chambers HF, et al. Practice guidelines for the diagnosis and management of skin and soft-tissue infections: 2014 Update by the Infectious Diseases Society of America. *Clin Infect Dis.* 2014;59:e10–e52. doi:10.1093/cid/ciu444.
16. Hatlen TJ, Miller LG. Staphylococcal skin and soft tissue infections. *Infect Dis Clin N Am.* 2021;35:81–105. doi:10.1016/j.idc.2020.10.003.
17. Bassetti M, Carnelutti A, Righi E. The role of methicillin-resistant *Staphylococcus aureus* in skin and soft tissue infections. *Curr Opin Infect Dis.* 2017;30:150–157. doi:10.1097/QCO.0000000000000353.
18. Kale P, Dhawan B. The changing face of community-acquired methicillin-resistant *Staphylococcus aureus. Indian J Med Microbiol.* 2016;34:275–285. doi:10.4103/0255-0857.188313.
19. Abetz JW, Adams NG, Mitra B. Skin and soft tissue infection management failure in the emergency department observation unit: A systematic review. *Emerg Med J.* 2018;35:56–61. doi:10.1136/emermed-2016-205950.
20. Centers for Disease Control and Prevention. Healthcare-Associated Infections—Community Interface Surveillance Report, Emerging Infections Program Network, Methicillin-Resistant Staphylococcus aureus, 2017. Available at: https://www.cdc.gov/hai/eip/pdf/2017-MRSA-Report508.pdf. Last accessed, September 28, 2021.
21. Gunderson CG. Overtreatment of nonpurulent cellulitis. *J Hosp Med.* 2016;11:587–590. doi:10.1002/jhm.2593.
22. Moffarah AS, al Mohajer A, Hurwitz BL, et al. Skin and soft tissue infections. *Microbiol Spectrum.* 2016;4:1–16. doi:10.1128/microbiolspec.DMIH2-0014-2015.
23. Yamamoto LG. Treatment of skin and soft tissue infections. *Pediatr Emerg Care.* 2017;33:49–55. doi:10.1097/PEC.0000000000001001.
24. Ricci JA, Bayer LR, Orgill DP. Evidence-based medicine: The evaluation and treatment of pressure injuries. *Plast Reconstr Surg.* 2017;139:275e–286e. doi:10.1097/PRS.0000000000002850.
25. Quirke M, Ayoub F, McCabe A, et al. Risk factors for nonpurulent leg cellulitis: A systematic review and meta-analysis. *Br J Dermatol.* 2017;177:382–394. doi:10.1111/bjd.15186.
26. Lipsky BA, Berendt AR, Cornia PB, et al. Infectious Diseases Society of America clinical practice guidelines for the diagnosis and treatment of diabetic foot infections. *Clin Infect Dis.* 2012;54:132–173. doi:10.1093/cid/cis346.
27. Liu C, Bayer A, Cosgrive SE, et al. Clinical practice guidelines by the Infectious Diseases Society of America for the treatment of methicillin-resistant *Staphylococcus aureus* infections in adults and children. *Clin Infect Dis.* 2011;52:1–38. doi:10.1093/cid/ciq146.
28. Rybak MJ, Le J, Lodise TP, et al. Therapeutic monitoring of vancomycin for serious methicillin-resistant Staphylococcus aureus infections: A revised consensus guideline and review by the American Society of Health-System Pharmacists, the Infectious Diseases Society of America, the Pediatric Infectious Diseases Society, and the Society of Infectious Diseases Pharmacists. *Clin Infect Dis.* 2020;71:1361–1364. *Am J Health Syst Pharm.* 2020;77:835-864. doi:10.1093/ajhp/zxaa036.
29. European Pressure Ulcer Advisory Panel, National Pressure Injury Advisory Panel and Pan Pacific Pressure Injury Alliance. Prevention and Treatment of Pressure Ulcers/Injuries: Clinical Practice Guideline. Quick Reference Guide. Emily Haesler (Ed.). 2019. Available at: http://www.internationalguideline.com/static/pdfs/Quick_Reference_Guide-10Mar2019.pdf. Last accessed, September 28, 2021.
30. Silverberg B. A structured approach to skin and soft tissue infections (SSTIs) in an ambulatory setting. *Clin Pract.* 2021;11:65–74. doi:10.3390/clinpract11010011.
31. Blackberg A, Trell K, Rasmussen M. Erysipelas: A large retrospective study of aetiology and clinical presentation. *BMC Infect Dis.* 2015;15:402–407. doi:10.1186/s12879-015-1134-2.
32. Kosar L, Laubscher T. Management of impetigo and cellulitis: Simple considerations for promoting appropriate antibiotic use in skin infections. *Canadian Fam Phys.* 2017;615–618.
33. Galli L, Venturini E, Bassi A, et al. Common community-acquired bacterial skin and soft tissue infections in children: An intersociety consensus on impetigo, abscess, and cellulitis treatment. *Clin Ther.* 2019;41:532–551.e17. doi:10.1016/j.clinthera.2019.01.010.
34. Johnson MK. Impetigo. *Adv Emerg Nurs J.* 2020;42:262–269. doi:10.1097/TME.0000000000000320.
35. Pasternak MS. Lymphadenitis and lymphangitis. In: Bennett JE, Dolin R, Blaser MJ, eds. *Mandell, Douglas, and Bennett's Principles and Practice of Infectious Diseases*. 9th ed. Philadelphia, PA: Elsevier, Inc.; 2020:1317–1329.e3.
36. Seelang K, Manning ML, Saks M, et al. Skin and soft tissue infection management, outcomes, and follow-up in the emergency department of an urban academic hospital. *Adv Emerg Nurs J.* 2014;36:348–359. doi:10.1097/TME.0000000000000039.
37. VanEperen A, Segreti J. Empirical therapy in methicillin-resistant *Staphylococcus aureus* infections: An up-to-date approach. *J Infect Chemother.* 2016;22:351–359. doi:10.1016/j.jiac.2016.02.012.
38. John J Jr. The treatment of resistant staphylococcal infections [version 1; peer review: 3 approved]. *F1000 Research.* 2020;9(F1000 Faculty Rev):150. doi:10.12688/f1000research.17718.1.
39. McClain SL, Bohan JG, Stevens DL. Advances in the medical management of skin and soft tissue infections. *BMJ.* 2016;355:i6004. doi:10.1136/bmj.i6004.
40. Bassetti M, Magnasco L, Del Puente F, et al. Role of new antibiotics in the treatment of acute bacterial skin and skin-structure infections. *Curr Opin Infect Dis.* 2020;33:110–120. doi:10.1097/QCO.0000000000000631.
41. Saeed K, Esposito S, Gould I, et al. Hot topics in necrotising skin and soft tissue infections. *Int J Antimicrob Agents.* 2018;52:1–10. doi:10.1016/j.ijantimicag.2018.02.012.
42. Stevens DL, Bryant AE. Necrotizing soft-tissue infections. *New Engl J Med.* 2017;377:2253–2265. doi:10.1056/NEJMra1600673.
43. Stevens DL, Bryant AE, Goldstein EJC. Necrotizing soft tissue infections. *Infect Dis Clin N Am.* 2021;35:135–155. doi:10.1016/j.idc.2020.10.004.
44. Peetermanns M, de Prost N, Eckmann C, et al. Necrotizing skin and soft tissue infections in the intensive care unit. *Clin Microbiol Infect.* 2020;26:8–17. doi: 10.1016/j.cmi.2019.06.031.
45. Oppegaard O, Rath E. Treatment of necrotizing soft tissue infections: Antibiotics. *AdvEx Med Biol.* 2020;1294:87–103. doi:10.1007/978-3-030-57616-5_7.
46. Boulton AJM, Armstrong DG, Hardman MJ, et al. Diagnosis and management of diabetic foot infections. Arlington, VA: American Diabetes Association; 2020. Available at https://www.ncbi.nlm.nih.gov/books/NBK554227/pdf/Bookshelf_NBK554227.pdf. Last accessed, September 28, 2021.
47. Lipsky BA, Uckay I. Treating diabetic foot osteomyelitis: A practical state-of-the-art update. *Medicina.* 2021;57:39. doi:10.3390/medicina57040339.
48. Ramirez-Acuna JM, Cardenas-Cadena SA, Marquez-Salas PA, et al. Diabetic foot ulcers: Current advances in antimicrobial therapies and emerging treatments. *Antibiotics (Basel).* 2019;8:193. doi:10.3390/antibiotics8040193.
49. Perez-Pavila A, Martinez-Fierro ML, Rodriguez-Lazalde JG, et al. Current therapeutic strategies in diabetic foot ulcers. *Medicina.* 2019;55:714. doi:10.3390/medicina55110714.
50. Thurber EG, Kisuula F, Humbyrd C, et al. Inpatient management of diabetic foot infections: A review of the guidelines for hospitalists. *J Hosp Med.* 2017;12:984–1000. doi:10.12788/jhm.2842.

51. Saeed K, Esposito S, Akram A, et al. Hot topics in diabetic foot infection. *Int J Antimicrob Agents.* 2020;55:1–9. doi:10.1016/j.ijantimicag.2020.105942.
52. Kwon KT, Armstrong DG. Microbiology and antimicrobial therapy for diabetic foot infections. *Infect Chemother.* 2018;50:11–20. doi:10.3947/ic.2018.50.1.11.
53. Manas AB, Taori S, Ahluwalia R, et al. Admission time deep swab specimens compared with surgical bone sampling in hospitalized individuals with diabetic foot osteomyelitis and soft tissue infection. *Int J Lower Extrem Wounds.* 2020;1–9. doi:10.1177/1534734620916386.
54. Pitocco D, Spanu T, Di Leo M, et al. Diabetic foot infections: A comprehensive overview. *Eur Rev Med Pharmacol Sci.* 2019;23(2 Suppl.):26–37. doi:10.26355/eurrev_201904_17471.
55. Zenelaj B, Bouvet C, Lipsky BA, et al. Do diabetic foot infections with methicillin-resistant Staphylococcus aureus differ from those with other pathogens? *Int J Lower Extrem Wounds.* 2014;13:263–272. doi:10.1177/1534734614550311.
56. Selva Olid A, Sola I, Barajas-Nava LA, et al. Systemic antibiotics for treating diabetic foot infections. *Cochrane Database Syst Rev.* 2015;9:CD009061. doi:10.1002/14651858.CD009061.pub2.
57. Jull AB, Cullum N, Dumville JC, et al. Honey as a topical treatment for wounds. *Cochrane Database Syst Rev.* 2015;3:CD005083. doi:10.1002/14651858.CD005083.pub4.
58. Atkinson RA, Cullum NA. Interventions for pressure ulcers: A summary of evidence for prevention and treatment. *Spinal Cord.* 2018;56:186–198. doi:10.1038/s41393-017-0054-y.
59. Roufogalis AL, Hutchinson ML. Best practices in pressure injury treatment. *Crit Care Nurs Clin N Am.* 2020; 32:501–520. doi:10.1016/j.cnc.2020.08.002.
60. Edberg LE, Black JM, Goldberg M, et al. Revised National Pressure Ulcer Advisory Panel pressure injury staging system. *J Wound Ostomy Continence Nurs.* 2016;43:585–597. doi:10.1097/WON.0000000000000281.
61. Hajhosseini B, Longaker MT, Gurtner GC. Pressure injury. *Ann Surg.* 2020;271:671–679. doi:10.1097/SLA.0000000000003567.
62. Dana AN, Bauman WA. Bacteriology of pressure ulcers in individuals with spinal cord injury: What we know and what we should know. *J Spinal Cord Med.* 2015;38:147–160. doi:10.1179/2045772314Y.0000000234.
63. Westby MJ, Dumville JC, Soares MO, et al. Dressings and topical agents for treating pressure ulcers. *Cochrane Database Syst Rev.* 2017;6:CD011947. doi:10.1002/14651858.CD011947.pub2.
64. Goldstein EJC, Abrahamian FM. Diseases transmitted by cats. *Microbiol Spectrum.* 2015;3:IOL5–0013. doi:10.1128/microbiolspec.IOL5-0013-2015.
65. Jacob J, Lorber B. Diseases transmitted by man's best friend: The dog. *Microbiol Spectrum.* 2015;3(4):IOL5-002-2015. doi:10.1128/microbiolspec.IOL5-0002-2015.
66. Centers for Disease Control and Prevention. Leading causes of nonfatal injury reports, 2000–2019. Available at https://webappa.cdc.gov/sasweb/ncipc/nfilead.html. Last accessed, September 28, 2021.
67. Greene SE, Fritz SA. Infectious complications of bite injuries. *Inf Dis Clin N Am.* 2021;35:219–236. doi:10.1016/j.idc.2020.10.005.
68. Murphy J, Qaisi M. Management of human and animal bites. *Oral Maxillofacial Surg Clin N Am.* 2021;33:373–380. doi:10.1016/j.coms.2021.04.006.
69. Savu AN, Schoenbrunner AR, Politi R, et al. Practical review of the management of animal bites. *Plast Reconstr Surg Glob Open.* 2021;9:e3778. doi:10.1097/GOX.0000000000003778.
70. Goldstein EJC, Abrahamian FM. Bites. In: Bennett JE, Dolin R, Blaser MJ, eds. *Mandell, Douglas, and Bennett's Principles and Practice of Infectious Diseases.* 9th ed. Philadelphia, PA: Elsevier, Inc.; 2020:3765–3770.e2.
71. Kennedy SA, Stoll LE, Lauder AS. Human and other mammalian bite injuries of the hand: Evaluation and management. *J Am Acad Ortho Surg.* 2015;23:47–57. doi:10.5435/JAAOS-23-01-47.
72. Rupprecht CE, Briggs D, Brown CM, et al. Use of a reduced (4-dose) vaccine schedule for postexposure prophylaxis to prevent human rabies: Recommendations of the Advisory Committee on Immunization Practices. *MMWR Recomm Rep.* 2010;59(RR02):1–9.
73. Centers for Disease Control and Prevention, U.S. Department of Health and Human Services. Updated guidelines for antiretroviral postexposure prophylaxis after sexual, injection-drug use, or other nonoccupational exposure to HIV—United States, 2016; Update 2018. Available at https://stacks.cdc.gov/view/cdc/38856. Last accessed, September 28, 2021.
74. Havers FP, Moro PL, Hunter P, et al. Use of Tetanus Toxoid, Reduced Diphtheria Toxoid, and Acellular Pertussis Vaccines: Updated Recommendations of the Advisory Committee on Immunization Practices—United States, 2019. *MMWR Morb Mortal Wkly Rep.* 2020;69:77–83. doi:http://dx.doi.org/10.15585/mmwr.mm6903a5.
75. Kroger AT, Pickering LK, Mawle A, et al. Immunization. In: Bennett JE, Dolin R, Blaser MJ, eds. *Mandell, Douglas, and Bennett's Principles and Practice of Infectious Diseases.* 9th ed. Philadelphia, PA: Elsevier, Inc.; 2020:3771–3812.e5.
76. Fooks AR, Cliquet F, Finke S, et al. Rabies. *Nat Rev Dis Primers.* 2017(Nov 30);3:17091. doi:10.1038/nrdp.2017.91.
77. Rabies vaccines: WHO position paper—April 2018. World Health Organization Weekly Epidemiological Record 2018;16(20 April):201-219. Available at https://www.who.int/publications/i/item/who-wer9316. Last accessed, September 28, 2021.

Bacteremia and Infective Endocarditis

134

Daniel B. Chastain

KEY CONCEPTS

1. Bacteremia, defined as detection of bacteria in the bloodstream, is most often caused by a focal (primary) source of infection and may be complicated by the development of secondary (metastatic) foci, including infective endocarditis.
2. Infective endocarditis usually occurs secondary to a bloodstream infection in adult patients with specific risk factors (eg, injection drug use, heart failure, valvular disease, and healthcare exposure) and those with implanted cardiac material (eg, prosthetic heart valves).
3. A wide variety of pathogens may cause bacteremia, which is dependent on the patient population, primary source of infection, and geographic region.
4. Three groups of organisms cause most cases of infective endocarditis: staphylococci, streptococci, and enterococci.
5. The clinical presentation of bacteremia and infective endocarditis is highly variable and non-specific, but ranges from asymptomatic to hemodynamic instability and organ dysfunction.
6. Diagnosis of bacteremia and infective endocarditis requires the integration of clinical, laboratory, and diagnostic findings.
7. In patients with suspected or confirmed bacteremia, empirical antibacterial therapy should target the usual pathogens at the site(s) of suspected primary source(s) of infection and then be deescalated based on organism identification and susceptibility testing.
8. Treatment of infective endocarditis involves isolation of the infecting pathogen and determination of antimicrobial susceptibilities, followed by parenteral antimicrobial therapy (in most cases) for an extended period.
9. Source control which may include drainage, debridement, device removal, and definitive reconstructive manners is a critical component in managing patients with bacteremia.
10. Identification and susceptibility testing of the pathogen should guide definitive therapy in patients with bacteremia or infective endocarditis, but in most cases, β-lactams, such as penicillin G (or ceftriaxone), nafcillin (or an alternative antistaphylococcal or penicillinase-resistant penicillin) and ampicillin (with or without gentamicin or ceftriaxone) remain the drugs of choice for streptococcal, staphylococcal, and enterococcal bacteremia and endocarditis, respectively.

BEYOND THE BOOK

A 35-year-old man with a medical history of diabetes mellitus and injection drug use but no known drug allergies was admitted with diabetic ketoacidosis and left foot cellulitis associated with purulent drainage for which he was started on IV vancomycin and ampicillin/sulbactam. His cellulitis progressed over the next 3 days prompting magnetic resonance imaging (MRI) to be performed which revealed an abscess within the skin and subcutaneous fat, along the dorsum of the foot involving the metatarsals and phalanges consistent with osteomyelitis. He was taken to the operating room for debridement. Operating room cultures and blood cultures obtained on each day of hospitalization grew methicillin-susceptible *Staphylococcus aureus* (MSSA). Postoperatively, he has clinically improved and is anxious to be discharged.

Vital signs and laboratory values from today:

Na 142mEq/L, Cl 101mEq/L, BUN 14mg/dL, Glucose 90mg/dL, K 3.7mEq/L, BUN 22mEq/L, SCr 1.0mg/dL, WBC 20.1K/mm^3, Hgb 12.2g/dL, Hct 40%, Plt 307K/mm^3
1.9 m, 89.6 kg
96.9°F (36.1 °C), 95 beats/min, 17 breaths/min, 100% on room air, 110/53 mm Hg

Q1. Do you agree with this antibacterial regimen? If not, what alternative antibacterial regimen (drug/dose/route/duration) and monitoring plan do you recommend? Please explain rationale.

Q2. What was this patient's most likely primary source of infection? Does this patient need any additional diagnostic tests prior to developing a final plan? If so, please identify and explain rationale.

Q3. Does this patient meet criteria for uncomplicated or complicated *S. aureus* bacteremia? Please explain rationale.

Q4. Assuming the next set of blood cultures are sterile, what antibacterial regimen (drug/dose/route/duration) and monitoring plan do you recommend for outpatient treatment? Please explain rationale.

INTRODUCTION

1 Bacteremia reflects the presence of bacteria in the bloodstream, an otherwise sterile environment, which is identified based on the detection of any true-positive blood culture (Chapter e126, "Laboratory Tests to Direct Antimicrobial Pharmacotherapy").[1] Introduction of bacteria into blood is frequently caused by a focal (primary) source of infection, such as respiratory tract infections

(Chapter 129, "Lower Respiratory Tract Infections"), intra-abdominal infections (Chapter 137, "Intra-abdominal Infections"), urinary tract infections (Chapter 139, "Urinary Tract Infections"), as well as bone and joint infections (Chapter 141, "Bone and Joint Infections"), but may also occur due to indwelling devices, medical procedures, or daily activities, such as oral hygiene. In select cases, a primary source cannot be identified. Bacteremia may be further complicated by the development of a systemic inflammatory response syndrome (SIRS) (Chapter 142, "Sepsis and Septic Shock"), or (metastatic) secondary foci, including infective endocarditis in 3% to 8% of cases.

Endocarditis is an inflammation of the endocardium, the membrane lining the chambers of the heart and covering the cusps of the heart valves.[2,3] More commonly, *infective endocarditis* refers to infection of the heart valves by various microorganisms after entry into the bloodstream. Although it typically affects native valves, it may also involve non-valvular areas or implanted material (eg, prosthetic heart valves, cardiac defibrillators, pacemakers, and vascular catheters). Bacteria primarily cause infective endocarditis, but fungi and a variety of other microorganisms can lead to the disease.[2,4] In most cases, infective endocarditis occurs secondary to a bloodstream infection, which originated from a primary source of infection (eg, bacterial endocarditis is secondary to a bacteremia originating from a primary source of infection).

Infective endocarditis is best classified based on the etiologic organism, anatomic site of infection, and pathogenic risk factors.[2,5,6] Infective endocarditis is often referred to as *acute* or *subacute* depending on the pace and severity of the clinical presentation. The acute, fulminating form is associated with high fevers and systemic toxicity. Virulent bacteria, such as *Staphylococcus aureus*, frequently cause this syndrome, and if untreated, death may occur within days to weeks. On the other hand, subacute infective endocarditis is more indolent, caused by less virulent organisms, such as viridans group streptococci, and usually occurs in patients with preexisting valvular heart disease. Infection may also occur following surgical insertion of a prosthetic heart valve, resulting in prosthetic valve infective endocarditis (PVE), or insertion of a cardiac implantable electronic device, resulting in cardiac device infective endocarditis (CDIE).[7,8]

TABLE 134-1 Risk Factors for Bacteremia

- Advanced age
- Chronic liver disease
- Diabetes mellitus
- End-stage renal disease on hemodialysis
- Functional or anatomic asplenia
- HIV infection
- Immunosuppressive medications
- Indwelling prostheses (eg, vascular catheters, surgically implanted materials, and orthopedic prostheses)
- Intravenous drug use
- Malignancies
- Malnutrition and hypoalbuminemia (less than 3 g/dL [30 g/L])
- Neutropenia
- Peripheral vascular disease
- Receipt of corticosteroids
- Recent procedures (eg, urogenital surgery, prostate biopsy, endoscopic retrograde cholangiopancreatography)
- Solid organ transplant
- Stem cell transplant
- Trauma or loss of skin integrity
- Urinary retention

Data from References 12–14

TABLE 134-2 Risk Factors for Infective Endocarditis

- Presence of a prosthetic valve (highest risk)
- Previous infective endocarditis (highest risk)
- Healthcare-related exposure (high risk)
- Congenital heart disease (CHD)
- Advanced age
- Chronic IV access
- Diabetes mellitus
- Acquired valvular dysfunction (eg, rheumatic heart disease)
- Cardiac implantable device
- Chronic heart failure
- Mitral valve prolapse with regurgitation
- Intravenous drug use
- HIV infection
- Poor dentition and/or oral hygiene

Data from References 5, 6, 8, 20, and 21.

EPIDEMIOLOGY

In the United States, the incidence of bacteremia ranges from 113 to 204 per 100,000 persons and is associated with high rates of morbidity and mortality.[1,9] The epidemiology of bacteremia is difficult to characterize due to differences in study design, definitions used for community- and healthcare-associated bacteremia, as well as the overlap with numerous clinical syndromes.[10] However, patient population, geographic region, and infection prevention practices affect the etiology and rate of bacteremia. For example, in the United States, the annual incidence of *Staphylococcus aureus* bacteremia ranges from 38 to 46 per 100,000 person-years compared to 10 to 30 per 100,000 person-years elsewhere.[11,12]

Risk factors for developing bacteremia are generally non-specific, but some are more specific for individual pathogens or groups of pathogens than others (Table 134-1).[13,14] For example, persons who inject drugs (PWID) have a significantly increased risk for invasive methicillin resistant *S. aureus* (MRSA) bacteremia compared to others. Alternatively, patients who undergo urogenital surgeries are at increased risk for developing gram-negative bacteremia postoperatively.

Though the overall incidence of infective endocarditis has remained stable in the United States, the prevalence of PWID has increased while the prevalence of patients with traditional risk factors has decreased.[15–17] Infective endocarditis is more common in men and primarily affects older patients likely due to an aging population with high rates of valvular disease and valve replacement surgery (increasing rates of healthcare-associated infective endocarditis). Most cases occur in individuals older than 60 years of age, and it is less common in children.[18–20] Native valve infective endocarditis (NVE) occurs in 71% to 78% of cases, whereas PVE and CDIE account for 13% to 17% and 3% to 5% of cases, respectively.[6,16,21] PWID are also at high risk and account for 5% to 13% of cases. Other conditions associated with a higher incidence of infective endocarditis include diabetes mellitus, long-term hemodialysis, and poor dental hygiene.[6,20]

2 Most persons with infective endocarditis have risk factors, such as preexisting cardiac valvular abnormalities. Many types of structural heart disease result in turbulent blood flow that increases the risk for infective endocarditis. A predisposing risk factor, however, may be absent in up to 25% of cases (Table 134-2).[5,6,8,20,21]

Rheumatic heart disease was a prevalent risk factor for infective endocarditis, but the incidence of this disease continues to decline. The risk of infective endocarditis in persons with mitral valve prolapse and regurgitation is small; however, because the condition is prevalent, it is an important contributor to the overall number of infective endocarditis cases.[22] The risk of PVE is highest in the first 3 months after valve replacement and occurs in 1% to 3% of patients during the first postoperative year.[20,23]

ETIOLOGY

3 *Escherichia coli*, *Klebsiella* spp., *Pseudomonas aeruginosa*, *S. aureus*, *Enterococcus* spp., and *Streptococcus pneumoniae* are most often identified in patients with bacteremia from high income countries with the addition of *Salmonella* spp. in developing regions.[10] Historically, the etiology differed by whether the onset is

community- or healthcare-acquired (eg, *S. pneumoniae* and *E. coli* are most often associated with community-acquired cases whereas *P. aeruginosa* is associated with healthcare-exposure) as well as the primary source of infection. However, a significant number of patients in the ambulatory care setting have frequent interaction with the healthcare system due to receipt of immunosuppressive medications, oftentimes necessitating vascular catheters, use of ambulatory surgery centers, and overall increasing age of the population. As a result, distinction between community- and healthcare-acquired has become less clear.[24] Alternatively, primary sources of infection differs, whereby urinary tract infections are more common in community-acquired cases while vascular catheters are more often implicated in patients who develop bacteremia in healthcare settings.[25]

4 Nearly every organism causing human disease may cause infective endocarditis, but three groups of organisms result in a majority of cases: staphylococci, streptococci, and enterococci (Table 134-3).[4-6,26] The incidence of staphylococci, particularly *S. aureus*, continues to increase primarily due to healthcare exposure and intravenous drug use, surpassing viridans group streptococci as the leading cause of infective endocarditis.[5,21,26] Staphylococci (*S. aureus* and coagulase-negative staphylococci) are the most common cause of PVE within the first year after valve surgery. In general, streptococci cause infective endocarditis in patients with community-acquired disease and underlying cardiac abnormalities, such as mitral valve prolapse or rheumatic heart disease. Enterococcal endocarditis tends to follow genitourinary manipulations or obstetric procedures.[23] Although polymicrobial infective endocarditis is uncommon, it is encountered most often in PWID.[5] There are many exceptions to the preceding generalizations; thus, isolation of the causative pathogen and determination of its antimicrobial susceptibilities offer the best chance for successful therapy.

The mitral and aortic valves are affected most commonly in cases involving a single valve. Subacute endocarditis tends to involve the mitral valve, whereas acute disease often involves the aortic valve. Up to 35% of cases involve concomitant infections of both the aortic and the mitral valves. Infection of the tricuspid valve is less common, with most of these cases occurring in PWID. It is rare for the pulmonic valve to be infected.[23,26]

Although outcomes for infective endocarditis have improved with rapid diagnosis, appropriate treatment (eg, antimicrobial therapy, surgery, or both), and prompt recognition of complications should they arise, in-hospital mortality remains approximately 20%, while 6-month mortality is 30%.[19] Factors associated with increased mortality include heart failure, increasing age, endocarditis caused by resistant organisms, such as gram-negative bacteria, or fungi, left-sided endocarditis caused by *S. aureus*, paravalvular complications, healthcare-acquired infection, and PVE.[5,6,26] The presence of heart failure has the greatest negative impact on the short-term prognosis.[5] For left-sided NVE, mortality rates range from 15% to 45%; lower rates (4%-16%) occur with community-acquired disease that is most commonly caused by viridans group streptococci, while higher rates (25%-45%) occur with healthcare-associated disease that is more commonly caused by enterococci and staphylococci. Even higher mortality rates are seen with unusually encountered organisms (eg, mortality rates greater than 80% for fungi).[5,6] The mortality rate for right-sided infective endocarditis in PWID is generally low (eg, less than 10%).[5] For those who relapse after treatment for infective endocarditis, most will do so within the first 2 months after discontinuation of antimicrobials. Relapse rates for viridans group streptococcus are generally low (2%), whereas relapse is more likely in those with enterococcal infection (8%-20%) and PVE (10%-15%).[23] Despite appropriate treatment and recovery, the risk of morbidity and mortality following infective endocarditis persists for years, with a 5-year mortality rate of approximately 45%.[27] Morbidity remains elevated because of a greater likelihood of recurrent infective endocarditis, heart failure, and embolism or, if a valve is replaced, the risk of anticoagulation, valve thrombosis, or additional valve surgery.[28]

PATHOPHYSIOLOGY

The pathophysiology of bacteremia is multifactorial and may result from numerous causes such as daily oral hygiene, medical procedures, injection drug use, or seeding the bloodstream from focal (primary) source of infection, but the risk varies considerably between syndromes (Tables 134-3 and 134-4).[1,29,30] As a result, bacteremia is frequently considered a secondary infection originating from the focal source (eg, respiratory tract, intra-abdominal tract), but approximately 10% of cases are categorized as primary bacteremia in which bacteria are directly introduced into the bloodstream without an obvious primary source (eg, injection drug use, vascular catheter insertion).[31] Identification of the primary source is critical to making therapeutic decisions.

TABLE 134-3 Etiologic Organisms in Infective Endocarditis[a]

Agent	Percentage of Cases
Staphylococci	30-70
S. aureus (coagulase positive)	20-68
Coagulase negative	3-26
Streptococci	9-38
Viridans group streptococci	10-28
Other streptococci	3-14
Enterococci	5-18
Gram-negative aerobic bacilli	1.5-13
Fungi	1-9
Miscellaneous bacteria	less than 5
Polymicrobial infections	1-2
"Culture negative"	5-17

[a]Values encompass community-acquired, healthcare-associated, native valve, and prosthetic valve infective endocarditis.

Data from References 4, 6, 17, and 26.

TABLE 134-4 Probability of Bacteremia in Various Clinical Scenarios

High (greater than 50%)	• Discitis and vertebral osteomyelitis • Epidural abscesses • Acute, non-traumatic native septic arthritis • Meningitis • Septic shock • Catheter-related bloodstream infections • Endovascular infections (eg, infective endocarditis, septic thrombophlebitis, vascular graft infections)
Moderate (21%-50%)	• Severe sepsis • Acute pyelonephritis • Cholangitis • Community acquired pneumonia, severe • Pyogenic liver abscesses • Rigors/chills in a febrile patient • Non-vascular shunt (eg, ventriculoperitoneal shunt) infections
Low to moderate (10%-20%)	• Cellulitis in patients with comorbidities • Ventilator-associated pneumonia
Low (less than 10%)	• Uncomplicated cellulitis • Cystitis • Prostatitis • Community acquired pneumonia, non-severe • Hospital-acquired pneumonia
Very low (less than 5%)	• Fever within 48 hours postoperatively • Isolated fever in general medicine patients

Data from References 1, 29, and 30.

Skin and mucosal membranes of the respiratory and gastrointestinal tract serve as the first barrier to defense against bacterial invasion into the bloodstream.[29] In some cases, the host immune response can eradicate bacteria that enter the bloodstream which results in a transient, benign condition. However, if bacteria are able to overcome the host immune response (patients with turbulent cardiac blood flow, foreign or prosthetic material, or when host defense mechanisms fail due to inherent or acquired immune deficits), bacteria can then disseminate throughout the body via hematogenous spread leading to a systemic infection and inducing an inflammatory response. Both transient and persistent bacteremia can lead to secondary metastatic infections involving the meninges, pericardium, kidneys, vertebrae, joints, as well as the heart valves resulting in infective endocarditis.

The development of infective endocarditis via hematogenous spread, the most common route, requires the sequential occurrence of several factors. These components are complex and not fully elucidated.[32,33]See figure 1 or reference 33 for a visual representation.

1. *The endothelial surface of the heart is damaged.* This injury occurs with turbulent blood flow associated with the valvular lesions previously described.
2. *Platelet and fibrin deposition occurs on the abnormal epithelial surface.* These platelet-fibrin deposits form a "sterile vegetation," which is referred to as *non-bacterial thrombotic endocarditis.*
3. *Bacteremia gives organisms access to the endocardial surface.* Transient bacteremia commonly follows certain dental, GI, urologic, and gynecologic procedures. Staphylococci, viridans group streptococci, and enterococci are most likely to adhere to non-bacterial thrombotic endocarditis, probably because of production of specific adherence factors such as adhesins for staphylococci and dextran by some oral streptococci. Gram-negative bacteria rarely adhere to heart valves and are uncommon causes of infective endocarditis.
4. *After colonization of the endothelial surface, a "vegetation" of fibrin, platelets, and bacteria forms.* As the vegetation matures, a protective cover of fibrin and platelets protects bacteria from host immune response. This allows unimpeded bacterial growth to concentrations as high as 10^9 to 10^{11} organisms per gram of tissue, in addition to biofilm formation.

The pathogenesis of early PVE or CDIE differs from infective endocarditis acquired by the hematogenous route because surgery may directly inoculate prosthetic material with bacteria from the patient's skin or operating room personnel.[26,34] In the case of early PVE, a recently placed non-endothelialized valve is more susceptible to bacterial colonization than are native valves. Bacteria also may colonize the new valve from contaminated bypass pumps, cannulas, and pacemakers or from a nosocomial bacteremia subsequent to an intravascular catheter.[8,23,26] The mechanism of bacterial colonization and pathogenesis in late PVE is similar to NVE.[23]

One or more vegetations, varying in size from a few millimeters to centimeters, may be seen in a patient with infective endocarditis. Bacteria within the vegetation grow slowly and are protected from antimicrobials and host defenses. The adverse effects of infective endocarditis and the resulting lesions can be far-reaching and include the following: local perivalvular damage, embolization of septic fragments with potential hematogenous seeding of remote sites, and formation of antibody complexes.[23,32]

Formation of vegetations may destroy valvular tissue, and continued destruction can lead to acute heart failure in 50% to 60% of cases via perforation of the valve leaflet, rupture of the chordae tendineae or papillary muscle, or, for patients with PVE, valve dehiscence.[35,36] Occasionally, valvular stenosis may occur. Abscesses can develop in the valve ring or in myocardial tissue itself, potentially involving cardiac conduction tissue. Even with resolution of the process, fibrosis of tissue with some residual dysfunction is possible.

Vegetations may be friable, and fragments may be released downstream. These infected particles, termed *septic emboli*, can result in organ abscess or infarction. Septic emboli from right-sided endocarditis commonly lodge in the lungs, causing pulmonary abscesses. Emboli from left-sided vegetations commonly affect organs with high blood flow such as the kidneys, spleen, and brain.[5,32]

Circulating immune complexes consisting of antigen, antibody, and complement may deposit in organs, producing local inflammation, and damage them (eg, glomerulonephritis in the kidneys). Other potential pathologic changes that result from immune-complex deposition or septic emboli include the development of "mycotic" aneurysms (although the aneurysm is usually bacterial in origin, not fungal), cerebral infarction, splenic infarction and abscess, and skin manifestations such as petechiae, Osler's nodes, and Janeway lesions.[23,32]

CLINICAL PRESENTATION

Bacteremia

5 Clinical manifestations of bacteremia vary but may involve fever, chills, rigors, altered hemodynamics, shock, coagulation disorders, cutaneous findings (eg, ulcerations), and a documented or suspected primary source of infection.[1,25] Patients with bacteremia may be normothermic with a normal white blood cell count as neither leukocytosis nor fever (≥ 38°C) alone or in combination predict the presence of bacteremia.[30] However, rigors and shaking chills increased the likelihood of bacteremia. Symptoms may reflect the primary focus of infection and depend on whether other organs or organ systems are involved. Past medical and surgical history may also impact patient complaints upon presentation. In some cases, bacteremia may evoke an inflammatory response resulting in sepsis, but not all cases of bacteremia progress to sepsis.

Infective Endocarditis

5 The clinical presentation of infective endocarditis is highly variable and non-specific. Fever is the most common finding, in more than 90% of patients, and is often accompanied by other vague symptoms (Clinical Presentation).[35,36] Heart murmurs are found in the majority of patients (approximately 85%), most often preexisting, with some documented as new or changing. Infective endocarditis usually begins insidiously and worsens gradually. Patients may present with non-specific findings such as fever, chills, weakness, dyspnea, cough, night sweats, weight loss, or malaise. In contrast, patients with acute disease, such as PWID and those with *S. aureus* infective endocarditis, may appear with classic signs of sepsis.

Splenomegaly is an uncommon finding in acute infective endocarditis, due to improved diagnostics and antimicrobial therapy, but it occurs more frequently in patients with subacute infective endocarditis. Other important clinical signs may include the following peripheral manifestations ("stigmata") of endocarditis[19,26,32]:

1. Osler's nodes: 2 to 15 mm painful, tender, purplish or erythematous subcutaneous papules or nodules on the pads of the fingers and toes due to embolism, immunologic phenomena, or both occurring in less than 5% of cases.
2. Janeway lesions: Hemorrhagic, painless plaques on the palms of the hands or soles of the feet due to embolism occurring in less than 5% of cases.
3. Splinter hemorrhages: Thin, linear hemorrhages found under the nail beds of the fingers or toes.

CLINICAL PRESENTATION Infective Endocarditis

General

- The clinical presentation of infective endocarditis is highly variable and non-specific

Symptoms

- The patient may complain of fever, chills, weakness, dyspnea, cough, night sweats, weight loss, and/or malaise

Signs

- Fever is common, as is a heart murmur (sometimes new or changing). The patient may have congestive heart failure, cardiac conduction abnormalities, cerebral manifestations, embolic phenomenon, splenomegaly, or skin manifestations (eg, Osler's no des, Janeway lesions)

Laboratory Tests

- The patient's white blood cell count may be normal or only slightly elevated
- Non-specific findings include anemia (normochromic, normocytic), thrombocytopenia, an elevated erythrocyte sedimentation rate or C-reactive protein, and altered urinalysis (proteinuria/microscopic hematuria)

Other Diagnostic Tests

- An electrocardiogram, chest radiograph or computed tomography, and echocardiogram are commonly performed. Echocardiography to determine the presence of valvular vegetations plays a key role in the diagnosis of infective endocarditis; it should be performed in all suspected cases

4. Petechiae: 1 to 2 mm in diameter, erythematous, painless, non-blanching, hemorrhagic lesions most often visualized on the anterior trunk, buccal mucosa and palate, and conjunctivae that resolve after a few days.
5. Clubbing of the fingers: Proliferative changes in the soft tissues about the terminal phalanges observed in long-standing endocarditis.
6. Roth's spots: Retinal infarct with central pallor and surrounding hemorrhage.
7. Emboli: Embolic phenomena occur in up to one-third of cases and may result in significant complications. Right-sided endocarditis may result in pulmonary emboli, causing pleuritic pain with hemoptysis. Left-sided endocarditis can result in renal artery emboli causing flank pain with hematuria, splenic artery emboli causing abdominal pain, and cerebral emboli, which may result in hemiplegia or alteration in mental status.

Patients with infective endocarditis typically have laboratory abnormalities; however, none of these changes is specific for the disease. Anemia (normochromic, normocytic), thrombocytopenia, and leukocytosis may be present. The white blood cell count is often normal or only slightly elevated, sometimes with a mild left shift. Acute bacterial endocarditis, however, may present with an elevated white blood cell count, consistent with a fulminant infection. The erythrocyte sedimentation rate (ESR) and C-reactive protein (CRP) may be elevated in approximately 60% of patients. Often the urinalysis shows proteinuria and microscopic hematuria, which may occur in 50% to 65% and 30% to 60% of patients, respectively.[32]

Diagnosis

Bacteremia

6 Bacteremia is diagnosed by detection of organism(s) from blood cultures (Chapter e126). Ideally, at least two sets of blood cultures, where each set consists of one aerobic bottle and one anaerobic bottle is obtained prior to administration of antibacterial therapy to lessen the risk of false-negative results (3 sets are necessary in cases of infective endocarditis).[5,37] Each set of blood cultures should be collected by a trained phlebotomist from separate venipuncture sites that have been disinfected rather than vascular catheters due to a decreased risk of contamination from normal skin flora. Upper extremity vessels are preferred over lower extremity vessels or those affected by dermatologic diseases.[38]

Interpretation of positive blood cultures represents a challenging task to determine the clinical significance of the organism(s) identified, especially in the case of normal skin flora which can cause bacteremia in the right clinical setting (eg, intravascular catheter infections). Single blood culture sets should be avoided due to decreased sensitivity as the cumulative yield of true pathogens increases with the number of blood cultures[39]. In addition, collection of blood cultures after receipt of antibacterial therapy significantly decreases the sensitivity of blood cultures.[37]

When assessing significance of positive blood cultures, the number of positive cultures and the total number of cultures obtained, organism(s) isolated, site(s) of collection, and likelihood of bacteremia must be considered.[38,40] Detection of certain organisms (eg, *S. aureus*, *S. pneumoniae*, Enterobacterales, yeast) should always be considered clinically significant, whereas other organisms may represent clinically significant pathogens or contaminants depending on the clinical status of the patient (Table 134-5).

TABLE 134-5 Interpretation of Positive Blood Cultures

True pathogens	• β-Hemolytic streptococci • *Bacteroides* spp. • Enterobacterales • *Fusobacterium* spp. • *Haemophilus influenzae* • *Listeria monocytogenes* • *Neisseria meningitidis* • *Pseudomonas aeruginosa* • *Staphylococcus aureus* • *Streptococcus pneumoniae* • Yeast
Possible pathogens	• *Clostridium* spp. • *Enterococcus* spp. • Viridans group streptococci
Unlikely pathogens	• *Bacillus* spp. • Coagulase-negative staphylococci[a] • *Corynebacterium* spp. • *Cutibacterium acnes* • *Micrococcus* spp.

[a]Probability of being a true pathogen increases in the setting of a vascular catheter

Data from References 38 and 40

Infective Endocarditis

6 The signs and symptoms of infective endocarditis are not specific, and the diagnosis is often unclear. The identification of infective endocarditis requires the integration of clinical, laboratory, and echocardiographic findings. The Modified Duke Criteria include major and minor variables (Table 134-6).[41,42] Based on the number of major and minor criteria that are fulfilled, patients suspected of infective endocarditis are categorized into three separate groups: definite infective endocarditis, possible infective endocarditis, or rejected infective endocarditis.[42]

TABLE 134-6 Diagnosis of Infective Endocarditis According to the Modified Duke Criteria

Definite IE

Pathological criteria
- Microorganisms demonstrated by culture or histological examination of a vegetation, a vegetation that has embolized, or an intracardiac abscess specimen; or pathological lesions; vegetation or intracardiac abscess confirmed by histological examination showing active endocarditis

Clinical criteria
- Two major criteria, or
- One major criteria and three minor criteria, or
- Five minor criteria

Possible IE

One major criterion and one minor criteria, or
Three minor criteria

Rejected IE

Firm alternative diagnosis explaining evidence of infective endocarditis, or
Resolution of infective endocarditis syndrome with antimicrobial therapy for four or fewer days, or
No pathological evidence of infective endocarditis at surgery or autopsy, with antimicrobial therapy for 4 or fewer days, or does not meet criteria for possible infective endocarditis, as above

Major Criteria

Blood culture positive for infective endocarditis

Typical microorganisms consistent with infective endocarditis from 2 separate blood cultures:
- Viridans streptococci, *S. gallolyticus*, HACEK group, *S. aureus*; or
- Community-acquired enterococci, in the absence of a primary focus; or

Microorganisms consistent with infective endocarditis from persistently positive blood cultures, defined as follows:
- At least two positive blood cultures drawn greater than 12 hours apart; or
- Three or a majority of 4 or more separate blood cultures (with first and last sample drawn at least 1 hr apart)

Single positive blood culture for *Coxiella* burnetii or antiphase I immunoglobulin G antibody titer >1:800

Evidence of endocardial involvement

Echocardiogram positive for infective endocarditis (transesophageal echocardiography recommended for patients with prosth etic valves, rated at least "possible infective endocarditis" by clinical criteria, or complicated infective endocarditis [paravalvul ar abscess]; transthoracic echocardiography as first test for other patients), defined as follows:
- Oscillating intracardiac mass on valve or supporting structures, in the path of regurgitant jets or on implanted material in the absence of an alternative anatomic explanation; or abscess; or
- New partial dehiscence of prosthetic valve

New valvular regurgitation (worsening or changing of preexisting murmur not sufficient)

Minor Criteria

Predisposition, predisposing heart condition, or injection drug use
Fever, temperature >38°C (100.4°F)
Vascular phenomena, major arterial emboli, septic pulmonary infarcts, mycotic aneurysm, intracranial hemorrhage, conjunctival hemorrhages, and Janeway lesions
Immunologic phenomena: glomerulonephritis, Osler's nodes, Roth's spots, and rheumatoid factor
Microbiologic evidence: positive blood culture but does not meet a major criterion as noted above or serologic evidence of active infection with organism consistent with infective endocarditis
Echocardiographic minor criteria eliminated

HACEK, Haemophilus species (*H. parainfluenzae, H. aphrophilus, H. paraphrophilus*), Aggregatibacter species, *Cardiobacterium hominis, Eikenella corrodens*, and *Kingella kingae*.

Data from References 41 and 42.

The hallmark of infective endocarditis is a continuous bacteremia caused by bacteria shedding from the vegetation into the bloodstream; 90% to 95% of patients with infective endocarditis have positive blood cultures.[2,5,23,43] In most cases, three sets of blood cultures, should be collected prior to starting antimicrobial therapy, with the first and last set drawn at least 1 hour apart. This allows expedient initiation of empirical antimicrobial therapy and can help guide early decisions regarding other potential interventions. Most cases of infective endocarditis are caused by easily cultivable pathogens that can be isolated from routine blood cultures within a 5-day incubation period. However, prolonged incubation of blood cultures or specialized testing may need to be performed (see "'culture-negative' infective endocarditis" below). In patients who undergo valve surgery, excised valve tissue should be submitted for microbiologic testing. Additionally, histopathologic evaluation should be performed to identify the presence of microorganisms and characteristics of inflammatory changes. Specialized testing (eg, polymerase chain reaction [PCR]) may also be performed on valve tissue to improve the likelihood of identifying the infectious etiology.

"Culture-negative" infective endocarditis describes a patient in whom a clinical diagnosis of infective endocarditis is likely, but blood cultures do not yield a pathogen. This condition is often the consequence of previous antimicrobial therapy, improperly collected blood cultures, or unusual organisms.[5] When blood cultures from patients suspected of having infective endocarditis do not grow after 48 to 72 hours, cultures should be held for up to a month to detect growth of fastidious organisms.[5] Specialized testing, such as serology or PCR, may be required to identify less common pathogens (eg, *Coxiella burnetii*, *Bartonella* spp., *Brucella* spp.).

An electrocardiogram, chest radiograph or computed tomography, and echocardiogram are performed for patients suspected of endocarditis. The electrocardiogram rarely shows important diagnostic findings but may reveal heart block, suggesting extension of the infection. The chest radiograph or computed tomography may provide more diagnostic information, such as identification of septic pulmonary emboli in a patient with right-sided endocarditis. Septic pulmonary emboli may occur, leading to multiple lung foci.

Echocardiography plays an important role in the diagnosis and management of infective endocarditis and should be performed for all patients suspected of this infection.[5,6] In addition to helping in the diagnosis of infective endocarditis, the echocardiogram allows the clinician to evaluate hemodynamic stability and the need for urgent surgical intervention; it also provides a rough estimate of the likelihood of embolism.[5] Typically, transthoracic echocardiography (TTE) is performed first due to the rapidity (eg, fasting state unnecessary) and accessibility (eg, 24-hour service available in most institutions) followed by transesophageal echocardiography (TEE). TEE is more sensitive for detecting vegetations (90%-100%) as compared with TTE (40%-66%), and TEE maintains good specificity (90%-100%).[2,6,19] However, TTE may be the only evaluation needed for children or adults in whom the clinical suspicion of infective endocarditis is relatively low.[5,43] An initial or follow-up TEE is recommended in high-risk patients such as those with CHD, previous endocarditis, new murmur, heart failure, or other stigmata of endocarditis.[5,28] For those patients with suspected PVE or CDIE, TEE should be considered mandatory. The lack of vegetation on echocardiogram does not exclude infection even if the transesophageal approach is used. In these cases, there is an evolving role for advanced imaging modalities such as three dimensional TEE, 18-F fluorodeoxyglucose (FDG) positron emission tomographic/computed tomographic (PET/CT), and single-photon emission computed tomography.[5,6]

TREATMENT

Desired Outcomes

The desired outcomes for treatment of bacteremias are to:

1. Eradicate the causative organism with optimal therapy while minimizing therapeutic failure and potential for resistance
2. Identify and manage the focal (primary) source of infection as well as any secondary foci (metastatic) of infections
3. Relieve the signs and symptoms associated with the infection including the bacteremia, primary source of infection, and if present, secondary metastatic infections
4. Decrease morbidity and mortality associated with the bacteremia and primary source of infection
5. Provide cost-effective antimicrobial therapy determined by the likely or identified pathogen, drug susceptibilities, hepatic and renal function, drug allergies, and anticipated drug toxicities

The desired outcomes for treatment and prophylaxis of infective endocarditis are to:

1. Relieve the signs and symptoms of the disease
2. Decrease morbidity and mortality associated with the infection
3. Eradicate the causative organism with minimal drug exposure
4. Provide cost-effective antimicrobial therapy determined by the likely or identified pathogen, drug susceptibilities, hepatic and renal function, drug allergies, and anticipated drug toxicities
5. Prevent infective endocarditis from occurring or recurring in high-risk patients with appropriate prophylactic antimicrobials

General Approach to Treatment

Bacteremia

7 Urgent initiation of appropriate antibacterial therapy is necessary in patients with bacteremia as delays are associated with increased morbidity and mortality.[44] Empirical parenteral therapy should be based on the usual pathogens at the site(s) of presumptive primary source(s) of infection. In the case of an unknown primary source of infection or primary bacteremia (those without an obvious source), selection of empirical parenteral antibacterial therapy is more challenging but should provide a broad spectrum of activity while additional diagnostic testing is performed to determine the site(s) of infection. Source control (eg, drainage, debridement) may be required depending on the primary source(s) or secondary metastatic of infections (eg, intra-abdominal infections [Chapter 137], bone and joint infections [Chapter 141]). Additional (double) coverage is unnecessary if the empirical therapy is likely to have activity against the potential pathogens but may prove beneficial if patient-specific risk factors for antimicrobial resistance are present or local resistance rates are high based on antibiogram data (Chapter e126).

Once microbiologic data from blood cultures are available, findings should then be interpreted to differentiate contamination from true bacteremia in conjunction with the patient's clinical history, physical findings, risk factors (Table 134-1), and diagnostic testing. However, if the significance of blood culture findings or antimicrobial selection is uncertain, consultation with an infectious diseases specialist should be performed.[44] Antibacterial therapy should be deescalated to target that specific pathogen based on microbiologic data including Gram's stain results from rapid diagnostic testing and antimicrobial susceptibility testing data. Though no general guideline exists for bacteremia, management often depends on the specific organism(s) identified, as well as primary source(s) or secondary metastatic infections to determine the appropriate non-pharmacological and pharmacological treatments. In most cases, treatment is initiated in the hospital, but can often be completed in the outpatient setting (termed outpatient antimicrobial therapy [OPAT]) once source control has been achieved and the patient has clinically improved. Patients considered for OPAT must be hemodynamically stable, compliant with therapy, have careful medical monitoring, understand the potential complications of the disease, and have immediate access to medical care. Advances in technology allow for the outpatient administration of complex antimicrobial regimens that significantly reduce the cost of therapy. Simple regimens, such as single daily doses of ceftriaxone or continuous infusions of penicillin, may improve patient convenience and potentially compliance. Although bacteremia and infective endocarditis are common in PWID and home healthcare would substantially reduce the cost of treatment, many clinicians are hesitant with outpatient IV therapy because central venous access is required. However, there are no significant differences in rates of vascular access complications between those who do and do not inject drugs.[45] Parenteral antibacterial therapy has been considered the standard of care, but emerging data support the use of oral antibacterial therapy in select patients.[46]

Infective Endocarditis

Empirical antimicrobial therapy should usually be initiated in most patients after presumptive or confirmed diagnosis of infective endocarditis.[5] However, in select patients, who are not acutely ill, empiric antimicrobial therapy can be withheld until the results of blood or tissue cultures or serologic tests are available. Due to the importance of identifying an infectious etiology, antimicrobial therapy should not be started until blood cultures have been obtained. Patient history, including past medical, surgical, social, and family, risk factors, and current and previous antimicrobial therapy should be considered when selecting empirical antimicrobial therapy (Table 134-2). Consultation with an infectious diseases specialist should occur to assist in selecting an optimal empirical therapy.

Specific treatment recommendations from the American Heart Association (AHA) and the European Society of Cardiology (ESC) provide guidance for the management of infective endocarditis.[5] Both provide important recommendations for the combination of early diagnosis, early antimicrobial therapy, and early surgery; but there are some subtle differences. The ESC guidelines recommend that an "endocarditis team," consisting of cardiologists, cardiac surgeons, and specialists in infectious diseases, manage patients with infective endocarditis. The AHA guidelines place more emphasis on a team-based approach when assessing the timing and need for surgical intervention.

The AHA and ESC guidelines use an evidence-based scoring system where recommendations are given a classification as well as level of evidence. Class I recommendations are conditions for which there is evidence, general agreement, or both that a given procedure or treatment is useful and effective. Class II recommendations are conditions for which there is conflicting evidence, a divergence of opinion, or both about the usefulness/efficacy of a procedure or treatment (IIa implies that the weight of evidence/opinion is in favor of usefulness/efficacy, whereas IIb implies that usefulness/efficacy is less well established by evidence/opinion). Class III recommendations are conditions for which there is evidence, general agreement, or both that the procedure/treatment is not useful/effective and in some cases may be harmful. Level of evidence is listed as A (data derived from multiple randomized clinical trials), B (data derived from a single randomized trial or non-randomized studies), and C (consensus opinion of experts).

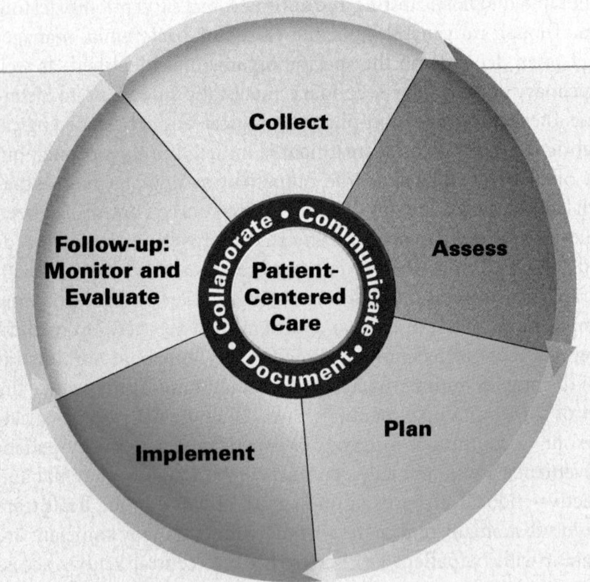

Patient Care Process for Bacteremia and Infective Endocarditis

The image shows the five fundamental steps included in The Pharmacist's Care Process endorsed by the Joint Commission for Pharmacy Practitioners (2014). The tagline of this process reads collaborate, communicate, and document. The five fundamental steps listed here are collect, assess, plan, implement, and follow-up: monitor and evaluate. All these steps are listed in a circular block diagram.

Collect

- Patient characteristics (eg, age, sex, height, weight, pregnancy status, allergies)
- Patient history (eg, past medical, surgical, family)
- Social history (eg, ethanol/IV drug use, recent travel, home residence, exposure to animals) and dietary habits, including intake of unpasteurized dairy products
- Current medication use, including prescription, nonprescription, and other substances, with emphasis on previous inpatient and outpatient antimicrobial use
- Objective data
  - Temperature, blood pressure, respiratory rate, complete blood count (eg, white blood cell count, red blood cell count, hemoglobin, platelets), chemistry panel (eg, serum creatinine), urinalysis
  - Results from blood and/or valve tissue cultures and specialized testing (eg, serology, polymerase chain reaction)
  - Diagnostic testing (eg, electrocardiograph, chest radiograph, echocardiography)

Assess

- Identify risk factors (eg, immunocompromised status, recent dental procedure, central venous catheter, IV drug abuse, dietary habits) (see Tables 134-1 and 134-2)
- Assess signs and symptoms (eg, temperature >100.4°F [38°C], [see Clinical Presentation box], radiographic evidence, pathogen identification, physical examination findings)
- Determine potential infectious etiologies and likely primary (focal) source of infection based on patient history, current and previous antimicrobial use, risk factors, microbiologic data, and diagnostic testing (See Table 134-4)
- Interpret positive blood cultures to determine whether the organism(s) is of clinical significance or contamination (see Table 134-5)
- Determine the need for source control (eg, drainage, debridement, device removal, and definitive reconstructive manners) in patients with bacteremia and surgical intervention (eg, heart failure, persistent bacteremia, persistent vegetation) in patients with infective endocarditis
- Identify patients with underlying high-risk cardiac complications that would be candidates for antimicrobial prophylaxis

Plan*

- Determine the most appropriate empirical antimicrobial therapy, including dose, route, and frequency, based on patient characteristics, history, risk factors, and current and previous antimicrobial therapy
- Deescalate empirical therapy to an evidence-based regimen, including dose, route, frequency, and duration (see Tables 134-8 to 134-13), based on microbiologic and specialized testing results
- Develop monitoring parameters to assess efficacy and safety (eg, toxicities)
- Select evidence-based prophylaxis, including dose, route, and frequency (see Table 134-14)

Implement

- Provide patient education regarding all elements of treatment plan
- Initiate and deescalate antimicrobial therapy as appropriate
- Select an appropriate duration of therapy based on microbiologic and specialized testing results
- Develop an outpatient antimicrobial therapy (OPAT) plan at hospital discharge, including dose, route, frequency, and any necessary laboratory tests

Follow-up: Monitor and Evaluate

- Monitor for resolution of signs and symptoms of bacteremia and infective endocarditis
- Monitor results from blood and/or valve tissue cultures and specialized testing
- Monitor for the presence of antimicrobial related-adverse effects and toxicities
- Provide patient education regarding antimicrobial prophylaxis for infective endocarditis

**Collaborate with patient, caregivers, and other healthcare professionals.*

8 The most important approach in the treatment of infective endocarditis is isolation of the infecting pathogen and determination of antimicrobial susceptibilities, followed by high-dose, antimicrobial therapy, most often administered via parenteral route, for an extended period.[5–7,32] Susceptibility testing is crucial given the increasing rate of antimicrobial resistance to commonly encountered pathogens. Treatment usually is started in the hospital, but for select patients it is often completed in the outpatient setting (OPAT). Large doses of parenteral antimicrobials, as opposed to oral antimicrobials, are recommended to achieve bactericidal concentrations within vegetations. An extended duration of therapy is required, even for susceptible pathogens, because microorganisms are enclosed within valvular vegetations and fibrin deposits. These barriers impair host defenses and protect microbes from phagocytic cells. In addition, high bacterial concentrations within vegetations may result in an inoculum effect that further resists killing (see Chapter e126 for additional discussion). Many bacteria are not actively dividing, further limiting the rate of bacterial death. For most patients, a minimum of 4 to 6 weeks of therapy is required.[5,6]

In the Partial Oral Treatment of Endocarditis (POET) trial, changing to oral antimicrobial therapy after at least 10 days of IV therapy was non-inferior to continuing IV antimicrobial therapy in patients with left-sided native or PVE caused by streptococci, *Enterococcus faecalis*, *S. aureus* (not MRSA), or coagulase-negative staphylococci.[47] All-cause mortality, unplanned cardiac surgery, embolic events, or relapse of bacteremia within 6 months, was similar between groups. Oral regimens included a combination of at least two of the following antimicrobials: moxifloxacin, amoxicillin, clindamycin, rifampicin, dicloxacillin, fusidic acid, and linezolid. Due to strict inclusion and exclusion criteria, frequent outpatient follow-up required, and use of oral antimicrobial agents that are unavailable or infrequently used in the United States, only a select group of patients with left-sided infective endocarditis with functioning GI tracts and a high likelihood for compliance may be candidates for combination oral antimicrobial therapy.

TABLE 134-7 Sources for Common Causes of Bacteremia

Enterobacterales (eg, *E. coli*, *Klebsiella* spp., *Enterobacter* spp., *Serratia* spp., *Citrobacter* spp.)	• Genitourinary tract • Gastrointestinal tract • Respiratory tract (in hospitalized patients) • Translocation from the gastrointestinal or genitourinary tract due to disruption or procedure • Vascular catheter-related (if applicable)
Pseudomonas aeruginosa	• Respiratory tract (in hospitalized patients) • Vascular catheter- or prostheses-related (if applicable) • Genitourinary tract • Wounds
Staphylococcus aureus	• Wounds • Vascular catheter- or prostheses-related (if applicable) • Post-surgical • Injection drug use
Coagulase negative staphylococci	• Vascular catheter- or prostheses-related (if applicable) • Post-surgical
Enterococcus spp.	• Translocation from the gastrointestinal tract due to disruption or procedure • Genitourinary tract (eg, UTI, prostatitis) • Vascular catheter- or prostheses-related (if applicable)
Viridans group streptococci	• Oral mucosa
Anaerobes	• Oral mucosa • Gastrointestinal tract • Genitourinary tract

Data from References 48

Non-pharmacologic Therapy

Bacteremia

1 Management of bacteremia requires identification and resolution of primary source(s) of infection via source control which is defined as a physical intervention aimed at removing or eliminating a focus of invasive infection (Table 134-7) and most often performed by a surgeon.[48] Source control may include one or more of the following: drainage, debridement, device removal, and definitive reconstructive manners. The ability to successfully complete source control depends on whether an anatomic diagnosis can be established and if the patient is stable enough to undergo the procedure(s).

In addition, echocardiography, a component of the Modified Duke Criteria, is frequently performed in patients with bacteremia, especially in those with suspected infective endocarditis. Though less clear for other causes of bacteremia, echocardiography should be performed in all patients with *S. aureus* bacteremia as the prevalence of infective endocarditis is approximately 25%.[49] However, significant variation exists as to which patients should undergo TEE following an unremarkable TTE. While TEE is preferred due to increased sensitivity, TTE may be sufficient in select patients without specific risk factors for infective endocarditis, such as those with nosocomial acquisition without intracardiac devices or dependence on hemodialysis.

Due to the high morbidity and mortality associated with bacteremia, evidence-based practices that include appropriate selection and duration of antimicrobial therapy, in addition to diagnostic testing to identify the primary source(s) or secondary metastatic infection(s), as well as infective endocarditis, are crucial. Unfortunately, these recommendations do not always translate into clinical practice. Consultation with infectious diseases providers to ensure adherence to these evidence-based practices, especially in patients with *S. aureus* or *Enterococcus* spp. bacteremia, has been associated with decreased risk of recurrence, fewer readmissions, and lower mortality rates.[50–53] Since consultation with infectious diseases providers may not be feasible in all healthcare settings, automated pharmacist and/or antimicrobial stewardship program interventions have been developed to increase adherence to evidence-based practices.[54]

Infective Endocarditis

Surgical intervention to remove the infectious foci and repair valves and/or valvular structures is an important adjunct in the management of both NVE and PVE and is now performed in up to 50% of patients.[21] In most surgical cases, valvectomy and valve replacement are performed to remove infected tissue and to restore hemodynamic function. Indications for surgery include heart failure, persistent bacteremia, persistent vegetation, an increase in vegetation size, or recurrent emboli despite prolonged antimicrobial treatment, valve dysfunction, paravalvular extension (eg, abscess), or endocarditis caused by difficult to treat or resistant organisms (eg, fungi or gram-negative bacteria).[5–7] More controversial is the appropriate timing of surgery as well as duration of antimicrobial therapy postoperatively. Additionally, studies evaluating postsurgical outcomes and associated mortality are limited such that a specific risk prediction system has not been established.[55–59] Early surgery (eg, within 48 hr) may be appropriate in patients with severe heart failure and large vegetations, whereas patients with septic shock, advanced age, or neurologic complications of infective endocarditis may have more detrimental outcomes.[55,57,60,61] The multiple factors that need to be considered in evaluating the need for and timing of surgery is why a multidisciplinary management approach (eg, “endocarditis team”) is critical.[5,6,32]

Pharmacologic Therapy

Bacteremia

Gram-Negative Bacilli Detection of gram-negative bacilli from blood cultures should always be considered significant and prompt initiation of empirical parenteral therapy based on the patient's history, comorbidities, previous microbiologic results, as well as whether the infection is community- or healthcare-acquired and local resistance patterns. Ceftriaxone, cefepime, or piperacillin/tazobactam should be added in cases where *P. aeruginosa* is an unlikely pathogen. While an anti-pseudomonal carbapenem (eg, meropenem) should be active, these broad-spectrum antibacterial agents are typically reserved for patients with a history of drug-resistant gram-negative organisms. The risks for *P. aeruginosa* bacteremia include hospital-onset gram-negative bacteremia, as well as healthcare exposures, hemodialysis, residence in a long-term care facility, recent antibacterial or chemotherapy treatment, or immunodeficiency. If *P. aeruginosa* is a concern (eg, hospital-onset gram-negative bacteremia), a single agent consisting of an anti-pseudomonal cephalosporin, anti-pseudomonal β-lactam/β-lactamase inhibitor (eg, piperacillin/tazobactam), or anti-pseudomonal carbapenem (eg, meropenem), is appropriate where less than 10% to 20% of *P. aeruginosa* isolates are resistant to the empiric therapy. Alternatively, double coverage consisting of an anti-pseudomonal cephalosporin (eg, ceftazidime, cefepime), anti-pseudomonal β-lactam/β-lactamase inhibitor (eg, piperacillin/tazobactam), or anti-pseudomonal carbapenem (eg, meropenem) combined with an aminoglycoside or anti-pseudomonal fluoroquinolone should be considered in patients with immunodeficiencies or risk factors for drug-resistant *P. aeruginosa* hospitalized at a facility where more than 10% to 20% of *P. aeruginosa* isolates are resistant to the empiric therapy.[62] Empiric antibacterial therapy against multidrug-resistant organisms (eg, extended spectrum β-lactamase [ESBL]- or carbapenem resistant is warranted in patients with a history of infection(s) caused multidrug-resistant organisms, areas with high local prevalence of multidrug-resistant organisms, and cases of breakthrough bacteremia in patients receiving antibacterial therapy for gram-negative organisms.

Once identification and susceptibility results are available, antibacterial therapy should be deescalated to the most narrow spectrum agent to target the specific pathogen(s) isolated and avoid unnecessary adverse events and inducing resistance.[62] Parenteral therapy has been considered the standard of care for gram-negative bacilli bacteremia. Many oral antimicrobial agents are highly bioavailable and provide therapeutic concentrations within the bloodstream and at the primary source of infection, which may achieve similar outcomes to patients treated exclusively with parenteral antimicrobial therapy, especially in patients with uncomplicated gram-negative bacteremia defined as no evidence of central nervous system, cardiovascular, osteoarticular, or other deep-seated infection.[63]

Similar 30-day mortality was observed in patients with uncomplicated Enterobacterales bacteremia from a urinary, intra-abdominal, vascular catheter, pulmonary, or skin and soft tissue source who switched to an oral antibacterial agent after a median 3 days of parenteral therapy compared to those who continued parenteral therapy for the entire duration.[46] The majority of patients in the oral therapy group were changed to a fluoroquinolone or trimethoprim/sulfamethoxazole, while the remainder received oral β-lactams. Oral β-lactams have not been frequently used for patients with uncomplicated Enterobacterales bacteremia due to limited bioavailability and variable bloodstream concentrations.[63] However, 30-day recurrent bacteremia and 30-day mortality were not significantly different with oral β-lactams compared with oral fluoroquinolones or trimethoprim/sulfamethoxazole among patients with *E. coli*, *Klebsiella* spp., or *Proteus* spp. bacteremia from a urinary source.[64] Patients were transitioned to oral fluoroquinolones or trimethoprim/sulfamethoxazole after a median 5 days of parenteral therapy compared to 4 days for those receiving oral β-lactams, which consisted of amoxicillin/clavulanate, cephalexin, and cefpodoxime proxetil. In most cases, patients with uncomplicated Enterobacterales bacteremia may be safely transitioned to oral antibacterial therapy after approximately 3 days of parenteral therapy. Selection of oral antibacterial therapy with high bioavailability and optimal dosing are necessary to ensure therapeutic concentrations within the bloodstream and at the primary source of infection.[65] However, parenteral therapy should be administered for the entire duration in cases where those criteria cannot be satisfied.

Traditionally, patients with uncomplicated gram-negative bacteremia received 14 days of parenteral antibacterial therapy, but treatment durations can be shortened to 7 days in most patients. A randomized trial comparing 7 to 14 days of antibacterial therapy in patients with uncomplicated gram-negative bacteremia found no significant differences in 14- or 28-day mortality between groups.[66] Additionally, a 9-day duration of antimicrobial therapy and a 16-day duration for uncomplicated *P. aeruginosa* bacteremia resulted in similar rates of recurrent infection or mortality within 30 days of antimicrobial cessation.[30]

Gram Positive

Staphylococcus aureus Empirical therapy in patients with suspected *S. aureus* bacteremia, prior to susceptibility results, should include activity against MRSA with either vancomycin or daptomycin in the majority of cases due to the increased rate of MRSA identified in hospital- and community-acquired bacteremias.[49] If the isolate is later identified as MSSA, therapy should be deescalated to an antistaphylococcal or penicillinase-resistant penicillin (eg, nafcillin, oxacillin) or cephalosporin (eg, cefazolin) as vancomycin is less effective than β-lactams against MSSA.[67] Though cefazolin may be considered in patients who report a hypersensitivity to penicillin not associated with anaphylactic features, treatment should be dictated by allergy history or skin testing. Alternatively, vancomycin or daptomycin (a respiratory source of bacteremia should be ruled out prior to starting daptomycin) should be administered to those unable to tolerate β-lactams. Vancomycin and daptomycin are considered first-line treatment of MRSA bacteremia. Though time to blood culture sterilization may be decreased with combination therapy compared to single-drug therapy, rates of morbidity and mortality remain unchanged.

Management of some patients with MRSA bacteremia may be complicated by persistent bacteremia, defined as inability to sterilize blood cultures after 3 to 7 days of active therapy.[68,69] Persistent *S. aureus* bacteremia is associated with higher rates of secondary metastatic infections and death and may warrant the use of salvage therapy consisting of daptomycin 8 to 10 mg/kg combined with a β-lactam such as ceftaroline.[70]

Establishing a duration of therapy requires differentiation of patients with uncomplicated or low-risk and complicated or high-risk *S. aureus* bacteremia.[49,68] To meet criteria for uncomplicated or low-risk *S. aureus* bacteremia, all of the following criteria must be met: 1) sterile repeat blood cultures 48 to 96 hours after the initial positive culture, 2) defervescence within 72 hr after initiation of active therapy, 3) exclusion of infective endocarditis/secondary metastatic infection, 4) no implanted prostheses (eg, prosthetic valves, cardiac devices, or arthroplasties), 5) not dependent on hemodialysis. Patients with uncomplicated *S. aureus* bacteremia require treatment for 2 weeks, whereas those with complicated *S. aureus* bacteremia should be treated for 4 to 6 weeks from the first negative blood culture or source control. Differentiating uncomplicated *S. aureus* bacteremia from complicated *S. aureus* bacteremia is challenging as almost 33% of patients initially classified as having uncomplicated *S. aureus* bacteremia were eventually diagnosed with complicated *S. aureus* bacteremia.[71] As a result, the majority of patients should receive 4 to 6 weeks of treatment. Parenteral therapy is considered standard of care in patients with uncomplicated and complicated *S. aureus* bacteremia, but successful use of oral therapies has been reported in patients with or uncomplicated *S. aureus* bacteremia.[72]

Coagulase negative Staphylococcus spp.

IV vancomycin should be started empirically in patients with suspected coagulase negative *Staphylococcus* spp. bacteremia due to high rates of methicillin resistance.[73] As with management of *S. aureus* bacteremia, an antistaphylococcal or penicillinase-resistant penicillin (eg, nafcillin, oxacillin) or cephalosporin (eg, cefazolin) should be administered if the isolate is methicillin susceptible, whereas vancomycin or daptomycin should be reserved for those infected with methicillin-resistant strains. Treatment duration varies, depending on catheter removal, from 5 to 7 days in patients with negative follow-up blood cultures, no evidence of secondary metastatic infection, and no intravascular prostheses to 7 to 14 days in patients with at least two positive blood cultures obtained more than 24 hours apart or intravascular prostheses.[74] However, treatment of *S. lugdunensis* bacteremia should be managed in a similar manner to that of *S. aureus* bacteremia due to similarities in virulence.

Streptococcus spp

β-Lactams remain first-line therapy for streptococcal bacteremias. However, combination empirical therapy with IV vancomycin and ceftriaxone should administered in patients with suspected *S. pneumoniae* bacteremia, pending susceptibilities, until central nervous system involvement can be ruled out. For empirical treatment of Group A streptococcal (*S. pyogenes*) bacteremia, IV penicillin should be combined with IV clindamycin to suppress toxin production, as well as decrease the risk of treatment failure and death.[75] IV clindamycin can be discontinued after 48 hr in patients without shock, organ failure, or necrotizing fasciitis. In most cases of streptococcal bacteremia, monotherapy with IV penicillin or ceftriaxone is appropriate once susceptibility results are available, although it is unclear if parenteral therapy is required for the entire duration of treatment.[76] Antibacterial therapy is typically administered for 14 days, but limited data are available evaluating optimal treatment duration.

Enterococcus spp.

Enterococcus spp. are usually of low virulence but inherently resistant to many classes of antibacterial agents.[5] *E. faecalis* is the most common clinical isolate (approximately 97%) of the two species.[74,77] Penicillins and glycopeptides are most active despite their inability to consistently kill these organisms. Ampicillin has greater in vitro activity than penicillin, although there are no clinical data to document differences in efficacy. IV ampicillin should be administered when the isolate is susceptible in non-critically ill patients with no evidence of infective endocarditis. Alternatively, IV vancomycin can be administered in patients who report hypersensitivity to penicillin and are unable to be desensitizied. Ampicillin-resistant, vancomycin-susceptible isolates can be treated with IV vancomycin or daptomycin. The incidence of vancomycin-resistant enterococci (VRE), primarily with *E. faecium*, is increasing. Vancomycin resistance occurs when the bacterium replaces the normal vancomycin target with a peptidoglycan precursor that does not bind vancomycin.[78] In cases of ampicillin-resistant enterococci and VRE, at least 10 mg/kg of daptomycin or linezolid should be administered.[79] Combination therapy, consisting of a β-lactam plus an aminoglycoside (IV ampicillin or IV penicillin plus gentamicin) or β-lactam combination (IV ampicillin plus ceftriaxone) should be used in critically ill patients or those with suspected infective endocarditis.[77] IV ampicillin plus ceftriaxone is preferred if the isolate displays high-level aminoglycoside resistance or to avoid potential aminoglycoside toxicities. Because the aminoglycoside cannot penetrate the bacterial cell in the absence of the penicillin, enterococci is resistant to aminoglycosides by routine susceptibility testing (low-level resistance). However, in the presence of an agent that disrupts the cell wall such as penicillin, the aminoglycoside can gain entry, attach to bacterial ribosomes, and cause rapid cell death. A combination of vancomycin plus gentamicin is also synergistic against enterococci and is an appropriate therapy for the penicillin-allergic patient.[78,80,81] Other aminoglycosides, such as tobramycin and amikacin, cannot be substituted routinely due to resistance. Use of two β-lactam antimicrobials results in saturation of the cell membrane penicillin-binding proteins producing synergistic bactericidal activity.[77] Though the optimal duration of treatment remains undefined, the majority of cases can be treated with 5 to 7 days of therapy.[74]

Anaerobes

In most situations, treatment of anaerobic bacteremia is usually empiric based on historical susceptibility patterns due to difficulties associated with isolating an organism and performing susceptibility tests.[82] Limited data are available describing treatment of anaerobic bacteremia as management depends on resolution of the primary source.

Infective endocarditis

In most cases, vancomycin should be included in the empirical regimen to cover the most common causes of infective endocarditis, staphylococci, streptococci, and enterococci. Ceftriaxone should be added to cover aerobic gram-negative bacilli in patients with acute presentations. In patients with subacute presentations, ampicillin/sulbactam should be included in the empirical regimen to provide coverage against *S. aureus*, viridans group streptococci, enterococci, and HACEK organisms. Once causative bacteria is identified from blood or tissue cultures or serologic tests, antimicrobial therapy should be deescalated to target that specific pathogen.

β-Lactam antimicrobials, such as penicillin G (or ceftriaxone), nafcillin (or oxacillin), and ampicillin, remain the drugs of choice for streptococcal, staphylococcal, and enterococcal infective endocarditis, respectively. Tables 134-8 to 134-11 summarize these recommendations, which are discussed in more detail in the following sections. Tables 134-12 and 134-13 list drug dosing and monitoring recommendations for adult and pediatric patients, respectively. Because these guidelines focus on common causes of infective endocarditis, readers are referred to other references for more in-depth discussion of unusually encountered organisms.[5,6,83,84]

8 For some pathogens, such as enterococci, the use of synergistic antimicrobial combinations (including an aminoglycoside) is essential to obtain a bactericidal effect. Combination antimicrobials may also decrease the emergence of resistant organisms during treatment (eg, PVE caused by coagulase-negative staphylococci) and hasten the pace of clinical and microbiologic response (eg, some streptococcal and staphylococcal infections). Occasionally, combination treatment will result in a shorter treatment course.

Streptococcal Endocarditis

Streptococci are a common cause of infective endocarditis, with most isolates being viridans group streptococci. Viridans group streptococci refers to many different species, such as *Streptococcus sanguinis, Streptococcus oralis, Streptococcus salivarius, Streptococcus mutans*, and *Gemella morbillorum*.[5] These bacteria are common inhabitants of the human mouth and gingiva, and they are especially common causes of NVE.[5,42] During dental surgery, and even when brushing the teeth, these organisms can cause a transient bacteremia. In susceptible individuals, this may result in infective endocarditis. Streptococcal endocarditis is usually subacute, and the response to medical treatment is very good. *Streptococcus gallolyticus* (formerly known as *Streptococcus bovis*) is not a viridans group

TABLE 134-8 Treatment options for native valve endocarditis caused by *Streptococcus* spp. and *Staphylococcus* spp.

Agent[a]	Duration	Strength of Recommendation	Comments
Highly Penicillin-Susceptible (MIC ≤ 0.12 μg/mL [mg/L]) Viridans Group Streptococci and *S. gallolyticus*			
Aqueous crystalline penicillin G sodium[b]	4 weeks	IIaB	2-week regimens are not intended for the following patients: • Most patients >65 years of age • Children • Impairment of the eighth cranial nerve function • Renal function with a creatinine clearance <20 mL/min (<0.33 mL/s) • Known cardiac or extracardiac abscess • Infection with *Abiotrophia, Granulicatella*, or *Gemalla* species
Ceftriaxone	4 weeks	IIaB	
Aqueous crystalline penicillin G sodium[b] plus gentamicin	2 weeks	IIaB	
Ceftriaxone plus gentamicin	2 weeks	IIaB	
Vancomycin	4 weeks	IIaB	Recommended only for patients unable to tolerate penicillin or ceftriaxone
Viridans Group Streptococci and *S. gallolyticus* Relatively Resistant to Penicillin (MIC >0.12 to ≤0.5 μg/mL [mg/L])			
Aqueous crystalline penicillin G sodium[b] plus gentamicin	4 weeks 2 weeks	IIaB	
Ceftriaxone plus gentamicin	4 weeks 2 weeks	IIbC	
Vancomycin	4 weeks	IIaB	Recommended only for patients unable to tolerate penicillin or ceftriaxone
Oxacillin-Susceptible Staphylococci[c]			
Nafcillin or oxacillin	6 weeks	IC	
Cefazolin	6 weeks	IB	For use in patients with non-anaphylactoid-type penicillin allergies; patients with an unclear history of immediate-type hypersensitivity to penicillin should be considered for skin testing
Vancomycin	6 weeks	IB	For use in patients with anaphylactoid-type hypersensitivity to penicillin and/or cephalosporins
Daptomycin	6 weeks	IIaB	For use in patients with immediate-type hypersensitivity reactions to penicillin
Oxacillin-Resistant Staphylococci			
Vancomycin	6 weeks	IC	
Daptomycin	6 weeks	IIbB	

[a]See Tables 134-9 and 134-10 for appropriate dosing, administration, and monitoring information.

[b]May use ampicillin in the event of a penicillin shortage.

[c]Regimens indicate treatment for left-sided endocarditis or complicated right-sided endocarditis; uncomplicated right-sided endocarditis may be treated for shorter durations and is described in the text. Please refer Table 134-7 for treatment of NVE caused by enterococci.

Data from References 5 and 6.

TABLE 134-9 Treatment options for prosthetic valve endocarditis (PVE) caused by *Streptococcus* spp. and *Staphylococcus* spp.

Agent[a]	Duration	Strength of Recommendation	Comments
Highly Penicillin-Susceptible (MIC ≤ 0.12 μg/mL [mg/L]) Viridans Group Streptococci and *S. gallolyticus*			
Aqueous crystalline penicillin G sodium[b] plus gentamicin	6 weeks 2 weeks	IIaB	Combination therapy with gentamicin has not demonstrated superior cure rates compared with monotherapy with a penicillin or cephalosporin and should be avoided in patients with CrCl <30 mL/min (<0.50 mL/s)
Ceftriaxone plus gentamicin	6 weeks 2 weeks	IIaB	
Vancomycin	6 weeks	IIaB	Recommended only for patients unable to tolerate penicillin or ceftriaxone
Relatively Resistant or Fully Resistant (MIC > 0.12 μg/mL [mg/L]) Viridans Group Streptococci and *S. gallolyticus*			
Aqueous crystalline penicillin G sodium[b] plus gentamicin	6 weeks	IIaB	
Ceftriaxone plus gentamicin	6 weeks	IIaB	
Vancomycin[c]	6 weeks	IIaB	Recommended only for patients unable to tolerate penicillin or ceftriaxone
Oxacillin-Susceptible Staphylococci			
Nafcillin or oxacillin plus rifampin plus gentamicin	≥6 weeks ≥6 weeks 2 weeks	IB	Cefazolin may be substituted for nafcillin or oxacillin in patients with non-immediate-type hypersensitivity

(continued)

TABLE 134-9 Treatment options for prosthetic valve endocarditis (PVE) caused by *Streptococcus* spp. and *Staphylococcus* spp.[c] (*Continued*)

Agent[a]	Duration	Strength of Recommendation	Comments
Vancomycin	≥6 weeks	IB	Recommended only for patients with anaphylactoid-type hypersensitivity to penicillin and/or cephalosporins
plus rifampin	≥6 weeks		
plus gentamicin	2 weeks		
Oxacillin-Resistant Staphylococci			
Vancomycin	≥6 weeks	IB	
plus rifampin	≥6 weeks		
plus gentamicin	2 weeks		

[a]See Tables 134-9 and 134-10 for appropriate dosing, administration, and monitoring information.

[b]May use ampicillin in the event of a penicillin shortage.

[c]The ESC 2015 guidelines recommend gentamicin (3 mg/kg/day) be administered with vancomycin for the initial 2 weeks of therapy in patients with relatively resistant strains to penicillin.

PVE, prosthetic valve endocarditis; MIC, minimum inhibitory concentration.

Please refer Table 134-3 for treatment of PVE caused by enterococci.

Data from References 5 and 6.

TABLE 134-10 Treatment Options for Native or Prosthetic Valve Endocarditis Caused by Enterococci

Agent[a]	Duration[b]	Strength of Recommendation	Comments
Ampicillin-, Penicillin-, and Vancomycin-Susceptible Strains			
Ampicillin plus gentamicin	4-6 weeks	IIaB	Native valve plus symptoms present for <3 months: use 4-week regimen
Aqueous crystalline penicillin G sodium plus gentamicin	4-6 weeks	IIaB	Prosthetic valve or native valve plus symptoms present for >3 months: use 6-week regimen
Ampicillin plus ceftriaxone	6 weeks	IIaB	Recommended regimen if creatinine clearance is <50 mL/min (<0.83 mL/s; at baseline or due to therapy with a gentamicin-containing regimen)
Vancomycin plus gentamicin	6 weeks	IIaB	Recommended only for patients unable to tolerate penicillin or ampicillin
Gentamicin-Resistant Strains			
If susceptible, use streptomycin in the place of gentamicin in the regimens listed above if creatinine clearance is >50 mL/min (>0.83 mL/s), cranial nerve VIII function is intact and there is laboratory capability for rapid streptomycin serum concentrations.			
Penicillin-Resistant Strains			
Ampicillin–sulbactam plus gentamicin (β-lactamase–producing strain)	6 weeks	IIbC	
Vancomycin plus gentamicin (intrinsic penicillin resistance[c])	6 weeks	IIbC	May also be used in patients with β-lactamase–producing strains who have known intolerance to ampicillin–sulbactam
***Enterococcus Faecium* Strains Resistant to Penicillin, Aminoglycosides, and Vancomycin[d]**			
Linezolid	>6 weeks	IIbC	Antimicrobial cure rates may be <50%; bacteriologic cure may only be achieved with cardiac valve replacement
Daptomycin	>6 weeks	IIbC	

[a]See Tables 134-9 and 134-10 for appropriate dosing, administration, and monitoring information.

[b]All patients with prosthetic valves should be treated for at least 6 weeks.

[c]Infectious diseases consult highly recommended.

[d]Patients should be managed by a multidisciplinary team that includes specialists in cardiology, cardiovascular surgery, infectious diseases, and clinical pharmacy.

Data from Reference 5.

streptococcus, but it is included in this treatment group because it is penicillin-susceptible and requires the same treatment. *S. gallolyticus* is a non-enterococcal group D streptococci that resides in the GI tract. Infective endocarditis caused by this organism is often associated with a GI pathology, especially colon carcinoma. Endocarditis caused by *Streptococcus pneumoniae, Streptococcus pyogenes*, and group B, C, and G streptococci are uncommon, and their treatment is not well defined.[5,6]

Antibacterial regimens for viridans group streptococci are well studied, and in uncomplicated cases, the cure rate is expected to be more than 95%.[5,6] Viridans group streptococci are penicillin-susceptible, although some are more susceptible than others. Most are highly susceptible to penicillin G and have minimum inhibitory concentrations (MICs) of less than 0.12 μg/mL (mg/L).[45]

Approximately 10% to 20% are moderately susceptible (MIC 0.12-0.5 μg/mL [mg/L]). This different in vitro susceptibility led to recommendations that the MIC be determined for all viridans group streptococci to guide therapy. Some streptococci are deemed tolerant to the killing effects of penicillin, where the minimum bactericidal concentration (MBC) exceeds the MIC by 32 times. A tolerant organism is inhibited but not killed by an antimicrobial normally considered bactericidal.[5] Bactericidal activity is preferred for successful treatment of infective endocarditis; therefore, infections with a tolerant organism may relapse after treatment. Tolerant strains do not respond as readily to

TABLE 134-11 Treatment Options for Culture-Negative Endocarditis and Endocarditis Caused by Gram-Negative Organisms[a]

Agent[b]	Duration[c]	Strength of Recommendation	Comments
HACEK[d] Microorganisms			
Ceftriaxone	4 weeks	IIaB	Other third- or fourth-generation cephalosporins may be used as an alternative
Ampicillin or Ampicillin–sulbactam	4 weeks	IIaB	Should only use if growth is adequate for in vitro susceptibility testing; otherwise, consider organism to be resistant
Ciprofloxacin	4 weeks	IIbC	Recommended for patients with known intolerance to cephalosporins or ampicillin; other fluoroquinolones may be used as an alternative
Culture-Negative Endocarditis, Native Valve[e]			
Vancomycin plus cefepime	4-6 weeks	IIaC	Recommended when onset is acute (days); *S. aureus*, β-hemolytic streptococci, and aerobic gram-negative bacilli should be covered
Vancomycin plus ampicillin–sulbactam	4-6 weeks	IIaC	Recommended when onset is subacute (weeks); *S. aureus*, viridans group streptococci, HACEK, and enterococci should be covered
Culture-Negative Endocarditis, Early (<1 Year) Prosthetic Valve[e]			
Vancomycin plus cefepime plus rifampin plus gentamicin	6 weeks	IIaC	Staphylococci, enterococci, and aerobic gram-negative bacilli should be covered
Culture-Negative Endocarditis, Late (>1 Year) Prosthetic Valve[e]			
Vancomycin plus ceftriaxone	6 weeks	IIaC	Staphylococci, viridans group streptococci, and enterococci should be covered
Suspected *Bartonella*, Culture-Negative			
Ceftriaxone	6 weeks	IIaB	
plus gentamicin	2 weeks		
with or without doxycycline	6 weeks		
Culture-Positive *Bartonella*			
Doxycycline plus gentamicin	6 weeks 2 weeks	IIaB	Rifampin is recommended as an alternative in patient who cannot be given gentamicin

[a]Infectious disease consult highly recommended.

[b]See Tables 134-9 and 134-10 for appropriate dosing, administration, and monitoring.

[c]All patients with prosthetic valves should be treated for 6 weeks.

[d]*Haemophilus* species (*H. parainfluenzae, H. aphrophilus*, and *H. paraphrophilus*), *Aggregatibacter* species, *Cardiobacterium hominis, Eikenella corrodens*, and *Kingella kingae*.

[e]Duration of therapy for culture-negative endocarditis may be variable and should be based on clinical course and recommendations from infectious diseases consult.

Data from References 5 and 6.

β-lactam therapy as non-tolerant ones, this phenomenon is primarily a laboratory finding with little clinical significance. Treatment for tolerant strains is identical to that for non-tolerant organisms, and measurement of the MBC is not recommended.

An assortment of regimens can be used to treat uncomplicated NVE caused by fully susceptible viridans group streptococci (see Table 134-5). Shorter-course antimicrobial regimens are advocated when possible. With susceptible streptococcal endocarditis (MIC ≤0.12 μg/mL [mg/L]), a 2-week regimen of high-dose parenteral penicillin G or ceftriaxone in combination with an aminoglycoside is as effective as 4 weeks of penicillin alone.[5]

Two single-drug regimens consist of high-dose parenteral penicillin G or ceftriaxone for 4 weeks. If short- term, 2-week therapy is desired, the guidelines suggest either high-dose parenteral penicillin G or ceftriaxone in combination with an aminoglycoside.[5] When used in select patients, this combination is as effective as 4 weeks of penicillin alone. Although streptomycin was listed in previous guidelines, gentamicin is the preferred aminoglycoside because serum drug concentrations are obtained easily, clinicians are more familiar with its use, and the few strains of streptococci resistant to the effects of streptomycin–penicillin remain susceptible to gentamicin–penicillin. Other aminoglycosides are not recommended. Whether extended-interval aminoglycoside dosing has a role in infective endocarditis continues to be debated. The combination of ceftriaxone (2 g daily) with gentamicin (3 mg/kg daily) for 2 weeks was compared with ceftriaxone (2 g daily) alone for 4 weeks for penicillin-susceptible streptococci and both regimens were safe and effective with similar clinical cure rates at 3 months following treatment.[85] Data support extended-interval dosing for the treatment of streptococcal infective endocarditis, and as compared with three-times- daily dosing this approach may have greater efficacy.[5]

The rationale for combination therapy against penicillin-susceptible viridans group streptococci is that enhanced activity against these organisms is usually observed in vitro when cell-wall-active agents are combined with aminoglycosides.[86] Combined treatment results in quicker sterilization of vegetations in animal models of endocarditis and probably explains the high response rates observed for patients treated for a total of 2 weeks.[5,85] The combined treatment, however, is not superior to penicillin alone.

The decision of which regimen to use depends on the perceived risk versus benefit. For example, a 2-week course of gentamicin in an elderly patient with renal impairment may be associated with ototoxicity, nephrotoxicity, or both. Furthermore, the 2-week regimen is not recommended for patients with known extracardiac infection. On the other hand, a 4-week course of penicillin alone generally entails greater expense, especially if the patient remains in the hospital. Monotherapy with once-daily ceftriaxone offers ease of administration, facilitates home healthcare treatment, and may be cost-effective.[5,6]

9 When a patient has a history of hypersensitivity with anaphylactic features to penicillin, vancomycin should be chosen for infective endocarditis caused by viridans group streptococci.

TABLE 134-12 Drug Dosing Table for Treatment of Infective Endocarditis[a]

Drug	Brand Name	Recommended Dose	Pediatric (Ped) Dose[b]	Additional Information
Ampicillin	NA	2 g IV every 4 hr	50 mg/kg every 4 hr or 75 mg/kg every 6 hr	24-hr total dose may be administered as a continuous infusion: 12 g IV every 24 hr
Ampicillin–sulbactam	Unasyn®	3 g IV every 6 hr	50 mg/kg every 4 hr or 75 mg/kg every 6 hr	
Aqueous crystalline penicillin G sodium	NA			
• MIC <0.12 μg/mL (mg/L) (native valve only)		3 million units IV every 4 hr or every 6 hr	50,000 units/kg IV every 6 hr	24-hr total dose may be administered as a continuous infusion: 12-18 million units IV every 24 hr (Ped: 200,000 units/kg IV/24 hours)
• All other indications		4 million units IV every 4 hr or 6 million units IV every 6 hr	50,000 units/kg IV every 4 hr or 75,000 units/kg IV every 6 hr	24 million units IV every 24 hr (Ped: 300,000 units/kg IV every 24 hr)
Cefazolin	N/A	2 g IV every 8 hr	33 mg/kg IV every 8 hr	
Cefepime	Maxipime®	2 g IV every 8 hr	50 mg/kg IV every 8 hr	
Ceftriaxone sodium	N/A	2 g IV or IM every 24 hr 2 g IV or IM every 12 hr	100 mg/kg IV or IM every 24 hr	
Ciprofloxacin	Cipro®	400 mg IV every 12 hr or 500 mg po every 12 hr	20-30 mg/kg IV or po every 12 hr	Avoid use if possible in patients <18 years of age
Daptomycin	Cubicin®	≥8 mg/kg IV every 24 hr	6 mg/kg IV every 24 hr	Doses as high as 10-12 mg/kg IV every 24 hr have been used in adults with enterococcus resistant to penicillin, aminoglycosides and vancomycin; doses should be calculated using actual body weight
Doxycycline	Vibramycin®	100 mg IV or po every 12 hr	1-2 mg/kg IV or po every 12 hr	
Gentamicin sulfate	NA	3 mg/kg IV or IM every 24 hr or 1 mg/kg IV or IM every 8 hr[c]	1 mg/kg IV or IM every 8 hr	Once-daily dosing is only recommended for treatment of streptococcal infections.
Linezolid	Zyvox®	600 mg IV or po every 12 hr	10 mg/kg IV every 8 hr	
Nafcillin or oxacillin	NA	2 g IV every 4 hr	50 mg/kg IV every 6 hr	24-hr total dose may be administered as a continuous infusion: 12 g IV every 24 hr'
Rifampin	Rifadin®	300 mg IV or po every 8 hr	5-7 mg/kg IV or po every 8 hr	
Streptomycin	NA	7.5 mg/kg IV or IM every 12 hr		
Vancomycin	Vancocin®	15-20 mg/kg IV every 8 hours or every 12 hr	15 mg/kg IV every 6 hr	A loading dose of 25-30 mg/kg may be administered in adults; doses should be calculated using actual body weight; single doses should not exceed 2 g

[a]All doses assume normal renal function.

[b]Should not exceed adult dosage.

[c]Actual body weight should be used when the full aminoglycoside dose is administered once daily; when administered in three divided doses, use ideal body weight or adjusted body weight when actual body weight is >120% ideal body weight.

When vancomycin is used, the addition of gentamicin is not recommended.[5] The published experience with penicillin is more extensive than with alternative regimens; consequently, a thorough allergy history and skin test, if available, must be obtained before a second-line therapy is administered.

For patients with complicated infections (eg, extracardiac foci) or when the streptococcus has an MIC of 0.12 to less than or equal to 0.5 μg/mL (mg/L), combination therapy with an aminoglycoside for the first 2 weeks and penicillin (higher dose) or ceftriaxone is recommended, followed by penicillin or ceftriaxone alone for an additional 2 weeks (see Table 134-9).[5] Some viridans group streptococci, previously referred to as nutritionally variant streptococci, have biologic characteristics that complicate diagnosis and treatment. For patients infected with nutritionally variant streptococci or when the *Streptococcus* spp. has an MIC of more than 0.5 μg/mL (mg/L), treatment should follow the enterococcal endocarditis treatment guidelines.

For patients with endocarditis of prosthetic valves or other prosthetic material caused by viridans group streptococci and *S. gallolyticus*, choices of treatment are similar to those without prosthetic material (eg, penicillin or ceftriaxone); however, treatment courses are extended to 6 weeks (see Table 134-9). For penicillin-susceptible isolates with an MIC of 0.12 μg/mL (mg/L) or less, high-dose parenteral penicillin G or ceftriaxone should be administered for 6 weeks with or without an aminoglycoside for the first 2 weeks. On the contrary, for isolates with an MIC greater than 0.12 μg/mL (mg/L), high-dose parenteral penicillin G or ceftriaxone combined with an aminoglycoside should be administered for the entire 6 weeks.

Staphylococcal Endocarditis

Endocarditis is most commonly caused by staphylococci, in particular *S. aureus*, mainly because of increased rates of injection drug use, more frequent use of vascular catheters, and increased frequency of valve replacement surgery.[19] Coagulase-negative staphylococci (usually *Staphylococcus epidermidis*) and *S. aureus* are prominent causes of PVE.

TABLE 134-13 Drug Monitoring of Select Agents

Drug	Major Adverse Drug Reactions	Monitoring Parameters	Comments
Daptomycin	Myopathy, rhabdomyolysis	CPK at least weekly; monitor for signs and symptoms of muscle pain	More frequent monitoring may be warranted in patients with renal dysfunction or receiving concomitant therapy with HMG-CoA reductase inhibitors; discontinue if symptomatic and CPK > 5 times ULN or if CPK ≥10 times ULN
Gentamicin	Nephrotoxicity, ototoxicity, neuromuscular blockade	When dosed three times daily: • Target peak serum concentrations of 3-4 μg/mL (mg/L; 6.3-8.4 μmol/L) and trough serum concentrations of <1 μg/mL (mg/L; <2.1 μmol/L)	Avoid concomitant use of other nephrotoxic agents such as diuretics, non-steroidal antiinflammatory drugs, and radiocontrast media. Avoid rapid IV administration
Linezolid	Thrombocytopenia, optic, or peripheral neuropathy	Platelet counts at baseline and weekly, visual changes	More common with prolonged therapy (≥2 weeks for thrombocytopenia, >28 days for visual symptoms); avoid concomitant myelosuppressive agents
Rifampin	Hepatotoxicity	Baseline liver function tests, and then at least every 2-4 weeks during therapy	Avoid concomitant medications that cause hepatotoxicity; may cause red or orange discoloration of bodily secretions (urine, sweat, tears)
Vancomycin	Nephrotoxicity, vancomycin infusion reaction	AUC-guided or trough-guided serum concentration monitoring	Vancomycin infusion reaction may be managed by prolonging the infusion time from 1 to 2 hr; administration of an antihistamine prior to loading or maintenance doses may also be considered

CPK, creatinine phosphokinase; ULN, upper limit of normal; AUC, area under the curve.

Staphylococcal endocarditis is not a homogeneous disease; appropriate management requires consideration of several questions: Is the organism methicillin resistant? Should combination therapy be used? Is the infection on a native or prosthetic valve? Does the patient have a history of injection drug use? Is the infection on the left or right side of the heart? Another consideration in staphylococcal endocarditis is that some organisms may exhibit tolerance to antimicrobials. Similar to streptococci, however, the concern for tolerance among staphylococci should not affect antimicrobial selection.[5]

The recommended therapy for patients with left-sided, native valve infective endocarditis caused by MSSA is 6 weeks of nafcillin or oxacillin; a longer duration of therapy may be needed for complicated infections (eg, presence of perivalvular abscess or septic metastases). From in vitro studies, the combination of an aminoglycoside and penicillinase-resistant penicillin or vancomycin enhances the activity of these drugs for MSSA. In animal models of endocarditis, combinations of penicillin with an aminoglycoside eradicate organisms from vegetations more rapidly than penicillins alone.[5,49] In most human studies, the addition of an aminoglycoside to nafcillin hastens the resolution of fever and bacteremia, but it does not affect survival or relapse rates and can increase nephrotoxicity.[49] As a result, the AHA and ESC guidelines no longer recommend the addition of gentamicin because clinical benefit has not been demonstrated and there is an increased risk of toxicity (see Table 134-8).

9 If a patient has a mild, delayed hypersensitivity to penicillin, cefazolin may be an effective alternative, but should be avoided for patients who report anaphylactic-type reactions to penicillins (see Table 134-8). The potential for a true immediate-type hypersensitivity should be assessed through a careful history or skin test, if available (Chapter e108). Vancomycin is an option for a patient with a positive skin test or a history of hypersensitivity with anaphylactic features to penicillin.

Vancomycin, however, kills *S. aureus* slowly and is inferior to antistaphylococcal or penicillinase-resistant penicillins (eg, nafcillin, oxacillin) or cephalosporins (eg, cefazolin).[5] Alternatively, patients with hypersensitivity to penicillin can be considered for penicillin desensitization or daptomycin, a lipopeptide antimicrobial approved for right-sided infective endocarditis and *S. aureus* bacteremia.[5,6] Unfortunately, left-sided infective endocarditis caused by *S. aureus* continues to have a poor prognosis, with a mortality rate between 25% and 40%.[5] For reasons discussed in the following section, those with infective endocarditis associated with injection drug use have a more favorable response to therapy.

9 During the past decade, staphylococci more commonly have become resistant to antistaphylococcal or penicillinase- resistant penicillins (eg, MRSA). Although vancomycin is still the most commonly selected antimicrobial in these cases (see Table 134-8), susceptibility reports with an MIC greater than 2 μg/mL (mg/L) and reports of vancomycin-resistant *S. aureus* strains are increasing.[68] Success with daptomycin or linezolid has been demonstrated for these patients.[87–89] Use of daptomycin in clinical practice may extend beyond the FDA-approved indication of right-sided NVE, and higher doses of daptomycin (greater than or equal to 8 mg/kg/day) should be used. Additionally, higher doses may be preferred by some experts due to favorable drug tolerability and potential for decreased treatment-emergent resistance, although prospective, randomized clinical trials are lacking.[90–92] To date, linezolid has not been approved by the FDA for use in endocarditis as most available data are based on case reports, and there is concern regarding use of a bacteriostatic agent for this condition.[68,87] The presence or lack of a prosthetic heart valve in patients with a methicillin-resistant organism guides therapy and determines whether vancomycin should be used alone or, if a prosthetic valve is present, combination therapy is necessary (Table 134-6).[5]

Staphylococcus Endocarditis: PWID

Infective endocarditis in PWID is frequently (60%-70%) caused by *S. aureus*, although other organisms may be common in certain geographic locations.[6,19] In this setting, the tricuspid valve is frequently infected, resulting in right-sided infective endocarditis. Most patients have no history of valve abnormalities, are usually otherwise healthy, and have a good response to medical treatment. Nonetheless, surgery may be required.

As previously mentioned, an uncomplicated, left-sided MSSA endocarditis may be treated sufficiently with 6 weeks of monotherapy with an antistaphylococcal or penicillinase-resistant penicillin.[5]

However, the clinical response with right- sided MSSA endocarditis in PWID is usually excellent and may be treated effectively (clinical and microbiologic cure exceeding 85%) with a 2-week course of nafcillin, oxacillin, or daptomycin.[5] Short 2-week courses of vancomycin for endocarditis in PWID are not recommended because of limited bactericidal activity, poor penetration into vegetations, and increased drug clearance in this population resulting in high rates of failure. If vancomycin is selected, the standard 6-week regimen should be used. Selection of a 2-week treatment duration may be appropriate for patients with MSSA right-sided endocarditis if they do not have signs of renal failure, extrapulmonary septic emboli, aortic or mitral valve involvement, or central nervous system infection, otherwise a 6-week regimen is indicated.[5]

Although previous guidelines emphasized combination therapy with an aminoglycoside for the 2-week duration based on earlier studies, the current recommendation for monotherapy is based on data showing that a 2-week regimen of an antistaphylococcal or penicillinase-resistant penicillin alone, without the addition of an aminoglycoside, is as effective as combined therapy in MSSA tricuspid valve endocarditis.[93] Combination treatment (daptomycin plus 4 days of gentamicin) was no different in success rates but had higher rates of renal toxicity compared to daptomycin monotherapy.

Alternative treatment approaches for staphylococcal endocarditis in PWID using oral antibacterial therapies (ciprofloxacin and rifampin) or long-acting lipoglycopeptides (eg, dalbavancin or oritavancin) have demonstrated efficacy.[94–96] However, concerns with resistance (eg, ciprofloxacin), patient adherence, and limited published data prohibit their routine use for the treatment of infective endocarditis in PWID.[5]

Staphylococcal Endocarditis: Prosthetic Valves

PVE accounts for 10% to 30% of all infective endocarditis cases.[6,15] Staphylococci (*S. aureus* and coagulase-negative staphylococci), gram-negative bacilli, and fungi are the main causes of early PVE, while the microbiology of late PVE mirrors that of NVE. An episode of PVE occurring within 2 months of surgery strongly suggests that the cause is staphylococci implanted during the procedure. Yet the risk of staphylococcal endocarditis remains elevated for up to 12 months after valve replacement.[97] Because this type of infective endocarditis is typically a nosocomial infection, methicillin-resistant organisms are common, and vancomycin is the cornerstone of therapy. Combination antimicrobials are recommended because of the high morbidity and mortality associated with PVE and its refractoriness to therapy.[5,68] Although the addition of rifampin to an antistaphylococcal or penicillinase-resistant penicillin or vancomycin does not result in predictable bacterial synergism, rifampin may have unique activity against staphylococcal infection that involves prosthetic material, where its addition results in a higher microbiologic cure rate.[5] Combination therapy also decreases the emergence of resistance to rifampin, which frequently occurs when it is used alone. For methicillin-resistant staphylococci (both MRSA and coagulase-negative staphylococci), vancomycin is recommended with rifampin for 6 weeks or more (Table 134-9). Due to the risk of developing on therapy resistance, rifampin should not be started until blood cultures have sterilized.[98] Gentamicin is added for the first 2 weeks if the organism is aminoglycoside susceptible; traditional dosing should be used as once-daily regimens have not been adequately evaluated in PVE and are not recommended.[5]

For MSSA, an antistaphylococcal or penicillinase-resistant penicillin is administered in place of vancomycin. PVE responds poorly to medical treatment and has a higher mortality compared with NVE. Valve dehiscence and incompetence can result in acute heart failure, and surgery is often a component of treatment.[5,60]

The use of anticoagulation is controversial in PVE. In general, those who require anticoagulation for a prosthetic valve should continue the anticoagulant cautiously during endocarditis therapy, unless a contraindication to therapy exists. It is recommended to hold all anticoagulation for at least 2 weeks for patients with *S. aureus* PVE if a recent CNS embolic event has occurred.[5]

Enterococcal Endocarditis

Enterococci are the third leading cause of infective endocarditis, but they are more resistant to therapy than staphylococci and streptococci.[78,80,99] Enterococci are noteworthy as no single antimicrobial is bactericidal. In addition, monotherapy with penicillin for infective endocarditis caused by enterococci results in relapse rates of 50% to 80%.[5,80,99] Thus, combination therapy consisting of a cell-wall–active agent such as a penicillin or vancomycin and an aminoglycoside (or cephalosporin with ampicillin) are necessary for bactericidal activity. Additionally, resistance to all available drugs is increasing.

Enterococcal endocarditis requires 4 to 6 weeks of IV ampicillin or IV penicillin G plus an aminoglycoside for cure (Table 134-10). IV ampicillin plus ceftriaxone is as effective and better tolerated as IV ampicillin plus gentamicin and should be considered as a treatment option.[5,6] A 6-week course is recommended for patients with symptoms lasting longer than 3 months and those with PVE. Streptomycin and gentamicin have similar efficacy, but gentamicin is preferred due to the inability to obtain streptomycin serum concentrations in most laboratories.[5,80] In the treatment of enterococcal endocarditis, relatively low serum concentrations of aminoglycosides appear adequate for successful therapy, such as a gentamicin peak concentration of approximately 3 to 4 μg/mL (mg/L; 6.3-8.4 μmol/L).[5,80,81] Treatment of enterococcal endocarditis does not have the high success rate seen with infective endocarditis caused by viridans group streptococci, presumably because the organism is more resistant to killing.

Although some data support the use of extended-interval aminoglycoside dosing for other types of endocarditis (eg, streptococci), the data are more vague regarding this strategy in enterococcal endocarditis.[80] Some studies suggest that extended-interval aminoglycoside dosing and short-interval (traditional) dosing are clinically equivalent, discordant studies imply otherwise.[77,81,100] Extended-interval dosing is appropriate in the setting of non-high-level aminoglycoside resistant (MIC <500 μg/mL [mg/L]) *E. faecalis* infective endocarditis and this strategy has been adopted by the new ESC Guidelines.[6,100] This recommendation differs from the current AHA guidelines, which continue to support traditional dosing.[5]

Resistance among enterococci to penicillins and aminoglycosides is increasing.[5] Enterococci that exhibit high-level resistance to streptomycin (MIC >2,000 μg/mL [mg/L]) are not synergistically killed by penicillin and streptomycin because the aminoglycoside either no longer binds to the ribosome or is inactivated by an aminoglycoside-modifying enzyme, streptomycin adenylase.[80] Because enterococci will appear resistant to aminoglycosides on routine susceptibility testing, the only way to distinguish high-level from low-level resistance is by performing special susceptibility tests using 500 to 2,000 μg/mL (mg/L) of the aminoglycoside.[78] High-level streptomycin-resistant enterococci occur with a frequency approaching 60%, and high-level resistance to gentamicin is now found in 10% to 50% of isolates. Although most gentamicin-resistant enterococci are resistant to all aminoglycosides (including amikacin), 30% to 50% remain susceptible to streptomycin.[80] The incidence of high-level aminoglycoside resistance is increasing; however, data on appropriate therapy are sparse, and therapeutic options are few.[77,80,81]

In addition to isolates with high-level aminoglycoside resistance, β-lactamase-producing enterococci (especially *E. faecium*) have been reported. If these organisms are discovered, use of vancomycin or ampicillin-sulbactam in combination with gentamicin should be considered. Treating multidrug-resistant enterococci, such as VRE, is difficult, and data on appropriate therapy are sparse. Guidelines suggest either linezolid or daptomycin (at least 10 mg/kg), although use of either agent has produced conflicting results.[5,6] Surgery and replacement of the infected cardiac valve may be the only cure.

HACEK Group

Fastidious gram-negative bacteria from the group of bacteria including *Haemophilus parainfluenzae*, *Haemophilus aphrophilus*, *Aggregatibacter* species, *Cardiobacterium hominis*, *Eikenella corrodens*, and *Kingella kingae* (HACEK group) account for 0.8% to 6% of infective endocarditis cases.[101] Frequently, these types of infective endocarditis present as subacute illnesses with large vegetations and emboli. These oropharyngeal organisms are slow growing and should be considered as possible causes of "culture-negative" endocarditis. With proper treatment, infectious endocarditis caused by HACEK organisms has a low mortality rate. β-Lactamase–producing organisms are occurring more often; hence, HACEK organisms should be considered resistant to ampicillin alone and should not be used unless in vitro susceptibility testing is adequate. Ceftriaxone, or an alternate third- or fourth-generation cephalosporin, is the preferred treatment in most cases. Ciprofloxacin may be considered as an option if a hypersensitivity to cephalosporins is present (Table 134-11).[5,6] Treatment is usually for 4 weeks, but it should be extended to 6 weeks in PVE caused by one of these organisms.

Less Common Types of Infective Endocarditis

Atypical Microorganisms

Endocarditis caused by organisms, such as *Bartonella* spp., *C. burnetii*, *Brucella* spp., *Candida* spp., and *Aspergillus* spp., *Legionella* spp., and gram-negative bacilli (eg, *Pseudomonas*), is relatively uncommon. Medical therapy for infective endocarditis caused by these organisms is usually unsuccessful.[5,6] Consultation with an infectious diseases expert is warranted when these microorganisms are identified.

In addition to *Pseudomonas* spp., other gram-negative bacilli that have been implicated include *Salmonella* spp., *E. coli*, *Citrobacter* spp., *Klebsiella* spp., *Enterobacter* spp., *Serratia marcescens*, *Proteus* spp., and *Providencia* spp. These infections have a poor prognosis, with mortality rates as high as 60% to 80%. Cardiac surgery in concert with an extended duration of combination antibacterial therapy is recommended (class IIa; level of evidence: B) for most patients with gram-negative bacillary infective endocarditis. Readers are referred to the AHA guidelines for more extensive review of treatment regimens for infective endocarditis due to *Pseudomonas* spp. and unusual gram-negative bacteria.[5]

Fungi cause less than 2% of endocarditis cases; most patients with fungal endocarditis have undergone recent cardiovascular surgery, are PWID, have received prolonged treatment with indwelling central venous catheters, or are immunocompromised.[102] *Candida* spp. and *Aspergillus* spp. are the most commonly involved, and the mortality rate is high (>80%) for the following reasons: (1) large, bulky vegetations that often form, (2) systemic septic embolization that may occur, (3) the tendency of fungi to invade the myocardium, (4) poor penetration of vegetations by antifungals, (5) the low toxic-to-therapeutic ratio of agents such as amphotericin B, and (6) the lack of consistent fungicidal activity of available antifungal agents.[5,6,102] When fungal infective endocarditis is identified, a combined medical–surgical approach is warranted. Because these infections occur infrequently, scant clinical data are available to make solid treatment recommendations. Amphotericin B with or without flucytosine or high dose echinocandin is the recommended pharmacologic approach for *Candida* spp. endocarditis while voriconazole is suggested for those with *Aspergillus* spp. endocarditis.[5,6,84,103] Greater than 6 weeks of therapy is usually recommended, followed by lifelong suppressive therapy with an oral azole in most cases.

C. burnetii (Q fever), an obligate intracellular bacterium, is most likely to be identified via serology or PCR testing since it cannot be isolated from routine blood cultures. It is a common cause of infective endocarditis in certain areas of the world where goat, cattle, and sheep farming are widespread. The most favorable therapy for Q fever is unknown but may include doxycycline with hydroxychloroquine, trimethoprim/sulfamethoxazole, rifampin, or fluoroquinolones for at least 18 months.[104] *Brucella* spp. are facultative intracellular gram-negative bacilli. Humans are infected by this organism after ingesting infected unpasteurized dairy products or undercooked meat, inhaling infectious aerosols, or contacting infected tissues. This type of infective endocarditis is more common in veterinarians and livestock handlers. Cure requires valve replacement and antimicrobial agents including doxycycline with streptomycin, gentamicin, or doxycycline with trimethoprim–sulfamethoxazole or rifampin for an extended period (6 weeks to months).[105]

Culture-Negative Endocarditis

Sterile blood cultures are reported in up to 40% of patients with infective endocarditis if strict diagnostic criteria are used.[2,6,41] This type of infective endocarditis may occur as a result of previous antimicrobial therapy (most common), unidentified subacute right-sided infective endocarditis, slow-growing fastidious organisms, non-bacterial etiologies (eg, fungi), non-infective endocarditis, and improperly collected blood cultures. When blood cultures from patients suspected of infective endocarditis show no growth after 48 to 72 hours, cultures should be held for up to a month and special testing techniques (eg, serological analysis, PCR) pursued to detect fastidious or non-bacterial organisms.[5,43]

The AHA guidelines provide general recommendations for culture-negative infective endocarditis (Table 134-11) and suggest that therapy should be guided based on the individual patient's medical history and epidemiological risks identified. Selection of treatment can be difficult, balancing the need to cover all likely organisms against potential toxic drug effects (eg, aminoglycosides). Antimicrobial selection should involve consultation with an infectious diseases specialist. Irrespective of the chosen treatment, extended antimicrobial therapy is required. The empirical approaches for culture-negative infective endocarditis highlight the need for proper collection and monitoring of blood cultures and an extensive medication history.

EVALUATION OF THERAPEUTIC OUTCOMES

The evaluation of patients treated for bacteremia or infective endocarditis includes assessment of disease signs and symptoms, blood cultures, microbiologic tests, inflammatory markers, serum drug concentrations, and other tests to evaluate organ function.

Signs and Symptoms

Time to clinical improvement in patients with bacteremia largely depends on the infectious etiology, primary source of infection, presence of secondary metastatic foci, and degree of source control. In general, patients with gram-negative bacteremia clinically improve at a faster rate than those with gram-positive bacteremia, especially *S. aureus*.[30]

Fever usually subsides within 1 week of initiating therapy for patients with infective endocarditis.[23] Persistence of fever may indicate ineffective antimicrobial therapy, emboli, right-sided endocarditis, intravascular catheter infections, or drug reactions. For some patients, fever may persist even with appropriate antimicrobial therapy. With defervescence, the patient should begin to feel better, and other symptoms, such as lethargy or weakness, should subside. Echocardiography, typically a TTE, should be performed when antimicrobial therapy has been completed to determine new baseline cardiac function (eg, ventricular size and function).[5]

Blood Cultures

After initiating antimicrobial therapy, follow-up blood cultures should be obtained every 24 to 48 hours until sterile in most patients as duration of bacteremia may impact duration of therapy.[30] With *S. aureus* bacteremia, positive follow-up blood cultures are associated with increased mortality.[106] Additionally, positive follow-up blood cultures, indicative of prolonged duration of bacteremia, may suggest that the antimicrobials are inactive against the pathogen, the doses are not producing adequate concentrations at the site of infection, or lack of source control in some patients.[107] In most situations, the duration of therapy should be determined beginning on the first day blood cultures were negative in patients with previously positive blood cultures. Alternatively, the duration of therapy should be counted from the first postoperative day in patients who undergo valve surgery with intraoperative findings of a paravalvular abscess or resultant positive culture from the valve tissue. During the remainder of therapy, frequent blood cultures are not necessary but should be obtained if fever recurs.[4]

However, positive follow-up blood cultures in gram-negative bacteremia are uncommon.[30,108] As a result, follow-up blood cultures may be unnecessary except in patients who remain febrile despite antimicrobial therapy, relapse, or lack source control. In these cases, duration of therapy should begin on the first day of active therapy based on antimicrobial susceptibility testing.

Microbiologic Tests

10 Identification and susceptibility testing should be performed on all organisms isolated from blood cultures to guide definitive therapy in patients with bacteremia or infective endocarditis.[5,49,65] The agent being used should be tested, as well as alternatives that may be required if intolerance, allergy, or resistance occurs. Occasionally, it is useful to determine whether synergy exists for antimicrobial combinations, although synergistic regimens usually can be predicted from the literature.

Inflammatory Markers

Inflammatory markers are commonly used in infectious diseases processes for diagnosing, monitoring of clinical outcomes, and assisting clinicians with evaluating the efficacy of antibacterial therapy. Only one inflammatory marker, rheumatoid factor (RF), is part of the Modified Duke Criteria for diagnosis. Other inflammatory markers, such as ESR, CRP, and procalcitonin (PCT), have all been investigated for evaluating the outcomes of patients with bacteremia and infective endocarditis.[109,110] While these markers may be beneficial in assessing clinical outcomes, further evidence is needed to establish routine use for infective endocarditis.

Serum Drug Concentrations

Of the agents used for bacteremia and infective endocarditis, therapeutic drug monitoring is routinely available for aminoglycosides (except streptomycin) and vancomycin. Few data, however, support attaining any specific serum concentrations for patients with infective endocarditis. In general, serum concentrations of the antibacterial should exceed the MIC of the organisms.

When aminoglycosides are administered for infective endocarditis caused by gram-positive cocci with a traditional three-times-daily regimen, peak serum concentrations are recommended to be on the low side of the traditional ranges (3-4 μg/mL [mg/L; 6.3-8.4 μmol/L] for gentamicin). If extended-interval dosing is used, which is only recommended in streptococcal infective endocarditis, the most appropriate method of monitoring has not been determined. When vancomycin is administered, the primary goal is to ensure adequate concentrations, based on area under the curve (AUC)-guided or trough-guided serum concentration monitoring.

PREVENTION

Antimicrobial prophylaxis is used as an attempt to prevent infective endocarditis for patients who are at the highest risk.[5-7] (Table 134-14) The use of antimicrobials for this purpose requires consideration of (1) cardiac conditions associated with endocarditis, (2) procedures causing bacteremia, (3) organisms likely to cause endocarditis, and (4) pharmacokinetics, spectrum, cost, adverse effects, and ease of administration of available antimicrobial agents. The objective of prophylaxis is to diminish the likelihood of infective endocarditis in high-risk individuals from procedures that result in bacteremia. Although there are no prospective, controlled human trials demonstrating that prophylaxis in high-risk individuals protects against the development of endocarditis during bacteremia-inducing procedures, animal studies suggest possible benefit.[7] Furthermore, many causes of infective endocarditis appear not to be secondary to an invasive procedure. Bacteremia as a consequence of daily activities may be the major culprit, and the value of antimicrobial prophylaxis before bacteremia-causing procedures has been questioned.

TABLE 134-14 Prophylaxis of Infective Endocarditis

Highest Risk Cardiac Conditions	Presence of a prosthetic heart valve Prosthetic material used for cardiac valve repair Prior diagnosis of infective endocarditis Cardiac transplantation with subsequent valvulopathy Congenital heart disease (CHD)[a]	
Types of procedures	Dental procedures that require perforation of the oral mucosa or manipulation of the periapical region of the teeth of gingival tissue Invasive respiratory procedures involving an incision or biopsy Invasive procedures involving infected skin, skin structures, or musculoskeletal tissue	
Antimicrobial Options	**Adult Doses[b]**	**Pediatric Doses[b] (mg/kg)**
Oral amoxicillin	2 g	50
IM or IV ampicillin[c]	2 g	50
IM or IV cefazolin or ceftriaxone[c–e]	1 g	50
Oral cephalexin[d–f]	2 g	50
Oral doxycycline[e]	100 mg	<45 kg, 4.4 mg/kg or >45 kg, 100 mg
Oral azithromycin or clarithromycin[e]	500 mg	15
IV vancomycin[b,c,e]	15 to 20 mg/kg (not to exceed 2 g per dose)	15 (maximum dose of 1 g)

[a]Includes only the following: unrepaired cyanotic CHD, prophylaxis within the first 6 months of implanting prosthetic material to repair a congenital heart defect, and repaired CHD with residual defects at or adjacent to prosthetic material.

[b]All one-time doses administered 30-60 minutes prior to initiation of the procedure except for IV vancomycin which should be administered 120 minutes prior to the procedure.

[c]For patients unable to tolerate oral medication.

[d]Should be avoided in patients with immediate-type hypersensitivity reaction to penicillin or ampicillin (eg, anaphylaxis, urticaria, or angioedema).

[e]Option for patients with non-immediate hypersensitivity reaction to penicillin or ampicillin.

[f]May substitute with an alternative first- or second-generation cephalosporin at an equivalent dose.

Data from References 7 and 111.

The effectiveness or ineffectiveness of antimicrobial prophylaxis has not been proven, and the common practice of using antimicrobial therapy in this setting remains controversial. The mechanism of a beneficial effect in humans is unclear, but antimicrobials may decrease the number of bacteria at the surgical site, kill bacteria after they are introduced into the blood, and prevent adhesion of bacteria to the valve.

Regardless of the controversy about whether prophylactic antimicrobials should be used, infective endocarditis prophylaxis is recommended in select situations in those with underlying high-risk cardiac conditions. The AHA released updated guidelines that better define who should and should not receive infective endocarditis prophylaxis.[7]

Key points are that (1) only a small number of cases of infective endocarditis might be prevented with antimicrobial prophylaxis for dental procedures, even if 100% effective; (2) infective endocarditis prophylaxis should be recommended only for patients with underlying cardiac conditions associated with the highest risk, which includes presence of a prosthetic heart valve, prosthetic material used for cardiac valve repair, prior diagnosis of infective endocarditis, cardiac transplantation with subsequent valvulopathy, CHD, for dental procedures involving manipulation of gingival tissue or the periapical region of teeth or perforation of the oral mucosa, invasive respiratory procedures involving an incision or biopsy, or invasive procedures involving infected skin, skin structures, or musculoskeletal tissue; (3) prophylaxis is not recommended based solely on an increased lifetime risk of acquisition of infective endocarditis; and (4) administration of antimicrobials solely to prevent endocarditis is not recommended for patients who undergo a gastrointestinal tract or genitourinary procedure.

To determine whether a patient should receive prophylactic antimicrobials, one needs to assess the patient's risk and whether he or she is undergoing a procedure resulting in bacteremia. When antimicrobial prophylaxis is appropriate, a single 2-g dose of amoxicillin is recommended for adult patients at risk, given 30 to 60 minutes before undergoing procedures associated with bacteremia. Because the duration of antimicrobial prophylaxis appears to be relatively short, guidelines do not advocate a second oral dose of amoxicillin, which was recommended previously. Alternative prophylaxis regimens for patients with hypersensitivity to penicillins or those unable to take oral medications are also provided. Clindamycin is no longer recommended for prophylaxis for dental procedures due to greater risk of adverse reactions compared to other prophylactic antimicrobials. A summary of guideline recommendations is available in Table 134-11. Refer the full AHA guideline for more detailed information.[7]

ABBREVIATIONS

AHA	American Heart Association
ANC	absolute neutrophil count
CDIE	cardiac device infective endocarditis
CHD	congenital heart disease
CPK	creatinine kinase
CRP	c-reactive protein
ESBL	extended spectrum β-lactamase
ESC	European Society of Cardiology
ESR	erythrocyte sedimentation rate
HACEK	the group of bacteria including *Haemophilus parai nfluenzae, Haemophilus aphrophilus, Aggregatibacter* species, *Cardiobacterium hominis, Eikenella corrodens*, and *Kingella kingae*
IE	infective endocarditis
MBC	minimum bactericidal concentration
MIC	minimum inhibitory concentration
MRSA	methicillin-resistant *Staphylococcus aureus*
MSSA	methicillin-susceptible *Staphylococcus aureus*
NVE	native valve endocarditis
OPAT	outpatient antimicrobial therapy
PCR	polymerase chain reaction
PCT	procalcitonin
PVE	prosthetic valve endocarditis
PWID	persons who inject drugs
RF	rheumatoid factor
SBT	serum bactericidal titer
TEE	transesophageal echocardiography
TTE	transthoracic echocardiography
ULN	upper limit of normal
VRE	vancomyc inresistant enterococcus

REFERENCES

1. Coburn B, Morris AM, Tomlinson G, Detsky AS. Does this adult patient with suspected bacteremia require blood cultures? *JAMA*. Aug 1 2012;308(5):502–511. doi:10.1001/jama.2012.8262.
2. Thuny F, Grisoli D, Cautela J, Riberi A, Raoult D, Habib G. Infective endocarditis: Prevention, diagnosis, and management. *Can J Cardiol*.Sep 2014;30(9):1046–1057. doi: 10.1016/j.cjca.2014.03.042.
3. Sandoe JAT, Watkin RW, Elliott TSJ, Dayer MJ. Infective endocarditis in the adult patient. *Medicine*. 2017;45(11):678–682. 2017/11/01. doi:https://doi.org/10.1016/j.mpmed.2017.08.004.
4. Fernández Guerrero ML, Álvarez B, Manzarbeitia F, Renedo G. Infective endocarditis at autopsy: A review of pathologic manifestations and clinical correlates. *Medicine (Baltimore)*. May 2012;91(3):152–164. doi: 10.1097/MD.0b013e31825631ea.
5. Baddour LM, Wilson WR, Bayer AS, et al. Infective endocarditis in adults: Diagnosis, antimicrobial therapy, and management of complications. *Circulation* 2015;132(15):1435–1486. doi: 10.1161/CIR.0000000000000296.
6. Habib G, Lancellotti P, Antunes MJ, et al. 2015 ESC Guidelines for the management of infective endocarditis: The Task Force for the Management of Infective Endocarditis of the European Society of Cardiology (ESC). Endorsed by: European Association for Cardio-Thoracic Surgery (EACTS), the European Association of Nuclear Medicine (EANM). *Eur Heart J*.Nov 21 2015;36(44):3075–3128. doi: 10.1093/eurheartj/ehv319.
7. Nishimura RA, Otto CM, Bonow RO, et al. 2017 AHA/ACC Focused Update of the 2014 AHA/ACC guideline for the management of patients with valvular heart disease: A report of the American College of Cardiology/American Heart Association Task Force on Clinical Practice Guidelines. *Circulation*. Jun 20 2017;135(25):e1159–e1195. doi: 10.1161/cir.0000000000000503.
8. Baddour LM, Epstein AE, Erickson CC, et al. Update on cardiovascular implantable electronic device infections and their management. *Circulation* 2010;121(3):458–477. doi: 10.1161/CIRCULATIONAHA.109.192665.
9. Kern WV, Rieg S. Burden of bacterial bloodstream infection—A brief update on epidemiology and significance of multidrug-resistant pathogens. *Clin Microbiol Infect* 2020;26(2):151–157. doi: 10.1016/j.cmi.2019.10.031.
10. Laupland KB, Church DL. Population-based epidemiology and microbiology of community-onset bloodstream infections. *Clin Microbiol Rev*. 2014;27(4):647–664. doi:10.1128/CMR.00002-14.
11. El Atrouni WI, Knoll BM, Lahr BD, Eckel-Passow JE, Sia IG, Baddour LM. Temporal trends in the incidence of *Staphylococcus aureus* bacteremia in Olmsted County, Minnesota, 1998 to 2005: A population-based study. *Clin Infect Dis*.Dec 15 2009;49(12):e130–e138. doi: 10.1086/648442.
12. Tong SY, Davis JS, Eichenberger E, Holland TL, Fowler VG Jr. Staphylococcus aureus infections: Epidemiology, pathophysiology, clinical manifestations, and management. *Clin Microbiol Rev*.Jul 2015;28(3):603–661. doi: 10.1128/cmr.00134-14.

13. Graff LR, Franklin KK, Witt L, et al. Antimicrobial therapy of gram-negative bacteremia at two university-affiliated medical centers. *Am J Med.* Feb 15 2002;112(3):204–211. doi:10.1016/s0002-9343(01)01092-0
14. Cervera C, Almela M, Martinez-Martinez JA, Moreno A, Miro JM. Risk factors and management of Gram-positive bacteraemia. *Int J Antimicrob Agents.* 2009;34(Suppl 4):S26–S30. doi:10.1016/S0924-8579(09)70562-X.
15. Pant S, Patel NJ, Deshmukh A, et al. Trends in infective endocarditis incidence, microbiology, and valve replacement in the United States from 2000 to 2011. *J Am Coll Cardiol.* May 19 2015;65(19):2070–2076. doi:10.1016/j.jacc.2015.03.518.
16. Toyoda N, Chikwe J, Itagaki S, Gelijns AC, Adams DH, Egorova NN. Trends in infective endocarditis in California and New York State, 1998-2013. *JAMA.*Apr 25 2017;317(16):1652–1660. doi: 10.1001/jama.2017.4287.
17. Talha KM, Dayer MJ, Thornhill MH, et al. Temporal trends of infective endocarditis in North America from 2000 to 2017 – A systematic review. *Open Forum Infect Dis* 2021;8(11)doi: 10.1093/ofid/ofab479.
18. Elder RW, Baltimore RS. The changing epidemiology of pediatric endocarditis. *Infect Dis Clin North Am.* Sep 2015;29(3):513–524. doi:10.1016/j.idc.2015.05.004.
19. Wang A, Gaca JG, Chu VH. Management considerations in infective endocarditis: A review. *JAMA.* Jul 3 2018;320(1):72–83. doi:10.1001/jama.2018.7596.
20. Chirouze C, Hoen B, Duval X. Infective endocarditis epidemiology and consequences of prophylaxis guidelines modifications: The dialectical evolution. *Curr Infect Dis Rep.* Nov 2014;16(11):440. doi:10.1007/s11908-014-0440-y.
21. Hoen B, Duval X. Infective endocarditis. *N Engl J Med.* Aug 22 2013;369(8):785. doi:10.1056/NEJMc1307282.
22. Katan O, Michelena HI, Avierinos JF, et al. Incidence and predictors of infective endocarditis in mitral valve prolapse: A population-based study. *Mayo Clin Proc.* Mar 2016;91(3):336–342. doi:10.1016/j.mayocp.2015.12.006.
23. Hill EE, Herijgers P, Herregods MC, Peetermans WE. Evolving trends in infective endocarditis. *Clin Microbiol Infect.* Jan 2006;12(1):5–12. doi:10.1111/j.1469-0691.2005.01289.x.
24. Yardena S-I, Boaz F, Ruth O-W, et al. Reappraisal of community-acquired bacteremia: A proposal of a new classification for the spectrum of acquisition of bacteremia. *Clin Infect Dis.* 2002;34(11):1431–1439. doi:10.1086/339809.
25. Rodríguez-Baño J, López-Prieto MD, Portillo MM, et al. Epidemiology and clinical features of community-acquired, healthcare-associated and nosocomial bloodstream infections in tertiary-care and community hospitals. *Clin Microbiol Infect.* 2010;16(9):1408–1413. doi:10.1111/j.1469-0691.2010.03089.x.
26. Benito N, Miró JM, de Lazzari E, et al. Health care-associated native valve endocarditis: Importance of non-nosocomial acquisition. *Ann Intern Med.* May 5 2009;150(9):586–594. doi:10.7326/0003-4819-150-9-200905050-00004.
27. Bin Abdulhak AA, Tleyjeh IM. Indications of surgery in infective endocarditis. *Curr Infect Dis Rep.* Mar 2017;19(3):10. doi:10.1007/s11908-017-0569-6.
28. Thuny F, Grisoli D, Collart F, Habib G, Raoult D. Management of infective endocarditis: challenges and perspectives. *Lancet.* Mar 10 2012;379(9819):965–975. doi:10.1016/s0140-6736(11)60755-1.
29. Christaki E, Giamarellos-Bourboulis EJ. The complex pathogenesis of bacteremia: From antimicrobial clearance mechanisms to the genetic background of the host. *Virulence.* Jan 1 2014;5(1):57–65. doi:10.4161/viru.26514.
30. Fabre V, Sharara SL, Salinas AB, Carroll KC, Desai S, Cosgrove SE. Does this patient need blood cultures? A scoping review of indications for blood cultures in adult nonneutropenic inpatients. *Clin Infect Dis.* Aug 22 2020;71(5):1339–1347. doi:10.1093/cid/ciaa039.
31. Siegman-Igra Y, Fourer B, Orni-Wasserlauf R, et al. Reappraisal of community-acquired bacteremia: A proposal of a new classification for the spectrum of acquisition of bacteremia. *Clin Infect Dis.* Jun 1 2002;34(11):1431–1439. doi:10.1086/339809.
32. Klein M, Wang A. Infective endocarditis. *J Intensive Care Med.* Mar 2016;31(3):151–163. doi:10.1177/0885066614554906.
33. Werdan K, Dietz S, Löffler B, et al. Mechanisms of infective endocarditis: Pathogen-host interaction and risk states. *Nat Rev Cardiol.* Jan 2014;11(1):35–50. doi:10.1038/nrcardio.2013.174.
34. Athan E, Chu VH, Tattevin P, et al. Clinical characteristics and outcome of infective endocarditis involving implantable cardiac devices. *JAMA.* Apr 25 2012;307(16):1727–1735. doi:10.1001/jama.2012.497.
35. Sexton DJ, Spelman D. Current best practices and guidelines. Assessment and management of complications in infective endocarditis. *Infect Dis Clin North Am.* Jun 2002;16(2):507–521, xii. doi:10.1016/s0891-5520(01)00011-3.
36. Habib G, Hoen B, Tornos P, et al. Guidelines on the prevention, diagnosis, and treatment of infective endocarditis (new version 2009): The Task Force on the Prevention, Diagnosis, and Treatment of Infective Endocarditis of the European Society of Cardiology (ESC). Endorsed by the European Society of Clinical Microbiology and Infectious Diseases (ESCMID) and the International Society of Chemotherapy (ISC) for Infection and Cancer. *Eur Heart J.* Oct 2009;30(19):2369–2413. doi:10.1093/eurheartj/ehp285.
37. Cheng MP, Stenstrom R, Paquette K, et al. Blood culture results before and after antimicrobial administration in patients with severe manifestations of sepsis: A diagnostic study. *Ann Intern Med.* Oct 15 2019;171(8):547–554. doi:10.7326/M19-1696.
38. Doern GV, Carroll KC, Diekema DJ, et al. Practical guidance for clinical microbiology laboratories: A comprehensive update on the problem of blood culture contamination and a discussion of methods for addressing the problem. *Clin Microbiol Rev.* Dec 18 2019;33(1). doi:10.1128/CMR.00009-19.
39. Lee A, Mirrett S, Reller LB, Weinstein MP. Detection of bloodstream infections in adults: How many blood cultures are needed? *J Clin Microbiol.* Nov 2007;45(11):3546–3548. doi:10.1128/JCM.01555-07.
40. Pien BC, Sundaram P, Raoof N, et al. The clinical and prognostic importance of positive blood cultures in adults. *Am J Med.* Sep 2010;123(9):819–828. doi:10.1016/j.amjmed.2010.03.021.
41. Durack DT, Lukes AS, Bright DK. New criteria for diagnosis of infective endocarditis: Utilization of specific echocardiographic findings. Duke Endocarditis Service. *Am J Med.* Mar 1994;96(3):200–209. doi:10.1016/0002-9343(94)90143-0.
42. Li JS, Sexton DJ, Mick N, et al. Proposed modifications to the Duke criteria for the diagnosis of infective endocarditis. *Clin Infect Dis.* Apr 2000;30(4):633–638. doi:10.1086/313753.
43. Liesman RM, Pritt BS, Maleszewski JJ, Patel R. Laboratory diagnosis of infective endocarditis. *J Clin Microbiol.* Sep 2017;55(9):2599–2608. doi:10.1128/jcm.00635-17.
44. Cunha BA. Empiric antimicrobial therapy for bacteremia: Get it right from the start or get a call from infectious disease. *Clin Infect Dis.* Oct 15 2004;39(8):1170–1173. doi:10.1086/424525.
45. Price CN, Solomon DA, Johnson JA, Montgomery MW, Martin B, Suzuki J. Feasibility and safety of outpatient parenteral antimicrobial therapy in conjunction with addiction treatment for people who inject drugs. *J Infect Dis.* Sep 2 2020;222(Suppl 5):S494–S498. doi:10.1093/infdis/jiaa025.
46. Tamma PD, Conley AT, Cosgrove SE, et al. Association of 30-day mortality with oral step-down vs continued intravenous therapy in patients hospitalized with enterobacteriaceae bacteremia. *JAMA Intern Med.* Mar 1 2019;179(3):316–323. doi:10.1001/jamainternmed.2018.6226.
47. Iversen K, Ihlemann N, Gill SU, et al. Partial oral versus intravenous antimicrobial treatment of endocarditis. *N Engl J Med.* Jan 31 2019;380(5):415–424. doi:10.1056/NEJMoa1808312.
48. Marshall JC. Principles of source control in the early management of sepsis. *Curr Infect Dis Rep.* Sep 2010;12(5):345–353. doi:10.1007/s11908-010-0126-z.
49. Holland TL, Arnold C, Fowler VG Jr. Clinical management of staphylococcus aureus bacteremia: A review. *JAMA.* 2014;312(13):1330–1341. doi:10.1001/jama.2014.9743.
50. Goto M, Schweizer ML, Vaughan-Sarrazin MS, et al. Association of evidence-based care processes with mortality in *Staphylococcus aureus* bacteremia at Veterans Health Administration Hospitals, 2003-2014. *JAMA Intern Med.* Oct 1 2017;177(10):1489–1497. doi:10.1001/jamainternmed.2017.3958.
51. Bai AD, Showler A, Burry L, et al. Impact of infectious disease consultation on quality of care, mortality, and length of stay in *Staphylococcus aureus* bacteremia: Results from a large multicenter cohort study. *Clin Infect Dis.* May 15 2015;60(10):1451–1461. doi:10.1093/cid/civ120.
52. Lee RA, Vo DT, Zurko JC, Griffin RL, Rodriguez JM, Camins BC. Infectious diseases consultation is associated with decreased mortality in enterococcal bloodstream infections. *Open Forum Infect Dis.* Mar 2020;7(3):ofaa064. doi:10.1093/ofid/ofaa064.
53. Walensky RP, McQuillen DP, Shahbazi S, Goodson JD. Where is the ID in COVID-19? *Ann Intern Med.* Oct 6 2020;173(7):587–589. doi:10.7326/M20-2684.
54. Wenzler E, Wang F, Goff DA, et al. An Automated, pharmacist-driven initiative improves quality of care for *Staphylococcus aureus* bacteremia. *Clin Infect Dis.* Jul 15 2017;65(2):194–200. doi:10.1093/cid/cix315.
55. Gelsomino S, Maessen JG, van der Veen F, et al. Emergency surgery for native mitral valve endocarditis: The impact of septic and cardiogenic

shock. *Ann Thorac Surg.* May 2012;93(5):1469–1476. doi:10.1016/j.athoracsur.2011.11.025.

56. Manne MB, Shrestha NK, Lytle BW, et al. Outcomes after surgical treatment of native and prosthetic valve infective endocarditis. *Ann Thorac Surg.* Feb 2012;93(2):489–493. doi:10.1016/j.athoracsur.2011.10.063.
57. Ramirez-Duque N, Garcia-Cabrera E, Ivanova-Georgieva R, et al. Surgical treatment for infective endocarditis in elderly patients. *J Infect.* Aug 2011;63(2):131–138. doi:10.1016/j.jinf.2011.05.021.
58. Kiefer T, Park L, Tribouilloy C, et al. Association between valvular surgery and mortality among patients with infective endocarditis complicated by heart failure. *JAMA.* Nov 23 2011;306(20):2239–2247. doi:10.1001/jama.2011.1701.
59. De Feo M, Cotrufo M, Carozza A, et al. The need for a specific risk prediction system in native valve infective endocarditis surgery. *Sci World J.* 2012;2012:307571. doi:10.1100/2012/307571.
60. Byrne JG, Rezai K, Sanchez JA, et al. Surgical management of endocarditis: The society of thoracic surgeons clinical practice guideline. *Ann Thorac Surg.* Jun 2011;91(6):2012–2019. doi:10.1016/j.athoracsur.2011.01.106.
61. Kang DH, Kim YJ, Kim SH, et al. Early surgery versus conventional treatment for infective endocarditis. *N Engl J Med.* Jun 28 2012;366(26):2466–2473. doi:10.1056/NEJMoa1112843.
62. Safdar N, Handelsman J, Maki DG. Does combination antimicrobial therapy reduce mortality in gram-negative bacteraemia? A meta-analysis. *Lancet Infect Dis.* Aug 2004;4(8):519–527. doi:10.1016/S1473-3099(04)01108-9.
63. Mogle BT, Beccari MV, Steele JM, Fazili T, Kufel WD. Clinical considerations for oral beta-lactams as step-down therapy for Enterobacteriaceae bloodstream infections. *Expert Opin Pharmacother.* Jun 2019;20(8):903–907. doi:10.1080/14656566.2019.1594774.
64. Sutton JD, Stevens VW, Chang NN, Khader K, Timbrook TT, Spivak ES. Oral beta-lactam antimicrobials vs fluoroquinolones or trimethoprim-sulfamethoxazole for definitive treatment of enterobacterales bacteremia from a urine source. *JAMA Network Open.* Oct 1 2020;3(10):e2020166. doi:10.1001/jamanetworkopen.2020.20166.
65. Al-Hasan MN, Rac H. Transition from intravenous to oral antimicrobial therapy in patients with uncomplicated and complicated bloodstream infections. *Clin Microbiol Infect.* Mar 2020;26(3):299–306. doi:10.1016/j.cmi.2019.05.012.
66. Yahav D, Franceschini E, Koppel F, et al. Seven versus 14 days of antimicrobial therapy for uncomplicated gram-negative bacteremia: A noninferiority randomized controlled trial. *Clin Infect Dis.* Sep 13 2019;69(7):1091–1098. doi:10.1093/cid/ciy1054.
67. Gentry CA, Rodvold KA, Novak RM, Hershow RC, Naderer OJ. Retrospective evaluation of therapies for *Staphylococcus aureus* endocarditis. *Pharmacotherapy.* Sep-Oct 1997;17(5):990–997.
68. Liu C, Bayer A, Cosgrove SE, et al. Clinical practice guidelines by the infectious diseases society of america for the treatment of methicillin-resistant *Staphylococcus aureus* infections in adults and children. *Clin Infect Dis.* Feb 1 2011;52(3):e18–e55. doi:10.1093/cid/ciq146.
69. Minejima E, Mai N, Bui N, et al. Defining the breakpoint duration of *Staphylococcus aureus* bacteremia predictive of poor outcomes. *Clin Infect Dis.* Feb 3 2020;70(4):566–573. doi:10.1093/cid/ciz257.
70. Rose W, Fantl M, Geriak M, Nizet V, Sakoulas G. Current paradigms of combination therapy in methicillin-resistant *Staphylococcus aureus* (MRSA) bacteremia: Does it work, which combination and for which patients? *Clin Infect Dis.* May 16 2021;doi:10.1093/cid/ciab452.
71. Holland TL, Raad I, Boucher HW, et al. Effect of algorithm-based therapy vs usual care on clinical success and serious adverse events in patients with staphylococcal bacteremia: A randomized clinical trial. *JAMA.* Sep 25 2018;320(12):1249–1258. doi:10.1001/jama.2018.13155.
72. Dagher M, Fowler VG Jr, Wright PW, Staub MB. A narrative review of early oral stepdown therapy for the treatment of uncomplicated *Staphylococcus aureus* bacteremia: Yay or nay? *Open Forum Infect Dis.* Jun 2020;7(6):ofaa151. doi:10.1093/ofid/ofaa151.
73. Diekema DJ, Pfaller MA, Schmitz FJ, et al. Survey of infections due to Staphylococcus species: Frequency of occurrence and antimicrobial susceptibility of isolates collected in the United States, Canada, Latin America, Europe, and the Western Pacific region for the SENTRY Antimicrobial Surveillance Program, 1997-1999. *Clin Infect Dis.* May 15 2001;32(Suppl 2):S114–S132. doi:10.1086/320184.
74. Mermel LA, Allon M, Bouza E, et al. Clinical practice guidelines for the diagnosis and management of intravascular catheter-related infection: 2009 Update by the Infectious Diseases Society of America. *Clin Infect Dis.* Jul 1 2009;49(1):1–45. doi:10.1086/599376.
75. Babiker A, Li X, Lai YL, et al. Effectiveness of adjunctive clindamycin in beta-lactam antimicrobial-treated patients with invasive beta-haemolytic streptococcal infections in US hospitals: A retrospective multicentre cohort study. *Lancet Infect Dis.* May 2021;21(5):697–710. doi:10.1016/S1473-3099(20)30523-5.
76. Arensman K, Shields M, Beganovic M, et al. Fluoroquinolone versus beta-lactam oral step-down therapy for uncomplicated streptococcal bloodstream infections. *Antimicrob Agents Chemother.* Oct 20 2020;64(11). doi:10.1128/AAC.01515-20.
77. Beganovic M, Luther MK, Rice LB, Arias CA, Rybak MJ, LaPlante KL. A review of combination antimicrobial therapy for *Enterococcus faecalis* bloodstream infections and infective endocarditis. *Clin Infect Dis.*Jul 2 2018;67(2):303–309. 10.1093/cid/ciy064.
78. O'Driscoll T, Crank CW. Vancomycin-resistant enterococcal infections: Epidemiology, clinical manifestations, and optimal management. *Infect Drug Resist.* 2015;8:217–230. doi: 10.2147/IDR.S54125.
79. Britt NS, Potter EM, Patel N, Steed ME. Comparative effectiveness and safety of standard-, medium-, and high-dose daptomycin strategies for the treatment of vancomycin-resistant enterococcal bacteremia among veterans affairs patients. *Clin Infect Dis.* Mar 1 2017;64(5):605–613. doi:10.1093/cid/ciw815.
80. Pericas JM, Zboromyrska Y, Cervera C, et al. Enterococcal endocarditis revisited. *Future Microbiol.* 2015;10(7):1215–1240. doi:10.2217/fmb.15.46.
81. Arias CA, Contreras GA, Murray BE. Management of multidrug-resistant enterococcal infections. *Clin Microbiol Infect.* Jun 2010;16(6):555–562. doi:10.1111/j.1469-0691.2010.03214.x.
82. Kim J, Lee Y, Park Y, et al. Anaerobic bacteremia: Impact of inappropriate therapy on mortality. *Infect Chemothe.* Jun 2016;48(2):91–98. doi:10.3947/ic.2016.48.2.91.
83. Tattevin P, Revest M, Lefort A, Michelet C, Lortholary O. Fungal endocarditis: Current challenges. *Int J Antimicrob Agents.* Oct 2014;44(4):290–294. doi:10.1016/j.ijantimicag.2014.07.003.
84. Pappas PG, Kauffman CA, Andes DR, et al. Clinical practice guideline for the management of candidiasis: 2016 update by the Infectious Diseases Society of America. *Clin Infect Dis.* Feb 15 2016;62(4):e1–e50. doi:10.1093/cid/civ933.
85. Sexton DJ, Tenenbaum MJ, Wilson WR, et al. Ceftriaxone once daily for four weeks compared with ceftriaxone plus gentamicin once daily for two weeks for treatment of endocarditis due to penicillin-susceptible streptococci. Endocarditis Treatment Consortium Group. *Clin Infect Dis.* Dec 1998;27(6):1470–1474. doi:10.1086/515038.
86. Falagas ME, Matthaiou DK, Bliziotis IA. The role of aminoglycosides in combination with a beta-lactam for the treatment of bacterial endocarditis: A meta-analysis of comparative trials. *J Antimicrob Chemother.* Apr 2006;57(4):639–647. doi:10.1093/jac/dkl044.
87. Falagas ME, Manta KG, Ntziora F, Vardakas KZ. Linezolid for the treatment of patients with endocarditis: A systematic review of the published evidence. *J Antimicrob Chemother.*Aug 2006;58(2):273–280. 10.1093/jac/dkl219.
88. Fowler VG Jr, Boucher HW, Corey GR, et al. Daptomycin versus standard therapy for bacteremia and endocarditis caused by *Staphylococcus aureus. N Engl J Med.* Aug 17 2006;355(7):653–665. doi:10.1056/NEJMoa053783.
89. Levine DP, Lamp KC. Daptomycin in the treatment of patients with infective endocarditis: Experience from a registry. *Am J Med.* Oct 2007;120(10 Suppl 1):S28–S33. doi:10.1016/j.amjmed.2007.07.011.
90. Wu G, Abraham T, Rapp J, Vastey F, Saad N, Balmir E. Daptomycin: Evaluation of a high-dose treatment strategy. *Int J Antimicrob Agents.* Sep 2011;38(3):192–196. doi:10.1016/j.ijantimicag.2011.03.006.
91. Durante-Mangoni E, Casillo R, Bernardo M, et al. High-dose daptomycin for cardiac implantable electronic device-related infective endocarditis. *Clin Infect Dis.* Feb 1 2012;54(3):347–354. doi:10.1093/cid/cir805.
92. Carugati M, Bayer AS, Miro JM, et al. High-dose daptomycin therapy for left-sided infective endocarditis: A prospective study from the international collaboration on endocarditis. *Antimicrob Agents Chemother.* Dec 2013;57(12):6213–6222. doi:10.1128/AAC.01563-13.
93. Yung D, Kottachchi D, Neupane B, Haider S, Loeb M. Antimicrobials for right-sided endocarditis in intravenous drug users: A systematic review. *J Antimicrob Chemother.* Nov 2007;60(5):921–928. doi:10.1093/jac/dkm324.
94. Dworkin RJ, Lee BL, Sande MA, Chambers HF. Treatment of right-sided *Staphylococcus aureus* endocarditis in intravenous drug users with ciprofloxacin and rifampicin. *Lancet.* Nov 4 1989;2(8671):1071–1073. doi:10.1016/s0140-6736(89)91083-0.
95. Heldman AW, Hartert TV, Ray SC, et al. Oral antimicrobial treatment of right-sided staphylococcal endocarditis in injection drug users: Prospective randomized comparison with parenteral therapy. *Am J Med.* Jul 1996;101(1):68–76. doi:10.1016/s0002-9343(96)00070-8.

96. Thomas G, Henao-Martinez AF, Franco-Paredes C, Chastain DB. Treatment of osteoarticular, cardiovascular, intravascular-catheter-related and other complicated infections with dalbavancin and oritavancin: A systematic review. *Int J Antimicrob Agents.* Sep 2020;56(3):106069. doi:10.1016/j.ijantimicag.2020.106069.
97. Casey JR, Kaur R, Friedel VC, Pichichero ME. Acute otitis media otopathogens during 2008 to 2010 in Rochester, New York. *Pediatr Infect Dis J.* Aug 2013;32(8):805–809. doi:10.1097/INF.0b013e31828d9acc.
98. Riedel DJ, Weekes E, Forrest GN. Addition of rifampin to standard therapy for treatment of native valve infective endocarditis caused by *Staphylococcus aureus*. *Antimicrob Agents Chemother.* Jul 2008;52(7):2463–2467. doi:10.1128/AAC.00300-08.
99. Reyes K, Zervos M. Endocarditis caused by resistant enterococcus: An overview. *Curr Infect Dis Rep.* Aug 2013;15(4):320–328. doi:10.1007/s11908-013-0348-y.
100. Miro JM, Pericas JM, del Rio A, Hospital Clinic Endocarditis Study G. A new era for treating *Enterococcus faecalis* endocarditis: Ampicillin plus short-course gentamicin or ampicillin plus ceftriaxone: That is the question!. *Circulation.* Apr 30 2013;127(17):1763–1766. 10.1161/CIRCULATIONAHA.113.002431.
101. Chambers ST, Murdoch D, Morris A, et al. HACEK infective endocarditis: Characteristics and outcomes from a large, multi-national cohort. *PLoS One.* 2013;8(5):e63181. doi:10.1371/journal.pone.0063181.
102. Pierrotti LC, Baddour LM. Fungal endocarditis, 1995-2000. *Chest.* Jul 2002;122(1):302–310. doi:10.1378/chest.122.1.302.
103. Baeten JM, Palanee-Phillips T, Brown ER, et al. Use of a vaginal ring containing dapivirine for HIV-1 prevention in women. *N Engl J Med.* Dec 1 2016;375(22):2121–2132. doi:10.1056/NEJMoa1506110.
104. Kersh GJ. Antimicrobial therapies for Q fever. *Expert Rev Anti Infect Ther.* Nov 2013;11(11):1207–1214. doi:10.1586/14787210.2013.840534
105. Solera J. Update on brucellosis: Therapeutic challenges. *Int J Antimicrob Agents.* Nov 2010;36(Suppl 1):S18–S20. doi:10.1016/j.ijantimicag.2010.06.015.
106. Lopez Dupla M, Martinez JA, Vidal F, et al. Clinical characterization of breakthrough bacteraemia: A survey of 392 episodes. *J Int Med.* Aug 2005;258(2):172–180. doi:10.1111/j.1365-2796.2005.01513.x.
107. Wiggers JB, Xiong W, Daneman N. Sending repeat cultures: Is there a role in the management of bacteremic episodes? (SCRIBE study). *BMC Infect Dis.* Jun 13 2016;16:286. doi:10.1186/s12879-016-1622-z.
108. Clemmons AB, Young HN, Bland CM, et al. Incidence and utility of follow-up blood cultures in cancer patients with gram-negative bacteremia. *Diagn Microbiol Infect Dis.* Oct 2021;101(2):115444. doi:10.1016/j.diagmicrobio.2021.115444.
109. Watkins R. The role for inflammatory markers in the diagnosis and management of infective endocarditis. *Infect Dis Clin Pract.* 03/01 2010;18. doi:10.1097/IPC.0b013e3181aba67c.
110. von Dach E, Albrich WC, Brunel AS, et al. Effect of C-reactive protein-guided antimicrobial treatment duration, 7-day treatment, or 14-day treatment on 30-day clinical failure rate in patients with uncomplicated gram-negative bacteremia: A randomized clinical trial. *JAMA.* Jun 2 2020;323(21):2160–2169. doi:10.1001/jama.2020.6348.
111. Wilson Walter R., Gewitz Michael, Lockhart Peter B., et al. Prevention of viridans group streptococcal infective endocarditis: A scientific statement from the American Heart Association. *Circulation* 2021;14310.1161/cir.0000000000000969.

135

Tuberculosis

Rocsanna Namdar and Charles A. Peloquin

KEY CONCEPTS

1. Tuberculosis (TB) is one of the most prevalent communicable infectious diseases on earth; and it remains out of control in many developing nations. These nations require medical and financial assistance from developed nations in order to control the spread of TB globally.
2. In the United States, TB disproportionately affects the foreign born and other ethnic minorities, reflecting immigration patterns and greater ongoing transmission in these communities. Additional TB surveillance and preventive treatments are required within these communities.
3. TB is the leading cause of death in human immunodeficiency virus (HIV) infection worldwide. Coinfection with HIV and TB accelerates the progression of both diseases, thus, requiring rapid diagnosis and treatment of both diseases.
4. Mycobacteria are slow-growing organisms; in the laboratory, they require special stains, special growth media, and long periods of incubation to isolate and identify.
5. TB can produce atypical signs and symptoms in infants, older adults, and immunocompromised hosts, and it can progress rapidly in these patients.
6. Latent TB infection (LTBI) can lead to reactivation disease years after the primary infection occurred.
7. The patient suspected of having active TB disease must be isolated until the diagnosis is confirmed and the patient is no longer contagious. Often, isolation takes place in specialized "negative-pressure" hospital rooms to prevent the spread of TB.
8. Isoniazid and rifampin are the two most important drugs in the treatment of TB. Organisms resistant to both these drugs (multidrug-resistant TB [MDR-TB]) are much more difficult to treat.
9. Directly observed treatment (DOT) should be used whenever possible to reduce treatment failures and the selection of drug-resistant isolates.
10. To avoid the development of resistance, never add a single drug to a failing TB treatment regimen.

BEYOND THE BOOK

Read and review the study questions in the Self-Study Module 6 on Tuberculosis: Managing Tuberculosis Patients and Improving Adherence located on the Centers for Disease Control and Prevention (CDC) website: Self-Study Modules - Continuing Education Activities | TB | CDC Module6.pdf (cdc.gov). Focus on the Adherence to Treatment section (pages 27-55). This module is designed to teach healthcare providers about methods to improve medication adherence in different types of patients with tuberculosis disease. Strategies to improve patient adherence are described including directly observed therapy, incentives, and education. The module is a useful tool for students to enhance their understanding of assessment and implementation steps in the patient care process.

INTRODUCTION

1 Tuberculosis (TB) remains a leading infectious killer globally. TB is caused by *Mycobacterium tuberculosis*, which can produce either a silent, latent infection, or a progressive, active disease.[1] Left untreated or improperly treated, TB causes progressive tissue destruction and, eventually, death. Because of renewed public health efforts, TB rates in the United States continue to decline. In contrast, TB remains out of control in many developing countries.[1] Given increasing drug resistance, it is critical that a major effort be made to control TB before the most potent drugs are no longer effective.

TB rates generally have risen with increasing urbanization and overcrowding because it is easier for an airborne disease to spread when people are living in closer proximity to each other. Hence, TB became a significant pathogen in Europe during the Middle Ages and peaked during the Industrial Revolution, when it caused significant mortality in Europe and in the United States.[1] This dire threat led to the rise of public health departments and to procedures such as the isolation of infected patients. Thus, TB was directly responsible for many of the healthcare practices that are used today. Unfortunately, in developing nations, some of these practices are not widely available, and TB continues to rage unabated (Fig. 135-1).

EPIDEMIOLOGY

Over one-fourth of the world's population is infected by *M. tuberculosis*.[1] In 2019, there were about 10 million new cases and 1.2 million deaths from TB reported.[1] In the United States, 9 million people are latently infected with *M. tuberculosis*, meaning that they are not currently sick but that they could fall ill with TB at any time.[2] In 2019, 8,916 new TB cases were reported in the United States.[2] A further drop occurred in 2020, driven largely by measures to prevent

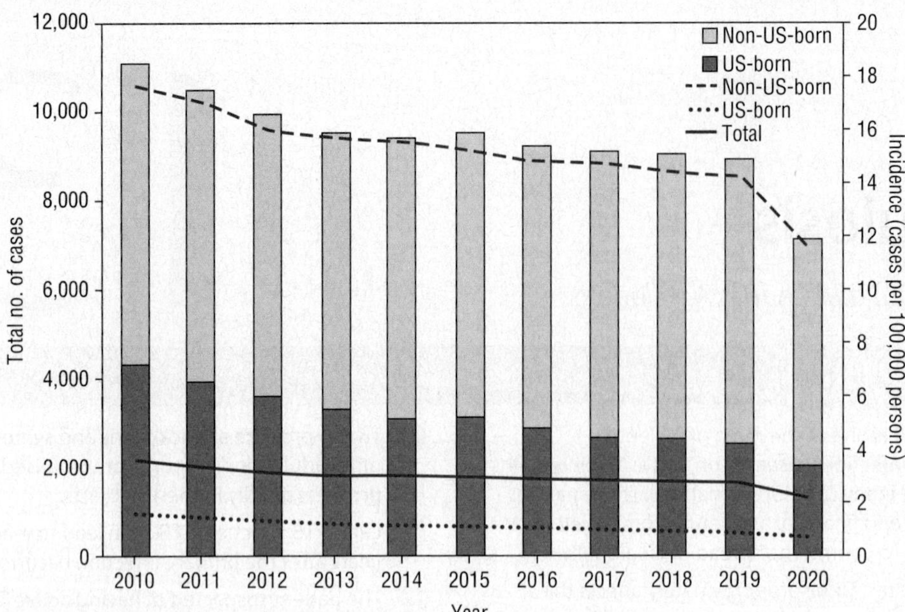

FIGURE 135-1 Reported tuberculosis cases in the United States. (Note: Number of tuberculosis cases among persons with unknown origin are not shown [range = 2-61]. Total rate includes cases among persons with unknown national origin. Rates for non–US-born and US-born persons were calculated by using midyear Current Population Survey estimates. Total rate was calculated by using midyear population estimates from the US Census Bureau.) *(Reprinted from reported Tuberculosis in the United States, 2017. Atlanta, GA: US Department of Health and Human Services, CDC; 2018.)*

another respiratory pathogen, COVID-19.[3] TB cases in the United States declined by approximately 5% per year from 1953 to 1983.[2] Starting in 1984, cases plateaued, and then rose from 1988 to 1992.[2] Since 1993, more effective infection control practices and treatment protocols have reduced TB rates significantly. However, the eradication of TB from the United States remains difficult because it is tied to immigration from high incidence countries.[1-3]

Risk Factors for Infection

Location and Place of Birth

California, Florida, New York, and Texas accounted for just over half of the TB cases reported nationally in 2019.[3] Within these states, TB is most prevalent in large urban areas and among those born outside the United States in high TB incidence countries.[3]

The percentage of foreign-born persons with TB in the United States has increased annually, reaching 71% in 2019.[3] In 2019, over half of foreign-born persons with TB originated from five countries: Mexico, the Philippines, India, Vietnam, and China.[3] Healthcare workers must consider TB when caring for patients from these countries who experience symptoms such as cough, fever, and weight loss. Furthermore, foreign-born persons account for almost 90% of the multidrug-resistant (MDR) TB cases in the United States.[3]

Close contacts of pulmonary TB patients such as family members, coworkers, or coresidents in places such as prisons, shelters, or nursing homes are most likely to become infected. The more prolonged the contact, the greater is the risk, with infection rates as high as 30%.[2,3] People with TB frequently have limited access to healthcare, live in crowded conditions, or are homeless.[2,3] Many have histories of alcohol use disorder or illicit drug use, and are coinfected with hepatitis B or HIV. These concurrent social and health problems make treating some TB patients particularly challenging.

Ethnicity and Age

2 In the United States, TB disproportionately affects the foreign-born and other ethnic minorities. In 2019, Asians accounted for 36% percentage of total TB cases; Hispanic/Latino people for 30%, and Blacks 20%.[3] Non–US-born persons had a TB rate 15.5 times greater than the rate among US-born persons.[3] These disparities are the result of a complex interplay of social and environmental factors including urbanization, access to healthcare, poverty, and migration.[3,4,43]

In 2019, the number of TB cases was highest in the 25- to 44-year and the 45- to 64-year-age groups, while the rate per 100,000 population was highest in those over 65 years of age.[3] The overall TB incidence was 2.7 per 100,000 population.[3]

Coinfection with Human Immunodeficiency Virus

3 In patients who have LTBI, human immunodeficiency virus (HIV) is the most important risk factor, especially for people between the ages of 25 and 44 years.[4] TB and HIV act synergistically within patients and across populations, making each disease worse than it might otherwise be. In 2019, 4.9% of TB patients with known HIV statues were coinfected, with about 7.8% in the 25- to 44-year age group.[3-5] HIV coinfection may not increase the risk of acquiring *M. tuberculosis* infection, but it does increase the likelihood of progression to active disease.[4] There are higher mortality rates in persons coinfected with HIV and MDR or and extensively drug-resistant (XDR) TB.[5]

Risk Factors for Disease

Once infected with *M. tuberculosis*, a person's lifetime risk of active TB is approximately 10%.[2-4] The greatest risk for active disease occurs during the first 2 years after infection. Children younger than 2 years and adults older than 65 years have two to five times greater risk for active disease compared with other age groups. Patients with underlying immune suppression (eg, renal failure, cancer, and immunosuppressive drug treatment) have 4 to 16 times greater risk than other patients.[5] HIV-infected patients with *M. tuberculosis* infection are 100 times more likely to develop active TB than normal hosts.[5] HIV-infected patients have an annual risk of active TB of approximately 10%, rather than a lifetime risk at that rate.[5] Therefore, all patients with HIV infection should be screened for TB infection, and those known to be infected with *M. tuberculosis* should be tested for HIV infection.

ETIOLOGY

M. tuberculosis is a slender bacillus with a waxy outer layer.[6] It is 1 to 4 μm in length, and under the microscope, it is either straight or slightly curved in shape.[6] It does not stain well with Gram stain, so the Ziehl–Neelsen stain or the fluorochrome stain must be used instead.[6] After Ziehl–Neelsen staining with carbol-fuchsin, mycobacteria retain the red color despite acid–alcohol washes. Hence, they are called *acid-fast bacilli* (AFB).[6] On culture, *M. tuberculosis* grows slowly, doubling about every 20 hours. This is slow compared with gram-positive and gram-negative bacteria, which double about every 30 minutes.

Culture and Susceptibility Testing

All clinical specimens suspected of containing mycobacteria should be cultured. Culture is required for species identification and for drug-susceptibility testing.

4 Direct susceptibility testing involves inoculating specialized media with organisms taken directly from a concentrated, smear-positive specimen.[6] This approach produces susceptibility results in 2 to 3 weeks. Culture-based phenotypic drug-susceptibility testing methods are the primary methods for drug-resistance detection. These methods are time consuming and require sophisticated laboratory infrastructure. Direct susceptibility testing uses critical concentrations of antituberculosis drugs to determine resistance of an isolate. A critical concentration is a previously established breakpoint separating "susceptible" from "resistant." Indirect susceptibility testing involves inoculating the test media with organisms obtained from a pure culture of the organisms, which can take several more weeks.[1,6]

The most common agar method has limitations which include length of time to obtain results, drug degradation during incubation, and a qualitative result (susceptible or resistant). The newer mycobacterial growth indicator tube (MGIT, Becton Dickson, Sparks, MD) systems use liquid media and detect live mycobacteria in as few as 9 to 14 days.[7,8]

Rapid identification tests are now available, but cost and care of equipment remain an issue in many parts of the world.[6-9] The Enhanced Amplified *Mycobacterium tuberculosis* Direct test has been approved for use by the US Food and Drug Administration (FDA) in AFB smear-positive and smear-negative specimen in patients with fewer than 7 days of antimycobacterial therapy and the Gene Xpert MTB/RIF assay in patients with fewer than 3 days of treatment.[9-11] The Amplicor *Mycobacterium tuberculosis* test has been approved for smear-positive samples.[7,8]

The Hain test, a line-probe assay that diagnoses resistance to isoniazid and rifampin by detecting several gene mutations responsible for drug resistance, has also entered into limited clinical use in the United States.[8] The Gene X-pert MTB/RIF test simultaneously identifies *M. tuberculosis* and rapidly determines if resistance to rifampin is present.[9-11] The test has excellent performance in both smear-positive and -negative patients, and high accuracy for determination of rifampicin resistance.[9,11] Colorimetric redox indicator and nitrate reduction assays for rapid detection of rifampicin and isoniazid resistance are both inexpensive and have rapid turnaround times of 1 week. Microscopic observation drug-susceptibility assay is a simple test using sputum samples to detect characteristic patterns of growth of *M. tuberculosis* and resistance patterns.[9,11] Time to diagnosis is 7 days and drug susceptibilities are available at the time of diagnosis.[11] Most patients with microscopic observation drug-susceptibility assays are diagnosed within 2 weeks, and it is similarly efficient irrespective of bacterial burden.[12]

Other tests are designed to detect common genetic changes associated with drug resistance, such as changes in the *katG* gene associated with isoniazid resistance and the *rpoB* gene associated with rifampin resistance.[8,13] Mutations that affect the *rpoB* gene alter the protein structure of the target so that rifampin cannot bind; thus, conferring resistance. Similarly, isoniazid-resistant isolates can be detected by sequencing the *inhA* gene which leads to overproduction of the drug target and mutations in *katG* gene which inhibits activation of isoniazid prodrug. Probe assays do not eliminate the need for conventional culture and susceptibility testing; conventional drug-susceptibility testing is needed to diagnose XDR-TB. The decision to use nucleic acid amplification tests should be individualized.[8,13] Advanced sequencing techniques continue to evolve.

Transmission

M. tuberculosis is transmitted from person to person by coughing or other activities that cause the organism to be aerosolized.[14] These particles, called *droplet nuclei,* contain one to three bacilli and are small enough (1-5 mm) to reach the alveolar surface.[15] Approximately 30% of individuals who experience prolonged contact with an infectious TB patient will become infected.[14]

A person with cavitary, pulmonary TB and a cough is considered infectious and may infect greater than 30% of contacts until that person is treated effectively, although this percentage and the absolute number can vary significantly. A person with the uncommon laryngeal form of TB can spread organisms even when talking, so the transmission rates can be even higher.[14,15]

The National TB Molecular Surveillance Center performs whole genome sequencing on isolates of *M. tuberculosis* gathered from newly diagnosed patients in the United States. Samples are submitted by contracted laboratories and then genotype results are loaded into the system to identify chains of transmission and outbreaks.[8] Public health interventions can be targeted and cases that are the same cluster are likely to be related and treated similarly.[8]

PATHOPHYSIOLOGY

Immune Response

T-lymphocyte responses are essential to controlling *M. tuberculosis* infections.[14,15] In the mouse model, two different T-cell responses—the T-helper type 1 (TH_1) response and the T-helper type 2 (TH_2) response—have been described. The TH_1 response is the preferred response to TB, and the TH_2 response, including the potentially subversive influence of interleukin (IL) 4, is undesirable.[14,15] This dichotomy is clearer in the mouse model, and in many humans, the T-cell response may be classified as TH_0 (elements of both TH_1 and TH_2).[14,15] In either case, T lymphocytes activate macrophages that, in turn, engulf and kill mycobacteria. T lymphocytes also destroy immature macrophages that harbor *M. tuberculosis* but are unable to kill the invaders.[14,15] CD4+ cells are the primary T cells involved, with contributions by $\gamma\ \delta$ T cells and CD8+ T cells.[14] CD4+ T cells produce INF-γ and other cytokines, including IL-2 and IL-10, that coordinate the immune response to TB.[14,15] Because CD4+ cells are depleted in HIV-infected patients, these patients are unable to mount an adequate defense to TB.[14,15]

Although B-cell responses and antibody production can be demonstrated in TB-infected mammals, these humoral responses may not contribute much to the control of TB within the host.[15] Tumor necrosis factor-α (TNF-α) and INF-γ are important cytokines involved in coordinating the host's cell-mediated response.[16] Rheumatoid arthritis patients treated with TNF-α inhibitors (such as infliximab) have high rates of reactivation TB.[16] Therefore, patients deficient in the activity of TNF-α or INF-γ should be screened for TB infection and offered appropriate treatment.

M. tuberculosis has several ways of evading or resisting the host immune response.[15] In particular, *M. tuberculosis* can inhibit the fusion of lysosomes to phagosomes inside macrophages, preventing the destructive enzymes found in the lysosomes from getting to the bacilli captured in the phagosomes. This inhibition of destructive mechanisms allows time for *M. tuberculosis* to escape into the cytoplasm. Virulent *M. tuberculosis* bacilli are able to multiply in the macrophage cytoplasm, thus perpetuating their spread. Finally, lipoarabinomannan (LAM), the principal structural polysaccharide of the mycobacterial cell wall, inhibits the host immune response.[15] LAM induces immunosuppressive cytokines, thus blocking macrophage activation; additionally, LAM scavenges O_2, thus preventing attack by superoxide anions, hydrogen peroxide, singlet oxygen, and hydroxyl radicals.[15] These survival mechanisms make *M. tuberculosis* a particularly difficult organism to control. Any defects in the host immune system make it likely that *M. tuberculosis* will not be controlled and that active disease will ensue.

Primary Infection

Primary infection usually results from inhaling airborne particles that contain *M. tuberculosis*.[15,17] The progression to clinical disease depends on three factors: (a) the number of *M. tuberculosis* organisms inhaled (infecting dose), (b) the virulence of these organisms, and (c) the host's cell-mediated immune response.[15,17] At the alveolar surface, the bacilli that were delivered by the droplet nuclei are ingested by pulmonary macrophages. If these macrophages inhibit or kill the bacilli, infection is aborted.[15] If the macrophages cannot do this, the organisms continue to multiply. The macrophages eventually rupture, releasing many bacilli, and these mycobacteria are then phagocytized by other macrophages. This cycle continues over several weeks until the host is able to mount a more coordinated response.[15,17] During this early phase of infection, *M. tuberculosis* multiplies logarithmically.[15]

Some of the intracellular organisms are transported by the macrophages to regional lymph nodes in the hilar, mediastinal, and retroperitoneal areas. The cycle of phagocytosis and cell rupture continues. During lymph node involvement, the mycobacteria may be held in check. More frequently, *M. tuberculosis* spreads throughout the body through the bloodstream.[14,15] When this intravascular dissemination occurs, *M. tuberculosis* can infect any tissue or organ in the body. Most commonly, *M. tuberculosis* infects the posterior apical region of the lungs. This may be so because of the high oxygen content or less vigorous immune response in this area.[14,17]

After about 3 weeks of infection, T lymphocytes are presented with *M. tuberculosis* antigens. These T cells become activated and begin to secrete INF-γ and the other cytokines noted earlier. The processes described in the "Immune Response" section above then begin to occur.[14] First, T lymphocytes stimulate macrophages to become bactericidal.[14,15] Large numbers of activated microbicidal macrophages surround the solid caseous (cheese-like) tuberculous foci (the necrotic area of infection).[14,15] This process of creating activated microbicidal macrophages is known as cell-mediated immunity.[15]

When cell-mediated immunity occurs, delayed-type hypersensitivity (DTH) also develops through the activation and multiplication of T lymphocytes. DTH refers to the cytotoxic immune process that kills nonactivated immature macrophages that are permitting intracellular bacillary replication.[15] These immature macrophages are killed when the T lymphocytes initiate Fas-mediated apoptosis (programmed cell death).[15] The bacilli released from the immature macrophages then are killed by the activated macrophages.[15]

After 3 weeks, in most recently infected individuals, macrophages have begun to form granulomas to contain the organisms. In a typical tuberculous granuloma, activated macrophages accumulate around a caseous lesion and prevent its further extension.[15] At this point, the infection is largely under control, and bacillary replication falls off dramatically. Depending on the inflammatory response, tissue necrosis and calcification of the infection site plus the regional lymph nodes may occur.

Over 1 to 3 months, activated lymphocytes reach an adequate number, and tissue hypersensitivity results. In practical terms, this is the reason why tests to diagnose LTBI, purified protein derivative (PPD) skin test, and the INF-γ release assays take between 2 and 12 weeks to become positive. Any remaining mycobacteria are believed to reside primarily within granulomas or within macrophages that have avoided detection and lysis, although some residual bacilli have been found in various types of cells.[6,14]

Approximately 90% of infected patients have no further clinical manifestations. Most patients only show a positive skin or blood test for immune response (70%), whereas some also have radiographic evidence of stable granulomas.[17] This radiodense area on chest radiograph is called a *Ghon's complex*. Approximately 5% of patients (usually children, older adults, and the immunocompromised) experience "progressive primary" disease that occurs before skin test conversion, which presents as a progressive pneumonia, usually in the lower lobes.[17] Disease frequently spreads, leading to meningitis and other severe forms of TB.[17,18] Because of this risk of severe disease, young, elderly, and immunocompromised patients, including those with HIV, should be evaluated and treated for latent or active TB.[17,18]

Reactivation Disease

6 Roughly 10% of infected patients develop reactivation disease at some point in their lives. Nearly half of these cases occur within 2 years of infection.[14,17] In the United States, most cases of TB result from reactivation. Reinfection is uncommon in the United States because of the low rate of exposure and because previously sensitized individuals possess some degree of immunity to reinfection.[14,17] Exceptions include patients coinfected with HIV who live in areas of higher exposure to *M. tuberculosis*.

The apices of the lungs are the most common sites for reactivation (85% of cases).[14,17] For reasons that are not entirely known (waning cellular immunity, loss of specific T-cell clones, blocking antibody), organisms within granulomas emerge and begin multiplying extracellularly.[14,17] The inflammatory response produces caseating granulomas, which eventually will liquefy and spread locally, leading to the formation of a hole (cavity) in the lungs.

The immune response contributes to the severity of the lung damage, and DTH allows for intracellular mycobacterial multiplication.[14,15] In addition, there is "innocent bystander" killing of host cells and locally thrombosed blood vessels.[14] The killing of mycobacteria, macrophages, and neutrophils that have entered the battle releases cytokines and lysozymes into the infectious foci. This toxic mixture can be too much for the surrounding alveoli and airway cells, causing regional necrosis and structural collapse.[14] These unstable foci liquefy, spreading the infection to neighboring areas of the lung, creating a cavity. Some of this necrotic material is coughed out, producing droplet nuclei. Bacterial counts in the cavities can be as high as 10^8 per milliliter (or 10^{11}/L) of cavitary fluid. Partial healing may result from fibrosis, but these lesions remain unstable and may continue to expand.[14] If left untreated, pulmonary TB continues to destroy the lungs, resulting in hypoxia, respiratory acidosis, and eventually death.

Extrapulmonary and Miliary Tuberculosis

Caseating granulomas at extrapulmonary sites can undergo liquefaction, releasing tubercle bacilli and causing symptomatic disease.[14] Extrapulmonary TB without concurrent pulmonary disease is uncommon in normal hosts but more common in HIV-infected patients. Because of these unusual presentations, the diagnosis of TB is difficult and often delayed in immunocompromised hosts.[14] Lymphatic and pleural diseases are the most common forms of extrapulmonary TB, followed by bone, joint, genitourinary, meningeal, and other forms.[14] Occasionally, a massive inoculum of organisms enters the bloodstream, causing a widely disseminated form of the disease known as *miliary TB*. It is named for the millet seed appearance of the small granulomas seen on chest radiographs, and it can be rapidly fatal.[14] Miliary TB is a medical emergency requiring immediate treatment.

Influence of Human Immunodeficiency Virus Infection on Pathogenesis

3 HIV infection is the strongest single risk factor for progressing to active TB.[14,17] As CD4+ lymphocytes multiply in response to the mycobacterial infection, HIV multiplies within these cells and selectively destroys them. In turn, the TB-fighting lymphocytes are depleted.[14,17] This vicious cycle puts HIV-infected persons at 100 times the risk of active TB compared with HIV-negative people.[19,20] In addition, the combination of HIV infection and certain social behaviors increases the risk of newly acquired TB. In select areas of the United States during the resurgence of TB during the early 1990s, up to 50% of new TB cases were the result of recent infection, particularly among HIV-infected individuals.[1,19,20]

As mycobacteria spread throughout the body, HIV replication accelerates in lymphocytes and macrophages. This leads to progression of HIV disease.[14,19,20] HIV-infected persons who are infected with TB deteriorate more rapidly unless they receive antimycobacterial chemotherapy.[19,20] Most clinicians now recommend integrated antiretroviral therapy beginning TB treatment first, and then beginning HIV treatment within 2 to 12 weeks.[21-23] However, the timing needs to be individualized based on degree of immunosuppression from HIV and the individual's tolerance of the treatment regimen. Immune reconstitution inflammatory syndrome or a paradoxical worsening of TB can occur, especially in persons with more severe immunosuppression; this results from a reinvigorated inflammatory response to TB.[21,23] HIV-positive persons should be screened for tuberculous infection or disease soon after they are shown to be HIV positive.[21]

CLINICAL PRESENTATION

The classical presentation of TB is weight loss, fatigue, a productive cough, fever, and night sweats. The onset of TB may be gradual, and the diagnosis may not be considered until a chest radiograph is performed. Unfortunately, many people do not seek medical attention until more dramatic symptoms, such as hemoptysis, occur. At this point, infected persons typically have large cavitary lesions in the lungs. These cavities are loaded with *M. tuberculosis*. Expectoration or swallowing of infected sputum may spread the disease to other areas of the body.[14,17,24] Physical examination is nonspecific but can be suggestive of progressive pulmonary disease.

Human Immunodeficiency Virus

5 Persons coinfected with HIV may have atypical presentations.[19-21,24] As their CD4+ counts decline, HIV-positive individuals are less likely to have positive skin tests, cavitary lesions, or fever. Pulmonary radiographic findings may be minimal or absent. HIV-positive persons have a higher incidence of extrapulmonary TB and are more likely to present with progressive primary disease. Because their symptoms are not specific to TB, a thorough workup for TB is essential.[20,21]

Extrapulmonary

Extrapulmonary TB typically presents as a slowly progressive decline in organ function.[14,17-19] Infected persons may have low-grade fever and other constitutional symptoms. Those with genitourinary TB may present with sterile pyuria and hematuria. Lymphadenitis often involves the cervical and supraclavicular nodes and may appear as a neck mass with spontaneous drainage. Tuberculous arthritis and osteomyelitis occur most commonly in the older adults and usually affect the lower spine and weight-bearing joints. TB of the spine is known as *Pott's disease*.[14] Abnormal behavior, headaches, or convulsions suggest tuberculous meningitis. Involvement of the peritoneum, pericardium, larynx, and adrenal glands also occurs.[14,18]

Older Adults

5 TB in the older adults is easily confused with other respiratory diseases. Many clinical findings are muted or absent altogether. Compared with younger patients, TB in the older adults is far less likely to present with positive skin tests, fevers, night sweats, sputum production, or hemoptysis.[14,17,24] Weight loss may occur but is nonspecific. In contrast, mental status changes are twice as common in older adults, and mortality is six times higher.[14,17] TB is a preventable cause of death in older adults that should not be overlooked.

Children

5 TB in children, especially those younger than 12 years, may present as a typical bacterial pneumonia and is called *progressive primary TB*.[17,18,24] Clinical disease often begins 1 to 2 months after exposure and precedes skin-test positivity. Unlike adults, pulmonary TB in children often involves the lower and middle lobes.[17,18] Dissemination to the lymph nodes, gastrointestinal (GI) and genitourinary tracts, bone marrow, and meninges is common. Because of

CLINICAL PRESENTATION Tuberculosis

Signs and Symptoms

- Patients typically present with cough, weight loss, fatigue, fever, and night sweats.[2,14,15]
- Frank hemoptysis usually occurs late in the course of disease but may present earlier.

Physical Examination

- Dullness to chest percussion, rales, and increased vocal fremitus are observed frequently on auscultation but a normal lung examination is common compared to the degree of radiological lung involvement.
- Patient is usually thin with evidence or recent weight loss.

Laboratory Tests

- Moderate elevations in the white blood cell count with a lymphocyte predominance.
- High platelet count (thrombocytosis) and mild-to-moderate anemia are common.

Diagnostic Considerations

- Positive-sputum smear
- Fiber-optic bronchoscopy (if sputum tests are inconclusive and suspicion is high)

Chest Radiograph

- Patchy or nodular infiltrates in the apical areas of the upper lobes or the superior segment of the lower lobes.[2,14,15]
- Cavitation that may show air–fluid levels as the infection progresses.

delays in recruitment of cellular immunity, cavitary disease is infrequent, and the number of organisms present typically is smaller than in an adult. Because cavitary lesions are uncommon, children do not spread TB readily. However, TB can be rapidly fatal in a child, and it requires prompt chemotherapy.

DIAGNOSIS

The following section focuses on diagnostic testing for infection with *M. tuberculosis*. If active disease is suspected based on clinical presentation, additional diagnostic tests are also reviewed to confirm active disease.

Diagnostic Testing

The key to stopping the spread of TB is early identification of infected individuals.[24] Table 135-1 lists the populations most likely to benefit from testing (column 1 persons are at highest risk for TB, followed by those in column 2). Members of these high-risk groups should be tested for TB infection and educated about the disease.

The Mantoux test is a quantitative TB skin test that uses tuberculin PPD. The standard 5-tuberculin-unit PPD dose is placed intracutaneously on the volar aspect of the forearm with a 26- or 27-gauge needle.[24,25] This injection should produce a small, raised, blanched wheal. An experienced professional should read the test in 48 to 72 hours. The area of induration (the "bump") is the important end point, not the area of redness. Table 135-1 lists the criteria for interpretation.[24,25] The Centers for Disease Control and Prevention (CDC) does not recommend the routine use of anergy panels.[24-27] Aplisol and tubersol 5-tuberculin-unit products are available commercially and are similar in sensitivity, specificity, and reactivity. It is important, however, to use one product and notify appropriate users when switching between products.[27]

The "booster effect" occurs for persons who do not respond to an initial skin test but show a positive reaction if retested about a week later or longer.[17,28] Persons with past *M. tuberculosis* infection and some with past immunization with bacillus Calmette-Guérin (BCG) vaccine or past infection with other mycobacteria may "boost" with a second skin test. Individuals who require periodic skin testing, such as healthcare workers, should receive a two-stage test initially.[17,28] Once they are shown to be skin-test negative, any positive skin test later shows recent infection, and this requires an evaluation to consider treatment.

The PPD skin test is an imperfect diagnostic tool. Up to 20% of persons with active TB are falsely skin-test negative, presumably because they may be immunocompromised.[25,26] False-positive results are more common in low-risk patients and those recently vaccinated with BCG. Despite BCG vaccination, one should not ignore a positive PPD result especially if the induration is more than 15 mm.[24] These individuals require careful evaluation for active disease, and they may be offered preventive treatment because many come from areas where TB infection is common.

Interferon-γ release assays (IGRA) measure the release of INF-γ in blood in response to the TB antigens.[29] They may provide quick and specific results for identifying *M. tuberculosis*. IGRAs do not trigger a booster effect and are more specific for testing *M. tuberculosis* than the PPD. The QuantiFERON-TB Gold test is an enzyme-linked immunosorbent assay and the T-SPOT.®TB is an enzyme-linked immunospot assay.[29] Both tests can be used for diagnosing LTBI and TB disease caused by *M. tuberculosis*. However, these are the tests designed to diagnose LTBI and are not to be used to confirm or reject a diagnosis of active TB disease. For active TB, the IGRAs provide supporting evidence for the diagnosis but need to be interpreted in light of other evidence of active TB disease such as epidemiological risk factors and other studies. The antigenic proteins are absent from BCG vaccine strains and from most non-TB mycobacteria. Therefore, QuantiFERON-TB Gold test does not trigger a booster effect and is more specific for testing of *M. tuberculosis* than the PPD. Although these tests can provide results to diagnose both latent infection and disease, they cannot differentiate between the two. Results are available within 24 hours, instead of the 2 to 3 days required for the traditional PPD skin test; and the patient does not have to return to the clinic as required by the PPD skin test. The CDC has approved the use of these tests in all circumstances

TABLE 135-1 Criteria for Tuberculosis Positivity

Reaction ≥5 mm of Induration	Reaction ≥10 mm of Induration	Reaction ≥15 mm of Induration
HIV-infected persons	Recent immigrants (ie, within the last 5 years) from high-prevalence countries	Persons with no risk factors for TB
A recent contact of a person with TB disease	Injection drug users	
Fibrotic changes on chest radiograph consistent with prior TB	Residents and employees[a] of the following high-risk congregate settings: prisons and jails, nursing homes and other long-term facilities for the elderly, hospitals and other healthcare facilities, residential facilities for patients with AIDS, and homeless shelters	
Patients with organ transplants and other immunosuppressed patients (receiving the equivalent of 15 mg/day or more of prednisone for 1 month or longer, taking TNF-α antagonists)[b]	Mycobacteriology laboratory personnel, persons with the following clinical conditions that place them at high risk: silicosis, diabetes mellitus, chronic renal failure, some hematologic disorders, other specific malignancies, gastrectomy, and jejunoileal bypass	
	Children younger than 5 years of age or infants, children, and adolescents exposed to adults at high risk	

Interpretation of IGRA Results

The interpretation of IGRAs is based on the amount of IFN-γ, in T-SPOT®.TB. An IGRA is recommended over a TST in persons at least 5 years of age who are likely to have *M. tuberculosis* infection; who are at low or moderate risk of the disease progressing; in whom it has been determined that LTBI testing is necessary; and who have been vaccinated against Calmette-Guérin or are not likely to return for follow-up after a TST. The TST is a viable second option in certain circumstances, such as if an IGRA is unavailable. Laboratories should provide both the qualitative and quantitative results.

- Qualitative results are reported positive, negative, indeterminate, or borderline.
- Quantitative results are reported as numerical values that include a response to the TB antigen and two controls, nil and mitogen.
- Quantitative results may be useful for clinical decision making in individual cases, in combination with risk factors.

[a]For persons who are otherwise at low risk and who are tested at the start of employment, a reaction of ≥15 mm induration is considered positive.

[b]Risk of TB for patients treated with corticosteroids increases with higher dose and longer duration.

AIDS, acquired immunodeficiency syndrome; TST, tuberculin skin tests.

Data from Centers for Disease Control and Prevention. Screening for tuberculosis and tuberculosis infection in high-risk populations: recommendations of the Advisory Council for the Elimination of Tuberculosis. M.M.W.R. 1995;44(No. RR-11):19–34.

Group	Testing Strategy	Considerations
Likely to Be Infected **High** Risk of Progression (TST ≥5mM)	**Adults** **Acceptable:** IGRA or TST Consider dual testing where a positive result from either result would be considered **positive** **Children ≤5 years of age** **Acceptable:** TST **Acceptable:** IGRA or TST Consider dual testing where a positive result from either result would be considered **positive**[a]	Prevalence of BCG vaccination Expertise of staff and/or laboratory Test availability Patient perceptions Staff perceptions Programmatic concerns
Likely to Be Infected **Low** to **Intermediate** Risk of Progression (TST ≥10 mM)	**Preferred:** IGRA where available **Acceptable:** IGRA or TST	
Unlikely to Be Infected (TST >15 mM)	**Testing for LTBI is not recommended** **If necessary:** **Preferred:** IGRA where available **Acceptable:** Either IGRA OR TST **For serial testing:** **Acceptable:** Either IGRA OR TST Consider repeat or dual testing where a negative result from either would be considered **negative**[b]	

FIGURE 135-2 Summary of recommendations for testing for latent tuberculosis infection (LTBI).
[a]Performing a second diagnostic test when the initial test is a negative is a strategy to increase sensitivity. This may reduce specificity, but the panel decided that this is an acceptable trade off in situations in which the consequences of missing LTBI exceed the consequences of inappropriate therapy.
[b]Performing a confirmatory test following an initial positive result is based upon both the evidence that false positive results are common among individuals who are unlikely to be infected with *Mycobacterium tuberculosis* and the committee's presumption that performing a second test on those patients whose initial test was positive will help identify initial false positive results. *(Adapted from Lewinsohn DM, Leonard MK, LoBue PA, et al. Official American Thoracic Society/Infectious Diseases Society/Centers for Disease Control and Prevention clinical practice guidelines: diagnosis of tuberculosis in adults and children. 2017;64:e1–e11.)*

in which the PPD is used. IGRAs may be preferred for testing in patients who are suspected not to return for follow-up PPD reads or in patients who have received the BCG vaccine.[29] IGRA is recommended over a TST or PPD in individuals 5 years or older who meet the following criteria: (1) are likely to be infected with *M. tuberculosis*, (2) have a low-to-intermediate risk of disease progression, (3) testing for LTBI is warranted, (4) history of BCG vaccination, and (5) are unlikely to return to have their PPD read.[29] IGRA rather than PPD is also suggested in all other individuals who are likely to be infected with *M. tuberculosis*, who have a low-to-intermediate risk of disease progression, and in whom testing for LTBI is warranted.[29] There are insufficient data to recommend a preference for either a PPD or IGRA as the first-line diagnostic test in patients likely to be infected with *M. tuberculosis*, who have a high risk of progression to disease, and in whom diagnostic testing is warranted.[29] Figure 135-2 summarizes the recommendations for testing for latent tuberculosis infections (LTBI).

The sensitivity for young children (younger than 5 years) and in immunocompromised individuals has not been clearly established.[30-32] A PPD test is recommended in healthy children (younger than 5 years) for whom diagnostic testing is warranted. The American Academy of Pediatrics recommends IGRAs in place of PPD skin test in immunocompetent children aged 5 years or older who have received BCG vaccination to confirm TB infection.[31] However, an increasing number of experts are using the IGRAs in children 3 years or older.

IGRAs perform similarly to the PPD in detecting TB in HIV-infected persons with LTBI. Both PPD and IGRA have suboptimal sensitivity for active TB especially in the severely immunocompromised.[33,34]

Culture and Staining

When active TB is suspected, attempts should be made to isolate *M. tuberculosis* from the site of infection.[17,24] Sputum collected in the morning usually has the highest yield.[17,24] Daily sputum collection over three consecutive days is recommended. Microscopic examination is the most rapid and inexpensive TB diagnostic tool. After staining, microscopic examination ("smear") detects about 8,000 to 10,000 organisms per milliliter (8×10^6/L to 10×10^6/L) of specimen, so a patient can be "smear-negative" but still grow *M. tuberculosis* on culture. Microscopic examination also cannot determine which of the more than 150 mycobacterial species is present or whether the organisms in the original samples were alive or dead.[17,24]

For persons unable to expectorate, sputum induction with aerosolized hypertonic saline may produce a diagnostic sample. Bronchoscopy, in older children, or aspiration of gastric fluid via a nasogastric tube, in children (5 years or younger), may be attempted for select individuals.[17] For persons with suspected extrapulmonary TB, samples of draining fluid, biopsies of the infected site, or both may be attempted. Blood cultures are positive occasionally, especially in persons with acquired immunodeficiency syndrome (AIDS).[17,19]

TREATMENT

Drugs used in the treatment of active disease are divided into first-line and second-line agents. First-line agents should be the preferred options unless susceptibility results dictate otherwise. Treatment in special populations is also addressed.

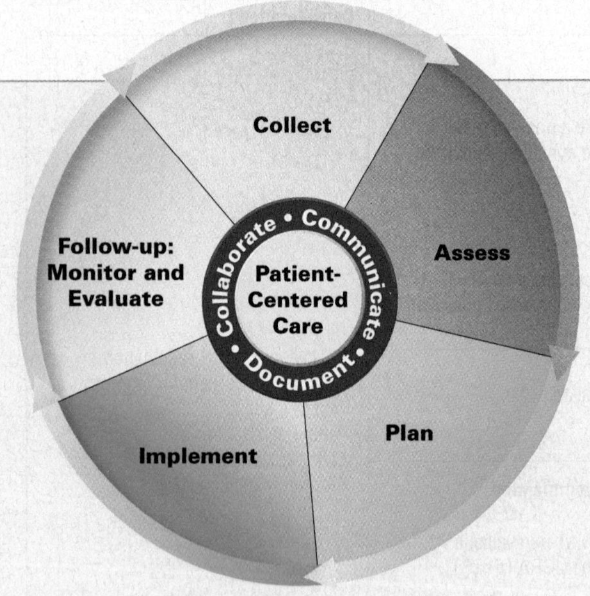

Patient Care Process for Active Tuberculosis

The image shows the five fundamental steps included in The Pharmacist's Care Process endorsed by the Joint Commission for Pharmacy Practitioners (2014). The tagline of this process reads collaborate, communicate, and document. The five fundamental steps listed here are collect, assess, plan, implement, and follow-up: monitor and evaluate. All these steps are listed in a circular block diagram.

Collect

- Patient characteristics (eg, age, sex, ethnicity)
- Patient medical history (medical risk factors, eg, immunocompromised, HIV, tobacco/ethanol/IV drug use)
- Social history (eg, living conditions, recent contacts)
- Current medications including prescription and nonprescription medicines, herbal products
- Information and history about patients adherence to medications
- History of clinical signs and symptoms (weight loss, cough, hemoptysis)
- Objective data
  - Sputum smears/culture
  - Chest x-ray
  - Tuberculin skin test (TST)/IGRA
  - Pertinent labs (white blood cell, platelets, serum creatinine, LFTs)

Assess

- Patient's potential for risk of transmission
- Risk of mycobacterial resistance
- Risk of drug malabsorption/drug interactions
- Need for therapeutic drug monitoring
- Immune status
- Ability/willingness to be adherent to prescribed regimen
- Psychological status to determine understanding and following instructions for adherence; need for directly observed therapy
- Ability/willingness to maintain follow-up

Plan*

- Devise a drug-therapy regimen with healthcare team to include most appropriate antituberculosis agents, dose, route, frequency, and duration (see Tables 135-3 and 135-4)
- Monitoring parameters including efficacy (eg, sputum smears) and safety (eg, LFTs, neuropathy); frequency and timing of follow-up (see Table 135-8)
- Patient education (eg, purpose of treatment, infection control, drug-specific information, importance of compliance/legal ramifications and risk of non-compliance)

Implement

- Provide patient education regarding all elements of treatment plan and goals
- Ensure patient understanding of risk of transmission and importance of adherence
- Schedule follow-up (eg, adherence assessment, adverse effects, response to treatment)

Follow-up: Monitor and Evaluate

- Monthly clinic evaluation
- Objective data
  - Sputum smears
  - Chest x-ray results
  - Pertinent labs
- Determine response to therapy
  - Clinical response (cough, fever, night sweats)
  - Culture results
- Need for therapeutic drug monitoring
- Presence of adverse effects
- Patient adherence to treatment plan
  - Tablet/Capsule counts for compliance or attending directly observed treatment

**Collaborate with patients, caregivers, and other healthcare professionals.*

Desired Outcome

The primary desired outcomes during the treatment of TB are:

1. Rapid identification of a new TB case.
2. Initiation of specific antituberculosis treatment.
3. Eradication of *M. tuberculosis* infection.
4. Achievement of a noninfectious state in the patient, thus ending isolation.
5. Prevention of the development of resistance.
6. Adherence to the treatment regimen by the patient.
7. Cure of the patient as quickly as possible (generally at least 6 months of treatment).

Patients with active disease should be isolated to prevent spread of the disease, and appropriate samples for smears and cultures should be collected. Secondary goals are identification of the index case that infected the individual, identification of all persons infected by both the index case and the new case of TB ("contact investigation"), and completion of appropriate treatments for those individuals.

General Approaches

Drug treatment is the cornerstone of TB management.[35] Monotherapy can be used only for infected persons who do not have active TB (latent infection, as shown by a positive skin test or positive IGRA). Once active disease is present, most patients receive four drugs.[35] The duration of treatment depends on the condition of the host, extent of disease, presence of drug resistance, and tolerance of medications. Most patients are treated for 6 months, and 18 to 24 months of treatment may be necessary for cases of MDR-TB.[35] Because the duration of treatment is so long and because many individuals feel better after a few weeks of treatment, careful follow-up is required. Directly observed therapy (DOT) by a healthcare worker is a cost-effective way to ensure completion of treatment and is considered the standard of care.[36,37]

Principles for Treating Latent Infection and for Treating Disease

Asymptomatic patients with tuberculous infection have a bacillary load of about 10^3 organisms, compared with 10^{11} organisms in a patient with cavitary pulmonary TB.[14] As the number of organisms increases, the likelihood of naturally occurring drug-resistant mutants also increases. Naturally occurring mutants that are resistant to antituberculosis drugs are found at rates of 1 in 10^6 to 1 in 10^8 organisms.[13] When treating asymptomatic latent infection with monotherapy, the risk of selecting out resistant organisms is low. In contrast, the risk of selecting out isoniazid-resistant organisms is unacceptably high for patients with cavitary TB. One can prevent selection of these resistant mutants by adding more drugs because the rates for resistance mutations to multiple drugs are additive functions of the individual rates. For example, only 1 in 10^{13} organisms would be naturally resistant to both isoniazid (1 in 10^6) and rifampin (1 in 10^7).[13,35] It is unlikely that such rare organisms are present in a previously untreated patient.

Combination chemotherapy is required for treating active TB disease. Generally, four drugs are given at the outset of treatment. Of the most commonly used four drugs, rifampin and isoniazid are the best drugs for preventing resistance.[38]

Three subpopulations of mycobacteria are proposed to exist within the body, and each appears to respond to certain drugs.[35,38] Most numerous are the extracellular, rapidly dividing bacteria, often found within cavities (about 10^7-10^9 so-called "log phase" organisms). These are killed most readily by isoniazid, followed by rifampin.[38,39] A second group resides within caseating granulomas (possibly 10^5-10^7 organisms). These organisms appear to be in a semidormant state, with occasional bursts of metabolic activity. Pyrazinamide, through its conversion within *M. tuberculosis* to pyrazinoic acid, appears most active against these so-called "acid phase" organisms. The third subset is the intracellular mycobacteria present within macrophages (10^4-10^6) and other "non-replicating persisters."[39] Rifampin, bedaquiline, and pretomanid appear to be most active against these "nonreplicating" persisters. While this model explains what happens during the treatment of TB, there is no practical way to quantitate these mycobacterial subpopulations within a given patient.

Nonpharmacologic Therapy

7 Nonpharmacologic interventions aim to: (a) prevent the spread of TB, (b) find where TB has already spread using contact investigation, and (c) replenish the weakened (consumptive) infected person to a state of normal weight and well-being. The first two items are performed by public health departments. Clinicians involved in the treatment of TB should verify that the local health department has been notified of all new cases of TB.

Workers in hospitals and other institutions must prevent the spread of TB within their facilities.[28] All such workers should learn and follow each institution's infection control guidelines. This includes using personal protective equipment, including properly fitted respirators, and closing doors to "negative-pressure" rooms. These hospital isolation rooms draw air in from surrounding areas rather than blowing air (and *M. tuberculosis*) into these surrounding areas. The air from the isolation room may be treated with ultraviolet lights and then vented safely outside. However, these isolation rooms work properly only if the door is closed.

Debilitated persons infected with TB may require therapy for other medical problems, including substance abuse and HIV infection, and some may need nutritional support. Therefore, clinicians involved in substance abuse rehabilitation and nutritional support services should be familiar with the needs of persons infected with TB. Surgery may be needed to remove destroyed lung tissue, space-occupying infected lesions (*tuberculomas*), and certain extrapulmonary lesions.[24] BCG is the only clinically relevant vaccine for TB in use today. Although it is one of the most commonly administered vaccines in history, it is of limited value, and cannot prevent infection by *M. tuberculosis*. BCG (discussed further) may prevent extreme forms of TB in infants.[24]

Pharmacologic Therapy

Treating Latent Infection

The treatment of LTBI has been called *prophylaxis*. The keys to successful treatment of LTBI are: (a) infection by a drug-susceptible isolate, (b) adherence to the regimen, and (c) no exogenous reinfection.[40] Table 135-2 lists the first-line treatment options for latent tuberculosis.

Because young children, older adults, and HIV-positive persons are at greater risk of active disease once infected with *M. tuberculosis*, they require careful evaluation. Once active TB is ruled out, they should receive treatment for latent infection.[40]

There are three recommended treatment regimens for LTBI: 3 months of once-weekly isoniazid plus rifapentine; 4 months of daily rifampin or 3 months of daily isoniazid plus rifampin. Table 135-2 outlines recommended starting doses. The CDC recommends the 12-week isoniazid/rifapentine regimen as an equal alternative to

TABLE 135-2 Doses Recommended for Latent Tuberculosis Treatment Regimens

Drug	Duration	Dose
Isoniazid and rifapentine	Once weekly for 3 months	Adults and children > 12 years: Isoniazid: 15 mg/kg Rifapentine: 10-14 kg: 300 mg 14.1-25 kg: 450 mg 25.1-32 kg: 600 mg 32.1-49.9 kg: 750 mg ≥50 kg: 900 mg Children 2-11 years: Isoniazid: 25 mg/kg Rifapentine: see above
Isoniazid and rifampin	Daily for 3 months	Adult: Isoniazid: 5 mg/kg Rifampin: 10 mg/kg Children: Isoniazid: 10-20 mg/kg Rifampin: 15-20 mg/kg
Rifampin	Daily for 4 months	Adults: 10 mg/kg Children: 15-20 mg/kg

Data from Sterling TR, Njie G, Zenner D, et al. Guidelines for the Treatment of Latent Tuberculosis Infection: Recommendations from the National Tuberculosis Controllers Association and CDC, 2020. MMWR Recomm Rep. 2020;69:1.

9 months of daily isoniazid for treating LTBI in otherwise healthy patients aged 12 years or older who have a predictive factor for a greater likelihood of developing active TB. These include recent exposure to contagious TB, conversion from negative to positive on an indirect test for infection (ie, IGRA or TST), radiographic findings of healed pulmonary TB, and untreated HIV infection.[40] Twelve weeks of once-weekly isoniazid and rifapentine by DOT was compared with daily self-administered isoniazid for 9 months in over 8,000 participants.[41] The isoniazid and rifapentine regimen was not inferior in efficacy to self-administered isoniazid, had a significantly higher completion rate (82% vs. 69%), and was associated with fewer grade 3 or 4 adverse reactions (1.6% vs. 3%).[41,42] Hypersensitivity reactions were more common with the isoniazid/rifapentine regimen and close clinical follow-up should be undertaken. These regimens are effective and safe.[42] The disadvantages of rifamycin-based regimens are the drug interactions. Rifabutin has less pronounced interactions than rifampin and may be used in place of rifampin due to contraindications or drug interactions. HIV-infected patients who are otherwise healthy and are not taking antiretroviral medications are also included in this category. The 3-month rifapentine and isoniazid combination is recommended for HIV-positive persons providing drug interactions allow.[40] Drug interactions with rifapentine vary with the frequency of the dose and the affected companion drug. Precautions should be taken as HIV-infected patients are more likely to have extrapulmonary TB or pulmonary TB with normal findings on chest radiograph.

Alternative options for treatment of LTBI include 6 or 9 months of isoniazid which carry a higher toxicity risk and lower treatment completion rates due to the longer length of therapy.[40] For recent skin-test converters of all ages, the risk of active TB outweighs the risk for drug toxicity.[40] Pregnant females, persons who misuse alcohol, and those with poor diets who are treated with isoniazid should receive pyridoxine (vitamin B6) 10 to 50 mg daily to reduce the incidence of central nervous system (CNS) effects or peripheral neuropathies. All patients who receive treatment of LTBI should be monitored monthly for adverse drug reactions and for possible progression to active TB. Newer regimens under investigation include 1 month of daily rifapentine plus isoniazid (tested in HIV-positive patients to date), and 6 weeks of rifapentine daily alone. When resistance to isoniazid and rifampin is suspected in the isolate causing infection, there are no randomized controlled trials to prove what regimen should be used to treat LTBI among contacts.[40]

Treating Active Disease

8 The treatment of active TB requires the use of multiple drugs. There are two primary antituberculosis drugs, isoniazid and rifampin.[36,38] Isoniazid and rifampin should be used together whenever possible. Typically, *M. tuberculosis* is either susceptible or resistant to a given drug. Theoretically, minimal inhibitory concentration results could be used to guide dosing in the treatment of moderately resistant *M. tuberculosis*, but this remains to be studied prospectively.[36,38]

Drug-susceptibility testing should be done on the initial isolate for all patients with active TB. These data should guide the selection of drugs over the course of treatment.[35,43] However, some patients are unable to provide a suitable specimen for laboratory testing. If susceptibility data are not available for a given patient, the drug susceptibility data for the suspected source case or regional susceptibility data should be used.[35,43]

Drug resistance should be expected for patients presenting for the retreatment of TB. These patients require retesting of drug susceptibility using freshly collected specimens. It is imperative to learn what drugs the patient received and for how long the patient received them.[35] A treatment history, often called a *drug-o-gram*, shows the start and stop dates of all antimycobacterial drugs on a horizontal bar graph.[35] A drug-o-gram should be constructed for all retreatment patients.

9 The standard TB treatment regimen is isoniazid, rifampin, pyrazinamide, and ethambutol for 2 months, followed by isoniazid and rifampin for 4 months, a total of 6 months of treatment.[35] If susceptibility to isoniazid, rifampin, and pyrazinamide is shown, ethambutol can be stopped. Without pyrazinamide, a total of 9 months of isoniazid and rifampin treatment is required. Table 135-3 shows the recommended treatment regimens for drug susceptible tuberculosis. When intermittent therapy is used, DOT is essential. Doses missed during an intermittent TB regimen decrease its efficacy and increase the relapse rate. HIV-positive patients should not receive highly intermittent regimens. In general, regimens given daily five times each week or three times weekly can be used for HIV-positive patients. Less frequent dosing is associated with higher failure and relapse rates and the selection of rifampin-resistant organisms.[35]

When a patient's sputum smears convert to a negative, the risk of the patient infecting others is greatly reduced, but it is not zero.[35,44] Such patients can be removed from respiratory isolation, but they must be careful not to cough on others and should meet with others only in well-ventilated places. Smear-negative patients still may be culture positive, so they still can transmit TB to others.

Patients who are slow to respond clinically, those who remain culture-positive at 2 months of treatment, those with cavitary lesions on chest radiograph, and perhaps HIV-positive patients should be treated for a total of 9 months and for at least 6 months from the time that they convert to smear and culture negativity.[35,44] Some authors recommend therapeutic drug monitoring (TDM), the use of serum drug concentrations, to optimize therapy for such patients.[39,45,46] When isoniazid and rifampin cannot be used, treatment durations often become 2 years or more regardless of immune status.[35,44] The most promising shorter regimens for MDR-TB may be the combination of bedaquiline, pretomanid and linezolid, generally for 6 months.[47] The treatment of MDR-TB will continue to evolve.

10 Adjustments to the regimen should be made once the susceptibility data are available.[35] If the organism is drug-resistant, careful consideration of the remaining therapeutic options must be made. Two or more drugs with in vitro activity against the patient's isolate and that the patient has not received previously should be added to the regimen, as needed.[35,43] In the United States, there is no standard regimen for MDR-TB.[35,43,47] Each patient's exposure history, treatment history (including toxicity and adherence issues), and current susceptibility data must be considered simultaneously. *It is critical to avoid monotherapy, and it is critical to never add a single drug to a failing regimen.*[38,39] Adding one drug at a time leads to the sequential selection of drug resistance until there are no drugs left. TB specialists should be consulted regarding cases of MDR-TB. It may take several months for a patient with MDR-TB to become culture-negative because the drugs used lack the potency of isoniazid and rifampin.[35,46] Consequently, prolonged respiratory isolation may be required.

Drug resistance should be considered in the following situations:

1. Patients who have received prior therapy for TB.
2. Patients from areas with a high prevalence of resistance (South Africa, Dominican Republic, Peru, Southeast Asia, the Baltic countries, and the former Soviet states).
3. Patients who are unhoused, institutionalized, or use IV drugs, or who are infected with HIV.
4. Patients who still have AFB-positive sputum smears after 1 to 2 months of therapy.
5. Patients who still have positive cultures after 2 to 4 months of therapy.
6. Patients who fail treatment or relapse after treatment.
7. Patients known to be exposed to MDR-TB cases.

TABLE 135-3 Drug Regimens for Microbiologically Confirmed Pulmonary Tuberculosis Caused by Drug Susceptible Organisms

	Initial Phase		Continuation Phase		
Regimen	Drugs	Interval and Doses[a]	Drugs	Interval and Doses[a]	Comments[b,c]
1	Isoniazid Rifampin Pyrazinamide Ethambutol	Daily for 8 weeks 7 days/week for 56 doses or 5 days/week for 40 doses[d]	Isoniazid/ Rifampin	7 days/week for 126 doses or 5 days/week for 90 doses	This is preferred regimen for patient with newly diagnosed pulmonary tuberculosis.
2	Isoniazid Rifampin Pyrazinamide Ethambutol	Daily for 8 weeks 7 days/week for 56 doses or 5 days/week for 40 doses[d]	Isoniazid/ Rifampin	Three times weekly for 54 doses	Preferred alternative regimen in situations in which more frequent DOT during continuation phase is difficult to achieve.
3	Isoniazid Rifampin Pyrazinamide Ethambutol	Three times weekly for 8 weeks Three times weekly for 24 doses	Isoniazid/ Rifampin	Three times weekly for 54 doses	Caution in patients with HIV and/or cavitary disease. Missed doses can lead to treatment failure, relapse, and acquired drug resistance.
4	Isoniazid Rifampin Ethambutol Pyrazinamide	Daily for 2 weeks, then twice weekly for 6 weeks 7 days/week for 14 doses, then twice weekly for 12 doses[e]	Isoniazid/ Rifampin	Twice weekly for 36 doses	Do not use twice weekly regimens in HIV-infected patients or patients with smear positive and/or cavitary disease. If doses are missed, then therapy is equivalent to once weekly, which is inferior.

RIF, rifampin.

[a]When DOT is used, drugs may be given 5 days/week and the necessary number of doses adjusted accordingly. Although there are no studies that compare 5 with 7 daily doses, extensive experience indicates this would be an effective practice. DOT should be used when drugs are administered <7 days/week.

[b]Based on expert opinion, patients with cavitation on initial chest radiograph and positive cultures at completion of 2 months of therapy should receive a 7-month (31-week) continuation phase.

[c]Pyridoxine (vitamin B6), 25 to 50 mg/day, is given with isoniazid to all persons at risk of neuropathy (eg, pregnant women; breastfeeding infants; persons with HIV; patients with diabetes, alcoholism, malnutrition, or chronic renal failure; or patients with advanced age). For patients with peripheral neuropathy, experts recommend increasing pyridoxine dose to 100 mg/day.

[d]Five-day-a-week administration is always given by DOT.

[e]Alternatively, some US tuberculosis control programs have administered intensive-phase regimens 5 days/week for 15 doses (3 weeks), then twice weekly for 12 dose.

Reprinted, with permission, from Nahid P, et al. Executive Summary: Official American Thoracic Society/Centers for Disease Control and Prevention/Infectious Diseases Society of America Clinical Practice Guidelines: Treatment of drug-susceptible tuberculosis. Clin Infect Dis. 1 October 2016;63(7):853–867.

Empirical therapy with four or more drugs may be needed for acutely ill patients.[35] These regimens may be altered when the susceptibility pattern becomes known. If the index case is known, then the same effective regimen should be employed for the new case, with help from specialists. *XDR-TB* refers to "extensively drug-resistant TB." Such organisms are resistant to at least isoniazid, rifampin, a fluoroquinolone, and either bedaquiline or linezolid; refer such cases to specialists.[48,49]

Special Populations

Tuberculous Meningitis and Extrapulmonary Disease

Patients with CNS TB usually are treated for longer periods (9-12 months instead of 6 months).[35] In general, isoniazid, pyrazinamide, ethionamide, cycloserine, and linezolid penetrate the cerebrospinal fluid readily, but rifampin, ethambutol, and amikacin have variable CNS penetration.[39] Of the quinolones, levofloxacin may be preferred. Extrapulmonary TB of the soft tissues can be treated with conventional regimens.[35] TB of the bone typically is treated for 9 months, occasionally with surgical debridement.[35]

Children TB in children may be treated with regimens similar to those used in adults, although some physicians still prefer to extend treatment to 9 months.[35] Pediatric doses of isoniazid and rifampin on a milligram-per-kilogram basis are higher than those used in adults (Table 135-4).[35]

Pregnancy Females with TB should be cautioned against becoming pregnant because the disease poses a risk to the fetus and to the mother. If already pregnant, the usual treatment is isoniazid, rifampin, and ethambutol for 9 months.[50] Isoniazid and ethambutol are relatively safe for use in pregnant females.[50] B vitamins are particularly important during pregnancy and should be provided to females being treated for TB. Rifampin is associated rarely with birth defects, including limb reduction and CNS lesions.[35,50] In general, rifampin is used in pregnant females with TB. Pyrazinamide has not been studied in large numbers of pregnant women, but anecdotal data suggest that it may be safe.[35]

Aminoglycoside use during pregnancy may lead to hearing loss in the newborn, including complete deafness. Aminoglycosides must be reserved for critical situations where alternatives do not exist.[35] Although the polypeptide capreomycin has not been studied, it probably carries the same risks.

Ethionamide may cause premature delivery and congenital deformities when used during pregnancy.[35,50] Down syndrome also has been reported with ethionamide, so it cannot be recommended in this setting. *p*-Aminosalicylic acid has been used safely in pregnancy, but specific data are lacking.[50] Cycloserine is known to cross the placenta, but the effects on the developing fetus are not known. Therefore, cycloserine generally cannot be recommended during pregnancy.[50]

Ciprofloxacin, levofloxacin, moxifloxacin, and the other quinolones are associated with permanent damage to cartilage in the weight-bearing joints of immature animals, especially dogs and rabbits.[50] Although these drugs do not frequently cause joint problems in humans, other antituberculosis agents should be used during pregnancy.

Pregnant females with LTBI are not at the same level of risk compared with those with active disease. Therapy for LTBI may be delayed until after pregnancy. However, in the case of recent infection documented by a skin-test conversion or a newly positive IGRA and in immunosuppressed females who are found to have LTBI

TABLE 135-4 Suggested Starting Doses[a] of First-Line Antituberculosis Drugs for Adults and Children[b,c]

			Typical Doses			
Drug	**Preparation**	**Adults/Children**	**Daily**	**1× Per Week**	**2× Per Week**	**3× Per Week**
First-Line Drugs						
Isoniazid	Tablets (50, 100, 300 mg); elixir (50 mg/5 mL); aqueous solution (100 mg/mL) for IV or intramuscular injection	Adults[c]	5 mg/kg	15 mg/kg	15 mg/kg	15 mg/kg
		Children[c]	10-15 mg/kg	—	20-30 mg/kg	—
Rifampin	Capsule (150, 300 mg); powder may be suspended for oral administration; aqueous solution for IV injection	Adults[d,e]	10 mg/kg	—	10 mg/kg	10 mg/kg
		Children[c]	10-20 mg/kg	—	10-20 mg/kg	—
Rifabutin	Capsule (150 mg)	Adult[d,e]	5 mg/kg	—	—	—
		Children	Appropriate dosing for children is unknown	Appropriate dosing for children is unknown	Appropriate dosing for children is unknown	Appropriate dosing for children is unknown
Rifapentine	Tablet (150 mg, film coated)	Adults[c]	20 mg per kg daily is now being used for active TB	—	—	—
		Children	The drug is not approved for use in children	The drug is not approved for use in children	The drug is not approved for use in children	The drug is not approved for use in children
Pyrazinamide	Tablet (500 mg, scored)	Adults[c]	Weight 40-55 kg: 1,000 mg	—	Weight 40-55 kg: 2,000 mg	Weight 40-55 kg: 1,500 mg
			Weight 56-75 kg: 1,500 mg	—	Weight 56-75 kg: 3,000 mg	Weight 56-75 kg: 2,500 mg
			Weight 76-90 kg: 2,000 mg	—	Weight 76-90 kg: 4,000 mg	Weight 76-90 kg: 3,000 mg
		Children[c]	15-30 mg/kg	—	50 mg/kg	—
Ethambutol	Tablet (100, 400 mg)	Adults[c]	Weight 40-55 kg: 800 mg	—	Weight 40-55 kg: 2,000 mg	Weight 40-55 kg: 1,200 mg
			Weight 56-75 kg: 1,200 mg	—	Weight 56-75 kg: 2,800 mg	Weight 56-75 kg: 2,000 mg
			Weight 76-90 kg: 1,600 mg	—	Weight 76-90 kg: 4,000 mg	Weight 76-90 kg: 2,400 mg
		Children[d,e]	15-20 mg/kg daily	—	50 mg/kg	—

Higher doses of rifampin and rifapentine are being studied. Rifabutin dose may need to be adjusted when there is concomitant use of protease inhibitors or non-nucleoside reverse transcriptase inhibitors.

[a]Dose per weight is based on ideal body weight. Children weighing more than 40 kg should be dosed as adults.

[b]For purposes of this document, adult dosing begins at age 15 years.

[c]The authors of this chapter do not agree with the use of maximum doses, since this arbitrarily caps doses for patients who otherwise might need larger doses. These maximum doses were not based on prospective studies in large or overweight individuals, and do not consider patients with documented malabsorption of their medications. Clinical judgment should be used in such circumstances.

[d]The drug can likely be used safely in older children but should be used with caution in children younger than 5 years, in whom visual acuity cannot be monitored. In younger children, ethambutol at the dose of 15 mg/kg/day can be used if there is suspected or proven resistance to isoniazid or rifampin.

[e]It should be noted that, although this is the dose recommended generally, most clinicians with experience using cycloserine indicate that it is unusual for patients to be able to tolerate this amount. Serum concentration measurements are often useful in determining the optimal dose for a given patient.

Data from Reference 36.

while pregnant, treatment for LTBI is started during the second trimester of pregnancy.[40,50] Although most antituberculosis drugs are excreted in breast milk, the amount of drug received by the infant through nursing is insufficient to cause toxicity. Quinolones should be avoided in nursing mothers.[51]

HIV Infection For drug-susceptible strains of tuberculosis, patients with AIDS and other immunocompromised hosts may be managed with chemotherapeutic regimens similar to those used in immunocompetent individuals, although treatment is often extended to 9 months (see Table 135-3).[23,35] The precise duration to recommend remains a matter of debate. Highly intermittent regimens (twice or once weekly) are not recommended for HIV-positive TB patients. Rifamycin-based treatments are most effective; however, agents should be selected based on susceptibility and HIV drug interactions. Prognosis has been particularly poor for HIV-infected patients infected with MDR-TB, so all efforts should be made to reduce the time between clinical presentation, diagnosis of TB, and start of appropriate treatment. Recommendations for management of HIV and TB published by the World Health Organization (WHO) and others have provided guidance on monitoring of treatment, side effects, and drug interactions of HIV and TB, MDR, and XDR-TB.[23,52] The timing for antiretroviral treatment in patients with TB and HIV is unclear. In patients with CD4 cell counts <200/mm³ (0.20 × 10⁹/L) or <50/mm³ (0.05 × 10⁹/L) reductions in mortality have been seen when antiretroviral treatment was initiated within 2 weeks of antituberculosis treatment.[52,53] Differentiation must be made between infection with *M. tuberculosis* and nontuberculous mycobacteria, such as *M. avium* complex, because the drugs used are different. While awaiting laboratory results, the patient can be treated empirically for TB if there is any doubt about the causative organism. Some patients with AIDS malabsorb their oral medications; this is discussed in the "Therapeutic Drug Monitoring" section below.[45]

Renal Failure For nearly all patients, isoniazid and rifampin do not require dose modification in renal failure. They are eliminated primarily by the liver.[39] In the unlikely event that peripheral neuropathies develop, the frequency of isoniazid dosing may be reduced. Pyrazinamide and ethambutol typically require a reduction in dosing frequency from daily to three times weekly (Table 135-5).[35,39]

Renally cleared TB drugs include the aminoglycosides (amikacin, kanamycin, and streptomycin), capreomycin, ethambutol, cycloserine, and levofloxacin.[35,39,54] Dosing intervals need to be extended for these drugs (Table 135-5). Moxifloxacin is approximately 50% cleared by the kidneys but may not require a change in dose from once daily, as used for TB. The metabolites of isoniazid, pyrazinamide, and *p*-aminosalicylic acid are cleared primarily by the kidneys. The role of these metabolites in causing toxicity is unknown, so their accumulation in renal failure may carry some risk.

Ethionamide and its sulfoxide metabolite are hepatically cleared, so dosing is unchanged.[35,54] *p*-Aminosalicylic acid is converted largely to metabolites prior to renal elimination; these metabolites may accumulate in renal failure.[54,55] For patients on hemodialysis, the usual 12-hour dosing interval for *p*-aminosalicylic acid granules seems to be safe. Dialysis will remove the metabolites. Serum concentration monitoring must be performed for cycloserine to avoid dose-related toxicities in renal failure patients.[55] Data regarding peritoneal dialysis are lacking. Ethambutol should be avoided in peritoneal dialysis patients, based on anecdotal evidence.

Hepatic Failure Antituberculosis drugs that rely on hepatic clearance for most of their elimination include isoniazid, rifampin, pyrazinamide, ethionamide, and *p*-aminosalicylic acid.[39] Moxifloxacin is approximately 50% cleared by the liver. Elevations of serum transaminase concentrations generally are not correlated with the residual capacity of the liver to metabolize drugs, so these markers cannot be used as guides for drug dosing. Furthermore, isoniazid, rifampin, pyrazinamide, and, to a lesser degree, ethionamide, *p*-aminosalicylic acid, and, rarely, ethambutol may cause hepatotoxicity.[35,38,39] For some patients with drug-susceptible TB, a "liver-sparing" regimen may include linezolid, amikacin, levofloxacin, or ethambutol, at least temporarily.[35,38,39] Because this regimen requires 18 or more months of treatment to be successful, patients usually are switched to isoniazid- and rifampin-containing regimens as soon as they are able.

Morbid Obesity Data are not available for dosing the TB drugs for patients with morbid obesity.[39] Relatively hydrophilic drugs (isoniazid, pyrazinamide, the aminoglycosides, capreomycin, *p*-aminosalicylic acid, and cycloserine) can be dosed initially based on ideal body weight. Low or high serum concentrations can be avoided by checking the serum concentrations.[45]

The TB Drugs

The interested reader is referred to several other publications for more detailed information regarding these drugs (see Table 135-4).[35,44,45] The "maximum" dose for a given patient is the dose that produces the desired response with an acceptable level of toxicity.[45] This can only be determined on a case-by-case basis. Artificially capping doses may deprive patients of needed drug.

Primary Antituberculosis Drugs

Isoniazid Isoniazid is one of the two most important TB drugs. It is highly specific for mycobacteria, with a minimal inhibitory concentration against *M. tuberculosis* of 0.01 to 0.25 mcg/mL (mg/L;

TABLE 135-5 Dosing Recommendations for Adult Patients with Reduced Renal Function and for Adult Patients Receiving Hemodialysis

Drug	Change in Frequency?	Recommended Dose and Frequency for Patients with Creatinine Clearance <30 mL/min (0.50 mL/s)[a,b,c,d]
Isoniazid	No change	300 mg once daily or 900 mg three times per week
Rifampin	No change	600 mg once daily or 600 mg three times per week
Pyrazinamide	Yes	25-35 mg/kg per dose three times per week (not daily)
Ethambutol	Yes	15-25 mg/kg per dose three times per week (not daily)
Levofloxacin	Yes	750-1,000 mg per dose three times per week (not daily)
Cycloserine	Yes	250 mg once daily, or 500 mg/dose three times per week[e]
Ethionamide	No change	250-500 mg/dose daily
p-Aminosalicylic acid	No change	4 g/dose, twice daily
Streptomycin	Yes	12-15 mg/kg per dose two or three times per week (not daily)
Capreomycin	Yes	12-15 mg/kg per dose two or three times per week (not daily)
Kanamycin	Yes	12-15 mg/kg per dose two or three times per week (not daily)
Amikacin	Yes	12-15 mg/kg per dose two or three times per week (not daily)

[a]Standard doses are given unless there is intolerance.

[b]The medications should be given after hemodialysis on the day of hemodialysis.

[c]Monitoring of serum drug concentrations should be considered to ensure adequate drug absorption, without excessive accumulation, and to assist in avoiding toxicity.

[d]Data are not available for patients receiving peritoneal dialysis. Until data become available, begin with doses recommended for patients receiving hemodialysis and verify adequacy of dosing, using serum concentration monitoring.

[e]The appropriateness of 250-mg daily doses has not been established. There should be careful monitoring for evidence of neurotoxicity.

Reprinted, with permission, from Nahid P, et al. Executive Summary: Official American Thoracic Society/Centers for Disease Control and Prevention/Infectious Diseases Society of America Clinical Practice Guidelines: Treatment of drug-susceptible tuberculosis. Clin Infect Dis. 1 October 2016;63(7):853–867.

0.07-1.82 μmol/L). It is bactericidal and is thought to inhibit mycolic acid synthesis and disruption of the cell wall in susceptible organisms.[56] Most nontuberculous mycobacteria such as *M. avium* are resistant to isoniazid, although *M. kansasii* and *M. xenopi* are susceptible. The most common mechanisms of resistance result from mutations in the *katG* or *inhA* genes.[56]

Isoniazid is readily absorbed from the GI tract and from intramuscular injection sites. It also can be given as a short IV infusion over 5 minutes if diluted in about 20 mL of normal saline.[57] Isoniazid should be given on an empty stomach whenever possible.[57] *N*-Acetyltransferase 2 forms the principal metabolite acetylisoniazid, which lacks antimycobacterial activity. The rate at which humans acetylate isoniazid is determined genetically; slow acetylation is an autosomal recessive trait and reflects a relative lack of *N*-acetyltransferase 2. Fast acetylators have isoniazid half-lives of less than 2 hours. Approximately 50% of Whites and Blacks and 80% to 90% of Asians and Native Alaskans are rapid acetylators. Slow acetylators have isoniazid half-lives of 3 to 4 hours and may be at an increased risk of neurotoxicity. The association of acetylator status and risk of hepatotoxicity, however, appears to be weak.[56] Poor absorption and rapid clearance of isoniazid for patients receiving highly intermittent therapy are associated with poor clinical outcomes.[56,58]

Transient elevations of the serum transaminases occur in 12% to 15% of patients receiving isoniazid and usually occur within the first 8 to 12 weeks of therapy.[35] Overt hepatotoxicity, however, occurs in only 1% of cases. Risk factors for hepatotoxicity include patient age, preexisting liver disease, excessive alcohol intake, pregnancy, coadministration of other medications that are potentially hepatotoxic, and the postpartum state. Isoniazid also may result in neurotoxicity, most frequently presenting as peripheral neuropathy or, in overdose, as seizures and coma. Patients with pyridoxine deficiency, such as pregnant females, persons who misuse alcohol, children, and the malnourished, are at increased risk. Isoniazid may inhibit the metabolism of phenytoin, carbamazepine, primidone, and warfarin.[38] Patients who are being treated with these agents should be monitored closely, and appropriate dose adjustments should be made when necessary.

Rifampin The introduction of rifampin into routine use during the 1970s allowed for true short-course treatment of TB (6-9 months).[35] Without rifampin, treatment is generally 18 months or longer. Drug resistance to rifampin is an ominous prognostic factor because it is frequently associated with isoniazid resistance and leaves the patient with few good therapeutic options. Clinicians *must* take care to protect susceptibility to rifampin by carefully treating their patients. Rifampin shows bactericidal activity against *M. tuberculosis* and several other mycobacterial species, including *M. bovis* and *M. kansasii*.[59] It is also active against a broad array of other bacteria. Alteration of the target site on RNA polymerase, primarily through changes in the *rpoB* gene, leads to most forms of rifampin resistance.[35,59]

Rifampin usually is given orally, but it also can be given as a 30-minute IV infusion.[59] Oral doses are best given on an empty stomach.[60] Patients with AIDS, diabetes, and other GI problems have difficulty absorbing rifampin after oral doses, and this has been associated with therapeutic failures in some cases.[35,59,61] Rifampin is metabolized to 25-desacetyl rifampin, which retains some of rifampin's activity; most of rifampin and its metabolite are cleared in the bile. Rifampin generally is given at 600 mg daily or intermittently, although this dose does not take full advantage of rifampin's concentration-dependent killing.[39,45] Higher doses (1,200-2,400 mg) are being considered based on clinical trials.[62]

Elevations in hepatic enzymes have been attributed to rifampin in 10% to 15% of patients, with overt hepatotoxicity occurring in less than 1%.[35,59] More frequent adverse effects of rifampin include rash, fever, and GI distress. Allergic reactions to rifampin have been reported and occur more frequently with intermittent rifampin doses 900 mg or more twice weekly. These reactions may take the form of a flu-like syndrome with development of fever, chills, headache, arthralgias, and, rarely, hypotension and shock.[36] Alternatively, hemolytic anemia or acute renal failure may occur, requiring permanent discontinuation.

Rifampin's potent induction of hepatic enzymes, especially cytochrome P450 3A4, may enhance the elimination of many other drugs, most notably the protease inhibitors used to treat HIV (Table 135-6). HIV-positive patients may benefit from the use of rifabutin instead of rifampin.[23,35,60] Furthermore, women who use oral contraceptives must use another form of contraception during therapy because increased clearance of the hormones may lead to unexpected pregnancies. Patient records should be reviewed for potential drug interactions before dispensing rifampin. Rifampin may turn urine and other secretions orange-red and may permanently stain some types of contact lenses.

Other Rifamycins Rifabutin is used for disseminated *M. avium* infection in AIDS patients and is quite active against *M. tuberculosis*. Most rifampin-resistant organisms are resistant to rifabutin. Because rifabutin is a less potent enzyme inducer than rifampin, it may be used for patients who are receiving HIV protease inhibitors.[36,50,61,62] For HIV-positive patients, the American Thoracic Society/CDC recommends regimens with three or more doses of the TB drugs per week (see Table 135-3). Rifapentine is a long-acting rifamycin that has been tested as part of a 4-month regimen that includes moxifloxacin for selected TB patients.[63] It is approximately as potent an enzyme inducer as rifampin, so similar drug interactions are likely.[52,64]

Pyrazinamide Adding pyrazinamide to the first 2 months of treatment with isoniazid and rifampin shortens the duration to 6 months for most patients.[35] Pyrazinamide may be bacteriostatic or bactericidal depending on the concentration and the susceptibility of the organism. It is usually well absorbed and displays a fairly long half-life.[39,65] The most common toxicities of pyrazinamide are GI distress, arthralgias, and elevations in the serum uric acid concentrations.[35,44] Most patients do not experience true gout. Hepatotoxicity is the major limiting adverse effect and is dose-related when pyrazinamide is given daily.

A fixed-combination product (rifater) of rifampin 120 mg, isoniazid 50 mg, and pyrazinamide 300 mg is designed to prevent drug resistance by keeping the self-medicating patient from using only one drug at a time. If the patient is receiving DOT, there is no particular advantage to this product. The typical dose of rifater will be five to six tablets daily. When pyrazinamide is discontinued after 2 months of treatment, the combination product rifamate (isoniazid 150 mg and rifampin 300 mg) can be substituted.

Ethambutol Ethambutol replaced *p*-aminosalicylic acid as a first-line agent in the 1960s because it was better tolerated by patients.[39] It is used as a fourth drug for TB while awaiting susceptibility data and its use is intended to prevent emergence of rifampin resistance.[35,44] If the organism is susceptible to isoniazid, rifampin, and pyrazinamide, ethambutol can be stopped. Ethambutol is active against most mycobacteria, by inhibiting synthesis of metabolites and impairing cell metabolism, and is generally bacteriostatic.

Ethambutol should not be given with antacids.[66,67] For patients with renal failure, the ethambutol dose should be reduced to three times per week.[68] Retrobulbar neuritis is the major adverse effect. Patients may complain of a change in visual acuity, the inability to see the color green, or both. They should be monitored monthly while on the drug using Snellen wall charts for visual acuity and Ishihara red-green color discrimination cards.[35]

Quinolones Levofloxacin and moxifloxacin are sometimes used to treat MDR-TB because of their excellent activity against

TABLE 135-6 Recommended Regimens for the Concomitant Treatment of TB and HIV Infection in Adults

Combined Regimen for Treatment of HIV and TB	Pharmacokinetic Effect of the Rifamycin	Tolerability/Toxicity	Antiviral Activity When Used with Rifamycin	Recommendations (Comments)
Efavirenz-based antiretroviral therapy[a] with rifampin-based TB treatment	Well-characterized, modest decrease in concentrations in some patients	Low rates of discontinuation	Excellent	Preferred (efavirenz should not be used during the first trimester of pregnancy)
PI-based antiretroviral therapy[a] with rifabutin-based TB treatment	Little effect of rifabutin on PI concentrations, but marked increases in rifabutin concentrations	Low rates of discontinuation (if rifabutin is appropriately dose-reduced)	Favorable, although published clinical experience is not extensive	Preferred for patients unable to take efavirenz[b] (caution to ensure patients who discontinue PI not to continue to receive reduced rifabutin dose)
Nevirapine-based antiretroviral therapy with rifampin-based TB treatment	Moderate decrease in concentrations	Concern about hepatotoxicity when used with isoniazid, rifampin, and pyrazinamide	Suboptimal when nevirapine is initiated using once-daily dosing largely favorable when nevirapine is given twice daily throughout cotreatment	Alternative for patients who cannot take efavirenz, though efavirenz is preferred (nevirapine should not be initiated among women with CD4 > 250 cells/μL [0.25 × 10^9/L] or men with CD4 > 400 cells/μL [0.40 × 10^9/L])
Raltegravir-based antiretroviral therapy with rifampin-based TB treatment	Significant decrease in concentrations with standard dosing	Limited experience	Limited published clinical experience	Alternative at higher doses for patients who cannot take efavirenz and who have baseline viral load <100,000 copies/mL (100 × 10^6/L)
Dolutegravir-based antiretroviral therapy with rifampin-based TB-treatment	Coadministration with rifampicin results in decreases in dolutegravir plasma exposure requiring increased dose of dolutegravir	Limited experience	Limited published clinical experience	Alternative for patients who cannot take efavirenz
Zidovudine/lamivudine/abacavir/tenofovir with rifampin-based TB treatment	50% decrease in zidovudine, possible effect on abacavir not evaluated	Anemia	No published clinical experience, but this regimen is less effective than efavirenz- or atazanavir-based regimens in persons not taking rifampin	Alternative for patients who cannot take efavirenz or nevirapine and if rifabutin not available
Zidovudine/lamivudine/tenofovir with rifampin-based TB treatment	50% decrease in zidovudine, no other effects predicted	Anemia	Favorable, but not evaluated in a randomized trial	Alternative for patients who cannot take efavirenz and abacavir and if rifabutin not available
Zidovudine/lamivudine/abacavir with rifampin-based TB treatment	50% decrease in zidovudine, possible effect on abacavir not evaluated	Anemia	Early favorable experience, but this combination is less effective than efavirenz- or nevirapine-based regimens in persons not taking rifampin	Alternative for patients who cannot take efavirenz and tenofovir and if rifabutin not available
Superboosted[c] lopinavir-based antiretroviral therapy or double dose lopinavir/ritonavir-based therapy with rifampin-based TB treatment	Moderate decrease in concentrations	Hepatitis	Early favorable experience of super-boosting among young children and double dose among adults already on antiretroviral drugs at the time of rifampin initiation	Alternative if rifabutin not available; double dose an option among adults already taking lopinavir-based antiretroviral therapy and virologically suppressed at the time of tuberculosis treatment initiation; super boosting has not been adequately tested in adults but may be effective

[a]With two nucleoside analogues.

[b]Includes patients with NNRTI-resistant HIV, those unable to tolerate efavirenz, and women during the first one to two trimesters of pregnancy.

[c]Super boosting of lopinavir is achieved by giving lopinavir 400 mg together with 400 mg ritonavir twice daily. Double dose lopinavir/ritonavir is lopinavir 800 mg plus ritonavir 200 mg twice daily.

Data from Managing Drug Interactions in the Treatment of HIV-Related Tuberculosis. 2013. Available at: https://www.cdc.gov/tb/publications/guidelines/tb_hiv_drugs/recommendations02.htm.

M. tuberculosis. Table 135-7 lists WHO proposed categories of drugs for treating MDR-TB and XDR-TB. Moxifloxacin is a possible replacement for certain first-line agents.[69,70] Moxifloxacin has been compared with isoniazid and ethambutol during the first 8 weeks of therapy for pulmonary TB. There was no significant increase in 8-week culture negativity when compared with isoniazid. However, shorter time to culture conversion was seen when compared with ethambutol.[70] Quinolones are useful because most are available in oral and IV dosage forms, so they can be used in critically ill patients. However, resistance of MTB to the fluoroquinolones is a major concern. Resistance is attributed to mutations in the gyrA and gyrB genes and can develop in a relatively short period of time.[59,71]

TABLE 135-7 The WHO Proposed Categories of Drugs for Treating MDR- and XDR-TB[a]

Groups and steps	Medicine
Group A: Include all three medicines	Levofloxacin or moxifloxacin
	Bedaquiline[b,c]
	Linezolid[d]
Group B: Add one or both medicines	Clofazimine
	Cycloserine or terizidone
	Ethambutol
	Delamanid[d]
	Pyrazinamide[f]
Group C: Add to complete the regimen and when medicines from Groups A and B cannot be used	Imipenem–cilastatin or meropenem[g]
	Amikacin (or streptomycin)[h]
	Ethionamide orprothionamide[i]
	P-aminosalicylic acidi

ECG: electrocardiogram; GDG: Guideline Development Group; IPD: individual patient data; LPA: line probe assay.

[a]This table is intended to guide the design of individualized, longer MDR-TB regimens medicines in Group C are ranked by decreasing order of usual preference for use, subject to other considerations.

[b]*Adapted from Nahid P, et al. Executive Summary: Official American Thoracic Society/Centers for Disease Control and Prevention/Infectious Diseases Society of America Clinical Practice Guidelines: Treatment of drug-susceptible tuberculosis. Clin Infect Dis. 1 October 2016;63(7):853–867.*

[c]In 2019, new evidence on the concurrent use of bedaquiline and delamanid was made available to the GDG. With regard to safety, the GDG concluded that the data suggest no additional safety concerns regarding concurrent use of bedaquiline and delamanid. Both medicines may be used concurrently in patients who have limited other treatment options available to them, provided that sufficient monitoring (including baseline and follow-up ECG and electrolyte monitoring) is in place. The data on the effectiveness of concurrent use of bedaquiline and delamanid were reviewed by the GDG, but owing to the limited evidence and potential residual confounding in the data, the GDG was unable to proceed with a recommendation on effectiveness.

[d]Use of linezolid for at least 6 months has been shown to increase effectiveness, although toxicity may limit use.

[e]Evidence on the safety and effectiveness of delamanid beyond 6 months and in children aged under 3 years was insufficient for review. The use of delamanid beyond these limits should follow best practices in "off-label" use.

[f]Pyrazinamide is counted as an effective agent only when confirmed susceptibility.

[g]Every dose of imipenem–cilastatin and meropenem is administered with clavulanic acid, which is available only in formulations combined with amoxicillin. Amoxicillin–clavulanic acid is not counted as an additional effective TB agent and should not be used without imipenem–cilastatin or meropenem.

[h]Amikacin and streptomycin are to be considered only when confirmed susceptibility, and if high-quality audiometry monitoring for hearing loss can be ensured. Streptomycin is to be considered only if amikacin cannot be used and confirmed susceptibility (ie, resistance to streptomycin is not detectable with second-line molecular LPAs and phenotypic drug-susceptibility testing is required). Kanamycin and capreomycin are no longer recommended for use in MDR-TB regimens.

[i]These agents showed effectiveness only in regimens without bedaquiline, linezolid, clofazimine, or delamanid, and are thus proposed only when other options to compose a regimen are not possible.

Bedaquiline Bedaquiline is a diarylquinoline that operates by a new mechanism which targets the ATP synthase pump and depletes cellular energy stores and does not demonstrate cross-resistance with existing TB drugs.[72,73] The WHO and CDC have issued recommendations stating that bedaquiline may be used at a dose of 400 mg daily for 2 weeks and then 200 mg three times a week for 22 weeks of treatment in adults with pulmonary MDR-TB when an effective treatment regimen cannot otherwise be provided.[74] Bedaquiline may be used on a case-by-case basis in children, HIV-infected persons, pregnant females, and in individuals with extrapulmonary TB. Patients treated with bedaquiline should be closely monitored every week for potential side effects and an electrocardiogram (QT monitoring) should be performed at baseline and at weeks 2, 12, and 24.[71,74] The QT monitoring is required due to a black box warning issued by the FDA as a result of increased rates of death due to QT prolongation in patients receiving bedaquiline.[72,73]

Linezolid Linezolid is a synthetic inhibitor of ribosomal translation that has been used for drug-resistant Gram-positive infections since 2000.[71] It has oral bioavailability near 100% that is not affected by food.[71,75] Clearance involves oxidation of the morpholine ring, and renal elimination of parent drug plus metabolites.[59,71,75] CSF concentrations are 57% of plasma.[75] The most frequently used dose for TB is 600 mg once daily. Higher doses appear to be more toxic.[35,74,76] Trough concentrations are associated with mitochondrial toxicity, leading to cytopenias and peripheral and ocular neuropathies.[71] Rifampin can reduce linezolid plasma exposure by about a third.[71] Linezolid is a weak inhibitor of monoamine oxidase and should usually not be used with MAOIs, SSRIs or triptans due to reports of serotonergic syndrome.[75]

Clofazimine Clofazimine is a drug with good activity against *M. leprae* and some activity against *M. tuberculosis* and *M. avium*. It is used in doses of 100 mg daily in advanced cases of MDR-TB or *M. avium* complex, especially when therapeutic options are limited.[35,39] The drug has a terminal elimination half-life that is weeks long. GI distress and skin discoloration are the most important adverse reactions. Although uncommon, severe GI pain may occur because of deposition of clofazimine crystals within the intestines; this may require surgical correction.[75]

Delamanid and Pretomanid Delamanid and Pretomanid are nitroimidazole derivatives that are chemically related to metronidazole and work through inhibiting mycolic acid synthesis.[75,77] These agents have potent in vitro and in vivo activity with low minimal inhibitory concentrations against *M. tuberculosis*.[78] Delamanid has centralized marketing authorization by the European Medicines Agency for use in the European Union.[78] Pretomanid is FDA-approved as part of a regimen including bedaquiline and linezolid, the so-called BPaL regimen. Food increases pretomanid absorption.[73,79] Pretomanid is metabolized by multiple reductive and oxidative pathways, with CYP3A4 responsible for approximately 20%.[70] Efavirenz reduces the AUC of pretomanid by 35%, and rifampin reduces the AUC by 66%.[73,79] Combinations of pretomanid with other antituberculosis drugs are also being investigated.

Beta-lactams: Imipenem, Meropenem, and Ceftazidime Imipenem and meropenem are synthetic carbapenems, and ceftazidime is a third-generation cephalosporin.[59,75] These antibiotics target penicillin-binding proteins which are involved in bacterial cell-wall synthesis.[59,75] Resistance occurs by enzymatic degradation. Specifically, *M. tuberculosis* possesses an extended spectrum class A β-lactamase (BlaC), which must be inactivated.[75] Clavulanic acid and avibactam are beta-lactamase inhibitors that prevent the enzymatic degradation caused by β-lactamase.[59,75,80] Clavulanic acid can be given orally (only in combination with amoxicillin); the other drugs are given intravenously.[71] Dosing has been empiric, and has not been established. Imipenem has been dosed at 1,000 mg 12 hours and meropenem at 1,000 mg 8 hours, intravenously.

Aminoglycosides Streptomycin, amikacin, and kanamycin are active against mycobacteria, and amikacin is preferred for TB. Aminoglycosides are given IM or IV and are renally cleared by glomerular filtration. They must be dosed appropriately in patients with renal dysfunction.[45,79]

Aminoglycosides occasionally cause nephrotoxicity, although it tends to be mild and reversible. They also cause ototoxicity (vestibular and cochlear), which may become permanent with continued use.[59,79] Older patients and those receiving long durations of treatment are most likely to experience hearing loss, whereas vestibular toxicity is highly unpredictable.[59]

Ethionamide Ethionamide shares structural features with two other antimycobacterial agents, isoniazid and thiacetazone, a drug not used in the United States. Prothionamide, the n-propyl derivative of ethionamide, is used in Europe. Ethionamide is only active against organisms of the genus *Mycobacterium*, and it should be considered primarily bacteriostatic because it is difficult to achieve serum concentrations that would be bactericidal.[39,59] GI toxicity is the dose-limiting adverse effect. The drug should be introduced gradually in 250-mg increments, as described earlier for cycloserine. Rarely will a patient tolerate more than 1,000 mg daily in divided oral doses. Ethionamide may be administered with a light snack or prior to bedtime to minimize GI intolerance. Food does not affect absorption significantly.[81] Little ethionamide is recovered in the urine, so doses remain the same in renal failure.[55] Ethionamide may cause goiter with or without hypothyroidism (especially when given with p-aminosalicylic acid), gynecomastia, alopecia, impotence, menorrhagia, and photodermatitis. The management of diabetes also may be more difficult for patients receiving ethionamide. Because of these problems, ethionamide only is used when necessary.

p-Aminosalicylic Acid In the United States, only the enteric-coated, sustained-release granule form (Paser) is available.[39,82] GI disturbances are the most common adverse effects from *p*-aminosalicylic acid. Diarrhea is usually self-limited, with symptoms improving after the first 1 to 2 weeks of therapy. Occasionally, a few doses of an opioid will resolve the problem. It also is important to tell the patient that the empty granules will appear in the stool. Although FDA-approved for three daily doses, pharmacokinetic data support twice-daily dosing.[83,84]

Various types of malabsorption, including steatorrhea, were reported with previous dosage forms of *p*-aminosalicylic acid. Hypersensitivity and, rarely, severe hepatitis may occur. *p*-Aminosalicylic acid is known to produce goiter, with or without myxedema, which seems to occur more frequently with concomitant ethionamide therapy.[39,59]

Other New Drugs and Delivery Systems Other new drugs in Phase II trials for treatment of TB include: Delpazolid (LCB01-0371) and sutezolid (PNU-100480) that target protein synthesis. SQ-109 is a new chemical class that targets MmpL3, an essential membrane transporter involved in the building of the mycolic acids as part of the outer membrane of mycobacteria. Macozinone (PBTZ-169) targets the flavoenzyme DprE1, blocking the synthesis of the cell wall precursor decaprenyl phosphoarabinose and provoking lysis of the *M. tuberculosis*. Liposomes are under investigation as delivery systems for various agents against mycobacteria, including isoniazid, rifampin, and the aminoglycosides. By changing the pharmacokinetic profile of such agents, their use in the treatment of mycobacterial infections could be enhanced greatly.

Corticosteroids Adjunctive therapy with corticosteroids may be of benefit for some patients with tuberculous meningitis or pericarditis to relieve inflammation and pressure.[35] They should be avoided in most other circumstances because they detract from the immune response to TB.

Bacille Calmette-Guérin Vaccine The BCG vaccine is an attenuated, hybridized strain of *M. bovis*. It was developed in 1921 and is used as a prophylactic vaccine against TB. Administration of BCG vaccine is compulsory in many developing countries and is officially recommended in many others. Vaccination with BCG produces a subclinical infection resulting in sensitization of T lymphocytes and cross-immunity to *M. tuberculosis*, as well as cutaneous hypersensitivity and, in many cases, a positive TST.

The efficacy of several different BCG preparations ranged from negative 56% (some patients did worse with the vaccine) to positive 80%.[36,85] The primary benefit of BCG vaccination appears to be the prevention of severe forms of TB in children.[86] The incidence of tuberculous meningitis and miliary TB is 52% to 100% lower and incidence of pulmonary TB is 2% to 80% lower in vaccinated children younger than 15 years than it was in unvaccinated controls.[86,87]

Side effects occur in 1% to 10% of vaccinated persons and usually include severe or prolonged ulceration at the vaccination site, lymphadenitis, and lupus vulgaris. Pregnant women and patients with impaired immune systems, including those with HIV infection, should avoid vaccination. The WHO had recommended, however, that in populations where the risk of TB is high, HIV-infected infants who are asymptomatic should receive BCG vaccine at birth or as soon as possible thereafter. Because BCG infection has occurred in AIDS patients given the vaccine, individuals with symptomatic HIV infection should not be vaccinated.[35]

THERAPEUTIC DRUG MONITORING

TDM, or applied pharmacokinetics, generally should be used if patients are failing appropriate treatment (no clinical improvement after 2-4 weeks or smear positive after 4-6 weeks).[45,79,88] Patients with AIDS, diabetes, obesity, cystic fibrosis, various GI disorders, or MDR-TB may be tested prospectively, before problems arise, to ensure adequate treatment. Blood samples collected at 2 and 6 hours after a dose have been used with some success, although they may not be the optimal sampling times for all the drugs.[89,90] Finally, TDM of the TB and HIV drugs is perhaps the most logical way to untangle the complex drug interactions that take place.[52,91]

EVALUATION OF THERAPEUTIC OUTCOMES

Monitoring of the Pharmaceutical Care Plan

The most serious problem with TB therapy is patient nonadherence to the prescribed regimens.[35] Unfortunately, there is no reliable way to identify such patients a priori. Noncompliance rates of up to 89% have been reported with TB therapy.[89,92] It is critical to the control of TB that such adherence rates be improved dramatically. The most effective way to achieve this end is with DOT.[35] Despite criticisms that it will cost more money, DOT is far cheaper in the long run to prevent the further spread of disease with DOT than to track down and treat additional cases of TB continuously.

The homeless and other underprivileged individuals are often assumed to constitute a group of patients considered "unreliable," and DOT should be reserved for them; it is also assumed that "responsible" patients cared for by private physicians may be treated with daily, unsupervised therapy. However, outcomes (sputum culture conversion to negative at 3 months) for patients with pulmonary TB who were treated by private physicians were compared with outcomes for patients treated via DOT in a city-run clinic. Three-month culture conversion occurred in only 40% of the private-care patients, compared with 90% in the city clinic-care patients.[89,92] Clearly, expansion of the use of DOT to nearly all patients with TB may be of benefit.

Patients who are AFB-smear positive should have sputum samples sent for AFB stains every 1 to 2 weeks until two consecutive smears are negative. This provides early evidence of a response to treatment.[35] Once on maintenance therapy, sputum cultures can be performed monthly until two consecutive cultures are negative, which generally occurs over 2 to 3 months. If sputum cultures continue to be positive after 2 months, drug-susceptibility testing should be repeated, and serum concentrations of the drugs should be checked.

TABLE 135-8 Antituberculosis Drug Monitoring Table

Drug	Adverse Effects	Monitoring
Isoniazid	Asymptomatic elevation of aminotransferases, clinical hepatitis, fatal hepatitis, peripheral neurotoxicity, CNS effects, lupus-like syndrome, hypersensitivity, monoamine poisoning, diarrhea	LFT monthly in patients who have preexisting liver disease or who develop abnormal liver function that does not require discontinuation of drug; dosage adjustments may be necessary in patients receiving anticonvulsants or warfarin
Rifampin	Cutaneous reactions, GI reactions (nausea, anorexia, abdominal pain), flu-like syndrome, hepatotoxicity, severe immunologic reactions, orange discoloration of bodily fluids (sputum, urine, sweat, tears), drug interactions due to induction of hepatic microsomal enzymes	Liver enzymes and interacting drugs as needed (eg, warfarin)
Rifabutin	Hematologic toxicity, uveitis, GI symptoms, polyarthralgias, hepatotoxicity, pseudojaundice (skin discoloration with normal bilirubin), rash, flu-like syndrome, orange discoloration of bodily fluids (sputum, urine, sweat, tears)	Drug interactions are less problematic than rifampin
Rifapentine	Similar to those associated with rifampin	Drug interactions are being investigated and are likely similar to rifampin
Pyrazinamide	Hepatotoxicity, GI symptoms (nausea, vomiting), nongouty polyarthralgia, asymptomatic hyperuricemia, acute gouty arthritis, transient morbilliform rash, dermatitis	Serum uric acid can serve as a surrogate marker for adherence; LFTs in patients with underlying liver disease
Ethambutol	Retrobulbar neuritis, peripheral neuritis, cutaneous reactions	Baseline visual acuity testing and testing of color discrimination; monthly testing of visual acuity and color discrimination in patients taking >15-20 mg/kg, having renal insufficiency, or receiving the drug for >2 months
Streptomycin	Ototoxicity, neurotoxicity, nephrotoxicity	Baseline audiogram, vestibular testing, Romberg's testing, and SCr Monthly assessments of renal function and auditory or vestibular symptoms
Amikacin/kanamycin	Ototoxicity, nephrotoxicity	Baseline audiogram, vestibular testing, Romberg's testing, and SCr; monthly assessments of renal function and auditory or vestibular symptoms
Capreomycin	Nephrotoxicity, ototoxicity	Baseline audiogram, vestibular testing, Romberg's testing, and SCr Monthly assessments of renal function and auditory or vestibular symptoms Baseline and monthly serum K^+ and Mg^{2+}
p-Aminosalicylic acid	Hepatotoxicity, GI distress, malabsorption syndrome, hypothyroidism, coagulopathy	Baseline LFTs and TSH TSH every 3 months
Moxifloxacin	GI disturbance, neurologic effects, cutaneous reactions	No specific monitoring recommended
Bedaquililne	GI disturbances, dizziness, headache, rash, arthralgia	Serum K, Ca, MgECG at baseline, weeks 2, 12, 24. Weekly ECG for persons taking other QTc prolonging drugs, history of arrhythmias, hypothyroidism, uncompensated heart failure, or have serum K, Ca, or Mg below normal

LFT, liver function test; SCr, serum creatinine; TSH, thyroid-stimulating hormone.

Data from Nahid P, et al. Executive Summary: Official American Thoracic Society/Centers for Disease Control and Prevention/Infectious Diseases Society of America Clinical Practice Guidelines: Treatment of drug-susceptible tuberculosis. Clin Infect Dis. 1 October 2016;63(7):853–867.

Serum chemistries, including blood urea nitrogen, creatinine, aspartate transaminase, and alanine transaminase, and a complete blood count with platelets should be performed at baseline and periodically thereafter, depending on the presence of other factors that may increase the likelihood of toxicity (eg, advanced age, alcohol abuse, pregnancy)[35] (Table 135-8). Hepatotoxicity should be suspected for patients whose serum transaminases exceed five times the upper limit of normal or whose total bilirubin concentration exceeds 3 mg/dL (51.3 μmol/L) and for patients with symptoms such as nausea, vomiting, or jaundice. At this point, the offending agent(s) should be discontinued. Sequential reintroduction of the drugs with frequent testing of liver enzymes is often successful in identifying the offending agent; other agents may be continued. Alternative agents should be selected as needed. Audiometric testing should be performed at baseline and monthly for patients who must receive aminoglycosides for more than 1 to 2 months. Vision testing (Snellen visual acuity charts and Ishihara color discrimination plates) should be performed on all patients who receive ethambutol. All patients diagnosed with TB should be tested for HIV infection.

ABBREVIATIONS

AFB	acid-fast bacillus
BCG	bacillus Calmette-Guérin
CDC	Centers for Disease Control and Prevention
CNS	central nervous system
DOT	directly observed treatment
DTH	delayed-type hypersensitivity
HIV	human immunodeficiency virus
IGRA	interferon-γ release assay
IL	interleukin
INF	interferon
LAM	lipoarabinomannan
LTBI	latent tuberculosis infection
MAC	*Mycobacterium avium* complex
MDR	multidrug-resistant
PPD	purified protein derivative
TB	tuberculosis
TDM	therapeutic drug monitoring

TH_1	T-helper type 1
TH_2	T-helper type 2
TNF	tumor necrosis factor
TST	tuberculin skin test
WHO	World Health Organization
XDR	extensively drug-resistant

REFERENCES

1. WHO. *Global Tuberculosis Report*. Geneva: World Health Organization; 2020.
2. Centers for Disease Control and Prevention (CDC). *Reported Tuberculosis in the United States 2020*. Atlanta, GA: US Department of Health and Human Services, CDC; 2020. Available at: https://www.cdc.gov/tb/statistics/reports/2019/default.htm.
3. Deutsch-Feldman M, Pratt RH, Price SF, Tsang CA, Self JL. Tuberculosis—United States, 2020. *MMWR Morb Mortal Wkly Rep.* 2021;70:409–414.
4. Schwartz NG, Price SF, Pratt RH, Langer AJ. Tuberculosis—United States, 2019. *MMWR Morb Mortal Wkly Rep.* 2020;69:286–289.
5. Global HIV/AIDS response. *Epidemic Update and Health Sector Progress Towards Universal Access*. Geneva: World Health Organization;2011.
6. Magee JG. Mycobacterium tuberculosis. In: Ollar RA, Connell ND, eds. *Molecular Mycobacteriology: Techniques and Clinical*. New York, NY: Marcel Dekker Inc.; 1999.
7. Issa R, Mohd Hassan NA, Abdul H, et al. Detection and discrimination of Mycobacterium tuberculosis complex. *Diagn Microbiol Infect Dis.* 2012;72:62–67.
8. Centers for Disease Control and Prevention (CDC). Updated guidelines for the use of nucleic acid amplification tests in the diagnosis of tuberculosis. *MMWR Morb Mortal Wkly Rep.* 2009;58:7–10.
9. Boehme CC, Nabeta P, Hillemann D, Nicol MP, et al. Rapid molecular detection of tuberculosis and rifampin resistance. *N Engl J Med.* 2010;363(11):1005.
10. Availability of an assay for detecting Mycobacterium tuberculosis, including rifampin-resistant strains, and considerations for its use—United States, 2013. Centers for Disease Control and Prevention. *MMWR Morb Mortal Wkly Rep.* 2013;62:821–827.
11. World Health Organization. Automated real-time nucleic acid amplification technology for rapid and simultaneous detection of tuberculosis and rifampicin resistance: Xpert MTB/RIF system. Policy statement. 2011. Available at: http://whqlibdoc.who.int/publications/2011/9789241501545_eng.pdf. Accessed September 13, 2021.
12. Wallis RS. Biomarkers and diagnostics for tuberculosis: Progress, needs, and translation into practice. *Lancet.* 2010;375:1845–1938.
13. Somoskovi A, Parsons LM, Salfinger M. The molecular basis of resistance to isoniazid, rifampin, and pyrazinamide in Mycobacterium tuberculosis. *Respir Res.* 2001;2:164–168.
14. Pathogenesis of tuberculosis. In: Heemskerk D, Caws M, Marais B, Farrar J, eds. *Tuberculosis in Adults and Children*. 1st ed. London: Springer; 2015;140.
15. Daniel TM, Boom WH, Ellner JJ. Immunology and susceptibility. In: Reichman LB, Hershfield ES, eds. *Tuberculosis: A Comprehensive International Approach*. 3rd ed. New York, NY: Marcel Dekker; 2006:157–185.
16. Long R, Gardam M. Tumor necrosis factor-α inhibitors and the reactivation of latent tuberculosis infection. *Can Med Assoc J.* 2003;168:1153–1156.
17. American Thoracic Society/Centers for Disease Control and Prevention. Diagnostic standards and classification of tuberculosis in adults and children. *Am J Respir Crit Care Med.* 2000;161:1376–1395.
18. Cruz AT, Stark JR. Clinical manifestations of tuberculosis in children. *Paediatr Respir Rev.* 2007;8:107–117.
19. Cain KP, McCarthy KD, Heilig CM, et al. An algorithm for tuberculosis screening and diagnosis in people with HIV. *N Engl J Med.* 2010;362(8):707–716.
20. Getahun H, Gunneberg C, Granich R, Nunn P. HIV infection–associated tuberculosis: The epidemiology and the response. *Clin Infect Dis.* 2010;50(Suppl 3):S201–S207. doi:10.1086/651492.
21. Panel on Opportunistic Infections in Adults and Adolescents with HIV. Guidelines for the prevention and treatment of opportunistic infections in adults and adolescents with HIV: Recommendations from the Centers for Disease Control and Prevention, the National Institutes of Health, and the HIV Medicine Association of the Infectious Diseases Society of America. Available at https://clinicalinfo.hiv.gov/sites/default/files/guidelines/documents/Adult_OI.pdf. Accessed September 30, 2021.
22. Naidoo K, Yende-Zuma N, Padayatch N, et al. The immune reconstitution inflammatory syndrome after antiretroviral therapy initiation in patients with tuberculosis: Findings from the SAPiT trial. *Ann Intern Med.* 2012;157:313.
23. Panel on Antiretroviral Guidelines for Adults and Adolescents. Guidelines for the Use of Antiretroviral Agents in Adults and Adolescents with HIV. Department of Health and Human Services. Available at: https://clinicalinfo.hiv.gov/sites/default/files/guidelines/documents/AdultandAdolescentGL.pdf. Accessed September 30, 2021.
24. Lewinsohn D, Leonard M, LoBue P, Cohn D, Daley C, et al. Official American Thoracic Society/Infectious Diseases Society/Centers for Disease Control and Prevention clinical practice guidelines: Diagnosis of tuberculosis in adults and children. 2017;64:e1–e11.
25. Centers for Disease Control and Prevention. Screening for tuberculosis and tuberculosis infection in high-risk populations: Recommendations of the Advisory Council for the Elimination of Tuberculosis. *MMWR.* 1995;44(No. RR-11):19–34.
26. Akolo C, Adetifa I, Sheppard S, Volmink J. Treatment of latent tuberculosis infection in HIV infected persons. *Cochrane Database Syst Rev.* 2010;(1):CD000171.
27. Centers for Disease Control and Prevention. Anergy skin testing and preventive therapy for HIV-infected persons: Revised recommendations. *MMWR Recomm Rep.* 1997;46:10.
28. Jensen PA, Lambert LA, Iademarco MF, Ridzon R, Centers for Disease Control and Prevention. Guidelines for preventing the transmission of Mycobacterium tuberculosis in health care settings. *MMWR Recomm Rep.* 2005;54(RR-17):1–141.
29. Mazurek GH, Jereb J, Varnon A, et al. Updated guidelines for interferon gamma release assay to detect Mycobacterium tuberculosis infection, United States. *MMWR Recomm Rep.* 2010;59(RR-5):1–25.
30. Starke JR, Committee on Infectious Diseases. Interferon-γ release assays for diagnosis of tuberculosis infection and disease in children. *Pediatrics.* 2014;134:e1763.
31. Bergamini BM, Losi M, Vaienti F, et al. Performance of commercial blood tests for the diagnosis of latent tuberculosis infection in children and adolescents. *Pediatrics.* 2009;123:e419–e424.
32. Lighter J, Rigaud M, Eduardo R, Peng CH, et al. Latent tuberculosis diagnosis in children by using the quantiferon-TB gold in tube test. *Pediatrics.* 2009;123:30–37.
33. Richeldi L, Losi M, D'Amico R, et al. Performance of tests for latent tuberculosis in different groups of immunocompromised patients. *Chest.* 2009;136:198–204.
34. Perry S, Catanzaro A. Use of clinical risk assessments in evaluation of nucleic acid amplification tests for HIV/tuberculosis. *Int J Tuberc Lung Dis.* 2000;4:S34.
35. Nahid P, Dorman SE, Alipanah N, Barry PM, Brozek JL, et al. American Thoracic Society/Centers for Disease Control/Infectious Disease Society of America. Treatment of drug susceptible tuberculosis. *CID.* 2016;1:1–49.
36. Fujiwara PI, Larkin C, Frieden TR. Directly observed therapy in New York City. *Clin Chest Med.* 1997;18:135–148.
37. Cruz AT, Starke JR. Increasing adherence for latent tuberculosis infection therapy with health department-administered therapy. *Pediatr Infect Dis J.* 2012;31:193.
38. Peloquin CA. Pharmacological issues in the treatment of tuberculosis. *Ann NY Acad Sci.* 2001;953:157–164.
39. Peloquin CA. Antituberculosis drugs: Pharmacokinetics. In: Heifets LB, ed. *Drug Susceptibility in the Chemotherapy of Mycobacterial Infections*. Boca Raton, FL: CRC Press; 1991:59–88.
40. Sterling TR, Njie G, Zenner D, et al. Guidelines for the Treatment of Latent Tuberculosis Infection: Recommendations from the National Tuberculosis Controllers Association and CDC, 2020. *MMWR Recomm Rep.* 2020;69:1.
41. Centers for Disease Control and Prevention. Recommendations for use of isoniazid–rifapentine regimen with direct observation to treat Mycobacterium tuberculosis infection. *MMWR Morb Mortal Wkly Rep.* 2011;60:1650–1653.
42. Alsultan A, Peloquin CA. Therapeutic drug monitoring in the treatment of tuberculosis: An update. *Drugs.* 2014;74:839–854.
43. Horsburgh CR Jr, Barry CE, Lange C. Treatment of Tuberculosis. *N Engl J Med.* 2015 November 26;373(22):2149–2160.
44. Heysell SK, Moore JL, Keller SJ, Houpt ER. Therapeutic drug monitoring for slow response to tuberculosis in a state control program. *Emerg Infect Dis.* 2010;16:1546–1553.

45. Zumla A, Abubaker I, Raviglione M, et al. Drug resistant tuberculosis—Current dilemmas, unanswered questions, challenges, and priority needs. *J Infect Dis.* 2012;205:S228–S240.
46. Conradie F, Diacon AH, Ngubane N, et al. Treatment of highly drug resistant pulmonary tuberculosis. *N Engl J Med.* 2020;382:893–902.
47. Seaworth BJ, Griffith DE. Therapy of multidrug resistant and extensively drug resistant tuberculosis. *Microbiol Specr.* 2017;5.
48. Mirzayev F, Viney K, Linh NN, et al. World Health Organization recommendations on the treatment of drug-resistant tuberculosis, 2020 update. *Eur Respir J.* 2021;57:2003300.
49. Miele K, Bamrah MS, Tepper NK. Tuberculosis in pregnancy. *Obstet Gynecol.* 2020;135:1444.
50. Briggs GG, Freeman RK, Yaffe SJ. *Drugs in Pregnancy and Lactation: A Reference Guide to Fetal and Neonatal Risk.* 7th ed. Philadelphia: Lippincott Williams & Wilkins; 2005.
51. Managing drug interactions in the treatment of HIV-related tuberculosis. Centers for Disease Control and Prevention. 2013. Available at: http://www.cdc.gov/tb/TB_HIV_Drugs/default.htm. Accessed September 1, 2021.
52. Abdool Karim SS, Naidoo K, Grobler A, et al. Timing of initiation of antiretroviral drugs during tuberculosis therapy. *N Engl J Med.* 25, 2010;362(8):697–706. doi:10.1056/NEJMoa0905848.
53. Malone RS, Fish DN, Spiegel DM, et al. The effect of hemodialysis on isoniazid, rifampin, pyrazinamide, and ethambutol. *Am J Respir Crit Care Med.* 1999;159:1580–1584.
54. Malone RS, Fish DN, Spiegel DM, et al. The effect of hemodialysis on cycloserine, ethionamide, para-aminosalicylate, and clofazimine. *Chest.* 1999;116:984–990.
55. Peloquin CA, Davies GR. The treatment of tuberculosis. *Clin Pharmacol and Therapeutics.* 2021;110(6):1455–1466.
56. Crabbe SJ. Drug InfoSearch—Intravenous isoniazid. *P&T.* 1990;15:1483–1484.
57. Peloquin CA, Namdar R, Dodge AA, Nix DE. Pharmacokinetics of isoniazid under fasting conditions, with food, and with antacids. *Int J Tuberc Lung Dis.* 1999;3:703–710.
58. Weiner M, Burman W, Vernon A, et al. Low isoniazid concentration associated with outcome of tuberculosis treatment with once-weekly isoniazid and rifapentine. *Am J Respir Crit Care Med.* 2003;167:1341–1347.
59. Peloquin CA, Namdar R, Singleton MD, Nix DE. Pharmacokinetics of rifampin under fasting conditions, with food, and with antacids. *Chest.* 1999;115:12–18.
60. Weiner M, Benator D, Burman W, et al. Association between acquired rifamycin resistance and the pharmacokinetics of rifabutin and isoniazid among patients with HIV and tuberculosis. *Clin Infect Dis.* 2005;40:1481–1491.
61. Velasques, GE, Brooks ME, Coit JM, et al. Efficacy and safety of high-dose rifampin in pulmonary tuberculosis. A randomized controlled trial. *Am J Respir Crit Care Med.* 2018;198:657–666.
62. Dorman SE, Nahid P, Kurbatova EV. Four month rifapentine regimens with or without moxifloxacin for tuberculosis. *N Engl J Med.* 2021;384:1705–1718.
63. Burman WJ, Gallicano K, Peloquin CA. Comparative pharmacokinetics and pharmacodynamics of the rifamycin antibiotics. *Clin Pharmacokinet.* 2001;40:327–341.
64. Peloquin CA, Jaresko GS, Yong CL, et al. Population pharmacokinetic modeling of isoniazid, rifampin, and pyrazinamide. *Antimicrob Agents Chemother.* 1997;41:2670–2679.
65. Peloquin CA, Bulpitt AE, Jaresko GS, et al. Pharmacokinetics of pyrazinamide under fasting conditions, with food, and with antacids. *Pharmacotherapy.* 1998;18:1205–1211.
66. Peloquin CA, Bulpitt AE, Jaresko GS, et al. Pharmacokinetics of ethambutol under fasting conditions, with food, and with antacids. *Antimicrob Agents Chemother.* 1999;43:568–572.
67. Summers KK, Hardin TC. Treatment of tuberculosis in hemodialysis patients. *J Infect Dis Pharmacother.* 1996;2:37–55.
68. WHO consolidated guidelines on tuberculosis. *Module 4: Treatment —Drug-Resistant Tuberculosis Treatment.* Geneva: World Health Organization; 2020.
69. CDC. Media Statement: Landmark TB Trial Identifies Shorter-Course Treatment Regimen. Oct. 22, 2020. Available at: https://www.cdc.gov/nchhstp/newsroom/2020/landmark-tb-trial-media-statement.html.
70. Peloquin CA, Davies GR. The treatment of tuberculosis. *Tutorial in Clinical Pharmacol and Therap.* 2020;1–10.
71. Chang KC, Nuermberger E, Sotgiu G, Leung CC. New drugs and regimens for tuberculosis. *Respirology.* 2018;23:978–990.
72. Ignatius EH, Dooley KE. New drugs for the treatment of tuberculosis. *Clin Chest Med.* 2019;40:811–827.
73. Friedman LR, Dedicoat M, Davies PD, eds. *Clinical Tuberculosis.* 6th ed. Boca Raton: CRC Press; 2020. https://www.taylorfrancis.com/books/e/9781351249980.
74. Boeree MJ, et al. High-dose rifampicin, moxifloxacin, and SQ109 for treating tuberculosis: A multi-arm, multi-stage randomized controlled trial. *Lancet Infect Dis.* 2017;17:39–49.
75. Safety and efficacy of various doses and treatment durations of linezolid plus bedaquiline and pretomanid in participants with pulmonary TB, XDR-TB; Pre XDR-TB or non-responsive/intolerant MDR-TB. Available at: https://clinicaltrials.gov/ct2/show/NCT03086486. Accessed September 20, 2021.
76. Zhu M, Nix DE, Adam RD, et al. Pharmacokinetics of cycloserine under fasting conditions, with orange juice, food, and antacids. *Pharmacotherapy.* 2001;21:891–897.
77. Liu Y et al. Delamanid: From discovery to its use for pulmonary multidrug-resistant tuberculosis (MDR-TB). *Tuberculosis (Edinb).* 2018; 111:20–30.
78. Märtson AG, Burch G, Ghimire S, Alffenaar JC, Peloquin CA. Therapeutic drug monitoring in patients with tuberculosis and concurrent medical problems. *Expert Opin Drug Metab Toxicol.* 2021 Jan;17(1):23–39.
79. Deshpande D, Srivastava S, Chapagain M, et al. Ceftazidime-avibactam has potent sterilizing activity against highly drug-resistant tuberculosis. *Sci Adv.* 2017;3:e1701102.
80. Zhu M, Namdar R, Stambaugh JJ, et al. Population pharmacokinetics of ethionamide in patients with tuberculosis. *Tuberculosis.* 2002;82:91–96.
81. Peloquin CA, Henshaw TL, Huitt GA, et al. Pharmacokinetic evaluation of p-aminosalicylic acid granules. *Pharmacotherapy.* 1994;14:40–46.
82. Peloquin CA, Berning SE, Huitt GA, et al. Once-daily and twice-daily dosing of *p*-aminosalicylic acid (PAS) granules. *Am J Respir Crit Care Med.* 1999;159:932–934.
83. Peloquin CA, Zhu M, Adam RD, et al. Pharmacokinetics of p-aminosalicylate under fasting conditions, with orange juice, food, and antacids. *Ann Pharmacother.* 2001;35:1332–1338.
84. The role of BCG vaccine in the prevention and control of tuberculosis in the United States. A joint statement by the Advisory Council for the Elimination of Tuberculosis and the Advisory Committee on Immunization Practices. *MMWR Recomm Rep.* 1996;45:1.
85. Roy A, Eisenhut M, Harris RJ, et al. Effect of BCG vaccination against Mycobacterium tuberculosis infection in children: Systematic review and meta-analysis. *BMJ.* 2014;349:g4643.
86. Colditz GA, Brewer TF, Berkey CS, et al. Efficacy of BCG vaccine in the prevention of tuberculosis. Meta-analysis of the published literature. *JAMA.* 1994;271:698.
87. Chaulk CP, Friedman M, Dunning R. Modeling the epidemiology and economics of directly observed therapy in Baltimore. *Int J Tuberc Lund Dis.* 2000;4:201–207.
88. Friedman LN, Dedicoat M, Davies PDO, eds. *Clinical Tuberculosis.* 6th ed. Boca Raton: CRC Press; 2020. https://www.taylorfrancis.com/books/e/9781351249980.
89. Tappero JW, Bradford WZ, Agerton TB, et al. Serum concentrations of antimycobacterial drugs in patients with pulmonary tuberculosis in Botswana. *Clin Infect Dis.* 2005;41:461–469.
90. Perlman DC, Segal Y, Rosenkranz S, et al. The clinical pharmacokinetics of rifampin and ethambutol in HIV-infected persons with tuberculosis. *Clin Infect Dis.* 2005;41:1638–1647.
91. Peloquin CA. Agents for tuberculosis. In: Piscitelli SC, Rodvold KA, eds. *Drug Interactions in Infectious Diseases.* Totowa, NJ: Humana Press, 2001:109–120.
92. Brudney K, Dobkin J. Resurgent tuberculosis in New York City: Human immunodeficiency virus, homelessness, and the decline of tuberculosis control programs. *Am Rev Respir Dis.* 1991;144:745–749.

Gastrointestinal Infections and Enterotoxigenic Poisonings

136

Andrew M. Roecker and Brittany N. Bates

KEY CONCEPTS

1. Infectious diarrhea is a disease that causes significant morbidity and mortality worldwide. Its etiology includes various bacteria, viruses, and protozoans, with viral causes being most predominant globally.
2. Two types of infectious diarrhea include watery or enterotoxigenic diarrhea and dysentery or bloody diarrhea. Common pathogens responsible for watery diarrhea are viruses and enterotoxigenic *Escherichia coli*. Common pathogens responsible for dysentery diarrhea are *Shigella* spp., *Campylobacter jejuni*, nontyphoid *Salmonella*, and enterohemorrhagic *E. coli*.
3. Fluid and electrolyte replacement is the cornerstone of therapy for diarrheal illnesses. Oral rehydration therapy is preferred in most cases of mild and moderate diarrhea.
4. The use of antibacterial therapy for infectious diarrhea is not commonly indicated due to the mild and self-limited nature of the infection, or viral etiology. Antibiotic therapy is recommended in cases of severe diarrhea, moderate-to-severe cases of traveler's diarrhea, most cases of febrile dysenteric diarrhea, and culture-proven bacterial diarrhea in high-risk patients.
5. Loperamide and diphenoxylate/atropine may offer symptomatic relief in patients with moderate watery diarrhea; however, use of antimotility agents should be avoided in patients with watery and dysentery diarrhea.
6. Diarrheal illness can be largely prevented by procedures to prevent contaminated food or water supplies and with appropriate personal hygiene.
7. Oral vancomycin or fidaxomicin are recommended as the initial therapy for patients with *Clostridioides difficile* infection.
8. Common traveler's diarrheal pathogens include enterotoxigenic *E. coli*, *Shigella* spp., *Campylobacter* spp., *Salmonella* spp., and viruses.
9. Patient education on prevention strategies and appropriate self-treatment of traveler's diarrhea is preferred, and prophylaxis with antibacterials is not recommended.
10. Pathogens commonly responsible for food poisoning include *Staphylococcus* spp., *Salmonella* spp., *Shigella* spp., and *Clostridioides* spp.

BEYOND THE BOOK

Perform a literature search to identify investigational drugs and therapies for *Clostridioides difficile* infection (CDI) not addressed in the book chapter. Create a document that describes the proposed mechanism of action for each agent.

INTRODUCTION

Gastrointestinal (GI) infections and enterotoxigenic poisonings encompass a wide variety of medical conditions characterized by inflammation of the GI tract. Inflammation-induced vomiting and diarrhea are responsible for much of the morbidity and mortality of these conditions. Diarrhea is defined as a decrease in consistency of bowel movements (ie, unformed stool) and an increase in frequency of stools to three or more per day.[1,2] Acute diarrheal disease is commonly associated with diarrhea lasting less than 7 days, prolonged diarrhea lasts 7 to 13 days, persistent diarrhea lasts 14 to 29 days, and chronic diarrhea lasts 30 days or longer.

This chapter focuses on infectious etiologies of acute GI infections and enterotoxigenic poisonings. A wide variety of viral, bacterial, and parasitic pathogens are responsible for these infections. Chapter e138, "Parasitic Diseases," discusses the common protozoans that cause gastroenteritis. This chapter will focus on pathogenesis and management of common viral and bacterial etiologies. Because the clinical consequences of dysenteric diarrhea can be more severe compared with cases of watery diarrhea, the chapter is organized accordingly. Epidemiology, clinical presentation, diagnosis, treatment, and prevention strategies are discussed for all GI infections generally, and further elaborated in subsequent sections for specific diseases such as *Clostridioides difficile* infection, traveler's diarrhea, and foodborne illnesses.

EPIDEMIOLOGY

Dehydration resulting from acute infectious diarrhea is the second leading cause of mortality in children younger than 5 years, killing 525,000 annually.[2] Globally, 1.7 billion cases of infectious diarrhea occur yearly and cause over 1.39 million deaths.[2,3] The incidence of diarrhea for all children younger than age 5 years is 2.9 episodes per child per year. The incidence of diarrhea is higher in younger children, with 4.5 episodes per child per year among children aged 6 to 11 months, compared with 2.3 episodes per child per year among children aged 24 to 59 months.[2,3] Younger children also have a higher risk of death from acute dehydrating diarrhea, and diarrheal disease is still the leading global cause of malnutrition in children younger than 5 years.[2] Although the incidence of childhood diarrhea has been declining, diarrhea remains a major health problem in children, especially in those younger than 1 year.

In the United States, 179 million episodes of acute gastroenteritis occur each year, resulting in nearly 500,000 hospitalizations and more than 5,000 deaths.[4-7] The highest mortality risk from infectious diarrhea in the United States occurs in the elderly, which contrasts to the developing world where the risk of death is highest among young children.[4] Twenty-five percent of all hospitalizations and 85% of all mortality associated with diarrhea involved the elderly (age 60 years and older).[4] In addition to children and the elderly, other groups at risk for GI infections include travelers and campers, patients in chronic care facilities, military personnel stationed abroad, and immunocompromised patients.

ETIOLOGY

1 The etiology of GI infections and enterotoxigenic poisonings includes a wide variety of viruses, bacteria, and parasites, although the specific incidence of each is difficult to quantify. Etiologic agents are rarely identified due to the infrequent collection of stool samples, or inability of many laboratories to detect the full range of pathogenic organisms. In this chapter, discussions of pathogens responsible for enterotoxigenic diarrhea focus on viral pathogens (rotavirus and norovirus), enterotoxigenic *Escherichia coli* (ETEC), and cholera. Common pathogens associated with dysenteric diarrhea discussed will be *Shigella* spp., *Salmonella* spp., *Campylobacter* spp., enterohemorrhagic *E. coli* (EHEC), *Yersinia enterocolitica*, and *C. difficile*. Characteristics of watery and dysenteric diarrhea and common pathogens responsible for them are outlined in Table 136-1.

Viruses are now the leading global cause of infectious diarrhea. Noroviruses, previously known as Norwalk-like viruses, account for greater than 90% of viral gastroenteritis among all age groups, and 50% of outbreaks worldwide. In the United States, noroviruses have been responsible for about 21% of all acute gastroenteritis cases in young children with outpatient visits, emergency department visits, and annual hospitalizations numbering 627,000, 281,000, and 14,000, respectively.[8] Outbreaks occur throughout the year and have been documented in families, healthcare systems, cruise ships, and college dormitories.

In infants and children, rotavirus, a double-stranded, wheel-shaped, RNA virus, is the most common cause of infectious diarrhea globally, and 1 million people die annually from the infection.[9] In the United States, approximately 3.5 million cases of diarrhea, 500,000 physician visits, 50,000 hospitalizations, and 20 deaths occur each year in children younger than 5 years. Rotavirus is a ubiquitous contagion, infecting the vast majority of children younger than 5 years. After the initial infection, 40% of children are protected against subsequent rotavirus infection, 75% are protected against subsequent gastroenteritis, and up to 88% are protected against severe gastroenteritis. After more extensive vaccination coverage for rotavirus in recent years, hospitalizations from this infection have significantly decreased.[9] Other viral etiologies include astrovirus, enteric adenovirus, pestivirus, coronavirus, and enterovirus. These viruses are increasingly identified as causative etiologies of diarrhea. Characteristics of viral pathogens causing gastroenteritis are outlined in Table 136-2.

2 Bacterial causes of acute gastroenteritis in the United States account for more than 5 million cases of diarrhea annually; however, these are vastly underreported and a causative pathogen is identified in less than 3% of cases.[4] FoodNet in 2019 identified 25,866 laboratory confirmed infections, resulting in 6,164 hospitalizations and 122 deaths from these infections.[4,10] Common pathogens responsible for watery diarrhea in the United States are norovirus and ETEC, while those most commonly associated with dysentery diarrhea are *Campylobacter* spp., EHEC, *Salmonella* spp., and *Shigella* spp. Other organisms that are responsible for dysentery include *Aeromonas* spp., noncholera *Vibrio*, and *Y. enterocolitica*. Characteristics of acute bacterial pathogens causing gastroenteritis are summarized in Table 136-3.

Cholera has been rare in the United States because of advanced water and sanitation systems, although slight increases in its incidence have occurred in recent years without clear causes. It is endemic on the Indian subcontinent and sub-Saharan Africa with five countries, Democratic Republic of the Congo, Haiti, Somalia, the United Republic of Tanzania, and Yemen, causing 80% of all cases.[11-13] *Vibrio cholerae* is a gram-negative bacillus sharing similar characteristics with the family Enterobacterales. Cholera is caused by toxigenic *V. cholerae* serogroups O1 or O139. Infections due to *V. cholerae* result in severe and voluminous diarrhea that can quickly result in dehydration. Approximately half of those persons infected with *V. cholerae* O1 are symptomatic, whereas only 1% to 5% of those infected with *V. cholerae* O139 manifest symptoms.[12,13] Vaccination is available to affected areas and to people traveling to those areas that might help in reducing prevalence and severity of disease.[13]

E. coli is a gram-negative bacillus commonly found in the human GI tract, and *E. coli*–associated diarrhea may be differentiated into several distinct categories based on pathogenic features of diarrheal disease: enteroaggregative *E. coli* (EAEC), EHEC, enteroinvasive *E. coli* (EIEC), enteropathogenic *E. coli* (EPEC), and ETEC. ETEC occurs most commonly, and accounts for about half of all cases of *E. coli* diarrhea. There are an estimated 79,000 cases of ETEC in the United States each year.[4] ETEC is also the most common cause of traveler's diarrhea and a common cause of food- and water-associated outbreaks. Infections with EIEC and EPEC are primarily a disease of children in developing countries.[14] EAEC strains are implicated in persistent diarrhea (≥14 days) in human immunodeficiency virus (HIV)-infected patients.[15] EHEC, also known as Shiga toxin–producing *E. coli* (STEC), causes watery diarrhea that becomes bloody in 1 to 5 days in 80% of patients.[14]

TABLE 136-1 Acute Infectious Diarrhea Clinical Syndromes: Watery Versus Dysentery

	Watery	Dysentery
Percentage of patients	90-95	5-10
Stools		
Appearance	Watery	Bloody
Volume	Increased: ++/+++	Increased: +/++
Number per day	<10	>10
Reducing substances	0 to +++	0
pH	5-7.5	6-7.5
Occult blood	Negative	Positive
Fecal polymorphonuclear cells	Absent or few	Many
Mechanisms	Toxins Reduced absorption	Toxins Mucosal invasion
Complications		
Dehydration	Could be severe	Mild
Others	Acidosis, shock, electrolyte imbalance	Tenesmus, rectal prolapse, seizures
Etiology	*Vibrio cholerae*	*Shigella* spp.
	Enterotoxigenic *Escherichia coli* (ETEC)	*Salmonella* spp.
	Rotaviruses	*Campylobacter* spp.
	Noroviruses	*Yersinia* spp.
		Enterohemorrhagic *E. coli* (EHEC)
		Clostridioides difficile

TABLE 136-2 Characteristics of Agents Responsible for Acute Viral Gastroenteritis

Virus	Peak Age of Onset	Time of Year	Duration	Mode of Transmission	Common Symptoms
Rotavirus	6 months to 2 years	October to April	3-7 days	Fecal–oral, water, food	Nausea, vomiting, diarrhea, fever, abdominal pain, lactose intolerance
Norovirus	All age groups	Peak in winter	2-3 days	Fecal–oral, food, water, environment	Nausea, vomiting, diarrhea, abdominal cramps, myalgia
Astrovirus	<7 years	Winter	1-4 days	Fecal–oral, water, shellfish	Diarrhea, headache, malaise, nausea
Enteric adenovirus	<2 years	Year-round	7-9 days	Fecal–oral	Diarrhea, respiratory symptoms, vomiting, fever
Pestivirus	<2 years	NR	3 days	NR	Mild
Coronavirus-like particles	<2 years	Fall and early winter	7 days	NR	Respiratory disease
Enterovirus	NR	NR	NR	NR	Mild diarrhea, secondary organ damage

NR, not reported.

TABLE 136-3 Characteristics of Acute Bacterial Gastroenteritis

Bacteria	Incubation Period	Duration	Mode of Transmission	Common Symptoms
Watery Diarrhea				
Vibrio cholerae	2-3 days	1-3 days	Contaminated food or water with human feces usually in areas of inadequate treatment of sewage and drinking water	Profuse watery diarrhea, vomiting, and leg cramps Death can occur within hours without treatment
Enteroaggregative *E. coli*	NR	NR	Contaminated food or water with animal or human feces	Chronic, watery, mucoid, secretory diarrhea with low-grade fever in immunocompromised persons (HIV infections)
Enteroinvasive *E. coli*	10-18 hours	NR	Contaminated food or water with animal or human feces	Watery diarrhea in young children in the developing world
Enteropathogenic *E. coli*	9-12 hours	NR	Contaminated food or water with animal or human feces	Acute onset of profuse watery diarrhea, vomiting, and low-grade fever in young children (<2 years of age) in the developing world
Enterotoxigenic *E. coli*	1-3 days	3-4 days	Contaminated food or water with animal or human feces	Watery diarrhea and abdominal cramping
Dysentery Diarrhea				
Campylobacter jejuni	2-5 days	5-7 days	Contaminated food (particularly poultry), water, or contact with infected animals	Diarrhea (often bloody), cramping, abdominal pain, and fever
Enterohemorrhagic *E. coli*	3-4 days	5-7 days	Contaminated food (particularly cattle) or water with animal or human feces	Severe stomach cramps, diarrhea (often bloody), and vomiting Approximately 5%-10% develop hemolytic uremic syndrome
Nontyphoid *Salmonella*	12-36 hours	1-5 days	Contaminated food, water, or contact with infected animals	Diarrhea (sometimes bloody), fever, and abdominal cramps
Shigella	1-3 days	1-7 days	Fecal–oral Contaminated food or water with infected human feces	Watery or bloody diarrhea (8-10 stools/day), severe abdominal pain, fever, and malaise
Yersinia	4-7 days	1-3 weeks	Contaminated food or water	Fever, abdominal pain, and diarrhea (often bloody)

NR, not reported.

EHEC is believed to be the major etiologic factor responsible for the development of hemorrhagic colitis and hemolytic uremic syndrome (HUS). The annual disease burden of STEC in the United States is more than 20,000 infections and as many as 250 deaths; however, the failure of many clinical laboratories to screen for this organism greatly complicates any estimates.[16] In the United States, STEC causes 50% to 60% of all EHEC infections, but in the southern hemisphere, including Argentina, Australia, Chile, and South Africa, non-STEC serotypes are often more prevalent. Non-STEC strains generally produce a lower frequency of dysentery than STEC-positive strains (62% vs 85%).

The *Campylobacter* spp. are flagellated, curved, gram-negative rods. Although there are 14 different species, *Campylobacter jejuni* is the species responsible for more than 99% of *Campylobacter*-associated gastroenteritis. Approximately 2.4 million persons are affected each year in the United States, involving almost 1% of the entire population.[4]

Salmonella enterica is a gram-negative bacilli belonging to the family Enterobacterales. The most prevalent *S. enterica* serotypes are Typhi and Paratyphi, which cause enteric fever. Gastroenteritis is caused by *S. enterica* serotypes Typhimurium or Enteritidis. In the United States, the largest burden of *Salmonella* infection is due to nontyphoidal serotypes, causing approximately 1.4 million cases of salmonellosis, 16,000 hospitalizations, and 600 deaths, occurring annually.[17]

Approximately 165 million cases of shigellosis occur worldwide with 450,000 cases from the United States annually.[18,19] *Shigella* spp. are gram-negative bacilli belonging to the family Enterobacterales. Four species most often associated with disease are *Shigella dysenteriae* type 1, *Shigella flexneri*, *Shigella boydii*, and *Shigella sonnei*.[18,19] *Shigella sonnei* and *S. flexneri* are the most common causes of gastroenteritis in the United States. The other two *Shigella* spp. are more commonly acquired during travel to developing countries. Poor sanitation or personal hygiene, inadequate water supply, malnutrition, and increased population density are associated with an increased risk of *Shigella* gastroenteritis epidemics.

Yersinia spp. are non–lactose-fermenting gram-negative coccobacilli that are widely distributed in nature. The genus *Yersinia* includes six species known to cause disease in humans. *Yersinia enterocolitica* and, to a lesser extent, *Y. pseudotuberculosis* are most likely associated with intestinal infection, but overall both are a relatively infrequent cause of diarrhea and abdominal pain. More than 50 serotypes of *Y. enterocolitica* exist; of these, serotypes 0:3, 0:8, and 0:9 are associated most frequently with enterocolitis.[20] Children are most likely to experience illness with *Y. enterocolitica* infection.

PATHOPHYSIOLOGY

Acute gastroenteritis and its resulting diarrhea are caused by altered movement of ions and water resulting in increased colonic secretion. Under normal conditions, the GI tract has tremendous capacity to absorb fluid and electrolytes, allowing only 100 to 200 mL of fluid to be excreted in the stool daily.[21] The classic enteric pathogen that causes secretary diarrhea is *V. cholerae*, but ETEC and rotavirus also cause watery diarrhea and are much more predominant etiologies in the United States.

V. cholerae is an enteric pathogen that causes classical secretory diarrhea due to changes in ion secretion and absorption. Among the toxins produced by *V. cholerae*, the most important is cholera toxin.[11] Cholera toxin consists of two subunits, A and B. The B subunits are responsible for delivery of the A subunit into the cell. The A subunit stimulates adenylate cyclase, which increases intracellular cyclic adenosine monophosphate (cAMP) and results in protein kinase A–mediated activation of cystic fibrosis transmembrane conductance regulator. This leads to increased chloride secretion and decreased sodium absorption producing the severe watery diarrhea characteristic of the disease.[21] The toxin likely acts along the entire intestinal tract, but most fluid loss occurs in the duodenum. The net effect of the cholera toxin is isotonic fluid secretion early in the intestinal tract that exceeds the absorptive capacity of the latter intestinal tract.

ETEC also causes watery diarrhea characterized by severe intestinal water secretion by producing plasmid-mediated enterotoxins: heat-labile toxin and heat-stable toxin. The heat-labile toxin has two subunits (A and B) that have similar antigenic properties and action on the gut mucosa as cholera toxin. Heat-labile toxins increase chloride secretion via activation of cAMP. The net effect is luminal accumulation of electrolytes that draws water into the intestine, and production of a cholera-like secretory diarrhea.[22] Heat-stable toxin is thought to be nonantigenic and produces watery diarrhea by acting on the small intestine.

Rotavirus induces changes in transepithelial fluid balance, and causes malabsorption as a consequence of destruction of the epithelial lining of intestine, and vascular damage and ischemia in villi. Once rotavirus infects small intestinal villus cells, viroplasms are formed and its toxin, nonstructural protein 4, is released. The viral enterotoxin increases intracellular calcium, and the increase in calcium disrupts microvillus cytoskeleton, as well as barrier function. Changes to the villi include shortening of villus height, crypt hyperplasia, and mononuclear cell infiltration of the lamina propria.[23]

Inflammatory diarrhea is caused by two groups of organisms—enterotoxin-producing, noninvasive bacteria (eg, EAEC, EHEC) or invasive organisms (eg, *Campylobacter* spp., *Salmonella* spp., *Shigella* spp.). The enterotoxin-producing organisms adhere to the mucosa, activate cytokines, and stimulate the intestinal mucosa to release inflammatory mediators. Invasive organisms, which can also produce enterotoxin, invade the intestinal mucosa to induce an acute inflammatory reaction, involving the activation of local and systemic cytokines and inflammatory mediators.

Ingestion of as few as 10 to 200 viable organisms of the *Shigella* spp. causes disease in healthy adults.[18,19] *Shigella* multiply and spread within the submucosa of the small bowel, but they rarely extend beyond the mucosa. Inflammatory diarrhea is caused by the pathogens invading the epithelial barrier through M cells where they encounter and eliminate macrophages. The destruction of macrophages after emergence from M cells causes an initial release of interleukin (IL)-1β. This initial inflammatory process is exacerbated by free bacteria binding to toll-like receptor that causes the production of IL-6 and IL-8. Both IL-1β and IL-8 attract polymorphonucleocytes.[24] Release of polymorphonucleocytes activates chloride secretion and subsequent diarrhea. Degranulation and release of toxic substances by neutrophils cause ulceration of the epithelium, distortion of the crypts, death to intestinal epithelium, sloughing of mucosal cells, bloody mucoid exudate into the gut lumen, and submucosal accumulation of inflammatory cells with microabscess formation.[25] Microabscesses eventually may coalesce, forming larger abscesses. *Shigella* will frequently affect the entire colon. In addition to the virulence characteristics of invasiveness, *S. dysenteriae* type 1 and, to a lesser degree, *S. flexneri* and *S. sonnei* produce a cytotoxin or Shiga toxin, which can lead to HUS.[14]

The pathogenicity of EHEC is related to the production of Shiga-like toxins, so named because of their resemblance to the Shiga toxin of *S. dysenteriae*.[21] The cytotoxic effect of Shiga-like toxins disrupts the mucosal integrity of the large intestine, causing diarrhea. In addition, the toxin is able to pass through the intestinal epithelium to reach the endothelial cells lining small blood vessels that supply the gut, kidney, and other viscera, causing the myriad metabolic events that could eventually lead to HUS.

CLINICAL PRESENTATION

Gastroenteritis is an illness characterized by diarrhea, which may be accompanied by nausea, vomiting, fever, and abdominal pain. For effective diagnosis and management, it is important to distinguish noninflammatory diarrhea that produces watery diarrhea from inflammatory diarrhea or dysentery. Most enteric pathogens produce acute diarrhea and pathogens associated with dysentery will often result in grossly bloody stools and mucus. Systemic symptoms of gastroenteritis, such as fever, are often associated with dysentery of infectious origin. Symptoms of enteric pathogens that cause watery and dysentery diarrhea are listed in Table 136-1.

A physical examination and careful history that includes information about symptoms and symptom duration, the number of individuals affected, and recent history of travel, diet, and medications are important factors in making a diagnosis. Infections with norovirus or ETEC will often result in mild, self-limiting disease, whereas cholera will commonly produce severe dehydrating diarrhea. Infections with enteric pathogens such as *Campylobacter* spp., EHEC, *Salmonella* spp., *Shigella* spp., and *Y. enterocolitica* can result in severe symptomatology due to dysentery. The utilization of serum C-reactive protein (CRP) in young adult patients with infectious diarrhea may be able to help differentiate between noninflammatory and inflammatory causes.[26] Assessing CRP could assist with diagnosis, prognosis, and treatment selection. The clinical presentation of acute viral and bacterial gastroenteritis is summarized in Tables 136-2 and 136-3, respectively.

Stool culture is an important tool in making an organism-specific diagnosis and determining susceptibility to antimicrobial agents. Due to the low yield, stool cultures are not recommended in most mild-to-moderate watery diarrhea. Instead, indications for stool cultures include dysenteric diarrhea, persistent diarrhea in immunocompromised patients (ie, persons aged 65 years and older with comorbid diseases, neutropenia, or HIV infection), and diarrhea where an outbreak is suggested.[1] An appropriately obtained stool culture identifies the presence of *Campylobacter*, *Salmonella*, and *Shigella* spp. The yield of stool cultures for other pathogens is increased if the test is ordered specifically based on history and physical examination. For dysenteric diarrhea, the laboratory should be instructed to evaluate for EHEC including STEC (*E. coli* O157:H7). In hospitalized patients who develop diarrhea 3 days after hospitalization or in those with recent exposure to antimicrobials or chemotherapy, stool specimen should be sent for *C. difficile* toxins A and B. In addition to stool cultures, microscopic examination for fecal polymorphonuclear cells, or a simple immunoassay for the neutrophil marker lactoferrin, can further provide evidence of an inflammatory process and increase the yield of cultures in patients presenting with dysenteric diarrhea.[1]

Complications

Complications associated with acute diarrhea most likely result from dehydration so treatment focuses primarily on rehydration therapy, regardless of the etiology. Dysenteric diarrhea is more likely to have severe complications, especially in children younger than 5 years and in elderly. Bacteremia is the most common complication of gastroenteritis and can be seen after infections with nontyphoid *Salmonella*, *C. jejuni* or *C. fetus*, and *Y. enterocolitica*.[16] Nontyphoid *Salmonella* is most common in children younger than 5 years, elderly, and patients with hemoglobinopathy, malaria, or immunosuppression. Bacteremia due to *Campylobacter* spp. has been reported in patients with HIV infection, malignancy, transplantation, and hypogammaglobulinemia. *Y. enterocolitica* bacteremia has been rarely reported, but has an increased prevalence in patients with diabetes mellitus, severe anemia, hemochromatosis, iron overload (frequent transfusion), cirrhosis, malignancy, and in the elderly.[27] Persistent bacteremia with these pathogens will commonly result in prolonged intermittent fever with chills. Potentially complicating the diagnosis, stool cultures frequently are negative and leukocyte counts are often within the normal range. Vascular complications such as seeding of atherosclerotic plaques or aneurysms in arterial vessels occur in 10% to 25% of adults with bacteremia. Localized infections involving bone, cysts, heart, kidney, liver, lungs, pericardium, and spleen develop in 5% to 10% of patients with bacteremia.

A severe complication in patients infected with EHEC is HUS. HUS is defined by the triad of acute renal failure, thrombocytopenia, and microangiopathic hemolytic anemia and is more commonly observed in children younger than 5 years and in the elderly.[28] Approximately 2% to 7% of cases infected with STEC strains are complicated by development of HUS, which increases mortality associated with this infection. *S. dysenteriae* type 1 can also cause HUS, although more rarely than observed with EHEC.[18]

Shigella infection may also lead to complications such as generalized seizures, sepsis, toxic megacolon, perforated colon, arthritis, and protein-losing enteropathy. Mortality is rare, but it may be more likely with *S. dysenteriae* type I. Less than 3% of persons who are infected with *S. flexneri* will later develop Reiter syndrome, characterized by pains in the joints, irritation of the eyes, and painful urination. This can lead to chronic arthritis.[29]

Infection with *C. jejuni* has been associated with Guillain-Barré syndrome (GBS), but the relationship is not well understood.[30] The risk of developing GBS after *C. jejuni* infection appears to be low (approximately 1 case of GBS per 1,000 *C. jejuni* infections). The weakness associated with GBS usually starts in the legs, with difficulty in walking, and may progress to a complete paralysis of all extremities that lasts several weeks and usually requires intensive care.

Approximately 10% to 30% of adult patients develop a reactive arthritis 1 to 2 weeks after recovery from gastroenteritis secondary to *S. flexneri*, *Salmonella* spp., *C. jejuni*, and *Y. enterocolitica*. This arthritis, involving the knees, ankles, toes, fingers, and wrists, usually resolves in 1 to 4 months but may persist in approximately 10% of patients.[30] This complication is more common in persons with the HLA-B27 antigen.

A general complication that could occur long after an infectious gastroenteritis, especially with dysentery and toxin-mediated dysentery, is postinfectious irritable bowel syndrome (IBS). This is classified as IBS symptoms for at least 3 months following an episode of gastroenteritis or traveler's diarrhea showing recurrent abdominal pain or discomfort.[31] Albeit rare, some long-term complications associated with these infections strengthen the need for appropriate diagnosis and treatment.

TREATMENT

Mortality associated with infectious diarrhea has declined substantially in the past two decades, especially among children younger than 1 year. Preventative measures including improved sanitation, breast-feeding and weaning practices, and increased use of oral rehydration therapy (ORT) for affected individuals are responsible for the decrease in case-fatality rates.

General Approach to Treatment

The cornerstone of management for all GI infections and enterotoxigenic poisonings is to prevent dehydration by correcting fluid and electrolyte imbalances. In mild, self-limiting acute gastroenteritis, a diet of oral fluids and easily digestible foods is recommended. In patients with severe dehydrating watery diarrhea and dysenteric diarrhea, IV rehydration therapy, antibiotics, and/or antimotility treatments are needed.

Rehydration Therapy

Initial assessment of fluid loss is essential for successful rehydration therapy and should include acute weight loss, as it is the most reliable means of determining the extent of water loss. However, if accurate baseline weight is not available, clinical signs are helpful in determining approximate deficits (Table 136-4). Physical assessment generally is more reliable in young children and infants than in adults.

3 Fluid replacement is the cornerstone of therapy for dehydration due to diarrhea regardless of etiology. For the treatment of mild-to-moderate dehydration, ORT is superior to administration of IV fluids. Oral replacement therapy reverses dehydration in nearly all patients with mild-to-moderate diarrhea with 94% to 97% efficacy.[1] It offers advantages of being inexpensive, noninvasive, and not requiring inpatient administration. Moreover, thirst drives use of ORT and provides a safeguard against overhydration. Replacement of ongoing losses as well as continuation of normal feeding should also be addressed.

The necessary components of oral rehydration solutions (ORS) include carbohydrates (typically glucose), sodium, potassium, chloride, and water. Using both salt and glucose in the ORS takes advantage of glucose-coupled sodium transport in the small bowel and enhances sodium and subsequently water transport across intestinal walls. The World Health Organization/United Nations Children's Fund (WHO/UNICEF) endorsed a reduced osmolarity solution (osmolarity ≤250

TABLE 136-4 Clinical Assessment of Degree of Dehydration in Children Based on Percentage of Body Weight Loss[a]

Variable	Minimal or No Dehydration (<3% Loss of Body Weight)	Mild-to-Moderate (3%-9% Loss of Body Weight)	Severe (≥10% Loss of Body Weight)
Blood pressure	Normal	Normal	Normal to reduced
Quality of pulses	Normal	Normal or slightly decreased	Weak, thready, or not palpable
Heart rate	Normal	Normal to increased	Increased (bradycardia in severe cases)
Breathing	Normal	Normal to fast	Deep
Mental status	Normal	Normal to listless	Apathetic, lethargic, or comatose
Eyes	Normal	Sunken orbits/decreased tears	Deeply sunken orbits/absent tears
Mouth and tongue	Moist	Dry	Parched
Thirst	Normal	Eager to drink	Drinks poorly; too lethargic to drink
Skin fold	Normal	Recoil in <2 seconds	Recoil in >2 seconds
Extremities	Warm, normal capillary refill	Cool, prolonged capillary refill	Cold, mottled, cyanotic, prolonged capillary refill
Urine output	Normal to decreased	Decreased	Minimal
Hydration therapy	None	ORS 50-100 mL/kg over 3-4 hours	Lactated Ringer's solution or normal saline 20 mL/kg over 15-30 minutes IV until mental status or perfusion improves Followed by 5% dextrose/0.45% sodium chloride IV at higher maintenance rates or ORS 100 mL/kg over 4 hours
Replacement of ongoing losses	For each diarrheal stool or emesis <10 kg body weight: 60-120 mL ORS >10 kg body weight: 120-240 mL ORS	Same as minimal dehydration	If unable to tolerate ORS, administer through nasogastric tube or administer 5% dextrose/0.45% sodium chloride with 20 mEq/L (mmol/L) potassium chloride IV

ORS, oral rehydration solution.

[a]Percentages vary among patients for each dehydration category; hemodynamic and perfusion status is most important; when unsure of category, therapy for more severe category is recommended.

TABLE 136-5 Comparison of Common Solutions Used in Oral Rehydration and Maintenance

Product	Na (mEq/L)[b]	K (mEq/L)[b]	Base (mEq/L)	Carbohydrate (mmol/L)	Osmolarity (mOsm/L)
WHO/UNICEF (2002)	75	20	30	75	245
Pedialyte	45	20	30	140	250
Infalyte	50	25	30	70	200
Oralyte	60	20	0	90	260
Rehydralyte	75	20	30	140	250
Cola[a]	2	0	13	700	750
Apple juice[a]	5	32	0	690	730
Chicken broth[a]	250	8	0	0	500
Sports beverage[a]	20	3	3	255	330

[a]These solutions should be avoided in dehydration.

[b]Concentration of monovalentions expressed in mEq/L is numerically equivalent to mmol/L concentration.

mOsm/L) as the use of these solutions reduced stool volume, shortened duration of diarrhea, and decreased need for unscheduled IV therapy when compared with previously used ORS more than or equal to 310 mOsm/L.[32] The newer formulation of ORS less than or equal to 250 mOsm/L was, however, more likely to cause hyponatremia (blood sodium levels <130 mEq/L [mmol/L]).[33] If commercial ORS are unavailable, one can be roughly duplicated by mixing ½ teaspoon of salt with 6 teaspoons of sugar in 1 L of water.[34]

In restoring fluid and electrolyte balance in cholera infections, polymer-based ORS may be more efficacious than glucose-based ORS. Polymer-based ORS contains rice, wheat, sorghum, or maize. This polymer-based ORS releases glucose more slowly after digestion and, when absorbed in the small bowel, enhances the reabsorption of water and electrolyte secreted into the bowel lumen during diarrhea. Polymer-based ORS reduces the duration of diarrhea in adults with cholera when compared with glucose-based ORS more than or equal to 310 and less than or equal to 270 mOsm/L.[35]

Guidelines for rehydration therapy based on the degree of dehydration and replacement of ongoing losses are outlined in Table 136-4. ORS should be given in small and frequent volumes (5 mL every 2 to 3 minutes in a teaspoon or oral syringe). Nasogastric administration of ORS is an alternative method of administration in a child with persistent vomiting. For breast-fed infants, nursing should be continued. The composition of commercial ORS and commonly consumed beverages is listed in Table 136-5. Clear fluids, such as soft drinks, sweetened fruit drinks, chicken broth, and sports drinks, should be avoided in the treatment of dehydration. These hyperosmolar solutions may cause an osmotic diarrhea.

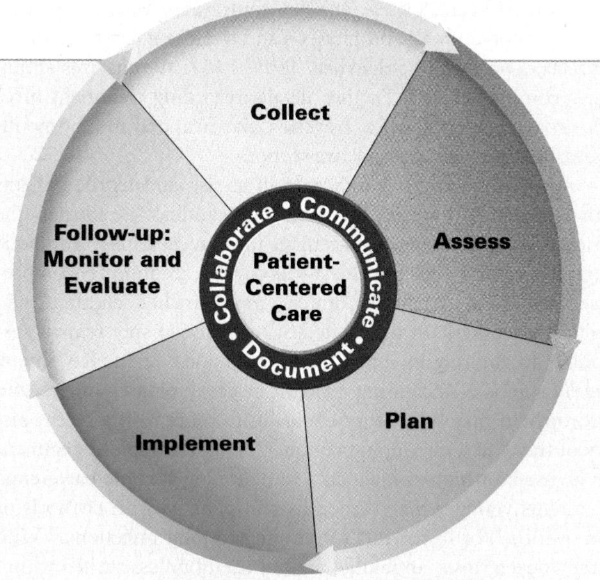

Patient Care Process for *Clostridioides difficile* Infections (CDI)

The image shows the five fundamental steps included in The Pharmacist's Care Process endorsed by the Joint Commission for Pharmacy Practitioners (2014). The tagline of this process reads collaborate, communicate, and document. The five fundamental steps listed here are collect, assess, plan, implement, and follow-up: monitor and evaluate. All these steps are listed in a circular block diagram.

Collect

- Patient characteristics (eg, age, sex)
- Patient medical history (personal and family), including any previous episodes of CDI
- Social history (eg, tobacco/ethanol use) and dietary habits
- Current medications including OTC, herbal products, dietary supplements, acid suppressive medication, and previous antibiotic use (within the past 3 months)
- Characteristics of diarrhea including onset, number of episodes per day, and presence of blood
- Objective data
  - Blood pressure (BP), heart rate (HR), respiratory rate (RR), height, weight, O_2-saturation
  - Labs including white blood cell count (WBC) and serum creatinine (SCr)
  - Stool sample to be tested for *C. difficile* toxins
  - Radiographic abdominal imaging if concern for ileus or megacolon

Assess

- Hemodynamic stability (eg, systolic BP <90 mm Hg, HR > 110 bpm, O_2-sat <90% [0.90], RR)
- Radiographic studies for the presence of ileus, megacolon, or perforation
- Presence of CDI risk factors (age, antibiotic use, recent healthcare exposure, chemotherapy, GI surgery, tube feeding, acid suppressive medications)
- Ability to stop offending antibiotic agent if applicable
- Ability/willingness to pay for first-line treatment options
- Ability/willingness to try investigational therapies such as fecal microbiota transplant (if applicable for recurrent disease)
- Ability/willingness to pay for adjunctive therapy with bezlotoxumab

Plan*

- Drug therapy regimen including specific antibiotic dose, route, frequency, and duration (see Table 136-7)
- Discontinuation of offending antibiotic agent if applicable
- Monitoring parameters, such as resolution of diarrhea; frequency and timing of follow-up
- Patient education (eg, purpose of treatment, drug-specific information, and prevention of disease transmission)
- Self-monitoring for resolution of diarrhea and when to seek emergency medical attention
- Referrals to other providers when appropriate (eg, infectious diseases, gasteroenterology)

Implement

- Provide patient education regarding all elements of treatment plan
- Use motivational interviewing and coaching strategies to maximize adherence
- Schedule follow-up

Follow-up: Monitor and Evaluate

- Resolution of diarrhea
- Presence of adverse effects (eg, CNS effects, metallic taste if metronidazole used; nausea, abdominal pain)
- Patient adherence to treatment plan using multiple sources of information
- Educate on limiting risk factors, such as antibiotic agents and acid suppressive medications

Collaborate with patient, caregivers, and other healthcare professionals.

In the treatment of severe dehydration, the primary goal of therapy is rapid restoration of fluid losses, correction of metabolic acidosis, and replacement of potassium deficiency. Severely dehydrated patients should be resuscitated initially with IV lactated Ringer solution or normal saline to restore hemodynamic stability. Lactated Ringer solution is preferred initially over normal saline because normal saline does not assist in correcting a metabolic acidosis. As GI and renal perfusion should be addressed aggressively, rapid IV administration is preferred over prolonged administration regimens for restoring extracellular fluids and electrolytes.[36] After rehydration, maintenance fluid is given based on accurate recording of intake and output volumes. ORT should be instituted as soon as it can be tolerated.

Early refeeding with age-appropriate unrestricted diet is recommended in children. Early refeeding during or immediately following the start of rehydration did not increase the risk of complications such as unscheduled IV fluids, vomiting, or development of persistent diarrhea compared with late refeeding that ranged from 20 to 48 hours after start of rehydration.[36] Initially, easily digested foods such as bananas, applesauce, and cereal should be introduced and foods high in fiber, sodium, and sugar should be avoided. One caveat would be that lactase deficiency may be exacerbated among known lactase-deficient patients and may persist up to 10 days.

Antimicrobial Therapy

4 The indiscriminate use of antimicrobial therapy produces increases in antimicrobial resistance, side effects of antimicrobial agents, and the threat of superinfections owing to eradication of normal flora. Increasing fluoroquinolone resistance in *Campylobacter* and multidrug resistance in *Salmonella* spp. worldwide reinforces the importance of judicious use of antibiotics and prudent infection control measures.[37,38] Antibiotic therapy is recommended in severe cases of diarrhea, moderate-to-severe cases of traveler's diarrhea, most cases of febrile dysenteric diarrhea, and culture-proven bacterial diarrhea. Antimicrobial therapy is not recommended in EHEC diarrhea as it may increase HUS risk.

Antibiotic therapy is recommended in severe cases of cholera and ETEC diarrhea. In cases of cholera, antibiotics shorten the duration of diarrhea, decrease fluid loss, and shorten the duration of the carrier state.[1,12] It is important to consider local susceptibility patterns in the selection of the antimicrobial regimen. In areas of high fluoroquinolone resistance, azithromycin has been effective in patients with cholera. In patients with ETEC diarrhea, empiric antibiotics reduce severity and duration of diarrhea. A short course of therapy with fluoroquinolones is the most commonly recommended therapy due to increased resistance among other drug classes.[39] Rifaximin has been effective for ETEC for travel in Mexico.[40] Further discussions of antibiotic prophylaxis and treatment can be found in the section on traveler's diarrhea. Table 136-6 summarizes antibiotic recommendations. Further details regarding treatment of *C. difficile*–associated diarrhea, traveler's diarrhea, and foodborne illnesses are discussed in respective sections.

Antibiotic therapy is indicated in at-risk and febrile patients with dysenteric diarrhea. In shigellosis, antibiotics shorten the period of fecal shedding and attenuate the clinical illness. Antibiotic therapy is reserved for the elderly, those who are immunocompromised, children in daycare centers, malnourished children, and healthcare workers. In the United States, *Shigella* spp. remain susceptible to fluoroquinolones. Fluoroquinolone resistance among *Shigella* spp. is of increasing concern in developing countries, and azithromycin may be a better choice in patients with a recent history of travel to a developing region.[1,18] Similar antibiotic regimens can be used for high-risk patients who develop *Yersinia* bacteremia (ie, infants younger than 3 months and patients with cirrhosis or iron overload) or in patients with bone and joint infections.[41] With Campylobacteriosis, antibiotics are not useful unless started within 4 days of the start of the illness because they do not shorten the duration or severity of diarrhea and only shorten the duration of bacterial excretion. Antibiotics are warranted in patients with high fevers, severe bloody diarrhea, prolonged illnesses (more than 1 week), pregnancy, and immunocompromised states, including HIV infection. Fluoroquinolone resistance among *Campylobacter* spp. has increased, and is now 10% to 13% in the United States and 41% to 88% in Europe and Asia. Resistance may be the result of the use of

TABLE 136-6 Recommendations for Antibiotic Therapy

Pathogen	Children	Adults
Watery Diarrhea		
Enterotoxigenic *Escherichia coli*	Azithromycin 10 mg/kg/day given orally once daily × 3 days; ceftriaxone 50 mg/kg/day given IV once daily × 3 days	Ciprofloxacin 750 mg orally once daily × 1-3 days. Alternatives: rifaximin 200 mg orally three times daily × 3 days; azithromycin 1,000 mg orally × 1 day *or* 500 mg orally daily × 3 days
Vibrio cholerae O1	Erythromycin 30 mg/kg/day divided every 8 hours orally × 3 days; azithromycin 10 mg/kg/day given orally once daily × 3 days	Doxycycline 300 mg orally × 1 day Alternatives: azithromycin 500 mg orally once daily × 3 days; ciprofloxacin 750 mg orally once daily × 3 days; ceftriaxone IV
Dysenteric Diarrhea		
Campylobacter species[a]	Azithromycin 10 mg/kg/day given orally once daily × 3-5 days; erythromycin 30 mg/kg/day divided into two to four doses orally × 3-5 days	Azithromycin 500 mg orally once daily × 3 days Alternatives: ciprofloxacin 750 mg orally once daily × 7 days
Salmonella Nontyphoidal[a]	Ceftriaxone 100 mg/kg/day divided IV every 12 hours × 7-10 days; azithromycin 20 mg/kg/day orally once daily × 7 days	Ceftriaxone 2 g IV/IM once; ciprofloxacin 750 mg orally once daily × 7-10 days; Alternatives: ampicillin 250-500 mg orally every 6 hours × 7 days; azithromycin 500 mg orally once daily × 7 days; Trimethoprim-sulfamethoxazole 160/800 mg twice daily × 7 days For immunocompromised patients, duration should be increased to 14 days for both fluoroquinolones and azithromycin
Shigella species[a]	Azithromycin 10 mg/kg/day given orally once daily × 3 days; ceftriaxone 50 mg/kg/day given IV once daily × 3 days	Azithromycin 500 mg orally once daily × 3 days; ceftriaxone 2 g IV/IM once; ciprofloxacin 750 mg orally once daily × 3 days; Alternatives: ampicillin 250-500 mg orally every 6 hours × 7 days; Trimethoprim-sulfamethoxazole 160/800 mg twice daily × 7 days
Yersinia species[a]	Treat as children with shigellosis	Trimethoprim-sulfamethoxazole 160/800 mg twice daily × 7 days Alternatives: cefotaxime IV or ciprofloxacin 750 mg orally once daily × 7 days
Traveler's Diarrhea		
Prophylaxis[a]		None recommended
Treatment		Azithromycin 1,000 mg orally × 1 day or 500 mg orally daily × 3 days, Ciprofloxacin 750 mg orally × 1 day or 500 mg orally twice daily × 3 days; levofloxacin 500 mg orally daily × 3 days, ofloxacin 400 mg twice daily × 1-3 days, rifamycin SV 388 mg twice daily × 3 days, rifaximin 200 mg three times daily × 3 days

[a]For high-risk patients only. See the preceding text for the high-risk patients in each infection.

fluoroquinolone antibiotics in poultry and other animal feed, and the frequent use of these agents internationally in treating enteric infections. Macrolides like azithromycin are recommended especially in patients with a recent history of travel to Asia.[39]

Nontyphoid *Salmonella* infection leads to bacteremia in approximately 8% of otherwise healthy adults. However, patients with increased risk of bacteremia should be treated with antibiotics if appropriate diagnosis is made. High-risk patients include neonates or infants younger than 1 year, persons older than 50 years, and patients with primary or secondary immunodeficiency such as acquired immunodeficiency syndrome (AIDS) or chemotherapy-induced inflammatory bowel disease, sickle cell disease, vascular abnormalities (prostatic heart valve or abdominal aneurysm), or prosthetic joints.[18] If cultures are positive for Salmonellosis and antibacterial therapy is warranted, susceptibility testing should be done for appropriate targeted therapy due to concern of resistance. *Salmonella enterica* serotype Typhi can cause enterocolitis and is a risk for typhoid fever. Although this pathogen is less prevalent, recent data have shown extensive drug resistance (susceptible to carbapenem or macrolide only), especially when travel to certain areas of the world (eg, Pakistan) were involved.[42] When treatment is required, it is important to take a full patient history to see if a patient may have a drug-resistant pathogen as the causative agent.

Outcomes of some bacterial diarrheal illnesses may be worsened by the use of antibacterials, therefore precluding their use. In patients infected with EHEC, use of a fluoroquinolone or trimethoprim-sulfamethoxazole may increase the risk of HUS by increasing the production of Shiga-like toxin.[1,41] Empiric antimicrobial therapy should be withheld when clinical suspicion is high due to the high local prevalence EHEC, patient clinical presentation suggestive of EHEC infection, or a known foodborne outbreak of dysentery with an incubation period of longer than 2 days. Antibiotics should not be given to infants or children due to a higher incidence of HUS in this population. Treatment of EHEC infection is primarily limited to supportive care, which may include fluid replacement therapy, hemodialysis, hemofiltration, transfusion red blood cells and/or platelets, and other interventions as indicated clinically. Severe disease may lead to chronic kidney failure and potential need of renal transplantation.

Antimotility Agents

5 Antimotility drugs such as diphenoxylate/atropine and loperamide offer symptomatic relief in patients with watery diarrhea by reducing the number of stools. However, in both enterotoxigenic and dysenteric diarrhea, slowing of fecal transit time with these agents is thought to result in extended toxin-associated damage, worsening symptomatology and leads to complications. Therefore, antimotility drugs should be avoided if possible and are not recommended in patients with toxin-mediated dysenteric diarrhea (ie, EHEC, pseudomembranous colitis, shigellosis). However, some evidence suggests that in adults with dysenteric diarrhea these agents do not appear to be harmful if given concomitantly with antibacterial therapy.[41]

Probiotics

Probiotics are preparations of microorganisms and most commercial products have been derived from food sources, particularly cultured milk products (ie, lactobacilli and bifidobacteria). When used in the treatment or prophylaxis of infectious diarrhea and antibiotic-associated diarrhea, efficacy is variable. Most individual studies have not shown significant benefit from the use of probiotics and meta-analyses have shown conflicting results, with one demonstrating efficacy when trials were assessed in aggregate[43] and another demonstrating no benefit.[44] Significantly decreased rates of CDI followed lactobacillus use in patients receiving 2 or more days of systemic antibacterials.[45] No serious adverse effects have been reported in otherwise healthy persons; however, there are data suggesting a rare but increased incidence of fungemia or bacterial sepsis with probiotic use. With confounding data both supporting and refuting the use of probiotics for prevention, the decision should be based upon patient-specific criteria.

Oral Zinc Supplementation

Zinc deficiency is largely due to inadequate dietary intake and is common in many developing countries where morbidity and mortality associated with acute diarrhea in children remains high. In children older than 6 months who demonstrate moderate signs of malnutrition, zinc supplementation may shorten the duration of diarrhea by approximately 27 hours (95% CI −14.62 to −39.34).[46] Therefore, oral zinc supplementation of 20 mg/day for 1 to 2 weeks may have an additional benefit over ORS alone in reducing childhood mortality in developing countries. Common side effects include metallic taste and vomiting. At high doses, zinc supplementation may cause epigastric pain, lethargy, and fatigue.

PREVENTION OF GASTROINTESTINAL INFECTIONS

6 Public health measures of improved water supply and sanitation facilities and the quality control of commercial products are important for the control of the majority of GI infections. In addition, following simple rules of personal hygiene and safe food preparation can prevent many diarrheal diseases. Hand washing with soap and running water is instrumental in preventing the spread of illness and should be emphasized for caregivers and persons with diarrheal illnesses. Safe food handling and preparation practices can significantly decrease the incidence of certain enteric infections.

Reporting suspected outbreaks and cases of notifiable illness to local health authorities is vital to investigation of threats of enteric infection arising from increasingly global and industrialized food supplies. The reporting of specific infectious diseases to the appropriate public health authorities is the cornerstone of public health surveillance, outbreak detection, and prevention and control efforts.

Vaccines are used to boost specific immune processes directed against the bacteria themselves or against adherence appendages, cytotoxins, or enterotoxins. Unfortunately, there are only a few vaccines available for prevention of gastroenteritis. Vaccines for typhoid fever are the parenteral Vi capsular polysaccharide vaccine (ViCPS) and the oral live-attenuated Ty21a vaccine.[47] Efficacy rates for both vaccines range from 50% to 80%. The ViCPS is indicated for children who are 2 years of age or older, and a booster dose is administered 2 years after the first. The Ty21a vaccine is indicated for children 6 years or older; one capsule should be swallowed whole every other day for a total of four doses at least 1 week before the potential exposure. A booster should be taken every 5 years if continued protection is needed.

In the United States, routine rotavirus vaccination is recommended for all infants beginning at age 2 months. There are two vaccines, RotaTeq (RV5) and Rotarix (RV1), available for reducing rotaviral gastroenteritis.[48] The RV5 vaccine is a live, oral vaccine that offers 74% efficacy against gastroenteritis of any severity and 98% efficacy against severe disease. This vaccine also decreased office visits by 86%, emergency department visits by 94%, and hospitalizations by 96%. The RV1 vaccine is a live-attenuated human rotavirus vaccine. This vaccine has clinical efficacy of 79% against gastroenteritis of any severity and 96% efficacy against severe rotavirus disease. Rotarix reduced hospitalizations by 100% and medically attended visits by 92% in the first rotavirus season, and reduced hospitalizations by 96% through two seasons.[48] The RV5 vaccine is administered orally in a three-dose series at ages 2, 4, and 6 months while the RV1 vaccine is administered orally in a two-dose series at ages 2 and

4 months. The first dose may be given between 6 weeks and 14 weeks and 6 days of age and all doses should be given before 8 months of age. The vaccines are contraindicated in infants with severe allergic reactions to vaccine components, diagnosed with severe combined immunodeficiency, and with history of intussusception.[49]

Although not available in the United States, two oral vaccines against diarrheal pathogens are available in other countries. Dukoral consists of killed *V. cholerae* O1 organisms and the cholera B subunit, and is licensed in over 60 countries. Shanchol consists of killed whole cells from a mix of pathogenic strains of *V. cholerae* (O1 and O139) and is licensed in India.[11,13] Both vaccines are given in two doses (three doses of Dukoral are required for children aged 2-5 years) and administered about 7 to 14 days apart (up to 42 days apart for Dukoral). Dukoral must be administered with a buffer that requires 75 to 150 mL of clean water while Shanchol does not require the buffer. Both vaccines demonstrated protective efficacy of 47% to 87% after two doses but almost none after a single dose. Protection is achieved in approximately 1 week following the last dose and persists for approximately 2 years. The common side effects of the vaccines were considered mild and included abdominal pain, headache, fever, and nausea. The WHO does not require vaccination for international travel to or from endemic areas because vaccines require two doses and provide incomplete protection for a relatively short period of time.[13]

There are vaccines in development for common enteric pathogens including ETEC and *Shigella* spp. with the potential for combining them in a single vaccine. These are still in preliminary and animal-based studies, but could significantly affect global public health if they come to fruition for human administration, especially in the infants and children.[50]

EVALUATION OF THERAPEUTIC OUTCOMES

Appropriate follow-up care of patients with acute diarrhea is based on successful restoration of fluid losses. The clinical signs and symptoms that lead to the diagnosis also can assess adequate rehydration, and should be monitored frequently. With ORT preferred, routine laboratory testing often is unnecessary. Electrolytes should be measured in those receiving IV fluids, when oral replacement fails, or when signs of hypernatremia or hypokalemia are present. Follow-up stool samples to ensure complete evacuation of the infecting pathogen may be necessary only in patients who are at high risk to initiate or contribute to a community outbreak. All patients should be monitored for complications associated with the infecting pathogen, resolution of the diarrhea, and adverse reactions to the pharmacologic agents used. Prompt discharge of hospitalized patients is recommended when rehydration is achieved, IV fluids have not been required, oral intake equals or exceeds losses, or adequate education and medical follow-up are ensured. For most patients, discharge can occur in 16 to 24 hours.

CLOSTRIDIOIDES DIFFICILE

Epidemiology

C. difficile is the most commonly recognized cause of infectious diarrhea in healthcare settings with high rates of disease in the elderly and those exposed to antibiotic agents. While almost all antibiotics have been implicated in *C. difficile* infection (CDI), those most commonly associated include fluoroquinolones, clindamycin, carbapenems, and third-/fourth-generation cephalosporins. CDI often occurs during or shortly after completion of antimicrobial therapy; however, disease onset can be delayed for 3 or more months.[51] Other risk factors for acquisition of *C. difficile* include recent healthcare exposure, chemotherapy, patients undergoing gastrointestinal surgery or receiving tube feeding, and potentially those receiving acid suppressive medications. While some studies show an association between *CDI* and acid suppressing medications, such as proton pump inhibitors (PPIs) and histamine-2 blockers, there is variability in the literature and a need for prospective randomized trials to confirm this link.[51,52]

Incidence of CDI was steadily rising in the early 2000s, appearing to peak around 2010 at approximately 500,000 cases annually in the United States and Europe. Growing concern for CDI, especially in the healthcare facilities, led to the creation of the Centers for Disease Control and Prevention (CDC) Emerging Infection Program (EIP) CDI tracking program. This program has been conducting population-based surveillance of *C. difficile* in 10 US cities since 2011 in order to estimate the national burden of CDI. While the epidemiology of CDI has remained relatively steady, trends indicate a decline in healthcare associated infecitons.[51,53] One confounding factor in the estimation of CDI incidence is the introduction of more sensitive tests, such as nucleic acid amplification tests (NAATs), which may lead to overdiagnosis.[53] Recurrent CDI is a major problem, with escalating risk of infection and increased mortality with subsequent infections.[51,52]

Etiology and Pathophysiology

C. difficile is a gram-positive spore-forming obligate anaerobic bacterium that may colonize the large intestine of healthy individuals, as well as those experiencing a symptomatic CDI. *C. difficile* is transmitted most commonly by the fecal-oral route through ingestion of *C. difficile* spores. Pathogenic CDI occurs when there is disruption of the bowel flora and/or an inadequate immune response. Two major toxins (toxin A [TcdA] and toxin B [TcdB]) are released and lead to a loss of integrity of colonic epithelial cells.[54] This mediates an inflammatory cascade that causes tissue damage and results in diarrhea. Initially, raised white and yellowish plaques form in the colon and the surrounding mucosa may become inflamed. With progression of disease, pseudomembranous plaques become enlarged and scattered over the colorectal mucosa resulting in pseudomembranous colitis.[51] The production of binary toxin, mutations causing hyperproduction of toxins, antibiotic resistance, increased sporulation, and mutations that increase adherence to the intestinal epithelium may contribute to the virulence and disease severity in the host. Some strains, such as BI/NAP1/027, express multiple mutations that make it hypervirulent and are a cause of significant clinical concern.[54]

CLINICAL PRESENTATION

Symptoms of CDI range from mild diarrhea to fulminant disease and toxic megacolon. The diarrhea is typically watery and nonbloody, and is often associated with abdominal discomfort, fever, and leukocytosis. Patients with new and unexplained diarrhea (>3 unformed stools in 24 hours) should be evaluated for CDI.

Diagnosis of CDI is confirmed by identification of *C. difficile* organisms/toxin in stool or by colonoscopic or histopathologic findings revealing pseudomembranous colitis.[51]

The optimal test for laboratory diagnosis remains controversial. Nucleic acid amplification tests (NAAT), such as PCR-based toxin testing, are very popular in the United States and have high sensitivity and specificity; however, they should only be used in patients with acute diarrhea due to the possibility of detecting the toxins in asymptomatic patients.[51,52] Alternatively, a stepwise approach uses screening for glutamate dehydrogenase (GDH) as the initial step. GDH assays detect a common antigen present in all isolates of *C. difficile*, including nontoxigenic strains, thus requiring combination with another test (typically a toxin test with or without NAAT). The stepwise approach may be preferred in institutions where there is no criteria for stool submission in order to minimize the false positive results that may result with NAAT alone. Utility of toxigenic culture or cell culture neutralization assays are limited due to delayed results and high cost. Use of toxin enzyme immunoassay (EIA) alone has a low sensitivity and has largely been replaced by NAAT testing or incorporated into multistep algorithms along with GDH assays.[51,55]

Treatment

Supportive care of CDI includes fluid and electrolyte replacement therapy, in addition to discontinuation of the offending antimicrobial if possible. Antimotility agents (such as diphenoxylate/atropine and loperamide) and exchange resins (such as cholestyramine and colestipol) have been used in CDI; however, in general their use is discouraged. Empiric therapy for CDI may be considered if the patient has a strong pre-test suspicion for CDI and is severely ill, or if there is an expected substantial delay in laboratory confirmation. Antibiotic therapy is based on disease severity and may vary for first episode or recurrent infection.[51] Table 136-7 outlines CDI disease severity and treatment regimens for initial episodes according to the IDSA/SHEA 2017 clinical practice guidelines. Differences exist among the available guidelines with regard to the definitions of nonsevere, severe, and fulminant or complicated CDI and slight treatment differences. There is a need for prospectively validated severity scores for patients with CDI.

7 In the United States, vancomycin and fidaxomicin are FDA approved for CDI. These treatments are well tolerated because they have minimal systemic absorption when administered orally; the main adverse effects are nausea and abdominal pain. The recommended treatment course is 10 days and repeat stool testing is not recommended as a test of cure.[51] For nearly three decades oral metronidazole was the drug of choice for mild-to-moderate CDI; however, it has fallen out of favor based on evidence showing it is significantly less effective than vancomycin or fidaxomicin. The IDSA/SHEA 2017 clinical practice guidelines recommended therapies for both nonsevere and severe CDI include oral vancomycin or fidaxomicin. However, based on emerging data demonstrating the sustained response and safety profile of fidaxomicin, it is now the preferred therapy for initial CDI episodes. Vancomycin represents an acceptable alternative if fidaxomicin is not available, which may be reasonable based on the cost and variable medical insurance coverage of fidaxomicin.[56] When used for CDI, vancomycin must be administered orally because IV vancomycin does not achieve adequate gut lumen concentrations for effective bacterial elimination. Vancomycin is available as a capsule and there are several reconstituted oral solution or suspensions commercially available. The IV formulation has also been compounded and administered orally as a cost-effective option.

In patients with severe/complicated or fulminant CDI the preferred regimen is combination therapy with IV metronidazole and vancomycin.[57] The route of vancomycin administration is patient-dependent; oral is preferred, but if ileus is present, rectal administration via retention enema is recommended at a dose of 500 mg in 100 mL of saline administered four times daily. Fidaxomicin has not been studied in complicated or fulminant disease, therefore is not recommended.[51] Some patients with fulminant disease may require surgical intervention with procedures such as diverting loop ileostomy or total colectomy.

Recurrent CDI (rCDI) is typically defined as an episode of CDI within 8 weeks from the previous episode. Approximately 15% to 35% of patients will have a recurrence and the rate nearly doubles after two or more recurrences.[58] Risk factors for recurrent CDI include increasing age, use of additional antimicrobials, gastric acid suppression, hypervirulent strains, and low antibody response to *C. difficile* toxins.[51,58] The preferred regimen for the first episode of rCDI is fidaxomicin standard dose or an extended-pulsed regimen (200 mg twice daily for 5 days, then once every other day for 20 days). Pulsed and tapered oral vancomycin is an alternative approach for the first recurrence. If metronidazole was used initially, then a standard vancomycin course can be utilized for the first recurrence. For patients with multiple recurrences fidaxomicin remains the preferred agent; however, pulsed/tapered vancomycin, vancomycin followed by rifaximin, or fecal microbiota transplantation (FMT) are acceptable alternatives.[56]

The importance of the gut microbiome and its relationship to primary and recurrent CDI has led to research on several emerging therapies for CDI. Multiple randomized controlled trials have shown efficacy of FMT with resolution rates up to 90%. The American College of Gastroenterology recommends FMT by colonoscopy or capsule formulation oral ingestion with rCDI.[58,59] Protocols that have been studied include stool suspension administered to the lower bowel (through colonoscopy, rectal tube, or enema) or the upper GI tract (through nasogastric or duodenal tube or gastroscope). Several microbiota products available in a capsule formulation are undergoing clinical trials and may be available for use in the near future.[6,60]

A monoclonal antibody, bezlotoxumab, that binds to and neutralizes toxin B is FDA approved as an adjunctive therapy to reduce the recurrence of CDI. The approved dose is 10 mg/kg IV as a single dose during antibacterial treatment for CDI. Bezlotoxumab is not an antibiotic and should not be used as monotherapy. For patients with rCDI within 6 months, IDSA/SHEA suggest bezlotoxumab use during the administration of standard of care antibiotics. There may be feasibility concerns, such as cost and logistics, with this approach. The benefit of adding bezlotoxumab to fidaxomicin is unknown at this time due to limited data with concurrent use of these agents.[56] While generally well tolerated, adverse effects were greater in patients with heart failure who were treated with bezlotoxumab; use in these patients should be considered carefully.[61]

Growing concern for CDI has led to an influx of new antibiotics targeting *C. difficile*. A common characteristic of many of the emerging therapies for CDI is a narrow spectrum of activity with the aim to minimize gut dysbiosis. As many of these agents complete phase III trials, it may change the treatment landscape for CDI in the future.[62]

TABLE 136-7 *Clostridioides difficile* Infection Severity and Treatment

Severity	Markers of Disease Severity	Recommended Treatment
Nonsevere	WBC ≤15,000 cells/mm³ (15 × 10⁹/L) SCr <1.5 mg/dL (133 μmol/L)	Vancomycin 125 mg orally four times daily for 10 days, OR Fidaxomicin[a] 200 mg orally twice daily for 10 days, OR Metronidazole[b]
Severe	WBC >15,000 cells/mm³ (15 × 10⁹/L) SCr >1.5 mg/dL (133 μmol/L)	Vancomycin 125 mg orally four times daily for 10 days, OR Fidaxomicin 200 mg orally twice daily for 10 days
Fulminant	Hypotension or shock Ileus and/or megacolon	Metronidazole 500 mg IV every 8 hours *PLUS* vancomycin 500 mg every 6 hours via NG or orally (if ileus present use rectally)

[a]Fidaxomicin is preferred over vancomycin for patients with an initial CDI per IDSA/SHEA 2021 Focused Update.

[b]Metronidazole is an alternative therapy if other agents are unavailable or too costly.

Data from References 51 and 56.

NG, nasogastric; SCr, serum creatinine; WBC, white blood cell.

Prevention of CDI involves both preventing the acquisition of the infection and stopping transmission of *C. difficile* spores to other patients. CDI has become the focus of antimicrobial stewardship efforts aimed at eliminating unnecessary antibiotics and reducing durations of therapy, which may be responsible for the plateau of CDI rates in recent years. The use of probiotics to prevent CDI remains controversial.[60,63] Some studies and meta-analyses have shown no benefit, while other evidence supports probiotic safety and efficacy in preventing CDI. Currently, there is insufficient evidence to recommend probiotics and they are not recommended by the American College of Gastroenterology.[1,51] Hand washing and contact precautions are imperative measures in preventing the spread of the organism. Alcohol is less effective at eliminating *C. difficile* spores compared to use of soap and water; however, there is no association between alcohol-based hand hygiene and increased CDI incidence. Nonetheless, the use of soap and water to prevent disease transmission is the preferred strategy. Proper environmental disinfecting measures in healthcare settings include use of sporicidal cleaning agents.[51,60,61,63]

TRAVELER'S DIARRHEA

Traveler's diarrhea describes the clinical syndrome manifested by malaise, anorexia, and abdominal cramps followed by the sudden onset of diarrhea that incapacitates many travelers. It interferes with planned activities or work in 30% of those affected. In particular, an increased risk lies with North Americans and Northern Europeans traveling to Latin America, southern Europe, Africa, and Asia. The highest risk is observed with patients with immunocompromised conditions, achlorhydria, inflammatory bowel disease, and people with chronic debilitating medical conditions. Overall, 30% to 70% of people traveling to high-risk areas will develop the illness.[39]

8 The onset of symptoms usually occurs during the first week of travel but can occur anytime during the visit or after returning home. Traveler's diarrhea is caused by contaminated food or water. The most common pathogens are bacterial and include ETEC, *Campylobacter* spp., *Shigella* spp., and *Salmonella* spp.[10] Viral causes occur in less than 10% of cases with 80% to 90% of cases resulting from bacterial etiologies.[39] Enterotoxigenic *E. coli* is predominantly pathogenic in Latin America, Africa, and South Asia. The invasive enteric pathogens (*Campylobacter* spp., *Salmonella* spp., and *Shigella* spp.) are more important causes of traveler's diarrhea in Asia.

The severity of the syndrome is determined by the number of stools per day and the presence of cramping, nausea, and vomiting. Mild diarrhea is defined as one to three loose stools per day that are associated with abdominal cramps lasting less than 14 days. Moderate diarrhea indicates more than four loose stools daily associated with dehydration, and severe diarrhea is defined as the presence of blood in stools or a fever. Traveler's diarrhea is rarely life-threatening and in most cases, symptoms resolve in several days without treatment. Travelers to high-risk areas should pack a kit that includes a thermometer, loperamide, antibiotics (3-day course) (see "Treatment" section below), ORS salts, and a water purification method.[39]

Prevention

9 Patient education in avoiding high-risk food and beverages should be the best method for minimizing the risk. High-risk foods and beverages include raw or undercooked meat and seafood, moist foods served at room temperature, fruits that cannot be peeled, vegetables, milk from a questionable source, hot sauces on the table, tap water, unsealed bottled water, iced drinks, and food from street vendors. Although education is readily available, the incidence of diarrhea was similar in travelers who followed advice and those who engaged in riskier eating habits.[64] Rationales for this include that cooking foods does not always kill pathogens and food should not be considered safe unless it is cooked until steaming hot. Nonetheless, advisement of avoidance measures regarding safe foods, beverages, and eating establishments is recommended to heighten awareness.

Bismuth subsalicylate 524 mg (two chewable tablets or 2 ounces) orally four times daily for up to 3 weeks is a commonly recommended prophylactic regimen.[39] Bismuth subsalicylate may inhibit enterotoxin activity and prevent diarrhea. Persons taking this regimen should be informed of adverse events, including temporary black discoloration of tongue and stools, and, rarely, tinnitus.

Although the efficacy of prophylactic antibiotics has been documented, their use is not recommended for most travelers due to the potential side effects of antibiotics (eg, photosensitivity), predisposition to other infections such as CDI or vaginal candidiasis, the increased risk of selection of drug-resistant organisms, cost, lack of data on the safety and efficacy of antibiotics given for more than 2 or 3 weeks, and availability of rapidly effective antibiotics for treatment. Prophylactic antibiotics are recommended only in high-risk individuals or in situations in which short-term illness could ruin the purpose of the trip, such as a military mission. A fluoroquinolone is the drug of choice when traveling to most areas of the world.[39] Due to fluoroquinolone resistance among *Campylobacter* spp., azithromycin can be considered when traveling to South and Southeast Asia.

Rrifaximin is a nonabsorbed oral rifamycin that has activity against enteric pathogens and may have a role in the prevention of traveler's diarrhea in select populations. Rrifaximin 200 mg once, twice, or three times daily with meals for 2 weeks resulted in equal protection of 72% for each of the three dosing regimens compared with placebo.[40] Since rifaximin is effective against traveler's diarrhea due to noninvasive strains of *E. coli*, this agent should be reserved for travel regions where *E. coli* predominates, such as Latin America and Africa. Rifaximin has a tolerability and safety profile comparable to that of placebo. The concern with the rifamycin class is the emergence of resistance when used as monotherapy.

Treatment

The goals of treatment are to avoid dehydration, reduce the severity and duration of symptoms, and prevent interruption of planned activities. Fluid and electrolyte replacement should be initiated at the onset of diarrhea. ORT is generally not required in otherwise healthy individuals; flavored mineral water offers a good source of sodium and glucose. In infants and young children, elderly, and those with chronic debilitating medical conditions, ORT is recommended. For symptom relief, loperamide is preferred because of its quicker onset and longer duration of relief relative to bismuth. Standard dosing of loperamide is 4 mg orally initially and then 2 mg with each subsequent loose stool to a maximum of 16 mg/day in patients without bloody diarrhea and fever. Loperamide should be discontinued if symptoms persist for more than 48 hours. Other symptomatic therapy in mild diarrhea includes bismuth subsalicylate 524 mg every 30 minutes for up to eight doses.[39] As previously discussed, there is insufficient evidence to warrant the recommendation of probiotics.

Since behavioral modification has limited efficacy and chemoprophylaxis is not recommended in most travelers, the current recommendation relies on self-treatment. A single dose of antibiotic and up to 3 days of treatment will improve the condition within 24 to 36 hours, shortening the duration of diarrhea by 1 to 2 days.[39] A single dose of fluoroquinolone is recommended initially and if diarrhea is improved within 12 to 24 hours, antibiotics should be discontinued. Otherwise, it can be continued for up to 3 days. A fluoroquinolone is recommended when traveling to most areas of the world. Where fluoroquinolone-resistant *Campylobacter* is common, such as in South and Southeast Asia, azithromycin should be used.[39] Azithromycin can also be used in pregnant women and children younger than age 16 years. Empiric treatment of young children should be instituted with caution.

Rifaximin was as effective as a 3-day course of ciprofloxacin in shortening the duration of diarrhea in noninvasive traveler's diarrhea. However, rifaximin was not as effective in patients with fever and bloody diarrhea and in those with invasive pathogens. Therefore, a 3-day course of rifaximin has been approved for the treatment of traveler's diarrhea caused by noninvasive strains of *E. coli* in people 12 years or older and can be considered when traveling to areas where *E. coli*–associated traveler's diarrhea is common, such as Mexico and Jamaica.[39]

For rapid improvement in symptoms, antibiotic therapy with adjunctive treatment with loperamide has shown benefit.[65] All clinical trials concluded that the combination therapy was safe, and the worsening of the disease with the use of antimotility treatment has not been encountered.

FOOD POISONING

10 Foodborne illnesses result from the ingestion of food containing pathogenic microorganisms that cause GI infections or preformed toxins that were produced by microorganisms that cause enterotoxigenic poisonings. In the United States, foodborne diseases cause approximately 76 million illnesses, 325,000 hospitalizations, and 5,200 deaths each year.[4] Foodborne transmission may account for up to 80% of acute gastroenteritis. However, the incidence and outbreaks of foodborne illness have declined in recent years.[66] Common enteric pathogens responsible for foodborne diseases have been discussed in the previous sections (*Campylobacter* spp., *E. coli*, norovirus, nontyphoidal *Salmonella*, *Shigella*). Common foodborne pathogens that cause enterotoxigenic poisonings include *Bacillus cereus*, *Clostridioides botulinum*, *Clostridioides perfringens*, and *Staphylococcus aureus*. Characteristics of pathogens responsible for foodborne illnesses are summarized in Table 136-8.

Because foodborne disease can appear as sporadic cases or outbreaks, the diagnosis should be suspected whenever two or more people present with acute GI or neurologic manifestations after sharing a meal within the previous 72 hours. Important clues about etiologic agents can be gathered from demographic information (age, gender, etc.), the clinical syndrome, incubation period, and medical history, type of foods consumed, seasonality, and geographic location of the outbreak.

Enterotoxigenic poisonings result from ingestion of food contaminated by preformed toxins. Therefore, symptoms are rapid in onset, but most cases of food poisoning are of short duration with recovery occurring within 1 to 2 days. *B. cereus* causes two different types of clinical syndromes. The first one is characterized by a short incubation period and vomiting. The second syndrome has a longer incubation period and is characterized by diarrhea. Foodborne *C. perfringens* infection may present as two distinct syndromes. Type A organisms are seen in Western Hemisphere nations and result in a 24-hour illness characterized by watery diarrhea and epigastric pain. Type C organisms can be found in undercooked pork and occur in underdeveloped tropical regions. They can produce a toxin-related syndrome called *enteritis necroticans*, which is a coagulative transmural necrosis of the intestinal wall.[67] This syndrome can result in intestinal perforation leading to sepsis and mortality in approximately 40% of victims.

Foodborne botulism results from the ingestion of food contaminated with preformed toxins or toxin-producing spores from

TABLE 136-8 Food Poisonings

Organism	Principal Foods	Peak Incidence (United States)	Time to Symptoms	Duration	Common Symptoms
Enterotoxigenic Poisonings					
Bacillus cereus	Fried rice, dairy products, spices, bean sprouts, vegetables	None	1-6 hours 6-24 hours	1 day 1 day	Nausea, vomiting Diarrhea
Clostridioides botulinum	Home-canned fruits, vegetables, meats, honey	None	18-36 hours		Double vision, blurred vision, drooping eyelids, slurred speech, difficulty swallowing, dry mouth, and muscle weakness
Clostridioides perfringens (type A)	Meats, poultry, gravies, dried or precooked foods	Fall, winter, spring	8-12 hours	1 day	Abdominal cramps, diarrhea
Staphylococcus aureus	Salad, pastries, ham, sandwiches, puddings, unpasteurized milk, cheese products	Summer	1-6 hours	1 day	Nausea, vomiting, abdominal cramps, diarrhea
GI Infections					
Campylobacter spp.	Poultry, dairy products, clams, water	Spring, summer	2-5 days	7 days	Diarrhea (may be bloody), cramping, abdominal pain, fever
Enteropathogenic *E. coli*	Water	None	1-3 days	5-7 days	Severe diarrhea, vomiting, dehydration
Enterotoxigenic *E. coli*	Water, ice, food	None	1-3 days	3-4 days	Profuse watery diarrhea, abdominal cramping
Salmonella spp.	Beef, poultry, water, eggs, dairy products	Summer	12-72 hours	4-7 days	Diarrhea (sometimes bloody), fever, abdominal cramps
Shigella spp.	Salad, water	Summer	1-2 days	5-7 days	Diarrhea (often bloody), fever, abdominal cramps
Vibrio cholerae	Water	None	2 hours to 5 days	2-3 days	Profuse watery diarrhea, vomiting, leg cramps
Vibrio parahemolyticus	Shellfish (oysters)	Spring, summer, fall	24 hours	3 days	Watery diarrhea, abdominal cramping, nausea, vomiting, fever, chills
Yersinia enterocolitica	Dairy products, raw or undercooked pork products	None	4-7 days	1-3 weeks	Fever, abdominal pain, diarrhea (often bloody)

C. botulinum. Poisoning from *C. botulinum* is rare; only 110 cases are reported per year in the United States. Botulism is almost always associated with improper preparation or storage of food. Seven distinct toxins (A to G) have been described. The toxins prevent the release of acetylcholine at the peripheral cholinergic nerve terminal. Toxin activity has prompted the use of minute locally injected doses to treat select spastic disorders, such as blepharospasm, hemifacial spasm, and certain dystonias. Foodborne botulism is suspected when patients present with acute GI symptoms concurrently or just prior to the onset of a symmetric descending paralysis without sensory or central nervous system involvement. Diagnosis is made by culturing *C. botulinum* from the stool. The clinical presentation may resemble GBS associated with *C. jejuni* infection. The difference lies in the onset of neurologic symptoms, which typically occur 1 to 3 weeks after the onset of *C. jejuni* infection, and the condition usually is manifested by an ascending paralysis in *C. jejuni*–associated GBS.

Treatment consists primarily of respiratory support and use of botulinum antitoxin. If evaluation is performed within several hours of ingestion, gastric lavage or induction of vomiting is suggested. Cathartics and enemas also can be used to remove residual toxin from the bowel, but they are contraindicated in cases of ileus. Botulinum antitoxin is a concentrated preparation of equine globulins obtained from horses immunized with toxins A, B, and E. Because trivalent antitoxin is equine in origin, patients should be tested for hypersensitivity before receiving the product intravenously. Newer and more effective methods of treatment and prevention are under development, including a botulinum toxin vaccine consisting of nontoxic botulinum fragments. Prevention always should be stressed. Botulinum toxins are heat labile and readily destroyed by 10 minutes of boiling. All home-canned foods should be processed according to directions and boiled, not just warmed, prior to consumption.

In foodborne illnesses, the cornerstone of therapy remains supportive care. ORT is preferred in replenishing and maintaining fluid and electrolyte balance, and IV fluid therapy should be reserved for those who are severely ill and cannot tolerate oral therapy. Antiemetics and antimotility agents offer symptomatic relief, but the latter should not be given in patients who present with high fever, bloody diarrhea, or fecal leukocytes. Antimicrobial therapy is not effective in the management of *S. aureus*, *C. perfringens*, or *B. cereus* food poisonings. In developed countries, many of the foodborne illnesses can be prevented with proper food selection, preparation, and storage. However, in developing countries, sanitation and clean water supply are larger concerns.

ABBREVIATIONS

AIDS	acquired immunodeficiency syndrome
cAMP	cyclic adenosine monophosphate
CDI	*Clostridioides difficile* infection
CRP	C-reactive protein
EAEC	enteroaggregative *Escherichia coli*
EHEC	enterohemorrhagic *Escherichia coli*
EIA	enzyme immunoassay
EIEC	enteroinvasive *Escherichia coli*
EPEC	enteropathogenic *Escherichia coli*
ETEC	enterotoxigenic *Escherichia coli*
FDA	Food and Drug Administration
FMT	fecal microbiota transplant
GBS	Guillain-Barré syndrome
GDH	glutamate dehydrogenase
HIV	human immunodeficiency virus
HUS	hemolytic uremic syndrome
IDSA	Infectious Diseases Society of America
IBS	irritable bowel syndrome
IL	Interleukin
IVIG	intravenous immune globulin
NAAT	nucleic acid amplification tests
NAP-1	North American pulsed-field type 1
ORS	oral rehydration solution
ORT	oral rehydration therapy
PKA	protein kinase A
PPI	proton pump inhibitor
SHEA	Society for Healthcare Epidemiology of America
STEC	Shiga toxin–producing *Escherichia coli*
UNICEF	United Nations Children's Fund
ViCPS	Vi capsular polysaccharide vaccine
WHO	World Health Organization

REFERENCES

1. Shane AL, Mody RK, Crump JA, et al. 2017 Infectious Diseases Society of America clinical practice guidelines for the diagnosis and management of infectious diarrhea. *Clin Infect Dis.* 2017;65(12):e45–e80.
2. World Health Organization. Diarrhoeal disease. Available at: http://www.who.int/mediacentre/factsheets/fs330/en/. Accessed June 6, 2018.
3. GBD Diarrhoeal Diseases Collaborators. Estimates of global, regional, and national morbidity, mortality, and aetiologies of diarrhoeal diseases: A systematic analysis for the Global Burden of Disease Study 2015. *Lancet Infect Dis.* 2017;17:909–948.
4. CDC . *Foodborne Diseases Active Surveillance Network (FoodNet): FoodNet 2015 Surveillance Report (Final Data).* Atlanta, GA: U.S. Department of Health and Human Services, CDC; 2017.
5. Scallan E, Griffin PM, Angulo FJ, Tauxe RV, Hoekstra RM. Foodborne illness acquired in the United States—Unspecified agents. *Emerg Infect Dis.* 2011;17(1):16–22.
6. Scallan E, Hoekstra RM, Angulo FJ, et al. Foodborne illness acquired in the United States—Major pathogens. *Emerg Infect Dis.* 2011;17(1):7–15.
7. Powell MR. Trends in reported foodborne illness in the United States; 1996-2013. *Risk Analysis.* 2016;36(8):1589–1598.
8. Payne DC, Vinje J, Szilagyi PG, et al. Norovirus and medically attended gastroenteritis in U.S. children. *N Eng J Med.* 2013;368:1121–1130.
9. Shah MP, Dahl RM, Parahar UD, et al. Annual changes in rotavirus hospitalization rates before and after rotavirus vaccine implementation in the United States. *PLoS ONE.* 2018;13(2):1–13.
10. Tack Danielle M, Ray Logan, Griffin Patricia M, et al. Preliminary Incidence and Trends of Infections with Pathogens Transmitted Commonly Through Food—Foodborne Diseases Active Surveillance Network, 10 U.S. Sites, 2016–2019. MMWR. Morbidity and Mortality Weekly Report 2020;69:509–514. 10.15585/mmwr.mm6917a1.
11. World Health Organization. Cholera, 2016. *Weekly Epidem Record.* 2017;92(36):521–536.
12. Leibovici-Weissman Y, Neuberger A, Bitterman R, et al. Antimicrobial drugs for treating cholera (review). *Cochrane Database Sys Rev.* 2014;6:1–181.
13. World Health Organization. Cholera vaccines: WHO position paper—August 2017. *Weekly Epidem Record.* 2017;92(34):477–500.
14. Fang FC, Patel R. 2017 Infectious Diseases Society of America infectious diarrhea guidelines: A view from the clinical laboratory. *Clin Infect Dis.* 2017;65(12):1974–1976.
15. Flores J, Okhuysen PC. Enteroaggregative *Escherichia coli* infection. *Curr Opin Gastroenterol.* 2009;25(1):8–11.
16. Pfeiffer ML, DuPont HL, Ochoa TJ. The patient presenting with acute dysentery—A systematic review. *J Infect.* 2012;64(4):374–386.
17. Voetsch AC, Van Gilder TJ, Angulo FJ, et al. FoodNet estimate of the burden of illness caused by nontyphoidal *Salmonella* infections in the United States. *Clin Infect Dis.* 2004;38(Suppl 3):S127–S134.
18. Toro C, Arroyo A, Sarria A, et al. Shigellosis in subjects with traveler's diarrhea versus domestically acquired diarrhea: Implications for antimicrobial therapy and human immunodeficiency virus surveillance. *Am J Trop Med Hyg.* 2015;93(3):491–496.
19. Switaj TL, Winter KJ, Christensen SR. Diagnosis and management of foodborne illness. *Am Fam Physician.* 2015;92(5):358–365.
20. Sabina Y, Rahman A, Ray RC, Montet D. *Yersinia enterocolitica*: Mode of transmission, molecular insights of virulence, and pathogenesis of infection. *J Pathog.* 2011;2011:429069.
21. Hodges K, Gill R. Infectious diarrhea: Cellular and molecular mechanisms. *Gut Microbes.* 2010;1(1):4–21.

22. Lucas ML. Enterocyte chloride and water secretion into the small intestine after enterotoxin challenge: Unifying hypothesis or intellectual dead end? *J Physiol Biochem.* 2008;64(1):69–88.
23. Trivedi TK, Desai R, Hall AJ, et al. Clinical characteristics of norovirus-associated deaths: A systematic literature review. *Am J Infect Control.* 2013;41:654–657.
24. Rallabhandi P, Awomoyi A, Thomas KE, et al. Differential activation of human TLR4 by *Escherichia coli* and *Shigella flexneri* 2a lipopolysaccharide: Combined effects of lipid A acylation state and TLR4 polymorphisms on signaling. *J Immunol.* 2008;180(2):1139–1147.
25. Fernandez MI, Sansonetti PJ. *Shigella* interaction with intestinal epithelial cells determines the innate immune response in shigellosis. *Int J Med Microbiol.* 2003;293(1):55–67.
26. Kim DH, Kang SH, Jeong WS, et al. Serum C-reactive protein (CRP) levels in young adults can be used to discriminate between inflammatory and non-inflammatory diarrhea. *Dig Dis Sci.* 2013;58:504–508.
27. Haverly RM, Harrison CR, Dougherty TH. *Yersinia enterocolitica* bacteremia associated with red blood cell transfusion. *Arch Pathol Lab Med.* 1996;120(5):499–500.
28. Freedman SB, Xie J, Neufeld MS, et al. Shiga toxin-producing *Escherichia coli* infection, antibiotics, and risk of developing hemolytic uremic syndrome: A meta-analysis. *Clin Infect Dis.* 2016;62(10):1251–1258.
29. Garg AX, Pope JE, Thiessen-Philbrook H, Clark WF, Ouimet J. Arthritis risk after acute bacterial gastroenteritis. *Rheumatology (Oxford).* 2008;47(2):200–204.
30. Allos BM. *Campylobacter jejuni* infections: Update on emerging issues and trends. *Clin Infect Dis.* 2001;32(8):1201–1206.
31. Connor BA, Riddle MS. Post-infectious sequelae of traveler's diarrhea. *J Travel Med.* 2013;20(5):303–312.
32. Hahn S, Kim S, Garner P. Reduced osmolarity oral rehydration solution for treating dehydration caused by acute diarrhoea in children. *Cochrane Database Syst Rev.* 2002;(1):CD002847.
33. Musekiwa A, Volmink J. Oral rehydration salt solution for treating cholera: </= 270 mOsm/L solutions vs >/= 310 mOsm/L solutions. *Cochrane Database Syst Rev.* 2011;(12):CD003754.
34. Barr W, Smith A. Acute diarrhea. *Am Fam Physician.* 2014;89(3):180–189.
35. Gregorio GV, Gonzales ML, Dans LF, Martinez EG. Polymer-based oral rehydration solution for treating acute watery diarrhoea. *Cochrane Database Syst Rev.* 2009;(2):CD006519.
36. Gregorio GV, Dans LF, Silvestre MA. Early versus delayed refeeding for children with acute diarrhoea. *Cochrane Database Syst Rev.* 2011;(7):CD007296.
37. Payot S, Bolla JM, Corcoran D, Fanning S, Megraud F, Zhang Q. Mechanisms of fluoroquinolone and macrolide resistance in *Campylobacter* spp. *Microbes Infect.* 2006;8(7):1967–1971.
38. Parry CM, Threlfall EJ. Antimicrobial resistance in typhoidal and nontyphoidal salmonellae. *Curr Opin Infect Dis.* 2008;21(5):531–538.
39. Connor BA. Traveler's diarrhea. CDC Yellow Book. Available at: https://wwwnc.cdc.gov/travel/yellowbook/2018/the-pre-travel-consultation/travelers-diarrhea. Accessed June 6, 2018.
40. DuPont HL, Jiang ZD, Okhuysen PC, et al. A randomized, double-blind, placebo-controlled trial of rifaximin to prevent travelers' diarrhea. *Ann Intern Med.* 2005;142(10):805–812.
41. Strand TA, Sharma PR, Gjessing HK, et al. Risk factors for extended duration of acute diarrhea in young children. *PLoS ONE.* 2012;7(5):1–6.
42. Centers for Disease Control and Prevention. Extensively drug-resistant *Salmonella typhi* infections among U.S. residents without international travel. Health Alert network. February 2021. https://emergency.cdc.gov/han/2021/han00439.asp. Accessed June 8, 2021.
43. Hempel S, Newberry SJ, Maher AR, et al. Probiotics for the prevention and treatment of antibiotic-associated diarrhea: A systemic review and meta-analysis. *JAMA.* 2012;307(18):1959–1969.
44. Allen SJ, Wareham K, Wang D, et al. Lactobacilli and bifidobacteria in the prevention of antibiotic-associated diarrhoea and *Clostridium difficile* diarrhoea in older patients (PLACIDE): A randomised, double-blind, placebo-controlled, multicentre trial. *Lancet.* 2013;382(9900):1249–1257.
45. Maziade PJ, Ship N, Sniffen JC, Goldstein EJC. Enhanced *Clostridioides difficile* infection prevention with a pharmacy-controlled policy that adds a three-strain *Lactobacillus* probiotic concomitantly to antibiotic therapy. *Clin Infect Dis.* May 09, 2021. https://academic.oup.com/cid/advance-article/doi/10.1093/cid/ciab414/6272833.
46. Lazzerini M, Ronfani L. Oral zinc for treating diarrhoea in children. *Cochrane Database Syst Rev.* 2012;6:CD005436.
47. Steinberg EB, Bishop R, Haber P, et al. Typhoid fever in travelers: Who should be targeted for prevention? *Clin Infect Dis.* 2004;39(2):186–191.
48. Cortese MM, Parashar UD. Prevention of rotavirus gastroenteritis among infants and children: Recommendations of the Advisory Committee on Immunization Practices (ACIP). *MMWR Recomm Rep.* 2009;58(RR-2):1–25.
49. Centers for Disease Control and Prevention. Addition of history of intussusception as a contraindication for rotavirus vaccination. *MMWR.* 2011;60(41):1427.
50. Walker RI. An assessment of enterotoxigenic *Escherichia coli* and *Shigella* vaccine candidates for infants and children. *Vaccine.* 2015;33:954–965.
51. McDonald LC, Gerding DN, Johnson S, et al. Clinical practice guidelines for *Clostridium difficile* infection in adults and children: 2017 update by the Infectious Diseases Society of America (IDSA) and the Society for Healthcare Epidemiology of America (SHEA). *Clin Infect Dis.* 2018;66(00):e1–e48.
52. Tariq Raseen, Singh Siddharth, Gupta Arjun, et al. Association of gastric acid suppression with recurrent *Clostridium difficile* infection. *JAMA Internal Medicine.* 2017;177:784. 10.1001/jamainternmed.2017.0212.
53. Guh Alice Y, Mu Yi, Winston Lisa G, et al. Trends in U.S. burden of *Clostridioides difficile* infection and outcomes. *N Eng J Med.* 2020;382:1320–1330. 10.1056/nejmoa1910215.
54. Abt Michael C, McKenney Peter T, Pamer Eric G. *Clostridium difficile* colitis: Pathogenesis and host defence. *Nat Rev Microbiol.* 2016;14:609–620. 10.1038/nrmicro.2016.108.
55. Bagdasarian N, Rao K, Malani PN. Diagnosis and treatment of *Clostridium difficile* in adults: A systematic review. *JAMA.* 2015;313:398–408.
56. Johnson S, Lavergne V, Skinner AM, et al. Clinical Practice Guideline by the Infectious Diseases Society of America (IDSA) and Society for Healthcare Epidemiology of America (SHEA): 2021 Focused Update Guidelines on management of *Clostridioides difficile* infection in adults. *Clin Infect Dis.* 2021;73:e1029–e1044. 10.1093/cid/ciab549.
57. Rokas EE, Johnson JW, Beardsley JR, Ohl CA, Luther VP, Willaimson JC. The addition of intravenous metronidazole to oral vancomycin is associated with improved mortality in critically ill patients with *Clostridium difficile* infection. *Clin Infect Dis.* 2015;61(6):934–941.
58. Song Jung Hoon, Kim You Sun. Recurrent *Clostridium difficile* infection: Risk factors, treatment, and prevention. *Gut Liver.* 2019;13:16–24. 10.5009/gnl18071.
59. Youngster I, Russell GH, Pindar C, Ziv-Baran T, Sauk J, Hohmann EL. Oral, capsulized, frozen fecal microbiota transplantation for relapsing *Clostridium difficile* infection. *JAMA.* 2014;312(17):1772–1778.
60. Kelly CR, Fischer M, Allegretti JR, et al. ACG Clinical Guidelines: Prevention, diagnosis, and treatment of *Clostridioides difficile* infections. *Am J Gastroenterol.* 2021;116:1124–1147. 10.14309/ajg.0000000000001278.
61. Kufel WD, Devanathan AS, Marx AH, et al. Bezlotoxumab: A novel agent for the prevention of recurrent *Clostridium difficile* infection. *Pharmacotherapy.* 2017;37(10):1298–1308.
62. Cho Janice M, Pardi Darrell S, Khanna Sahil. Update on treatment of *Clostridioides difficile* infection. *Mayo Clin Proc.* 2020;95:758–769. 10.1016/j.mayocp.2019.08.006.
63. Goldenberg JZ, Yap C, Lytvyn L, et al. Probiotics for the prevention of *Clostridium difficile*–associated diarrhea in adults and children. *Cochrane Database Sys Rev.* 19,2017;12:CD006095. doi: 10.1002/14651858.
64. Shlim D. Looking for evidence that personal hygiene precautions prevent traveler's diarrhea. *Clin Infect Dis.* 2005;41(Suppl 8):S531–S535.
65. Riddle MS, Arnold S, Tribble DR. Effect of adjunctive loperamide in combination with antibiotics on treatment outcomes in traveler's diarrhea: A systematic review and meta-analysis. *Clin Infect Dis.* 2008;47(8):1007–1014.
66. Imanishi M, Manikonda K, Murthy BP, Gould LH. Factors contributing to decline in foodborne disease outbreak reports, United States. *Emerg Infect Dis.* 2014;20(9):1551–1553.
67. Sobel J, Tucker N, Sulka A, McLaughlin J, Maslanka S. Foodborne botulism in the United States, 1990–2000. *Emerg Infect Dis.* 2004;10(9):1606–1611.

137

Intra-Abdominal Infections

Alan E. Gross, Jamie L. Wagner, and Keith M. Olsen

KEY CONCEPTS

1. Most intra-abdominal infections are caused by a defect in the gastrointestinal (GI) tract and are best treated by surgical drainage, resection, and/or repair.
2. Primary peritonitis is generally caused by a single organism (*Staphylococcus aureus* in patients undergoing chronic ambulatory peritoneal dialysis [CAPD] or *Escherichia coli* in patients with cirrhosis).
3. Secondary peritonitis is usually caused by a mixture of bacteria, including enteric gram-negative bacilli and anaerobes, which enhance the pathogenic potential of the bacteria.
4. For peritonitis, early and effective IV fluid resuscitation and electrolyte replacement therapy are essential. A common cause of early death is tissue hypoperfusion precipitated by inadequate intravascular volume.
5. Treatment is generally initiated on a "presumptive" or empirical basis and should be based on the likely pathogen(s), local resistance patterns, and severity of illness.
6. Antimicrobial regimens for secondary peritonitis, determined by the severity of illness and microbiology data, include: (a) third-generation cephalosporin (ceftriaxone) with metronidazole, (b) piperacillin/tazobactam, (c) a carbapenem (imipenem, meropenem, or ertapenem), or (d) a quinolone (levofloxacin or ciprofloxacin) plus metronidazole or moxifloxacin alone.
7. Treatment of patients with peritoneal dialysis-associated peritonitis should include an antistaphylococcal antimicrobial, such as a first-generation cephalosporin (cefazolin) or vancomycin, as well as an agent with significant gram-negative bacterial activity such as a third-generation cephalosporin or aminoglycoside; intraperitoneal administration is preferred.
8. The duration of antimicrobial treatment should be 4 days after achievement of source control for most secondary peritonitis infections.
9. Patients treated for intra-abdominal infections should be assessed for the occurrence of drug-related adverse effects, particularly hypersensitivity reactions (β-lactam antimicrobials), diarrhea (most agents), fungal infections (most agents), and nephrotoxicity (aminoglycosides).

BEYOND THE BOOK

Activity 1:

Answer the questions for the case below on the basis of the information contained within the chapter and develop a treatment plan following the patient care process.

Case: A 59-year-old woman with history of cirrhosis secondary to alcohol abuse is admitted from an outside hospital for altered mental status and concern for hepatic encephalopathy. The patient lives at home, and the day before admission, the patient told her spouse that her stomach was hurting. The spouse expresses concern that the patient was not receiving lactulose for the past 1.5 weeks and missed her recent liver clinic appointment. The patient was initially admitted for less than 24 hours to an outside hospital and received unknown antibiotics before transfer to the current hospital. On exam, the patient is drowsy and not very responsive to questions. Patient appears jaundiced and is complaining of abdominal pain. No nausea, vomiting, or shortness of breath is observed.

Home medications:
Folic acid 1 mg orally every day
Lactulose 10 g orally twice a day
Magnesium oxide 400 mg orally twice a day
Pantoprazole 40 mg orally every day
Potassium chloride 20 mEq orally twice a day
Hydrochlorothiazide 25 mg orally every day
Spironolactone 25 mg orally every day
ALL: NKDA
Pertinent Labs:
Total bilirubin 11.5 mg/dL (197 μmol/L)
Direct bilirubin 3.9 mg/dL (67 μmol/L)
Alkaline phosphatase 68 U/L (1.13 μkat/L)
AST/ALT 65/27 U/L (1.08/0.45 μkat/L)

Albumin 2.3 g/dL (23 g/L)
Creatinine 0.7 mg/dL (62 μmol/L)
WBC 14.8 × 10^9/L (14,800/μL)
Hemoglobin 8.9 g/dL (89 g/L; 5.52 mmol/L)
Platelets 92 × 10^9/L (92,000/μL)
INR 3.2
No significant culture history
Vitals: Pulse 106 BPM, Respiratory rate 24 BPM, BP 145/65 mm Hg, O_2 Saturation 96% (0.96) on room air, Tmax 38°C
Diagnostic paracentesis on admission: Ascites fluid cell count/differential; Color: Yellow, cloudy; WBC: 8,080 cells/μL (8.08 × 10^9/L); RBC: 5,280 cells/μL (5.28 × 10^9/L); Neutrophil: 74% (0.74); Gram stain: negative

1. How do you classify this patient's infection?
   A. Cholecystitis
   B. Cholangitis
   C. Spontaneous bacterial peritonitis
   D. Secondary bacterial peritonitis
2. What laboratory data and patient symptoms support the diagnosis above?
3. What are the likely pathogens that could cause this syndrome?
4. What empiric therapy do you initiate?
   A. Cefepime
   B. Cefepime + metronidazole
   C. Ceftriaxone
   D. Ceftriaxone + metronidazole
   E. Meropenem

Answers to Postclass Beyond the Book Activity 1 exercise:

1. C.
2. The patient has liver cirrhosis, which is a risk factor for spontaneous bacterial peritonitis (SBP). They present with fever, abdominal pain, and an ascitic fluid with >250/μL (0.25 × 10^9/L) PMN, which is suggestive of SBP. Although the Gram stain of the ascitic fluid was negative, the Gram stain is often negative with low inoculum infections and/or in patients who have received antibiotic therapy.
3. SBP is typically monomicrobial. The most common pathogens are *Streptococcus* species and Enterobacterales such as *Escherichia coli* and *Klebsiella* spp. Notably, anaerobes are not a common cause of SBP.
4. C. Ceftriaxone is the correct response, given it provides adequate empiric activity for the pathogens listed in question 3. Furthermore, it does not provide unnecessary broad coverage for anaerobes (responses B, D, and E are incorrect) or *Pseudomonas* (responses A, B, and E are incorrect).

Activity 2: Watch the video entitled "Diverticulosis and Diverticulitis Assessment" by Picmonic (https://www.picmonic.com/pathways/nursing/courses/standard/medical-surgical-nursing-pathophysiology-296/inflammatory-intestinal-disorders-1421/diverticulosis-and-diverticulitis-assessment_1147). This 1.5-minute video provides a general overview of diverticulosis and diverticulitis. The video is useful to enhance student understanding regarding the COLLECT and ASSESS steps in the patient care process.

INTRODUCTION

Intra-abdominal infections are those contained within the peritoneal cavity or retroperitoneal space. The peritoneal cavity extends from the undersurface of the diaphragm to the floor of the pelvis and contains the stomach, small bowel, large bowel, liver, gallbladder, and spleen. The duodenum, pancreas, kidneys, adrenal glands, great vessels (aorta and vena cava), and most mesenteric vascular structures reside in the retroperitoneum. Intra-abdominal infections may be generalized or localized, complicated or uncomplicated, and community- or healthcare-associated. Uncomplicated intra-abdominal infections are confined within visceral structures, such as the liver, gallbladder, spleen, pancreas, kidney, or female reproductive organs, and do not extend into the peritoneum, while complicated intra-abdominal infections involve anatomical disruption, extend beyond a single organ, and yield peritonitis and/or abscess.

Community-acquired intra-abdominal infections are usually caused by the patient's own microflora, are present within 48 hours of admission to the hospital, and occur in patients that do not have significant history of healthcare exposure (ie, presence of an invasive device; known methicillin-resistant *Staphylococcus aureus* [MRSA] infection or colonization; or healthcare facility residence, dialysis, or surgery in the prior 12 months). Healthcare-associated intra-abdominal infections can be classified as either community-onset or hospital-onset. Community-onset infection occurs in patients presenting from the community with the aforementioned healthcare exposure risk factors, while hospital-onset infection is defined by infection occurring after 48 hours of hospitalization.[1]

Peritonitis is defined as the acute inflammatory response of the peritoneal lining to microorganisms, chemicals, or foreign-body injury. This chapter deals only with peritonitis of infectious origin. An *abscess* is a purulent collection of fluid separated from surrounding tissue by a wall consisting of inflammatory cells and adjacent organs. It usually contains necrotic debris, bacteria, and inflammatory cells. These processes differ considerably in presentation and approach to treatment.

EPIDEMIOLOGY

Peritonitis may be classified as primary, secondary, or tertiary. Primary peritonitis, also called *spontaneous bacterial peritonitis*, is an infection of the peritoneal cavity without an evident source in the abdomen. Bacteria may be transported from the bloodstream to the peritoneal cavity, where the inflammatory process begins. In secondary peritonitis, a focal disease process is evident within the abdomen. Secondary peritonitis may involve perforation of the gastrointestinal (GI) tract (possibly because of ulceration, ischemia, or obstruction), postoperative peritonitis, or posttraumatic peritonitis (blunt or penetrating trauma). Tertiary peritonitis occurs in critically ill patients, and it persists or recurs at least 48 hours after attempted management of primary or secondary peritonitis.[2,3]

1 Primary peritonitis occurs in both children and adults, although the incidence and mortality rates in both populations have been declining.[4] Primary peritonitis develops in up to 10% to 30% of patients with alcoholic cirrhosis.[4-7] Patients undergoing chronic ambulatory peritoneal dialysis (CAPD) average one episode of peritonitis every 20 to 33 months.[8,9] Secondary peritonitis may be caused by perforation of a peptic ulcer; traumatic perforation of the stomach, small or large bowel, uterus, or urinary bladder; appendicitis; pancreatitis; diverticulitis; bowel infarction; inflammatory bowel disease; cholecystitis; operative contamination of the peritoneum; or diseases of the female genital tract, such as septic abortion, postoperative uterine infection, endometritis, and salpingitis. Diverticulitis is the eighth most frequent diagnosis for outpatients in the United States and is responsible for over 216,000 hospital admissions in 2012.[10] Appendicitis is also a common cause of intra-abdominal infections. More than 300,000 appendectomies are performed in the United States for suspected appendicitis each year.[11] Most healthcare-associated intra-abdominal infections occur as complications following intra-abdominal surgeries.

TABLE 137-1 Causes of Bacterial Peritonitis

Primary (spontaneous) bacterial peritonitis
Cirrhosis with ascites
Nephrotic syndrome
Peritoneal dialysis (may be secondary to catheter site infection)
Secondary bacterial peritonitis
Miscellaneous causes
Diverticulitis
Appendicitis
Inflammatory bowel diseases
Salpingitis
Biliary tract infections
Necrotizing pancreatitis
Neoplasms
Intestinal obstruction
Perforation
Mechanical GI problems
Any cause of small bowel obstruction (adhesions, hernia)
Vascular causes
Mesenteric arterial or venous occlusion (atrial fibrillation)
Mesenteric ischemia without occlusion
Trauma
Blunt abdominal trauma with rupture of intestine
Penetrating abdominal trauma
Iatrogenic intestinal perforation (endoscopy)
Intraoperative events
Solid organ transplant in the abdomen
Peritoneal contamination during abdominal operation
Leakage from GI anastomosis

GI, gastrointestinal.

ETIOLOGY

Primary peritonitis in adults occurs most commonly in association with alcoholic cirrhosis, especially in its end stage, or with ascites caused by postnecrotic cirrhosis, chronic active hepatitis, acute viral hepatitis, congestive heart failure, malignancy, systemic lupus erythematosus, or nephritic syndrome. It may also result from the use of a peritoneal catheter for dialysis or CNS ventriculoperitoneal shunting for hydrocephalus. Rarely, primary peritonitis occurs without apparent underlying disease.

Potential causes of bacterial peritonitis include inflammatory processes of the GI tract or abdominal organs, bowel obstruction, vascular occlusions that may lead to gangrene of the intestines, and neoplasia that may cause intestinal perforation or obstruction (Table 137-1). Other possible causes include those resulting from traumatic injuries, postoperative infections, or solid organ transplant in the abdomen.

Diverticulitis arises from inflammation of diverticula, intestinal protrusions into the surrounding muscle layer, and can be considered as both uncomplicated and complicated intra-abdominal infections. Risk factors for diverticulitis include smoking, physical inactivity, obesity, diets low in fiber and high in processed carbohydrates and red meat, and use of nonsteroidal anti-inflammatory drugs (NSAIDs).[10]

Abscesses are the result of chronic inflammation and may occur without preceding generalized peritonitis. They may be located within one of the spaces of the peritoneal cavity or within one of the visceral organs and may range from a few milliliters to a liter or more in volume. These collections often have a fibrinous capsule and may take from a few weeks to years to form.

The causes of intra-abdominal abscess overlap those of peritonitis and, in fact, may occur sequentially or simultaneously. Appendicitis is the most frequent cause of abscesses. Other potential causes of intra-abdominal abscess include pancreatitis, diverticulitis, lesions of the biliary tract, genitourinary tract infections, perforation in the abdomen, trauma, and leaking intestinal anastomoses. In addition, pelvic inflammatory disease in women may lead to formation of a tubo-ovarian abscess. For some diseases, such as appendicitis and diverticulitis, abscesses occur more frequently than generalized peritonitis. Protein–calorie malnutrition, antecedent steroid therapy, and diabetes mellitus may also contribute to the formation of an intra-abdominal abscess.

Microflora of the Gastrointestinal Tract and Female Genital Tract

A full appreciation of intra-abdominal infections requires an understanding of the normal microflora within the GI tract. There are striking differences in bacterial species and concentrations of flora within the various segments of the GI tract (Table 137-2), and this bacterial environment usually determines the severity of infectious processes in the abdomen. Generally, the low gastric pH eradicates bacteria that enter the stomach. With achlorhydria, bacterial counts may rise to 10^5 to 10^7 organisms/mL (10^8 to 10^{10}/L). The normally low bacterial count may also increase by 1,000- or 10,000-fold with gastric outlet obstruction, hemorrhage, gastric cancer, and in patients receiving histamine 2 (H2)-receptor antagonists, proton pump inhibitors, or antacids.[12,13] A two- to threefold increase in spontaneous bacterial peritonitis has been demonstrated with the use of proton pump inhibitors.[12]

The biliary tract (gallbladder and bile ducts) is sterile in most healthy individuals, but in people older than 70 years, those with acute cholecystitis, jaundice, or common bile duct stones, it is likely to be colonized by aerobic gram-negative bacilli (particularly *E. coli* and *Klebsiella* spp.) and enterococci.[14,15] Patients with biliary tract bacterial colonization are at greater risk of intra-abdominal infection.

In the distal ileum, bacterial counts of aerobes and anaerobes are quite high. In the colon, there may be 500 to 600 different types of

TABLE 137-2 Usual Microflora of the GI Tract

Site	Commonly Found Bacteria	Approximate Concentration (No. of Organisms/mL [×10³/L]) Aerobes	Anaerobes
Stomach[a]	*Streptococcus, Lactobacillus*	10-100	Rare
Biliary tract	Normally sterile (*Escherichia coli, Klebsiella*, or enterococci in some patients)	0	0
Proximal small bowel	*Streptococcus* (including enterococci), *E. coli, Klebsiella, Lactobacillus*, diphtheroids	100	Few
Distal ileum	*E. coli, Klebsiella, Enterobacter*, enterococci, *Bacteroides fragilis, Clostridium*, peptostreptococci	10^4-10^6	10^5-10^7
Colon	*Bacteroides* spp., peptostreptococci, *Clostridium, E. coli, Klebsiella*, enterococci, *Enterobacter, Candida*, and many others	10^5-10^8	10^9-10^{11}

GI, gastrointestinal.

[a]With achlorhydria, acid suppressive therapy, gastric cancer, or gastric outlet obstruction, bacterial counts may rise to 10^5/mL (10^8/L).

bacteria in stool, with concentrations often reaching 10^{11} organisms/mL (10^{14}/L), and anaerobic bacteria outnumbering aerobic bacteria by more than 1,000 to 1.[16,17] Fortunately, most colonic bacteria are not pathogens because they cannot survive in environments outside the colon. Perforation of the colon results in the release of large numbers of anaerobic and aerobic bacteria into the peritoneum.

The colonic flora generally remains the same unless exposed to a broad spectrum of antimicrobials or a GI infectious process. In either case, the flora may change due to the antibiotic or infectious process and is often replaced by more pathogenic bacteria. Depending on the type of antibiotic and spectrum, the duration of use, route of administration, and distribution to the GI tract, antibiotics can cause shifts in the normal GI microflora leading to increased drug resistance.[18]

The lower female genital tract is generally colonized by a large number of aerobic and anaerobic bacteria. Anaerobes may number 10^9 organisms/mL (10^{12}/L) and often include lactobacilli, eubacteria, clostridia, anaerobic streptococci, and, less frequently, *Bacteroides fragilis*. Aerobic bacteria most often are streptococci and *Staphylococcus epidermidis*, and these may number 10^8 organisms/mL (10^{11}/L).

PATHOPHYSIOLOGY

Intra-abdominal infection results from bacterial entry into the peritoneal or retroperitoneal spaces or from bacterial collections within intra-abdominal organs. In primary peritonitis, bacteria may enter the abdomen via the bloodstream or the lymphatic system by transmigration through the bowel wall, through an indwelling peritoneal dialysis catheter, or via the fallopian tubes in females. Hematogenous bacterial spread (through the bloodstream) occurs more frequently with tuberculosis peritonitis or peritonitis associated with cirrhotic ascites. When peritonitis results from peritoneal dialysis, skin surface flora is introduced via the peritoneal catheter. In secondary peritonitis, bacteria most often enter the peritoneum or retroperitoneum as a result of perforation of the GI or female genital tracts caused by diseases or traumatic injuries. In addition, peritonitis or abscesses may result from contamination of the peritoneum during a surgical procedure or from an anastomotic leak. In diverticulitis, it is postulated that stool particles accumulate within the diverticula to either erode into the abdominal cavity or form an abscess.[10]

The physiologic characteristics of the peritoneal cavity determine the nature of the response to infection or inflammation within it. The peritoneum is lined by a highly permeable serous membrane with a surface area approximately that of skin. The peritoneal cavity is lubricated with less than 100 mL of sterile, clear yellow fluid, normally with fewer than 250 WBC cells/μL (0.25×10^9/L), a specific gravity below 1.016, and protein content below 3 g/dL (30 g/L).[4,19] These conditions change drastically with peritoneal infection or inflammation, as described below.

After bacteria are introduced into the peritoneal cavity, there is an immediate response to contain the invasion. Humoral and cellular defenses respond first, then the omentum adheres to the affected area. A limited bacterial inoculum is handled rapidly by defense mechanisms, including complement activation and a leukocyte response. Under certain conditions, bacteria are not contained and disseminate throughout the peritoneal cavity, resulting in peritonitis. This is more likely to occur in the presence of a foreign body, hematoma, dead tissue, a large bacterial inoculum, continuing bacterial contamination, and contamination involving a mixture of synergistic organisms.

When bacteria become dispersed throughout the peritoneum, the inflammatory process involves most of the peritoneal lining. There is an outpouring into the peritoneum of fluid containing leukocytes, fibrin, and other proteins that form exudates on the inflamed peritoneal surfaces and begin to form adhesions between peritoneal structures. This process, combined with a paralysis of the intestines (ileus), may result in confinement of the contamination to one or more locations within the peritoneum. Fluid also begins to collect in the bowel lumen and wall, and distension may result.

The fluid and protein shift into the abdomen (called *third-spacing*) may be so dramatic that circulating blood volume is decreased, which may cause a decrease in cardiac output leading to hypovolemic shock. Accompanying fever, vomiting, or diarrhea may worsen the fluid imbalance. A reflex sympathetic response, manifested by perspiration, tachycardia, and vasoconstriction, may be evident. With an inflamed peritoneum, bacteria and endotoxins are absorbed easily into the bloodstream (translocation), and this may result in septic shock.[4,5,19] Other foreign substances present in the peritoneal cavity potentiate peritonitis. These adjuvants, notably feces, dead tissues, barium, mucus, bile, and blood, have detrimental effects on host defense mechanisms, particularly on bacterial phagocytosis.

Many of the manifestations of intra-abdominal infections, particularly peritonitis, result from cytokine activity. Inflammatory cytokines, such as tumor necrosis factor-α (TNF-α), interleukin (IL) 1, IL-6, IL-8, and interferon-γ (INF-γ), are produced by macrophages and neutrophils in response to bacteria and bacterial products or in response to tissue injury resulting from the surgical incision.[4,19] These cytokines produce wide-ranging effects on the vascular endothelium of organs, particularly the liver, lungs, kidneys, and heart. With uncontrolled activation of these mediators, sepsis may result (see Chapter 142, "Sepsis and Septic Shock").[20-22]

Peritonitis may result in death because of the effects on major organ systems. Fluid shifts, cytokines, and microorganism toxins may result in hypovolemia, hypoperfusion, and shock. Hypoalbuminemia may result from protein loss into the peritoneum, exacerbating intravascular volume loss. Pulmonary function may be compromised by the inflamed peritoneum, producing splinting (muscle rigidity caused by pain) that inhibits adequate diaphragmatic movement leading to atelectasis and pneumonia. Increased lung vascular permeability and resulting shunting of blood may induce onset of acute respiratory distress syndrome and associated hypoxemia and hypercarbia. With fluid loss and hypotension, renal and hepatic perfusion may be compromised, and acute renal and hepatic failures are potential threats.

If peritoneal contamination is localized but bacterial elimination is incomplete, an abscess results. This collection of necrotic tissue, bacteria, and WBCs may be at single or multiple sites and may be within one of the spaces of the peritoneal cavity or in one of the visceral organs. The location of the abscess is often related to the site of primary disease. For example, abscesses resulting from appendicitis tend to appear in the right lower quadrant or the pelvis; those resulting from diverticulitis tend to appear in the left lower quadrant or pelvis.

An abscess begins by the combined action of inflammatory cells (such as neutrophils), bacteria, fibrin, and other inflammatory mediators. Bacteria may release heparinases that cause local thrombosis and tissue necrosis or fibrinolysins, collagenases, or other enzymes that allow extension of the process into surrounding tissues. Neutrophils gathered in the abscess cavity die in 3 to 5 days, releasing lysosomal enzymes that liquefy the core of the abscess. A mature abscess may have a fibrinous capsule that isolates bacteria and the liquid core from antimicrobials and immunologic defenses.

Within the abscess, the oxygen tension is low, and anaerobic bacteria thrive; thus, the size of the abscess may increase because it is hypertonic, resulting in an additional influx of fluid. Hypertonicity promotes the formation of L-form bacteria, which are resistant to antimicrobial agents that disrupt cell walls. Abscess formation may continue and mature for long periods of time and may not be readily evident to either patient or physician. In some instances, the abscess may resolve spontaneously, and, infrequently, it may erode into adjacent organs or rupture and cause diffuse peritonitis. If the abscess erodes through the skin, it may result in an enterocutaneous fistula, connecting the peritoneum to skin, or in a draining sinus tract.

The overall outcome of an intra-abdominal infection depends on key factors: patient-specific risk factors, inoculum size, virulence of the contaminating organisms, the presence of adjuvants within the peritoneal cavity that facilitate infection, the adequacy of host defenses, source control, and the adequacy of initial treatment.[23-25]

Microbiology of Intra-Abdominal Infection

2 The prevalence of pathogens has not appreciably changed in community-onset intra-abdominal infection, although susceptibility to antibiotics has decreased over time. Primary bacterial peritonitis is often caused by a single organism. In children, the pathogen is usually group A *Streptococcus*, *E. coli*, *Streptococcus pneumoniae*, or *Bacteroides* species.[26-29] When peritonitis occurs in association with cirrhotic ascites, *E. coli* is isolated most frequently. Other potential pathogens are: *Haemophilus influenzae*, *Klebsiella* spp., *Pseudomonas* spp., anaerobes, and *S. pneumoniae*.[30] Occasionally, primary peritonitis may be caused by *Mycobacterium tuberculosis*. Peritonitis in patients undergoing peritoneal dialysis is caused most often by common skin organisms, such as coagulase-negative staphylococci, *S. aureus*, streptococci, and enterococci. Gram-negative bacteria associated with peritoneal dialysis infections include *E. coli*, *Klebsiella* spp., and *Pseudomonas* spp.[9] The mortality rate from primary peritonitis caused by gram-negative bacteria is much greater than that from gram-positive bacteria.[4,5]

3 Because of the diverse bacteria present in the GI tract, secondary intra-abdominal infections are often polymicrobial.[16] The mean number of different bacterial species isolated from infected intra-abdominal sites ranged from 2.9 to 3.7, including an average of 1.3 to 1.6 aerobes and 1.7 to 2.1 anaerobes.[30,31] With proper anaerobic specimen collection, anaerobic organisms are isolated in most patients. In one report of patients with gangrenous and perforated appendicitis, an average of 10.2 different organisms was isolated from each patient, including 2.7 aerobes and 7.5 anaerobes.[32] Purely aerobic or anaerobic infections are uncommon, as are infections caused by fungi. Table 137-3 gives the frequencies with which specific bacteria were isolated from patients with peritonitis and other intra-abdominal infections.[33,34] Nosocomial infections tend to have a more diverse array of pathogens, are more likely to involve *Pseudomonas* spp., and have a higher likelihood of multidrug-resistance compared with isolates from community-acquired infections.[35]

TABLE 137-3 Pathogens Isolated from Patients with Intra-Abdominal Infection

	Secondary Peritonitis[33,35] (%)	Community-Acquired Infection[35] (%)	Nosocomial Infection[35] (%)
Gram-Negative Bacteria			
Escherichia coli	32-61	29	22.5
Enterobacter	8-26	5.2	8.0
Klebsiella	6-26	2.8	4.5
Proteus	4-23	1.7	2.4
Pseudomonas	5-13	5	13
Gram-Positive Bacteria			
Enterococcus	18-24	10.6	18
Streptococcus	6-55	13.7	10
Staphylococcus	6-16	3.1	4.8
Anaerobic Bacteria			
Bacteroides	25-80	13.7	10.3
Clostridium	5-18	3.5	3.4
Fungi	2-5	3	4

Visceral organ abscesses differ in character from the typical intra-abdominal abscess. Hepatic abscesses may be polymicrobial (involving *E. coli*, *Klebsiella* spp., and anaerobes) or occasionally may be caused by amoeba.[17] Pancreatic abscesses are often polymicrobial, involving enteric bacteria that ascend through the biliary system. Splenic abscesses usually result from hematogenous dissemination of bacteria, such as *E. coli*, *S. aureus*, *Proteus mirabilis*, *Enterococcus* spp., and *Klebsiella pneumoniae*, as well as anaerobes.[17] Pelvic inflammatory disease is associated initially with *Neisseria gonorrhoeae* or *Chlamydia trachomatis*. However, tubo-ovarian abscesses are usually polymicrobial, having a mix of gram-positive and gram-negative aerobes and anaerobes.

Bacterial Synergism

The size of the bacterial inoculum and the number and types of bacterial species present in intra-abdominal infections influence patient outcome. The combination of aerobic and anaerobic organisms appears to greatly increase the severity of infection. In animal studies, combinations of aerobic and anaerobic bacteria were much more lethal than infections caused by aerobes or anaerobes alone.

Facultative bacteria may provide an environment conducive to the growth of anaerobic bacteria.[16] Although many bacteria isolated in mixed infections are nonpathogenic by themselves, their presence may be essential for the pathogenicity of the bacterial mixture.[23] The role of facultative bacteria in mixed infections can include (a) promotion of an appropriate environment for anaerobic bacterial growth through oxygen consumption, (b) production of nutrients necessary for anaerobes, and (c) production of extracellular enzymes that promote tissue invasion by anaerobes.

Rat models of intra-abdominal infection demonstrate that uncontrolled infection with an implanted mix of aerobes and anaerobes leads to a two-stage (biphasic) infectious process. There is an early peritonitis phase with a high mortality rate and isolation of *E. coli* from blood and a late abscess formation phase in all survivors with isolation of anaerobes such as *B. fragilis* and *Fusobacterium varium*. These experiments and others support the concept that aerobic enteric organisms and anaerobes are pathogens in intra-abdominal infections. Aerobic bacteria, particularly *E. coli*, appear responsible for the early mortality from peritonitis, whereas anaerobic bacteria are major pathogens in abscesses, with *B. fragilis* predominating.[36]

Enterococcus can be isolated from many intra-abdominal infections in humans, but its role as a pathogen is not clear. Enterococcal infection occurs more commonly in postoperative peritonitis, in the presence of specific risk factors indicating failure of the host's defenses (immunocompromised patients), or with the use of broad-spectrum antibiotics.[37,38]

CLINICAL PRESENTATION

Intra-abdominal infections have a wide spectrum of clinical features often depending on the specific disease process, the location and magnitude of bacterial contamination, and concurrent host factors. Peritonitis is usually recognized easily, but intra-abdominal abscesses may often continue for considerable periods of time, either going unrecognized or being attributed to an unrelated disease process. Patients with primary and secondary peritonitis present quite differently (Table 137-4).[4,5,19,39-41]

TABLE 137-4 Clinical Presentation of Peritonitis

Primary Peritonitis
General
The patient may not be in acute distress, particularly with peritoneal dialysis
Signs and symptoms
The patient may complain of loss of appetite, bloating, nausea, vomiting (sometimes with diarrhea), and abdominal tenderness
Temperature may be only mildly elevated or not elevated in patients undergoing peritoneal dialysis
Bowel sounds are hypoactive
The cirrhotic patient may have worsening encephalopathy
Cloudy dialysate fluid with peritoneal dialysis
Laboratory tests
The patient's WBC count may be only mildly elevated
Ascitic fluid usually contains greater than 250 leukocytes/mm^3 (0.25 × 10^9/L), and bacteria may be evident on Gram stain of a centrifuged specimen
In 60%-80% of patients with cirrhotic ascites, the Gram stain is negative
Other diagnostic tests
Culture of peritoneal dialysate or ascitic fluid is typically positive, particularly if collected prior to initiation of antibiotics
In conjunction with clinical findings, procalcitonin may be helpful for limiting duration of antibiotic therapy in secondary and tertiary peritonitis
Secondary Peritonitis
Signs and symptoms
Generalized abdominal pain
Tachypnea
Tachycardia
Nausea and vomiting
Temperature is normal initially then increases to 37.8-38.9°C (100-102°F) within the first few hours and may continue to rise for the next several hours
Hypotension, hypoperfusion, and shock if volume is not restored
Decreased urine output due to vascular volume depletion
Physical examination
Voluntary abdominal guarding changing to involuntary guarding and a "board-like abdomen"
Abdominal tenderness and distension
Faint bowel sounds that cease over time
Laboratory tests
Leukocytosis (15,000-20,000 WBC/mm^3 [15 × 10^9 to 20 × 10^9/L]), with neutrophils predominating and an elevated percentage of immature neutrophils (bands)
Elevated hematocrit and blood urea nitrogen because of dehydration
Patient progresses from early alkalosis because of hyperventilation and vomiting to metabolic acidosis
Other diagnostic tests
Abdominal radiographs may be useful because free air in the abdomen (indicating intestinal perforation) or distension of the small or large bowel is often evident

WBC, white blood cell.

Primary peritonitis can develop over a period of days to weeks and is usually a more indolent process than secondary peritonitis. The first sign of peritonitis may be a cloudy dialysate in patients undergoing peritoneal dialysis or worsening encephalopathy in a cirrhotic patient.

The patient with generalized bacterial peritonitis presents most often in acute distress. The patient lies still, usually on his or her back, possibly with the hips slightly flexed. Any movement of the patient, including rocking the bed or breathing, worsens the generalized abdominal pain.

If peritonitis continues untreated, the patient may experience hypovolemic shock from third-space fluid loss into the peritoneum, bowel wall, and lumen. This may be accompanied by sepsis because the inflamed peritoneum absorbs bacteria and toxins into mesenteric blood vessels and lymph nodes, initiating production of inflammatory cytokines. Hypovolemic shock is the major factor contributing to mortality in the early stage of peritonitis.

Intra-abdominal abscesses may pose a difficult diagnostic challenge because the symptoms are neither specific nor dramatic. The patient may complain of abdominal pain or discomfort, but these symptoms are not reliable. Fever is usually present; often it is low grade, but it may be high, with a spiking pattern. The patient may have a paralytic ileus and abdominal distension. The abdominal examination is unreliable; tenderness and pain may be present, and a mass may be palpated.

Peritonitis may result from an abscess that ruptures, spreading bacteria and toxins throughout the peritoneum. In other patients, the entry of bacterial toxins into the systemic circulation from the abscess may lead to sepsis and progressive multisystem organ failure (eg, renal, hepatic, pulmonary, or cardiovascular).

Laboratory studies are not generally helpful in the diagnosis of intra-abdominal abscesses, although most patients will have leukocytosis. C-reactive protein has been suggested, but due to its lack of specificity, it is not very useful. Procalcitonin has been postulated to be of use, but its exact utility still must be determined. Some patients may have positive blood cultures, whereas others, particularly patients with diabetes, may have hyperglycemia. The finding of *Bacteroides* or enteric bacteria in the bloodstream is often indicative of an intra-abdominal infectious process.

Radiographic methods are used to make the diagnosis of an intra-abdominal abscess. Plain radiographs may show air–fluid levels or a shift of normal intra-abdominal contents by the abscess mass. GI contrast studies may also demonstrate this displacement of abdominal structures. Both of these modalities provide indirect evidence of abscess presence but are not generally helpful in precisely locating the abscess.

Ultrasound is the primary diagnostic method used when an intra-abdominal abscess is suspected. The procedure may be done at the bedside, which is particularly helpful when the patient is in the intensive care unit.

Computed tomography (CT) scanning is the preferred modality used to evaluate the abdomen for the presence of an abscess and is the imaging study of greatest value. If not contraindicated, an oral radiocontrast agent should be given to allow differentiation of the abscess from the bowel. IV radiocontrast material will be taken up preferentially in the wall of the abscess, creating a unique radiographic appearance, so-called rim enhancement. Magnetic resonance imaging offers no significant advantage when compared with CT scanning.

Intra-abdominal infection caused by disease processes at specific sites often produces characteristic manifestations that are helpful in diagnosis. For example, a patient with diverticulitis may exhibit stabbing left-lower-quadrant abdominal pain and constipation. Fever and leukocytosis are frequently present, and a tender mass is sometimes palpable. With appendicitis, the findings may be inconsistent, but many patients have a sudden onset of periumbilical or epigastric pain that is usually colicky and later shifts to the right lower quadrant. The location of pain may vary because the appendix can be in many locations (eg, retrocecal or pelvic) in the abdomen. A mass may be palpable on abdominal, pelvic, or rectal examination. The patient's temperature is generally mildly elevated early and then increases. If perforation and peritonitis occur, findings would include diffuse abdominal pain, rigidity, and sustained fever. More often, however, appendiceal perforation results in a local abscess.

TREATMENT

Desired Outcome

The primary goals of treatment are correction of the intra-abdominal disease processes or injuries that have caused infection and the drainage of purulent collections (abscesses). A secondary objective is to achieve a resolution of infection without major organ system complications (pulmonary, hepatic, cardiovascular, or renal failure) or adverse drug effects. Ideally, the patient should be discharged from the hospital after treatment with full function for self-care and routine daily activities.

General Approach to Treatment

The treatment of intra-abdominal infection most often requires hospitalization and the coordinated use of three major modalities: (a) prompt surgical control and drainage of the infected site, (b) hemodynamic resuscitation and support of vital organ functions, and (c) early administration of appropriate antimicrobial therapy to treat infection not eradicated by surgery.[16]

Antimicrobials are an important adjunct to drainage procedures in the treatment of secondary intra-abdominal infections; however, the use of antimicrobial agents without surgical source control is usually inadequate. For most cases of primary peritonitis, drainage procedures may not be required, and antimicrobial agents become the mainstay of therapy.

4 In the early phase of serious intra-abdominal infections, attention should be given to the maintenance of organ system functions. With generalized peritonitis, initial large volumes of IV fluids are required to restore vascular volume, to improve cardiovascular function, and to maintain adequate tissue perfusion and oxygenation. Adequate urine output should be maintained to ensure adequate resuscitation and proper renal function. Respiratory function can be assisted by a variety of methods, including oxygen therapy, pulmonary physiotherapy, and ventilatory support in severely ill patients. Often the critically ill patient with intra-abdominal infection will require intensive care management, particularly if there is cardiovascular or respiratory instability. In addition, isolation procedures may be required if the infectious process poses a threat to other hospitalized patients.

An important component of therapy is nutrition. Intra-abdominal infections often involve the GI tract or disrupt its function (ie, paralytic ileus). The return of GI motility may take days, weeks, and, occasionally, months. In the interim, enteral or parenteral nutrition, as indicated, facilitates improved immune function and wound healing to ensure recovery. Additional information pertaining to enteral and parenteral nutrition can be found elsewhere in this book (Chapters 165 and 166).

Nonpharmacologic Treatment

Drainage Procedures

Primary peritonitis is treated with antimicrobials and rarely requires drainage. Secondary peritonitis requires surgical correction of the underlying pathology. The drainage of the purulent material is the critical component of management of an intra-abdominal abscess. Without adequate drainage of the abscess, antimicrobial therapy and fluid resuscitation can be expected to fail.

Secondary peritonitis is treated surgically; this is often called *source control*, which refers to all the physical measures undertaken to eradicate the focus of infection.[5,16] At the time of laparotomy (surgical opening and exploration of the abdomen), attempts are made to correct the cause of the peritonitis. This may include patching a perforated ulcer with omentum, removal of a segment of perforated colon, or excision of a portion of gangrenous small intestine. In addition, the surgeon may elect to leave the abdomen open after the laparotomy, plan a re-laparotomy at a later time regardless of the patient's condition, or perform re-laparotomy if the patient develops reinfection.[5,16] The goal of all these procedures is to repair or remove the inflamed or gangrenous tissue and to prevent further bacterial contamination. The presence of active inflammation increases the difficulty of the surgical procedure, which results in a higher morbidity and mortality rate than if the same procedures were performed in an elective setting without inflammation. Electing to leave the abdomen open after surgery is usually to prevent abdominal compartment syndrome; however, this is unnecessary when fluid collections can be removed with percutaneous catheter drainage.[42]

The presence of active inflammation may make it technically impossible to perform the definitive surgical procedure. In this situation, attempts are made to provide drainage of the infected or gangrenous structures. If an intra-abdominal abscess, separate from any intra-abdominal organ, is discovered during an exploratory laparotomy, it may be debrided, excised, or drained. If the intra-abdominal abscess involves an abdominal structure, then a resection of part or of the entire organ may be required. An example of this situation is an abscess associated with diverticular disease of the colon. Management may include drainage of the abscess and resection of the involved part of the colon. All foreign material, necrotic tissue, feces, blood, or purulent material should be removed from the operative field, and the peritoneum should be copiously irrigated with 0.9% sodium chloride to decrease the concentrations of bacteria or other noxious substances.

After an abscess is located, it must be drained. This may be performed surgically or with percutaneous, image-guided techniques.[5,16,43] Typically, image-guided techniques use ultrasonography or CT scanning. The management of an intra-abdominal abscess with percutaneous catheter drainage may be sufficient to resolve the infection. Some patients may require a subsequent procedure to treat the underlying GI conditions; however, a significant advantage is obtained by first draining the abscess percutaneously. This allows the surgical procedure to be performed on a patient who is no longer suffering from the systemic manifestations of uncontrolled infection. Drainage techniques may be performed using endoscopy or laparoscopy. These minimal-access techniques may offer advantages when compared with traditional surgery but will probably be used less often than radiologically assisted percutaneous drainage techniques.

The most valuable microbiologic information may be obtained at the time of percutaneous or operative abscess drainage. If purulent material or presumably infected fluid is found, it is best to aspirate 2 to 3 mL into a syringe, remove any air, and tightly cap the syringe. The specimen should be promptly delivered to the microbiology laboratory, where a Gram stain should be performed immediately, and cultures prepared for identification of aerobic and anaerobic bacteria. If no fluid is available for collection, culture swab devices may be applied to the infected area; however, anaerobic organisms often are not isolated from swabs.

Fluid Therapy

4 Patients should be evaluated for signs of hypovolemia, hypoperfusion, and shock. Initial effective fluid repletion and management

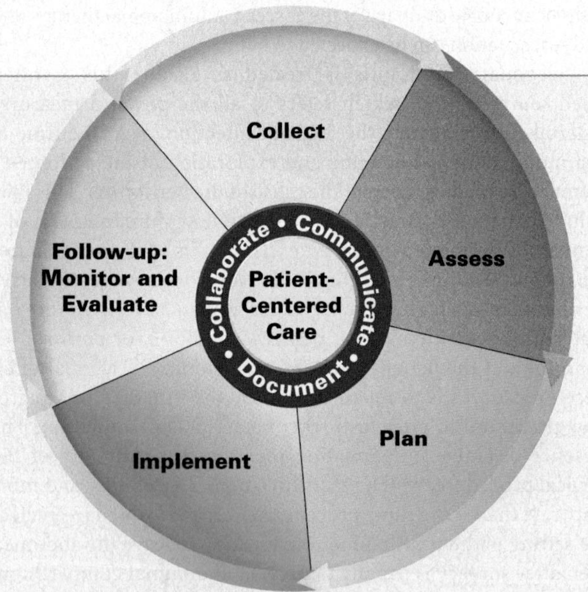

Patient Care Process for Treatment of Intra-Abdominal Infections

The image shows the five fundamental steps included in The Pharmacist's Care Process endorsed by the Joint Commission for Pharmacy Practitioners (2014). The tagline of this process reads collaborate, communicate, and document. The five fundamental steps listed here are collect, assess, plan, implement, and follow-up: monitor and evaluate. All these steps are listed in a circular block diagram.

Collect

- Patient characteristics (eg, age, sex, weight, body mass index)
- Patient history (past medical, family, social—dietary habits, tobacco use, alcohol use, substance abuse) and surgical operations (site, date, procedure)
- Medication history at hospital admission (prescription and non-non-prescription medications and supplements), drug allergies, and intolerances; previous antibiotic use, inpatient and outpatient, dose and duration
- Microbiologic results from blood, intra-abdominal fluids, and other sources, and obtain susceptibility results when they are available
- Laboratory results for infection, major organ function (particularly kidney and liver), and immune status

Assess

- Hemodynamic status (eg, MAP, HR)
- Estimate creatinine clearance for drug dosing
- Review all culture results and consider anaerobic bacteria even though they may not be isolated in cultures

Plan*

- Determine initial empiric treatment and monitoring plan
- Establish antimicrobial monitoring goals for microbiologic and clinical outcomes
- Consider other medications that may be needed during treatment or post-surgery (ie, fluids, analgesics, medications for nausea and vomiting, thrombosis prevention)
- Check for drug interactions and dose adjustments based on end-organ function

Implement

- Initiate an empiric antimicrobial regimen, modify therapy once microbiologic data is available, and establish a tentative stop date
- De-escalate antimicrobial therapy as appropriate based on response and microbiologic data
- Discontinue adjunct medications when not needed or indicated
- Assess patient as needed for response to surgical control, medications, and other treatments
- Use measures to minimize adverse events to medications and assess for occurrence of adverse events
- Assess pain control and progress of gastrointestinal function
- Change to oral medications when appropriate after patient resumes oral feeding

Follow-up: Monitor and Evaluate

- Determine whether patient shows improvement with signs and symptoms of infection within 2 to 3 days after antimicrobials are initiated and surgical source control is completed
- The patient should be reassessed continually to determine the success or failure of therapies
- Monitor for emergence of resistant bacterial isolates in blood or other sources and change antimicrobials if needed
- Monitor for occurrence of secondary infections such as respiratory and urinary tract
- Upon hospital discharge, determine which medications the patient should be discharged with and provide counseling; discontinue unnecessary medications

Collaborate with patient, caregiver(s), and other healthcare professionals.

are required for successful management of intra-abdominal infections. Fluid therapy is instituted for the purposes of achieving or maintaining intravascular volume to ensure adequate cardiac output, tissue perfusion, and correction of acidosis. Loss of fluid through vomiting, diarrhea, or nasogastric suction contributes to fluid depletion. A more thorough discussion of sepsis and septic shock, including fluid resuscitation, is presented elsewhere in this book (Chapters e42 and 142).

In patients with peritonitis, hypovolemia is often accompanied by metabolic acidosis. Although serum lactate is not a direct measure of tissue perfusion, it may serve as a surrogate marker representing tissue hypoxia and is therefore recommended by the Surviving Sepsis Campaign 2021 update to guide fluid administration. In those patients with sepsis hypoperfusion or septic shock, IV fluids should consist of a 30 mL/kg bolus of crystalloids with additional fluids targeting predefined therapeutic goals.[44-46]

Initial fluid resuscitation should be completed within 3 hours of hypoperfusion recognition. Thereafter, fluids may be required at a rate of 1 L/hr or higher. Once targeted therapeutic goals are reached, judicious use of fluids should be used, as a sustained positive fluid balance after initial resuscitation may be harmful.[16,47] Maintenance fluids should be instituted with 0.9% sodium chloride, 5% dextrose, and 0.45% sodium chloride, or a balanced crystalloid solution.[48] The administration rate should be based on estimated daily fluid loss through urine and nasogastric suction, including 0.5 to 1 L for insensible fluid loss. Potassium can be included in maintenance fluids if the patient is experiencing vomiting, diarrhea, or has nasogastric suction.

Pharmacologic Treatment

Antimicrobial Therapy

The goals of antimicrobial therapy are: (a) to eliminate the intra-abdominal infection and prevent the establishment of metastatic foci of infection or bacteremia, (b) to reduce suppurative complications (eg, abscess formation) after bacterial contamination, and (c) to prevent local spread of existing infection. After suppuration has occurred, a cure by antibiotic therapy alone is very difficult to achieve; antimicrobials may serve to improve the results obtained with surgery.

5 An empirical antimicrobial regimen should be started as soon as the presence of intra-abdominal infection is suspected. The Surviving Sepsis Campaign Guidelines recommend that antimicrobial therapy is administered immediately and within 1 hour of the recognition of sepsis or septic shock.[46] Therapy must be initiated based on the likely pathogens, potential resistance, and severity of patient illness. Resistance is common among gram-negative pathogens to fluoroquinolones and ampicillin/sulbactam; this emphasizes the importance of using local susceptibility data to guide empiric therapy and tailoring the antibiotic regimen based on susceptibility results.[49] Predominant pathogens, as discussed in the preceding section, vary depending on the site of intra-abdominal infection and the underlying disease process. Table 137-5 lists the likely pathogens against which antimicrobial agents should be directed.

TABLE 137-5 Likely Intra-Abdominal Pathogens

Type of Infection	Aerobes	Anaerobes
Primary (Spontaneous) Bacterial Peritonitis		
Children	Group A *Streptococcus*, *E. coli*, pneumococci	—
Cirrhosis	*E. coli*, *Klebsiella*, pneumococci (many others)	—
Peritoneal dialysis	*Staphylococcus*, *Streptococcus*, *E. coli*, *Klebsiella*, *Pseudomonas*	—
Secondary Bacterial Peritonitis		
Gastroduodenal	*Streptococcus*, *E. coli*	—
Biliary tract	*E. coli*, *Klebsiella*, enterococci	*Clostridium* or *Bacteroides* (infrequent)
Small or large bowel	*E. coli*, *Klebsiella*, *Proteus*	*B. fragilis* and other *Bacteroides*, *Clostridium*
Appendicitis	*E. coli*, *Pseudomonas*	*Bacteroides*
Abscesses	*E. coli*, *Klebsiella*, *Streptococcus*, enterococci	*B. fragilis* and other *Bacteroides*, *Clostridium*, anaerobic cocci
Liver	*E. coli*, *Klebsiella*, *Streptococcus*, enterococci, *Staphylococcus*, amoeba	*Bacteroides* (infrequent)
Spleen	*Staphylococcus*, *Streptococcus*, *E. coli*, *Salmonella*	

Antimicrobial Experience Many studies have been conducted evaluating or comparing the effectiveness of antimicrobials for the treatment of intra-abdominal infections. Substantial differences in patient outcomes between specific agents have not generally been demonstrated.[50]

Important findings from over 20 years of clinical trials regarding selection of antimicrobials for intra-abdominal infections are the following:

1. Antimicrobial regimens used for secondary infections should cover a broad spectrum of aerobic and anaerobic bacteria from the GI tract. The local epidemiology of resistant pathogens, patient-specific risk factors for resistant pathogens, and patient severity of illness should guide empiric treatment.
2. Resistance is prevalent among *B. fragilis* to clindamycin and Enterobacterales to ampicillin/sulbactam and quinolones, and therefore these agents should not be routinely used empirically for complicated intra-abdominal infections.[51,52]
3. If the causative pathogens are susceptible and the patient has clinically responded, antimicrobial treatment can be completed orally with amoxicillin/clavulanate, metronidazole with either ciprofloxacin or levofloxacin, or moxifloxacin.[53]
4. Four days of antimicrobial treatment after adequate source control is sufficient for most intra-abdominal infections.[16,54,55]

Intra-abdominal infections present in many different ways and with a wide spectrum of severity. The regimen employed and duration of treatment depends on the specific clinical circumstances (ie, the nature of the underlying disease process, severity of illness, and risk of resistant pathogens).

6 **Recommendations** For most intra-abdominal infections, the antimicrobial regimen should be effective against both aerobic and anaerobic bacteria.[55,56] When initial antimicrobial therapy is inactive, morbidity and mortality rates are higher than when initially active therapy is used.[55] Generally, agents with activity against enteric gram-negative bacilli, such as *E. coli* and *Klebsiella* spp., and anaerobes, including *B. fragilis,* should be administered. If most of the organisms can be eliminated through drainage or antimicrobials, the synergistic effect may be removed, and the patient's defenses may be able to resolve the remaining infection.

Table 137-6 lists the agents recommended by the Infectious Diseases Society of America (IDSA) and the Surgical Infection Society (SIS) for the treatment of community-acquired complicated intra-abdominal infections.[16,55] These recommendations were formulated using an evidence-based approach. Table 137-7 lists additional evidence-based recommendations for the treatment of complicated intra-abdominal infections. Choosing empiric antibiotic therapy based on these recommendations within the IDSA/SIS guidelines has been associated with a decreased time to active therapy for patients with community-onset complicated intra-abdominal infection.[57] Although most community-acquired infections are of mild-to-moderate severity, healthcare-associated infections tend to be more severe, more difficult to treat, and more common due to resistant pathogens. Table 137-8 presents guidelines for treatment and alternative regimens for specific situations. These are general guidelines; such a table cannot incorporate many factors, including local resistance patterns to commonly used agents such as quinolones.

TABLE 137-6 Recommended Agents for the Treatment of Community-Acquired Complicated Intra-Abdominal Infections in Adults

Agents Recommended for Mild-to-Moderate Infections	Agents Recommended for High Severity Infections
Single Agent	
Cefoxitin[a]	Piperacillin/tazobactam
Moxifloxacin[b]	Imipenem/cilastatin,[c] meropenem,[c] meropenem/vaborbactam,[d] imipenem/relebactam[d]
Ertapenem[c]	
Eravacycline[d]	
Combination Regimens	
Cefazolin,[a] cefuroxime,[a] ceftriaxone, or cefotaxime each in combination with metronidazole	Cefepime, ceftazidime, cefiderocol,[d] ceftazidime/avibactam,[d] or ceftolozane/tazobactam[d] each in combination with metronidazole
Ciprofloxacin[b] or levofloxacin[b] each in combination with metronidazole	Ciprofloxacin[b] or levofloxacin[b] each in combination with metronidazole

[a]Empiric first- and second-generation cephalosporin use should be avoided unless local antibiograms show >80% to 90% susceptibility of *E. coli* to these agents.

[b]Use of quinolones may be associated with treatment failure due to increasing resistance of enteric pathogens including *E. coli*. Empiric quinolone use should be avoided unless local antibiograms show >80% to 90% susceptibility of *E. coli* to quinolones.

[c]Carbapenems should be reserved for settings where there is a high risk of resistance to other agents (ie, extended-spectrum β-lactamase [ESBL]-producing pathogens).

[d]These broad-spectrum agents should be reserved for patients infected with Enterobacterales that are resistant to all other β-lactams. Ceftazidime/avibactam, meropenem/vaborbactam, and imipenem/relebactam are preferred for KPC-producing pathogens. Ceftolozane/tazobactam may have activity against multidrug-resistant *Pseudomonas;* however, susceptibility must be confirmed.

Data from References 16, 55, 58, and 59.

Most patients with severe intra-abdominal infection, sepsis, or healthcare-associated infection should be placed on piperacillin/tazobactam, cefepime with metronidazole, or a carbapenem with *Pseudomonas* activity such as imipenem, or meropenem. In patients with IgE-mediated allergic reactions to β-lactams (hives/urticaria, bronchospasm, angioedema, or anaphylaxis), a combination therapy with aztreonam, vancomycin, and metronidazole may be used. The benefits of systemic preemptive antifungal therapy (with fluconazole or an echinocandin) as a means to prevent invasive candidiasis in patients with intra-abdominal infection have not been established.[61] However, patients with intra-abdominal infections are often at high risk for systemic candidiasis, given multiple risk factors may be present such as recent abdominal surgery, the presence of a central line, parenteral nutrition, and broad-spectrum antibiotic use.[16,55,62] When invasive candidiasis is suspected, generally an echinocandin should be used empirically because these patients are often severely ill and may be at risk for infection with a fluconazole-resistant *Candida* species.[62] As noted in Table 137-7, *Candida* should be treated if isolated from cultures in patients with high-severity, community-acquired or healthcare-associated infection.[16,62] If the *Candida* spp. is fluconazole susceptible and the patient is clinically improving, it is reasonable to de-escalate from an echinocandin to fluconazole.

Aminoglycoside-based treatment regimens are not routinely recommended due to their narrow therapeutic index (nephrotoxicity, ototoxicity) relative to the recommended agents such as β-lactams.[63,64] Aminoglycosides are reserved primarily for infections due to presumed or proven multidrug-resistant pathogen(s).[50,55]

If an aminoglycoside is required, the initial dosage should be determined based on the patient's weight and renal function. Traditionally, gentamicin and tobramycin were administered multiple times daily with specific peak (6-10 mcg/mL [mg/L; 13-21 μmol/L]) and trough (less than 1-2 mcg/mL [mg/L; less than 2-4 μmol/L]) serum

TABLE 137-7 Evidence-Based Recommendations for Treatment of Complicated Intra-Abdominal Infections

	Grade of Recommendation[a]
Elements of Appropriate Intervention	
An appropriate source control procedure to drain infected foci, control ongoing peritoneal contamination by diversion or resection, and restore anatomic and physiological function to the extent feasible is recommended for nearly all patients with intra-abdominal infections	B-2
Community-Acquired Infections of Mild-to-Moderate Severity in Adults	
Antibiotics used for empiric treatment of community-acquired intra-abdominal infections should be active against enteric gram-negative aerobic and facultative bacilli and enteric gram-positive streptococci	A-1
For patients with mild-to-moderate, community-acquired infections, regimens with substantial anti-pseudomonal activity are not required (Table 137-6)	A-1
Empiric coverage of *Enterococcus* is not necessary in patients with mild-to-moderate community-acquired intra-abdominal infection	A-1
The use of agents listed as appropriate for high-severity, community-acquired infection and healthcare-associated infection is not recommended for patients with mild-to-moderate, community-acquired infection, because such regimens may carry a greater risk of toxicity and facilitate acquisition of more resistant organisms	B-2
High-Severity, Community-Acquired Infections in Adults[b]	
The empiric use of antimicrobial regimens with broad-spectrum activity against gram-negative organisms including *Pseudomonas* spp., such as meropenem, imipenem/cilastatin, piperacillin–tazobactam, ciprofloxacin or levofloxacin in combination with metronidazole, or ceftazidime or cefepime in combination with metronidazole, is recommended for patients with high-severity, community-acquired intra-abdominal infection (Table 137-6)	A-1
Aztreonam plus metronidazole is an alternative, but addition of an agent effective against gram-positive cocci is recommended	B-3
Healthcare-Associated Infections in Adults[c]	
Empiric antibiotic therapy for healthcare-associated intra-abdominal infections should be driven by local microbiologic results	A-2
To achieve empiric coverage of likely pathogens, multidrug regimens that include agents with expanded spectra of activity against gram-negative aerobic and facultative bacilli may be needed. These agents include meropenem, imipenem/cilastatin, piperacillin/tazobactam, or metronidazole combined with either cefepime or ceftazidime. For multidrug-resistant aerobic gram-negative pathogens, aminoglycosides, colistin, polymyxin B, meropenem/vaborbactam, imipenem/relebactam, eravacycline, cefiderocol, ceftazidime/avibactam, or ceftolozane/tazobactam may be required	B-3
Antimicrobial Agents Not Recommended	

(continued)

TABLE 137-7 Evidence-Based Recommendations for Treatment of Complicated Intra-Abdominal Infections (*Continued*)

	Grade of Recommendation[a]
Ampicillin/sulbactam is not recommended for use because of high rates of resistance to this agent among community-acquired *E. coli*	B-2
Quinolone-resistant *E. coli* have become common in some communities, and quinolones should not be used unless hospital surveys indicate 90% susceptibility of *E. coli* to quinolones	A-2
Clindamycin is not recommended for use because of increasing prevalence of resistance to these agents among *Bacteroides fragilis*	B-2
Because of the availability of less toxic agents demonstrated to be at least equally effective, aminoglycosides are not recommended for routine use in adults with community-acquired intra-abdominal infections	B-2
Oral Completion Therapy	
For adults recovering from an intra-abdominal infection, completion of the antimicrobial course with oral forms of moxifloxacin, ciprofloxacin plus metronidazole, levofloxacin plus metronidazole, an oral cephalosporin with metronidazole, or amoxicillin/clavulanic acid is acceptable in patients able to tolerate an oral diet and in patients in whom susceptibility studies do not demonstrate resistance	B-2
Duration of Therapy	
Antimicrobial therapy of established infection should be limited to 4 days, unless it is difficult to achieve adequate source control. Longer durations of therapy have not been associated with improved outcome	A-1
For acute stomach and proximal jejunum perforations, in the absence of acid-reducing therapy or malignancy and when source control is achieved within 24 hours, prophylactic anti-infective therapy directed at aerobic gram-positive cocci for 24 hours is adequate	B-2
Bowel injuries attributable to penetrating, blunt, or iatrogenic trauma that are repaired within 12 hours and any other intraoperative contamination of the operative field by enteric contents should be treated with antibiotics for ≤24 hours	A-1
Acute appendicitis without evidence of perforation, abscess, or local peritonitis requires only prophylactic administration of narrow spectrum regimens active against aerobic and facultative and obligate anaerobes; treatment should be discontinued within 24 hours	A-1
The administration of prophylactic antibiotics to patients with severe necrotizing pancreatitis prior to the diagnosis of infection is not recommended	A-1
Anaerobic Coverage	
Coverage for obligate anaerobic bacilli should be provided for distal small bowel, appendiceal, and colon-derived infection and for more proximal GI perforations in the presence of obstruction or paralytic ileus	A-1
Antifungal Therapy	
Antifungal therapy for patients with high-severity community-acquired or healthcare-associated infection is recommended if *Candida* is grown from intra-abdominal cultures	B-2
Anti-MRSA Therapy	
Empiric antimicrobial coverage directed against MRSA should be provided to patients with healthcare-associated intra-abdominal infection who are known to be colonized with the organism or who are at risk of having an infection due to this organism because of prior treatment failure and significant antibiotic exposure	B-2
Vancomycin is recommended for treatment of suspected or proven intra-abdominal infection due to MRSA	A-3
Antienterococcal Therapy	
Antimicrobial therapy for enterococci should be given when enterococci are recovered from patients with high-severity community-acquired or healthcare-associated infection	B-III
Empiric antienterococcal therapy is recommended for patients with high-severity community-acquired infections and healthcare-associated intra-abdominal infections, particularly those with postoperative infection, those who have previously received cephalosporins or other antimicrobial agents selected for *Enterococcus* species, immunocompromised patients, and those with valvular heart disease or prosthetic intravascular materials	B-II
Initial empiric antienterococcal therapy should be directed against *Enterococcus faecalis*. Antibiotics that can potentially be used against this organism, on the basis of susceptibility testing of the individual isolate, include ampicillin, ampicillin/sulbactam, piperacillin/tazobactam, imipenem/cilastatin, and vancomycin	B-III
Empiric therapy directed against vancomycin-resistant *Enterococcus faecium* is not recommended unless the patient is at very high risk for an infection due to this organism, such as a liver transplant recipient with an intra-abdominal infection originating in the hepatobiliary tree or a patient known to be colonized with vancomycin-resistant *E. faecium*	B-III

[a]Strength of recommendations: A, B, C = good, moderate, and poor evidence to support recommendation, respectively. Quality of evidence: 1 = Evidence from ≥1 properly randomized, controlled trial. 2 = Evidence from ≥1 well-designed clinical trial without randomization, from cohort or case-controlled analytic studies, from multiple time series, or from dramatic results from uncontrolled experiments. 3 = Evidence from opinions of respected authorities, based on clinical experience, descriptive studies, or reports of expert communities.

[b]Criteria for high-severity community-acquired infection: sepsis or septic shock, APACHE II score ≥15, delay in initial intervention >24 hours, advanced age, comorbidity and degree of organ dysfunction, low albumin level, poor nutritional status, degree of peritoneal involvement or diffuse peritonitis, inability to achieve adequate debridement or control of drainage, and presence of malignancy.

[c]Criteria for classification of intra-abdominal infections as healthcare-associated infection vary. However, patients who develop an infection after surgery, reside in a long-term care facility, who were recently hospitalized, or who have other significant healthcare exposure can be considered to have a healthcare-associated intra-abdominal infection.

MRSA, methicillin-resistant *Staphylococcus aureus*.

Data from References 16, 55, and 58.

concentration targets. Because aminoglycosides have concentration-dependent killing and have a relatively long postantibiotic effect for aerobic gram-negative bacilli, extended-interval dosing of aminoglycosides is possible. For most patients and indications, extended-interval aminoglycoside dosing (ie, 5-7 mg/kg once daily for tobramycin or gentamicin, 15-20 mg/kg once daily for amikacin) has replaced traditional dosing, given equivalent efficacy and decreased nephrotoxicity.[65-67]

Antimicrobial resistance continues to increase worldwide.[68-70] Enterobacterales producing extended-spectrum β-lactamases (ESBL) have been increasingly isolated from intra-abdominal

TABLE 137-8 Guidelines for Empiric Antimicrobial Agents for Intra-Abdominal Infections

	Primary Agents	Alternatives
Primary (Spontaneous) Bacterial Peritonitis		
Cirrhosis	Ceftriaxone, cefotaxime	1. Piperacillin/tazobactam, carbapenems 2. Aztreonam combined with an agent active against *Streptococcus* spp. (eg, vancomycin) or quinolones with significant *Streptococcus* spp. activity (levofloxacin, moxifloxacin)
Peritoneal dialysis	Initial empiric regimens should be active against both gram-positive (including *S. aureus*) and gram-negative pathogens: gram-positive agent (first-generation cephalosporin or vancomycin) plus a gram-negative agent (third-generation cephalosporin or aminoglycoside)	1. Cefepime or carbapenems may be used alone 2. Aztreonam or an aminoglycoside may be used in place of ceftazidime or cefepime as long as combined with a gram-positive agent 3. Quinolones may be used in place of gram-negative agents if local susceptibilities allow
	1. *Staphylococcus* spp.: oxacillin/nafcillin or first-generation cephalosporin	1. Vancomycin should be used for methicillin-resistant *Staphylococcus* spp. 2. May consider addition of rifampin for 5-7 days with vancomycin
	2. *Streptococcus* or *Enterococcus*: ampicillin	1. Daptomycin or linezolid should ideally be used to treat vancomycin-resistant *Enterococcus* spp. not susceptible to ampicillin
	3. Aerobic gram-negative bacilli: ceftazidime or cefepime	1. The regimen should be based on in vitro sensitivity tests
	4. *Pseudomonas aeruginosa*: two agents with differing mechanisms of action, such as an intraperitoneal ceftazidime or cefepime each combined with either tobramycin or oral ciprofloxacin	
Secondary Bacterial Peritonitis		
Perforated peptic ulcer	First-generation cephalosporins	1. Ceftriaxone, cefotaxime, or antianaerobic cephalosporins[a]
Other	Third- or fourth-generation cephalosporin with metronidazole, piperacillin–tazobactam or carbapenem	1. Ciprofloxacin[b] or levofloxacin[b] each with metronidazole or moxifloxacin[b] alone 2. Aztreonam with vancomycin and metronidazole 3. Antianaerobic cephalosporins[a]
Abscess		
General	Third- or fourth-generation cephalosporin with metronidazole or piperacillin/tazobactam	1. Imipenem/cilastatin, meropenem, or ertapenem 2. Ciprofloxacin[b] or levofloxacin[b] each with metronidazole or moxifloxacin alone
Liver	As above	Use metronidazole if amoebic liver abscess is suspected
Spleen	Ceftriaxone or cefotaxime	Moxifloxacin[b] or levofloxacin[b]
Other Intra-Abdominal Infections		
Appendicitis	Same management as for community-acquired complicated intra-abdominal infections as listed in Table 137-6[44]	
Community-acquired acute cholecystitis	Ceftriaxone or cefotaxime	Severe infection, piperacillin/tazobactam, antipseudomonal carbapenem, aztreonam with metronidazole
Cholangitis	Ceftriaxone or cefotaxime each with or without metronidazole	Vancomycin with aztreonam with or without metronidazole
Acute contamination from abdominal trauma	Antianaerobic cephalosporins[a] or metronidazole with either ceftriaxone or cefotaxime	1. Piperacillin/tazobactam or a carbapenem 2. Ciprofloxacin[b] or levofloxacin[b] each with metronidazole or moxifloxacin alone
Diverticulitis	Cefazolin, cefuroxime, or ceftriaxone with metronidazole or ampicillin/sulbactam	Ciprofloxacin[b] or levofloxacin[b] each with metronidazole or moxifloxacin alone

[a]Cefoxitin or ceftizoxime; these agents should be avoided empirically unless local antibiograms show >80% to 90% susceptibility of *E. coli* to these agents.

[b]Use of quinolones may be associated with treatment failure due to increasing resistance of enteric pathogens including *E. coli*. Empiric quinolone use should be avoided unless local antibiograms show >80% to 90% susceptibility of *E. coli* to quinolones.

Data from References 55 and 60.

cultures.[49,51] For patients with ESBL-producing pathogens, carbapenems are typically the drugs of choice. With the increased use of carbapenems, pathogens have continued to evolve with the development of β-lactamases that hydrolyze carbapenems (eg, *Klebsiella pneumoniae* carbapenemase [KPC]), multidrug-resistant *Pseudomonas* spp., and carbapenem-resistant *Acinetobacter* spp. Especially in patients with healthcare-associated intra-abdominal infections, these multidrug-resistant pathogens have forced clinicians to use more toxic and potentially less effective agents such as the polymyxins, tigecycline, and aminoglycosides. For example, the product labeling for tigecycline carries a Black Box Warning, as it has been associated with an increased risk of mortality relative to comparator agents, which is based on pooled data collected from randomized controlled trials including patients with intra-abdominal infections, skin and skin structure infections, and ventilator-associated pneumonia.[71-73] Accordingly, the 2017 SIS guidelines recommend against the use of tigecycline except potentially as part of a combination regimen for multidrug-resistant pathogens.[16] Three potential therapeutic options for multidrug-resistant pathogens, ceftolozane/tazobactam, ceftazidime/avibactam, and eravacycline have been FDA-approved for the treatment of complicated intra-abdominal infections in combination with metronidazole.[66,67,74] Ceftolozane/tazobactam may be active against multidrug-resistant pathogens, particularly *Pseudomonas* spp., while ceftazidime/avibactam is active against KPC-producing Enterobacterales.

These agents may be more effective than colistin-based regimens for infections due to KPC-producing Enterobacterales.[59,75-77] However, it is not uncommon for organisms that are resistant to all other β-lactams to also be resistant to these three new agents, and so susceptibility must be confirmed. Despite this, these agents are highly valuable in terms of their activity against multidrug-resistant pathogens, and as such, their use should be reserved for patients with a suspected or confirmed infection due to a pathogen resistant to all other β-lactams. The limited safe-and-effective therapeutic options for resistant organisms highlight the need, from an individual patient and public health standpoint, for pharmacists and other clinicians to ensure that antimicrobials are selected appropriately, at the optimal dose, and for the correct duration.

With intra-abdominal contamination from the upper GI tract (perforation of a peptic ulcer or biliary tract disease), anaerobes such as *B. fragilis* are uncommon pathogens, and therefore other empiric agents such as ampicillin, penicillin, or first-generation cephalosporins are reasonable. Anaerobic coverage is also not necessary for primary peritonitis associated with cirrhosis, and cefotaxime or ceftriaxone remain the treatments of choice.[78]

Empiric coverage of *Enterococcus* in mild-to-moderate, community-acquired intra-abdominal infections is not recommended.[55] The failure of host defenses may be a critical factor in the pathogenicity of enterococci. In patients with high-severity, community-acquired intra-abdominal infections or patients with healthcare-associated infection, coverage of *Enterococcus faecalis* should be included in the initial regimen.[16,55] Ampicillin remains the drug of choice for this indication because it is active against the vast majority of *E. faecalis*. Notably, piperacillin/tazobactam and imipenem/cilastatin both have activity against ampicillin-susceptible *E. faecalis*, and therefore these may be elegant choices for empiric therapy of high-severity community-acquired or healthcare-associated intra-abdominal infections. Vancomycin may also be active against enterococci; however, rates of vancomycin-resistant enterococci are increasing, especially in select patient populations (eg, liver transplantation, immunocompromised patients).[79] Agents, including linezolid or daptomycin, are commonly used for vancomycin-resistant *Enterococcus* infections. Table 137-7 lists additional evidence-based recommendations for *Enterococcus* spp. coverage.

7 Intraperitoneal administration of antibiotics is preferred over IV therapy in the treatment of peritonitis that occurs in patients undergoing CAPD.[60,80] The International Society of Peritoneal Dialysis guidelines for the diagnosis and pharmacotherapy of peritoneal dialysis-associated infections provide antimicrobial dosing recommendations based on the modality of dialysis (continuous or intermittent).[60]

Given the peritoneal catheter exit site and tunnel is frequently the source of peritoneal dialysis-related peritonitis, prophylaxis with topic antibiotic cream or ointment to the catheter exit site reduces infections caused by *S. aureus* and gram-negative bacilli, including *Pseudomonas* spp.[81] When infection occurs, antimicrobial agents effective against both gram-positive skin flora (including *S. aureus*) and gram-negative organisms should be used for initial intraperitoneal empiric therapy. The most important factors to take into consideration for initial antimicrobial selection are the dialysis center's and the patient's history of infecting organisms and their sensitivities. For empiric intraperitoneal therapy, cefazolin or vancomycin in cases of high prevalence of MRSA or β-lactam allergy may be used for gram-positive coverage. Glycopeptide-containing regimens (vancomycin) were more likely to achieve complete cure compared to first-generation cephalosporins.[80,82] When vancomycin is used, it is preferred that it be given intraperitoneally via intermittent dosing (15-30 mg/kg every 5-7 days) and serum concentrations should be maintained above 15 mcg/mL (mg/L; 10.4 μmol/L).[83] When administered via intermittent dosing, generally the antibiotic should dwell for at least 6 hours. One of these gram-positive agents should be combined with a gram-negative agent such as ceftazidime or an aminoglycoside. If an aminoglycoside is used, it is preferred that it be given intraperitoneally via intermittent dosing (eg, gentamicin 0.6 mg/kg/day). Long durations of aminoglycoside therapy should be avoided if possible to mitigate the risk of ototoxicity and loss of residual renal function. Another option is monotherapy with cefepime or imipenem/cilastatin. If patients have significant residual renal function, increased antimicrobial doses may not be necessary.[60,83] As with other intra-abdominal infections, source control should be prioritized; in patients with an ongoing catheter exit site or tunnel infection, catheter removal with reinsertion should be strongly considered. If peritonitis relapses or recurs, the catheter should be promptly removed. Antimicrobial therapy should typically be continued for 14 to 21 days. The reader is referred to recent guidelines for additional information.[60,81]

After acute bacterial contamination, such as with abdominal trauma where GI contents spill into the peritoneum, antibiotics should be administered. If the patient is seen soon after injury (within 2 hours) and surgical measures are instituted promptly, an anti-anaerobic cephalosporin (such as cefoxitin), a third-generation cephalosporin (such as ceftriaxone) with metronidazole, or piperacillin/tazobactam is effective in preventing most infectious complications. Antimicrobials should be administered as soon as possible after injury.[84]

8 For appendicitis, the antimicrobial regimen used should depend on the appearance of the appendix at the time of operation, which may be normal, inflamed, gangrenous, or perforated. It is advisable to begin antimicrobial agents before the appendectomy is performed. Reasonable regimens would be antianaerobic cephalosporins or, if the patient is seriously ill, piperacillin/tazobactam, or an anti-pseudomonal carbapenem. If, at operation, the appendix is normal or inflamed, postoperative antimicrobials are not required. If the appendix is gangrenous or perforated, a treatment course of 3 to 4 days with the agents listed in Table 137-6 is appropriate.[11,85] For uncomplicated appendicitis (defined as the absence of perforation, abscess, appendicolith, CT consistent with possible tumor, peritonitis, severe systemic illness) confirmed by CT, a nonsurgical approach of antibiotic therapy alone may also be considered.[11,86,87] Patients who received initial appendectomy (mostly open procedures), instead of antibiotics alone, experienced greater pain, a longer duration of sick leave from work, and more complications such as surgical site infections and delayed healing.[11] In addition, 27% of patients managed nonsurgically required an appendectomy within 1 year of their index hospitalization. In over 1,500 adults with appendicitis, antibiotics were found to be non-inferior to appendectomy at 30 days based on a quality of life questionaire.[87] However, complications were more common in the antibiotics groups and 29% required an appendectomy within 90 days. Similarly, a smaller randomized study also demonstrated that 27.3% of adult patients receiving antibiotics alone required an appendectomy within 1 year,[11] and 39.1% were at an increased risk of late recurrence of uncomplicated acute appendicitis within 5 years.[88] Conversely, another smaller randomized study found that adult patients who received a supportive care only for CT-confirmed uncomplicated appendicitis experienced similar treatment failure rates within 19 months compared to those who received 4 days of antibiotic therapy.[89] In children, nonoperative

management of uncomplicated appendicitis with 7 days of antibiotics had a success rate of 67.1% and had significantly fewer disability days at 1 year compared to those who underwent surgery.[90] Despite these limitations, the risks and benefits of surgery versus antibiotics alone should be considered along with the patient's own preferences.

Treatment of diverticulitis varies based on disease severity. For mild, acute uncomplicated diverticulitis, antibiotics are not necessary with appropriate follow-up in immunocompetent adults[91]; however, if antibiotics are prescribed, amoxicillin/clavulanate or an oral cephalosporin with metronidazole is recommended.[92] Oral antibiotics (ciprofloxacin with metronidazole) are as effective as intravenous antibiotics for uncomplicated diverticulitis.[93] In adults who present with complicated diverticulitis with an abscess, antibiotics that cover gram-negative aerobic bacilli and anaerobes should be combined with drainage of the abscess; however, once source control is achieved, antibiotics are no longer needed. In immunocompromised adults, early elective resectional surgery is recommended due to the risk for early, frequent, and severe relapses of complicated acute diverticulitis managed with antibiotics alone. In general, 15% to 30% of patients admitted for management of acute diverticulitis required surgery during that admission.[94] When surgery is required, laparoscopic surgery is preferred to open colectomy due to shorter lengths of hospital stay, fewer complications, and lower in-hospital mortality.[95]

Acute intra-abdominal contamination, such as after a traumatic injury, may be treated with a short antimicrobial course (24 hours).[84] For established infections (ie, peritonitis or intra-abdominal abscess), an antimicrobial course limited to 4 days after source control is appropriate.[16,54] This allows eradication of bacteria remaining in the peritoneum after a surgical procedure that may enter the peritoneum through healing suture lines. Under certain conditions, therapy for longer than 4 days would be justified (eg, when the focus of infection in the abdomen is still present). For some abscesses, such as pyogenic liver abscess, antimicrobials may be required for a month or longer. If definitive source control is not possible, then a duration of 5 to 7 days of antibiotic therapy may be considered based on the patient's clinical stability including resolution or improvement in leukocytosis, fever, GI function.[16] These patients should be closely monitored for clinical worsening after cessation of antibiotics; a source control intervention may need to be reconsidered or antibiotics may need to be reinitiated.

Intraperitoneal irrigation of antimicrobial agents for the prevention of surgical site infection, abscess development, and other complications in patients with peritonitis has been studied; however, the quality of the data is limited and precludes a definitive determination of efficacy.[96,97] Possibly the most important aspect of peritoneal irrigation is the dilutional effect on bacteria and adjuvants that promote infection (intestinal contents and hemoglobin), and elimination of debris and gross contamination. Most systemically administered antimicrobials easily cross the peritoneal membrane so that peritoneal fluid concentrations are similar to serum. Confined areas, such as an abscess, can be expected to attain much lower antimicrobial concentrations. Given the unclear benefit of antibiotic irrigation, irrigation with crystalloid fluid alone is recommended.[16]

EVALUATION OF THERAPEUTIC OUTCOMES

Whichever antimicrobial regimen is chosen, the patient should be reassessed continually to determine the success or failure of therapies. The clinician should recognize that there are many reasons for poor patient outcomes with intra-abdominal infections, improper antimicrobial administration is only one. The patient may be immunocompromised, which decreases the likelihood of successful outcome with any regimen. There may be surgical reasons for poor patient outcome. Failure to identify all intra-abdominal foci of infection or leaks from a GI anastomosis may cause continued infection. Finally, antimicrobial resistance may contribute to treatment failure as isolates from intra-abdominal infections are increasingly drug resistant.[49,98]

The outcome from intra-abdominal infection is not determined solely by what transpires in the abdomen. Unsatisfactory outcomes in patients with intra-abdominal infections may result from complications that arise in other organ systems, including renal or respiratory failure. Furthermore, pneumonia is a complication that is commonly associated with mortality after intra-abdominal infection.[99] Other nosocomial infections including catheter-related bacteremia and urinary tract infection are also independent predictors of mortality in patients with intra-abdominal infections.[100]

9 Once antimicrobials are initiated and the other important therapies described earlier are used, most patients should show improvement within 2 to 3 days. Usually, temperature will return to near normal, vital signs should stabilize, and the patient should not appear in distress, with the exception of recognized discomfort and pain from incisions, drains, and the nasogastric tube. Within 24 to 72 hours, aerobic bacterial culture results should return. If a suspected pathogen is not sensitive to the antimicrobial agents being given, the regimen should be changed to active therapy. If the isolated pathogen is susceptible to a narrower spectrum agent, therapy should be de-escalated.

With anaerobic culturing techniques and the slow growth of these organisms, anaerobes are often not identified until 4 to 7 days after culture. A report indicating that anaerobes were not isolated should not be the sole justification for discontinuing antianaerobic drugs because anaerobic bacteria that were present in the infectious process may not have been collected or maintained in anaerobic conditions which can lead to cell death in vitro.

Reasons for antimicrobial failure may not always be apparent. Even when antimicrobial susceptibility tests indicate that an organism is susceptible in vitro to the antimicrobial agent, therapeutic failures may occur. Possibly there is poor penetration of the antimicrobial agent into the focus of infection, or bacterial resistance may develop after initiation of antimicrobial therapy. In addition, it is possible that an antimicrobial regimen may encourage the development of infection by organisms not susceptible to the regimen being used. Superinfection in patients being treated for intra-abdominal infection can be caused by *Candida*; however, enterococci or opportunistic gram-negative bacilli such as *Pseudomonas* may be involved.

Treatment regimens for intra-abdominal infection can be judged as successful if the patient recovers from the infection without recurrent peritonitis or intra-abdominal abscess and without the need for additional antimicrobials. A regimen can be considered unsuccessful if a significant adverse drug reaction occurs, reoperation or percutaneous drainage is necessary, or patient improvement is delayed beyond 1 or 2 weeks. The costs of treatment can be significantly reduced if parenteral antimicrobials can be switched to oral agents for completion of therapy.[101]

ABBREVIATIONS

APACHE	acute physiology and chronic health evaluation
CAPD	chronic ambulatory peritoneal dialysis
CNS	central nervous system
CT	computed tomography
CVP	central venous pressure
ESBL	extended-spectrum β-lactamase
IDSA	Infectious Diseases Society of America
IL	interleukin
INF	interferon
KPC	*Klebsiella pneumoniae* carbapenemase

LD	loading dose
MAP	mean arterial pressure
MD	maintenance dose
MRSA	methicillin-resistant *Staphylococcus aureus*
SIS	Surgical Infection Society
TNF	tumor necrosis factor
WBC	white blood cell

REFERENCES

1. Silva-Nunes J, Cardoso T. Intra-abdominal infections: the role of different classifications on the selection of the best antibiotic treatment. *BMC Infect Dis.* 2019;19:980.
2. Pericleous M, Sarnowski A, Moore A, Fijten R, Zaman M. The clinical management of abdominal ascites, spontaneous bacterial peritonitis and hepatorenal syndrome: a review of current guidelines and recommendations. *Eur J Gastroenterol Hepatol.* 2016;28:e10–e18.
3. Jalan R, Fernandez J, Wiest R, et al. Bacterial infections in cirrhosis: a position statement based on the EASL Special Conference 2013. *J Hepatol.* 2014;60:1310–1324.
4. Levison ME, Bush LM. Peritonitis and intraperitoneal abscesses. In: Bennett JE, Dolin R, Blaser MJ, eds. *Mandell, Douglas, and Bennett's Principles and Practice of Infectious Diseases.* 8th ed. Philadelphia: Saunders; 2015:935–959[chapter 76].
5. Sartelli M, Chichom-Mefire A, Labricciosa FM, et al. The management of intra-abdominal infections from a global perspective: 2017 WSES guidelines for management of intra-abdominal infections. *World J Emerg Surg.* 2017;12:29.
6. Wiest R, Krag A, Gerbes A. Spontaneous bacterial peritonitis: recent guidelines and beyond. *Gut.* 2012;61:297–310.
7. Schmidt ML, Barritt AS, Orman ES, Hayashi PH. Decreasing mortality in patients hospitalized with cirrhosis in the United States from 2002 through 2010. *Gastroenterology.* 2015;148:967–977.
8. Niu B, Kim B, Limketkai BN, Sun J, Li Z, Woreta T, Chen PH. Mortality from spontaneous bacterial peritonitis among hospitalized patients in the USA. *Dig Dis Sci.* 2018;63(5):1327–1333.
9. Piraino B, Bernardini J. Catheter-related peritonitis. *Perit Dial Int.* 2013;33:592–595.
10. Young-Fadok TM. Diverticulitis. *N Engl J Med.* 2018;379:1635–1642.
11. Salminen P, Paajanen H, Rautio T, et al. Antibiotic therapy vs appendectomy for treatment of uncomplicated acute appendicitis: the APPAC randomized clinical trial. *JAMA.* 2015;313(23):2340–2348.
12. Min YW, Lim KS, Min BH, Gwak GY, Paik YH, Choi MS, et al. Proton pump inhibitor use significantly increases the risk of spontaneous bacterial peritonitis in 1965 patients with cirrhosis and ascites: a propensity score matched cohort study. *Aliment Pharmacol Ther.* 2014;40(6):695–704.
13. Ratelle M, Perreault S, Villeneuve JP, Tremblay L. Association between proton pump inhibitor use and spontaneous bacterial peritonitis in cirrhotic patients with ascites. *Can J Gastroenterol Hepatol.* 2014;28:330–334.
14. Toloza EM, Wilson SE. Cholecystitis and cholangitis. In: Fry DE, ed. *Surgical Infections.* Boston: Little, Brown; 1995:254–263.
15. Sartelli M, Catena F, Di Saverio S, et al. The challenge of antimicrobial resistance in managing intra-abdominal infections. *Surg Infect (Larchmt).* 2015;16:213–220.
16. Mazuski JE, Tessler JM, May AK, et al. The Surgical Infection Society revised guidelines on the management of intra-abdominal infection. *Surg Infect (Larchmt).* 2017;18(1):1–76.
17. Brook I. Microbiology and management of abdominal infections. *Dig Dis Sci.* 2008;53:2585–2591.
18. Jernberg C, Lofmark S, Edlund C, Jansson JK. Long-term impacts of antibiotic exposure on the human intestinal microbiota. *Microbiology.* 2010;156:3216–3223.
19. Shirah GR, O'Neill PJ. Intra-abdominal infections. *Surg Clin North Am.* 2014;94:1319–1333.
20. Riche FC, Cholley BP, Panis YH, et al. Inflammatory cytokine response in patients with septic shock secondary to generalized peritonitis. *Crit Care Med.* 2000;28:433–437.
21. Solomkin JS, Mazuski J. Intra-abdominal sepsis: newer interventional and antimicrobial therapies. *Infect Dis Clin North Am.* 2009;23:593–608.
22. Schietroma M, Piccione F, Carlei F, Sista F, Cecilia EM, Amicucci G. Peritonitis from perforated peptic ulcer and immune response. *J Invest Surg.* 2013;26:294–304.
23. Dever JB, Sheikh MY. Spontaneous bacterial peritonitis—diagnosis, treatment, and prevention. *Aliment Pharmacol Ther.* 2015;41:1116–1131.
24. Sartelli M, Weber DG, Ruppé E, et al. Antimicrobials: a global alliance for optimizing their rational use in intra-abdominal infections (AGORA). *World J Emerg Surg.* 2016;11:33.
25. Herzog T, Chromic AM, Uhl W. Treatment of complicated intra-abdominal infections in the era of multidrug resistant bacteria. *Eur J Med Res.* 2010;15:525–532.
26. Thompson AE, Marshall JC, Opal SM. Intra-abdominal infections in infants and children: descriptions and definitions. *Pediatr Crit Care Med.* 2005;6:S30–S35.
27. Rangel SJ, Rice-Townsend SE, Karki M, Moss RL. Peritonitis. In: Long SS, Prober CG, Fischer M, eds. *Principles and Practice of Pediatric Infectious Diseases.* 5th ed. Elsevier, Inc; 2018.
28. Guillet-Caruba C, Cheikhelard A, Guillet M, et al. Bacteriologic epidemiology and empirical treatment of pediatric complicated appendicitis. *Diagn Microbiol Infect Dis.* 2011;69:376–381.
29. Lee SL, Islam S, Cassidy LD, et al. Antibiotics and appendicitis in the pediatric population: an American Pediatric Surgical Association outcomes and Clinical Trials Committee systematic review. *J Pediatr Surg.* 2010;45:2181–2185.
30. Nanchal RS, Ahmad S. Infections in liver disease. *Crit Care Clin.* 2016;32(3):411–424.
31. Brook I, Frazier EH. Aerobic and anaerobic microbiology of retroperitoneal abscesses. *Clin Infect Dis.* 1998;26:9384941.
32. Bennion RS, Baron EJ, Thompson JE, et al. The bacteriology of gangrenous and perforated appendicitis—revisited. *Ann Surg.* 1990;211:165–171.
33. Marshall JC, Innes M. Intensive care unit management of intra-abdominal infection. *Crit Care Med.* 2003;31:2228–2237.
34. Sawyer RG, Rosenlof LK, Adams RB, et al. Peritonitis into the 1990s: changing pathogens and changing strategies in the critically ill. *Am Surg.* 1992;58:82–87.
35. Montravers P, Lepape A, Dubreuil L, et al. Clinical and microbiological profiles of community-acquired and nosocomial infections: results of the French prospective, observational EBIIA study. *J Antimicrob Chemother.* 2009;63:785–794.
36. Onderdonk AB, Bartlett JG, Louie T, et al. Microbial synergy in experimental intra-abdominal abscess. *Infect Immun.* 1997;13:22–26.
37. Donskey CJ, Chowdhry TK, Hecker MT, et al. Effect of antibiotic therapy on the density of vancomycin-resistant enterococci in the stool of colonized patients. *Ann Surg.* 2000;343:1925–1932.
38. Sitges-Serra A, Lopez MJ, Girvent M, et al. Postoperative enterococcal infection after treatment of complicated intra-abdominal sepsis. *Br J Surg.* 2002;89:361–367.
39. Yang SK, Xiao L, Zhang H, et al. Significance of serum procalcitonin as biomarker for detection of bacterial peritonitis: a systematic review and meta-analysis. *BMC Infect Dis.* 2014;14:452.
40. Mahmutaj D, Krasniqi S, Braha B, Limani D, Neziri B. The predictive role of procalcitonin on the treatment of intra-abdominal infections. *Open Access Maced J Med Sci.* 2017;5(7):909–914.
41. Covino M, Fransvea P, Rosa F, et al. Early procalcitonin assessment in the emergency department in patients with intra-abdominal infection: an excess or a need?. *Surg Infect.* 2021;epub ahead of print. doi:10.1089/sur.2020.373.
42. Boldingh QJJ, de Vries FEE, Boermeester MA. Abdominal sepsis. *Curr Opin Crit Care.* 2017;23(2):159–166.
43. Leppäniemi A, Kimball EJ, De Laet I, et al. Management of abdominal sepsis: a paradigm shift. *Anesthesiol Inten Ther.* 2015;47:400–408.
44. Rhodes A, Evans LE, Alhazzani W, et al. Surviving Sepsis Campaign: international guidelines for management of sepsis and septic shock 2016. *Crit Care Med.* 2017;43:304–377.
45. Rivers E, Nguyen B, Havstad S, et al. Early goal-directed therapy in the treatment of severe sepsis and septic shock. *N Engl J Med.* 2001;345:1368–1377.
46. Evans LE, Rhodes A, Alhazzani W, et al. Surviving Sepsis Campaign: international guidelines for management of sepsis and septic shock 2021. *Crit Care Med.* Nov 1;49(11):e1063–e1143.
47. Brotfain E, Koyman L, Toledan R, et al. Positive fluid balances as a major predictor of clinical outcomes with sepsis/septic shock after ICU discharge. *Am J Emerg Med.* 2016;34:2122–2126.
48. Semler MW, Kellum JA. Balanced crystalloid solutions. *Am J Respir Crit Care Med.* 2019;199(8):952–960.
49. Hackel MA, Badal RE, Bouchillon SK, Biedenbach DJ, Hoban DJ. Resistance rates of intra-abdominal isolates from intensive care units and non-intensive care units in the United States: the study for monitoring antimicrobial resistance trends 2010–2012. *Surg Infect (Larchmt).* 2015;16(3):298–304.

50. Wong PF, Gilliam AD, Kumar S, et al. Antibiotic regimens for secondary peritonitis of gastrointestinal origin in adults. *Cochrane Database Syst Rev*. 2007;2:CD004539.
51. Hoban DJ, Bouchillon SK, Hawser SP, Badal RE, Labombardi VJ, DiPersio J. Susceptibility of gram-negative pathogens isolated from patients with complicated intra-abdominal infections in the United States, 2007–2008: results of the Study for Monitoring Antimicrobial Resistance Trends (SMART). *Antimicrob Agents Chemother*. 2010;54:3031–3034.
52. Snydman DR, Jacobus NV, McDermott LA, et al. Lessons learned from the anaerobe survey: historical perspective and review of the most recent data (2005–2007). *Clin Infect Dis*. 2010;50(Suppl 1):S26–S33.
53. Hawser SP, Bouchillon SK, Hoban DJ, Badal RE. In vitro susceptibilities of aerobic and facultative anaerobic Gram-negative bacilli from patients with intra-abdominal infections worldwide from 2005–2007: results from the SMART study. *Int J Antimicrob Agents*. 2009;34:585–588.
54. Sawyer RG, Claridge JA, Nathens AB, et al. Trial of short-course antimicrobial therapy for intra-abdominal infection. *N Engl J Med*. 2015;372:1996–2005.
55. Solomkin JS, Mazuski JE, Bradley JS, et al. Diagnosis and management of complicated intra- abdominal infection in adults and children: guidelines by the Surgical Infection Society and the Infectious Diseases Society of America. *Clin Inf Dis*. 2010;50:133–164.
56. Gauzit R, Pean Y, Mistretta F, Lalaude O. Epidemiology, management, and prognosis of secondary non-postoperative peritonitis: a French prospective observational multicenter study. *Surg Infect*. 2009;10:119–127.
57. Huang LL, Van Schooneveld TC, Huang RD, et al. Guideline-concordant versus discordant antimicrobial therapy in patients with community-onset complicated intra-abdominal infections. *Infect Control and Hosp Epidemiol*. 2016;37:855–858.
58. Leone S, Damiani G, Pezone I, et al. New antimicrobial options for the management of complicated intra-abdominal infections. *Eur J Clin Microbiol Infect Dis*. 2019;38:819–827.
59. Tamma PD, Aitken SL, Bonomo RA, Mathers AJ, van Duin D, Clancy CJ. Infectious Diseases Society of America Antimicrobial Resistant Treatment Guidance: Gram-Negative Bacterial Infections. Available at: https://www.idsociety.org/globalassets/idsa/practice-guidelines/amr-guidance/idsa-amr-guidance.pdf. Accessed May 25, 2021.
60. Li PK, Szeto CC, Piraino B, et al. ISPD peritonitis recommendations: 2016 update on prevention and treatment. *Perit Dial Int*. 2016;36(5):481–508.
61. Knitsch W, Vincent J-L, Utzolino S, et al. A randomized, placebo-controlled trial of preemptive antifungal therapy for the prevention of invasive candidiasis following gastrointestinal surgery for intra-abdominal infections. *Clin Infect Dis*. 2015;61:1671–1678.
62. Pappas PG, Kauffman CA, Andes DR, et al. Clinical practice guideline for the management of candidiasis: 2016 update by the Infectious Diseases Society of America. *Clin Inf Dis*. 2016;62(4):e1–e50.
63. Hooker KD, DiPiro JT, Wynn JJ. Aminoglycoside combinations versus single β-lactams for penetrating abdominal trauma: a meta-analysis. *J Trauma*. 1991;31:1155–1160.
64. Solomkin JS, Dellinger EP, Christou NV, et al. Results of a multicenter trial comparing imipenem/cilastatin to tobramycin/clindamycin for intra-abdominal infections. *Ann Surg*. 1990;212:581–591.
65. Nicolau DP, Freeman CD, Belliveau PP, Nightingale CH, Ross JW, Quintiliani R. Experience with a once-daily aminoglycoside program administered to 2184 adult patients. *Antimicrob Agents Chemother*. 1995;39:650–655.
66. Rybak MJ, Abate BJ, Kang SL, Ruffing MJ, Lerner SA, Drusano GL. Prospective evaluation of the effect of an aminoglycoside dosing regimen on rates of observed nephrotoxicity and ototoxicity. *Antimicrob Agents Chemother*. 1999;43:1549–1555.
67. Olsen KM, Rudis MA, Rebuck JA, et al. Effect of once-daily dosing vs. multiple daily dosing of tobramycin on enzyme markers of nephrotoxicity. *Crit Care Med*. 2004;32(8):1678–1682.
68. Boucher HW, Talbot GH, Bradley JS, et al. Bad bugs, no drugs: no ESKAPE! an update from the Infectious Diseases Society of America. *Clin Infect Dis*. 2009;48(1):1–12.
69. Centers for Disease Control and Prevention. Antibiotic resistance threats in the United States; 2013. Available at: http://www.cdc.gov/drugresistance/threat-report-2013/. Accessed April 4, 2018.
70. World Health Organization. Antimicrobial resistance: global report on surveillance. Geneva: Switzerland; 2014. Available at: http://www.who.int/drugresistance/documents/surveillancereport/en/. Accessed April 4, 2018.
71. Tasina E, Haidich AB, Kokkali S, Arvanitidou M. Efficacy and safety of tigecycline for the treatment of infectious diseases: a meta-analysis. *Lancet Infect Dis*. 2011;11(11):834–844.
72. Prasad P, Sun J, Danner R, Natanson C. Excess deaths associated with tigecycline after approval based on non-inferiority trials. *Clin Infect Dis*. 2012;54:1699–1709.
73. US Food and Drug Administration. FDA drug safety communication: increased risk of death with Tygacil (tigecycline) and approved new boxed warning. US Food and Drug Administration; September 27, 2013. Available at: http://www.fda.gov/Drugs/DrugSafety/ucm369580.htm. Accessed April 4, 2018.
74. Eravacycline Package Insert. Watertown, MA: Tetraphase Pharmaceuticals, Inc.; August 2018.
75. Ceftazidime/avibactam Package Insert. Cincinnati, OH: Forest Pharmaceuticals; September 2015.
76. Ceftolozane/tazobactam Package Insert. Lexington, MA: Cubist; May 2015.
77. van Duin D, Lok JJ, Easley M, et al. Colistin versus ceftazidime-avibactam in the treatment of infections due to carbapenem-resistant Enterobacteriaceae. *Clin Infect Dis*. 2018;66:163–171.
78. Runyon BA. Management of adult patients with ascites due to cirrhosis: Update 2012. Available at: http://www.aasld.org/publications/practice-guidelines-0. Accessed April 4, 2018.
79. Deshpande LM, Fritsche TR, Moet GJ, Biedenbach DJ, Jones RN. Antimicrobial resistance and molecular epidemiology of vancomycin-resistant enterococci from North America and Europe: a report from the SENTRY antimicrobial surveillance program. *Diagn Microbiol Infect Dis*. 2007;58:163–170.
80. Ballinger AE, Palmer SC, Wiggins KJ, et al. Treatment for peritoneal dialysis-associated peritonitis. *Cochrane Database Syst Rev*. 2014;(4):CD005284.
81. Szeto CC, Li PKT, Johnson DW, et al. ISPD catheter-related infection recommendations: 2017 update. *Perit Dial Int*. 2017;37(2):141–154.
82. Flanigan MJ, Lim VS. Initial treatment of dialysis associated peritonitis: a controlled trial of vancomycin versus cefazolin. *Perit Dial Int*. 1991;11:31–37.
83. Fish R, Nipah R, Jones C, Finney H, Fan SL. Intraperitoneal vancomycin concentrations during peritoneal dialysis-associated peritonitis: correlation with serum levels. *Perit Dial Int*. 2012;32:332–338.
84. Bozorgzadeh A, Pizzi WF, Barie PS, et al. The duration of antibiotic administration in penetrating abdominal trauma. *Am J Surg*. 1999;172:125–135.
85. van Rossem CC, Schreinemacher MH, van Geloven AA, et al. Antibiotic duration after laparoscopic appendectomy for acute complicated appendicitis. *JAMA Surg*. 2016;151(4):323–329.
86. Sallinen V, Ak EA, You JJ, et al. Meta-analysis of antibiotics versus appendicectomy for non-perforated acute appendicitis. *Br J Surg*. 2016;103(6):656–667.
87. Flum DR, Davidson GH, Monsell SE, et al. A randomized trial comparing antibiotics with appendectomy for appendicitis. *N Engl J Med*. 2020;383(20):1907–1919.
88. Salminen P, Tuominen R, Paajanen H, et al. Five-year follow-up of antibiotic therapy for uncomplicated acute appendicitis in the APPAC randomized clinical trial. *JAMA*. 2018;320(12):1259–1265.
89. Park HC, Kim MJ, Lee BH. Randomized clinical trial of antibiotic therapy for uncomplicated appendicitis. *Br J Surg*. 2017;104(13):1785–1790.
90. Minneci PC, Hade EM, Lawrence AE, et al. Association of nonoperative management using antibiotic therapy vs laparoscopic appendectomy with treatment success and disability days in children with uncomplicated appendicitis. *JAMA*. 2020;324(6):581–593.
91. Francis NK, Sylla P, Abou-Khalil M, et al. EAES and SAGES 2018 consensus conference on acute diverticulitis management: evidence-based recommendations for clinical practice. *Surg Endosc*. 2019;33(9):2726–2741.
92. Stollman N, Smalley W, Hirano I, AGA Institute Clinical Guidelines Committee. American Gastroenterological Association institute guideline on the management of acute diverticulitis. *Gastroenterology*. 2015;149(7):1944–1949.
93. Ridgway PF, Latif A, Shabbir J, et al. Randomized controlled trial of oral vs intravenous therapy for the clinically diagnosed acute uncomplicated diverticulitis. *Colorectal Dis*. 2009;11(9):941–946.
94. Wilkins T, Embry K, George R. Diagnosis and management of acute diverticulitis. *Am Fam Physician*. 2013;87(9):612–620.
95. Guller U, Jain N, Hervey S, Purves H, Pietrobon R. Laparoscopic vs open colectomy: outcomes comparison based on large nationwide databases. *Arch Surg*. 2003;138(11):1179–1186.
96. Schein M, Gecelter G, Freinkel W, et al. Peritoneal lavage in abdominal sepsis: a controlled clinical study. *Arch Surg*. 1990;125:1132–1135.
97. Norman G, Atkinson RA, Smith TA, et al. Intracavity lavage and wound irrigation for prevention of surgical site infection. *Cochrane Database Syst Rev*. 2017;10:CD012234.

98. Baquero F, Hsueh P, Paterson DL, et al. In vitro susceptibilities of aerobic and facultatively anaerobic gram-negative bacilli isolated from patients with intra-abdominal infections worldwide: 2005 results from study for monitoring antimicrobial resistance trends. *Surg Infect.* 2009;10:99–104.
99. Merlino JI, Yowler CJ, Malangoni MA. Nosocomial infections adversely affect the outcomes of patients with serious intra-abdominal infections. *Surg Infect (Larchmt).* 2004;5:21–27.
100. Christou NV, Barie PS, Dellinger EP, et al. Surgical Infection Society intra-abdominal infection study. *Arch Surg.* 1993;128:193–199.
101. Paladino JA, Gilliland-Johnson KK, Adelman MH, Coohn SM. Pharmacoeconomics of ciprofloxacin plus metronidazole vs. piperacillin–tazobactam for complicated intra-abdominal infections. *Surg Infect.* 2008;9:325.

Parasitic Diseases

e138

Alireza FakhriRavari, Ana Elizabeth Markez, and Jason M. Cota

KEY CONCEPTS

1. Single-dose tinidazole is the preferred treatment for giardiasis treatment.
2. HIV-infected patients with cryptosporidiosis must receive antiretroviral therapy as the mainstay of therapy in addition to antiparasitic therapy.
3. *Entamoeba histolytica*-specific immunoassays are required to diagnose amebiasis because stool sample microscopy does not distinguish between *E. histolytica* and the nonpathogenic *Entamoeba*.
4. Metronidazole and tinidazole are tissue-acting agents against *Entamoeba*, whereas paromomycin and iodoquinol are luminal amebicides.
5. Benznidazole is recommended for treatment of Chagas disease in all patients without established cardiomyopathy.
6. Atovaquone and azithromycin combination therapy is recommended for treatment of babesiosis.
7. Patients with noncalcified parenchymal neurocysticercosis should initially receive symptomatic therapy with corticosteroids and antiepileptic drugs followed by antihelminthic therapy.
8. For head lice, either nonprescription 1% permethrin or pyrethrins plus piperonyl butoxide topical preparations are agents of choice unless local resistance to these agents is documented.
9. A single application of 5% permethrin results in cure rates in more than 90% of subjects with scabies at 14 and 28 days, but a second dose should be applied 1 week later because its ovicidal efficacy remains unclear.
10. Chemoprophylaxis with non-chloroquine antimalarial drugs such as atovaquone-proguanil and doxycycline retain effectiveness in areas where chloroquine-resistant *Plasmodium falciparum* exposure is likely.

BEYOND THE BOOK

Review the figures depicting the life cycle of each of the following parasites on the Centers for Disease Control and Prevention (CDC) Website. Identify the primary way in which each parasite enters the human host and propose at least one strategy to prevent infection from that parasite. The parasites below are listed in order of least to most complex life cycle.

Head Lice (https://www.cdc.gov/parasites/lice/head/biology.html)

Giardiasis (https://www.cdc.gov/parasites/giardia/pathogen.html)

Cryptosporidiosis (https://www.cdc.gov/parasites/crypto/pathogen.html)

Cysticercosis (https://www.cdc.gov/parasites/cysticercosis/biology.html)

Chagas Disease (https://www.cdc.gov/parasites/chagas/biology.html)

Malaria (https://www.cdc.gov/dpdx/malaria/)

This activity is intended to help learners propose risk factors for parasitic infections and nonpharmacologic measures that can be implemented to prevent disease transmission.

INTRODUCTION

Parasitic diseases remain a significant global health problem causing approximately 1 million deaths per year and affecting more than 1.7 billion people worldwide.[1-4] In the United States, immunocompromised patients, ethnic/racial minorities, immigrants, those with recent travel to developing regions, individuals living in poor sanitary conditions, and people who lack access to basic healthcare services appear to be at the highest risk for developing parasitic diseases.[5,6] However, people in every income and social strata can become infected. In fact, the CDC has referred to five diseases as neglected parasitic infections and has prioritized these for increased public health action.[6] They include Chagas disease, cysticercosis, toxocariasis, toxoplasmosis, and trichomoniasis.

Host–Parasite Relationship

General prevention and treatment principles of parasitic infections are based on the host–parasite relationship. *Symbiosis* describes an essential biological relationship between two species. *Parasitism* is a symbiotic relationship in which one species (the host) is injured through the activities of the other (the parasite). The life cycle of a parasite may occur solely in human hosts or in one or more hosts before it causes human disease. *Definitive hosts* are those in which parasites undergo sexual reproduction, whereas *intermediate hosts* allow larval or asexual stages of development to occur. Determining what part of a parasite's life cycle occurs in human hosts is important for antiparasitic drug development.

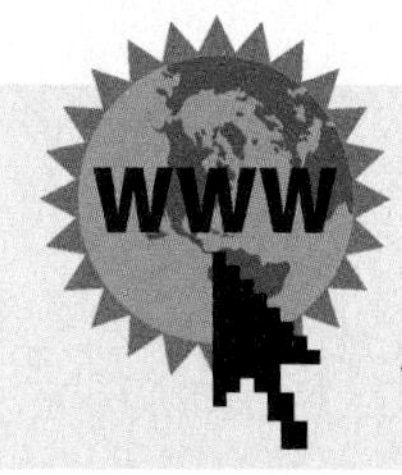

The complete chapter, learning objectives, and other resources can be found at **www.pharmacotherapyonline.com.**

139

Urinary Tract Infections

Julianna M. Fernandez and Elizabeth A. Coyle

KEY CONCEPTS

1 Urinary tract infections (UTIs) can be classified as uncomplicated and complicated. *Uncomplicated* refers to an infection in an otherwise healthy, premenopausal female who lacks structural or functional abnormalities of the urinary tract. Most often complicated infections are associated with a predisposing lesion of the urinary tract; however, the term may be used to refer to all other infections, except for those in the otherwise healthy, premenopausal adult female.

2 Recurrent UTIs are considered either reinfections or relapses. Reinfection usually happens more than 2 weeks after the last UTI and is treated as a new uncomplicated UTI. Relapse usually happens within 2 weeks of the original infection and is a relapse of the original infection because of unsuccessful treatment of the original infection, a resistant organism, or anatomical abnormalities.

3 The majority (75%-90%) of uncomplicated UTIs are caused by *Escherichia coli* and the remainder are caused primarily by *Staphylococcus saprophyticus*, *Proteus* spp., and Klebsiella spp. Complicated infections may be associated with other gram-negative organisms and *Enterococcus faecalis.*

4 Symptoms of lower UTIs include dysuria, urgency, frequency, nocturia, and suprapubic heaviness, whereas upper UTIs involve more systemic symptoms such as fever, nausea, vomiting, and flank pain.

5 Significant bacteriuria has been defined as bacterial counts of greater than 10^5 organisms (colony-forming unit [CFU])/mL (10^8 CFU/L) of a midstream clean catch urine. However, this is too general and significant bacteriuria in patients with symptoms of UTI may be defined as greater than 10^2 organisms (CFU)/mL (10^5 CFU/L).

6 The goals of treatment of UTIs are to eradicate the invading organism(s), prevent or treat systemic consequences of infections, prevent the recurrence of infection, and prevent antimicrobial resistance.

7 Uncomplicated UTIs can be managed most effectively with short-course therapy (3 days) with either trimethoprim–sulfamethoxazole, one dose of fosfomycin, or 5 days of nitrofurantoin. Fluoroquinolones should be reserved for suspected pyelonephritis or complicated infections.

8 When choosing appropriate antibiotic therapy, practitioners need to be cognizant of antibiotic resistance patterns, particularly to *E. coli*. Trimethoprim–sulfamethoxazole has diminished activity against *E. coli* in some areas of the country, with reported resistance in some areas greater than 20%.

9 Acute bacterial prostatitis can be managed with many agents that have activity against the causative organism. Chronic prostatitis requires prolonged therapy with an agent that penetrates the prostatic tissue and secretions. Therapy with fluoroquinolone or trimethoprim–sulfamethoxazole is preferred for up to 6 weeks.

BEYOND THE BOOK

EY, a 28-year-old pregnant female presents to her OB clinic for a routine week 18 appointment. Her past medical history is unremarkable except for seasonal allergies. In the clinic, she is hemodynamically stable with a BP 130/72 mm Hg, HR 78 BPM, RR 16, and temperature 97.5°F (36.4°C). Her home medications include a daily maternal multivitamin and diphenhydramine PRN. The patient denies any dysuria, urinary frequency, costovertebral angle tenderness, or suprapubic pain.

1. Should this patient be screened for urinary tract infection?
2. Which of the following clinical or laboratory features places this patient at an increased risk of a complicated UTI?
   a. Age
   b. Pyuria
   c. Pregnancy
   d. Positive leukocyte esterase
3. Which of the following would be most appropriate in managing EY's bacteriuria?
   a. Ciprofloxacin 500 mg orally twice daily for 3 days
   b. Antibiotics not indicated now
   c. Trimethoprim/sulfamethoxazole 800/160 mg twice daily for 10 days

d. Nitrofurantoin 100 mg orally twice daily for 7 days.

4. Three days later, EY calls the clinic because she has a low-grade fever (99.5°F [37.5°C]) and is complaining of having pyuria, frequent urination, and intermittent back pain. She has been busy the past few days and has not had a chance to pick up her prescription. The culture from the urinalysis from 3 days ago has grown out *E. coli* that is sensitive to ciprofloxacin, nitrofurantoin, fosfomycin, and trimethoprim/sulfamethoxazole. Which of the following is the best recommendation for EY now?
   a. Trimethoprim/sulfamethoxazole 800/160 mg twice daily for 14 days
   b. Start the prescription from 3 days ago
   c. Levofloxacin 250 mg orally daily for 7 days
   d. Piperacillin/tazobactam 3.375 g IV every 6 hours for 7 days

INTRODUCTION

Infections of the urinary tract represent a wide variety of syndromes, including urethritis, cystitis, prostatitis, and pyelonephritis. Urinary tract infections (UTIs) are the most commonly occurring bacterial infections and one of the most common reasons for antibiotic exposure, especially in females of childbearing age.[1-3] Approximately 60% of females will develop a UTI during their lifetime with about one-fourth having a recurrence within a year.[2] Infections in males occur much less frequently until the age of 65 years at which point the incidence rates in males and females are similar.

UTI is defined as the presence of microorganisms in the urinary tract that cannot be accounted for by contamination. The organisms present have the potential to invade the tissues of the urinary tract and adjacent structures. Infection may be limited to the growth of bacteria in the urine, which frequently may not produce symptoms. UTI can present as several syndromes associated with an inflammatory response to microbial invasion and can range from asymptomatic bacteriuria (ASB) to pyelonephritis with bacteremia or sepsis.

UTIs are classified as lower and upper UTIs. Typically, they have been described by anatomic site of involvement. Lower tract infections correspond to cystitis (bladder), and pyelonephritis (an infection involving the kidneys) represents upper tract infection.

1 Also, UTIs are designated as uncomplicated or complicated. Uncomplicated infections occur in individuals who lack structural or functional abnormalities of the urinary tract which interfere with the normal flow of urine or voiding mechanism. These infections occur in premenopausal females of childbearing age (15-45 years) who are otherwise normal, healthy individuals. Infections in males generally are not classified as uncomplicated because these infections are rare and most often represent a structural or neurologic abnormality.

Complicated UTIs are usually the result of a predisposing lesion of the urinary tract, such as a congenital abnormality or distortion of the urinary tract, a stone, indwelling catheter, prostatic hypertrophy, obstruction, or neurologic deficit that interferes with the normal flow of urine and urinary tract defenses. Complicated infections occur in both genders and frequently involve the upper and lower urinary tract.

2 Recurrent UTIs in healthy nonpregnant females—two or more UTIs occurring within 6 months or three or more UTIs within 1 year—are a common problem. They are characterized by multiple symptomatic infections with asymptomatic periods occurring between each episode and may be either reinfections or relapses. Reinfections are caused by a different organism than originally isolated and account for the majority of recurrent UTIs. Relapses are the development of repeated infections with the same initial organism and usually indicate a persistent infectious source.[2]

ASB is a common finding, particularly among those 65 years of age and older when there is significant bacteriuria (more than 10^5 bacteria/mL [10^8/L] of urine) in the absence of signs or symptoms.

TABLE 139-1 Diagnostic Criteria for Significant Bacteriuria

≥10^2 CFU coliforms/mL (10^5 CFU/L) or ≥10^5 CFU noncoliforms/mL (10^8 CFU/L) in a symptomatic female
≥10^4 CFU bacteria/mL (10^7 CFU/L) in a symptomatic male
≥10^5 CFU bacteria/mL (10^8 CFU/L) in asymptomatic individuals on two consecutive specimens
Any growth of bacteria on suprapubic catheterization in a symptomatic patient
≥10^{2-5} CFU bacteria/mL (10^{5-8} CFU/L) in a catheterized patient

CFU, colony-forming unit.

Symptomatic abacteriuria or acute urethral syndrome consists of symptoms of frequency and dysuria in the absence of significant bacteriuria. This syndrome is commonly associated with *Chlamydia* infections.

Significant abacteriuria is a term used to distinguish the presence of microorganisms that represent true infection versus contamination of the urine as it passes through the distal urethra prior to collection. Historically, bacterial counts equal to or greater than 100,000 organisms/mL (10^8/L) of urine in a "clean-catch" specimen were judged to indicate true infection.[4-6] Counts less than 100,000 organisms/mL (10^8/L) of urine, however, may represent true infection in certain situations, for example, with concurrent antibacterial drug administration, rapid urine flow, low urinary pH, or upper tract obstruction.[6] Table 139-1 lists the clinical definitions of significant bacteriuria, which are dependent on the clinical setting and the method of specimen collection.[6] These criteria allow for more appropriate specificity and sensitivity in documenting infection under differing clinical circumstances.

EPIDEMIOLOGY

The prevalence of UTIs varies with age and gender. In newborns and infants up to 6 months of age, the prevalence of abacteriuria is approximately 1% and is more common in boys. Most of these infections are associated with structural or functional abnormalities of the urinary tract and also have been correlated with noncircumcision.[7] Between the ages of 1 and 6 years, UTIs occur more frequently in females. The prevalence of abacteriuria in females and males of this age group is 3% to 7% and 1% to 2%, respectively.[7,8] Infections occurring in preschool boys usually are associated with congenital abnormalities of the urinary tract. These infections are difficult to recognize because of the age of the patient, but they often are symptomatic. In addition, the majority of renal damage associated with UTI develops at this age.[7,8]

Through grade school and before puberty, the prevalence of UTI is approximately 1%, with 5% of females reported to have significant bacteriuria prior to leaving high school. This percentage increases dramatically to 1% to 4% after puberty in nonpregnant females primarily as a result of sexual activity. Approximately one in five women will suffer a symptomatic UTI at some point in their lives. Many females have recurrent infections with a significant proportion having a history of childhood infections. In contrast, the prevalence of bacteriuria in adult males is low (less than 0.1%).[9]

In the older adults, the ratio of bacteriuria in women and men is dramatically altered and is approximately equal in persons older than 65 years. The overall incidence of UTI increases substantially in this population with the majority of infections being asymptomatic. The rate of infection increases further for older adults who are residing in nursing homes, particularly those who are hospitalized frequently. A variety of factors increase the risk of infection including structural and anatomical changes such as benign prostatic hypertrophy in males and prolosapse in women resulting in either urinary retention or incontinence, respectively. Patients suffering from fecal incontinence as a complication of advanced dementia or neuromuscular disease including strokes are also at increased risk. Urinary instrumentation (catheterization) along with some medications such as the sodium-glucose co-transporter inhibitors also creates an environment that is more supportive of UTIs.[10]

ETIOLOGY

3 The bacteria causing UTIs usually originate from bowel flora of the host. Although virtually every organism is associated with UTIs, certain organisms predominate as a result of specific virulence factors. The most common cause of uncomplicated UTIs is *Escherichia coli*, which accounts for 80% to 90% of community-acquired infections. Additional causative organisms in uncomplicated infections include *Staphylococcus saprophyticus*, *Klebsiella pneumoniae*, *Proteus* spp., *Pseudomonas aeruginosa*, and *Enterococcus* spp.[11] Because *S. epidermidis* is frequently isolated from the urinary tract, it should be considered initially a contaminant. Repeat cultures should be performed to help confirm the organism as a real pathogen.

Organisms isolated from individuals with complicated infections are more varied and generally are more resistant than those found in uncomplicated infections. *E. coli* is a frequently isolated pathogen, but it accounts for less than 50% of infections. Other frequently isolated organisms include *Proteus* spp., *K. pneumoniae*, *Enterobacter* spp., *P. aeruginosa*, staphylococci, and enterococci. Enterococci represent the second most frequently isolated organisms in hospitalized patients.[11-13] In part, this finding may be related to the extensive use of third-generation cephalosporin antibiotics, which are not active against the enterococci. Vancomycin-resistant *E. faecalis* and *E. faecium* (vancomycin-resistant enterococci) have become more widespread, especially in patients with long-term hospitalizations or underlying malignancies. Vancomycin-resistant enterococci are major therapeutic and infection control issues because these organisms are susceptible to few antimicrobials.[12,13] *S. aureus* infections may arise from the urinary tract, but they are more commonly a result of bacteremia producing metastatic abscesses in the kidney. *Candida* spp. are common causes of UTI in the critically ill and chronically catheterized patient. Most UTIs are caused by a single organism; however, in patients with stones, indwelling urinary catheters, or chronic renal abscesses, multiple organisms may be isolated. Depending on the clinical situation, the recovery of multiple organisms may represent contamination and a repeat evaluation should be done.

PATHOPHYSIOLOGY

Route of Infection

Organisms typically gain entry into the urinary tract via three routes: the ascending, hematogenous (descending), and lymphatic pathways. The female urethra usually is colonized by bacteria believed to originate from the fecal flora. The short length of the female urethra and its proximity to the perirectal area make colonization of the urethra likely. Other factors that promote urethral colonization include the use of spermicides and diaphragms as methods of contraception.[2,3] Although there is evidence in females that bladder infections follow colonization of the urethra, the mode of ascent of the microorganisms is incompletely understood. Massage of the female urethra and sexual intercourse allow bacteria to reach the bladder.[14] Once bacteria have reached the bladder, the organisms quickly multiply and can ascend the ureters to the kidneys. This sequence of events is more likely to occur if vesicoureteral reflux (reflux of urine into the ureters and kidneys while voiding) is present. UTIs are more common in females than in males because the anatomic differences in location and length of the urethra tend to support the ascending route of infections as the primary acquisition route.

Infection of the kidney by hematogenous spread of microorganisms usually occurs as the result of dissemination of organisms from a distant primary infection in the body. Infections via the descending route are uncommon and involve a relatively small number of invasive pathogens. Bacteremia caused by *S. aureus* may produce renal abscesses. Additional organisms include *Candida* spp., *Mycobacterium tuberculosis*, *Salmonella* spp., and enterococci. Of particular interest, it is difficult to produce experimental pyelonephritis by IV administration of common gram-negative organisms such as *E. coli* and *P. aeruginosa*. Overall, less than 5% of documented UTIs results from hematogenous spread of microorganisms.

There appears to be little evidence supporting a significant role for renal lymphatics in the pathogenesis of UTIs. There are lymphatic communications between the bowel and kidney, as well as between the bladder and kidney. There is no evidence, however, that microorganisms are transferred to the kidney via this route. After bacteria reach the urinary tract, three factors determine the development of infection: the size of the inoculum, the virulence of the microorganism, and the competency of the natural host defense mechanisms. Most UTIs reflect a failure in host defense mechanisms.

Host Defense Mechanisms

The normal urinary tract generally is resistant to invasion by bacteria and is efficient in rapidly eliminating microorganisms that reach the bladder. The urine under normal circumstances is capable of inhibiting and killing microorganisms. The factors thought to be responsible include a low pH, extremes in osmolality, high urea concentration, and high organic acid concentration. Bacterial growth is further inhibited in males by the addition of prostatic secretions.[14,15]

The introduction of bacteria into the bladder stimulates micturition with increased diuresis and efficient emptying of the bladder. These factors are critical in preventing the initiation and maintenance of bladder infections. Patients who are unable to void urine completely are at greater risk of developing UTIs and frequently have recurrent infections. Also, patients with even small residual amounts of urine in their bladder respond less favorably to treatment than patients who are able to empty their bladders completely.[16]

An important virulence factor of bacteria is their ability to adhere to urinary epithelial cells resulting in colonization of the urinary tract, bladder infections, and pyelonephritis. Various factors that act as anti-adherence mechanisms are present in the bladder preventing bacterial colonization and infection. The epithelial cells of the bladder are coated with a urinary mucus or slime called *glycosaminoglycan*. This thin layer of surface mucopolysaccharide is hydrophilic and strongly negatively charged. When bound to the uroepithelium, it attracts water molecules and forms a layer between the bladder and urine. The anti-adherence characteristics of the glycosaminoglycan layer are nonspecific and when the layer is removed by dilute acid solutions, rapid bacterial adherence results.[17]

In addition, the Tamm–Horsfall protein is a glycoprotein produced by the ascending limb of Henle and distal tubule that is secreted into the urine and contains mannose residues. These mannose residues bind *E. coli* that contain small surface-projecting organelle on their surfaces called *pili* or *fimbriae*. Type 1 fimbriae are mannose-sensitive, and this interaction prevents the bacteria from binding to similar receptors present on the mucosal surface of the bladder. Other factors that possibly prevent adherence of bacteria include immunoglobulins (Ig) G and A, which are synthesized systemically and in the kidney with upper tract infections. The role of Igs in preventing bladder infection is less clear. Patients with reduced urinary levels of secretory IgA are, however, at increased risk of infections of the urinary tract.

After bacteria have invaded the bladder mucosa, an inflammatory response is stimulated with the mobilization of polymorphonuclear leukocytes (PMNs) and resulting phagocytosis. PMNs are primarily responsible for limiting the tissue invasion and controlling the spread of infection in the bladder and kidney. They do not play a role in preventing bladder colonization or infections and actually contribute to renal tissue damage.

Other host factors that may play a role in the prevention of UTIs are the presence of *Lactobacillus* in the vaginal flora and circulating estrogen levels. In premenopausal women, circulating estrogen supports the vaginal tract growth of lactobacilli, which produce lactic acid to help maintain a low vaginal pH, thereby preventing *E. coli* vaginal colonization.[18] Topical estrogens are used for the prevention of UTI in postmenopausal women who have more than three recurrent UTI episodes per year and are not on oral estrogens.[19]

Bacterial Virulence Factors

Pathogenic organisms have differing degrees of pathogenicity (virulence), which play a role in the development and severity of infection. Bacteria that adhere to the epithelium of the urinary tract are associated with colonization and infection. The mechanism of adhesion of gram-negative bacteria, particularly *E. coli*, is related to bacterial fimbriae that are rigid, hair-like appendages of the cell wall.[9] These fimbriae adhere to specific glycolipid components on epithelial cells. The most common type of fimbriae is type 1, which binds to mannose residues present in glycoproteins. Glycosaminoglycan and Tamm–Horsfall protein are rich in mannose residues that readily trap those organisms that contain type 1 fimbriae, which are then washed out of the bladder.[20] Other fimbriae are mannose-resistant and are associated more frequently with pyelonephritis, such as P fimbriae, which bind avidly to specific glycolipid receptors on uroepithelial cells. These bacteria are resistant to washout or removal by glycosaminoglycan and are able to multiply and invade tissue, especially the kidney. In addition, PMNs, as well as secretory IgA antibodies, contain receptors for type 1 fimbriae, which facilitate phagocytosis, but are lacking receptors for P fimbriae.

Other virulence factors include the production of hemolysin and aerobactin.[21] Hemolysin is a cytotoxic protein produced by bacteria that lyses a wide range of cells, including erythrocytes, PMNs, and monocytes. *E. coli* and other gram-negative bacteria require iron for aerobic metabolism and multiplication. Aerobactin facilitates the binding and uptake of iron by *E. coli*; however, the significance of this property in the pathogenesis of UTIs remains unknown.[22]

PREDISPOSING FACTORS TO INFECTION

The normal urinary tract typically is resistant to infection and colonization by pathogenic bacteria. In patients with underlying structural abnormalities of the urinary tract, the typical host defenses previously discussed usually are lacking or compromised. There are several known abnormalities of the urinary tract system that interfere with its natural defense mechanisms, the most important of which is obstruction. Obstruction can inhibit the normal flow of urine disrupting the natural flushing and voiding effect in removing bacteria from the bladder and resulting in incomplete emptying. Common conditions that result in residual urine volumes include prostatic hypertrophy, urethral strictures, calculi, tumors, bladder diverticula, and drugs such as anticholinergic agents. Additional causes of incomplete bladder emptying include neurologic malfunctions associated with stroke, diabetes, spinal cord injuries, tabes dorsalis, and other neuropathies. Vesicoureteral reflux represents a condition in which urine is forced up the ureters to the kidneys. Urinary reflux is associated not only with an increased incidence of UTIs and pyelonephritis but also with renal damage.[8,16] Reflux may be the result of a congenital abnormality or, more commonly, bladder overdistension from obstruction. Other risk factors include urinary catheterization, mechanical instrumentation, pregnancy, and the use of spermicides and diaphragms.

CLINICAL PRESENTATION

4 The presenting signs and symptoms of UTIs in adults are recognized easily. Females frequently will report gross hematuria. Systemic symptoms, including fever, typically are absent in this setting. Unfortunately, large numbers of persons with significant bacteriuria are asymptomatic. These individuals may be normal, healthy persons, older adults, children, pregnant persons, and persons with indwelling catheters. Attempts at differentiating upper tract from lower tract infections on the basis of symptoms alone are not reliable.

Older adults frequently do not experience specific urinary symptoms, but they will present with altered mental status, change in eating habits, or gastrointestinal (GI) symptoms. In addition, patients with indwelling catheters or neurologic disorders commonly will not have lower tract symptoms. Instead, they may present with flank pain and fever. Many of the aforementioned patients, however, frequently will develop upper tract infections with bacteremia and no or minimal urinary tract symptoms.

Symptoms alone are unreliable for the diagnosis of bacterial UTIs. The key to the diagnosis of UTI is the ability to demonstrate significant numbers of microorganisms in an appropriate urine specimen to distinguish contamination from infection. The type and extent of laboratory examination required depends on the clinical situation.

CLINICAL PRESENTATION Urinary Tract Infections in Adults

Signs and Symptoms

- Lower UTI: Dysuria, urgency, frequency, nocturia, and suprapubic heaviness
- Gross hematuria
- Upper UTI: Flank pain, fever, nausea, vomiting, and malaise

Physical Examination

- Upper UTI: Costovertebral tenderness

Laboratory Tests

- Bacteriuria
- Pyuria (WBC count more than 10/mm^3 [10 × 10^6/L])
- Nitrite-positive urine (with nitrite reducers)
- Leukocyte esterase-positive urine
- Antibody-coated bacteria (upper UTI)

Urine Collection

Examination of the urine is the cornerstone of laboratory evaluation for UTIs. There are three acceptable methods of urine collection. The first is the *midstream clean-catch method*. After cleaning the urethral opening area in both men and women, 20 to 30 mL of urine is voided and discarded. The next part of the urine flow is collected and should be processed immediately (refrigerated as soon as possible). Specimens that are allowed to sit at room temperature for several hours may result in falsely elevated bacterial counts. The midstream clean-catch is the preferred method for the routine collection of urine for culture. When a routine urine specimen cannot be collected or contamination occurs, alternative collection techniques must be used.

The two acceptable alternative methods include catheterization and suprapubic bladder aspiration. Catheterization may be necessary for patients who are uncooperative or who are unable to void urine. If catheterization is performed carefully with the aseptic technique, the method yields reliable results. However, the introduction of bacteria into the bladder may result and the procedure is associated with infection in 1% to 2% of patients. Suprapubic bladder aspiration involves inserting a needle directly into the bladder and aspirating the urine. This procedure bypasses the contaminating organisms present in the urethra and any bacteria found using this technique generally are considered to represent significant bacteriuria.[23-26] Suprapubic aspiration is a safe and painless procedure that is most useful in newborns, infants, paraplegics, seriously ill patients, and others in whom infection is suspected and routine procedures have provided confusing or equivocal results.

Bacterial Count

5 The diagnosis of UTI is based on the isolation of significant numbers of bacteria from a urine specimen. Microscopic examination of a urine sample is an easy-to-perform and reliable method for the presumptive diagnosis of bacteriuria. The examination may be performed by preparing a Gram stain of unspun or centrifuged urine. The presence of at least one organism per oil-immersion field in a properly collected uncentrifuged specimen correlates well with more than 100,000 CFU/mL (10^5 CFU/mL or 10^8 CFU/L) of urine. For detecting smaller numbers of organisms, a centrifuged specimen is more sensitive. Such examinations detect more than 10^5 bacteria (CFU)/mL (10^8 CFU/L) with a sensitivity of greater than 90% and a specificity of greater than 70%.[23,24] A quantitative count of greater than or equal to 10^5 CFU/mL (10^8 CFU/L) is considered indicative of a UTI; however, up to 50% of women will present with clinical symptoms of a UTI with lower counts (10^3 CFU/mL) (10^6 CFU/L).[4]

Pyuria, Hematuria, and Proteinuria

Microscopic examination of the urine for leukocytes is used to determine the presence of pyuria. The presence of pyuria in a symptomatic patient correlates with significant bacteriuria.[25] Pyuria is defined as a white blood cell (WBC) count of greater than 10 WBC/mm^3 (10×10^6/L) of urine. A count of 5 to 10 WBC/mm^3 (5×10^6 to 10×10^6/L) is accepted as the upper limit of normal. It should be emphasized that pyuria is nonspecific and signifies only the presence of inflammation and not necessarily infection. Thus, patients with pyuria may or may not have infection. Sterile pyuria has long been associated with urinary tuberculosis, as well as chlamydial and fungal urinary infections. Hematuria, microscopic or gross, is frequently present in patients with UTI, but is nonspecific. Hematuria may indicate the presence of other disorders, such as renal calculi, tumors, or glomerulonephritis. Proteinuria is found commonly in the presence of infection.

Chemistry

Several biochemical tests have been developed for screening urine for the presence of bacteria. A common dipstick test detects the presence of nitrite in the urine, which is formed by bacteria that reduce nitrate normally present in the urine. False-positive tests are uncommon. False-negative tests are more common and are frequently caused by the presence of gram-positive organisms or *P. aeruginosa* that do not reduce nitrate.[26] Other causes of false tests include low urinary pH, frequent voiding, and dilute urine.

The leukocyte esterase dipstick test is a rapid screening test for detecting the presence of pyuria. Leukocytes esterase is found in primary neutrophil granules and indicates the presence of WBCs. The leukocyte esterase test is a sensitive and highly specific test for detecting more than 10 WBC/mm^3 (10×10^6/L) of urine. When the leukocyte esterase test is used with the nitrite test, the reported positive predictive value and specificity are 79% and 82%, respectively, for the detection of bacteriuria.[27,28] These tests can be useful in the outpatient evaluation of uncomplicated UTIs. However, urine culture is still the "gold standard" test in determining the presence of UTIs.

Culture

The most reliable method of diagnosing UTI is by quantitative urine culture. Urine in the bladder is normally sterile making it possible to differentiate contamination of the urine from infection by quantifying the number of bacteria present in a urine sample. This criterion is based on a properly collected midstream clean-catch urine specimen. Patients with infection usually have greater than 10^5 bacteria/mL (10^8/L) of urine. However, as many as one-third of females with symptomatic infection have less than 10^5 bacteria/mL (10^8/L). Also, a significant portion of patients with UTIs, either symptomatic or asymptomatic, have less than 10^5 bacteria/mL (10^8/L) of urine.

Several laboratory methods are used to quantify bacteria present in the urine. The most accurate method is the pour-plate technique. This method is unsuitable for a high-volume laboratory because it is expensive and time-consuming. The streak-plate method is an alternative that involves using a calibrated-loop technique to streak a fixed amount of urine on an agar plate. This method is used most commonly in diagnostic laboratories because it is simple to perform and less costly.

After identification and quantification are complete, the next step is to determine the susceptibility of the organism. There are several methods by which bacterial susceptibility testing may be performed. Knowledge of bacterial susceptibility and achievable urine concentration of the antibiotics puts the clinician in a better position to select an appropriate agent for treatment.

Infection Site

History and physical examination are of little value in predicting the site of infection. The most direct method to determine the location of infection within the urinary system and differentiate upper tract from lower tract involvement is a ureteral catheterization procedure as described by Stamey and colleagues.[29] The method involves the passage of a catheter into the bladder and then into each ureter, where quantitative cultures are obtained. Although this method provides direct quantitative evidence for UTI, it is invasive, technically difficult, and expensive. The Fairley bladder washout technique is a modification of the Stamey procedure that involves Foley catheterization only.[30] After the catheter is passed into the bladder, bladder samples are obtained, and the bladder is washed out with culture samples taken at 10, 20, and 30 minutes. The procedure shows that up to 50% of patients have renal involvement, regardless of signs and symptoms. Other investigators found 10% to 20% of tests to be equivocal.[30]

Noninvasive methods of localization may be more acceptable for routine use; however, they have limited clinical value. Patients with pyelonephritis can have abnormalities in urinary concentrating ability. The use of concentrating ability for localization of UTIs, however, is associated with high false-positive and false-negative responses and is not useful clinically.[26] The antibody-coated bacteria test is an immunofluorescent method that detects bacteria coated with Ig in freshly voided urine indicating upper UTI. The sensitivity and specificity of this test to localize the site of infection are reported to average 88% and 76%, respectively.[31] Because of the high incidence of false-positive and false-negative results, antibody-coated bacteria testing is not used routinely in the management of UTIs.

Virtually all patients with uncomplicated lower tract infections can be cured with a short course of antibiotic therapy and this assumption sometimes can be used to distinguish between patients with lower and upper tract infections. Patients who do not respond or who relapse may do so because of upper tract involvement. It is rarely necessary to localize the site of infection to direct the clinical management of such patients.

TREATMENT

Desired Outcomes

6 The goals of UTI treatments are (a) to eradicate the invading organism(s), (b) to prevent or to treat systemic consequences of infection, (c) to prevent the recurrence of infection, and (d) to decrease the potential for collateral damage with too broad of antimicrobial therapy.

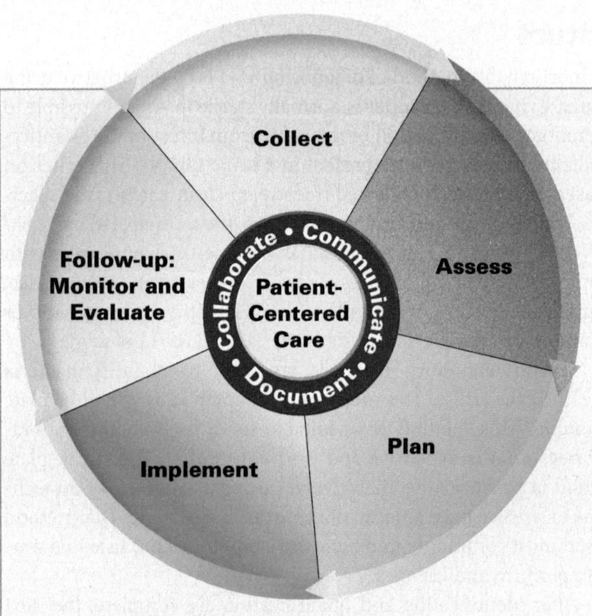

Patient Care Process for Urinary Tract Infection

An illustration shows that patient-centered care includes collaboration, communication, and documentation. The actions associated with the care are collect, assess, plan, implement, and follow-up by monitoring and evaluating.

Collect

- Patient characteristics (eg, age, sex, pregnant, immunocompetent)
- Patient symptoms (see Clinical Presentation box)
- Patient medical history (including history of past UTIs)
- Social history (eg, sexually active) and dietary habits
- Current medications including nonprescription and/or herbal products, dietary supplements
- Objective data
  - o Vital signs: blood pressure (BP), heart rate (HR), respiratory rate (RR), height, weight, O_2 saturation, temperature
  - o Labs including white blood cell count (WBC), serum creatinine (SCr)
  - o Urinalysis (eg, nitrite or leukocyte esterase +) +/− culture and sensitivity data
  - o Urine dipstick test
  - o Physical exam (eg, abdominal tenderness, costovertebral tenderness)

Assess

- Hemodynamic stability (eg, systolic BP <90 mm Hg >110 bpm)
- Mental status
- Urinary catheter present

Plan

- Drug therapy regimen including drug name, dose, route, frequency, and duration (see Tables 134-2, 134-3, and 134-4)
- Monitoring parameters including efficacy (eg, afebrile, WBC, urinalysis, resolution of symptoms), decrease in urinary discomfort and safety (eg, signs and symptoms of antibiotic hypersensitivity, SCr, WBC, hemodynamics)
- Patient education (eg, purpose of treatment, personal hygiene, drug-specific information, medication administration instructions, when to follow-up if no improvement observed; see Table 139-3)
- Self-monitoring for resolution of symptoms (eg, urinary discomfort, flank pain, fever, mental status changes)
- Referrals to other providers when appropriate (eg, urologist)

Implement*

- Provide patient education regarding all elements of treatment plan
- Use motivational interviewing and coaching strategies to maximize adherence
- Schedule follow-up if necessary

Follow-up: Monitor and Evaluate

- Resolution of urinary symptoms (eg, burning, discomfort during urination, flank pain, tenderness)
- Normalization of labs (eg, WBC, SCr)
- Urinalysis presence of adverse effects (eg, rash, diarrhea)
- Patient adherence to treatment plan using multiple sources of information
- Reevaluate if patient does not respond adequately to treatment

Collaborate with patient, caregivers, and other healthcare professionals.

Management

The management of a patient with a UTI includes initial evaluation, selection of an antibacterial agent, and duration of therapy and follow-up evaluation. The initial selection of an antimicrobial agent for the treatment of UTI is based primarily on the severity of the presenting signs and symptoms, the site of infection and whether the infection is determined to be uncomplicated or complicated. Other considerations include antibiotic susceptibility, side-effect potential, cost, current antimicrobial exposure, and the comparative inconvenience of different therapies.[1]

Various pharmacologic factors may affect the action of antibacterial agents. Certainly, the ability of the agent to achieve appropriate concentrations in the urine is of utmost importance. Factors that affect the rate and extent of excretion through the kidney include the patient's glomerular filtration rate and whether or not the agent is actively secreted. Filtration depends on the molecular size and degree of protein binding of the agent. Agents such as sulfonamides, tetracyclines, and aminoglycosides enter the urine via filtration. As the glomerular filtration rate is reduced, the amount of drug that enters the urine is reduced. Most β-lactam agents and quinolones are filtered and are actively secreted into the urine. For this reason, most of these agents achieve high urinary concentrations despite unfavorable protein-binding characteristics or the presence of renal dysfunction.

The ability to eradicate bacteria from the urine is related directly to the sensitivity of the microorganism and the achievable concentrations of the antimicrobial agent in the urine. Unfortunately, most susceptibility testing is directed at achievable concentrations in the blood. There is a poor correlation between achievable blood concentrations of antimicrobial agents and the eradication of bacteria from the urine.[32] In the treatment of lower tract infections, plasma concentrations of antibacterial agents may not be important, but achieving appropriate plasma concentrations appears critical in patients with bacteremia and renal abscesses.

Nonspecific therapies have been advocated in the treatment and prevention of UTIs. Fluid hydration has been used to produce rapid dilution of bacteria and removal of infected urine by increased voiding. A critical factor appears to be the amount of residual volume remaining after voiding. As little as 10 mL of residual urine can alter the eradication of infection significantly.[16] Paradoxically, increased diuresis also may promote susceptibility to infection by diluting the normal antibacterial properties of the urine. Often in clinical practice, the concentrations of antimicrobial agents in the urine are so high that dilution has little effect on efficacy.

The antibacterial activity of the urine is related to the low pH, which is the result of high concentrations of various organic acids. Large volumes of cranberry juice increase the antibacterial activity of the urine and prevent the development of UTIs.[3,33] Apparently, the fructose and other unknown substances (condensed tannins, proanthocyanidin) in cranberry juice may act to interfere with adherence mechanisms of some pathogens, thereby preventing infection or reinfection. Acidification of the urine by cranberry juice does not appear to play a significant role. Although there are a number of favorable studies, the benefit of ingested cranberry juice appears to be minimal and larger studies involving oral tablets or capsules need to be done to prove effectivness.[35-38] Females with repeated UTIs who receive the recommended 36 mg/d of proanthocyanidins (found in cranberry products) may gain some benefit but studies remain largely inconclusive.[36-40] The use of other agents (ascorbic acid) to acidify the urine to try to hinder bacterial growth does not achieve significant enough acidification. Consequently, attempts to acidify urine with systemic agents are not recommended. Lactobacillus potentially helps keep the vaginal pH in the normal range (pH 4-4.5); therefore, regulating genitourinary bacteria aiding in the prevention of UTIs.[41] In addition, *Lactobacillus* probiotics may aid in the prevention of female UTIs by decreasing the vaginal pH, thereby decreasing *E. coli* colonization.[19,33,34] In postmenopausal women, estrogen replacement may be of help in the prevention of recurrent UTIs. After 1 month of topical estrogen replacement, vaginal *Lactobacillus* as well as vaginal pH and *E. coli* colonization decrease.[18,33]

Phenazopyridine hydrochloride is nonprescription urinary anesthetic/analgesic that can be used for symptom relief in UTIs. It is frequently used by patients as self-medication to alleviate the dysuria associated with UTIs. The use of phenazopyridine in the treatment of UTIs is controversial. It has no antimicrobial properties and has a number of adverse effects such as red-orange discoloration of body fluids, rash, anaphylaxis, and rare effects such as hemolytic anemia, methemoglobinemia, and acute renal failure. In addition, its use can mask the symptoms of an untreated or inappropriately treated UTI. Unfortunately, there are not any guidelines for its role in the treatment of UTIs; however, experts agree that if phenazopyridine is used, only use the recommended dose (maximum 200 mg three times a day) and limited to 1 to 2 days for symptomatic relief of the dysuria with UTIs.[41,42] In addition, it should be used with the combination of appropriate antibiotic therapy.

Pharmacologic Therapy

Ideally, the antimicrobial agent chosen should be well tolerated, well absorbed, achieve high urinary concentrations, and have a spectrum of activity limited to the known or suspected pathogen(s). Table 139-2 lists the most common agents used in the treatment of UTIs along with comments concerning their general use. Table 139-3 presents an overview of various therapeutic options for outpatient therapy of UTI. Table 139-4 describes empirical treatment regimens for selected clinical situations.

8 The therapeutic management of UTIs is best accomplished by first categorizing the type of infection: acute uncomplicated cystitis, symptomatic abacteriuria, ASB, complicated UTIs, recurrent infections, or prostatitis. In choosing the appropriate antibiotic therapy, aware of the increasing resistance of *E. coli* and other pathogens to many frequently prescribed antimicrobials.[44] Resistance to *E. coli* is as high as 37% for amoxicillin and ampicillin.[1,45] Most *E. coli* remain susceptible to trimethoprim–sulfamethoxazole, although resistance is continuing to increase and has been reported as high as 27%.[46] Although resistance to the fluoroquinolones remains low, these agents are being used more frequently and the incidence of fluoroquinolone-resistant *E. coli* is increasingly being reported and is of great concern.[45-51] Current or recent antibiotic exposure is the most significant risk factor associated with *E. coli* resistance and with the extensive use of the fluoroquinolones and trimethoprim–sulfamethoxazole for various infections, including UTIs, resistance will continue to increase.[45-50] In addition, broad-spectrum antimicrobials such as fluoroquinolones and broad-spectrum cephalosporins have a high impact on GI flora, increasing the risk of collateral damage (term used to refer to ecological adverse effects of antibiotic therapy) or the selection of resistant *E. coli* pathogens.[45-48,51,52] In light of rising resistance and in order to decrease the overuse of broad-spectrum antimicrobials, agents such as nitrofurantoin and fosfomycin are now considered first-line treatments along with trimethoprim–sulfamethoxazole in acute uncomplicated cystitis. Both nitrofurantoin and fosfomycin have little effects on the gut flora and *E. coli* susceptibility still remains high.[52-56] With the increased use of nitrofurantoin and fosfomycin since the 2010 guidelines, clinicians are starting to evaluate the success rate of resolution of uncomplicated lower UTIs in women when single-dose fosfomycin versus nitrofurantoin are used. More research will need to be done to establish that one therapy is more effective than the other.[57] Antibiotic therapy should be determined based on the geographic resistance patterns, as well as the patient's recent history of antibiotic exposure.

Acute Uncomplicated Cystitis

Acute uncomplicated cystitis is the most common form of UTI. These infections typically occur in females of childbearing age and often are

TABLE 139-2 Commonly Used Antimicrobial Agents in the Treatment of UTIs

Drug	Adverse Drug Reactions	Monitoring Parameters	Comments
Oral Therapy			
Trimethoprim–sulfamethoxazole	Rash, Stevens–Johnson Syndrome, renal failure, photosensitivity, hematologic (neutropenia, anemia, etc.)	Serum creatinine, BUN, electrolytes, signs of rash, and CBC	This combination is highly effective against most aerobic enteric bacteria except *P. aeruginosa*. High urinary tract tissue concentrations and urine concentrations are achieved, which may be important in complicated infection treatment. Also effective as prophylaxis for recurrent infections
Nitrofurantoin	GI intolerance, neuropathies, and pulmonary reactions	Baseline serum creatinine and BUN	This agent is effective as both a therapeutic and prophylactic agent in patients with recurrent UTIs. Main advantage is the lack of resistance even after long courses of therapy
Fosfomycin trometamol	Diarrhea, headache, and angioedema	No routine tests recommended	Single-dose therapy for uncomplicated infections, low levels of resistance, use with caution in patients with hepatic dysfunction
Fluoroquinolones			
Ciprofloxacin Levofloxacin	Hypersensitivity, photosensitivity, GI symptoms, dizziness, confusion, and tendonitis (black box warning)	CBC, baseline serum creatinine, and BUN	The fluoroquinolones have a greater spectrum of activity, including *P. aeruginosa*. These agents are effective for pyelonephritis and prostatitis. Avoid in pregnancy and children. Moxifloxacin should not be used owing to inadequate urinary concentrations
Penicillins			
Amoxicillin–clavulanate	Hypersensitivity (rash, anaphylaxis), diarrhea, superinfections, and seizures	CBC, signs of rash, or hypersensitivity	Due to increasing *E. coli* resistance, amoxicillin–clavulanate is the preferred penicillin for uncomplicated cystitis
Cephalosporins			
Cefaclor Cefpodoxime-proxetil	Hypersensitivity (rash, anaphylaxis), diarrhea, superinfections, and seizures	CBC, signs of rash, or hypersensitivity	There are no major advantages of these agents over other agents in the treatment of UTIs, and they are more expensive. These agents are not active against enterococci
Parenteral Therapy			
Aminoglycosides			
Gentamicin Tobramycin Amikacin	Ototoxicity, nephrotoxicity	Serum creatinine and BUN, serum drug concentrations, and individual pharmacokinetic monitoring	These agents are renally excreted and achieve good concentrations in the urine. Amikacin generally is reserved for multidrug-resistant bacteria
Penicillins			
Ampicillin–sulbactam Piperacillin–tazobactam	Hypersensitivity (rash, anaphylaxis), diarrhea, superinfections, and seizures	CBC, signs of rash, or hypersensitivity	These agents generally are equally effective for susceptible bacteria. The extended-spectrum penicillins are more active against *P. aeruginosa* and enterococci and often are preferred over cephalosporins. They are useful in renally impaired patients or when an aminoglycoside is to be avoided
Cephalosporins			
Ceftriaxone Ceftazidime Cefepime Ceftozolane/tazaobactam Ceftazidime/avabactam	Hypersensitivity (rash, anaphylaxis), diarrhea, superinfections, and seizures	CBC, signs of rash, or hypersensitivity	Second- and third-generation cephalosporins have a broad spectrum of activity against gram-negative bacteria, but are not active against enterococci and have limited activity against *P. aeruginosa*. Ceftazidime and cefepime are active against *P. aeruginosa*. They are useful for nosocomial infections and urosepsis due to susceptible pathogens
Carbapenems/monobactams			
Imipenem–cilistatin Meropenem Meropenem/vaborbactam Doripenem Ertapenem Aztreonam	Hypersensitivity (rash, anaphylaxis), diarrhea, superinfections, and seizures	CBC, signs of rash, or hypersensitivity	Carbapenems have a broad spectrum of activity, including gram-positive, gram-negative, and anaerobic bacteria. Imipenem, meropenem, and doripenem are active against *P. aeruginosa* and enterococci, but ertapenem is not. Aztreonam is a monobactam that is only active against gram-negative bacteria, including some strains of *P. aeruginosa*. Generally useful for nosocomial infections when aminoglycosides are to be avoided and in penicillin-sensitive patients
Fluoroquinolones			
Ciprofloxacin Levofloxacin	Hypersensitivity, photosensitivity, GI symptoms, dizziness, confusion, and tendonitis (black box warning)	CBC, baseline serum creatinine, and BUN	These agents have broad-spectrum activity against both gram-negative and gram-positive bacteria. They provide urine and high-tissue concentrations and are actively secreted in reduced renal function

BUN, blood urea nitrogen; CBC, complete blood count; GI, gastrointestinal; UTIs, urinary tract infections.

TABLE 139-3 Overview of Outpatient Antimicrobial Therapy for Lower Tract Infections in Adults

Indications	Antibiotic	Oral Dose	Interval[a]	Duration
Lower tract infections				
Uncomplicated	Trimethoprim–sulfamethoxazole	1 DS tablet	Twice a day	3 days
	Nitrofurantoin monohydrate	100 mg	Twice a day	5 days
	Fosfomycin trometamol	3 g	Single dose	1 day
	Ciprofloxacin	250 mg	Twice a day	3 days
	Levofloxacin	250 mg	Once a day	3 days
	Amoxicillin–clavulanate	500 mg	Every 8 hours	5-7 days
	Pivmecillinam	400 mg	Twice a day	3 days
Complicated	Trimethoprim–sulfamethoxazole	1 DS tablet	Twice a day	7-10 days
	Ciprofloxacin	250-500 mg	Twice a day	7-10 days
	Levofloxacin	250 mg	Once a day	10 days
		750 mg	Once a day	5 days
	Amoxicillin–clavulanate	500 mg	Every 8 hours	7-10 days
Recurrent infections	Nitrofurantoin	50 mg	Once a day	6 months
	Trimethoprim–sulfamethoxazole	1/2 SS tablet	Once a day	6 months
Acute pyelonephritis	Trimethoprim–sulfamethoxazole	1 DS tablet	Twice a day	14 days
	Ciprofloxacin	500 mg	Twice a day	14 days
		1,000 mg ER	Once a day	7 days
	Levofloxacin	250 mg	Once a day	10 days
		750 mg	Once a day	5 days
	Amoxicillin–clavulanate	500 mg	Every 8 hours	14 days

DS, double strength; SS, single strength.

[a]Dosing intervals for normal renal function.

TABLE 139-4 Evidence-Based Empirical Treatment of UTIs and Prostatitis

Diagnosis	Pathogens	Treatment Recommendation	Comments
Acute uncomplicated cystitis	*Escherichia coli*, *Staphylococcus saprophyticus*	1. Nitrofurantoin × 5 days (A,I)[m] 2. Trimethoprim–sulfamethoxazole × 3 days (A,I)[a] 3. Fosfomycin trometamol × 1 dose (A,I)[a] 4. Fluoroquinolone × 3 days (A,I)[a] 5. β-Lactams × 3-7 days (B,I)[a] 6. Pivmecillinam × 3-7 days (A,I)	Short-course therapy more effective than single dose Reserve fluoroquinolones as alternatives to development of resistance (A-III)[a] β-Lactams as a group are not as effective in acute cystitis then trimethoprim–sulfamethoxazole or the fluoroquinolones, do not use amoxicillin or ampicillin[a] Pivmecillinam not available in the United States
Pregnancy	As above	1. Amoxicillin–clavulanate × 7 days 2. Cephalosporin × 7 days 3. Trimethoprim–sulfamethoxazole × 7 days	Avoid trimethoprim–sulfamethoxazole during the third trimester
Acute pyelonephritis			
Uncomplicated	*E. coli*	1. Quinolone × 7 days (A,I)[a] 2. Trimethoprim–sulfamethoxazole (if susceptible) × 14 days (A,I)[a]	Can be managed as outpatient
	Gram-positive bacteria	1. Amoxicillin or amoxicillin–clavulanic acid × 14 days	
Complicated	*E. coli* *P. mirabilis* *K. pneumoniae* *P. aeruginosa* *Enterococcus faecalis*	1. Quinolone × 14 days 2. Extended-spectrum penicillin plus aminoglycoside	Severity of illness will determine duration of IV therapy; culture results should direct therapy Oral therapy may complete 14 days of therapy
Prostatitis	*E. coli* *K. pneumoniae* *Proteus* spp. *P. aeruginosa*	1. Trimethoprim–sulfamethoxazole × 4-6 weeks 2. Quinolone × 4-6 weeks	Acute prostatitis may require IV therapy initially Chronic prostatitis may require longer treatment periods or surgery

UTI, urinary tract infection.

[a]Strength of recommendations: A, good evidence for; B, moderate evidence for; C, poor evidence for and against; D, moderate against; E, good evidence against. Quality of evidence: I, at least one proper randomized, controlled study; II, one well-designed clinical trial; III, evidence from opinions, clinical experience, and expert committees.

Data from Reference 1.

related to sexual activity. Although the presence of dysuria, frequency, urgency, and suprapubic discomfort frequently is associated with lower tract infection, a significant number of patients have upper tract involvement as well.[3] Because these infections are predominantly caused by *E. coli*, antimicrobial therapy initially should be directed against this organism. Other common causes include *S. saprophyticus* and occasionally *K. pneumoniae* and *Proteus mirabilis*. Because the causative organisms and their susceptibility generally are known, many clinicians advocate a cost-effective approach to management. This approach includes a urinalysis and initiation of empirical therapy without a urine

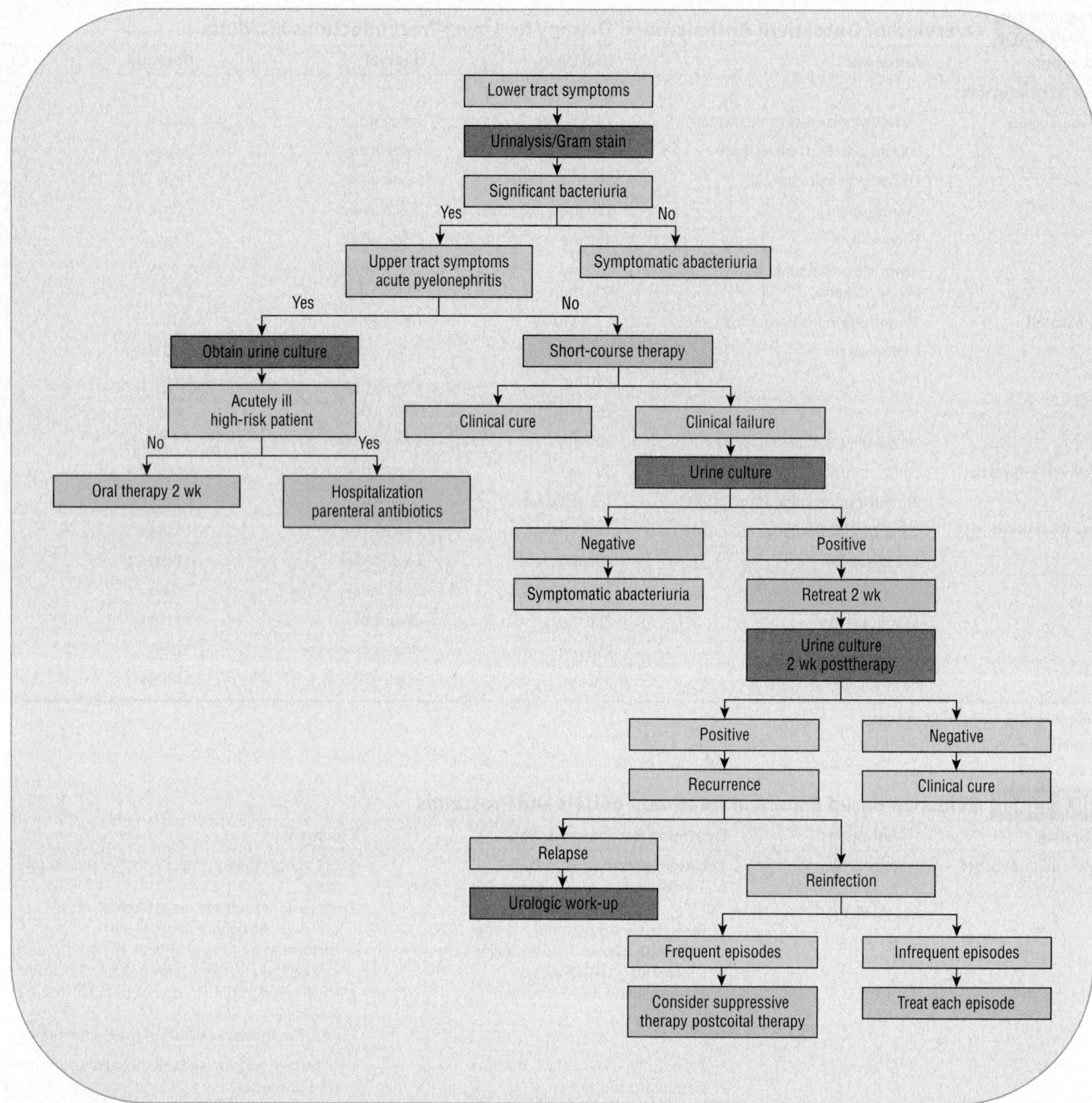

FIGURE 139-1 Management of urinary tract infections in females.

culture (Fig. 139-1).[1] Therefore, the susceptibility patterns of the geographic area drive the choice of empiric therapy.

The goal of treatment for uncomplicated cystitis is to eradicate the causative organism and to reduce the incidence of recurrence caused by relapse or reinfection. The ability to reduce the chance of recurrence depends on the agent's efficacy in eradicating the uropathogenic bacteria from the vaginal and GI reservoir. In the past, conventional therapy consisted of an effective oral antibiotic administered for 7 to 14 days. However, acute cystitis is a superficial mucosal infection that can be eradicated with much shorter courses of therapy (3 days). Advantages of short-course therapy include increased adherence, fewer side effects, decreased cost, and less potential for the development of resistance.

7 Three-day courses of trimethoprim–sulfamethoxazole or a fluoroquinolone (eg, ciprofloxacin or levofloxacin, not moxifloxacin) are superior to single-dose therapies.[55,58-60] Although the fluoroquinolones have shown excellent efficacy in acute cystitis, the guidelines recommend reserving these agents for patients with suspected or possible pyelonephritis due to the collateral damage risk. Instead, a 3-day course of trimethoprim–sulfamethoxazole, a 5-day course of nitrofurantoin, or a one-time dose of fosfomycin should be considered as first-line therapy.[1,53-61] In areas where there is more than 20% resistance of *E. coli* to trimethoprim–sulfamethoxazole, nitrofurantoin or fosfomycin should be used. Amoxicillin or ampicillin should not be used due to the high incidence of resistant *E. coli*. Instead, if a β-lactam must be used, amoxicillin–clavulanate, cefdinir, cefaclor, or cefpodoxime proxetil for 3 to 7 days are the preferred choices. For most adult females, short-course therapy is the treatment of choice for uncomplicated lower UTIs. Short-course therapy is inappropriate for patients who have had previous infections caused by resistant bacteria, for male patients, and for patients with complicated UTIs. If symptoms recur or do not respond to therapy, a urine culture should be obtained and conventional therapy with a suitable agent instituted.[1]

Symptomatic Abacteriuria

Symptomatic abacteriuria or acute urethral syndrome represents a clinical syndrome in which females present with dysuria and pyuria, but the urine culture reveals less than 10^5 bacteria/mL (10^8/L) of urine. Acute urethral syndrome accounts for more than half the complaints of dysuria seen in the community today. Infections typically involve small numbers of coliform bacteria, including *E. coli*, *Staphylococcus* spp., or *Chlamydia trachomatis*. Additional causes include *Neisseria gonorrhoeae*, *Gardnerella vaginalis*, and *Ureaplasma urealyticum*.

Most patients presenting with pyuria will, in fact, have infection that requires treatment. If antimicrobial therapy is ineffective, a culture should be obtained. If the patient reports recent sexual activity, therapy for *C. trachomatis* should be considered. Chlamydial treatment should consist of 1 g azithromycin or doxycycline 100 mg twice daily for 7 days. Often, concomitant treatment of all sexual partners is required to cure chlamydial infections and prevent reacquisition (see Chapter 140, "Sexually Transmitted Diseases").

Asymptomatic Bacteriuria

ASB is the finding of two consecutive urine cultures with more than 10^5 organisms/mL (10^8/L) of the same organism in the absence of urinary symptoms. Most patients with ASB are older females. Also, pregnant females frequently present with ASB. Although these individuals typically respond to treatment, relapse and reinfection are common and chronic ASB is difficult to eradicate.

The management of ASB depends on the age of the patient and whether or not the person is pregnant. In children, because of a greater risk of developing renal scarring and long-standing renal damage, treatment should consist of the same conventional courses of therapy as used for symptomatic infection. The greatest risk of renal damage occurs during the first 5 years of life.[62-63] In nonpregnant females, therapy is controversial; however, treatment has little effect on the natural course of infections. Two groups characterize ASB in the elderly: those with persistent bacteriuria and those with intermittent bacteriuria.

Several studies in hospitalized older adults, however, have not found antimicrobial therapy to be efficacious for abacteruria.[64-67] Thorough investigation of other causes of acute functional or cognitive changes or decline that may point to possible infection is encouraged in order to avoid unnecessary use of antibiotics which may lead to adverse consequences. However, persons with bacteriuria along with other systemic signs suggesting severe infection should be treated empirically with broad spectrum antimicrobial therapy until other causes are ruled out.[64] A number of questions remain unanswered due to limited data. For example: What is the effect of eradication of bacteriuria on life expectancy? What are the cost-effectiveness and risk-to-benefit ratio of therapy? What is the effect on morbidity? Certainly with the information available and the high adverse reaction rate in the elderly, vigorous treatment and screening programs cannot be advocated.

Complicated Urinary Tract Infections

Acute Pyelonephritis

A presentation of high-grade fever (more than 38.3°C [100.9°F]) and severe flank pain should be treated as acute pyelonephritis and warrants aggressive management. Severely ill patients with pyelonephritis should be hospitalized and IV antimicrobials administered initially (see Table 139-4). However, milder cases may be managed with orally administered antibiotics in an outpatient setting. Signs and symptoms of nausea, vomiting, and dehydration may require hospitalization.

At the time of presentation, a Gram stain of the urine should be performed along with a urinalysis, culture, and sensitivity tests. The Gram stain should indicate the morphology of the infecting organism(s) and help direct the selection of an appropriate antibiotic. However, the precise identity and susceptibility of the infecting organism(s) will be unknown initially, warranting empirical therapy. The goals of treatment include the achievement of therapeutic concentrations of an antimicrobial agent in the bloodstream and urinary tract to which the invading organism is susceptible and sufficient therapy to eradicate residual infection in the tissues of the urinary tract.

In the mild-to-moderate symptomatic patient in whom oral therapy is considered, an effective agent should be administered for 7 to 14 days, depending on the agent used.[1,68-73] Oral antibiotics that are highly active against the probable pathogens and that are sufficiently bioavailable are preferred. Fluoroquinolones (ciprofloxacin or levofloxacin) orally for 7 to 10 days are the first-line choice in mild-to-moderate pyelonephritis. Other options include trimethoprim–sulfamethoxazole for 14 days. If amoxicillin–clavulanate or an oral cephalosporin is used, it is recommended to give an initial long-acting parenteral antimicrobial such as ceftriaxone first and continue the oral agent for 10 to 14 days. If a Gram stain reveals gram-positive cocci, *Enterococcus faecalis* should be considered and treatment directed against this potential pathogen (ampicillin). Close follow-up of outpatient treatment is mandatory to ensure success.

In the seriously ill patient, parenteral therapy should be administered initially. Therapy should provide a broad spectrum of coverage and should be directed toward bacteremia or sepsis, if present. A number of antibiotic regimens have been used as empirical therapy, including an IV fluoroquinolone, an aminoglycoside with or without ampicillin, and extended-spectrum cephalosporins with or without an aminoglycoside and carbapenems.[1,74] Other options include aztreonam, the β-lactamase inhibitor combinations (eg, ampicillin–sulbactam, piperacillin–tazobactam, cetazidime/avabactam and cefetolozone/tazobactam), carbapenems (eg, imipenem, meropenem, doripenem, or ertapenem), novel boronic acid-based beta-lactamase inhibitor (eg, meropenem-vaborbactam), and IV trimethoprim–sulfamethoxazole.[74-76] If the patient has been hospitalized within the past 6 months, has a urinary catheter, or is a nursing home resident, the possibility of *P. aeruginosa* and enterococci, as well as multiple resistant organisms, should be considered. In this setting, broader spectrum coverage is recommended such as an extended spectrum beta-lactam/beta-lactamase inhibitor or carbapenem. Ertapenem should not be used in this situation owing to its inactivity against enterococci and *P. aeruginosa*.[72]

Effective therapy should stabilize the patient within 12 to 24 hours. A significant reduction in urine bacterial concentrations should occur in 48 hours. If bacteriologic response has not occurred, an alternative agent should be considered based on susceptibility testing. If the patient fails to respond clinically within 3 to 4 days or has persistently positive blood or urine cultures, further investigation is needed to exclude bacterial resistance, possible obstruction, papillary necrosis, intrarenal or perinephric abscess, or some other disease process. Usually by the third day of therapy, the patient is afebrile and significantly less symptomatic. In general, after the patient has been afebrile for 24 hours, parenteral therapy may be discontinued and oral therapy instituted to complete a 2-week course. Follow-up urine cultures should be obtained 2 weeks after completion of therapy to ensure a satisfactory response and detect possible relapse.

Urinary Tract Infections in Males

The management of UTIs in males is distinctly different and often more difficult than in females. Infections in male patients are considered to be complicated because endogenous bacteria in the presence of functional and/or structural abnormalities that disrupt the normal defense mechanisms of the urinary tract cause them. The incidence of infections in males younger than 60 years is much less than the incidence in females. During the adult years, the occurrence of infection can be related directly to some manipulation of the urinary tract. The most common causes are instrumentation of the urinary tract, catheterization, and renal and urinary stones. Uncomplicated

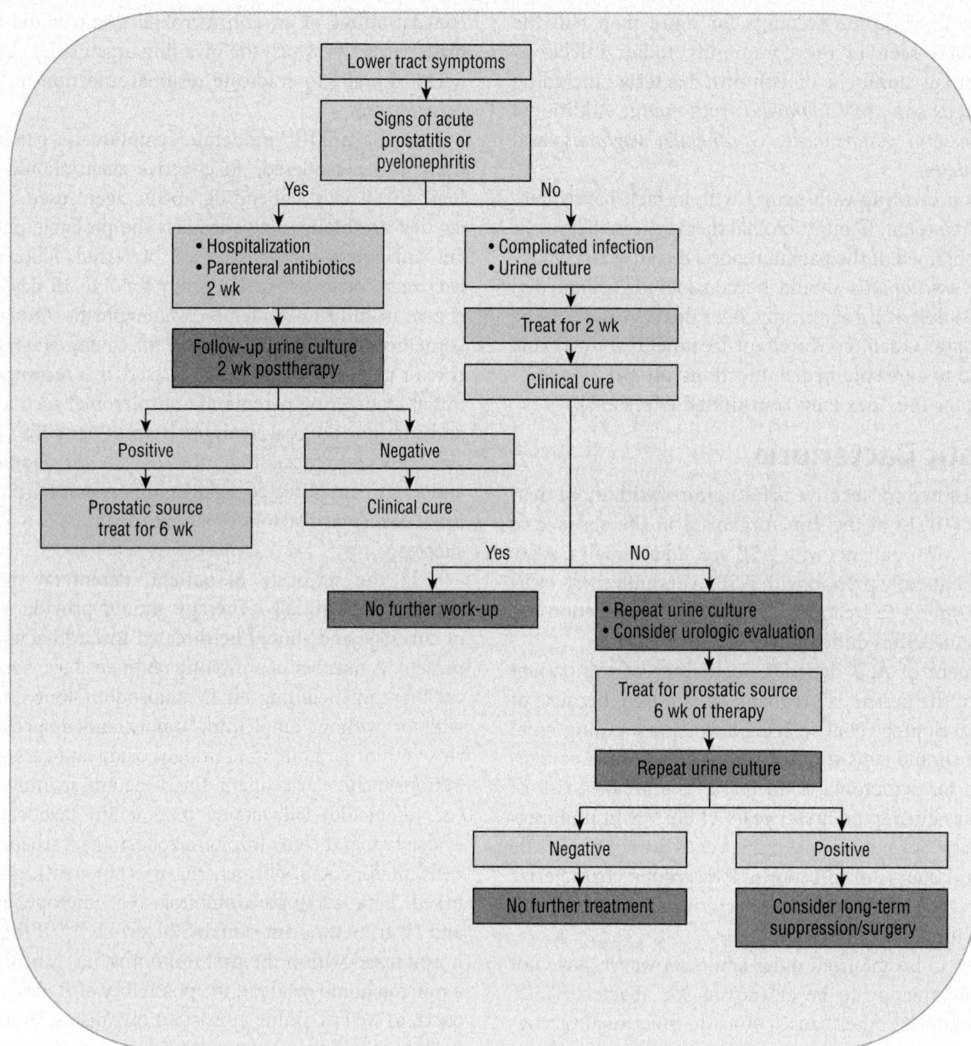

FIGURE 139-2 Management of urinary tract infections in males.

infections are rare, but they may occur in young males as a result of homosexual activity, noncircumcision, and having sex with partners who are colonized with uropathogenic bacteria. As the patient ages, the most common cause of infection is related to bladder outlet obstruction because of prostatic hypertrophy. In addition, the prostate gland may become infected and provide a nidus for recurrent infection in males.

The conventional view is that therapy in males requires prolonged treatment (Fig. 139-2). A urine culture should be obtained before treatment because the cause of infection in males is not as predictable as in females. Single-dose or short-course therapy is not recommended in males. Considerably fewer data are available comparing various antimicrobial agents in males as compared with females. If gram-negative bacteria are presumed, trimethoprim–sulfamethoxazole or the quinolone antimicrobials should be considered because these agents achieve high renal tissue, urine, and prostatic concentrations.[77]

Initial therapy should be for 10 to 14 days. Factors associated with treatment success are isolation of a single organism, the absence of significant obstruction or anatomic abnormalities, a normally functioning urinary tract, and the absence of prostatic involvement. Parenteral therapy may be required in certain situations, such as in severely ill patients, in the presence of acute prostatitis or epididymitis and in patients who cannot tolerate oral medications. A comparison of 2-week versus 6-week therapy in males with recurrent infections who were given trimethoprim–sulfamethoxazole had cure rates of 29% and 62%, respectively.[78] Other investigators advocate longer treatment periods in males, as well.[79] Follow-up cultures at 4 to 6 weeks after treatment are important in males to ensure bacteriologic cure. Many patients require longer periods of treatment and possible alterations in antibiotics, depending on culture and sensitivity results and clinical response.

Recurrent Infections

Recurrent episodes of UTI account for a significant portion of all UTIs. Of the individuals suffering from recurrent infections, 80% can be considered reinfections, that is, the recurrence of infection by an organism different from the organism isolated from the preceding infection. These persons most commonly are females and recurrence develops in approximately 20% of females with cystitis. Reinfections can be divided into two groups: those with less than three episodes per year and those who develop more frequent infections. Treatment strategies are continuing to develop, as well as, an understanding of the role of the microbiome.[80,81] An excellent overview of the various treatment modalities for recurrent UTI in females has been published.[81]

Management strategies depend on predisposing factors, number of episodes per year, and the person's preference. Factors commonly associated with recurrent infections include sexual intercourse and diaphragm or spermicide use for birth control. Therapeutic options include self-administered therapy, postcoital therapy, and continuous low-dose prophylaxis. In persons with infrequent infections (less than three infections per year), each episode may be treated as a separately occurring infection. Short-course therapy is appropriate in this setting. Many females have been treated successfully with self-administered short-course therapy at the onset of symptoms.[43,83]

In persons with more frequent symptomatic infections and no apparent precipitating event, long-term prophylactic antimicrobial therapy may be instituted. Prophylactic therapy reduces the frequency of symptomatic infections in older males and females, and children. In females, most studies show a reinfection rate of two to three per patient-year reduced to 0.1 to 0.2 per patient-year with treatment.[83] Before prophylaxis is initiated, individuals should be treated conventionally with an appropriate agent. Trimethoprim–sulfamethoxazole (one-half of a single-strength tablet), trimethoprim (100 mg daily), fluoroquinolone (levofloxacin 500 mg daily), and nitrofurantoin (50 or 100 mg daily) all reduce the rate of reinfection as the single-agent therapy.[83] Full-dose therapy with these agents is unnecessary and single daily doses can be used. Therapy generally is prescribed for a period of 6 months, during which time urine cultures are followed monthly. If symptomatic episodes develop, the patient should receive a full course of therapy with an effective agent and then resume prophylactic therapy. Therapy with methenamine hippurate for short-term use may be beneficial, but its overall utility is not well documented, especially for long-term prophylaxis.[84] In females who experience symptomatic reinfections in association with sexual activity, voiding after intercourse may help prevent infection. Also, single-dose prophylactic therapy with trimethoprim–sulfamethoxazole taken after intercourse reduces the incidence of recurrent infection significantly.[83]

In postmenopausal females with recurrent infections, the lack of estrogen results in changes in the bacterial flora of the vagina, resulting in increased colonization with uropathogenic *E. coli.* Topically administered estrogen cream reduces the incidence of infections in this population.[18,19]

The remaining 20% of recurrent UTIs are relapses, that is, persistence of infection with the same organism after therapy for an isolated UTI. The recurrence of symptomatic or ASB after therapy usually indicates that the person has renal involvement, a structural abnormality of the urinary tract or chronic bacterial prostatitis. In the absence of structural abnormalities, relapse often is related to renal infection and requires a long duration of treatment. Females who relapse after short-course therapy should receive a 2-week course of therapy. In patients who relapse after 2 weeks of therapy, therapy should be continued for another 2 to 4 weeks. If relapse occurs after 6 weeks of therapy, urologic evaluation should be performed and any obstructive lesion should be corrected. If this is not possible, therapy for 6 months or longer may be considered. Asymptomatic adults who have no evidence of urinary obstruction should not receive long-term therapy.

In males, relapse usually indicates bacterial prostatitis, the most common cause of persistent bacteriuria. Although many agents have been used for long-term therapy of relapses, trimethoprim–sulfamethoxazole and the fluoroquinolones appear to be highly effective.

Special Conditions

Urinary Tract Infections in Pregnancy

During pregnancy, significant physiologic changes occur to the entire urinary tract that dramatically alter the prevalence of UTIs and pyelonephritis. Severe dilation of the renal pelvis and ureters, decreased ureteral peristalsis, and reduced bladder tone occur during pregnancy.[86] These changes result in urinary stasis and reduced defenses against reflux of bacteria to the kidneys. In addition, increased urine content of amino acids, vitamins, and nutrients encourages bacterial growth. All of these factors increase the incidence of bacteriuria resulting in symptomatic infections, especially during the third trimester.

ASB occurs in 4% to 7% of pregnant persons. Of whom, 20% to 40% will develop acute symptomatic pyelonephritis during pregnancy. If untreated, ASB has the potential to cause significant adverse effects, including prematurity, low birth weight, and stillbirth.[86,87] Because pyelonephritis is associated with significant adverse events during pregnancy, routine screening tests for bacteriuria should be performed at the initial prenatal visit and again at 28 weeks of gestation. In persons with significant bacteriuria, symptomatic or asymptomatic, treatment is recommended so as to avoid possible complications. Organisms associated with bacteriuria are the same as those seen in uncomplicated UTIs with *E. coli* isolated most frequently.

Therapy should consist of an agent administered for 7 days that has a relatively low adverse effect potential and is safe for the mother and baby. The administration of amoxicillin, amoxicillin–clavulanate, or cephalexin is effective in 70% to 80% of patients. Nitrofurantoin has been used in pregnancy; however, it must be used with caution as occurrences of birth defects have been reported. Tetracyclines should be avoided because of teratogenic effects and sulfonamides should not be administered during the third trimester because of the possible development of kernicterus and hyperbilirubinemia. In addition, fluoroquinolones should not be given because of their potential to inhibit cartilage and bone development in the newborn. A follow-up urine culture 1 to 2 weeks after completing therapy and then monthly until gestation is complete is recommended. Optimal treatment for preventing recurrent UTI and ASB has yet to be defined.[89]

Catheterized Patients

The use of an indwelling catheter frequently is associated with infection of the urinary tract and represents the most common cause of hospital-acquired infection. The incidence of catheter-associated infection is related to a variety of factors, including method and duration of catheterization, the catheter system (open or closed), the care of the system, the susceptibility of the patient, and the technique of the healthcare personnel inserting the catheter. Catheter-related infections are reasonably preventable infections and are now considered one of the hospital-acquired complications chosen by the Centers for Medicare and Medicaid Services in which hospitals will no longer receive reimbursement for the treatment.[90,91]

Bacteria may enter the bladder in a number of ways. During the catheterization, bacteria may be introduced directly into the bladder from the urethra. Once the catheter is in place, bacteria may pass up the lumen of the catheter by the movement of air bubbles, motility of the bacteria, or capillary action. In addition, bacteria may reach the bladder from around the exudative sheath that surrounds the catheter in the urethra. Cleaning the periurethral area thoroughly and applying an antiseptic (povidone-iodine) can minimize infection occurring during insertion of the catheter. The use of closed drainage systems has reduced significantly the ability of bacteria to pass up the lumen of the catheter and cause infection. A bacterium passing around the catheter sheath in the urethra is probably the most important pathway for infection. Avoiding manipulation of the catheter and trauma to the urethra and urethral meatus can minimize this path of acquisition.

Persons with indwelling catheters acquire UTIs at a rate of 5% per day.[90-92] The closed systems are capable of preventing bacteriuria in most patients for up to 10 days with appropriate care. After 30 days of catheterization, however, there is a 78% to 95% incidence of bacteriuria, despite use of a closed system.[91,93] Unfortunately, UTI symptoms in a catheterized person are not clearly defined. Fever, peripheral leukocytosis, and urinary signs and symptoms may be of little predictive value.[90,91] When bacteriuria occurs in the asymptomatic, short-term catheterized person (less than 30 days), the use of systemic antibiotics should be withheld and the catheter should be removed as soon as possible. If the person becomes symptomatic, the catheter should be removed and treatment as described for complicated infections started. The optimal duration of therapy is unknown. In the long-term catheterized person (more than 30 days), bacteriuria is inevitable.[90,91] The administration of systemic antibiotics active against the infecting organism will sterilize the urine; however, reinfection occurs rapidly in more than 50% of persons. In addition, resistant organisms recolonize the urine. Symptomatic individuals must be treated because they are at the risk of developing pyelonephritis and bacteremia. Bacteria adhere to the catheter and produce a biofilm consisting of bacterial glycocalyces, Tamm–Horsfall protein, as well as apatite and struvite salts, that act to protect the bacteria from antibiotics.[92] Biofilm mechanisms and their treatment continue to be examined and more fully understood.[93,94] Recatheterization with a new sterile unit should be performed in symptomatic individuals, if the existing catheter has been in place for more than 2 weeks.

Various methods have been proposed to prevent the development of bacteriuria and infection in the patient with an indwelling catheter (see Table 139-4). The success of these methods depends on the type of catheter and the length of time it is in place. The use of constant bladder irrigation with antiseptic or antibacterial solutions reduces the incidence of infection in those with open drainage systems, but this approach has no advantage in those with closed systems. The use of prophylactic systemic antibiotics in persons with short-term catheterization reduces the incidence of infection over the first 4 to 7 days.[91,93] With long-term catheterization, however, antibiotics only postpone the development of bacteriuria and lead to the emergence of resistant organisms. Therefore, antibiotic prophylaxis should not be utilized in short-term or long-term catheterized patients.

PROSTATITIS

Bacterial prostatitis is an inflammation of the prostate gland and surrounding tissue as a result of infection. It is classified as either acute or chronic. By definition, pathogenic bacteria and significant inflammatory cells must be present in prostatic secretions and urine to make the diagnosis of bacterial prostatitis. Prostatitis occurs rarely in young males, but it is commonly associated with recurrent infections in persons older than 30 years. As many as 50% of all males develop some form of prostatitis at some period in their life.[95-97] The acute form typically is an acute infectious disease characterized by a sudden onset of fever, tenderness, and urinary and constitutional symptoms. Chronic prostatitis presents with few symptoms related to the prostate but rather symptoms of urinating difficulty, low back pain, perineal pressure, or a combination of these. It represents a recurring infection with the same organism that results from incomplete eradication of bacteria from the prostate gland.

Pathogenesis and Etiology

The exact mechanism of bacterial infection of the prostate is not well understood. The possible routes of infection are the same as those for UTIs. Reflux of infected urine into the prostate gland is thought to play an important role in causing infection. Intraprostatic reflux of urine occurs commonly and results in direct inoculation of infected urine into the prostate.[95-97] In addition, intraprostatic reflux of sterile urine can result in a chemical prostatitis and may be the cause of nonbacterial prostatitis. Sexual intercourse may contribute to infection of the prostate gland because prostatic secretions from males with chronic prostatitis and vaginal cultures from their sexual partners grow identical organisms. Other known causes of bacterial prostatitis include indwelling urethral and condom catheterization, urethral instrumentation, and transurethral prostatectomy in patients with infected urine.

Physiologic factors are believed to contribute to the development of prostatitis. Functional abnormalities found in bacterial prostatitis include altered prostate secretory functions. Prostatic fluid obtained from normal males contains prostatic antibacterial factor. This heat-stable, low-molecular-weight cation is a zinc-complexed polypeptide that is bactericidal to most urinary tract pathogens.[98] The antibacterial activity of prostatic antibacterial factor is related directly to the zinc content of prostatic fluid. Prostate fluid zinc levels and prostatic antibacterial factor activity also appear diminished in persons with prostatitis, as well as in older males.[98] Whether these changes are a cause or effect of prostatitis remains to be determined.

The pH of prostatic secretions in patients with prostatitis is altered.[99] Normal prostatic secretions have a pH in the range of 6.6 to 7.6. With increasing age, the pH tends to become more alkaline. With inflammation of the prostate, prostatic secretions may have an alkaline pH in the range of 7 to 9. These changes suggest a generalized secretory dysfunction of the prostate that not only can affect the pathogenesis of prostatitis but also can influence the mode of therapy.

Gram-negative enteric organisms are the most frequent pathogens in acute bacterial prostatitis.[95-97] *E. coli* is the predominant organism, occurring in 75% of cases. Other gram-negative organisms frequently isolated include *K. pneumoniae*, *P. mirabilis*, and less frequently, *P. aeruginosa*, *Enterobacter* spp., and *Serratia* spp. Infrequently, cases of gonococcal and staphylococcal prostatitis occur. *E. coli* most commonly causes chronic bacterial prostatitis with other gram-negative organisms isolated less frequently. The importance of gram-positive organisms in chronic bacterial prostatitis remains controversial. *S. epidermidis*, *S. aureus*, and diphtheroids have been isolated.

Clinical Presentation

Acute bacterial prostatitis presents similarly to other acute infections with fever, chills, myalgias, and other typical signs and symptoms. Massage of the prostate will express a purulent discharge that will readily grow the pathogenic organism. Prostatic massage is contraindicated in acute bacterial prostatitis, however, because of the risk of inducing bacteremia and the associated local pain. The diagnosis of acute bacterial prostatitis can be made from the clinical presentation, abdominal, genital, and digital rectal examination, and the presence of significant bacteriuria. As with other UTIs, the infecting organism can be isolated from a midstream specimen.

In contrast, chronic bacterial prostatitis is more difficult to diagnose and treat. Chronic bacterial prostatitis typically is characterized by recurrent UTIs with the same pathogen and is the most common cause of recurrent UTI in males. The patient's clinical presentation can vary widely. Many adults, however, are asymptomatic.

Because physical examination of the prostate is often normal, urinary tract localization studies are critical to the diagnosis of chronic bacterial prostatitis. The method of quantitative localization culture, as described by Meares and Stamey,[15,100] remains the diagnostic standard (Fig. 139-3). The method compares the bacterial

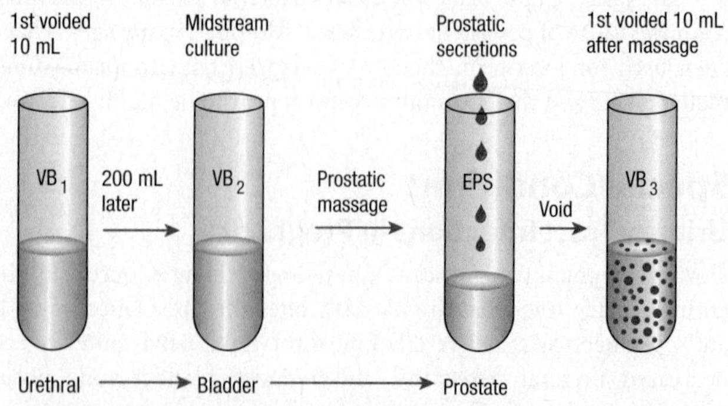

FIGURE 139-3 Segmented cultures of the lower tract in men. (EPS, expressed prostatic secretions; VB_1, voiding bladder 1; VB_2, voiding bladder 2; VB_3, voiding bladder 3.)

CLINICAL PRESENTATION Bacterial Prostatitis

Signs and Symptoms

- Acute bacterial prostatitis: High fever, chills, malaise, myalgia, localized pain (perineal, rectal, sacrococcygeal), frequency, urgency, dysuria, nocturia, and retention
- Chronic bacterial prostatitis: Voiding difficulties (frequency, urgency, dysuria), low back pain, and perineal and suprapubic discomfort

Physical Examination

- Acute bacterial prostatitis: Swollen, tender, tense, or indurated gland
- Chronic bacterial prostatitis: Boggy, indurated (enlarged) prostate in most patients

Laboratory Tests

- Bacteriuria
- Bacteria in EPSs

growth in sequential urine and prostatic fluid cultures obtained during micturition. The first 10 mL of voided urine is collected (voiding bladder 1, or VB_1) and constitutes urethral urine. After approximately 200 mL of urine has been voided, a 10-mL midstream sample is collected (VB_2). This specimen represents bladder urine. After the person voids, the prostate is massaged and expressed prostatic secretions (EPS) are collected. After prostatic massage, the patient voids again and 10 mL of urine is collected (VB_3).

The diagnosis of bacterial prostatitis is made when the number of bacteria in EPS is 10 times that of the urethral sample (VB_1) and midstream sample (VB_2). If no EPS is available, the urine sample following massage (VB_3) should contain a bacterial count 10-fold greater than that of VB_1 or VB_2. If significant bacteriuria is present, ampicillin, cephalexin, or nitrofurantoin should be given for 2 to 3 days to sterilize the urine prior to performing the localization study.

Treatment

9 The goals for the management of bacterial prostatitis are the same as those for UTIs. Acute bacterial prostatitis responds well to appropriate antimicrobial therapy that is directed at the most commonly isolated organisms. Prostatic penetration of antimicrobials occurs because the acute inflammatory reaction alters the cellular membrane barrier between the bloodstream and the prostate. Most patients can be managed with oral antimicrobial agents, such as trimethoprim–sulfamethoxazole and the fluoroquinolones (eg, ciprofloxacin, levofloxacin) (see Table 139-4). Other effective agents in this setting include cephalosporins and β-lactam–β-lactamase combinations. Although IV therapy is rarely necessary for total treatment, IV to oral sequential therapy with trimethoprim–sulfamethoxazole or the fluoroquinolones is appropriate. Most patients will become afebrile within 36 hours of antibiotic treatments.[96] The conversion to an oral antibiotic can be considered after the patient is afebrile for 48 hours or after 3 to 5 days of IV therapy. The total course of antibiotic therapy should be 4 weeks in order to reduce the risk of development of chronic prostatitis, although in some cases 2 weeks may be sufficient. Therapy may be prolonged with chronic prostatitis (6-12 weeks). Long-term suppressive therapy also may be initiated for recurrent infections, such as three times weekly ciprofloxacin, trimethoprim–sulfamethoxazole regular-strength tablet daily, or nitrofurantoin 100 mg daily.[100]

Chronic bacterial prostatitis often presents a more vexing situation because cures are obtained rarely. Despite high serum concentrations of antibacterial drugs in excess of the minimal inhibitory concentrations of the infecting organisms, bacteria persist in prostatic fluid. Most likely the failure to eradicate sensitive bacteria is caused by the inability of antibiotics to reach sufficient concentrations in the prostatic fluid and cross the prostatic epithelium.

Several factors that determine antibiotic diffusion into prostatic secretions were delineated from the canine model. Lipid solubility is a major determinant in the ability of drugs to diffuse from plasma across epithelial membranes. The degree of ionization in plasma also affects the diffusion of drugs. Only unionized molecules can cross the lipid barrier of prostatic cells, and the drug's pK_a (negative logarithm of acid ionization constant) directly determines the fraction of unchanged drug.

The pH gradient across the membrane has an influence on tissue penetration, as well. A pH gradient of at least one pH unit between separate compartments allows for ion trapping. As the unionized drug crosses the epithelial barrier into prostatic fluid, it becomes ionized allowing less drug to diffuse back across the lipid barrier. In early studies with the canine model, the prostatic pH was acidic (6.4).[99] In humans, however, the pH of prostatic secretions from an inflamed prostate is actually basic (8.1-8.3).[99]

The choice of antibiotics in chronic bacterial prostatitis should include agents that are capable of reaching therapeutic concentrations in the prostatic fluid and which possess the spectrum of activity to be effective. Agents that achieve therapeutic prostatic concentrations include trimethoprim and the fluoroquinolones. Sulfamethoxazole penetrates poorly and probably contributes little to trimethoprim activity when used in combination. The fluoroquinolones appear to provide the best therapeutic options in the management of chronic bacterial prostatitis. Therapy should be continued for 4 to 6 weeks initially. Longer treatment periods may be necessary in some cases. If therapy fails with these regimens, chronic suppressive therapy may be used or surgery considered.

ANSWERS FOR BEYOND THE BOOK

1. **Correct answer:** Yes, pregnant females should be screened for ASB and treated if it is present. *(Reference: Asymptomatic Bacteriuria Guidelines)*

2. **Correct answer C:** Pyuria and leukocyte esterase can be found in the urinalysis of patients with or without a urinary tract infection but do not increase their risk for a complicated UTI. Age is not a specific risk factor associated with an increase in complicated UTI. Pregnancy does increase the risk of complicated UTI due to anatomical changes and host factors during pregnancy.

3. **Correct answer D:** Ciprofloxacin is not appropriate due to concerns about safety and risk to fetus during pregnancy. Not treating is inappropriate due to potential complications of urinary tract infections in pregnancy, specifically pyelonephritis, premature birth, and low birth weight. Trimethoprim/Sulfamethoxazole would be an appropriate choice, especially since she is in her second trimester, but the treatment

would only be for 3 days. Nitrofurantoin has clinical experience and is relatively safe in pregnancy, especially after the first trimester.

4. **Correct answer A:** The patient is now showing signs of pyelonephritis with the fever and back pain, so longer treatment would be necessary. Therefore, longer treatment would be required than the 7 days of nitrofurantoin. In addition, pyelonephritis is not isolated in the bladder so you would need an agent that gets blood and tissue concentrations. Levofloxacin like ciprofloxacin is a fluoroquinolone and is therefore inappropriate due to concerns about safety and risk to fetus during pregnancy. The patient can be treated with oral therapy in an outpatient setting, so piperacillin/tazobactam intravenous would not be appropriate and is too broad spectrum for this sensitive *E. coli*. Trimethoprim/Sulfamethoxazole would be an appropriate choice, especially since she in in her second trimester, and is given orally for outpatient therapy. Fourteen days would be the appropriate length of treatment.

ABBREVIATIONS

ASB	asymptomatic bacteriuria
CFU	colony-forming unit
EPS	expressed prostatic secretions
GI	gastrointestinal
PMN	polymorphonuclear leukocyte
UTI	urinary tract infection
WBC	white blood cell

REFERENCES

1. Gupta K, Hooton TM, Naber KG, et al. International clinical practice guidelines for the treatment of acute uncomplicated cystitis and pyelonephritis in women: A 2010 update by the Infectious Diseases Society of America and the European Society for Microbiology and Infectious Diseases. *Clin Infect Dis.* 2011;52(5):e103–e120.
2. Naber KG, Cho YH, Matsumoto T, Schaeffer AJ. Immunoactive prophylaxis of recurrent urinary tract infections: A meta-analysis. *Int J Antimicrob Agents.* 2009;33(2):111–119.
3. Kallen AJ, Welch HG, Sirovich BE. Current antibiotic therapy for isolated urinary tract infections in women. *Arch Intern Med.* 2006;166(6):635–639. doi: 10.1001/archinte.166.6.635.
4. Nicolle LE. Uncomplicated urinary tract infection in adults including uncomplicated pyelonephritis. *Urol Clin North Am.* 2008;35(1):1–12,v. doi: 10.1016/j.ucl.2007.09.004.
5. Little P, Turner S, Rumsby K, et al. Developing clinical rules to predict urinary tract infection in primary care settings: Sensitivity and specificity of near patient tests (dipsticks) and clinical scores. *Br J Gen Pract.* 2006;56(529):606–612.
6. Platt R. Quantitative definition of bacteriuria. *Am J Med.* 1983;75(1b):44–52. doi: 10.1016/0002-9343(83)90072-4.
7. Alper BS, Curry SH. Urinary tract infection in children. *Am Fam Physician.* 2005;72(12):2483–2488.
8. Okarska-Napierała M, Wasilewska A, Kuchar E. Urinary tract infection in children: Diagnosis, treatment, imaging: Comparison of current guidelines. *J Pediatr Urol.* 2017;13(6):567–573. doi: 10.1016/j.jpurol.2017.07.018. Epub 2017 Sep 19.
9. Sobel J, Kaye D. *Urinary Tract Infections.* 7th ed. Philadelphia, PA: Churchill Livingstone/Elsevier; 2010.
10. Cortes-Penfield NW, Trautner BW, Jump RLP. Urinary tract infection and asymptomatic bacteriuria in older adults. *Infect Dis Clin North Am.* 2017;31(4):673–688. doi: 10.1016/j.idc.2017.07.002 PMID: 29079155. PMCID: PMC5802407.
11. Nicolle L, Anderson PA, Conly J, et al. Uncomplicated urinary tract infection in women. Current practice and the effect of antibiotic resistance on empiric treatment. *Can Fam Physician.* 2006;52:612–618.
12. Shigemura K, Arakawa S, Tanaka K, Fujisawa M. Clinical investigation of isolated bacteria from urinary tracts of hospitalized patients and their susceptibilities to antibiotics. *J Infect Chemother.* 2009;15(1): 18–22. doi: 10.1007/s10156-008-0652-x. Epub 2009 Mar 12.
13. Heintz BH, Halilovic J, Christensen CL. Vancomycin-resistant enterococcal urinary tract infections. *Pharmacotherapy.* 2010;30(11):1136–1149. doi: 10.1592/phco.30.11.1136.
14. Stamatiou C, Bovis C, Panagopoulos P, et al. Sex-induced cystitis—patient burden and other epidemiological features. *Clin Exp Obstet Gynecol.* 2005;32(3):180–182.
15. Stamey TA, Fair WR, Timothy MM, Chung HK. Antibacterial nature of prostatic fluid. *Nature.* 1968;218(5140):444–447. doi: 10.1038/218444a0.
16. Shand DG, Nimmon CC, O'Grady F, Cattell WR. Relation between residual urine volume and response to treatment of urinary infection. *Lancet.* 1970;760(1):1305–1306. doi: 10.1016/s0140-6736(70)91907-0.
17. Parsons CL, Shrom SH, Hanno PM, Mulholland SG. Bladder surface mucin. Examination of possible mechanisms for its antibacterial effect. *Invest Urol.* 1978;16(3):196–200.
18. Raz R, Stamm WE. A controlled trial of intravaginal estriol in postmenopausal women with recurrent urinary tract infections. *N Engl J Med.* 1993;329(11):753–756. doi: 10.1056/NEJM199309093291102
19. Stamm WE. Estrogens and urinary-tract infection. *J Infect Dis.* 2007;195(5):623–624. 10.1086/511526. Epub 2007 Jan 18.
20. Orskov I, Ferencz A, Orskov F. Tamm-horsfall protein or uromucoid is the normal urinary slime that traps type 1 fimbriated *Escherichia coli*. *Lancet.* 1980;1(8173):887. doi: 10.1016/s0140-6736(80)91396-3.
21. Measley RE Jr, Levison ME. Host defense mechanisms in the pathogenesis of urinary tract infection. *Med Clin North Am.* 1991;75(2):275–286. doi: 10.1016/s0025-7125(16)30453-9.
22. Flores-Mireles AL, Walker JN, Caparon M, Hultgren SJ. Urinary tract infections: Epidemiology, mechanisms of infection and treatment options. *Nat Rev Microbiol.* 2015;13(5):269–284. doi: 10.1038/nrmicro3432. Epub 2015 Apr 8.
23. Jenkins RD, Fenn JP, Matsen JM. Review of urine microscopy for bacteriuria. *JAMA.* 1986;255(24):3397–3403.
24. Pezzlo M. Detection of urinary tract infections by rapid methods. *Clin Microbiol Rev.* 1988;1(3):268–280. doi: 10.1128/CMR.1.3.268.
25. Stamm WE. Measurement of pyuria and its relation to bacteriuria. *Am J Med.* 1983;75(1b):53–58. doi: 10.1016/0002-9343(83)90073-6.
26. Pappas PG. Laboratory in the diagnosis and management of urinary tract infections. *Med Clin North Am.* 1991;75(2):313–325. doi: 10.1016/s0025-7125(16)30456-4.
27. St John A, Boyd JC, Lowes AJ, Price CP. The use of urinary dipstick tests to exclude urinary tract infection: A systematic review of the literature. *Am J Clin Pathol.* 2006;126(3):428–436. doi: 10.1309/C69RW1BT7E4QAFPV.
28. Nys S, van Merode T, Bartelds AI, Stobberingh EE. Urinary tract infections in general practice patients: Diagnostic tests versus bacteriological culture. *J Antimicrob Chemother.* 2006;57(5):955–958. doi: 10.1093/jac/dkl082. Epub 2006 Mar 22.
29. Stamey TA, Govan DE, Palmer JM. The localization and treatment of urinary tract infections: The role of bactericidal urine levels as opposed to serum levels. *Medicine (Baltimore).* 1965;44:1–36. doi: 10.1097/00005792-196501000-00001.
30. Fairley KF, Bond AG, Brown RB, Habersberger P. Simple test to determine the site of urinary-tract infection. *Lancet.* 1967;2(7513): 427–428. doi: 10.1016/s0140-6736(67)90849-5.
31. Thomas VL, Forland M. Antibody-coated bacteria in urinary tract infections. *Kidney Int.* 1982;21(1):1–7. doi: 10.1038/ki.1982.1.
32. Stamey TA, Fair WR, Timothy MM, et al. Serum versus urinary antimicrobial concentrations in cure of urinary-tract infections. *N Engl J Med.* 1974;291(22):1159–1163. doi: 10.1056/NEJM197411282912204.
33. Barrons R, Tassone D. Use of lactobacillus probiotics for bacterial genitourinary infections in women: A review. *Clin Ther.* 2008;30(3):453–468. doi: 10.1016/j.clinthera.2008.03.013.
34. Zelenitsky SA, Zhanel GG. Phenazopyridine in urinary tract infections. *Ann Pharmacother.* 1996;30(7-8):866–868. doi: 10.1177/106002809603000727.
35. Stapleton AE, Dziura J, Hooton TM, et al. Recurrent urinary tract infection and urinary *Escherichia coli* in women ingesting cranberry juice daily: A randomized controlled trial. *Mayo Clin Proc.* 2012;87(2):143–150. doi: 10.1016/j.mayocp.2011.10.006.
36. Jepson RG, Williams G, Craig JC. Cranberries for preventing urinary tract infections. *Cochrane Database Syst Rev.* 2012;10:CD001321. doi: 10.1002/14651858.CD001321.pub5.
37. Stapleton AE. Cranberry-containing products are associated with a protective effect against urinary tract infections. *Evid Based Med.* 2013;18(3):110–111.. doi: 10.1136/eb-2012-100984. Epub 2012 Nov 2.
38. Singh I, Gautam LK, Kaur IR. Effect of oral cranberry extract (standardized proanthocyanidin-A) in patients with recurrent UTI by pathogenic *E. coli*: A randomized placebo-controlled clinical research study. *Int Urol Nephrol.* 2016;48(9):1379–1386. doi: 10.1007/s11255-016-1342-8. Epub 2016 Jun 17.
39. Jepson R, Craig J, Williams G. Cranberry products and prevention of urinary tract infections. *JAMA.* 2013;310(13):1395–1396. doi: 10.1001/jama.2013.277509.

40. Howell AB, Botto H, Combescure C, et al. Dosage effect on uropathogenic *Escherichia coli* anti-adhesion activity in urine following consumption of cranberry powder standardized for proanthocyanidin content: A multicentric randomized double blind study. *BMC Infect Dis*. 2010;10:94. doi: 10.1186/1471-2334-10-94.
41. Stapleton AE, Au-Yeung M, Hooton TM, et al. Randomized, placebo-controlled phase 2 trial of a Lactobacillus crispatus probiotic given intravaginally for prevention of recurrent urinary tract infection. *Clin Infect Dis*. 2011;52(10):1212–1217. doi: 10.1093/cid/cir183. Epub 2011 Apr 14.
42. Gaines KK. Phenazopyridine hydrochloride: The use and abuse of an old standby for UTI. *Urol Nurs*. 2004;24(3):207–209.
43. Masson P, Matheson S, Webster AC, Craig JC. Meta-analyses in prevention and treatment of urinary tract infections. *Infect Dis Clin North Am*. 2009;23(2):355–385. doi: 10.1016/j.idc.2009.01.001
44. Chen YH, Ko WC, Hsueh PR. Emerging resistance problems and future perspectives in pharmacotherapy for complicated urinary tract infections. *Expert Opin Pharmacother*. 2013;14(5):587–596. doi: 10.1517/14656566.2013.778827.
45. Olson RP, Harrell LJ, Kaye KS. Antibiotic resistance in urinary isolates of *Escherichia coli* from college women with urinary tract infections. *Antimicrob Agents Chemother*. 2009;53(3):1285–1286. doi: 10.1128/AAC.01188-08. Epub 2008 Dec 22.
46. Colgan R, Johnson JR, Kuskowski M, Gupta K. Risk factors for trimethoprim-sulfamethoxazole resistance in patients with acute uncomplicated cystitis. *Antimicrob Agents Chemother*. 2008;52(3): 846–851. doi: 10.1128/AAC.01200-07. Epub 2007 Dec 17.
47. Bergman M, Nyberg ST, Huovinen P, et al. Association between antimicrobial consumption and resistance in *Escherichia coli*. *Antimicrob Agents Chemother*. 2009;53(3):912–917. doi: 10.1128/AAC.00856-08. Epub 2008 Dec 22.
48. Talan DA, Krishnadasan A, Abrahamian FM, et al. Prevalence and risk factor analysis of trimethoprim-sulfamethoxazole- and fluoroquinolone-resistant *Escherichia coli* infection among emergency department patients with pyelonephritis. *Clin Infect Dis*. 2008;47(9):1150–1158. doi: 10.1086/592250.
49. Paterson DL. "Collateral damage" from cephalosporin or quinolone antibiotic therapy. *Clin Infect Dis*. 2004;38(Suppl 4):S341–S345. doi: 10.1086/382690.
50. Karlowsky JA, Hoban DJ, Decorby MR, et al. Fluoroquinolone-resistant urinary isolates of *Escherichia coli* from outpatients are frequently multidrug resistant: Results from the North American Urinary Tract Infection Collaborative Alliance-Quinolone Resistance Study. *Antimicrob Agents Chemother*. 2006;50(6):2251–2254. doi: 10.1128/AAC.00123-06.
51. Johnson L, Sabel A, Burman WJ, et al. Emergence of fluoroquinolone resistance in outpatient urinary *Escherichia coli* isolates. *Am J Med*. 2008;121(10):876–884. doi: 10.1016/j.amjmed.2008.04.039.
52. Wagenlehner FM, Weidner W, Naber KG. An update on uncomplicated urinary tract infections in women. *Curr Opin Urol*. 2009;19(4):368–374. doi: 10.1097/MOU.0b013e32832ae18c.
53. Kashanian J, Hakimian P, Blute M Jr, et al. Nitrofurantoin: The return of an old friend in the wake of growing resistance. *BJU Int*. 2008;102(11):1634–1637. doi: 10.1111/j.1464-410X.2008.07809.x. Epub 2008 Jul 24.
54. Knottnerus BJ, Nys S, Ter Riet G, et al. Fosfomycin tromethamine as second agent for the treatment of acute, uncomplicated urinary tract infections in adult female patients in the netherlands? *J Antimicrob Chemother*. 2008;62(2):356–359. doi: 10.1093/jac/dkn177. Epub 2008 Apr 19.
55. Tice AD. Short-course therapy of acute cystitis: A brief review of therapeutic strategies. *J Antimicrob Chemother*. 1999;43(Suppl A):85–93.
56. Stein GE. Comparison of single-dose fosfomycin and a 7-day course of nitrofurantoin in female patients with uncomplicated urinary tract infection. *Clin Ther*. 1999;21(11):1864–1872. doi: 10.1016/S0149-2918(00)86734-X.
57. Huttner A, Kowalczyk A, Turjeman A, et al. Effect of 5-day nitrofurantoin vs single-dose fosfomycin on clinical resolution of uncomplicated lower urinary tract infection in women: A randomized clinical trial. *JAMA*. 2018;319(17):1781–1789. doi: 10.1001/jama.2018.3627.
58. Cox CE, Marbury TC, Pittman WG, et al. A randomized, double-blind, multicenter comparison of gatifloxacin versus ciprofloxacin in the treatment of complicated urinary tract infection and pyelonephritis. *Clin Ther*. 2002;24(2):223–236. doi: 10.1016/s0149-2918(02)85019-6.
59. Iravani A, Klimberg I, Briefer C, et al. A trial comparing low-dose, short-course ciprofloxacin and standard 7 day therapy with co-trimoxazole or nitrofurantoin in the treatment of uncomplicated urinary tract infection. *J Antimicrob Chemother*. 1999;43(Suppl A): 67–75.
60. Stass H, Kubitza D. Pharmacokinetics and elimination of moxifloxacin after oral and intravenous administration in man. *J Antimicrob Chemother*. 1999;43(Suppl B):83–90. doi: 10.1093/jac/43.suppl_2.83.
61. Gupta K, Hooton TM, Roberts PL, Stamm WE. Short-course nitrofurantoin for the treatment of acute uncomplicated cystitis in women. *Arch Intern Med*. 2007;167(20):2207–2212. doi: 10.1001/archinte.167.20.2207.
62. Chang SL, Shortliffe LD. Pediatric urinary tract infections. *Pediatr Clin North Am*. 2006;53(3):379–400. doi: 10.1016/j.pcl.2006.02.011.
63. Korbel L, Howell M, Spencer JD. The clinical diagnosis and management of urinary tract infections in children and adolescents. *Paediatr Int Child Health*. 2017;37(4):273–279. doi: 10.1080/20469047.2017.1382046. Epub 2017 Oct 5.
64. Nicolle LE, Gupta K, Bradley SF, et al. Clinical practice guideline for the management of asymptomatic bacteriuria: 2019 Update by the Infectious Diseases Society of America. *Clin Infect Dis*. 2019;68(10):e83–e110. doi: 10.1093/cid/ciy1121 PMID: 30895288.
65. Lin K, Fajardo K; U.S. Preventive Services Task Force. Screening for asymptomatic bacteriuria in adults: U.S. Preventive services task force reaffirmation recommendation statement. *Ann Intern Med*. 2008;149(1):43–47. doi: 10.7326/0003-4819-149-1-200807010-00009.
66. Juthani-Mehta M, Quagliarello V, Perrelli E, et al. Clinical features to identify urinary tract infection in nursing home residents: A cohort study. *J Am Geriatr Soc*. 2009;57(6):963–970. doi: 10.1111/j.1532-5415.2009.02227.x.
67. Nicolle LE, Bjornson J, Harding GK, MacDonell JA. Bacteriuria in elderly institutionalized men. *N Engl J Med*. 1983;309(23):1420–1425. doi: 10.1056/NEJM198312083092304.
68. Neal DE Jr. Complicated urinary tract infections. *Urol Clin North Am*. 2008;35(1):13–22. doi: 10.1016/j.ucl.2007.09.010.
69. Talan DA, Stamm WE, Hooton TM, et al. Comparison of ciprofloxacin (7 days) and trimethoprim-sulfamethoxazole (14 days) for acute uncomplicated pyelonephritis pyelonephritis in women: A randomized trial. *JAMA*. 2000;283(12):1583–1590. doi: 10.1001/jama.283.12.1583.
70. van Nieuwkoop C, van't Wout JW, Assendelft WJ, et al. Treatment duration of febrile urinary tract infection (futirst trial): A randomized placebo-controlled multicenter trial comparing short (7 days) antibiotic treatment with conventional treatment (14 days). *BMC Infect Dis*. Aug 19, 2009;9:131. doi: 10.1186/1471-2334-9-131.
71. Katchman EA, Milo G, Paul M, et al. Three-day vs longer duration of antibiotic treatment for cystitis in women: Systematic review and meta-analysis. *Am J Med*. 2005;118(11):1196–1207. doi: 10.1016/j.amjmed.2005.02.005.
72. Peterson J, Kaul S, Khashab M, et al. A double-blind, randomized comparison of levofloxacin 750 mg once-daily for five days with ciprofloxacin 400/500 mg twice-daily for 10 days for the treatment of complicated urinary tract infections and acute pyelonephritis. *Urology*. 2008;71(1):17–22. doi: 10.1016/j.urology.2007.09.002.
73. Brown P, Ki M, Foxman B. Acute pyelonephritis among adults: Cost of illness and considerations for the economic evaluation of therapy. *Pharmacoeconomics*. 2005;23(11):1123–1142. doi: 10.2165/00019053-200523110-00005.
74. Curran M, Simpson D, Perry C. Ertapenem: A review of its use in the management of bacterial infections. *Drugs*. 2003;63(17):1855–1878. doi: 10.2165/00003495-200363170-00006.
75. Wagenlehner FM, Wagenlehner C, Redman R, et al. Urinary bactericidal activity of doripenem versus that of levofloxacin in patients with complicated urinary tract infections or pyelonephritis. *Antimicrob Agents Chemother*. 2009;53(4):1567–1573. doi: 10.1128/AAC.01133-08. Epub 2009 Feb 2.
76. van Duin D, Bonomo RA. Ceftazidime/Avibactam and Ceftolozane/Tazobactam: Second-generation β-Lactam/β-Lactamase inhibitor combinations. *Clin Infect Dis*. 2016;63(2):234–241. doi: 10.1093/cid/ciw243. Epub 2016 Apr 20.
77. Coker TJ, Dierfeldt DM. Acute bacterial prostatitis: Diagnosis and management. *Am Fam Physician*. 2016;93(2):114–20. PMID: 26926407.
78. Gleckman R, Crowley M, Natsios GA. Therapy of recurrent invasive urinary-tract infections of men. *N Engl J Med*. 1979;301(16):878–880. doi: 10.1056/NEJM197910183011607.
79. Lipsky BA. Urinary tract infections in men. Epidemiology, pathophysiology, diagnosis, and treatment. *Ann Intern Med*. 1989;110(2):138–150. doi: 10.7326/0003-4819-110-2-138.
80. Whiteside SA, Razvi H, Dave S, et al. The microbiome of the urinary tract: A role beyond infection. *Nat Rev Urol*. 2015;12(2):81–90. doi: 10.1038/nrurol.2014.361. Epub 2015 Jan 20.
81. O'Brien VP, Hannan TJ, Schaeffer AJ, Hultgren SJ. Are you experienced? Understanding bladder innate immunity in the context of recurrent urinary tract infection. *Curr Opin Infect Dis*. 2015;28(1): 97–105. doi: 10.1097/QCO.0000000000000130.

82. Geerlings SE, Beerepoot MA and Prins JM. Prevention of recurrent urinary tract infections in women: Antimicrobial and nonantimicrobial strategies. *Infect Dis Clin North Am.* 2014;28(1): 135–147. doi: 10.1016/j.idc.2013.10.001. Epub 2013 Dec 7.
83. Cortes-Penfield NW, Trautner BW, Jump RLP. Urinary tract infection and asymptomatic bacteriuria in older adults. *Infect Dis Clin North Am.* 2017;31(4):673–688. doi: 10.1016/j.idc.2017.07.002 PMID: 29079155. PMCID: PMC5802407.
84. Lee BS, Bhuta T, Simpson JM, Craig JC. Methenamine hippurate for preventing urinary tract infections. *Cochrane Database Syst Rev.* 2012;10:CD003265. doi: 10.1002/14651858.CD003265.pub3.
85. Renard J, Ballarini S, Mascarenhas T, et al. Recurrent lower urinary tract infections have a detrimental effect on patient quality of life: A prospective, observational study. *Infect Dis Ther.* 2015;Mar 4(1): 125–135. doi: 10.1007/s40121-014-0054-6.
86. Kalinderi K, Delkos D, Kalinderis M, Athanasiadis A, Kalogiannidis I. Urinary tract infection during pregnancy: Current concepts on a common multifaceted problem. *J Obstet Gynaecol.* 2018;38(4): 448–453. doi: 10.1080/01443615.2017.1370579 PMID: 29402148.
87. Christensen B. Which antibiotics are appropriate for treating bacteriuria in pregnancy? *J Antimicrob Chemother.* 2000;46(Suppl 1): 29–34.
88. McDermott S, Daguise V, Mann H, et al. Perinatal risk for mortality and mental retardation associated with maternal urinary-tract infections. *J Fam Pract.* 2001;50(5):433–437.
89. Schneeberger C, Geerlings SE, Middleton P, Crowther CA. Interventions for preventing recurrent urinary tract infection during pregnancy. *Cochrane Database Syst Rev.* 2012;11:CD009279. doi: 10.1002/14651858.CD009279.pub2.
90. Saint S, Meddings JA, Calfee D, et al. Catheter-associated urinary tract infection and the medicare rule changes. *Ann Intern Med.* 2009;150(12):877–884. doi: 10.7326/0003-4819-150-12-200906160-00013.
91. Hooton TM, Bradley SF, Cardenas DD, et al. Diagnosis, prevention, and treatment of catheter-associated urinary tract infection in adults: 2009 international clinical practice guidelines from the infectious diseases society of america. *Clin Infect Dis.* 2010;50(5):625–663. doi: 10.1086/650482.
92. Ohkawa M, Sugata T, Sawaki M, et al. Bacterial and crystal adherence to the surfaces of indwelling urethral catheters. *J Urol.* 1990;143(4):717–721. doi: 10.1016/s0022-5347(17)40071-1.
93. Chenoweth CE, Gould CV, Saint S. Diagnosis, management, and prevention of catheter-associated urinary tract infections. *Infect Dis Clin North Am.* 2014;28(1):105–19. doi: 10.1016/j.idc.2013.09.002 PMID: 24484578.
94. Kostakioti M, Hadjifrangiskou M, Hultgren SJ. Bacterial biofilms: Development, dispersal, and therapeutic strategies in the dawn of the postantibiotic era. *Cold Spring Harb Perspect Med.* 2013;3(4):a010306. doi: 10.1101/cshperspect.a010306.
95. Murphy AB, Macejko A, Taylor A, Nadler RB. Chronic prostatitis: Management strategies. *Drugs.* 2009;69(1):71–84. doi: 10.2165/00003495-200969010-00005.
96. Coker TJ, Dierfeldt DM. Acute bacterial prostatitis: Diagnosis and management. *Am Fam Physician* 2016;93(2):114–20. PMID: 26926407.
97. Lipsky BA, Byren I, Hoey CT. Treatment of bacterial prostatitis. *Clin Infect Dis.* 2010;50(12):1641–1652. doi: 10.1086/652861.
98. Fair WR, Couch J, Wehner N. Prostatic antibacterial factor. Identity and significance. *Urology.* 1976;7(2):169–177. doi: 10.1016/0090-4295(76)90305-8.
99. Pfau A, Perlberg S, Shapira A. The pH of the prostatic fluid in health and disease: Implications of treatment in chronic bacterial prostatitis. *J Urol.* 1978;119(3):384–387. doi: 10.1016/s0022-5347(17)57497-2.
100. Wagenlehner FM, Naber KG. Current challenges in the treatment of complicated urinary tract infections and prostatitis. *Clin Microbiol Infect.* 2006;12(Suppl 3):67–80. doi: 10.1111/j.1469-0691.2006.01398.x.

Sexually Transmitted Infections 140

Yvonne J. Burnett and Humberto R. Jimenez

KEY CONCEPTS

1. A single dose of ceftriaxone is recommended for uncomplicated gonococcal infections. Antimicrobial stewardship concerns over the impact on the microbiome, increasing rates of azithromycin resistance and continued low ceftriaxone resistance rates, led to the move away from dual drug therapy. If chlamydial infection cannot be excluded, doxycycline should be added.
2. Chlamydia genital tract infections represent the most frequently reported communicable disease in the United States. Females are frequently asymptomatic or minimally symptomatic and, if left untreated, may develop complications such as pelvic inflammatory disease (PID), ectopic pregnancy, or infertility. All sexually active females younger than 25 years and women with multiple sexual partners should be screened annually.
3. A 7-day course of metronidazole is the preferred treatment for trichomoniasis in women, with single dose tinidazole as an alternative. Single-dose metronidazole remains the recommended therapy for men.
4. PID treatment should target gonorrhea and chlamydia, with the addition of anaerobic coverage.
5. Parenteral penicillin is the treatment of choice for all syphilis infections. Alternative therapies for penicillin-allergic patients are usually suboptimal, have insufficient data, require prolonged oral courses, and/or are not recommended for specific populations. When allergies are reported, clarification of the type of reaction is critical to ensure optimal therapy. For true penicillin allergies, penicillin desensitization protocols are available when penicillin is required.
6. Oral acyclovir, famciclovir, and valacyclovir are effective in reducing viral shedding, duration of symptoms, and time to healing of first-episode genital herpes infections, with maximal benefits seen when therapy is initiated at the earliest stages of infection. Patient-initiated, episodic antiviral therapy started within 1 day of lesion onset or during the prodromal stage preceding an outbreak offers an alternative to continuous suppressive therapy of recurrent infection in some individuals.
7. Human papilloma virus (HPV) vaccination reduces complications associated with HPV infection, including development of genital warts and HPV-related cancers. Adolescent vaccination, prior to onset of sexual activity is recommended. Despite robust safety and efficacy data, vaccination rates remain below 80% in target populations.

BEYOND THE BOOK

Obtaining a relevant and culturally sensitive sexual history is an important part of ensuring an individual's optimal health. Patient interviews should include the five Ps: partners, practices, protection, past STIs, and prevention of pregnancy strategies.

Watch the following videos that focus on the importance of collecting a sexual history and understanding at-risk populations. These videos are useful to enhance student understanding regarding the Collect and Assess steps in the patient care process.

https://www.cdc.gov/std/be-smart-be-well/letstalk.htm

https://www.youtube.com/watch?v=WUsebbT39C4

INTRODUCTION

Sexually transmitted infections (STIs) encompass a wide variety of pathogens (Table 140-1), diverse presentations, and continually evolving diagnosis, treatment and prevention strategies. STIs impact short- and long-term health of millions in the United States, yet continue to be underfunded, stigmatized, and devalued as a public health priority. Since 2000, rates continue to rise, with chlamydia doubling, gonorrhea increasing 40%, and primary and secondary syphilis cases soaring fivefold.[1,2] In 2018, one in five people in the United States had an STI.[2] Almost half of the 26 million new infections in 2018 were acquired by teens and young adults (15-24 years old).[1] Besides in youth, STIs rates are disproportionally higher in marginalized groups, specifically sexual and gender minorities (encompassing lesbian, gay, bisexual, and transgender communities), Black, Latinx, American Indian/Alaska Native, and Native Hawaiian/other Pacific Islander people.[1] Furthermore, the financial impact of STIs are substantial, costing the U.S. healthcare system an estimated $16 billion in direct lifetime medical costs.[3]

STI health consequences range from urogenital discomfort to encephalitis. Women are especially susceptible to complications, many of which center around reproductive health. Pregnancy-related morbidity is often devastating, including stillbirth and fetal or newborn transmission. Men can also experience reproductive sequelae. Extragenital manifestations, such as neurosyphilis and septic arthritis, can be classic findings or present with non-specific symptoms.

While the terms sexually transmitted diseases (STDs) and STIs are often used interchangeably, there has been a global shift toward using the term STI. Many infections are asymptomatic, with some clearing spontaneously. An STD is a recognizable disease or condition that develops from an STI. Thus, the term STI is more accurate, more inclusive, and carries less stigma than STD.[4]

The risk of acquiring and transmitting an STI varies based on pathogen, host characteristics, local epidemiology, individual behavior, sexual networks, and broader social and structural factors.

TABLE 140-1 Sexually Transmitted Infections

Disease	Associated Pathogens
Bacterial	
Gonorrhea	*Neisseria gonorrhoeae*
Syphilis	*Treponema pallidum*
Chancroid	*Haemophilus ducreyi*
Granuloma inguinale	*Klebsiella granulomatis*
Enteric disease	*Salmonella* spp., *Shigella* spp., *Campylobacter* spp.
Campylobacter infection	*Campylobacter jejuni*
Bacterial vaginosis	*Gardnerella vaginalis, Mycoplasma hominis, Bacteroides* spp., *Mobiluncus* spp.
Chlamydial	
Nongonococcal urethritis	*Chlamydia trachomatis*
Lymphogranuloma venereum	*C. trachomatis*, type L
Viral	
Acquired immunodeficiency syndrome	Human immunodeficiency virus
Herpes genitalis	Herpes simplex virus, types 1 and 2
Viral hepatitis	Hepatitis A, B, C, and D viruses
Condylomata acuminata	Human papillomavirus
Mycoplasmal	
Nongonococcal urethritis	*Mycoplasma genitalium*
Protozoal	
Trichomoniasis	*Trichomonas vaginalis*
Fungal	
Vaginal candidiasis	*Candida albicans*

Age-specific STI rates are historically higher in men versus women; however, reported rates may not represent true gender differences and may reflect ease of detection in men. In recent years, male-to-female ratios for most STIs have declined or reversed, reflecting improved STI screening. Rates of some STIs, such as syphilis and HIV, are disproportionately greater in men who have sex with men (MSM).[1] The risks of acquiring select STIs are elevated among racial and ethnic minorities in the United States, particularly, chlamydia, gonorrhea, and (primary and secondary) syphilis rates among Black versus White Americans.[5] Multiple or anonymous sex partners, condomless sex, and sex while under the influence of drugs or alcohol can increase STI (and HIV) acquisition risks.[6] Limited access and reduced engagement with medical care, living in areas with high prevalence, high-risk sexual networks, and marginalized and/or stigmatized communities are broader factors that can increase STI risk.[7]

The national strategy toward addressing STIs has historically centered on screening, treating, and preventing infections based on individual risks and/or behaviors. These tactics, combined with the complexities of the US healthcare system, societal discomfort discussing sexuality and sexual health, and structural inequities, have led to some of the highest STI rates among higher income nations. Healthcare provider's implicit bias and systemic discriminatory policies have also hampered efforts to reduce STIs through suboptimal screening initiatives and limited engagement of affected individuals within the healthcare system.[8,9] The Committee on Prevention and Control of STIs in the United States encourages a new approach, centered around the understanding that sexual health is a "state of physical, emotional, mental, and social well-being in relation to sexuality; it is not merely the absence of disease, dysfunction or infirmity," as stated by World Health Organization (WHO).[10] Efforts should be more holistic, addressing principal drivers of health inequities, such as social determinants of health and structural bias and acknowledging how social networks and prevalence variations impact STI risk. To expand the STI workforce, the Centers for Disease Control and Prevention (CDC) encourages primary care providers help close STI screening and treatment gaps.[9,11]

Other than complete abstinence, the most effective way to prevent STI transmission is by maintaining a mutually monogamous sexual relationship between uninfected partners. Short of this, use of barrier contraceptive methods provide varying degrees of protection. Reducing the number of partners and increased testing can also lower risk. Obtaining a relevant and culturally sensitive sexual history is important to perform an accurate risk assessment. Even when providers ask about sexual and STI history, less often are number or gender of sex partners, or types of sexual practices collected. Patient interviews should include the five Ps: partners, practices, protection, past STIs, and prevention of pregnancy strategies.[11]

Treating STIs appropriately and early is important to curb transmission and prevent complications. Ensuring screening and/or treatment of sex partners is a critical facet of STI management. Partner referral can be initiated by the index patient or provider.[12] Expedited partner therapy (EPT) is another option when partners cannot receive a medical evaluation. In EPT, a partner's prescription is provided to the index patient for the dual benefit of treating the partner(s) and preventing reinfection of the index patient. Although legal status of EPT has not always been explicitly clear, the CDC and the Center for Law and the Public's Health have found that EPT is permissible or potentially allowable in all states and other US territories. Increased awareness and education are needed to remove barriers that continue to limit this practice.[12]

With the exception of human immunodeficiency virus (HIV) infection, reviewed in detail in Chapter 148, the most frequently occurring STIs in the United States are discussed in this chapter. The varied spectrum of clinical syndromes produced by common STIs is determined not only by the etiologic pathogen(s) but also by differences in anatomy and reproductive physiology. For many STIs, signs and symptoms overlap sufficiently to prevent accurate diagnosis without microbiologic confirmation. Frequently, symptoms are minimal or absent despite the presence of infection. Table 140-2 lists common clinical syndromes associated with STIs.[4]

First, STIs commonly presenting with urethritis or vaginal discharge and associated complications are discussed, followed by STIs commonly associated with genital ulcers or lesions. Several STIs not included in this chapter warrant mention, including increased awareness of proctitis among MSM caused by gram-negative bacteria normally present in the gut microbiota, such as *Campylobacter* and *Shigella* species, as well as atypical organisms, such as herpes simplex virus (HSV). Outbreak concerns and growing viral hepatitis rates led to updates in screening recommendations. The most current information on the epidemiology, diagnosis, and treatment of these and other STIs can be obtained at the CDC Website (http://www.cdc.gov).

GONORRHEA

Epidemiology and Etiology

Gonorrhea is the second most commonly reported notifiable disease in the United States.[1,4] Since the mid-1990s through early 2000s, rates of reported cases in the United States remained relatively stable. However, since a historic low in 2009, rates of gonorrhea have increased 92% with 616,392 cases reported to the CDC in 2019 equating to 188.4 cases/100,000 persons compared to 98.1 cases/100,000 persons in 2009.[1] Of growing concern are substantial numbers of infections that remain undiagnosed and unreported,

TABLE 140-2 Selected Syndromes Associated with Common Sexually Transmitted Pathogens

Syndrome	Commonly Implicated Pathogens	Common Clinical Manifestations[a]
Urethritis	*C. trachomatis*, herpes simplex virus, *N. gonorrhoeae*, *T. vaginalis*, *Ureaplasma spp.*, *M. genitalium*	Urethral discharge, dysuria
Epididymitis	*C. trachomatis*, *N. gonorrhoeae*, Enterobacterales	Scrotal pain, inguinal pain, flank pain, urethral discharge
Cervicitis/vulvovaginitis	*C. trachomatis*, *G. vaginalis*, herpes simplex virus, human papillomavirus, *N. gonorrhoeae*, *T. vaginalis*	Abnormal vaginal discharge, vulvar itching/irritation, dysuria, dyspareunia
Genital ulcers (painful)	*H. ducreyi*, herpes simplex virus	Usually multiple vesicular/pustular (herpes) or papular/pustular (*H. ducreyi*) lesions that can coalesce; painful, tender lymphadenopathy[b]
Genital ulcers (painless)	*T. pallidum*	Usually single papular lesion, usually painless
Genital/anal warts	Human papillomavirus	Multiple lesions ranging in size from small papular warts to large exophytic condylomas
Pharyngitis	*C. trachomatis*, herpes simplex virus, *N. gonorrhoeae*	Symptoms of acute pharyngitis, cervical lymphadenopathy, fever[c]
Proctitis	*C. trachomatis*, herpes simplex virus, *N. gonorrhoeae*, *T. pallidum*	Constipation, anorectal discomfort, tenesmus, mucopurulent rectal discharge
Salpingitis	*C. trachomatis*, *N. gonorrhoeae*	Lower abdominal pain, purulent cervical or vaginal discharge, adnexal swelling, fever[d]

[a]For some syndromes, clinical manifestations can be minimal or absent.

[b]Recurrent herpes infection can manifest as a single lesion.

[c]Most cases of pharyngeal gonococcal infection are asymptomatic.

[d]Salpingitis increases the risk of subsequent ectopic pregnancy and infertility.

thereby perpetuating spread of disease. Reported cases among males increased 112% compared to 42% among females from 2012 to 2019. Higher rates in males may be representative of increased transmission, detection via extra-genital screening among MSM, or both.[1]

In 2013, the CDC identified drug-resistant *Neisseria gonorrhoeae* as a top three pathogen presenting an urgent level threat, posing an immediate health threat requiring urgent and aggressive action.[13] The 2019 update maintains the urgent threat level, showcasing increasing resistance over time and doubling of infections from 2013 to 2019.[14] Additionally, the WHO identified drug-resistant *N. gonorrhoeae* as a high priority organism for new antibiotic development.[15] Due to rising resistance, large numbers of asymptomatic infections, and ease of transmission, gonorrhea is difficult to control. Additionally, HIV infection is more easily transmitted in patients coinfected with gonorrhea.[4]

Pathophysiology

N. gonorrhoeae, the causative agent of gonorrhea infections, a gram-negative diplococcus, does not have any animal or environmental reservoirs and humans are the only known host. *N. gonorrhoeae* infects mucosa of the urethra, endocervix, anorectum, pharynx, and conjunctiva. After mucosal damage is established, polymorphonuclear (PMN) leukocytes invade tissue and form submucosal abscesses, resulting in purulent exudates.[4,16]

Gonorrhea is highly transmissible via sexual contact. Female risk of acquisition after a single episode of vaginal intercourse with an infected male partner is 50% to 70%; however, risk of female-to-male transmission following a single act is 20%.[17,18] With repeated exposure, risk of female-to-male transmission increases to 60% to 80%.[17] Although transmission rates for other types of sexual contact are not quantified, anal intercourse is likely more efficient while oral sex is less efficient than penile-vaginal sex.[16]

Clinical Presentation

Individuals infected with gonorrhea can be symptomatic or asymptomatic and have infections involving several anatomic sites. Interestingly, most untreated symptomatic patients become asymptomatic within 6 months, with only a few becoming asymptomatic carriers of disease.[4,16] In settings where sexually active women are routinely screened for subclinical infections, most diagnosed with gonorrhea are asymptomatic. Up to 50% of women experience nonspecific symptoms, including mucopurulent vaginal discharge or post-intercourse vaginal bleeding. In comparison, 90% of males experience symptoms within 2 to 6 days following exposure, most commonly mucopurulent penile discharge or dysuria.[1,19] The most common clinical features of gonococcal infections are presented in Table 140-3.

Complications associated with untreated gonorrhea appear more pronounced in women, likely a result of a high percentage who experience nonspecific or minimal symptoms. As a result, many women do not seek treatment until after development of serious complications, such as pelvic inflammatory disease (PID). Approximately 10% to 20% of women with gonorrhea develop PID.[1,6,20] Left untreated, PID can cause infertility and ectopic pregnancies. Previous reports indicate 0.5% to 3% of gonorrhea infections result in disseminated gonococcal infection (DGI), but the risk may be less given declining prevalence of strains prone to dissemination.[21–23] Usual clinical manifestations of DGI are tender necrotic skin lesions, tenosynovitis, and monoarticular arthritis, or rarely meningitis or endocarditis.[4,16]

Diagnosis

Obtaining specific microbiologic diagnosis is recommended to reduce complications, reinfections, and transmission versus clinical diagnosis. Diagnosis of gonococcal infections can be made by Gram-stained smears, culture, or detection of cellular components (eg, enzymes, antigens, or DNA).[4]

Nucleic acid detection tests replaced culture or Gram stain in most settings as the primary diagnostic or screening test. These offer increased sensitivity and/or specificity over traditional diagnostic methods and provide more rapid results versus culture.[4,24]

Nucleic acid amplification tests (NAATs) are the most widely used and employ techniques and have high sensitivity for detecting *N. gonorrhoeae* using noninvasive specimens (eg, self-collected

TABLE 140-3 Presentation of Gonorrhea Infections

	Males	Females
General	Incubation period: 1-14 days	Incubation period: 1-14 days
	Symptom onset in 2-8 days	Symptom onset in 10 days
Site of infection	Most common: urethra	Most common: endocervical canal
	Others: rectum (usually caused by rectal intercourse in MSM), oropharynx, eye	Others: urethra, rectum (usually caused by perineal contamination), oropharynx, eye
Symptoms	Commonly symptomatic, may be asymptomatic	Can be asymptomatic or minimally symptomatic
	Urethral infection: dysuria and urinary frequency	Endocervical infection: usually asymptomatic or mildly symptomatic
	Anorectal infection: asymptomatic to severe rectal pain	Urethral infection: dysuria, urinary frequency
	Pharyngeal infection: asymptomatic to mild pharyngitis	Anorectal and pharyngeal infection; symptoms same as for men
Signs	Purulent urethral or rectal discharge can be scant to profuse Anorectal: pruritus, mucopurulent discharge, bleeding	Abnormal vaginal discharge or uterine bleeding; purulent urethral or rectal discharge can be scant to profuse
Complications	Rare (epididymitis, prostatitis, inguinal lymphadenopathy, urethral stricture)	PID and associated complications (ie, ectopic pregnancy, infertility)
	Disseminated gonorrhea	Disseminated gonorrhea

urine specimens, vaginal swabs). A NAAT is recommended by the CDC for detection of gonorrhea[4,24] and are approved for endocervical (women), urethral (men), and urine specimens. Extragenital diagnostic NAAT testing is now available for pharyngeal and rectal samples, in combination with testing for *Chlamydia trachomatis*.[25] A major drawback of NAATs is their inability to provide resistance data. In cases of documented treatment failure, culture and antimicrobial susceptibility testing is recommended.[4,24]

While NAATs are most commonly used in clinical practice, Gram stains can be used to make a presumptive diagnosis of gonorrhea infections. A Gram stain performed on purulent male urethral discharge is diagnostic for infection when gram-negative diplococci are identified within PMN leukocytes. However, due to lower sensitivity, Gram-stained smears are not recommended for diagnosis of endocervical, rectal, pharyngeal, and asymptomatic male urethral infections. Because of the pharyngeal presence of nonpathogenic *Neisseria* spp., Gram stain is not useful in pharyngeal infection diagnosis.[4,16]

Bacterial cultures are highly sensitive and specific, provide opportunity for susceptibility testing, and can be performed on a variety of specimens. Prolonged turnaround times, decreased sensitivity compared to NAATS, and additional laboratory requirements preclude widespread usage. With the expansion of FDA-approval of NAATs on various specimen types, culture is primarily reserved for cases of suspected or documented treatment failures, as a test of cure (TOC) following use of alternative treatment regimens, or when evaluating for DGI.[4]

Routine screening for *N. gonorrhoeae* is recommended in certain populations to reduce burden of disease and morbidity associated with gonococcal infection. As females are more commonly asymptomatic, the CDC and US Preventative Services Task Force (USPSTF) recommend routine annual screening for gonococcal infection for all sexually active women younger than 25.[4,26] For those 25 years and older, annual screening is recommended for those at increased risk of gonococcal infection (eg, multiple or new sexual partners, partners with an STI, inconsistent condom use, transactional sex, or history of STI[s]). Pregnant women should be screened for gonorrhea at the first prenatal visit and again during the third trimester, for those at continued risk. The CDC also recommends that MSM should be screened at least annually, regardless of condom use, testing sites involved with sexual activity.[4]

TREATMENT

1 *N. gonorrhoeae* has developed resistance to all antibiotics previously used for treatment, including sulfonamides, penicillins, tetracyclines, fluoroquinolones, and early generation macrolides and cephalosporins. In 2020, the CDC issued updated gonorrhea treatment recommendations.[27]

A single 500 mg ceftriaxone dose is recommended for treatment of uncomplicated gonococcal infections. Previously, dual antibiotic therapy with different mechanisms of action (ceftriaxone plus azithromycin or doxycycline) was recommended to delay further development of cephalosporin resistance. However, rising incidence of azithromycin resistance, antimicrobial stewardship concerns regarding microbiome harm, pharmacokinetic and pharmacodynamic considerations, and continued low ceftriaxone resistance, influenced the recommendation to current single-drug regimen. Single-dose intramuscular (IM) ceftriaxone remains the only recommended agent for treating gonorrhea as ceftriaxone-based regimens have well-documented efficacy in the treatment of urethral, cervical, rectal, and pharyngeal infections.[4,27,28] (Table 140-4). To optimize pharmacokinetic and pharmacodynamic properties of ceftriaxone, the dose of ceftriaxone was increased from previous recommendations. Additionally, patients weighing 150 kg or more should receive ceftriaxone 1 g.[4]

An 800 mg oral dose of cefixime may be substituted if ceftriaxone is unavailable or not feasible, but due to reduced bactericidal levels and efficacy, especially in pharyngeal infections, this regimen is not preferred. Note that based on pharmacokinetic and pharmacodynamic properties, the dose of cefixime was optimized to 800 mg compared to the previous dose of 400 mg.[4,27] Additionally, only ceftriaxone is effective in treating pharyngeal gonorrhea as oral cephalosporins do not reliably cure these infections.[27,28]

Because coexisting chlamydial infections are common, documented in up to 50% of women and 20% of men with gonorrhea, and symptoms may be similar to that of gonorrhea, for those where concurrent chlamydial infection has not been ruled out, chlamydia treatment should be added.[27,29] Doxycycline 100 mg orally twice daily for 7 days is preferred to azithromycin 1 g orally as a single dose.[27] Where previously azithromycin and doxycycline were both considered first-line therapy, this change was based on data suggesting lower efficacy rates when treating chlamydial with azithromycin compared with doxycycline, with increased concern regarding rectal chlamydia.[30–32]

Despite resistance concerns, to date, ceftriaxone treatment failure in the United States has not been reported. If cephalosporins cannot be used, due to allergy or concern for resistance, the recommended alternate regimen is a single dose of 240 mg IM gentamicin in combination with 2 g oral azithromycin. While azithromycin as a single 2 g dose appears highly effective in eradicating both gonorrhea and chlamydia, it is not recommended as a preferred alternative due to concerns regarding resistance. GI side effects are common with the 2 g dose of azithromycin.[27,33]

Parenteral ceftriaxone is the recommended therapy for DGI, including meningitis and endocarditis, and any type of gonococcal infection in children. In DGI, patients should be hospitalized and treated with ceftriaxone or an alternative parenteral cephalosporin (see Table 140-4). Although marked improvement is usually noted within 48 hours of initiating therapy, treatment should be continued for at least 7 days, with longer durations necessary for serious infections, such as meningitis and endocarditis.[4] Gonococcal ophthalmia is highly contagious in adults and neonates and requires ceftriaxone therapy. Single, but higher, dose therapy is adequate for gonococcal conjunctivitis, although some physicians recommend continuing therapy until cultures are negative at 48 to 72 hours. Topical antibiotics are not effective when used alone for ocular infections and are unnecessary with appropriate systemic therapy. Infants with any evidence of ocular infection should be evaluated for signs of DGI.[4,34]

Treatment of gonorrhea during pregnancy is essential to prevent ophthalmia neonatorum. Pregnant women infected with *N. gonorrhoeae* should be treated with a single intramuscular dose of ceftriaxone 500 mg, with the addition of 1 g of oral azithromycin if chlamydia has not been ruled out. Fluoroquinolones and tetracyclines are contraindicated in pregnancy. Gonococcal infection in newborns results primarily from passage through an infected birth canal, but may be transmitted in utero. Conjunctival involvement, characterized by intense, bilateral conjunctival inflammation with chemosis, usually develops within 7 days of delivery. If not treated promptly, corneal ulceration and blindness can develop. Because the law in most states requires neonatal prophylaxis with topical ocular antimicrobials, gonococcal ophthalmia neonatorum is rare in the United States. The CDC recommends erythromycin (0.5%) ophthalmic ointment be instilled in each conjunctival sac immediately postpartum.[4,27,34]

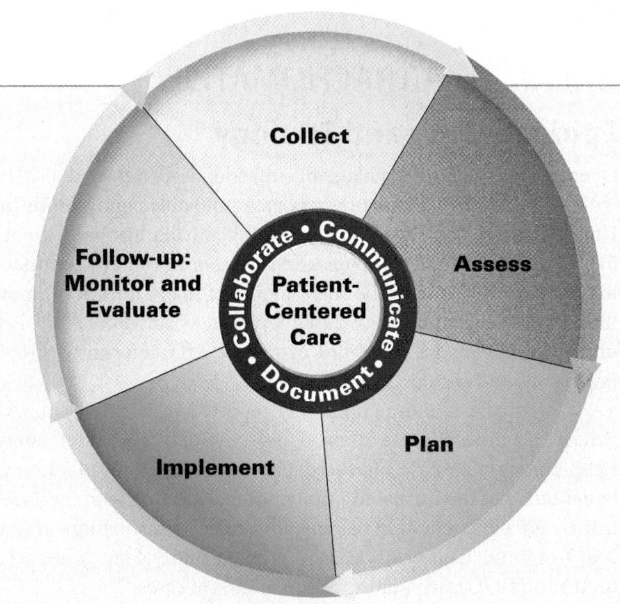

Patient Care Process for Genital Infection due to *Neisseria gonorrhoeae*

Collect

- Patient characteristics (eg, age, gender, pregnancy status)
- Patient medical history (personal and family)
- Social history, including sexual history
- Current medications
- Objective data
  - Blood pressure (BP), heart rate (HR), respiratory rate (RR), height, weight
  - Laboratory data including urine NAATs for gonorrhea and chlamydia, and/or urethral or vaginal cultures
  - Signs and symptoms consistent with gonorrhea (dysuria, mucopurulent urethral or vagina discharge)

Assess

- Presence of additional STIs (chlamydia, syphilis, HIV, etc.)
- Presence of extra-genital infection
- Ability/willingness to obtain follow-up testing as needed
- Ability/willingness to notify sexual partners
- Emotional status (eg, presence of anxiety, depression)

Plan

- Drug therapy regimen including, dose, route, frequency, and duration (Table 140-4)
- Monitoring parameters including efficacy (eg, retest 3 months after treatment) and safety, frequency and timing of follow-up
- Patient education (eg, purpose of treatment, notification of sexual partners, safe sexual practices, drug-specific information)
- Self-monitoring for resolution of gonorrhea symptoms, and seeking follow-up for a reevaluation if not resolved
- Referrals to other providers when appropriate (eg, HIV care, behavioral health)

Implement*

- Provide patient education regarding all elements of treatment plan
- Use motivational interviewing and coaching strategies to maximize adherence
- Schedule follow-up (eg, retest 3 months after treatment)
- Offer expedited partner therapy for patient's sexual partner(s) and partner education

Follow-up: Monitor and Evaluate

- Resolution of symptoms (eg, dysuria, mucopurulent urinary or vaginal discharge); in absence of symptom resolution after treatment, assess for resistance by obtaining culture and susceptibilities Presence of adverse effects (eg, rash or gastrointestinal [GI] upset)
- Patient adherence to treatment plan
- Reevaluation of laboratory tests in specific time frames (eg, retest after 3 months for retest)

Collaborate with patient, caregivers, and other healthcare professionals.

TABLE 140-4 Treatment of Gonorrhea

Type of Infection	Recommended Regimens[a]	Alternative Regimens[a]
Uncomplicated infections of the cervix, urethra, and rectum in adults	Ceftriaxone 500 mg IM once[b,c]	Gentamicin 240 mg IM[d] *plus* Azithromycin 2 g orally once *or* When ceftriaxone administration is not feasible, cefixime 800 mg orally once[c]
Uncomplicated infections of the pharynx	Ceftriaxone 500 mg IM once[b,c]	Consult with infectious disease expert
DGI in adults (>45 kg)	Ceftriaxone 1-2 g IM or IV every 12-24 hours[c,e]	Cefotaxime 1 g IV every 8 hours[c,e] or ceftizoxime 1 g IV every 8 hours[c,e]
Gonococcal conjunctivitis in adults	Ceftriaxone 1 g IM once[f]	
Ophthalmia neonatorum	Ceftriaxone 25-50 mg/kg IV or IM once (not to exceed 250 mg)	
Infants born to mothers with gonococcal infection (prophylaxis)	Erythromycin (0.5%) ophthalmic ointment in a single application[g] Ceftriaxone 25-50 mg/kg IM or IV once (not to exceed 125 mg)	

[a]Recommendations are those of the CDC.

[b]For patients weighing > 150 kg, a 1 g dose of ceftriaxone is recommended.

[c]If chlamydial infection cannot be ruled out, treatment for chlamydia should be administered. Preferred therapy is doxycycline 100 mg orally twice daily × 7 days. Azithromycin 1 g orally once may be used as an alternative. Tetracyclines are contraindicated during pregnancy. Pregnant women should be treated with recommended cephalosporin-based combination therapy. In severe cephalosporin allergy, consultation with an infectious diseases expert is recommended.

[d]For patients with severe cephalosporin allergy.

[e]Parenteral treatment duration should be determined in consultation with an infectious diseases expert. Gonococcal meningitis should be treated with ceftriaxone 2 g IV every 12 hours. Parenteral therapy for meningitis should be continued for at least 10 to 14 days and at least 4 weeks in endocarditis.

[f]A single lavage of the infected eye with normal saline should be considered; empiric therapy for *C. trachomatis* is recommended.

[g]Efficacy in preventing chlamydial ophthalmia is unclear.

Evaluation of Therapeutic Outcomes

Persistent symptoms following treatment with a recommended regimen often indicate reinfection rather than treatment failure, reflecting the need for improved patient education and sex partner referral. If reinfection is most likely, retreatment with the initial regimen is recommended. However, reinfection can no longer be assumed due to increased rates of drug resistance and subsequent treatment failure. True treatment failure should be considered in persons whose symptoms do not resolve within 3 to 5 days after appropriate treatment or who failed a TOC (positive culture 72 hours after or positive NAAT at least 7 days after receiving treatment) and abstained from sexual contact during the posttreatment 7-day follow-up period. The CDC recommends all treatment failures receive culture and sensitivity testing. Persistent symptoms may also be due to other infectious causes, such as *C. trachomatis*.[4,16,27]

While the CDC does not recommend a TOC for patients with uncomplicated urogenital or rectal gonorrhea treated, any patient treated for pharyngeal gonorrhea should return 7 to 14 days after treatment for a TOC. The TOC test may be either culture or NAAT; however, if the NAAT is positive, confirmatory culture should be obtained prior to retreatment. Antimicrobial susceptibilities should be obtained for all TOC positive cultures. Patients who require retreatment should receive TOC 7 to 14 days following the second regimen. Additionally, as reinfection within 12 months occurs in 7% to 12% of persons treated for gonorrhea, all patients who receive treatment for gonorrhea should be retested 3 months after treatment or when the patient next presents for medical care in the following 12 months.[4,35,36]

Recent sex partners (within 60 days of preceding onset of symptoms or diagnosis) should be referred for evaluation and treatment. The recommended EPT regimen for uncomplicated gonorrhea infections is a single oral dose of cefixime 800 mg, with the addition of oral doxycycline 100 mg twice daily for 7 days if chlamydia cannot be ruled out.[27] Patients and sex partners should abstain from unprotected sexual intercourse for 7 days after both have completed treatment and symptoms have resolved.[4] EPT is contraindicated for females experiencing signs or symptoms of PID and should seek prompt medical care. EPT should be used with caution among MSM due to high rates of co-infection of HIV and syphilis, and inadequate data regarding the EPT efficacy due to concerns of cefixime resistance rates in this population.

CHLAMYDIA TRACHOMATIS

Epidemiology and Etiology

Over 1.8 million cases of chlamydia infection were reported in 2019, making it the most frequently reported notifiable condition in the United States since 1994.[1] Since 2000, chlamydia has been a notifiable condition in all 50 states and infection rates have continued to rise. However, due to the silent nature of many infections, more than double the number of cases reported occur annually.[1,2] Left untreated, chlamydia infections can cause PID, infertility, ectopic pregnancy, and chronic pelvic pain.[4,37]

Chlamydia is more commonly reported in females, approximately 1.75 times the rate in males, reflective of increased screening. Rates among men have increased 32% from 2015 to 2019 and may be reflective of the increased number of male testing with increased urine and extragenital screening, increased transmission among MSM, or both.[1] Chlamydia is also a primary cause of nongonococcal urethritis (NGU), accounting for up to 40% of cases.[4,38,39]

Coinfection with chlamydia occurs in a substantial number of individuals with gonorrhea and all individuals diagnosed with *N. gonorrhoeae* should be assumed to have *C. trachomatis* present, until chlamydial infection has been ruled out.[4] Chlamydial infections, especially rectal infections, are associated with significantly increased risk of acquiring HIV infection.[40] In addition to genital infections, ocular infections in adults (via autoinoculation) and infants (via vaginal delivery through an infected birth canal) are reported. Pharyngeal and rectal infections may develop secondary to orogenital or receptive anal intercourse, respectively, with an infected individual.[4,37]

Pathophysiology

C. trachomatis is an obligate intracellular bacterium that exclusively infects humans, via infection of mucosal epithelial cells. Like viruses, chlamydiae require cellular material from host cells for replication and eventually lead to host cell death. *C. trachomatis* shares a similar outer membrane and ribosomes to gram-negative bacteria, but lacks cell-wall peptidoglycan, and cannot be detected via Gram staining. Their complex two-stage lifecycle includes an infectious and noninfectious forms, and even after treatment, nonviable and noninfectious organisms may persist within cells for up to 3 weeks.[37]

Risk of chlamydia transmission after exposure is not well described, but is believed to be less than that of *N. gonorrhoeae*. The risk of male-to-female and female-to-male transmission is 39% and

TABLE 140-5 Presentation of Chlamydia Infections

	Males	Females
General	Incubation period: 7-35 days Symptom onset: 7-21 days	Incubation period: 7-35 days Symptom onset: 7-21 days
Site of infection	Most common: urethra Others: rectum (receptive anal intercourse), oropharynx, eye	Most common: endocervical canal Others: urethra, rectum (usually caused by perineal contamination), oropharynx, eye
Symptoms	More than 50% of urethral and rectal infections are asymptomatic Urethral infection: mild dysuria, discharge Pharyngeal infection: asymptomatic to mild pharyngitis	More than 66% of cervical infections are asymptomatic Urethral infection: usually subclinical; dysuria and frequency uncommon Rectal and pharyngeal infection: symptoms same as for men
Signs	Scant to profuse, mucoid to purulent urethral or rectal discharge Rectal infection: pain, discharge, bleeding	Abnormal vaginal discharge or uterine bleeding, purulent urethral or rectal discharge can be scant to profuse
Complications	Epididymitis, Reiter's syndrome (rare)	PID and associated complications (ie, ectopic pregnancy, infertility) Reiter's syndrome (rare)

32%, respectively.[41] The rate of transmission per-act is 10%, increasing to 55% with multiple encounters between sexual partners.[42]

Clinical Presentation

Chlamydia causes a range of clinical syndromes, including urethritis, cervicitis, proctitis, and conjunctivitis. In comparison with gonorrhea, chlamydial genital tract infections are more frequently asymptomatic, and when present, symptoms tend to be less noticeable. Urethral discharge is usually less profuse and more mucoid or watery than that associated with gonorrhea.[4,37,38] Many cases of chlamydia in asymptomatic or minimally symptomatic women are diagnosed as a result of screening. Table 140-5 summarizes usual clinical presentations of chlamydial infections.

Chlamydia can be transmitted to an infant during contact with infected cervicovaginal secretions. Nearly two-thirds of infants acquire chlamydial infection after endocervical exposure, with primary morbidity associated with seeding of the infant's eyes, nasopharynx, rectum, or vagina. In exposed infants, neonatal conjunctivitis develops in as many as 50%, and pneumonia develops in up to 16%. Inclusion conjunctivitis in newborns is usually self-limited, but can result in scarring and micropannus of the cornea. Interstitial pneumonitis occurring secondary to carriage in the nasopharynx typically is mild, but it can be severe and require hospitalization.[4,37,43]

Diagnosis

Laboratory confirmation of chlamydial infection is important because of the relative lack of symptom specificity when present.[4] Cell culture is the reference standard against which all other diagnostic tests are measured. Because chlamydiae are obligate intracellular organisms, specimens for culture must be obtained from endocervical (women) or urethral (men) epithelial cell scrapings rather than from urine or urethral discharges. Although tissue culture techniques have close to 100% specificity, the sensitivity is as low as 70%. Because of the technical demands of specimen collection, transport, processing, expense, and prolonged time until results (3-7 days), culture is not widely used for diagnostic purposes. However, culture remains the diagnostic standard in medicolegal cases, such as sexual assault and child abuse because of its high specificity and ability to detect only viable organisms.[4,37]

Similar to gonorrheal testing, NAATs can be used to detect small amounts of chlamydial DNA or RNA, and are highly sensitive and specific for detecting infection in urine, urogenital, and anal specimens. As such, they are recommended for detecting chlamydia infection.[4] In 2019, NAATs were approved for diagnosis of chlamydial infection in extragenital sites including the pharynx and rectum.[26] Use of self-collected vaginal or anal specimens or first-void urine samples offers greater patient acceptability. Because NAATs can detect as little as a single-gene copy in a specimen, whether it is live or a nonviable organism, nucleic acid residues that persist following successful antibiotic therapy can result in a false-positive test for several weeks following cure. Molecular tests that do not use nucleic amplification are no longer recommended for diagnosis of *C. trachomatis* because of their poor sensitivity in comparison to NAATs.[4,25]

Because of the high rate of asymptomatic disease and the high prevalence of chlamydial infection in sexually active females 25 years of age or younger and sexually active women with new sex partners or multiple sex partners, the CDC and USPSTF recommends routine annual screening in these individuals.[4,27] Additionally, the CDC recommends routine, at least annual, chlamydia screening of genital and rectal sites in MSM populations. Screening for rectal chlamydia among MSMs may also be a cost-effective intervention for HIV prevention.[44] Pregnant women are recommended to be screened at the first prenatal visit and during the third trimester if at continued risk.[4]

TREATMENT

Many antimicrobials, including tetracyclines, macrolides, and some fluoroquinolones, display good *in vitro* and *in vivo* activity against *C. trachomatis*. In most clinical trials, cure rates exceed 90% for these agents.[4,36,37] Treatment of *C. trachomatis* is limited based on the organism's unique life cycle. Antibiotics must target the intracellular active form, requiring medications with good intracellular penetration. Additionally, to maintain concentrations throughout the organisms life-cycle (up to 48 hours), selection of an antibiotic with long half-life or prolonged course of therapy is important.

Previously, single-dose azithromycin 1 g orally and doxycycline 100 mg orally twice daily for 7 days was equally considered regimens of choice for treatment of uncomplicated urogenital chlamydia infections (Table 140-6).[4] Because of its prolonged serum and tissue half-life, azithromycin is the only single-dose therapy effective in treating *C. trachomatis*. Both therapies clear over 97% of urogenital infections; however, there are concerns regarding azithromycin efficacy in rectal chlamydia.[30-32,45-47] As rectal chlamydia may occur by autoinoculation from the vaginal tract and cannot be predicted by sexual activity, doxycycline is now preferred as first line. Additionally, doxycycline demonstrates better *in vitro* activity against *C. trachomatis*.[48] For those patients with adherence concerns, azithromycin may be used, but TOC after treatment is recommended. Although some fluoroquinolones have activity against *C. trachomatis*, high dosages have not consistently eradicated chlamydial infections.[4,37,38]

For pregnant women, treatment can significantly reduce the risk of pregnancy complications and newborn transmission. Because tetracyclines and fluoroquinolones are contraindicated during pregnancy, azithromycin is recommended (see Table 140-6). Due to concerns regarding persistence of chlamydia infections after exposure to penicillin-class antibiotics, amoxicillin is an alternative therapy

TABLE 140-6 Treatment of Chlamydia Infections

Infection	Recommended Regimens[a]	Alternative Regimens[a]
Uncomplicated urethral, endocervical, or rectal infection in adults	Doxycycline 100 mg orally twice daily for 7 days	Azithromycin 1 g orally once[b], *or* levofloxacin 500 mg orally once daily for 7 days
Urogenital infections during pregnancy	Azithromycin 1 g orally as a single dose	Amoxicillin 500 mg orally three times daily for 7 days
Conjunctivitis of the newborn or pneumonia in infants	Erythromycin base or ethylsuccinate 50 mg/kg/day orally in four divided doses for 14 days[c,d]	Azithromycin suspension 20 mg/kg/day orally once daily for 3 days[c]

[a]Recommendations are those of the CDC.

[b]Azithromycin may be used if there are concerns for nonadherence. Test after treatment is recommended due to reduced efficacy in rectal chlamydia.

[c]An association between oral erythromycin and azithromycin and infantile hypertrophic pyloric stenosis (IHPS) has been reported in infants aged <6 weeks. Infants treated with either of these antimicrobials should be followed for signs and symptoms of IHPS.

[d]Topical therapy alone is inadequate for ophthalmia neonatorum and is unnecessary when systemic therapy is administered. Effectiveness of erythromycin treatment is approximately 80%; therefore, a second course of therapy may be required.

only in pregnant women. When compliance with a multiday regimen is a concern, azithromycin is the preferred treatment in women, regardless of pregnancy status, and directly observed single-dose administration ensures adherence. TOC 3 to 4 weeks after completion should be obtained for pregnant patients treated for chlamydial infections.[4]

C. trachomatis transmission during perinatal exposure can result in neonatal or infant infections of the eye, oropharynx, lungs, urogenital tract, and rectum. Despite efficacy in preventing gonococcal ophthalmia, topical erythromycin ointment (0.5%) appears less effective in preventing chlamydial ophthalmia and has no effect on nasal carriage or colonization, so the potential for other infections, including pneumonia, remains. Because of high percentage of treatment failures, topical therapy is not recommended to treat ophthalmia caused by *C. trachomatis*. Instead, an oral erythromycin regimen is recommended.[4]

Evaluation of Therapeutic Outcomes

Treatment of chlamydial infections with recommended regimens is highly effective; therefore, posttreatment laboratory testing for therapeutic failure is not recommended unless symptoms persist or there are specific concerns (eg, regimen nonadherence or pregnancy). However, due to high risk of reinfection, all patients treated for chlamydia should be retested approximately 3 months after treatment. Posttreatment tests should not be performed for at least 3 weeks following completion of therapy due to false positives with continued presence of nonviable organisms.[4] When posttreatment tests are positive, suspect noncompliance, failure to treat sexual partners, or laboratory error rather than inadequate therapy or resistance. Infants with pneumonitis should receive follow-up testing, and sometimes subsequent courses of therapy, because erythromycin is only 80% effective.[4,37]

Sex partners of patients with *C. trachomatis* infections should be examined, tested for other STIs, and counseled on prevention. EPT may also be offered with either azithromycin or doxycycline-based regimens. Patients, and sex partners, should abstain from unprotected sexual intercourse for 7 days after both have completed treatment and symptoms have resolved.[4]

TRICHOMONIASIS

Epidemiology and Etiology

2 In 2018, 6.9 million people developed trichomoniasis in the United States, making it the most common nonviral STI. The prevalence is approximately 2.6 million, with 2.1% of US women aged 14 to 59 years infected at a given time.[2,5,49] The distribution of trichomoniasis is varied; women are six times more likely to be infected than men, with disproportionate infection among women 40 years of age or older (11%) and Black women (13%).[49] Men who have sex with women are at greater risk of trichomoniasis compared to MSM exclusively and are usually asymptomatic. The causative organism, *Trichomonas vaginalis*, is primarily transmitted through sexual contact although acquisition from inanimate objects is a theoretical possibility since the organism can survive for up to 3 hours in a wet environment.[50] Neonatal infections may also occur. Coinfection with other STIs is not unusual, and the inflammatory response produced by trichomoniasis increases the risk of acquiring HIV by at least 50%.[4,50–54]

Pathophysiology

Trichomonads typically infect the squamous epithelium of the genital tract. Extragenital sites are epidemiologically important because infection can persist and result in reinfection. After attachment to vaginal or urethral mucosa, trichomonads elicit an inflammatory response that manifests as discharge containing large numbers of PMNs.[50]

Clinical Presentation

Trichomonal infections are reported more commonly in women than in men. Most patients experience minimal or no symptoms, with untreated infections lasting years. The clinical presentation of trichomoniasis in males and females is presented in Table 140-7. Trichomoniasis is one of the principal infectious causes of vaginal discharge (in addition to bacterial vaginosis and vulvovaginal candidiasis). In both genders, trichomoniasis can manifest as urethral discharge and dysuria and should be considered in NGU. Rarely, *T. vaginalis* can lead to epididymitis, prostatitis, and/or infertility in men and PID in women. During pregnancy, it can cause preterm rupture of membranes, premature delivery, endometritis, and low-birth-weight neonates.[4,50]

Diagnosis

Testing for *T. vaginalis* should be performed on all women presenting with vaginal discharge and at least annually in women with HIV. Screening may be considered in settings of high prevalence (eg, STI clinic, correctional facilities) and for persons at increased risk for infection (eg, recent STI diagnosis, multiple sexual partners, transactional sex). *T. vaginalis* produces nonspecific symptoms that may be indistinguishable from bacterial vaginosis, which can be concomitantly present. Because *T. vaginalis* requires a pH range of 4.9 to 7.5 for survival, a vaginal discharge pH of greater than 5 usually indicates the presence of either *T. vaginalis* or *Gardnerella vaginalis*, a common cause of bacterial vaginosis. The simplest means of diagnosis is a wet mount of vaginal discharge where *T. vaginalis* is visualized via bright-field microscopy. Trichomoniasis is confirmed if characteristic pear-shaped, flagellated, motile organisms are observed. This technique is still readily used given its relative convenience for experienced personnel and low cost. However, the wet mount is only 51% to 65% sensitive, with lower sensitivities in men and women with low-grade, subacute, or chronic infections. Culture was the gold standard for trichomoniasis and is highly specific; however, these tests are labor intensive, expensive, not widely available, and have a long turnaround.[4,50,52–54]

TABLE 140-7 Presentation of Trichomonas Infections

	Males	Females
General	Incubation period: 3-28 days Organism can be detectable within 48 hours after exposure to infected partner	Incubation period: 3-28 days
Site of infection	Most common: urethra Others: rectum (usually caused by rectal intercourse in MSM), oropharynx, eye	Most common: endocervical canal Others: urethra, rectum (usually caused by perineal contamination), oropharynx, eye
Symptoms	Can be asymptomatic (more common in males than females) or minimally symptomatic Urethral discharge (clear to mucopurulent) Dysuria, pruritus	Can be asymptomatic or minimally symptomatic Scant to copious, typically malodorous vaginal discharge (50%-75%) and pruritus (worse during menses) Dysuria, dyspareunia (pain with sexual intercourse)
Signs	Urethral discharge	Vaginal discharge Vaginal pH 4.5-6 Inflammation/erythema of vulva, vagina, and/or cervix Urethritis
Complications	Epididymitis and chronic prostatitis (uncommon) Male infertility (decreased sperm motility and viability)	PID and associated complications (ie, ectopic pregnancy, infertility) Premature labor, premature rupture of membranes, and low-birth-weight neonates (neonatal infection risk is low) Cervical neoplasia

TABLE 140-8 Treatment of Trichomoniasis

Type	Recommended Regimens[a]	Alternative Regimens[d]
Symptomatic and asymptomatic infections	Women Metronidazole 500 mg orally twice daily for 7 days[a,b,c] Men Metronidazole 2 g orally in a single dose[b,c]	Tinidazole 2 g orally in a single dose
Persistent or recurrent infections	Metronidazole 2 g orally once daily for 7 days *or* timidazole 2 g orally once daily for 7 days	
Treatment in pregnancy[e]	Metronidazole 500 mg orally twice daily for 7 days[c]	

[a]Recommendations are those of the CDC.

[b]Randomized controlled trial comparing metronidazole 500 mg twice daily for 7 days and a single 2 g dose in women found fewer treatment failures in the 7-day regimen.

[c]Metronidazole labeling approved by the FDA does not include this regimen. Dosage regimens for treatment of trichomoniasis included in the product labeling are the single 2 g dose; 250 mg three times daily for 7 days; and 375 mg twice daily for 7 days. The 250-mg and 375-mg dosage regimens are currently not included in the CDC recommendations.

[d]For men, data are lacking for alternative treatment regimens and regimens for persistent infection. Consult an infectious diseases specialist.

[e]Symptomatic pregnant women can be treated with this regimen at any stage of pregnancy.

Newer diagnostic tests are now widely available, with the sensitivities approaching those of culture techniques. NAAT are FDA-approved for *T. vaginalis* detection in vaginal, endocervical or urine specimens in women and is three to five times more sensitive than wet mount microscopy (95%-100%). In men, urethral swab specimens may yield a higher sensitivity than urine.[50,55] Rapid point of care tests are also readily available, allowing for office-based testing. Sensitivity among these tests can vary and might be higher in symptomatic women.[4,52–55]

TREATMENT

3 Recommended and alternative treatment regimens for *T. vaginalis* include either metronidazole or tinidazole (Table 140-8).[4] Metronidazole 500 mg twice daily for 7 days was more effective than 2 g single-dose regimen.[56] Increasing the dose for either agent to 2 g once daily for 7 days cures persistent infections. Adding topical metronidazole or tinidazole may improve efficacy during persistent infection. Tinidazole 2 g orally as a single dose is an alternative for women. Single-dose therapy with 2 g of metronidazole or tinidazole are recommended for men with trichomoniasis. To achieve maximal cure rates and prevent relapse, simultaneous treatment of infected sexual partners for presumed infection is recommended.[4,52–54]

In patients who fail to respond to an initial course of metronidazole therapy, a second course of therapy with metronidazole 500 mg twice daily for 7 days is recommended. Infections refractory to a second course of treatment often respond to a 2 g daily 7-day regimen of either agent.[4,57] Tinidazole should be considered after failure to a 7-day metronidazole regimen given its longer half-life, greater serum concentrations, and a lower minimum lethal concentration demonstrated in 60% of *T. vaginalis* isolates compared to metronidazole.[58] The combination of oral and intravaginal administration improves cure rates in refractory cases. There are higher rates of resistance with metronidazole (4%-10%) versus tinidazole (1%); however, resistance testing is not routinely performed by most laboratories. In persistent cases, consultation with the CDC is recommended for treatment and resistance testing.[53,59]

Metronidazole is associated with a risk of a disulfiram-like reaction, although published data have not supported this claim. *In vitro* and animal data described a possible inhibition of aldehyde dehydrogenase and subsequent increase in acetaldehyde levels, which can cause facial flushing, nausea, vomiting, and other symptoms. Although there are considerable human data describing disulfiram-like reactions after concomitant metronidazole and alcohol use, these manifestations may be attributed directly to alcohol. Most controlled studies failed to find an association between metronidazole with alcohol use and disulfiram-like reactions.[60] The updated CDC guidelines do not link metronidazole use with the potential for a disulfiram-like reaction in those that consume alcohol concurrently.[4]

The CDC recommends testing all symptomatic pregnant women for *T. vaginalis*, regardless of pregnancy stage, and to consider treatment. Concerns regarding the use of metronidazole in pregnant women and breastfeeding have been raised. Some clinicians prefer to delay treatment in women in the first trimester; however, metronidazole is pregnancy category B and may be used for treatment in any trimester. Tinidazole is pregnancy category C and should be avoided. Both agents are secreted in breast milk, although metronidazole is indicated for use in neonates and infants. Metronidazole concentrations in breast milk were deemed compatible with breastfeeding when the mother was given 500 mg three times daily, while 2-g dose warrants a 12 to 24 hour breastfeeding pause. Careful monitoring of breastfed child is recommended with metronidazole treatment of the mother. Breastfeeding should be deferred for 72 hours after a 2-g dose of tinidazole.[4,52]

Evaluation of Therapeutic Outcomes

Retesting for *T. vaginalis* is recommended for all sexually active women within 3 months following initial treatment due to high rates of reinfection. If retesting with NAAT is clinically warranted without reexposure (eg, third trimester), the optimal timing to prevent a false-positive is 3 weeks. Concurrent treatment of all sex partners is critical to ensure relief of symptoms and prevent reinfection and transmission. When patients remain symptomatic, it is important to ensure patient adherence and to determine if reinfection has occurred. In these cases, a repeat course of therapy, including sexual partner(s) is indicated. In situations where reinfection can be excluded, a relative resistance to metronidazole or tinidazole should be assumed, and an alternative regimen prescribed. Culture and sensitivity are warranted for infections unresponsive to alternative regimens.[4]

ASSOCIATED COMPLICATIONS

Mycoplasma Genitalium

Of notable importance is *Mycoplasma genitalium* infection, a common cause of NGU. The CDC has identified *M. genitalium* infections as an emerging issue due to the increasing rates of resistance and lack of diagnostic assays.[4,19,61,62]

M. genitalium is a known colonizer of the genital tract in both males and females; however, it is an emerging cause of urogenital infections.[4,19,61,62] While *C. trachomatis* accounts for a majority of NGU cases, *M. genitalium* is the causative pathogen in up to 20% of NGU cases and 25% of nonchlamydial NGU. Rates are even higher in persistent or recurrent NGU, constituting approximately 30% of cases.[4] The relationship between *M. genitalium* and other male anogenital tract infections, like epididymitis or clinical proctitis, is not well defined. The pathogenic role is even less defined in women, as infections are commonly asymptomatic, but has been isolated in up to 30% of cervical infections. However, women infected with *M. genitalium* are at a 2 to 2.5-fold increased risk of cervicitis, PID, infertility, and preterm delivery.[61] Many infections go undiagnosed, but *M. genitalium* should be suspected in persistent or recurrent urethritis or proctitis and considered in persistent or recurrent cervicitis or PID.[4,19,61,62] There are no current recommendations for routine screening in asymptomatic individuals.

M. genitalium lacks a cell wall and is a slow growing, fastidious organism. It is not readily cultured in a laboratory and, when able to grow, may take up to 6 months to isolate. NAATs are the preferred method to detect *M. genitalium*.[19,63]

The 7-day doxycycline regimen, a primary treatment option for NGU, is largely ineffective for treatment of *M. genitalium* urethritis, with a median cure rate of 31%.[4] A 1 g single dose of azithromycin was significantly more effective than doxycycline, and has been the mainstay of therapy for *M. genitalium* infections.[4,19,61,62] Unfortunately, resistance to azithromycin is rapidly emerging, with 50% of all *M. genitalium* infections caused by organisms already resistant to azithromycin. The overuse of macrolides to treat respiratory tract infections, like community acquired pneumonia, may play a role in azithromycin resistance seen in *M. genitalium*. Moxifloxacin, 400 mg daily for 7, 14, or 21 days, has been successfully used to eradicate *M. genitalium* infections.[61,62] To optimize chance of treatment success, CDC STI guidelines recommend doxycycline 100 mg twice daily for 7 days followed by moxifloxacin 400 mg daily for 7 days.[4,64] Macrolide susceptibility testing is unavailable in the United States. If macrolide susceptibility is known, a regimen of doxycycline 100 mg twice daily for 7 days followed by azithromycin 1 g and then 500 mg daily for 3 days is an alternative option. For those with unknown or known macrolide resistance, the doxycycline-moxifloxacin regimen is preferred.

As with all STIs, patients are recommended to abstain from unprotected sexual activity until both partners have completed treatment and are asymptomatic. Additionally, patients and their sexual partners should be screened for other STIs and counseled on risk of transmission and consequences of untreated infections. If a patient's sexual partner is not tested, the same treatment may be offered to both.[62]

Pelvic Inflammatory Disease

PID is an inflammatory disorder of the upper female genital tract and can include any combination of endometritis, salpingitis, tubo-ovarian abscess, and pelvic peritonitis that may result in long-term reproductive damage, including infertility, ectopic pregnancy, and chronic pelvic pain. It is most often caused by ascending infection of the vagina and cervix, most commonly with STI pathogens. Microorganisms that colonize the vaginal canal may also play a role, including anaerobes or causes of bacterial vaginitis, as well as enteric gram-negative rods. The microbiologic etiology of acute PID is not well known. Where gonorrhea or chlamydia were once thought to be the primary cause, <50% of women with acute PID test positive for one of these organisms. The role of *M. genitalium* is unclear, but testing was unavailable for this organism until recently and may be considered in persistent cases.[4,20]

Acute PID is difficult to diagnose as many patients may be asymptomatic or have subtle, nonspecific symptoms. PID is often diagnosed based on clinical findings and confirmed with more invasive testing. Delays in diagnosis and treatment likely contribute to inflammatory sequelae and long-term reproductive damage. The hallmark sign of PID is sudden onset pelvic and lower abdominal pain, notably after menses. Additional signs may include abnormal vaginal discharge, intermenstrual or postcoital bleeding, dyspareunia, and dysuria. All patients with suspected PID should undergo cervical or vaginal NAAT testing for gonorrhea or chlamydia. Vaginal fluid may also be evaluated for signs of bacterial vaginosis. Negative endocervical screening does not rule out upper reproductive tract infections, but positive results may help guide therapy.[4,20]

4 Treatment for PID is targeted toward empiric coverage for *N. gonorrhoeae* and *C. trachomatis* and anaerobic bacteria. Patients with suspected PID should be initiated on treatment with ceftriaxone 1 g IV daily (or cefotetan 2 g IV every 12 hours or cefoxitin 2 g IV every 6 hours) plus doxycycline 100 mg orally twice daily for 14 days and metronidazole 500 mg orally twice daily for 14 days.[65] The addition of metronidazole resulted in reduced pelvic pain and was associated with higher clinical improvement compared to ceftriaxone and doxycycline alone. This is an update from the previous guideline recommendations and aligns with current gonorrhea and chlamydia treatment recommendations.[4] Patients who require hospitalization for PID should be initiated on a parenteral regimen. Once the patient is clinically stable and can tolerate oral medications, they can be switched to oral formulations to complete two weeks of therapy. Ampicillin-sulbactam 3 g IV every 6 hours plus doxycycline can be used as an alternative. Clindamycin 900 mg IV every 8 hours plus gentamicin IV is another alternative treatment regimen, but provides suboptimal coverage for anaerobic organisms.[4,66,67]

Clinical improvement (defervescence, reduction in abdominal/pelvic pain) should occur within 3 days of initiation of therapy. Intrauterine contraceptive devices (IUD) have not been associated with PID, outside of the initial 3 months after insertion. If an IUD user is diagnosed with PID, the IUD does not need to be removed, but may be considered if the patient does not show clinical improvement within 72 hours.[4] All patients with confirmed gonorrheal or chlamydial PID should be retested 3 months after treatment. Recent sex partners should also be evaluated and presumptively treated for chlamydia and gonorrhea, regardless of the etiology of PID.

EPT may be offered and partners should be instructed to abstain from sexual intercourse until both partners have been treated and symptoms have resolved. Approximately one-third of women report chronic pelvic pain after treatment and resolution of PID. Infertility may occur in up to 20% of patients and ectopic pregnancy in <1%.[68] Routine screening for gonorrhea and chlamydia as recommended by the USPSTF and CDC, and early recognition of symptoms may help reduce the burden of disease.[4,27]

SYPHILIS

Epidemiology and Etiology

Syphilis is a chronic bacterial infection that presents through various stages. Although nearly eradicated in 2000, cases of syphilis have increased 400% in the United States from 2000 to 2019, with an annual total of primary and secondary syphilis diagnoses of around 39,000. While the rise of newly diagnosed cases are primarily attributed to males, a majority of whom identify as MSM, a 179% increase was observed in women during the years 2015 to 2019.[1] This increase among women has been accompanied by a threefold rise in congenital syphilis during the same period.[69] In 2018, one-third of congenital syphilis cases in live-born infants were symptomatic, while 6% of maternal syphilis cases resulted in stillbirth.[69]

Rates of coinfection with HIV have remained high, particularly among MSM. Similar to other STIs, syphilis can increase the risk of acquiring HIV in exposed individuals. In addition, immunologic defects in HIV-infected individuals can produce an atypical serologic response to syphilis. In particular, the possibility of delayed seroreactivity, markedly elevated serologic titers, and increased false-positive results could complicate the diagnosis, as well as assessment of treatment efficacy in HIV-positive individuals infected with syphilis. As a result of this association, the CDC recommends that all patients diagnosed with syphilis be tested for HIV infection.[4,70]

Pathophysiology

The causative organism is *Treponema pallidum* subspecies *pallidum*, a spirochete. The primary mode of transmission is through sexual contact, with the organism penetrating through intact mucous membrane or a break in the cornified epithelium. The spirochetes replicate locally, followed by widespread dissemination through the lymphatic and intravascular systems. Transmissibility varies based on the stage of the infection, with the highest rates early in the course of disease. *T. pallidum* can also cross the placenta during any time of the pregnancy and during any stage of infection. Despite the limited risk of transmission after the first few years, approximately one-third of those are untreated will develop further clinical manifestations and irreversible complications, such as neurological and cardiovascular complications.[70]

Clinical Presentation

The clinical presentation of syphilis is varied with progression through multiple stages possible in untreated or inadequately treated patients (Table 140-9).

TABLE 140-9 Presentation of Syphilis Infections

General	
Primary	Incubation period: 10-90 days (mean, 21 days)
Secondary	Develops 2-8 weeks after initial infection in untreated or inadequately treated individuals
Latent	Develops 4-10 weeks after secondary stage in untreated or inadequately treated individuals; risk of secondary stage relapse within the first year
Neurosyphilis	Neuroinvasion can occur at any stage (weeks to years)
Tertiary	Develops in approximately 28% of untreated or inadequately treated individuals 10-30 years after initial infection
Site of Infection	
Primary	Genital or external genitalia area (perineum, mouth, throat)
Secondary	Multisystem involvement secondary to hematogenous and lymphatic spread
Neurosyphilis	Meninges, cerebral vasculature, brain parenchyma, eyes, ears
Tertiary	CNS, heart, bones, and joints
Signs and Symptoms	
Primary	Single, painless, indurated lesion (chancre) that erodes, ulcerates, and eventually heals (typical); regional lymphadenopathy is common; multiple, painful, purulent and/or multiple lesions possible
Secondary	Pruritic or nonpruritic rash (may involve the palms and soles), mucocutaneous lesions, flu-like symptoms, lymphadenopathy
Latent	Asymptomatic
Neurosyphilis	Meningitis (headache, photophobia, stiff neck), general paresis, stroke, dementia, ocular (blindness, blurred vision, eye pain) and otic (deafness, imbalance) complications
Tertiary	Cardiovascular syphilis (aortitis or aortic insufficiency), gummatous lesions involving any organ or tissue

CNS, central nervous system.

Primary Syphilis

The primary stage, characterized by a chancre on cutaneous or mucocutaneous tissue exposed to the organism, is highly infectious. Lesions are usually painless, solitary and indurated, although they may be painful and/or present as multiple lesions. Regional lymphadenopathy may accompany the chancre. Syphilis should be considered with atypical presentations as lesions can mimic other infectious or noninfectious etiologies. As such, appropriate diagnostic testing is important. Chancres heal within 4 to 6 weeks, while lymphadenopathy may persist longer.[70–72]

Secondary Syphilis

Often referred to as the "great imitator" due to its florid and diverse differential diagnosis, the secondary stage of syphilis is characterized by a variety of mucocutaneous eruptions resulting from widespread hematogenous and lymphatic spread of *T. pallidum*. Skin lesions are often maculopapular and are usually nonpruritic, developing first on trunk and proximal arms and disseminating bilaterally. Secondary syphilis lesions typically involve the palms and soles, can present as mucous patches, and/or can have a wart-like appearance (condylomata lata). Patchy alopecia is another finding periodically seen.

Constitutional symptoms often accompany secondary syphilis, such as malaise, low-grade fever, pharyngitis, headache, anorexia, and generalized lymphadenopathy. Subclinical hepatitis, renal dysfunction, and neurologic findings may also be present. If untreated, secondary syphilis disappears spontaneously within 1 to 6 months.[70–72]

Latent Syphilis

Persons with an absence of mucocutaneous lesions or other evidence of disease are in a latency period, which can only be diagnosed with positive serologic tests for syphilis. Prior to the availability of effective treatment, 25% of those infected developed secondary syphilis relapses, 90% of which occurred within the first year.[73] These individuals are thus deemed potentially infectious during this early period. By CDC terminology for the latent infection, the first year after acquisition is designated as early latent (or non primary, non secondary) syphilis.[74] Those with asymptomatic infection established to be over 12 months from exposure, or when a duration cannot be determined, are classified as late latent syphilis (or late or unknown duration syphilis). If left untreated, syphilis can slowly produce an inflammatory reaction in virtually any organ in the body. Most patients with late syphilis will have no further sequelae. However, approximately 28% will develop further disease years after the initial infection.[70-72]

Neurosyphilis

Neurologic manifestations, including ocular and otic, may present at any stage of syphilis. Central nervous system (CNS) invasion by treponemes can lead to cerebrospinal fluid abnormalities (eg, pleocytosis, elevated protein levels) in up to half of the individuals with early infections, with the majority being devoid of symptoms (asymptomatic neurosyphilis). Some patients will have meningeal symptoms (eg, headache, photophobia, stiff neck) present in early infection. Meningovascular (eg, stroke, seizures) or parenchymal (eg, dementia, aphasia) are other complications of neuroinvasion, which at times may overlap. The latter manifestations are more apt to occur years after infection, although strokes have been described early in disease. Ocular findings, especially uveitis, can be part of the neurological presentation. Hearing loss and/or vestibular dysfunction (eg, dizziness, vertigo) are rare, although syphilis should be considered for patients presenting with these complaints.[70,71]

Tertiary Syphilis

Non neurologic manifestations of late syphilis include benign gumma formation and cardiovascular syphilis. Gummas, nonspecific granulomatous lesions, are the classic lesions of late syphilis and can infiltrate any organ or tissue. Gummas of critical organs, such as the heart or brain, can be fatal. Cardiovascular disease often manifests as aortic insufficiency, ascending aortic aneurysm or myocarditis. Treatment of all patients with latent syphilis is essential, as there is no way to predict which patients will experience disease progression.[70]

Congenital Syphilis

In pregnant women with syphilis, *T. pallidum* can cross the placenta at any time during pregnancy. The risk of fetal infection is greatest in pregnant women with primary and secondary syphilis and declines in pregnant women with late disease. Transmission of syphilis during pregnancy occurs primarily transplacentally and can result in fetal death, prematurity, or congenital syphilis. Symptoms vary based on onset, with early congenital manifestations appearing from 2 weeks to 2 years, and late syphilis symptoms appearing after 2 years throughout adolescence. Manifestations of early congenital syphilis resemble those of secondary syphilis, in addition to other findings, notably hemolytic anemia, hepatic dysfunction, intrauterine growth retardation, bone deformities, or nephrotic syndrome. Deformities of the nose (saddle nose) and lower extremities (anterior bowing) are examples of untreated late syphilis complications.[70,72]

Diagnosis

Syphilis is diagnosed through a combination of clinical and/or laboratory criteria and is stage-dependent. Techniques used to directly visualize *T. pallidum*, such as darkfield microscopy, are now only performed by select facilities (eg, STI specialty clinics). Polymerase chain reaction (PCR)–based tests are used by some institutions despite not being commercially available in the United States. Unlike other methods, PCR does not require specimens from fresh lesions or tissue samples. Real-time PCR can detect *T. pallidum* DNA when primary syphilis is highly suspected, even when darkfield microscopy is negative.[75] PCR is also useful for detection in other bodily fluids and tissues.[70,71]

Serologic tests are the mainstay in the diagnosis and are based on two distinct antibody responses elicited by syphilis. Tests are categorized as nontreponemal or treponemal based on the type of antibodies they detect. Nontreponemal tests identify immunoglobulin released by inflamed tissues and/or *T. pallidum* by forming immune complexes with the reagent. Rapid plasma reagin (RPR) card test is the most common nontreponemal test. The Venereal Disease Research Laboratory (VDRL) slide test, another nontreponemal test, is almost exclusively used for CSF specimens. A positive RPR test can indicate the presence of any stage of syphilis or congenital syphilis if taken at least 3 weeks after exposure. RPR tests are simple and inexpensive, but require manual manipulation and interpretation.[70]

Beyond their screening role, RPR tests help monitor syphilis progression, treatment success, and identify reinfection as they measure *T. pallidum* antibody titers. Higher titers (eg, 1:512) correlate with a greater spirochetal burden and stage of infection. In 1% to 2% of secondary syphilis cases, the high concentrations of antibodies prevent the antigen–antibody complex from forming, leading to a false-negative. This phenomenon is called the "prozone" effect. Titers generally decline by at least fourfold after effective treatment (eg, 1:64 → 1:16), with only 20% of individuals failing to serorevert to a nonreactive test. Thus, strategic sequential RPR tests are an integral part of syphilis management. Access to previous diagnosis and treatment history is often necessary to determine if reinfection has occurred.[4,70,71,75]

In diagnosing all stages of syphilis, treponemal tests are more sensitive and specific than nontreponemal tests. Cost has contributed to their role as confirmatory tests rather than screening tools. Treponemal tests detect antibodies specific against *T. pallidum* antigens, which persist throughout a person's lifetime after infection. This test cannot distinguish between a new or past infection, nor treatment status. They can identify syphilis 6 to 14 days after a chancre develops, earlier than RPR tests (10-15 days). For many years, the fluorescent treponemal antibody absorption (FTA-ABS) test or the *T. pallidum* particle agglutination assay (TPPA) were the most frequently used treponemal tests. However, enzyme-linked immunoassays (EIAs) and chemiluminescent immunoassays (CIAs) are increasingly utilized as these processes are cheaper and allow for automated testing and interpretation. Advances in point of care could further remove challenges for screening and diagnosing syphilis, especially in rural and resource-limited areas.[4,70,71,75]

The traditional algorithm for diagnosing syphilis involves an initial RPR test, followed by a treponemal test for confirmation if the RPR was reactive. For individuals with a previously treated infection, presenting with new clinical suspicion of syphilis (or being screened due to high risk of re-exposure), a new RPR test should be collected. RPR results should be compared to their last titer. A fourfold or greater increase would suggest reinfection.[4,70,72,76]

For many laboratories with high volumes and programs screening large numbers (eg, prenatal screening), a reverse sequence algorithm is now a viable option. This strategy uses a treponemal test for the initial screen, with a positive test reflexively followed by an RPR test. If there is discordance with the RPR test, a second treponemal test distinct from the initial product would resolve the discrepancy. The availability of EIAs/CIAs for high throughput at increasingly lower costs have made this algorithm more attractive economically and logistically. Products testing for multiple pathogens, such as a point of care dual syphilis and HIV-1 test, have been approved and are in development.

False-positive tests occur more commonly with non treponemal tests than treponemal ones, and can cause anxiety, stigmatization and unnecessary treatment. Acute febrile illnesses, after immunizations, pregnancy, injection drug use, hepatitis C infection, HIV, and autoimmune disease (particularly lupus erythematosus) can induce these false-positives. Regardless of which test is used initially, confirmation with the other type is necessary for the diagnosis. If the nontreponemal test is negative after a positive treponemal test during a reverse algorithm screening, a second treponemal test based on a different antigen than the original test should be performed to adjudicate the results.[4,70,72,76]

Taking an accurate and careful history is important when considering a syphilis diagnosis, particularly when lesions are not present or missed early in disease. Missed identification of primary lesions delay diagnosis and may lead to uncertainty when patients present in later stages, particularly given the wide range of syphilis manifestations. In latent disease, early non primary, non secondary syphilis can be differentiated from late or unknown duration syphilis if within the past 12 months an individual: had a negative RPR result, recent primary or secondary syphilis without current symptoms, a sex partner diagnosed with primary or secondary syphilis or a fourfold increase in RPR titers from a previously treated infection.[4,70]

A lumbar puncture is recommended for those with neurologic findings at any stage. A confirmatory diagnosis in those with a reactive VDRL from a CSF specimen of a patient with consistent clinical picture. However, a probable diagnosis can be made if there are neurologic symptoms, a positive serum RPR test and CSF abnormalities. A lumbar puncture is not required for diagnosis of ocular and otic syphilis as it yields an unremarkable CSF result in 30% and 90% of ocular and otic syphilis, respectively. For tertiary syphilis, diagnosis requires a clinically compatible case with microbiologic identification or a positive treponemal test.[4,70]

Maternal and congenital screening recommendations vary by state, with most requiring testing at the first prenatal visit. Some states mandate testing at the third trimester and/or delivery, whereas others recommend testing only for women at increased risk (eg, recreational drug use, STI diagnosis during pregnancy, high prevalence areas, or partner(s) with HIV). Additional maternal risk factors include multiple partners (regardless of HIV status), engaging in transactional sex, late or no prenatal care, incarceration, and unstable housing or homelessness. A congenital syphilis diagnosis can be made if the mother has untreated or inadequately treated syphilis at delivery or a reactive treponemal result of the infant/child with clinical findings or a positive RPR test.[4,69,70]

TREATMENT

Table 140-10 presents the CDC's treatment recommendations.[3] 5 Parenteral penicillin G is the treatment of choice for all stages of syphilis. Because *T. pallidum* multiplies slowly, single doses of short- or intermediate-acting penicillins do not provide the prolonged, low-level exposure to penicillin required for treponeme eradication. As a result, benzathine penicillin G is the only penicillin effective for single-dose therapy.[4,70]

The recommended treatment for syphilis of less than 1 year's duration is benzathine penicillin G 2.4 million units as a single IM dose. In patients with late syphilis (including those with tertiary syphilis) or of unknown duration, benzathine penicillin G is administered weekly for three successive doses.[4] There is limited data regarding the questionable benefit of additional doses of benzathine penicillin G (or any other antibiotics) for later stages of syphilis.

Neurosyphilis requires more intensive therapy. The preferred regimen is 18 to 24 million units of IV penicillin G per day, administered as 3 to 4 million units every 4 hours or by continuous infusion, for 10 to 14 days. Intramuscular procaine penicillin G 2.4 million units once daily plus probenecid 500 mg orally four times daily is another option when IV administration is not feasible, such as outpatient treatment requiring a peripherally inserted central catheter (PICC) placement. Benzathine penicillin G alone in standard weekly doses does not consistently provide treponemicidal levels in the CSF, resulting in treatment failures. Because *T. pallidum* penicillin resistance has not emerged, the primary need for alternative drugs in treating syphilis is for penicillin-allergic patients.[4]

Alternative regimens recommended for penicillin-allergic patients are doxycycline 100 mg orally twice daily or tetracycline 500 mg orally four times daily for 2 to 4 weeks depending on the duration of syphilis infection. Parenteral ceftriaxone is another option, particularly because there is a low propensity of cross-reactivity between penicillin and cephalosporins. Ceftriaxone 1 g IV for 10 days was superior to two weekly doses of benzathine penicillin G.[77] In neurosyphilis, ceftriaxone 2 g daily for at least 10 days was as effective as IV penicillin G.[78] Clinicians may avoid ceftriaxone if the penicillin reaction was IgE-mediated or life-threatening (eg, Stevens Johnson Syndrome). Various other beta-lactams have been successfully used to treat syphilis; however, none offer significant advantage over benzathine penicillin G. Azithromycin 2 g as a single dose is no longer recommended due to increasing and unpredictable rates of resistance. Tetracyclines and ceftriaxone should be reserved for cases of documented penicillin allergy and, given concerns regarding patient compliance with these regimens, follow-up serologic testing is particularly important.[4]

For pregnant patients, penicillin is the treatment of choice at the dosage recommended for adults with that particular stage of syphilis. Some clinicians administer an additional IM dose of benzathine penicillin G 2.4 million units 1 week after completion of the recommended regimen, although there is no literature supporting this practice. In women allergic to penicillin, safe and effective alternatives are not available; therefore, skin testing should be performed to confirm a penicillin allergy. Women with positive penicillin skin tests may undergo penicillin desensitization and receive the appropriate treatment regimen for their stage of disease.[4]

Patients treated for primary and secondary syphilis may experience an acute reaction characterized by flu-like symptoms, such as transient headache, fever, chills, malaise, arthralgia, myalgia, tachypnea, peripheral vasodilation, and aggravation of syphilitic lesions, called the Jarisch-Herxheimer reaction. It usually begins within 6 to 8 hours of initiating therapy and lasts 12 to 24 hours. The exact mechanism of the reaction is unknown, although proposed etiologies, including immunologic mechanisms and release of endotoxin or other toxic treponemal products, are not substantiated. The Jarisch-Herxheimer reaction is independent of the drug and dose used and should not be confused with penicillin allergy. Most reactions can be managed symptomatically with analgesics, antipyretics, and rest. Steroids and antihistamines have been administered prior to initiation of syphilitic therapy, but are of limited value.[4,70]

Evaluation of Therapeutic Outcomes

Table 140-10 lists the CDC recommendations for serologic follow-up of patients treated for syphilis.[4] Quantitative nontreponemal tests (eg, RPR) should be performed at 6 and 12 months in all patients treated for primary, secondary, and early non-primary, non-secondary syphilis and at 6, 12, and 24 months for late disease or when duration is unknown. In general, the time to reach seronegativity is proportional to the duration of the disease. Serologic cure is defined by a drop in nontreponemal titers by at least fourfold by 12 months in those treated within a year of infection and by 24 months if the time of exposure cannot be determined or treatment 12 months after infection. Table 140-10 also includes specific testing recommendations for other stages of syphilis. Despite appropriate therapy, about 15% to 20% of patients fail to mount a sufficient antibody titer response. There is limited guidance on the best course of action when this occurs. If the titers were initially low at the time of treatment (eg, 1:2, 1:4), a twofold decline or no change may dictate additional serologic follow-up without retreatment.[4,70,72]

When retreatment is indicated, individuals should receive three weekly treatments of 2.4 million units of IM benzathine penicillin G, excluding neurosyphilis. Retreatment may be indicated when an alternate treatment was used initially, such as doxycycline in a

TABLE 140-10 Drug Therapy and Follow-up of Syphilis

Stage/Type of Syphilis	Recommended Regimens[a,b]	Follow-up Serology
Primary, secondary, or early latent syphilis (<1 year's duration)	Adults: Benzathine penicillin G 2.4 million units IM in a single dose Children: Benzathine penicillin G 50,000 units/kg IM in a single dose, up to 2.4 million units	Quantitative nontreponemal tests at 6 and 12 months, with failure if titer does not decrease at least fourfold in 12 months[c]
Late latent syphilis (>1 year's duration), syphilis of unknown duration, tertiary syphilis or retreatment after failure	Adults: Benzathine penicillin G 2.4 million units IM once a week for 3 successive weeks (7.2 million units total) Children: Benzathine penicillin G 50,000 units/kg IM once a week for 3 successive weeks, up to 7.2 million units total	Quantitative nontreponemal tests at 6, 12, and 24 months, with failure if titer does not decrease at least fourfold in 24 months[c]
Neurosyphilis, including ocular or otic involvement	Aqueous crystalline penicillin G 18-24 million units IV (3-4 million units every 4 hours or by continuo us infusion) for 10-14 days[d,f] *or* Aqueous procaine penicillin G 2.4 million units IM daily plus probenecid 500 mg orally four times daily, both for 10-14 days	Repeat CSF examination is no longer required at 6 months if adequate RPR response (decrease by fourfold or greater)
Congenital syphilis (infants with proven or highly probable disease)	Aqueous crystalline penicillin G 50,000 units/kg/dose IV every 12 hours during the first 7 days of life and every 8 hours thereafter for a total of 10 days *or* Procaine penicillin G 50,000 units/kg IM daily for 10 days[d]	Serologic follow-up only recommended if antimicrobials other than penicillin are used
Penicillin-Allergic Patients[e,f]		
Primary, secondary, or early latent syphilis	Doxycycline 100 mg orally two times daily for 14 days *or* Tetracycline 500 mg orally four times daily for 14 days *or* Ceftriaxone 1-2 g IM or IV daily for 10-14 days	Same as for non–penicillin-allergic patients
Late latent syphilis (>1 year's duration) or syphilis of unknown duration	Doxycycline 100 mg orally twice a day for 28 days *or* Tetracycline 500 mg orally four times daily for 28 days	Same as for non–penicillin-allergic patients

[a]Recommendations are those of the CDC.

[b]The CDC recommends that all patients diagnosed with syphilis be tested for HIV infection.

[c]No specific recommendations exist for tertiary syphilis because of the lack of available data.

[d]Some experts administer benzathine penicillin G 2.4 million units IM once per week for up to 3 weeks after completion of the neurosyphilis regimens to provide a total duration of therapy comparable to that used for late syphilis in the absence of neurosyphilis.

[e]For nonpregnant patients; pregnant patients should be treated with penicillin after desensitization.

[f]Growing data support ceftriaxone efficacy, although the optimal dosage and treatment duration are unclear; in neurosyphilis, 2 g IV daily for at least 10 days found to be as effective as intravenous penicillin G in a recent study.

CSF, cerebrospinal fluid.

patient without a penicillin-allergy. This differs from treatment of a repeat infection diagnosed within 1 year of exposure, which warrants a single IM dose of benzathine penicillin 2.4 million units. For women treated during pregnancy, monthly quantitative nontreponemal tests are recommended in those at high risk of reinfection. Recent sex partners (within 90 days) of anyone diagnosed should be treated presumptively if serologic tests are not immediately available.[4]

GENITAL HERPES

Epidemiology and Etiology

Genital herpes infections are the predominate cause of genital ulceration in the United States and globally. These infections are primarily attributed to HSV-2, with a prevalence of 11.9% among 14- to 49-year-olds and approximately 572,000 new infections annually.[2,79] The number of individuals with genital herpes is magnified by rising infections caused by HSV-1, usually associated with oropharyngeal disease (eg, "cold sores").[80] Most persons with HSV-2 are unaware of their infection.[81] Only 30% of those with HSV-1 infection experience clinically recognized outbreaks. HSV-2 rates among women are almost twice that of men. The incidence of HSV-2 is strongly correlated with the start of sexual activity, with rates decreasing gradually in subsequent age groups. Alternatively, HSV-1 is usually acquired earlier in childhood and is inversely proportional to socioeconomic status. Although the number of lifetime sexual partners, age of sexual debut, and STI history correlate with HSV-2 infection, it is commonly transmitted through long-term relationships rather than casual sexual relationships.[82,83]

Genital herpes is of major public health importance, despite most individuals having limited or no manifestations of disease. Although the risk of HSV is higher during clinical outbreaks, most transmission occurs during periods of asymptomatic shedding, hampering prevention efforts. Serious complications, particularly among those with immunosuppression, during pregnancy, and neonates born to mothers with HSV, may occur. For people who experience symptoms, episodes are often recurrent, causing painful ulcers and generalized discomfort for days at a time. A diagnosis of genital herpes may impact sexual relationships, cause social stigma, and lead to psychological distress. For various reasons, the CDC does not recommend screening for HSV in the general population.[3] Similar to syphilis and other STDs, the presence of genital herpes lesions is associated with an increased risk of acquiring HIV following exposure.[4,83–85]

Pathophysiology

HSV-1 and 2 are two members of the Herpesvirus family. Humans are the sole known reservoir for HSV. Each virus is capable of causing clinically indistinguishable infections, although the likelihood of causing disease in a specific anatomic area differs. Infection is transmitted via inoculation of virus from infected secretions onto mucosal surfaces (eg, urethra, oropharynx, cervix, and conjunctivae) or through abraded skin.[4,83–85]

The cycle of HSV infection occurs in five stages: initial mucosal or dermal infection, ganglia infection, establishment of latency, reactivation, and recurrent infection. After cell entry, transportation and replication occurs via viral spread from peripheral sensory nerves to contiguous cells and ganglia, most commonly the sacral nerve root ganglia if genital entry and the trigeminal ganglia if oropharyngeal entry. Chronic infection is established at this time, with clinical latency occurring for the majority of the person's life. Latency does not mean dormancy, as viral replication occurs in infected neurons and peripheral nerve endings, despite lack of symptoms. These reactivation periods are highly variable among patients. Stress, illness, and sun exposure (UV light) are identified as precipitating factors.[83,84]

Clinical Presentation

The signs and symptoms of genital herpes infection are influenced by many factors, including previous exposure to HSV, viral type, and host factors, such as age and site of infection. Because a high percentage of initial and recurrent infections are asymptomatic, and viral shedding can occur in the absence of apparent lesions or symptoms, identification and education of individuals with genital herpes is essential in controlling transmission. A summary of the clinical presentation of genital herpes is provided in Table 140-11. Those who experience symptoms usually develop multiple painful ulcers, at times accompanied by itching, discomfort, paresthesias, and local lymphadenopathy. These symptoms are typically more severe, involve neurologic complaints (fever, headache, malaise, myalgias), and persist longer in the first episode, especially if they occur during primary infection. Lesions may present at various stages in addition to ulcers, such as vesicles, pustules, and crusting. Frequency of genital herpetic recurrences differ among the HSV types after the first episode, with 90% of those infected with HSV-2 experiencing within the first year in comparison to 55% of HSV-1-infected individuals.[4,83–85]

Recurrent episodes are usually more localized, have fewer lesions, are shorter in duration, and present with milder symptoms. About half of recurrent ulcers are preceded by prodomal symptoms (mild burning, itching, tingling, or shooting pains), which could extend to the buttocks or leg. Prodromal symptoms may also occur in the absence of genital lesions. Mucocutaneous HSV is detected in these prodromal states, solidifying the evidence that viral reactivation is linked to the symptom presentation. HSV as the cause of atypical presentations can be missed and warrant HSV testing when the clinical picture is uncertain. Education on signs and symptoms of genital herpes to those who were unaware of their seropositivity have resulted in a 48% to 62% observation of classic lesions within the following months, highlighting the knowledge gap among the general public. HSV-1 is associated with a lower rate of asymptomatic and symptomatic recurrence, while HSV-2 is characterized by more frequent recurrences and subclinical shedding.[4,83–85]

TABLE 140-11 Presentation of Genital Herpes Infections

General	Incubation period: 2-14 days (mean, 4 days) Can be caused by either HSV-1 or HSV-2
Classification of infection	
First-episode primary	Initial genital infection in individuals lacking antibody to either HSV-1 or HSV-2
First-episode nonprimary	Initial genital infection in individuals with clinical or serologic evidence of prior HSV (usually HSV-1) infection
Recurrent	Appearance of genital lesions at some time following healing of first-episode infection
Signs and symptoms	
First-episode infections	Most primary infections are asymptomatic or minimally symptomatic Multiple painful pustular or ulcerative lesions on external genitalia developing over a period of 7-10 days; lesions heal in 2-4 weeks (mean, 21 days) Flu-like symptoms (eg, fever, headache, malaise) during first few days after appearance of lesions Others—local itching, pain, or discomfort; vaginal or urethral discharge, tender inguinal adenopathy, paresthesias, urinary retention Severity of symptoms greater in females than in males Symptoms are less severe (eg, fewer lesions, more rapid lesion healing, fewer or milder systemic symptoms) with nonprimary infections Symptoms more severe and prolonged in the immunocompromised On average viral shedding lasts approximately 11-12 days for primary infections and 7 days for non-primary infections
Recurrent	Prodrome seen in approximately 50% of patients prior to appearance of recurrent lesions; mild burning, itching, or tingling are typical prodromal symptoms Compared to primary infections, recurrent infections associated with (1) fewer lesions that are more localized, (2) shorter duration of active infection (lesions heal within 7 days), and (3) milder symptoms Severity of symptoms greater in females than in males Symptoms more severe and prolonged in the immunocompromised On average viral shedding lasts approximately 4 days Asymptomatic viral shedding is more frequent during the first year after infection with HSV
Therapeutic implications of HSV-1 vs HSV-2 genital infection	Primary infections caused by HSV-1 and HSV-2 virtually indistinguishable Recurrent infections and subclinical viral shedding are less frequent with HSV-1 Recurrent infections with HSV-2 tend to be more severe
Complications	Secondary infection of lesions; extragenital infection because of autoinoculation; disseminated infection (primarily in immunocompromised patients); meningitis or encephalitis; neonatal transmission

HSV-1, herpes simplex virus type 1; HSV-2, herpes simplex virus type 2.

Complications

Complications from genital herpes infections resulting from both local autoinoculation and extragenital spread commonly to the eye, rectum, pharynx, and fingers. CNS involvement is seen occasionally and can take several forms, including encephalitis, aseptic meningitis, and transverse myelitis. HSV-2 is more likely to cause aseptic meningitis than HSV-1, while HSV-1 is the most commonly identified cause of acute viral encephalitis.

A major concern is the effect of genital herpes on neonates exposed during pregnancy. Neonatal herpes is associated with a high mortality and significant morbidity. It is transmitted to the newborn primarily through exposure in the birth canal but, in rare cases, transplacentally. The risk of transmission during birth appears much greater for first-episode primary infections than for recurrent infections. Neonatal herpes infection has a case-fatality rate of approximately 50%, with a large proportion of surviving infants experiencing significant morbidity, including permanent neurologic damage. Morbidity and mortality caused by HSV in immunocompromised transplant recipients or those receiving cancer chemotherapy has dramatically reduced by the inclusion of antiviral prophylaxis into most therapeutic plans.[4,83,84]

Diagnosis

Confirmation of genital herpes infection can be made only with laboratory testing. Viral culture and HSV DNA detection with PCR assays are primary modalities used to confirm the diagnosis of first-episode genital herpes as the antibodies produced early in infection may not be detected (complete seroconversion can take months). These tests can also be used when recurrent lesions are present. Although viral culture is highly specific, it is relatively insensitive in detecting HSV in ulcers in the latter stages of healing and in recurrent infections, in part due to reduced viral load. Viral culture is expensive, time-consuming, and improper collection or transport of specimens can result in false-negative results, but may be helpful when acyclovir resistance is suspected. In most situations, HSV isolation from culture takes 48 to 96 hours.[4,83]

PCR assays are the preferred diagnostic tests due to greater sensitivity (in active lesions or asymptomatic viral shedding), significantly faster turnaround, and wider availability. Subtyping should be sought once HSV is detected. Although some PCR tests can differentiate serotype, not all have that capability. Serologic testing plays a role in diagnosing HSV infection in select scenarios: (1) recurrent genital symptoms present with negative PCR/culture; (2) patients with clinical signs of HSV infection without laboratory confirmation; (3) when the partner has documented genital herpes. Type-specific serology can distinguish between HSV-1 and HSV-2 based on HSV-specific glycoprotein G-1 and glycoprotein G-2, respectively. The sensitivity of these tests can vary from 80% to 98%, with false-negatives more likely to occur early in disease. EIAs are the most commonly used tests, which at low index values (1.1-3.0) have high rates of false-positivity. A confirmatory test with another method, such as the Biokit or a western blot, should be performed before interpretation of an EIA, particularly when with low index values.[4,83,84]

TABLE 140-12 Treatment of Genital Herpes

Type of Infection	Recommended Regimens[a,b]	Alternative Regimens
First clinical episode of genital herpes[c]	Acyclovir 400 mg orally three times daily for 7-10 days,[d] *or* Famciclovir 250 mg orally three times daily for 7-10 days,[d] *or* Valacyclovir 1 g orally twice daily for 7-10 days[d]	Acyclovir 5-10 mg/kg IV every 8 hours for 2 -7 days or until clinical improvement occurs, followed by high-dose oral therapy (valcyclovir 1 g thrice daily) to complete 10-14 days of total therapy[e]
Recurrent infection		
Episodic therapy[f]	Acyclovir 800 mg orally twice daily for 5 days, *or* Acyclovir 800 mg orally three times daily for 2 days, *or* Famciclovir 125 mg orally twice daily for 5 days, *or* Famciclovir 1 g orally twice daily for 1 day, *or* Famciclovir 500 mg orally once, followed by 250 mg orally twice daily for 2 days, *or* Valacyclovir 500 mg orally twice daily for 3 days, *or* Valacyclovir 1 g orally once daily for 5 days	
Suppressive therapy[g]	Acyclovir 400 mg orally twice daily, *or* Famciclovir 250 mg orally twice daily,[h] *or* Valacyclovir 500 mg or 1 g orally once daily[i]	

[a]Recommendations are those of the CDC.

[b]HIV-infected patients can require more aggressive therapy.

[c]Primary or nonprimary first episode.

[d]Treatment duration can be extended if healing is incomplete after 10 days.

[e]Only for patients with severe symptoms or complications that necessitate hospitalization. HSV encephalitis requires 14-21 days of IV therapy.

[f]Requires initiation of therapy within 24 hours of lesion onset or during the prodrome that precedes some outbreaks.

[g]Consider discontinuation of treatment after one year to assess frequency of recurrence.

[h]Famciclovir appears less effective for suppression of viral shedding.

[i]Valacyclovir 500 mg appears less effective than other valacyclovir and acyclovir regimens in patients with 10 or more recurrences per year.

IV, intravenous.

TREATMENT

Management goals for genital herpes include symptom relief, reducing the clinical course to prevent complications and recurrences, and minimizing disease transmission. The CDC recommended genital herpes treatments include the antiviral agents acyclovir, valacyclovir, and famciclovir (Table 140-12). The overall efficacy of these agents is comparable, although patient compliance can be improved with less frequent dosing regimens.[4]

First-Episode Infections

6 Oral formulations of acyclovir, famciclovir, and valacyclovir have demonstrated efficacy in reducing viral shedding, duration of symptoms, and time to healing of first-episode genital herpes infections, with maximal benefits seen when therapy is initiated at the earliest stages of infection. Table 140-12 lists the recommended regimens for first-episode infections. The CDC recommends all patients with first episodes genital herpes receive systemic antiviral therapy to prevent severe or prolonged symptoms associated with newly acquired infections. Additionally, topical antiviral therapy offers minimal clinical benefit and is not recommended. In immunocompromised patients, or those with severe symptoms or complications necessitating hospitalization, parenteral acyclovir is recommended, but has been associated with renal, GI, bone marrow, and CNS toxicity, particularly in patients with renal dysfunction receiving high doses. No antiviral regimen is known to prevent latency or alter the subsequent frequency and severity of recurrences in humans.[4,83–85]

Recurrent Infections

Mild and infrequent recurrences can be managed without pharmacologic therapy. When therapy is warranted or desired, there are two approaches: episodic or chronic suppressive therapy. Episodic therapy is initiated early during the course of the recurrence, preferably within 6 to 12 hours of the onset of prodromal symptoms, but within 24 hours after lesions first appear. Timely episodic therapy can decrease the duration of lesions by 1 to 2 days. Valacyclovir and famciclovir have improved pharmacokinetic profiles versus acyclovir, allowing for reduced dosing frequency and shorter courses. For optimal therapy, providers should prescribe the regimen of choice ahead of recurrences to allow the patient to initiate treatment at home at the first sign of symptoms.[4,83–85]

Table 140-12 lists the recommended suppressive regimens. Daily suppressive therapy may yield a benefit for patients with frequent episodes (≥6 per year), severe recurrences, those who wish to reduce transmission risk to a partner, and to ease anxiety over unpredictable recurrences. Suppressive therapy reduces the frequency and severity of clinical episodes and asymptomatic shedding in 70% to 80% of patients experiencing frequent recurrences. The extent to which suppressive therapy decreases disease transmission to sexual partners remains to be determined. Because the frequency of recurrences tends to diminish over time, periodic "drug holidays" are advocated to assess changes in the underlying recurrence rate and determine if continued suppressive therapy is warranted.[4,83,84]

Selected Populations

Immunocompromised patients are at greatest risk for severe and recurrent HSV infections. Acyclovir, valacyclovir, and famciclovir have been used to prevent reactivation of infection in patients seropositive for HSV who undergo transplantation procedures or induction chemotherapy. Immunocompromised individuals, such as patients with acquired immunodeficiency syndrome (AIDS), who fail treatment or prophylaxis with recommended antiviral doses frequently demonstrate improved response with higher doses. Resistant isolates are a concern in this immunocompromised population, mediated by alterations in viral thymidine kinase. Resistance is conferred to acyclovir, valacyclovir, and, commonly, famciclovir. If resistance is suspected or confirmed with recommended first-line antivirals, foscarnet is usually effective. However, foscarnet is associated with a greater risk of serious adverse effects. Intravenous cidofovir or topical imiquimod may be effective alternatives to forscarnet. Lesional application of an extemporaneous compounded cidofovir (1%) gel or trifluridine ophthalmic solution appears to offer some benefits.[4,83–85]

The safety of famciclovir and valacyclovir during pregnancy is not well established. Acyclovir has been used in pregnant patients and has produced no evidence of teratogenicity. However, levels in amniotic fluid are similar to infants treated with acyclovir, of which 20% develop neutropenia. Because of the high maternal and infant morbidity associated with first-episode primary genital infections or severe recurrent infections at or near term, many clinicians advocate the use of systemic acyclovir as the standard of care in such cases.[4,85,86]

Evaluation of Therapeutic Outcomes

Antivirals can reduce morbidity and improve patient quality of life. Outside of serious conditions, like encephalitis and neonatal infection, these agents are palliative. CDC guidelines suggest discontinuation of suppressive therapy after 1 year should be considered to assess for possible changes in the patient's intrinsic pattern of recurrence. In most patients, decreases in recurrence rates and severity of symptoms occur over time. However, some clinicians prefer to continue suppressive therapy indefinitely because it significantly reduces asymptomatic viral shedding, reducing the risk of disease transmission to uninfected sexual partners.[4]

Education on the natural course of the infection, reinforcing accurate information, and dispelling misconceptions can significantly improve a patient's experience with HSV. Descriptions of typical and atypical presentations can empower patients to initiate therapy early and minimize anxiety. Prevention strategies should be emphasized, highlighting disclosure to partner(s), abstaining from sexual activity when active lesions are present, condom use, and antiviral therapy.[83,84]

HUMAN PAPILLOMAVIRUS INFECTIONS

Epidemiology and Etiology

In 2018, the CDC estimated there were 43 million HPV infections in the United States, 13 million of which were new infections.[5] However, as HPV is not a reportable condition, the incidence is likely much higher. HPV accounts for approximately 50% of new STIs each year.[2] Over 40% of women have evidence of HPV infection, with incidence peaking in teens and early twenties, aligning with initiation of sexual activity.[5] Additionally, lifetime risk of acquiring an HPV infection is over 80%, and risk increases with number of sexual partners.[86] Since the introduction of the HPV vaccine, incidence of HPV infections in teen girls and women in their early twenties have decreased.[87] Persistent infection with some HPV types can cause genital warts and cancer, and reinfection is common, especially in young, sexually active populations.

More than 125 HPV types have been characterized and over 40 are associated with genital tract lesions. Of these, infection with types 6 and 11 most commonly develop low-grade dysplasia manifested as genital warts. Infection with several HPV types, particularly HPV-16 and HPV-18, is associated with cervical neoplasma, the second most common cancer in women worldwide and accounts for approximately 66% cervical cancers in the United States.[4,5,88] The WHO estimates that 84% of HPV lesions are represented as cervical cancers worldwide.[89] Persistent carriers of oncogenic HPV strains, in combination with a variety of other factors including immunosuppression, smoking, chlamydial infection, may all play a role in promotion of viral persistence and cancer.[88] Additionally, women living with HIV are six times more likely to develop cervical cancer compared to women without HIV.[90,91]

Pathophysiology

HPV is a double-stranded DNA virus that targets basal epithelial cells. It enters cells through a break in the epithelium, and replicates within basal cells as it differentiates and progresses to the epithelial surface. Virus is shed with dead keratinocytes and infection is transmitted via contact dead keratinocyte or free virions. In a wart, viral replication is associated with excessive proliferation of all epidermal layers, except the basal layer, whereas malignant HPV disease is associated with proliferation of basal cells. HPV is transmitted by sexual intercourse, including oral sex, and may also be spread by touching an infected partner's genitalia.[88,89]

Clinical Presentation

In most individuals, genital infection with HPV is subclinical and self-limited, clearing within 6 to 9 months. HPV can infect genitalia of both women and men, as well as perianal, anal, and oropharynx regions in both genders. Approximately 1% of all infected individuals develop genital warts. When present, genital warts can be large and multifocal, producing variable degrees of discomfort. Appearance of genital warts may differ based on gender and anatomic site. For example, penile warts may be slightly raised with a rough pigmented surface, while vulvar warts are usually soft and whitish. Based on HPV DNA detection methods, most warts will regress spontaneously within 1 to 2 years of their initial appearance. HPV, while known for links to cervical cancer, can also cause cancer of the anus, penis, vulva, vagina, and oropharynx, but are less common.[4,88,89]

Diagnosis

Anogenital warts are diagnosed clinically and confirmed by biopsy in cases where the diagnosis is uncertain, when warts do not respond to standard treatment, or the patient is immunocompromised. The Papanicolaou smear (Pap smear) is the most frequently used and cost-effective diagnostic test for detecting clinical and subclinical HPV in women. However, Pap smears are neither specific for HPV nor useful in detecting latent infections. Various tests for detecting HPV DNA, RNA, or capsid protein also are available, and unlike the Pap smear do not require subjective interpretation of the results. The HPV-specific tests are only approved in women with abnormal Pap smears or women older than 30 years. However, use of HPV

DNA testing as a routine screening test in lieu of Pap smears is expected in the near future. In women identified to have high-risk HPV strain infections, follow-up cytology is performed. HPV tests are not approved for use in men and are not indicated as a screening tool for STIs.[4,88,89]

Routine screening for cervical cancer is recommended for all persons with a cervix, regardless of gender identity or partner preference. Age recommendations vary by organization. The USPSTF and the American College of Obstetricians and Gynecologists (ACOG) recommend routine cervical cancer screening every 3 years for all persons with a cervix ages 21 to 65 regardless of vaccination status. For women 30 to 65, screening can also include one of several FDA-approved oncogenic or high-risk HPV tests. The American Cancer Society recommends cervical screening of any persons with a cervix, regardless of gender identity, ages 25 to 65 by combining a Pap test with an HPV test or a Pap test alone every 3 years.[91–93] Data are insufficient to recommend routine anal cancer screening. An annual digital anorectal exams (DARE) may be useful in high-risk patient populations for early detection of HPV. The updated CDC STI Guidelines provide a table detailing the screening recommendations from various organizations.[4]

TREATMENT

No consensus exists regarding the best treatment approach for patients with genital HPV infection, particularly because most cases appear to be transient with spontaneous regression of lesions. A number of treatments are recommended (see Table 140-13), but none are clearly superior. Treatment is directed toward patients with manifestations of genital warts, with the goal of removing or destroying lesions and grossly infected surrounding tissue. Shared decision making between patient and provider determine the decision to treat and utilization of patient or provider applied therapy. Type of therapy is depended upon lesion location, provider experience, patient preference, and availability. Provider-applied therapies, cryotherapy and surgical removal, are options for any site, while acid treatments are options for vaginal, cervical, and intra-anal warts. Many patients will require multiple courses of therapy. Because such treatments neither stop viral expression in surrounding tissue nor eliminate viral latency, recurrence of lesions is common.[4]

Vaccination

7 As lesions are difficult to successfully treat, high incidence of reinfection, and concern for malignancy with persistent infections, the focus of HPV treatment is primarily on prevention. The only way to avoid acquiring HPV is to abstain from any type of sexual activity; however, barrier contraceptive methods may help decrease the risk of HPV transmission. Therefore, three HPV vaccines are licensed in the United States and endorsed by the CDC and Advisory Committee on Immunization Practices (ACIP).[94] The vaccines cover the most common and virulent HPV strains. Cervarix (a bivalent vaccine for HPV-16 and 18), Gardasil (a quadrivalent vaccine (4vHPV) for HPV-6, 11, 16, and 18), and Gardasil 9 (a 9-valent (9vHPV) vaccine for HPV-6, 11, 16, 18, 31, 33, 45, 52, and 58) are all indicated for preventing cervical precancers and cervical cancer in females 9 to 26 years of age. The 9vHPV vaccine offers protection against seven oncogenic strains of HPV, which accounts for approximately 80% of cervical cancers.[95] In addition, 4vHPV and 9vHPV are indicated in unvaccinated males 9 to 26 years of age.[94]The FDA extended approval for use of the 9vHPV for women and men ages 27 to 45 years and in 2019 ACIP recommended that adults in that age group discuss receiving the HPV vaccine with their provider through shared decision making.[94] For women and men ages 30 to 45 years, the cost-effectiveness of HPV vaccination should be considered as vaccination may provide limited health benefit at the population level.[96] All three vaccines are equally recommended by the ACIP; however, only 9vHPV vaccine is available for sale within the United States.[94,95]

Although it is ideal to vaccinate patients prior to the onset of sexual activity, those infected with one or more HPV types may still receive protection from vaccination.[4] Additionally, while the vaccine indication is cervical cancer prevention, males are included in the recommendations to reduce spread of asymptomatic disease and reduce risk of HPV-related malignancies.

Previously, all vaccines were administered as a three-dose series over 6 months, but in 2016 ACIP recommendation changed for patients less than 15 years to a two-dose schedule at 0 and 6 to 12 months. Data in women aged 16 to 26 years support the use of a two-dose schedule in those 9 to 14 years old, instead of the three-dose schedule, as antibody response with two doses was non inferior to three doses. All other age groups are recommended to receive the three-dose series at 0, 2, and 6 months.[94,96–99]

The safety profile of the HPV vaccines has been well established over the past decade.[99–102] The CDC and FDA continuously monitor the safety of vaccines via program such as Vaccine Adverse Event Reporting System (VAERS), Vaccine Safety Data link, and Clinical Immunization Safety Assessment Project.[100] The most common adverse events are related to injection site reactions, including pain, redness, or swelling. Additionally, patients may also report fever, headache, asthenia, nausea, or muscle or joint pain. Early VAERS data showed high rates of syncope. Syncope is a known adverse event after any injectable vaccination, and adolescents are also more likely to experience syncope after a medical procedure, including vaccination. In response, the FDA, CDC, and ACIP recommend to observe all patients for 15 minutes after administration of the vaccine to monitor for syncope, taking appropriate precautions to prevent falls and injuries from fainting. Over 90% of health events reported to VAERS were classified as nonserious.[1,100] HPV vaccination has not been linked to new autoimmune diseases or neurologic disorders.[99–101]

The main goal of HPV vaccination is to prevent HPV-associated malignancies; however, time from HPV infection to cervical cancer may exceed 20 years, so effects of the vaccine may not be seen for some time.[88,100] Although the ability to measure effect of the vaccine on malignancies is limited, introduction of the vaccines has substantially reduced HPV prevalence and HPV-related diseases.[5,103] There was substantially reduced risk of cervical cancer among Swedish girls ages 10 to 30 vaccinated with the quadrivalent HPV vaccine.[103] There have also been concerns regarding the long-term effect of the vaccine given the young age at which it is recommended to be administered. Antibody titers maintain appropriate levels for approximately 10 years and there is no evidence to suggest that protection decreases with time.[86] Patients should be vaccinated prior to onset of sexual activity to gain the greatest protection from the vaccine for the duration of time when they are at highest risk. As mentioned, the vaccine may still be protective even after patients have become sexually active.

Despite CDC and ACIP recommendations, the number of adolescents receiving the vaccine is below the desired threshold of 80%.[7,102,104,105] However, numbers are increasing. In girls aged 13 to 17, 70% received at least one dose of the vaccine and 54% received the entire series. The numbers are lower for boys, with 66% receiving at least one dose and 49% receiving all three.[102] Rates of vaccine implementation may increase with interventions, such as patient education and reminders, but a barrier still exists introducing this vaccine into a nontraditional target population.[105,106]

Other STIs

Several STIs other than those just discussed occur with varying frequency in the United States and throughout the world. Although an in-depth discussion of these diseases is beyond the scope of this chapter, Table 135-13 lists recommended treatment regimens.[4]

TABLE 140-13 Treatment Regimens for Miscellaneous STIs

Infection	Recommended Regimens[a]	Alternative Regimens
Cervicitis[b]	Doxycycline 100 mg orally twice daily for 7 days	Azithromycin 1 g orally in a single dose
Epididymitis		
Acute infection most likely caused by *C. trachomatis* or *N. gonorrhoeae*	Ceftriaxone 500 mg IM in a single dose PLUS doxycycline 100 mg orally twice daily for 7 days	
Acute infection most likely caused by *C. trachomatis, N. gonorrhoeae,* or enteric organisms (men who practice insertive anal sex)	Ceftriaxone 500 mg IM in a single dose PLUS levofloxacin 500 mg orally daily for 10 days	
Acute infection most likely caused by enteric organisms only	Levofloxacin 500 mg orally daily for 10 days	
Lymphogranuloma venereum	Doxycycline 100 mg orally twice daily for 21 days[c]	Azithromycin 1 g weekly for 3 weeks or erythromycin base 500 mg orally four times daily for 21 days[c,d]
Nongonococcal urethritis (NGU)	Doxycycline 100 mg orally twice daily for 7 days	Azithromycin 1 g orally in a single dose or 500 mg orally in a single dose followed by 250 mg daily for 4 days
NGU (persistent or recurrent or due to *M. genitalium*)	Doxycycline 100 mg orally twice daily for 7 days followed by moxifloxacin 400 mg orally daily for 7 days	If azithromycin resistance can be ruled out, moxifloxacin may be substituted with oral azithromycin 1 g and then 500 mg daily for 3 days
HPV infection		
External genital/perianal warts	*Provider-Administered Therapies:* Cryotherapy (eg, liquid nitrogen or cryoprobe); repeat weekly as necessary, *or* TCA 80%-90% *or* BCA 80%-90% applied to warts; repeat weekly as necessary, *or* Surgical removal (tangential scissor excision, tangential shave excision, curettage, or electrosurgery) *Patient-Applied Therapies:* Podofilox 0.5% solution or gel applied twice daily for 3 days, followed by 4 days of no therapy; cycle is repeated as necessary for up to four cycles. Imiquimod 3.75% or 5% cream applied at bedtime three times weekly for up to 16 weeks,[e,f] *or* Sinecatechins 15% ointment applied three times daily for up to 16 weeks	
Vaginal and anal warts	Cryotherapy with liquid nitrogen, or TCA or BCA 80%-90% as for external HPV warts; repeat weekly as necessary Surgical removal (not for vaginal or urethral meatus warts)	
Urethral meatus warts	Cryotherapy with liquid nitrogen, or surgical removal	
Prevention (ages 9-14 years)[f]	Gardasil9® (HPV 9-valent [type s 6, 11, 16, 18, 31, 33, 45, 52, 58]) recombinant vaccine 0.5 mL IM on day 1; a second dose administered 6-12 months following the first dose	
Prevention (age ≥15-26 years)[f]	Gardasil (HPV 9-valent [types 6, 11, 16, 18, 31, 33, 45, 52, 58]) recombinant vaccine 0.5 mL IM on day 1; a second and third dose are administered 1 and 6 months following the first dose	

[a]Recommendations are those of the CDC.

[b]Consider concurrent treatment for gonorrhea infection if the patient is at risk for gonorrhea.

[c]Pregnant patients should be treated with erythromycin.

[d]If NGU is due to *C. trachomatis*, refer to treatment in Table 140-6 . If NGU not due to *C. trachomatis*, consider HSV, trichomoniasis, *M. genitalium*, or HPV as potential causes of NGU and perform testing when appropriate.

[e]Safety during pregnancy is not established.

[f]CDC recommendations: vaccination is recommended in adolescents 11-12 years of age, and can be given as early as age 9. Catch up vaccination is recommended through age 26 years for those who either were not previously vaccinated, or who did not complete the vaccination series. Vaccination for adults ages 27-45 can be considered.

BCA, bichloracetic acid; HPV, human papillomavirus; TCA, trichloroacetic acid.

ABBREVIATIONS

ACIP	Advisory Committee on Immunization Practices
BCA	bichloracetic acid
CDC	Centers for Disease Control and Prevention
CNS	central nervous system
CSF	cerebrospinal fluid
DGI	disseminated gonococcal infection
DNA	deoxyribonucleic acid
EIA	enzyme immunoassay
EPT	expedited partner therapy
FDA	Food and Drug Administration
GI	gastrointestinal
HIV	human immunodeficiency virus
HPV	human papillomavirus
HSV	herpes simplex virus

HSV-1	herpes simplex virus type 1
HSV-2	herpes simplex virus type 2
IM	intramuscular
IUD	intrauterine contraceptive device
IV	intravenous
MSM	men who have sex with men
NAATs	nucleic acid amplification tests
NGU	nongonococcal urethritis
Pap	Papanicolaou smear
PCR	polymerase chain reaction
PID	pelvic inflammatory disease
RPR	rapid plasma reagin
STD	sexually transmitted disease
STI	sexually transmitted infection
TCA	trichloroacetic acid
TOC	test of cure
USPSTF	US Preventative Services Task Force
VAERS	Vaccine Adverse Event Reporting System

REFERENCES

1. Centers for Disease Control and Prevention. Sexually Transmitted Disease Surveillance 2019. Atlanta: U.S. Department of Health and Human Services; 2021. Available at: https://www.cdc.gov/std/statistics/2019/default.htm. Accessed May 15, 2021.
2. Kreisel KM, Spicknall IH, Gargano JW, et al. Sexually transmitted infections among US women and men: Prevalence and incidence estimates, 2018. *Sex Transm Dis.* 2021;48(4):208–214. doi:10.1097/OLQ.0000000000001355
3. Chesson HW, Spicknall IH, Bingham A, et al. The estimated direct lifetime medical costs of sexually transmitted infections acquired in the United States in 2018. *Sex Transm Dis.* 2021;48(4):215–221. doi:10.1097/OLQ.0000000000001380
4. Workowski KA, achman LH, Chant PA et al . Sexually transmitted infections treatment guidelines, 2021. *MMWR Recomm Rep* 2021;70:1–187.
5. Centers for Disease Control and Prevention. Sexually Transmitted Disease Surveillance 2018. Atlanta: U.S. Department of Health and Human Services; 2019. doi:10.15620/cdc.79370.
6. Centers for Disease Control and Prevention. HIV/AIDS & STIDs Detailed Fact Sheet. 2021. Available at: https://www.cdc.gov/std/hiv/stdfact-std-hiv-detailed.htm. Accessed May 15, 2021.
7. U.S. Department of Health and Human Services, Office of Disease Prevention and Health Promotion. Healthy People 2020: Sexually Transmitted Diseases. Available at: https://www.healthypeople.gov/2020/topics-objectives/topic/sexually-transmitted-diseases. Accessed May 15, 2021.
8. U.S. Department of Health and Human Services. 2020. Sexually Transmitted Infections National Strategic Plan for the United States: 2021–2025. Washington, DC.
9. National Academies of Sciences, Engineering, and Medicine 2021. Sexually Transmitted Infections: Adopting a Sexual Health Paradigm. Washington, DC: The National Academies Press. https://doi.org/10.17226/25955.
10. World Health Organization. Defining sexual health: Report of a technical consultation on sexual health, 28-31 January 2002. Geneva: World Health Organization; 2006.
11. Barrow RY, Ahmed F, Bolan GA, Workowski KA Recommendations for providing quality sexually transmitted diseases clinical services. *MMWR Recomm Rep* 2020;68(No. RR-5):1–20. doi: http://dx.doi.org/10.15585/mmwr.rr6805a1externalicon 2020.
12. Centers for Disease Control and Prevention. Sexually Transmitted Diseases: Expedited Partner Therapy. 2021. Available at: https://www.cdc.gov/std/ept/default.htm. Accessed May 15, 2021.
13. Centers for Disease Control and Prevention. *Antibiotic Resistance Threats in the United States, 2013.* Atlanta, GA: U.S. Department of Health and Human Services; 2013.
14. Centers for Disease Control and Prevention. Antibiotic Resistance Threats in the United States, 2019. Atlanta, GA: U.S. Department of Health and Human Services, CDC; 2019. http://dx.doi.org/10.15620/cdc:82532.
15. World Health Organization. *Prioritization of Pathogens to Guide Discovery, Research, and Development of New Antibiotics for Drug-Resistant Bacterial Infections, Including Tuberculosis.* Geneva, Switzerland: World Health Organization; 2017.
16. Marrazzo JM, Apicella MA. *Neisseria gonorrhoeae.* In: Bennett JE, Dolin R, Blaser MJ, eds. *Mandell, Douglas, and Bennett's Principles and Practice of Infectious Diseases.* 9th ed. [*electronic version*]; Clinical Key, 2021. Philadelphia, PA: Elsevier. Accessed January 21, 2021.
17. Hooper RR, Renolds GH, Jones OG, et al. Cohort study of venereal disease, I: The risk of gonorrhea transmission from infected women to men. *Am J Epidemiol.* 1978;108:136–144.
18. Lin JS, Donegan Sp, Heeren TC, et al. Transmission of *Chlamydia trachomatis* and *Neisseria gonorrhoeae* among men with urethritis and their female sex partners. *J Infect Dis.* 1998;178:1707–1712.
19. Babu TM, Urban MA, Augebraun MH. Urethritis. In: Bennet JE, Dolin R, Blaser MJ, eds. *Mandell Douglas, and Bennett's Principles and Practice of Infectious Diseases,* 9th ed. [*electronic version*]; Clinical Key, 2021. Philadelphia, PA: Elsevier. Accessed January 12, 2021.
20. Brunham RC, Gottlieb SL, Paavonen J. Pelvic inflammatory disease. *N Engl J Med.* 2015;372(21):2039–2048.
21. Bleich AT, Sheffield JS, Wendel GD, et al. Disseminated gonococcal infections in women. *Obstet Gynecol.* 2012;119:597–602.
22. Belkacem A, Caumes E, Ouanich J, et al. Working Group FRA-DGI. Changing patterns of disseminated gonococcal infection in France: Cross-sectional data 2009-2011. *Sex Transm Infect.* 2013;89:613–615.
23. Nettleton WD, Kent JB, Macomber K, et al. Ongoing cluster of highly related disseminated gonococcal infections—Southwest Michigan. *MMWR.* 2019;69(12):353–354 2020.
24. Centers for Disease Control and Prevention. Recommendations for the laboratory-based detection of *Chlamydia trachomatis* and *Neisseria gonorrhoeae*—2014. *MMWR Recomm Rep.* 2014;63:1–19.
25. U.S. Food and Drug Administration. FDA clears first diagnostic tests for extragenital testing for chlamydia and gonorrhea. FDA news release. May 23, 2019. Available at: https://www.fda.gov/news-events/press-announcements/fda-clears-first-diagnostic-tests-extragenital-testing-chlamydia-and-gonorrhea. Accessed May 15, 2021.
26. LeFevre ML, U.S. Preventive Services Task Force. Screening for Chlamydia and gonorrhea: U.S. Preventive Services Task Force recommendation statement. *Ann Intern Med.* 2014;161:902–910.
27. St. Cyr S, Barbee L, Workowski KA, et al. Update to CDC's treatment guidelines for gonococcal infection. *MMWR Morb Mortal Wkly Rep.* 2020;69:1911–1916.
28. Centers for Disease Control and Prevention. Update to CDC's sexually transmitted diseases treatment guidelines, 2010: Oral cephalosporins no longer a recommended treatment for gonococcal infections. *MMWR Morb Mortal Wkly Rep.* 2012;61(31):590–594.
29. Lyss SB, Kamb ML, Peterman TA, et al. *Chlamydia trachomatis* among patients infected with and treated for *Neisseria gonorrhoeae* in sexually transmitted disease clinics in the United States. *Ann Intern Med.* 2003;139:178–185.
30. Lau A, Kong FYS, Fairley CK, et al. Azithromycin or doxycycline for asymptomatic rectal *Chlamydia trachomatis. N Engl J Med.* 2021;24;384(25):2418–2427. 10.1056/NEJMoa2031631.
31. Kong FY, Tabrizi SN, Fairley CK, et al. The efficacy of azithromycin and doxycycline for the treatment of rectal chlamydia infection: A systematic review and meta-analysis. *J Antimicrob Chemother.* 2015;70:1290–7.
32. Kong FY, Tabrizi SN, Law M, et al. Azithromycin versus doxycycline for the treatment of genital chlamydia infection: A meta-analysis of randomized controlled trials. *Clin Infect Dis.* 2014;59:193–205.
33. Kirkcaldy RD, Weinstock HS, Moore PC, et al. The efficacy and safety of gentamicin plus azithromycin and gemifloxacin plus azithromycin as treatment of uncomplicated gonorrhea. *Clin Infect Dis.* 2014;59:1083–1091.
34. Woods CR. Gonococcal infections in neonates and young children. *Semin Pediatr Infect Dis.* 2005;16:258–270.
35. Fung M, Scott KC, Kent CK, Klausner JD. Chlamydial and gonococcal reinfection among men: A systematic review of data to evaluate the need for retesting. *Sex Transm Infect.* 2007;83:304–309.
36. Hosenfield CB, Workowski KA, Berman S, et al. Repeat infection with chlamydia and gonorrhea among females: A systematic review of the literature. *Sex Transm Dis.* 2009;36:478–489.
37. Batteiger BE, Tan M. *Chlamydia trachomatis* (trachoma, genital infections, perinatal infections, lymphogranuloma venereum). In: Bennett JE, Dolin R, Blaser MJ, eds. *Mandell, Douglas, and Bennett's Principles and Practice of Infectious Diseases,* 8th ed. [*electronic version*]; Clinical Key, 2021. Philadelphia, PA: Elsevier. Accessed January 21, 2021.
38. O'Connell CM, Ferone ME. *Chlamydia trachomatis* genital infections. *Microbial Cell.* 2016;3:390–403.

39. Bachmann LH, Manhart LE, Martin DH, et al. Advances in the understanding and treatment of male urethritis. *Clin Infect Dis.* 2015;61 Suppl 8:S763–S769. doi:10.1093/cid/civ755
40. Bernstein KT, Marcus JL, Nieri G, et al. Rectal gonorrhea and chlamydia reinfection is associated with increased risk of HIV seroconversion. *J Acquir Immune Defic Syndr.* 2010;53:537–543.
41. Katz BP, Caine VA, Jones RB, et al. Estimation of transmission probabilities for chlamydial infections. In: Bowie WR, Caldwell HD, Jones RP, eds. *Chlamydial Infections.* Cambridge, UK: Cambridge University Press; 1990;567–570.
42. Althaus CL, Turner KM, Mercer CH, et al. Effectiveness and cost-effectiveness of traditional and new partner notification technologies for curable sexually transmitted infections: Observational study, systematic reviews and mathematical modelling. *Health Technol Assess.* 2014;18:1–100.
43. Zar HJ. Neonatal chlamydial infections: Prevention and treatment. *Paediatr Drugs.* 2005;7:103–110.
44. Chesson HW, Bernstein KT, Gift TL, Marcus JL, Pipkin S, Kent CK. The cost-effectiveness of screening men who have sex with men for rectal chlamydial and gonococcal infection to prevent HIV Infection. *Sex Transm Dis.* 2013;40:366–71.
45. Geisler WM, Uniyal A, Lee JY, et al. Azithromycin versus doxycycline for urogenital *Chlamydia trachomatis* infection. *N Engl J Med.* 2015;373:2512–21.
46. Lau CY, Qureshi AK. Azithromycin versus doxycycline for genital chlamydial infections: A meta-analysis of randomized clinical trials. *Sex Transm Dis.* 2002;29:497–502.
47. Elgalib A, Alexander S, Tong CY, White JA. Seven days of doxycycline is an effective treatment for asymptomatic rectal *Chlamydia trachomatis* infection. *Int J STD AIDS.* 2011;22:474–7.
48. Reveneau N, Crane DD, Fischer E, Caldwell HD. Bactericidal activity of first-choice antibiotics against gamma inter-feron-induced persistent infection of human epithelial cells by *Chlamydia trachomatis. Antimicrob Agents Chemother.* 2005;49:1787–93.
49. Flagg EW, Meites E, Phillips C, Papp J, Torrone EA. Prevalence of *Trichomonas vaginalis* among civilian, noninstitutionalized male and female population aged 14 to 59 years: United States, 2013 to 2016. *Sex Transm Dis.* 2019Oct;46(10):e93–e96.
50. Abdallah M, Augenbraun MH, McCormack W. Vulvovaginitis and cervicitis. In: Bennett JE, Dolin R, Blaser MJ, eds. Mandell, Douglas, and Bennett's Principles and Practice of Infectious Diseases, 8th ed. [*electronic version*]; Clinical Key, 2021. Philadelphia, PA: Elsevier. Accessed January 12, 2021.
51. Masha SC, Cools P, Sanders EJ, Vaneechoutte M, Crucitti T. *Trichomonas vaginalis* and HIV infection acquisition: A systematic review and meta-analysis. *Sex Transm Infect.* 2019;95(1):36–42. doi: 10.1136/sextrans-2018-053713.
52. Meites E, Gaydos CA, Hobbs MM, et al. A review of evidence-based care of symptomatic trichomoniasis and asymptomatic *Trichomonas vaginalis* infections. *Clin Infect Dis.* 2015;61(S8):S837–848.
53. Kissinger P. *Trichomonas vaginalis*: A review of epidemiologic, clinical and treatment issues. *BMC Infect Dis.* 2015;15(307):1–8.
54. Bouchemal K, Bories C, Loiseau PM. Strategies for prevention and treatment of *Trichomonas vaginalis* infections. *Clin Microbiol Rev.* 2017;30:811–825.
55. Dize L, Agreda P, Quinn N, et al. Comparison of self-obtained penile meatal swabs to urine for the detection of *C. trachomatis, N. gonorrhoeae* and *T. vaginalis. Sex Transm Infect.* 2013;89:305–7.
56. Kissinger P, Muzny CA, Mena LA, et al. Single-dose versus 7-day-dose metronidazole for the treatment of trichomoniasis in women: An open-label, randomised controlled trial. *Lancet Infect Dis.* 2018;18(11):1251–1259. doi:10.1016/S1473-3099(18)30423-7.
57. Alessio C, Nyirjesy P. Management of resistant trichomoniasis. *Curr Infect Dis Rep.* 2019;21(9):31. Published 2019 Aug 6. doi:10.1007/s11908-019-0687-4
58. Kirkcaldy RD, Augostini P, Asbel LE, et al. *Trichomonas vaginalis* antimicrobial drug resistance in 6 US cities, STD Surveillance Network, 2009-2010. *Emerg Infect Dis.* 2012;18:939–943.
59. Seña AC, Bachmann LH, Hobbs MM, et al. Persistent and recurrent *Trichomonas vaginalis* infections: epidemiology, treatment and management considerations. *Expert Rev Anti Infect Ther.* 2014;12(6):637–685. https://doi.org/10.1586/14787210.2014.887440.
60. Mergenhagen KA, Wattengel BA, Skelly MK, Clark CM, Russo TA. Fact versus fiction: A review of the evidence behind alcohol and antibiotic interactions. *Antimicrob Agents Chemother.* 2020;64(3):e02167-19. Published 2020 Feb 21. doi:10.1128/AAC.02167-19
61. Sethi S, Zaman K, Jain N. *Mycoplasma genitalium* infections: Current treatment options and resistance issues. *Infect Drug Resist.* 2017;10:283–292.
62. Decker CF. Emerging sexually transmitted diseases: Hepatitis C, lymphogranuloma venereum (LGV), and *Mycoplasma genitalium* infections. *Dis Mon.* 2016;62:314–318.
63. U.S. Food and Drug Administration. FDA permits marketing of first test to aid in the diagnosis of a sexually-transmitted infection known as *Mycoplasma genitalium*. FDA news release. January 23, 2019. Available at: https://www.fda.gov/news-events/press-announcements/fda-permits-marketing-first-test-aid-diagnosis-sexually-transmitted-infection-known-mycoplasma. Accessed May 15, 2021.
64. Durukan D, Read TRH, Murray G, et al. Resistance-guided antimicrobial therapy using doxycycline-moxifloxacin and doxycycline-2.5 g azithromycin for treatment of *Mycoplasma genitalium* infection: Efficacy and tolerability. *Clin Infect Dis.* 2020;71(6):1461–1468.
65. Wiesenfeld HC, Meyn LA, Darville T, et al. A randomized controlled trial of ceftriaxone and doxycycline, with or without metronidazole, for the treatment of acute pelvic inflammatory disease. *Clin Infect Dis.* 2021;72(7):1181–1189.
66. McGregor JA, Crombleholme WR, Newton E, et al. Randomized comparison of ampicillin-sulbactam to cefoxitin and doxycycline or clindamycin and gentamicin in the treatment of pelvic inflammatory disease or endometritis. *Obstet Gynecol.* 1994;83(6):998–1004. doi:10.1097/00006250-199406000-00020.
67. Sweet RL. Treatment of acute pelvic inflammatory disease. *Infect Dis Obstet Gynecol.* 2011;2011:561909. doi:10.1155/2011/561909
68. Ness RB, Trautmann G, Richter HE, et al. Effectiveness of treatment strategies of some women with pelvic inflammatory disease: A randomized controlled trial. *Obstet Gynecol.* 2005;106:573–580.
69. Kimball A, Torrone E, Miele K, et al. Missed opportunities for prevention of congenital syphilis—United States, 2018. *MMWR Morb Mortal Wkly Rep.* 2020;69:661–665. doi: http://dx.doi.org/10.15585/mmwr.mm6922a.
70. Radolf JD,Tramont EC, Salazar JC. Syphilis (*Treponema pallidum*). In: Bennett JE, Dolin R, Blaser MJ, eds. *Mandell, Douglas, and Bennett's Principles and Practice of Infectious Diseases*, 9th ed. [*electronic version*]; Clinical Key, 2021. Philadelphia, PA: Elsevier. Accessed January 12, 2021.
71. Hook EW. Syphilis. *Lancet.* 2017;389(10078):1550–1557. doi: 10.1016/S0140-6736(16)32411-4. 2019 March 9, 393(10175):986.
72. Markewitz R, Pauli D, Wandinger KP. The modern epidemic of syphilis. *N Engl J Med.* 2020;382(24):2379–2380. 10.1056/NEJMc2006129.
73. Clark EG, Danbolt N. The Oslo study of the natural history of untreated syphilis; an epidemiologic investigation based on a restudy of the Boeck-Bruusgaard material; a review and appraisal. *J Chron Dis.* 1955;2:311–344.
74. Centers for Disease Control and Prevention. Syphilis (*Treponema* pallidum): 2018 case definition. 2018. https://wwwn.cdc.gov/nndss/conditions/syphilis/case-definition/2018/. Accessed May 15, 2021.
75. Gayet-Ageron A, Lautenschlager S, Ninet B, Perneger TV, Combescure C. Sensitivity, specificity and likelihood ratios of PCR in the diagnosis of syphilis: A systematic review and meta-analysis. *Sex Transm Infect.* 2013;89(3):251–256. doi: 10.1136/sextrans-2012-050622.
76. Ortiz DA, Shukla MR, Loeffelholz MJ. The traditional or reverse algorithm for diagnosis of syphilis: Pros and cons. *Clin Infect Dis.* 2020;71(Suppl 1):S43–S51. doi: 10.1093/cid/ciaa307.
77. Cao Y, Su X, Wang Q, et al. A multicenter study evaluating ceftriaxone and benzathine penicillin G as treatment agents for early syphilis in Jiangsu, China. Clin Infect Dis 2017; 65:1683–88.
78. Bettuzzi T, Jourdes A, Robineau O, et al. Ceftriaxone compared with benzylpenicillin in the treatment of neurosyphilis in France: A retrospective multicentre study. *Lancet Infect Dis.* 2021[epub ahead of print]. https://doi.org/10.1016/S1473-3099(20)30857-4.
79. McQuillan G, Kruszon-Moran D, Flagg EW, Paulose-Ram R. Prevalence of herpes simplex virus type 1 and type 2 in persons aged 14–49: United States, 2015–2016. *NCHS Data Brief, no 304.* 2018(304):1–18.
80. Xu F, Sternberg MR, Kottiri BJ, et al. Trends in herpes simplex virus type 1 and type 2 seroprevalence in the United States. *JAMA.* 2006;296(8):964–973.
81. Fanfair RN, Zaidi A, Taylor LD, Xu F, Gottlieb S, Markowitz L. Trends in seroprevalence of herpes simplex virus type 2 among non-Hispanic blacks and non-Hispanic whites aged 14 to 49 years—United States, 1988 to 2010. *Sex Transm Dis.* 2013;40(11):860–864.

82. Centers for Disease Control and Prevention. Genital herpes – CDC fact sheet (detailed). Last updated: January 19, 2021. Available at: https://www.cdc.gov/std/herpes/stdfact-herpes-detailed.htm. Accessed May 30, 2021.
83. Schiffer JT, Corey l. Herpes simplex virus. *Mandell, Douglas, and Bennett's Principles and Practice of Infectious Diseases*, 9th ed. [*electronic version*]; Clinical Key, 2021. Philadelphia, PA: Elsevier. Accessed January 12, 2021.
84. Gnann JW, Whitley RJ. Genital herpes. *New Engl J Med.* 2016;375:666–674.
85. Corey L, Wald A. Maternal and neonatal herpes simplex virus infections. *N Engl J Med.* 2009;361:1375–1385.
86. Bogani G, Maggiore ULR, Signorelli M, et al. The role of human papillomavirus vaccines in cervical cancer: Prevention and treatment. *Crit Rev Oncol Hematol.* 2018;122:92–97.
87. Markowitz LE, Hariri S, Lin C, et al. Reduction in human papillomavirus (HPV) prevalence among young women following HPV vaccine introduction in the United States, National Health and Nutrition Examination Surveys, 2003-2010. *J Infect Dis.* 2013;208:385–93.
88. Bonnez W. Papillomaviruses. In: Bennett JE, Dolin R, Blaser MJ, eds. *Mandell, Douglas, and Bennett's Principles and Practice of Infectious Diseases* [*electronic version*]; Clinical Key, 2020. 9th ed. Philadelphia, PA: Elsevier. Accessed January 12, 2021.
89. WHO. Human papillomavirus vaccines: WHO position paper, May 2017—Recommendations. *Vaccine.* 2017;35:5753–5755.
90. Stelzle D, Tanaka LF, Lee KK, et al. Estimates of global burden of cervical cancer associated with HIV. *Lancet Glob Health.* 2021;9:e161–169.
91. Committee on Practice Bulletins—Gynecology. Practice Bulletin No. 168: Cervical cancer screening and prevention. *Obstet Gynecol.* 2016;128:e111–30.
92. U.S. Preventive Services Task Force. Screening for Cervical Cancer: US Preventative Services Task Force Recommendation Statement. *JAMA.* 2018;320(7):674–686. 10.1001/jama.2018.10897.
93. Saslow D, Solomon D, Lawson HW, et al. American Cancer Society, American Society for Colposcopy and Cervical Pathology, and American Society for Clinical Pathology screening guidelines for the prevention and early detection of cervical cancer. *Am J Clin Pathol.* 2012;137:516–42.
94. Meites E, Szilagyi PG, Chesson HW, et al. Human papillomavirus vaccination for adults: Updated recommendations of the Advisory Committee on Immunization Practices. *MMWR Morb Mortal Wkly Rep.* 2019;68(32):698–702.
95. Petrosky E, JA Jr, Hariri S, et al. Use of 9-valent human papillomavirus (HPV) vaccine: Updated HPV vaccination recommendations of the advisory committee on immunization practices. *MMWR Morb Mortal Wkly Rep.* 2015;64:300–304.
96. Kim JJ, Simms KT, Killen J, et al. Human papillomavirus vaccination for adults aged 30 to 45 years in the United States: A cost-effectiveness analysis. *PLoS Med.* 2021;18(3):e1003534. Published 2021 Mar 11. doi:10.1371/journal.pmed.1003534.
97. Meites E, Kempe A, Markowitz LE. Use of a 2-dose schedule for human papillomavirus vaccination—updated recommendations of the Advisory Committee on Immunization Practices. *MMWR Morb Mortal Wkly Rep.* 2016;65:1405–1408.
98. Markowitz LE, Meites E, Unger ER. Two vs three doses of human papillomavirus vaccine: New policy for the second decade of the vaccination program. *JAMA.* 2016;316:2370–2372.
99. Markowitz LE, Gee J, Chesson H, Stokley S. Ten years of human papillomavirus vaccination in the United States. *Acad Pediatr.* 2018;18:S3–S10.
100. Centers for Disease Control and Prevention. Human papillomavirus (HPV) vaccine safety. Available at: https://www.cdc.gov/vaccinesafety/vaccines/hpv-vaccine.html. Accessed May 15, 2021.
101. Shimabukuro TT, Su JR, Marquez PL, et al. Safety of the 9-valent human papilloma virus. Pediatrics. 2019;144(6):e20191791. doi: 10.1542/peds.2019-1791.
102. Stokley S, Jeyaraja J, Yankey D, et al. Human papillomavirus vaccination coverage among adolescents, 2007-2013, and postlicensure vaccine safety monitoring, 2006-2014— United States. *MMWR Morb Mortal Wkly Rep.* 2014;63:620–624.
103. Lei J, Ploner A, Elfstrom KM, et al. HPV Vaccination and the risk of invasive cervical cancer. *N Engl J Med.* 2020;383(14):1340–1348.
104. Walker TY, Evans LD, Yankey D, et al. National, regional, state, and selected local area vaccination coverage among adolescents aged 13–17 years—United States, 2018. *MMWR Morb Mortal Wkly Rep.* 2019;68(33):718–723.
105. Bloom P, Ogbuanu I. Vaccination to prevent human papillomavirus infections: From promise to practice. *PLoS Med.* 2017;14:e1002325.
106. Henriksen R, Sogaard PE, Grennert L, et al. Autoimmune antibodies and pregnancy outcome in women with false-positive syphilis test results. A retrospective controlled investigation of women from 5170 deliveries. *Acta Obstet Gynecol Scand.* 1989;68:537–540.

141

Bone and Joint Infections

Bryan T. Alexander and Scott J. Bergman

KEY CONCEPTS

1. The most common cause of osteomyelitis (particularly that acquired by hematogenous spread) and infectious arthritis is *Staphylococcus aureus* (*S. aureus*).
2. Culture and susceptibility information are essential as a guide for antimicrobial treatment of osteomyelitis and infectious arthritis.
3. Joint aspiration and examination of synovial fluid are extremely important to evaluate the possibility of infectious arthritis.
4. The most important treatment modality of acute osteomyelitis is the administration of appropriate antibiotics in adequate doses for a sufficient length of time.
5. Antibiotics generally are given in high doses so that adequate antimicrobial concentrations are reached within the infected bone and joints.
6. Oral antimicrobial therapies can be used for osteomyelitis to follow a parenteral regimen in children who have a good clinical response to IV antibiotics and in adults without diabetes mellitus or peripheral vascular disease when the organism is susceptible to the oral antimicrobial, a suitable oral agent is available, and adherence is ensured.
7. The standard duration of antimicrobial treatment for acute osteomyelitis is 4 to 6 weeks.
8. The three most important therapeutic approaches to the management of infectious arthritis are appropriate antibiotics, joint drainage, and joint rest.
9. Monitoring of antibiotic therapy is important and typically involves noting clinical signs of inflammation, periodic white blood cell (WBC) counts, C-reactive protein, and erythrocyte sedimentation rate (ESR) determinations.

BEYOND THE BOOK

Activity #1 The long-acting lipoglycopeptide antibiotics, dalbavancin and oritavancin, are potentially useful treatments for bone and joint infections because of their infrequent dosing and gram-positive spectrum of activity. Conduct a literature search to identify one primary research report published on these agents in the last 2 years. If the manuscript provides data on the safety or effectiveness of these drugs in treating deep-seated infection for longer than 2 weeks, reflect on the advantages and disadvantages for this type of treatment strategy.

Activity #2 The OVIVA trial, as discussed in the chapter, was a practice changing study for many clinicians and has significantly motivated the process of shifting more treatment courses for bone and joint infections away from IV agents, which require OPAT, toward appropriate oral regimens. However, the results of this trial aren't applicable to all clinical situations that arise. Review the OVIVA study methods, results, and conclusions (https://www.nejm.org/doi/full/10.1056/NEJMoa1710926) and make a list of the clinical situations and oral regimens for which these study results may apply. This will help you advocate for the use of oral therapy in the most appropriate circumstances.

INTRODUCTION

Bone and joint infections are comprised of two disease processes known, respectively, as *osteomyelitis* and *septic* or *infectious arthritis*. They are unique and separate infectious entities with different signs and symptoms and infecting organisms. Prosthetic joint infections, resulting from the advancement of modern technology, are distinct and blend attributes of each disease. Despite therapy, these infections all cause significant morbidity from residual damage with chronic or recurring infections. Emphasis on initiating antibiotic therapy, targeted to the most likely pathogens, as soon as possible is important in reducing long-term complications.

EPIDEMIOLOGY

Osteomyelitis

(1) Osteomyelitis has historically been an uncommon disease. One classic publication reported that 247 patients had osteomyelitis in a prominent American teaching hospital during a 4-year period.[1] In Spain there were more than 500 cases of osteoarticular infections per year over the course of a decade.[2] Over that time, the incidence increased from 11.4 to 24.4 cases per 100,000 person-years.[3] Acute osteomyelitis has an annual incidence of 0.4 per 1,000 children. Osteomyelitis cases have been rising in adults due to an aging population having more cases of diabetic foot infections and prosthetic joint replacements. Osteomyelitis can be caused by contiguous spread, including postoperative contamination, direct puncture from trauma, or associated with adjacent soft tissue infections, which is the most common source. *Hematogenous osteomyelitis* comprises 19% of infections, and osteomyelitis occurring in patients with significant peripheral vascular disease comprises 34% of infections.

The bacteriology of hematogenous osteomyelitis is unique, in that one pathogen, *S. aureus*, is responsible for more than 80% of these infections. Streptococci and *Escherichia coli* (*E. coli*) make up the remainder in most of the population. One exception is in children 3 months to 4 years of age. With the advent of molecular diagnostics, *Kingella kingae* (*K. kingae*), an organism that is part of the oral microbiota, has been identified as a common cause of preschool osteoarticular infections.[4] After children reach the age of 4 years, *S. aureus* again accounts for nearly 80% of infections. *Haemophilus influenzae* type b used to be an important pathogen but has been almost completely eliminated with the use of the conjugate vaccine. Osteomyelitis in neonates can result from organisms transferred from the mother at birth such as Group B Streptococcus, and *E. coli*, but is most commonly from infection with *S. aureus*.

Vertebral osteomyelitis occurs through hematogenous spread and has several unique features, being most common in adults over 50 years of age and often misdiagnosed initially. It typically presents with recalcitrant back pain unresponsive to usual symptomatic therapies, elevated inflammatory markers, and sometimes fever.[5] The lumbar and thoracic regions are the locations of most infections. Infections are most likely to develop in the vascular areas near the subchondral plate region of the vertebral body. These infections are typically monomicrobial and are caused principally by staphylococci.[5] Gram-negative organisms, most commonly the Enterobacterales, *E. coli* and *Klebsiella pneumoniae,* that originate within the urinary tract or intra-abdominal cavity are more common in older patients.[7] *Mycobacterium tuberculosis* and fungi also are known to cause infections in the spine, albeit rarely. Skin and respiratory tract infections are other sources of infection known to lead to vertebral infections.

Contiguous-spread disease has several important differences compared with hematogenous osteomyelitis. Although *S. aureus* is still the most common organism isolated, polymicrobial infections occur more often than with hematogenous osteomyelitis. *Streptococcus spp., Staphylococcus epidermidis, E. coli, Pseudomonas aeruginosa* (*P. aeruginosa*), and anaerobes can also be isolated.

Patients with diabetes mellitus frequently have infections that involve the foot. Cases extending to the bone may result in mixed infection, including with gram-negative bacilli. Puncture injuries to the foot, causing osteochondritis, are another reason for gram-negative infection, sometimes caused by *P. aeruginosa*. *S. aureus* remains a significant pathogen in these patients due to its prevalence on the skin. When anaerobes are grown from cultures, they usually are found in association with other organisms, including aerobic bacteria. *Bacteroides fragilis* comprises the majority of anaerobic isolates. Predisposing factors in patients who have anaerobic osteomyelitis include vascular disease, peripheral neuropathy, trauma, bites, or contiguous infections such as abscess.

Infectious Arthritis

Infectious or septic arthritis is an inflammatory reaction within the joint space. Septic arthritis is one of the most common causes of new cases of arthritis. The incidence of proven or likely septic arthritis is 4 to 10 cases per 100,000 patient-years. The incidence of septic arthritis increases 10-fold among patients that have rheumatoid arthritis.[8]

Although relatively infrequent, neonates can have infectious arthritis because of a broad range of organisms similar to osteomyelitis, with *S. aureus*, Group B *Streptococcus*, and *E. coli* being most common. *K. kingae* is now considered predominant in those 6 months to 4 years old, while *S. aureus* is the most common pathogen in children 4 years of age and older.[9] Pneumococcal arthritis is decreasing in incidence as a result of conjugate pneumococcal vaccine administration to infants.[10] If the child has not been fully vaccinated or is immunocompromised, *S. pneumoniae* or *H. influenzae* type b may be a cause.

Some organisms, such as *S. aureus* and *Neisseria gonorrhoeae*, are especially likely to infect a joint during bacteremia. Gonococcal arthritis is a common manifestation of disseminated gonococcal infection, occasionally with associated osteomyelitis.[11] Gonococcal arthritis is now uncommon in North America and Europe, although it remains an important concern in developing countries.

Within the adult population, *S. aureus* is responsible for the majority of arthritis cases.[12] Streptococcal infections are the second most common, followed by gram-negative organisms. Among the latter, *E. coli* is the most common; however, *P. aeruginosa* can be seen in special situations such as in people who inject drugs (PWID) or nosocomial infections.

Although rare, infectious arthritis can be caused by fungi, mycobacteria, or viruses such as varicella-zoster, rubella, or parvovirus.[13] Penetrating injury of the joint can result in an infection due to *Pasteurella* or *Capnocytophaga* from dog or cat bites, *Eikanella* in human bites, or *Pantoea* when the injury is induced by a thorn.

ETIOLOGY

Osteomyelitis

The most common method of classifying osteomyelitis is based on the mode of acquisition of the bone infection. Disease that results from spread through the bloodstream is termed *hematogenous osteomyelitis,* while that reaching the bone from an adjoining soft tissue infection is termed *contiguous osteomyelitis.* Patients with peripheral vascular disease are at risk for the development of contiguous osteomyelitis, and they present unique management features so are sometimes classified separately. Osteomyelitis that results from direct inoculation, such as from trauma, puncture wounds, or surgery, generally is also classified as inoculation osteomyelitis.

Osteomyelitis also can be classified based on the duration of the disease. Acute osteomyelitis describes infections of recent onset, with symptoms usually present about one week, whereas chronic infections are those of a longer duration. Some authors describe chronic infections as those with symptoms for more than one month before therapy, while other authors define chronic infections as any relapse of an initial infection. Hematogenous osteomyelitis almost always involves one bone, whereas contiguous osteomyelitis can present in multiple bones, especially when vascular insufficiency is an underlying risk factor.

Infectious Arthritis

Most infecting organisms produce an infection in a single joint, termed *monoarticular infection*; however, infections also can involve two or more joints, especially when associated with bacteremia. As with osteomyelitis, joint infections also can be classified according to the mechanisms by which the infecting organism reaches the joint. Infectious arthritis can result by spread from an adjacent bone infection, direct contamination of the joint space through trauma or surgery, or hematogenous dissemination. Hematogenous spread of the disease comprises the majority of infections; spread from osteomyelitis and direct inoculation are much less frequent. Septic arthritis is most prevalent in children and the elderly. Approximately, one-third of people with septic arthritis are children younger than 2 years of age.[8]

Unlike children, adults often have significant systemic diseases that predispose them to septic arthritis, such as diabetes mellitus, immunosuppressive states (eg, cancer or liver disease), or preexisting joint disease, particularly rheumatoid arthritis. Additional risk factors associated with adult septic arthritis (more than one factor may be present) are systemic corticosteroid use, arthrocentesis, distant infection, or trauma. PWID and individuals with intravascular infections such as endocarditis also are prone to develop septic arthritis.

PATHOPHYSIOLOGY

Osteomyelitis

Hematogenous Osteomyelitis

Hematogenous osteomyelitis is typically a disease of the growing bone in children, but occurs primarily in vertebrae of adults. Table 141-1 summarizes the primary characteristics of osteomyelitis.

TABLE 141-1 Types of Osteomyelitis, Age Distribution, Common Sites, and Risk Factors

Type of Osteomyelitis	Typical Age (years)	Site(s) Involved	Risk Factors
Hematogenous	<1	Long bones and joints	Prematurity, umbilical or other central venous catheter or venous cut-down, respiratory distress syndrome, and perinatal asphyxia
	1-20	Long bones (femur, tibia, and humerus)	Infection (pharyngitis, cellulitis, and respiratory infections), trauma, and sickle cell disease
	Older than 50	Vertebrae	Diabetes mellitus, blunt trauma to spine, and urinary tract infection
Contiguous	Older than 50	Femur, tibia, and mandible	Hip fractures and open fractures, soft tissue infections or abscesses
Direct Inoculation	<18	Feet and hands	Puncture injury to extremity or other trauma
Vascular insufficiency	Older than 50	Feet and toes	Diabetes mellitus, peripheral vascular disease, and pressure sores

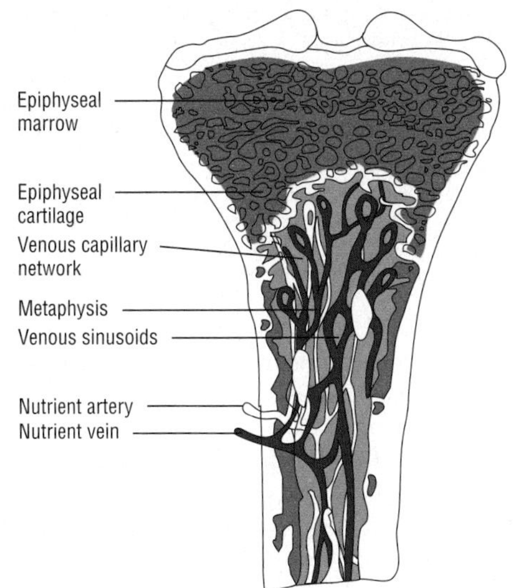

FIGURE 141-1 Cross-section of normal bone.

Unique features of the anatomy and vascular supply of long bones appear to predispose them to become infected.[14] Bacteria are seeded within the metaphysis (Fig. 141-1) as the nutrient arteries of the long bones divide within the medullary canal of the bone into small arterioles. These end in hairpin turns near the growth plate and flow into veins, of much wider diameter, that drain the medullary cavity.[1] The infection is initiated within the bend of arterioles where there is considerable slowing of blood flow in the hairpin capillary loops. This sludging of blood flow allows bacteria present within the bloodstream to settle and initiate an inflammatory response. They have access to the bone by gaps in the endothelium and the absence of a basement membrane. In addition to these structural features, phagocytosis is less active within the metaphysis. After the bacteria settle in the bone, avascular necrosis can occur from occlusion of the nutrient vessels and release of bacterial enzymes. Once the infection is initiated, exudate begins to form within the bone marrow and the fluid accumulates under increased pressure. The age of the patient largely determines the next stage in the pathophysiology.

Neonatal infections commonly involve multiple bones. The vascular supply of long bones in neonates has unique anatomic characteristics that affect their clinical presentation. Bridging blood vessels go across the epiphyseal plate from the metaphysis into the epiphysis, thus enabling an infection that started within the metaphyseal area to spread easily to involve the epiphyses and then break into the joint. Therefore, in infants, not only can the infection spread under the periosteum or break through the periosteum and the shaft as in older children, but the infection also can spread directly through the bridging blood vessels to involve the joint.

In children older than 12 to 18 months, hematogenous osteomyelitis typically involves a single bone and has a predilection for involvement of the long bones, such as the femur, tibia, humerus, and fibula. The infection that started in the metaphysis of a long bone is prevented from spreading into the epiphysis and the adjacent joint space because of the epiphyseal growth plate which acts as a physical barrier; however, the exudate often dissects from the medulla through the soft cortex to the subperiosteal space as the periosteum in these children is loosely attached to the underlying cortex. The periosteum is thick and not easily ruptured; thus, the subperiosteal space retains the pus, sometimes forming a subperiosteal abscess. If there is significant damage to the periosteum, the pus can decompress into a soft tissue abscess. The cortex obtains most of its blood supply from the periosteum and a subperiosteal abscess can impair the blood flow to the outer portion of the cortical bone resulting in a devitalized piece of dead bone termed a *sequestrum*. The elevated periosteum remains viable because its blood supply, derived from the overlying muscle, is unaffected. The raised periosteum will continue to produce bone; however, this new bone is now separated from the cortex because the periosteum has been raised from the infection. This new bone that is deposited under the periosteum is termed *involucrum*. In addition to these anatomic and functional features, there is some evidence that trauma is associated with developing an infection in specific bones. Children who develop hematogenous osteomyelitis may report some type of trauma before the onset of their symptoms, and animal data indicate that traumatized bone is more likely to become infected than normal bone.

In adults, the periosteum is tightly bound to the cortex which is thick. These anatomic features generally cause the infections to remain intramedullary. As expected, subperiosteal abscess formation is less common in this population. The infection can spread to subperiosteal structures through the Haversian and Volkmann canals.

Osteomyelitis of the vertebrae is also acquired hematogenously and this occurs most frequently in patients older than 50 years of age.[5] Vertebral disease in younger adults and children usually involves the disk space and the two vertebral facets adjoining it because of the nature of the vascular supply of the vertebrae at that age. This syndrome is known as diskitis.

Direct Inoculation Osteomyelitis

This category of osteomyelitis includes infections caused by direct entrance of organisms from a source outside the body. Penetrating wounds (eg, trauma), open fractures, and various invasive orthopedic procedures can result in direct inoculation of organisms into the bone. More than 80% of cases of postoperative osteomyelitis are known to occur following open reduction of fractures. Specifically, these infections occur most commonly after internal fixation of a hip, femoral, or tibial shaft fracture. Inoculation osteomyelitis can also occur as a result of penetrating foreign bodies, most commonly nail puncture injuries to the foot.

Contiguous Spread Osteomyelitis

Osteomyelitis secondary to spread from an adjacent soft tissue infection is called *contiguous osteomyelitis*. It can result from pressure ulcers (typically from laying in the decubitus position) or from adjacent soft tissue infections that most often involves the distal extremities (eg, diabetic foot infection). Less commonly, infection can spread from infected teeth to involve the mandible, or occur secondary to sinus infections by spreading through the mucosal lining of the sinuses into the vascular system surrounding the bone.

Contiguous-spread osteomyelitis occurs most commonly in patients older than age 50, likely because predisposing factors, such as diabetes mellitus, vascular diseases, or hip fractures, exist more often in this age group.

Patients with osteomyelitis in association with severe vascular insufficiency are extremely difficult to manage.[15] Frequently, patients with vascular disease develop osteomyelitis in their toes or even their fingers, and there is typically an adjacent area of infection, such as cellulitis or dermal ulcers. Importantly, infections in these patients can be polymicrobial, usually including *Staphylococcus* and *Streptococcus*, or a combination of those and Enterobacterales. Enterococci and anaerobic organisms also can be involved, but not as often.

Chronic Osteomyelitis

Chronic osteomyelitis is more likely to occur if large segments of bone become avascular and necrotic. It is common in inadequately managed foot infections of patients with diabetes. This results in a piece of devitalized bone to which antimicrobial delivery is impaired. As a result, the infection is prone to exacerbations and may lead to weakening of that bone or to the formation of draining sinuses to the skin.

Infectious Arthritis

Infectious arthritis usually is acquired by hematogenous spread. The synovial tissue is highly vascular and does not have a basement membrane, so organisms in the blood can easily reach the synovial fluid. Table 141-2 summarizes the characteristics of acute infectious arthritis.

Preexisting abnormal joint architecture, joint trauma, and surgery are risk factors because chronic inflammation or trauma makes the joint more susceptible to infection. Individuals with rheumatoid arthritis can be prone to bacterial infection because of an inherent phagocytic defect, as well as concomitant corticosteroid therapy, biologic response modifier, or other immunosuppressants. Patients infected with disseminated or untreated *N. gonorrhoeae* are at risk of gonococcal arthritis.

In addition to hematogenous spread, organisms can gain access to the joint from a deep-penetrating wound injury, intra-articular steroid injections, arthroscopy, prosthetic joint surgery, or spread to the joint from a contiguous focus of osteomyelitis. After bacteria gain access to the joint, the organisms begin to multiply and produce a purulent exudate within the joint. If this joint effusion is present beyond 7 days, chronic and sometimes irreversible damage can occur to the bone and joint as a result of proteolytic enzymes and pressure necrosis. Purulent effusions can promote cartilage destruction by increasing leukocyte enzyme activity. In conjunction with the development of the effusion, almost all patients will develop a hot, swollen, and painful joint.

CLINICAL PRESENTATION

Osteomyelitis

The clinical presentation of acute *hematogenous osteomyelitis* is summarized in Table 141-3. Although neonatal *hematogenous osteomyelitis* can spread rapidly to involve the joint, often there are few associated systemic symptoms.[14] A joint effusion is present in 60% to 70% of neonatal infections. Decreased limb motion or edema over the affected area may be the only signs from which to suspect the diagnosis. While it is sometimes acute in onset, the disease is often insidious in children.

Vertebral osteomyelitis produces nonspecific symptoms, such as constant back pain, fever or night sweats, and weight loss.[5] The pain typically is present at rest and increases in severity with movement. Serious neurologic complications can occur if the infection extends and compresses the spinal cord.

The presentation of osteomyelitis after surgery or trauma depends on the precipitating cause. If the infection follows surgery or bone trauma, the symptoms usually are noted within 1 month. The most frequent symptom is pain in the area of infection. Less commonly, patients also can develop a fever and elevated WBC count.

With contiguous-spread osteomyelitis there is often an area of localized tenderness, warmth, edema, and erythema over the infected site. Patients with significant vascular insufficiency usually have less pronounced local symptoms, such as pain, swelling, and redness. Less commonly, they also can have fever and elevated WBC count.

Infectious Arthritis

Patients with nongonococcal bacterial arthritis almost always present with a fever, and 50% of patients have an elevated WBC count

TABLE 141-2 Characteristics of Acute Infectious Arthritis

Feature	Finding
Peak incidence	Children younger than 16 years Adults older than 50 years
Clinical findings	Fever of 38-40°C (100.4-104°F) in children; painful swollen joint in the absence of trauma Physical examination: Effusion, restriction of joint motion, tenderness, redness, and warmth of joint
Most commonly affected joints	Knee, hip, ankle, elbow, wrist, and shoulder
Laboratory findings	
Erythrocyte sedimentation rate	Elevated in 90% of cases
White blood cell count	Elevated in 30%-60% of cases
Left shift	Seen in two-thirds of patients
Blood culture	Positive in 40% of cases
Needle aspiration of joint	Gram-stain diagnostic in 30%-50% of cases. Synovial fluid cultures are positive in 60%-80% of cases. Synovial fluid yields an elevated white blood cell count with a high percentage of neutrophils. Synovial fluid glucose decreased relative to serum glucose. Lactic acid levels elevated in nongonococcal infectious arthritis, but not in gonococcal infectious arthritis

TABLE 141-3 Clinical Presentation of Hematogenous Osteomyelitis

Signs and symptoms
Significant tenderness of the affected area, pain, swelling, fever, chills, decreased motion, and malaise

Laboratory tests
Elevated erythrocyte sedimentation rate, C-reactive protein, and white blood cell count 50% of patients will have positive blood cultures

Diagnostic studies
Bone changes observed on radiographs 10-14 days after the onset of infection. Magnetic resonance imaging and technetium scans positive as early as 1 day after the onset of infection

(see Table 141-2). Nongonococcal bacterial arthritis is almost always monoarticular. The knee is the most commonly involved joint, but infections also can occur in the shoulder, wrist, hip, ankle, interphalangeal joints, and elbow joints. Sometimes, the initial focus of infection that acted as the portal of entry can be identified. Common routes for bacterial entrance include infections of the respiratory tract, skin, and urinary tract or which led to subsequent bacteremia; often no specific source can be identified. Blood cultures are important in these patients because they can be positive in 50% of patients.

The most frequent initial sign of disseminated gonococcal infections is the triad of dermatitis, tenosynovitis (inflammation and swelling of a tendon), and migratory polyarthralgia or polyarthritis. Women are more prone to develop disseminated gonococcal infections than men by a ratio of 4:1. The second and third trimesters of pregnancy and the time of menses appear to be the times of greatest risk for developing gonococcal bacteremia, hypothesized to be associated with mucosal vascularity. Common joints involved include the knee, wrist, elbow, and ankle. Presentation varies slightly depending on whether or not the woman is pregnant. In nonpregnant women, duration of symptoms are longer, presence of joint effusion is more likely, and white blood cells are more often present within the synovial fluid.[16]

Another type of infectious arthritis occurs following prosthetic joint surgery. The most common symptom is pain. Local signs of inflammation and fever are common in acute infections but chronic infections present in a more subtle fashion, typically with pain alone and often loosening of the prosthesis. With these infections, the C-reactive protein (CRP) typically is elevated, although a leukocytosis often is absent. Infections from intra-operative contamination usually become apparent within 1 year of surgery. Those that present early (<3 months) are usually *S. aureus,* but occasionally gram-negative, anaerobic, or polymicrobial infections are also seen. Less virulent skin organisms such as *S. epidermidis, Enterococcus,* or the anaerobic gram-positive bacillus, *Cutibacterium* (formerly *Propionibacterium*) *acnes* present later, often 3 to 12 months from surgery. After 1 year, hematogenous spread becomes a risk factor for *S. aureus* infection again.

Radiologic and Laboratory Tests

Osteomyelitis

2 The evaluation of a patient who may have osteomyelitis has several unusual aspects. Radiographs of the involved area should be obtained to rule out other processes such as a fracture. Bone changes characteristic of osteomyelitis appear late and are not typically seen until at least 10 to 14 days after the onset of the infection, as more than 50% of the bone matrix must be decalcified before the lesions can be detected radiologically. Magnetic resonance imaging (MRI) is the most sensitive and commonly used diagnostic imaging modality in those without metal hardware. It offers the advantage of better anatomic definition, especially of abscesses or joint effusions, compared to plain radiograph or traditional computed topography (CT) scan. Radionuclide bone scanning (with technetium or gallium) CT or positron emission tomography (PET) scanning can be useful in identifying the focus of osteomyelitis in patients unable to have an MRI.[17]

Despite the seriousness of osteomyelitis, often there are few laboratory abnormalities. The erythrocyte sedimentation rate (ESR), CRP, and WBC count may be the only laboratory abnormalities. The degree of abnormality of these laboratory findings does not correlate with the disease outcome; however, these inflammatory markers are useful for monitoring therapy. CRP is generally the more sensitive marker of response to therapy and often increases and decreases before the ESR.

When a clinical assessment of osteomyelitis is suspected, it is important to establish a bacteriologic diagnosis by culture of the infected bone and blood. Accurate culture information is especially important as a guide for treatment of osteomyelitis in this era of increasing antimicrobial resistance. Bone aspiration or bone biopsy is valuable in determining an accurate bacteriologic diagnosis. In addition, they help determine whether or not there is an abscess present. If an abscess is identified, it must be drained and the pus cultured with a Gram stain performed. Aspirates of subperiosteal pus or metaphyseal fluid yield a pathogen in 70% of cases. Cultures should be done for both aerobic and anaerobic bacteria. A Gram-stain result from the aspirate can be useful in initiating appropriate empirical antibiotic therapy.

If a specimen is obtained from a previously undrained or unopened wound abscess, the true etiologic pathogen usually can be identified. In chronic osteomyelitis, however, identification can be more difficult. Open wounds and draining sinuses frequently are contaminated with colonizing organisms and thus provide inaccurate culture information. They cannot be relied on to reflect the true etiologic pathogen unless consecutive deep sinus tract cultures reveal the same pathogens.[15] Cultures of loculated pus aspirates in the area of orthopedic devices removed from infected bone can be trusted, however, to identify the true etiologic organism. The preferable time to obtain culture material in a patient with a chronic draining sinus is at the time of open surgical debridement.

In addition to performing cultures from the involved bone, it also is important to obtain cultures from any site believed to be the primary source of a bacteremia. Approximately 50% of patients with hematogenous osteomyelitis will have positive blood cultures and may obviate the need for bone aspiration in these patients.

Infectious Arthritis

3 Radiographs of infected joints often reveal distension of the joint capsule with soft tissue swelling in the adjacent space. MRI can be helpful in identifying an infected joint, especially the shoulder and hip. In patients who have developed an infected prosthetic joint, loosening of the prosthesis can be seen radiographically.

When evaluating the possibility of a patient having infectious arthritis, immediate joint aspiration with analysis of the synovial fluid is extremely important. The presence of purulent fluid usually indicates the presence of a septic joint, although other inflammatory arthritic conditions such as rheumatoid arthritis or gout can also demonstrate purulence. The synovial fluid WBC count and percentage of neutrophils found are important factors in defining an infectious etiology. The specific values best predictive of infection are variable based on multiple factors, including whether a native or prosthetic joint is being sampled, and exist along a continuum of sensitivity and specificity, as illustrated in Table 141-4. As with osteomyelitis, most patients will have an elevated CRP concentration and ESR. However, serum WBC, ESR, and CRP may not be useful acutely in septic arthritis.[18] Approximately half of patients

TABLE 141-4 Synovial Fluid Analysis Associated with Infectious Arthritis

Native Joint Fluid	
WBC >50,000 cells/μL (50 × 10^9/L) >90% (0.90) neutrophil count	Sensitivity 62%, Specificity 92%, Sensitivity 73%, Specificity 79%.
Prosthetic Joint Fluid	
Knee	
Acute (<6 weeks from arthroplasty) WBC >8100 cells/μL (8.1 × 10^9/L) *Chronic (>6 months from arthroplasty)* WBC >1700 cells/μL (1.7 × 10^9/L) OR >65% (0.65) neutrophil count	Sensitivity 86%, Specificity 89%, Sensitivity ≈95%, Specificity ≈90%.
Hip	
WBC >4200 cells/μL (4.2 × 10^9/L)	Sensitivity 84%, Specificity 93%.

Data from References 60-63.

with an infected native joint have a low synovial glucose level, usually less than 40 mg/dL (2.2 mmol/L). Both blood and joint fluid should be cultured aerobically and anaerobically in a patient suspected of having an infected joint. These cultures or Gram stains of joint fluid demonstrate bacteria in > 50% of patients with septic arthritis; however, such results are positive in only 25% of patients with gonococcal arthritis. Pharyngeal, rectal, cervical, or urethral smears and cultures, as well as cultures of cutaneous lesions, should be performed if a disseminated gonococcal infection is considered. Nucleic acid–based assays should also be used for the diagnosis of genital gonococcal infection.

TREATMENT

Desired Outcome

Osteomyelitis

The goals of treatment are resolution of the infection and prevention of long-term sequelae. The ultimate outcome of osteomyelitis depends on the acute or chronic nature of the disease and how rapidly appropriate therapy including surgical drainage where appropriate is initiated. Patients with acute osteomyelitis have the best prognosis.

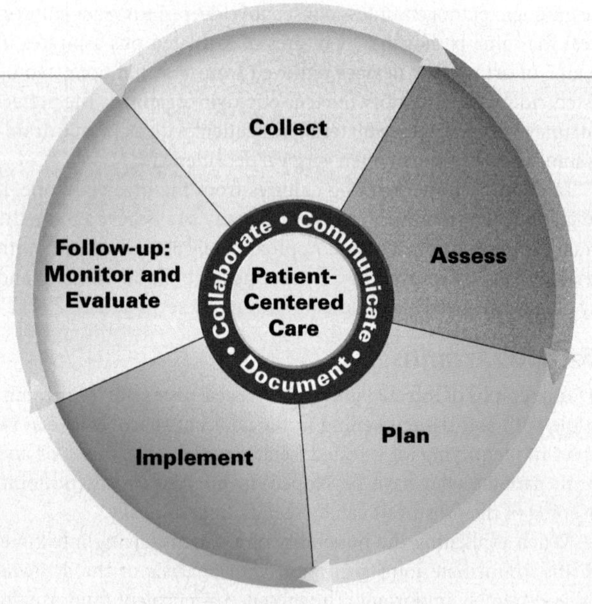

Patient Care Process for Bone and Joint Infections

The image shows the five fundamental steps included in The Pharmacist's Care Process endorsed by the Joint Commission for Pharmacy Practitioners (2014). The tagline of this process reads collaborate, communicate, and document. The five fundamental steps listed here are collect, assess, plan, implement, and follow-up: monitor and evaluate. All these steps are listed in a circular block diagram.

Collect

- Patient characteristics (eg, age, sex, pregnancy status)
- Patient medical history
- Social history (eg, ethanol or injection drug use) and living conditions
- Current medications and recent antibiotic use
- Objective data
  - Culture of bone, synovial fluid, or deep tissue (not superficial)
  - Labs including white blood cells (WBC), serum creatinine (SCr), and C-reactive protein (CRP) or erythrocyte sedimentation rate (ESR)
  - Imaging for infection

Assess

- Risk factors for bone and joint infections (Table 141-1)
- Markers of infection (Tables 141-2 and 141-3)
- Culture results and antimicrobial susceptibilities
- Ability/willingness to adhere to treatment regimen, including self-administration of outpatient parenteral therapy or travel to infusion center
- Ability/willingness to pay for treatment options (eg, home health, infusion center visits, and/or prescriptions from pharmacy)
- Ability/willingness to obtain laboratory monitoring tests (eg, WBC, SCr, serum drug concentrations)
- Emotional status (eg, presence of anxiety, depression)

Plan*

- Drug therapy regimen including specific antibiotic dose, route, frequency, and duration (see Table 141-6)
- Monitoring parameters including efficacy (eg, WBC, CRP or ESR, pain, limb swelling) and safety (eg, complete blood count, SCr, diarrhea); frequency and timing of follow-up (Table 141-7)
- Patient education (eg, purpose of treatment, invasive procedures, drug-specific information, medication administration/injection technique)
- Self-monitoring for resolution of symptoms, occurrence of adverse effects, when to seek emergency medical attention
- Referrals to other providers when appropriate (eg, infectious diseases specialist, orthopedic surgeon, vascular surgeon, endocrine/diabetes specialist)

Implement*

- Provide patient education regarding all elements of treatment plan
- Use motivational interviewing and coaching strategies to maximize adherence
- Schedule follow-up (2-4 weeks)

Follow-up: Monitor and Evaluate

- Resolution of symptoms (eg, pain, limb/joint swelling, instability)
- Presence of adverse effects (eg, cytopenias, diarrhea, hypersensitivity reactions)
- Patient adherence to treatment plan using multiple sources of information
- Reevaluate again at the end of therapy

Collaborate with patient, caregivers, and other healthcare professionals.

Cure rates exceeding 80% can be expected for patients with acute osteomyelitis who have surgery when indicated and receive appropriate antibiotics for 4 to 6 weeks. When the growth plate is involved in children, discrepancies in the growth of bones or angular bone deformities can result. The infection is almost never fatal.

In contrast, patients with chronic osteomyelitis have a much poorer prognosis. Dead bone and other necrotic material from the infection act as a bacterial reservoir and make the infection very difficult to eliminate. Adequate surgical debridement to remove all the dead bone and necrotic material, combined with prolonged administration of antibiotics, provides the best chance to obtain a cure. The inability to remove all the dead bone can allow residual infection and require suppressive antibiotics to control the infection. Amputation, declines in quality of life, and recurrent infection are not uncommon with chronic osteomyelitis.

Infectious Arthritis

While many patients who develop infectious arthritis recover with no long-term sequelae, 50% are left with decreased joint function or mobility. Gonococcal arthritis usually resolves rapidly with antibiotics and has fewer sequelae. Individuals at greatest risk for long-term sequelae are those who have symptoms present for more than 7 days before starting therapy and those with infections occurring within the hip joint and infections caused by gram-negative organisms. Common long-term residual effects following infectious arthritis are limited joint motion and persistent pain.

During the initial phase of the infection, weight bearing such as walking on the joint should be avoided. Passive range-of-motion exercises should be initiated when the pain begins to subside to maintain joint mobility. Approximately one-third of patients with bacterial arthritis have a poor joint outcome, such as severe functional deterioration. Poor joint outcomes are associated with older patients, those with preexisting joint disease, and patients with an infected joint containing synthetic material.

General Approach to Treatment

Osteomyelitis

4 Following completion of the steps needed to determine the infecting organism, the most important treatment modality of acute osteomyelitis is the administration of appropriate antibiotics in adequate doses for a sufficient length of time. It is important to stress that early antibiotic therapy can mitigate the need for surgery, subsequent sepsis, chronic infection, disruption of longitudinal bone growth, and angular deformity of the bone. A long delay in treatment can allow bone necrosis to occur and make eradication of the infection much more difficult. In these patients with chronic osteomyelitis, exacerbations of the infection can result if all necrotic tissue or infected indwelling hardware are not removed surgically and all microorganisms eliminated. Chronic suppressive antimicrobial therapy and adjunctive treatment with hyperbaric oxygen or antibiotic-impregnated implants during surgery also have been used.

If a patient with hematogenous osteomyelitis does not respond by having a decrease in fever, local swelling, redness, and pain following the initiation of adequate antibiotic therapy, the patient should undergo surgical debridement of the infected area. It is important to emphasize the priority of starting antibiotics immediately after the cultures have been obtained for best microbiological yield and outcomes.[19]

Infectious Arthritis

Patients with infectious arthritis are typically admitted to the hospital to obtain synovial fluid and blood cultures and initiate antimicrobial therapy. An attempt to decrease bacterial burden in the joint space is made by performing either open or arthroscopic debridement. Empiric antibiotics are started as soon as culture specimens are collected. As with osteomyelitis, early initiation of antibiotic therapy is important to avoid complications such as avascular necrosis, limb-length discrepancy, and pathologic fractures. Staphylococci and streptococci are the most common organisms found in septic arthritis, accounting for approximately 70% to 85% of all cases, so treatment should be directed accordingly.[20,21]

In patients with prosthetic joint devices, orthopedic surgeons must work alongside infectious disease practitioners to determine the best course of action.[22] The gold standard treatment method includes resection of the implant, placement of a temporary antibiotic-impregnated cement spacer, and delayed component reimplantation. Retention of the implant may be necessary in patients who will receive irrigation and debridement in addition to antibiotic therapy, or antibiotic therapy alone in patients unable to tolerate surgical procedures.[23]

Pharmacologic Therapy

Osteomyelitis

Antibiotic Selection A critical component in the management of osteomyelitis is the selection of appropriate antibiotics. Empiric therapy must be selected on the basis of the most likely infecting organism while the results of culture and susceptibility data are pending. Once culture and susceptibility results are obtained, the antimicrobial therapy should be tailored. Table 141-5 summarizes empiric therapy recommendations.

With *Staphylococcus* being the most common bacteria in osteomyelitis, resistance patterns must be considered when deciding on an empiric agent. For communities showing low evidence of resistant strains of *S. aureus*, oxacillin or nafcillin has historically been the drug of choice, although cefazolin is now being used more often to treat susceptible strains due to ease of dosing, lower cost, and fewer adverse effects compared to anti-staphylococcal penicillins.[22-24] Clindamycin can be used in less severe cases, in patients with severe beta-lactam allergies or where methicillin-resistant *Staphylococcus aureus* (MRSA) rates are unknown.[25,26] Clindamycin is used more commonly in children because MRSA is more likely to be community-acquired and susceptible to clindamycin in this population. If 10% or more of *S. aureus* isolates are methicillin resistant in the surrounding community, then an agent active against MRSA should be selected empirically. Vancomycin is the treatment of choice in this scenario and in adults since they often have risk factors for hospital-associated MRSA.[25,26] Daptomycin is an effective alternate in patients where mitigation of the adverse effects associated with vancomycin or a more convenient dosing strategy are prioritized.[27]

In the setting of vertebral osteomyelitis, empiric therapy should be initiated in conjunction with culture if the patient is hemodynamically unstable, septic, or experiencing neurologic compromise; otherwise, it is recommended empiric therapy be held while awaiting culture results.[5] Vancomycin in combination with a fluoroquinolone or third/fourth-generation cephalosporin such as ceftriaxone is a reasonable empiric regimen.

5 **Antibiotic Bone Concentration** Antibiotics used in the management of acute osteomyelitis generally are given in high doses (adjusted for weight, renal function, hepatic function, or both) so that adequate antimicrobial concentrations are reached within the infected bone and joint.[23,28] Table 141-6 summarizes antibiotic doses that have been successful in the treatment of osteomyelitis.

6 **Oral Antibiotic Therapy** Criteria for the use of oral outpatient antibiotic therapy for osteomyelitis include all of the following:

- Confirmed osteomyelitis
- Initial positive clinical response to parenteral antibiotics
- A suitable oral agent is available
- Adherence is ensured

TABLE 141-5 Empiric Treatment of Osteomyelitis

Patient Subtype	Likely Infecting Organism	Antibiotic[a]	Recommendation Grades[b]
Newborn	*Staphylococcus aureus*, Group B *Streptococcus Escherichia coli*	Cefazolin 50-150 mg/kg/day IV	B-3
Children 3 years of age or younger	1. If vaccinated for *Haemophilus influenzae* type b: *K. kingae, S. aureus* or streptococci 2. If not vaccinated against *H. influenzae* type b (*or Streptococcus pneumoniae)*	1. Cefazolin 100-150 mg/kg/day IV 2. Cefuroxime 150 mg/kg/day IV Alternatives are ceftriaxone 75 mg/kg/day IV or amoxicillin-clavulanate 40-45 mg/kg/day orally	B-3 B-3
Children 4 years of age and older	*S. aureus*	Vancomycin 60 mg/kg/day IV, clindamycin 40 mg/kg/day, or cefazolin 100-150 mg/kg/day IV	A-3
Adults	*S. aureus*	Vancomycin 15 mg/kg every 12 hours or cefazolin 2 g IV every 8 hours	A-3
Persons who inject drugs	*S. aureus, Pseudomonas*	Vancomycin 15 mg/kg every 12 hours plus ciprofloxacin 750 mg orally twice daily, ceftazidime or cefepime 2 g IV every 8 hours	B-3
Postoperative or posttrauma patients	Gram-positive and gram-negative organisms	Vancomycin 15 mg/kg IV every 12 hours plus ceftazidime or cefepime 2 g IV every 8 hours	B-3
Patients with vascular insufficiency	Gram-positive and gram-negative organisms	Vancomycin 15 mg/kg IV every 12 hours plus ceftriaxone 2 g every 24 hours	B-3
	If anaerobes suspected (e.g. necrosis)	Add metronidazole 500 mg every 8 hours or clindamycin 900 mg IV every 8 hours or substitute ertapenem for ceftriaxone	C-3

IV, intravenous.

[a]Dosage should be adjusted for some agents in patients with renal and/or hepatic dysfunction.

[b]Strength of recommendations: A, B, C = good, moderate, and poor evidence to support recommendation, respectively. Quality of evidence: 1 = Evidence from more than one properly randomized, controlled studies or multiple time series; or dramatic results from uncontrolled experiments. 2 = Evidence from more than one well-designed clinical trial with randomization, from cohort or case-controlled analytic studies. 3 = Evidence from opinions of respected authorities, based on clinical experience, descriptive studies, or reports of expert communities.

TABLE 141-6 Antimicrobial Agents and Typical Doses for the Treatment of Bone and Joint Infections

Antimicrobial	Dose[a]	Comments
Amoxicillin	Adult: 1 g orally every 8 hours Children: 80-90 mg/kg/day divided every 12 hours	500-875 mg orally twice daily to 500 mg three times daily may be used for chronic suppression in adults
Amoxicillin/Clavulanate	Adult: 2,000/125 mg orally every 12 hours Children: 80-90 mg/kg/day of amoxicillin divided every 12 hours	875/125 mg orally twice daily or 500/125 mg three times daily may be used for step-down therapy or chronic suppression
Ampicillin	Adult: 2 g IV every 4 hours[21] Children: 150-200 mg/kg/day in four equal doses (max 8-12 g daily) VO: 12 g IV every 24 hours, continuous, or in six divided doses	May add IV aminoglycoside or ceftriaxone when treating *Enterococcus* spp. Continue adjunct therapy for 4-6 weeks in patients with infective endocarditis
Ampicillin/Sulbactam	Adult: 3 g IV every 6 hours	3-g dose equals 2-g ampicillin and 1-g sulbactam
Anti-staphylococcal penicillins (nafcillin, oxacillin, dicloxacillin)	Adult: Nafcillin or oxacillin 2 g IV every 4 hours Children: ≤200 mg/kg/day in four equal doses (max dose 8-12 g daily) VO: Nafcillin or oxacillin 2 g IV every 4 hours or continuous infusion	Adverse effects and cost are higher than cefazolin Dicloxacillin 500 mg three or four times daily may be used for suppression in adults
Aztreonam	Adult: 2 g IV every 8 hours	Use for patients with severe penicillin allergy and quinolone-resistant strains
Cefepime	Adult: 2 g IV every 8-12 hours	For Enterobacterales, 2 g IV every 12 hours
Cefotetan	Adult: 2 g IV every 12 hours	
Ceftazidime	Adult: 2 g IV every 8 hours	
Ceftriaxone	Adult: 2 g IV every 24 hours Children: 80-100 mg/kg/dose every 12-24 hours	
Ciprofloxacin	Adult: 400 IV every 8-12 hours or 500-750 mg orally every 12 hours	Should not be used as monotherapy for *Staphylococcus* infection, but may be combined with rifampin. Higher dose for *Pseudomonas*.
Clindamycin	Adult: 600 mg IV every 6 hours or 300-600 mg orally every 6 hours Children: 40 mg/kg/day in four equal doses (max dose 3 g daily) VO: 600-900 mg IV every 8 hours, or 300-450 mg orally four times daily	Recommended as second line for sensitive staphylococcal infection. 300 mg twice daily or three times daily may be used for suppression in adults.
Daptomycin	Adult: 6-8 mg/kg IV every 24 hours	
Doxycycline	Adult: 100 mg orally twice daily	Can be used in addition to rifampin for Brucella infection

(Continued)

TABLE 141-6 Antimicrobial Agents and Typical Doses for the Treatment of Bone and Joint Infections (*Continued*)

Antimicrobial	Dose[a]	Comments
Ertapenem	Adult: 1 g IV every 24 hours Children: 15 mg/kg every 12 hours	
First-generation cephalosporin (Cefazolin, Cephalexin)	Adult: Cefazolin 2 g IV every 8 hours Children: 100-150 mg/kg/day in 3 equal doses (max dose 6 g daily)	Cephalexin 500 mg orally every 6 hours or 1 g orally every 8 hours for step-down treatment.[21] Cephalexin 500 mg twice or three times daily may be used for suppression
Imipenem/cilastatin	Adult: 500 mg IV every 6 hours	Can add IV aminoglycoside empirically for treatment of *P. aeruginosa*
Levofloxacin	Adult: 500-750 mg IV once daily or 750 mg orally once daily	Add rifampin for treatment of *S. aureus*
Linezolid	Adult: 600 mg IV or orally every 12 hours Children: 30 mg/kg/day in three equal doses (max dose 1.2 g for no more than 28 days)	Long-term use can lead to cytopenias
Meropenem	Adult: 1 g IV every 8 hours	
Metronidazole	Adult: 500 mg orally or IV every 8 hours	Drug of choice for *Bacteroides* species and other susceptible anaerobes
Minocycline	Adult: 200 mg orally initially, then 100 mg orally twice daily	
Moxifloxacin	Adult: 400 mg orally once daily	For streptococci, Enterobacterales, and other susceptible gram-negative organisms. Not recommended for staphylococcal infection unless combined with rifampin.
Penicillin G	Adult: 3-4 million units IV every 4 hours or 20 million units IV continuous every 24 hours	For *Enterococcus*, add 4-6 weeks of aminoglycoside therapy in patients with infective endocarditis
Piperacillin/Tazobactam	Adult: 4.5 g IV every 6-8 hours	Every 6 hours or extended infusion (over 4 hours) for *P. aeruginosa*
Rifampin	Adult: 300 mg orally twice daily Children: 10 mg/kg/day orally divided twice daily	Only to be used in combination with another antimicrobial
Trimethoprim–Sulfamethoxazole	Adult: 1-2 double-strength tablets orally twice daily or 1 double-strength tablet orally three times a day	Second-line agent for Enterobacterales and other susceptible aerobic gram-negative organisms.
Vancomycin	Adult: 15 mg/kg IV every 12 hours Children: 60 mg/kg/day in four equal doses	Adjust based on patient and pharmacokinetic parameters. Target trough of 15 mcg per milliliter (mg/L; 10.4 μmol/L) or area under the concentration-curve of 400-600. Consider loading dose for MRSA. For *Enterococcus*, add 4-6 weeks of aminoglycoside therapy in patients with infective endocarditis. If bacteria is known, use only if resistant to beta-lactams or patient is allergic to first-line options

IV, intravenous; MRSA, methicillin resistant *Staphylococcus aureus*; VO, vertebral osteomyelitis.

[a]Dosage should be adjusted for some agents in patients with renal and/or hepatic dysfunction.

Suitable candidates are children with good clinical response to intravenous therapy and adults without diabetes mellitus or peripheral vascular disease.

The use of oral antibiotics is well studied in children.[29-31] Typically, injectable antibiotics are used initially and then switched to oral antibiotics when the patient is afebrile and there is a decrease in the signs of inflammation.[19] If pus is obtained on the initial needle aspirate, or if a reduction in fever, local swelling, and tenderness does not occur despite adequate rest, immobilization, and intensive antibiotic therapy, patients undergo surgical drainage. The patients enrolled in oral antibiotic trials generally had disease of recent onset, identification of a specific infecting organism, enforced adherence, and surgery as indicated. In patients who meet these criteria, oral antibiotics appear to offer a great advantage in the treatment of osteomyelitis. Patients not meeting these criteria may have a higher risk of developing chronic osteomyelitis if oral therapy is inappropriate or not strictly adhered to. In adults, oral antibiotics are used more conservatively due to more limited blood flow to the bones, but evidence is emerging that oral therapy can be effective for adult osteomyelitis and septic arthritis.[32-34] Ciprofloxacin and levofloxacin are well-studied oral primary therapy due to their high bioavailability and great distribution into bone.[35] Fluoroquinolones (with the exception of delafloxacin) are not reliably effective against staphylococci on their own as resistance develops rapidly and should not be used alone empirically. They have successfully been combined with rifampin when isolates are susceptible to both classes of drugs.[36] Rifampin is particularly useful for treating infections with biofilms that have a propensity to grow on smooth surfaces such as bone, and especially prosthetic devices.[37] However, rifampin has a multitude of drug interactions, and caution should be used when adding to a regimen.

Duration of Antibiotic Therapy

7 Following debridement, bone takes 3 to 4 weeks to revascularize, which becomes the basis of treatment duration. The specific duration of antibiotic therapy needed in the management of osteomyelitis and septic arthritis has traditionally been 4 to 6 weeks and 3 to 4 weeks, respectively.[38] For adults, those durations of treatment are still recommended but newer studies in children have explored shorter durations along with more liberal transitions to oral antibiotics. For children with *septic arthritis*, a course as short as 10 days is sufficient as long as the CRP level normalizes.[39] French guidelines recommend treatment for a minimum of 3 weeks in children with osteomyelitis as failure rates approaching 20% have been observed with antibiotics administered for less than that.[40] This is based on studies showing that improvement in the patient's clinical signs and symptoms in addition to normalization of the CRP level or ESR is an important parameter for predicting efficacy.[41,42] Treatment failures

may be due to the presence of residual bacteria in necrotic bone or infected hardware (wires, plates, screws, and rods) that could not be removed.[35] If signs or symptoms are still present at the end of therapy, treatment should be extended. For adults, guidelines from the Infectious Diseases Society of America (IDSA) recommend therapy for 8 weeks in adults with osteomyelitis from MRSA,[43] particularly in patients with vertebral osteomyelitis at high risk of relapse such as those with end-stage renal disease or undrained paravertebral/psoas abscesses.[44] In some cases of chronic osteomyelitis, lifelong suppressive therapy might be the most appropriate option, particularly when prosthetic devices remain.[45] The goal in chronic suppressive therapy is to avoid readmissions from exacerbation of established infection; however, the use of this approach must be balanced with the risk for development of antimicrobial resistance and toxicity over extended periods.[46] Often specific dosing regimens of oral therapies are utilized in this situation (see Table 141-6).[46]

Duration of antibiotic administration for vertebral osteomyelitis can vary depending on the infecting organism, extent of bone destruction, or presence of abscesses. The IDSA guidelines recommend a minimum of 6 weeks of either parenteral therapy or highly bioavailable oral therapy.[3] This is necessary because of the outcomes in older patients with degenerative bone disease that have reduced blood flow to the site of infection and are most at risk of the disease. With gram-negative bacteria a longer duration (8 weeks or greater) is associated with less rates of recurrence compared to shorter durations (4-6 weeks).[7] One prospective trial compared 6 and 12 weeks of treatment for patients with pyogenic vertebral osteomyelitis (most commonly *S. aureus*) and found the longer duration to be no better.[47] However, patients with prosthetic joint infections have benefited from 12 weeks of antibiotic therapy.[48] For patients with retained hardware following prosthetic joint infection, 3 to 6 months of therapy is often necessary.[45] Many questions remain on the optimal duration for bone infections in adults and whether it is safe to use shorter courses.[35]

Special Populations

Osteomyelitis in PWID has unique features. More than 50% of such infections involve the vertebral column and up to 20% of infections are located in either the sternoarticular or pelvic girdle. Infections are much less frequent within the extremities. They also have an unusual spectrum of organisms. Although *Staphylococcus* and *Streptococcus* are sometimes cultured, with MRSA being more common than in the general population, gram-negative bacteria are responsible for many infections. In one outbreak *P. aeruginosa*, either singly or in combination with other organisms, was cultured in 78% of all such infections. *Klebsiella*, *Enterobacter*, and *Serratia* species also can be less commonly identified. Spinal infections are caused predominately by *S. aureus*.[49]

Patients with sickle cell anemia and related hemoglobinopathies also represent a unique population, in that two-thirds of bone infections in these patients are caused by *Salmonella* species, while the rest are usually caused by staphylococci and other gram-negative organisms.[50] Bowel infarctions from sickle cell disease can facilitate the entry of salmonellae from the colon into the bloodstream with resultant hematogenous spread to the bone. Osteomyelitis in patients with sickle cell disease may occur in any bone, but it most commonly involves the medullary cavity of long or tubular bones. Because of the difficulty in separating bone pain during a sickle cell crisis from that of an infection, osteomyelitis can be relatively advanced in these patients by the time the diagnosis is made.

Infectious Arthritis

Antibiotic Selection

8 The three most important treatments for infectious arthritis are appropriate antibiotics, joint drainage, and joint rest. Smears of the synovial fluid can be useful to select appropriate antibiotic therapy initially.[8] If bacteria are not observed on the Gram stain in a patient who has a purulent joint effusion, antibiotics still should be initiated because of the low sensitivity of the Gram stain. A delay in initiating antibiotics significantly increases the likelihood for long-term complications. The specific antibiotic selected depends on the most likely infecting organism, but it should typically target *Staphylococcus* spp. (eg, vancomycin, daptomycin, or clindamycin). When staphylococci infect prosthetic hardware that cannot be removed, rifampin is recommended to be added to the therapy for its effects on biofilm, but drug–drug interactions should always be evaluated with use of this agent.[45]

Antibiotic Joint Space Concentration

The antibiotics selected usually are administered parenterally to achieve sufficient concentrations within the synovial fluid, and thus intra-articular antibiotic injections are unnecessary.

In prosthetic joint infections, antimicrobial cement spacers are often used to aid in delivery of the antimicrobial to the site of infection. The most common antimicrobials used include vancomycin and aminoglycosides (tobramycin or gentamicin).[51] However, the doses of each agent are widely variable and it is uncertain whether the placement of antimicrobial cement spacers adds outcome benefit to systemic therapy.[51,52] The idea that antimicrobial cement spacers provide only beneficial local exposure of the antimicrobial agent without systemic consequences has been questioned.[53] The incidence of acute kidney injury in patients receiving treatment with antimicrobial cement spacers was 4.8%, with the incidence ranging from 2% to 17% based on the definition of acute kidney injury used.[54]

Similar to osteomyelitis, once the infection is confirmed and initial response to parenteral therapy is achieved, culture susceptibilities have resulted, and adherence is ensured, then selected oral antibiotics can be used for the treatment of infectious arthritis.

Home Antibiotic Therapy

Because the management of bone and joint infections frequently requires prolonged parenteral antibiotics, administration of intravenous treatment in the home or a clinic is commonly performed. This is called outpatient parenteral antimicrobial therapy (OPAT).[55] Although acute osteomyelitis is one of the more common infectious diseases that can be treated with long-term intravenous antibiotics outside the hospital, not all patients are acceptable candidates for home administration. Patients must be screened to include those who are receiving a stable treatment, are interested and motivated in participating, who have good venous access, often have support from family members or caregivers, and safe and stable housing including refrigerated drug storage capability. Certain exclusion criteria also must be considered. Patients are not eligible if their eyesight or dexterity prevent them from attaching the admixture to their catheter when they do not have a caregiver that can help them daily. Although many providers are leery about allowing patients to receive parenteral antibiotics at home if they have any recent history of intravenous drug use, this bias is inappropriate in the setting of a structured therapy program for opioid use disorder which can lead to better outcomes for both disease states.[56] In addition to meeting these initial screening criteria, patients complete training before hospital discharge. Understanding of aseptic technique, proper catheter care, and correct administration techniques must be documented. Complications in patients receiving outpatient courses of parenteral antibiotics are fairly common (18%), and often lead to readmission when they occur.[57,58] Patients without adequate insurance or the support at home necessary to administer intravenous antibiotics may choose to come to an infusion center for each treatment. Others may need to be admitted to a skilled nursing facility for the duration of their therapy. A midline or central intravenous catheter is often required for long-term venous access. This is most commonly accomplished with a peripherally inserted central catheter (PICC).

The specific antibiotic regimen characteristics must also be considered when evaluating a patient for home antibiotics. After susceptibility of the microbiologic culture, the number of required daily antimicrobial doses is important. Most skilled nursing facilities are only able to accommodate infusions once each day. The stability of the antibiotic at room temperature is relevant when considering a continuous infusion (that can ideally be exchanged once daily), and shelf life can determine the required frequency of deliveries. Aminoglycosides and vancomycin have unique requirements for monitoring of the regimen, such as more frequent serum creatinine and drug-level monitoring. Although an organism can be susceptible to several antimicrobial agents, the use of the most practically simple regimen may often take precedence in OPAT over antimicrobial stewardship principles of selecting the most narrow spectrum agent.[58]

Individualized Therapy

Individualized therapy is important in the treatment of osteomyelitis and infectious arthritis. Patient quality of life may be significantly diminished in the short term from an inconvenient treatment regimen, but the long-term sequelae of inadequately treated infection can be much worse, such as impaired joint motion-draining sinus tracts, or even amputation, if it is required. Patient demographics, infection characteristics (eg, infecting organism and its susceptibility patterns), treatment cost, and quality-of-life issues all play a major role in evaluating individualized treatment alternatives (oral therapy or OPAT) rather than requiring patients to remain hospitalized to receive 4 to 6 weeks of intravenous antibiotics. Although serious adverse reactions are uncommon, in one study 85.7% of children receiving vancomycin had some form of adverse drug events and 42.9% of patients required the drug be discontinued.[59] Monitoring is important to ensure that personalized therapy is effective to both cure the infection and minimize the risk for complications.

EVALUATION OF THERAPEUTIC OUTCOMES

Monitoring of the Pharmaceutical Care Plan

9 Patients with bone and joint infections must be monitored closely. Table 141-7 summarizes a pharmaceutical care monitoring protocol. An assessment of a therapy's success or failure is based on the patient's clinical findings and laboratory values. The clinical signs of inflammation, such as swelling, tenderness, pain, redness, and fever, should resolve relatively quickly with appropriate therapy. Initially, the clinical signs are assessed daily until improvement and then periodically thereafter. Elevations in the CRP or ESR may not return to normal until after several weeks of therapy. The WBC count usually is obtained once (or twice) per week until it returns to the normal range and then is monitored for myelosuppression along with other blood cells. If by the end of the 4- to 6-week antibiotic course the clinical findings of osteomyelitis are no longer present and the CRP and ESR are within normal limits, the patient can be considered a clinical cure. Patients can relapse, however, after initially appearing to be cured. No relapse for 1 year generally is considered a complete cure.

If a patient fails to resolve the clinical signs and symptoms of inflammation after appropriate empirical antibiotics, suspicion for an abscess should be raised. Additional imaging and surgical debridement may be needed, particularly in situations where there was retained hardware or incompletely resected infection. In addition, the patient might have a resistant or an atypical infecting organism that may require a modification of the antibiotic therapy. It is especially important to identify the infecting organism and its susceptibility pattern. Follow-up cultures at subsequent debridements can be useful to assess the antibiotic therapy in patients with unresolved infection.

Despite apparently adequate surgery and antibiotics, some patients can fail therapy and have relapses in their infection. This scenario is more common in those having chronic osteomyelitis, especially with peripheral vascular disease. These patients can require long-term oral suppressive antimicrobial therapy to keep the infection under control.

TABLE 141-7 Monitoring Protocol

Parameter	Frequency	Notes
Culture and susceptibility	At initiation of treatment	No need to repeat unless clinical failure or original was not from a deep culture site (surgical sample)
Basic or complete metabolic laboratory panel	Weekly	Monitoring for electrolyte abnormalities and renal function
C-reactive protein or erythrocyte sedimentation rate	At initiation and completion of treatment	Although some providers will obtain weekly, this is often unnecessary as levels may not normalize until several weeks of therapy are complete
Therapeutic drug monitoring	Weekly	Agents such as vancomycin, aminoglycosides, and some antifungal therapies require ongoing monitoring for efficacy, toxicity, or both
Clinical signs of inflammation (redness, pain, swelling, tenderness, and fever)	Daily during initiation of therapy	
Adherence of outpatient therapy	Reinforce before starting therapy and with each healthcare visit	Adherence is critical if treatment is to be successful
Complete blood count	Weekly	White blood cell count is monitored for normalization to indicate efficacy. Certain antimicrobial agents may cause blood dyscrasias when used for long-term therapy (eg, linezolid, trimethoprim–sulfamethoxazole, as well as vancomycin and beta-lactams to a lesser extent)

ABBREVIATIONS

CRP	C-reactive protein
CT	computed tomography
ESR	erythrocyte sedimentation rate
IDSA	Infectious Diseases Society of America
MRI	magnetic resonance imaging
MRSA	methicillin-resistant *Staphylococcus aureus*
OPAT	outpatient parenteral antimicrobial therapy
PET	positron emission tomography
PICC	peripherally inserted central catheter
PWID	person who injects drugs
WBC	white blood cell
VO	vertebral osteomyelitis

REFERENCES

1. Waldvogel FA, Medoff G, Swartz MN. Osteomyelitis: A review of clinical features, therapeutic considerations and unusual aspects. *N Engl J Med.* 1970;282(4):198–206.
2. Titecat M, Senneville E, Wallet F, et al. Bacterial epidemiology of osteoarticular infections in a referent center: 10-year study. *OrthopTraumatol Surg Res.* 2013;99(6):653–658.
3. Kremers HM, Nwojo ME, Ransom JE, Wood-Wentz CM, Melton LJ 3rd, Huddleston PM 3rd. Trends in the epidemiology of osteomyelitis: A population-based study, 1969 to 2009. *J Bone Joint Surg Am.* 2015;97(10):837–845.
4. Juchler C, Spyropoulou V, Wagner N, et al. The contemporary bacteriologic epidemiology of osteoarticular infections in children in Switzerland. *J Pediatr.* 2018;194:190–196.e1.
5. Berbari EF, Kanj SS, Kowalski TJ, et al. Executive summary: 2015 Infectious Diseases Society of America (IDSA) clinical practice guidelines for the diagnosis and treatment of native vertebral osteomyelitis in adults. *Clin Infect Dis.* 2015;61(6):859–863.
6. Desoutter S, Cottier JP, Ghout I, et al. Susceptibility pattern of microorganisms isolated by percutaneous needle biopsy in nonbacteremic pyogenic vertebral osteomyelitis. *Antimicrob Agents Chemother.* 2015;59(12):7700–7706.
7. Kim DY, Kim UJ, Yu Y, et al. Microbial etiology of pyogenic vertebral osteomyelitis according to patient characteristics. *Open Forum Infect Dis.* 2020;7(6):ofaa176. https://doi.org/10.1093/ofid/ofaa176.
8. Ross JJ. Septic arthritis of native joints. *Infect Dis Clin N Am.* 2017; 31:203–218. https://doi.org/10.1016/j.idc.2017.01.001.
9. Hernandez-Ruperez MB, Suarez-Arrabal MD, Villa-Garcia A, et al. Kingellakingae as the main cause of septic arthritis: Importance of molecular diagnosis. *Pediatr Infect Dis J.* 2018;37(12):1211–1216.
10. Olarte L, Romero J, Barson W, et al. Osteoarticular infections caused by streptococcus pneumoniae in children in the post-pneumococcal conjugate vaccine era. *Pediatr Infect Dis J.* 2017;36(12):1201–1204.
11. Russ-Friedman C, Coates K, Torabi M, et al. Neisseria gonorrhoeae septic arthritis with acute osteomyelitis. *Sex Transm Dis.* 2020; 47(9): e36–e38. doi: 10.1097/OLQ.0000000000001212
12. Mathews CJ, Weston VC, Jones A, Field M, Coakley G. Bacterial septic arthritis in adults. *Lancet.* 2010;375(9717):846–855.
13. Marks M, Marks JL. Viral arthritis. *Clin Med (Lond).* 2016; 16(2): 129–134. 10.7861/clinmedicine.16-2-129
14. Funk SS, Copley LA. Acute hematogenous osteomyelitis in children: Pathogenesis, diagnosis, and treatment. *Orthop Clin North Am.* 2017;48(2):199–208.
15. Lipsky BA, Berendt AR, Cornia PB, et al. 2012 Infectious Diseases Society of America clinical practice guideline for the diagnosis and treatment of diabetic foot infections. *Clin Infect Dis.* 2012;54(12): e132–e173.
16. Bleich AT, Sheffield JS, Wendel GD Jr, Sigman A, Cunningham FG. Disseminated gonococcal infection in women. *Obstet Gynecol.* 2012;119(3):597–602.
17. Manz N, Krieg AH, Heininger U, Ritz N. Evaluation of the current use of imaging modalities and pathogen detection in children with acute osteomyelitis and septic arthritis. *Eur J Pediatr.* 2018;177(7):1071–1080.
18. Long B, Koyfman A, Gottlieb M. Evaluation and management of septic arthritis and its mimics in the emergency department. *West J Emerg Med.* 2019; 20(2): 331–341. https://doi.org/10.5811/westjem.2018.10.40974.
19. Spruiell MD, Searns JB, Heare TC, et al. Clinical care guideline for improving pediatric acute musculoskeletal infection outcomes. *J Pediatric Infect Dis Soc.* 2017;6(3):e86–e93.
20. Murillo O, Gomez-Junyent J, Grau I, et al. Clinical findings of bacteremic septic arthritis according to the site of acquisition: The overlap between health care-related and community- and nosocomial-acquired cases. *Eur J Intern Med.* 2016;28:38–42.
21. Ascione T, Pagliano P, Balato G, Mariconda M, Rotondo R, Esposito S. Oral therapy, microbiological findings, and comorbidity influence the outcome of prosthetic joint infections undergoing 2-stage exchange. *J Arthroplasty.* 2017;32(7):2239–2243.
22. Lee B, Tam I, Weigel B 4th, et al. Comparative outcomes of beta-lactam antibiotics in outpatient parenteral antibiotic therapy: Treatment success, readmissions and antibiotic switches. *J Antimicrob Chemother.* 2015;70(8):2389–2396.
23. DeRonde KJ, Girotto JE, Nicolau DP, et al. Management of pediatric acute hematogenous osteomyelitis, part I: Antimicrobial stewardship approach and review of therapies for methicillin-susceptible *Staphylococcus aureus*, streptococcus pyogenes, and Kingellakingae. *Pharmacotherapy.* 2018;38(9):947–966.
24. Youngster I, Shenoy ES, Hooper DC, Nelson SB. Comparative evaluation of the tolerability of cefazolin and nafcillin for treatment of methicillin-susceptible *Staphylococcus aureus* infections in the outpatient setting. *Clin Infect Dis.* 2014;59(3):369–375.
25. Kaplan SL. Recent lessons for the management of bone and joint infections. *J Infect.* 2014;68(Suppl 1):S51–S56.
26. Pendleton A, Kocher MS. Methicillin-resistant *Staphylococcus aureus* bone and joint infections in children. *J Am Acad Orthop Surg.* 2015;23(1):29–37.
27. Byren I, Rege S, Campanaro E, et al. Randomized controlled trial of the safety and efficacy of daptomycin versus standard-of-care therapy for management of patients with osteomyelitis associated with prosthetic devices undergoing two-stage revision arthroplasty. *Antimicrob Agents Chemother.* 2012;56(11):5626–5632.
28. Thabit AK, Fatani DF, Bamakhrama MS, et al. *Int J Infect Dis.* 2019. 81: 128–136. https://doi.org/10.1016/j.ijid.2019.02.005
29. Zaoutis T, Localio AR, Leckerman K, Saddlemire S, Bertoch D, Keren R. Prolonged intravenous therapy versus early transition to oral antimicrobial therapy for acute osteomyelitis in children. *Pediatrics.* 2009;123(2):636–642.
30. Keren R, Shah SS, Srivastava R, et al. Comparative effectiveness of intravenous vs oral antibiotics for postdischarge treatment of acute osteomyelitis in children. *JAMA Pediatr.* 2015;169(2):120–128.
31. Alcobendas R, Remesal A, Murias S, Nunez E, Calvo C. Outpatients with acute osteoarticular infections had favourable outcomes when they received just oral antibiotics without intravenous antibiotics. *Acta Paediatr.* 2018;107(10):1792–1797.
32. Daver NG, Shelburne SA, Atmar RL, et al. Oral step-down therapy is comparable to intravenous therapy for *Staphylococcus aureus* osteomyelitis. *J Infect.* 2007;54(6):539–544.
33. Babouee Flury B, Elzi L, Kolbe M, et al. Is switching to an oral antibiotic regimen safe after 2 weeks of intravenous treatment for primary bacterial vertebral osteomyelitis? *BMC Infect Dis.* 2014;14:226.
34. Li HK, Rombach I, Zambellas R, Walker AS, McNally MA, et al. Oral versus intravenous antibiotics for bone and joint infection. *New Engl J Med.* 2019;380:425–36.
35. Spellberg B, Lipsky BA. Systemic antibiotic therapy for chronic osteomyelitis in adults. *Clin Infect Dis.* 2012;54(3):393–407.
36. Coiffier G, Albert JD, Arvieux C, Guggenbuhl P. Optimizing combination rifampin therapy for staphylococcal osteoarticular infections. *Joint Bone Spine.* 2013;80(1):11–17.
37. Zimmerli W, Sendi P. Orthopaedic biofilm infections. *APMIS.* 2017;125(4):353–364.
38. White CN, Rolston KV. Osteomyelitis: Drug bioavailability and bone penetration are key. *JAAPA.* 2012;25(7):21–27.
39. Peltola H, Paakkonen M, Kallio P, Kallio MJ, Osteomyelitis-Septic Arthritis (OM-SA) Study Group. Prospective, randomized trial of 10 days versus 30 days of antimicrobial treatment, including a short-term course of parenteral therapy, for childhood septic arthritis. *Clin Infect Dis.* 2009;48(9):1201–1210.
40. Lorrot M, Gillet Y, Gras Le Guen C, Launay E, Cohen R, Grimprel E. Antibiotic therapy of bone and joint infections in children: Proposals of the French pediatric infectious disease group. *Arch Pediatr.* 2017;24(12S):S36–S41.
41. Peltola H, Paakkonen M, Kallio P, Kallio MJ; Osteomyelitis-Septic Arthritis Study Group. Short- versus long-term antimicrobial treatment for acute hematogenous osteomyelitis of childhood: Prospective,

randomized trial on 131 culture-positive cases. *Pediatr Infect Dis J.* 2010;29(12):1123–1128.
42. Paakkonen M, Peltola H. Simplifying the treatment of acute bacterial bone and joint infections in children. *Expert Rev Anti Infect Ther.* 2011;9(12):1125–1131.
43. Liu C, Bayer A, Cosgrove SE, et al. Clinical practice guidelines by the Infectious Diseases Society of America for the treatment of methicillin-resistant *Staphylococcus aureus* infections in adults and children. *Clin Infect Dis.* 2011;52(3):e1855.
44. Park KH, Cho OH, Lee JH, et al. Optimal duration of antibiotic therapy in patients with hematogenous vertebral osteomyelitis at low risk and high risk of recurrence. *Clin Infect Dis.* 2016;62(10):1262–1269.
45. Osmon DR, Berbari EF, Berendt AR, et al. Diagnosis and management of prosthetic joint infection: Clinical practice guidelines by the Infectious Diseases Society of America. *Clin Infect Dis.* 2013;56(1):e1e25.
46. Sigueira M, Saleh A, Klika A, et al. Chronic Suppression of Periprosthetic Joint Infections with Oral Antibiotics Increases Infection-Free Survivorship. *J Bone Joint Surg.* 2015;97(15):1220–1232. doi: 10.2106/JBJS.N.00999
47. Bernard L, Dinh A, Ghout I, et al. Antibiotic treatment for 6 weeks versus 12 weeks in patients with pyogenic vertebral osteomyelitis: An open-label, non-inferiority, randomised, controlled trial. *Lancet.* 2015;385(9971):875–882.
48. Bernard L, Arvieux C, Brunschweiler B, et al. Antibiotic Therapy for 6 or 12 Weeks for Prosthetic Joint Infection. *N Engl J Med.* 2021;384: 1991–2001. https://doi.org/10.1056/NEJMoa2020198.
49. Ziu M, Dengler B, Cordell D, Bartanusz V. Diagnosis and management of primary pyogenic spinal infections in intravenous recreational drug users. *Neurosurg Focus.* 2014;37(2):E3.
50. Marti-Carvajal AJ, Agreda-Perez LH. Antibiotics for treating osteomyelitis in people with sickle cell disease. *Cochrane Database Syst Rev.* 2016;11:CD007175.
51. Iarikov D, Demian H, Rubin D, Alexander J, Nambiar S. Choice and doses of antibacterial agents for cement spacers in treatment of prosthetic joint infections: Review of published studies. *Clin Infect Dis.* 2012;55(11):1474–1480.
52. Athans V, Veve MP, Davis SL. Trowels and tribulations: Review of antimicrobial-impregnated bone cements in prosthetic joint surgery. *Pharmacotherapy.* 2017;37(12):1565–1577.
53. Edelstein AI, Okroj KT, Rogers T, Della Valle CJ, Sporer SM. Systemic absorption of antibiotics from antibiotic-loaded cement spacers for the treatment of periprosthetic joint infection. *J Arthroplasty.* 2018;33(3):835–839.
54. Luu A, Syed F, Raman G, et al. Two-stage arthroplasty for prosthetic joint infection: A systematic review of acute kidney injury, systemic toxicity and infection control. *J Arthroplasty.* 2013;28(9):1490–1498.e1.
55. Norris AH, Shrestha NK, Allison GM, et al. 2018 Infectious Diseases Society of America Clinical Practice Guideline for the management of outpatient parenteral antimicrobial therapy. *Clin Infect Dis.* 2019; 68(1):e1–e35.
56. Outpatient parenteral antimicrobial therapy among people who inject drugs: A review of the literature. *Open Forum Infect Dis.* 2018; 5(9): ofy194, https://doi.org/10.1093/ofid/ofy194.
57. Keller SC, Williams D, Gavgani M, et al. Rates of and risk factors for adverse drug events in outpatient parenteral antimicrobial therapy. *Clin Infect Dis.* 2018;66(1):11–19.
58. Mahoney MV, Ryan KL, and Alexander BT. Evaluation of OPAT in the Age of Antimicrobial Stewardship. *Curr Treat Opt Infect Dis.* 2020;12: 158–177.
59. Faden D, Faden HS. The high rate of adverse drug events in children receiving prolonged outpatient parenteral antibiotic therapy for osteomyelitis. *Pediatr Infect Dis J.* 2009;28(6):539–541.
60. Margaretten ME, Kohlwes J, Moore D, Bent S. Does this adult patient have septic arthritis?. *JAMA.* 2007;297(13):1478–1488.
61. Sukhonthamarn K, Tan TL, Xu C, et al. Determining diagnostic thresholds for acute postoperative periprosthetic joint infection. *J Bone Joint Surg Am.* 2020;102(23):2043–2048.
62. Trampuz A, Hanssen AD, Osmon DR, et al. Synovial fluid leukocyte count and differential for the diagnosis of prosthetic knee infection. *Am J Med.* 2004;117(8):556–562.
63. Schinsky MF, Della Valle CJ, Sporer SM, Paprosky WG. Perioperative testing for joint infection in patients undergoing revision total hip arthroplasty. *J Bone Joint Surg Am.* 2008;90(9):1869–1875.

Sepsis and Septic Shock

142

S. Lena Kang-Birken and Sul R. Jung

KEY CONCEPTS

1. Gram-negative organisms are isolated in 44% to 59% in sepsis or septic shock, followed by gram-positive bacteria in 37% to 52%, and fungi in 4% to 10%. *Candida albicans* remains the most prevalent *Candida* species: however, non-*albicans Candida* species collectively is more frequently isolated.
2. Pathogenesis of sepsis is complex and multifactorial consisting of causative pathogen, host characteristics, and the inflammatory responses during which the interactions between pro- and anti-inflammatory cytokines, procoagulant state, and decreased fibrinolysis occur simultaneously.
3. The highest mortality is reported in patients with complicated intra-abdominal infections, chronic kidney disease, renal replacement therapy, multiple organ dysfunction, candidemia, and septic shock.
4. Initial resuscitation from sepsis-induced hypoperfusion should begin with at least 30 mL/kg of IV crystalloid fluid. Dynamic fluid responsiveness assessment by examining cardiac output with fluid bolus is essential to avoid fluid overload.
5. Prompt initiation of empiric broad-spectrum intravenous (IV) antibiotics within 1 hour of recognition of sepsis or septic shock improves survival, and the regimen should be assessed daily for potential de-escalation.
6. Norepinephrine is the preferred vasopressor in fluid-resuscitation refractory septic shock, and vasopressin may be added to achieve and maintain mean arterial pressure (MAP) goal of at least 65 mm Hg.
7. Implementation of a performance improvement program encompassing sepsis screening for high-risk patients and immediate treatment including fluid resuscitation, antimicrobial agents, treatment includes echinocandins, triazoles, or a formulation of amphotericin B and faster transition to vasopressor to meet MAP goal improves patient outcomes.
8. Intravenous hydrocortisone is recommended for patients with septic shock who require ongoing norepinephrine to maintain target MAP.
9. Initiate insulin therapy at a glucose level of greater than 180 mg/dL (10 mmol/L) with a target range between 144 and 180 mg/dL (8-10 mmol/L) to reduce potential hypoglycemia and associated mortality.

BEYOND THE BOOK

Watch the video entitled "Four Ways to Get Ahead of Sepsis" by the Centers for Disease Control and Prevention (CDC), https://www.youtube.com/watch?v=5JvGiAFLels. This 2-minute video provides an overview of manifestation of sepsis especially among individuals who are at high risk of infection. It highlights the importance of prevention, recognition of the signs and symptoms of sepsis, and awareness of sepsis as medical emergency. This video will enhance the students' understanding regarding the COLLECT and ASSESS steps in the patient care process. In a small group, create your own treatment summary pocket card for sepsis and septic shock based on the 2021 Surviving Sepsis Campaign international guidelines. Name the preferred initial treatment regimen and monitoring plan for the following: fluid resuscitation, antimicrobial therapy, vasopressor, and adjunct therapy including glucose control, corticosteroid, venous thromboembolism prophylaxis and stress ulcer prophylaxis. This activity will enhance the student understanding of key treatment elements of the PLAN step in the patient care process.

INTRODUCTION

Sepsis is a medical emergency when left untreated has a high probability of death. It has a unique disease process where it may impact multiple organ systems. The inflammatory response with the release of numerous cytokines will directly affect the vasculature causing a capillary leak, hypovolemia, decreased cardiac output, and hypotension leading to renal failure, heart failure, brain failure, also puts stress on our endocrine system, etc. Due to the potential expansive downward spiral, sepsis requires a prompt recognition, efficient assessment, and aggressive treatment.

The sepsis guidelines published in 2016 (Sepsis-3) derived new categorization and definition of the sepsis continuum.[1] However, it is still important to recognize the old definitions related to the spectrum of sepsis and how they were utilized in the clinical trials and guidelines prior to the 2016 revision. Periods of bacteremia, systemic inflammatory response syndrome (SIRS), sepsis, severe sepsis, septic shock, or multiple organ dysfunction syndrome often overlap, and they signify an important continuum of progressive physiologic decline. *Severe sepsis* was defined in patients with an acute organ dysfunction, such as acute renal failure or respiratory failure in 2012 guidelines (Sepsis-2).[2] Sepsis-induced hypotension is defined as a systolic BP less than 90 mm Hg or MAP less than

TABLE 142-1 Comparison of Definitions from Sepsis-2 and Sepsis-3 Guidelines

Sepsis-2 Guideline (2012)	Sepsis-3 Guideline (2016)
Systemic inflammatory response syndrome (SIRS) to infectious or noninfectious insults is defined as having two or more of the following: • Temperature >38°C or <36°C • Heart rate >90 beats/minute • Respiratory rate >20 breaths/minute • WBC >12,000/mm^3 (12 × 10^9/L) or <4,000 cells/mm^3 (4 × 10^9/L) or >10% (0.10) immature bands **Sepsis**: SIRS + probable or documented infection **Severe sepsis**: Sepsis + one or more organ dysfunction or hypoperfusion **Septic shock**: Sepsis + refractory hypotension despite fluid resuscitation (30 mL/kg) or serum lactate >9 mg/dL (1 mmol/L)	**Sepsis**: Life-threatening organ dysfunction caused by a dysregulated host response to infection • Acute change in total SOFA score ≥2 points **Septic shock**: Sepsis + persistent hypotension requiring vasopressor use and serum lactate >18 mg/dL (2 mmol/L) despite adequate fluid resuscitation

SOFA, sequential organ failure assessment; WBC, white blood cell.
Data from References 1 and 2.

70 mm Hg (Table 142-1).[2] *Septic shock* refers to sepsis patients with sepsis-induced hypotension that is refractory to adequate fluid resuscitation, thus requiring vasopressor administration. Sepsis-induced tissue hypoperfusion is defined as infection-induced hypotension, elevated lactate, or oliguria.[2,3] Sepsis-3 redefined sepsis by combining sepsis and severe sepsis from Sepsis-2 guideline as "life-threatening organ dysfunction caused by a dysregulated host response to infection."[1] The definition of septic shock is when a septic patient has persistent hypotension (MAP <65 mm Hg) requiring vasopressor along with continued elevated serum lactate (≥18 mg/dL [2 mmol/L]) post adequate fluid resuscitation defined as 30 mL/kg of crystalloids.

EPIDEMIOLOGY

Sepsis continues to pose a major healthcare burden. The US Nationwide Inpatient Sample reported a significant increase in the hospitalizations due to sepsis from 1.2% in 2005 to 2.7% in 2014.[4] Despite aggressive, prompt medical care and advances, overall in-hospital deaths remain approximately 15%, but the mortality rate may be as high as 50.7% in septic shock.[4-6] In addition, the total cost of hospitalization due to sepsis increased from $22.2 to $38.1 billion between 2005 and 2014, making it the most expensive condition to be treated in US hospitals.[4] Given the public health and financial burden, there is a vital need for clinicians to comprehend the pathophysiology and optimal management approaches for acutely ill patients with sepsis or septic shock.

ETIOLOGY

Risk Factors for Infection

Pathogenesis of sepsis is multifactorial, which begins with the patient's specific predisposition to infection. Advanced or young age, and preexisting conditions including heart failure, diabetes, chronic obstructive pulmonary disease, cirrhosis, alcohol dependence, end-stage renal disease, and other immunosuppressive diseases such as neoplasm and human immunodeficiency virus (HIV) predispose patients at risk for infection.[4,7] Male sex has been associated with a higher incidence of sepsis in prior studies; however, the difference between the sexes is diminishing.[7,8] Once the infection occurs, the risk factors for developing sepsis and organ dysfunction have not been well described. However, multiple factors including patients' risk factors for infection, site of infection, etiologic microorganism, and a specific organ dysfunction as well as the number of organs contribute to poor prognosis.[7,9]

Pathogens

1 Among the microorganisms isolated from blood cultures, gram-negative organisms were isolated in 44% to 59% of patients with sepsis or septic shock, gram-positive bacteria in 37% to 52%, anaerobic organisms in 5%, and fungi in 4% to 10%.[8-12] However, in the majority (approximately 70%) of sepsis cases, a specific causal microorganism was not documented.[8,10]

The most common anatomic source of infection that leads to sepsis is the lung (40%-42%), followed by intra-abdominal space (31%-34%) and genitourinary tract (11%-15%).[9-11]

Gram-Negative Bacteria

Escherichia coli is by far the most commonly isolated gram-negative microorganism in sepsis (55%-60%), followed by *Klebsiella* species, *Proteus* species, *Enterobacter* species, and *Pseudomonas aeruginosa*.[9,11,13,14] *P. aeruginosa* and *Acinetobacter* species are more likely to be associated with prior antibiotic exposure and usually exhibit multidrug resistance.[14,15]

Mortality increases significantly with increasing severity of sepsis (3.5% for sepsis, 9.9% in severe sepsis, and 29% in septic shock), especially in the presence of *P. aeruginosa*.[14] Furthermore, the severity of underlying conditions is a major factor associated with the negative outcome of gram-negative sepsis. For example, patients with severe or fatal conditions, such as acute leukemia, aplastic anemia, cirrhosis, or HIV, have a significantly worse prognosis than those patients with nonfatal underlying conditions such as diabetes mellitus or chronic renal insufficiency.[7]

Gram-Positive Bacteria

The most common gram-positive organisms are *Staphylococcus aureus*, followed by coagulase-negative *Staphylococci*, *Enterococcus* species, and *Streptococcus pneumoniae*.[9,11,13] Higher mortality in *S. aureus* bacteremia was reported in older age, shock, preexisting renal failure, and the presence of a rapidly fatal underlying disease. Enterococci are most commonly isolated from blood cultures following a prolonged hospitalization and treatment with broad-spectrum cephalosporins.

Anaerobic Bacteria

Anaerobic bacteria, most commonly *Bacteroides fragilis* and *Clostridium* species, are usually considered low-risk organisms for the development of sepsis. If present, anaerobes are often found together with other pathogenic bacteria that are commonly found in sepsis. Polymicrobial infections accounted for 5% to 39% of sepsis, especially in cases of intra-abdominal infections.[7,11,13] Mortality rates associated with polymicrobial infections are similar to sepsis caused by a single organism.

Fungi

Candidemia is among the most common fungal etiologic causes of bloodstream infections. *Candida albicans* remains the most prevalent *Candida* species from blood isolates (38%-61%), but there are increasing incidences of invasive infections due to non-*albicans* species.[9,12,16-18] Non-*albicans Candida* species include *C. glabrata* (16%-28%), *C. parapsilosis* (14%-17%), *C. tropicalis* (7.5%-17%), and *C. krusei* (4.1%). Traditionally, risk factors for fungal infection include abdominal surgery, poorly controlled diabetes mellitus, prolonged granulocytopenia, use of broad-spectrum antibiotics or corticosteroids, prolonged hospitalization, central venous catheter, total parenteral nutrition, hematologic malignancy, and chronic indwelling bladder (Foley) catheter. Patients with candidemia and severe sepsis and septic shock were more likely to have been admitted from nursing homes or transferred from outside hospitals.[12]

The use of azoles in response to the rising incidences of *Candida* bloodstream infection has led to fluconazole-resistant *Candida* species. Resistance to fluconazole occurs in 17% of *C. albicans*, 58% of *C. parapsilosis*, 33% of *C. glabrata*, and 100% of *C. krusei* among critically ill patients with invasive candidiasis.[17]

Patients with septic shock due to candidemia had a 30-day mortality rate of 54%. A higher in-hospital mortality of 61% was reported among patients with healthcare-associated candidemia. The mortality rate was 53% in patients with *C. krusei* candidemia; *C. parapsilosis* candidemia was associated with the lowest 12-week mortality rate of 24%.[19]

PATHOPHYSIOLOGY

2 The cascade leading to the development of sepsis is complex and multifactorial, involving causative pathogen (virulence and organism load), host characteristics (comorbidities and immunosuppression), and the inflammatory responses (Fig. 142-1). The inflammatory responses lead to damage to host tissue, and the anti-inflammatory response causes leukocytes to activate. If the balance to control the local inflammatory process and to eradicate the invading pathogens is lost, systemic inflammatory response occurs which may lead to sepsis and septic shock.

Cellular Components for Initiating the Inflammatory Process

The pathophysiologic focus of gram-negative sepsis has been on the lipopolysaccharide component of the gram-negative bacterial outer cell membrane. Commonly referred to as endotoxin, this substance is generally released with bacterial lysis. Upon its release, it forms a complex with an endogenous protein called a lipopolysaccharide-binding protein. Lipid A is the innermost region of the lipopolysaccharide and is highly immunoreactive. Its predominant effect is to activate macrophages through the CD14 receptor located on the macrophage. This endotoxin-lipopolysaccharide–binding protein complex is responsible for most of the toxic effects—the release of cytokine mediators which triggers the inflammatory cascade that is critical in the progression to sepsis and/or septic shock.[20]

In gram-positive sepsis, the exotoxin peptidoglycan on the cell wall surface exhibits pro-inflammatory activity. Similar to lipid A component of gram-negative bacteria, the exotoxin peptidoglycan binds to the CD14 receptors of the macrophages. However, the potency of exotoxin peptidoglycan is less than that of endotoxin.[20] Clinically important exotoxins are those produced by *S. aureus* and *Streptococcus pyogenes* in septic shock.

Pro- and Anti-Inflammatory Mediators

A complex interaction between pro-inflammatory and anti-inflammatory mediators plays a major role in the pathogenesis of sepsis. In general, pro-inflammatory reactions are directed at eliminating invading pathogens and the anti-inflammatory reactions limit local and systemic tissue injury. The key pro-inflammatory mediators are tumor necrosis factor (TNF) and interleukin (IL)-1, IL-6, and IL-12, which are released by activated macrophages and endothelial cells. The TNF level is highly elevated early in the inflammatory response in the majority of patients with sepsis, which leads to activation of other cytokines such as IL-1 and IL-6, associated with cellular damage. There is a correlation between the plasma TNF levels and the severity of sepsis and poor prognosis. In addition, higher levels of IL-6 have been reported in patients with septic shock than in those with SIRS.[21] TNF also stimulates the release of cyclooxygenase-derived arachidonic acid metabolites (thromboxane A_2 and prostaglandins) that contribute to vascular endothelial damage.

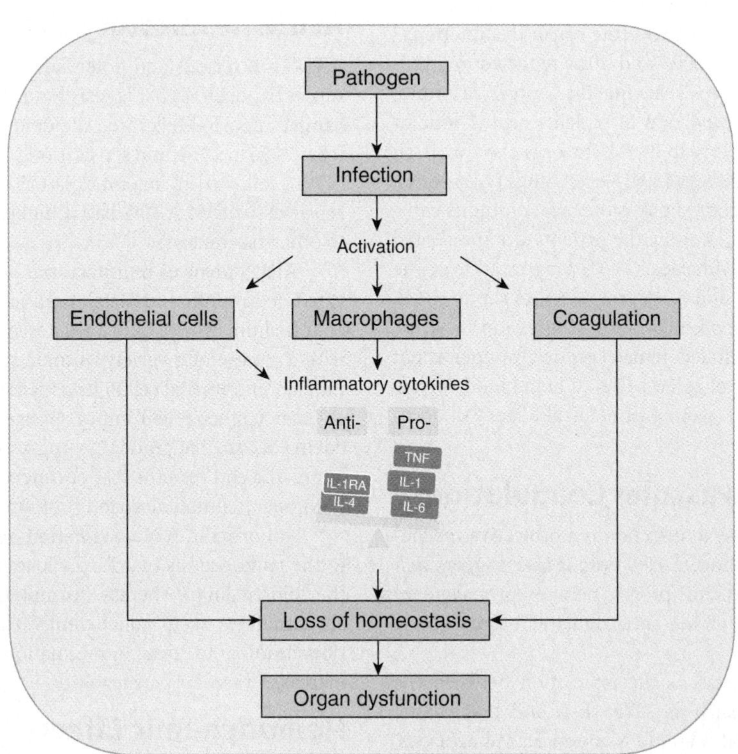

FIGURE 142-1 Pathophysiology of sepsis.

The significant anti-inflammatory mediators include interleukin-1 receptor antagonist (IL-1RA) IL-4, and IL-10. IL-1RA binds to IL-1, blocking its activity. Furthermore, anti-inflammatory cytokines inhibit the production of the pro-inflammatory cytokines and down-regulate some inflammatory cells. Levels of IL-10 and IL-1RA are higher in septic shock than in sepsis, and higher levels are found among nonsurviving patients than in survivor.[21,22]

The activation and secretion of pro- and anti-inflammatory mediators in septic shock occur as a simultaneous immune response as early as the first 24 hours of diagnosis, but the balance between pro- and anti-inflammatory mechanisms determines the degree of inflammation, ranging from local antibacterial activity to systemic tissue toxicity, organ failure, shock, or death (Fig. 142-1).

Cascade of Sepsis

Macrophages and endothelial cells produce a variety of cytokines that mediate a primary mechanism of injury in sepsis. When injured, endothelial cells allow circulating cells such as granulocytes and plasma constituents to enter inflamed tissues, which can result in organ damage.

The microcirculation is also affected by sepsis-induced inflammation. The arterioles become less responsive to either vasoconstrictors or vasodilators. The capillaries are less perfused even at the early phases of septic shock, and there is neutrophil infiltration and protein leakage into the venules.[23]

The inflammatory process in sepsis is also directly linked to the coagulation system. Pro-inflammatory mechanisms that promote sepsis are also procoagulant and antifibrinolytic, whereas fibrinolytic mechanisms can be anti-inflammatory.[24] A key endogenous substance involved in inflammation of sepsis is activated protein C, which enhances fibrinolysis and inhibits inflammation. Levels of protein C are generally reduced in patients with sepsis.[24]

COMPLICATIONS

Sepsis may lead to several complications including disseminated intravascular coagulation (DIC) and multiple organ dysfunctions, which are important predictors of patient outcome. Among the patients admitted to US hospitals between 2009 and 2014 due to sepsis, approximately half had at least two acute organ dysfunctions.[5] National inpatient data between 2005 and 2014 reported approximately 20% of patients with sepsis having three-organ dysfunction, and an increase in the proportion of patients having four or more organ dysfunction from 16% to 24%.[4] The organ dysfunction occurred most frequently in kidneys (39%-49%), lungs (24%-43%), and heart (28%-40%).[4,5,8,25,26] Septic shock is the most ominous complication associated with sepsis. Among the patients who presented to the emergency department with sepsis, 3.6% progressed to septic shock within the first 4 hours, and 8.4% progressed to septic shock between 4 and 48 hours.[27] The predictors for progression to septic shock in the latter group included female gender, nonpersistent hypotension, band neutrophils of at least 10% (0.1) in blood, lactate of at least 36 mg/dL (4 mmol/L), and past medical history of coronary artery disease.[27]

Disseminated Intravascular Coagulation

The host inflammatory response to infection is a protective mechanism against the infecting pathogen. However, it also triggers disturbances in coagulation. A dynamic process between procoagulant mechanisms and naturally occurring anticoagulants occurs nearly universally in septic patients.

The initial procoagulant state is the interaction between the pro-inflammatory cytokines, such as TNF, IL-1, and IL-6, tissue factor expression by endothelial cells and mononuclear phagocytes, and platelet-activating factor, which together contributes to hypercoagulopathy in the early inflammatory state.[28] Simultaneously, antithrombin synthesis is down-regulated, allowing ongoing thrombin formation. This acute phase interaction of the pro-inflammatory and hypercoagulative state is believed to sequester bacteria as part of compartmentalization.[28] Coagulation abnormalities consisting of excessive fibrin formation, compromised fibrin removal from a depressed fibrinolytic system, and endothelial injury may manifest as a small reduction in platelet count and subclinical clotting time prolongation or in more severe cases, DIC.

Simultaneous widespread microvascular thrombosis and profuse bleeding from various sites characterize DIC. Consumption of clotting factors from ongoing thrombosis eventually leads to a hypocoagulable state. Various degrees of coagulation abnormalities may be present in 50% to 70% of septic patients. However, about 35% will progress to DIC.[28] Complications of DIC vary and depend on the affected organ and the severity of the coagulopathy. DIC can produce acute renal failure, hemorrhagic necrosis of the gastrointestinal (GI) mucosa, liver failure, acute pancreatitis, acute respiratory distress syndrome (ARDS), and pulmonary failure. As the procoagulant state is the key to the ignition of the pathogenesis to DIC and multiple organ dysfunction, coagulation dysfunction and organ dysfunction often coexist in sepsis.

Acute Kidney Injury

The acute kidney injury (AKI), defined as an absolute increase in serum creatinine of 0.3 mg/dL (27 mmol/L) or more within a 48-hour period, not only affects survival but also leads to worsening of chronic kidney disease or failure requiring renal replacement therapy. Sepsis-induced AKI has been reported up to 49% and was associated with hypoperfusion, leading to renal ischemia. However, normal or even increased renal blood flow may be present in sepsis-induced AKI, providing an explanation for lack of beneficial evidence with the use of dopamine, a renal vasodilator in the treatment of AKI in septic patients. Rather, AKI develops from a complex relationship between the activation of inflammation and pro-inflammatory molecules causing renal tubular injury and tubular epithelial dysfunction.[29] Subsequently, the injured kidney is unable to regulate the blood flow, making it more vulnerable to changes in blood flow as BP varies and ultimately lead to progression to multiple organ dysfunction.

Acute Respiratory Distress Syndrome

ARDS is a serious and potentially fatal condition, characterized by severe hypoxemia that is resistant to oxygen. The National Inpatient Sample reported increased incidence of ARDS in the United States from 2006 to 2014, and sepsis is one of the most common risk factors (47%), followed by pneumonia (45%) and shock (44%). Moreover, sepsis-associated ARDS had a higher mortality rate in comparison to other risk factors.

ARDS involves multifactorial processes which begin with activated neutrophils and platelets adhering to the pulmonary capillary endothelium which then initiates multiple inflammatory cascades with a release of a variety of toxic substances. There is diffuse pulmonary endothelial cell injury, increased capillary permeability, and alveolar epithelial cell injury. Consequently, interstitial pulmonary edema occurs that gradually progresses to alveolar flooding and collapse. The end result is loss of functional alveolar volume, impaired pulmonary compliance, and profound hypoxemia.[30]

Abnormalities of coagulation and fibrinolysis are also integral to the pathogenesis of ARDS. Coagulation is locally upregulated in the injured lung, whereas fibrinolytic activity is depressed. These abnormalities occur concurrently, but favor alveolar fibrin deposition, leading to local inflammation, macrophage migration, and increased vascular permeability.

Hemodynamic Effects

Sepsis and septic shock are associated with excessive sympathetic outflow, high plasma catecholamine levels, myocardial depression, vascular hyporeactivity, and autonomic dysfunction. The hallmark of the hemodynamic effect of sepsis is the hyperdynamic state characterized by low systemic vascular resistance (SVR) and high cardiac output with tachycardia and arterial hypotension.[23,31]

Sepsis-induced myocardial dysfunction, defined as the intrinsic myocardial systolic and diastolic dysfunction of both the left and right sides of the heart, occurs from excessive adrenergic stress.[32] Sepsis from overwhelming inflammation may cause direct myocardial damage (eg, cardiomyopathy and tachyarrhythmia). Simultaneously, the heart, as part of the circulatory system responding to peripheral hemodynamics, may be responding to alterations in preload, afterload, and microcirculation during sepsis. The microvasculature system, consisting of arterioles, capillaries, venules, and microlymphatics, is a functional system that responds promptly to changes in blood flow to the tissues and metabolic demand. It regulates adequate blood flow to tissues, ensuring adequate oxygen delivery and meet the oxygen demand. During sepsis and septic shock, massive pro-inflammatory cytokines are released, targeting the endothelium, the key component of this microvascular blood flow. Consequently, microvascular impairment leads to loss of ability to regulate oxygen distribution within the capillary network.[23] The severity of microcirculatory abnormalities and their persistence are associated with organ dysfunction. The combination of decreased preload, reduced afterload, myocardial dysfunction, microcirculatory impairments, and blood flow redistribution between organs lead to hemodynamic alterations during sepsis.

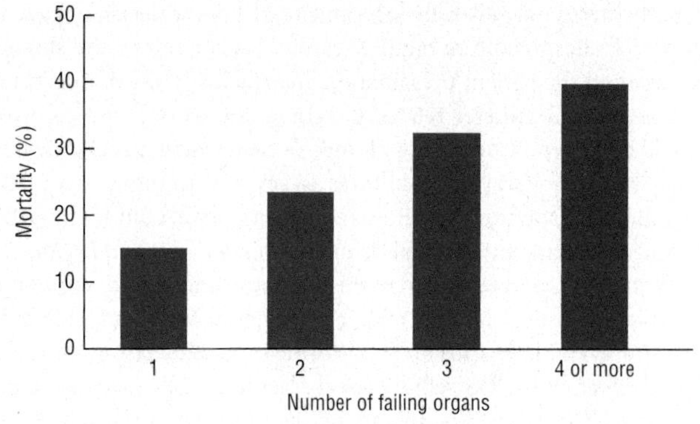

FIGURE 142-2 Mortality related to the number of failing organs.

Septic Shock

There are four different types of shock syndrome: hypovolemic, cardiogenic, obstructive, and vasodilatory/distributive. Septic shock falls under the vasodilatory/distributive shock. Distributive shock results from overall systemic vasodilation leading to hypoperfusion. Hallmark signs and symptoms of distributive shock include a decrease in BP, an increase in heart rate in response to a decrease in SVR, and pulmonary capillary wedge pressure. The cardiac output is typically normal after adequate fluid resuscitation in vasodilatory shock unlike other syndromes which are expected to have a low cardiac output. Details of the different shock syndromes are discussed in Chapter e42, "Shock Syndromes."

Prognostic Factors

3 The highest mortality was reported in patients with intra-abdominal infection secondary to ischemic bowel (75%), whereas obstructive uropathy-associated urinary tract infection was associated with the lowest hospital mortality (26%).[10] In-hospital mortality rate with AKI in sepsis was two- to threefold higher in patients with stage 3 kidney disease compared to those without kidney disease. Furthermore, the mortality rate was significantly higher in patients receiving renal replacement therapy than those without (40% vs 22%, respectively).[33] Associated mortality rates were also high in patients with severe sepsis and ARDS and DIC (36% and 29%, respectively).[26] As the number of failing organs increased from one to four or more, the mortality rate increased from 15% to 40% (Fig. 142-2).[5] Patients with candidemia generally have septic shock, and the associated mortality is significantly higher in comparison to patients with bacteremia (47% vs 28%, respectively).[12]

An elevated serum lactate concentration of more than 36 mg/dL (4 mmol/L) upon initial presentation and persistent elevation in lactate for more than 24 hours were associated with an increased mortality rate.[34] Furthermore, the 28-day mortality rate was the highest (45%) among patients with septic shock and hyperlactatemia of more than 23 mg/dL (2.5 mmol/L), followed by hyperlactatemia without vasopressor need (35%), and no hyperlactatemia with vasopressor need (28%). Hyperlactatemia increased the risk of 28-day mortality independent of vasopressor need.[35]

Diagnosis

Identification of Pathogens

The presence of clinical features suggesting sepsis should prompt further evaluation of the patient. In addition to obtaining a careful history of any underlying conditions and recent travel, injury, animal exposure, infection, or use of antibiotics, a complete physical examination should be performed to determine the source of the infection.

A collection of specimens should be sent for culture prior to initiating any antimicrobial therapy to increase the yield of cultures, making identification of a pathogen more likely. Minimally, two sets of blood cultures (both aerobic and anaerobic bottles) should be collected without temporal separation between the sets.[2] Culturing of

CLINICAL PRESENTATION Sepsis and Septic Shock

The clinical presentation of sepsis varies significantly depending on the site of the infection (ie, pulmonary versus urinary tract), host response to the infection based on the patient's underlying health status and risk factors, and organ dysfunction. The initial presentations may include general malaise or myalgia and nonspecific signs such as fever (or hypothermia), chills, tachycardia, tachypnea, or change in mental status. As uncontrolled sepsis progresses, the presentation varies again depending on the specific organ system dysfunction. Arterial hypotension can be present, which may compromise organ perfusion, leading to oliguria. Hyperventilation can occur, causing impaired gas exchange which can then lead to respiratory alkalosis. Altered glucose metabolism, including impaired gluconeogenesis and excessive insulin release, is evidenced by either hyperglycemia or hypoglycemia. Increased glycolysis with impaired clearance of lactate by the hypoperfused liver and kidneys result in elevated lactate levels which then contributes to metabolic acidosis.

all body sites is not generally recommended, but the decision regarding which sites to culture requires careful consideration and should be based on the patient presentation and the likely site of infection. With suspected catheter-related infection, one set of blood cultures should be drawn through every lumen of each vascular access device along with peripheral blood cultures. In severe community-acquired pneumonia, respiratory secretions along with blood cultures must be obtained. Urinary antigen detection of *S. pneumoniae* and *Legionella* serogroup 1 is recommended to yield identification. To document a soft tissue infection, a Gram stain and bacterial culture of any obvious wound exudates should be performed. A needle aspiration of a closed infection such as cellulitis or abscess may be needed for Gram stain and bacterial culture. In abdominal infections, fluid collections identified by imaging studies should be aspirated for Gram stains and aerobic and anaerobic cultures. Implementation of accurate and rapid molecular diagnostic testing has demonstrated a positive impact on prescribing appropriate therapy in bloodstream infections such as methicillin-resistant *S. aureus* (MRSA) and *Candida* species.[2,36,37]

A lumbar puncture is indicated in altered mental status, severe headache, or a seizure, assuming there are no focal cranial lesions identified by computed tomography scan. Further tests may be indicated to assess any systemic organ dysfunction caused by severe sepsis. The laboratory tests should include WBC with differential, hemoglobin, platelet count, complete chemistry profile, coagulation parameters, serum lactate, and arterial blood gases. The potential role of biomarkers such as PCT levels or C-reactive protein for diagnosis of infection in patients with sepsis remains undefined as there is no definitive way to discriminate the acute inflammatory pattern of sepsis from other generalized inflammation.[2]

Assessment of Acutely Ill, High-Risk Patients

Sepsis-3 redefined sepsis to "life-threatening organ dysfunction caused by a dysregulated host response to infection" based on the evidence of greater in-hospital mortality among patients with sequential sepsis-related organ failure.[1,38] As such, early recognition of sepsis using a formal screening tool is critical. Organ dysfunction can be evaluated by using the SOFA scoring system. SOFA encompasses various organ systems such as pulmonary, coagulation, hepatic, cardiovascular, renal, and neurological and gives a score ranging from 0 to 4 for each system to characterize a septic patient's prognosis (Table 142-2). Higher total score is associated with an increased probability of mortality. A SOFA score of 2 or more is associated with an increased risk of mortality by 10% in hospitalized patients with presumed infection.[1] One of the difficulties in using the SOFA score is that clinicians need laboratory results such as platelets, bilirubin, and creatinine, which may not be available initially. Quick SOFA (qSOFA), on the other hand, utilizes three data elements: respiratory rate ≥22 breaths/min, altered mental status, and systolic BP ≤100 mm Hg. qSOFA of ≥2 or SOFA score change of ≥2 can serve as an indication for higher vigilance and potentially quicker escalation of care. If baseline SOFA score is unknown, then score of zero is used as baseline. If a patient has all three mentioned elements, in-hospital mortality can be as high as 40% to 50%.[1] However, the 2021 Surviving Sepsis Campaign guideline recommends that qSOFA should not be used as a single screen tool since it is less sensitive than having two of four SIRS criteria in identifying sepsis-induced organ dysfunction.[39]

TABLE 142-2 Abbreviated Sepsis-Related Sequential Organ Failure Assessment

Organ System	Measured Variables for Scoring System
Pulmonary	PaO_2/FiO_2 (<200 to ≥400 mm Hg [26.6-53.2 kPa])
Coagulation	Platelets (<50 to ≥150 × 10^3/mm^3 [50 × 10^9 - 150 × 10^9/L])
Liver	Bilirubin (<1.2-11.9 mg/dL [20.5-203.5 μmol/L])
Cardiovascular	MAP (<70 with or without vasopressor to ≥70 mm Hg)
Central nervous system	Glasgow Coma Scale (6-15)
Renal	Serum creatinine (<1.2-4.9 mg/dL [106-433 μmol/L]), urine output (<500 mL/d)

FiO_2, fraction of inspired oxygen; MAP, mean arterial pressure; PaO_2, partial pressure of oxygen.

Data from Reference 1.

TREATMENT

Since publication of the Surviving Sepsis Campaign in 2003, key concepts have changed the way we recognize and treat septic patients over the decades.[40] In 2001, early goal-directed therapy (EGDT) with resuscitation targets was introduced, and it heavily influenced the Sepsis-2 guideline.[2,41] The 2016 guideline (Sepsis-3) incorporated the data from the Protocolized Care for Early Septic Shock (ProCESS), Australasian Resuscitation in Sepsis Evaluation (ARISE), and Protocolized Management in Sepsis (ProMISe) trials which failed to confirm the survival advantage of protocolized EGDT.[42-44] In addition, Sepsis-3 not only changed the definition of classifying categories of sepsis but also emphasized the use of dynamic resuscitation markers.

It is important to discuss EGDT since the 2001 trial put the emphasis in early recognition of sepsis and a protocolized, quantitative approach to patient care for this disease state.[41] This was a single center, prospective, randomized study that included 263 patients who met the SIRS criteria and systolic BP ≤90 mm Hg or lactate ≥36 mg/dL (4 mmol/L). Specific resuscitation targets (ie, central venous pressure [CVP] of 8 to 12 mm Hg, MAP ≥65, hematocrit of ≥30% [0.30], and central venous oxygen saturation [$Scvo_2$] ≥70% [0.70]) were evaluated for reducing mortality. When EGDT and standard therapy were compared, the standard therapy led to significantly higher 28-day mortality rate. Subsequently, EGDT was quickly adopted and redefined the early, aggressive resuscitation of patients with sepsis and septic shock for the next decade. Notably, the ProCESS (1,341 subjects), ProMISe (1,234 subjects), and ARISE (1,588 subjects) investigators failed to confirm the survival benefits of protocolized targets for CVP and hemoglobin between EGDT and usual care.[42-44] However, these investigators were able to recognize the disease early allowing for quicker admission of patients from the emergency department to the inpatient care setting which may assist in overall mortality benefit in both standard therapy and EGDT.[45]

Desired Outcomes

In addition to timely recognition and diagnosis of sepsis, other primary goals include prompt hemodynamic support, rapid identification of the pathogen, source control either medically and/or surgically, early initiation of appropriate IV antimicrobial therapy, and avoidance of complications such as organ failure and septic shock. Supportive care such as stress ulcer prophylaxis and venous thromboembolism prophylaxis is important to prevent complications during the stay in the ICU. Table 142-3 describes the selected treatment recommendations from the surviving sepsis campaign.

Initial Resuscitation

4 Once the patient is recognized for sepsis and septic shock, early effective fluid resuscitation is crucial for preventing further sepsis-induced tissue hypoperfusion. The guidelines recommend at least 30 mL/kg of IV crystalloid fluid within the first 3 hours. The patient

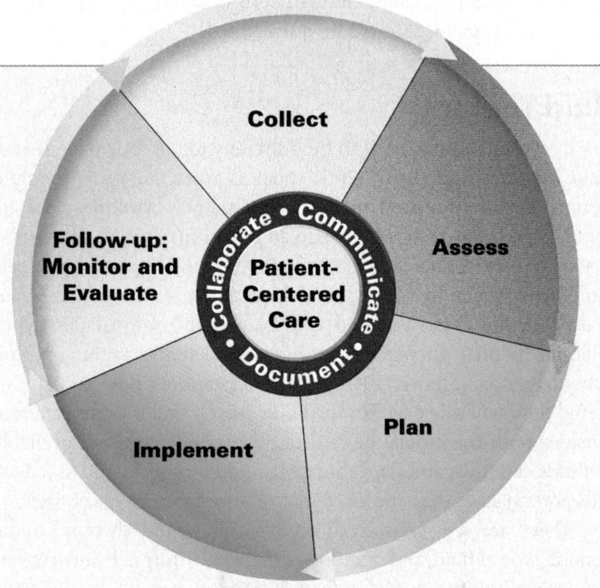

Patient Care Process for Sepsis and Septic Shock

The image shows the five fundamental steps included in patient care process for Sepsis and Septic shock. The tagline of this process reads collaborate, communicate, and document. The five fundamental steps listed here are collect, assess, plan, implement, and follow-up: monitor and evaluate. All these steps are listed in a circular block diagram.

Collect

- Patient characteristics (eg, age, sex)
- Patient medical history (including recent hospitalization and infection within last 6 months)
- Social history (eg, tobacco/ethanol use/intravenous drug user/place of residence)
- Current medications (prescription and nonprescription; including recent history of antibiotic usage within last 6 months)
- Subjective data (including general constitutional and infection-site specific, onset)
- Objective data
  - Temperature, blood pressure (BP), heart rate, respiratory rate, mean arterial pressure (MAP), O_2-saturation, height, and weight
  - Labs including white blood cell (WBC) count with differential, hemoglobin, platelet count, complete serum chemistry including serum creatinine, and bilirubin, lactate, procalcitonin (PCT), coagulation panel including prothrombin time and activated partial thromboplastin time, and arterial blood gas including pH, $PaCO_2$, PaO_2, and HCO_3
  - Objective parameters for sequential organ failure assessment (see sequential organ failure assessment [SOFA]; Table 142-2)
  - Microbiology data (including Gram stain, culture, rapid diagnostic testing)

Assess

- Mental status
- Systemic inflammatory response (SIRS) criteria (Table 142-1)
- Hemodynamic stability (eg, systolic BP >100 mm Hg, MAP >65 mm Hg)
- Presence of organ dysfunction (lactate >18 mg/dL (2 mmol/L), baseline; SOFA/qSOFA; Table 142-2)
- Identification of pathogen and antibiotic susceptibility
- Risk of multidrug-resistant bacterial pathogen (recent hospitalization, infection, antibiotic-resistant organism, broad-spectrum antibiotic usage)
- Risk of fungal pathogen (recent usage of broad-spectrum antibiotics/corticosteroids/total parenteral nutrition, abdominal surgery, etc.)

Plan*

- Initiate 1-hour performance improvement bundle (Table 142-7)
- Initial fluid resuscitation with intravenous (IV) balanced crystalloid for hypotension
- Begin antimicrobial therapy regimen based on site of infection (Table 142-5)
- Perform passive leg raise to assess response to fluid resuscitation (increase in stroke volume by 10%-15%)
- Initiate vasopressor if MAP <65 mm Hg with adequate fluid resuscitation (Table 142-6)
- Administer IV hydrocortisone if ongoing requirement for vasopressor to maintain MAP
- Initiate adjunct therapy including glucose control, venous thromboembolism prophylaxis, and stress ulcer prophylaxis
- Monitoring parameters: including efficacy (eg, signs and symptoms of infection, mental status, MAP, lactate, WBC with differential) and safety

Implement*

- Management of vasopressor selection after initial norepinephrine
- Daily assessment for opportunities to de-escalate antimicrobial therapy
- Design tapering schedule of IV hydrocortisone
- Coordination of treatment plan during transitioning from the ICU to a medicine unit

Follow-up: Monitor and Evaluate

- Resolution of symptoms of infection
- PCT levels along with clinical evaluation to determine the antimicrobial treatment duration
- Normalization of lactate and MAP >65 mm Hg for discontinuation of vasopressors
- Presence of adverse effects of antimicrobial agents and vasopressors

Collaborate with other healthcare professionals.

TABLE 142-3 Evidence-Based Treatment Recommendations and Best Practice Statements

Recommendations	Recommendation Grades
Fluid therapy	
Initial resuscitation from sepsis-associated hypotension with at least 30 mL/kg of IV crystalloid fluid within 1 hour	Strong recommendation, low evidence
Balanced crystalloids instead of normal saline for additional fluids guided by frequent assessment of dynamic measures	Weak recommendation, low evidence
Antimicrobial therapy	
IV broad-spectrum antibiotic within 1 hour of diagnosis of sepsis and septic shock against likely bacterial/fungal pathogens	Strong recommendation, moderate evidence
Empiric MRSA coverage for patients at high risk for MRSA	Best practices statement
Reassess antibiotic therapy daily with microbiology and clinical data to narrow coverage (de-escalation)	Best practices statement
Combination therapy for patients at high risk for multidrug-resistant bacterial pathogens	Weak recommendation, low quality evidence
Optimize dosing strategies based on pharmacokinetics/pharmacodynamics parameters	Best practices statement (PS)
Empiric antifungal therapy for patients at high risk of fungal infection	Weak recommendation, low evidence
Shorter duration of treatment duration using clinical evaluation and procalcitonin	Weak recommendation, low evidence
Vasopressors	
Initiate vasopressor therapy to maintain MAP ≥65 mm Hg	Strong recommendation, moderate evidence
Norepinephrine as the first-choice vasopressor	Strong recommendation, moderate evidence
Add vasopressin to norepinephrine instead of increasing norepinephrine dose to achieve adequate MAP	Weak recommendation, moderate evidence
Corticosteroids	
IV hydrocortisone for septic shock with ongoing requirement for vasopressor	Weak recommendation, low evidence
Hydrocortisone should be tapered when vasopressors are no longer required	Weak recommendation, low evidence
Glucose control	
Use insulin dosing protocol when two consecutive blood glucose levels are >180 mg/dL (10 mmol/L), targeting an upper blood glucose <180 mg/dL (10 mmol/L)	Strong recommendation, high-level evidence
Venous thomboembolism prophylaxis	
Use daily low-molecular-weight heparin (LMWH) over unfractionated heparin	Strong recommendation, moderate evidence
Stress ulcer prophylaxis	
Stress ulcer prophylaxis should be given to patients who have bleeding risk factors	Strong recommendation, low evidence
Either proton pump inhibitors or H2 receptor blockers	Weak recommendation, low evidence

MAP, mean arterial pressure; MRSA, Methicillin-resistant *Staphylococcus aureus*.
Data from Reference 46.

should be reassessed for hemodynamic status by measurements with better diagnostic accuracy at predicting those who are likely to respond to additional fluid.[39,46] It also recommends target MAP of 65 mg Hg to assess the need for vasopressors. While MAP indicates degree of tissue perfusion, elevated serum lactate represents tissue hypoxia and therefore should be normalized.

Fluid Therapy

Initial resuscitation effort with fluid therapy for a septic patient with tissue hypoperfusion or in septic shock is a key therapy.[47] The fluid therapy is closely related to the inflammatory cytokines that are released by the body in response to an infection. The pro-inflammatory cytokines lead to capillary leak. As the fluid travels more freely from intravascular to extravascular space, there is an overall increase in fluid in the extravascular space leading to intravascular hypovolemia. In turn, this causes end-organ edema, dysfunction, and ultimately organ failure. Therefore, understanding how the administered fluid will move within the body is essential. It is important to consider both the indication and the contraindications of available IV fluids carefully, and fluid therapy should be considered as a drug with potential benefits and risks that require frequent assessment.

There are few considerations regarding fluid therapy: initial amount, type of fluid, and duration of therapy.[48] The guidelines recommend the administration of at least 30 mL/kg crystalloids within the first 3 hours. This 30 mL/kg dose was based on observational study. Despite the lack of a robust quality of evidence this dose has been widely used in many landmark trials such as the ProCESS, ARISE, and ProMISe.[42-44] However, this amount of fluid is to be given judiciously within 3 hours. For example, if an 80-kg patient requires 30 mL/kg fluid resuscitation, the complete 2.4 L should not be administered as a single bolus dose, but as needed based on the proper assessment of fluid status and fluid responsiveness. To reduce fluid overload associated with static measurements using an invasive placement of a central venous catheter, dynamic assessment of fluid responsiveness has been used with goal-directed therapy.[49] Dynamic assessment was defined as an increase in stroke volume of more than 10% to 15% after a fluid challenge of 250 to 500 mL of crystalloids or from endogenous source by using the passive leg raise. Passive leg raise is performed by laying the patient in a supine position and raising both legs 45° at the same time. This will allow the blood from the leg to act as a bolus back to the heart. Using the passive leg raise test to check for fluid responsiveness intermittently leads to decreased use of IV fluids, especially for patients who are no longer responding adequately to IV fluid alone. Fluid therapy guided by dynamic assessment of fluid responsiveness by examining cardiac output was associated with decreased mortality compared to standard care.[49] Furthermore, the use of a dynamic assessment also decreased the length of stay in the ICU and the duration of mechanical ventilation.[50]

Guidelines recommend using ideal body weight in fluid resuscition.[39,46] However, the optimal dosing strategy for obese patients with septic shock is unknown. Dosing based on adjusted body weight was associated with improved mortality compared to actual body weight and ideal body weight.[51] Further prospective studies are needed to confirm the optimal fluid dosing in obese patients.

The type of fluid administered (ie, crystalloids such as dextrose, sodium chloride, lactated ringer, and Plasma-Lyte) or colloid (ie, albumin) serves as an important factor in resuscitation (Table 142-4). Ideally, the fluid should expand the intravascular volume without providing excess free water leading to tissue edema.[52] The Saline versus Albumin Fluid Evaluation (SAFE) trial found similar safety but no significant benefit in length of stay in ICUs and mortality between crystalloids and albumin.[53] Based on cost and accessibility, the guidelines recommend a crystalloid product (balanced solution such as lactated ringers and Plasma-Lyte or normal saline) as first-line fluid for resuscitation. Colloid (ie, albumin) can be utilized in patients who have already received considerable amount of crystalloids and continue to require fluid.[46] Hetastarch products should be avoided at all times as they increase the risk of renal failure, requiring renal replacement therapy and death in multiple studies.[46]

TABLE 142-4 Comparison of IV Fluids–Crystalloids and Colloid

		Crystalloids				Colloid
	Human Plasma	Dextrose 5%	Sodium chloride 0.9%	Lactated ringers	Plasma-Lyte 148	Albumin 5%
pH	7.35-7.45	4	5	6.5	5.5	7.4
Osmolarity (mOsmol/L)	291	252	308	273	294	330
Sodium (mEq/L or mmol/L)	135-145	–	154	130	140	–
Chloride (mEq/L or mmol/L)	96-106	–	154	109	98	–
Potassium (mEq/L or mmol/L)	3.5-5	–	–	4	5	–
Bicarbonate (mEq/L or mmol/L)	23-27	–	–	28 (lactate)	27 (acetate)	–
Calcium (mg/dL [mmol/L])	8.5-10.5 [2.13-2.63]	–	–	2.7	–	–
Magnesium (mEq/L [mmol/L])	1.8-2.4 [0.9-1.2]	–	–	–	3	–
Glucose (mg/dL [mmol/L])	70-100 [3.9-5.6]	50	–	–	–	–
Tonicity[a]		Isotonic[b]	Isotonic	Isotonic	Isotonic	Isotonic

[a]Tonicity is based on comparison of osmolarity of the product and human plasma. Hypotonic is defined as osmolarity <250 mOsmol/L, isotonic is between 250 and 375 mOsmol/L, and hypertonic is >375 mOsmol/L.

[b]Dextrose 5% acts as hypotonic solution in body. It can also increase CO_2 and lactate production.

Data from Reference 52.

Among crystalloid solutions, there is increasing evidence of potential harm in developing hyperchloridemic metabolic acidosis from excessive administration of normal saline and subsequent increased renal failure and mortality in comparison to balanced salt solutions.[54-56] The 2021 Surviving Sepsis Campaign guideline updated their nonspecific fluid recommendation to favoring balanced crystalloid over normal saline for resuscitation.[39,54,55,57]

Lastly, the total duration of fluid therapy is based on the four phases of septic shock: ROSE—resuscitation, optimization, stabilization, and evacuation.[48] *Resuscitation* phase occurs within minutes and the patient will most likely have a positive fluid balance especially after the 30 mL/kg bolus. During the second phase of optimization (within hours), the goal is to keep a neutral fluid balance between intake and output. During this time, the clinician should consider the source of infection as well as any potential organ dysfunction when deciding volume and end point in fluid administration. For instance, a patient with peritonitis-related septic shock will most likely require more fluid than pneumonia-associated septic shock. Also, it is important to avoid fluid overload to decrease the risk of ARDS and other consequences such as intra-abdominal hypertension. During the third phase, *stabilization,* which usually occurs in days, the focus should be on organ support and keeping fluid balance neutral to net negative. During this time, the patient would most likely need maintenance doses (30 mL/kg/day) of fluid only. Finally, the *evacuation* phase occurs in days to weeks, and it is suggested to keep fluid balance negative. While attempting to achieve negative balance, careful deliberation to avoid excess fluid removal is crucial. Another hypotensive event in a recovering septic shock patient can lead to a further damage.

Infection Source Control

Once the anatomic site of infection is identified, prompt efforts to eradicate that source should be made as source control has been associated with increased survival. In sepsis and septic shock, the infectious foci should be controlled once the patient is stabilized after initial resuscitation, but optimally no more than 6 to 12 hours after diagnosis. With an infected intravascular catheter, the catheter should be removed and cultured. However, infected central venous catheters without septic shock or fungemia may be treated with prolonged antimicrobial therapy if catheter removal is not practical. Urinary tract catheters should be removed if association with sepsis is suspected. Suspicion of soft tissue infections such as cellulitis or wound infection or bone involvement should lead to aggressive debridement of the affected area. Evidence of an abscess or sepsis associated with any intra-abdominal pathology (ie, GI perforation, ischemic bowel, cholecystitis, infected pancreatic necrosis) should prompt surgical intervention. Reduced survival with delayed surgical source control was reported in observational studies, and as such, the Surgical Infection Society guidelines on the management of intra-abdominal infections suggest earlier source control, allowing only a short delay for rapid resuscitation in patients who are hemodynamically unstable with sepsis.[39,46,58]

Antimicrobial Therapy

5 Empiric IV antibiotics should be administered immediately after initial recognition of sepsis or septic shock as a strong correlation has been reported between time to antimicrobials and mortality.[39,46,47,59]

In addition to the timing of the empiric antibiotic, administration of appropriate antibiotic, especially for multidrug-resistant bacteria, has a great impact in reducing mortality.[14,15,34,60] Inappropriate initial antimicrobial therapy occurred in about 20% of patients with septic shock, and was associated with a fivefold reduction in survival in comparison to those who received appropriate therapy (52% vs 10%, respectively).[61] Early and appropriate antibiotic administration improves the mortality in patients with sepsis and septic shock.[62] Therefore, the guidelines recommend immediate administration of IV antimicrobials, ideally within 1 hour in patients with possible septic shock or a high likelihood for sepsis, but administration within 3 hours may be reasonable in patients with possible sepsis without shock.[39]

Septic shock caused by *C. albicans* demonstrated 25% survival with initial appropriate therapy but only 4.6% survival without.[61] Among the patients with candidemia, delayed appropriate antifungal treatment, especially in the presence of septic shock and failure to achieve timely source control, was independently associated with a greater risk of hospital mortality.[18,63,64] Hence, accurate and rapid

TABLE 142-5 Empiric Antimicrobial Regimens in Sepsis

Infection (site or type)	Antimicrobial regimen		Additional considerations
	Community-acquired	Hospital-acquired	
Urinary tract	Ceftriaxone or ciprofloxacin or levofloxacin	Ceftriaxone or ceftazidime or ciprofloxacin or levofloxacin	
Respiratory tract	Levofloxacin[a] or moxifloxacin or ceftriaxone + clarithromycin or azithromycin	Piperacillin or tazobactam or ceftazidime or cefepime or carbapenem[b] + levofloxacin or ciprofloxacin or aminoglycoside	± Vancomycin or linezolid
Intra-abdominal	Ertapenem or ciprofloxacin or levofloxacin + metronidazole or Ceftriaxone + metronidazole	Carbapenem[b] or Piperacillin or tazobactam or Ceftazidime or cefepime + metronidazole	
Skin/soft tissue	Vancomycin or linezolid or daptomycin	Vancomycin + piperacillin/tazobactam	
Catheter-related		Vancomycin	
Unknown	Piperacillin/tazobactam or carbapenem[b]	Carbapenem[b]	

[a]750 mg once daily.

[b]Imipenem and meropenem.

identification of candidemia is critical in prompt initiation of appropriate therapy.[37,46]

Selection of Antimicrobial Agents

The selection of an optimal empiric regimen requires assessment of several factors. Key patient factors include age, concomitant underlying diseases, chronic organ dysfunction (ie, liver or renal failure), presence of immunosuppression (ie, active cancer, neutropenia, or uncontrolled HIV infection), or presence of indwelling devices (ie, central venous lines or urinary catheter). Interviewing the patient or the patient's representative for recent hospitalization, recent history or colonization with specific pathogens, and the receipt of antimicrobials within the previous 3 months is helpful in assessing risk for infection with multidrug-resistant pathogens. Infection factors include type or anatomic site of infection, the most likely pathogens, acquisition of the organism from the community or healthcare institution, and the usual antibiotic susceptibility and resistance profile of the prevalent pathogens at the institution.

Table 142-5 lists specific empiric antimicrobial regimens for the anatomic site of infection based on the most likely pathogens.[46,58,65-68] However, general suggestions can be made when treating critically ill patients with sepsis or septic shock.

For patients at risk for sepsis or septic shock with MRSA, an anti-MRSA agent should be initiated empirically.[40] Risk factors for MRSA include prior history of MRSA infection or colonization, recent IV antibiotics or hospitalization, history of recurrent skin infections, presence of invasive devices, and hemodialysis. Vancomycin remains the mainstay of therapy for MRSA-associated infections.[69] Revised therapeutic monitoring of vancomycin guideline recommends monitoring area under the curve (AUC) over 24 hours in place of monitoring trough levels based on efficacy and nephrotoxicity data in patients with serious infections due to MRSA.[70] The 2016 Infectious Diseases Society of America (IDSA) guidelines recommend either vancomycin or linezolid for hospital-acquired/ventilator-associated pneumonia.[65] Linezolid has better lung penetration into epithelial lining fluids than vancomycin. However, linezolid was not superior to vancomycin in microbiological and clinical cure rates in patients with nosocomial pneumonia due to MRSA.[69]

Daptomycin is a cyclic lipopeptide that exhibits rapid bactericidal activity against gram-positive microorganisms including MRSA and vancomycin-resistant enterococci (VRE).[71] Daptomycin resulted in a 70% success rate for critically ill septic patients with bacteremia due to MRSA, VRE, *E. faecium* or coagulase-negative staphylococci.[71] The daptomycin cohort had significantly lower clinical failure for MRSA bacteremia when matched with vancomycin cohort patients (29% vs 45%) and lower all-cause 30-day mortality (6.1% vs 15.3%).[72]

Bloodstream infections caused by extended-spectrum beta-lactamases (ESBL)-producing Enterobacterales are associated with high rates of morbidity and mortality of up to 44% in patients with sepsis or septic shock.[73] Mortality was especially high with a delay in appropriate antimicrobial therapy.[73,74] The appropriate empiric antibiotic therapy in critically ill patients with sepsis or septic shock is crucial. Carbapenems remain active and have been regarded as the treatment of choice for serious infections due to ESBL pathogens. However, increased use of carbapenems has led to the emergence of carbapenem-resistant Enterobacterales which represents a greater threat. Piperacillin/tazobactam has been evaluated in observational studies as carbapenem-sparing therapy with conflicting results.[74,75] In a meta-analysis of 25 observational studies describing 3,824 participants who received either beta-lactam/beta-lactamase inhibitor or carbapenem as empiric or definitive therapy for ESBL-producing bacterial bloodstream infections, 30-day mortality was not significantly different.[74] However, all-cause 30-day mortality was 12.3% in the piperacillin/tazobactam group and 3.7% in the meropenem group (absolute risk difference of 8.6%) in hospitalized patients who received definitive treatment for bloodstream infections due to ceftriaxone-resistant *Escherichia coli* or *Klebsiella pneumoniae.*[76] Piperacillin/tazobactam should no longer be considered an alternative to meropenem for definitive treatment of bloodstream infection due to ESBL-producing gram-negative pathogens.

Combination therapy does not appear to be more effective than monotherapy in reducing organ failure or mortality in low-risk patients including sepsis without shock.[13] However, multidrug resistance in sepsis due to gram-negative bacteremia was strongly associated with the receipt of inappropriate empiric therapy and a threefold increase in the risk of hospital mortality.[15] The guidelines suggest using two antimicrobial agents in patients at risk of multidrug-resistant pathogens.[39] Risk factors include recent history of infection due to antibiotic-resistant organism, hospital-acquired infection, and recent history of hospitalization or use of broad-spectrum antibiotics. Once the pathogen and its susceptibilities are reported, double gram-negative coverage is no longer necessary except for highly resistant organisms. The greatest benefit of combination therapy appeared to be in patients with septic shock due to *Pseudomonas* or multidrug-resistant gram-negative bacteremia such as *Acinetobacter* and in neutropenic patients with sepsis or septic shock.[77-79] Combination therapy consisting of antibiotics from two different classes increases the probability of at least one active agent. For instance, if *P. aeruginosa* infection is suspected, beta-lactam antipseudomonal agents (ceftazidime or cefepime), antipseudomonal fluoroquinolone (ciprofloxacin or levofloxacin), or an aminoglycoside should be included in the regimen.[65]

Antifungal Therapy

Patients with candidemia are generally sicker based on their higher Acute Physiology and Chronic Health Evaluation (APACHE) II scores and have a higher mortality rate than those with bacteremia.[12] However, the use of empiric antifungal in all critically ill patients is not supported.[80] As such, clinicians should consider empiric antifungal therapy based on the risk factors for invasive *Candida* infections and no other known cause of fever.[39] The risk factors include febrile neutropenic patients after 4-7 days of broad-spectrum antibiotics, immunocompromised status, dialysis, prolonged invasive vascular devices, total parental nutrition, necrotizing pancreatitis, major surgery especially abdominal, corticosteroids, prolonged ICU stay, or fungal colonization.[39,81]

Invasive candidiasis remains the most common form of fungal infections, and empiric parenteral treatment includes echinocandins, triazoles, or a formulation of amphotericin B.[81,82] The selection depends on the clinical status of the patient, the local susceptibility of the most prevalent *Candida* species, recent exposure to antifungal agents, relative drug toxicity, and the presence of organ dysfunction or shock that would affect drug clearance. Recent exposure to antibiotics and fluconazole has been associated with fluconazole-resistant *Candida* species.[83] Fluconazole resistance among *Candida* species from bloodstream infections ranges between 12% and 28%.[16,17] *C. glabrata* was the only species that may exhibit resistance to both triazoles and echinocandins. Among the 180 isolates of *C. glabrata* isolated from nosocomial bloodstream infections, 62% were nonsusceptible to caspofungin.[16]

Triazoles (fluconazole, voriconazole) are recommended in hemodynamically stable patients who have not had previous triazole exposure and not known to be colonized with azole-resistant *Candida* species.[81] However, preferred empiric therapy for suspected invasive candidiasis in nonneutropenic patients in the ICU is an echinocandin (anidulafungin, micafungin, or caspofungin). Ecinocandins exhibit potent activity against all *Candida* species, including *C. krusei* that is typically resistant to an azole, as well as *Aspergillus* species. Empiric use of an echinocandin should be considered in most patients, despite the severity of illness including septic shock, who have been treated with other antifungal agents or suspected *C. glabrata* or *C. krusei* infection.[81]

Resistance to fluconazole, caspofungin, and amphotericin B was reported in 28%, 2.9%, and 3.1%, respectively, of adults admitted to ICUs with invasive candidiasis who received antifungal therapy empirically.[17] Approximately 20% of the antifungal agents were changed primarily based on *Candida* susceptibility, followed by inadequate clinical response. Hospital mortality was comparable between echinocandin (caspofungin/anidulafungin) and fluconazole (56% vs 58%, respectively). Micafungin 100 mg daily was noninferior to liposomal amphotericin B 3 mg/kg daily or caspofungin 70 mg followed by 50 mg daily for the treatment of invasive candidiasis in patients with or without neutropenia. Overall treatment success was numerically lower in patients with neutropenia than those without (64% vs 73%).[84] All three echinocandins appear to be comparable in terms of efficacy, pharmacology, and adverse effects, and the guidelines do not make a distinction or recommend a preferred agent.[81]

There was no difference in treatment efficacy or mortality outcomes in critically ill patients with invasive candidiasis receiving an amphotericin B formulation compared with those receiving an echinocandin or voriconazole.[82] However, amphotericin B was poorly tolerated. Liposomal formulation of amphotericin B (3-5 mg/kg daily) remains as an alternative to echinocandins in patients with echinocandin intolerance or toxicity.

Pharmacokinetics and Pharmacodynamic Principles of Antimicrobial Agents in Sepsis

Physiologic changes during sepsis including unstable hemodynamics, increased cardiac output, variable kidney, and hepatic perfusions, or hypoalbuminemia can dramatically alter antimicrobial pharmacokinetics.[85] Initially, high creatinine clearance can be seen in patients with normal serum creatinine because of increased renal preload. Reduced serum albumin leads to altered drug binding. Volume of distribution may be increased because of fluid accumulation from leaky capillaries into the extracellular space from aggressive fluid resuscitation. Consequently, some antimicrobial agents especially hydrophilic antimicrobials including aminoglycosides, beta-lactams, carbapenems, and vancomycin can result in suboptimal serum concentrations with standard doses. Hence, optimal dosing strategies based on pharmacokinetic and pharmacodynamic principles targets are recommended in critically ill patients.[39]

Inadequate vancomycin trough plasma concentrations in relation to the MIC of the pathogen has been associated with clinical failure in septic shock due to MRSA.[86] Trough concentrations of 15 to 20 mg/L (10.4-13.8 μmol/L) and AUC/MIC higher than 400 were associated with improved survival. The revised vancomycin dosing guideline recommends a target AUC/MIC of 400 to 600 in serious MRSA infections.[70]

Daptomycin plasma concentrations after a dose of 6 to 8 mg/kg/day for primarily staphylococcal-related infections were lower in critically ill patients than healthy volunteers.[87] Daptomycin clearance did not change significantly in patients with or without sepsis. However, volume of distribution appeared to be larger. Consequently, weight-based daptomycin dose of at least 10 mg/kg/day was recommended.[87]

The time the plasma drug concentration remains above the pathogen MIC in relation to the dosing interval (T > MIC) best describes the pharmacodynamics of beta-lactams. A minimum T > MIC of 60% of the dosing interval generally provides a good clinical response. However, sepsis or septic shock may require longer duration of T > MIC.[88] Extended infusion or continuous infusion rather than the standard 30 minutes to achieve longer T > MIC as well as a loading dosing prior to the prolonged infusion to achieve effective beta-lactam concentration without delay optimizes the pharmacokinetics and pharmacodynamics of beta-lactam antibiotics. A prolonged infusion of beta-lactams after an initial bolus dose is preferred in place of a short intermittent infusion.[39,89,90] Continuous infusion of meropenem was associated with improved clinical cure rate in patients with sepsis, greater microbiological eradication, and decreased hospital mortality compared with a standard 30-minute intermittent infusion.[91]

Based on its concentration-depending killing activity, the Sepsis-3 guidelines recommend once daily dosing of 5-7 mg/kg daily gentamicin or an equivalent aminoglycoside in patients without severely reduced renal function. This high dosing strategy yielded comparable clinical efficacy but decreased renal toxicity compared to the multiple daily dosing regimens.[46] However, suboptimal aminoglycoside concentrations may occur in the early phase of therapy in critically ill patients, suggesting higher dosing of 8 mg/kg gentamicin may be required for optimal effect.[92] Target trough concentrations of below 2 mg/L (4.18 μmol/L) should be monitored to detect potential renal toxicity.

As sepsis progresses, organ perfusion decreases because of significant myocardial depression and leads to multiple organ dysfunction. Consequently, clearance of antimicrobial agents is decreased, prolonging the elimination half-life and accumulation of metabolites. Dosing strategies need to be assessed and modified continuously through the course of treatment for optimal efficacy.

De-escalation

Empiric antimicrobial agents should be initiated immediately after the diagnosis of sepsis and septic shock is suspected due to the serious nature of the disease, but the antimicrobial regimen should be reassessed daily based on the microbiological and clinical data. This creates a potential de-escalation opportunity as part of good antibiotic stewardship to narrow down the spectrum once the pathogen has been identified to avoid unnecessary use of antimicrobials.[39,46,93] De-escalation may also prevent drug toxicities and the development of nosocomial super infections with *Candida* species, *Clostridioides*, or VRE. Improved patient care outcomes have been demonstrated with such de-escalation of antibiotic therapy. The hospital mortality rate among patients admitted to the ICU with severe sepsis or septic shock was 27% in whom therapy was de-escalated, 33% in the category of no change, and 43% in the escalation group.[94]

The data on timing or precise criteria to de-escalate in case of negative cultures is lacking. However, antimicrobial regimens should still be assessed daily for opportunity for de-escalation in response to clinical improvement including shock resolution or decrease in vasopressor requirement and/or evidence of infection resolution by biomarkers, especially PCT.[39,46]

EVALUATION OF THERAPEUTIC OUTCOMES

PCT is a serum biomarker that increases in response to endotoxins and inflammatory cytokines that are released during systemic bacterial infections, and it rises early in severe sepsis by pneumonia and bloodstream infections. Measurements of PCT concentrations may assist in determining the duration of antimicrobial therapy in sepsis.[39,46] The use of PCT concentration in critically ill patients was associated with reduced daily doses of antimicrobials, duration of antimicrobial treatment, and mortality.[95]

Duration of Therapy

The average duration of antimicrobial therapy in a patient with sepsis is 7 to 10 days in the absence of source control issues, and fungal infections can require 10 to 14 days.[46,81] However, the duration can be longer in patients with a compromised immune status, slow clinical response, large infection site, undrainable focus of infection, bacteremia with *S. aureus*, multidrug-resistant gram-negative pathogens.

However, over the past two decades, clinical trials have demonstrated that shorter courses are as efficacious as longer courses, especially with successful source control and are associated with fewer adverse events.[96,97] A 7-day course of therapy for both hospital-acquired and ventilator-associated pneumonia is recommended.[65] A short course of antimicrobial treatment (median duration of 4 days) for patients with complicated intra-abdominal infection and adequate source control had similar surgical site infection, recurrent intra-abdominal infection, or death as the control group with a median of 8 days of antibiotics whose antibiotic duration was based on symptoms (ie, fever, leukocytosis, and ileus).[97] The Surgical Infection Society recommends no more than 4 full days of antimicrobial therapy for patients with adequate source control and no more than 5 to 7 days in patients in whom a definitive source control was not performed.[58]

Once adequate source control is achieved, the guidelines suggest shorter duration of antimicrobial therapy in place of historically longer duration.[39] However, when optimal duration of therapy is unclear especially in the absence of identifiable causative pathogen, PCT along with clinical evaluation is suggested in determining the antimicrobial treatment duration.

Hemodynamic Support with Vasopressors

The Surviving Sepsis Campaign guidelines recommend a target MAP of at least 65 mm Hg (MAP = [SBP + 2*DBP]/3).[39,46] Achievement of a high (MAP of 80-85 mm Hg) or low (MAP of 65-70 mm Hg) target did not result in significant difference in mortality at 28 and 90 days.[98] Among the patients with preexisting hypertension, those in the high target group had less renal dysfunction and need for renal replacement therapy. However, the incidence of newly diagnosed atrial fibrillation was significantly higher in the high target group. The number needed to treat was 9.5 to prevent one patient from necessitating renal replacement therapy.[99]

Vasopressors should be used to achieve and maintain MAP goal in fluid-resuscitation refractory shock, and they are titrated up carefully to an end point of adequate organ perfusion. There are several adrenergic receptors that are the key to understanding the mechanism of action of various vasopressors (Table 142-6). Alpha-adrenergic receptors are located in the vascular wall and in the heart, and the alpha-receptor agonists induce peripheral vasoconstriction as well as increase the duration of contraction in the heart. Beta-adrenergic receptors are primarily found in the heart. Stimulation of the beta receptors causes inotropic and chronotropic effect. Dopamine receptors are in the renal, splanchnic, coronary, and cerebral vascular beds. Dopamine receptor agonists cause vasodilation of the renal and splanchnic vessels. As dopamine is a precursor to epinephrine and norepinephrine, it affects both alpha-1 and beta-1 receptors, causing peripheral vasoconstriction and inotropy. There are three types of vasopressin receptors: V1, V2, and V3 receptors. Vasopressin works on the V1 and V2 receptors, which are in vascular smooth muscles and basolateral membrane of the collecting

TABLE 142-6 Mechanism of Action and Hemodynamic Effects of Vasopressors in Septic Shock

	Receptor affinity				Physiologic outcome			
Drug	**Dopamine**	**Alpha-1**	**Beta-1**	**Beta-2**	**HR**	**SV**	**SVR**	**CO**
Dopamine (0.5-2)[a]	+++	–	+	–	↔ or ↑	↑	↔ or ↑	↑
Dopamine (5-10)[a]	++	+	+++	+	↑	↑	↔ or ↑	↑↑
Dopamine (10-20)[a]	++	+++	++	–	↑	↑	↑↑	↑
Epinephrine	–	++++	++++	+++	↑	↑	↑↑	↑↑
Norepinephrine	–	++++	++	+	↔ or ↑	↔	↑↑	↑
Phenylephrine	–	+++	–	–	↔ or ↓	–	↑↑	↔
Vasopressin	V1 receptor				↔ or ↓	–	↑↑	↔ or ↓
Angiotensin II	AT receptor				↑	–	↑	↑

CO, cardiac output; HR, heart rate; SV, stroke volume; SVR, systemic vascular resistance; V1, vasopressin receptor 1; V2, vasopressin receptor 2.

[a]mcg/kg/min.

Data from Reference 100.

duck, respectively. Vasopressin contracts vascular smooth muscle mainly through the V1 receptor and retains water via V2 receptors.

6 The guidelines recommend norepinephrine as the first-line agent for patients with septic shock.[40] Norepinephrine, a potent alpha-adrenergic agent with less pronounced beta-adrenergic activity than epinephrine, is the preferred vasopressor to correct hypotension in fluid refractory septic shock.[39,46,100] It increases MAP and SVR via vasoconstrictive effects on peripheral vascular beds with little changes in heart rate and less increase in stroke volume compared to dopamine. Norepinephrine is more potent than dopamine in refractory septic shock. Norepinephrine was associated with lower risk of mortality and lower risk of arrhythmia compared to dopamine.[101]

Dopamine may be considered as an alternative agent to norepinephrine in a small subset of patients who have bradycardia or are at low risk of developing arrhythmia.[46,99] Dopamine increases MAP and cardiac output by increasing the heart rate and cardiac contractility, making it potentially useful for patients with compromised systolic function. However, it is arrhythmogenic and can cause tachycardia, limiting its role in maintaining MAP.[101]

Epinephrine is a nonspecific alpha- and beta-adrenergic agonist (Table 142-6). Overall mortality at 90 days between norepinephrine and epinephrine was not significantly different in patients with septic shock.[101] However, there are several adverse effects associated with epinephrine including tachycardia, lactic acidosis, and impaired blood flow to the splanchnic system.

Optimal dosing of norepinephrine among obese patients with septic shock is important to consider as many drug studies do not include obese patients and therefore leave clinicians to extrapolate pharmacokinetic parameters from nonobese patients at bedside. Weight-based dosing of norepinephrine in obese adult patients (body mass index [BMI] >30 kg/m^2) did not achieve goal MAP earlier than the non-WBD group, and there was no difference in mortality (23.6% vs 23.1%, respectively).[102] However, morbidly obese (BMI >40 kg/m^2) patients had significantly higher cumulative norepinephrine use in the WBD group compared to the non-WBD group, and higher cumulative dose was identified as an independent risk factor for mortality during hospitalization and at 1 year.[103] Further studies are needed to assess appropriate norepinephrine dosing strategies.

Vasopressin, also known as antidiuretic hormone, is produced in the hypothalamus and released from pituitary. In a healthy individual, it controls osmolality by stimulating the V2 receptors in the kidneys, but has little effect on BP. However, in a state of distributive shock, vasopressin binds to V1 receptors in vascular smooth muscle, which leads to vasoconstriction, thereby increasing BP. In contrast, after the initial rise in vasopressin concentration in septic shock, vasopressin level decreases to normal range due to the combination of depletion of vasopressin stores and inhibition of synthesis and release.[99] A synthetic formulation of vasopressin is dosed at 0.03 U/min without titration unlike most vasopressors, as higher doses of vasopressin have been associated with cardiac, digital, and splanchnic ischemia.

The role of vasopressin as a single vasoactive agent or in combination with norepinephrine remains controversial. The VANISH trial compared vasopressin to norepinephrine in patients with septic shock and reported no significant difference between the two groups in 28-day mortality or kidney injury.[104] The VASST trial comparing norepinephrine alone and norepinephrine with low dose (0.01-0.03 U/min) vasopressin in patients with septic shock showed similar mortality rates (39% vs 35%, respectively). When the investigators reevaluated the VASST trial, using the new definition of septic shock from the Sepsis-3 guidelines, the sample size decreased by half, and the 28-day mortality rates were increased by about 10% for both groups.[105] Patients with less severe sepsis who received norepinephrine less than 15 mcg/min had improved survival in the combination group than in the norepinephrine alone group (36% vs 27%, respectively). Combination therapy of vasopressin with norepinephrine reduced mortality in comparison to norepinephrine alone (RR 0.91; 95% CI 0.83-0.99).[105] There was no difference in risks for digital ischemia or arrythmias. Adding vasopressin to norepinephrine is recommended (dose ranging from 0.25-0.5 mcg/kg/min) rather than increasing the norepinephrine dose to achieve adequate MAP.

The first synthetic angiotensin II was approved for the use in vasopressor refractory septic shock. In the setting of decreased renal perfusion, the angiotensinogen from liver and renin produced by the kidney come together to form angiotensin I which is then transformed to angiotensin II by angiotensin-converting enzyme. Angiotensin II ultimately increases BP by increasing sympathetic activity that stimulates pituitary gland to increase antidiuretic hormone secretion to promote sodium, chloride, and water reabsorption in the kidneys. It also continues to promote aldosterone secretion from the adrenal gland, where aldosterone will carry on the sodium and water reabsorption in the distal tubule and collecting duct of the kidney via sodium-potassium pump. Angiotensin II was evaluated in adult patients with persistent hypotension despite adequate fluid resuscitation and received >0.2 ng/kg/min norepinephrine equivalent vasopressor use (ATHOS-3 trial).[106] A greater response in MAP was reported in 321 patients who received angiotensin II versus placebo (69.9% vs 23.4%). Patients in the ATHOS-3 trial who had AKI requiring renal replacement therapy (RRT) at initiation of angiotensin II had significantly higher 28-day survival (53% vs 30%) and discontinuation of RRT in the angiotension II group (38% vs 15%) compared with placebo.[107] Based on limited clinical experience in sepsis and safety data, synthetic angiotensin II's place of therapy in septic shock remains unclear.

Sepsis-induced myocardial dysfunction can exacerbate hemodynamic instability which may lead to worse outcomes in septic shock. Inotropic agents such as dobutamine and epinephrine have been used in patients with persistent hypoperfusion despite adequate fluid resuscitation. However, no randomized comparative trials have been conducted in this population. There was no clear reduction in mortality in dobutamine combined with norepinephrine to norepinephrine alone or between dobutamine and epinephrine.[108] Hence, the guidelines provided a weak recommendation to use either drug only in selected situations of persistent hypoperfusion despite adequate fluid resuscitation and arterial BP.[39,46]

Performance Improvement Bundle

The Surviving Sepsis Campaign recommends implementation of hospital-based performance improvement efforts such as a core set of recommendation ("bundle") because they have been associated with improved patient outcomes.[2,46] While the details of each institution's performance improvement bundle may be different, there is a common theme of improved management of patients with sepsis and septic shock.[109] Hospital mortality rates dropped 0.7% per site for every 3 months of participation. Hospital and ICU lengths of stay decreased by 4% for every 10% increase in site compliance in a 7.5-year study.[110]

7 The Sepsis-3 guidelines described a 1-hour care, consisting of three major components of initial treatment immediately after early recognition of sepsis: administration of fluid, administration of parenteral antibiotics, and use of vasopressor agents (Table 142-7).[47] Resolution of serum lactate is desired to indicate adequate tissue perfusion and therefore should be repeated within 2 to 4 hours of the initial level. The interpretation of repeat lactate requires careful consideration especially in patients with concomitant hepatic and/or renal failure as metabolism and elimination of lactate may be decreased in this setting. The guidelines endorse using a performance improvement program including sepsis screening and prompt initial treatment considered as standard of care for sepsis and septic shock.[39]

TABLE 142-7 Sepsis-3 (2016) Performance Improvement Checklist for Bundle-Care Compliance

One-hour bundle
• Measure initial lactate
• Repeat in 2 hours if initial lactate >18 mg/dL (2 mmol/L)
• Obtain cultures (blood, urine, sputum, etc.) prior to administration of antibiotics
• Administer broad-spectrum IV antibiotics within 1 hour
• Initial fluid resuscitation of 30 mL/kg crystalloid for hypotension or lactate ≥36 mg/dL (4 mmol/L)
• Vasopressors if MAP <65 mm Hg during or after completion of fluid resuscitation
Outcome measurements
• Length of stay in ICU and hospital
• Rate of organ dysfunction
• Mortality rate

MAP, mean arterial pressure.

Data from References 46 and 47.

Adjunctive Therapies

Sepsis and septic shock present multitudes of complications in a relative short span of time. In addition to prompt initiation of a performance improvement bundle, several adjunctive therapies including transfusions of blood products, oxygen supplement, mechanical ventilation, or RRT may be required. Key pharmacological adjunctive therapies are described below.

8 In Sepsis-3 guidelines, IV hydrocortisone is recommended for adult patients with septic shock who are hemodynamically unstable after initial resuscitation with IV fluids and vasopressors.[46] Cortisol levels vary widely in patients with septic shock, and an increased mortality has been associated with both low and high serum cortisol levels. Data on the benefits of corticosteroids as adjunct therapy in patients with sepsis and septic shock are conflicting with regards to reduction of overall mortality.[111-117] A significant shock reversal and reduction in mortality were reported in patients with septic shock unresponsive to fluid resuscitation and vasopressors for more than an hour and had relative adrenal insufficiency who received prolonged courses (>5 days) of low-dose corticosteroid therapy compared to placebo (38% vs 44%; relative risk 0.84).[111] The Corticosteroid Therapy of Septic Shock (CORTICUS) found no survival benefit for patients who were unresponsive to adequate fluid replacement and required vasopressors, with or without adrenal insufficiency.[112] However, CORTICUS included patients with septic shock regardless of their responsiveness to vasopressor therapy. Subsequent meta-analyses and systematic reviews continue to present conflicting data. Low-dose corticosteroids reduced 28-day mortality, increased shock reversal, and reduced organ injury based in an analysis of 22 randomized controlled trials.[113] Another systematic review of 35 trials of sepsis detected no significant benefit on mortality.[114]

After publication of the Sepsis-3 guidelines, two large, randomized, blinded, multicenter, controlled trials of low-dose corticosteroids use in patients with septic shock did not confirm or refute previously published data on reduction of mortality.[115,116] However, these landmark studies offer other practical benefits of low-dose corticosteroids. Both trials clearly defined adequate fluid resuscitation, vasopressor-dependent shock, and appropriate antimicrobial therapy. The 90-day mortality in the Adjunctive Corticosteroid Treatment in Critically Ill Patients with Septic Shock (ADRENAL) trial was similar between continuous infusion of hydrocortisone 200 mg/day for maximum of 7 days and placebo (27.9% vs 28.8%, respectively).[115,117] The 90-day mortality in the Activated Protein C and Corticosteroids for Human Septic Shock (APROCCHSS) trial was 43% with hydrocortisone 50 mg IV bolus every 6 hours plus fludrocortisone 50 mcg tablet via a nasogastric tube once daily for 7 days and 49% with placebo.[116] The dramatic difference in the mortality data may rise from the patients' severity of illness. The patients from the APROCCHSS trial may have been more seriously ill based on their SOFA and APACHE II scores and had higher proportions of patients who required RRT or who had bacteremia. Regardless, both trials showed significantly faster resolution of shock and increase in vasopressor-free days, providing reassurance of short-term benefits of low-dose hydrocortisone in selected patients even if there is not clear benefit for short- or long-term mortality.[115-118]

The 2021 guidelines updated the recommendation to adding low dose hydrocortisone 200 mg/day for patients with septic shock who require ongoing norepinephrine dose of >0.25 mcg/kg/min at least 4 hours to maintain the target MAP.[39] Continuous infusion of hydrocortisone may prevent a significant increase in blood glucose associated with repetitive bolus injections. Steroid should be tapered when vasopressors are no longer required as hemodynamic and immunologic rebound effects have been reported with abrupt cessation of corticosteroids.[46]

9 Hyperglycemia and insulin resistance are frequently associated with sepsis regardless of the presence of diabetes prior to sepsis, and more severe hyperglycemia is associated with higher morbidity and mortality.[2,46] The NICE-SUGAR trial, the largest study to date on glucose control in ICU patients, reported a higher incidence of mortality at 90 days with intensive insulin therapy (target glucose range of 81-108 mg/dL [4.5-6.0 mmol/L]) than with conventional therapy (target of <180 mg/dL [10.0 mmol/L]).[119] Intensive insulin therapy targeting blood glucose of 80 to 110 mg/dL (4.4 to 6.1 mmol/L) in septic patients did not improve overall mortality and was associated with a higher incidence of hypoglycemia (blood glucose less than 40 mg/dL [2.2 mmol/L]).[120] The Sepsis-3 guidelines recommended initiating insulin when two consecutive blood glucose levels are greater than 180 mg/dL (10.0 mmol/L) based on the NICE-SUGAR trial. However, the guidelines do not give a specific target glucose range other than monitoring glucose of less than 180 mg/dL (10 mmol/L) every 1 to 2 hours until the glucose levels and insulin requirements are stable to avoid hypoglycemia.[46]

A meta-analysis of 35 randomized controlled trials compared four blood glucose targets (180 mg/dL [10 mmol/L]) and risks of hospital mortality and hypoglycemia.[121] There were no significant differences in mortality among the groups. However, lower target ranges (less than 110 [6.1 mmol/L] and 110-144 mg/dL [6.1-8 mmol/L]) were associated with a four- to ninefold increased risk of hypoglycemia in comparison to the higher target ranges. No significant difference in risk of hypoglycemia was noted between a range of 144-180 mg/dL (8-10 mmol/L) and greater than 180 mg/dL (10 mmol/L). The current recommendation remains to initiate insulin therapy at a glucose level of greater than 180 mg/dL (10 mmol/L) with a target range between 144 and 180 mg/dL (8-10 mmol/L).[39]

Pharmacologic venous thromboembolism (VTE) prophylaxis should be initiated in all patients admitted to the ICU with sepsis and septic shock.[39,46]

Overall, the incidence of VTE in the ICU is approximately 10%. However, the incidence was much higher (37.2%) in patients with sepsis and septic shock which may increase the length of stay in ICU (18.2 vs 13.4 days, respectively).[122]

There is limited data comparing low molecular weight heparin to unfractionated heparin in VTE prophylaxis among septic patients. However, the overall rate of VTE and pulmonary embolism was lower in critically ill patients receiving LMWH in comparison to unfractionated heparin administered twice daily, and overall mortality was also reduced, albeit not significant.[123] The guideline continues to recommend LMWH over unfractionated heparin for VTE prophylaxis in patients with sepsis or septic shock.[39] If pharmacologic prophylaxis is contraindicated, mechanical prophylactic measures should be considered.[125]

An international prospective cohort study reported clinically important GI bleeding occurred in 2.6% in critically ill adult patients.[124] Prophylaxis with either a proton pump inhibitor (PPI) or histamine 2 receptor antagonist reduced the risk of GI bleeding in comparison to no prophylaxis.[124] The use of pantoprazole versus placebo did not demonstrate any effect on mortality.[126] However, PPI use did reduce GI bleeding. A higher risk of *C. difficile* infections was noted with PPI use.[39]

The guidelines continue to recommend stress ulcer prophylaxis should be initiated in all patients with sepsis and septic shock who have risk factors for GI bleeding.[39] Risk factors for clinically relevant GI bleeding include shock, coagulopathy, and chronic liver disease.[125] The selection of agent should also consider patient's renal, liver, hematologic dysfunction, as dose adjustments may be necessary. Although preventing clinically significant GI bleeding is important, it also must be balanced with potential adverse events from decreasing pH of the stomach such as possibility of developing *C. difficile* infection.[46]

ABBREVIATIONS

AKI	acute kidney injury
APACHE	acute physiology and chronic health evaluation
ARDS	acute respiratory distress syndrome
AUC	area under the curve
BMI	body mass index
BP	blood pressure
CVP	central venous pressure
DIC	disseminated intravascular coagulation
EGDT	early goal-directed therapy
ESBL	extended-spectrum beta-lactamases
GI	gastrointestinal
HIV	human immunodeficiency virus
H2RA	histamine 2 receptor antagonist
ICU	intensive care unit
IV	intravenous
IL	interleukin
IL-1RA	interleukin-1 receptor antagonist
LMWH	low-molecular-weight heparin
MAP	mean arterial pressure
MIC	minimum inhibitory concentration
MRSA	methicillin-resistant *Staphylococcus aureus*
PCT	procalcitonin
PPI	proton pump inhibitor
RRT	renal replacement therapy
$Scvo_2$	central venous oxygen saturation
SIRS	systemic inflammatory response syndrome
SOFA	sequential organ failure assessment
SVR	systemic vascular resistance
T > MIC	time above minimum inhibitory concentration
TNF	tumor necrosis factor
qSOFA	quick sequential organ failure assessment
VRE	vancomycin-resistant enterococci
VTE	venous thromboembolism
WBC	white blood cell
WBD	weight-based dosing

REFERENCES

1. Singer M, Deutschman CS, Seymour CW, et al. The third international consensus definitions for sepsis and septic shock (Sepsis-3). *JAMA.* 2016;315:801–810.
2. Dellinger RP, Levy MM, Rhodes A, et al. Surviving sepsis campaign: International guidelines for management of severe sepsis and septic shock. *Crit Care Med.* 2013;41:580–637.
3. Levy MM, Fink MP, Marshall JC, et al. 2001 SCCM/ESICM/ACCP/ATS/SIS International Sepsis Definitions Conference. *Crit Care Med.* 2003;31:1250–1256.
4. Rubens M, Saxena A, Ramamoorthy V, et al. Increasing sepsis rates in the United States: Results from national inpatient sample, 2005 to 2014. *J Intensiv Care Med.* 2020;35:858–868:885066618794136. doi:10.1177/0885066618794136.
5. Rhee C, Dantes R, Epstein L, et al. Incidence and trends of sepsis in US hospitals using clinical vs claims data, 2009–2014. *JAMA.* 2017;318:1241–1249.
6. Vincent J-L, Jones G, David S, et al. Frequency and mortality of septic shock in Europe and North America: A systematic review and meta-analysis. *Critical Care.* 2019;2310.1186/s13054-019-2478-6.
7. Walkey AJ, Lagu T, Lindenauer PK. Trends in sepsis and infection sources in the United States. A population-based study. *Ann Am Thorac Soc.* 2015;12:216–220.
8. Paoli C, Reynolds M, Sinha M, et al. Epidemiology and costs of sepsis in the United States—An analysis based on timing of diagnosis and severity level. *Crit Care Med.* 2018;46:1889–1897.
9. Herrán-Monge R, Muriel-Bombín A, García-García MM., et al. Epidemiology and changes in mortality of sepsis after the implementation of surviving sepsis campaign guidelines. *J Intensive Care Med.* 2017;34:740–750. 10.1177/0885066617711882.
10. Leligdowicz A, Dodek PM, Norena M, et al. Association between source of infection and hospital mortality in patients who have septic shock. *Am J Resp Crit Care Med.* 2014;189:1204–1212.
11. Thomas-Ruddel DO, Poidinger B, Kott M, et al. Influence of pathogen and focus of infection on procalcitonin values in sepsis patients with bacteremia or candidemia. *Crit Care.* 2018;22:128. doi:10.1186/s13054-018-2050-9.
12. Guillamet CV, Vazquez R, Micek ST, et al. Development and validation of a clinical prediction rule for candidemia in hospitalized patients with severe sepsis and septic shock. *J Crit Care.* 2015;30:715–720.
13. Brunkhorst FM, Oppert M, Marx G, et al. Effect of empirical treatment with moxifloxacin and meropenem vs meropenem on sepsis-related organ dysfunction in patients with severe sepsis. *JAMA.* 2012;307:2390–2399.
14. Burnham JP, Lane MA, Kollef MH. Impact of sepsis classification and multidrug-resistance status on outcome among patients treated with appropriate therapy. *Crit Care Med.* 2015;43:1580–1586.
15. Martinez-Nadal Gemma, Puerta-Alcalde Pedro, Gudiol Carlota, et al. Inappropriate empirical antibiotic treatment in high-risk neutropenic patients with bacteremia in the era of multidrug resistance. *Clinical Infectious Diseases.* 201910.1093/cid/ciz319.
16. Wisplinghoff H, Ebbers J, Geurtz L, et al. Nosocomial bloodstream infections due to Candida spp. in the USA: Species distribution, clinical features and antifungal susceptibilities. *Int J Antimicrob Agents.* 2014;43:78–81.
17. Al-Dorzi HM, Sakkijha H, Khan R, et al. Invasive candidiasis in critically ill patients: A prospective cohort study in two tertiary care centers. *J Intensive Care Med.* 2018. doi:10.1177/0885066618767835.
18. Kato Hideaki, Yoshimura Yukihiro, Suido Yoshihiro, et al. Mortality and risk factor analysis for Candida blood stream infection: A multicenter study. *J Infect Chemother.* 2019;25:341–345. 10.1016/j.jiac.2019.01.002.
19. Diekema D, Arbefeville S, Boyken L, et al. The changing epidemiology of healthcare-associated candidemia over three decades. *Diagn Microb Infect Dis.* 2012;73:45–48.
20. Tamayo E, Fernandez A, Almansa R, et al. Pro- and anti-inflammatory responses are regulated simultaneously from the first moments of septic shock. *Eur Cytokine Network.* 2011;22:82–87.
21. Chousterman BG, Swirski FK, Weber GF. Cytokine storm and sepsis disease pathogenesis. *Semin Immunopathol.* 2017;39:517–528.
22. Carlyn C, Andersen N, Baltch A, et al. Analysis of septic biomarker patterns: Prognostic value in predicting septic state. *Diagn Microb Infect Dis.* 2015;83:312–318.
23. De Backer D, Ricottilli F, Ospina-Tascón GA. Septic shock: A microcirculation disease. *Curr Opin Anaesthesiol.* 2021;34:85–91. 10.1097/aco.0000000000000957.
24. Fourrier F. Severe sepsis, coagulation, and fibrinolysis: Dead end or one way? *Crit Care Med.* 2012;40:2704–2708.
25. Hatfield K, Dantes R, Baggs J, et al. Assessing variability in hospital-level mortality among U.S. Medicare beneficiaries with hospitalizations for severe sepsis and septic shock. *Crit Care Med.* 2018;46:1753–1760.
26. Kudo D, Kushimoto S, Miyagawa N, et al. The impact of organ dysfunctions on mortality in patients with severe sepsis: A multicenter prospective observational study. *J Crit Care.* 2018;45:178–183. 10.1016/j.jcrc.2018.03.011.
27. Capp R, Horton CL, Takhar SS, et al. Predictors of patients who present to the emergency department with sepsis and progress to septic shock

between 4 and 48 hours of emergency department arrival. *Crit Care Med.* 2015;43:983–988.
28. Simmons J, Pittet J. The coagulopathy of acute sepsis. *Curr Opin Anaesthesiol.* 2015;28:227–236.
29. Bellomo R, Kellum JA, Ronco C, et al. Acute kidney injury in sepsis. *Intensive Care Med.* 2017;43:816–828. 10.1007/s00134-017-4755-7.
30. Kim W, Hong S. Sepsis and acute respiratory distress syndrome: Recent update. *Tuberc Respir Dis.* 2016;79:53–57.
31. Pulido JN, Afessa B, Masaki M, et al. Clinical spectrum, frequency, and significance of myocardial dysfunction in severe sepsis and septic shock. *Mayo Clin Proc.* 2012;87:620–628.
32. Lv X, Wang H. Pathophysiology of sepsis-induced myocardial dysfunction. *Mil Med Res.* 2016;3:30–38.
33. Peters E, Antonelli M, Wittebole X, et al. A worldwide multicenter evaluation of the influence of deterioration or improvement of acute kidney injury on clinical outcome in critically ill patients with and without sepsis at ICU admission: Results from the Intensive Care Over Nations audit. *Crit Care.* 2018;22:188–198.
34. Londoño J, Nino C, Arichila A, et al. Antibiotic has more impact on mortality than other early goal-directed therapy components in patients with sepsis: An instrumental variable analysis. *J Crit Care.* 2018;48:191–197.
35. Thomas-Rueddel D, Poidinger B, Weiss M, et al. Hyperlactatemia is an independent predictor of mortality and denotes distinct subtypes of severe sepsis and septic shock. *J Crit Care.* 2015;30:439.e1–439.e6.
36. Davies J, Gordon CL, Tong SY, et al. Impact of results of a rapid Staphylococcus aureus diagnostic test on prescribing of antibiotics for patients with clustered gram-positive cocci in blood cultures. *J Clin Microbiol.* 2012;50:2056–2058.
37. Aittakorpi A, Kuusela P, Koukila-Kahkola P, et al. Accurate and rapid identification of Candida spp. frequently associated with fungemia by using PCR and the microarray-based prove-it sepsis assay. *J Clin Microbiol.* 2012;50:3635–3640.
38. Seymour CW, Liu VX, Iwashyna TJ, et al. Assessment of clinical criteria for sepsis for the third international consensus definitions for sepsis and septic shock (Sepsis-3). *JAMA.* 2016;315:762–774.
39. Evans Laura, Rhodes Andrew, Alhazzani Waleed, et al. Surviving sepsis campaign: international guidelines for management of sepsis and septic shock 2021. *Intensive Care Med.* 2021;47:1181–1247. 10.1007/s00134-021-06506-y.
40. Dellinger R, Carlet J, Masur H, et al. Surviving sepsis campaign guidelines for management of severe sepsis and septic shock. *Crit Care Med.* 2004;32:858–873.
41. Rivers E, Nguyen B, Havastad S, et al. Early goal-directed therapy in the treatment of severe sepsis and septic shock. *N Engl J Med.* 2001;345:1368–1377.
42. The ProCESS Investigators. A randomized trial of protocol-based care for early septic shock. *N Engl J Med.* 2014;370:1683–1693.
43. The ARISE Investigators and the ANZICS Clinical Trials Group. Goal-directed resuscitation for patients with early septic shock. *N Engl J Med.* 2014;371:1496–1506.
44. Mouncey PR, Osborn TM, Power GS, et al. Trial of early, goal-directed resuscitation for septic shock. *N Engl J Med.* 2015;372:1301–1311.
45. Nguyen HB, Jaehne AK, Jayaprakash N, et al. Early goal-directed therapy in severe sepsis and septic shock: Insights and comparison to ProCESS, ProMISe, and ARISE. *Crit Care.* 2016;20:160. doi:10.1186/s13054-016-1288-3.
46. Rhodes A, Evans LE, Alhazzani W, et al. Surviving sepsis campaign: International guidelines for management of sepsis and septic shock: 2016. *Crit Care Med.* 2017;45:486–552.
47. Levy MM, Evans LE, Rhodes A. The surviving sepsis campaign bundle: 2018 update. *Crit Care Med.* 2018;46:997–1000.
48. Malbrain MLNG, van Regenmortel N, Saugel B, et al. Principles of fluid management and stewardship in septic shock: It is time to consider the four D's and the four phases of fluid therapy. *Ann Intensive Care.* 2018;8:66. doi:10.1186/s13613-018-0402-x.
49. Bednarczyk JM, Fridfinnson JA, Kumar A, et al. Incorporating dynamic assessment of fluid responsiveness into Goal-Directed Therapy: A systematic review and meta-analysis. *Crit Care Med.* 2017;45:1538–1545.
50. Douglas IS, Alapat PM, Corl KA, et al. Fluid response evaluation in sepsis hypotension and shock. *Chest* 2020;158:1431–1445. 10.1016/j.chest.2020.04.025.
51. Taylor SP, Karvetski CH, Templin MA, et al. Initial fluid resuscitation following adjusted body weight dosing is associated with improved mortality in obese patients with suspected septic shock. *J Crit Care* 2018;43:7–12. 10.1016/j.jcrc.2017.08.025.
52. Brown RM, Semler MW. Fluid management in sepsis. *J Intensive Care Med.* 2018. doi:10.1177/0885066618784861.
53. Finfer S, Belloma R, Boyce N, et al. A comparison of albumin and saline for fluid resuscitation in the intensive care unit. *N Engl J Med.* 2004;350:2247–2256.
54. Semler MW, Self WH, Wanderer JP, et al. Balanced crystalloids versus saline in critically ill adults. *N Engl J Med.* 2018;378:829–839.
55. Filis C, Vasileiadis I, Koutsoukou A. Hyperchloraemia in sepsis. *Ann Intensive Care.* 2018;8:43. doi:10.1186/s13613-018-0388-4.
56. Brown Ryan M., Wang Li, Coston Taylor D., et al. Balanced Crystalloids versus Saline in Sepsis. A secondary analysis of the SMART Clinical Trial. *Am J Resp Crit Care Med.* 2019;200:1487–1495. 10.1164/rccm.201903-0557oc.
57. Self WH, Semler MW, Wanderer JP, et al. Balanced crystalloids versus saline in noncritically ill adults. *N Engl J Med.* 2018;378:819–828.
58. Mazuski JE, Tessier JM, May AK, et al. The surgical infection society revised guidelines on the management of intra-abdominal infection. *Surg Infect.* 2017;18:1–76.
59. Rothrock SG, Cassidy DD, Barneck M, et al. Outcome of immediate versus early antibiotics in severe sepsis and septic shock: A systematic review and meta-analysis. *Ann Emerg Med.* 2020;76:427–441. 10.1016/j.annemergmed.2020.04.042.
60. Liu VX, Fielding-Singh V, Greene JD, et al. The timing of early antibiotics and hospital mortality in sepsis. *Am J Respir Crit Care Med.* 2017;196:856–863.
61. Kumar A, Ellis P, Arabi Y, et al. Initiation of inappropriate antimicrobial therapy results in a fivefold reduction of survival in human septic shock. *Chest.* 2009;136:1237–1248.
62. Sherwin R, Winters M, Vike G, et al. Does early and appropriate antibiotic administration improve mortality in emergency department patients with severe sepsis or septic shock? *J Emerg Med.* 2017;53:588–595.
63. Grim SA, Berger K, Teng C, et al. Timing of susceptibility-based antifungal drug administration in patients with Candida bloodstream infection: Correlation with outcomes. *J Antimicrob Chemother.* 2012;67:707–714.
64. Kollef M, Micek S, Hampton N, et al. Septic shock attributes to Candida infection: Importance of empiric therapy and source control. *Clin Infect Dis.* 2012;54:1739–1746.
65. Kalil AC, Metersky ML, Klompas M, et al. Management of adults with hospital-acquired and ventilator-associated pneumonia: 2016 clinical practice guidelines by the Infectious Diseases Society of America and the American Thoracic Society. *Clin Infect Dis.* 2016;63:e61–e111.
66. Stevens DL, Bisno AL, Chambers HF, et al. Practice guidelines for the diagnosis and management of skin and soft tissue infections: 2014 update by the Infectious Disease Society of America. *Clin Infect Dis.* 2014;59:147–159.
67. Wagenlehner FME, Tandogdu Z, Bjerklund Johansen TE. An update on classification and management of urosepsis. *Curr Opin Urol.* 2017;27:133–137.
68. Metlay JP, Waterer GW, Long AC, et al. Diagnosis and treatment of adults with community-acquired pneumonia. An Official Clinical Practice Guideline of the American Thoracic Society and Infectious Diseases Society of America. *Am J Resp Crit Care Med.* 2019;200:e45–e67. 10.1164/rccm.201908-1581st.
69. Liu C, Bayer A, Cosgrove SE, et al. Clinical practice guidelines by the Infectious Disease Society of America for the treatment of methicillin-resistant *Staphylococcus aureus* infections in adults and children. *Clin Infect Dis.* 2011;52:1–38.
70. Rybak Michael J, Le Jennifer, Lodise Thomas P, et al. Therapeutic monitoring of vancomycin for serious methicillin-resistant Staphylococcus aureus infections: A revised consensus guideline and review by the American Society of Health-System Pharmacists, the Infectious Diseases Society of America, the Pediatric Infectious Diseases Society, and the Society of Infectious Diseases Pharmacists. *Am J Health Syst Pharm.* 2020;77:835–864. 10.1093/ajhp/zxaa036.
71. Brown JE, Fominaya C, Christensen KJ, et al. Daptomycin experience in critical care patients: Results from a registry. *Ann Pharmacother.* 2012;46:495–502.
72. Claeys KC, Zasowski EJ, Casapao AM, et al. Daptomycin improves outcomes regardless of vancomycin MIC in a propensity-matched analysis of methicillin-resistant *Staphylococcus aureus* bloodstream infections. *Antimicro Agents Chemother.* 2016;60:5841–5848.
73. Russo A, Falcone M, Gutierrez-Gutierrez B, et al. Predictors of outcome in patients with severe sepsis or septic shock due to extended-spectrum beta-lactamase-producing Enterobacteriaceae. *Int J Antimicrob Agents.* 2018;52:577–585.

74. Sfeir MM, Askin G, Christos P. Beta-lactam/beta-lactamase inhibitors versus carbapenem for bloodstream infections due to extended-spectrum beta-lactamase-producing Enterobacteriaceae: Systematic review and meta-analysis. *Int J Antimicrob Agents.* 2018;52:554–570.
75. Son S, Lee N, Ko J, et al. Clinical effectiveness of carbapenems versus alternative antibiotics for treating ESBL-producing Enterobacteriaceae bacteraemia: A systematic review and meta-analysis. *J Antimicrob Chemother.* 2018;73:2631–2642.
76. Harris P, Tambyah P, Lye D, et al. Effect of piperacillin-tazobactam vs meropenem on 30-day mortality for patients with *E. coli* or *Klebsiella pneumoniae* bloodstream infection and ceftriaxone resistance. *JAMA.* 2018;320:984–994.
77. Vasquez-Grande G, Kumar A. Optimizing antimicrobial therapy of sepsis and septic shock: Focus on antibiotic combination therapy. *Semin Respir Crit Care Med.* 2015;36:154–166.
78. Bass SN, Bauer SR, Neuner EA, et al. Impact of combination antimicrobial therapy on mortality risk for critically ill patients with carbapenem-resistant bacteremia. *Antimicrob Agents Chemother.* 2015;59:3748–3753.
79. Poulikakos P, Tansarli GS, Falgas ME. Combination antibiotic treatment versus monotherapy for multidrug-resistant, extensively drug-resistant, and pandrug-resistant Acinetobacter infections: A systematic review. *Eur J Clin Microbiol Infect Dis.* 2014;33:1675–1685.
80. Timsit Jean-Francois, Azoulay Elie, Schwebel Carole, et al. Empirical micafungin treatment and survival without invasive fungal infection in adults with ICU-acquired sepsis, Candida colonization, and multiple organ failure. *JAMA* 2016;316:1555. 10.1001/jama.2016.14655.
81. Pappas PG, Kauffman CA, Andes DR, et al. Clinical practice guideline for the management of Candidiasis: 2016 update by the Infectious Diseases Society of America. *Clin Infect Dis.* 2016;62:e1–e50.
82. Keane S, Geoghegan P, Povoa P, et al. Systematic review on the first line treatment of amphotericin B in critically ill adults with candidemia or invasive candidiasis. *Expert Rev Anti Infect Ther.* 2018;16:839–847.
83. Ben-Ami R, Olshtain-Pops K, Krieger M, et al. Antibiotic exposure as a risk factor for fluconazole-resistant Candida bloodstream infection. *Antimicrob Agents Chemother.* 2012;56:2518–2523.
84. Chandrasekar P, Sirohi B, Seibel N, et al. Efficacy of micafungin for the treatment of invasive candidiasis and candidaemia in patients with neutropenia. *Mycoses.* 2018;61:331–336.
85. Fujii Motoki, Karumai Toshiyuki, Yamamoto Ryohei, et al. Pharmacokinetic and pharmacodynamic considerations in antimicrobial therapy for sepsis. *Expert Opin Drug Metab Toxicol.* 2020;16:415–430. 10.1080/17425255.2020.1750597.
86. Zelenitsky S, Rubinstein E, Ariano R, et al. Vancomycin pharmacodynamics and survival in patients with methicillin-resistant *Staphylococcus aureus*-associated septic shock. *Int J Antimicrob Agents.* 2013;41:255–260.
87. D'Avolio A, Pensi D, Baietto L, et al. Daptomycin pharmacokinetics and pharmacodynamics in septic and critically ill patients. *Drugs.* 2016;76:1161–1174.
88. Masich A, Heavner M, Gonzales J, et al. Pharmacokinetic/pharmacodynamic considerations of beta-lactam antibiotics in adult critically ill patients. *Curr Infect Dis Rep.* 2018;20:9. doi:10.1007/s11908-018-0613-1.
89. Roberts J, Abdul-Aziz M, Lipman J, et al. Individualised antibiotic dosing for patients who are critically ill: Challenges and potential solutions. *Lancet Infect Dis.* 2014;14:498–509.
90. Vardakas Konstantinos Z, Voulgaris Georgios L, Maliaros Athanasios, et al. Prolonged versus short-term intravenous infusion of antipseudomonal β-lactams for patients with sepsis: A systematic review and meta-analysis of randomised trials. *Lancet Infect Dis.* 2018;18:108–120. 10.1016/s1473-3099(17)30615-1.
91. Chen P, Chen F, Lei jiexin, et al. Clinical outcomes of continuous vs intermittent meropenem infusion for the treatment of sepsis: A systematic review and meta-analysis. *Adv Clin Exp Med.* 2020;29:993–1000. 10.17219/acem/121934.
92. Heavner M, Claeys K, Masich A, et al. Pharmacokinetic and pharmacodynamic considerations of antibiotics of last resort in treating gram-negative infections in adult critically ill patients. *Curr Infect Dis Rep.* 2018;20:10. doi:10.1007/s11908-018-0614-0.
93. Barlam TF, Cosgrove SE, Abbo LM, et al. Implementing an antibiotic stewardship program: Guidelines by the Infectious Disease Society of America and the Society for Healthcare Epidemiology of America. *Clin Infect Dis.* 2016;62:e51–e77.
94. Garnacho-Montero J, Gutierrez-Pizarraya A, Escoresc-Ortega A, et al. De-escalation of empirical therapy is associated with lower mortality in patients with severe sepsis and septic shock. *Intensive Care Med.* 2014;40:32–40.
95. Huang HB, Peng JM, Weng L, et al. Procalcitonin-guided antibiotic therapy in intensive care unit patients: A systematic review and meta-analysis. *Ann Intensive Care.* 2017;7:114.
96. Chotiprasitsakul D, Han JH, Cosgrove SE, et al. Comparing the outcomes of adults with Enterobacteriaceae bacteremia receiving short-course versus prolonged-course antibiotic therapy in a multicenter, propensity score-matched cohort. *Clin Infect Dis.* 2018;66:172–177.
97. Sawyer RG, Claridge JA, Nathens AB, et al. Trial of short-course antimicrobial therapy for intra-abdominal infection. *N Engl J Med.* 2015;372:1996–2005.
98. Asfar P, Meziani F, Hamel JF, et al. High versus low blood-pressure target in patients with septic shock. *N Engl J Med.* 2014;370:1583–1593.
99. Gelinas JP, Russell JA. Vasopressors during sepsis: Selection and targets. *Clin Chest Med.* 2016;37:251–262.
100. Van Diepen S, Katz JN, Albert JM, et al. Contemporary management of cardiogenic shock. *Circulation.* 2017;136:e232–e268.
101. Avni T, Lador A, Lev S, et al. Vasopressors for the treatment of septic shock: Systematic review and meta-analysis. *PLoS One.* 2015;10:e0129305.
102. Vadiei N, Daley MJ, Murthy MS, et al. Impact of norepinephrine weight-based dosing compared with non-weight based dosing in achieving time to goal mean arterial pressure in obese patients with septic shock. *Ann Pharmacother.* 2017;51:194–202.
103. Kotecha AA, Vallabhajosyula S, Apala DR, et al. Clinical outcomes of weight-based norepinephrine dosing in underweight and morbidly obese patients: A propensity-matched analysis. *J Intensive Care Med.* 2018. doi:10.1177/0885066618768180.
104. Gordon AC, Mason AJ, Thirunavukkarasu N, et al. Effect of early vasopressin vs norepinephrine on kidney failure in patients with septic shock. *JAMA.* 2016;316:509. 10.1001/jama.2016.10485.
105. Russell JA, Lee T, Singer J, et al. The septic shock 3.0 definition and trials: A vasopressin and septic shock trial experience. *Crit Care Med.* 2017;45:940–948.
106. Khanna A, English SW, Wang XS, et al. Angiotensin II for the treatment of vasodilatory shock. *N Engl J Med.* 2017;377:419–430.
107. Tumlin JA, Murugan R, Deane AM, et al. Outcomes in patients with vasodilatory shock and renal replacement therapy treated with intravenous angiotensin II. *Crit Care Med.* 2018;46:949.
108. Belletti Alessandro, Benedetto Umberto, Biondi-Zoccai Giuseppe, et al. The effect of vasoactive drugs on mortality in patients with severe sepsis and septic shock. A network meta-analysis of randomized trials. *J Crit Care.* 2017;37:91–98. 10.1016/j.jcrc.2016.08.010.
109. Damiani E, Donati A, Serafini G, et al. Effect of performance improvement programs on compliance with sepsis bundles and mortality: A systematic review and meta-analysis of observational studies. *PLoS One.* 2015;10:e0125827.
110. Levy M, Thodes A, Phillips GS, et al. Surviving sepsis campaign: Association between performance metrics and outcomes in a 7.5-year study. *Crit Care Med.* 2015;43:3–12.
111. Annane D, Bellissant E, Bollaert PE, et al. Corticosteroids in the treatment of severe sepsis and septic shock in adults: A systematic review. *JAMA.* 2009;301:2362–2375.
112. Sprung CL, Annane D, Keh D, et al. Hydrocortisone therapy for patients with septic shock. *N Engl J Med.* 2008;358:111–124.
113. Annane D, Ellissant E, Bollaert PE, et al. Corticosteroids for treating sepsis. *Cochrane Database Syst Rev.* 2015:CD002243. doi:10.1002/14651858.CD002243.
114. Volbeda M, Wetterslev J, Gluud C, et al. Glucocorticosteroids for sepsis: Systematic review with meta-analysis and trial sequential analysis. *Intensive Care Med.* 2015;41:1220–1234.
115. Venkatesh B, Finfer S, Cohen J, et al. Adjunctive glucocorticoid therapy in patients with septic shock. *N Engl J Med.* 2018;378:797–808.
116. Annane D, Renault A, Brun-Buisson C, et al. Hydrocortisone plus fludrocortisone for adults with septic shock. *N Engl J Med.* 2018;378:809–818.
117. Venkatesh B, Finfer S, Myburgh J. Long term outcomes of the ADRENAL trial. *N Engl J Med.* 2018;378:1744–1745.
118. Rygård SL, Butler E, Granholm A, et al. Low-dose corticosteroids for adult patients with septic shock: A systematic review with meta-analysis and trial sequential analysis. *Intensive Care Med.* 2018;44:1003–1016. 10.1007/s00134-018-5197-6.
119. Finfer S, Liu B, Chittock DR, et al. Hypoglycemia and risk of death in critically ill patients. *N Engl J Med.* 2012;367:1108–1118.

120. Song F, Zhong LJ, Han L, et al. Intensive insulin therapy for septic patients: A meta-analysis of randomized controlled trials. *Biomed Res Int.* 2014. doi:10.1155/2014/698265.
121. Yatabe T, Inoue S, Sakaguchi M, et al. The optimal target for acute glycemic control in critically ill patients: A network meta-analysis. *Intensive Care Med.* 2016;43:16–28. 10.1007/s00134-016-4558-2.
122. Kaplan D, Casper C, Elliott G, et al. VTE incidence and risk factors in patients with severe sepsis and septic shock. *Chest.* 2015;148:1224–1230.
123. Beitland S, Sandven I, Kjaervik LK, et al. Thromboprophylaxis with low molecular weight heparin versus unfractionated heparin in intensive care patients: A systematic review with meta-analysis and trial sequential analysis. *Intensive Care Med.* 2015;41:1209–1219.
124. Krag M, Perner A, Wetterslev J, et al. Prevalence and outcome of gastrointestinal bleeding and use of acid suppressants in acutely ill adult intensive care patients. *Intensive Care Med.* 2015;41:833–845.
125. Krag Mette, Marker Søren, Perner Anders, et al. Pantoprazole in Patients at Risk for Gastrointestinal Bleeding in the ICU. *New Engl J Med.* 2018;379:2199–2208. 10.1056/nejmoa1714919.
126. Granholm Anders, Zeng Linan, Dionne J, et al. Predictors of gastrointestinal bleeding in adult ICU patients: A systematic review and meta-analysis. *Intensive Care Med.* 2019;45:1347–1359. 10.1007/s00134-019-05751-6.

Superficial Fungal Infections

143

Thomas E. R. Brown and Linda D. Dresser

KEY CONCEPTS

1. Vulvovaginal candidiasis (VVC) is a fungal infection of the vagina that can be classified as uncomplicated or complicated. This classification is useful in determining appropriate pharmacotherapy.
2. *Candida albicans* is the major pathogen responsible for VVC. The number of cases of non–*C. albicans* species appears to be increasing.
3. Signs and symptoms of VVC are not pathognomonic, and reliable diagnosis must be made with laboratory tests including vaginal pH, saline microscopy, and 10% potassium hydroxide (KOH) microscopy.
4. *C. albicans* is the predominant species causing all forms of mucosal candidiasis. Important host and exogenous risk factors have been identified that predispose an individual to the development of mucosal candidiasis. In oropharyngeal and esophageal candidiasis, the key risk factor is impaired host immune system.
5. A topical antimycotic agent is the first choice for treating oropharyngeal candidiasis. Systemic therapy can be used in patients who are not responding to an adequate trial of topical treatment or are unable to tolerate topical agents and in those at high risk for systemic candidiasis. Fluconazole and itraconazole are the most effective azole antimycotic agents.
6. For esophageal candidiasis, topical agents are not of proven benefit; oral fluconazole or itraconazole solution is the first choice.
7. Optimal antiretroviral therapy is important for the prevention of recurrent and refractory candidiasis in patients with human immunodeficiency virus (HIV) infection.
8. Primary or secondary prophylaxis of fungal infection is not recommended routinely for HIV-infected patients; use of secondary prophylaxis should be individualized for each patient.
9. Topical antimycotic agents are first-line treatment for fungal skin infections. Oral therapy is preferred for the treatment of extensive or severe infection and those with tinea capitis or onychomycosis.
10. Oral antimycotic agents such as terbinafine and itraconazole are first-line treatment for toenail and fingernail onychomycosis.

BEYOND THE BOOK

Watch the YouTube video entitled "Watch and Learn KOH preparation" by Richard Usatine, MD. This 4-minute video demonstrates the quickest and most accurate way to diagnose fungal skin infections. The video is useful in visualizing fungal elements such as hyphae and pseudohyphae.

INTRODUCTION

Superficial mycoses are among the most common infections in the world and the second most common vaginal infections in North America. Mucocutaneous candidiasis can occur in three forms—oropharyngeal, esophageal, and vulvovaginal disease—with oropharyngeal and vulvovaginal disease being the most common. Over the past 15 to 20 years, the occurrence rates of some fungal infections have increased dramatically. The prevalence of fungal skin infections varies throughout different parts of the world, from the most common causes of skin infections in the tropics to relatively rare disorders in the United States.

VULVOVAGINAL CANDIDIASIS

1 *Vulvovaginal candidiasis* (VVC) refers to infections in individuals with or without symptoms who have positive vaginal cultures for *Candida* species. Depending on episodic frequency, VVC can be classified as either sporadic or recurrent.[1] This classification is essential to understanding the pathophysiology, as well as the pharmacotherapy, of VVC. Furthermore, VVC may be defined as uncomplicated, which refers to sporadic infections that are susceptible to all forms of antifungal therapy regardless of the duration of treatment, or complicated, in which consideration of factors affecting the host, microorganism, and pharmacotherapy all have an essential role in successful treatment.[1] Complicated VVC includes recurrent VVC, severe disease, non–*C. albicans* candidiasis, and host factors, including diabetes mellitus, immunosuppression, and pregnancy.[1]

Epidemiology

There is minimal information on the incidence and prevalence of VVC. Healthcare workers are not required to report cases of VVC; therefore, estimates are derived from self-reported histories. Epidemiologic data are limited because VVC usually is diagnosed without microscopy and/or cultures, and antifungal nonprescription preparations are available for self-treatment.[1] Fifty to 72% of females will have had at least one episode of VVC.[1] It is rare before menarche and increases dramatically at about 20 years of age, with the peak incidence between age 30 and 40 years. It is associated with the initial act of sexual intercourse. Between 40% and 50% of females who experience one episode of VVC experience a second episode, and 5% experience recurrent VVC.[2] The incidence after menopause remains unknown. However, healthy postmenopausal females with vulvar conditions taking hormone replacement therapy (HRT) were more prone to developing VVC than those who were not taking HRT (culture-positive, clinical VVC in 49% on HRT vs 1% on those not on HRT).[3]

Costs from VVC can be direct (medical visits and self-treatment) and indirect (nonmedical expenses, eg, time losses from work, costs of travel, and time required in obtaining treatment). There are 6 million visits to healthcare providers each year, resulting in more than $1 billion spent annually on these medical visits and self-treatment.[4] Nonprescription sales for feminine itch and yeast treatments were $302 million in the United States in 2017.[5]

Pathophysiology

2 *C. albicans* is the major pathogen responsible for VVC, accounting for 80% to 92% of symptomatic episodes. The remainder are caused by non–*C. albicans* species, with *Candida glabrata* dominating.[6] The number of cases of non–*C. albicans* candidiasis appears to be increasing, possibly related to the use of nonprescription vaginal antifungal preparations and short-course therapy and/or the increased use of long-term maintenance therapy in preventing recurrent infections.[1]

Candida species can act as commensal members of the vaginal flora. Asymptomatic colonization with *Candida* species occurs in 10% to 20% of females of reproductive age.[6,7] *Candida* organisms are dimorphic; blastospores are responsible for colonization (transmission and spread), whereas germinated *Candida* forms are associated with tissue invasion and symptomatic infections.[8] To colonize the vagina, *Candida* species must be able to attach to the mucosa. The attachment process is complex. Not only are candidal surface structures important for attachment, but appropriate receptors for attachment must be present in the epithelial tissue. Not all females have the same range of receptors, which may explain variation in colonization.[7] Changes in the host's vaginal environment or response are necessary to induce a symptomatic infection. Unfortunately, in most cases of symptomatic VVC, no precipitating factor can be identified.[8]

Risk Factors

Several factors predispose a woman to VVC. VVC is not considered to be a sexually transmitted disease, although sexual factors can be important. There is a dramatic increase in the frequency of VVC when females become sexually active. In addition, oral-genital contact can increase the risk.[1] However, the treatment of asymptomatic partners is not recommended.[6] Contraceptive agents, including the diaphragm with spermicide, the contraceptive sponge, and the intrauterine device, increase the risk of VVC.[9] *Candida* species are capable of adhering to the contraceptive vaginal ring.[9] Oral contraceptive users demonstrated increased risk of candidiasis; however, these reports were with the higher-dose oral contraceptive pills, and the risk may not be as great with the lower-estrogen-dose oral contraceptives.[8]

Antibiotic use can increase the risk of VVC, but it is significant in only a small number of females. The mechanism by which antibiotics can increase the risk of VVC is unknown; colonization, however, is a prerequisite.[1] Three days of antibiotics increased the prevalence of asymptomatic vaginal colonization of *Candida* and the incidence of symptomatic VVC.[10] Diet (excess refined carbohydrates), douching, and tight-fitting clothing often are listed as important risk factors; however, no association has been established between these factors and increased risk of VVC.[1]

CLINICAL PRESENTATION

3 The clinical presentation of VVC is given in Table 143-1.[1,6] These signs and symptoms are not pathognomonic, and a reliable diagnosis cannot be made without laboratory tests. The value of self-diagnosis and the success of self-treatment is limited. Self-diagnosis has a sensitivity of 35%, a specificity of 89%, and a positive predictive value of 62%. Only 30% to 40% of females that complained of vaginal itching had VVC.[8] The American College of Obstetricians and Gynecologists (ACOG) recommends that whenever possible females requesting treatment for VVC should be examined and evaluated. They only recommend self-diagnosis in compliant females with multiple confirmed prior cases of VVC who report the same symptoms. They further recommend that if these individuals fail to improve on a short course of therapy, they be evaluated for a further diagnosis.[11] Therefore, in most instances the diagnosis should be based on both clinical presentation and investigations, including vaginal pH, saline microscopy, and 10% potassium hydroxide (KOH) microscopy of vaginal discharge. The vaginal pH remains normal in VVC, and microscopic investigations should detect blastospores or pseudohyphae. *Candida* cultures usually are not required in the diagnosis of uncomplicated VVC. However, they are recommended when an individual presents with classic signs and symptoms of VVC, has a normal vaginal pH, but microscopy is inconclusive or recurrence is suspected.[6]

TABLE 143-1 Clinical Presentation of Vulvovaginal Candidiasis

General	Often involves both the vulva and the vagina
Symptoms	Intense vulvar itching, soreness, irritation, burning on urination, and dyspareunia
Signs	Erythema, fissuring, curdy "cheese"-like discharge, satellite lesions, edema
Laboratory tests	Vaginal pH—normal, saline, and 10% KOH microscopy—blastospores or pseudohyphae
Other diagnostic tests	*Candida* cultures not recommended unless classic signs and symptoms with normal vaginal pH and microscopy are inconclusive or recurrence is suspected

KOH, potassium hydroxide.

TREATMENT

Goals of Therapy

The goal of therapy is complete resolution of symptoms in patients who have symptomatic VVC. A test of the cure is not necessary if symptoms resolve.[6] Antimycotic agents used in the treatment of VVC do not meet the definition of being fungicidal agents because of their slower killing rate. At the end of therapy, the number of viable organisms drops below the detectable range. However, by 6 weeks after a course of therapy, 25% to 40% of females will have positive yeast cultures and remain asymptomatic.[1] Asymptomatic colonization with *Candida* species does not require therapy.

General Approaches to Treatment

The approach to therapy is to remove or improve any predisposing factors if they can be identified. An effective antimycotic agent should have limited local and systemic side effects, a high cure rate, and easy administration. Additionally, it would be advantageous to use a treatment that resolves symptoms within 24 hours, has broad antimycotic activity (to cover increasing rates on non–*C. albicans* species), prevents recurrence, and can be used over a shortened period of time, such as 1 to 3 days. Many topical azoles antifungals (such as clotrimazole and miconazole) are available without a prescription, and although this may increase public access to these medications, there is concern that having them available without a prescription may lead to inappropriate use. A study conducted using 10 actors as simulated patients who visited 60 pharmacies found that vaginal antimycotics were more likely to be appropriately provided to individuals as more information was exchanged, if interactions involved a pharmacist, and if questions regarding specific symptoms were used.[12]

Patients should be advised to avoid harsh soaps and perfumes that can cause or worsen vulvar irritation. The genital area must be kept clean and dry by avoiding constrictive clothing and frequent or prolonged exposure to hot tub use.[13] Douching is not recommended for either prevention or treatment.[8] Cool baths can soothe the skin.[13] The value of oral use of lactobacillus remains unclear, and according to a systematic review the use of lactobacilli containing vaginal products does not hold much promise. There was no evidence of vaginal colonization after probiotic use.[14]

Treatment of VVC will be considered to have positive outcomes if the symptoms of VVC are resolved within 24 to 48 hours and no adverse medication events are experienced. Self-assessment of symptom relief is appropriate for most cases of VVC. If symptoms remain unresolved or recur, then further testing and treatment can be required.

Pharmacologic Treatments

Uncomplicated Vulvovaginal Candidiasis

Uncomplicated VVC is an infection in females who are not immunocompromised, do not have diabetes, and are not pregnant. There are many different products, routes, and durations of treatment. No product route or duration of treatment is superior to any other. Cure rates for uncomplicated VVC are between 80% and 95% with topical or oral azoles and between 70% and 90% with nystatin preparations. Table 143-2 lists many available topical and oral preparations for the treatment of uncomplicated VVC. There are no significant differences in in vitro activity or clinical efficacy among the topical azole agents.[1,6,11,13] Some topical products can cause vaginal burning, stinging, or irritation; conversely, the vehicle used in topical creams or gels can provide initial symptomatic relief.[1] Of note, most topical preparations can decrease the efficacy of latex condoms and diaphragms.

TABLE 143-2 Treatment for Uncomplicated Vulvovaginal Candidiasis

Active Ingredient	Preparation	Regimen
Nonprescription/Topical Vaginal Products		
Butoconazole	2% cream	One applicator × 3 days
Clotrimazole	1% cream	One applicator × 1 day
	100 mg tablet	One 100 mg tablet × 7 days
	2% cream	One applicator × 1 day
	200 mg tablet	One 200 mg tablet × 3 days
	10% cream	One applicator × 1 day
	500 mg tablet	One 500 mg tablet × 1 day
Miconazole[a]	2% cream	One applicator × 1 day
	100 mg suppository	One 100 mg suppository × 7 days
	200 mg suppository	One 200 mg suppository × 3 days
	1,200 mg ovule	One ovule × 1 day
Ticonazole	2% cream	One applicator × 3 days
	6.5% cream	One applicator × 1 day
Prescription/Topical		
Nystatin	100,000 unit tablet	One tablet × 14 days
Terconazole	0.4% cream	One applicator × 7 days
	0.8% cream	One applicator × 3 days
Oral Products		
Fluconazole	150 mg	One tablet × 1 day

[a]The FDA warns of the possible increase in the anticoagulant effects of warfarin with concomitant use.

Oral azoles (such as fluconazole or itraconazole) have been used in the treatment of VVC and are therapeutically equivalent to topical therapies.[1] Patients may prefer oral therapy because of its convenience.[15] There were no differences between the routes in short-term mycologic cure rates. There was a significant difference between long-term cure rates in favor of long-term follow-up; however, the clinical significance of this finding is uncertain.[16]

In the treatment of uncomplicated VVC, the duration of therapy is not critical. Cure rates with different lengths of treatment have not demonstrated that one duration of therapy is significantly better.[15-17] Shorter-duration therapies (eg, clotrimazole 1-day therapy) consist of higher concentrations of azoles that maintain the local therapeutic effect for up to 72 hours and allow for resolution of signs and symptoms.[18] There was less than 7% difference in short-term cure rates or improvement between any two treatments in any two studies and no significant differences in short- or long-term clinical cure rates among 1-day regimens.[17] There are many options for the treatment of uncomplicated VVC, and selection of an azole antimycotic agent should be based primarily on an individual patient's preference and past experience.[17]

Complicated Vulvovaginal Candidiasis

Complicated VVC occurs in patients who are immunocompromised or have uncontrolled diabetes mellitus or are pregnant.[1] Unlike with uncomplicated VVC, product selection is important in these individuals. The duration of therapy and/or route of administration is important. Immunocompromised females or those with uncontrolled diabetes mellitus need a more aggressive treatment plan and treatment should be lengthened to 10 to 14 days regardless of the route of administration.[11] Therapeutic options include those listed in Table 143-2; however, regimens should be continued for 10 to 14 days. Cure rates increased from 67% with single-dose oral fluconazole therapy in females with complicated VVC therapy to 80% when the 150 mg dose of fluconazole was repeated 72 hours after the initial dose.[19]

VVC during pregnancy can be considered complicated because consideration of host factors such as hormonal changes that can affect normal flora are essential in selecting therapeutic regimens. Topical agents are considered to be safe throughout pregnancy. Imidazole topical agents (such as fluconazole) were more effective than nystatin for VVC during pregnancy and treatment for 7 days was more effective than treatments of 4 days or less.[20] Oral therapy is not recommended as larger doses of fluconazole have been linked to birth defects.[8] Instead, the ACOG recommends a topical imidazole therapy for 7 days.[11]

Recurrent Vulvovaginal Candidiasis

Recurrent vulvovaginal candidiasis (RVVC) is defined as having more than four episodes of VVC within a 12-month period. Fewer than 5% of females develop RVVC, and its pathogenesis is poorly understood. A proper diagnosis should be obtained to rule out other infections or nonmycotic contact dermatitis. RVVC is best treated in two stages: an initial intensive stage followed by prolonged antifungal therapy to achieve mycologic remission (with 150 mg oral fluconazole daily for 10 days followed by 6 months of fluconazole 150 mg weekly). Ninety percent of females receiving 10-day initial and 6-month prolonged treatments were symptom free for the 6 months following initial treatment, and there were 50% fewer symptomatic episodes in the 6 months (compared with placebo treatment after the initial 10 days).[21] The Infectious Diseases Society of America recommends 10 to 14 days of induction therapy with a topical or oral azole, followed by 150 mg of fluconazole once weekly for 6 months for recurring *Candida* VVC.[22,23]

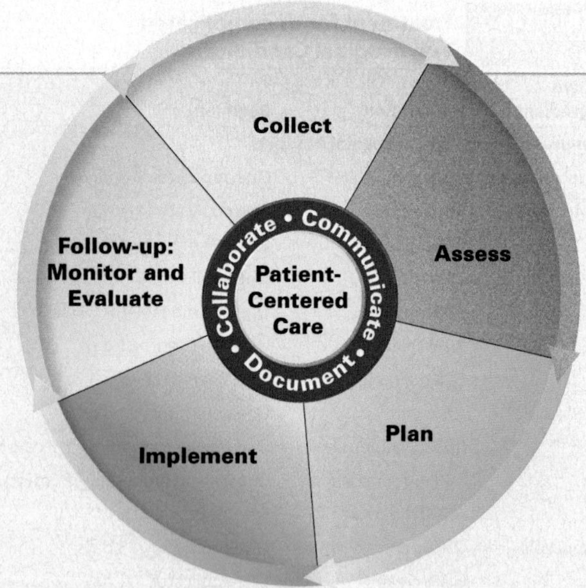

Patient Care Process for Vulcovaginal Candidiasis

The image shows the five fundamental steps included in The Pharmacist's Care Process endorsed by the Joint Commission for Pharmacy Practitioners (2014). The tagline of this process reads collaborate, communicate, and document. The five fundamental steps listed here are collect, assess, plan, implement, and follow-up: monitor and evaluate. All these steps are listed in a circular block diagram.

Collect

- Patient characteristics (age, pregnancy status)
- Patient medical history (previous vaginal infections, diabetes mellitus)
- Social history (sexual activity)
- Current meds (oral contraceptives, antibiotics)

Assess

- Symptoms consistent with VVC (itching, clumpy white vaginal discharge)
- Absence of fever, pelvic pain, colored or foul smelling vaginal discharge
- Possibility of sexually transmitted disease
- Recurrence of symptoms from previous vaginal infection

Plan*

- Remove predisposing risk factors if possible
- Select a drug therapy regimen including specific antifungal(s) dose, route, frequency, and duration (Table 143-2)
- Education of the patient regarding causes of VVC and the selected treatment
- Refer to other healthcare providers if complicated or recurrent VVC or risk factors for sexually transmitted disease

Implement

- Provide patient counselling (avoid harsh soaps, perfumes, hot tub use, contraceptive use)
- Keep vaginal area clean and dry, avoid constrictive clothing
- Self-assessment of symptom relief is appropriate

Follow-up: Monitor and Evaluate

- Monitor for complete resolution of symptoms within 24-48 hours of initiation of therapy (itching, clumpy white discharge)
- Determine the presence of adverse effects (nausea, abdominal discomfort, vaginal irritation)
- Refer to other healthcare providers if symptoms do not resolve despite adherence

Collaborate with patient, caregivers, and other healthcare professionals.

Antifungal-Resistant Vulvovaginal Candidiasis

Resistance to azole antimycotics should be considered in individuals who have persistently positive yeast cultures and fail to respond to therapy despite adherence to prescribed regimens.[1] These infections can be treated with boric acid or 5-flucytosine.[24] Boric acid is administered as a 600 mg intravaginal capsule daily for 14 days of induction therapy, followed by a maintenance regimen of one capsule intravaginally twice weekly. Boric acid should not be administered orally, as it is toxic. Flucytosine cream is administered vaginally, 1,000 mg inserted nightly for 7 days. The prevalence of *C. glabrata* is higher in those with diabetes. In a study of patients with diabetes and VVC, 68% had isolates for *C. glabrata* compared with 28.8% for *C. albicans*. Those with *C. glabrata* had significantly higher mycological cure rates with 600 mg of boric acid suppositories for 14 days compared with a single dose of fluconazole 150 mg.[25]

OROPHARYNGEAL AND ESOPHAGEAL CANDIDIASIS

Oropharyngeal and esophageal candidiasis are common and localized infections that occur in patients with human immunodeficiency virus (HIV) infection, diabetes, leukemia, and other malignancies. These infections are also associated with antimicrobial therapy, steroid use, radiation therapy, and denture use.

Oropharyngeal candidiasis (OPC), often referred to as *thrush*, is caused by the yeast *Candida*. *C. albicans*, a common oral commensal organism, is the most frequent infecting species. OPC is also referred to as *candidiasis* (or the more correct but less commonly used term *candidosis*). The infection may extend into the esophagus, causing esophageal candidiasis.

Epidemiology and Etiology

Candida is a commensal fungus found in the oral cavity in up to 65% of healthy individuals with higher prevalence in healthy children and young adults.[26,27] *Candida* carriage increases in immunocompromised and hospitalized patients.[27] Even in the era of highly active antiretroviral therapy (AART) up to 80% of HIV-infected persons may demonstrate oral yeast colonization.[28] The organism is capable of transition to a pathogen causing symptomatic mucosal infections in association with predisposing host factors.[27] *C. albicans* is the predominant colonizing *Candida* species (70%-80%), but any of the non–*C. albicans* species such as *C. glabrata* and *C. tropicalis*, which may account for 5% to 8%, respectively, can be colonizers. Colonization rates are influenced by the severity and nature of the underlying medical illness and the duration of hospitalization, as well as age (highest in infants younger than 18 months of age and in adults older than 60 years of age). A variety of host and exogenous factors (Table 143-3) can lead to the transformation of asymptomatic colonization to symptomatic disease, such as oropharyngeal and esophageal candidiasis. *C. albicans* is the most common species causing all forms of mucosal candidiasis in humans. Less frequently, non–*C. albicans* species can be pathogenic and cause disease. These include *C. glabrata, C. tropicalis, C. krusei,* and *C. parapsilosis.*[28,29] *C. krusei,* although relatively uncommon, generally is recovered from mucosal surfaces of neutropenic patients with hematologic malignancies.[29] *Candida dubliniensis* has been identified in both HIV-infected and noninfected patients, and may cause ~15% of infections previously ascribed to *C. albicans.*[29] In patients with cancer, non–*C. albicans* species account for almost half of all *Candida* infections.

Oropharyngeal candidiasis remains the most common opportunistic infection in patients with HIV disease, and it may be the first clinical manifestation of the HIV infection in the majority of untreated patients. OPC occurs in 50% to 90% of HIV-infected patients if the disease progresses to acquired immunodeficiency syndrome (AIDS).[26,28,29] The use of effective antiretroviral therapy has led to a significant reduction in the primary incidence and ultimately refractory disease. The absolute CD4 T-cell count is the primary risk factor for development of OPC with the greatest risk at CD4 T-cell levels <200 cells/mm^3 (0.2 × 10^9/L). Also, the HIV viral load is a predictor of OPC development; OPC increases with HIV viral loads >10,000 copies/mL (10 × 10^6/L). This finding correlates with the observation that initiation of antiretroviral therapy and subsequent increase in CD4 T-cell counts does not fully account for the decrease in OPC incidence.[28] Regardless of the CD4 T-cell count, or HIV viral load, OPC is predictive for the development of AIDS-related illnesses if left untreated.[26,29]

In non-HIV diseases, such as cancer, the incidence of OPC varies depending on the type of malignant neoplastic disease, level of immune suppression, and type and duration of treatment, but it is less common than in HIV-infected patients. OPC was initially reported in ~25% of patients with solid tumors and up to 60% in those with hematologic malignancies or bone marrow transplant recipients.[30] Rates of OPC have decreased significantly in these patients because

TABLE 143-3 Risk Factors for the Development of Oropharyngeal and/or Esophageal Candidiasis

Local Factors	Potential Mechanisms
Use of steroids and antibiotics	Suppression of cellular immunity and inhibition of phagocytosis by steroids, including chronic use of inhaled and topical steroids
	Alteration of endogenous oral flora by broad-spectrum antibiotics, especially when used with steroids, creates a milieu for proliferation of *Candida* species because of reduced environmental and nutritional competition
Dentures	Enhanced adherence of *Candida* species to the acrylic material of dentures, reduced saliva flow under surfaces of denture fittings, improperly fitted dentures, and poor oral hygiene provide a milieu conducive to the survival of microorganisms
Xerostomia caused by drugs (eg, tricyclic antidepressants and phenothiazine), chemotherapy, radiotherapy to the head/neck, and various diseases (eg, Sjögren's syndrome, HIV, and cancer of the head/neck), as well as bone marrow transplant recipients	Reduced dilutional and cleansing effect caused by low secretion rate and low pH in saliva: Saliva and mucosa secretions have defense factors, such as lactoferrin, sialoperoxidase, isozyme, histidine-rich polypeptide, secretory IgA antibodies, and specific anti-*Candida* antibodies, that help prevent adhesion and overgrowth of *Candida* species
Smoking	
Disruption of oral mucosa caused by chemotherapy and radiotherapy, ulcers, endotracheal intubation trauma, and burns	Oral mucositis induced by radiation and breaks in the physical barrier of the oral epithelium, which is protective against invasion by microorganisms; altered rate of mucosa regeneration by cancer chemotherapy, which increases vulnerability to infection
Systemic Factors	**Potential Mechanisms**
Drugs (eg, cytotoxic agents, corticosteroids, and immunosuppressants after organ transplant), omeprazole, and environmental chemicals (eg, benzene and pesticides)	Reduced immunity because of drug-induced neutropenia or cell-mediated immunity; potent inhibition of gastric acid by PPIs can facilitate the growth of *Candida* species; PPIs also can inhibit the cytotoxic effect of lymphocytes and reduce salivary secretion
Neonates or the elderly	Immature immune system of neonates who usually acquire infection during birth to a mother with vaginal candidiasis or from exposure to infected bottle nipples or to skin of adult caregiver
	Elderly—unclear if this is the direct effect of age per se or contribution from dentures or underlying comorbidity
HIV infection/AIDS	Depletion of CD4 T lymphocytes especially below 200-300 cells/mm^3 (0.2 × 10^9 to 0.3 × 10^9/L); anti-*Candida* protective mechanism of T lymphocytes at a mucosal level is unclear but can be caused by altered cytokines, especially interferon-γ, that inhibit transformation of *Candida* blastoconidia to the more invasive hyphal phase
Diabetes	Higher than normal numbers of *C. albicans* cultured from saliva of diabetic patients; can be related to the elevated glucose levels and reduced chemotactic factor in saliva, altered neutrophil function, and reduced saliva volume and flow
Malignancies (eg, leukemia and head/neck cancer)	Use of intensive radiotherapy and chemotherapy can disrupt oral mucosa and cause xerostomia; prolonged use of broad-spectrum antibiotics in neutropenic patients can alter the normal oral flora; because of the prolonged neutropenia, the principal immune defect, seen especially in leukemic patients, the initial oropharyngeal candidiasis can become systemic or invasive
Nutritional deficiencies (eg, iron, folate, and vitamins B1, B2, B6, B12, and C)	Can be related to dietary restriction or GI absorption problems; deficiencies can serve to enhance the pathogenic potential of the *Candida* inhabitants, alter host defense mechanisms, or change epithelial barrier integrity

AIDS, acquired immunodeficiency syndrome; GI, gastrointestinal; HIV, human immunodeficiency virus; IgA, immunoglobulin A; PPI, proton pump inhibitor.

of widespread use of antifungal prophylaxis. Incidence in other patient populations predisposed to OPC such as the hospitalized patient administered broad-spectrum antibiotics or denture and other oral appliance users is not well quantified. However, it does represent at-risk individuals where the clinical pharmacist has an important patient-care role.[27,30]

OPC can predispose patients to develop more invasive disease, including esophageal candidiasis.[30] The esophagus is the second most common site of gastrointestinal (GI) candidiasis. The prevalence of esophageal candidiasis increased mainly due to the emergence of AIDS, as well as the increased numbers of other severely immunocompromised patients, especially those with hematologic malignancies.[29] The mean incidence of esophageal candidiasis among HIV-infected patients is less than OPC and ranges from 15% to 20%.[29] The risk of esophageal candidiasis is increased in HIV-infected patients when the CD4 T-cell count has dropped below 100 to 200 cells/mm^3 (0.1×10^9 to 0.2×10^9/L), as well as in those with OPC.[30,31] However, the absence of OPC does not necessarily exclude the possibility of esophageal disease. Like OPC, the presence of esophageal candidiasis can help predict HIV disease progression and prognosis.[30] The incidence of esophageal candidiasis in non–HIV-infected immunocompromised patients is not well established. *C. albicans* is the most common cause of esophageal candidiasis, accounting for ~80% of cases, with the rest being caused by non–*C. albicans* species.[28] However, the widespread use of the azole agents for treatment and prophylaxis has led to an emergence of refractory infections that are more challenging to treat.

Pathogenesis and Host Defenses

The pathogenesis of OPC is most clearly elucidated in the setting of HIV infection. There appear to be several levels of immune defense against the development of OPC in HIV-infected persons, and they involve both systemic and local immunity. The primary line of host defense against *C. albicans* is cell-mediated immunity (CMI) at the mucosal surfaces, which is mediated by CD4 T cells.[26] The efficacy of the CD4 T cells is reduced when the number of cells drops below a protective threshold, and protection against infection becomes dependent on secondary or local immune mechanisms.[26,28] When the number of CD4 T cells drops too low, recruitment of these cells to the oral cavity is impaired. The CD4 T-cell count is the hallmark predictor for development of OPC. However, HIV viral load may have a stronger association with OPC than CD4 cell number.[28,32] The possibility that HIV plays a strong role in susceptibility to infection is supported by the observation that OPC is more common in HIV-infected persons than in those with similar immunosuppression, such as lymphoma and bone marrow transplant. When the primary line of defense fails, the secondary host defenses become crucial. These include the CD8 T cells, salivary cytokines, and other innate immune cells, such as the neutrophils, macrophages, and epithelial cells (with anti-*Candida* activity). Deficiencies or dysfunction in any of these can result in increased susceptibility to OPC. The problem with the CD8 T cells is caused more by a dysfunction of the microenvironment, specifically reduction in the E-cadherin adhesion molecule that promotes migration of the cells through mucosal tissues.[29] The role of humoral immunity by antibodies as a protective mechanism is unclear and controversial. The changeover of the role of *Candida* species from commensal to pathogenic in the human host usually occurs when breakdown in these host defenses occurs. The pathogenesis of OPC is still not completely understood. It is important to develop a better understanding of the pathogenesis and role of host defenses, including the mechanism of CD8 T-cell activity, reduced adhesion molecules, and whether other cofactors, such as HIV viral load, AART, and injection drug use, play a role. Immunotherapeutic modalities can then be developed to eliminate the susceptibility factors and significantly reduce OPC in the at-risk populations.

Significant differences exist in the virulence among *Candida* species in mucosal candidiasis. One virulence factor is the ability of the organism to adapt and survive in response to changes in the host environment.[28] The genes required for virulence are regulated in response to the environmental signals indigenous to the host environment (eg, temperature, pH, osmotic pressure, iron and calcium ion concentrations, oxygenation, and carbon and nitrogen availability). The ability of *C. albicans* to undergo reversible morphologic transition between the budding pseudohyphal and the more invasive hyphal growth forms is also a determinant of virulence, and genes are recognized to play a role.[26] Other virulence factors are the adhesive ability of *C. albicans* to epithelial cells and proteins and its ability to invade host cells by means of phospholipase and proteinase enzymes. This may be one of the factors leading to OPC in non–HIV-infected individuals. Other components of the pathogenesis in the absence of HIV are the ability of the *Candida* species to adhere to buccal epithelial cells.[33] This may be a key element in the development of OPC in patients with altered microflora, including those receiving broad-spectrum antimicrobial therapy.

Risk Factors

4 Several host and exogenous factors contribute to the ability of *Candida* species to cause infection (see Table 143-3). Local and systemic factors, as well as characteristics of the organism itself, can increase the susceptibility of an individual to *Candida* infections.[26] Endocrine disorders besides diabetes mellitus, such as hypothyroidism, hypoparathyroidism, and hypoadrenalism, also can predispose patients to *Candida* species overgrowth. Patients with primary immune deficiencies such as lymphocytic abnormalities, phagocytic dysfunction, immunoglobulin A (IgA) deficiency, viral-induced immune paralysis, and severe congenital immunodeficiencies are also at risk for oropharyngeal candidiasis as well as disseminated candidiasis. Oral mucosal disease, such as lichen planus, can be preexistent causes of candidiasis. Smoking has been suggested as a predisposing risk factor. In many cases, multiple concurrent predisposing factors to candidiasis can exist, for example, xerostomia with mucositis and a break in the epithelial surface or immunosuppression, such as might occur in a leukemic patient receiving radiation and chemotherapy. The severity and extent of *Candida* infections increase with the number and severity of predisposing risk factors.[27]

CLINICAL PRESENTATION AND DIAGNOSIS

Oropharyngeal candidiasis can manifest in several major forms (Table 143-4).[26,27] The clinical signs and symptoms of OPC and the locations of the lesions can be quite diverse (Table 143-5). A presumptive diagnosis of OPC usually is made by the characteristic appearance on the oral mucosa, with resolution of signs and symptoms after antifungal therapy. Pseudomembranous candidiasis, commonly known as *oral thrush,* is the classic and most common form seen in immunosuppressed and immunocompetent hosts. Erythematous and hyperplastic candidiasis and angular cheilitis occur less commonly in the HIV-infected population. Dysphagia, odynophagia, and retrosternal chest pain are common complaints of esophageal candidiasis, which is usually, but not always, accompanied by the presence of OPC. Clinical symptomatology, along with a therapeutic trial of antifungal, can provide a reliable presumptive diagnosis of esophageal candidiasis. If antifungal therapy does not lead to resolution, more invasive tests such as upper GI endoscopy can be undertaken.

TREATMENT

Desired Outcomes

The primary desired outcome in the management of OPC is a clinical cure, that is, elimination of clinical signs and symptoms. Even

TABLE 143-4 Clinical Classification of Oropharyngeal Candidiasis

Types	Population at Risk	Clinical Signs and Appearance
Pseudomembranous (thrush)	Neonates, patients with HIV or cancer, the debilitated elderly, patients on broad-spectrum antibiotics or steroid inhalers, patients with dry mouth from various causes, and smokers	Classic "cottage cheese" appearance, yellowish white, soft plaques (or milk curds) overlying areas of erythema on the buccal mucosa, tongue, gums, and throat; plaques are easily removed by vigorous rubbing but can leave red or bleeding sites when removed; lesions on the tongue dorsum give it a bald, depapillated appearance
Erythematous (atrophic)	Patients with HIV, patients on broad-spectrum antibiotics or steroid inhalers	Sensitive and painful erythematous mucosa with few, if any, white plaques; lesions are generally on the dorsal surface of the tongue or the hard palate, occasionally on the soft palate, but any part of the mucosa can be involved; appear as flat red patches on the palate or atrophic patches on the tongue dorsum with loss of papillae. Can be acute or chronic
Hyperplastic (candidal leukoplakia)	Smokers; uncommon in patients with HIV	Thick white and adherent keratotic plaques commonly seen on the buccal mucosa and lateral border of the tongue; can also be seen on the lips and the bottom of the mouth; plaques cannot be easily scraped off or only partially removed; this condition is distinct from oral hairy leukoplakia, and it can progress to severe dysplasia or malignancy
Angular cheilitis	Patients with HIV, denture wearers	Painful red, ulcerative, cracking, or fissuring lesion at one or both corners of the mouth because of an inflammatory reaction; usually lesions are small and rather punctate, but occasionally they can extend in a linear fashion from the angles onto the facial skin
Denture stomatitis (chronic atrophic)	Denture wearers who tend to be elderly and have poor oral hygiene	Red, flat lesions on the mucosa beneath the denture and extend right up to the denture border; more commonly located beneath a maxillary denture, although they can be encountered beneath a mandibular denture
Central papillary atrophy (median rhomboid glossitis)	Uncommon (<1% prevalence), males more commonly infected than females (3:1)	Rhomboid-shaped hypertrophic or atrophic plaque in the mid-dorsal tongue. Lesions may not resolve completely

HIV, human immunodeficiency virus.

TABLE 143-5 Clinical Presentation of Oropharyngeal and Esophageal Candidiasis

Oropharyngeal Candidiasis	Esophageal Candidiasis
General	**General**
The clinical features can be quite diverse (see Table 143-4)	This usually occurs as an extension of OPC; however, the esophagus can be the only site involved; the distal two-thirds, rather than the proximal one-third, is the most common site
Symptoms	**Symptoms**
Symptoms are diverse and range from none to a sore, painful mouth, burning tongue, metallic taste, and dysphagia and odynophagia with involvement of the hypopharynx	Typically, the symptoms are dysphagia, odynophagia, and retrosternal chest pain but can be asymptomatic in some patients; although rare, epigastric pain can be the dominant symptom
Signs	**Signs**
Signs are variable and can include diffuse erythema and white patches on the surfaces of the buccal mucosa, throat, tongue, or gums; constitutional signs are absent	Constitutional signs, including fever, occasionally occur; physical findings can range from a few to numerous white or beige plaques of variable size Plaques can be hyperemic or edematous, with ulceration in more severe cases Most advanced cases can occur with increased mucosal friability and narrowing of lumen Uncommon complications include perforation and aortic–esophageal fistula formation
Laboratory tests	**Laboratory tests**
Scraping of an active lesion for microscopic examination can help confirm the diagnosis (presence of pseudohyphae and budding yeast) but is usually not necessary Cultures are not necessary because isolation of *Candida* species does not distinguish between colonization and true infection; cultures can be taken in patients responding poorly to therapy to determine the infecting species and to predict likely drug resistance	The best test is upper GI endoscopy (more useful than barium swallow); helps exclude other causes of esophagitis (eg, viral, aphthous ulcers); diagnosis is confirmed by the histologic presence of *Candida* species in biopsy lesions taken during endoscopy Cultures to look for drug-resistant *Candida* species are warranted in patients who require endoscopy

GI, gastrointestinal; OPC, oropharyngeal candidiasis.

when the patient is relatively asymptomatic, it is important to treat the initial episode of OPC to avoid progression to more extensive disease. In the most severe cases, the patient's quality of life can be impaired; this can result in decreased fluid and nutritional intake. Lack of appropriate treatment of OPC can lead to more extensive oral disease, especially in patients who are immunocompromised. The most serious complication of untreated OPC is extension of the infection to esophageal candidiasis which is more debilitating with greater impact on the patient's quality of life. Appropriate antifungal therapy should be initiated for both OPC and esophageal candidiasis. Preventing or minimizing the number of future recurrences of both types of candidiasis is an equally important outcome. The approach depends largely on the underlying predisposing conditions. Mycologic cure is not a necessary treatment outcome because it may not be feasible or realistic, given that *Candida* species exist commonly as part of the normal mouth flora.

Minimizing toxicities and drug-drug interactions of systemic antifungal agents and maximizing adherence by ensuring that the patient understands the importance of therapy and the directions to take the medication appropriately are important secondary outcomes of therapy.

General Approach to Treatment

The management of OPC should be individualized for each patient, taking into consideration the underlying immune status, other concurrent mucosal and medical diseases, concomitant medications, and exogenous infectious sources. Generally, topical therapy is used in mild forms of infections that have limited ability to spread. Systemic therapies are reserved for more moderate infection which may lead to dissemination of the infection.[27,28,34]

Whenever feasible, it is desirable to minimize all predisposing factors, such as administration of corticosteroids, chemotherapeutic agents, and antimicrobials, as well as to institute proper oral hygiene and resolve concurrent conditions, such as denture stomatitis. Selection of an appropriate antifungal agent for treatment of candidiasis requires consideration of several factors, including the patient's drug adherence, adequate saliva for dissolution of solid topical medications, risk of caries from sucrose- or dextrose-containing preparations, potential drug interactions, coexisting medical conditions (eg, liver disease), location and severity of the infection, and the need for long-term maintenance therapy.

5 Topical antimycotic therapies should be the first choice for milder forms of infections.[34] The efficacy of antimycotic agents for OPC varies in different patient populations. Until the polyene antimycotic agents became available in the 1950s, gentian violet, an aniline dye, was used to treat OPC. Problems with gentian violet include fungal resistance, skin irritation, and especially the unaesthetic staining of the oral mucosa. In resource limited areas gentian violet remains a therapeutic option. Gentian violet solution of 0.00165% does not stain the oral mucosa and has potent antifungal activity.[35] Topical agents, such as nystatin and clotrimazole, are the standard of treatment for uncomplicated OPC and generally are effective for treatment in otherwise healthy adults and infants with no underlying immunodeficiencies. Topical agents are available in an assortment of formulations, including oral rinses (suspension), troches, powder, vaginal tablets, creams, and most recently as a mucoadhesive tablet[30,34,36] (Table 143-6).

Topical agents require frequent applications because of the short contact time with the oral mucosa; the ideal contact time is 20 to 30 minutes. Sufficient saliva is needed to dissolve clotrimazole troches, and this can be problematic for patients with xerostomia. Also, the rough surface of the tablet can become irritating to the oral soft tissue. Troches also contain dextrose, which has cariogenic potential. Nystatin suspension might be a better choice for patients with xerostomia, but it is difficult to maintain adequate contact time with the oral mucosa. Some patients complain of the unpleasant taste of nystatin, which can cause nausea and vomiting; this is especially problematic in cancer patients experiencing chemotherapy-induced nausea. The high sucrose content of nystatin suspension is cariogenic in dentate patients, and it should be used with caution in diabetic patients.[27,30] Miconazole 50 mg mucoadhesive tablets are a buccal adherent miconazole product approved for the local treatment of OPC in adults and adolescents older than age 16 years.[37] This product offers the advantage of a once-daily formulation that is tasteless, odorless, and sugar free.[36] Topical creams, such as clotrimazole, ketoconazole, miconazole, and nystatin (usually mixed with a steroid), are more appropriate for application three times daily to the corners of the mouth in treating angular cheilitis, the inflammation, drying, and cracking of the corners of the mouth.[34]

Systemic therapy is necessary in patients with OPC that is refractory to topical treatment, those who cannot tolerate topical agents, have moderate-to-severe disease, and those at high risk for disseminated systemic or invasive candidiasis. Effective treatment of esophageal candidiasis generally requires the use of systemic antifungal agents. However, these agents have the disadvantage of producing more side effects (see Table 143-6) and drug-drug interactions (see Chapter 144, "Invasive Fungal Infections"). Fluconazole is inexpensive and generally well tolerated, and its absorption is unaffected by food or gastric acidity. Ketoconazole requires gastric acidity for absorption, which can be problematic and this agent is not recommended today with the availability of more effective triazoles. Itraconazole capsules also have the same absorption problem and are no longer recommended. In contrast, itraconazole solution has enhanced absorption and is best taken in a fasting state; in addition, the solution provides the benefit of both topical effects to the oral mucosa and systemic effects and is beneficial to patients with mucositis or swallowing problems. Whenever possible, it is generally beneficial to limit the use of systemic azole agents to prevent unnecessary drug exposure and to minimize the potential for occurrence of drug-resistant candidiasis, particularly from fluconazole resistance.

Oropharyngeal Candidiasis: Human Immuodeficiency Virus–Infected Patients

Treatment for initial or recurrent episodes of OPC should be started with topical agents, provided that clinical symptoms are not severe and that there is minimal risk of esophageal involvement.[29,34] Clinical responses with the resolution of signs and symptoms generally occur within 5 to 7 days of initiating treatment. Clotrimazole appears to be the most effective topical agent and demonstrates comparable clinical response rates with both fluconazole and itraconazole.[29,34] However, topical therapy is associated with more frequent relapses than with fluconazole.[31,34] This may be of limited clinical significance in patients receiving effective AART because of their decreased susceptibility to opportunistic infection. In practice, nystatin suspension is still used frequently in initial episodes of OPC, although it is the least effective agent and is associated with frequent treatment failures and early relapses, especially in patients with advanced HIV disease or neutropenia.[27,30] Miconazole mucoadhesive tablets 50 mg once daily (MMT) were non-inferior to clotrimazole troches 10 mg five times daily for the treatment of OPC in HIV-infected patients. Safety and tolerability was also similar between treatment groups.[37]

Systemic oral azoles should be reserved for use in the more severe episodes of OPC unresponsive to topical agents or in patients with concurrent esophageal involvement.[30,34] In clinical practice, fluconazole usually is the systemic azole agent of choice because of its proven efficacy, favorable absorption, safety, and drug-interaction profiles, and it is relatively inexpensive. Fluconazole is superior to ketoconazole and itraconazole capsules.[30,34] Fluconazole should be given 100 to 200 mg/day for 7 to 14 days.[34] A single dose of fluconazole 750 mg orally was as effective as fluconazole 150 mg orally for 14 days, which warrants further evaluation, given the potential advantages of adherence and cost-effectiveness.[38] Itraconazole oral solution with an improved absorption profile compared with the capsule formulation is as effective as fluconazole, with comparable clinical and mycologic response and relapse rates.[30,34] However, it carries a higher risk of drug interactions because it is a potent inhibitor of the cytochrome P450 enzymes, and it is associated with more nausea than fluconazole. Posaconazole is an extended-spectrum triazole with potent in vitro activity against both *C. albicans* and non–*C. albicans* species. It is equivalent to fluconazole in terms of efficacy, safety, and tolerability.[39] Posaconazole, itraconazole solution, and voriconazole are the azole alternatives to fluconazole in the management of moderate-to-severe OPC.[33] Other agents that are effective are amphotericin B and the echinocandins (caspofungin, micafungin, and anidulafungin). They are reserved for refractory OPC, however, because of their greater toxicity. They are also more expensive and are less convenient to use.

TABLE 143-6 Therapeutic Options for Mucosal Candidiasis (With Strength of Recommendation and Quality of Evidence)

Initial Episodes of OPC[a]: Treat for 7-14 Days	Common/Significant Side Effects
Clotrimazole 10 mg troche: hold 1 troche in mouth for 15-20 minutes for slow dissolution five times daily (B-2)	Altered taste, mild nausea, vomiting
Nystatin 100,000 units/mL suspension: 5 mL swish and swallow orally four times daily (B-2)	Mild nausea, vomiting, diarrhea
Miconazole 50 mg mucoadhesive buccal tablets 50 mg orally daily (A-1)	Diarrhea, headache, nausea, dysgeusia, upper abdominal pain, and vomiting
Fluconazole 100 mg tablets[b]: 100-200 mg orally daily (A-1)	GI upset, hepatitis not common
Itraconazole 10 mg/mL solution[c]: 200 mg orally daily (A-2)	GI upset, not common: hepatotoxicity, CHF, pulmonary edema with long-term use[d]
Posaconazole 40 mg/mL suspension: 400 mg orally daily with a full meal (A-2)	GI upset, fever, headache, increased hepatic transaminases not common
Fluconazole-Refractory OPC: Treat for ≥14 Days	
Itraconazole 10 mg/mL solution: 200 mg orally daily (A-3)	See above
Voriconazole 200 mg tablets: 200 mg orally twice daily (>40 kg), taken on empty stomach (A-3)	GI upset, rash, reversible visual disturbance (altered light perception, photopsia, chromatopsia, photophobia), increased hepatic transaminases, hallucinations, or confusion
Posaconazole 40 mg/mL suspension: 400 mg orally twice daily × 3 days, then 400 mg daily × 28 days (A-2)	See above
Amphotericin B 100 mg/mL suspension[e]: 1-5 mL swish and swallow orally four times daily (B-2)	Oral: nausea, vomiting, diarrhea with higher dose
Amphotericin B deoxycholate 50 mg injection: 0.3–0.7 mg/kg/day IV daily (B-2)	IV: fever, chills, sweats, nephrotoxicity, electrolyte disturbances, bone marrow suppression
Caspofungin 50 mg IV daily (B-2)	Fever, headache, infusion-related reactions (<5%) (eg, rash, facial swelling, pruritus, vasodilation), hypokalemia, increased hepatic transaminases, anemia, neutropenia
Micafungin 150 mg IV daily (B-2)	Similar to caspofungin
Anidulafungin 200 mg IV daily (B-2)	Similar to caspofungin
Esophageal Candidiasis[a]: Treat for 14-21 Days	
Fluconazole 100 mg tablets: 200-400 mg orally (3-6 mg/kg) daily (A-1)	See above
Echinocandin: see above (B-2)	See above
Amphotericin B deoxycholate 50 mg injection: 0.3-0.7 mg/kg/day IV daily (B-2)	See above
Posaconazole 40 mg/mL suspension: 400 mg orally twice daily (A-3)	See above
Itraconazole 10 mg/mL solution[c]: 200 mg orally daily (A-3)	See above
Voriconazole 200 mg tablets: 200 mg orally twice daily (>40 kg) (A-3)	See above
Voriconazole IV and echinocandins (A-1): generally reserved for refractory cases	See above
Fluconazole-Refractory EC: Treat for 21-28 Days	
Itraconazole 10 mg/mL solution: 200 mg orally daily (A-2)	See above
Posaconazole 40 mg/mL suspension: 400 mg orally twice daily (A-3)	See above
Voriconazole 200 mg tablets: 200 mg orally twice daily (>40 kg), taken on empty stomach (A-3)	See above
Caspofungin 50 mg IV daily (B-2)	See above
Micafungin 150 mg IV daily (B-2)	Similar to caspofungin
Anidulafungin 100 mg IV on day 1, then 50 mg IV daily (B-2)	Similar to caspofungin
Amphotericin B deoxycholate: 0.3-0.7 mg/kg/day IV, or lipid-based amphotericin 3-5 mg/kg/day IV (B-2)	See above

CHF, congestive heart failure; GI, gastrointestinal; OPC, oropharyngeal candidiasis.

[a]Initial episodes of OPC can be adequately treated first with topical agents before resorting to systemic therapy (B-2), but systemic therapy is required for effective treatment of esophageal candidiasis. (A-2) Suppressive therapy is recommended for patients with frequent or severe recurrences (A-1).

[b]Fluconazole is more effective than ketoconazole (A-1).

[c]Solution is more effective than capsule (A-1); solution is better taken on an empty stomach.

[d]Suspension is not marketed; can be prepared extemporaneously by pharmacy.

[e]See discussion under onychomycosis.

Recommendation grades: Strength of recommendation: **A**—Both strong evidence for efficacy and substantial clinical benefit to support recommendation for use. *Should always be offered.* **B**—Moderate evidence for efficacy but only limited clinical benefit, to support recommendation for use. *Should generally be offered.* **C**—Evidence for efficacy is insufficient to support recommendation for or against use; or evidence for efficacy might not outweigh adverse consequences or cost of the treatment under consideration. *Optional.* **D**—Moderate evidence for lack of efficacy or adverse outcome supports a recommendation against use. *Should generally not be offered.* Quality of evidence: **1**—Evidence from at least one properly designed randomized, controlled trial. **2**—Evidence from at least one well-designed trial without randomization, from cohort or case-controlled analytic studies (preferably from more than one center), or from multiple time-series studies, or dramatic results from uncontrolled experiments. **3**—Evidence from opinions of respected authorities based on clinical experience, descriptive studies, or reports of expert committees. (UR) Evidence currently unrated.

Oropharyngeal Candidiasis: Non-Human Immunodeficiency Virus–Infected Patients

This patient population includes patients with hematologic malignancy (eg, leukemias) or blood and bone marrow transplantation (BMT) with a long duration of neutropenia and chronic graft-versus-host disease, patients with solid tumors, patients with solid-organ transplants who are receiving immunosuppressive therapy, and patients with diabetes mellitus, as well as patients on prolonged courses of antibiotics or corticosteroids and the debilitated elderly.

Specific antifungal therapy can be unnecessary for asymptomatic patients at relatively low risk for disseminated candidiasis, such as those who are not granulocytopenic or who are expected to have a short duration of granulocytopenia.[34] Many of these infections will clear spontaneously after recovery of the granulocytes or discontinuation of antibiotic and/or immunosuppressive therapy. However, antifungal therapy usually is required for patients who have persistent infection or significant symptoms, usually pain, or who are granulocytopenic with a relatively high risk of fungal dissemination. Topical agents first can be given a therapeutic trial depending on the severity of infection and the degree of immunosuppression. Although both nystatin and clotrimazole can be effective in treating OPC, nystatin suspension does not effectively reduce the incidence of either oropharyngeal or systemic *Candida* infections in immunocompromised patients receiving chemotherapy or radiation; its use often is associated with treatment failures and early relapses.[34] Clotrimazole appears to be more effective in reducing colonization and treating acute episodes in cancer patients who are immunocompromised. MMTs were superior to miconazole oral gel in patients with head and neck cancer in achieving a complete response to therapy.[40] MMT has not been studied against clotrimazole in this patient population specifically but is approved for use in adults with OPC.

Topical therapy with clotrimazole or nystatin for 7 days is usually adequate for treating mucocutaneous candidiasis in most solid-organ transplant patients.[30] Use of topical therapy will reduce the number of systemic drugs that these patients receive and hence minimize the risk of drug-drug interactions. Failure to respond to topical agents warrants the use of fluconazole. Low-dose amphotericin B solution as "swish and swallow" (100 mg/mL, 1 mL four times daily) for 7 to 10 days is reserved for the unusual cases of treatment failure as it is not readily available and requires compounding.

Patients who develop OPC because of prolonged antibiotic use or aerosolized corticosteroids use can be managed successfully by discontinuation of the offending agent, and the infection usually will resolve. If there is a strong desire to treat because of discomfort or need to hasten symptom resolution or an inability to stop the offending agent, therapy with a topical agent, either MMT, clotrimazole, or nystatin, is effective in most cases. The advantage of systemic azoles is the convenience of less frequent dosing. Symptoms usually improve in 3 or 4 days. Infants should be given smaller amounts more frequently (eg, nystatin 100,000 units every 2-3 hours) to ensure better contact time. For denture-related OPC, or candidal stomatitis, effective therapy requires treatment of both the mouth and the dentures to avoid relapse. The dentures must be brushed vigorously and disinfected every night by soaking in antiseptic solution, such as chlorhexidine gluconate 0.25% or a commercial denture disinfectant product.[30,34] Topical antifungal therapy of the oral cavity is required. Consistent proper oral hygiene and care of the dentures can help prevent relapse.

Systemic azole agents are used for treating OPC in patients who have failed or who are unable to take topical therapy.[30,34,39] The preceding discussion on the relative efficacy of fluconazole, itraconazole, and ketoconazole in HIV-infected patients can be extrapolated to the non–HIV-infected population. Oral fluconazole 100 to 200 mg daily is used more commonly because of more extensive experience with its use, and it is more effective and has a more favorable absorption and side-effect profile compared with other available azoles.[34] If the oral route is not feasible for reasons such as severe chemotherapy-induced mucositis, fluconazole can be administered IV. In patients unresponsive to azoles, IV amphotericin B in relatively low doses of 0.1 to 0.3 mg/kg/day can be tried.[34] Because of the higher risk for dissemination in patients who are severely neutropenic (<100 neutrophils/mm^3 [0.1×10^9/L]) or clinically unstable (hypotensive or febrile), some clinicians prefer to initiate therapy with IV amphotericin B at 0.6 mg/kg/day, with therapy continued until the neutropenia has resolved, or an echinocandin.[34] The echinocandins caspofungin, micafungin, and anidulafungin are all effective for the treatment of OPC, thus offering other options, with fewer adverse effects in the patient with refractory disease.[34]

Esophageal Candidiasis: Human Immunodeficiency Virus–Infected Patients

6 Treatment of esophageal candidiasis has not been as well studied as OPC. Because of the significant morbidity of esophageal candidiasis and the absence of evidence supporting the efficacy of topical antifungals, treatment requires systemic antifungal agents.[26,28] Fluconazole is superior to ketoconazole and itraconazole capsules with respect to endoscopic cure and clinical response and usually produces a more rapid onset of action and resolution of symptoms. Fluconazole is as effective as itraconazole solution, with reported response rates of >80% to 90%.[31,34] However, itraconazole solution causes more nausea and drug interactions because of inhibition of the cytochrome P450 enzymes. Amphotericin B, voriconazole, posaconazole, and the echinocandins are also effective in esophageal candidiasis, but they are generally reserved for patients with advanced or inadequately controlled HIV disease where the candidiasis tends to recur or becomes refractory to azole therapy.[41-43]

Esophageal Candidiasis: Non-Human Immunodeficiency Virus–Infected Patients

As in the case of HIV-infected patients, treatment of esophageal candidiasis requires systemic therapy. Patients can be started on oral fluconazole 200 to 400 mg/day for 14 to 21 days.[34] Higher fluconazole doses (up to 400 mg/day) have been suggested for patients with severe symptoms or those who are neutropenic.[44] Other agents recommended if fluconazole is not an option are an echinocandin or IV amphotericin B at 0.3 to 0.7 mg/kg. Itraconazole solution, posaconazole, and voriconazole are effective alternatives that may be considered for those not responding adequately to fluconazole. An echinocandin or IV amphotericin B may be selected over fluconazole for initial therapy in neutropenic patients who present with severe symptoms or who are at high risk for dissemination of *Candida* species, such as those receiving other aggressive immunosuppressive therapy (eg, corticosteroids, total-body irradiation, or antithymocyte globulin) and who have documented evidence of esophageal candidiasis or who have failed an initial empirical trial of oral nonabsorbable agents or systemic azoles.[34] Therapy should be continued at least until the neutropenia resolves. For patients whose symptoms have resolved and who are afebrile and clinically stable, therapy should be discontinued, and the patients should be monitored closely for infection recurrence. In high-risk patients, particularly those with persistent fever and neutropenia, the potential presence of clinically occult, diffuse GI or disseminated candidiasis should be considered. The echinocandins and newer azole agents (voriconazole and posaconazole) offer less toxic alternatives or oral agents and are preferred in patients who are intolerant of amphotericin B deoxycholate or who have preexisting renal impairment.[30,44,45]

Antifungal-Refractory Oral Mucosal Candidiasis

Treatment failure is generally defined as persistence of signs and symptoms of OPC or esophageal candidiasis after an appropriate trial of antifungal therapy.[29] Treatment of refractory oral mucosal candidiasis is frequently unsatisfactory, and clinical response is usually short-lived, with rapid and periodic recurrences. The key risk factors for occurrence of refractory candidiasis are advanced stage of AIDS with low CD4 cell counts (<50 cells/mm^3 [0.05 × 10^9/L]) and repeated or prolonged courses of various systemic antifungal agents, in particular systemic azoles.[30,34] Frequent or prolonged use of fluconazole can be associated with fluconazole-refractory candidiasis because of selection of more resistant non–*C. albicans* species. An important initial management strategy is to assess and optimize the antiretroviral therapy of the patient with refractory OPC to help improve the immune function. With the widespread use of AART, fluconazole-refractory OPC is now less commonly encountered. It is also important to identify and rectify potentially correctable causes of clinical failures of mucosal candidiasis, such as poor drug adherence, adequate dosing, reduced drug absorption associated with hypochlorhydria, and drug-drug interactions.

Few controlled studies have assessed the effectiveness of antifungal agents. Doubling of the fluconazole dosage to 400 or 800 mg/day can be effective in some patients with infection caused by *Candida* species of intermediate resistance, although the response may be only transient.[31] Fluconazole oral suspension can be beneficial in some patients because of increased salivary concentrations obtained when the suspension is taken with the swish and swallow technique.[34] Patients with fluconazole-refractory mucosal candidiasis can be treated with itraconazole oral suspension because it can be effective in 64% to 80% of patients; however, the benefit is short-lived if chronic suppressive therapy is not maintained.[29,34] Posaconazole suspension was successful in ~74% of patients with refractory oral or esophageal candidiasis; voriconazole may also be efficacious in these patients. Amphotericin B oral suspension is another alternative for azole-refractory patients.[31,34] It has broad-spectrum activity against many fungal species and low likelihood of *Candida* species resistance. Amphotericin B suspension is no longer available commercially in the United States, but it can be prepared extemporaneously by the pharmacy.[46]

IV amphotericin B deoxycholate has been the alternative for patients with endoscopically proven disease who have failed fluconazole or itraconazole therapy. Patients with severe disease unresponsive to other agents require IV amphotericin B 0.3 to 0.7 mg/kg/day for 7 to 10 days to achieve clinical response; higher dose or longer treatment duration can be needed in more severe disease.[31,34] After response, suppressive therapy with amphotericin B is required to increase disease-free intervals. Patients who fail to respond to amphotericin B and require >1 mg/kg/day might be candidates for liposomal amphotericin B preparations because of renal and/or bone marrow toxicities, although at a markedly higher cost. Flucytosine usually is not used as monotherapy because of rapid development of resistance but can be used in combination with an azole or amphotericin B.[31] Less toxic agents that are also effective are voriconazole and the echinocandins.[44,45] Voriconazole, a triazole antifungal available in both oral and IV preparations, is as effective as fluconazole for esophageal candidiasis, and has shown success in treatment of fluconazole-refractory disease.[43] However, voriconazole has more side effects and multiple pharmacokinetic drug interactions compared to fluconazole.[43] Caspofungin is the first of the echinocandins to be approved for esophageal candidiasis. Micafungin and anidulafungin have been approved for this indication. All three echinocandins have similar efficacy and tolerability profile as fluconazole, although higher relapse has been reported with caspofungin and anidulafungin compared with fluconazole.[34,45] Because the echinocandins require IV administration and are expensive, they are primarily used in patients who are refractory to the triazoles or have serious triazole-related adverse effects. As a class, the echinocandins have a favorable adverse effect profile. They are less toxic than amphotericin B (see Table 143-6) and have less impact on the cytochrome P450 enzymes than either itraconazole or voriconazole. Immunomodulation with adjunctive granulocyte-macrophage colony-stimulating factor and interferon have been used for refractory oral candidiasis in limited numbers of patients.[34]

Antifungal Prophylaxis

7 Ensuring that the HIV-infected patient is receiving appropriate antiretroviral therapy to enhance the immune system is perhaps the most important measure in preventing future episodes of mucosal candidiasis (oropharyngeal, esophageal, and vulvovaginal).[34] Initial success of treatment often is followed by symptomatic recurrences, especially in patients with advanced or poorly controlled HIV disease. Long-term suppressive therapy with fluconazole is effective in preventing recurrences or new infections of OPC in HIV disease and in patients with cancer.[34] However, the indications for antifungal prophylaxis and the best long-term management strategy still have not been well established. Fluconazole does not provide complete protection, and breakthrough infections can occur.[31] The reduced risk of recurrence of OPC does not improve survival. In addition, chronic exposure to azole therapy might lead to the development of refractory disease or emergence of azole resistance.[34] However, in a randomized trial of continuous versus episodic fluconazole therapy, continuous therapy did not result in a higher rate of refractory OPC or esophageal disease.[47] HIV specialists do not recommend primary or secondary prophylaxis for OPC.[31] The rationale includes effectiveness of therapy for acute episodes of OPC, low incidence of serious invasive fungal disease, low mortality associated with mucosal candidiasis, potential for drug interactions, potential for emergence of drug resistance, and the prohibitive long-term cost of prophylaxis.

8 The decision to use secondary prophylaxis should be individualized for each patient. Secondary prophylaxis can be considered in patients with multiple recurrent episodes of symptomatic OPC or when the disease is sufficiently severe and affecting the quality of life.[31] Patients with a history of one or more episodes of documented esophageal candidiasis and a CD4 T-cell count still <200 cells/mm^3 (0.2 × 10^9/L) despite being on AART are candidates for secondary prophylaxis. Oral fluconazole 100 mg three times weekly is the regimen recommended by the Infectious Diseases Society of America for patients deemed in need of chronic suppressive therapy.[22] Itraconazole solution 200 mg daily orally is an alternative as suppressive therapy for OPC.[34]

Patients with malignant neoplastic diseases who are receiving irradiation, cytotoxic, and/or immunosuppressive therapy are at high risk for fungal infections in addition to bacterial and viral infections. Prophylaxis of *Candida* infection is controversial, and the results of studies have been conflicting and difficult to evaluate. In the hematopoietic stem cell transplant (HSCT) population, fluconazole prophylaxis is recommended prior to engraftment. Cross-resistance to other azoles may occur among *Candida* species; this should be a treatment consideration in a patient who develops a breakthrough fungal infection. Micafungin is an alternative to fluconazole prophylaxis of candidiasis.[48] The value of antifungal prophylaxis in these patients needs to be considered in the broader context of not only reducing colonization and the risk of superficial candidiasis but also, more importantly, reducing the risk for invasive candidiasis and improving survival. Management of these infections in this patient population is discussed further in Chapter 145, "Infections in Immunocompromised Patients."

TABLE 143-7 Patient Counseling Tips for Managing Oropharyngeal Candidiasis

1. Clean the oral cavity prior to administering the topical antifungal agent. Daily fluoride rinses can help reduce the risk of caries when using an agent containing sucrose or dextrose.
2. Use the topical antifungal agent after meals, as saliva flow and mouth movements can reduce the contact time.
3. Troches should be slowly dissolved in the mouth, not chewed or swallowed whole, over 15-20 minutes, and the saliva swallowed.
4. Suspension should be swished around the mouth in the oral cavity to cover all areas for as long as possible, ideally at least 1 minute, then gargled and swallowed.
5. Remove dentures while medication is being applied to the oral tissues.
6. Use a suspension or buccal mucoadhesive tablet instead of a troche if xerostomia is present; if a troche is preferred, the patient should rinse or drink water prior to dosing. For xerostomia, suggest nonpharmacologic measures for symptomatic relief (eg, ice chips, sugarless gum or hard candy, citrus beverages).
7. Dentures should be removed and disinfected overnight using an antiseptic solution (eg, chlorhexidine 0.12%-0.2%). Disinfect oral tissues in addition to dental prosthesis.
8. Complete treatment course even though symptomatic improvement can occur in 48-72 hours.
9. Maintain good oral hygiene. Brush teeth daily (twice daily) and floss, rinse mouth, or brush teeth after eating sweets.
10. Stop smoking; avoid alcohol.

Data from Reference 42.

Evaluation of Therapeutic Outcomes

Efficacy end points for oropharyngeal and esophageal candidiasis include rapid relief of symptoms and prevention of complications without early relapse after completion of the course of therapy.[31,34] Sterilization of the oral cavity is not a feasible end point because mycologic eradication is rarely achievable, especially in HIV-positive patients. Symptomatic relief of presenting signs and symptoms (see Table 143-5) generally occurs within 48 to 72 hours of starting therapy, with complete resolution by 7 to 10 days. Patients should be advised about the time course and told to return for reassessment when signs and symptoms recur. It is usually unnecessary for the patient to be reassessed soon after finishing the treatment course. However, HIV patients should be questioned and examined for the occurrence of mucosal candidiasis as part of their regular follow-up. The frequency of monitoring can be more often in neutropenic patients because of concern for dissemination of candidiasis. During the period of neutropenia, temperature should be monitored daily, as well as signs of dissemination.

Efficacy of the antifungal agent is partly influenced by patient adherence to the medication regimen. Patients must be counseled on proper administration and dosing, in particular for topical agents (Table 143-7).[44] Safety end points include monitoring for occurrence of the relevant drug side effects and drug interactions (see Table 143-6). Mild GI intolerance can occur with topical therapy, but serious adverse effects are rare. It is prudent to monitor for hypersensitivity reactions, especially rash and pruritus that might occur with any medication. GI intolerance is more associated with the oral azoles. Hepatotoxicity can occur when azole therapy is prolonged beyond 7 to 10 days or high doses are used. Periodic monitoring of liver enzymes (alanine transaminase and aspartate amino-transferase) should be considered, especially if prolonged therapy (longer than 21 days) is anticipated. Patients who are receiving IV amphotericin B require daily monitoring by a pharmacist.

MYCOTIC INFECTIONS OF THE SKIN, HAIR, AND NAILS

Superficial cutaneous mycoses affect up to 20% to 25% of the population globally.[49] The usual pathogens are the dermatophytes classified by genera: *Trichophyton*, *Epidermophyton*, and *Microsporum*.[50] Less frequently infection is caused by nondermatophyte fungi (eg, *Malassezia furfur*) and *Candida* species. Dermatophytes can penetrate keratinous structures of the body and therefore infections are limited to hair, nails, and skin. These infections affect both males and females and all races. Reservoirs of mycotic infections include humans, animals, and soil.[50,51] Individuals can develop an infection if they come in contact with a reservoir in addition to having a conducive environment for mycotic growth (ie, moist conditions). Risk factors for the development of an infection include prolonged exposure to sweat or soaking in water, maceration, intertriginous folds, sharing personal belongings such as combs, and close living quarters (dormitories, barracks).[51]

Mycotic infections of the skin have a classic appearance that consists of a central clearing surrounded by an advancing red, scaly, elevated border, also referred to as an "active" border.[52] The central clearing of the lesion may distinguish dermatophytoses from other skin eruptions such as psoriasis or lichen planus that have a more uniform inflammatory presentation.[52] Infections of the nail can appear chalky and dull yellow or white and become brittle and crumbly.

Diagnosis usually is based on patient history, as well as the physical examination.[53,54] Diagnostic tests include direct microscopic examination of a specimen after the addition of KOH or fungal cultures. The KOH test is quick, inexpensive, and easy to perform, whereas cultures are more expensive and take longer to obtain results. Diagnostic tests are recommended when systemic therapy is likely to be prescribed.[53,54]

9 A general approach to treatment of superficial mycotic infections includes keeping the infected area dry and clean and limiting exposure to the infected reservoir. Topical agents generally are considered to be first-line therapy for infections of the skin. Oral therapy is preferred when the infection is extensive or severe or when treating tinea capitis or onychomycosis.[55,56] Table 143-8 lists specific treatments for each mycotic infection. Superficial mycotic infections are categorized by the pattern and site of infection.[50] The most commonly occurring infections in North America are detailed in the following sections.

Tinea Pedis

Tinea pedis is the most common dermatophytoses (affecting ~70% of adults). It is better known as "athlete's foot" and occurs in hot weather, with exposure to surface reservoirs (locker room floors), and with use of occlusive footwear.[51] Tinea pedis has three common presentations. The most common is the interdigital form which is characterized by fissuring, maceration, and scaling of the spaces between the toes (most frequently the fourth and fifth toes). Patients often complain of itching and burning. The "moccasin-like" distribution presentation is usually caused by *Trichophyton rubrum*. In this form the plantar surface becomes chronically scaly and thickened with accompanying erythema of the soles, heels, and sides of the foot. The third presentation, vesiculobulous tinea pedis, is characterized by the formation of vesicles, pustules, and occasionally bullae typically on the soles of the foot. Contact dermatitis, pustular psoriasis, and eczema would be in the differential diagnosis. Disruption of skin integrity with tinea pedis is a risk factor for streptococcal cellulitis as a complication. Treatment with topical therapy for 2 to 4 weeks often is adequate for mild infections; however, severe infections or involvement of the nails require oral therapy[51] (see Table 143-8). Recurrence of infection occurs in up to 70% of individuals especially if there is concomitant onychomycosis. Prolonged treatment with either topical or systemic therapy may be required.[50,55] Other nonpharmacologic measures such as disinfecting footwear, avoidance of walking barefoot in public places, controlling hyperhidrosis, wearing absorbent socks, and nonocclusive shoes should be advised.

TABLE 143-8 Treatment of Mycoses of the Skin, Hair, and Nails

	Topical[a,b]	Oral Regimen[c]
Tinea pedis	Butenafine, daily Sertaconazole, twice daily Luliconazole, daily Naftifine cream daily, gel daily	Fluconazole 150 mg 1 per week × 1-4 weeks
Tinea manuum	Ciclopirox, twice daily	Ketoconazole 200 mg daily × 4 weeks
Tinea cruris	Clotrimazole, twice daily Luliconazole, daily Naftifine cream, daily	Itraconazole 200-400 mg/day × 1 week
Tinea corporis	Econazole, daily	Terbinafine 250 mg/day × 2 weeks
	Haloprogin, twice daily	
	Ketoconazole cream, daily Luliconazole daily	
	Miconazole, twice daily	
	Naftifine cream, daily	
	Oxiconazole, twice daily	
	Sulconazole, twice daily	
	Terbinafine, twice daily	
	Tolnaftate, twice daily	
	Triacetin cream, solution, three times daily	
	Undecylenic acid, various preparations: apply as directed	
Tinea capitis	Shampoo only in conjunction with oral therapy **or** for treatment of asymptomatic carriers	Terbinafine 250 mg/day × 4-8 weeks
Tinea barbae	Ketoconazole twice weekly × 4 weeks	Ketoconazole 200 mg daily × 4 weeks
	Selenium sulfide daily × 2 weeks	Itraconazole 100-200 mg/day × 4-6 weeks
		Griseofulvin 500 mg/day × 4-6 weeks
Pityriasis versicolor	Clotrimazole, twice daily	Ketoconazole
	Econazole, daily	
	Haloprogin, twice daily	Fluconazole
	Ketoconazole, daily	
	Miconazole, twice daily	Itraconazole 200 mg daily × 3-7 days
	Oxiconazole cream only, twice daily	
	Sulconazole, twice daily	
	Tolnaftate, three times daily	
Onychomycosis	Ciclopirox 8% nail lacquer: apply solution at night for up to 48 weeks (fingernails and toenails) Efinaconazole 10% topical solution daily for 48 weeks (toenails) Tavaborole 5% topical solution daily for 48 weeks (toenails)	Terbinafine 250 mg/day × 6 weeks (fingernail), 12 weeks (toenail) Itraconazole 200 mg twice daily × 1 week/month for 2 months (fingernail); 200 mg daily × 12 weeks (toenail) Fluconazole 50 mg daily or 300 mg once weekly for ≥6 months (fingernail) or 12 months (toenail)

[a]Other products are available, including combination products.

[b]Length of therapy depends on mycotic sensitivity and severity of infection.

[c]Only capsule formulation studied; give with food for increased absorption.

Tinea Manuum

Tinea manuum is a superficial fungal infection of one or infrequently both hands, and can involve the feet (tinea pedis). The infection presents with dry and hyperkeratotic palmar surface of the hand. The fingernails, when involved, may present with vesicles and scaling. Contact dermatitis, eczema, psoriasis, and callus formation should be in the differential diagnosis. Treatment of this infection is similar to tinea pedis (see Table 143-8). Emollients that contain lactic acid also can be useful.[51] Relapse or recurrence is frequent especially if tinea pedis or onychomycosis is present.

Tinea Cruris

Tinea cruris is an infection of the proximal thighs and buttocks.[56] It is referred to as "jock itch" and is more common in males. Tinea cruris and tinea pedis often occur concurrently. High humidity and warm temperatures along with wet or tight-fitting clothes contribute to the development of tinea cruris. The scrotum and penis often are spared from infection. The lesions are red, scaling with raised borders. Pustules or vesicles and maceration are usually found along the active border. Itching and burning are the most common patient complaint. The differential diagnosis would include candida infection, erythrasma, mechanical intertrigo, psoriasis, and seborrheic dermatitis.[52] Treatment with topical therapy is recommended and should continue for 1 to 2 weeks after symptom resolution. Severe infections can require oral therapy (see Table 143-8). Relief of pruritus and burning can be facilitated with short-term (2 or 3 days) topical steroids (2.5% hydrocortisone).[51] The feet of the patient should also be examined as a source of infection. Nonpharmacological measures such as keeping the area dry or avoiding prolonged exposure to moisture are important patient counselling points.

Tinea Corporis

Tinea corporis, also known as ringworm, is an infection of the glabrous skin of the trunk, extremities, or face.[52] Lesions of tinea corporis may be singular or multiple and appear as round, scaly lesions with central clearing and a raised border with sharp margination. The border may exhibit pustules. The degree of pruritis is variable. The differential diagnosis includes nummular eczema, contact dermatitis, psoriasis, pityriasis rosea, tinea versicolor, granuloma annulare, and Lyme disease.[52] Prior use of topical corticosteroid preparations may alter the appearance such that the central clearing and raised borders are no longer apparent impacting diagnosis. Diagnosis should be confirmed with KOH examination of skin scrapings of the edge of the lesion. Therapy is similar to that for tinea pedis, tinea manuum, and tinea cruris (see Table 143-8). If the infection is widespread, systemic antifungal therapy may be necessary.

Tinea Capitis

Tinea capitis is a mycotic infection involving the scalp, hair follicles, and adjacent skin that primarily affects children.[57,58] Treatment should consist of oral therapy, as well as the cleaning of combs and brushes, which can be contaminated (see Table 143-8). Daily shampooing is recommended for removal of scales. Some children and adults can be asymptomatic carriers, thereby facilitating spread of the infection.[58] Terbinafine had the highest cure rates at 75%-78% when compared with griseofluvin, ketoconazole, itraconazole, and fluconazole.[59] Family members who culture positive for *Trichophyton tonsurans* should be treated with an antifungal shampoo (eg, ketoconazole, selenium sulfide, or povidone-iodine).[58]

Tinea Barbae

Tinea barbae affects the hairs and follicles of beards and mustaches.[58] Treatment is similar to that for tinea capitis (see Table 143-8). Removal of the beard or mustache is recommended.[51]

Pityriasis Versicolor

Hyper- and hypopigmented scaly patches characterize pityriasis versicolor, which is also known as *tinea versicolor*. It is caused by yeasts of the *Malassezia* genus that, with the exception of *Malassezia pachydermatis*, are all lipophilic. The seborrheic areas (scalp, face, back and front of the trunk) of the human body are always colonized by one or more *Malassezia* spp., such as *M. globosa*, *M. sympodialis*, *M. sloffiae*, and *M. restricta* are the most common colonizers; *M. globosa* and *M. furfur* are most frequent clinical infection isolates. The lesions are found on the trunk, face, and extremities.[50] It is more common in adults and in areas with tropical ambient temperatures. Topical treatment usually is adequate unless there is extensive involvement, recurrent infections, or failure of topical therapy.[60] Ketoconazole 2% shampoo was significantly more effective than selenium sulfide 2.5% shampoo (89% vs 35% cure rate).[60] Recurrence of infection after cessation of treatment may be as high as 60% in the first year and 80% the second year. Suppressive maintenance therapy either orally or topically may be used in these cases.[49]

Onychomycosis (Tinea Unguium)

Onychomycosis is a fungal infection of the nail apparatus and is the most common single cause of nail dystrophy, affecting up to 8% of the general population and accounting for up to 50% of all nail problems.[60-63] Onychomycosis more commonly affects the toenails (2%-14% of adults), ~4 to 19 times more frequently than fingernails, with prevalence increasing with age.[62] This can be because of the slower growth of toenails (three times slower than fingernails), making it easier for fungi to establish infection. Onychomycosis has a significant impact on quality of life, both functional and psychosocial. In addition, the affected nails can disrupt the integrity of the surrounding skin, potentially increasing the risk of secondary bacterial infections.[62]

Onychomycosis is due to infection by dermatophytes (tinea unguium), yeasts, and nondermatophyte fungi.[64] Dermatophytes are the most frequent causes of onychomycosis (~90% in toenail and ~50% in fingernail infections).[65] The dermatophytes responsible for causing >90% of cases of onychomycosis are *Trichophyton rubrum* (71%) and *Trichophyton mentagrophytes* (20%).[57,58] Less common fungi causing onychomycosis are the nondermatophytic molds (2.3%-11%) and yeasts (5.6%). *C. albicans* is the most commonly isolated yeast and typically affects fingernails rather than toenails.[60,66] Risk factors for dermatophytic onychomycosis are increasing age (especially older than 40 years), family history and genetic factors, immunodeficiency (eg, HIV, renal transplant, immunosuppressive therapy, and defective polymorphonuclear chemotaxis), diabetes mellitus, psoriasis, peripheral vascular disease, smoking, prevalence of tinea pedis, frequent nail trauma, and sporting activities such as swimming.[66,67] These risk factors also appear to apply to recurrence of onychomycosis. Mold onychomycosis does not seem to be associated with systemic or local predisposing factors, but there is a risk of systemic dissemination in immunosuppressed patients.[66] *Candida* onychomycosis seems to always occur in immunosuppressed patients.[66]

Onychomycosis can present in four or five different major clinical forms, of which lateral distal subungual onychomycosis is the most common type.[60,66,68] In distal subungual onychomycosis, the nail plate, the nail bed, and, in advanced cases, the matrix are all affected, and *T. rubrum* is the most common etiologic cause. The worst case of onychomycosis is progression of the infection to total dystrophic onychomycosis, characterized by almost complete destruction of the nail plate. White superficial onychomycosis is usually caused by *T. mentagrophytes*, where the infection is localized to the surface of the nail plate. In proximal subungual onychomycosis, the fungi (usually *T. rubrum*) invade the nail through the proximal nail fold and spread to the nail plate and matrix. Although proximal subungual onychomycosis is relatively uncommon in the general population, it occurs most frequently in severely immunocompromised patients and is often considered a marker for AIDS.[66,68] Because of the multifactorial etiology of onychomycosis, it is important to differentiate onychomycosis from other causes of nail dystrophies so that the patient receives appropriate therapy and is not subjected to prolonged treatment with unnecessary drugs. Besides clinical history and physical examination, proper diagnosis of onychomycosis can include the combination of direct microscopy of scrapings from the appropriate nail area to look for fungal hyphae and fungal cultures, and, if necessary, histologic examination.[62,69,70] Table 143-9 provides a differential diagnosis for fungal nail diseases.[71]

TREATMENT

General Approach

In general, onychomycosis of the toenail is more difficult to treat than fingernails, requires longer treatment duration, and is associated with a higher recurrence. The treatment options for onychomycosis include oral and topical therapies, mechanical or chemical nail avulsion, or a combination of these. Onychomycosis merits proper assessment and treatment consideration because it is a debilitating disease and can exert a negative impact on quality of life (eg, cosmetic and psychosocial effects, pain, discomfort, and decreased ambulation).[62,64,66,72] It is reasonable to not treat persons with minimal toenail involvement and no associated symptoms.[71] Although definitive data are lacking regarding the risk of progression of untreated disease, it can lead to complications such as cellulitis or reduced mobility, which can further compromise peripheral circulation in those with diabetes or peripheral vascular disease; additionally, infected nails can serve as a source of transmission of

TABLE 143-9 Differential Diagnosis of Fungal Nail Infections

Diagnosis	Features Consistent with Diagnosis
Psoriasis	Nail pitting, rash elsewhere on body, family history of psoriasis
Lichen planus	Nail atrophy, scarring at proximal aspect of the nail
Periungual squamous cell carcinoma	Single nail affected, pain, warty nail fold change, or ooze from the edge of nail
Yellow nail syndrome	Multiple nails turn yellow, grow slowly, increased longitudinal and transverse curvature, intermittent pain and shedding, associated with chronic sinusitis, bronchiectasis, lymphedema
Trauma	Single nail affected, homogeneous alteration of nail color and altered shape of nail

Reprinted, with permission, from de Berker D. Clinical practice. Fungal nail disease. N Engl J Med. 2009;360:2108–2116. Copyright © 2009 Massachusetts Medical Society. All rights reserved.

TABLE 143-10 Factors That May Impact Treatment Decisions and Outcomes

- Type and severity of onychomycosis
- Causative organism—dermatophyte vs molds or yeast
- Infection of the finger vs toenail
- Extent of disease—involvement of matrix, one or two lateral edges, number of nails
- Thickness of nail plate
- Other sites of mycotic infection (palms, soles, toe webs)
- Other nail alterations affecting outcome (onycholysis, paronychia, dermatophytoma, etc.)
- Other nail diseases and symptoms
- Age and underlying medical conditions (diabetes, poor perfusion, immunocompromised)
- Drug interactions and adverse effects
- Cost of therapy

Data from References 67, 69, and 70.

fungi to other areas of the body, as well as to other people, such as close household contacts, or in communal bathing places.[63,64,66,72,73] Treatment decisions should be made on an individual basis. The primary end point of treatment is eradication of the organism, with secondary end points being clinical cure and improvement.[63] Assessment of clinical success (cure or improvement) requires follow-up for several months after the end of treatment because of the slow growth rate of nails, especially toenails (1 mm/month).[62,66] Successful eradication of the fungus does not always result in normalization of the nails because they can have been dystrophic prior to infection. This can cause patient dissatisfaction, especially if this is not explained before starting treatment.[68] There are several factors that must be taken into account on a patient-by-patient basis to ensure appropriate treatment decisions (Table 143-10). The impact of patient adherence on the success of treatment cannot be overemphasized. Patients need to be educated about their disease, expectations of treatment, and prevention of recurrence, and various strategies have been suggested to improve treatment success.[70]

Topical Therapy

10 Conventional topical antifungal products are available as creams, ointments, powders, and solutions.[64,66,73] Mycological cure rates in open labeled trials are between 45% and 65%; however, cure rates in high quality studies are low (2%-10%). Despite this, most experts consider topical therapy a feasible option when the infection is superficial involving the nail plate without matrix involvement, such as white superficial onychomycosis, involves a partial area of the nail plate not exceeding 50% (owing to difficulty of applying treatment to the margin of the nail), is limited to a few (three or four) nails, is in the early stages of distal subungual onychomycosis when infection is still confined to the distal edge of the nail, or when systemic therapy is contraindicated.[62,66,72] Four products demonstrated cure rates between 2% and 10% after 48 weeks of treatment.[74] The highest quality of evidence was with efinconazole, an azole antifungal agent. Moderate quality evidence was with tavaborole, an oxaborole antifungal, and ciclopirox hydrolacquer. The poorest quality was with ciclopirox 8% lacquer. Amoroline 5% nail lacquer was not included in the review. In separate studies amorolfine produced higher mycologic and treatment cure rates than ciclopirox 8% lacquer.[64,72] Nail lacquers contain a volatile vehicle, used to deliver the drug, evaporates and leaves an occlusive film with a high-drug concentration on the nail surface.[66,73] These insolble therapies require nail filing before application. The ciclopirox hyprolacquer is a water soluble product that does not require nail filing for absorption into the nail.[62,66,72] Combining topical therapy with debridement of the affected nail (thus diminishing the amount of nail requiring treatment) may increase the likelihood of successful treatment, although there is no strong supporting evidence.[71] Topical therapy is not associated with systemic adverse effects or drug interactions. Any adverse effect will be localized to the application site, such as mild erythema in the adjacent skin area.

Systemic Therapy

Oral antifungal therapy is considered to be more effective than topical for treating onychomycosis. Terbinafine and itraconazole (capsule), the first-line agents for treatment, have yielded higher efficacy rates using shorter treatment periods (generally 3 months or shorter) for toenail and fingernail onychomycosis compared with the traditional agents, such as griseofulvin and ketoconazole, which are rarely used nowadays. Terbinafine, an allylamine, exerts fungicidal activity and demonstrates the greatest in vitro activity against dermatophytes compared with the other oral antifungals; it has good activity against nondermatophyte molds and only marginal activity against *Candida* species.[62,73] Like other azoles, itraconazole is fungistatic, has a broad antifungal spectrum, and is active against dermatophytes, nondermatophytes, and *Candida* species.[62,73] Both agents have lipophilic and keratinophilic properties, which explains their excellent penetration (appearing in the nail plate within days of treatment initiation) and accumulation in the nails, achieving concentrations far exceeding the minimal inhibitory concentration (MIC) of most dermatophytes. Nail terbinafine concentrations are detected within 1 week of starting therapy, whereas itraconazole can be detected 1 (fingernails) to 2 weeks (toenails) after starting therapy.[66] Both drugs are slowly eliminated from the nail, with effective drug concentrations persisting in nails for 30 to 36 weeks after completion of treatment with terbinafine and for 27 weeks with itraconazole.[68] The persistence of drug in the nails explains in part the long-term protection against relapses after the end of treatment and also permits use of intermittent (pulse) dosing.

The treatment of toenail onychomycosis requires a 12-week course, whereas a 6-week course is adequate for fingernail onychomycosis with either drug (see Table 143-8).[63,68,75] Terbinafine is the first-line agent for onychomycosis; itraconazole is the alternative. Terbinafine is more effective than itraconazole either by continuous or pulse dosing.[62,72,73] Mycologic cure rates for terbinafine range from 77% to 100% depending on the study.[66,76,77] Continuous terbinafine was the most effective therapy for toenail onychomycosis.[78-81] In addition, terbinafine was reported to achieve high cure rates in high-risk immunosuppressed patients, such as diabetics and organ transplant recipients, comparable to the immunocompetent population, with no significant adverse effects or drug interactions. It also appears to be effective in HIV patients and nondermatophyte infections.[75,81,82] Itraconazole pulse therapy is the preferred method over continuous dosing for fingernail infections, and it is licensed as twice-daily dosing for a 1-week cycle per month for two consecutive months (ie, two pulses), or as daily therapy for 6 weeks (see Table 143-8).[68,75] Although itraconazole pulse therapy is not approved by the US Food and Drug Administration (FDA), three or four pulses are effective for toenail infections; otherwise, half the dose is taken daily for 3 months (see Table 143-8).[68,75] In addition to lower drug cost, the potential advantages of itraconazole pulse therapy compared with continuous therapy are a lower risk of adverse drug effects and improved patient adherence.

Terbinafine was the most cost-effective therapy in terms of highest success rate, lowest relapse rate, and highest number of disease-free days for both fingernail and toenail infections.[83] The cost per cure with the use of oral terbinafine (based on cure rates from clinical trials) ranged from $2,439 to $7,944, depending on disease severity.[84] Compared with the amount of money a patient would consider reasonable to spend on treatment, the expense for a course of systemic therapy is considerably higher.[84,85]

Both terbinafine and itraconazole generally are well tolerated. The more common adverse effects reported with terbinafine are GI (eg, diarrhea, dyspepsia, nausea, and abdominal pain), dermatologic (eg, rash, urticaria, and pruritus), and headache; less common adverse effects are taste disturbances, fatigue, inability to concentrate, and asymptomatic liver enzyme abnormalities.[68,72,75] Terbinafine can cause transient decrease in absolute lymphocyte counts; hence, monitoring of complete blood counts can be useful, especially in immunocompromised patients.[75] Although uncommon, severe adverse effects have been reported with terbinafine, including erythema multiforme, Stevens-Johnson's syndrome, toxic epidermal necrolysis, pancytopenia, lupus erythematosus, psoriasis, hair loss, and hepatotoxicity. Severe hepatotoxicity is rare.[86] Terbinafine thus is not recommended for patients with chronic or active liver disease, although hepatotoxicity can occur in patients with no preexisting liver disease or serious underlying medical condition. Prior to initiating terbinafine treatment, it is recommended to obtain appropriate nail specimens for laboratory testing to confirm the diagnosis of onychomycosis. Liver function parameters (serum transaminases) should be assessed at baseline and periodically during treatment with terbinafine.[75,86]

The common adverse effects of itraconazole are similar to those of terbinafine, such as GI disturbance, dermatologic disorders, and headache; less common adverse effects include dizziness, fatigue, fever, decreased libido, and asymptomatic liver enzyme abnormalities (1%-5% with continuous dosing and ~2% with pulse dosing).[68,72,87] Although still considered rare, 24 serious cases of liver failure, including transplantation and death, have been reported with the use of itraconazole.[86] Some of these patients did not have preexisting liver disease or serious underlying medical conditions, and some developed within the first week of treatment. Itraconazole should be avoided in patients with elevated liver enzymes or active liver disease or in those who have experienced other drug-induced liver toxicity. Liver function parameters (serum transaminases) should be assessed prior to and periodically during treatment. However, some experts have suggested that frequent monitoring is not as necessary if pulse therapy is used because symptomatic hepatotoxicity has not been reported with pulse therapy.[87] In addition, there is risk of developing congestive heart failure (CHF) associated with the use of itraconazole, possibly related to its potential negative inotropic effect.[63,76] Therefore, itraconazole should not be used in patients with evidence of ventricular dysfunction, such as CHF. Symptomatic assessment for the development of CHF also should be included as part of therapy monitoring. Before a patient is subjected to several months of itraconazole treatment, it is important to confirm the diagnosis of onychomycosis.

In contrast to the azoles, terbinafine does not inhibit the cytochrome P450 (CYP)3A4 isoenzymes, but it is a potent inhibitor of the CYP2D6 isoenzymes, which are responsible for metabolism of tricyclic antidepressants and other psychotropic drugs.[63,68,75] The most significant drug interactions with terbinafine are decreased clearance of 33% by cimetidine and increased clearance of 100% by rifampin. Other drug interactions of variable clinical significance are tricyclic antidepressants, cyclosporine, caffeine, theophylline, and terfenadine. Itraconazole and its major metabolite can inhibit the CYP3A4 isoenzymes and result in numerous clinically significant drug interactions where coadministration with several drugs are contraindicated (eg, alprazolam, midazolam, triazolam, pimozide, lovastatin, simvastatin, cisapride, and terfenadine).[62,68,75]

Fluconazole is also active against dermatophytes, *Candida* species, and some nondermatophytes[68,72]; however, it does not have FDA approval for treatment of onychomycosis. The overall mycologic cure rate of fluconazole is 48%, which is lowest compared with all other oral agents.[78] The most effective dose and treatment duration have not been clearly established, with a variety of dosing regimens used, ranging from 50 mg daily to 300 mg once weekly for 6 to 12 months (see Table 143-8).[68,75] The advantages of fluconazole include a relatively good safety profile and fewer drug interactions compared with itraconazole.[68,75]

These three oral antifungal agents have superseded the use of griseofulvin and ketoconazole as treatments of choice for onychomycosis.[62,72,73] Griseofulvin has a narrow antifungal spectrum, low clinical efficacy, especially for toenail infections, high relapse rates, and the need for prolonged treatment duration (up to 12-18 months for toenails). Use of ketoconazole is also associated with high relapse rates, and the prolonged treatment duration carries an increased risk of hepatotoxicity.

Treatment Response and Recurrence

Treatment failures and recurrence rates of infection following initial cure are high, ranging from 20% to 50%.[63,71] Recurrence could be either a relapse (original infection not completely cured) or reinfection (new infection after achieving a cure of the original). Factors associated with poor response to systemic therapy include a compromised immune system (AIDS), reduced blood flow (diabetes, peripheral vascular disease, vasculitis, connective tissue disease, and CHF), coexisting nail disease (psoriasis), nail factors (slow growth, thick nails, and severe disease), drug-resistant organisms because of extensive prior drug exposure, and reduced bioavailability (absorption problems, poor compliance, and drug interactions).[68,71] To improve treatment outcomes and reduce recurrence, patients should be counseled on the importance of proper foot hygiene, for example, wearing breathable footwear and 100% cotton socks with frequent changes, keeping the nails short and clean, keeping the feet dry, protecting the feet in shared bathing areas, treating tinea pedis, and controlling other predisposing medical conditions.[71]

The use of combination therapy (topical–oral or oral–oral agents) can improve cure rates and shorten treatment duration, as this approach provides complementary mechanisms of attack.[71,72] Favorable results were achieved with itraconazole or terbinafine combined with amorolfine.[71,72] To date, no specific combination has been approved or endorsed for use. Other novel approaches include giving supplemental therapy and use of boosted therapy.[71,72] The efficacy and role of either approach remain to be defined.

ABBREVIATIONS

ACOG	American College of Obstetricians and Gynecologists
AIDS	acquired immune deficiency syndrome
BMT	bone marrow transplantation
CHF	congestive heart failure
CMI	cell-mediated immunity
CYP	cytochrome P450
FDA	Food and Drug Administration

GI	gastrointestinal
HAART	highly active antiretroviral therapy
HIV	human immunodeficiency virus
HRT	hormone replacement therapy
HSCT	hematopoietic stem cell transplant
IgA	immunoglobulin A
KOH	potassium hydroxide
MIC	minimum inhibitory concentration
MMT	miconazole mucoadhesive tablet
OPC	oropharyngeal candidiasis
RVVC	recurrent vulvovaginal candidiasis
VVC	vulvovaginal candidiasis

REFERENCES

1. Sobel JD, Faro S, Force R, et al. Vulvovaginal candidiasis: Epidemiologic, diagnostic and therapeutic considerations. *Am J Obstet Gynecol.* 1998;178:203–211.
2. Center for Disease Control and Prevention. Vaginal Discharge-STD Treatment Guidelines. 2006. Available at: www.cdc.gov/std/treatment/2006/vaginaldischarge.htm.
3. Fischer G, Bradford J. Vulvovaginal candidiasis in postmenopausal women: The role of hormone replacement therapy. *J Low Genit Tract Dis.* 2011;15:263–237.
4. Lipsky MS, Waters T, Sharp LK. Impact of vaginal antifungal products on utilization of health care services: Evidence from physician visits. *J Am Board Fam Pract.* 2000;13:178–182.
5. Consumers Healthcare Products Association. OTC sales by category 2014–2017. Available at: www.chpa.org/OTCsCategory.aspx. Accessed May 2018.
6. Gonçalves B, Ferreira C, Alves CT, et al. Vulvovaginal candidiasis: Epidemiology, microbiology and risk factors. *Crit Rev Microbiol.* 2015;42:905–927. 10.3109/1040841x.2015.1091805.
7. Sustr V, Foessleitner P, Kiss H, et al. Vulvovaginal candidosis: Current concepts, challenges and perspectives. *J Fungi.* 2020;6:267. 10.3390/jof6040267.
8. Farr A, Effendy I, Frey Tirri B, et al. Guideline: Vulvovaginal candidosis (AWMF 015/072, level S2k). *Mycoses.* 2021;64:583–602. 10.1111/myc.13248.
9. Camacho DP, Consolaro ME, Patussi EV, Donatti L, Gasparetto A, Svidzinski TL. Vaginal yeast adherence to the combined contraceptive vaginal ring (CCVR). *Contraception.* 2007;76:439–443.
10. Xu J, Schwartz K, Bartoces M, Monsur J, Severson RK, Sobel JD. Effect of antibiotics on vulvovaginal candidiasis: A MetroNet study. *J Am Board Fam Med.* 2008;21:261–268.
11. ACOG practice bulletin: Clinical management guidelines for obstetrician-gynecologists. *Obstet Gynecol.* 2006;107:1195–1206.
12. Watson MC, Bond CM, Grimshaw J, Johnston M. Factors predicting the guideline compliant supply (or non-supply) of non-prescription medicines in the community pharmacy setting. *Qual Saf Health Care.* 2006;15:53–57.
13. Haefner HK. Current evaluation and management of vulvovaginitis. *Clin Obstet Gynecol.* 1999;42:184–195.
14. Wijgert JHHM, Verwijs MC. Lactobacilli-containing vaginal probiotics to cure or prevent bacterial or fungal vaginal dysbiosis: A systematic review and recommendations for future trial designs. *BJOG: Int J Obst Gynaecol.* 2019;127:287–299. 10.1111/1471-0528.15870.
15. Sobel J. Factors involved in patient choice of oral or vaginal treatment for vulvovaginal candidiasis. *Patient Prefer Adher.* 2014;8:31–34. 10.2147/ppa.s38984.
16. Nurbhai M, Grimshaw J, Watson M, Bond CM, Mollison JA, Ludbrook A. Oral versus intravaginal imidazole and triazole antifungal treatment of uncomplicated vulvovaginal candidiasis (thrush). *Cochrane Database Syst Rev.* 2007;4:CD002845. doi:10.1002/14651858.CD002845.pub2.
17. Edelman DA, Grant S. One-day therapy for vaginal candidiasis. A review. *J Reprod Med.* 1999;44:543–547.
18. Mendling W, Plempel M. Vaginal secretion levels after 6 days, 3 days and 1 day of treatment with 100-, 200-, 500-mg vaginal tablets of clotrimazole and their therapeutic efficacy. *Chemotherapy.* 1982;28(suppl 1):43–47.
19. Sobel JD, Kapernick PS, Zervos M, et al. Treatment of complicated candida vaginitis: Comparison of single and sequential doses of fluconazole. *Am J Obstet Gynecol.* 2001;185:363–369.
20. Young G, Jewell D. Topical treatment for vaginal candidiasis (thrush) in pregnancy. *Cochrane Database Syst Rev.* 2001;4:CD000225. doi:10.1002/14651858.CD000225.
21. Sobel JD, Wiesenfeld HC, Martens M, et al. Maintenance fluconazole therapy for recurrent vulvovaginal candidiasis. *N Engl J Med.* 2004;351:363–369.
22. Pappas PG, Kauffman CA, Andes DA, et al. Clinical practice guidelines for the management of candidiasis: 2016 Update by the Infectious Diseases Society of America. *Clin Infect Dis.* 2016;62(4):e1–e50.
23. Edwards JE, Schwartz MM, Schmidt CS, et al. A fungal immunotherapeutic vaccine (NDV-3A) for treatment of recurrent vulvovaginal candidiasis—A phase 2 randomized, double-blind, placebo-controlled trial. *Clin Infect Dis.* 2018;66:1928–1936. 10.1093/cid/ciy185.
24. Sobel JD, Chiam W, Nagappan V, Leaman D. Treatment of vaginitis caused by *Candida glabrata*: Use of topical boric acid and flucytosine. *Am J Obstet Gynecol.* 2003;189:1297–1300.
25. Ray D, Goswami R, Banerjee U, Dadhawl V, et al. Prevalence of *Candida glabrata* and its response to boric acid vaginal suppositories in comparison with oral fluconazole in patients with diabetes and vulvovaginal candidiasis. *Diabetes Care.* 2007;30:312–317.
26. Leigh JE, Shetty K, Fidel PL Jr. Oral opportunistic infections in HIV-positive individuals: Review and role of mucosal immunity. *AIDS Patient Care STDS.* 2004;18:443–456.
27. Farah CS, Lynch N, McCullough MJ. Oral fungal infections: An update for the general practitioner. *Aust Dent J.* 2010;55(1 suppl):48–54.
28. Thompson GR III, Patel PK, Kirkpatrick WR, et al. Oropharyngeal candidiasis in the era of antiretroviral therapy. *Oral Surg Oral Med Oral Pathol Oral Radiol Endod.* 2010;109:488–495.
29. Delgado ACD, de Jesus PR, Aoki FH, et al. Clinical and microbiological assessment of patients with long-term diagnosis of human immunodeficiency virus infection and *Candida* oral colonization. *Clin Microbiol Infect.* 2009;15:364–371.
30. Laudenbach JM, Epstein JB. Treatment strategies for oropharyngeal candidiasis. *Expert Opin Pharmaocother.* 2009;10(9):1413–1421.
31. Benson CA, Kaplan JE, Masur H, et al. Treating opportunistic infections among HIV-infected adults and adolescents: Recommendations from CDC, the National Institutes of Health, and the HIV Medicine Association/Infectious Diseases Society of America. *Clin Infect Dis.* 2004;40:S131–S235.
32. Mercante DE, Leigh JE, Lilly EA, et al. Assessment of the association between HIV viral load and CD4 cell count on the occurrence of oropharyngeal candidiasis in HIV-infected patients. *J Acquir Immune Defic Syndr.* 2006;42:578–583.
33. Soysa NS, Samaranayake LP, Ellepola ANB. Antimicrobials as a contributory factor in oral candidosis: A brief overview. *Oral Dis.* 2008;14:138–143.
34. Pappas PG, Kauffman CA, Andes D, et al. Guidelines for management of candidiasis: 2009 update by the Infectious Diseases Society of America. *Clin Infect Dis.* 2009;48:503–535.
35. Jurevic RJ, Traboulsi RS, Mukherjee PK, et al. Identification of gentian violet concentration that does not stain oral mucosa, possesses anti-candidal activity and is well tolerated. *Eur J Clin Microbiol Infect Dis.* 2011;30(5):629–633.
36. Lalla RV, Bensadoun RJ. Miconazole mucoadhesive tablet for oropharyngeal candidiasis. *Expert Rev Anti Infect Ther.* 2011;9(1):13.
37. Vazquez JA, Patton LL, Epstein JB, et al. Randomized, comparative, double-blind, double-dummy, multicenter trial of miconazole buccal tablet and clotrimazole troches for the treatment of oropharyngeal candidiasis: Study of Miconazole Lauriad® Efficacy and Safety (SMiLES). *HIV Clin Trials.* 2010;11(4):186–196.
38. Hamza OJM, Matee MIN, Bruggemann RJM, et al. Single-dose fluconazole versus standard 2-week therapy for oropharyngeal candidiasis in HIV-infected patients: A randomized, double-blind, double-dummy trial. *Clin Infect Dis.* 2008;47:1270–1276.
39. Vasquez JA, Skiest DJ, Nieto L, et al. A multicenter randomized trial evaluating posaconazole versus fluconazole for the treatment of oropharyngeal candidiasis in subjects with HIV/AIDS. *Clin Infect Dis.* 2006;42:1179–1186.
40. Bensadoun RJ, Daoud J, El Gueddari B, et al. Comparison of the efficacy and safety of miconazole 50 mg mucoadhesive buccal tablets with miconazole 500 mg gel in the treatment of oropharyngeal candidiasis: A prospective, randomized, single-blind, multicenter, comparative, phase III trial in patients treated with radiotherapy for head and neck cancer. *Cancer.* 2008;112(1):204–211.
41. Arathoon EG, Gotuzzo E, Noriega LM, et al. Randomized, double-blind, multicenter study of caspofungin versus amphotericin B for treatment of oropharyngeal and esophageal candidiasis. *Antimicrob Agents Chemother.* 2002;46:451–457.

42. Villanueva A, Gotuzzo E, Arathoon EG, et al. A randomized, double-blind study of caspofungin versus fluconazole for the treatment of esophageal candidiasis. *Am J Med.* 2002;113:294–299.
43. Deresinski SC, Stevens DA. Caspofungin. *Clin Infect Dis.* 2003;36:1445–1457.
44. Akpan A, Morgan R. Oral candidiasis. *Postgrad Med J.* 2002;78:455–459.
45. Morris MI, Villmann M. Echinocandins in the management of invasive fungal infections, part 1. *Am J Health Syst Pharm.* 2006;63:1693–1703.
46. Grim SA, Smith KM, Romanelli F, Ofotokun I. Treatment of azole-resistant oropharyngeal candidiasis with topical amphotericin B. *Ann Pharmacother.* 2002;36:1383–1386.
47. Goldman M, Cloud GA, Wade KD, et al. A randomized study of the use of fluconazole in continuous versus episodic therapy in patients with advanced HIV infection and a history of oropharyngeal candidiasis: AIDS clinical trials group study 323/mycoses study group 40. *Clin Infect Dis.* 2005;41:1473–1480.
48. Marr KA, Bow E, Chiller T, et al. Fungal Infection prevention after hematopoietic cell transplantation. *Bone Marrow Transplant.* 2009;44:483–487.
49. Routt ET, Jim On SC, Zeichner JA, Kircik LH. What is new in fungal pharmacotherapeutics? *J Drugs Dermatol.* 2014;13(4): 391–395.
50. Schwartz RA. Superficial fungal infections. *Lancet.* 2004;364:1173–1182.
51. Mendez-Tovar LJ. Pathogenesis of dermatophytosis and tinea versicolor. *Clin Dermatol.* 2010;28:185–189.
52. Hainer BL. Dermatophyte infections. *Am Fam Physician.* 2003;67:101–108.
53. Drake LA, Dinehart SM, Farmer ER, et al. Guidelines of care for superficial mycotic infections of the skin: Tinea corporis, tinea cruris, tinea faciei, tinea manuum, and tinea pedis. *J Am Acad Dermatol.* 1996;34:282–286.
54. Sahoo AK, Mahajan R. Management of tinea corporis, tinea cruris and tinea pedis. A comprehensive review. *Dermatol Online J.* 2016;7:77–86.
55. Gupta AK, Chow M, Daniel CR, Aly R. Treatments of tinea pedis. *Dermatol Clin.* 2003;21:431–462.
56. Gupta AK, Chaudhry M, Elewski B. Tinea corporis, tinea cruris, tinea nigra, and piedra. *Dermatol Clin.* 2003;21:395–400.
57. Higgins EM, Fuller LC, Smith CH. Guidelines for the management of tinea capitis. *Br J Dermatol.* 2000;143:53–58.
58. Hay RJ. Tinea capitis: Current status. *Mycopathologia.* 2016;182:87–93. 10.1007/s11046-016-0058-8.
59. Gupta AK, Bamimore MA, Renaud HJ, et al. A network meta-analysis on the efficacy and safety of monotherapies for tinea capitis, and an assessment of evidence quality. *Pediatr Dermatol.* 2020;37:1014–1022. 10.1111/pde.14353.
60. Ansarun H, Ghaffarpour G. Comparison of effectiveness between ketoconazole 2% and selenium sulfide 2% shampoos in the treatment of tinea versicolor. *Iranian J Derm.* 2005;8:21–25.
61. Effendy I, Lecha M, Feuilhade de Chauvin M, et al. Epidemiology and clinical classification of onychomycosis. *J Eur Acad Dermatol Venereol.* 2005;19(supp 11):8–12.
62. Roberts DT, Taylor WD, Boyle J. Guidelines for treatment of onychomycosis. *Br J Dermatol.* 2003;148:402–410.
63. Nunley KS, Cornelius L. Current management of onychomycosis. *J Hand Surg.* 2008;33A:1211–1214.
64. Welsh O, Vera-Cabrera L, Welsh E. Onychomycosis. *Clin Dermatol.* 2010;28:151–159.
65. Kaur R, Kashyap B, Bhalla P. Onychomycosis—Epidemiology, diagnosis and management. *Indian J Med Microbiol.* 2008;26(2):108–116.
66. Baran R, Kaoukhov A. Topical antifungal drugs for the treatment of onychomycosis: An overview of current strategies for monotherapy and combination therapy. *J Eur Acad Dermatol Venereol.* 2005;19:21–29.
67. Tosti A, Hay R, Arenas-Guzman R. Patients at risk of onychomycosis—Risk factor identification and active prevention. *J Eur Acad Dermatol Venereol.* 2005;19(suppl 1):13–16.
68. Iorizzo M, Piraccini BM, Rech G, Tosti A. Treatment of onychomycosis with oral antifungal agents. *Expert Opin Drug Deliv.* 2005;2:435–440.
69. Feuilhade de Chauvin M. New diagnostic techniques. *J Eur Acad Dermatol Venereol.* 2005;19(suppl 1):20–24.
70. Gupta AK, Tu LQ. Onychomycosis therapies: Strategies to improve efficacy. *Dermatol Clin.* 2006;24:381–386.
71. de Berker D. Fungal nail disease. *N Engl J Med.* 2009;360:2108–2116.
72. Lecha M, Effendy I, Feuilhade de Chauvin M, et al. Treatment options—Development of consensus guidelines. *J Eur Acad Dermatol Venereol.* 2005;19(suppl 1):25–33.
73. Gupta AK, Tu LQ. Therapies for onychomycosis: A review. *Dermatol Clin.* 2006;24:375–379.
74. Foley K, Gupta AK, Versteeg S, et al. Topical and device-based treatments for fungal infections of the toenails. *Cochrane Database Syst Rev.* 2020;(1):CD012093. 10.1002/14651858.cd012093.pub2.
75. Gupta AK, Ryder JE, Skinner AR. Treatment of onychomycosis: Pros and cons of antifungal agents. *J Cutan Med Surg.* 2004;8:25–30.
76. Sigurgeirsson B, Elewski EE, Rich PA, et al. Intermittent versus continuous terbinafine in the treatment of toenail onychomycosis: A randomized, double-blind, comparison. *J Dermatol Treat.* 2006;17:38–44.
77. Warshaw EM, Fett DD, Bloomfield HE, et al. Pulse verus continuous terbinafine for onychomycosis: A randomized, double-blind, controlled trial. *J Am Acad Dermatol.* 2005;53:578–584.
78. Gupta AK, Ryder JE, Johnson AM. Cumulative meta-analysis of systemic antifungal agents for the treatment of onychomycosis. *Br J Dermatol.* 2004;150:537–544.
79. Haugh M, Helou S, Boissel JP, Cribier BJ. Terbinafine in fungal infections of the nails: A meta-analysis of randomized clinical trials. *Br J Dermatol.* 2002;147:118–121.
80. Crawford F, Young P, Godfrey C, et al. Oral treatments for toenail onychomycosis: A systematic review. *Arch Dermatol.* 2002;138:811–816.
81. Cribier BJ, Bakshi R. Terbinafine in the treatment of onychomycosis: A review of its efficacy in high-risk populations and in patients with nondermatophyte infections. *Br J Dermatol.* 2004;150:414–420.
82. Gupta AK, Lynch LE, Kogan N, et al. The use of intermittent terbinafine for the treatment of dermatophyte toenail onychomycosis. *J Eur Acad Dermatol Venereol.* 2009;23:256–262.
83. Casciano J, Amaya K, Doyle J, et al. Economic analysis of oral and topical therapies for onychomycosis of the toenails and fingernails. *Manag Care.* 2003;12:47–54.
84. Schram SE, Warshaw EM. Costs of pulse versus continuous terbinafine for onychomycosis. *J Am Acad Dermatol.* 2007;56:525–527.
85. Cham PM, Chen SC, Grill JP, et al. Reliability of self-reported willingness-to-pay and annual income in patients treated for toenail onychomycosis. *Br J Dermatol.* 2007;156:922–928.
86. Food and Drug Administration. FDA issues health advisory regarding the safety of Sporanox products and Lamisil tablets to treat finger nail infections. 2001. Available at: www.fda.gov/cder/drug/advisory/sporanox-lamisil/advisory.htm.
87. Gupta AK, Chwetzoff, Del Rosso J, Baran R. Hepatic safety of itraconazole. *J Cutan Med Surg.* 2002;6:210–213.

144

Invasive Fungal Infections

Peggy L. Carver and Gregory A. Eschenauer

KEY CONCEPTS

1. Systemic mycoses can be caused by pathogenic fungi and include histoplasmosis, coccidioidomycosis, cryptococcosis, blastomycosis, paracoccidioidomycosis, and sporotrichosis, or infections by opportunistic fungi such as *Candida albicans*, *Aspergillus* species, *Trichosporon*, *Candida glabrata*, *Fusarium*, *Alternaria*, and *Mucor*.
2. The diagnosis of fungal infection is accomplished by careful evaluation of clinical symptoms, results of serologic tests, and histopathologic examination and culture of clinical specimens. Rapid, accurate diagnostic laboratory tests are currently under development.
3. Histoplasmosis is caused by *Histoplasma capsulatum* and is endemic in parts of the central United States along the Ohio and Mississippi River valleys, and in Central and South America. Although most patients experience asymptomatic infection, some can experience chronic, disseminated disease.
4. Asymptomatic patients with histoplasmosis are not treated, while patients with evident disease are treated with either oral itraconazole or an IV amphotericin B lipid formulation.
5. Blastomycosis is caused by *Blastomyces dermatitidis*. In the immunocompetent host, acute pulmonary blastomycosis can be mild and self-limited and may not require treatment. However, consideration should be given to treating all infected individuals to prevent extrapulmonary dissemination. All persons with moderate-to-severe pneumonia, disseminated infection, or those who are immunocompromised require antifungal therapy.
6. Coccidioidomycosis is caused by *Coccidioides immitis* and *Coccidioides posadasii* and is endemic in some parts of the southwestern United States. It can cause nonspecific symptoms, acute pneumonia, or chronic pulmonary or disseminated disease. Primary pulmonary disease (unless severe) frequently is not treated, whereas disseminated and meningeal disease is treated with fluconazole.
7. Cryptococcosis is caused by *Cryptococcus neoformans*, which occurs primarily in immunocompromised patients, and *Cryptococcus gattii*, which occurs primarily in nonimmunocompromised patients. Patients with acute meningitis are treated with lipid formulations of amphotericin B with flucytosine. Patients infected with human immunodeficiency virus (HIV) often require long-term suppressive therapy with fluconazole or itraconazole.
8. A variety of *Candida* species (including *C. albicans*, *C. glabrata*, *Candida tropicalis*, *Candida parapsilosis*, and *Candida krusei*) can cause diseases such as mucocutaneous, oral, esophageal, vaginal, and hematogenous candidiasis, as well as candiduria. Candidemia can be treated with a variety of antifungal agents; the optimal choice depends on previous patient exposure to antifungal agents, potential drug interactions and toxicities of each agent, and local epidemiology of intensive care unit (ICU) or hematology–oncology centers.
9. Aspergillosis can be caused by a variety of *Aspergillus* species that can cause superficial infections, pneumonia, allergic bronchopulmonary aspergillosis (BPA), or invasive infection. Voriconazole has emerged as the drug of choice of most clinicians for primary therapy of most patients with invasive aspergillosis (IA). Combination therapy may be considered in cases of severe infection, especially in patients with persistent neutropenia.

BEYOND THE BOOK

Watch the following two videos, which provide a brief (9:48) overview of the epidemiology, diagnosis, and treatment of candidemia

Candida: Systemic Candidiasis Treatment & Prevention. https://tinyurl.com/u22fqmt

INTRODUCTION

1 Advances in medical technology including organ and bone marrow transplantation, cytotoxic chemotherapy, the widespread use of indwelling IV catheters, and the increased use of potent broad-spectrum antimicrobial agents all have contributed to the dramatic increase in the incidence of fungal infections worldwide.[1-3] Problems remain in the diagnosis, prevention, and treatment of fungal infections.[1,4-6] The Infectious Diseases Society of America (IDSA) publishes guidelines regarding the prophylaxis and treatment of many commonly encountered fungal infections.[7-12]

MYCOLOGY

Fungi are eukaryotic organisms with a defined nucleus enclosed by a nuclear membrane; a cytoplasmic membrane containing lipids, glycoproteins, and sterols, mitochondria, golgi apparatus, and ribosomes bound to endoplasmic reticulum; and a cytoskeleton with microtubules, microfilaments, and intermediate filaments. Fungi have rigid cell walls composed of chitin, cellulose, or both that stain with Gomori methenamine silver or periodic acid–Schiff reagent. Most fungi, except *Candida* species, are too weakly gram-positive to

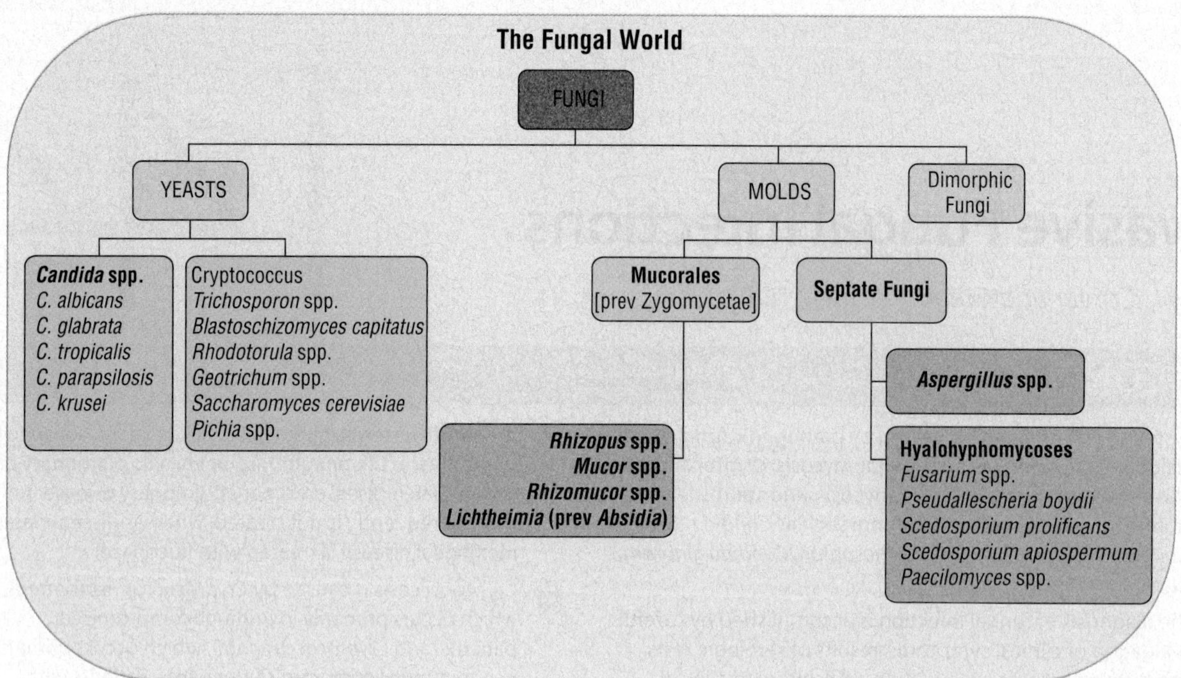

FIGURE 144-1 Morphologically, pathogenic fungi can be grouped as either filamentous molds or unicellular yeasts. Molds grow as multicellular branching, thread-like filaments (hyphae) that are either septate (divided by transverse walls) or coenocytic (multinucleate without crosswalls).

be seen well on Gram stain. *Cryptococcus neoformans* has a polysaccharide capsule surrounding the cell wall.[1]

Morphologically, pathogenic fungi can be grouped as either filamentous molds or unicellular yeasts (Fig. 144-1). *Molds* grow as multicellular branching, threadlike filaments (hyphae) that are either septate (divided by transverse walls) or coenocytic (multinucleate without crosswalls). Yeasts are oval or spherically shaped unicellular forms that generally produce pasty or mucoid colonies on agar medium similar to those observed with bacterial cultures. Yeasts have rigid cell walls and reproduce by budding, a process in which daughter cells arise from pinching off a portion of the parent cell.

Many pathogenic fungi, including the etiological agents of histoplasmosis, coccidioidomycosis, blastomycosis, paracoccidioidomycosis, and sporotrichosis, are termed *dimorphic fungi.* These pathogens can exist as either a yeast or a mold, depending on the pathogen, ambient CO_2, the production of host 17-beta-estradiol, the site of growth (in the host or in the laboratory setting), and temperature. Temperature shifts provoke reversible conversions between the hyphal (22-25°C) and yeast (37°C) phases. Dimorphic fungi can infect humans with either normal or impaired host immune defenses. Usually, yeasts are the parasitic form that invades human or animal host tissue, whereas molds are the free-living form found in the environment.[13]

Clinical Versus Microbial Resistance

Host factors contribute greatly to clinical outcome. A patient may respond clinically to treatment with an antifungal agent despite resistance to that agent in vitro because the patient's own immune system may eradicate the infection, or the agent may reach the site of infection in high concentrations. Thus, in vitro susceptibility does *not* necessarily equate with in vivo clinical success, and in vitro resistance might *not* always correlate with treatment failure.[6]

It is important to distinguish between clinical resistance and microbial resistance. *Clinical resistance* refers to failure of an antifungal agent in the treatment of a fungal infection that arises from factors other than microbial resistance, such as failure of the antifungal agent to reach the site of infection or inability of a patient's immune system to eradicate a fungus whose growth is retarded by an antifungal agent.[14]

Microbial resistance can refer to *primary* or *secondary* resistance, as determined by in vitro susceptibility testing using standardized methodology. *Primary* or *intrinsic resistance* refers to resistance recorded prior to drug exposure in vitro or in vivo. *Secondary* or *acquired resistance* develops on exposure to an antifungal agent and can be either reversible, owing to transient adaptation, or acquired as a result of one or more genetic alterations.[14]

Susceptibility Testing of Antifungal Agents

Most laboratories do not routinely perform susceptibility tests on fungal isolates, but standardized methods for performing these tests are being developed and are now available for testing selected yeasts. As the prevalence of nosocomial and community-acquired fungal infections become more prominent, the need for in vitro susceptibility testing increases. Susceptibility testing is occasionally indicated, for example, in a patient with prolonged fungemia with a presumed susceptible isolate, and is most helpful in dealing with infections caused by non-*albicans* species of *Candida.*[5-7]

Clinical breakpoints (CBPs) are antimicrobial concentrations (MICs) obtained from susceptibility testing, which are used to define isolates as susceptible, intermediate, or resistant. No CBPs have been established for posaconazole, isavuconazole, or amphotericin B versus *Candida*, or for antifungal agents and filamentous fungi such as *Aspergillus.*[6] CBPs can be used to differentiate strains for which there is a high likelihood of treatment success (organisms that are clinically susceptible [S]), from those for which treatment is more likely to fail (clinically resistant [R]) (Tables 144-1–144-3). A clinically intermediate (I) or susceptible dose-dependent (SDD) category can be assigned to pathogens for which the level of antimicrobial agent activity is associated with uncertain therapeutic effect, implying that infections due to the isolate may be appropriately treated in body sites where the drugs are

TABLE 144-1 General Patterns of In Vitro Susceptibility of *Candida* Species

	Patterns of Susceptibility						
	Azoles					Echinocandins	Amphotericin B
Candida species	Fluconazole	Itraconazole	Voriconazole	Posaconazole	Isavuconazole	Caspofungin Anidulafungin Micafungin	
C. albicans	Yes	Yes	Yes	Yes	Yes	Yes	Yes
C. tropicalis	Yes	Yes	Yes	Yes	Yes	Yes	Yes
C. parapsilosis	Yes	Yes	Yes	Yes	Yes	Yes[a]	Yes
C. glabrata	Variable[b]	Variable[b]	Variable[b]	Variable[b]	Variable[b]	Yes	Yes
C. krusei	No	Yes	Yes	Yes	Yes	Yes	Yes
C. lusitaniae	Yes	Yes	Yes	Yes	Yes	Yes	Variable[c]

[a]Most isolates of *C. parapsilosis* have reduced susceptibility to echinocandins.

[b]Approximately 15% of *C. glabrata* isolates are resistant to fluconazole; *C. glabrata* generally exhibits cross-resistance across the azole class.[15]

[c]Although frank resistance to amphotericin B is not observed in all isolates, it is well described for isolates of *C. lusitaniae.*

Data from Reference 7.

TABLE 144-2 General Patterns of In Vitro Susceptibility of Non-*Candida* Fungal Pathogens

	Patterns of Susceptibility						
	Azoles					Echinocandins	Amphotericin B
Pathogen	Fluconazole	Itraconazole	Voriconazole	Posaconazole	Isavuconazole	Caspofungin Anidulafungin Micafungin	Yes
Aspergillus fumigatus/ flavus	No	Yes	Yes	Yes	Yes	Yes	Yes
Aspergillus terreus	No	Yes	Yes	Yes	Yes	Yes	No
Fusarium	No	No	Variable	Variable	Variable	No	Variable
Scedosporium	No	No	Yes	Variable	Variable	No	No
Lomentospora	No	No	Variable	No	No	No	No
Mucorales[a]	No	No	No	Variable	Variable	No	Yes
Cryptococcus	Yes	Yes	Yes	Yes	Yes	No	Yes
Histoplasma	Yes	Yes	Yes	Yes	Yes	No[b]	Yes
Coccidioides	Yes	Yes	Yes	Yes	Yes	No[b]	Yes

[a]Includes *Rhizopus*, *Mucor*, and *Absidia* species.

[b]While the echinocandins display activity against the mycelial forms of endemic fungi such as *Histoplasma* spp., *Blastomyces* spp., and *Coccidioides* spp., they display significantly higher MIC values against the yeast forms of these organisms, and should not be used to treat these infections.

Data from References 9, 10, 12, and 16.

TABLE 144-3 Clinical Breakpoints for *Candida* Species and Azole Antifungals

Drug[a]	Species	Interpretive Clinical Breakpoints (mg/L)			
		S	I	SDD	R
Fluconazole	*C. albicans*	≤2	---	4	≥8
	C. glabrata	---	---	≤32	≥64
	C. krusei	---	---	---	---
	C. parapsilosis	≤2	---	4	≥8
	C. tropicalis	≤2	---	4	≥8
Voriconazole	*C. albicans*	≤0.12	0.25-0.5	---	≥1
	C. glabrata	---	---	---	---
	C. krusei	≤0.5	1	---	≥2
	C. parapsilosis	≤0.12	0.25-0.5	---	≥1
	C. tropicalis	≤0.12	0.25-0.5	---	≥1

[a]Clinical breakpoints have not been established for isavuconazole by CLSI.

S, susceptible; I, intermediate; SDD, susceptible-dose dependent; R, resistant; ---, not defined or not applicable.

Data from Reference 6.

physically concentrated or when a high dosage of drug can be used. Although CBPs are designed to guide therapy, they do not distinguish between fungal isolates with or without resistance mechanisms, nor do they always allow for early detection of resistant isolates.[6] Table 144-3 shows the currently approved interpretive CBPs for *Candida* species.

Resistance to Antifungal Agents

Understanding mechanisms of resistance is an important process in the optimization of antifungal therapy. The most exhaustive and definitive accounts of antifungal resistance have been described in *Candida* species, in particular *C. albicans* and, to a lesser extent, *C. glabrata*, *C. tropicalis*, and *Candida krusei*, as well as in a few *C. neoformans* isolates.[14] *C. glabrata* isolates are increasingly resistant to both azole and echinocandin antifungal agents.

There are four different mechanisms that result in azole resistance: (a) mutations or upregulation of *ERG11* (an enzyme involved in the ergosterol biosynthesis pathway), (b) expression of multidrug efflux transport pumps that decrease antifungal drug accumulation within the fungal cell, (c) alteration of the structure or concentration of antifungal drug target proteins,

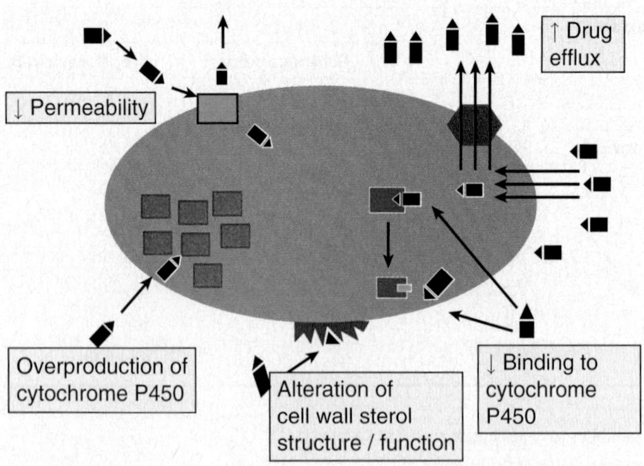

FIGURE 144-2 Mechanisms of azole resistance. Four different mechanisms result in azole resistance: (a) mutations or upregulation of *ERG11*, the target enzyme of azoles, (b) expression of multidrug efflux transport pumps that decrease antifungal drug accumulation within the fungal cell, (c) alteration of the structure or concentration of antifungal drug target proteins, and (d) alteration of membrane sterol proteins.

and (d) alteration of membrane sterol proteins (Fig. 144-2). Although detailed analysis of each of the elucidated mechanism of resistance is beyond the scope of this chapter, interested readers are referred to a publication that has comprehensively summarized this topic.[14]

The most commonly reported mechanisms of azole resistance among *C. albicans* isolates include reduced permeability of the fungal cell membrane to azoles, modification or overproduction of the target fungal enzymes (cytochrome P450, CYP) resulting in decreased binding of the azole to the target site, alterations in sterol synthesis, and activation of efflux pumps capable of actively pumping azoles from the target pathogen. Fluconazole resistance is observed most frequently in *C. glabrata*, which is often resistant, and in *C. krusei*, for which fluconazole resistance is universal.[5,14] With the increase in echinocandin use, there has been an increase in the number of reports of echinocandin-resistant isolates from patients failing therapy. Echinocandin exposure and previous episodes of *C. glabrata* are predictors of FKS gene mutations in *Candida*.[17,18]

Although, to date, the rate of amphotericin B resistance remains low, the exact incidence remains difficult to quantify and the response to antifungal agents difficult to characterize.[6] As such, no consensus for therapy has been formulated at this time, although clinicians should keep in mind that *C. glabrata, Candida guilliermondii, C. krusei*, and *Candida lusitaniae* may have a higher propensity to developing resistance than other species.

Acquired resistance of *Aspergillus* species during long-term azole exposure, while still relatively uncommon, is emerging, and varies widely between geographic centers. Acquisition of primary-resistant isolates is also increasing, due to the agricultural use of azoles.[19] Cross-resistance of azole-resistant strains of *Aspergillus* to amphotericin B has not been described. Azole resistance among *Aspergillus* spp. (specifically *Aspergillus fumigatus*) is predominantly mediated by specific point mutations in TR/L98H in the CYP51A gene promoter region, causing amino acid changes and tandem repeats, and often results in cross-resistance with azole antifungals.[19]

EPIDEMIOLOGY AND PATHOGENESIS

Systemic mycoses caused by primary or pathogenic fungi include histoplasmosis, coccidioidomycosis, cryptococcosis, blastomycosis, paracoccidioidomycosis, and sporotrichosis. Primary pathogens can cause disease in both healthy and immunocompromised individuals, although disease generally is more severe or disseminated in the immunocompromised host.[1] *Candida* species are commensals in humans, and most infections are iatrogenic.[20] Mycoses caused by opportunistic fungi such as *Aspergillus* species, *Fusarium*, *Alternaria*, and *Mucor* are found only in the immunocompromised host.[1]

Most fungal infections are acquired as a result of accidental inhalation of airborne conidia. For example, *Histoplasma capsulatum* is found in soil contaminated by bat, chicken, or starling excreta, and *C. neoformans* is associated with pigeon droppings. Although some fungi, including *C. neoformans*, and *Aspergillus* species, are ubiquitous pathogens with worldwide distribution, other fungi have regional distributions associated with specific geographic environments.[1]

Invasive fungal infections (IFIs) are a major cause of morbidity and mortality in the immunocompromised patient.[21,22] Patients with decreased neutrophil counts or decreased neutrophil function are at higher risk of infections, particularly infections caused by *Candida* and *Aspergillus* species. In patients with hematologic malignancies and following hematopoietic stem cell transplantation (HSCT), there has been a shift in the most commonly encountered IFIs from *Candida* spp. to *Aspergillus* spp.[23,24]

Nosocomially acquired fungal infections can arise from either exogenous or endogenous flora. Endogenous flora can include normal commensal organisms of the skin, GI, genitourinary, or respiratory tract. *C. albicans* is found as a normal commensal of the GI tract in 20% to 30% of humans. A complex interplay of host and pathogen factors influences the acquisition and development of fungal infections. Intact skin or mucosal surfaces serve as primary barriers to infection. Alterations in the balance of normal flora caused by the use of antibiotics or alterations in nutritional status can allow the proliferation of fungi such as *Candida*, increasing the likelihood of systemic invasion and infection.[20] *Candida* species are the fourth most commonly isolated bloodstream isolate.[25]

Diagnosis and Rapid Diagnostic Tests

2 The diagnosis of IFIs is accomplished by careful evaluation of clinical symptoms, results of serologic tests, and histopathologic examination and culture of clinical specimens. While direct microscopy, culture and histological techniques constitute the "gold standard" for diagnosis, obtaining biopsies from sterile body sites for these studies is a highly invasive approach that may not be possible in severely ill patients. Also, histopathology lacks sensitivity and selectivity, as several filamentous fungi may exhibit undistinguishable morphologies. Further, the finding of a positive culture from a sterile site may indicate transient colonization and not true infection, especially for opportunistic fungi. Fungi may require special laboratory conditions, with additional time (up to 4 days) required in order to obtain species identification and the results of susceptibility testing. Some species, such as *C. glabrata*, tend to grow more slowly; initial identification of yeast from blood averages 100 hours (~4 days) in most institutions.[27] Several rapid, accurate diagnostic laboratory tests, including matrix-assisted laser desorption ionization time-of-flight mass spectrometry (MALDI-TOF), peptide nucleic acid (PNA) in situ hybridization (PNA-FISH), PCR, galactomannan, and T2 magnetic resonance assays, have the potential to enhance sensitivity and speed of diagnosis of IFIs.[28,29]

New laboratory methods that allow for early differentiation of IFIs due to *Aspergillus* species versus zygomycetes and other molds would be helpful in allowing clinicians in the earlier initiation of appropriate antifungal therapy. These underscore the need for rapid diagnosis and identification of clinically significant isolates to species level, and the need for susceptibility testing.[28]

Risk Factors for Fungal Infections

Increasing use of aggressive and intensive cancer chemotherapeutic regimens, immunosuppressive therapy for autoimmune disorders, and transplantation have led to an increase in the number of susceptible hosts, contributing to the changing epidemiology of fungal infections. Infection epidemiology can drastically vary depending on patients' underlying concomitant conditions, comorbidities, confounding risk factors, and geographical area.[20]

A clinical indicator for a patient's immunologic status is the quantitation of absolute neutrophil count (ANC). Neutropenia, defined as an ANC $\leq$ 500/mm^3 (0.5 $\times$ 10^9/L), dramatically escalates the risk of acquiring and opportunistic infection. Major risk factors for *Candida* bloodstream infections (BSIs) in ICU patients include the use of central venous catheters (CVCs), receipt of multiple antibiotics or parenteral nutrition (PN), extensive surgery and burns, renal failure and hemodialysis, mechanical ventilation, and prior fungal colonization.[26]

TREATMENT

Invasive Mycoses

Strategies for the prevention or treatment of invasive mycoses can be classified broadly as prophylaxis, early empirical therapy, empirical therapy, and secondary prophylaxis or suppression. In patients undergoing cytotoxic chemotherapy, antifungal therapy is directed primarily at the prevention or treatment of infections caused by *Candida* and *Aspergillus* species.

Prophylactic therapy with oral or IV antifungal agents is administered prior to and throughout periods of granulocytopenia (absolute neutrophil count < 1,000 cells/μL [1 $\times$ 10^9/L]) or other immunosuppressive events (such as development of graft-versus-host disease [GvHD] in hematopoietic stem cell transplant recipients). The potential benefits of prophylactic therapy must be weighed against the potential risks inherent in each regimen, including safety, efficacy, cost, the prevalence of infection, and the potential consequences (eg, resistance) of widespread use.[23,24]

Empirical therapy is the administration of systemic antifungal agents in patients with signs and symptoms of fungal infection, but without confirmation of infection. For example, empirical therapy with systemic antifungal agents is administered to granulocytopenic patients with persistent or recurrent fever despite the administration of appropriate antimicrobial therapy.[30,31]

Secondary prophylaxis (or *suppressive therapy*) is the administration of systemic antifungal agents (generally prior to and throughout the period of granulocytopenia) to prevent relapse of documented IFI.[32]

HISTOPLASMOSIS

In humans, histoplasmosis is caused by inhalation of dust-borne microconidia of the dimorphic fungus *H. capsulatum*. Although there exist two dimorphic varieties of *H. capsulatum*, the small-celled (2-5 μm) form (var. *capsulatum*) occurs globally, whereas the large-celled (8-15 μm) form (var. *duboisii*) is confined to the African continent and Madagascar. In tissues stained by conventional techniques, *H. capsulatum* appears as an oval or round, narrow-pore, budding, unencapsulated yeast.[33]

Epidemiology

3 Although histoplasmosis is found worldwide, certain areas of North, Central, and South America are recognized as highly endemic areas. In the United States, most disease is localized along the Ohio and Mississippi River valleys, where more than 90% of residents may be affected. However, due to differences in reporting requirements, variable diagnostic methodologies and capabilities, and a lack of adequate surveillance, particularly in low-resource settings, infections occur in other areas. Infections have been increasingly identified in some classically "non-endemic" areas of the United States, including the Rocky Mountain states (Montana and Idaho), the southeast (Florida and South Carolina), and the North Central states of Minnesota and North Dakota. Additional cases are being reported in Africa, Asia, and worldwide, in patients with HIV or those receiving immunosuppressive agents.[34]

Precise reasons for this endemic distribution pattern are unknown but are thought to include moderate climate, humidity, and soil characteristics. *H. capsulatum* is found in nitrogen-enriched soils, particularly those heavily contaminated by avian or bat guano, which accelerates sporulation. Blackbird or pigeon roosts, chicken coops, and sites frequented by bats, such as caves, attics, or old buildings, serve as "microfoci" of infections; once contaminated, soils yield *Histoplasma* for many years. Although birds are not infected because of their high body temperature, bats (mammals) may be infected and can pass yeast forms in their feces, allowing the spread of *H. capsulatum* to new habitats. Air currents carry the spores for great distances, exposing individuals who were unaware of contact with the contaminated site.[33]

Pathophysiology

At ambient temperatures, *H. capsulatum* grows as a mold. The mycelial phase consists of septate branching hyphae with terminal micro- and macroconidia that range in size from 2 to 14 μm in diameter. When soil is disturbed, these conidia become aerosolized and reach the bronchioles or alveoli.[33]

Animal studies demonstrate that within 2 to 3 days after reaching lung tissue, the conidia germinate, releasing yeast forms that begin multiplying by binary fission. During the next 9 to 15 days, organisms are ingested but not destroyed by large numbers of macrophages that are recruited to the infected site, resulting in small infiltrates. Infected macrophages migrate to the mediastinal lymph nodes and other sites within the mononuclear phagocyte system, particularly the spleen and liver. At this time, the onset of specific T-cell immunity in the nonimmune host activates the macrophages, rendering them capable of fungicidal activity. Tissue granulomas form, many of which develop central caseation and necrosis over the next 2 to 4 months. Over a period of several years, these foci become encapsulated and calcified, often with viable yeast trapped within the necrotic tissue.[33]

Cellular immunity, as measured by histoplasmin skin-test reactivity, wanes in the absence of occasional reexposure. Although exposure to heavy inocula can overcome these immune mechanisms, resulting in severe disease, reinfection occurs frequently in endemic areas. In the immune individual, the reactions of acquired immunity begin 24 to 48 hours after the appearance of yeast forms, resulting in milder forms of illness and little proliferation of organisms. Although viable organisms can be found within granulomas years after initial infection, the organisms appear to have little ability to proliferate within the fibrous capsules, except in immunocompromised patients.[33]

Clinical Presentation

The outcome of infection with *H. capsulatum* depends on a complex interplay of host, pathogen, and environmental factors.[10,33] Host factors include the degree of immunosuppression and the presence of immunity (from prior infection). Environmental factors include inoculum size, exposure within an enclosed area, and duration of exposure. Hematogenous dissemination from the lungs to other tissues probably occurs in all infected individuals during the first

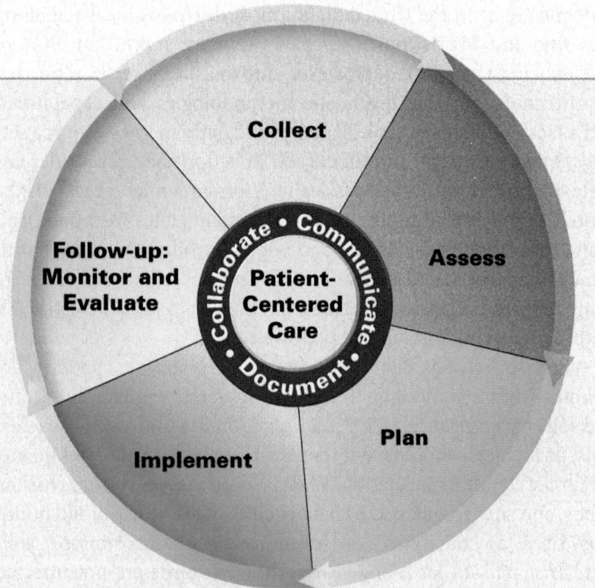

Patient Care Process for Candidemia

Collect

- Patient characteristics (eg, age, sex, pregnant)
- Patient medical history (personal and family)
- Social history (eg, intravenous drug use)
- Current medications including non-prescription aspirin/NSAID use, herbal products, dietary supplements, and prior antifungal therapy
- Prior antifungal therapy (if applicable)
- Objective data
  - Blood pressure (BP), heart rate (HR), respiratory rate (RR), height, weight, O_2-saturation
  - Laboratory findings including white blood cells (WBC) with differential, hemoglobin (Hgb), platelets, serum creatinine (SCr), liver function tests (LFTs), blood cultures and susceptibility data
  - Objective confirmation of candidemia (+ blood cultures)

Assess

- Hemodynamic stability (eg, systolic BP 110 bpm, O_2-sat <90% [0.90], RR)
- Presence of
  - Ability/willingness to pay for antifungal agents
  - Ability/willingness to obtain laboratory monitoring tests
- Emotional status (eg, presence of anxiety, depression)

Plan*

- Empiric drug therapy regimen including specific antifungal agent(s), dose, route, frequency, and duration (see Table 144-9); and plan for step-down antifungal therapy, if appropriate, based on blood culture results (*Candida* species) of susceptibility testing, patient-specific factors (eg, LFTs, SCr, prior antifungal therapy, severity of illness)
- Monitoring parameters including efficacy including signs and symptoms of infection, temperature, BP, HR, WBC, daily blood cultures until negative cultures are obtained, transthoracic or transesophageal echocardiogram (TTE or TEE), ophthalmological examination, and safety (eg, LFTs, SCr, rash)
- Patient education (eg, purpose of treatment, drug-specific information)
- Referrals to other providers when appropriate (eg, ophthalmology)

Implement*

- Provide patient education regarding all elements of treatment plan
- Schedule follow-up (eg, labs, susceptibility data)

Follow-up: Monitor and Evaluate

- Resolution of symptoms (eg, shortness of breath, chest pain, limb swelling, redness, pain)
- Presence of adverse effects (three- to fivefold increase in LFTs, increased SCr, presence of rash)
- Patient adherence to treatment plan using multiple sources of information
- Reevaluate antifungal agent(s) to assess need for specific therapy (pathogen-directed, based on results of blood cultures) including step-down antifungal therapy, once final blood cultures and the results of susceptibility testing are available
- Reevaluate duration of therapy as blood culture and other laboratory data become available after the start of therapy (see text)

Collaborate with patient, caregivers, and other healthcare professionals.

2 weeks of infection before specific immunity has developed but is nonprogressive in most cases, which leads to the development of calcified granulomas of the liver and/or spleen. Progressive pulmonary infection is common in patients with underlying centrilobular emphysema.

Acute and chronic manifestations of histoplasmosis appear to result from unusual inflammatory or fibrotic responses to the pathogen, including pericarditis and rheumatologic syndromes during the first year after exposure, with chronic mediastinal inflammation or fibrosis, broncholithiasis, and enlarging parenchymal granulomas later in the course of disease.

In the vast majority of patients, low-inoculum exposure to *H. capsulatum* results in mild or asymptomatic pulmonary histoplasmosis. However, in Africa, infection with *H. capsulatum* var. *duboisii* results primarily in skin and soft tissue infection and only rarely in pulmonary disease.[34] The course of disease generally is benign, and symptoms usually abate within a few weeks of onset. Patients exposed to a higher inoculum during an acute primary infection or reinfection can experience an acute, self-limited illness with flu-like pulmonary symptoms, including fever, chills, headache, myalgia, and a nonproductive cough. Patients with diffuse pulmonary histoplasmosis can have diffused radiographic involvement, become hypoxic, and require ventilatory support. A low percentage of patients present with arthritis, erythema nodosum, pericarditis, or mediastinal granuloma.

Chronic pulmonary histoplasmosis generally presents as an opportunistic infection imposed on a preexisting structural

TABLE 144-4 Clinical Manifestations and Therapy of Histoplasmosis

Type of Disease and Common Clinical Manifestations	Therapy/Comments
Acute pulmonary histoplasmosis	
Asymptomatic or mild-to-moderate disease	*Asymptomatic, mild, or symptoms <4 weeks:* No therapy is generally required. Itraconazole[a] orally (200 mg three times daily for 3 days and then 200 mg once or twice daily for 6-12 weeks) is recommended for patients who continue to have symptoms for greater than 1 month
Moderately severe to severe diffuse pulmonary disease	Lipid amphotericin B 3-5 mg/kg/day IV for 1-2 weeks followed by itraconazole orally 200 mg orally three times daily for 3 days then twice daily for a total of 12 weeks of therapy; methylprednisolone (0.5-1 mg/kg daily IV) during the first 1-2 weeks of antifungal therapy is recommended for patients who develop respiratory complications, including hypoxemia or significant respiratory distress
CNS histoplasmosis	Amphotericin B should be used as initial therapy (lipid formulations at 5 mg/kg/day IV, for a total dosage of 175 mg/kg for 4-6 weeks, followed by itraconazole orally 200 mg two or three times daily for at least a year; some patients may require lifelong therapy; response to therapy should be monitored by repeat lumbar punctures to assess *Histoplasma* antigen levels, WBC, and CSF antibody titers
Progressive histoplasmosis	*Moderately severe to severe:* Liposomal amphotericin B (3 mg/kg daily) IV, amphotericin B lipid complex (ABLC, 5 mg/kg daily) IV, or deoxycholate amphotericin B (0.7-1 mg/kg daily) for 1-2 weeks IV, followed by itraconazole orally (200 mg twice daily for at least 12 months) *Mild to moderate:* Itraconazole (200 mg orally twice daily for at least 12 months). Immunosuppressed patients may require lifelong suppressive therapy with itraconazole 200 mg daily

[a]Itraconazole plasma concentrations should be measured during the second week of therapy to ensure that detectable concentrations have been achieved. If the concentration is below 1 mcg/mL (mg/L; 1.4 μmol/L), the dose may be insufficient or drug interactions can be impairing absorption or accelerating metabolism, requiring a change in dosage. If plasma concentrations are greater than 10 mcg/mL (mg/L; 14 μmol/L), the dosage can be reduced.

Data from References 10 and 33.

abnormality, such as lesions resulting from emphysema. Patients demonstrate chronic pulmonary symptoms and apical lung lesions that progress with inflammation, calcified granulomas, and fibrosis. Patients with early, non-cavitary disease often recover without treatment. Progression of disease over a period of years, seen in 25% to 30% of patients, is associated with cavitation, bronchopleural fistulas, extension to the other lung, pulmonary insufficiency, and often death.

In patients exposed to a large inoculum and in immunocompromised hosts, successful containment of the organism within macrophages may not occur, resulting in a progressive illness characterized by yeast-filled phagocytic cells and an inability to produce granulomas. This disease, termed *disseminated histoplasmosis*, is characterized by persistent parasitization of macrophages. The clinical severity of the diverse forms of disseminated histoplasmosis (Table 144-4) generally parallels the degree of macrophage parasitization observed.

Acute (infantile) disseminated histoplasmosis is characterized by massive involvement of the mononuclear phagocyte system by yeast-engorged macrophages. Typically, this severe type of infection is seen in infants and young children and (rarely) in adults with Hodgkin's disease or other lymphoproliferative disorders. In infants or children, acute disseminated histoplasmosis is characterized by unrelenting fever, anemia, leukopenia or thrombocytopenia, enlargement of the liver, spleen, and visceral lymph nodes, and GI symptoms, particularly nausea, vomiting, and diarrhea. The chest roentgenogram often demonstrates remnants of the initiating acute pulmonary lesion. Untreated disease is uniformly fatal in 1 to 2 months. A less severe "subacute" form of the disease, which occurs in both infants and immunocompetent adults, is characterized by focal destructive lesions in various organs, weight loss, weakness, fever, and malaise. Untreated disease is fatal in approximately 10 months.

Most adults with disseminated histoplasmosis demonstrate a mild, chronic form of the disease. Untreated patients often are ill for 10 to 20 years, demonstrating long asymptomatic periods interrupted by relapses of clinical illness characterized primarily by weight loss, weakness, and fatigue. Chronic disseminated histoplasmosis can be seen in patients with lymphoreticular neoplasms (Hodgkin's disease) and patients undergoing immunosuppressant chemotherapy for organ transplantation or for rheumatic diseases. Although CNS involvement occurs in 10% to 20% of patients with severe underlying immunosuppressive conditions, focal organ involvement is uncommon. The disease is characterized by the development of focal granulomatous lesions, often with bone marrow involvement resulting in thrombocytopenia, anemia, and leukemia. Fever, hepatosplenomegaly, and GI ulceration are common.

Histoplasmosis in HIV-Infected Patients

Adult patients with AIDS demonstrate an acute form of disseminated disease that resembles the syndrome seen in infants and children. Progressive disseminated histoplasmosis (PDH), which is defined as a clinical illness that does not improve after at least 3 weeks of observation and that is associated with physical or radiographic findings and/or laboratory evidence of involvement of extrapulmonary tissues, can occur as the direct result of initial infection or because of the reactivation of dormant foci. In endemic areas, 50% of AIDS patients demonstrate PDH as the first manifestation of their disease. PDH is characterized by fever (75% of patients), weight loss, chills, night sweats, enlargement of the spleen, liver, or lymph nodes, and anemia. Pulmonary symptoms occur in only one-third of patients and do not always correlate with the presence of infiltrates on chest roentgenogram. A clinical syndrome resembling septicemia is seen in approximately 25% to 50% of patients.[10]

Diagnosis

The diagnosis of histoplasmosis is made on the basis of histopathology, cultures, antigen detection, and serologic tests for *Histoplasma*-specific antibodies. Detection of single, ovoid cells 2 to 5 μm in diameter with narrow-based budding by direct examination or by histologic study of blood smears or tissues should raise strong suspicion of infection with *H. capsulatum* because colonization does not occur as with *Aspergillus* or *Candida* infection. In patients with acute self-limited histoplasmosis, extensive testing to verify the diagnosis may not be necessary.[33]

In most patients, serologic evidence (complement fixation test or immunodiffusion testing) remains the primary method in the diagnosis of histoplasmosis. Detection of *Histoplasma* antigen by enzyme immunoassay (EIA) in the urine, blood, or bronchoalveolar lavage fluid of infected patients provides rapid diagnostic information and is particularly useful in patients who are severely ill. The highest sensitivity is obtained by testing both urine and serum.[33] *Histoplasma* EIA has also been used to monitor the course of therapy and to detect relapses in patients with AIDS, and the clearance of antigen from serum and urine correlates with clinical efficacy during maintenance therapy.[33]

Treatment

4 Table 144-4 summarizes the recommended therapy for the treatment of histoplasmosis. In general, asymptomatic or mildly ill patients and patients with sarcoid-like disease do not benefit from antifungal therapy. In the vast majority of patients, low-inoculum exposure to *H. capsulatum* results in *mild* or *asymptomatic* pulmonary histoplasmosis. The course of disease generally is benign, and symptoms usually abate within a few weeks of onset. Therapy can be helpful in symptomatic patients whose conditions have not improved during the first month of infection. Fever persisting more than 3 weeks can indicate that the patient is developing progressive disseminated disease, which can be aborted by antifungal therapy. Whether antifungal therapy hastens recovery or prevents complications is unknown because it has never been studied in prospective trials. The goals of therapy are resolution of clinical abnormalities, prevention of relapse, and eradication of infection whenever possible, although chronic suppression of infection can be adequate in immunosuppressed patients, including those with HIV disease.[10] Such patients may also require longer durations of therapy and lifelong suppressive therapy if immunosuppression cannot be reduced.

Fluconazole remains a second-line agent for the treatment of histoplasmosis due to inferior outcomes as compared to itraconazole in patients with and without AIDS. Clinical data regarding the use of newer azoles are limited. *Histoplasma* isolates from patients who have relapsed following therapy with fluconazole retain susceptibility to itraconazole, posaconazole, and isavuconazole, but not voriconazole. Voriconazole was clinically inferior to itraconazole as an initial or step-down therapeutic regimen.[35,36] While both have activity against *Histoplasma*, posaconazole appears to be more active than itraconazole in the immune compromised and non-immune compromised mouse model of infection. Both agents have been used successfully in a few patients. Of note, the echinocandins have no activity against *Histoplasma*.

In regions experiencing high rates of histoplasmosis (>5 cases/100 patient-years), itraconazole 200 mg/day orally is recommended as prophylactic therapy in HIV-infected patients. Fluconazole is not an acceptable alternative because of its inferior activity against *H. capsulatum* and its lower efficacy for the treatment of histoplasmosis.[10]

Although patients receiving secondary prophylaxis (chronic maintenance therapy) might be at low risk for recurrence of systemic mycosis when their $CD4^+$ T lymphocyte counts increase to greater than 100 cells/μL (0.1×10^9/L) in response to highly active antiretroviral therapy (HAART), the number of patients who have been evaluated is insufficient to warrant a recommendation to discontinue prophylaxis.

Evaluation of Therapeutic Outcomes

Response to therapy should be measured by resolution of radiologic, serologic, and microbiologic parameters and by improvement in signs and symptoms of infection. Although investigators are limited by the lack of standardized criteria to quantify the extent of infection, degree of immunosuppression, or treatment response, response rates (based on resolution or improvement in presenting signs and symptoms) of greater than 80% have been reported in case series in AIDS patients receiving varied dosages of amphotericin B. Rapid responses are reported, with the resolution of symptoms in 25% and 75% of patients by days 3 and 7 of therapy, respectively.

After the initial course of therapy for histoplasmosis is complete, lifelong suppressive therapy in some patients with oral azoles is recommended because of the frequent recurrence of infection. Relapse rates in AIDS patients not receiving maintenance therapy range from 50% to 90%.[10] Antigen testing can be useful for monitoring therapy since concentrations decrease with therapy and increase with relapse.

BLASTOMYCOSIS

Blastomycosis is a systemic fungal infection primarily caused by the *Blastomyces dermatitidis* complex, a dimorphic fungus that infects primarily the lungs. Patients, however, can present with a variety of pulmonary and extrapulmonary clinical manifestations. Pulmonary disease can be acute or chronic and can mimic infection with tuberculosis, pyogenic bacteria, other fungi, or malignancy. Blastomycosis can disseminate to virtually every other body organ, and approximately 40% of patients with blastomycosis present with skin, bone and joint, or genitourinary tract involvement without any evidence of pulmonary disease.[8,37]

Pulmonary infection probably occurs by inhalation of conidia, which convert to the yeast form in the lung. A vigorous inflammatory response ensues, with neutrophilic recruitment to the lungs followed by the development of cell-mediated immunity and the formation of non-caseating granulomas.

Epidemiology

The *Blastomyces dermatitidis* complex includes *B. dermatitidis* and *B. gilchristii*, although they are often referred to solely as *B. dermatitidis*. *B. dermatitidis* has been isolated from soil containing decayed vegetation, decomposed wood, and pigeon manure, frequently in association with warm, moist soil of wooded areas near fresh water. *B. dermatitidis* is endemic to the southeastern and south central states of the United States (especially those bordering on the Mississippi and Ohio River basins) and the Midwestern states and Canadian provinces bordering the Great Lakes and St. Lawrence River. Infection due to other rarer species occurs outside this endemic region, such as *B. helicus* in the western United States.[8,37] Although initial review of sporadic cases suggested that males with outdoor occupations that exposed them to soil were at greatest risk for blastomycosis, there is no sex, age, or occupational predilection for blastomycosis.[8,37]

Pathophysiology and Clinical Presentation

Colonization does not occur with *Blastomyces*.[8,37] *Pulmonary blastomycosis* is the most common manifestation, and can range from asymptomatic infection to acute pneumonia with or without respiratory failure to chronic disease. Typical symptoms of acute pulmonary infection include fever, shaking chills, and productive, purulent cough, with or without hemoptysis. The clinical presentation can be difficult to differentiate from other respiratory infections, including bacterial pneumonia, on the basis of clinical symptoms alone. Development of the acute respiratory distress syndrome (ARDS) is associated with high mortality.

Sporadic pulmonary blastomycosis can present as a more chronic or subacute disease, with low-grade fever, night sweats, weight loss, and productive cough that resembles tuberculosis rather than bacterial pneumonia. *Chronic pulmonary blastomycosis* is characterized by fever, malaise, weight loss, night sweats, chest pain, and productive cough. Patients often are thought to have tuberculosis and frequently have evidence of disseminated disease that can appear 1 to 3 years after the primary pneumonia has resolved. Reactivation of disease can occur in the lungs or as the focus of new infection in other organs.

In approximately 15% to 50% of patients, dissemination occurs, with the most common sites including the skin and bony skeleton, although less commonly the prostate, oropharyngeal mucosa, and abdominal viscera are involved. CNS disease, while exceedingly uncommon, is associated with the highest mortality rate.

Laboratory and Diagnostic Tests

The simplest and most successful method of diagnosing blastomycosis is by direct microscopic visualization of the large,

TABLE 144-5 Therapy of Blastomycosis

Type of Disease	Preferred Treatment
Pulmonary[a]	
Moderately severe to severe disease	Lipid formulation of amphotericin B 3-5 mg/kg IV daily or amphotericin B[b] 0.7-1 mg/kg IV daily (total dose 1.5-2.5 g) × 1-2 weeks or until improvement is noted, followed by itraconazole[c] 200 mg orally three times daily for 3 days, then 200 mg twice daily, × total of 6-12 months
Mild-to-moderate disease	Itraconazole[b] 200 mg orally three times daily for 3 days, then 200 mg twice daily, for a total of 6 months[b]
CNS disease	*Induction:* Lipid formulation of amphotericin B 5 mg/kg IV daily × 4-6 weeks, followed by an oral azole as consolidation therapy *Consolidation:* Fluconazole 800 mg orally daily, or itraconazole[c] 200 mg two or three times orally daily, or voriconazole 200-400 mg orally twice daily, for ≥12 months and until resolution of CSF abnormalities
Disseminated or Extrapulmonary Disease	
Moderately severe to severe disease	Lipid formulation of amphotericin B 3-5 mg/kg IV daily or amphotericin B[b] 0.7-1 mg/kg IV daily × 1-2 weeks or until improvement is noted, followed by itraconazole[c] 200 mg orally three times daily for 3 days, then 200 mg twice daily × 6-12 months. Treat osteoarticular disease with 12 months of antifungal therapy Most clinicians prefer to step down to itraconazole[c] therapy once the patient's condition improves
Mild to moderate	Itraconazole[c] 200 mg orally three times daily for 3 days, then 200 mg once or twice daily × ≥12 months. Treat osteoarticular disease with 12 months of antifungal therapy
Immunocompromised Host (Including Patients with AIDS, Transplants, or Receiving Chronic Glucocorticoid Therapy)	
Acute disease	Lipid formulation of amphotericin B 3-5 mg/kg IV daily or amphotericin B[a] 0.7-1 mg/kg IV daily × 1-2 weeks or until improvement is noted, then give suppressive therapy for a total of at least 12 months of therapy
Suppressive therapy	Itraconazole[c] 200 mg orally three times daily for 3 days, then 200 mg twice daily for a total of at least 12 months of therapy; lifelong suppressive therapy with oral itraconazole[c] 200 mg daily may be required for immunosuppressed patients in whom immunosuppression cannot be reversed, and in patients who experience relapse despite appropriate therapy

[a]In the immunocompetent host, acute pulmonary blastomycosis can be mild and self-limited and may not require treatment.

[b]Desoxycholate amphotericin B.

[c]Serum levels of itraconazole should be determined after the patient has received itraconazole for ≥2 weeks, to ensure adequate drug exposure.

[d]Azoles should not be used during pregnancy.

AIDS, acquired immunodeficiency syndrome.

Data from Reference 8.

multinucleated yeast with single, broad-based buds in sputum or other respiratory specimens following staining.[8,37] Culture growth is slow and can require up to 30 days to isolate and identify a small inoculum.

No reliable skin test exists to determine the incidence and prevalence of disease in endemic populations, and reliable serologic diagnosis of blastomycosis is not available. Quantitative antigen testing is available, with highest sensitivity from urine samples, although cross-reactivity with other endemic fungi (including *H. capsulatum*) results in a low specificity.[37]

Treatment

Non-HIV-Infected Patient

5 In the immunocompetent host, acute pulmonary blastomycosis can be mild and self-limited and may not require treatment. However, consideration should be given to treating all infected individuals to prevent extrapulmonary dissemination. All individuals with moderate-to-severe pneumonia, disseminated infection, or those who are immunocompromised require antifungal therapy.

In patients with mild-to-moderate pulmonary blastomycosis, itraconazole is effective; however, in patients with moderately severe to severe pulmonary disease, the clinical presentation of the patient, the immune competence of the patient, and the toxicity of the antifungal agents are the main determinants of the choice of antifungal therapy (Table 144-5). In the case of disease limited to the lungs, cure might have occurred without treatment before the diagnosis is made. Regardless of whether or not the patient receives treatment, however, he or she must be followed carefully for many years for evidence of reactivation or progressive disease.[8,37]

Some authors recommend azole therapy for the treatment of self-limited pulmonary disease, with the hope of preventing late extrapulmonary disease; however, data supporting the efficacy of these regimens are lacking.[8,37] Itraconazole 200 to 400 mg/day demonstrated 90% efficacy as a first-line agent in the treatment of non-life-threatening non-CNS blastomycosis, and for compliant patients who completed at least 2 months of therapy, a success rate of 95% was noted. No therapeutic advantage was noted with the higher (400 mg) dosage as compared with patients treated with 200 mg.[38]

All patients with disseminated blastomycosis, as well as those with extrapulmonary disease, require therapy. Amphotericin B is recommended for patients with overwhelming or life-threatening disease, CNS infection, and treatment failures.[8,37] Lipid preparations of amphotericin B have largely replaced conventional amphotericin B for treatment of blastomycosis, despite their higher cost, due to their decreased renal toxicity. Surgery has only a limited role in the treatment of blastomycosis.

HIV-Infected Patient

For unclear reasons, blastomycosis is an uncommon opportunistic disease among immunocompromised individuals, including AIDS patients; however, blastomycosis can occur as a late (CD4 lymphocytes < 200 cells/mm^3 [0.2 × 10^9/L]) and frequently fatal complication of HIV infection. In this population, overwhelming disseminated disease with frequent involvement of the CNS is common.[8,37] Following induction therapy with amphotericin B (total cumulative dose of 1 g), HIV-infected patients should receive chronic suppressive therapy with an oral azole antifungal for at least a year and until they are on effective antiretroviral therapy with a CD4+ T-cell count > 150 cells/μL (0.15 × 10^9/L).[8,37]

COCCIDIOIDOMYCOSIS

Epidemiology

Coccidioidomycosis is caused by infection with *Coccidioides immitis* and *Coccidioides posadasii,* dimorphic fungi found in the southwestern and western United States, as well as in parts of Mexico and South America. In North America, the endemic regions encompass the semiarid areas of the southwestern United States from California to Texas known as the Lower Sonoran Zone, where there is scant annual rainfall, hot summers, and sandy, alkaline soil. *Coccidioides* grows in the soil as a mold, and mycelia proliferate during the rainy season. During the dry season, resistant arthroconidia form and become airborne when the soil is disturbed.

Although generally considered to be a regional disease, coccidioidomycosis has increased in importance in recent years

TABLE 144-6 Factors for Severe, Disseminated Infection with Coccidioidomycosis

Race (Filipino and African American ancestry)
Pregnancy (especially when infection is acquired or reactivated in the second or third trimester)
Male gender
Neonates
Compromised cellular immune system, including
• AIDS patients
• Patients receiving corticosteroids, immunosuppressive agents, or chemotherapy

AIDS, acquired immune deficiency syndrome.

Data from Reference 39.

because of the increased tourism and population in endemic areas, the increased use of immunosuppressive therapy in transplantation and oncology, and the AIDS epidemic. Although there is no racial, hormonal, or immunologic predisposition for acquiring primary disease, these factors affect the risk of subsequent dissemination of disease (Table 144-6).[39]

Pathophysiology

When individuals come in contact with contaminated soil during ranching, dust storms, or proximity to construction sites or archeological excavations, arthroconidia are inhaled into the respiratory tree, where they transform into spherules, which reproduce by cleavage of the cytoplasm to produce endospores. The endospores are released when the spherules reach maturity. Similar to histoplasmosis, an acute inflammatory response in the tissue leads to infiltration of mononuclear cells, ultimately resulting in granuloma formation.[39]

Clinical Presentation

Coccidioidomycosis encompasses a spectrum of illnesses ranging from primary uncomplicated respiratory tract infection that resolves spontaneously to progressive pulmonary or disseminated infection.[39] Initial or primary infection almost always involves the lungs. Although approximately one-third of the population in endemic areas is infected, the average incidence of symptomatic disease is only approximately 0.43%.

Signs and Symptoms

Primary Coccidioidomycosis ("*Valley Fever*"): Approximately 60% of infected patients have an asymptomatic, self-limited infection without clinical or radiological manifestations. Most of the remaining 40% of patients exhibit non-specific symptoms that are often indistinguishable from ordinary upper respiratory infections, including fever, cough, headache, sore throat, myalgias, and fatigue that occur 1 to 3 weeks after exposure to the pathogen. More commonly, a diffuse, mild erythroderma or maculopapular rash is observed. Patients can have pleuritic chest pain and peripheral eosinophilia.

A fine, diffuse rash can appear during the first few days of the illness. Primary pneumonia can be the first manifestation of disease, characterized by a productive cough that can be blood-streaked, as well as single or multiple soft or dense homogeneous hilar or basal infiltrates on chest roentgenogram. *Chronic, persistent pneumonia, or persistent pulmonary coccidioidomycosis* (primary disease lasting more than 6 weeks) is complicated by hemoptysis, pulmonary scarring, and the formation of cavities or bronchopleural fistulas.

Necrosis of pulmonary tissue with drainage and cavity formation occurs commonly. Most parenchymal cavities close spontaneously or form dense nodular scar tissue that can become superinfected with bacteria or spherules of *Coccidioides*. These patients often have persistent cough, fevers, and weight loss.

Disseminated disease occurs in less than 1% of infected patients. The most common sites for dissemination are the skin, lymph nodes, bone, and meninges, although spleen, liver, kidney, and adrenal gland also can be involved. Occasionally, miliary coccidioidomycosis occurs with rapid, widespread dissemination, often in concert with positive blood cultures for *Coccidioides*. Patients with AIDS frequently present with miliary disease. Coccidioidomycosis in AIDS patients appears to be caused by reactivation of disease in most patients. Dissemination also is more likely if infection occurs during pregnancy, especially during the third trimester or in the immediate postpartum period.[39]

CNS infection occurs in approximately 16% of patients with disseminated coccidioidomycosis. Patients can present with meningeal disease without previous symptoms of primary pulmonary infection, although disease usually occurs within 6 months of the primary infection. The signs and symptoms are often subtle and non-specific, including headache, weakness, changes in mental status (lethargy and confusion), neck stiffness, low-grade fever, weight loss, and occasionally, hydrocephalus. Space-occupying lesions are rare, and the main areas of involvement are the basilar meninges.

The diagnoses of coccidioidomycosis generally utilizes identification or recovery of *Coccidioides* spp. from clinical specimens and detection of specific anticoccidioidal antibodies in serum or other body fluids.

TREATMENT

Goals of Therapy

Desired outcomes of treatment are resolution of signs and symptoms of infection, reduction of serum concentrations of anticoccidioidal antibodies, and return of function of involved organs. It would also be desirable to prevent relapse of illness on discontinuation of therapy, although current therapy is often unable to achieve this goal.

General Approach

6 Therapy for coccidioidomycosis is difficult, and the results are unpredictable. Guidelines[11] are available for treatment of this disease; however, optimal treatment for many forms of this disease still generates debate. The efficacy of antifungal therapy for coccidioidomycosis often is less certain than that for other fungal etiologies, such as blastomycosis, histoplasmosis, or cryptococcus, even when in vitro susceptibilities and the sites of infections are similar. The refractoriness of coccidioidomycosis can relate to the ability of *Coccidioides* spherules to release hundreds of endospores, maximally challenging host defenses.[39] Fortunately, only approximately 5% of infected patients require therapy.

Specific Agents Used for the Treatment of Coccidioidomycosis

Although there is continued disagreement among experts in endemic areas whether antifungal therapy in patients with uncomplicated early coccidioidal infection might shorten the course of illness or reduce the development of more serious complications, prospective randomized trials addressing this question are lacking. The excellent tolerability of oral azoles has lowered the threshold for deciding to treat primary infection, and clinicians should treat patients with significantly debilitating illness, those with extensive pulmonary disease, and with who are frail due to advanced age, concurrent diabetes or comorbidities.[11]

Azole antifungals, primarily fluconazole and itraconazole, have replaced amphotericin B as initial therapy for most chronic pulmonary or disseminated infections. Amphotericin B is now usually reserved for patients with respiratory failure because of infection with *Coccidioides* species, those with rapidly progressive coccidioidal infections, or women during pregnancy. Therapy often ranges from many months to years in duration, and in some patients, lifelong suppressive therapy is needed to prevent relapses. Specific antifungals (and their usual dosages) for the treatment of coccidioidomycosis include IV lipid formulations of amphotericin B (3-5 mg/kg/day), IV or oral fluconazole (usually 400-800 mg/day, although dosages as high as 1,200 mg/day have been used without complications), and itraconazole (200-300 mg orally twice daily or three times daily, as capsules or solution).[39] If itraconazole is used, measurement of serum concentrations can be helpful to ascertain whether oral bioavailability is adequate.

Given the efficacy and superior tolerability profile of the triazole antifungals, amphotericin B products are generally only recommended for patients refractory to or intolerant of other agents, or in those with rapid deterioration. Compared to amphotericin B deoxycholate, the lipid formulations of amphotericin B have not been studied extensively in coccidioidal infection but can offer a means of giving more drug with less toxicity. Fluconazole probably is the most frequently used medicine given its tolerability, although high relapse rates have been reported in some studies. Itraconazole therapy resulted in superior response in patients with skeletal infection, and relapse rates in the overall study population were lower with itraconazole therapy than with fluconazole.[39,40] Posaconazole was effective treatment in patients with refractory infections. Its efficacy relative to other triazole antifungals is unknown.

Combination therapy with members of different classes of antifungal agents has not been evaluated in patients, and there is a hypothetical risk of antagonism. However, some clinicians feel that outcome in severe cases is improved when amphotericin B is combined with an azole antifungal. If the patient improves, the dosage of amphotericin B can be slowly decreased while the dosage of azole is maintained.[39]

Primary Respiratory Infection

Although most patients with symptomatic primary pulmonary disease recover without therapy, management should include follow-up visits for 1 to 2 years to document resolution of disease or to identify as early as possible evidence of pulmonary or extrapulmonary complications.

Patients with a large inoculum, severe infection, or concurrent risk factors (eg, HIV infection, organ transplant, pregnancy, or high doses of corticosteroids) probably should be treated, particularly those with high CF titers, in whom incipient or occult dissemination is likely. Because some racial or ethnic populations have a higher risk of dissemination, some clinicians advocate their inclusion in the high-risk group. Common indicators that are used to judge the severity of infection include weight loss (greater than 10%), intense night sweats persisting more than 3 weeks, infiltrates involving more than one-half of one lung or portions of both lungs, prominent or persistent hilar adenopathy, CF antibody titers of greater than 1:16, failure to develop dermal sensitivity to coccidioidal antigens, inability to work, or symptoms that persist for more than 2 months.[39]

Commonly prescribed therapies include currently available oral azole antifungals at their recommended doses for courses of therapy ranging from 3 to 6 months.[39] In patients with diffuse pneumonia with bilateral reticulonodular or miliary infiltrates, therapy usually is initiated with amphotericin B; several weeks of therapy are required to produce clear evidence of improvement. Consolidation therapy with oral azoles can be considered at that time. The total duration of therapy should be at least 1 year, and in patients with underlying immunodeficiency, oral azole therapy should be continued as secondary prophylaxis.

Infections of the Pulmonary Cavity

Many pulmonary infections that are caused by *Coccidioides* are benign in their course and do not require intervention. In the absence of controlled clinical trials, evidence of the benefit of antifungal therapy is lacking, and asymptomatic infections generally are left untreated. Symptomatic patients can benefit from oral azole therapy, although recurrence of symptoms can be seen in some patients once therapy is discontinued. Surgical resection of localized cavities provides resolution of the problem in patients in whom the risks of surgery are not too high.[39]

Extrapulmonary (Disseminated) Disease

Nonmeningeal Disease

Almost all patients with disease located outside the lungs should receive antifungal therapy, which is usually initiated with 400 mg/day of an oral azole. Amphotericin B is an alternative therapy and can be necessary in patients with worsening lesions or with disease in particularly critical locations such as the vertebral column. Approximately 50% to 75% of patients treated with amphotericin B for nonmeningeal disease achieve a sustained remission, and therapy usually is curative in patients with infections localized strictly to skin and soft tissues without extensive abscess formation or tissue damage. The efficacy of local injection into joints or the peritoneum, as well as intra-articular or intradermal administration, remains poorly studied. Amphotericin B appears to be most efficacious when cell-mediated immunity is intact (as evidenced by a positive coccidioidin or spherulin skin test or low CF antibody titer). However, controlled trials that document these clinical impressions are lacking.[39]

Meningeal Disease

Fluconazole has become the drug of choice for the treatment of coccidioidal meningitis. A minimum dose of 400 mg/day orally leads to a clinical response in most patients and obviates the need for intrathecal amphotericin B. Some clinicians will initiate therapy with 800 or 1,000 mg/day, and itraconazole dosages of 400 to 600 mg/day are comparably effective. It is also clear, however, that fluconazole only leads to remission rather than cure of the infections; thus suppressive therapy must be continued for life. Ketoconazole cannot be recommended routinely for the treatment of coccidioidal meningitis because of its poor CNS penetration following oral administration. Patients who do not respond to fluconazole or itraconazole therapy are candidates for intrathecal amphotericin B therapy with or without continuation of azole therapy. The intrathecal dose of amphotericin B ranges from 0.01 to 1.5 mg given at intervals ranging from daily to weekly. Therapy is initiated with a low dosage and is titrated upward as patient tolerance develops.[39]

CRYPTOCOCCOSIS

Epidemiology

Cryptococcosis is a noncontagious, systemic mycotic infection caused by the ubiquitous encapsulated soil yeast *Cryptococcus*, which is found in soil, particularly in pigeon droppings, although disease occurs throughout the world, even in areas where pigeons are absent. Infections caused by *C. neoformans* var. *grubii* (serotype A) are seen worldwide among immunocompromised hosts, followed by *C. neoformans* var. *neoformans* (serotype D). On the other hand, *Cryptococcus gattii* (serotypes B and C) is geographically more restricted and in contrast to *C. neoformans*, rarely infects immunosuppressed patients, is not associated with HIV infection, and the infections are more difficult to treat. *C. gattii* is not associated with birds; its main reservoir was thought to be limited to certain species of eucalyptus tree. Until recently, it was most common in tropical and subtropical areas, such as Australia, South America, Southeast Asia, and central Africa, with the highest incidence in Papua New Guinea and Northern Australia, although infections occur in nontropical areas such as North America and Europe. *C. gattii* emerged on Vancouver Island, British Columbia, Canada, in 1999, and subsequently spread to the Vancouver lower mainland, Washington state, and Oregon.[41,42]

Infection is acquired by inhalation of the organism. Immunocompromised patients are at elevated risk, including those with malignancies, diabetes mellitus, chronic renal failure, and organ transplants and those receiving immunosuppressive agents. In most developed countries, widespread use of HAART has significantly decreased the incidence of cryptococcosis; however, the incidence and mortality of this infection are still extremely high in areas with limited access to HAART and a high incidence of HIV.[9,42]

Disease can remain localized in the lungs or can disseminate to other tissues, particularly the CNS, although the skin also can be affected. Hematogenous spread generally occurs in the immunocompromised host, although it also has been seen in individuals with intact immune systems.

Clinical Presentation

Primary cryptococcosis in humans almost always occurs in the lungs, although the pulmonary focus usually produces a subclinical infection. Symptomatic infections usually are manifested by cough, rales, and shortness of breath that generally resolve spontaneously. Cryptococcus can present as part of an immune reconstitution inflammatory syndrome (IRIS), a paradoxical worsening of preexisting infectious processes following the initiation of HAART in HIV-infected individuals. The symptoms of cryptococcal meningitis are nonspecific. Headache, fever, nausea, vomiting, mental status changes, and neck stiffness are generally observed. Less common symptoms include visual disturbances (photophobia and blurred vision), papilledema, seizures, and aphasia. Intracerebral mass lesions (cryptococcomas) are more common in *C. gattii* than in *C. neoformans*, presumably due to their different host immune responses.[42]

Laboratory Tests

With cryptococcal meningitis, the CSF opening pressure is elevated. There is a CSF pleocytosis (usually lymphocytes), leukocytosis, a decreased glucose concentration, and an elevated CSF protein concentration. There is also a positive cryptococcal antigen (detected by LA). The test is rapid, specific, and extremely sensitive, but false-negative results can occur. False-positive tests can result from cross-reactivity with rheumatoid factor and *Trichosporon beigelii*. *C. neoformans* can be detected in approximately 60% of patients by India ink smear of CSF, and it can be cultured in more than 96% of patients. Occasionally, large volumes of CSF are required to confirm the diagnosis.

The CSF parameters in patients with AIDS are similar to those seen in non-AIDS patients, with the exception of a decreased inflammatory response to the pathogen, resulting in a strikingly low number of leukocytes in CSF and extraordinarily high cryptococcal antigen titers.[42]

Treatment

The choice of treatment for disease caused by *C. neoformans* depends on both the anatomic sites of involvement and the host's immune status, and thus, treatment recommendations are divided into three specific risk groups: (a) HIV-infected individuals, (b) transplant recipients, and (c) non–HIV-infected and nontransplant hosts (Table 144-7).[9] The management of cryptococcosis includes systemic antifungal therapy, control of elevated intracranial pressure (ICP), and supportive care. When possible, immune defects should be addressed. Although no randomized clinical trials have been performed to address this, outcomes of treatment for CNS cryptococcosis (without mass lesions or hydrocephalus) appear to be similar for disease due to either *C. neoformans* or *C. gattii*.[41]

Non-immunocompromised Patients

7 Prior to the introduction of amphotericin B, cryptococcal meningitis was an almost uniformly fatal disease; approximately 86%

TABLE 144-7 Therapy of Cryptococcosis[a,b]

Type of Disease and Common Clinical Manifestations	Therapy/Comments
Non-immunocompromised Patients (Non–HIV-Infected, Nontransplant)	
Meningoencephalitis *without* neurological complications, in patients in whom CSF yeast cultures are negative after 2 weeks of therapy	*Induction:* Amphotericin B[c,d] IV 0.7-1 mg/kg/day *plus* flucytosine 100 mg/kg/day orally in four divided doses × ≥4 weeks
Meningoencephalitis with neurological complications	*Induction:* Same as for patients without neurologic complications, but consider extending the induction therapy for a total of 6 weeks.
Follow all regimens with suppressive therapy	*Consolidation:* Fluconazole 400-800 mg orally daily × 8 weeks *Maintenance:* Fluconazole 200 mg orally daily × 6-12 months
Mild-to-moderate pulmonary disease (Nonmeningeal disease)	Fluconazole 400 mg orally daily × 6-12 months
Severe pulmonary cryptococcosis	*Same as CNS disease × 12 months*
Cryptococcemia (non-meningeal, non-pulmonary disease)	*Same as CNS disease × 12 months*
HIV-infected Patients	
Primary therapy; induction and consolidation[e]	*Preferred regimen: Induction: Amphotericin B[d] IV 0.7-1 mg/kg IV daily plus flucytosine 100 mg/kg/day orally in four divided doses for ≥2 weeks. Alternative regimens, in order of preference: Amphotericin B[d] IV 0.7-1 mg/kg IV daily × 4-6 weeks or liposomal amphotericin B 3-4 mg/kg IV daily[f] × 4-6 weeks or ABLC 5 mg/kg IV daily × 4-6 weeks or Amphotericin B[c] IV 0.7 mg/kg IV daily, plus fluconazole 800 mg (12 mg/kg) orally daily × 2 weeks, followed by fluconazole 800 mg (12 mg/kg) orally daily × ≥8 weeks or fluconazole ≥800 mg (1,200 mg/day is preferred) orally daily plus flucytosine 100 mg/kg/day orally in four divided doses × 6 weeks or fluconazole 800-1,200 mg/day orally daily × 10-1 2 weeks (a dosage ≥1,200 mg/day is preferred when fluconazole is used alone)[g]*
Follow all regimens with suppressive therapy	*Consolidation:* Fluconazole 400 mg (6 mg/kg) orally daily × ≥8 weeks *Maintenance[h]:* Fluconazole 200 mg orally daily x ≥ 1 year[i]
Organ Transplant Recipients	
Mild-to-moderate non-CNS disease or mild-to-moderate symptoms without diffuse pulmonary infiltrates	Fluconazole 400 mg (6 mg/kg) orally daily × 6-12 months
CNS disease, moderately severe or severe CNS disease or disseminated disease without CNS disease, or severe pulmonary disease without evidence of extrapulmonary or disseminated disease	*Induction:* Liposomal amphotericin B 3-4 mg/kg IV daily,[f] or ABLC 5 mg/kg IV daily *plus* flucytosine 100 mg/kg/day orally in four divided doses × ≥2 weeks If induction therapy does not include flucytosine, consider a lipid formulation of amphotericin B for ≥4-6 weeks of induction therapy. Consider the use of a lipid formulation of amphotericin B lipid formulation (6 mg/kg IV daily) in patients with a high-fungal burden disease or relapse of disease

TABLE 144-7 Therapy of Cryptococcosis[a,b]

Type of Disease and Common Clinical Manifestations	Therapy/Comments
Follow all regimens with suppressive therapy	*Consolidation:* Fluconazole 400-800 mg (6-12 mg/kg) per day orally for 8 weeks *Maintenance:* Fluconazole 200-400 mg per day orally for 6-12 months

[a]When more than one therapy is listed, they are listed in order of preference.

[b]See the text for definitions of induction, consolidation, suppressive/maintenance therapy, and prophylactic therapy.

[c]Deoxycholate amphotericin B.

[d]In patients with, or at risk of renal disease, lipid formulations of amphotericin B can be substituted for deoxycholate amphotericin B. Doses are liposomal amphotericin B 3-4 mg/kg IV daily, or amphotericin B lipid complex (ABLC) 5 mg/kg IV daily.

[e]Initiate HAART therapy 2-10 weeks after commencement of initial antifungal treatment.

[f]Liposomal amphotericin B has been given safely up to 6 mg/kg daily; could be considered in treatment failure or in patients with a high fungal burden.

[g]Or until cerebrospinal fluid (CSF) cultures are negative.

[h]Consider discontinuing suppressive therapy during HAART in patients with a CD4 cell count ≥100 cells/μL (0.1×10^9/L) and an undetectable or very low HIV RNA level sustained for ≥3months (with a minimum of 12 months of antifungal therapy). Consider reinstitution of maintenance therapy if the CD4 cell count decreases to <100 cells/μL (0.1×10^9/L).

[i]Drug level monitoring is strongly advised.

HIV, human immunodeficiency virus; IT, intrathecal.

Data from Reference 9.

of patients died within 1 year. The use of large (1-1.5 mg/kg) daily doses of amphotericin B resulted in cure rates of approximately 64%. When amphotericin B is combined with flucytosine, a smaller dose of amphotericin B can be employed because of the in vitro and in vivo synergy between the two antifungal agents.[43] Resistance develops to flucytosine in up to 30% of patients treated with flucytosine alone, limiting its usefulness as monotherapy.[42] Combination therapy with amphotericin B and flucytosine has become standard therapy, will sterilize the CSF within 2 weeks of treatment in 60% to 90% of patients, and most immunocompetent patients will be treated successfully with 6 weeks of combination therapy.[43] Lipid formulations of amphotericin B are preferred because they increase the likelihood of completing the full course of therapy.[42] However, because of the need for prolonged IV therapy and the potential for renal and hematologic toxicity with this regimen, alternative regimens utilizing shorter (2 weeks) courses of amphotericin B followed by consolidation therapy with fluconazole for 8 weeks, then maintenance therapy with a lower dosage of fluconazole for 6 to 12 months has been advocated.[9]

For asymptomatic, immunocompetent hosts with isolated mild-to-moderate pulmonary disease and no evidence of CNS disease, careful observation can be warranted; in the case of symptomatic infection, fluconazole for 6 to 12 months is warranted. Patients with severe pulmonary disease should be treated with the same regimens as for CNS disease. Additionally, patients with non-CNS, nonpulmonary cryptococcosis, such as cryptococcemia, usually have disseminated disease and treatment regimens similar to those as for CNS disease are recommended.[9]

Despite low CSF concentrations of amphotericin B (2%-3% of those observed in plasma), the use of intrathecal amphotericin B is not recommended for the treatment of cryptococcal meningitis except in very ill patients or in patients with recurrent or progressive disease despite aggressive therapy with IV amphotericin B.[9]

The recommended management of raised ICP in cryptococcal meningitis (without hydrocephalus, a mass lesion, or a shift on computed tomography [CT] scan) has been repeated CSF removal by spinal tap. Those who do not respond and have ongoing raised ICP should have ophthalmologic monitoring for possible vision loss, and should be considered for ventriculoperitoneal shunt surgery. Neither corticosteroids (in the absence of IRIS) nor acetazolamide is recommended for management of raised ICP. Symptomatic, medically refractory mass lesions that may be compressing vital structures should be considered for surgical therapy.[9]

Immunocompromised Patients

Immunocompromised hosts with isolated severe pulmonary and extrapulmonary disease (including cryptococcemia) without CNS disease should be treated similar to non-immunocompromised patients with CNS disease. Induction regimens as short as 2 weeks in HIV-infected patients with CNS disease are effective. However, continuation of combination induction therapy is recommended in patients who have not improved or are deteriorating, or in those with anticipated/proven persistent positive CSF cultures. Non-HIV immunocompromised patients with CNS infection, such as solid organ transplant recipients, are generally managed with regimens similar to those recommended for patients with HIV.[9]

Organ Transplant Recipients

Cryptococcosis has been documented in an average of 2.8% of solid-organ transplant recipients. The median time to disease onset is 21 months after transplantation; 68.5% of the cases occur greater than 1 year after transplantation.

Induction therapy for solid organ transplant recipients with cryptococcal meningoencephalitis consists of liposomal amphotericin B or amphotericin B lipid complex (ABLC) plus flucytosine for at least 2 weeks. Fluconazole consolidation therapy should be administered for 8 weeks, and maintenance therapy should be continued for at least 6 to 12 months. Immunosuppressive management should include sequential or stepwise reduction of immunosuppressants, with consideration of lowering the corticosteroid dose first. Amphotericin B should be used with caution in transplant recipients and is not recommended as first-line therapy in this patient population due to the risk of nephrotoxicity in this population that frequently has reduced renal function. If used, the tolerated dosage of amphotericin B is uncertain, but 0.7 mg/kg daily is suggested with frequent renal function monitoring. Regardless of the agent utilized, all antifungal dosages need to be carefully monitored.[9]

HIV-Infected Patients

Primary antifungal prophylaxis for cryptococcosis is not routinely recommended in HIV-infected patients in the United States and Europe. However, in areas with limited HAART availability, high levels of antiretroviral drug resistance, and a high burden of disease, clinicians may wish to consider the use of either prophylactic therapy or a preemptive strategy with serum cryptococcal antigen testing for asymptomatic antigenemia.[9]

Early studies confirmed the benefit of early high-dose amphotericin B use, the usefulness of flucytosine added to amphotericin B for induction therapy, and the slight superiority of fluconazole over itraconazole for consolidation therapy.[43]

Amphotericin B formulations combined with flucytosine during the 2-week induction phase of therapy is the initial treatment of choice, as this regimen has been repeatedly validated in clinical trials.[44-46] Amphotericin B plus fluconazole and flucytosine plus fluconazole are non-preferred alternatives. In patients who cannot tolerate flucytosine, amphotericin B alone for 4 to 6 weeks is an alternative. After the initially successful 2-week induction period, consolidation therapy with fluconazole can be administered for 8 weeks. In patients in whom fluconazole cannot be given, itraconazole is an acceptable, albeit less effective, alternative.[9]

In HIV-infected patients, mortality is highly associated with elevated ICP (CSF opening pressure greater than 250 mm H_2O [2.5 kPa]). At the initiation of antifungal therapy, lumbar drainage should remove enough CSF to normalize the opening pressure. Patients initially should undergo daily lumbar punctures to maintain CSF opening pressure in the normal range. When the CSF pressure is normal for several days, the procedure can be suspended.[9] Adjunctive steroid treatment is not recommended.[47] Similarly, neither mannitol nor acetazolamide therapy provides any clear benefit in the management of elevated ICP.[9]

Suppressive (Maintenance) Therapy for Cryptococcal Meningitis in HIV-Infected Patients

Relapse of *C. neoformans* meningitis occurs in approximately 50% of AIDS patients after completion of primary therapy. Persistence of asymptomatic urinary *C. neoformans* has been documented in a high percentage of AIDS patients despite seemingly adequate courses of therapy for primary meningeal disease. The prostate appears to act as a sequestered reservoir of infection in these patients, resulting in systemic relapse.

Patients appear to be at low risk for recurrence of cryptococcosis when they have successfully completed a course of initial therapy for cryptococcosis, remain asymptomatic with regard to signs and symptoms of cryptococcosis, have received antifungal therapy for greater than 3 of the previous 6 months, have a serum cryptococcal antigen titer less than 1:512, or have a sustained increase (eg, greater than 6 months) in their $CD4^+$ T-lymphocyte counts to greater than 100 to 200 cells/μL (0.1×10^9-0.2×10^9/L) and an HIV viral load of less than 50 copies/mL (50×10^3/L).

After the completion of induction/consolidation phases of therapy, long-term chronic suppression with fluconazole (200 mg orally daily) should be continued for a minimum of 1 year. Maintenance therapy can be discontinued after 1 year in patients who have successfully completed primary therapy, are free of symptoms and signs of active cryptococcosis, and have been receiving HAART with a sustained CD4 cell count greater than 100 cells/mL (0.100×10^6/L) and an undetectable viral load sustained for at least 3 months.[9,43] One consideration regarding the initiation of HAART involves concern for immune reconstitution inflammatory syndrome (IRIS) in patients with AIDS not on antiretroviral therapy. In such patients, initiation of HAART may provoke an exuberant inflammatory response resulting in new/worsened symptoms, including possibly increasing intracranial pressure. Therefore, the initiation of HAART should be withheld during the induction phase of treatment, and started 2 to 10 weeks after the start of antifungal therapy. Corticosteroids may be necessary for major complications.[9,42]

CANDIDA INFECTIONS

Candida species are yeasts that exist primarily as small (4-6 μm), unicellular, thin-walled, ovoid cells that reproduce by budding. On agar medium, they form smooth, white, creamy colonies resembling staphylococci. Although there are more than 150 species of *Candida*, eight species—*C. albicans*, *C. tropicalis*, *Candida parapsilosis*, *C. krusei*, *Candida dublinensis*, *C. guilliermondii*, *C. lusitaniae*, and *C. glabrata*—are regarded as clinically important pathogens in human disease. Yeast forms, hyphae, and pseudohyphae can be found in clinical specimens.[48]

Pathophysiology

8 *C. albicans* is a normal commensal of the skin, female genital tract, and entire GI tract of humans. Therefore, the mere presence of hyphae or pseudohyphae in a clinical specimen is insufficient for the diagnosis of invasive disease. The majority of infections with *C. albicans* are acquired endogenously, although human-to-human transmission also can occur. Although the term *fungemia* refers to the presence of fungi in the blood, the most commonly isolated organism is *C. albicans*. Candidiasis can cause mucocutaneous or systemic infection, including endocarditis, peritonitis, arthritis, and infection of the CNS (mucocutaneous infections caused by *Candida* are discussed in further detail in Chapter 143).

Adherence of *C. albicans* is important in the pathogenesis of oral candidiasis and subsequent colonization of the GI tract. Because evidence suggests that the GI tract is often the portal of entry for *Candida* in disseminated disease, factors that alter the adherence of *Candida* are crucial in the development of local and systemic infection. *C. tropicalis* adheres to intravascular catheters at a higher rate than *C. albicans*, a factor that may help to account for the increased incidence of systemic infections caused by this pathogen.

CANDIDEMIA AND ACUTE HEMATOGENOUSLY DISSEMINATED CANDIDIASIS

Epidemiology

Candidemia is the fourth most common BSI in US hospitals.[25] It is associated with high mortality, increased length of hospital stay, and significant economic burden.[49] Although patients with neutropenia are at high risk for IFIs, the use of antifungal prophylaxis and prompt initiation of antifungal therapy in persistently febrile patients with neutropenia who do not respond to antibiotics has resulted in a reduction in the frequency of *Candida* BSIs in this population.[7]

The most commonly encountered clinical species of *Candida* include *C. albicans, C. glabrata, C. tropicalis, C. parapsilosis, C. lusitaniae, C. krusei*, and *C. guilliermondii*. While *C. albicans* is still the most common species of *Candida* causing candidemia, its relative frequency is decreasing, while the frequency of the other, non-*albicans* species, especially *C. glabrata*, has increased.[15] The change in species is of concern clinically, as certain pathogens, such as *C. krusei* and *C. glabrata*, are intrinsically more resistant to commonly used triazole drugs.[15] Although risk factors for the development of *Candida* BSIs in ICU patients can be identified, factors that lead to the acquisition of specific species are still unclear.[26] The emergence of infections caused by *Candida auris*, a novel, pathogenic *Candida* species associated with a high (40%-60%) mortality is concerning. Several outbreaks of *C. auris*, which first appeared in 2009, have been reported in the United Kingdom and Spain. Most infections appear in patients with previous exposure to antifungals and has high potential for interhuman transmission.[50]

Patients' characteristics influence the distribution of *Candida* species: *C. krusei* and *C. tropicalis* in patients with hematologic malignancies, while *C. parapsilosis* is most common in children, neonates, and patients with central lines and receiving parenteral nutrition. Fungemia caused by *C. glabrata* is observed more commonly in adults older than 65 years of age, perhaps due to an increased rate of oral colonization with *C. glabrata* in the elderly, and also associated with antimicrobial use and severity of underlying illness.[15]

Pathophysiology

Candida is acquired via the GI tract, although organisms also can enter the bloodstream via indwelling IV catheters. Immunosuppressed patients, including those with lymphoreticular or hematologic malignancies, diabetes, and immunodeficiency diseases and those receiving immunosuppressive therapy with high-dose corticosteroids, immunosuppressants, antineoplastic agents, or broad-spectrum antimicrobial agents, are at high risk for IFIs (Table 144-8). Major risk factors include the use of CVCs, total PN, receipt of multiple antibiotics, extensive surgery and burns, renal failure and hemodialysis, mechanical ventilation, and prior fungal colonization. Patients who have undergone surgery (particularly surgery of the GI tract) are increasingly susceptible to disseminated candidal infections.[15,26,48]

TABLE 144-8 Risk Factors for Invasive Candidiasis

Colonization
Corrected colonization index (CCI) ≥0.4[a]
Colonization index (CI) ≥0.8[a]
Candida spp. cultured from sites other than blood
Candiduria
Antibiotic use
Number of antibiotics prior to infection (per additional antibiotics)
Use of two or more antibiotics
Use of broad-spectrum antibiotics in previous 10 days
Surgery
Surgery on ICU admission
Gastro-abdominal surgery
Abdominal drainage
Elective surgery
Cardiopulmonary bypass time >120 minutes Hickman catheter
Foreign devices
Central venous catheter
Triple lumen catheter in patients who have undergone surgery
Bladder catheter
Renal failure and dialysis
Prior hemodialysis
Hemofiltration procedures
Increased serum creatinine[b]
New-onset hemodialysis within 3 days of admission to ICU
Acute renal failure
Underlying disease/baseline characteristics
Total parenteral nutrition
Diabetes mellitus Apache II (per point)
Signs of severe sepsis
Diarrhea at any time
Mechanical ventilation ≥10 days
Hospital-acquired bacterial infection
Bacterial peritonitis by ICU day 11
GI disease
ICU length of stay
Transferred from other hospital
Use of corticosteroids
Profound neutropenia (ANC <100/mm^3 [0.100 × 10^9/L])

[a]CI = the ratio of number of nonblood distinct body sites (dbs) heavily colonized with identical strains to the total number of dbs; CCI = the product of the CI and the ratio of the number of dbs showing heavy growth (≥10^5 CFU/mL [10^8 CFU/L]) to the total of dbs growing *Candida* spp.

[b]Serum creatinine >1.2 mg/dL (106 μmol/L) in females, >1.6 mg/dL (141 μmol/L) in males.

Data from Reference 26.

Clinical Presentation of Hematogenous Candidiasis

Dissemination of *C. albicans* can result in infection in single or multiple organs, particularly the kidney, brain, myocardium, skin, eye, liver, spleen, bone, and joints.[48]

Laboratory Tests

The interpretation of positive surveillance cultures of the skin, mouth, sputum, feces, or urine is hampered by their occurrence as commensal pathogens and in distinguishing colonization from invasive disease. A rapid presumptive identification of *C. albicans* can be made by incubation of *Candida* in serum; formation of a germ tube (the beginning of hyphae, which arise as perpendicular extensions from the yeast cell, with no constriction at their point of origin) within 1 to 2 hours offers a positive identification of *C. albicans*. Unfortunately, *C. dubliniensis* also can produce a germ tube, and a negative germ tube test does not rule out the possibility of *C. albicans*, but further biochemical tests must be performed to differentiate between other non-*albicans* species.

Several rapid diagnostic methods are available at many hospitals, which can result in much more rapid identification of pathogens, including specific species, than with the use of traditional microbiological techniques. Matrix-assisted laser desorption/ionization time-of-flight intact cell mass spectrometry (MALDI-TOF-ICMS), a multiplex polymerase chain reaction (PCR) panel that includes five *Candida* species, and T2 Magnetic Resonance Assays provide rapid detection and identification of pathogenic *Candida* species.[48,51] Also available is the PNA fluorescence in situ hybridization (FISH) method, which uses fluorescein-labeled PNA probes that target *C. albicans* 26S rRNA for the identification of *C. albicans*, and a multiplex polymerase chain reaction (PCR) panel. The test has excellent sensitivity (99%-100%) and specificity (100%) in the direct identification of *C. albicans* from blood cultures.[52]

Treatment

The list of risk factors for invasive candidiasis in critically ill patients is extensive, and trying to decipher which patients may benefit from antifungal prophylaxis or empirical therapy based on risk factors in an ICU is exceedingly difficult. In addition, the number of risk factors present in ICU patients changes over time, and the majority of ICU patients will have more than one risk factor. Clinically useful, practical predictive algorithms and "scoring systems" to identify high-risk patients early during their ICU admission have not proved successful thus far. To maximize its clinical utility as a decision-making tool, the ideal algorithm would identify high-risk populations (ones with a rate of invasive candidiasis of 10%-15%), providing clinicians with a means of administering prophylaxis to a minimal number of patients, while preventing the maximal number of invasive candidiasis cases.[26]

Although it is common practice in today's standard of care to place indwelling catheters in patients for the administration of medications and parenteral nutrition (TPN), catheter-related infections are a common complication. These foreign bodies (especially triple lumen catheters) double as entry ports for normal skin flora or other nosocomial pathogens, and they provide a readily available site for the binding of pathogens via microbiotic biofilms. Their subsequent role as a source of BSIs is facilitated by frequent use, TPN, and the potential for contamination of catheters by medical staff who are colonized with *Candida* species. Most consensus recommendations urge removal of all existing tunneled CVCs and implantable devices, particularly in patients with fungemia caused by *C. parapsilosis*, which is frequently associated with catheters, as it has been associated with reduced mortality in adults, and a shorter duration of candidemia.[7] Arguments against the removal of all catheters in patients with candidemia include the prominent role of the gut as a source for disseminated candidiasis, the significant cost and potential for complications, and the problems that can be encountered in patients with difficult vascular access. However, in an individual patient it is often difficult to determine the relative contribution of gut versus catheter as the primary source of fungemia. The evidence for this recommendation is weakest in cancer patients with severe neutropenia and mucositis (eg, acute leukemia, stem cell transplant), in whom candidemia is almost always primarily of gut origin, and removal of CVCs is least likely to have an impact on mortality.[7]

Hematogenous Candidiasis

There is a high rate of mortality in non-neutropenic patients with fungal blood cultures. Delays in the initiation of antifungal therapy may significantly increase mortality.[53,54] Treatment of candidiasis should be guided by knowledge of the infecting species, the clinical status of the patient, and when available, the antifungal susceptibility of the infecting isolate. Therapy should be continued for 2 weeks after documented clearance of blood cultures, with resolution of all signs and symptoms of infection. All patients should undergo dilated fundoscopic examination within the first week of therapy. Susceptibility testing of the infecting isolate is a useful adjunct to species identification during selection of a therapeutic approach, since it can be used to identify isolates that are unlikely to respond to fluconazole or amphotericin B.[7] However, this is not currently available at many institutions.

Non-immunocompromised Patient

Prophylaxis In ICUs, the use of fluconazole for prophylaxis or empirical therapy is common.[55] However, studies that demonstrated benefit in the prevention of invasive candidal BSIs did so either by using highly selective criteria or by studying patients in an unusually high-risk ICU setting, and the role of antifungal prophylaxis in the surgical ICU remains extremely controversial. For a study to demonstrate efficacy in clinical trials, the baseline rate of invasive candidiasis must be greater than 10%, and that prophylaxis must result in greater than fourfold reduction of disease. Although ICU-specific, greater than 10% rate of invasive candidiasis is generally found only in the setting of high-risk transplant patients (eg, patients undergoing liver transplantation), or in patients with a constellation of risk factors.[26] However, a significant benefit to prophylaxis in such high-risk, non-transplant patients has not been established.[56,57] Prophylactic antifungals may be indicated in patients with recurrent intestinal perforations and/or anastomotic leaks as these patients may be at high risk for invasive candidiasis and the use of empiric fluconazole may significantly decrease the incidence of infection.[58]

"Empirical" Therapy (Also Known as Preemptive Therapy) The term "preemptive" antifungal therapy is often used to describe early antifungal therapy given to high-risk patients with persistent signs and symptoms and clinical, laboratory, or radiologic surrogate markers of infection but without mycological evidence of infection, or those heavily colonized with *Candida*.[26] Few data are available for assessing the role of antifungals as empirical therapy for *suspected* candidiasis in patients who do not yet exhibit a positive culture. The empiric use of fluconazole in one study, and micafungin in another, did not significantly improve outcomes; thus, preemptive/empiric use is not recommended at this time.[30,59]

Initial Antifungal Therapy in Non-Neutropenic Patients with Documented Candidemia, in Whom the Species Is Not Yet Identified and Results of Antifungal Susceptibility Testing Are Not Known Azoles (fluconazole or voriconazole) and deoxycholate amphotericin B are similarly effective for the therapy of documented candidemia in non-neutropenic patients; however, fewer adverse effects are observed with azole therapy.[60,61] Echinocandins are at least as effective as amphotericin B, fluconazole, or isavuconazole in (primarily non-neutropenic) adult patients with candidemia.[62-66] Both fluconazole and the echinocandins are associated with fewer drug-related adverse events than amphotericin B preparations. Among the lipid-associated formulations of amphotericin B, liposomal amphotericin B (AmBisome) and ABLC (Abelcet) have been approved for use in proven cases of candidiasis. The lipid-associated formulations are less toxic but as effective as amphotericin B deoxycholate. Although the use of combination therapy (high-dose fluconazole plus amphotericin B) was superior to treatment with fluconazole alone, it was associated with a higher rate of nephrotoxicity, and the routine use of combination therapy in this patient population is not yet recommended.[67]

For empiric therapy in non-neutropenic adults, IDSA guidelines (Table 144-9) recommend use of an echinocandin or fluconazole (intravenous or oral) as initial therapy. Echinocandins are recommended for patients with moderately severe to severe illness, and patients with recent azole exposure. Patients may be transitioned to fluconazole (intravenous or oral) if their *Candida* isolates are known/likely to be susceptible to fluconazole (eg, *C. albicans*, *C. parapsilosis*) in patients who are clinically stable, and in whom repeat negative blood cultures have been obtained. Fluconazole may be used initially in patients who are less critically ill, with no recent azole exposure, who are not at high risk for *C. glabrata* or with central nervous system or endocardial disease.[7]

Antifungal Therapy for Specific *Candida* Species

Since *C. glabrata* often demonstrate reduced susceptibility to fluconazole, treatment with echinocandins is recommended as initial therapy (pending the results of susceptibility testing), although there are successful treatment outcomes reported in response to fluconazole therapy of 6 to 12 mg/kg/day, and may be suitable in less critically ill patients.[7,69,70]

Regardless of the species of *Candida*, in the absence of metastatic complications of disease, antifungal therapy should be continued for 2 weeks after the last positive blood culture, and until there is resolution of signs and symptoms of infection. It is important to note when counting days of therapy that the days of treatment "begin" on the first day of documented clearance of *Candida* species from bloodstream, with the use of an effective antifungal agent to which the species is susceptible. As such, blood cultures should be repeated until negative. Existing central venous catheters should be removed when feasible, and all patients should undergo dilated retinal examination (preferably by an ophthalmologist) to rule out *Candida* endopthalmitis.[7]

In non-neutropenic adults, once the species of *Candida* has been identified, echinocandin therapy is recommended for the management of systemic *C. krusei* infections. *C. tropicalis* and *C. parapsilosis* may be treated with fluconazole at 6 mg/kg/day. Candidemia due to *C. parapsilosis* has increased in frequency among pediatric populations and appears to be associated with a lower mortality rate than other species of *Candida*. Since many, but not all isolates of *C. lusitaniae* are resistant to amphotericin B, fluconazole at 6 mg/kg/day is the preferred agent for treatment of this species. In patients with *C. parapsilosis* candidemia,[7] fluconazole is recommended, since MICs of echinocandins tend to be higher for *C. parapsilosis*. However, overall treatment success of candidemia or invasive candidiasis with echinocandins versus other agents was similar, and there was no difference in 30-day mortality between patients treated with fluconazole or an echinocandin.[71] The in vitro susceptibility of *C. auris* to antifungal agents is variable. However, while most isolates are susceptible to echinocandins, most are resistant to fluconazole, and ~40% of isolates are resistant to more than 2 classes of antifungal agents. An echinocandin is recommended as first-line therapy, with the addition of amphotericin B recommended in case of persistent fungemia or lack of clinical response.[50]

Expert opinion is divided regarding the optimal therapy of infections caused by *C. glabrata*. Guidelines recommend the use of an echinocandin until susceptibility is proven.[7] The severity of illness and choice of antifungal predict response in patients with *C. glabrata* fungemia, and the choice of antifungal (fluconazole or an echinocandin) does not influence mortality.[66,69] When fluconazole is dosed appropriately (Table 144-9), *C. glabrata* fluconazole susceptibility breakpoints are predictive of clinical and microbiological response.[70] Echinocandin therapy is independently associated with treatment success, but not survival, in invasive candidiasis due to *C. glabrata*.[66,69]

Immunocompromised Patients

In immunocompromised patients, the optimal agent, dose, and duration of therapy are unclear, and patients must be monitored carefully with serial blood cultures and careful physical examinations, particularly of the retina. Treatment guidelines in neutropenic patients generally approximate those from non-neutropenic hosts. Patients who experience prolonged neutropenia and persistent candidemia may benefit from administration of a recombinant cytokine (granulocyte colony-stimulating factor) that accelerates recovery from neutropenia.[7]

TABLE 144-9 Antifungal Therapy of Invasive Candidiasis

Type of Disease and Common Clinical Manifestations	Therapy/Comments
Prophylaxis of Candidemia	
Non-neutropenic patients	Not recommended except for severely ill/high-risk patients in whom fluconazole IV/oral 400 mg daily should be used (see the text)
Neutropenic patients[a]	Fluconazole IV/oral 400 mg daily *or* itraconazole solution 2.5 mg/kg every 12 hours orally *or* micafungin 50 mg (1 mg/kg in patients under 50 kg) IV daily. The optimal duration of therapy is unclear but at a minimum should include the period at risk for neutropenia.
Solid-organ transplantation, liver transplantation	*Patients with key risk factors[b]:* Fluconazole 400 mg orally daily is preferred
Empirical (Preemptive) Antifungal Therapy	
Suspected disseminated candidiasis in febrile non-neutropenic patients	None recommended; data are lacking defining subsets of patients who are appropriate for therapy (see the text)
Suspected candidiasis in febrile neutropenic patients	A lipid formulation of amphotericin B, caspofungin, micafungin, voriconazole, isavuconazole, posaconazole, or itraconazole for duration of neutropenia
Initial Antifungal Therapy of Documented Candidemia and Acute Hematogenously Disseminated Candidiasis, Unknown Species	
Patients who are less critically ill and who have had no recent azole exposure	*Remove existing central venous catheters when feasible plus fluconazole IV (loading dose of 800 mg [12 mg/kg], then 400 mg [6 mg/kg] daily) or an echinocandin.[c]* Treatment duration: 2 weeks after the last positive blood culture and resolution of signs and symptoms of infection
Patients with recent azole exposure, moderately severe or severe illness, or who are at high risk of infection due to *C. glabrata* or *C. krusei*	An echinocandin[c] Transition from an echinocandin to fluconazole IV/oral is recommended for patients who are clinically stable and have isolates (eg, *C. albicans*) likely to be susceptible to fluconazole
Antifungal Therapy of Specific Pathogens	
C. albicans, C. tropicalis, and *C. parapsilosis*	Fluconazole IV/oral 6 mg/kg/day *or* an echinocandin[c]; transition to fluconazole is recommended in patients who are clinically stable and whose isolates are likely to be susceptible to fluconazole (eg, *C. albicans*); voriconazole IV (400 mg [6 mg/kg] twice daily × two doses then 200 mg [3 mg/kg] twice daily thereafter) is efficacious, but offers little advantage over fluconazole; it may be utilized as step-down oral therapy for selected cases of candidiasis due to *C. krusei* or voriconazole-susceptible *C. glabrata* *Patients intolerant or refractory to other therapy*: Amphotericin B lipid complex IV 3-5 mg/kg/day Liposomal amphotericin B IV 3-5 mg/kg/day
C. krusei	An echinocandin[c]
C. lusitaniae	Fluconazole IV/orally 6 mg/kg/day
C. glabrata	An echinocandin[c] (transition to fluconazole or voriconazole therapy is not recommended without confirmation of isolate susceptibility)
Urinary candidiasis	*Asymptomatic disease:* Generally no therapy is required *Symptomatic or high-risk patients[d]*: Removal of urinary tract instruments, stents, and Foley catheters, +7-14 days therapy with fluconazole 200 mg orally daily *or* amphotericin B IV 0.3-1 mg/kg/day

[a]Patients at significant risk for invasive candidiasis include those receiving standard chemotherapy for acute myelogenous leukemia, allogeneic bone marrow transplants, or high-risk autologous bone marrow transplants. However, among these populations, chemotherapy or bone marrow transplant protocols do not all produce equivalent risk, and local experience should be used to determine the relevance of prophylaxis.

[b]Risk factors include re-transplantation, re-operation, renal failure requiring hemodialysis, transfusion of ≥40 units of cellular blood products including platelets, packed red blood cells, and auto transfusion; choledochojejunostomy, and Candida colonization in the perioperative period.[68]

[c]Echinocandin = caspofungin 70 mg loading dose, then 50 mg IV daily maintenance dose, or micafungin 100 mg daily, or anidulafungin 200 mg loading dose, then 100 mg daily maintenance dose.

[d]Patients at high risk for dissemination include neutropenic patients, low-birth-weight infants, and patients who will undergo urologic manipulation.

PO, orally.

Data from Reference 7.

Prophylaxis Recognition of the role of the GI tract in invasive *Candida* infections has led to efforts to decrease infections by prophylactic administration of topical or systemically absorbed antifungal agents in immunocompromised patients. The use of systemically absorbable agents such as azole antifungal agents appears to decrease the risk of IFIs.[7,72]

Several antifungal agents, including oral fluconazole (400 mg/day), posaconazole (200 mg three times daily), IV micafungin or caspofungin (50 mg daily) administered from the start of the conditioning regimen until day 75, can reduce the frequency of invasive *Candida* infections and decrease mortality in patients undergoing allogeneic bone marrow transplantation.[7,72]

Similarly, in less risk-selected patients with hematologic malignancies who are undergoing remission-induction chemotherapy, fluconazole, posaconazole, or caspofungin, during induction chemotherapy for the duration of neutropenia, are effective in preventing systemic infection and death caused by *Candida* species.[7,72]

For solid-organ transplant recipients, fluconazole or an echinocandin is recommended as postoperative antifungal prophylaxis for liver, pancreas, and small bowel transplant recipients at high risk of candidiasis.[7,68]

Widespread use of prophylactic fluconazole in all ICU patients is not warranted and may lead to an increase in resistance and adverse events. If utilized, prophylactic fluconazole should target high-risk patients with a presumed risk of invasive candidiasis of 10% to 15%.[7,26]

Empirical Therapy for Febrile Neutropenic Patients

In patients who have not been receiving antifungal prophylaxis, *Candida* spp. are the most likely cause of IFI. In patients receiving fluconazole prophylaxis, fluconazole-resistant *Candida* spp. (eg, *C. glabrata* and *C. krusei*) and invasive mold infections, particularly *Aspergillus* spp., are the most likely causes. A lipid formulation of amphotericin B, caspofungin, micafungin, voriconazole, isavuconazole, posaconazole, or itraconazole are recommended as suitable options for empiric antifungal therapy in neutropenic patients.[72] Guidelines recommend adding empiric antifungal therapy after 4 or more days of fever despite empiric antibiotic therapy in patients who are not receiving prophylaxis with mold-active agents and who are at high risk for mold infections (duration of neutropenia >10 days, allogeneic HSCT recipients, and high-dose corticosteroid treatment).[72]

For persistently febrile patients who have been receiving anti-mold prophylaxis, a different class of antifungal agent with activity against molds should be used for empiric therapy. The choice of the initial antifungal agent may vary based on an institution's experience (ie, epidemiology and susceptibility patterns) and patient risks for specific mold infections (eg, *Aspergillus* vs infections caused by the Mucorales). In patients with pulmonary nodules or nodular pulmonary infiltrates, invasive mold infection should be strongly suspected and treated. As fluconazole lacks activity against filamentous fungi, its use in patients at high risk for these pathogens should be avoided. In addition, clinicians need to consider that echinocandins are not active against *Cryptococcus* spp., *Trichosporon* spp., and filamentous molds other than *Aspergillus* spp. (eg, *Fusarium* spp.), nor are they active against the endemic fungi (*Histoplasma, Blastomyces,* and *Coccidioides* spp.).[73]

CANDIDURIA

Within the urinary tract, most common lesions are either *Candida* cystitis or hematogenously disseminated renal abscesses. *Candida* cystitis often follows catheterization or therapy with broad-spectrum antimicrobial agents. The diagnosis of *Candida* cystitis can be problematic because of the frequent presence of *Candida* pseudohyphae and yeast cells in urine specimens secondary to urethral colonization. The usefulness of urine colony counts or antibody coating techniques is questionable. The recovery of 10,000 organisms or visualization of both yeast and pseudohyphae from fresh midstream urine or from bladder urine obtained by single catheterization (not indwelling) is suggestive of genitourinary candidiasis. In most patients, the infection is asymptomatic and clears spontaneously without specific antifungal therapy.[7]

Initial therapy of candidal cystitis should focus on removal of urinary catheters whenever possible. Changing the catheter will eliminate candiduria in only 20% of patients, whereas discontinuation will eradicate *Candida* in 40% of patients. Asymptomatic candiduria rarely requires therapy. Therapy should be used in neutropenic patients, very low-birth-weight infants (<1500 g), and those who will undergo urologic manipulation, because of the risk of dissemination.[7]

Oral fluconazole 200 mg/day for 14 days hastens the time to a negative urine culture as compared with placebo treatment, but 2 weeks after the end of therapy, the frequency of a negative urine culture remains the same with both treatments.[74] Treatment should include removal of catheters and stents whenever possible plus 7 to 14 days of therapy. Bladder irrigation with amphotericin B (50 mg in 500 mL sterile water instilled twice daily into the bladder via a three-way catheter) is only transiently effective. Minimal quantities (less than 3%) of amphotericin B are absorbed systemically from the bladder.[7]

ASPERGILLOSIS

Saprophytic molds belonging to the *Aspergillus* spp. can be found around the world, of which, *Aspergillus fumigatus* is the most commonly observed pathogen, followed by *Aspergillus flavus*.

Invasive aspergillosis (IA) is the second most common IFI, with increasing incidence over the last 20 years along with the advances in the treatment of hematological malignancies. The infection most commonly affects immunocompromised patients and patients with acute myeloid leukemia (AML) and those who undergo allogeneic HSCT who develop GvHD are at highest risk. In the highest risk group, IA rates can reach 25%. The frequency of IA and infections caused by other molds have increased over the past 2 decades. Despite heightened awareness of the profiles of patients at risk for *Aspergillus* infections, and despite the advent of liposomal formulations of amphotericin B, IA continues to be associated with extremely high mortality rates. The crude mortality approaches 75% in patients with AIDS and bone marrow transplant patients. Major target sites for primary invasive disease include the lungs and sinuses; frequently, secondary infections involve the central nervous system. The appropriate duration of treatment is based on the extent of the infection, response to therapy, and host factors.[75]

Epidemiology

Aspergillus is a ubiquitous mold that grows well on a variety of substrates, including soil, water, decaying vegetation, moldy hay or straw, and organic debris. Although more than 300 species of *Aspergillus* have been characterized, three species are most commonly pathogenic: *A. fumigatus*, *A. flavus*, and *A. niger*. The varying degrees of pathogenicity of each species depend on their relative geographic prevalence, conidial size and shape, thermotolerance, and production of mycotoxins. For example, transport of *A. fumigatus* conidia into the lungs is facilitated by their smaller diameter in comparison with *A. flavus* and *A. niger*.

9 The term *aspergillosis* may be broadly defined as a spectrum of diseases attributed to allergy, colonization, or tissue invasion caused by members of the fungal genus *Aspergillus*. A single satisfactory classification system for these disease entities is difficult because different populations of patients can develop the same type of infection. For example, osteomyelitis can result from local trauma or hematogenous dissemination in an immunocompromised host. Colonization in normal hosts can lead to allergic diseases ranging from asthma to allergic bronchopulmonary aspergillosis (BPA) or, rarely, invasive disease.[75]

Pathophysiology

Aspergillosis is acquired by inhalation of airborne conidia that are small enough (2.5-3 μm) to reach alveoli or the paranasal sinuses. Each conidiophore releases 10^4 conidia that remain suspended for long periods and are viable for months in dry locations. Although some authors advocate monitoring of hospital air for *Aspergillus* conidia, guidelines for interpreting results are not available. The use of high-efficiency particulate air (HEPA) filters in operating rooms and laminar flow rooms and removal of immunocompromised patients from hospital renovation sites can be helpful in preventing infection in this population.

Superficial or locally invasive infections of the ear, skin, or appendages often can be managed with topical antifungal therapy. Skin infections in patients with burn wounds, although uncommon, can progress to deep-tissue invasion despite the use of topical or parenteral antifungal agents. Risk factors for deep infection include extensive thermal injuries, malnutrition, cirrhosis, and previous infection with *Pseudomonas aeruginosa*.

Allergic manifestations of *Aspergillus* range in severity from mild asthma to allergic BPA. BPA, which is almost always caused by *A. fumigatus*, is characterized by severe asthma with wheezing, fever, malaise, weight loss, chest pain, and a cough productive of blood-streaked sputum. Following recurrent episodes of severe asthma, the disease usually progresses to fibrosis and bronchiectasis with granuloma formation. When *Aspergillus* conidia become trapped in the viscous mucus of asthmatic patients, BPA develops. The fungus grows, releasing toxins and antigens. The resulting host sensitization results in a variety of immune reactions. Early in the course of disease, an immunoglobulin E (IgE)-mediated (type I) immune reaction results in bronchospasm, eosinophilia, and immediate skin reactivity. The ensuing fibrosis and pulmonary infiltrates appear to be mediated by circulating or precipitating antibody complexes of IgG antibody, followed by granuloma formation and mononuclear infiltration because of a type IV delayed hypersensitivity reaction. Therapy is aimed at minimizing the quantity of antigenic material released in the tracheobronchial tree. Management of acute asthma attacks minimizes trapping of *Aspergillus* by bronchial secretions, and administration of corticosteroids clears lung infiltrates.[75] Antifungal therapy generally is not indicated in the management of allergic manifestations of aspergillosis, although some patients have demonstrated a decrease in their corticosteroid dose following therapy with itraconazole.[12]

Aspergilloma

Pulmonary aspergillomas are fungus balls arising in preexisting cavities because of tuberculosis, histoplasmosis, lung tumors, or radiation fibrosis, although occasionally no previous pulmonary disease is present. The diagnosis of aspergilloma generally is made on the basis of chest radiographs, on which aspergillomas appear as a solid rounded mass, sometimes mobile, of water density within a spherical or ovoid cavity and separated from the wall of the cavity by an airspace of variable size and shape. Patients generally experience chest pain, dyspnea, and sputum production. Hemoptysis is observed in 50% to 80% of patients, probably because of ulceration of the epithelial lining of the cavity with formation of granulation tissue, and hemoptysis is the cause of death in up to 26% of patients with aspergilloma. A poor prognosis is associated with increasing size or number of aspergillomas, immunosuppression (including corticosteroids), increasing *Aspergillus*-specific titers, underlying sarcoidosis, and HIV infection. Although *Aspergillus* can be cultured in only 50% to 60% of patients, precipitating antibodies are positive in virtually 100% of patients.

Invasive disease occurs rarely, and therapy therefore is controversial. There are no controlled clinical trials with which to guide therapy, and recommendations for treatment have been generated from uncontrolled trials and case reports. Concern regarding the risk of severe hemorrhage has led some clinicians to use aggressive surgical excision of aspergillomas or pulmonary resection in patients with hemoptysis. Complications, including bronchopulmonary fistulas, hemorrhage, empyema, and persistent airspace problems, have led to the recommendation that surgical intervention be reserved for patients with severe (greater than 500 mL per 24 hours) hemoptysis, however. Bronchial artery embolization has been used to occlude the vessel that supplies the bleeding site in patients experiencing hemoptysis. Unfortunately, bronchial artery embolization generally is unsuccessful or only temporarily effective. Collateral circulation eventually develops, supplying blood flow to the affected area, and hemoptysis often recurs; consequently, reembolization is often unsuccessful. Bronchial artery embolization should be used as a temporizing procedure in a patient with life-threatening disease who might respond to more definitive therapy if hemoptysis is stabilized. Mild-to-moderate hemoptysis should be managed conservatively. Patients with spillage during surgery are recommended to receive a minimum of 4 weeks of therapy post-operatively. Hemoptysis generally ceases when the aspergilloma is eradicated.[12,75]

Invasive Aspergillosis

IA remains a disease of very high mortality: for example, in HSCT recipients with a diagnosis of invasive aspergillosis, the 3-month post HSCT mortality rate is 50% for autologous transplant recipients but approaches 75% for allogeneic HSCT recipients.[75]

Although exposure to *Aspergillus* conidia is nearly universal, impaired host defenses are required for the development of invasive disease. Phagocytes (neutrophils, monocytes, and macrophages) rather than antibodies or lymphocytes constitute the primary host defense system against invasive disease with aspergillosis. Macrophages prevent germination of conidia and also eradicate conidia, providing the first line of defense against invasive disease. Administration of corticosteroids appears to impair the killing of conidia by macrophages and to impair mobilization of neutrophils. Neutrophils halt hyphal growth and dissemination and kill mycelia, constituting a second line of defense. Prolonged neutropenia appears to be the most important predisposing factor to the development of IA, accounting for the high frequency of disease in patients with acute leukemia.[75]

Invasive disease with *Aspergillus* can arise de novo or from any of the allergic or colonizing forms of aspergillosis. Predisposing factors to the development of IA include glucocorticoid therapy, particularly following chronic administration or with higher dosages (30-200 mg/day of prednisone), cytotoxic agents, and recent or concurrent therapy with broad-spectrum antimicrobial agents. Patients with chronic hepatitis, alcoholism, diabetes mellitus, chronic granulomatous disease, leukopenia (less than 1,000 cells/mm^3 [1 × 10^9/L]), leukemia (particularly acute lymphocytic or myelogenous leukemia), lymphoma, and acute rejection of an organ transplant are also at a higher risk of invasive disease. Although rare, IA has been reported in apparently normal hosts.[75] For example, hospitalized patients with severe influenza, or more recently, SARS-CoV-2 infection, may develop superinfection due to *Aspergillus*.[76] Aspergillosis is an uncommon fungal infection in patients with AIDS, usually associated with other risk factors for infection, such as corticosteroid use and neutropenia.[12]

Clinical Presentation

The lung is the most common site of invasive disease. In the immunocompromised host, aspergillosis is characterized by vascular invasion leading to thrombosis, infarction, necrosis of tissue, and dissemination to other tissues and organs in the body. If bone marrow function returns, cavitation of the pulmonary lesion generally occurs, and the spread of infection can be halted. The progressive nature of the disease and its refractoriness to therapy are, in part, caused by the organism's rapid growth and its tendency to invade blood vessels.[75]

Clinical Presentation: Aspergillosis

Signs and Symptoms

Patients with invasive pulmonary aspergillosis (IPA) generally have blunted or non-specific signs and symptoms of infection due to impaired inflammatory responses. Patients often present with classic signs and symptoms of acute pulmonary embolus: pleuritic chest pain, fever, hemoptysis, and friction rubs. The CNS, liver, spleen, heart, GI tract, pericardium, and other body sites are involved in a substantial minority of cases. In neutropenic patients with *Aspergillus* pneumonia, hyphae invade the walls of bronchi and surrounding parenchyma, resulting in an acute necrotizing, pyogenic pneumonitis. As a result, patients often present with classic signs and symptoms of acute pulmonary embolus: pleuritic chest pain, fever, hemoptysis, and friction rubs.[75]

Diagnosis

The diagnosis of aspergillosis is complicated by the presence of *Aspergillus* as a normal commensal in the human GI tract and respiratory secretions, and establishment of a definitive diagnosis of disease is difficult. The likelihood of IFIs is assessed on a scale of probability (possible, probable, proven) based upon host factors, clinical and microbiological criteria.[29] Demonstration of *Aspergillus* by repeated culture and microscopic examination of tissue provides the most firm diagnosis. A definitive diagnosis of IPA can be made by obtaining a biopsy of lung tissue; however, thrombocytopenia often limits clinicians' ability to perform this procedure. The appearance of *Aspergillus* in tissues varies with increasing host resistance from the normal vegetative hyphae found with necrotic tissue and exudate in the alveoli of immunocompromised hosts to the compact, tangled filaments (*granules*) observed in fungal balls. Identification of *Aspergillus* generally is based on the appearance of 2- to 4-μm-wide septate hyphae that are dichotomously branched at 45° angles. Sporulation is observed rarely in tissue. Although growth on Sabouraud dextrose or brain-heart infusion agar can be used for primary culture, bronchoscopy or bronchoalveolar lavage cultures are positive in only 40% of histopathologically identified specimens. Blood, CSF, and bone marrow cultures are rarely positive for *Aspergillus*.

The diagnosis is determined with the use of high resolution CT, in which IPA will manifest early on as "halo sign" (an area of low attenuation surrounding a nodular lung lesion, caused by edema or bleeding surrounding an ischemic area). In late IA nodular lesions, diffuse pulmonary infiltrates, consolidation, or ground glass opacities can be observed, and CT scans may demonstrate the crescent sign (an air crescent near the periphery of a lung nodule caused by contraction of infarcted tissue), while chest radiographs can demonstrate wedge-shaped, pleural-based infiltrates or cavities. These signs are not specific to IPA, however, as bacteria and other fungal infections may produce similar findings. CT abnormalities are best documented in neutropenic marrow transplant recipients and commonly precede plain chest radiograph abnormalities.[75]

Laboratory Tests

The diagnosis of aspergillosis, and other invasive mold infections, remains difficult. New laboratory methods that allow for early differentiation of IFIs due to *Aspergillus* species versus zygomycetes and other molds would be helpful in allowing clinicians in the earlier initiation of appropriate antifungal therapy. Although PCR-based testing is being performed in some centers, and appears promising, no FDA-approved method is commercially available.

The galactomannan test is an enzyme-linked immunosorbent assay (ELISA) (Platelia *Aspergillus* EIA test; Bio-Rad Laboratories) that detects galactomannan, an antigen released from *Aspergillus* hyphae upon invasion of host tissue. The clinical utility of this assay has been assessed in the clinical setting by sampling serum, BAL fluid, cerebrospinal fluid (CSF), and pleural fluid; however, the currently approved test is performed on serum. Additionally, while FDA-approved for use in the diagnosis of IA in HSCT recipients and in patients with leukemia; its usefulness in solid-organ transplant and pediatric populations needs to be established. In most patients, circulating antigen can be detected at a mean of 8 days before diagnosis by other means. The test has a sensitivity ranging from 40% to 90% and a specificity of approximately 90%; however, the sensitivity of the assay is decreased in patients receiving mold-active drugs on the day of sampling. False positives can occur, particularly in patients with other IFIs (including histoplasmosis and blastomycosis), receiving antibiotics such as amoxicillin–clavulanate, and in neonates. False negatives can occur during the concomitant use of antifungals, presumably because the level of galactomannan is related to the fungal burden. In addition, it is important to note that the utility of galactomannan testing in the setting of prophylaxis has not been defined.[12,75]

1,3-β-D-Glucan is a component of fungal cell walls that can be detected colorimetrically in clinical samples, including blood and bronchoalveolar lavage specimens, using a chromogenic variant of the limulus amoebocyte lysate assay. However, the current FDA-approved test (Fungitell; Associates of Cape Cod) is performed only on serum, and is nonspecific for *Aspergillus*. The 1,3-β-D-glucan test can be used to detect most fungi, with the exception of *Mucorales*. False positives are problematic with the test, with many processes and products associated with elevated levels, including hemodialysis with cellulose membranes, intravenous immune globulin or serum albumin administration, gastrointestinal surgery, and in other cases for unclear reasons.[77]

TREATMENT

Invasive Aspergillosis

Therapy for IA is far from optimal at this time in part because of the difficulties in establishing a diagnosis and in part because of a lack of truly effective antifungal agents. Administration of amphotericin B appears to decrease mortality from more than 90% to approximately 45%. These data, however, are difficult to interpret because many patients were diagnosed postmortem, or amphotericin B therapy was not administered until the patient had very advanced disease. Although early diagnosis and administration of antifungal therapy can result in higher response rates, correction of underlying immune deficits (in particular, return of neutrophil counts) is of paramount importance in eradication of infection.[75]

Until the diagnosis of aspergillosis can be determined more rapidly and definitively, empirical therapy must be instituted when invasive disease is suspected. In patients at highest risk for invasive disease (acute leukemia and bone marrow transplant recipients), the most important predisposing factors include prolonged severe neutropenia (less than 100 cell/μL [0.1×10^9/L] for more than 1 week), graft rejection, chronic administration of corticosteroids, and tissue damage from preexisting infection.[75]

Prophylaxis As noted above in the discussion of prophylaxis for *Candida* infections in immunocompromised hosts, prophylaxis with azoles or echinocandins can reduce the incidence of aspergillosis in select high-risk populations. The incidence of IFIs following solid organ transplantation varies with the organ being transplanted and the epidemiology at individual centers. *Candida* and *Aspergillus* species are the leading causative agents, with the median time to onset following transplantation depending on the type of transplant. Several organizations have developed guidelines for the prevention of IFIs in patients with malignancies and in those undergoing solid organ or hematopoietic stem cell transplantation.[68,72,78]

Specific Therapy

The outcome of invasive aspergillosis (IA) continues to be associated with significant attributable mortality, especially in patients with hematological malignancies and in HSCT recipients. Older azole antifungal agents (miconazole, ketoconazole, and fluconazole) possess poor in vitro activity against *Aspergillus* species; however, newer triazoles (itraconazole, voriconazole, posaconazole, and isavuconazole) demonstrate improved activity both in vitro and in animal models of infection. Antifungal agents with in vitro activity against *Aspergillus* species include amphotericin B, the echinocandins, and the azoles itraconazole, voriconazole, posaconazole, and isavuconazole. Historically, high dosages (1-1.5 mg/kg/day) of deoxycholate amphotericin B were utilized for the treatment of suspected or proven invasive aspergillosis. Lipid formulations of amphotericin B are overall less nephrotoxic and at least as effective as amphotericin B, and they can be effective when amphotericin B is not.[79] Initial dosing of 10 mg/kg/day and 3 mg/kg/day of liposomal amphotericin B were equally effective, but there was decreased nephrotoxicity with the use of 3 mg/kg/day.[80]

Voriconazole has emerged as the drug of choice of most clinicians for primary therapy of most patients with IA, based on a pivotal study in which a randomized comparison of voriconazole and deoxycholate amphotericin B followed by other licensed antifungal agents for primary therapy for invasive aspergillosis demonstrated superior antifungal efficacy and improved survival at week 12 in the voriconazole arm.[81] Subsequently, isavuconazole has been approved for the primary treatment of aspergillosis, based upon the results of a double-blind, randomized, multinational trial in subjects with proven or probable invasive fungal disease caused by *Aspergillus* spp. or other filamentous fungi. Isavuconazole was well tolerated, with fewer drug-related adverse effects than voriconazole.[82] Posaconazole was shown to be non-inferior to voriconazole for the treatment of aspergillosis in a prospective, double-blind randomized trial.[83] In patients who are unable to tolerate or are not responding to azole therapy, or who are infected with azole-resistant isolates, amphotericin B can be used, with response measured by defervescence and radiographic clearing. To treat microfoci, therapy should be continued after resolution of clinical and radiographic abnormalities until cultures (if they can be obtained) are negative, and reversible underlying predispositions have abated.

Clinical response rather than any arbitrary total dose should guide duration of therapy. The optimal dosage or duration of treatment of invasive disease is unknown and dependent on the extent of disease, the response to therapy, and the patient's underlying disease(s) and immune status. Response to therapy is largely related to the extent of aspergillosis at the time of diagnosis, and host factors, such as resolution of neutropenia and the return of neutrophil function, lessening immunosuppression, and the return of graft function from a bone marrow or organ transplant.[12]

Although caspofungin (and other echinocandins) have in vitro activity against *Aspergillus* species, echinocandins are unable to completely kill or inhibit *Aspergillus* species. Comparative randomized prospective trial data are not available for the echinocandins. Caspofungin is approved by the FDA for use as salvage therapy in patients who are refractory to or intolerant of other therapies such as conventional amphotericin B, lipid formulations of amphotericin B, and/or itraconazole.[12] However, for primary therapy of aspergillosis, response rates are lower with caspofungin than those obtained with voriconazole and amphotericin B.[84]

Given the continued high mortality of aspergillosis, combination therapy has been explored. However, while the advantages of combination therapy include the possibility of more rapid, synergistic killing, disadvantages include the possibility of antagonism, as well as increased cost and the increased risk of drug interactions and adverse effects. Combination therapy with voriconazole plus anidulafungin versus voriconazole alone was explored in a randomized, double-blind, placebo-controlled trial of patients with invasive aspergillosis. Combination therapy demonstrated a trend toward decreased 6-week survival compared to monotherapy, but did not achieve statistical significance (mortality rates 19.3% vs 27.5%, respectively).[85] Thus, there are as yet no firm recommendations regarding the use of combination therapy.[12]

Secondary Prophylaxis

The use of prophylactic antifungal therapy to prevent primary infection or reactivation of aspergillosis during subsequent courses of chemotherapy is recommended.[12] In granulocytopenic patients who recover from an episode of IA, the risk of relapse of aspergillosis during subsequent courses of chemotherapy is greater than 50%. Voriconazole reduced the incidence of invasive fungal function infection (mostly aspergillosis) to 6.7% when used as secondary prophylaxis in allogeneic stem cell transplant recipients with prior infection.[32]

Treatment Options for Emerging Pathogens

The increased frequency of fungal pathogens that were once rare is gaining attention from the medical community. Mucormycosis, fusariosis, lomentosporiosis, and scedosporiosis are the most frequent cause of non-*Aspergillus* mold infections.[16]

Mucorales Infections

Mucormycosis, previously known as zygomycosis, is a term describing infections caused by fungi belonging to the order Mucorales. Permissive environmental conditions, selective antifungal pressure, and increased numbers of immunosuppressed patients have led to increased numbers of infections caused by the Mucorales, which include *Rhizomucor* spp., *Lichtheimia* spp. (formerly Absidia spp.), *Rhizopus* spp., *Mucor* spp., and *Cunninghamella* spp. Prompt initiation of antifungal therapy is crucial, as treatment delays are associated with increased mortality.[86]

Of currently available systemic antifungals, only amphotericin B (including the lipid formulations) displays reliable activity against the Mucorales, while posaconazole and isavuconazole display variable activity, with wide MIC ranges.[16,87] Therapy with a liposomal or lipid-complex formulation of amphotericin B at a dosage of greater than or equal to 5 mg/kg/day, in addition to surgical debridement, is advocated by experts.[86,88]

Fusarium, Scedosporium, and *Lomentospora*

Unfortunately, the early presentation of *Fusarium, Scedosporium,* and *Lomentospora* infections often mimics that of aspergillosis. On histopathology, *Scedosporium* species resembles *Aspergillus* species with dichotomously branching, septate hyphae and has a tendency for invasion of vascular structures. These pathogens often demonstrate intrinsic to variable resistance to amphotericin B and are associated with high mortality rates. Interpretive CBPs for antifungal MICs and these pathogens are not available, and the optimal choice and duration of therapy is unknown. Global guidelines recommend the following strategies: for fusariosis, voriconazole (with or without a lipid amphotericin B product); for lomentosporosis, voriconazole plus terbinafine; and for scedosporiosis, voriconazole.[16,89]

Antifungal Therapy

Clinicians must have working knowledge of mechanism of action, spectrum of activity, dosing, and adverse effects of antifungals in order to provide appropriate recommendations for therapy. Dosing adjustments are needed for many antifungal agents in the setting of renal or hepatic dysfunction. A summary of the most common adverse effects of systemic antifungal agents are summarized in Fig. 144-3 and described in the text below.

The antifungal armamentarium for the treatment of IFIs includes (a) inhibitors of the fungal cell membrane such as polyenes (eg, amphotericin B) and azole antifungals, (b) inhibitors of DNA (5-flucytosine), and (c) inhibitors of cell wall biosynthesis (echinocandins).

Antifungal therapy generally includes one or more antifungal agents, depending on the severity of infection and the patients' immune status. Rarely are the agents used in combination. Often therapy is initiated with an IV agent such as an echinocandin or amphotericin B, and therapy is changed to an oral (azole) regimen as the patient's clinical status improves and oral therapy is tolerated.

Antifungal stewardship, particularly with integration of real-time decision support for the results of rapid diagnostic testing methods such as MALDI-TOF, may improve diagnosis and quality of care, while decreasing mortality and the cost of antifungal therapy.[93]

Amphotericin B

Amphotericin B remains the therapy of choice for many systemic fungal infections despite a lack of controlled clinical trials documenting the optimal dosage, duration of therapy, or relative efficacy of this agent in comparison with newer azole antifungal agents. During pregnancy, amphotericin B remains the treatment of choice for most fungal infections because azole antifungals are teratogenic.[94] The side effects of amphotericin B generally are categorized

Adverse Effect	Polyenes	Azoles					Echino-candins
	AmB	Flucon	Itra	Vori	Posa	Isavu	Micafungin Anidulafungin caspofungin
Nephrotoxicity	✓	✗	✗ (possible with IV)	✗ (possible with IV)	✗	✗	✗
Abdominal discomfort	✗	✓	✓	✓	✓	✓	✗
↑ Hepatic transaminases	✓	✓	✓	✓	✓	✓	✓
Rash, photosensitivity	✗	✓	✓	✓ Can lead to malignancy	✓	✓	✓
Infusion-related reactions/ histamine release	✓	✗	✗	✗	✗	✗	✓
CNS & visual disturbances	✗	✗	✗	✓	✗	✗	✗
Cardiomyopathy (itra), ↑ QT (azoles), ? echinos	✗	✓	✓	✓	✓	↓QT	?

FIGURE 144-3 Adverse effects of systemic antifungal agents. *Data from References 90-92.*

as acute (infusion-related) or long term. Amphotericin B commonly causes renal functional impairment, including decreased glomerular filtration rate, hypokalemia, hypomagnesemia, metabolic acidosis due to distal (or type 1) renal tubular acidosis (RTA), and polyuria due to nephrogenic diabetes insipidus. The nephrotoxicity associated with amphotericin B is usually reversible with discontinuation of therapy. However, recurrent renal dysfunction can occur if treatment is reinstituted. The risk of amphotericin B nephrotoxicity is increased by higher daily doses and concurrent therapy with other nephrotoxins, such as an aminoglycoside or cyclosporine. Salt loading (eg, 500-1,000 mL normal saline infusion) prior to dosing ameloriates/delays the onset of nephrotoxicity, and close monitoring and repletion of potassium and magnesium are necessary.[12,95]

Lipid Formulations of Amphotericin B

The use of deoxycholate amphotericin B is frequently associated with the development of induced nephrotoxicity. In an attempt to decrease the incidence of nephrotoxicity, three lipid formulations of amphotericin B have been developed and approved for use in humans: ABLC (Abelcet; Enzon Pharmaceuticals), ABCD (Amphotec; Intermune Pharmaceuticals), and liposomal amphotericin B (AmBisome; Gilead Pharmaceuticals). In these preparations, amphotericin B is incorporated into the phospholipid bilayer membrane rather than in the enclosed aqueous phase.[96]

The various lipid formulations of amphotericin B exhibit markedly different pharmacokinetics; however, whether these differences result in different outcomes in the treatment of specific types of infections (eg, CNS infections) is unclear. Although larger doses of these preparations are required to achieve similar pharmacologic effects as the deoxycholate form of amphotericin B, the toxicity appears to be much lower. Although the FDA-approved dosages of these agents are 5 mg/kg/day (ABLC), 3 to 6 mg/kg/day (ABCD), and 3 to 5 mg/kg/day (liposomal amphotericin B), the agents appear generally equipotent.[96] The optimal dose of these compounds for serious *Candida* infections is unknown; however, dosages of 3 to 5 mg/kg/day appear reasonable.[7]

Lipid formulations of amphotericin B, especially liposomal amphotericin B and amphotericin B lipid complex, are generally preferred over amphotericin B deoxycholate in clinical practice guidelines given their reduced potential for nephrotoxicity. There is up to a 6.6-fold increase in mortality in patients with amphotericin B–induced nephrotoxicity, and lipid formulations result in a significantly decreased incidence and severity of nephrotoxicity; liposomal amphotericin B may be less nephrotoxic than the ABLC.[96] Liposomal amphotericin B also results in significantly fewer infusion-related reactions than amphotericin B deoxycholate.[96,97]

Flucytosine

Flucytosine (also known as 5-flucytosine) is a fluorinated pyrimidine analog that is highly water-soluble. Patients with creatinine clearances of less than 40 mL/min (0.67 mL/s) should receive careful dosage adjustments. Peak serum concentrations (2 hours after an oral dose) should be monitored in all patients to maintain peak serum concentrations between 20 and 100 mg/L (155 and 775 μmol/L).[98,99]

Flucytosine generally is associated with few side effects in patients with normal renal, GI, and hematologic function, although rash, GI discomfort, diarrhea (5%-10%), and reversible elevations in hepatic enzymes are observed occasionally. In patients with renal dysfunction or concomitant amphotericin B therapy, leukopenia, thrombocytopenia, and (rarely) enterocolitis can occur. Myelotoxicity is well correlated with peak concentrations >100 mg/L (775 μmol/L).[98,99] Flucytosine is rapidly converted to 5-fluorouracil, which is toxic to mammalian cells, once taken up by fungal cells. Patients treated with flucytosine have detectable amounts of 5-fluorouracil in their serum and urine, although the mechanism of flucytosine toxicity is still incompletely understood. Flucytosine may be secreted into the GI tract, deaminated by intestinal bacteria, and reabsorbed as 5-fluorouracil.[98]

Flucytosine is used in combination with amphotericin B or fluconazole in the treatment of cryptococcosis or (less commonly) candidiasis. The rapid development of resistance to flucytosine, however, precludes its use as single-agent therapy. Mechanisms for drug resistance can include loss of deaminase and decreased permeability to the drug.[98]

Echinocandins

The echinocandins (caspofungin, micafungin, and anidulafungin) act as concentration-dependent, non-competitive inhibitors of BG synthase, an essential component of the cell wall of susceptible filamentous fungi that is absent in mammalian cells.

All echinocandins display linear pharmacokinetics following administration of IV dosages, and are degraded primarily by the liver (also in the adrenals and spleen) by hydrolysis and *N*-acetylation. Following initial distribution, echinocandins are taken up by red blood cells (micafungin) and the liver (caspofungin and micafungin) where they undergo slow degradation to mainly inactive metabolites, although two uncommon metabolites of micafungin possess antifungal activity. Degradation products are excreted slowly over many days, primarily through the bile. Among the echinocandins, anidulafungin is unique in being eliminated almost exclusively by slow chemical degradation rather than undergoing hepatic metabolism.

Echinocandins are available only as parenteral formulations, are not dialyzable, and do not require dosage adjustment in patients with renal insufficiency. They have minimal CSF penetration, largely because of their high protein binding and large molecular weights, although the clinical relevance of these findings can be disputed, given that several other antifungal agents (amphotericin B and itraconazole) are effective for the treatment of fungal meningitis despite low CSF concentrations. The echinocandins are well tolerated, although some patients may report histamine release resulting in rash, facial swelling, and itchiness.[100]

Azole Antifungal Agents

Adverse effects of azoles include GI disturbances (primarily nausea, vomiting, epigastric pain, and diarrhea), which appear to be more common in patients receiving ketoconazole and the solution formulation of itraconazole.[12] Although cyclodextrin is not absorbed following oral administration, use of the IV formulations of posaconazole and voriconazole is not recommended by the manufacturers because of concerns for potential nephrotoxicity secondary to accumulation of the cyclodextrin vehicle. This concern is likely not clinically relevant.[101] Fluconazole is well tolerated; intestinal complaints are the most frequently reported, followed by headaches and rash. Unlike ketoconazole, fluconazole does not inhibit testicular or adrenal steroidogenesis in healthy volunteers or hospitalized patients. Reversible alopecia occurs not infrequently and usually appears after several months of treatment with higher doses of fluconazole.[91] Azoles are potentially teratogenic and should be avoided in pregnant women.[94]

Azole antifungals have been implicated in idiosyncratic drug-induced liver injury with the incidence and pattern of injury varying between specific agents. The exact mechanism of toxicity has not been elucidated and there is varying level of evidence with regards to the effect of dose on the development of the toxicity. It is recommended that baseline liver function tests (LFTs) be obtained for patients being started on therapy with these agents and periodically monitored. In general, hepatotoxicity can occur at any time after initiation of the antifungal with most cases occurring in the first month of therapy. The liver injury is usually reversible with discontinuation of the offending agent. Substitution of the offending azole antifungal with a different azole antifungal can occur without impacting resolution of the toxicity.[91] Isavuconazole is less hepatotoxic than voriconazole.[82]

Azole antifungals are associated with QT prolongation as the result of cardiac hERG-mediated potassium channel blockade. However, azoles alone are not considered significant risk factors for serious drug-induced QT prolongation. Instead, the combination of azoles with other risk factors, such as other QT-prolonging medications, electrolyte abnormalities, and heart disease, is necessary to yield risk for serious QT prolongation. Isavuconazole is unique amongst the azoles in that it shortens the QT interval, and so is an option in cases of azole-induced QT prolongation.[92]

Itraconazole

Itraconazole is triazole antifungal with a broad spectrum of antifungal activity. Despite its marked structural similarity to ketoconazole, itraconazole differs in several important respects. Itraconazole appears to have greater specificity against fungal versus mammalian CYP, resulting in greater potency and a decrease in CYP-mediated side effects. In addition, itraconazole possesses in vitro activity against *Aspergillus* and *Sporothrix* species.

Like ketoconazole, the capsule formulation of itraconazole depends on the availability of low gastric pH for dissolution and absorption. Administration with food appears to enhance significantly the bioavailability of itraconazole capsules. Because itraconazole exhibits pH-dependent dissolution and absorption, absorption of the capsule formulation is impaired in patients receiving antacids or H_2-receptor antagonists and in patients with achlorhydria. Plasma concentrations of itraconazole following a single oral dose (capsules) in HIV-infected patients are approximately 50% lower than concentrations observed in healthy volunteers. The capsule formulation of itraconazole exhibits unpredictable oral bioavailability, particularly in subjects with hypochlorhydria and in patients with enteropathy caused by mucositis or GvHD of the gut. An oral suspension formulation of itraconazole was subsequently developed that uses cyclodextrin as a solubilizing vehicle to increase the solubility of the drug. The oral bioavailability of the solution is unaffected by alterations in gastric pH (such as concomitant omeprazole use) or in patients with enteropathy. The bioavailability of the oral solution is optimized in the fasting state.[102,103] A novel capsule formulation was developed which may result in more rapid and consistent attainment of therapeutic concentrations.[104]

Fluconazole

Fluconazole is a triazole antifungal agent with markedly different pharmacologic features than other marketed azole antifungals. The small molecular weight, low protein binding, and increased water solubility of fluconazole result in rapid, essentially complete absorption of drug following oral administration. Because fluconazole is excreted primarily (greater than 80%) as unchanged drug in the urine, dosage adjustments are necessary in patients with renal dysfunction.[90]

Voriconazole

The hepatic biotransformation of voriconazole is fairly complex and involves CYP2C19, CYP3A4, and CYP2C9, with most metabolism mediated through CYP2C19. Two of the CYPs involved in voriconazole metabolism (CYP2C19 and CYP2C9) exhibit genetic polymorphism; variability in the CYP2C19 genotype accounts for approximately 30% of the overall between subject variability in voriconazole pharmacokinetics. About 3% to 5% of white and African human populations are poor metabolizers, while 15% to 20% of Asian populations are poor metabolizers. Drug levels can be as much as fourfold greater in poor metabolizers than in individuals who are homozygous extensive metabolizers. Coadministration of voriconazole with drugs that are potent CYP450 enzyme inducers can significantly reduce voriconazole levels. Voriconazole drug interactions are dose-dependent, as they exhibit unpredictable nonlinear pharmacokinetics; thus, drug interactions are more difficult to predict and manage.[92] Voriconazole is uniquely associated with phototoxicity. In addition, patients receiving long-term voriconazole are risk for development of skin cancer (primarily squamous cell carcinoma) and periostitis.[91,92]

The most common side effect of voriconazole is a reversible disturbance of vision (photopsia), which occurs in approximately 30% of patients but rarely leads to discontinuation of the drug. Symptoms tend to occur during the first week of therapy and decrease or disappear despite continued therapy. Patients experience altered color discrimination, blurred vision, the appearance of bright spots and wavy lines, and photophobia. Patients should be cautioned that driving can be hazardous because of the risk of visual disturbances. The visual effects are associated with changes in electroretinogram tracings, which revert to normal when treatment with the drug is stopped; no permanent damage to the retina has been demonstrated. Less common are visual and/or auditory hallucinations, which are associated with concentrations >5.5 μg/mL (mg/L; 15.7 μmol/L).[92]

Posaconazole

Posaconazole has a broad spectrum of antifungal activity, including *Aspergillus* and *Candida* species and variable activity against the Mucorales. Posaconazole was initially developed as an oral suspension for the prevention of IFIs in immunocompromised patients, including hematologic malignancy patients with prolonged neutropenia from chemotherapy as well as HSCT patients with GvHD.[23,24] However, to ensure adequate absorption, the suspension formulation had to be administered two to three times daily, with a high fat meal or a nutritional supplement. Most patients with GvHD, and many with chemotherapy-associated nausea or vomiting, mucositis or diarrhea, were unable to comply with the requirement for a fatty meal, resulting in decreased plasma concentrations of posaconazole and an increased risk of breakthrough fungal infection. The development of IV and delayed-release tablet formulations of posaconazole has circumvented these absorption issues and allows once daily oral administration of posaconazole following administration of a twice daily loading dose on the first day of therapy.[92]

Isavuconazole

Isavuconazole, available both orally and IV, has a broad spectrum of activity against a number of clinically important yeasts and molds, including *Candida* spp., *Aspergillus* spp., *C. neoformans*, *Trichosporon* spp., and variable activity against the Mucorales. The most commonly reported adverse events, which are mild and limited in nature, include nausea, diarrhea, and elevated liver function tests. The potential advantage of this agent over other currently available broad-spectrum azole antifungals is a clinically useful alternative to voriconazole for the treatment of invasive aspergillosis, due to its lack of genetically determined variability in plasma levels, and more favorable and predictable drug interaction profile.[92]

Drug Interactions with Antifungal Agents

The interaction of azole antifungal agents with other CYP-metabolized drugs is well recognized. All azoles are inhibitors of the CYP3A4 enzyme system, and voriconazole and fluconazole additionally are inhibitors of CYP2C8/9 and CYP2C19. Apart from fluconazole (a substrate of CYP3A4 but mostly eliminated in the urine as unchanged drug) and posaconazole (metabolized by uridine diphosphate glucuronidation), the azoles appear to be metabolized

TABLE 144-10 Plasma Concentration Monitoring of Antifungal Agents

	Serum Concentration Monitoring Necessary?	Target Concentration Range	Timing of Sample
Echinocandins	No	NA	NA
Amphotericin B (including lipids)	No	NA	NA
Fluconazole	No	NA	NA
Isavuconazole	Unclear; appears to demonstrate limited pharmacokinetic variability and no clear thresholds for efficacy or toxicity have been elucidated	NA	NA
Itraconazole	Yes, to ensure absorption and efficacy	*Efficacy:* Prophylaxis: >0.5 μg/mL (mg/L; 0.7 μmol/L) Treatment: >1 μg/mL (mg/L; 1.4 μmol/L) *Toxicity:* <5 μg/mL (mg/L; 7 μmol/L)	Trough 7 days after initiation of therapy
Voriconazole	Probably yes—in all patients treated for IFI, altered liver function, potential drug-drug interactions, lack of response *Low* concentrations are associated with poor outcome; *high* concentrations are associated with adverse effects Variable metabolism due to non-linear PK and genetic variability in CYP2C19 → unpredictable dose-exposure relationship	*Efficacy:* Prophylaxis: trough >0.5-2 μg/mL (mg/L; 1.4-5.7 μmol/L) Treatment: trough >1-2 μg/mL (mg/L; 2.9-5.7 μmol/L) Concentrations >2.0 μg/mL (mg/L; 5.7 μmol/L) are associated with improved outcome; 2-5.5 μg/mL (mg/L; 5.7-15.7 μmol/L) is probably the best target *Toxicity:* concentrations >5.5 μg/mL (mg/L; 15.7 μmol/L) are associated with ↑ risk of neurotoxicity	Trough after 5-7 days therapy if no loading dose administered; 48 hours after administration of loading dose in critically ill patient (time to steady state is unpredictable due to nonlinear metabolism)
Posaconazole delayed release tablets	Maybe Outcomes (but not adverse events) correlate with higher plasma concentrations in prophylaxis and possibly treatment	*Efficacy:* Prophylaxis: >0.7 μg/mL (mg/L; 1 μmol/L) Treatment: Not well studied; concentrations >1.25 μg/mL (mg/L; 1.78 μmol/L) *Toxicity:* Correlation with toxicity poorly defined	Random level at SS (>7 days therapy). The long $t_{1/2}$ ensures little fluctuation in peaks and troughs at SS
Flucytosine	Yes—high concentrations are associated with toxicity	*Toxicity:* "Peak" <80-100 μg/mL (mg/L; 620-775 μmol/L) *Efficacy:* Peak >20 μg/mL (mg/L; 155 μmol/L)	2 hours postdose "peak", 3-5 days after initiation of therapy

NA, not applicable.

Data from References 12,92, and 99.

almost entirely via the CYP3A4 subfamily. As expected, numerous clinically significant interactions have been documented with azole antifungals and a variety of other drugs. In most cases, the azole interferes with the metabolism of the other CYP-metabolized drug. Relative to ketoconazole and itraconazole, fluconazole appears to be intermediate in its ability to inhibit human cytochromes P450. The magnitude of fluconazole-induced inhibition of cyclosporine metabolism depends on the dosage of fluconazole. Isavuconazole appears to be a more modest inhibitor of CYP3A4 compared to voriconazole and posaconazole.[92,105]

Predictably, drugs such as rifampin, rifabutin, isoniazid, phenytoin, and carbamazepine, which are known to induce the activity of cytochromes P450, result in increased metabolism of the azole antifungals and can result in therapeutic failures. Increased dosages of azole antifungals can be required in patients receiving these combinations of drugs.[105]

Itraconazole is an inhibitor of intestinal Pgp. Significant increases in digoxin (a Pgp substrate) have been observed in patients receiving both agents concurrently. Interactions with other substrates of Pgp would be expected to occur.[105]

Echinocandins are not inducers of CYP enzymes, nor do they interact with Pgp, and are considered poor substrates of CYP3A4. Nevertheless, drug interactions are noted with caspofungin and cyclosporine and tacrolimus; the mechanism for these interactions is not yet known. Rifampin both inhibits (acutely) and induces (after chronic administration) caspofungin metabolism, and a dosage increase is recommended in patients receiving other enzyme inducers, such as efavirenz, nevirapine, phenytoin, dexamethasone, and carbamazepine. Although micafungin does not significantly affect the clearance (or area under the plasma-concentration vs time curve [AUC]) of tacrolimus, it increases the AUCs of sirolimus and nifedipine and decreases the clearance of cyclosporine.[100]

Therapeutic Drug Monitoring of Antifungal Agents

There is insufficient data to justify the routine use of therapeutic drug monitoring (TDM) for the prophylaxis or treatment of fungal infections with all antifungal agents. In addition, logistics, cost, and incorporation of TDM have yet to be worked out in modern prophylactic algorithms. However, under certain circumstances, serum or plasma concentration monitoring of select agents is warranted. Given the tremendous interpatient and intrapatient variability in voriconazole metabolism, TDM is warranted in most patients. Also, given the poor oral bioavailability of itraconazole capsules and posaconazole solution, monitoring is recommended, particularly in patients with GvHD of the gut, mucositis, or diarrhea, or poor oral intake or those receiving concomitant therapy with proton-pump inhibitors. Although the use of posaconazole tablets may result in a decreased need for TDM, patients with a higher weight and those experiencing diarrhea are more likely to have lower levels. Additional settings include patients susceptible to flucytosine toxicity, to document adequate oral absorption of poorly bioavailable azoles in cases of suspected treatment failure or concern about compliance or absorption, solubility and finally, when drug interactions that might reduce or accelerate the metabolism of azoles is suspected.[92,99] The need for isavuconazole TDM is undefined, as clinical experience has demonstrated limited pharmacokinetic variability and no clear correlations between concentrations and response or toxicity.[92] Recommendations regarding plasma concentration monitoring of antifungals are summarized in Table 144-10.

ABBREVIATIONS

AIDS	acquired immunodeficiency syndrome
ABCD	amphotericin B colloid dispersion
ABLC	amphotericin B lipid complex
AUC	area under the plasma-concentration versus time curve
BG	(1,3)-β-D-glucan
BPA	bronchopulmonary aspergillosis
BSI	bloodstream infection
CBP	clinical breakpoint
CT	computed tomography
CVC	central venous catheter
CSF	cerebrospinal fluid
CYP	cytochrome P450
ELISA	enzyme-linked immunosorbent assay
FISH	fluorescence in situ hybridization
GvHD	graft-versus-host disease
HEPA	high-efficiency particulate air
HAART	highly active antiretroviral therapy
HSCT	hematopoietic stem cell transplantation
IA	invasive aspergillosis
ICP	intracranial pressure
ICUs	intensive care units
IDSA	Infectious Diseases Society of America
IPA	invasive pulmonary aspergillosis
IRIS	immune reconstitution inflammatory syndrome
LFT	liver function test
MALDI-TOF-ICMS	matrix-assisted laser desorption ionization time-of-flight mass spectrometry
NSAID	non-steroidal antiinflammatory drug
PDH	progressive disseminated histoplasmosis
PN	parenteral nutrition
PNA	peptide nucleic acid
RR	respiratory rate
SDD	susceptible dose-dependent
TDM	therapeutic plasma drug concentration monitoring
TEE	transesophageal echocardiogram
TTE	transthoracic echocardiogram
WBC	white blood cell

REFERENCES

1. JE B. Introduction to mycoses. In: Bennett JE DR, Blaser MJ, eds. *Mandell, Douglas, and Bennett's Principles and Practice of Infectious Diseases*. Elsevier; 2020:3082–86.
2. Pfaller MA, Jones RN, Messer SA, Edmond MB, Wenzel RP. National surveillance of nosocomial blood stream infection due to species of Candida other than Candida albicans: frequency of occurrence and antifungal susceptibility in the SCOPE Program. SCOPE Participant Group. Surveillance and Control of Pathogens of Epidemiologic. *Diagn Microbiol Infect Dis.* Feb 1998;30(2):121–9.
3. Pfaller MA, Jones RN, Doern GV, et al. International surveillance of blood stream infections due to Candida species in the European SENTRY Program: species distribution and antifungal susceptibility including the investigational triazole and echinocandin agents. SENTRY Participant Group (Europe). *Diagn Microbiol Infect Dis.* Sep 1999;35(1):19–25.
4. Pfaller MA, Diekema DJ. Progress in antifungal susceptibility testing of Candida spp. by use of Clinical and Laboratory Standards Institute broth microdilution methods, 2010 to 2012. *J Clin Microbiol.* Sep 2012;50(9):2846–56. doi:10.1128/JCM.00937-12.
5. Pfaller MA, Andes D, Diekema DJ, Espinel-Ingroff A, Sheehan D, Testing CSfAS. Wild-type MIC distributions, epidemiological cutoff values and species-specific clinical breakpoints for fluconazole and Candida: time for harmonization of CLSI and EUCAST broth microdilution methods. *Drug Resist Updat.* Dec 2010;13(6):180–95. doi:10.1016/j.drup.2010.09.002.
6. Eschenauer GA, Carver PL. The evolving role of antifungal susceptibility testing. *Pharmacotherapy.* May 2013;33(5):465–75. doi:10.1002/phar.1233.
7. Pappas PG, Kauffman CA, Andes DR, et al. Clinical Practice Guideline for the Management of Candidiasis: 2016 Update by the Infectious

Diseases Society of America. *Clin Infect Dis.* Feb 15 2016;62(4):e1–50. doi:10.1093/cid/civ933.

8. Chapman SW, Dismukes WE, Proia LA, et al. Clinical practice guidelines for the management of blastomycosis: 2008 update by the Infectious Diseases Society of America. *Clin Infect Dis.* Jun 15 2008;46(12):1801–12. doi:10.1086/588300.
9. Perfect JR, Dismukes WE, Dromer F, et al. Clinical practice guidelines for the management of cryptococcal disease: 2010 update by the Infectious Diseases Society of America. *Clin Infect Dis.* Feb 1 2010;50(3):291–322. doi:10.1086/649858.
10. Wheat LJ, Freifeld AG, Kleiman MB, et al. Clinical practice guidelines for the management of patients with histoplasmosis: 2007 update by the Infectious Diseases Society of America. *Clin Infect Dis.* Oct 1 2007;45(7):807–25. doi:10.1086/521259.
11. Galgiani JN, Ampel NM, Blair JE, et al. 2016 Infectious Diseases Society of America (IDSA) Clinical Practice Guideline for the Treatment of Coccidioidomycosis. *Clin Infect Dis.* Jul 27 2016;63(6):e112–46. doi:10.1093/cid/ciw360.
12. Patterson TF, Thompson GR 3rd, Denning DW, et al. Practice Guidelines for the Diagnosis and Management of Aspergillosis: 2016 Update by the Infectious Diseases Society of America. *Clin Infect Dis.* Aug 15 2016;63(4):e1–60. doi:10.1093/cid/ciw326.
13. Gauthier GM. Fungal dimorphism and virulence: molecular mechanisms for temperature adaptation, immune evasion, and in vivo survival. *Mediators Inflamm.* 2017;2017:8491383. doi:10.1155/2017/8491383.
14. Cowen LE, Sanglard D, Howard SJ, Rogers PD, Perlin DS. Mechanisms of antifungal drug resistance. *Cold Spring Harb Perspect Med.* Jul 2014;5(7):a019752. doi:10.1101/cshperspect.a019752.
15. Pfaller MA, Diekema DJ. Epidemiology of invasive candidiasis: a persistent public health problem. *Clin Microbiol Rev.* Jan 2007;20(1):133–63. doi:10.1128/CMR.00029-06.
16. Lamoth F, Kontoyiannis DP. Therapeutic challenges of non-aspergillus invasive mold infections in immunosuppressed patients. *Antimicrob Agents Chemother.* 2019;63(11). doi:10.1128/AAC.01244-19.
17. Alexander BD, Johnson MD, Pfeiffer CD, et al. Increasing echinocandin resistance in Candida glabrata: clinical failure correlates with presence of FKS mutations and elevated minimum inhibitory concentrations. *Clin Infect Dis.* Jun 2013;56(12):1724–32. doi:10.1093/cid/cit136.
18. Shields RK, Nguyen MH, Press EG, et al. The presence of an FKS mutation rather than MIC is an independent risk factor for failure of echinocandin therapy among patients with invasive candidiasis due to Candida glabrata. *Antimicrob Agents Chemother.* Sep 2012;56(9):4862–9. doi:10.1128/AAC.00027-12.
19. Vermeulen E, Lagrou K, Verweij PE. Azole resistance in Aspergillus fumigatus: a growing public health concern. *Curr Opin Infect Dis.* Dec 2013;26(6):493–500. doi:10.1097/qco.0000000000000005.
20. Sardi JCO, Scorzoni L, Bernardi T, Fusco-Almeida AM, Mendes Giannini MJS. Candida species: current epidemiology, pathogenicity, biofilm formation, natural antifungal products and new therapeutic options. *J Med Microbiol.* Jan 2013;62(Pt 1):10–24. doi:10.1099/jmm.0.045054-0.
21. McCoy D, Depestel DD, Carver PL. Primary antifungal prophylaxis in adult hematopoietic stem cell transplant recipients: current therapeutic concepts. *Pharmacotherapy.* Nov 2009;29(11):1306–25. doi:10.1592/phco.29.11.1306.
22. Eschenauer GA, Lam SW, Carver PL. Antifungal prophylaxis in liver transplant recipients. *Liver Transpl.* Aug 2009;15(8):842–58. doi:10.1002/lt.21826.
23. Ullmann AJ, Lipton JH, Vesole DH, et al. Posaconazole or fluconazole for prophylaxis in severe graft-versus-host disease. *N Engl J Med.* Jan 2007;356(4):335–47. doi:10.1056/NEJMoa061098.
24. Cornely OA, Maertens J, Winston DJ, et al. Posaconazole vs. fluconazole or itraconazole prophylaxis in patients with neutropenia. *N Engl J Med.* Jan 2007;356(4):348–59. doi:10.1056/NEJMoa061094.
25. Wisplinghoff H, Bischoff T, Tallent SM, Seifert H, Wenzel RP, Edmond MB. Nosocomial bloodstream infections in US hospitals: analysis of 24,179 cases from a prospective nationwide surveillance study. *Clin Infect Dis.* Aug 1 2004;39(3):309–17. doi:10.1086/421946.
26. Lam SW, Eschenauer GA, Carver PL. Evolving role of early antifungals in the adult intensive care unit. *Crit Care Med.* May 2009;37(5):1580–93. doi:10.1097/CCM.0b013e31819dec9b.
27. Fernandez J, Erstad BL, Petty W, Nix DE. Time to positive culture and identification for Candida blood stream infections. *Diagn Microbiol Infect Dis.* Aug 2009;64(4):402–7. doi:10.1016/j.diagmicrobio.2009.04.002.
28. Schelenz S, Barnes RA, Barton RC, et al. British Society for Medical Mycology best practice recommendations for the diagnosis of serious fungal diseases. *Lancet Infect Dis.* Apr 2015;15(4):461–74. doi:10.1016/s1473-3099(15)70006-x.
29. Donnelly JP, Chen SC, Kauffman CA, et al. Revision and Update of the Consensus Definitions of Invasive Fungal Disease From the European Organization for Research and Treatment of Cancer and the Mycoses Study Group Education and Research Consortium. *Clin Infect Dis.* Sep 2020;71(6):1367–76. doi:10.1093/cid/ciz1008.
30. Schuster MG, Edwards JE Jr, Sobel JD, et al. Empirical fluconazole versus placebo for intensive care unit patients: a randomized trial. *Ann Intern Med.* Jul 15 2008;149(2):83–90.
31. Walsh TJ, Pappas P, Winston DJ, et al. Voriconazole compared with liposomal amphotericin B for empirical antifungal therapy in patients with neutropenia and persistent fever. *N Engl J Med.* Jan 2002;346(4):225–34. doi:10.1056/NEJM200201243460403.
32. Cordonnier C, Rovira M, Maertens J, et al. Voriconazole for secondary prophylaxis of invasive fungal infections in allogeneic stem cell transplant recipients: results of the VOSIFI study. *Haematologica.* Oct 2010;95(10):1762–8. doi:10.3324/haematol.2009.020073.
33. Jr DGS. Histoplasma capsulatum (Histoplasmosis). In: JE B, R D, MJ B, eds. *Mandell, Douglas, And Bennett's Principles and Practice of Infectious Diseases.* 9th ed. Elsevier; 2020:3162–76.
34. Ashraf N, Kubat RC, Poplin V, et al. Re-drawing the maps for endemic mycoses. *Mycopathologia.* Oct 2020;185(5):843–65. doi:10.1007/s11046-020-00431-2.
35. Hendrix MJ, Larson L, Rauseo AM, et al. Voriconazole versus itraconazole for the initial and step-down treatment of histoplasmosis: a retrospective cohort. *Clin Infect Dis.* Oct 2020; doi:10.1093/cid/ciaa1555.
36. Spec A, Connolly P, Montejano R, Wheat LJ. In vitro activity of isavuconazole against fluconazole-resistant isolates of Histoplasma capsulatum. *Med Mycol.* Oct 2018;56(7):834–7. doi:10.1093/mmy/myx130.
37. M GG, S KB. Blastomycosis. In: JE B, R D, MJ B, eds. *Mandell, Douglas, And Bennett's Principles and Practice of Infectious Diseases.* 9th ed. Elsevier; 2020:3177–89.
38. Dismukes WE, Bradsher RW, Cloud GC, et al. Itraconazole therapy for blastomycosis and histoplasmosis. NIAID Mycoses Study Group. *Am J Med.* Nov 1992;93(5):489–97. doi:10.1016/0002-9343(92)90575-v.
39. N GJ. Coccidioidomycosis (Coccidioides Species). In: JE B, R D, MJ B, eds. *Mandell, Douglas, And Bennett's Principles and Practice of Infectious Diseases.* 9th ed. Elsevier; 2020:3190–3200.
40. Graybill JR, Stevens DA, Galgiani JN, Dismukes WE, Cloud GA. Itraconazole treatment of coccidioidomycosis. NAIAD Mycoses Study Group. *Am J Med.* Sep 1990;89(3):282–90. doi:10.1016/0002-9343(90)90339-f.
41. Hoang LMN, Philips P, Galanis E. Cryptococcus gattii: a review of the epidemiology, clinical presentation, diagnosis, and management of this endemic Yeast in the Pacific Northwest. *Clinical Microbiology Newsletter.* 2011;33(24):187–95. doi:10.1016/j.clinmicnews.2011.11.003.
42. R PJ. Cryptococcosis (Cryptococcus neoformans and Cryptococcus gattii). In: JE B, R D, MJ B, eds. *Mandell, Douglas, and Bennett's Principles and Practice of Infectious Diseases.* 9th ed. Elsevier; 2020:3146–61.
43. Dismukes WE. Antifungal therapy: lessons learned over the past 27 years. *Clin Infect Dis.* May 2006;42(9):1289–96. doi:10.1086/503043.
44. van der Horst CM, Saag MS, Cloud GA, et al. Treatment of cryptococcal meningitis associated with the acquired immunodeficiency syndrome. National Institute of Allergy and Infectious Diseases Mycoses Study Group and AIDS Clinical Trials Group. *N Engl J Med.* Jul 3 1997;337(1):15–21. doi:10.1056/nejm199707033370103.
45. Brouwer AE, Rajanuwong A, Chierakul W, et al. Combination antifungal therapies for HIV-associated cryptococcal meningitis: a randomised trial. *Lancet.* May 2004;363(9423):1764–7. doi:10.1016/S0140-6736(04)16301-0.
46. Day JN, Chau TT, Lalloo DG. Combination antifungal therapy for cryptococcal meningitis. *N Engl J Med.* Jun 2013;368(26):2522–3. doi:10.1056/NEJMc1305981.
47. Beardsley J, Wolbers M, Kibengo FM, et al. Adjunctive dexamethasone in HIV-associated cryptococcal meningitis. *N Engl J Med.* Feb 2016;374(6):542–54. doi:10.1056/NEJMoa1509024.
48. MS L, JE E. Candida Species. In: JE B, R D, MJ B, eds. *Mandell, Douglas, and Bennett's Principles and Practice of Infectious Diseases.* 9th ed. Elsevier; 2020:3087–3102:chap 256.
49. Horn DL, Neofytos D, Anaissie EJ, et al. Epidemiology and outcomes of candidemia in 2019 patients: data from the prospective antifungal

therapy alliance registry. *Clin Infect Dis.* Jun 2009;48(12):1695–703. doi:10.1086/599039.

50. Lamoth F, Kontoyiannis DP. The Candida auris alert: facts and perspectives. *The Journal of Infectious Diseases.* Jan 30 2018;217(4):516–20. doi:10.1093/infdis/jix597.
51. Halliday CL, Kidd SE, Sorrell TC, Chen SC. Molecular diagnostic methods for invasive fungal disease: the horizon draws nearer? *Pathology.* Apr 2015;47(3):257–69. doi:10.1097/pat.0000000000000234.
52. Alexander BD, Ashley ED, Reller LB, Reed SD. Cost savings with implementation of PNA FISH testing for identification of Candida albicans in blood cultures. *Diagn Microbiol Infect Dis.* Apr 2006;54(4):277–82. doi:10.1016/j.diagmicrobio.2005.10.011.
53. Morrell M, Fraser VJ, Kollef MH. Delaying the empiric treatment of candida bloodstream infection until positive blood culture results are obtained: a potential risk factor for hospital mortality. *Antimicrob Agents Chemother.* Sep 2005;49(9):3640–5. doi:10.1128/AAC.49.9.3640-3645.2005.
54. Kludze-Forson M, Eschenauer GA, Kubin CJ, Della-Latta P, Lam SW. The impact of delaying the initiation of appropriate antifungal treatment for Candida bloodstream infection. *Med Mycol.* Mar 2010;48(2):436–9. doi:10.3109/13693780903208256.
55. Garey KW, Neuhauser MM, Bearden DT, et al. Evaluation of antifungals in the surgical intensive care unit: a multi-institutional study. *Mycoses.* May 2006;49(3):226–31. doi:10.1111/j.1439-0507.2006.01222.x.
56. Knitsch W, Vincent JL, Utzolino S, et al. A randomized, placebo-controlled trial of preemptive antifungal therapy for the prevention of invasive candidiasis following gastrointestinal surgery for intra-abdominal infections. *Clin Infect Dis.* Dec 2015;61(11):1671–8. doi:10.1093/cid/civ707.
57. Ostrosky-Zeichner L, Shoham S, Vazquez J, et al. MSG-01: A randomized, double-blind, placebo-controlled trial of caspofungin prophylaxis followed by preemptive therapy for invasive candidiasis in high-risk adults in the critical care setting. *Clin Infect Dis.* May 2014;58(9):1219–26. doi:10.1093/cid/ciu074.
58. Eggimann P, Francioli P, Bille J, et al. Fluconazole prophylaxis prevents intra-abdominal candidiasis in high-risk surgical patients. *Crit Care Med.* Jun 1999;27(6):1066–72.
59. Timsit JF, Azoulay E, Schwebel C, et al. Empirical micafungin treatment and survival without invasive fungal infection in adults with ICU-acquired sepsis, Candida Colonization, and multiple organ failure: The EMPIRICUS randomized clinical trial. *JAMA.* Oct 2016;316(15):1555–64. doi:10.1001/jama.2016.14655.
60. Kullberg BJ, Sobel JD, Ruhnke M, et al. Voriconazole versus a regimen of amphotericin B followed by fluconazole for candidaemia in non-neutropenic patients: a randomised non-inferiority trial. *Lancet.* Oct 22-28 2005;366(9495):1435–42. doi:10.1016/S0140-6736(05)67490-9.
61. Rex JH, Bennett JE, Sugar AM, et al. A randomized trial comparing fluconazole with amphotericin B for the treatment of candidemia in patients without neutropenia. Candidemia Study Group and the National Institute. *N Engl J Med.* Nov 1994;331(20):1325–30. doi:10.1056/NEJM199411173312001.
62. Reboli AC, Rotstein C, Pappas PG, et al. Anidulafungin versus fluconazole for invasive candidiasis. *N Engl J Med.* Jun 2007;356(24):2472–82. doi:10.1056/NEJMoa066906.
63. Kuse ER, Chetchotisakd P, da Cunha CA, et al. Micafungin versus liposomal amphotericin B for candidaemia and invasive candidosis: a phase III randomised double-blind trial. *Lancet.* May 2007;369(9572):1519–27. doi:10.1016/S0140-6736(07)60605-9.
64. Kullberg BJ, Viscoli C, Pappas PG, et al. Isavuconazole versus caspofungin in the treatment of Candidemia and other invasive Candida infections: the ACTIVE trial. *Clin Infect Dis.* 05 2019;68(12):1981–89. doi:10.1093/cid/ciy827.
65. Mora-Duarte J, Betts R, Rotstein C, et al. Comparison of caspofungin and amphotericin B for invasive candidiasis. *N Engl J Med.* Dec 2002;347(25):2020–9. doi:10.1056/NEJMoa021585.
66. Andes DR, Safdar N, Baddley JW, et al. Impact of treatment strategy on outcomes in patients with candidemia and other forms of invasive candidiasis: a patient-level quantitative review of randomized trials. *Clin Infect Dis.* Apr 2012;54(8):1110–22. doi:10.1093/cid/cis021.
67. Rex JH, Pappas PG, Karchmer AW, et al. A randomized and blinded multicenter trial of high-dose fluconazole plus placebo versus fluconazole plus amphotericin B as therapy for candidemia and its consequences in nonneutropenic subjects. *Clin Infect Dis.* May 15 2003;36(10):1221–8. doi:10.1086/374850.
68. Aslam S, Rotstein C, Practice AIDCo. Candida infections in solid organ transplantation: Guidelines from the American Society of Transplantation Infectious Diseases Community of Practice. *Clin Transplant.* 2019;33(9):e13623. doi:10.1111/ctr.13623.
69. Eschenauer GA, Carver PL, Lin SW, et al. Fluconazole versus an echinocandin for Candida glabrata fungaemia: a retrospective cohort study. *J Antimicrob Chemother.* Apr 2013;68(4):922–6. doi:10.1093/jac/dks482.
70. Eschenauer GA, Carver PL, Patel TS, et al. Survival in patients with Candida glabrata bloodstream infection is associated with fluconazole dose. *Antimicrob Agents Chemother.* 2018;62(6). doi:10.1128/AAC.02566-17. PMC5971561. https://www.ncbi.nlm.nih.gov/pubmed/29581112. Accessed Jun.
71. Chiotos K, Vendetti N, Zaoutis TE, et al. Comparative effectiveness of echinocandins versus fluconazole therapy for the treatment of adult candidaemia due to Candida parapsilosis: a retrospective observational cohort study of the Mycoses Study Group (MSG-12). *Journal of Antimicrobial Chemotherapy.* December 1, 2016 2016;71(12):3536–39. doi:10.1093/jac/dkw305.
72. National Comprehensive Cancer Network. Prevention and Treatment of Cancer-Related Infections (Version 2.2020). https://www.nccn.org/professionals/physician_gls/pdf/infections.pdf. Accessed February 15, 2021.
73. Lionakis MS, Lewis RE, Kontoyiannis DP. Breakthrough invasive mold infections in the hematology patient: current concepts and future directions. *Clin Infect Dis.* 10 2018;67(10):1621–30. doi:10.1093/cid/ciy473.
74. Sobel JD, Kauffman CA, McKinsey D, et al. Candiduria: a randomized, double-blind study of treatment with fluconazole and placebo. The National Institute of Allergy and Infectious Diseases (NIAID) Mycoses Study Group. *Clin Infect Dis.* Jan 2000;30(1):19–24. doi:10.1086/313580.
75. GR T, TF P. *Aspergillus* species. In: JE B, R D, MJ B, eds. *Mandell, Douglas, and Bennett's Principles and Practice of Infectious Diseases.* 9th ed. Elsevier; 2020.
76. Verweij PE, Rijnders BJA, Brüggemann RJM, et al. Review of influenza-associated pulmonary aspergillosis in ICU patients and proposal for a case definition: an expert opinion. *Intensive Care Med.* Aug 2020;46(8):1524–35. doi:10.1007/s00134-020-06091-6.
77. Finkelman MA. Specificity influences in (1→3)-β-d-glucan-supported diagnosis of invasive fungal disease. *J Fungi (Basel).* Dec 2020;7(1). doi:10.3390/jof7010014.
78. Husain S, Camargo JF. Invasive Aspergillosis in solid-organ transplant recipients: Guidelines from the American Society of Transplantation Infectious Diseases Community of Practice. *Clin Transplant.* 2019;33(9):e13544. doi:10.1111/ctr.13544.
79. Walsh TJ, Hiemenz JW, Seibel NL, et al. Amphotericin B lipid complex for invasive fungal infections: analysis of safety and efficacy in 556 cases. *Clin Infect Dis.* Jun 1998;26(6):1383–96.
80. Cornely OA, Maertens J, Bresnik M, et al. Liposomal amphotericin B as initial therapy for invasive mold infection: a randomized trial comparing a high-loading dose regimen with standard dosing (AmBiLoad trial). *Clin Infect Dis.* May 2007;44(10):1289–97. doi:10.1086/514341.
81. Herbrecht R, Denning DW, Patterson TF, et al. Voriconazole versus amphotericin B for primary therapy of invasive aspergillosis. *N Engl J Med.* Aug 8 2002;347(6):408–15. doi:10.1056/NEJMoa020191.
82. Maertens JA, Raad II, Marr KA, et al. Isavuconazole versus voriconazole for primary treatment of invasive mould disease caused by Aspergillus and other filamentous fungi (SECURE): a phase 3, randomised-controlled, non-inferiority trial. *Lancet.* Feb 20 2016;387(10020):760–9. doi:10.1016/S0140-6736(15)01159-9.
83. Maertens JA, Rahav G, Lee DG, et al. Posaconazole versus voriconazole for primary treatment of invasive aspergillosis: a phase 3, randomised, controlled, non-inferiority trial. *Lancet.* Feb 2021;397(10273):499–509. doi:10.1016/S0140-6736(21)00219-1.
84. Viscoli C, Herbrecht R, Akan H, et al. An EORTC Phase II study of caspofungin as first-line therapy of invasive aspergillosis in haematological patients. *J Antimicrob Chemother.* Dec 2009;64(6):1274–81. doi:10.1093/jac/dkp355.
85. Marr KA, Schlamm HT, Herbrecht R, et al. Combination antifungal therapy for invasive aspergillosis: a randomized trial. *Ann Intern Med.* Jan 20 2015;162(2):81–89. doi:10.7326/m13-2508.
86. DP K, RE L. Agents of mucormycosis and entomophthoramycosis. In: JE B, R D, MJ B, eds. *Mandell, Douglas, and Bennett's Principles and Practice of Infectious Diseases.* 9th ed. Elsevier; 2020:3117–3130.
87. Marty FM, Ostrosky-Zeichner L, Cornely OA, et al. Isavuconazole treatment for mucormycosis: a single-arm open-label trial and case-control analysis. *Lancet Infect Dis.* Jul 2016;16(7):828–37. doi:10.1016/S1473-3099(16)00071-2.
88. Cornely OA, Alastruey-Izquierdo A, Arenz D, et al. Global guideline for the diagnosis and management of mucormycosis: an initiative of the European Confederation of Medical Mycology in cooperation with the Mycoses Study Group Education and Research Consortium. *Lancet Infect Dis.* 2019;19(12):e405–21. doi:10.1016/S1473-3099(19)30312-3.

89. Hoenigl M, Salmanton-García J, Walsh TJ, et al. Global guideline for the diagnosis and management of rare mould infections: an initiative of the European Confederation of Medical Mycology in cooperation with the International Society for Human and Animal Mycology and the American Society for Microbiology. *Lancet Infect Dis*. Feb 2021;doi:10.1016/S1473-3099(20)30784-2.
90. Lewis RE. Current concepts in antifungal pharmacology. *Mayo Clin Proc*. Aug 2011;86(8):805–17. doi:10.4065/mcp.2011.0247.
91. Benitez LL, Carver PL. Adverse effects associated with long-term administration of azole antifungal agents. *Drugs*. 2019;79(8):833–53. doi:10.1007/s40265-019-01127-8.
92. Klatt ME, Eschenauer GA. Review of pharmacologic considerations in the use of azole antifungals in lung transplant recipients. *J Fungi (Basel)*. Jan 2021;7(2). doi:10.3390/jof7020076.
93. Eschenauer GA. Antifungal stewardship: Still catching up? Commentary on "Variability in antifungal stewardship strategies among Society for Healthcare Epidemiology of America (SHEA) Research Network facilities." *Infect Control Hosp Epidemiol*. 2020;41(5):590–91. doi:10.1017/ice.2020.85
94. Cottreau JM, Barr VO. A review of antiviral and antifungal use and safety during pregnancy. *Pharmacotherapy*. 2016;36(6):668–78. doi:10.1002/phar.1764.
95. Llanos A, Cieza J, Bernardo J, et al. Effect of salt supplementation on amphotericin B nephrotoxicity. *Kidney Int*. Aug 1991;40(2):302–8. doi:10.1038/ki.1991.214.
96. Hamill RJ. Amphotericin B formulations: a comparative review of efficacy and toxicity. *Drugs*. Jun 2013;73(9):919–34. doi:10.1007/s40265-013-0069-4.
97. Walsh TJ, Finberg RW, Arndt C, et al. Liposomal amphotericin B for empirical therapy in patients with persistent fever and neutropenia. National Institute of Allergy and Infectious Diseases Mycoses Study Group. *N Engl J Med*. Mar 1999;340(10):764–71. doi:10.1056/NEJM199903113401004.
98. Vermes A, Guchelaar HJ, Dankert J. Flucytosine: a review of its pharmacology, clinical indications, pharmacokinetics, toxicity and drug interactions. *J Antimicrob Chemother*. Aug 2000;46(2):171–9. doi:10.1093/jac/46.2.171.
99. Andes D, Pascual A, Marchetti O. Antifungal therapeutic drug monitoring: established and emerging indications. *Antimicrob Agents Chemother*. Jan 2009;53(1):24–34. doi:10.1128/AAC.00705-08.
100. Eschenauer G, Depestel DD, Carver PL. Comparison of echinocandin antifungals. *Ther Clin Risk Manag*. Mar 2007;3(1):71–97.
101. Turner RB, Martello JL, Malhotra A. Worsening renal function in patients with baseline renal impairment treated with intravenous voriconazole: a systematic review. *Int J Antimicrob Agents*. Oct 2015;46(4):362–6. doi:10.1016/j.ijantimicag.2015.05.023.
102. De Beule K, Van Gestel J. Pharmacology of itraconazole. *Drugs*. 2001;61(Suppl 1):27–37. doi:10.2165/00003495-200161001-00003.
103. Johnson MD, Hamilton CD, Drew RH, Sanders LL, Pennick GJ, Perfect JR. A randomized comparative study to determine the effect of omeprazole on the peak serum concentration of itraconazole oral solution. *J Antimicrob Chemother*. Feb 2003;51(2):453–7. doi:10.1093/jac/dkg089.
104. Lindsay J, Sandaradura I, Wong K, et al. Serum levels, safety and tolerability of new formulation SUBA-itraconazole prophylaxis in patients with haematological malignancy or undergoing allogeneic stem cell transplantation. *J Antimicrob Chemother*. Dec 2017;72(12):3414–19. doi:10.1093/jac/dkx295.
105. Saad AH, DePestel DD, Carver PL. Factors influencing the magnitude and clinical significance of drug interactions between azole antifungals and select immunosuppressants. *Pharmacotherapy*. Dec 2006;26(12):1730–44. doi:10.1592/phco.26.12.1730.

Infections in Immunocompromised Patients

145

Scott W. Mueller and Douglas N. Fish

KEY CONCEPTS

1. An *immunocompromised host* is a patient with defects in host immune defenses that predispose to infection. Risk factors include neutropenia, immune system defects from disease or immunosuppressive drug therapy, compromise of natural host defenses, environmental contamination, and changes in normal flora of the host.
2. Immunocompromised patients are at high risk for a variety of bacterial, fungal, viral, and protozoal infections. Bacterial infections caused by gram-positive cocci (staphylococci and streptococci) occur most frequently, followed by gram-negative bacterial infections caused by Enterobacterales and *Pseudomonas aeruginosa.* Fungal infections caused by *Candida* and *Aspergillus*, as well as certain viral infections (herpes simplex virus [HSV], cytomegalovirus [CMV]), are also important causes of morbidity and mortality.
3. Risk of infection in patients with neutropenia is associated with both the severity and duration of neutropenia. Patients with severe neutropenia (absolute neutrophil count less than 500 cells/mm^3 [0.5×10^9/L]) for greater than 7 to 10 days are considered to be at high risk of infection.
4. Fever (single oral temperature of greater than or equal to 38.3°C [100.9°F], or a temperature of greater than or equal to 38°C [100.4°F] for greater than or equal to 1 hour) is the most important clinical finding in patients with neutropenia and is usually the stimulus for further diagnostic workup and initiation of antimicrobial treatment. Infection should be considered as the cause of fever until proven otherwise. Usual signs and symptoms of infection may be altered or absent in patients with neutropenia. Appropriate empiric broad-spectrum antimicrobial therapy must be rapidly instituted to prevent excessive morbidity and mortality.
5. Empiric antimicrobial regimens for neutropenic infections should be based on patients' individual risk factors, as well as institutional infection and susceptibility patterns. The significant morbidity and mortality associated with gram-negative infections require that initial empiric regimens for treatment of febrile neutropenia have good activity against *P. aeruginosa* and Enterobacterales. Parenteral regimens most commonly recommended for initial inpatient treatment include monotherapy with an antipseudomonal β-lactam, or a combination regimen consisting of an antipseudomonal β-lactam plus an aminoglycoside. Low-risk patients may be successfully treated with oral antibiotics (fluoroquinolone plus amoxicillin-clavulanate), with the treatment setting determined by the patient's clinical status.
6. Patients with neutropenia who remain febrile after 3 to 5 days of initial antimicrobial therapy should be reevaluated to determine whether treatment modifications are necessary. Common antimicrobial modifications include addition of vancomycin (if not already administered) and antifungal therapy (amphotericin B, an echinocandin, or fluconazole). Therapy should be directed at causative organisms, if identified, but broad-spectrum regimens should be maintained during neutropenia.
7. The optimal duration of therapy for febrile neutropenia is controversial. The decision to discontinue antimicrobials is based on resolution of neutropenia, defervescence, culture results, and clinical stability of the patient.
8. Prophylactic antimicrobials are administered to patients with cancer who are expected to experience prolonged neutropenia, as well as to hematopoietic cell and solid-organ transplant recipients. Prophylactic regimens may include antibacterial, antifungal, antiviral, or antiprotozoal agents, or a combination of these, selected according to risk of infection with specific pathogens. Optimal prophylactic regimens should consider individual patient risk for infection and institutional infection and susceptibility patterns.
9. Patients undergoing hematopoietic cell transplant (HCT, previously referred to as hematopoietic stem cell transplant) are at an extremely high risk of infection because of prolonged neutropenia following intensive chemotherapy with or without irradiation, while solid-organ transplant (SOT) recipients are at high risk because of prolonged administration of immunosuppressive drugs. Fungal (*Aspergillus*) and viral (CMV) infections are particularly troublesome in these populations, and prophylactic regimens directed against these pathogens are commonly used. When documented, these infections must be treated aggressively to optimize patient outcomes. Nevertheless, mortality rates are often high despite appropriate and aggressive antimicrobial therapy.
10. Immunocompromised patients must be continuously assessed for evidence of infection and response to antimicrobial therapy. Because a large number of antimicrobials may potentially be used, the occurrence of drug-related adverse effects must also be carefully assessed. Efforts should be directed at designing cost-effective treatment strategies that promote optimal patient outcomes.

BEYOND THE BOOK

Refer to "Chapter 143: Infection in an Immunocompromised Patient: Making a Rash Decision Level II" in Pharmacotherapy Casebook: A Patient-Focused Approach, 11e (may be obtained online through AccessPharmacy). After studying the patient presentation, briefly answer Questions 1 through 5 and the Follow-up Case Questions 1 through 3 regarding patient Scarlet Hives's febrile neutropenia following hematopoietic cell transplant. The purpose of this exercise is to gain experience in applying knowledge regarding assessment of possible infection in immunocompromised patients and development of an appropriate therapeutic plan based on clinical presentation, patient characteristics, type and severity of potential infection, past treatment history, and potential causative pathogens.

INTRODUCTION

An immunocompromised host is a patient with intrinsic or acquired defects in host immune defenses that predispose to infection. Advances in modern medicine have created more immunocompromised hosts than ever before. Historically, many of these patients died of their underlying diseases. Dramatic improvements in survival have been achieved by more aggressive therapy of underlying diseases and improved supportive care. However, because such aggressive therapy often renders patients profoundly immunosuppressed for long periods, opportunistic infections remain important causes of morbidity and mortality. This chapter focuses on risk factors for infection, common pathogens and infection sites, and prevention and management of suspected or documented infections in patients with cancer (including hematopoietic cell transplant [HCT] patients) and solid-organ transplant (SOT) recipients. Chapter 148, "Human Immunodeficiency Virus," discusses infectious complications associated with human immunodeficiency virus (HIV) infection.

RISK FACTORS FOR INFECTION/ EPIDEMIOLOGY

Numerous factors, such as underlying disease, immunosuppressive drug therapy, and antimicrobial administration, determine the immunocompromised host's risk of developing infection (see Table 145-1). These same factors may also influence the epidemiology of the associated infections. Multiple risk factors are present concomitantly in many patients.

TABLE 145-1 Risk Factors and Common Pathogens in Immunocompromised Patients

Risk Factor	Patient Conditions	Common Pathogens
Neutropenia	Acute leukemia Chemotherapy	Bacteria: *Staphylococcus aureus*, *Staphylococcus epidermidis*, *Escherichia coli*, *Klebsiella pneumoniae*, *Pseudomonas aeruginosa*, streptococci, enterococci Fungi: *Candida*, *Aspergillus*, Mucorales (*Mucor*) Viruses: Herpes simplex
Impaired cell-mediated immunity	Lymphoma Immunosuppressive therapy (steroids, cyclosporine, chemotherapy, CAR-T)	Bacteria: *Listeria*, *Nocardia*, *Legionella*, Mycobacteria Fungi: *Cryptococcus neoformans*, *Candida*, *Aspergillus*, *Histoplasma capsulatum* Viruses: Cytomegalovirus, varicella-zoster, herpes simplex Protozoa: *Pneumocystis jirovecii*
Impaired humoral immunity	Multiple myeloma Chronic lymphocytic leukemia Splenectomy Immunosuppressive therapy (steroids, chemotherapy, CAR-T)	Bacteria: *S. pneumoniae*, *H. influenzae*, *N. meningitidis*
Loss of protective skin barriers	Venipuncture, bone marrow aspiration, urinary catheterization, vascular access devices, radiation, biopsies	Bacteria: *S. aureus*, *S. epidermidis*, *Bacillus* spp., *Corynebacterium jeikeium* Fungi: *Candida*
Mucous membranes	Respiratory support equipment, endoscopy, chemotherapy, radiation	Bacteria: *S. aureus*, *S. epidermidis*, streptococci, Enterobacterales, *P. aeruginosa*, *Bacteroides* spp., *Clostridioides difficile* Fungi: *Candida* Viruses: Herpes simplex
Surgery	Solid-organ transplantation	Bacteria: *S. aureus*, *S. epidermidis*, Enterobacterales, *P. aeruginosa*, *Bacteroides* spp., *C. difficile* Fungi: *Candida* Viruses: Herpes simplex
Alteration of normal microbial flora	Antimicrobial therapy Chemotherapy Hospital environment	Bacteria: Enterobacterales, *P. aeruginosa*, *Legionella*, *S. aureus*, *S. epidermidis*, *C. difficile* Fungi: *Candida*, *Aspergillus*
Blood products, donor organs	Bone marrow transplantation Solid-organ transplantation	Fungi: *Candida* Viruses: Cytomegalovirus, Epstein–Barr virus, hepatitis B, hepatitis C Protozoa: *Toxoplasma gondii*

CAR-T, chimeric antigen receptor T cell.

Neutropenia

1 2 3 Neutropenia is defined as an abnormally reduced number of neutrophils circulating in peripheral blood. Although exact definitions of neutropenia can vary, an absolute neutrophil count (ANC) of less than 1,000 cells/mm^3 (1.0×10^9/L) indicates a reduction sufficient to predispose patients to infection.[1-3] ANC is the sum of the absolute numbers of both mature neutrophils (polymorphonuclear cells [PMNs], also called *polys* or *segs*) and immature neutrophils (*bands*). The absolute number of PMNs and bands is determined by dividing the total percentage of these cells (obtained from the white blood cell [WBC] differential) by 100 and then multiplying the quotient obtained by the total number of WBCs.

The degree or severity of neutropenia, rate of neutrophil decline, and duration of neutropenia are important risk factors for infection.[1-5] All patients with neutropenia are considered to be at risk for infection, but those with ANC less than 500 cells/mm^3 (0.5×10^9/L) are at greater risk than those with ANCs of 500 to 1,000 cells/mm^3 (0.5×10^9 to 1.0×10^9/L). Most treatment guidelines use ANC less than 500 cells/mm^3 (0.5×10^9/L) as the critical value in making therapeutic decisions regarding the management of suspected or documented infections.[1-5] Risk of infection and death are greatest among patients with less than 100 neutrophils/mm^3 (0.1×10^9/L) ("profound neutropenia").[1-6] In patients with chemotherapy-induced neutropenia, the risk of infection is also increased according to both the rapidity of ANC decline and duration of neutropenia. Patients with severe neutropenia of more than 7 to 10 days' duration are considered to be at especially high risk for serious infections.[1-4] The duration of chemotherapy-induced neutropenia varies considerably among subsets of patients with cancer according to the specific chemotherapeutic agents used and the intensity of treatment. Patients undergoing HCT may have no detectable granulocytes in peripheral blood for up to 3 to 4 weeks and are at particular risk for severe infections with a variety of pathogens.[4-8]

Bacteria and fungi commonly cause infections in patients with neutropenia. Gram-negative bacilli (*Escherichia coli, Klebsiella pneumoniae, P. aeruginosa*) historically were the most common causes of bacterial infection and remain frequent pathogens.[3,5,7-12] During the 1980s gram-positive cocci (*Staphylococcus aureus, Staphylococcus epidermidis,* and other coagulase-negative staphylococci, streptococci, and enterococci) emerged as the most common cause of acute bacterial infections among patients with neutropenia, accounting for up to 80% of all bloodstream infections.[5] This shift was likely due to widespread use of prophylaxis with fluoroquinolones, aggressive chemotherapy regimens associated with severe mucositis, and more frequent use of central venous catheters.[5,7,9,10,13] However, gram-negative infections are again increasing in incidence and now account for approximately half of all bacterial infections.[4-7,10-12] Gram-negative infections are associated with significant morbidity and mortality, in large part due to increasing antibiotic resistance.[10-12] Patients who are neutropenic for extended periods and who receive broad-spectrum antibiotics are at high risk for fungal infections, usually due to *Candida* or *Aspergillus* spp.[1-7,13] Viral infections, although not as common as bacterial and fungal infections, also may cause severe infection in patients with neutropenia.[1,4,6,7] Successful treatment of infections in patients with neutropenia is highly dependent on resolution of neutropenia.[1-6,8]

Immune System Defects

Although not as readily quantifiable, abnormalities may exist in granulocyte function as well as in cell numbers. In addition to neutropenia, defects in T-lymphocyte and macrophage function (cell-mediated immunity), B-cell function (humoral immunity), or both predispose patients to infection.[3-5,7] Cellular immune dysfunction is the result of underlying disease or immunosuppressive drug therapy or radiation; these defects result in a reduced ability of the host to defend against intracellular pathogens. Patients with malignancies and transplant patients receiving a wide variety of immunosuppressive agents, such as cyclosporine, tacrolimus, sirolimus, mycophenolate, corticosteroids, azathioprine, antineoplastic agents, and chimeric antigen receptor T cell (CAR-T) therapy, are at risk for a wide variety of infections (Table 145-1). Although some of these pathogens are associated with only asymptomatic or mild disease in normal hosts, they may cause disseminated, life-threatening infections in immunocompromised hosts.

Underlying disease also frequently causes defects in humoral immune function. Patients with multiple myeloma and chronic lymphocytic leukemia have progressive hypogammaglobulinemia that results in defective humoral immunity. Splenectomy performed as a part of the staging process for Hodgkin's disease places patients at risk for infectious complications. Disease states with humoral immune dysfunction predispose the patient to serious, life-threatening infection with encapsulated organisms such as *Streptococcus pneumoniae, Haemophilus influenzae,* and *Neisseria meningitidis.*

Destruction of Protective Barriers

Loss of protective barriers is a major factor predisposing immunocompromised patients to infection. Damage to skin and mucous membranes by surgery, venipuncture, IV and urinary catheters, radiation, and chemotherapy disrupts natural host defense systems, leaving patients at high risk for infection. Chemotherapy-induced mucositis may erode mucous membranes of the oropharynx and gastrointestinal (GI) tract and establish a portal for subsequent infection by bacteria, herpes simplex virus (HSV), and *Candida.*[1-6] Medical and surgical procedures, such as transplant surgery, indwelling IV catheter placement, bone marrow aspiration, biopsies, and endoscopy, further damage the integument and predispose patients to infection. Infections resulting from disruption of protective barriers usually are a result of skin flora, such as *S. aureus, S. epidermidis,* and streptococci.[3-5]

Environmental Contamination/Alteration of Microbial Flora

Infections in immunocompromised patients are caused by organisms either colonizing the host or acquired from the environment. Microorganisms may be easily transferred from patient to patient on the hands of hospital personnel unless strict infection prevention policies are followed. Contaminated equipment, such as nebulizers or ventilators, and contaminated water supplies have been responsible for outbreaks of *P. aeruginosa* and *Legionella pneumophila* infections, respectively. Foods, such as fruits and green leafy vegetables, which often are colonized with gram-negative bacteria and fungi, are sources of microbial contamination in immunocompromised hosts.[1,6]

Most infections in patients with cancer are caused by organisms colonizing body sites, such as the skin, oropharynx, and GI tract, and are therefore caused by the patient's own endogenous flora.[4-7] The GI tract is a common site from which infections in immunocompromised hosts originate. Periodontitis, pharyngitis, esophagitis, colitis, perirectal cellulitis, and bacteremias are caused predominantly by normal flora of the gut; bloodstream infections are thought to arise from microbial translocation across injured GI mucosa.[1,6,7] Normal flora may be significantly disrupted and altered; oropharyngeal flora rapidly change to primarily gram-negative bacilli in hospitalized patients. Many patients with cancer may already be colonized with gram-negative bacilli on admission as a result of frequent prior hospitalizations and clinic visits. In hospitalized patients with cancer, however, many infections are caused by colonizing organisms acquired after admission.[1]

Although hospitalization and severity of illness are important risk factors for colonization by gram-negative bacilli, administration of broad-spectrum antimicrobial agents has the greatest impact on flora of immunocompromised hosts. Use of these agents disrupts GI tract flora and predisposes patients to infection with more virulent or resistant pathogens. Antineoplastic drugs (eg, cyclophosphamide, doxorubicin, and fluorouracil) and acid-suppressive therapy (eg, H_2-receptor antagonists, proton-pump inhibitors, and antacids) also may result in changes in GI flora and possibly predispose patients to infection.[1,4,5]

ETIOLOGY OF INFECTIONS IN PATIENTS WITH NEUTROPENIA AND CANCER

2 Infection remains a significant cause of morbidity and mortality in neutropenic patients with cancer. Febrile neutropenia occurs in 10% to 50% of patients with solid tumors and 80% to 100% of those with hematological malignancies.[1,2,5] More than 50% of patients with febrile neutropenia have an established or occult infection, but causative pathogens are microbiologically documented in only 30% to 40% of cases. Infections can be documented clinically (but not microbiologically) in another 30% to 40% of patients, with the remaining 20% to 40% of patients manifesting infection only by fever.[2-5] Bloodstream infections account for approximately 10% to 25% of all febrile episodes during neutropenia.[1,4,5,9] Patients with profound neutropenia are at greatest risk for systemic infection, with at least 20% of these individuals developing bacteremia.[1-6] Areas of impaired or damaged host defenses, such as the oropharynx, lungs, skin, sinuses, and GI tract, are common sites of infection. These local infections may progress to cause systemic infection and bacteremia.[4,5,8,9]

Table 145-1 lists organisms commonly infecting immunocompromised patients. Bacteremic episodes in patients with cancer are caused by gram-positive organisms in 45% to 75% of cases, these rates being highly institution specific.[1,3,5,7,9-11,13] Important risk factors for these infections include frequent use of indwelling central and peripheral IV catheters, frequent use of broad-spectrum antibiotics with excellent gram-negative activity but often relatively poor gram-positive coverage, high rates of mucositis caused by aggressive cancer treatments, and prophylaxis with trimethoprim–sulfamethoxazole or fluoroquinolones.[1,3,5,7-11,14] Staphylococci (especially *S. epidermidis*) account for most infections, but *Bacillus* spp. and *Corynebacterium jeikeium* are also important pathogens.[1,4,5,7,13] Rates of infection due to methicillin-resistant *S. aureus* (MRSA) have increased in the hospital and community settings.[4-6,13,14,16] Viridans streptococci, which may be resistant to β-lactams, also have emerged as important pathogens, particularly in patients with chemotherapy-induced mucositis of the oropharynx.[3-6,12] Enterococci, including vancomycin-resistant strains, also may be problematic in many institutions.[4,6,13,14,16] Bacteremia caused by vancomycin-resistant enterococci (VRE) in patients with neutropenia is associated with a mortality rate up to 30%.[3,10,13,14,16,17]

Gram-positive infections are not always immediately life-threatening and are associated with somewhat lower mortality rates overall (approximately 5%-10%) compared with gram-negative infections.[1,4,10] However, increasing rates of antibiotic resistance have made treatment of gram-positive infections in immunocompromised patients more challenging.[4,7,10,13,14] MRSA infections are associated with increased morbidity, mortality, and hospital costs compared with susceptible organisms.[10,13,18] Methicillin resistance among coagulase-negative staphylococci, which may cause 40% to 80% of infections in certain populations, is common (70%-90% of isolates).[1,4,6,7,10,13,14] Vancomycin-resistant organisms such as VRE are increasing in importance.[1,3,4,10,13,17] Thus, prevention and timely diagnosis and treatment of gram-positive infections are clearly of great importance in the management of patients with neutropenia and cancer.

Gram-negative infections remain important causes of morbidity and mortality (approximately 10%-30%) in immunocompromised patients with cancer.[5,10] However, the relative frequency of gram-negative infections caused by specific pathogens has been changing. *E. coli* and *Klebsiella* remain the most common isolates at many centers.[4,5,7] However, strains of Enterobacterales producing extended-spectrum β-lactamases (ESBLs) that hydrolyze cephalosporins, and carbapenemases that inactivate carbapenems, have emerged and are a cause for concern.[1,4,5,7,10,14] The global spread of carbapenem-resistant Enterobacterales (CRE) is especially concerning. The frequency of infections resulting from other gram-negative organisms, such as *Klebsiella-Enterobacter*, *Serratia*, and *Citrobacter*, has also been increasing.[1,4,5] Infections with these particular organisms may be difficult to treat because of the ease of β-lactamase induction and the more frequent development of resistance to multiple antibiotics.[1,4,5,7,10-12,14]

P. aeruginosa has long been an important pathogen in patients with cancer. *P. aeruginosa* infection rates are decreasing in patients with solid tumors but not in patients with hematologic malignancies.[3,7,10] Infections caused by *P. aeruginosa* are associated with significant morbidity and mortality in patients with neutropenia, with reported mortality rates of 31% to 75%.[1,5,10] The frequency of infection caused by difficult-to-treat organisms such as *Stenotrophomonas maltophilia* appears to be increasing at many centers, probably because of selective pressures of broad-spectrum antimicrobial use.[7,11] As with gram-positive organisms, antibiotic resistance among gram-negative organisms has continued to increase at alarming rates and has made appropriate antibiotic selection for treatment of febrile neutropenia more difficult.[1,5,14,16] Mortality rates of up to 40% to 70% have been reported in patients with infection caused by multidrug-resistant gram-negative pathogens.[5,14] Although the GI tract is a common site of bacterial infection, severe infections caused by anaerobic organisms are relatively infrequent. Anaerobes are found most frequently in mixed infections, such as perirectal cellulitis and mucositis-associated oropharyngeal infections.[4,7]

In addition to bacterial infections, neutropenic cancer patients are at risk for invasive fungal infections. Patients with extended periods of profound neutropenia who have been receiving broad-spectrum antibiotics, corticosteroids, or both are at the highest risk for invasive fungal infection. Up to one-third of patients with febrile neutropenia who do not respond to 1 week of broad-spectrum antibiotic therapy will have a systemic fungal infection.[1,4,11] Large autopsy studies have documented a change over time in invasive fungal infections. Whereas from 1989 to 2003 over 30% of autopsies of patients with hematologic malignancies found deep fungal infection (75% of which were undiagnosed prior to death), this number decreased to 19% from 2004 to 2008 (49% undiagnosed prior to death). These improvements may be due to improved awareness, diagnostic techniques, and treatments. One single center estimated the average prevalence of invasive fungal infections was 30% in those autopsied over a 20-year period. Causative pathogens were usually either *Aspergillus* spp., *Candida* spp., or Mucorales fungi (such as *Mucor* spp.).[16] Mortality rates in patients with invasive fungal infections are highly dependent on pathogens, sites of infection, and underlying risk factors but often exceed 30% overall.[17]

Candida albicans is a common fungal pathogen in neutropenic cancer patients, especially those with solid tumors.[1,3,4,15,19,21] However, non-*albicans* species of *Candida* including *Candida glabrata*, *C. tropicalis*, *C. parapsilosis*, and *C. krusei* are being isolated with increasing frequency and are more common than *C. albicans* infections in some studies.[15,21] Increased infections caused by pathogens such as *Trichosporon* spp., *Fusarium* spp., and *Curvularia* spp. have also been reported.[15,19,22] The shift toward more frequent infection with non-*albicans Candida* is important because of significantly decreased rates of azole susceptibility among many of these strains.[19] Because *Candida* spp. are normal flora, alteration of body host defenses is an important risk factor for the development of these infections. Oral thrush is the most common clinical manifestation of fungal infection. Mucous membranes damaged from chemotherapy and radiation serve as areas of *Candida* surface colonization and subsequent entry into the bloodstream; disease then may disseminate throughout the body. Organs such as the liver, spleen, kidney, and lungs are commonly involved in disseminated disease.[1,4,19] Hepatosplenic candidiasis is a particularly important infection in patients with hematologic malignancies.[7,19,21] In patients with invasive candidiasis, overall attributable mortality is as high as 35% to 50%.[3,13,15,18,21]

Invasive infections caused by *Aspergillus* spp. are a serious complication of neutropenia. Mortality rates have historically approached 80% in patients with prolonged neutropenia and/or patients undergoing allogeneic HCT; however, mortality is now reported as low as 30%.[3,20,22,24] These infections are particularly prevalent and more common in patients with hematologic malignancies and in patients undergoing HCT; invasive aspergillosis may occur in up to 10% of these patients.[3,15,19,22,24,25] Infections resulting from *Aspergillus* species (including *A. fumigatus*, *A. terreus*, *A. flavus*, and *A. niger*) usually are acquired via inhalation of airborne spores. After colonizing the lungs, *Aspergillus* invades the lung parenchyma and pulmonary vessels, resulting in hemorrhage, pulmonary infarcts, and a high mortality rate. Invasive pulmonary disease is the dominant manifestation of infection in patients with neutropenia. However, *Aspergillus* also may cause other infections, including sinusitis, cutaneous infection, and disseminated disease involving multiple organs, including the CNS.[19,25] Prolonged neutropenia is the primary risk factor for invasive pulmonary aspergillosis in patients with acute leukemia; use of corticosteroids also may predispose patients to disease.[21] Invasive aspergillosis should be suspected in neutropenic cancer patients colonized with *Aspergillus* (in sputum and/or nasal cultures) who remain persistently febrile despite at least 1 week of broad-spectrum antibiotic therapy.[1,4,25] Increased infections caused by other yeasts (such as *Trichosporon*) and molds (such as Mucorales, *Fusarium*, and *Curvularia*) have also been reported.[13,15,16,19,22]

Chemotherapy-induced mucous membrane damage may predispose neutropenic cancer patients to reactivation of HSV, manifesting as gingivostomatitis or recurrent genital infections. Untreated oropharyngeal HSV infections may spread to involve the esophagus and often coexist with *Candida* infections. Clinical disease resulting from HSV occurs most often in patients with serologic evidence (eg, serum antibodies to HSV) of prior infection. Both HSV-seropositive HCT recipients and HSV-seropositive patients with leukemia receiving intensive chemotherapy are at high risk for recurrent HSV disease during periods of immunosuppression.[3,4,6]

Pneumocystis jirovecii and *Toxoplasma gondii* are the most common parasitic pathogens found in immunocompromised cancer patients. Patients with hematologic malignancies and those receiving high-dose corticosteroids as part of chemotherapy regimens are at the greatest risk of infection.[3,4,6] Routine use of trimethoprim–sulfamethoxazole prophylaxis has substantially reduced the incidence of these infections.[1,4,6]

Because the majority of infecting organisms in patients with cancer are from the host's own flora, some centers have used routine surveillance cultures in an attempt to prospectively identify causes of fever and suspected infection. In a typical surveillance culture program, cultures of the nose, mouth, axillae, and perirectal area are performed twice weekly, and culture results are correlated with the clinical status of the patient. Because these cultures are costly and have low diagnostic yield, the utility of surveillance culture programs is believed to be limited.[1,4] However, surveillance cultures are useful as research tools and in patients with prolonged profound neutropenia, and in institutions that have high rates of antimicrobial resistance or have problems with pathogens such as *P. aeruginosa* or *Aspergillus* spp. Surveillance cultures should be limited to the anterior nares for detecting colonization with MRSA, *Aspergillus*, and penicillin-resistant pneumococci and to the rectum for detecting VRE, *P. aeruginosa*, and multiple-antibiotic-resistant gram-negative bacilli (such as CRE).[1,4]

Knowledge of infection rates and local susceptibility patterns is essential for guiding optimal management of febrile neutropenia. These parameters must be monitored closely because the spectrum of infectious complications is related to multiple factors, including cancer chemotherapy regimens and antimicrobial therapy used for treatment and prophylaxis.

CLINICAL PRESENTATION

4 The most important clinical finding in the patient with neutropenia is fever. Because of the potential for significant morbidity and mortality associated with infection in these patients, fever should be considered to be the result of infection until proved otherwise.[1,2,4,5,7] At the first appearance of fever, the patient should be evaluated carefully for other signs and symptoms of infection. The use of biomarkers such as procalcitonin (PCT) has been extensively investigated for their utility in helping diagnose infections in patients with febrile neutropenia. Although elevated PCT levels (typically ≥0.5 ng/mL [mcg/L]) have been associated with a significantly greater likelihood of bacterial infection in the febrile patient, lack of elevated PCT levels does not necessarily correspond to lack of infection and should not be used as the sole rationale for withholding or stopping initial antibiotic therapy.[22]

TREATMENT

Management of patients with febrile neutropenia, including both prophylaxis and treatment of infectious complications, can be extremely challenging. Although published guidelines are available, the most optimal clinical management of these patients remains unclear in many aspects.

Desired Outcomes

4 5 The goals of therapy in neutropenic cancer patients with new fever are the following: (a) protect the neutropenic patient from early death caused by undiagnosed infection; (b) prevent breakthrough bacterial, fungal, viral, and protozoal infections during periods of neutropenia; (c) effectively treat established infections; (d) reduce morbidity and allow for continued administration of optimal antineoplastic therapy; (e) avoid unnecessary use of antimicrobials that contribute to increased resistance; and (f) minimize toxicities and cost of antimicrobial therapy while increasing patient quality of life. Empirical broad-spectrum antibiotic therapy is effective at reducing early mortality.[1,2,4,9,10]

General Approach to Treatment

General guidelines for management of febrile episodes and documented infections in patients with neutropenia are shown in Figs. 145-1 and 145-2.[1] Although many controversies remain regarding optimal management of these patients, updated evidence-based guidelines from the Infectious Diseases Society of America (IDSA) for the management of febrile neutropenia were published in 2010 and, regarding outpatient management, in 2018.[1,2] Similarly, the National Comprehensive Cancer Network (NCCN) published updated clinical practice guidelines for the prevention and treatment of cancer-related infections in 2021.[4] Selected specific recommendations are discussed in the following sections of this chapter, and their associated evidence-based rankings are summarized in Table 145-2.

Fever in the neutropenic cancer patient is considered to be caused by infection until proved otherwise. High-dose broad-spectrum bactericidal, usually parenteral, empirical antibiotic

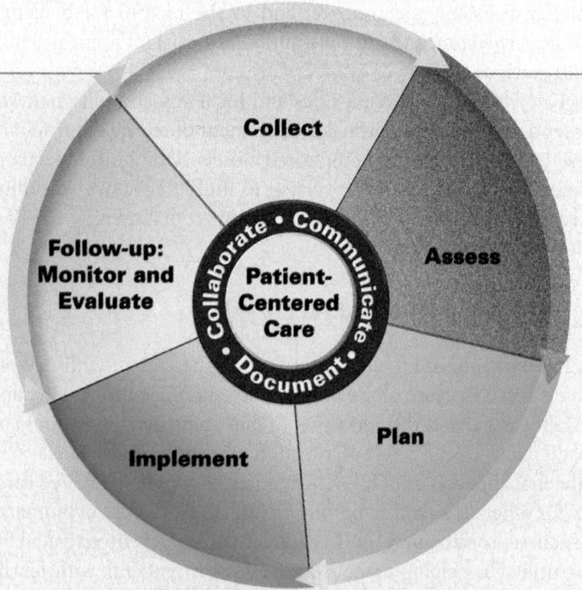

Patient Care Process for the Treatment of Suspected Infection in an Immunocompromised Host

Collect

- Patient characteristics (eg, age, sex, height, weight)
- Patient medical history (oncologic, surgical, vaccines, previous infections, time since transplant/engraftment/last oncologic regimen or transplant engraftment)
- Social history (eg, drug/ethanol use), travel history (eg, endemic exposures)
- Current medications (eg, antimicrobial prophylaxis/treatment, immunomodulating agents [immunosuppressive or immunostimulatory])
- Prior medications (eg, antimicrobial, oncologic, immunomodulating) and future planned medications (eg, life-saving oncologic or immunomodulating regimens)
- Objective Data
  - Mean arterial blood pressure (MAP), heart rate (HR), respiratory rate (RR), O_2-saturation, altered mental status (AMS), urine output (UO), skin turgor/integrity
  - Labs including white blood cells (WBC) with differential, absolute neutrophil count (ANC) and trends, serum creatinine (SCr), lactate, liver function tests (LFT), blood glucose
  - Culture data (eg, bacterial, fungal, viral), microbiologic diagnostic tests (eg, procalcitonin, galactomannan, β-D-glucan, viral polymerase chain reaction tests, infectious serologies)
  - Presence of central, peripheral, urinary catheters, and indwelling ports

Assess

- For febrile neutropenia: assess risk of infectious complications for possible outpatient management (see Table 145-3) including logistical barriers (eg, access to care, compliance, support)
- Hemodynamic/clinical stability and evidence of organ malperfusion (eg, MAP <65 mm Hg, HR >100 bpm, RR>22, AMS, decreased UO, renal dysfunction)
- Evidence of infection at common sites (see Clinical Presentation boxes: "Febrile Neutropenia" and "Infection in Solid Organ Transplant Patients")
- Assess risk of infection based on duration/degree of neutropenia or magnitude of immunosuppression
- Assess need for colony-stimulating factors (CSF) (see Table 145-8)
- Assess risk for infection with specific pathogens (see Table 145-1)
- Assess contraindications to specific antimicrobial therapy (eg, allergies, drug-drug/disease interactions)
- Assess previous and current culture results and susceptibilities

Plan*

- Antimicrobial regimen including specific antimicrobial(s), dose, route, frequency, and duration (see Figs. 145-1, 145-2; Tables 145-4, 145-5, and 145-7)
- Monitoring parameters including efficacy (eg, resolution of infectious symptoms, fever, ANC) and safety (eg, antimicrobial side effects, *Clostridioides difficile*, CNS toxicity)
- Patient education if treated outpatient (eg, self-monitoring, when/how to seek help, adherence)
- Referrals to other providers when appropriate (eg, infectious disease specialist)

Implement*

- Provide patient and caregiver education regarding when/how to seek advance medical attention
- Provide integrated health professionals, patient and family education (eg, expected outcomes/goals of therapy, therapeutic drug monitoring, avoidance of exposures)

Follow-up: Monitor and Evaluate*

- De-escalation of empiric antimicrobial regimens to targeted therapy (see Table 145-7)
- Resolution of infectious symptoms (see also Figs. 145-1 and 145-2)
- Presence of adverse effects specific to the antimicrobial regimen
- Presence of drug-drug interactions potentially requiring changes in drug regimens or additional therapeutic drug monitoring
- Patient adherence to outpatient antimicrobial plan
- Therapeutic drug levels to adjust antimicrobial therapy (see Table 145-6)

**Collaborate with patient, caregivers, and other healthcare professionals.*

CLINICAL PRESENTATION Febrile Neutropenia[1-7]

General

- Due to high risk for serious infections, frequent (at least daily) careful clinical assessments must be performed to search for possible evidence of infection
- Physical assessment should include examination of all common sites of infection, including mouth/pharynx, nose and sinuses, respiratory tract, GI tract, urinary tract, skin, soft tissues, perineum, and intravascular catheter insertion sites

Symptoms

- Usual signs and symptoms of infection may be absent or altered in patients with neutropenia owing to low numbers of leukocytes and an inability to mount an inflammatory response (eg, no infiltrate on chest x-ray film, urinary tract infection without pyuria)
- Pain may be present at the infection site(s)

Signs

- Fever in this setting is defined as a single oral temperature ≥38.3°C (100.9°F) in the absence of other causes or temperature ≥38°C (100.4°F) for 1 hour or more. Other causes of fever unrelated to infection in this patient population include reactions to blood products, chemotherapeutic agents (and other drugs, including biologics), cell lysis, and underlying malignancy
- Usual signs of infection may be absent or altered; patients with bacteremia commonly exhibit no signs of infection other than fever

Laboratory Tests

- Neutropenia (ANC ≤1,000 cells/mm^3 [1.0 × 10^9/L])
- Blood cultures (two or more sets, including vascular access devices) for bacteria and fungi; cultures of other suspected infection sites (infection can be documented microbiologically in only about 30% of cases, about half of which are due to bacteremia)
- Other cultures should be obtained as indicated clinically according to the presence of signs or symptoms
- Recent surveillance cultures (nasal, rectal) should be reviewed, if available
- Complete blood count and blood chemistries should be obtained frequently to monitor neutropenia, plan supportive care, guide drug dosing, and assess patient's overall status

Other Diagnostic Tests

- Chest x-ray
- Aspiration, biopsy of skin lesions
- Procalcitonin is indicative of bacterial infection when elevated, but negative test does not rule out infection
- Other diagnostic tests as indicated clinically on the basis of physical examination and other assessments

therapy should be initiated at the onset of fever or at the first signs or symptoms of infection. Withholding antibiotic therapy until an organism is isolated results in unacceptably high mortality rates. Undiagnosed infection in immunocompromised patients can rapidly disseminate and result in death if left untreated or if treated improperly. For example, failure to initiate appropriate antibiotic therapy for *P. aeruginosa* bacteremia at the onset of fever in neutropenic cancer patients resulted in mortality rates of 15%, 48%, and 70% within 12, 24, and 48 hours, respectively.[1,4,27] Appropriate empirical antibiotic therapy is 70% to 90% effective at reducing early morbidity and mortality.[1,4,10] Therapy must be appropriate and initiated promptly, ideally within 1 hour after initial onset of fever. Antimicrobial therapy must likewise be initiated promptly in neutropenic patients with cancer who are afebrile but with other clinical signs and symptoms of possible infection.

When designing optimal empirical antibiotic regimens, clinicians must consider infection patterns and antimicrobial susceptibility trends in their respective institutions. Patient factors such as risk for infection, drug allergies, concomitant nephrotoxins, and previous antimicrobial exposure (including prophylaxis) must be considered.[1-4] Assessment of the patient's risk of infection will help determine the appropriate route and setting (eg, inpatient versus outpatient) for antibiotic administration (Fig. 145-1). Patients with neutropenia and fever can be divided into low- and high-risk groups for complications of severe infection. Risk stratification drives both type and setting of antimicrobial therapy. The Multinational Association for Supportive Care in Cancer (MASCC) risk-index score is recommended by many clinical guidelines to assess a patient's risk of complications.[1,2,4] Additional evaluation tools including Talcott groups and the Clinical Index of Stable Febrile Neutropenia (CISNE) score are also recommended.[2] These tools are provided in Table 145-3.

Most experts agree that, in general, low-risk patients have an anticipated duration of neutropenia less than or equal to 7 days, are clinically stable, and have no or few comorbidities, and have no bacterial focus or systemic signs of infection other than fever. In contrast, high-risk patients are those with an anticipated duration of neutropenia greater than 7 days or profound neutropenia, are clinically unstable or have comorbid medical problems (eg, focal or systemic signs of infection, GI symptoms, nausea, vomiting, diarrhea, hypoxemia, and chronic lung disease), or have a high-risk cancer (eg, acute leukemia) and/or have undergone high intensity chemotherapy. High-risk patients (eg, MASCC less than 21, Talcott Groups I through III, CISNE ≥3) should be hospitalized for parenteral antibiotics whereas low-risk patients may be candidates for oral or outpatient antibiotics. Scoring tools such as MASCC must be used in conjunction with, not as a replacement for, careful clinical assessment of patients when selecting low-risk patients for oral outpatient management. Many additional patient factors (eg, worsening renal function, altered mental status, severe anemia, or thrombocytopenia) may increase risk of complications and potentially exclude patients from outpatient management of febrile neutropenia (see also "Oral Antibiotic Therapy for Management of Febrile Neutropenia" section below).[1,2,4,28]

The optimal antibiotic regimen for empirical therapy in febrile neutropenia remains controversial, but it is clear that no single regimen can be recommended for all patients. Because of their frequency and relative pathogenicity, *P. aeruginosa* and other gram-negative bacilli and staphylococci remain the primary targets of

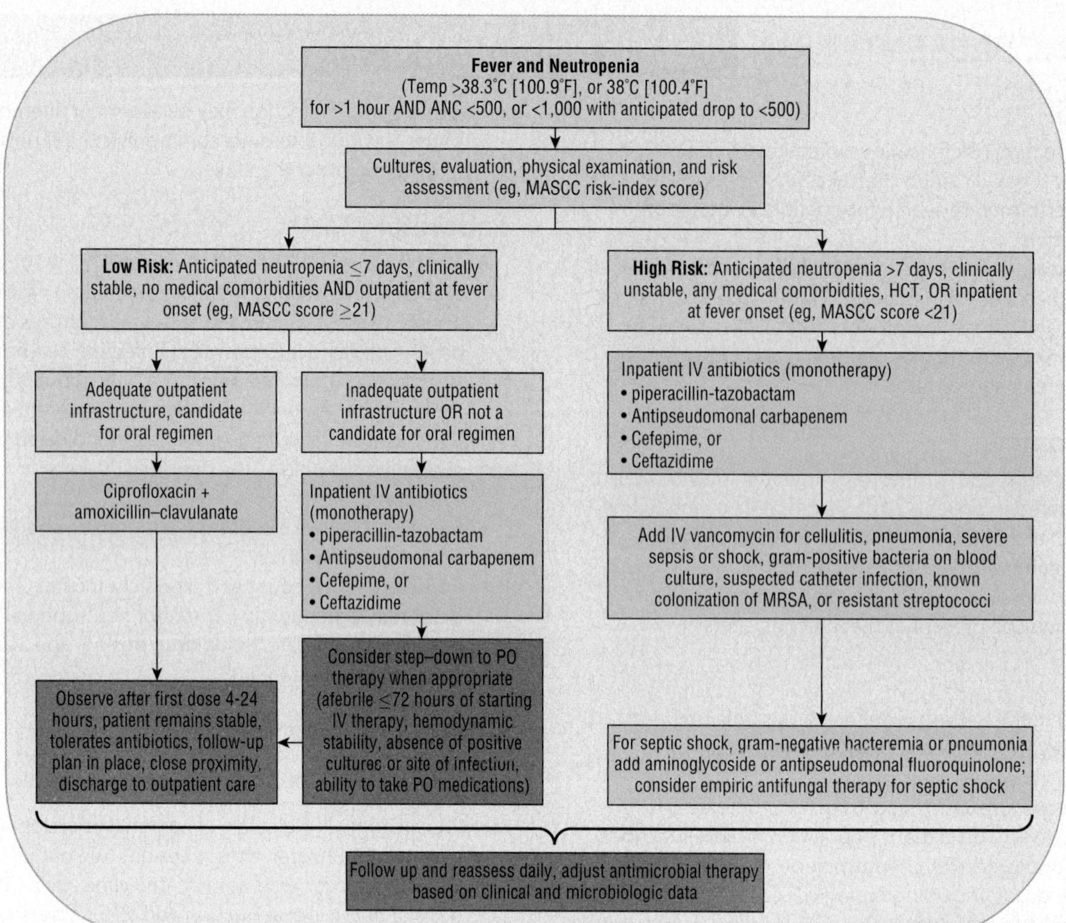

FIGURE 145-1 Initial management of febrile episodes in patients with neutropenia. (ANC, absolute neutrophil count [expressed as cells/mm^3]; HCT, hematopoietic cell transplantation; MASCC, Multinational Association for Supportive Care in Cancer; PO, oral.)

empirical antimicrobial therapy.[1,2,4] Although *P. aeruginosa* may be documented in fewer than 5% of bloodstream infections in the population of hospitalized patients, adequate antipseudomonal antibiotic coverage still must be included in empirical regimens because of the significant morbidity and mortality associated with this pathogen.[1,3,16] All empirical regimens must be carefully monitored and appropriately revised on the basis of documented infections, susceptibilities of bacterial isolates, development of more defined clinical signs and symptoms of infection, or a combination of these factors.

Although there are some differences among them, consensus guidelines generally recognize three different types of empirical parenteral antibiotic regimens: (a) monotherapy with an antipseudomonal β-lactam such as a cephalosporin (cefepime or ceftazidime), a carbapenem (imipenem–cilastatin or meropenem), or piperacillin–tazobactam; (b) two-drug combination therapy with an antipseudomonal β-lactam plus either an aminoglycoside or an antipseudomonal fluoroquinolone (ciprofloxacin or levofloxacin); and (c) monotherapy or two-drug combination therapy as above, plus the addition of vancomycin (Fig. 145-1).[1,4] Each of these regimens has advantages and disadvantages, which are summarized in Table 145-4. There is no overwhelming evidence that any one of these regimens is superior to the others. The overall response to empirical antibiotic regimens in febrile neutropenic patients with cancer is approximately 70% to 90% regardless of whether a pathogen is isolated or which antimicrobial regimen is used.[1,3,4,10] Additionally, other alternative regimens may also be appropriate based on specific patient characteristics or susceptibilities of suspected pathogens within a specific institution.

β-Lactam Monotherapy

Monotherapy with an antipseudomonal β-lactam is recommended by IDSA 2010 and NCCN 2021 guidelines as initial parenteral therapy for management of febrile neutropenia without suspected or proven resistant organisms or complications (eg, pneumonia, hypotension, and vascular access infection).[1,4] β-Lactam antibiotics that have been evaluated as monotherapy for management of febrile episodes in neutropenic cancer patients include antipseudomonal cephalosporins (ceftazidime and cefepime), piperacillin–tazobactam, and antipseudomonal carbapenems (imipenem–cilastatin and meropenem).[1,4] Three different meta-analyses assessing as many as 46 clinical trials involving more than 7,600 patients found no significant differences overall between monotherapy and combination therapy (β-lactam/aminoglycoside) in rates of survival, treatment response, and bacterial/fungal superinfections.[4,29] Monotherapy with antipseudomonal β-lactams is therefore recommended by treatment guidelines and routinely used for initial treatment.[1,4] Institutional susceptibility patterns and patient characteristics should drive drug selection for the management of individual patients with febrile neutropenia.[1,4]

Ceftazidime-avibactam, ceftolozane-tazobactam, and meropenem-vaborbactam, and cefiderocol have appropriate overall spectrum of antibacterial activity with good activity against *P. aeruginosa* and other gram-negative organisms as well as many gram-positive pathogens. Neither the 2021 NCCN nor the 2010 IDSA consensus guidelines specifically recommend these agents due to a lack of supportive clinical evidence at the time the guidelines were written.[1,4]

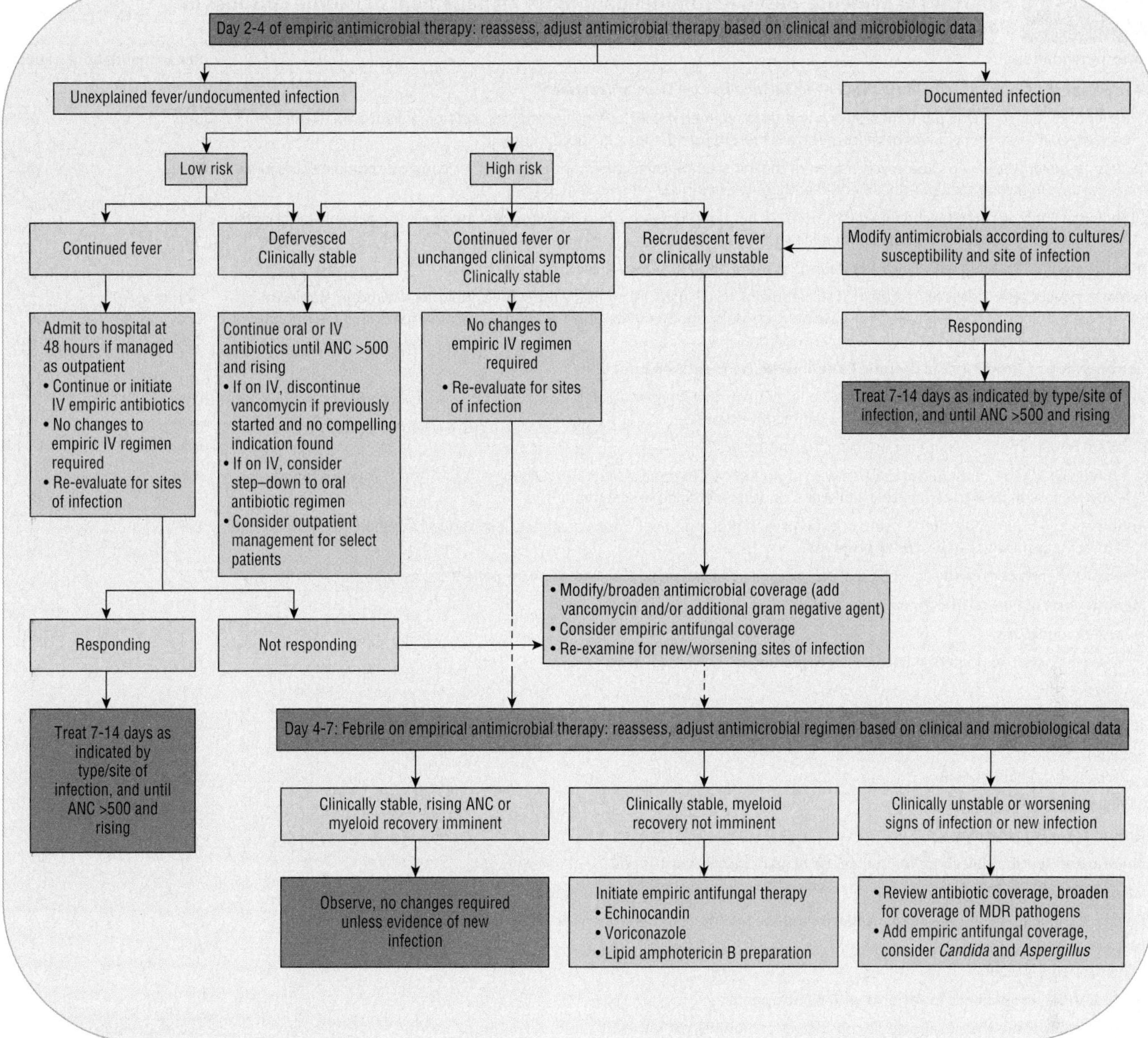

FIGURE 145-2 Subsequent management of febrile episodes in patients with neutropenia who have already received empirical antimicrobial therapy for 2 to 4 days. (ANC, absolute neutrophil count [expressed as cells/mm^3 or x 10^6/L; MDR, multidrug-resistant; PO, oral.)

TABLE 145-2 Summary of Evidence-Based Recommendations for Management of Febrile Episodes in Patients with Neutropenia

Recommendations	Recommendation Grades[a]
The first dose of empirical antibiotic therapy should be administered within 1 hour after triage from initial presentation	Strong, low
Oral antibiotics are feasible for treatment of carefully selected patients at low risk for complications	A-1
Clinical judgment and consideration of multiple patient factors should be used when selecting candidates for outpatient management	Moderate, low
The MASCC index, Talcott's rules, and CISNE are recommended tools for identifying patients who may be candidates for outpatient management	Moderate, intermediate
Patients who are eligible for outpatient management must meet appropriate psychosocial and logistical requirements	Moderate, low
For outpatient management, first doses of antibiotics should be administered in the clinic, emergency department, or hospital	Moderate, low
Monotherapy with appropriate antibiotics is as effective as combination regimens for initial empirical treatment of febrile neutropenic episodes	A-1
Patients at high risk for serious life-threatening infections must be initially treated with IV antibiotics. Patients at low risk can be treated with either IV or oral drugs (see text for risk stratification criteria)	A-2
Oral therapy with a fluoroquinolone (ciprofloxacin or levofloxacin) plus amoxicillin-clavulanate is appropriate for initial outpatient treatment	Moderate, intermediate
Patients who become afebrile within 2-4 days of beginning initial empirical antibiotic therapy and in whom specific organisms have been identified should be treated for ≥7 days (until cultures are negative and patient has clinically recovered). Low-risk patients in whom no organism is identified can be switched to oral antibiotics if desired, whereas patients originally classified as high risk should continue on IV antibiotics	B-2

(continued)

TABLE 145-2 Summary of Evidence-Based Recommendations for Management of Febrile Episodes in Patients with Neutropenia (*Continued*)

Recommendations	Recommendation Grades[a]
Management of Patients with Persistent Fever During First 2-4 Days of Treatment	
In patients initially receiving monotherapy or a two-drug regimen *not* including vancomycin, addition of vancomycin can be considered if any criteria for use of vancomycin are present (see the text for specific criteria)	B-3
In patients *already* receiving vancomycin as part of the initial empirical regimen, withdrawal of vancomycin should be considered after 2 days in the absence of a documented pathogen requiring continued therapy	A-2
Other initial antibiotics can be continued if the disease has not progressed, or switched to oral therapy if the patient was classified as low risk even in the presence of continued fever	A-1
Management of Patients with Fever Persisting for More Than 2-4 Days After Initial Treatment	
Reassess patient after 2 days of treatment. If still febrile by day 4, then: (a) continue the same antibiotics if clinically stable; (b) change antibiotics if any evidence of disease progression or antibiotic toxicities; or (c) add an antifungal drug if the duration of neutropenia is expected to be more than 5-7 additional days	Option a: A-1 Option b: A-3 Option c: A-3
Continuation of Antibiotics in Afebrile Patients with No Identified Infection	
Antibiotic therapy can be discontinued after 3 days of treatment if patient is afebrile for ≥48 hours and absolute neutrophil count (ANC) is ≥500 cells/mm^3 (0.5 × 10^9/L) for 2 consecutive days	A-2
If patient remains neutropenic, continue IV or oral antibiotics	A-2
Antibiotics should be continued in patients with profound neutropenia (ANC <100 cells/mm^3 [0.1 × 10^9/L]), mucous membrane lesions of mouth or GI tract, unstable vital signs, or other identified risk factors	A-2
Antibiotics can be stopped after 2 weeks in patients with prolonged neutropenia of unclear continued duration, no identified site of infection, and who can be closely observed	C-3
Alternatively, antibiotics can be discontinued after 4 days if no infection is documented and the patient shows no response to therapy	C-3
Management of Fungal Infections	
Suspected candidiasis:	
Lipid-associated amphotericin B (LAMB) or caspofungin[b]	A-1
Voriconazole	B-1
Fluconazole or itraconazole	B-1
Candidemia:	
An echinocandin[b] or LAMB	A-2
Fluconazole or voriconazole	B-3
Granulocyte Transfusions	
There are no specific indications for routine use of granulocyte transfusions	C-2
Colony-Stimulating Factors	
Colony-stimulating factors are not indicated for routine treatment of neutropenia in either febrile or afebrile patients	B-2
Prophylactic use of colony-stimulating factors should be considered for patients in whom the anticipated risk of fever and neutropenia is ≥20%	A-2
Antimicrobial Prophylaxis in Patients with Neutropenia	
Fluoroquinolone prophylaxis should be considered for high-risk patients with profound neutropenia (ANC <100 cells/mm^3 [0.1 × 10^9/L]) expected to last 7-10 days	Moderate, high
Antibacterial prophylaxis is not required in routinely recommended in low-risk patients who are expected to be neutropenic <7 days	A-3
Prophylaxis with trimethoprim–sulfamethoxazole should be administered to all patients at high risk for *Pneumocystis jirovecii* pneumonia, regardless of whether they are neutropenic	Strong, high
Prophylaxis with an oral triazole or parenteral echinocandin is recommended in high-risk patients, starting with induction chemotherapy and continued for duration of neutropenia	Moderate, intermediate
In HCT, prophylaxis with fluconazole, micafungin,[b] posaconazole, itraconazole, voriconazole, or LAMB is recommended during the period of risk of neutropenia	A-1 for fluconazole and micafungin,[b] all others B-2
In HCT recipients with graft-versus-host disease, or patients with neutropenia with hematologic malignancies, prophylaxis with posaconazole is recommended for prevention of invasive fungal infections	A-1
HSV-seropositive patients undergoing HCT or leukemia induction therapy should receive acyclovir prophylaxis during neutropenia, and for at least 30 days after HCT	Strong-high for prophylaxis, A-2 for duration
In HCT, prophylaxis with acyclovir should be administered during neutropenia and for at least 1 year afterward to prevent VZV infection or reactivation	A-2

[a]Cited evidence-based guidelines utilize different systems for grading the strengths of recommendation and quality of the associated evidence. Letter/number-based recommendations are from references 1 and 2; qualitative (descriptive) recommendations are from the other cited guidelines. Readers are advised to consult the original documents for full explanations of the grading systems and definitions used in individual guidelines.

[b]Expert opinion indicates all echinocandins are likely interchangeable and equally effective.

Strength of recommendations: A, B, C = good, moderate, and poor evidence to support recommendation for use, respectively; D = moderate evidence to support a recommendation against use. *Quality of evidence*: 1 = evidence from ≥1 properly randomized, controlled trial; 2 = evidence from ≥1 well-designed clinical trial without randomization, from cohort or case–control analytic studies, from multiple time series, or from dramatic results from uncontrolled experiments; 3 = evidence from opinions of respected authorities, based on clinical experience, descriptive studies, or reports of expert committees.

Qualitative (descriptive) recommendations: *Strong, high*: strong recommendation based on high-quality evidence; *Strong, moderate*: strong recommendation based on moderate-quality evidence; *Strong, low*: strong recommendation based on low-quality evidence; *Moderate, high*: moderate recommendation based on high-quality evidence; *Moderate, intermediate*: moderate recommendation based on intermediate-quality evidence; *Moderate, low*: moderate recommendation based on low-quality evidence; *Weak, moderate*: weak recommendation, moderate quality evidence from RCTs with important limitations or exceptionally strong evidence from unbiased observational studies; *Weak, low*: weak recommendation, low-quality evidence for at least one critical outcome from observational studies, RCTs with serious flaws, or indirect evidence.

Data from references 1, 2, 4, 6, 22, 23, and 25.

TABLE 145-3 Tools for Evaluating Febrile Neutropenia and Identifying Low-Risk Individuals for Outpatient Management

	Patient Characteristic	Score or Group
MASCC		
	Burden of febrile neutropenia: no or mild symptoms *OR* moderate symptoms	5 points 3 points
	No hypotension (systolic blood pressure >90 mm Hg)	5 points
	No chronic obstructive pulmonary disease	4 points
	Solid tumor or hematologic malignancy with no previous fungal infection	4 points
	No dehydration requiring parenteral fluids	3 points
	Outpatient status	3 points
	Age <60 years	2 points
	Maximum total score = 26 points; score ≥21 points indicates low risk for medical complications	
Talcott		
	Inpatients at time of fever onset	Group I
	Outpatients with acute comorbidity requiring, by itself, hospitalization	Group II
	Outpatients without comorbidity but with uncontrolled cancer	Group III
	Outpatients with cancer controlled and without comorbidity	Group IV
	Groups I-III = high risk; Group IV = low risk	
CISNE		
	Eastern Cooperative Oncology Group performance status ≥2	2 points
	Stress-induced hyperglycemia	2 points
	Chronic obstructive pulmonary disease	1 point
	Chronic cardiovascular disease	1 point
	National Cancer Institute Common Toxicity Criteria mucositis of grade ≥2	1 point
	Monocytes <200/μL (0.2 × 10^9/L)	1 point

Maximum total score = 8 points; 0 points = low risk; 1-2 points = intermediate risk; ≥3 points = high risk. Suggested for use with patients with solid tumors who have undergone mild-to-moderate intensity chemotherapy and who appear to be clinically stable. Patients with CISNE score 0-2 would be considered candidates for outpatient management.

Data from References 2 and 4.

TABLE 145-4 Comparative Advantages and Disadvantages of Various Antibiotic Regimens for Empiric Therapy of Febrile Neutropenic Patients with Cancer

Regimen	Potential Advantages	Potential Disadvantages
β-Lactam monotherapy (ceftazidime, cefepime, piperacillin–tazobactam, imipenem–cilastatin, or meropenem)	Efficacy comparable to combination regimens; decreased drug toxicities; ease of administration; possibly less expensive	Possibly less efficacy in profound neutropenia or prolonged neutropenia; limited gram-positive activity; no potential for additive/synergistic effects; increased selection of resistant organisms; increased colonization and superinfection rates
Antipseudomonal β-lactam plus aminoglycoside (eg, gentamicin or tobramycin + cefepime, ceftazidime, or piperacillin–tazobactam)	Traditional regimen, broad-spectrum coverage; optimal therapy of *Pseudomonas aeruginosa*; rapidly bactericidal; synergistic activity; decreased bacterial resistance; reduction of superinfections	Limited gram-positive activity; potential for nephrotoxicity; need for therapeutic monitoring of aminoglycoside concentrations
Antipseudomonal β-lactam plus fluoroquinolone (ciprofloxacin or higher-dose levofloxacin + ceftazidime, cefepime, or piperacillin–tazobactam)	Efficacy similar to other regimens when used in combination therapy; no cross-resistance with β-lactams; possibility for oral administration; may be useful in patients with renal impairment in whom aminoglycosides are undesirable	Marginal gram-positive activity; fluoroquinolones not recommended as monotherapy; resistance may develop rapidly
Empirical regimens containing vancomycin (added to antipseudomonal β-lactam ± aminoglycoside or fluoroquinolone)	Early effective therapy of gram-positive infections	No demonstrated benefit of vancomycin empirical therapy versus addition of vancomycin if needed later; increased risk of selection for vancomycin-resistant enterococci; risk of toxicities; excessive cost; need for therapeutic monitoring of vancomycin concentrations
Oral antibiotic regimens (eg, ciprofloxacin or levofloxacin + amoxicillin–clavulanate or clindamycin)	Efficacy comparable with parenteral therapy in low-risk patients; less expensive; reduced exposure of patients to nosocomial pathogens	Least studied treatment approach; less potent than parenteral antibiotics; requires compliant patient with 24-hour access to medical care should clinical instability develop

Data from references 1-5, 10, 27, and 28.

These agents are also considered to be too broad-spectrum and expensive for routine empiric use. However, they may be considered reasonable treatment options in selected patients at high risk for, or with previous history of, infection with multidrug-resistant (MDR) pathogens or in institutions with high rates of infection with MDR pathogens in certain high-risk patients.

Use of monotherapy has several potential advantages and disadvantages (see Table 145-4). Perhaps the most common concerns are those regarding the selection of resistant strains of organisms, such as *P. aeruginosa*, *Klebsiella-Enterobacter* group, and *Serratia* spp., through expression of ESBL and type 1 β-lactamases, especially with ceftazidime.[1,4,10,14] Activity against gram-positive organisms such as coagulase-negative staphylococci, MRSA, enterococci (including VRE), penicillin-resistant *S. pneumoniae*, and some strains of viridans streptococci is poor with some single β-lactams, but cefepime and antipseudomonal carbapenems have good activity against most viridans streptococci and pneumococci.[1,4] Although ceftazidime has been widely studied and used for treatment of febrile neutropenia, newer agents may be more effective owing to ceftazidime's susceptibility to β-lactamase induction and lower activity against gram-positive organisms.[1,4,10,14,30] Ertapenem, a carbapenem, and ceftaroline, a cephalosporin active against MRSA, have excellent activity against many gram-negative organisms but should not be routinely used in the empirical treatment of febrile neutropenia due to their weak activity against *P. aeruginosa*. For the same reason, broad-spectrum tetracycline derivatives (eg, tigecycline, eravacycline, omadacycline) are not acceptable options for empiric monotherapy in most patients.

As with all empirical antibiotic regimens, patients receiving monotherapy should be monitored closely for treatment failure, secondary infections, and development of resistance. Use of monotherapy may not be appropriate in institutions with high rates of gram-positive infections or infections caused by relatively resistant gram-negative pathogens such as *P. aeruginosa* and *Klebsiella-Enterobacter*. The carbapenems are less susceptible to inducible β-lactamases and often may be used effectively in these institutions. Overall, similar efficacy has been observed with monotherapy with antipseudomonal β-lactams compared to aminoglycoside combination therapy for treatment of *P. aeruginosa* infections.[1,4,29]

Aminoglycoside Plus Antipseudomonal β-Lactam

Regimens consisting of an aminoglycoside plus an antipseudomonal β-lactam traditionally have been the most commonly used for empirical treatment of febrile neutropenia, although many such regimens may lack adequate gram-positive activity (see Table 145-4).[1,4] This relative lack of activity remains a concern because of the increasing frequency of gram-positive infections. The choice of aminoglycoside and β-lactam for inclusion in empirical regimens should be based on institutional epidemiology and antimicrobial susceptibility patterns. Similar efficacy is observed with an antipseudomonal β-lactam in combination with an aminoglycoside.[1,4,29]

Combinations of broad-spectrum β-lactams and aminoglycosides may provide improved activity (eg, synergy activity against bacteria commonly involved in neutropenic infections). The exact role of synergy in the outcome of patients with febrile neutropenia treated with empirical antibiotic therapy is somewhat controversial, particularly in light of the efficacy of single-drug regimens and nephrotoxicity associated with aminoglycosides.[29,30] Nevertheless, combinations of antibiotics appear to be beneficial in patients with persistent profound neutropenia.

Aminoglycoside toxicity may be a concern in patients receiving these regimens who are already receiving other nephrotoxic drugs, such as cisplatin and cyclosporine. Administration of aminoglycosides in large single daily doses (once-daily dosing) may be as effective, less costly, and no more toxic than conventional dosing methods. Although once-daily aminoglycoside dosing regimens appear to be safe and effective in these patients, standard dosing regimens are recommended for infections where data are not sufficient to recommend once-daily dosing (eg, endocarditis).[1,4]

Fluoroquinolones as a Component of Empirical Regimens

Because the fluoroquinolone antibiotics have broad-spectrum activity (particularly against gram-negative pathogens), rapid bactericidal activity, and favorable pharmacokinetic and toxicity profiles, these agents have been investigated as empirical therapy for febrile neutropenia. Ciprofloxacin is the preferred agent for use in this clinical setting because of its relatively better activity against *P. aeruginosa* and more extensive evidence-based support for its use.[1,4] Response rates to quinolone-containing combination regimens are comparable to those obtained with the other regimens described previously.[1,3,4] Ciprofloxacin is not recommended for monotherapy, however, because of its relatively poor activity against gram-positive pathogens, particularly streptococci, and variable response rates in clinical studies.[1,4] Although delafloxacin has a spectrum of antibacterial activity that seems favorable for febrile neutropenia, no data currently exist for this indication and its use is not recommended. Fluoroquinolones should also not be used as empirical therapy in patients who have received quinolones as infection prophylaxis because of the risk of drug resistance.[1,4] Rates of fluoroquinolone resistance are increasing, and streptococcal treatment failures are a concern.[12,14,16] Although fluoroquinolones are not generally considered first-line empirical therapy for inpatient use, they may be useful as one component of combination regimens in patients with allergies or other contraindications to first-line agents.[1,4]

Empirical Regimens Containing Vancomycin

The inclusion of vancomycin in initial empirical therapy of febrile neutropenic patients with cancer is not currently recommended by IDSA 2010 or NCCN 2021 guidelines unless the patient has specific risk factors; however, this remains an ongoing debate. This controversy continues because of the high incidence of gram-positive infections in this population, particularly MRSA. One approach is to include vancomycin in the initial empirical antibiotic regimen, thereby providing early effective treatment of possible gram-positive infections. Inclusion of vancomycin in initial empirical regimens may be appropriate because of higher rates of MRSA infections as well as aggressive chemotherapy regimens causing significant mucosal damage that increases the risk for streptococcal infections. Decreased mortality from penicillin-resistant viridans streptococcal infections has been observed when vancomycin was included in initial therapy.[1,6,30] A second approach is to withhold vancomycin from initial empirical regimens, later adding the drug if gram-positive organisms are isolated from cultures or if there is clinical deterioration. Support for both these approaches can be found in the medical literature.[1,4,30,31] Prospective studies and multiple meta-analyses have failed to document increased response rates or decreased mortality with the routine addition of vancomycin to initial empirical regimens, provided that vancomycin can be added later as needed.[1,4,30,31] In addition to increased costs of therapy, vancomycin was also associated with increased adverse effects, including nephrotoxicity.[4] Finally, concerns remain regarding selection of resistant gram-positive bacteria such as VRE with excessive vancomycin use.[1,4,26,32]

Vancomycin is recommended for inclusion in initial empirical regimens only in patients at high risk for gram-positive infection, particularly due to MRSA and coagulase-negative staphylococci (including patients with evidence of infection of central venous catheters and other indwelling lines), high risk for viridans streptococcal infection due to severe mucositis, or pneumonitis or soft tissue infection in hospitals with high rates of MRSA infections.[1,4,10,30] Rates of β-lactam resistance among viridans streptococci range up to 25%.[1,4] Empirical vancomycin use may be justified in institutions using empirical or prophylactic antibiotic regimens without good activity against streptococci (eg, ciprofloxacin) and in patients known to be colonized with MRSA or β-lactam–resistant pneumococci. In patients with preliminary culture results indicating gram-positive infection, empirical vancomycin is appropriate while the susceptibility results are pending. Lastly, empirical use of vancomycin may be recommended in patients with hypotension or other evidence of cardiovascular impairment or sepsis without an identified pathogen.[1,4] If empirical vancomycin therapy is initiated and no evidence of gram-positive infection is found after 48 to 72 hours, the drug should be discontinued.[1,4] Continuing vancomycin when not warranted results in higher costs, more toxicities, and greater risk of development of VRE.[1,4,32] Of note, augmented renal clearance occurs with some frequency (approximately 16%) in patients with febrile neutropenia and has been associated with significantly higher rates of subtherapeutic vancomycin concentrations.[33] Clinicians should be alert to the need for therapeutic drug monitoring of vancomycin in patients with febrile neutropenia and should carefully monitor patient response to therapy in those receiving vancomycin or other renally excreted antimicrobials.[27,33,34]

Other antimicrobial agents, such as quinupristin–dalfopristin, linezolid, daptomycin, telavancin, and ceftaroline, should be reserved for documented infections caused by multiresistant gram-positive pathogens that are not susceptible to, or are unresponsive to, vancomycin. The role of these drugs in the routine treatment of febrile neutropenia is undetermined, and linezolid is associated with risk of myelosuppression.[1,4]

Oral Antibiotic Therapy for Management of Febrile Neutropenia

An individual patient's risk for complications of severe infection determines appropriate antibiotic therapy and the proper setting for administration (see Table 145-4).[1-3,5] Risk stratification is based on several parameters (eg, MASCC score or other tools previously mentioned) as well as response to empirical antimicrobial therapy if IV therapy is initially given.[1] Benefits of oral therapy on an outpatient basis include increased convenience and quality of life for patients and caregivers and reduced exposure to multidrug-resistant institutional pathogens.[1,2,4] Outpatient therapy of low-risk patients is common practice in most institutions. Careful patient selection obviously is required for such management strategies. Important criteria include patient and provider comfort, a history of protocol and medication compliance, caregiver support and transportation available 24 hours per day, and close proximity (less than 1 hour or less than 30 miles [48 km]) to appropriate medical care in the event of failure to respond to outpatient antibiotic therapy.[2] If a patient qualifies for oral therapy based on clinical and other factors, the first dose of oral regimen should be given in the clinic or hospital and the patient observed for at least 4 hours to ensure tolerance and clinical stability.

Because of the excellent spectrum of activity and favorable pharmacokinetics of currently available oral antibiotics, particularly the fluoroquinolones, oral antibiotics have an important role in the management of selected patients. In patients at low risk for severe or complicated bacterial infection, empirical therapy with broad-spectrum oral antibiotic agents achieves similar patient outcomes as parenteral antibiotics, with response rates of 77% to 95%.[1,3,4,28] Patients judged to be low risk with reliable follow-up may thus be appropriate candidates for oral antibiotic therapy administered on an outpatient basis.[1-4,28] Ciprofloxacin or levofloxacin in combination with amoxicillin–clavulanate (or clindamycin for penicillin-allergic patients) for enhanced gram-positive coverage has been most commonly studied for outpatient therapy in low-risk patients and is recommended by IDSA and NCCN guidelines.[1,2,4] In general, monotherapy with ciprofloxacin should be avoided due to relatively poor gram-positive activity. Levofloxacin has been used as monotherapy for outpatient treatment of low-risk patients, due to enhanced gram-positive activity, and is formally recommended by NCCN guidelines, although the IDSA guidelines recommend only combination therapy initially. If used, only the higher-dose levofloxacin 750 mg regimen should be administered in order to provide adequate activity against organisms such as *S. aureus* and *P. aeruginosa*.[1,4] Moxifloxacin has also been endorsed as a monotherapy option by NCCN guidelines; however, the lack of *P. aeruginosa* activity warrants special consideration.[4]

In patients at low risk for severe bacterial infection who were initiated on IV antibiotics, oral antibiotics may play a role in step-down therapy. Carefully selected patients with neutropenia may be safely switched from broad-spectrum parenteral therapy to oral antibiotic regimens with response rates comparable to patients remaining on IV therapy.[1,2,4,28] Patient selection criteria generally include defervescence within 72 hours of initiation of parenteral therapy, hemodynamic stability, absence of positive cultures or a discernible site of infection, and ability to take oral medications. Many of these patients are able to complete their course of therapy at home.[1,2,4,28] Changing parenteral antimicrobials to oral regimens in carefully selected patients is an acceptable practice and allows for less expensive hospitalizations and earlier patient discharges.[2]

Antimicrobial Therapy After Initiation of Empirical Therapy

6 After initiation of empirical antimicrobial therapy (Table 145-5), judicious assessment of febrile neutropenic patients with cancer is mandatory to evaluate response, clinical status, laboratory data, and potential need for therapy adjustments. After 2 to 4 days of empirical antimicrobial therapy, the clinical status and culture results should be reevaluated to determine whether therapeutic modifications are necessary (Fig. 145-2). Modifications of antimicrobial therapy should be based on clinical and laboratory data; antibiotic therapy should be optimized based on culture results. However, during periods of neutropenia, patients generally should continue to receive broad-spectrum therapy because of risk of secondary infections or breakthrough bacteremias when antimicrobial coverage is too narrow.[1,4] The treatment duration for a documented infection should be appropriate for the particular organism and site, and should continue for at least the duration of neutropenia (until ANC greater than or equal to 500 cells/mm^3 [0.5×10^9/L]) or longer if clinically necessary.

In patients who become afebrile after 2 to 4 days of therapy with no infection identified, it is generally optimal to continue antibiotic therapy until neutropenia has resolved (ANC greater than or equal to 500 cells/mm^3 [0.5×10^9/L]). Some clinicians switch therapy to an oral regimen (eg, ciprofloxacin plus amoxicillin–clavulanate) after 2 days of IV therapy in low-risk patients who become afebrile and have no evidence of infection. In high-risk patients, parenteral antibiotic regimens should be continued until resolution of neutropenia.[1,4] However, in afebrile patients with prolonged neutropenia but no signs or symptoms of infection, consideration can be given to discontinuing antibiotic therapy or switching to fluoroquinolone prophylaxis (discussed in "Prophylaxis of Infections in Neutropenic Patients with Cancer" below), provided that patients can be observed carefully and have ready access to medical care.

The optimal management of patients who remain febrile in the absence of microbiologic or clinical documentation of infection remains highly controversial. Persistently febrile patients should be evaluated carefully, but modifications generally are not made to initial antimicrobial regimens within the first 2 to 4 days of therapy

TABLE 145-5 Drug Dosing Table

Drug	Brand Name	Usual Dosing Regimen	Special Population Dose	Other
Amoxicillin–clavulanate	Augmentin®	875 mg orally every 12 hours		In combination with ciprofloxacin for outpatient treatment
Ceftazidime	Fortaz®	2 g IV every 8 hours		
Ceftazidime–avibactam	Avycaz®	2.5 g IV every 8 hours, administered over 2 hours		Not studied in febrile neutropenia, but spectrum is appropriate if high rates of MDR gram-negative bacteria (esp. CRE)
Cefepime	Maxipime®	2 g IV every 12 hours		
Ceftaroline	Teflaro®	600 mg IV every 12 hours		Activity against methicillin-resistant *S. aureus*
Ceftolozane–tazobactam	Zerbaxa®	1.5 g IV every 8 hours		Not studied in febrile neutropenia, but spectrum is appropriate if high rates of MDR gram-negative bacteria
Piperacillin–tazobactam	Zosyn®	3.375-4.5 g IV every 6 hours		
Imipenem–cilastatin	Primaxin®	500 mg IV every 6 hours		
Meropenem	Merrem®	1 g IV every 8 hours		
Meropenem–vaborbactam	Vabomere®	4 g IV every 8 hours, administered over 3 hours		Not studied in febrile neutropenia, but spectrum is appropriate if high rates of MDR gram-negative bacteria (esp. CRE)
Doripenem	Doribax®	500 mg IV every 8 hours		
Tobramycin	Nebcin®	Traditional: 2 mg/kg loading dose, followed by 1.5 mg/kg IV every 8 hours. Alternative: 5-7 mg/kg IV once daily		Traditional dosing: Guided by measured serum concentrations
Gentamicin	Garamycin®	Traditional: 2 mg/kg loading dose, followed by 1.5 mg/kg IV every 8 hours. Alternative: 5-7 mg/kg IV once daily		Traditional dosing: Guided by measured serum concentrations
Amikacin	Amikin®	Traditional: 7.5 mg/kg IV every 12 hours. Alternative: 15-20 mg/kg IV once daily		Traditional dosing: Guided by measured serum concentrations
Ciprofloxacin	Cipro®	400 mg IV every 8 hours	Outpatient treatment: 750 mg orally every 12 hours	May be given orally in low-risk patients in combination with amoxicillin–clavulanate
Levofloxacin	Levaquin®	750 mg IV once daily	Outpatient treatment: 750 mg orally once daily	May be given orally in low-risk patients
Moxifloxacin	Avelox®	400 mg IV/orally once daily	Outpatient treatment: 400 mg orally once daily	For select outpatient use, lacks *P. aeruginosa* activity
Delafloxacin	Baxdela®	300 mg IV or 450 mg orally every 12 hours		Activity includes methicillin-resistant *S. aureus* and *P. aeruginosa*; not studied in febrile neutropenia, but spectrum is appropriate
Vancomycin	Vancocin®	30-40 mg/kg/day IV in two divided doses administered every 12 hours		For methicillin-resistant *S. aureus* infection; dosing guided by serum concentrations to achieve trough of 15-20 mg/L (10-14 µmol/L)
Nafcillin	Nafcil®	1-2 g IV every 6 hours		For methicillin-susceptible *S. aureus* infection
Daptomycin	Cubicin®	Skin/soft tissue infections: 4 mg/kg IV once daily; bacteremia: 6 mg/kg IV once daily		For infection (esp. bacteremia) due to methicillin-resistant *S. aureus*, vancomycin-resistant enterococci
Linezolid	Zyvox®	600 mg IV or orally every 12 hours		For infection due to vancomycin-resistant enterococci
Ampicillin	Omnipen®, Polycillin®, Principen®	1-2 g IV every 4 hours		In combination with gentamicin for *Listeria* infection
Erythromycin	E-mycin®, Erythrocin®	1-2 g IV every 4-6 hours		For *Legionella* infection
Clotrimazole	Mycelex Troche®	10 mg orally five times daily		Administered as oral troche; dissolve in mouth
Nystatin	Nystatin Oral®	100,000 units orally every 4-6 hours		Administered as suspension; swish and swallow

TABLE 145-5 Drug Dosing Table

Drug	Brand Name	Usual Dosing Regimen	Special Population Dose	Other
Fluconazole	Diflucan®	800 mg IV or orally once, then 400-800 mg IV or orally once daily	Prophylaxis of *Candida* infection: 400 mg IV or orally once daily	
Itraconazole	Sporanox®	200-400 mg/day orally divided twice daily	Prophylaxis of *Candida* infection: 200 mg orally twice daily	Therapeutic drug monitoring recommended
Voriconazole	Vfend®	6 mg/kg IV every 12 hours for two doses, then 4 mg/kg IV or 200 mg orally every 12 hours	Prophylaxis in high-risk patients: 200 mg orally twice daily	Therapeutic drug monitoring recommended
Posaconazole	Noxafil®	Suspension: 800 mg/day orally in two to four divided doses Oral DR or IV: 300 mg every 12 hours × 2 doses, then 300 mg daily	Prophylaxis in high-risk patients: 200 mg orally three times daily	DR formulation has improved bioavailability, administered with food. Suspension: administer with full meal or enteral nutritional supplements. Therapeutic drug monitoring recommended
Isavuconazonium	Cresemba®	372 mg IV/oral every 8 hours × 6 doses, then 372 mg daily		Limited clinical experience
Lipid-associated amphotericin B (LAMB)	AmBisome®, Abelcet®	3-5 mg/kg IV once daily	Prophylaxis in high-risk patients: 1 mg/kg IV once daily	
Flucytosine	Ancobon®	25 mg/kg/day orally every 6 hours		In combination with LAMB for cryptococcal meningitis. Therapeutic drug monitoring recommended
Caspofungin	Cancidas®	70 mg IV once, then 50 mg IV once daily		
Micafungin	Mycamine®	100 mg IV once daily	Prophylaxis in high-risk patients: 50 mg IV once daily	
Anidulafungin	Eraxis®	200 mg IV once, then 100 mg IV once daily		
Acyclovir	Zovirax®	5-10 mg/kg IV every 8 hours, or 800 mg orally two to five times daily	Prophylaxis of HSV or VZV: 800-1,600 mg orally twice daily; CMV prophylaxis in allogeneic HCT: 800 mg orally four times daily; HSV or VZV encephalitis: 10 mg/kg IV every 8 hours	
Valacyclovir	Valtrex®	1 g orally every 8 hours	Prophylaxis of HSV or VZV: 500 mg orally two or three times daily; CMV prophylaxis in allogeneic HCT: 2 g orally four times daily	
Ganciclovir	Cytovene®	CMV treatment or preemptive therapy: 5 mg/kg IV every 12 hours	CMV prophylaxis: 5-6 mg/kg IV daily 5 days/wk	
Valganciclovir	Valcyte®	CMV preemptive therapy: 900 mg orally every 12 hours for 2 weeks	CMV prophylaxis: 450-900 mg orally daily	
Foscarnet	Foscavir®	CMV treatment: 90 mg/kg IV every 12 hours for 2 weeks; CMV preemptive therapy: 60 mg/kg IV every 12 hours for 2 weeks	CMV prophylaxis: 60 mg/kg IV two or three times daily for 7 days, then 90-120 mg/kg IV daily	
Letermovir	Prevymis®	480 mg IV or orally once daily		For prophylaxis of CMV infection and disease in CMV-seropositive allogeneic HCT recipients, used through day 100 post-transplant
CMV hyperimmune globulin	Cytogam®	400 mg/kg IV every other day for three to five doses		Consider as adjunct to ganciclovir or foscarnet for treatment of CMV pneumonia; IVIG considered equally effective
Trimethoprim–sulfamethoxazole	Bactrim®, Cotrimoxazole®	Treatment of *P. jirovecii*: 15-20 mg/kg/day IV divided every 6 hours[b]	Prophylaxis of *P. jirovecii*: 160 mg/800 mg orally daily or three times per week	
Atovaquone	Mepron®	Treatment of *P. jirovecii*: 750 mg orally every 12 hours	Prophylaxis of *P. jirovecii*: 1,500 mg/day orally in one or two divided doses every 12 hours	
Pentamidine	Pentam®	Treatment of *P. jirovecii*: 4 mg/kg IV once daily	Prophylaxis of *P. jirovecii*: 300 mg by inhalation once monthly	

(continued)

TABLE 145-5 Drug Dosing Table (*Continued*)

Drug	Brand Name	Usual Dosing Regimen	Special Population Dose	Other
Clindamycin	Cleocin®	450-600 mg orally every 6 hours		In combination with primaquine for *P. jirovecii*, or with pyrimethamine for toxoplasmosis
Primaquine	Aralen®, Primaquine®	15 mg orally once daily		In combination with clindamycin for *P. jirovecii*
Dapsone	Dapsone®	100 mg orally once daily		In combination with trimethoprim for *P. jirovecii*
Trimethoprim	Triprim®	15-20 mg/kg/day orally divided every 6 hours		In combination with dapsone for *P. jirovecii*
Pyrimethamine	Daraprim®	50-100 mg orally once daily[c]		In combination with sulfadiazine for toxoplasmosis
Sulfadiazine	Sulfadiazine®	1 g orally every 4-6 hours		In combination with pyrimethamine for toxoplasmosis
Thiabendazole	Mintezol®	25 mg/kg orally every 12 hours (maximum 3 g/day)		For *Strongyloides* and other intestinal worm infections

unless there is evidence of clinical deterioration (see Fig. 145-1).[1,3,4] It is important to note that the persistence of fever does not necessarily mean failure of a given antimicrobial regimen; up to 25% of patients with neutropenia have fever due to noninfectious causes.[7] This is particularly true if patients are otherwise clinically stable. Fever after two or more days of antibiotic therapy can be due to a number of causes, including nonbacterial infection, resistant bacterial infection or infection slow to respond to therapy, emergence of a secondary infection, inadequate drug concentrations, drug fever, infection at an avascular site (eg, catheter infection or abscess), or noninfectious causes such as tumor or administration of blood products.[1,3,4] Patients with documented infection who are receiving appropriate antimicrobial therapy (based on in vitro susceptibility tests) often remain febrile until resolution of neutropenia occurs. Therefore, the same antibiotic regimen can be continued in patients who remain febrile despite 2 to 4 days of antibiotic therapy but are otherwise clinically stable, especially if neutropenia is expected to resolve within 1 week. However, antibiotic regimens may require modification in patients experiencing toxicities (Table 145-6) as well as in patients with evidence of progressive disease, clinical instability, or documentation of an organism not covered by the initial regimen.[1,3,4] If not already part of the regimen, vancomycin should be considered as warranted by clinical and laboratory findings. However, if vancomycin was included in the initial empirical regimen and the patient is still febrile after 2 to 3 days of therapy without isolating a gram-positive pathogen, discontinuation of vancomycin should be considered to reduce the risk of toxicities or resistance.[1,4]

Initiation of Antifungal Therapy

Patients with neutropenia who remain febrile despite more than 4 to 7 days of broad-spectrum antibiotic therapy are candidates for antifungal therapy. A high percentage of febrile patients who die during prolonged neutropenia have evidence of invasive fungal infection on autopsy, even though many had no evidence of fungal disease before death.[16] Persistence of fever or development of a new fever during broad-spectrum antibiotic therapy may indicate the presence of a fungal infection, most commonly due to *Candida* or *Aspergillus* spp.[15,19,22] Blood cultures are positive in fewer than 50% of patients with neutropenia and invasive fungal infections.[21,22] Rapid, sensitive diagnostic tests for fungi such as serum β-D-glucan, galactomannan, or fungal DNA assays are available and may be considered in higher-risk patients, however, delaying initiation of antifungal therapy pending results of these tests or isolation of fungal organisms may be associated with high morbidity and mortality. The empirical addition of antifungal therapy is thus justified in this clinical setting.[1,4] Empirical antifungal therapy should be initiated after 4 to 7 days of broad-spectrum antibiotic therapy in persistently febrile patients if the duration of continued neutropenia is expected to be greater than 1 week. Administered doses must be adequate to treat undiagnosed fungal infection and prevent fungal superinfection in high-risk patients with febrile neutropenia.[1,4,21]

Evidence-based recommendations from published guidelines for management of suspected or documented fungal infections in patients with neutropenia are summarized in Table 145-2.[21,25,34] Empirical coverage for both *Candida* spp. and *Aspergillus* should be considered because these organisms are responsible for more than 90% of fungal infections in patients with neutropenia and cancer.[6,15,19,22] *Aspergillus* is also particularly common in patients with hematologic malignancies and in patients undergoing HCT. In the setting of febrile neutropenia, lipid-associated amphotericin B (LAMB) products are almost exclusively recommended over conventional amphotericin B due to reduced toxicities despite significantly higher cost without clear improvement in efficacy.[1,4,20,21,25,34] Although the use of higher doses of LAMB has been advocated in an effort to improve efficacy, lower doses (3 mg/kg) of liposomal amphotericin B may be as efficacious as higher doses (10 mg/kg) with lower cost and fewer toxicities.[4] Although LAMB products are recommended for empiric therapy of neutropenic fever when antifungal agents are desired, they are not preferred agents in patients with presumed or documented invasive fungal infections.[4,18,21]

The azole compounds are also used in the management of febrile neutropenia.[1,4,21,25,34] The azoles have replaced LAMB as preferred antifungals for many patients with FN due to the increased cost and toxicities of LAMB.[4] However, concerns regarding the emergence of *Candida* strains with decreased azole susceptibility and unclear efficacy advantages have prevented these agents from replacing amphotericin B as the clear gold standard in patients with persistent febrile neutropenia.[20,25,34] Fluconazole has good efficacy against *C. albicans* but lacks activity against molds such as *Aspergillus*. The use of fluconazole as an alternative to amphotericin B for empirical antifungal therapy is thus perhaps most appropriate in hospitals in which infections due to *Aspergillus* or non-*albicans* strains of *Candida* are not common.[1,4,20,34] If fluconazole is used as antifungal prophylaxis in patients with cancer, it should not be included in empirical antifungal regimens. Voriconazole is the preferred agent in the treatment of documented invasive fungal infections and is recommended as a reliable option for febrile neutropenia.[1,4,34] Despite failing to meet noninferiority criteria when compared against LAMB for empiric therapy in patients with febrile neutropenia, voriconazole is a preferred agent for invasive aspergillosis

TABLE 145-6 Drug Monitoring of Selected Antimicrobials for Febrile Neutropenia, HCT, and SOT

Drug	Adverse Reaction	Monitoring Parameters	Comments
Antibacterial Agents			
Aminoglycosides (Tobramycin, Gentamicin, Amikacin)	Nephrotoxicity	Serum creatinine, urine output, serum concentrations	Extended-interval ("once daily") dosing potentially associated with less renal toxicity, similar efficacy to traditional dosing. Goal trough concentration <1 mcg/mL (mg/L; 2 μmol/L) during extended-interval dosing
Imipenem–cilastatin	CNS toxicities, seizures	Serum creatinine, mental status, CNS function	Increased incidence with higher dose, failure to adjust dose/interval for reduced renal function. Increased risk compared to meropenem or doripenem
Linezolid	Myelosuppression, thrombocytopenia, optic/peripheral neuropathy, serotonin syndrome	CBC, vision changes, serum lactate, heart rate, blood pressure, temperature, myoclonus	Myelosuppression and neuropathy more common with prolonged use. Short course unlikely to affect marrow recovery in HCT. Weak MAO inhibitor, serotonin syndrome possible with other serotonergic drugs such as SSRIs and SNRIs
Nafcillin	Interstitial nephritis	Serum creatinine, urine output	Reversible, requires switch to alternative β-lactam
Vancomycin	Nephrotoxicity, infusion reactions	Serum creatinine, urine output, blood pressure, heart rate, serum concentrations	Dose adjustment required for renal dysfunction. Pretreatment and slow infusion may decrease incidence of infusion reaction. Goal trough concentration 15-20 mcg/mL (mg/L; 10-14 μmol/L) for serious infections
Antifungal Agents			
Amphotericin B (lipid-associated)	Nephrotoxicity, hepatotoxicity, electrolyte disturbances, infusion reactions	Serum creatinine, electrolytes, LFTs, blood pressure, heart rate	Liposomal preparations associated with less renal toxicity, similar efficacy to standard preparation. Electrolyte disturbances occur before creatinine alterations. Pretreatment and slow infusion may decrease incidence of infusion reaction
Flucytosine	Myelosuppression, GI toxicities	CBC, GI symptoms, serum creatinine, flucytosine serum concentrations	Dose adjustment required for renal dysfunction. Goal serum concentrations are peak <100 mcg/mL (mg/L; 775 μmol/L) and trough 20-40 mcg/mL (mg/L; 155-310 μmol/L)
Posaconazole	Hepatotoxicity, rash; interactions with CYP450 3A4	LFTs, skin, posaconazole serum concentrations	Poor absorption with suspension, goals of >1 mcg/mL (mg/L; 1.4 μmol/L) for treatment and >0.7 mcg/mL (mg/L; 1 μmol/L) for prophylaxis. Parenteral formulation contains SBECD, not recommended for patients with CrCL<50 mL/min (0.83 mL/s). Multiple interactions with drugs metabolized by CYP 3A4, including immunosuppressants; close monitoring needed
Voriconazole	Mental status changes, headache, hallucinations, visual disturbances, hepatotoxicity, QTc prolongation; interactions with CYP450 2C9, 2C19, and 3A4	Mental status, visual function, LFTs, ECG, voriconazole serum concentrations	Mental status/visual changes associated with elevated troughs >5.5 mcg/mL (mg/L; 16 μmol/L); goal trough 1-5.5 mcg/mL (mg/L; 3-16 μmol/L) for treatment and prophylaxis, target trough of >2 mcg/mL (mg/L; 6 μmol/L) in disease with poor prognosis. Parenteral formulation contains SBECD, not recommended for patients with CrCL<50 mL/min (0.83 mL/s). Multiple interactions with drugs metabolized by CYP enzymes, including immunosuppressants; close monitoring needed
Antiviral Agents			
Foscarnet	Nephrotoxicity, hypocalcemia	Serum creatinine, electrolytes	IV hydration prior to administration. Dose adjustment required for renal dysfunction
Ganciclovir, valganciclovir	Myelosuppression, thrombocytopenia	CBC, serum creatinine	Dose adjustment required for renal dysfunction
Antiprotozoal/Antiparasitic Agents			
Dapsone	Hemolytic anemia, hypersensitivity (fever, jaundice, eosinophilia), peripheral neuropathy	CBC, bilirubin, LFTs, muscle strength, G6PD testing before use	Higher incidence of hemolytic anemia in G6PD-deficient patients
Pentamidine (IV)	Nephrotoxicity, leukopenia, hypotension, QTc prolongation, pancreatitis, hypo/hyperglycemia	Serum creatinine, serum blood glucose, blood urea nitrogen, CBC, blood pressure, heart rate; ECG	Adequate hydration recommended
Primaquine	Hemolytic anemia	CBC, bilirubin, G6PD testing before use	Avoid use in G6PD-deficient patients (hemolytic anemia)
Pyrimethamine	Bone marrow suppression	CBC	Folinic acid 5-10 mg/day often used for prevention of bone marrow toxicity
Trimethoprim–sulfamethoxazole	Myelosuppression, hyperkalemia, rash	Serum creatinine, electrolytes, CBC, skin	Dose adjustment required for renal dysfunction

CBC, complete blood count; ECG, electrocardiogram; G6PD, glucose-6-phosphate dehydrogenase; HCT; hematopoietic cell transplantation; LFT, liver function test; MAO, monoamine oxidase; PFT, pulmonary function test; QTc, corrected Q-T interval; SBECD, sulfobutylether-β-cyclodextrin; SOT, solid-organ transplantation; SSNRI, selective serotonin–norepinephrine reuptake inhibitor; SSRI, selective serotonin reuptake inhibitor.

Therapeutic drug monitoring recommendations from Reference 30.

(especially pulmonary) due to improved survival and less toxicity when compared to amphotericin B.[1,4,20,25,34-36] Isavuconazonium, the prodrug of isavuconazole, has activity against invasive aspergillosis and mucormycosis that is generally comparable to voriconazole and posaconazole. Isavuconazonium has shown reductions in mortality and overall treatment success similar to voriconazole in a largely neutropenic patient population with hematologic malignancies and suspected invasive fungal infections including a subgroup of proven or probable aspergillosis.[37,38] The most recent guidelines recommend isavuconazonium as an alternative to voriconazole in the treatment of invasive aspergillosis, although there are few data related to use as empiric therapy of febrile neutropenia.[4,21,34] Posaconazole has extended activity against some Mucorales and rare molds in addition to *Candida* and *Aspergillus*, but is only approved for prophylaxis of fungal infections in patients with neutropenia. The improved bioavailability of the delayed-release tablets and availability of a parenteral dosage form make posaconazole an attractive option; although clinical data are relatively limited, the most recent guidelines also recommend posaconazole as an alternative to voriconazole for presumed or documented invasive disease.[21,34] Itraconazole has similar efficacy as amphotericin B, with fewer toxicities. However, current lack of a parenteral dosage form, erratic oral absorption, numerous potential drug-drug interactions, and availability of many other antifungal options limit the use of itraconazole for empiric therapy.[21,34,35] Therapeutic drug monitoring has been recommended for some azole antifungals given potential for interpatient variability, therapeutic failure associated with subtherapeutic concentrations, and toxicities associated with supratherapeutic concentrations (Table 145-6).[4,18,21,28,31,34,39]

The echinocandin antifungals (caspofungin, micafungin, and anidulafungin) are attractive agents for treatment of febrile neutropenia because of their broad spectrum of antifungal activity and favorable adverse effect profiles. Caspofungin is as effective as, and also generally better tolerated than, liposomal amphotericin B for empirical treatment of patients with neutropenia with persistent fever.[1,4] Therefore, caspofungin is considered an appropriate alternative to LAMB and voriconazole.[1,4,20,21,25] Micafungin and anidulafungin have not been as well studied specifically in this setting; however, most experts consider them likely as effective and all echinocandins are recommended.[1,4,21,25]

Initiation of Antiviral Therapy

Patients with febrile neutropenia associated with vesicular or ulcerative skin or mucosal lesions should be evaluated carefully for infection due to HSV or varicella-zoster virus (VZV). Mucosal lesions from viral infections provide a portal of entry for bacteria and fungi during periods of immunosuppression. If viral infection is presumed or documented, patients with neutropenia should receive aggressive antiviral therapy to aid healing of primary lesions and prevent disseminated disease. Acyclovir traditionally has been used in this population. However, the newer antivirals valacyclovir and famciclovir have better oral absorption and more convenient dosing schedules. Routine use of antiviral agents in the management of patients without mucosal lesions or other evidence of viral infection generally is not recommended.[1,4] Treatment recommendations for viral infections are given in Table 145-7.

Duration of Antimicrobial Therapy

7 The optimal duration of antimicrobial therapy in patients with cancer and neutropenia remains controversial. Decisions regarding discontinuation of empirical antimicrobial therapy often are more difficult and complex than those regarding initiation of therapy (see Figs. 145-1). One point on which experts agree, however, is that the most important determinant of the total duration of antibiotic therapy is the patient's ANC.[1,4] If ANC is greater than or equal to 500 cells/mm^3 (0.5 × 10^9/L) for 2 consecutive days, if the patient is afebrile and clinically stable for 48 hours or more, and if no pathogen has been isolated, then antibiotics can be discontinued. Some clinicians advocate that patients with ANC less than 500 cells/mm^3 (0.5 × 10^9/L) be maintained on antibiotic therapy until resolution of neutropenia, even if they are afebrile. However, prolonged antibiotic use has been associated with superinfections resulting from resistant bacteria and fungi and increases the risk of antibiotic-related toxicities.[1,4] If low-risk patients are clinically stable with negative cultures but the ANC still is less than 500 cells/mm^3 (0.5 × 10^9/L), antibiotics may be discontinued after a total of 5 to 7 afebrile days. However, patients with profound neutropenia (ANC greater than 100 cells/mm^3 [0.1 × 10^9/L]), mucosal lesions, or unstable vital signs or other risk factors should continue to receive antibiotics until ANC has increased greater than or equal to 500 cells/mm^3 (0.5 × 10^9/L) and the patient is clinically stable.[1,4]

Patients who are persistently neutropenic and febrile, but who are stable clinically with no active site of infection, often can be successfully discontinued from antimicrobials after at least 2 weeks of therapy. However, these patients must be monitored carefully because reinstitution of antibiotics may be necessary.[1,4] An alternative approach is to place these patients on antimicrobial prophylaxis (discussed in the section "Prophylaxis of Infections in Neutropenic Patients with Cancer" below). Patients with documented infections should receive antimicrobial therapy until the infecting organism is eradicated and signs and symptoms of infection have resolved (at least 10-14 days of therapy).

Consensus guidelines provide useful information regarding the management of febrile episodes in patients with cancer and neutropenia.[1,4] However, therapy (including initial empirical regimens, modifications, and duration of treatment) must be individualized based on specific patient parameters and response to therapy.

Colony-Stimulating Factors

Because resolution of neutropenia is arguably the most important determinant of patient outcome from both febrile episodes and documented infections, numerous studies have evaluated hematopoietic colony-stimulating factors (CSFs) (sargramostim [granulocyte-macrophage colony-stimulating factor] and filgrastim [granulocyte colony-stimulating factor]) as adjunct therapy to antimicrobial treatment of febrile neutropenic patients with cancer. A meta-analysis found that use of CSFs is associated with reduced total duration and severity of chemotherapy-related neutropenia, reduced duration of antibiotic use, fewer hospitalizations, and decreased hospital length of stay.[40] However, this meta-analysis failed to demonstrate a benefit of CSFs in relation to important outcomes such as decreased overall mortality or infection-related mortality.[40] Evidence-based guidelines from the IDSA, American Society of Clinical Oncology (ASCO), and the NCCN recommend that CSFs should not be routinely initiated in patients with uncomplicated fever and neutropenia.[1,4,41,42] However, CSFs should be considered in patients who are at high risk for infection-associated complications, or who have factors that are predictive of poor clinical outcomes.[4,41,42] These factors are summarized in Table 145-8. Patients with prolonged neutropenia and documented severe infections who are not responding to appropriate antimicrobial therapy may also benefit from treatment with CSFs.[41,42] Clinical judgment must be exercised in determining which patients may benefit from judicious use of these expensive agents.

Direct transfusion of neutrophils has also been studied for treatment of febrile neutropenia or documented infections.[5,43] Routine use of neutrophil transfusions is not generally supported by data demonstrating improved clinical outcomes. However, use may be considered in patients with profound prolonged neutropenia with severe documented infections and in whom causative organisms have not been eradicated with appropriate antimicrobial therapy in combination with CSFs.[4] At present, the use of

TABLE 145-7 Infectious Complications During Neutropenia, and After Hematopoietic Cell and Solid-Organ Transplantation: Syndromes of Disease and Treatment Guidelines

Pathogen	Syndromes of Disease	Recommended Treatment
Bacterial		
Gram-negative aerobic bacilli (Enterobacterales, *Pseudomonas aeruginosa*, *Haemophilus influenzae*)	Blood, urinary tract, pulmonary, abdomen	*Empiric:* Ceftazidime ± aminoglycoside,[a,b] cefepime ± aminoglycoside[a,b]; piperacillin–tazobactam; imipenem–cilastatin ± aminoglycoside[a,b] *Definitive:* According to culture and sensitivity results
Gram-positive cocci (*Staphylococcus aureus*, *Staphylococcus epidermidis*, *Streptococcus pneumoniae*, *Enterococcus faecalis*)	Skin, blood, urinary tract, pulmonary, abdomen	*Empiric:* Nafcillin; vancomycin *Definitive:* According to culture and sensitivity results
Legionella spp.	Pulmonary	Erythromycin; azithromycin; ciprofloxacin; levofloxacin
Listeria monocytogenes	CNS	Ampicillin with gentamicin[a]; trimethoprim–sulfamethoxazole
Nocardia spp.	Skin, pulmonary, CNS	Sulfadiazine; trimethoprim–sulfamethoxazole
Fungal		
Candida spp.[c]	Blood, urinary tract, mucous membranes, skin, disseminated disease	Clotrimazole; nystatin; fluconazole; itraconazole; amphotericin B ± flucytosine; lipid-associated amphotericin B (LAMB); caspofungin; micafungin; anidulafungin
Aspergillus spp.[d]	Skin, pulmonary, CNS	Voriconazole; LAMB; caspofungin; micafungin; posaconazole; itraconazole; isavuconazole
Cryptococcus neoformans	Skin, pulmonary, CNS	LAMB + flucytosine; fluconazole
Mucorales (*Mucor*)	Rhinocerebral disease	LAMB; posaconazole
Viral		
Herpes simplex virus	Skin, CNS, mucous membranes, pulmonary	Acyclovir; foscarnet
Human herpesvirus-6	CNS, hepatic, bone marrow	Ganciclovir; foscarnet
Cytomegalovirus	Pulmonary, blood, urinary tract, GI tract	Ganciclovir; foscarnet; immunoglobulin
Varicella-zoster virus	Skin, disseminated disease	Acyclovir; foscarnet
Epstein–Barr virus	Lymphoproliferative disease	Rituximab
Papovaviruses (BK, JC)	Skin, CNS	No effective treatment
Protozoal/Parasitic		
Pneumocystis jirovecii	Pulmonary	Trimethoprim–sulfamethoxazole; atovaquone; pentamidine; dapsone + trimethoprim; clindamycin + primaquine
Toxoplasma gondii	CNS	Pyrimethamine + sulfadiazine; pyrimethamine + clindamycin
Strongyloides stercoralis	Pulmonary, CNS	Thiabendazole

[a]Choice of specific agent determined according to institutional susceptibilities to individual drugs.

[b]For penicillin-allergic adults, use aztreonam or ciprofloxacin + an aminoglycoside.

[c]Refer to the Clinical Practice Guidelines of the Infectious Diseases Society of America (*Reference 21*) for selection and dosing of antifungal agents for specific infections.

[d]Refer to the Clinical Practice Guidelines by the Infectious Diseases Society of America (*Reference 25*) for selection and dosing of antifungal agents for specific infections.

neutrophil transfusions is not recommended for routine management of patients with febrile neutropenia.[4]

Prophylaxis of Infections in Neutropenic Patients with Cancer

8 Owing to the potential morbidity and mortality of infections in neutropenic cancer patients, environmental modifications and prophylactic antimicrobial regimens have been implemented to prevent these complications. The overall goal of antimicrobial prophylaxis in patients with cancer is to decrease the number and severity of systemic infections during prolonged periods of neutropenia. As with febrile neutropenia, patient risk factors for development of infection and complications should be assessed prior to initiation of prophylaxis (Table 145-9).

General Measures

Because approximately 50% of pathogens infecting neutropenic cancer patients are acquired in the hospital, reducing acquisition of infectious organisms from the environment is a basic component in controlling nosocomial infections.[1,4,6] Patients with neutropenia should be placed in reverse isolation (isolation to protect patients from contracting infections after exposure to others) with standard barrier precautions, and strict adherence to infection prevention guidelines by hospital personnel.[1,4,6] Plants and fresh or dried flowers are usually prohibited as part of standard neutropenic precautions in order to minimize risk of exposure to pathogenic bacteria. Proper handwashing and respiratory hygiene by hospital personnel are simple yet effective infection prevention measures.[44] Most patients with neutropenia do not require specific room ventilation; however, HCT recipients should be placed in a private positive-pressure room with greater than 12 air exchanges per hour and HEPA filtration.[1,4,6]

Bacterial Infections

Combinations of oral nonabsorbable antibiotics, such as gentamicin, nystatin, vancomycin, polymyxin B, and colistin, have been widely studied as a means of reducing colonization of the GI tract with virulent pathogens. Although selective intestinal decontamination with oral nonabsorbable antibiotics successfully reduces infections, these

TABLE 145-8 Recommendations for Use of Colony-Stimulating Factors in the Management of Patients with Cancer and Those Undergoing Stem Cell Transplantation

Primary prophylaxis of febrile neutropenia
1. Colony-stimulating factors (CSFs) (filgrastim, pegfilgrastim, or sargramostim) may be considered in patients who have a high risk of febrile neutropenia (>20% incidence) based on myelotoxicity of the planned chemotherapy regimen.
2. When risk of febrile neutropenia is 10%-20%, CSFs may be considered in the presence of certain patient and clinical factors predisposing to increased complications from prolonged neutropenia, including patient age >65 years; poor performance status; extensive prior treatment including large radiation ports; administration of combined chemoradiotherapy; cytopenias due to bone marrow involvement by tumor; poor nutritional status; presence of open wounds or active infections; previous surgery; poor renal function; liver dysfunction, particularly when evidenced by increased bilirubin; and lack of antibiotic prophylaxis.
Secondary prophylaxis of febrile neutropenia
1. CSFs (filgrastim, pegfilgrastim, or sargramostim) recommended for patients who experienced neutropenic complications from prior cycles of chemotherapy, and in which a reduced dose may compromise disease-free or overall survival or treatment outcome.
Therapeutic use in febrile neutropenia
1. CSFs should not be routinely used for patients with neutropenia who are afebrile.
2. CSFs (filgrastim or sargramostim only) may be considered in patients with febrile neutropenia who are at high risk for infection-associated complications, or who have prognostic factors that are predictive of poor clinical outcomes, including profound neutropenia (absolute neutrophil count <100 cells/mm^3 [0.1 × 10^9/L]); expected prolonged period of neutropenia (>10 days); patient age >65 years; uncontrolled primary disease; sepsis syndrome, or severe infection manifest by hypotension and multiorgan dysfunction; pneumonia; invasive fungal infection; other clinically documented infection; hospitalized at the time of the development of fever; or severe complications during previous episode of febrile neutropenia.
Reduction in duration of neutropenia in HCT
1. CSFs are recommended to mobilize peripheral-blood progenitor cells (PBPC) prior to chemotherapy and to reduce the duration of neutropenia after autologous PBPC transplantation.

Data from References 4, 39, and 40.

regimens are not routinely recommended for prophylaxis because of problems that include unpalatability, cost, frequent adverse effects (eg, nausea, vomiting, and diarrhea), and development of resistance.[1-6]

Prophylaxis with orally administered, systemically available antibiotics such as trimethoprim–sulfamethoxazole and fluoroquinolones is effective at reducing gram-negative infections.[1,4] Although trimethoprim–sulfamethoxazole is effective as prophylaxis against *P. jirovecii*, its lack of activity against *P. aeruginosa* is worrisome when used as prophylaxis against bacterial infection, particularly in institutions where pseudomonal infections are frequent.[1] Other concerns with trimethoprim–sulfamethoxazole prophylaxis include selection of resistant organisms, predisposition to development of oral fungal infections, and delay in bone marrow recovery resulting in prolonged neutropenic episodes.[1,4,6]

Fluoroquinolones are more effective than placebo in preventing febrile episodes and gram-negative infections in neutropenic cancer patients and, in some studies, have decreased all-cause mortality and infection-related mortality.[1,4,6,45] However, there are several potential limitations to their use. In particular, ciprofloxacin may lack adequate gram-positive activity and may not be the preferred fluoroquinolone for this reason. Although fluoroquinolone prophylaxis has been associated with colonization and infection with fluoroquinolone-resistant gram-negative organisms, these findings have not been consistent in various studies.[1,4,11,45] The risk of colonization or infection with strains resistant to the prophylactic agent is also lower with fluoroquinolones compared to trimethoprim–sulfamethoxazole.[36] However, patients experiencing breakthrough infection during fluoroquinolone prophylaxis should not be subsequently placed on a fluoroquinolone-containing empirical antibiotic regimen.[1,4] Although studies have not consistently documented increased fluoroquinolone resistance in association with prophylaxis, other potentially unfavorable outcomes such as increased risk of *Clostridioides difficile* infection should also be considered in weighing the potential benefits of fluoroquinolone prophylaxis.[1,4,11,36,45]

Although the benefits of prophylaxis with fluoroquinolones outweigh the potential risks in patients with neutropenia who are at intermediate to high risk for infection (Table 145-9), antibacterial prophylaxis in general remains somewhat controversial due to continued concerns regarding the potential for development of resistant bacteria, high cost, and lack of consistent benefits related to patient survival.[1,4,11] Therefore, antibacterial prophylaxis is not recommended routinely for all patients with neutropenia. Prophylaxis with ciprofloxacin or levofloxacin generally is indicated for intermediate- to high-risk patients expected to be profoundly neutropenic for more than 1 week as shown in Table 145-9.[1,4,6,44] Fluoroquinolone prophylaxis is not routinely recommended for patients with solid tumors.[23,27,44] High-dose levofloxacin may be preferred by some clinicians due to enhanced gram-positive activity. An oral cephalosporin (cefpodoxime) may be considered for patients intolerant of fluoroquinolones.[44] Neutrophil recovery eliminates the need for continued prophylaxis, and recovery may be facilitated by use of CSFs.[41] CSFs have also been formally recommended by ASCO and NCCN for primary prevention of FN in high-risk patients (see Table 145-8).[1,4]

Fungal Infections

Because patients with neutropenia are at risk for mucocutaneous and invasive fungal infections that are difficult to diagnose and treat, antifungal prophylaxis can be considered in intermediate- to high-risk patients at institutions where fungal infections in patients with cancer occur frequently.[1,4] The goal of antifungal prophylaxis is to prevent development of invasive fungal infections during periods of risk, thereby reducing morbidity and mortality. Similar to antibacterial prophylaxis, prophylaxis against fungal infection is specifically recommended for patients who are at risk for profound, protracted neutropenia (Table 145-9).[4,6,23,44]

Antifungal prophylaxis with an oral triazole agent (fluconazole, itraconazole, voriconazole, posaconazole, isavoconazole), parenteral echinocandin, or LAMB is recommended in select patients starting at the time of induction chemotherapy.[4,44] Fluconazole prophylaxis has been particularly well studied and reduces the incidence of both superficial and systemic fungal infections; it also significantly decreases mortality from fungal infections in patients with leukemia and HCT recipients.[4,38] However, use of fluconazole prophylaxis has contributed to the emergence of infections caused by *C. krusei* and *C. glabrata*, pathogens that frequently are resistant to fluconazole and other azole-type antifungal agents.[4,23] When compared to prophylaxis with mold-active agents, patients on fluconazole have a higher rate of aspergillosis and invasive fungal-related mortality but lower rate of adverse events leading to discontinuation.[37] The choice of a specific agent should be determined by the types of fungal isolates at individual institutions and risk for invasive mold infection compared to invasive candidiasis.[1,4,21,44,46] After initiation, antifungal prophylaxis should be continued until resolution of neutropenia or the need for institution of antifungal therapy for suspected/documented infection.[4,18,21,23,44]

Other Infections

Use of trimethoprim–sulfamethoxazole prophylaxis in patients with cancer at risk for *P. jirovecii* pneumonia has substantially reduced the incidence of this infection. Trimethoprim–sulfamethoxazole is therefore recommended for use in patients receiving

TABLE 145-9 Risk-Based Prophylactic Strategies for Patients with Neutropenia

Risk Group	Patient Characteristics	Prophylactic Strategies
High risk	*Neutropenia:* Severe (absolute neutrophil count <100/mm^3 [0.1 × 10^9/L]) and/or prolonged (≥10 days) *Malignancy/treatment:* Hematologic malignancy (acute leukemia), allogeneic HCT, GVHD with high-dose steroids (≥20 mg prednisone equivalents daily for ≥1 month), or use of alemtuzumab or purine-containing regimens	Consider bacterial prophylaxis with fluoroquinolone for duration of neutropenia. Give fungal prophylaxis with product and duration based on patient-specific factors. Give/consider viral prophylaxis with product and duration based on patient-specific factors. Consider protozoal prophylaxis with product and duration based on patient-specific factors
Moderate risk	*Neutropenia:* Moderate duration (7-10 days) *Malignancy/treatment:* Autologous HCT, multiple myeloma, lymphoma, chronic lymphocytic leukemia, purine analog therapy	Consider bacterial prophylaxis with fluoroquinolone for duration of neutropenia. Consider fungal prophylaxis with product and duration based on patient-specific factors. Give/consider viral prophylaxis with product and duration based on patient-specific factors. Consider protozoal prophylaxis with product and duration based on patient-specific factors
Low risk	*Neutropenia:* Short duration (≤7 days) *Malignancy/treatment:* Solid tumor treated with conventional chemotherapy	Antibacterial and antifungal prophylaxis not indicated. Viral prophylaxis considered during neutropenia if patient has prior HSV episode

GVHD, graft versus host disease; HCT, hematopoietic cell transplant; HSV, herpes simplex virus.

Data from References 1, 4, 6, 27, 37, and 42.

higher-risk chemotherapeutic regimens (see Table 145-9).[1,4,44] Antiviral prophylaxis with acyclovir, valacyclovir, or famciclovir is recommended to reduce the risk of HSV reactivation in patients with acute leukemia undergoing intensive chemotherapy.[4,44] Prophylaxis with a nucleoside reverse transcriptase inhibitor such as entacavir or tenofovir is recommended for patients at high risk of HBV reactivation.[4,44] Finally, patients should be assessed for indications for administration of vaccines such pneumococcal, influenza, varicella, and varicella zoster in order to provide protection from vaccine-preventable infections that commonly occur in patients with neutropenia and immunosuppression.[38] Many vaccines will be most effective when administered to patients prior to beginning immunosuppressive chemotherapy regimens, while inactivated influenza vaccine may also be administered to already immunocompromised patients.[38]

When considering use of antimicrobial (antibacterial, antifungal, and antiviral) prophylaxis in patients with neutropenia and cancer, the risks and benefits of prophylaxis must be weighed against issues with development of resistance, toxicities, and other concerns.

Evaluation of Therapeutic Outcomes

10 Close monitoring of patients with febrile neutropenia, including both clinical and laboratory parameters, is essential for early detection and treatment of infectious complications. Three general therapeutic outcomes have been defined in the setting of febrile neutropenia: (a) success (survival during the febrile episode until resolution of neutropenia by judicious selection of empirical antimicrobial therapy), (b) success with modification (same as [a] but with additions/modifications to empirical therapy), and (c) failure (death during febrile neutropenia).[1] Because many of the drugs that can be used in this setting (eg, aminoglycosides and amphotericin B) have significant toxicity potential, careful attention must be paid to prevention and management of drug-related adverse effects. Evaluations of the parameters given in the Clinical Presentation are appropriate to help monitor and guide therapy. In addition, the NCCN guidelines for febrile neutropenia provide comprehensive recommendations on clinical/laboratory monitoring parameters, including schedules.[4] The reader is referred to individual chapters within this book for more detailed discussions of monitoring parameters related to specific types of infections (eg, pneumonia and urinary tract infections).

INFECTIONS IN PATIENTS UNDERGOING HCT

1 Infection remains a major barrier to successful HCT.[47-50] Recipients of HCT are at enhanced risk for infection because of prolonged periods of neutropenia. In addition, patients receiving allogeneic transplants (related, matched unrelated, or cord blood) receive prolonged immunosuppressive drug therapy for prevention and treatment of graft-versus-host disease (GVHD) following engraftment. Allogeneic HCT recipients are generally slower to engraft when compared to autologous HCT recipients.[4] Intensive pretransplant conditioning regimens (high-dose chemotherapy and total-body irradiation), as well as GVHD itself, often disrupt protective barriers, such as mucous membranes, skin, and the GI tract, placing patients at further risk of infection.[4,48,49] Although infectious complications are still associated with considerable morbidity and mortality, studies have documented significant reduction in mortality after HCT in association with reductions in disease caused by bacterial, fungal, and viral infections.[4] As the number of HCTs performed increases and patients live longer, the population of HCT recipients is expected to continue to grow exponentially.[42]

Etiology and Clinical Presentation of Infections

2 10 The timing with which specific types of infections typically occur following HCT is shown in Fig. 145-3, but the relative incidence and importance of specific pathogens vary greatly according to the specific type of HCT performed. Patients receiving allogeneic transplants are at greatest risk for infection after HCT and are predisposed to earlier and more severe infections with opportunistic pathogens such as *Aspergillus*. The presence of GVHD also has an impact on the incidence and timing of various infections, including invasive fungal infections.

After administration of intensive conditioning regimens to eliminate malignant cells and prevent rejection of donor cells, patients may remain profoundly neutropenic for 3 to 4 weeks. During this pre-engraftment period, patients are at risk for the same types of infectious complications that occur in other granulocytopenic patients with cancer (eg, bacterial and fungal infections) and should be managed accordingly (see Table 145-1).[4] Table 145-7 lists regimens for treatment of specific infections.

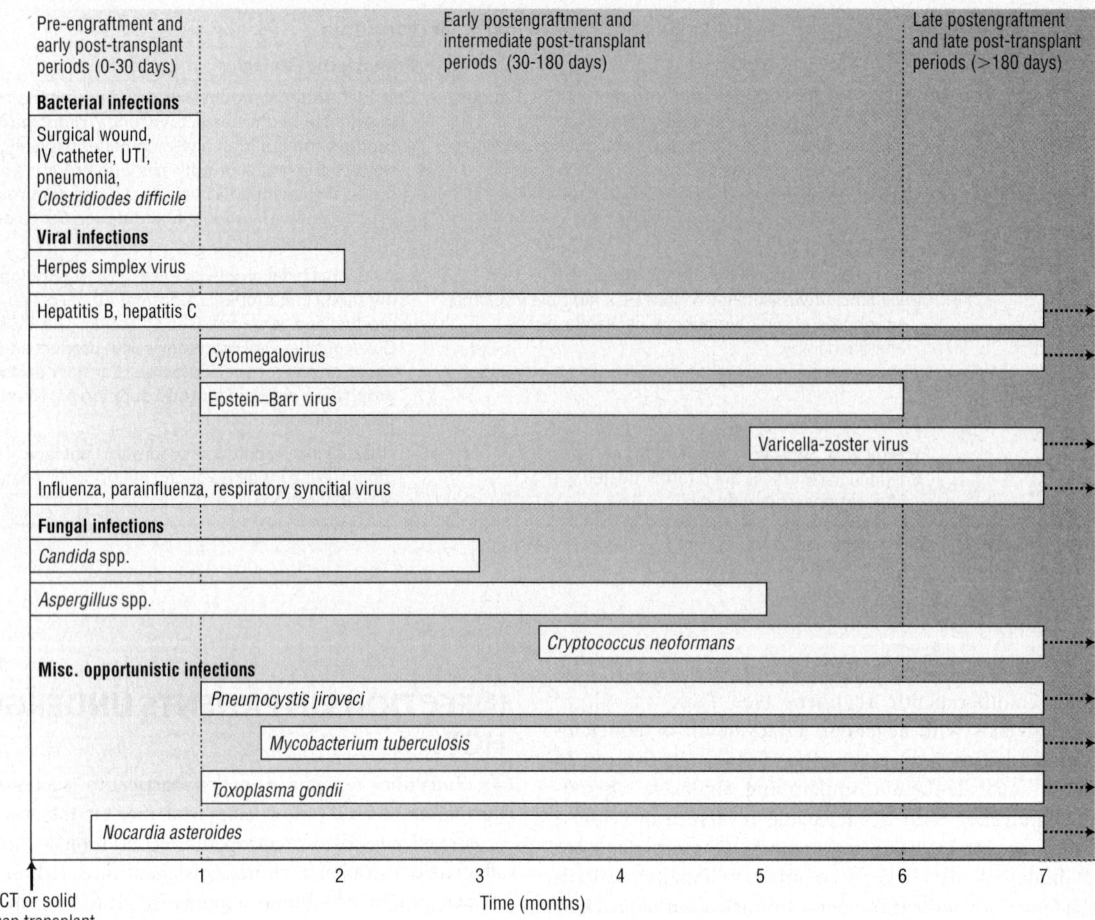

FIGURE 145-3 Timetable for the occurrence of infections in hematopoietic cell transplantation (HCT) and solid-organ transplant patients. (UTI, urinary tract infection.)

HCT recipients remain at high risk for infection after bone marrow engraftment has occurred.[4] Significant defects in neutrophil function and cell-mediated and humoral immunity, persisting for several months after transplantation, predispose patients to infectious complications. Furthermore, specific medications, regimens, and therapies utilized are associated with added risk or a prolonged risk of various infections (alemtuzumab, anti-CD20 antibodies, fludarabine, steroids, asplenia, etc.).[4] Acute and chronic GVHD following allogeneic HCT also results in prolonged periods of immunosuppression.[4,48,49] Those who experience acute GVHD had a 60% higher infection rate and higher risk of developing serious or fatal infections compared to allogeneic HCT recipients without acute GVHD.[49] Even in the absence of active GVHD, 10% to 20% of all deaths are attributable to infection after year two in allogeneic HCT recipients.[51]

HCT recipients are at significant risk for serious bacterial infections at various sites.[4,50] Bacteremia is particularly concerning following allogeneic HCT as those with GVHD have a three-fold increased risk.[48] Bacteremia has been reported in up to half of HCT recipients with gram-positive and gram-negative bacteremia occurring at similar rates.[48,50,52] However gram-negative bacteremia remains of significant clinical importance because mortality rates may reach 45% for increasingly common multidrug resistant strains.[11] *Clostridioides difficile* has become a common and important cause of gastrointestinal infections.[4,41,50]

Fungal infections, especially those caused by *Candida* and *Aspergillus* spp., are serious and often result in fatal complications. Fungi remain a serious cause of infection, particularly in allogeneic HCT recipients, for up to 1 to 2 years following transplantation and may occur in as many as 20% of patients.[4,52,54] Significant mortality is associated with invasive aspergillosis (up to 60%) and mucormycosis infections.[4] HCT recipients are also at risk for serious viral infections, particularly HSV and cytomegalovirus (CMV). HSV infections may include gingivostomatitis, esophagitis, genital lesions, and, rarely, pneumonia during the first month after transplant.[4,55] Clinical disease is more common in patients with serologic evidence of prior exposure and latent HSV infection pretransplant. Therefore, reactivation of latent disease during periods of immunosuppression is the most common etiology of HSV infection. Without prophylaxis, as many as 80% of HSV-seropositive patients experience mucocutaneous disease after intensive chemotherapy compared with less than 25% of seronegative patients.[4,55] HSV infections often coexist with *Candida* infection and mucositis secondary to chemotherapy, radiation, or both.[4,55] Painful swallowing associated with these conditions often makes it difficult for patients to take oral medications and maintain adequate nutritional intake. Because of the considerable morbidity associated with HSV reactivation after transplantation, the HSV serologic status of patients should be determined prior to transplant.

HCT recipients are at high risk for CMV infections during the early postengraftment period. Infections range in severity from asymptomatic infection with viral shedding (urine, throat, and lungs), to life-threatening disseminated disease and interstitial pneumonia.[4,55] As with HSV, patients seropositive for CMV before transplantation are at high risk for reactivation of infection during periods of immunosuppression; up to 60% of seropositive patients develop reactivation after transplantation compared with only 3% of seronegative patients.[4,55] Other risk factors for CMV infection in HCT recipients include advanced age, human lymphocyte antigen mismatch, total-body irradiation, multiagent conditioning regimens, and presence of GVHD.[4,55] Patients without evidence of latent CMV infection (CMV-seronegative) before transplantation may develop primary CMV infection after receiving bone marrow or blood products from CMV-seropositive donors. Although the typical onset of both primary and recurrent CMV infection is 1 to 2 months after transplantation, late-onset infections may occur more than 100 days after transplantation.[4,55,56] Patients receiving allogeneic transplants are at highest risk for CMV reactivation, with progression to clinical disease in approximately 10% to 30% of patients.[4,55] The most serious clinical manifestation of CMV disease is interstitial pneumonia, which is associated with a mortality rate greater than 50% even when treated.[45] Interstitial pneumonia also may result from other infectious (*P. jirovecii*, VZV) and noninfectious causes (pulmonary damage by radiation and chemotherapy).[4,55] This clinical syndrome manifests as fever, dyspnea, hypoxia, nonproductive cough, and diffuse pulmonary infiltrates. As many as 40% of allogeneic HCT recipients will develop some form of interstitial pneumonia; it is a leading cause of infectious death in HCT recipients and a significant proportion are viral in etiology.[45]

During the late postengraftment period (beginning approximately 180 days after transplantation), infections remain a major problem in patients suffering from chronic GVHD. Infections common during the late postengraftment period include those caused by encapsulated bacteria, such as *S. pneumoniae* and *H. influenzae*, fungi, and viruses, including CMV and VZV.[4,54] Patients not undergoing allogeneic transplantation or suffering from chronic GVHD generally have few infections in this period.

Up to 60% of allogeneic patients with a history of VZV who survive up to 10 months after transplantation will develop VZV disease.[4,54,55] Infection with VZV is most common in allogeneic HCT recipients with acute or chronic GVHD.[54,55] Both primary (varicella) and recurrent disease (herpes zoster) usually present as skin lesions, most of which remain contained to local areas; however, 30% of these infections may disseminate to other cutaneous areas or body organs, causing severe morbidity or mortality.[4,45,55,57]

Prevention and Treatment

Desired Outcomes

The goals of therapy in managing HCT recipients from the neutropenic period through the late postengraftment period are: (a) protect the patient from early death caused by undiagnosed infection; (b) employ effective prophylactic therapy to prevent common bacterial, fungal, viral, and protozoal/parasitic infections; (c) effectively and aggressively treat established infections; (d) avoid unnecessary use of antimicrobials that contribute to increased resistance; and (e) minimize toxicities and cost while increasing patient quality of life.

Prophylaxis and Management of Infections in Recipients of HCT

8 9 The overall goal of prophylaxis and treatment of infection in HCT recipients is prevention of infectious morbidity and mortality. Specific goals of antimicrobial use in HCT recipients include (a) prevention of bacterial, fungal, viral, and protozoal infections during pre-engraftment and postengraftment periods and (b) effective treatment of established infections. These goals must be achieved at the lowest possible toxicity and cost. Prophylactic therapy should be aimed specifically at pathogens known to cause a high incidence of infection within the HCT population in general and within the specific institution. In addition, prophylactic therapy should be limited to regimens proved to be effective through well-designed clinical trials.

Appropriate immunizations should be a primary consideration in the prevention of infections in HCT recipients. Immunizations against common bacterial and viral pathogens are timed to avoid periods of severe immunosuppression following HCT when the protective response to vaccination potentially would be decreased.[4,58] Recommended vaccines for immunization of HCT recipients include three doses each of diphtheria–pertussis–tetanus (or diphtheria–tetanus), inactivated polio, conjugated *H. influenzae* type b, and conjugated 13-valent pneumococcal; two doses each of hepatitis A and HBV; and one dose of meningococcal conjugate vaccine 6 to 12 months post-transplant. One dose of the 23-valent pneumococcal vaccine should follow after 12 months. The influenza vaccine should be resumed at least 4 to 6 months after transplantation, and continued annually for life. Family members, close contacts, and healthcare providers of HCT recipients also should be vaccinated annually against influenza. The injectable inactivated influenza vaccine is preferred both before and after HCT due to severe underlying illnesses pretransplant and contraindication of the live-attenuated intranasal product post-transplant.[4,54,58] Finally, the live-attenuated measles–mumps–rubella vaccine should be administered no sooner than 24 months after HCT if the patient is considered to be immunocompetent.[44,48,54,58]

The live-attenuated varicella vaccine may be considered in patients seronegative for VZV owing to the risk of primary VZV infection, but if administered should be given no sooner than 24 months after transplant.[4,54,58] Shingrix® (recombinant zoster vaccine) is approved for immunocompetent adults and is effective at preventing herpes zoster, post-herpetic neuralgia, and herpes zoster–related complications and related hospitalizations.[49] Shingrix® is also currently recommended by the Centers for Disease Control for prevention of zoster in immunocompromised individuals and may also be considered for patients undergoing HCT.[50]

Bacterial Infections

Prophylaxis of infections in HCT recipients is similar in many ways to that used in other patients with neutropenia. Oral antibacterial prophylaxis is used commonly; considerations are the same as those discussed in the "Prophylaxis of Infections in Neutropenic Patients with Cancer" section. Although rates of bacteremia and other bacterial infections after HCT are decreased with prophylaxis, overall mortality rates have not been consistently reduced.[2,4,54,61] Therefore, routine use of prophylactic antibiotics in HCT is somewhat controversial but should be considered in patients at moderate-to-high risk of infection (Table 145-9). Fluoroquinolones are the most frequently used agents, with levofloxacin preferred over ciprofloxacin due to enhanced gram-positive activity.[4] For those intolerant to a fluoroquinolone, cefpodoxime or trimethoprim–sulfamethoxazole may be considered.[2,4] These regimens usually are started either within 72 hours of beginning the chemotherapy conditioning regimens or on the day of hematopoietic cell infusion and continued throughout the neutropenic period. Patients who become febrile while receiving prophylaxis should be managed according to general guidelines for febrile neutropenia.

Antibiotic prophylaxis against bacterial infection is also recommended in the late postengraftment period (greater than 100 days after transplantation) in certain high-risk patients, specifically allogeneic HCT recipients with chronic GVHD.[4] Antibiotics should be targeted against encapsulated bacteria, particularly *S. pneumoniae*, and should be selected based on local susceptibility patterns for these organisms; penicillin is preferred in areas with low rates of penicillin-resistant pneumococci.[4] Patients receiving trimethoprim–sulfamethoxazole for prophylaxis of other opportunistic infections may be adequately protected and do not necessarily require an additional antibiotic, though the addition of penicillin may be considered.[4]

Prophylaxis should be continued as long as the chronic GVHD is being actively treated.

Viral Infections

Prophylaxis of recurrent HSV infection is recommended for all HSV-seropositive patients undergoing HCT.[2,4,55] Approximately 0% to 10% of HSV-seropositive patients receiving acyclovir experienced viral shedding, clinical symptoms of viral reactivation, or both compared with 60% to 80% of patients receiving placebo.[4,55] Many patients eventually require IV acyclovir because of the development of severe mucositis from conditioning regimens. However, oral acyclovir, valacyclovir, or famciclovir is effective and considerably less expensive in patients who can take oral medications. Valacyclovir has replaced acyclovir as first-line therapy in current guidelines. The antiviral agent usually is started at the time of the conditioning regimen and continued until bone marrow engraftment or resolution of mucositis (approximately 30 days after HCT), although longer durations of prophylaxis should be considered in allogeneic HCT recipients with GVHD or frequent HSV reactivations before transplantation.[2,4,55] In addition to preventing recurrence of HSV disease, acyclovir prophylaxis may reduce the incidence of CMV reactivation.[4,54] Patients receiving ganciclovir or foscarnet for prophylaxis or treatment of CMV infection do not need additional antiviral therapy for prevention of HSV or VZV.[4,55] Patients developing active HSV or VZV infection should be treated with high-dose acyclovir.[4,45,55-57]

Oral acyclovir or valacyclovir given for up to 12 months after transplantation also significantly reduces reactivation of VZV infections and prevents the occurrence of severe VZV disease.[2,4] Patients receiving either allogeneic or autologous HCT may therefore be considered for long-term (up to 1 year after transplantation) prophylaxis against VZV.[2,4] Immunocompromised, nonimmune patients exposed to chickenpox or shingles should receive varicella-zoster immunoglobulin 625 units intramuscularly within 10 days (ideally as soon as possible) after close contact with persons with chickenpox or shingles for prevention of VZV-related disease.[52]

Acyclovir-resistant HSV has been reported occasionally in HCT recipients receiving acyclovir prophylaxis. Foscarnet is a drug of choice for treatment of documented infection with acyclovir-resistant HSV and should be reserved for this use.[4,45,55]

Prevention of CMV disease is a well-accepted indication for prophylaxis in HCT recipients because of the high associated infectious morbidity and mortality. If possible, CMV-seronegative patients should receive donor cells and supportive blood products from seronegative donors only; however, CMV-seropositive patients are not at significant additional risk by receiving blood or donor cells from seropositive donors.[57] Although acyclovir has relatively poor in vitro activity against CMV, a decrease in CMV infection and an improvement in overall survival were reported in HSV- and CMV-seropositive allogeneic HCT recipients receiving IV acyclovir.[4,45,55]

Ganciclovir has been well studied for prophylaxis with HCT because of its superior activity against CMV compared with acyclovir.[4,54] Oral valganciclovir has excellent pharmacokinetics, produces serum levels of ganciclovir that are at least similar to those achieved after IV administration, and is routinely used in many centers due to the convenience of oral dosing in certain patients.[4,54,55] Although administration of prophylactic valganciclovir to CMV-seropositive patients may significantly decrease the occurrence of CMV viremia, there is no clear survival benefit compared to a preemptive approach (ie, initiating IV ganciclovir or valganciclovir only after detecting a specific threshold of CMV copies from blood or bronchoalveolar fluid), and ganciclovir-related bone marrow suppression is frequently problematic.[53] Therefore, a preemptive approach is generally preferred over a ganciclovir prophylaxis strategy.[4,54,55] Preemptive therapy with ganciclovir and valganciclovir remains a current standard of therapy.[4,54,55] Detection of CMV is typically done by quantitative polymerase chain reaction (PCR)-based tests. Preemptive therapy significantly reduces the occurrence of CMV disease (including CMV pneumonia) and significantly improves survival up to 180 days after transplantation.[4] Because CMV viremia and PCR-positive bronchoalveolar lavage are highly predictive of subsequent CMV disease, preemptive ganciclovir or valganciclovir therapy should be considered for autologous HCT recipients within the first 100 days after transplantation or in allogeneic HCT recipients at any time after transplantation.[4] The doses of ganciclovir or valganciclovir for preemptive therapy are the same as those used for prophylaxis. Foscarnet can also be used for either prophylaxis or preemptive therapy of CMV disease in patients intolerant of ganciclovir or in the setting of ganciclovir resistant CMV.

CMV prophylaxis (rather than preemptive therapy) may be considered for specific allogeneic HCT recipients for the first 100 days after transplantation.[44] Letermovir is a highly active inhibitor of CMV replication approved for prophylaxis (but not treatment) of CMV infection and disease in CMV-seropositive recipients undergoing allogeneic HCT. In allogeneic HCT recipients assigned to letermovir or placebo, letermovir prophylaxis for a median of 82 days posttransplant substantially reduced CMV infections and disease within the first 6 months after transplant. Unlike ganciclovir, letermovir is not associated with bone marrow suppression and is therefore becoming an agent of choice for CMV prophylaxis in high-risk HCT recipients.[46] Clinical practice guidelines recommend that letermovir may be considered for primary prophylaxis of CMV disease in CMV-seropositive allogeneic HCT recipients.

Prophylaxis of CMV disease with either IV immunoglobulin (IVIG) or CMV hyperimmune globulin (CMVIG) has demonstrated variable and inconclusive benefits, and their use is not currently recommended.[4]

Ganciclovir and valganciclovir are the drugs of choice for treatment of active CMV infection in HCT recipients (see Table 145-6). Foscarnet also may be used for treatment or prevention of infections in HCT recipients as an alternative to ganciclovir/valganciclovir because of its relative lack of bone marrow toxicity or in cases of resistant CMV. Foscarnet-related nephrotoxicity is often problematic, however, especially in the post-transplant period when patients may be receiving other nephrotoxic agents. Cidofovir has not been well studied in HCT recipients and is also associated with nephrotoxicity, but this agent may also be considered for preemptive therapy or treatment of active disease as a third-line option.[4]

Numerous combination treatments such as interferon plus ganciclovir have been used unsuccessfully for treatment for CMV pneumonitis. However, the combination of high-dose IVIG and ganciclovir may decrease the mortality of the syndrome from 85% to 30% to 50%.[4,64] Ganciclovir plus CMVIG also is considered effective for treatment of CMV disease, although this regimen has not been studied as extensively in the HCT population in a controlled fashion. However, CMVIG was not more effective than IVIG; therefore, ganciclovir plus IVIG is considered as the treatment regimen of choice for severe or life-threatening CMV disease based on benefit-versus-risk considerations rather than definitive clinical data.[4,55,64] The potential for ganciclovir-associated bone marrow suppression prior to marrow engraftment and in patients who are just recovering from granulocytopenia remains a concern, especially in patients with unstable renal function. CSFs are beneficial in this setting (Table 145-7), providing benefits similar to those noted in patients with neutropenia and acquired immunodeficiency syndrome receiving ganciclovir therapy for CMV retinitis.[4]

Fungal Infections

Prophylaxis with antifungal agents is efficacious and generally recommended for prevention of mucocutaneous and disseminated fungal infections in high-risk HCT recipients (Tables 140-2 and 140-9).[2,4] Patients specifically recommended for prophylaxis with fluconazole or an echinocandin include all allogeneic recipients and autologous transplant recipients with extensive mucositis.[2,4] Fluconazole remains the most commonly used agent; it is started on the day of transplantation and continued until resolution of neutropenia or, in allogeneic HCT, for at least 75 days after transplantation.[4] The variable activity of fluconazole against non-*albicans* species of *Candida* may be problematic in this population, as is lack of activity against *Aspergillus*.[4] Prophylaxis with fluconazole effectively reduced colonization, infection, and infection-related mortality due to *Candida* spp. in some HCT populations, but has not consistently reduced overall mortality or invasive infections such as aspergillosis in all types of HCT recipients.[4] Micafungin was more efficacious than fluconazole in the prevention of early-onset *Candida* infections in HCT recipients with neutropenia prior to engraftment, and also showed a trend to fewer episodes of invasive aspergillosis.[4] Posaconazole was also more effective than fluconazole in the late prevention of invasive *Aspergillus* and other fungal infections in HCT recipients with GVHD receiving additional immunosuppressive therapy.[4] In a meta-analysis, prophylaxis with agents active against *Aspergillus* were associated with a 33% reduction in mortality related to invasive fungal infections compared to fluconazole.[37] Fluconazole and micafungin are both supported by a high level of evidence for fungal prophylaxis and either are appropriate following HCT with local fungal ecology, risk factors, and cost being appropriate determinants for specific populations.[4] Most experts consider caspofungin and anidulafungin reasonable alternatives to micafungin and current guidelines do not differentiate among echinocandins.[4] Voriconazole, posaconazole, LAMB products, and to a lesser extent itraconazole may be used for prophylaxis of fungal infections in HCT recipients but do not carry the same strength of recommendation due to less favorable side-effect profiles or lack of positive comparative studies.[4] Posaconazole is the preferred agent in high-risk HCT recipients with severe GVHD due to the risk of invasive mold infections (Table 145-2).[2,4] When the risk of invasive aspergillosis infection is >6%, prophylaxis with a mold-active triazole such as posaconazole (voriconazole or isavuconazonium as alternatives) is appropriate.[2] Isavuconazonium has not been well studied for prophylaxis in HCT recipients and, although recommended as an option in some clinical guidelines, it has not been recommended in others.[2,4]

Therapeutic drug monitoring for some azole antifungals remains important (Table 145-6). Furthermore, use of azole antifungals as prophylaxis introduces the potential for pharmacokinetic (CYP450 inhibition) and pharmacodynamic (eg, QTc prolongation with most azoles and fluoroquinolones) drug-drug interactions that vary in duration and severity. Drug half-lives, potential therapeutic benefit (eg, infection-free mortality), potential harm, and future oncologic plans must be assessed when initiating, continuing, adjusting, or discontinuing a potentially interacting medication. An alternative prophylaxis regimen (echinocandin) may be preferred to an azole when the risk of a drug interaction is too great (eg, proteasome inhibitors, tyrosine kinase inhibitors, or vinca alkaloids). Consideration should be given to the mechanism of drug interaction and drug half-life before initiating therapy.[4]

Pulmonary infection with *P. jirovecii* is a relatively infrequent complication of HCT that is associated with high rates of mortality, especially in patients with GVHD.[4,50,54] Therefore, prophylaxis is recommended for a period of 3 to 6 months after autologous HCT, and for at least 6 months and while receiving immunosuppressive therapy after allogeneic HCT. Exposure to specific immunosuppressing medications (eg, >20 mg of prednisone daily for >4 weeks) also warrants prophylaxis. Prophylaxis with trimethoprim–sulfamethoxazole significantly reduces the incidence of *P. jirovecii* as well as *P. jirovecii*–related mortality so effectively that desensitization should be considered for intolerant reactions before switching to an alternative (eg, dapsone, atovaquone, or pentamidine).[4,44,54] Trimethoprim–sulfamethoxazole should also prevent *Toxoplasma gondii*, a rare but often fatal infection.[4,54]

Use of Colony-Stimulating Factors

Filgrastim, pegfilgrastim, and sargramostim have been studied in HCT recipients in an effort to speed bone marrow recovery, reduce the period of neutropenia, and decrease infectious complications. CSFs appear effective as well as safe following autologous HCT and should be utilized. Although increased rates of GVHD and mortality with use of CSFs following allogeneic HCT have been reported by retrospective studies, a meta-analysis found no increased risk and CSFs may be given to allogeneic HCT recipients to reduce the duration of severe neutropenia.[41] The use of CSFs is now routinely recommended to mobilize blood progenitor cells and reduce the period of neutropenia in autologous transplants (Table 145-7).[33,41,42]

Evaluation of Therapeutic Outcomes

10 Close monitoring of HCT recipients, including clinical and laboratory data, is essential for early detection and treatment of infectious complications. In addition, because many of the drugs commonly used in this setting (eg, ganciclovir, amphotericin B, and trimethoprim–sulfamethoxazole) have significant toxicity potential in HCT recipients, careful attention must be paid to prevention and management of drug-related adverse effects as well as drug-drug interactions. Monitoring parameters related to specific types of infections (eg, pneumonia and urinary tract infections) should be applied as appropriate. The reader is referred to other chapters within this book for more specific information.

Infections in Solid-Organ Transplant Recipients

Solid-organ transplantation (SOT) is an established mode of treatment for end-stage diseases of the heart, lungs, kidney, liver, pancreas, and small bowel. More than 39,000 organs were transplanted in the United States in 2020, and nearly 900,000 organs have been transplanted in the United States since 1988.[55] Patient and allograft survival rates have greatly improved due to improvements in immunosuppressive drug therapy, candidate selection, and transplant surgery techniques as well as more experience in the management of complications (including infection) in these patients. Despite advances in diagnostic techniques and antimicrobial therapy, infectious complications remain important causes of morbidity and mortality after SOT.

Risk Factors

1 Many risk factors for infection are present in SOT recipients (see Table 145-1). The most important risk factor in this population is immunosuppressive drug therapy for prevention and treatment of allograft rejection. Risk of infection depends on specific immunosuppressive drug regimens as well as the intensity (numbers and doses/exposure of drugs) and duration of immunosuppression. Most opportunistic infections in transplant patients occur during the first 6 months after transplantation, when the intensity and total cumulative exposures to immunosuppressive therapy are very high.[56,57,65,66]

Immunosuppressive drugs, often in escalated doses, are used to treat episodes of graft rejection and include immunoglobulins directed against T cells (eg, antithymocyte globulin), antibodies against interleukin 2 receptors (basiliximab), T-cell–depleting antibodies (alemtuzumab), B-lymphocyte depleting antibodies (rituximab), and high-dose corticosteroids. Rejection episodes often occur during the period 2 to 4 months posttransplant when the overall cumulative dose or net state of immunosuppression is high. Therefore, patients already at risk for infection are placed at even higher risk if additional immunosuppressive therapy is needed to treat one or more episodes of graft rejection.[65,67] Immunosuppressive drug therapy must be evaluated carefully when infections occur because, in many cases, immunosuppression may have to be reduced or altered to allow patients to survive the infectious episode, at the expense of increased risk of graft rejection. Risk of increased infectious complications from immunosuppressive therapy used to treat rejection episodes is determined, at least in part, by the specific therapy used.[56,65,68]

The organ type, organ donor status, surgical technique, recipient status, and underlying illness of the recipients are also critical determinants of infection risk and possible etiologies. These considerations are extremely important within the first 3 months following SOT and may provide heightened suspicion leading to specific prophylaxis, preemptive strategies, and earlier appropriate and targeted treatment of infectious complications.[58,59,67-69]

Etiology

2 As in patients with cancer, microorganisms infecting SOT recipients are present before transplantation or are acquired from exogenous sources. Although opportunistic viral, fungal, and protozoal infections may occur commonly, bacterial infections remain the most frequent infectious complications after transplantation in all allograft recipients.[65,70,71] Liver, small bowel, and lung transplant recipients are at high risk for serious gram-negative bacterial infections as a result of the technically difficult surgical procedures and precolonization.[70,72] All transplant recipients are at risk for mucocutaneous candidiasis from species colonizing body sites. Invasive fungal infection is less common following kidney and pancreas transplantation but may occur in up to 30% to 60% of heart, lung, liver, and small bowel transplant recipients. Invasive fungal infections following lung, liver, and small bowel transplantation are associated with mortality rates up to 60% to 80%.[73,74] *Candida* spp. is the most common of all systemic fungal infections in transplant recipients.[74-76] Abdominal surgery, especially the more complex procedures required for liver and small bowel transplantation, predispose patients to serious fungal disease, most likely as a consequence of entering an area of the body already colonized with *Candida* spp.[64] Lung and heart transplant recipients are particularly at risk for invasive aspergillosis; these infections may occur in up to 35% of patients and in lung transplant recipients may be more common than infections caused by *Candida* spp.[63,64,73,77]

Organisms present as latent tissue infections may reactivate and cause clinical disease with administration of immunosuppressive drug therapy. Disease resulting from infection reactivation has been noted with viruses (HSV, human herpesvirus-6, CMV, VZV, Epstein–Barr virus [EBV]), protozoa (*T. gondii*), and mycobacteria (*Mycobacterium tuberculosis*).[65-68] Serologic or immunologic tests are performed prior to transplantation to assess the risk for reactivation infection and identify other subclinical infections (eg, HBV, hepatitis C virus [HCV], *Legionella*). Many patients with reactivated infection have no clinical symptoms; often the only evidence of active infection is a rise in antibody titer from the pretransplant baseline, positive culture, increasing viral replication, or histologic evidence. Reactivation of latent infection may result in severe life-threatening disease in immunosuppressed hosts.[56,58,66,67]

Exogenous sources of infection in transplant patients include environmental contamination and transmission of microorganisms via transplanted organs and blood products. Environmental sources of infection are similar to those noted in other immunocompromised hosts, such as patients with cancer. Airborne pathogens, especially fungi such as *Aspergillus* and *Cryptococcus neoformans*, may cause infections in transplant patients; environmental exposure is an established risk factor for invasive mold infections among lung transplant patients.[63] Travel to areas of geographically endemic mycoses (eg, *Coccidioides immitis*, *Histoplasma capsulatum*, *Blastomyces dermatitidis*) or animal exposures may broaden infectious risk.[56] SOT recipients are also at high risk for nosocomial infections (MRSA, *P. aeruginosa*, *Acinetobacter*). Optimal prevention and management of nosocomial infections in transplant patients require knowledge of the current epidemiology of infections and susceptibility patterns within an institution.[56,57,60,61]

Infections transmitted via donor organs or blood products are major causes of morbidity and mortality in transplant patients and may include HSV, *T. gondii*, HBV, and HCV. The most important infections transmitted from the donor, however, are caused by CMV.[67-69] These infections may cause serious disease, predispose patients to other opportunistic infections, and contribute to acute and chronic allograft dysfunction or rejection, post-transplant lymphoproliferative disorders (particularly associated with EBV), and cardiac complications and atherosclerosis in heart transplant recipients.[67-69] In contrast to reactivation disease, transplant patients contracting primary CMV disease are at increased risk for serious life-threatening infections.[56,58,67-69] The most important source of primary CMV infection in transplant patients is the donor organ. Efforts are made to avoid transplanting organs from CMV-seropositive donors into CMV-seronegative recipients because of the potentially severe consequences. With the relative scarcity of suitable organs and the rapidity with which transplant decisions often must be made, however, this is not always possible. The consequences of transplanting an organ from a CMV-seropositive donor into an already CMV-seropositive recipient are less clear. CMV reinfection (as well as reactivation) syndromes may occur in these patients and antilymphocyte immunosuppression may increase the risk of complications.[56,59,67,69] Conversely, mammalian target of rapamycin (mTOR) inhibitors as part of a chronic immunosuppressive regimen may decrease the risk of CMV infection and related disease.[67,69] CMV serostatus, net immunosuppression, and organ type (among others factors) inform the practitioner of risk to determine an appropriate preventative strategy.[56,59,67,69] Furthermore, primary CMV disease may be transmitted from seropositive blood products. The availability of leukoreduced and CMV-seronegative blood products has decreased the risk of transmission but has not eliminated it.

Organs from donors seropositive for *T. gondii* or HSV generally are not withheld from seronegative patients as effective prophylaxis is common. Organs from known HIV-infected donors may now be used for transplantation in HIV-infected recipients (the HIV Organ Policy Equity Act) and outcomes of a limited number of transplanted patients have been favorable thus far.[70] Center-specific and HIV-specific criteria often apply, but in general those stable on antiretroviral therapy with well-controlled disease may be considered for SOT (as well as HCT) without prohibitively high risk for acceleration of HIV disease or opportunistic infections beyond what would be expected in other transplant recipients. The impact of protease inhibitors and highly active antiretroviral therapy on long-term outcome of HIV-infected patients following transplantation is believed to have improved the overall feasibility of transplanting these individuals.[70,71] Similarly, with highly effective therapies now available, organs from HCV-infected donors may be used for transplantation in HCV-infected recipients (and in some cases HCV-negative recipients).[70,72]

Timing of Infections After Transplantation

As with HCT, the overall time course for infections can be divided into three general periods after transplantation (see Fig. 145-3).[56,57] Although risk of infection with specific pathogens varies with the type of transplant, the time course of infections is similar in all transplant recipients. During the early post-transplant period (within the first month after transplantation), patients are at risk for infections already present and brought forward from the pretransplant period (eg, HBV, HCV, HIV); postoperative infections, such as surgical wound and catheter infections; infection resulting from colonized donor organs (pneumonia following lung transplant);

and reactivation of HSV.[56,57,67] In the intermediate post-transplant period (1-6 months after transplant), risk is highest for viral infections, including CMV, EBV, HBV, and HCV. The combination of these "immunomodulating" viruses plus sustained immunosuppressive therapy leads to a high risk for opportunistic infections with pathogens such as *P. jirovecii*, *Aspergillus*, and *Nocardia asteroides*.[56-58] In the late post-transplant period (greater than 6 months after transplant), patients are at risk for persistent infections (particularly viral) from earlier post-transplant periods, reactivation of VZV and *Cryptococcus neoformans*, and routine infections affecting the general population.[56,57] In addition, patients who required additional immunosuppression therapy for acute or chronic rejection are at continued high risk for opportunistic infections (*Aspergillus* and *P. jirovecii*).[56,57] Although Fig. 145-3 illustrates infection patterns common to all solid-organ transplants, the relative incidence and importance of a particular pathogen vary according to the type of transplant, immunosuppression, and prophylaxis measures.

Types of Infections and Clinical Presentation

10 Transplant patients are at risk for infections occurring at a variety of sites, including skin, surgical wound, urinary tract, lungs, blood, abdomen, and CNS. However, most infections occur at or near the site of the transplanted organ. For example, heart transplant and heart-lung transplant recipients most often are infected within the lungs or thoracic cavity. Urinary tract infections remain an important cause of morbidity in renal transplant patients, especially in the early posttransplant period. Administration of prophylactic antibiotics (eg, trimethoprim–sulfamethoxazole) to these patients has reduced the incidence and severity of urinary tract infections.[4,69] Serious bacterial and fungal infections originating from the abdomen and GI tract are most common after liver transplantation and are related to variables such as length of surgery and surgical procedures performed. Risk of bacteremia, usually originating from the gut, is high in liver transplant patients. Renal transplant recipients are at the lowest risk for infections and infectious deaths, whereas patients receiving heart, lung, and liver transplants are at the highest risk for infection-related morbidity and mortality.[61,73]

In contrast to patients with febrile neutropenia, the threshold for initiating empirical antimicrobial therapy is higher in febrile transplant patients. Appropriate therapy for the large numbers of pathogens that may cause infections in transplant patients varies greatly from organism to organism (Table 145-6). Therefore, careful attempts at definitive diagnosis of suspected infections must be made. If comprehensive workup reveals no source of infection, careful observation of the febrile transplant patient (rather than empirical therapy) is common practice. Surveillance cultures and weekly quantitative amplification nucleic acid testing of CMV may be useful during the first 3 to 4 months for detecting CMV infections if the patient is not receiving prophylaxis.[56,67,69] Management and monitoring of documented infections are similar to that in other types of patients.

Prevention and Treatment

Desired Outcomes

The goals of therapy in managing SOT recipients are similar to those in HCT and include : (a) protect the patient from early death caused by undiagnosed infection, from the surgical procedure through the late postengraftment period; (b) prevent common bacterial, fungal, viral, and protozoal/parasitic infections; (c) effectively and aggressively treat established infections; (d) avoid unnecessary use of antimicrobials; and (e) minimize toxicities and cost while increasing patient quality of life and avoiding harm to the engrafted organ(s).

Prevention of Infection in Solid-Organ Transplantation

8 The goals of antimicrobial drug use in solid-organ transplant recipients are (a) prevention of infectious complications in the immediate postoperative period, (b) prevention of late infectious complications associated with prolonged periods of immunosuppression, and (c) effective treatment of established infections in order to prevent graft dysfunction and rejection and decrease patient morbidity and mortality. All of these goals must be achieved at the lowest possible toxicity and cost.

Prevention of infection in the transplant patient can be accomplished in several ways. First, risk of environmental contamination should be minimized.[56] Patients should be protected from institutional infectious outbreaks. Efforts should be made to vaccinate organ transplant candidates prior to transplantation whenever possible for vaccine preventable disease based on age and anticipated risk factors post-transplant. Live vaccines should be given more than 4 weeks in advance from the time of anticipated transplantation.[48] Transplant recipients should receive influenza vaccination annually, pneumococcal (PCV13 and/or PPSV23 separated by 8 weeks), hepatitis A and B vaccination series (if indicated, ideally started pre-transplant), HPV series (if indicated), zoster series, and Tdap generally 2 months or greater following transplantation; however, their immunologic responses to these vaccines may be suboptimal due to immunosuppressive therapy.[48] Timing of reinstitution of regular vaccinations in relation to transplantation is not absolute, but live-attenuated vaccines (varicella, zoster, MMR) should be avoided early post transplantation, if not altogether, similar to recommendations for HCT.[48] An exception is made for varicella seronegative pediatric liver and kidney transplant recipients who are on low levels of immunosuppression without recent graft rejection.[48]

Because the most important source of primary CMV infection is an infected donor organ, CMV serostatus should be evaluated in all recipients and donors. Two standard strategies to manage CMV in SOT recipients have been recommended. Preemptive therapy is effective for some populations (eg, kidney transplant) but requires weekly monitoring, close follow-up and appropriate risk stratification of patients for CMV-related complications. Prophylaxis is effective and easy to administer without the need for careful discrimination of suitable patients; but, universal prophylaxis results in unnecessary exposure (toxicities) and cost to low-risk patients (CMV serostatus donor negative, recipient negative).[67,69] The best approach to preventing CMV disease remains controversial and does require risk stratification as either preemptive therapy or prophylaxis can be appropriate depending on patient specific factors (including immunosuppressive strategy). Most experts agree that CMV prophylaxis is not required in donor negative, recipient negative SOT patients. These patients may qualify for antiviral prophylaxis targeted against other herpes infections (eg, acyclovir) or preemptive therapy.[56,60,69]

CMV prophylaxis is commonly recommended in high-risk patients (ie, seronegative patients receiving seropositive organs). Oral valganciclovir and IV ganciclovir prophylaxis are effective for reducing the incidence of both primary and reactivated CMV infection in SOT.[67,69] Prophylaxis is recommended as a preferred strategy in many CMV-seropositive SOT recipients partly due to a lack of well-designed studies comparing prophylaxis to preemptive therapy in all SOT types.[67,69] Additional risk factors for CMV disease, the associated clinical impact of "indirect effects" of CMV, and logistical barriers should be considered on an individual basis when designing a strategy. For example, valganciclovir prophylaxis has been recommended for all CMV positive lung transplant recipients in part due to very high risk of CMV disease and associated severe consequences of direct and indirect effects on the graft.[56,69] The duration of CMV prophylaxis is typically 3 to 12 months depending on donor and recipient CMV serology status, immunosuppressive regimen, and

CLINICAL PRESENTATION Infections in Solid-organ Transplant Patients

General

- Because transplant patients are at high risk for serious infections, frequent (at least daily), careful clinical assessments must be performed to search for evidence of infection
- Clinical presentation of infection is variable and depends on the type and site of infection, type of transplant, time after transplantation, immune status of the host, and dose and duration of immunosuppressive therapy
- Primary viral disease usually is more symptomatic and severe than disease caused by reactivation
- Physical assessment should include examination of all common sites of infection, including mouth/pharynx, nose and sinuses, respiratory tract, GI tract, urinary tract, skin, soft tissues, perineum, and intravascular catheter insertion sites

Symptoms

- Usual signs and symptoms of infection may be absent or altered in patients receiving intensive immunosuppressive regimens owing to an inability to mount a typical inflammatory response (eg, no infiltrate on chest x-ray film, urinary tract infection without pyuria)
- Pain may be present at infection site(s)

Signs

- Fever is the single most important clinical sign indicating the presence of infection, though it may not be present in all infected patients. Other causes of fever unrelated to infection in this patient population include reactions to blood products, drugs, embolic events, and ischemic injury
- Usual signs of infection may be absent or altered
- Signs of allograft dysfunction may be related to infection. Distinguishing fever caused by allograft rejection from that caused by infection often is difficult and frequently requires allograft biopsy

Laboratory Tests

- Blood cultures (at least two sets, including vascular access devices) for bacteria and fungi; cultures of other suspected or potential infection sites (urine, lungs, surgical wounds, and soft tissue infections)
- Other cultures should be obtained as clinically indicated according to the presence of signs or symptoms
- Complete blood count and chemistries should be obtained frequently to monitor allograft function, plan supportive care, guide drug dosing, and assess patient's overall status
- Surveillance testing for CMV and HSV may be useful during first 3 months after transplantation for early detection of infection

Other Diagnostic Tests

- Chest x-ray
- Aspiration, biopsy of skin lesions
- Other diagnostic tests as indicated clinically on the basis of physical examination and other assessments

type of organ transplanted.[56,67,69] Because CMV replication and disease occurs in up to one-third of donor-positive/recipient-negative SOT recipients within 3 to 6 months after stopping prophylaxis (termed postprophylaxis delayed-onset CMV disease), continued surveillance after discontinuation of prophylaxis should be considered based on patient-specific risk stratification.[56,67,69] Ganciclovir or valganciclovir prophylaxis also may significantly reduce reactivation of CMV infection in seropositive patients receiving antithymocyte globulin for treatment of acute rejection.[67,69]

Prophylactic high-dose oral acyclovir or valacyclovir effectively reduces the incidence of CMV infection and disease following renal transplantation. However, acyclovir is less active against CMV and may be less efficacious in some high-risk renal or other nonrenal transplant patients; therefore, valganciclovir is generally preferred if prophylaxis is required.[56,67,69] Acyclovir prophylaxis may be recommended for targeting other herpes viruses when the risk of CMV is low and should not be used to treat active CMV replication.[69,74]

Preemptive IV ganciclovir or valganciclovir is an effective strategy in many SOT recipients, but requires appropriate monitoring and a reliance on patient compliance. Additionally, no established thresholds have been clearly defined as a "cut-point" for initiation of preemptive valganciclovir when monitoring quantitative CMV copies (eg, absolute value, viral load kinetics, or viral doubling time).[67,69] Neither preemptive nor prophylaxis strategies are perfect for each situation. Therefore, it is imperative that each SOT center develop a method based on patient risk, logistics, and cost and continually assess patient risk with cumulative net immunosuppression in mind when prescribing a CMV preventative strategy.[67,69] Since ganciclovir-related bone marrow suppression is not as problematic in SOT recipients as in HCT recipients and valganciclovir is relatively well tolerated, many centers in the United States opt for a prophylactic strategy while also extending either duration or preemptive monitoring when additional risk factors (eg, intensified immunosuppression) are encountered.

The additional benefit of CMVIG compared to standard CMV prophylaxis in high risk heart, lung, and small bowel transplant recipients is controversial. Cohort-level evidence suggests some possible benefit and therefore some experts will add monthly infusions in special circumstances; however, the optimal role of CMVIG has yet to be established.[56,67,69]

The use of mTOR inhibitors (sirolimus, everolimus) as part of an immunosuppressive regimen in SOT recipients may be useful in prevention of CMV disease. mTOR inhibitors exert a marked anti-CMV effect through reduction in viral replication and/or potent immunomodulating properties.[75] In a meta-analysis, patients receiving immunosuppressant regimens containing mTOR inhibitors (with or without a calcineurin inhibitor [CNI]) displayed a nearly threefold reduction in CMV infections compared to patients receiving CNI alone.[75] Although mTOR inhibitors are associated with significantly lower CMV infection rates in most SOT recipients, CMV disease with related complications is only one of many factors that must be considered when designing an immunosuppressive regimen.[67,69]

Although use of prophylactic acyclovir in HSV-seropositive patients undergoing HCT is well accepted, prophylaxis in SOT recipients remains controversial. Reactivation disease caused by HSV occurs in approximately 25% of HSV-seropositive patients who are not receiving prophylaxis.[74] Mucocutaneous disease is the most common presentation, but nonmucocutantious HSV disease also is seen occasionally and is associated with significant morbidity and high mortality (eg, HSV pneumonitis).[74] Acyclovir is therefore used at some centers because of the high incidence of clinical HSV infection after transplantation. Acyclovir prophylaxis of HSV infection may be considered in patients following a preemptive strategy for management of CMV infection, but would not be necessary in patients receiving ganciclovir or valganciclovir for CMV prophylaxis.[56,74]

Prophylactic antimicrobial agents are also of benefit to SOT recipients in certain other clinical situations. Antibiotic prophylaxis, with agents such as cefazolin started perioperatively and continued for less than 24 hours, is considered to effectively reduce wound infection rates following renal transplantation.[62,73] Although the benefits of perioperative prophylaxis have not been well studied in other types of transplantation procedures, surgical prophylaxis usually is considered mandatory for pancreas, liver, heart, lung, or small bowel transplant patients because of the high risk of perioperative bacterial infections.[62,73] High rates of infection have been reported following liver and intestinal transplant often resulting from intra-abdominal pathogens (eg, gram-negative bacteria, *Enterococcus*, *Candida*, anaerobes) depending on patient, donor, and surgical risk factors. Broader surgical prophylaxis such as a third-generation cephalosporin plus ampicillin, ampicillin/sulbactam, or piperacillin/tazobactam have been recommended for liver transplant. An even broader approach with the addition of vancomycin and fluconazole has been suggested for intestinal transplant given the high risk of multidrug resistant and polymicrobial infection.[62] Pulmonary infections are particularly common in lung and heart-lung transplant recipients. They often are caused by bacteria colonizing the airways of the diseased organs prior to transplantation. Therefore, perioperative antibiotics for lung and heart-lung procedures often are selected based on pretransplant sputum cultures and/or known colonizations of the patient (including assist devices [eg, ventricular assist device or extracorporeal membrane oxygenation circuit]).[62]

Post-transplant antibiotic prophylaxis is effective in decreasing the number of bacterial infections in renal transplant patients. Prophylactic trimethoprim–sulfamethoxazole traditionally has been used because it is inexpensive and well tolerated; other antibiotics, such as the fluoroquinolones, also have been evaluated.[56] Administration of oral low-dose trimethoprim–sulfamethoxazole (one double-strength tablet, either daily or three times/week) for 6 to 12 months for prevention of *P. jirovecii* infection following heart and lung transplantation is common, although the efficacy and optimal duration are somewhat controversial.[56] Selective bowel decontamination with nonabsorbable antibiotics in combination with a low-bacterial diet (no fresh fruits and vegetables) may reduce oropharyngeal and GI colonization with gram-negative aerobes and *Candida* in liver transplant patients; however, conclusive evidence of benefit is lacking and this practice is not recommended routinely.[62,73] Similarly, prebiotics and probiotics cannot be currently recommended.[62]

Because immunosuppressed transplant recipients are at risk for mucocutaneous fungal infections, prophylactic oral or topical antifungal agents may be indicated in these patients. Liver, pancreas, and small bowel transplant recipients are clearly at high risk for invasive fungal infections and should receive prophylaxis with fluconazole though the optimal duration remains unclear.[62,66] Antifungal prophylaxis has also been suggested for lung and heart-lung transplant recipients due to the high incidence of invasive fungal infections in these patients (up to 35% of patients, with mortality rates up to 60%).[64] Prophylaxis targeting *Aspergillus* spp. with inhaled amphotericin B or LAMB, or systemic regimens active against *Candida* and *Aspergillus* spp. such as itraconazole, voriconazole, posaconazole, and echinocandins have all been reported; however, data from well-designed trials supporting either the general recommendation for prophylaxis or choice of specific agent are largely lacking and center-to-center variability is great.[63,65,74] Oral voriconazole or inhaled LAMB for a period of 3 to 6 months post-transplant are most often recommended for prophylaxis of invasive fungal infection in lung and heart-lung transplant recipients.[63,64] However, prophylaxis out to a year or longer is not uncommon with oral triazole agents.[63,64] Concentrations of immunosuppressant drugs should be monitored closely in transplant patients receiving azole-type antifungal agents (fluconazole, itraconazole, and voriconazole).

Transplant patients, especially heart and heart-lung recipients, without serologic evidence of prior exposure to *T. gondii* who receive organs from seropositive donors are at high risk for toxoplasmosis.[56] Many of these patients will be receiving trimethoprim–sulfamethoxazole for prophylaxis of *P. jirovecii* infection; this agent will also provide effective prophylaxis against *T. gondii* as well as *N. asteroides*. Although prophylaxis specifically for *T. gondii* is not given routinely at all centers, this therapy for a period of up to 12 months may be justified in high-risk patients because of the delays in diagnosis and serious infections associated with toxoplasmosis.[56,71]

ABBREVIATIONS

ANC	absolute neutrophil count
ASCO	American Society of Clinical Oncology
CAR-T	chimeric antigen receptor T cell
CDI	*Clostridioides difficile* infection
CISNE	Clinical Index of Stable Febrile Neutropenia
CMV	cytomegalovirus
CMVIG	cytomegalovirus hyperimmune globulin
CNT	calcineurin inhibitor
CRE	carbapenem-resistant Enterobacterales
CSF	colony-stimulating factor
EBV	Epstein–Barr virus
ESBL	extended-spectrum β-lactamases
GI	gastrointestinal
GVHD	graft-versus-host disease
HBV	hepatitis B virus
HCV	hepatitis C virus
HIV	human immunodeficiency virus
HCT	hematopoietic cell transplantation
HSV	herpes simplex virus
IDSA	Infectious Diseases Society of America
IVIG	intravenous immunoglobulin
LAMB	lipid-associated amphotericin B
MASCC	Multinational Association for Supportive Care in Cancer
MDR	multidrug resistant
MRSA	methicillin-resistant *Staphylococcus aureus*
NCCN	National Comprehensive Cancer Network
PCR	polymerase chain reaction
PCT	procalcitonin
PMN	polymorphonuclear leukocyte
SOT	solid-organ transplantation
VRE	vancomycin-resistant enterococci
VZV	varicella-zoster virus
WBC	white blood cell

REFERENCES

1. Freifeld AG, Bow EJ, Sepiowitz KA, et al. Clinical practice guideline for the use of antimicrobial agents in neutropenic patients with cancer: 2010 Update by the Infectious Disease Society of America. *Clin Infect Dis.* 2011;52(4):e56–e93. 10.1093/cid/cir073.
2. Taplitz RA, Kennedy EB, Bow EJ, et al. Outpatient management of fever and neutropenia in adults treated for malignancy: American Society of Clinical Oncology and Infectious Diseases Society of America clinical practice guideline update. *J Clin Oncol.* 2018;36:1443–1453. doi:10.1200/JCO.2017.77.6211.
3. Lyman GH, Abella E, Pettengell R. Risk factors for febrile neutropenia among patients with cancer receiving chemotherapy: A systematic review. *Clin Rev Oncol Hematol.* 2014;90:190–199. doi:10.1016/j.critrevonc.2013.12.006.
4. National Comprehensive Cancer Network. Prevention and treatment of cancer-related infections. NCCN Clinical Practice Guidelines in Oncology (NCCN Guidelines®), v.1.2021. July 2, 2021. Available at: https://www.nccn.org/professionals/physician_gls/pdf/infections.pdf. Accessed October 2, 2021.
5. Gustinetti G, Mikulska M. Bloodstream infections in neutropenic cancer patients: A practical update. *Virulence.* 2016;7:280–297. doi:10.1080/21505594.2016.1156821.
6. Logan C, Koura D, Taplitz R. Updates in infection risk and management in acute leukemia. *Hematol.* 2020;1:135–139. doi:10.1182/hematology.2020000098.
7. Marin M, Gudiol C, Ardanuy C, et al. Factors influencing mortality in neutropenic patients with haemotologic malignancies or solid tumours with bloodstream infection. *Clin Microbiol Infect.* 2015;21:583–590. doi:10.1016/j.cmi.2015.01.029.
8. Cesar-Arce A, Volkow-Fernandez P, Valero-Saldana LM, et al. Infectious complications and multidrug-resistant bacteria in patients with hematopoietic stem cell transplantation in the first 12 months after transplant. *Transplant Proc.* 2017;49:1444–1448. doi:10.1016/j.transproceed.2017.03.081.
9. Rolston KV. Neutropenic fever and sepsis: Evaluation and management. *Cancer Treat Res.* 2014;161:181–202. 10.1007/978-3-319-04220-6_6.
10. Dumford D, Skalweit MJ. Antibiotic-resistant infections and treatment challenges in the immunocompromised host. An update. *Infect Dis Clin N Am.* 2020;34:821–847. 10.1016/j.idc.2020.08.005.
11. Trecarichi EM, Tumbarello M. Antimicrobial-resistant gram-negative bacteria in febrile neutropenic patients with cancer: Current epidemiology and clinical impact. *Curr Opin Infect Dis.* 2014;27:200–210. doi:10.1097/QCO.0000000000000038.
12. Zhang S, Wang Q, Ling Y, et al. Fluoroquinolone resistance in bacteremic and low risk febrile neutropenic patients with cancer. *BMC Cancer.* 2015;15:42–46. doi:10.1186/s12885-015-1063-x.
13. Seagle EE, Williams SL, Chiller TM. Recent trends in epidemiology of fungal infections. *Infect Dis Clin N Am.* 2021;35:237–260. doi:10.1016/j.idc.2021.03.001.
14. Hidron A, Edwards JR, Patel J, et al. Antimicrobial-resistant pathogens associated with healthcare-associated infections: Summary of data reported to the National Healthcare Safety Network at the Centers for Disease Control and Prevention, 2011–2014. *Infect Control Hosp Epidemiol.* 2016;37:1288–1301. doi:10.1017/ice.2016.174.
15. Nelson RE, Jones M, Lie CF, et al. The impact of healthcare-associated methicillin-resistant *Staphylococcus aureus* infections on post-discharge healthcare costs and utilization. *Infect Control Hosp Epidemiol.* 2015;36(5):534–542. 10.1017/ice.2015.22.
16. Lewis RE, Cahyame-Zuniga L, Leventakos K, et al. Epidemiology and site of involvement of invasive fungal infections in patients with haematological malignancies: A 20-year autopsy study. *Mycoses.* 2013;56:638–645. doi:10.1111/myc.12081.
17. Chen K, Wang Q, Pleasants RA, et al. Empiric treatment against invasive fungal diseases in febrile neutropenic patients: A systematic review and network meta-analysis. *BMC Infect Dis.* 2017;17:159–170. doi:10.1186/s12879-017-2263-6.
18. Pappas PG, Kauffman CA, Andes DR, et al. Clinical practice guideline for the management of candidiasis: 2016 Update by the Infectious Diseases Society of America. *Clin Infect Dis.* 2016:62:e1–e50. doi:10.1093/cid/civ933.
19. Wu P-F, Liu W-L, Hsieh M-H, et al. Epidemiology and antifungal susceptibility of candidemia isolates of non-*albicans Candida* species from cancer patients. *Emerg Microbes Infect.* 2017;6:e87. doi:10.1038/emi.2017.74.
20. van de Peppel RJ, Visser LG, Dekkers OM, et al. The burden of invasive aspergillosis in patients with haemotological malignancy: A meta-analysis and systematic review. *J Infect.* 2018;76:550–562. doi:10.1016/j.jinf.2018.02.012.
21. Patterson TF, Thompson GR, Deming DW, et al. Practice guidelines for the diagnosis and management of aspergillosis: 2016 Update by the Infectious Diseases Society of America. *Clin Infect Dis.* 2016;63:e1–e60. doi:10.1093/cid/ciw326.
22. Wu C-W, Wu J-Y, Chen C-K, et al. Does procalcitonin, C-reactive protein, or interleukin-6 test have a role in the diagnosis of severe infection in patients with febrile neutropenia? A systematic review and meta-analysis. *Support Care Cancer.* 2015;23:2863–2872. doi:10.1007/s00520-015-2650-8.
23. Taplitz RA, Kennedy EB, Bow EJ, et al. Antimicrobial prophylaxis for adult patients with cancer-related immunosuppression: ASCO and IDSA clinical practice guideline update. *J Clin Oncol.* 2018;36:3043–3054. doi:10.1200/JCO.18.00374.
24. Kim YJ, Jun YH, Kim YR, et al. Risk factors for mortality with *Pseudomonas aeruginosa* bacteremia; retrospective study of impact of combination antimicrobial therapy. *BMC Infect Dis.* 2014;14:161–167. doi:10.2147/IDR.S268744.
25. Beyar-Katz O, Dickstein Y, Borok S, et al. Empirical antibiotics targeting gram-positive bacteria for the treatment of febrile neutropenic patients with cancer. *Cochrane Database Syst Rev.* 2017;6(6):CD003914. doi:10.1002/14651858.
26. Gouliouris T, Warne B, Cartwright EJP, et al. Duration of exposure to multiple antibiotics is associated with increased risk of VRE bacteraemia: A nested case-control study. *J Antimicrob Chemother.* 2018;73:1692–1699. 10.1093/jac/dky075.
27. Hirai K, Ishii H, Shimoshikiryo T, et al. Augmented renal clearance in patients with febrile neutropenia is associated with increased risk for subtherapeutic vancomycin concentrations. *Ther Drug Monit.* 2016;38:706–710. doi:10.1097/FTD.0000000000000346.
28. Ruhnke M, Cornely OA, Schmidt-Hieber M, et al. Treatment of invasive fungal diseases in cancer patients—Revised 2019 recommendations of the Infectious Diseases Working Party (AGIHO) of the German Society of Hematology and Oncology (DGHO). *Mycoses.* 2020;63:653–682. 10.1111/myc.13082.
29. Blyth CC, Gilroy NM, Guy SD, et al. Consensus guidelines for the treatment of invasive mould infections in haematological malignancy and haemopoietic stem cell transplantation, 2014. *Intern Med J.* 2014;44(12b):1333–1349. doi:10.1111/imj.12598.
30. Omrani AS, Almaghrabi RS. Complications of hematopoietic stem cell transplantation: Fungal infections. *Hematol Oncol Stem Cell Ther.* 2017;10:239–244. doi:10.1016/j.hemonc.2017.05.013.
31. John J, Loo A, Mazur S, et al. Therapeutic drug monitoring of systemic antifungal agents: A pragmatic approach for adult and pediatric patients. *Expert Opin Drug Metab Toxicol.* 2019;15:881–895. 10.1080/17425255.2019.1671971.
32. Mhaskar R, Clark OA, Lyman G, et al. Colony-stimulating factors for chemotherapy-induced febrile neutropenia. *Cochrane Database Syst Rev.* 2014;10:CD003039. doi:10.1002/14651858.CD003039.pub2.
33. Smith TJ, Bohlke K, Lyman GH, et al. Recommendations for the use of WBC growth factors: American Society of Clinical Oncology clinical practice guideline update. *J Clin Oncol.* 2015;33:3199–3212. doi:10.1200/JCO.2015.62.3488.
34. National Comprehensive Cancer Network. Hematopoietic growth factors. NCCN Clinical Practice Guidelines in Oncology (NCCN Guidelines®), v.4.2021; May 20, 2021. Available at: http://www.nccn.org/professionals/physician_gls/pdf/growthfactors.pdf. Accessed October 6, 2021.
35. Cugno C, Deola S, Filippini P, et al. Granulocyte transfusions in children and adults with hematological malignancies: Benefits and controversies. *J Transl Med.* 2015;13:362–378. doi:10.1186/s12967-015-0724-5.
36. Gafter-Gvili A, Fraser A, Paul M, et al. Antibiotic prophylaxis for bacterial infections in afebrile neutropenic patients following chemotherapy. *Cochrane Database Syst Rev.* 2014;1:CD004386. doi:10.1002/14651858.CD004386.pub3.
37. Ethier MC, Science M, Beyene J, et al. Mould-active compared with fluconazole prophylaxis to prevent invasive fungal diseases in cancer patient receiving chemotherapy or haematopoietic stem-cell transplantation: A systematic review and meta-analysis of randomized controlled trials. *Br J Cancer.* 2012;106:1626–1637. doi:10.1038/bjc.2012.147.
38. Rubin LG, Levin MJ, Ljungman P, et al. 2013 IDSA clinical practice guidelines for vaccination of the immunocompromised host. *Clin Infect Dis.* 2014;58:e44–e100. doi:10.1093/cid/cit816.
39. Dandoy CE, Ardura MI, Papnicalaou GA, Auletta JJ. Bacterial bloodstream infections in the allogeneic hematopoietic cell transplant patient: New considerations for a persistent nemesis. *Bone Marrow Transpl.* 2017;52:1091–1106. doi:10.1038/bmt.2017.14.
40. Miller HK, Braun TM, Stillwell T, et al. Infectious risk after allogeneic hematopoietic cell transplantation complicated by acute

graft-versus-host disease. *Biol Blood Marrow Transplant.* 2017;23:522–528. doi:10.1016/j.bbmt.2016.12.630.

41. Schuster MG, Cleveland AA, Dubberke ER, et al. Infections in hematopoietic cell transplant recipients: Results from the organ transplant infection project, a multicenter, prospective, cohort study. *Open Forum Infect Dis.* 2017;4(2):ofx050. 10.1093/ofid/ofx050.
42. Battiwalla M, Tichelli A, Majhail NS. Long-term survivorship after hematopoietic cell transplantation: Roadmap for research and care. *Biol Blood Marrow Transplant.* 2017;23:184–192. doi:10.1016/j.bbmt.2016.11.004.
43. Misch EA, Andes DR. Bacterial infections in the stem cell recipient and hematologic malignancy patient. *Infect Dis Clin N Am.* 2019;33:399–445. doi:10.1016/j.idc.2019.02.011.
44. Ullmann AJ, Schmidt-Hieber M, Bertz H, et al. Infectious diseases in allogeneic haematopoietic stem cell transplantation: Prevention and prophylaxis strategy guidelines 2016. *Ann Hematol.* 2016;95:1435–1455. doi:10.1007/s00277-016-2711-1.
45. Lin R, Liu Q. Diagnosis and treatment of viral diseases in recipients of allogeneic hematopoietic stem cell transplantation. *J Hematol Oncol.* 2013;6:94. doi:10.1186/1756-8722-6-94.
46. Marty FM, Ljungman P, Chemaly RF, et al. Letermovir prophylaxis for cytomegalovirus in hematopoietic-cell trans-plantation. *N Engl J Med.* 2017;377:2433–2444. doi:10.1056/NEJMoa1706640.
47. Neofytos D. Antimicrobial prophylaxis and preemptive approaches for the prevention of infections in the stem cell transplant recipient, with analogies to the hematologic malignancy patient. *Infect Dis Clin N Am.* 2019;33:361–380. doi:10.1016/j.idc.2019.02.002.
48. Chong PP, Avery RK. A comprehensive review of immunization practices in solid organ transplant and hematopoietic stem cell transplant recipients. *Clin Ther.* 2017;39:1581–1598. doi:10.1016/j.clinthera.2017.07.005.
49. Shingles (herpes zoster vaccination information for healthcare providers. Available at: https://www.cdc.gov/vaccines/vpd/shingles/hcp/shingrix/recommendations.html. Accessed October 3, 2021.
50. Winston DJ, Mullane KM, Cornely OA, et al. Inactivated varicella zoster vaccine in autologous haemopoietic stem-cell transplant recipients: An international, multicentre, randomised, double-blind, placebo-controlled trial. *Lancet.* 2018;391:2116. doi:10.1016/S0140-6736(18)30631-7.
51. Averbuch D, Tridello G, Hoek J, et al. Antimicrobial resistance in gram-negative rods causing bacteremia in hematopoietic stem cell transplant recipients: Intercontinental prospective study of the Infectious Diseases Working Party of the European Bone Marrow Transplantation Group. *Clin Infect Dis.* 2017;65:1819–1828. 10.1093/cid/cix646.
52. Centers for Disease Control and Prevention. Updated recommendations for use of VariZIG: United States, 2013. *MMWR.* 2013;62(28):574–576.
53. Boeckh M, Nichols WG, Chemaly RF, et al. Valganciclovir for the prevention of complications of late cytomegalovirus infection after allogeneic hematopoietic cell transplantation: A randomized trial. *Ann Intern Med.* 2015;162:1–10. doi:10.7326/M13-2729.
54. Britt WJ. Cytomegalovirus. In: Bennett JE, Dolin R, Blaser MJ, eds. *Mandell, Douglas, and Bennett's Principles and Practice of Infectious Diseases.* 9th ed. Philadelphia, PA: Elsevier, Inc.; 2020:1857–1871.e3.
55. United States Department of Health & Human Services Organ Procurement and Transportation Network. Available at: https://optn.transplant.hrsa.gov/data/view-data-reports/national-data/#. Accessed October 10, 2021.
56. Fishman JA. Infection in organ transplantation. *Am J Transplant.* 2017;17:856–879. doi:10.1111/ajt.14208.
57. Guenette A, Husain S. Infectious complications following solid organ transplantation. *Crit Care Clin.* 2019;35:151–168. doi:10.1016/j.ccc.2018.08.004.
58. Hosseini-Moghaddam SM, Shokoohi M, Singh G, et al. A multi-center case-control study of the effect of acute rejection and cytomegalovirus infection on pneumocystis pneumonia (PCP) in solid organ transplant recipients. *Clin Infect Dis.* 2018; doi:10.1093/cid/ciy682.
59. Fischer SA, Lu K. American Society of Transplantation Infectious Disease Community of Practice. Screening of donor and recipient in solid organ transplantation. *Am J Transplant.* 2013;13:9–21. doi:10.1111/ajt.12094.
60. Gagliotti C, Morsillo F, Moro ML, et al. Infectious in liver and lung transplant recipients: A national prospective cohort. *Eur J Clin Microbiol Infect Dis.* 2018;37:399–407. doi:10.1007/s10096-018-3183-0.
61. Hamandi B, Husain S, Grootendorst P, Papadimitropoulos EA. Clinical and microbiological epidemiology of early and late infectious complications among solid-organ transplant recipients requiring hospitalization. *Transpl Int.* 2016;29:1029–1038. doi:10.1111/tri.12808.
62. Anesi JA, Blumberg EA, Abbo LM. Perioperative antibiotic prophylaxis to prevent surgical site infections in solid organ transplantation. *Transplantation.* 2018;102:21–34. doi:10.1097/TP.0000000000001848.
63. Kennedy CC, Razonable RR. Fungal infections after lung transplantation. *Clin Chest Med.* 2017;38:511–520. doi:10.1016/j.ccm.2017.04.011.
64. Kabir V, Maertens J, Kuypers D. Fungal infections in solid organ transplantation: An update on diagnosis and treatment. *Transplant Rev.* 2019;33:77–86. 10.1016/j.trre.2018.12.001.
65. Schwartz IS, Patterson TF. The emerging threat of antifungal resistance in transplant infectious disease. *Curr Infect Dis Rep.* 2018;20:2. doi:10.1007/s11908-018-0608-y.
66. Andes DR, Safdar N, Baddley JW, et al. The epidemiology and outcomes of invasive *Candida* infections among organ transplant recipients in the United States: Results of the Transplant-Associated Infection Surveillance Network (TRANSNET). *Transpl Infect Dis.* 2016;18:921–931. 10.1111/tid.12613.
67. Kotton CN, Kumar D, Caliendo AM, et al. The third international consensus guidelines on the management of cytomegalovirus in solid organ transplantation. *Transplantation.* 2018;102(6):900–931. doi:10.1097/TP.0000000000002191.
68. Razonable RR, Humar A. Cytomegalovirus in solid organ transplant recipients—Guidelines of the American Society of Transplantation Infectious Diseases Community of Practice. *Clin Transplant.* 2019;33:e13512. 10.1111/ctr.13512.
69. Martin-Gandul C, Mueller NJ, Pascual M, Manuel O. The impact of infection on chronic allograft dysfunction and allograft survival after solid organ transplantation. *Am J Transplant.* 2015;15:3024–3040. doi:10.1111/ajt.13486.
70. Boyarsky BJ, Strauss AT, Segev DL. Transplanting organs from donors with HIV or hepatitis C: The viral frontier. *World J Surg.* 2021;45:3503–3510. 10.1007/s00268-020-05924-1.
71. Muller E, Barday Z, Mendelson M, et al. HIV-positive-to-HIV-positive kidney transplantation—Results at 3 to 5 years. *N Engl J Med.* 2015;372(7):613–620. 10.1056/NEJMoa1408896.
72. Levitsky J, Formica RN, Bloom RD, et al. The American Society of Transplantation Consensus Conference on the user of hepatitis C viremic donors in solid organ transplantation. *Am J Transplant.* 2017;17:2790–2802. 10.1111/ajt.14381.
73. Kritkos A, Manuel O. Bloodstream infections after solid-organ transplantation. *Virulence.* 2016;7(3):329–340. doi:10.1080/21505594.2016.1139279.
74. Martin-Gandul C, Stampf S, Héquet D, et al. Preventive strategies against cytomegalovirus and incidence of α-herpesvirus infections in solid organ transplant recipients: A nationwide cohort study. *Am J Transplant.* 2017;17:1813–1822. doi:10.1111/ajt.14192.
75. Andrassy J, Hoffmann VS, Rentsch M, et al. Is cytomegalovirus prophylaxis dispensable in patients receiving an mTOR inhibitor-based immunosuppression? A systematic review and meta-analysis. *Transplantation.* 2012;94:1208–1217. doi:10.1097/TP.0b013e3182708e56.

Antimicrobial Prophylaxis in Surgery

146

Salmaan Kanji

KEY CONCEPTS

1. Prophylactic antibiotic therapy differs from presumptive and therapeutic antibiotic therapy, in that the latter involves treatment regimens for presumed or documented infections, whereas the goal of prophylactic therapy is to prevent infections in high-risk patients or procedures.
2. The risk of a surgical site infection (SSI) is determined from both the type of surgery and the patient-specific risk factors; however, most commonly used classification systems account for only procedure-related risk factors.
3. The timing of antimicrobial prophylaxis is of paramount importance. Antibiotics should be administered within 1 hour before surgery to ensure adequate drug levels at the surgical site prior to the initial incision.
4. Antimicrobial agents with short half-lives (eg, cefazolin) may require intraoperative redosing during procedures that last more than 3 hours or 2.5 half-lives of the antimicrobial used.
5. The type of surgery, intrinsic patient risk factors, most commonly identified pathogenic organisms, institutional antimicrobial resistance patterns, and cost must be considered when choosing an antimicrobial agent for prophylaxis.
6. Single-dose prophylaxis is appropriate for many types of surgery. First-generation cephalosporins (eg, cefazolin) are the mainstay for prophylaxis in most surgical procedures because of their spectrum of activity, safety, and cost.
7. Vancomycin as a prophylactic agent should be limited to patients with a documented history of life-threatening β-lactam hypersensitivity or those in whom the incidence of infections with organisms resistant to cefazolin (eg, methicillin-resistant *Staphylococcus aureus*) is documented or high enough to justify use.

BEYOND THE BOOK

Watch the video entitled "WHO: Prevention of surgical site infections (WHO Global Guidelines 2016)" at https://tinyurl.com/yyocdygz. In 2017, the World Health Organization (WHO) published global recommendations for the prevention of surgical site infections and produced this promotional video. After viewing the video, read the official press release at https://tinyurl.com/zttj3s9. These two media releases highlight the global impact of surgical site infections and the need for a world-wide approach to prevention.

INTRODUCTION

According to the National Center for Health Statistics and the National Hospital Discharge Survey, nearly 57 million outpatient and 51 million inpatient surgical procedures are performed annually in the United States.[1,2] Infection is the most common complication of surgery.[3] Surgical site infections (SSIs) occur in approximately 3% to 6% of patients and prolong hospitalization by an average of 7 days at a direct annual cost of $5 billion to $10 billion.[4,5] SSIs that involve a prosthetic joint or antimicrobial-resistant organism can cost in excess of $90,000.[6] SSIs are now the most common cause of nosocomial infections among hospitalized patients (20% of all hospital-acquired infections).[7] Incidence rates are likely under-reported, as approximately 50% of SSIs occur after hospital discharge and the Centers for Disease Control and Prevention (CDC) defines SSI as an infection affecting the surgical incision or deep tissue at the operation site that occurs up to 30 days after surgery or even up to a year after surgery for patients receiving implants.[8] Prophylactic administration of antibiotics decreases the risk of infection after many surgical procedures and represents an important component of care for this population.

Antibiotics administered prior to the contamination of previously sterile tissues or fluids are called prophylactic antibiotics. The goal of prophylaxis is to prevent an infection from developing. Although eradication of distal (preexisting, unrelated to surgery) infections lowers the risk for subsequent postoperative infections, it does not per se constitute a prophylactic regimen. In fact, surgical prophylaxis should be prescribed concurrently under these circumstances because of important antimicrobial spectrum- and timing-related concerns. Both SSIs and hospital-acquired infections not directly related to the surgical site (eg, urinary tract infections and pneumonia) are termed *nosocomial*. Prevention of hospital-acquired infections is a major goal of antibiotic prophylaxis.

1 Presumptive antibiotic therapy is administered when an infection is suspected but not yet proven. Clinical scenarios where presumptive therapy is used commonly include acute cholecystitis, open compound fractures, and acute appendicitis of less than 24-hour duration. In these situations, if signs of perforation, contamination, or infection are absent during surgery, then routine prophylactic treatment rather than presumptive therapy is warranted. An operative finding of a gangrenous gallbladder or a perforated appendix, however, is suggestive of an established infectious process, and a therapeutic antibiotic regimen is required.[4]

According to the CDC's National Nosocomial Infections Surveillance System (NNIS),[4,7] SSIs can be categorized as either incisional (eg, cellulitis of the incision site) or organ/space (eg, meningitis; Fig. 146-1). Incisional SSIs are subcategorized into superficial (involving only the skin or subcutaneous tissue) and deep (fascial and muscle layers) infections. Organ/space SSIs can involve any anatomic area other than the incision site. For example, a patient who develops bacterial peritonitis after bowel surgery has an organ/space SSI.

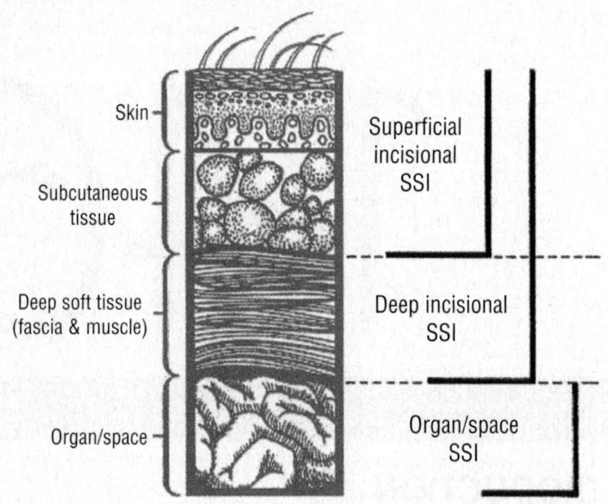

FIGURE 146-1 Cross-section of abdominal wall depicting Centers for Disease Control and Prevention classifications of surgical site infections (SSI). (*Reprinted, with permission, from Alexander JW, Solomkin JS, Edwards MJ. Updated recommendations for control of surgical site infections. Ann Surg. 2011; 253:1082–1093.*)

Although microbiologic testing of surgical drainage material or sites may help to guide care, the specificity of a negative culture is poor and generally does not rule out an SSI.[4,7] Clinical signs or symptoms of SSI may include localized heat, erythema, swelling, fever, and purulent drainage from the wound.

RISK FACTORS FOR SURGICAL SITE INFECTIONS

2 SSI incidence depends on both procedure- and patient-related factors. The risk for SSIs has been stratified by surgical procedure in a classification system developed by the National Research Council (NRC; Table 146-1). The NRC classification system proposes that the risk of an SSI depends on the microbiology of the surgical site, the presence of a preexisting infection, the likelihood of contaminating previously sterile tissue during surgery, and the events during and after surgery.[8,9] A patient's NRC procedure classification is the primary determinant of whether antibiotic prophylaxis is warranted. However, because a patient's NRC wound classification is influenced by surgical findings (eg, gangrenous gallbladder) and perioperative events (eg, major technique breaks), categorization generally occurs intraoperatively.[10] Colon surgery has the highest rates of SSI followed by gall bladder, cardiac, gynecologic, orthopedic, and spinal surgery. Minimally invasive approaches to surgery, when available, tend to be associated with lower rates of SSI when compared to traditional approaches to the same surgery.[8]

Inherent Patient Risk

The NRC classification system does not account for the influence of underlying patient risk factors for SSI development, instead categorizing the risks for SSIs simply based on a specific surgical procedure. Certain disease states and conditions (listed in Table 146-2) are known to increase SSI risk by either increasing the length or complexity of the surgery (eg, obesity) or reducing the immune response (eg, diabetes). Preexisting distal infections increase SSI rates and should be resolved prior to surgery whenever possible. Diabetic patients have an increased risk for SSIs, especially those with uncontrolled perioperative blood sugars where risk is doubled.[11] Preoperative smoking is an independent risk factor for SSI because of the deleterious effects of nicotine on wound healing.

TABLE 146-2 Patient and Operation Characteristics That May Influence the Risk of Surgical Site Infection

Patient	Operation
Age	Duration of surgical scrub
Nutritional status (preoperative albumin <3.5 g/dL [35 g/L])	Preoperative skin preparation
Diabetes and preoperative glycemic control	Preoperative shaving
Smoking and alcohol use	Duration of operation
Obesity	Antimicrobial prophylaxis
Coexisting infections at distal body sites	Operating room ventilation
Colonization with resistant microorganisms	Sterilization of instruments
	Implantation of prosthetic materials
Altered immune response	
Length of preoperative stay	Surgical drains
	Surgical technique

Reprinted, with permission, from Alexander JW, Solomkin JS, Edwards MJ. Updated recommendations for control of surgical site infections. *Ann Surg.* 2011;253:1082–1093.

TABLE 146-1 National Research Council Wound Classification, Risk of Surgical Site Infection, and Indication for Antibiotics

	SSI Rate (%)			
Classification	Preoperative Antibiotics	No Preoperative Antibiotics	Criteria	Antibiotics
Clean	0.8	5.1	No acute inflammation or transection of GI, oropharyngeal, genitourinary, biliary, or respiratory tracts; elective case, no technique break	Not indicated unless high-risk procedure[a]
Clean–contaminated	1.3	10.1	Controlled opening of aforementioned tracts with minimal spillage/minor technique break; clean procedures performed emergently or with major technique breaks	Prophylactic antibiotics indicated
Contaminated	10.2	21.9	Acute, nonpurulent inflammation present; major spillage/technique break during clean–contaminated procedure	Prophylactic antibiotics indicated
Dirty	N/A	N/A	Obvious preexisting infection present (abscess, pus, or necrotic tissue present)	Therapeutic antibiotics required

N/A, not applicable; SSI, surgical site infection.

[a]High-risk procedures include implantation of prosthetic materials and other procedures where SSI is associated with high morbidity (see the text).

Data from References 5 and 8.

Preoperative immunosuppression, including corticosteroid use, may also increase infection risk. Patients coinfected with human immunodeficiency virus (HIV) and hepatitis C are at approximately double the risk of SSI as the general population.[12] Malnutrition is a well-described risk factor for postoperative complications, including SSI, impaired wound and colonic anastomosis healing, and prolonged hospital stay. Although enteral feeding during the perioperative period can reduce bacterial translocation by maintaining the integrity of the intestinal mucosa, nutritional supplementation does not decrease the incidence of infection.[13] Some patient-related risk factors are potentially modifiable (glycemic control, alcohol and smoking status, preoperative albumin, and obesity). These represent opportunities for optimization prior to elective surgical procedures.[7]

Colonization of the nares with *S. aureus* is a well-described SSI risk factor.[4] A large multicenter study involving more than 38,000 patients undergoing more than 42,000 cardiac and orthopedic procedures showed that preoperative screening for carriers of *S. aureus* followed by intranasal mupirocin administration and chlorhexidine bathing for 5 days before surgery significantly reduced *S. aureus* SSI from 0.36% to 0.2%.[11] Although the absolute risk difference is small, this represents a 44% relative risk reduction.[8] The potential impact on patient outcomes and health resource utilization is large, given the number of surgeries performed annually. However, the logistics and cost of prescreening and treatment of colonized patients represent a challenge. Other factors shown to increase the risk of SSI are age, length of preoperative hospital stay, and obesity.[4]

Identifying SSI Risk

Two large epidemiologic studies have objectively quantified SSI risk based on specific patient- and procedure-related factors. The Study on the Efficacy of Nosocomial Infection Control (SENIC) analyzed more than 100,000 surgery cases to identify and validate risk factors for SSI.[14] Abdominal operations, operations lasting longer than 2 hours, contaminated or "dirty" procedures (as per NRC classification), and more than three underlying medical diagnoses each was associated with an increased incidence of SSI. When NRC classification was stratified by the number of SENIC risk factors present, SSI incidence varied by as much as a factor of 15 within the same NRC operative category (Table 146-3).[15]

In a subsequent analysis of more than 84,000 surgical cases, the NNIS attempted to simplify and refine the SENIC system by quantifying intrinsic patient risk using the American Society of Anesthesiologists' (ASA) preoperative assessment score (Table 146-4).[16,17] An ASA score greater than or equal to 3 was a strong predictor for the development of an SSI. Other factors associated with increased SSI incidence are contaminated or "dirty" operations (NRC criteria) and surgical procedures lasting longer than average. As in the SENIC study, the SSI rate was linked to the number of risk factors present and varied considerably within NRC class. The NNIS basic SSI risk index is composed of the following criteria: ASA score = 3, 4, or 5; wound class; and duration of surgery. Overall, for 34 of the 44 NNIS procedure categories, SSI rates increased proportionally with the number of risk factors present.[8] The SSI rate was generally lower when the procedure was done laparoscopically.

While these tools are able to broadly predict SSI risk, a more individualized approach to quantifying a patient's risk of developing an SSI is possible using the Surgical Site Infection Risk Score (SSIRS) which is a validated scoring system that incorporates both patient- and procedure-related risk factors.[18] Although evidence-based recommendations for antimicrobial prophylaxis during surgery are best established using the results of randomized clinical trials, many studies have small sample sizes and do not stratify patients according to overall SSI risk. Future studies, particularly those involving clean procedures, should be stratified by SSI risk so that the subset of high-risk patients who might benefit the most from prophylaxis is clearly established.

TABLE 146-3 Surgical Site Infection Incidence (%) Stratified by NRC Wound Classification and SENIC Risk Factors[a]

Number of SENIC Risk Factors	Clean	Clean–Contaminated	Contaminated	Dirty
0	1.1	0.6	N/A	N/A
1	3.9	2.8	4.5	6.7
2	8.4	8.4	8.3	10.9
3	15.8	17.7	11.0	18.8
4	N/A	N/A	23.9	27.4

[a]Study on the Efficacy of Nosocomial Infection Control (SENIC) risk factors include abdominal operation, operations lasting >2 hours, contaminated or dirty procedures by National Research Council (NRC) classification, and more than three underlying medical diagnoses.

N/A, not applicable; NRC, National Research Council; SENIC, Study on the Efficacy of Nosocomial Infection Control.

Data from Reference 15.

TABLE 146-4 American Society of Anesthesiologists' Physical Status Classification

Class	Description
1	Normal healthy patient
2	Mild systemic disease
3	Severe systemic disease that is not incapacitating
4	Incapacitating systemic disease that is a constant threat to life
5	Not expected to survive 24 hours with or without operation

Data from Reference 17.

BACTERIOLOGY

The most important consideration when choosing antibiotic prophylaxis is the bacteriology of the surgical site. Organisms involved in an SSI are acquired by one of two ways: endogenously (from the patient's own normal flora) or exogenously (from contamination during the surgical procedure). Based on the type and anatomic location of the procedure and the NRC classification (see Table 146-1), resident flora can be predicted and appropriate antibiotic choices made. According to NNIS data, *S. aureus*, coagulase-negative staphylococci, enterococci, *Escherichia coli*, and *Pseudomonas aeruginosa* are the pathogens most commonly isolated (Table 146-5).[16] With

TABLE 146-5 Major Pathogens in Surgical Wound Infections

Pathogen	Percent of Infections[a]
Staphylococcus aureus	20
Coagulase-negative staphylococci	14
Enterococci	12
Escherichia coli	8
Pseudomonas aeruginosa	8
Enterobacter species	7
Proteus mirabilis	3
Klebsiella pneumoniae	3
Other *Streptococcus* species	3
Candida albicans	3
Group D streptococci	2
Other gram-positive aerobes	2
Bacteroides fragilis	2

[a]Data reported by the National Nosocomial Infections Surveillance System from January 1992 through June 2004.

Data from Reference 5.

the widespread use of broad-spectrum antibiotics, however, *Candida* species and methicillin-resistant *Staphylococcus aureus* (MRSA) are becoming more prevalent.[16]

Factors affecting the ability of an organism to induce an SSI depend on organism count, organism virulence, and host immunocompetency. Organisms in the commensal flora generally are not pathogenic. These organisms often serve the host as a form of protection against invasive organisms that otherwise would colonize the surgical site. Opportunistic organisms usually are kept in check by normal flora and rarely are problematic unless they are present in large numbers. The loss of normal flora through the use of broad-spectrum antibiotics can destabilize homeostasis, allowing pathogenic bacteria to proliferate and infection to occur.[5]

Normal flora translocated to a normally sterile tissue site or fluid during a surgical procedure can become pathogenic. For example, *S. aureus* or *Staphylococcus epidermidis* may be translocated from the surface of the skin to deeper tissues or *E. coli* from the colon to the peritoneal cavity, bloodstream, or urinary tract. Studies in animals and healthy volunteers have shown bacterial virulence to be an important determinant in the development of secondary infections.[19,20] Whereas more than one million *S. aureus* per square centimeter or gram of tissue are required to produce infection in animals, less than 100,000 *Streptococcus pyogenes* per square centimeter or gram of tissue are required at the same site.[20,21]

Impaired host defense reduces the number of bacteria required to establish an infection. A breach of normal host defenses through surgical intervention (eg, insertion of a prosthetic device) may enable organisms to cause infection. In addition, the loss of specific immune factors, such as complement activation, tissue-derived inhibitors (eg, proinflammatory cytokines), cell-mediated response (eg, T-cell function), and granulocytic or phagocytic function (eg, neutrophils or macrophages), can greatly increase the risk for SSI development.[22] Vascular occlusive states related to the surgical procedure or those occurring from hypovolemic shock can greatly affect blood flow to the surgical site, thus diminishing host defense mechanisms against microbial invasion. Traumatized tissue, hematomas, and the presence of foreign material also lead to more infections. When a foreign body is introduced during a surgical procedure, fewer than 100 bacterial colony-forming units are required to cause an SSI.[23] Studies examining *S. aureus*-contaminated wound infections on the skin of healthy volunteers demonstrate a 10,000-fold reduction in the number of organisms required to establish a wound infection if sutures are not present.[19]

ANTIMICROBIAL RESISTANCE AND STEWARDSHIP

Colonization of the host with antibiotic-resistant hospital flora prior to or during surgery may lead to an SSI that is unresponsive to routine antibiotic therapy. The most common cause of nosocomially acquired multiresistant organisms is transmission from hospital personnel.[24] Patients treated with broad-spectrum antibiotic therapy are at increased risk for colonization with hospital flora.

With cephalosporins established as first-line agents for prophylaxis, organisms resistant to cephalosporins represent the majority of pathogens causing SSIs. MRSA and coagulase-negative staphylococci have emerged as the most common pathogens in patients who develop SSIs despite prophylaxis with cephalosporins particularly in cardiothoracic, vascular, orthopedic, and neurologic surgery. Methicillin resistance not only limits the treatment/-prophylaxis options available, but it also is associated with increased mortality, longer hospital lengths of stay, and increased costs. Although the use of vancomycin for prophylaxis may be appropriate for some operations performed in hospitals with a high rate of infection due to MRSA, there is little guidance on what constitutes a "high rate" of MRSA infection and whether providing prophylaxis with vancomycin alone will result in fewer SSIs.[25] A more effective strategy would be to screen elective surgical candidates for MRSA colonization preoperatively. MRSA colonization is predictive of MRSA SSI and thus effective prophylaxis with vancomycin is then reserved for carriers only. Some single center studies evaluating the decolonization of MRSA carriers preoperatively (ie, with intranasal mupirocin, chlorhexidine showers) have yielded mixed results and may not be cost-effective.[25]

The increase in frequency of fungal infections in surgical patients has drawn concern. In hospitalized patients, the incidence of nosocomial *Candida* infections nearly doubled from 1992 to 2004.[16,26] Overzealous use of broad-spectrum antibiotics is the most likely cause for this increase. A study of patients undergoing cardiovascular surgery identified female sex, length of stay in the ICU, and duration of central venous catheterization as risk factors for postoperative *Candida* infections. Although presurgical *Candida* colonization is associated with a higher risk of fungal SSIs, routine preoperative use of prophylactic antifungal agents is not being advocated at this time.[26]

Antimicrobial stewardship programs are typically run by multidisciplinary teams in hospitals to promote responsible antimicrobial use and optimize antimicrobial therapy through multimodal educational and clinical interventions with an aim to reduce antimicrobial resistance and infection-related morbidity and mortality. Systematic reviews suggest that these programs are effective in reducing the development of antimicrobial resistance and hospital-acquired infections.[27] Typically antimicrobial stewardship programs target areas of the hospital where there is high use of antimicrobials but surgical units and operating rooms are often overlooked. Given that approximately 15% of all antimicrobials prescribed in hospital are for surgical prophylaxis and the opportunity to improve the outcomes of surgical patients with respect to SSIs, surgical units would benefit from antimicrobial stewardship programs and surgeons should be part of the multidisciplinary team.[28]

SCHEDULING ANTIBIOTIC ADMINISTRATION

3 4 The following principles must be considered when providing antimicrobial surgical prophylaxis: (a) the agents should be delivered to the surgical site prior to the initial incision, and (b) bactericidal antibiotic concentrations should be maintained at the surgical site throughout the surgical procedure. Although animal and human models have demonstrated the efficacy of a single dose of an antibiotic administered just prior to bacterial contamination, long operations often require intraoperative doses of antibiotics to maintain adequate concentrations at the surgical site for the duration of surgery.[29] Antibiotic administration should be completed within 60 minutes prior to the initial incision, preferably at the time of anesthetic induction. Since the administration duration varies between antimicrobials, this needs to be considered when determining when to start the infusion. Administration of antibiotics too early may result in concentrations below the minimum inhibitory concentration (MIC) toward the end of the operation, and administration too late leaves the patient unprotected at the time of initial incision. In a study examining the timing of antibiotic administration to 2,847 patients receiving prophylaxis, Classen et al.[29] evaluated patients who received prophylaxis early (2-24 hours before surgery), preoperative prophylaxis (0-2 hours prior to surgery), perioperative prophylaxis (up to 3 hours after first incision), and postoperative prophylaxis (greater than 3 hours after the first incision). The risk of infection was lowest (0.6%) for patients who received preoperative prophylaxis, moderate (1.4%) for those who received perioperative antibiotics, and greatest for those who received postoperative antibiotics (3.3%)

or preoperative antibiotics too early (3.8%). The risk for an SSI increases dramatically with each hour from the time of initial incision to the time when antibiotics are eventually administered. For these reasons, prophylactic antibiotics should not be prescribed to be given "on call to the operating room (OR)," which can occur two or more hours prior to the initial incision, nor should concurrent therapeutic antibiotics be relied on to provide adequate protection. In both situations, the chance for improperly timed doses is high. Although the landmark study by Classen et al.[29] confirmed that antimicrobial prophylaxis should be administered within 2 hours prior to the initial incision, administration immediately prior to the incision may not allow enough time for the drug to distribute throughout the tissues involved in the surgery.

In a large randomized controlled trial in Switzerland, hospitalized surgical patients were randomized to early (in the anesthesia room) or late (in the operating room) prophylactic antimicrobials.[30] A total of 2,589 patients in the early group received their antimicrobials a median of 42 minutes prior to the incision while 2,586 patients in the late group received their antimicrobials a median of 16 minutes prior to the incision. All patients received cefuroxime (plus metronidazole for colorectal surgery) as a single dose except for long operations where the cefuroxime (and metronidazole for colorectal surgery) was readministered every 4 hours during the operation. SSIs were 5% in both groups suggesting that the current recommendation to administer surgical prophylaxis within 60 minutes prior to the incision is adequate.

Despite the importance of appropriately timed prophylactic antibiotic therapy, many patients receive antibiotics outside of the optimal time window in relation to surgery. Potential barriers include antibiotics ordered after the patient has arrived in the OR, delayed antibiotic preparation or delivery, and use of antibiotics that require long infusion times. One retrospective study assessed the timing of prophylactic antibiotics in more than 32,000 patients and found that 91.9% of patients received an antibiotic dose within 60 minutes of the initial surgical incision.[31]

Although most studies comparing single versus multiple doses of prophylactic antibiotics have failed to show a benefit of multidose regimens, the duration of operations in these studies may not be as long as that frequently observed in clinical practice. Proponents of administering a second antibiotic dose during lengthy operations suggest that the risk for SSI is just as great at the end of surgery (during wound closing) as it is during the initial incision. One study of patients undergoing clean–contaminated operations suggests that procedures longer than 3 hours require a second intraoperative dose of cefazolin or substitution of cefazolin with a longer-acting antimicrobial agent.[5] A second study of patients undergoing elective colorectal surgery suggests that low serum antimicrobial concentrations at the time of surgical closure is the strongest predictor of postoperative SSI.[32] Studies of patients undergoing cardiac surgery also have demonstrated a higher infection rate among patients with undetectable antibiotic serum concentrations at the conclusion of the procedure.[33] Ideally antibiotic prophylaxis should be repeated when surgeries last longer than two half-lives of chosen antibiotic (ie, 4 hours for cefazolin) or if intraoperative blood loss exceeds 1.5 L.[7]

One strategy to ensure appropriate redosing of prophylactic antibiotics during long operations is use of a visual or auditory reminder system. One hospital reported its experience with such a system, finding that an automated reminder improved compliance and reduced SSIs. However, even with the reminder system, intraoperative redosing was done in only 68% of eligible patients.[34] Although optimizing the efficacy of antimicrobial prophylaxis is often the main focus of guideline documents, equal emphasis should be placed on avoidance of harms associated with unnecessary or prolonged courses of prophylactic antibiotics. A recent cohort study of more than 79,000 patients suggests that prolonged courses of prophylactic antibiotics (eg, more than 24-hour post–skin closure) was associated with higher risks of acute kidney injury and *C. difficile* infection without further reducing the rates of SSIs.[35]

ANTIMICROBIAL CHOICE

5 The choice of prophylactic antibiotic depends on the type of surgical procedure, the most frequent pathogens seen with this procedure, safety and efficacy profiles of the antimicrobial agent, current literature evidence supporting its use, and cost. Although most SSIs involve the patient's normal flora, antimicrobial selection also must take into account the susceptibility patterns of nosocomial pathogens within each institution. Typically, gram-positive coverage should be included in the choice of surgical prophylaxis because organisms such as *S. aureus* and *S. epidermidis* are encountered commonly as skin flora. The decision to broaden antibiotic prophylaxis to agents with gram-negative and anaerobic spectra of activity depends on both the surgical site (eg, upper respiratory, GI, or genitourinary tract) and whether the operation will transect a hollow viscous or mucous membrane that may contain resident flora.[4]

Although antimicrobial prophylaxis can be administered through a variety of routes (eg, oral, topical, or intramuscular), the parenteral route is favored because of the reliability by which adequate tissue concentrations may be acheived.[36] Cephalosporins are the most commonly prescribed agents for surgical prophylaxis because of their broad antimicrobial spectrum, favorable pharmacokinetic profile, low incidence of adverse side effects, and low cost. First-generation cephalosporins, such as cefazolin, are the preferred choice for surgical prophylaxis, particularly for clean surgical procedures.[4,5,10] In cases where broader gram-negative and anaerobic coverage is desired, antianaerobic cephalosporins, such as cefoxitin and cefotetan, are appropriate choices. Although third-generation cephalosporins (eg, ceftriaxone) have been advocated for prophylaxis because of their increased gram-negative coverage and prolonged half-lives, their inferior gram-positive and anaerobic activity and high cost have discouraged the widespread use of these agents.[4,5,10]

Allergic reactions are the most common side effects associated with cephalosporin use. Reactions can range from minor skin manifestations at the site of infusion to rash, pruritus, and rarely anaphylaxis (less than 0.02%). The structural similarity between penicillins and cephalosporins (each contains a β-lactam ring) has led to considerable confusion about the cross-allergenicity between these two classes of drugs. Twenty percent of the general population is labeled "penicillin allergic," yet of these patients, only 10% to 20% have positive results of a penicillin skin test.[37] The rate of cross-reactivity with cephalosporins is approximately 2%, but as only 20% of all "penicillin-allergic" patients truly are penicillin allergic, the true incidence of cross-reactivity likely is less than 1%. Routine penicillin skin testing is not cost-effective.[37] The administration of cephalosporins is both safe and cost-effective for many patients who are labeled "penicillin allergic," and they can be used by patients who have not experienced an immediate or type I penicillin allergy.

Vancomycin can be considered for prophylactic therapy in surgical procedures involving implantation of a prosthetic device in which the rate of MRSA is high.[38] If the risk of MRSA is low, and a β-lactam hypersensitivity exists, clindamycin can be used for many procedures instead of cefazolin to limit vancomycin use. Infusion-related side effects, such as thrombophlebitis and hypotension, particularly with vancomycin, usually can be controlled by adequate dilution and slower administration rates.

Pseudomembranous colitis secondary to cephalosporins is uncommon and generally easily treated with a short course of oral metronidazole. Although infrequent, bleeding abnormalities related to cephalosporin use have been reported.[39] The primary hematologic effect appears to be inhibition of vitamin K–dependent clotting factors that results in prolongation of the prothrombin time. The mechanism for this effect, most commonly seen with cefotetan, is related to the methylthiotetrazole side chain of the β-lactam molecule. Patients at greatest risk for this hypoprothrombinemic effect have received a prolonged course of these agents and have underlying risk factors for vitamin K deficiency, such as malnutrition.

Because inappropriate prophylactic antibiotic use not only can induce antibiotic resistance but also can negatively affect an institution's antibiotic budget, initiatives to curtail inappropriate antibiotic use have become the focus of many drug use evaluation efforts. Potential sources of inappropriate antibiotic prophylaxis include the use of broad-spectrum antimicrobials when a narrow-spectrum agent is warranted, extending prophylaxis for durations beyond that recommended in published guidelines, and using expensive antibiotics when equivalent, less expensive agents are available. Individualized institutional guidelines that take into account the best literature evidence, institution-based antibiotic susceptibility data, and surgeon preference are important tools for rationalizing antibiotic prophylaxis use.[40] This also highlights a potential role for antimicrobial stewardship.

RECOMMENDATIONS FOR SPECIFIC TYPES OF SURGERY

Guidelines for surgical prophylaxis usually are structured according to the tissues affected during an operation. Although many different surgical procedures may be performed at any one anatomic site, this method of categorization still is optimal because the factors related to the success of a prophylactic regimen, such as the endogenous flora that are expected and the pharmacokinetics, pharmacodynamics, and spectrum of selected antimicrobials, generally, are constant for a particular surgical site (see the discussion above). The choice of antimicrobial prophylaxis is always best evaluated using the results of properly conducted clinical trials. In the absence of studies specific to the procedure in question, extrapolation from data on regimens for different procedures in the same anatomic site in question usually can be made. Subsequent modifications to each prophylactic regimen should be based on intraoperative findings or events.

6 A comprehensive review of the surgical prophylaxis literature is beyond the scope of this chapter, but important factors are reviewed here for common types/sites of surgery. Specific recommendations are summarized in Table 146-6. The reader is referred to published guidelines and review articles.[3-5,10,36,41]

Gastrointestinal Surgery

GI surgery can be categorized according to surgical site and infectious risk. Gastroduodenal surgery and hepatobiliary surgery generally are considered to be clean or clean–contaminated surgeries, with SSI rates generally less than 5%. Colorectal surgery, including appendectomies, is considered contaminated because of the large quantities and polymicrobial nature of bacterial flora within the colon. SSI rates for these types of surgeries generally range from 15% to 30%. Emergent abdominal surgery involving bowel perforation or peritonitis is considered a dirty surgical procedure, associated with a greater than 30% risk of SSI, and should be treated with therapeutic rather than prophylactic antibiotics.[4]

Gastroduodenal Surgery

Insignificant numbers of bacteria usually are found in the stomach and duodenum because of their acidity. The rate of SSIs in gastroduodenal surgery generally is low, so procedures in this region can be classified as clean. The risk for an SSI in this population increases with any condition that can lead to bacterial overgrowth, such as obstruction, hemorrhage, or malignancy, or increasing the pH of gastroduodenal secretions with concomitant acid suppression therapy. Antimicrobial prophylaxis is of clinical benefit only in this high-risk population. In most cases, a single IV dose of cefazolin will provide adequate prophylaxis.[10] Antimicrobial prophylaxis is indicated in esophageal surgery only in the presence of obstruction. Postoperative therapeutic antibiotics may be indicated if perforation is detected during surgery, depending on whether an established infection is present.

Use of antibiotic prophylaxis for percutaneous endoscopic gastrostomy placement is also warranted. Postoperative peristomal infection can occur in up to 30% of patients and a systematic review of 12 trials involving 1,271 patients found a significant reduction in peristomal infections with antimicrobial prophylaxis (OR 0.36, 95% CI 0.26-0.50).[42] A single dose of cefazolin given 30 minutes preoperatively is preferred over longer regimens.

There are few well-designed clinical trials of antimicrobial prophylaxis in bariatric surgery (ie, Roux en Y gastric bypass, gastric banding, sleeve gastrectomy). However, given that obesity is a consistently identified risk factor for SSIs, guidelines do promote antimicrobial prophylaxis with cefazolin as this is the agent that has been most studied.[43] Dosing is still controversial, but at higher doses is generally recommended based on greater volumes of distribution in morbidly obese patients.[10] Pharmacokinetic studies suggest that 2 g of cefazolin provided adequate tissue levels for 4.8 hours.[43]

Hepatobiliary Surgery

Although bile normally is sterile, and the SSI rate after biliary surgery is low, antibiotic prophylaxis is of benefit in this population. Bile contamination (bactobilia) can increase the frequency of SSIs and is present in many patients (eg, those with acute cholecystitis or biliary obstruction and those of advanced age).[41] In general, however, the correlation between bactobilia in surgical specimens and the subsequent pathogens implicated in an SSI is poor. The most frequently encountered organisms are *E. coli*, *Klebsiella* species, and enterococci. *Pseudomonas* is an uncommon finding in the absence of cholangitis. Most of the SSI literature on biliary tract surgery pertains to cholecystectomy while more recent trials pertain to laparoscopic procedures which have eclipsed the traditional open cholecystectomy because of a reduction in recovery time and hospital stay. The evidence in open cholecystectomy strongly supports the use of antimicrobial prophylaxis while the evidence for laparoscopic procedures is less impressive.[10] Trials comparing first-, second-, and third-generation cephalosporins have not demonstrated benefit over single-dose cefazolin prophylaxis even in high-risk patients (eg, age greater than 60 years, previous biliary surgery, acute cholecystitis, jaundice, obesity, diabetes, and common bile duct stones).[44] Ciprofloxacin and levofloxacin are effective alternatives for β-lactam-allergic patients undergoing open cholecystectomy.[45,46] In fact, oral levofloxacin appears to provide similar intraoperative gallbladder tissue concentrations.[46] For patients undergoing elective laparoscopic cholecystectomy, antibiotic prophylaxis has traditionally not been recommended but newer trials and systematic reviews are conflicting and assessments of current practice are reflective of this.[47,48] Detection of an active infection during surgery (eg, gangrenous gallbladder and suppurative cholangitis) is an indication for a course of postoperative therapeutic antibiotics. The risk for SSIs in cirrhotic patients undergoing transjugular intrahepatic portosystemic shunt surgery may be reduced with a single prophylactic dose of ceftriaxone,[49] but not with single doses of shorter-acting cephalosporins.[50]

Appendectomy

Acute appendicitis can be broadly categorized as complicated (evidence of perforation, gangrene, peritonitis, or abscess formation) or uncomplicated. Complicated appendicitis should be treated as an active intra-abdominal infection. While appendectomy for uncomplicated appendicitis is more common it has been associated with SSI rates of 9% to 30% in the absence of antimicrobial prophylaxis. Randomized controlled trials do suggest that preoperative

TABLE 146-6 Most Likely Pathogens and Specific Recommendations for Surgical Prophylaxis

Type of Operation	Likely Pathogens	Recommended Prophylaxis Regimen[a]	Comments	Grade of Recommendation[b]
GI Surgery				
Gastroduodenal	Enteric gram-negative bacilli, gram-positive cocci, oral anaerobes	Cefazolin 1 g × 1	High-risk patients only (obstruction, hemorrhage, malignancy, acid suppression therapy, morbid obesity)	IA
Bariatric surgery	Enteric gram-negative bacilli, gram-positive cocci, oral anaerobes	Cefazolin 2 g x 1	Intraoperative redosing required for procedures longer than 4 hours	IB
Cholecystectomy	Enteric gram-negative bacilli, anaerobes	Cefazolin 1 g × 1 for high-risk patients; Laparoscopic: controversial	High-risk patients only (open biliary tract procedures, acute cholecystitis, common duct stones, previous biliary surgery, jaundice, age >60 years, obesity, diabetes mellitus)	IA
Transjugular intrahepatic portosystemic shunt (TIPS)	Enteric gram-negative bacilli, anaerobes	Ceftriaxone 1 g × 1	Longer-acting cephalosporins preferred	IA
Appendectomy	Enteric gram-negative bacilli, anaerobes	Cefoxitin or cefotetan 1 g × 1 or cefazolin 1 g plus metronidazole 1 g × 1	Second intraoperative dose of cefoxitin may be required if procedure lasts longer than 3 hours	IA
Colorectal	Enteric gram-negative bacilli, anaerobes	Orally: neomycin 1 g + erythromycin base 1 g at 1, 2, and 11 PM 1 day preoperatively plus mechanical bowel preparation IV: cefoxitin or cefotetan 1 g × 1	Role of mechanical bowel preparation is controversial. It is widely used despite evidence suggesting it may have no effect on SSI or other clinical outcomes	IA
GI endoscopy	Variable, depending on procedure, but typically enteric gram-negative bacilli, gram-positive cocci, oral anaerobes	Orally: amoxicillin 2 g × 1 IV: ampicillin 2 g × 1 or cefazolin 1 g × 1	Recommended only for high-risk patients undergoing high-risk procedures (see the text)	IA
Urologic Surgery				
Prostate resection, shock-wave lithotripsy, ureteroscopy	*E. coli*	Ciprofloxacin 500 mg orally or Trimethoprim–sulfamethoxazole 1 DS tablet	All patients with positive preoperative urine cultures should receive a course of antibiotic treatment	IA–IB
Removal of external urinary catheters, cystography, urodynamic studies, simple cystourethroscopy	*E. coli*	Ciprofloxacin 500 mg orally or Trimethoprim–sulfamethoxazole 1 DS tablet	Should be considered only in patients with risk factors (see the text)	IB
Gynecological Surgery				
Cesarean section	Enteric gram-negative bacilli, anaerobes, group B streptococci, enterococci	Cefazolin 1 g × 1 (<80 kg), Cefazolin 2 g x 1 (>80 kg). Add azithromycin 500 mg IV × 1 if non-elective procedure	Antimicrobial administration should be prior to the initial incision as opposed to after umbilical cord clamping	IA
Hysterectomy	Enteric gram-negative bacilli, anaerobes, group B streptococci, enterococci	Vaginal: cefazolin 2 g × 1 (3 g if >120 kg) Abdominal: cefotetan 1 g × 1 or cefazolin 2 g × 1	Metronidazole 1 g IV × 1 is recommended alternative for penicillin allergy	IA
Head-and-Neck Surgery				
Maxillofacial surgery	*Staphylococcus aureus*, streptococci spp., oral anaerobes	Cefazolin 2 g or clindamycin 600 mg	Repeat intraoperative dose for operations longer than 4 hours	IA
Head-and-neck cancer resection	*S. aureus*, streptococci spp., oral anaerobes	Clindamycin 600 mg at induction and every 8 hours × 2 more doses	Ampicillin/sulbactam 3 g for clean–contaminated procedures	IA

(continued)

TABLE 146-6 Most Likely Pathogens and Specific Recommendations for Surgical Prophylaxis (*Continued*)

Type of Operation	Likely Pathogens	Recommended Prophylaxis Regimen[a]	Comments	Grade of Recommendation[b]
Cardiothoracic Surgery				
Cardiac surgery	*S. aureus*, *S. epidermidis*, *Corynebacterium*	Cefazolin 1 g every 8 hours × 48 hours Intranasal mupirocin twice daily for 5 days preoperatively for patients colonized with *S. aureus*	Patients >80 kg (176 lb) should receive 2 g of cefazolin instead; in areas with high prevalence of *S. aureus* resistance, vancomycin should be considered	IA
Thoracic surgery	*S. aureus*, *S. epidermidis*, *Corynebacterium*, enteric gram-negative bacilli	Cefuroxime 750 mg IV every 8 hours × 48 hours	First-generation cephalosporins are deemed inadequate, and shorter durations of prophylaxis have not been adequately studied	IA
Vascular Surgery				
Abdominal aorta and lower extremity vascular surgery	*S. aureus*, *S. epidermidis*, enteric gram-negative bacilli	Cefazolin 1 g at induction and every 8 hours × 2 more doses	Although complications from infections may be infrequent, graft infections are associated with significant morbidity	IB
Orthopedic Surgery				
Joint replacement	*S. aureus*, *S. epidermidis*	Cefazolin 1 g × 1 preoperatively, then every 8 hours × 2 more doses. Intranasal mupirocin twice daily for 5 days preoperatively for patients colonized with *S. aureus*	Vancomycin reserved for penicillin-allergic patients or where institutional prevalence of methicillin-resistant *S. aureus* warrants use	IA
Hip fracture repair	*S. aureus*, *S. epidermidis*	Cefazolin 1 g × 1 preoperatively, then every 8 hours for 48 hours	Compound fractures are treated as if infection is presumed	IA
Open/compound fractures	*S. aureus*, *S. epidermidis*, gram-negativebacilli, polymicrobial	Cefazolin 1 g × 1 preoperatively, then every 8 hours for a course of presumed infection	Gram-negative coverage (ie, gentamicin) often indicated for severe open fractures	IA
Neurosurgery				
CSF shunt procedures	*S. aureus*, *S. epidermidis*	Cefazolin 1 g every 8 hours × 3 doses or ceftriaxone 2 g × 1	No agents have been shown to be better than cefazolin in randomized comparative trials	IA
Spinal surgery	*S. aureus*, *S. epidermidis*	Cefazolin 1 g × 1	Limited number of clinical trials comparing different treatment regimens	IB
CSF shunt procedures	*S. aureus*, *S. epidermidis*	Cefazolin 1 g every 8 hours × 3 doses or ceftriaxone 2 g × 1	No agents have been shown to be better than cefazolin in randomized comparative trials	IA
Craniotomy	*S. aureus*, *S. epidermidis*	Cefazolin 1 g × 1 or cefotaxime 1 g × 1	Vancomycin 1 g IV × 1 can be substituted for patients with penicillin allergy	IA

CSF, cerebrospinal fluid; DS, double strength.

[a]One-time doses are optimally infused at induction of anesthesia except as noted. Repeat doses may be required for long procedures. See the text for references.

[b]Strength of recommendations:

Category IA: Strongly recommended and supported by well-designed experimental, clinical, or epidemiologic studies.

Category IB: Strongly recommended and supported by some experimental, clinical, or epidemiologic studies and strong theoretical rationale.

Category II: Suggested and supported by suggestive clinical or epidemiologic studies or theoretical rationale.

antimicrobials are effective at reducing this risk and should be administered in all cases.[51] Numerous antibiotic regimens, all with activity against gram-positive and gram-negative aerobes and anaerobic pathogens, are effective in reducing SSI incidence.[41] A cephalosporin with antianaerobic activity, such as cefoxitin or cefotetan, is recommended as first-line therapy; however, a comparative trial of cefoxitin and cefotetan suggests that cefotetan may be superior, possibly because of its longer duration of action.[52] Alternatively, cefazolin in combination with metronidazole is also effective. In patients with β-lactam allergy, metronidazole in combination with gentamicin is an effective regimen. Broad-spectrum antibiotics covering nosocomial pathogens (eg, *Pseudomonas*) do not further reduce SSI risk and instead may increase the cost of therapy and promote bacterial resistance. Although single-dose therapy with cefotetan is adequate, prophylaxis with cefoxitin may require intraoperative redosing if the procedure extends beyond 3 hours.

Colorectal Surgery

In the absence of adequate prophylactic therapy, the risk for SSI after colorectal surgery is high (5.4%-23.2%) because of the significant bacterial counts in fecal material present in the colon (frequently greater than 10^9 per gram).[53] Anaerobes and gram-negative aerobes predominate, but gram-positive aerobes also may play an important role. Reducing this bacterial load with a thorough bowel preparation regimen (4 L of polyethylene glycol solution or 90 mL of sodium phosphate solution administered orally the day before surgery) is controversial; however, 99% of US surgeons in a survey routinely use mechanical preparation.[54] The presumed value of a mechanical bowel preparation goes beyond its effect on SSIs as it is also thought to facilitate bowel manipulation, enable safe passage of surgical instruments, and allow for intraoperative colonoscopy if needed. A randomized trial of 380 patients undergoing elective colorectal surgery suggests that SSIs are not reduced by preoperative mechanical bowel preparation.[55] This finding was confirmed in two meta-analyses showing that mechanical bowel preparation does not reduce the risk of anastomotic leakage or other complications, including postoperative infection.[56,57] Despite this new evidence, mechanical bowel preparations continue to be a standard of practice prior to elective bowel surgery.

Risk factors for SSIs include age over 60 years, hypoalbuminemia, poor preoperative bowel preparation, corticosteroid therapy, malignancy, and operations lasting longer than 3.5 hours.[10] Antimicrobial prophylaxis reduced mortality from 11.2% to 4.5% in a pooled analysis of trials comparing antimicrobial prophylaxis with no prophylaxis for colon surgery.[58] Effective antibiotic prophylaxis consisting of an oral and IV regimen reduces even further the risk for an SSI. A Cochrane review comparing oral, IV, and combination regimens found that while each one was more effective at reducing SSI than placebo, combination therapy (oral and IV) was superior to oral regimens alone (OR 0.52 [0.35, 0.76]) and IV regimens alone (OR 0.55 [0.43, 0.71]).[59] This finding was confirmed by a systematic review of 14 trials, and now clinical practice guidelines from the American Society of Colon and Rectal Surgeons recommends the combination of oral antibiotics and mechanical bowel preparation preoperatively in addition to intravenous antibiotics at the time of surgery.[53,60]

Several oral regimens designed to reduce bacterial counts in the colon have been studied.[41] The combination of 1-g neomycin and 1-g erythromycin base given orally 19, 18, and 9 hours preoperatively is the regimen most commonly used in the United States.[60] Neomycin is poorly absorbed but provides intraluminal concentrations that are high enough to effectively kill most gram-negative aerobes. Oral erythromycin is only partially absorbed but still produces concentrations in the colon that are sufficient to suppress common anaerobes. If surgery is postponed, the antibiotics must be readministered to maintain efficacy. Optimally, the bowel preparation regimen (if used) should be completed prior to starting the oral antibiotic regimen. This is of particular concern because most procedures now are performed electively on a "same-day surgery" basis. In this case, the bowel preparation regimen is self-administered by the patient at home on the day prior to hospital admission, and compliance cannot be monitored carefully.

Single-dose cephalosporins are the most used and studied preoperative IV antimicrobial. Cefoxitin or cefotetan is used most commonly, but other second- and some third-generation cephalosporins also are effective.[61] The role of metronidazole in combination with cephalosporin therapy is unclear. Only retrospective evidence suggests that the addition of metronidazole to a cephalosporin or extended-spectrum penicillin provides additional benefit.[62] Until this finding is confirmed in prospective studies, metronidazole should be reserved for combination therapy with cephalosporins with poor anaerobic coverage (eg, cefazolin). At this time, the evidence recommending the addition of metronidazole to cephalosporins with anaerobic activity (eg, cefotaxime, cefoxitin, and ceftriaxone) is insufficient.[63] For β-lactam-allergic patients, perioperative doses of gentamicin and metronidazole have been used. Postoperative antibiotics generally are unnecessary in the absence of any untoward events or findings during surgery. IV antibiotics are required for colostomy reversal and rectal resection because enterally administered antibiotics will not reach the distal segment that is to be reanastomosed or resected.[64]

Gastrointestinal Endoscopy

Despite the large number of endoscopic procedures performed each year, the rate of postprocedural infection is relatively low. The highest bacteremia rates have been reported in patients undergoing esophageal dilation for stricture or sclerotherapy for management of esophageal varices. Although postprocedural bacteremia can occur in as many as 22% of patients, the bacteremia usually is transient (less than 30 minutes) and rarely results in clinically significant infection. Therefore, antimicrobial prophylaxis is routinely recommended only for high-risk patients (eg, patients with prosthetic heart valves, a history of endocarditis, systemic-pulmonary shunt, synthetic vascular graft less than 1-year-old, complex cyanotic congenital heart disease, obstructed bile duct, or liver cirrhosis, as well as immunocompromised patients) undergoing high-risk procedures (eg, stricture dilation, variceal sclerotherapy, and endoscopic retrograde cholangiopancreatography, ERCP).[65] Single-dose preprocedural regimens similar to those for endocarditis prophylaxis are most common (amoxicillin for patients who can tolerate oral premedication or either IV ampicillin or cefazolin). A meta-analysis of antimicrobial prophylaxis for endoscopic placement of percutaneous feeding tubes also suggests that a single preoperative dose of antibiotics reduces the risk of postoperative infection compared with no antibiotic (6.4% vs 24%).[66] Consensus guidelines have adopted this recommendation and suggest a single dose of cefazolin within 30 minutes prior to the procedure.[65]

Urologic Surgery

Preoperative bacteriuria is the most important risk factor for development of an SSI after urologic surgery. All patients should have a preoperative urinalysis and should receive therapeutic antibiotics if bacteriuria is detected. Patients undergoing clean urologic procedures with sterile urine preoperatively are at low risk for developing an SSI, and antimicrobial prophylaxis is not recommended.[10] Antibiotic prophylaxis is recommended for all patients undergoing transurethral resection of the prostate or bladders tumors, shockwave lithotripsy, percutaneous renal surgery, or ureteroscopy.[67] The exact incidence of SSIs in this population is obscured by the frequent use of postoperative urinary catheters and the subsequent risk of bacteriuria. *E. coli* is the most frequently encountered organism. Routine use of broad-spectrum antibiotics, such as third-generation cephalosporins and fluoroquinolones, does not decrease SSI rates more than cefazolin, but the ability to administer fluoroquinolones orally rather than IV makes antimicrobial prophylaxis with ciprofloxacin easier and less expensive.[68] First- or second-generation cephalosporins are considered the antimicrobial agents of choice for patients undergoing open or laparoscopic procedures involving entry into the urinary tract and any urologic surgical procedures involving the intestine, rectum, vagina, or implanted prosthesis.[67] The evidence supporting antimicrobial prophylaxis for the removal of external urinary catheters, cystography, urodynamic studies, simple cystourethroscopy, and open or laparoscopic urologic procedures that do not involve entry into the urinary tract is not as evident. Only patients considered to have risk factors (patients of advanced age; those with anatomic anomalies, poor nutritional history, externalized catheters, colonized endogenous/exogenous material, or distant coexistent infection; smokers; immunocompromised patients; and those who are hospitalized for a prolonged stay) should receive antimicrobial prophylaxis.[67]

Obstetric and Gynecologic Surgeries

Cesarean Section

Cesarean section is the most frequently performed surgical procedure in the United States.[10] Prophylactic antibiotics are given to prevent endometritis, the most commonly occurring SSI. In the past, antibiotics were recommended for only high-risk patients, including those with premature membrane rupture or those not receiving prenatal care. Several large trials, as well as a meta-analysis of 95 trials, have shown benefit in administering prophylactic antibiotics to all women undergoing emergent or elective cesarean section regardless of their underlying risk factors.[69] Cefazolin remains the drug of choice despite the wide spectrum of potential pathogens, and a single 2-g dose for patients weighing 80 kg or more and a single 1-g dose for patients weighing less than 80 kg is recommended.[70] For patients with a β-lactam allergy, preoperative metronidazole is an acceptable alternative.[69] In women undergoing nonelective cesarean section, a composite outcome of endometritis, wound infection, or other infection occurring within 6 weeks was 6.1% in women who received extended spectrum coverage with azithromycin plus cefazolin versus 12% in those who received cefazolin alone.[71] This study makes a strong argument for extending the spectrum of coverage with azithromycin in addition to the standard cephalosporin regimen for patients undergoing nonelective cesarean section.

During a cesarean section, unlike other surgical procedures, the most appropriate timing of antibiotic administration has been a source of controversy. Traditionally, antimicrobials were administered after the initial incision and when the umbilical cord was clamped in an attempt to minimize infant drug exposure, which theoretically could mask the signs of infection and induce antimicrobial resistance. The most recent CDC guidelines suggest that high-quality evidence supports antimicrobial administration at the time of the initial incision instead of at the time of umbilical cord clamping.[4] A meta-analysis of seven randomized controlled trials reports a 43% reduction in postpartum endometritis without an increase in neonatal sepsis or antimicrobial resistance.[4]

Hysterectomy

The most important factor affecting the incidence of SSI after hysterectomy is the type of procedure performed. Vaginal hysterectomies are associated with a high rate of postoperative infection when performed without the benefit of prophylactic antibiotics because of the polymicrobial flora normally present at the operative site.[72] As with cesarean sections, cefazolin is the drug of choice for vaginal hysterectomies despite the wide spectrum of possible pathogens.[72] The American College of Obstetricians and Gynecologists (ACOG) recommends a single dose of either cefazolin or cefoxitin.[73] For patients with a β-lactam allergy, a single preoperative dose of either metronidazole or doxycycline also is effective.[73]

Prophylactic antibiotics are recommended for abdominal hysterectomy despite the lack of bacterial contamination from the vaginal flora. Single-dose cefotetan was superior to single-dose cefazolin,[74] and the investigators suggested that cefotetan should be the drug of choice for abdominal hysterectomies. However, other investigators suggested that either agent is appropriate, provided 24 hours of antimicrobial coverage is not exceeded.[10] The ACOG guidelines suggest that first- (such as cefazolin), second- (such as cefotetan), or third-generation cephalosporins can be used for prophylaxis.[73] Metronidazole plus an aminoglycoside or fluoroquinolone is also effective and can be used if patients are allergic to β-lactam antibiotics. Antibiotic prophylaxis may not be required in laparoscopic gynecologic surgery or tubal microsurgery.[75] As with other surgical procedures, perioperative events and findings may require the use of therapeutic antibiotics after surgery.

Head-and-Neck Surgery

The use of prophylactic antibiotics during head-and-neck surgery depends on the procedure type. Clean procedures (per NRC definition), such as thyroidectomy, lymph node excision, and simple tooth extraction, are associated with a low incidence of SSI. Antimicrobial prophylaxis is not recommended for these procedures. Head-and-neck surgeries involving an incision through a mucosal layer are associated with a higher risk for SSI but antimicrobial prophylaxis is not always associated with a reduction in SSI (ie, adenoidectomy, tonsillectomy, and septoplasty).[10] The normal flora of the mouth is polymicrobial; both anaerobes and gram-positive aerobes predominate. Although typical doses of cefazolin usually are ineffective for anaerobic infections, a 2-g dose produces concentrations high enough to inhibit these organisms. A single dose of clindamycin is adequate for prophylaxis in maxillofacial surgery unless the procedure lasts longer than 4 hours, when a second dose should be administered intraoperatively.[76] The greatest evidence for antimicrobial prophylaxis is in head-and-neck cancer resection surgeries. For most head-and-neck cancer resection surgeries, including free-flap reconstruction, 24 hours of clindamycin is appropriate, and no additional benefit of extending therapy beyond 24 hours is seen. Ampicillin/sulbactam is preferred to clindamycin to cover aerobic, anaerobic, and gram-negative bacteria in clean–contaminated oncologic surgery.[77] Topical therapy with clindamycin, amoxicillin–clavulanate, and ticarcillin–clavulanate has been described in small trials, but the exact role of topical antibiotics is not defined.[78] Antimicrobial prophylaxis is not indicated for endoscopic sinus surgery without nasal packing.[36]

Cardiothoracic Surgery

Although cardiac surgery generally is considered a clean procedure, antibiotic prophylaxis lowers SSI incidence.[41] The substantial morbidity related to an SSI in this population, coupled with the routine implementation of prosthetic devices, further justifies the routine use of prophylaxis.[79] Patients who develop SSIs after coronary artery bypass graft surgery have a mortality rate of 22% at 1 year compared with 0.6% for those who do not develop an SSI.[80] Risk factors for developing an SSI after cardiac surgery include obesity, renal insufficiency, connective tissue disease, reexploration for bleeding, and poorly timed administration of antibiotics.[79] Skin flora pathogens predominate; gram-negative organisms are rare.

Cefazolin has been studied extensively and is considered the drug of choice. Although several studies and a meta-analysis advocate the use of second-generation cephalosporins (eg, cefuroxime) rather than cefazolin, various methodologic flaws in these studies have limited the extrapolation of these results to practice. Cefazolin was as effective as cefuroxime in a large, randomized trial of 702 patients undergoing open heart surgery and thus remains the standard of care.[81] Both patient weight and timing of cefazolin administration relative to surgery must be considered when developing a dosing strategy. Patients weighing greater than 80 kg (176 lb) should receive 2-g cefazolin rather than 1 g. Doses should be administered no earlier than 60 minutes before the first incision and no later than the beginning of induction.[77] Extending therapy beyond 48 hours does not further reduce SSI rates. Single-dose cefazolin therapy may be sufficient but is not recommended by the Society of Thoracic Surgeons at this time pending further study.[82]

7 Routine vancomycin administration may be justified in hospitals having a high incidence of MRSA or when sternal wounds are to be explored surgically for possible mediastinitis. However, a large comparative trial enrolling almost 900 patients in a single center with a high prevalence of MRSA infections found that both cefazolin and vancomycin had similar efficacy in preventing SSI in patients undergoing cardiac surgery that required sternotomy.[83] Mediastinitis constitutes a failure of a prior prophylactic regimen. Continued postoperative vancomycin should be guided by culture and sensitivity data.[37] Subsequent antibiotic therapy is guided by intraoperative findings.

Since *S. aureus* is routinely identified as the most common pathogen in SSIs after cardiac surgery, several studies have investigated alternative methods for preoperative eradication including nasal mupirocin administration (ie, twice daily for 5 days preoperatively) and chlorhexidine body wash (ie, daily preoperatively for up to 5 days). A bundled approach (ie, more than one intervention implemented together) in addition to preoperative antimicrobials appears to further reduce the risk of postoperative SSI in both cardiac and orthopedic surgeries.[11,84]

Pulmonary resection is associated with significant SSI risk, and prophylactic antibiotics have an established role in preventing postoperative infectious morbidity. Pleuropulmonary infections are much more common than wound infections, and pathogenic organisms likely migrate from the oral cavity or pharynx.[85] First-generation cephalosporins are inadequate; 48 hours of cefuroxime is preferred. A regimen of ampicillin–sulbactam is superior to first-generation cephalosporins, but further studies are required before this agent can be recommended as first-line prophylactic therapy.[86]

Vascular Surgery

Vascular surgery, like cardiac surgery, generally is considered clean by NRC criteria. Although vascular graft infections occur infrequently (3%-5%), the associated morbidity and mortality are extensive because treatment often requires surgical graft removal along with therapeutic antibiotic therapy.[87] Prophylactic antibiotics are of benefit, particularly for procedures involving the abdominal aorta, lower extremities, or the implantation of prosthetic devices. Cefazolin is regarded as the drug of choice. Twenty-four hours of prophylaxis with cefazolin is adequate; longer courses may lead to bacterial resistance.[88] For patients with β-lactam allergy, 24 hours of oral ciprofloxacin was effective.[87]

Orthopedic Surgery

Most orthopedic surgery is clean by definition; thus, prophylactic antibiotics generally are indicated only when prosthetic materials (eg, pins, plates, and artificial joints) are implanted.[23] A late-occurring infectious complication in this surgical population can result in substantial morbidity and may lead to prosthesis failure and subsequent removal. Staphylococci species are the most frequently encountered pathogens; gram-negative aerobes are infrequent. The use of cefazolin is supported by substantial evidence in the literature and therefore is the prophylactic agent of choice. Vancomycin, although effective, is not recommended for routine use unless a patient has a documented history of a serious allergy to β-lactams, or the propensity for MRSA infections at a particular institution necessitates its use. The current recommended duration of prophylaxis for joint replacement and hip fracture surgery is 24 hours.[10] Antibiotic-impregnated cement and beads have been used to lower SSI rates, but conclusive data regarding their efficacy are lacking.[23]

Duration of prophylaxis for the surgical repair of long bone fractures depends on the nature of the fracture. Multiple doses of prophylactic antibiotics offer no advantage over a single preoperative dose for repair of closed bone fractures and is more cost effective.[89,90] Patients suffering open (compound) fractures are particularly susceptible to infection because bacterial contamination almost always has occurred already. Under these circumstances, the use of antibiotics is presumptive. In this setting, cefazolin often is combined with an aminoglycoside, but controlled trials are lacking.[91] A clinical trial comparing clindamycin and cloxacillin suggests that clindamycin is superior and may be appropriate as monotherapy for Gustilo type I and II open fractures but not for type III fractures, for which added gram-negative activity is recommended.[92] Duration of antibiotic therapy is highly variable and depends on surgical findings during debridement, results of intraoperative cultures, and clinical status. A prospective trial and subsequent systematic review comparing short (less than 24 hours) and long (greater than 24 hours) courses of antimicrobial prophylaxis for severe trauma suggests that longer courses of antibiotics do not offer additional benefit and may be associated with the development of resistant infections.[93] However, established joint infections and osteomyelitis require an extended course of therapeutic antibiotics.

As in cardiac surgery, there is evidence to support the use of preoperative intranasal mupirocin and chlorhexidine body wash for patients colonized with *S. aureus*. For elective procedures, patients would be instructed to administer these at home in the days prior to the surgery. This bundled approach appears to further reduce the risk of postoperative SSI in addition to preoperative antimicrobials.[11,84]

Neurosurgery

The rates of SSI after clean neurosurgical operations (ie, craniotomy, spinal procedures) are low; however, the morbidity and mortality of central nervous system SSI, should they occur, are high. Preoperative antibiotics are effective at reducing SSI rates and are recommended even in clean procedures.[94,95] While many antimicrobials have been studied, a single dose of cefazolin is what is recommended.[10]

Procedures involving cerebrospinal fluid (CSF) shunt placement should be considered separately because this procedure involves placement of a foreign body and is associated with higher infection rates. A study of 780 patients undergoing neurosurgical procedures that included shunt surgery reported that single doses of cefotaxime and trimethoprim–sulfamethoxazole were equally effective in preventing SSIs.[96] Most studies of procedures involving a shunt have been small in size and do not consistently show lower infection rates with antibiotic prophylaxis, although the results of a systematic review and meta-analysis suggest that a significant improvement in the incidence of shunt infection with 24 hours of systemic antibiotics (ie, cefazolin) and the use of antibiotic-impregnated catheters independently.[97]

SSIs associated with spinal surgery are rare but devastating when they occur. The use of antimicrobial prophylaxis in this setting is warranted and recommended.[93] Large randomized, controlled trials are lacking, but cefazolin is the antibiotic recommended most commonly. Cephalosporin penetration into the vertebral disk has been questioned. Some small studies suggest that the addition of gentamicin, which has better penetration, might be warranted; however, there is a paucity of clinical trials comparing these two regimens.[98]

NONPHARMACOLOGIC INTERVENTIONS

Strategies other than antimicrobial and aseptic technique for reducing postoperative infections have been investigated in different types of surgeries. The most commonly cited and practiced interventions include intraoperative maintenance of normothermia, provision of supplemental oxygen in the perioperative period, and aggressive perioperative glucose control. Although interventions to maintain normothermia intraoperatively provide supplemental oxygen in the perioperative period, and aggressively control perioperative glucose show a significant reduction in SSI, they cannot be generalized to all types of surgeries. However, given the simplicity and low cost of these interventions, many clinicians consider applying these measures outside of the studied population(s).

Core body temperature can fall by 1°C to 1.5°C intraoperatively in patients under general anesthesia. Intraoperative hypothermia has been associated with impaired immune function, decreased blood flow to the surgical site, decreased tissue oxygen tension, and an increased risk of SSI. Efforts to maintain intraoperative normothermia should be exercised and may include the use of warming blankets and IV fluid warmers to maintain core body temperature between 36°C and 38°C. One prospective trial of 200 patients undergoing colorectal surgery found that maintenance of normothermia reduced postoperative infection rates along with other morbidity parameters, including length of stay.[99] CDC guidelines promote maintaining normothermia with strong recommendation based on moderate- to high-quality evidence.[4]

Low oxygen tension in the tissues that make up the surgical site increases the risk of bacterial colonization and subsequent SSI by decreasing the efficiency of neutrophil activity. Administration of high concentrations of oxygen (80% via ventilator or 12 L/min via a nonrebreather mask) reduced postoperative infection rates significantly in a multicenter randomized trial of 500 patients undergoing colorectal surgery.[100] Supplemental oxygen during the intraoperative and immediate postoperative periods is recommended even in patients with normal pulmonary function.[4]

Diabetes and poor glucose control are well-known risk factors for SSI. The increased risk of infection is thought to be due to both macrovascular (vasculopathy and venoocclusive disease) and microvascular (subtle immunologic deficiencies, including neutrophil dysfunction and reduced complement and antibody activity) complications. Aggressive control of perioperative blood glucose not only decreases the incidence of SSI in diabetics and nondiabetics but is also a better predictor of SSI risk than long-term glucose control (eg, as measured by hemoglobin A1C).[7,101] Perioperative blood glucose levels should be checked in all patients regardless of diabetes status and glucose targets of 6.1-8.3 mmol/L (110-150 mg/dL) are recommended.[4] In cardiac surgery the recommended target is <10 mmol/L (180 mg/dL).[7]

Prophylactic antibiotics are only effective when therapeutic concentrations in the surgical field are maintained for the entire duration of the surgery. While consideration of drug half-life in the context of the duration of surgery has been discussed earlier in this chapter, other patient-related factors may influence the effectiveness of antibiotic prophylaxis and warrant consideration when choosing a prophylactic regimen (Table 146-7).

Obese patients require larger doses of prophylactic antibiotics to maintain therapeutic drug levels when compared to nonobese patients. Patients with a body mass index greater than 40 kg/m^2 are more likely to have subtherapeutic concentrations at the end of surgery with cefazolin 1 g preoperatively (and intraoperative for surgeries greater than 3 hours) and thus should receive 2 g doses.[102] Underlying disease states that may affect antibiotic metabolism and/or elimination should be considered when developing a prophylactic regimen. For example, patients with thermal burn and spinal cord injuries eliminate certain classes of antibiotics, primarily the aminoglycosides and β-lactams, at unusually high rates compared with controls and will need more frequent intraoperative dosing. Conversely, individuals with renal failure may need less frequent dosing of renally cleared antibiotics. For example, while intraoperative dosing for cefazolin should be every 3 to 4 hours in patients with normal renal function, this interval should be extended to 8 hours for patients with creatinine clearances of less than 50 mL/min (0.83 mL/s). Individuals who are aggressively fluid resuscitated pre- or intraoperatively or those undergoing cardiac bypass may have altered antibiotic disposition related to increased volume of distribution and reduced total body clearance and may need larger doses (ie, 2-g cefazolin).

TABLE 146-7 Strategies for Implementing an Institutional Program to Ensure Appropriate Use of Antimicrobial Prophylaxis in Surgery

1. **Educate:** Develop an educational program that enforces the importance and rationale of timely antimicrobial prophylaxis. Make this educational program available to all healthcare practitioners involved in the patient's care.
2. **Standardize the ordering process:** Establish a protocol (eg, a preprinted order sheet) that standardizes antibiotic choice according to current published evidence, formulary availability, institutional resistance patterns, and cost.
3. **Standardize the delivery and administration process:** Use system that ensures antibiotics are prepared and delivered to the holding area in a timely fashion. Standardize the administration time to <1 hour preoperatively. Designate responsibility and accountability for antibiotic administration. Provide visible reminders to prescribe/administer prophylactic antibiotics (eg, checklists). Develop a system to remind surgeons/nurses to readminister antibiotics intraoperatively during long procedures.
4. **Provide feedback:** Follow up with regular reports of compliance and infection rates.

EVALUATION OF THERAPEUTIC OUTCOMES

When evaluating the outcome of surgical antibiotic prophylaxis, it is important to differentiate any potential SSI from other postoperative infection or complication. Although fever and leukocytosis are common in the immediate postoperative period, they typically resolve with prompt ambulation, timely removal of invasive devices, prevention and/or resolution of atelectasis through optimal respiratory care, and effective analgesia. It is important to remember that the emergence of distal infections, such as pneumonia, does not constitute a failure of surgical prophylaxis. Prophylaxis should be as short as possible because prolonged prophylactic regimens may contribute to the selection of resistant organisms and may make any infection more difficult to treat.

Surgical site appearance is the most important determinant of the presence of an infection. Drainage of pus from the incision accompanied by redness, warmth, and pain or tenderness is highly suggestive of an SSI. By definition, any surgical site that requires incision and drainage by the surgeon is considered infected regardless of appearance. Failure to heal and wound dehiscence also are seen with SSIs, although the surgical technique and nutritional status may be important contributing factors.

The presentation of signs and symptoms consistent with an SSI in relation to previous surgery is an important consideration when evaluating therapeutic outcomes after surgical prophylaxis. Many SSIs will not be evident during acute hospitalization. In fact, SSIs may not become evident until up to 30 days later or, in the case of prosthesis implantation, up to 1 year later. Thus, the true incidence of SSI can be determined only by completing comprehensive postdischarge surveillance. All studies investigating the efficacy of surgical prophylaxis must include adequate postdischarge follow-up to be able to thoroughly assess the success of any prophylactic regimen.

ABBREVIATIONS

ACOG	American College of Obstetricians and Gynecologists
ASA	American Society of Anesthesiologists
CDC	Centers for Disease Control and Prevention
CSF	cerebrospinal fluid
MRSA	methicillin-resistant *Staphylococcus aureus*
MSSA	methicillin-sensitive *Staphylococcus aureus*
NNIS	National Nosocomial Infections Surveillance System
NRC	National Research Council
SENIC	Study on the Efficacy of Nosocomial Infection Control
SSI	surgical site infection
WHO	World Health Organization

REFERENCES

1. Hollingsworth JM, Krein SL, Ye Z, et al. Opening of ambulatory surgery centers and procedure use in elderly patients: data from Florida. *Arch Surg* 2011;146:187–193.
2. National Hospital Discharge Survey. Available at: ftp://ftp.cdc.gov/pub/Health_Statistics/NCHS/Datset_Documentation/NHDS/NHDS_2010_Documentation.pdf. Accessed October 19, 2015.
3. Alexander JW, Solomkin JS, Edwards MJ. Updated recommendations for control of surgical site infections. *Ann Surg.* 2011;253:1082–1093.
4. Berríos-Torres SI, Umscheid CA, Bratzler DW, et al. Centers for Disease Control and Prevention Guideline for the Prevention of Surgical Site Infection, 2017. *JAMA Surg.* 2017;152(8):784–791. 10.1001/jamasurg.2017.0904.28467526.
5. Hendrick TL, Anastacio MM, Sawyer RG. Prevention of surgical site infection. *Expert Rev Anti Infect Ther.* 2006;4:223–233.
6. Kurtz SM, Lau E, Watson H, Schmier JK, Parvizi J. Economic burden of periprosthetic joint infection in the United States. *J Arthroplasty.* 2012;27(8 Suppl):61–5.e1. 10.1016/j.arth.2012.02.022.22554729.
7. Ban KA, Minei JP, Laronga C, et al. American College of Surgeons and Surgical Infection Society: Surgical Site Infection Guidelines, 2016 Update. *J Am Coll Surg.* Jan 2017;224(1):59–74. 10.1016/j.jamcollsurg.2016.10.029.27915053.
8. Stryja J, Sandy-Hodgetts K, Collier M et al. Surgical site infection: preventing and managing surgical site infection across health care sectors. *J Wound Care.* 2020;29(2)(Suppl 2b):S1–S69.
9. Cruse PJE, Foord R. A five-year prospective study of 23,649 surgical wounds. *Arch Surg.* 1973;107:206–210.
10. Bratzler DW, Dellinger EP, Olsen KM, et al. Clinical practice guidelines for antimicrobial prophylaxis in surgery. *Am J Health Syst Pharm.* 2013;70:195–283.
11. Martin ET, Kaye KS, Knott C et al. Diabetes and risk of surgical site infection: a systematic review and meta-analysis. *Infect Control Hosp Epidemiol.* 2016;37(1):88–99. https://doi.org/10.1017/ice.2015.249.
12. Drapeau CMJ, Pan A, Bellacosa C, et al. Surgical site infections in HIV-infected patients: results from an Italian prospective multicenter observational study. *Infection.* 2009;37:455–460.
13. Dionigi R, Rovera F, Dionigi G, et al. Risk factors in surgery. *J Chemother.* 2001;13:6–11.
14. Haley RW, Culver DH, Morgan WM, et al. Identifying patients at high risk of surgical wound infection: a simple multivariate index of patient susceptibility and wound contamination. *Am J Epidemiol.* 1985;127:206–215.
15. Wilson AP, Hodgson B, Liu M, et al. Reduction in wound infection rates by wound surveillance with postdischarge follow-up and feedback. *Br J Surg.* 2006;93:630–638.
16. NNIS. National Nosocomial Infections Surveillance (NNIS) System Report, data summary from January 1992 through June 2004 issued October 2004. *Am J Infect Control.* 2004;32:470–485.
17. Owens WD, Felts JA, Spitznagel EL. ASA physical status classifications: a study of consistency of ratings. *Anesthesiology.* 1978;49:239–243.
18. van Walraven C, Musselman R, et al. The Surgical Site Infection Risk Score (SSIRS): A model to predict the risk of surgical site infections. *PLoS ONE.* 2013;8(6):e67–167. https://doi.org/10.1371/journal.pone.0067167.
19. Elek SD, Conen PE. The virulence of *Staphylococcus pyogenes* for man: A study of the problems of wound infection. *Br J Exp Pathol.* 1958;38:573–586.
20. Burke JF. Identification of the sources of staphylococci contaminating the surgical wound during operation. *Ann Surg.* 1963;158:898–904.
21. Kaiser AB, Kernodle DS, Parker RA. Low-inoculum model of surgical wound infection. *J Infect Dis.* 1992;166:393–399.
22. Esposito S. Immune system and surgical site infection. *J Chemother.* 2001;13:12–16.
23. De Lalla F. Antibiotic prophylaxis in orthopedic prosthetic surgery. *J Chemother.* 2001;13:48–53.
24. Halwani M, Solaymani-Dodaran M, Grundman H, et al. Cross transmission of nosocomial pathogens in an adult intensive care unit: incidence and risk factors. *J Hosp Infect.* 2006;63:39–46.
25. Kim DH, Spencer M, Davidson SM, et al. Institutional prescreening for detection and eradication of methicillin-resistant *Staphylococcus aureus* in patients undergoing elective orthopaedic surgery. *J Bone Joint Surg Am.* 2010;92:1820–1826.
26. Munoz P, Burrillo A, Bouza E. Criteria used when initiating antifungal therapy against *Candida* spp. in the intensive care unit. *Int J Antimicrob Agents.* 2000;15:83–90.
27. Davey P, Marwick CA, Scott CL, et al. Interventions to improve antibiotic prescribing practices for hospital inpatients. *Cochrane Database Syst Rev.* Feb 9, 2017;2:CD003543. 10.1002/14651858.CD003543.pub4.28178770.
28. Sartelli M, Duane TM, Catena F, et al. Antimicrobial stewardship: a call to action for surgeons. *Surg Infect (Larchmt).* Dec 2016;17(6):625–631. 10.1089/sur.2016.187.27828764.
29. Classen DC, Evans RS, Pestotnik SL, et al. The timing of prophylactic administration of antibiotics and the risk of surgical wound infection. *N Engl J Med.* 1992;326:281–286.
30. Weber WP, Mujagic E, Zwahlen M, et al. Timing of surgical antimicrobial prophylaxis: a phase 3 randomised controlled trial *Lancet Infect Dis.* Jun 2017;17(6):605–614. 10.1016/S1473-3099(17)30176-728385346.
31. Hawn MT, Richman JS, Vicks CC, et al. Timing of surgical antibiotic prophylaxis and the risk of surgical site infection. *JAMA Surg.* 2013;148:649–657.
32. Zelenitzky SA, Ariano RE, Harding GKM, et al. Antibiotic pharmacodynamics in surgical prophylaxis: an association between intraoperative antibiotic concentrations and efficacy. *Antimicrob Agents Chemother.* 2002;46:3026–3030.
33. Goldman DA, Hopkins CC, Karchmer AW. Cephalothin prophylaxis in cardiac valve surgery: a prospective, double-blind comparison of two-day and six-day regimen. *J Thorac Cardiovasc Surg.* 1977;73:470–479.
34. Zanetti G, Flanagan HL Jr, Cohn LH, et al. Improvement of intraoperative antibiotic prophylaxis in prolonged cardiac surgery by automated alerts in the operating room. *Infect Control Hosp Epidemiol.* 2003;24:79.
35. Branch-Elliman W, O'Brien W, Strymish J, Itani K, Wyatt C, Gupta K. Association of duration and type of surgical prophylaxis with antimicrobial-associated adverse events. *JAMA Surg.* 2019;154(7):590–598. doi:10.1001/jamasurg.2019.0569.
36. Weed HG. Antimicrobial prophylaxis in the surgical patient. *Med Clin North Am.* 2003;27:59–75.
37. Salkind AR, Cuddy PG, Foxworth JW. The rational clinical examination: is this patient allergic to penicillin? An evidence-based analysis of the likelihood of penicillin allergy. *JAMA.* 2001;285:2498–2505.
38. Gemmel CG, Edwards DI, Fraise AP, et al. Guidelines for the prophylaxis and treatment of methicillin *Staphylococcus aureus* (MRSA) infections in the UK. *J Antimicrob Chemother.* 2006;57:589–608.
39. Wong RS, Cheng G, Chang NP, et al. Use of cefoperazone still needs a caution for bleeding from induced vitamin K deficiency. *Am J Hematol.* 2006;81:76.
40. Frighetto L, Marra CA, Stiver HG, et al. Economic impact of standardized orders for antimicrobial prophylaxis program. *Ann Pharmacother.* 2000;34:154–160.
41. Bratzler DW, Houck PM. Antimicrobial prophylaxis for surgery: an advisory statement from the National Surgical Infection Prevention Project. *Clin Infect Dis.* 2004;38:1706–1715.
42. Lipp A, Lusardi G. Systemic antimicrobial prophylaxis for percutaneous endoscopic gastrostomy. *Cochrane Database Syst Rev.* 2013;11:CD005571.
43. Ferraz AAB, Santa-Cruz F, Edmiston CE Jr., et al. Antibiotic prophylaxis in bariatric surgical procedures: is there an ideal antimicrobial agent? *Surg Infect* 2020;Oct:654–658.
44. Jewesson PJ, Stiver G, Wai A, et al. Double-blind comparison of cefazolin and ceftizoxime for prophylaxis against infections following elective biliary tract surgery. *Antimicrob Agents Chemother.* 1996;40:70–74.

45. Agrawal CS, Sehgal R, Singh RK, Gupta AK. Antibiotic prophylaxis in elective cholecystectomy: a randomized, double-blinded study comparing ciprofloxacin and cefuroxime. *Ind J Physiol Pharmacol.* 1999;43:501–504.
46. Swoboda S, Oberdorfer K, Klee F, et al. Tissue and serum concentrations of levofloxacin 500 mg administered intravenously or orally for antibiotic prophylaxis in biliary surgery. *J Antimicrob Chemother.* 2003;51:459–462.
47. Matsui Y, Satoi S, Hirooka S, Kosaka H, Kawaura T, Kitawaki T Reappraisal of previously reported meta-analyses on antibiotic prophylaxis for low-risk laparoscopic cholecystectomy: an overview of systematic reviews. *BMJ Open.* Mar 16, 2018;8(3):e016666. 10.1136/bmjopen-2017-01666629549197.
48. Gomez-Ospina JC, Zapata-Copete JA, Bejarano M, García-Perdomo HA. Antibiotic prophylaxis in elective laparoscopic cholecystectomy: a systematic review and network meta-analysis. *J Gastrointest Surg.* Mar 19, 2018. 10.1007/s11605-018-3739-429556974.
49. Gulberg V, Deibert P, Ochs A, et al. Prevention of infectious complications after transjugular intrahepatic portosystemic shunt in cirrhotic patients with a single dose of ceftriaxone. *Hepatogastroenterology.* 1999;46:1126–1130.
50. Deibert P, Schwartz S, Olschewski M, et al. Risk factors and prevention of early infection after implantation or revision of transjugular intrahepatic portosystemic shunts: results of a randomized study. *Dig Dis Sci.* 1998;43:1708–1713.
51. Andersen BR, Kallehave FL, Andersen HK. Antibiotics versus placebo for prevention of postoperative infection after appendicectomy. *Cochrane Database Syst Rev.* 2005;3:CD001439.
52. Liberman MA, Greason KL, Frame S, Ragland JJ. Single-dose cefotetan or cefoxitin versus multiple-dose cefoxitin as prophylaxis in patients undergoing appendectomy for acute nonperforated appendicitis. *J Am Coll Surg.* 1995;180:77–80.
53. Migaly J, Bafford AC, Francone TD, Clinical Practice Guidelines Committee of the American Society of Colon and Rectal Surgeons. The American Society of Colon and Rectal Surgeons clinical practice guidelines for the use of bowel preparation in elective colon and rectal surgery. *Dis Colon Rectum.* Jan 2019;62(1):3–8.
54. Zmora O, Wexner SD, Hajjar L, et al. Trend in preparation for colorectal surgery: survey of the members of the American Society of Colon and Rectal Surgeons. *Am Surg.* 2003;69:150–154.
55. Zmora O, Mahajna A, Bar-Zakai B, et al. Colon and rectal surgery without mechanical bowel preparation: a randomized, prospective trial. *Ann Surg.* 2003;237:363–367.
56. Cao F, Li J, Li F. Mechanical bowel preparation for elective colorectal surgery: updated systematic review and meta-analysis. *Int J Colorectal Dis.* 2012;27:803–810.
57. Dahabreh IJ, Steele DW, Shah N, Trikalinos TA. Oral Mechanical Bowel Preparation for Colo-rectal Surgery. Comparative Effectiveness Review No. 128. Rockville, MD: Agency for Healthcare Research and Quality; April 2014. AHRQ Publication No. 14-EHC018-EF. Available at: www.effectivehealthcare.ahrq.gov/reports/final.cfm. Accessed October 19, 2015.
58. Baum ML, Anish DS, Chalmers TC, et al. A survey of clinical trials of antibiotic prophylaxis in colon surgery: evidence against further use of no-treatment controls. *N Engl J Med.* 1981;305:795–799.
59. Nelson RL, Gladman E, Barbateskovic M. Antimicrobial prophylaxis for colorectal surgery. *Cochrane Database Syst Rev.* 2014;5:CD001181.
60. Battersby CLF, Hajibandeh S, Hajibandeh S. Oral antibiotics as adjunct to systemic antibiotics and mechanical bowel preparation for prevention of surgical site infections in colorectal surgery. Do we really need more trials? *Dis Colon Rectum.* Jun 2018;61(6):e341–e342.
61. Fujita S, Saito N, Yamada T, et al. Randomized, multicenter trial of antibiotic prophylaxis in elective colorectal surgery: single dose vs 3 doses of a second-generation cephalosporin without metronidazole and oral antibiotics. *Arch Surg.* 2007;142:657–661.
62. Mittelkotter U. Antimicrobial prophylaxis for abdominal surgery: is there a need for metronidazole? *J Chemother.* 2001;13:27–34.
63. Kobayashi M, Mohri Y, Tonouchi H, et al. Randomized clinical trial comparing intravenous antimicrobial prophylaxis alone with oral and intravenous antimicrobial prophylaxis for the prevention of a surgical site infection in colorectal cancer surgery. *Surg Today.* 2007;37:383–388.
64. Ghorra SG, Rzeczycki TP, Natarajan R, Pricolo VE. Colostomy closure: impact of preoperative risk factors on morbidity. *Am Surg.* 1999;65:266–269.
65. ASGE Standards of Practice Committee. Antibiotic prophylaxis for GI endoscopy. *Gastrointest Endosc.* 2015;81:81–89.
66. Sharma VK, Howden CW. Meta-analysis of randomized, controlled trials of antibiotic prophylaxis before percutaneous endoscopic gastrostomy. *Am J Gastroenterol.* 2001;96:1951–1952.
67. Wolf Jr JS, Bennett CJ, Dmochowski RR, Hollenbeck BK, Pearles MS, Schaeffer AJ. Best practice policy statement on urologic surgery antimicrobial prophylaxis. *J Urol.* 2008;179:1379–1390.
68. Christiano AP, Hollowell CM, Kim H, et al. Double-blind, randomized comparison of single-dose ciprofloxacin versus intravenous cefazolin in patients undergoing outpatient endourologic surgery. *Urology.* 2000;55:182–185.
69. Smaill FM, Grivell R. Antibiotic prophylaxis versus noprophylaxis for preventing infection after cesarean section. *Cochrane Database System Rev.* 2014;100.1002/14651858. Art. No.: CD007482.
70. Committee on Practice Bulletins-Obstetrics. ACOG Practice Bulletin No. 199: Use of prophylactic antibiotics in labor and delivery. *Obstet Gynecol.* Sep2018;132(3):e103–e119.
71. Tita AT, Szychowski JM, Boggess K, et al. Adjunctive azithromycin prophylaxis for cesarean delivery. *N Engl J Med.* Sep 29, 2016;375(13):1231–1241. 10.1056/NEJMoa160204427682034.
72. Guaschino S, De Santo D, De Seta F. New perspectives in antibiotic prophylaxis for obstetric and gynaecological surgery. *J Hosp Infect.* 2002;50(suppl A):S13–S16.
73. ACOG Practice Bulletin No. 195: Prevention of infection after gynecologic procedures. *Obstet Gynecol.* Jun2018;131(6):e172–e189.
74. Hemsell DL, Johnson ER, Hemsell PG, et al. Cefazolin is inferior to cefotetan as single dose prophylaxis for women undergoing elective total abdominal hysterectomy. *Clin Infect Dis.* 1995;20:677–684.
75. Sturlese E, Retto G, Pulia A, et al. Benefits of antibiotic prophylaxis in laparoscopic gynaecological surgery. *Clin Exp Obstet Gynecol.* 1999;26:217–218.
76. Meuller SC, Henkel KO, Neumann J, et al. Perioperative antibiotic prophylaxis in maxillofacial surgery: penetration of clindamycin into various tissues. *J Craniomaxillofac Surg.* 1999;27:172–176.
77. Van der Poorten V, Uyttebroek S, Robbins KT, et al. Perioperative antibiotics in clean-contaminated head and neck surgery: a systematic review and meta-analysis. *Adv Ther.* Apr2020;37(4):1360–1380.
78. Grandis JR, Vickers RM, Rihs JD, et al. Efficacy of topical amoxicillin plus clavulanate–ticarcillin plus clavulanate and clindamycin in contaminated head and neck surgery: effect of antibiotic spectra and duration of therapy. *J Infect Dis.* 1994;170:729–732.
79. Roy MC. Surgical-site infections after coronary artery bypass graft surgery: discriminating site-specific risk factors to improve prevention efforts. *Infect Control Hosp Epidemiol.* 1998;19:229–233.
80. Hollenbeak CS, Murphy DM, Koenig S, et al. The clinical and economic impact of deep chest surgical site infections following coronary artery bypass graft surgery. *Chest.* 2000;118:397–402.
81. Curtis JJ, Boley TM, Walls JT, et al. Randomized, prospective comparison of first- and second-generation cephalosporins as infection prophylaxis for cardiac surgery. *Am J Surg.* 1993;166:734–737.
82. Edwards FH, Egleman RM, Houck P, et al. The society of thoracic surgeons practice guidelines series: antibiotic prophylaxis in cardiac surgery, part 1: duration. *Ann Thorac Surg.* 2006;81:397–404.
83. Finkelstein R, Rabino G, Masiah T, et al. Vancomycin versus cefazolin prophylaxis for cardiac surgery in the setting of a high prevalence of methicillin-resistant staphylococcal infections. *J Thorac Cardiovasc Surg.* 2002;123:326–332.
84. Schweizer ML, Perencevich E, McDaniel J, et al. Effectiveness of a bundled intervention of decolonization and prophylaxis to decrease Gram positive surgical site infections after cardiac or orthopedic surgery: systematic review and meta-analysis. *BMJ.* 2013;346:f2743.
85. Sok M, Dragas AZ, Erzen J, et al. Sources of pathogens causing pleuropulmonary infections after lung cancer resection. *Eur J Cardiothorac Surg.* 2002;22:23–27.
86. Boldt J, Piper S, Uphus D, et al. Preoperative microbiologic screening and antibiotic prophylaxis in pulmonary resection operations. *Ann Thorac Surg.* 1999;68:208–211.
87. Pratesi C, Russo D, Dorigo W, et al. Antibiotic prophylaxis in clean surgery: Vascular surgery. *J Chemother.* 2001;13:123–128.
88. Terpstra S, Noorkhoek GT, Voesten HG, et al. Rapid emergence of resistant coagulase-negative staphylococci on the skin after antibiotic prophylaxis. *J Hosp Infect.* 1999;43:195–202.
89. Slobogean GP, Kennedy SA, Davidson D, et al. Single- versus multiple-dose antibiotic prophylaxis in the surgical treatment of closed fractures: a meta-analysis. *J Orthop Trauma.* 2008;22:264–269.
90. Slobogean PG, O'Brien PJ, Brauer CA. Single-dose versus multiple-dose antibiotic prophylaxis for the surgical treatment of closed fractures: a cost-effective analysis. *Acta Orthop.* 2010;81:256–262.

91. Gillespie WJ, Walenkamp G. Antibiotic prophylaxis for surgery for proximal femoral and other closed long bone fractures. *Cochrane Database Syst Rev.* 2001;1:CD000244.
92. Vasenius J, Tulikoura I, Vainionpaa S, Rokkanen P. Clindamycin versus cloxacillin in the treatment of 240 open fractures: a randomized, prospective study. *Ann Chir Gynaecol.* 1998;87:224–228.
93. Shaffer WO, Baisden JL, Fernand R, Matz PG. An evidence-based clinical guideline for antibiotic prophylaxis in spine surgery. *Spine J.* Oct 2013;13(10):1387–1392. 10.1016/j.spinee.2013.06.030.23988461.
94. Barker FG II. Efficacy of prophylactic antibiotics against meningitis after craniotomy: a meta-analysis. *Neurosurgery.* 2007;60:887–894.
95. Watters WC 3rd, Baisden J, Bono CM, et al. Antibiotic prophylaxis in spine surgery: an evidence-based clinical guideline for the sue of prophylactic antibiotics in spine surgery. *Spine J.* 2009;9:142–146.
96. Whitby M, Johnson BC, Atkinson RL, et al. The comparative efficacy of intravenous cefotaxime and trimethoprim/sulfamethoxazole in preventing infection after neurosurgery: a prospective, randomized study. Brisbane Neurosurgical Infection Group. *Br J Neurosurg.* 2000;14:13–18.
97. Ratilal B, Costa J, Sampaio C. Antibiotic prophylaxis for surgical introduction of intracranial ventricular shunts: a systematic review. *J Neurosurg Pediatr.* 2008;1:48–56.
98. Riley LH 3rd. Prophylactic antibiotics for spine surgery: description of a regimen and its rationale. *J South Orthop Assoc.* 1998;7:212–217.
99. Kurz A, Sessler DI, Lenhardt R. Perioperative normothermia to reduce the incidence of surgical-wound infection and shorten hospitalization. Study of Wound Infection and Temperature Group. *N Engl J Med.* 1996;334:1209–1215.
100. Greif R, Akca O, Horn EP, et al. Supplemental perioperative oxygen to reduce the incidence of surgical-wound infection. Outcomes Research Group. *N Engl J Med.* 2000;342:161–167.
101. Kao LS, Meeks D, Moyer VA, Lally KP. Peri-operative glycaemic control regimens for preventing surgical site infections in adults. *Cochrane Database Syst Rev.* 2009;3:CD006806.
102. Ho VP, Nicolau DP, Dakin GF, et al. Cefazolin dosing for surgical prophylaxis in morbidly obese patients. *Surg Infect (Larchmt).* 2012;13:33–37.

Vaccines and Immunoglobulins 147

Mary S. Hayney

KEY CONCEPTS

1. Live vaccines may confer life-long immunity but cannot be administered to immunosuppressed patients.
2. Inactivated and subunit vaccines and toxoids often require multiple doses to protect from infection, and generally booster doses are needed following the primary series.
3. Children less than 2 years of age are unable to mount T-cell–independent immune responses that are elicited by polysaccharide vaccines.
4. Severely immunocompromised individuals should not receive live vaccines, and their responses to inactivated, polysaccharide, toxoid, and recombinant vaccines may be poor.
5. The childhood and adult immunization schedules are updated frequently and published annually. These documents can be used to develop an immunization plan.
6. Immunoglobulin (Ig) provides short-term, rapid postexposure protection from measles, hepatitis A, varicella, and other infections.
7. Ig adverse effects are often secondary to infusion rate. Slowing the IV infusion rate ameliorate chills, nausea, and fever that may develop during administration.
8. Rh_0(D) Ig prevents Rh-negative mothers from mounting an immune response against the Rh(D) antigen on the red blood cells of the fetus that results in hemolytic disease of the newborn.

BEYOND THE BOOK

Devise immunization recommendations for the below mentioned cases.

1. A 56-year-old male with newly diagnosed type 2 diabetes who has not received any vaccines in the past 12 years.
2. A 26-year-old patient who was fully immunized prior to kidney transplant 6 years ago.
3. A 52-year-old male who smokes a pack of cigarettes every day and has not received any vaccines as an adult.
4. A healthy 5 month old child who has not received any vaccines.

Use the immunization schedules found at https://www.cdc.gov/vaccines/schedules

INTRODUCTION

Immunization provides protection from infectious diseases. Immunity to an infectious agent can be acquired by exposure to the disease, by transfer of antibodies from mother to fetus, through administration of immunoglobulin (Ig), and from vaccination. Immunization is the process of introducing an antigen into the body to induce protection against the infectious agent without causing disease. An *antigen* is a substance that induces an immune response. An *antibody* produced by the humoral arm of the immune system usually is the response that is measured as evidence of successful vaccination. However, cellular immune responses, which are more difficult to measure, are also an important aspect of vaccine responses. This chapter introduces the clinical use of vaccines and immunoglobulins. Agents with a limited use, such as agents for bioterrorism or travel, are beyond the scope of this chapter.

PRODUCTS USED TO IMMUNIZE

1 2 3 Vaccines induce active immunity—that is, immunity generated by a natural immunologic response to an antigen. Vaccines can be live-attenuated or inactivated. Inactivated vaccines may consist of whole or part of the pathogen that induces a protective immune response. Live-attenuated vaccines induce an immunologic response similar to that occurring with natural infection. Because the organisms in live-attenuated vaccines undergo limited replication in the vaccinated individual after administration, they may confer lifelong immunity with one dose (as does a natural infection). Viral vector vaccines are transfected with the gene for the antigen to which immunization is desired. The viral vector which can be further engineered to not replicate, is just the carrier for the gene. The viral vector enters the cell inducing an immune response to the target infection when the inserted gene is expressed during the course of the "infection." With an mRNA vaccine, the mRNA is protected by a liposome from degradation and facilitates its entry into cells, then uses cellular machinery to transcribe the mRNA. Following transcription, the antigen is expressed as a protein on the cell surface which initiates an immune response. Multiple doses of inactivated vaccines usually are needed to induce long-lasting, effective immunity. Additional doses at varying time intervals (booster doses) often are required to maintain immunity. Booster doses of such vaccines elicit memory responses from the B cells that produce immunoglobulin G (IgG). The immune system already has developed an array of antibodies to the antigen. Upon restimulation with a booster dose, the B cells, which produce the most specific antibodies against the antigen, are selected and maintained in the "immunologic memory." Thus, the booster dose results in a rapid, intense antibody response that is long-lasting. Inactivated vaccines can also differ in immunity potential, depending on their composition. For example, polysaccharide vaccines tend to be poorly immunogenic in infants, whereas protein–polysaccharide conjugated vaccines of the same antigen tend to be highly immunogenic (eg, pneumococcal polysaccharide vaccine vs pneumococcal conjugated vaccine). T-cell–independent immune response is made to polysaccharide antigens that stimulate B cells directly.[1] There is no maturation or booster response with a T-cell–independent immune response, and children younger than

2 years cannot make this type of response. Protein–polysaccharide conjugate vaccines stimulate T cells and promote interactions between T cells and B cells when producing the protective immune responses consisting of immunologic memory and high-affinity IgG. Toxoids are inactivated bacterial toxins that stimulate the production of antibodies against the bacterial toxins rather than the infecting bacterial pathogens.

Immunoglobulins (Igs) are sterile solutions containing antibody derived from human (Ig) sources. Igs are derived from donor pools of blood plasma and are processed using cold ethanol fractionation in order to inactivate known potential pathogens. These products are indicated for induction of passive immunity (temporary immunity to infection as a result of administration of antibodies not produced by the host; see other immunoglobulins below).

In addition to the active component in a vaccine, other active and inert ingredients are often present. Some inactivated vaccines contain adjuvants which are chemicals that stimulate a strong, but short-lived inflammatory response which strengthens the immune response to the antigen. These adjuvants also increase local tissue irritation when injected. Suspending agents, such as water, saline, or complex fluids containing proteins (eg, albumin), are used as the vehicle for the vaccines. Preservatives, stabilizers, and antibiotics may be added to help maintain the integrity of the product. Immunized individuals may respond with allergic reactions not to the agent itself but to the other components of the pharmaceutical preparation. Different manufacturers of the vaccines have different active and inert ingredients or different quantities of these ingredients in their products.

Some vaccines manufactured by different companies are considered interchangeable. Hepatitis A, hepatitis B, and *Haemophilus influenzae* type b (Hib) conjugate vaccines from different manufacturers used for the primary series of three doses are considered interchangeable. It is preferable to use diphtheria, tetanus toxoids, and acellular pertussis (DTaP) vaccine from the same manufacturer to complete the entire primary series. However, immunization should not be delayed if the particular type of vaccine administered for the initial doses cannot be ascertained easily or the vaccine provider does not have the product available.[1]

FACTORS AFFECTING RESPONSE TO IMMUNIZATION

Various factors are known to affect response to vaccines. Viability of the live antigen is an important factor as discussed previously. Total dose also is important because there seems to exist a threshold dose above which no further increase in immune response is seen. The interval between immunization doses, number of doses given, or both may change immune response to an agent. Among hepatitis B vaccine nonresponders, a significant proportion of individuals mount a vaccine response when given additional doses of vaccine.[2] In contrast, additional doses of influenza vaccine are minimally effective in individuals with chronic illness.[3] Generally, intervals longer than those recommended between vaccine doses do not affect immune response.[1]

The route and site of administration of the immunobiologic are important. This is best illustrated by the hepatitis B vaccine, which elicits a satisfactory antibody response when given in the deltoid muscle but not a consistent response when administered in the gluteal area. Injections should be administered at a site with little likelihood of site damage. Vaccines containing adjuvants should be given into a muscle mass because they can cause irritation when given subcutaneously or intradermally.[1]

Host factors influence vaccine response. Immunocompromise, increasing age, underlying disease, and genetic background have been associated with poor response rates.[1–6]

VACCINE ADMINISTRATION

Subcutaneous injections should be administered into the thigh of infants and in the upper arm area over the triceps of older children and adults. A ⅝-in., 25-gauge needle (0.508 mm × 1.6 cm) should be used, taking care not to administer the dose intradermally or intramuscularly (IM). For IM injection, the anterolateral aspect of the upper thigh (infants and toddlers) or the deltoid muscle of the upper arm (children and adults) should be used. Appropriate needle size and length are important to both vaccine immune response and safety (TABLE 147-1). The buttock should not be used because of the potential for inadequate immunologic response and the potential risk of injury to the sciatic nerve. When the buttock must be used (as for large doses of Ig), only the upper outer quadrant should be used with the needle inserted anteriorly.

The rotavirus vaccines are administered orally. The tube of vaccine should be squeezed inside the infant's mouth toward the inner cheek until the dosing tube is empty. If the infant regurgitates or spits out the vaccine, readministration is not recommended.[7]

Live-attenuated influenza vaccine is administered intranasally.[3] A specially designed sprayer is inserted just inside the nostril, and the dose is sprayed by rapidly depressing the plunger of the sprayer. The clip is removed from the plunger so that the second half of the dose can be administered into the other nostril. The vaccinated individual should breathe normally. The dose does not need to be repeated if the individual sneezes during or shortly after administration.

Questions often arise concerning the simultaneous administration of vaccines. In general, inactivated and live-attenuated vaccines can be administered simultaneously at separate sites. If two or more inactivated

TABLE 147-1 Needle Length and Injection Site for Intramuscular Vaccine Administration

Age Group	Needle Length	Injection Site
Neonates (0-28 days)	5/8 in. (16 mm)[a]	Anterolateral thigh
Infants (1-12 months)	1 in. (25 mm)	Anterolateral thigh
Toddlers (1-2 years)	1-1.25 in. (25-32 mm)	Anterolateral thigh[b]
	5/8-1 in. (16-25 mm)	Deltoid muscle
Children (3-10 years)	5/8-1 in. (16-25 mm)	Deltoid muscle[b]
	1-1.25 in. (25-32 mm)	Anterolateral thigh
Children (11-18 years)	5/8-1 in. (16-25 mm)	Deltoid muscle[b]
	1-1.5 in. (25-38 mm)	Anterolateral thigh
Adults (>19 years)		
Men and women < 60 kg (130 lb)	1 in. (25 mm)[c]	Deltoid muscle
Men 70-118 kg (152-260 lb)	1-1.5 in. (25-38 mm)	Deltoid muscle
Women 70-90 kg (152-200 lb)		
Men >118 kg (260 lb)	1.5 in. (38 mm)	Deltoid muscle
Women >90 kg (200 lb)		

[a]Skin should be stretched without bunching of subcutaneous tissue.

[b]This table is not intended for determining the correct indications and dosages for using antibody-containing products. Unvaccinated persons might not be fully protected against measles during the entire recommended interval, and additional doses of Ig or measles vaccine might be indicated after measles exposure. Concentrations of measles antibody in an Ig preparation can vary by manufacturer's lot. Rates of antibody clearance after receipt of an Ig preparation also might vary. Recommended intervals are extrapolated from an estimated half-life of 30 days for passively acquired antibody and an observed interference with the immune response to measles vaccine for 5 months after a dose of 80 mg IgG/kg.

[c]Some experts recommend 5/8 in. (16 mm) needle, but skin must be stretched without bunching of subcutaneous tissue.

Adapted from Kroger A, Bahta L, Hunter P. General Best Practice Guidelines for Immunization. Best Practices Guidance of the Advisory Committee on Immunization Practices (ACIP).

TABLE 147-2 Recommended Intervals Between Administration of Immunoglobulin and Measles- or Varicella-Containing Vaccine[a]

Product/Indication	Dose, Including mg Immunoglobulin G(IgG)/kg Body Weight	Recommended Interval before Measles or Varicella-containing[b] Vaccine Administration
RSV monoclonal antibody (Synagis®)[c]	15 mg/kg IM	None
TIG	250 units (10 mg IgG/kg) IM	3 months
Hepatitis A Ig		
Contact prophylaxis	0.02 mL/kg (3.3 mg IgG/kg) IM	3 months
International travel	0.06 mL/kg (10 mg IgG/kg) IM	3 months
HBIG	0.06 mL/kg (10 mg IgG/kg) IM	3 months
RIG	20 IU/kg (22 mg IgG/kg) IM	4 months
Measles prophylaxis Ig		
Standard (ie, nonimmunocompromised) contact	0.5 mL/kg (40 mg IgG/kg) IM	6 months
Blood transfusion		
RBCs, washed	10 mL/kg negligible IgG/kg IV	None
RBCs, adenine-saline added	10 mL/kg (10 mg IgG/kg) IV	3 months
Packed RBCs (Hct 65%) [0.65][d]	10 mL/kg (60 mg IgG/kg) IV	6 months
Whole blood (Hct 35%-50%) (0.35-0.50)[d]	10 mL/kg (80-100 mg IgG/kg) IV	6 months
Plasma/platelet products	10 mL/kg (160 mg IgG/kg) IV	7 months
Cytomegalovirus IV immunoglobulin (IGIV)	150 mg/kg maximum	6 months
IVIG		
Replacement therapy for immune deficiencies[e]	300-400 mg/kg Iv[d]	8 months
Immune thrombocytopenic purpura treatment	400 mg/kg IV	8 months
Immune thrombocytopenic purpura treatment	1 g/kg IV	10 months
Postexposure varicella prophylaxis[f]	400 mg/kg IV	8 months
Varicella Ig	125 units/kg (60-200 mg IgG/kg) IM maximum 625 units	5 months

HBIG, hepatitis B Ig; RBCs, red blood cells; RIg, rabies Ig; TIG, tetanus Ig.

[a]This table is not intended for determining the correct indications and dosages for using antibody-containing products. Unvaccinated persons might not be fully protected against measles during the entire recommended interval, and additional doses of Ig or measles vaccine might be indicated after measles exposure. Concentrations of measles antibody in an Ig preparation can vary by manufacturer's lot. Rates of antibody clearance after receipt of an Ig preparation also might vary. Recommended intervals are extrapolated from an estimated half-life of 30 days for passively acquired antibody and an observed interference with the immune response to measles vaccine for 5 months after a dose of 80 mg IgG/kg.

[b]Varicella-containing vaccine, as used here, does not include zoster vaccine. Zoster vaccine may be given without regard to antibody-containing blood products.

[c]Contains antibody only to respiratory syncytial virus (RSV).

[d]Assumes a serum IgG concentration of 16 mg/mL (g/L).

[e]Measles and varicella vaccinations are recommended for children with asymptomatic or mildly symptomatic human immunodeficiency virus (HIV) infection but are contraindicated for persons with severe immunosuppression from HIV or any other immunosuppressive disorder.

vaccines cannot be administered simultaneously, they can be administered without regard to spacing between doses. Inactivated and live vaccines can be administered simultaneously or, if they cannot be administered simultaneously, at any interval between doses. If live vaccines are not administered simultaneously, their administration should be separated by at least 4 weeks. Live viral vaccines may interfere with purified protein derivative response; thus, tuberculin testing should be postponed for 4 to 6 weeks after administration of live-virus vaccine.[1]

Simultaneous administration of Ig and live-attenuated vaccines may interfere with host antibody response. A dose relationship exists between administration of Ig and inhibition of immune response to a vaccine (TABLE 147-2). Whole blood and other blood products containing antibodies may interfere with the response to the measles, mumps, rubella, and varicella vaccines. In any individual, if vaccination with MMR or varicella is followed by emergency Ig administration, the vaccine can be repeated or seroconversion to viral antigens can be confirmed after sufficient time has elapsed (see TABLE 147-2). Ig does not interfere with the response to oral vaccines. Inactivated vaccines and Igs may be administered simultaneously using separate anatomical sites.[1]

VACCINE STORAGE

Appropriate storage is critical to maintaining the integrity of vaccines. Refrigerator temperature is defined as between 2°C and 8°C (36°F to 46°F) and freezer temperature as 50°C (−58°F) to −15°C (5°F). Inactivated vaccines are stored refrigerated. Varicella and COVID-19 (Moderna) vaccine must be stored frozen. MMR vaccine can be stored in either the freezer or refrigerator. The Pfizer COVID-19 vaccine requires ultra-cold temperatures (−80°C to −60°C; −112°F to −76°F) for long-term storage. Live-attenuated influenza vaccine is stored in the refrigerator. Specific storage conditions for individual vaccines can be found in the package insert.

IMMUNIZATION OF SPECIAL POPULATIONS

Groups of individuals may have precautions to vaccines. Many precautions are temporary, and vaccines can be administered later.

Infants

The age of the recipient is an important determining factor in vaccine response. In the first few months of life, passively transferred maternal antibodies acquired during the third trimester of gestation protect an infant. However, the maternal antibodies also inhibit the immune response to live vaccines because the circulating antibodies neutralize the vaccine before the infant has the opportunity to mount an immune response. For this reason, MMR and varicella vaccines are not administered until maternal antibodies have waned, generally by infant age 12 months.

Premature infants should be vaccinated at the same chronologic age using the same schedule and precautions for full-term infants. The full recommended doses of vaccines should be used, regardless of age or birth weight. Breastfed infants should be vaccinated according to standard pediatric schedules.

Pregnant Females and Postpartum Immunization

The benefit of most vaccines outweighs the risk for administration to those who are pregnant. As with most drugs, a lack of information regarding risks to the fetus exists rather than any actual known risk.[1] For example, no cases of congenital rubella syndrome from inadvertent administration of rubella vaccine to a pregnant person have ever been reported. Universal influenza immunization is recommended for individuals who will be or are pregnant during influenza season. Tdap should be administered during the late second trimester or third trimester of pregnancy.[8] Although live vaccines generally are avoided because of the theoretical risk of transmission of the vaccine organism to the fetus, inactivated vaccines may be administered when the benefits outweigh the risks.[1] Insufficient evidence is available for the human papillomavirus (HPV) series during pregnancy, so it should be deferred.[1]

Administration of live vaccines, such as rubella or varicella, is deferred until pregnancy is completed and is routinely recommended for those who do not have evidence of immunity prior to hospital discharge. These live vaccines can be administered without regard to administration of Rh_o(D) Ig in the postpartum period. Additionally, Tdap is recommended for all new mothers who have not received a Tdap before because household contacts are frequently implicated as the source of pertussis infection in a young infant.[8]

Immunocompromised Hosts

4 Immunization of individuals with chronic disease, such as immunocompromise, diabetes or connective tissue disease, alcoholism, or those with cancer or HIV disease, must be individualized based on the disease state and its treatment. In general, severely immunocompromised individuals should not receive live vaccines. Administration of other vaccines may be indicated, but responses may be lower than those mounted by healthy individuals, but may still confer protection.[4]

Patients with chronic pulmonary, renal, hepatic, or metabolic disease who are not receiving immunosuppressants can receive both live-attenuated and killed vaccines and toxoids. Generally, immunization should be considered early in the course of the disease in an attempt to induce immunity at a point when the disease is less severe.

Patients with active malignant disease can receive killed vaccines or toxoids but should not be given live vaccines. The MMR vaccine is not contraindicated for close contacts, however. Live-virus vaccines can be administered to persons with leukemia who have not received chemotherapy for at least 3 months. Vaccines should be timed so that they do not coincide with the start of chemotherapy or radiation therapy.[3] Annual influenza vaccine should be administered 2 weeks prior to chemotherapy or between cycles.[3] If vaccines cannot be given at least 2 weeks before the start of these therapies, immunization should be postponed until 3 months after the therapy has been completed. Passive immunization with Ig can be used in place of active immunization regardless of the history of immunization.

Glucocorticoids may cause suppressed responses to vaccines. For the purposes of immunization, the immunosuppressing dose of corticosteroids is prednisone 20 mg or more daily or 2 mg/kg daily, or an equivalent dose of another steroid, for at least 2 weeks. Patients receiving long-term, alternate-day steroid therapy with short-acting agents, administration of maintenance physiologic doses of steroids (eg, 5-10 mg/day of prednisone) topical, aerosol, intra-articular, bursal, or tendon steroid injections require no special consideration for immunization. If patients have been receiving high-dose corticosteroids or have had a course lasting longer than 2 weeks, then at least 1 month should pass before immunization with live-virus vaccines.[1]

Patients with HIV infection may have suboptimal immune responses to live and inactivated vaccines. The routinely recommended vaccines should be administered to children. MMR should be administered to anyone older than 12 months of age without evidence of immunity and who are not severely immunocompromised (CD4% greater than 15% [or CD4 fraction >0.15] and CD4 count greater than 200 lymphocytes/mm^3 [0.2×10^9/L] for at least 6 months) and repeat MMR series should be considered if vaccinated prior to initiation of combination antiretroviral therapy.[9] Two doses of varicella vaccine separated by 3 months are recommended for those with no evidence of immunosuppression. Adults should receive routinely recommended vaccines. Zoster vaccine may be administered to individuals with HIV infection who do not have clinical manifestations of AIDS and have CD4 counts greater than 200/mm^3 (0.2×10^9/L).[1]

Solid Organ Transplant Patients

Organ transplantation has become routine treatment of end-stage organ disease of many causes. Solid organ transplant patients remain on immunosuppressive regimens for the rest of their lives. These immunosuppressive regimens result in a higher risk of infection and decrease the protection conferred by immunization.[10]

Whenever possible, transplant patients should be immunized prior to transplantation. Live vaccines generally are not given after transplantation. Posttransplantation diphtheria, tetanus, pneumococcal, and influenza vaccine responses are unpredictable. Decreased immune response has been documented following hepatitis B vaccine series.

Patients with Hematopoietic Stem Cell Transplant

Patients with hematopoietic stem cell transplantation receive therapy that almost eliminates hematopoietic cells and may require immunosuppressive medications post-transplant for graft-versus-host disease. Therefore, reimmunization with inactivated vaccines should begin approximately 6 months after hematopoietic stem cell transplantation. Annual influenza immunization may begin as soon as 6 months after successful engraftment. Hematopoietic stem cell transplant recipients are at increased risk for fulminant infection with encapsulated bacteria, so pneumococcal vaccines, meningococcal vaccines, and Hib vaccines are recommended. MMR and varicella vaccines can be administered at 24 months. Immunization of household contacts and healthcare workers also is necessary.[1,11]

CONTRAINDICATIONS AND PRECAUTIONS

There are few contraindications to the use of vaccines except those outlined earlier. The contraindications include a history of anaphylactic reactions to the vaccine or a component of the vaccine.

Unexplained encephalopathy occurring within 7 days of a dose of pertussis vaccine is a contraindication to future doses of pertussis vaccines. Immunosuppression and pregnancy are temporary contraindications to live vaccines. An interval of time must elapse based on the dose of Ig before a live vaccine can be administered (see TABLE 147-2). A personal or family history of seizures is a precaution for receiving the combination MMR–varicella (MMRV) vaccine. Immunizers should use MMR and varicella vaccines separately.[1] Generally, mild-to-moderate local reactions, mild acute illnesses, concurrent antibiotic use, prematurity, family history of adverse events, diarrhea, and lactation or breastfeeding are not contraindications to immunization.

OBTAINING AN IMMUNIZATION HISTORY

An immunization history should be obtained from every patient, regardless of the reason for the healthcare visit. State-based or other public health jurisdiction-based immunization information systems, also called immunization registries, have been developed to improve immunization coverage by allowing healthcare providers access to records at any contact with the healthcare system. If an official written record is not available, patient characteristics (eg, military service, travel history, and occupation) may provide clues to the immunization history. Serologic testing for immunity has a limited role in documenting immunization history but is done in selected circumstances (eg, employment in a healthcare facility). If a written record does not exist, one should be generated at the time of initiation of immunization. Patients without a written record should be considered susceptible, and an immunization program started and completed unless a serious adverse reaction occurs. As a general rule, the risks associated with overimmunization are minimal relative to the risks associated with contracting vaccine-preventable diseases.[1]

Every healthcare visit, regardless of its purpose, should be viewed as an opportunity to review a patient's immunization status and to administer needed vaccines. Immunization is perhaps the most cost-effective health intervention available. Each visit should include assessment of individuals' vaccine needs, administration of indicated vaccines, and documentation of immunization histories. The outcome measurement of what percentage of patients in a particular practice site is completely immunized is extremely important because the benefits of optimal vaccine use extend beyond the individual patient to the public as a whole.

VACCINE SAFETY

The United States has a robust vaccine safety monitoring system. Healthcare providers must report all events requiring medical attention within 30 days of vaccination to the Vaccine Adverse Event Reporting System (VAERS), which serves as a central depot for vaccine-related adverse effects. Only a temporal association between the adverse event and vaccine administration is required. No adverse event rates can be determined because only the number of adverse events reported is known; the number of vaccines administered is not known. This database can be used to survey for changes in the frequencies of adverse events, to evaluate risk factors for adverse events, and to find rare adverse events.[11] VAERS reports can be made online at https://vaers.hhs.gov/reportevent.html. In addition to VAERS, the Vaccine Safety Datalink connects the Centers for Disease Control and Prevention (CDC) and large healthcare systems to actively monitor vaccine safety, and the Clinical Immunization Safety Assessment Project is a partnership between the CDC and academic medical centers to provide expert consultation and conduct research on vaccine safety.[13] The Institute of Medicine is an independent body that studies and reports on vaccine safety.[14]

The National Childhood Vaccine Injury Act of 1986 offers a no-fault alternative means to compensate individuals for injury following vaccination. The program offers liability protection to manufacturers and an efficient means of recovering damages for individuals potentially injured by vaccines. The types of vaccine-related injuries that are considered for compensation are outlined in the Health Resources and Services Administration's Vaccine Injury table (https://vaers.hhs.gov/docs/VAERS_Table_of_Reportable_Events_Following_Vaccination.pdf).

USE OF VACCINES

The Advisory Committee on Immunization Practices (ACIP) is composed of medical and public health experts who make recommendations for vaccine use.[15] They consider burden of disease, vaccine efficacy and safety, and cost effectiveness of vaccines. Other professional organizations, for example, the American Academy of Pediatrics, the American Academy of Family Physicians, or the American College of Obstetrics and Gynecology, publish guidelines. Usually, these guidelines are the same as those issued by the ACIP or the groups try to reconcile their recommendations.

5 The latest vaccine schedules can be found at https://www.cdc.gov/vaccines/schedules/hcp/index.html. All states require children to be fully immunized prior to entering elementary school; however, optimal protection is achieved by immunizing at the recommended ages, which requires special attention to children younger than 2 years. Adults and adolescents also require vaccination and often are unaware of this need. An early adolescent preventive health visit at age 11 to 12 years is recommended. This visit is an opportunity to catch up on missed immunizations and to administer meningococcal conjugate, Tdap, and HPV vaccines. Additionally, another visit at age 16 is recommended during which time the second meningococcal conjugate vaccine can be administered and a discussion regarding the need for meningococcal serogroup B vaccine series can occur. All individuals older than 6 months of age should receive an annual seasonal influenza vaccine. Adults should receive routine tetanus–diphtheria (Td) or Tdap boosters and be immune to MMRV by either immunization or history of infection. Adults need zoster vaccine after age 50 years, and pneumococcal vaccines after age 65 years. Certain individuals with conditions or lifestyles that put them at high risk for vaccine-preventable diseases also should be immunized as described in the following text and outlined in the immunization schedules in the appendices.

VACCINES

Diphtheria Toxoid Adsorbed

Diphtheria is an acute illness caused by the toxin released by a *Corynebacterium diphtheriae* infection. The toxin inhibits cellular protein synthesis, and membranes form on mucosal surfaces. Systemic toxemia can result in myocarditis, neuritis, and thrombocytopenia. Membrane formation can cause respiratory obstruction, and significant toxin absorption can lead to severe illness and death.

Diphtheria toxoid adsorbed is a sterile suspension of modified toxins of *C. diphtheriae* that induces immunity against the exotoxin of this organism. Two strengths of diphtheria toxoid are available in the United States: pediatric strength (D) and adult strength (d), which contains less antigen. The widespread use of diphtheria toxoid essentially has eliminated diphtheria from the United States.

Primary immunization with diphtheria toxoid (D) is indicated for children older than 6 weeks. The toxoid is given in combination with tetanus toxoid and acellular pertussis vaccine (as DTaP or in combination with additional childhood vaccines that have been licensed to decrease the number of injections required to complete the childhood immunization recommendations) at age 2, 4, and

6 months. Additional doses are given at age 15 to 18 months and again at age 4 to 6 years.[8] Booster doses should be given every 10 years.

For unimmunized adults, a complete three-dose series of diphtheria toxoid should be administered, with the first two doses given at least 4 weeks apart and the third dose given 6 to 12 months after the second. One of the vaccine doses in this series should be Tdap. The combined Td preparation is used for adults because it contains less diphtheria toxoid than the pediatric dose and is associated with fewer reactions to the diphtheria component. All adults should receive booster doses of Td or Tdap every 10 years.[8] Adverse effects of diphtheria toxoid include mild-to-moderate tenderness, erythema, and induration at the injection site. Systemic reactions occur rarely.

Haemophilus Influenzae Type b Vaccines

Before 1995, Hib was responsible for thousands of cases of serious illnesses (eg, meningitis, epiglottitis, pneumonia, sepsis, and septic arthritis). The incidence of Hib disease has declined more than 99% since the introduction of the conjugate vaccines based on the organism's capsular substance, polyribosylribitol phosphate (PRP).[16]

Hib conjugate vaccines are indicated for routine use in all infants and children younger than 5 years. Multiple products in various combinations are available for use in infants and children of different ages. The primary series of Hib vaccination consists of a 0.5-mL IM dose at ages 2, 4, and 6 months. The series should not be initiated in an infant younger than 6 weeks. Although use of one product for the entire primary series is desirable, adequate protection is achieved even when different products are used during the initial series. Following the primary series, a booster dose is recommended at age 12 to 15 months. Any of the Hib conjugate vaccines are suitable for the booster dose regardless of which conjugate was used for the primary series of doses.[16]

Schedules are more complex for infants who do not begin Hib immunization at the recommended age or who have fallen behind in the immunization schedule. For infants 7 to 11 months of age who have not been vaccinated, three doses of Hib vaccine should be given: two doses spaced 4 weeks apart and then a booster dose at age 12 to 15 months (but at least 8 weeks since the second dose). For unvaccinated children ages 12 to 14 months, two doses should be given, with an interval of 2 months between doses. In a child older than 15 months, a single dose of any of the vaccine preparations is indicated.[16]

Vaccines for Hib are recommended for routine use only for children up to age 59 months; beyond this age, the incidence of invasive Hib disease is low. Patients with certain underlying conditions (eg, children with HIV infection, sickle cell disease, splenectomy, and hematopoietic stem cell transplants and young children receiving chemotherapy for malignancies) are at higher than normal risk for Hib infection, and use of at least one dose of vaccine in these patients should be considered.[16] Adverse reactions to the Hib vaccine are uncommon. Erythema and induration at the injection site occur in approximately 5% to 30% of children and resolve within 12 to 24 hours. Fever, diarrhea, and vomiting are reported occasionally.[16]

Hepatitis Vaccines

Information on vaccination for viral hepatitis is given in Chapter 58.

Human Papillomavirus Vaccine

HPV infections are the most common sexually transmitted infections, with the highest prevalence of infection in sexually active young adults. Although more than 120 different HPV types have been identified, at least 40 different types of HPV infect the anogenital tract. These 40 different viruses are grouped into low-risk and high-risk types. Low-risk types can cause genital warts and mild abnormalities on Papanicolaou (Pap) tests. Ninety percent of all cases of genital warts and the majority of respiratory papillomatosis are caused by types 6 and 11. As many as 18 types are considered high risk as they have the ability to penetrate the nucleus of an epithelial cell to transform it to a precancerous cell. They cause abnormal Pap test results and may lead to cancer of the cervix, vulva, vagina, anus, penis, or oropharynx. Types 16 and 18 cause about 70% of all cervical cancers. Another 10% of HPV-related cancers are caused by types 31, 33, 45, 52, and 58. Men who have sex with men (MSM) are at a higher risk for infection with HPV, genital warts, and anal cancer.[17] The incidence of cancers associated with HPV is higher among MSM, and the rate of anal cancer among MSM continues to rise. High-risk HPV infections are necessary but not sufficient for the development of cervical cancer and for the majority of other anogenital and oral squamous cell cancers.

A 9-valent HPV vaccine against types 6 and 11 and 16, 18, 31, 33, 45, 52, and 58 is licensed for the prevention of HPV. ACIP recommends HPV vaccine for the prevention of HPV-related disease in individuals aged 9 to 26 years. Individuals who start the HPV series between the ages of 9 and 14 years should receive two doses separated by 6 months. This vaccine is administered as a three-dose series using a schedule of 0, 1 to 2, and 6 months for individuals who start the series at age 15 years or older. The vaccines are recommended for adolescents aged 11 to 12 years and catch-up immunization for individuals aged 13 to 26 years. The ACIP recommended shared clinical decision making for HPV vaccine for individuals aged 27 to 45 years.[17]

The vaccine is well tolerated, with injection-site reactions and systemic reactions (eg, headache and fatigue) occurring as commonly in immunized individuals as in the groups receiving placebo. Although syncope is possible with any immunization, the target population of adolescents and young adults has a higher incidence of syncope, including with administration of the HPV vaccine.[17]

Influenza Virus Vaccine

Information on vaccination for influenza is given in Chapter 131.

Measles Vaccine

Measles (rubeola) is a highly contagious viral illness characterized by rash and high fever. Complications of measles infections include severe diarrhea, otitis media, pneumonia, and encephalitis. Measles results in one to two deaths per 1,000 cases, with a much higher death rate in developing countries. With widespread vaccination, measles has been eliminated from the Western Hemisphere.

The measles vaccine is a live-attenuated viral vaccine that produces a subclinical, noncommunicable infection. Approximately 95% of vaccine recipients mount a protective immune response after a single dose, and most individuals are protected for life.[9] Most persons who do not respond to the first dose of measles vaccine will respond after receiving a second dose, and this forms the basis for the two-dose vaccine strategy that was implemented in the United States in 1989.

The measles vaccine is administered subcutaneously as a 0.5-mL dose in the arm (or in the thigh if the patient is younger than 15 months). The vaccine is administered routinely for primary immunization to persons 12 to 15 months of age. Two combinations of measles containing vaccines are available: measles, mumps, rubella (MMR) or measles, mumps, rubella, varicella (MMRV). The measles vaccine is not administered earlier than 12 months (except in certain outbreak circumstances or for travel) because persisting maternal antibody that was acquired transplacentally late in gestation can neutralize the vaccine virus before the vaccinated person can mount an immune response. A second dose of measles-containing vaccine is recommended when children are 4 to 6 years old.[9] The second dose of vaccine results in response in up to 99% of individuals.

Measles-containing vaccine should not be given to pregnant females or immunosuppressed individuals. An exception is HIV-infected patients, who are at high risk for severe complications if they develop measles. Adults with HIV infection who have no evidence of measles immunity should be immunized as long as they are not severely immunocompromised (CD4 greater than 200 lymphocytes/mm^3 [0.2×10^9/L] for at least 6 months). The second dose should be given 1 month later.[8] Children with HIV who are not severely immunocompromised can be immunized according to the childhood immunization schedule at 12 months and 4 to 6 years of age.[9]

Administration of Ig interferes with measles vaccine response, so the recommended interval between the Ig and vaccine is determined by the dose of Ig (see TABLE 147-2).[1] Live vaccines not administered during the same visit must be delayed for at least 4 weeks following measles or MMR vaccine.[1]

Measles vaccine is indicated in all persons born after 1956 or in those who lack documentation of wild-virus infection by either history or antibody titers. Two doses of a measles-containing vaccine separated by at least one month are required for children, college students, and healthcare workers who were born in 1957 or later.[9]

The measles vaccine has an excellent safety record. The most common side effect following vaccination is fever, which occurs in 5% to 15% of vaccinees. Transient generalized rash may occur in approximately 5% of vaccine recipients. These reactions generally appear 5 to 12 days postvaccination and last 2 to 5 days. Other adverse effects, such as headache, cough, sore throat, eye pain, malaise, and transient thrombocytopenia, occur less frequently.[9]

Meningococcal Vaccines

N. meningitidis is a leading cause of meningitis and sepsis in children and young adults in the United States. Five serotypes, A, B, C, W-135, and Y, cause almost all infections in humans. The infection is transmitted by respiratory droplets from infected individuals and asymptomatic carriers. Symptoms include severe headache, sensitivity to light, stiff neck, nausea and vomiting, and high fever. Mortality occurs in 24 to 48 hours following onset of symptoms in 10% to 13% of infected individuals.[18] Immunization is recommended for high-risk populations, such as those exposed to the infection, those in the midst of uncontrolled outbreaks, travelers to areas with epidemic or hyperendemic meningococcal disease, and individuals who have terminal complement component deficiencies or asplenia.

MenACWY Conjugate

Two meningococcal (MenACWY) conjugate vaccines combining the same serotypes are licensed for use in individuals aged 9 months to 55 years old (Menactra®, Sanofi-Pasteur) or 2 months to 55 years old (Menveo®, Novartis).

The meningococcal conjugate vaccine is recommended for adolescents at ages 11 to 12 years with a second dose at age 16 years. Reimmunization at 5-year interval is recommended for individuals who are at high risk.[18]

Injection-site reactions are the most common adverse effects following administration of either the meningococcal conjugate or polysaccharide vaccine.

MenB vaccines

Meningococcal serogroup B (MenB) vaccines use recombinant antigens from the bacterial capsule, specifically factor H binding protein, Neisseria adhesin A, neisserial heparin binding antigen, and outer membrane vesicles. The ACIP recommends either of the two MenB vaccines, Trumenba® or Bexsero®, for individuals at high risk for invasive meningococcal disease.[17] Additionally, MenB vaccine use should be considered through shared clinical decision-making for adolescents and young adults. Trumenba® requires two or three dose series administered at 0 and 6 months or 0, 2, and 6 month intervals. (The three-dose series should be used for high-risk individuals and during an outbreak.) Bexsero® requires two doses with at least one month between doses. Both vaccines were licensed based upon antibody response studies.[18] The most common adverse events after MenB vaccines are pain at the injection site, fatigue, headache, myalgia, and chills.

Mumps Vaccine

Mumps is a viral illness that classically causes bilateral parotitis 16 to 18 days after exposure. Fever, headache, malaise, myalgia, and anorexia may precede the parotitis. Serious complications are rare but more common in adults.

The mumps vaccine is a live-attenuated vaccine. The vaccine is available in combinations with measles, rubella (as MMR), and varicella (MMRV) vaccines.

The vaccine is administered as a 0.5-mL subcutaneous injection in the upper arm. Dosing recommendations coincide with those for measles vaccine, with the first dose administered at age 12 to 15 months and the second dose prior to the child's entry into elementary school. Two doses of mumps-containing vaccine are recommended for school-aged children, international travelers, students in post–high school educational institutions, and healthcare workers born after 1956.[9] A single dose of vaccine is acceptable documentation of immunity to mumps for other adults considered at lower risk of mumps infection, including adults born after 1956 and those with an uncertain history of wild-virus infection. Mumps vaccine should not be given to pregnant women or immunosuppressed patients.[1] A third dose of mumps vaccine should be considered for individuals at risk for infection during an outbreak.[19]

Serious adverse reactions to the vaccine are reported rarely. Fever, parotitis, rash, and lymphadenopathy occur rarely. Local reactions, including soreness, burning, and stinging, may occur at the injection site.[9]

Pertussis Vaccine

Pertussis is caused by a bacterial infection with *Bordetella pertussis*. The infection starts with signs and symptoms of an acute respiratory infection, called the catarrhal stage. The coughing spells manifest about a week later. Typically, young children will have the characteristic whoop as they struggle to inhale while coughing. Adolescents and adults are more likely to have prolonged periods of coughing. Pertussis can affect any age group, but young infants are at much higher risk for pneumonia, seizures, brain damage, and death. Their rate of hospitalization is much higher than for other age groups. The individual is contagious during the catarrhal stage and the first 2 weeks of the cough.[8]

Acellular pertussis vaccines contain components of the *B. pertussis* organism. All acellular vaccines contain pertussis toxin, and some contain one or more additional bacterial components (eg, filamentous hemagglutinin, pertactin, and fimbriae types 2 and 3). Acellular pertussis vaccine is recommended for all doses of the pertussis schedule at 2, 4, 6, and 15 to 18 months of age. A fifth dose of pertussis vaccine is given to children 4 to 6 years of age.[20] Pertussis vaccine is administered in combination with diphtheria and tetanus (DTaP). Administration of an acellular pertussis-containing vaccine (Tdap) is also recommended for adolescents once between ages 11 and 18 years and a single dose of Tdap should be administered to all adults.[19] Additional doses of acellular pertussis-containing vaccine for adults are acceptable, as the ACIP considers Td and Tdap interchangeable.[20] Special attention is warranted for the immunization of individuals who have close contact with young infants. Tdap should be administered to pregnant individuals in their late second or third trimester of pregnancy. Tdap should also be administered to all close contacts, including household contacts and out of home care providers.[8]

Local administration site reactions are relatively common. Systemic reactions, such as moderate fever, occur in 3% to 5% of vaccinees. Rarely, high fever, febrile seizures, persistent crying spells, and hypotonic hyporesponsive episodes occur following vaccination. Encephalopathy without known cause within 7 days of a pertussis vaccine are contraindications to future doses of this vaccine.[1]

Pneumococcal Vaccines

Streptococcus pneumoniae is a common pathogen with a range of manifestations, including asymptomatic upper respiratory tract colonization, sinusitis, acute otitis media, pharyngitis, pneumonia, meningitis, and bacteremia. Rates of invasive infections are highest in children younger than 2 years and in the elderly.[21,22] The majority of invasive pneumococcal infection deaths occur in the elderly or in those with underlying medical conditions. Four pneumococcal vaccine preparations, PCV13, PCV15, PCV20 and 23-valent pneumococcal polysaccharide vaccine (PPSV23) are available. The vaccines have different indications and are not interchangeable. The vaccines have different indications and are not interchangeable.

Pneumococcal Polysaccharide Vaccine

Pneumococcal polysaccharide vaccine (Pneumovax 23) is a mixture of highly purified capsular polysaccharides from 23 of the most prevalent or invasive types of *S. pneumoniae* seen in the United States. These 23 types represent 85% to 90% of all blood isolates and 85% of pneumococcal isolates from other generally sterile sites. The vaccine is administered IM or subcutaneously as a single 0.5-mL dose. [24]

Pneumococcal Conjugate Vaccine

Pneumococcal conjugate vaccines were initially developed to protect infants and young children from invasive pneumococcal disease. In clinical use, the vaccine is associated with a dramatic decline in invasive disease not only in immunized young children but also in individuals in all age groups. Conjugate vaccines are also used to protect adults with high risk medical conditions and those aged 65 years and older.[23]

Immunization of Children PCV13 or PCV15 is administered as a 0.5-mL IM injection at 2, 4, and 6 months of age and between 12 and 15 months of age. A single dose of PCV13 or PCV15 should be administered to children aged 6 to 18 years with sickle cell disease or splenic dysfunction, HIV infection, immunocompromising conditions, cochlear implant, or cerebral spinal fluid leak. PPSV23 can be used in conjunction with PCV13 or PCV15. PPSV23 should be administered after age 2 years and at least 2 months after the last dose of PCV13 or PCV15.

Immunization of Adults The ACIP recommended PCV20 or PCV15 followed by PPSV23 in 8 weeks for adults with immunocompromising conditions (TABLE 147-3).[25] Either PCV15 or PCV20 should be administered with at least a year interval in those adults for whom it has been recommended and have already received one or more doses of PPSV23.

For adults aged 65 years and older who are not immunocompromised, either PCV20 or PCV15 followed by PPSV23 in one year is recommended. If PCV15 is used for an individual aged 65 years or older who is immunocompromised (Table 142-3), PPSV23 should be administered 8 weeks later.[23]

TABLE 147-3 Pneumococcal Vaccines Use in Adults

Vaccine naive adults
PCV15 followed by PPSV23 or PCV20
PCV13-immunized adults
Conjugate vaccine should not be repeated
PPSV23-immunized adults
PCV15 or PCV 20 at least 1 year after last dose of PPSV23
Indications for PCV20 or PCV15 followed by PPSV23 for adults 19 years and older
Immunocompromising conditions*
Functional or anatomic asplenia
Sickle cell disease or other hemaglobinopathies
Congenital or acquired immunodeficiencies HIV infection
Chronic renal failure or nephrotic syndrome Leukemias, lymphomas, Hodgkin's lymphoma Generalized malignancy
Diseases requiring treatment with immunosuppressive drugs, including long-term systemic corticosteroids or radiation therapy
Diseases requiring treatment with immunosuppressive drugs, including long-term systemic corticosteroids or radiation therapy
Solid organ transplantation
Multiple myeloma
High risk medical conditions**
Chronic heart disease
Chronic liver disease
Chronic lung disease
Diabetes mellitus
Alcoholism
Cigarette smoking

CV20, 20-valent pneumococcal conjugate vaccine; PCV15, 15-valent pneumococcal conjugate vaccine; PPSV23, 23-valent pneumococcal polysaccharide vaccine.

*If PCV15 is used for immunocompromising conditions, administer PPSV23 8 weeks later.

**If PCV15 is used for those with high risk medical conditions, administer PPSV23 12 months later.

Data from Reference 23.

Poliovirus Vaccines

Poliomyelitis is a contagious viral infection that usually causes asymptomatic infection; however, in its serious form it causes acute flaccid paralysis. Poliovirus is spread via the fecal–oral route. The virus replicates in the upper respiratory tract, GI tract, and local lymphatics. The vast majority of polio infections are subclinical and asymptomatic. Polio has been eliminated from the United States since 1979, and the last case in Western Hemisphere was reported in 1991. Global eradication efforts are entering the final stages, and the eradication of polio should be accomplished in the next few years.

An inactivated vaccine developed by Jonas Salk was licensed for use in 1955. In 1987, an enhanced-potency inactivated polio vaccine (IPV) was introduced and that replaced the original inactivated vaccine. A live-attenuated oral polio vaccine (OPV) was developed by Albert Sabin in 1962. OPV was the primary immunizing agent for poliovirus infection. Widespread OPV use is responsible for the elimination of wild-type polio in most of the world. However, with no poliovirus circulation in the United States for years, IPV is the recommended vaccine for the primary series and booster dose for children.[26] OPV will continue to be used in areas of the world that have circulating poliovirus. The CDC maintains a stockpile of OPV to be used only in case of an outbreak.

The IPV series is administered routinely to children at ages 2, 4, and 6 to 18 months, and 4 to 6 years.[26] Primary polio immunization is recommended for all children up to age 18 years. Primary immunization of adults over age 18 years is not recommended routinely because a high level of immunity already exists in this age group, and the risk of exposure in developed countries is exceedingly small. However, unimmunized adults who are at increased risk for exposure because of travel, residence, or occupation should receive IPV series.

No serious side effects are attributable to IPV. Pregnant women should be given IPV only if there is a clear need, such as women who will be traveling or living in an area with endemic or epidemic poliovirus.

Rabies Vaccine and Immunoglobulin

Rabies is a virtually universally fatal infection in humans. Although all mammals are susceptible to rabies, carnivorous mammals are reservoirs of the virus and responsible for persistence of the virus in nature. In the United States, most human cases of rabies are from exposure to rabid bats, but raccoons, foxes, skunks, and coyotes are also associated with possible exposure. Worldwide, canines are the primary vectors. Transmission of rabies can occur via percutaneous, permucosal, or airborne exposure to the rabies virus. Circumstances favoring such transmission include animal bites and attacks and contamination of scratches, cuts, abrasions, and mucous membranes with saliva or other infectious material (brain tissue). Unprovoked attacks and daytime attacks by nocturnal animals are considered highly suspect. A few cases of person-to-person transmission have been reported.

Symptoms of rabies are nonspecific during the prodromal stage—fever, headache, malaise, irritability, nausea, and vomiting. The acute neurologic phase is characterized by hyperexcitability, hyperactivity, hallucinations, salivation, a fear of water, and air. Patients die within 5 days of presentation with these neurologic symptoms.

Human diploid cell vaccine, and purified chick embryo cell rabies vaccine are killed vaccines used for preexposure and postexposure rabies virus prophylaxis. Preexposure indications for rabies vaccine include persons whose vocation or avocation place them at high risk for rabies exposure, such as veterinarians, animal handlers, laboratory workers in rabies research or diagnostic laboratories, cavers, wildlife officers where animal rabies is common, and anyone who handles bats. Travelers who will be in a country or area of a country where there is a constant threat of rabies, whose stay is likely to extend beyond 1 month, and who may not have readily available medical services (eg, Peace Corps workers and missionaries) should be considered for preexposure prophylaxis. Rabies immunization of immunocompromised individuals should be postponed until the immunosuppression has resolved, or activities should be modified to minimize the potential exposure to rabies. If the vaccine is used in immunocompromised persons, antibody titers should be checked postimmunization. Pregnancy is not a contraindication if the risk of rabies is great. Both vaccine preparations can be administered for preexposure prophylaxis as a three-dose series of 1 mL IM on days 0 and 7 and once between days 21 and 3 years later.[26] Individuals with ongoing risk of exposure—either continuous risk (eg, research laboratory staff or those involved in rabies biologics production) or individuals with frequent exposures (eg, those involved with rabies diagnosis, spelunkers, veterinarians, animal control workers, and wildlife workers in rabies-enzootic areas)—should undergo serologic testing every 6 months and 2 years, respectively, to monitor rabies antibody concentrations. A booster dose is recommended if the complete virus neutralization is less than 1:5 serum dilution by the rapid fluorescent focus inhibition test.[27]

Preexposure prophylaxis does not eliminate the need for postexposure therapy. Persons previously immunized with rabies vaccine or those who previously received postexposure prophylaxis should receive two 1-mL IM doses of rabies vaccine on postexposure days 0 and 3.[27] Rabies Ig should not be given to this group.

Postexposure prophylaxis should be given after percutaneous or permucosal exposure to saliva or other infectious material from a high-risk source. Each case must be considered individually. Consideration needs to be given to the geographic area, species of animal, circumstances of the incident, and type of exposure. Local or state health departments should be contacted for assistance. Thorough cleansing of the wound with soap and water followed by irrigation with a virucidal agent such as povidone–iodine solution is an extremely important part of the management of rabies-prone wounds. Individuals who have not been immunized previously should receive the recommended regimen of rabies Ig (see Rabies Immunoglobulin below) and four doses of rabies vaccine 1 mL IM on days 0, 3, 7, and 14 after exposure. However, a fifth dose in a series should be considered if the exposed individual is immunocompromised. Vaccine response for these immunocompromised individuals should be checked.[28] Rabies vaccine must be administered in the deltoid muscle in adults and in the anterolateral thigh in children. The gluteal region should not be used.[1,27]

Adverse reactions to rabies biologicals are less common and less serious with the currently available vaccines compared with previously used preparations. Local or mild systemic symptoms can typically be managed with anti-inflammatory medications or antihistamines. Systemic allergic reactions ranging from hives to anaphylaxis occur in a small number of subjects. Given the lack of alternative therapy and the fact that rabies infection is almost always fatal, persons exposed to rabies who do have adverse reactions should continue the vaccine series in a setting with medical support services.[27]

Human rabies Ig is used in conjunction with rabies vaccine as part of postexposure rabies management for previously unvaccinated individuals. The product is derived from plasma obtained from donors who have been hyperimmunized with rabies vaccine and have high titers of circulating antibody.

In persons who previously have not been immunized against rabies, rabies Ig is given simultaneously with rabies vaccine to provide optimal coverage in the interval before immune response to the vaccine occurs. The efficacy of this regimen has been clearly demonstrated as it provides virtually complete protection from rabies when administered with the vaccine series promptly following exposure.[27] Rabies Ig does not interfere with vaccine-induced antibody formation. Its use is not recommended beyond 8 days after initiation of the vaccine series nor in persons previously immunized to rabies.

Human rabies Ig is administered in a dose of 20 international units/kg (0.133 mL/kg). If anatomically feasible, the entire dose should be infiltrated around the wound(s). Any remaining volume should be administered IM at a site distant from the rabies vaccination site. This product should never be administered by the IV route. Because other antibodies in the rabies Ig may interfere with the response to live-virus vaccines (MMR and varicella), it is recommended that these immunizations be delayed for 3 months.[1]

Side effects are rare but may include local soreness at the wound or IM injection site and mild temperature elevations. Pregnancy is not a contraindication to its use.

Rotavirus Vaccine

Rotavirus infection is virtually universal by age 5 years. Rotavirus can cause severe dehydrating diarrhea primarily among children aged 4 months to 23 months. The virus is usually transmitted fecal-orally and has a seasonal pattern with infection most likely in winter. In the pre-vaccine era, about 50% of hospitalizations for diarrhea among children were attributed to rotavirus.

Two vaccines for infants are available in the United States. A pentavalent human-bovine reassortment vaccine is administered orally at ages 2, 4, and 6 months. The monovalent human rotavirus vaccine is administered orally at ages 2 and 4 months. If brands of vaccines are changed during the series, a three-dose series should be used. The infant should be younger than 15 weeks of age for dose 1, and the maximum age for the last dose of the vaccine is 8 months.[7]

Rotavirus vaccination confers a small increased risk of intussusception following vaccine administration. Intussusception is a condition in which the bowel folds in itself in a telescoping fashion which can lead to inflammation, ischemia, or bowel obstruction. A history of intussusception is a contraindication to rotavirus vaccine. Severe combined immunodeficiency is also a contraindication.[28]

Rubella Vaccine

Rubella (German measles) is characterized by an erythematous rash, lymphadenopathy, arthralgia, and low-grade fever. The most important consequence of rubella infection occurs during pregnancy, particularly during the first trimester. Congenital rubella syndrome is associated with auditory, ophthalmic, cardiac, and neurologic defects. Rubella infection during pregnancy can also result in miscarriage or stillbirth. The primary goal of rubella immunization is to prevent congenital rubella syndrome. Rubella is no longer endemic in the United States, but high immunization rates are necessary to prevent rubella outbreaks from imported cases.[9]

Rubella vaccine contains live-attenuated rubella virus. The vaccine is available in combinations with measles and mumps (as MMR), or varicella (MMRV) vaccines.

Rubella vaccine induces antibodies that are protective against wild-virus infection. A second dose is recommended, at the same time measles vaccine is administered (as a second dose of MMR). The vaccine is indicated for children older than 1 year of age. Individuals born before 1957 are assumed to be immune to rubella except for females who could become pregnant. Therefore, all females of childbearing potential should have documentation of receiving at least one dose of a rubella-containing vaccine or laboratory evidence of immunity. The vaccine should not be given to immunosuppressed individuals, although MMR vaccine should be administered to individuals with HIV infection without evidence of immunity (see section "Measles Vaccine").[9] Adverse effects of the rubella virus vaccine tend to increase with the age of the recipient. Mild symptoms are similar to wild-virus infection and include lymphadenopathy, rash, urticaria, fever, malaise, sore throat, headache, myalgias, and paresthesias of the extremities. These symptoms occur 7 to 12 days after vaccination and last 1 to 5 days. Joint symptoms occur more often in susceptible postpubertal females. Arthralgia occurs in 25% of vaccinees, and 10% have arthritis-like symptoms. These symptoms usually begin 1 to 3 weeks after vaccination, persist for 1 day to 3 weeks, and rarely recur.[9]

The rubella vaccine has never been associated with congenital rubella syndrome, but its use during pregnancy is contraindicated. However, routine pregnancy testing prior to vaccination is not recommended. Females should be counseled not to become pregnant for 4 weeks following vaccination.[9]

Tetanus Toxoid Adsorbed and Tetanus Immunoglobulin

Tetanus is a severe acute illness caused by the exotoxin of *Clostridium tetani*. Tetanus is the only vaccine-preventable disease that is not contagious as it is acquired from the environment. Tetanus toxin interferes with neurotransmitters that promote muscle relaxation, leading to continuous muscle spasms that are characteristic of tetanus. Death can be due to the tetanus toxin itself or secondary to a complication such as aspiration pneumonia, dysregulation of the autonomic nervous system, or pulmonary embolism.

Tetanus toxoid is an adjuvanted suspension of the toxoid derived from *C. tetani*. A series of three 0.5-mL doses of tetanus toxoid elicits protection in virtually all individuals. Primary vaccination provides protection for at least 10 years.[8] Additional doses of tetanus toxoid (combined with diphtheria toxoid, ie, Td) are recommended as part of wound management if a patient has not received a dose of tetanus toxoid within the preceding 5 years. For minor or clean wounds, no dose is given (TABLE 147-4). Tetanus Ig should be given to individuals who have received fewer than three doses of tetanus toxoid and have more serious wounds. It can be administered with tetanus toxoid, provided that separate syringes and separate injection sites are used.

In children, primary immunization against tetanus usually is offered in conjunction with diphtheria and pertussis vaccination (using DTaP or a combination vaccine that includes other antigens used to decrease the number of injections to complete the childhood immunization schedule) at age 2, 4, 6, and 15 to 18 months.[8] In children 7 years and older and in adults who have not been immunized previously, a series of three 0.5-mL doses of a tetanus toxoid-containing vaccine is administered IM initially. The first two doses are given 1 to 2 months apart, and the third dose is recommended at 6 to 12 months after the second dose. Boosters are recommended every 10 years, and unless there is contraindication to diphtheria toxoid, Td or Tdap should be used.[8]

Adverse reactions to tetanus toxoid include mild-to-moderate local reactions at the injection site, such as warmth, erythema, and induration. Occasionally, a nodule at the injection site develops and remains for a few weeks. This type of reaction is indicative of high preexisting antibody concentrations, and additional doses of toxoid should not be given any sooner than 10 years. Local reactions do not limit the use of the toxoid for further dosing.

Tetanus Ig is a sterile, concentrated, nonpyrogenic solution of Igs prepared from hyperimmunized humans. It is used to provide passive immunity to tetanus after the occurrence of traumatic wounds in nonimmunized or suboptimally immunized persons (see TABLE 147-4).[8] A dose of 250 to 500 units IM should be administered. When administered with tetanus toxoid, separate sites for administration should be used. Tetanus Ig also is used for treatment of tetanus. In this setting, a single dose of 3,000 to 6,000 units IM is administered.

Adverse effects of tetanus Ig include pain, tenderness, erythema, and muscle stiffness at the injection site, which may persist for several hours. Systemic reactions occur rarely. IV administration has been associated with severe adverse reactions and is not recommended.

TABLE 147-4 Tetanus Prophylaxis

Vaccination History	Clean, Minor Wounds		All Other Wounds	
	Td[a]	TIG	Td or Tdap[a]	TIG
Unknown or fewer than three doses	Yes	No	Yes	Yes
Three or more doses	No[a,b]	No	No[a,c]	No

[a]A single dose of Tdap should be used for the next dose of tetanus–diphtheria toxoid for individuals aged >10 years.

[b]Yes, if more than 10 years since the last dose.

[c]Yes, if more than 5 years since the last dose.

Data from Reference 8.

Varicella and Zoster Vaccines

Varicella is a highly contagious disease caused by varicella-zoster virus. The clinical illness is characterized by the appearance of successive waves of pruritic vesicles that rapidly crust over. Malaise and fever are common and last for 2 to 3 days. The virus remains dormant in the dorsal ganglia and reactivates as herpes zoster, also known as *shingles*. Although the exact stimulus for reactivation is unknown, a decrease in varicella-specific cell-mediated immunity associated with age or immunosuppression appears to be necessary but not sufficient for reactivation.

Varicella Vaccine

Live-attenuated varicella vaccine contains the Oka/Merck strain of varicella virus. Varicella vaccine must be kept frozen and protected from light. Once reconstituted, it must be administered subcutaneously within 30 minutes.[29] The varicella vaccine is recommended for all children at 12 to 15 months of age, with a second dose prior to entering school between ages 4 and 6 years.[29] Two doses separated by 4 to 8 weeks should be administered to anyone who lacks immunity to varicella. Because the varicella vaccine is a live vaccine, it is contraindicated during pregnancy and in immunocompromised individuals. An exception is children with asymptomatic or mildly symptomatic HIV infection, who should receive two doses of varicella vaccine 3 months apart. In addition, children with humoral immune deficiencies may be immunized. Persons who have received blood, plasma, or Ig products in the recent past should not receive varicella vaccine because of concern that passively acquired antibody will interfere with response to the vaccine. The recommended time interval between antibody-containing products and varicella vaccine depends on the dose of Ig (see TABLE 147-2).[1] Although no adverse events associated with salicylate use after vaccination have been reported, salicylates should be avoided for 6 weeks after vaccination because of the association of salicylate use and Reye syndrome following varicella infection.[35]

Common adverse events include local swelling, and erythema at the injection site occur in up to 32% of patients and fever in 10%

to 15%. A varicella-like rash occurs in approximately 4% of vaccinees, accompanied by few, if any, systemic symptoms. The rash may be localized at the injection site or generalized. Lesions usually are few in number (2-10) and often papular rather than vesicular. Transmission of vaccine virus to susceptible close contacts has occurred but is rare and believed to occur only when the vaccinee develops a rash. Because the risk of vaccine virus transmission is low and primary infection can be severe, vaccination of household contacts of immunocompromised patients is recommended to prevent introduction of varicella into the household.[29] Varicella vaccine is contraindicated in immunosuppressed individuals and those who are pregnant. Aspirin should be avoided for 6 weeks following varicella vaccine administration because of its association with Reye syndrome. Also, a caution in those with a personal or family history of seizures exists for the use of MMRV. Consider using the MMR and varicella vaccines separately.[29]

Zoster Vaccine

After the primary infection with varicella-zoster virus manifested as chicken pox, the virus remains latent in the dorsal ganglia. Herpes zoster, also called *shingles*, occurs upon reactivation of varicella-zoster virus associated with waning cellular immunity to the virus. Herpes zoster can occur at any age, but the incidence dramatically increases with age. The rate of disease increases sharply after age 50 years. The disease rate in individuals older than 80 years of age is 15 cases per 1,000 person-years. Patients with HIV, cancer, or other conditions associated with immunosuppression are at increased risk for disease.[30]

The clinical presentation of herpes zoster usually is a vesicular eruption limited to one dermatome. The most common complication is postherpetic neuralgia, which is pain that persists for weeks to years after the skin lesions have healed. The risk of postherpetic neuralgia increases with age. Virtually no risk of developing postherpetic neuralgia with herpes zoster exists prior to age 50 years, but the risk increases to 50% to 75% after ages 60 and 75 years, respectively.[31]

A recombinant zoster vaccine (RZV) with an adjuvant is recommended by the ACIP for use in individuals aged 50 years and older and immunocompromised individuals aged 19 years and older as a two-dose series at 0 and 2 to 6 months.[30] The vaccine is approximately 91% effective for the prevention of zoster in those aged 50 years and older though effectiveness is lower in immunocompromised populations.[41] Although the incidence of serious adverse effects were similar in the vaccine and placebo groups, the incidence of injection site and systemic adverse events were much higher in the vaccine group. Almost 80% of those who receive RZV report injection site pain with 9% of those reporting injection site reactions that interfere with their normal activities. No difference in the incidence of injection site reactions were found when comparing dose 1 to dose 2.[30]

Varicella-Zoster Immunoglobulin

Varicella-zoster Ig is used after exposure to varicella for passive immunization of susceptible immunodeficient patients or other susceptible individuals at particularly high risk for complications of varicella infection. Postexposure prophylaxis with varicella-zoster Ig is indicated for the following susceptible individuals: (a) immunocompromised patients without evidence of immunity, (b) neonates whose mothers develop varicella within 5 days before or 2 days after delivery, (c) hospitalized premature infants (more than 28 weeks of gestation) whose mothers have no evidence of immunity, (d) hospitalized preterm infants (less than 28 weeks' gestation or weight less than 1,000 g), and (e) susceptible pregnant individuals.[29] If varicella is prevented, vaccination should be offered at a later date. Exposure to varicella is defined as direct indoor contact for more than 1 hour with an infectious person. A negative history of clinical disease is not a reliable indicator of varicella susceptibility. Most people with a negative clinical history will have detectable antibody on laboratory testing.

For maximum effectiveness, varicella-zoster Ig must be given as soon as possible and not more than 10 days following exposure.[29] Because this agent may only attenuate infection, patients who receive varicella-zoster Ig still may have a period of communicability, and varicella-zoster Ig may prolong the incubation period to 28 days. Antiviral therapy can be initiated if signs and symptoms of varicella infection become apparent.

Administration of varicella-zoster Ig is by the IM route at doses of 125 plaque-forming units per 10 kg of body weight up to 625 units (five vials) for patients weighing more than 40 kg. The dose for newborn infants is 125 units.[29]

OTHER IMMUNOBIOLOGICS

Immunoglobulin

Ig is available as both intramuscular immunoglobulin (IMIG) and IV immunoglobulin (IVIG) preparations. These products contain a wide spectrum of IgG antibodies to the pathogens prevalent in the area from which the donors were obtained. IMIG typically contains 15% to 18% protein and not less than 90% IgG. A number of IVIG preparations are available commercially in the United States. Generally, these preparations contain greater than 90% IgG monomers and trace to small amounts of IgA. Because different processes are used in the preparation of IMIG and IVIG products, they are not interchangeable.

When administered either IV or IM, Ig distributes in approximately 5% of the body weight of the recipient. The plasma half-life of Ig ranges from 18 to 32 days. This range of half-life probably is attributable to the variation in the half-life of IgG subclasses. Peak serum concentrations occur immediately with IVIG but within 2 days with IMIG. After the initial period of equilibration, circulating IgG levels are superimposable between IV and IM equivalent dosages. No dosage adjustment is necessary in patients with renal insufficiency, hepatic insufficiency, or both, dialysis patients, or geriatric patients.

6 Ig is indicated in a wide variety of circumstances to provide passive immunity to individuals. The indications for IMIG differ from those for IVIG. IMIG is indicated for providing passive immunity in patients with hepatitis A infections in those for whom IMIG is recommended in addition to immunization, hepatitis B exposures (however, hepatitis B Ig is significantly more effective), measles, varicella, and primary immunodeficiency diseases. Although IMIG is indicated for the treatment of primary immunodeficiency, IVIG is better tolerated and is more effective. IMIG is not indicated for prevention of rubella, mumps, or poliomyelitis. TABLE 147-5 lists the suggested dosages of IMIG for prevention or attenuation of various infectious diseases.

TABLE 147-5 Indications and Dosage of Intramuscular Immunoglobulin in Infectious Diseases

Primary immunodeficiency states	1.2 mL/kg IM then 0.6 mL/kg every 2-4 weeks
Hepatitis A exposure	0.02 mL/kg IM within 2 weeks if <1 year or >39 years of age
Hepatitis A prophylaxis	0.02 mL/kg IM for exposure <3 months' duration
	0.06 mL/kg IM for exposure up to 5 months' duration
Hepatitis B exposure	0.06 mL/kg (HBIG preferred in known exposures)
Measles exposure	0.5 mL/kg (maximum dose 15 mL) as soon as possible

There are many licensed indications, as well as off-label uses, for IVIG.[43] The therapeutic dose of IVIG is set empirically at 2 g/kg, often given as five daily doses of 400 mg/kg each. Mechanisms of IVIG action for treatment of these conditions have been hypothesized.

1. *Primary Immunodeficiency States.*[32,33] In primary immunodeficiency states, monthly doses of between 100 and 800 mg/kg are administered; the average dose is 200 to 400 mg/kg. The immunodeficiency states for which IVIG is indicated include both antibody deficiencies and combined immune deficiencies. Significant reactions can occur in patients with low intrinsic levels of IgA given IVIG with greater amounts of IgA. An IVIG product with low amounts of IgA should be used for these patients.
2. *Immune Thrombocytopenia.*[34] For the treatment of hemorrhage associated with immune thrombocytopenia (ITP), doses of 1 g/kg daily for 2 to 3 days plus high-dose methylprednisolone are indicated. Adults tend to respond less well to IVIG than do children. IVIG is acceptable for treatment of both chronic and acute ITP, and IVIG has been used for ITP associated with pregnancy without adverse effects on the fetus. Corticosteroids remain the drugs of choice for adult ITP. In thrombotic thrombocytopenia purpura, IVIG is reported to be effective in patients who do not respond to plasmapheresis. Other platelet disorders in which IVIG may be useful include neonatal immune thrombocytopenia, perinatal autoimmune thrombocytopenia, drug-induced thrombocytopenia, thrombocytopenia secondary to infection, and transfusion-refractory thrombocytopenia; however, the data supporting these uses are minimal.
3. *Chronic Lymphocytic Leukemia.*[35] IVIG is used as a prophylactic measure in patients with chronic lympocytic leukemia who have had a serious bacterial infection.
4. *Kawasaki Disease.*[36] This disease, which generally occurs in children, carries the hallmark of development of coronary artery abnormalities. Generally, the American Academy of Pediatrics recommends that if the strict criteria for Kawasaki disease are met, an IVIG dose of 400 mg/kg/day for four consecutive days be used or, preferably, 2 g/kg as a single dose. The dose should be administered within 10 days of disease onset. Aspirin therapy also should be initiated.
5. *Pediatric HIV infection.*[37] IVIG prevents serious bacterial infections in children with HIV infection. However, in the era of highly active anti-retroviral therapy, its use has waned.
6. *Allogeneic bone marrow transplantation.*[38]
7. *Chronic inflammatory demyelinating polyneuropathy.*[38] This disabling neuropathy often responds to corticosteroids, IVIG, or plasmapheresis.
8. *Multifocal motor neuropathy*[39] IVIG is considered first-line therapy.
9. *Kidney transplantation involving a recipient with high antibody concentrations or an ABO-incompatible donor.*[40] Some transplant recipients have antibody concentrations that present an immunological barrier to transplantation. Desensitization can be accomplished using IVIG.

Many other uses of IVIG have been identified. These uses are off-label but may be generally accepted in the medical community for routine treatment.[32]

7 Adverse effects of Ig vary with the route of administration. Following IMIG, pain, tenderness, and muscle stiffness persisting for hours or days are common. Repeat courses may cause sensitization with resulting allergic reactions. Chills, fever, nausea, and vomiting often are related to the rate of the infusion.[41] Infusion should be given at a rate of 0.01 to 0.02 mL/kg/min for 30 minutes. If no reactions occur, then the rate can be increased to 0.02 to 0.04 mL/kg/min. If reactions do occur, the infusion should be stopped for 30 minutes and restarted at a lower rate. Although recommendations for infusion rate vary slightly depending on the preparation, the guidelines presented can be followed for the various IV preparations.

Most adverse reactions are mild and transient. Arthralgia, myalgia, fever, pruritus, nausea, vomiting, chest tightness, palpitations, diaphoresis, dizziness, pallor, and respiratory distress have been reported. Rarely, aseptic meningitis has occurred from a few hours to 2 days after high-dose infusion. The syndrome resolves within days without sequelae. Acute renal failure has been reported, primarily in individuals with underlying renal dysfunction, diabetes, sepsis, volume depletion, or other nephrotoxic drugs or in patients older than 65 years. To minimize the risk, ensure adequate hydration prior to infusion and choose an IVIG product that does not contain high-sucrose concentrations for individuals at high risk.[41]

Ig products are derived from human blood. Precautions such as donor screening and fractionation procedures and solvent–detergent treatment during the manufacturing process render the IVIG products free of HIV and hepatitis B and C viruses. Although no manufacturing process can guarantee no viral contamination, the potential infection risk from Ig preparations is very small.

Rh_o(D) Immunoglobulin

8 Second only to the ABO blood group system, Rhesus antigen D [Rh_o(D)] is an important antigen in human blood. The Rh_o(D) locus encodes this antigen, but this locus is absent in approximately 15% of the population. Individuals lacking the Rh_o(D) locus are Rh_o(D) negative and have the potential to mount an antibody response to erythrocytes with the Rh_o(D) present. Rh_o(D) incompatibility during pregnancy can lead to sensitization of the mother. The maternal antibodies developed following normal fetal leakage of erythrocytes to the mother can cause hemolytic disease of the newborn during subsequent pregnancies.

Rh_o(D) Ig is a sterile solution of Igs prepared from human sera with high titers of Rh_o(D) antibody. Rh_o(D) Ig suppresses the antibody response and formation of anti-Rh_o(D) in Rh_o(D)-negative individuals exposed to Rh_o(D)-positive blood. Administration of Rh_o(D) Ig prevents hemolytic disease of the newborn in subsequent pregnancies with a Rh_o(D)-positive fetus. When administered within 72 hours of delivery of a full-term infant, Rh_o(D) Ig reduces active antibody formation from 1% to about 0.2%. The reduction in antibody formation is lower when Rh_o(D) Ig is given beyond 72 hours postpartum. Smaller doses of Rh_o(D) Ig are used after abortion, miscarriage, amniocentesis, or abdominal trauma. In addition, Rh_o(D) Ig is used in the case of a premenopausal female who is Rh_o(D) negative and has inadvertently received Rh_o(D)-positive blood or blood products.[42]

The dosage of Rh_o(D) Ig varies with the indication. A standard dose of 300 mcg is given within 72 hours of a term delivery. Occasionally, when the fetus is known to be Rh_o(D) positive, a 300-mcg dose is given at 28 weeks' gestation and within 72 hours after delivery. For postpregnancy termination occurring up to 13 weeks' gestation, one microdose (50 mcg) vial is given within 72 hours. For pregnancy termination after 13 weeks, one standard dose (300 mcg) is given within 72 hours. In other circumstances, such as in abdominal trauma, amniocentesis, or transfusion accidents, the dosage (number of standard dose vials) is based on the estimated packed red blood cell volume of fetal/maternal hemorrhage divided by 15. Rh_o(D) Ig is administered IM only.

Adverse reactions to Rh_o(D) Ig include injection-site tenderness and fever. Rh_o(D) may minimally interfere with response to rubella or varicella vaccine. Rubella- or varicella-seronegative females should be immunized with MMR or MMRV at hospital discharge even if they received Rh_o(D) Ig postpartum.[1]

Vaccine Hesitancy

Vaccine confidence is the trust that individuals and providers have in recommended vaccines, in those who administer vaccines, and the policies and processes by which vaccines are developed, manufactured, licensed, and recommended.[43] Vaccine hesitancy is a global threat to protection conferred by strong immunization programs. A variety of justifications for choosing not to vaccinate exist. The Strategic Advisory Group of Experts (SAGE), a working group under the World Health Organization (WHO), defined three overarching drivers for vaccine hesitancy: complacency, convenience, and confidence.[44] This "3 Cs Model" defined complacency as a low perceived risk of contracting vaccine-preventable diseases, and therefore low necessity to receive vaccines. Convenience is based on socioeconomic factors such as availability, accessibility, affordability, and ability to understand, such as language barriers or low health literacy. Confidence stems from trust in various aspects of healthcare, such as the vaccine itself, healthcare professionals administering vaccines, or policy-makers who advocate for vaccination and determine their need.

Communication is key to relaying a vaccine message starting with empathy and understanding. Healthcare providers should assume that individuals want to be vaccinated and make a strong recommendation for vaccines. Healthcare workers must be prepared to share facts that address misinformation and respond to patient questions. An active discussion of expected side effects is associated with patient confidence. Finally, the conversation can be concluded by encouraging the individual to take action to get the vaccine.[45]

VACCINE INFORMATION RESOURCES

The field of vaccinology is developing rapidly, with numerous changes in recommendations for vaccine use made each year. Keeping up to date with the current recommendations can be a challenge. The childhood and adult immunization schedules are updated frequently and published annually. Recommendations for the use of influenza vaccine are issued annually. Healthcare providers involved in primary care and immunization delivery must keep themselves abreast of these changes in a systematic way. Reading electronic newsletters and browsing reliable websites are efficient methods for obtaining information (TABLE 147-6). Although several excellent, reliable, and timely websites exist, hundreds of sites with misleading and incorrect information also exist. Many of these sites are targeted at parents.

TABLE 147-6 Web Resources for Vaccine Information

Recommended Internet Sites for Vaccine Information	
http://www.cdc.gov/vaccines/	Vaccines & Immunizations Centers for Disease Control and Prevention
www.immunize.org	Immunization Action Coalition
www.nfid.org/	National Foundation for Infectious Diseases
www.cdc.gov/mmwr/	Morbidity and Mortality Weekly Report
http://www.nationalacademies.org/hmd/	The National Academies of Sciences, Engineering, and Medicine. Health and Medicine Division
http://www.hrsa.gov/vaccinecompensation/	Vaccine Injury Compensation Program
http://www.chop.edu/centers-programs/vaccine-education-center/	Vaccine Education Center Children's Hospital of Philadelphia
https://vaers.hhs.gov/index.html	Vaccine Adverse Event Reporting System
Recommended Electronic Newsletters	
www.immunize.org/express	The Immunization Action Coalition's newsletter
www.cdc.gov/mmwr/	Morbidity and Mortality Weekly Report

Parents and patients often have questions regarding vaccine safety. The Vaccine Education Center at the Children's Hospital of Philadelphia has several documents that may answer those questions (http://www.chop.edu/centers-programs/vaccine-education-center). The CDC is another source of information for parents (https://www.cdc.gov/vaccines/parents/vaccine-decision/index.html). Vaccines are the only class of medications to which nearly every patient is exposed. Knowledge of these agents is critical to providing pharmaceutical care. Dramatic progress in public health has been made through the appropriate use of immunization. Additional improvements in quality of life and mortality can be made through continued increases in vaccination coverage with careful attention to this aspect of care by all healthcare providers.

ABBREVIATIONS

ACIP	Advisory Committee on Immunization Practices
CDC	Centers for Disease Control and Prevention
DTaP	diphtheria, tetanus toxoids, and acellular pertussis
Hib	*Haemophilus influenzae* type b
HPV	human papillomavirus
Ig	immunoglobulin
IMIG	intramuscular immunoglobulin
IPV	inactivated polio vaccine
ITP	idiopathic (immune) thrombocytopenic purpura
IVIG	IV immunoglobulin
MenB	meningococcal serogroup B
MMR	measles, mumps, rubella vaccine
MMRV	measles, mumps, rubella, varicella vaccine
MSM	men who have sex with men
OPV	oral polio vaccine
PCV	pneumococcal conjugate vaccine
PPSV23	23-valent pneumococcal polysaccharide vaccine
RZV	recombinant zoster vaccine
Td	tetanus–diphtheria
Tdap	tetanus, diphtheria, acellular pertussis
TIG	Tetanus immune globulin
VAERS	Vaccine Adverse Event Reporting System

REFERENCES

1. Kroger A, Bahta L, Hunter P. General Best Practice Guidelines for Immunization. Best Practices Guidance of the Advisory Committee on Immunization Practices (ACIP). Available at: www.cdc.gov/vaccines/hcp/acip-recs/general-recs/downloads/general-recs.pdf. Accessed on October 7, 2022.
2. Centers for Disease Control and Prevention. Prevention of hepatitis B virus infection in the United States: Recommendations of the Advisory Committee on Immunization Practices. *MMWR Morb Mortal Wkly Rep.* 2018;67:1–31.
3. Grohskopf LA, Alyanak E, Broder KR, et al. Prevention and control of seasonal influenza with vaccines: Recommendations of the Advisory Committee on Immunization Practices—United States, 2020-21 influenza season. *MMWR Morb Mortal Wkly Rep.* 2020;69(RR-# 8):1–24.
4. McGrath B, Broadhurst M, Roman C. Infectious disease considerations in immunocompromised patients. *JAAPA.* 2020;33:16–25.
5. Kennedy RB, Ovsyannikova IG, Palese P, Poland GA. Current challenges in vaccinology. *Front Immunol.* Jun 25, 2020;11:1181. doi: 10.3389/fimmu.2020.01181.
6. Weinberger B. Vaccines for the elderly: Current use and future challenges. *Immun Ageing.* 2018;15:3.
7. Centers for Disease Control and Prevention. Prevention of rotavirus gastroenteritis among infants and children. Recommendations of the Advisory Committee on Immunization Practices (ACIP). *MMWR Morb Mortal Wkly Rep.* 2009;58:1–24.

8. Liang JL, Tiwari T, Moro P., et al. Prevention of pertussis, tetanus and diphtheria with vaccines in the United States: Recommendations of the Advisory Committee on Immunization Practices. *MMWR Morb Mortal Wkly Rep.* 2018;67(No. RR#2):1–44.
9. Centers for Disease Control and Prevention. Prevention of measles, rubella, congenital rubella syndrome, and mumps, 2013: Summary recommendations of the Advisory Committee on Immunization Practices (ACIP). *MMWR Morb Mortal Wkly Rep.* 2013;62:1–33.
10. Danziger-Isakov L, Kumar D. Vaccination of solid organ transplant candidates and recipients: Guidelines from the American Society of Transplantation Infectious Diseases Community of Practice. *Clin Transplant.* 2019;33:e13563.
11. Chong PP, Avery RK. A comprehensive review of immunization practices in solid organ transplant and hematopoietic stem cell transplant recipients. *Clin Ther.* 2017;39:1581–1598.
12. Centers for Disease Control and Prevention. Immunization Information Systems (IIS). https://www.cdc.gov/vaccines/programs/iis/. Accessed on October 7, 2022.
13. Centers for Disease Control and Prevention. Vaccine Safety. Available at: https://www.cdc.gov/vaccinesafety/index.html. Accessed on October 7, 2022.
14. National Academy of Medicine. Institute of Medicine for Vaccine Safety. Available at: https://www.vaccinesafety.edu/IOM-Reports.htm. Accessed on October 7, 2022.
15. Centers for Disease Control and Prevention. Advisory Committee on Immunization Practices. Available at: https://www.cdc.gov/vaccines/acip/committee/index.html. Accessed on October 7, 2022.
16. Oliver SE, Moro P, Blain AE. Chapter 8 *Haemophilus influenzae*. In: Hamborsky J, Kroger A, Wolfe C, eds. *Epidemiology and Prevention of Vaccine-Preventable Diseases.* 14th ed. Washington, DC: Public Health Foundation; 2021.
17. Meites E, Gee J, Unger E, Markowitz L. Chapter 11 Human papillomavirus. In: Hamborsky J, Kroger A, Wolfe C, eds. *Epidemiology and Prevention of Vaccine-Preventable Diseases.* 14th ed. Washington, DC: Public Health Foundation; 2021.
18. Mbaeyi SA, Bozio CH, Duffy J., et al. Meningococcal vaccination: Recommendations of the Advisory Committee on Immunization Practices, United States 2020. *MMWR Morb Mortal Wkly Rep.* 2020;69(No. RR#9):1–41.
19. Marin M, Marlow M, Moore KL, Patel M. Recommendation of the advisory committee on immunization practices for use of a third dose of mumps virus–containing vaccine in persons at increased risk for mumps during an outbreak. *MMWR Morb Mortal Wkly Rep* 2018;67:33–38.
20. Havers FP, Moro PL, Hunter P, Hariri S, Bernstein H. Use of tetanus toxoid, reduced diphtheria toxoid, and acellular pertussis vaccines: Updated recommendations of the Advisory Committee on Immunization Practices — United States, 2019. *MMWR Morb Mortal Wkly Rep.* 2020;69:77–83.
21. Palmu AA, De Wals P, Toropainen M, et al. Similar impact and replacement disease after pneumococcal conjugate vaccine introduction in hospitalised children with invasive pneumococcal disease in Europe and North America. *Vaccine.* Mar 12, 2021;39(11):1551–1555. doi: 10.1016/j.vaccine.2021.01.070. Epub 2021 Feb 18.
23. Kobayashi M, Farrar JL, Gierke R, et al. Use of 15-Valent Pneumococcal Conjugate Vaccine Among U.S. Children: Updated Recommendations of the Advisory Committee on Immunization Practices — United States, 2022. MMWR Morb Mortal Wkly Rep 2022;71:1174–1181. doi: http://dx.doi.org/10.15585/mmwr.mm7137a3.
24. Kobayashi M, Farrar JL, Gierke R, et al. Use of 15-Valent Pneumococcal Conjugate Vaccine and 20-Valent Pneumococcal Conjugate Vaccine Among U.S. Adults: Updated Recommendations of the Advisory Committee on Immunization Practices — United States, 2022. MMWR Morb Mortal Wkly Rep 2022;71:109–117. doi: http://dx.doi.org/10.15585/mmwr.mm7104a1external icon.
25. Childs L, Kobayashi M, Farrar JL, Pilishvili T. The efficacy and effectiveness of pneumococcal vaccines against pneumococcal pneumonia among adults: a systematic review and meta-analysis. *Open Forum Infect Dis.* 2021;8(Suppl 1):S130–S131. http://doi.org/10.1093/ofid/ofab466.215.
26. Estivariz CF, Link-Gelles R, Shimabukuro T. Chapter 18. Poliomyelitis. (updated November 2020) In: Hamborsky J, Kroger A, Wolfe C, eds. *Epidemiology and Prevention of Vaccine-Preventable Diseases.* 13th ed. Washington, DC: Public Health Foundation; 2015.
27. Rao AK, Briggs D, Moore SM, et al. Use of a Modified Preexposure Prophylaxis Vaccination Schedule to Prevent Human Rabies: Recommendations of the Advisory Committee on Immunization Practices — United States, 2022. MMWR Morb Mortal Wkly Rep 2022;71:619–627. doi: http://dx.doi.org/10.15585/mmwr.mm7118a2.
28. Centers for Disease Control and Prevention. Addition of history of intussusception as a contraindication for rotavirus vaccination. *MMWR Morb Mortal Wkly Rep.* 2011;60(41):1427.
29. Lopez A, Harrington T, Marin M. Chapter 22. Varicella, eds. Hamborsky J, Kroger A, Wolfe C. eds. *Epidemiology and Prevention of Vaccine-Preventable Diseases.* 14th ed. Washington, DC: Public Health Foundation; 2021.
30. Dooling KL, Guo A, Patel M, et al. Recommendations of the Advisory Committee on Immunization Practices for Use of Herpes Zoster Vaccines. *MMWR Morb Mortal Wkly Rep.* 2018;67:103–108.
31. Forbes HJ, Thomas SL, Smeeth L, et al. A systematic review and meta-analysis of risk factors for postherpetic neuralgia. *Pain.* Jan 2016;157(1):30–54. doi: 10.1097/j.pain.0000000000000307.
32. Robert P, Hotchko M. Polyvalent immune globulin usage by indication in the United States, 2012: A quantitative analysis of the use of polyvalent immune globulin (intravenous and subcutaneous) by medical indication in the United States in 2012. *Transfusion.* 2015;55:S6–S12.
33. Krivan G, Jolles S, Granados EL, et al. New insights in the use of immunoglobulins for the management of immune deficiency (PID) patients. *Am J Clin Exp Immunol.* 2017;6:76–83.
34. Audia S, Bonnotte B. Emerging therapies in immune thrombocytopenia. *J Clin Med.* Mar 2, 2021;10(5):1004. doi: 10.3390/jcm10051004.
35. Legendre P, Chahwan D, Marjanovic Z, et al. Utilization of intravenous or subcutaneous immunoglobulins in secondary immune deficiency (ULTIMATE): A retrospective multicenter study. *Clin Immunol.* Jun 2020;215:108419. doi: 10.1016/j.clim.2020.108419. Epub 2020 Apr 11.
36. Sadeghi P, Izadi A, Mojtahedi SY, et al. A 10-year cross-sectional retrospective study on Kawasaki disease in Iranian children: Incidence, clinical manifestations, complications, and treatment patterns. *BMC Infect Dis.* Apr 19, 2021;21(1):368. doi: 10.1186/s12879-021-06046-2.
37. Perez EE. Immunoglobulin use in immune deficiency and autoimmune disease states. *Am J Manag Care.* Jun 2019;25(6 Suppl):S92–S97.
38. Foster JH, Cheng WS, Nguyen NY, Krance R, Martinez C. Immunoglobulin prophylaxis in pediatric hematopoietic stem cell transplant. *Pediatr Blood Cancer.* Dec2018;65(12):e27348. doi: 10.1002/pbc.27348. Epub 2018 Sep 11.
39. Briani C, Cocito D, Campagnolo M, Doneddu PE, Nobile-Orazio E. Update on therapy of chronic immune-mediated neuropathies. *Neurol Sci.* Jan 16, 2021. doi: 10.1007/s10072-020-04998-y. Epub ahead of print.
40. Songsaroj P, Kahwaji J, Vo A, Jordan SC. Modern approaches to incompatible kidney transplantation. *World J Nephrol.* 2015;4:354–362.
41. Späth PJ, Granata G, La Marra F, Kuijpers TW, Quinti I. On the dark side of therapies with immunoglobulin concentrates: The adverse events. *Frontiers Immunol.* 2015;6:11.
42. Committee on Practice Bulletins-Obstetrics. Practice Bulletin No. 181: Prevention of Rh D alloimmunization. *Obstet Gynecol.* 2017;130:e57–e70.
43. Centers for Disease Control and Prevention. Vaccinate with confidence. Strategy to reinforce confidence in COVID-19 vaccines. Available at: https://www.cdc.gov/vaccines/covid-19/vaccinate-with-confidence.html
44. Macdonald NE. Vaccine hesitancy: Definition, scope and determinants. *Vaccine.* 2015;33(34):4161–4164.
45. Centers for Disease Control and Prevention. Building confidence in COVID-19 vaccines among your patients. Tips for the healthcare team. Available at: https://www.cdc.gov/vaccines/covid-19/downloads/VaccinateWConfidence-TipsForHCTeams_508.pdf

148

Human Immunodeficiency Virus Infection

Peter L. Anderson, Kristina M. Brooks, and Courtney V. Fletcher

KEY CONCEPTS

1. Infection with human immunodeficiency virus (HIV) occurs through three primary routes: sexual, parenteral, and perinatal. Sexual intercourse, primarily receptive anal and vaginal intercourse, is the most common method for transmission.
2. HIV infects cells expressing cluster of differentiation 4 (CD4) receptors, such as T-helper lymphocytes, monocytes, macrophages, dendritic cells, and brain microglia. Infection occurs via an interaction between glycoprotein 160 (gp160) on HIV with CD4 (primary interaction) and chemokine coreceptors (secondary interactions) present on the surfaces of these cells.
3. The hallmark of untreated HIV infection is profound CD4 T-lymphocyte depletion and severe immunosuppression (Acquired Immunodeficiency Syndrome [AIDS]) that puts persons with HIV at significant risk for infectious diseases caused by opportunistic pathogens. Opportunistic infections (OIs) in settings without access to antiretroviral drugs are the chief cause of morbidity and mortality associated with HIV infection.
4. The current goal of combination antiretroviral therapy (ART) is to achieve maximal and durable suppression of HIV replication, measured as the level of HIV-RNA in plasma (viral load) less than the lower limit of quantitation, usually 20 to 50 copies/mL (20×10^3–50×10^3/L). Another equally important outcome is an increase in CD4 lymphocytes because this closely correlates with the risk for developing OIs.
5. General principles for the management of OIs include preventing or reversing immunosuppression with ART, preventing exposure to pathogens, vaccination, prospective immunologic monitoring, primary chemoprophylaxis, treatment of acute episodes, secondary chemoprophylaxis, and discontinuation of prophylaxes following ART and subsequent immune recovery.
6. Clinical use of antiretroviral agents is complicated by drug-drug interactions. Some interactions are beneficial and used purposely; others may be harmful, leading to dangerously elevated or inadequate drug concentrations. For these reasons, clinicians involved in the pharmacotherapy of HIV infection must exercise constant vigilance and maintain a current knowledge of drug interactions.
7. Recommendations for the initial treatment of HIV advocate a minimum of two or three active antiretroviral agents from at least two drug classes. The typical regimen consists of two nucleoside/nucleotide analogs with an integrase strand transfer inhibitor (InSTI).
8. Inadequate suppression of viral replication allows HIV to select for antiretroviral-resistant HIV variants, a major factor limiting the ability of antiretroviral drugs to inhibit virus replication. Recommendations for treating drug-resistant HIV include choosing at least two drugs (preferably three) of different classes to which the patient's virus is susceptible. Susceptibility can be assessed using either genotypic or phenotypic resistance testing.
9. The reduction of viral load with ART lowers the risk of transmission to others. Additionally, pre- and post-exposure prophylaxis with antiretroviral agents in at-risk persons lowers HIV acquisition risk.
10. The longer life span conferred by ART has given rise to other medical issues. A wide spectrum of complications associated with older age have become common, some of which overlap with adverse effects from antiretroviral drugs. Medical management of these contemporary HIV complications is constantly evolving.

BEYOND THE BOOK

Review and complete the "HIV Infection: The Antiretroviral-Naïve Patient Level II" patient case in the *Pharmacotherapy Casebook: A Patient-Focused Approach.*

INTRODUCTION

Acquired immunodeficiency syndrome (AIDS) was first recognized in a cohort of young, previously healthy men who have sex with men (MSM) with new-onset profound immunologic deficits, *Pneumocystis carinii* (now *Pneumocystis jirovecii*) pneumonia (PCP), and/or Kaposi's sarcoma. A retrovirus, human immunodeficiency virus type 1 (HIV-1), is the major cause of AIDS. A second retrovirus, HIV-2, is also recognized to cause AIDS, although it is less virulent, transmissible, and prevalent than HIV-1. These retroviruses are transmitted primarily by sexual contact and by contact with infected blood or blood products. Several risk behaviors for the acquisition of HIV infection have been identified in the United States, most notably the practice of anorectal intercourse and the sharing of blood-contaminated needles by injection-drug users. In many resource-limited countries, the majority of HIV transmission occurs via heterosexual intercourse and from childbearing people to their offspring. Initially, the medical management of HIV consisted of repeated treatments for opportunistic infections (OIs) and eventual palliative care. In the mid-1990s, a new era in the pharmacotherapy for HIV, known as *combination antiretroviral therapy* (ART), was born. ART consists of combinations of antiretroviral agents with different mechanisms of action that potently and durably suppress HIV replication, delay the onset of AIDS, reverse HIV-associated immunologic deficits, reduce HIV transmission, and significantly prolong survival. Modern antiretroviral drugs and ART regimens have improved tolerability and efficacy. Nevertheless, therapeutic challenges remain in the present ART era including the need for continuous adherence to medications and care, drug-drug interactions, drug-resistant HIV, acute and long-term drug toxicities, and other complications associated with a prolonged life span. Despite progress in the treatment access for this disease, large numbers of persons with HIV remain outside of care, nationally and globally. Significant efforts to develop an HIV vaccine have not been fruitful. However, prophylactic use of antiretroviral drugs effectively prevents HIV infection in persons at high risk of exposure and those exposed to the virus.

EPIDEMIOLOGY

The epidemiologic characteristics of HIV infection differ according to geographic region and depend upon the mode of transmission, governmental prevention efforts and resources, and cultural factors.[1,2]

1 Infection with HIV occurs through three primary modes: sexual, parenteral, and perinatal. Sexual intercourse, primarily anal and vaginal intercourse, is the most common method for transmission. The probability of HIV transmission depends on the type of sexual exposure. The highest risk is from receptive anorectal intercourse at about 1.4 transmissions per 100 sexual acts.[3] Transmission risk is lower for receptive vaginal intercourse, and insertive sex acts have lower risk than receptive acts. Condom use reduces risk of transmission by approximately 80%.[3] Other factors that affect the probability of infection include the stage of HIV disease and viral load in the index partner. For example, transmission is significantly higher when the index partner has early or late HIV compared with asymptomatic HIV, as these disease stages are associated with higher viral loads.[3] Individuals with genital ulcers or sexually transmitted infections are at greater risk for contracting HIV. HIV incidence and prevalence are lower in cultures that advocate male circumcision, which reduces risk of male acquisition of HIV approximately 50%.[3] Casual contact with persons with HIV is not a significant risk factor for HIV transmission.

Prevention of sexual transmission has focused primarily on education that encourages safer sex practices such as use of condoms and reduction of high-risk behavior (eg, intercourse or promiscuity with partners of unknown HIV status).[4] A powerful tool for HIV prevention is combination ART for the infected individual, as this dramatically lowers viral replication and infectiousness, significantly reducing the risk of transmission to others.[3,5] In fact, the HIV scientific community has endorsed the notion that "U = U," which means undetectable (plasma HIV-RNA) = untransmittable (no HIV transmissions).[6] Another effective prevention tool is chemoprophylaxis with antiretroviral drugs, as this significantly reduces HIV acquisition risk among uninfected individuals.[7-9] A combined approach has been advocated for optimal prevention.[10] Prevention strategies under investigation include HIV vaccines and topical vaginal/rectal microbicides, such as vaginal rings containing antiretroviral drugs.[11,12]

Parenteral transmission of HIV broadly encompasses infections due to infected blood exposure from needle sticks, IV injection with used needles, receipt of blood products, and organ transplants. Use of contaminated needles or other injection-related paraphernalia by drug abusers has been the main cause of parenteral transmissions. The risk of HIV transmission from sharing needles is approximately 0.67 per 100 episodes.[3,13] Prevention strategies include stopping drug use, obtaining needles from credible sources (eg, pharmacies), never reusing or sharing any paraphernalia, using sterile procedures in all injecting activities, and safely disposing of used paraphernalia.[10]

Before widespread screening, HIV was readily transmitted in blood products.[13] However, blood and tissue products in the healthcare system are now rigorously screened for HIV. The estimated risk for receiving contaminated blood or blood products in the United States is well below 1:2,300,000 and that for receiving a contaminated tissue transplant is 1:55,000.[14,15] Healthcare workers have a small but definite occupational risk of contracting HIV through accidental exposure. Most cases of occupationally acquired HIV have been the result of a percutaneous needle stick injury, which carries an estimated 0.3% risk of transmitting HIV.[3,16] Mucocutaneous exposures (eg, blood splash in eyes, mouth, or nose) carries a transmission risk of approximately 0.09%.[16] Significant risk factors for seroconversion with a needle stick include deep injury, injury with a device visibly contaminated with blood, and advanced HIV disease in the index patient (high viral load). The risk of transmission from a healthcare worker with HIV to a patient is extremely remote. Comprehensive medical guidelines, including antiretroviral drug prophylaxis, have been developed to minimize the hazard of HIV transmission for healthcare workers and persons exposed by rape or other means.[13,16]

Perinatal infection, or vertical transmission, is the most common cause of pediatric HIV infection. Most infections occur during or near to the time of birth, although a fraction can occur in utero.[2] The risk of mother-to-child transmission is approximately 25% in the absence of ART. Factors that increase the likelihood of vertical transmission include prolonged rupture of membranes, chorioamnionitis, genital infection during pregnancy, preterm delivery, vaginal delivery, birth weight less than 2.5 kg, illicit drug use and cigarette smoking during pregnancy, and high maternal viral load.[17] Breast-feeding in the absence of ART can also transmit HIV. The frequency of breast milk transmission is approximately 5% to 10% in the first 6 months and 15% to 20% through 18 to 24 months without interventions to reduce transmission.[18] High levels of virus in breast milk and in the mother are associated with higher risk of transmission. Formula feeding prevents breast milk transmission of HIV but may not improve mortality from other causes early in life in resource limited settings.[19] In the United States, mothers with HIV are recommended not to breastfeed.[19] A separate and comprehensive set of medical guidelines including antiretroviral drug prophylaxis have been developed to minimize the risk of mother-to-child HIV transmission.[19]

Persons with HIV infection are broadly categorized as those living with HIV and those with an AIDS diagnosis (stage 3). An AIDS diagnosis is made when the presence of HIV is laboratory-confirmed and the CD4 (T-helper cell) count drops below 200 cells/mm^3 (0.2×10^9/L) for those aged 6 years or older, or after an AIDS indicator condition is diagnosed.[20] Further distinctions regarding the stage of HIV and AIDS (stage 3) are given in the revised Centers for Disease Control and Prevention (CDC) surveillance case definition (Table 148-1).[20] In the United States, the CDC estimates HIV epidemiology using models that rely on surveillance data from state and local health departments.[10] Using these models about 1.2 million individuals are living with HIV (all stages) in the United States.[10] Approximately 13% of persons with HIV are unaware of their infection and only approximately 50% of those who are aware of their infection are consistently retained in care. Therefore, about half of persons with HIV are not receiving ART regularly, which significantly contributes to the ongoing transmission of HIV infection in the United States, totaling 36,800 new infections per annum.[21,22]

The epidemic in the United States was initially established in MSM, and this population continues to be prominently affected by HIV, accounting for 65% of new cases.[21]

TABLE 148-1 Surveillance Case Definition for HIV Infection Stage Based on CD4+ T-lymphocyte Counts, United States, 2014

	Age on date of CD4+ T-lymphocyte test					
	<1 year		1-5 years		≥6 years	
Stage	**Cells/μL ($\times 10^6$/L)**	**%**	**Cells/μL ($\times 10^6$/L)**	**%**	**Cells/μL ($\times 10^6$/L)**	**%**
1	≥1,500	≥34	≥1,000	≥30	≥500	≥26
2	750-1,499	26-33	500-999	22-29	200-499	14-25
3 (AIDS)	<750	<26	<500	<22	<200	<14

AIDS-defining conditions

Bacterial infections, multiple or recurrent (specific to children <6 years)	
Candidiasis of bronchi, trachea, or lungs	Lymphoma, Burkitt
Candidiasis, esophageal	Lymphoma, immunoblastic
Cervical cancer, invasive (specific to adults, adolescents, children >6 years)	Lymphoma, primary, or brain
Coccidioidomycosis, disseminated or extrapulmonary	*Mycobacterium avium* complex or *Mycobacterium kansasii*, disseminated or extrapulmonary
Cryptococcosis, extrapulmonary	*Mycobacterium tuberculosis*, any site (pulmonary or extrapulmonary)
Cryptosporidiosis, chronic intestinal (duration >1 month)	*Mycobacterium*, other species or unidentified species, disseminated or extrapulmonary
Cytomegalovirus disease (other than liver, spleen, or nodes), onset at age >1 month	*Pneumocystis jirovecii* pneumonia (PCP)
Cytomegalovirus retinitis (with loss of vision)	Pneumonia, recurrent (specific to adults, adolescents, children >6 years)
Encephalopathy, HIV-related	Progressive multifocal leukoencephalopathy
Herpes simplex: chronic ulcer(s) (duration >1 month); or bronchitis, pneumonitis, or esophagitis, onset at age >1 month	*Salmonella* septicemia, recurrent Toxoplasmosis of brain, onset at age >1 month Wasting syndrome due to HIV
Histoplasmosis, disseminated or extrapulmonary Isosporiasis, chronic intestinal (duration >1 month) Kaposi's sarcoma	

Data from Reference 20.

Heterosexual transmissions accounted for approximately 23% of new cases and approximately 65% of these are women. Injection-drug use makes up about 7% of new cases. For women, the main risk factor for transmission is heterosexual intercourse (~85% of cases) and injection-drug use (~15% of cases). For men, the main risks are MSM (~81%), heterosexual sex (~10%), and injection-drug use (~10%).[21] Black and Hispanic communities are disproportionately affected by HIV infection. Of new infections in recent years, 42% were in Black persons and 29% were in Hispanic persons, although these populations only make up 12% and 18% of the US population, respectively. A relatively large proportion of these populations are not well linked to appropriate prevention, care, and treatment services, which represents a significant public health challenge.[10]

The number of individuals living with HIV globally has risen to 37.6 million persons.[1,23] Increases are due to longer lifespans due to wider implementation of ART worldwide. This has reduced the death rate and new infection rate. For example, the peak number of new infections was 3 million per year in 1997 and this has declined to 1.5 million in 2020. New infections in children (mostly due to perinatal transmission) have declined by 52% between 2010 and 2020, and overall deaths have declined by approximately 59% since 2004. Nevertheless, approximately 690,000 people succumbed to HIV in 2019 and HIV is still a major contributor to the global burden of disease.[1,23] The highest concentration of HIV cases in the world is in sub-Saharan Africa, where approximately 26 million people are infected. However, new infections have declined there by approximately 25% to 38% since 2010, depending on the region. Heterosexual transmission is the most common mode of transmission in sub-Saharan Africa and worldwide. Women in sub-Saharan Africa and resource-limited countries are at disproportionately high risk for acquiring HIV because of biological and cultural factors that foster HIV transmission, such as limited ability to negotiate condom use. Other important epidemiologic features of the HIV epidemic include growing incidence among injection-drug users in North Africa and the Middle East, as well as some regions of Eastern Europe and Central Asia (eg, Russia and Ukraine).[23]

ETIOLOGY

HIV is an enveloped single-stranded RNA virus and a member of the Lentivirinae (*lenti*, meaning "slow") subfamily of retroviruses. Lentiviruses are characterized by their indolent infectious cycle. There are two related but distinct types of HIV: HIV-1 and HIV-2. HIV-2, found mostly in western Africa, consists of seven phylogenetic lineages designated as subtypes (clades) A through G. Four groups of HIV-1 are recognized: M (main or major), N (non-M, non-O), O (outlier), and P (pending the identification of further cases).[2] The nine subtypes of HIV-1 group M are identified as A through D, F through H, J, and K. Mixtures of subtypes are referred to as *circulating recombinant forms.* Group M, subtype B, is primarily responsible for the epidemic in North America and western Europe.[24]

HIV in humans was the result of a cross-species transmission (zoonosis) from primates infected with simian immunodeficiency virus (SIV).[24] Phylogenetic and geographic relationships suggest that HIV-2 arose from SIV that infects sooty mangabeys, and HIV-1 groups M and N arose from SIVcpz, a virus that infects chimpanzees (*Pan troglodytes troglodytes*). Groups O and P may have arisen from an SIV variant that infects wild gorillas. Cultural practices, such as preparation and eating of bush meat or keeping animals as pets, may have allowed the virus to cross from primates to humans. The earliest known human infection with HIV has been traced to central Africa in 1959, but cross-species transmissions probably date back to the early 1900s.[24] Modern transportation, promiscuity, and drug use have caused the rapid and continued spread of the virus within the United States and throughout the world. This chapter focuses on HIV-1 group M, which is the predominant strain likely to be encountered in the western world.

PATHOGENESIS

2 Understanding the life cycle of HIV (Fig. 148-1) is necessary because the current strategies used for HIV treatment target points in this cycle. Once HIV enters the human body, the outer glycoprotein (gp160) on its surface, which is composed of two subunits (gp120 and gp41), has affinity for CD4 receptors, which are proteins present on the surface of T-helper lymphocytes, monocytes, macrophages, dendritic cells, and brain microglia. The gp120 subunit is responsible for CD4 binding. Once initial binding occurs, the intimate association of HIV with the cell is enhanced by further binding to chemokine coreceptors. The two major chemokine receptors used by HIV are chemokine (C–C motif) receptor 5 (CCR5) and chemokine (C–X–C motif) receptor 4 (CXCR4). HIV isolates may contain a mixture of viruses that target one or the other of these coreceptors, and some viral strains may be dual-tropic (ie, can use both coreceptors). The HIV strain that preferentially uses CCR5, referred to as R5 viruses, is macrophage-tropic and typically implicated in most cases of sexually transmitted HIV.[25] Individuals with a common 32-base-pair deletion in the CCR5 gene are protected from progression of HIV disease, and those who are homozygous for the 32-base-pair deletion have a degree of resistance to acquisition of HIV-1.[26] The HIV strain that targets CXCR4, designated X4 virus, is T-cell-tropic and often is predominant in the later stage of disease. CD4 and coreceptor attachment of HIV to the cell promotes membrane fusion, which is mediated by gp41, and finally internalization of the viral genetic material and enzymes necessary for replication.

After internalization, the viral protein shell surrounding the nucleic acid (capsid) undergoes a disassembly process in preparation for replication.[27] The genetic material of HIV is positive-sense single-stranded RNA; the virus must transcribe this RNA into DNA (transcription normally occurs from DNA to RNA; HIV works backward, hence the name *retrovirus*). To do so, HIV is equipped with the unique enzyme RNA-dependent DNA polymerase (reverse transcriptase). HIV reverse transcriptase first synthesizes a complementary strand of DNA using the viral RNA as a template. The RNA portion of this DNA-RNA hybrid is then partially removed by ribonuclease H (RNase H), allowing HIV reverse transcriptase to complete the synthesis of a double-stranded DNA molecule. The fidelity of HIV reverse transcriptase is poor, and many mistakes are made during the process. These errors in the final DNA product contribute to the rapid mutation of the virus, which enables the virus to evade the immune response (thus complicating vaccine development), and promotes the evolution of drug resistance during partially suppressive therapy. Following reverse transcription, the final double-stranded DNA product migrates into the nucleus and is integrated into the host cell chromosome by integrase, another enzyme unique to HIV.

The integration of HIV into the host chromosome is critically important. Most notably, HIV can establish a persistent, latent infection, particularly in long-lived cells of the immune system such as memory T lymphocytes. The virus is effectively hidden in these cells until the cells become activated, and this characteristic has greatly complicated efforts to cure HIV infection.[28] It also necessitates continuous ART therapy because virus reemerges from this reservoir if therapy is suspended.

After integration, HIV preferentially replicates in activated cells. Activation by antigens, cytokines, or other factors stimulates the cell to produce nuclear factor kappa B (NF-κB), an enhancer-binding protein. NF-κB normally regulates the expression of T-lymphocyte genes involved in growth but also can inadvertently activate replication of HIV.[28] HIV encodes six regulatory and accessory proteins,

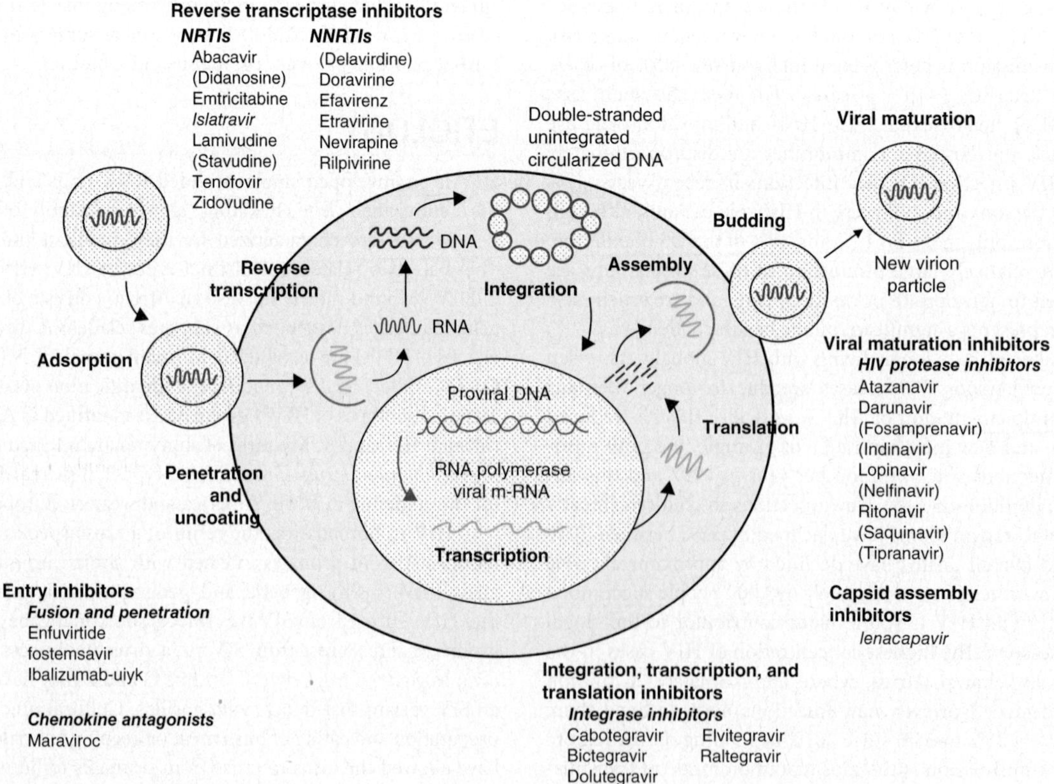

FIGURE 148-1 Life cycle of human immunodeficiency virus with potential targets where replication may be interrupted. Italicized compounds were in development at the time of this writing. Parentheses indicate medications that are no longer used in clinical practice.

such as Tat, Nef, Rev, Vpu, Vif, and Vpr, which enhance replication and inhibit innate immunity. For example, the Tat protein is a potent amplifier of HIV gene expression; it binds to a specific RNA sequence of HIV that initiates and stabilizes transcription elongation.[28] Vif is a viral protein that binds human APOBEC 3G, a cytidine deaminase that disrupts the virus' genetic code by converting viral RNA cytosine to uracil, thereby providing innate cellular immunity.[29] Vpu inhibits tetherin, a human cellular membrane protein that prevents release of virus particles after budding from infected cells. Assembly of new viral particles occurs in a stepwise manner beginning with the coalescence of HIV proteins beneath the host cell lipid bilayer. The nucleocapsid is subsequently formed with viral single-stranded RNA and other components packaged inside. Once packaged, the virion then buds through the plasma membrane, acquiring the characteristics of the host lipid bilayer. After the virus buds, the maturation process begins. Within the virion, protease, another enzyme unique to HIV, cleaves large precursor polypeptides (gag and gag-pol) into functional proteins (capsid, protease, reverse transcriptase, and integrase) that are necessary to produce a complete and infectious virus. Without this enzyme, the virion is immature and unable to infect other cells. Capsid is key to this final maturation process, as well as many other roles in the HIV life-cycle such as facilitating reverse transcription, intracellular transport, nuclear entry, and integration.[30] Thus, potent capsid inhibitors are under development and soon will join the antiretroviral armamentarium.

The natural history of HIV infection exhibits three general phases: acute, chronic, and terminal (AIDS). Initial rounds of HIV replication during acute infection take place largely in the mucosal CD4+, CCR5+ T-cell pools in the gut, resulting in a massive CD4 T-cell depletion in these tissues.[31] Cells are destroyed by various mechanisms, including cell lysis from newly budding virions, cytotoxic T-lymphocyte-induced cell killing, and induction of apoptosis. Following this destruction of the mucosal CD4 T-cell pool, which lasts for 2 to 3 weeks, a state of heightened immune activation ensues during the chronic infection phase, which can last for several years. The activated state is characterized by high levels of activation markers on circulating T cells (eg, HLA-DR and CD38) and proinflammatory cytokines, and may result from HIV antigen as well as translocation of microbial antigens from the T-cell-depleted gut mucosa. Heightened activation enables further HIV replication and ultimately leads to continued depletion of CD4+, CCR5+ T cells. HIV-1 exhibits a high turnover rate during this chronic phase, with an estimated 10 billion new viruses produced each day.[32] More than 99% of these viruses are produced in newly infected activated cells. Nevertheless, for much of the chronic phase, the immune system is able to operate well enough to prevent overt OIs that herald AIDS. However, the depletion of CD4 cells and continuous cellular activation eventually lead to a final collapse of the immune system, or AIDS. HIV may use the CXCR4 coreceptor during this last phase of infection, and these viruses infect a broader range of CD4 cells (naïve and central-memory) speeding the disease progression. It is this unrelenting destruction of CD4 cells that causes the profoundly compromised immune system and AIDS.

DIAGNOSIS

Detection of HIV and Surrogate Markers of Disease Progression

HIV is diagnosed through a multi-step process.[33] The presence of HIV infection is screened with an enzyme-linked immunosorbent assay (ELISA), which detects antibodies against HIV-1. Although ELISA has been the mainstay of HIV screening for decades, the technology has been evolving to detect infection earlier in the time course of the disease.[34] Older ELISA tests detected IgG (second-generation tests), but more modern tests detect IgG and IgM (third-generation tests) and may further include detection of p24 antigen, an early marker of infection (fourth-generation tests). These technological advances enable earlier detection of HIV by as much as 15 to 20 days compared with older second-generation tests. ELISA tests are generally highly sensitive (greater than 99%) and highly specific (greater than 99%), but rare false-positive results can occur particularly in those with autoimmune disorders.[33] False-negative results also occur and may be attributed to the "window period" before adequate production of antibodies or antigen. This "window period" between HIV acquisition and detection of HIV with fourth- and third-generation tests is approximately 2 and 3 weeks, respectively.[33] Positive screening tests are confirmed with another enzyme immunoassay to specify if the antibodies are to HIV-1 versus HIV-2 (although HIV-2 is rare in the United States, this step ensures proper diagnosis and treatment). If this follow-up assay is indeterminant or negative, an HIV nucleic acid test is performed for definitive diagnosis. HIV-RNA is the earliest indicator of infection, detectable ~10 days from acquisition and about 1 week before fourth-generation tests.[34] Several point-of-care screening kits are available for serum, plasma, whole blood, or oral fluids. While oral fluid tests are convenient, they are not as sensitive as blood assays, which may result in false-negatives early in infections; this is a particular disadvantage in the setting of HIV testing prior to initiating or continuing preexposure prophylaxis (PrEP).[34] Clinicians should be aware that HIV acquisition during PrEP may be associated with prolonged HIV suppression and delayed antibody expression.[35] HIV testing is recommended when HIV infection is suspected because of symptoms and/or high-risk behavior.[36] Additionally, the CDC recommends routine HIV screening at least once in all healthcare settings in all persons 13 to 64 years, a policy called "opt-out" testing.[37] A focus of the recommendations is to screen persons at high risk of HIV infection (eg, MSM) at least annually and to screen pregnant women while they are in care. The policy states that consent for medical care will imply consent for HIV testing; however, the person must be informed of the test and can opt out of taking it. Because states may have different HIV consent laws, the local requirements for HIV testing should be consulted. The rationale for the opt-out strategy is to diagnose those who unknowingly carry HIV so as to initiate ART early, leading to improved prognosis and reduced forward transmissions.

Once diagnosed, HIV disease is monitored primarily by two surrogate biomarkers, viral load and CD4 cell count.[38] The viral load test quantifies the degree of viremia by measuring the number of copies of viral RNA (HIV-RNA) in the plasma. Methods for determining HIV-RNA include reverse-transcription polymerase chain reaction (RT-PCR), branched-chain DNA, transcription-mediated amplification, and nucleic acid sequence-based assay. RT-PCR is used more widely than the other techniques.[34] Irrespective of the method used, viral load is reported as the number of viral RNA copies per milliliter of plasma. Each assay has its own lower limit of quantitation, and results can vary from one assay method to the other; therefore, the same assay method should be used consistently for each patient. Reductions in viral load often are reported in base 10 logarithm. For example, if a patient presents initially with a viral load of 100,000 copies/mL (10^5 copies/mL or 10^8 copies/L) and subsequently has a viral load of 10,000 copies/mL (10^4 copies/mL or 10^7 copies/L), the decrease is 1 $\log_{10}$. Given that HIV-RNA varies within a patient, a perceptible clinical response is generally considered when the decline in viral load is more than 0.5 $\log_{10}$.[38] Viral load is a major prognostic factor for disease progression, CD4 count decline, and death.[38] It is also the predominant way to assess the effectiveness of treatment.

Because HIV attacks and leads to the destruction of cells bearing the CD4 receptor, the number of CD4 lymphocytes (T-helper cells) in the blood is a critical surrogate marker of disease progression and immune system status.[38] The normal adult CD4 lymphocyte count ranges from 500 to 1,600 cells/mm³ (0.5×10^9–1.6×10^9/L), or 40% to 70% (0.4-0.7) of total lymphocytes. CD4 counts in children are age dependent, with younger children having higher CD4 counts (see Table 148-1). The hallmark of HIV disease is depletion of CD4 cells and the associated development of OIs and malignancies, especially at lower CD4 cell counts.

CLINICAL PRESENTATION

3 Clinical presentation of primary HIV infection varies, but most patients (50%-90%) have an acute retroviral syndrome or mononucleosis-like illness, presumably due to the host immune response to the virus (ie, "cytokine storm").[39] Although many of these symptoms are nonspecific (eg, fever, headache, fatigue, lymphadenopathy, pharyngitis, rash), the presence of aseptic meningitis, oral or genital ulcers, and leukopenia should raise suspicion of acute HIV infection in the setting of a potential exposure. Symptoms often last 2 weeks, and hospitalization may be required for a small fraction of patients. Primary infection is associated with a high viral load (more than 10^6 copies/mL [10^9/L]) and a precipitous drop in CD4 cells. After several weeks, an immune response is mounted, the amount of HIV-RNA in plasma falls substantially, CD4 cells rebound slightly, and symptoms resolve gradually. However, as described above, this clinically latent period is not virologically latent because HIV replication is continuous (~10 billion viruses per day) and immune system destruction is ongoing. A steady decrease in CD4 cells (~50 cells/μL [0.05×10^9/L] per year) is the most measurable aspect of this immune system deterioration during the asymptomatic phase. Plasma viral load, on the other hand, is stabilized at a particular level or "set point." The set point correlates strongly with the CD4 cell decline and time to AIDS and morbidity. For example, prior to ART, the Multicenter AIDS Cohort Study measured viral load in 1,604 HIV-positive men and followed them for as long as 11 years. The CD4 cell count decline was approximately twice as fast in those with HIV-RNA above 30,000 copies/mL (30×10^6/L) compared with those with HIV-RNA less than or equal to 500 copies/mL (500×10^3/L) and mortality rates (within 6 years) were 69.5% versus 0.9%, respectively.[40] Thus, a higher viral set point is associated with faster disease progression and poorer prognosis. Not all individuals infected with HIV progress to AIDS—these so-called "long-term nonprogressors" (also known as "elite controllers") may be infected with a defective virus (eg, Nef-deficient HIV) or may have an intrinsic ability to resist infection (eg, CCR5 mutation).

Most children born with HIV are asymptomatic. On physical examination, children often present with nonspecific signs, such as lymphadenopathy, hepatomegaly, splenomegaly, failure to thrive, weight loss or unexplained low birth weight (in prenatally exposed infants), and fever of unknown origin.[41] Laboratory findings include anemia, hypergammaglobulinemia (primarily IgA and IgM), altered mononuclear cell function, and altered T-cell subset ratios. Of note, the normal range for CD4 cell counts in young children is much different from the range in adults (Table 148-1). Children have different susceptibility and/or exposures to OIs compared with adults. Bacterial infections, including *Streptococcus pneumoniae*, *Salmonella* spp., and *Mycobacterium tuberculosis*, may be more prevalent in children with AIDS than in adults with the disease. Kaposi's sarcoma is rare in children. Children with HIV infection may develop lymphocytic interstitial pneumonitis without evidence of *P. jirovecii* or other pathogens on lung biopsy.

Some children (~25%) will progress to AIDS rapidly within the first year of life. A presentation of serious OIs such as *P. jirovecii* pneumonia, encephalopathy, failure to thrive, and a precipitous drop in CD4 cells are common in these infants. General management of children with HIV involves principles similar to those used for adults: ART, treatment and prophylaxis of OIs, and supportive care.[42,43]

TREATMENT

Desired Outcomes

4 The central goals of ART are to decrease morbidity and mortality, improve quality of life, restore and preserve immune function, and prevent further transmission.[38] The most important and effective way to achieve these goals is maximal and durable suppression of HIV replication, which is interpreted as plasma HIV-RNA less than the lower limit of quantitation (ie, undetectable; usually less than 20 or 50 copies/mL [20×10^3 or 50×10^3/L]). Such a profound reduction in HIV-RNA is associated with reduced transmissions and long-term response to therapy (ie, durability), as well as increases in CD4 lymphocytes that closely correlate with a reduced risk for developing OIs. While undetectable HIV-RNA almost always corresponds with a rise in CD4 lymphocytes, some patients respond virologically or immunologically without the other.

General Approach to Treatment

5 Contemporary combinations of two or three active antiretroviral agents from two pharmacologic classes potently inhibit HIV replication to undetectable plasma levels, prevent and reverse immune deficiency, and substantially decrease morbidity and mortality—constituting the modern ART era.[44] Principles that serve as a guide for the clinical use of antiretroviral agents include[45]:

1. Ongoing HIV replication leads to immune system damage and progression to AIDS. HIV infection is always harmful, and true long-term survival free of clinically significant immune dysfunction is unusual.
2. Plasma HIV-RNA levels indicate the magnitude of HIV replication and its associated rate of CD4 cell destruction, whereas CD4 cell counts indicate the extent of HIV-induced immune damage already suffered.
3. Use of potent combination ART to suppress HIV replication to below the levels of detection of sensitive plasma HIV-RNA assays limits the potential for selection of antiretroviral-resistant HIV variants, the major factor limiting the ability of antiretroviral drugs to inhibit virus replication and delay disease progression. Therefore, maximum achievable suppression of HIV replication should be the goal of therapy.
4. The most effective means for accomplishing durable suppression of HIV replication is simultaneous initiation of combinations of effective anti-HIV drugs with which the patient has not been treated previously and that are not cross-resistant with antiretroviral agents with which the patient has been treated previously.
5. Each of the antiretroviral drugs used in combination therapy regimens always should be used according to optimal schedules and dosages.
6. The available effective antiretroviral drugs are limited in number and mechanism of action, and cross-resistance between specific drugs has been documented. Therefore, any change in ART increases future therapeutic constraints.
7. People of child-bearing potential should receive optimal ART regardless of pregnancy status.
8. The same principles of ART apply to both children and adults with HIV, although treatment of children with HIV involves unique pharmacologic, virologic, and immunologic considerations.
9. Persons with acute primary HIV infections should be treated with combination ART to suppress virus replication to levels below the limit of detection of sensitive plasma HIV-RNA assays.

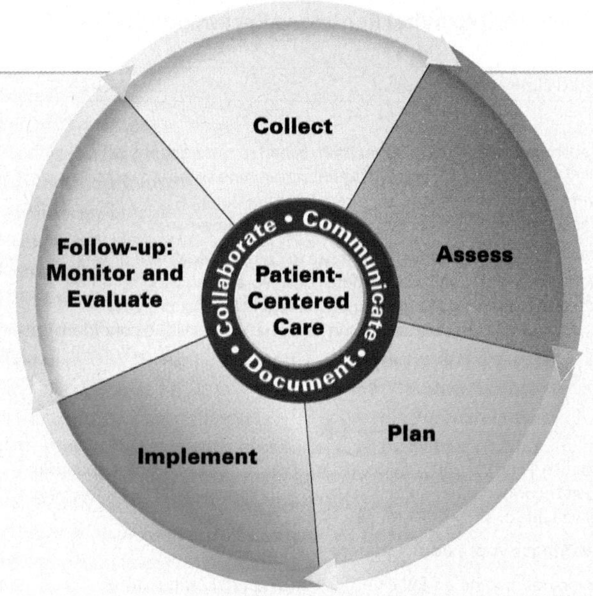

Patient Care Process for Human Immunodeficiency Virus (HIV)

Collect

- Patient characteristics (eg, age, sex at birth, gender identity, race, ethnicity, contraception methods, or pregnancy intentions)
- Patient medical history (eg, HBV, HCV, STIs, other chronic/acute illnesses)
- Previous HIV history (mode of transmission, date of diagnosis, nadir CD4$^+$ T-cell count, history of previous opportunistic infections, history of antiretroviral resistance)
- Social history (eg, drug use, sexual history, high-risk behaviors)
- Current prescription and nonprescription medications including herbal products, dietary supplements, and any previous antiretroviral regimens
- Objective data
  - HIV screening and confirmatory tests
  - HIV-RNA and CD4$^+$ cell count
  - Baseline antiretroviral resistance testing
  - HLA-B*5701 testing
  - Complete blood count, basic metabolic panel, liver function panel, sexually transmitted infection screening

Assess

- Understanding of disease state and goals of treatment
- Access to ART (ie, insurance and co-pays)
- Willingness to start and adhere to ART
- Potential drug-drug interactions
- Any contraindications or concerns related to recommended ART regimens (eg, chronic kidney disease, ART resistance, HLA-B*5701 genotype, history of cardiovascular disease, hyperlipidemia, uncontrolled psychiatric illness, pregnancy or desire to become pregnant, history of multiple bone fractures, or severe osteoporosis)
- Need for opportunistic infection prophylaxis (ie, CD4$^+$ cell count)

Plan*

- ART regimen including specific agents, dose, frequency, administration (eg, food requirements), drug-drug interactions (see Tables 148-2 and 148-3)
- Monitoring parameters including efficacy (eg, HIV-RNA, CD4$^+$ cell count) and safety (eg, adverse effects, SCr, LFTs, CBC)
- Follow-up every 3 months until HIV-RNA is undetectable
- Patient education (eg, purpose of treatment, importance of adherence, transmission risk, drug-specific information; see Table 148-3)
- Referrals to other providers when appropriate (eg, behavioral health, social work)

Implement*

- Provide patient education regarding all elements of treatment plan
- Emphasize need for adherence to ART regimen and provide resources that can be used to maximize adherence
- Schedule follow-up for assessment of ART efficacy, safety, and adherence

Follow-up: Monitor and Evaluate

- Therapeutic efficacy (ie, reduction in HIV-RNA) and safety
- Restoration of immune function (ie, increasing CD4$^+$ cell count)
- Presence of adverse effects (eg, GI upset, headache, nausea)
- Renal and hepatic function
- Patient access and adherence to ART

Collaborate with patient, caregivers, and other healthcare professionals.

The extent to which these principles will continue to stand the test of time is unknown; new information on the pathogenesis and treatment of HIV accrues constantly. As of October 2021, 34 antiretroviral compounds have been approved by the FDA; six (amprenavir, delavirdine, didanosine, indinavir, stavudine, and zalcitabine) have since been removed from the US market. Table 148-2 presents the state of the art for treatment of persons with HIV as of October 2021.[38] Treatment is recommended for all persons with HIV regardless of CD4 lymphocyte count, as long as the patient is ready to adhere to therapy. Urgent indications for therapy include pregnancy, history of AIDS-defining illness, CD4 counts below 200 cells/mm^3 (0.2×10^9/L), HIV-associated nephropathy, HIV/hepatitis C virus coinfection, and/or HIV/hepatitis B virus coinfection.

The optimal time to initiate therapy in chronic HIV infection was a matter of debate. The main arguments for postponing therapy were the concern for cumulative drug toxicity and trepidation for drug resistance and loss of therapeutic options. These concerns were well-founded when older drugs such as lopinavir/ritonavir, stavudine, zidovudine, indinavir, and efavirenz were the mainstay of therapy. Today, the availability of newer medications with different mechanisms of action (eg, InSTIs) significantly improved adverse event profiles, and the convenience of single tablet regimens helps

TABLE 148-2 Treatment of Human Immunodeficiency Virus Infection: Antiretroviral Regimens Recommended as Initial Therapy for Persons with HIV

	Regimen	Selected Limitations
Recommended Initial Regimens for Most Persons with HIV		
InSTI based	Bictegravir + tenofovir alafenamide fumarate + emtricitabine (coformulated) (AI)	Not recommended if CrCl <30 mL/min (0.5 mL/s); interactions with polyvalent cations; bictegravir inhibits creatinine secretion increasing serum creatinine (distinguish vs renal dysfunction); CNS/psychiatric side effects (primarily in those with preexisting conditions)
	Dolutegravir + abacavir + lamivudine (coformulated) (AI)	Only if HLA-B*5701 negative; do not use in chronic hepatitis B infection; interactions with polyvalent cations; dolutegravir inhibits creatinine secretion increasing SCr (distinguish vs renal dysfunction); CNS/ psychiatric side effects (primarily in those with preexisting conditions)
	Dolutegravir + (tenofovir disoproxil fumarate or tenofovir alafenamide fumarate)[a] + (emtricitabine or lamivudine)[b] (AI)	Same as above without HLA-B*5701 negative requirement
	Dolutegravir + lamivudine (AI)	Do not use if HIV VL ≥500,000 copies/mL (500 × 10^6/L), chronic hepatitis B infection or hepatitis B infection status is unknown, or if HIV genotype is unavailable or shows resistance to either component
Recommended initial regimens in certain clinical situations (some potential disadvantages vs previous category)		
InSTI based	Elvitegravir + cobicistat + tenofovir disoproxil fumarate + emtricitabine (coformulated) (BI)	Initiation not recommended if CrCl <70 mL/min (1.17 mL/s); food requirement; interactions with polyvalent cations; CYP3A4 drug interactions; cobicistat inhibits creatinine secretion increasing SCr (distinguish vs renal dysfunction); CNS/psychiatric side effects (primarily in those with preexisting conditions)
	Elvitegravir + cobicistat + tenofovir alafenamide fumarate + emtricitabine (coformulated) (BI)	Not recommended if CrCl <30 mL/min (0.5 mL/s); otherwise, same as above
	Raltegravir + (tenofovir disoproxil fumarate or tenofovir alafenamide) + (emtricitabine or lamivudine) (BI for tenofovir disoproxil fumarate+ (emtricitabine or lamivudine)[b]; BII for tenofovir alafenamide + emtricitabine)	Raltegravir can be dosed once or twice daily depending on the formulation; interactions with polyvalent cations; creatine kinase increases; TDF/ FTC not recommended if CrCl <50 mL/min (0.83 mL/s) and TAF/FTC not recommended if CrCl <30 mL/min (0.5 mL/s); CNS/psychiatric side effects (primarily in those with preexisting conditions)
HIV PI based[c]	Atazanavir + ritonavir (or cobicistat) + (tenofovir disoproxil fumarate or tenofovir alafenamide fumarate)[a] + (emtricitabine or lamivudine) (BI)	GI side effects; food requirement; CYP3A4 drug interactions; hyperbilirubinemia leading to drug discontinuation, especially in those with Gilbert's syndrome. use of cobicistat with TDF/FTC not recommended if CrCl <70 mL/min (1.17 mL/s); use of TAF/FTC not recommended if CrCl <30 mL/min (0.5 mL/s); cobicistat inhibits creatinine secretion increasing SCr (distinguish vs renal dysfunction)
	Darunavir + (ritonavir or cobicistat) + (tenofovir disoproxil fumarate or tenofovir alafenamide)[a] + (emtricitabine or lamivudine)[b] (AI)	Rash (darunavir has sulfonamide moiety); GI side effects; food requirement; CYP3A4 drug interactions; use of cobicistat with TDF/ FTC not recommended if CrCl <70 mL/min (1.17 mL/s); use of TAF/FTC not recommended if CrCl <30 mL/min (0.5 mL/s); cobicistat inhibits creatinine secretion increasing serum creatinine (distinguish vs renal dysfunction)
	Darunavir + ritonavir (or cobicistat) + abacavir + lamivudine (BII)	Only if HLA-B*5701 negative; see issues above
NNRTI based	Doravirine + tenofovir disoproxil fumarate + lamivudine (coformulated) (BI)	Not recommended if CrCl <50 mL/min (0.83 mL/s); CNS side effects
	Doravirine + tenofovir alafenamide + emtricitabine (BIII)	TAF/FTC not recommended if CrCl <30 mL/min (0.5 mL/s); CNS side effects
	Efavirenz + tenofovir disoproxil fumarate + (emtricitabine or lamivudine)[b] (coformulated) (BI)	CNS side effects with efavirenz; CYP450 drug interactions; empty stomach dosing before bed; not recommended if CrCl <50 mL/min (0.83 mL/s)
	Efavirenz + tenofovir alafenamide + emtricitabine (BII)	CNS side effects with efavirenz; CYP450 drug interactions; empty stomach dosing before bed; TAF/FTC not recommended if CrCl <30 mL/min (0.5 mL/s)
	Rilpivirine + (tenofovir disoproxil fumarate or tenofovir alafenamide)[a] + emtricitabine (coformulated) (BI for TDF and BII for TAF)	Not recommended when HIV-RNA >100,000 copies/mL (100 × 10^6/L) or CD4 <200 cells/μL (0.2 × 10^9/L); no proton-pump inhibitors (rilpivirine); food requirement; antacid interactions
If abacavir and tenofovir cannot be used	Dolutegravir + lamivudine (AI)	Do not use if HIV VL ≥500,000 copies/mL (500 × 10^6/L), chronic hepatitis B infection or hepatitis B infection status is unknown, or if HIV genotype is unavailable or shows resistance to either component
	Darunavir + ritonavir + raltegravir (CI)	Only if HIV-RNA <100,000 copies/mL (100 × 10^6/L) and CD4 >200 cells/mm^3 (0.2 × 10^9/L); raltegravir must be dosed twice daily; do not use in chronic hepatitis B infection
	Darunavir + ritonavir + lamivudine (CI)	Do not use in chronic hepatitis B infection

(Continued)

TABLE 148-2 Treatment of Human Immunodeficiency Virus Infection: Antiretroviral Regimens Recommended as Initial Therapy for Persons with HIV (*Continued*)

Regimen	Selected Limitations
Selected regimens or components that should not be used at any time	
Regimen or component	**Comment**
Monotherapy with any single agent (AI)	Inferior virologic efficacy; risk of virologic rebound and resistance
Any NRTI only regimen (AI)	Inferior virologic efficacy
Unboosted PIs (ie, darunavir) (AII)	Inadequate bioavailability
Etravirine + unboosted PIs (AII)	Possible induction of PI metabolism, doses not established
Nevirapine in ARV naïve with higher CD4 counts (>250 cells/μL [0.25 × 10^9/L] for women, >400 cells/μL [0.4 × 10^9/L] for men) (BI)	High incidence of symptomatic hepatotoxicity

[a]TAF and TDF are pro drugs of tenofovir with differing pharmacology and safety profiles. Safety, cost, and access should be considered when deciding between which form to use.

Evidence-based rating definition. Rating strength of recommendation—A: Strong recommendation. B: Moderate recommendation. C: Optional recommendation. Rating Quality of Evidence Supporting the Recommendation—I: Evidence from randomized, controlled trials. II: Evidence from at least one well-designed clinical trial without randomization or observational cohorts with long-term clinical outcomes. III: Expert opinion. Lamivudine and emtricitabine are considered interchangeable endpoints.

[b]Emtricitabine and lamivudine are interchangeable.

[c]Boosted darunavir is generally preferred over boosted atazanavir.

Data from Reference 38.

to mitigate these issues. Two large randomized controlled trials helped address the issue of whether initiating therapy immediately or waiting for a lower CD4 count provided clinical benefit.[46,47] In the START trial, immediate ART resulted in significantly fewer serious AIDS events (HR 0.28, 95% CI 0.15-0.50) and non-AIDS events (HR 0.61, 0.38-0.97) as compared with delaying ART until CD4 count fell below 350 cells/μL (0.35 × 10^9/L).[46] The TEMPRANO study also found that immediate ART resulted in fewer deaths or severe HIV-related illnesses as compared with deferred ART (HR among patients with a baseline CD4 greater than or equal to 500 cells/μL [0.5 × 10^9/L], 0.56; 95% CI, 0.33-0.94).[47] Immediate ART and subsequent suppressed viral load is also known to substantially prevent ongoing HIV transmissions compared with delayed ART.[48] Taken together, these studies provide high-quality evidence that untreated HIV is harmful even at high CD4 counts and immediate ART confers individual- and population-level benefit compared with delayed ART. Major policy-makers, including the WHO and US Department of Health and Human Services (DHHS), now recommend immediate ART regardless of CD4 count.[38,49]

More recent efforts have shifted toward immediate or rapid ART initiation, meaning that antiretroviral therapy is started on the same day or within a few days to weeks of HIV diagnosis. This strategy generally increases ART uptake, improves engagement and retention in HIV care, reduces time to viral suppression, and improves overall rates of those on ART with viral suppression. Several randomized controlled studies in resource-limited settings have shown marked improvements in these outcomes,[50] and prospective observational studies within the United States have shown similar patterns.[51] However, this approach requires the alignment of several resources within a short time frame and thus may be logistically challenging to implement in some settings.

An excellent source of information on updated treatment guidelines is available at https://clinicalinfo.hiv.gov/en/guidelines. Healthcare professionals involved in the care of persons with HIV are urged to consult the most current literature on the principles and strategies for ART therapy.

Pharmacologic Therapy

Several methods of therapeutic intervention have been evaluated against HIV, including systemic antiretroviral drugs (the focus of this chapter) for direct inhibition of chronic viral replication or prevention of HIV acquisition; vaccination; immunomodulators to help stimulate and restore the immune system; and topical antiretroviral drugs or virucides (chemicals that destroy intact viruses) to prevent HIV infection. Antiretroviral medications are the only FDA-approved options for HIV treatment, and the latter three approaches are now investigational. Several approaches for an HIV vaccine are in development, including whole killed virus, subunit and peptide vaccination, recombinant live vector, naked DNA delivery, adenovirus vectors, and mRNA. Historically, vaccine progress has been slow. Genetic variability in HIV and a nascent understanding of the role of the immune system in suppressing viral replication are significant barriers to the development of an effective HIV vaccine with long-lasting and protective immunity. Efforts are underway to understand the correlates of protection from various studies to inform the vaccine field going forward.[52,53] Immunomodulators have also been investigated as a way to restore immune function (eg, aldesleukin) and to potentially cure HIV through "shock and kill" strategies (activate the immune system to bring HIV out of latency, then suppress its replication).[54] Topical virucidal or antiretroviral drug formulations for vaginal or rectal use to prevent sexual transmission of HIV are in various phases of development.[11] Collectively, these agents have demonstrated modest efficacy and are discussed in more depth in the PrEP section.

Antiretroviral Agents Systemic delivery of antiretroviral agents for direct inhibition of viral replication has been the most successful strategy for both treatment and prophylaxis. Five general classes of drugs are available: entry inhibitors (fusion inhibitors, CD4 post-attachment inhibitors, gp120 attachment inhibitors, and chemokine receptor antagonists), nucleos(t)ide reverse transcriptase inhibitors (N(t)RTIs), non-nucleoside reverse transcriptase inhibitors (NNRTIs), integrase strand transfer inhibitors (InSTIs), and HIV PIs (Table 148-3).[38] Newer agents exhibit significant advantages over first-generation drugs in terms of pharmacokinetics, tolerability, safety, and efficacy. This section will highlight specific advantages of newer agents over first-generation drugs and will focus the discussion on agents used most often. Updated drug information is available in the DHHS guidelines including common adverse events and dosing recommendations for hepatic and renal insufficiency for

TABLE 148-3 Selected Pharmacologic Characteristics of Selected Antiretroviral Compounds for HIV Treatment

Drug	F (%)	$t_{1/2}$[a]	Adult Dosing Recommendation[b] (doses/day)	Plasma C_{max}/C_{min} (ng/mL or mcg/L)	Distinguishing Adverse Effects
Integrase inhibitors (InSTI)					
Bictegravir	?	17.3 hr	50 mg orally once daily	6,150/2,610	Diarrhea, nausea, headache, weight gain
Cabotegravir		41 hr	Oral lead-in: 30 mg orally once daily × 28 days	8,000/4,600	Headache, nausea, abnormal dreams, anxiety, insomnia, depressive disorders, hepatotoxicity
Cabotegravir LA	N/A	6-12 weeks (absorption-limited)	600 mg/3 mL IM × 1 (loading) 400 mg/2 mL every 4 weeks (continuation) *Or* 600 mg/3 mL every 8 weeks (continuation)	8,000/1,500 4,200/2,800	IM only: injection site reactions
Dolutegravir	?	14 hr	50 mg orally once daily *Or* 50 mg orally twice daily	3,670/1,110 4,150/2,120	Insomnia, headache, depression, and suicidal ideation (rare—usually patients with preexisting psychiatric conditions), weight gain, hepatotoxicity, hypersensitivity reactions including rash (can be severe)
Elvitegravir (coformulated with cobicistat)	?	13 hr	150 mg orally once daily	2,100/290	Diarrhea, nausea, depression and suicidal ideation (rare—usually patients with preexisting psychiatric conditions)
Raltegravir	?	9 hr	400 mg orally twice daily *Or* 1,200 mg orally once daily	2,171/68.5 7,575/51.6	Rash (can be severe), nausea, headache, diarrhea, pyrexia, creatine phosphokinase increases, weight gain, insomnia, depression, and suicidal ideation (rare—usually patients with preexisting psychiatric conditions)
Nucleoside (nucleotide) reverse transcriptase inhibitors (NRTIs)					
Abacavir	83	1.5/20 hr	300 mg orally twice daily *Or* 600 mg orally once daily	3,000/20 4,260[c]	Hypersensitivity (HLA-B*5701 test to predict); possible increased risk of MI with recent or current use but studies vary
Emtricitabine	93	10/39 hr	200 mg orally once daily	1,800/90	Rarely pigmentation on soles and palms in non-White populations
Lamivudine	86	5/22 hr	150 mg orally twice daily *Or* 300 mg orally once daily	1,400/370 2,410/110	Headache
Tenofovir alafenamide	?	0.4 (TAF) and 35/150 hr TAF and tenofovir components	25 mg orally once daily *Or* 10 mg orally once daily (when coformulated with cobicistat)	160 and 30/ NA[c] and 10	Diarrhea, nausea, headache; increased lipids and weight gain vs TDF; less renal and bone toxicity vs TDF
Tenofovir disoproxil fumarate	25	17/150 hr(tenofovir component)	300 mg orally once daily	299/115	Renal dysfunction (proximal tubulopathy), bone demineralization
Zidovudine	85	2/7 hr	200 mg orally three times daily *Or* 300 mg orally twice daily	1,020/100 2,290/20	Anemia, neutropenia, myopathy
Nonnucleoside reverse transcriptase inhibitors (NNRTIs)					
Doravirine	64	15 hr	100 mg orally once daily	962/396	Nausea, dizziness, abnormal dreams
Efavirenz	43	48 hr	600 mg orally once daily *Or* 400 mg orally once daily	4,072/1,768	CNS disturbances, rash, serum transaminase elevations, hiperlipidemia, QT prolongation
Etravirine	?	41 hr	200 mg orally twice daily	736/161	Rash (including SJS), nausea, hypersensitivity reactions
Nevirapine	93	25 hr	200 mg orally twice daily[d] *Or* 400 mg orally once daily	5,400/3,730 6,658/2,929	Potentially serious rash (including SJS) and symptomatic hepatotoxicity
Rilpivirine	?	50 hr	25 mg orally once daily	280/120	Rash, depression, insomnia, headache, hepatotoxicity, QT prolongation

(*Continued*)

TABLE 148-3 Selected Pharmacologic Characteristics of Selected Antiretroviral Compounds for HIV Treatment (*Continued*)

Drug	*F* (%)	$t_{1/2}$[a]	Adult Dosing Recommendation[b] (doses/day)	Plasma C_{max}/C_{min} (ng/mL or mcg/L)	Distinguishing Adverse Effects
Rilpivirine LA		13-28 weeks	900 mg/3 mL IM × 1 (loading) 600 mg/2 mL IM every 4 weeks (continuation) *Or* 900 mg/3 mL IM every 8 weeks (continuation)	139/37.2 116/82.2	IM only: injection site reactions
Protease inhibitors (PIs)					
Atazanavir	68	7 hr	400 mg orally once daily *Or* 300 mg orally once daily[f]	2,298/120 4,420/636	Unconjugated hyper bilirubinemia, cholelithiasis, nephrolithiasis, serum transaminase elevations
Darunavir	82	15 hr	800 mg orally once daily[f] *Or* 600 mg orally twice daily[f]	7,070/3,860	Hepatotoxicity, rash, metabolic side effects
Lopinavir[g]	?	5.5 hr	800 mg orally once daily *Or* 400 mg orally twice daily	9,800/7,100	Hyperlipidemia, GI intolerance, metabolic side effects
Pharmacoenhancers					
Cobicistat	?	3-4 hr	150 mg orally once daily	990/30	SCr increases
Ritonavir	60	3-5 hr	100 mg orally once daily *Or* 100 mg orally twice daily		GI intolerance, hyperlipidemia
Fusion inhibitors					
Enfuvirtide	84	3.8 hr	90 mg/1 mL SQ twice daily	5,000/3,300	Injection-site reactions, rare hypersensitivity reactions
CCR5 antagonists					
Maraviroc	33	15 hr	300 mg orally twice daily[h]	618/33.6	Hepatotoxicity, abdominal pain, cough, dizziness
CD4 post-attachment inhibitors					
Ibalizumab-uiyk	N/A	79 hr	2,000 mg IV loading dose, then 800 mg every 2 weeks	567,000/230	Diarrhea, dizziness, nausea, rash, infusion reactions
Gp120 attachment inhibitors					
Fostemsavir	27	11 hr	600 mg orally twice daily	1,770/478	Nausea; QTc prolongation; transaminase and transient bilirubin elevations; sleep disturbance, dizziness

C_{max}, maximum plasma concentration; C_{min}, minimum plasma concentration; *F*, bioavailability; IM, intramuscular; IV, intravenous; NA, not applicable; PO, by mouth; SQ, subcutaneous; $t_{1/2}$, elimination half-life; LA, long acting.

[a]NtRTIs: Plasma NtRTI $t_{1/2}$/intracellular (peripheral blood mononuclear cells) NtRTI-triphosphate $t_{1/2}$; plasma $t_{1/2}$ only for other classes.

[b]Dose adjustment may be required for treatment-experienced patients with resistance mutations, weight, renal or hepatic disease, and drug interactions.

[c]C_{min} concentration typically below the limit of quantification.

[d]Initial dose escalation recommended to minimize side effects.

[e]Must be boosted with low doses of ritonavir (100-200 mg once or twice daily).

[h]Dose adjustment required with the concomitant use of medications that inhibit or induce CYP3A4.

[f]Available as coformulation 4:1 lopinavir to ritonavir.

Data from Reference 38 and individual package inserts.

all antiretroviral drugs.[38] There are other antiviral medications that exhibit modest, non-suppressive anti-HIV activity against HIV, such as the anti-herpes and anti-hepatitis B antivirals acyclovir, adefovir, entecavir, foscarnet, and interferon-alpha. These therapies should not be used as alternative options for HIV treatment but can be used in the setting of suppressive ART.

Reverse transcriptase inhibitors consist of two classes: those that are chemical derivatives of purine- and pyrimidine-based nucleosides and nucleotides (nucleoside/nucleotide reverse transcriptase inhibitors [NRTIs]) and those that are not (nonnucleoside reverse transcriptase inhibitors [NNRTIs]). Recommended NRTIs include the thymidine analog zidovudine (AZT or ZDV); the deoxycytidine analogs emtricitabine (FTC) and lamivudine (3TC); the deoxyguanosine analog abacavir sulfate (ABC); and tenofovir, which is a deoxyadenosine-monophosphate nucleotide analog (a nucleotide is a nucleoside with one or more phosphates). **Note that drug abbreviations are provided here and below for reference, but their use is discouraged because they may lead to prescribing or administration errors.**

As a class, the NRTIs require phosphorylation in cells to the 5′-triphosphate moiety to become pharmacologically active. Intracellular phosphorylation occurs by cytoplasmic or mitochondrial kinases and phosphotransferases (not viral kinases). The 5′-triphosphate moiety acts in two ways: (1) it competes with endogenous deoxyribonucleotides for the catalytic site of reverse transcriptase, and (2) if taken up and incorporated by reverse transcriptase, it prematurely terminates DNA elongation, as it lacks the requisite 3′-hydroxyl for sugar-phosphate linking. NRTIs are active against both HIV-1 and HIV-2.[38] Emtricitabine, lamivudine, and tenofovir are also active against hepatitis B virus, and a combination of these agents should be used when possible in HIV–hepatitis B coinfected patients.

Tenofovir comes in two pro drug formulations, tenofovir disoproxil fumarate (TDF) and tenofovir alafenamide (TAF). Tenofovir disoproxil fumarate is an ester pro drug that releases tenofovir upon absorption and first pass metabolism, producing relatively high systemic concentrations of tenofovir, which confers some risk of proximal tubulopathy and bone demineralization (both usually mild and reversible). Tenofovir alafenamide contains a different pro drug configuration such that more of the intact pro drug reaches the systemic circulation and penetrates lymphoid cells. Once in lymphoid cells, tenofovir is released via hydrolysis by cathepsin A in lymphoid tissues or in hepatic cells via carboxylesterase 1. This strategy results in higher intracellular concentrations in cells of interest, but lower systemic tenofovir concentrations and less change in markers of proximal tubulopathy and bone demineralization.[55] However, TAF has been associated with weight gain and lipid abnormalities in comparison to TDF.[56,57]

Although NRTI triphosphates (or diphosphate for tenofovir) are specific for HIV reverse transcriptase, their adverse effects may be caused in part by inhibition of mitochondrial DNA or RNA synthesis.[38] It is largely this problem that differentiates the first-generation drugs (didanosine, stavudine, and zidovudine) from the agents used most often (tenofovir disoproxil fumarate, tenofovir alafenamide, emtricitabine, lamivudine, and abacavir). The mitochondrial toxicities associated with first-generation drugs include peripheral neuropathy, pancreatitis, lipoatrophy (subcutaneous fat loss), myopathy, anemia, and rarely life-threatening lactic acidosis with fatty liver. The newer agents exhibit less potential to cause these toxicities, but they still have their own adverse event profiles to be considered (see Table 148-3).

Most of the newer NRTIs are eliminated by the kidney, and dose adjustments are required for renal insufficiency; abacavir is an exception as it is metabolized in the liver and should not be used in advanced hepatic impairment. Resistance has been reported for all NRTIs, including cross-resistance within the class as multiple and/or specific mutations in the viral genome accrue.[58]

NNRTIs are a chemically heterogeneous group of agents that bind noncompetitively to reverse transcriptase adjacent to the catalytic site, forcing a conformation change to the enzyme. Unlike NRTIs, NNRTIs do not require intracellular activation, do not compete against endogenous deoxyribonucleotides, and do not have intrinsic antiviral activity against HIV-2. Recommended NNRTIs include doravirine (DOR), efavirenz (EFV), etravirine (ETR), nevirapine (NVP), and rilpivirine (RPV).[38] As a class, the NNRTIs are generally associated with rash and hepatotoxicity, including rare life-threatening cases, particularly for nevirapine.[38] The use of first-generation NNRTIs (nevirapine and efavirenz) are on the decline largely because of tolerability and/or safety concerns. However, some patients have remained on efavirenz-based therapy and both efavirenz and nevirapine are still used in certain regions of the world. NNRTIs tend to have long plasma half-lives and they are mainly cleared by liver and/or gut-mediated metabolism through the cytochrome P450 (CYP) enzyme system. Rilpivirine is the only NNRTI available in both an immediate release oral and a long-acting injectable formulation. Caution should be used for those with advanced hepatic insufficiency (nevirapine should not be used in moderate or advanced hepatic insufficiency). NNRTIs can be perpetrators of drug-drug interactions, most often induction of CYP metabolism. Exceptions to this are doravirine and rilpivirine, which do not induce or inhibit CYP metabolism. The older NNRTIs were unique in that a single mutation was needed to confer high-level cross-resistance for the class (not including etravirine and doravirine). This has been termed a *low-genetic barrier* to resistance.[58]

Recommended HIV PIs include atazanavir (ATV), darunavir (DRV), and lopinavir (LPV). Ritonavir (RTV) is also an older PI that is now used as a pharmacoenhancer for this class of drugs. HIV PIs competitively inhibit the cleavage of the gag-pol polyprotein, which is a crucial step in the viral maturation process, thereby resulting in the production of immature, noninfectious virions. HIV PIs have activity against HIV-1 and HIV-2 (particularly darunavir and lopinavir).[38] HIV PIs are generally associated with GI distress and metabolic changes, such as increased lipids, insulin insensitivity, and changes in body fat distribution. Some of these issues can be traced to formulation problems due to limited aqueous solubility, requiring high levels of excipients and large pill burdens. The first-generation HIV PIs (eg, indinavir, nelfinavir, saquinavir, lopinavir) exhibited poor solubility leading to erratic absorption (nelfinavir, saquinavir), crystallization of drug in urine (indinavir), gastrointestinal distress (nelfinavir, lopinavir), and hyperlipidemia (lopinavir). Generally, the newer HIV PIs, darunavir and atazanavir, improve upon, but do not eliminate, these issues. HIV PIs are cleared by liver- and gut-mediated metabolism (mainly CYP3A), and dose adjustments may be required in hepatic insufficiency. HIV PIs are almost always used with low doses of CYP3A inhibitors, ritonavir or cobicistat, to increase the plasma concentrations of the HIV PI of interest. Thus, CYP3A- and P-gp-mediated drug interactions with concomitant medications are important considerations for PIs. Resistance to the HIV PIs generally requires the buildup of multiple mutations, termed a *high-genetic barrier* to resistance. Multiple mutations can lead to cross-resistance.[58]

There are four drugs that block HIV entry and these are generally reserved for treatment-experienced patients. Enfuvirtide (T20) is a synthetic 36-amino-acid peptide that binds gp41, inhibiting envelope fusion of HIV-1 with the target cell. It does not have activity against HIV-2. Subcutaneous injection is the preferred route of administration and injection-site reactions (pain, erythema, nodules) are the most common adverse effects, nearing 100% incidence. Enfuvirtide is cleared via protein catabolism and amino acid recycling.[38] Maraviroc is a CCR5 antagonist with activity against HIV-1 and HIV-2. The long-term consequences of blocking CCR5 (a human receptor) are unknown but may include increased susceptibility to disease by flaviviruses (eg, West Nile virus and tickborne encephalitis virus).[59] One advantage of targeting a human receptor is that resistance to CCR5 antagonists may be more difficult to develop. Because CCR5 antagonists are only effective against R5 virus and not X4 virus, a viral tropism assay must be performed prior to using a CCR5 antagonist. Maraviroc is a CYP3A and P-glycoprotein substrate and is therefore susceptible to drug-drug interactions and caution should be used in those with advanced hepatic insufficiency. Maraviroc has been associated with rash and hepatotoxicity. Resistance mutations have been identified for enfuvirtide, which has a low-genetic barrier to resistance, but assays for maraviroc resistance have not been developed other than the R5 versus X4 tropism test.[38,58] Ibalizumab-uiyk is a recombinant humanized monoclonal antibody with activity against HIV-1 that binds to domain 2 of the CD4 receptor on host cells. The binding of ibalizumab-uiyk to the CD4 receptor does not affect its ability to bind gp120 on viral particles, but it interferes with the post-attachment steps necessary for the entry of HIV-1 into host cells. Ibalizumab-uiyk is administered by infusion and is indicated for heavily treatment-experienced adults with multidrug-resistant HIV-1 infection who are failing their current antiretroviral regimen.[60] It has activity against R5-tropic, X4-tropic, and dual-tropic viruses. The most common adverse effects associated with ibalizumab-uiyk include diarrhea, dizziness, nausea, and rash. Decreased susceptibility to ibalizumab-uiyk has been seen in some subjects, but the clinical significance of this is not well understood. There is no evidence of cross-resistance between ibalizumab-uiyk and any other antiretroviral class. Fostemsavir is an oral pro-drug of temsavir, which is an attachment inhibitor that binds near the CD4 receptor binding site to prevent conformational changes in gp120, thus preventing HIV from entering CD4 cells.[61] This medication is indicated as salvage therapy in heavily treatment-experienced patients. Temsavir is metabolized by esterases and CYP3A4 and is susceptible to drug-drug interactions with CYP3A4 inducers. Temsavir caused QTc prolongation at doses multiple-fold higher than those used clinically. Caution is advised in patients with a history of QTc prolongation or associated cardiac diseases, or in combination with other medications that may cause Torsades de Pointes.

InSTI options include bictegravir (BIC), cabotegravir (CAB), dolutegravir (DTG), elvitegravir (EVG), and raltegravir (RAL). Cabotegravir is the only InSTI available in both immediate release oral and long acting injectable forms. InSTIs bind to HIV integrase while it is in a specific complex with viral DNA and inhibit the strand transfer that incorporates the proviral DNA into the chromosomal DNA. InSTIs are active against HIV-1 and HIV-2. Cabotegravir, dolutegravir, and raltegravir are primarily glucuronidated by UGT1A1 and are not susceptible to major CYP-mediated drug interactions, although other kinds of interactions are important (Table 148-2). In particular, polyvalent cation containing antacids and mineral supplements bind InSTIs in the gut leading to reduced bioavailability. Recommendations vary on how to mitigate these interactions, including temporal separation (eg, elvitegravir and raltegravir), simultaneous administration with food (eg, bictegravir and dolutegravir), or consideration of an antacid with a different mechanism of action (eg, histamine-2 receptor antagonists or proton pump inhibitors). Bictegravir is metabolized by both UGT1A1 and CYP3A4 and is susceptible to interactions through both enzymatic pathways. Elvitegravir is extensively metabolized by CYP3A and is coformulated with cobicistat, a potent CYP3A inhibitor, to optimize drug exposure and enable once-daily dosing. InSTIs are relatively well tolerated with adverse events that include rash, nausea, and headache. This class of medications, particularly dolutegravir, has also been associated with CNS and psychiatric side effects (eg, insomnia, depression, and increased risk of suicidality) with a higher risk among those with a history of psychiatric conditions. InSTIs may also cause more weight gain than PIs or NNRTIs, with the greatest weight gain with bictegravir and dolutegravir.[62,63] InSTIs should be used with caution in advanced hepatic insufficiency. Multiple mutations have been identified conferring resistance to InSTIs, including cross-resistance as mutations accrue. Bictegravir and dolutegravir have a higher genetic barrier to resistance compared with elvitegravir and raltegravir.[58]

Novel antiviral agents in the classes listed above and agents in new drug classes that exploit other steps in the HIV life cycle (see Fig. 148-1) are in development, with a focus on long-lasting activity and/or high activity against drug-resistant virus.[64] Capsid inhibitors are a novel drug class in development, with the potential to interfere with multiple different steps in the HIV replication cycle. The capsid inhibitor lenacapavir is being evaluated in long-acting formulations of up to six months duration for both HIV treatment and prevention. Islatravir is a potent nucleoside analog reverse transcriptase/translocation inhibitor (translocation is the repositioning of reverse transcriptase after incorporating a nucleotide so it is ready to accept the next incoming nucleotide). Islatravir is being studied in long-acting formulations for up to six months duration as well. Long-acting antiretroviral therapy is emerging as a new treatment paradigm.

Drug Interactions 6 Medical use of antiretroviral agents is complicated by clinically significant drug-drug interactions that can occur with many of these agents.[38,65] Some interactions are beneficial and used purposely (eg, ritonavir and cobicistat as pharmacokinetic enhancers); others may be harmful, leading to dangerously elevated (eg, toxic) or inadequate drug concentrations (non-suppressive). Clinicians involved in the pharmacotherapy of HIV must understand the mechanistic basis for these interactions and maintain a current knowledge of drug interactions for these reasons.

Antiretroviral-associated drug interactions encompass a variety of mechanisms, including but not limited to: CYP3A-associated first-pass metabolism, efflux and uptake drug transporters, and systemic clearance. The newer HIV PIs, NNRTIs (doravirine, etravirine, and rilpivirine), the CCR5 antagonist maraviroc, and the InSTI elvitegravir are extensively metabolized by CYP3A. In general, efavirenz, etravirine, and nevirapine are inducers of CYP3A, whereas the PIs and their pharmacoenhancers inhibit CYP3A. Ritonavir is a potent mechanism-based inhibitor of CYP3A-mediated metabolism and is now used exclusively at lower doses as a pharmacokinetic enhancer of other HIV PIs. Similarly, cobicistat, which is an analog of ritonavir without antiretroviral activity, is also a potent mechanism-based inhibitor of CYP3A activity and is used in a similar fashion. However, the interaction profiles for ritonavir and cobicistat differ and thus when switching between these agents, similar interactions cannot be assumed.[66] PIs and pharmacoenhancers also inhibit efflux (eg, P-glycoprotein and breast cancer resistance protein [BCRP]) and uptake transporters (eg, organic anion transporting polypeptide [OATP]), which contributes to the overall drug-drug interaction profile including certain statins (eg, rosuvastatin)[67] and the direct oral anticoagulant, dabigatran etexilate.[68] Some PIs including ritonavir induce transporters, making drug-drug interactions difficult to predict.

Darunavir and lopinavir must be taken with ritonavir or cobicistat to achieve optimal plasma concentrations. Atazanavir is also primarily used with ritonavir or cobicistat for the same reason, though it can be used without a pharmacoenhancer if dose adjusted. Many potential concomitant drugs on the market are substrates for CYP3A and drug transporters, and are therefore susceptible to clinically relevant drug interactions with HIV PIs, NNRTIs, and pharmacoenhancers. Agents with narrow therapeutic indices and/or that exhibit major changes in pharmacokinetics with inhibitors or inducers of enzymes and/or transporters for which they are substrates are most important in this regard. Examples include, but are not limited to, simvastatin, lovastatin, corticosteroids (including inhaled, intranasal, and intraarticular), ergot derivatives, some antiarrhythmics, some erectile dysfunction drugs, some anticoagulants, and some anti-cancer agents.

The drug interaction potential of antimycobacterium agents, specifically the rifamycins, are particularly relevant, given the high potential for such infections in persons with HIV.[65] Rifampin and rifapentine, potent inducers of CYP3A metabolism and conjugation enzymes, are contraindicated with the use of HIV PIs, most NNRTIs, bictegravir, cabotegravir (oral and injectable), elvitegravir, and maraviroc because antiretroviral concentrations are reduced substantially even with ritonavir enhancement. Efavirenz should be administered as a 600 mg dose with rifampin; the 400 mg dose should not be used.[38] The usual dose of efavirenz can be used with rifapentine; dose adjustment is not required, which may be due in part to the concomitant use of isoniazid.[69] Raltegravir and dolutegravir doses should be increased in the presence of rifampin, with raltegravir dosing doubled and dolutegravir being administered twice daily. Dolutegravir and raltegravir do not require dose adjustment with once-weekly rifapentine, but should not be coadministered if rifapentine is administered once daily. The use of tenofovir alafenamide, a P-gp substrate, with rifamycins is also discouraged unless benefits outweigh risks and virologic response is closely monitored.[38,70,71] Tenofovir disoproxil fumarate does not require dose adjustment and may be a suitable alternative in these cases. Ritonavir enhancement generally allows coadministration of HIV PIs with rifabutin.[38,65] In such cases, the rifabutin dose will require adjustment, given its CYP3A-mediated clearance. Similarly, the herbal product St. John's wort (*Hypericum perforatum*) is a potent inducer of metabolism and is contraindicated with PIs, NNRTIs, INSTIs, tenofovir alafenamide, and maraviroc.[38] The pharmacology of CYP3A interactions may be complicated by simultaneous induction/inhibition of drug transporter–mediated (eg, P-glycoprotein) bioavailability or clearance and/or other phase I (eg, CYP 2B6 for RTV) or phase II enzymes.

Some antiretroviral drugs require acidic environments for optimal absorption leading to interactions with antacids, particularly proton-pump inhibitors (eg, atazanavir, rilpivirine). On the other hand, some antiretroviral agents chelate polyvalent cations in antacids or mineral supplements, reducing absorption following coadministration (eg, InSTIs). Other potential mechanisms for drug interactions include inhibition of renal tubule secretion (eg, tenofovir and OAT inhibitors; inhibition of MATE and/or OCT2 by dolutegravir, bictegravir, and cobicistat), and antagonistic phosphorylation for NRTIs of the same nucleobase (eg, lamivudine and emtricitabine). This list of drug interactions and mechanisms for drug interactions is not complete. Clinicians who treat HIV must monitor for, and stay abreast of, antiretroviral drug interaction data. Websites are available that catalog and regularly update HIV drug-interaction information (http://www.hiv-druginteractions.org/), and the DHHS guidelines for antiretroviral use provide, and regularly update, excellent summaries of known clinically relevant drug interactions.[38]

Landmarks in the Evolution of Antiretroviral Therapy

7 ART has undergone major changes over the past decades. Illustrating these changes is important for a thorough understanding of current treatment strategies. The first landmark in this evolution was the availability of zidovudine, the first antiretroviral agent, which conferred a survival benefit in persons with AIDS, when given as monotherapy. A combination of two NRTIs was superior to zidovudine monotherapy in immunologic and virologic parameters, as well as survival benefit. Later, triple therapy (two NRTIs with an HIV PI or NNRTI) was associated with reduced incidence of OIs and improved survival, establishing the current paradigm of ART. Triple drug therapy has since evolved to include new drug classes (eg, INSTI), coformulations, and better tolerated agents. This has in turn led to improvements in convenience, tolerability, safety, and virologic efficacy—enabling two drug therapy in some circumstances.

7 Taken together, these landmarks established that HIV should not be treated with single or dual NRTIs alone. Recommendations for initial treatment of most people with HIV now advocate a minimum of two active antiretroviral agents provided at least one in the regimen has a high barrier to resistance (eg, dolutegravir or boosted darunavir). Recommended initial regimens for most people with HIV comprise an InSTI with 1 to 2 NRTIs, and include bictegravir with tenofovir alafenamide plus emtricitabine; dolutegravir with tenofovir (as either tenofovir disoproxil fumarate or tenofovir alafenamide) plus emtricitabine; dolutegravir plus abacavir/lamivudine (abacavir can only be used in patients who are HLA-B*5701 negative); and dolutegravir with lamivudine (except in persons with baseline HIV viral loads >500,000 copies/mL (500×10^6/L), hepatitis B coinfection, or when antiretroviral therapy is to be initiated prior to the availability of hepatitis B serologic testing or HIV genotypic resistance testing). Multiple alternative regimens are also safe and effective, but have some disadvantages compared with those recommended for most persons with HIV such as dosing convenience (eg, the use of multiple tablets or twice daily administration), drug-drug interactions, weaker virologic responses with high viral loads, lower tolerability, or greater risk of long-term toxicities. Recommended antiretroviral regimens for initial therapy are listed in Table 148-2. Recommended first-line ART regimens constantly evolve and clinical controversies may emerge as data and clinical experience accrue and new strategies come under consideration, thus it is always advised to review the DHHS guidelines for the most updated ART recommendations.

Adherence The simplest definition of adherence is the patient's follow-through on taking medication as directed. As with any chronic therapy, variable adherence to ART is common, and significantly impacts virologic response. Factors associated with poor adherence include major psychiatric illnesses, active substance use, unstable social circumstances, adverse events, and poor adherence with clinic visits.[38] Most, but not all, modern ART regimens consist of coformulations and long half-life drugs allowing for once-daily dosing (sometimes without food restrictions), which facilitates improved adherence compared with multiple dose units, multiple doses per day, and food restrictions with dosing. Average adherence rates are approximately 80% with antiretroviral regimens. Longer dosing "holidays" increase the risk of breakthrough viremia; however, newer regimens are more forgiving.[72] As clinicians, it is critical to establish a relationship of trust with the patient and to communicate to the patient the importance of proper medication taking. Education should be aimed at understanding the disease process, monitoring, goals of therapy, and consequences of poor adherence. An individual's "readiness" to take medications should be clearly established before treatment is initiated.[38] Help from caregivers, friends, and/or family members should be leveraged by the patient because social and psychological support are among the most important factors that influence adherence in this patient population. Strategies to encourage adherence, such as pill boxes, alarms, and setting a routine schedule should be discussed. Pharmacological approaches are among strategies being used to assess adherence objectively.[73]

Efficacy Based on clinical trial data, more than 90% of patients will achieve undetectable viral loads with preferred and alternative ART regimens.[74-76] Given high efficacy across modern ART regimens, side effect profiles can help distinguish preferred versus alternative regimens. Starting with the nucleos(t)ide analog backbones, several studies have compared tenofovir alafenamide against tenofovir disoproxil fumarate, which have generally shown similar efficacy rates. Tenofovir disoproxil fumarate is associated with greater renal toxicity and bone demineralization, especially with the concomitant use of pharmacoenhancers,[77] whereas tenofovir alafenamide has been associated greater weight gain and lipid increases.[56] Abacavir–lamivudine combined with dolutegravir exhibits superior efficacy rates regardless of baseline viral load compared with efavirenz–tenofovir disoproxil fumarate–emtricitabine,[76] and similar efficacy rates to other InSTI combinations recommended for most people with HIV.[75] Together, these studies established recommendations for tenofovir disoproxil fumarate–emtricitabine or lamivudine, tenofovir alafenamide–emtricitabine, or abacavir–lamivudine as initial NRTI components of therapy. As mentioned above, if abacavir is to be used in any regimen, a test for the presence of HLA-B*5701 must be done as its presence has been strongly correlated with the development of abacavir hypersensitivity. Should this test be positive, an abacavir allergy should be added to the patient's medical record and abacavir should not be used in the patient, as the hypersensitivity reaction can be life-threatening.

The third active agent of ART regimens has also evolved based on large, randomized, controlled trials. Efavirenz and PIs maintained a long history as the recommended third active agent until comparative trials demonstrated poorer tolerability and more therapy discontinuations for efavirenz and PIs versus InSTIs.[76,78] Together, these and other studies support recommendations for InSTIs as third active agents for initial ART in most people with HIV. Many agents are available for inclusion in regimens recommended in certain clinical situations, including NNRTIs (eg, doravirine, efavirenz, or rilpivirine) or PIs (darunavir and atazanavir boosted with either cobicistat or ritonavir).[38] Dual ART therapy may also be considered in situations where the use of tenofovir disoproxil fumarate, tenofovir alafenamide, or abacavir are not optimal choices. Dual ART regimens for initial therapy include more potent agents (dolutegravir plus lamivudine[79] and darunavir/ritonavir plus either lamivudine or raltegravir) and have evidence supporting their use in patients who are not ideal candidates for other recommended ART regimens. Clinicians are urged to consult the most recommended preferred and alternative regimens, as they are continuously updated with new studies and as longer-term follow-up data accrue.

Regimen Simplification and Long-Acting Therapies Patients with sustained undetectable HIV-RNA taking out-of-date drug regimens may be candidates for simplification to one of the recommended regimens as previously described, or a more desirable alternative regimen based on past treatment history and other patient-specific factors. There are two additional dual antiretroviral combinations that may be considered in participants who are suppressed: dolutegravir with rilpivirine,[80] and long-acting intramuscular injectable cabotegravir with rilpivirine. As these drugs do not have activity against hepatitis B, they should be avoided in persons with HIV and hepatitis B coinfection. Screening for drug-drug interactions and avoiding use in individuals with resistance mutations to individual drug components is also critical to avoid therapeutic failure. Dolutegravir with rilpivirine is available as a coformulated tablet, and this regimen has shown high rates of continued virologic suppression following ART switch.

Cabotegravir with rilpivirine represents the first long-acting injectable combination approved for this indication. Studies with intramuscular cabotegravir/rilpivirine demonstrated noninferiority to oral ART.[81] This combination is only recommended in persons with HIV who have been suppressed and on stable ART for at least 3 to 6 months.[38] Cabotegravir with rilpivirine also cannot be used in pregnant or breastfeeding women until additional data supporting its use are available in this population. An oral lead-in period for 28 days is optional to ensure tolerability before starting the injections. The first intramuscular injection of cabotegravir with rilpivirine is given as a loading dose on the last day of oral therapy (600 mg [3 mL] of cabotegravir and 900 mg [3 mL] of rilpivirine), and then is administered as a maintenance dose (400 mg [2 mL] of cabotegravir and 600 mg [2 mL] of rilpivirine) every 4 weeks thereafter. Injections are administered intramuscularly into the gluteal muscle. Alternatively, 600 mg [3 mL] of cabotegravir and 900 mg [3 mL] can be given as a maintenance dose every 8 weeks. A window period of 7 days is allowed around scheduled doses for unforeseen circumstances, but gaps beyond 7 days may require bridging with oral therapy to ensure that subtherapeutic exposures do not occur. The most common side effects are mild-moderate injection site reactions (>80%) that generally decrease over time. Despite the high rates of injection site reactions, over 90% of participants in clinical trials still preferred long-acting injectable options over daily oral ART. Other long-acting therapies in development such as lenacapavir and islatravir hold great promise to further expand options for people living with HIV.[64]

Resistance 9 Regimen failure may be associated with antiretroviral resistance, and testing for such resistance is a useful clinical tool.[38,58] The two types of resistance tests available are phenotype and genotype. A phenotype test determines the concentration of antiretroviral agent necessary to inhibit replication of the patient's viral isolate by 50% (inhibitory concentration of 50% [IC_{50}]) in a recombinant in vitro viral assay. Results usually are expressed as a fold change in susceptibility (IC_{50}) compared with a wild-type laboratory strain virus. Generally, the fold-change in IC_{50} increases as HIV accumulates additional mutations that confer resistance to a particular drug. However, a single mutation may confer a high fold-change in IC_{50} for some drugs (eg, lamivudine, emtricitabine, efavirenz, nevirapine), rendering them ineffective after a single mutation. Although small-to-moderate increases in the fold change suggest reduced susceptibility to that antiretroviral agent, resistance may not be absolute, and partial susceptibility may remain. Theoretically, drug concentrations may be increased to overcome reduced susceptibility. The strength of phenotypic testing is to provide resistance information for complex mutation patterns, but it is also associated with higher cost, limited number of commercial providers, and slower turnaround time for results. Genotyping assesses genetic mutations and associated codon changes in gp41, reverse transcriptase, integrase, or protease in the patient's virus and compares it with the wild-type sequence. Certain mutations are known to confer resistance to specific drugs. An updated list of drug resistance mutations can be found at https://www.iasusa.org/resources/hiv-drug-resistance-mutations/, and the Stanford HIVdb Program also has useful tools for analyzing HIV drug resistance mutations: https://hivdb.stanford.edu/. Mutations are listed by the wild-type amino acid followed by the position in the protein or enzyme and end with the mutation found in the patient's virus. For example, a common mutation caused by lamivudine and emtricitabine is the M184V mutation: a substitution of valine (V) for methionine (M) at the 184 position of reverse transcriptase. Mutations can confer varying degrees of antiretroviral drug resistance and in some cases, weighting algorithms have been developed to predict the relative impact of mutation combinations on antiretroviral activity. Algorithms have also been developed to predict a phenotype from a genotype test (ie, virtual phenotype). Resistance mutations may not be purely detrimental, for example, while M184V confers significant resistance to lamivudine and emtricitabine, it is also associated with a less fit virus. Interpretation of genotype resistance tests is complex; the reader is encouraged to obtain expert advice and consult the most recent guidelines on HIV resistance testing.

Treatment of Special Populations

Pregnancy Several considerations are relevant to the treatment of pregnant persons, including the health of the mother, prevention of HIV transmission to the fetus, potential for teratogenicity, and drug dosing issues based on pharmacokinetic changes during pregnancy. Treatment recommendations should be consulted to address the specific requirements for pregnant people with HIV and the prevention of vertical transmission.[19] Generally, pregnant people should be treated as would nonpregnant people, with the goal of maximally suppressing HIV-RNA. Pregnant people already on a suppressive regimen may remain on their current therapy unless there are known safety or efficacy concerns with the combination that they are taking. Preferred initial regimens for HIV treatment during pregnancy include a dual NRTI backbone (abacavir/lamivudine or tenofovir disoproxil fumarate/emtricitabine or lamivudine) with either an InSTI (dolutegravir or raltegravir) or boosted PI (atazanavir/ritonavir or darunavir/ritonavir). Alternative options include tenofovir alafenamide/emtricitabine or zidovudine/lamivudine for a dual NRTI backbone, and efavirenz or rilpivirine with one of the recommended NRTI backbones.

Efavirenz was historically avoided in persons planning to become pregnant due to concerns of neural tube defects, but a large-scale clinical study and ongoing monitoring of the Antiretroviral Pregnancy Registry (http://www.apregistry.com/HCP.aspx) have since shown no increased risk of birth defects with efavirenz in comparison to other ART options or background rates in pregnant people without HIV. Dolutegravir use at the time of conception was also associated with a higher rate of neural tube defects in infants in a preliminary analysis from the Tsepamo study. Long-term follow-up with additional women showed lower rates and the difference was no longer statistically significant, and other studies have not shown a signal.[19] Nonetheless, the potential risks and known benefits of dolutegravir treatment should be discussed with people of child-bearing potential. Cobicistat-containing regimens should be avoided in pregnancy as exposures to cobicistat and coformulated medications (ie, atazanavir, darunavir, and elvitegravir) are significantly reduced during pregnancy, which may increase the risk of treatment failure and perinatal HIV transmission.[19,82] If a person becomes pregnant while on one of these regimens, consideration should be given toward switching therapy, which may also carry its own risk of breakthrough, or more frequent viral load monitoring may be performed. Infants born to people with HIV require prophylaxis to prevent HIV transmission, and the exact recommendations vary depending on the maternal viral load, treatment history, and level of risk for transmission. Zidovudine is recommended intrapartum depending on the mother's viral load (more than 1,000 copies/mL [1×10^6/L] or unknown), based on early studies demonstrating clear prophylactic effectiveness as well as extensive familiarity with the side effect profile.[19] Infants considered low risk for perinatal HIV transmission (ie, maternal viral load suppressed at delivery and no adherence concerns) should receive zidovudine prophylaxis for 4 weeks after birth. Infants considered high risk (ie, mother received either no antepartum or intrapartum ART, only intrapartum ART, or antepartum ART but did not achieve viral suppression) should receive presumptive HIV treatment with zidovudine/lamivudine and either nevirapine or raltegravir from birth through 6 weeks of age. Perinatal HIV transmission has been reduced to less than 0.5% for pregnant people who are treated with ART and when infant prophylaxis is used. Breastfeeding is not recommended in the United States, but in resource-limited settings where lack of clean water makes breastfeeding a more favorable option, infants should receive additional prophylaxis.[49]

Preventing HIV Transmission

HIV treatment is a necessary component of reducing HIV-associated morbidity and mortality. However, it is also critical for preventing new HIV transmissions from occurring. There are several approaches for preventing new HIV transmissions as detailed in this section. Pharmacists play an important role in both treating and preventing HIV, and some states now allow pharmacists to prescribe and dispense HIV pre- and postexposure prophylaxis (PEP) in recognition of the critical role that pharmacists play in this cascade.

Undetectable Equals Untransmittable (U=U) Undetectable equals untransmittable ("U=U," or Treatment as Prevention [TasP]) refers to the concept that people with HIV who achieve and maintain suppressed or undetectable viral loads (meaning viral loads <200 copies/mL [200×10^3/L)) do not sexually transmit HIV to others.[6] This was demonstrated through multiple clinical studies that evaluated serodiscordant (ie, one partner with HIV and one without HIV) heterosexual and male-male couples. No linked HIV transmissions occurred between couples when the partner with HIV maintained a suppressed viral load. U=U requires persons with HIV to remain adherent to their prescribed ART and thus maintain suppression (exact length varies by duration of therapy and confirmation of viral suppression).[38,83] Individuals should be counseled on the need to remain adherent with routine viral load monitoring if solely following the U=U strategy and should still undergo routine STI screening. Partners without HIV should still be offered PrEP, particularly if unsure whether their partner's viral load is undetectable, if they have multiple sexual partners, or if they feel more comfortable taking PrEP. PEP should also be offered in cases where the partner with HIV has been inconsistently taking ART or is no longer suppressed. Condom use can help prevent other STIs. U=U does not cover other routes of HIV transmission, such as breastfeeding, sharing of drug injection equipment, or needlestick injuries.

Postexposure Prophylaxis (PEP) Protection of people from potential HIV exposure is an important concern. The CDC has issued guidelines governing antiretroviral PEP of occupational (oPEP) and other non-occupational HIV exposures (nPEP) that should be consulted for updates as the knowledge in this field evolves.[13,16] Occupational exposures are those that happen in a work setting, most commonly needlestick injuries in healthcare workers, whereas non-occupational exposures occur outside of work, such as condomless intercourse or injection drug use. The principles are to assess the exposure risk and treat as soon as possible after high-risk exposures to prevent HIV infection. Assessing the exposure risk requires knowledge of the HIV-infection status of the source individual, which may be difficult to ascertain. The HIV status of the source should be determined as soon as possible with a rapid HIV test, whenever feasible. However, providers may have to rely on reasonable suspicion when this is not possible, so provider expertise is essential. PEP should not be delayed while waiting on the HIV status of the source if reasonable suspicion is present. PEP should be considered an urgent medical situation. The guidelines as of October 2021 recommend conventional ART regimens as summarized in Table 148-4, initiated as soon as possible and within a maximum of 72 hours of the potential exposure. Animal studies show reduced PEP efficacy when initiated 72 hours or more after the exposure.[16] The optimal duration of treatment is unknown, but at least 4 weeks

TABLE 148-4 Recommended Regimens for Occupational and Non-occupational Postexposure Prophylaxis

Population	Ranking	Regimen
Occupational postexposure prophylaxis (oPEP)[16]		
Healthcare workers	Preferred	Tenofovir disoproxil fumarate 300 mg/emtricitabine 200 mg once daily + raltegravir 400 mg twice daily
	Alternative	Consult guidelines
Non-occupational postexposure prophylaxis (nPEP)		
Adults and adolescents ≥13 years, including pregnant persons, and normal renal function (CrCl ≥60 mL/min [1.0 mL/s])	Preferred	Tenofovir disoproxil fumarate 300 mg/emtricitabine 200 mg once daily + raltegravir 400 mg twice daily *OR* dolutegravir 50 mg once daily
	Alternative	Tenofovir disoproxil fumarate 300 mg/emtricitabine 200 mg once daily + darunavir 800 mg/ritonavir 100 mg once daily
Adults and adolescents ≥13 years, including pregnant persons, and renal dysfunction (CrCl <60 mL/min [1.0 mL/s])	Preferred	Zidovudine/lamivudine (dose-adjusted per CrCl) + raltegravir 400 mg twice daily *OR* dolutegravir 50 mg once daily
	Alternative	Zidovudine/lamivudine (dose-adjusted per CrCl) + darunavir 800 mg/ritonavir 100 mg once daily

Data from References 13 and 16.

TABLE 148-5 Recommended Regimens for Preexposure Prophylaxis

PrEP Option	Emtricitabine with Tenofovir Disoproxil Fumarate	Emtricitabine with Tenofovir Alafenamide	Cabotegravir
Initial FDA approval	2012	2019	2021
Administration route	Oral	Oral	IM injection
	Persons at risk through sex or injection drug use[a]	Persons weighing at least 35 kg (77 lb) who are at risk through sex, excluding people at risk through receptive vaginal sex.	Persons at-risk through sex
Dosing	Emtricitabine 200 mg/tenofovir disoproxil fumarate 300 mg	Emtricitabine 200 mg/enofovir alafenamide fumarate. 25 mg	Oral: 30 mg IM injection: 600 mg (3 mL)
	On-demand strategy also possible ("2-1-1")[b]	On-demand strategy not recommended (no data)	On-demand strategy not recommended (no data)
Dosing frequency	Once daily	Once daily	Oral lead-in: once daily IM injection: once monthly × first 2 months then every 2 months thereafter
HIV monitoring[c]	Every 3 months	Every 3 months	Month 1 visit and every 2 months thereafter
Safety monitoring	Renal[d] Optional: bone density	Renal[d], lipids Optional: bone density	None
Side effects	"Start-up syndrome" during 1st month; headache, abdominal pain, weight loss	"Start-up syndrome" during 1st month; diarrhea, weight gain	Injection site reactions, headache, fever, fatigue, myalgia, rash
Use in renal impairment	CrCl ≥60 mL/min (1.0 mL/s)	CrCl ≥30 mL/min (0.5 mL/s)	Can be used; no restrictions

[a]Only TDF has been studied in persons who inject drugs, but this population is expected to benefit from all systemic PrEP forms.

[b]Only MSM: 2 pills 2-24 hours before sex (closer to 24 hours preferred), 1 pill 24 hours after first dose, 1 pill 48 hours after first dose. If sex occurs the day after completing the 2-1-1 series, continue taking 1 pill daily until 48 hours after the last sexual event. If sex occurs <7 days from the last 2-1-1 dose, resume 1 pill daily. If sex occurs ≥7 days between the last pill and next sexual event, reinitiate with 2 pills.

[c]Consists of laboratory testing (antigen, antibody, and HIV-1 RNA [PCR]) and assess for signs/symptoms of acute HIV infection.

[d]Renal function should be assessed every 6 months for persons ≥50 years of age or with CrCl <90 mL/min (1.5 mL/s) and every 12 months in all other patients.

Data from References 36 and 103.

of therapy is advocated. Expert consultation is needed when exposure to drug-resistant virus is suspected or confirmed to optimize the PEP regimen, but this should not delay initial initiation of PEP.

Preexposure Prophylaxis (PrEP) Preexposure prophylaxis (PrEP) involves the use of antiretroviral medications to prevent HIV. There are now three FDA-approved options for use in persons without HIV and at risk of HIV acquisition, to prevent infection should an HIV-exposure occur. These include oral emtricitabine with tenofovir (either in the form of tenofovir disoproxil fumarate or tenofovir alafenamide) and long-acting injectable cabotegravir. PrEP is effective in MSM, sero-discordant couples, and heterosexual men and women, including those who inject drugs, though the exact PrEP combinations that are approved in each of these populations vary based on available data (see Table 148-5).[36,84]

All sexually active adults and adolescents should be informed about PrEP. Prior to initiating PrEP, a negative HIV test should be documented, including negative symptoms of acute HIV infection. Reports of drug resistance from oral PrEP failures were mostly among individuals who initiated PrEP during acute HIV infection, in the window period before the rapid HIV test could detect infection. HIV acquisition during PrEP (especially for cabotegravir) can be challenging to diagnose because of prolonged HIV suppression and delayed antibody expression. HIV testing should be repeated at least every 3 months for those on oral PrEP, and for persons on cabotegravir, HIV testing is recommended at the month 1 visit (second injection) and then every 2 months thereafter (beginning with the third injection). Promotion of adherence and screening for potential drug-drug interactions is critical for PrEP effectiveness. It is also critical to continue routinely screening for STIs (all persons on PrEP) and hepatitis C virus (MSM, transgender women, and persons who inject drugs) as PrEP does not protect against these infections.

The most up-to-date PrEP guidelines should be consulted, as new PrEP strategies are under evaluation. Topical virucidal or antiretroviral drug formulations for use vaginally or rectally to prevent sexual transmission of HIV are in various phases of development. Use of a dapivirine ring resulted in a ~30% reduction in HIV acquisition, leading to review by the European Medicines Agency (EMA) for HIV prevention in women.[11]

EVALUATION OF THERAPEUTIC OUTCOMES

Two laboratory tests are used to evaluate response to ART: the plasma HIV-RNA and CD4 cell counts.[38] These tests should be performed at baseline, along with a medical history and physical, urinalysis, hematology, chemistries, serologies for coinfections, and patient education about HIV infection. An HIV resistance test is recommended upon initiation of care. After therapy is initiated, patients are generally monitored at 3-month intervals until HIV-RNA reaches undetectable levels. An assessment at 2 to 8 weeks is warranted to document early response. Monitoring may be increased to every 6 months in stabilized patients.

The two main indications for a change in therapy are significant toxicity and treatment failure. Should a single agent be responsible for an intolerable side effect that agent often can be singly changed out of the regimen. For example, the patient who experiences intolerable CNS disturbances during initiation of efavirenz can switch to a boosted PI or InSTI without changing the dual NRTI backbone. Maintaining virologic suppression is an important goal for switching therapy due to adverse events. Caution must be exercised when drugs in the regimen have overlapping toxicities, which makes changing a single agent problematic. Serious and life-threatening toxicities warrant cessation of the whole regimen before deciding upon a subsequent therapy.

As a general guide, the inability to achieve and maintain less than 200 copies/mL (200×10^3/L) of HIV-RNA represents treatment failure and should prompt consideration for changing therapy. This includes the inability to achieve less than 200 copies/mL (200×10^3/L) by 24 weeks of therapy initiation (repeat testing is suggested to confirm), or, after HIV-RNA suppression, repeated detection of greater than 200 copies/mL (200×10^3/L) of HIV-RNA.

Therapeutic Failure

9 The most important measure of therapeutic failure is suboptimal suppression of viral replication. Many reasons may underlie suboptimal suppression of viral replication such as pre-ART disease factors (eg, high viral load or preexisting drug resistance), nonadherence to medication, development of new drug resistance, intolerance to one or more medications, adverse drug-drug or drug-food interactions, or pharmacokinetic-pharmacodynamic variability.[38] In cases of suboptimal suppression of viral replication, these potential causes should be investigated and addressed, if possible. As a general rule, drug resistance develops for regimens that do not maximally suppress HIV replication. Drug resistance testing is recommended while the patient is undergoing the failing regimen or within 4 weeks after stopping the regimen as long as the HIV-RNA count is greater than 500 copies/mL (500×10^3/L), which is the threshold for most resistance assays (~500-1,000 copies/mL [$\sim 500 \times 10^3$–1.0×10^6/L]). Virus may revert to wild type if more than 4 to 6 weeks has elapsed between regimen discontinuation and the resistance test. Most clinicians use the genotype assay because it is less expensive and results typically are available sooner compared with the phenotype assay. Resistance results usually require expert interpretation.

Treating patients who have drug-resistant HIV utilizes the same general treatment approaches described for initial therapy above. Several antiretroviral drugs are well-suited for drug-resistant HIV. The drugs in the newer classes (ie, InSTIs, entry inhibitors) are also active against NRTI-, NNRTI-, and PI-resistant viruses in highly treatment-experienced patients in controlled trials.[38] Patients should be treated with at least two (preferably three) fully active antiretroviral drugs from different mechanistic classes based on medication history and resistance tests. The goal of therapy is to suppress HIV-RNA to undetectable levels. In cases when undetectable HIV-RNA cannot be attained, maintenance on the regimen is preferred over drug discontinuation so as to prevent rapid immunological and clinical decline.

Prior to the availability of new drugs and drug classes, other strategies were studied to help manage therapeutic failure including drug holidays, structured or strategic treatment interruptions, and structured intermittent therapy. The overall premise of these strategies was similar: stop all antiretrovirals to spare the patient from drug toxicities and to allow the virus to revert to wild type. Reinitiation of therapy was intended to reestablish control of viral replication, as wild-type virus would be expected to predominate, although it was known that resistant virus was archived in long-lived cells, so viral suppression was short lived. Patients randomized to episodic therapy (drug-sparing) guided by the CD4 experienced significantly increased risk of opportunistic disease or death from any cause, including non-AIDS causes.[85,86] Viral replication is damaging to the immune system and end organs and drug-sparing approaches are not advocated.

HIV CURE RESEARCH

In 2007, the "Berlin patient," a person with HIV and new-onset acute myeloid leukemia, underwent an allogeneic bone marrow transplant with homozygous CCR5delta32 stem cells.[87] Following a complicated clinical course, including graft versus host disease and second transplant, he was found to be free of HIV infection, as no virus could be detected in any sample tested in 2009. This was deemed a sterilizing cure and his case gave hope to researchers and patients alike for curing HIV infection. In 2019, a second person, the "London Patient," has been reported as cured of HIV infection. Replicating these individuals treatment and clinical course, however, is not a practical or safe strategy for most persons living with HIV infection. Developing a cure will be particularly challenging because HIV integrates its genome into host cells, creating a latent reservoir. Thus, researchers have begun focusing on creating "functional cures," where new treatments might allow patients to stop ART without disease progression. Ongoing clinical trials are evaluating such approaches.

COMPLICATIONS OF HIV INFECTION AND AIDS

3 In the pre-ART era, the major therapeutic focus was prevention and treatment of OIs associated with uncontrolled HIV replication and the steady decline in CD4 cells. Uncontrolled HIV is an insidious disease; persons often present with OIs, a consequence of the weakened immune system rather than HIV per se. Most OIs are caused by organisms that are common in the environment and often represent the reactivation of quiescent, hidden infections common in the population. The probability of developing specific OIs is closely related to CD4 count thresholds (Fig. 148-2). These CD4 thresholds serve as a basis for initiating primary OI chemoprevention.

5 In the ART era, the main principle in the management of OIs is treating HIV infection to enable CD4 cell recovery and maintenance above protective levels.[65] Additional important principles regarding management of OIs are as follows:

1. Prevent exposure to opportunistic pathogens
2. Vaccinate to prevent first-episode disease (consult HIV-specific guidelines)
3. Use primary chemoprophylaxis at certain CD4 thresholds to prevent first-episode disease
4. Treat emergent OI
5. Use secondary chemoprophylaxis to prevent disease recurrence
6. Discontinue prophylaxes with sustained ART-associated immune recovery

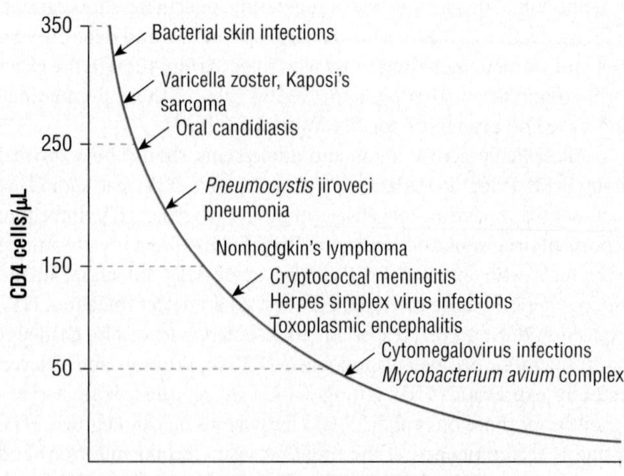

FIGURE 148-2 Natural history of opportunistic infections associated with human immunodeficiency virus infection. CD4 counts expressed as cells/μL can be converted into SI units by multiplying by 10^6/L.

Several considerations are required for the patient who presents with an OI and is simultaneously diagnosed with HIV and who thus needs both OI and ART treatment. Immediate initiation of ART is indicated for OIs that respond to CD4 recovery, such as cryptosporidiosis, progressive multifocal leukoencephalopathy (JC virus), and mild-to-moderate Kaposi's sarcoma (HHV8 virus). Rapid initiation of ART (within days to weeks) is also indicated in the setting of other OIs such as tuberculosis, *Mycobacterium avium* complex (MAC), and PCP, but several potential issues need consideration. First, drug-drug interactions and the complexity of adhering to concomitant ART and OI regimens can be daunting. Careful review of potential interactions and adherence support should be provided. Second, clinicians must be cognizant of potentially overlapping drug toxicities (eg, rash) that create problems when attempting to stop the perceived culprit drug. Third, an immune reconstitution inflammatory syndrome (IRIS) has been associated with initiation of ART in the presence of underlying OIs. IRIS is generally characterized by fever and worsening of OI manifestations in the first few weeks to months after initiating ART despite evidence of treatment efficacy. Risk factors for IRIS are a low CD4 count (eg, less than 50 cells/μL [0.050×10^9/L]) and a high antigenic burden. An ART-associated rapid-onset immune reconstitution against the smoldering OI infection, and resulting proinflammatory cytokine cascade, is the mechanism of IRIS. The most serious IRIS reactions involve neurological OIs such as cryptococcal meningitis, where IRIS can lead to increased morbidity and mortality. For cryptococcal meningitis, it may be prudent to delay ART until completion of the induction or induction/consolidation phase of antifungal therapy (up to 10 weeks). Generally, treatment of IRIS is supportive and may include corticosteroids and/or NSAIDs, depending on the OI. Expert consultation should be used in the management of ART initiation in patients with advanced HIV infection and OIs, and the most up-to-date guidelines should be consulted.

The epidemiology of specific OIs can depend upon geographical region.[49,65] For instance, TB is particularly endemic on the African continent and is considered a major OI in that region, but the incidence of TB is relatively uncommon in the United States. Major OIs in the United States include PCP, toxoplasmosis, MAC, cytomegalovirus retinitis, and cryptococcal meningitis. All have decreased substantially in incidence with the advent of ART. Furthermore, primary and secondary chemoprophylaxis for specific OIs have contributed to the same decreases. Nevertheless, opportunistic diseases continue to be complications of HIV disease and occur at low CD4 lymphocyte counts in patients who are unaware of their HIV infection, or who have not responded to ART therapy or OI prophylaxis because of adherence issues or inadequate engagement with the healthcare system.

Selected OIs and recommended first-line regimens for OI treatment are given in Table 148-6. Recommended therapies for primary OI prophylaxis are given in Table 148-7.[65] These recommendations are representative and not as extensive as in the published guidelines, which include multiple additional treatment considerations and alternatives, as well as coverage of less common OIs. The following brief discussion of PCP provides a more in-depth overview of the epidemiology, diagnosis, clinical manifestations, and results of treatment and serves as an illustration for the principles discussed above.

Pneumocystis jirovecii Pneumonia

5 *Pneumocystis jirovecii* (*carinii*) pneumonia (PCP) is the most common life-threatening OI in patients with AIDS.[88] *P. jirovecii* was formerly named *P. carinii*; the name change was made to distinguish the organism that infects humans (*P. jirovecii*) from the strain that infects rodents (*P. carinii*). Nevertheless, the acronym PCP is still used today. PCP was common early in the AIDS epidemic, but the incidence of PCP has fallen markedly since the advent of ART and effective prophylaxis for PCP. It still occurs in persons unaware of their HIV infection, and breakthrough PCP can occur in those with variable adherence to ART and/or prophylaxis.

P. jirovecii is a fungus that has protozoan characteristics as well.[88] Exposure to *P. jirovecii* is widespread; two-thirds of the population have developed serum antibodies by age 2 to 4 years. The organism resides without consequence in humans unless the host becomes immunologically impaired.[88] Disease associated with immunosuppression probably occurs from both new acquisition and reactivation. Ninety percent of PCP cases in AIDS patients occurred in those with CD4 counts less than 200 cells/mm³ (0.2×10^9/L).[65] Other risk factors include oral thrush, recurrent bacterial pneumonia, unintentional weight loss, and high-plasma HIV-RNA. Past episodes of PCP increase risk for future episodes, which provides the basis for secondary chemoprophylaxis, as described below.

The presentation of PCP in AIDS often is insidious.[88] Characteristic symptoms include fever and dyspnea. Clinical signs are tachypnea with or without rales or rhonchi and a nonproductive or mildly productive cough occurring over a period of weeks, although more fulminant presentations can occur. Chest radiographs may show florid or subtle interstitial and bilateral infiltrates but occasionally are normal. Arterial blood gases may show minimal hypoxia (PaO_2, 80-95 mm Hg [10.6-12.6 kPa]) but in more advanced disease may be markedly abnormal. The diagnosis of PCP usually is made by identification of the organism in induced sputum or in specimens obtained from bronchoalveolar lavage. Less commonly, transbronchial or open lung biopsy is used to locate the organism. The stain used for organism identification affects the sensitivity and specificity of the respiratory samples. Many laboratories prefer direct immunofluorescent staining using monoclonal antibodies. PCR is an alternative diagnostic method that is highly sensitive and specific for detecting *Pneumocystis*. Unfortunately, PCR does not distinguish whether the presence of the organism is due to colonization or disease. 1,3-β-D-glucan is a component of *Pneumocystis* cell walls that is elevated in patients with PCP. The assay for 1,3-β-D-glucan has a high sensitivity for those with PCP and can therefore be used to rule out PCP, but it is nonspecific because elevation may also be due to various causes, including other fungal infections.[65]

Untreated PCP has a mortality rate of nearly 100%. Several potential treatments are available for PCP, but the treatment of choice is trimethoprim–sulfamethoxazole (also called cotrimoxazole), which is associated with a response rate of 60% to 100%.[65] Parenteral pentamidine is equally efficacious but significantly more toxic. Trimethoprim–sulfamethoxazole is also the regimen of choice for primary and secondary prophylaxis of PCP in patients with and without HIV.[65] Additional drugs, such as echinocandins, and vaccines are in development for PCP.[89]

When used for treatment of PCP, the dose of trimethoprim–sulfamethoxazole is 15 to 20 mg/kg/day (based on the trimethoprim component) as three to four divided doses. Treatment duration typically is 21 days but also must be based on clinical response. Trimethoprim–sulfamethoxazole is usually initiated by the IV route, although oral therapy may suffice in mildly ill and reliable outpatients or for completion of a course of therapy after a response has been achieved with IV administration.[65,89] Patients with moderate-to-severe PCP (eg, PaO_2 more than 70 mm Hg [9.3 kPa]) should be treated with corticosteroids as soon as possible after starting PCP therapy and certainly within 72 hours, in order to blunt the deterioration seen just after initiation of PCP therapy. Alternative regimens include primaquine with clindamycin or IV pentamidine for moderate-to-severe disease, and dapsone with trimethoprim, primaquine with clindamycin, or atovaquone for mild-to-moderate PCP.[65] Early initiation of ART (within 2 weeks) is recommended, keeping in mind the potential issues described earlier.

Adverse reactions to trimethoprim–sulfamethoxazole and pentamidine are common, occurring in 20% to 85% of patients

TABLE 148-6 Selected Therapies for Common Opportunistic Pathogens in HIV-Infected Individuals

Clinical Disease	Preferred Initial Therapies for Acute Infection in Adults (Strength of Recommendation in Parentheses)	Common Drug- or Dose-Limiting Adverse Reactions
Fungi		
Candidiasis, oral	Fluconazole 100 mg orally for 7-14 days (AI)	Elevated liver function tests, hepatotoxicity, nausea, and vomiting
	Or	
	Nystatin 500,000 units oral swish (~5 mL) four times daily for 7-14 days (BII)	Taste, patient acceptance
Candidiasis, esophageal	Fluconazole 100-400 mg orally or IV daily for 14-21 days (AI)	Same as above
	Or	
	Itraconazole 200 mg/day orally for 14-21 days (AI)	Elevated liver function tests, hepatotoxicity, nausea, and vomiting
Pneumocystis jirovecii pneumonia	*Moderate to severe episodes* Trimethoprim–sulfamethoxazole IV or orally 15-20 mg/kg/day as trimethoprim component in three to four divided doses for 21 days[a] (AI) moderate or severe therapy should be started IV *Mild-to-moderate episodes* Trimethoprim–sulfamethoxazole 15-20 mg/kg/day as trimethoprim component orally in three divided doses or trimethoprim–sulfamethoxazole double strength tablets, two tablets three times daily	Skin rash, fever, leucopenia Thrombocytopenia
Cryptococcal meningitis	Liposomal amphotericin B 3-4 mg/kg/day IV with flucytosine 100 mg/kg/day orally in four divided doses for a minimum of 2 weeks (AI) *followed by*	Nephrotoxicity, hypokalemia, anemia, fever, chills Bone marrow suppression
	Fluconazole 800 mg/day, orally for 8 weeks. (AI)[a] Doses can be reduced to 400 mg orally once daily in clinically stable patients with negative CSF cultures. (AIII)[a]	Same as above
Histoplasmosis	Liposomal amphotericin B 3 mg/kg/day IV for 2 weeks (AI) *followed by*	Same as above
	Itraconazole 200 mg orally thrice daily for 3 days then twice daily, for 12 months (AII)[a]	
Coccidioidomycosis	Amphotericin B deoxycholate 0.7-1.0 mg/kg IV daily (AII) or lipid formulation amphotericin B 4-6 mg/kg IV daily (AIII) until clinical improvement, then switch to an azole (BIII)	Same as above
	Or	
	Fluconazole 400-800 mg IV or PO once daily (meningeal disease) (AII)[a]	Same as above
Protozoa		
Toxoplasmic encephalitis	Pyrimethamine 200 mg orally once, followed by weight-based therapy: • If <60 kg, pyrimethamine 50 mg orally once daily • If >60 kg, pyrimethamine 75 mg orally once daily	Bone marrow suppression
	Plus • If <60 kg, sulfadiazine 1 g orally four times daily • If >60 kg, sulfadiazine 1.5 g orally four times daily And Leucovorin 10-25 mg orally daily for 6 weeks (AI)[a]	Rash, drug fever
Isosporiasis	Trimethoprim and sulfamethoxazole: 160 mg trimethoprim and 800 mg sulfamethoxazole orally or IV four times daily for 10 days (AII)[a]	Same as above
Bacteria		
Mycobacterium avium complex	Clarithromycin 500 mg orally twice daily, *plus* ethambutol 15 mg/kg/day orally (AI) for at least 12 months	GI intolerance, optic neuritis, peripheral neuritis, elevated liver tests
Salmonella enterocolitis or bacteremia	Ciprofloxacin 500-750 mg orally (or 400 mg IV) twice daily for 14 days (longer duration for bacteremia or advanced HIV) (AIII)	GI intolerance, headache, dizziness
Campylobacter enterocolitis (mild to moderate)	Ciprofloxacin 500-750 mg orally (or 400 mg IV) twice daily for 7-10 days (or longer with bacteremia) (BIII)	Same as above
Shigella enterocolitis	Ciprofloxacin 500-750 mg orally (or 400 mg IV) twice daily for 7-10 days (*Or* >14 days for bacteremia) (AIII)	Same as above
Viruses		
Mucocutaneous herpes simplex	Acyclovir 5 mg/kg IV every 8 hr until lesions regress, then acyclovir 400 mg orally three times daily until complete healing (famciclovir or valacyclovir is alternative) (AIII)	GI intolerance, crystalluria
Primary varicella-zoster	Acyclovir 10-15 mg/kg every 8 hr IV for 7-10 days (severe cases), then switch to oral valacyclovir 1 g three times daily after defervescence if no evidence of visceral involvement (famciclovir or acyclovir is alternative) (AIII)	Obstructive nephropathy, CNS symptoms
Cytomegalovirus (retinitis)	Ganciclovir 5 mg/kg IV every 12 hr or valganciclovir 900 mg orally twice daily for 14-21 days (AI) with or without: Intravitreal ganciclovir (2 mg) or foscarnet (2.4 mg) for 1-4 doses over 7-10 days (for sight threatening lesions) *plus* valganciclovir 900 mg twice daily for 14-21 days then once daily until immune recovery from ART (AIII)[a]	Neutropenia, thrombocytopenia

(*Continued*)

TABLE 148-6 Selected Therapies for Common Opportunistic Pathogens in HIV-Infected Individuals (*Continued*)

Clinical Disease	Preferred Initial Therapies for Acute Infection in Adults (Strength of Recommendation in Parentheses)	Common Drug- or Dose-Limiting Adverse Reactions
Cytomegalovirus esophagitis or colitis	Ganciclovir 5 mg/kg IV every 12 hr for 21-42 days; may switch to valganciclovir 900 mg orally every 12 hr when oral therapy can be tolerated (BI)	Same as above

[a]Maintenance therapy is recommended.

ART, antiretroviral therapy; CSF, cerebrospinal fluid; HIV, human immunodeficiency virus.

See Table 126-3 for levels of evidence-based recommendations.

Data from Reference 66.

TABLE 148-7 Therapies for Prophylaxis of Select First-Episode Opportunistic Diseases in Adults and Adolescents

Pathogen	Indication	First Choice (Strength of Recommendation in Parentheses)
I. Standard of care		
Pneumocystis jirovecii	CD4⁺ count <200/mm³ (<0.2 × 10⁹/L) *or* oropharyngeal candidiasis	Trimethoprim–sulfamethoxazole, one double-strength tablet orally once daily (AI) or one single-strength tablet orally once daily (AI)
Histoplasma capsulatum	CD4⁺ count <150/mm³ (<0.15 × 10⁹/L) endemic geographic area and high risk for exposures	Itraconazole 200 mg orally once daily (BI)
Mycobacterium tuberculosis		
Isoniazid-sensitive	(Active TB should be ruled out): + test for latent TB infection with no prior TB treatment history (AI) *Or* – test for latent TB infection, but close contact with case of active tuberculosis (AII)	*Rifapentine (weight-based) orally plus isoniazid 900 mg orally plus pyridoxine 50 mg orally once weekly for 12 weeks (AII) Rifapentine Weekly Dose: • 32.1-49.9 kg: 750 mg • >50 kg: 900 mg *Or* Isoniazid 300 mg plus rifampin 600mg plus pyridoxine 25–50 mg orally daily for 3 months (AI) *Rifapentine only recommended for persons receiving RAL-, EFV-or once daily DTG- based ART regimen
For exposure to drug-resistant TB	Consult public health authorities	
Toxoplasma gondii	Immunoglobulin G antibody to *Toxoplasma* and CD4⁺ count <100/mm³ (<0.1 × 10⁹/L)	Trimethoprim–sulfamethoxazole one double-strength tablet orally once daily (AII)
Mycobacterium avium complex	CD4⁺ count <50/mm³ (<0.05 × 10⁹/L)	Azithromycin 1,200 mg orally once weekly (AI) or 600 mg orally twice weekly (BIII) *Or* clarithromycin 500 mg orally twice daily (AI)
Varicella zoster virus (VZV)	Preexposure: CD4 ≥200/mm³ (≥0.2 × 10⁹/L), no history of varicella vaccination or infection, or, if available, negative antibody to VZV Postexposure: Significant exposure to chicken pox or shingles for patients who have no history of vaccination or either condition or, if available, negative antibody to VZV	Varicella vaccination; two doses, 3 months apart (BIII) Varicella-zoster immune globulin, 125 IU per 10 kg (maximum of 625 IU) IM, as soon as possible and within 10 days after exposure (AIII)
Streptococcus pneumoniae	Any individual regardless of CD4 count	13-valent polysaccharide vaccine, 0.5 mL intramuscularly once (AI) followed by 23-valent polysaccharide vaccine 0.5 mL 8 weeks later (CIII) Re-vaccinate with PPV23 0.5 mL IM one time (BII) if the following: • Aged 19-64 years and >5 years since first PPV23 dose • Final dose to be given at >65 years, and if >5 years since the previous PPV23 dose • Typically, no more than 3 doses of PPV23 in a lifetime
Hepatitis B virus	All susceptible patients	HBV vaccine IM (Engerix-B 20 µg/mL or Recombivax HB 10 µg/mL), 0, 1, and 6 months (AII) Anti-HBs should be obtained 1 month after the vaccine series completion (BIII)
Influenza virus	All patients (annually, before influenza season)	Inactivated trivalent influenza virus vaccine (annual): 0.5 mL intramuscularly (AIII) (live-attenuated vaccine is contraindicated in all persons with HIV)
Hepatitis A virus	All susceptible (anti-hepatitis A virus–negative) patients at increased risk for hepatitis A infection (eg, chronic liver disease, injection drug users, men who have sex with men)	Hepatitis A vaccine: two doses at 0 and 6-12 months (AII) antibody response should be assessed 1 month after vaccination; with revaccination as needed when CD4 >200 cells/µL (>0.2 × 10⁹/L)(BIII)
Human papillomavirus (HPV) infection	Target age for vaccination: 11-12 years (AIII) Vaccination through age 26 is recommended but vaccine effectiveness is lower if vaccination occurs after onset of sexual activity (BII)	HPV recombinantvaccine 9 valent intramuscularly at months 0, 1-2, and 6 (BIII)

See Table 126-3 for levels of evidence-based recommendations.

Data from Reference 66.

in this setting.[65] The more common adverse reactions seen with trimethoprim–sulfamethoxazole are rash (rarely including Stevens-Johnson syndrome), fever, leukopenia, elevated serum transaminase levels, and thrombocytopenia. The incidence of these adverse reactions is higher in persons with HIV than in those not infected with HIV. Mild rashes should be watched closely for progression to more severe reactions but are not an absolute contraindication to continuing therapy. This highlights the need for thoughtful consideration of ART components because of overlapping toxicities with some antiretrovirals such as NNRTIs, which are also associated with rash and hypersensitivity, including life-threatening cases. Alternative treatments can have their own side effect profiles to consider. Dosage modification or pharmacokinetic monitoring can reduce the toxicity of trimethoprim–sulfamethoxazole. Early addition of adjunctive corticosteroid therapy to anti-PCP regimens decreases the risk of respiratory failure and improves survival. The adverse effects associated with corticosteroid use for this scenario are minimal, primarily an increased incidence of herpetic lesions, although some concerns exist about the potential for reactivation of tuberculosis or cytomegalovirus and/or long-term effects on bones.

Prevention of PCP is clearly a preferable treatment strategy. Primary prophylaxis is recommended for any person with HIV who has a CD4 lymphocyte count less than 200 cells/mm^3 (0.2×10^9/L) (or CD4 percentage of total lymphocytes less than 14% [0.14]) or a history of oropharyngeal candidiasis.[65,88] Secondary PCP prophylaxis is recommended for all persons with HIV who have had a previous episode of PCP. Trimethoprim–sulfamethoxazole is the most effective and least expensive agent and is the preferred therapy for both primary and secondary prophylaxis of PCP in adults and adolescents.[65,88] It also confers cross-protection against toxoplasmosis and many bacterial infections. The recommended dose in adults and adolescents is one double-strength tablet daily, although other regimens, such as one double-strength tablet thrice weekly or one single-strength tablet daily and gradual dose escalation using liquid trimethoprim–sulfamethoxazole, have been used to reduce the incidence of adverse reactions and improve adherence. Alternative prophylactic regimens are available if trimethoprim–sulfamethoxazole cannot be tolerated.

In the ART era, the profound reduction in HIV replication and restoration in CD4 cell count to levels rarely associated with the development of OIs provides a basis for the discontinuation of primary and secondary prophylaxis.[65] For PCP, primary prophylaxis should be discontinued in patients receiving and responding to ART who have a CD4 cell count greater than 200 cells/mm^3 (0.2×10^9/L) sustained for at least 3 months, but should be reinstated if the CD4 count drops to less than 200 cells/mm^3 (0.2×10^9/L). The same criteria apply for both discontinuation and reinitiation of secondary prophylaxis of PCP. However, continued secondary prophylaxis should be considered when the original PCP episode occurred at a CD4 count greater than 200 cells/mm^3 (0.2×10^9/L).

Comprehensive recommendations are available for management of PCP and other OIs in the context of HIV infection, including prophylaxis, treatment, and removal of prophylaxis with the control of HIV infection.[65] Readers are advised that data continue to emerge on new OI therapies, the safety of stopping primary and secondary prophylaxis, as well as criteria for when to restart secondary prophylaxis. The most current guidelines should always be consulted. Similar OI guidelines specific to children have been developed and are updated regularly.[43]

The Aging HIV Population

9 Given the life-prolonging effects of ART, approximately half of persons with HIV are over 50 years of age in resource-rich countries.[90] Along with older age come higher rates of well-known chronic and acute illnesses such as osteoporosis and osteopenia, renal and hepatic insufficiency, metabolic syndrome, neurocognitive decline, atherosclerotic disease, frailty, and non-AIDS malignancies. Many of these illnesses occur at higher than expected rates in older persons with HIV in the ART era.[91,92] The cause(s) of these higher rates is the focus of intense study. Initially, adverse events from antiretroviral medications such as hyperlipidemia were thought to contribute significantly to these conditions but ongoing inflammation and viral persistence play a critical role. Therefore, ART generally protects against non-AIDS events and it is universally recommended to manage these emerging complications. Additionally, persons with HIV should adopt healthy habits to slow the aging process including healthy diets, regular exercise, and adequate sleep.

One-third of deaths in people living with HIV are attributed to cancer.[93] While contemporary ART has reduced the incidence of HIV-related cancers such as Kaposi's sarcoma and non-Hodgkin's lymphoma, other non-AIDS-related malignancies impact persons with HIV at significantly elevated rates such as Hodgkin's lymphoma and anal, lung, skin, and hepato-carcinoma. Part of this risk may be attributed to elevated exposures or susceptibilities to human papillomavirus (oral and anal cancer), smoking (lung carcinoma), and chronic hepatitis B and/or C coinfection (liver cancer), which are modifiable risk factors. For example, guidelines advocate HPV vaccination for younger persons with HIV, as well as increased screening for anal cancer in those with existing genital or anal warts.[65] Antiretroviral drugs may contribute directly to these increased cancer rates, as some agents have been associated with cancers in observational studies.[94] However, persisting immunosuppression may be an underlying cause of higher cancer rates in persons with HIV.[91] While the approach to treatment of non-AIDS-related malignancies in persons with HIV is similar to that in persons without HIV, treatment is complicated by drug-drug interactions or additive toxicities that may exist between the antiretrovirals and the oncolytics.[95]

Cardiovascular disease has also emerged as a major concern for persons with HIV. Persons with HIV are at higher risk of cardiovascular disease compared with persons without HIV, including persons with viral suppression.[91] This increased risk is similar in magnitude to other well-established risk factors such as hypertension and hyperlipidemia. Elevated systemic inflammation and its impact on endothelial structure and function and the clotting cascade is thought to underlie much of this risk, as elevations in circulating C-reactive protein and IL-6 correlate with clinical outcomes. Statins are beneficial in persons with HIV and dyslipidemia, in part because of their anti-inflammatory effects. In this population, pitavastatin reduced markers of arterial inflammation and immune system activation.[96] Antiretroviral drugs themselves may also contribute to cardiovascular risk, given the well-known relationships between PIs, efavirenz, and certain NRTIs with dyslipidemia (increased triglycerides and low-density lipoproteins [LDL] and decreased high-density lipoproteins [HDL]) and abnormal glucose homeostasis (insulin resistance and impaired glucose tolerance).[91] Retrospective studies have found an association between myocardial infarction and abacavir use, but other studies have not, so this association is controversial and highlights the difficulty in using observational and retrospective data to attribute risk to these emerging medical conditions. Tenofovir alafenamide has been associated with lipid increases in comparison to tenofovir disoproxil,[56] though it is unclear whether tenofovir disoproxil has lipid-lowering properties or if tenofovir alafenamide is involved in mechanistically causing these increases.[91] Metabolic abnormalities in persons with HIV on ART, such as hyperlipidemia and hyperglycemia, should be reviewed with consideration given toward optimizing ART where possible to minimize side effects and avoid drug-drug interactions.

Another relevant problem for persons with HIV is body fat abnormalities. Older ART was associated with changes in body fat distribution[97] and newer ART options, such as InSTIs and tenofovir alafenamide, have been associated with weight gain. The thymidine analogs, particularly stavudine, were associated with lipoatrophy of the subcutaneous fat in the extremities and face, and these agents and older PIs were associated with hypertrophy of the deep abdominal fat depot. Collectively these fat abnormalities were termed HIV lipodystrophy. Newer agents are less associated with lipodystrophy compared with older agents, which provides a basis for switching therapy to newer regimens or initiating therapy with preferred regimens. The best management of body fat changes is prevention through initiation of preferred regimens less likely to cause such changes (see current recommendations for initial therapy, Table 148-2).[65] The weight gain with InSTIs and tenofovir alafenamide is a separate issue from lipodystrophy seen with older ARV medications. The greatest weight gain was with InSTIs (dolutegravir ~ bictegravir > raltegravir > elvitegravir), followed by PIs, and then NNRTIs.[62,63] Tenofovir alafenamide has also been associated with greater weight gain than tenofovir disoproxil fumarate,[56] and this effect is more pronounced when combined with dolutegravir. A clear underlying mechanism has not been established, and some studies have also failed to identify associations.

Functional declines of end organs such as kidney, liver, skeletal muscle (frailty), and brain (cognition) are other important considerations for older persons with HIV. These declines are expected with aging but are related with HIV itself.[91] However, certain drugs may also exacerbate these issues. The NNRTI efavirenz, for instance, is commonly associated with central nervous system perturbations including somnolence, attention deficits, and psychiatric issues. These effects exacerbate neurocognitive impairment, although this is controversial and difficult to disentangle from the effects of HIV. Similarly, integrase inhibitors have been associated with neuropsychiatric side effects, such as insomnia, worsening depression, and increased suicidality, particularly among those with preexisting psychiatric conditions. These effects have primarily been analyzed with dolutegravir, with risk factors including preexisting conditions, age over 60 years, female sex, and the concomitant use of abacavir.[98] The most important defense against HIV-associated neurocognitive decline is durable suppression of viral replication.[99]

HIV also causes a nephropathy (termed HIV-associated nephropathy, or HIVAN), most commonly a glomerulopathy that can lead to end-stage renal disease in the absence of ART.[100] The incidence of this condition has declined by approximately 60% in the ART era, demonstrating that ART is the most important intervention against HIVAN. Black people are more likely to experience HIVAN compared with White people. Some antiretroviral drugs impact renal health and these may exacerbate the effects of HIV. For example, atazanavir and lopinavir may crystallize in urine leading to obstruction, whereas tenofovir may injure the proximal tubule leading to Fanconi syndrome in rare cases.[101] The newer tenofovir alafenamide pro-drug is less likely to cause proximal tubulopathy because plasma concentrations of tenofovir are lower compared with tenofovir disoproxil.[74] Renal function should be monitored routinely in all persons with HIV, including consideration for more frequent monitoring for patients receiving the drugs mentioned above.[38]

Persons with HIV experience coinfection with hepatitis B (HBV) and hepatitis C virus (HCV) relatively commonly, and this can drive declines in hepatic function in this population.[65] For example, up to 30% of persons with HIV in the United States have HIV-HCV (~300,000 individuals) including as many as 90% of persons who use injection drugs and 90% of persons with hemophilia. HIV worsens the prognosis of HCV by reducing the chance of HCV clearance and accelerating HCV progression. With chronic HCV infection, progression to fibrosis, cirrhosis, and liver failure is several-fold faster in HIV-HCV patients versus HCV-monoinfected patients. ART reduces progression to hepatic decompensation and, among HIV-HCV coinfected population on ART, progression is faster in those who do not fully suppress HIV replication. For these reasons, ART is recommended for HIV-HCV coinfected persons and HCV therapy should be offered according to HCV guidelines.[102] The most important consideration for co-treatment is potential drug-drug interactions between ART and HCV therapies. Again, the most recent information should be consulted in reviewing potential interactions.[38,102]

The same general principles extend to HIV-HBV coinfected patients, who comprise approximately 10% of the HIV population.[65] However, two unique considerations are relevant for HIV-HBV coinfection. First, the ART regimen should include tenofovir (in the form of tenofovir disoproxil or alafenamide) plus either lamivudine or emtricitabine, given the HBV activity of these agents. Second, hepatic flares and decompensation has been reported when tenofovir-based therapy was interrupted or discontinued. If discontinuation is necessary, close monitoring of hepatic function is indicated.

Despite these issues in the contemporary ART era, the pharmacotherapy of HIV infection has steadily improved over the past 30 years, such that HIV is now a chronic but manageable condition. Whether the patient will ultimately mount a durable response to ART depends upon adherence, convenience/tolerability, and pharmacologic effectiveness. As discussed throughout this chapter, a large number of considerations go into choosing the optimal ART for a given patient. These factors include pre-ART disease characteristics (eg, resistance testing, viral load, and CD4 count), ART characteristics (eg, coformulations, food requirements, drug-drug interactions), comorbid conditions (eg, preexisting renal dysfunction), potential for pregnancy, HLA-B*5701 and/or tropism testing (if abacavir or maraviroc are being considered), and co infections (eg, TB infection). The clinician's knowledge and application of HIV pathophysiology and pharmacologic principles of ART will ultimately guide therapeutic success.

ACKNOWLEDGMENTS

The authors wish to thank Drs. Thomas Kakuda and Jenna Yager for their invaluable contributions and efforts on previous editions of this chapter and Cecilia Nguyen for help with the OI tables. This work was supported by Grants K08 AI152942, R01 AI122298, UM1 AI06701, R01 HD085887, and R01 AI124965 from the National Institute of Allergy and Infectious Disease.

ABBREVIATIONS

AIDS	acquired immunodeficiency syndrome
ART	antiretroviral therapy
CCR5	chemokine (C–C motif) receptor 5
CD	cluster of differentiation
CDC	Centers for Disease Control and Prevention
CXCR4	chemokine (C–X–C motif) receptor 4
CYP	cytochrome P450
DHHS	Department of Health and Human Services
ELISA	enzyme-linked immunosorbent assay
FDA	Food and Drug Administration
gp	glycoprotein
HCV	hepatitis C virus
HDL	high-density lipoprotein
HIV	human immunodeficiency virus
HIVAN	HIV-associated nephropathy
HLA	human leukocyte antigen
IC_{50}	concentration of antiretroviral agent necessary to inhibit 50% of viral replication
Ig	immunoglobulin
InSTI	integrase strand transfer inhibitor
IRIS	immune reconstitution inflammatory syndrome
LDL	low-density lipoprotein
LTR	long-terminal repeat
MAC	*Mycobacterium avium* complex

MSM	men who have sex with men
NNRTI	nonnucleoside reverse transcriptase inhibitor
NRTI	nucleoside/nucleotide reverse transcriptase inhibitor
OI	opportunistic infection
PCP	*Pneumocystis jirovecii* (*carinii*) pneumonia
PCR	polymerase chain reaction
PI	protease inhibitor
PEP	postexposure prophylaxis
PrEP	preexposure prophylaxis
RT-PCR	reverse-transcription polymerase chain reaction
SIV	simian immunodeficiency virus
TB	tuberculosis
TAF	tenofovir alafenamide
TDF	tenofovir disoproxil fumarate
WHO	World Health Organization

REFERENCES

1. Henry J Kaiser Family Foundation. The Global HIV/AIDS Epidemic. 2021. Available at https://www.kff.org/global-health-policy/fact-sheet/the-global-hivaids-epidemic/.
2. Maartens G, Celum C, Lewin SR. HIV infection: Epidemiology, pathogenesis, treatment, and prevention. *Lancet.* 2014;384(9939):258–271.
3. Patel P, Borkowf CB, Brooks JT, et al. Estimating per-act HIV transmission risk: A systematic review. *AIDS.* 2014;28(10):1509–1519.
4. Centers for Disease Control and Prevention: US Public Health Service: Preexposure prophylaxis for the prevention of HIV infection in the United States—2021 Update: a clinical practice guideline. https://www.cdc.gov/hiv/pdf/risk/prep/cdc-hiv-prep-guidelines-2021.pdf.
5. Cohen MS, Chen YQ, McCauley M, et al. Antiretroviral therapy for the prevention of HIV-1 transmission. *N Engl J Med.* 2016;375(1):830–839.
6. Eisinger RW, Dieffenbach CW, Fauci AS. HIV viral load and transmissibility of HIV infection: Undetectable equals untransmittable. *JAMA.* 2019;321(5):451–452.
7. Baeten JM, Donnell D, Ndase P, et al. Antiretroviral prophylaxis for HIV prevention in heterosexual men and women. *N Engl J Med.* 2012;367(5):399–410.
8. Chasela CS, Hudgens MG, Jamieson DJ, et al. Maternal or infant antiretroviral drugs to reduce HIV-1 transmission. *N Engl J Med.* 2010;362(24):2271–2281.
9. Grant RM, Lama JR, Anderson PL, et al. Preexposure chemoprophylaxis for HIV prevention in men who have sex with men. *N Engl J Med.* 2010;363(27):2587–2599.
10. Centers for Disease Control and Prevention. Monitoring selected national HIV prevention and care objectives by using HIV surveillance data—United States and 6 dependent areas, 2016. *HIV Surveillance Supplemental Report.* 2018;23(4).
11. Baeten JM, Palanee-Phillips T, Brown ER, et al. Use of a vaginal ring containing dapivirine for HIV-1 prevention in women. *N Engl J Med.* 2016;375(22):2121–2132.
12. Esparza J. A brief history of the global effort to develop a preventive HIV vaccine. *Vaccine.* 2013;31(35):3502–3518.
13. Domiguez KL, Smith DK, Thomas V, et al. Updated guidelines for antiretroviral postexposure prophylaxis after sexual, injection drug use, or other nonoccupational exposure to HIV—United States: Recommendations from the U.S. Department of Health and Human Services. 2016. Available at https://stacks.cdc.gov/view/cdc/38856.
14. Dodd RY, Crowder LA, Haynes JM, Notari EP, Stramer SL, Steele WR. Screening blood donors for HIV, HCV, and HBV at the American Red Cross: 10-Year trends in prevalence, incidence, and residual risk, 2007 to 2016. *Transfus Med Rev.* 2020;34(2):81–93.
15. Zou S, Dodd RY, Stramer SL, et al. Probability of viremia with HBV, HCV, HIV, and HTLV among tissue donors in the United States. *N Engl J Med.* 2004;351(8):751–759.
16. Kuhar DT, Henderson DK, Struble KA, et al. Updated US Public Health Service Guidelines for the management of occupational exposures to human immunodeficiency virus and recommendations for postexposure prophylaxis. *Infection Control and Hospital Epidemiology.* 2013;34(9):875–892.
17. Magder LS, Mofenson L, Paul ME, et al. Risk factors for in utero and intrapartum transmission of HIV. *J Acquir Immune Defic Syndr.* 2005;38(1):87–95.
18. World Health Organization. HIV Transmission through Breastfeeding. 2007. Available at http://apps.who.int/iris/bitstream/10665/43879/1/9789241596596_eng.pdf.
19. Panel on Treatment of HIV-Infected Pregnant Women and Prevention of Perinatal Transmission. Recommendations for the Use of Antiretroviral Drugs in Pregnant Women with HIV Infection and Interventions to Reduce Perinatal HIV Transmission in the United States. Available at https://clinicalinfo.hiv.gov/en/guidelines/perinatal/whats-new-guidelines.
20. Revised surveillance case definition for HIV infection—United States, 2014. *MMWR Recomm Rep* 2014;63(RR-03):1–10.
21. Centers for Disease Control and Prevention. HIV/AIDS Basic Statistics 2021 [updated 10-01-2021]. Available at http://www.cdc.gov/hiv/basics/statistics.html.
22. Li Z, Purcell DW, Sansom SL, Hayes D, Hall HI. Vital signs: HIV transmission along the continuum of care—United States, 2016. *MMWR Morb Mortal Wkly Rep.* 2019;68(11):267–272.
23. AIDS U. Global HIV & AIDS statistics—Fact sheet. 2021.
24. Sharp PM, Hahn BH. Origins of HIV and the AIDS pandemic. *Cold Spring Harb Perspect Med.* 2011;1:1.
25. Shaw GM, Hunter E. HIV transmission. *Cold Spring Harb Perspect Med.* 2012;2(11).
26. McLaren PJ, Fellay J. HIV-1 and human genetic variation. *Nat Rev Genet.* 2021;22(10):645–657.
27. Tang H, Kuhen KL, Wong-Staal F. Lentivirus replication and regulation. *Annu Rev Genet.* 1999;33:133–170.
28. Chan JK, Greene WC. Dynamic roles for NF-κB in HTLV-I and HIV-1 retroviral pathogenesis. *Immunol Rev.* 2012;246(1):286–310.
29. Cullen BR. Role and mechanism of action of the APOBEC3 family of antiretroviral resistance factors. *J Virol.* 2006;80(3):1067–1076.
30. Carnes SK, Sheehan JH, Aiken C. Inhibitors of the HIV-1 capsid, a target of opportunity. *Curr Opin HIV AIDS.* 2018;13(4):359–365.
31. Siewe B, Landay A. Key concepts in the early immunology of HIV-1 infection. *Curr Infect Dis Rep.* 2012;14(1):102–109.
32. Ho DD, Neumann AU, Perelson AS, et al. Rapid turnover of plasma virions and CD4 lymphocytes in HIV-1 infection. *Nature.* 1995;373(6510):123–126.
33. Centers for Disease Control and Prevention. Laboratory testing for the diagnosis of HIV infection: Updated recommendations. 2014. Available at https://stacks.cdc.gov/view/cdc/23447.
34. Branson BM. HIV diagnostics: Current recommendations and opportunities for improvement. *Infect Dis Clin North Am.* 2019;33(3):611–628.
35. Marzinke MA, Grinsztejn B, Fogel JM, et al. Characterization of HIV infection in cisgender men and transgender women who have sex with men receiving injectable cabotegravir for HIV prevention: HPTN 083. *J Infect Dis.* 2021.
36. Saag MS, Gandhi RT, Hoy JF, et al. Antiretroviral drugs for treatment and prevention of HIV infection in adults: 2020 Recommendations of the International Antiviral Society—USA Panel. *JAMA.* 2020;324(16):1651–1669.
37. Branson BM, Handsfield HH, Lampe MA, et al. Revised recommendations for HIV testing of adults, adolescents, and pregnant women in health-care settings. *MMWR Recomm Rep.* 2006;55(RR-14):1–17.
38. Panel on Antiretroviral Guidelines for Adults and Adolescents. Guidelines for the Use of Antiretroviral Agents in Adults and Adolescents Living with HIV: Department of Health and Human Services. Available at https://clinicalinfo.hiv.gov/en/guidelines/adult-and-adolescent-arv/whats-new-guidelines.
39. Richey LE, Halperin J. Acute human immunodeficiency virus infection. *American Journal of Medical Sciences.* 2013;345(2):136–142.
40. Mellors JW, Munoz A, Giorgi JV, et al. Plasma viral load and CD4+ lymphocytes as prognostic markers of HIV-1 infection. *Ann Intern Med.* 1997;126(12):946–954.
41. Khoury M, Kovacs A. Pediatric HIV infection. *Clin Obstet Gynecol.* 2001;44(2):243–275.
42. Panel on Antiretroviral Therapy and Medical Management of HIV-Infected Children. Guidelines for the Use of Antiretroviral Agents in Pediatric HIV Infection. Available at https://clinicalinfo.hiv.gov/en/guidelines/pediatric-arv/whats-new-guidelines.
43. Panel on Opportunistic Infections in HIV-Exposed and HIV-Infected Children. Guidelines for the Prevention and Treatment of Opportunistic Infections in HIV-Exposed and HIV-Infected Children: Department of Health and Human Services. Available at https://clinicalinfo.hiv.gov/en/guidelines/pediatric-opportunistic-infection/whats-new.
44. Walensky RP, Paltiel AD, Losina E, et al. The survival benefits of AIDS treatment in the United States. *J Infect Dis.* 2006;194(1):11–19.

45. NIH Panel to Define Principles of Therapy of HIV Infection. Report of the NIH panel to define principles of therapy of HIV infection. 1997.
46. INSIGHT START Study Group, Lundgren JD, Babiker AG, et al. Initiation of antiretroviral therapy in early asymptomatic HIV infection. *N Engl J Med.* 2015;373(9):795–807.
47. The TEMPRANO ANRS 12136 Study Group, Danel C, Moh R, et al. A trial of early antiretrovirals and isoniazid preventive therapy in Africa. *N Engl J Med.* 2015;373(9):808–822.
48. Cohen MS, Chen YQ, McCauley M, et al. Prevention of HIV-1 infection with early antiretroviral therapy. *N Engl J Med.* 2011;365(6):493–505.
49. Organization WH. Consolidated guidelines on HIV prevention, testing, treatment, service delivery and monitoring: Recommendations for a public health approach. 2021.
50. Mateo-Urdiales A, Johnson S, Smith R, Nachega JB, Eshun-Wilson I. Rapid initiation of antiretroviral therapy for people living with HIV. *Cochrane Database Syst Rev.* 2019;6:CD012962.
51. Coffey S, Halperin J, Rana AI, Colasanti JA. Rapid antiretroviral therapy: Time for a new standard of care. *Clin Infect Dis.* 2021;73(1):134–136.
52. Hargrave A, Mustafa AS, Hanif A, Tunio JH, Hanif SNM. Current status of HIV-1 vaccines. *Vaccines (Basel).* 2021;9(9).
53. Kim JH, Excler J-L, Michael NL. Lessons from the RV144 Thai Phase III HIV-1 vaccine trial and the search for correlates of protection. *Ann Rev Med.* 2015;66(1):423–437.
54. Kula-Pacurar A, Rodari A, Darcis G, Van Lint C. Shocking HIV-1 with immunomodulatory latency reversing agents. *Semin Immunol.* 2021;51:101478.
55. Mills A, Crofoot GJ, McDonald C, et al. Tenofovir alafenamide versus tenofovir disoproxil fumarate in the first protease inhibitor–based single-tablet regimen for initial HIV-1 therapy: A randomized phase 2 study. *J Acquir Immune Defic Syndr.* 2015;69(4):439–445.
56. Surial B, Mugglin C, Calmy A, et al. Weight and metabolic changes after switching from tenofovir disoproxil fumarate to tenofovir alafenamide in people living with HIV: A cohort study. *Ann Intern Med.* 2021;174(6):758–767.
57. Mallon PW, Brunet L, Hsu RK, et al. Weight gain before and after switch from TDF to TAF in a U.S. cohort study. *J Int AIDS Soc.* 2021;24(4):e25702.
58. Wensing AM, Calvez V, Ceccherini-Silberstein F, et al. 2019 update of the drug resistance mutations in HIV-1. *Top Antivir Med.* 2019;27(3):111–121.
59. Telenti A. Safety concerns about CCR5 as an antiviral target. *Curr Opin HIV AIDS.* 2009;4(2):131–135.
60. Emu B, Fessel J, Schrader S, et al. Phase 3 study of ibalizumab for multidrug-resistant HIV-1. *N Engl J Med.* 2018;379:645–654.
61. Seval N, Frank C, Kozal M. Fostemsavir for the treatment of HIV. *Expert Rev Anti Infect Ther.* 2021;19(8):961–966.
62. Ruderman SA, Crane HM, Nance RM, et al. Brief report: Weight gain following ART initiation in ART-naive people living with HIV in the current treatment era. *J Acquir Immune Defic Syndr.* 2021;86(3):339–343.
63. Eckard AR, McComsey GA. Weight gain and integrase inhibitors. *Curr Opin Infect Dis.* 2020;33(1):10–19.
64. Thoueille P, Choong E, Cavassini M, Buclin T, Decosterd LA. Long-acting antiretrovirals: A new era for the management and prevention of HIV infection. *J Antimicrob Chemother.* 2021.
65. Panel on Guidelines for the Prevention and Treatment of Opportunistic Infections in Adults and Adolescents with HIV. Guidelines for the Prevention and Treatment of Opportunistic Infections in HIV-infected Adults and Adolescents: Recommendations from the Centers for Disease Control and Prevention, the National Institutes of Health, and the HIV Medicine Association of the Infectious Diseases Society of America. Available at https://clinicalinfo.hiv.gov/en/guidelines/adult-and-adolescent-opportunistic-infection/.
66. Tseng A, Hughes CA, Wu J, Seet J, Phillips EJ. Cobicistat versus ritonavir: Similar pharmacokinetic enhancers but some important differences. *Ann Pharmacother.* 2017;51(11):1008–1022.
67. Kiser JJ, Gerber JG, Predhomme JA, Wolfe P, Flynn DM, Hoody DW. Drug/Drug interaction between lopinavir/ritonavir and rosuvastatin in healthy volunteers. *J Acquir Immune Defic Syndr.* 2008;47(5):570–578.
68. Kumar P, Gordon LA, Brooks KM, et al. Differential influence of the antiretroviral pharmacokinetic enhancers ritonavir and cobicistat on intestinal P-glycoprotein transport and the pharmacokinetic/pharmacodynamic disposition of dabigatran. *Antimicrob Agents Chemother.* 2017;61(11).
69. Podany AT, Bao Y, Swindells S, et al. Efavirenz pharmacokinetics and pharmacodynamics in HIV-infected persons receiving rifapentine and isoniazid for tuberculosis prevention. *Clin Infect Dis.* 2015;61(8):1322–1327.
70. Cerrone M, Alfarisi O, Neary M, et al. Rifampicin effect on intracellular and plasma pharmacokinetics of tenofovir alafenamide. *J Antimicrob Chemother.* 2019;74(6):1670–1678.
71. Martin TCS, Hill LA, Tang ME, Balcombe SM. Tenofovir alafenamide and rifabutin co-administration does not lead to loss of HIV-1 suppression: A retrospective observational study. *Int J Infect Dis.* 2020;100:470–472.
72. Parienti JJ, Fournier AL, Cotte L, et al. Forgiveness of dolutegravir-based triple therapy compared with older antiretroviral regimens: A prospective multicenter cohort of adherence patterns and HIV-RNA replication. *Open Forum Infect Dis.* 2021;8(7):ofab316.
73. Spinelli MA, Haberer JE, Chai PR, Castillo-Mancilla J, Anderson PL, Gandhi M. Approaches to objectively measure antiretroviral medication adherence and drive adherence interventions. *Curr HIV/AIDS Rep.* 2020;17(4):301–314.
74. Sax PE, Wohl D, Yin MT, et al. Tenofovir alafenamide versus tenofovir disoproxil fumarate, coformulated with elvitegravir, cobicistat, and emtricitabine, for initial treatment of HIV-1 infection: Two randomised, double-blind, phase 3, non-inferiority trials. *Lancet.* 2015;385(9987):2606–2615.
75. Sax PE, Pozniak A, Montes ML, et al. Coformulated bictegravir, emtricitabine, and tenofovir alafenamide versus dolutegravir with emtricitabine and tenofovir alafenamide, for initial treatment of HIV-1 infection (GS-US-380-1490): A randomised, double-blind, multicentre, phase 3, non-inferiority trial. *Lancet.* 2017;390:2073–2082.
76. Walmsley SL, Antela A, Clumeck N, et al. Dolutegravir plus abacavir-lamivudine for the treatment of HIV-1 infection. *N Engl J Med.* 2013;369(19):1807–1818.
77. Pilkington V, Hughes SL, Pepperrell T, et al. Tenofovir alafenamide vs. tenofovir disoproxil fumarate: An updated meta-analysis of 14 894 patients across 14 trials. *AIDS.* 2020;34(15):2259–2268.
78. Molina JM, Clotet B, van Lunzen J, et al. Once-daily dolutegravir versus darunavir plus ritonavir for treatment-naïve adults with HIV-1 infection (FLAMINGO): 96 week results from a randomized, open-label, phase 3b study. *Lancet HIV.* 2015;2(4):e127–e136.
79. Cahn P, Madero JS, Arribas JR, et al. Durable efficacy of dolutegravir plus lamivudine in antiretroviral treatment-naive adults with HIV-1 infection: 96-Week results from the GEMINI-1 and GEMINI-2 randomized clinical trials. *J Acquir Immune Defic Syndr.* 2020;83(3):310–318.
80. Aboud M, Orkin C, Podzamczer D, et al. Efficacy and safety of dolutegravir-rilpivirine for maintenance of virological suppression in adults with HIV-1: 100-Week data from the randomised, open-label, phase 3 SWORD-1 and SWORD-2 studies. *Lancet HIV.* 2019;6(9):e576–e587.
81. Rizzardini G, Overton ET, Orkin C, et al. Long-acting injectable cabotegravir + rilpivirine for HIV maintenance therapy: Week 48 pooled analysis of phase 3 ATLAS and FLAIR trials. *J Acquir Immune Defic Syndr.* 2020;85(4):498–506.
82. Boyd SD, Sampson MR, Viswanathan P, Struble KA, Arya V, Sherwat AI. Cobicistat-containing antiretroviral regimens are not recommended during pregnancy: Viewpoint. *AIDS.* 2019;33(6):1089–1093.
83. Blackstock O, Myers J, Kobrak P, Daskalakis D, Committee icwtMCC. U=U Guidance for Implementation in Clinical Settings. 2020.
84. Delany-Moretlwe S, Hughes JP, Bock P, et al. Cabotegravir for the prevention of HIV-1 in women: results from HPTN 084, a phase 3, randomised clinical trial. Lancet. 2022 May 7; 399(10337): 1779-1789. Epub 2022 Apr 1.
85. El-Sadr WM, Lundgren J, Neaton JD, et al. CD4+ count-guided interruption of antiretroviral treatment. *N Engl J Med.* 2006;355(22):2283–2296.
86. Phillips AN, Neaton J, Lundgren JD. The role of HIV in serious diseases other than AIDS. *AIDS.* 2008;22(18):2409–2418.
87. Brown TR. I am the Berlin patient: A personal reflection. *AIDS Res Hum Retroviruses.* 2015;31(1):2–3.
88. Krajicek BJ, Thomas CF Jr, Limper AH. Pneumocystis pneumonia: Current concepts in pathogenesis, diagnosis, and treatment. *Clin Chest Med.* 2009;30(2):265–278.
89. Gingerich AD, Norris KA, Mousa JJ. Pneumocystis pneumonia: Immunity, vaccines, and treatments. *Pathogens.* 2021;10(2).
90. Falutz J, Branas F, Erlandson KM. Frailty: The current challenge for aging people with HIV. *Curr Opin HIV AIDS.* 2021;16(3):133–140.
91. McGettrick P, Barco EA, Mallon PWG. Ageing with HIV. *Healthcare (Basel).* 2018;6(1).
92. Gabuzda D, Jamieson BD, Collman RG, et al. Pathogenesis of aging and age-related comorbidities in people with HIV: Highlights from the HIV ACTION Workshop. *Pathog Immun.* 2020;5(1):143–74.

93. Brickman C, Palefsky J. Cancer in the HIV-infected host: Epidemiology and pathogenesis in the antiretroviral era. *Current HIV/AIDS Reports*. 2015;12(4):388–396.
94. Bruyand M, Ryom L, Shepherd L, et al. Cancer risk and use of protease inhibitor or nonnucleoside reverse transcriptase inhibitor-based combination antiretroviral therapy: The D: A: D study. *J Acquir Immune Defic Syndr.* 2015;68(5):568–577.
95. Mounier N, Katlama C, Costagliola D, et al. Drug interactions between antineoplastic and antiretroviral therapies: Implications and management for clinical practice. *Crit Rev Oncol/Hematol.* 2009;72(1):10–20.
96. Toribio M, Fitch KV, Sanchez L, et al. Effects of pitavastatin and pravastatin on markers of immune activation and arterial inflammation in HIV. *AIDS.* 2017;31(6):797–806.
97. Stanley TL, Grinspoon SK. Body composition and metabolic changes in HIV-infected patients. *J Infect Dis.* 2012;205(Suppl 3):S383–S390.
98. Hoffmann C, Llibre JM. Neuropsychiatric adverse events with dolutegravir and other integrase strand transfer inhibitors. *AIDS Rev.* 2019;21(1):4–10.
99. Zayyad Z, Spudich S. Neuropathogenesis of HIV: From initial neuroinvasion to HIV-associated neurocognitive disorder (HAND). *Curr HIV/AIDS Rep.* 2015;12(1):16–24.
100. Rosenberg AZ, Naicker S, Winkler CA, et al. HIV-associated nephropathies: Epidemiology, pathology, mechanisms and treatment. *Nature Reviews Nephrology*. 2015;11(3):150–160.
101. Bagnis CI, Stellbrink HJ. Protease inhibitors and renal function in patients with HIV infection: A systematic review. *Infect Dis Ther.* 2015.4(1):15–50.
102. AASLD and IDSA. HCV Guidance: Recommendations for testing, managing, and treating hepatitis C. Available at http://www.hcvguidelines.org/.
103. Preexposure Prophylaxis for the Prevention of HIV Infection in the United States – 2021 Update Clinical Practice Guideline. US Public Health Service. Available at https://www.cdc.gov/hiv/pdf/risk/prep/cdc-hiv-prep-guidelines-2021.pdf.

Cancer: The Disease and Treatment

149

Lisa M. Cordes and Sandra Cuellar

KEY CONCEPTS

1. Carcinogenesis is a multistep process that includes initiation, promotion, conversion, and progression.
2. Cancer cells demonstrate unique traits that distinguish them from normal cells. Cancer cells can stimulate their own growth, resist inhibitory signals, avoid programmed cell death, grow new blood vessels (angiogenesis), invade local tissues, and spread to distant sites (ie, metastases).
3. Screening programs are designed to detect cancers in asymptomatic people who are at risk of a specific cancer.
4. Diagnosis and staging inform the treatment goals and help select the most appropriate anticancer therapy. The treatment goal may be cure, control, or palliation. The therapy may include a combination of surgery, radiation therapy, or systemic anticancer agents. Systemic anticancer agents include chemotherapy, targeted agents, and immunotherapy.
5. Chemotherapy inhibits cancer growth by killing rapidly proliferating cells. These agents can be categorized as either cell-cycle phase-specific, targeting one specific phase of the cell cycle, or cell-cycle phase-nonspecific, targeting all proliferating cells regardless of their place in the cell cycle. Cell-cycle phase-specific chemotherapy is generally administered more frequently or as a continuous infusion, and cell-cycle phase-nonspecific chemotherapy is usually administered less frequently.
6. Small-molecule targeted agents inhibit kinases or enzymes responsible for activating various proteins involved in intracellular signaling cascades. These agents treat cancer by correcting a dysregulated signaling pathway.
7. A monoclonal antibody (mAb) is a type of targeted therapy that recognizes an antigen preferentially expressed on cancer cells or immune cells or that targets growth factors responsible for cancer growth. These antibodies can also be used to deliver drugs, radioisotopes, or toxins to the antigen-expressing cells.
8. Immunotherapies are anticancer treatments that simulate or restore the immune system to recognize and eliminate cancer cells. Immune checkpoint inhibitors, cytokines, therapeutic vaccines, and chimeric antigen receptor (CAR) T-cell therapies are types of immunotherapies.
9. Various factors can affect the response and adverse drug reactions a patient may experience with anticancer therapy. When determining the optimal therapy, the health professional should carefully consider patient-specific factors, tumor-specific factors, and treatment goals.

BEYOND THE BOOK

Patient Case

RM is a 64-year-old individual with newly diagnosed stage IV renal cell carcinoma (clear cell histology) who presents to clinic for initiation of anticancer treatment. Given her poor prognostic risk group, the oncologist recommends a vascular endothelial growth factor receptor (VEGFR) inhibitor and/or immunotherapy. Of the first-line therapy options provided in the National Comprehensive Cancer Network, or NCCN, guidelines, her insurance will cover the following: cabozantinib monotherapy; axitinib + pembrolizumab; cabozantinib + nivolumab; ipilimumab + nivolumab; and lenvatinib + pembrolizumab. The oncologist is requesting your assistance with treatment planning and implementation.

- PMH: HTN diagnosed 1.5 years ago, gastrointestinal perforation diagnosed 6 weeks ago, metastatic clear cell, renal cell carcinoma diagnosed 4 weeks ago
- Vitals: O_2 sat: 98% (0.98) RA; HR 82 bpm; BP 179/103 mm Hg; 37.4°C
- Labs:
  - Sodium 137 mEq/L (136-145 mEq/L [mmol/L])
  - Potassium 3.9 mEq/L (3.4-5.1 mEq/L [mmol/L])
  - Chloride 99 mEq/L (98-107 mEq/L [mmol/L])
  - Glucose 96 mg/dL (74-99 mg/dL) (5.3 mmol/L [4.1-5.5 mmol/L])
  - Albumin 4.1 g/dL (3.5-5.2 g/dL) (41 g/L [35-52 g/L])

- Calcium 10.4 mg/dL (8.6-10.2 mg/dL) (2.60 mmol/L [2.15-2.55 mmol/L])
- Magnesium 1.7 mg/dL (1.6-2.6 mg/dL) (0.70 mmol/L [0.66-1.07 mmol/L])
- Creatinine 0.94 mg/dL (CrCl ~80 mL/min) (83 μmol/L [CrCl ~1.33 mL/s])
- Phosphorous 2.8 mg/dL (2.5-4.5 mg/dL) (0.90 mmol/L [0.81-1.45 mmol/L])
- ALT 28 U/L (0-33 U/L) (0.47 μkat/L [0-0.55 μkat/L])
- AST 23 U/L (0-32 U/L) (0.38 μkat/L [0-0.53 μkat/L])
- T Bili 0.02 mg/dL (0.00-1.2 mg/dL) (0.3 μmol/L [0-20.5 μmol/L])
- Hgb 10.2 g/dL (11.2-15.7 g/dL) 102 g/L [112-157 g/L]; 6.33 mmol/L [6.95-9.74 mmol/L])
- Platelets 225 × 10^3/mm^3 (173 × 10^3 − 369 × 10^3/mm^3) (225 × 10^9/L [173 × 10^9 − 369 × 10^9/L])
- ANC 3.02 × 10^3/mm^3 (1.56 × 10^3 − 6.13 × 10^3/mm^3) (3.02 × 10^9/L [1.56 × 10^9 − 6.13 × 10^9/L])
- LDH 215 U/L (125 – 220 U/L) (3.58 μkat/L [2.08 – 3.67 μkat/L])

Allergies: NKDA

Medication List: lisinopril 5 mg PO daily

Questions

1. Given all the first-line treatment options for clear cell renal cell carcinoma are covered by the patient's insurance, what treatment option would you recommend for RM at this time?
2. When counseling RM prior to treatment initiation, what adverse drug reactions should be discussed?
3. What monitoring parameters should be considered for the selected treatment regimen?

Answers

INTRODUCTION

Cancer is a group of many different diseases characterized by uncontrolled cellular growth, local tissue invasion, and distant metastases. It is the second leading cause of death in Americans. In the United States, nearly 1.9 million cases of cancer are projected to occur in 2022, with an estimated 600,000 deaths.[1] Figure 149-1 shows the estimated incidence of common cancers and cancer-related deaths. The most common cancers are prostate, breast, and lung cancer. The most common cause of cancer-related death in the United States is lung cancer, accounting for approximately 130,000 deaths each year. These cancers are discussed in further detail in subsequent chapters.

Health professionals treating patients with cancer should have a thorough understanding of the pharmacokinetic, pharmacodynamic, and pharmacogenomic properties of all available anticancer agents, in addition to the reported safety and efficacy of each agent in each cancer population. Health professionals should critically evaluate, summarize, and communicate the essential information to other health professionals, patients, and caregivers. This chapter defines the etiology, pathology, diagnosis, staging, and screening; introduces anticancer therapies and their related adverse drug reactions; and provides general information on how to administer systemic anticancer agents safely.

ETIOLOGY OF CANCER

Normal healthy cells are strictly regulated, with stimulatory and inhibitory signals in a delicate balance. For normal cells to become cancer cells, it is believed that a physical, chemical, or biological agent must damage the cell and cause a genetic and/or epigenetic alteration that is subsequently propagated during cell division. Cancer cells eventually acquire multiple alterations, and these alterations lead to uncontrolled proliferation, invasion, and metastases.

Carcinogenesis

1 The mechanisms by which cancers occur are incompletely understood. A cancer is thought to develop from a cell in which the normal mechanisms that control cell growth and proliferation are altered. Current evidence supports the concept of carcinogenesis as a multistage process that is genetically regulated.[2,3] The first step in this process is *initiation*, which requires exposure of normal cells to carcinogens. These carcinogens produce genetic alterations that, if not repaired, result in irreversible cellular changes. The changed cell may subsequently have an altered response to their environment that provides a selective growth advantage and permits the development of a clonal population of cancer cells. During the second step, known as *promotion*, carcinogens or other factors alter the environment to favor growth of the altered cell population compared to normal cells. Promotion could be affected by chemoprevention strategies (strategies to lower cancer risk), including changes in lifestyle and diet. At some point, the altered cell becomes cancerous (*conversion* or *transformation*). Depending on the cancer, 5 to 20 years may elapse between the initiation and the development of a clinically detectable cancer. The final stage, called *progression*, involves further genetic alterations that lead to increased cell proliferation. The critical elements of this phase include invasion into local tissues and the development of metastases.

Substances that may act as carcinogens include a myriad of chemical, physical, and biologic agents. Chemical exposures may occur by occupational and environmental means or by lifestyle habits. Some chemicals associated with cancer include aniline dye, asbestos, and benzene. Aniline dye is a known cause of bladder cancer; benzene is a known cause of leukemia, and asbestos is a known cause of mesothelioma. As shown in Table 149-1, some medications and hormones used for therapeutic purposes are also classified as carcinogens.[4] Physical agents that act as carcinogens include ionizing radiation and ultraviolet light; radiation induces mutations by forming free radicals that damage deoxyribonucleic acid (DNA)

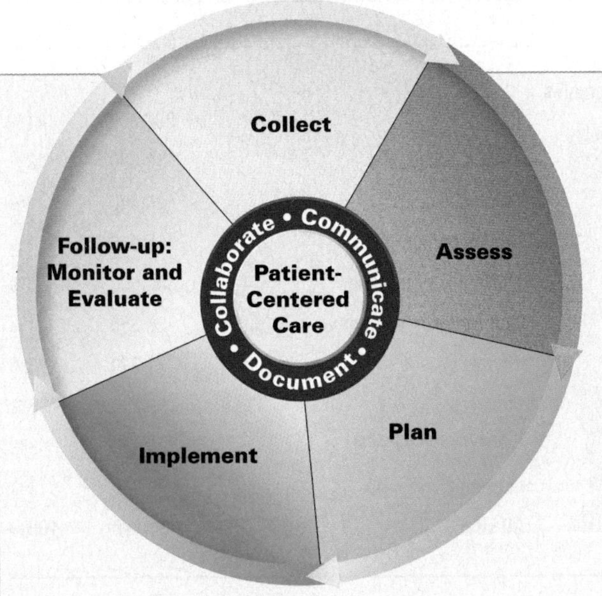

Patient Care Process for Cancer

Collect

- Patient characteristics (eg, age, biological sex)
- Patient medical history (eg, comorbidities, prior anticancer therapies)
- Family history, social history, lifestyle factors, and dietary habits
- Current medications and allergies
- Objective data
  - Imaging (eg, PET scan, CT scan, MRI)
  - Tumor characteristics (eg, histology, mutations, stage)
  - Vital signs and laboratory values, including chemistries, organ function, CBC with differential, pregnancy status, hepatitis B serologies, and medication-specific assessments (eg, left ventricular ejection fraction for anthracyclines)
  - Physical exam
  - Pharmacogenomics, if applicable

Assess

- Performance status (see Table 149-8)
- Goals of care (eg, palliation)
- Treatment history (eg, type of treatment, response, tolerability)
- Desire for fertility preservation
- Immunization status
- Barriers to treatment (eg, transportation, insurance, compliance, health literacy)
- Role for nonmedication treatment measures (eg, radiation, surgery)
- Need for genetics counseling, if applicable

Plan

- Anticancer therapy regimen and supportive care
- Monitoring parameters (see Table 149-7)
- Patient education (eg, goals of care, drug-specific information, calendar for cyclic regimens, contraception requirements)
- Restaging timepoints to assess response
- Administration requirements (eg, central venous catheter)

Implement

- Administer immunizations prior to chemotherapy initiation, if possible
- Provide patient education regarding all elements of the treatment plan
- Obtain consent for anticancer therapy
- Schedule follow-up for response and toxicity assessments

Follow-up: Monitor and Evaluate

- Assess adverse drug reactions and supportive care measures
- Assess patient adherence, if applicable
- Assess tumor response to treatment (eg, CT scan)
- Reevaluate goals of care
- Determine adherence to treatment plan

and other cellular components. Biologic agents that are associated with certain cancers include natural compounds (ie, viruses) or pollutants. The Epstein-Barr virus may be an important factor in the initiation of Burkitt lymphoma. Similarly, infection with the human papilloma virus (HPV) is a cause of cervical and head-and-neck cancers. Hereditary factors, age, and gender may also contribute to the development of cancer.

Genetic Alterations

In recent years, there has been marked progress in our understanding of the genetic changes that lead to the development of cancer.[2,3] Two types of genes play an important role in the development of cancer: oncogenes and tumor suppressor genes. Figure 149-2 illustrates the acquired capabilities of cancer cells that differ from normal cellular function.[5]

Oncogenes

Oncogenes develop from normal genes, called proto-oncogenes. Proto-oncogenes are present in all cells and are essential regulators of normal cellular functions. Genetic alterations of the proto-oncogene through point mutation, chromosomal rearrangement, or gene amplification can activate the oncogene. Carcinogens may cause these genetic alterations (somatic mutations), or these alterations may be inherited (germline mutations). After activation, the oncogene produces either excessive amounts of the normal gene product or an abnormal gene product. The result is dysregulation of normal cell growth and proliferation, which imparts a distinct growth advantage to the cell and increases the probability of transformation. For example, the erythroblastic leukemia viral oncogene (*ErbB*) family members are oncogenes that mediate cell proliferation and differentiation through activation of intracellular signaling pathways. As an oncogene, the *ErbB* gene product is typically mutated, overexpressed, or amplified, resulting in excessive cellular proliferation, invasion, and metastasis in several cancers. Table 149-2 lists examples of oncogenes by their cellular function.

Tumor Suppressor Genes

Tumor suppressor genes regulate and inhibit inappropriate cellular growth and proliferation.[2] Genetic alterations result in loss of

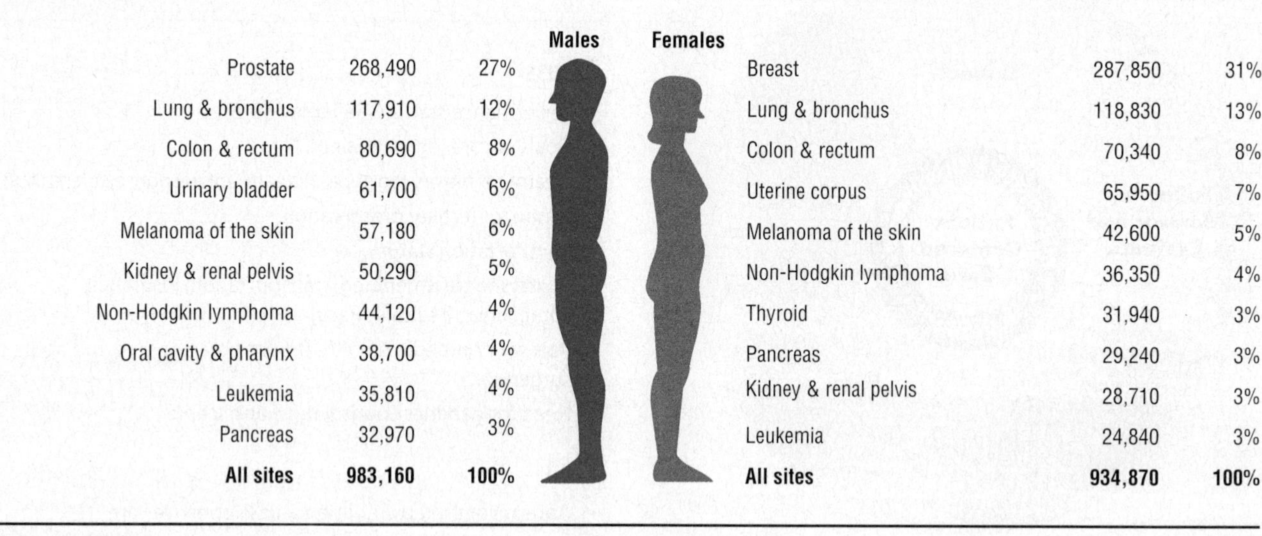

Estimated New Cases

Males			Females		
Prostate	268,490	27%	Breast	287,850	31%
Lung & bronchus	117,910	12%	Lung & bronchus	118,830	13%
Colon & rectum	80,690	8%	Colon & rectum	70,340	8%
Urinary bladder	61,700	6%	Uterine corpus	65,950	7%
Melanoma of the skin	57,180	6%	Melanoma of the skin	42,600	5%
Kidney & renal pelvis	50,290	5%	Non-Hodgkin lymphoma	36,350	4%
Non-Hodgkin lymphoma	44,120	4%	Thyroid	31,940	3%
Oral cavity & pharynx	38,700	4%	Pancreas	29,240	3%
Leukemia	35,810	4%	Kidney & renal pelvis	28,710	3%
Pancreas	32,970	3%	Leukemia	24,840	3%
All sites	**983,160**	**100%**	**All sites**	**934,870**	**100%**

Estimated Deaths

Males			Females		
Lung & bronchus	68,820	21%	Lung & bronchus	61,360	21%
Prostate	34,500	11%	Breast	43,250	15%
Colon & rectum	28,400	9%	Colon & rectum	24,180	8%
Pancreas	25,970	8%	Pancreas	23,860	8%
Liver & intrahepatic bile duct	20,420	6%	Ovary	12,810	4%
Leukemia	14,020	4%	Uterine corpus	12,550	4%
Esophagus	13,250	4%	Liver & intrahepatic bile duct	10,100	4%
Urinary bladder	12,120	4%	Leukemia	9,980	3%
Non-Hodgkin lymphoma	11,700	4%	Non-Hodgkin lymphoma	8,550	3%
Brain & other nervous system	10,710	3%	Brain & other nervous system	7,570	3%
All sites	**322,090**	**100%**	**All sites**	**287,270**	**100%**

FIGURE 149-1 Estimated 2022 cancer incidences (top) and deaths (bottom) in the United States for males and females. Estimates are rounded to the nearest 10 and exclude basal cell and squamous cell skin cancers and in situ carcinoma except urinary bladder. *(Reprinted, with permission, from Siegel RL, Miller KD, Fuchs HE, et al. Cancer Statistics. CA Cancer J Clin. 2022;72(1):7-33.)*

control over normal cell growth. *Retinoblastoma* 1 and *TP53* are examples of tumor suppressor genes. Mutation of *TP53* is one of the most common genetic alterations associated with cancer. The normal gene product of *TP53* is responsible for negative regulation of the cell cycle (ie, a series of cellular events that lead to the division and duplication of a cell), allowing the cell cycle to halt for repairs, corrections, and responses to other external signals. Inactivation of *TP53* following a genetic alteration removes this checkpoint, allowing genetic alterations to accumulate within a cell. Mutation of *TP53* is linked to a variety of cancers. For example, a germline mutation in which an individual has only one functional copy of *TP53* is associated with Li-Fraumeni syndrome, a syndrome characterized by multiple cancers by early adulthood. Another important function of *TP53* may be modulation of cytotoxic drug effects; loss of *TP53* is associated with anticancer drug resistance.

DNA Repair Genes

Another important type of gene that plays a role in cancer development is the DNA repair gene. Their normal function is to repair DNA damaged by environmental factors or errors in DNA that occur during replication.[2] If not corrected, these errors can result in alterations that activate oncogenes or inactivate tumor suppressor genes. Subsequently, more genetic alterations accumulate within a cell, and the risk for transformation increases for the altered cell population. Specifically, DNA repair genes can affect mismatch repair, single-strand break repair, and double-strand break repair. For example, poly ADP ribose polymerase (PARP) is a family of proteins responsible for DNA repair and programmed cell death by affecting multiple repair mechanisms.[6] PARP1 is a member of the PARP family that plays a role in repairing single-strand DNA breaks. Deficiencies in DNA repair genes have been discovered in breast, colon, and ovarian cancers.

Accumulation of Genetic Alterations

It has become evident that a single genetic alteration is probably insufficient to initiate cancer. Most cancers acquire multiple somatic genetic alterations; some alterations may make no contribution to the development of cancer (eg, passenger mutations), while other

TABLE 149-1 Selected Drugs and Hormones Known to Cause Cancer in Humans

Drug or Hormone	Type of Cancer
Alkylating agents (eg, chlorambucil, mechlorethamine, melphalan, procarbazine, and nitrosoureas)	Leukemia
Anabolic steroids	Liver
Anthracyclines (eg, doxorubicin)	Leukemia
Antiestrogens (tamoxifen)	Endometrium
Antithymocyte globulin	Lymphoma
BRAF inhibitors (dabrafenib, encorafenib, vemurafenib)	Primary malignancies
BTK inhibitors (acalabrutinib, ibrutinib, zanubrutinib)	Second primary malignancies
Cisplatin	Leukemia
Coal tars (topical)	Skin
Cobimetinib	Primary cutaneous malignancies
Elotuzumab	Second primary malignancies
Filgrastim	Leukemia
Isatuximab	Second primary malignancies
Lenalidomide	Second primary malignancies
PARP inhibitors (olaparib, niraparib, talazoparib)	MDS/AML
Pioglitazone	Bladder
Steroidal estrogens (estrogen replacement therapy, oral contraceptives)	Endometrium, breast, liver
Epipodophyllotoxins (etoposide)	Leukemia
Immunosuppressive drugs (cyclosporine, azathioprine)	Lymphoma, skin
Oxazaphosphorines (cyclophosphamide, ifosfamide)	Urinary bladder, leukemia
Tacrolimus	Lymphoma
Tazemetostat	Second malignancy
TNF-α inhibitors	Leukemia, skin
Voriconazole	Skin

FDA-approved package inserts. *Data from References 4, 58, and 59.*

alterations likely support the ongoing survival of cancer (eg, driver mutations). Scientists postulate that combinations of alterations are required for carcinogenesis and that the next generation of cells inherits each alteration. Thus, several detectable genetic alterations may be present in cancer. Although early alterations are found in premalignant lesions and established cancers, later alterations are found only in established cancer. This theory of sequential genetic alteration has been demonstrated in colon cancer. In colon cancer, the initial genetic alteration is believed to be loss of the *APC, or adenomatous polyposis coli* gene, which results in the formation of a small benign polyp (ie, abnormal tissue growth in a mucus membrane). An oncogenic mutation of ras genes is often the next step, leading to enlargement of the polyp. Loss of function of DNA mismatch repair enzymes may occur at many points during the transformation. Loss of *TP53* and another gene, believed to be the *deleted in colorectal cancer, or DCC,* gene, completes the transformation. Loss of *TP53* may be a late event in the development and progression of colon cancer and other cancers.

Four genes have been associated with DNA mismatch repair: *mutL homologue 1, mutS homologue 2, mutS homologue 6*, and *post-meiotic segregation increased 2.* When one or more of these proteins is mutated or missing, mistakes made during DNA replication may not be recognized or repaired. As a result, the tumor cell has a higher frequency of mutations known as mismatch repair deficient (dMMR). Tumors with a defective mismatch repair system may contain thousands of somatic mutations.[7] When a high number of these mutations accumulate within microsatellites (short repeating sequences of DNA), the tumor is characterized as microsatellite instability-high (MSI-H). As discussed later in the chapter, dMMR and MSI-H tumors are more susceptible to immune checkpoint inhibitors.

Epigenetic Alterations

Epigenetics refers to changes in gene expression that occur without altering the DNA sequence. The two most common mechanisms of epigenetic regulation include methylation and histone modification. DNA methylation commonly occurs at CpG dinucleotides (or islands) and is catalyzed by DNA methyltransferases (DNMTs). Histones are basic proteins associated with DNA in the nucleosome. These proteins may be modified by acetylation, methylation, or phosphorylation on their N-terminal tail. These modifications play a role in transcriptional regulation. For example, histone deacetylases (HDAC) repress transcription, and histone acetylases activate transcription. Epigenetic changes may be involved in the development of cancer by either priming the cell or making it susceptible to genetic alterations associated with the development of cancer. For example, hypermethylation at CpG dinucleotides found near tumor suppressor genes can switch these genes off and promote cancer development. Anticancer agents, identified as inhibitors of DNMT or HDAC, target these modifications. Figure 149-3 shows the effects of these inhibitors on methylation, chromatin formation, and transcription.

An oncometabolite is a metabolite whose abnormal accumulation may result in epigenetic dysregulation and carcinogenesis. Isocitrate dehydrogenase (IDH) 1 and 2 are enzymes involved in cellular metabolism through the conversion of isocitrate to alpha-ketoglutarate (αKG).[8] Mutations in *IDH1* and *IDH2* have been identified in gliomas and acute myeloid leukemia (AML) and result in the conversion of αKG to D-2-hydroxyglutarate. Elevated levels of D-2-hydroxyglutarate, an oncometabolite, inhibit αKG-dependent histone and DNA demethylases, which have been associated with impaired cellular differentiation. Anticancer agents have been developed to inhibit the mutant variants of IDH1 and 2 enzymes, thereby restoring myeloid differentiation.

PATHOLOGY OF CANCER

2 Cancer cells demonstrate several characteristics that differentiate them from normal cells. These traits include uncontrolled proliferation in which the cell cycle is no longer strictly regulated. Genetic alterations permit activation of multiple oncogenes and suppression of various tumor suppressor genes, releasing the cancer cells from the strict regulation observed with healthy cells. The cancer cells subsequently undergo multiple cell divisions, allowing the tumor size to increase exponentially. Cancer cells also resist programmed cell death by inhibiting apoptosis and senescence (aging). Lastly, cancer cells grow new blood vessels, invade new local tissue, and spread to distant sites.

Cell Cycle

The cell cycle incorporates a series of events by which normal and cancer cells divide and make new cells. This process is strictly regulated in healthy cells. Oncogenes and tumor suppressor genes provide the stimulatory and inhibitory signals that regulate the cell cycle. These signals converge on a molecular system in the nucleus known as the cell-cycle clock. The function of the

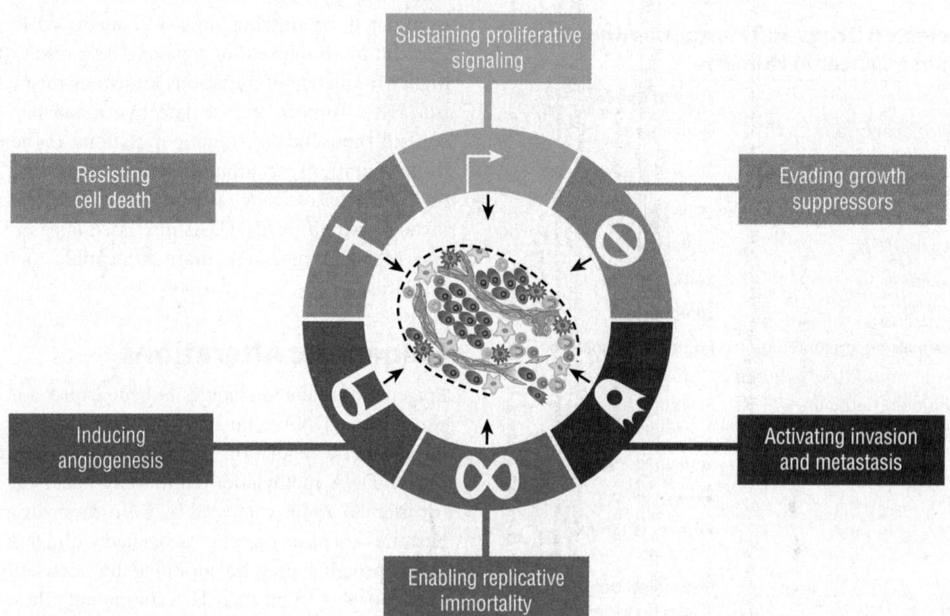

FIGURE 149-2 Functional capabilities acquired by cancer cells, including angiogenesis, self-proliferation, insensitivity to antigrowth signals and limitless growth potential, metastasis, and antiapoptotic effects. It is thought that most, if not all, cancer cells acquire these functions through a variety of mechanisms, including activation of oncogenes and mutations in tumor suppressor genes. *(Reprinted from Cuellar S, Haaf CM. Neoplastic Diseases. In: Tisdale J, Miller D, eds. Drug-Induced Diseases. 3rd ed. ASHP; 2018. Reprinted from Cell, Vol 144(5), Hanahan D, Weinberg RA, The Hallmarks of Cancer: The Next Generation, Copyright © 2011, with permission from Elsevier)*

TABLE 149-2 Examples of Oncogenes and Tumor Suppressor Genes

Gene	Associated Human Cancer
Oncogenes	
ALK	Lung cancer, lymphomas, neuroblastoma, and ovarian cancer
BCR-ABL	ALL, CML
BCL-2	B-cell lymphomas, myeloid leukemia
BRAF	Colon cancer, lung cancer, melanoma, ovarian cancer, thyroid cancer
ERBB1	Colon cancer, glioblastoma multiforme, lung cancer
ERBB2	Breast cancer, gastric cancer, lung cancer
FLT3	AML, colorectal cancer
KIT (CD117)	Acute leukemia, GIST
MET	Lung cancer, colon cancer, melanoma, endometrial cancer
MYC	AML, breast cancer, lung cancer, pancreatic cancer, retinoblastoma, B- and T-cell lymphomas
PI3KCA	Lung cancer, ovarian cancer, breast cancer, lymphoma
RAS (NRAS, HRAS, KRAS)	Colon cancer, melanoma, ovarian cancer, thyroid cancer
ROS1	Lung cancer, cholangiocarcinoma
RET	Lung cancer, thyroid cancer
Tumor Suppressor Genes	
APC	Colon cancer, thymus cancer
BRCA1, BRCA2	Breast cancer, ovarian cancer, prostate cancer
MSH2, MLH1, PMS1, PMS2, MSH6	Colon cancer
NF1, NF2	Leukemias, melanoma
TP53	Multiple cancers
PTEN	Lung cancer, ovarian cancer
RB1	Bladder cancer, retinoblastoma, sarcoma
VHL	Renal cell cancer

Data from My Cancer Genome. Available at http://www.mycancergenome.org/

clock in healthy cells is to integrate the signal input and determine if the cell cycle should proceed. The clock is composed of a series of interacting proteins, the most important of which are cyclins and cyclin-dependent kinases (CDKs). Cyclins and CDKs promote entry into the cell cycle and are overexpressed in several cancers. CDK inhibitors have been identified as important negative regulators of the cell cycle.

The cell cycle proceeds from one cell division to the next. The cycle involves five phases: DNA replication (S phase), cell division (M phase), two resting phases (G_1 and G_2), and a nondividing state (G_0 phase). In the first resting phase, G_1, the cell grows in size and decides to commit to the cell cycle or remain in a resting state. If the cell is normal, the cell will move into the S phase to synthesize its DNA. Next, the cell enters the second resting phase, G_2, in which the cell prepares to divide. In the M phase, the cell enters mitosis and yields two daughter cells. If the cell is not healthy, the cell can stop dividing and initiate apoptosis. Figure 149-4 depicts the cell cycle and the phases of activity for some chemotherapy agents.

Four checkpoints exist within the cell cycle, one in each phase of the cell cycle, and serve as quality control checkpoints. The cell will not proceed to the next phase unless all requirements for the current phase are met. Complexes of cyclin and CDK regulate these checkpoints. These complexes lead to the activation of other proteins that are responsible for the specific events of each phase of the cell cycle. The first checkpoint is called the restriction site. *Retinoblastoma* complexed to a transcription factor called E2F controls the restriction site. The presence of this complex prevents cell-cycle progression. A cell can proceed beyond the G_1 restriction site and continue into the S phase when cyclin–CDK complexes phosphorylate *Retinoblastoma* and target it for degradation. A cell may alternatively withdraw into the G_0 phase in the presence of antimitogenic or the absence of mitogenic factors.

Defense Systems

When the normal regulatory mechanisms for cell growth fail, backup defense systems may be activated. The secondary defenses

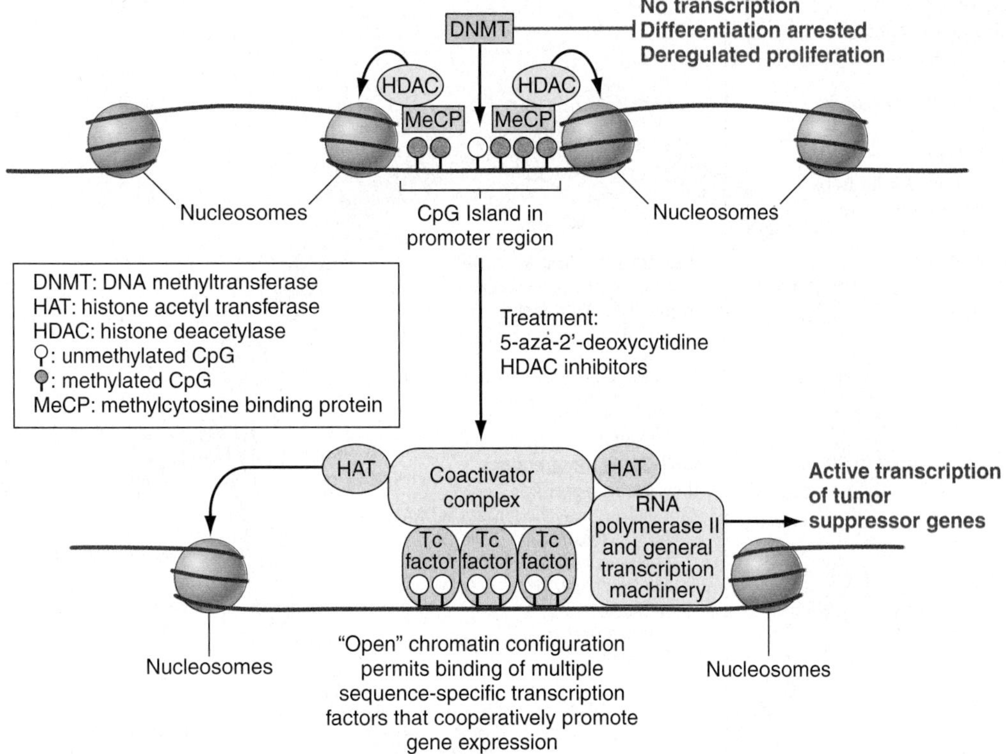

FIGURE 149-3 Epigenetic regulation of gene expression in cancer cells. CpG islands within the promoter and enhancer regions of the gene are methylated, resulting in the complexes with HDAC activity. Chromatin is in a condensed conformation that inhibits transcription (upper figure). Inhibitors of DNMT with inhibitors of HDAC confer a chromatin structure that allows transcription (lower figure). *(Reproduced, with permission, from Longo DL. Cancer cell biology and angiogenesis. In: Longo DL, Fauci AS, Kasper DL, et al., eds. Harrison's Principles of Internal Medicine. 18th ed. New York, NY: McGraw Hill; 2012.)*

include apoptosis (programmed cell death or suicide) and cellular senescence. Apoptosis is a normal mechanism of cell death required for tissue homeostasis. This process is regulated by oncogenes and tumor suppressor genes and is also a mechanism of cell death after exposure to cytotoxins. Overexpression of oncogenes responsible for apoptosis may produce an "immortal" cell, which has increased potential for malignancy. For example, *B-cell lymphoma 2* (*BCL-2*) is normally located on chromosome 18, but it may be translocated to chromosome 14 in proximity to the immunoglobulin heavy chain gene. This translocation leads to overexpression of *BCL-2* in lymphoid malignancies, which decreases apoptosis and confers a survival advantage. As another example, loss of *TP53* disrupts normal apoptotic pathways, imparting a survival advantage. Apoptosis may also play an important role as a mechanism of inherent resistance to some chemotherapy agents.

Cellular senescence is another important defense mechanism.[2] Laboratory studies demonstrate that after a cell population has undergone a preset number of doublings, growth stops and the cells die. This is known as senescence, a process that is regulated by telomeres. Telomeres are the DNA segments or caps at the ends of chromosomes. They are responsible for protecting the end of the DNA from damage. With each replication, the length of the telomeres is shortened. After the telomeres are shortened to a critical length, senescence is triggered. In this way, telomeres tally and limit the number of cell doublings. In cancer cells, the function of telomeres is overcome by overexpression of an enzyme known as telomerase. Telomerase replaces the portion of the telomeres lost with each cell division, thereby avoiding senescence and permitting an infinite number of cell doublings.

Immune Evasion

Immunosurveillance, a key feature of the host immune system, is recognizing and eliminating abnormal cells, including malignant cells. Antitumor immunity depends on T-cell identification of tumor antigens: a process regulated in part by various receptor-ligand interactions. Cytotoxic T-lymphocyte–associated antigen-4 (CTLA-4) and programmed death-1 (PD-1) are inhibitory receptors expressed on activated T-cells that serve as immune checkpoints. Checkpoints are critical in maintaining self-tolerance and preventing autoimmunity. When these T-cell receptors bind to their respective ligands on tumor cells, B7-1 and PD-ligand-1 (PD-L1), T-cell downregulation occurs and the tumor is able to evade immunosurveillance. These ligands are overexpressed on multiple types of tumors, and this process represents one of the multiple mechanisms that tumors evade immune elimination. Immune checkpoint inhibitors block the receptor-ligand interactions, reverse the immune downregulation, and allow for tumor cell elimination.

Cancer Growth

The study of cancer growth forms the foundation for many of the basic principles of modern chemotherapy. The growth of cancerous tumors is based on Gompertzian kinetics (see Fig. 149-5).[2] Gompertz was an insurance actuary who described the relationship between age and expected death. This mathematical model also approximates cancer cell proliferation. In the early stages, cancer growth is exponential, which means that cancer takes a constant amount of time to double its size. During this early phase, most cancer cells are actively dividing. This population of cells is called the growth

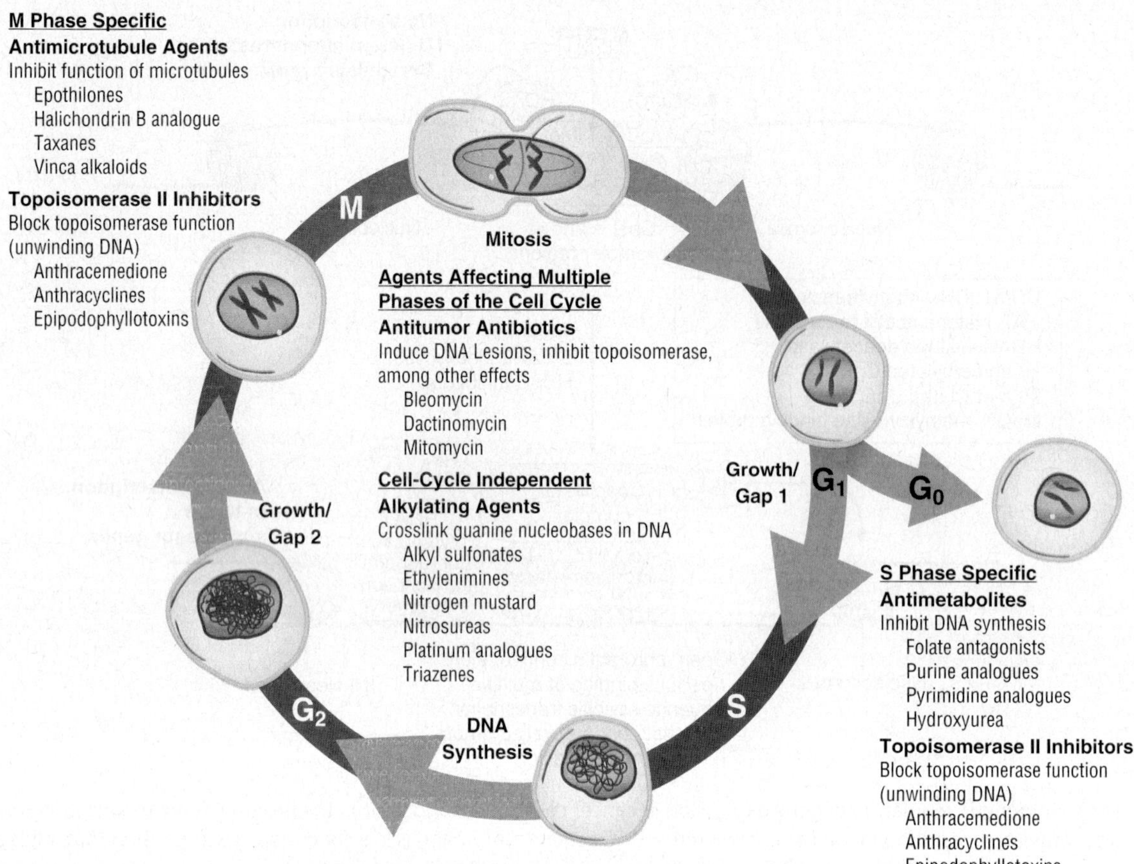

FIGURE 149-4 Cell-cycle activity for chemotherapy. Cell-cycle phase-specific chemotherapy is most active during a particular phase. Cell-cycle phase-nonspecific chemotherapy may have activity in more than one phase. In many cases, it is likely that chemotherapy cytotoxicity involves multiple intracellular sites of action and may not be linked to specific cell-cycle events.

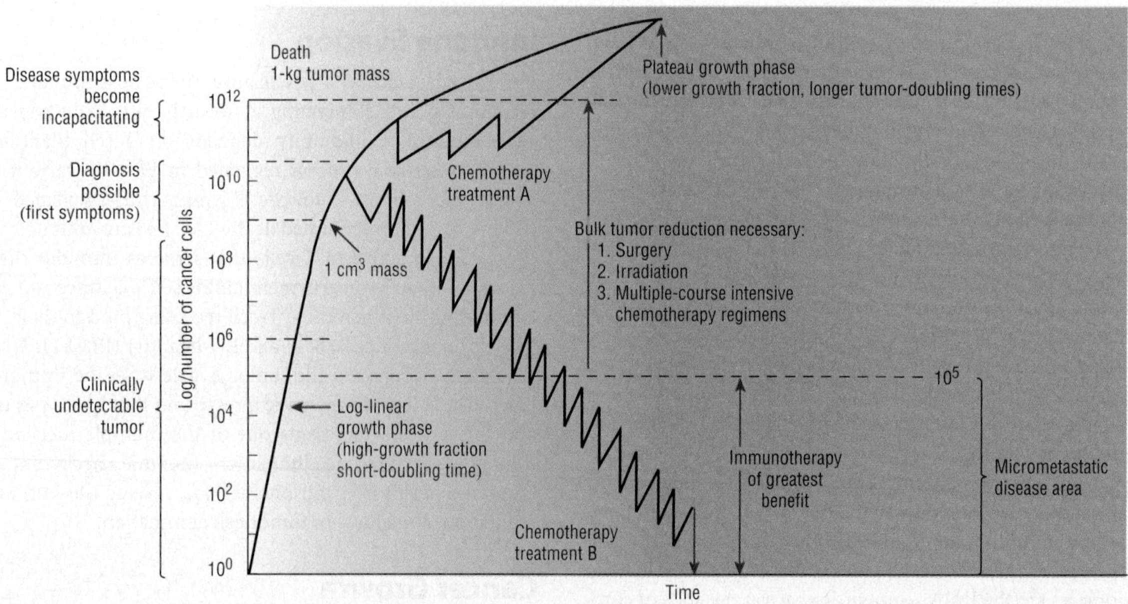

FIGURE 149-5 Gompertzian kinetics tumor-growth curve: relationship to symptoms, diagnosis, and various treatment regimens. *(Reproduced, with permission, from Buick RN. Cellular basis of chemotherapy. In: Dorr RT, Von Hoff DD, eds. Cancer Chemotherapy Handbook. 2nd ed. New York, NY: Appleton & Lange/McGraw Hill; 1994:3-14.)*

fraction. The doubling time, or time required for cancer to double in size, is very short. Because cytotoxic chemotherapy agents typically have a greater effect on rapidly dividing cells, cancers are most sensitive to their effects when the cancer is small, and the growth fraction is high. As cancer grows, the doubling time is slowed. The growth fraction decreases, probably owing to cancer outgrowing its blood and nutrient supply or the inability of blood and nutrients to diffuse throughout the mass. Wide variability exists in measured doubling times for different cancers. The doubling time of most solid tumors is about 2 to 3 months, but some cancers have doubling times of only days (eg, aggressive non-Hodgkin lymphoma [NHL]).[9]

Tumor burden impacts diagnosis and treatment (see Fig. 149-5). It takes about 10^9 cancer cells (1 g mass, 1 cm in diameter) for cancer to be clinically detectable by palpation or radiography. A cancer of this size has likely undergone about 30 doublings in cell number. It only takes 10 additional doublings for this 1 g mass to reach 1 kg in size. Cancer possessing 10^{12} cells (1 kg mass) is considered lethal. Thus, a cancer is clinically undetectable for most of its life span. Tumor burden also impacts treatment. The cell kill hypothesis states that a certain percentage of cells will be killed with each course of cytotoxic chemotherapy. For example, if cancer consists of 1,000 cells and the first treatment kills 90% of the cells, then 10% or 100 cells remain. The second treatment kills another 90% of cells, and again only 10% or 10 cells remain. According to this hypothesis, the tumor burden will never reach zero. Cancers consisting of less than 10^4 cells are believed to be small enough for elimination by host factors, including immunosurveillance. The limitations of this theory are that it assumes all cancers are equally responsive to treatment and that resistance to anticancer agents and the development of metastases do not occur.[2]

Invasion and Metastasis

As cancer grows, cancer cells break away or shed from the primary site to invade surrounding tissue and metastasize to distant sites. Metastatic disease is associated with a poorer prognosis and shortened survival compared to earlier disease. The cancer cells invade adjacent tissue or metastasize to distant sites by hematogenous or lymphatic spread, but not all shedded cells result in a metastatic lesion. The shed cells must first find an environment suitable for growth. The onset and time course for metastasis development depends largely on the individual cancer, as illustrated by the diverse patterns of metastasis observed for different cancers. Breast cancer, for example, tends to metastasize very early. Prostate cancer commonly metastasizes to bone, and colon cancer commonly metastasizes to the liver. Other less common modes of disease spread include dissemination via cerebrospinal fluid and transabdominal spread within the peritoneal cavity.

For a cancer cell to break away from the primary tumor site, the shed cell and surrounding host tissue must first secrete substances that stimulate angiogenesis. The shed cells must then detach from the primary tumor by expressing proteins that degrade the extracellular matrix, such as matrix metalloproteases, and invade surrounding blood and lymph vessels. The cells must then attach to the vascular endothelium. The cells may proliferate within the lumen of the vessel but most commonly extravasate into the surrounding tissue. The local microenvironment may provide growth factors that can serve as fertilizer to potentiate the development of a metastatic site. At every step, the potential metastatic cell must fight the host immune system. Finally, the metastasis must again initiate angiogenesis to ensure continued growth and proliferation.

Angiogenesis is the development of new blood vessels. This process becomes unregulated in several cancers and supports growth, invasion, and metastasis. Angiogenesis is regulated by pro- and antiangiogenic growth factors, which are released in response to hypoxia and other stresses to the cell. Proangiogenic growth factors include vascular endothelial growth factor (VEGF), fibroblast growth factor, platelet-derived growth factor (PDGF), and tumor necrosis factor-alpha (TNF-α). Antiangiogenic growth factors include interleukin-12, or IL-12, interferon, and tissue inhibitors of metalloproteinases. The best-studied proangiogenic factor is VEGF, whose elevated levels have been associated with a poor prognosis and an increased risk of metastases in many cancers, including breast cancer, non-small cell lung cancer (NSCLC), ovarian cancer, and colon cancer. Similar to other growth factors, VEGF binds to specific receptors located on the extracellular domain: VEGF-receptor (VEGFR)-1, -2, and -3. VEGFR-1 and VEGFR-2 are expressed primarily in endothelial cells and some cancer cells and mediate the biologic effects of VEGF. Each of the receptors induces a different signal transduction pathway. These pathways eventually result in the generation of proteases necessary for the breakdown of the extracellular matrix. Inhibiting the development of new blood vessels can limit or prevent tumor growth.

DIAGNOSIS OF CANCER

Tumors may be either benign or malignant. Benign tumors are noncancerous growths that are often encapsulated, localized, and indolent. Benign tumors are named for the cell or tissue of origin, followed by the suffix-oma. The tumor cells resemble the cells from which they developed. These masses seldom metastasize and rarely recur after being removed. In contrast to benign tumors, malignant tumors invade and destroy the surrounding tissue. The cancer cells are genetically unstable, and loss of normal cell architecture results in cells that are atypical of their tissue or cell of origin. These cells lose the ability to perform their usual functions. This loss of structure and function is called anaplasia. Cancers tend to metastasize, and consequently, recurrences are common after removal or destruction of the primary tumor. Cancers arising from epithelial cells are called carcinomas, and those arising from muscle or connective tissue are called sarcomas. Table 149-3 lists common nomenclature by tissue type.[10]

TABLE 149-3 Tumor Classification by Tissue Type

Tissue of Origin	Benign	Malignant
Epithelial Tissues		
Stratified squamous	Papilloma	Carcinoma (squamous, epidermoid)
Glandular tissue	Adenoma	Adenocarcinoma
Connective tissue		
Fibrous tissue	Fibroma	Fibrosarcoma
Bone	Osteoma	Osteosarcoma
Fat	Lipoma	Liposarcoma
Cartilage	Chondroma	Chondrosarcoma
Muscle		
Smooth muscle	Leiomyoma	Leiomyosarcoma
Striated muscle	Rhabdomyoma	Rhabdomyosarcoma
Blood and lymphoid cells		
	"Myeloproliferative disorders"	Leukemias
Lymphoid tissue	Plasmacytosis	Plasmacytoma; multiple myeloma; Hodgkin and NHL
Neural tissue		
Glial tissue	"Benign" gliomas	Glioblastoma multiforme; astrocytoma
Nerve sheath	Neurofibroma	Neurofibrosarcoma
Meninges	Meningioma	Malignant meningioma
Other cells		
Pigment-producing cells	Nevus	Melanoma

Adapted from National Cancer Institute: SEER Training Modules Tumor List [cited 2021 July 18]. Available at: https://training.seer.cancer.gov/disease/categories/tumors.html.

Screening

3 Because cancers are most curable before they metastasize, early detection and treatment have obvious potential benefits. Cancer screening programs are designed to detect cancers in individuals who have not yet developed symptoms. Still screening is only available for a few cancers, such as colon, prostate, breast, lung, and cervical cancers. Available screening tools include a cytology test, the Papanicolaou, or Pap, smear test for cervical cancer, and mammography for breast cancer. Limitations of the available screening tests include false-negative test results (related to the sensitivity of the test), false-positive test results (related to the specificity), and overdiagnosis (true positives not likely to become clinically significant). For example, most abnormal test results identified by screening mammography are false-positive, although the specificity of a mammogram exceeds 90%. For most cancers, a lack of effective screening method and inaccessible anatomic site limits the potential impact of a screening program. Public education on the early warning signs of common cancers is therefore extremely important for facilitating early detection. The American Cancer Society and other organizations publish guidelines for routine screening examinations (see Table 149-4).[11,12]

Clinical Presentation

4 The presenting signs and symptoms vary widely and depend on the type of cancer. The presentation in adults may include any of the seven warning signs listed in Table 149-5, as well as headaches, weight loss, chronic pain, fatigue, or anorexia.[13] The warning signs of cancer in pediatrics are different and reflect the cancers more common in this population (see Table 149-6). The definitive diagnosis of cancer relies on procuring a tissue sample and pathologic assessment of this sample. This sample can be obtained by numerous methods, including an excisional, core, or needle aspiration biopsy. A tissue diagnosis is essential because many benign tumors can masquerade as cancers and most tumors are not cancer. Depending on the tumor type, the diagnosis may include evaluating genetic alterations such as hormone receptor status in breast cancer or epidermal growth factor receptor (EGFR) status in NSCLC. Multiple companion or complementary tests are available and are indicated to detect

TABLE 149-5 Cancer's Seven Warning Signs

Change in bowel or bladder habits
A sore that does not heal
Unusual bleeding or discharge
Thickening or lump in the breast or elsewhere
Indigestion or difficulty in swallowing
Obvious change in wart or mole
Nagging cough or hoarseness
If YOU have a warning signal, see your doctor!

Data from Reference 13.

TABLE 149-4 American Cancer Society Screening Guidelines for Early Detection of Cancer in Average-Risk Asymptomatic Individuals

Cancer	Population	Age (years)	Test or Procedure	Frequency
Breast	Women	40-44	Mammography	Every year, optional
		45-54		Every year
		≥55		Every 1-2 years; depending on life expectancy
Cervical	Individuals with a cervix	25-65	Primary HPV test alone[a]	Every 5 years (preferred)
			Co-testing (cytology [Papanicolaou, or Pap, smear test] and HPV test) every 5 years	Every 5 years; acceptable if access to primary HPV testing is not available
			Cytology (Papanicolaou, or Pap, smear test) alone	Every 3 years; acceptable if access to primary HPV testing is not available
		>65	Options as above	Options as above should be continued until criteria for cessation are met[b]
Colorectal	All	45-75	Fecal immunochemical test	Annual
			High-sensitivity guaiac-based fecal occult blood test	Annual
			Multitarget stool DNA test	Every 3 years
			CT colonography	Every 5 years
			Flexible sigmoidoscopy	Every 5 years
			Colonoscopy	Every 10 years
		76-85	Options as above	Options as above; depending on patient history, preferences, and life expectancy
Lung	Current or former smokers, ≥30-pack-year history	55-74	Low-dose helical CT	Annual[c]
Prostate	Individuals with a prostate	≥50	Prostate-specific antigen test with or without digital rectal examination	Option if at least a 10-year life expectancy to make informed decision with their healthcare provider whether to be screened

[a]Use an FDA-approved HPV test for primary screening.

[b]Adequate negative prior screening is two consecutive negative primary HPV tests, or two negative cotests, or three negative cytology tests within the last 10 years, with the most recent occurring within the last 3-5 years.

[c]In adults who currently smoke or have quit within the last 15 years and have at least a 30-pack-year history and receive evidence-based smoking cessation counseling if they are current smokers and have undergone a process of informed/shared decision making that included information about the potential benefits, limitations, and harms of screening with low-dose CT and have access to a high-volume, high-quality lung cancer screening and treatment center.

Data from References 11 and 12.

TABLE 149-6 Cancer's Warning Signs in Children

Continued, unexplained weight loss
Headaches with vomiting in the morning
Increased swelling or persistent pain in bones or joints
Lump or mass in abdomen, neck, or elsewhere
Development of a whitish appearance in the pupil of the eye
Recurrent fevers not caused by infections
Excessive bruising or bleeding
Noticeable paleness or prolonged tiredness

a select mutation associated with a specific tumor type or identify hundreds of genetic mutations in any solid tumor.

Staging

Following a pathologic diagnosis, cancers should be staged to determine the extent of the disease (ie, tumor location and size) before starting treatment. Staging provides information on prognosis and guides treatment selection. A staging workup may involve physical examination, biopsy, imaging tests (ie, computed tomography [CT] scans, magnetic resonance imaging [MRI], and positron emission tomography [PET] scans), and laboratory tests. The laboratory tests may include tumor markers, antigens, or other substances produced by cancer. However, tumor markers are often nonspecific and may be elevated in many different cancers or patients with nonmalignant conditions. As a result, tumor markers are generally more useful for monitoring response and detecting recurrence than diagnostic tools. For example, human chorionic gonadotropin, or hCG, and alpha-fetoprotein, or AFP, in testicular cancer or prostate-specific antigen, or PSA, in prostate cancer are useful markers to monitor response or recurrence. After starting treatment, the staging workup is usually repeated at regular intervals to evaluate the effectiveness of the treatment.

The most common staging system for solid tumors is the TNM system that describes the tumor (T), nodes (N), and metastases (M). A numerical value is assigned to each letter to indicate the size or extent of disease. The T describes the size of the primary tumor and spread to adjacent tissues; the N specifies the size, location, and number of regional lymph nodes affected by cancer; and the M describes the presence or absence of metastases. Each letter is followed by an Arabic number that uniquely describes that tumor, node, or metastases. After the individual T, N, and M are determined, their values are combined to provide an overall stage identified using Roman numerals ranging from stage I to stage IV. For example, stage $T_3N_1M_0$, which describes a moderate-to-large primary mass with regional lymph node involvement and no distant metastases, is typically a stage III cancer. This simplified staging system allows healthcare professionals to identify the extent of disease easily. For example, stage I usually indicates localized cancer, stages II and III typically indicate local and regional disease, and stage IV typically indicates distant metastases. The criteria for classifying disease extent are quite specific for each different cancer. Alternative staging systems are used in clinical practice for leukemias and lymphomas, as discussed in subsequent chapters.

TREATMENT MODALITIES

Three main modalities are used to treat cancer: surgery, radiation, and systemic anticancer agents. These modalities may be used alone but are typically given sequentially or concurrently to treat a specific cancer. The timing of the different modalities relative to one another is based on the outcomes of a clinical trial.

Surgery is the oldest treatment modality, and it plays a major role in diagnosis and treatment. It may be curative if the primary cancer has not metastasized. Surgery remains the treatment of choice for most early stage cancers, such as breast and colon cancers. Surgery typically involves the removal of the primary tumor and adjacent lymph nodes. This modality may also be used to remove isolated metastases and relieve symptoms associated with metastatic disease. For example, hepatic metastases may be removed for patients with colon cancer.

Radiation therapy can be used alone for localized cancer or cancer that may encompass a single radiation field. It was first used to treat cancer in the late 1800s and remains a mainstay of treatment for some cancers. Radiation therapy may also be used to alleviate symptoms associated with vena cava syndrome, bone metastases, spinal cord compression, and brain tumors. This modality typically damages normal tissue surrounding the cancer, but the normal tissue typically repairs itself more readily than the cancer cells. Several different types of radiation therapy are available, including external beam radiation therapy, stereotactic radiation, brachytherapy, and radioisotopes. Both early and late toxicities associated with radiation therapy are dependent on the organs within the radiation field. For example, mucositis is commonly observed in patients receiving radiation for head-and-neck cancer. Secondary cancers are a devastating late toxicity that can occur following radiation therapy.

Systemic anticancer agents include chemotherapy, targeted therapy, and immunotherapy. Hormonal therapy is used for the treatment of cancer and is discussed in other chapters. Multiple radiopharmaceuticals are also now available. In general, systemic anticancer agents are developed to destroy cancer cells while minimizing effects on healthy cells. Specific agents will be discussed later in this chapter.

Combined Modality Treatment

As stated earlier in the chapter, a cancer may be treated with multiple modalities. For example, systemic anticancer agents are often administered to patients with local disease (ie, early stage) following surgery or radiation therapy. Because many patients with local disease have undetectable metastatic disease (ie, micrometastases) at diagnosis, localized anticancer treatment alone may fail to eliminate the cancer completely. *Adjuvant* therapy is systemic therapy administered to eradicate micrometastatic disease after surgery or radiation. The goal of adjuvant therapy is to reduce recurrence rates and prolong long-term survival. Thus, adjuvant therapy is given to patients with potentially curable cancers who have no clinically detectable disease after surgery or radiation. Because adjuvant therapy is given when the cancer is undetectable (ie, no measurable disease), its effectiveness is evaluated by recurrence rates and survival. *Neoadjuvant* (ie, preoperative or preradiation) therapy may be given to patients before surgery or radiation therapy to reduce tumor burden and destroy micrometastases. For example, neoadjuvant therapy has been given to patients with breast cancer to reduce the primary tumor size and allow for a less invasive surgical procedure.

The management of hematologic malignancies typically involves systemic anticancer therapies and radiation therapy since these cancers are systemic diseases that cannot be effectively treated with localized modalities. Systemic therapy that is administered to eradicate the cancer cells is called *induction* therapy. When a complete remission (the disappearance of all signs of cancer) is documented, postremission, or *consolidation*, therapy is administered. These therapies are designed to eradicate any remaining disease, similar to adjuvant therapy for solid tumors, and can include systemic therapy, a hematopoietic stem cell transplant (HSCT), or radiation therapy. *Maintenance* therapy is sometimes administered after consolidation therapy. The goal of this therapy is to prevent cancer from recurring or to maintain a response. Not all treatment phases are employed for all hematologic malignancies.

Goals of Care

The goals of care depend on the cancer stage and patient factors, such as comorbidities. When an anticancer agent is administered to patients with local or regional disease, the treatment (eg, adjuvant therapy) is often administered to cure the patient and may be labeled as *curative* therapy. When cancer has metastasized to distant sites, a cure is usually not possible, with rare exceptions, including testicular cancer. Anticancer therapy may be administered to patients with metastatic disease to slow cancer progression and prolong survival by months to years. If anticancer therapy is given to patients with the goal of reducing symptoms, the treatment is often called *palliative* therapy.

SYSTEMIC THERAPY

Chemotherapy

Chemotherapy was first administered in 1941 when Goodman and Gilman gave nitrogen mustard to patients with lymphoma. As discussed later in the chapter, a chemotherapy agent is typically given as part of a combination regimen, in which multiple anticancer agents with different mechanisms of action and toxicities are given together. Most chemotherapy agents target rapidly proliferating cells (both normal and cancer cells), and these agents might act at one or more phases of the cell cycle. A chemotherapy agent that demonstrates major activity in a particular phase of the cell cycle is known as a cell-cycle phase-specific agent. For example, antimetabolites exert their effect during the S phase. Cell-cycle phase-specific agents may be less active in other phases of the cell cycle. A cell-cycle phase-nonspecific agent has significant activity in multiple phases. Alkylating agents, such as nitrogen mustards, are examples of cell-cycle phase-nonspecific agents. Despite this classification, it is believed that most chemotherapy agents provide cytotoxic effects following interactions with other intracellular activities, not just specific cell-cycle events. Knowledge of cell-cycle specificity has been used to optimize treatment schedules. For example, a cell-cycle phase-specific chemotherapy agent is typically administered as a continuous infusion or in multiple repeated fractions to maximize the number of cancer cells in the sensitive cell-cycle phase. Thus, a cell-cycle phase-specific chemotherapy agent is also termed "schedule dependent." In contrast, cell-cycle phase-nonspecific chemotherapy is active in many phases, and consequently, these agents are not schedule dependent. The activity of these chemotherapy agents depends on the dose, so these chemotherapies are termed "dose-dependent." Chemotherapy agents are typically given in a defined repeating schedule called a cycle. The cycle length typically depends on the toxicities associated with the chemotherapy agent, such that sufficient time elapses between doses to allow a patient to adequately recover from a serious adverse drug reaction (eg, neutropenia). The number of cycles depends, in part, on the treatment goals. The number of cycles is typically defined by prior clinical trials for early stage disease. In contrast, the number of cycles is generally determined by individualized treatment response and tolerability for locally advanced or metastatic disease.

Targeted Agents

Targeted anticancer agents, including small-molecule inhibitors and mAbs, stop cancer progression by blocking aberrant intracellular signaling pathways that govern cell responses, movement, and division. Some of these agents can cause cancer cell death by inducing apoptosis or stimulating the immune system to destroy the cancer cells.

The first small-molecular targeted agent was developed in the late 1980s. Small-molecule targeted agents have a low molecular weight (less than 1,000 Da) and have been specifically designed to interfere with intracellular signaling pathways. These agents are typically given orally once or twice daily until disease progression or unacceptable toxicity occurs. Since resistance commonly develops with small-molecule targeted agents, they may be administered concurrently with other anticancer agents.

Similar to small-molecule targeted agents, most mAbs are administered with other anticancer treatments. Both mAbs and targeted agents have been developed to interfere with intracellular signaling. Although small-molecule targeted agents typically inhibit intracellular kinases, mAbs target the extracellular receptors or their natural ligands and prevent ligand binding to the receptor. The net effect of both strategies is to interfere with intracellular signal transduction and decrease cell proliferation (see Fig. 149-6). Some common receptors and pathways affected by available small-molecule targeted agents and mAbs include ErbB2 family, mitogen-activated protein kinase (MAPK) pathway, and phosphatidylinositide 3-kinase (PI3K) pathway.

The ErbB family of receptors contains four known members: ErbB1 (also known as EGFR), ErbB2 (human EGFR 2 [HER2]), ErbB3, and ErbB4. EGFR and HER2 are overexpressed in several cancers, including breast, lung, gastric, and colon cancers. The roles of the other receptors in cancer growth and proliferation are still under investigation. Members of this family are inactive by themselves and must form a dimer (a molecule composed of two subunits) either with a member of the same family (homodimer) or with a member of a different ErbB family (heterodimer). Dimerization of the receptor leads to kinase phosphorylation and subsequent activation of downstream pathways required to activate signal transduction and cell growth.

Well-described intracellular signaling pathways include PI3K, Janus kinase–signal transducers (JAK) and activators of transcription (STAT), and MAPK. When these pathways are activated, they promote cell proliferation and survival. These pathways consist of a chain of proteins that ultimately communicate a signal from a cell surface receptor to the DNA found in the nucleus. A protein within a signaling pathway communicates by adding a phosphate group to its neighboring protein; the phosphate groups act as an "on" or "off" switch for the pathway. In cancer, a mutated protein permits the pathway to remain in the "on" or "off" position. The downstream effectors of these pathways also initiate cell-cycle progression by promoting the expression of cyclins and repressing the expression of CDK inhibitors.

The MAPK signaling pathway regulates many fundamental cellular processes, including cell differentiation, proliferation, and senescence. These pathways relay the intracellular signals through a series of ras, raf, MEK (MAPK-extracellular signal-regulated kinase), and extracellular signal-regulated kinase (ERK) proteins that subsequently phosphorylate and regulate nuclear and cytoplasmic structures. Some of these proteins are commonly altered in pancreatic, melanoma, colorectal, hepatocellular, and other solid tumors.

The PI3K signaling pathway also regulates cell proliferation, growth, survival, and mobility. PI3K becomes activated in response to growth hormones. It ultimately activates protein kinase B (known as AKT), a serine-threonine kinase that serves as a master switch for the cell-cycle progression. Fully activated protein kinase B translocates to the nucleus, inhibiting proapoptotic signals and activating antiapoptotic substrates. It can also phosphorylate mammalian target of rapamycin (mTOR). After

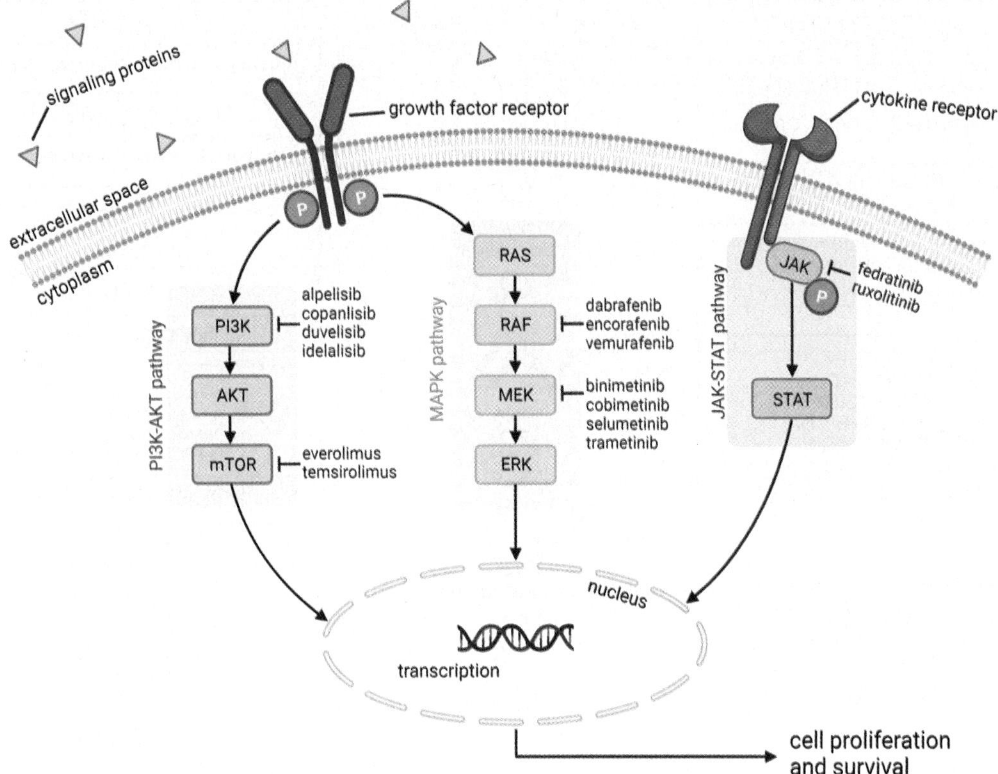

FIGURE 149-6 Common intracellular signaling pathways and targeted therapies that inhibit these pathways. Activation of the PI3K-AKT pathway, the MAPK pathway, or the JAK/STAT pathway leads to downstream signaling and ultimately cell proliferation and survival. (*Image created with BioRender.*)

being activated, mTOR stimulates protein synthesis by phosphorylating translation regulators. mTOR also contributes to protein degradation and angiogenesis. Phosphatase and tensin homolog, or *PTEN* is a tumor suppressor gene that blocks intracellular signaling through this pathway and is frequently inactivated in several solid tumors.

The JAK-STAT signaling pathway helps regulate the immune system. This pathway contains three main components: extracellular receptors, JAKs, and STAT. The pathway is initiated when cytokines or growth factors bind to the receptor, activate JAK, and subsequently recruit STAT. The STAT proteins then translocate to the nucleus and modify gene expression. Altered JAK signaling has been associated with JAK mutations in patients with myelofibrosis.

Immunotherapy

Immunotherapy works by boosting the natural defenses of the host immune system to eradicate tumor cells. These agents work in two main ways: training the individual's immune system to attack cancer directly or by administering immune components that result in a more general stimulation of the immune system. Agents classified as immunotherapies include cytokines, CAR T-cell therapies, immune checkpoint inhibitors, and therapeutic vaccines.

Combination Therapy

Although a single anticancer agent may be administered to a patient, the more common approach to systemic therapy is to administer multiple agents known as a regimen. Initially, this approach was based on the Goldie-Coldman hypothesis, which addresses cancer cell heterogeneity and the inevitable development of drug resistance. The individual agents selected for combination therapy should have different mechanisms of action and adverse drug reaction profiles. For example, myelosuppressive agents may be combined with non-myelosuppressive agents to minimize myelosuppression. The individual agents should each have significant activity against the cancer, and the combination therapy should have known clinical benefit in the cancer to be treated. Combination regimens that include multiple chemotherapy agents with or without a targeted agent or immunotherapy have been used to successfully manage many cancers for decades. Predictive biomarkers, such as HER2 and BRAF, may be used to identify which patients may benefit from targeted therapy.

CHEMOTHERAPY

5 Since all chemotherapy agents interfere with the cellular synthesis of DNA, ribonucleic acid (RNA), or proteins, chemotherapy agents are commonly categorized by their mechanism of action. For example, alkylators exert their effects on DNA and protein synthesis by binding to DNA and preventing the unwinding of the DNA molecule. As another example, antimetabolites resemble nucleotide bases or inhibit enzymes involved in synthesizing DNA and proteins. Figure 149-7 shows the sites of action of common categories of anticancer agents.

The following sections discuss the biochemical classification system and the individual agents within each classification. The clinical uses, mechanisms of action, common adverse drug reactions, and practical patient management for most available chemotherapy

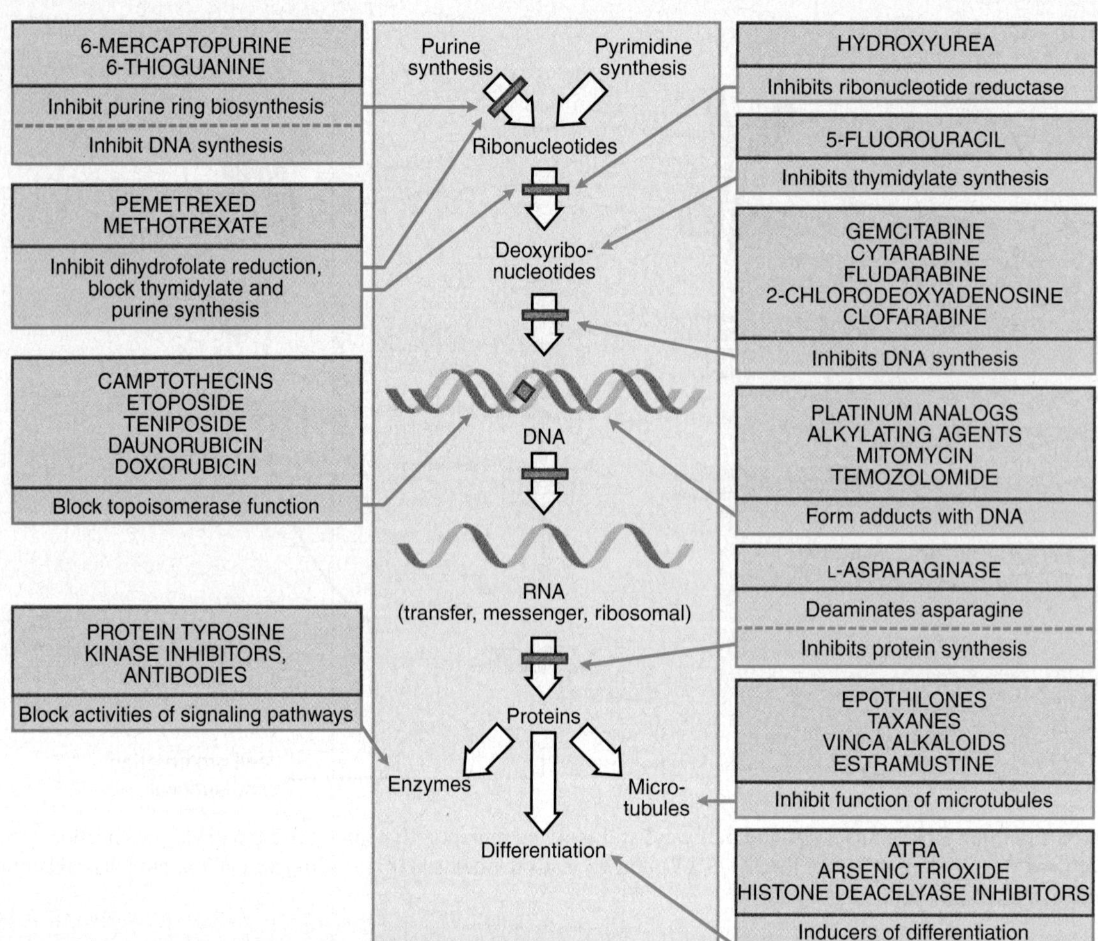

FIGURE 149-7 Mechanisms of action of commonly used anticancer agents (all-trans-retinoic acid). *(Reproduced, with permission, from Chabner BA. General principles of chemotherapy. In: Brunton LL, Chabner BA, Knollman BC, eds. Goodman & Gilman's The Pharmacologic Basis of Therapeutics. 12th ed. New York, NY: McGraw Hill; 2010.)*

agents are also discussed. Table 149-7 summarizes monitoring parameters of individual anticancer agents.

Antimetabolites

Antimetabolites are similar to the nucleotides that make up DNA and RNA. The body mistakes these chemotherapy agents for the naturally occurring nucleotide bases and metabolizes these agents as the natural nucleotides. These chemotherapy agents ultimately disrupt replication and cell division by interfering with the production of nucleic acids, DNA, and RNA. Unfortunately, these compounds are not selective for cancer cells, and rapidly dividing normal cells may be affected. The most common toxicities associated with the antimetabolites are secondary to their effect on rapidly dividing normal cells, such as bone marrow and gastrointestinal tract cells. The three major classes of antimetabolites include pyrimidine analogues, purine analogues, and folate antagonists. Hypomethylating agents are also considered antimetabolites.

Pyrimidine Analogues

Cytarabine Cytarabine is a cytidine analogue commonly used to treat AML, acute lymphoblastic leukemia (ALL), and NHL. It is phosphorylated to its active phosphates within cancer cells and inhibits DNA polymerase, an enzyme responsible for strand elongation. It is also incorporated directly into DNA, where it inhibits DNA replication and acts as a chain terminator to prevent DNA elongation. Deaminase enzymes, particularly cytidine deaminase, degrade cytarabine and other cytidine analogues.

Cytarabine may be given intravenously or intrathecally. Intrathecal administration allows for cytotoxic concentrations of cytarabine to be maintained in the central nervous system (CNS) for several hours. It may be given to patients with leukemia.

The dose-limiting toxicities are leukopenia and thrombocytopenia. Other common toxicities include nausea, vomiting, mucositis, and diarrhea. Following administration of high-dose cytarabine (greater than 1 g/m^2 per dose), cerebellar syndrome may occur presenting with dysarthria, nystagmus, and ataxia. The risk of cerebellar syndrome is strongly correlated with advanced age and renal dysfunction. Renal dysfunction permits accumulation of high levels of triphosphate, which is believed to be neurotoxic. Hepatic dysfunction, high cumulative doses, and bolus dosing may also increase the risk of neurotoxicity. Conjunctivitis or keratitis is another common toxicity associated with high-dose cytarabine. Prophylactic corticosteroid or saline eye drops should be administered with high-dose cytarabine to minimize irritation. Allopurinol may be given with high-dose cytarabine to minimize the risk of tumor lysis syndrome (TLS), a group of metabolic complications that can occur following the breakdown of dying cancer cells.

Fluoropyrimidines Fluorouracil (sometimes referred to as 5-FU) is a fluorinated uracil analogue initially synthesized in the late 1950s. It acts as a false pyrimidine and undergoes sequential phosphorylation to a mono-, di-, and triphosphate similar to natural nucleotide bases. In the presence of folates, the monophosphate binds tightly to and interferes with the function of thymidylate synthase. The

TABLE 149-7 Monitoring of Anticancer Drugs[a]

Agent	Notable Adverse Drug Reactions	Monitoring Parameters	Comments
Chemotherapeutic Agents			
Antimetabolites			
Capecitabine	Diarrhea, PPE, mild nausea and vomiting, mucositis	Stool count, hands and feet for early signs of skin breakdown, CBC, liver function, renal function	Adjust dose for renal impairment Oral prodrug of fluorouracil Warfarin results in increased anticoagulant effects May require phenytoin dose reduction Deficiency of DPD correlates with increased toxicity
Cladribine	Myelosuppression, fever, immunosuppression, severe opportunistic infections occur	CBC, signs of infection	Risk of opportunistic infections necessitate prophylactic antibiotics for PJP and other infections
Cytarabine	*General toxicities:* myelosuppression, nausea and vomiting, diarrhea, mucositis, TLS, flu-like syndrome, rash *High-dose toxicities:* worsening of above, cerebellar toxicity, conjunctivitis	CBC, uric acid, signs of infection, renal function, neurologic examinations (signs of confusion)	High-dose infusions should be administered over 2-3 hours to decrease risk of CNS toxicity Use corticosteroid eye drops during treatment and for 48 hours after treatment to prevent conjunctivitis with high-dose cytarabine Increased risk of neurotoxicity with high-dose cytarabine in setting of renal impairment Use preservative-free preparations for IT preparations: occasionally combined with hydrocortisone & methotrexate
Fludarabine	Myelosuppression, immunosuppression, diarrhea, rare CNS toxicity (somnolence, seizures, altered mental status), hearing and visual changes, pulmonary toxicity, TLS	CBC, uric acid, signs of infection, renal function, neurologic examinations	Adjust dose for renal impairment Risk of opportunistic infections necessitates prophylactic antibiotics for PJP and HSV
Fluorouracil	Mucositis, diarrhea, PPE, myelosuppression, hyperpigmentation, photosensitivity, ocular toxicity, myocardial ischemic symptoms	CBC, stool count, hands and feet for early signs of skin breakdown	Deficiency of DPD correlates with increased toxicity Drug interaction with warfarin: increased anticoagulant effect
Gemcitabine	Myelosuppression, flu-like syndrome, rash, elevations in liver transaminases	CBC, liver function	Fixed dose rate (10 mg/m^2/minute) may be used in lymphoma and sarcoma settings, associated with increased myelosuppression
Mercaptopurine	Myelosuppression, dry skin, rash, hepatotoxicity, hyperbilirubinemia	CBC, liver function	Allopurinol increases the toxicity of mercaptopurine by interfering with metabolism Mercaptopurine reduces anticoagulant effects of warfarin Consider pharmacogenomic testing for TPMT and NUDT15
Methotrexate	Myelosuppression, mucositis, renal failure at high doses, nausea and vomiting, CNS toxicity (more severe with IT administration), hepatotoxicity	CBC, liver function, renal function, urine pH, methotrexate drug levels with high-dose therapy	Adjust dose or avoid use with renal impairment, avoid drugs that decrease renal excretion of methotrexate (eg, NSAIDs, PPIs, sulfas, penicillins) Distributes readily into third-space fluids (ascites, pleural effusions), prolonging exposure and increasing toxicity; may be contraindication for use Monitor methotrexate levels with high-dose administration; these must include leucovorin rescue to prevent excessive myelosuppression; sodium bicarbonate given for high-dose therapy to prevent nephrotoxicity (maintain urine pH >7) Use preservative-free preparations for IT and high-dose administration; occasionally combined with hydrocortisone & cytarabine IT
Pemetrexed	Myelosuppression, stomatitis, pharyngitis, rash, desquamation, fatigue	CBC, renal function, skin examinations	Avoid with renal impairment Avoid NSAIDs during administration Supplement with folic acid (400-1,000 mcg PO daily starting 1 week before first dose, continued 21 days after last dose) and vitamin B_{12} (1,000 mcg IM 7 days prior to first dose and every 3 cycles thereafter) to decrease myelosuppression Premedicate with dexamethasone (day before, the day of, and day after) to decrease incidence of rash
Pentostatin	Myelosuppression, rash, renal toxicity, hepatic toxicity, pulmonary toxicity, CNS toxicity	CBC, renal function, hepatic function, lung function, sign of neurotoxicity	Hydration pre/post pentostatin administration Risk of opportunistic infections necessitate prophylactic antibiotics for PJP and HSV
Trifluridine and tipiracil	Myelosuppression, asthenia/fatigue, decreased appetite, diarrhea, nausea and vomiting, abdominal pain, pyrexia	CBC, renal function	Adjust dose for moderate renal impairment

(Continued)

TABLE 149-7 Monitoring of Anticancer Drugs[a] (*Continued*)

Agent	Notable Adverse Drug Reactions	Monitoring Parameters	Comments
Microtubule-Targeting Drugs			
Cabazitaxel	Myelosuppression, hypersensitivity reactions, diarrhea, asthenia, nausea and vomiting, peripheral neuropathy, alopecia	CBC, signs of infection, stool count, signs of hypersensitivity reactions, liver function	Avoid with hepatic impairment Premedicate with H_1 and H_2 antagonist plus dexamethasone to decrease risk of hypersensitivity
Docetaxel	Myelosuppression, fluid retention (edema, pleural effusions, ascites), alopecia, rash, peripheral neuropathy, hypersensitivity reactions, nail toxicity	CBC, liver function, signs/symptoms of fluid retention	Contraindicated with hepatic impairment (hyperbilirubinemia, elevated transaminases, or elevated alkaline phosphatase) Premedicate with dexamethasone to lower risk of fluid retention
Eribulin	Myelosuppression, peripheral neuropathy, asthenia, alopecia, nausea, constipation	CBC, liver function, renal function, potassium and magnesium levels	Dose reduce for Child-Pugh class A or B hepatic impairment and moderate renal impairment May cause QTc prolongation in patients with electrolyte or congenital abnormalities (avoid other drugs that may prolong QTc interval)
Ixabepilone	Myelosuppression, peripheral neuropathy, hypersensitivity reactions, asthenia, arthralgias, alopecia	CBC, signs of hypersensitivity reactions, liver function	Avoid or adjust dose with hepatic impairment CYP3A4 substrate, levels may be effected by inducers or inhibitors, avoid use or dose adjustment to ixabepilone may be necessary Premedicate with H_1 and H_2 antagonist
Paclitaxel and nab-paclitaxel	Myelosuppression, hypersensitivity reactions, peripheral neuropathy, myalgias or arthralgias, mucositis, cardiac arrhythmias, alopecia	CBC, signs of hypersensitivity reactions, liver function	Avoid or adjust dose with hepatic impairment Premedicate with dexamethasone, H1 and H2 antagonist before paclitaxel; nab-paclitaxel is associated with minimal risk of hypersensitivity reactions and does not require premedication Neurotoxicity may require discontinuation or dose reduction Products are not interchangeable
Vinblastine and vinorelbine	Myelosuppression, mucositis, neurotoxicity (less common than with vincristine), myalgias, SIADH (rarely), vesicant	CBC, liver function	Adjust dose with elevated bilirubin Treat extravasation injury with warm soaks and injection of hyaluronidase
Vincristine	Peripheral neuropathy (highest of vinca alkaloids); motor, sensory, autonomic, and cranial nerves may be affected (paresthesias, ileus, urinary retention, facial palsies) and can be irreversible; SIADH; vesicant	Signs of neurotoxicity (tingling in extremities, constipation, CNS toxicity), liver function	Adjust dose with elevated bilirubin Treat constipation aggressively to prevent ileus Doses are commonly capped at 2 mg to minimize neurotoxicity LETHAL if administered IT Treat extravasation similar to vinblastine
Topoisomerase Inhibitors			
Irinotecan and liposomal irinotecan	Diarrhea: acute (during or immediately after infusion, related to cholinergic effects) and delayed (>24 hours after administration) Nausea and vomiting, myelosuppression, alopecia, fatigue, increased liver enzymes, pulmonary toxicity	CBC, liver function, stool count, fluid status, electrolytes	Acute diarrhea is treated or prevented with atropine, delayed diarrhea is managed with antimotility agents Consider dose adjustment with elevated total bilirubin or UGT1A1 deficiency Products are not interchangeable and have different indications
Topotecan	Myelosuppression, alopecia, diarrhea	CBC, renal function	Adjust dose for renal impairment
Daunorubicin	Myelosuppression, mucositis, nausea and vomiting, alopecia, vesicant Cardiac toxicities: acute (not related to cumulative dose, arrhythmias, pericarditis); chronic (cumulative injury to myocardium with total dose >250 mg/m^2)	CBC, LVEF, liver function	Adjust dose for elevated bilirubin LVEF should be >50% to administer safely Extravasation managed with dexrazoxane
Doxorubicin and liposomal doxorubicin	Similar to daunorubicin, cardiac toxicity associated with cumulative doses >250 mg/m^2, radiation recall reactions	CBC, LVEF, liver function	Adjust dose for elevated bilirubin LVEF should be >50% to administer safely May discolor urine (red-orange) Liposomal form: decreased risk of cardiac and vesicant toxicities
Epirubicin	Similar to daunorubicin, cardiac toxicity associated with cumulative doses >450 mg/m^2	CBC, LVEF, liver function	Adjust dose for elevated bilirubin LVEF should be >50% to administer safely
Etoposide	Myelosuppression, nausea and vomiting (may be worse with oral and high-dose regimens), alopecia, mucositis, hypotension (infusion rate–related), hypersensitivity reactions	CBC, blood pressure	Adjust dose for renal impairment Requires large volumes of fluid for IV administration because of limited solubility (maximum concentration 0.4 mg/mL) Available orally in liquid-filled gelatin capsules; ~50% bioavailability but absorption is variable and greater at lower oral doses

TABLE 149-7 Monitoring of Anticancer Drugs[a]

Agent	Notable Adverse Drug Reactions	Monitoring Parameters	Comments
Idarubicin	Similar to daunorubicin, total cumulative dose not well established; >150 mg/m² reported to be associated with decreased LVEF	CBC, LVEF, liver function	Adjust dose for elevated bilirubin LVEF should be >50% to administer safely
Mitoxantrone	Myelosuppression, nausea and vomiting, mucositis, alopecia, less cardiotoxic than the anthracyclines	CBC, LVEF, liver function	Not a vesicant (may cause vein irritation but not associated with severe tissue injury such as anthracyclines) May discolor urine blue-green
Alkylating Agents			
Bendamustine	Myelosuppression, infection, dermatologic reactions including Stevens-Johnson syndrome, TLS, infusion reactions	CBC, signs of infection, signs of dermatologic toxicity, uric acid	Allopurinol may increase risk for Stevens-Johnson syndrome
Busulfan	General toxicities: myelosuppression, skin hyperpigmentation, pulmonary fibrosis, gynecomastia, adrenal insufficiency High (HSCT) dose toxicities: seizures, hepatic veno-occlusive disease, severe nausea and vomiting	CBC, pulmonary status, liver function, signs of edema (weight gain, fluid status)	Bone marrow recovery may be delayed (3-6 weeks), pulmonary fibrosis associated with >3-year exposure and/or prior chest radiation Seizure prophylaxis with HSCT doses Pharmacokinetic monitoring is required with IV busulfan IV and oral preparations are not interchangeable Put tablets in gelatin capsules for easier administration with high doses
Carboplatin	Myelosuppression (thrombocytopenia), nausea and vomiting (acute and delayed), risk of hypersensitivity reactions at higher cumulative doses (frequently results in cross-hypersensitivity to cisplatin)	CBC, renal function	Calvert formula used to dose carboplatin Lower incidence of nephrotoxicity, neurotoxicity, nausea and vomiting than cisplatin
Chlorambucil	Myelosuppression, increased liver enzymes, skin rash, menstrual irregularities, pulmonary toxicity, risk of secondary malignancies, infertility and sterility, teratogenic	CBC, liver function, pulmonary function	Administer on an empty stomach, food decreases absorption May be dosed in low daily-dosing regimens, higher dose (ie, pulse), or intermittent dosing schedules administered biweekly or monthly; pulse dosing may require patients to take several tablets (eg, 10-20 tablets) per dose
Cisplatin	Nephrotoxicity, potassium and magnesium wasting, severe nausea and vomiting (acute or delayed onset), peripheral neuropathy that is cumulative and dose related, ototoxicity, anemia seen with chronic dosing	Renal function, potassium and magnesium levels, GI symptoms (nausea and vomiting)	Avoid with renal impairment IV hydration required before and after administration; ensure good urine output; potassium and magnesium sulfate in IV fluid to replace losses; consider carboplatin with impaired renal function Aggressive antiemetics required pretreatment and after treatment to prevent delayed nausea and vomiting Doses should not exceed 100 mg/m² (maximum single dose and per-cycle dose)
Cyclophosphamide	Hemorrhagic cystitis, nausea and vomiting (acute and delayed), myelosuppression, alopecia, SIADH (typically with high doses of >2 g/m²), risk of secondary malignancies, infertility and sterility	CBC, renal function, urinalysis	Adjust dose for renal impairment Hydration needed to prevent hemorrhagic cystitis (PO or IV); mesna may be required with high-dose regimens (see ifosfamide) Instruct patients to take oral tablets in the morning to allow for elimination of toxic metabolite Absorbed through skin: avoid spills Drug interactions: CYP450 inducers (eg, barbiturates) may increase formation of toxic metabolites; CYP450 inhibitors may increase myelosuppression
Ifosfamide	Hemorrhagic cystitis, nephrotoxicity, myelosuppression, CNS effects (somnolence, confusion, disorientation, cerebellar symptoms that are dose related), nausea and vomiting (acute and delayed), alopecia	CBC, urinalysis, renal function	Adjust dose for renal impairment 3-4 L/day fluid for hydration; potassium, magnesium, and phosphate may be required to replace losses Mesna is always given (typically 60%-100% of ifosfamide dose); may be delivered in same IV bag CNS toxicity, nausea, and vomiting may be more severe with rapid infusion Methylene blue is controversial for CNS toxicity
Lurbinectedin	Myelosuppression, nausea and vomiting, hepatotoxicity	CBC, liver function, magnesium	Avoid coadministration with strong or moderate CYP3A inducers or inhibitors
Mechlorethamine	Myelosuppression, severe nausea and vomiting, vesicant, secondary malignancies, sterility and infertility	CBC, GI symptoms (nausea and vomiting)	Antidote for extravasation is sodium thiosulfate

(Continued)

TABLE 149-7 Monitoring of Anticancer Drugs[a] (*Continued*)

Agent	Notable Adverse Drug Reactions	Monitoring Parameters	Comments
Melphalan	Myelosuppression, nausea and vomiting, diarrhea, mucositis, secondary malignancies, hypersensitivity reactions	CBC, renal function, electrolytes, liver function	Complete administration of IV dose should occur within 60 min of reconstitution for Alkeran formulation Melphalan is NOT interchangeable with melphalan flufenamide
Melphalan flufenamide	Myelosuppression, nausea and vomiting, secondary malignancies	CBC, uric acid, ECG	Prophylactic antiviral for HSV and PJP Melphalan flufenamide is NOT interchangeable with melphalan
Nitrosoureas (carmustine and lomustine)	Myelosuppression, severe nausea and vomiting, cumulative nephrotoxicity, pulmonary fibrosis, facial flushing during infusion	CBC, renal function, pulmonary function	Bone marrow recovery may require 6-8 weeks Carmustine is a vein irritant Facial flushing may be related to alcohol vehicle Also available in wafer form for implantation into brain tumor cavities after resection Lomustine is administered orally
Oxaliplatin	Pharyngolaryngeal dysesthesias, nausea and vomiting, anaphylaxis risk Peripheral neuropathy >50% patients: acute form (<14 days, rapid onset, reversible, exacerbated by cold); chronic form (onset >14 days and may be permanent)	CBC, renal function, acute and chronic neuropathies	Adjust dose for renal impairment Avoid exposure to cold
Procarbazine	Myelosuppression, diarrhea, neurotoxicity, neuropathy, flu-like syndrome, infertility and sterility, secondary malignancies	CBC	Administer as a single daily dose on an empty stomach Drug interactions: MAOIs that interact with tyramine-rich foods and may precipitate hypertensive crisis; TCAs and SSRIs; sympathomimetics; disulfiram-like reaction with alcohol
Thiotepa	Myelosuppression, nausea and vomiting, mucositis, pruritus and dermatitis	CBC, dermatologic toxicities	Most commonly used in HSCT preparative regimens
Trabectedin	Myelosuppression, rhabdomyolysis, hepatotoxicity, nausea and vomiting, diarrhea or constipation, cardiomyopathy	CBC, CPK, liver function	Extravasation may lead to tissue necrosis
Triazenes (dacarbazine and temozolomide)	Myelosuppression, severe nausea and vomiting, increased liver enzymes, flu-like syndrome (may last for several days after dacarbazine administration), facial flushing, photosensitivity	CBC, liver function	Dispense in a light-proof bag Temozolomide crosses the blood-brain barrier, may cause lymphosuppression and requires PJP prophylaxis when given with radiation therapy
DNA Methyltransferase Inhibitors			
Azacitidine and decitabine	Myelosuppression and infection, constitutional symptoms, musculoskeletal symptoms (arthralgias), cough, dyspnea	CBC, infection	Oral formulation decitabine/cedazuridine available
Immunomodulatory Imide Drugs			
Lenalidomide	Teratogen, fatigue, peripheral neuropathy, neutropenia and thrombocytopenia, thromboembolic events	CBC, signs of thrombosis, signs of peripheral neuropathies, pregnancy status	REMS program for fetal toxicity Adjust dose for renal impairment Prophylactic anticoagulation may be required
Pomalidomide	Teratogen, neutropenia, hepatotoxicity, thromboembolic events	Same as for lenalidomide	REMS program for fetal toxicity Adjust dose for renal and hepatic impairment Prophylactic anticoagulation may be required
Thalidomide	Teratogen, somnolence, constipation, dizziness or orthostatic hypotension, rash, peripheral neuropathy, thromboembolic events, increased HIV viral load	Same as for lenalidomide	REMS program for fetal toxicity Prophylactic anticoagulation may be required
Retinoids			
Bexarotene	Peripheral edema, insomnia, headache, fever, increased triglycerides and cholesterol, hypothyroidism, leukopenia and anemia, dry skin, increased liver enzymes, pancreatitis, photosensitivity	CBC, liver function, cholesterol and triglyceride levels, thyroid function	Avoid gemfibrozil to treat elevated triglycerides Limit vitamin A supplements May cause hypoglycemia in patients receiving insulin, sulfonylureas, or metformin Teratogenic, contraindicated in pregnancy, patients should be educated about proper contraceptive measures
Tretinoin	Headache, differentiation syndrome (consisting of pulmonary symptoms, fever, hypotension, and pleural effusions), dry skin and mucous membranes, mucositis, increases in liver enzymes and bilirubin	CBC, liver function, signs of differentiation syndrome	Differentiation syndrome must be treated promptly with corticosteroids Teratogenic, contraindicated in pregnancy, patients should be educated about proper contraceptive measures

TABLE 149-7 Monitoring of Anticancer Drugs[a]

Agent	Notable Adverse Drug Reactions	Monitoring Parameters	Comments
Miscellaneous Agents			
Arsenic trioxide	Differentiation syndrome (pulmonary infiltrates, respiratory distress, fever, and hypotension), QTc prolongation, electrolyte abnormalities (hypokalemia, hyperkalemia, hypomagnesemia), hyperglycemia, rash, lightheadedness, fatigue, musculoskeletal pain	ECG, serum electrolytes (calcium, magnesium, potassium), renal function	Differentiation syndrome must be treated promptly with corticosteroids Do not give if QTc >500 msec Replace electrolytes before therapy
Asparaginase	Anaphylaxis, thrombosis, pancreatitis, glucose intolerance, hemorrhage, hepatotoxicity	Pancreatic enzymes, liver function, glucose, coagulation parameters (fibrinogen, PT, PTT), hypersensitivity reactions, blood glucose, CBC	FDA-approved products include L-asparaginase, recombinant asparaginase (*Erwinia*), pegaspargase, and calaspargase pegol
Bleomycin	Anaphylaxis and hypersensitivity reactions, fever and flu-like symptoms, mucositis, pulmonary fibrosis	Obtain PFTs before use and if signs of pulmonary toxicity develop, monitor for anaphylactic reactions	Adjust dose for renal impairment Test dose (1 unit) is recommended but controversial; premedicate for subsequent doses with acetaminophen Pulmonary toxicity associated with cumulative dose >400 units and preexisting pulmonary disease
Hydroxyurea	Myelosuppression, rash, skin hyperpigmentation, TLS, secondary leukemias	CBC, uric acid	Dose may need to be adjusted with renal impairment (use with caution) Used to decrease white blood cell counts rapidly to prevent adverse effects of leukocytosis
Lanreotide	Abdominal pain, musculoskeletal pain, vomiting, headache, injection site reaction, hypertension, glucose abnormalities	Glucose, thyroid function, heart rate	Cholelithiasis and complications of cholelithiasis May need to adjust anti-diabetic medications in diabetic patients May decrease heart rate, use with caution in at-risk patients
Mitomycin	Myelosuppression (delayed and prolonged), mucositis, nausea and vomiting, vesicant, pulmonary fibrosis, hemolytic anemia and uremic syndrome	CBC, renal function, pulmonary function	Apply ice or cold packs to site for extravasation May be given intravenously or by intravesical administration; also available as a ureteral gel formulation
Omacetaxine	Myelosuppression (thrombocytopenia including increased risk of hemorrhage, anemia, neutropenia), diarrhea, nausea, fatigue, asthenia, injection site reaction, pyrexia, infection, lymphopenia, hyperglycemia	CBC, blood glucose	
Targeted Agents: Small Molecules			
Anaplastic Lymphoma Kinase (ALK) Inhibitors			
Alectinib	Fatigue, bradycardia, hepatotoxicity, anemia, constipation, edema, myalgia, visual disturbances	CBC, liver function, heart rate, CPK	Administer with food
Brigatinib	ILD and pneumonitis, hypertension, bradycardia, visual disturbances, CPK elevation, pancreatic enzyme elevation, hyperglycemia	HR, BP, pulmonary symptoms, CPK, pancreatic enzymes	Dose escalation required to decrease early-onset pulmonary symptoms Avoid strong CYP3A inhibitors and inducers; may affect hormonal contraceptives
Ceritinib	Gastrointestinal toxicity, increases in liver enzymes, fatigue, visual disturbances, QTc prolongation, bradycardia, hyperglycemia	CBC, renal function, liver function, blood glucose, pancreatic enzymes, cardiac monitoring, electrolytes	Administer on an empty stomach
Crizotinib	Nausea and vomiting, diarrhea, constipation, fatigue, increases in liver enzymes, visual disorders, edema, ILD, QTc prolongation, bradycardia	CBC, renal function, liver function, HR, BP, cardiac monitoring, electrolytes, pulmonary symptoms	Visual disorders (visual impairment, blurred vision, and photopsia) occur in approximately 50% of patients
Lorlatinib	Hepatotoxicity, CNS toxicity, hyperlipidemia, atrioventricular block, ILD and pneumonitis	Liver function, lipids, ECG	Strong CYP3A inducers are contraindicated, avoid strong CYP3A4 inhibitors and CYP3A4 substrates
B-Cell Lymphoma 2 (BCL-2) Inhibitors			
Venetoclax	TLS, myelosuppression, diarrhea, upper respiratory tract infection	CBC, uric acid, electrolytes	Ramp-up dose required Premedicate with anti-hyperuricemics and ensure adequate hydration Contraindicated with strong CYP3A inhibitors during initiation and ramp-up Avoid strong and moderate CYP3A inhibitors, strong or moderate CYP3A inducers, P-gp inhibitors, or narrow therapeutic substrates Avoid live-attenuated vaccines Administer with a meal

(Continued)

TABLE 149-7 Monitoring of Anticancer Drugs[a] (*Continued*)

Agent	Notable Adverse Drug Reactions	Monitoring Parameters	Comments
Breakpoint Cluster Region-Abelson (BCR-ABL) Inhibitors			
Bosutinib	Nausea and vomiting, edema, pleural effusions and ascites, myelosuppression, CHF, arthralgias, rash, diarrhea, increased liver enzymes, hypophosphatemia	CBC, liver function, electrolytes, Philadelphia chromosome levels, signs of edema	Adjust dose for hepatic impairment Avoid antacids and PPIs Maintenance dose based on CBC Administer with food
Dasatinib	Nausea and vomiting, edema, pleural effusions and ascites, myelosuppression, CHF, arthralgias, fatigue, rash, diarrhea, increased liver enzymes, QTc prolongation, hypophosphatemia, hypocalcemia	CBC, liver function, electrolytes, signs of edema, Philadelphia chromosome levels	Avoid antacids, H_2 antagonists, and PPIs Maintenance dose based on CBC
Imatinib	Nausea and vomiting, edema, pleural effusions and ascites, myelosuppression, CHF, arthralgias, rash, diarrhea, increased liver enzymes, hypophosphatemia	CBC, liver function, electrolytes, Philadelphia chromosome levels, signs of edema	Dose adjustments should be considered with severe liver and moderate renal impairment May increase warfarin effects Maintenance dose based on CBC Take with meals and a full glass of water
Nilotinib	Nausea and vomiting, edema, myelosuppression, increased lipase, hyperglycemia, arthralgias, rash, diarrhea, increased liver enzymes, QTc prolongation	CBC, liver function, serum lipase, serum glucose, electrolytes, Philadelphia chromosome levels	Adjust dose for hepatic impairment Take on an empty stomach CYP3A4 substrate: avoid inhibitors Maintenance dose based on CBC Avoid PPIs, stagger administration with H_2 antagonists and antacids if use is necessary
Ponatinib	Myelosuppression, hypertension, rash, abdominal pain, fatigue, headache, dry skin, constipation, arthralgia, nausea, pyrexia, thromboembolic events, hepatotoxicity, CHF, pancreatitis, hemorrhage (secondary to thrombocytopenia), fluid retention	Cardiac monitoring (CHF, arrhythmias), BP, pancreatic enzymes, fluid retention, CBC, liver function	May need to decrease dose or hold therapy if hepatotoxicity develops Avoid antacids and drugs that decrease gastric pH
BRAF Inhibitors			
Dabrafenib	Papilloma, arthralgia, alopecia, fatigue, headache, PPE, pyrexia	CBC, serum glucose, electrolytes, renal function, dermatologic evaluations	Take on an empty stomach
Encorafenib	Cutaneous and noncutaneous malignancies, hemorrhage, uveitis, QTc prolongation	Visual symptoms, ophthalmologic evaluations, ECG, electrolytes	Avoid strong and moderate CYP3A inhibitors, strong inducers, and sensitive CYP3A substrates Use nonhormonal contraceptives
Vemurafenib	Papilloma, arthralgia, alopecia, fatigue, headache, photosensitivity reaction, hypersensitivity reactions, QTc prolongation	Liver function, electrolytes, cardiac monitoring, dermatologic evaluations	Radiation sensitization/recall
Bruton's Tyrosine Kinase (BTK) Inhibitors			
Acalabrutinib	Infections, secondary primary malignancies, atrial flutter and fibrillation	CBC, cardiac monitoring	Avoid strong CYP3A inhibitors, strong CYP3A inducers Avoid PPIs, stagger administration with H_2 antagonists and antacids if use is necessary
Ibrutinib	Diarrhea, fatigue, musculoskeletal pain, nausea, rash, atrial fibrillation, hemorrhage, TLS, myelosuppression	CBC, renal function, liver function, uric acid levels, electrolytes, cardiac monitoring	Reduce dose with hepatic impairment Dose modifications for use with CYP3A inhibitors or inducers
Zanubrutinib	Myelosuppression, infections, secondary malignancies, cardiac arrhythmias, hemorrhage, rash, bruising, diarrhea, cough	CBC, liver function	Dose modifications for use with CYP3A inhibitors or inducers
Cyclin-Dependent Kinase (CDK) Inhibitors			
Abemaciclib	Diarrhea, neutropenia, hepatotoxicity, venous thromboembolism	CBC, electrolytes, liver function	Avoid moderate and strong CY3A inducers Dose reduce with moderate and strong CYP3A inhibitors Reduce dose with severe hepatic impairment
Palbociclib	Thromboembolic events, infection, bone marrow suppression, gastrointestinal toxicity	CBC, infection	Administer with food
Ribociclib	QTc prolongation, hepatobiliary toxicity, neutropenia	ECG, electrolytes, liver function, CBC	Avoid drugs known to prolong QTc interval, strong CYP3A inhibitors, strong CYP3A inducers, sensitive CYP3A substrates

TABLE 149-7 Monitoring of Anticancer Drugs[a]

Agent	Notable Adverse Drug Reactions	Monitoring Parameters	Comments
Colony-Stimulating Factor-1 Receptor (CSF-1R) Inhibitors			
Pexidartinib	Hepatotoxicity, hair color change, rash, dysgeusia, edema of eyelid, fatigue	Liver function, creatinine clearance	REMS program for liver toxicity Dose adjustment for renal and hepatic impairment Take on empty stomach Acid-reducing agents: Administer pexidartinib 2 hours before or 2 hours after locally-acting antacids; administer pexidartinib ≥2 hours before or 10 hours after a H2-receptor antagonist; avoid concomitant administration of pexidartinib with PPIs
Epidermal Growth Factor Receptor (EGFR) Inhibitors			
Afatinib	Rash, diarrhea, ILD, keratitis, stomatitis	Liver function, renal function, dermatologic evaluations, electrolytes, LVEF in patients with cardiac risk factors, pulmonary symptoms	Administer on an empty stomach
Dacomitinib	ILD, diarrhea, dermatologic toxicity	Pulmonary symptoms, skin	Avoid PPIs and sensitive CYP2D6 inhibitors Initiate use of moisturizers and appropriate measures to limit sun exposure
Erlotinib	Rash, diarrhea, ILD, hepatic and renal failure reported	Liver function, renal function, electrolytes, pulmonary symptoms, dermatologic evaluations	Dose reductions or delays may be required for rash but supportive care should be attempted first Major interaction with warfarin (may lead to increased bleeding risk) H_2 antagonists, PPIs, and antacids may decrease drug levels Administer on an empty stomach as food increases absorption and possibly toxicity
Gefitinib	Similar to erlotinib	Liver function, renal function, electrolytes, pulmonary symptoms, dermatologic evaluations	Similar precautions and drug interactions as with erlotinib
Osimertinib	Gastrointestinal toxicity, dermatologic toxicity, ILD/pneumonitis, pneumonia, pulmonary embolism, cardiomyopathy, QTc prolongation	Cardiac monitoring (LVEF, QTc), pulmonary symptoms, dermatologic evaluations	Avoid strong CYP3A4 inhibitors and inducers Avoid drugs that prolong QTc
Enhancer of Zeste Homolog 2 (EZH2) Inhibitors			
Tazemetostat	Myelosuppression, fatigue, nausea and vomiting, secondary malignancies	CBC	Avoid moderate/strong CYP3A4 inhibitors or inducers
Fibroblast Growth Factor Receptor (FGFR) Inhibitors			
Erdafitinib and Pemigatinib	Ocular disorders, hyperphosphatemia, stomatitis, creatinine increased, PPE, elevated liver enzymes	Ophthalmological exams, phosphate levels	Avoid moderate/strong CYP2C9 or CYP3A4 inhibitors and inducers Increased phosphate levels are a pharmacodynamic effect
FMS-Like Tyrosine Kinase-3 (FLT3) Inhibitors			
Gilteritinib	PRES, QTc prolongation, pancreatitis, hypersensitivity	ECG, electrolytes	Avoid dual P-gp and CYP3A inducers and strong CYP3A inhibitors
Midostaurin	Pulmonary toxicity	ECG	Administer with food Avoid strong CYP3A inducers
Hedgehog Inhibitors			
Glasdegib	QTc prolongation, teratogenic effects	Pregnancy status, ECG	Boxed warning for severe birth defects and embryo-fetal death; advise females to use contraception during treatment and for 20 months after the last dose; advise males to use condoms during treatment and for at least 8 months after the last dose; do not donate blood during treatment and for 30 months after the last dose; do not donate sperm during treatment and for 8 months after the last dose

(Continued)

TABLE 149-7 Monitoring of Anticancer Drugs[a] (Continued)

Agent	Notable Adverse Drug Reactions	Monitoring Parameters	Comments
Sonidegib	Fatigue, alopecia, amenorrhea, musculoskeletal toxicity, teratogenic effects	Pregnancy status, CPK, renal function, liver function	Boxed warning for severe birth defects and embryo-fetal death; advise females to use contraception during treatment and for 20 months after the last dose; advise males to use condoms during treatment and for at least 8 months after the last dose; do not donate blood during treatment and for 20 months after the last dose; do not donate sperm during treatment and for 8 months after the last dose Avoid strong and moderate CYP3A modulators; moderate CYP3A inhibitors may be used for short term
Vismodegib	Muscle spasms, alopecia, dysgeusia, fatigue, nausea and vomiting, diarrhea, decreased appetite, constipation, arthralgias, teratogenic effects	Pregnancy status	Boxed warning for severe birth defects and embryo-fetal death; patients should not donate blood or blood products while receiving vismodegib and for at least 7 months after the last dose; verify pregnancy status within 7 days prior to treatment initiation; do not donate sperm during treatment and for 3 months after the last dose
Human Epidermal Growth Factor Receptor 2 (HER2) Inhibitors			
Lapatinib	Diarrhea, rash, nausea, vomiting, fatigue, decreases in LVEF, hepatotoxicity, QTc prolongation, ILD	Liver function, cardiac monitoring (LVEF, QTc), electrolytes, pulmonary symptoms	Adjust dose for severe hepatic impairment Administer on empty stomach Avoid strong CYP3A4 inhibitors (if unavoidable, consider dose reduction), avoid strong CYP3A4 inducers (if unavoidable, consider gradual dose increases)
Neratinib	Diarrhea, hepatotoxicity	Liver function, electrolytes	Use prophylactic antidiarrheals Lower starting dose for hepatic impairment Avoid PPIs, strong and moderate CYP3A inhibitors, strong and moderate CYP3A inducers, and sensitive P-gp substrates
Tucatinib	Diarrhea, hepatotoxicity	Liver function, Child-Pugh score, stool count	Dose adjustment recommended for hepatic impairment
Histone Deacetylase (HDAC) Inhibitors			
Belinostat	Pyrexia, nausea, fatigue, anemia, hepatotoxicity, infection, TLS	Liver function, renal function, CBC, uric acid levels	Empiric dose reduction in patients known to be homozygous for UGT1A1*28 allele
Panobinostat	Cardiotoxicity, nausea and vomiting, diarrhea, hemorrhage, infection, hepatotoxicity	Cardiac monitoring, electrolytes, CBC, liver function, pregnancy status	Boxed warnings for cardiovascular events and gastrointestinal events
Romidepsin	Myelosuppression, infection, nausea and vomiting, fatigue, anorexia, ECG T-wave changes	CBC, cardiac monitoring (ECG), electrolytes	Monitor INR with concurrent use of warfarin
Vorinostat	Diarrhea, fatigue, nausea, thrombocytopenia, anorexia, dysgeusia, thromboembolic events, hyperglycemia	CBC, electrolytes, serum glucose, renal function	Avoid or adjust dose for hepatic impairment Increase in INR with concomitant warfarin Severe thrombocytopenia and GI bleeding have been reported with concomitant use with vorinostat and other HDAC inhibitors (eg, valproic acid)
Isocitrate Dehydrogenase (IDH) Inhibitors			
Enasidenib	Differentiation syndrome, TLS, myelosuppression, hepatotoxicity, nausea and vomiting	CBC, electrolytes, signs of differentiation syndrome	Differentiation syndrome may be life-threatening. If suspected, initiate oral or intravenous corticosteroids and hemodynamic monitoring until improvement Decrease dosage of OATP1B1, OATP1B3, BCRP, and P-gp substrates with coadministration
Ivosidenib	Differentiation syndrome, QTc prolongation, Guillain-Barré Syndrome, TLS	CBC, chemistries, CPK, ECG, electrolytes, signs of differentiation syndrome	Differentiation syndrome may be life-threatening. If suspected, initiate oral or intravenous corticosteroids and hemodynamic monitoring until improvement Reduce ivosidenib dose with strong CYP3A4 inhibitors Avoid strong CYP3A inducers; sensitive CYP3A substrates; drugs that prolong QTc interval Avoid high-fat meal

TABLE 149-7 Monitoring of Anticancer Drugs[a]

Agent	Notable Adverse Drug Reactions	Monitoring Parameters	Comments
Janus Kinase (JAK) Inhibitors			
Fedratinib	Encephalopathy, thrombocytopenia, anemia, nausea and vomiting, diarrhea, hepatotoxicity, amylase/lipase elevations	CBC, liver function, thiamine, symptoms of encephalopathy, pancreatic enzymes	Assess and replete thiamine at baseline and periodically Avoid coadministration with strong and moderate CYP3A4 inducers; avoid dual CYP3A4 and CYP2C19 inhibitors; and reduce fedratinib dose with strong CYP3A4 inhibitors Reduce dose for severe renal impairment, avoid use with severe hepatic impairment
Ruxolitinib	Thrombocytopenia, anemia, bruising, dizziness, headache, infections, cardiovascular abnormalities	CBC, renal function, liver function, cardiac monitoring	Consider dose adjustment for renal and hepatic impairment
Mitogen-Activated Protein Kinase-Extracellular Signal-Regulated Kinase (MEK) Inhibitors			
Binimetinib	Cardiomyopathy, venous thromboembolism, ILD, hepatotoxicity, rhabdomyolysis, hemorrhage, ophthalmic events	LVEF, ophthalmologic evaluation, liver function, CPK, renal function	Reduce dose for moderate and severe hepatic impairment
Cobimetinib and Selumetinib	Dermatologic toxicity, nausea and vomiting, pyrexia, hemorrhage, new primary malignancies, cardiomyopathy, ophthalmic events, hepatotoxicity, rhabdomyolysis	CBC, liver function, dermatologic evaluation, ophthalmologic evaluation, LVEF, CPK, electrolytes	Avoid coadministration with strong or moderate CYP3A inducers or inhibitors Selumetinib capsules contain vitamin E which may result in increased vitamin E levels and risk of bleeding
Trametinib	Diarrhea, lymphedema, hemorrhage, venous thromboembolism, febrile reactions, cardiomyopathy, dermatologic toxicity, hyperglycemia, hypertension, ophthalmic events	CBC, liver function, LVEF, ophthalmologic evaluation, dermatologic evaluation, BP	Capsules are stored refrigerated Administer on an empty stomach
Mesenchymal-Epithelial Transition (MET) Inhibitors			
Tepotinib and Capmatinib	Edema, fatigue, hepatotoxicity, dyspnea, musculoskeletal pain	Liver function, pulmonary symptoms	Modify dose for hepatotoxicity during treatment Take tepotinib with food
Mammalian Target of Rapamycin (mTOR) Inhibitors			
Everolimus	Rash, asthenia, stomatitis, nausea, edema, anorexia, anemia, pneumonitis, hyperglycemia, hyperlipidemia, hypertriglyceridemia, hypophosphatemia, elevated liver enzymes, elevated creatinine, lymphopenia, thrombocytopenia, leukopenia, infection	Metabolic toxicities, CBC, renal function, liver function, electrolytes, pulmonary symptoms	Adjust dose for hepatic impairment Cholesterol or diabetic medications may need to be initiated or dosages increased CYP3A4 and P-gp substrate; may require dose adjustment based on concurrent medication
Temsirolimus	Similar to everolimus with addition of infusion-related reactions	Similar to everolimus, infusion reactions	Adjust dose for hepatic impairment Requires diphenhydramine premedication
Nuclear Export Inhibitors			
Selinexor	Myelosuppression, nausea and vomiting, hyponatremia, diarrhea, weight loss, loss of appetite, neurotoxicity	CBC, electrolytes, volume status, weight	Dose adjustment for hyponatremia Maintain adequate fluid and caloric intake throughout treatment and consider IV hydration in patients at risk of dehydration
Poly ADP Ribose Polymerase (PARP) Inhibitors			
Niraparib	MDS/AML, myelosuppression, cardiovascular toxicity	CBC, liver function, BP, HR	Dose adjust for hepatic impairment and myelosuppression
Olaparib	MDS/AML, fatigue, musculoskeletal pain, dermatitis, nausea and vomiting, upper respiratory infections, anemia, pneumonitis	CBC, pulmonary symptoms	Reduce dose for renal impairment
Rucaparib	MDS/AML, nausea and vomiting	CBC	Adjust dose of CYP1A2, CYP3A, CYP2C9, or CYP2C19 substrates, if clinically indicated. If coadministration with warfarin cannot be avoided, consider increasing the frequency of INR monitoring
Talazoparib	MDS/AML, myelosuppression	CBC, renal function	Reduce starting dose for renal impairment Reduce dose with certain P-gp inhibitors
Platelet-Derived Growth Factor Receptor-alpha (PDGFR-α) Inhibitors			
Avapritinib	Edema, hair color change, rash, abdominal pain, fatigue, excessive tear production, anemia, CNS toxicity	Liver function, CBC	Dose adjustment for hepatic impairment Dose adjustment for concomitant CYP3A4 inhibitors Take on empty stomach

(Continued)

TABLE 149-7 Monitoring of Anticancer Drugs[a] (*Continued*)

Agent	Notable Adverse Drug Reactions	Monitoring Parameters	Comments
Ripretinib	Arthralgia/myalgia, hypertension, LV dysfunction, dermatologic toxicity, alopecia, abdominal pain, constipation, diarrhea, nausea and vomiting	LVEF, BP, dermatologic evaluation	Withhold for at least 1 week prior to elective surgery; do not administer for at least 2 weeks following major surgery and until adequate wound healing
Phosphatidylinositide 3-Kinase (PI3K) Inhibitors			
Alpelisib	Dermatologic reactions, severe diarrhea, pneumonitis, hyperglycemia, severe hypersensitivity reactions	Blood glucose, dermatologic evaluation, pulmonary symptoms	Avoid strong CYP3A inducers, closely monitor with concurrent CYP2C9 substrates (eg, warfarin)
Copanlisib	Infections, hyperglycemia, hypertension, pneumonitis, neutropenia, dermatologic reactions	CBC, blood glucose, BP	Reduce dose with strong CYP3A inhibitors; avoid strong CYP3A inducers Consider PJP prophylaxis
Duvelisib	Infections, neutropenia, fatal/serious diarrhea, dermatologic reactions, pneumonitis, hepatotoxicity	CBC, liver function, dermatologic evaluation, pulmonary symptoms, GI symptoms	REMS program for infections, diarrhea/colitis, cutaneous reactions, and pneumonitis Avoid strong CYP3A inducers; reduce moderate and strong CYP3A inhibitors PJP prophylaxis required; consider antiviral prophylaxis for CMV
Idelalisib	Fatal/serious diarrhea, intestinal perforation, hepatotoxicity, pneumonitis, infections, neutropenia, dermatologic reactions, anaphylaxis	Liver function, CBC, dermatologic evaluation, pulmonary symptoms, GI symptoms	REMS program for hepatotoxicity, diarrhea/colitis, pneumonitis, infections, intestinal perforation PJP prophylaxis required
Umbralisib	Increased serum creatinine, infections, dermatologic reactions, decreased potassium, myelosuppression, hepatotoxicity, abdominal pain, decreased appetite, diarrhea, nausea and vomiting	CBC, liver function, symptoms of infection, dermatologic evaluations	PJP prophylaxis required Consider prophylactic antivirals to prevent CMV
Proteasome Inhibitors			
Bortezomib	Fatigue or malaise, nausea and vomiting, diarrhea, anorexia, constipation, myelosuppression (especially thrombocytopenia), hyponatremia, hypokalemia, peripheral neuropathy (cumulative and dose-related), fever	CBC, thyroid function, symptoms of neuropathy, electrolytes	Adjust dose for hepatic impairment Administer IV or subcutaneous (subcutaneous administration has been shown to decrease neuropathies); increased risk of severe neuropathy with preexisting neuropathy Coadministration with strong CYP3A4 inhibitors can increase bortezomib concentrations
Carfilzomib	Fatigue, anemia, thrombocytopenia, nausea, diarrhea, dyspnea, pyrexia, infusion-related reactions, rare reports of cardiac arrest, CHF, and MI	Pulmonary symptoms, CBC, liver function, cardiac monitoring, infusion reactions	Premedicate with dexamethasone before all cycle 1 doses then as needed for future cycles to reduce the incidence of infusion reactions
Ixazomib	Gastrointestinal toxicity, thrombocytopenia, peripheral neuropathy, edema, cutaneous reactions, hepatotoxicity	CBC, liver function, dermatologic evaluation	Administer on an empty stomach Reduce starting dose for hepatic or renal impairment Avoid use with strong CYP3A4 inducers Consider antiviral prophylaxis
Ras Inhibitors			
Sotorasib	Hepatotoxicity, interstitial lung disease, diarrhea, musculoskeletal pain, fatigue, cough	Pulmonary symptoms, liver function	Avoid coadministration with PPIs and H2 antagonists Avoid coadministration with strong CYP3A4 inducers, CYP3A4 substrates, and P-gp substrates
Rearranged during Transfection (RET) Inhibitors			
Pralsetinib	Edema, constipation, diarrhea, hepatotoxicity, musculoskeletal pain, cough, fatigue, hypertension	Liver function, BP	Take on empty stomach Avoid use with strong CYP3A4 inducers and inhibitors Withhold at least 5 days prior to elective surgery. Do not administer for at least 2 weeks after surgery and until adequate wound healing
Selpercatinib	Thrombocytopenia, hemorrhage, hypertension, QTc prolongation, rash, constipation, diarrhea, xerostomia, impaired wound healing	CBC, liver function, BP, QTc	Avoid moderate/strong CYP3A inhibitors Avoid PPIs, H2 antagonists, and antacids Dose adjustment with hepatic impairment Withhold for at least 1 week prior to elective surgery; do not administer for at least 2 weeks following major surgery and until adequate wound healing
Tropomyosin Receptor Kinase (TRK) Inhibitors			
Entrectinib	Cardiotoxicity, CNS toxicity, hepatotoxicity, vision disorders, skeletal fractures	CBC, liver function, uric acid, ECG, electrolytes	Avoid strong CYP3A inhibitors, if coadministration cannot be avoided, dose adjust entrectinib

TABLE 149-7 Monitoring of Anticancer Drugs[a]

Agent	Notable Adverse Drug Reactions	Monitoring Parameters	Comments
Larotrectinib	Neurotoxicity, hepatotoxicity	Liver function	Avoid strong CYP3A inhibitors and inducers; avoid sensitive CYP3A substrates Reduce starting dose in moderate or severe hepatic impairment
Vascular Endothelial Growth Factor Receptor (VEGFR) Multikinase Inhibitors			
Axitinib	Diarrhea, rash, PPE, bleeding, thrombotic events, hypertension, hepatotoxicity, hypothyroidism, proteinuria, GI perforation, fatigue, rare reports of RPLS	CBC, liver function, BP, thyroid function, urine protein, neurologic evaluation, dermatologic evaluation	Blood pressure should be well-controlled prior to administration Hold for at least 2 days prior to elective surgery and do not administer for at least 2 weeks following major surgery and until adequate wound healing Adjust dose for hepatic impairment Substrate of CYP3A4, may require dose adjustment based on concurrently administered medication
Cabozantinib	Diarrhea, stomatitis, PPE, decreased weight, decreased appetite, nausea, fatigue, oral pain, hair color changes, dysgeusia, hypertension, abdominal pain, constipation, increased liver enzymes, proteinuria, lymphopenia, neutropenia, thrombocytopenia, hypocalcemia, hypophosphatemia, GI perforations and fistulas, hemorrhage	BP, urine protein, CBC, liver function, thyroid function, electrolytes, dermatologic evaluation	Blood pressure should be well-controlled prior to administration Hold for at least 3 weeks prior to elective surgery and do not administer for at least 2 weeks following major surgery and until adequate wound healing Adjust dose for hepatic impairment Substrate of CYP3A4, may require dose adjustment based on concurrently administered medication
Lenvatinib	Hypertension, fatigue, diarrhea, proteinuria, stomatitis, PPE, hypothyroidism, hepatotoxicity, thromboembolic events, renal toxicity, hypocalcemia, GI perforation	Liver function, renal function, thyroid function, BP, electrolytes	Blood pressure should be well-controlled prior to administration Hold for at least 1 week prior to elective surgery and do not administer for at least 2 weeks following major surgery and until adequate wound healing Adjust dose for severe hepatic and renal impairment Weight-based dosing for HCC
Pazopanib	Diarrhea, hypertension, hair/skin hypopigmentation, nausea, anorexia, vomiting, decreased weight, fatigue, musculoskeletal pain, dysgeusia, dyspnea, hypothyroidism, proteinuria, fatal hepatotoxicity, thromboembolic events	Liver function, cardiac monitoring (ECG), BP, thyroid function, urine protein, dermatologic evaluation	Blood pressure should be well-controlled prior to administration Hold for at least 1 week prior to elective surgery and do not administer for at least 2 weeks following major surgery and until adequate wound healing Adjust dose for hepatic impairment Take on empty stomach Reduce dose when administered with strong CYP3A4 inhibitors, avoid CYP3A4 inducers, concomitant use with simvastatin increases liver enzymes
Regorafenib	Asthenia, fatigue, decreased appetite, PPE, diarrhea, mucositis, weight loss, infection, hypertension, dysphonia, hepatotoxicity, hemorrhage	Liver function, BP, dermatologic evaluation	Blood pressure should be well-controlled prior to administration Hold for at least 2 weeks prior to elective surgery and do not administer for at least 2 weeks following major surgery and until adequate wound healing Administer with food (low-fat breakfast that contains <30% fat) Monitor INR closely with concomitant warfarin because of an increased risk of hemorrhage
Sorafenib	Diarrhea, rash, PPE, fatigue, hypertension, prolonged QTc interval, cardiac events (including MI), hepatitis	BP, liver function, cardiac monitoring, electrolytes, dermatologic evaluation	Blood pressure should be well-controlled prior to administration Hold for at least 10 days prior to elective surgery and do not administer for at least 2 weeks following major surgery and until adequate wound healing Administer on an empty stomach May increase the anticoagulation effects of warfarin
Sunitinib	Diarrhea, rash, bleeding, CHF and cardiac effects, QTc prolongation, fatigue, hypertension, hepatotoxicity, thyroid dysfunction	CBC, liver function, BP, thyroid function, cardiac monitoring (CHF, ECG), electrolytes	Blood pressure should be well-controlled prior to administration Hold for at least 3 weeks prior to elective surgery and do not administer for at least 2 weeks following major surgery and until adequate wound healing CYP3A4 substrate, may require dose adjustment based on concurrent medications

(*Continued*)

TABLE 149-7 Monitoring of Anticancer Drugs[a] (*Continued*)

Agent	Notable Adverse Drug Reactions	Monitoring Parameters	Comments
Tivozanib	Diarrhea, hypertension, decrease appetite, stomatitis, thyroid dysfunction, proteinuria, thromboembolic events	BP, liver function, proteinuria, thyroid function	Blood pressure should be well-controlled prior to administration Hold for at least 24 days prior to elective surgery and do not administer for at least 2 weeks following major surgery and until adequate wound healing Avoid strong CYP3A4 inducers Dose adjustment for hepatic impairment
Vandetanib	Diarrhea, rash, acne, nausea, hypertension, headache, fatigue, upper respiratory tract infections, decreased appetite, abdominal pain, QTc prolongation, torsades de pointes and sudden death, ILD, hemorrhage, increased liver enzymes	Liver function, electrolytes, cardiac monitoring (ECG), BP, pulmonary symptoms, dermatologic evaluation	Hold for at least 1 month prior to elective surgery and do not administer for at least 2 weeks following major surgery and until adequate wound healing REMS program for QTc prolongation and sudden death; avoid other medications that prolong the QTc interval Adjust dose for renal impairment Advise patients to wear sunscreen and protective clothing when exposed to sun
Targeted Agents: mAbs & ADCs			
Antibodies That Target BCMA (B-Cell Maturation Antigen)			
Belantamab mafodotin	Myelosuppression, ocular toxicity, infusion-related reactions, electrolyte abnormalities, transaminitis	CBC, complete metabolic panel, infusion-related reactions, ophthalmic evaluations	ADC with payload MMAF (a microtubule disrupting agent) REMS program because of risk of ocular toxicity Patients should use preservative-free lubricant eye drops at least 4 times a day, starting with the initial infusion and continuing until the end of therapy; avoid contact lenses unless otherwise directed
Antibodies That Target CD19			
Loncastuximab tesirine	Myelosuppression, edema, dermatologic toxicity, musculoskeletal pain	CBC, infection, skin evaluation	ADC with payload SG3199 (an alkylating agent) Premedicate with dexamethasone
Tafasitamab	Myelosuppression, infusion-related reactions, edema, decrease appetite, diarrhea, fatigue, fever	CBC, infusion-related reactions, infection	Premedication (may include acetaminophen, an H1 receptor antagonist, an H2 receptor antagonist, and/or glucocorticoids) for initial infusion, may discontinue for subsequent infusions
Antibodies That Target CD20			
Obinutuzumab	Infusion-related reactions, myelosuppression, nausea, diarrhea, PML, HBV reactivation	CBC, hepatitis B screening at baseline, renal function, electrolytes, infusion-related reactions, fluid status	Patients should be screened for hepatitis B before therapy initiation Antimicrobial, antiviral, and antifungal prophylaxis in select patients Anti-hyperuricemic prophylaxis and hydration if risk for TLS Premedicate with acetaminophen, an antihistamine, and a glucocorticoid
Ofatumumab	Neutropenia, pneumonia, pyrexia, cough, diarrhea, anemia, fatigue, dyspnea, rash, nausea, bronchitis, upper respiratory infection	Infusion-related reactions, CBC, hepatitis B screening at baseline	Patients should be screened for hepatitis B before therapy initiation Premedicate with acetaminophen, antihistamine, and corticosteroid Infusion rate-escalation required
Rituximab	Hypersensitivity reactions and infusion-related reactions, TLS (especially with large tumor burden), myelosuppression and infection, rare reports of PML, severe skin reactions, myalgias, tachycardia	Infusion-related reactions, CBC, neurologic examination, hepatitis B screening at baseline, electrolytes, HR, BP	Patients should be screened for hepatitis B before therapy initiation Infusion-related reactions may be severe; increase rate of infusion gradually and premedicate with acetaminophen and diphenhydramine Rituximab and hyaluronidase available for subcutaneous injection after 1 full dose of IV rituximab
Antibodies That Target CD22			
Inotuzumab ozogamicin	Myelosuppression, infusion-related reactions, QTc interval prolongation, hepatotoxicity	CBC, ECG, infusion-related reactions, liver function	ADC with a calicheamicin derivative payload Premedicate with a corticosteroid, antipyretic, and antihistamine
Antibodies That Target CD30			
Brentuximab vedotin	Neutropenia, peripheral neuropathy, fatigue, nausea and vomiting, anemia, diarrhea, rash, thrombocytopenia, infusion-related reactions, TLS, rare reports of PML	CBC, symptoms of neuropathy, infusion-related reactions, uric acid levels, electrolytes	ADC with payload MMAE (a microtubule disrupting agent) Adjust dose for renal and hepatic impairment

TABLE 149-7 Monitoring of Anticancer Drugs[a]

Agent	Notable Adverse Drug Reactions	Monitoring Parameters	Comments
Antibodies That Target CD33			
Gemtuzumab ozogamicin	Hypersensitivity and infusion-related reactions, hemorrhage	Infusion-related reactions	ADC with a calicheamicin derivative payload Premedicate with a corticosteroid, antihistamine, and acetaminophen
Antibodies That Target CD38			
Daratumumab	Infusion-related reactions, pyrexia, fatigue, upper respiratory tract infection, nausea, myelosuppression	CBC, acute or delayed infusion-related reactions	Type and screen patients prior to starting treatment as daratumumab may interfere with cross-matching and red blood cell antibody screening Premedicate with corticosteroids, antipyretics, and antihistamines; administer post-infusion medications Available as subcutaneous injection in combination with hyaluronidase
Isatuximab	Myelosuppression, infusion-related reactions, hypertension, diarrhea, infection, secondary malignancies	CBC, infusion-related reactions, BP	Premedicate with acetaminophen, H1 and H2 antagonist; also administer dexamethasone prior to administration Antiviral prophylaxis recommended
Antibodies That Target CD52			
Alemtuzumab	Myelosuppression and immunosuppression, autoimmune conditions, infection, infusion-related reactions, nausea and vomiting, fever, hypotension, rash, headache, fatigue, secondary malignancies	CBC, infusion-related reactions, CMV, $CD4^+$ counts, HR, BP, autoimmune symptoms, symptoms of infection	Restricted distribution Patients should be started on antiviral and PJP prophylaxis during and for 6 months post-treatment
Antibodies That Target CD79B			
Polatuzumab vedotin	Peripheral neuropathy, infusion-related reactions, myelosuppression, infections, TLS, hepatotoxicity	CBC, symptoms of neuropathy, infusion-related reactions, uric acid levels, electrolytes, liver function	ADC with payload MMAE (a microtubule disrupting agent) Premedicate with an antihistamine and antipyretic
Antibodies That Target Chemokine Receptor			
Mogamulizumab	Dermatologic reactions, infusion-related reactions, infections, autoimmune complications, complications of allogeneic HSCT	Infusion-related reactions	Administer diphenhydramine and acetaminophen for the first infusion
Antibodies That Target GD2 Receptor			
Dinutuximab	Infections, infusion-related reactions, hypokalemia, hypotension, capillary leak syndrome, neurological ocular toxicity, pain, bone marrow suppression, hemolytic uremic syndrome	CBC, electrolytes, renal function, BP, infusion-related reactions	Premedicate with IV analgesics (such as morphine), an antihistamine, acetaminophen, antiemetics, and IV hydration
Naxitamab	Edema, hypertension, tachycardia, dermatologic toxicity, diarrhea, nausea and vomiting, headache, peripheral neuropathy, anxiety, irritability, cough, fever, infusion-related reactions	BP, HR, infusion-related reactions	Premedications and supportive medications (pain management): 5 days prior to the first infusion in each cycle, initiate a 12-day course (day-4 through day 7) of prophylactic medication for neuropathic pain (eg, gabapentin); give oral opioids 45 to 60 minutes prior to initiation of each infusion with additional IV opioids as needed for breakthrough pain during infusion; consider ketamine for pain not adequately controlled by opioids
Antibodies That Target Nectin-4			
Enfortumab vedotin	Myelosuppression, peripheral neuropathy, ocular toxicity, dermatologic toxicity, alopecia, diarrhea, dysgeusia, decreased appetite, hyperglycemia	CBC, blood glucose, liver function, Child-Pugh score	ADC with payload MMAE (a microtubule disrupting agent) Dose capped at 125 mg Avoid use in Child-Pugh classes B and C
Antibodies That Target EGFR			
Cetuximab, necitumumab, and panitumumab	Rash, paronychial cracking in fingers or toes, asthenia, abdominal pain, nausea, constipation, diarrhea, infusion and hypersensitivity reactions, electrolyte wasting, cardiopulmonary arrest	Electrolytes, infusion-related reactions, dermatologic evaluation	Dose reductions or delays may be required for rash but supportive care should be attempted first Decreased risk of infusion-related reactions with panitumumab and does not appear to be cross-reactive (ie, a patient may receive panitumumab if they react to cetuximab) Monitor patients during treatment for hypomagnesemia, hypocalcemia, and hypokalemia, and for at least 8 weeks following the completion of therapy

(*Continued*)

TABLE 149-7 Monitoring of Anticancer Drugs[a] (*Continued*)

Agent	Notable Adverse Drug Reactions	Monitoring Parameters	Comments
Antibodies That Target EGFR and MET			
Amivantamab	Pulmonary toxicity, rash, paronychia, ocular toxicity, infusion-related reactions, nausea and vomiting	Infusion-related reactions, pulmonary symptoms, dermatologic evaluations	A bispecific antibody that binds both EGFR and MET The first two infusions should be administered via peripheral line Premedication is required
Antibodies That Target HER2			
Ado-trastuzumab emtansine	Cardiac toxicity, thrombocytopenia, hemorrhage, hepatotoxicity, infusion-related reactions, peripheral neuropathy, ILD, embryo-fetal toxicity	CBC, liver function, pregnancy status, cardiac monitoring (LVEF), pulmonary symptoms	ADC with payload DM1 (a microtubule inhibitor) Ado-trastuzumab emtansine is NOT interchangeable with other antibodies that target HER2
Fam-trastuzumab deruxtecan	Myelosuppression, decrease LVEF, ILD, constipation, diarrhea, decrease appetite, nausea and vomiting	CBC, LVEF, liver function, pulmonary symptoms, fever	ADC with payload DXd (a topoisomerase I inhibitor) Fam-trastuzumab deruxtecan is NOT interchangeable with other antibodies that target HER2
Margetuximab	Alopecia, cardiac toxicity (hypertension and decrease LVEF), abdominal pain, diarrhea, nausea and vomiting, headache, fatigue, fever, infusion-related reactions	LVEF, BP, infusion-related reactions	Consider premedications (including antihistamines, corticosteroids, and antipyretics) with future cycles if a mild to moderate infusion reaction occurs
Pertuzumab	Diarrhea, nausea, alopecia, rash, neutropenia, fatigue, peripheral neuropathy, embryo-fetal toxicity, left ventricular dysfunction, infusion-related reactions	LVEF, infusion-related reactions, pregnancy status	Available in combination with trastuzumab and hyaluronidase as a single subcutaneous injection
Trastuzumab	Cardiac toxicity (congestive cardiomyopathy, usually reversible with medical management), infusion-related reactions, pulmonary toxicity, embryo-fetal toxicity	Infusion-related reactions, cardiac monitoring (LVEF)	Do not administer with anthracyclines because of increased cardiotoxicity Trastuzumab is NOT interchangeable with other antibodies that target HER2 Trastuzumab with hyaluronidase available for subcutaneous injection
Antibodies That Target SLAMF7 (Signaling Lymphocytic Activation Molecule Family 7)			
Elotuzumab	Fatigue, pyrexia, diarrhea or constipation, respiratory infections, peripheral neuropathy, hepatotoxicity, infusion-related reactions, secondary primary malignancies	Liver function, infusion-related reactions, infections	May interfere with the assay used to monitor M-protein which can impact the determination of complete response Premedicate with dexamethasone, diphenhydramine, an H2 antagonist, and acetaminophen
Antibodies That Target TROP2 (Trophoblast Cell-Surface Antigen 2)			
Sacituzumab govitecan	Myelosuppression, nausea and vomiting, alopecia, rash, abdominal pain, fatigue, hypersensitivity reaction	CBC, infusion-related reactions	ADC with payload SN-38 (a topoisomerase I inhibitor) Premedication with corticosteroids, an H1 and H2 antagonist Patients who are homozygous for the UGT1A1*28 allele are at increased risk of toxicity
Antibodies That Target VEGFR			
Bevacizumab	GI perforation, impaired wound healing, hypertension, proteinuria, thrombotic events, hemorrhage, rare reports of RPLS	BP, urine protein, neurologic examination, signs of GI perforation, symptoms of thromboembolism	Withhold 28 days prior to elective surgery. Do not administer for at least 2 weeks following a major surgical procedure and until adequate wound healing
Ramucirumab	GI perforation, impaired wound healing, hypertension, proteinuria, thyroid dysfunction, thromboembolic events, hemorrhage	BP, urine protein, thyroid function, liver function	Withhold 28 days prior to elective surgery. Do not administer for at least 2 weeks following a major surgical procedure and until adequate wound healing
Bispecific T-Cell Engagers			
Blinatumomab	Infusion-related reactions, cytokine release syndrome, neurologic toxicities, infections, fever, headache, peripheral edema, rash, TLS, hepatotoxicity, bone marrow suppression	CBC, liver function, neurological examination, uric acid levels, electrolytes	Premedicate with dexamethasone prior to the first dose of each cycle, prior to a step dose or when restarting therapy after an interruption >4 hours Administered as a continuous intravenous infusion over 28 days
Fusion Proteins			
Moxetumomab pasudotox	Renal toxicity, infusion-related reactions, electrolyte abnormalities, hemolytic uremic syndrome	Renal function, electrolytes, infusion-related reactions	Premedicate with acetaminophen, an antihistamine, and an H2 antagonist Consider low-dose aspirin on days 1-8 of each cycle

TABLE 149-7 Monitoring of Anticancer Drugs[a]

Agent	Notable Adverse Drug Reactions	Monitoring Parameters	Comments
Ziv-aflibercept	Myelosuppression, diarrhea, proteinuria, increases in liver enzymes, stomatitis, fatigue, hypertension, weight decreased, decreased appetite, epistaxis, abdominal pain, dysphonia, increased serum creatinine, headache, hemorrhage, GI perforation, compromised wound healing, arterial thromboembolic events, fistula formation	BP, urine protein, signs and symptoms of hemorrhage, CBC, liver function, renal function	Hold at least 4 weeks before elective surgery and restart at least 4 weeks after major surgery and after the surgical wound is fully healed
Immunotherapy			
Immune Checkpoint Inhibitors			
Ipilimumab	Fatigue, irAEs (eg, enterocolitis, dermatitis, endocrinopathy, hepatitis), infusion-related reactions (rare)	Thyroid function, electrolytes, liver function, renal function, dermatologic evaluations, GI symptoms, consider CBC	Treat severe irAEs with corticosteroids
Atezolizumab, avelumab, cemiplimab, dostarlimab, durvalumab, nivolumab, and pembrolizumab	Fatigue, irAEs (eg, pneumonitis, colitis, hepatitis, thyroid dysfunction)	Liver function, renal function, thyroid function, GI symptoms	Treat severe irAEs with corticosteroids For avelumab, premedicate with an antihistamine and acetaminophen prior to the first four infusions
Cytokines			
Interleukin-2	Flu-like syndrome (fevers, chills, malaise), vascular or capillary leak syndrome (hypotension, pulmonary and peripheral edema), nausea and vomiting, diarrhea, nephrotoxicity, myelosuppression (thrombocytopenia and leukopenia), bacterial infections, CNS toxicities (somnolence and confusion), arrhythmias, rash, itching	Intense monitoring required, electrolytes, liver function, renal function, CBC, thallium stress test, pulmonary function tests, cardiac monitoring during administration, BP, HR	Vasopressor support and fluid resuscitation may be necessary during treatment because of hypotension Pulmonary edema can be managed with cautious use of diuretics; short courses of albumin may also be beneficial Itching may respond to treatment with antihistamines; emollient skin creams or occlusive agents are effective for dry, peeling skin Avoid corticosteroids because they may counteract the antitumor effects of interleukin-2 Patients on beta-blockers will need to be tapered off before initiation of interleukin-2
Therapeutic Vaccines			
Sipuleucel-T	Infusion-related reactions, chills, fatigue, back pain, nausea, joint ache, headache, thromboembolic events have occurred	Infusion-related reaction	Physicians and patients must be registered Premedicate with an antihistamine and acetaminophen For autologous use only
Talimogene laherparepvec	Fatigue, chills, pyrexia, nausea, influenza-like illness, injection-site pain, cellulitis, risk of herpetic infection	Herpetic infections, injection-site complications, immune-mediated events	Administered directly into the cutaneous, subcutaneous, and/or nodal lesion(s) Precautions for accidental exposure of healthcare workers and close contacts Acyclovir and other antiviral medications may interfere with the efficacy
Chimeric Antigen Receptor (CAR) Therapies			
Axicabtagene ciloleucel, brexucabtagene autoleucel, idecabtagene vicleucel, lisocabtagene maraleucel, tisagenlecleucel	Hypersensitivity, myelosuppression, hypogammaglobulinemia, secondary malignancies, neurologic toxicities, cytokine release syndrome	CBC, infection, cytokine release syndrome, neurologic examinations	For autologous use only REMS program to mitigate the risk of cytokine release syndrome and neurological toxicities

[a]Only approximate guidelines can be given. Consult current references before dispensing as not all dose adjustments and monitoring parameters are provided in the table.

Data from Reference 59.

BP, blood pressure; CBC, complete blood count; CHF, congestive heart failure; CMV, cytomegalovirus; CPK, creatinine phosphokinase; CYP, cytochrome P450 isoenzyme; DXd, DX-8951 derivative; GI, gastrointestinal; H1 and H2, histamine 1 and 2; HCC, hepatocellular carcinoma; HHV-8, human herpes virus 8; HIV, human immunodeficiency virus; HR, heart rate; ILD, interstitial lung disease; IM, intramuscular; INR, international normalized ratio; IT, intrathecal; IV, intravenous; MAOI, monoamine oxidase inhibitor; MI, myocardial infarction; MMAE, monomethylauristatin E; PFTs, pulmonary function tests; PJP, pneumocystis jirovecii pneumonia; PML, progressive multifocal leukoencephalopathy; PPIs, proton pump inhibitors; PRES, posterior reversible encephalopathy syndrome; PT, prothrombin time; PTT, partial thromboplastin time; RPLS, reversible posterior leukoencephalopathy syndrome; SIADH, syndrome of inappropriate secretion of antidiuretic hormone; SSRI, selective serotonin reuptake inhibitor; TCA, tricyclic antidepressant.

triphosphate metabolite is incorporated into RNA as a false base and interferes with its function. The interference with both thymidine formation and RNA function contributes to its cytotoxic effects. Fluorouracil is commonly used to treat gastrointestinal tract and head-and-neck cancers.

The dosage and administration influence both the mechanism of action and toxicity profile. With continuous-infusion regimens, the inhibition of thymidylate synthesis plays a greater role, and dose-limiting toxicities include palmar-plantar erythrodysesthesia (PPE) and diarrhea. Comparatively, the incorporation into RNA plays a greater role with intermittent bolus schedules. The dose-limiting toxicity commonly associated with a bolus administration is myelosuppression.

Several pharmacologic strategies have been attempted to increase its cytotoxicity against cancer cells and decrease its toxicity to normal cells. The most common strategy combines fluorouracil with the reduced folate leucovorin. Folates increase the reduced folate pool, stabilize the monophosphate–thymidylate synthase complex, and prolong the inhibition of thymidylate synthase. Clinical trials suggest that combining reduced folates with fluorouracil provides greater anticancer activity and improves tolerability.

Dihydropyrimidine dehydrogenase (DPD) is a pyrimidine catabolic enzyme responsible for about 80% of the catabolism of fluorouracil. Reduced expression of this enzyme has been associated with drug accumulation and serious adverse drug reactions. DPD deficiency is an autosomal recessive genetic disorder, with genetic variation in the *DPYD* gene associated with reduced enzyme activity. DPD deficiency occurs in up to 5% of the overall population. Fluorouracil is contraindicated in patients with known DPD deficiency.

Capecitabine is an oral pyrimidine uracil analogue used to treat breast and colon cancers. Because capecitabine is enzymatically converted to fluorouracil, it shares the same mechanisms of action. Capecitabine is typically taken twice daily with food for the first 14 days of a 21-day treatment cycle. Since chronic twice-daily oral dosing produces sustained fluorouracil levels similar to those observed with continuous infusions, PPE and diarrhea are the dose-limiting toxicities.

Uridine triacetate is a pro-drug of uridine and competitively inhibits fluorouracil-mediated cell damage. It is approved for the emergency treatment of adult and pediatric patients following a fluorouracil or capecitabine overdose, regardless of symptoms. It is also indicated for patients who have received fluorouracil or capecitabine and exhibit early onset, severe, or life-threatening cardiac or CNS toxicity and/or early onset unusually severe adverse drug reactions within 96 hours following exposure. It is not recommended for nonemergent treatment of adverse drug reactions. The safety and efficacy have not been established when more than 96 hours have elapsed following the end of fluorouracil or capecitabine administration. Few adverse drug reactions have been reported, but the most common are vomiting, nausea, and diarrhea.

Gemcitabine Gemcitabine is a fluorine-substituted deoxycytidine analogue structurally related to cytarabine and is used to treat pancreatic cancer, NSCLC, breast cancer, and urothelial cancer. Its activation and mechanism of action are similar to those of cytarabine. Gemcitabine is incorporated into DNA, where it inhibits DNA polymerase activity. It also inhibits ribonucleotide reductase, which is the enzyme required to convert ribonucleotides into the deoxyribonucleotides needed for DNA synthesis and repair. Compared with cytarabine, gemcitabine achieves intracellular concentrations about 20 times higher, secondary to increased penetration of cell membranes and greater affinity for the activating enzyme deoxycytidine kinase. Gemcitabine that is incorporated into DNA has a prolonged intracellular half-life. Its stereoconfiguration causes another normal base pair to be added next to the fraudulent gemcitabine base pair in the DNA strand. This "masked chain termination" protects the gemcitabine from excision and elimination. Flu-like symptoms, myelosuppression, liver enzyme abnormalities, and dermatologic toxicities are commonly associated with gemcitabine.

Trifluridine and Tipiracil Trifluridine and tipiracil are combined in a molar ratio of 1:0.5 in one tablet approved for the treatment of metastatic colorectal and gastric cancers. Trifluridine is a thymidine-based nucleoside analogue, and tipiracil is a thymidine phosphorylase inhibitor. Following uptake into cancer cells, trifluridine is incorporated into DNA, interferes with DNA synthesis, and inhibits cell proliferation. Inclusion of tipiracil increases trifluridine exposure by inhibiting its metabolism by thymidine phosphorylase. The dose-limiting toxicity is myelosuppression; patients older than 65 years of age may be at greater risk. Other common toxicities include asthenia/fatigue, nausea, decreased appetite, diarrhea, vomiting, abdominal pain, and pyrexia.

Purine Analogues

Cladribine and Pentostatin Cladribine and pentostatin are purine nucleoside analogues with slightly different mechanisms of action. Both agents are used to treat hairy cell leukemia. Cladribine is resistant to inactivation by adenosine deaminase and is triphosphorylated to an active form incorporated into DNA that inhibits DNA synthesis and early chain termination. Its anticancer activity is unusual for an antimetabolite, in that it affects both actively dividing and resting cancer cells. Pentostatin is a potent inhibitor of adenosine deaminase. Adenosine deaminase is an enzyme critical in purine base metabolism and is found in high concentrations in lymphatic tissue. Both agents have immunosuppressive effects that place patients at risk for serious opportunistic infections and require the administration of prophylactic antibiotics.

Fludarabine Fludarabine is an adenine analogue used to treat chronic lymphocytic leukemia (CLL) and indolent NHL. Similar to cytarabine, fludarabine interferes with DNA polymerase, causing chain termination. Fludarabine also incorporates into RNA, resulting in inhibition of transcription. Fludarabine is immunosuppressive; it has been associated with the development of opportunistic infections, secondary to its effect on T cells and subsequent decrease in CD4 counts. It is often given as part of a conditioning regimen prior to HSCT. Prophylactic antibiotics and antiviral medications are recommended and should continue until CD4 counts normalize.

Mercaptopurine and Thioguanine 6-Mercaptopurine and its analogue thioguanine are oral antimetabolites used for the treatment of ALL. These antimetabolites are rapidly converted to ribonucleotides that inhibit purine biosynthesis or undergo purine interconversion reactions needed to supply purine precursors to synthesize nucleic acids. Clinical cross-resistance is generally observed. Both antimetabolites are metabolized by thiopurine methyltransferase (TPMT) and hypoxanthine phosphoribosyl transferase to produce multiple metabolites that contribute to the observed anticancer activity, hepatotoxicity, and myelosuppression. Additionally, nucleoside diphosphate-linked moiety X (nudix)-type motif 15 (NUDT15) catalyzes the conversion of the cytotoxic metabolite into a less toxic compound. Certain genetic alterations within the *TPMT* or *NUDT15* gene can lead to a reduction or loss of enzyme activity. Therefore, patients who are homozygous or heterozygous for a genetic alteration that affects TPMT or NUDT15 activity may experience an accumulation of toxic metabolites and an increased risk of severe myelosuppression. The Clinical Pharmacogenetics Implementation Consortium provides primary dosing recommendations for patients with *TPMT* or *NUDT15* alterations.

6-Mercaptopurine depends on xanthine oxidase for an initial oxidation step. Its metabolism is markedly decreased by coadministration with a xanthine oxidase inhibitor (eg, allopurinol), which may lead to serious adverse drug reactions. If allopurinol is given concurrently with 6-mercaptopurine to minimize TLS, the dose of 6-mercaptopurine must be reduced.

Folate Antagonists

Methotrexate Methotrexate is commonly used to treat ALL and some lymphomas. It inhibits dihydrofolate reductase (DHFR), which results in the depletion of intracellular pools of reduced folates (tetrahydrofolates) essential for thymidylate and purine synthesis. Folates are essential cofactors for DNA and RNA synthesis and, thus, lack of either thymidine or purines prevents DNA or RNA synthesis.

Chemotherapy regimens may contain low-, intermediate- or high-dose methotrexate and may incorporate methotrexate administered orally, intravenously, or intrathecally. High-dose, defined as doses greater than 500 mg/m^2/dose given intravenously as prophylaxis or treatment of CNS disease, can cause severe myelosuppression and gastrointestinal toxicity. The development of these toxicities is related to both the maximal concentrations and the time that concentrations remain above 0.02 mg/L (50 nmol/L). These effects may be neutralized by exogenously supplying reduced folates, such as leucovorin (folinic acid), which bypasses the metabolic block induced by DHFR inhibitors. Leucovorin should be administered until methotrexate levels fall below the threshold and various dosing algorithms are available. Vigorous hydration and sodium bicarbonate to alkalinize the urine should be given to decrease the risk of renal failure. Patients with third space fluids may require prolonged leucovorin rescue since these fluids influence methotrexate volume of distribution and elimination half-life.

Glucarpidase is approved for the treatment of toxic plasma methotrexate concentrations in patients with delayed methotrexate clearance because of impaired renal function. It is important to note that methotrexate concentrations within 48 hours after glucarpidase administration can only be reliably measured by chromatographic methods. Immunoassays can overestimate methotrexate concentration because of interference from metabolites.

Methotrexate is highly protein bound, and drugs such as sulfonamides, salicylates, phenytoin, and tetracyclines may displace methotrexate from albumin. Increased toxicity may be observed. Nonsteroidal anti-inflammatory drugs and vitamin C may also affect methotrexate disposition and prolong methotrexate elimination half-life. Although the exact mechanism is uncertain, proton pump inhibitors are thought to inhibit methotrexate elimination and potentially increase methotrexate toxicity.

Pemetrexed Pemetrexed is a multitargeted antifolate that is used to treat nonsquamous NSCLC and mesothelioma. It inhibits at least three biosynthetic pathways in thymidine and purine synthesis. In addition to inhibiting DHFR, it also inhibits thymidine synthase and glycinamide ribonucleotide formyltransferase, decreasing the risk of the development of drug resistance. Severe hematologic toxicity and deaths associated with neutropenic sepsis have been reported in clinical trials: elevated baseline cystathionine or homocysteine concentrations correlate with this unexpected toxicity. Routine supplementation of folic acid and vitamin B_{12} before the initiation of pemetrexed and throughout treatment reduces levels of these substances and lowers the risk of mortality related to neutropenic sepsis. Dexamethasone should be given with pemetrexed to minimize the risk of dermatologic toxicities.

Pralatrexate Pralatrexate is an antifolate drug approved for patients with relapsed or refractory peripheral T-cell lymphoma. It competitively inhibits DHFR and polyglutamylation by the enzyme folylpolyglutamyl synthetase. This inhibition results in the depletion of thymidine and other synthesis of biological molecules that depends on single carbon transfer. The most common adverse drug reactions resulting in dose reductions are pyrexia, mucositis, febrile neutropenia, sepsis, and thrombocytopenia.

Hypomethylating Agents

Azacitidine and decitabine are nucleoside analogues that demonstrate dose-dependent effects. These analogues exert their effects at lower doses by directly incorporating into DNA and inhibiting DNMT, which leads to cellular differentiation and apoptosis.[14] At higher doses, these agents might cause the formation of covalent adducts between DNMT and the active drug being incorporated into DNA, particularly in cells actively dividing. Hypomethylation also normalizes the function of genes that control cell differentiation and proliferation, promoting normal cell maturation.[14] Decitabine is also available in combination with cedazuridine, a cytidine deaminase inhibitor that impedes the degradation of decitabine and allows for improved systemic exposure following oral administration.

These inhibitors slow the progression of myelodysplastic syndrome (MDS) to AML, reduce transfusion requirements, and allow for the improvement of normal hematopoiesis over time. Azacitidine tablets are approved for the maintenance treatment of AML in patients who achieve complete remission following intensive induction chemotherapy and cannot complete intensive curative treatment. The primary toxicity is myelosuppression, particularly during early phases of treatment as the malignant clone driving the MDS is cleared from the bone marrow, and normal hematopoiesis is slowly restored. As a result, infections occur frequently.

Microtubule-Targeting Drugs

Microtubules are an integral part of the cytoskeleton and help maintain the shape of a cell. These structures are also involved in chromosome separation during mitosis and form the mitotic spindle responsible for separating chromosomes during cell replication. Several chemotherapy agents affect microtubule function, including taxanes, vinca alkaloids, epipodophyllotoxins, epitholones, and macrolides.

Taxanes

Paclitaxel and docetaxel are taxane plant alkaloids with antimitotic activity used to treat many different solid tumors. Paclitaxel and docetaxel both act by binding to tubulin, but they do not interfere with tubulin assembly. Instead, the taxanes promote microtubule assembly and interfere with microtubule disassembly. They induce tubulin polymerization, resulting in formation of inappropriately stable, nonfunctional microtubules. The stability of the microtubules damages cells by disrupting the dynamics of microtubule-dependent structures required for mitosis and other cellular functions. Taxanes also have some nonmitotic actions that can promote cancer cell death, such as inhibition of angiogenesis.

Resistance to the antitumor effects of the taxanes is attributable to alterations in tubulin or tubulin-binding sites or to P-glycoprotein (P-gp)-mediated multidrug resistance. Although paclitaxel and docetaxel have very similar mechanisms of action, cross-resistance between the two chemotherapy agents is incomplete. Myelosuppression and peripheral neuropathy frequently occur with both docetaxel and paclitaxel. Fluid retention is more common with docetaxel, and hypersensitivity reactions may be more frequent with conventional paclitaxel. Both require premedication to decrease the likelihood of hypersensitivity reactions; docetaxel's premedication also reduces fluid retention.

Two paclitaxel formulations are available. The original product (ie, conventional paclitaxel) contains Cremophor and ethanol. The subsequent product (nab-paclitaxel) contains paclitaxel bound to albumin and does not include the Cremophor excipient believed to contribute to hypersensitivity reactions. In clinical trials, nab-paclitaxel has shown comparable activity to conventional paclitaxel with a lower incidence of hypersensitivity reactions. Peripheral neuropathy remains a common adverse event with nab-paclitaxel. Nab-paclitaxel is approved for the treatment of metastatic breast cancer, NSCLC, and pancreatic cancer. The products are not interchangeable, and the doses are not comparable on a mg-to-mg basis.

Cabazitaxel is a semisynthetic derivative of docetaxel that has demonstrated anticancer activity in castrate-resistant prostate cancer that has progressed following treatment with docetaxel-based chemotherapy. Despite having the same mechanism of action, the lack of affinity for P-gp allows cabazitaxel to remain inside the cancer cells, partially accounting for its benefit in the refractory setting. Toxicities and premedications are similar to docetaxel.

Vinca Alkaloids

Vincristine, vinblastine, and vinorelbine are natural alkaloids derived from the periwinkle (vinca) plant. These agents act as mitotic inhibitors or spindle poisons. Although these alkaloids have a very similar structure, they have different activities and patterns of toxicity. These agents are used to treat different cancers. For example, vinblastine may be used to treat testicular cancer and Hodgkin lymphoma; vincristine may be used to treat NHL and Hodgkin lymphoma; and vinorelbine may be used to treat NSCLC and breast cancer. Vinorelbine and vinblastine are associated with dose-limiting myelosuppression, while vincristine is associated with dose-limiting neurotoxicity, including constipation and paralytic ileus. All vinca alkaloids are vesicants upon extravasation; local heat application allows dispersal or dilution of the alkaloid to minimize tissue damage. Vinca alkaloids should never be administered intrathecally, and accidental overdose is associated with a very high mortality rate.

Vinca alkaloids bind to tubulin and disrupt the normal balance between polymerization and depolymerization of microtubules, inhibiting the assembly of microtubules and disrupting microtubule dynamics. This interferes with the formation of the mitotic spindle and causes cells to accumulate in mitosis. These agents also disturb a variety of microtubule-related processes in cells and induce apoptosis. Resistance to the vinca alkaloids develops primarily from P-gp-mediated multidrug resistance, decreasing drug accumulation and retention within cancer cells.

Miscellaneous Antimicrotubule Agents

Eribulin is a fully synthetic antimicrotubule analogue of the macrolide halichondrin B. Eribulin inhibits tubulin polymerization by inhibiting microtubule growth, but it does not shorten or promote microtubule depolymerization. Additionally, eribulin only binds to the β-tubulin subunit and has demonstrated the ability to overcome taxane resistance conferred by β-tubulin mutations. The most common toxicities are similar to other microtubule inhibitors, but eribulin demonstrates a decreased incidence of neuropathy than vincristine and taxanes. Eribulin is approved for the treatment of metastatic breast cancer and unresectable or metastatic liposarcoma.

Ixabepilone is a synthetic epothilone approved for the treatment of metastatic breast cancer. Its binding to microtubules appears distinct from other microtubule inhibitors such as the taxanes. Thus, it has demonstrated activity in taxane-resistant cells. Dose-limiting toxicities are leukopenia and neuropathy, consistent with other microtubule inhibitors. Other toxicities include anemia, thrombocytopenia, diarrhea, myalgia, and alopecia. Premedication with antihistamines must be administered to reduce the risk of hypersensitivity reactions.

Topoisomerase Inhibitors

Topoisomerases (I and II) are essential enzymes involved in maintaining DNA topologic structure during replication. These enzymes cleave DNA strands and form intermediates with the strands during replication, producing a gap through which DNA strands can pass and then reseal the strand breaks. Topoisomerase I produces single-strand breaks, and topoisomerase II produces double-strand breaks. Several important anticancer agents interact with topoisomerase enzymes: camptothecins, anthracyclines, and podophyllotoxins.

Camptothecins

Topotecan and irinotecan, through an active metabolite SN-38, inhibit topoisomerase I enzyme activity. Topoisomerase I enzymes stabilize DNA single-strand breaks and inhibit strand resealing. Topotecan is available for oral and intravenous administration, and it is used to treat ovarian cancer and small cell lung cancer (SCLC). Irinotecan is used for the treatment of colorectal cancer and other gastrointestinal malignancies. SN-38 undergoes metabolism in part by uridine diphosphate-glucuronosyl transferase 1A1 (UGT1A1). Although variant tandem repeats in the promoter of this gene have been associated with a higher risk of diarrhea and neutropenia, genotyping has not been widely adopted in clinical practice. A starting dose reduction should be considered for patients known to be homozygous for the UGT1A1*28 allele, but specific dosing recommendations have yet to be determined. All patients receiving irinotecan are at risk of developing early and/or late diarrhea. Early diarrhea (ie, within 24 hours of irinotecan administration) is a cholinergic effect and may be prevented or treated with atropine, whereas late diarrhea is typically treated with loperamide.

In combination with fluorouracil and leucovorin, liposomal irinotecan is approved for the treatment of patients with metastatic adenocarcinoma of the pancreas whose disease has progressed following gemcitabine-based therapy. The common toxicities associated with irinotecan have been observed with liposomal irinotecan, including gastrointestinal toxicity and myelosuppression.

Anthracyclines

The anthracyclines include doxorubicin, daunorubicin (daunomycin), idarubicin, and epirubicin. These agents share a common, four-membered anthracene ring complex with an attached aglycone or sugar portion. The ring complex is a chromophore and accounts for the intense colors of these derivatives.[15] Anthracyclines are sometimes classified as antitumor antibiotics, but they have multiple mechanisms of action, including intercalation into DNA and inhibition of topoisomerase II. The production of free radicals following their metabolism may also contribute to their anticancer activity. These agents are used to treat many cancers, including leukemias, lymphomas, and multiple solid tumors.

Although the dose-limiting toxicity is myelosuppression, development of cardiomyopathy is a significant concern with these agents. All patients should have a baseline study to evaluate left ventricular ejection fraction (LVEF). Since the probability of congestive heart failure increases with the cumulative dose, a maximum cumulative dose has been suggested for each anthracycline. The relatively low level of defensive enzymes found in cardiac muscle that scavenge against oxygen-free radicals may account for the relative risk of cardiomyopathy compared to toxicity in other organs. Oxygen-free-radical formation likely contributes to extravasation injury associated with these agents, as well. When extravasated (ie, leaked from the intravascular space into the surrounding tissues), anthracyclines are vesicants known to cause significant tissue damage, including blistering and necrosis. Other common toxicities include nausea, vomiting, and alopecia. Doxorubicin also causes a red discoloration of the urine. Resistance to anthracyclines is usually secondary to P-gp-mediated multidrug resistance, but altered topoisomerase II activity may also contribute to the development of resistance.

Liposomal formulations of both doxorubicin and daunorubicin were developed to improve the safety profile of these agents while maintaining their efficacy. A liposomal combination product containing daunorubicin and cytarabine is also available in a fixed 1:5 molar ratio, which is approved for the treatment of AML.

Mitoxantrone has been identified as an anthracendione. It was synthesized to develop a chemotherapy agent with comparable antitumor activity to doxorubicin but with an improved safety profile. Similar to the anthracyclines, mitoxantrone is an intercalating topoisomerase II inhibitor, but its potential for free-radical formation is much less than that of the anthracyclines. This decreased tendency for free-radical formation may explain the reduced risks of cardiac toxicity and ulceration after extravasation. Mitoxantrone may be used with other anticancer agents to treat leukemias and lymphomas. Common toxicities include nausea, vomiting, alopecia, and blue discolored urine.

Etoposide

Etoposide is a semisynthetic podophyllotoxin derivative that binds to tubulin and interferes with microtubule formation. Etoposide also damages cancer cells by causing strand breakage through inhibition of topoisomerase II. Resistance may be caused by differences in topoisomerase II levels, increased cell ability to repair strand breaks, or increased levels of P-gp. Etoposide is cell-cycle phase-specific and arrests cells in the S or early G_2 phase. As a result, activity is much greater when administered in divided doses over several days rather than in large single doses. Etoposide may be used to treat testicular cancer and SCLC. Toxicities include dose-limiting myelosuppression, as well as nausea, vomiting, and alopecia.

Alkylating Agents

The alkylating agents are among the oldest and most widely used class of chemotherapy agents. Their clinical use evolved from the observation of myelosuppression and lymph node shrinkage in soldiers exposed to sulfur mustard gas warfare during World War I. In an effort to develop similar agents that might be useful in treating lymphomas, less reactive derivatives were synthesized. Clinical trials confirmed their anticancer activity in the mid-1940s.

All alkylating agents work by covalently bonding to highly reactive alkyl groups or substituted alkyl groups with nucleophilic groups of proteins and nucleic acids. Some agents react directly with biologic molecules, but others form an intermediate compound that reacts with these molecules. The most common binding site for alkylating agents is the seven-nitrogen group of the DNA base guanine. These covalent interactions result in cross-linking between two DNA strands or between two bases in the same DNA strand and prevent the separation of DNA strands that need to occur during replication. Reactions between DNA and RNA and between drugs and proteins may also occur. Alkylating agents are cell-cycle phase-nonspecific, but their greatest effect is seen in rapidly dividing cells.

As a class, alkylators are cytotoxic, mutagenic, teratogenic, carcinogenic, and myelosuppressive. Resistance to these chemotherapies can occur from increased DNA repair capabilities, decreased entry into or accelerated exit from cells, increased inactivation inside cells, or lack of cellular mechanisms to result in cell death after DNA damage. They are inactivated by hydrolysis, making spontaneous degradation an important component of their elimination.[16]

Nitrogen Mustards

Bendamustine Bendamustine is an alkylating agent with a benzimidazole ring that demonstrates only partial cross-resistance in vitro with other alkylating agents.[17] It is used primarily to treat lymphoid malignancies, such as CLL and NHL. Bendamustine is incompatible with polycarbonate or acrylonitrile-butadiene-styrene found in syringes and adapters and has been shown to minimize the integrity of these supplies. Typical adverse drug reactions associated with alkylating agents have been observed with bendamustine, but it appears to cause less alopecia.

Cyclophosphamide and Ifosfamide Cyclophosphamide and ifosfamide are nitrogen mustard derivatives and are widely used to treat solid tumors and hematologic malignancies. These mustards are closely related in structure, clinical use, and toxicity. Neither agent is active in its parent form and must be activated by cytochrome P450 enzymes. The cytochrome P450-mediated metabolites 4-hydroxycyclophosphamide and 4-hydroxyifosfamide are also cytotoxic compounds. Acrolein, a metabolite of cyclophosphamide and ifosfamide, has little anticancer activity but is responsible for hemorrhagic cystitis associated with ifosfamide and high-dose cyclophosphamide. Mesna is used to reduce the incidence of hemorrhagic cystitis by supplying a free thiol group that binds to and deactivates acrolein. Encephalopathy after ifosfamide can occur within 48 to 72 hours after the infusion and is generally reversible once the infusion is stopped. Methylene blue has been suggested to manage neuropathy, but data is lacking to support its routine use. The increased production of dechloroethylated metabolites after administering ifosfamide compared with cyclophosphamide may explain the increased risk of CNS toxicity associated with ifosfamide.

Melphalan Originally approved in the 1960s, melphalan is one of the oldest chemotherapy agents still used in clinical practice. It is indicated for the palliative treatment of patients with multiple myeloma and as a high-dose conditioning regimen before HSCT. Over 50 years after melphalan's approval, melphalan flufenamide became the first peptide-drug conjugate approved by the US Food and Drug Administration (FDA). The lipophilic properties of melphalan flufenamide allow for passive distribution into cells where it is hydrolyzed to melphalan.[18] Melphalan flufenamide is given in combination with dexamethasone and is approved for patients with relapsed or refractory multiple myeloma but is not indicated as part of a conditioning regimen. Serious adverse drug reactions include myelosuppression, infections, and secondary malignancies.

Nitrosoureas

Carmustine and Lomustine Carmustine and lomustine are characterized by their lipophilicity and ability to cross the blood-brain barrier; both agents are used to treat brain cancers. Carmustine is also used to treat multiple myeloma and lymphoma and in preparation for an HSCT. It is available as an intravenous preparation and a drug-impregnated biodegradable wafer for direct application to the tumor cavity after surgical resection of brain tumors. Both agents cause dose-limiting myelosuppression, but the nadir is typically delayed to 4 to 6 weeks after administration. The nitrosoureas decompose to reactive alkylating metabolites and isocyanate compounds that have several effects on reproducing cells.[19]

Nonclassic Alkylating Agents

Several other chemotherapy agents appear to act as alkylators, although their structures do not include the classic alkylating groups. These agents are capable of binding covalently to cellular components and include procarbazine, dacarbazine, temozolomide, and platinum analogues.[19]

Dacarbazine and Temozolomide Dacarbazine and temozolomide are commonly classified as triazenes and undergo demethylation to the same active intermediate (monomethyl triazeno-imidazole-carboxamide, or MTIC) that interrupts DNA replication by causing methylation of guanine. Unlike dacarbazine, temozolomide does not require the liver for activation and is chemically degraded to monomethyl triazeno-imidazole-carboxamide at physiologic pH. Both agents inhibit DNA, RNA, and protein synthesis.[19]

Important pharmacokinetic differences exist between these two agents. Dacarbazine is poorly absorbed and must be administered by intravenous infusion. Temozolomide is rapidly absorbed after oral administration; it demonstrates nearly 100% bioavailability under fasted conditions. Dacarbazine penetrates the CNS poorly, but temozolomide readily crosses the blood-brain barrier, achieving therapeutically active concentrations in cerebrospinal fluid and brain tumor tissues. Temozolomide is approved for the treatment of glioblastoma, and dacarbazine used to treat Hodgkin lymphoma. Common adverse drug reactions include nausea and vomiting, alopecia, and myelosuppression.

Platinum Analogues The platinum derivatives—cisplatin, carboplatin, and oxaliplatin—are chemotherapy agents with remarkable usefulness in cancer treatment. Recognition of cisplatin's cytotoxic activity resulted from a serendipitous observation that bacterial growth in culture was altered when an electric current was delivered to the media through platinum electrodes. The growth change was noted to be similar to that produced by alkylating agents and radiation. It was found that a platinum–chloride complex, now known as cisplatin, generated by the current was responsible for the changes. Carboplatin is a structural analogue of cisplatin in which a carboxycyclobutane moiety replaces the chloride groups of the parent compound. It shares a similar spectrum of clinical activity with cisplatin, and cross-resistance is common. Oxaliplatin is an organoplatinum compound in which the platinum is complexed with an oxalate ligand as the leaving group and to diaminocyclohexane. Its spectrum of activity differs substantially from the other platinum compounds and includes notable activity against colorectal cancers.

The cytotoxicity of the platinum derivatives depends on platinum binding to DNA and the formation of intrastrand cross-links or adducts between neighboring guanines. These intrastrand links cause a major bending of the DNA. These agents may cause cellular damage by distorting the normal DNA conformation and preventing bases normally paired from lining up with each other. Interstrand cross-links also occur.

The aquated species differ among these platinum compounds, but all of these species contribute to anticancer activity. The cytotoxic form of cisplatin is the aquated species in which hydroxyl groups or water molecules replace the two chloride groups. This reaction occurs readily in low chloride concentrations, such as the concentrations present within cells, and produces a positively charged compound that can react with DNA. The aquated species is responsible for both the efficacy and toxicity of cisplatin. Carboplatin also undergoes aquation but at a slower rate. Oxaliplatin becomes active when the oxalate ligand is displaced in physiologic solutions.[19]

Resistance to the therapeutic effects of platinum compounds may occur through several mechanisms. The ability to repair platinum-induced DNA damage may be increased, or the compounds may be inactivated by increased intracellular glutathione levels, metallothioneins, or other thiol-containing proteins. Altered uptake into cells may also affect sensitivity to platinum compounds.

The dose-limiting toxicities differ substantially among these compounds. Cisplatin can cause serious nephrotoxicity, ototoxicity, peripheral neuropathy, emesis, and anemia, but its significant anticancer activity in many tumors makes it a valuable agent despite these toxicities. Most of these toxicities can be prevented or managed with aggressive supportive care measures. Intravenous hydration, mannitol, and diuretics have been used to minimize the risk of nephrotoxicity, but it appears intravenous hydration alone is adequate. In contrast, carboplatin administration is limited by hematologic toxicity. Patients with compromised renal function require dose reductions to limit myelosuppressive toxicity. The most widely used dosage schema, the Calvert formula, uses a target area-under-the-curve and renal and nonrenal parameters to estimate the carboplatin dose. Carboplatin's potential to cause renal damage, peripheral neuropathy, and ototoxicity is much less than comparable cisplatin doses. Oxaliplatin is not nephrotoxic or ototoxic, but it can cause peripheral neuropathies and unique cold-induced neuropathies. Intravenous calcium and magnesium were commonly used to minimize the risk of neuropathy. Still these measures do not appear to decrease the risk of acute neurotoxicity or cumulative sensory neurotoxicity based on the results of a controlled trial.[20] All of the platinum derivatives have the potential to cause hypersensitivity reactions, including anaphylaxis after a threshold exposure is reached. Desensitization protocols may be successful in reestablishing tolerance to these agents.

Trabectedin and Lurbinectedin Both trabectedin and lurbinectedin (an analogue of trabectedin) are alkylating agents that bind guanine residues in the minor groove of DNA. Subsequently, adducts form and cause a bending of the DNA helix toward the major groove. Trabectedin is approved for the treatment of patients with unresectable or metastatic soft tissue sarcoma who have received a prior anthracycline-containing regimen, whereas lurbinectedin is indicated for metastatic SCLC following progression with platinum-based therapy. Warnings associated with both agents include myelosuppression, hepatotoxicity, and embryo-fetal toxicity. Additionally, trabectedin has been associated with rhabdomyolysis, cardiomyopathy, and capillary leak syndrome.

Endocrine Therapies

Endocrine therapies are perhaps the earliest successful approach to target the growth processes of cancer cells. Endocrine manipulation is an option for managing cancers in which growth is under gonadal hormonal control, such as breast, prostate, and endometrial cancers. These cancers may regress if the feeding hormone is eliminated or antagonized. Major organ system toxicity is uncommon from endocrine therapies. These therapies are discussed in detail in Chapters 151, "Breast Cancer," and 154, "Prostate Cancer."

Corticosteroids

Corticosteroids are also useful anticancer therapies because of their lymphotoxic effects. These agents are primarily used to treat hematologic malignancies and are also given in combination with chemotherapy for prostate cancer. In addition to their cytotoxic effects, corticosteroids have many other applications as part of supportive care measures and management of oncologic emergencies. Short-term corticosteroid regimens are generally well tolerated.

Therapeutic Radiopharmaceuticals

An oncology therapeutic radiopharmaceutical is an agent that contains a radionuclide and is used to treat cancer or palliate tumor-associated symptoms. Radioisotopes can emit either alpha or beta particles as their payload.[21] Alpha emitters have high energy and travel only the length of a few cell diameters resulting in double-strand DNA breaks of adjacent cells. In contrast, beta emitters have lower energy and travel the length of hundreds of cell diameters. As a result, these agents affect the cancer cells they bind and other cells within the path length of the radioisotope's emissions (ie, bystander effect). Additionally, some radioisotopes emit gamma radiation with no mass or charge and can travel further than alpha or beta particles.

Ibritumomab Tiuxetan

Ibritumomab tiuxetan is a radioimmunoconjugate that consists of the murine anticluster of differentiation (CD)20 antibody ibritumomab and a linker chelator tiuxetan that allows the attachment of yttrium-90 (active radiotherapy). This therapeutic radiation isotope selectively delivers beta particles to B-cells that express the CD20 antigen. Consequently, ibritumomab tiuxetan can induce cell death in CD20-positive and -negative cancer cells while also inducing antibody-dependent cell-mediated cytotoxicity (ADCC), complement-dependent cytotoxicity (CDC), and apoptosis. These processes are described later in the chapter. Ibritumomab tiuxetan is indicated for the treatment of low-grade or follicular B-cell NHL. The therapeutic regimen consists of two steps: rituximab is administered on day 1, and about 1 week later (day 7, 8, or 9), an additional dose of rituximab is administered, followed by yttrium-90-ibritumomab within 4 hours after completion of the rituximab infusion.

Adverse drug reactions include severe infusion-related reactions and myelosuppression. Ibritumomab tiuxetan results in prolonged thrombocytopenia and neutropenia, and dose modifications are necessary based on baseline neutrophil and platelet blood counts. The median duration of thrombocytopenia and neutropenia were 24 and 22 days, respectively. Monitoring and managing cytopenias and their complications is necessary for up to 3 months after completing treatment.

Iobenguane I 131

Iobenguane is a molecule structurally similar to norepinephrine and is therefore involved in the same uptake pathways. Labeled with I 131, this agent targets the norepinephrine transporter and is a beta emitter. Two rare tumors, pheochromocytoma and paraganglioma, express high levels of norepinephrine on their cell surfaces. When iobenguane I 131 is administered, it accumulates in these tumor cells allowing the radioisotope to cause cell death and tumor necrosis. Of note, this agent is only approved for patients with an iobenguane positive scan.

Before administration of iobenguane I 131, patients should receive thyroid-blocking medication. Additionally, medications that reduce catecholamine uptake or deplete stores should not be administered concurrently with iobenguane I 131 as they may interfere with the efficacy. The most common toxicities include myelosuppression, fatigue, hypertension, nausea, and vomiting.

Lutetium Lu 177 Dotatate

Lutetium Lu 177 dotatate is a radiolabeled somatostatin analogue that emits beta and gamma radiation and is approved for the treatment of somatostatin receptor-positive gastroenteropancreatic neuroendocrine tumors (GEP-NET). After binding to somatostatin receptor-expressing cells, such as GEP-NET cells, lutetium Lu 177 is taken up into the cell where the beta emission induces cellular damage.

Special precautions should be taken with the administration of somatostatin analogues before lutetium Lu 177. An amino acid solution must be administered before, during, and after lutetium Lu 177 to decrease reabsorption of the radiopharmaceutical through the proximal tubules, thereby reducing the radiation exposure to the kidneys. In addition, patients must be advised on minimizing exposure to contacts. Reported adverse drug reactions include increased hepatic enzymes, hyperglycemia, hypokalemia, nausea, and vomiting. Patients should also be monitored for neuroendocrine hormonal crisis.

Radium Ra 223 dichloride

Radium Ra 223 dichloride (ie, radium-223) is an alpha emitter, which is indicated for the treatment of patients with castration-resistant prostate cancer who have symptomatic bone metastases and no known visceral metastatic disease. Radium-223 mimics calcium and forms complexes with hydroxyapatite at areas of increased bone turnover, such as bone metastases. Alpha particles are then emitted, resulting in DNA breaks and an antitumor effect. Toxicities of radium-223 include bone marrow suppression, gastrointestinal adverse drug reactions, dehydration, and potentially increased risk of fractures in select patients.

Miscellaneous Agents

Arsenic Trioxide

Arsenic is an organic element and a well-known poison that is an effective treatment for acute promyelocytic leukemia, or APL. As an anticancer agent, arsenic trioxide acts as a differentiating agent, inducing the growth progression of cancer cells into mature, more normal cells. It also induces apoptosis. Notable adverse drug reactions associated with arsenic trioxide include QTc prolongation, hepatotoxicity, and differentiation syndrome. Previously known as "retinoic acid syndrome," differentiation syndrome is a potentially fatal complication of arsenic trioxide. It has been reported with other agents, including tretinoin, enasidenib, ivosidenib, and gilteritinib, which are discussed later in the chapter. This syndrome, which is thought to be caused by a rapid release of cytokines, may present with fever, difficulty breathing, edema, weight gain, and hypotension and must be rapidly treated with corticosteroids.

Asparaginase

L-Asparaginase is unique among anticancer agents in its unusual mechanism of action, source, and patterns of toxicity. It is an enzyme produced by *Escherichia coli* or *Erwinia chrysanthemi*. L-Asparagine is a nonessential amino acid that can be synthesized by most mammalian cells except cells with certain lymphoid malignancies, which have no or limited synthetase levels required for L-asparagine formation. L-Asparagine is degraded by the enzyme L-asparaginase, which depletes existing supplies and inhibits protein synthesis.

Multiple asparaginase products are commercially available. Recombinant asparaginase (*Erwinia*) is produced by fermentation of a genetically engineered *Pseudomonas* bacterium. Pegaspargase and calaspargase pegol are modified versions of L-asparagine conjugated to monomethoxypolyethylene glycol which permits a longer half-life and therefore less frequent administration. All of these products are approved to treat patients with ALL when used as part of a combination chemotherapy regimen. Additionally, recombinant asparaginase (*Erwinia*) is approved to treat patients with lymphoblastic lymphoma. Increased L-asparagine synthetase activity within cancer cells causes treatment resistance. Severe toxicities include anaphylaxis, thrombosis, pancreatitis, glucose intolerance, hemorrhage, and hepatotoxicity.

Bleomycin

Bleomycin is an antitumor antibiotic used with other anticancer agents to treat Hodgkin lymphoma and testicular cancer. It is also used for pleurodesis to prevent a pleural effusion recurrence. Bleomycin is a mixture of peptides from fungal *Streptomyces* species. Its strength is expressed in units of drug activity, and one unit is roughly equal to 1 mg of polypeptide protein. The predominant peptide is bleomycin A2, which makes up about 70% of the commercial drug product. Its cytotoxicity is secondary to DNA strand breakage, which it produces via free-radical formation. Cytotoxicity depends on the binding of the bleomycin–iron complex to DNA. The bleomycin–iron complex then reduces molecular oxygen to free oxygen radicals that cause primarily single-strand breaks in DNA. Bleomycin has greatest effect on cells in the G2 and M phases of the cell cycle.

Bleomycin is inactivated within cells by the enzyme aminohydrolase. This enzyme is widely distributed but is present in only low concentrations in the skin and the lungs, explaining the predominant toxicities of bleomycin to those sites. Therefore, baseline pulmonary function tests and monitoring for pulmonary toxicity are necessary. The risk of pulmonary toxicity increases with age over 70 years and cumulative lifetime bleomycin doses 400 units or higher. The presence of hydrolase enzymes in cancer cells is the primary mechanism of resistance to bleomycin. As a result, cells can also become resistant by repairing the DNA breaks produced by bleomycin.

Hydroxyurea

Hydroxyurea is a unique drug that inhibits ribonucleotide reductase. Cells accumulate in the S phase because DNA synthesis is inhibited, and only abnormally short DNA strands are produced. This anticancer agent was used to treat chronic myeloid leukemia (CML) because of its ability to cause a rapid decline in white blood cells.

Lanreotide

As an octapeptide analogue of somatostatin, the mechanism of lanreotide is believed to be similar to that of natural somatostatin through the inhibition of neuroendocrine functions. Somatostatin analogues are commonly used to treat hypersecretion syndromes associated with neuroendocrine tumors, but only recently have been proven to have an antitumor effect associated with prolonged progression-free survival. Lanreotide is approved for the treatment of unresectable, well or moderately differentiated, locally advanced, or metastatic GEP-NET. Common toxicities include abdominal pain, musculoskeletal pain, vomiting, headache, injection site reaction, and hypertension. In addition, patients should be monitored for hypoglycemia, hyperglycemia, and gallstones.

Mitomycin

Mitomycin, also known as mitomycin C, is a natural product classified as an antitumor antibiotic. It has similarities to nitrogen mustards and may function as an alkylating agent, although its toxicity pattern differs from conventional alkylating agents. Mitomycin may be given intravenously in combination with other chemotherapy agents to treat gastric or pancreatic cancer. When given by this route of administration, delayed myelosuppression may occur, so treatment is typically given every 6 weeks. Mitomycin may also be given as an instillation directly into the bladder (ie, intravesical instillation) for the treatment of localized bladder cancer. Additionally, a ureteral gel formulation is available, which is administered via a ureteral catheter or nephrostomy tube to treat upper tract urothelial cancer.

Omacetaxine Mepesuccinate

Omacetaxine mepesuccinate is a natural ester of the alkaloid cephalotaxine. It inhibits protein translation and thus prevents the initial elongation step of protein synthesis. It is given subcutaneously for treatment of patients with CML who have failed two or more approved therapies for this disease. Additionally, synergy with these approved therapies has been demonstrated in a few clinical studies, and additional combination trials are ongoing. Adverse drug reactions include myelosuppression, hemorrhage, and hyperglycemia.

Retinoids

Three retinoids are available to treat patients with cancer. Tretinoin (all-trans-retinoic acid), a naturally occurring derivative of vitamin A (retinol), is used to treat acute promyelocytic leukemia. Other retinoids indicated for the treatment of cancers include alitretinoin (9-cis-retinoic acid) gel for topical management of Kaposi's sarcoma lesions and bexarotene gel or capsules for treatment of cutaneous T-cell lymphoma.

Retinoids are classified as morphogens, small molecules released from one type of cell that can affect the growth and differentiation of neighboring cells. Their normal roles in the human body are to induce differentiation of some cells, stop the differentiation of others, and both suppress and induce apoptosis in different cell types. Their diverse actions come from the diversity of their receptors. The two classes of retinoid receptors are retinoid X receptors and retinoic acid receptors. Retinoid X receptors are versatile; they bind to retinoic acid receptors and to other nuclear receptors, such as thyroid hormone receptors. After being activated, the receptors act as transcription factors that regulate the expression of genes that control cellular growth and differentiation.

Tretinoin binds primarily to the retinoic acid-α receptors. Alitretinoin is considered a pan-agonist, which means that it binds to all known retinoid receptors, producing diverse regulatory effects. Bexarotene is synthetic and is classed as a rexinoid. It is the first retinoid X receptor–selective retinoid agonist.

The common adverse drug reactions differ for these three agents. Tretinoin may be associated with differentiation syndrome. Alitretinoin is associated with pain, itching, and rash, and bexarotene is associated with skin reactions, thyroid disorders, hypercholesterolemia, and hyperlipidemia.

Thalidomide, Lenalidomide, and Pomalidomide

Thalidomide, the infamous drug that caused severe limb deformities when used by pregnant individuals as a nonprescription sedative in the 1960s, is approved to treat leprosy and multiple myeloma. Thalidomide is a glutamic acid derivative and is broadly classified as an immunomodulatory drug. Lenalidomide and pomalidomide are analogues of thalidomide with similar therapeutic activity but different adverse drug reaction profiles. Lenalidomide is approved for the treatment of multiple myeloma, transfusion-dependent anemia caused by MDS with a specific mutation, follicular lymphoma, marginal zone lymphoma, and mantle cell lymphoma. Pomalidomide is approved for the treatment of multiple myeloma and Kaposi sarcoma.

These drugs have many potential mechanisms of action, but the most important is angiogenesis inhibition, which is also linked to their teratogenic effects. Other possible mechanisms include direct inhibition of cancer cells, free radical oxidative damage to DNA, interference with adhesion of cancer cells, inhibition of TNF-α production, or alteration of cytokine secretion that affects the growth of cancer cells.

The most common toxicities for thalidomide include somnolence, constipation, dizziness, orthostatic hypotension, rash, and peripheral neuropathies. In contrast, lenalidomide is associated with much less somnolence and neuropathies compared with thalidomide. Neutropenia, thrombocytopenia, and thrombotic events are common with thalidomide, lenalidomide, and pomalidomide. To avoid embryo-fetal exposure and inform healthcare professionals and patients of the teratogenic potential, these agents are only available through a risk evaluation and mitigation strategy (REMS) program.

TARGETED AGENTS: SMALL MOLECULES

6 Small-molecule targeted agents (molecular weight less than 1,000 Da) are typically identified as kinase inhibitors. Kinases are enzymatic proteins that constitute the intracellular signaling pathways, such as the JAK-STAT and MAPK/ERK pathways described earlier. Following ligand binding to an extracellular receptor, kinases transmit signals to the cell interior that stimulates activation of the pathway. The small-molecule targeted agents turn off or inhibit these pathways by inhibiting the adenosine triphosphate (ATP) binding domain of the kinases. Most of the approved kinase inhibitors inhibit more than one kinase. The binding to multiple kinases typically leads to off-target effects or toxicities; some toxicities are attributed to specific kinase families. Although most inhibitors are given orally continuously for months to years, their anticancer activity is typically limited by the development of resistance. Before initiating therapy, some targeted drugs require identification of the target within the tumor using a companion or complementary diagnostic test. Of note, most kinase inhibitors and mAbs are associated with a warning for embryo-fetal toxicity. The individual product labeling should be referenced for contraception guidelines in females of reproductive potential and males with female partners of reproductive potential.

Anaplastic Lymphoma Kinase (ALK) Inhibitors

Crizotinib

Crizotinib binds to the ATP intracellular domain of activated ALK, thereby inhibiting phosphorylation and subsequent downstream signaling. ALK rearrangements were first identified in large cell lymphomas and later in NSCLC. In NSCLC, the most common rearrangement involves inversion of chromosome 2p that is primarily fused to the echinoderm microtubule-like protein 4 (EML4), which forms the ALK-EML4 oncogene fusion protein. This rearrangement leads to the activation of downstream signaling pathways and inhibition of apoptosis. ALK-EML4 has a higher prevalence in younger patients, never or light smokers, and adenocarcinoma histology. Crizotinib also inhibits other kinases, such as ROS1, RON, and mesenchymal-epithelial transition (MET). Crizotinib is approved for the treatment of patients with metastatic NSCLC that is ALK or ROS1-positive and for ALK-positive anaplastic large cell lymphoma.

The most common toxicities reported in patients taking crizotinib include nausea, vomiting, diarrhea, constipation, fatigue, and elevated transaminases. Visual disorders occur in about half of patients and usually occur within the first weeks of therapy. Edema is also commonly seen and is most likely attributed to the inhibition of MET. Crizotinib has been associated with interstitial lung disease/pneumonitis, hepatotoxicity, QTc interval prolongation, and bradycardia.

Many patients with ALK-positive NSCLC initially respond to crizotinib. Still most patients will develop resistance possibly related to the development of brain metastases or genetic alterations in ALK. The L1196M mutation has been recently identified as a mechanism of crizotinib resistance.

Alectinib, Brigatinib, and Ceritinib

Alectinib, brigatinib, and ceritinib are second-generation ALK inhibitors approved for the treatment of patients with metastatic ALK-positive NSCLC. Similar to crizotinib, these agents inhibit autophosphorylation of ALK and subsequent downstream signaling. In addition to ALK, ceritinib also inhibits insulin-like growth factor 1 receptor, although to a lesser extent.[22]

Toxicities that are seen with both alectinib and ceritinib include fatigue, bradycardia, and hepatotoxicity. Additional adverse drug reactions seen in patients taking alectinib include anemia, constipation, edema, and myalgia. Brigatinib has been associated with pulmonary toxicities and bradycardia. Patients taking ceritinib should be monitored for QTc interval prolongation, gastrointestinal toxicity, pancreatitis, and hyperglycemia. Visual disturbances have been reported with second-generation ALK inhibitors, although to a much lesser extent. While crizotinib and brigatinib may be taken without regard to food, alectinib should be taken with food. Of note, ceritinib was previously recommended at a higher dose administered on an empty stomach, but the currently approved dose is lower and is to be taken with food to improve gastrointestinal tolerability. To decrease the risk of early onset pulmonary toxicities, a dose-escalation approach must be used with brigatinib.

Lorlatinib

A third-generation ALK and ROS1-inhibitor, lorlatinib, is approved for the treatment of ALK-positive NSCLC. It has demonstrated activity in the first-line setting and following progression on one or more ALK inhibitors.[23] Similar to other agents in this category, lorlatinib is associated with hepatotoxicity and interstitial lung disease/pneumonitis. CNS toxicities, hyperlipidemia, and atrioventricular block have also been reported.

BCL-2 Inhibitor

Venetoclax is a selective inhibitor of BCL-2, an antiapoptotic protein overexpressed in CLL. Permeabilization of the mitochondrial membrane, with the help of mediators BAX and BAK, is the last step in the apoptosis pathway. BCL-2 constrains BAX and BAK, resulting in CLL cells resistant to apoptosis.[24] Venetoclax binds directly to the BCL-2 protein restoring the apoptotic process. It is approved for the treatment of patients with CLL, small lymphocytic lymphoma, and newly diagnosed AML in adults who are unable to receive intensive induction chemotherapy (eg, age 75 years or older). Reported toxicities associated with venetoclax include myelosuppression, fatigue, diarrhea, cough, and upper respiratory tract infection. To reduce the risk of TLS, a weekly dose escalation over the first 5 weeks is required, and patients should receive antihyperuricemic agents and hydration. Oral administration of venetoclax should be with food.

Breakpoint Cluster Region-Abelson (BCR-ABL) Inhibitors

Imatinib

Imatinib is a selective inhibitor of the *bcr-abl* fusion gene, the product of the Philadelphia chromosome (Ph). The Ph chromosome is the hallmark finding of CML, and it is a translocation of genetic material between chromosomes 9 and 22. Imatinib binds to the kinase-binding site of the *bcr-abl* gene, competitively blocking access to ATP. This prevents tyrosine-kinase phosphorylation of the gene and downstream activation of cellular proliferation. An additional effect of imatinib is its ability to inhibit stem-cell factor receptor (KIT) and PDGF receptor (PDGFR).

Imatinib is a standard treatment option for newly diagnosed Ph positive (Ph^+) CML and gastrointestinal stromal tumors (GIST). A major advantage of imatinib is that it can eliminate the Ph, resulting in cytogenetic responses (ie, elimination of the genetic defect). Imatinib and other BCR-ABL inhibitors are further discussed in Chapter 158, "Chronic Leukemias." Imatinib is also approved for the treatment of Ph^+ALL and other rare diseases.

Potential serious adverse drug reactions observed with imatinib include fluid retention and rash. Severe fluid retention (ie, pleural effusion, pericardial effusion, and ascites) occurs in fewer than 10% of patients taking imatinib, but patients should be monitored regularly for early signs and symptoms of fluid retention and instructed to call their health professionals when symptoms first develop. Additionally, a rash may require early intervention because Stevens-Johnson syndrome has been reported.

Dasatinib, Nilotinib, and Bosutinib

The second-generation kinase inhibitors dasatinib, nilotinib, and bosutinib share the same binding site on the BCR-ABL kinase ATP-binding domain with imatinib. These inhibitors maintain clinical activity in patients with CML with some mutations in the BCR-ABL binding site that confer imatinib resistance. Still, none of these inhibitors are active against the genetic alteration identified as T315I. Dasatinib is approved for the treatment of Ph^+CML and Ph^+ALL. Nilotinib and bosutinib are approved for the treatment of Ph^+CML. Both bosutinib and dasatinib also inhibit a family of kinases called sarcoma kinases that are believed to mediate cellular differentiation, proliferation, and survival; sarcoma kinases have been implicated in modulating multiple oncogenic signal transduction pathways.

These second-generation agents have a toxicity profile similar to that of imatinib, with myelosuppression, nausea, vomiting, headache, and fluid retention being commonly reported. Bosutinib does not inhibit KIT or PDGFR, which may account for its reported decrease in the incidence of myelosuppression.

Ponatinib

As mentioned earlier, the T315I mutation, often referred to as the gatekeeper mutation, confers resistance to the above BCR-ABL inhibitors. Ponatinib, a third-generation agent, was developed to inhibit this mutated conformation of BCR-ABL and provide an effective treatment for this traditionally resistant tumor. Ponatinib is approved for the treatment of Ph^+ALL and Ph^+CML in patients for whom no other kinase inhibitors are indicated, such as those with a T315I mutation. Common toxicities are similar to other BCL-ABL inhibitors, such as hypertension, rash, headache, constipation, fever, and nausea. Arterial thrombosis and hepatotoxicity have also been observed.

BRAF Inhibitors

BRAF is mutated in a variety of solid tumors, with most mutations occurring at codon 600. This codon is in the activation loop of BRAF and increases downstream activity at MEK then ERK, which results in proliferation and survival of cancer cells. BRAF is altered in approximately 65% of papillary thyroid carcinomas, 35% of melanomas and anaplastic thyroid carcinomas, 11% of colorectal cancers, and 5% of NSCLC.[25] The most common BRAF mutations in melanomas are the V600E mutation, which replaces valine with glutamic acid at codon 600 (~80% of cases), and the V600K mutation, which replaces valine with lysine (~8% of cases). Dabrafenib, encorafenib, and vemurafenib inhibit BRAF V600, thereby blocking the MAPK pathway in BRAF-mutated cells.

For patients with BRAF-mutated melanoma, combination therapy with a BRAF and MEK inhibitor has been associated with improved outcomes, so doublet therapy is given in clinical practice: dabrafenib with trametinib, encorafenib with binimetinib, and vemurafenib with cobimetinib. Dabrafenib is approved for V600E and V600K mutated melanoma, V600E NSCLC, and V600E anaplastic thyroid cancer. Vemurafenib is approved for melanoma with a V600E mutation and for the treatment of Erdheim-Chester disease with a V600 mutation. Encorafenib is approved for melanoma with a V600E or V600K mutation (in combination with binimetinib) and for patients with colorectal cancer with a BRAF V600E mutation (in combination with cetuximab).

Toxicities associated with all BRAF inhibitors either as monotherapy or in combination with a MEK inhibitor include uveitis, arthralgia, fatigue, and nausea. Patients should be monitored for the development of new cutaneous malignancies and noncutaneous squamous cell carcinoma associated with the dabrafenib-, encorafenib-, and vemurafenib-induced paradoxical activation of the MAPK pathway.[26] PPE and pyrexia are commonly seen with dabrafenib, whereas QTc prolongation is more commonly reported with encorafenib and vemurafenib. Vemurafenib is also associated with severe dermatologic reactions and photosensitivity.

Bruton's Tyrosine Kinase (BTK) Inhibitors

BTK is involved in the B-cell receptor signaling pathway that leads to B-cell proliferation and differentiation upon its activation. In B-cell malignancies, the B-cell receptor signaling pathway promotes disease progression, although the exact mechanism of B-cell receptor stimulation has not been determined. The first-generation BTK inhibitor, ibrutinib, forms an irreversible covalent bond with a cysteine residue of BTK, resulting in the inhibition of malignant B-cell proliferation and survival. Ibrutinib is approved for the treatment of chronic graft-versus-host disease and the following B-cell malignancies: Waldenstrom's macroglobulinemia; mantle cell lymphoma; marginal zone lymphoma; and CLL. Acalabrutinib is approved for both CLL and mantle cell lymphoma while zanubrutinib is only approved for mantle cell lymphoma. Although the frequency of adverse drug reactions varies between BTK inhibitors, patients should generally be monitored for hemorrhage, infections, cytopenias, cardiovascular effects (eg, atrial fibrillation), and TLS. Additional common toxicities include diarrhea, fatigue, musculoskeletal pain, nausea, and rash.

CDK Inhibitors

As discussed earlier in this chapter, CDKs play an important role in cell-cycle progression. Specifically, CDK 4/6 and cyclin D1 regulate transition from the G_1 phase to the S phase by phosphorylating the retinoblastoma protein. Palbociclib, ribociclib, and abemaciclib inhibit CDK 4/6, resulting in the blockade of retinoblastoma protein hyperphosphorylation and ultimately G_1 arrest.[27] In breast cancer, it has been demonstrated that cyclin D1 expression and subsequent retinoblastoma protein phosphorylation can be maintained despite estrogen receptor (ER) antagonism. Therefore, inhibiting CDK 4/6 may overcome acquired resistance to hormonal therapy observed in ER-positive breast cancer.[27]

Palbociclib, ribociclib, and abemaciclib are approved for use in ER-positive, HER2-negative advanced, or metastatic breast cancer in combination with an aromatase inhibitor in postmenopausal patients. Additionally, palbociclib and abemaciclib are approved in combination with fulvestrant after failure of endocrine therapy, and abemaciclib is approved as monotherapy in this population following progression on endocrine therapy and chemotherapy. Patients receiving these agents should be monitored for hematologic toxicities, infections, and pulmonary embolisms. Ribociclib has been associated with concentration-dependent QTc prolongation, so electrocardiograms (ECGs) and electrolytes should be regularly monitored.

Colony-Stimulating Factor-1 Receptor Inhibitors

Tenosynovial giant cell tumors are rare malignancies that often arise from the joints, bursae, or tendon sheaths and may be associated with significant morbidity and functional limitations.[28] These tumors are characterized by the overexpression of colony-stimulating factor–1 receptor ligand that promotes cell proliferation and accumulation in the synovium. Pexidartinib inhibits colony-stimulating factor–1 receptor and is approved for the treatment of select patients with tenosynovial giant cell tumors. However, due to the severe risk of hepatotoxicity, pexidartinib is only available through a REMS program. Pexidartinib is also associated with many known drug-drug interactions.

EGFR Inhibitors

Erlotinib

Erlotinib is an oral first-generation selective EGFR kinase inhibitor. By competing with ATP for its binding site on the EGFR kinase cytosolic domain, it blocks intracellular downstream signaling and ultimately interferes with the proliferation and growth of cancer cells. Erlotinib is approved for patients with metastatic NSCLC whose tumors have EGFR exon 19 deletions or exon 21 (L858R) substitution mutations detected by an FDA-approved test. Erlotinib is also approved for use in pancreatic cancer in combination with gemcitabine.

The most common adverse drug reactions that occur with erlotinib result from the abundance of EGFR in skin and mucosa and include acneiform rash and diarrhea. Some studies suggest that the development of a rash may be predictive of a response to therapy and correlates with clinical benefit.[29] Interstitial lung disease is a rare adverse drug reaction reported in patients taking erlotinib.

Afatinib and Dacomitinib

Unlike erlotinib which reversibly binds to EGFR, afatinib and dacomitinib irreversibly block all kinases of the ErbB family by covalently binding to the intracellular kinase domain which subsequently inhibits tumor growth. Afatinib is approved for the treatment of patients with EGFR mutation-positive NSCLC and previously treated squamous NSCLC. Dacomitinib is approved for the first-line treatment of patients with metastatic NSCLC harboring an EGFR exon 19 deletion or exon 21 (L858R) substitution mutation. Adverse drug reactions observed with afatinib and dacomitinib are similar to those reported with erlotinib.

Gefitinib

Gefitinib similarly blocks the promotion of the development of lung cancer cells with specific EGFR mutations (exon 19 deletions and exon 21 substitution). It is approved for the first-line treatment of metastatic NSCLC, whose tumors harbor specific EGFR gene mutations, based on the results of a clinical trial that demonstrated an improvement in response in this specific population. Gefitinib has similar adverse drug reactions compared to other EGFR inhibitors, including diarrhea and skin reactions.

Osimertinib

Osimertinib is approved for the treatment of patients with metastatic NSCLC whose tumors harbor EGFR exon 19 deletions or exon 21 L858R mutations, as detected by an FDA-approved test. It is also indicated for EGFR T790M mutation-positive NSCLC after disease progression on or after an EGFR inhibitor. The T790M mutation, also referred to as the EGFR gatekeeper mutation, occurs in about 50% of patients who develop acquired resistance to first-line therapy with erlotinib or gefitinib.[30] Gastrointestinal and dermatologic toxicities are commonly reported with osimertinib. Serious adverse drug reactions include interstitial lung disease/pneumonitis, pneumonia, and pulmonary embolism.

Enhancer of Zest Homolog 2 (EZH2) Inhibitors

EZH2 is overexpressed or mutated in many malignancies, including follicular lymphoma and various solid tumors. Tazemetostat, a selective inhibitor of histone methyltransferase EZH2, is approved for the treatment of patients with epithelioid sarcoma. It is also indicated for patients with follicular lymphoma that is EZH2 mutation-positive or for those with no satisfactory alternative treatment options. It is commonly associated with fatigue and gastrointestinal adverse drug reactions. Secondary malignancies, including T-cell lymphoblastic lymphoma, MDS, and AML, have also been associated with the use of tazemetostat.

Fibroblast Growth Factor Receptor (FGFR) Inhibitors

The FGFR pathway regulates numerous physiological processes, including embryogenesis, wound healing, inflammation, and angiogenesis.[31] Alterations occur in approximately 7% of solid tumors, and multiple oral FGFR inhibitors are currently approved for use. Erdafitinib is a pan-FGFR inhibitor (FGFR1-4) approved for the treatment of patients with urothelial carcinoma with a susceptible FGFR3 or FGFR2 alteration. Infigratinib, also a pan-FGFR inhibitor, is indicated for the treatment of patients with cholangiocarcinoma with an FGFR2 fusion. Pemigatinib inhibits FGFR1, 2, and 3, and is approved for the treatment of patients with cholangiocarcinoma with an FGFR2 fusion. Serious ocular disorders have been reported with all agents. Interestingly, elevated phosphate levels are common with FGFR inhibitors as the FGFR pathway is involved in a sodium-dependent phosphate cotransporter in the proximal renal tubule. Monitor phosphate levels closely and adjust or hold treatment according to the guidance provided in the prescribing information.

FMS-Like Tyrosine Kinase-3 (FLT3) Inhibitors

FLT3 is one of the most common mutations in AML and is known to play a role in the normal growth and differentiation of hematopoietic precursor cells. FLT3 mutations can be divided into internal tandem duplications or point mutations of the activation loop of the tyrosine kinase domain.

Midostaurin inhibits multiple receptors, including FLT3 mutant kinases, resulting in apoptosis of leukemic cells. It is indicated in combination with cytotoxic chemotherapy for the treatment of FLT3-positive AML. Other indications include mast cell leukemia and systemic mastocytosis. Adverse drug reactions reported with midostaurin include pulmonary toxicity, febrile neutropenia, gastrointestinal toxicities, fatigue, and hyperglycemia.

Similarly, gilteritinib inhibits multiple receptors including FLT3. It is a second-generation agent indicated for the treatment of adult patients who have relapsed or refractory AML with an FLT3 mutation. Patients taking gilteritinib must be monitored for differentiation syndrome, QTc prolongation, pancreatitis, posterior reversible encephalopathy syndrome, and creatine phosphokinase elevation. Other common adverse drug reactions include edema, stomatitis, rash, and elevated serum transaminases. Both midostaurin and gilteritinib are oral agents; midostaurin should be administered with food, whereas gilteritinib may be administered without regard to food. Fedratinib is another FLT3 inhibitor but will be discussed later in the chapter with the JAK inhibitors.

HDAC Inhibitors

The mechanism of HDAC inhibitors was discussed earlier in the chapter. Belinostat is an HDAC inhibitor that is approved for the treatment of relapsed or refractory peripheral T-cell lymphoma. The most common toxicities reported with belinostat include pyrexia, nausea, fatigue, and anemia.

Panobinostat is an HDAC inhibitor that has been shown to improve progression-free survival with bortezomib and dexamethasone in patients with multiple myeloma who have received at least two prior regimens, including bortezomib and an immunomodulatory agent.[32] Since severe cardiac toxicities and QTc prolongation have been reported with panobinostat, an ECG and electrolytes should be monitored at baseline and during treatment. Nausea, vomiting, and severe diarrhea are often seen with panobinostat.

Similar to belinostat and panobinostat, romidepsin and vorinostat inhibit HDAC. Romidepsin is approved for the treatment of cutaneous or peripheral T-cell lymphoma who have received at least one prior therapy, and vorinostat is approved for patients with cutaneous T-cell lymphoma who have received at least two prior therapies. Patients receiving romidepsin should be monitored for myelosuppression, ECG changes, and infections. Reactivation of DNA viruses, including Epstein Barr virus and hepatitis B virus (HBV), have been reported with romidepsin. Additional serious adverse drug reactions reported with vorinostat include venous thromboembolism (VTE), dose-related thrombocytopenia, and anemia.

Hedgehog Inhibitors

Sonidegib, vismodegib, and glasdegib are oral inhibitors of the Hedgehog signaling pathway that is abnormally activated in basal cell carcinoma, medulloblastoma, and leukemias. Through binding to smoothened, or SMO receptor, these agents prevent downstream signaling and activation of the Hedgehog pathway leading to the inhibition of tumor growth.

The Hedgehog pathway is essential for early embryogenesis. Therefore, sonidegib, vismodegib, and glasdegib can cause embryotoxicity, fetotoxicity, and teratogenicity. The approved labeling for these drugs contains specific recommendations regarding contraception for patients of child-bearing potential and for patients with a pregnant partner or a partner of child-bearing potential, as well as limitations regarding blood and sperm donation during treatment and for several months following the last dose.

Vismodegib is approved for metastatic or locally advanced basal cell carcinoma, while sonidegib is approved only for locally advanced disease. Vismodegib is generally well tolerated, and toxicities include muscle spasm, alopecia, dysgeusia, fatigue, and nausea. Sonidegib is associated with an increased risk of serious musculoskeletal toxicities, and the probability of developing this adverse drug reaction appears to rise with increasing sonidegib exposure. Grades 3 and 4 serum lipase and creatine kinase elevations have also been reported. Sonidegib uniquely has a very long elimination half-life of 28 days compared to vismodegib and other small-molecular targeted agents.

Glasdegib is given in combination with low-dose cytarabine and is indicated for the treatment of newly diagnosed AML in patients 75 years of age or older or for those with comorbidities that preclude intensive induction chemotherapy. Similar to vismodegib and sonidegib, muscle spasms and fatigue have been reported with glasdegib. QTc prolongation may occur so ECGs and electrolytes should be monitored while on treatment.

HER2 Inhibitors

Lapatinib is a 4-anilinoquinazoline kinase inhibitor that inhibits the intracellular kinase domains of both EGFR (ErbB1) and HER2 (ErbB2). It has demonstrated clinical activity with capecitabine in patients with previously treated breast cancer whose tumors overexpress HER2. Lapatinib is also approved for use with letrozole in postmenopausal patients for the treatment of hormone receptor–positive metastatic breast cancer that overexpresses HER2. Warnings associated with lapatinib include reduced LVEF, interstitial lung disease, diarrhea, rash, and QTc prolongation in addition to a boxed warning for hepatotoxicity. Two specific mutations observed in the HLA-DQA and HLA-DRB genes have been associated with an increased risk of hepatotoxicity.[33]

In addition to EGFR and HER2, neratinib irreversibly inhibits HER4 and is approved for HER2-positive breast cancer. Diarrhea is the most common toxicity associated with neratinib, and antidiarrheal prophylaxis is recommended during the first two treatment cycles. Patients should be monitored for gastrointestinal toxicities, fatigue, dehydration, and hepatotoxicity.

Unlike lapatinib and neratinib, tucatinib is selective for HER2 inhibition but has minimal effects on EGFR. It is approved for HER2-positive breast cancer in combination with trastuzumab and capecitabine. Serious adverse drug reactions associated with tucatinib are similar to lapatinib and neratinib and include diarrhea and hepatotoxicity. Additionally, tucatinib may cause a "false" elevation in serum creatinine resulting from the inhibition of proximal tubule transporters which reduces creatinine secretion. This increase in serum creatinine does not affect glomerular filtration and is reversible upon treatment discontinuation.

IDH Inhibitors

As discussed earlier in the chapter, IDH mutations are associated with impaired cellular differentiation in about 15% to 20% of patients with AML. Ivosidenib and enasidenib are approved for the treatment of AML with a susceptible IDH1 or IDH2 mutation, respectively. Nausea, vomiting, diarrhea, and elevated serum bilirubin have been reported with enasidenib. Common toxicities associated with ivosidenib include nausea, mucositis, rash, and leukocytosis. Warnings for ivosidenib include QTc prolongation and Guillain-Barré syndrome. Differentiation syndrome, as discussed above with arsenic trioxide, is a potentially fatal complication associated with both IDH inhibitors.

JAK Inhibitors

Ruxolitinib is an oral inhibitor of JAK1 and JAK2 of the JAK-STAT signaling pathway; these kinases are involved in the regulation of blood and immunologic functioning. In myelofibrosis and polycythemia vera, JAK1 and JAK2 activity is dysregulated. Ruxolitinib has been shown to modulate the affected JAK1 and JAK2 activity resulting in clinical responses and symptomatic improvement. Approved indications for ruxolitinib include the treatment of intermediate- or high-risk myelofibrosis and the treatment of polycythemia vera in patients who have had an inadequate response to or are intolerant of hydroxyurea. It is also approved for acute, corticosteroid-refractory graft-versus-host disease. The most common toxicities include thrombocytopenia, anemia, bruising, dizziness, and headache. Caution must be used when stopping ruxolitinib as severe cases of withdrawal syndrome have been reported.

While ruxolitinib inhibits both JAK1 and JAK2, fedratinib has a higher affinity for JAK2. Fedratinib is approved for myelofibrosis. The product labeling includes a boxed warning for encephalopathy so thiamine should be assessed and repleted at baseline and periodically throughout treatment. Additional adverse drug reactions associated with fedratinib include hematologic toxicities, gastrointestinal toxicities, and hepatotoxicity.

MEK Inhibitors

Reported resistance mechanisms of the BRAF inhibitors dabrafenib, encorafenib, and vemurafenib include reactivation of the MAPK pathway. The combination of BRAF and MEK inhibition has demonstrated delayed resistance in melanoma and decreased incidence of secondary cancers. MEK inhibitors, including binimetinib, cobimetinib, and trametinib, are given in combination with a BRAF inhibitor, and their indications in BRAF V600 mutated tumors are discussed above. Severe toxicities associated with MEK inhibitors include cardiomyopathy and hemorrhage. Rhabdomyolysis and hepatotoxicity have been reported with binimetinib and cobimetinib. Additionally, VTE and interstitial lung disease have been associated with binimetinib and trametinib.

Unlike the other agents in this class, selumetinib has not demonstrated success in early trials with BRAF-mutated tumors. However, selumetinib has shown tumor shrinkage and clinical benefit in children with neurofibromatosis type 1, a rare genetic disorder associated with peripheral-nerve sheath tumors known as plexiform neurofibromas.[34] Inhibition of MEK has proven successful since overactivation of the RAS pathway has been associated with neurofibromatosis type 1. Common toxicities are similar to other MEK inhibitors and include nausea, vomiting, diarrhea, increased creatine phosphokinase, rash, and paronychia. Interestingly, selumetinib capsules contain vitamin E, and, therefore, its use comes with a warning regarding increased vitamin E levels and risk of bleeding.

MET Inhibitors

The MET gene is a proto-oncogene associated with tumor cell growth and survival. MET Exon 14 skipping results in aberrant downstream signaling from the MET receptor resulting in tumor invasion, migration, and metastasis. Alterations in MET are reported in approximately 3% of solid tumors, including NSCLC. Both capmatinib and tepotinib inhibit the MET signaling pathway and are approved for patients with NSCLC harboring a MET Exon 14 skipping alteration. Hepatotoxicity and interstitial lung disease have been reported in clinical trials with capmatinib and tepotinib. Additionally, capmatinib has been associated with photosensitivity so patients should be instructed to limit ultraviolet exposure during treatment.

mTOR Inhibitors

Temsirolimus and its primary active metabolite, sirolimus, bind to the intracellular protein 12-kilodalton FK506 binding protein 12 and this protein-drug complex inhibits mTOR by blocking its kinase activity. mTOR inhibition suppresses the production of proteins that regulate progression through the cell cycle resulting in G_1-phase arrest. Temsirolimus is administered via IV infusion and is approved for the treatment of advanced renal cell carcinoma.

The most common adverse drug reactions with temsirolimus are rash, asthenia, mucositis, nausea, edema, and anorexia. Infusion reactions may occur and pretreatment with an antihistamine is recommended. Metabolic abnormalities are common with temsirolimus, including hyperglycemia and hyperlipidemia. Rare but potentially serious toxicities include interstitial lung disease, immunosuppression, and renal failure.

Similar to temsirolimus, everolimus is an mTOR inhibitor that reduces protein synthesis and cell proliferation by binding to FK506 binding protein 12. Everolimus is administered orally and has the following indications: advanced renal cell carcinoma; hormone receptor–positive, HER2-negative breast cancer with exemestane in postmenopausal patients; subependymal giant cell astrocytoma with tubular sclerosis complex; renal angiomyolipoma with tubular sclerosis complex; and pancreatic, gastrointestinal, and lung neuroendocrine tumors. Dosage forms for everolimus include traditional oral tablets and tablets for oral suspension, but it is important to note that the indications differ depending on formulation. Stomatitis is one of the most common toxicities with everolimus, and other adverse drug reactions are similar to those of temsirolimus.

Nuclear Export Inhibitor

Selinexor is a first-in-class nuclear export inhibitor approved for patients with treatment-refractory diffuse large B-cell lymphoma and multiple myeloma. Through binding to exportin-1, selinexor inhibits nuclear export resulting in the retention of tumor suppressor proteins in the nucleus and the prevention of oncoprotein messenger RNA translation.[35] Exportin-1 is overexpressed in many cancer cells and has been associated with the development of resistance to anticancer agents.

Patients receiving selinexor should be monitored for thrombocytopenia, neutropenia, gastrointestinal toxicities, and hyponatremia. Additionally, infections are commonly reported and may include upper respiratory infection, pneumonia, and sepsis. Patients should be counseled on the potential neurotoxicity associated with selinexor, which may include syncope, hallucinations, amnesia, and mental status changes, among others.

PARP Inhibitors

PARP is essential for the repair of single-stranded DNA breaks through the base-excision-repair pathway. Tumors with breast cancer gene 1 (*BRCA1*) or *BRCA2* mutations are highly sensitive to the accumulation of single-strand DNA breaks because they exhibit a compromised ability to repair double-strand DNA breaks. Typically, double-strand DNA breaks are repaired through the homologous recombination repair pathway which involves proteins such as *BRCA1* and *BRCA2*. When tumors have deficiencies in homologous recombination repair (through a *BRCA* or other mutation), they lack the ability to repair DNA damage and are therefore more susceptible to the effects of PARP inhibition. This concept is known as *synthetic lethality* and occurs when there is a lethal synergy between two nonlethal events.[2] Four PARP inhibitors are currently available and their corresponding FDA-approved indications are as follows: niraparib is approved for ovarian, fallopian tube, or primary peritoneal cancers; olaparib is approved for *BRCA*-mutated, HER2-negative breast cancer, *BRCA*-mutated ovarian cancer, homologous recombination deficient-positive ovarian cancer, *BRCA*-mutated pancreatic cancer, and homologous recombination repair gene-mutated prostate cancer; rucaparib is approved for *BRCA*-mutated ovarian cancer and *BRCA*-mutated prostate cancer; and talazoparib is approved for *BRCA*-mutated, HER2-negative locally advanced or metastatic breast cancer.

As a class, these agents are commonly associated with anemia, fatigue, and nausea. Secondary malignancies of MDS/AML have been reported. Similar to tucatinib described earlier in the chapter, olaparib and rucaparib are commonly associated with a "false" elevation in serum creatinine. Niraparib is more often associated with thrombocytopenia and hypertension, whereas transaminase elevation is most commonly seen with rucaparib and talazoparib. Talazoparib is also associated with myelosuppression.

PDGFR-α Inhibitors

PDGFR-α belongs to a family of growth factors that act as mitogens (peptides that induce cell division) for cells of mesenchymal origin and is a hallmark of GIST. Signaling of this pathway results in differentiation, growth, and angiogenesis. Ripretinib and avapritinib are oral PDGFR-α inhibitors. Ripretinib is approved for the treatment of refractory GIST and avapritinib is approved for the treatment of GIST harboring a PDGFR-α Exon 18 mutation and advanced systemic mastocytosis. In addition to inhibiting PDGFR, ripretinib also inhibits BRAF and VEGFR, which are reflected in its toxicity profile. Ripretinib has been associated with cutaneous malignancies (including squamous cell carcinoma and melanoma), hypertension, cardiac dysfunction, PPE, and impaired wound healing. Warnings for avapritinib include intracranial hemorrhage and CNS effects.

PI3K Inhibitors

Malignant B-cell proliferation and survival depend on PI3K signaling. The p110δ isoform is highly expressed in malignant lymphoid B-cells and plays a direct role in activation of the PI3K pathway. The four PI3K inhibitors that are approved for hematologic indications have different affinities for the PI3K isoforms: idelalisib primarily inhibits p110δ; duvelisib inhibits p110δ and p110γ; copanlisib preferentially targets p110α and p110δ; and umbralisib primarily targets p110δ.[36,37] Idelalisib is an oral agent approved for the treatment of relapsed CLL (in combination with rituximab), follicular B-cell NHL, and small lymphocytic lymphoma. Duvelisib is an oral agent indicated for relapsed or refractory CLL, small lymphocytic lymphoma, and follicular lymphoma. Copanlisib, the only intravenously administered PI3K inhibitor, is indicated for relapsed follicular lymphoma. Umbralisib, the most recently approved oral PI3K inhibitor, also inhibits casein kinase 1 epsilon (thought to be involved in the pathogenesis of lymphoid malignancies) and is indicated for the treatment of relapsed or refractory follicular lymphoma and marginal zone lymphoma. In solid tumors, mutations in the p110α subunit of PI3K result in dysregulation of the PI3K/mTOR pathway.[38] Alpelisib, an oral PI3Kα-selective inhibitor, is the only PI3K inhibitor approved for the treatment of a solid tumor: PI3KCA-mutated, hormone receptor–positive, HER2-negative breast cancer (in combination with fulvestrant).

Serious adverse drug reactions are associated with these agents. Duvelisib has a REMS program to increase awareness and mitigate the risks of infections, diarrhea/colitis, cutaneous reactions, and pneumonitis. Similarly, idelalisib has a REMS program for hepatotoxicity, diarrhea/colitis, pneumonitis, and intestinal perforation. *P. jirovecii* pneumonia prophylaxis should be administered during treatment with duvelisib, idelalisib, umbralisib, and considered for patients receiving copanlisib. Antiviral prophylaxis to prevent cytomegalovirus infection should also be considered in select patients. Both alpelisib and copanlisib have been associated with hyperglycemia. Serious hypertension, including infusion-related hypertension, has been commonly reported with copanlisib. Umbralisib holds a warning for allergic-type reactions due to Yellow No. 5 which is contained in the dosage form.

Proteasome Inhibitors

The proteasome is an enzyme complex that is responsible for degrading proteins that control the cell cycle. Some of the proteins degraded by proteasomes regulate critical functions for cancer growth, such as regulation of the cell cycle, transcription factors, apoptosis, angiogenesis, and cell adhesion.

Bortezomib reversibly inhibits the 26S proteasome resulting in accumulation of IκB, an inhibitor of the major transcription factor nuclear factor κB (NF-κB). NF-κB induces transcription of genes that block cell death pathways and promote cell proliferation. Its activity depends on its release from its inhibitory partner protein, IκB, in the cytoplasm and its move to the nucleus. When IκB fails to degrade, through the actions of bortezomib, NF-κB remains in the cytoplasm, preventing it from transcribing the genes that promote cancer growth. Bortezomib is approved for the treatment of multiple myeloma and mantle cell lymphoma.

The most commonly reported toxicities with bortezomib include fatigue, nausea, diarrhea, thrombocytopenia, and fever. Peripheral neuropathy may develop or worsen with the use of bortezomib. Subcutaneous administration of bortezomib has been associated with a lower incidence of severe peripheral neuropathy when compared with intravenous administration. Caution should be used when treating patients with existing heart disease as cardiac failure has been reported. Patients should also be monitored for hypotension and acute respiratory syndrome. At least 72 hours should elapse between consecutive doses of bortezomib to minimize cumulative toxicity by permitting the restoration of proteasome function between doses. Proteasome inhibitors are associated with herpes reactivation so antiviral prophylaxis should be considered.

Carfilzomib is a second-generation, irreversible inhibitor of the 20S proteasome and is approved for relapsed or refractory multiple myeloma. As a result of its irreversible inhibition, carfilzomib produces more sustained inhibition of the proteasome. Carfilzomib is a more potent and selective inhibitor of the chymotrypsin-like activity of the proteasome and immunoproteasome and has demonstrated the ability to overcome bortezomib resistance in cell lines. Compared to bortezomib, carfilzomib is associated with a lower incidence of peripheral neuropathy, but serious cardiovascular and renal adverse drug reactions have been reported.

Ixazomib is an oral 20S proteasome inhibitor approved with lenalidomide and dexamethasone for the treatment of patients with multiple myeloma. Common adverse drug reactions are gastrointestinal toxicity, thrombocytopenia, peripheral neuropathy, peripheral edema, and back pain. Ixazomib has a unique administration schedule for an oral agent (given on days 1, 8, and 15 of a 28-day cycle) and should be taken on an empty stomach.

Ras Inhibitors

The Kirsten ras (KRAS) oncogene is the most prevalent genomic driver in NSCLC and activating mutations occur in 25% to 30% of nonsquamous NSCLC tumors.[39] In response to extracellular stimuli, KRAS cycles between active guanosine triphosphate-bound and inactive guanosine diphosphate-bound states. The KRAS G12C mutation is the most frequent KRAS variant and, when present, favors active guanosine triphosphate resulting in increased cell signaling. Sotorasib binds to the switch II region only found on the inactive configuration, locking it in the inactive state and preventing downstream activation.[39] Patients taking sotorasib should be monitored for hepatotoxicity and interstitial lung disease. Common adverse drug reactions include diarrhea, musculoskeletal pain, fatigue, and cough.

Rearranged During Transfection (RET) Inhibitors

RET is a proto-oncogene with downstream signaling pathways of MAPK and PI3K-AKT. Activating mutations are associated with medullary thyroid cancer, and oncogenic kinase fusions have been discovered in NSCLC. Pralsetinib and selpercatinib are both oral RET inhibitors approved for the treatment of the following RET fusion-positive solid tumors: metastatic NSCLC; advanced or metastatic medullary thyroid cancer; and advanced or metastatic thyroid cancer refractory to radioactive iodine.

Although approved for the same indications, pralsetinib and selpercatinib have different off-target effects: pralsetinib inhibits FLT3, JAK1-2, VEGFR, PDGFR, and FGFR, whereas selpercatinib inhibits VEGFR and FGFR. Their toxicity profile is reflective of their inhibition of VEGFR. Notably, more hematologic adverse drug reactions have been reported with pralsetinib. Selpercatinib has been associated with concentration-dependent QTc prolongation, which is not common with pralsetinib.

Tropomyosin Receptor Kinase (TRK) Inhibitors

Chromosomal rearrangements involving in-frame fusions of neurotrophic tyrosine receptor kinase (*NTRK*) genes with various partners can result in constitutively activated chimeric TRK fusion proteins that can act as oncogenic drivers. Larotrectinib is an inhibitor of TRK proteins and has received a tissue/site agnostic approval. It is indicated for the treatment of adult and pediatric patients with solid tumors that have an *NTRK*-gene fusion. Adverse drug reactions include fatigue, nausea, dizziness, vomiting, transaminitis, cough, constipation, and diarrhea. Warnings with larotrectinib include neurotoxicity and hepatotoxicity.

Similar to larotrectinib, entrectinib is a TRK inhibitor approved for the treatment of solid tumors with an *NTRK*-gene fusion. Entrectinib also inhibits ROS1 and ALK and is indicated for the treatment of ROS1-positive NSCLC. Patients receiving entrectinib should be monitored for cardiac toxicities (including QTc prolongation), CNS effects, fractures, hepatotoxicity, hyperuricemia, and vision disorders.

VEGFR Multikinase Inhibitors

Most small-molecule kinase inhibitors are promiscuous; significant off-target activity is associated with these agents due to the inhibition of multiple kinases. The oral multikinase inhibitors described in this section all inhibit VEGFR and, thus, angiogenesis. However, their activity and adverse drug reaction profile may differ because of off-target effects. Inhibiting downstream signaling from the VEGFR results in class toxicities, including hypertension, proteinuria, wound healing complications, bleeding, VTE, and gastrointestinal perforations/fistulas. Hypertension must be well-controlled prior to therapy initiation. Additionally, patients with recent serious cardiovascular events (eg, myocardial infarction), hemorrhage, or gastrointestinal perforation/fistula should avoid VEGFR inhibitors. Due to altered wound healing, VEGFR inhibitors should be held before elective surgery and after major surgery until adequate wound healing.

Sorafenib and Sunitinib

First-generation inhibitors, sunitinib and sorafenib, inhibit multiple growth factor receptors (eg, VEGFR-2 and PDGFR), cell surface proteins (eg, KIT), and cytokine receptors (eg, FLT3), and, thus, disrupt multiple aberrant intracellular signaling pathways. In addition, sorafenib inhibits Raf, which is part of the MAPK signaling pathway. Sunitinib is approved for GIST, pancreatic neuroendocrine tumors, and renal cell carcinoma; and sorafenib is approved for unresectable hepatocellular carcinoma, advanced renal cell carcinoma, and differentiated thyroid carcinoma refractory to radioactive iodine treatment.

In addition to the traditional VEGFR inhibitor toxicities listed above, sunitinib is uniquely associated with a yellow discoloration of the skin or hair which is related to the yellow color of the active drug. Although this adverse drug reaction is benign, patients who develop a yellowing of the skin must be evaluated for hepatotoxicity which has also been reported with sunitinib.

Axitinib, Pazopanib, and Tivozanib

The next-generation inhibitors axitinib, pazopanib, and tivozanib inhibit VEGFR-1, -2, -3, KIT, and PDGFR. However, axitinib and tivozanib have enhanced potency and selectivity to all VEGFR kinases with minor activity against PDGFR and KIT. All three agents are indicated for the treatment of advanced renal cell carcinoma. Pazopanib has an additional indication for the treatment of patients with advanced soft tissue sarcoma who have received prior chemotherapy.

Cabozantinib

Cabozantinib is a small-molecule inhibitor of numerous receptor kinases, most importantly RET, VEGFR-2, and MET. As described earlier, MET is required for several important processes during embryogenesis (eg, angiogenesis) and leads to abnormal growth and proliferation of several tumors. Medullary thyroid cancers express mutated RET as well as VEGFR-2 and MET. Cabozantinib is approved for the treatment of metastatic medullary thyroid cancer, renal cell carcinoma, and hepatocellular carcinoma. Toxicities reported in clinical trials include diarrhea, PPE, electrolyte abnormalities, transaminitis, and stomatitis. Of note, cabozantinib is available as both an oral capsule and tablet, which are not bioequivalent and therefore not interchangeable.

Lenvatinib

Lenvatinib primarily inhibits VEGFR-1, -2, and -3, but it can also inhibit other kinases including FGFR, PDGFR, KIT, and RET. Lenvatinib is approved for the following indications: as a single agent for the treatment of radioactive iodine-refractory differentiated thyroid cancer; as a single agent for the treatment of unresectable hepatocellular carcinoma; in combination with everolimus for the treatment of renal cell carcinoma; and in combination with pembrolizumab for patients with advanced endometrial carcinoma. Common toxicities seen with lenvatinib include fatigue, diarrhea, stomatitis, and PPE.

Regorafenib

Regorafenib is a multikinase inhibitor that blocks the activity of several protein kinases, including those involved in the regulation of tumor angiogenesis (VEGFR-1, -2, and -3), oncogenes and downstream targets (KIT, RET, RAF1, and BRAF), as well as PDGFR and FGFR. Many of these targets are important in gastrointestinal carcinomas, and regorafenib has demonstrated activity in these tumors. FDA-approved indications include colorectal cancer, GIST, and hepatocellular carcinoma. Serious adverse drug reactions reported with regorafenib include hepatotoxicity and reversible posterior leukoencephalopathy syndrome. Common adverse drug reactions with regorafenib include asthenia, mucositis, gastrointestinal toxicities, and PPE. To improve tolerability, a weekly dose-escalation strategy has been proposed.[40] Regorafenib should be given orally with a low-fat evening meal, as the toxicities appear minimized when given at night.

Vandetanib

Vandetanib is a small-molecule inhibitor of RET, VEGFR-2 and -3, and EGFR. It is approved for the treatment of metastatic medullary thyroid cancer. Toxicities observed with vandetanib include diarrhea and rash. Vandetanib can prolong the QTc interval, and cases of Torsades de pointes and sudden death have been reported. Because of this risk, vandetanib is only available through a REMS program where prescribers and pharmacies must be certified through the program before prescribing or dispensing vandetanib.

TARGETED AGENTS: ANTIBODIES

7 Biologic therapies are a diverse group of agents that include cytokines, mAbs, and growth factors. Biologics are generally large and complex molecules that are manufactured in a microorganism or other living system. The mAb is the most common biologic therapy available to treat patients with solid tumors and hematologic malignancies.

Biosimilars

Due to the complex process associated with manufacturing biologics, "generic" biologic products are not approved in the same manner as small-molecule pharmaceuticals. Unlike generic small-molecule agents that must demonstrate bioequivalence to a branded product, biosimilars must be "highly similar" to the reference product. Biosimilars must demonstrate that no clinically meaningful differences in safety, purity, and potency exist between it and the reference product. Some biosimilar agents undergo additional evaluation and testing to meet the requirements of an "interchangeable product." An interchangeable product is expected to produce the same clinical result as the reference product and can generally be substituted without consulting the prescriber.[41] Of note, some institutions have a therapeutic interchange list that permits substitutions of biosimilars based on policies developed by the local Pharmacy and Therapeutics Committee.

Monoclonal Antibodies

A mAb is designed to target a pathway critical for the survival and proliferation of cancer cells resulting in selective destruction of the malignant cells while minimizing toxicities to healthy tissues. The mAb can bind to either the extracellular receptor or its natural ligand and prevent the activation of downstream intracellular signaling. Additionally, some immunotherapies (eg, immune checkpoint inhibitors) are mAbs that target a specific pathway to allow for immune activation.

Each mAb consists of immunoglobulin sequences that are known to recognize a specific antigen or protein on the surface of cells. There are five classes of immunoglobulins, but IgG is the most commonly used therapeutically. Similar to endogenous antibodies, the Fab portion is composed of heavy and light chains that are responsible for binding to antigens, and the constant region determines the effector function of the antibody. The mAb may be naked (unconjugated) or conjugated to a toxin (immunotoxin), chemotherapy agent (antibody-drug conjugate [ADC]), or radioactive particle (radioimmunoconjugate).

In 2017, the standard nomenclature for mAbs was revised. As before, mAbs receive a random prefix, an infix indicating the target, and the suffix "-mab." However, the prior requirement to include the source (ie, -o-, -u-, -xi-, and -zu- to indicate murine, human, chimeric, and humanized, respectively) has been removed. The nonproprietary name of a mAb consists of a core name (eg, trastuzumab) and a distinguishing suffix composed of four lowercase letters (eg, trastuzumab-dkst). If the product is conjugated, a separate word is added to identify the toxin, chemotherapy, or radioactive particle. For example, the ADC ado-trastuzumab emtansine consists of the mAb trastuzumab plus emtansine which identifies the name of the cytotoxic payload and linker. The prefix "ado" was added to reduce the potential for confusion between the ADC and the unconjugated mAb.

The first mAbs used in humans were murine, but most of the antibodies used today are humanized or human. These agents differ in the amount of foreign component. Hypersensitivity and infusion-related reactions, with or without the development of antiproduct antibodies, are generally greatest with murine antibodies and least with humanized antibodies. The severity of these reactions can range from mild (eg, fever, chills, nausea, and rash) to severe, life-threatening anaphylaxis with cardiopulmonary collapse. Patients with a hypersensitivity or infusion-related reaction may also experience chest or back pain during the infusion. Patients with circulating cancer cells in the bloodstream are at highest risk for more severe reactions. Patients must be monitored closely during infusion. The reactions tend to be more severe with the initial few treatments and subside with subsequent infusions. Some mAbs require premedication, including antihistamines, acetaminophen, or corticosteroids, to minimize hypersensitivity reactions. Recommended infusion rates may be longer for the initial dose, with incremental increases as tolerated. For patients experiencing signs or symptoms of infusion-related reactions, the infusion should be interrupted, and prompt treatment with antihistamines, corticosteroids, and other supportive measures should be initiated. Other adverse drug reactions are typically determined by the selectivity of the target antigen. mAbs against antigens found on normal and cancer cells are expected to have increased toxicity compared with tumor-specific antigens found only on malignant tissues.

Unconjugated mAbs that target antigens on the cell surface of cancer cells may induce death of cancer cells by several mechanisms. These mAbs could directly mediate cell killing through CDC, ADCC, or inhibiting intracellular signaling. CDC occurs when the Fc portion of the antibody activates the complement system, leading to tumor cell lysis. ADCC occurs when effector cells that contain Fc receptors bind to the Fc portion of the antibody and either lyses or phagocytizes the antibody-containing cell. Natural killer cells, monocytes, and macrophages are all capable of mediating ADCC. Finally, antibody binding may result in the transmission of signals that induce apoptosis or programmed cell death in the targeted cell.

Immunoconjugates deliver a payload, typically a chemotherapy agent, toxin, or radioactive particle to a cell targeted by the antibody. After the antibody binds the target antigen, the payload is internalized by the target cell and kills cancer cells through traditional mechanisms of action. In addition to killing the target cell, radioimmunoconjugates are capable of killing antigen-negative cancer cells, sometimes termed the "bystander effect." Theoretically, immunoconjugates deliver therapy to specific sites of disease while limiting systemic exposure to the chemotherapy, radiation, or toxin. The mAb might also contribute to the observed anticancer effects.

Antibody-Drug Conjugates

ADCs were developed to exploit the selectivity and binding properties of mAbs to deliver cytotoxic chemotherapy directly to the targeted cell. These agents consist of three components: the antibody, the linker, and the cytotoxic payload. To cause cancer cell death, the antibody must first bind to the target antigen, and then the complex must be internalized into the cell through receptor-mediated endocytosis. The antibody-drug complex is then degraded, the cytotoxic payload is released, and cancer cell death occurs. Theoretical benefits of conjugates are a result of the delivery of cytotoxic chemotherapy directly to the target site resulting in decreased toxicity.

Antibodies That Target B-Cell Maturation Antigen

The B-cell maturation antigen, or BCMA, is overexpressed on multiple myeloma cells and is thought to play a role in cell survival. Belantamab mafodotin, an ADC that targets B-cell maturation antigen, is approved for the treatment of multiple myeloma. Monomethyl auristatin phenylalanine is a microtubule-disrupting agent that is attached via a linker to the mAb. Belantamab mafodotin is available through a REMS program to manage the risk of ocular toxicity and it requires registration of patients and providers. Severe vision loss, corneal ulcer, blurred vision, and dry eye have been associated with belantamab mafodotin. Although the mechanism of ocular toxicity is still under investigation, it is theorized that an uptake of the ADC into the corneal epithelial tissue may be the culprit.[42] Other common toxicities include thrombocytopenia and infusion-related reactions.

Antibodies That Target CD19

The CD19 antigen is a cell surface protein expressed on B-cell lymphocytes and B-cell malignancies. Overexpression leads to tumor cell proliferation. Destruction of CD19-expressing malignant cells may be accomplished through a bispecific T-cell engager (eg, blinatumomab) or through CAR T-cell therapy (eg, axicabtagene ciloleucel, brexucabtagene autoleucel, lisocabtagene maraleucel, tisagenlecleucel) which are discussed later in the chapter.

Tafasitamab is a humanized mAb that targets CD19 and mediates ADCC, antibody-dependent cellular phagocytosis, and direct cytotoxicity.[43] It has demonstrated synergistic activity in combination with lenalidomide and is approved for the treatment of relapsed or refractory diffuse large B-cell lymphoma in patients who are not eligible for autologous HSCT. Patients receiving tafasitamab should be monitored for infusion-related reactions, myelosuppression, and infections.

Loncastuximab tesirine is an ADC-targeting CD19, and the cytotoxic payload is an alkylating agent (SG3199). It is approved for the treatment of patients with large B-cell lymphoma. Patients receiving loncastuximab tesirine must be monitored for effusions and edema, myelosuppression, infections, and cutaneous reactions. Photosensitivity reactions have also been reported so patients should be counseled to minimize or avoid exposure to sunlight.

Antibodies That Target CD20

Rituximab

Rituximab is a chimeric antibody directed against the CD20 antigen found on the surface of normal and cancerous B-cells. The Fab domain of rituximab binds to the CD20 antigen on B lymphocytes and the Fc domain recruits immune effector functions to mediate B-cell lysis. The mechanisms of its anticancer effect include CDC and ADCC of malignant B-cells and possibly a direct apoptotic effect.

Rituximab is approved for the treatment of low-grade or follicular, CD20-positive, B-cell NHL in multiple settings and for the treatment of CD20-positive CLL with standard chemotherapy. Rituximab is also indicated for the treatment of a variety of immune-mediated diseases, including rheumatoid arthritis, granulomatosis with polyangiitis, and microscopic polyangiitis. It is administered as an intravenous infusion.

Infusion-related reactions associated with rituximab primarily occur during the first infusion and are components of an infusion-related complex secondary to the amount of circulating B-cells. After the first infusion, the incidence and the severity of these reactions decrease dramatically. Premedication and additional supportive care medications may be required depending on indication. The most common reactions with the infusion-related complex are transient fever, chills, nausea, asthenia, and headache. Additionally, rituximab and other mAbs targeting CD20 may cause HBV reactivation and should not be administered in patients with severe, active infections.

Rituximab is also available in combination with hyaluronidase, which is administered via subcutaneous injection. When mAbs are administered subcutaneously, hyaluronidase is a necessary component because it degrades hyaluronan and allows for a more permeable extracellular matrix providing greater diffusion capacity and bioavailability of the mAb. All patients must receive at least one full dose of a rituximab product by intravenous infusion without experiencing severe adverse drug reactions before starting treatment with rituximab/hyaluronidase. The combination product is approved for follicular lymphoma, diffuse large B-cell lymphoma, and CLL.

Obinutuzumab

Obinutuzumab is a type II humanized anti-CD20 mAb approved for CLL and follicular lymphoma. When compared with the type I anti-CD20 antibodies such as rituximab, type II agents exhibit a different elbow hinge angle and therefore bind CD20 in a different orientation. Furthermore, the Fc portion of obinutuzumab has been glycoengineered to reduce fucosylation resulting in improved receptor affinity and enhanced ADCC potency.[44]

Adverse drug reactions associated with obinutuzumab include infusion-related reactions, myelosuppression, nausea, and diarrhea. HBV reactivation and progressive multifocal leukoencephalopathy have also been reported with obinutuzumab.

Ofatumumab

Ofatumumab is a type I human mAb that also targets the CD20 antigen. Its mechanism of action is similar to that of rituximab, but ofatumumab targets a different epitope than rituximab, has greater affinity for the antigen, and dissociates from the epitope slower than rituximab. Specifically, ofatumumab binds to two regions of the CD20 antigen, the small extracellular loop and the N-terminal region of the large extracellular loop. As a result, anticancer activity has been demonstrated in patients who have progressed on rituximab in a variety of B-cell cancers. Ofatumumab is approved for the treatment of CLL. Adverse drug reactions are similar to rituximab with fewer infusion-related reactions and a higher rate of infectious complications.

Antibodies That Target CD22

CD22 is expressed on over 90% of leukemic blasts in patients with B-cell ALL. Inotuzumab ozogamicin is an ADC-targeting CD22 on B-cells. This agent consists of an IgG4 antibody linked to calicheamicin (an antitumor antibiotic) and is approved for the treatment of relapsed or refractory B-cell precursor ALL in adults. Prescribing information for inotuzumab ozogamicin warns of the risk for increased post-HSCT nonrelapse mortality rate. Potentially severe toxicities include hepatotoxicity, myelosuppression, infusion-related reactions, and QTc prolongation.

Antibodies That Target CD30

Brentuximab vedotin is an ADC that targets the CD30 antigen found on cancer cells. Upon binding to the CD30 antigen, brentuximab vedotin is internalized by endocytosis and the dipeptide bond that links the naked mAb to the chemotherapy monomethylauristatin E (also known as MMAE) is cleaved. Monomethylauristatin E then binds to microtubules and acts as an inhibitor of microtubule polymerization. It may also induce apoptosis by inhibiting NF-κB. Brentuximab vedotin is indicated for Hodgkin lymphoma, anaplastic large cell lymphoma, peripheral T-cell lymphoma, and mycosis fungoides. Infusion-related reactions, peripheral neuropathy, and neutropenia are common toxicities seen with brentuximab vedotin administration; these toxicities are common with other microtubule inhibitors.

Antibodies That Target CD33

Consisting of an IgG4 kappa antibody linked to a calicheamicin derivative, gemtuzumab ozogamicin is an ADC-targeting CD33, which is expressed on leukemic cells in AML. Gemtuzumab ozogamicin has a unique approval history. In 2000, gemtuzumab ozogamicin received an accelerated approval for the treatment of patients with AML but was removed from the market soon thereafter due to lack of benefit and excessive toxicity. However, since then, multiple studies have been completed using a modified dosing scheme resulting in the reapproval of gemtuzumab ozogamicin for the treatment of CD33-positive AML. Warnings associated with the use of this agent include hepatotoxicity (including veno-occlusive disease), infusion-related reactions, and hemorrhage. Other common toxicities are infection, fever, nausea, vomiting, constipation, headache, rash, and mucositis.

Antibodies That Target CD38

Daratumumab is a mAb that inhibits CD38-expressing tumor cells by inducing apoptosis directly through Fc-mediated cross-linking and immune-mediated tumor cell lysis through CDC, ADCC, and antibody-dependent cellular phagocytosis. Myeloid-derived suppressor cells and a subset of regulatory T-cells express CD38. Daratumumab is administered as an intravenous infusion and is also available in combination with hyaluronidase for subcutaneous injection. Both formulations are approved for the treatment of patients with multiple myeloma and are typically given in combination with other anticancer agents.

The most frequently reported adverse drug reactions are infusion-related reactions, fatigue, nausea, back pain, pyrexia, cough, upper respiratory tract infection, and myelosuppression. Premedications (corticosteroid, antipyretic, and an antihistamine) and a postinfusion medication (corticosteroid) are recommended to prevent acute and delayed infusion reactions. Daratumumab interferes with blood bank cross-matching by binding to CD38 on red blood cells possibly resulting in a positive indirect Coombs test. It is therefore recommended that a type and screen be performed prior to treatment initiation. If a blood transfusion is necessary, inform the blood bank that the patient has received daratumumab.

Isatuximab is a mAb-targeting CD38 that is indicated for the treatment of multiple myeloma in combination with dexamethasone and either pomalidomide or carfilzomib. Warnings associated with isatuximab are similar to those with daratumumab including infusion-related reactions and a false-positive indirect Coombs test. Additionally, patients receiving isatuximab are at risk of developing a second primary malignancy, such as skin cancer. In one study, the overall incidence of a second primary malignancy was 3.9% in patients receiving isatuximab, pomalidomide, and dexamethasone versus 0.7% in patients receiving only pomalidomide and dexamethasone.[45]

Daratumumab, isatuximab, and all other mAbs approved for the treatment of multiple myeloma (regardless of target) are associated with a warning for interference with the M-protein assay which is used for the clinical monitoring of patients with multiple myeloma. The interference is related to the assay being unable to distinguish between M-proteins and mAbs.

Antibodies That Target CD52

Alemtuzumab is a recombinant humanized mAb that is directed against CD52. CD52 is expressed on the surface of B and T lymphocytes, natural killer cells, monocytes, and macrophages. Its anticancer activity comes from binding to the CD52 antigen present on leukemic lymphocytes and inducing cell lysis and death. Alemtuzumab is indicated as a single agent for the treatment of B-cell CLL.

Alemtuzumab is associated with severe infusion-related reactions, hematologic toxicity, and opportunistic infections. Hematologic toxicity consisting of severe prolonged neutropenia and thrombocytopenia occurs in most patients. Health professionals should monitor complete blood counts before each dose to determine the need for dose modification. Since CD52 is expressed on lymphocytes, alemtuzumab can induce profound lymphopenia including a decrease in CD4 and CD8 counts. Patients should receive prophylaxis for *Pneumocystis jirovecii* pneumonia and herpes virus, which should be continued for a minimum of 2 months after completing alemtuzumab therapy or until recovery of CD4 counts. Alemtuzumab is only available through a restricted distribution program that allows access for patients deemed appropriate for treatment.

Antibodies That Target CD79B

While CD79B is present on the surface of most malignant B-cells, its expression on mature B-cells is restricted, thus making it an attractive target.[46] Polatuzumab vedotin is an ADC consisting of monomethylauristatin E conjugated to an anti-CD79B mAb. It is given in combination with bendamustine and rituximab for the treatment of diffuse large B-cell lymphoma. Toxicities include peripheral neuropathy, infusion-related reactions requiring premedications, myelosuppression, infections, multifocal leukoencephalopathy, TLS, and hepatotoxicity.

Antibodies That Target Chemokine Receptor

Mogamulizumab is a recombinant humanized IgG1 kappa mAb that targets CC chemokine receptor 4–expressing cells. CC chemokine receptors are a subfamily of chemokine receptors that possess four cysteine residues; chemokines are chemoattractants that facilitate the migration of cells. CC chemokine receptor 4 is involved in the trafficking of lymphocytes to various organs. Mogamulizumab is indicated for relapsed or refractory mycosis fungoides or Sézary syndrome. The most common adverse drug reactions are rash, infusion-related reactions, fatigue, diarrhea, musculoskeletal pain, and upper respiratory tract infection.

Antibodies That Target GD2

Glycolipid GD2 is expressed primarily on the cell surface of neuroblastoma cells and on normal tissues, including neurons and peripheral sensory nerve fibers.[47] The function of the GD2 carbohydrate antigen is not completely understood, but it is thought to play a role in the attachment of tumor cells to extracellular matrix proteins.[47] Dinutuximab is a chimeric mAb that binds GD2, thereby inducing cell lysis through ADCC and CDC. This activity is thought to be enhanced when dinutuximab is given with granulocyte-macrophage colony-stimulating factor (GM-CSF) and interleukin-2. Dinutuximab is approved to be given with GM-CSF, interleukin-2, and 13-cis-retinoic acid for the treatment of pediatric patients with high-risk neuroblastoma. Serious toxicities associated with dinutuximab include infusion-related reactions and neurotoxicities. Patients should be monitored for infections, hypokalemia, hypotension, and capillary leak syndrome. Severe neuropathic pain occurs in most patients and intravenous opioids are required prior to, during, and immediately following administration.

Similar to dinutuximab, naxitamab binds to cell surface GD2 and induces ADCC and CDC. Naxitamab is indicated in combination with GM-CSF for the treatment of pediatric and adult patients with high-risk neuroblastoma. Serious toxicities include infusion-related reactions, neurotoxicity, and hypertension. To manage severe neuropathic pain, patients should receive a 12-day course of a neuropathic pain medication (eg, gabapentin) starting 4 days before initiation in addition to opioids before the start of the infusion.

Antibodies That Target Nectin-4

Using the microtubule-disrupting agent monomethylauristatin E as its payload, enfortumab vedotin is an ADC-targeting nectin-4 that is approved for the treatment of urothelial carcinoma. Nectin-4 is an adhesion protein on cell surfaces that is highly expressed in urothelial cancer and also reported in breast, lung, and pancreatic cancer. Serious adverse drug reactions associated with enfortumab vedotin include skin reactions, peripheral neuropathy, hyperglycemia, and ocular disorders. Patients, particularly those with diabetes mellitus, should monitor blood glucose levels closely, and enfortumab vedotin should be held if blood glucose is greater than 250 mg/dL (13.9 mmol/L). Patients should be monitored for vision changes, and prophylactic artificial tears may be considered for dry eyes.

Antibodies That Target EGFR

Cetuximab

Cetuximab is a chimeric mAb that binds specifically to the extracellular domain of EGFR on both normal and cancer cells, and competitively inhibits the binding of epidermal growth factor and other ligands, such as transforming growth factor-α. Binding of cetuximab to the EGFR inhibits cell growth, induces apoptosis, and inhibits VEGF production. Cetuximab is indicated for the treatment of metastatic KRAS wild-type (ie, without mutation) colorectal cancer and for squamous cell head-and-neck cancer. Acneiform rash and skin reactions occur in most patients receiving cetuximab, as observed with other agents that inhibit EGFR. Multiple follicular or pustular lesions generally appear within the first 2 weeks of therapy and usually resolve after cessation of treatment. Resolution can be slow, continuing beyond 28 days in nearly half of cases. In patients who develop a severe rash, dose modifications may be necessary. Interestingly, a trend for improved responses with increasing severity of skin reactions has been suggested but additional research is required to confirm this association.[29]

Additionally, patients receiving cetuximab should be monitored for other serious adverse drug reactions including infusion-related reactions and electrolyte abnormalities. Hypomagnesemia may be severe and can occur within days or months after treatment. Cardiopulmonary arrest and sudden death have also been reported.

Panitumumab

Panitumumab, the first human mAb approved to treat cancer, is an IgG2 antibody that binds to the cell surface EGFR. It is approved to treat RAS wild-type metastatic colon cancer. Adverse drug reactions are similar to cetuximab, although severe infusion-related reactions appear to be less common because panitumumab does not have a murine component.

Both cetuximab and panitumumab are more effective in patients with tumors that are RAS wild-type compared to tumors that are RAS mutation-positive. Therefore, patients with metastatic colorectal cancer should not receive anti-EGFR antibody therapy if a RAS mutation is detected. Genetic testing of colorectal cancers is discussed in further detail in Chapter 153, "Colorectal Cancer."

Necitumumab

Necitumumab is a next-generation mAb that binds to the human EGFR and blocks the binding of EGFR to its ligands. It is approved for the treatment of patients with metastatic *squamous* NSCLC in combination with gemcitabine and cisplatin. Serious and clinically significant adverse drug reactions include cardiopulmonary arrest, hypomagnesemia, thromboembolic events, dermatologic toxicities, and infusion reactions. Since increased toxicity and mortality was observed when necitumumab was given with pemetrexed and cisplatin for the treatment of nonsquamous NSCLC, patients with metastatic nonsquamous NSCLC should not receive necitumumab.

Antibodies That Target EGFR and MET

Amivantamab is a bispecific antibody that binds both EGFR and MET. It is approved for the treatment of patients with NSCLC that harbors an EGFR exon 20 insertion mutation. These mutations are associated with de novo EGFR inhibitor resistance and a poor patient prognosis.[48] Due to the high incidence of amivantamab infusion-related reactions, the prescribing information recommends premedications and peripheral administration of the first two infusions. Other serious adverse drug reactions include interstitial lung disease, dermatologic toxicities, and ocular toxicities.

Antibodies That Target HER2

HER2-Targeting mAbs

Trastuzumab is a humanized mAb that selectively binds to HER2. HER2 is overexpressed in about 33% of breast cancers, in about 22% of gastroesophageal junction and gastric cancers, and to varying degrees in other malignancies. Trastuzumab inhibits cell-cycle progression by decreasing cells entering the S phase of the cell cycle, which leads to downregulation of HER2 receptors on cancer cells and decreased cell proliferation. Trastuzumab also leads to ADCC and CDC and directly induces apoptosis in cells overexpressing HER2. In addition, synergy between trastuzumab and chemotherapy has been demonstrated, resulting in trastuzumab often being used in combination regimens. Trastuzumab is administered via intravenous infusion and is approved for the treatment of HER2-positive breast cancer and metastatic gastric or gastroesophageal junction adenocarcinoma. The tumor should overexpress HER2 as measured by diagnostic tests that can quantify gene amplification or protein expression. Additionally, a trastuzumab and hyaluronidase subcutaneous injection formulation has been approved for the treatment of HER2-positive breast cancer.

The most serious adverse drug reactions associated with trastuzumab include cardiomyopathy, hypersensitivity reactions, and increased myelosuppression. An evaluation of cardiac function should be performed before administration and extreme caution should be exercised in patients with preexisting cardiac dysfunction and in those who have received prior anthracyclines. In patients who develop a clinically significant decrease in LVEF (defined as greater than 16% decrease in ejection fraction from pretreatment levels or an ejection fraction below normal limits and greater than 10% decrease from baseline), discontinuation of therapy should be considered. Myelosuppression is infrequent with trastuzumab alone, but the incidence of neutropenia and febrile neutropenia is higher when trastuzumab is given with myelosuppressive chemotherapy.

Pertuzumab is a humanized mAb that targets the HER2 receptor. It is synergistic with trastuzumab and is effective in tumors that have developed resistance to trastuzumab. Pertuzumab binds to the extracellular domain II of HER2, a site distinct from trastuzumab, and inhibits its ligand-dependent HER2–HER3 dimerization, which subsequently decreases tumor proliferation and resistance pathways. Dual targeting of the HER2 receptor allows for increased efficacy against variant forms of the HER2 receptor, including truncated HER2 receptors. Similar to trastuzumab, it appears to induce ADCC in cancer cells. Pertuzumab is approved to treat HER2-overexpressed breast cancer in combination with trastuzumab and chemotherapy. Warnings and precautions are similar to those of trastuzumab, including a boxed warning for cardiotoxicity.

Because pertuzumab and trastuzumab are often administered as part of the same regimen in clinical practice, a subcutaneous formulation of these agents in combination with hyaluronidase was developed for the treatment of breast cancer. Warnings associated with this agent include cardiomyopathy, pulmonary toxicity, exacerbation of chemotherapy-induced neutropenia, and administration-related reactions.

Margetuximab, another HER mAb, binds to the same extracellular domain of HER2 as trastuzumab, but has a modified Fc region. The modified Fc is thought to allow for increased binding to the activating receptor and decreased binding to the inhibitory receptor, thus leading to greater ADCC compared to trastuzumab.[49] Margetuximab is approved for the treatment of HER2-positive metastatic breast cancer in combination with chemotherapy in patients who have received two or more prior anti-HER2 regimens. Similar to other agents in this class, the margetuximab product labeling contains a warning for left ventricular dysfunction.

HER2-Targeting ADCs

Ado-trastuzumab emtansine (sometimes referred to as T-DM1) is indicated for the treatment of HER2-positive breast cancer, whereas fam-trastuzumab deruxtecan is approved for the treatment of patients with HER2-positive breast cancer and gastric cancer. Ado-trastuzumab emtansine is an ADC that consists of the humanized anti-HER2 mAb trastuzumab covalently linked to the microtubule inhibitory drug derivative of maytansine 1. The adverse drug reactions associated with ado-trastuzumab emtansine are similar to those reported with trastuzumab and microtubule inhibitors.

Fam-trastuzumab deruxtecan is an ADC that consists of an anti-HER2 mAb covalently linked to DX-8951 derivative, a topoisomerase I inhibitor. Warnings on the product labeling include pneumonitis, neutropenia, and left ventricular dysfunction. Unlike most ADCs, nausea and vomiting are common with fam-trastuzumab deruxtecan, and it is associated with a moderate emetic risk. It is important to note that ado-trastuzumab emtansine, fam-trastuzumab deruxtecan, and trastuzumab are not interchangeable and should not be substituted for one another.

Monoclonal Antibodies That Target Signaling Lymphocytic Activation Molecule Family 7 (SLAMF7)

Elotuzumab is an IgG mAb directed against SLAMF7. SLAMF7 is expressed on multiple myeloma cells, natural killer cells, and other immune cells. The antitumor effects of elotuzumab are a result of ADCC and through blocking multiple myeloma and stromal cell interaction but it is not thought to induce CDC.[50] Elotuzumab is approved in combination with lenalidomide and dexamethasone for the treatment of patients with multiple myeloma. The most common adverse drug reactions reported include fatigue, diarrhea, constipation, pyrexia, peripheral neuropathy, decreased appetite, cough, and respiratory infections. Patients should also be monitored for infusion-related reactions, infections, second primary malignancies, and hepatotoxicity.

Antibodies That Target Trophoblast Cell-Surface Antigen 2 (TROP2)

Sacituzumab govitecan is an ADC-targeting TROP2, which is a transmembrane calcium signal transducer overexpressed in many epithelial cancers. The cytotoxic payload of sacituzumab govitecan is SN-38 which, as described above, is the active metabolite of the topoisomerase I inhibitor irinotecan. Therefore, precautions and adverse drug reactions are similar between these agents. Boxed warnings for sacituzumab govitecan include neutropenia and diarrhea. The management strategy for diarrhea is similar to that of irinotecan: atropine is used for acute diarrhea, whereas loperamide is the best option for delayed diarrhea. Patients homozygous for the UGT1A1*28 allele are at increased risk of neutropenia, febrile neutropenia, and anemia. Sacituzumab govitecan is approved for the treatment of triple negative breast cancer and urothelial carcinoma.

Antibodies That Target VEGF

Bevacizumab

Bevacizumab is a humanized mAb directed against circulating VEGF. It binds to all biologically active circulating isoforms of VEGF and prevents the activation and promotion of angiogenesis. Bevacizumab is approved for the treatment of patients with multiple types of solid tumors including the following: cervical cancer; colorectal cancer; glioblastoma; nonsquamous NSCLC; ovarian, fallopian tube, or primary peritoneal cancer; and renal cell carcinoma. A bevacizumab biosimilar, bevacizumab-awwb, was the first biosimilar approved for the treatment of cancer.

Several serious adverse drug reactions have been associated with bevacizumab, including hypertension, bleeding, and thrombotic events. Hypertension is more common in patients with a history of uncontrolled blood pressure, and it responds to oral antihypertensive medications. Although the most common bleeding episodes are transient epistaxis, fatal CNS and gastrointestinal hemorrhages have been reported. The product labeling includes warnings regarding the risk of gastrointestinal perforation, wound dehiscence, and hemorrhage. Bevacizumab is not recommended for use within 28 days of major surgery and patients should be instructed to report abdominal pain (an initial sign of gastrointestinal hemorrhage) to their health professionals immediately. Paradoxically, bevacizumab also has been associated with thrombotic events, including deep vein thrombosis, pulmonary embolism, and myocardial infarction, especially in elderly patients with a history of cardiac events. Another potentially serious adverse drug reaction associated with bevacizumab is proteinuria/nephrotic syndrome, and patients should be monitored for the development or worsening of proteinuria with serial urine dipsticks.

Ramucirumab

Ramucirumab is a human mAb that binds to VEGFR-2 resulting in the inhibition of ligand-induced proliferation. While bevacizumab binds the circulating ligand (ie, VEGF), ramucirumab inhibits angiogenesis through the specific blockade of VEGFR-2. Ramucirumab is approved for the treatment of advanced gastric or gastroesophageal junction adenocarcinoma as a single agent or with paclitaxel. Other indications include the following: treatment of metastatic NSCLC in combination with erlotinib or docetaxel; treatment of hepatocellular carcinoma in patients who have an AFP of ≥400 ng/mL (mcg/L) following treatment with sorafenib; and for the treatment of metastatic colorectal cancer in the second-line setting. When administered as a single agent, the most common toxicities associated with ramucirumab are hypertension and diarrhea. Patients should also be monitored for thromboembolic events, hypertension, proteinuria, and thyroid dysfunction.

Bispecific T-Cell Engagers

Blinatumomab is a bispecific T-cell engaging antibody directed against a B-lymphocyte-specific molecule CD19. Through the formation of a synapse, blinatumomab serves as a linker between CD19 on malignant B-cells and CD3 on T-cells, thereby potentiating T-cell–induced cytotoxic cell killing. Blinatumomab is indicated for the treatment of CD19-positive B-cell precursor ALL.

Due to its short half-life (~2 hours) and mechanism of action, blinatumomab is administered as a continuous intravenous infusion over 28 days. In addition to possible decreased efficacy, early trials that utilized shorter infusion durations also reported a higher rate of neurologic toxicities and cytokine release syndrome (CRS). Patients receiving blinatumomab are usually hospitalized for initiation of cycles 1 and 2 to monitor for infusion-related reactions. Patients should also be monitored for CRS, neurological toxicities, and infections. Other common adverse drug reactions include fever, headache, peripheral edema, and rash.

Fusion Proteins

Moxetumomab pasudotox is a CD-22-directed cytotoxin that is composed of a recombinant murine immunoglobulin variable domain fused to a truncated form of *Pseudomonas* exotoxin. It is approved for the treatment of relapsed or refractory hairy cell leukemia. The most common adverse drug reactions include infusion-related reactions, edema, nausea, headache, pyrexia, constipation, anemia, and diarrhea. Most patients develop anti-moxetumomab binding and neutralizing antibodies.

Ziv-aflibercept is a soluble recombinant fusion protein that was designed to block multiple signals that stimulate the angiogenic process. It was developed by fusing sections of the VEGFR-1 and VEGFR-2 immunoglobulin domains to the Fc portion of human IgG1. Ziv-aflibercept blocks VEGFA, VEGFB, and phosphatidylinositol-glycan biosynthesis class F by "trapping" the ligands before they get to the native transmembrane receptors and thus decreasing pro-angiogenic signaling and tumor growth. It is approved with chemotherapy for resistant or progressive metastatic colorectal cancer and has toxicities similar to other anti-VEGF therapies.

IMMUNOTHERAPY

Immune Checkpoint Inhibitors

8 As discussed earlier in the chapter, immune checkpoint inhibitors (including PD-1, PD-L1, and CTLA-4 inhibitors) reverse immune down-regulation, thereby unleashing T-cells to eliminate malignant cells. PD-L1 is overexpressed on multiple types of tumors, and it has been suggested that PD-L1 expression is associated with increased tumor aggressiveness. Unlike cytotoxic chemotherapy, which can elicit cell death immediately after administration, immune checkpoint inhibitors may have a slower onset based on their inherent mechanism of action. Furthermore, durable responses are more common with checkpoint inhibitors compared to cytotoxic chemotherapy as immune activation against the tumor may continue months after administration. Given their potential to activate the immune system, immune-related adverse events (irAEs) may occur. Immune checkpoint inhibitors should be avoided in patients with underlying autoimmune conditions or a history of transplant—see more details in Chapter 150 "Supportive Care."

CTLA-4 Inhibitor

Ipilimumab is a human mAb that blocks CTLA-4 and was the first FDA-approved immune checkpoint inhibitor. CTLA-4 acts as a negative regulator of T-cell function, decreasing the ability of the immune system to mount an antitumor response. By binding to CTLA-4, ipilimumab allows for enhanced T-cell stimulation, proliferation, and antitumor activity. Based on its ability to produce an enhanced immune response, ipilimumab has been associated with several severe and fatal irAEs including enterocolitis, hepatitis, dermatitis, neuropathies, and endocrinopathies. Infusion-related reactions may occur. Ipilimumab is often administered in combination with nivolumab and is indicated for the treatment of MSI-H or dMMR colorectal cancer, melanoma, NSCLC, mesothelioma, hepatocellular carcinoma, and renal cell carcinoma.

PD-1 Inhibitors

As described earlier in the chapter, PD-1 inhibitors bind to the PD-1 receptor and block the interaction of its ligand resulting in the restoration of T-cell activity. The toxicity profile of all four medications in this class is similar and includes fatigue and irAEs, Common irAEs include dermatologic conditions and endocrine dysfunction. Patients should also be monitored for potentially fatal irAEs including colitis, pneumonitis, nephritis, hepatitis, myocarditis, and neurologic events.

Cemiplimab is a recombinant human IgG4 mAb approved for the treatment of advanced cutaneous squamous cell carcinoma, basal cell carcinoma, and NSCLC. Dostarlimab is a humanized IgG4 mAb approved for the treatment of dMMR recurrent or advanced endometrial cancer.

Nivolumab and pembrolizumab are IgG4 mAbs approved for Hodgkin lymphoma and for the treatment of numerous solid tumors. Both agents were originally studied in patients with metastatic cancer, but their use is now expanding to earlier in the disease course (eg, adjuvant setting). Depending on the indication, these agents may be given alone or in combination with chemotherapy or targeted therapy. Additionally, nivolumab is approved to be given in combination with ipilimumab, as described above.

Pembrolizumab received the FDA's first tissue/site agnostic approval for the treatment of MSI-H or dMMR solid tumors. It is also approved for tumor mutational burden-high cancer (≥10 mutations/megabase) in patients who have progressed following prior treatment and have no satisfactory alternate options. Tumor mutational burden is a measure of somatic mutations in a tumor and may help identify patients that may benefit from immunotherapy.[51]

PD-L1 Inhibitors

Unlike the PD-1 inhibitors which bind to the receptor, PD-L1 inhibitors bind to the associated ligand resulting in immune activation. Since PD-1 and PD-L1 inhibitors target the same pathway, adverse drug reactions and monitoring are the same.

Atezolizumab is an IgG1 mAb indicated for the treatment of SCLC, triple-negative breast cancer, NSCLC, hepatocellular carcinoma, melanoma, and urothelial carcinoma. Durvalumab, a human IgG1 mAb, is approved for patients with NSCLC and SCLC. Avelumab is a human IgG1 mAb approved for the treatment of Merkel cell carcinoma, urothelial carcinoma, and in combination with axitinib for renal cell carcinoma.

Unlike the other PD-L1 inhibitors, infusion-related reactions are common with avelumab, and premedications are required prior to the first four infusions at minimum. The development of antidrug antibodies has been shown to reduce avelumab exposure, and exploratory analyses suggest that the development of these antidrug antibodies may reduce the effectiveness in some populations. The development of antidrug antibodies does not appear to affect the incidence or severity of adverse drug reactions.

Cytokines

Interleukin-2 (Aldesleukin)

Interleukin-2 is a cytokine produced by recombinant DNA technology that promotes B- and T-cell proliferation and differentiation and initiates a cytokine cascade with multiple interacting immunologic effects. The interleukin-2 receptor is expressed in increased amounts on activated T-cells and mediates most of the effects of aldesleukin. Anticancer activity depends on proliferation of cytotoxic immune cells that can recognize and destroy cancer cells without damaging normal cells. Some of these cytotoxic cells are natural killer cells, lymphokine-activated killer cells, and tumor-infiltrating lymphocytes. Aldesleukin is approved for the treatment of metastatic renal cell carcinoma and melanoma.

Aldesleukin is a toxic therapy that requires vigorous supportive care under the supervision of experienced healthcare professionals. The most common dose-limiting toxicities are hypotension, fluid retention, and renal dysfunction. Aldesleukin decreases peripheral vascular resistance, producing peripheral vasodilation, tachycardia, and hypotension. A characteristic vascular or capillary leak syndrome produces fluid retention, which in turn can cause respiratory compromise. These toxicities require administration of vasopressors in most patients, judicious use of fluid support and diuretics, and supplemental oxygen. Patients with underlying cardiovascular or renal abnormalities are more susceptible to these toxicities, making careful patient selection important. Most patients treated with aldesleukin experience thrombocytopenia, anemia, eosinophilia, reversible cholestasis, and skin erythema with burning and pruritus; some patients have neuropsychiatric changes, hypothyroidism, and bacterial infections. In general, the toxicities from aldesleukin reverse quickly after therapy is stopped and can be managed or prevented by careful monitoring and supportive care.

Therapeutic Vaccines

Sipuleucel-T was the first therapeutic vaccine approved by the FDA. It is classified as an autologous cellular immunotherapy and is indicated for the treatment of asymptomatic or minimally symptomatic metastatic castrate-resistant prostate cancer. Through leukapheresis, a patient's dendritic cells are collected and isolated, then cultured ex-vivo. The fusion protein is composed of prostate acid phosphatase, or PAP, and GM-CSF. Prostate acid phosphatase is selectively expressed on prostatic tissues and GM-CSF is included to enhance the immune response. Antigen-presenting cells take up this antigen and are then reinfused into the donor patient to stimulate a T-cell response.

Treatment with sipuleucel-T consists of three infusions separated by approximately 2 weeks. Due to the leukapheresis, ex-vivo cell manipulation, and reinfusion, treatment with sipuleucel-T can be logistically challenging. Premedication consisting of acetaminophen and an antihistamine should be given prior to each infusion to decrease the risk of an infusion-related reaction. Common toxicities include chills, fatigue, back pain, nausea, joint ache, and headache.

Talimogene laherparepvec is an oncolytic viral therapy based on a modified herpes simplex virus type 1. Talimogene laherparepvec is modified through the deletion of two herpes simplex virus genes, ICP34.5 and ICP47, and is designed to lyse tumor cells and promote antitumor immunity. It is indicated for the local treatment of unresectable cutaneous, subcutaneous, and nodal lesions in patients with melanoma recurrent after initial surgery and is injected directly into the lesion. The most common toxicities are fatigue, chills, pyrexia, nausea, influenza-like illness, and injection site pain. Pyrexia, chills, and influenza-like illness can occur any time during treatment but are more frequent during the first 3 months. Cellulitis is the most commonly reported serious adverse drug reaction.

CAR T-Cell Therapies

CAR T-cell therapies were the first FDA-approved genetically modified autologous T-cell immunotherapies and are also known as adoptive T-cell therapies. Peripheral blood mononuclear cells are harvested from a patient via apheresis. The T-cells are then reprogrammed with a transgene encoding a CAR, which consists of a binding domain and signaling domains. Following lymphodepletion with a conditioning regimen (often fludarabine and cyclophosphamide), the CAR T-cells are then reinfused into the patient.

The design of CAR T-cells has evolved over the years primarily to improve the signaling capability. Four anti-CD19 CARs are currently FDA-approved: axicabtagene ciloleucel (second-generation agent) for the treatment of follicular lymphoma and large B-cell lymphoma; brexucabtagene autoleucel (second-generation agent) for the treatment of mantle cell lymphoma; tisagenlecleucel (second-generation agent) for the treatment of ALL and diffuse large B-cell lymphoma; and lisocabtagene maraleucel (third-generation agent) for the treatment of large B-cell lymphoma. Binding the CD19-expressing cell activates downstream signaling through the costimulatory signaling domains, resulting in cytokine and chemokine secretion and ultimate destruction of the B-cell. Although all four agents are similar in mechanism, they differ in their costimulatory signaling domains. Axicabtagene ciloleucel and brexucabtagene autoleucel both include a CD28 and CD3-zeta signaling domain, whereas tisagenlecleucel contains a 4-1BB and CD3-zeta domain. Lisocabtagene maraleucel is considered a next-generation CAR T-cell because it contains multiple costimulatory domains, including CD28 and 4-1BB in addition to CD3-zeta.

Additionally, idecabtagene vicleucel, a second-generation CAR therapy targeting B-cell maturation antigen, is approved for the treatment of relapsed or refractory multiple myeloma. Similar to tisagenlecleucel, the idecabtagene vicleucel CAR construct contains signaling domains 4-1BB and CD3-zeta. After binding to the B-cell maturation antigen, the signaling domains will activate cytokine and chemokine secretion, resulting in destruction of the targeted cell.

Toxicities associated with CAR T-cell therapies can be severe and life-threatening. As a result, a REMS program has been implemented which, among other requirements, mandates hospitals and clinics be certified before administering these agents.

Cytokine-associated toxicities are common and include CRS, which manifests with hypotension, tachycardia, fever, and hypoxia. Organ dysfunction may also be present. The typical time to onset of CRS is 2 to 3 days and the usual duration is 7 to 8 days.[52] Immune effector cell-associated neurotoxicity syndrome, or ICANS, is the terminology used for neurotoxicities associated with CAR T-cell treatment. CAR T-cell-related neurotoxicities can be fatal or life-threatening. The typical time to onset is 4 to 10 days after treatment, and symptoms last approximately 14 to 17 days.[52] Common neurotoxicities include encephalopathy, headache, tremor, dizziness, and aphasia, but serious events, such as seizures and cerebral edema, have also been reported. See Chapter 150 "Supportive Care" for management of CRS and ICANS.

RESPONSE CRITERIA

The response to anticancer agents and other treatment modalities could be described as a cure; complete response, or CR; partial response, or PR; stable disease, or SD; or progression. A cure implies that the patient is entirely free of disease and has the same life expectancy as a cancer-free individual. Because of our inability to detect small numbers of cancer cells, we can never be absolutely certain that an individual patient is cured. Cancers that are curable with treatment are characterized by a stable plateau in the survival curve where the risk of relapse is very low. For most curable cancers, the survival curve has plateaued by about 5 years. Therefore, patients with a curable cancer who are alive 5 years from the time of diagnosis without disease recurrence are often considered "cured," but patients with some malignancies, such as breast cancer and melanoma, are still at significant risk for relapse after 5 years.

Response Criteria for Solid Tumors

In an attempt to simplify and unify response definitions in clinical practice, clinical trials, and published reports, the response evaluation criteria in solid tumors (RECIST) criteria were developed in 2000 and revised in 2009 (RECIST 1.1).[53] At baseline, overall tumor burden and measurable disease is assessed. Target lesions are identified and measured at baseline and are later re-evaluated to determine objective tumor response. Nontarget lesions are also assessed. A CR means disappearance of all target lesions and any pathological lymph nodes must be reduced in short axis to less than 10 mm. A PR is defined as a 30% or greater decrease in the sum of diameters of target lesions from baseline. Overall, objective response rates for a given treatment are calculated by adding the CR and PR rates. Progressive disease is defined as a 20% or greater increase in the sum of diameters of target lesions when compared to the smallest sum since treatment initiation. The development of one or more new lesions while receiving treatment is also considered progressive disease. A patient whose tumor size neither grows nor shrinks by the above criteria is termed to have stable disease. Some patients may experience subjective improvement in cancer-related symptoms without a defined response. Although clinically important, this does not indicate an objective response. RECIST 1.1 is the most widely accepted criteria for the assessment of tumor response in solid tumors but it does not come without shortcomings. The modified RECIST, or mRECIST, assessment may be more accurate for the evaluation of tumor burden in some cancers.[54]

Furthermore, the emergence of immunotherapy in oncology has led to the need for revised response criteria that accounts for the mechanism of immunotherapeutic agents. RECIST neglects to take into account pseudoprogression (ie, "flare") associated with these agents, which may inadvertently result in the premature discontinuation of an effective therapy. Pseudoprogression refers to apparent tumor growth on imaging, resulting from an immunotherapy treatment-related effect rather than malignant cell proliferation. The apparent progression is thought to be a result of immune infiltrates and is followed by tumor regression. Immune-related response criteria, or irRC, and immune-related RECIST, or irRECIST, have been proposed to overcome the challenges of RECIST 1.1 with immunotherapy.[55,56]

Response Criteria for Hematologic Malignancies

The response definitions described above are applicable to solid tumors, but leukemias and multiple myeloma are not characterized by discrete, measurable masses. Responses in these cancers are measured by elimination of abnormal cells (eg, return to normal hematology parameters and normal bone marrow in leukemia), return of tumor markers to normal levels (eg, normal serum protein electrophoresis in multiple myeloma), or improved function of affected organs (eg, improved renal function after obstructive uropathy). Cytogenetic markers and molecular techniques have an increasingly important role in determining whether all cancer has been truly eliminated. For example, in CML, the Ph can be detected by polymerase chain reaction techniques even when no leukemia is evident in the bone marrow or bloodstream. Patients without evidence of the Ph are classified as having a complete cytogenetic response. Measuring cytogenetic responses is increasingly common in patients with known cytogenetic abnormalities, and the absence of a complete cytogenetic response may be predictive of disease relapse. Minimal residual disease (MRD) is a prognostic factor used to guide treatment in ALL and AML. Data regarding MRD is still emerging, but it is now recommended that MRD be monitored in patients with AML as MRD positivity is associated with higher relapse rates and shorter survival.[57]

FACTORS AFFECTING TREATMENT RESPONSE

9 Factors affecting response include tumor burden, cancer cell heterogeneity, drug resistance, dose intensity, and patient-specific factors, such as pharmacogenomics. The significance of tumor burden was discussed earlier in the chapter. Tumors consist of a heterogeneous population of cells. Because of the genetic instability of cancer cells compared with normal cells, genetic alterations commonly occur during cell division. Large tumors have therefore undergone many cell divisions and express multiple genetic alterations, resulting in genetically varied populations. In 1979, Goldie and Coldman proposed that these cytogenetic changes were not completely random and were highly associated with the ability of tumors to develop drug resistance. The probability of developing resistant cell populations increases as tumor size increases. It is believed that a small percentage of resistant cancer cells may survive initial therapy. Resistant populations later proliferate and eventually become the dominant population, which could explain the common pattern of an initial response to therapy followed by progressive tumor regrowth despite continuing the same treatment.

Drug Resistance

Drug resistance may be either acquired or inherited. Mechanisms of drug resistance include altered drug transport systems, metabolism, and target enzymes; ability to repair drug-induced damage; and insensitivity to drug-induced apoptosis.[2] For example, multidrug resistance has been observed with natural chemotherapies (eg, anthracyclines, vinca alkaloids, epipodophyllotoxins, taxanes), and it occurs when some cancer cells are exposed to increasing concentrations of a specific chemotherapy. Surprisingly, these same cells also become resistant to other structurally unrelated chemotherapies and are therefore considered multidrug resistant. The resistant cancer cells may overexpress the drug transporter P-gp, which enhances the export of these chemotherapies. Other potential mechanisms of drug resistance include inactivation of chemotherapy by glutathione metabolism, upregulation of drug targets, alternative intracellular signaling pathways, and decreased apoptosis. The last mechanism can be mediated by overexpression of BCL-2 or loss of TP53, as discussed earlier in the chapter.

Dose Intensity

The relationship between dose and response has been extensively explored for chemotherapy agents, because dose is believed to be a critical factor in determining response for many cancers. Dose intensity is defined as the dose delivered to the patient over a specified period of time. The three main variables that determine delivered dose intensity are the dose per course, the interval between doses, and the total cumulative dose. Dose density refers to shortening of the usual interval between doses (eg, every 2 weeks instead of every 3 weeks) and is designed to maximize the effects of therapy on tumor growth kinetics. This strategy has been extensively studied in breast cancer. The delivery of optimal dose intensity is often compromised by the toxicities of the anticancer agent. Treatment cycles are commonly delayed because of inadequate recovery from toxicity, especially myelosuppression. Subsequent doses of the anticancer agents are often reduced to prevent or minimize the severity of these toxicities. The impact on patient outcome has been proven in studies showing reduced rates of response and survival in individuals receiving less-than-optimal doses. Understanding the pathophysiology of toxicities has led to the development of more effective agents to prevent and manage these toxicities. The development of chemoprotective agents has facilitated application of dose-intensity principles. For example, CSFs minimize neutropenia and permit delivery of dose-intensive or dose-dense regimens that are myelosuppressive. The concept of dose intensity is particularly important in the setting of high-dose chemotherapy with autologous hematopoietic stem cell support. Although lethal myelosuppression is avoided through HSCT, other severe end-organ toxicities emerge as doses of the anticancer agents are increased.

Molecular Biomarkers

A molecular biomarker is a molecular characteristic of the tumor that influences prognosis or predicts response to a specific therapy. Many of these molecular biomarkers are somatic mutations that contribute to the development of the cancer. Prognostic biomarkers inform the risk of clinical outcomes such as disease progression or recurrence. Numerous tests are currently available that measure tumor gene expression and may provide information on a patient's risk of recurrence. For example, the Oncotype Dx® Breast Cancer Assay measures 21 genes associated with breast cancer recurrence and chemotherapy benefit in select patients with breast cancer. A predictive biomarker predicts response to a specific therapeutic intervention. For example, EGFR and ALK mutations predict response to EGFR and ALK inhibitors in NSCLC. Similarly, HER2 overexpression predicts response to trastuzumab in breast cancer. Molecular testing of cancer at the time of diagnosis allows for personalized therapy with targeted agents.

Patient-Specific Factors

Patient-specific factors create unpredictable variability in response to anticancer therapy. For example, interindividual variations in absorption, distribution, or elimination could lead to sub- or supratherapeutic levels of anticancer agents and their metabolites. The genetic alterations that resulted in the cancer can also affect response. For example, breast cancers that overexpress HER2 are often sensitive to anthracycline-based regimens. As a result, both efficacy and tolerability can be affected. Healthcare professionals in oncology may preemptively modify doses based on variations in body size, blood counts, and organ function to optimize the effectiveness of therapy and minimize toxicity. However, more specific tools are becoming available as we learn how to identify and apply genetic differences. Pharmacogenomics is the study of the role of inheritance in individual variation of drug response. In oncology, several clinically relevant genetic polymorphisms or variations have been identified that can affect pharmacokinetics and pharmacodynamics. Examples include polymorphisms in genes responsible for the activity of the enzymes DPD (responsible for fluorouracil metabolism), TPMT and NUDT15 (responsible for thiopurine metabolism), UGT1A1 (responsible for irinotecan metabolism), and cytochrome P450 2D6 (responsible for tamoxifen metabolism). Patients with deficiencies in these enzymes can experience significant and possibly life-threatening toxicity. Identifying these genetic variants could permit individualization of regimens to reduce toxicity. Furthermore, pharmacokinetic and pharmacodynamic modeling is associated with improved responses and decreased toxicity in children with ALL.

The presence of other disease states (eg, comorbidities) may also affect response to treatment by limiting treatment options. The overall functional status of a patient may be assessed using performance status scales, such as the Karnofsky Performance Status and the Eastern Cooperative Oncology Group or ECOG scales (see Table 149-8). These scales can be used to predict patient tolerance of anticancer therapy and to assess the effects of therapy on the patient's level of activity and quality of life. For many cancers, performance status at diagnosis is the most important prognostic indicator.

Today's oncology healthcare professionals have a wealth of information to consider when designing a personalized treatment approach. Patient-specific factors (eg, performance status, comorbidities, organ function, and pharmacogenomics), tumor-specific

TABLE 149-8 Assessing the Performance Status of Patients with Cancer

Eastern Cooperative Oncology Group (ECOG) Performance Status Scale		Karnofsky Performance Scale	
Grade	**Description**	**Percent**	**Description**
0	Fully active, able to carry on all pre-disease performance without restriction.	100	Normal, no complaints, no evidence of disease.
		90	Able to carry on normal activity; minor signs or symptoms of disease.
1	Restricted in physically strenuous activity, but ambulatory and able to carry out work of a light or sedentary nature (eg, light housework, office work).	80	Normal activity with effort; some signs or symptoms of disease.
		70	Cares for self; unable to carry on normal activity or to do active work.
2	Ambulatory and capable of all self-care, but unable to carry out any work activities. Up and about more than 50% of waking hours.	60	Requires occasional assistance but is able to care for most of personal needs.
		50	Requires considerable assistance and frequent medical care.
3	Capable of only limited self-care, confined to bed or chair more than 50% of waking hours.	40	Disabled, requires special care and assistance.
		30	Severely disabled, hospitalization indicated. Death not imminent.
4	Completely disabled. Cannot carry on any self-care. Totally confined to bed or chair.	20	Very ill, hospitalization and active supportive care necessary.
		10	Moribund.
5	Dead.	0	Dead.

Adapted from ECOG-ACRIN Cancer Research Group. ECOG Performance Status [cited 2021 July 18]. Available at: https://ecog-acrin.org/resources/ecog-performance-status.

factors (eg, pathology, stage, and biomarkers), and treatment goals (eg, palliation and cure) are all considered when determining the best treatment option. Treatment cost can also be an important consideration.

DRUG ADMINISTRATION

Dosage and Administration

Healthcare professionals should monitor all clinical and laboratory values that are affected by a specific anticancer agent at baseline and periodically during treatment. For example, a complete blood count should be evaluated weekly or before each cycle while receiving anticancer agents associated with myelosuppression. In general, an absolute neutrophil count, or ANC of 1,500 cells/mm^3 (1.5 × 10^9/L) or above, and a platelet count of 100,000 cells/mm^3 (100 × 10^9/L) or above are usually required before administering myelosuppressive agents. In addition, a chemistry panel is drawn to assess organ function, especially for agents eliminated or metabolized via those routes.

Anticancer agents might be dosed based on body size (such as body weight or body surface area [BSA]) or as a fixed (ie, flat) dose. Cytotoxic chemotherapy is generally dosed based on BSA. BSA is commonly used as an estimate of cardiac output and subsequent distribution to the liver and kidneys, the primary determinants of drug elimination. The most common methods used to determine BSA are the Mosteller and DuBois formulas. Traditionally, body-sized dosing has been used for mAbs but some agents, such as some immune checkpoint inhibitors, may use a flat dose. In contrast, most oral targeted agents are based on a fixed-dose approach.

Other dosing methods are being used to improve tolerability and anticancer activity. For example, carboplatin is dosed based on the patient's estimated glomerular filtration rate or GFR. This method is known as the Calvert formula and has been demonstrated to achieve adequate levels of carboplatin while minimizing excessive toxicity.

Molecular diagnostic tests are required prior to administration of some targeted agents (eg, trastuzumab, vemurafenib, and crizotinib), which are indicated only for patients whose tumors express a specific protein or gene. Additionally, health professionals must know how to interpret the findings from the various diagnostic tests. For example, some tests may identify if a tumor is mutation positive or negative, whereas other tests may identify the specific genetic alteration present in the tumor.

Safety and Handling

All anticancer agents regardless of the route of administration should be handled with care to avoid inadvertent exposure to healthcare professionals and caregivers. Consequently, all healthcare facilities should have written procedures for safely handling these agents, and all personnel should be oriented to these procedures. Healthcare professionals should provide information about safe handling and disposal to patients and their families when a patient is prescribed an oral anticancer agent. Patients should be informed of proper methods for disposing of potentially contaminated body excreta and cytotoxic waste. Safe handling includes avoiding skin contact and inhalation, but patient-centered guidelines regarding safe handling of oral anticancer agents have not been developed.

The United States Pharmacopeia regulates the preparation of extemporaneously compounded sterile preparations and should be used by healthcare professionals that prepare intravenous chemotherapy. Chapter 800 provides standards for the safe handling of hazardous agents in the healthcare setting. The most common avenue of exposure is via inhalation or skin absorption. Individuals preparing intravenous chemotherapy should work in an International Organization for Standardization, or ISO Class 5 biologic safety cabinet and wear appropriate personal protective equipment including a gown, face mask, eye protection, hair covers, shoe covers, and double sterile chemotype gloves. Closed-system vial-transfer devices should be used when possible. Negative-pressure techniques should be used in drug preparation to minimize aerosolization. Health professionals administering chemotherapy should take similar precautions to avoid exposure. Double chemotherapy-tested gloves, protective gowns, and protective eyewear (if there is potential for splashing) should be worn whenever handling or administering hazardous drugs. Kits for cleaning up chemotherapy spills should be located in all areas where chemotherapy is handled and cytotoxic waste should be disposed of properly.

ABBREVIATIONS

ADC	antibody-drug conjugate
ADCC	antibody-dependent cell-mediated cytotoxicity
ALL	acute lymphoblastic leukemia
ALK	anaplastic lymphoma kinase
αKG	alpha-ketoglutarate
AML	acute myeloid leukemia
ATP	adenosine triphosphate
BCL-2	B-cell lymphoma 2
BCR-ABL	breakpoint cluster region-Abelson
BRCA	breast cancer gene
BTK	Bruton's tyrosine kinase
CAR	chimeric antigen receptor
CD	cluster of differentiation
CDC	complement-dependent cytotoxicity
CDK	cyclin-dependent kinase
CLL	chronic lymphocytic leukemia
CML	chronic myeloid leukemia
CNS	central nervous system
CRS	cytokine release syndrome
CT	computed tomography
CTLA-4	cytotoxic T-lymphocyte–associated antigen 4
DHFR	dihydrofolate reductase
dMMR	mismatch repair deficient
DNA	deoxyribonucleic acid
DNMT	DNA methyltransferase
DPD	dihydropyrimidine dehydrogenase
ECG	electrocardiogram
EGFR	epidermal growth factor receptor
EML4	echinoderm microtubule-like protein 4
ER	estrogen receptor
ErbB	erythroblastic leukemia viral oncogene
ERK	extracellular signal-regulated kinase
FDA	Food and Drug Administration
FGFR	fibroblast growth factor receptor
FLT3	FMS-like tyrosine kinase 3
GEP-NET	gastroenteropancreatic neuroendocrine tumors
GIST	gastrointestinal stromal tumor
HBV	hepatitis B virus
HDAC	histone deacetylase
HER2	human epidermal growth factor receptor 2
HPV	human papilloma virus
HSCT	hematopoietic stem cell transplant
IDH	isocitrate dehydrogenase
irAE	immune-related adverse event
JAK	Janus kinase
KIT	stem-cell factor receptor
KRAS	kirsten ras
LVEF	left ventricular ejection fraction
mAb	monoclonal antibody
MAPK	mitogen-activated protein kinase
MDS	myelodysplastic syndrome

MEK	mitogen-activated protein kinase—extracellular signal-regulated kinase
MET	mesenchymal-epithelial transition
MRD	measurable residual disease
MSI-H	microsatellite instability-high
mTOR	mammalian target of rapamycin
NF-κB	nuclear factor-κB
NHL	non-Hodgkin lymphoma
NSCLC	non-small cell lung cancer
NTRK	neurotrophic receptor tyrosine kinase
NUDT15	nudix (nucleoside diphosphate linked moiety X)-type motif 15
PARP	poly ADP ribose polymerase
PD-1	programmed death-1
PD-L1	programmed death ligand-1
PDGF	platelet-derived growth factor
PDGFR	platelet-derived growth factor receptor
P-gp	p-glycoprotein
Ph	Philadelphia chromosome
Ph^+	Philadelphia chromosome-positive
PI3K	phosphatidylinositide 3-kinases
PPE	palmar-plantar erythrodysesthesia
RECIST	response evaluation criteria in solid tumors
REMS	risk evaluation and mitigation strategy
RET	rearranged during transfection
RNA	ribonucleic acid
SCLC	small cell lung cancer
SLAMF7	signaling lymphocytic activation molecule family 7
STAT	signal transducers and activators of transcription
TLS	tumor lysis syndrome
TNF-α	tumor necrosis factor-alpha
TPMT	thiopurine methyltransferase
TRK	tropomyosin receptor kinase
TROP2	trophoblast cell-surface antigen 2
UGT1A1	uridine diphosphate-glucuronosyl transferase 1A1
VEGF	vascular endothelial growth factor
VEGFR	vascular endothelial growth factor receptor
VTE	venous thromboembolism

REFERENCES

1. Siegel RL, Miller KD, Fuchs HE, et al. Cancer Statistics. *Ca Cancer J Clin.* 2022;72(1):7–33. 10.3322/caac.21708.
2. Clark JW, Longo DL. Cancer cell biology. In: Jameson J, Fauci A, Kasper D, Hauser S, Longo D, Loscalzo J, eds. *Harrison's Principles of Internal Medicine.* 20th ed. McGraw Hill; 2018.
3. Moasser MM, Ai WZ. Neoplasia. In: Hammer G, McPhee S, eds. *Pathophysiology of Disease: An Introduction to Clinical Medicine.* 8th ed. McGraw Hill; 2019.
4. Cuellar S, Haaf CM. Neoplastic Diseases. In: Tisdale J, Miller D, eds. *Drug-Induced Diseases.* 3rd ed. ASHP; 2018.
5. Hanahan D, Weinberg RA. Hallmarks of cancer: The next generation. *Cell.* 2011;144(5):646–674. doi:10.1016/j.cell.2011.02.013.
6. Chan CY, Tan KV, Cornelissen B. PARP inhibitors in cancer diagnosis and therapy. *Clin Cancer Res.* 2021;27:1585–1594. doi:10.1158/1078-0432.CCR-20-2766.
7. Le DT, Uram JN, Wang H, et al. PD-1 blockade in tumors with mismatch-repair deficiency. *N Engl J Med.* 2015;372. doi:10.1056/NEJMoa1500596.
8. Clark O, Yen K, Mellinghoff IK. Molecular pathways: Isocitrate dehydrogenase mutations in cancer. *Clin Cancer Res.* 2016;22(8):1837–1842. doi:10.1158/1078-0432.CCR-13-1333.
9. Stricker TP, Kumar V. Neoplasia. In: Kumar V, Abbas A, Aster J, Fausto N, eds. *Robbins and Cotran Pathologic Basis of Disease.* 8th ed. Philadelphia, PA: Saunders; 2010:259–330.
10. National Cancer Institute. Training Modules Tumor List [cited 2021 July 18]. Available at: https://training.seer.cancer.gov/disease/categories/tumors.html.
11. Smith RA, Andrews KS, Brooks D, et al. Cancer screening in the United States, 2019: A review of current American Cancer Society guidelines and current issues in cancer screening. *Ca Cancer J Clin.* 2019;69(3):184–210.
12. Fontham ETH, Wolf AMD, Church TR, et al. Cervical cancer screening for individuals at average risk: 2020 Guideline update from the American Cancer Society. *CA Cancer J Clin.* 2020;70(5):321–346. doi:10.3322/caac.21628.
13. American Cancer Society study communicating cancer information through mass distribution leaflets: An American Cancer Society study. *Ca Cancer J Clin.* 1967;17:291–293.
14. Saliba AN, John AJ, Kaufmann SH. Resistance to venetoclax and hypomethylating agents in acute myeloid leukemia. *Cancer Drug Resist.* 2021;4:125–142. doi:10.20517/cdr.2020.95.
15. Rubin EH, Hait WN. Drugs that target DNA topoisomerase. In: Waun K, Bast R, Hait W, eds. *Cancer Medicine.* 8th ed. Shelton, CT: People's Medical Publishing House-USA; 2010:645–654.
16. Colvin M. Alklating agents and platinum antitumor compounds. In: Waun K, Bast R, Hait W, eds. *Cancer Medicine.* 8th ed. Shelton, CT: People's Medical Publishing House-USA; 2010:633–644.
17. Kost SEF, Bouchard EDJ, LaBossiere E, et al. Cross-resistance and synergy with bendamustine in chronic lymphocytic leukemia. *Leuk Res* 2016;50:63–71. 10.1016/j.leukres.2016.09.016.
18. Richardson PG, Oriol A, Larocca A, et al. Melflufen and dexamethasone in heavily pretreated relapsed and refractory multiple myeloma. *J Clin Oncol.* 2021;39(7):757–767. doi:10.1200/JCO.20.02259.
19. Colvin M. Alkylating agents and platinum antitumor compounds. In: Waun K, Bast R, Hait W, eds. *Cancer Medicine.* 8th ed. Shelton, CT: People's Medical Publishing House_USA; 2010:633–644.
20. Loprinzi CL, Qin R, Dakhil SR, et al. Phase III randomized, placebo-controlled, double-blind study of intravenous calcium and magnesium to prevent oxaliplatin-induced sensory neurotoxicity. *J Clin Oncol.* 2014;32(10):997–1005. doi:10.1200/JCO.2013.52.0536.
21. Turck R. Radio-pharmaceuticals for cancer treatment: Are they ready for prime time yet. *Ann Oncol.* 2018;29(7):1594–1597. doi:10.1093/annonc/mdy142.
22. Shaw AT, Kim D, Mehra R, et al. Ceritinib in ALK-rearranged non-small-cell lung cancer. *N Engl J Med.* 2014;370:1189–1197. doi:10.1056/NEJMoa1311107.
23. Solomon BJ, Besse B, Bauer TM, et al. Lorlatinib in patients with ALK-positive non-small-cell lung cancer: Results from a global phase 2 study. *Lancet Oncol.* 2018;19(12):1654–1667. doi:10.1016/S1470-2045(18)30649-1.
24. Anderson MA, Deng J, Seymour JF, et al. The BCL2 selective inhibitor venetoclax induces rapid onset apoptosis of CLL cells in patients via a TP53-independent mechanism. *Blood.* 2016;127(25):3215–3224. doi:10.1182/blood-2016-01-688796.
25. My Cancer Genome. Biomarkers/BRAF. Vanderbilt-Ingram Cancer Center; [cited 2021 July 21]. Available at: https://www.mycancergenome.org/content/gene/braf/.
26. Long GV, Stroyakovskiy D, Gogas H, et al. Combined BRAF and MEK inhibition versus BRAF inhibition alone in melanoma. *N Engl J Med.* 2014;371:1877–1888. 10.1056/NEJMoa1406037.
27. Finn RS, Crown JP, Lang I, et al. The cyclin-dependent kinase 4/6 inhibitor palbociclib in combination with letrozole versus letrozole alone as first-line treatment of oestrogen receptor-positive, HER2-negative, advanced breast cancer (PALOMA-1/TRIO-18): A randomised phase 2 study. *Lancet Oncol.* 2015;16(1):25–35. doi:10.1016/S1470-2045(14)71159-3.
28. Tap WD, Gelderblom H, Palmerini E, et al. Pexidartinib versus placebo for advanced tenosynovial giant cell tumour (ENLIVEN): A randomised phase 3 trial. *Lancet.* 2019;394(10197):478–487. doi:10.1016/S0140-6736(19)30764-0.
29. Li T, Perez-Soler R. Skin toxicities associated with epidermal growth factor receptor inhibitors. *Target Oncol.* 2009;4(2):107–119. doi:10.1007/s11523-009-0114-0.
30. Ricordel C, Friboulet L, Facchinetti F, et al. Molecular mechanisms of acquired resistance to third-generation EGFR TKIs in EGFR T790M-mutant lung cancer. *Ann Oncol* 2018;29:i28–i37. 10.1093/annonc/mdx705.
31. Patani H, Bunney TD, Thiyagarajan N, et al. Landscape of activating cancer mutations in FGFR kinases and their differential responses to inhibitors in clinical use. *Oncotarget.* 2016;7(17):24252–24268. doi:10.18632/oncotarget.8132.
32. San-Miguel JF, Hungria VTM, Yoon S, et al. Panobinostat plus bortezomib and dexamethasone versus placebo plus bortezomib and dexamethasone in patients with relapsed or relapsed and refractory multiple myeloma: A multicentre, randomised, double-blind

phase 3 trial. *Lancet Oncol.* 2014;15(11):1195–1206. doi:10.1016/S1470-2045(14)70440-1.

33. Schaid DJ, Spraggs CF, McDonnel SK, et al. Prospective validation of HLA-DRB1*07:01 allele carriage as a predictive risk factor for lapatinib-induced liver injury. *J Clin Oncol.* 2014;32(22):2296–2303. doi:10.1200/JCO.2013.52.9867.
34. Gross AM, Wolters PL, Dombi E, et al. Selumetinib in children with inoperable plexiform neurofibromas. *N Engl J Med.* 2020;382:1430–1442. doi:10.1056/NEJMoa1912735.
35. Grosicki S, Simonova M, Spicka I, et al. Once-per-week selinexor, bortezomib, an dexamethasone versus twice-per-week boretzomib and dexamethasone in patients with multiple myeloma (BOSTON): A randomised, open-label, phase 3 trial. *Lancet.* 2020;396(10262):1563–1573. doi:10.1016/S0140-6736(20)32292-3.
36. Paul J, Soujon M, Wengner AM, et al. Simultaneous inhibition of PI3Kδ and PI3Kα induces ABC-DLBCL regression by blocking BCR-dependent and -independent activation of NF-κB and AKT. *Cancer Cell.* 2017;31(1):64–78. 10.1016/j.ccell.2016.12.003.
37. Fowler NH, Samaniego F, Jurczak W, et al. Umbralisib, a dual PI3Kδ/CK1ε inhibitor in patients with relapsed or refractory indolent lymphoma. *J Clin Oncol.* 2021;39(15):1609-1618. doi:10.1200/JCO.20.03433.
38. Juric D, Rodon J, Tabernero J, et al. Phosphatidylinositol 3-kinase α-selective inhibition with alpelisib (BYL719) in PI3KCA-altered solid tumors: Results from the first-in-human study. *J Clin Oncol.* 2018;36(13):1291–1299. doi:10.1200/JCO.2017.72.7107.
39. Skoulidis F, Li BT, Dy GK, et al. Sotorasib for lung cancers with KRAS p.G12C mutation. *N Engl J Med.* 2021;384:2371–2381. doi:10.1056/NEJMoa2103695.
40. Bekaii-Saab TS, Ou F, Ahn DH, et al. Regorafenib dose-optimisation in patients with refractory metastatic colorectal cancer (ReDOS): A randomised, multicentre, open-label, phase 2 study. *Lancet Oncol.* 2019;20(8):1070–1082. doi:10.1016/S1470-2045(19)30272-4.
41. U.S. Food and Drug Administration. Biosimilars and interchangeable products [cited 2018 December 18]. Available at: https://www.fda.gov/Drugs/DevelopmentApprovalProcess/HowDrugsareDevelopedandApproved/ApprovalApplications/TherapeuticBiologicApplications/Biosimilars/ucm580419.htm.
42. Dolgin E. Specter of eye toxicity looms over BCMA-targeted therapy. *Nat Biotechnol.* 2020;38:1363–1365. doi:10.1038/s41587-020-00757-8.
43. Salles G, Duell J, Barca EG, et al. Tafasitamab plus lenalidomide in relapsed or refractory diffuse large B-cell lymphoma (L-MIND): A multicentre, prospective, single-arm, phase 2 study. *Lancet Oncol.* 2020;21(7):978–988. doi:10.1016/S1470-2045(20)30225-4.
44. Tobinai K, Klein C, Oya N, et al. A review of Obinutuzumab (GA101), a Novel Type II Anti-CD20 Monoclonal Antibody, for the treatment of patients with B-cell malignancies. *Adv Ther.* 2017;34:324–356. doi:10.1007/s12325-016-0451-1.
45. Attal M, Richardson PG, Rajkumar SV, et al. Isatuximab plus pomalidomide and low-dose dexamethasone versus pomalidomide and low-dose dexamethasone in patients with relapsed and refractory multiple myeloma (ICARIA-MM): A randomized, multicentre, open-label, phase 3 study. *Lancet.* 2019;394:2096–2107. doi:10.1016/S0140-6736(19)32556-5.
46. Palanca-Wessels MC, Czuczman M, Salles G, et al. Safety and activity of the anti-CD79B antibody-drug conjugate polatuzumab vedotin in relapsed or refractory B-cell non-Hodgkin lymphoma and chronic lymphocytic leukaemia: A phase 1 study. *Lancet Oncol.* 2015;16(6):704–715. doi:10.1016/S1470-2045(15)70128-2.
47. Nazha B, Inal C, Owonikoko TK. Disialoganglioside GD2 expression in solid tumors and role as a target for cancer therapy. *Front Oncol.* 2020;10:1000. doi:10.3389/fonc.2020.01000.
48. Vyse S, Huang PH. Targeting EGFR exon 20 insertion mutations in non-small cell lung cancer. *Sig Transduct Target Ther.* 2019;4(5). doi:10.1038/s41392-019-0038-9.
49. Rugo HS, Im S, Cardoso F, et al. Efficacy of margetuximab vs trastuzumab in patients with pretreated ERBB2-positive advanced breast cancer. *JAMA Oncol.* 2021;7(4):573–584. doi:10.1001/jamaoncol.2020.7932.
50. van de Donk NW, Moreau P, Plesner T, et al. Clinical efficacy and management of monoclonal antibodies targeting CD38 and SLAMF7 in multiple myeloma. *Blood.* 2016;127(6):681–695. doi:10.1182/blood-2015-10-646810.
51. McNamara MG, Jacobs T, Lamarca A, et al. Impact of high tumor mutational burden in solid tumors and challenges for biomarker application. *Cancer Treat Rev.* 2020;89:102084. 10.1016/j.ctrv.2020.102084.
52. The NCCN Clinical Practice Guidelines in Oncology: Management of Immunotherapy-Related Toxicities (version 3.2021). National Comprehensive Cancer Network. Available at: https://www.nccn.org/professionals/physician_gls/pdf/immunotherapy.pdf. [cited May 16, 2021].
53. Eisenhauer EA, Therasse P, Bogaerts J, et al. New response evaluation criteria in solid tumours: Revised RECIST guideline (version 1.1). *Eur J Cancer.* 2009;45(2):228–247. doi:10.1016/j.ejca.2008.10.026.
54. Lencioni R, Llovet JM. Modified RECIST (mRECIST) assessment for hepatocellular carcinoma. *Semin Liver Dis.* 2010;30(1):52–60. 10.1055/s-0030-1247132.
55. Wolchok JD, Hoos A, O'Day S, et al. Guidelines for the evaluation of immune therapy activity in solid tumors: Immune-related response criteria. *Clin Cancer Res.* 2009;15(23):7412–7420. doi:10.1158/1078-0432.CCR-09-1624.
56. Bohnsack O, Hoos A, Ludajic K. Adaptation of the immune related response criteria: irRECIST. Abstract presented at: ESMO 2014 Congress; 2014 September 26-30; Madrid, Spain.
57. Schuurhuis GJ, Heuser M, Freeman S, et al. Minimal/measurable residual disease in AML: A consensus document from the European LeukemiaNet Working Party. *Blood.* 2018;131(12):1275–1291. doi:10.1182/blood-2017-09-801498.
58. Compagni A, Christofori G. Recent advances in research on multistage tumorigenesis. *Br J Cancer.* 2000;83:1–5.
59. FDA U.S. Food and Drug Administration. Drugs@FDA: FDA-Approved Drugs. Available at: https://www.accessdata.fda.gov/scripts/cder/daf/.

150

Supportive Care in Cancer

Amber B. Clemmons and Ashley E. Glode

KEY CONCEPTS

1. Myelosuppression (low blood counts), a common dose-limiting toxicity for numerous anticancer agents, is managed with blood product transfusions, colony-stimulating factors (CSFs), and/or anticancer therapy dose reduction or delay.
2. Prevention of chemotherapy-induced nausea/vomiting (CINV) throughout the entire risk period is based on emetic risk of regimen, patient risk factors, and response. Management of chemotherapy-induced mucositis and diarrhea uses supportive care measures.
3. Tumor lysis syndrome (TLS) is one of the most common oncologic emergencies and warrants prophylaxis with hydration and either allopurinol or rasburicase depending on risk stratification and TLS management requires ongoing monitoring to correct electrolyte disturbances to prevent clinical sequelae, such as renal impairment, cardiac events, or seizures. Extravasation of intravenous (IV) chemotherapy requires prompt intervention, which may include antidote administration.
4. Immunotherapies are associated with unique immune-related adverse effects (irAEs) managed with immunosuppression (commonly corticosteroids) and dose delay or permanent discontinuation if necessary. Dose reduction is not a strategy used to manage irAEs.
5. Anticancer treatments which capitalize on the immune system, such as chimeric antigen receptor T cell (CAR-T) therapy, can cause cytokine release syndrome (CRS) and neurotoxicity, requiring close monitoring and prompt intervention with the anti-interleukin-6 agent tocilizumab and corticosteroid, respectively.
6. Dermatologic toxicities from cancer treatment are broad in presentation, and accurate identification is important to determine appropriate supportive care interventions. Patients may experience endocrine, cardiovascular, and ocular toxicities as a complication of cancer treatment; prompt identification and management are key to minimizing long-lasting adverse drug reactions (ADRs).
7. Osteopenia or osteoporosis from anticancer treatment or bone fractures and pain from malignancy metastasizing to bone are common. Prevention of skeletal-related complications is important to maintaining patient quality of life.
8. Venous thromboembolisms (VTEs) can be caused by malignancy, treatment, implanted devices (catheters or ports), and comorbidities, and both prevention and treatment are unique in patients with cancer. Routine prophylaxis is recommended in some scenarios, treatment of VTE should continue for at least 3 months or as long as the patient has active cancer or is receiving anticancer therapy, and only certain agents are recommended for prophylaxis and treatment.
9. Patients with cancer may be impacted by pain from various causes, including their disease or complications of cancer treatment and at different time points during their treatment.
10. Numerous long-term physical and psychological complications can occur after cancer treatment. Patients should be educated about potential risk for infertility and secondary malignancies from anticancer treatments.

BEYOND THE BOOK

Activity

Immune checkpoint inhibitors have revolutionized the treatment of patients with cancer. However, their unique toxicity profile brings a new challenge to the health professional. Oncologic societies have published multiple guidelines to aid in managing immune-related adverse events (irAEs). Please review the *National Comprehensive Cancer Network (NCCN) Clinical Practice Guidelines in Oncology* (NCCN Guidelines) for the "Management of Immunotherapy-Related Toxicities"[1] (https://www.nccn.org/professionals/physician_gls/pdf/immunotherapy.pdf). Based on these guidelines and the *National Cancer Institute (NCI) Common Terminology Criteria for Adverse Events (CTCAE) v5.0* guidelines[2] (https://ctep.cancer.gov/protocoldevelopment/electronic_applications/docs/CTCAE_v5_Quick_Reference_8.5x11.pdf), please provide your recommendations on the case below.

This activity is helpful to enhance student understanding of the Assess, Plan, Implement, and Follow-up steps in the patient care process.

Patient Case

AD is a 64-year-old patient with metastatic melanoma who presents to the clinic for cycle 5, day 1 of pembrolizumab. The chief complaint is a 3-day history of severe abdominal pain and "profuse diarrhea," which is estimated to be about 10 bowel movements

(continued)

per day (baseline = 1 bowel movement/day). There is tenderness to palpation on examination, but overall, you feel the symptoms are not life-threatening, afebrile and the patient denies blood in their stool. Based on vital signs and laboratory assessments, the patient is admitted to the inpatient oncology service. Workup suggests an inflammatory process in the colon, which you attribute to pembrolizumab.

PMH: Hypertension (HTN) diagnosed 3 years ago, metastatic melanoma diagnosed 5 months ago

Vitals: O_2sat: 98% (0.98) RA; HR 82 bpm; BP 99/51 mm Hg; 37.4°C

Labs: sodium 138 mEq/L (mmol/L; 136-145 mEq/L [mmol/L]); potassium 2.9 mEq/L (mmol/L; 3.4-5.1 mEq/L [mmol/L]); chloride 99mEq/L(mmol/L;98-107mEq/L[mmol/L]);glucose98mg/dL(74-99mg/dL)(5.4mmol/L[4.1-5.5mmol/L]);albumin3.6g/dL(3.5-5.2g/dL) 36 g/L [35-52 g/L]); calcium 9.28 mg/dL (8.60-10.2 mg/dL) (2.32 mmol/L [2.15-2.55 mmol/L]); magnesium 1.34 mg/dL (1.61-2.60 mg/dL) (0.55 mmol/L [0.66-1.07 mmol/L]); phosphorous 2.0 mg/dL (2. 5-4.5 mg/dL) (0.65 mmol/L [0.81-1.45 mmol/L]); creatinine 0.94 mg/dL (83 μmol/L; CrCl ~80 mL/min [1.33 mL/s]); ALT 28 U/L (0-33 U/L) (0.47 μkat/L [0 -0.55 μkat/L]); ALT 23 U/L (0-32 U/L) (0.38 μkat/L [0-0.53 μkat/L]); T Bili 0.02 mg/dL (0-1.2 mg/dL) (0.3 μmol/L [0-20.5 μmol/L])

Allergies: NKDA

Medication List: lisinopril 10 mg PO once daily; pembrolizumab 200 mg IV every 3 weeks

- Q1. Using NCI CTCAE v5.0, what grade of colitis is AD experiencing?
- Q2. Based on the NCCN guidelines, what is your initial treatment recommendation for this patient? Include any pharmacotherapy interventions and affiliated supportive care measures as well as plan for the current anticancer regimen.
- Q3. After 72 hours of treatment with your initial recommendation, AD's symptoms have not improved. What is your recommendation for the treatment of refractory colitis?

INTRODUCTION

Anticancer treatments can result in numerous adverse drug reactions (ADRs), many of which may be life-threatening if not appropriately managed. ADRs (or toxicities) often relate to the agent's mechanism of action or "off-target" effects. Cytotoxic chemotherapy acts on rapidly dividing cells, often resulting in myelosuppression, gastrointestinal (GI) effects (mucositis, diarrhea, etc.), alopecia, and infertility. Biologic therapies and targeted small molecule agents have various ADRs, depending on the altered intracellular signaling, for example, rash with epidermal growth factor receptor (EGFR) inhibitors and hemorrhage or thrombosis with vascular endothelial growth factor (VEGF) inhibitors. Immunotherapies have a unique ADR profile, including autoimmune toxicities related to the modulation of the immune system. In general, toxicities are commonly graded via the Common Terminology Criteria for Adverse Events (CTCAE) scale from 0 (no toxicity) to 5 (death).[2] The principles of preventing and managing some of the most common and severe ADRs associated with anticancer therapies are detailed below.

HEMATOLOGIC TOXICITIES: ANEMIA, NEUTROPENIA, AND THROMBOCYTOPENIA

Normal hematopoiesis consists of several well-orchestrated steps. Pluripotent stem cells differentiate, proliferate, and maturate to allow the formation of the blood cells seen in the peripheral circulation. Specifically, myeloid stem cells give rise to erythrocytes, platelets, monocytes, basophils, neutrophils, and eosinophils. In contrast, lymphoid stem cells give rise to B-lymphocytes, T-lymphocytes, and natural killer cells (Fig. 150-1).

1 Myelosuppression, depressed bone marrow function resulting in low blood counts—anemia, neutropenia, and thrombocytopenia—can occur due to cancer invasion in bone marrow or after various anticancer therapies. Myelosuppression is typically not an immediate effect because the circulating blood cells must first be killed by the anticancer treatment or used by the body. For example, neutropenia typically occurs first because white blood cells (WBCs) have a short lifespan of 6 to 12 hours, followed by thrombocytopenia as platelets have a lifespan of 5 to 10 days. Anemia typically occurs late since erythrocytes have a relatively long lifespan of 120 days. The lowest blood cell count (or nadir) typically occurs 10 to 14 days after cytotoxic chemotherapy administration, with a recovery in cell counts occurring by 3 to 4 weeks after administration, or later depending on the agent (eg, nitrosoureas and radiolabeled monoclonal antibodies at 4-6 weeks). Patients with leukemia or receiving a hematopoietic stem cell transplantation (HSCT) typically have a more rapid nadir of approximately 5 to 7 days due to the intensity of therapy utilized in these conditions and the nature of the disease. In many scenarios, subsequent doses should be delayed until minimum suggested blood counts (eg, absolute neutrophil count [ANC] ≥1,000-1,500 cells/mm^3 [1×10^9 - 1.5×10^9/L], platelets ≥100,000/μL [100×10^9/L]) are achieved to minimize additional toxicity and morbidity. Dose reductions may be considered empirically based on baseline myelosuppression or, more commonly, during treatment based on either prolonged recovery of counts or severe myelosuppression warranting intervention (transfusions/occurrence of neutropenic fever). However, clinicians must balance dose reduction with treatment goals since reduced treatment intensity can compromise efficacy in certain disease states (eg, breast cancer, lymphoma). Clinicians accept some myelosuppression if it is not compromising the patient's quality of life, and the cancer is responding to therapy. In patients where cure is commonly the goal, the empiric use of hematopoietic growth factor products (also called colony-stimulating factors [CSFs]) provides an alternative to dose reduction.

Neutropenia

Neutropenia is associated with an increased risk of infection, the probability of which increases when ANC is <500 cells/mm^3 (0.5×10^9/L) or when the duration of neutropenia is prolonged (>7-10 days). Other risk factors for infection include alteration in the integrity of physical defense barriers and the functional integrity of the leukocytes, which can be affected by underlying cancer, anticancer agent, or radiation therapy (RT).

Infections are difficult to identify in the neutropenic patient since usual signs and symptoms of infection (eg, purulent drainage) are often absent. Therefore, clinicians heavily rely on fever as an indicator of infection in these patients. Prompt initiation of empiric antibiotics, based on likely organisms from patient presentation

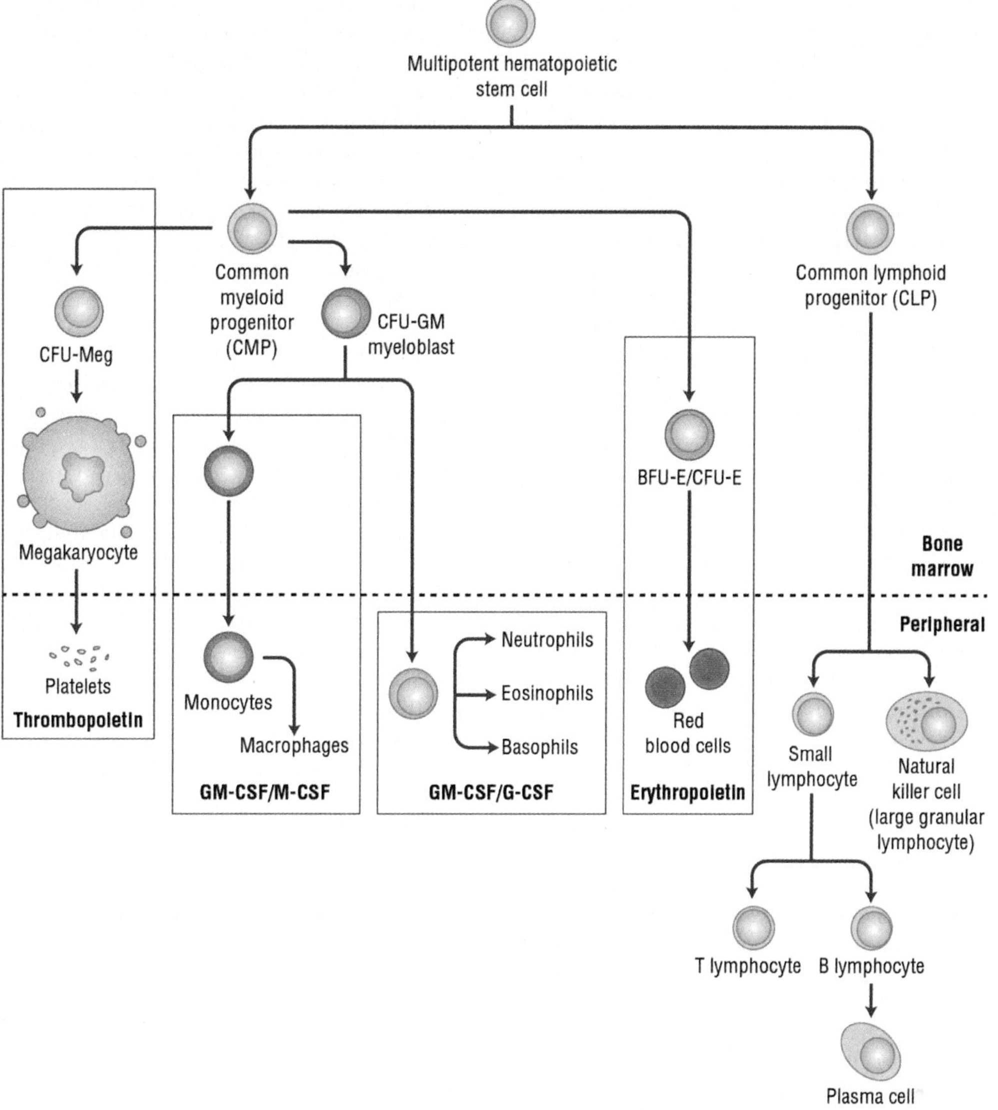

FIGURE 150-1 Schematic of hematopoiesis with site of action of targetable hematopoietic growth factors. Multipotent hematopoietic stem cells (HSCs) differentiate in the bone marrow into common myeloid or lymphoid progenitors (CMP, CLP) which ultimately generate all mature blood cells. In the lymphoid lineage, the CLP gives rise to B cells, T cells, and natural killer (NK) cells. In the myeloid lineage, the CMP gives rise to several colony forming units (CFUs) and burst forming units (BFUs) that result in the creation of platelets (also called thrombocytes), red blood cells (also called erythrocytes), and myeloblast cells (which further give rise to neutrophils, basophils, eosinophils) as well as monocytes (which become macrophages). Numerous hematopoietic growth factors influence the self-sustaining HSCs to differentiate into these various cells; notably, further differentiation of myeloblasts, megakaryocytes, and erythrocytes can be stimulated by granulocyte colony-stimulating factor (G-CSF) or monocyte/macrophage-stimulating factor (M-CSF), thrombopoietin, and erythropoietin, respectively.

and history and local antibiogram, is paramount to prevent mortality. The most common source of infection in these patients is self-infection with body flora, which includes both gram-positive and gram-negative bacteria. Specific treatment of infections in immunocompromised hosts is discussed in Chapter 145, "Infections in Immunocompromised Patients."

CSF products may minimize the severity of neutropenia and subsequently reduce the risk of infection. These products provide proteins essential for the normal growth and maturation of blood cell components (Fig. 150-1). Filgrastim stimulates the production of neutrophilic granulocytes, and sargramostim promotes the proliferation of granulocytes (neutrophils and eosinophils), monocytes, and macrophages. Although sargramostim stimulates megakaryocytes, no consistent effect on platelet production has been observed in trials, and this agent is not commonly used in clinical practice. Both CSFs initially enhance demargination and mobilization of mature cells from the marrow and then provide constant stimulation of stem cell progenitors. Pegfilgrastim is a pegylated form of filgrastim with a substantially longer half-life allowing for single-dose administration compared to daily doses of filgrastim. A pegfilgrastim device is available, which can be placed immediately after the end of chemotherapy to auto-inject the dose of pegfilgrastim 24 hours later. Several biosimilar CSF products are also available and generally considered interchangeable.[3]

For optimal efficacy, CSFs should be started between 24 and 72 hours after chemotherapy. Filgrastim and sargramostim can be stopped the day before chemotherapy, whereas pegfilgrastim should not be administered within 12 days before the next dose of chemotherapy due to its extended half-life.[3] CSFs should not be administered within 14 days of chimeric antigen receptor T cell (CAR-T) due to increased risk of cytokine release syndrome (CRS).[3] Subcutaneous administration is preferred for CSFs. Because of the high cost of these agents, doses of filgrastim are commonly rounded to the nearest product vial size to minimize waste.

CSFs are generally well tolerated, with the most common ADR being bone pain, which can be mitigated with routine concomitant use of an antihistamine, such as loratadine and/or pain medications such as nonsteroidal anti-inflammatory agent naproxen, if no contraindicating factor exists, for the week after CSF administration.[3] Other ADRs include constitutional symptoms (low-grade fever, myalgia, headache, etc.), injection site reactions, and generalized maculopapular rash, with a rare but serious ADR of splenic rupture.

Guidelines exist regarding appropriate use of CSFs for prophylaxis of neutropenia based on the propensity of a regimen to cause febrile neutropenia (FN), which can also be determined from safety results in clinical trial reports.[3,4] Primary prophylaxis, the prevention of neutropenia with the first cycle of chemotherapy, is recommended for patients receiving a chemotherapy regimen with ≥20% risk of FN.[3,4] Most dose-dense chemotherapy regimens require CSF support to maintain dose intensity and schedule.[3] Additionally, primary prophylaxis can be considered for patients with at least one risk factor who are receiving a chemotherapy regimen with a 10% to 20% risk of FN (intermediate risk). Patient risk factors include age at least 65 years receiving full chemotherapy dose intensity, previous chemotherapy or RT, persistent neutropenia, bone marrow involvement of tumor cells, recent surgery and/or open wounds, liver dysfunction, and renal dysfunction. Secondary prophylaxis refers to the prevention of recurrent neutropenia in patients who had experienced a neutropenic complication (eg, FN) with the prior cycle of chemotherapy. Secondary prophylaxis is generally reserved for patients with chemosensitive cancers where a dose reduction or delay may affect survival. In other scenarios, dose reduction or delay in chemotherapy may be utilized instead of CSFs. Re-evaluation of FN risk is warranted after each cycle and at changes in therapy. CSFs are not recommended for neutropenic patients who are afebrile or routinely for management of FN. However, they may be considered for high-risk patients based on clinical judgment and patient-specific risk factors.[3,4] The use of CSFs in pediatric oncology patients is guided by clinical protocol.

Regarding patients with myeloid malignancies, since myeloid blast cells have receptors for granulocyte CSF and granulocyte-macrophage CSF, some experts were initially concerned that the use of CSFs would stimulate the regrowth of leukemia. Although subsequent studies have addressed these concerns and CSFs can be considered after initial induction therapy (although beneficial impact is deemed to be modest), many clinicians do not initiate filgrastim until an initial remission is achieved. CSFs are used following consolidation therapy in adult patients with acute leukemia. Notably, the use of CSFs can interfere with the interpretation of the day 14 bone marrow examination in this population (ie, may see immature myeloid forms erroneously suggesting residual disease); therefore, CSFs should be discontinued at least 7 days before a bone marrow biopsy.[5] Growth factors are not recommended in patients with acute promyelocytic leukemia during induction therapy due to increased risk of differentiation syndrome.[5]

Other uses for CSFs include peripheral blood stem cell mobilization protocols (notably, higher doses than used for prophylaxis) and the management of congenital or idiopathic neutropenia. In patients undergoing HSCT, CSFs have also proven effective in accelerating engraftment and treating graft failure; therefore, they are recommended postautologous HSCT and can be considered postallogeneic HSCT.[4] CSFs should be used with caution in patients receiving concomitant chemotherapy and RT, especially if the RT involves the mediastinum, as these patients appear to experience more significant thrombocytopenia.

Trilaciclib is a first-in-class myeloprotective agent approved for patients with extensive stage small cell lung cancer with ongoing trials for patients diagnosed with other malignancies. When administered before chemotherapy, trilaciclib arrests hematopoietic stem and progenitor cells in the G1 phase to prevent cellular damage from the cytotoxic chemotherapy. It is administered intravenously on each day of chemotherapy administration. The most common adverse effects are fatigue, hepatotoxicity, and electrolyte imbalances (calcium, potassium, and phosphate). Trilaciclib has several drug-drug interactions, including with cisplatin which may result in increased risk of nephrotoxicity.[6]

Anemia

Anemia is a common complication after cytotoxic chemotherapy and various tyrosine kinase inhibitors (TKIs), such as those targeting EGFR, human epidermal growth factor receptor 2 (HER2), and VEGF. Incidence varies by cancer type and stage as well as dose and duration of therapy. Further, patient-specific factors may contribute to nutritional deficiencies (ie, iron, folate, vitamin B12), receipt of RT, renal dysfunction, and anemia of chronic disease. Fatigue is the most common symptom of anemia, with some patients reporting other symptoms such as shortness of breath. Other causes of fatigue should be considered, such as insomnia, depression, unrelieved pain, and underlying malignancy.

The mainstay of treatment of symptomatic or severe chemotherapy-induced anemia is red blood cell transfusion. Transfusions of packed red blood cells (PRBCs) are generally indicated for hemoglobin <8 g/dL (80 g/L; 4.97 mmol/L) or higher if the patient is experiencing extreme fatigue or dyspnea, tachycardia, or chest pain. Erythropoiesis-stimulating agents (ESAs; epoetin alfa, darbepoetin alfa) may be considered in patients with underlying kidney disease and those receiving palliative treatment who have a hemoglobin <10 g/dL (100 g/L; 6.21 mmol/L). ESAs are restricted to these populations due to serious ADRs, including thrombosis and myocardial infarction, and increased risk of mortality in patients with cancer. Other ADRs of ESAs include injection site reactions, rash, flu-like symptoms, and HTN . Therefore, the risks and benefits of ESA use must be discussed with patients in advance. Generally, these ADRs occurred when the target hemoglobin of 12 g/dL (120 g/L; 7.45 mmol/L) is exceeded or hemoglobin rises too rapidly. Evaluation for iron deficiency is advised before initiating ESA with appropriate ongoing laboratory monitoring. If ESAs are utilized, the goal is to achieve the minimum hemoglobin needed to avoid transfusions. ESAs should not be used for nonchemotherapy-induced anemia, except for select patients with myelodysplastic syndrome. Clinical practice guidelines for cancer and chemotherapy-induced anemia are available.[3,7]

Thrombocytopenia

Thrombocytopenia associated with chemotherapy increases the risk for significant bleeding. The mainstay of management is platelet transfusion which is administered to patients with platelet count <10,000 cells/mm^3 (10 × 10^9/L) or higher if patient is experiencing active bleeding, undergoing an invasive procedure, has coagulation abnormalities (eg, acute promyelocytic leukemia), or has fever/documented infection.[8] Alloimmunization rarely occurs due to antibodies against human leukocyte antigen (HLA) antigens; in these scenarios, histocompatible donors must be utilized.

GI TOXICITIES: DIARRHEA, MUCOSITIS, AND NAUSEA/VOMITING

Diarrhea

Mucosal damage can occur at any point along the entire length of the GI tract. In the lower portion of the GI tract, this usually manifests as diarrhea and abdominal pain although onset of symptoms varies by inciting agent (eg, generally within a few days of cytotoxic chemotherapy versus delayed after immunotherapy). Monitoring includes stool count per day, electrolytes, and fluid balance since supplementation may be necessary. After infectious causes have been ruled out, mild-to-moderate diarrhea can safely be treated with loperamide (up to 2 mg every 2 hours), with oral antibiotics and/or octreotide for persistent diarrhea (≥48 hours). Adjunctive diphenoxylate/atropine (diphenoxylate 5 mg four times a day; maximum 20 mg per day) can also be used. Nonpharmacologic interventions include cessation of products containing lactose, alcohol, or high-osmolar supplements with addition of clear liquids and small frequent meals; the BRAT diet (banana, rice, applesauce, toast) may also be considered. Severe or complicated diarrhea (dehydration, hypotension, bleeding, fever, neutropenia, severe cramping, unresponsive to intervention, etc.) warrants hospital admission with hydration, antibiotics, and the somatostatin analog octreotide; notably, anticancer treatment often needs to be held.[9]

Certain anticancer agents are known to commonly cause diarrhea. Irinotecan and sacituzumab govitecan can cause both acute diarrhea, occurring in first 24 hours and managed with atropine to counteract the underlying cholinergic mechanism, and delayed diarrhea, which occurs after 24 hours, and is managed supportively as per above. Other agents that commonly induce diarrhea are 5-fluorouracil, capecitabine, certain targeted chemotherapy agents (eg, imatinib and EGFR, HER2, VEGF, phosphoinositide-3 kinase [PI3K], cyclin-dependent kinase, or CDK4/6, inhibitors), and immune checkpoint inhibitors (ICIs); see "Immune-Related Adverse Events" section. Management of diarrhea may vary by agent and its route of administration.

Mucositis

Due to rapid cellular turnover, the GI mucosa is a common site of toxicity associated with anticancer therapy, particularly cytotoxic chemotherapy agents (eg, fluorouracil, methotrexate) and agents, such as multikinase and mammalian target of rapamycin (mTOR) inhibitors. The subsequent inflammation (mucositis) can lead to painful ulcerations and an inability to eat, drink, or swallow. Disruption of the GI mucosal barrier may also provide an avenue for systemic microbial invasion and infection.

Prevention of mucositis is mainly through good oral hygiene. High-risk patients (poor dentition, high-dose chemotherapy, or RT involving the oropharynx) should undergo a dental evaluation before starting therapy and use mouth rinses (baking soda and salt water or plain saline rinses) during therapy.[10] Oral cryotherapy is recommended before certain chemotherapy, such as high-dose melphalan and 5-fluorouracil, to provide vasoconstriction in prevention of drug delivery to mucosal tissue. Prevention with palifermin, a keratinocyte growth factor, can be considered for patients receiving specific HSCT regimens.[11] Dexamethasone mouthwash can be utilized for mTOR-associated mucositis.[12]

After mucositis has developed, treatment is mainly supportive, including use of topical or systemic analgesics. Despite insufficient data, numerous formulations of "magic mouthwash" are commonly used in clinical practice. There are commercially available products, or a compound can be made often including ingredients of viscous lidocaine, diphenhydramine, and liquid antacid. Severe mucositis may lead to dehydration and require IV hydration and opioid analgesics, with prolonged severe cases also warranting evaluation for IV nutrition. Local infections caused by *Candida* species and herpes simplex virus (HSV) can occur; therefore, suspicious lesions should be cultured and appropriate antifungal or antiviral treatment initiated. Mild infections (ie, thrush) may be treated with topical antifungal therapy, such as clotrimazole troches or nystatin oral suspension, whereas more severe oral or esophageal fungal infections require systemic antifungal treatment (see Chapter 144, "Invasive Fungal Infections").

Nausea/Vomiting

Introduction

Chemotherapy-induced nausea/vomiting (CINV) is the nausea/vomiting (N/V) associated with the administration of chemotherapy, which is a physiologic and psychological process. The impact of CINV on quality of life is substantial. Unless adequately prevented and managed, CINV can lead to adverse outcomes such as metabolic derangements, nutritional depletion, anorexia, weight loss, premature withdrawal of anticancer treatment, and/or degeneration of self-care and functional ability.[13]

Antiemetic prophylaxis is based on emetogenicity, the likelihood an agent will induce N/V,[14] although this can be tailored by patient risk factors (age <50 years, female, history of motion or morning sickness, prior poor CINV control, and depression or anxiety) and prior lack of response to antiemetics.[13] Guidelines divide IV anticancer therapies into four risk categories: highly emetogenic chemotherapy (HEC), moderately emetogenic chemotherapy (MEC), low emetogenic chemotherapy (LEC), and minimally emetogenic, which causes CINV in >90%, 30% to 90%, 10% to 30%, and <10% of patients, respectively.[13] Oral anticancer therapy is classified as minimal-to-low if <30% risk or moderate-to-high risk if ≥30% risk.[13]

Pathophysiology and Definitions Chemotherapy damages enterochromaffin cells lining the GI tract which releases serotonin. This process is the peripheral pathway, originating outside the central nervous system (CNS) and occurs within 24 hours of chemotherapy administration (acute CINV). Secondarily, chemotherapy alters the modulation of dopamine and substance P in the CNS. This process is the central pathway that originates within the CNS and occurs within 24 to 72 hours after chemotherapy administration (delayed CINV)[15] (see Chapter 53, "Nausea and Vomiting," Fig. 53-1). CINV can also be classified as anticipatory (conditioned response occurring before chemotherapy begins), breakthrough (occurs within 5 days of prophylactic antiemetics and requires rescue therapy), refractory, or chronic.

Presentation and Evaluation/Monitoring

Clinical presentation of CINV can include more than just emesis and/or nausea. Patients may also present with poor oral intake, malnutrition, weight loss, abdominal discomfort, dehydration, and dizziness. Monitoring should include laboratory markers of serum electrolytes and renal function as well as assessment of fluid status (input and output), blood pressure (BP; orthostatic hypotension), and medication history.

When evaluating CINV, providers must rule out other potential causes of N/V. The differential diagnosis may include fluid and electrolyte abnormalities, volume depletion, hypercalcemia, drug-/opiate-induced, GI obstruction, increased intracranial pressure, brain or meningeal involvement, uremia, and infection.[15] Ongoing monitoring should include emesis count, nausea score (usually a visual analog scale, or VAS), electrolytes, fluid balance, oral intake, and medication use.

Prevention and Treatment

Several antiemetic guidelines exist (American Society of Clinical Oncology [ASCO], National Comprehensive Cancer Network [NCCN]); however, variations exist across guidelines, which may partially be due to the information available at the time of guideline publication. Some examples of differences across guidelines are with respect to the classification of emetic risk (eg, carboplatin AUC ≥4), preference for 5-hydroxytryptamine/serotonin receptor antagonist (5-HT3-RA) agent in MEC doublet, strength of recommendation for four-drug prophylaxis in HEC and HSCT, duration of dexamethasone in certain regimens, olanzapine dose, management of breakthrough CINV, and recommendation for adjunctive agents.[13,14] Therefore, clinicians should consider these variations when implementing recommendations in practice.

2 Antiemetic prophylaxis is determined by risk category: HEC, quadruplet (or triplet, per NCCN); MEC, doublet (or triplet, per NCCN); LEC, monotherapy; minimal, no prophylaxis (Table 150-1). The primary goal of prevention is no vomiting and no nausea throughout the risk period. The duration of emetic risk is 2 days for MEC and 3 days for HEC—antiemetics should be initiated before any chemotherapy with ≥10% risk (generally 30 minutes before) and administered through risk period.

Patients receiving multiday chemotherapy regimens should be provided antiemetics appropriate for the agent with highest emetogenicity on each day chemotherapy is administered and for the risk period after completion of the regimen, which depends on emetogenicity of last agent(s) administered. For example, a triplet antiemetic therapy is used for 4- to 5-day cisplatin regimens. In patients undergoing HSCT conditioning regimens, triplet or quadruplet antiemetic therapy is recommended.[14]

Oral Anticancer Therapy-Induced N/V

The antiemetic risk of oral anticancer therapies is divided into two categories: moderate-to-high risk (≥30%) versus minimal-to-low risk (<30%). Prophylaxis for moderate-to-high risk is a 5-HT3-RA given 30 minutes before anticancer therapy each day. Prophylaxis for minimal-to-low risk is an as-needed antiemetic agent (5-HT3-RA, prochlorperazine, or metoclopramide). Although if CINV does occur, a scheduled antiemetic before anticancer therapy is recommended.[13] Practical issues must be taken into consideration when choosing a prophylaxis regimen for oral anticancer therapy regimens including setting (inpatient versus outpatient) and available route(s) of administration, overlap with IV regimens, duration of risk period and antiemetic duration of efficacy, tolerability of prolonged antiemetic use, and adherence. Administration of prophylaxis and associated oral anticancer therapy at nighttime may be considered to improve tolerability.

Radiation-Induced N/V

The prevention of radiation-induced N/V is also based on emetogenic risk, which is dependent on the anatomic site of RT.[14] The optimal medication, dosing, and duration of prophylaxis regimen is unknown. Highly emetogenic RT includes total body irradiation (TBI), for which ondansetron or granisetron plus dexamethasone prophylaxis is recommended. For moderate risk, such as RT to the upper abdomen or craniospinal region, ondansetron or granisetron before each fraction as well as dexamethasone before the first five fractions is recommended. For minimal and low risk RT, rescue therapy is recommended.[14]

Regarding those receiving concomitant RT and chemotherapy, antiemetic prophylaxis is based on the emetogenic risk of the chemotherapy regimen, unless the emetogenic risk level of RT is higher, and continuing prophylaxis appropriate for RT if it continues beyond the end of chemotherapy prophylaxis period.[13,14]

Anticipatory CINV

Anticipatory N/V is often a result of prior negative experience. Patient education is critical: first, educate on what prophylaxis is being offered to alleviate fear; second, educate on specific management strategies for coping with CINV. For example, behavioral therapy can be employed and if benzodiazepine is prescribed; this can be administered 30 minutes before arriving to ambulatory care treatment center or before meals, depending on association of event/food with onset of nausea. Often, lorazepam 0.5 to 2 mg oral (PO)/IV every 4 to 6 hours or pre-meals is utilized in clinical practice.

Management of Breakthrough and Refractory CINV

All patients should be provided with breakthrough (PRN) medication and instructed to take as soon as feel nauseated or have emesis. Choice of breakthrough agent may vary in practice, although selecting an agent not previously given as prophylaxis and consideration of toxicities of antiemetics are key considerations. Options include olanzapine, phenothiazine, metoclopramide, dronabinol, scopolamine patch, haloperidol, 5-HT3-RA, dexamethasone, or benzodiazepine.

TABLE 150-1 CINV Prophylaxis for IV Chemotherapy Regimens

CINV Prophylaxis Regimen Definitions

Quadruplet Therapy	Triple Therapy	Doublet Therapy	Monotherapy
5-HT3-RA + steroid + NK1-RA + olanzapine	5-HT3-RA + steroid + NK1-RA *or* olanzapine	5-HT3-RA + steroid Optional: triplet regimen based on patient-specific risk factors (ie, NK1-RA- or olanzapine-based triplet)	5-HT3-RA *or* dexamethasone (per ASCO) *or* metoclopramide *or* prochlorperazine (per NCCN) All ONCE Doses

CINV Prophylaxis Recommendations for IV Chemotherapy[14]

Risk	Phase	Prophylaxis
HEC	Acute Phase	Quadruplet: 5-HT3-RA + dexamethasone + NK1-RA + olanzapine
	Delayed Phase	Olanzapine on days 2-4 If used on day 1, oral aprepitant continues days 2-3 If regimen other than AC, dexamethasone continues days 2-3 (dose varies by which NK1 utilized)
MEC	Acute Phase	Doublet: 5-HT3-RA + dexamethasone
	Delayed Phase	Dexamethasone 8 mg PO/IV on days 2-3 only if patients receiving therapies with known potential for delayed CINV
LEC	Acute Phase	Monotherapy: 5-HT3-RA or dexamethasone
	Delayed Phase	None
Minimal	Acute Phase	None
	Delayed	None

AC, anthracycline + cyclophosphamide; NK1-RA, neurokinin-1 receptor antagonist.

Notes: Per ASCO guideline,[14] carboplatin with AUC ≥4 specifically warrants prophylaxis in acute phase with 5-HT3-RA + Dex + NK1-RA and none in delayed phase. When given at equipotent doses, oral and IV serotonin receptor antagonists are equivalent in efficacy.

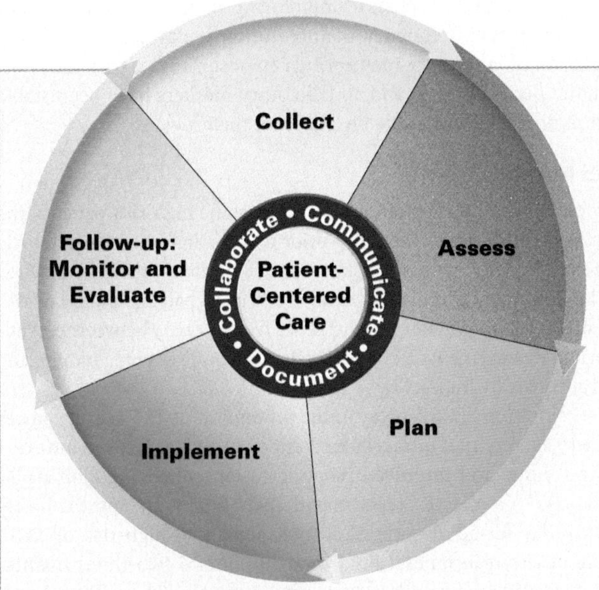

Patient Care Process for Supportive Care in Cancer

The patient care process for tumor lysis syndrome (TLS). See "Oncologic Emergencies: TLS and Extravasation" section and Table 150-2.

Collect

- Patient demographic factors including concomitant medications, cancer diagnosis, and current/impending anticancer treatment intervention(s) along with their affiliated TLS risk category
- Laboratory markers: potassium, SCr, calcium, phosphorus, and uric acid

Assess

- Urine output and hydration status
- Presence of cardiac arrhythmias or seizure activity (ie, obtain ECG and EEG if warranted)
- Presence of symptoms of hyperkalemia (eg, muscle cramps), hypocalcemia (eg, paresthesia), hyperphosphatemia (eg, lethargy), and/or hyperuricemia (eg, oliguria/anuria)

Plan*

- Drug therapy regimen to include hydration with allopurinol for intermediate-risk or rasburicase for high risk. Additionally, add interventions for specific laboratory TLS as indicated (eg, phosphorus binder for hyperphosphatemia)
- Monitoring above laboratory parameters as per risk level

Implement

- Patient education on symptoms of clinical TLS
- Schedule follow-up laboratory monitoring as per risk level

Follow-up: Monitor and Evaluate

- Ongoing laboratory monitoring (at least daily or more frequently if intermediate to high risk or active clinical TLS)
- Resolution of any signs/symptoms and ongoing clinical assessment for renal, cardiac, and/or neurologic changes

**Collaborate with patient, caregivers, and other healthcare professionals.*

If breakthrough occurs, future cycles should be adjusted (ie, increase prophylaxis).[13] Specifically, if olanzapine was not previously included in prophylaxis, it should be added.[14]

ONCOLOGIC EMERGENCIES: TLS AND EXTRAVASATION

Oncologic emergencies are a diverse group of acute complications associated with cancer pathophysiology itself and/or the initiation of anticancer treatments. These situations may be the presenting reason for acute hospitalization whereby a diagnosis of cancer is made or may occur at any time during a patient's course of management. Prompt identification and adequate initial treatment are critical to prevent morbidity and mortality. Many complications are considered oncologic emergencies, including TLS and extravasation, which are detailed below. (3) Other oncologic emergencies are beyond the scope of this chapter but include hypersensitivity reaction (see Chapter e108, "Drug Allergy"), FN (see Chapter 145, "Infections in Immunocompromised Patients"), hypercalcemia of malignancy (see Chapter 69, "Calcium and Phosphorus Homeostasis"), malignant spinal cord compression, superior vena cava syndrome, malignant pericardial effusion, malignant airway obstruction, disseminated intravascular coagulopathy, hyponatremia, hyperviscosity syndrome, and leukocytosis.[16,17]

Tumor Lysis Syndrome

TLS is the most common disease-related oncologic emergency. TLS occurs due to the rapid destruction of cells either spontaneously from cancer progression or due to effects of antineoplastic therapy.[18] The lysis of cells releases intracellular contents leading to catabolism of nucleic acids, which results in hyperuricemia while the release of potassium and phosphorus leads to hyperkalemia, hyperphosphatemia, and secondary hypocalcemia. Urate or phosphorus-calcium crystals can cause renal insufficiency, hyperkalemia can cause cardiac disturbances, and hyperphosphatemia can lead to seizures. Laboratory TLS is defined by the Cairo-Bishop Criteria[73] (Table 150-2) while clinical TLS is the presence of laboratory TLS plus at least one of the following: renal impairment (serum creatinine [SCr] $\geq 1.5 \times$ ULN), cardiac arrhythmias, or seizures. Cairo-Bishop grading scale for TLS evaluates level of renal impairment, cardiac arrhythmia, and seizure activity on a grade 0 to 5 scale.[18] Risk factors are patient-related (preexisting conditions such as dehydration, hypotension, acidosis, renal or cardiac disease) and disease-related (cancer diagnosis, tumor burden – bulky tumor >10 cm or WBC $>25 \times 10^3/\mu L$ ($25 \times 10^9/L$), elevated lactate dehydrogenase, high proliferation rate, chemotherapy sensitivity). While lactate dehydrogenase is a surrogate marker for cell turnover rate and can therefore be a component in risk assessment, it is not part of the diagnosis of TLS.[19] TLS occurs most commonly in patients with aggressive hematologic malignancies, such as high-grade lymphomas or acute leukemias. Incidence varies widely depending on cancer and treatment type. Notably, TLS can occur not just after traditional cytotoxic IV chemotherapy, but also after RT, oral chemotherapy, or targeted therapy (eg, monoclonal antibodies).[20] TLS often occurs within

TABLE 150-2 **Tumor Lysis Syndrome: Definition, Presentation, and Management**

Laboratory TLS[a]	Symptoms/Signs	Management Strategies
Uric acid ≥8 mg/dL (476 μmol/L) or >25% ↑ from baseline	• Obstructive uropathy, hematuria, flank pain, lethargy, oliguria, or anuria	• Prevention: hydration, allopurinol (or potentially febuxostat); consider for low risk and optional for intermediate risk • Management: continue hydration; rasburicase optional for intermediate risk and recommended for high risk; allopurinol for those unable to receive rasburicase
Calcium ≤7 mg/dL (1.75 mmol/L) or >25% ↓ from baseline	• Muscle cramp/spasms, tetany, paresthesia, neurologic (confusion, hallucination, seizure), arrhythmia, bradycardia, cardiac failure, death	• First, manage hyperphosphatemia • If symptomatic, IV calcium may be administered
Potassium ≥6 mEq/L (mmol/L) or >25% ↑ from baseline	• GI (nausea, diarrhea, anorexia), muscle weakness/cramps, ECG abnormalities, sudden death	• Loop diuretic • IV insulin + dextrose • Inhaled albuterol • If mild/moderate – oral resin binder • If ECG changes – IV calcium • If acidotic – IV sodium bicarbonate
Phosphorous ≥4.5 mg/dL (1.45 mmol/L) in adults or ≥6.5 mg/dL (2.1 mmol/L) in children (>25% ↑ from baseline)	• GI (nausea, diarrhea), lethargy, seizures	• Reduce phosphorus intake • Phosphorus binders

[a]Two or more of the laboratory changes must be observed within 3 days before or 7 days after cytotoxic therapy.

Data from References 17 and 73.

12 to 72 hours of initiation of antineoplastic therapy, although it can occur later depending on the antineoplastic agent's onset of activity or spontaneously prior to treatment initiation.

TLS Monitoring

TLS Monitoring includes laboratory markers (uric acid, potassium, calcium, phosphorus), renal function, urine output, fluid status, and if needed assessment for arrhythmias (electrocardiogram [ECG]) or seizure activity (electroencephalogram [EEG]). At a minimum, daily assessment during period of risk is required, but more frequent monitoring may be warranted. For example, patients with intermediate risk warrant monitoring every 8 to 12 hours while those classified as high risk and those with active laboratory or clinical TLS may warrant up to every 4- to 8-hour laboratory monitoring.[21] Further, certain cytotoxic therapies have specific guidance regarding required monitoring and management of TLS for patients receiving those agents (eg, venetoclax).[22]

Clinicians should consider trends in laboratory markers (ie, levels and time between any changes in levels), patient risk stratification, and time point around chemotherapy when making recommendations for monitoring and interventions. Adjustment of laboratory monitoring should occur based on patient response to interventions (ie, increase monitoring if optimal response not achieved, reduce frequency of monitoring if not TLS occurring). Cessation of laboratory monitoring can occur once a patient is outside the period of risk, and all laboratory markers have been stable within normal limits at the discretion of the provider.

TLS Management

Prevention of TLS is paramount. First, in some high-risk patients, the oncologist may opt to "de-bulk" prior to initiating intensive cytotoxic chemotherapy to reduce the risk of severe TLS often with agents, such as cyclophosphamide or hydroxyurea.[23] Second, all patients should be risk stratified, which dictates prophylaxis. Overlap exists between prevention and management of TLS as all patients require ongoing monitoring and adequate hydration (Table 150-2).

Hydration is a mainstay in the prevention of TLS as it enhances urinary excretion of intracellular components via increased intravascular volume and improved renal perfusion enhancing glomerular filtration.[24] Guidelines recommend hydration with approximately 3 L/m^2/day for adult patients at intermediate-to-high risk of TLS[25] while others recommend fluid intake of one to two times maintenance requirements with a goal urine output of 80 to 100 mL/m^2/hr.[24] Although specific fluid types or hydration rates are not standardized, typical fluids are isotonic saline or dextrose containing products as potassium additives or fluids containing potassium (ie, Lactated Ringer's) should be avoided given the risk of hyperkalemia.[25] While diuretics may be used to enhance excretion, caution is warranted, and providers must first ensure no obstruction or hypovolemia exists. No benefit is seen with the addition of alkalinization (ie, sodium bicarbonate); therefore, this strategy is no longer recommended.[25] Hydration should be continued during management of TLS.

Prevention and Management of Hyperuricemia

Hyperuricemia occurs due to the breakdown of nucleic acids released from cells. As uric acid is poorly soluble, it can precipitate leading to obstructive uropathy and acute kidney injury. To prevent and manage hyperuricemia, patients at low risk may receive allopurinol, those with intermediate risk can receive either allopurinol or rasburicase, and those at high risk are recommended to receive rasburicase.

Allopurinol is a xanthine oxidase inhibitor which prevents the conversion of xanthine to uric acid. Therefore, this intervention is preventative with a slow onset of action and should ideally be initiated at least a day before starting chemotherapy. Notably, xanthine itself can accumulate and lead to crystallization, although the precise impact on TLS is not well characterized. Recommended dose of allopurinol is 300 mg/m^2/day PO in one to three divided doses rounded to tablet size (available in 100 mg and 300 mg tablets), with a maximum of 800 mg/day; intravenous (IV) administration is available with different dosing for those unable to take oral medications. Renal dose adjustment is necessary. Allopurinol may cause GI ADRs, rash, as well as hypersensitivity reactions particularly in Asian populations due to a higher frequency of HLA-B*58:01 allele associated with more severe cutaneous drug reaction.[19] Febuxostat is another xanthine oxidase inhibitor which may be used as an alternative to allopurinol.[26] This agent does not require renal dose adjustment and is associated with lower risk of hypersensitivity reactions.

In patients with hyperuricemia before anticancer treatment begins, xanthine oxidase inhibitors are unlikely to be effective. Therefore, rasburicase, a recombinant urate oxidase that converts uric acid into more soluble allantoin, is warranted for the management of hyperuricemia. A fixed dose of rasburicase (6 mg IV once)[27] is recommended for adult patients as a cost-saving measure. Pediatric protocols may require weight-based dosing. Peak activity occurs around 4 hours, and it is generally well tolerated, although GI ADRs, headache, and rash may occur. Notably, pregnant patients and those with glucose-6-phosphate dehydrogenase (G6PD), deficiency are at risk for hemolysis and methemoglobinemia; therefore, assessment in those of certain ethnic background (African American, Mediterranean, or Southeast Asian) who are more likely to exhibit G6PD deficiency is warranted before administration if feasible. Further, blood samples drawn after administration of rasburicase must be immediately placed on ice for transport to laboratory, otherwise the drug continues to act on the blood sample and can lead to falsely low readings.

Management of Electrolyte Disturbances

Rapid treatment of hyperkalemia can be achieved with loop diuretics or intracellular shift of potassium via the administration of 10 units of IV insulin (0.1 unit/kg for pediatric patients) followed by dextrose (generally 25-50 mL of 50% dextrose for adults) or inhalation of albuterol. For mild hyperkalemia not necessitating rapid treatment, cation exchange resins, such as sodium polystyrene sulfate 15 to 30 g PO once, with repeat doses as needed based on repeat potassium levels, can be utilized to remove potassium through the GI tract. Slow infusion of calcium gluconate (1 g IV for adults) can be administered to patients with ECG changes as it can stabilize myocardial membranes, while sodium bicarbonate (50 mEq IV for adults) can be administered if metabolic acidosis is present. Potassium level of 7 mEq/L (mmol/L) or greater or a widening QRS complex warrants immediate attention with aggressive interventions and close monitoring.[19]

Treatment of hyperphosphatemia includes minimization of dietary phosphorus intake and use of phosphorus binders (ie, sevelamer, calcium acetate, aluminum hydroxide), although caution is warranted for aluminum-based products in patients with renal dysfunction while calcium carbonate products should be avoided in those with hypercalcemia.

Hypocalcemia should not be directly managed unless the patient is symptomatic, due to the risk of furthering the calcium phosphate deposition in renal tubules. First, hyperphosphatemia should be corrected. If hypocalcemia is symptomatic, a slow infusion of calcium gluconate may be administered with ECG monitoring for resolution of symptoms and not necessarily correction to normal value.

Patients with congestive heart failure (HF), renal insufficiency (eg, anuria), calcium-phosphorus product of 70 mg^2/dL^2 (5.6 $mmol^2/L^2$) or more, or TLS refractory to aforementioned interventions may need dialysis to manage electrolyte disturbances.[19] Further details on electrolyte management can be found in Chapter 69, "Calcium and Phosphorous Homeostasis" and Chapter 70, "Potassium and Magnesium Homeostasis."

Extravasation

Extravasation is the unintentional leakage of drug from the injection site into surrounding subcutaneous or subdermal healthy tissue where uptake of the drug may result in cell death. Symptoms and signs of extravasation may include pain, redness, or swelling as well as difficulty with utilization of the IV line such as resistance to infusion or lack of blood return.[28] While fairly infrequent (incidence <7%), it can lead to negative patient outcomes and morbidity.[29] Prevention methods include but are not limited to proper vascular access, the use of a central IV line (eg, port, peripherally inserted central catheter, also known as PICC), and adherence to chemotherapy administration guidelines.[30] Cytotoxic chemotherapy can be classified as exfoliants (cause tissue peeling/inflammation without cell death), inflammitants (cause inflammation/erythema/flare reaction without pain), irritants (cause inflammation/pain without tissue damage), or vesicants (cause tissue necrosis/blisters).[30]

Management of extravasation of a vesicant is specific to the chemotherapy agent and may include administration of a certain antidote (Table 150-3). Dimethyl sulfoxide administered topically neutralizes free radicals and promotes absorption as well as possesses anti-inflammatory, anesthetic, and vasodilatory properties. Hyaluronidase administered subcutaneously (SQ) promotes drug diffusion and absorption by degrading hyaluronic acid, which breaks down subcutaneous tissue bonds. Sodium thiosulfate administered SQ can neutralize mechlorethamine into nontoxic thioesters and neutralizes via the creation of an alkaline-rich environment where the vesicant can bind sodium thiosulfate.[28,30] Dexrazoxane is an IV agent, Food and Drug Administration (FDA) approved for the management of extravasation of anthracyclines due to its proposed mechanism of preventing free radical formation through binding of iron and reduction in oxidative stress. Precise dosing and administration information for each antidote agent can be found in product labeling and tertiary drug information resources.

TABLE 150-3 Management of Extravasation

Chemotherapy Agent/ Vesicant	Potential Antidote(s)	Compress Recommendation	
		Cool	Warm
Anthracycline agents	Dexrazoxane	X	
	Dimethyl sulfoxide		
Cisplatin	Sodium thiosulfate	X	
	Dimethyl sulfoxide		
Antitumor antibiotics			
Dactinomycin	--	X	
Mitomycin	Dimethyl sulfoxide	X	
Mitoxantrone	Dimethyl sulfoxide	X	
Docetaxel	Hyaluronidase	X	
Mechlorethamine	Sodium thiosulfate	--	--
Oxaliplatin	Sodium thiosulfate	Controversial/ unknown	
Paclitaxel	Hyaluronidase	X	
Vinca alkaloids	Hyaluronidase	Avoid	X

Data from References 28 and 30.

Nonpharmacologic interventions are standard for any extravasation and include immediate cessation of the chemotherapy agent, aspiration, avoidance of flushing the IV line as this may further potentiate the extravasation, and elevation of the limb for ~48 hours to promote drainage.[28,30] Compresses generally applied for ~20 minutes four times a day for 24 to 48 hours are recommended. While a cool compress is recommended for extravasation of most agents to localize the vesicant by providing vasoconstriction to avoid further spread of the drug, only warm compresses should be used for the extravasation of vinca alkaloids to avoid further tissue damage and promote drug absorption and redistribution.[28,30] Moist compresses and occlusive dressings should be avoided.[31]

IMMUNE-RELATED ADVERSE EVENTS

The use of ICIs (ie, cytotoxic T-lymphocyte-associated protein 4 [CTLA4], programmed cell death protein 1 [PD-1], and programmed death-ligand 1 [PD-L1] inhibitors) in cancer care has exploded at a rapid pace. These agents work by activating the immune system, but ICIs can also attack healthy cells causing a unique group of toxicities called irAEs. Although irAEs are the most notable toxicities seen with ICIs, fatigue is the most common ADR. The most commonly affected organ systems are skin, gut, endocrine, lung, and musculoskeletal system, whereas cardiovascular, hematologic, renal, neurologic, and ocular irAEs are rare. The onset of irAEs is delayed and varies by organ system affected and specific ICI administered. Rash/dermatitis presents first, about 2 to 3 weeks following first ICI dose, while diarrhea/colitis typically presents around week 5, and hepatotoxicity and hypophysitis around week 7.[32] The incidence rate of any grade irAEs ranges from 15% to 90%.[1] CTLA4 inhibitors are associated with a higher rate of irAEs than PD-1/PD-L1 inhibitors, and severe irAEs result in treatment delay or discontinuation in 0.5% to 13% of patients. Combination treatment of ipilimumab and nivolumab is associated with the highest rate of severe irAEs and often requires treatment delay or discontinuation. Fortunately, irAEs are typically reversible, with the exception of endocrine-related irAEs.

The prompt recognition and management of irAEs is key to keeping patients on therapy. Several clinical practice guidelines to manage irAEs have been published by various professional organizations including the Society for Immunotherapy of Cancer,[33] the European Society for Medical Oncology,[34] the NCCN,[1] and ASCO.[32] The majority of irAEs that occur are mild to moderate, and patients may typically continue on ICI therapy. Notably, ICI therapy is not dose-reduced for toxicities, only held/delayed. (4) Management varies slightly by the organ system affected, but first-line therapy is commonly systemic corticosteroids with doses ranging from 0.5 to 2 mg/kg/day of oral prednisone. If corticosteroids are indicated for irAE management, ICI therapy should be held until the irAE is grade ≤1 and the patient has tapered off corticosteroids. Patients who present with severe irAEs are treated with IV methylprednisolone at 1 to 2 mg/kg/day initially and typically require ICIs to be held or permanently discontinued. If no response to corticosteroids within 48 to 72 hours, occurs additional immunosuppression is recommended based on evidence for treating autoimmune diseases for the respective organ system affected. Commonly employed immunosuppressive agents include tumor necrosis factor (TNF) inhibitors (ie, infliximab, etanercept), vedolizumab, mycophenolate, IV immunoglobulin, or IVIG, and rituximab.

Patients on prolonged corticosteroid require additional interventions, including monitoring for hyperglycemia, H2-receptor antagonists or proton pump inhibitors to prevent gastritis, anti-infective prophylaxis (eg, consider prophylaxis against herpes zoster), and vitamin D and calcium supplementation (see "Bone Health" section). Patients receiving prednisone equivalent of ≥20 mg for ≥4 weeks require PJP (*Pneumocystis jirovecci pneumonia*) prophylaxis as well as fungal prophylaxis (eg, fluconazole) if it is continued for ≥6 weeks. In patients requiring anti-TNF therapy, testing for hepatitis B and C virus should be conducted prior to administration if possible, but should not delay initiation of TNF inhibitor treatment. TNF inhibitors should be avoided in patients with immune-related hepatitis due to the risk for hepatotoxicity.

Patients at higher risk of developing irAEs or experiencing an exacerbation of underlying comorbidities include those with autoimmune diseases. These patients may experience a flare of their underlying condition; therefore, immunosuppression for their preexisting autoimmune condition should be optimized prior to ICI initiation. Ideally, patients who are on prednisone for their autoimmune condition would be controlled on <10 mg of prednisone daily (or equivalent) prior to starting ICI. Caution is also utilized in patients who were prior organ transplant recipients as they are at risk for graft failure and transplant organ loss. In patients who received an allogeneic stem cell transplant, graft-versus-host disease (GVHD) is a risk.

ICIs are a significant advancement in the treatment of cancer; however, they are associated with unique toxicities called irAEs. These toxicities are delayed in presentation and have a prolonged duration. irAEs may occur months and even years after ICI discontinuation requiring clinicians to remain vigilant in monitoring patients. irAEs are commonly managed with immunosuppression, typically corticosteroids. Patients with mild-to-moderate irAEs can often remain on therapy, but patients who require corticosteroids or have severe irAEs often need to have treatment held or permanently discontinued. Additional supportive care interventions are required in patients on prolonged courses of corticosteroids or who require additional immunosuppressive therapy beyond corticosteroids.

CELLULAR IMMUNOTHERAPY ADRs: CRS AND NEUROTOXICITY

While immune activation directly leads to the efficacy of therapies that engage T cells, the subsequent massive release of various cytokines can lead to clinically significant ADRs, namely CRS and neurotoxicity. These events can occur after infusions of any cellular immunotherapy product, such as CAR-T therapy (eg, tisagenlecleucel and axicabtagene ciloleucel) or bispecific T-cell engaging therapy (BiTE; eg, blinatumomab). These ADRs require prompt identification and accurate grading to provide optimal management. (5) However, their grading and management may differ by product as delineated below. Ongoing studies are evaluating optimal prevention and management of these ADRs.

CAR-T

CRS is caused by endogenous or infused immune effector cells, such as T cells, leading to a supraphysiologic and rapid release of cytokines.[35] CRS grading is based on symptoms, which includes fever at onset and may also include hypotension and/or hypoxia.[35] Symptoms can be progressive, and end-organ damage may occur. CRS typically presents in the first 2 weeks with median onset of approximately 3 days after CAR-T infusion and median duration of about 1 week necessitating monitoring of vital signs (temperature, BP, and oxygen saturation) twice daily during this time.[1] Treatment of CRS includes antipyretics for fever with fluid and/or oxygen supplementation as clinically necessary. Tocilizumab, an anti-interleukin-6 agent, is FDA-approved for moderate to severe cases (eg, grade 2 and higher CRS) dosed as 8 mg/kg IV (maximum dose: 800 mg) with up to three repeat doses in 24 hours. Dexamethasone 10 mg IV up to every 6 hours is recommended for persistent refractory grade 2 (eg, nonresponse to 1-2 doses of tocilizumab) and for grade 3-4 CRS. For refractory grade 4, methylprednisolone 1,000 mg/day for up to three doses IV can be utilized with escalation to every 12 hours if refractory.[1,36]

Neurotoxicity after cellular immunotherapy was specifically termed immune effector cell-associated neurotoxicity syndrome (ICANS).[35] ICANS is thought to be due to diffusion of either the immune effector cells and/or cytokines through blood-brain barrier into the CNS. ICANS typically occurs within the first 4 weeks of cellular infusion with median onset of approximately 7 days and duration of about 14 days.[1] Signs and symptoms of ICANS can vary among patients and may include aphasia, impairment in cognition, reduced level of consciousness, seizures, motor weakness, or cerebral edema. ICANS grading requires the assessment of five domains: level of consciousness, seizure activity, motor findings, cerebral edema/elevated intracranial pressure, as well as the 10-point Immune Effector Cell-Associated Encephalopathy, or ICE Score, which should all be assessed twice daily during the at-risk period.[1] Notably, the Cornell Assessment of Pediatric Delirium (CAPD) is used instead of ICE Score for pediatric patients under the age of 12 years with further specific guidance available for interpreting actions in patients under 2 years.[35] Management of ICANS includes supportive care with aspiration precautions as well as anti-epileptics and interventions to manage elevated intracranial pressure as needed. Further, corticosteroids are the mainstay of management of ICANS of grade 2 or higher[36] with dexamethasone (grade 2: 10 mg IV and may repeat; grade 3: 10 mg IV q 6 hours or methylprednisolone 1 mg/kg IV q12 hours; grade 4: high-dose steroid regimen such as methylprednisolone 1,000 mg/day or twice daily × 3 days with a rapid taper over approximately 1 week).[1]

Bispecific T-Cell Engaging (BiTE)—Blinatumomab

Blinatumomab is a BiTE antibody construct that links CD3 T cells to the targeted malignant cells (CD19 B cells) for destruction in patients with B-cell acute lymphoblastic leukemia, or ALL. Unlike CAR-T therapy, which once infused is active within the body, due to short half-life blinatumomab is administered as a continuous infusion which allows for the management of ADRs via holding drug or discontinuation.

CRS is less common and often less severe after blinatumomab than CAR-T, most often low grade and occurring in the first cycle or at dose escalation.[37,38] Prevention of CRS includes cytoreduction for high-risk patients, initiation of blinatumomab with dose escalation inpatient for monitoring, and routine prophylactic dexamethasone.[38,39] The CTCAE is utilized for grading CRS after blinatumomab. Management of CRS from blinatumomab includes utilization of dexamethasone, dose interruption, or discontinuation[38] and potentially off-label use of tocilizumab for severe CRS.[37] Notably, the use of corticosteroids has not been shown to impact efficacy.[40]

Neurotologic events are common after blinatumomab (~50%-65% of patients), most frequently occurring within 1 to 2 weeks of the first cycle.[37] Severe (grade 3 or higher) events occur in approximately 10% to 20% of patients which necessitates holding therapy and resumption at a lower rate with permanent discontinuation for grade 4 neurotoxicity, if >1 seizure, or if recurs when a patient is receiving reduced infusion rate.[38] Precise management may vary by institution or research protocol,[41] including the use of dexamethasone or tocilizumab for severe symptoms (encephalopathy, aphasia).[37,39,41] Anti-epileptics are warranted for patients with seizure activity, although prophylaxis is not routinely utilized.[39]

DERMATOLOGIC TOXICITIES

6 Anticancer treatment can cause a variety of dermatologic toxicities affecting a patient's skin, hair, and nails. These toxicities may result in dose reductions or treatment discontinuation, which affects patient outcomes. It is important to be able to accurately recognize, prevent, and manage these ADRs.

Skin

Dry Skin (Xerosis) and Pruritus

Dry skin is reported in up to 84% of patients on anticancer treatment and can negatively impact their quality of life and lead to infections, sensitization to allergens and pruritus.[42-44] Dry skin and pruritus are reported more commonly with targeted therapies. Skin can be more sensitive to ultraviolet radiation and more prone to skin pigmentation. Counseling points on prevention measures include avoiding alcohol-containing lotions and irritating products, limiting shower time, using gentle cleansers, routinely applying emollients and sun-protective measures. Treatment of mild-to-moderate pruritis can include a topical antipruritic agent containing menthol 0.5% or a topical corticosteroid (mometasone furoate 0.1% ointment or betamethasone valerate 0.1% ointment) and oral antihistamines, in particular nonsedating second-generation agents. Second-line options include antiepileptic agents (pregabalin and gabapentin), doxepin, aprepitant, and short-term, systemic corticosteroids (0.5-2 mg/kg/day).

Acneiform RASH

Acneiform rash or papulopustular eruption is characterized by an eruption of papules and pustules commonly appearing on the face, scalp, upper chest, and back.[43] It is the most common ADR in patients treated with EGFR inhibitors (all grade: 75%-90%, grade 3/4: 10%-20%) and commonly seen in patients on MEK (mitogen-activated protein kinase) inhibitors (all grade: 74%-85%, grade 3/4: 5%-10%). It begins within the first few days to weeks following treatment initiation, and patients report pruritus, stinging, and pain. Prevention and management strategies for this rash are detailed in Table 150-4 and commonly include a good skin care routine, avoidance of sun exposure, topical corticosteroids, and oral antibiotics.

Hand-Foot Syndrome and Hand-Foot Skin Reaction

Hand-foot syndrome (HFS) also known as palmar-plantar erythrodysesthesia syndrome, acral erythema, or toxic erythema, is characterized by redness, marked discomfort, swelling, and tingling in the palms of the hands and soles of the feet.[43] Common chemotherapy causes include 5-fluorouracil, capecitabine, doxorubicin, pegylated liposomal doxorubicin, docetaxel, and cytarabine. It may be severe (grade 3/4) in 5% to 10% of patients, and the incidence increases with the use of multiple causative agents. Hand-foot skin reaction (HFSR) differs from HFS in presentation with well-defined painful hyperkeratosis. Multikinase VEGFR inhibitors such as sorafenib, cabozantinib, sunitinib, and regorafenib are a common cause. HFSR is less common with lenvatinib, pazopanib, and sunitinib and is grade 3/4 in 5% to 20% of patients.

The onset of this reaction is usually within days to weeks, but may take up to 6 months to appear. With HFS, the first symptoms are dysesthesia of the palms and soles with a tingling that develops into burning pain, swelling, and erythema followed by hyperkeratosis. Lesions can progress to blisters, desquamation, erosions, ulcerations, and bleeding associated with discomfort and moderate to severe pain. HFSR more commonly affects the soles, and blisters occur followed by callus-like hyperkeratosis at pressure-bearing areas. Table 150-4 includes prevention and management strategies for HFS and HFSR.

Pigmentary Changes

Hyperpigmentation may occur at different sites and in different patterns.[42] It can present within days to months after treatment and usually fades months after therapy discontinuation. Some of the agents associated with hyperpigmentation include busulfan, bleomycin, methotrexate, capecitabine, 5-fluourouracil, docetaxel, doxorubicin, ifosfamide, and thiotepa. C-kit inhibitors (eg, imatinib) can cause diffuse or localized hypopigmentation, as c-kit is involved in the regulation of melanocyte function. It is usually reversible with dose reductions or discontinuation. Patients, especially those with melanoma, on immunotherapy may experience vitiligo-like lesions.

Other Rashes

Many treatments may cause a nonspecific maculopapular rash or morbilliform eruption that starts gradually with mild symptoms including pruritus weeks after treatment.[42] Management includes antihistamines and when localized topical corticosteroids or when more diffuse short-term oral corticosteroids. Up to 50% of patients on rapidly accelerated fibrosarcoma (RAF)/ v-raf murine sarcoma viral oncogene homolog B1 (BRAF) inhibitors may experience a maculopapular rash that appears early and spreads quickly.[45] Approximately 20% of patients on these therapies also develop non-melanoma skin cancer that should be excised. Less commonly, rash occurs in patients treated with gemcitabine, pemetrexed, and liposomal doxorubicin.[45] Up to 95% of patients may experience acute or chronic RT dermatitis, and patients receiving concurrent chemotherapy are at higher risk.[46] A delayed recall reaction may occur weeks to years following RT and present as a new rash that appears after treatment with a precipitating drug. Common offending agents include taxanes, doxorubicin, and gemcitabine. Prevention and management strategies include instructing the patient to wear loose fitting clothing to avoid friction, avoid sun exposure and exposure to extremes of temperature, and not use cosmetic or irritating products to the radiated skin. Patients should use a good emollient during treatment, and topical corticosteroids may be added. Anticancer

TABLE 150-4 Acneiform Rash/HFS/HFSR

Toxicity	Prevention	Treatment
Acneiform rash (Papulopustular exanthema)	• Avoid frequent washing with hot water • Avoid skin irritants, including OTC anti-acne medications containing benzoyl peroxide, solvents, or disinfectants • Use alcohol-free[a] OTC moisturizing creams or ointments BID, preferably with urea-containing (5%-10%) moisturizers to the body • Avoid excessive sun exposure • Apply sunscreen (SPF) ≥15 to exposed areas of body and reapply every 2 hours when outside • Oral antibiotics for 6 weeks at start of therapy (doxycycline 100 mg PO BID or minocycline 100 mg PO daily; if unable to tolerate/allergy cephadroxil 500 mg PO BID or trimethoprim-sulfamethoxazole 160/80 mg PO BID), with or without topical low/moderate-strength steroid to face and chest BID	Grade 1/2: • Continue anticancer treatment • Continue or initiate: oral antibiotic for 6 weeks AND topical low/moderate steroid • Reassess after 2 weeks; if no improvement or worsening escalate therapy Grade ≥3: • Interrupt anticancer treatment until grade 0/1 • Obtain bacterial/viral/fungal cultures if infection is suspected • Continue or initiate: oral antibiotic for 6 weeks AND topical low/moderate steroid, systemic corticosteroids (eg, prednisone 0.5-1 mg/kg × 7 days) • Reassess after 2 weeks; if no improvement or worsening may need to discontinue treatment
HFS and HFSR	• Avoid irritation to hands and feet; long walks, heavy carrying without protection • Avoid chemical stress; skin irritants, solvents, or disinfectants • Treat predisposing factors before anticancer therapy • Apply 10% urea cream TID • For taxane-based therapy: use skin cooling gloves or socks • For capecitabine-based therapy: may consider celecoxib 200 mg PO BID	• Anticancer treatment interruption and dose reduction commonly required; initiation of topical agents (HFS and HFSR) or cooling (HFS) may allow for continued dosing • Hyperkeratosis: treat with keratolytics (topical creams or ointments with 5%-10% salicylic acid or 10%-40% urea) • Inflammation: high-potency topical corticosteroids (eg, clobetasol proprionate 0.05%) • Erosions and ulcerations: antiseptic solutions (eg, silver sulfadiazine 1%, polyhexanide 0.02%-0.04%) • Pain: lidocaine 5% cream or patches • Reassess after 2 weeks; if no improvement or worsening escalate therapy

BID, two times daily; OTC, over the counter; SPF, sun protection factor; TID, three times daily.

[a]Avoid SD alcohol 40, denatured alcohol, ethanol, and isopropyl alcohol.

Data from Reference 43.

treatment can cause photosensitivity, phototoxic, or photoallergic reactions. Inflammatory rashes occur on photo-exposed areas in patients treated with 5-fluorouracil and taxanes. Vemurafenib and vandetanib are associated with ultraviolet A (UVA) sensitivity, and preventive sun measures are required.[42]

Hair

Alopecia

Alopecia is one of the more distressing and well-known dermatologic toxicities mainly caused by chemotherapy but is also reported with targeted agents and hormone therapy.[42,43] Chemotherapy-induced alopecia (CIA) typically results in diffuse complete hair loss on the entire scalp, but patients may have diffuse partial alopecia, or patchy, unevenly distributed alopecia. It may also involve eyebrows, eyelashes, and body hair. CIA typically begins 1 to 3 weeks after treatment, and hair will start regrowing 2 to 3 months after completion. Hair loss severity is dependent upon the type, dose, method of administration, and time between treatments. Cyclophosphamide, doxorubicin, irinotecan, and taxanes are associated with a high risk of CIA. Endocrine therapy-induced alopecia usually does not result in complete hair loss and is located primarily on the crown of the scalp, with recession of the frontal and bitemporal hairline. It is more common in postmenopausal women receiving aromatase inhibitors and is most noticeable between 6 and 18 months after treatment initiation. Scalp cooling is the only proven method to prevent CIA, but efficacy is only 50% to 80%. Scalp cooling causes vasoconstriction and reduced biochemical activity in the scalp and hair follicles. These techniques are contraindicated in patients whose cancer can metastasize to the scalp, such as leukemia and lymphoma. To treat alopecia following anticancer treatment, patients may use topical minoxidil 5%. Patients may also consider taking biotin to stimulate hair growth. Patients are informed about potential alopecia prior to initiating treatment, and a discussion regarding hats, scarfs, or wigs to protect the scalp should occur.

Other Hair Changes

Patients on targeted therapies may report changes in hair quality, texture, and growth pattern starting months 2 or 3 of treatment.[42] Excessive hair growth in androgen-dependent areas of the body may occur in women on endocrine therapies. Trichomegaly, or longer, thicker, and often curled eyelashes and hypertrichosis are associated with EGFR inhibitors. Patients may need to trim their eyelashes to prevent eye irritation. The hypopigmentation associated with c-KIT inhibitors, such as pazopanib, also impacts the hair presenting as white hair growth.

Nails

Nail changes are common during treatment and usually disappear following the completion of therapy.[42] Cytotoxic chemotherapy usually results in melanonychia (black or brown discoloration that is diffuse, transverse, or longitudinal), leukonychia (white spots), onycholysis (nail detachment from the nail bed), Beau's lines (indentations across the nail), onychomadesis (proximal separation of the nail plate from the nail matrix), and onychorrhexis (brittle nails). Patients receiving a taxane may experience painful subungual hemorrhage followed by onycholysis and occasional abscess. Chemotherapy and targeted therapy may cause brittle nails, nail cracking, and splitting. Preventive strategies include decreased exposure to water, use of cotton gloves, and nail hydration with thick emollients. Patients may consider oral biotin to help with nail growth and nail lacquers. Asymptomatic splinter subungual hemorrhages of black, red, or brown are common in patients treated with

VEGFR inhibitors. EGFR inhibitors are associated with the risk of paronychia occurring two or more months after treatment initiation on finger and toenails. Similar lesions are reported less frequently with MEK inhibitors and mTOR inhibitors.[43] Additional prevention methods include the use of comfortable shoes, adequate nail trimming, and use of antiseptic solutions. If fissuring occurs, protective covering should be applied.

ENDOCRINE TOXICITIES

The endocrine system is complex and composed of a series of glands that produce and secrete hormones used by the body for a variety of functions. Anticancer treatment can impact these glands resulting in dysfunction in hormone production.

Hypothalamic-Pituitary Dysfunction

RT is a common cause of hypothalamic-pituitary dysfunction in patients with cancer. The onset and severity are dose-dependent and may occur years later. Symptoms are nonspecific and include fatigue and weakness. Management includes hormone replacement as necessary.[47] Although rare, ICI can cause hypophysitis, inflammation of the pituitary gland which is delayed in onset and also managed with hormone replacement as well as ICI dose delays and discontinuation if necessary[1] (see Chapter e98, "Pituitary Gland Disorders").

Thyroid Dysfunction

Thyroid function can be affected by a variety of anticancer treatments including RT, targeted therapy, and cytokines.[48] Hypothyroidism is more common than hyperthyroidism. Patients on multitargeted TKIs and ICIs should have their thyroid function (thyroid-stimulating hormone [TSH] and free thyroxine or T4) monitored at baseline and periodically while on treatment. Hypothyroidism is common in patients on sunitinib, with a variable onset, most commonly 4 weeks. Other TKIs associated with hypothyroidism include sorafenib, imatinib, dasatinib, nilotinib, and axitinib. Drug-induced hypothyroidism can persist following TKI discontinuation. Patients on thyroid hormones prior to treatment initiation often need dose increases while on TKI treatment. ICIs are associated with both hyper- and hypothyroidism, with hypothyroidism being more common. Hyperthyroidism also often transitions into hypothyroidism. Patients can typically continue on ICI but need lifelong thyroid supplementation.[1] RT to the neck is associated with primary hypothyroidism, especially when treated during childhood. Five years after treatment nearly half of patients develop hypothyroidism, with a median onset of 1.5 years posttreatment[48] (see Chapter 96, "Thyroid Disorders").

Hyperglycemia

Hyperglycemia is a common toxicity seen in patients with cancer. Glucocorticoids are likely the most common cause of hyperglycemia. They are used as an antiemetic, for edema from brain metastasis, prevention of transplant rejection, treatment of GVHD, and irAEs, and even in some anticancer treatment regimens.[49] Agents that inhibit the phosphoinositide-3 kinase (PI3:K)/protein kinase B (also known as AKT)/mTOR pathway are associated with hyperglycemia due to the interruption of intracellular response to insulin, resulting in decreased glucose transport, decreased glycogen synthesis, and increased glycolysis.[50] The PI3K inhibitors (eg, alpelisib) and mTOR inhibitors (eg, everolimus) are associated with grade 3 to 4 hyperglycemia in approximately 10% of patients. ICIs can rarely cause hyperglycemia, pancreatitis, and new-onset type I diabetes. L-asparaginase can induce hyperglycemia through both direct and indirect effects inhibition of insulin production and release, and pancreatitis, respectively.[49]

Patients should be periodically screened for diabetes by fasting plasma glucose, oral glucose test, hemoglobin A1c, random plasma glucose levels, or pre- or postprandial glucose testing. Management of hyperglycemia should consider glycemic variability of the agent administered, and commonly includes oral anti-hyperglycemic agents and insulin. Patients may require treatment interruption or discontinuation if hyperglycemia cannot be controlled[49,50] (see Chapter 94, "Diabetes Mellitus").

BONE HEALTH

7 Cancer and its treatment can have a significant impact on bone health. Patients may be at risk for osteoporosis and metastatic bone disease, which can significantly affect quality of life.

Osteoporosis

Osteoporosis is a common complication of anticancer treatment, especially hormonal therapy.[51] Additionally, chronic inflammation associated with cancer can promote increased bone loss via altered systemic bone remodeling, increased bone resorption, and impaired bone formation. Rates of bone loss from anticancer treatment can be more than sevenfold greater than that of normal aging. Patients with the following conditions may be considered for bone-modifying treatment: premenopausal women receiving gonadotropin-releasing hormone (GnRH) therapies causing ovarian suppression, premenopausal women with chemotherapy-induced ovarian failure or who have had an oophorectomy, postmenopausal women who are receiving aromatase inhibitors, men who have received or are receiving androgen deprivation therapy, patients undergoing or with a history of bone marrow transplantation, or patients with chronic (>3-6 months) glucocorticoid treatment. Assessment and treatment of bone loss is similar to other patients at risk for osteoporosis (see Chapter 112, "Osteoporosis" for more detail).

Bone Metastases

Metastatic bone disease is common in multiple myeloma, prostate, breast, lung, and kidney cancer.[52] Bone metastases commonly affect the axial skeleton and lead to skeletal-related events (SREs): pathological fracture, need for RT to the bone, surgery to bone, spinal cord compression, and hypercalcemia of malignancy. Bone pain is the result of structural damage and will be discussed in more detail (see "Bone Pain (Not Oncologic Emergency)" section). Preventing SREs is important as they are associated with loss of mobility, decreased social functioning, reduced quality of life, increased health care expenditure, and poor survival.

The pathophysiology of bone metastases is not completely understood.[52] Disseminated tumor cells enter the bone marrow microenvironment and may stay dormant for years before causing damage. Proliferating tumor cells can produce a variety of cytokines and growth factors, which increase osteoblast production of receptor activator of nuclear factor kappa-B ligand, or RANKL, that then leads to the activation of osteoclasts and disruption of normal bone formation and bone resorption. Multiple skeletal sites are typically involved. Patients report pain and boney tenderness. Imaging modalities (eg, computed tomography [CT] scan, magnetic resonance imaging [MRI], bone scan, positron emission tomography [PET]) are used for diagnosis and monitoring every 3 to 6 months.

The goal of treatment is to prevent disease progression and palliate symptoms.[52] Treatment varies by the underlying malignancy. Local external beam RT is effective at relieving painful bone metastasis with overall response rates of 70% to 80%. Approximately one-third of patients report complete pain relief. Targeted RT with systemic radioisotopes may be used to spare normal tissues in patients will multiple metastatic sites in some malignancies. Radium-223 (^{223}Ra) is a bone-seeking alpha particle-emitting radiopharmaceutical approved for use in bone-predominant metastatic castration-resistant prostate cancer (see Chapter 154, "Prostate Cancer"). Surgical intervention may be recommended to maintain

TABLE 150-5 BMA Dosing for Bone Metastases

Medication	Brand Name[a]	Dose
Denosumab	Xgeva	120 mg SQ every 4 weeks
Pamidronate	Aredia	90 mg IV over 2 hours every 3-4 weeks
Zoledronic acid	Zometa	4 mg IV over 15 minutes every 3-4 weeks[b]

[a]Note: unique brand names, dosing, and schedule for this indication.
[b]May be dosed every 12 weeks after treatment for 3-6 months.
Data from Reference 52.

TABLE 150-6 Lifetime Cumulative Anthracycline Dose Conversion and Maximums

Anthracycline	Conversion Factor	Maximum Recommended Cumulative Dose (mg/m²)
Doxorubicin	1	550
Daunorubicin	1	550 (no CV risk factors)
	0.7	400 (chest irradiation or CV risk factors)
Epirubicin	1.6	900
Idarubicin	0.3	150
Mitoxantrone	0.25	140

CV, cardiovascular.
Data from Reference 60.

patient function and mobility by relieving pain, preventing impending fractures and/or neural compression, or stabilizing a pathological fracture.

Bone-modifying agents (BMA; eg, zoledronic acid, pamidronate, and denosumab; Table 150-5), potent inhibitors of bone resorption, are also used to relieve pain and reduce the risk of and time to the development of SREs. Patient factors including the risk for an SRE and overall disease control help to determine which BMA is used. Denosumab is preferred when considering efficacy, convenience, and renal health. However, generic bisphosphonates are more cost-effective and not associated with a risk of rebound osteolysis. Once a patient develops bone metastases, it is common to initiate therapy and continue indefinitely. Use in specific cancers will be discussed in their respective chapters (see Chapter 151, "Breast Cancer"; Chapter 154, "Prostate Cancer"; and Chapter 159, "Multiple Myeloma"). BMAs are generally well tolerated; however, they may cause hypocalcemia due to the inhibition of bone resorption. Calcium and vitamin D levels should be monitored at baseline and throughout treatment.[52,53] Patients who are vitamin D deficient should be repleted and then maintained with daily supplements of 800 to 2,000 units/day. To maintain an adequate daily calcium intake, supplementation of 1,000 to 1,200 mg/day should be recommended. With prolonged BMA administration, it is important to monitor for osteonecrosis of the jaw and for patients to have a thorough dental exam prior to initiation if possible.

Spinal cord compression is a medical emergency that requires an urgent MRI to confirm the diagnosis.[52] Patients with spinal cord compression should receive 16 to 24 mg of dexamethasone/day to decrease inflammation and preserve function. This should be tapered over 2 weeks if possible. Patients with a single area of compression and good performance status may be amenable to surgery followed by RT. Patients unable to tolerate surgery should receive RT alone.

OTHER TOXICITIES

Ocular Toxicities

A broad spectrum of ocular toxicities may be seen with anticancer treatment. Common ocular toxicities reported include blurred vision, photophobia, conjunctivitis, cataracts, abnormal lacrimation, dry eye, keratitis, optic neuropathy, and retinopathy.[54-56] Ocular toxicities are typically mild (grade 1-2) but may progress to severe and result in blindness. For agents associated with more severe toxicities, routine ophthalmic surveillance and baseline assessment are recommended. Follow-up appointments with the cancer care team should include an assessment of eye pain, redness, and changes in vision. Some specific management strategies for ocular toxicities include artificial tears and lubricants for dry eyes and keratitis, steroid eye drops for conjunctivitis (especially from high-dose cytarabine), and systemic diuretics to manage periorbital edema (that is common with BCR-ABL TKIs like imatinib). Patients who experience photophobia and flashing lights from anaplastic lymphoma kinase (ALK) inhibitors tend to have symptoms improve over time.

Cardiovascular Toxicities

Patient-related and treatment-related factors contribute to cardiovascular toxicities experienced by patients with cancer.[57] Cardiovascular toxicity may be a short- or long-term complication, asymptomatic or symptomatic, as well as reversible or irreversible. Patients may experience HF, HTN, QT prolongation, arrhythmias, myocarditis, and other cardiac abnormalities from systemic treatment, RT, CAR-T therapy, or HSCT. A thorough cardiac workup should be conducted before initiating any potential cardiotoxic treatment, and any conditions identified should be well controlled according to current cardiovascular guidelines before treatment. A baseline risk assessment should include cardiac history, anticancer treatment history, cardiovascular risk factors, BP, hemoglobin A1c, cholesterol profile, cardiac biomarkers (troponin and natriuretic peptides), ECG, and echocardiogram (ECHO).

Left Ventricular Dysfunction/Heart Failure

Anthracyclines, HER2-targeted therapy, VEGFR inhibitors, and some proteasome inhibitors (eg, carfilzomib) may cause left ventricular dysfunction (LVD).[58] Anthracyclines are associated with type I LVD, which is a result of cellular loss, and is irreversible.[59] Anthracycline-induced cardiotoxicity can be categorized as acute, occurring immediately after the infusion (<1% of patients); early-onset progressive, occurring during therapy or within the first year of treatment (~2%); or late-onset chronic, occurring at least 1 year after therapy (1.6%-5%). Risk factors include cumulative dose, IV bolus administration, higher single dose, history of prior RT, use of other concomitant cardiotoxic drugs (cyclophosphamide, trastuzumab, paclitaxel), female gender, underlying cardiovascular disease, age (young and older adult), increased time since completion of chemotherapy, and increase in cardiac biomarkers (troponin, natriuretic peptides) during and after treatment. The risk of cardiotoxicity is cumulative, whereby patients are at risk for cardiotoxicity when they have reached the cumulative lifetime doses of anthracyclines. Patients who have received more than one type of anthracycline should have their cumulative lifetime dose converted to doxorubicin equivalents (Table 150-6).[60] Type II cardiotoxicity results from cellular dysfunction (mitochondrial and protein alterations) and is usually temporary, without injury marker release, and cardiac function returns to baseline. HER2-targeted agents and VEGF inhibitors are common examples of agents that cause type II LVD. When these agents are given in combination with anthracyclines, the risk of cardiovascular toxicity increases; therefore, trastuzumab should not be given in combination with anthracyclines. Type II LVD is not dose-related or cumulative.

Quantitative assessment with an ECHO or multigated acquisition (MUGA) of LV ejection fraction (LVEF) and diastolic function prior to cardiotoxic treatment may help to identify patients at high risk of cardiovascular complications.[58] It also serves to establish a baseline should symptoms occur during treatment. Patients should have routine monitoring with an ECHO or MUGA while on therapy (for HER2 therapy every 3 months; for anthracyclines after cumulative doxorubicin dose of 250 mg/m^2 or its equivalent, or after each additional 100 mg/m^2) and following treatment completion to evaluate for delayed onset cardiovascular toxicity.

Patients receiving treatment known to cause cardiotoxicity should be considered to have stage A HF (see Chapter 36, "Chronic Heart Failure"). Patients may be considered for prophylactic angiotensin converting enzyme inhibitors (ACEIs), angiotensin receptor blockers (ARBs), or selected beta-blockers (BBs) to decrease the risk of cardiotoxicity. Dexrazoxane may be used as a cardioprotectant in certain patients receiving >300 mg/m^2 cumulative anthracycline-based treatment, or at anthracycline treatment initiation in patients with preexisting cardiomyopathy. Because dexrazoxane has the potential to decrease anthracycline efficacy due to its free radical scavenging activity, it is not widely used.

Asymptomatic patients treated with anthracyclines who have a decrease in LVEF of ≥10% from baseline to 50% or a decrease to ≥40% and <50%, initiation of cardioprotective agents (ACEIs, ARBs, or BBs), if not already prescribed, and a cardiology (cardio-oncology specialist) consultation should occur. A benefit-risk discussion for continued anthracycline use versus changing to non-anthracycline treatment should occur. Patients may benefit from the use of dexrazoxane or liposomal doxorubicin, if appropriate. Patients on trastuzumab who experience the same impact in LVEF should also have a cardiology consultation and cardioprotective treatments started. If mild asymptomatic reductions in LVEF occur, trastuzumab therapy may be continued. If trastuzumab is stopped, LVEF can be reassessed within 3 to 6 weeks and restarted if LVEF is >50%. In patients on other therapy associated with LVD, if LVEF decreases, cardioprotective treatment and repeat LVEF assessment should occur every 3 months. Patients who have LVD and are diagnosed with HF should be managed according to the American College of Cardiology/American Heart Association guidelines.

Hypertension

HTN is a risk factor for chemotherapy-induced cardiotoxicity. Several cancer treatments are associated with the risk of HTN, most notably the VEGF inhibitors. BP increases usually occur within 1 day of treatment initiation and stabilizes within 6 to 10 days. Possible predictors of HTN include age ≥ 60 years, body mass index ≥25 kg/m^2, and pre-HTN. Resting BP should be monitored daily during the first cycle of VEGF inhibitor treatment, and once BPs are stabilized, it can be extended to every 2 to 3 weeks while on treatment. More frequent monitoring is recommended in patients with preexisting HTN and those at a higher cardiac risk. Potential contributors to BP elevation include obstructive sleep apnea, excessive alcohol consumption, nonsteroidal anti-inflammatory drugs (NSAIDs), adrenal steroids, erythropoietin, oral contraceptives, and sympathomimetics (methylphenidate). Management of HTN should follow the American College of Cardiology/American Heart Association guidelines (see Chapter 30, "Hypertension"). It is important to be mindful of potential drug-anticancer treatment interactions when selecting antihypertensive therapy. Once VEGF inhibitor therapy is stopped, HTN management should be modified and stopping antihypertensive therapy may be necessary to avoid hypotension.

QT Prolongation

Several anticancer therapies have a known potential to cause QT prolongation including arsenic trioxide, midostaurin, histone deacetylase inhibitors, TKIs and cyclin-dependent kinase 4/6 inhibitors.[58] Some agents with warnings for serious or life-threatening risks for QT interval prolongation include sunitinib, sorafenib, vandetanib, crizotinib, vemurafenib, dasatinib, lapatinib, and nilotinib. Agents associated with QT interval prolongation should be used with caution in patients with hypokalemia or hypomagnesemia, genetic long QT syndrome, and those on other QT prolonging medications. Electrolyte abnormalities should be corrected prior to initiation and during therapy. ECGs should be conducted at baseline and periodically to assess for QT prolongation and arrhythmia.

Others

Atrial fibrillation (AF) can also occur with some anticancer agents (eg, ibrutinib, anthracyclines, immunomodulatory agents).[61] Management of AF from anticancer treatment considers rhythm versus rate control and thromboembolic prophylaxis. There is no valid risk assessment in patients with active cancer, so several cardiovascular and oncology-related factors are considered, including the CHADS-VASC score; HAS_BLED score; thromboembolic and bleeding risk of the malignancy; platelet count; and life expectancy (see Chapter 40, "Arrhythmias"). Anticoagulant selection should consider potential drug interactions with anticancer therapy. Rate control is typically preferred over rhythm control, particularly if the agent causing AF is continued. BB is commonly used due to the lack of drug-drug interactions. Cardiac ischemia is a rare cardiovascular toxicity from anticancer treatment.[59] Anti-microtubule agents (ie, taxanes and vinca alkaloids), anti-metabolites (ie, fluorouracil, capecitabine), platinum compounds (ie, cisplatin), and some VEGF inhibitors have been linked to ischemic events.[62] Baseline ECG and frequent vital sign monitoring are recommended for early detection.

SPECIAL CONSIDERATIONS

VTE Prevention and Management

8 VTE, which includes deep VTE (DVT) and pulmonary embolism (PE), is a common cause of cancer-associated morbidity and mortality. Potential pathophysiological causes for VTE in patients with cancer include known hypercoagulability (pro-coagulants expressed by cancer cells), vessel wall damage, and vessel stasis from direct tumor compression.[62] Several factors place patients at a higher risk of VTE, including the malignancy type and stage, systemic treatment used, surgery, RT, and use of indwelling catheters. Patient factors such as advanced age, comorbidities, previous VTE, hereditary thrombophilia, and immobilization and hospitalization also contribute to VTE risk. The risk of a patient with cancer developing a VTE is four- to sevenfold greater than the general population and is reported in up to 15% of patients each year.[63] Patients with cancer are also more likely to have higher rates of VTE recurrence and bleeding complications during VTE treatment.[63]

Prophylaxis

Routine prophylaxis is not recommended in all patients with cancer but is indicated in certain scenarios.[62,63] Patients with an active malignancy who are hospitalized should be offered thromboprophylaxis with unfractionated heparin (UFH) or low-molecular-weight heparin (LMWH) in the absence of bleeding or other contraindications. Patients who have major surgery for their cancer should receive thromboprophylaxis for at least 7 to 10 days. Patients who have a high-risk abdominal or pelvic cancer surgery should have VTE prophylaxis continued for up to 4 weeks postoperatively. Patients who are ambulatory receiving chemotherapy should be assessed for VTE risk utilizing the Khorana prediction model. Patients identified to have a high risk (Khorana score ≥2; see NCCN guidelines for score calculation) should be offered prophylaxis with apixaban, rivaroxaban, or LMWH for up to 6 months or longer if the risk persists.

Patients diagnosed with multiple myeloma who are receiving treatment with immunomodulatory drugs may be indicated to receive VTE prophylaxis based upon their SAVED and IMPEDE VTE Score (see NCCN guidelines for score algorithms). Patients determined to be high risk should be offered enoxaparin, dalteparin, warfarin, or apixaban prophylaxis, while low risk patients may be offered no intervention or aspirin prophylaxis. Refer to the NCCN and ASCO guidelines for specific drug dosing recommendations.

Treatment

Once a patient is diagnosed with a VTE, treatment should be continued for at least 3 months or as long as the patient has active cancer or is receiving anticancer therapy.[62] For noncatheter associated clots, patients should be on anticoagulation indefinitely while the cancer is active, while they are receiving treatment, or if risk factors for recurrence persist. For a catheter-associated clot, patients should be on anticoagulation as long as the catheter is in place. The agent used for VTE treatment should be selected based upon a variety of factors: renal failure, hepatic disease, inpatient or outpatient status, FDA approval, cost, patient preference, ease of administration, monitoring, bleeding risk, and ability to reverse anticoagulation, if needed. Direct oral anticoagulants (DOACs), LMWHs, fondaparinux, and UFH are available options for initial treatment. Warfarin is not recommended as first-line therapy in patients with cancer, as LMWHs have been associated with a lower risk of recurrent VTE without an increased risk of major bleeding, but may be used for long-term anticoagulation in certain circumstances. DOACs are absorbed primarily in the stomach and proximal bowel (apixaban is partially absorbed in the colon) and may not be good options for patients who have had significant resections of these areas. DOACs should be used with caution in patients with genitourinary or GI tract lesions, pathology or instrumentation, since they have been associated with an increased risk of GI bleeding and possibly genitourinary tract bleeding. LMWH is preferred in these patients. Refer to the NCCN and ASCO guidelines for specific drug dosing recommendations.

Unique Considerations

Thrombocytopenia is a common complication of anticancer treatment and can place patients on anticoagulation at an increased risk of bleeding. Generally, anticoagulation is considered safe to use in patients with a platelet count of 50×10^9/L (50,000/mm^3) or more. The NCCN guidelines provide guidance for prophylactic and treatment dosing of anticoagulation in patients who are thrombocytopenic.[62] Some additional contraindications to anticoagulation include active bleeding, indwelling neuraxial catheters, neuraxial anesthesia/lumbar puncture, interventional spine, and pain procedures. The NCCN guidelines also offer further guidance on potential relative contraindications to anticoagulation and recommendations for holding anticoagulation around surgeries and procedures, including lumbar punctures. Patients with cancer are at risk for recurrent VTE and anticoagulation failure. Patients may require a change in dose, schedule, or agent. The NCCN guidelines also provide recommendations if this occurs.

Pain Management

9 Pain is one of the most common symptoms experienced by patients with cancer. It can be acute or chronic, and has multiple possible etiologies such as the disease itself (eg, tumor invasion, organ obstruction), treatment (eg, chemotherapy, RT, and surgical incisions), or diagnostic procedures (eg, biopsy). Nociceptive and neuropathic are the two most predominant mechanisms of pain pathophysiology. To ensure proper management, a comprehensive pain assessment should be completed at the initial evaluation, at each subsequent contact, and at the start of a new therapy. The goals of pain management are to optimize patient treatment outcomes in five dimensions, also known as the 5A's of pain management outcomes: analgesia (optimize, analgesia), activities (optimize activities of daily living), adverse effects (minimize ADRs), aberrant drug-taking (avoid aberrant drug-taking), and affect (relationship between pain and mood). Treatment must be individualized considering clinical circumstances and patient wishes, with the goal of maximizing function and quality of life (see Chapter 79, "Pain Management" for more information).

It is important to determine if pain is related to an oncologic emergency, which is a life-threatening event directly or indirectly related to a patient's cancer or anticancer treatment. This includes pain due to bone fracture or impending fracture of weight-bearing bone, epidural or leptomeningeal metastases, pain associated with infection, or obstructed or perforated viscus. Oncologic emergency-related pain should be treated immediately while concurrently treating the underlying condition. Patients with pain not related to an oncologic emergency may be treated with a combination of pharmacologic analgesics; nonopioids (eg, NSAIDs or acetaminophen), opioids, and adjuvant analgesics (eg, antidepressants, anticonvulsants, topical agents, and corticosteroids) or nonpharmacologic integrative interventions (eg, physical, cognitive modalities, spiritual).

Adult cancer pain can be categorized by level of pain intensity (0-no pain, 10-worst pain; mild [1-3], moderate [4-7], and severe [8-10]) which can be used to help guide treatment decisions (Table 150-7). For patients with severe pain, pain crisis, or uncontrolled pain, hospital or inpatient hospice may be required for treatment due to the frequent need to reassess and adjust opioid dosing to achieve adequate pain control (Fig. 150-2). See Chapter 79, "Pain Management" and NCCN Adult Cancer Pain guidelines[64] for medication dosing, ADRs, drug interaction, and contraindication information. Patients may experience inadequate pain relief despite

TABLE 150-7 Cancer-Related Pain Treatment Recommendations

Pain Intensity (Numerical Rating Score)	Opioid-naïve	Opioid-tolerant
Mild (1-3)	• Nonopioid analgesics + adjuvant analgesics	• Nonopioid analgesics + adjuvant analgesics • Re-evaluate need for opioid analgesics and initiate gradual dose reductions if indicated
Moderate (4-6)	• Nonopioid analgesics + adjuvant analgesics + short-acting opioids as needed • Titrate every 3-4 hours • If ≥4 doses are needed/day, consider addition of long-acting opioid based on TDD	• Nonopioid analgesics + adjuvant analgesics + short-acting opioids as needed • Titrate short-acting opioids with goal of increasing TDD by 30%-50% until pain relief is achieved • If ≥4 doses are needed/day, consider addition or increase in dose of long-acting opioid based on TDD
Severe (7-10)	• Consider hospital or inpatient hospice admission • IV or oral short-acting opioids	

TDD, total daily dose.

Data from Reference 64.

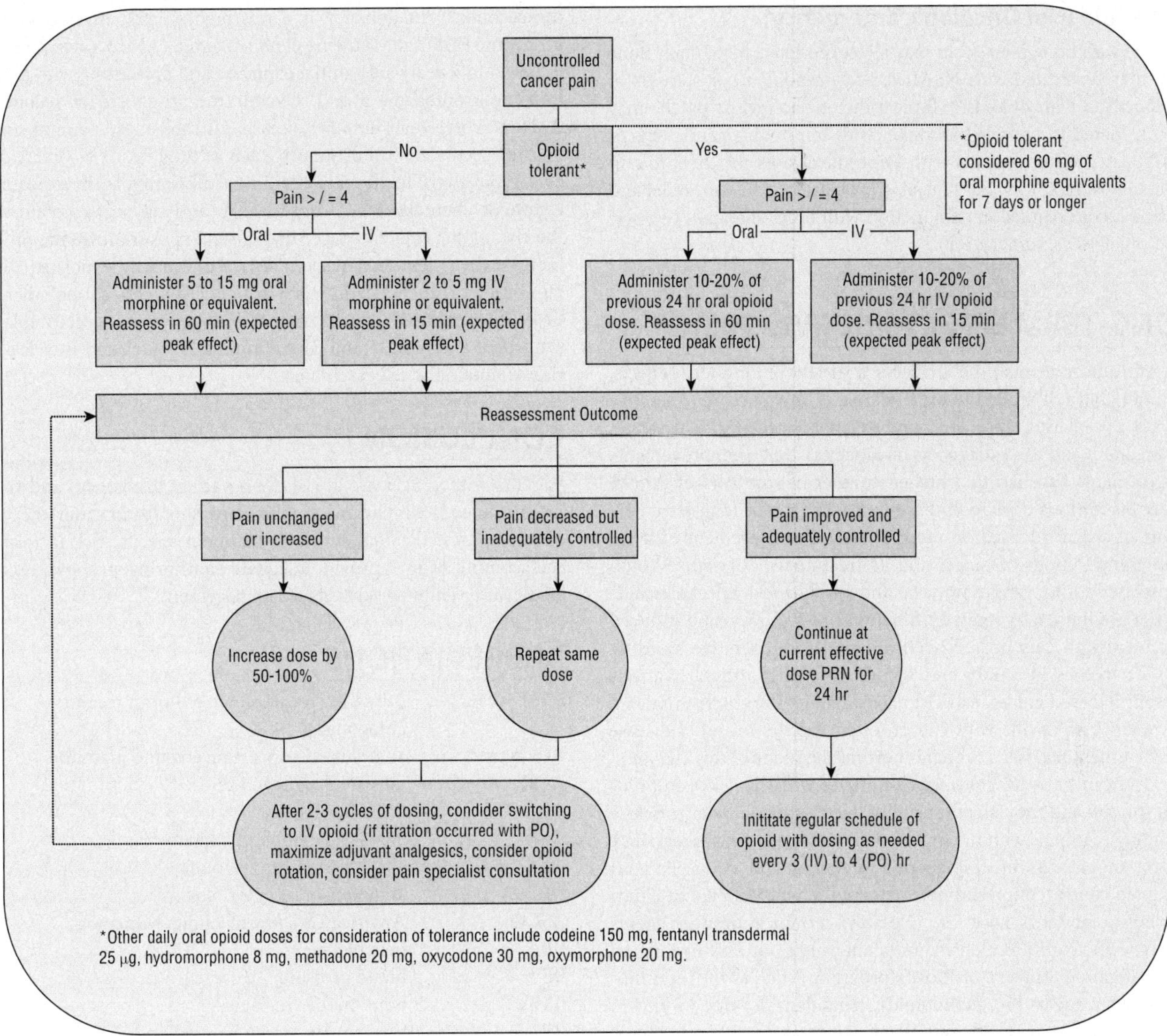

FIGURE 150-2 Treatment algorithm for cancer pain crisis. Patients should first be assessed for opioid tolerance and then managed according to their pain score on the 0-10 numeric rating scale. Patients in pain crisis require frequent monitoring and reassessment of their pain score to determine if redosing of opioids are needed to achieve adequate pain control. (Data from NCCN Clinical Practice Guidelines in Oncology [NCCN Guidelines®]. Adult Cancer Pain V.2.2021. National Comprehensive Cancer Network, Inc. Accessed July 29, 2021.)

pharmacologic therapy or may not tolerate opioid titration due to ADRs. In these scenarios, interventional therapies may be appropriate to eliminate or significantly reduce pain levels, and/or may allow a significant decrease in systemic analgesics. Some useful interventional therapies include nerve blocks, vertebral augmentation, regional infusion of analgesics, radiofrequency ablation, and others.[64]

Additional interventions may be needed for treatment in specific scenarios. Some specific cancer pain syndromes with unique treatment considerations include neuropathic pain, bone pain (not associated with an oncologic emergency), and pain from mucositis, pharyngitis and esophagitis (see "GI Toxicities: Diarrhea, Mucositis, and Nausea/Vomiting" section).

Neuropathic Pain

Cancer-related neuropathic pain can be caused by the cancer itself, or the acute or chronic effects of anticancer treatment.[64] Many chemotherapy agents including taxanes, platinums, vinca alkaloids, epothilones, eribulin, and bortezomib cause treatment-related neuropathy.[65] No agents are recommended for the prevention of chemotherapy-induced peripheral neuropathy (CIPN). Patients who develop intolerable neuropathy and/or functional impairment may require dose delays, reductions, substitutions of treatment, or discontinuations. Adjuvant analgesics commonly used to manage neuropathic pain include anticonvulsants (eg, pregabalin, gabapentin), antidepressants (eg, tricyclic antidepressants, serotonin-norepinephrine reuptake inhibitors), and topical treatments (eg, gel or patch lidocaine).[64] The ASCO CIPN guidelines support the use of duloxetine for patients with established painful CIPN[65]; however, the NCCN guidelines recommend antidepressants and anticonvulsants first-line.[64] Corticosteroids may also be used, particularly in the setting of radiculopathies from vertebral body compression fractures (see "Bone Health" section for more information). See Chapter 79, "Pain Management" and NCCN Adult Cancer Pain guidelines for medication dosing, ADRs, and interaction and contraindication information.

Bone Pain (Not Oncologic Emergency)

Patients with bone metastases may also experience bone pain. Bone pain may be treated with NSAIDs, acetaminophen, or steroids in combination with opioids.[64] Topical diclofenac (gel or patch) may be considered to provide pain relief with minimal systemic effects. BMAs are used in patients with bone metastases for their role in reducing overall SREs, but they also provide modest pain relief and may be recommended in conjunction with other therapies (eg, systemic analgesics, surgery, RT).

LONG-TERM EFFECTS/SURVIVORSHIP

10 Anticancer agents pose a risk for a variety of long-term effects, including but not limited to organ damage, impact on reproductive organs, as well as immunologic and psychological effects. Advances in screening and early diagnosis of cancer as well as improvements in treatments have led to a higher number of survivors of cancer. Many institutions have multidisciplinary clinics for long-term survivors of cancer focused on monitoring and management of long-term complications of cancer and its treatments. Survivors should be assessed for long-term physical and psychosocial effects, including but not limited to organ dysfunction (eg, anthracycline-induced cardiotoxicity), pain or neuropathy, depression, cognitive dysfunction, as well as infertility and secondary malignancies.[66] Various consensus-based guidelines exist regarding long-term screening and follow-up for patients with cancer, often specific to initial disease and treatment regimens, which is beyond the scope of this chapter.[67]

Anticancer treatments may be affiliated with the risk of embryo-fetal toxicity and the risk of infertility due to gonadotoxicity. Before initiating regimens with the risk of embryo-fetal toxicity, pregnancy testing of patients of childbearing potential and counseling on adequate contraception to both male and female patients of childbearing potential is necessary. Notably, certain anticancer agents have specific contraception requirements and even Risk Evaluation and Mitigation Strategy, or REMS, programs, such as the immunomodulatory agents (eg, thalidomide, lenalidomide) due to known teratogenicity. In men, chemotherapy can produce oligospermia or azoospermia, as well as infertility; however, serum testosterone levels are rarely altered unless the patient is receiving hormonal therapy aimed at lowering testosterone (eg, androgen deprivation therapy). The recovery of spermatogenesis after completing therapy is unpredictable. Age, total dose, duration of therapy, combination chemotherapy, and the chemotherapy mechanisms are other important variables. In women, toxic effects on the ovaries result clinically in amenorrhea, vaginal epithelial atrophy, and menopausal symptoms. These effects are related to dose and age. Younger patients are more resistant to the effects on the ovaries. As with men, the recovery of fertility is unpredictable, but women younger than 25 years of age appear to have the best outcomes. The effects of the alkylating agents on fertility have been extensively studied finding profound and consistently detrimental effects on reproductive function. The risk of infertility with other anticancer agents is largely unknown. The risk of infertility should be discussed with all patients of childbearing potential (ie, informed consent and counseling) before they receive anticancer agents, and they should be informed about options for fertility preservation to allow for referral to fertility specialists if deemed desirable by the patient.[68,69]

Secondary cancers induced by anticancer agents or RT are serious long-term consequences.[70] For curable cancers, the relatively small risk for the occurrence of secondary malignancies is far outweighed by the benefits of survival. The risk of secondary malignancies is of particular concern in patients receiving adjuvant chemotherapy. The risk of secondary malignancies is highest after receiving certain cytotoxic chemotherapy agents, such as alkylating agents, anthracyclines, and epipodophyllotoxins. Most commonly the secondary malignancy is a treatment-related myelodysplastic syndrome (MDS) or acute myeloid leukemia (AML), often approximately 5 to 7 years after initial exposure and presenting with a deletion in chromosome 5 or 7. Overall, the prognosis for secondary AML is worse than *de novo* disease. Further, these patients are at risk for secondary solid tumors, such as lung, skin, or breast cancers, typically 10 to 20 years after initial alkylating agent exposure.[70] Cytotoxic chemotherapy is not the only anti-cancer treatment with the risk of subsequent cancer diagnosis. Exposure to radiation can increase the risk of secondary cancers. Additionally, exposure to certain oral anticancer agents, such as poly (ADP-ribose) polymerase, or PARP, inhibitors, which can increase the risk of myelodysplastic syndrome and AML,[71] and BRAF inhibitors which can increase the risk of squamous cell carcinoma.[72]

CONCLUSION

Patients with cancer are at risk for a variety of disease- and treatment-induced complications. Clinicians should consider the type of cancer as well as patient- and treatment-specific risk factors for each complication to provide adequate monitoring, prophylaxis, and evidence-based interventions for management.

ABBREVIATIONS

5-HT3-RA	5-hydroxytryptamine/serotonin receptor antagonist
ACEIs	angiotensin converting enzyme inhibitors
ADR	adverse drug reaction
AF	atrial fibrillation
ALK	anaplastic lymphoma kinase
ANC	absolute neutrophil count
ARBs	angiotensin receptor blockers
ASCO	American Society of Clinical Oncology
BB	beta blocker
BP	blood pressure
BMA	bone-modifying agent
BRAF	v-raf murine sarcoma viral oncogene homolog B1
CAR-T	chimeric antigen receptor T cell
CIA	chemotherapy-induced alopecia
CINV	chemotherapy-induced nausea and vomiting
CIPN	chemotherapy-induced peripheral neuropathy
CNS	central nervous system
CRS	cytokine release syndrome
CSF	colony-stimulating factor
CT	computed tomography
CTCAE	common toxicity criteria for adverse events
CTLA4	cytotoxic T-lymphocyte-associated protein 4
DOAC	direct oral anticoagulant
ECG	electrocardiogram
ECHO	echocardiogram
EEG	electroencephalogram
EGFR	epidermal growth factor receptor
ESA	erythropoiesis-stimulating agent
FDA	Food and Drug Administration
FN	febrile neutropenia
G6PD	glucose-6-phosphate dehydrogenase
GI	gastrointestinal
GnRH	gonadotropin-releasing hormone
HSCT	hematopoietic stem cell transplantation
HEC	highly emetogenic chemotherapy
HER2	human epidermal growth factor receptor 2
HF	heart failure
HFS	hand-foot syndrome
HFSR	hand-foot skin reaction

HTN	hypertension
HLA	human leukocyte antigen
ICANS	immune effector cell-associated neurotoxicity syndrome
ICI	immune checkpoint inhibitor
IrAE	immune-related adverse event
IV	intravenous
LEC	low emetogenic chemotherapy
LMWH	low-molecular-weight heparin
LVD	left ventricular dysfunction
LVEF	left ventricular ejection fraction
MEC	moderately emetogenic chemotherapy
MEK	mitogen-activated protein kinase
mTOR	mammalian target of rapamycin
MUGA	multigated acquisition
NCCN	National Comprehensive Cancer Network
NCI	National Cancer Institute
NSAIDs	nonsteroidal anti-inflammatory drugs
N/V	nausea/vomiting
PD-1	programmed cell death protein 1
PD-L1	programmed death-ligand 1
PI3K	phosphoinositide-3 kinase
PO	oral
PRN	as needed
RT	radiation therapy
SCr	serum creatinine
SQ	subcutaneously
SRE	skeletal-related event
TLS	tumor lysis syndrome
TNF	tumor necrosis factor
TKI	tyrosine kinase inhibitor
UFH	unfractionated heparin
ULN	upper limit of normal
VEGF	vascular endothelial growth factor
VTE	venous thromboembolism
WBC	white blood cell

REFERENCES

1. National Comprehensive Cancer Network (NCCN) Clinical Practice Guidelines in Oncology. Management of immunotherapy related toxicities. v3.2021. Available at: https://www.nccn.org/professionals/physician_gls/pdf/immunotherapy.pdf. Accessed July 29, 2021.
2. Common Terminology Criteria for Adverse Events (CTCAE). Published online 2017:155.
3. National Comprehensive Cancer Network (NCCN) Clinical Practice Guidelines in Oncology. Hematopoietic Growth Factors. v4.2021. Available at: https://www.nccn.org/professionals/physician_gls/pdf/growthfactors.pdf. Accessed July 29, 2021.
4. Smith TJ, Bohlke K, Lyman GH, et al. Recommendations for the use of WBC growth factors: ASCO clinical practice guideline update. *J Clin Oncol.* 2015;33(28):3199–3212. doi:10.1200/JCO.2015.62.3488.
5. National Comprehensive Cancer Network (NCCN) Clinical Practice Guidelines in Oncology. Acute Myeloid Leukemia. v3.2021. Available at: https://www.nccn.org/professionals/physician_gls/pdf/aml.pdf. Accessed July 29, 2021.
6. Trilaciclib. Prescribing information. G1 Therapeutics, Inc.; 2021. Available at: https://www.accessdata.fda.gov/drugsatfda_docs/label/2021/214200s000lbl.pdf. Accessed August 4, 2021.
7. Bohlius J, Bohlke K, Castelli R, et al. Management of cancer-associated anemia with erythropoiesis-stimulating agents: ASCO/ASH clinical practice guideline update. *J Clin Oncol.* 2019;37(15):1336–1351. doi:10.1200/JCO.18.02142.
8. Schiffer CA, Bohlke K, Delaney M, et al. Platelet transfusion for patients with cancer: American Society of Clinical Oncology Clinical Ppractice Guideline Update. *J Clin Oncol.* 2018;36(3):283–299. doi:10.1200/JCO.2017.76.1734.
9. Benson AB, Ajani JA, Catalano RB, et al. Recommended guidelines for the treatment of cancer treatment-induced diarrhea. *J Clin Oncol.* 2004;22(14):2918–2926. doi:10.1200/JCO.2004.04.132.
10. Hong CHL, Gueiros LA, Fulton JS, et al. Systematic review of basic oral care for the management of oral mucositis in cancer patients and clinical practice guidelines. *Support Care Cancer.* 2019;27(10):3949–3967. doi:10.1007/s00520-019-04848-4.
11. Bowen JM, Gibson RJ, Coller JK, et al. Systematic review of agents for the management of cancer treatment-related gastrointestinal mucositis and clinical practice guidelines. *Support Care Cancer.* 2019;27(10):4011–4022. doi:10.1007/s00520-019-04892-0.
12. Brown TJ, Gupta A. Management of cancer therapy–associated oral mucositis. *JCO Oncol Pract.* 2020;16(3):103–109. doi:10.1200/JOP.19.00652.
13. National Comprehensive Cancer Network (NCCN) Clinical Practice Guidelines in Oncology. Antiemesis. v1.2021. Available at: https://www.nccn.org/professionals/physician_gls/pdf/antiemesis.pdf. Accessed July 29, 2021.
14. Hesketh PJ, Kris MG, Basch E, et al. Antiemetics: ASCO guideline update. *J Clin Oncol.* 2020;38(24):2782–2797. doi:10.1200/JCO.20.01296.
15. Navari RM, Qin R, Ruddy KJ, et al. Olanzapine for the prevention of chemotherapy-induced nausea and vomiting. *N Engl J Med.* 2016;375(2):134–142. doi:10.1056/NEJMoa1515725.
16. Lewis MA, Hendrickson AW, Moynihan TJ. Oncologic emergencies: Pathophysiology, presentation, diagnosis, and treatment. *CA Cancer J Clin.* Published online 2011:n/a-n/a. doi:10.3322/caac.20124.
17. Pi J, Kang Y, Smith M, Earl M, Norigian Z, McBride A. A review in the treatment of oncologic emergencies. *J Oncol Pharm Pract.* 2016;22(4):625–638. doi:10.1177/1078155215605661.
18. Rahmani B, Patel S, Seyam O, et al. Current understanding of tumor lysis syndrome. *Hematol Oncol.* 2019;37(5):537–547. doi:10.1002/hon.2668.
19. Williams SM, Killeen AA. Tumor lysis syndrome. *Arch Pathol Lab Med.* 2019;143(3):386–393. doi:10.5858/arpa.2017-0278-RS.
20. Howard SC, Trifilio S, Gregory TK, Baxter N, McBride A. Tumor lysis syndrome in the era of novel and targeted agents in patients with hematologic malignancies: A systematic review. *Ann Hematol.* 2016;95(4):563–573. doi:10.1007/s00277-015-2585-7.
21. McBride A, Trifilio S, Baxter N, Gregory T, Howard S. Managing tumor lysis syndrome in the era of novel cancer therapies. *J Adv Pract Oncol.* 2017;8(7). doi:10.6004/jadpro.2017.8.7.4.
22. Venetoclax. Prescribing information. AbbVie Inc.; 2020. Available at: https://www.rxabbvie.com/pdf/venclexta.pdf. Accessed July 29, 2021.
23. Zafrani L, Canet E, Darmon M. Understanding tumor lysis syndrome. *Intensive Care Med.* 2019;45(11):1608–1611. doi:10.1007/s00134-019-05768-x.
24. Coiffier B, Altman A, Pui C-H, Younes A, Cairo MS. Guidelines for the management of pediatric and adult tumor lysis syndrome: An evidence-based review. *J Clin Oncol.* 2008;26(16):2767–2778. doi:10.1200/JCO.2007.15.0177.
25. Jones GL, Will A, Jackson GH, Webb NJA, Rule S, the British Committee for Standards in Haematology. Guidelines for the management of tumour lysis syndrome in adults and children with haematological malignancies on behalf of the British Committee for Standards in Haematology. *Br J Haematol.* 2015;169(5):661–671. doi:10.1111/bjh.13403.
26. Bellos I, Kontzoglou K, Psyrri A, Pergialiotis V. Febuxostat administration for the prevention of tumour lysis syndrome: A meta-analysis. *J Clin Pharm Ther.* Published online April 10, 2019:jcpt.12839. doi:10.1111/jcpt.12839.
27. Yu X, Liu L, Nie X, et al. The optimal single-dose regimen of rasburicase for management of tumour lysis syndrome in children and adults: A systematic review and meta-analysis. *J Clin Pharm Ther.* 2017;42(1):18–26. doi:10.1111/jcpt.12479.
28. Boschi R, Rostagno E. Extravasation of antineoplastic agents: Prevention and treatments. *Pediatr Rep.* 2012;4(3):28. doi:10.4081/pr.2012.e28.
29. Harrold K, Gould D, Drey N. The management of cytotoxic chemotherapy extravasation: A systematic review of the literature to evaluate the evidence underpinning contemporary practice. *Eur J Cancer Care (Engl).* 2015;24(6):771–800. doi:10.1111/ecc.12363.
30. Kreidieh FY. Overview, prevention and management of chemotherapy extravasation. *World J Clin Oncol.* 2016;7(1):87. doi:10.5306/wjco.v7.i1.87.
31. Pluschnig U, Haslik W, Bartsch R, Mader RM. Extravasation emergencies: State-of-the-art management and progress in clinical research. *Memo - Mag Eur Med Oncol.* 2016;9(4):226–230. doi:10.1007/s12254-016-0304-2.
32. Brahmer JR, Lacchetti C, Schneider BJ, et al. Management of immune-related adverse events in patients treated with immune checkpoint

inhibitor therapy: American Society of Clinical Oncology Clinical Practice Guideline. *J Clin Oncol.* 2018;36(17):1714–1768. doi:10.1200/JCO.2017.77.6385.
33. Puzanov I, Diab A, Abdallah K, et al. Managing toxicities associated with immune checkpoint inhibitors: Consensus recommendations from the Society for Immunotherapy of Cancer (SITC) Toxicity Management Working Group. *J Immunother Cancer.* 2017;5(1):95. doi:10.1186/s40425-017-0300-z.
34. Haanen JBAG, Carbonnel F, Robert C, et al. Management of toxicities from immunotherapy: ESMO Clinical Practice Guidelines for diagnosis, treatment and follow-up. *Ann Oncol.* 2017;28:iv119–iv142. doi:10.1093/annonc/mdx225.
35. Lee DW, Santomasso BD, Locke FL, et al. ASTCT consensus grading for cytokine release syndrome and neurologic toxicity associated with immune effector cells. *Biol Blood Marrow Transplant.* 2019;25(4):625–638. doi:10.1016/j.bbmt.2018.12.758.
36. Neelapu SS. Managing the toxicities of CAR T-cell therapy. *Hematol Oncol.* 2019;37(S1):48–52. doi:10.1002/hon.2595.
37. Stein AS, Schiller G, Benjamin R, et al. Neurologic adverse events in patients with relapsed/refractory acute lymphoblastic leukemia treated with blinatumomab: Management and mitigating factors. *Ann Hematol.* 2019;98(1):159–167. doi:10.1007/s00277-018-3497-0.
38. Blinatumomab. Prescribing information. Amgen; 2020. https://www.pi.amgen.com/~/media/amgen/repositorysites/pi-amgen-com/blincyto/blincyto_pi_hcp_english.pdf. Accessed July 29, 2021.
39. Jain T, Litzow MR. Management of toxicities associated with novel immunotherapy agents in acute lymphoblastic leukemia. *Ther Adv Hematol.* 2020;11:204062071989989. doi:10.1177/2040620719899897.
40. Aldoss I, Khaled SK, Budde E, Stein AS. Cytokine release syndrome with the novel treatments of acute lymphoblastic leukemia: Pathophysiology, prevention, and treatment. *Curr Oncol Rep.* 2019;21(1):4. doi:10.1007/s11912-019-0753-y.
41. Crist M, Emadi A, Duffy A. Real-world experience managing blinatumomab toxicities in adults with relapsed/refractory acute lymphoblastic leukemia. *J Oncol Pharm Pract.* 2020;26(5):1080–1085. doi:10.1177/1078155219881680.
42. Cury-Martins J, Eris APM, Abdalla CMZ, Silva G de B, Moura VPT de, Sanches JA. Management of dermatologic adverse events from cancer therapies: Recommendations of an expert panel. *An Bras Dermatol.* 2020;95(2):221–237. doi:10.1016/j.abd.2020.01.001.
43. Lacouture ME, Sibaud V, Gerber PA, et al. Prevention and management of dermatological toxicities related to anticancer agents: ESMO Clinical Practice Guidelines☆. *Ann Oncol.* 2021;32(2):157–170. doi:10.1016/j.annonc.2020.11.005.
44. Hallquist Viale, RN, MS, CNS, ANP - 2016 - Management of Dermatologic Toxicities Associated W.pdf.
45. Lacouture ME. Management of dermatologic toxicities. *J Natl Compr Canc Netw.* 2015;13(5S):686–689. doi:10.6004/jnccn.2015.0204.
46. Leventhal J, Young M. Radiation dermatitis: Recognition, prevention, and management. *Oncology (Williston Park).* 2017;31(12):855–857, 894-899.
47. Hong W, Bast R Jr, Hait W, et al. *Holland-Frei Cancer Medicine 8.* 8th ed. People's Medical Publishing House, USA Ltd.; 2010.
48. Hartmann K. Thyroid disorders in the oncology patient. *J Adv Pract Oncol.* 2015;6(2). doi:10.6004/jadpro.2015.6.2.2.
49. Hwangbo Y, Lee EK. Acute hyperglycemia associated with anti-cancer medication. *Endocrinol Metab.* 2017;32(1):23. doi:10.3803/EnM.2017.32.1.23.
50. Goldman JW, Mendenhall MA, Rettinger SR. Hyperglycemia associated with targeted oncologic treatment: Mechanisms and management. *The Oncologist.* 2016;21(11):1326–1336. doi:10.1634/theoncologist.2015-0519.
51. Shapiro CL, Van Poznak C, Lacchetti C, et al. Management of osteoporosis in survivors of adult cancers with nonmetastatic disease: ASCO clinical practice guideline. *J Clin Oncol.* 2019;37(31):2916–2946. doi:10.1200/JCO.19.01696.
52. Coleman R, Hadji P, Body J-J, et al. Bone health in cancer: ESMO Clinical Practice Guidelines. *Ann Oncol.* 2020;31(12):1650–1663. doi:10.1016/j.annonc.2020.07.019.
53. Pittman K, Antill YC, Goldrick A, Goh J, de Boer RH. Denosumab: Prevention and management of hypocalcemia, osteonecrosis of the jaw and atypical fractures. *Asia Pac J Clin Oncol.* 2017;13(4):266–276. doi:10.1111/ajco.12517.
54. Harman LE. Ophthalmic complications related to chemotherapy in medically complex patients. *Cancer Control.* 2016;23(2):150–156. doi:10.1177/107327481602300209.
55. Fu C, Gombos DS, Lee J, et al. Ocular toxicities associated with targeted anticancer agents: An analysis of clinical data with management suggestions. *Oncotarget.* 2017;8(35):58709–58727. doi:10.18632/oncotarget.17634.
56. Sharma D. Ophthalmic complications of targeted therapies: A review. *Delta J Ophthalmol.* 2017;18(3):117. doi:10.4103/DJO.DJO_23_17.
57. Lyon AR, Dent S, Stanway S, et al. Baseline cardiovascular risk assessment in cancer patients scheduled to receive cardiotoxic cancer therapies: A position statement and new risk assessment tools from the Cardio-oncology study group of the Heart Failure Association of the European Society of Cardiology in collaboration with the International Cardio-oncology Society. *Eur J Heart Fail.* 2020;22(11):1945–1960. doi:10.1002/ejhf.1920.
58. Curigliano G, Lenihan D, Fradley M, et al. Management of cardiac disease in cancer patients throughout oncological treatment: ESMO consensus recommendations. *Ann Oncol.* 2020;31(2):171–190. doi:10.1016/j.annonc.2019.10.023.
59. Curigliano G, Cardinale D, Suter T, et al. Cardiovascular toxicity induced by chemotherapy, targeted agents and radiotherapy: ESMO Clinical Practice Guidelines. *Ann Oncol.* 2012;23(suppl 7):vii155–vii166. doi:10.1093/annonc/mds293.
60. Blake L, Palumbo A, Diaz A, Bubalo J. Anthracycline-induced cardiotoxicity in adults. *J Hematol Oncol Pharm.* 2018;8(4):4.
61. Alexandre J, Cautela J, Ederhy S, et al. Cardiovascular toxicity related to cancer treatment: A pragmatic approach to the American and European Cardio-Oncology Guidelines. *J Am Heart Assoc.* 2020;9(18). doi:10.1161/JAHA.120.018403.
62. National Comprehensive Cancer Network (NCCN) Clinical Practice Guidelines in Oncology. Cancer-associated venous thromboembolic disease. v1.2021. Available at: https://www.nccn.org/professionals/physician_gls/pdf/vte.pdf. Accessed July 29, 2021.
63. Key NS, Khorana AA, Kuderer NM, et al. Venous thromboembolism prophylaxis and treatment in patients with cancer: ASCO clinical practice guideline update. *J Clin Oncol.* 2020;38(5):496–520. doi:10.1200/JCO.19.01461.
64. National Comprehensive Cancer Network (NCCN) Clinical Practice Guidelines in Oncology. Adult Cancer Pain. v2.2021. Available at: https://www.nccn.org/professionals/physician_gls/pdf/pain.pdf. Accessed July 29, 2021.
65. Loprinzi CL, Lacchetti C, Bleeker J, et al. Prevention and management of chemotherapy-induced peripheral neuropathy in survivors of adult cancers: ASCO guideline update. *J Clin Oncol.* 2020;38(28):3325–3348. doi:10.1200/JCO.20.01399.
66. Shapiro CL. Cancer survivorship. Longo DL, ed. *N Engl J Med.* 2018;379(25):2438–2450. doi:10.1056/NEJMra1712502.
67. National Comprehensive Cancer Network (NCCN) Clinical Practice Guidelines in Oncology. Survivorship. v2.2021. Available at: https://www.nccn.org/professionals/physician_gls/pdf/survivorship.pdf. Accessed July 29, 2021.
68. Salama M, Woodruff TK. Anticancer treatments and female fertility: Clinical concerns and role of oncologists in oncofertility practice. *Expert Rev Anticancer Ther.* 2017;17(8):687–692. doi:10.1080/14737140.2017.1335199.
69. Oktay K, Harvey BE, Partridge AH, et al. Fertility preservation in patients with cancer: ASCO Clinical Practice Guideline Update. *J Clin Oncol.* 2018;36(19):1994–2001. doi:10.1200/JCO.2018.78.1914.
70. Chabner B, Long D, eds. *Cancer Chemotherapy and Biotherapy: Principles and Practice.* 5th ed. Wolters Kluwer Health/Lippincott Williams & Wilkins; 2011.
71. Morice P-M, Leary A, Dolladille C, et al. Myelodysplastic syndrome and acute myeloid leukaemia in patients treated with PARP inhibitors: A safety meta-analysis of randomised controlled trials and a retrospective study of the WHO pharmacovigilance database. *Lancet Haematol.* 2021;8(2):e122–e134. doi:10.1016/S2352-3026(20)30360-4.
72. Peng L, Wang Y, Hong Y, et al. Incidence and relative risk of cutaneous squamous cell carcinoma with single-agent BRAF inhibitor and dual BRAF/MEK inhibitors in cancer patients: A meta-analysis. *Oncotarget.* 2017;8(47):83280–83291. doi:10.18632/oncotarget.21059.
73. Cairo MS, Bishop M. Tumour lysis syndrome: New therapeutic strategies and classification. *Br J Haematol.* 2004;127(1):3–11. 10.1111/j.1365-2141.2004.05094.x 15384972.

151

Breast Cancer

Bonnie Lin Boster, Neelam K. Patel, and Jaime Kaushik

KEY CONCEPTS

1. Breast cancer is usually diagnosed in the early stages when it is highly curable.
2. Although controversial, regular screening mammography in women younger than 50 years of age is beneficial, and many studies demonstrate that annual or biennial screening mammography in women aged 50 to 74 years reduces the breast cancer mortality rate.
3. Local therapy of early-stage breast cancer consists of modified radical mastectomy or lumpectomy plus external-beam radiation therapy. The surgical approach to the ipsilateral axilla may consist of a lymph node mapping procedure with sentinel lymph node biopsy or a full-level I/II axillary lymph node dissection. Breast conserving therapy (BCT) includes lumpectomy, surgical evaluation of the lymph node basin, and radiation.
4. The goal of adjuvant and neoadjuvant chemotherapy is cure while the goal of chemotherapy in the metastatic setting is palliation.
5. Adjuvant endocrine therapy reduces the rates of relapse and death in patients with hormone receptor–positive early breast cancer. Adjuvant chemotherapy reduces the rates of relapse and death in all patients with early-stage breast cancer.
6. The choice of the most appropriate chemotherapy, endocrine therapy, and human epidermal growth factor receptor-2 (*HER2*) targeted therapy regimen is complex and rapidly changes as results from ongoing randomized clinical trials are reported.
7. Neoadjuvant chemotherapy and biotherapy are appropriate for selected patients with early breast cancer and most patients with locally advanced and inflammatory breast cancer (IBC) followed by local therapy and further adjuvant systemic therapy as indicated.
8. About 55% of women with metastatic breast cancer (MBC) will respond to chemotherapy regimens; anthracycline- and taxane-containing regimens are the most active.
9. Initial therapy of MBC in most women with hormone receptor–positive tumors should include endocrine therapy.
10. *HER2*-targeted therapies and other biologic or targeted agents (eg, everolimus, cyclin-dependent kinase [CDK] inhibitors) in combination with chemotherapy or endocrine therapy are options for patients with MBC.

BEYOND THE BOOK

Activity #1

Learners are encouraged to review "Breast Cancer: An Opportunity Lost Level II" in the *Pharmacotherapy Casebook: A Patient-Focused Approach* to practice applying their knowledge to develop a patient-centered care plan for a patient with breast cancer.

INTRODUCTION

In this chapter, the terms "women" and "men" are used to reflect gender identified in previous research studies and other literature on breast cancer and to recognize the biological sex of individuals at birth. In doing so, we recognize that not all patients with breast cancer identify as females or males at the time of diagnosis and treatment of breast cancer. Breast cancer is the most common cancer and is second only to lung cancer as a cause of cancer death in American women. About 284,200 new cases of breast cancer were diagnosed and 44,130 people died of breast cancer in 2021.[1] In addition to invasive breast cancers, 49,290 cases of noninvasive, ductal carcinoma in situ (DCIS), cancer were diagnosed among women in the United States in 2021.[1]

Breast cancer incidence rates increased in the 1980s and decreased starting in 2000. The decreased incidence is thought to be related to decreased use of menopausal hormone therapy, also known as hormone replacement therapy (HRT), in postmenopausal individuals.[2] The incidence of DCIS also increased during the 1980s, due to the increased use of screening mammography.[2] Since 2004, breast cancer has slowly increased by about 0.3% per year, and during 2012 to 2016, DCIS has decreased by about 2.1% per year.[2] The increase in breast cancer incidence has been attributed to increases in body mass index (BMI) and declines in the average number of births per individual.[2]

Breast cancer incidence rates vary considerably across racial and ethnic groups in the United States. For example, the average annual age-adjusted incidence rate from 2012 to 2016 was 130.8 cases per 100,000 among non-Hispanic White women, 126.7 cases among non-Hispanic Black women, 94.7 cases in American Indian/Alaska Native women, 93.7 cases in Hispanic women, and 93.2 cases among Asian/Pacific Islander women.[2] The higher incidence rates in White women than in other racial and ethnic groups may be related to differences in reproductive and lifestyle factors and access to and use of screening.

(1) For all racial and ethnic groups, most breast cancers are diagnosed at an early stage when tumors are small and localized. Unfortunately, breast cancer mortality is higher among Black women compared to White women despite the lower incidence. The cause of

this disparity between White and Black women is widely debated and multifactorial, and proposed explanations include differences in stage at diagnosis, tumor characteristics, obesity, comorbidities, access to care, early detection, and treatment.[2] Overall breast cancer mortality rates in the United States have declined since 1990; this decline has been attributed to improvements in early detection and treatment.[2]

The median age at diagnosis for breast cancer is 62 years.[2] Although lung cancer is the leading cause of cancer deaths for women regardless of age, breast cancer is the leading cause of cancer deaths for women between the age of 20 and 59 years.[1]

EPIDEMIOLOGY AND ETIOLOGY

The two variables most strongly associated with the occurrence of breast cancer are biological sex and age. Although one commonly thinks of breast cancer as a disease confined to women, about 2,650 cases of breast cancer are estimated to be diagnosed in men in the United States in 2021.[1] Men are more likely to have more advanced disease at the time of diagnosis. Men also have lower unadjusted rates of overall survival than women with breast cancer. This difference is not only due to advanced disease at diagnosis but also older age at diagnosis as well as shorter life expectancy in general.[3] Treatment of breast cancer is similar regardless of sex or gender.

The incidence of breast cancer increases with advancing age. A frequently quoted breast cancer statistic is that one in eight women will develop breast cancer during her lifetime. It should be emphasized that this is a cumulative lifetime risk of developing the disease from birth to death. The one-in-eight women figure is often misinterpreted by women who assume that it translates into one in eight women being diagnosed with breast cancer each year. A more useful method of presenting the risk data is based on age intervals. For example, the 10-year probability of breast cancer diagnosis of a 20-year-old individual is 1 in 1,479, but this risk changes to 1 in 28 for a 60-year-old individual.

A number of calculators are available to estimate a woman's risk of developing breast cancer. The National Cancer Institute (NCI) has an online version of the Breast Cancer Risk Assessment Tool (https://bcrisktool.cancer.gov/calculator.html). This tool is based on a statistical model known as the Gail model, derived from a mammography screening project conducted in the 1970s. It was designed for health professionals to project an individualized risk for invasive breast cancer over a 5-year period and over their lifetime. This model has been shown to provide accurate estimates in several racial and ethnic groups, but it has not been validated for those with genetic risk factors, a previous history of in situ or invasive breast cancer, or for certain subgroups. Other risk assessment models also exist, each taking into account different risk factors.

Endocrine Factors

Many endocrine factors have been associated with the risk of breast cancer. Many of these relate to the total duration of menstrual life. Early menarche, generally defined as menstruation beginning before age of 11 years, increases the cumulative lifetime risk of breast cancer development. Similarly, a late age of natural menopause (age 55 years or later) increases the risk of breast cancer development.[2] Conversely, bilateral oophorectomy before the age of 45 years reduces the risk of developing breast cancer.[4] Nulliparity and a late age at first birth (greater than or equal to 30 years) are reported to increase the lifetime risk of developing breast cancer.[2] Investigators postulate that international differences in age of menarche, age at menopause, and childbearing may account for a substantial part of the international differences in the incidence of breast cancer.

Many studies have evaluated the relationship between exogenous hormones and the development of breast cancer. The Women's Health Initiative (WHI) is a series of clinical trials designed to investigate the risks and benefits of treatment strategies that could affect women's health issues, such as breast cancer. The estrogen plus progestin trial reported an increased risk of breast cancer in women taking combined estrogen and progestin. In the estrogen alone trial, which included postmenopausal women with prior hysterectomy, the incidence of breast cancer was lower in those who received estrogen alone compared with those who received placebo.[2] Unresolved issues remain as to whether lower doses or short-term use of estrogen or estrogen–progestin for menopausal symptoms can be safe and effective. A longer duration of HRT and concurrent use of progestins contribute to breast cancer risk. In addition, the impact of HRT use on breast cancer risk also varies according to BMI and breast density.[2] The use of postmenopausal HRT in individuals with a history of breast cancer is generally contraindicated. Individuals who are considering HRT should carefully consider the risks versus benefits (see Chapter 102, "Hormone Therapy in Women" for a detailed discussion of HRT).

Epidemiologic studies of oral contraceptives do not show a consistent relationship between the use and breast cancer risk. Results are conflicting, and assessment of the studies should consider the particular oral contraceptive products involved, daily and cumulative doses of the hormones administered, and latency period for development of breast cancer. It is also important to note that oral contraceptives are known to reduce the risk of ovarian and endometrial cancers.[5] Benefits and risk associated with oral contraceptives should be considered and discussed with each patient.

Genetic Factors

Both personal and family histories influence a woman's risk of developing breast cancer. A personal history of breast cancer is associated with an increased risk of developing contralateral breast cancer. Cancers of the uterus and ovary are also associated with an increased risk of developing breast cancer. Several cancer family syndromes include breast cancer in association with other types of cancers.

About 10% of all breast cancers in the US population can be attributed to family history. Empirical estimates of the risks associated with particular patterns of family history of breast cancer indicate the following[2,4]:

1. Having any first-degree relative with breast cancer increases a woman's risk of breast cancer about 50%. Risk increases with increasing numbers of affected first-degree relatives.
2. The risk is affected by both the woman's age and the age of the relative when diagnosed. A higher risk is seen when a woman and her relative at diagnosis are younger than 50 years.
3. The risk associated with having any second-degree relative with breast cancer is complex and depends on other family history patterns. The risk is generally lower than that of first-degree relatives.
4. Affected family members on both the maternal and the paternal sides are important to consider in the evaluation of risk.

Although individuals with a family history of breast cancer are at increased risk for the disease, the diagnosis of breast cancer is still uncommon in young individuals even with a positive family history.

Germline mutations in either *BRCA1* or *BRCA2* are associated with an increased risk for breast and ovarian cancer. These genes function as tumor suppressor genes, maintaining genomic integrity and DNA repair. Compared with an average individual's 10% lifetime risk of developing breast cancer, the probability of developing breast cancer by the age of 80 years in individuals with a *BRCA1* or *BRCA2* mutation is estimated to be 70%.[2]

The probability of being a *BRCA* gene mutation carrier is related to ethnicity and family history. Ashkenazi (Eastern European) Jewish descendants have an unusually high (2.5%) carrier rate of germline mutations in *BRCA1* and *BRCA2* compared with the rest of the US population.[2] Conversely, clinically significant *BRCA* mutations occur at a frequency of about one in 400 persons in the general, non-Jewish US population.[2] Testing for *BRCA1* and *BRCA2* mutations is now widely available, but it is generally recommended only when there is personal or family history suggestive of hereditary cancer, when the test results can be adequately interpreted, and when results will assist with diagnosis and management. The decision to test an individual for a genetic mutation related to breast cancer risk is complex, and several organizations have published recommendations on genetic susceptibility testing for individuals who meet the criteria for increased risk.[6]

Although most genetic causes of breast cancer are attributed to *BRCA1* and *BRCA2,* other genes that have been associated with hereditary breast cancer include *TP53, CHEK2, PALB2, PTEN, ATM, STK11, CDH1*, and others.[6]

Environmental and Lifestyle Factors

Breast cancer incidence rates vary considerably among countries, which suggests that environmental and lifestyle factors play an important role. See Table 151-1 for details.

Several endocrine, genetic, environmental, and lifestyle factors are associated with the development of breast cancer to varying degrees. Some factors are modifiable, but others are not. The impact of individual risk factors may vary depending on other confounding variables such as age, family history, estrogen use, and menopausal status. Further studies are needed to confirm the importance of factors that are associated with the risk of developing breast cancer.

PREVENTION AND EARLY DETECTION

Current efforts at breast cancer prevention are directed toward the identification and removal of risk factors often referred to as risk-reducing strategies. Prophylactic bilateral mastectomies or bilateral salpingo-oophorectomy are considered for individuals who are at high risk for the development of breast or ovarian cancer, particularly if the breast tissue is difficult to evaluate by both physical examination and mammography and if the individual have persistent disabling fears that they will be diagnosed with cancer. Guidelines for the incorporation of surgical risk-reducing strategies are largely based on genetics and other known risk factors for the development of breast (or ovarian) cancer.

Numerous agents are available for pharmacologic risk reduction, including the selective estrogen receptor modulators (SERMs), tamoxifen and raloxifene, and aromatase inhibitors (AIs), anastrozole and exemestane. Tamoxifen (20 mg/day × 5 years) reduces the risk of invasive and noninvasive estrogen receptor (ER)-positive breast cancers in individuals with a high risk for breast cancer by about 50%.[4] Tamoxifen has been shown to be a relatively safe drug with an acceptable toxicity profile when used to treat pre- or postmenopausal patients with breast cancer. Toxicities associated with tamoxifen are described in the "Endocrine Therapy" section under Curative Breast Cancer. Similarly, raloxifene (60 mg/day × 5 years), reduces the rates of noninvasive and invasive breast cancers in high-risk, postmenopausal individuals, but not to the same degree as tamoxifen does. Both agents increased thromboembolic events while only tamoxifen increases rates of endometrial cancer.[4] Although the benefits of raloxifene have decreased compared to tamoxifen, it may still be the treatment of choice when considering toxicities.[4]

A similar reduction in the risk of contralateral primary breast cancers was demonstrated with the AIs, exemestane and anastrozole. Both exemestane (25 mg/day × 3 years) and anastrozole (1 mg/day × 5 years) reduce rates of invasive breast cancers in high-risk, postmenopausal individuals and have tolerable adverse drug reactions. AIs have not been compared to SERMs and both classes of agents are appropriate options.[4] Although neither exemestane nor anastrozole is Food and Drug Administration (FDA)-approved for breast cancer risk reduction, the American Society of Clinical Oncology, or ASCO, and National Comprehensive Cancer Network (NCCN) guidelines include AIs as acceptable options for risk reduction in postmenopausal women.[4,7] Any decision to use tamoxifen, raloxifene, or the AIs for risk reduction should be made after a thorough discussion of the woman's risk of breast cancer, the potential benefits, and the potential serious adverse drug reactions.

The rationale for early detection of breast cancer is based on the relationship between the stage of breast cancer at diagnosis and the probability of cure. If all breast cancer cases could be detected at an early stage of the disease (ie, small primary tumor and negative lymph nodes), then more patients theoretically could be cured of their disease. Screening guidelines for early detection of breast cancer in women at average risk have been developed by several organizations, including but not limited to the American Cancer Society (ACS), the United States Preventive Services Task Force (USPSTF), and the NCCN (see Table 151-2).[8-10] The ACS guidelines are most commonly cited. However, it is important to note that the expert panels developing these guidelines often differ in their approach and analysis of the available data, as is evident in the different recommendations in the guidelines.

2 The most controversial screening recommendation for breast cancer is annual mammography. Although screening mammography clearly decreases mortality from breast cancer, the controversies surround the balance of benefits and harms associated with a less than perfect screening test in individuals of different ages at average risk of developing breast cancer. The largest benefit for the number needed to invite for screening to prevent one breast cancer death was seen for women aged 60 to 69 years old.[11] Incorporation of this information into national guidelines differs with each organization (Table 151-2).

Other radiologic methods of breast imaging are also being investigated (eg, digital mammography [two-dimensional, 2D], digital breast tomosynthesis [also known as tomosynthesis or three-dimensional mammography], ultrasonography, and magnetic resonance imaging [MRI]). Recommendations regarding these other

TABLE 151-1 Environmental and Lifestyle Factors

Factor	Comments
Elevated Risk	
Alcohol consumption	Some evidence that consumption before first pregnancy may affect risk; women who have 2-3 alcoholic drinks per day have a 20% higher risk compared to non-drinkers
Tobacco	Slight increase, notably in long-term, heavy smokers who started smoking before first pregnancy
Radiation exposure	Exposure particularly if before 10-30 years of age, eg, Hodgkin lymphoma
Reduced Risk	
Diet: Fruit and vegetable intake	Limited but increased evidence
Physical activity	Has protective effect independent of BMI
No Association	
Diet: Fat intake	No association based on recent meta-analysis
Mixed Results	
Diet: Soy	Reduced risk in Asian women but not the case with Western populations
Excess body weight/ weight gain	Reduced risk in premenopausal women but elevated risk in postmenopausal women

Data from Reference 2.

TABLE 151-2 Breast Cancer Screening Guidelines

Risk Category	ACS	USPSTF	NCCN
Average Risk			
BSE	Not recommended but encourages breast awareness	Not recommended	Age ≥25 years: breast awareness
CBE	Evidence does not support	Insufficient evidence	Age ≥25-39 years: every 1-3 years
			Age ≥40 years: annually
Mammography	Age 40-44 years: opportunity annually	Age 40-50 years: individualized decision	Age ≥40 years: annually; consider tomosynthesis
	Age 45-54 years: annually	Age 50-74 years: biennial	
	Age ≥55 years: biennially or opportunity annually (as long as in good health and at least 10-year life expectancy)	Age >75 years: insufficient evidence	
High Risk[a,b]			
BSE	NA	NA	All ages: breast awareness
CBE	NA	NA	All ages: every 6-12 months
Mammography	Age ≥30 years: annually with MRI	NA	Prior RT or strong family history or genetic predisposition, age ≥25 years: annually (+ CBE); consider tomosynthesis
			All other categories: annually (+ CBE); consider tomosynthesis
Breast MRI	Age ≥30 years: annually with mammogram	NA	Annually with mammogram + CBE for (a) prior RT, age ≥25 years; (b) lifetime risk >20%; (c) consider MRI if history of LCIS or ADH/ALH and lifetime risk >20%

ACS, American Cancer Society; ADH, atypical ductal hyperplasia; ALH, atypical lobular hyperplasia; BSE, breast self-examination; CBE, clinical breast examination by a healthcare professional; LCIS, lobular carcinoma in situ; MRI, magnetic resonance imaging; NA, not addressed; NCCN, National Comprehensive Cancer Network; RT, thoracic radiation therapy; USPSTF, United States Preventive Services Task Force.

[a]High risk is defined by the ACS as women with (1) a known *BRCA1/2* gene mutation; (2) untested woman with first-degree relative with a known *BRCA1/2* gene mutation; (3) lifetime risk of breast cancer of 20%-25% or greater using a risk-assessment tool based largely on family history; (4) radiation therapy to the chest between the ages of 10 and 30 years; (5) LiFraumeni syndrome, Cowden syndrome, or Bannayan-Riley-Ruvalcaba syndrome or have first-degree relatives with one of these syndromes.

[b]High risk is defined by the NCCN as women with (1) prior thoracic radiation therapy before age 30 years, (2) 5-year risk of ≥1.7% of invasive breast cancer in women ≥35 years old, (3) lifetime risk of >20% as defined by models that are largely based on family history, (4) strong family history or genetic predisposition, (5) LCIS or ADH/ALH and lifetime risk of >20%, (6) prior history of breast cancer.

Data from References 2, and 8-10.

radiologic methods vary among the national guidelines and definitions of "high risk" also vary among the guidelines (Table 151-2). It should also be noted that any screening procedure has risks and they should be discussed with patients so they are able to make an informed decision regarding these procedures. The risks involved with screening mammograms include false-negative results, false-positive results, overdiagnosis (true positives that will not become clinically significant), and radiation risk. The rate of false-negative results with the current technology is about 20%.[12] Although the specificity of mammography is quite high (90%), most abnormal examinations are false-positive results, leading to additional biopsies and psychological distress.[11] The term "overdiagnosis" refers primarily to the increased detection of DCIS from screening mammography (see "Noninvasive Carcinoma" section for a detailed discussion of DCIS).

CLINICAL PRESENTATION

A painless lump is the initial sign of breast cancer in most women. The typical malignant mass is solitary, unilateral, solid, hard, irregular, and nonmobile. In small numbers of cases, stabbing or aching pain is the first symptom. Less commonly, nipple discharge, retraction, or dimpling may herald the onset of the disease. In more advanced cases, prominent skin edema, redness, warmth, and induration of the underlying tissue may be observed.

The breast is a complex organ composed of skin, subcutaneous tissue, fatty tissue, and branching ductal and glandular structures (Fig. 151-1). Various diseases that affect these structures can produce a palpable mass. In addition, the physiologic changes associated with the menstrual cycle can cause normal breast changes. Common causes of breast masses in young individuals are fibroadenoma, fibrocystic disease, carcinoma, and fat necrosis.

Breast cancer that is confined to a localized breast lesion is often referred to as *early*, *primary*, *localized*, or *curable*. Breast cancer that has spread to local–regional lymph nodes is still considered early stage (see Fig. 151-2). Unfortunately, breast cancer cells often spread by contiguity, through lymph channels, and through the blood to distant sites. When breast cancer cells can be detected clinically or radiologically in sites distant from the breast, the disease is referred to as *advanced* or *metastatic* breast cancer (MBC). Tissues most commonly involved with distant metastases are lymph nodes (other than local–regional lymph nodes), skin, bone, liver, lungs, and brain. Symptoms of bone pain, difficulty breathing, abdominal enlargement, jaundice, and mental status changes may herald the clinical presentation of MBC. A small percentage of women have signs and symptoms of distant metastases when they first seek treatment. In virtually all of them, a neglected breast mass has been present for several months to years. In addition, 20% to 30% of all patients who initially present with early breast cancer will eventually develop signs and symptoms of MBC.[13]

DIAGNOSIS

The initial workup for a woman presenting with a breast mass or symptoms suggestive of breast cancer should include a careful history, physical examination of the breast, three-dimensional diagnostic mammography, and possibly other breast imaging techniques such as ultrasonography or MRI. Most breast cancers can be

CLINICAL PRESENTATION Breast Cancer

General

- The patient may not have any symptoms because breast cancer may be detected in asymptomatic patients through routine screening mammography.

Local Signs and Symptoms

- A painless, palpable lump is most common.
- Less common: pain; nipple discharge, retraction, or dimpling; skin edema, redness, or warmth.
- Palpable local–regional lymph nodes may also be present.

Signs and Symptoms of Systemic Metastases

- Varies depending on the site of metastases, but may include bone pain, difficulty breathing, abdominal pain or enlargement, jaundice, or mental status changes.

Laboratory Tests

- Tumor markers such as cancer antigen 15-3, or CA 15-3, or carcinoembryonic antigen, or CEA, may be elevated in patients with metastatic disease.
- Alkaline phosphatase or liver function test results may be elevated in patients with metastatic disease.

Other Diagnostic Tests

- Mammography (with or without ultrasonography, breast MRI, or both).
- Biopsy for pathology review and determination of tumor ER, progesterone receptor (PR), and *HER2* status.
- Systemic staging tests may include chest radiography, chest computed tomography (CT), bone scan, abdominal CT or ultrasonography, or MRI.

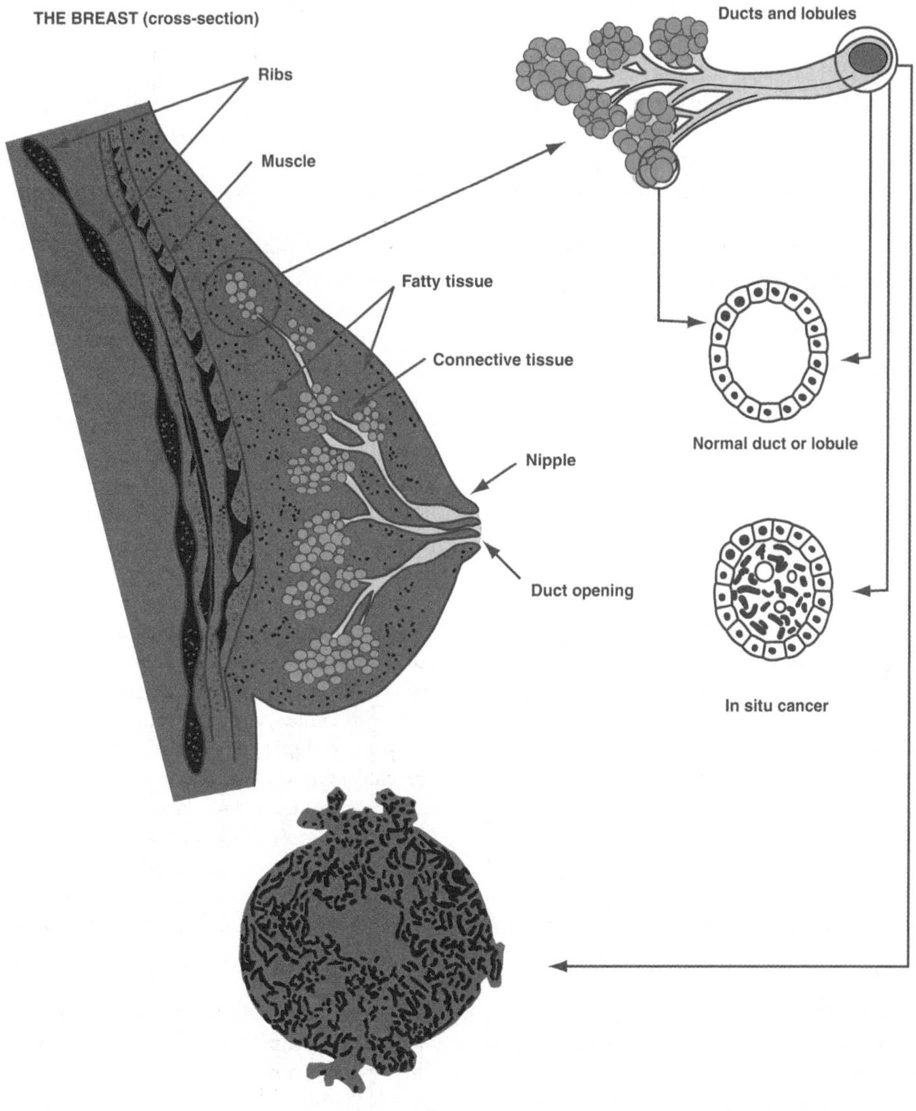

FIGURE 151-1 Breast anatomy. An illustration shows the cross-section of the breast. The breast lies posterior to the ribs and muscles and consists of fatty tissues and connective tissues. The ducts in the breast lead to the opening in the nipple. A normal duct or lobule is hollow, while the one with cancer is blocked.

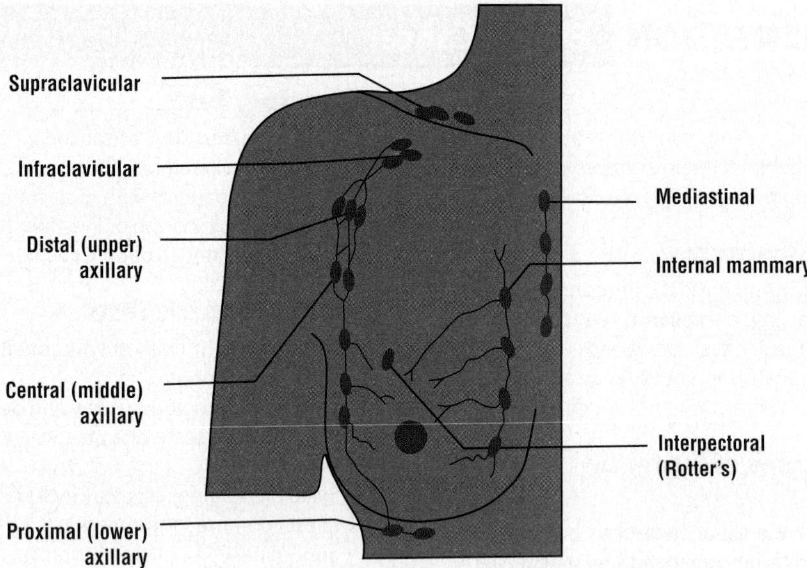

FIGURE 151-2 Lymph node anatomy. An illustration shows that the position of nodes as follows: supraclavicular, mediastinal, internal mammary, interpectoral or Rotter's, proximal or lower axillary, central or middle axillary, distal or upper axillary, and supraclavicular.

visualized on a mammogram as a mass, a cluster of calcifications, or a combination of these findings. One major factor that affects the ability of mammography to detect cancer includes breast density, which may be affected by age, menopausal status, and HRT use. Ultrasonography, MRI, digital mammography, and tomosynthesis are alternate breast imaging methods that are being investigated for women with dense breasts or other specific subsets of patients with breast cancer (eg, MRI in patients with IBC).[14] The technical quality of the examination and the expertise of the radiologist are also important factors affecting reliability.

Breast biopsy is indicated for a mammographic abnormality that suggests malignancy or for a palpable mass on physical examination. Three techniques are available: fine-needle aspiration, core-needle biopsy, and excisional biopsy.[14] Excisional biopsy completely removes the abnormal tissue. Needle biopsies are performed percutaneously and include both core-needle biopsy (which removes a core of tissue) and fine-needle aspiration (which removes cells from the suspicious site). Core-needle biopsy is the preferred biopsy method for mammographically detected, nonpalpable abnormalities.[14] Core-needle biopsy offers a more definitive histologic diagnosis, avoids inadequate samples, and can distinguish invasive from in situ breast cancer (which fine-needle biopsy cannot). After confirmation of malignancy via core-needle biopsy, subsequent surgical procedures are performed (either before or after systemic therapy) to assure complete removal of the abnormal tissue.

PATHOPHYSIOLOGY

The pathologic evaluation of breast tissue serves to establish the histologic diagnosis and to confirm the presence or absence of other factors believed to influence prognosis.

Invasive Carcinoma

Invasive breast cancers are a histologically heterogeneous group of lesions. Most breast cancers are adenocarcinomas and are classified on the basis of their microscopic appearance as ductal or lobular, corresponding to the ducts and lobules of the normal breast (see Fig. 151-1). The various histologic types of breast cancer have different prognoses, but it is unknown whether their response to therapy differs because patients in therapeutic trials are not typically stratified according to histologic type. The five most common types of invasive breast cancer are briefly described below.

Invasive or *infiltrating ductal carcinoma* is the most common histology, accounting for about 75% of all invasive breast cancers. These tumors commonly spread to the axillary lymph nodes, and their prognosis is poorer than for some other histologic types. *Invasive or infiltrating lobular carcinoma* accounts for 15% of breast tumors.[2] Both clinical and radiologic findings for these tumors may be quite subtle. The typical presentation is an area of ill-defined thickening in the breast in contrast to a prominent lump characteristic of infiltrating ductal carcinoma (IDC). *Infiltrating lobular carcinoma* (ILC) can also be more difficult to detect by mammography. Overall, ILC and IDC have similar likelihoods of axillary node involvement and disease recurrence and death, but the sites of metastases may differ. While IDC more frequently metastasizes to the bone or to the liver, lung, or brain, ILC tends to metastasize to the leptomeninges, peritoneal surfaces, retroperitoneum, gastrointestinal tract, reproductive organs, and other unusual sites.

The most common special types of invasive cancer are *cribriform, mucinous, tubular,* and *papillary*. The prognosis may be more favorable with these rare and unusual histologies.[2] Special situations seen clinically and histologically include Paget's disease of the breast, phyllodes tumors, and IBC. Paget's disease of the breast is characterized by neoplastic cells in the nipple areolar complex. The patient presents clinically with eczematous changes in the nipple with itching, burning, oozing, bleeding, or some combination of these. Phyllodes tumors of the breast are rare tumors with subtypes that range from benign to malignant. These tumors often enlarge rapidly, are painless, and can appear as fibroadenomas.[14] IBC is rare, aggressive, and characterized clinically by prominent skin edema, redness and warmth, and induration of the underlying tissue. Biopsies of the involved skin reveal cancer cells in the dermal lymphatics. IBC typically has a rapid onset and is often mistaken for infectious cellulitis or mastitis. The prognosis of patients with IBC is poor even if the disease is apparently localized.[14]

Noninvasive Carcinoma

As with invasive carcinoma, the noninvasive lesions may be divided broadly into ductal and lobular categories. The development of malignancy is a multistep process and invasive breast cancer has a pre-invasive (ie, in situ) phase. During the carcinoma in situ phase, normal epithelial cells undergo genetic alterations that result in malignant transformation. Transformed epithelial cells proliferate and pile up within lobules or ducts but lack the required genetic alterations that enable the cells to penetrate the basement membrane. Carcinoma in situ is diagnosed when malignant transformation of cells has occurred, but the basement membrane is intact.

The widespread use of screening mammography with subsequent biopsy and greater recognition of noninvasive breast carcinoma by pathologists has resulted in a significant increase in the diagnosis of in situ breast cancer. An estimated 49,290 new cases of female noninvasive DCIS were diagnosed in 2021.[1] The natural history of these disorders is not well described, and thus the debate continues whether carcinoma in situ is a pre-invasive cancer or simply a marker of unstable epithelium that represents an increased risk for the development of subsequent aggressive cancer. DCIS is more frequently diagnosed than lobular carcinoma in situ (LCIS). Most cases of DCIS today are found by biopsies performed for clustered microcalcifications seen on screening mammography, a hallmark of this disorder.

TREATMENT

The ultimate goal of treatment for noninvasive carcinomas is to prevent the development of invasive disease. If left untreated, 15% to 50% of DCIS lesions will progress to invasive breast cancer.[15] Therefore, more than 50% of these tumors do not progress to invasive disease, but identifying this group of patients is not yet possible and all diagnoses should be treated.

Locoregional treatment of DCIS depends on its location, size, and pathology.[14] Treatment options include surgery (mastectomy or lumpectomy), radiation therapy, and adjuvant endocrine therapy if hormone receptor-positive. Axillary lymph node dissection (ALND) is generally not indicated, although sentinel lymph node biopsy (SLNB) (see the "Curative Breast Cancer" section) may be considered in selected patients.[14]

Cytotoxic chemotherapy has no role in the treatment of patients with pure DCIS. It is important to determine hormone receptor status on the cancer cells. Tamoxifen treatment for 5 years may be considered in premenopausal and postmenopausal women with hormone receptor–positive DCIS. Anastrozole for 5 years may also be considered in postmenopausal women with hormone receptor–positive DCIS, particularly if they are less than 60 years.[14]

Unlike DCIS, LCIS is a microscopic diagnosis; generally no palpable mass and no specific clinical abnormality exists. LCIS does not generally demonstrate calcifications on mammography and the diagnosis is usually an incidental finding in biopsy specimens obtained because of symptoms or mammography findings consistent with benign lesions. It is unclear whether LCIS is a precursor lesion or serves as a marker of risk for developing invasive carcinoma in the breast. The 10-year incidence of developing invasive carcinoma is 13.9%.[16] The risk for the development of breast cancer is equally high in either breast, which makes the management of LCIS controversial. Some experts favor a program of observation, with physical examination every 6 to 12 months, annual mammography, and consideration of annual breast MRI or ultrasound.[10] In selected women with high-risk genetic mutations or strong family history and in women who are anxious about the development of cancer, bilateral mastectomies may be considered.[4] Radiation and systemic chemotherapy have no role in the management of LCIS. The use of chemoprevention with tamoxifen in premenopausal women or tamoxifen, raloxifene, anastrozole, or exemestane in postmenopausal women may also be considered for risk reduction (see the "Prevention and Early Detection" section for details).[4] These decisions are often difficult to discuss with patients because these treatments have toxicities. Nonetheless, a discussion regarding the risks and benefits is warranted.

STAGING AND PROGNOSIS

The natural history of breast cancer varies among patients, with some having extremely aggressive disease that progresses rapidly and others following a more indolent course. The ability to predict prognosis is extremely important in designing personalized treatment recommendations. Several pathologic prognostic and predictive factors have been identified. Prognostic factors are characteristics or measurements available at diagnosis or at the time of surgery that in the absence of neoadjuvant or adjuvant systemic therapy are associated with recurrence rate, death rate, or other clinical outcomes. Predictive factors are measurements available at diagnosis that are associated with response to a specific therapy. Prognostic and predictive factors fall into these general categories: (a) patient characteristics that are independent of the disease, such as age; (b) cancer characteristics, such as tumor size or histologic type; (c) other biomarkers that are measurable parameters in tissues, cells, or fluids, such as hormone-receptor status; and (d) genetic variables. The use of prognostic and predictive factors can personalize treatment to patients, increase the likelihood of clinical benefit, and reduce the risk of unnecessary toxicities.

Age at diagnosis and ethnicity can affect prognosis. Some younger patients, particularly those younger than 35 years, have more aggressive forms of breast cancer and a worse prognosis. Younger patients are more likely to present with poor prognostic features, such as affected lymph nodes, large tumor size, and tumors negative for hormone receptors. Black individuals have decreased survival compared with White individuals. The cause of this racial disparity is widely debated, with possible explanations including access to care, socioeconomic status, cultural differences, higher stage at diagnosis, and more aggressive biologic features.

Potentially modifiable prognostic factors include alcohol use, dietary factors, weight, and exercise. Agencies such as the ACS have recognized that physical activity, weight control, and diet are potentially modifiable risk factors for reducing the risk of recurrent breast cancer and other comorbidities (eg, heart disease, diabetes).[17]

Tumor size and the number of involved lymph nodes are established independent factors that influence the risk for breast cancer recurrence and subsequent metastatic disease. The number of affected lymph nodes is directly related to the risk of disease recurrence. The staging system for breast cancer recognizes the absolute number of positive nodes as a prognostic factor (see Table 151-3 for further details).[18] The relationship between tumor size and lymph node status is complex and is not a simple grouping.

Certain histologic subtypes and clinical presentation of breast cancer have prognostic importance. As mentioned earlier, treatment recommendations may differ because women with pure *tubular* or *mucinous* tumors have more favorable outcomes than those with *invasive ductal carcinomas*.[14] IBC, a clinical designation and not a distinct histologic subtype, is associated with a poor prognosis.[14]

Nuclear grade and tumor (histologic) differentiation are also independent prognostic indicators. Several histologic grading systems have been developed, most of which grade tumors with a score from 1 to 3: grade 1, well differentiated; grade 2, moderately differentiated; and grade 3, poorly differentiated. Grading is incorporated as part of the staging system (see Table 151-4 for details regarding grading).[18] Higher grade tumors are associated with higher rates of distant metastasis and poorer survival. This factor aids in making treatment decisions, particularly for patients with small tumors and negative lymph nodes. Additional factors may include lymphovascular invasion and proliferation indices.

TABLE 151-3 Definitions for Tumor, Node, Metastasis

TX	Primary tumor cannot be assessed	
T0	No evidence of primary tumor	
Tis (DCIS)	Ductal carcinoma in situ	
Tis (Paget)	Paget's disease of the nipple NOT associated with invasive carcinoma or carcinoma in situ	
T1	Tumor ≤2 cm in greatest dimension	
	T1mi	<0.1 cm; microinvasion
	T1a	>0.1 cm ≤0.5 cm
	T1b	>0.5 cm ≤1 cm
	T1c	>1 cm ≤2 cm
T2	Tumor >2 cm ≤5 cm	
T3	Tumor >5 cm	
T4	Tumor of any size with direct extension to the chest wall and/or to the skin	
	T4a	Extension to the chest wall; invasion or adherence to pectoralis muscle in the absence of invasion of chest wall structures
	T4b	Ulceration and/or ipsilateral macroscopic satellite nodules and/or edema (including peau d'orange) of the skin that does not meet the criteria of inflammatory carcinoma
	T4c	Both T4a and T4b present
	T4d	Inflammatory carcinoma
Regional Lymph Nodes: Clinical (cN)		
cNX	Regional lymph nodes cannot be assessed	
cN0	No regional lymph node metastases	
cN1	Metastases to movable ipsilateral level 1, II axillary lymph node(s)	
	cN1mi	Micrometastases (approximately 200 cells, >0.02 cm <0.2 cm)
cN2	Metastases in ipsilateral level I, II axillary lymph nodes that are clinically fixed or matted; or in ipsilateral internal mammary nodes in the absence of axillary lymph node metastases	
	cN2a	Metastases in ipsilateral level I, II axillary lymph nodes fixed to one another (matted) or to other structures
	cN2b	Metastases only in ipsilateral internal mammary nodes in the absence of axillary lymph node metastases
cN3	Metastases in ipsilateral infraclavicular (level III axillary) lymph node(s) with or without level I, II axillary lymph node involvement; or in ipsilateral internal mammary lymph node(s) with level I, II axillary lymph node metastases; or metastases in ipsilateral supraclavicular lymph node(s) with or without axillary or internal mammary lymph node involvement	
	cN3a	Metastases in ipsilateral infraclavicular lymph node(s)
	cN3b	Metastases in ipsilateral internal mammary lymph node(s) and axillary lymph node(s)
	cN3c	Metastases in ipsilateral supraclavicular lymph node(s)
Regional Lymph Nodes: Pathologic (pN)		
pNX	Regional lymph nodes cannot be assessed	
pN0	No regional lymph node metastasis identified or ITCs only	
	pN0(i+)	ITCs only, no larger than 0.02 cm in regional lymph nodes
	pN0(mol+)	Positive molecular findings by reverse transcriptase polymerase chain reaction; no ITCs detected
pN1	Micrometastases; or metastases in 1-3 axillary lymph nodes; and/or clinically negative internal mammary nodes with micrometastases or macrometastases by sentinel lymph node biopsy	
	pN1mi	Micrometastases, (approximately 200 cells, >0.02 cm <0.2 cm)
	pN1a	Metastases in ipsilateral internal mammary sentinel nodes, excluding ITCs
	pN1c	pN1a and pN1b combined
pN2	Metastases in 4-9 axillary lymph nodes; or positive ipsilateral internal mammary lymph nodes by imaging in the absence of axillary lymph node metastases	
	pN2a	Metastases in 4-9 lymph nodes (at least one deposit >0.2 cm)
	pN2b	Metastases in clinically detected internal mammary lymph nodes with or without microscopic confirmation; with pathologically negative axillary nodes
pN3	Metastases ≥10 or more axillary lymph nodes; or in infraclavicular (level III axillary) lymph nodes; or positive ipsilateral internal mammary lymph nodes by imaging in the presence ≥1 positive level I, II axillary lymph nodes; or in >3 axillary lymph nodes and micrometastases or macrometastases by sentinel lymph node biopsy in clinically negative ipsilateral internal mammary lymph nodes; or in ipsilateral mammary lymph nodes	
	pN3a	Metastases in ≥10 axillary lymph nodes (at least one tumor deposit >0.2 cm) or metastatses to infraclavicular (level III axillary lymph) nodes
	pN3b	pN1a or pN2a in the presence of cN2b (positive internal mammary nodes by imaging) or pN2a in presence of pN1b
	pN3c	Metastases in ipsilateral supraclavicular lymph nodes
Distant Metastasis (M)		
M0	No clinical or radiographic evidence of distant metastases	
	cM0(i+)	No clinical or radiographic evidence of distant metastases in the presence of tumor cells or deposits <0.02 cm detected microscopically or by molecular techniques in circulating blood, bone marrow, or other nonregional nodal tissue in a patient without symptoms or signs of metastases
cM1	Distant metastases detected by clinical and radiographic means	
pM1	Any histologically proven metastases in distant organs; or if in nonregional nodes, metastases >0.02 cm	

ITCs, isolated tumor cells.

Reproduced, with permission, from Hortobagyi GN, Connolly JL, D'Orsi CJ, et al. Breast. In: Amin EB, Edge SB, Gress DM, et al., AJCC Cancer Staging Manual. 8th Ed. Chicago, IL: Springer. 2017:589–638.

Hormone receptors are not strong prognostic markers but are used clinically to predict responses to endocrine therapy. Determination of both ER and PR status is an established procedure that is important in the management of breast cancer. Most patients with primary or MBC have hormone receptor–positive tumors. Hormone receptor positivity, more common in postmenopausal individuals, is associated with a higher response to endocrine therapy and longer disease-free survival.

The *HER2* protein is normally expressed at low levels in the epithelial cells of normal breast tissue. *HER2* overexpression occurs in

TABLE 151-4 Clinical Staging System

TNM	Grade	HER2	ER	PR	Stage	TNM	Grade	HER2	ER	PR	Stage
Tis N0 M0	Any	Any	Any	Any	0						
T1[a] N0 M0	G1[b]	Positive	Positive	Positive	IA	T0 N1[c] M0	G1	Positive	Positive	Positive	IB
T0 N1mi M0				Negative		T1[a] N1[c] M0				Negative	IIA
T1[a] N1mi M0			Negative	Positive		T2 N0 M0			Negative	Positive	
				Negative						Negative	
		Negative	Positive	Positive				Negative	Positive	Positive	IB
				Negative						Negative	IIA
			Negative	Positive					Negative	Positive	
				Negative	IB					Negative	
	G2[d]	Positive	Positive	Positive	IA		G2	Positive	Positive	Positive	IB
				Negative						Negative	IIA
			Negative	Positive					Negative	Positive	
				Negative						Negative	
		Negative	Positive	Positive				Negative	Positive	Positive	IB
				Negative						Negative	IIA
			Negative	Positive					Negative	Positive	
				Negative	IB					Negative	IIB
	G3[e]	Positive	Positive	Positive	IA		G3	Positive	Positive	Positive	IB
				Negative						Negative	IIA
			Negative	Positive					Negative	Positive	
				Negative						Negative	
		Negative	Positive	Positive				Negative	Positive	Positive	
				Negative	IB					Negative	IIB
			Negative	Positive					Negative	Positive	
				Negative						Negative	
T2 N1[f] M0	G1	Positive	Positive	Positive	IB	T0 N2 M0	G1	Positive	Positive	Positive	IIA
T3 N0 M0				Negative	IA	T1[a] N2 M0				Negative	IIIA
			Negative	Positive		T2 N2 M0			Negative	Positive	
				Negative	IIB	T3 N1[f] M0				Negative	
		Negative	Positive	Positive	IIA	T3 N2 M0		Negative	Positive	Positive	IIA
				Negative	IIB					Negative	IIIA
			Negative	Positive					Negative	Positive	
				Negative						Negative	IIIB
	G2	Positive	Positive	Positive	IB		G2	Positive	Positive	Positive	IIA
				Negative	IIA					Negative	IIIA
			Negative	Positive					Negative	Positive	
				Negative	IIB					Negative	
		Negative	Positive	Positive	IIA			Negative	Positive	Positive	IIA
				Negative	IIB					Negative	IIIA
			Negative	Positive					Negative	Positive	
				Negative	IIIB					Negative	IIIB
	G3	Positive	Positive	Positive	IB		G3	Positive	Positive	Positive	IIB
				Negative	IIB					Negative	IIIA
			Negative	Positive					Negative	Positive	
				Negative						Negative	
		Negative	Positive	Positive				Negative	Positive	Positive	
				Negative	IIIA					Negative	IIIB
			Negative	Positive					Negative	Positive	
				Negative	IIIB					Negative	IIIC

(Continued)

TABLE 151-4 Clinical Staging System (*Continued*)

TNM	Grade	HER2	ER	PR	Stage	TNM	Grade	HER2	ER	PR	Stage
T4 N0 M0	G1	Positive	Positive	Positive	IIIA	Any T Any N M1	Any	Any	Any	Any	IV
T4 N1[f] M0				Negative	IIIB						
T4 N2 M0			Negative	Positive							
Any T N3 M0				Negative							
		Negative	Positive	Positive							
				Negative							
			Negative	Positive							
				Negative	IIIC						
	G2	Positive	Positive	Positive	IIIA						
				Negative	IIIB						
			Negative	Positive							
				Negative							
		Negative	Positive	Positive							
				Negative							
			Negative	Positive							
				Negative	IIIC						
	G3	Positive	Positive	Positive	IIIB						
				Negative							
			Negative	Positive							
				Negative							
		Negative	Positive	Positive							
				Negative	IIIC						
			Negative	Positive							
				Negative							

[a]T1 includes T1mi.

[b]N1 does not include N1mi. T1N1miM0 and T0N1miM0 are included for prognostic staging with T1N0M0 cancers of the same prognostic factor status.

[c]N1 includes N1mi, T2, T3, and T4 cancers and N1mi are included for prognostic staging with T2N1, T3N1, and T4N1, respectively.

[d]G1 Low combined histologic grade (favorable), SBR (Scarf-Bloom Richardson grading system, Nottingham Modification) score of 3-5 points.

[e]G2 Intermediate combined histologic grade (moderately favorable), SBR score of 6-7 points.

[f]G3 High combined histologic grade (unfavorable), SBR score of 8-9 points.

Reproduced, with permission, from Hortobagyi GN, Connolly JL, D'Orsi CJ, et al. Breast. In: Amin EB, Edge SB, Gress DM, et al., AJCC Cancer Staging Manual. 8th Ed. Chicago, IL: Springer. 2017:589–638.

about 15% to 20% of breast cancers and is associated with increased tumor aggressiveness, increased rates of recurrence, and increased mortality rates.[2,19] *HER2* overexpression is associated with poor prognosis and is measured by fluorescence in situ hybridization (FISH) and immunohistochemistry (IHC). Tumors that are either IHC 3+ or FISH positive are considered to be positive for *HER2*.[14] *HER2*-positive status clearly predicts response to *HER2*-targeted therapy. Patients with *HER2*-positive MBC treated with trastuzumab, a monoclonal antibody (mAb) directed against the extracellular domain of the *HER2* receptor, have improved survival rates compared to patients with *HER2*-negative MBC or patients with *HER2*-positive MBC who do not receive trastuzumab.

Genetic profiling is also being used to provide prognostic and predictive information on clinical outcomes of breast cancer.[14] Further details on these assays are available in the "Genomic Testing" section under Curative Breast Cancer.

Breast cancer stage is based on the primary tumor extent and size, presence and extent of lymph node involvement, and presence or absence of distant metastases (Fig. 151-2, Tables 151-3 and 151-4). Although many possible combinations of T and N are possible within a given stage, simplistically, stage 0 represents carcinoma in situ (Tis) or disease that has not invaded the basement membrane of the breast tissue. Stage I represents a small primary invasive tumor without lymph node involvement or with micrometastatic nodal involvement, and stage II disease usually involves regional lymph nodes. Stages I and II are often referred to as *early breast cancer*. It is in these early stages that the disease is highly curable (99% 5-year survival in patients with disease confined to the breast, node negative).[2] Stage III, also referred to as *locally advanced disease*, usually represents a large tumor with extensive nodal involvement in which either node or tumor is fixed to the chest wall. A wide variety of clinical scenarios can be seen within this group of patients, including neglected tumors that have spread locally to IBCs that are a unique clinical entity. IBC is associated with similar clinical findings compared with neglected, locally advanced breast tumors (eg, erythema representing skin involvement). The distinction between the two diagnoses lies in the rapidity of onset of symptoms. Many locally advanced breast cancers are diagnosed in patients who have had symptoms for months to years and have neglected to seek medical attention. Although these women have a poor prognosis because of the delay in diagnosis, they are not classified as IBC. Stage IV disease is characterized by the presence of metastases to organs distant from the primary tumor and is often referred to as *advanced or metastatic disease* as described earlier (27% 5-year survival rate in patients with distant metastases).[2] Most individuals with breast cancer in the United States present in early stages where the prognosis is favorable

(91% of newly diagnosed patients have disease confined to the breast or local lymph nodes).[2]

Staging for breast cancer is separated into clinical and pathologic staging. Clinical stage is assigned before surgery and is based on physical examination (assessment of tumor size and presence of axillary lymph nodes), imaging (eg, mammography, ultrasonography), and pathologic examination of tissues (eg, biopsy results). Pathologic staging occurs after surgery and adds data from surgical exploration and resection. The American Joint Committee for Cancer (AJCC) publishes staging criteria for cancers.

TREATMENT

Curative Breast Cancer (Stage I-III)

Desired Outcomes

In the curative setting, through the use of different modalities of treatment—surgery, radiation, and systemic therapy, the desired outcome is cure of disease. This differs significantly from the desired outcomes when treating metastatic disease. Locoregional and systemic therapy and their roles in curing breast cancer are discussed below. While the desired outcome is the same for patients with stage I-III breast cancer, the terminology and sequence of therapies may differ. For example, *locally advanced breast cancer (stage III)* generally refers to breast carcinomas with significant primary tumor and nodal disease but in which distant metastases cannot be documented. In this setting, neoadjuvant systemic therapy may be administered to decrease tumor size prior to surgery and/or to allow for breast conserving surgery if desired by the patient. This approach to systemic therapy also allows for assessment of response to therapy. In contrast, the intent of adjuvant systemic therapy is to eradicate micrometastatic disease. A predetermined number of cycles or duration of systemic therapy is given in the neoadjuvant and adjuvant settings. Clinicians and patients must weigh the short- and long-term effects of systemic therapy against the benefits of lowering the risk of breast cancer recurrence.

Locoregional Therapy

3 Most patients presenting with breast cancer have an *in situ* tumor (stage 0), a small invasive tumor with negative lymph nodes (stage I), or a small invasive tumor with axillary lymph node involvement (stage II). Surgery alone can cure most, if not all, patients with in situ cancers: 70% to 80% of patients with stage I and about half of patients with stage II cancers. The choice of surgical procedures has changed drastically over the past 50 years, which is related to an increased understanding of the biology of breast cancer and the results of a series of well-conducted clinical trials performed over this time period.

Most patients diagnosed with breast cancer can be treated with BCT, a less extensive surgery than mastectomy (complete removal of the breast) that maintains acceptable cosmetic results and rates of local and distant recurrence and mortality.[14] BCT includes removal of part of the breast, surgical evaluation of the axillary lymph node basin, and radiation therapy to the breast. The amount of breast tissue removed as a part of BCT varies from removing the cancerous "lump" (ie, lumpectomy) with a small margin of adjacent normal-appearing tissue to removing the "lump" with a wider excision of adjacent normal-appearing tissue (ie, wide local excision) to removing the entire quadrant of the breast that includes the cancerous "lump" (ie, quadrantectomy). All these techniques are referred to as segmental or partial mastectomy. Overall survival rates are similar to BCT compared with mastectomy; however, a small increase in the risk of locoregional recurrence occurs with BCT.[14]

Several factors should be considered in selecting patients for BCT, such as younger age, family history, and genetic predisposition. The NCCN guidelines recommend that women who carry a known *BRCA1* or *BRCA2* mutation undergo mastectomy and consider additional risk reduction strategies (eg, bilateral mastectomies).[6] Bilateral total mastectomy and oophorectomy reduce the risk of breast cancer recurrence in patients with *BRCA1* or *BRCA2* mutations. Multiple sites of cancer within the breast and the inability to attain negative pathologic margins on the excised breast specimen are indications for mastectomy. Other relative contraindications may need to be considered when making the decision for the type of surgery. Local recurrence after BCT has not been consistently associated with an increased mortality rate, but it can be distressing to the patient and requires surgical removal of the remaining breast tissue. Other considerations include previous radiation to the breast, expected cosmetic result, and extent of local disease. The availability of an external-beam radiation facility and the patient's willingness to comply with the prescribed course of radiotherapy must also be considered. Radiotherapy after BCT reduces the 10-year risk of first recurrence by 16% and the 15-year risk of breast cancer death by 4% as compared with no radiotherapy.[14] External-beam radiation therapy after BCT usually involves 3 to 5 weeks of radiation therapy directed to the entire breast tissue to eradicate residual disease. Local tumor control is similar with shorter courses versus longer courses of radiation, and toxicities, such as breast shrinkage, telangiectasias, and breast edema are less common with shorter regimens. The NCCN guidelines recommended radiation course is 40 to 42.5 Gy in 15 to 16 fractions or 46 to 50 Gy in 23 to 25 fractions.[14] Complications associated with radiation therapy to the breast are generally minor and include reddening and erythema of the breast tissue and subsequent shrinkage of the total breast mass beyond that predicted on the basis of breast tissue removal.

Postmastectomy radiation therapy to the chest wall and regional lymph nodes (if indicated) may also be required in certain situations when tumors are large or the number of positive axillary lymph nodes is high. Post-mastectomy radiation is recommended for patients with ≥4 positive axillary lymph nodes and should be considered in situations where the tumor is ≤5 cm with negative axillary lymph nodes and margins <1 mm, the tumor is >5 cm with negative lymph nodes, 1 to 3 lymph nodes are positive, and if there are positive margins.[14]

The optimal sequence of radiation therapy and chemotherapy is somewhat controversial, but it is common to begin radiation after completion of chemotherapy when chemotherapy is recommended. If chemotherapy is not indicated, radiation is administered after surgery (see the "Biologic or Targeted Therapy" section under Curative Breast Cancer for a discussion of sequencing trastuzumab).

Accurate assessment of the spread of breast cancer cells to the axillary lymph nodes is critical for prognosis and personalizing local and systemic treatments. The number of positive axillary lymph nodes remains the most powerful predictor of breast cancer recurrence and survival, but other benefits may include a therapeutic effect of removing the lymph nodes and obtaining information to guide treatment selection. However, axillary dissection is associated with significant morbidity, including lymphedema, arm pain or numbness, and reduced quality of life.[14] About 60% of patients with early-stage breast cancer (ESBC) present with lymph node–negative disease, which indicates that many women would derive no therapeutic benefit but would be exposed to the complications from the full ALND.

For these reasons, a procedure involving lymphatic mapping and SLNB is recommended for patients with clinically negative lymph nodes.[20] The sentinel lymph node(s) is the first lymph node(s) that receives lymph drainage from the primary tumor. Injection of a vital blue dye, a radiocolloid, or both, around the primary breast tumor identifies the sentinel lymph node(s) in most patients, and the status of this lymph node(s) predicts the status of the remaining nodes in the nodal basin. Patients with lymph nodes that are

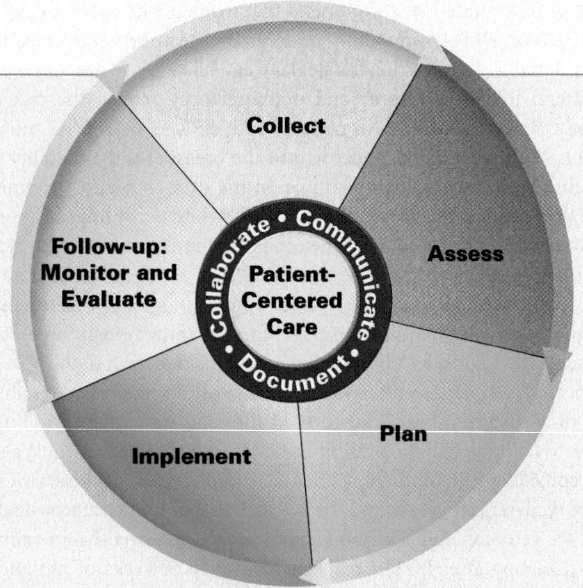

Patient Care Process for Breast Cancer

An illustration shows that patient-centered care includes collaboration, communication, and documentation. The actions associated with the care are collect, assess, plan, implement, and follow-up by monitoring and evaluating.

Collect

- Patient characteristics (eg, age, biological sex)
- Physical examination, including clinical breast examination (if appropriate) and general examination to evaluate for MBC
- Patient medical history (personal and family history for breast and ovarian cancers, start of menstruation, time of menopause, surgical history [eg, hysterectomy, oophorectomy])
- Social history (eg, tobacco/ethanol use) and dietary habits
- Current medications including OTC use, herbal products, birth control, and dietary supplements
- Objective data
  - Height, weight
  - Laboratory findings including complete blood count with differential, SCr, total bilirubin, AST, ALT, alkaline phosphatase
  - Staging
  - Tumor genomics if appropriate (eg, Oncotype DX, MammaPrint, Prosigna). For other details, see "Genomic Testing" under Systemic Therapy section
  - For other details, see section "Clinical Presentation"

Assess

- Comorbidities
- Current medications and medication adherence
- Ability/willingness to pay for treatment options, insurance coverage
- Emotional status (eg, presence of anxiety, depression)
- Type of and response to prior treatment(s) and need for dose reductions and/or supportive care
- For other details, see section "Clinical Presentation"

Plan*

- Drug therapy regimen including specific chemotherapy, endocrine therapy, or targeted therapy and include dose, route, frequency, duration, and supportive care (see Fig. 151-3, Tables 151-5–151-8 and 151-10 in "Curative Breast Cancer" and "Metastatic Breast Cancer" sections)
- Monitoring parameters including efficacy (eg, staging studies such as CT chest, abdomen/pelvis, bone scan, CT/MRI brain in the cases of metastatic disease; ultrasound in the cases of neoadjuvant therapy), adverse drug reaction management (eg, nausea/vomiting, mucositis, neutropenia, hot flashes, myalgias), and safety (eg, CBC with differential, SCr, total bilirubin, AST/ALT, DEXA scan for bone health); frequency and timing of follow-up
- Patient education (eg, goal of treatment, dietary and lifestyle modification, drug-specific information; see "Curative Breast Cancer" and "Metastatic Breast Cancer" sections and Table 151-9)
- Self-monitoring for resolution of nausea/vomiting, mucositis, fever, when to seek emergency medical attention
- Referrals to other providers when appropriate (eg, dietician, supportive care services, psychiatry, bone health, cardiology, genetics)

Implement*

- Provide patient education regarding all elements of the treatment plan. If patient has completed curative therapy, review survivorship care plan (ie, frequency of clinic visits)
- Use motivational interviewing and coaching strategies to maximize adherence
- Schedule follow-up (eg, labs, staging scans, monitoring tests [eg, ECHO/MUGA, DEXA scan, ultrasound])

Follow-up: Monitor and Evaluate

- Resolution of adverse drug reactions (eg, nausea/vomiting, mucositis, myalgia)
- Presence of adverse drug reactions (eg, constipation, diarrhea)
- Patient adherence to treatment plan using multiple sources of information
- Re-evaluate duration of therapy, depending on specific regimen

**Collaborate with patient, caregivers, and other healthcare professionals.*

suspicious for cancer involvement either by physical examination or imaging should have a biopsy performed to exclude lymph node involvement.[14] Historically, patients with positive sentinel nodes have proceeded to a level I and II ALND. However, ALND after SLNB in women with clinically node-negative tumors smaller than 5 cm, fewer than three involved sentinel lymph nodes, and undergoing BCT with subsequent breast irradiation results in higher morbidity, no improvement in local recurrence, and no difference in disease-free or overall survival as compared with SLNB alone.[21] Therefore, the ASCO and NCCN guidelines do not recommend

ALND for women with ESBC with one or two positive sentinel lymph nodes who will receive BCT followed by radiation.[14,20] Women undergoing mastectomy with positive sentinel lymph nodes should be offered ALND.

Systemic Therapy

As stated previously, the desired therapeutic outcome of curative systemic therapy for breast cancer differs significantly from that of metastatic disease. Systemic therapy—chemotherapy, biologic or targeted therapy, and endocrine therapy—in this setting is administered with curative intent. For patients with inflammatory or locally advanced/unresectable breast cancer, neoadjuvant chemotherapy is considered the treatment of choice.[22]

Genomic Testing Intensive research efforts have been directed toward identifying characteristics of the primary tumor (eg, pathologic or molecular prognostic factors) that may predict for a higher or lower likelihood of distant metastases and death in node-negative patients. Although many prognostic factors continue to be investigated, no single factor or combination of factors sufficiently identifies those at risk of metastases or is sufficiently standardized to be reproducibly applicable to all patients. Several multigene expression assays are commercially available as decision-support tools for adjuvant chemotherapy.[23] Oncotype DX® is one test that screens for expression of 21 genes with reverse transcription polymerase chain reaction (RT-PCR), and reports a recurrence score that correlates with the risk of distant recurrence or death from breast cancer in women with ER-positive, node-negative, invasive breast cancer. This test was initially validated in node-negative invasive breast cancer. A low recurrence score (≤15) indicates a low risk of recurrence with endocrine therapy alone indicating that perhaps adjuvant chemotherapy could be avoided. A high recurrence score (≥26) indicates a high risk of recurrence despite endocrine therapy, suggesting a need for adjuvant chemotherapy followed by endocrine therapy. For premenopausal patients with a score of 16 to 25, chemotherapy followed by endocrine therapy may be considered.[14,24] Postmenopausal patients with ER-positive, node-positive (1-3 positive lymph nodes) with a recurrence score of <26 may receive only endocrine therapy in the adjuvant setting. Premenopausal patients with a risk score less than 26 may derive benefit from chemotherapy followed by endocrine therapy and should be considered based on other factors. Patients with 1 to 3 positive lymph nodes and a recurrence score of ≥26 should be offered chemotherapy regardless of menopausal status.[14] Other commercially available multigene assays include MammaPrint® and Prosigna®. MammaPrint® screens the tumor for 70 genes with microarray technology in breast cancer patients with ESBC, regardless of hormone-receptor status. The assay reports the predicted rates of recurrence as high or low. PAM50 (Prosigna®) is a multigene test that screens the tumor for 50 genes (plus 5 control genes) to predict distant relapse-free survival and likelihood of recurrence at 10 years in postmenopausal women with ER-positive breast cancer treated with endocrine therapy regardless of nodal status.[23]

Cytotoxic Chemotherapy *Systemic adjuvant therapy* is defined as the administration of systemic therapy after definitive local therapy (surgery, radiation, or both) when there is no evidence of metastatic disease but a high likelihood of disease recurrence. By the time breast cancers become clinically detectable, they have likely been present for a number of years and have had an opportunity to establish distant micrometastases. Micrometastatic disease can travel from the primary breast tumor and spread to distant organs through several different routes (eg, hematogenous spread through blood vessels, lymphangitic spread through lymph channels, local extension to surrounding structures). Local therapies, such as breast surgery and irradiation, do not eradicate distant micrometastases; therefore, systemic therapy is required to target these tumor cells that may have escaped the local area of the breast. The risk of micrometastatic disease is one factor used to identify patients with a high risk of recurrence who would require systemic adjuvant therapy. Chemotherapy, endocrine therapy, targeted therapy, or some combination of these agents improves disease-free and/or overall survival for high-risk patients in specific prognostic subgroups (eg, nodal involvement, menopausal status, hormone-receptor status, or *HER2* status) based on the results of several hundred randomized clinical trials.

The benefit of adjuvant chemotherapy has been studied and established through several clinical trials over the years. With the evolution of chemotherapy regimens to the current standard, disease-free survival is increased with the addition of chemotherapy regardless of ER/PR status. A 12.4% increase in 5-year disease-free survival is seen when taxanes are added to anthracycline chemotherapy.[25] Five-year overall survival is increased with the addition of chemotherapy, but longer follow-up may be needed to solidify this benefit. Adjuvant chemotherapy is recommended in most women with lymph node metastases or with primary breast cancers larger than 1 cm in diameter (both node-negative and node-positive).[29]

6 Several international and national groups have developed guidelines for the treatment of ESBC based on specific patient and disease characteristics and as newer data are available. The four most commonly referenced guidelines are the St. Gallen International Expert Consensus Conference, European Society of Medical Oncology, or ESMO, the American Society of Clinical Oncology (ASCO), and the NCCN guidelines.[14,26-28] These guidelines are updated annually to every 2 years or more frequently based on available evidence. Recommendations from the NCCN guidelines for patients with tumors 1 cm or larger or positive lymph nodes are summarized in Fig. 151-3. For patients with tumors smaller than 1 cm, micrometastatic lymph node involvement, or negative lymph nodes, treatment is highly individualized and based on multiple patient- and tumor-related factors, including hormone-receptor status, *HER2* status, comorbidities, and patient preferences. Specific treatment recommendations are complex and readers are referred to the guidelines for further details.

7 The use of neoadjuvant systemic therapy is the standard of care for patients with locally advanced breast cancer and IBC and represents an important treatment option for patients with ESBC. This approach to therapy usually consists of chemotherapy, either alone or combined with biologic or targeted therapy, but in special circumstances may also include endocrine therapy (eg, in inoperable patients with significant comorbidities or in tumors with high sensitivity to endocrine therapy). Advantages of preoperative systemic therapy include a decrease in tumor size to minimize surgery, determination of response to chemotherapy or hormone therapy (an important prognostic indicator), and other theoretical advantages (eg, delivery of chemotherapy through an intact vascular system). Preoperative chemotherapy has similar disease-free or overall survival rates compared with adjuvant chemotherapy (the same chemotherapy and the same number of cycles), but is associated with higher rates of BCT.[14] Patients who receive neoadjuvant chemotherapy may experience a pathological complete response (defined as no tumor left at surgery [pCR]) after chemotherapy. Patients who achieve a pCR have a significantly longer disease-free and overall survival compared to patients who do not achieve a pCR.[14] The use of preoperative systemic therapy in patients with ESBC is generally recommended because of the ability to assess the response to therapy as well as the potential to decrease the size of the tumor, allowing for less radical surgery and better cosmetic results.

The most common cytotoxic drugs that have been used alone and in combination as adjuvant therapy for breast cancer include doxorubicin, epirubicin, cyclophosphamide, methotrexate, fluorouracil, carboplatin, paclitaxel, and docetaxel. Combination chemotherapy regimens (polychemotherapy) are more effective than

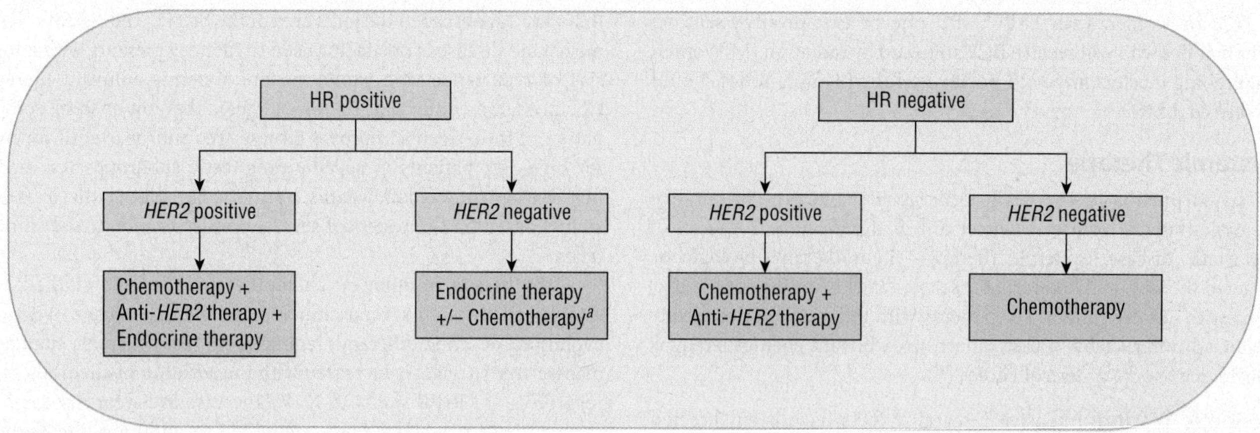

FIGURE 151-3 Treatment of patients with breast cancers larger than 1 cm or with positive lymph nodes. Refer to the text for definitions of HR and *HER2* positivity. Refer to the text for the management of patients with tumors smaller than 1 cm, micrometastatic lymph node involvement, or negative lymph nodes.
[a]Oncotype DX® may identify patients who derive little benefit from chemotherapy (see the "Genomic Testing" section under Curative Breast Cancer for details). (HR, hormone receptor; *HER2*, human epidermal growth factor receptor-2.)

single-agent chemotherapy. Table 151-5 lists the most common combination chemotherapy regimens used.

Anthracyclines (doxorubicin or epirubicin) and taxanes (paclitaxel or docetaxel) have become the cornerstones of modern chemotherapy for the adjuvant treatment of breast cancer. Anthracycline-containing chemotherapy regimens decrease the 10-year risk of recurrence from 47% to 39% and 10-year overall mortality from 40% to 35%. As mentioned previously, the addition of taxanes to anthracycline-based chemotherapy has a modest added benefit in disease-free survival.[25,29] Proportional reductions in recurrence and breast cancer mortality were largely independent of age, nodal status, tumor size, tumor differentiation, or ER status. Most of these trials enrolled node-positive patients only, but some high-risk node-negative patients were also included.[29,30]

Cytotoxic chemotherapy is a particularly important treatment modality for patients with tumors that do not express ER or PR and do not overexpress *HER2* (often referred to as triple-negative breast cancer [TNBC]).[31] TNBC represents an uncommon subtype (10%-15%) and has a relatively poor prognosis.[32] Patients with TNBC treated with anthracycline- and taxane-based chemotherapy have significantly decreased survival compared to patients with other breast cancer subtypes. Ironically, this patient subgroup is more likely to respond to neoadjuvant chemotherapy. Furthermore, patients with TNBC who achieve a pCR have excellent long-term survival, but those who have residual disease at the time of surgery have a worse prognosis than non-TNBC patients. The optimal type and duration of chemotherapy for patients with TNBC is unknown. More recently, the addition of carboplatin to a neoadjuvant anthracycline- and taxane-based chemotherapy regimen resulted in a higher pCR rate as compared to chemotherapy without carboplatin, but with increased toxicity.[31] Identification of actionable molecular targets for this aggressive breast cancer subtype is needed and ongoing (eg, epidermal growth factor receptor [EGFR] and poly-ADP ribose polymerase [PARP]). Adjuvant capecitabine for 6 to 8 cycles may be offered because it improves disease-free and overall survival as compared to those who did not receive additional chemotherapy.[33]

Although the optimal duration of chemotherapy administration is unknown, it takes between 12 and 24 weeks and depends on the regimen being used. Optimally, chemotherapy should be initiated within 12 weeks of surgical removal of the primary tumor.[34] "Dose intensity" and "dose density" are critical factors in achieving optimal outcomes in adjuvant breast cancer therapy. *Dose intensity* is defined as the amount of drug administered per unit of time and is typically reported in milligrams per square meter of body surface area per week (mg/m²/week). Increasing dose, decreasing time between doses, or both can increase dose intensity. *Dose density* is one way of achieving dose intensity but not by increasing the amount

TABLE 151-5 Selected Neo/Adjuvant Chemotherapy Regimens for Breast Cancer

Dose-Dense AC → Paclitaxel[a]	**AC → Paclitaxel**
Doxorubicin 60 mg/m² IV bolus, day 1	Doxorubicin 60 mg/m² IV, day 1
Cyclophosphamide 600 mg/m² IV, day 1	Cyclophosphamide 600 mg/m² IV, day 1
Repeat cycles every 14 days for 4 cycles (must be given with growth factor support)	Repeat cycles every 21 days for 4 cycles
Followed by:	*Followed by:*
Paclitaxel 80 mg/m² IV weekly	Paclitaxel 80 mg/m² IV weekly
Repeat cycles every 7 days for 12 cycles	Repeat cycles every 7 days for 12 cycles
TC[a]	
Docetaxel 75 mg/m² IV, day 1	
Cyclophosphamide 600 mg/m² IV, day 1	
Repeat cycles every 21 days for 4 cycles	
Dose-Dense AC → Dose Dense Paclitaxel[a]	
Doxorubicin 60 mg/m² IV bolus, day 1	
Cyclophosphamide 600 mg/m² IV, day 1	
Repeat cycles every 14 days for 4 cycles (must be given with growth factor support)	
Followed by:	
Paclitaxel 175 mg/m² IV over 3 hours	
Repeat cycles every 14 days for 4 cycles (must be given with growth factor support)	

AC, Adriamycin (doxorubicin), Cytoxan (cyclophosphamide); TC, Taxotere (docetaxel), cyclophosphamide.

[a]Designated as a preferred regimen in the NCCN Breast Cancer Guidelines.

Data from Reference 14.

of drug given, as occurs with dose escalation, but instead by decreasing the time between treatment cycles. Dose reductions for standard treatment regimens should be avoided unless necessitated by severe toxicity. Increasing doses beyond those contained in standard treatment regimens does not appear to be beneficial and may be harmful.

The short-term toxicities of chemotherapy used in the adjuvant setting are generally well tolerated. Supportive therapy of patients receiving systemic adjuvant chemotherapy has improved over the past decades. More effective antiemetics have become available to manage chemotherapy-induced nausea and vomiting, and myeloid growth factors can prevent febrile neutropenia, particularly in elderly patients and patients receiving dose-dense chemotherapy regimens. The use of myeloid growth factors to support some adjuvant chemotherapy regimens may be required (eg, with dose-dense regimens), but these are not routinely used with adjuvant chemotherapy regimens. Many other adverse drug reactions are common with the chemotherapy regimens used for the treatment of ESBC, and patients should be appropriately counseled regarding the likelihood of alopecia, weight gain, fatigue, peripheral neuropathy, and myelosuppression. Patients who are menstruating often experience a cessation of menses that may not return; cessation of menses may be accompanied by signs and symptoms of menopause. Leukemia and other hematologic disorders have long been associated with the alkylating agents (eg, cyclophosphamide) and the topoisomerase II inhibitors (eg, doxorubicin and epirubicin; see Chapter 150, "Supportive Care in Cancer" for more information).

Cardiomyopathy induced by doxorubicin occurs in fewer than 1% to 2% of individuals whose total dose of anthracycline is less than 300 mg/m^2 of doxorubicin equivalents.[35] This risk may be further decreased by the use of continuous infusion or weekly doxorubicin. It should be noted that epirubicin in the adjuvant setting is usually given at a dose of 100 mg/m^2.[14] At this dose, epirubicin has an equal risk of cardiomyopathy as standard doxorubicin doses when both agents are given as bolus or short infusions. Taxanes are often associated with hypersensitivity reactions, peripheral neuropathy, or myalgias and arthralgias for a few days after the infusion.

It is currently not possible to accurately predict who will attain this survival benefit. Genetic prognostic tools, such as Oncotype DX®, can help to identify patients who may derive little or no benefit from chemotherapy. However, these tests are only appropriate in specific subsets of patients. Many adjuvant chemotherapy regimens are available, but most of these regimens have not been directly compared in randomized clinical trials. NCCN guideline recommendations are purposefully vague, and they do not differentiate between patients with node-positive or -negative breast cancer. The NCCN guidelines have designated preferred chemotherapy regimens, as listed in Table 151-5, although detailed information is not provided regarding the rationale behind these designations.

Biologic or Targeted Therapy Therapies directed at molecular targets through novel mechanisms are often referred to as targeted therapy. Many of the targeted therapies are also biologic therapies because they are mAbs. Trastuzumab is a mAb targeted against the *HER2*-receptor protein. Trastuzumab in combination with or sequentially after adjuvant chemotherapy is recommended for patients with early-stage, *HER2*-positive breast cancer, resulting in a 48% reduction in the risk of recurrence as well as superior disease-free and overall survival, compared with chemotherapy alone (Table 151-6).[14] Although the benefit of adding trastuzumab to these regimens is clear, the optimal trastuzumab-based regimen is less clear because the type of chemotherapy, sequence of administration, and duration of trastuzumab differed among the trials.

Most of the regimens investigated in these adjuvant trials included an anthracycline and a taxane given concurrently with trastuzumab or sequentially before trastuzumab. Administration of a taxane with trastuzumab may be more effective than trastuzumab administered after chemotherapy. Sequential and concomitant use of trastuzumab with chemotherapy prolongs disease-free survival as compared with chemotherapy alone. Concomitant trastuzumab also improves overall survival, but sequential trastuzumab does not.[14] The adjuvant use of trastuzumab without an anthracycline provides similar benefit with diminished cardiac adverse drug reactions as compared with traditional anthracycline-containing adjuvant trastuzumab regimens.[14] The optimal duration of trastuzumab therapy is unknown, although the majority of data support the use of trastuzumab for a total of 52 weeks (range, 9-104 weeks). The most

TABLE 151-6 Selected Regimens for HER2-Positive Early-Stage Breast Cancer

Neo/Adjuvant Regimen	Drugs	Doses	Frequency	Cycles
PH → H[a]	Paclitaxel	80 mg/m^2 IV over 1 hour	Every 7 days	12 weeks
	Trastuzumab	4 mg/kg IV → 2 mg/kg IV	Every 7 day	12 weeks
	Followed by			
	Trastuzumab	6 mg/kg IV	Every 21 days	Complete 1 year
TCH[a]	Docetaxel	75 mg/m^2 IV	Every 21 days	6
	Carboplatin	AUC 6 IV	Every 21 days	6
	Trastuzumab	4 mg/kg IV → 2 mg/kg IV	Every 7 days	18 weeks
	Followed by			
	Trastuzumab	6 mg/kg IV	Every 21 days	Complete 1 year
TCHP[a]	Docetaxel	75 mg/m^2 IV	Every 21 days	6
	Carboplatin	AUC 6 IV	Every 21 days	6
	Trastuzumab	8 mg/kg IV → 6 mg/kg IV	Every 21 days	6
	Pertuzumab	840 mg IV → 420 mg IV	Every 21 days	6
	Followed by			
	Trastuzumab	6 mg/kg IV	Every 21 days	Complete 1 year
	Pertuzumab	420 mg IV	Every 21 days	Complete 1 year

PH (paclitaxel, trastuzumab); TCH (docetaxel, carboplatin, trastuzumab); TCHP (docetaxel, carboplatin, trastuzumab, pertuzumab).

[a]Designated as a preferred regimen in the NCCN Breast Cancer Guidelines.

Data from Reference 14.

commonly used trastuzumab-based neo/adjuvant chemotherapy regimens are listed in Table 151-6.

The addition of mAb pertuzumab is another important treatment option for patients with *HER2*-positive breast cancer in the neoadjuvant setting.[36] The addition of pertuzumab to trastuzumab and chemotherapy produces high rates of pCR at the time of surgery in patients with tumors larger than 2 cm or positive lymph nodes (see Table 151-6 for details regarding the most commonly used regimens). Additionally, an approximately 1% absolute benefit in invasive disease-free survival at 3 years that continues for at least 6 years as well as an improvement in overall survival can occur with the addition of pertuzumab. The FDA added an indication for pertuzumab in combination with trastuzumab in the adjuvant setting for high-risk *HER2*-positive breast cancer based on this trial.[37] A newer formulation containing pertuzumab, trastuzumab, and hyaluronidase-zzxf injection for subcutaneous use is approved for the treatment of *HER2*-positive breast cancer in all settings.[38]

The incidence of adverse cardiac drug reactions associated with the addition of trastuzumab increases when an anthracycline is included in the regimen before administration of trastuzumab. The risk of symptomatic heart failure with adjuvant trastuzumab ranges from 0.5% to 4%.[39] The higher risk of cardiac complications may be acceptable in many patients, given the significant reductions in breast cancer recurrence and death. Sequential administration of trastuzumab after chemotherapy produces a lower incidence of cardiac toxicity. Also, the use of a non-anthracycline–based regimen (see Table 151-6) is associated with a low incidence of symptomatic heart failure as compared with other regimens.[14] Concurrent administration of trastuzumab with an anthracycline is controversial because of potentially higher rates of cardiac dysfunction (see the "HER2-Targeted Agents" section under MBC [Stage IV] for more toxicity details) and not generally recommended outside of a clinical trial.

Patients who received concurrent radiation therapy with adjuvant trastuzumab do not experience a significant increase in cardiac events or acute radiation-related adverse drug reactions.[40] Therefore, if radiation therapy is clinically indicated, trastuzumab is typically administered concomitantly with radiation.

Many questions remain regarding the optimal use of trastuzumab in the adjuvant or neoadjuvant therapy of ESBC. The use of trastuzumab with chemotherapy in the adjuvant or neoadjuvant setting is now considered to be the standard of care for patients with node-positive and high-risk node-negative *HER2*-positive breast cancer.[14] The use of *HER2*-targeted therapy in patients with small, *HER2*-positive, node-negative tumors is controversial. A single arm, nonrandomized clinical trial demonstrated an excellent 3-year disease-free survival (98.7%) in patients who received weekly paclitaxel and trastuzumab for 12 weeks, followed by trastuzumab every 3 weeks for a total of 1 year in patients with lymph-node negative, *HER2*-positive, breast cancers smaller than 3 cm.[41] Seven-year follow-up data reported disease-free survival of 93% and an overall survival of 97% which confirms the benefit of this regimen in small, *HER2*-positive, node-negative tumors.[42] The NCCN guidelines recommend consideration of this regimen for patients who have pathologic T1N0M0 *HER2*-positive breast cancer.[14] Neratinib (240 mg by mouth daily for 1 year), an oral tyrosine kinase inhibitor of EGFR, *HER2*, and *HER4*, is indicated for extended adjuvant therapy after completion of trastuzumab (within previous 2 years) based on small improved disease-free survival. The most common adverse drug reactions of neratinib include diarrhea, which requires aggressive management, as well as nausea, fatigue, and vomiting. Neratinib may be an option for extended adjuvant therapy in some patients at higher risk of recurrence.[43]

The use of ado-trastuzumab emtansine (also known as T-DM1) in the adjuvant setting following neoadjuvant therapy when residual disease is found at the time of surgery is the standard of care because it improves invasive disease-free survival at 3 years compared with trastuzumab (88% vs 77%).[14,44] Patients should be counseled on adverse drugs reactions of ado-trastuzumab emtansine that are different than trastuzumab. Ado-trastuzumab emtansine is associated with peripheral neuropathy, thrombocytopenia, and liver dysfunction.

Endocrine Therapy 5 Endocrine therapies that have been studied in the treatment of primary or early-stage breast cancer include tamoxifen, toremifene, oophorectomy, ovarian irradiation, luteinizing hormone–releasing hormone (LHRH) agonists, and AIs. The choice of agent(s) depends on menopausal status of the individual.

If chemotherapy and radiation therapy are not indicated, adjuvant endocrine therapy is generally initiated shortly after surgery or as soon as pathology results are known. When adjuvant chemotherapy is also indicated, endocrine therapy should be administered after chemotherapy is completed.[14] Some clinicians also recommend the initiation of endocrine therapy after completion of radiation therapy, but this recommendation is controversial because few trials have addressed the issue of concurrent versus sequential endocrine therapy and radiation therapy.

Tamoxifen is historically considered as the gold standard adjuvant endocrine therapy and has been used in this setting for several decades. Tamoxifen is antiestrogenic in breast cancer cells, but it has estrogenic properties in other tissues and organs.[45] More recent studies show that tamoxifen, and other similar drugs, have many estrogenic and antiestrogenic effects that depend on the tissue and the gene in question, and they are more appropriately considered SERMs. Women receiving adjuvant tamoxifen therapy have reduced risk of recurrence and mortality compared with women not receiving adjuvant tamoxifen therapy.[45] In the United States, tamoxifen is generally considered the adjuvant endocrine therapy of choice for premenopausal women, although newer data also support the use of LHRH agonists or oophorectomy in combination with AIs.

The pharmacologic disposition of tamoxifen in humans is complex (see Fig. 151-4). Tamoxifen is considered a prodrug. Although the parent compound has significant clinical activity, tamoxifen is metabolized through multiple enzymes, including cytochrome P450 (CYP)3A4, CYP2C19, CYP2D6, and others, to metabolites that are more active than the parent compound.[45] The active metabolites 4-hydroxytamoxifen (4OH-tamoxifen) and 4-hydroxy-*N*-desmethyltamoxifen (endoxifen) have nearly a 100-fold higher affinity for the ER as compared with tamoxifen. Endoxifen is present in the serum at a 6- to 12-fold higher concentration as compared with 4OH-tamoxifen, and is considered to be the most important metabolite for the clinical activity of tamoxifen. Polymorphisms in CYP2D6 can increase or decrease the formation of endoxifen and may improve or diminish clinical outcomes, respectively. Although some studies have reported an association between certain CYP2D6 polymorphisms and poorer disease-free or relapse-free survival in patients receiving tamoxifen, other studies report either no relationship or the opposite effect between clinical outcomes and CYP2D6 polymorphisms. Multiple commercially available CYP2D6 assays are available, but widespread testing for patients receiving tamoxifen is not currently recommended based on available evidence.[14] Potent inhibitors of CYP2D6, such as paroxetine and fluoxetine, may decrease endoxifen levels in patients receiving tamoxifen.[14] The clinical outcomes related to such drug-drug interactions in an individual patient are largely unknown and may depend on their underlying CYP2D6 genetic status (eg, poor metabolizer, extensive metabolizer). Although high-quality evidence on strong CYP2D6 inhibitors and breast cancer outcomes in patients receiving tamoxifen is limited, many experts recommend avoidance of known strong inhibitors of CYP2D6, if possible, in patients receiving tamoxifen.

The duration of tamoxifen therapy in the adjuvant setting is 5 to 10 years. Results of several studies suggest that a longer duration

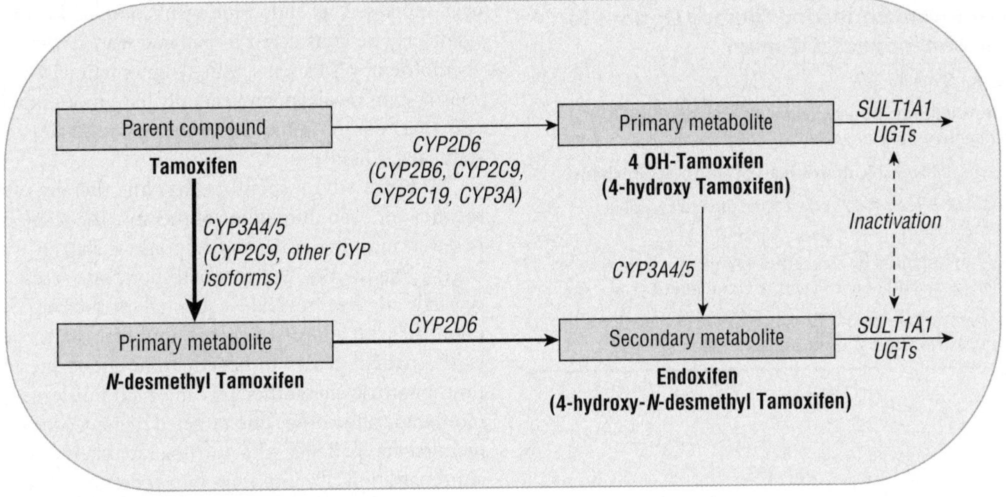

FIGURE 151-4 Tamoxifen metabolism. Widths of the arrows approximate the allocation of parent compound to various metabolites. An equation shows the metabolism of tamoxifen. The parent compound tamoxifen forms primary metabolite 4 OH-tamoxifen or 4-hydroxy tamoxifen in the presence of CYP2D6, CYP2B6, CYP2C9, CYP2C19, and CYP3A, and forms primary metabolite *N*-desmethyl tamoxifen in the presence of CYP3A45 or CYP2C9 and other CYP isoforms. Secondary metabolite endoxifen or 4-hydroxy-*N*-desmethyl tamoxifen is formed from 4 OH-tamoxifen in the presence of CYP3A4 5 and from *N*-desmethyl tamoxifen in the presence of CYP2D6. SULT1A1 and UGTs inactivate 4 OH-tamoxifen and endoxifen.

(eg, 10 years vs 5 years) of tamoxifen may be more effective in some patients. Some studies showed improved disease-free survival (ATLAS trial, aTTom trial) and improved overall survival (ATLAS trial), whereas other trials showed detrimental effects.[14,46] Increased adverse drug reactions occur with 10 years of tamoxifen therapy, including an increased risk of developing endometrial cancer (ATLAS and aTTom trials) and pulmonary embolism (ATLAS trial only) compared with those receiving tamoxifen for 5 years.[14] Based on these data, the administration of tamoxifen for 10 years can be considered in women with a higher risk of breast cancer recurrence.

The most reliable information regarding the adverse drug reactions of tamoxifen comes from the NSABP Breast Cancer Prevention Trial (P-1).[4] This trial randomized women 35 years of age or older who were at increased risk for breast cancer to placebo or to 20 mg/day of tamoxifen for 5 years. Although the primary finding of this study is that tamoxifen reduces the risk of invasive breast cancer by 49%, this study also provides comprehensive data on the risk of adverse drug reactions associated with tamoxifen. The only symptomatic differences noted between the placebo and tamoxifen group were related to hot flashes and vaginal discharge, both of which occurred more often in the tamoxifen group. No important differences between the two groups were observed in the various self-reported instruments (eg, depression scale, a global quality-of-life, and a sexual function scale). Tamoxifen did not increase the risk of ischemic heart disease but did reduce the risk of hip radius and spine fractures. The risks of stroke, pulmonary embolism, and deep vein thrombosis were higher in the tamoxifen group, particularly in women aged 50 years or older. The rate of endometrial cancer was also increased in the tamoxifen group, and this increased risk occurred primarily in women aged 50 years or older. The increased risk of endometrial carcinoma is similar in magnitude to that associated with postmenopausal estrogen replacement therapy and is likely related to an estrogenic effect of tamoxifen on the endometrium. Some experts argue that this risk is acceptable because endometrial cancer induced by tamoxifen is low stage, low grade, easily treated with surgery and does not pose a life-threatening risk to women. Tamoxifen was also associated with an increased risk of uterine sarcomas (a more aggressive form of endometrial cancer), but this risk is lower than the more common endometrial cancers identified in the study. Routine endometrial biopsy is not currently recommended for women receiving tamoxifen therapy. However, women receiving tamoxifen therapy should be counseled to have regular gynecologic examinations and immediately report unusual vaginal bleeding to their primary clinicians for further evaluation.[4]

In premenopausal women, the use of LHRH agonists (ovarian suppression) or ovarian ablation provides benefit in the adjuvant setting. Agents used to suppress ovarian function in this setting include goserelin, triptorelin, and leuprolide. A benefit was observed with goserelin as compared with CMF (cyclophosphamide, methotrexate, fluorouracil) chemotherapy in patients with hormone-sensitive premenopausal breast cancer but not in patients with hormone-receptor–negative tumors.[14] It is not clear whether the benefit of chemotherapy in this population is a result of the antitumor activity of chemotherapy or the endocrine effects of chemotherapy-induced amenorrhea. Consequently, some studies have investigated the benefits of adding ovarian ablation or suppression to chemotherapy either with or without tamoxifen. Results from these studies clearly indicate a benefit from ceasing menses regardless of whether this is caused by chemotherapy or ovarian ablation or suppression.[14] The optimal duration of adjuvant LHRH agonist use is unknown, with trials ranging from 18 months to 5 years of treatment. Two published clinical trials evaluated an LHRH agonist combined with tamoxifen or an AI in premenopausal women. In the Tamoxifen and Exemestane Trial (TEXT), premenopausal patients with hormone receptor–positive ESBC were randomized to receive 5 years of tamoxifen or exemestane, both concomitantly with triptorelin for ovarian suppression. In the Suppression of Ovarian Function Trial (SOFT), premenopausal patients with hormone receptor–positive ESBC were randomized to receive 5 years of tamoxifen alone, tamoxifen with triptorelin, or exemestane with triptorelin. Combined results of the tamoxifen/triptorelin arms and exemestane/triptorelin arms from SOFT and TEXT showed significantly prolonged 5-year disease-free survival with exemestane as compared to tamoxifen.[47] In a subsequent analysis of SOFT, the estimated 5-year disease-free survival

TABLE 151-7 Adjuvant Endocrine Therapy Options for Postmenopausal Women

Aromatase inhibitor for 5 years
Tamoxifen for 2-3 years followed by aromatase inhibitor to complete 5 years of endocrine therapy
Tamoxifen for 2-3 years followed by up to 5 years of aromatase inhibitor
Aromatase inhibitor for 2-3 years followed by tamoxifen to complete 5 years of endocrine therapy
Tamoxifen for 4.5-6 years followed by aromatase inhibitor for 5 years *or* consider tamoxifen for an additional 5 years to complete 10 years
If contraindication to aromatase inhibitors, patients who decline or are intolerant of aromatase inhibitors, tamoxifen for 5 years ≤10 years

Data from Reference 14.

rate was similar with tamoxifen alone versus tamoxifen with ovarian suppression.[48] As expected, patients who received tamoxifen with ovarian suppression experienced more menopausal symptoms such as hot flushes, sweating, and vaginal dryness as compared to patients who received tamoxifen alone. Based on these data, the combination of ovarian suppression and an AI is recommended in premenopausal women with hormone receptor–positive ESBC. Tamoxifen is still considered an option for adjuvant endocrine therapy in certain patients (eg, low-risk of recurrence and/or intolerance to ovarian suppression plus AI).[14]

In postmenopausal women, AIs are the standard of care in the adjuvant setting. Four different approaches to therapy have been undertaken with these agents as outlined in Table 151-7.

Most national and international guidelines currently recommend incorporation of an AI into the adjuvant endocrine therapy regimen for all postmenopausal, hormone-sensitive breast cancers.[14] The NCCN guidelines consider the three available AIs (anastrozole, letrozole, and exemestane) to have similar antitumor efficacy and toxicity profiles. AIs are generally well tolerated. Adverse drug reactions include bone loss or osteoporosis, hot flashes, myalgias or arthralgias, vaginal dryness or atrophy, mild headaches, and diarrhea. Bone modifying agents, which are often coadministered with AIs in the metastatic setting, may also be beneficial in patients treated with AIs in the adjuvant setting (see Chapter 112, "Osteoporosis" for more detail). Other worrisome adverse drug reactions include questionable effects on the cardiovascular system (eg, hypercholesterolemia), cognitive functioning, and joint health.

All patients with ER/PR-positive breast cancer should be offered adjuvant endocrine therapy determined by their menopausal status and risk of recurrence.

Metastatic Breast Cancer (MBC, Stage IV)

Treatment of MBC with cytotoxic, endocrine, or targeted therapy often results in regression of disease and improvements in quality of life. More recent advances have also improved overall survival with the addition of biologic or targeted therapies. The choice of therapy for metastatic disease is based on the presence or absence of certain tumor characteristics. The most important predictive factors are *HER2*, estrogen, and progesterone receptors in the primary or metastatic tumor tissue. Tumors overexpressing *HER2* receptor protein are more likely to benefit from *HER2*-targeted therapy. Regimens that combine *HER2*-targeted therapy with chemotherapy are preferred first-line therapy for these patients.[49] Tumors expressing high levels of ER, PR, or both are more likely to respond to endocrine therapy. The addition of targeted therapies that overcome endocrine resistance are first-line regimens in this patient population. For TNBC, tumors expressing programmed death-ligand (PD-L1) benefit from the addition of immunotherapy to cytotoxic chemotherapy. For cases where hormone receptors and *HER2* receptors are over-expressed, an endocrine agent combined with a *HER2*-targeted agent may be considered in patients who cannot tolerate cytotoxic chemotherapy.[49] Patients with symptomatic visceral or central nervous system involvement generally have more rapidly growing cancers that require initial chemotherapy regardless of tumor marker status (eg, ER/PR).

Patients who respond to first-line therapy often respond to a second- (or even third-) line of therapy. The response rate, however, is lower and the duration of response is shorter with second- (and third-) line therapy. Patients with hormone receptor-positive MBC typically receive several sequential endocrine therapy regimens (alone or with a targeted agent) until their tumors cease to respond or the patient ceases to benefit from endocrine therapy, at which time cytotoxic chemotherapy can be administered. Subsequent chemotherapy after endocrine/targeted therapy combinations is recommended for patients who can tolerate chemotherapy. Concurrent administration of more than one endocrine therapy or combining chemotherapy plus endocrine therapy is generally avoided in the setting of MBC because of increased toxicity and no substantial improvement in overall survival. Women with hormone receptor–negative tumors; or those with rapidly progressive or symptomatic lung, liver, or bone marrow involvement (a visceral crisis); or progressive disease while on initial endocrine therapy (with or without a targeted agent) are treated with cytotoxic chemotherapy.[14] If a patient's disease progresses while on the first-line chemotherapy regimen or if the patient is unable to tolerate the regimen due to toxicities, a subsequent regimen is selected.

All breast cancer patients with bone metastases should be considered for treatment with a bone-modifying agent (eg, pamidronate, zoledronic acid, or denosumab) because these agents decrease the risk of skeletal-related events, such as fractures, spinal cord compression, and pain, and the need for radiation to the bones or surgery.[50] These agents do not act as anticancer agents and should be co-administered with other therapies targeting the cancer cells. The frequency of administration is dependent on the agent selected and could be every month versus every 3 months. See Chapter 150, "Supportive Care in Cancer" for more information.

Desired Outcomes

4 MBC is currently incurable and palliation is the goal of treatment. However, some patients live for many years with metastatic disease, making this a chronic disease requiring long-term management strategies that improve or maintain quality of life. Therefore, sequential single-agent chemotherapy is often chosen over combination chemotherapy regimens, but specific clinical situations may require more rapid responses in which combination chemotherapy may be indicated. Endocrine therapy is generally better tolerated than chemotherapy and may be a more appropriate option for patients with hormone receptor–positive breast cancer. Tumor response to a particular treatment regimen may be measured by changes in laboratory tests, diagnostic imaging, and physical signs and symptoms. The patient usually continues treatment with the regimen, unless the patient cannot tolerate the regimen or the cancer is progressing at a rate that will cause symptoms (or is causing symptoms already). Optimizing quality of life is an important therapeutic end point in the treatment of patients with MBC and eventually requires discontinuation of active cancer therapy and a shift to supportive care with hospice services. Oncology clinicians, in close collaboration with their patients, consider these tradeoffs between quantity and quality of life when making treatment decisions.

Chemotherapy

8 Cytotoxic chemotherapy is eventually required in most patients with MBC. Most patients with MBC have tumors that lack *HER2*-overexpression. Hormone receptor–positive tumors that fail to respond to initial endocrine/targeted therapy regimens or become

refractory to endocrine therapy require chemotherapy. Patients with TNBC require chemotherapy as initial therapy of metastases.

Combination chemotherapy results in an objective response in about 47% to 55% of unselected, chemotherapy-naïve patients.[14] The clinical use of biomarkers and genetic panels to assist treatment decisions is relatively new. In the absence of predictive biomarkers, chemotherapy is chosen based on overall efficacy, the risk of toxicity, performance status and presence of comorbidities in the patient, aggressiveness of disease (eg, indolent vs visceral crisis), and patient preferences related to schedules, dosing route (eg, oral vs intravenous), and frequency (eg, weekly vs every 3 weeks) of the chemotherapy.

While response rates are high with combination chemotherapy, sequential use of single-agent therapies is also an effective strategy that may be preferred due to decreased rates of adverse drug reactions. In the palliative setting, when efficacy is similar, the least toxic approach is preferred. In clinical practice, patients who require a rapid response (eg, those with symptomatic bulky metastases or a visceral crisis) should receive combination chemotherapy despite the added toxicity. This decision is complex and should be made on an individual patient basis.

Most patients experience partial responses to chemotherapy. The median duration of response is highly variable, ranging from 3 to 15 months. Some patients with small volume metastatic disease will have an excellent response to an initial course of chemotherapy and may live 5 to 10 years or longer without evidence of disease. The median overall survival for patients after commonly used chemotherapy combinations ranges between 10 and 33 months. After a chemotherapy regimen has been initiated, it is usually continued until progressive disease or intolerable adverse drug reactions occur.[51] Table 151-8 lists some selected chemotherapy agents used in the metastatic setting.

Factors associated with an increased likelihood of response to chemotherapy include good performance status, a limited number (one to two) of disease sites (or involved organ systems), and prolonged previous response to chemotherapy or hormonal therapy (ie, long disease-free interval). Patients who develop progressive disease during chemotherapy have a lower likelihood of response to subsequent chemotherapy. However, this is not necessarily true for patients who are given chemotherapy after a treatment-free interval of substantial duration (eg, more than 1 year). Contrast to this, TNBC is an aggressive phenotype and is associated with poor prognosis because duration of response to chemotherapy is often short.

Many chemotherapeutic agents have demonstrated activity in the treatment of breast cancer, including doxorubicin (conventional and liposomal), epirubicin, paclitaxel (conventional and albumin-bound), docetaxel, capecitabine, fluorouracil, cyclophosphamide, methotrexate, vinblastine, vinorelbine, gemcitabine, ixabepilone, eribulin, carboplatin, cisplatin, mitomycin, thiotepa, and melphalan. The most active classes of chemotherapy in MBC are the anthracyclines and the taxanes, producing response rates as high as 50% in patients who have not received prior chemotherapy for metastatic disease.[14] Doxorubicin (conventional and liposomal) and epirubicin are generally considered therapeutically equivalent when dosed appropriately. Administration of these agents is limited by their cumulative cardiotoxicity. Paclitaxel, docetaxel, and albumin-bound paclitaxel are also FDA-approved for the treatment of MBC and are generally considered therapeutically equivalent but lack complete cross-resistance. Taxane administration is limited by cumulative peripheral neuropathy. Most patients will likely receive each of these agents at some point in the course of their MBC.

Many patients with MBC have been exposed to adjuvant chemotherapy consisting of an anthracycline and a taxane. If metastases are found within 6 to 12 months of completing treatment with these agents, many clinicians will choose a treatment from a different chemotherapy class. If it has been a long time since their adjuvant therapy, then retreating with the same agents may be considered. However, given the cardiotoxicity associated with the anthracyclines, the use of these agents in the metastatic setting has been generally avoided until the availability of liposomal anthracyclines. Pegylated liposomal doxorubicin is associated with less cardiotoxicity and similar efficacy compared with conventional doxorubicin and is a viable option for women who recur more than 1 year after their adjuvant anthracycline-containing chemotherapy regimen.[51]

Weekly administration of paclitaxel and albumin-bound paclitaxel results in higher response rates, time-to-progression, and survival and a more favorable adverse drug reaction profile compared

TABLE 151-8 Selected Regimens for *HER2*-Negative Metastatic Breast Cancer

Single Agent Chemotherapy	
Paclitaxel[a]	**Vinorelbine[a]**
Paclitaxel 175 mg/m^2 IV Repeat cycle every 21 days *or* Paclitaxel 80 mg/m^2/week IV Repeat dose every 7 days	Vinorelbine 25 mg/m^2/week IV Repeat dose every 7 days
Capecitabine[a]	**Gemcitabine[a]**
Capecitabine 1,000-1,250 mg/m^2 orally twice daily for 14 days Repeat cycle every 21 days	Gemcitabine 800-1,200 mg/m^2/week IV, days 1, 8, and 15 Repeat cycle every 28 days
Eribulin[a]	**Liposomal Doxorubicin[a]**
Eribulin 1.4 mg/m^2 IV, days 1 and 8 Repeat cycle every 21 days	Liposomal doxorubicin 50 mg/m^2 IV Repeat cycle every 28 days
Combination Chemotherapy Regimens	
Gemcitabine + Carboplatin	**Docetaxel + Capecitabine**
Gemcitabine 1,000 mg/m^2 IV, days 1 and 8 Carboplatin AUC 2 IV, days 1 and 8 Repeat cycle every 21 days	Docetaxel 75 mg/m^2 IV, day 1 Capecitabine 950 mg/m^2 orally twice daily for 14 days Repeat cycle every 21 days
Additional Targeted Therapies	
Olaparib[a]	**Talazoparib[a]**
Olaparib tablet 300 mg orally twice daily Repeat cycle every 28 days	Talazoparib tablet 1 mg orally daily Repeat cycles every 28 days
Atezolizumab + albumin bound paclitaxel[a]	**Pembrolizumab + chemotherapy (albumin-bound paclitaxel, paclitaxel, or gemcitabine + carboplatin)[a]**
Atezolizumab 840 mg IV, days 1 and 15 Albumin-bound paclitaxel 100 mg/m^2 IV, days 1, 8, and 15 Repeat cycle every 28 days	Pembrolizumab 200 mg IV, day 1 (given every 21 days) Albumin-bound paclitaxel 100 mg/m^2 IV, days 1, 8, and 15 (given every 28 days) *OR* Paclitaxel 90 mg/m^2 IV, days 1, 8, and 15 (given every 28 days) *OR* Pembrolizumab 200 mg IV, day 1 Gemcitabine 1,000 mg/m^2 IV, days 1 and 8 Carboplatin AUC 2 IV, days 1 and 8 Repeat cycle every 21 days

[a]Designated as a preferred regimen in the NCCN Breast Cancer Guidelines.

Data from Reference 14.

with administration every 3 weeks.[14] With weekly administration, the toxicity profile of paclitaxel changes with less myelosuppression and delayed onset of peripheral neuropathy but slightly more fluid retention and skin and nail changes. Although the risk of hypersensitivity reactions is also slightly less at these lower doses (requiring fewer premedications), it remains at about 3% despite the incorporation of all available preventive measures. The most appropriate weekly dose of albumin-bound paclitaxel in the metastatic setting is not clear. Doses of 100 to 150 mg/m^2/week administered on days 1, 8, and 15 of a 28-day cycle have been investigated, demonstrating some evidence of a dose-response relationship. In the metastatic palliative setting, a lower dose is generally given to minimize toxicity while not significantly compromising efficacy. Docetaxel is most appropriately dosed on an every 3-week schedule for MBC. Weekly dosing did not produce improvements in disease response and was associated with significantly more toxicities than the every 3-week dosing strategy.

After patients have been treated with an anthracycline and a taxane, single-agent capecitabine, vinorelbine, or gemcitabine have resulted in response rates of 20% to 30%.[14] Of these agents, only capecitabine is FDA-approved as a single agent for MBC. Gemcitabine is only FDA-approved in combination with paclitaxel for MBC. However, all of these are included in most national and international guidelines as appropriate therapy for MBC. Decisions regarding which agent to choose are based on patient characteristics, expected toxicities, and previous exposure to chemotherapy.

Other antimicrotubule agents have also been approved for the management of MBC, demonstrating significant benefits in patients who have had prior exposure to other chemotherapy agents. Ixabepilone is an epothilone with a similar but distinct mechanism of action from the taxanes, binding to β-microtubulin in a unique manner but ultimately leading to microtubule stabilization and cell death, similar to the taxanes. It is approved for use in combination with capecitabine and as a single agent. Eribulin is another antimicrotubule agent with a unique mechanism of action. The first synthetic analogue of halochondrin B, eribulin inhibits polymerization of tubulin into microtubules and suppresses the microtubule growth phase, similar to the vinca alkaloids. The mechanism of action for eribulin differs from the vinca alkaloids, in that eribulin does not appear to have any effect on the microtubule shortening phase. These subtle differences may be important for eribulin's efficacy in patients who have been exposed to multiple therapies, including other antimicrotubule agents. It is approved for use as a single agent who have received at least two prior chemotherapies for their MBC.[14] Both of these agents are associated with similar toxicities compared with the taxanes and vinca alkaloids, respectively (eg, myelosuppression, neuropathy, myalgias or arthralgias, alopecia, and skin and nail changes with ixabepilone and myelosuppression and neuropathy with eribulin). Hypersensitivity is occasionally seen with ixabepilone because it is also solubilized in Cremophor-EL, the likely causative agent in paclitaxel-associated hypersensitivity. However, eribulin has not been associated with hypersensitivity reactions and is not formulated in a complex solvent system that may predispose patients to allergic-type reactions. Neuropathy may become problematic in patients who have received numerous sequential neurotoxic chemotherapy agents.

Sacituzumab govitecan-hziy, an antibody-drug conjugate (ADC), is approved for adult patients with metastatic TNBC who received at least two prior therapies for metastatic disease. This ADC is combined with a topoisomerase I inhibitor (SN-38) that allows the antibody to target trophoblast cell surface antigen, or Trop-2, expressing cancer cells and then release the topoisomerase I inhibitor. The most common adverse drug reactions are nausea, diarrhea, and myelosuppression.[52]

Endocrine Therapy

9 Endocrine therapy should be considered in combination with a targeted agent as first-line therapy for patients with hormone-positive MBC, when feasible. The choice of endocrine therapy is based on the menopausal status of the patient, prior therapies and previous response, duration of response, or disease-free interval. Combinations of targeted therapies with endocrine agents may not be appropriate for all patients, and individual decisions should consider other comorbidities, the complexity of the regimen, expected adverse drug reactions, and drug or disease interactions.

The pharmacologic goal of endocrine therapy for breast cancer is to either (a) decrease circulating levels of estrogen or (b) prevent the effects of estrogen on breast cancer cells by blocking the hormone receptors or downregulating the presence of these receptors. The first goal depends on the menopausal status of the patient while the second goal is independent of menopausal status. Combinations of endocrine therapy with different mechanism of action have not demonstrated benefits over single-agent endocrine therapy and are generally not recommended outside the context of a clinical trial.

Several different classes of targeted agents are now approved in combination with endocrine therapy. These combinations address de novo or acquired resistance with endocrine therapy alone and have demonstrated efficacy over single agents in specific patient populations. However, combination therapy is generally associated with increased toxicity compared with single agent endocrine therapy. Optimal subsequent therapy after progression on initial targeted-endocrine treatment is largely unknown and the subject of ongoing clinical trials. However, most patients with hormone-positive MBC will receive several lines of targeted-endocrine combination regimens or endocrine therapy alone sequentially before chemotherapy is considered.

Outside of regimens that include novel targeted agents, little evidence exists that the survival benefit from one endocrine therapy is clearly superior to that achieved with other therapies in women with MBC. Prior to the availability of targeted agents, randomized controlled trials comparing different endocrine therapies (eg, antiestrogens, AIs, progestins, estrogens, androgens) and surgical procedures (eg, oophorectomy, adrenalectomy, and hypophysectomy) showed similar overall survival in patients with MBC. Therefore, the choice of a particular endocrine therapy was based primarily on the mechanism of action, toxicity, and patient preference (see Tables 151-9 and 151-10). Based on these criteria, AIs, tamoxifen or toremifene, and fulvestrant are the preferred initial agents in MBC except when the patient's cancer recurs during or within 1 year of adjuvant therapy with the same class of agent. In these cases, therapies from a different pharmacologic class were indicated.

In postmenopausal women, the main source of estrogen is derived from the peripheral conversion of androstenedione produced by the adrenal gland into estrone and estradiol. This conversion requires the enzyme aromatase. Aromatase also catalyzes the conversion of androgens to estrogens in the ovary in premenopausal women and in extraglandular tissues (eg, the breast and breast cancer cells) in postmenopausal women. Therefore, AIs effectively reduce the levels of estrogens in circulation and in the target organ. Third-generation AIs include anastrozole, letrozole, and exemestane. A major advantage of these specific compounds is their toxicity profile, which consists mainly of bone loss and osteoporosis, mild nausea, hot flashes, arthralgias/myalgias, and mild fatigue. Anastrozole and letrozole are nonsteroidal triazole compounds that reversibly and competitively inhibit aromatase; they have no intrinsic hormonal activity. Exemestane is a steroidal compound that binds irreversibly to aromatase, forming a covalent bond. Although this mechanism may have theoretical advantages to the reversible binding of the nonsteroidal agents, no clinical evidence that this drug is superior to other agents in this class exists. AIs should only be used in postmenopausal women. Pre- or perimenopausal women, whose ovaries are functioning, are not appropriate candidates for these therapies, but the use of AIs in addition to ovarian ablation or suppression (eg, oophorectomy or LHRH agonists) is appropriate and acceptable.

TABLE 151-9 Drug Monitoring for Endocrine Therapies

Drug	Adverse Drug Reaction	Monitoring Parameters	Comments
Aromatase inhibitors	• Hot flashes • Arthralgias or myalgias • Osteoporosis • Hypercholesterolemia	• Patient assessment • BMD • Lipid panel	• Interval of monitoring controversial
Antiestrogens: SERMs[a]	• Hot flashes • Endometrial hyperplasia or cancer • Venous thromboembolism • Osteopenia (premenopausal women only)	• Patient assessment • Annual gynecologic assessment • Consider BMD for premenopausal women	• Routine transvaginal ultrasonography and endometrial biopsies are not recommended in the absence of symptoms
Antiestrogens: SERDs[a]	• Hot flashes • Injection-site reactions	• Patient assessment	
LHRH agonists	• Hot flashes • Injection-site reactions • Osteoporosis	• Patient assessment • BMD	

BMD, bone mineral density.

[a]Liver function tests obtained periodically to screen for changes in hepatic elimination, hepatotoxicity and the presence of hepatic metastases.

TABLE 151-10 Therapies Used for Hormone Receptor–Positive Metastatic Breast Cancer

Drug	Initial Dose	Special Population Dose	Comments
Aromatase Inhibitors: Nonsteroidal			
Anastrozole	1 mg orally daily		
Letrozole	2.5 mg orally daily	Caution in severe liver impairment[a]	
Aromatase Inhibitor: Steroidal			
Exemestane	25 mg orally daily		Take after meals
Antiestrogens: SERMs			
Tamoxifen	20 mg orally daily	See text regarding *CYP2D6*	
Toremifene	60 mg orally daily		
Antiestrogen: SERD			
Fulvestrant	500 mg IM every 28 days (after loading days 1, 15, 29)	Moderate liver impairmenta administer 250 mg IM every 28 days (after loading days 1, 15, 29)	
LHRH Agonists			
Goserelin	3.6 mg SC every 28 days	Premenopausal women only	
Leuprolide	3.75 mg IM every 28 days	Premenopausal women only	Not FDA-approved for breast cancer; other formulations are administered differently
Triptorelin	3.75 mg IM every 28 days	Premenopausal women only	Not FDA-approved for breast cancer
Biologic/Targeted Therapies			
Abemaciclib (+/− Letrozole or Fulvestrant)	Single agent 200 mg orally twice a day continuously **OR** Combination 150 mg orally twice a day continuously	Adjust dose for diarrhea, myelosuppression, and/or severe hepatic impairment. Monitor for hepatotoxicity and thromboembolism. Avoid concomitant strong inhibitors of *CYP3A4* and moderate/strong inducers of *CYP3A4*	Do not split tablets
Palbociclib (+ Letrozole or Fulvestrant)	125 mg orally daily × 21 days, followed by 7 days off, repeated every 28 days	Adjust dose for myelosuppression and severe hepatic impairment. Monitor for nausea, diarrhea, and hepatotoxicity. Avoid concomitant strong inhibitors of *CYP3A4* and moderate/strong inducers of *CYP3A4*	Do not split tablets Take with meals (capsules only)
Ribociclib (+ Letrozole or Fulvestrant)	600 mg orally daily × 21 days, followed by 7 days off, repeated every 28 days	Adjust dose for myelosuppression and/or severe hepatic or renal impairment. Monitor for hepatotoxicity and QT prolongation. Avoid concomitant strong inhibitors of *CYP3A4* and moderate/strong inducers of *CYP3A4*	Do not split tablets
Alpelisib (+ Fulvestrant)	300 mg orally daily	Adjust dose for dermatologic toxicity, hyperglycemia and diarrhea. Monitor for hyperglycemia and dermatologic toxicity. Avoid concomitant strong inducers of *CYP3A4*	Take after meals. Do not split tablets
Everolimus (+ Exemestane or Fulvestrant or Tamoxifen)	10 mg orally daily	Adjust dose in mild, moderate and severe liver impairment; also monitor for myelosuppression, hyperglycemia, dyslipidemia, renal dysfunction. May need to adjust dose with concomitant CYP3A4 inhibitors/inducers	Do not split tablets

IM, intramuscular; SC, subcutaneous.

[a]Severe liver impairment: Child-Pugh class C; moderate liver impairment: Child-Pugh class B; minor liver impairment: Child-Pugh class A.

Antiestrogens bind to ERs, which inhibit receptor-mediated gene transcription and therefore block the effect of estrogen on the end target. This class of agents is subdivided into two pharmacologic categories, SERMs and selective estrogen receptor downregulators (SERDs). SERMs include tamoxifen and toremifene (and raloxifene for breast cancer–risk reduction in high-risk women) and demonstrate tissue-specific activity, both estrogenic and antiestrogenic, as described previously. The agonist activity is thought to be responsible for many of the adverse reactions seen with these agents, including the increased risk of endometrial cancer, and has led to the development of pure ER antagonists that lack estrogen agonist activity. SERDs are also referred to as pure antiestrogens. These molecules bind to ER, inhibit estrogen binding, and degrade the drug–ER complex, thus decreasing the amount of ER expressed. Fulvestrant is currently the only pure antiestrogen currently commercially available in the United States.

The most commonly utilized SERM in the treatment of breast cancer is tamoxifen. The toxicities of tamoxifen are described in the "Endocrine Therapy" section under Curative Breast Cancer. The only additional toxicity that may be observed in the setting of MBC (specifically bone metastases) is a tumor flare or hypercalcemia, which occurs in about 5% of patients after the initiation of any SERM therapy and is not an indication to discontinue the drug. It is generally accepted that this reaction is associated with response to endocrine therapy, but patients who do not experience such a reaction may still respond. This reaction is seen less frequently with the concurrent use of bisphosphonates as a result of their inhibition of osteoclasts, subsequently preventing the release of calcium from the bone.

Toremifene is another commercially available SERM for the treatment of breast cancer. It exhibits similar efficacy and tolerability compared with tamoxifen in the metastatic setting. Cross-resistance to toremifene has been demonstrated in patients with tamoxifen-refractory disease. Details regarding its metabolism are available and indicate it may be an alternative to tamoxifen in settings where there are concerns regarding drug interactions. However, toremifene use in the United States is minimal.[53] Raloxifene, another SERM, was originally approved for the prevention of osteoporosis in postmenopausal women. Available data with raloxifene as a treatment for breast cancer show low response rates and no significant clinical benefit. Consequently, the use of this agent for breast cancer treatment should be discouraged. The clinical benefits of raloxifene for breast cancer risk reduction in high-risk postmenopausal women have been discussed (see the "Prevention and Early Detection" section).

Fulvestrant, an SERD, is approved for the second-line therapy of postmenopausal patients with hormone receptor–positive tumors either alone or in combination with targeted therapy. When combined with ovarian suppression or ablation, fulvestrant is an appropriate therapy in premenopausal women. It is unique, in that it is given as an intramuscular injection. Adverse drug reactions related to fulvestrant include injection-site reactions, hot flashes, asthenia, and headaches.

In premenopausal women, one of the goals of endocrine therapy is to reduce estrogen production which can be accomplished with surgery, radiation, or medication. While radiotherapeutic ablation of the ovaries is effective, this approach is typically not used in the United States because of its morbidity. Medical ovarian suppression with LHRH analogs is increasingly used instead of oophorectomy in premenopausal women. Because the effects of the LHRH analogs are reversible, the administration of these agents may also determine how a patient will tolerate estrogen deprivation. If the patient tolerates this therapy, then an oophorectomy may be recommended as a permanent therapeutic intervention.

The activity of LHRH analogs is related to its ability to downregulate LHRH receptors in the pituitary and decrease luteinizing hormone levels, which subsequently decreases circulating estrogen to suppressed/ablated levels. Therefore, the effect of LHRH analogs on circulating estrogen levels in premenopausal breast cancer is similar to an oophorectomy. The three agents available in the United States are leuprolide, goserelin, and triptorelin, but only goserelin is FDA-approved for the treatment of MBC. These agents are administered as an injection every 4 weeks (all products have extended formulations, lasting 3 months to 1 year, but they are not recommended for the initial treatment of breast cancer) and are associated with minimal adverse drug reactions, including amenorrhea, bone loss or osteoporosis, hot flashes, and occasional nausea (see Table 151-9). LHRH analogs may also produce a flare response because of an initial surge in luteinizing hormone and estrogen production lasting 2 to 4 weeks. This flare response is similar to that seen with tamoxifen, and patients with high-volume, bulky disease should be monitored for increasing pain and hypercalcemia during the initiation period.

Biologic or Targeted Therapy

10 Therapies directed at molecular targets through novel mechanisms are often referred to as targeted therapy. Many of the targeted therapies are also biologic therapies because they are mAbs. For breast cancer, several agents are directed at targets that are differentially expressed in breast cancer cells and play a critical role in their proliferation and survival.

CDK Inhibitors CDK, in coordination with their regulatory cyclin partners, form CDK-cyclin heterodimer complexes that control cell cycling. CDK-4 and -6 are critical components of this process. In some breast cancer cell lines, these complexes are responsible for phosphorylating the retinoblastoma tumor suppressor gene product, or RB, thus inactivating the suppression of cell division and allowing unregulated progression through the cell cycle. Three CDK-inhibitors have an FDA-approved indication for MBC (abemaciclib, palbociclib, and ribociclib). These agents selectively inhibit CDK-4 and -6, effectively preventing retinoblastoma tumor suppressor gene product phosphorylation and leaving it in an active state that is able to appropriately regulate cell division. CDK inhibitors have improved progression-free survival in combination with AIs (as first-line therapy) and fulvestrant (as first- and second-line therapy) (see Table 151-10). A CDK inhibitor-containing regimen should be considered as first-line therapy in newly diagnosed patients with *HER2*-negative, hormone receptor–positive MBC. The addition of the CDK inhibitor to endocrine therapy increases the toxicity of the regimen. Neutropenia (all grades) is the dose-limiting toxicity of palbociclib and ribociclib and is also fairly common with abemaciclib. However, low rates of neutropenic fever and other infections have been reported. The dose-limiting adverse drug reaction with abemaciclib is diarrhea and occurs in nearly all patients. Diarrhea is typically managed with dose reductions and medical interventions, allowing most patients to continue therapy. Ribociclib also has a warning in its labeling for QT prolongation and requires electrocardiogram monitoring for the first two cycles.[54]

Mammalian Target of Rapamycin (mTOR) Inhibitors The phosphatidylinositol 3-kinase (PI3K)/protein kinase-B (also called Akt) pathway includes many different proteins, of which one of the most important is the mTOR tyrosine kinase. mTOR is an important mediator for cell proliferation and regulation of apoptosis, angiogenesis, and cellular metabolism. Everolimus, an oral mTOR inhibitor, improved progression-free survival when given in combination with either exemestane, fulvestrant, or tamoxifen and should be considered in patients with hormone receptor–positive MBC whose disease has progressed within a year of or while receiving endocrine therapy (see Table 151-10). The choice of endocrine therapy depends on what endocrine therapy the patient received previously.

The most common serious (grade 3 or 4) adverse drug reactions reported in the combination everolimus/exemestane trial were stomatitis, anemia, dyspnea, and pneumonitis. Adverse metabolic effects can be seen and monitoring should include fasting glucose, hemoglobin A1C, and lipid panel.

PI3K Inhibitors PI3Ks play a critical role in regulating many biological functions including cell growth, proliferation, and survival.[55] Alpelisib, a PI3K inhibitor, is approved in combination with fulvestrant for postmenopausal women and men, with hormone receptor–positive, *HER2*-negative, PIK3CA-mutated, advanced or metastatic breast cancer as detected by an FDA-approved test following progression on or after an endocrine-based regimen.

Several important toxicities associated with alpelisib require close monitoring and may lead to dose reductions due to intolerability. Hyperglycemia, including ketoacidosis, may occur with alpelisib and patients' fasting glucose should be monitored closely especially upon initiation of this agent. Many patients will require medical intervention with antidiabetic medications. Other adverse drug reactions that may be significant include rash and diarrhea. Antihistamine administration prior to rash onset may decrease rash incidence/severity and should be considering upon initiation of alpelisib.

Poly (ADP-Ribose) Polymerase (PARP) Inhibitors PARP is a family of enzymes partially responsible for repairing single-strand DNA breaks. Patients who harbor a germline mutation in *BRCA1* or *BRCA2* have impaired ability to repair double-strand DNA breaks. TNBC is strongly associated with germline mutations in the *BRCA1* gene.[56] These patients are candidates for therapy with the PARP inhibitors. Olaparib and talazoparib, given as single agents, improve progression-free survival compared with single-agent chemotherapy in patients with *HER2*-negative MBC who had a germline mutation in *BRCA1* or *BRCA2*. Rates of severe adverse drug reactions (grade 3 or higher) are less common with the PARP inhibitors compared with chemotherapy. Commonly reported adverse drug reactions of PARP inhibitors include anemia, nausea, vomiting, diarrhea, and fatigue.[57]

***HER2*-Targeted Agents** *HER2* is an important protein for maintenance of breast cancer cell proliferation and survival. The *HER2*-targeted agents currently available in the United States are trastuzumab, pertuzumab, ado-trastuzumab emtansine, fam-trastuzumab deruxtecan, margetuximab, lapatinib, neratinib, and tucatinib. To date, no benefit has been observed with the administration of trastuzumab to patients with *HER2*-negative tumors (IHC score of 0-1+, or FISH negative) and a questionable benefit has been observed with administration of trastuzumab to women with tumors that are 2+ for *HER2* by IHC staining alone. As mentioned previously, trastuzumab is a mAb targeted against the *HER2*-receptor protein. Pertuzumab is also a mAb but binds to a different epitope on *HER2* and prevents protein dimerization and subsequent cell signaling. Ado-trastuzumab emtansine and fam-trastuzumab deruxtecan are ADC with a trastuzumab backbone linked to cytotoxic chemotherapy. In the case of ado-trastuzumab, the chemotherapy portion is a potent tubulin inhibitor and in fam-trastuzumab deruxtecan, a topoisomerase inhibitor. Lapatinib, neratinib, and tucatinib are small-molecule tyrosine kinase inhibitors targeted against the *HER2* protein, leading to cell signaling blockade and decreased cell proliferation.

First-line therapy with a pertuzumab-trastuzumab-taxane combination is the preferred option for *HER2*-overexpressing MBC in patients who have not received pertuzumab in the neoadjuvant or adjuvant setting. Docetaxel administered every 3 weeks in combination with trastuzumab and pertuzumab (both administered every 3 weeks) has the most evidence to support its use in this setting. Substitution of docetaxel with weekly paclitaxel may be used if patients cannot tolerate docetaxel.[58]

Ado-trastuzumab emtansine is the recommended second-line *HER2*-targeted therapy for MBC after a patient progresses on or can no longer tolerate first-line therapy. Subsequent therapy (third-line) for *HER2*-positive MBC is controversial. Choice of regimen may depend on the presence of brain metastases, organ function, and residual toxicities from previous regimens. Possible options include fam-trastuzumab deruxtecan, tucatinib + trastuzumab + capecitabine, a lapatinib combination regimen, a chemotherapy + trastuzumab combination, margetuximab-cmkb + chemotherapy, or neratinib + capecitabine. For patients with tumors that are hormone receptor-positive, endocrine therapy, either alone or with trastuzumab or lapatinib, is an option.

Brain metastases are common in patients with *HER2*-positive MBC, with over 50% of patients experiencing brain metastases over their lifetime. This statistic is somewhat misleading because the brain is an uncommon site of first recurrence in patients with ESBC (1%-3%); this observation is related to the overall success of *HER2*-targeted therapy at extracranial sites and the ability of the blood-brain barrier to prevent *HER2*-targeted mAb from accessing these tissues, creating a sanctuary site for breast cancer cells. Nonetheless, responses in the brain have been reported with the large, *HER2*-targeted antibodies and are likely due to disruptions in the blood-brain barrier from disease or prior local therapy (surgery or radiation). The small molecule tyrosine kinase inhibitors, particularly tucatinib, have shown efficacy in patients with brain metastases, but local therapies tend to offer the best approach in combination with systemic therapy. Local therapy including surgery, whole-brain radiation, stereotactic radiosurgery, or some combination of these approaches is considered as initial therapy. Systemic therapy is continued if the other metastatic sites are stable. If extracranial metastases are progressing, a change in the *HER2*-targeted therapy according to guidelines is appropriate. If local therapy fails to control disease in the brain, best supportive or palliative care may be indicated, depending on the status of their extracranial sites of disease and their overall performance status.[59]

Adverse drug reactions of *HER2*-targeted therapies are primarily related to the heart. All therapies in this class, regardless of their exact mechanism of receptor blockade, have some degree of cardiotoxicity. Heart failure associated with trastuzumab is somewhat reversible with pharmacologic management, and some patients have continued therapy with trastuzumab after their left ventricular ejection fraction has returned to normal with medical management and/or a pause in therapy. Close monitoring for clinical signs and symptoms of heart failure and routine echocardiography are recommended in order to intervene with appropriate cardiac treatments for all patients on *HER2*-targeted agents. Rare QT prolongation has also been reported with lapatinib, but the clinical significance of this effect is unclear. Concurrent administration of drugs that increase systemic exposure to lapatinib or have similar effects on QT interval may predispose patients to this rare complication and warrant closer monitoring.

Infusion-related reactions (primarily fever and chills) are associated with mAbs and are seen with trastuzumab, pertuzumab, ado-trastuzumab emtansine, fam-trastuzumab deruxtecan, and margetuximab. These reactions can range depending on the agent but may occur in up to 40% of patients receiving trastuzumab.[39] Postmarketing surveillance data have identified pulmonary toxicity and anaphylaxis as rare but potentially life-threatening reactions associated with trastuzumab. Other infusion-related reactions may include mild nausea, pain at tumor sites, rigors, headaches, dizziness, hypotension, rash, and asthenia, which are much less common. If patients experience mild hypersensitivity reactions, they may require the addition of premedications to mitigate this response. If the reaction is more severe, they may be unable to safely receive subsequent doses.

Several *HER2*-targeted therapies, particularly fam-trastuzumab deruxtecan, have been associated with interstitial lung disease. Drug-induced interstitial lung disease includes conditions like pulmonary fibrosis and inflammation that may be life-threatening.[60] Treatment for this toxicity may include corticosteroids and depending on severity may require patient to discontinue therapy with the agent.

Other adverse drug reactions associated with *HER2*-targeted therapies may include rash and diarrhea. Diarrhea is more significant for patients treated with pertuzumab and when *HER2* TKIs are used in combination with chemotherapy (eg, neratinib plus capecitabine). This adverse drug reaction is generally manageable with aggressive antidiarrheal therapy or dose reductions. Other rare effects have been reported (QT prolongation, hepatotoxicity) and patients should be counseled regarding these effects. Drug-drug and drug-food interactions are particularly important with the *HER2* TKIs because of their metabolism through CYP enzymes and other pharmacokinetic and pharmacodynamic issues. Many of the adverse drug reactions listed previously may be exacerbated by drug or food interactions, and careful review of patients' medication lists and education regarding these issues is extremely important.

Immunotherapy

While mAbs against programmed cell death protein 1 (PD-1) and programmed death-ligand (PD-L1) have failed to demonstrate antitumor activity as single agents in MBC, combining these agents with traditional chemotherapy have proven effective in certain patient populations. Most recently, several chemotherapy-immunotherapy combinations have been FDA-approved for treatment of patients with metastatic TNBC whose tumors express PD-L1. Pembrolizumab (mAb against PD-1) is approved in combination with albumin-bound paclitaxel, paclitaxel, or the combination of carboplatin + gemcitabine. Atezolizumab (mAb against PD-L1) is approved in combination with albumin-bound paclitaxel (see Table 151-8). Adverse drug reactions reported with the addition of immune therapies to traditional chemotherapy can be substantial and require close monitoring. Immune-related toxicities may include rash, colitis, hepatitis, hyper/hypothyroidism, and pneumonitis.

Radiation Therapy

Radiation is an important modality in the treatment of symptomatic MBC. The most common indication for treatment with radiation therapy is painful bone metastases or other localized sites of disease refractory to systemic therapy. Radiation therapy provides significant pain relief to about 90% of patients who are treated for painful bone metastases. Radiation is also an important modality in the palliative treatment of metastatic brain lesions and spinal cord lesions, which respond poorly to systemic therapy, as well as eye or orbit lesions and other sites where significant accumulation of tumor cells occurs. Skin and lymph node metastases confined to the chest wall area may also be treated with radiation therapy for palliation (eg, open wounds or painful lesions). Chemotherapy may also be added to radiation for sensitization purposes in certain circumstances.

EVALUATION OF THERAPEUTIC OUTCOMES

The desired therapeutic outcome for ESBC differs significantly from that of MBC. Surgery, radiation, neoadjuvant/adjuvant therapy—chemotherapy, biologic or targeted therapy, and endocrine therapy—is conducted and administered, respectively, with curative intent. Adjuvant therapy is intended to eradicate micrometastases and thus cure the patient of breast cancer. Neoadjuvant therapy is administered to reduce the tumor size prior to surgery and/or to allow breast conserving surgery if the patient desires. In addition, neoadjuvant therapy allows assessment of response or sensitivity to chemotherapy and/or biologic/targeted therapy. In the neoadjuvant setting, local imaging, such as mammogram or ultrasound, is done to assess tumor response to chemotherapy, biologic or targeted therapy, or endocrine therapy. The overall goal of neoadjuvant and adjuvant therapy is to cure the disease, which cannot be fully evaluated for years after initial diagnosis and treatment. Patients are recommended to have a history and physical every 3 to 6 months for the first 3 years after completion of primary therapy, every 6 months for the following 2 years, and then yearly thereafter. Routine laboratory tests or imaging are not recommended unless there is suspicion of recurrence or metastatic disease.[61]

Palliation is the therapeutic outcome in the treatment of MBC. Optimizing benefits and minimizing toxicity are general therapeutic goals of any therapy administered in this setting. Careful consideration of quality of life is important in this setting. Tumor response to a particular treatment regimen may be measured by changes in laboratory tests, diagnostic imaging, or physical signs or symptoms. The patient usually continues treatment with the regimen, unless the patient cannot tolerate the regimen or the cancer is progressing at a rate that will cause symptoms (or is causing symptoms already). Optimizing quality of life is an important therapeutic end point in the treatment of patients with MBC and eventually requires discontinuation of active cancer therapy and a shift to supportive care with hospice services.

ABBREVIATIONS

ACS	American Cancer Society
ADC	antibody-drug conjugate
AI	aromatase inhibitor
ALND	axillary lymph node dissection
ASCO	American Society of Clinical Oncology
BCT	breast-conserving therapy
BMI	body mass index
CDK	cyclin-dependent kinases
CT	computed tomography
CYP	cytochrome P450 enzyme
DCIS	ductal carcinoma in situ
EGFR	epidermal growth factor receptor; also known as HER1
ER	estrogen receptor
ESBC	early-stage breast cancer
FDA	Food and Drug Administration
FISH	fluorescence in situ hybridization
HER2	human epidermal growth factor receptor-2
HRT	hormone replacement therapy
IBC	inflammatory breast cancer
IDC	infiltrating ductal carcinoma
IHC	immunohistochemistry
ILC	infiltrating lobular carcinoma
LCIS	lobular carcinoma in situ
LHRH	luteinizing hormone–releasing hormone
MBC	metastatic breast cancer
mAb	monoclonal antibody
MRI	magnetic resonance imaging
mTOR	mammalian target of rapamycin
NCCN	National Comprehensive Cancer Network
PARP	poly-ADP ribose polymerase
pCR	pathological complete response
PD-1	programmed cell death protein 1
PD-L1	programmed death-ligand 1
PI3K	phosphatidylinositol 3-kinase
PR	progesterone receptor
SERD	selective estrogen receptor downregulator
SERM	selective estrogen receptor modulators
SLNB	sentinel lymph node biopsy
TNBC	triple negative breast cancer
USPSTF	United States Preventive Services Task Force
WHI	Women's Health Initiative

REFERENCES

1. Siegel RL, Miller KD, Fuchs HE, et al. Cancer statistics, 2021. *CA Cancer J Clin.* 2021;71:7–33. doi:10.3322/caac.21654.
2. American Cancer Society. *Breast Cancer Facts and Figures 2019–2020.* Atlanta: American Cancer Society, Inc; 2019.
3. Giordano SH. Breast cancer in men. *N Engl J Med.* 2018;378:2311–2320. 10.1056/NEJMra1707939.
4. NCCN Clinical Practice Guidelines in Oncology (NCCN Guidelines) for Breast Cancer Risk Reduction V1.2021. National Comprehensive Cancer Network, Inc 2021. All rights reserved. Last accessed, June 12, 2021.
5. Del Pup L, Codacci-Pisanelli G, Peccatori F. Breast cancer risk of hormonal contraception: Counselling considering new evidence. *Crit Rev Oncol Hematol.* 2019;137:123–130. doi:10.1016/j.critrevonc.2019.03.001.
6. NCCN Clinical Practice Guidelines in Oncology (NCCN Guidelines) for Genetic/Familial High-Risk Assessment: Breast, Ovarian, and Pancreatic Cancer V2.2021. National Comprehensive Cancer Network, Inc 2021. All rights reserved. Last accessed, June 12, 2021.
7. Visvanathan K, Fabian CJ, Bantug E, et al. Use of endocrine therapy for breast cancer risk reduction: ASCO clinical practice guideline update. *J Clin Oncol.* 2019;37:3152–3165. 10.1200/jco.19.01472.
8. Smith RA, Andrews KS, Brooks D, et al. Cancer screening in the United States, 2019: A review of current American Cancer Society guidelines and current issues in cancer screening. *CA Cancer J Clin.* 2019;69:184–210. doi:10.3322/caac.21557.
9. Siu AL. Screening for Breast Cancer: U.S. Preventive Services Task Force Recommendation Statement. *Ann Intern Med.* 2016;164:279–296. doi:10.7326/m15-2886.
10. NCCN Clinical Practice Guidelines in Oncology (NCCN Guidelines) for Breast Cancer Screening and Diagnosis V1.2021. National Comprehensive Cancer Network, Inc 2021. All rights reserved. Last accessed, June 12, 2021.
11. Breast Cancer Screening (PDQ) Health Professional Version was originally published by the National Cancer Institute. https://www.cancer.gov/types/breast/hp/breast-screening-pdq#cit/section_1.9. Last accessed June 12, 2021.
12. Mammograms was originally published by the National Cancer Institute. https://www.cancer.gov/types/breast/mammograms-fact-sheet. Last accessed June 12, 2021.
13. Claessens AKM, Ibragimova KIE, Geurts SME, et al. The role of chemotherapy in treatment of advanced breast cancer: An overview for clinical practice. *Crit Rev Oncol Hematol.* 2020;153:102988. doi:10.1016/j.critrevonc.2020.102988.
14. NCCN Clinical Practice Guidelines in Oncology (NCCN Guidelines) for Breast Cancer V4.2021. National Comprehensive Cancer Network, Inc 2021. All rights reserved. Last accessed, June 12, 2021.
15. Hwang ES, Solin L. De-escalation of locoregional therapy in low-risk disease for DCIS and early-stage invasive cancer. *J Clin Oncol.* 2020;38:2230–2239. 10.1200/jco.19.02888.
16. Wong SM, King T, Boileau J, et al. Population-based analysis of breast cancer incidence and survival outcomes in women diagnosed with lobular carcinoma in situ. *Ann Surg Oncol.* 2017;24:2509–2517. doi:10.1245/s10434-017-5867-6.
17. Demark-Wahnefried W, Rogers LQ, Alfano CM, et al. Practical clinical interventions for diet, physical activity, and weight control in cancer survivors. *CA Cancer J Clin.* 2015;65:167–189. doi:10.3322/caac.21265.
18. Hortobagyi GN, Connolly JL, D'Orsi CJ, et al. Breast. In: Amin EB, Edge SB, Gress DM, et al., *AJCC Cancer Staging Manual.* 8th Ed. Chicago, IL: Springer. 2017:589–638.
19. Loibl S, Gianni L. HER2-positive breast cancer. *Lancet.* 2017;389:2415–2429. doi:10.1016/S0140-6736(16)32417-5.
20. Lyman GH, Temin S, Edge SB, et al. Sentinel lymph node biopsy for patients with early-stage breast cancer: American Society of Clinical Oncology clinical practice guideline update. *J Clin Oncol.* 2014;32:1365–1383. doi:10.1200/jco.2013.54.1177.
21. Giuliano AE, Ballman KV, McCall L, et al. Effect of axillary dissection vs no axillary dissection on 10-year overall survival among women with invasive breast cancer and sentinel node metastasis: The ACOSOG Z0011 (Alliance) Randomized Clinical Trial. *JAMA.* 2017;318:918–926. doi:10.1001/jama.2017.11470.
22. Korde LA, Somerfield MR, Carey LA, et al. Neoadjuvant chemotherapy, endocrine therapy, and targeted therapy for breast cancer: ASCO Guideline. *J Clin Oncol.* 2021;39:1485–1505. doi:10.1200/jco.20.03399.
23. Adaniel C, Jhaveri K, Heguy A, et al. Genome-based risk prediction for early stage breast cancer. *Oncologist.* 2014;19:1019–1027. doi:10.1634/theoncologist.2014-0124.
24. Sparano JA, Gray RJ, Makower DF, et al. Adjuvant chemotherapy guided by a 21-gene expression assay in breast cancer. *N Engl J Med.* 2018;379:111–121. doi:10.1056/NEJMoa1804710.
25. Goldvaser H, Ribnikar D, Majeed H, et al. Absolute benefit from adjuvant chemotherapy in contemporary clinical trials: A systemic review and meta-analysis. *Cancer Treat Rev.* 2018;71:68–75. doi:10.1016/j.ctrv.2018.10.010.
26. Burstein HJ, Curigliano G, Thürlimann B, et al. Customizing local and systemic therapies for women with early breast cancer: The St. Gallen International Consensus Guidelines for treatment of early breast cancer 2021. *Ann Oncol.* 2021: doi:10.1016/j.annonc.2021.06.023.
27. Cardoso F, Kyriakides S, Ohno S, et al. Early breast cancer: ESMO Clinical Practice Guidelines for diagnosis, treatment and follow-up. *Ann Oncol.* 2019;30:1194–1220. doi:10.1093/annonc/mdz173.
28. Denduluri N, Somerfield MR, Chavez-MacGregor M, et al. Selection of optimal adjuvant chemotherapy and targeted therapy for early breast cancer: ASCO Guideline Update. *J Clin Oncol.* 2021;39:685–693. doi:10.1200/jco.20.02510.
29. Shah AN, Gradishar WJ. Adjuvant anthracyclines in breast cancer: What Is Their Role?. *Oncologist.* 2018;23(10):1153–1161. doi:10.1634/theoncologist.2017-0672.
30. Blum JL, Flynn PJ, Yothers G, et al. Anthracyclines in early breast cancer: The ABC Trials-USOR 06-090, NSABP B-46-I/USOR 07132, and NSABP B-49 (NRG Oncology). *J Clin Oncol.* 2017;35:2647–2655. doi:10.1200/jco.2016.71.4147.
31. Kumar P, Aggarwal R. An overview of triple-negative breast cancer. *Arch Gynecol Obstet.* 2015: doi:10.1007/s00404-015-3859-y.
32. SEER Cancer Stat Facts: Female breast cancer subtypes. https://seer.cancer.gov/statfacts/html/breast-subtypes.html. Last accessed, June 13, 2021.
33. Masuda N, Lee SJ, Ohtani S, et al. Adjuvant capecitabine for breast cancer after preoperative chemotherapy. *N Engl J Med.* 2017;376:2147–2159. doi:10.1056/NEJMoa1612645.
34. Chavez-MacGregor M, Clarke CA, Lichtensztajn DY, et al. Delayed initiation of adjuvant chemotherapy among patients with breast cancer. *JAMA Oncol.* 2016;2(3):322–329. doi:10.1001/jamaoncol.2015.3856.
35. Doxorubicin Hydrochloride. Prescribing information. Pfizer Labs; 2020. Accessed September 4, 2021. http://labeling.pfizer.com/showlabeling.aspx?id=530.
36. Jhaveri K, Esteva FJ. Pertuzumab in the treatment of HER2+ breast cancer. *J Natl Compr Canc Netw.* 2014;12:591–598. doi:10.6004/jnccn.2014.0059.
37. von Minckwitz G, Procter M, de Azambuja E, et al. Adjuvant pertuzumab and trastuzumab in early HER2-positive breast cancer. *N Engl J Med.* 2017;377:122–131. doi:10.1056/NEJMoa1703643.
38. Gao JJ, Osgood CL, Gong Y, et al. FDA approval summary: Pertuzumab, trastuzumab, and hyaluronidase–zzxf injection for subcutaneous use in patients with HER2-positive breast cancer. *Clin Cancer Res.* 2021;27:2126–2129. doi:10.1158/1078-0432.ccr-20-3474.
39. Herceptin (trastuzumab). Prescribing information. Genetech; 2021. Accessed July 1, 2021. https://www.gene.com/download/pdf/herceptin_prescribing.pdf.
40. Mignot F, Ajgal Z, Xu H, et al. Concurrent administration of anti-HER2 therapy and radiotherapy: Systematic review. *Radiother Oncol.* 2017;124(2):190–199. doi:10.1016/j.radonc.2017.07.006.
41. Tolaney SM, Barry WT, Dang CT, et al. Adjuvant paclitaxel and trastuzumab for node-negative, HER2-positive breast cancer. *N Engl J Med.* 2015;372:134–141. doi:10.1056/NEJMoa1406281.
42. Tolaney SM, Guo H, Pernas S, et al. Seven-year follow-up analysis of adjuvant paclitaxel and trastuzumab trial for node-negative, human epidermal growth factor receptor 2-positive breast cancer. *J Clin Oncol.* 2019;37:1868–1875. doi:10.1200/jco.19.00066.
43. Chan A, Delaloge S, Holmes FA, et al. Neratinib after trastuzumab-based adjuvant therapy in patients with HER2-positive breast cancer (ExteNET): A multicentre, randomised, double-blind, placebo-controlled, phase 3 trial. *Lancet Oncol.* 2016;17:367–377. doi:10.1016/S1470-2045(15)00551-3.
44. von Minckwitz G, Huang CS, Mano MS, et al. Trastuzumab emtansine for residual invasive HER2-positive breast cancer. *N Engl J Med.* 2019;380:617–628. doi:10.1056/NEJMoa1814017.
45. Soltamox (tamoxifen). Prescribing information. Midatech Pharma US; 2018. Accessed September 4, 2021. https://www.accessdata.fda.gov/drugsatfda_docs/label/2018/021807s005lbl.pdf.
46. Tremont A, Lu J, Cole JT. Endocrine therapy for early breast cancer: Updated review. *Ochsner J.* 2017;17(4):405–411.
47. Pagani O, Regan MM, Walley BA, et al. Adjuvant exemestane with ovarian suppression in premenopausal breast cancer. *N Engl J Med.* 2014;371:107–118 doi:10.1056/NEJMoa1404037.

48. Francis PA, Regan MM, Fleming GF, et al. Adjuvant ovarian suppression in premenopausal breast cancer. *N Engl J Med.* 2015;372:436–446. doi:10.1056/NEJMoa1412379.
49. Giordano SH, Temin S, Chandarlapaty S, et al. Systemic therapy for patients with advanced human epidermal growth factor receptor 2-positive breast cancer: ASCO Clinical Practice Guideline Update. *J Clin Oncol.* 2018;36:2736–2740. doi:10.1200/JCO.2018.79.2697.
50. Van Poznak C, Somerfield MR, Moy B. Role of bone-modifying agents in metastatic breast cancer: An American Society of Clinical Oncology-Cancer Care Ontario Focused Guideline Update Summary. *J Oncol Pract.* 2017;13:822–824. doi:10.1200/JOP.2017.027672.
51. Partridge AH, Rumble RB, Carey LA, et al. Chemotherapy and targeted therapy for women with human epidermal growth factor receptor 2-negative (or unknown) advanced breast cancer: American Society of Clinical Oncology Clinical Practice Guideline. *J Clin Oncol.* 2014;32:3307–3329. doi:10.1200/JCO.2014.56.7479.
52. Bardia A, Hurvitz SA, Tolaney SM, et al. Sacituzumab govitecan in metastatic triple-negative breast cancer. *N Engl J Med.* 2021;384:1529–1541. doi:10.1056/NEJMoa2028485.
53. Vogel CL, Johnston MA, Capers C, et al. Toremifene for breast cancer: A review of 20 years of data. *Clin Breast Cancer.* 2014;14:1–9. doi:10.1016/j.clbc.2013.10.014.
54. Hecht KA, Selby C. Review of cyclin-dependent kinase 4/6 inhibitors for the treatment of hormone receptor-positive advanced breast cancer. *Ann Pharmacother.* 2018:1060028018793656. doi:10.1177/1060028018793656.
55. Ellis H, Ma CX. PI3K inhibitors in breast cancer therapy. *Curr Oncol Rep.* 2019;21:110. doi:10.1007/s11912-019-0846-7.
56. Tong CWS, Wu M, Cho WCS, et al. Recent advances in the treatment of breast cancer. *Front Oncol.* 2018;8:227. doi:10.3389/fonc.2018.00227.
57. Litton JK, Rugo HS, Ettl J, et al. Talazoparib in patients with advanced breast cancer and a germline BRCA mutation. *N Engl J Med.* 2018;379:753–763. doi:10.1056/NEJMoa1802905.
58. Giordano SH, Temin S, Davidson NE. Systemic therapy for patients with advanced human epidermal growth factor receptor 2-positive breast cancer: ASCO Clinical Practice Guideline Update Summary. *J Oncol Pract.* 2018;14:501–504. doi:10.1200/JOP.18.00290.
59. Ramakrishna N, Temin S, Chandarlapaty S, et al. Recommendations on disease management for patients with advanced human epidermal growth factor receptor 2-positive breast cancer and brain metastases: American Society of Clinical Oncology clinical practice guideline. *J Clin Oncol.* 2014;32:2100–2108. doi:10.1200/JCO.2018.79.2713.
60. Hackshaw MD, Danysh HE, Singh J, et al. Incidence of pneumonitis/interstitial lung disease induced by HER2-targeting therapy for HER2-positive metastatic breast cancer. *Breast Cancer Res Treat.* 2020;183:23–39. doi:10.1007/s10549-020-05754-8.
61. Runowicz CD, Leach CR, Henry NL, et al. American Cancer Society/American Society of Clinical Oncology Breast Cancer Survivorship Care Guideline. *CA Cancer J Clin.* 2016;66:43–73. doi:10.3322/caac.21319.

152

Lung Cancer

Keith A. Hecht and Eve M. Segal

KEY CONCEPTS

1. Lung cancer is the leading cause of cancer deaths in both men and women in the United States. The overall 5-year survival rate for all types of lung cancer is approximately 22%.
2. Cigarette smoking is responsible for most lung cancers. Smoking cessation should be encouraged, particularly in those receiving curative treatment (ie, Stages I to IIIA non-small cell lung cancer [NSCLC] and limited-stage small cell lung cancer [SCLC]).
3. NSCLC is the most commonly diagnosed type of lung cancer (about 80%). NSCLC typically has a slower growth rate and doubling time than SCLC.
4. Annual screening with low-dose computed tomography (LDCT) imaging is recommended to identify lung cancer in high-risk individuals.
5. The treatment goals for lung cancer are cure (early-stage disease), prolonged survival, and maintenance of, or improved quality of life through alleviation of symptoms. Early-stage lung cancer has the highest cure rates, following surgical resection of the tumor with or without chemotherapy for NSCLC and chemoradiotherapy for SCLC.
6. Treatment decisions for NSCLC are guided by the stage of disease, histology (squamous or nonsquamous), targetable mutations such as epidermal growth factor (EGFR) exon 19 deletion or L858R, EGFR exon 20 insertion, Kirsten rat sarcoma viral oncogene homologue (KRAS), anablastyic lymphoma kinase (ALK), B-rapidly accelerated fibrosarcoma (BRAF), neurotrophic receptor kinase (NTRK), rearranged during transfection (RET), mesenchymal epithelial transition factor (MET), and receptor tyrosine kinase (ROS1), and programmed death ligand (PD-L1) expression levels of the tumor. Patient-specific factors (eg, performance status, comorbid conditions) must also be considered when developing a treatment plan.
7. Targeted therapies for advanced-stage NSCLC are preferred over platinum-based doublets or immunotherapy as first-line therapy in patients whose tumors harbor targetable genetic mutations such as EGFR exon 19 deletions or exon 21 (L858R) substitution mutations, EGFR exon 20 insertion mutations, or mutations in ALK, BRAF, NTRK, KRAS, MET, RET, or ROS1.
8. For patients without a targetable mutation, immunotherapy with anti-programmed-death 1 (PD-1) targeting monoclonal antibody is recommended as first-line treatment of metastatic NSCLC that is PD-L1 positive (tumor proportion score [TPS] ≥50%). Immunotherapy can be added to a platinum doublet in patients with tumors that do not have a targetable genetic mutation and/or are PD-L1 negative. Patients with extensive-stage SCLC may receive immunotherapy either with a platinum doublet as first-line therapy or alone as second-line therapy.
9. In the treatment of limited stage SCLC, thoracic radiation is always combined with chemotherapy and the regimen of choice is etoposide and cisplatin. Prophylactic cranial irradiation is added in patient who achieve a completion response.
10. Treatment approach for patients who experience relapsed SCLC include repeating initial chemotherapy regimen (if >6 months since end of therapy) or second-line therapy with topotecan or lurbinectidin.
11. Optimal patient care includes the management of adverse drug reactions from drug therapy. Adverse drug reactions may cause delays in treatment administration, increase morbidity, and contribute to treatment failure.

BEYOND THE BOOK

"View the video "Lung Cancer Screening". Detect Lung Cancer early" (https://www.youtube.com/watch?v=2cZWXC077L8&t=143s) regarding the use of low-dose computed tomography (CT) scans for early detection in patients at an increased risk of lung cancer. What are some consequences of lung cancer screening in patients who are not at high risk for the disease? Consider the process for low-dose CT scan and the characteristics of appropriate candidates for screening. What are some difficulties patients may have while undergoing this exam? The information is useful to enhance understanding regarding the COLLECT and ASSESS steps in the patient care process.

INTRODUCTION AND EPIDEMIOLOGY

1 Lung cancer is a leading cause of morbidity and mortality. It has reached epidemic proportions in many industrialized countries and is the most common cause of cancer-related death in the world. About 236,740 new cases of lung cancer were diagnosed in the United States in 2022.[1] This represents a continued decline in new lung cancer diagnoses that began more than 30 years ago. Despite major advances in the understanding and management of lung cancer, the overall 5-year survival rate for lung cancer remains low at only 22%. In the United States, lung cancer accounts for about 12% of newly diagnosed cancers and is the leading cause of cancer death in adult men and women, with about 130,180 deaths in 2022. The incidence and mortality related to lung cancer are declining, which

has been attributed to decreased tobacco use over the last 50 years as well as the development of new therapies. The incidence of lung cancer increases with age, with 61% of deaths occurring between ages 65 and 85 years.[1] Lung cancer incidence and mortality are higher in Black men and slightly lower in Black women compared to White counterparts.[1] The cure rate is highest with early-stage disease treated with surgical resection; however, most patients present with metastatic disease.[1]

Two leading oncology groups in the United States have published clinical practice guidelines for the treatment of lung cancer. The National Comprehensive Cancer Network (NCCN) has developed consensus-based guidelines that provide recommendations regarding the screening, staging, and treatment of both non-small cell lung cancer (NSCLC) and small cell lung cancer (SCLC).[2,3] The American Society of Clinical Oncology (ASCO) publishes several evidence-based guidelines that are regularly updated regarding the care of patients with lung cancer.[4,5] ASCO also has endorsed the guidelines of other organizations including guidelines on the use of molecular testing for NSCLC[6] and guidelines on the treatment of SCLC.[7]

ETIOLOGY

Lung carcinomas arise from normal bronchial epithelial cells that have acquired multiple genetic lesions and express a variety of phenotypes.[8] Important advances have been made in our understanding of the molecular genetic changes involved in lung cancer pathogenesis.[8] A large variety of molecular lesions result in the abrogation of key cellular regulatory and growth control pathways. Mutations cause activation of proto-oncogenes, inhibition of tumor suppressor genes, and production of autocrine (self-stimulatory) growth factors contributing to cellular proliferation and malignant transformation.[8]

Many of these molecular alterations are common to both SCLC and NSCLC, but certain mutations are found more frequently in specific subtypes of lung cancer and can be potentially treated with targeted interventions. In autocrine loop abnormalities, SCLC frequently overexpresses C-KIT, a protein tyrosine kinase receptor that is specific for stem cell factor. For NSCLC, multiple mutations have been identified that can drive tumor growth and survival. These biomarkers serve as targets of drug therapy. Multiple targetable mutations have been identified in NSCLC including EGFR, ALK, KRAS, BRAF, NTRK, MET, RET, ROS1, and HER2.[8-10]

2 Smoking is a major cause of lung cancer, with about 80% of lung cancer deaths in the United States directly attributed to tobacco use. Tobacco smoke contains many substances, including tumor promoters, carcinogens, and cocarcinogens.[11] The association between environmental tobacco smoke (ETS; also referred to as passive smoking) and lung cancer risk in nonsmokers is clear. Studies show that spouses of smokers have a 25% higher risk of lung cancer than spouses of nonsmokers. In addition, workplace exposure to ETS increases the risk of lung cancer by about 17%. ETS contributes to about 3,000 lung cancers annually. Although these studies are observational, they consistently show a dose-risk relationship, with no safe level of exposure.[11] Smoking cessation is associated with a gradual decrease in the risk, but more than 5 years is necessary before an appreciable decline in risk occurs and the risk never returns to that of a nonsmoker.[11] Because of the public health implications, the United States has several tobacco control efforts, including anti-smoking campaigns, increased tobacco taxes, and smoke-free areas in many public areas. Although the prevalence of cigarette smoking has slowly decreased, it remains at about 14% in 2019.[12]

Although most cases of lung cancer are attributable to cigarette smoking, less than 20% of smokers develop lung cancer, suggesting other risk factors are relevant. An increased risk of lung cancer has been associated with exposure to other environmental respiratory carcinogens (eg, asbestos, benzene, and arsenic). Genetic risk factors are also important, with an increased risk of lung cancer observed in those with first-degree relatives diagnosed with the disease. Lung cancer risk is associated with polymorphisms that affect the expression and/or function of enzymes regulating the metabolism of tobacco carcinogens, DNA repair, or inflammation. Patients with a history of chronic obstructive airway disease and adults with asthma are at an increased risk of lung cancer.[8,10]

HISTOLOGIC CLASSIFICATION

Before treatment begins, it is critical that an experienced lung cancer pathologist reviews the pathologic material to confirm malignancy, characterize the tumor histology, and identify targetable molecular characteristics of the tumor.

3 NSCLC is diagnosed in most (80%) lung cancer patients. NSCLC typically has a slower growth rate and doubling time than SCLC. The histologic classification of NSCLC is well defined and widely accepted (Table 152-1).[13] Histologic types, subtypes, and identifiable variants provide information about the prognosis and can influence therapeutic decisions.[13,14]

Four major cell types of carcinomas (squamous cell, adenocarcinoma, large cell, and small cell) account for more than 90% of lung tumors. Early studies with localized disease demonstrated that radiation could cure SCLC, while surgery could not. Studies with the other histologic types demonstrated better outcomes with surgery

TABLE 152-1 Histologic Classification of Non-Small Cell Lung Carcinomas

1. Squamous cell carcinoma
   - Papillary
   - Clear cell
   - Small cell
   - Basaloid
2. Adenocarcinoma
   - Minimally invasive adenocarcinoma
   - Invasive adenocarcinoma
   - Lepidic predominant (previously classified as bronchioalveolar carcinoma)
   - Acinar predominant
   - Papillary predominant
   - Micropapillary predominant
   - Solid predominant with mucin
   - Variants of invasive adenocarcinoma
   - Invasive mucinous adenocarcinoma (previously classified as bronchioalveolar carcinoma)
   - Colloid
   - Fetal (low and high grade)
   - Enteric
3. Large cell carcinoma
   - Large cell neuroendocrine carcinoma
   - Combined large cell neuroendocrine carcinoma
   - Basaloid carcinoma
   - Lymphoepithelioma-like carcinoma
   - Clear cell carcinoma
   - Large cell carcinoma with rhabdoid phenotype
4. Adenosquamous carcinoma
5. Sarcomatoid carcinomas
   - Pleomorphic carcinoma
   - Spindle cell carcinoma
   - Giant cell carcinoma
   - Carcinosarcoma
   - Pulmonary blastoma
   - Other
6. Carcinoid tumor
   - Typical carcinoid
   - Atypical carcinoid
7. Carcinomas of salivary gland type
   - Mucoepidermoid carcinoma
   - Adenoid cystic carcinoma
   - Epimyoepithelial carcinoma

Adapted from 2004 WHO classification and the 2011 IASCL/ATS/ERS classification.

than with radiation, which provided the basis for the general classification of SCLC and NSCLC. Historically, systemic treatment for NSCLC histologies was the same and resulted in a similar overall prognosis, which supported a general classification of SCLC and NSCLC. Incorporation of genetics in NSCLC and the availability of targeted therapies have led to personalized treatment. Optimal therapy requires knowledge of histology, immunotherapy marker expression, and genetic mutational status.[6,8]

Squamous cell carcinoma, one of the most common histologies of all lung cancers, now represents less than 30% of cases. It has a much higher incidence in males and smokers, with a strong dose-response relationship to tobacco exposure. Studies of the natural history of lung cancer in show a relatively constant tumor volume doubling time (104-122 days).[15] Squamous cell tumors are slower to metastasize with eventual spread to the hilar and mediastinal lymph nodes, liver, adrenal glands, kidneys, bone, and gastrointestinal tract.

Other histologies occurring in NSCLC are collectively referred to as nonsquamous NSCLC. Adenocarcinoma accounts for half of lung cancers and is increasing in frequency. It is the most common histology in nonsmoking patients. The natural history of adenocarcinoma in the lung shows that small tumors discovered through screening are relatively slow growing and tumor doubling time increases as they enlarge. Doubling time of tumors discovered with screening is about 576 days, while those found only with routine patient care grew more rapidly, doubling in size every 169 days.[15] This histology is likely to metastasize from a relatively small tumor (often before diagnosis) and spread widely to distant sites, including the contralateral lung, liver, bone, adrenal glands, kidneys, and CNS. Table 152-1 shows several subclassifications and variants of adenocarcinoma. Large cell carcinomas are infrequently occurring, undifferentiated epithelial tumors, which tend to be large and bulky tumors arising in the periphery of the lung. Large cell carcinomas have a propensity to metastasize in a pattern like adenocarcinomas and are associated with a similar prognosis.[3,10]

SCLCs account for 15% of all lung tumors. They are distinguished by their appearance as small cells with round to oval nuclei. Historically, SCLC was referred to as "oat cell" carcinoma due to its appearance. These tumors occur in major bronchi and the periphery of the lung. SCLC is aggressive and rapidly growing, with 60% to 70% of patients initially presenting with disease outside the hemithorax. SCLC commonly expresses neuroendocrine differentiation, which may account for some of the paraneoplastic syndromes frequently associated with this disease. SCLC secretes gastrin-releasing peptide that acts as an autocrine growth factor. The secretion of other peptide hormones, cytogenetic abnormalities, and amplification and increased expression of oncogenes are also common. SCLC typically metastasizes to the lymph nodes, opposite lung, liver, adrenal glands and other endocrine organs, bone, bone marrow, and CNS.[2,9] Unlike NSCLC, SCLC treatment is not guided by specific biomarkers due to their lack of clinical data demonstrating efficacy with targeted agents. However, genetic studies may be performed should new targeted therapies be developed.

Lung tumors can exhibit more than one cell type (eg, adenosquamous). Mixed histology tumors should also undergo genetic testing.[6,8] Patients can have multiple lung nodules arising in different lobes or the contralateral lung. This is referred to as synchronous tumors, and the nodules can be the same or different cell types. Synchronous tumors worsen overall prognosis.[3]

CLINICAL PRESENTATION

At the time of diagnosis, 16% of lung cancers are localized, 22% have regional spread, and 57% have distant metastases (some patients are not staged). Location and extent of the tumor determine presenting signs and symptoms. A lesion in the central portion of the bronchial tree is more likely to cause symptoms at an earlier stage as compared with a lesion in the periphery of the lung, which may remain asymptomatic until the lesion is large or has spread. The most common initial signs and symptoms include cough, dyspnea, and chest pain or discomfort, with or without hemoptysis.[10] Many patients with lung cancer also have chronic pulmonary and/or cardiovascular diseases (usually related to smoking), and such symptoms may go unnoticed or be attributed to concomitant diseases. Many patients also exhibit systemic symptoms of malignancy such as anorexia, weight loss, and fatigue. Disseminated disease can cause extrapulmonary signs and symptoms such as neurologic deficits resulting from CNS metastases, bone pain or pathological fractures secondary to bone metastases, or liver dysfunction resulting from tumor involvement in the liver.[10]

Paraneoplastic syndromes are signs and symptoms that occur at sites away from the tumor location(s) and are not associated with

CLINICAL PRESENTATION Lung Cancer

Local signs and symptoms

- Cough
- Hemoptysis
- Dyspnea
- Rust-streaked or purulent sputum
- Chest, shoulder, or arm pain
- Wheeze and stridor
- Superior vena cava obstruction
- Pleural effusion or pneumonitis
- Dysphagia (secondary to esophageal compression)
- Hoarseness (secondary to laryngeal nerve paralysis)
- Horner's syndrome
- Phrenic nerve paralysis
- Pericardial effusion/tamponade
- Tracheal obstruction

Extrapulmonary signs and symptoms

- Bone pain and/or pathologic fractures
- Liver dysfunction
- Neurologic deficits
- Spinal cord compression

Paraneoplastic syndromes

- Weight loss
- Cushing's syndrome
- Hypercalcemia (most commonly in squamous cell lung cancer)
- Syndrome of inappropriate secretion of antidiuretic hormone (most commonly in SCLC)
- Pulmonary hypertrophic osteoarthropathy
- Clubbing
- Anemia
- Eaton-Lambert myasthenic syndrome
- Hypercoagulable state

direct tumor involvement. They may be caused by the production of biologically active substances (eg, peptide hormones) or antibodies or by other undefined mechanisms. Paraneoplastic syndromes occur more frequently with lung cancer than with any other tumor, and more frequently with SCLC than with NSCLC. These syndromes may be the first signs of a tumor and may prompt the search for an underlying malignancy.[9]

SCREENING AND PREVENTION

4 Most patients with lung cancer have advanced disease at the time of diagnosis, which contributes to the poor prognosis associated with this disease. Surgery and radiation are the most effective treatment modalities in NSCLC and SCLC, respectively. Only patients diagnosed in early clinical stage can be cured with these treatment modalities alone.[2,3,16,17] The need to diagnose lung cancer earlier provides rationale for screening.

The survival benefits of screening with low-dose computed tomography (LDCT) were first documented in the National Lung Cancer Screening Trial, which enrolled more than 54,000 high-risk smokers. Screening discovered 70% of tumors at stage I or II, when they were potentially curable with surgical resection. The study reported a decrease in overall mortality (7% vs 7.5%) and lung cancer-specific mortality (1.3% vs 1.7%) with LDCT versus control.[18]

The evidence-based recommendation is to offer annual screening with LDCT to high-risk individuals, defined as aged 50 to 80 years with a 20-pack-year history who are still smoking or have quit for less than 15 years.[19] This recommendation comes with a few caveats, including the fact that the most important step is for current smokers to quit. Follow-up trials to the National Lung Cancer Screening Trial validated the earlier onset of screening[20] and the pack year criteria.[21]

Chemoprevention (the use of prophylactic medications to prevent the development of cancer) has failed to show benefit for lung cancer. Many studies of potential chemopreventive agents, including nonsteroidal anti-inflammatory drugs, retinoids, inhaled glucocorticoids, vitamin E, selenium, and green tea extracts, have been conducted, but none have been successful.[22] In summary, the most effective prevention/early intervention approach is to avoid tobacco, maintain a healthy diet with high amounts of fruits and vegetables, and offer screening to high-risk individuals.

DIAGNOSIS

A patient suspected of having lung cancer should undergo a diagnostic evaluation. Diagnosis of lung cancer requires visualization of the cancerous lesion and tissue sampling for pathologic assessment. Patients must have a thorough history and physical examination with emphasis on detecting signs and symptoms of the primary tumor, regional spread, distant metastases, and paraneoplastic syndromes. Performance status should be assessed to determine if a patient is a candidate for aggressive therapy.[2,3,9,10]

Visualization of suspected tumor(s) provides information necessary to choose the most appropriate sampling technique. Computed tomography (CT) scans of the chest and upper abdomen are the most common initial radiologic evaluations. The staging workup can include an endobronchial ultrasound, positron emission tomography (PET) scan, or other tests.[9,10] The use of integrated CT-PET technology has been reported to improve the diagnostic accuracy in the staging of NSCLC over either test alone.[10]

Once located, pathologic examination of tumor tissue is necessary to establish the diagnosis of lung cancer. Tissue is usually obtained through the least invasive method most likely to result in an adequate sample; methods include sputum cytology, tumor biopsy by bronchoscopy, mediastinoscopy, percutaneous needle biopsy, or open lung biopsy. The tissue sample not only confirms malignancy, it is also necessary to determine the specific tumor type and to provide tissue for molecular analysis including testing for PD-L1 and genetic mutations that drive tumor growth.[4,5] Once the diagnosis is established, additional radiologic tests may be required to evaluate lymph nodes and potential metastatic sites for complete staging.[2,3,9,10]

STAGING

Once the diagnosis of lung cancer is confirmed, the extent of disease must be determined to estimate prognosis and guide therapy. For NSCLC, tumor growth and spread are staged with the American Joint Committee on Cancer, tumor, node, and metastasis (TNM) staging system. SCLC is typically staged with the Veterans Administration Lung Cancer Study Group method.[13,23]

Non-Small Cell Lung Cancer

Clinical staging of NSCLC with the TNM system incorporates the size of the tumor, extent of nodal involvement, and presence of metastatic sites.[13] Clinical stages and associated survival rates are described in Table 152-2. For comparison of various therapeutic modalities, a simpler stage grouping system is used in which stage I refers to tumors confined to the lung without lymphatic spread, stage II refers to large tumors with ipsilateral peribronchial or hilar lymph node involvement, stage III includes other lymph node and regional involvement that may or may not involve both lungs, and stage IV includes tumor with distant metastases. Local disease is associated with the highest cure and survival rates, while advanced disease results in 5-year survival of less than 5%. Once evidence of metastatic disease has been identified, further evaluation is not necessary.

Small Cell Lung Cancer

The most commonly used system of staging SCLC was developed originally by the Veterans Administration Lung Cancer Study Group.[23] This system categorizes SCLC into two stages: limited and extensive disease. When evidence of the tumor is confined to a single hemithorax and can be encompassed by a single radiation field, the disease is considered limited. Progression beyond this point is extensive disease. About 60% to 70% of patients initially present with extensive-stage disease. The initial pretreatment evaluation of an SCLC patient should include a medical history, a clinical examination, and laboratory survey, as well as a CT scan of the chest, abdomen, and head. The typical approach is to identify tumor spread that would demonstrate extensive stage, at which time the workup can stop. For patients without extrathoracic disease, a bone scan and bone marrow biopsy should be performed to confirm limited-stage disease.[2,9]

TREATMENT

Desired Outcomes

5 The treatment goals for lung cancer include cure, prolonged survival when cure is not possible, and maintenance of/improved quality of life through symptom alleviation. The ability to achieve these goals depends on tumor histology, extent of disease, and patient characteristics such as age, history, and performance status.[2,3] Stages I and II (NSCLC) or limited-stage (SCLC) diseases are commonly referred to as early-stage disease, while stages III and IV (NSCLC) or extensive-stage (SCLC) diseases are referred to as advanced-stage disease. In patients with early-stage disease who can tolerate aggressive treatment, a definitive cure is the desired outcome of treatment. In patients with advanced-stage disease who can tolerate aggressive therapy, the desired outcome is prolongation of survival.

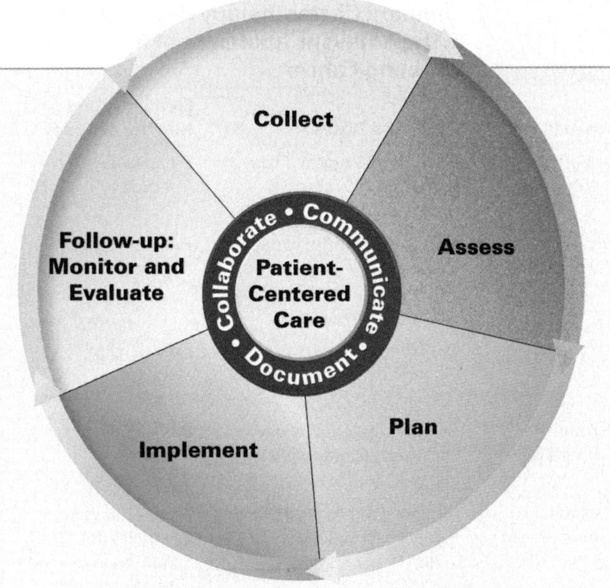

Patient Care Process for Lung Cancer

Collect

- Patient characteristics (eg, age, ancestry)
- Patient history (past medical, family, social—dietary habits, tobacco use)
- Current medications and any prior anticancer therapy
- Symptoms of pain, pain score, pain management
- Clinical and objective evaluation of tumor status
- Objective data
  - BP, HR, height, weight, respiratory rate
  - Labs (eg, serum electrolytes, complete blood count, Scr, BUN)
  - Imaging scans (CT scan, endobrachial ultrasound)
  - Biopsy to obtain histology (Table 152-1) and biomarkers (PD-1, EGFR, ALK, etc.)

Assess

- Type of and response to any prior treatments
- Stage of tumor (Table 152-2)
- Anticancer treatment options based on the cancer's histology, stage, and biomarkers
- Need for any dose adjustments (renal/hepatic function, drug interaction)
- Adverse drug reactions from current anticancer regimen if this is second dose or second cycle
- Barriers to adherence for oral anticancer regimens
- Emotional status (eg, presence of anxiety, depression)

Plan*

- Goals of treatment (curative or palliative)
- Drug therapy regimen including drugs, dose, route, frequency, and duration (Tables 152-3 to 152-7)
- Supportive care plan (eg, antiemetics, premedications, infection prophylaxis, and medications for specific drugs [eg, folic acid and vitamin B_{12} for pemetrexed])
- Patient education (eg, treatment plan and schedule, adverse drug reactions and how to manage them)
- Provide tools to support adherence to anticancer treatments and supportive care medications
- Encourage use of a diary to track pain medication and diarrhea/constipation medications

Implement*

- Provide patient education regarding all elements of the treatment plan
- Use motivational interviewing and coaching strategies to maximize adherence
- Schedule follow-up for assessment of adverse drug reactions and timing of next cycle

Follow-up: Monitor and Evaluate

- Presence of adverse drug reactions
- Measure appropriate laboratory values to determine the presence of serious adverse drug reactions that warrant dose adjustments, delays, or discontinuation at the next cycle
- Assess for signs/symptoms of infection
- Inquire about pain symptoms
- Verify patient adherence to the treatment plan

**Collaborate with patient, caregivers, and other healthcare professionals.*

Regardless of treatment goals, all therapies should improve quality of life. Patients should carefully weigh the potential benefits of treatment against the significant toxicities associated with an aggressive approach. Treatment decisions must include the healthcare team and an informed, well-counseled patient.

Non-Small Cell Lung Cancer

6 If left untreated, patients with advanced NSCLC will die within months.[10] Surgery, radiation, and systemic therapies with cytotoxic chemotherapy, immunotherapy, or targeted therapies are used in the management of NSCLC. The applications of these treatment modalities are determined by stage- and patient-specific factors.[3,10]

Local Disease (Stage I-II)

Local disease is associated with a favorable prognosis and the treatment goal is cure. A multimodal approach involving surgery, radiation, and systemic treatments is utilized for early-stage disease. Surgery is the primary treatment and may be used alone or in combination with radiation and/or systemic therapy.[3] Patients who are not surgical candidates or refuse surgical interventions can be treated with radiation, although cure rates are lower. Stage IA and IB tumors are treated with surgery.[3,24] If surgical margins are positive, re-resection is recommended. Alternatively, patients may receive radiotherapy with or without chemotherapy. Although controversial, patients with IB tumors and high-risk features (eg, poorly differentiated tumors, vascular invasion, large tumors, visceral pleural involvement) may also receive adjuvant chemotherapy.[3,24,25]

The primary treatment of stage IIA and IIB diseases is surgery followed by adjuvant chemotherapy, typically for four cycles. The optimal adjuvant chemotherapy regimen is not clear. Positive clinical trials used platinum-based regimens, with arguably the best clinical

TABLE 152-2 Tumor (T), Node (N), Metastasis (M) Staging for Non-Small Cell Lung Cancer

Primary Tumor (T)		Description
T_1		Tumor ≤3 cm in diameter, surrounded by lung or visceral pleura, without invasion more proximal than lobar bronchus
	T_{1mi}	Minimally invasive adenocarcinoma: adenocarcinoma (≤3 cm in diameter) with a predominately lepidic pattern
	T_{1a}	Tumor ≤1 cm in diameter
	T_{1b}	Tumor >1 cm but ≤2 cm in diameter
	T_{1c}	Tumor >2 cm but ≤3 cm in diameter
T_2		Tumor >3 cm but ≤5 cm, or tumor with any of the following features: - Involves main bronchus, without involvement of the carina - Invades visceral pleura - Associated with atelectasis or obstructive pneumonitis that extends to the hilar region, involving part or all of the lung
	T_{2a}	Tumor >3 cm but ≤4 cm
	T_{2b}	Tumor >4 cm but ≤5 cm
T_3		Tumor >5 cm but ≤7 cm or directly invading the parietal pleura, chest wall, phrenic nerve, parietal pericardium, or with separate tumor nodule(s) in the same lobe as the primary tumor
T_4		Tumor >7 cm or tumor of any size that invades the diaphragm, mediastinum, heart, great vessels, trachea, recurrent laryngeal nerve, esophagus, vertebral body, carina, or with separate tumor nodules in a different ipsilateral lobe
Regional Lymph Nodes (N)		
N_0		No regional lymph node metastases
N_1		Metastasis in ipsilateral peribronchial and/or ipsilateral hilar lymph nodes and intrapulmonary nodes, including involvement by direct extension
N_2		Metastasis in ipsilateral mediastinal and/or subcarinal lymph node(s)
N_3		Metastasis in contralateral mediastinal, contralateral hilar, ipsilateral or contralateral scalene, or supraclavicular lymph node(s)
Distant Metastasis (M)		
M_0		No distant metastasis
M_1		Distant metastasis
	M_{1a}	Separate tumor nodule(s) in a contralateral lobe; tumor with pleural or pericardial nodules, or malignant pleural or pericardial effusion
	M_{1b}	Single extrathoracic metastasis in a single organ (including involvement of a single nonregional node)
	M_{1c}	Multiple extrathoracic metastases

Stage	T	N	M	5-Year Survival (%)
IA1	T_{mi}-T_{1a}	N_0	M_0	92%
IA2	T_{1b}	N_0	M_0	83%
IA3	T_{1c}	N_0	M_0	77%
IB	T_{2a}	N_0	M_0	68%
IIA	T_{2b}	N_0	M_0	60%
IIB	T_{1a}, T_{1b}, T_{1c}, T_{2a}, T_{2b}	N_1	M_0	53% (all IIB)
	T_3	N_0	M_0	
IIIA	T_{1a}, T_{1b}, T_{1c}, T_{2a}, T_{2b}	N_2	M_0	36% (all IIIA)
	T_3	N_1	M_0	
	T_4	N_0, N_1	M_0	
IIIB	T_{1a}, T_{1b}, T_{1c}, T_{2a}, T_{2b}	N_3	M_0	26% (all IIIB)
	T_3, T_4	N_2	M_0	
IIIC	T_3, T_4	N_3	M_0	13%
IVA	Any T	Any N	M_{1a} or M_{1b}	10%
IVB	Any T	Any N	M_{1c}	<1%

TABLE 152-3 Common Chemotherapy Regimens Used in the Adjuvant Treatment of Non-Small Cell Lung Cancer

Regimen	Drugs and Doses	Frequency and Number of Cycles
Cisplatin/etoposide	Cisplatin 100 mg/m² IV day 1 Etoposide 100 mg/m² IV daily on day 1, 2, and 3	Every 28 days for 4 cycles
Cisplatin/vinorelbine	Cisplatin 50 mg/m² IV day 1 and 8 Vinorelbine 25 mg/m² IV day 1, 8, 15, and 22	Every 28 days for 4 cycles
	Cisplatin 100 mg/m² IV day 1 Vinorelbine 30 mg/m² IV day 1, 8, 15, and 22	Every 28 days for 4 cycles
Carboplatin/paclitaxel	Carboplatin AUC 6 IV day 1 Paclitaxel 200 mg/m² IV day 1	Every 21 days for 4 cycles
Cisplatin/pemetrexed	Cisplatin 75 mg/m² IV day 1 Pemetrexed 500 mg/m² IV day 1	Every 21 days for 4 cycles (for nonsquamous histology only)

trial data coming from cisplatin–vinorelbine (Table 152-3).[14] The absolute benefit in 5-year overall survival ranges from no benefit to 15%, with a recent systematic review reporting an absolute difference of 4%. The analysis suggested little effect of the chemotherapy regimen.[14] Although genetics and histology influence systemic treatment and outcomes in advanced disease, this approach has not been tested in large, randomized trials of adjuvant chemotherapy.

The benefits of adjuvant targeted therapy in patients who have undergone a complete resection of their NSCLC has been identified. In patients with stage Ib to IIIa disease whose tumors test positive for sensitizing EGFR mutations, the kinase inhibitor, osimertinib, improved 2-year disease-free survival from 52% to 89% compared to placebo.[26] Benefit was demonstrated in patients regardless of chemotherapy use after surgery. The study was planned for a 3-year duration of treatment; however, it was stopped early due to clinical benefit, leaving the optimal duration of therapy in the adjuvant setting unknown. In patients whose tumors have a PD-L1 expression of at least 1%, 1 year of adjuvant therapy with the PD-L1 inhibitor, atezolizumab, following complete resection and chemotherapy for the treatment of stage II-IIIA NSCLC, resulted in improved disease-free survival at 2 years (74.6% vs 61.0%) and at 3 years (60% vs 48.2%).[27] It is important to note atezolizumab is not approved for use in patients with stage IB disease. Targeted therapies are discussed in further detail in the section of this chapter covering treatment of advanced stage and relapsed NSCLC, information on proper dosing can be found in Tables 152-4, 152-5, and 152-6.

Some patients with early-stage NSCLC receive neoadjuvant therapy, therapy before surgery. Such patients could include those with tumors that are considered operable but may be difficult to resect due to the tumors size, location, involvement of other structures, or extent of lymph node involvement. Typically, these patients would receive the same regimens used in the adjuvant setting, but given before surgery. The addition of immunotherapy to chemotherapy in this setting improves outcomes. In patients with resectable NSCLC with a tumor size greater than 4 cm or having positive lymph node involvement, adding the PD-L1 inhibitor nivolumab to standard chemotherapy every 3 weeks for 3 cycles improves the median event free survival (31.6 vs 20.8 months) and rate of pathologic complete response prior to surgery (24% vs 2.2%).[28] The use of adjuvant targeted therapy in patients received neoadjuvant nivolumab has not been studied.

TABLE 152-4 Selected Regimens for the First-Line Treatment of Advanced-Stage Non-Small Cell Lung Cancer

	Nonsquamous		Squamous	
Place in Therapy	PD-L1 ≥50%	PD-L1 1%-49%	PD-L1 ≥50%	PD-L1 1%-49%
First Line	Pembrolizumab 200 mg IV on day 1 every 21 days or 400 mg IV on day 1 every 42 days Repeat until disease progression or unacceptable toxicity for a maximum of 2 years	Platinum + pemetrexed + pembrolizumab Cisplatin 75 mg/m² or Carboplatin AUC 5 IV on day 1 Pemetrexed 500 mg/m² IV on day 1 Pembrolizumab 200 mg IV on day 1 Repeat cycle every 3 weeks × 4 cycles—Pembrolizumab maintenance up to 31 additional doses or until progression	Pembrolizumab 200 mg IV on day 1 every 21 days or 400 mg IV on day 1 every 42 days Repeat until disease progression, or unacceptable toxicity for a maximum of 2 years	Carboplatin + paclitaxel + pembrolizumab Carboplatin AUC 6 IV on day 1 Paclitaxel 200 mg/m² IV on day 1 or nab-paclitaxel 100 mg/m² IV on day 1, 8, and 15 Pembrolizumab 200 mg IV on day 1 Repeat cycle every 3 weeks × 4 cycles–Pembrolizumab maintenance up to 31 additional doses or until progression
	Atezolizumab 840 mg IV on day 1 repeat every 14 days or 1,200 mg IV on day 1 repeat every 21 days or 1,680 mg IV on day 1 repeat every 28 days Continue until disease progression or unacceptable toxicity	Atezolizumab + carboplatin + paclitaxel + bevacizumab Atezolizumab 1,200 mg IV on day 1 Carboplatin AUC 6 IV on day 1 Paclitaxel 200 mg/m² IV on day 1 Bevacizumab 15 mg/kg IV on day 1 Repeat cycle every 3 weeks × 6 cycles Atezolizumab and bevacizumab maintenance until progression	Carboplatin + taxane + pembrolizumab Carboplatin AUC 6 IV on day 1 Paclitaxel 200 mg/m² IV on day 1or nab-paclitaxel 100 mg/m² IV on day 1, 8, and 15 Pembrolizumab 200 mg IV on day 1 Repeat cycle every 3 weeks × 4 cycles Pembrolizumab maintenance up to 31 additional doses or until progression	Nivolumab + ipilimumab + carboplatin + paclitaxel Nivolumab 360 mg IV on day 1 and 22 Ipilimumab 1 mg/kg IV on day 1 Paclitaxel 200 mg/m² on day 1 and 22 Carboplatin AUC 6 IV on day 1 and 22 Followed by nivolumab and ipilimumab maintenance every 42 days until disease progression or unacceptable toxicity for a maximum of 2 years
	Cemiplimab 350 mg IV on day 1 Repeat every 21 days until disease Continue until disease progression or unacceptable toxicity	Nivolumab + ipilimumab + platinum + pemetrexed Nivolumab 360 mg IV on days 1 and 22 Ipilimumab 1 mg/kg IV on day 1 Pemetrexed 500 mg/m² on days 1 and 22 Carboplatin AUC 6 IV or cisplatin 75 mg/m² on day 1 and 22 Followed by nivolumab and ipilimumab maintenance every 42 days until disease progression or unacceptable toxicity for a maximum of 2 years	Atezolizumab 840 mg IV on day 1 repeat every 14 days or 1,200 mg IV on day 1 repeat every 21 days or 1,680 mg IV on day 1 repeat every 28 days Continue until disease progression or unacceptable toxicity	Nivolumab + ipilimumab Nivolumab 3 mg/kg IV on day 1, 15, and 29 Ipilimumab 1 mg/kg IV on day 1 Repeat every 42 days until disease progression or unacceptable toxicity for a maximum of 2 years
	Platinum + pemetrexed + pembrolizumab Cisplatin 75 mg/m² or carboplatin AUC 5 IV on day 1 Pemetrexed 500 mg/m² IV on day 1 Pembrolizumab 200 mg IV on day 1 Repeat cycle every 3 weeks × 4 cycles Pembrolizumab maintenance up to 31 additional doses or until progression	Nivolumab + ipilimumab Nivolumab 3 mg/kg IV on day 1, 15, and 29 Ipilimumab 1 mg/kg IV on day 1 Repeat every 42 days until disease progression or unacceptable toxicity for a maximum of 2 years	Cemiplimab 350 mg IV on day 1 Repeat every 21 days until disease progression or unacceptable toxicity	Pembrolizumab 200 mg IV on day 1 every 21 days or 400 mg IV on day 1 every 42 days Repeat until disease progression, or unacceptable toxicity for a maximum of 2 years
First-line: Contraindications to PD-1 or PD-L1 Inhibitors	Carboplatin + pemetrexed Carboplatin AUC 5 IV on day 1 Pemetrexed 500 mg/m² IV on day 1 Repeat cycle every 3 weeks × 4 or 6 cycles followed by pemetrexed maintenance		Gemcitabine + cisplatin Gemcitabine 1,000 mg/m² IV on day 1, 8, and 15 Cisplatin 100 mg/m² IV on day 1 Repeat cycle every 28 days	

TABLE 152-5 Selected Regimens for the Second-Line Treatment of Advanced-Stage Non-Small Cell Lung Cancer

Second Line: No previous checkpoint inhibitor	Nivolumab 240 mg IV on day 1 repeat every 14 or 480 mg IV on day 1 repeat every 28 days Continue until disease progression or unacceptable toxicity
	Atezolizumab 840 mg IV on day 1 repeat every 14 days or 1,200 mg IV on day 1 repeat every 21 days or 1,680 mg IV on day 1 repeat every 28 days Continue until disease progression or unacceptable toxicity
	Pembrolizumab 200 mg IV on day 1 every 21 days or 400 mg IV on day 1 every 42 days Repeat until disease progression, or unacceptable toxicity
Second Line: Other recommend	Docetaxel + ramucirumab Docetaxel 75 mg/m^2 IV day 1 Ramucirumab 10 mg/kg IV day 1 Repeat every 21 days

Adjuvant radiation should generally be avoided in patients with local disease who have complete resection and clean margins as it does not improve survival. However, radiation, or more commonly chemoradiotherapy, can be indicated in specific situations. Patients who are medically inoperable should receive chemoradiotherapy if they can tolerate the combined modality. Patients who have positive margins after resection should ideally undergo "re-resection"; if that is not possible, then radiation to the positive margin(s) with or without chemotherapy can be given. Concurrent rather than sequential administration of chemotherapy and radiation therapy is preferred when both are used.[3] Recommended regimens combined with radiation include cisplatin with either gemcitabine or docetaxel for patients with squamous histology or cisplatin combined with pemetrexed in patients with nonsquamous histology. Carboplatin may be substituted in patients who cannot tolerate cisplatin.

Locally Advanced Disease (Stage III)

Patients with more advanced local disease have large tumors, multiple tumors, and/or nodal involvement. This group of patients is heterogeneous, and few large clinical trials are available to guide treatment. Treatment is best planned by a multidisciplinary team where individual features and patient preferences are considered. Optimal outcomes are achieved with multimodality therapy that typically includes systemic chemotherapy. For patients with stage III disease (large tumor [T_3 or T_4] or mediastinal node positive), radiation in the adjuvant or neoadjuvant setting with or without chemotherapy is recommended. Patients with operable disease should be considered for surgery preceded or followed by systemic chemotherapy. Adjuvant chemotherapy after surgery prolongs overall survival in patients with completely resected stage III disease (Table 152-3).[3,14] Two meta-analyses have reported that neoadjuvant chemotherapy improves 5-year survival by 5% compared to surgery alone.[29,30] The stage most likely to benefit, what regimen is best, or how it would compare to surgery followed by adjuvant therapy were not evaluated. The potential benefit of reducing tumor size to make the surgery more feasible is attractive for patients with large tumors. A trial of neoadjuvant versus adjuvant therapy has not been reported; however, both approaches are equivalent and superior to surgery alone.[3] If neoadjuvant chemotherapy is to be utilized in stage III disease, consideration should be given to the inclusion of nivolumab as described earlier.

Radiation may be given in place of surgery as the local treatment modality combined with chemotherapy. Although a large definitive trial has not been performed to compare radiation and surgery in this subset of patients, several small randomized trials have shown no difference in outcomes, such as overall survival, event-free survival and local failure rates.[31,32] Therefore, it is recommended that patients with resectable stage IIIA NSCLC be treated with chemotherapy followed by surgery or radiation, depending on patient and tumor features.[3,24] As with local disease, the use of targeted therapy with atezolizumab or osimertinib with appropriate biomarker expression is recommended for patients with resectable stage IIIa disease.

Patients with stage IIIA disease who are not surgical candidates are typically treated with both a platinum-containing regimen and concurrent radiotherapy. Patients with tumors that cannot fit safely in a radiation field may receive induction chemotherapy followed by chemoradiotherapy. Responding patients may then become surgical candidates.

Stage IIIB and IIIC NSCLC are generally considered unresectable. These patients should receive induction therapy with chemoradiation. Patients who respond to chemoradiation (about 80% of patients) should then receive consolidation therapy with the PD-L1 inhibitor, durvalumab, for 1 year. In a large clinical trial, durvalumab demonstrated significantly sustained benefits over placebo in progression-free survival (16.9 vs 5.6 months) and overall survival (47.5 vs 29.1 months).[33] Durvalumab should not be used if a patient undergoes surgical resection. Patients with stage III disease who are not candidates for radiation are treated like those with stage IV disease.[3-5,24]

Advanced (Stage IV) and Relapsed Disease

About 56% of NSCLC patients have advanced disease (stage IV) at diagnosis.[1,3,10] Typically, these patients are not surgical candidates; however, those who harbor a single metastatic site may undergo resection of the primary tumor and the metastatic site.[4,5] Chemoradiotherapy can be considered for patients with a tumor that fits in a tolerable radiation field. However, for most patients systemic therapy is the primary treatment modality.

The treatment approach for NSCLC that has relapsed after initial treatment of localized disease is like the approach used for patients who have stage IV disease at diagnosis. The goal of initial therapy is to palliate symptoms, improve quality of life, and increase survival. Therapy for advanced-stage NSCLC depends on patient-specific factors and tumor characteristics.

TABLE 152-6 Selected Oral Targeted Therapies for Advanced, Mutation-Driven NSCLC

Drug and Dosing	Adverse Reactions: Common	Adverse Reactions: Rare but Serious	Monitoring Parameters	Comments
EGFR Exon 19 Deletion or *EGFR l858R* Mutation				
Osimertinib 80 mg (1 × 80 mg tablet) once daily	• Anorexia • Dermatologic reactions including dry skin and rash • Diarrhea • Fatigue • Myelosuppression • Paronychia • Stomatitis	• Cardiomyopathy • Interstitial lung disease • Keratitis • QTc interval prolongation	• Signs and symptoms of interstitial lung disease (dyspnea, cough, and fever) • Skin exam • CMP at baseline and periodically • Ophthalmic exam periodically and at the onset of any vision changes • CBC at baseline and periodically • ECG periodically in patients with congenital long QTc syndrome, heart failure, electrolyte abnormalities, or concomitantly receiving other QT prolonging agents • Ejection fraction at baseline and periodically in patients at risk for developing heart failure or if patients develop cardiac symptoms	• Can be taken without regard to meals • Increase dose by 50% if patient taking strong cytochrome P4503A4 inducer • Activity not effected by T790M mutation • Improved CNS activity compared to other EGFR targeting agents • Can be used in patients who have progressed while receiving earlier generation inhibitors (erlotinib, gefitinib, dacomitinib)
Erlotinib 150 mg (1 × 150 mg tablet) once daily	• Anorexia • Cough • Fatigue • Diarrhea • Dyspnea • Nausea and vomiting • Rash	• Cerebrovascular accident • Gastrointestinal perforation • Hemolytic anemia with thrombocytopenia • Hepatotoxicity including hepatorenal syndrome • Interstitial lung disease • Ocular disorders including corneal perforation, ulceration, or severe keratitis • Severe rash, including Stevens-Johnson syndrome and toxic epidermal necrolysis	• Signs and symptoms of interstitial lung disease • Skin exam • CMP at baseline and periodically • Ophthalmic examinations periodically and at the onset of any changes in vision • Signs and symptoms of hemorrhage if patients receiving warfarin	• Should be taken 1 hour before or 2 hours after meals • Best absorbed in acidic gastric environment • Cytochrome P450 3A4 substrate, use with caution with 3A4 inducers/inhibitors • Increased hemorrhage risk with warfarin • Resistance caused by T790M mutation • Has been studied in combination with bevacizumab or ramucirumab
Afatinib 40mg (1 × 40 mg tablet) once daily	• Anorexia • Dermatologic reactions including dry skin and rash • Diarrhea • Nausea and vomiting • Paronychia • Pruritus • Stomatitis	• Hepatotoxicity • Interstitial lung disease • Keratitis • Renal impairment from dehydration due to diarrhea • Severe rash, including Stevens-Johnson syndrome and toxic epidermal necrolysis	• Signs and symptoms of interstitial lung disease • Skin exam • CMP at baseline and periodically • Ophthalmic examinations periodically and at onset of any changes in vision	• Should be taken 1 hour before or 2 hours after meals • Dose reduction recommended for severe renal impairment • Diarrhea can be severe and require dose reductions • Pharmacokinetics may be affected by P-glycoprotein inhibitors and inducers • Resistance caused by T790M mutation • Patients with reduced ejection fraction excluded from clinical trials
ALK Rearrangement				
Alectinib 600 mg (4 × 150 mg capsules) twice daily	• Anemia • Constipation • Edema • Fatigue • Hepatotoxicity • Leukopenia • Myalgia • Photosensitivity	• Bradycardia • Endocarditis • Gastrointestinal perforation • Increased creatine kinase • Interstitial lung disease • Pulmonary embolism • Renal impairment	• Signs and symptoms of interstitial lung disease • CMP at baseline and periodically • CBC with differential monthly • Liver function tests every 2 weeks for the first 3 months of treatment then monthly • Heart rate and blood pressure should be monitored regularly • CPK every 2 weeks for the first month of treatment and with patient reports of unexplained muscle pain, tenderness, or weakness	• Should be taken with meals • Counsel regarding appropriate precautions to protect from UVA/UVB exposure

(*Continued*)

TABLE 152-6 Selected Oral Targeted Therapies for Advanced, Mutation-Driven NSCLC (*Continued*)

Drug and Dosing	Adverse Reactions: Common	Adverse Reactions: Rare but Serious	Monitoring Parameters	Comments
Brigatinib 90 mg (1 × 90 mg tablet) orally once daily for 7 days then increase to 180 mg (1 × 180 mg tablet) daily if tolerated	• Cough • Diarrhea • Fatigue • Hyperglycemia • Increased creatine kinase • Increased serum lipase and amylase • Nausea	• Bradycardia • Hypertension • Interstitial lung disease • Pneumonitis, including pneumonia • Visual disturbances	• Signs and symptoms of interstitial lung disease • Ophthalmic examinations periodically and at the onset of any changes in vision • Blood pressure should be monitored after 2 weeks then monthly • Heart rate and blood pressure should be monitored regularly • CPK levels should be monitored regularly • Fasting serum glucose at baseline and regularly • Lipase and amylase levels monitored regularly	• Can be taken without regard to meals • Dose reduction recommended for severe renal or hepatic impairment • Cytochrome P450 3A4 substrate, should not be used with moderate-to-strong inhibitors or inducers of 3A4
Lorlatinib 100 mg (1 × 100 mg tablet) once daily	• Arthralgia • Diarrhea • Dyslipidemia • Dyspnea • Edema • Fatigue • Peripheral neuropathy • Weight gain	• Atrioventricular block • CNS effects such as mood disorders or seizures • Hepatotoxicity • Hyperglycemia • Hypertension • Interstitial lung disease	• Signs and symptoms of interstitial lung disease • Blood pressure should be monitored after 2 weeks then monthly • Heart rate and blood pressure should be monitored regularly • Fasting serum glucose at baseline and regularly • Serum cholesterol and triglycerides at baseline, 1 month and 2 months after initiation then periodically • ECG at baseline and periodically	• Can be taken without regard to meals • Dose reduction recommended for severe renal impairment • Has demonstrated efficacy after the failure of previous ALK targeted therapies • Patients with severe psychiatric illness excluded from clinical trials
ROS1 Rearrangement				
Crizotinib 250 mg (1 × 250 mg capsule) twice daily	• Anorexia • Constipation • Diarrhea • Dizziness • Edema • Fatigue • Hepatotoxicity • Lymphopenia and neutropenia • Nausea and vomiting • Neuropathy • Upper respiratory infection, including possible pneumonia • Vision disorders	• Bradycardia • Interstitial lung disease • Pulmonary embolism • QTc interval prolongation	• Signs and symptoms of interstitial lung disease • CMP at baseline and periodically • Ophthalmic evaluation in patients with new-onset vision changes • CBC with differential monthly • ECG should be monitored periodically in patients with heart failure, bradyarrhythmias, electrolyte abnormalities, or concomitantly receiving other QT prolonging agents • Heart rate and blood pressure should be monitored regularly	• Can be taken without regard to meals • Dose reduction recommended for severe renal or hepatic impairment • Cytochrome P450 3A4 substrate, should not be used with strong inhibitors or inducers of 3A4 • Fatal hepatotoxicity has occurred • Ocular toxicity can lead to severe vision loss
Entrectinib 600 mg (3 × 200 mg capsules) once daily	• Arthralgia/myalgia • Constipation • Edema • Fatigue • Nausea/vomiting/diarrhea • Vision disorders • Weight gain	• Fractures • Heart failure • Hepatoxicity • Hyperuricemia • Mood disorder • QT prolongation	• Liver function tests every 2 weeks for the first month of therapy then monthly • Uric acid level at baseline and periodically • CMP at baseline and periodically to anticipate risk of QT prolongation • Ejection fraction at baseline and periodically	• Also indicated for *NTRK* mutation positive NSCLC • Can be taken without regard to meals
BRAF V600E Mutation				
Trametinib 2 mg (1 × 2 mg tablet) once daily	• Edema • Fatigue • Fever • Nausea/vomiting/diarrhea • Rash	• Cutaneous or other malignancy • Hemorrhagic events • Cardiomyopathy • Colitis with or without perforation • Hyperglycemia • Interstitial lung disease • Ocular toxicity • Venous thromboembolism	• Signs and symptoms of interstitial lung disease • Fasting serum glucose at baseline and regularly • Dermatologic evaluations at baseline and every 2 months • Ejection fraction at baseline, 1 month after initiation of therapy then every 2-3 months • Ophthalmic evaluation at baseline and within 24 hours of any visual disturbances	• Should be used with dabrafenib • Can be taken without regard to meals • Permanently discontinue if symptomatic cardiomyopathy or decrease in ejection fraction by greater than 20% (0.20)

TABLE 152-6 Selected Oral Targeted Therapies for Advanced, Mutation-Driven NSCLC (*Continued*)

Drug and Dosing	Adverse Reactions: Common	Adverse Reactions: Rare but Serious	Monitoring Parameters	Comments
Dabrafenib 150 mg (2 × 75 mg capsules) twice daily	• Edema • Fatigue • Fever • Nausea/vomiting/ diarrhea • Rash	• Cardiomyopathy • Cutaneous or other malignancy • Hemorrhagic events • Hyperglycemia • Uveitis	• Fasting serum glucose at baseline and regularly • Dermatologic evaluations at baseline and every 2 months • Ejection fraction at baseline, 1 month after initiation of therapy then every 2-3 months	• Should be used with trametinib • Should be taken 1 hour before or 2 hours after meals • Permanently discontinue if symptomatic cardiomyopathy or decrease in ejection fraction by greater than 20% (0.20) • Hemolytic anemia can occur if patient has glucose-6-phosphate dehydrogenase deficiency
MET exon 14 Mutation				
Capmatinib 400 mg (2 × 200 mg tablets) twice daily	• Edema • Decreased appetite • Dyspnea • Fatigue • Nausea/vomiting	• Hepatotoxicity • Interstitial lung disease • Photosensitivity	• Signs and symptoms of interstitial lung disease • Liver function tests at baseline then every 2 weeks for 3 months, then monthly	• Can be taken without regard to meals • Avoid coadministration of strong CYP3A inducers or inhibitors • Patients should be counseled regarding appropriate precautions to protect from ultraviolet light A/B exposure
Tepotinib 450 mg (2 × 225 mg tablets) once daily	• Dyspnea • Edema • Fatigue • Myalgias • Nausea/diarrhea	• Hepatoxicity • Interstitial lung disease	• Signs and symptoms of interstitial lung disease (dyspnea, cough, and fever) • Liver function tests at baseline then every 2 weeks for 3 months, then monthly	• Should be taken with meals
RET Rearrangement				
Selpercatinib 160 mg (2 × 80 mg capsules) twice daily	• Diarrhea • Edema • Fatigue • Hepatotoxicity • Hyperglycemia • Hypertension • Hypocalcemia • Leukopenia • Rash • Thrombocytopenia • Xerostomia	• Hemorrhage • Hypersensitivity • Impaired wound healing QT prolongation • Tumor lysis syndrome	• Liver function tests at baseline then every 2 weeks for 3 months, then monthly • Electrolytes, including calcium, at baseline and periodically • Blood pressure at baseline, 1 week after therapy initiation, then monthly • ECG at baseline and periodically	• Can be taken without regard to meals • Dose reduce to 120 mg if patient is less than 50 kg • Dose reduction recommended for severe hepatic impairment • Patients should watch for signs/symptoms of hypersensitivity • Hold therapy for planned surgical procedures
Pralsetinib 400 mg (4 × 100 mg capsules) once daily	• Constipation • Edema • Fatigue • Hepatotoxicity • Hypertension • Musculoskeletal pain • Myelosuppression	• Hemorrhage • Impaired wound healing • Interstitial lung disease • Tumor lysis syndrome	• Signs and symptoms of interstitial lung disease • Liver function tests at baseline then every 2 weeks for 3 months, then monthly • Blood pressure at baseline, 1 week after therapy initiation, then monthly	• Should be taken 1 hour before or 2 hours after meals • Dosing modifications required if used concomitantly with strong P-glycoprotein inhibitors or strong CYP3A inhibitors or inducers • Hold therapy for planned surgical procedures
NTRK Gene Fusion Positive				
Larotrectinib 100 mg (1 × 100 mg capsule) twice daily	• Constipation or diarrhea • Dizziness • Fatigue • Hepatotoxicity • Hypocalcemia • Musculoskeletal pain • Myelosuppression • Nausea/Vomiting	• CNS effects including cognitive impairment or mood disorders • Fractures	• Liver function tests at baseline then every 2 weeks for 1 month, then monthly	• Can be taken without regard to meals • Dosing modification required if used concomitantly with strong CYP3A4 inhibitors or inducers • Dose reduction recommended for patients with severe hepatic impairment • Inform patients to report signs/symptoms of possible fracture

(*Continued*)

TABLE 152-6 Selected Oral Targeted Therapies for Advanced, Mutation-Driven NSCLC (*Continued*)

Drug and Dosing	Adverse Reactions: Common	Adverse Reactions: Rare but Serious	Monitoring Parameters	Comments
KRAS G12C Mutation				
Sotorasib 960 mg (8 × 120 mg tablets) once daily	• Diarrhea • Fatigue • Hepatotoxicity • Musculoskeletal pain • Nausea	• Interstitial lung disease	• Signs and symptoms of interstitial lung disease • Liver function tests at baseline then every 3 weeks for 3 months, then monthly	• Can be taken without regard to meals • Avoid administration with drugs that decrease gastric acid • Has only been evaluated after progression on other therapies for advanced disease

The most important patient-specific factor is performance status, as described in Chapter 149, "Cancer: The Disease and Treatment." Patients with an Eastern Cooperative Oncology Group (ECOG) performance status of 0 to 2 are most likely to derive benefit from intensive treatment. Patients with significant comorbidities should be considered for less intensive therapy (eg, single-agent therapy). Patients with poor ECOG performance status (3 or 4) do not respond well to chemotherapy and have a high likelihood of toxicity and should receive best supportive care and palliative radiation when necessary.[4,5]

Three pathways have been identified for advanced NSCLC: (1) targetable genetic mutation-driven, which is further divided based on the sensitizing mutation (eg, EGFR, ALK), (2) immune sensitive (PD-L1+), and (3) nonbiomarker-driven therapy treatment, which is further classified as squamous histology or nonsquamous histology due to drug toxicity and efficacy (Fig. 152-1). Unlike tumors of nonsquamous histology, tumors of squamous histology do not usually harbor targetable genetic mutations. Testing for these mutations in squamous tumors is encouraged, but optional. However, like other histologies of NSCLC, squamous histology tumors should have PD-L1 testing to determine sensitivity to first-line immunotherapy.[3,8,10]

PD-L1 expression is tested with an immunohistochemistry assay; as it relates to treatment selection, a tumor is PD-L1+ if 1% or more of the viable tumor cells stain positive for PD-L1 expression (TPS ≥1%). Testing for targetable genetic mutations identifies tumors that harbor sensitizing mutations that respond to targeted therapies. Selected treatments for each group are listed in Table 152-4.

Targetable Genetic Mutation 7 Patients with advanced lung cancer with confirmed positive for targetable genetic driver mutation have several treatment options based on the specific mutation: EGFR, KRAS, ALK, ROS1, $BRAF^{V600E}$, METex14 skipping, NTRK, or RET-fusion. Genetic testing of tumors should be performed at the time of diagnosis in all patients, including those with localized disease.[3,5] Adverse drug reactions and monitoring parameters of select oral targeted therapies used in NSCLC are included in Table 152-6.

Tumors should be tested for mutations in the kinase domain of EGFR (exon 18–exon 24). Deletion mutations in exon 19 and point mutations in exon 21 comprise 90% of EGFR mutations. The only mutation associated with resistance to EGFR inhibitors is an insertion mutation in exon 20, which results in steric hindrance that prevents the drug from binding to the kinase. The prevalence of EGFR mutations varies depending on tumor histology, ethnicity, sex, and smoking history. The highest prevalence occurs in adenocarcinomas, patients of Asian descent, biological females, and nonsmokers. The overall prevalence is 32% of NSCLC patients worldwide.[34]

Patients with a tumor that harbors an activating mutation in the EGFR receptor should receive a first-line EGFR kinase inhibitor.[5] In prospective randomized trials, first-generation EGFR inhibitors (erlotinib and gefitinib) provide superior progression-free survival compared with chemotherapy. Erlotinib has been evaluated in combination with recombinant monoclonal antibodies targeting VEGF. Erlotinib in combination with bevacizumab or ramucirumab has demonstrated improved progression-free survival compared to erlotinib alone. However, this modest improved survival comes with more adverse drug reactions including hypertension and liver toxicities.[35,36] The second-generation inhibitor afatinib has also been shown to be better than chemotherapy as first-line therapy. Meta-analysis comparing EGFR inhibitors (erlotinib, gefitinib, and afatinib) suggests that these three agents have similar overall progression-free survival results (about 11 months) and response rates that are about two times higher than chemotherapy. The meta-analysis also showed that prognosis with exon 19 deletion is better than exon 21 L858R mutation.[37] Dacomitinib, another second-generation irreversible inhibitor, has been compared to gefitinib in this population. In a clinical trial, patients who were randomized to dacomitinib reported improved progression-free survival (14.7 vs 9.2 months) and overall survival (34.1 vs 26.8 months) compared with gefitinib.[38]

Osimertinib, a third-generation EGFR tyrosine kinase inhibitor, shows the most impressive activity in EGFR-positive tumors. The FLAURA trial evaluated patients with EGFR-positive NSCLC to receive first-line osimertinib or prescriber's choice of gefitinib or erlotinib. Patients receiving osimertinib had significantly longer median progression-free survival (18.9 vs 10.2 months) and median overall survival also favored osimertinib (38.6 vs 31.8 months).[39] Two other endpoints in this trial that favored osimertinib were the improved CNS response rate and lower rate of CNS disease defining progression, which is consistent with the improved CNS penetration of osimertinib. This finding is important for NSCLC patients because more than half will develop CNS metastasis during their disease course.[40] Osimertinib is also better tolerated than the first-generation agents, which is consistent with the lower affinity for wild-type EGFR. These characteristics make osimertinib the preferred agent to target EGFR-mutation positive tumors.[3]

Subsequent therapy after progression during treatment with an EGFR inhibitor depends on initial treatment and further genetic evaluation. Many clinicians will repeat tumor genetic testing to identify other targetable mutations before starting new therapy. If patients received initial therapy with a first- or second-generation agent, testing for the acquired T790M mutation should be conducted. If the tumor tests positive for T790M, osimertinib is the drug of choice. If the patient received initial therapy with osimertinib, systemic therapy is recommended.

Patients with exon 20 insertions tend to be resistant to treatment with EGFR kinase inhibitors. New treatment options have

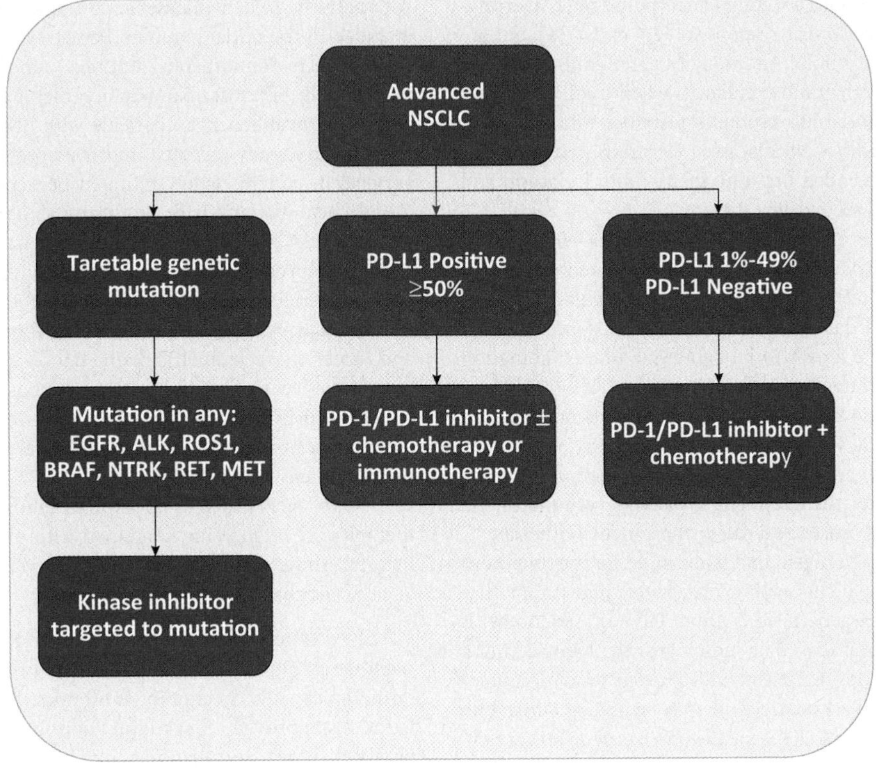

FIGURE 152-1 Algorithm for initial treatment of advanced-stage NSCLC.

emerged for these patients. Amivantamab is a bispecific antibody targeted to EGFR and MET. Overall response rate was 40% with a medium duration of response of 11.1 months in patients who progressed after platinum-based chemotherapy.[41] Mobocertinib is a kinase inhibitor administered orally that irreversibly binds and inhibits EGFR exon 20 insertion mutations at lower concentrations than wild type EGFR. This selective inhibition for mutant EGFR leads to a more favorable adverse drug reaction profile compared to other EGFR inhibitors.[42] It also is effective after platinum-based chemotherapy (overall response rate, 28% median duration of response, 17.5 months).[43]

In summary, patients with advanced NSCLC that harbors an EGFR mutation of exon 19 or L858R should be treated with first-line osimertinib. Upon progression, patients can be retested for an additional targetable mutation/amplification. Most patients will proceed to a platinum doublet with or without immunotherapy. Patients with exon 20 insertions who have progressed on platinum-based chemotherapy should be treated with amivantamab or mobocertinib.

KRAS point mutations are another type of frequently occurring oncogenic mutation, occurring in 25% of patients with adenocarcinomas.[3] This mutation is more commonly associated with cigarette smoking and carriers a poor prognosis.[44] Since the discovery of this therapeutic target, finding an effective treatment for patients with KRAS mutations has been elusive. The KRAS inhibitor, sotorasib, is effective in patients with KRAS G12C mutated advanced NSCLC who were previously treated with standard therapies. Objective response was observed in 37.1% of patients and was durable (median duration of response, 11.1 months).[45]

The presence of an ALK rearrangement represents another therapeutic target for patients with NSCLC. The ALK mutation is less common than EGFR mutations, occurring in 2% to 5% of lung cancer patients.[46] Several ALK inhibitors have been approved for use. First-generation ALK inhibitors crizotinib and ceritinib established ALK inhibition as superior to chemotherapy. Each has shown improvement in median progression-free survival compared to chemotherapy (crizotinib: 10.9 vs 7 months; ceritinib 16.6 vs 8.1 months).[47,48] Second-generation inhibitors alectinib and brigatinib have higher activity than their first-generation counterparts and have demonstrated a dramatic improvement in outcomes compared with crizotinib therapy (median progression-free survival: alectinib, 34.8 vs 10.9 months and brigatinib, 24 vs 11 months).[49,50] The third-generation inhibitor lorlatinib has built on the success of its predecessors with improved potency and improved penetration of the blood-brain barrier. The CROWN trial demonstrated superiority of lorlatinib over crizotinib in a head-to-head comparison (median progression-free survival, not yet reached, [exceeding 33 months] vs 9.3 months).[51] It is important to note that of the second- and third-generation ALK inhibitors, only alectinib has shown improved overall survival compared to crizotinib.[48] Based on this evidence, patients with ALK-positive advanced NSCLC should receive initial treatment with a second (alectinib or brigatinib) or third (lorlatinib)-generation ALK inhibitor.[3]

Patients who relapse while receiving initial ALK-targeted therapy may be treated with an advanced-generation ALK inhibitor. Patients who initially received crizotinib can receive second- or third-generation inhibitors, while patients initially treated with a second-generation inhibitor should be offered lorlatinib. Lorlatinib is able to produce complete responses, even in patients with CNS disease.[52] Patients already receiving lorlatinib who have limited relapse can be treated with local therapy (such as radiation) and continuation of lorlatinib. Patients with widespread relapsed disease should be considered for the nonbiomarker-driven pathway.[3,5]

Mutation in ROS1 is a rare genetic driver of NSCLC occurring in 1% of patients. It has proven to be a highly active target for drug therapy. In patients with metastatic, ROS1-positive NSCLC, regardless of prior chemotherapy for metastatic disease, crizotinib has a

72% response rate, including a 6% complete response rate.[53] Certinib and entrecitinib produce similar responses (62% and 77%), but are better tolerated than crizotinib.[3] Additionally, entrecitinb has better CNS penetration than crizotinib. Similar to when used in patients with ALK mutations, lorlatinib produces response rate was 36%, including in patients with CNS disease.[52] Ceritinib, crizotinib, or entrecitinib are recommended first-line agents, with lorlatinib and entrecitinib as potential second-line therapy.

For the 1% to 2% of patients with metastatic adenocarcinoma who have the BRAF^{V600E} mutation, the combined use of trametinib, a mitogen-activated extracellular signal-regulated kinase, or MEK, inhibitor, and dabrafenib, an inhibitor of some mutated BRAF kinases, has been shown to be beneficial. The combination of trametinib and dabrafenib produces response rate of 63% to 64%, including complete responses in 6% of patients and median progression-free survival times of 9.7 to 10.9 months, in patients with or without prior chemotherapy.[54,55] This combination of kinase inhibitors is approved for the treatment of patients with metastatic BRAF^{V600E}-positive lung cancer, regardless of prior chemotherapy.[3]

Larotrectinib is a novel agent that is approved for the treatment of adult and pediatric patients with a metastatic solid tumor that is positive for an NTRK gene fusion. About 0.2% of patients with NSCLC have this genetic driver of tumor growth. Larotrectinib's approval is based on a study of patients with a variety of solid tumors, including NSCLC.[56] Similarly, entrectinib may be used as a first-line treatment for patients with NTRK gene fusions, based on an accelerated approval of three ongoing phase 1 or 2 clinical trials of patients with advanced or metastatic NTRK fusion-positive solid tumors.[57]

Other less common mutations that occur in NSCLC that have specific targeted agents available include METex14 skipping mutation and RET fusions, both of which occur in about 1% to 2% of all NSCLC patients.[3] Capmatinib is a tyrosine kinase inhibitor that inhibits several MET mutations, including METex14 skipping mutation.[58] Tepotinib can also be used in patients with METex14 skipping mutations.[59] In patients with RET gene rearrangements, selective RET inhibitors, selpercatinib and pralsetinib can be used, resulting in positive response in patients who have progressed on chemotherapy and patients who are treatment naïve.[60,61]

After options targeting genetic mutations have been exhausted, other systemic therapies may be considered with most patients proceeding down the "nonbiomarker-driven" pathway.[3]

Chemotherapy for PD-L1+ and Nonbiomarker Tumors

Cytotoxic chemotherapy with a platinum-based doublet backbone is considered the standard of care for managing NSCLC without targetable genetic mutation. A variety of combinations have been evaluated, but the most used doublets consist of either cisplatin or carboplatin combined with paclitaxel (or nab-paclitaxel) or pemetrexed.[3,4] In general, carboplatin and paclitaxel have less toxicity for patients with squamous cell NSCLC.[62] For patients with nonsquamous NSCLC, a combination of a platinum agent with pemetrexed is widely considered the preferred chemotherapy regimen. This was seen in a pivotal phase III trial of NSCLC patients compared six cycles of cisplatin and either gemcitabine or pemetrexed. When overall survival was analyzed by histology, cisplatin and pemetrexed was superior to other platinum combinations in patients with nonsquamous NSCLC. Furthermore, cisplatin and pemetrexed had less neutropenia, anemia, and thrombocytopenia but more nausea compared to other regimens.[63]

Maintenance therapy is the ongoing use of one or more agents after a positive tumor response to four to six cycles of an initial chemotherapy regimen until disease progression.[3] Several studies show that continuation or switch maintenance therapy improves survival of NSCLC patients with nonsquamous histology.[4] In continuation maintenance therapy, patients receive ongoing treatment with at least one of the agents used in the initial chemotherapy regimen. Alternatively, switch maintenance therapy starts a new agent not included in the initial regimen. Pemetrexed is the most established maintenance chemotherapy option. A meta-analysis showed that pemetrexed, given as maintenance therapy, provided a consistent overall survival benefit in patients with nonsquamous NSCLC.[64] A retrospective study reported improved progression-free and overall survival in patients who continued bevacizumab after completing initial chemotherapy with bevacizumab. A meta-analysis of trials of combined pemetrexed and bevacizumab maintenance therapy showed improved progression-free survival. However, no difference in overall survival was observed and the combination resulted in more toxicity.[65] Because of concerns about efficacy (pemetrexed) and safety (bevacizumab), maintenance with these agents is not recommended for patients with squamous NSCLC. Based on the benefit of maintenance therapy, trials of immunotherapy included maintenance therapy with the monoclonal antibody components of their regimens.

Novel agents such as checkpoint inhibitors and other targeted therapies are often being combined with platinum doublet chemotherapy. These regimens and their survival benefits are described later in this chapter.

PD-L1+ Tumors 8 Patients who have PD-L1+ tumors and no sensitizing mutations are eligible for a variety of first-line immunotherapies with checkpoint inhibitors. Food and Drug Administration approved checkpoint inhibitors for NSCLC include pembrolizumab, atezolizumab, nivolumab, and cemiplimab. These immune checkpoint inhibitors either bind to the PD1 receptor on T cells (pembrolizumab, nivolumab, cemiplimab) or the PD-1 ligand (PD-L1) on tumor cells (atezolizumab, durvalumab). Checkpoint inhibitors are associated with improved overall survival compared to patients receiving cytotoxic chemotherapy.[3] These agents may be used alone, in combination with chemotherapy, or a CTLA-4 inhibitor, ipilimumab. Certain patients may be contraindicated to treatment with checkpoint inhibitors. These include patients with a history of autoimmune diseases, on concomitant treatment with immunosuppressive agents, or those who harbor driver mutations. Presently, recommended treatments are guided by a patient's PD-L1 positivity status or TPS threshold. Patients are divided into three distinct categories: TPS ≥50%, TPS 1%-49%, and TPS <1%.

PD-L1 ≥50% Treatment Recommendations Regardless of histology, single-agent checkpoint inhibitor is recommended as initial treatment in patients with metastatic NSCLC with PD-L1 expression levels of at least 50%, and who are negative for sensitizing oncogenic mutations. This recommendation came from a pivotal phase III trial that showed both improved median progression-free (10.3 vs 6 months) and overall survival (30 vs 14.2 months).[66,67] In addition to pembrolizumab, atezolizumab and cemiplimab have significantly prolonged overall survival and improved tolerability compared to platinum chemotherapy in the first-line setting for patients with metastatic PD-L1+ ≥50% NSCLC tumors.[3,68,69] All three agents are designated as preferred first-line therapies in this setting. The selection of which agent to use is often made by the ordering clinician.

Although patients with NSCLC who are PD-L1 of more than 50% benefit from immunotherapy monotherapy, a variety of other treatment strategies may be utilized to enhance clinical benefit or due to immunotherapy contraindications. Alternatives to immunotherapy monotherapy include chemoimmunotherapy, dual immunotherapy, or chemotherapy alone. These treatment modalities are described in more detail below.

PD-L1 1%-49% Treatment Recommendations Combination therapy that consists of a checkpoint inhibitor and chemotherapy is recommended as the preferred first-line treatment in patients with metastatic NSCLC, regardless of PD-L1 expression levels and histology.

For adenocarcinoma NSCLC, combination therapy with pembrolizumab plus chemotherapy is preferred because it improves overall 1-year survival rates (69.2% vs 49.4%).[70] Different treatment regimens are utilized for patients with a diagnosis of squamous NSCLC. For this histology, a combination of pembrolizumab plus carboplatin and either paclitaxel (or albumin-bound paclitaxel) is preferred as initial treatment regardless of PD-L1 expression levels because it improves overall survival (15.9 vs 11.3 months).[3,71] Refer to Table 152-4 for additional treatment options for patients with squamous NSCLC.

Since the approval of pembrolizumab in combination with chemotherapy, the management of both squamous and nonsquamous NSCLC has substantially changed. At the time of this writing, over seven first-line treatments are now being utilized. Therefore, management has shifted from a defined algorithm of platinum doublet chemotherapy into one where there are multiple competing first-line strategies. The advantages of this paradigm shift are that treatment regimens can be individualized to a patient's treatment goal, preferences, specific factors, and/or performance status. One possible treatment strategy is to use a chemotherapy-free regimen of nivolumab and the cytotoxic T-cell lymphocyte associated protein 4, or CTLA-4, inhibitor, ipilimumab, which improves outcomes compared with chemotherapy alone in patients with metastatic NSCLC with a PD-L1 expression level of 1% or higher.[72] Dual immunotherapy is therefore an option for patients who are contraindicated to chemotherapy (eg, renal impairment.)[3] Another alternative treatment strategy is the concept of limited chemotherapy. The advantage of using a limited-chemotherapy strategy is that effective disease control and improved overall survival can be achieved without suppressing any immunogenicity.[73] This was demonstrated in a landmark phase III double-blind trial who received nivolumab/ipilimumab and two cycles of platinum-doublet chemotherapy followed by nivolumab/ipilimumab maintenance compared to four cycles of chemotherapy alone. Overall survival was improved with chemoimmunotherapy (nivolumab/ipilimumab) and two cycles of platinum-doublet chemotherapy followed by nivolumab/ipilimumab maintenance compared to four cycles of chemotherapy alone (15.8 months vs 11 months, respectively).[74] This treatment strategy may be ideal for a patient who requires a limited-chemotherapy option or is contraindicated to receiving ongoing chemotherapy maintenance.

Furthermore, single-agent immunotherapy with pembrolizumab may also be used. This recommendation was based from a randomized phase III trial comparing first-line pembrolizumab to chemotherapy in patients with NSCLC with a PD-L1 expression of 1% or more (TPS of ≥1%).[75] Patients with the highest level of PDL-1 expression (TPS ≥50%) had a median overall survival of 20 months versus 12 months in the chemotherapy arm, respectively. The survival benefit decreased as PD-L1 expression decreased, but survival was higher for the pembrolizumab in all groups. In certain circumstances, such as poor ECOG performance status or those who cannot tolerate or refuse platinum-based chemotherapy, single-agent checkpoint inhibitors may be used in patients who have expression levels of 1%-49%. Other first-line treatment strategies may be utilized and can be seen in Table 152-4.

Nonbiomarker Driven Approximately, half of the NSCLC patient population have PD-L1 TPS scores <1% or are PD-L1 negative.[76,77] Due to the lack of randomized clinical trials for this patient population, there are no defined or optimal treatment strategies that have been identified now. Therefore, patients who are PD-L1 <1%, a performance status of 0-2, and negative for actionable oncogenes are treated similarly to patients with TPS scores of 1% to 49% with pembrolizumab in combination with chemotherapy being the preferred initial treatment.[3]

For patients with metastatic NSCLC who are not candidates for targeted therapies or have progressed despite targeted therapies and are candidates for further therapy, combination chemotherapy in the form of a platinum doublet is the preferred treatment option. Targeted therapies have also been incorporated to various platinum doublet regimens. The benefit of adding the VEGF inhibitor, bevacizumab to a platinum doublet chemotherapy regimen leads to longer median progression-free survival (6.2 vs 4.5 months) and overall survival times (12.3 vs 10.3).[78] Therefore, the addition of bevacizumab to chemotherapy is recommended for patients with advanced NSCLC. However, due to the bleeding risk associated with bevacizumab, eligible patients must have nonsquamous histology, no recent hemoptysis, no CNS metastasis, and are not receiving therapeutic anticoagulation.[3] Cisplatin and pemetrexed have not been directly compared with carboplatin, paclitaxel, and bevacizumab and both regimens are listed as treatment options in nonsquamous NSCLC.

The most recent treatment advancement is using chemoimmunotherapy which was described earlier in this chapter. However, for patients with driver mutations, the use of chemoimmunotherapy is controversial. Patients with driver mutations like EGFR and ALK do not have the same responsiveness to immunotherapy compared to patients without driver mutations.[79] Furthermore, second-line trials have also demonstrated that these subsets of patients do not derive an overall survival benefit with checkpoint blockade.[80,81] When checkpoint inhibitors are combined with anti-angiogenic agents (eg, VEGF inhibitors), it is possible to overcome the tumor resistance seen in EGFR and ALK positive tumors. This may be due to VEGF inhibitors augmenting chemoimmunotherapy by suppressing antigen presentation and potentiating PD-L1 blockade.[81] This mechanism of action hypothesis was confirmed in the IMpower150 study which evaluated the addition of atezolizumab to treatment with carboplatin, pemetrexed, and bevacizumab (ABCP) in patients with nonsquamous NSCLC.[82] ABCP resulted in significantly longer median progression-free survival for all patients (8.3 vs 6.8 months) as well as those with EGFR or ALK mutations (9.7 vs 6.1 months). ABCP remains the first chemoimmunotherapy regimen to show a benefit in patients with driver mutations. Clinical guidelines recommend the combination of checkpoint inhibitors with a VEGF inhibitor, and chemotherapy as first-line therapy for patients with nonbiomarker-driven NSCLC.[3]

Relapsed Disease Inevitably, patients with metastatic NSCLC will experience disease progression. For patients without driver mutations or patients who have exhausted available targeted therapies, systemic chemotherapy or immunotherapy remain the treatment of choice.

Monotherapy with nivolumab, pembrolizumab, atezolizumab, docetaxel, or pemetrexed are the most commonly considered options for second-line therapy in patients with a good performance status who progress during or after first-line chemotherapy.[3-5] Nivolumab and pembrolizumab, and atezolizumab, are options in the second-line setting for patients who have not previously received immunotherapy. A meta-analysis of randomized trials of PD-1 inhibitors found that these agents significantly improved survival outcomes as compared to single-agent chemotherapy.[83] This benefit was seen regardless of histology. Clinical benefit from PD-1 inhibitors is superior compared to docetaxel regardless of the level of PD-1 expression. However, patients with higher levels of PD-1 expression received an even greater benefit than those patients with low-level expression.

For patients who have failed initial treatment with immunotherapy, second-line treatment would be chemotherapy. Docetaxel was the first chemotherapy to receive Food and Drug Administration approval for the treatment of advanced NSCLC after failure of a platinum-based chemotherapy regimen. Docetaxel, at the 75 mg/m^2 dose, was superior to best supportive care in terms of time-to-disease progression (10.6 vs 6.7 weeks), median survival (7.5 vs 4.6 months), and 1-year survival (37% vs 11%).[84] The efficacy of docetaxel has been improved with the addition of ramucirumab. A large, randomized trial of docetaxel with or without ramucirumab reported longer progression-free survival (4.5 vs 3 months) and overall survival (10.5 vs 9.1 months) favoring the ramucirumab arm.[85] Response by histology was not analyzed, but ramucirumab appeared to be active in all histologies. Due to the relatively modest improvement in survival, clinicians must decide if the benefit outweighs the risks in adverse drug reactions and cost. Although ramucirumab binds to the VEGF receptor, it is important to note that safety concerns (serious and fatal bleeding) like those seen with bevacizumab and chemotherapy in squamous histology were not reported.

The second chemotherapy agent approved as second-line treatment is pemetrexed. When compared to docetaxel, there were no difference in efficacy outcomes but there were significantly fewer adverse drug reactions in patients receiving pemetrexed, including lower rates of hospitalizations due to toxicities.[86] Pemetrexed is a preferred chemotherapy option based on this study, but it is not appropriate as second-line therapy when it is used as maintenance therapy. It is also important to note that pemetrexed should not be used for patients with squamous NSCLC.

The comparative trials indicate that pemetrexed and docetaxel are equally effective, and docetaxel plus ramucirumab is superior to docetaxel alone. Similarly, nivolumab, pembrolizumab, and atezolizumab are superior to docetaxel alone.[87] All five monotherapies and ramucirumab-docetaxel are acceptable regimens, but checkpoint inhibitors are preferred in patients who are naïve to this modality due to an impressive durability of response.[3] It is not clear, if a platinum doublet should be used or a single cytotoxic agent. If a platinum doublet is selected, then the regimen would be selected based on histology (as described below for tumors that are PD-L1 negative and have no targetable genetic mutations). If single-agent chemotherapy is selected, pemetrexed is preferred for nonsquamous cell tumors and docetaxel with or without ramucirumab for squamous cell tumors (Table 152-5). However, since most patients with relapsed metastatic disease are heavily pretreated and are more likely to experience significant adverse drug reactions, single-agent chemotherapy tends to be preferred.

Third-line therapy (and beyond) is reasonable for patients who have a good performance status and can tolerate another agent. Monotherapy with an active agent would typically be used in this setting. For patients who received a PD-L1 guided therapy, docetaxel would be an option with or without ramucirumab. For those who received second-line docetaxel with or without ramucirumab, an immune checkpoint inhibitor would be an option. For patients who want treatment beyond third line, a single agent could be used.[3-5] The best agent(s) has not been determined in clinical trials. Therapeutic decisions are based on patient-specific factors including prior therapies and potential contraindications to specific agents. The most common treatment option is monotherapy with an agent known to have activity in clinical trials.

Older Patients and Poor-Performance Status Single-agent chemotherapy is an alternative in older patients (>65 years old) or those with an ECOG performance status of 2 or greater. First-line, single-agent chemotherapy has objective response rates of 5% to 25% with no significant effect on overall survival. Rarely, complete responses occur and tend to have limited durations.[88] The most active cytotoxic chemotherapy agents are cisplatin, carboplatin, docetaxel, paclitaxel, etoposide, gemcitabine, ifosfamide, irinotecan, topotecan, mitomycin, vinblastine, vinorelbine, and pemetrexed.[3] Targeted therapies are also active as a single agent and should be considered in patients with a mutation-positive tumor.

Historically, patients with an ECOG performance status 2 were excluded from NSCLC trials because of excessive toxicity with minimal benefit from combination cytotoxic therapy. Updated ASCO guidelines state that available data support the use of single-agent and combination chemotherapy but are relatively weak and incorporate older patients or poor patients with a poor performance status. They emphasize the need to individualize this decision.[4,5] A recent meta-analysis shows that patients with performance status 2 benefit from treatment. The NCCN guidelines list both single agents and combinations for patients with a performance status of 2, and best supportive care for patients with a performance status of 3 or 4 unless they have a mutation or gene rearrangement where they can receive a tyrosine kinase inhibitor.[3]

Evaluation of Therapeutic Outcomes

For patients who have undergone surgical resection, a physical examination and chest radiography are recommended every 3 to 4 months for the first 2 years, then every 6 months for 3 years, and then annually. In addition, a low-dose spiral chest CT scan is recommended annually to monitor for evidence of local recurrence. Suspicious symptoms or physical findings (eg, bone pain, visual abnormalities, headache, or elevated liver function tests) should prompt an evaluation to rule out distant metastases.[3-5]

Tumor response to chemotherapy is generally evaluated at the end of the second or third cycle and at the end of every second cycle thereafter. Patients with stable disease, with an objective response, or with a measurable decrease in tumor size (complete or partial response) should continue until four to six cycles have been administered. Patients with nonsquamous histology tumors who respond (ie, nonprogressive disease) should be considered for maintenance therapy with pemetrexed. Following initial therapy for NSCLC, patients must be monitored for evidence of disease progression.[3-5] Second-line therapy and beyond is traditionally given until progression. The immune checkpoint inhibitors can display a different response pattern than traditional chemotherapy or targeted therapy. It can take some time for the immune system to become activated and then the tumor will initially be infiltrated with cytotoxic lymphocytes that can appear radiographically as progression prior to a response. The median time-to-response for immune checkpoint inhibitors is 10 to 12 weeks. Although the registry trials continue to assess response based on Response Evaluation Criteria in Solid Tumors (RECIST) criteria, an immune response criterion has been proposed where progression needs to be documented on two consecutive assessments at least 4 weeks apart.[89]

Small Cell Lung Cancer

Small cell lung cancer is a rapidly dividing malignancy that spreads early in the disease course. Consequently, about 60% to 70% of patients present with extensive-stage disease. When patients with SCLC are not treated, the disease quickly becomes fatal. Fortunately, SCLCs are responsive to chemotherapy and radiation. Chemotherapy with or without radiotherapy is the treatment of choice for most patients. Even after a complete response to therapy, the cancer usually recurs within 6 to 8 months, and survival time following recurrence is typically short (about 4 months). With treatment, median survival rates for patients with limited and extensive disease are 14 to 20 and 9 to 11 months, respectively. Treatment planning starts with stage of disease (ie, limited vs extensive stage), but must also consider other factors, including performance status (treatment usually restricted to performance status 0 or 1), patient age, comorbid conditions (eg, renal failure), and patient desire to receive treatment.[2,16]

Limited Disease

9 When a single SCLC mass is found, local therapy with radiation or surgery is considered, although the use of surgery in SCLC is limited to solitary nodules, without evidence of metastasis to lymph nodes. One of the differences between SCLC and NSCLC is that radiation is preferred for treatment of local disease over surgery. Radiation is always combined with chemotherapy in limited-stage SCLC, and the regimen of choice is etoposide and cisplatin (ie, EP

TABLE 152-7 Chemotherapy Regimens Used in the Treatment of SCLC

	Regimen	Drugs and Doses
First Line	Etoposide/cisplatin (EP)	Cisplatin 75 mg/m² IV on day 1 Etoposide 100 mg/m² IV on days 1-3; repeat cycle every 3 weeks for 4-6 cycles or Cisplatin 60 mg/m² IV on day 1 Etoposide 120 mg/m² IV on days 1-3; repeat cycle every 3 weeks for 4-6 cycles
	Etoposide/carboplatin (EC)	Carboplatin AUC 5-6 IV on day 1 Etoposide 100 mg/m² IV on days 1-3; repeat cycle every 3 weeks for 4-6 cycles
	EC + atezolizumab[a]	Carboplatin AUC 5 IV on day 1 Etoposide 100 mg/m² IV on days 1-3 Atezolizumab 1,200 mg IV on day 1; repeat cycle every 3 weeks for 4 cycles followed by Atezolizumab 1,200 mg every 3 weeks or 1680 mg every 4 weeks as maintenance
	EP + durvalumab[a]	Carboplatin AUC 5-6 IV on day 1 Etoposide 80-100 mg/m² IV on days 1-3 Durvalumab 1,500 mg IV on day 1; repeat cycle every 3 weeks for 4 cycles followed by Durvalumab 1,500 mg every 4 weeks as maintenance
	EC + durvalumab[a]	Cisplatin 75-80 mg/m² IV on day 1 Etoposide 80-100 mg/m² IV on days 1-3 Durvalumab 1,500 mg IV on day 1; repeat cycle every 3 weeks for 4 cycles followed by Durvalumab 1,500 mg every 4 weeks as maintenance
Second Line	Topotecan	Topotecan 1.5 mg/m²/day IV days 1-5; repeat every 3 weeks
	Lurbinectedin	Lurbinectedin 3.2 mg/m²/day IV day 1; repeat every 3 weeks

[a]Extensive stage only.

regimen). Carboplatin may be substituted for cisplatin to reduce nausea and vomiting, nephrotoxicity, or neurotoxicity, although increased thrombocytopenia may result.[90] Alternative regimens have failed to demonstrate improved outcomes compared to EP plus concurrent radiation and typically have more toxicity. Guidelines recommend that the EP regimen be used with concurrent radiotherapy.[2,16] Regimens used in the treatment of SCLC can be found in Table 152-7. Because patients with SCLC commonly have a recurrence in the CNS, trials have been performed to evaluate the benefit of prophylactic cranial irradiation (PCI). A pivotal study showed that PCI reduces the incidence of brain metastasis and increases 3-year survival from 15% to 21%.[91] Therefore, patients who achieve a complete response with treatment should be offered PCI.

Extensive Disease

Historically, platinum regimens have been the treatment of choice in extensive disease as studies have failed to show superiority to the EP regimen as first-line treatment. As in limited disease, carboplatin is an acceptable substitute for cisplatin in EP.

8 Programmed death inhibition with either atezolizumab or durvalumab when added to standard chemotherapy in patients with extensive stage SCLC has been shown to improve overall survival. The addition of atezolizumab to standard chemotherapy improved median progression free survival (2 vs 4.3 months) and overall survival (12.3 vs 10.3 months).[92] Durvalumab demonstrated similar benefit, improving median overall survival from 10.3 to 13 months.[93] The complete regimens used in the studies are shown in Table 152-7.

Concurrent radiotherapy is not used routinely in extensive disease. However, a randomized study of extensive-stage patients responding to chemotherapy comparing observation or PCI reported that PCI decreased the 1-year risk of brain metastasis (14.6% vs 40.4%), and prolonged 1-year survival (27.1% vs 13.3%).[94] A more recent Japanese study reported that PCI reduced the risk of brain metastases but did not improve overall survival. The results of these studies led to guideline revisions recommending PCI for patients with extensive disease responding to chemotherapy.[2,16]

Relapsed Disease

Patients with SCLC who relapse or progress after first-line chemotherapy have a median survival of 4 to 5 months. Unfortunately, recurrent disease is usually less sensitive to chemotherapy.

10 Treatment approach for patients who experience relapsed SCLC often depends on the length of time between completion of the initial chemotherapy regimen and relapse. If this interval is less than 3 months, the patient has refractory SCLC and is unlikely to respond to second-line therapy and should receive best supportive care or be enrolled in a clinical trial. For those with greater than a 3-month time interval between first-line chemotherapy and relapse, the expected response rate to treatment is about 20%, and second-line therapy should be considered.[2,16] Based on limited evidence, if the interval between completion of initial chemotherapy and relapse is 6 months or greater, retreating the patient with the initial chemotherapy regimen may be considered.[2] Topotecan (intravenous and oral) is approved as second-line therapy for SCLC and has been considered standard second-line treatment of SCLC based on a trial that randomized patients to intravenous topotecan or to cyclophosphamide, doxorubicin, and vincristine (CAV) regimen.[95] The response rates, time-to-disease progression, and overall survival were not different between groups. The proportion of patients experiencing symptom improvement was higher in the topotecan arm. There were fewer dose reductions for topotecan (1% vs 11%) due to improved adverse drug reaction rates except for more anemia and thrombocytopenia from topotecan. Oral topotecan is similar in terms of dosing, toxicity, and effectiveness compared to intravenous topotecan.[96]

Lurbinectedin, an alkylating drug that binds guanine residues in deoxyribonucleic acid (DNA) inhibiting oncogenic transcription and causing apoptosis, is another effective second-line agent in relapsed SCLC and an alternative to topotecan.[97] In a single arm trial, it produced an overall response rate of 35.2% lasting a median of 5.3 months. Common adverse drug reactions include myelosuppression, fatigue, and elevations in serum creatinine and liver function tests. Other agents recommended in national guidelines include single-agent PD-L1 inhibitor, irinotecan, gemcitabine, paclitaxel, docetaxel, oral etoposide, temozolomide, and vinorelbine; CAV regimen; and participation in a clinical trial.[2,16]

Evaluation of Therapeutic Outcomes

The effectiveness of first-line therapy is evaluated after two to three cycles of treatment. If the patient achieves a complete or partial response, therapy is continued for four to six cycles of therapy. If the patient has evidence of progressive disease, therapy is discontinued or changed to a non–cross-resistant regimen. In the case of SCLC, responding patients benefit from the addition of PCI following initial therapy. After recovery from first-line therapy, follow-up visits should occur every 3 months for years 1, 2, and 3, then every 4 to 6 months for years 4 and 5, and then annually for patients with either a partial or complete response.[2,3]

Complications and Supportive Care

Patients with lung cancer frequently have numerous concurrent medical problems. Such problems may be related to invasion of the primary tumor and its metastases, paraneoplastic syndromes (see "Clinical Presentation" earlier), chemotherapy and radiotherapy toxicity, or concomitant disease states (eg, cardiac disease, renal dysfunction, chronic obstructive pulmonary disease, asthma, or diabetes). Depression is also common and sometimes persistent in patients with SCLC and NSCLC and should be treated. Identification, diagnosis, and treatment of the whole patient may improve the patient's overall quality of life and tolerance to cancer treatments.

11 The chemotherapy regimens used in the management of lung cancer are intensive and are associated with a wide variety of toxic effects. Nausea and vomiting may be severe. Cisplatin-containing regimens require the use of aggressive acute and delayed antiemetic regimens containing agents, such as serotonin antagonists, dexamethasone, and neurokinin-1 receptor antagonist, and olanzapine.[98] Patients experiencing protracted nausea and vomiting may require intravenous hydration and nutritional support. Myelosuppression is often the dose-limiting toxicity associated with chemotherapy. Granulocytopenia places patients at high risk for serious infections. Other toxic effects associated with these chemotherapy regimens include mucositis, anemia, nephrotoxicity, peripheral neuropathies, and ototoxicity. In multiple phase II clinical trials, trilaciclib, a cyclin-dependent kinase 4/6 inhibitor, has demonstrated efficacy in decreasing the incidence and severity of chemotherapy-induced myeylosuppression when administered prior to chemotherapy for extensive stage small cell lung cancer.[99] Its utility in other settings, or in comparison/combination with colony stimulating factors, has not been established.

About 30% to 65% of advanced-stage NSCLC patients will develop bone metastases, which may lead to significant bone pain, pathologic fractures, spinal cord compression, and hypercalcemia. A large meta-analysis determined denosumab, a RANK-ligand inhibitor and zoledronic acid (bisophosphonate) decrease the incidence of skeletal-related events such as fractures. Additionally, both agents have been shown to delay the onset of first event. The meta-analysis also found that denosumab has been shown to prolong overall survival compared to no treatment for bone metastases. Zoledronic acid was not determined to affect survival.[100]

Patients receiving radiation therapy may experience complications including severe esophagitis, fatigue, radiation pneumonitis, and cardiac toxicity. These toxicities are usually more common and severe when radiation is combined with chemotherapy. The patient's baseline performance status and the degree of pulmonary dysfunction (eg, chronic obstructive pulmonary disease from years of tobacco use) must be considered in decisions concerning radiation dosage and fractionation.

Patients who receive an immune checkpoint inhibitor can develop immune-related adverse events, which frequently include the gastrointestinal tract, skin, and pneumonitis. Holding therapy and intervening with steroids can blunt the progression of these toxicities. The other key point is that responses to immune checkpoint inhibitors can be delayed in onset.[101] A new response criterion has been developed for immunotherapies, which differs from RECIST criteria by requiring documentation of significant tumor grown on two occasions at least 4 weeks apart to be defined as progression.

Lung cancer patients frequently receive complex pharmacologic regimens that include chemotherapeutic agents, immune checkpoint inhibitors, antiemetics, antibiotics, analgesics, anticoagulants, bronchodilators, corticosteroids, anticonvulsants, and cardiovascular agents. Such regimens necessitate intensive therapeutic monitoring to avoid drug-related and radiotherapy-related toxic effects and to optimize therapeutic outcomes for individual patients.

CONCLUSION

Lung cancers remain the leading cause of cancer-related mortality in the United States. Early detection of lung cancer through appropriate screening methods, along with decreased use of tobacco products have helped lower lung cancer incidence and mortality. Advances in targeted therapies, such as inhibitors of the programmed death pathway and oral kinase inhibitors targeting specific mutations found in tumor cells, have had significant impact on the survival of patients with lung cancer.

ABBREVIATIONS

ALK	anaplastic lymphoma kinase
ASCO	American Society of Clinical Oncology
AUC	area under the curve
BRAF	B-rapidly accelerated fibrosarcoma
CAV	cyclophosphamide, doxorubicin, and vincristine
CBC	complete blood count
CMP	comprehensive medical panel
CNS	central nervous system
CPK	creatine phosphokinase
CT	computed tomography
DNA	deoxyribonucleic acid
EC	etoposide and carboplatin
ECG	electrocardiogram
ECOG	Eastern Cooperative Oncology Group
EGFR	epidermal growth factor receptor
EP	etoposide and cisplatin
ETS	environmental tobacco smoke
HER2	human epidermal growth factor
IP	irinotecan and cisplatin
KRAS	Kirsten rat sarcoma viral oncogene homologue
LDCT	low-dose computed tomography
MET	mesenchymal epithelial transition factor
MIA	minimally invasive adenocarcinoma
NCCN	National Comprehensive Cancer Network
NSCLC	non-small cell lung cancer
NTRK	neurotrophic receptor kinase
PCI	prophylactic cranial irradiation
PD-1	programmed death-1
PD-L1	programmed death ligand-1
PET	positron emission tomography
RECIST	response evaluation criteria in solid tumors
RET	rearranged during transfection
ROS1	receptor tyrosine kinase 1
SCLC	small cell lung cancer
TKI	tyrosine kinase inhibitor
TNM	tumor, node, and metastasis
TPS	tumor proportion score

REFERENCES

1. Siegel RL, Miller KD, Fuchs HE, Jemal A. Cancer statistics, 2022. *CA Cancer J Clin.* 2022;72(1):7–33. 10.3322/caac.21708.
2. National Comprehensive Cancer Network. Small Cell Lung Cancer v 1.2022. Published online December 7, 2021. Accessed December 21, 2021. https://www.nccn.org/professionals/physician_gls/pdf/sclc.pdf
3. National Comprehensive Cancer Network. Non-Small Cell Lung Cancer v 5.2021. Published online June 15, 2021. Accessed September

21, 2021. https://www.nccn.org/professionals/physician_gls/pdf/nscl.pdf

4. Hanna NH, Schneider BJ, Temin S, et al. Therapy for stage IV non-small-cell lung cancer without driver alterations: ASCO and OH (CCO) joint guideline update. *J Clin Oncol.* 2020;38(14):1608–1632. doi:10.1200/JCO.19.03022
5. Hanna NH, Robinson AG, Temin S, et al. Therapy for stage IV non–small-cell lung cancer with driver alterations: ASCO and OH (CCO) joint guideline update. *J Clin Oncol.* 2021;39(9):1040–1091. doi:10.1200/JCO.20.03570
6. Kalemkerian GP, Narula N, Kennedy EB, et al. Molecular testing guideline for the selection of patients with lung cancer for treatment with targeted tyrosine kinase inhibitors: American Society of Clinical Oncology endorsement of the College of American Pathologists/International Association for the Study of Lung Cancer/Association for Molecular Pathology clinical practice guideline update. *J Clin Oncol.* 2018;36(9):911–919. doi:10.1200/JCO.2017.76.7293
7. Simone CB, Bogart JA, Cabrera AR, et al. Radiation therapy for small cell lung cancer: An ASTRO clinical practice guideline. *Pract Radiat Oncol.* 2020;10(3):158–173. doi:10.1016/j.prro.2020.02.009
8. Larsen JE, Minna JD. The molecular biology of lung cancer. In: DeVita VT, Lawrence TS, Rosenberg SA, eds. *DeVita, Hellman, and Rosenberg's cancer: Principles & practice of oncology.* 11th ed. Wolters Kluwer; 2019:607–617.
9. Hann CL, Wu A, Rekhtman N, Rudin CM. Small cell and neuroendocrine tumors of the lung. In: DeVita VT, Lawrence TS, Rosenberg SA, eds. *DeVita, Hellman, and Rosenberg's cancer: Principles & practice of oncology.* 11th edition. Wolters Kluwer; 2019:671–699.
10. Chiang A, Detterbeck FC, Stewart T, Decker RH, Tanoue L. Non-small-cell lung cancer. In: DeVita VT, Lawrence TS, Rosenberg SA, eds. *DeVita, Hellman, and Rosenberg's cancer: Principles & practice of oncology.* 11th edition. Wolters Kluwer; 2019:618–670.
11. National Center for Chronic Disease Prevention and Health Promotion (US) Office on Smoking and Health. *The Health Consequences of Smoking—50 Years of Progress: A Report of the Surgeon General.* Centers for Disease Control and Prevention (US); 2014. Accessed June 29, 2021. http://www.ncbi.nlm.nih.gov/books/NBK179276/
12. Cornelius ME. Tobacco product use among adults—United States, 2019. *MMWR Morb Mortal Wkly Rep.* 2020;69. doi:10.15585/mmwr.mm6946a4
13. Amin MB, Edge S, Greene F, et al., eds. *AJCC cancer staging manual.* 8th ed. Springer International Publishing; 2017. Accessed June 29, 2021. https://www.springer.com/gp/book/9783319406176
14. Burdett S, Pignon JP, Tierney J, et al. Adjuvant chemotherapy for resected early-stage non-small cell lung cancer. *Cochrane Database Syst Rev.* 2015;(3). doi:10.1002/14651858.CD011430
15. Couraud S, Cortot AB, Greillier L, et al. From randomized trials to the clinic: Is it time to implement individual lung-cancer screening in clinical practice? A multidisciplinary statement from French experts on behalf of the French intergroup (IFCT) and the groupe d'Oncologie de langue francaise (GOLF). *Ann Oncol.* 2013;24(3):586–597. doi:10.1093/annonc/mds476
16. Rudin CM, Ismaila N, Hann CL, et al. Treatment of small-cell lung cancer: American Society of Clinical Oncology endorsement of the American College of Chest Physicians Guideline. *J Clin Oncol.* 2015;33(34):4106–4111. doi:10.1200/JCO.2015.63.7918
17. Bezjak A, Temin S, Franklin G, et al. Definitive and adjuvant radiotherapy in locally advanced non-small-cell lung cancer: American Society of Clinical Oncology Clinical Practice Guideline endorsement of the American Society for Radiation Oncology evidence-based clinical practice guideline. *J Clin Oncol.* 2015;33(18):2100–2105. doi:10.1200/JCO.2014.59.2360
18. National Lung Screening Trial Research Team, Aberle DR, Adams AM, et al. Reduced lung-cancer mortality with low-dose computed tomographic screening. *N Engl J Med.* 2011;365(5):395–409. doi:10.1056/NEJMoa1102873
19. US Preventive Services Task Force, Krist AH, Davidson KW, et al. Screening for lung cancer: US Preventive Services Task Force recommendation statement. *JAMA.* 2021;325(10):962–970. doi:10.1001/jama.2021.1117
20. de Koning HJ, van der Aalst CM, de Jong PA, et al. Reduced lung-cancer mortality with volume CT screening in a randomized trial. *N Engl J Med.* 2020;382(6):503–513. doi:10.1056/NEJMoa1911793
21. Meza R, Jeon J, Toumazis I, et al. Evaluation of the benefits and harms of lung cancer screening with low-dose computed tomography: Modeling study for the US Preventive Services Task Force. *JAMA.* 2021;325(10):988–997. doi:10.1001/jama.2021.1077
22. Keith RL, Miller YE. Lung cancer chemoprevention: Current status and future prospects. *Nat Rev Clin Oncol.* 2013;10(6):334–343. doi:10.1038/nrclinonc.2013.64
23. Micke P, Faldum A, Metz T, et al. Staging small cell lung cancer: Veterans Administration Lung Study Group versus International Association for the Study of Lung Cancer—what limits limited disease? *Lung Cancer.* 2002;37(3):271–276. doi:10.1016/s0169-5002(02)00072-7
24. Kris MG, Gaspar LE, Chaft JE, et al. Adjuvant systemic therapy and adjuvant radiation therapy for stage I to IIIA completely resected non-small-cell lung cancers: American Society of Clinical Oncology/Cancer Care Ontario clinical practice guideline update. *J Clin Oncol.* 2017;35(25):2960–2974. doi:10.1200/JCO.2017.72.4401
25. Indini A, Rijavec E, Bareggi C, Grossi F. Novel treatment strategies for early-stage lung cancer: The oncologist's perspective. *J Thorac Dis.* 2020;12(6):3390–3398. doi:10.21037/jtd.2020.02.46
26. Wu YL, Tsuboi M, He J, et al. Osimertinib in resected EGFR-mutated non-small-cell lung cancer. *N Engl J Med.* 2020;383(18):1711–1723. doi:10.1056/NEJMoa2027071
27. Felip E, Altorki N, Zhou C, et al. Adjuvant atezolizumab after adjuvant chemotherapy in resected stage IB–IIIA non-small-cell lung cancer (IMpower010): A randomised, multicentre, open-label, phase 3 trial. *Lancet.* 2021;398(10308):1344–1357. doi:10.1016/S0140-6736(21)02098-5
28. Forde PM, Spicer J, Lu S, et al. Neoadjuvant nivolumab plus chemotherapy in resectable lung cancer. *N Eng J Med.* 2022. 10.1056/nejmoa2202170.
29. Felip E, Rosell R, Maestre JA, et al. Preoperative chemotherapy plus surgery versus surgery plus adjuvant chemotherapy versus surgery alone in early-stage non-small-cell lung cancer. *J Clin Oncol.* 2010;28(19):3138–3145. doi:10.1200/JCO.2009.27.6204
30. Westeel V, Quoix E, Puyraveau M, et al. A randomised trial comparing preoperative to perioperative chemotherapy in early-stage non-small-cell lung cancer (IFCT 0002 trial). *Eur J Cancer.* 2013;49(12):2654–2664. doi:10.1016/j.ejca.2013.04.013
31. van Meerbeeck JP, Kramer GWPM, Van Schil PEY, et al. Randomized controlled trial of resection versus radiotherapy after induction chemotherapy in stage IIIA-N2 non-small-cell lung cancer. *J Natl Cancer Inst.* 2007;99(6):442–450. doi:10.1093/jnci/djk093
32. Pless M, Stupp R, Ris HB, et al. Induction chemoradiation in stage IIIA/N2 non-small-cell lung cancer: A phase 3 randomised trial. *Lancet.* 2015;386(9998):1049–1056. doi:10.1016/S0140-6736(15)60294-X
33. Spigel DR, Faivre-Finn C, Gray JE, et al. Five-year survival outcomes with durvalumab after chemoradiotherapy in unresectable stage III NSCLC: An update from the PACIFIC trial. *J Clin Oncol.* 2021;39(15_suppl):8511. doi:10.1200/JCO.2021.39.15_suppl.8511
34. Zhang YL, Yuan JQ, Wang KF, et al. The prevalence of EGFR mutation in patients with non-small cell lung cancer: A systematic review and meta-analysis. *Oncotarget.* 2016;7(48):78985–78993. doi:10.18632/oncotarget.12587
35. Nakagawa K, Garon EB, Seto T, et al. Ramucirumab plus erlotinib in patients with untreated, EGFR-mutated, advanced non-small-cell lung cancer (RELAY): A randomised, double-blind, placebo-controlled, phase 3 trial. *Lancet Oncol.* 2019;20(12):1655–1669. doi:10.1016/S1470-2045(19)30634-5
36. Saito H, Fukuhara T, Furuya N, et al. Erlotinib plus bevacizumab versus erlotinib alone in patients with EGFR-positive advanced non-squamous non-small-cell lung cancer (NEJ026): Interim analysis of an open-label, randomised, multicentre, phase 3 trial. *Lancet Oncol.* 2019;20(5):625–635. doi:10.1016/S1470-2045(19)30035-X
37. Kuan FC, Kuo LT, Chen MC, et al. Overall survival benefits of first-line EGFR tyrosine kinase inhibitors in EGFR-mutated non-small-cell lung cancers: A systematic review and meta-analysis. *Br J Cancer.* 2015;113(10):1519–1528. doi:10.1038/bjc.2015.356
38. Mok TS, Cheng Y, Zhou X, et al. Improvement in overall survival in a randomized study that compared dacomitinib with gefitinib in patients with advanced non-small-cell lung cancer and EGFR-activating mutations. *J Clin Oncol.* 2018;36(22):2244–2250. doi:10.1200/JCO.2018.78.7994
39. Ramalingam SS, Vansteenkiste J, Planchard D, et al. Overall survival with osimertinib in untreated, *EGFR*-mutated advanced NSCLC. *N Engl J Med.* 2020;382(1):41–50. doi:10.1056/NEJMoa1913662
40. Shin DY, Na II, Kim CH, Park S, Baek H, Yang SH. EGFR mutation and brain metastasis in pulmonary adenocarcinomas. *J Thorac Oncol.* 2014;9(2):195–199. doi:10.1097/JTO.0000000000000069
41. Park K, Haura EB, Leighl NB, et al. Amivantamab in EGFR exon 20 insertion–mutated non–small-cell lung cancer progressing on platinum chemotherapy: Initial results from the CHRYSALIS phase I study. *J Clin Oncol.* Published online August 2, 2021:JCO.21.00662. doi:10.1200/JCO.21.00662

42. Gonzalvez F, Vincent S, Baker TE, et al. Mobocertinib (TAK-788): A targeted inhibitor of EGFR exon 20 insertion mutants in non–small cell lung cancer. *Cancer Discov.* 2021;11(7):1672–1687. doi:10.1158/2159-8290.CD-20-1683
43. Ramalingam SS, Zhou C, Kim TM, et al. Mobocertinib (TAK-788) in EGFR exon 20 insertion (ex20ins)+ metastatic NSCLC (mNSCLC): Additional results from platinum-pretreated patients (pts) and EXCLAIM cohort of phase 1/2 study. *J Clin Oncol.* 2021;39(15_suppl):9014. doi:10.1200/JCO.2021.39.15_suppl.9014
44. Slebos RJC, Kibbelaar RE, Dalesio O, et al. K-ras oncogene activation as a prognostic marker in adenocarcinoma of the lung. *N Engl J Med.* 1990;323(9):561–565. doi:10.1056/NEJM199008303230902
45. Skoulidis F, Li BT, Dy GK, et al. Sotorasib for lung cancers with KRAS p.G12C mutation. *N Engl J Med.* 2021;384(25):2371–2381. doi:10.1056/NEJMoa2103695
46. Chia PL, Mitchell P, Dobrovic A, John T. Prevalence and natural history of ALK positive non-small-cell lung cancer and the clinical impact of targeted therapy with ALK inhibitors. *Clin Epidemiol.* 2014;6:423–432. doi:10.2147/CLEP.S69718
47. Solomon BJ, Mok T, Kim DW, et al. First-line crizotinib versus chemotherapy in ALK-positive lung cancer. *N Engl J Med.* 2014;371(23):2167–2177. doi:10.1056/NEJMoa1408440
48. Soria JC, Tan DSW, Chiari R, et al. First-line ceritinib versus platinum-based chemotherapy in advanced ALK-rearranged non-small-cell lung cancer (ASCEND-4): A randomised, open-label, phase 3 study. *Lancet.* 2017;389(10072):917–929. doi:10.1016/S0140-6736(17)30123-X
49. Mok T, Camidge DR, Gadgeel SM, et al. Updated overall survival and final progression-free survival data for patients with treatment-naive advanced ALK-positive non-small-cell lung cancer in the ALEX study. *Ann Oncol.* 2020;31(8):1056–1064. doi:10.1016/j.annonc.2020.04.478
50. Camidge DR, Kim HR, Ahn MJ, et al. Brigatinib versus crizotinib in advanced ALK inhibitor-naive ALK-positive non-small cell lung cancer: Second interim analysis of the phase III ALTA-1L trial. *J Clin Oncol Off J Am Soc Clin Oncol.* 2020;38(31):3592–3603. doi:10.1200/JCO.20.00505
51. Shaw AT, Bauer TM, de Marinis F, et al. First-line lorlatinib or crizotinib in advanced ALK-positive lung cancer. *N Engl J Med.* 2020;383(21):2018–2029. doi:10.1056/NEJMoa2027187
52. Solomon BJ, Besse B, Bauer TM, et al. Lorlatinib in patients with ALK-positive non-small-cell lung cancer: Results from a global phase 2 study. *Lancet Oncol.* 2018;19(12):1654–1667. doi:10.1016/S1470-2045(18)30649-1
53. Shaw AT, Ou SHI, Bang YJ, et al. Crizotinib in ROS1-rearranged non–small-cell lung cancer. *N Engl J Med.* 2014;371(21):1963–1971. doi:10.1056/NEJMoa1406766
54. Planchard D, Smit EF, Groen HJM, et al. Dabrafenib plus trametinib in patients with previously untreated BRAFV600E-mutant metastatic non-small-cell lung cancer: An open-label, phase 2 trial. *Lancet Oncol.* 2017;18(10):1307–1316. doi:10.1016/S1470-2045(17)30679-4
55. Planchard D, Besse B, Groen HJM, et al. Dabrafenib plus trametinib in patients with previously treated BRAF(V600E)-mutant metastatic non-small cell lung cancer: An open-label, multicentre phase 2 trial. *Lancet Oncol.* 2016;17(7):984–993. doi:10.1016/S1470-2045(16)30146-2
56. Drilon A, Laetsch TW, Kummar S, et al. Efficacy of larotrectinib in TRK fusion-positive cancers in adults and children. *N Engl J Med.* 2018;378(8):731–739. doi:10.1056/NEJMoa1714448
57. Doebele RC, Drilon A, Paz-Ares L, et al. Entrectinib in patients with advanced or metastatic NTRK fusion-positive solid tumours: Integrated analysis of three phase 1–2 trials. *Lancet Oncol.* 2020;21(2):271–282. doi:10.1016/S1470-2045(19)30691-6
58. Wolf J, Seto T, Han JY, et al. Capmatinib in *MET* exon 14–mutated or *MET*-amplified non–small-cell lung cancer. *N Engl J Med.* 2020;383(10):944–957. doi:10.1056/NEJMoa2002787
59. Paik PK, Felip E, Veillon R, et al. Tepotinib in non–small-cell lung cancer with *MET* exon 14 skipping mutations. *N Engl J Med.* 2020;383(10):931–943. doi:10.1056/NEJMoa2004407
60. Drilon A, Oxnard GR, Tan DSW, et al. Efficacy of selpercatinib in *RET* fusion–positive non–small-cell lung cancer. *N Engl J Med.* 2020;383(9):813–824. doi:10.1056/NEJMoa2005653
61. Gainor JF, Curigliano G, Kim DW, et al. Pralsetinib for RET fusion-positive non-small-cell lung cancer (ARROW): A multi-cohort, open-label, phase 1/2 study. *Lancet Oncol.* 2021;22(7):959–969. doi:10.1016/S1470-2045(21)00247-3
62. Schiller JH, Harrington D, Belani CP, et al. Comparison of four chemotherapy regimens for advanced non-small-cell lung cancer. *N Engl J Med.* 2002;346(2):92–98. doi:10.1056/NEJMoa011954
63. Scagliotti G, Brodowicz T, Shepherd FA, et al. Treatment-by-histology interaction analyses in three phase III trials show superiority of pemetrexed in nonsquamous non-small cell lung cancer. *J Thorac Oncol.* 2011;6(1):64–70. doi:10.1097/JTO.0b013e3181f7c6d4
64. Kulkarni S, Vella ET, Coakley N, et al. The use of systemic treatment in the maintenance of patients with non-small cell lung cancer: A systematic review. *J Thorac Oncol.* 2016;11(7):989–1002. doi:10.1016/j.jtho.2016.03.007
65. Shan F, Zhang B, Sun L, Xie L, Shen M, Ruan S. The role of combination maintenance with pemetrexed and bevacizumab for advanced stage nonsquamous non-small cell lung cancer: A systematic review and meta-analysis. *BioMed Res Int.* 2018;2018:5839081. doi:10.1155/2018/5839081
66. Reck M, Rodríguez-Abreu D, Robinson AG, et al. Pembrolizumab versus chemotherapy for PD-L1-positive non-small-cell lung cancer. *N Engl J Med.* 2016;375(19):1823–1833. doi:10.1056/NEJMoa1606774
67. Reck M, Rodríguez-Abreu D, Robinson AG, et al. Updated analysis of KEYNOTE-024: Pembrolizumab versus platinum-based chemotherapy for advanced non–small-cell lung cancer with PD-L1 tumor proportion score of 50% or greater. *J Clin Oncol.* 2019;37(7):537–546. doi:10.1200/JCO.18.00149
68. Herbst RS, Giaccone G, de Marinis F, et al. Atezolizumab for first-line treatment of PD-L1-selected patients with NSCLC. *N Engl J Med.* 2020;383(14):1328–1339. doi:10.1056/NEJMoa1917346
69. Sezer A, Kilickap S, Gümüş M, et al. Cemiplimab monotherapy for first-line treatment of advanced non-small-cell lung cancer with PD-L1 of at least 50%: A multicentre, open-label, global, phase 3, randomised, controlled trial. *The Lancet.* 2021;397(10274):592–604. doi:10.1016/S0140-6736(21)00228-2
70. Gandhi L, Rodríguez-Abreu D, Gadgeel S, et al. Pembrolizumab plus chemotherapy in metastatic non-small-cell lung cancer. *N Engl J Med.* 2018;378(22):2078–2092. doi:10.1056/NEJMoa1801005
71. Paz-Ares L, Luft A, Vicente D, et al. Pembrolizumab plus chemotherapy for squamous non-small-cell lung cancer. *N Engl J Med.* 2018;379(21):2040–2051. doi:10.1056/NEJMoa1810865
72. Hellmann MD, Paz-Ares L, Bernabe Caro R, et al. Nivolumab plus ipilimumab in advanced non–small-cell lung cancer. *N Engl J Med.* 2019;381(21):2020–2031. doi:10.1056/NEJMoa1910231
73. Deng H, Zhou C. From CheckMate 227 to CheckMate 9LA: Rethinking the status of chemotherapy in the immunotherapy era—chemo-free or chemo-reform? *Transl Lung Cancer Res.* 2021;10(4). doi:10.21037/tlcr-21-179
74. Reck M, Ciuleanu TE, Cobo M, et al. First-line nivolumab (NIVO) plus ipilimumab (IPI) plus two cycles of chemotherapy (chemo) versus chemo alone (4 cycles) in patients with advanced non-small cell lung cancer (NSCLC): Two-year update from CheckMate 9LA. *J Clin Oncol.* 2021;39(15_suppl):9000. doi:10.1200/JCO.2021.39.15_suppl.9000
75. Mok TSK, Wu YL, Kudaba I, et al. Pembrolizumab versus chemotherapy for previously untreated, PD-L1-expressing, locally advanced or metastatic non-small-cell lung cancer (KEYNOTE-042): A randomised, open-label, controlled, phase 3 trial. *Lancet.* 2019;393(10183):1819–1830. doi:10.1016/S0140-6736(18)32409-7
76. Dietel M, Savelov N, Salanova R, et al. Real-world prevalence of programmed death ligand 1 expression in locally advanced or metastatic non-small-cell lung cancer: The global, multicenter EXPRESS study. *Lung Cancer.* 2019;134:174–179. doi:10.1016/j.lungcan.2019.06.012
77. Peng L, Liang WH, Mu DG, et al. First-line treatment options for PD-L1–negative non-small cell lung cancer: A Bayesian network meta-analysis. *Front Oncol.* 2021;11:2371. doi:10.3389/fonc.2021.657545
78. Sandler A, Gray R, Perry MC, et al. Paclitaxel-carboplatin alone or with bevacizumab for non-small-cell lung cancer. *N Engl J Med.* 2006;355(24):2542–2550. doi:10.1056/NEJMoa061884
79. Bodor JN, Boumber Y, Borghaei H. Biomarkers for immune checkpoint inhibition in non-small cell lung cancer (NSCLC). *Cancer.* 2020;126(2):260–270. doi:10.1002/cncr.32468
80. Lee CK, Man J, Lord S, et al. Checkpoint inhibitors in metastatic EGFR-mutated non-small cell lung cancer-a meta-analysis. *J Thorac Oncol.* 2017;12(2):403–407. doi:10.1016/j.jtho.2016.10.007
81. Calles A, Riess JW, Brahmer JR. Checkpoint blockade in lung cancer with driver mutation: Choose the road wisely. *Am Soc Clin Oncol Educ Book.* Published online May 18, 2020. doi:10.1200/EDBK_280795
82. Socinski MA, Nishio M, Jotte RM, et al. IMpower150 final overall survival analyses for atezolizumab plus bevacizumab and chemotherapy in first-line metastatic nonsquamous NSCLC. *J Thorac Oncol.* Published online July 2021:S1556086421023224. doi:10.1016/j.jtho.2021.07.009
83. Ramos-Esquivel A, van der Laat A, Rojas-Vigott R, Juárez M, Corrales-Rodríguez L. Anti-PD-1/anti-PD-L1 immunotherapy versus

docetaxel for previously treated advanced non-small cell lung cancer: A systematic review and meta-analysis of randomised clinical trials. *ESMO Open*. 2017;2(3):e000236. doi:10.1136/esmoopen-2017-000236
84. Shepherd FA, Dancey J, Ramlau R, et al. Prospective randomized trial of docetaxel versus best supportive care in patients with non-small-cell lung cancer previously treated with platinum-based chemotherapy. *J Clin Oncol*. 2000;18(10):2095–2103. doi:10.1200/JCO.2000.18.10.2095
85. Garon EB, Ciuleanu TE, Arrieta O, et al. Ramucirumab plus docetaxel versus placebo plus docetaxel for second-line treatment of stage IV non-small-cell lung cancer after disease progression on platinum-based therapy (REVEL): A multicentre, double-blind, randomised phase 3 trial. *Lancet*. 2014;384(9944):665–673. doi:10.1016/S0140-6736(14)60845-X
86. Hanna N, Shepherd FA, Fossella FV, et al. Randomized phase III trial of pemetrexed versus docetaxel in patients with non-small-cell lung cancer previously treated with chemotherapy. *J Clin Oncol*. 2004;22(9):1589–1597. doi:10.1200/JCO.2004.08.163
87. Borghaei H, Paz-Ares L, Horn L, et al. Nivolumab versus docetaxel in advanced nonsquamous non-small-cell lung cancer. *N Engl J Med*. 2015;373(17):1627–1639. doi:10.1056/NEJMoa1507643
88. Ramalingam SS, Dahlberg SE, Langer CJ, et al. Outcomes for elderly, advanced-stage non small-cell lung cancer patients treated with bevacizumab in combination with carboplatin and paclitaxel: Analysis of Eastern Cooperative Oncology Group Trial 4599. *J Clin Oncol Off J Am Soc Clin Oncol*. 2008;26(1):60–65. doi:10.1200/JCO.2007.13.1144
89. Goffin J, Lacchetti C, Ellis PM, et al. First-line systemic chemotherapy in the treatment of advanced non-small cell lung cancer: Asystematic review. *J Thorac Oncol*. 2010;5(2):260–274. doi:10.1097/JTO.0b013e3181c6f035
90. Rossi A, Di Maio M, Chiodini P, et al. Carboplatin- or cisplatin-based chemotherapy in first-line treatment of small-cell lung cancer: The COCIS meta-analysis of individual patient data. *J Clin Oncol*. 2012;30(14):1692–1698. doi:10.1200/JCO.2011.40.4905
91. Aupérin A, Arriagada R, Pignon JP, et al. Prophylactic cranial irradiation for patients with small-cell lung cancer in complete remission. Prophylactic Cranial Irradiation Overview Collaborative Group. *N Engl J Med*. 1999;341(7):476–484. doi:10.1056/NEJM199908123410703
92. Horn L, Mansfield AS, Szczęsna A, et al. First-line atezolizumab plus chemotherapy in extensive-stage small-cell lung cancer. *N Engl J Med*. 2018;379(23):2220–2229. doi:10.1056/NEJMoa1809064
93. Paz-Ares L, Dvorkin M, Chen Y, et al. Durvalumab plus platinum-etoposide versus platinum-etoposide in first-line treatment of extensive-stage small-cell lung cancer (CASPIAN): A randomised, controlled, open-label, phase 3 trial. *Lancet*. 2019;394(10212):1929–1939. doi:10.1016/S0140-6736(19)32222-6
94. Slotman BJ, Mauer ME, Bottomley A, et al. Prophylactic cranial irradiation in extensive disease small-cell lung cancer: Short-term health-related quality of life and patient reported symptoms: Results of an international Phase III randomized controlled trial by the EORTC Radiation Oncology and Lung Cancer Groups. *J Clin Oncol*. 2009;27(1):78–84. doi:10.1200/JCO.2008.17.0746
95. von Pawel J, Schiller JH, Shepherd FA, et al. Topotecan versus cyclophosphamide, doxorubicin, and vincristine for the treatment of recurrent small-cell lung cancer. *J Clin Oncol*. 1999;17(2):658–667. doi:10.1200/JCO.1999.17.2.658
96. Eckardt JR, von Pawel J, Pujol JL, et al. Phase III study of oral compared with intravenous topotecan as second-line therapy in small-cell lung cancer. *J Clin Oncol*. 2007;25(15):2086–2092. doi:10.1200/JCO.2006.08.3998
97. Trigo J, Subbiah V, Besse B, et al. Lurbinectedin as second-line treatment for patients with small-cell lung cancer: A single-arm, open-label, phase 2 basket trial. *Lancet Oncol*. 2020;21(5):645–654. doi:10.1016/S1470-2045(20)30068-1
98. Hesketh PJ, Kris MG, Basch E, et al. Antiemetics: American Society of Clinical Oncology clinical practiceguideline update. *J Clin Oncol*. 2017;35(28):3240–3261. doi:10.1200/JCO.2017.74.4789
99. Weiss J, Goldschmidt J, Andric Z, et al. Effects of trilaciclib on chemotherapy-induced myelosuppression and patient-reported outcomes in patients with extensive-stage small cell lung cancer: Pooled results from three phase II randomized, double-blind, placebo-controlled studies. *Clin Lung Cancer*. 2021;22(5):449–460. doi:10.1016/j.cllc.2021.03.010
100. Bozzo A, Deng J, Abbas U, et al. Which bone-modifying agent is associated with better outcomes in patients with skeletal metastases from lung cancer? A systematic review and network meta-analysis. *Clin Orthop Relat Res*. 2021;479(9):2047–2057. doi:10.1097/CORR.0000000000001749
101. Wolchok JD, Hoos A, O'Day S, et al. Guidelines for the evaluation of immune therapy activity in solid tumors: Immune-related response criteria. *Clin Cancer Res*. 2009;15(23):7412–7420. doi:10.1158/1078-0432.CCR-09-1624

153

Colorectal Cancer

Lisa M. Holle, Jessica M. Clement, and Lisa E. Davis

KEY CONCEPTS

1. Advancing age, high-risk adenomatous polyps, inherited and acquired genetic susceptibilities, inflammatory bowel disease, diabetes mellitus, and lifestyle factors are associated with colorectal cancer risk.
2. Regular use of aspirin and other nonsteroidal anti-inflammatory drugs reduces the risk of colorectal cancer, but it is not recommended for routine cancer prevention, nor are any other therapies.
3. Effective colorectal cancer detection programs incorporate routine screening starting at the age of 45 years for average-risk individuals. Colorectal adenomas can progress to cancer and should be removed.
4. The treatment goal for stages I, II, and III colon cancer is cure; surgery should be offered to all eligible patients. Six months of fluoropyrimidine-based adjuvant systemic therapy reduces the risk of cancer recurrence and overall mortality in patients with stage III and select patients with stage II colon cancer; 3 months may be considered in select patients with stage II and III colon cancer. An oxaliplatin-containing regimen further reduces risk as compared with fluoropyrimidine alone in stage III patients.
5. Adverse drug reactions with the most common drugs used in the treatment of colorectal cancer include fluorouracil/capecitabine: palmar-plantar erythrodysesthesia, stomatitis, diarrhea, leukopenia; oxaliplatin: acute and persistent peripheral neuropathies; irinotecan: diarrhea, neutropenia. Deficiencies in dihydropyrmidine dehydrogenase (DPD) and uridine diphosphate-glucuronosyltransferase (UGT1A1) may increase adverse drug reactions with fluorouracil/capecitabine and irinotecan, respectively.
6. Combined modality neoadjuvant therapy consists of fluoropyrimidine-based chemosensitized radiation therapy (XRT) and surgery for patients with stage II or III cancer of the rectum and is considered the standard of care to decrease risk of local and distant disease recurrence.
7. Chemotherapy is palliative for metastatic disease. A fluoropyrimidine with oxaliplatin or irinotecan improves survival compared to fluoropyrimidine monotherapy and should be offered to patients who are candidates for aggressive treatment. The ability for patients to receive all active cytotoxic agents (eg, fluoropyrimidine, oxaliplatin, and irinotecan) during the course of their disease improves their overall survival.
8. Bevacizumab plus fluoropyrimidine-based chemotherapy as initial therapy for metastatic disease is considered standard of care and provides a survival benefit compared with combination chemotherapy alone. Hypertension, proteinuria, and impaired wound healing are common adverse drug reactions.
9. The addition of an epidermal growth factor receptor (EGFR) inhibitor (cetuximab or panitumumab) to initial treatment for *RAS* and *BRAF* wild-type, left-sided advanced or metastatic disease may improve tumor response rates (RRs) and survival. Papulopustular skin rashes, diarrhea, and hypomagnesemia are common, and infusion-related reactions may also occur.
10. Immune checkpoint inhibitors can provide benefit to patients with metastatic colorectal cancer when a deficiency in DNA mismatch-repair (MMR) genes or high microsatellite instability (MSI) is present. These agents are associated with immune-mediated adverse drug reactions.

BEYOND THE BOOK

For each of the available antiangiogenic inhibitor and EGFR inhibitors, describe when in the treatment of colorectal cancer (ie, neoadjuvant, adjuvant, first-line metastatic, second- or greater-line metastatic treatment) it is appropriate to use the drug, including the rationale and whether the drugs within a class are interchangeable. This activity is useful to enhance student understanding of the ASSESS, PLAN, and FOLLOW-UP steps in the patient care process.

INTRODUCTION

Colorectal cancer involves the colon, rectum, and anal canal. It is one of the three most common cancers in adult men and women in the United States.[1] In 2021, an estimated 149,500 new cases were diagnosed, of which 104,270 involves the colon and 45,230 involves the rectum. An additional 9,090 new cases of cancer involve the anus, anal canal, or anorectum. For both adult men and women, colorectal cancer is the third leading cause of cancer-related death in the United States. An estimated 52,980 deaths from cancer of the colon or rectum occurred during 2021.

Colorectal cancer mortality and incidence rates in the United States have decreased steadily over the past two decades. Incidence rates vary worldwide, with the highest incidence rates in countries with a high human development index (HDI).[2] The decline in colorectal cancer mortality rates is likely due to increased screening and/or improved treatments, but mortality rates continue to increase in low-income and middle-income countries in eastern Europe, Asia, and South America.

Multiple factors are associated with the development of colorectal cancer, including inherited susceptibility, lifestyle factors, and certain disease states. About 73% of affected individuals are diagnosed at an early stage of disease, which can potentially be cured with surgery alone or surgery followed by adjuvant XRT, chemotherapy, or both.[3] Five-year survival rates are about 91% for persons with early stages of colon and rectal cancer. Once the tumor has spread regionally to adjacent lymph nodes or tissues, the 5-year survival rate drops to 72% for both colon and rectal cancer. Five-year survival for individuals with metastatic disease is about 15%.

Treatment modalities for colorectal cancer include surgery, XRT, chemotherapy, targeted molecular therapies (eg, angiogenesis inhibitors and EGFR inhibitors), and immune checkpoint inhibitors. Surgery is the definitive procedure associated with cure. XRT can improve curability following surgical resection in rectal cancer and can reduce symptoms and complications associated with advanced disease. Chemotherapy is used in the adjuvant setting to increase cure rates and in treatment for advanced stages of disease to prolong survival. Some patients with metastatic disease who receive aggressive preoperative chemotherapy and targeted therapies experience higher resection rates and can be potentially cured. Much progress has been made in the treatment of advanced disease and the availability of active drug regimens that improve patients' survival.

EPIDEMIOLOGY

Colorectal cancer is the third most common diagnosed malignancy worldwide and the fourth most common cause of cancer-related deaths, accounting for about 1.9 million new cases and 935,000 deaths annually.[2] Although the highest incidence and mortality rates are found in economically developed countries, such as the United States, Australia, New Zealand, and Western Europe, where the HDI is highest, rates have stabilized or are decreasing. This is in contrast to countries with a medium-to-high HDI, such as Eastern Europe, Asia, and South America, where colorectal cancer incidence and mortality rates are increasing rapidly. These increases are believed to be associated with an increased prevalence of risk factors associated with westernization, such as unhealthy diet, obesity, and smoking. The lowest incidence rates are observed in less-developed areas such as sub-Saharan Africa and South Central Asia.

The incidence of invasive colon cancer is greatest among men, who have an age-adjusted incidence rate of 29.1 per 100,000, as compared with women for whom the rate is 24.3 per 100,000.[3] Invasive cancer of the rectum occurs less frequently, with an incidence rate of 14.1 and 9.0 per 100,000 for men and women, respectively. Differences in colorectal cancer incidence exist among ethnic groups in the United States, where incidence is highest among non-Hispanic Black individuals followed by American Indian/Alaska Native individuals, non-Hispanic White individuals, Hispanic individuals, and Asian/Pacific Islander individuals. Cultural and genetic factors as well as disparities in access to healthcare services may influence risk among population groups.

The overall incidence of colon and rectal cancers in the United States has steadily decreased since the mid-1980s, with an annual decline by 3.7% among individuals aged 65 years and older from 2009 to 2018.[3] However, the incidence rate increased by 1% per year in adults between 50 and 64 years of age and in adults younger than 50, the incidence of colorectal cancer increased by 2.2% annually. The incidence of colorectal cancer in adults younger than 55 has been increasing since the mid-1990s, with the most rapid increase in metastatic disease.[4]

Cancer incidence rates have been declining among every broadly defined racial/ethnic group since the mid-1990s, except in American Indian/Alaska Natives, for whom cancer incidence rates remain stable.[3]

Cancer of the colon and rectum accounts for about 8% of all cancer deaths in the United States.[1] The median age for death from cancer of the colon or rectum is 72 years. An estimated 52,980 individuals died of colorectal cancer in the United States in 2021, which represents a continued decline in overall combined mortality for both colon and rectal cancer. Overall mortality rates are highest among non-Hispanic Black individuals, although a steep rate of decline began in the late 1990s.[3] Colorectal cancer death rates are decreasing among all ethnic groups, but mortality rates are not lower in American Indian/Alaska Native individuals. Factors contributing to the overall decline in colorectal cancer mortality include decreasing incidence rates, screening programs with early polyp removal, and more effective and better tolerated treatments. Differences among different world geographic regions, and in population groups in the United States, may also reflect more unfavorable tumor characteristics, late stage at diagnosis, decreased access to screening programs, comorbidities, and lower availability or utilization of effective treatments.

ETIOLOGY AND RISK FACTORS

The development of colorectal cancer is related to both uncontrollable and modifiable risk factors. Age, family history, and clinical and genetic susceptibilities cannot be controlled by individuals. Modifiable lifestyle factors are responsible for more than half of the colorectal cancers.[4,5]

Personal Medical History

Age

1 An individual's risk of developing cancer of the colon or rectum increases with advancing age, rising progressively after age 50.[4] The median age at colon cancer diagnosis is 67 years in men and 71 years in women and 62 years in men and 63 years in women for rectal cancer. The proportion of individuals diagnosed with colorectal cancer who were younger than 50 increased from 6% to 11% between 1990 and 2013, with the majority of cases diagnosed in adults in their 40s.[3] The increase in colorectal cancer incidence in younger adults may reflect trends in obesity and detrimental lifestyle factors, but the role of modifiable and non-modifiable risk factors in early-onset colorectal cancer remains unclear.

Adenomatous Polyps or Colorectal Cancer

A prior history of high-risk adenomatous polyps, particularly multiple adenomas or size 1 to 2 cm or more, is associated with an increased risk of colorectal cancer.[4,5] Individuals with a prior diagnosis of colon or rectal cancer have a greater risk of developing a new malignancy at another area in their colon or rectum as compared to individuals without a prior history of colorectal cancer.

Inflammatory Bowel Disease

Individuals with chronic inflammatory bowel disease, such as ulcerative colitis or Crohn's disease, have about a twofold greater risk of developing colorectal cancer than the average individual.[4-6] This risk rises with increasing extent, duration, and severity of disease, a familial history of colorectal cancer, and coexistent primary sclerosing cholangitis. Persons diagnosed with chronic inflammatory bowel disease constitute about 1% to 2% of all new cases of colorectal cancer each year.

Diabetes Mellitus

Individuals with type 2 diabetes mellitus have an increased risk of developing colorectal cancer, independent of body mass size and physical activity level. Epidemiologic studies show that diabetes is associated with 26% to 53% increase in risk of colorectal cancer, as well as a higher risk of colorectal cancer-related and all-cause mortality.[7] Metformin use may improve survival outcomes in patients with colorectal cancer and diabetes, but further study is needed.

Family History and Inherited Genetic Risk

Colorectal Cancer or Adenomatous Polyps

Three specific patterns of colon cancer occurrence are generally observed: sporadic, familial, and recognized hereditary syndromes. Although most cases of colorectal cancer are sporadic in nature, about 30% of patients who develop colorectal cancer will have a family history of colorectal cancer that is not associated with an inherited syndrome.[4,5] First-degree relatives of patients diagnosed with colorectal cancer have an increased risk of the disease (two times the risk), which is higher if the relative was diagnosed at age 45 or younger (three to six times higher). Similarly, parents and siblings of relatives diagnosed with adenomatous polyps are at increased risk for developing colorectal cancer.

Hereditary Syndromes

Colorectal cancer is a consequence of several well-defined genetic syndromes.[4,5] The two most common forms of hereditary colon cancer are familial adenomatous polyposis (FAP) and Lynch syndrome, historically known as *hereditary nonpolyposis colorectal cancer* (HNPCC). Both forms result from a specific germline mutation. FAP is a rare autosomal dominant trait caused by inactivating mutations of the adenomatous polyposis coli (*APC*) gene and accounts for about 1% of all colorectal cancers. The disease is manifested by hundreds to thousands of tiny sessile adenomatous polyps that carpet the colon and rectum, typically arising during adolescence. The polyps continue to proliferate throughout the colon, with eventual transformation to malignancy. The risk of developing colorectal cancer for individuals with untreated FAP is virtually 100%; most will develop colorectal cancer by the fourth and fifth decades of life.

Lynch syndrome is an autosomal dominant inherited syndrome and is the most common hereditary predisposition for colorectal cancer.[4,5] Patients with Lynch syndrome are predisposed to many types of cancer (eg, endometrial, stomach, and ovarian), but the risk of colorectal cancer is the highest.[4] Germline mutations in one of the DNA mismatch-repair (MMR) genes, most commonly *MLH1*, *MSH2*, *MSH6*, or *PMS2*, or rarely, epithelial cell adhesion molecule (*EpCAM*), are responsible for Lynch syndrome, which accounts for 3% to 5% of overall colorectal cancer cases.[4,8] The estimated lifetime risk of developing colorectal cancer for carriers of germline MMR mutations is about 13% to 57%, depending on the specific affected gene.[8] Multiple generations within a family are affected, and colorectal cancer develops early in life, with a mean age at the time of diagnosis of about 44 to 61 years.[5] If Lynch syndrome is suspected in a patient diagnosed with colorectal cancer, typically due to early age at diagnosis or family cancer history, the tumor is examined for evidence of deficient MMR to distinguish between sporadic or germline genetic mutations. Clinicians should identify carriers of these MMR mutations so that they can be counseled and followed appropriately.[4,8]

Lifestyle Factors

Nonsteroidal Anti-inflammatory Drug and Aspirin Use

2 Several lifestyle factors influence colorectal cancer risk (Table 153-1). Regular (at least two doses/week) nonsteroidal anti-inflammatory drug (NSAID) and aspirin use is associated with a reduced risk of colorectal cancer. In an average-risk individual, regular aspirin use is associated with a 20% to 40% reduction in the risk of colorectal adenoma and colorectal cancer.[9]

Benefit is also seen with NSAID and cyclooxygenase-2 inhibitor (COX-2) use. NSAID use over a 10- to 15-year period is associated with protection against adenomas and colorectal cancer, with a 30% to 45% reduction in the risk of colorectal cancer.[9] The protective effects of these agents are related to their inhibition of COX-2, which is overexpressed and elevated in up to 50% of colorectal adenomas and 85% of sporadic colon carcinomas.[10] Inhibition of COX-2 also downregulates the phosphatidylinositol 3-kinase (PI3K) signaling pathway, which plays an important role in carcinogenesis and cancer cell resistance to apoptosis.[11]

TABLE 153-1 Lifestyle Factors Associated with Colorectal Cancer Risk

Factor	Comments
Elevated Risk	
Physical inactivity	Sedentary lifestyle associated with a 25%-50% increased risk of colorectal cancer compared with the risk in physically active individuals
Obesity	Elevated BMI, waist circumference, and waist-to-hip ratio directly associated with increased cancer risk
Alcohol intake	Moderate and heavy alcohol consumption associated with 20% or greater cancer risk compared to light drinking (<1 drink/day)
Smoking	Prolonged tobacco smoking increases risk of large adenomas and carcinoma; higher colorectal cancer mortality in current smokers; risk persists after smoking cessation
Western diet	High red meat, processed meat, and saturated fat dietary consumption increases cancer risk; cancer risk lower with diets high in whole fiber grains and cereals, fruits, and vegetables
Reduced Risk	
Aspirin and non-aspirin NSAID use	Regular aspirin or NSAID use associated with 20%-45% reduction in adenoma recurrence and colorectal cancer risk. Benefit in risk reduction may require at least 5-10 years of use
Postmenopausal hormone use	Exogenous hormone intake decreases the risk of adenomas, colon, and rectal cancer by about 35%
Calcium and vitamin D intake	Vitamin D 400 international units and calcium intake of 1,000 mg/day (adults <50 years) or 1,200 mg/day (adults >50 years) may help reduce colorectal cancer risk but data remain unclear

BMI, body mass index.

Postmenopausal Hormone Replacement Therapy

Exogenous postmenopausal oral hormone replacement therapy is associated with a significant reduction in colorectal cancer risk.[9,12] Risk reduction is seen in postmenopausal individuals receiving combined estrogen and progestin therapy and persists for about 10 years after therapy is discontinued. However, because of the harmful risks associated with postmenopausal hormone replacement therapy, its use is not recommended to prevent colorectal cancer.

Obesity and Physical Inactivity

1 Physical inactivity and elevated BMI are associated with an elevated risk of colon adenoma, colon cancer, and rectal cancer.[4,5,9] Compared to physically active individuals, physically inactive people have up to a 50% higher risk of developing colorectal cancer.[5]

Elevated BMI and higher general and abdominal body fatness are risk factors for colorectal cancer in adults, although the associations are weaker and less consistent for women.[4] The risk of colon cancer is about 50% higher in obese men, who also have a 25% higher risk of rectal cancer as compared to men of normal body weight. Obese women have about 10% increased risk of colon cancer, and even a higher body weight within the normal range appears to be associated with an increased risk of early onset colorectal cancer.

The relationship between physical inactivity and cancer risk is incompletely understood, but may be related to oxidative stress and immune dysfunction.[13] Obesity promotes insulin resistance, chronic inflammation, elevated insulin-like growth factor-1 levels, and altered levels of circulating sex hormones, which can contribute to tumorigenesis.[5,13]

Alcohol and Tobacco Use

1 Moderate and heavy alcohol consumption is a major risk factor for colorectal adenomas and colorectal cancer.[4,5,14] Individuals with an intake of two to three alcoholic beverages per day have a 21% higher risk of developing colorectal cancer, and heavier drinking further increases cancer risk.[4,14] This association is stronger in men than in women, perhaps due to differences in drinking patterns or alcohol metabolism.

An estimated 12% of colorectal cancer deaths are attributed to cigarette smoking.[4,5] Cigarette smoking is associated with an increased risk of colorectal cancer (about 38% and 18% in current and former smokers, respectively) and mortality than in nonsmokers.[15] The risk of colorectal cancer development increases with longer duration of smoking and number of cigarettes consumed daily, and persists after smoking cessation.

Gut Microbiota

The gut microbiota could play an important role in the development of colorectal adenomas and adenoma progression to colorectal cancer.[4,5] The gut microbiome is involved in absorption and metabolism of nutrients, drug metabolism, elimination of xenobiotics, and immune cell function.[5] Certain bacterial species, such as *Fusobacterium nucleatum* and *Bacteroides fragilis*, produce bacterial metabolites that promote and sustain local inflammation, cause DNA damage, alter the immune response, and affect pro-tumorigenic cell signaling pathways.[16] Factors that alter the composition and function of normal gut microbiota, such as diet, lifestyle, obesity, and drug therapy (eg, antimicrobials, antacids, and proton pump inhibitors), may be associated with increased risk of colorectal cancer.

Dietary Intake and Nutrients

1 Epidemiologic studies of worldwide incidence of colorectal cancer suggest economic development and dietary habits strongly influence its development. Dietary characteristics of economically developed countries and increased colorectal cancer risk include higher intake of red and processed meat, fat, and refined grains, and a lower intake of fruit, vegetables, and whole grains.

Many large epidemiologic studies have identified a positive association of a high consumption of red and processed meat with the risk of developing colorectal cancer.[4,5] Potential underlying mechanisms for this association include carcinogenic chemicals formed during the cooking process or the presence of specific fatty acids in red meat.[5] Processed meat products may increase exposure to carcinogenic nitrates and *N*-nitroso compounds.[5]

Worldwide, high-fiber dietary patterns have been associated with a low incidence of colorectal cancer.[2,5,9] Foods that are high in fiber include fruit, vegetables, whole grains, and cereals. Fruit and vegetables are rich in soluble fiber, vitamins, minerals, flavonoids, and other micronutrients that may be protective for colorectal cancer risk. However, the role of dietary fiber with regard to amount, source, and type and colorectal cancer risk has not been defined.

Dietary and supplemental calcium consumption is associated with a decreased risk of adenomas and colorectal cancer.[2,4,5,17] The protective effects of calcium may be due to antiproliferative, proapoptotic actions, and reduced colonic epithelial cell exposure to mutagens.[5,9] High levels of circulating 25-hydroxyvitamin D_3 are also associated with a reduced risk of colorectal cancer.[4,5,18] Vitamin D has antiproliferative, anti-inflammatory, and immune regulatory effects.[5,9,18] Vitamin D and calcium appear to interact synergistically to protect against adenoma recurrence and colorectal cancer, but large clinical trials have yet to confirm that supplementation with calcium and vitamin D in individuals with adequate dietary calcium and vitamin D intake reduces colorectal cancer risk.[4,5,9]

An association between folate intake through diet or supplements and colorectal cancer is complex, as data have shown both protective and tumor promoting effects.[4,9,19] However, the underlying basis for this is complex, particularly because alcohol use, smoking, genetic variants of the *methylenetetrahydrofolate reductase* gene, and other factors can interfere with folate metabolism. Thus, an adequate dietary folate intake may be enough to lower the risk of colorectal cancer, and exceeding normal intake may not be beneficial.

Deficiencies in other dietary micronutrients and antioxidants, including vitamin B_6, selenium, vitamin C, vitamin E, and carotenoids, may increase colorectal cancer risk, but there is no convincing evidence that the risk of colorectal cancer is greater in patients with low serum levels than in patients with adequate levels.[17,19]

PATHOPHYSIOLOGY

Anatomy and Bowel Function

The large intestine consists of the cecum; the ascending, transverse, descending, and sigmoid colon; and the rectum (Fig. 153-1). In adults, it extends about 1.5 m and has a diameter ranging from 8 cm in the cecum to 2 cm in the sigmoid colon. Absorption of fluid and solutes occurs in the right colon or the segments proximal to the middle of the transverse colon, with movement and storage of fecal material in the left colon and distal segments of the colon. Mucus secretion from goblet cells into the intestinal lumen lubricates the mucosal surface and facilitates movement of the dehydrated feces. It also serves to protect the luminal wall from bacteria and colonic irritants such as bile acids.

Four major tissue layers, from the lumen outward, form the large intestine: the mucosa, submucosa, muscularis propria, and serosa (Fig. 153-2). Embedded in the submucosa and muscularis propria is a rich lymphatic capillary system. Lymphatic channels do not extend into the mucosa. The muscularis propria consists of circular smooth muscle and outer longitudinal smooth muscle bands. Contraction of these muscle groups moves colonic material toward the anal canal. The outermost layer of the colon, the serosa, secretes a fluid that allows the colon to slide easily over nearby structures within the peritoneum. The serosa covers only the anterior and lateral aspects of the upper third of the rectum. The lower third lies completely extraperitoneal and is surrounded by fibrofatty tissue as well as adjacent organs and structures.

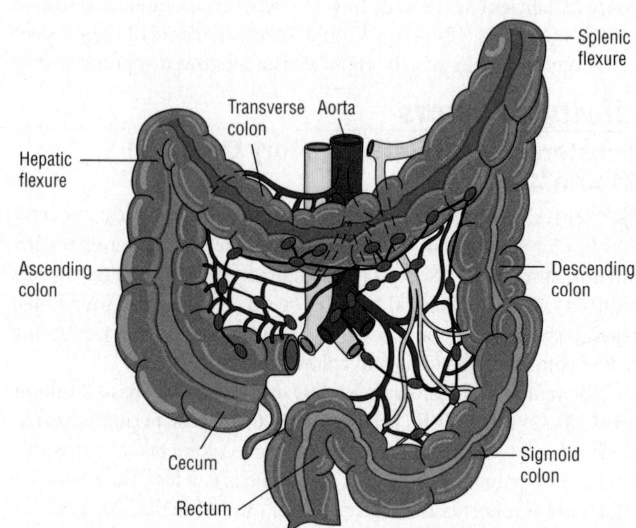

FIGURE 153-1 Colon and rectum anatomy.

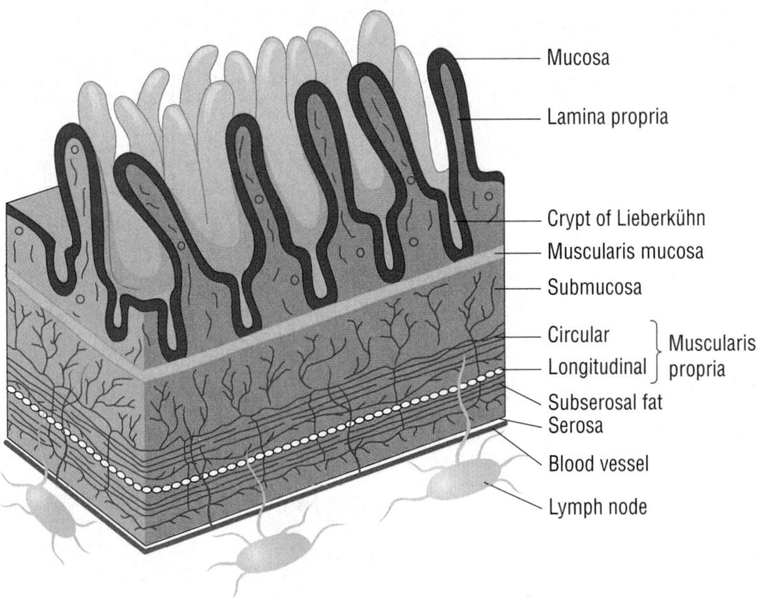

FIGURE 153-2 Cross-section of bowel wall.

The surface epithelium of the colonic mucosa undergoes continual renewal, and complete replacement of epithelial cells occurs every 4 to 8 days. Cell replication normally takes place within the lower third of the crypts, the tubular glands located within the intestinal mucosa. The cells then mature and differentiate to either goblet or absorptive cells as they migrate toward the bowel lumen. The total number of epithelial cells remains relatively constant as the number of cells migrating from the crypts is balanced by the rate of exfoliation of cells from the mucosal surface. This two-phase process is critical to the malignant transformation of the epithelial cells. The number of dysplastic and hyperplastic aberrant crypt foci increases with increasing age; as the mass of abnormal cells accumulates at the top of the crypt and starts to protrude into the stream of fecal matter, their contact with fecal mutagens can lead to further cell mutations and eventual adenoma formation.

Colorectal Tumorigenesis

The development of a colorectal neoplasm is a multistep process involving several genetic and phenotypic alterations of normal bowel epithelium structure and function, leading to dysregulated cell growth, proliferation, and tumor development. Because most colorectal cancers develop sporadically, with no inherited or familial disposition, efforts have been directed toward identifying these alterations and learning whether detection of such changes may lead to improved cancer detection or treatment outcomes.

Features of colorectal tumorigenesis include genomic instability, activation of oncogene pathways, mutational inactivation or silencing of tumor-suppressor genes, genes associated with DNA repair, and activation of growth factor pathways.[20] During the early stages of tumorigenesis, emerging tumor cells expressing tumor antigens are eliminated by the immune system, which serves as an initial barrier to cancer progression.[21] These cells eventually escape immune surveillance as the tumor microenvironment becomes progressively immunosuppressive.

Genetic models have been proposed for colorectal tumorigenesis that describe a process of transformation from adenoma to carcinoma (Fig. 153-3).[20,22,23] The adenoma to carcinoma sequence of tumor development reflects an accumulation of mutations within colonic epithelium that confers a selective growth advantage to the affected cells. Key elements of this process include hyperproliferation of epithelial cells to form a small benign neoplasm or adenoma in conjunction with acquisition of various genetic mutations and epigenetic alterations that promote transformation to adenocarcinoma.[5,20,22]

Two discrete adenoma to carcinoma progression sequences have been described, a traditional adenoma-carcinoma pathway (referred to as the chromosomal instability pathway) and the serrated neoplasia pathway.[5,22] Although both pathways share several genetic alterations, each has unique molecular and phenotypic characteristics. Table 153-2 lists important genetic mutations that are associated with colorectal cancers.[20,22,23]

Genomic Instability

Genomic instability is a hallmark of colorectal carcinogenesis, and presents as chromosomal instability (CIN) or MSI.[20] Three molecular pathways that lead to genomic instability are CIN, MSI, and CpG island methylator phenotype (CIMP) pathways. The CIN pathway accounts for about 85% of colorectal cancers, and typically follows genomic events initiated by a sporadic APC mutation, with subsequent activation of *RAS* or loss of *P53*.[22] Features of CIN include a high frequency of gene DNA amplifications/gains or deletions/losses and copy number alterations. Important consequences of CIN include imbalanced chromosome number (aneuploidy), chromosomal gene amplification, and loss of a wild-type allele of a tumor-suppressor gene, also referred to as loss of heterozygosity (LOH).

Up to 15% of colorectal cancers arise though the MSI pathway, which is caused by a disruption of DNA repair genes.[22] Microsatellites are a series of repeat nucleotide sequences that are spread out across the entire genome. Microsatellite replication errors within tumor DNA occur frequently, and mutations of the MMR genes that recognize and regulate DNA MMR errors contribute to MSI and colorectal tumorigenesis. Mutations in MMR genes can be inherited or developed by somatic causes. Germline mutation of MMR genes is an important characteristic of Lynch syndrome.

Alterations in gene expression or function in the absence of DNA sequence alterations are referred to as epigenetic changes, and these are usually due to methylation of DNA gene promoter regions or histone modifications.[22] The serrated neoplasia pathway

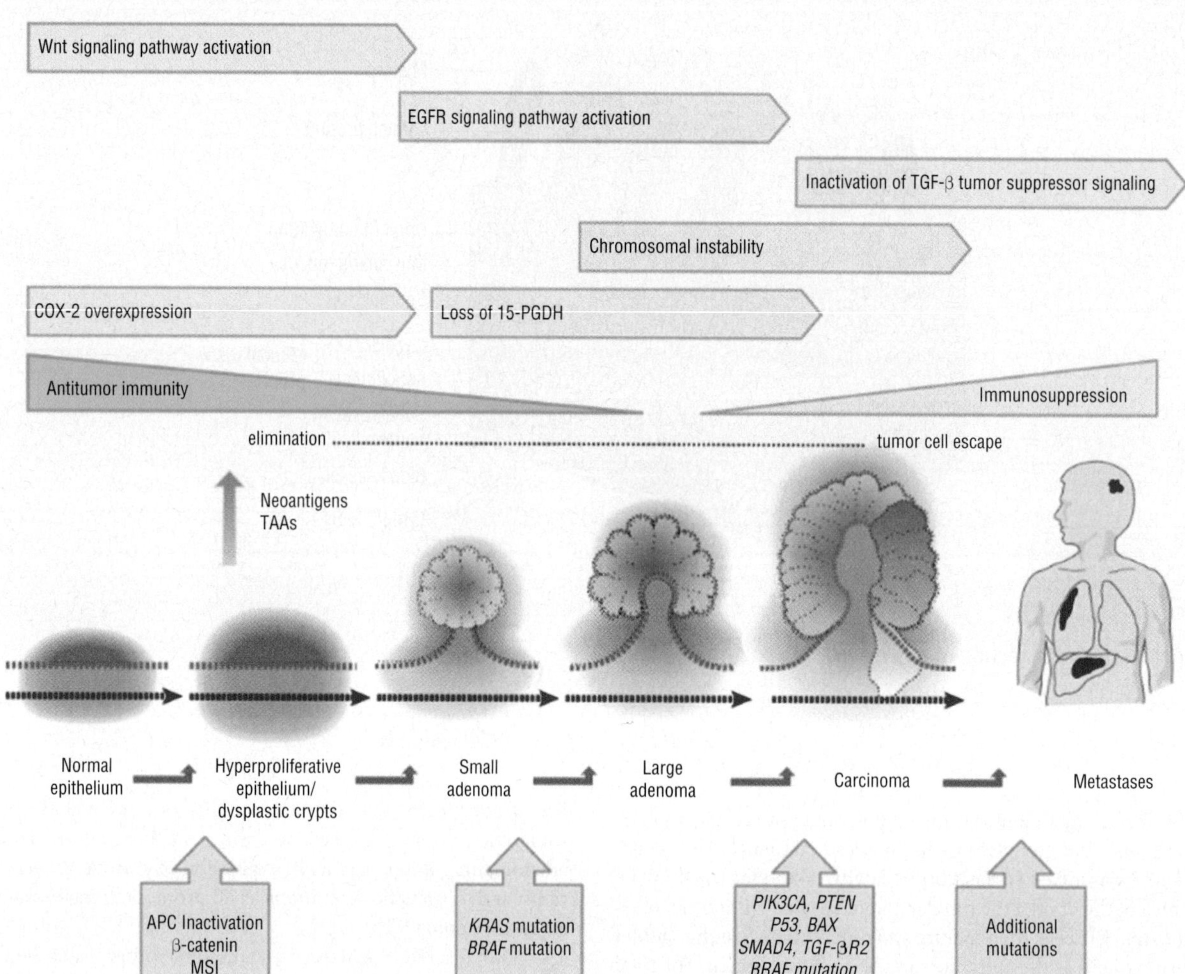

FIGURE 153-3 Genetic changes associated with the adenoma–carcinoma sequence in colorectal cancer. The accumulation of genetic changes in the pathogenesis of colorectal cancer includes initiated by aberrant DNA methylation or MMR gene mutation with subsequent disruption in transforming growth factor-β receptor type II (TGF-β2R) and BAX signaling; mutation in the *APC* gene or abnormalities in β-catenin leading to inappropriate activation of the Wnt signaling pathway; mutational activation of COX-2 and impaired prostaglandin degradation from loss of 15-prostaglandin dehydrogenase (15-PGDH); *KRAS, PIK3CA,* or *BRAF* oncogene activation; increased EGFR signaling; and deletions or mutations of tumor suppressor genes *SMAD4, PTEN, P53.* Chromosomal instability (CIN) is a common feature of sporadic disease, but causative factors are not defined. Tumor-associated antigens (TAAs) expressed by emerging tumor cells are eliminated by the immune system during early tumorigenesis but eventually escape immune surveillance. The sequence of molecular events may differ between somatic and inherited genetic alterations. *(Data from References 20,22, and 23.)*

(also referred to as the CIMP pathway) can lead to microsatellite stable and instable cancers. It accounts for 10%-20% of colorectal cancers, and is associated with epigenetic instability, *RAS* and *RAF* mutations. CIMP is characterized by hypermethylation of a panel of multiple genes that are associated with gene silencing and subsequent loss of tumor suppressor gene function.[5]

Growth Factor Signaling Pathways

Aberrant signaling of growth factor pathways plays an important role in colorectal tumorigenesis. Activation of prostaglandin signaling is an early step in the adenoma to carcinoma transformation process and is induced by upregulated expression of COX-2 and inflammation.[24] COX-2 mediates the synthesis of prostaglandin E2, which stimulates cancer growth. Furthermore, 80% of colorectal cancers have loss of 15-prostaglandin dehydrogenase, or 15-PGDH, the rate-limiting enzyme responsible for prostaglandin degradation. Dysregulated intracellular signal transduction from EGFR, a transmembrane glycoprotein involved in signaling pathways that affects cell growth, differentiation, proliferation, and angiogenesis, plays a key role in colorectal cancer pathogenesis and immune evasion in colorectal cancer. *EGFR* activation enables downstream signaling through the mitogen-activated protein kinase (MAPK)/RAS/RAF/MEK/ERK and PI3K/AKt/mTOR pathways, thereby promoting tumor differentiation, proliferation, progression, and survival.[22,24] EGFR is overexpressed in most colorectal cancers and high tumor EGFR overexpression is associated with a worse prognosis.[24] These mechanisms are relevant because of the availability of pharmacologic agents that can influence these signaling pathways and affect cell growth.

Oncogene and Tumor Suppressor Gene Alterations

Mutation or loss of the *APC* tumor suppressor gene is a key factor involved in tumor formation through constitutive activation of

TABLE 153-2 Genetic Mutations Associated with Colorectal Cancer

Type of Mutation	Disease	Genes	Comments
Germline	FAP	*APC*	Multiple adenomas and carcinomas in colon and rectum
	MYH-associated polyposis	*MYH*	Autosomal recessive syndrome; wide spectrum of degree of polyposis; frequent *KRAS* mutations
	Lynch syndrome	DNA MMR genes: *MSH2, MLH1, MSH6, PMS2, EpCAM*	Colorectal cancer in the absence of extensive polyposis; predisposition for endometrial, ovarian, gastric, hepatobiliary, urothelial, pancreatic, brain, and skin cancers
Somatic	Sporadic colorectal cancer	Oncogenes	
		KRAS	Mutations found in about 30%-50% of cancers
		NRAS	Mutations found in <5% of cancers
		BRAF	*BRAF* V600E mutation found in 5%-15% of cancers
		PIK3CA	Activating mutations found in 10%-20% of cancers
		EGFR	Gene upregulation in 30%-70% of cancers
		c-MYC	Elevated expression in 70%-80% with gene amplification/rearrangement in 10%-30% of cancers
		ERBB2 (known as HER2)	Gene amplification or mutation in 2%-7% of cancers
		SRC	Gene deregulated in up to 80% of cancers
		Tumor suppressor genes	
		P53	Loss or mutation in up to 60% of cancers
		SMAD4	Mutations in 3%-18% of cancers
		APC	Inactivated in up to 80% of sporadic cancers
		TGF-βR2	Inactivating mutations present in 20% of cancers; mutations in more than 90% of cancers with MSI
		PTEN	Frequency of inactivating mutations about 10% but loss of PTEN protein expression evident in 15%-20% of cancers

HER-2, human epidermal growth factor receptor 2; TGF-βR2, transforming growth factor-β receptor type II.

Data from References 20, 22, and 23.

the Wnt signaling pathway, a mediator of cell-cycle progression, cell proliferation, differentiation, and apoptosis.[22] The *APC* gene encodes for APC protein that binds to and degrades cytoplasmic β-catenin, a downstream component of the Wnt signaling pathway. Inactivation of the *APC* gene is the single gene defect responsible for FAP and is frequently an initiating event in sporadic colorectal cancer.

Mutational inactivation of *P53* represents a frequent and key step in colorectal tumorigenesis, occurring in the majority of colorectal cancers.[22] Normal *P53* gene expression is important for G_1 cell-cycle arrest to facilitate DNA repair during replication and to induce apoptosis. An additional step in tumor progression is the mutational inactivation of the transforming growth factor-β (TGF-β) signaling pathway, which facilitates adenoma transition to high-grade dysplasia or carcinoma and also inactivates *SMAD4*. In normal epithelium, TGF-β has an antiproliferative role and induces growth arrest and apoptosis. Alterations in *SMAD4* or TGF-β receptors lead to a loss of the normal growth inhibitory response to TGF-β.

Several oncogene-activating mutations play an important role in promoting colorectal cancer.[22] Mutations in members of the *RAS* gene family—*KRAS, HRAS,* and *NRAS*—in addition to *BRAF*, activate the MAPK signaling pathway, which stimulates cell proliferation and other activities that promote carcinogenesis. *HER2* gene amplification/overexpression occurs infrequently in colorectal cancer, although *RAS* and *BRAF* wild-type tumors have a greater likelihood of having HER2 overexpression.[24] Mutations of *PIK3CA*, which encodes the catalytic subunit of the PI3K survival pathway, increase production of phosphatidylinositol-3,4,5-triphosphate, which influences cell growth, proliferation, and survival. Mutation or loss of *PTEN*, a tumor suppressor gene that antagonizes PI3K signaling, produces similar effects. Multiple additional genetic alterations contribute to carcinoma formation and metastases by altering cellular growth, metabolism, migration, and invasive capabilities, and angiogenesis.[22,24]

Histology

Adenocarcinomas account for about 92% of tumors of the large intestine and about 7% are classified mucinous adenocarcinoma.[4] The other histologic types, such as signet-ring adenocarcinoma, squamous cell carcinoma, and neuroendocrine carcinomas, are rare. Adenocarcinomas are assigned one of the three tumor grade designations based on the degree of cellular differentiation, the degree to which the tumor resembles the structure, and the function of its cell of origin. The most differentiated adenocarcinomas are low-grade tumors, whereas high-grade tumors are the most undifferentiated, and have frequently lost the characteristics of mature normal cells. Poorly differentiated tumors are associated with a worse prognosis than those that are relatively better differentiated.

Mucinous adenocarcinomas possess the same basic structure as adenocarcinomas but differ in that they secrete an abundant quantity of extracellular mucus. They tend to be frequent in patients with MMR tumor mutations. Signet-ring adenocarcinomas also have a characteristic appearance but are uncommon. Signet-ring histology occurs more frequently in individuals younger than 50 years of age, patients with ulcerative colitis, and tends to be present at a more advanced stage of disease at diagnosis. Both mucinous and signet-ring adenocarcinoma histologies confer a poor prognosis. Patients with neuroendocrine tumors and squamous cell carcinoma often present with distant metastases and also have a poor prognosis.

PREVENTION AND SCREENING

Cancer prevention efforts can be either primary or secondary. Primary prevention strategies aim to prevent the development of colorectal cancer in a population at risk. Secondary prevention approaches are undertaken to prevent malignancy in a population that has already manifested an initial disease process.

Chemoprevention

2 Several agents have been evaluated as chemoprevention strategies for colorectal cancer, including prospective population-based screening trials of dietary fiber intake, and randomized controlled trials of calcium, vitamin D, and folate supplementation.[25-27] However, findings do not support their use now. Additional intervention trials of various micronutrients, epigenetic modulators, and other chemopreventive agents have been completed or are ongoing.[9,21,26,28-30] In addition, the most widely studied agents for the chemoprevention of colorectal cancer are aspirin, non-aspirin NSAIDs, and COX-2 selective inhibitors, but only aspirin is recommended for chemoprevention in some patients.[10,27,29] The effectiveness of these agents has been studied in high-risk individuals and within the general population.

In individuals with FAP, celecoxib, NSAIDs, and aspirin have been studied to delay the development of adenomatous polyps and to reduce polyp recurrence following colectomy with a retained rectum, but they are not viewed as alternatives to surgery.[25,26,29] In randomized controlled trials, celecoxib 400 mg orally twice daily as an adjunct to usual care significantly reduced the mean size and number of colorectal polyps after 6 to 9 months of treatment. However, the US Food and Drug Administration (FDA) approval for celecoxib was withdrawn because of lack of data showing long-term benefit. Sulindac induces adenoma regression but does not appear to delay or prevent malignancy. The benefits of these agents are transient because polyps increase in size and number within a few months after discontinuing treatment. These agents may be useful to reduce adenoma recurrence following surgery, but they are not recommended for chemoprevention.

2 Non-aspirin NSAIDs and COX-2 inhibitors reduce the risk of sporadic and recurrent colorectal adenomas in cohort and case-control studies, and COX-2 inhibitors were also effective in controlled trials.[31] Celecoxib is associated with a 34% relative risk reduction in adenoma recurrence and 55% risk reduction in the incidence of advanced adenomas.[29,31] Optimal dosing, agents, and duration of treatment remain to be determined, and cardiovascular events in addition to the risk of gastric ulceration and bleeding with these agents are of concern. Although NSAIDs may be appropriate for selected individuals at high risk for colorectal cancer but low risk for cardiovascular disorders, the US Preventive Services Task Force (USPSTF) has concluded that potential harms associated with NSAID use (other than aspirin) outweigh benefits for prevention of colorectal cancer in the general population.[32]

The use of aspirin as both a primary and a secondary chemopreventive agent remains controversial. In patients with prior adenomas or diagnosis of colorectal cancer, regular daily aspirin use reduces colorectal adenoma recurrence, and colorectal cancer incidence and mortality.[29,30]

Aspirin reduces the risk of sporadic and recurrent adenomas by about 17% and advanced adenomas by 28%.[29,31] Higher aspirin doses reduced the risk of colorectal cancer over a 23-year follow-up period by 26% among the general population, but lower doses (75-300 mg) of daily aspirin for 5 years were also associated with a reduction in the risk of colorectal cancer and in 20-year mortality from colorectal cancer by 34%.[29,30] Individuals with Lynch syndrome who received aspirin 600 mg daily for at least 2 years experienced a 59% reduction in colorectal cancer risk that became evident 5 years after the aspirin was first started and had been discontinued.[29]

Although the optimal aspirin dose and treatment durations are unknown, increasing evidence supports a chemoprotective effect of aspirin in select high-risk individuals and in the general population. The extent of risk reduction appears to be inversely related to the duration of therapy and the chemopreventive effects of aspirin may be delayed by 5 to 10 years. However, the balance of risks and benefits with long-term aspirin use is unclear, and aspirin is only recommended for chemoprevention in some patients. The USPSTF guidelines endorse daily low-dose aspirin for at least 10 years in adults aged 50 to 59 years with a ≥10% 10-year cardiovascular disease risk, a life expectancy of at least 10 years, and who are not at risk for bleeding, for primary prevention of both cardiovascular disease and colorectal cancer.[32] Adults of age 60 to 69 years may also receive low-dose-daily aspirin for at least 10 years if the benefits outweigh the risks, and an individual risk calculation model could be useful to identify those individuals who would benefit most.[33] *PIK3CA* mutations, which are present in up to 20% of colorectal cancers, may also be a useful biomarker.[29] Among aspirin users with a history of colorectal cancer, those with tumor *PIK3CA* mutations experienced longer survival times compared to individuals without *PIK3CA*-mutated tumors.

Randomized controlled trials of calcium, vitamin D, and folate supplementation as chemoprevention have also been conducted, but findings do not support their use now.[28-30] Despite data from epidemiologic and preclinical studies that suggest a benefit from calcium and vitamin D supplementation, data from randomized clinical trials have been inconsistent. Individuals with adequate vitamin D levels and no known increased risk of colorectal cancer do not appear to benefit from calcium or vitamin D supplementation.[29] In two trials, folate supplementation was associated with a nonsignificant increase in adenoma recurrence. Based on these results, the use of folate supplementation to reduce colorectal cancer risk is not recommended now.[26]

Newer preventive strategies include metformin chemoprevention and gut microbiota modulation using prebiotics, probiotics, and other approaches. Metformin reduced risk of adenoma and colorectal cancer in patients with type 2 diabetes, but definitive randomized clinical trials are needed to establish its effects among populations with different risk.[29] Findings from two randomized, controlled trials of prebiotics and probiotics have shown beneficial alterations in colorectal cancer biomarkers, and further studies are warranted to confirm clinical benefit in colorectal cancer prevention.[34]

Surgical Resection

Surgical resection remains an option to prevent colon cancer in individuals at extremely high risk for its development.[35] Despite the effects of NSAIDs and COX-2 selective inhibitors on adenoma development and recurrence in individuals with FAP, their effects are incomplete, and surgical resection is necessary for cancer prevention for these high-risk individuals. Individuals with FAP who have polyposis on lower endoscopy screening examinations should undergo colectomy or proctocolectomy, typically starting around the age of 20 years. Because of the high incidence of metachronous (ie, consecutive development) cancers (45%) in patients with Lynch syndrome, prophylactic subtotal colectomy is recommended for individuals who are not candidates for routine close follow-up. Colonoscopic polypectomy, removal of polyps detected during screening colonoscopy, is considered the standard of care for all individuals to prevent the progression of premalignant adenomatous polyps to adenocarcinomas.

Screening

Colorectal cancer screening decreases mortality by detecting cancers at an early, curable stage, and by detecting and removing adenomatous polyps. Effectiveness of screening programs relies on participation, which is influenced by test access, costs, risk of complications, technical aspects, expected and perceived burden of the test, and the socioeconomic status and cultural beliefs of the participating individual.[33] Multiple screening recommendations for early detection of colorectal cancer have been established; differences exist in specific screening guidelines published by various organizations.[36-41] Structural (visual) tests detect colorectal polyps and cancer while fecal-based tests detect early cancer. This section reviews available screening techniques for colon and rectal cancer.

Colonoscopy

Colonoscopy facilitates examination of the entire large bowel to the cecum in most patients and allows for simultaneous removal of premalignant lesions. Although no randomized trials show that colonoscopy directly decreases colorectal cancer mortality, observational studies show that screening colonoscopy and polypectomy reduces the incidence in colorectal cancer by about 80%, with a 50% to 60% reduction in colorectal mortality.[25,39] Colonoscopy allows for greater visualization of the colon, but it involves sedation, complete bowel preparation, and is associated with greater risk and inconvenience to patients. Colonoscopy is considered the gold standard for colorectal screening because of its ability to detect and remove lesions in the proximal as well as distal colon.[25,39,42]

Flexible Sigmoidoscopy

Flexible sigmoidoscopy (FSIG) uses a 60-cm flexible sigmoidoscope to examine the lower half of the bowel to the splenic flexure for most patients and is thus capable of detecting 50% to 60% of cancers.[39] According to some randomized trials, FSIG may decrease colorectal cancer incidence and mortality by 23% and 31%, respectively.[36,39] The combination of FSIG and a fecal-based test appears to improve sensitivity for lesions that will be missed by sigmoidoscopy alone, but the true benefit of this approach to general practice has not been established.[39] FSIG offers the advantage of not requiring sedation or extensive bowel preparation, but the entire colon cannot be examined with FSIG and suspicious lesions must be evaluated by colonoscopy.[42]

Computed Tomography Colonography

Computed tomography colonography, also referred to as *virtual colonoscopy*, is an imaging procedure that creates two- or three-dimensional images of the colon by combining multiple helical computed tomography (CT) scans.[36] Sedation is not required and initial tests show high sensitivity and specificity for detecting adenomas of at least 6 mm in size. However, the procedure requires complete bowel preparation and is associated with radiation exposure, and colonoscopy will still be necessary to remove detected lesions.[39,42] Individuals may find this method as a more acceptable option to colonoscopy or sigmoidoscopy, although the insufflation procedure can be associated with some discomfort.[5]

Fecal Occult Blood Tests

Fecal occult blood tests (FOBTs) detect occult blood in the stool that may be associated with bleeding adenomas or cancer. Results from randomized controlled trials of annual FOBT screening show a reduction in colorectal cancer mortality by 33%.[39] Unlike structural tests, FOBTs are noninvasive and do not require bowel preparation. However, they will not detect most polyps and may produce false-positive or false-negative results.[36,39] Two main methods are available to detect occult blood in the feces: guaiac-based FOBT (gFOBT) and fecal immunochemical tests (FITs), also known as immunochemical FOBT. gFOBTs detect pseudoperoxidase activity of heme in human blood. Because gFOBTs detect blood from any sources and some foods affect peroxidase activity, patients are instructed to avoid NSAIDs, red meat, vitamin C, and large amounts of citrus for at least 3 days before and through the testing period.

Several limitations associated with gFOBT screening are of concern. Many early-stage tumors do not bleed, or bleed intermittently, and therefore the false-negative rates can be high and are variable depending on the gFOBT product used. In addition, the test results may not be valid because the test is often poorly performed both in the home and in physician office settings.[36,39] However, these concerns are addressed by testing three successive stool samples. False-positive results can prove to be very expensive and inconvenient for a patient because of the follow-up tests required to confirm a positive result. Annual screening, preferably using a high-sensitivity gFOBT (eg, Hemoccult SENSA), is an acceptable option for individuals at average risk for colorectal cancer. It should be noted that FOBT conducted in conjunction with a digital rectal exam during an office visit is not considered adequate colorectal screening.

FITs were developed to reduce false-positive and false-negative test results associated with the gFOBT. FIT uses antibodies to detect the globin protein portion of human hemoglobin. Since globin is degraded by enzymes in the upper gastrointestinal tract, FIT is more specific for lower gastrointestinal bleeding. Also, no diet or medication restrictions are necessary and testing involves a single stool sample collection annually.[38] FIT is more accurate than gFOBT for detecting cancer and advanced adenomas, although colonoscopy identifies more adenomas.[39,42]

Stool DNA Screening Tests

Molecular screening strategies analyze stool samples for the presence of potential markers of malignancy in cells that are shed from premalignant polyps or adenocarcinomas in the bowel.[36,39] Adenomas and carcinomas can contain certain DNA mutations and markers of MSI that can be detected using multi-target stool DNA (mt-sDNA) testing. A combined FIT and mt-sDNA test is available that has improved sensitivity for advanced adenomas and sessile serrated polyps, but lower specificity compared to FIT.[33,36,39] The optimal appropriate screening interval is unclear, although it may be less frequent than annual FIT.[39] Like other stool-based tests, patients with positive test results should be followed up with a colonoscopy.

Capsule Colonography

Capsule colonography (CapC) is not approved for screening average-risk patients, but it is approved for colorectal imaging in patients who are not candidates for sedation or colonoscopy or who had a previous incomplete colonoscopy.[37,39] This procedure uses a wireless capsule device that is swallowed by the patient to examine the gastrointestinal tract, thereby avoiding risks associated with sedation and colonoscopy.

Serology Test

A *SEPT9* DNA methylated polymerase chain reaction (PCR)-based blood test is approved for colorectal cancer screening but is not recommended in US cancer screening guidelines. Methylated *SEPT9* DNA is a form of the *SEPT9* gene that distinguishes colorectal cancer from normal tissue and is found in circulating plasma with some colorectal cancers.[36] Although the test has low sensitivity for detecting colorectal cancer, it may be an alternative for individuals who refuse to undergo other screening tests.[39]

Screening Summary

3 Table 153-3 shows US screening guidelines for early detection of colorectal cancer with the goal of cancer prevention.[36-41] In recognition of the increasing incidence of colorectal cancer in adults younger than 50 years, the American Cancer Society, the National

TABLE 153-3 Guidelines for Colorectal Cancer Screening in the United States for Individuals at Average Risk, 45-50 Years of Age and Older[a,b]

	ACS	USPSTF	USMSTF	NCCN	ACP	ACG
Fecal-based Tests						
FIT	Annually	Annually	Annually	Annually	Every 2 years	Annually
gFOBT	Annually	Annually	Not recommended	Annually	Every 2 years	Not recommended
mt-sDNA	Every 3 years	Every 1 to 3 years (with FIT)	Every 3 years	Interval uncertain but every 3 years suggested	Not recommended	Every 3 years
Structural (visual) Tests						
Colonoscopy	Every 10 years	Every 10 years	Every 10 years	Every 10 years	Every 10 years	Every 10 years
CTC	Every 5 years	Every 5 years	Every 5 years	Every 5 years	Not recommended	Every 5 years
FSIG	Every 5 years	Every 5 years	Every 5-10 years	Every 5-10 years	Not recommended	Every 5-10 years
Others	------------	FSIG every 10 years + FIT *annually*	CapC every 5 years if patient declines other options	--------------	FSIG every 10 years + FIT every 2 years	CapC every 5 years if patient declines other options

[a]Starting at the age of 45 years (ACS, USPSTF, NCCN).

[b]Starting at the age of 45 years if Black individual (USMSTF).

ACP, American College of Physicians; ACG, American College of Gastroenterology; ACS, American Cancer Society; CapC, capsule colonography; CTC, computed tomography colonography; USMSTF, US Multi-Society Task Force on Colorectal Cancer; USPSTF, US Preventive Services Task Force.

Data from References 36-41.

Comprehensive Cancer Network (NCCN), and the USPSTF recommend initiating colorectal cancer screening for individuals at average risk for colorectal cancer (their only risk factor is age greater than or equal to 45 years) at the age of 45 years.[36,38,39,42] Recommended programs for regular screening include a colonoscopy every 10 years, annually with a high-sensitivity gFOBT or FIT, or an FSIG every 5 years. Recommendations for screening procedures and schedules vary among organizations. The US Multi-Society Task Force on Colorectal Cancer, the American College of Gastroenterology, and the American College of Physicians recommend colorectal cancer screening in adults at average risk beginning at the age of 50 years, except in Black individuals, for whom evidence supports screening starting at the age of 45 years.[37,40,41]

Several screening methods are available, which have the potential to reduce colorectal cancer mortality, and because each method is associated with different benefits and potential harms, patient preferences and available resources should be considered for individual patients.[36,42] More aggressive (usually starting at an earlier age) screening recommendations are given for moderate-to-high risk individuals and colonoscopy is generally preferred for initial screening and surveillance following polyp removal in this population.[5,39] Most organizations recommend discontinuing screening and surveillance in populations when risk may outweigh benefit. Routine colorectal cancer screening is recommended for individuals up to the age of 75 years with a life expectancy ≥10 years, with individualized screening decisions made for individuals aged 76 to 85 years and discontinuing screening in adults older than 85 years.[36-42]

CLINICAL PRESENTATION AND DIAGNOSIS

Signs and Symptoms

The signs and symptoms associated with colorectal cancer can be extremely varied and nonspecific. Patients with early-stage colorectal cancer are often asymptomatic, and lesions are usually found through screening studies. Any change in bowel habits (eg, constipation, diarrhea, alteration in size or shape of stool), abdominal pain, or distension may be warning signs of a malignant process. Obstructive symptoms and changes in bowel habits frequently develop with tumors located in the transverse and descending colon. Rectal cancer may be associated with tenesmus, though bleeding is the most common symptom. Bleeding may be acute or chronic and can appear as bright red blood mixed with stool or melena. Iron-deficiency anemia, presenting as weakness and fatigue, can develop from chronic occult blood loss.

About 20% of patients with colorectal cancer present with metastatic disease.[1] Metastatic spread occurs in the setting of direct tumor invasion of the peritoneum or by lymphatic or hematogenous spread. The venous drainage of the colon and rectum influences the pattern of metastases most commonly seen. The most common site of metastasis is the liver followed by the lungs, and then bones, specifically the sacrum, coccyx, pelvis, and lumbar vertebrae. Liver metastases are present in 25% of patients at presentation, with another 25% to 30% of patients developing liver metastases in the following 2 to 3 years from diagnosis.[43]

Workup

When a patient is suspected of having colorectal carcinoma, a complete history and physical examination should be performed. The patient history should include a past medical history and family history, especially noting the presence of inflammatory bowel disease, colorectal cancer, polyps, and familial clustering of cancers to assess risk for an inherited colorectal cancer syndrome, as well as a full medication history, including prescription, over-the-counter (OTC), and complementary or alternative therapies. A complete physical examination includes careful abdominal examination for the presence of masses or ascites, a rectal examination, and an assessment for possible hepatomegaly and lymphadenopathy. A breast and pelvic examination is recommended in all women.

Evaluation of the entire large bowel requires a total colonoscopy, which allows for tissue collection for histologic evaluation to provide a tissue diagnosis following the procedure. Patients with invasive cancer of the colon or rectum require a complete staging workup, which includes laboratory testing and imaging of the abdomen, pelvis, and chest. Baseline laboratory tests should be obtained and include a complete blood cell count, platelet count, international normalized ratio, prothrombin time, activated partial

CLINICAL PRESENTATION Colorectal Cancer

General

- Patient symptoms are usually nonspecific and can vary drastically among patients.
- Most patients are asymptomatic.

Symptoms

- Change in bowel habits (generally an increase in frequency) or rectal bleeding.
- Constipation, depending on the location of the tumor.
- Nausea, vomiting, and abdominal discomfort.
- Fatigue may be present if anemia is severe.

Signs

- Blood in the stool is the most common sign in symptomatic patients.
- Hepatomegaly and jaundice in advanced disease.
- Leg edema is a consequence of lymph node involvement, thrombophlebitis, fistula formation, weight loss, and pain in the lower back or radiating down the legs may be indicative of widespread disease.

Laboratory Tests

- Positive guaiac stool test and anemia (iron deficiency) from blood loss.
- Elevated carcinoembryonic antigen (CEA; more likely in patients with higher stages at presentation).
- Elevated liver enzymes may be present with metastatic disease.

thromboplastin time, liver chemistries, renal function tests, and CEA level. Abnormal liver chemistry test results may suggest liver involvement with tumor, though normal levels do not preclude metastatic involvement. Iron studies (eg, serum ferritin, serum iron, and total iron-binding capacity) may identify iron deficiency in patients with anemia.

CEA belongs to a group of cell-surface glycoproteins termed *oncofetal proteins*, which are expressed during embryonic development and re-expressed on the cell surfaces of many carcinomas, particularly those originating from the gastrointestinal tract. CEA concentrations can be measured in the blood and can, therefore, potentially serve as a marker for colorectal cancer. Elevated CEA levels are more frequent in patients with metastatic disease, but not all colorectal cancers produce CEA. Several concomitant disease states are associated with an elevated CEA: liver diseases, gastritis, peptic ulcer disease, diverticulitis, chronic obstructive pulmonary disease, chronic or acute inflammatory conditions, and diabetes.[44] Most commercially available assays list a value of less than 5 ng/mL (μg/L) as the upper limit of normal. Although CEA measurement is too insensitive and nonspecific to be used as a screening test for early-stage colorectal cancer, it is the surrogate marker of choice for monitoring colorectal cancer response to treatment, particularly if the pretreatment concentration is elevated.[44] The CEA test may have preoperative prognostic implications because it correlates with the size and degree of differentiation of the carcinoma. Elevated preoperative CEA levels correlate with poor survival and may predict the likelihood of recurrence, regardless of tumor stage at diagnosis. However, it should not be used as an indication for adjuvant therapy. After a potentially curative resection, CEA levels should return to normal within 4 to 6 weeks. Persistently elevated CEA levels may indicate residual disease, while elevations after normalization may indicate relapsed disease.

Radiographic imaging studies are used to evaluate the extent of disease involvement for initial staging, and subsequently to monitor disease response to therapy. Contrast dye-enhanced CT scans of the chest, abdomen, and pelvis are performed to evaluate pulmonary, hepatic, and retroperitoneal involvement as well as occult abdominal and pelvic disease. In certain cases, such as patients with contrast dye allergies, magnetic resonance imaging (MRI) of the abdomen and pelvis may be substituted. A glucose analog [^{18}F]-fluorodeoxyglucose-positron emission tomography (PET) scan may also be performed as the primary imaging modality or to confirm metastatic disease if findings from CT or MRI scans are not conclusive. PET imaging may provide functional information to assist in discriminating between benign and malignant disease by detecting tumor-related metabolic alterations in affected tissues. PET scans are commonly used for the detection of recurrent colorectal cancer in patients with rising CEA levels and inconclusive findings on standard imaging studies. A PET scan is often performed in conjunction with a CT scan for anatomical localization of a lesion(s). For initial rectal cancer staging, assessment of the extent of tumor spread into the surrounding mesorectum and depth of invasion within the bowel wall may be performed using MRI or endorectal ultrasound.

Because of the increased likelihood of Lynch syndrome in patients diagnosed with colorectal cancer younger than the age of 50 years, MMR protein testing on the cancer specimen is recommended. The level of MMR protein expression can be determined by immunohistochemistry, which is decreased with MMR gene mutations. Gene sequencing can also be performed to detect MSI. If immunohistochemical analysis of the tumor reveals the absence of MLHI protein expression, *BRAF* gene mutation testing is recommended to distinguish between somatic and germline *MLH1* gene mutation. Individuals with abnormal MMR protein expression or MSI should be referred for genetic counseling as additional testing and cancer susceptibility risk assessment may be appropriate for themselves and family members.

Staging

Staging examinations determine the extent of disease, which allows the clinician to develop treatment plans and estimate overall prognosis. The same TNM classification system is used for both cancers of the colon and rectum since the categories reflect similar survival outcomes.[44,45] This classification assesses three aspects of cancer growth: T (tumor size or penetration), N (lymph node involvement), and M (presence or absence of metastases). The TNM classification also allows for various subdivisions within each of the three categories, which is then used to determine the disease stage. Table 153-4 summarizes the staging definitions used in the TNM system and corresponding 5-year survival rates.[44-46] Figure 153-4 shows the various

TABLE 153-4 Colon Cancer by TNM Classification and Associated 5-Year Survival Rate

Stage	T	N	M	Survival (%)
0	T_{is}	N_0	M_0	95.6
I	T_1	N_0	M_0	97.4
	T_2	N_0	M_0	96.8
IIA	T_3	N_0	M_0	87.5
IIB	T_{4a}	N_0	M_0	79.6
IIC	T_{4b}	N_0	M_0	58.4
IIIA	T_1-T_2	N_1/N_{1c}	M_0	71.1
	T_1	N_{2a}	M_0	68.5
IIIB	T_3-T_{4a}	N_1/N_{1c}	M_0	60.6-68.7
	T_2-T_3	N_{2a}	M_0	53.4-81.7
	T_1-T_2	N_{2b}	M_0	62.4
IIIC	T_{4a}	N_{2a}	M_0	40.9
	T_3-T_{4a}	N_{2b}	M_0	21.8-37.3
	T_{4b}	N_1-N_2	M_0	15.7
IVA	Any T	Any N	M_{1a}	11.5[a]
IVB	Any T	Any N	M_{1b}	11.5[a]
IVC	Any T	Any N	M_{1c}	11.5[a]

Primary Tumor (T)

T_{is}, Carcinoma in situ: intraepithelial or invasion of lamina propria with no extension through muscularis mucosae.

T_1, Tumor invades submucosa through the muscularis mucosa but not into the muscularis propria.

T_2, Tumor invades muscularis propria.

T_3, Tumor invades through the muscularis propria into pericolorectal tissues.

T_{4a}, Tumor invades through the visceral peritoneum, including bowel perforation through tumor and invasion of tumor through inflammatory surface of visceral peritoneum.

T_{4b}, Tumor directly invades or is adherent to other organs or structures.

Lymph Nodes (N)

N_0, no regional lymph node metastasis.

N_1, metastasis in 1-3 lymph nodes.

N_{1a}, metastasis in 1 lymph node.

N_{1b}, metastasis in 2-3 lymph nodes.

N_{1c}, tissue tumor deposits without lymph node metastasis.

N_2, metastasis in 4 or more lymph nodes.

N_{2a}, metastasis in 4-6 lymph nodes.

N_{2b}, metastasis in more than 7 lymph nodes.

Distant Metastasis (M)

M_0, no distant metastasis

M_{1a}, metastasis confined to one site or organ without peritoneal metastasis.

M_{1b}, metastasis in two or more sites or organs without peritoneal metastasis.

M_{1c}, metastasis to the peritoneal surface with/without metastasis to another site or organ.

[a]Survival for Stage IVA-C.

Data from References 44-46.

stages of cancer based on cancer penetration through the bowel wall and extension to regional lymph nodes. An individual patient's stage is determined at the time of the initial diagnosis and does not change with progression of disease or recurrence. For example, if a patient is diagnosed with stage II colon cancer and later recurs with metastases to the liver, that patient is in stage II now with metastatic disease to the liver, not stage IV.

Prognosis

The stage of colorectal cancer upon diagnosis is the most important independent prognostic factor for survival and disease recurrence. Five-year survival is about 90% for individuals who present with a localized tumor stage at diagnosis as compared with about 14% for individuals with metastatic disease at diagnosis.[1]

Clinical factors present at the time of diagnosis that are associated with a poor prognosis and decreased survival include bowel obstruction or perforation, high preoperative CEA level, distant metastases, and location of the primary tumor in the rectum or rectosigmoid area.[47] Along with resection of the primary tumor, a minimum of 12 lymph nodes must be examined to accurately determine regional lymph node involvement and predict lymph node-negative disease. The pathologic assessment also includes determination of TNM stage, tumor type, and histologic grade, presence of venous, and lymphatic invasion, and whether the resected margins are free of tumor.[44] Consideration of these factors plays an important role in determining optimal strategies for treatment and appropriate follow-up. Additional morphologic tumor features that have been associated with adverse clinical outcome include infiltrative tumor border configuration, evidence of perineural invasion, extranodal tumor deposits, and presence of tumor budding, characterized by clusters of cells that possess properties of malignant stem cells and are associated with increased risk of local and distant spread.

Certain molecular markers, particularly MSI, 18q/*DCC* mutation or LOH, *BRAF V600E* mutation, and *RAS* mutations, are also associated with colorectal cancer prognosis, although the pathologic stage of disease remains the primary prognostic assessment.[44,48] Colorectal cancers with allelic LOH on chromosome 18q or absent DCC protein are associated with a worse prognosis within stages II and III disease, but data are insufficient to warrant use of this test in practice now.[49] MSI can be determined through DNA sequencing or by immunohistochemistry staining for protein products of the MMR genes. Colorectal cancers that demonstrate MSI-H appear to be associated with a more favorable outcome and do not benefit from adjuvant fluoropyrimidines for early-stage disease. Tumor DNA *BRAF* and *RAS* mutation status appears to be associated with overall survival but is not used to determine prognosis.

Although multiple prognostic biomarkers for colorectal cancer have been identified, single molecular tests other than MSI are not used routinely in clinical practice. However, several multigene assays have been developed that provide prognostic information to assist in identifying individuals at high risk for cancer recurrence from early-stage disease.[44,48] The Onco*type* DX colon cancer assay is commercially available and has been validated in several trials as a prognostic test for stages II and III colon cancer.[50,51] Gene expression profiles classify risk of recurrence as low, intermediate, or high, and these scores are prognostic for recurrence, disease-free survival, and overall survival. The ColoPrint gene expression assay characterizes the risk of recurrence as low or high, and is undergoing further validation in clinical trials.[44] The ability for these and other gene signature assays in development to predict which patients may benefit from adjuvant chemotherapy has not been well established.

TREATMENT

Desired Outcomes

Treatment goals for cancer of the colon or rectum are based on the stage of disease at presentation. Stages I, II, and III disease are considered potentially curable and the goal of management is to eradicate potential micrometastases after surgical resection. Based on the numbers and site(s) of metastases, about 20% to 30% of patients with metastatic colorectal cancer may be cured, if their metastases are considered resectable.[44] Most patients with stage IV disease are not curable, and treatments for metastatic disease are considered palliative to reduce symptoms, avoid disease-related complications,

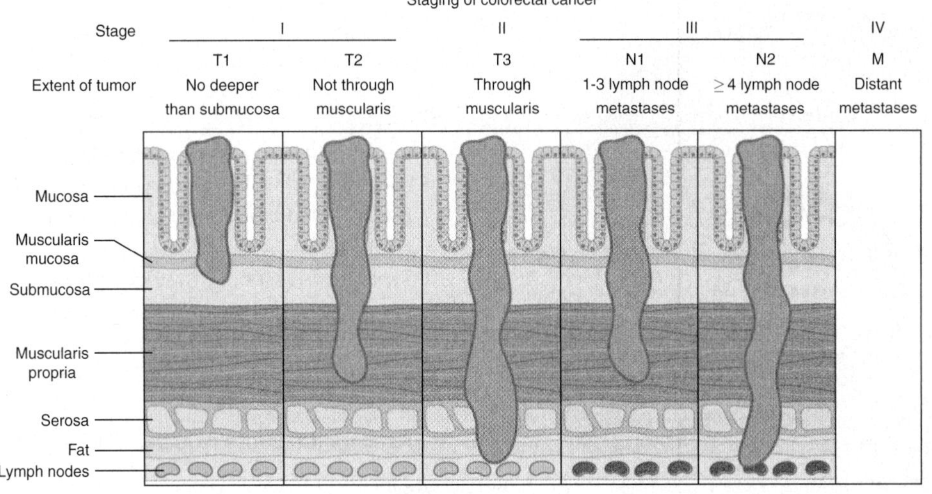

FIGURE 153-4 TNM staging for colorectal cancer. *(Reproduced with permission from Mayer RJ. Lower Gastrointestinal Cancers. In: Jameson J, Fauci AS, Kasper DL, et al., eds. Harrison's Principles of Internal Medicine, 20e. McGraw Hill; 2018.)*

and prolong survival. However, special attention should be given to those with oligometastatic lesions in the liver or lung since potential cure is still possible for some of these patients.

General Approach

Performance status, concomitant disease states, lifestyle factors, patient preferences, and patient age (although advanced age is not an absolute contraindication for aggressive therapies) must be considered in the treatment planning process. Special or emergent conditions, such as bowel obstruction or perforation, severe pain, anemia, or other symptomatic problems, need to be addressed acutely, after which time a more long-term disease-specific plan can be developed. The treatment approaches for cancer of the colon or rectum reflect two primary treatment goals: curative therapy for localized disease and palliative therapy for metastatic cancer.

For patients for whom treatment intent is curative, surgical resection of the primary tumor is the most important component of therapy. Depending on the extent of disease and whether the tumor originated in the colon or rectum, further adjuvant chemotherapy or chemotherapy plus XRT (chemoradiation) may be appropriate. For selected patients with resectable metastases, surgical resection may be an option. However, for most patients with metastases, systemic chemotherapy is the mainstay of treatment; XRT may also be useful for disease palliation of localized symptoms. Patients with metastatic disease who are asymptomatic may benefit from initiation of therapy and continuous treatment should be considered.

Operable Disease

Surgery

4 Individuals with operable—stages I, II, and III—cancer of the colon or rectum should undergo complete surgical resection of the primary tumor mass with regional lymphadenectomy as a curative approach for their disease.[33] The surgical approach for colon cancer generally involves complete resection of the tumor with at least a 5-cm margin of tumor-free bowel and regional lymphadenectomy of at least 12 lymph nodes.

The preferred surgical procedure for rectal cancer is total excision of the mesorectum, the surrounding tissue containing perirectal fat and draining lymph nodes.[33,45] If the distal margin clear of tumor is at least 1 cm, sphincter-preserving surgery may be possible for patients with cancers in the middle and lower portion of the rectum. Individuals who are not candidates for sphincter-sparing resections or have extensive local spread of tumor will require an abdominoperineal resection. This involves removal of the distal sigmoid colon, rectosigmoid colon, rectum, and anus with the establishment of a permanent sigmoid colostomy.

Colectomies for colon cancer can be performed as open procedures or laparoscopically. Laparoscopic colectomy has become an accepted procedure for colon cancer.[44] This technique appears to produce similar results to conventional surgery, with the benefits of a smaller surgical incision, shorter hospital stay, shorter duration of ileus, and reduced pain. Complications associated with colorectal surgery include infection, anastomotic leakage, obstruction, adhesion formation, sexual dysfunction, and malabsorption syndromes, depending on the site and extent of resection. Complications affecting bowel function associated with surgery for rectal cancer increase as the level of anastomosis approaches the anus.

Neoadjuvant XRT for Colon Cancer

XRT has a limited role in colon cancer because most recurrences are extrapelvic and occur in the abdomen. A subset of patients with recurrent disease or with T_4 tumors that have penetrated fixed structures may benefit from neoadjuvant (preoperative) fluorouracil-based chemoradiation to improve resectability.[44] Adverse reactions associated with XRT in colon cancer can be acute or chronic. Acute effects primarily include hematologic depression, dysuria, diarrhea, abdominal cramping, and proctitis. Chronic symptoms that sometimes persist for months following discontinuation of XRT include persistent diarrhea, proctitis or enteritis, small bowel obstruction, perineal tenderness, sexual dysfunction, and impaired wound healing.

Adjuvant Chemotherapy for Colon Cancer

Adjuvant chemotherapy in colorectal cancer is administered after complete tumor resection in an attempt to eliminate residual micrometastatic disease, thereby decreasing tumor recurrence and improving survival rates. Patients should start adjuvant therapy as soon as they are medically stable following surgery because each 4-week delay results in a 14% decrease in overall survival.[44] Because more than 90% of patients with stage I colon cancer are cured by surgical resection alone, adjuvant therapy is not indicated.

Patients with stage II disease who are at higher risk for relapse should be offered adjuvant therapy, with a detailed discussion regarding the potential benefits versus treatment-related toxicities.[44] High-risk features include those with inadequate lymph node

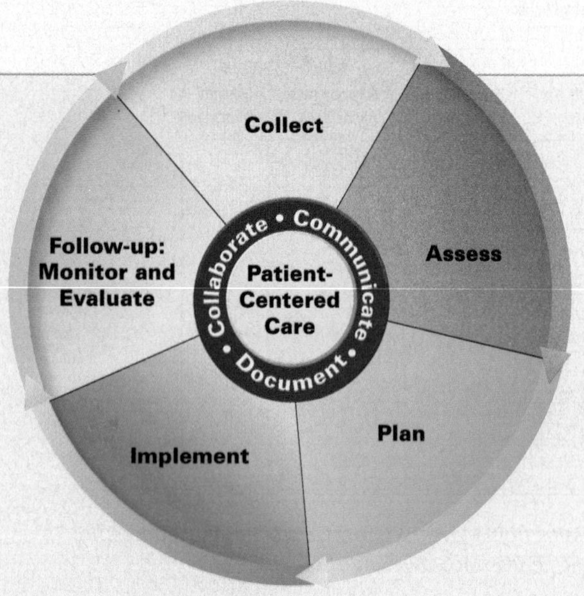

Patient Care Process for Colorectal Cancer

An illustration shows that patient-centered care includes collaboration, communication, and documentation. The actions associated with the care are collect, assess, plan, implement, and follow-up by monitoring and evaluating.

Collect

- Patient characteristics (eg, age, race, sex)
- Patient history (lifestyle factors—alcohol use, tobacco use, physical activity)
- Patient characteristics (eg, social history/situation, insurance coverage) and treatment preferences
- Patient medical and family history (eg, performance status, concurrent disease states [inflammatory bowel disease, colorectal cancer, polyps])
- Clinical presentation signs and symptoms (see Clinical Presentation box)
- Current signs and symptoms and evaluation of tumor growth (for follow-up visits)
- Current medications (prescription, over-the-counter, and complementary alternative)
- Objective data
    - BP, heart rate (HR), height, weight, and BSA
    - Labs (eg, serum electrolytes, renal function, liver chemistries, complete blood count, coagulation studies, carcinoembryonic antigen [CEA] level—see Workup)
    - Physical examination data (eg, hepatomegaly, lymphadenopathy, ascites)
    - Colorectal cancer staging (see Table 153-4)
    - Colorectal tumor genomics (eg, *KRAS*, *NRAS*, MMR/MSI, *BRAF*, *PIK3CA*, *NTRK*)

Assess

- Risk factors for treatment-related toxicities (eg, *UGT1A1*28* genotype, DPD deficiency, poor nutritional intake, uncontrolled blood pressure or hypertension, baseline peripheral neuropathy)
- Type of and response to prior treatments
- Potential for disease responsiveness to specific agents and risk factors for disease recurrence
- Potential problems with medication adherence to oral treatment regimens
- Need for drug dose reductions or supportive care

Plan*

- Goals of treatment
- Drug therapy regimen including specific anticancer agent(s), dose, route, frequency, and duration (see Tables 153-5, 153-6, and 153-7)
- Supportive care plan (eg, antiemetics, prophylactic antidiarrheals, infusion reaction prophylaxis)
- Monitoring parameters including efficacy (eg, cancer imaging studies-chest, abdominal, and/or pelvic CT scans and radiographs, CEA if previously elevated, symptoms of recurrence), safety (medication-specific adverse drug reactions, including major-dose limiting toxicities), and time frame (see Tables 153-5, 153-6, and 153-7)
- Patient education (eg, goals of treatment, expected and potential serious toxicities, drug therapy, monitoring and management plan)

Implement*

- Provide patient education regarding all elements of treatment plan
- Survivorship care plan (eg, primary prevention of other diseases, such as infections, and other cancers; support systems for maintaining healthy lifestyle choices and BMI)

Follow-up: Monitor and Evaluate

- Determine disease response to treatment (see "Evaluation of Therapeutic Outcomes" section) and occurrence of disease progression or recurrence (cancer imaging studies, CEA if previously elevated)
- Presence of adverse drug reactions (see "Evaluation of Therapeutic Outcomes" section and Tables 153-5, 153-6, and 157-7)
- Patient adherence to treatment plan using multiple sources of information (eg, patient self-report, medication administration records or refill data)
- Patient's satisfaction with treatment, including understanding of adherence

**Collaborate with patient, caregivers, and other healthcare professionals.*

sampling, perforation of the bowel at presentation, poorly differentiated tumors, lymphovascular invasion, perineural invasion, inadequately sampled lymph nodes (<12 evaluated), T_4 lesions (stage IIB/IIC), and lesions with localized perforation or close or indeterminate margins. Individuals with MSI-H tumors have a better prognosis compared to those with MSI-L and may not benefit or even be harmed from adjuvant chemotherapy.

The presence of lymph node involvement with tumor places patients with stage III colon cancer at high risk for recurrence, and the risk of death within 5 years of surgical resection alone is as high

TABLE 153-5 Chemotherapy Regimens for the Adjuvant Treatment of Colorectal Cancer

Regimen	Agents	Comments
FOLFOX[52,53]	Oxaliplatin 85 mg/m² IV on day 1 Leucovorin 400 mg/m² IV on day 1 Fluorouracil 400 mg/m² IV bolus, after leucovorin on day 1, then 1,200 mg/m²/day × 2 days CIV (total 2,400 mg/m² over 46-48 hr) Repeat every 2 weeks × 24 weeks[a,b]	Preferred regimen for stage III colon and rectal cancer high-risk stage colon cancer; common toxicities: sensory neuropathy, neutropenia
CAPEOX[53,54]	Oxaliplatin 130 mg/m² IV day 1 Capecitabine 1,000 mg/m² twice daily orally days 1 through 14 Each cycle lasts 3 weeks × 24 weeks[a,b]	Improved DFS in patients with stage III colon cancer compared to capecitabine alone or Roswell Park Regimen; common dose-limiting toxicities: neuropathies and hand-foot syndrome. A preferred regimen for adjuvant rectal therapy
Capecitabine[55]	Capecitabine 1,000 mg/m² to 1,250 mg/m² PO twice daily on days 1 through 14 Each cycle lasts 14 days and is repeated every 3 weeks × 24 weeks	Hand-foot syndrome common, useful for patients without vascular access or who have difficulties with travel to infusion center
Roswell Park Regimen[56]	Leucovorin 500 mg/m² IV day 1 over 2 hr Fluorouracil 500 mg/m² IV bolus 1 hr after leucovorin Repeat weekly for 6 of 8 weeks × 4 cycles	Leukopenia common dose-limiting toxicity, diarrhea, and stomatitis common
Simplified Biweekly[44]	Leucovorin 400 mg/m² per day IV Fluorouracil 400 mg IV bolus, after leucovorin, then 1,200 mg/m²/day days 1 and 2 (total 2,400 mg/m² over 46-48 hr) for 2 consecutive days Repeat every 2 weeks × 12 cycles	Hand-foot syndrome common

[a]Known as mFOLFOX6; survival benefit has not been demonstrated for patients 70 years and older.

[b]In patients with low-risk stage III (T1-3, any N), 3 months of CAPEOX is non-inferior to 6 months of CAPEOX for DFS but this has not been proven for FOLFOX. In patients with high-risk stage III disease (T4, N1-2, or any T, N2), 3 months of FOLFOX is inferior to 6 months of FOLFOX for DFS, but this has not been proven with CAPEOX. Grade 3 neuropathy is lower with 3 months of CAPEOX or FOLFOX.

CIV, continuous intravenous infusion; DFS, disease-free survival; OS, overall survival; PO, by mouth.

Data from References 44 and 52-56.

as 70%, depending on the number of lymph nodes involved.[4] In this group of patients, adjuvant chemotherapy significantly decreases risk of cancer recurrence and death and is standard of care.

4 Standard adjuvant chemotherapy regimens include a fluoropyrimidine (fluorouracil [with leucovorin] or capecitabine) in combination with oxaliplatin (FOLFOX or CAPEOX) or administered alone (Table 153-5).[52-56] The addition of oxaliplatin is superior to fluoropyrimidines alone in stage III colon cancer, but this benefit has not been observed in stage II colon cancer.[44]

Fluorouracil Plus Oxaliplatin Regimens 4 NCCN guidelines recommend the FOLFOX (fluorouracil/leucovorin and oxaliplatin) regimen as the preferred treatment for patients with stage III colon cancer who can tolerate combination therapy.[44] These recommendations are based on results from the Multicenter International Study of Oxaliplatin/5-Fluorouracil/Leucovorin in the Adjuvant Treatment of Colon Cancer (MOSAIC) trial, where the addition of oxaliplatin resulted in a 20% risk reduction in disease recurrence and increased 5-year disease-free survival (73% vs 67%) as compared with fluorouracil plus leucovorin alone.[52] With a median follow-up of 82 months, the addition of oxaliplatin resulted in an absolute 6-year overall survival difference of 2.5%. FOLFOX was associated with increased risk of paresthesia, neutropenia, and gastrointestinal toxicity (nausea, vomiting, and diarrhea) but toxicities were manageable with supportive care. This initial trial was performed with FOLFOX4 dosing schedule. Studies have further modified the regimen to improve tolerability and mFOLFOX6 regimen is now used.[44] A survival benefit has not been demonstrated for FOLFOX in patients with stage II colon cancer, but it is often used in stage II patients with multiple high-risk factors.[57]

5 Toxicity associated with fluorouracil differs based on the dose, route, and schedule of administration. Leukopenia is the primary dose-limiting toxicity of IV bolus fluorouracil, although diarrhea, stomatitis, and nausea and vomiting can also occur.[58] The incidence and severity of stomatitis can be significantly reduced with the use of oral cryotherapy. In this approach, the patient is instructed to chew and hold ice chips in the mouth during the period between 5 minutes prior to and 30 minutes following the bolus injection of fluorouracil. The protective effects of this procedure are probably related to the local vasoconstriction caused by the ice chips, which temporarily reduces blood flow to the oral mucosa, thereby reducing drug exposure to the oral mucosa.

5 Although continuous IV infusion fluorouracil is generally well tolerated, dose-limiting toxicities can be substantial. A distinct toxicity, palmar–plantar erythrodysesthesia ("hand-foot syndrome" or PPE), and stomatitis occur most frequently with this route of administration.[58] Hand-foot syndrome occurs in 24% to 40% of patients receiving extended continuous IV infusions and is characterized by painful swelling and erythroderma of the soles of the feet, palms of the hands, and distal fingers. The skin toxicity is fully reversible on interruption of therapy or dose reduction and is not life-threatening, but it can be significant and acutely disabling. The risk of stomatitis, diarrhea, and hematologic toxicity is not substantial at standard doses, but it increases with increasing fluorouracil doses. No significant difference is noted in the incidence of mucositis, diarrhea, nausea and vomiting, or alopecia between continuous and bolus IV fluorouracil administration.

5 An additional determinant of fluorouracil toxicity, regardless of the method of administration, is related to its catabolism and pharmacogenomic factors. DPD is the main enzyme responsible for the catabolism of fluorouracil to inactive metabolites. A rare pharmacogenetic disorder characterized by complete or near-complete deficiency of this enzyme has been identified in patients with cancer. Patients with this enzyme deficiency develop severe toxicity, including death, after fluorouracil administration. Molecular studies have identified a relationship between allelic variants in the *DPYD* gene (the gene that encodes DPD) and a deficiency in DPD activity.[44] An approved genetic test for *DPYD* polymorphisms is available to

identify patients who would require lower fluorouracil doses to avoid severe toxicity, but pretreatment DPYD genotyping is not recommended.

The addition of leucovorin to fluorouracil regimens increases the binding affinity of the active fluorouracil metabolite to thymidylate synthase (TS), thus enhancing its cytotoxic activity. Leucovorin administration prior to fluorouracil is the most effective approach to enable intracellular-reduced folates to accumulate prior to fluorouracil administration. When leucovorin is unavailable, levoleucovorin, the active isomer of racemic leucovorin, can be substituted as an alternative. The recommended levoleucovorin dose is 50% of the leucovorin dose.[59]

5 Oxaliplatin has minimal renal toxicity, myelosuppression, and nausea and vomiting when compared with other platinum-based drugs. Oxaliplatin is associated with both acute and persistent neuropathies.[60] The acute neuropathies occur within 1 to 2 days of dosing and resolve within 2 weeks. The neuropathies usually occur peripherally, but may also occur in the jaw and tongue. A rare acute syndrome of pharyngolaryngeal dysesthesia (1%-2% of patients) is characterized by subjective sensations of difficulty in swallowing and shortness of breath. Overall, acute neuropathies occur in about 90% of patients, and are precipitated or exacerbated by exposure to cold temperatures or cold objects. Thus, patients should be instructed to avoid cold drinks and use of ice, and to cover skin before exposure to cold environments or cold objects. Several prophylactic and treatment strategies have been studied with varying degrees of success. Persistent neuropathy is typically a cumulative adverse drug reaction occurring after 8 to 10 cycles. The neuropathy is characterized by paresthesia, dysesthesia, and hypoesthesia, but may also include deficits in proprioception that can interfere with daily activities (eg, writing, buttoning, swallowing, and difficulty walking as a result of impaired proprioception). Persistent neuropathy occurs in about one-half of patients receiving oxaliplatin but may improve or resolve with dosage reductions or cessation of oxaliplatin therapy.[44,60] Prophylaxis with calcium and magnesium infusions has not been proven effective. A "stop-and-go" approach where oxaliplatin is temporarily discontinued after 3 months of therapy (or sooner with significant neuropathic symptoms) with the other drugs continued reduces neurotoxicity without compromising antitumor activity and has been advocated.[44] Oxaliplatin can be reinitiated at disease progression in those patients who experience near complete resolution of neurotoxicity. Duloxetine may be used to treat painful neuropathy.

Fluorouracil/Leucovorin Regimens The efficacy of bolus and continuous infusion schedules generally favor continuous infusion of fluorouracil, which is probably related to its short plasma half-life and S-phase specificity for optimal TS inhibition. Continuous IV infusions also permit increased fluorouracil dose intensity, which may account for the higher response rates observed with prolonged infusions of fluorouracil. Most commonly, fluorouracil is administered by both IV bolus injection and continuous IV infusion (eg, FOLFOX and simplified biweekly regimens; see Table 153-5).

Capecitabine Regimens 4 Capecitabine can be used as an alternative for fluorouracil in an attempt to improve the safety and ease of administration of the chemotherapy regimen. Capecitabine is converted to fluorouracil through a three-step activation process, the final step being activation by thymidine phosphorylase, which is present in greatest concentrations at the tumor site. These activation steps lead to about a threefold increase in tumor fluorouracil levels. CAPEOX prolonged 3-year disease-free survival (71% vs 67%) as compared to bolus fluorouracil alone in patients with stage III disease, but did not prolong overall survival.[61] Capecitabine is non-inferior to bolus fluorouracil and leucovorin in patients with stage III colon cancer.[55] Disease-free survival between the groups was equivalent, and safety was improved with capecitabine.

5 The toxicities differ for the two regimens, with increased risks of neuropathies and hand-foot syndrome with CAPEOX and increased risk of neutropenia/neutropenic fever with fluorouracil-based regimens. The incidence of diarrhea and stomatitis is also decreased with capecitabine. Doses may need to be reduced in patients who experience adverse drug reactions. Patients with renal dysfunction can accumulate drug and often require dose modification. Capecitabine-based regimens are recommended when patients are unable to tolerate fluorouracil-based therapy.[44]

Selection of an Adjuvant Regimen Selecting a specific regimen from those listed in Table 153-5 requires an assessment of several patient-specific factors, including the performance status of the patient, comorbid conditions that may exist, and patient preferences for treatment based on lifestyle factors that are important to the patient. If a clinical trial is not an option, most patients with a good performance status will receive FOLFOX. Some patients prefer to not receive IV chemotherapy and may choose CAPEOX. Single-agent capecitabine may be the preferred option for patients with preexisting neuropathies, such as diabetic patients, or those patients wishing not to receive IV chemotherapy for any other reason. Fluorouracil and leucovorin have limited use now but are an acceptable option for patients, with low risk or average-risk stage II disease or those who cannot receive oxaliplatin and are unable to tolerate or take oral capecitabine. For example, patients who develop severe hand-foot syndrome may tolerate IV bolus fluorouracil/leucovorin because the risk of this toxicity is minimal with this administration method.

Patient age should also be considered when selecting an appropriate regimen. Subset analysis of the MOSAIC and National Surgical Adjuvant Breast and Bowel Project (NSABP)-C07 trials have demonstrated no overall survival benefit from adding oxaliplatin to patients older than 70 years and these patients may be appropriate for fluoropyrimidine-based therapy alone.[52,62]

The usual length of adjuvant therapy is 6 months. Non-inferiority studies have compared 3 versus 6 months of therapy in an effort to minimize long-term toxicities, particularly neuropathy associated with FOLFOX and CAPEOX. According to the results of two meta-analyses, 3 months of CAPEOX is non-inferior to 6 months of CAPEOX in terms of disease-free survival in patients with low-risk stage III disease, but the same results have not been proven for FOLFOX and overall survival results were not evaluated.[53] In patients with high-risk stage III disease, 6 months of FOLFOX is superior to 3 months (3-year disease-free survival 76% vs 72%; hazard ratio [HR] 1.27; 95% confidence interval [CI], 1.07-1.51), but this has not been evaluated with CAPEOX.[63] The incidence of grade 3 neuropathy is lower with 3 months of CAPEOX or FOLFOX. Therefore, it remains controversial whether 3 months of adjuvant therapy is appropriate for all individuals.

Adjuvant and Neoadjuvant Therapy for Rectal Cancer

6 Rectal cancer involves those tumors found below the peritoneal reflection in the most distal 15 cm of the large bowel, and as such it is distinct from colon cancer in that it has a propensity for both local and distant recurrence. The higher incidence of local failure and overall poorer prognosis associated with rectal cancer is a result of anatomic limitations in excising adequate radial margins around the rectal tumor. Most patients with stage II or III rectal cancer should receive combined-modality therapy consisting of chemoradiation and fluoropyrimidine-based chemotherapy perioperatively for a total of 6 months.[45]

6 Perioperative treatment can be accomplished with the use of neoadjuvant (preoperative) chemoradiation followed by surgery and adjuvant (postoperative) chemotherapy or total neoadjuvant therapy (fluoropyrimidine-based chemotherapy

followed by chemo XRT [or vice versa) followed by surgery]. FOLFOX or CAPEOX are the preferred fluoropyrimidine-based chemotherapy regimens, but fluorouracil and leucovorin combination regimens and capecitabine can be used.[45] Neoadjuvant chemoradiation significantly reduces local recurrence and has fewer toxicities, and improved sphincter-preserving surgeries as compared to postoperative chemoradiation.[45,64] However, some patients are unable to tolerate a typical 5- to 6-week chemoradiation regimen and may be more appropriate candidates for a short course of preoperative XRT alone.[45] Chemotherapy combined with XRT typically involves continuous infusion fluorouracil, oral capecitabine, or bolus fluorouracil and leucovorin; the addition of oxaliplatin to either fluoropyrimidine was associated with increased toxicities without clear improvements in complete remission rates or survival benefit.[45,64]

Metastatic Disease: Initial Therapy

Patients are generally classified as having resectable, potentially resectable, or unresectable metastatic disease. Surgery and XRT are used to manage isolated sites of tumor. Chemotherapy is used for disseminated disease and the primary treatment modality for unresectable metastatic colorectal cancer. Patients with resectable or potentially resectable metastases are candidates for multimodality therapy.[44,45] Tumor genotyping for *RAS* (*KRAS* and *NRAS*) and *BRAF* mutation status, *HER2* amplification, and determination of tumor MMR or MSI status (if not previously done) are recommended for patients at the time when metastatic disease is diagnosed to identify appropriate treatment options. Testing can also be performed on archived tissue samples obtained when the cancer was initially diagnosed.

Resectable (or Potentially Resectable) Metastatic Colorectal Cancer

7 Patients present with metastatic disease isolated to the liver or lung and who undergo resection of all metastatic and primary lesions (metastasectomy) have an increased probability of survival compared with those whose metastatic lesions remain unresected.[44] Therefore, strategies to increase the success rate of these resections (or convert unresectable lesions to resectable) are used in these patients. Neoadjuvant chemotherapy, also referred to as conversional chemotherapy, is the primary method to increase complete resection rates in both patients with resectable or potentially resectable liver or lung lesions. In some cases, individuals with metastatic disease initially deemed unresectable may achieve significant tumor regression following neoadjuvant chemotherapy to then be considered for surgery.

The optimal sequencing of chemotherapy for patients with initially resectable metastatic disease is controversial, as treatment options include surgery followed by chemotherapy or perioperative (pre- and postoperative) chemotherapy with surgery.[44,45] Because of the high risk of recurrence following resection of metastases, postoperative chemotherapy is always recommended. Administration of both pre- and postoperative chemotherapy is common practice, but the risk of hepatotoxicity associated with preoperative chemotherapy should be considered. Irinotecan-containing regimens can cause steatohepatitis and oxaliplatin-containing regimens can cause vascular sinusoidal obstructive liver injury.[44] Therefore, surgery is performed as soon as possible after the disease becomes resectable and preoperative chemotherapy is limited to a 2- to 3-month time period while patients undergo close monitoring.

The choice of neoadjuvant therapy depends on patient-specific factors and includes regimens such as FOLFOX, CAPEOX, FOLFIRI (infusional fluorouracil, leucovorin, and irinotecan), or FOLFOXIRI (infusional fluorouracil, leucovorin, oxaliplatin, and irinotecan). It is typically administered for 2 to 3 months before surgery. Adjuvant chemotherapy (preferably FOLFOX or CAPEOX) should be administered to patients to complete a total of 6 months of chemotherapy (pre- and postoperative).[44]

Patients with unresectable lesions are eligible for the same chemotherapy regimens. However, because the primary goal is surgical resection whenever possible, patients should be evaluated for possible resection after every 2 months of therapy. If resection occurs, adjuvant chemotherapy should be administered to complete a total of 6 months of chemotherapy.

Hepatic-Directed Therapies Hepatic-directed therapy, in addition to or as an alternative to surgical resection, can be considered in individuals with liver-only or liver-predominant metastatic disease. Hepatic artery infusion involves the placement of a permanent access catheter to the hepatic artery through which chemotherapy can be infused directly into the liver.[44] This approach offers the advantage of delivering high drug concentrations to tumors locally, thereby limiting systemic toxicities. Floxuridine with dexamethasone and fluorouracil with or without leucovorin are the most commonly used agents. Hepatic artery infusion is associated with potential biliary toxicity and the technical expertise required warrants use in selected patients by experienced practitioners. XRT can also be given to sites of hepatic tumor with external beam XRT or percutaneous arterial injection of micron-sized embolic particles loaded with a radioisotope (radioembolization). Other less common methods include tumor ablation procedures using radiofrequency ablation or microwave energy to generate heat that destroys localized tumor cells. Cryoablation can also be used, which includes placement of a cryoprobe into the tumor, either percutaneously or intraoperatively, and then lowering the probe temperature to −20°C to −40°C and rewarming it in cycles, resulting in formation of an ice ball that causes tumor destruction. These strategies may be useful for patients who have very small hepatic lesions and are unable to undergo liver resection surgery, but they are less successful than surgical interventions.

Unresectable Metastatic Colorectal Cancer

Unless the primary tumor is causing an obstruction, surgery in patients with established unresectable disease is rarely indicated. XRT may be useful to control localized symptoms in patients with metastatic colorectal cancer. Systemic chemotherapy palliates symptoms and improves survival in patients with unresectable disease. Common treatment regimens include combination of cytotoxics and a biologic agent.

Chemotherapy 7 Several chemotherapy regimens are acceptable for initial treatment of metastatic colorectal cancer.[44] The goals of therapy, history of prior chemotherapy, tumor genotype status, performance status/comorbidities, and risk of drug-related toxicities should be considered when an appropriate management strategy is defined for each individual. Treatment regimens are the same for metastatic cancer of the colon and rectum. Table 153-6 lists common initial chemotherapeutic regimens for metastatic disease.[44,45]

Most metastatic colorectal cancers are incurable, and treatment goals are to control cancer growth, reduce patient symptoms, improve quality of life, and extend survival. The benefit of palliative chemotherapy for metastatic colorectal cancer as compared to observation or supportive care alone with regard to these treatment goals has been established. According to results from multiple randomized trials and meta-analyses, chemotherapy prolongs life and improves quality of life of patients with metastatic colorectal cancer.[33,44,45]

Most first-line chemotherapy regimens for metastatic colorectal cancer incorporate a fluoropyrimidine. Irinotecan or oxaliplatin added to a fluoropyrimidine-based regimen significantly improves response rates, progression-free survival, and median survival.[44,45] The addition of the targeted anti-angiogenesis agent bevacizumab

TABLE 153-6 Initial Chemotherapeutic Regimens for Metastatic Colorectal Cancer[a]

Regimen	Agents	Major-Dose Limiting Toxicities	Comments
Patients Appropriate for Intensive Therapy with *RAS* Mutations			
FOLFOX +/− bevacizumab	Oxaliplatin 85 mg/m² IV day 1 Leucovorin 400 mg/m² IV day 1 Fluorouracil 400 mg/m² IV bolus, after leucovorin day 1, then 1,200 mg/m²/day × 2 days CIV (total 2,400 mg/m² over 46-48 hr) Repeat every 2 weeks +/− Bevacizumab 5 mg/kg IV day 1 before FOLFOX Repeat cycle every 2 weeks	FOLFOX: sensory neuropathy, neutropenia Bevacizumab: hypertension, thrombosis, proteinuria	Most commonly used first-line regimen
CAPEOX +/− bevacizumab	Oxaliplatin 130 mg/m² IV day 1 Capecitabine 1,000 mg/m² orally twice a day, days 1-14 Repeat cycle every 3 weeks +/− Bevacizumab 7.5 mg/kg IV day 1 Repeat cycle every 3 weeks	CAPEOX: diarrhea, hand-foot syndrome, neuropathies Bevacizumab: hypertension, thrombosis, proteinuria	Reduced capecitabine dose better tolerated; patient must be able to be adherent and report adverse drug reactions in a timely fashion
FOLFIRI +/− bevacizumab	Irinotecan 180 mg/m² IV day 1 Leucovorin 400 mg/m² IV day 1 Fluorouracil 400 mg/m² IV bolus, after leucovorin day 1, then 1,200 mg/m²/day × 2 days CIV (total 2,400 mg/m² over 46-48 hr) +/− Bevacizumab 5 mg/kg IV day prior to FOLFIRI Repeat cycle every 2 weeks	FOLFIRI: diarrhea, mucositis, neutropenia Bevacizumab: hypertension, thrombosis, proteinuria	May be preferred in patients who have preexisting neuropathy or those in which neuropathy may be debilitating to their line of work (eg, musician)
FOLFOXIRI +/− bevacizumab	Irinotecan 165 mg/m² IV day 1 prior to oxaliplatin Oxaliplatin 85 mg/m² IV prior to leucovorin day 1 Leucovorin 400 mg/m² IV day 1 prior to fluorouracil Fluorouracil 1,200 mg/m²/day × 2 days CIV (total 2,400 mg/m² over 48 hr) Repeat cycle every 2 weeks +/− Bevacizumab 5 mg/kg IV day 1 before FOLFOXIRI Repeat cycle every 2 weeks	FOLFOXFIRI: neutropenia, diarrhea, stomatitis, peripheral neurotoxicity, thrombocytopenia Bevacizumab: hypertension, thrombosis, proteinuria	[b]More neutropenia and peripheral neurotoxicity compared to FOLFIRI; often used in medically fit individuals with diffuse aggressive disease to palliate symptoms and as potential conversion therapy
Patients Appropriate for Intensive Therapy with *RAS* or *BRAF* Wild-Type and Left-Sided Colon Tumors			
FOLFOX + cetuximab or panitumumab	FOLFOX regimen + cetuximab (400 mg/m² IV loading dose, then cetuximab 250 mg/m² IV weekly thereafter OR cetuximab 500 mg/m² IV every 2 weeks) before FOLFOX OR FOLFOX regimen + panitumumab 6 mg/kg IV day 1 before FOLFOX Repeat cycle every 2 weeks	FOLFOX: sensory neuropathy, neutropenia Cetuximab: Papulopustular and follicular rash, asthenia, constipation, diarrhea, allergic reactions, hypomagnesemia Panitumumab: rash, diarrhea, hypomagnesemia	Only *RAS* or *BRAF* wild-type and left-sided tumor
FOLFIRI + cetuximab or panitumumab	FOLFIRI + cetuximab (400 mg/m² IV loading dose, then cetuximab 250 mg/m² IV weekly thereafter OR cetuximab 500 mg/m² IV every 2 weeks) before FOLFIRI OR FOLFIRI + panitumumab 6 mg/kg IV day 1 before FOLFIRI Repeat cycle every 2 weeks	FOLFIRI: diarrhea, mucositis, neutropenia Cetuximab: papulopustular and follicular rash, asthenia, constipation, diarrhea, allergic reactions, hypomagnesemia Panitumumab: rash, diarrhea, hypomagnesemia	Only *RAS* or *BRAF* wild-type and left-sided tumor; preferred for patients with preexisting neuropathy or those in whom neuropathy may be debilitating to their line of work (eg, musician)
Patients NOT Appropriate for Intensive Therapy with *RAS* Mutations			
Infusional fluorouracil + leucovorin +/− bevacizumab	Fluorouracil 400 mg/m² IV bolus, after leucovorin on day 1, then 1,200 mg/m²/day × 2 days CIV (total 2,400 mg/m² over 46-48 hr) Repeat cycle every 2 weeks +/− Bevacizumab 5 mg/kg IV day 1 prior to fluorouracil and leucovorin Repeat cycle every 2 weeks	Infusional fluorouracil/leucovorin: neutropenia, diarrhea Bevacizumab: hypertension, bleeding, proteinuria	Infusional fluorouracil/leucovorin regimen preferred to bolus fluorouracil regimen
Capecitabine +/− bevacizumab	Capecitabine 850-1,250 mg/m² orally twice a day, days 1-14 +/− Bevacizumab 7.5 mg/kg IV day 1 Repeat cycle every 3 weeks	Capecitabine: hand-foot syndrome, diarrhea, hyperbilirubinemia Bevacizumab: hypertension, thrombosis, proteinuria	

(Continued)

TABLE 153-6 Initial Chemotherapeutic Regimens for Metastatic Colorectal Cancer[a] (*Continued*)

Regimen	Agents	Major-Dose Limiting Toxicities	Comments
Patients NOT Appropriate for Intensive Therapy with *RAS* or *BRAF* Wild-Type and Left-Sided Tumors			
Cetuximab[c]	Cetuximab 400 mg/m² IV loading dose, then cetuximab 250 mg/m² IV weekly thereafter Or Cetuximab 500 mg/m² IV every 2 weeks	Papulopustular and follicular rash, asthenia, constipation, diarrhea, allergic reactions, hypomagnesemia	Only *RAS* or *BRAF* wild-type and left-sided tumor
Panitumumab[c]	6 mg/kg IV over 60 minutes every 2 weeks	Rash, diarrhea hypomagnesemia, rare allergic reactions	Only *RAS* or *BRAF* wild-type and left-sided tumor
Patients with dMMR or MSI-H			
Pembrolizumab	2 mg/kg IV every 2 weeks or 200 mg IV every 3 weeks or 400 mg IV every 6 weeks[d]	Immune-mediated adverse drug reactions (most common: skin, liver, kidney, gastrointestinal tract, lung and endocrine systems)	Only in MMR-d or MSI-H tumors. Patients should be closely monitored for adverse drug reactions and report any adverse drug reactions immediately as interruption of treatment or initiation of corticosteroids may be needed
Nivolumab +/- ipilimumab	Nivolumab 3 mg/kg IV over 30 minutes and ipilimumab 1 mg/kg IV over 30 minutes every 3 weeks × 4 doses, then nivolumab 3 mg/kg IV or nivolumab 240 mg IV every 2 weeks or 480 mg IV every 4 weeks[d]	Immune-mediated adverse drug reactions (most common: skin, liver, kidney, gastrointestinal tract, lung and endocrine systems)	Only in MMR-d or MSI-H tumors. Patients should be closely monitored for adverse drug reactions and report any adverse drug reactions immediately as interruption of treatment or initiation of corticosteroids may be needed
Patients NOT Appropriate for Intensive Therapy with *HER*-Amplified and *RAS* and *BRAF* WT			
Trastuzumab + (pertuzumab or lapatinib) or fam-trastuzumab deruxtecan-nxki	Trastuzumab 8 mg/kg IV day 1 of cycle 1 then 6 mg/kg IV every 21 days + pertuzumab 840 mg IV day 1 of cycle 1 then 420 mg IV every 21 days OR trastuzumab 4 mg/kg IV day of cycle 1 then 2 mg/kg IV weekly + lapatinib 1,000 mg po daily OR fam-trastuzumab deruxtecan-nxki 6.4 mg/kg IV on day 1 every 21 days	Trastuzumab + pertuzumab: hypokalemia, abdominal pain, diarrhea, fatigue, nausea; trastuzumab + lapatinib: fatigue, elevated liver enzymes, diarrhea, and rash; fam-trastuzumab deruxtecan-nxki, interstitial pneumonitis	Only in *HER*-amplified and *RAS* and *BRAF* WT tumors. Evaluate all patients for left ventricular ejection fraction at baseline and monitor closely throughout therapy. Do not substitute conventional or biosimilar trastuzumab with ado-trastuzumab emastine, fam-trastuzumab deruxtecan or trastuzumab/hyaluronidase

[a]NCCN Guideline recommendations for initial therapy. All recommendations are category 2A unless otherwise noted. Category 2A: based on lower-evidence, there is uniform NCCN consensus that intervention is appropriate.

[b]Original dosing was 1,600 mg/m²/day but it is recommended that US patients use this dose as they do not tolerate fluorouracil as well.

[c]NCCN Category 2B: based upon lower-evidence, there is NCCN consensus that this intervention is appropriate.

[d]Flat dosing is preferred.

Data from References 44 and 45.

further improves response rate and survival. Patients considered appropriate for initial intensive chemotherapy usually receive an oxaliplatin or irinotecan-containing regimen with infusional fluorouracil plus leucovorin and bevacizumab (unless contraindicated) or an EGFR inhibitor (if their tumors are left-sided and express *RAS* and *BRAF* wild-type). Capecitabine can be substituted for fluorouracil and leucovorin. If the patient has dMMR or MSI-H, they may receive immunotherapy. Patients who are not appropriate candidates for initial intensive therapy may be treated with fluoropyrimidine monotherapy with or without bevacizumab, EGFR inhibitor monotherapy (if their tumors are left-sided and express *RAS* and *BRAF* wild-type) immunotherapy if they have dMMR or MSI-H, or trastuzumab + pertuzumab or lapatinib or fam-trastuzumab deruxtecan-nxki (if their tumors have human epidermal growth factor receptor-2 [HER2] amplification and *RAS* and *BRAF* wild-type), as appropriate.[44] Patients may receive multiple different regimens; the sequence of drugs used appears less important than exposure to all active agents during the course of cancer treatments. Please refer to "Adjuvant Chemotherapy for Colon Cancer" section for more information on the toxicities of the regimens used in both the adjuvant and metastatic settings.

Fluorouracil can be administered as an IV bolus, a continuous infusion, or a combination of the two in the metastatic setting. Continuous IV infusion fluorouracil regimens increase the duration of drug exposure during the S-phase of the cell cycle, increase cytotoxicity, and are better tolerated than bolus administration. When combined with irinotecan or oxaliplatin, infusional fluorouracil is recommended because of improved efficacy.[44]

Unlike in the adjuvant setting, irinotecan added to fluorouracil plus leucovorin as initial therapy for metastatic disease improves tumor response rates, time-to-progression, and overall survival.[65] 5 The most common adverse drug reactions of irinotecan in these regimens are diarrhea, neutropenia, nausea and vomiting, dehydration, asthenia, abdominal pain, and alopecia; diarrhea and neutropenia are dose limiting. Two distinct patterns of diarrhea have been described. Early-onset diarrhea occurs during or within 2 to 6 hours after irinotecan administration and is characterized by lacrimation, diaphoresis, abdominal cramping, flushing, and/or diarrhea. These cholinergic symptoms, thought to be caused by inhibition of acetylcholinesterase, respond to atropine 0.25 to 1 mg given IV or subcutaneously. About 10% of patients experience acute symptoms during or shortly following the irinotecan. More commonly, late-onset diarrhea occurs 1 to 12 days after irinotecan administration and may last for 3 to 5 days. Late-onset diarrhea may require hospitalization or discontinuation of therapy, and fatalities have been reported. The risk of late-onset diarrhea can be decreased with aggressive antidiarrheal intervention. Aggressive intervention with high-dose loperamide therapy should consist of 4 mg taken at the first sign of soft or watery stools, followed by 2 mg orally every 2 hours until symptom-free for 12 hours; this regimen can be modified to 4 mg taken orally every 4 hours during the night.

5 The severity of delayed diarrhea is correlated with the systemic exposure (ie, area under the concentration-vs-time curve) of irinotecan and SN-38 (irinotecan's active metabolite) and with genetic polymorphisms in the enzyme UGT1A1, which is responsible for the glucuronidation of SN-38 to inactive metabolites. Reduced or deficient levels of the UGT1A1 enzyme are observed in Gilbert syndrome, a familial hyperbilirubinemia disorder, and correlate with irinotecan-induced diarrhea and neutropenia.[66] FDA-approved testing to determine *UGT1A1* genotype is commercially available. Although some individuals advocate testing *UGT1A1* genotype prior to starting irinotecan, widespread testing has not been adopted.[44,67] The prescribing information recommends considering a reduced dose of irinotecan in patients with *UGT1A1*28* genotype.

Oxaliplatin, in combination with infusional fluorouracil plus leucovorin, is FDA-approved for use in first-line and salvage regimens for metastatic colorectal cancer. Oxaliplatin incorporation into fluorouracil-based regimens as first-line therapy for metastatic colorectal cancer is associated with higher response rates and prolonged progression-free survival, with variable effects on overall survival.[68] Oxaliplatin is not effective as a single agent in colorectal cancer and is therefore only used in combination regimens.

To further improve survival rates achieved with FOLFOX and FOLFIRI regimens, a four-drug regimen (FOLFOXIRI) was developed and has been compared with FOLFIRI. FOLFOXIRI improved progression-free survival and overall survival compared to FOLFIRI, and a higher proportion of patients receiving FOLFOXIRI were able to undergo radical resection of metastases.[44] As expected, FOLFOXIRI causes more neutropenia, neurotoxicity, diarrhea, and alopecia, but may be appropriate for medically fit individuals with diffuse aggressive disease to palliate symptoms and as potential conversion therapy.

Capecitabine is an oral, tumor-activated, and tumor-selective fluoropyrimidine carbamate. Capecitabine can be administered alone or in combination with oxaliplatin (CAPEOX, also known as XELOX). When administered alone, it has higher response rates but comparable time-to-progression and median survival to fluorouracil/leucovorin. CAPEOX has similar progression-free and overall survival when compared with FOLFOX.[69] Hand-foot syndrome is common with capecitabine, while grades 3 or 4 neutropenia and stomatitis are more common with fluorouracil plus leucovorin. The convenience of oral administration and different toxicity profile make capecitabine a useful alternative to infusional fluorouracil in regimens for metastatic disease.

Targeted Therapy Guidelines and clinical practice recommend the addition of targeted therapy to one of the chemotherapy backbones mentioned earlier.[44]

8 Bevacizumab is a recombinant, humanized monoclonal antibody that inhibits vascular endothelial growth factor (VEGF). A modest increase in progression-free and overall survival benefit occurs when bevacizumab is combined with chemotherapy as compared with chemotherapy alone.[44] However, bevacizumab results in higher treatment-related mortality than chemotherapy alone (relative risk 1.33; 95% CI, 1.02-1.73) because of hemorrhage (24%), neutropenia (12%), and gastrointestinal perforation (7%).[70]

Hypertension is also common with bevacizumab.[44] The hypertension is easily managed with oral antihypertensive agents. Bleeding, thromboembolism, and proteinuria can also occur with bevacizumab. Proteinuria is monitored with urine dipsticks regularly during therapy, and the therapy is withheld in patients with 2+ protein or more, confirmed with a 24-hour urine collection. The risk of gastrointestinal perforation is increased by the addition of bevacizumab and extensive prior intra-abdominal surgery. Patients complaining of abdominal pain associated with vomiting or constipation should be evaluated for this rare but potentially fatal complication. Bevacizumab is also associated with a twofold increased risk of arterial thrombotic events, with patients who are older than 65 years or who have a prior history of arterial thrombotic events at greatest risk. Since bevacizumab can also interfere with wound healing, there should be at least a 6- to 8-week interval between the last dose of bevacizumab and elective surgery and wait at least 6 to 8 weeks to reinitiate bevacizumab after surgery. Necrotizing fasciitis can occur following wound healing or gastrointestinal perforation.

9 Cetuximab and panitumumab are monoclonal antibodies directed against EGFR. EGFR inhibitors may be used in combination with first-line chemotherapy regimens FOLFOX or FOLFIRI, or administered as single agents, but should not be combined with bevacizumab because of increased toxicity and no efficacy benefit.[44] The benefit of EGFR inhibitors, however, is limited to patients with wild-type *RAS* and *BRAF* tumors and they should not be used in patients with tumor *RAS* or *BRAF* mutations. Furthermore, patients with left-sided primary tumors have improved overall survival when treated with EGFR inhibitors while those with right-sided tumors (cecum to hepatic flexure) do not. Because fewer than 60% of patients with wild-type *KRAS* tumors respond to cetuximab or panitumumab, additional factors downstream of *RAS* signaling have been explored for their ability to predict response to EGFR inhibitors, including *BRAF* V600E mutation, and mutation or loss of *PTEN* or *PIK3CA*. Tumors with wild-type *KRAS*/*NRAS* and *BRAF* V600E mutation do not respond to anti-EGFR antibodies. The only situation where this might be beneficial is if the EGFR is administered in combination with a BRAF inhibitor, but now this has only been recommended after failure of the first-line setting (see "Metastatic Disease: Second-Line and Subsequent Therapy" section).

Severe infusion reactions, including anaphylaxis, can occur with cetuximab (3%) and panitumumab (1%).[44] Administration of panitumumab seems feasible in those who experienced a reaction with cetuximab.[71] Skin toxicity is also a common adverse drug reaction with these drugs and is not part of the infusion reaction. The presence of papulopustular skin rash correlates with response and survival. It most commonly occurs within 2 to 4 weeks of therapy initiation and preventative therapy with topical corticosteroids with moisturizer, sunscreen, and oral doxycycline is recommended unless contraindications exist.[72] Both these agents have also been associated with diarrhea and hypomagnesemia, which can occur even after discontinuation of the drug.

Trastuzumab and pertuzumab are monoclonal antibodies directed against HER2. Fam-trastuzumab deruxtecan-nxki is, an antibody drug conjugate with a trastuzumab backbone, linked to cytotoxic chemotherapy. Lapatinib is an oral tyrosine kinase inhibitor of both HER2 and EGFR1 receptors. A two-drug combination, trastuzumab + pertuzumab or lapatinib, or fam-trastuzumab deruxtecan-nxki alone is recommended as an option for patients with HER2 amplification and wild-type *RAS* and *BRAF* tumors.[44,45] Typically, they are reserved for second-line or subsequent therapy unless the patients cannot tolerate intensive therapy in the first-line setting (see "Metastatic Disease: Second-Line and Subsequent Therapy" section).

Immunotherapy 10 Immunotherapy is effective in dMMR tumors because these tumors encode mutant proteins and have the potential to be recognized and targeted by the immune system. Because the immune system can become suppressed when programmed death-ligands 1 and 2 (PD-L1 and PD-L2) on tumor cells bind to programmed cell death protein (PD-1) receptors on T cells, the use of PD-1 inhibitor drug therapy is reasonable in these tumors. The PD-1 inhibitor nivolumab has also been evaluated in combination with ipilimumab, a cytotoxic-T-lymphocyte-associated protein 4 (CTLA4) inhibitor; these drugs act synergistically to promote T-cell antitumor activity.[73] For more information about these therapies, see "Metastatic Disease: Second-Line and Subsequent Therapy" section.

Selection of an Initial Metastatic Regimen Several factors should be considered when selecting first-line therapy for metastatic colorectal cancer when disease palliation is the primary treatment goal. The first consideration is whether intensive therapy is appropriate for the patient. Those with multiple comorbidities or low performance status would likely better tolerate less-intensive therapy. The second consideration is *RAS* and *BRAF* status and side of tumor involvement. Those with wild-type *RAS* and *BRAF* and left-sided tumors can receive an EGFR inhibitor therapy. Patients with dMMR or MSI-H tumors could receive immunotherapy as first-line therapy. Also, patients with wild-type *RAS* and *BRAF* tumors, HER2-amplification, and are not appropriate for intensive therapy can receive HER2 inhibitor therapy. Once these factors are known, the selection of the appropriate regimen is based on the toxicity profile and convenience of administration for the patient. Based on the comparable results of FOLFIRI versus FOLFOX, either of these regimens is considered the reference standard in metastatic colorectal cancer. Most patients will receive first- and second-line regimens and patient preference for either sequence of treatments based on their different toxicity profiles is important. FOLFIRI may be chosen initially in patients with preexisting neuropathies, whereas FOLFOX may be chosen in patients with increased bilirubin or known UGT1A1 deficiency (known risk factors for delayed diarrhea). Alopecia occurs much more frequently with irinotecan compared to oxaliplatin combinations. Because FOLFOX can cause persistent neuropathy, a rationale for starting with FOLFIRI is that time-to-progression is longer with first-line treatment than in second line. Therefore, the time to death during which some patients will have to live with neuropathy may be shorter. Capecitabine is an appropriate substitute for IV fluorouracil in oxaliplatin combination regimens. Because of a higher response rate and modest survival benefit with FOLFOXIRI, this four-drug combination may be useful for patients with initially aggressive and symptomatic disease. Select patients who are candidates for FOLFOXIRI may benefit from the addition of bevacizumab, but the incidence of moderate or severe toxicities is increased.

Metastatic Disease: Second-Line and Subsequent Therapy

Systemic chemotherapy represents the mainstay of therapy for patients who have progressive disease following initial treatment for metastatic disease. Table 153-7 lists treatment options for relapsed/refractory metastatic disease.[44,45] Treatment options are based on the type of and response to prior treatments, the site and extent of disease, and patient factors and treatment preferences.

Systemic Chemotherapy

On disease progression following standard initial therapy, appropriate treatment options depend primarily on the type of prior therapy received (see Table 153-7). Because most patients will have received a combination of a fluoropyrimidine with either irinotecan or oxaliplatin, second-line therapy with the alternate regimen should be considered. Patient survival can exceed 2 years with this approach and it is important for patients to receive all traditional chemotherapy options if possible. Targeted agents can either be added to the regimens or used as single agents.

Irinotecan Irinotecan improves overall survival as compared to either best supportive care or continuous-infusion fluorouracil in patients who had progressed within 6 months of treatment with fluorouracil.[44] However, this approach is rarely used since single-agent fluorouracil is rarely given as first-line therapy.

The use of the FOLFIRI regimen after progression with first-line FOLFOX demonstrated an objective response rate of 4% with a median progression-free survival of 2.5 months.[44] These results are consistent with observations that demonstrate improved outcomes in those patients who are able to receive all active cytotoxic agents during the course of their disease.

Based on these results, irinotecan-based therapy should be considered standard second-line therapy for patients with disease

TABLE 153-7 Second-Line and Salvage Chemotherapy Regimens for Metastatic Colorectal Cancer

Disease Progression with First-Line Regimen	Comments
Second-line options	
FOLFIRI or irinotecan	After previous oxaliplatin-based regimen (without irinotecan) (ie, FOLFOX, CAPEOX); use with caution in patients with elevated bilirubin
FOLFIRI + bevacizumab or ziv-afilbercept or ramucirumab	After previous oxaliplatin-based regimen (without irinotecan) (ie, FOLFOX, CAPEOX); use with caution in patients with elevated bilirubin; bevacizumab is preferred antiangiogenic agent based on toxicity and cost
FOLFOX or CAPEOX ± bevacizumab	After previous irinotecan-based regimen (without oxaliplatin) (ie, FOLFIRI); bevacizumab FDA-approved to continue with second-line options
FOLFOX + cetuximab or panitumumab	After previous irinotecan-based regimen (without oxaliplatin) (ie, FOLFIRI); only if *RAS* wild-type and *BRAF* wild-type
Irinotecan + bevacizumab or ziv-afilbercept or ramucirumab	After previous oxaliplatin-based regimen (without irinotecan) (ie, FOLFOX, CAPEOX); use with caution in patients with elevated bilirubin; bevacizumab is preferred antiangiogenic agent based on toxicity and cost
FOLFIRI + cetuximab or panitumumab	After previous oxaliplatin-based regimen (without irinotecan) (ie, FOLFOX, CAPEOX); only if *RAS* wild-type and *BRAF* wild-type; if neither previously given; use with caution in patients with elevated bilirubin
Irinotecan ± cetuximab or panitumumab	Only if *RAS* wild-type and *BRAF* wild-type; if neither previously given; use with caution in patients with elevated bilirubin
Encorafenib + (cetuximab or panitumumab)	Only if *BRAF V600E* mutation positive
Nivolumab ± ipilimumab	Only if dMMR/MSI-H
Dostarlimab	Only if dMMR/MSI-H
Pembrolizumab	Only if dMMR/MSI-H
Trastuzumab + (pertuzumab or lapatinib) or fam-trastuzumab deruxtecan-nxki	Only if *HER2*-amplified and *RAS* and *BRAF* wild-type
Therapy After Second Progression or Third Progression (can use any of the previous recommendations)	
Regorafenib	Used after progressed through all available regimens
Trifluridine/tipiracil ± bevacizumab	Used after progressed through all available regimens
Clinical trial	If available and only if patient eligible
Best supportive care	Appropriate for patients who do not want to pursue treatment, or not eligible for cancer-directed therapy, or if quality of life is expected to decrease

CAPEOX, capecitabine plus oxaliplatin; dMMR, DNA mismatch repair deficiency; FOLFIRI, fluorouracil plus leucovorin plus irinotecan; FOLFOX, fluorouracil plus leucovorin plus oxaliplatin; MSI-H, high microsatellite instability.

Data from References 44 and 45.

progression with first-line treatment with oxaliplatin-containing regimens. Continuous-infusion fluorouracil with leucovorin and irinotecan (FOLFIRI), with or without targeted therapy, is most commonly given.

Oxaliplatin Oxaliplatin plus fluorouracil and leucovorin should be considered for patients who received primary treatment with irinotecan plus fluorouracil.[44] The combination of oxaliplatin plus fluorouracil and leucovorin is also effective as salvage therapy after initial treatment with irinotecan plus fluorouracil and leucovorin, with a similar response rate. Although irinotecan can be used effectively as a single agent in colorectal cancer, it should be noted that oxaliplatin does not have substantial activity alone, and should only be given in combination regimens.

Trifluridine/Tipiracil Trifluridine is a thymidine-based nucleoside analog that is incorporated into DNA and inhibits cell proliferation. The addition of tipiracil increases trifluridine exposure by inhibiting its metabolism by thymidine phosphorylase. This combination chemotherapy product has activity in both *RAS* mutant and wild-type tumors. Trifluridine/tipiracil is FDA-approved for treatment of metastatic colorectal cancer patients who have been previously treated with a fluoropyrimidine-, oxaliplatin-, and irinotecan-containing regimens, an anti-VEGF targeted therapy, and an anti-EGFR monoclonal antibody if *RAS* wild-type.[74] Trifluridine/tipiracil improves overall survival by approximately 2 months. This chemotherapy product is administered 35 mg/m^2 orally twice daily within 1 hour of completing morning and evening meals on days 1 through 5 and days 8 through 12 of a 28-day cycle. Common adverse drug reactions include myelosuppression, fatigue, diarrhea, nausea/vomiting, abdominal pain, and pyrexia.

Targeted Therapy

The addition of targeted therapy to chemotherapy in second and subsequent therapies does improve outcomes, but typically also increases toxicity. EGFR inhibitors may be administered in combination with other regimens in second-line and subsequent therapies. Angiogenesis inhibitors can also be used in second-line and subsequent therapy in combination with other regimens, even when they were used in first-line therapy.

EGFR Inhibitors 9 Patients with wild-type *RAS* and wild-type *BRAF* tumors who experience progression on therapies that do not contain an EGFR inhibitor may benefit from the combination of cetuximab or panitumumab and irinotecan, FOLFOX, or FOLFIRI.[44] However, further treatment is not recommended in those who had progressed while receiving an EGFR inhibitor. The combination of cetuximab and irinotecan significantly improves response rates (16% vs 4%) and progression-free survival (4 vs 2.6 months), but not overall survival when compared with irinotecan alone.[75] Panitumumab in combination with FOLFIRI also improves response rates (35% vs 10%) and progression-free survival (5.9 vs 3.9 months), but did not improve overall survival.[76]

BRAF Inhibitors In patients with *BRAF V600E* mutations, a two-drug regimen of encorafenib (a BRAF inhibitor) and an EGFR inhibitor (cetuximab or panitumumab) is recommended to improve overall outcomes in second- and subsequent-line therapies for metastatic disease. This regimen produces overall response rates of 20% and a median overall survival time of 9.3 months.[77] The most common adverse drug reactions with this doublet regimen are acneiform rashes and diarrhea.

Angiogenesis Inhibitors Angiogenesis inhibitors including VEGF inhibitors bevacizumab, ramucirumab, and ziv-aflibercept and the multikinase inhibitor regorafenib may be used in patients who have progressed on other therapies (see Table 153-7). VEGF inhibitors may be used as second- or subsequent-line therapies, whereas regorafenib is indicated for to third- or subsequent-line use. The NCCN guidelines recommend bevacizumab over ramucirumab and ziv-aflibercept based on toxicity and cost. Continuation of bevacizumab as second-line therapy provides a modest improvement in overall survival based on several clinical trials.[44] Bevacizumab may also be added to another second-line therapy in patients who did not receive it as part of their initial therapy, also resulting in a modest improvement in overall survival (12.1 vs 10.8 months).[78] Single-agent bevacizumab is not recommended because it is inferior to combination therapy.[44]

Ziv-aflibercept is a soluble recombinant fusion protein designed to block the angiogenic process. The agent was developed by fusing sections of the VEGFR-1 and VEGFR-2 immunoglobulin domains to the F_c portion of human immunoglobulin G1 and blocks VEGF-A, VEGF-B, and placental growth factor (PIGF) by "trapping" the ligands before they get to the native transmembrane receptors. In a phase III randomized trial, FOLFIRI plus ziv-aflibercept modestly, but significantly improves overall survival (13.5 vs 12.1 months) compared to FOLFIRI after progression on an oxaliplatin-based regimen.[79] It is dosed at 4 mg/kg as an IV infusion over 1 hour every 2 weeks and is associated with similar adverse drug reactions as bevacizumab.

Ramucirumab is a human monoclonal antibody that binds directly to the ligand-binding pocket of VEGFR-2 to block binding of VEGF-A, VEGF-C, and VEGF-D. A phase III randomized placebo-controlled trial of patients who progressed on an oxaliplatin-based regimen and bevacizumab were randomized to receive FOLFIRI with or without ramucirumab.[80] A modest but significant improvement in overall survival (13.3 vs 11.7 months) and progression-free survival (5.7 vs 4.5 months) were observed. Ramucirumab is administered as 8 mg/kg IV over 1 hour every 2 weeks and is associated with similar adverse drug reactions as bevacizumab.

The addition of ziv-aflibercept or ramucirumab to oxaliplatin regimens has not been evaluated and therefore is not recommended.[44] Additionally, the use of either of these drugs following failure of a bevacizumab-containing regimen has not been evaluated. Therefore, ziv-aflibercept and ramucirumab should only be used in patients naïve to antiangiogenic regimens and only with irinotecan-containing regimens.

Regorafenib, a small-molecule inhibitor of tumor angiogenesis (VEGFR-1, VEGFR-2, and VEGFR-3) and other downstream targets (FGF receptors, PDGF receptors, BRAF, KIT, and RET), is approved for the third- or fourth-line treatment of metastatic colorectal cancer. This oral agent is dosed 160 mg once daily for the first 21 days of each 28-day cycle, although it is common to start at a lower dose (80 or 120 mg) and titrate as tolerated.[44] In a phase III trial of patients with metastatic colorectal cancer and progression during or within 3 months of last chemotherapy, regorafenib demonstrated a 1.4-month improvement in overall survival when compared to placebo.[81] Patients with mutant or wild-type *RAS* may receive this therapy. Because this is an oral-only regimen, patients must be counseled on its use and potential toxicity. Regorafenib should be taken with a low-fat breakfast and may interact with CYP450 3A4 inducers and inhibitors. Toxicities include hypertension, hand-foot syndrome, diarrhea, and hepatotoxicity.

***HER2* Inhibitors** *HER2*, a member of the same kinase family as EGFR, is rarely overexpressed in colorectal cancer.[44] However, *HER2* overexpression/amplification is more common in *RAS* and *BRAF* wild-type tumors. MyPathway, a basket trial, showed that in patients with HER2 amplified metastatic colorectal cancer, the combination of trastuzumab and pertuzumab (HER2 monoclonal antibodies) produced response rates of 32%.[82] The most common adverse drug reactions are diarrhea, fatigue, and nausea. According to HERACLES study, trastuzumab and lapatinib (a *HER2* inhibitor) produced responses in patients with refractory *RAS* wild type colorectal cancer, who typically are refractory to therapy, producing a 30% response rate.[83] Adverse drug reactions of *HER2* inhibitors include fatigue, skin rash, and bilirubin increases.[82] *HER2* inhibitor therapy can be an option for those with tumor *HER2* overexpression when other options have failed.

Immunotherapy

10 Pembrolizumab, a humanized, IgG4 monoclonal antibody that binds to programmed cell death ligand-1, or PD-L1, with high affinity, is effective in metastatic colorectal cancer with dMMR or high tumor mutational burden. When used as first-line therapy in patients with metastatic colorectal cancer with dMMR, pembrolizumab has improved response rates and progression-free survival times compared with chemotherapy.[84] Nivolumab, another humanized IgG4 monoclonal antibody PD-1 inhibitor, has also been evaluated with or without ipilimumab in patients with metastatic colorectal cancer who have dMMR/MSI-H tumors. As first-line therapy, nivolumab and ipilimumab also improve response rates and progression-free survival times compared with chemotherapy alone.[85] Immunotherapy (dostarlimab, pembrolizumab, nivolumab +/− ipilimumab) may also be used as subsequent-line therapy if patients who have not previously received immunotherapy.

Immune checkpoint inhibitors are generally well tolerated. The adverse drug reactions are typically immune-mediated and commonly affect the skin, liver, kidneys, gastrointestinal tract, lung, and endocrine systems. Immune-mediated pneumonitis is an uncommon but serious adverse drug reaction. Close monitoring for these adverse drug reactions is important to allow for prompt identification and treatment to minimize morbidity and mortality. Treatment includes temporary treatment suspension and corticosteroid treatment. Refractory cases may require infliximab or immunotherapies.[86]

EVALUATION OF THERAPEUTIC OUTCOMES

The goal of monitoring is either to evaluate whether the patient is receiving any benefit from the management of the disease or to detect recurrence for those who have completed curative intent therapy. During treatment for active disease, patients should undergo monitoring for measurable tumor response, progression, or new metastases; these tests may include chest, abdominal or pelvic CT scans, or other imaging modalities, depending on known sites of disease and previous imaging results, and CEA measurements every 3 months if the CEA is or was previously elevated. These radiologic tests and other selected laboratories should also be evaluated with the development of any new symptoms or significant change in disease status. Patients should be evaluated during every treatment visit for the presence of anticipated adverse drug reactions, which generally include loose stools or diarrhea, nausea or vomiting, mouth sores, fatigue, and fever, as well as other adverse drug reactions such as neuropathy (oxaliplatin) and skin rash (EGFR inhibitors). In addition, a complete blood cell count should be obtained prior to each course of chemotherapy administration to ensure that hematologic indices are adequate. Baseline liver function tests and an assessment of renal function should be evaluated prior to and periodically during therapy. Hepatotoxicity may be seen with regorafenib, and in addition to neuropathy, oxaliplatin may cause renal injury. Serum electrolytes, including magnesium, should be monitored during treatment with EGFR inhibitors. Patients receiving bevacizumab, ziv-aflibercept, or regorafenib should be evaluated for hypertension and proteinuria.

Symptoms of recurrence such as pain syndromes, changes in bowel habits, rectal or vaginal bleeding, pelvic masses, anorexia, and weight loss develop in less than 50% of patients. Recurrences can be detected in asymptomatic patients because of increased serum CEA levels that lead to further examination. Although the value of CEA monitoring for disease recurrence is controversial because of its cost and emotional stress associated with false-positive elevations, CEA monitoring plays an important role in postoperative follow-up studies. A PET scan can identify sites of metastatic disease when a rising CEA level suggests metastatic disease but CT scans and other imaging studies are negative.

Patients who undergo curative surgical resection, with or without adjuvant therapy, require close follow-up based on the premise that early detection and treatment of recurrence could still render them cured. In addition, early treatment for asymptomatic metastatic colorectal cancer appears to be superior to delayed therapy. Specific practice guidelines for postoperative surveillance examinations following successful treatment for stage II or III disease were developed by NCCN and include history, physical examination, and CEA test every 3 to 6 months for the first 2 years, then every 6 months for a total of 5 years; chest and abdominal and pelvic CT scans every 6 to 12 months for up to 5 years following primary therapy; and colonoscopy at about 1 year after surgery. If an obstructing lesion prevented preoperative colonoscopy, it should be done within 3 to 6 months. Repeat colonoscopies are recommended at 3 years, unless findings of polyps warrant closer follow-up. PET/CT is not routinely indicated. Less intensive surveillance is recommended for patients treated for stage I disease because of low risk of recurrence.[44]

Posttreatment surveillance should also include a survivorship care plan with immunizations for vaccine-preventable diseases, early detection of second primary cancers, and support systems that encourage smoking cessation, establish regular exercise and maintain a healthy BMI, and encourage healthy lifestyle and dietary choices.[44] In addition, if there is a strong family history of colorectal cancer or related malignancies or clinicopathologic findings in an individual consistent with a hereditary syndrome, a consultation with a genetic counselor is indicated. Advances in the treatment for colorectal cancer now offer the potential to improve patient survival, but for many patients, improved disease-free and progression-free survival represent equally important therapeutic outcomes. Although treatment approaches for metastatic colorectal cancer have been historically assessed by their ability to produce a measurable objective tumor response, which is generally believed necessary for any treatment to improve survival, the effects of therapies on survival are clinically more meaningful than their ability to induce a tumor response. However, with the availability of multiple active treatments for metastatic disease, and the likelihood that patients will receive more than one during the course of their treatment, improvements in overall survival with new therapies will be increasingly difficult to determine.

In the absence of the ability of a specific treatment to demonstrate improved overall survival, important outcome measures should include the effects of the treatment on patient symptoms, daily activities, performance status and other quality-of-life indicators, progression-free survival, and time-to-treatment failure. Because most metastatic colorectal cancers are incurable, a specific decision regarding an individual patient's care will ultimately be required. This decision should be based on a careful assessment of the balance between risks associated with treatment (or lack thereof) and benefits of treatment. Efforts should also be made to ensure that the costs of screening, diagnostic tests, treatments, and procedures for colorectal cancer are consistent with their value in improving patient outcomes.

CONCLUSION

Colorectal cancer is a common cancer diagnosed in adults, but can be detected early through routine screening starting at the age of 45 years. Early-stage cancers can be cured with surgery. The addition of chemotherapy with a fluroropyrmdine-based regimen in some individuals with stage II and all individuals with stage III colorectal cancer is recommended following surgery to improve outcomes. In patients with rectal cancer, neoadjuvant chemotherapy and chemosensitized XRT followed by surgery is recommended to decrease the likelihood of recurrence. In patients with advanced colorectal cancer, chemotherapy is palliative and all active cytotoxic agents are administered to improve survival. The addition of targeted therapy in subsequent-line treatments is beneficial and depends upon specific patient factors. Unlike some other solid tumors, immunotherapy is only beneficial in a small subset of patients, but the benefit can be substantial in eligible patients.

ABBREVIATIONS

APC	adenomatous polyposis coli (gene)
BMI	body mass index
CAPEOX	capecitabine plus oxaliplatin
CEA	carcinoembryonic antigen
CI	confidence interval
CIN	chromosomal instability
CIMP	CpG island methylator phenotype
COX-2	cyclooxygenase-2
CT	computed tomography
DPD	dihydropyrimidine dehydrogenase
EGFR	epidermal growth factor receptor
EpCAM	epithelial cell adhesion molecule
FAP	familial adenomatous polyposis
FDA	Food and Drug Administration
FIT	fecal immunochemical test
FOBT	fecal occult blood test
FOLFIRI	fluorouracil, leucovorin, and irinotecan
FOLFOX	fluorouracil, leucovorin, and oxaliplatin
FOLFOXIRI	fluorouracil and leucovorin, oxaliplatin, irinotecan
FSIG	flexible sigmoidoscopy
gFOBT	guaiac-based fecal occult blood test
HDI	human development index
HR	hazard ratio
LOH	loss of heterozygosity
MAPK	mitogen-activated protein kinase
MMR	mismatch-repair
MRI	magnetic resonance imaging
MSI	microsatellite instability
mt-sDNA	multi-target stool DNA
NCCN	National Comprehensive Cancer Network
NSAID	non-steroidal anti-inflammatory drug
PD-1	programmed cell death protein
PD-L2	programmed cell death ligand-2
PET	positron emission tomography
PI3K	phosphatidylinositol 3-kinase
TGF-β	transforming growth factor-β
TS	thymidylate synthase
UGT1A1	uridine diphosphate-glucuronosyltransferase
USPSTF	United States Preventive Services Task Force
VEGF	vascular endothelial growth factor
VEGFR	vascular endothelial growth factor receptor
XELOX	capecitabine plus oxaliplatin
XRT	radiation therapy

REFERENCES

1. American Cancer Society. *Cancer Facts & Figures 2021*. Atlanta: American Cancer Society; 2021.
2. Lu B, Li N, Luo C-Y, et al. Colorectal cancer incidence and mortality: the current status, temporal trends and their attributable risk factors in 60 countries in 2000–2019. *Chinese Med J.* 2021; doi:10.1097/CM9.0000000000001619.
3. Howlader N, Noone AM, Krapcho M eds, et al. SEER Cancer Statistics Review, 1975–2018. Bethesda, MD: National Cancer Institute; 2021. https://seer.cancer.gov/csr/1975_2018/, based on November 2020 SEER data submission, posted to the SEER website, April 2021.
4. American Cancer Society. *Colorectal Cancer Facts & Figures 2020–022.* Atlanta: American Cancer Society; 2020.
5. Sawicki T, Ruszkowska M, Danielewicz, et al. A review of colorectal cancer in terms of epidemiology, risk factors, development, symptoms, and diagnosis. *Cancers.* 2021;13, 2025. https://doi.org/10.3390/cancers13092025.
6. Kim E, Change DK. Colorectal cancer in inflammatory bowel disease: the risk, pathogenesis, prevention and diagnosis. *World J Gasteroenterol.* 2014;20:9872–9881.
7. Cheng HC, Chang TK, Su WC, et al. Narrative review of the influence of diabetes mellitus and hyperglycemia on colorectal cancer risk and oncological outcomes. *Transl Oncol.* 2021;14:101089. doi:10.1016/j.tranon.2021.101089. Epub 2021 Apr 7.
8. Signorile ML, Disciglio V, Di Carlo G, et al. From genetics to histomolecular characterization: an insight into colorectal carcinogenesis in Lynch syndrome. *Int J Mol Sci.* 2021;22:6767. doi: 10.3390/ijms22136767.
9. Teixeria MC, Braghiroli MI, Sabbaga J, Hoff PM. Primary prevention of colorectal cancer myth or reality. *World J Gastoenterol.* 2014;20:1506015069.
10. Thun MJ, Jacobs EJ, Patrono C. The role of aspirin in cancer prevention. *Nat Rev Clin Oncol.* 2012;9:259–267.
11. Belayneh YM, Amare GG, Meharie BG. Updates on the molecular mechanisms of aspirin in the prevention of colorectal cancer: review. *J Oncol Pharm Pract.* 2021;27:954–961.
12. Gartlehner G, Patel SV, Feltner C, et al. Hormone therapy for the primary prevention of chronic conditions in postmenopausal women: evidence report and systematic review for the US Preventive Services Task Force. *JAMA.* 2017;318:2234–2249.
13. Friedenreich CM, Ryder-Burbidge C, McNeil J. Physical activity, obesity and sedentary behavior in cancer etiology: epidemiologic evidence and biologic mechanisms. *Mol Oncol.* 2021;15:790–800.
14. Rossi M, Anwar MJ, Usman A, et al. Colorectal cancer and alcohol consumption-populations to molecules. *Cancers (Basel).* 2018;10:38.
15. Fagunwa IO, Loughrey MB, Coleman HG. Alcohol, smoking and the risk of premalignant and malignant colorectal neoplasms. *Best Pract Res Clin Gastroenterol.* 2017;31:561–568.
16. Sánchez-Alcoholado L, Ramos-Molina B, Otero A, et al. The role of the gut microbiome in colorectal cancer development and therapy response. *Cancers.* 2020, 12, 1406; doi:10.3390/cancers12061406.
17. Veettil SK, Wong TY, Loo YS, et al. Role of diet in colorectal cancer incidence. Umbrella review of meta-analyses of prospective observational studies. *JAMA Network Open.* 2021;4(2):e2037341. doi:10.1001/jamanetworkopen.2020.37341.
18. Boughanem H, Canudas S, Hernandez-Alonso P, et al. Vitamin D intake and the risk of colorectal cancer: an updated meta-analysis and systematic review of case-control and prospective cohort studies. *Cancers.* 2021;13:2814. doi:10.3390/cancers13112814.
19. Song M, Garrett WS, Chan AT. Nutrients, foods, and colorectal cancer prevention. *Gastroenterology.* 2015;148:12441260.e16.
20. Li J, Ma X, Chakravarti D, et al. Genetic and biological hallmarks of colorectal cancer. *Genes & Dev.* 2021;35:787–820. doi:10.1101/gad.348226.120.
21. Fletcher R, Wang YJ, Schoen RE, et al. Colorectal cancer prevention: immune modulation taking the stage. *Biochimica et Biophysica Acta (BBA)—Reviews on Cancer.* 2018;1869:138148.
22. Harada S, Morlote D. Molecular pathology of colorectal cancer. *Adv Anat Pathol.* 2020;27:20–26.
23. Lai E, Liscia N, Donisi C, et al. Molecular-biology-driven treatment for metastatic colorectal cancer. *Cancers.* 2020;12, 1214; https://doi.org/10.3390/cancers12051214.
24. Rassol S, Rasool V, Naqvi T, Ganai BA, Shah BA. Genetic unraveling of colorectal cancer. *Tumor Biol.* 2014;35:5067–5082.
25. Stoffel EM. Updates on translational research on prevention of polyps and colorectal cancer. *Clin Colon Rectal Surg* 2018;31:153–160.
26. Waluga M, Zorniak M, Fichina J, et al. Pharmacological and dietary factors in prevention of colorectal cancer. *J Physiol Pharmacol.* 2018;69:325–336.
27. Kunzmann AT, Coleman HG, Huang WY, et al. Dietary fiber intake and risk of colorectal cancer and incident and recurrent adenoma in the Prostate, Lung, Colorectal, and Ovarian Cancer Screening Trial. *Am J Clin Nutr.* 2015;102:881–890.

28. Costea T, Hudită A, Ciolac OA, et al. Chemoprevention of colorectal cancer by dietary compounds. *Int J Mol Sci.* 2018;19:3787. 10.3390/ijms19123787.
29. Katona BW, Weiss JM. Chemoprevention of colorectal cancer. *Gastroenterol.* 2020;158:368–388.
30. Chapelle N, Martel M, Toes-Zoutendijk E, et al. Recent advances in clinical practice: colorectal cancer chemoprevention in the average-risk population. *Gut.* 2020;69:2244–2255. 10.1136/gutjnl-2020-320990.
31. Veettil SK, Lim KG, Ching SM, et al. Effects of aspirin and non-aspirin nonsteroidal anti-inflammatory drugs on the incidence of recurrent colorectal adenomas: a systematic review with meta-analysis and trial sequential analysis of randomized clinical trials. *BMC Cancer.* 2017;17(1):763. doi:10.1186/s12885-017-3757-8.
32. Bibbins-Domingo K, U.S. Preventive Services Task Force. Aspirin use for the primary prevention of cardiovascular disease and colorectal cancer: U.S. Preventive Services Task Force Recommendation Statement. *Ann Intern Med.* 2016;164:836–845.
33. Dekker E, Tanis PJ, Vleugels JLA, et al. Colorectal cancer. *Lancet.* 2019;394:1467–1480.
34. Fong W, Li Q, Yu J. Gut microbiota modulation: a novel strategy for prevention and treatment of colorectal cancer. *Oncogene* 2020;39:4925–4943.
35. NCCN Clinical Practice Guidelines in Oncology—Genetic/Familial High-Risk Assessment: Colorectal v1.2021. 2021. Available at: http://www.nccn.org/professionals/physician_gls/pdf/genetics_colon.pdf.
36. Wolf AMD, Fontham ETH, Church TR, et al. Colorectal cancer screening for average-risk adults: 2018 Guideline update from the American Cancer Society. *CA Cancer J Clin.* 2018;68:250–281.
37. Rex DK, Boland CR, Dominitz JA, et al. Colorectal cancer screening: recommendations for physicians and patients from the U.S. Multi-Society Task Force on Colorectal Cancer. *Gastroenterology.* 2017;153:307–323.
38. US Preventive Services Task Force. Screening for colorectal cancer. US Preventive Services Task Force Recommendation Statement. *JAMA.* 2021;325:1965–1977.
39. NCCN Clinical Practice Guidelines In Oncology—Colorectal Cancer Screening v.2.2021. 2021. Available at: http://www.nccn.org/professionals/physician_gls/pdf/colorectal_screening.pdf.
40. Shaukat A, Kahi CJ, Burke CA, et al. ACG clinical guidelines: colorectal cancer screening 2021. *Am J Gastroenterol.* 2021;116:458–479.
41. Qaseem A, Crandall CJ, Mustafa RA, et al. Screening for colorectal cancer in asymptomatic average-risk adults: a guidance statement from the American College of Physicians. *Ann Intern Med.* 2019;171:643–654.
42. Montminy EM, Jang A, Conner M, Karlitz JJ. Screening for colorectal cancer. *Med Clin N Am.* 2020;104:1023–1036.
43. Hadden WJ, de Reuver PR, Brown K, et al. Resection of colorectal liver metastases and extra-hepatic disease: a systematic review and proportional meta-analysis of survival outcomes. *HPB (Oxford).* 2016;18:209-220.
44. NCCN Clinical Practice Guidelines in Oncology—Colon Cancer v.3.2021. 2021. Available at: http://www.nccn.org/professionals/physician_gls/pdf/colon.pdf.
45. NCCN Clinical Practice Guidelines in Oncology—Rectal Cancer v.2.2021. 2021. Available at: http://www.nccn.org/professionals/physician_gls/pdf/rectal.pdf.
46. Amin MB, Greene FL, Edge SB, et al. Colon and rectum. *AJCC Cancer Staging Manual.* 8th ed. New York: Springer; 2017.
47. Libutti KS, Saltz LB, Willett CG. Cancers of the gastrointestinal tract: Cancer of the colon. In: DeVita VT, Lawrence TS, Rosenberg SA, eds. *Cancer: Principles and Practice of Oncology.* 10th ed. Philadelphia, PA: Lippincott Williams & Wilkins; 2015:1084–1126.
48. Sepulveda AR, Hamilton SR, Allegra CJ. Molecular biomarkers for the evaluation of colorectal cancer: guideline summary from the American Society for Clinical Pathology, College of American Pathologists, Association for Molecular Pathology, and American Society of Clinical Oncology. *J Oncol Pract.* 2017;13:333–337.
49. Bockelman C, Engelmann BE, Kaprio T, et al. Risk of recurrence in patients with colon cancer stage II and III: a systematic review and meta-analysis of recent literature. *Acta Oncol.* 2015;54:516.
50. Venook AP, Niedzwiecki D, Lopatin M, et al. Biologic determinants of tumor recurrence in stage II colon cancer: validation study of the 12-gene recurrence score in cancer and leukemia group B (CALGB) 9581. *J Clin Oncol.* 2013;31:1775–1781.
51. Yamanaka T, Oki E, Yamazaki K, et al. 12-Gene recurrence score assay stratifies the recurrence risk in stage II/III colon cancer with surgery alone: the SUNRISE study. *J Clin Oncol.* 2016;34:2906–2913.
52. Andre T, Boni C, Navarro M, et al. Improved overall survival with oxaliplatin, fluorouracil, and leucovorin as adjuvant treatment in stage II or III colon cancer in the MOSAIC trial. *J Clin Oncol.* 2009;27:3109–3116.
53. Grothey A, Sobrero AF, Shields AF, et al. Duration of adjuvant chemotherapy for stage III colon cancer. *N Engl J Med.* 2018;378:1177–1188.
54. Schmoll HJ, Cartwright T, Tabernero J, et al. Phase III trial of capecitabine plus oxaliplatin as adjuvant therapy for stage III colon cancer: a planned safety analysis in 1,864 patients. *J Clin Oncol.* 2007;25:102–109.
55. Twelves C, Scheithauer W, McKendrick J, et al. Capecitabine versus 5-fluorouracil/folinic acid as adjuvant therapy for stage III colon cancer: final results from the X-ACT trial with analysis by age and preliminary evidence of a pharmacodynamic marker of efficacy. *Ann Oncol.* 2012;23:1190–1197.
56. Haller DG, Catalano PJ, Macdonald JS, Mayer RJ. Phase III study of fluorouracil, leucovorin and levamisole in high risk stage II and III colon cancer: a final report of Intergroup 0089. *J Clin Oncol.* 2005;23:8671–8678.
57. Touringand C, Andre T, Bonnetain F, et al. Adjuvant therapy with fluorouracil and oxaliplatin in stage II and elderly patients (between ages 70–75 years) with colon cancer: subgroup analyses of the multicenter international study of oxaliplatin, fluorouracil, and leucovorin in the adjuvant treatment of colon cancer trial. *J Clin Oncol.* 2012;30:3353–3360.
58. Meta-Analysis Group in Cancer. Toxicity of fluorouracil in patients with advanced colorectal cancer: effect of administration schedule and prognostic factors. *J Clin Oncol.* 1998;16:3537–3541.
59. Chuang VTG, Suno M. Levoleucovorin as replacement for leucovorin in cancer treatment. *Ann Pharmacother.* 2012;46:1349–1357.
60. Weikhardt A, Wells K, Messersmith W. Oxaliplatin-induced neuropathy in colorectal cancer. *J Oncol.* 2011. doi:10.1155/2011/201593.
61. Haller DG, Tabernero J, Maroun J, et al. Capecitabine plus oxaliplatin compared with fluorouracil and folinic acid as adjuvant therapy for stage III colon cancer. *J Clin Oncol.* 2011;29:1465–1471.
62. Yothers G, O'Connell MJ, Allegra CJ, et al. Oxaliplatin as adjuvant therapy for colon cancer: updated results of NSABP C-07 trial, including survival and subset analyses. *J Clin Oncol.* 2011;29:3768–3774.
63. Andre T, Vernerey D, Mineur L, et al. Three versus six months of oxaliplatin-based adjuvant chemotherapy for patients with stage III colon cancer: disease-free survival results from a randomized, open-label, international duration evaluation of adjuvant (IDEA) France, phase III trial. *J Clin Oncol.* 2018;36:1469–1477.
64. Phillips JG, Hong TS, Ryan DP. Multidisciplinary management of early-stage rectal cancer. *J Natl Compr Canc Netw.* 2012;10:1577–1585.
65. Douillard J, Cunningham D, Roth A, et al. Irinotecan combined with fluorouracil compared with fluorouracil alone as first-line treatment for metastatic colorectal cancer: a multicentre randomised trial. *Lancet.* 2000;355:1041–1047.
66. Liu X, Cheng D, Kuang Q, et al. Association of UGT1A1*28 polymorphisms with irinotecan-induced toxicities in colorectal cancer: a meta-analysis in Caucasians. *Pharmacogenomics J.* 2014;14:120–129.
67. Lin PS, Semrad TJ. Molecular testing for the treatment of advanced colorectal cancer: an overview. *Methods Mol Bio.* 2018;1765:281–297.
68. de Gramont A, Figer A, Seymour M, et al. Leucovorin and fluorouracil with or without oxaliplatin as first-line treatment in advanced colorectal cancer. *J Clin Oncol.* 2000;18:2938–2947.
69. Twelves C. Capecitabine as first-line treatment in colorectal cancer. *Eur J Cancer.* 2002;38:1520.
70. Ranpura V, Hapani S, Wu S. Treatment-related mortality with bevacizumab in cancer patients: a meta-analysis. *JAMA.* 2011;305:487–494.
71. Resch G, Schaberl-Moser R, Kier P, et al. Infusion reactions to the chimeric EGFR inhibitor cetuximab—change to the fully human anti-EGFR monoclonal antibody panitumumab is safe. *Ann Oncol.* 2011;22:486–487.
72. Lacotoure ME, Anadkat MJ, Bensadoun RJ, et al. Clinical practice guidelines for the prevention and treatment of EGFR inhibitor-associated dermatologic toxicities. *Support Care Cancer.* 2011;19:1079–1095.
73. Overman MJ, Lonardi S, Wong WYM, et al. Durable clinical benefit with nivolumab plus ipilimumab in DNA mismatch repair-deficient/microsatellite instability-high metastatic colorectal cancer. *J Clin Oncol.* 2018;36:773–779.
74. Mayer RJ, Van Cutsem E, Falcone A, et al. Randomized trial of TAS-102 for refractory metastatic colorectal cancer. *N Engl J Med.* 2015;372:1909–1919.

75. Sobrero AF, Maurel J, Fehrenbacher L, et al. EPIC: Phase III trial of cetuximab plus irinotecan after fluoropyrimidine and oxaliplatin failure in patients with metastatic colorectal cancer. *J Clin Oncol.* 2008;26:2311–2319.
76. Peeters M, Price TJ, Cervantes A, et al. Randomized phase III study of panitumumab with fluorouracil, leucovorin, and irinotecan (FOLFIRI) compared with FOLFIRI alone as second-line treatment in patients with metastatic colorectal cancer. *J Clin Oncol.* 2010;23:4706–4713.
77. Kopetz S, Grothey A, Yaeger R, et al. Encorafenib, binimetinib, and cetuximab in *BRAF* V600E-mutated colorectal cancer. *N Engl J Med.* 2019;381:1632–1643.
78. Giantonio BJ, Catalano PJ, Meropol NJ, et al. Bevacizumab in combination with oxaliplatin, fluorouracil, and leucovorin (FOLFOX4) for previously treated metastatic colorectal cancer: results from the Eastern Cooperative Oncology Group Study E3200. *J Clin Oncol.* 2007;25:1539–1544.
79. Van Cutsem E, Tabernero J, Lakomy R, et al. Addition of afilbercept to fluorouracil, leucovorin, and irinotecan improves survival in a phase III randomized trial in patients with metastatic colorectal cancer previously treated with an oxaliplatin-based regimen. *J Clin Oncol.* 2012;30:3499–3506.
80. Tabernero J, Yoshino T, Cohn AL, et al. Ramucirumab versus placebo in combination with second-line FOLFIRI in patients with metastatic colorectal carcinoma that progressed during or after first-line therapy with bevacizumab, oxaliplatin, and a flucurropyrimidine (RAISE): a randomised, double-blind, multicentre, phase 3 study. *Lancet Oncol.* 2015;16:499–508.
81. Grothey A, Van Cutsem E, Sobreror A, et al. Regorafenib monotherapy for previously treated metastatic colorectal cancer (CORRECT): an international, multicenter, randomized, placebo-controlled, phase 3 trial. *Lancet.* 2013;381:303–312.
82. Meric-Bernstam F, Hurwitz H, Raghav KPS, McWilliams RR, Fakih M, VancerWalde A. Pertuzumabplus trastuzumab for HER2-amplified metastatic colorectal cancer (MyPathway): an updated report from a multicentre, open-label, phase 2a, multiple basket study. *Lancet Oncol.* 2019;20:518–530.
83. Sartore-Bianchi A, Trusolino L, Martino C, Bencardino K, Lonardi S, Bergamo F. Dual-targeted therapy with trastuzumab and lapatinib in treatment-refractory, KRAS codon 12/13 wild-type, HER2-positive metastatic colorectal cancer (HERACLES): a proof-of-concept, multicentre, open-label, phase 2 trial. *Lancet Oncol.* 2016;17:738–743.
84. Andre T, Shiu KK, Kim TW, et al. Pembrolizumab in microsatellite-instability-high advanced colorectal cancer. *N Engl J Med.* 2020;383:2207–2218.
85. Lenz H-J, van Cutsem E, Limon ML, et al. First-line nivolumab plus low-dose iplimumab for microsatellite instability-high/mismatch repair deficient metastatic colorectal cancer the phase 2 CheckMate 142 study. *J Clin Oncol.* 2022;10:161-170.
86. NCCN Clinical Practice Guidelines in Oncology—Management of Immunotherapy-Related Toxicities v.3.2021. 2021. Available at: http://www.nccn.org/professionals/physician_gls/pdf/immunotherapy.pdf.

154

Prostate Cancer

Daniel J. Crona and Amber B. Cipriani

KEY CONCEPTS

1. Prostate cancer is the most frequent cancer in men in the United States. The risk of prostate cancer is higher in those with increased age, Black individuals, and those with a family history of prostate cancer.
2. Screening is not universally recommended and individuals should discuss with their provider about risks versus benefits of screening. Digital rectal examination (DRE) and prostate-specific antigen (PSA) may be incorporated into individualized screening plans.
3. The prognosis for patients with prostate cancer depends on the histologic grade, the tumor size, and the disease stage. More than 85% of patients with localized disease, but less than 1% of those with metastatic disease can be cured.
4. Androgen deprivation therapy (ADT) with a luteinizing hormone-releasing hormone (LHRH) agonist plus an antiandrogen should be used in addition to radiation therapy for patients with locally advanced prostate cancer to improve outcomes over radiation therapy alone.
5. Systemic therapy for nonmetastatic castration-naïve disease that has not been treated with ADT may include either orchiectomy, LHRH agonist with or without an antiandrogen, gonadotropin-releasing hormone (GnRH) antagonist, or observation.
6. In metastatic castration-naïve disease, the addition of the following therapies to ADT improves survival: docetaxel, abiraterone, enzalutamide, or apalutamide.
7. Prostate cancer that has progressed despite androgen deprivation is called castration-resistant prostate cancer. First-line treatment options for nonmetastatic castration-resistant prostate cancer include apalutamide, darolutamide, and enzalutamide.
8. In metastatic castration-resistant prostate cancer, first-line treatment options include docetaxel with prednisone, abiraterone with prednisone, and enzalutamide. ADT is continued in all cases.
9. Germline genetic testing is recommended in patients with high-risk prostate cancer and/or a relevant family history. Somatic tumor genetic testing is recommended in metastatic disease to identify genetic variants that can be targeted with drug therapy.
10. Pembrolizumab may be considered in men whose tumors show deficiencies in deoxyribonucleic acid (DNA) mismatch repair (dMMR), test high for microsatellite instability (MSI-H), or have a tumor mutation burden greater than or equal to 10 mutations per megabase (TMB $\geq$10 mut/Mb).
11. Poly (ADP ribose) polymerase (PARP) inhibitors, including olaparib and rucaparib, can be considered in men with metastatic castration-resistant prostate cancer who have specific somatic or germline alterations in genes involved in homologous recombination (HR), such as *BRCA1* and *BRCA2*.

BEYOND THE BOOK

Review the following case and answer the questions based on the information provided in the chapter:

A 60-year-old male presents to the ED with worsening back pain over the past 2 months. His lab reports were notable for a decreased hemoglobin of 10.1 g/dL (101 g/L; 6.27 mmol/L), a blood glucose of 280 mg/dL (15.5 mmol/L), and an alkaline phosphatase of 324 IU/L (5.4 μkat/L). A CT scan of the chest, abdomen, and pelvis revealed diffuse spine masses and bilateral rib masses suspicious for malignancy. A biopsy of a pelvic bone mass was consistent with prostate adenocarcinoma. Other relevant information is as follows:

- Past medical history: HTN, Afib, T2DM
- Family history: Father died of a myocardial infarction at the age of 57 years, mother died of breast cancer at the age of 47 years
- Medications: apixaban 5 mg BID, metoprolol 50 mg BID, nifedipine ER 60 mg daily, simvastatin 40 mg qHS, metformin 1,000 mg PO BID, empagliflozin 10 mg daily
- Vitals: BP 130/80, HR 81, Ht 176 cm, Wt 103.2 kg
- Lab reports:
  - PSA 132 ng/mL (mcg/L)
  - Testosterone 350 ng/dL (12.1 nmol/L)

Questions for self-assessment:

1. How would you classify this patient's prostate cancer? Describe if the cancer is metastatic or nonmetastatic and the castration status of the patient.
2. What treatment options are available to this patient to treat his cancer (based on your classification above)?
3. Perform a drug interaction screen for the available agents being considered to treat this patient's prostate cancer. Are there any contraindications? What changes to the patient's current medication regimen would you recommend if any of the agents were to be initiated? (Hint: It might be helpful to make a table of the available options to treat prostate cancer and then consider these options with each of the drugs on the patient's current medication list.)
4. Would this patient be eligible for genetic testing? (You can review the detailed recommendations for genetic testing in prostate cancer by accessing the current NCCN® Guidelines at: http://nccn.org)
5. Bonus question: Using resources outside of the chapter, suggest a possible cause of the patient's elevated alkaline phosphatase.

INTRODUCTION

In this chapter, the term "male" is used only to reflect the biological sex of individuals at birth and not the gender identified by the patient. Moreover, we recognize that not all patients with prostate cancer identify as "men" at the time of diagnosis and treatment of this condition. Prostate cancer is the most commonly diagnosed cancer in biological males in the United States.[1] For most, prostate cancer has an indolent course, and treatment options for early disease include expectant management, surgery, or radiation. With expectant management, patients are monitored for disease progression or development of symptoms. Localized prostate cancer can be cured by surgery or radiation therapy, but advanced and metastatic prostate cancers are not yet curable. Treatments for advanced and metastatic prostate cancers can provide significant disease palliation for many patients for several years after diagnosis. The endocrine dependence of this tumor is well documented, and hormonal manipulation aimed at decreasing circulating androgens remains the basis for the treatment of advanced and metastatic disease.

EPIDEMIOLOGY

1 Prostate cancer is the most frequent cancer among biologically male individuals in the United States and represents the second leading cause of cancer-related deaths in biological males.[1] In the United States alone, it is estimated that 268,490 new cases of prostate cancer were diagnosed and more than 34,500 individuals died from this disease in 2022.[1] Although the incidence of prostate cancer increased during the late 1980s and early 1990s related to widespread PSA screening, the incidence declined rapidly from 2007 to 2014 because of recommendations against routine PSA screening. Deaths from prostate cancer have declined since 1993.[1] The slowing decline in prostate cancer mortality between 2013 and 2019 is probably related to the decrease in PSA screening and an increase in advanced-stage diagnoses.[1]

ETIOLOGY

Table 154-1 summarizes the possible risk factors associated with prostate cancer.[2-4] The widely accepted risk factors for prostate cancer are age, race/ethnicity, and family history of prostate cancer. The disease is rare in those younger than 40 years, but the incidence sharply increases with each subsequent decade of life. The increased risk can likely be attributed to cumulative lifetime exposure to testosterone, which is a known growth signal for the prostate.

Race and Ethnicity

The incidence of clinical prostate cancer varies across geographic regions. Scandinavian countries and the United States report the highest incidence of prostate cancer, while the disease is relatively rare in Japan and other Asian countries.[5] Black individuals from the United States have the highest rate of prostate cancer in the world, and prostate cancer mortality among them is more than twice that seen in White populations in the United States.[1] Hormonal, dietary, and genetic differences, and differences in access to healthcare may contribute to the altered susceptibility to prostate cancer in these populations.[2,3]

In addition, genetic variations in the androgen receptor gene (*AR*) exist. *AR* activation is inversely associated with CAG trinucleotide repeat length. Under normal circumstances, a CAG trinucleotide, consisting of the DNA building blocks cytosine, adenine and guanine, is repeated 10 to 35 times within a given gene. However, shorter CAG repeat sequences in *AR* have been found in Black individuals, and a meta-analysis demonstrated that carriers of a short CAG repeat had a 20% increased risk of prostate cancer when compared to individuals with long CAG repeats.[2]

Genetics and Family History

Approximately 5% to 10% of prostate cancers are believed to be inherited, but individuals with a brother or father with prostate cancer have twice the risk for developing prostate than the rest of the population.[6] Familial clustering of prostate cancer syndrome has been reported, and genome-wide scans have identified potential prostate cancer susceptibility candidate genes. Carriers of germline polymorphisms in one of 16 DNA damage repair genes (eg, *BRCA1*, *BRCA2*, and *CHEK2*) have been associated with an increased risk of developing aggressive prostate cancer.[4,5] Germline genetic testing to evaluate for inherited cancer susceptibility genes is now recommended in patients who are diagnosed with prostate cancer and have a relevant family history, or those who are diagnosed with advanced/high-risk disease.[7] Other genes implicated in hereditary prostate cancer are *MSH2* and *HOXB13*.[6] In addition to inherited genetics, common exposure to environmental and other risk factors may contribute to increased risk among patients with first-degree relatives with prostate cancer.[5]

Diet

The overall dietary factor associated with the lowest risk of developing prostate cancer appears to be adherence to a Mediterranean diet.[8] The typical Mediterranean diet is high in fruits, vegetables, legumes, fish, olive oil, and red wine, with low-to-moderate amounts of red meat, poultry, and dairy. In a meta-analysis that included

TABLE 154-1 Risk Factors Associated with Prostate Cancer

Factor	Possible Relationship
Probable Risk Factors	
Age	Greater than 70% of cases are diagnosed in men older than 65 years
Race/Ethnicity	Black individuals in the United States have a higher incidence and death rate
Genetic	Familial prostate cancer is inherited in an autosomal dominant manner
	Germline mutations in *ATM, ATR, BRCA1, BRCA2, BRIP1, CHEK2, FAM175A, FH, GEN1, HOXB13, MRE11A, MSH2, MSH6, NBN, PALB2, PMS2, RAD51C*, or *RAD51D* are more common in metastatic/high-risk prostate cancer compared to localized/low-risk
	Inherited polymorphisms (eg, CAG repeat length) that lead to increased androgen receptor (AR) activation
Possible Risk Factors	
Environmental	Incidence varies worldwide
	Nationalized individuals adopt intermediate incidence rates between those of the United States and their native country
Occupational	Increased risk associated with cadmium exposure
Diet	Mediterranean diet associated with reduced risk
	Increased risk associated with high-red meat and high-fat diets
	Decreased intake of 25-dihydroxyvitamin D, lycopene, and β-carotene increases risk

approximately 1.5 million subjects, adherence to a Mediterranean diet was associated with a small, but significantly reduced risk of prostate cancer.[8]

Many individual dietary factors have been assessed to ascertain their role in the development or prevention of prostate cancer.[9] Green tea and lycopene are considered the most useful, and at least not harmful. Green tea consumption was associated with a reduced risk of prostate cancer in a small casecontrol study. Lycopene, obtained primarily from tomatoes, has been associated with a decreased risk of prostate cancer in small cohort studies, although a meta-analysis failed to show benefit for high tomato consumption.[9]

Consistent with the beneficial effects of the Mediterranean diet, red meat, and high milk intake have been clearly and consistently associated with an increased risk of prostate cancer in epidemiological studies.[9]

Other Factors

Benign prostatic hyperplasia (BPH) is a common problem among geriatric patients, affecting greater than 40% of men older than 70 years (see Chapter 104, "Benign Prostatic Hyperplasia"). BPH results in the urinary symptoms of increased hesitancy and frequency. Because prostate cancer affects a similar age group, and often has similar presenting signs and symptoms, the presence of BPH often complicates prostate cancer diagnoses. But importantly, a BPH diagnosis does not appear to increase the risk of developing prostate cancer.[3]

Interestingly, smoking has not been validated as a risk factor for developing prostate cancer. However, smokers with prostate cancer have almost a two-times greater risk of prostate cancer-related mortality when compared with nonsmokers with prostate cancer.[3] In addition, both clinical and translational study results did not detect an association between alcohol consumption and prostate cancer development.[10,11]

CHEMOPREVENTION

The use of 5-α-reductase inhibitors, finasteride and dutasteride, to prevent prostate cancer has been debated for more than a decade.[12-15] These drugs inhibit 5-α-reductase, an enzyme that converts testosterone to its more active form, dihydrotestosterone (DHT), which is involved in prostate epithelial proliferation. Both finasteride and dutasteride can falsely lower PSA by about 50% in patients, and this must be considered when one interprets PSA in patients on these medications.[16] Although a number of large chemoprevention trials demonstrated a decreased risk of prostate cancer in patients who received 5-α-reductase inhibitors, this was coupled with an increased risk of developing more aggressive tumors. A survival benefit from chemoprevention with 5-α-reductase inhibitors has not been confirmed, although more contemporary analyses have called into question the association of 5-α-reductase inhibitors with the development of higher grade tumors.[17] Patients treated with 5-α-reductase inhibitors can experience adverse drug reactions, including gynecomastia, decreased libido, and erectile dysfunction.[13] Based on the concern for the development of more aggressive tumors, lack of survival benefit, and increased risk of adverse drug reactions, neither finasteride nor dutasteride is approved or recommended for preventing prostate cancer.[14,18]

Selenium and vitamin E, either alone or in combination, were evaluated as possible chemopreventive agents in the Selenium and Vitamin E Cancer Prevention Trial (SELECT), a clinical trial of healthy individuals. The results of this trial showed that selenium or vitamin E taken alone or together did not prevent prostate cancer. Furthermore, with a longer follow-up of that trial, dietary supplementation with vitamin E was found to significantly increase the risk of prostate cancer by 17%.[19] Other agents, including lycopene, green tea, nonsteroidal anti-inflammatory agents, isoflavones, and statins, have been evaluated for prostate cancer prevention, but none are recommended for routine use outside of a clinical trial.[20]

SCREENING

(2) Screening is not routinely recommended for all individuals at risk for prostate cancer. Rather, it is recommended that the individual discusses with their provider about risks versus benefits of screening. If prostate cancer screening is performed, the PSA test is the method of choice. PSA is a kallikrein-like serine protease, which liquefies seminal secretions and is produced by the prostate epithelial cells. Although PSA is specific for the prostate, it is not specific for cancer, and low specificity is a major limitation of the test. PSA may be elevated in patients with acute urinary retention, acute prostatitis, and prostatic ischemia or infarction, as well as BPH.[18,21] PSA elevations between 4.1 and 10 ng/mL (μg/L) cannot distinguish between BPH and prostate cancer, which limits the utility of the PSA test alone for the early detection of prostate cancer. Additionally, many patients with clinically significant prostate cancer do not have a serum PSA outside the reference range.[22]

Early detection of potentially curable prostate cancers is the goal of prostate cancer screening. For cancer screening to be beneficial, it must reliably detect cancer at an early stage, when intervention would decrease mortality. Whether prostate cancer screening fits these criteria is debatable.[23-26] The European Randomized Study of Screening for Prostate Cancer study demonstrated that compared to no PSA testing, PSA testing every 4 years decreased prostate cancer deaths in the screened group by about 1 per 1,000 men. However, the false-positive rate was 76% in the group that underwent PSA screening, which resulted in more than 13,000 unnecessary biopsies.[27] In the United States, the Prostate, Lung, Colon, and Ovarian Screening study showed no reduction in prostate cancer death between the annual screening group (PSA and DRE) and the usual care group, which is not surprising given the small reduction in death expected, and that about one-half of the patients in the usual care groups had PSA and/or DRE screening performed.[28] An updated systematic review found similar results in that PSA screening for prostate cancer may reduce the risk of prostate cancer mortality, but is associated with harms including false-positive results, biopsy complications, and over diagnosis in 20% to 50% of screen-detected prostate cancers. Early, active treatment for screen-detected prostate cancer may reduce the risk of metastatic disease, although the long-term impact of early, active treatment on prostate cancer mortality remains unclear. Active treatments for prostate cancer are frequently associated with sexual and urinary difficulties and thus can decrease quality of life for many patients.[29]

The US Preventive Services Task Force recommended that biologically male individuals aged 55 to 69 years make an individual decision about prostate cancer screening with their clinician (recommendation grade C) and recommended against routine screening for those aged 70 and older (recommendation grade D).[29] The American Urological Association does not recommend routine screening in biologic males between the ages of 40 and 54 years of average risk, but they recommend that the risks and benefits of prostate cancer screening are discussed with individuals aged 55 to 69 years.[23] For biologic males who elect to be screened, the frequency should be no more than 2 years, and screening every 5 years may be adequate. The American Society of Clinical Oncology recommends that asymptomatic biologically male individuals who have at least a 10-year life expectancy have an opportunity to make an informed decision about prostate cancer screening, including discussion of the uncertainties, risks, and potential benefits associated with screening.[26]

PATHOPHYSIOLOGY

The prostate gland is a solid, rounded, heart-shaped organ positioned between the neck of the bladder and the urogenital diaphragm (Fig. 154-1). The normal prostate is composed of acinar secretory cells arranged in a radial shape and surrounded by a foundation of supporting tissue. The size, shape, or presence of acini is almost always altered in the gland that has been invaded by prostatic carcinoma. Adenocarcinoma, the major pathologic cell type, accounts for more than 95% of prostate cancer cases.[30,31] Much rarer tumor types include small cell neuroendocrine cancers, sarcomas, and transitional cell carcinomas.

Prostate cancer can be graded systematically according to the histologic appearance of the malignant cell and then grouped into well, moderately, or poorly differentiated grades.[31,32] Approximately 8 to 15 core biopsies are used to examine gland architecture and assess for malignancy. If malignancy is found then it is rated on a scale of 1 (well differentiated) to 5 (poorly differentiated). The two most common scores are added to give the Gleason pattern, with the most prevalent pattern represented as the first number (ie, 3+4 or 4+3). The biopsies are further classified into five Gleason groups, which are used to aid in prognosis, with Gleason Group 1 representing a

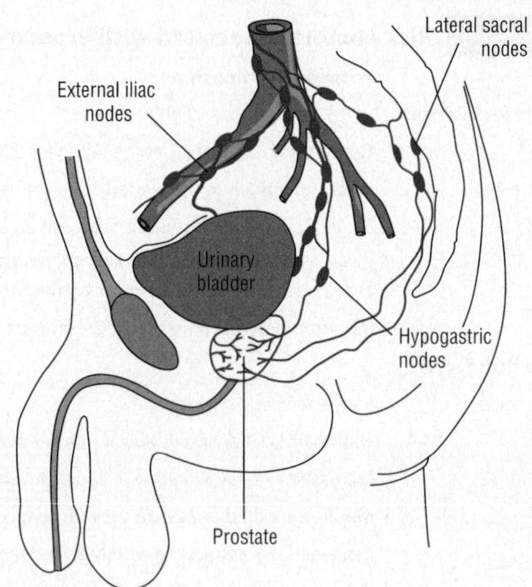

FIGURE 154-1 The prostate gland within the male genitourinary system.

Gleason score of ≤6 and Gleason Group 5 representing poorly differentiated disease with a Gleason score of 9 to 10. Poorly differentiated tumors grow rapidly (poor prognosis), while well-differentiated tumors grow slowly (better prognosis).

Metastatic spread can occur by local extension, lymphatic drainage, or hematogenous dissemination.[32,33] Lymph node metastases are more common in patients with large, undifferentiated tumors that invade the seminal vesicles. The pelvic and abdominal lymph node groups are the most common sites of lymph node involvement (see Fig. 154-1). Skeletal metastases from hematogenous spread are the most common sites of distant spread. Typically, the bone lesions are osteoblastic or a combination of osteoblastic and osteolytic. The most common site of bone involvement is the lumbar spine. Other sites of bone involvement include the proximal femur, pelvis, thoracic spine, ribs, sternum, skull, and humerus. The lung, liver, brain, and adrenal glands are the most common sites of visceral involvement, although these organs are not usually initially involved. About 25% to 35% of patients will have evidence of lymphangitic or nodular pulmonary infiltrates at autopsy. The prostate is rarely a site for metastatic involvement from other solid tumors.

Normal growth and differentiation of the prostate depend on the presence of androgens, specifically DHT.[33,34] The testes and the adrenal glands are the major sources of circulating androgens. Hormonal regulation of androgen synthesis is mediated through a series of biochemical interactions between the hypothalamus, pituitary, adrenal glands, and testes (Fig. 154-2). LHRH released from the hypothalamus stimulates the release of luteinizing hormone (LH) and follicle-stimulating hormone (FSH) from the anterior pituitary gland. LH complexes with receptors on the Leydig cell testicular membrane, and stimulates the production of testosterone and small amounts of estrogen. FSH acts on the Sertoli cells within the testes to promote the maturation of LH receptors and to produce an androgen-binding protein. Circulating testosterone and estradiol influence the synthesis of LHRH, LH, and FSH by a negative feedback loop operating at the hypothalamic and pituitary level.[35] Prolactin, growth hormone, and estradiol areimportant accessory regulators for prostatic tissue permeability, receptor binding, and testosterone synthesis.

Testosterone, the major androgenic hormone, accounts for 95% of the androgen concentration. The primary source of testosterone is the testes, but 3% to 5% of the testosterone concentration is derived from direct adrenal cortical secretion of testosterone or C19 steroids

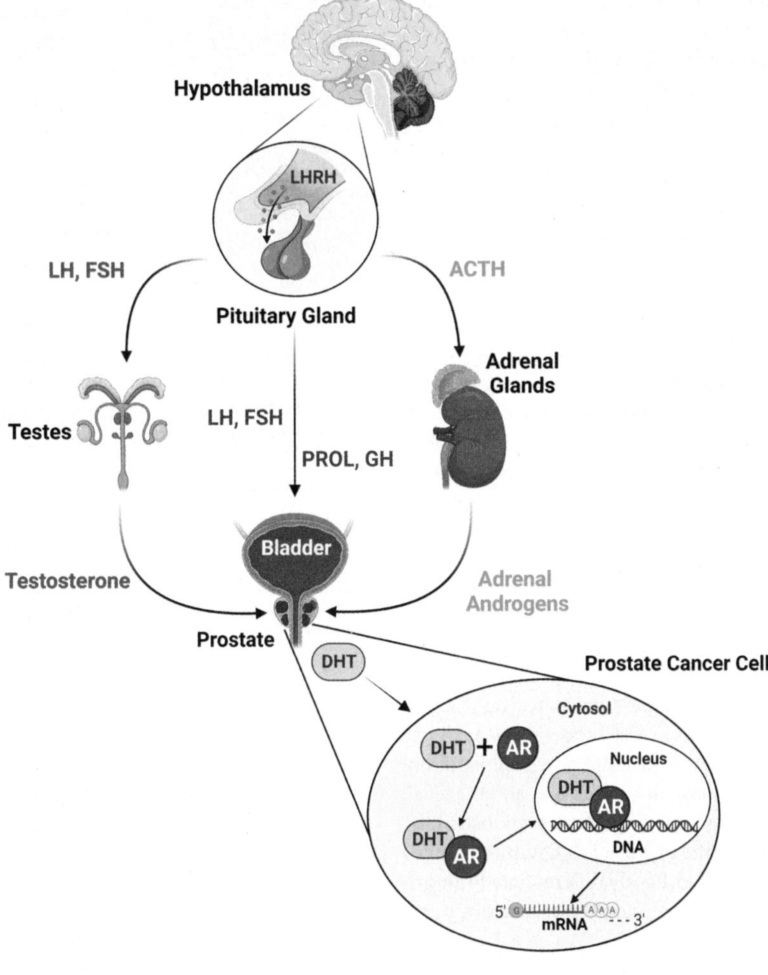

FIGURE 154-2 Hormonal regulation of the prostate gland. ACTH, adrenocorticotropic hormone; DNA, deoxyribonucleic acid; GH, growth hormone; mRNA, messenger ribonucleic acid; PROL, prolactin.

such as androstenedione.[32-34] 5α-reductase converts testosterone to DHT. When DHT is not bound to the AR, the AR remains inactive within the cytoplasm where it is bound to chaperone proteins (eg, heat shock protein 90 or HSP90).[36] However, when the AR is activated by DHT, the AR disassociates from heat shock protein 90, dimerizes, and then translocates into the nucleus where it binds to androgen response elements. AR binding to the androgen response elements regulates transcription of genes that regulate prostate cancer proliferation and cell survival (Fig. 154-2).[36,37]

In early-stage prostate cancers, aberrant tumor cell proliferation is promoted by the presence of androgens. For these tumors, the blockade of androgens induces tumor regression in most patients. Hormonal manipulations to ablate or reduce circulating androgens can occur through several mechanisms (Table 154-2).[33,34] The organs responsible for androgen production can be removed surgically (ie, orchiectomy, hypophysectomy, or adrenalectomy). Hormonal pathways that modulate prostatic growth can be interrupted at several steps (Fig. 154-2). Interference with LHRH or LH can reduce testosterone secretion by the testes.

Isolation of the naturally occurring hypothalamic decapeptide hormone, LHRH (also known as gonadotropin-releasing hormone or GnRH) has provided another group of effective agents for advanced prostate cancer treatment. The physiologic response to LHRH depends on both the dose and the mode of administration. Intermittent pulsed LHRH administration, which mimics the endogenous release pattern, causes sustained release of both LH and FSH, whereas high-dose or continuous intravenous administration of LHRH inhibits gonadotropin release due to receptor downregulation.[27] Structural modification of the naturally occurring LHRH and innovative delivery have produced a series of LHRH agonists that cause a similar downregulation of pituitary receptors and a decrease in testosterone production.[35]

Androgen synthesis can also be inhibited in the testes or in the adrenal gland. Antiandrogens inhibit the formation of the DHT-receptor complex and therefore interfere with androgen activity at the cellular level.[35] In advanced stages of disease, prostate cancer cells may survive and proliferate without the signals normally provided

TABLE 154-2 Hormonal Manipulations in Prostate Cancer

Androgen source ablation	**Androgen synthesis inhibitors**
Adrenalectomy	Abiraterone acetate
Orchiectomy	Ketoconazole
Hypophysectomy	
	First-generation antiandrogens
LHRH agonists	Bicalutamide
Goserelin	Flutamide
Leuprolide	Nilutamide
Triptorelin	
	Second-generation antiandrogens
LHRH/GnRH antagonists	Apalutamide
Degarelix	Darolutamide
Relugolix	Enzalutamide

by circulating androgens.[35] When this occurs, the tumor is no longer sensitive to therapies that depend on androgen blockade. These tumors are often referred to as hormone refractory, androgen independent, or castration-resistant. Re-exposure to androgens can still cause these castration-resistant tumors to proliferate, but they have developed resistance mechanisms to androgen suppression alone. Thus, ADT must be continued in patients with castration-resistant disease (in addition to therapies with other mechanisms of action), despite evidence that the prostate cancer is no longer sensitive to ADT when used alone.

CLINICAL PRESENTATION

Before the implementation of routine screening, prostate cancers were frequently diagnosed after the onset of symptoms, including urinary hesitancy, retention, painful urination, hematuria, and erectile dysfunction. With the introduction of screening, most prostate cancers are now identified before the development of symptoms, although this may change as routine screening is no longer the norm.

DIAGNOSIS AND STAGING

The information obtained from the diagnostic tests is used to stage the patient (Table 154-3). The eighth edition of the formal international classification system is the American Joint Committee on Cancer (AJCC) system (tumor, node, metastases [TNM]) (Table 154-4).

3 The prognosis for patients with prostate cancer depends on the histologic grade (ie, Gleason score), the tumor size, and the local extent of the primary tumor.[31] The most important prognostic factor is the histologic grade because the degree of differentiation ultimately determines the stage of disease. Poorly differentiated tumors are highly associated with both regional lymph node involvement and distant metastases.[28]

Data from 2011 to 2017 showed that among all patients with prostate cancer, 5-year overall survival was estimated to be >99% when the disease is localized at diagnosis, and the 5-year survival rate for all stages combined is 98%. However, for individuals who are diagnosed initially with metastatic prostate cancer, 5-year survival drops to 30%. These same 2011 to 2017 data also showed that 5-year overall survival rates were estimated at 98% in White individuals and 96% in Black individuals.[1] For almost the same period, the survival rates for localized or regional disease and distant disease were also approximately the same in White and Black individuals in the United States.[1]

TABLE 154-3 Diagnostic and Staging Workup for Prostate Cancer

Initial tests	DRE
	PSA level
	Biopsy
Staging tests	Gleason score on biopsy specimen
	Bone imaging
	Pelvic/abdominal imaging (mpMRI)
	Complete blood count
	Liver function tests
	Serum phosphatases (acid/alkaline)
Additional staging tests (depends on tumor classification, PSA, and Gleason score)	Obtain family cancer history/assess risk of germline genetic mutations
	Estimate life expectancy
	Somatic tumor mutation testing
	Lymph node evaluation
	Pelvic computed tomography
	PMSA-targeted PET-CT imaging (eg, Ga 68 PSMA-11 and piflufolastat F 18)

CT, computed tomography; mpMRI, multi-parametric magnetic resonance imaging; PET, positron emission tomography; PMSA, prostate-specific membrane antigen.

TREATMENT

Desired Outcomes

The desired outcome in early-stage prostate cancer is to minimize morbidity and mortality caused by prostate cancer.[7,38] The most appropriate therapy of early-stage prostate cancer is controversial. Early-stage disease may be treated with surgery, radiation, or expectant management. While surgery and radiation are curative, they are associated with significant morbidity and even mortality. Because the overall goal is to minimize morbidity and mortality associated with the disease, watchful waiting is appropriate in selected individuals. Advanced prostate cancer is not curable, and treatment should provide symptom relief and maintain quality of life. The mainstay of treatment for advanced prostate cancer is ADT, with a goal of reducing testosterone to castrate levels, with either surgical (eg, orchiectomy) or pharmacologic modalities (eg, LHRH agonist or LHRH/GnRH antagonist).

General Approach to Treatment

The initial treatment for prostate cancer depends primarily on the disease stage, the Gleason score, the presence of symptoms, and the life expectancy of the patient.[7] Prostate cancer is usually initially diagnosed by PSA and DRE, and then confirmed by a biopsy where the Gleason score is assigned. Asymptomatic patients with a low risk of recurrence may be managed by observation, radiation, or radical prostatectomy (Table 154-5). As patients with asymptomatic early-stage disease generally have an excellent 10-year survival, immediate morbidities of treatment must be balanced with the lower likelihood of dying from prostate cancer. More aggressive treatment of early-stage prostate cancer is generally reserved for younger individuals, although patient preference is a major consideration in all treatment decisions. In a patient with a normal life expectancy of less than 10 years, observation or radiation therapy may be offered. In those with

CLINICAL PRESENTATION Prostate Cancer

Localized Disease

- Usually asymptomatic

Locally Invasive Disease

- Ureteral dysfunction, frequency, hesitancy, and dribbling
- Impotence

Advanced Disease

- Back pain
- Spinal cord compression
- Lower extremity edema
- Pathologic fractures
- Anemia
- Weight loss

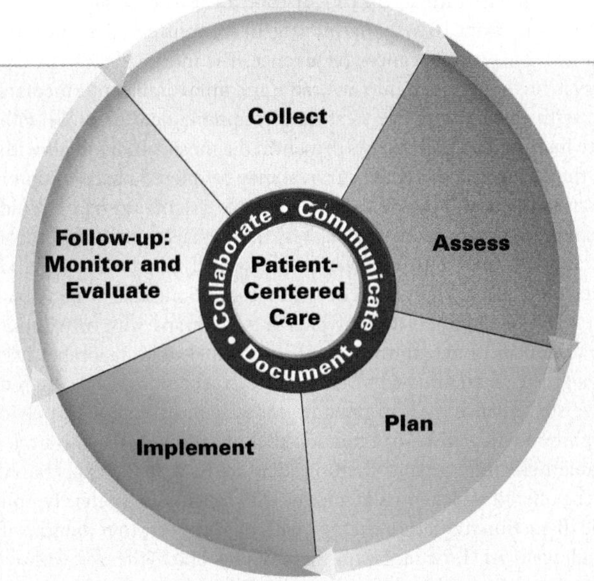

Patient Care Process for Prostate Cancer

Collect

- Patient characteristics (eg, age, race/ethnicity)
- Patient history (past medical, family, social, dietary habits)
- Family cancer history (to determine eligibility for and to interpret germline genetic testing)
- Current signs and symptoms (eg, frequency of urination, dribbling, hesitancy, pain, fatigue, weight loss, shortness of breath)
- Thorough medication history (including prescription, nonprescription medications, and other substances), drug allergies, and intolerances
- Objective data (see Table 154-3)
  - BP, heart rate, height, and weight
  - Labs (PSA level, complete blood count, serum electrolytes, renal function, liver function tests)
  - Physical examination (DRE, edema, breath sounds, ascites)
  - Imaging (see Table 154-3)
  - Pathology (Gleason score, determine number of positive biopsy cores)
  - Genetic testing (germline and/or somatic [tumor] based on risk factors)

Assess

- Determine the stage and risk category of disease based on, laboratory testing, imaging, and biopsy information (Table 154-4)
- Estimate life expectancy of the patient (can use Social Security Administration Life Insurance calculator)
- Evaluate current medication regimen and past medical history for potential drug-drug interactions or treatment contraindications
- Consider comorbidities that may impact therapy choice (cardiovascular risk, diabetes, seizure disorders)
- Address symptoms that require palliative management (ie, pain, impotence, fatigue, nausea)
- Identify concerns for medication access and medication adherence that could influence treatment choice
- Discuss short-term and long-term goals of care with the patient

Plan*

- Drug therapy regimen including drug(s), dose(s), route, frequency, and duration (see Table 154-7)
- Supportive care plan (antiemetics, premedication for chemotherapy, pain control, hot flash management)
- Monitoring parameters for adverse drug reactions (eg, complete blood count, liver function tests, subjective symptom assessments) and efficacy (eg, PSA levels, repeat imaging, symptom assessments)
- Patient education (self-monitoring for adverse drug reactions, expected timeframe for benefit and onset of adverse drug reactions, action needed for adverse drug reactions, monitoring schedule)
- Referrals to other providers when appropriate (eg, dietician, palliative care, urology)

Implement*

- Provide patient education regarding all elements of the treatment plan
- Use motivational interviewing and coaching strategies to maximize adherence
- Mitigate financial toxicity of drug therapy to ensure adherence
- Schedule follow-up

Follow-up: Monitor and Evaluate

- Presence of adverse drug reactions
- Monitoring response to treatment (eg, PSA, imaging studies depending on location of disease)
- Patient adherence to the treatment plan using multiple sources of information
- Patient satisfaction with the treatment plan
- New comorbidities or medications that may impact the treatment plan and patient treatment goals

**Collaborate with patient, caregivers, and other healthcare professionals.*

a normal life expectancy of equal to or greater than 10 years, either active surveillance, radiation (external beam or brachytherapy), or radical prostatectomy with a pelvic lymph node dissection may be offered. Radiation therapy and radical prostatectomy are generally considered therapeutically equivalent for localized prostate cancer, although neither has been proven to be better than observation alone in those with low risks of recurrence.[39]

A systematic review of 18 randomized trials and 473 observational studies compared the effectiveness and potential complications across prostate cancer treatment modalities. However, the analysis revealed that a paucity of high-quality available evidence limited comparisons of effectiveness between radiation, radical prostatectomy, and ADT. While the adverse drug reaction profiles were similar, the severity varied among the treatments.[40] Because radiation and prostatectomy have significant and immediate mortality when compared with expectant management alone, many patients may elect to postpone therapy until symptoms develop.

TABLE 154-4 Staging and Classification System for Prostate Cancer

AJCC 8th edition Classification

$T_xN_xM_x$ (cannot be assessed)

$T_0N_0M_0$ (nonpalpable)

T: Tumor

T_0: No evidence of primary tumor

T_1: Clinically inapparent tumor not palpable

- T_{1a}: Tumor incidental histologic finding in 5% or less of tissue resected
- T_{1b}: Tumor incidental histologic finding in 5% or more of tissue resected
- T_{1c}: Tumor identified by needle biopsy found in one or both sides, but not palpable

T_2: Tumor is palpable confined within the prostate

- T_{2a}: Tumor involves one-half of one side or less
- T_{2b}: Tumor involves more than one-half of one side, but not both sides
- T_{2c}: Tumor involves both sides

T_3: Extraprostatic tumor that is not fixed or does not invade adjacent structures

- T_{3a}: Extraprostatic extension (unilateral or bilateral)
- T_{3b}: Tumor invades seminal vesicle(s)

T_4: Tumor is fixed or invades adjacent structures other than the seminal vesicles such as external sphincter, rectum, bladder, levator muscles, and/or pelvic wall

N: Regional Lymph Nodes

N_0: No positive regional lymph nodes

N_1: Metastasis in regional lymph nodes

M: Distant Metastasis

M_0: No distant metastasis

M_{1a}: Nonregional lymph node(s)

M_{1b}: Bone(s)

M_{1c}: Other site(s) with or without bone disease

Individuals with T_{2b} and T_{2c} disease, a Gleason Group 2-3, or a PSA ranging from 10 to 20 ng/mL (μg/L) are considered at intermediate risk for prostate cancer recurrence. The intermediate-risk category is further divided into favorable and unfavorable intermediate risk, with more aggressive treatment recommended for those with more intermediate risk factors present at diagnosis.[7] Individuals with less than a 10-year expected survival may be offered observation or radiation therapy. Individuals with favorable risk may also be offered brachytherapy alone. In some cases, individuals with unfavorable risk and less than a 10-year expected survival may be also offered either radiation therapy with or without 4 to 6 months of neoadjuvant ADT, or radiation therapy plus brachytherapy with or without 4 to 6 months of neoadjuvant ADT. Individuals with favorable risk and a greater than or equal to 10-year life expectancy may be offered active surveillance, radical prostatectomy, with or without a pelvic lymph node dissection, or radiation therapy. Individuals with unfavorable risk and a greater than or equal to 10-year life expectancy may be offered radical prostatectomy, with or without a pelvic lymph node dissection, radiation therapy with or without 4 to 6 months of neoadjuvant ADT, or radiation therapy plus brachytherapy with or without 4 to 6 months of neoadjuvant ADT (Table 154-5).[7]

The treatment of patients at high or very-high risk of recurrence (stage T_3, a Gleason score ranging from 8 to 9, or a PSA value greater than 20 ng/mL [μg/L]) may be treated with ADT for 1.5 to 3 years combined with radiation therapy with or without brachytherapy (Table 154-5). Selected individuals with a low tumor volume may receive a radical prostatectomy with a pelvic lymph node dissection and additional therapy based on pathological evaluation. Docetaxel, in addition to radiation and ADT, can also be considered for patients in this risk recurrence group.[7]

4 Patients with T_{3b} and T_4 disease have a very-high risk of recurrence and are usually not candidates for radical prostatectomy because of extensive local spread of disease.[7] ADT with an LHRH

TABLE 154-5 Initial Management of Prostate Cancer Based on Expected Survival and Recurrence Risk

Recurrence Risk		Expected Survival (Years)	Initial Therapy
Very Low			
Has all of the following: • T_{1c} • Gleason group 1 • PSA less than 10 ng/mL (mcg/L) • Fewer than 3 prostate biopsies positive, ≤50% cancer in each core • PSA density <0.15 ng/mL/g (mcg/L/g)		<10 10-20 20 or more	Observation Active surveillance Active surveillance or radical prostatectomy or radiation therapy
Low			
Has all of the following but does not qualify for very low risk: • T_1-T_{2a} • Gleason Group 1 • PSA less than 10 ng/mL (mcg/L)		10 or more	Active surveillance or radical prostatectomy or radiation therapy
		<10	Observation
Intermediate			
• Has no high-risk group features • Intermediate risk factors (IRFs): • T_{2b}-T_{2c} • Gleason Group 2-3 • PSA10-20 ng/mL (mcg/L)			
Favorable Intermediate risk	Has all of following: • Only 1 intermediate risk factor • Gleason Grade Group 1-2 • <50% biopsy cores positive	10 or more	Active surveillance or radical prostatectomy +/− pelvic lymph node dissection or radiation therapy

(continued)

TABLE 154-5 Initial Management of Prostate Cancer Based on Expected Survival and Recurrence Risk (*Continued*)

Recurrence Risk		Expected Survival (Years)	Initial Therapy
		<10	Observation or Radiation therapy or Brachytherapy
Unfavorable intermediate risk	Has one or more of the following: • 2 or 3 intermediate risk factors • Gleason Grade Group 3 • ≥50% biopsy cores positive	10 or more	Radical prostatectomy +/− pelvic lymph node dissection or radiation therapy + ADT[a,b] or radiation therapy + brachytherapy +/− ADT
		<10	Observation or radiation therapy + ADT[a,b] or radiation therapy + brachytherapy +/− ADT
High Has no very-high risk features and has exactly ONE high-risk feature: • T_{3a} or • Gleason Grade Group 4-5 or 8 • PSA >20 ng/mL (mcg/L)		5 or more	Radiation therapy + ADT +/− docetaxel or radiation therapy + ADT + brachytherapy or radical prostatectomy and pelvic lymph node dissection
Very High Has at least one of the following: • T_{3b}-T_4 • Primary Gleason pattern 5 • 2 or 3 high-risk features • 4 cores with Gleason Grade Group 4 or 5		5 or more	Radiation therapy + ADT +/− docetaxel or radiation therapy + ADT + brachytherapy or radical prostatectomy and pelvic lymph node dissection
Locally Advanced/Metastatic disease			
Any T, N_1		5 or more	ADT +/− abiraterone and prednisone or radiation therapy + ADT +/− with or without abiraterone and prednisone)
Any T, Any N, M_1			ADT alone or in addition to: Apalutamide Abiraterone with prednisone Docetaxel Enzalutamide

[a]ADT therapy to achieve serum testosterone levels <50 ng/dL (1.7 nmol/L).

[b]LHRH agonists, LHRH/GnRH antagonists, or surgical castration are equivalent.

agonist plus an antiandrogen should be used either prior to, concurrent with, or following radiation therapy for patients with locally advanced prostate cancer to improve outcomes over radiation therapy alone in patients with localized prostate cancer. Androgen ablation should be instituted at diagnosis rather than waiting for symptomatic disease or progression to occur. In a randomized clinical trial of 500 patients with locally advanced prostate cancer who were randomized to either immediate initiation of ADT (either surgical or pharmacologic) or deferred hormonal therapy, patients who received immediate therapy had a median actuarial cause-specific survival of 7.5 years for immediate treatment as compared with 5.8 years for deferred treatment.[41]

5 Systemic therapy for nonmetastatic, castration-naïve disease, where the disease has not yet become resistant to ADT therapy, may include either orchiectomy, LHRH agonist with or without a first-generation antiandrogen (ie, combined androgen blockade [CAB]), GnRH antagonist, or observation. In patients with lymph node involvement (N_1) disease, abiraterone with a corticosteroid (eg, prednisone) can be used in addition to ADT (Table 154-6).[7]

6 ADT in addition to one of the following: docetaxel (six cycles), abiraterone with a corticosteroid (eg, prednisone), enzalutamide, or apalutamide are recommended options for patients with metastatic castration-naïve disease (Table 154-6).[7]

TABLE 154-6 First-Line Systemic Treatment Options for Advanced and Metastatic Prostate Cancer in Treatment-Naïve Patients

	Locally Advanced/ Non-metastatic	Metastatic
Castration-naïve (ADT initiated to achieve testosterone <50 ng/mL [mcg/L] in all cases)	• ADT • ADT + abiraterone + corticosteroid[a]	• ADT • ADT + abiraterone + corticosteroid[a] • ADT + apalutamide • ADT + docetaxel • ADT + enzalutamide
Castration-resistant (ADT continued to maintain testosterone <50 ng/mL [mcg/L] in all cases)	• Apalutamide • Darolutamide • Enzalutamide	• Abiraterone + corticosteroid[b] • Enzalutamide • Docetaxel + prednisone • Radium-223 (if symptomatic bone metastases) • Sipuleucel-T

[a]Treatment-naïve refers to those who have not received novel hormone therapy or docetaxel.

[b]Choice of corticosteroid is dependent on multiple factors, including abiraterone formulation.

Data from Reference 7.

When patients progress despite adequate androgen suppression, their disease is considered castration-resistant. Importantly, patients may progress on initial therapy without evidence of disease on scans. An increase in PSA or a rapid PSA doubling time (generally less than 10 months), could be indicative of progression and a biochemical recurrence. The development of new symptoms should also prompt a workup for disease progression. Importantly, further therapy is determined by the presence of symptomatic disease, or whether the metastatic progression is manifested as only a rising PSA (Table 154-6).[7]

7 For patients with nonmetastatic (M_0) castration-resistant disease, observation plus continued ADT is preferred if PSA doubling time is greater than 10 months. However, for patients with nonmetastatic castration-resistant prostate cancer who have a PSA doubling time less than or equal to 10 months, systemic therapy is recommended. Preferred systemic therapies for these patients include continuing ADT to maintain serum levels of testosterone less than 50 ng/dL (1.7 nmol/L) and a second-generation antiandrogen (eg, apalutamide, darolutamide, or enzalutamide) (Table 154-6).[7]

Patients with metastatic (M_1) castration-resistant prostate cancer should receive best supportive care in addition to other treatments (Fig. 154-3). ADT should continue, and initiating denosumab or an intravenous bisphosphonate should be considered in patients with bone metastases (see the discussion of LHRH agonists in the "Pharmacotherapy" section for more information). Palliative radiation therapy to bony metastases is also an option that may be utilized in these patients to provide relief of symptoms. When it comes to treatment selection for patients with metastatic castration-resistant prostate cancer, consideration should be given to previous lines of

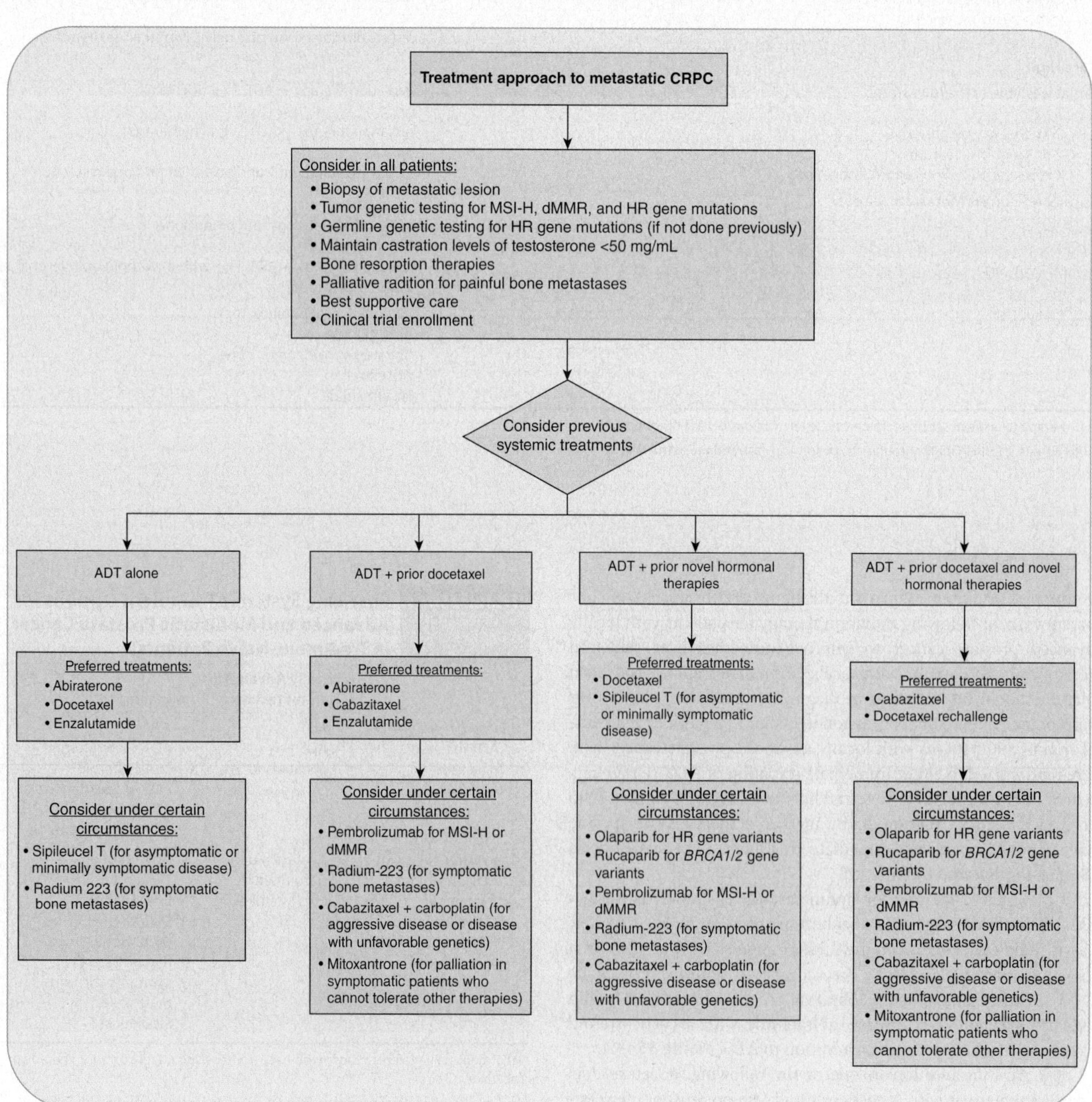

FIGURE 154-3 Treatment of metastatic castration-resistant prostate cancer. (*Data from Reference 7.*)

treatment, and providers should strive to choose an agent with a mechanism of action different from any therapies that the patient has failed (Fig. 154-3). Preferred first-line treatments (in conjunction with continuing ADT) include docetaxel plus prednisone, enzalutamide, or abiraterone. Sipuleucel-T, an immunotherapeutic, is also an option for patients without visceral metastases and who are clinically asymptomatic. Radium-223, an alpha emitter, is recommended for patients with bony metastases (and without evidence of visceral disease) (Table 154-6).[7]

8 In castration-resistant prostate cancer, genetic testing on tumor tissue (along with germline genetic testing if not already completed) is recommended to detect MSI-H, dMMR, or HR gene mutations (eg, *BRCA1/2*) is recommended. Those whose tumors test positive for MSI-H, dMMR, or TMB greater than or equal to 10 mut/Mb are eligible for treatment with the programmed cell death receptor 1, or PD1, inhibitor pembrolizumab. Evidence of pathogenic gene mutations in genes involved in HR indicates eligibility for olaparib, while the presence of pathogenic *BRCA1/2* mutations specifically indicates eligibility for rucaparib. Other agents include cabazitaxel, which can be used if the patient has failed docetaxel, or mitoxantrone, which can be considered when patients present with visceral metastases and cannot tolerate other therapies (Fig. 154-3).[7]

Nonpharmacologic Therapy

Observation/Active Surveillance

Observation is a treatment approach utilized in men with a shorter life expectancy and lower risk of disease. Observation involves monitoring the course of disease with laboratory testing and imaging, and starting palliative treatment if the cancer progresses. The advantages of observation are avoiding the adverse drug reactions associated with definitive therapies, such as radiation and radical prostatectomy, and minimizing the risk of unnecessary therapies. The major disadvantage of observation is the risk that cancer progresses and requires more intensive therapy. Active surveillance is similar to observation, although it may involve more invasive surveillance prostate biopsies. Those receiving active surveillance would generally be eligible for more aggressive treatment approaches upon progression.[7]

Orchiectomy

Bilateral orchiectomy, or surgical removal of the testes, is a form of ADT that rapidly reduces circulating androgens to castrate levels (less than 50 ng/dL [1.7 nmol/L]).[25] However, many patients are not surgical candidates because of advanced age, and other patients find this procedure psychologically unacceptable.[30] Orchiectomy is the preferred initial treatment in patients with impending spinal cord compression or ureteral obstruction, given their rapid onset.

Radiation

The two commonly used methods for radiation therapy are external beam radiotherapy and brachytherapy.[7] In external beam radiotherapy, doses of 70 to 75 Gy (7,000-7,500 rad) are delivered in 35 to 41 fractions in patients with low-grade prostate cancer and 75 to 80 Gy (7,500-8,000 rad) for those with intermediate- or high-grade prostate cancer. Brachytherapy involves the permanent implantation of radioactive beads of 145 Gy (14,500 rad) ^{125}iodine or 124 Gy (12,400 rad) ^{103}palladium and is generally reserved for individuals with low-risk cancers. Radiation therapy may also be given after surgery in patients with localized disease. Acute complications from radiation therapy include cystitis, proctitis, hematuria, urinary retention, penoscrotal edema, and impotence (30% incidence).[21,31] Chronic complications include proctitis, diarrhea, cystitis, enteritis, impotence, urethral stricture, and incontinence.[30,31] Because radiation therapy and radical prostatectomy have significant and immediate adverse effects compared with observation alone, many patients elect to postpone therapy until prostate cancer symptoms develop.

Radical Prostatectomy

Radical prostatectomy involves surgical removal of the prostate. Complications from radical prostatectomy include blood loss, stricture formation, incontinence, lymphocele, fistula formation, anesthetic risk, and impotence. Nerve-sparing radical prostatectomy can be performed in many patients; 50% to 80% regain sexual potency within the first year. However, even in patients with good preoperative sexual health, many do not return to baseline after surgery even with the assistance of erectile dysfunction treatments.[42] Nerve-sparing radical prostatectomy can be performed in many patients; 50% to 80% regain sexual potency within the first year. The surgery can be accompanied by a pelvic lymph node dissection to determine if the disease has spread to any regional nodes.

Pharmacotherapy

LHRH Agonists

LHRH agonists are a reversible method of androgen ablation and are as effective as orchiectomy in treating prostate cancer.[7,43] Currently available LHRH agonists include leuprolide, leuprolide depot, leuprolide implant, triptorelin depot, triptorelin implant, and goserelin acetate implant (Table 154-7). The leuprolide depot formulation contains leuprolide acetate in coated pellets. The dose is administered intramuscularly, and the coating dissolves at different rates to allow sustained leuprolide levels throughout the dosing interval. Goserelin acetate implant contains goserelin acetate dispersed in a plastic matrix of D,L-lactic, and glycolic acid copolymer and is administered subcutaneously. Hydrolysis of the copolymer material provides continuous release of goserelin over the dosing period.

Several randomized trials have demonstrated that leuprolide, goserelin, and triptorelin are effective agents when used alone in patients with advanced prostate cancer. Response rates of around 80% have been reported.[34] The currently available LHRH agonists or the dosage formulations have not been directly compared in clinical trials, but a meta-analysis showed no significant differences in efficacy or toxicity between leuprolide, goserelin, and orchiectomy.[44] Triptorelin is a more recent approval that is generally considered equally effective. Therefore, the choice between the three agents is usually made based on cost and patient and physician preference for a dosing schedule.

The most common adverse drug reactions reported with LHRH agonist therapy include a disease flare during the first week of therapy for patients with metastatic disease, hot flashes, erectile impotence, decreased libido, and injection-site reactions.[34] The disease flare is caused by an initial induction of LH and FSH by the LHRH agonist leading to an initial phase of increased testosterone production, and manifests clinically as either increased bone pain or increased urinary symptoms.[35] This flare reaction usually resolves after 2 weeks and has a similar onset and duration pattern for the depot LHRH products.[44,45] Tumor flare can be minimized by initiating an antiandrogen before the administration of the LHRH agonist and continuing for 2 to 4 weeks.[35] LHRH agonist monotherapy can be used as initial therapy, with response rates similar to those for orchiectomy. Caution should be exercised if initiating LHRH agonist therapy in patients with widely metastatic disease involving the spinal cord or having the potential for ureteral obstruction because irreversible complications may occur.

Another potentially serious complication of ADT is a decrease in bone mineral density leading to an increased risk for osteoporosis, osteopenia, and skeletal fractures. During initial therapy, bone mineral density of the hip and spine decreases by 2% to 3%.[46] Additionally, ADT has been associated with a 21% to 45% relative increase in fracture risk.[47-49] Therefore, most clinicians recommend that patients with increased risk for fracture based on the Fracture Assessment Tool, or FRAX, who are starting long-term ADT should have a baseline bone mineral density assessment performed, and all

TABLE 154-7 Hormonal Therapies for Prostate Cancer

Drug	Usual Dose	Adverse Drug Reactions	Hepatic/Renal Adjustments	Monitoring Parameters	Drug Interactions	Administration
First-Generation Antiandrogens						
Bicalutamide	50 mg/day PO (up to 150 mg/day unlabeled use)	Gynecomastia Hot flashes Gastrointestinal disturbances (diarrhea) Decrease libido LFT abnormalities Breast tenderness	Discontinue if ALT >2 times upper limit of normal or patient develops jaundice	Serum transaminases should be monitored prior to start of therapy and monthly for the first 4 months, then periodically thereafter Periodic monitoring of CBC, EKG, echocardiograms, serum testosterone, luteinizing hormone, and PSA	Inhibits CYP3A4 May increase the concentration of vitamin K antagonists	May be taken with or without food
Flutamide	750 mg/day PO	Gynecomastia Hot flashes Gastrointestinal disturbances (diarrhea) Loss of libido LFT abnormalities Breast tenderness Methemoglobinemia	Contraindicated in patients with hepatic impairment No dosage adjustment necessary in chronic renal impairment	Serum transaminases should be monitored prior to start of therapy and monthly for the first 4 months, then periodically thereafter Monitor for tumor reduction, PSA, testosterone/estrogen, and phosphatase serum levels	Substrate of CYP1A2 and CYP3A4	Administered orally in three divided doses; capsule may be opened into applesauce, pudding, or other soft foods
Nilutamide	300 mg/day PO for first month then 150 mg/day	Gynecomastia Hot flashes Gastrointestinal Disturbances (constipation) LFT abnormalities Breast tenderness Visual disturbances (impaired dark adaptation) Alcohol intolerance Interstitial pneumonitis	Contraindicated in patients with hepatic impairment Discontinue if ALT >2 times upper limit of normal or patient develops jaundice	Serum transaminases should be monitored prior to start of therapy and monthly for the first 4 months, then periodically thereafter Chest x-ray at baseline and consideration of pulmonary function testing (at baseline), PSA periodically	Substrate of CYP2C19 and weak inhibitor of CYP2C19	May be taken with or without food
Second-Generation Antiandrogens						
Apalutamide	240 mg/day PO	Gastrointestinal disturbances (diarrhea, nausea) Hot flashes Fatigue Hyperthyroidism Hypertension Rash Decreased weight Falls and fractures Peripheral edema Seizures	No adjustment necessary for renal or hepatic impairment	Complete blood counts baseline and periodically LFTs baseline and periodically TSH at baseline and every 4 months, PSA periodically	Strong inducer of CYP3A4 and CYP2C19, and a weak inducer of CYP2C9	May be taken with or without food
Darolutamide	1,200 mg/day PO	Fatigue Gastrointestinal disturbances (diarrhea, constipation, nausea) Rash Musculoskeletal disorders (back pain, arthralgias, pain in an extremity) Falls, including accidents/bone fractures Hypertension Seizures	For moderate hepatic impairment or severe renal impairment (not on dialysis): dose should be reduced to 600 mg/day	Complete blood counts baseline and periodically LFTs baseline and periodically, PSA periodically	BCRP transporter Inhibitor Darolutamide inhibits OATP1B1 and OATP1B3	Take with food

(continued)

TABLE 154-7 Hormonal Therapies for Prostate Cancer (*Continued*)

Drug	Usual Dose	Adverse Drug Reactions	Hepatic/Renal Adjustments	Monitoring Parameters	Drug Interactions	Administration
Enzalutamide	160 mg/day PO	Gastrointestinal disturbances (diarrhea) Musculoskeletal disorders (back pain, arthralgias, muscle pain, weakness) Asthenia Peripheral edema CNS (headache, dizziness) Seizures LFT abnormalities	No adjustment necessary for renal or hepatic impairment	Complete blood counts baseline and periodically LFTs baseline and periodically, PSA periodically	Strong CYP3A4 and moderate CYP2C9 and CYP2C19 inducer; avoid CYP3A4, CYP2C9, and CYP2C19 sensitive substrates. CYP2C8 substrate, avoid strong inducers and inhibitors of CYP2C8 If vitamin K antagonists are necessary, conduct additional INR monitoring	May be taken with or without food
Androgen Synthesis Inhibitor						
Abiraterone acetate	Abiraterone acetate: 1,000 mg/day PO + prednisone 5 mg daily PO (castration-naïve) or BID PO (CRPC). Micronized abiraterone: 500 mg daily PO + methylprednisolone 4 mg BID PO (CRPC)	Gastrointestinal disturbances (diarrhea) Edema Hypokalemia Hypophosphatemia LFT abnormalities Hypertriglyceridemia	250 mg daily for Child Pugh Class B; avoid use in Child Pugh Class C Withhold treatment if LFTs >5 times the ULN or bilirubin >3 ULN	Serum transaminases should be monitored prior to start of therapy, every 2 weeks for 3 months, then monthly thereafter Monitor for signs and symptoms of adrenocorticoid insufficiency; monthly for hypertension, hypokalemia, and fluid retention, PSA periodically	Substrate of CYP3A4 Use with caution with CYP3A4 inhibitors and inducers Inhibits CYP1A2, CYP2C19, CYP2C8, CYP2C9, CYP2D6, CYP3A4, and P-glycoprotein Use sensitive substrates with caution	For standard abiraterone, administer on an empty stomach, at least 1 hour before and 2 hours after food (micronized abiraterone can be given regardless of food)
Luteinizing-Hormone Releasing Hormone Agonists						
Goserelin	3.6 mg SQ implant every month 10.8 mg SQ implant every 3 months	Hot flashes Decreased libido Gynecomastia Osteoporosis Fatigue Weight gain	No adjustment necessary for renal or hepatic impairment	Monitor bone mineral density, serum calcium, and cholesterol/lipids, PSA periodically	May diminish the effects of antidiabetic agents	Vary injection site
Leuprolide	7.5 mg IM every month 22.5 mg IM every 3 months 30 mg IM every 4 months 45 mg IM every 6 months	Hot flashes Decreased libido Gynecomastia Osteoporosis Fatigue Weight gain	No adjustment necessary for renal or hepatic impairment	Serum testosterone ~4 weeks after initiation, PSA, blood glucose, and $HgbA_{1c}$ prior to initiation and periodically thereafter, PSA periodically	May diminish the effects of antidiabetic agents	Vary injection site
Triptorelin	3.75 mg IM every month 11.25 mg IM every 3 months 22.5 mg IM every 6 months	Hot flashes Decreased libido Gynecomastia Osteoporosis Fatigue Weight gain	No adjustment necessary for renal or hepatic impairment	Monitor serum testosterone levels and PSA periodically	May diminish the effects of antidiabetic agents	Vary injection site
Luteinizing-Hormone Releasing Hormone/Gonadotropin-Releasing Hormone Receptor Antagonists						
Degarelix	240 mg SQ loading dose 80 mg SQ every 28 days (following 28 days after loading dose)	Hot flashes Decreased libido Gynecomastia Osteoporosis Fatigue Weight gain	Use with caution with CL_{cr} <50 mL/min (0.83 mL/s) Do not use in patients with severe hepatic impairment	PSA periodically, serum testosterone monthly until castration achieved then every other month, LFTs at baseline in addition to serum electrolytes and bone mineral density	Use with caution with agents that may increase QTc interval	Vary injection site

(*continued*)

TABLE 154-7 Hormonal Therapies for Prostate Cancer (*Continued*)

Drug	Usual Dose	Adverse Drug Reactions	Hepatic/Renal Adjustments	Monitoring Parameters	Drug Interactions	Administration
Relugolix	360 mg PO followed by 120 mg PO daily	Hot flashes, Hypergylcemia, Hypertrigylceridemia, Musculoskeletal pain, Fatigue	No adjustment necessary for renal or hepatic impairment	PSA periodically, LFTs and serum electrolytes at baseline and periodically; bone mineral density periodically	Use with caution with agents that may increase QTc interval. Use with caution with CYP3A4 inhibitors and P-glycoprotein inhibitors	May be taken with or without food

ALT, alanine aminotransferase; BID, twice daily; BRCP, breast cancer resistance protein; CBC, complete blood count; CL_{cr}, creatinine clearance; CNS, central nervous system; CRPC, castrate-resistant prostate cancer; CYP, cytochrome P450; EKG, electrocardiogram; $HgbA_{1c}$, hemoglobin $A1_c$; IM, intramuscular injection; INR, international normalized ratio; LFT, liver function test; PO, oral administration; PSA, prostate surface antigen; QTc, corrected QT interval; SQ, subcutaneous injection; TSH, thyroid stimulating hormone; ULN, upper limit of normal.

Data from References 55-65 and 71.

patients should have a bone mineral density assessment performed 1 year after initiating ADT. These individuals should also be initiated on a calcium and vitamin D supplement, based on the same guidance for the general population from the National Osteoporosis Foundation guidelines (see Chapter 112, "Osteoporosis," for more information).[7,35]

In addition, an antiresorptive agent, either zoledronic acid, alendronate, or denosumab should be initiated in men with osteoporosis at the same schedule and doses used in the treatment of the general population with osteoporosis (see Chapter 112, "Osteoporosis," for more information).[7] In men with metastatic castration-resistant prostate cancer and bone metastases, zoledronic acid or denosumab should be considered to reduce skeletal-related events (SREs). A meta-analysis combined data from three identically designed double-blind randomized controlled trials that compared the efficacy and safety of denosumab at a dose of 120 mg every 4 weeks with that of zoledronic acid at a dose of 4 mg administered IV every 4 weeks.[50] Almost 6,000 patients with breast and prostate cancer and multiple myeloma were included in the meta-analysis. Denosumab is superior to zoledronic acid in reducing the risk of first skeletal-related event (SRE) by 17% and prolonging the median time-to-first SRE was 8 months. The benefits were consistent across tumor types evaluated, and the incidence of adverse drug reactions was not significantly different between the denosumab and zoledronic acid groups.[50]

ADT has also been associated with a higher incidence of metabolic effects. In a landmark population-based trial, patients treated with an ADT using an LHRH agonist had a greater risk of new-onset diabetes, coronary artery disease, and myocardial infarctions.[51] However, it is not clear whether ADT increases the risk of cardiovascular death. A published meta-analysis of eight trials with 4,141 patients treated with ADT evaluated prostate cancer-specific mortality and all-cause mortality.[52] The trials included patients with nonmetastatic disease who were treated with immediate predominantly LHRH agonist–based ADT versus no immediate ADT (control group). The risk of cardiovascular death for ADT versus control was not significantly different, and these results suggest that ADT does not increase cardiovascular mortality. Patients receiving ADT should be screened for cardiovascular disease and diabetes and appropriate interventions to prevent and treat these complications should be initiated.[7]

LHRH/GnRH Antagonists

An alternative to LHRH agonists are the approved GnRH antagonists, degarelix, and relugolix. Degarelix and relugolix work by binding reversibly to GnRH receptors in the pituitary gland, which reduces the production of testosterone to castrate levels. The major advantage of the GnRH antagonists over LHRH agonists is the rapidity at which they reduce testosterone levels. Castration levels are achieved in 7 days or less with both degarelix and relugolix, as compared with 28 days with leuprolide. Tumor flare does not occur with either GnRH antagonist, and antiandrogens are not required.

Degarelix is equivalent to leuprolide in lowering testosterone levels for up to 1 year. Degarelix is available as 40 and 20 mg/mL vials for subcutaneous injection, and the starting dose is 240 mg followed by 80 mg every 28 days. The starting dose should be divided into two 120 mg injections.[53] Degarelix has not been studied in combination with antiandrogens, and routine use of the combination is not recommended. The most frequently reported adverse reactions are mild to moderate in nature and include transient injection site reactions, including pain, and erythema, and hot flashes. Other adverse drug reactions include elevations in liver function tests, which occur in about 10% of patients. These individuals should also be initiated on a calcium and vitamin D supplement, based on the same guidance for the general population from the National Osteoporosis Foundation guidelines (see Chapter 112, "Osteoporosis," for more information).[7,35,53]

Relugolix is an oral LHRH antagonist. In a phase 3 trial, patients administered relugolix (120 mg once daily after a single 360 mg oral loading dose) was evaluated against leuprolide. Relugolix demonstrated similar testosterone suppression to leuprolide, but in contrast to leuprolide, testosterone suppression was quickly reversible for those receiving relugolix, underscoring the need for adherence. But most importantly, in contrast to the other FDA-approved LHRH agonists and GnRH antagonists, there does not seem to be an increased cardiovascular risk with relugolix. In patients with pre-existing cardiovascular disease the incidence of major cardiovascular events was lower in patients treated with relugolix than patients treated with leuprolide (3.6% vs 17.8%).[54] Hot flashes, hypergylcemia, hypertrigylceridemia, musculoskeletal pain, fatigue were common toxicities, and providers should use with caution with medications that increase QTc interval, or are inhibitors of cytochrome P450 (CYP) 3A4 or the p-glycoprotein (P-gp) efflux transporter (Table 154-7).[55-59]

Antiandrogens

The first-generation antiandrogens include flutamide, bicalutamide, and nilutamide. Three second-generation antiandrogens, apalutamide, enzalutamide, and darolutamide, are currently available (Table 154-7).[55-65] Antiandrogens have been used as monotherapy in previously untreated patients, but a meta-analysis showed that monotherapy with antiandrogens is less effective than LHRH agonists.[44] Therefore, for advanced prostate cancer, flutamide, bicalutamide, and nilutamide are indicated only in combination with ADT. Flutamide and bicalutamide are indicated in combination with an LHRH agonist, and nilutamide is indicated in combination with orchiectomy.[66] Antiandrogens can reduce the symptoms from the flare phenomenon associated with LHRH agonist therapy in patients with metastatic disease.[7,35,66]

As with first-generation antiandrogens, second-generation antiandrogens do not lower androgen levels, but inhibit androgen receptor signaling by competitively inhibiting androgen binding without stimulation of the androgen receptor. Second-generation antiandrogens may have an advantage over the currently available first-generation antiandrogen agents because they inhibit AR nuclear translocation and AR binding to DNA and coactivator recruitment, which leads to a reduction of AR-mediated transcription of genes known to promote prostate cancer proliferation (Fig. 154-2). Enzalutamide also has a greater affinity for the AR, and has shown activity in patients resistant to first-generation antiandrogens. Initially approved only after docetaxel failure, enzalutamide may be used in the first-line setting to delay the initiation of chemotherapy in nonmetastatic castration-resistant prostate cancer, as well as metastatic castration-naïve and metastatic castration-resistant disease.[7,67] Apalutamide and darolutamide are also second-generation antiandrogens. Apalutamide is approved for the treatment of nonmetastatic castration-resistant prostate cancer and metastatic castration-naïve prostate cancer.[68] The most common adverse drug reactions associated with apalutamide are fatigue and rash, and apalutamide requires thyroid-stimulating hormone monitoring. The adverse drug reactions of apalutamide and enzalutamide are similar to those of the other antiandrogens, but they both have an increased risk of seizures. Darolutamide is a structurally distinct second-generation antiandrogen, consisting of two pharmacologically active diastereomers,[69,70] which lowers penetration past the blood–brain barrier and results in low binding affinity for γ-aminobutyric acid type A receptors. As a result, darolutamide may cause fewer and less severe adverse drug reactions (eg, less fatigue, and also potentially lower risk for seizures) than enzalutamide and apalutamide despite similar metastasis-free survival rates. Darolutamide is approved for nonmetastatic castration-resistant prostate cancer. The most common antiandrogen-related adverse drug reactions are listed in Table 154-7.

Combined Androgen Blockade

Although up to 80% of patients with advanced prostate cancer will respond to initial hormonal manipulation, almost all patients will progress within 2 to 4 years after initiating therapy.[30] Two mechanisms have been proposed to explain this tumor resistance. The tumor could be heterogeneously composed of cells that are hormone-dependent and hormone-independent, or the tumor could be stimulated by extratesticular androgens that are converted intracellularly to DHT. The rationale for CAB is to interfere with multiple hormonal pathways to completely eliminate androgen action. Antiandrogen therapy should precede, or be co-administered with LHRH agonists, and should be continued for at least 7 days for patients with overt metastases who are at high risk of developing symptoms associated with a testosterone flare that can occur with LHRH agonist therapy alone.[7] Studies of short term (4-6 months) and long term (2-3 years) of CAB in those patients with locally advanced disease with intermediate-, high-, and very-high-risk features have all assessed in the neoadjuvant and adjuvant settings, or even concurrently with radiation therapy.[7] Whether the addition of an antiandrogen to ADT is necessary requires further study, but any survival advantage for patients treated with CAB, if present, is small.[72,73] While controversy remains around the appropriate clinical use of CAB, clinicians should recognize that the consequences of financial toxicity and increased side effects must be weighed against modest survival benefit.[72]

Alternative Drug Treatments

Secondary or salvage therapies for patients who progress after their initial therapy depend on what was used for initial management.[7] For patients initially diagnosed with localized prostate cancer, radiotherapy can be used in the case of failed radical prostatectomy. Alternatively, ADT can be used in patients who progress after either radiation therapy or radical prostatectomy.

Abiraterone Abiraterone is an androgen synthesis inhibitor that targets CYP17A1, which results in a decrease in circulating levels of testosterone.[71] Abiraterone is indicated in patients with metastatic castration-naïve prostate cancer or metastatic castration-resistant prostate cancer.[35] In both metastatic castration-naïve prostate cancer and castration-resistant prostate cancer, abiraterone improves overall survival.[7,74] Hypertension, hypokalemia, and edema may occur due to abiraterone-induced hypoadrenalism that is secondary to CYP17A1 inhibition. Corticosteroids (eg, prednisone) are prescribed concurrently with abiraterone to mitigate these potential adverse drug reactions. Abiraterone is available as the prodrug, abiraterone acetate, and should be taken on an empty stomach as food increases bioavailability by up to 10-fold.[71] A micronized formulation with improved bioavailability is available and can be taken with or without food and at a lower daily dose.[7] Monitoring of liver function tests is recommended at baseline, every 2 weeks for the first 3 months, and then monthly thereafter. Since abiraterone is an inhibitor of CYP2D6, medication profiles should be reviewed for potential drug interactions before initiation of abiraterone therapy.[71]

Chemotherapy 8 Chemotherapy with docetaxel improves survival in patients with metastatic castration-naïve and metastatic castration-resistant prostate cancer and is considered a first-line therapy option (see Table 154-8).[7,75-81] Docetaxel 75 mg/m² every 3 weeks combined with prednisone 5 mg twice a day was first studied in castration-resistant prostate cancer and shown to improve survival in this setting.[82] Subsequently, docetaxel 75 mg/m² every 3 weeks, without prednisone, was studied in the castration-sensitive setting and again shown to improve survival.[83] The most common adverse drug reactions with this regimen are nausea, alopecia, and bone marrow suppression. Other adverse drug reactions of docetaxel include fluid retention (premedication with corticosteroids can minimize) and peripheral neuropathy. Docetaxel is metabolized in the liver; patients with hepatic impairment may not be eligible for treatment with docetaxel because of an increased risk for toxicity (see Table 154-8).[81]

Cabazitaxel is a taxane with demonstrated activity in docetaxel-resistant cell lines and animal models.[80] Cabazitaxel has a lower affinity for the P-gp efflux transporter than docetaxel, which may explain why cabazitaxel is active in the setting of docetaxel resistance. In patients previously treated with docetaxel and prednisone, cabazitaxel 25 mg/m² every 3 weeks with prednisone 10 mg daily significantly improved progression-free and overall survival over mitoxantrone and prednisone, but a reduced cabazitaxel dose of 20 mg/m² every 3 weeks (with prednisone) has been FDA-approved based on evidence of similar efficacy but better tolerability.[84,85] The addition of carboplatin (AUC 4 mg/mL per min) to cabazitaxel 25 mg/m² demonstrated improved progression-free survival versus cabazitaxel alone.[86] As result, guidelines suggest the use of this combination in high-risk metastatic castration-resistant prostate cancer patients who have been pretreated with docetaxel.[7] Neutropenia, febrile neutropenia, neuropathy, and diarrhea are the most significant toxicities. Hypersensitivity reactions may occur and premedication with an antihistamine, a corticosteroid, and an H_2 antagonist is recommended. Cabazitaxel is extensively metabolized in the liver and should be avoided in patients with hepatic dysfunction (Table 154-8).[80] Mitoxantrone plus prednisone has not demonstrated a survival improvement after failure of docetaxel, but remains a palliative

TABLE 154-8 Chemotherapy, Immunotherapy, and Targeted Therapy for Prostate Cancer

Drug	Usual Dose	Toxicities	Hepatic/Renal Adjustments	Monitoring Parameters	Drug Interactions	Administration
Antimicrotubule Agents						
Cabazitaxel	25 mg/m² IV every 3 weeks	Fluid retention, constipation, mucositis, myelosuppression, hypersensitivity	Discontinue if ALT >2 times upper limit of normal or patient develops jaundice	CBC weekly during the first cycle, then prior to each treatment, PSA periodically, Monitor for hypersensitivity	Avoid concomitant use of CYP3A4 inducers and inhibitors	Administer IV infusion over 1 hour
Docetaxel	75 mg/m² IV every 3 weeks	Fluid retention, alopecia, mucositis, myelosuppression, hypersensitivity	AST/ALT >1.5 times the upper limit of normal and alkaline phosphatase >2.5 times the upper limit of normal do not administer	CBC with differential, LFTs, bilirubin, alkaline phosphatase, renal function, PSA periodically Monitor for hypersensitivity reactions	Avoid concomitant use of CYP3A4 inhibitors	Administer IV infusion over 1 hour Premedication with corticosteroids for 3 days beginning the day before
Immunotherapy						
Pembrolizumab	200 mg IV every 3 weeks or 400 mg IV every 6 weeks	Fatigue and immune-mediated (eg, diarrhea, pneumonitis, hepatitis, thyroiditis)	No adjustment needed for baseline renal/hepatic impairment; treat as immune-mediated toxicity if occurs during treatment	CBC, LFTs, renal function, thyroid function, glucose at baseline and during therapy, PSA periodically	Immunosuppressants may decrease therapeutic effect	Administer over 30 minutes
Sipuleucel-T	Each injection contains >50 million autologous CD54+ cells (obtained through leukapheresis) activated with PAP-GM-CSF Dose is given every 2 weeks for 3 total doses	Hypersensitivity, chills, fatigue, fever, headache, myalgias	No dosage adjustment necessary for renal or hepatic dysfunction	No specific laboratory monitoring recommended, PSA periodically	Immunosuppressants may decrease the therapeutic effects of sipuleucel-T	Administer IV infusion over 1 hour Observe the patient for 30 minutes after the completion of the infusion Premedicate with acetaminophen and an antihistamine 30 minutes prior to administration
Targeted Therapy						
Olaparib	300 mg PO BID	Anemia, nausea, fatigue, decreased appetite, venous thromboembolism	Reduce dose for moderate renal impairment	CBC at baseline and monthly, renal function periodically, PSA periodically	Avoid CYP3A4 inhibitors and inducers; reduce olaparib dose if using CYP3A4 inhibitor	Administer with or without food
Rucaparib	600 mg PO BID	Fatigue, nausea, anemia, hepatotoxicity, decreased appetite	None	CBC at baseline and monthly, PSA periodically	Inhibits CYP1A2, CYP2C19, CYP2C9, and CYP3A4	Administer with or without food
Nuclear Medicine						
Radium-223	50 kBq/kg (1.35 μCi) administered every 4 weeks for 6 injections	Nausea, vomiting, diarrhea, peripheral edema, anemia, lymphocytopenia, thrombocytopenia, and neutropenia	None	CBC should be monitored prior to every injection, PSA periodically	None	Administer radium-223 by slow IV injection over 1 minute

ALT, alanine aminotransferase; AST, asparate aminotransferase; BID, twice daily; CBC, complete blood count; CYP, cytochrome P450; IV, intravenous administration; LFT, liver function test; PAP-GM-CSF, prostatic acid phosphatase granulocyte-macrophage colony-stimulating factor; PO, oral administration; PSA, prostate surface antigen.

Data from References 75-81.

therapeutic option, specifically in patients with evidence of visceral metastases and who are not candidates for cabazitaxel or radium-223 therapy.[7]

Immunotherapy Sipuleucel-T is a novel autologous cellular immunotherapy FDA-approved for the treatment of asymptomatic or minimally symptomatic metastatic castration-resistant prostate cancer.[79] Alternative treatment options for this patient population are secondary hormonal therapy, including antiandrogen therapy, withdrawal of antiandrogen therapy, ketoconazole, abiraterone acetate, enzalutamide, corticosteroids, estrogen, or enrollment on a clinical trial, although none of these options has been shown to improve overall survival. No clinical trials have compared sipuleucel-T to secondary hormonal therapies. Patients treated with sipuleucel-T undergo leukapheresis on day 1 to collect peripheral blood mononuclear cells, the cellular fraction that includes immune effector cells. These cells are incubated with the prostatic acid phosphatase-granulocyte macrophage colony-stimulating factor, or PAP-GM-CSF, fusion protein. Prostatic acid phosphatase, or PAP, is the specific tumor antigen, and granulocyte-macrophage colony-stimulating factor, or GM-CSF, is the immune cell activator. The cellular product is then infused intravenously into the patient on day 3 or 4, providing an autologous infusion of activated cells. Each course of sipuleucel-T consists of three infusions of activated cells, given every 2 weeks. Sipuleucel-T prolongs overall survival by approximately 4 months.[79,87] Adverse drug reactions related to sipuleucel-T are generally mild.

9 Somatic and germline HR mutations are common in men with metastatic castration-resistant prostate cancer.[88] Germline genetic testing is recommended in patients with high-risk prostate cancer and/or a relevant family history. Somatic tumor genetic testing is recommended in metastatic disease to identify genetic variants that can be targeted with drug therapy. Pembrolizumab is a monoclonal antibody that inhibits the programmed cell death receptor–1 that is broadly FDA-approved for patients with metastatic solid tumors who have documented MSI-H, dMMR by molecular testing or TMB greater than or equal to 10 mut/Mb, who have progressed on prior treatment, and who have no alternative treatment options (Fig. 154-3).[78] Like other immune checkpoint inhibitors, pembrolizumab works by inhibiting signals that lead to T-cell senescence, and thereby increases the immune response to cancer (Table 154-8). MSI-H and dMMR are estimated to occur in approximately 5% to 12% metastatic castration-resistant prostate cancer patients, which makes pembrolizumab a viable treatment option.[88]

Targeted Therapy 9 11 PARP enzymes are involved in normal repair of both single-stand and double-strand DNA breaks. The combination of PARP enzyme inhibition by pharmacotherapy and inactivating HR gene mutations results in synthetic lethality that increases genetic instability and induces prostate cancer cell death. Olaparib has been proven effective in metastatic castration-resistant prostate cancer patients harboring pathogenic germline or somatic HR mutations (eg, *ATM*, *BRCA1/2*, *BRCA2*, *BARD*, *BRIP1*, *CDK12*, *CHEK1/2*, *FANCL*, *PALB2*, and *RAD51*) who had progressed on enzalutamide or abiraterone, by improving radiologic progression-free survival.[77] However, pre-specified subgroup analyses suggest that improvement is primarily observed in patients with *BRCA2* mutations.[89] A second PARP inhibitor, rucaparib, obtained FDA-accelerated approval in patients with metastatic castration-resistant prostate cancer. Rucaparib has been proven effective in metastatic castration-resistant prostate cancer patients who harbor germline or somatic mutations in *BRCA1/2*, and who have progressed after both second-generation antiandrogens or abiraterone- and taxane-based chemotherapy.[76] In this population, the overall response rate is approximately 44%, a majority of patients (56%) have a response duration >6 months, and progression-free survival is approximately 9 months.[90] Fatigue (including asthenia), nausea, vomiting, diarrhea, anemia, thrombocytopenia, and decreased appetite are the most common toxicities for these two PARP inhibitors. Both olaparib and rucaparib are CYP3A4 substrates. While olaparib doses should be adjusted when concomitantly with CYP3A4 inhibitors, doses of rucaparib do not require adjustments. However, rucaparib inhibits several CYP enzymes (including CYP3A4), and caution should be used with substrates of those enzymes concomitantly with rucaparib (Table 154-8).[76,77]

Nuclear Medicine Radium-223, an alpha emitter, can be administered to target specific bone metastases with alpha particles in patients with metastatic castration-resistant prostate cancer. Radium-223 administered every 4 weeks improved overall survival by 2.8 months in patients who had already received, were not eligible for, or had declined docetaxel therapy. Improvements in skeletal pain, pain-related outcomes, and quality of life were also significant. Opioid needs were decreased in patients who received radium-223 (36% vs 50%). The most common adverse drug reactions of radium-223 include nausea, diarrhea, vomiting, peripheral edema, and bone marrow suppression.[75,91] Radium-223 may be used in first-, second-, or third-line therapy in patients with metastatic castration-resistant prostate cancer with symptomatic primary bone metastases. Radium-223 has not been approved for use with concomitant abiraterone, second-generation antiandrogens, chemotherapy, immunotherapy, or targeted therapy.

EVALUATION OF THERAPEUTIC OUTCOMES

Monitoring of prostate cancer depends on the grade and the stage of the cancer.[35] When definitive, and curative therapy is attempted, objective parameters should be assessed to evaluate tumor response. These include assessment of the primary tumor size and evaluation of involved lymph nodes through imaging studies, as well as the response of tumor markers, such as PSA, for recurrence or progression. For patients on active surveillance, PSA levels should be checked every 6 months and combined with annual DRE. Following definitive therapy with intent to cure, PSA levels should be checked every 6 to 12 months for the first 5 years and then annually thereafter. For patients at high risk of recurrence, every 3-month PSA testing can be considered.[7] Local recurrence in the absence of a rising PSA may occur, so annual DRE and radiologic studies based on patient-reported symptoms are also performed. In the castration-naïve setting, the response to ADT, radiation, or both dictates monitoring frequency; however, PSA measurement and physical examination every 3 to 6 months can be considered. In the metastatic setting, treatments that directly target the AR signaling axis, traditional cytotoxic chemotherapies, immunotherapies and targeted therapies have demonstrated that they increase survival.

Clinical efficacy is measured with imaging studies (typically CT scans of abdomen/pelvis and bone scans), performance status, symptom scores, weight changes, quality of life, analgesic requirements, and PSA response. However, because PSA is such a robust and reliable biomarker of clinical efficacy in most prostate cancer patients, imaging studies are routine but not performed as often as they are for other solid tumors. When using PSA as a surrogate for disease progression, it is important to consider not only the degree of elevation, but also the velocity at which the marker changes. A rapid PSA velocity has been associated with an increased risk of all-cause mortality, and should warrant consideration of therapeutic intervention.

Monitoring for adverse drug reactions is different for each treatment modality but is similarly important. Monitoring parameters and a review of common adverse drug reactions are provided for hormonal therapies (Table 154-7), as well as chemotherapies, immunotherapies and target therapies (Table 154-8). For pembrolizumab, clinicians and patients should monitor for signs and symptoms of immune-mediated adverse drug reactions (eg, colitis, endocrinopathies, hepatitis, nephritis, or pneumonitis). For sipuleucel-T, clinicians should recognize that traditional markers of benefit (eg, PSA decline or evidence of improvement by imaging studies) may not be present.[7] For orally administered treatments (eg, abiraterone, second-generation antiandrogens, PARP inhibitors, and relugolix), medication adherence is also an important monitoring parameter to evaluate at each clinic visit.

CONCLUSION

Prostate cancer is the most commonly diagnosed cancer in biologic males in the United States (greater than 20% of the new cases), but the death rate from prostate cancer has declined over the past three decades and only approximately 10% of the cancer-related deaths are attributed to prostate cancer among biologic males in the United States. This shows that for most prostate cancer patients, the disease has an indolent course, and treatment options for localized disease are often effective. While localized prostate cancer can be cured by surgery or radiation therapy, advanced and metastatic prostate cancer are not yet curable. Advanced and metastatic prostate cancer have a consistent pattern of progression, and are fatal. Advances over the past two decades, focusing on improved treatments directly targeting the AR signaling axis, chemotherapies, immunotherapies, and targeted therapies have extended survival for many patients with advanced and metastatic prostate cancer. An understanding of when to initiate early treatment before progression to advanced or metastatic disease continues to evolve (eg, the emergence of novel PMSA-based imaging modalities). Moreover, future research will help clinicians to understand how to combine or sequence treatments for castration-resistant prostate cancer, and continued development of novel therapeutics will prolong survival in patients with the most deadly forms of metastatic prostate cancer (eg, treatment-resistant castration-resistant prostate cancer and neuroendocrine prostate cancer).

ABBREVIATIONS

ADT	androgen deprivation therapy
AJCC	American Joint Committee on Cancer
AR	androgen receptor
BPH	benign prostatic hyperplasia
CAB	combined androgen blockade
CAG	cytosine, adenine and guanine trinucleotide repeat
CYP	cytochrome P450
DHT	dihydrotestosterone
dMMR	deficient mismatch repair
DNA	deoxyribonucleic acid
DRE	digital rectal examination
FDA	United States Food and Drug Administration
FSH	follicle-stimulating hormone
GnRH	gonadotropin-releasing hormone
HR	homologous recombination
LH	luteinizing hormone
LHRH	luteinizing hormone–releasing hormone
MSI-H	microsatellite instability high
PARP	poly-ADP ribose polymerase
PMSA	prostate-membrane specific antigen
PSA	prostate-specific antigen
SRE	skeletal-related event
TMB	tumor mutation burden
TNM	tumor, node, metastasis
US	United States

REFERENCES

1. Siegel RL, Miller KD, Fuchs HE, Jemal A. Cancer Statistics, 2022. *CA Cancer J Clin.* 2022;72(1):7–33. 10.3322/caac.21708.
2. Sun J-H, Lee S-A. Association between CAG repeat polymorphisms and the risk of prostate cancer: A meta-analysis by race, study design and the number of (CAG)n repeat polymorphisms. *Int J Mol Med.* 2013;32(5):1195–1203. doi:10.3892/ijmm.2013.1474.
3. Hsieh K, Albertsen PC. Populations at high risk for prostate cancer. *Urol Clin North Am.* 2003;30(4):669–676. doi:10.1016/s0094-0143(03)00058-2.
4. Abida W, Armenia J, Gopalan A, et al. Prospective genomic profiling of prostate cancer across disease states reveals germline and somatic alterations that may affect clinical decision making. *JCO Precis Oncol.* 2017 Jul;2017:PO.17.00029. doi:10.1200/PO.17.00029.
5. Pritchard CC, Mateo J, Walsh MF, et al. Inherited DNA-repair gene mutations in men with metastatic prostate cancer. *N Engl J Med.* 2016;375(5):443–453. doi:10.1056/NEJMoa1603144.
6. Maia S, Cardoso M, Paulo P, et al. The role of germline mutations in the *BRCA1/2* and mismatch repair genes in men ascertained for early-onset and/or familial prostate cancer. *Fam Cancer* 2016;15(1):111–121. 10.1007/s10689-015-9832-x.
7. NCCN Clinical Practices Guidelines in Onocology (NCCN Guidelines®). Prostate cancer, v03.2022. [Internet]. National Comprehensive Cancer Network. [cited 2021 Nov 15]. Available from: https://www.nccn.org/professionals/physician_gls/pdf/prostate.pdf
8. Schwingshackl L, Hoffmann G. Adherence to Mediterranean diet and risk of cancer: A systematic review and meta-analysis of observational studies. *Int J Cancer.* 2014;135(8):1884–1897. doi:10.1002/ijc.28824.
9. Mandair D, Rossi RE, Pericleous M, Whyand T, Caplin ME. Prostate cancer and the influence of dietary factors and supplements: A systematic review. *Nutr Metab (Lond).* 2014;11:30. eCollection 2014. doi:10.1186/1743-7075-11-30.
10. Brunner C, Davies NM, Martin RM, et al. Alcohol consumption and prostate cancer incidence and progression: A Mendelian randomisation study. *Int J Cancer.* 2017;140(1):75–85. doi:10.1002/ijc.30436.
11. Zuccolo L, Lewis SJ, Donovan JL, Hamdy FC, Neal DE, Smith GD. Alcohol consumption and PSA-detected prostate cancer risk—A case-control nested in the ProtecT study. *Int J Cancer.* 2013;132(9):2176–2185. doi:10.1002/ijc.27877.
12. Thompson IM, Goodman PJ, Tangen CM, et al. The influence of finasteride on the development of prostate cancer. *N Engl J Med.* 2003;349(3):215–224. doi:10.1056/NEJMoa030660.
13. Wilt TJ, Macdonald R, Hagerty K, et al. 5-α-Reductase inhibitors for prostate cancer chemoprevention: an updated Cochrane systematic review. *BJU Int.* 2010;106(10):1444–1451. doi:10.1111/j.1464-410X.2010.09714.x.
14. Lacy JM, Kyprianou N. A tale of two trials: The impact of 5α-reductase inhibition on prostate cancer. *Oncol Lett.* 2014;8(4):1391–1396. doi:10.3892/ol.2014.2388.
15. Andriole GL, Bostwick DG, Brawley OW, et al. Effect of dutasteride on the risk of prostate cancer. *N Engl J Med.* 2010;362(13):1192–1202. doi:10.1056/NEJMoa0908127.
16. D'Amico AV, Roehrborn CG. Effect of 1 mg/day finasteride on concentrations of serum prostate-specific antigen in men with androgenic alopecia: A randomised controlled trial. *Lancet Oncol.* 2007;8(1):21–25. doi:10.1016/S1470-2045(06)70981-0.
17. Chau CH, Figg WD. Revisiting 5α-reductase inhibitors and the risk of prostate cancer. *Nat Rev Urol.* 2018;15(7):400–401. doi:10.1038/s41585-018-0018-9.
18. Kramer BS, Hagerty KL, Justman S, et al. Use of 5alpha-reductase inhibitors for prostate cancer chemoprevention: American Society of Clinical Oncology/American Urological Association 2008 Clinical Practice Guideline. *J Urol.* 2009;181(4):1642–1657. doi:10.1016/j.juro.2009.01.071.
19. Klein EA, Thompson IM, Tangen CM, et al. Vitamin E and the risk of prostate cancer: The Selenium and Vitamin E Cancer Prevention Trial (SELECT). *JAMA.* 2011;306(14):1549–1556. doi:10.1001/jama.2011.1437.
20. Thompson IM, Tangen CM, Goodman PJ, Lucia MS, Klein EA. Chemoprevention of prostate cancer. *J Urol.* 2009;182(2):499–507; discussion 508. doi:10.1016/j.juro.2009.04.015.
21. Cuzick J, Thorat MA, Andriole G, et al. Prevention and early detection of prostate cancer. *Lancet Oncol.* 2014;15(11): e484–e492. doi:10.1016/S1470-2045(14)70211-6.
22. Thompson IM, Pauler DK, Goodman PJ, et al. Prevalence of prostate cancer among men with a prostate-specific antigen level < or =4.0 ng per milliliter. *N Engl J Med.* 2004;350(22):2239–2246. doi:10.1056/NEJMoa031918.

23. Carter HB, Albertsen PC, Barry MJ, et al. Early detection of prostate cancer: AUA Guideline. *J Urol.* 2013;190(2):419–426. doi:10.1016/j.juro.2013.04.119.
24. Shteynshlyuger A, Andriole GL. Prostate cancer: To screen or not to screen? *Urol Clin North Am.* 2010;37(1):1–9. doi:10.1016/j.ucl.2009.11.004.
25. Sammon JD, Abdollah F, Choueiri TK, et al. Prostate-specific antigen screening after 2012 US Preventive Services Task Force Recommendations. *JAMA.* 2015;314(19):2077–2079. doi:10.1001/jama.2015.7273.
26. Basch E, Oliver TK, Vickers A, et al. Screening for prostate cancer with prostate-specific antigen testing: American Society of Clinical Oncology Provisional Clinical Opinion. *J Clin Oncol.* 2012;30(24):3020–3025. doi:10.1200/JCO.2012.43.3441.
27. Schröder FH, Hugosson J, Roobol MJ, et al. Prostate-cancer mortality at 11 years of follow-up. *N Engl J Med.* 2012;366(11):981–990. doi:10.1056/NEJMoa1113135.
28. Andriole GL, Crawford ED, Grubb RL, et al. Prostate cancer screening in the randomized Prostate, Lung, Colorectal, and Ovarian Cancer Screening Trial: Mortality results after 13 years of follow-up. *J Natl Cancer Inst.* 2012;104(2):125–132. doi:10.1093/jnci/djr500.
29. Fenton JJ, Weyrich MS, Durbin S, Liu Y, Bang H, Melnikow J. Prostate-Specific Antigen-Based Screening for Prostate Cancer: Evidence Report and Systematic Review for the US Preventive Services Task Force. *JAMA.* 2018;319(18):1914–1931. doi:10.1001/jama.2018.3712.
30. Khauli RB. Prostate cancer: Diagnostic and therapeutic strategies with emphasis on the role of PSA. *J Med Liban.* 2005;53(2):95–102.
31. Iczkowski KA. Current prostate biopsy interpretation: Criteria for cancer, atypical small acinar proliferation, high-grade prostatic intraepithelial neoplasia, and use of immunostains. *Arch Pathol Lab Med.* 2006;130(6):835–843. doi:10.5858/2006-130-835-CPBICF.
32. De Marzo AM, Meeker AK, Zha S, et al. Human prostate cancer precursors and pathobiology. *Urology.* 2003;62(5 Suppl 1):55–62. doi:10.1016/j.urology.2003.09.053.
33. Culig Z. Role of the androgen receptor axis in prostate cancer. *Urology.* 2003;62(5 Suppl 1):21–26. doi:10.1016/s0090-4295(03)00698-8.
34. Marks LS. Luteinizing hormone-releasing hormone agonists in the treatment of men with prostate cancer: Timing, alternatives, and the 1-year implant. *Urology.* 2003;62(6 Suppl 1):36–42. doi:10.1016/j.urology.2003.10.029.
35. Sharifi N, Gulley JL, Dahut WL. Androgen deprivation therapy for prostate cancer. *JAMA.* 2005;294(2):238–244. doi:10.1001/jama.294.2.238.
36. Jentzmik F, Azoitei A, Zengerling F, Damjanoski I, Cronauer MV. Androgen receptor aberrations in the era of abiraterone and enzalutamide. *World J Urol.* 2016;34(3):297–303. doi:10.1007/s00345-015-1624-2.
37. van Royen ME, van Cappellen WA, de Vos C, Houtsmuller AB, Trapman J. Stepwise androgen receptor dimerization. *J Cell Sci.* 2012;125(Pt 8):1970–1979. doi:10.1242/jcs.096792.
38. Scher HI. Prostate carcinoma: Defining therapeutic objectives and improving overall outcomes. *Cancer.* 2003;97(3 Suppl):758–771. doi:10.1002/cncr.11151.
39. Ganz PA, Barry JM, Burke W, et al. National Institutes of Health State-of-the-Science Conference: Role of active surveillance in the management of men with localized prostate cancer. *Ann Intern Med.* 2012;156(8):591–595. doi:10.7326/0003-4819-156-8-201204170-00401.
40. Wilt TJ, MacDonald R, Rutks I, Shamliyan TA, Taylor BC, Kane RL. Systematic review: Comparative effectiveness and harms of treatments for clinically localized prostate cancer. *Ann Intern Med.* 2008;148(6):435–448. doi:10.7326/0003-4819-148-6-200803180-00209.
41. Immediate versus deferred treatment for advanced prostatic cancer: Initial results of the Medical Research Council Trial. The Medical Research Council Prostate Cancer Working Party Investigators Group. *Br J Urol.* 1997;79(2):235–246. doi:10.1046/j.1464-410x.1997.d01-6840.x.
42. Dalkin BL, Christopher BA. Potent men undergoing radical prostatectomy: A prospective study measuring sexual health outcomes and the impact of erectile dysfunction treatments. *Urol Oncol.* 2008;26(3):281–285. doi:10.1016/j.urolonc.2007.02.012.
43. Novara G, Galfano A, Secco S, Ficarra V, Artibani W. Impact of surgical and medical castration on serum testosterone level in prostate cancer patients. *Urol Int.* 2009;82(3):249–255. doi:10.1159/000209352.
44. Seidenfeld J, Samson DJ, Hasselblad V, et al. Single-therapy androgen suppression in men with advanced prostate cancer: A systematic review and meta-analysis. *Ann Intern Med.* 2000;132(7):566–577. doi:10.7326/0003-4819-132-7-200004040-00009.
45. Hedlund PO, Henriksson P. Parenteral estrogen versus total androgen ablation in the treatment of advanced prostate carcinoma: Effects on overall survival and cardiovascular mortality. The Scandinavian Prostatic Cancer Group (SPCG)-5 Trial Study. *Urology.* 2000;55(3):328–333. doi:10.1016/s0090-4295(99)00580-4.
46. Smith MR, Finkelstein JS, McGovern FJ, et al. Changes in body composition during androgen deprivation therapy for prostate cancer. *J Clin Endocrinol Metab.* 2002;87(2):599–603. doi:10.1210/jcem.87.2.8299.
47. Smith MR, Lee WC, Brandman J, Wang Q, Botteman M, Pashos CL. Gonadotropin-releasing hormone agonists and fracture risk: A claims-based cohort study of men with nonmetastatic prostate cancer. *J Clin Oncol.* 2005;23(31):7897–7903. doi:10.1200/JCO.2004.00.6908.
48. Smith MR, Boyce SP, Moyneur E, Duh MS, Raut MK, Brandman J. Risk of clinical fractures after gonadotropin-releasing hormone agonist therapy for prostate cancer. *J Urol.* 2006;175(1):136–139; discussion 139. doi:10.1016/S0022-5347(05)00033-9.
49. Shahinian VB, Kuo Y-F, Freeman JL, Goodwin JS. Risk of fracture after androgen deprivation for prostate cancer. *N Engl J Med.* 2005;352(2):154–164. doi:10.1056/NEJMoa041943.
50. Lipton A, Fizazi K, Stopeck AT, et al. Superiority of denosumab to zoledronic acid for prevention of skeletal-related events: A combined analysis of 3 pivotal, randomised, phase 3 trials. *Eur J Cancer.* 2012;48(16):3082–3092. doi:10.1016/j.ejca.2012.08.002.
51. Keating NL, O'Malley AJ, Smith MR. Diabetes and cardiovascular disease during androgen deprivation therapy for prostate cancer. *J Clin Oncol.* 2006;24(27):4448–4456. doi:10.1200/JCO.2006.06.2497.
52. Nguyen PL, Je Y, Schutz FAB, et al. Association of androgen deprivation therapy with cardiovascular death in patients with prostate cancer: A meta-analysis of randomized trials. *JAMA.* 2011;306(21):2359–2366. doi:10.1001/jama.2011.1745.
53. Klotz L, Boccon-Gibod L, Shore ND, et al. The efficacy and safety of degarelix: A 12-month, comparative, randomized, open-label, parallel-group phase III study in patients with prostate cancer. *BJU Int.* 2008;102(11):1531–1538. doi:10.1111/j.1464-410X.2008.08183.x.
54. Shore ND, Saad F, Cookson MS, et al. Oral relugolix for androgen-deprivation therapy in advanced prostate cancer. *N Engl J Med.* 2020;382(23):2187–2196. doi:10.1056/NEJMoa2004325.
55. Orogovyx (relugolix) [package insert]. Brisbane, CA: Myovant Sciences, Inc., 2020.
56. Firmagon (degarelix) [package insert]. Parsippany, NJ: Ferring Pharmaceuticals, 2020.
57. Trelstar (triptorelin) [package insert]. Parsippany, NJ: Actavis Pharma, Inc., 2014.
58. Zoladex (goserelin) [package insert]. Wilmington, DE:AstraZeneca Pharmaceuticals LP, 2012.
59. Lupron Depot (leuprolide) [package insert]. North Chicago, IL: AbbVie Inc, 2014.
60. Eulexin (flutamide) [package insert]. Kenilworth, NJ: Schering Corporation, 2000.
61. Casodex (bicalutamide) [package insert]. Wilmington, DE: AstraZeneca Pharmaceuticals LP, 2008.
62. Nilandron (nilutamide) [package insert].St. Michael, Barbados: Concordia Pharmaceuticals, Inc, 2015.
63. Xtandi(enzalutamide) [package insert]. Northbrook, IL: Astellas Pharma, 2020.
64. Erleada(apalutamide) [package insert]. Horsham, PA: Janssen Pharmaceuticals, 2018.
65. Nubeqa (darolutamide) [package insert]. Whippany, NJ: Bayer Healthcare, Pharmaceuticals, Inc., 2019.
66. Akaza H. Combined androgen blockade for prostate cancer: Review of efficacy, safety and cost-effectiveness. *Cancer Sci.* 2011;102(1):51–56. doi:10.1111/j.1349-7006.2010.01774.x.
67. Beer TM, Armstrong AJ, Rathkopf DE, et al. Enzalutamide in metastatic prostate cancer before chemotherapy. *N Engl J Med.* 2014;371(5):424–433. doi:10.1056/NEJMoa1405095.
68. Smith MR, Saad F, Chowdhury S, et al. Apalutamide treatment and metastasis-free survival in prostate cancer. *N Engl J Med.* 2018;378(15):1408–1418. doi:10.1056/NEJMoa1715546.
69. Moilanen A-M, Riikonen R, Oksala R, et al. Discovery of ODM-201, a new-generation androgen receptor inhibitor targeting resistance mechanisms to androgen signaling-directed prostate cancer therapies. *Sci Rep.* 2015;5:12007. doi:10.1038/srep12007.
70. Fizazi K, Shore N, Tammela TL, et al. Darolutamide in nonmetastatic, castration-resistant prostate cancer. *N Engl J Med.* 2019;380(13):1235–1246. doi:10.1056/NEJMoa1815671.
71. Abiraterone [package insert]. Horsham, PA: Janssen Biotech, 2020.

72. Lukka H, Waldron T, Klotz L, et al. Maximal androgen blockade for the treatment of metastatic prostate cancer—A systematic review. *Curr Oncol.* 2006;13(3):81–93.
73. Vitzthum LK, Straka C, Sarkar RR, et al. Combined androgen blockade in localized prostate cancer treated with definitive radiation therapy. *J Natl Compr Canc Netw.* 2019;17(12):1497–1504. doi:10.6004/jnccn.2019.7335.
74. de Bono JS, Logothetis CJ, Molina A, et al. Abiraterone and increased survival in metastatic prostate cancer. *N Engl J Med.* 2011;364(21):1995–2005. doi:10.1056/NEJMoa1014618.
75. Xofigo (radium 223) [package insert]. Whippany, NJ: Bayer HealthCare Pharmaceuticals, Inc., 2019.
76. Rubraca (rucaparib) [package insert]. Boulder, CO: Clovis Oncology, Inc., 2020.
77. Lynparza (olaparib) [package insert]. Wilmington, DE: AstraZeneca Pharmaceuticals LP, 2021.
78. Keytruda (pembrolizumab) [package insert]. Whitehouse Station, NJ: Merck & Co, Inc., 2021.
79. Sipuleucel-T [package insert]. Seal Beach, CA: Dendreon Corporation, 2014.
80. Jevtana (cabazitaxel) [package insert]. Bridgewater, NJ: Sanofi-Aventis, 2021.
81. Taxotere (docetaxel) [package insert]. Bridgewater, NJ: Sanofi-Aventis, 2020.
82. Tannock IF, de Wit R, Berry WR, et al. Docetaxel plus prednisone or mitoxantrone plus prednisone for advanced prostate cancer. *N Engl J Med.* 2004;351(15):1502–1512.
83. Sweeney CJ, Chen Y-H, Carducci M, et al. Chemohormonal therapy in metastatic hormone-sensitive prostate cancer. *N Engl J Med.* 2015;373(8):737–746. doi:10.1056/NEJMoa1503747.
84. de Bono JS, Oudard S, Ozguroglu M, et al. Prednisone plus cabazitaxel or mitoxantrone for metastatic castration-resistant prostate cancer progressing after docetaxel treatment: A randomised open-label trial. *Lancet.* 2010;376(9747):1147–1154. doi:10.1016/S0140-6736(10)61389-X.
85. Eisenberger M, Hardy-Bessard A-C, Kim CS, et al. Phase III study comparing a reduced dose of cabazitaxel (20 mg/m^2) and the currently approved dose (25 mg/m^2) in post-docetaxel patients with metastatic castration-resistant prostate cancer-PROSELICA. *J Clin Oncol.* 2017;35(28):3198–3206. doi:10.1200/JCO.2016.72.1076.
86. Corn PG, Heath EI, Zurita A, et al. Cabazitaxel plus carboplatin for the treatment of men with metastatic castration-resistant prostate cancers: A randomised, open-label, phase 1-2 trial. *Lancet Oncol.* 2019;20(10):1432–1443. doi:10.1016/S1470-2045(19)30408-5.
87. Kantoff PW, Higano CS, Shore ND, et al. Sipuleucel-T immunotherapy for castration-resistant prostate cancer. *N Engl J Med.* 2010;363(5):411–422. doi:10.1056/NEJMoa1001294.
88. Sartor O, de Bono JS. Metastatic prostate cancer. *N Engl J Med.* 2018;378(7):645–657. doi:10.1056/NEJMra1701695.
89. de Bono J, Mateo J, Fizazi K, et al. Olaparib for metastatic castration-resistant prostate cancer. *N Engl J Med.* 2020;382(22):2091–2102. doi:10.1056/NEJMoa1911440.
90. Abida W, Patnaik A, Campbell D, et al. Rucaparib in men with metastatic castration-resistant prostate cancer harboring a *BRCA1* or *BRCA2* gene alteration. *J Clin Oncol.* 2020;38(32):3763–3772. 10.1200/JCO.20.01035.
91. Parker C, Nilsson S, Heinrich D, et al. Alpha emitter radium-223 and survival in metastatic prostate cancer. *N Engl J Med.* 2013;369(3):213–223. doi:10.1056/NEJMoa1213755.

155

Lymphomas

Alexandre Chan, Chia J. Tan, and Shawn P. Griffin

KEY CONCEPTS

1. With all stages and risk groups of Hodgkin lymphoma, restaging PET-CT following 8 to 12 weeks of chemotherapy will further guide the patient-specific treatment plan.
2. Patients with early-stage Hodgkin lymphoma should be treated with combination chemotherapy with or without involved-site radiation.
3. Combination chemotherapy with doxorubicin (adriamycin®), bleomycin, vinblastine, and dacarbazine (ABVD) is the primary treatment for patients with advanced-stage Hodgkin lymphoma. Patients with advanced unfavorable disease may be treated with more aggressive regimens, which are associated with a higher risk of secondary malignancies.
4. Some patients with Hodgkin lymphoma will be refractory to initial therapy or will have a recurrence following complete remission. Response to salvage therapy depends on the extent and site of recurrence, previous therapy, and duration of initial remission. High-dose chemotherapy and autologous hematopoietic stem cell transplantation (HSCT) should be considered in patients with refractory or relapsed disease.
5. The current classification system for non-Hodgkin lymphoma (NHL) is the World Health Organization (WHO) classification system, which classifies NHLs into specific disease entities, defined by a combination of morphology, immunophenotype, genetic features, and clinical features.
6. As compared with Hodgkin lymphoma, the clinical presentation of NHL is more variable because of disease heterogeneity and more frequent extranodal involvement.
7. The Ann Arbor staging system correlates poorly with prognosis in NHL because the disease does not spread through contiguous lymph nodes and often involves extranodal sites.
8. Several prognostic models have been developed to estimate prognosis in patients with NHL. The International Prognostic Index (IPI) score is a well-established model for patients with aggressive NHL. The Follicular Lymphoma International Prognostic Index (FLIPI) is a similar model for patients with follicular and other indolent lymphomas.
9. The clinical behavior and degree of aggressiveness can be used to categorize NHL into indolent and aggressive lymphomas. Patients with indolent lymphoma usually have relatively long survival, with or without aggressive chemotherapy. Although these lymphomas respond to a wide range of therapeutic approaches, few if any of these patients are cured of their disease. In contrast, aggressive lymphomas are rapidly growing tumors and patients have a short survival if appropriate therapy is not initiated. Most patients with aggressive lymphomas respond to intensive chemotherapy and many are cured of their disease.
10. Patients with localized follicular lymphoma can be cured with radiation therapy alone. Advanced follicular lymphoma is not curable, and many treatment options are available, including watchful waiting, radiation therapy, anti-CD20 monoclonal antibodies, chemoimmunotherapy, lenalidomide, PI3K inhibitors, an EZH2 inhibitor, CAR T-cell therapy, and high-dose chemotherapy with HSCT.
11. Patients with localized aggressive lymphomas can be cured with several cycles of R-CHOP (rituximab, cyclophosphamide, doxorubicin [Hydroxydaunorubicin], vincristine [Oncovin®], prednisone) chemotherapy and involved-field irradiation. Patients with bulky stage II, stage III, or stage IV aggressive lymphomas can be cured of their disease with R-CHOP chemotherapy.
12. Conventional-dose salvage therapy can induce responses in patients with aggressive lymphomas who relapse, but long-term survival and cure are uncommon. Some patients with aggressive lymphoma who relapse and respond to salvage therapy can be cured with high-dose chemotherapy and autologous HSCT.

BEYOND THE BOOK

1. Read the patient information sheets from the American Society of Clinical Oncology at Cancer.Net on the diagnosis of Hodgkin and non-Hodgkin lymphoma (https://tinyurl.com/y2rr48nq and https://tinyurl.com/wm8emum). These information sheets briefly describe the various procedures used to diagnose lymphoma and will help students to understand how lymphoma is diagnosed.
2. Search the database of FDA-approved drug products and identify drugs that have been approved by the FDA in the last 12 months for lymphoma. Select one drug and compare the mechanism of action and its role in therapy with existing treatments that carry the same indication. Discuss advantages of this new drug over current therapies and challenges posed when using this new medication.

INTRODUCTION

Lymphomas are a heterogeneous group of malignancies that arise from malignant transformation of immune cells that reside predominantly in lymphoid tissues. They most commonly present as a solid tumor but can sometimes present as circulating tumor cells in peripheral blood. The differing histology of lymphoma cells has led to classification of Hodgkin lymphoma (Reed–Sternberg cells) or non-Hodgkin lymphoma (NHL) (B- or T-cell lymphocyte markers). NHLs are further classified into distinct clinical entities, which are defined by a combination of morphology, immunophenotype, genetic features, and clinical features. Chemotherapy is the mainstay of treatment in patients with lymphoma, especially those with widespread disease. Overall cure rates are high for many subtypes of lymphomas, even when patients present with advanced disease.

HODGKIN LYMPHOMA

Hodgkin lymphoma is one of the most curable forms of cancer. Although initial reports of Hodgkin lymphoma demonstrated the disease to be uniformly fatal, an impressive 80% of patients can be cured today with recommended treatments.[1] Some of the keys to the success of the treatments for Hodgkin lymphoma include the appropriate use of multidrug chemotherapy regimens with differing mechanisms of action and toxicities and treatment with full doses of chemotherapy and on schedule whenever possible. It is also common to use radiation therapy in the treatment schema. However, the success of treatment has not been without cost. The treatment programs are intense, technically demanding, and associated with considerable acute toxicity and long-term complications. The long-term effects, particularly secondary malignancies, account for higher cumulative mortality than Hodgkin lymphoma 15 to 20 years after treatment. Long-term toxicities with standard chemotherapy regimens have been more fully documented in recent years and are shaping future therapies.[2,3]

Hodgkin lymphoma is named after Thomas Hodgkin, who first described seven cases of a mysterious disease of the lymph system in 1832. Although Hodgkin lymphoma was not the first cancer to be described, it was one of the first cancers to have methodical investigational treatments that ultimately lead to successful outcomes.[3]

Since many factors influence the prognosis of patients with Hodgkin lymphoma, treatment plans must be personalized for each patient. The staging for Hodgkin lymphoma uses the Ann Arbor Staging Classification where the "A" refers to the absence of B symptoms, and "B" refers to the presence of B symptoms. Beyond the stage of the disease, certain factors have been associated with a poor prognosis (unfavorable risk). Several research groups have defined these unfavorable factors, and the International Prognostic Score (IPS) is used clinically to predict an individual's risk of recurrence.

Epidemiology and Etiology

Hodgkin lymphoma represents less than 1% of all known cancers in the United States. About 8,540 new cases of Hodgkin lymphoma were diagnosed in the United States in 2022, and 920 deaths associated with Hodgkin lymphoma will occur during this same period.[4] Hodgkin lymphoma occurs slightly more frequently in males than in females. It exhibits bimodal distribution in industrialized countries; the first peak occurs in young adults and the second smaller peak occurs after the age of 50 years.[2,3] The 5-year overall survival for all stages of Hodgkin lymphoma is about 85%.[1] Death from recurrent Hodgkin lymphoma is less than those from all other causes 15 years after treatment.

The etiology of Hodgkin lymphoma is unknown, but laboratory and epidemiologic evidence supports infectious exposure as a potential cause.[2,3] Studies suggest an increased risk of Hodgkin lymphoma in patients who have been infected with the Epstein-Barr virus (EBV), and many patients experience EBV activation even before the onset of Hodgkin lymphoma. EBV is found in about 40% of all classical Hodgkin lymphoma cases, and it is frequently observed in cases of mixed cellularity and lymphocyte-depleted Hodgkin lymphoma. Reed–Sternberg cells (large, bilobate, multinuclear cells looking like "owl eyes"), the malignant cells in Hodgkin lymphoma, are linked to EBV. Individuals who are immunosuppressed, such as patients with congenital immunosuppression, solid-organ transplant recipients, and human immunodeficiency virus (HIV)-infection, are also at much higher risk of developing Hodgkin lymphoma. Although the risk of developing Hodgkin lymphoma is up to 25-fold greater in patients with HIV, the CD4 level may be low or within the normal range at diagnosis. Almost all cases of Hodgkin lymphoma in HIV-infected individuals are EBV positive and are most commonly the lymphocyte-deplete subtype of Hodgkin lymphoma. Hodgkin lymphoma is not an AIDS-defining illness.

Genetic factors are also associated with an increased risk of Hodgkin lymphoma. The strongest evidence comes from identical twin studies, which show that the unaffected identical twin has almost a 100-fold increase in risk.

Pathophysiology

Hodgkin lymphoma is a clonal malignant lymphoid disease of transformed B-lymphocytes. The malignant cell in Hodgkin lymphoma is the Reed–Sternberg cell, named after Dorothy Reed and Carl Sternberg, who were credited with the first definitive microscopic description of Hodgkin lymphoma.[2] Single-cell polymerase chain reaction and DNA microarray analyses indicate that nearly all classic Hodgkin lymphoma cases and all nodular lymphocyte-predominant Hodgkin lymphomas (NLPHLs) have immunoglobulin gene rearrangements, which indicates a germinal center or postgerminal center of B-cell origin. Interestingly, nearly all Reed–Sternberg cells of classical Hodgkin lymphoma fail to express B-cell specific cell surface proteins.

B-cell transcriptional processes are disrupted during malignant transformation, which prevents B-cell surface marker expression and production of immunoglobulin messenger ribonucleic acid. The normal cellular consequence of failure to express immunoglobulin is apoptosis, but because of alterations in the normal apoptotic pathways, cell survival and proliferation are favored. Reed–Sternberg cells overexpress nuclear factor-κB, which is associated with cell proliferation and antiapoptotic signals. Infections with viral and bacterial pathogens upregulate nuclear factor-κB and consequently are hypothesized to be involved with the etiology of Hodgkin lymphoma.[2] This hypothesis is supported by the presence of EBV in many Hodgkin lymphoma tumors, but not all tumors are associated with EBV. Another signaling pathway, Janus kinase–signal transduction and transcription (JAK–STAT), is also active in Hodgkin lymphoma.[2] As molecular techniques continue to improve, our understanding of the pathophysiology of Hodgkin lymphoma will also improve.

The histopathologic classification of Hodgkin lymphoma has undergone numerous changes over the past three decades. The current classification system is the 2016 World Health Organization (WHO) classification (Table 155-1).[5] This classification divides Hodgkin lymphoma into two major groups: classical Hodgkin lymphoma and NLPHL, which constitute about 95% and 5% of cases, respectively. Classic Hodgkin lymphoma is further divided into four subtypes: nodular sclerosis, mixed cellularity, lymphocyte-depleted, and lymphocyte-rich. The subtypes in these classifications are based on characteristics of the Reed–Sternberg cell, the surrounding cells, and the tissue. Nodular sclerosis has features that make it distinct from the other three subtypes, which represent a continuum of background cellularity, with lymphocyte-predominance being the most cellular and lymphocyte-depletion being the least cellular. Typical immunophenotype for classical Hodgkin lymphoma

TABLE 155-1 WHO Classification of the Mature B-Cell, T-Cell, and NK-Cell Neoplasms (2016)

B Cell	Mature T and NK Cells	Hodgkin Lymphoma
B-cell chronic lymphocytic leukemia/small lymphocytic lymphoma	T-cell prolymphocytic leukemia	Nodular lymphocyte-predominant Hodgkin lymphoma
B-cell prolymphocytic leukemia	T-cell granular lymphocytic leukemia	Classical Hodgkin lymphoma
Lymphoplasmacytic lymphoma	Aggressive NK-cell leukemia	Nodular sclerosis classical Hodgkin lymphoma
Splenic marginal zone B-cell lymphoma (± villous lymphocytes)	Adult T-cell leukemia/lymphoma (HTLV-I+)	Lymphocyte-rich classical Hodgkin lymphoma
Hairy cell leukemia	Extranodal NK/T-cell lymphoma, nasal type	Mixed cellularity classical Hodgkin lymphoma
Plasma cell myeloma/plasmacytoma	Enteropathy-associated T-cell lymphoma	Lymphocyte-depleted classical Hodgkin lymphoma
Extranodal marginal zone B-cell lymphoma of MALT type	Hepatosplenic $\gamma\delta$ T-cell lymphoma	
Mantle cell lymphoma	Subcutaneous panniculitis-like T-cell lymphoma	
Follicular lymphoma	**Mycosis fungoides/Sézary syndrome**	
Nodal marginal zone B-cell lymphoma (± monocytoid B cells)	**Anaplastic large cell lymphoma, primary cutaneous type**	
Diffuse large B-cell lymphoma (DLBCL)	**Peripheral T-cell lymphoma, not otherwise specified (NOS)**	
Germinal center B-cell type	**Angioimmunoblastic T-cell lymphoma**	
Activated B-cell type	**Anaplastic large cell lymphoma, primary systemic type**	
Burkitt lymphoma		

HTLV, human T-cell lymphotropic virus; MALT, mucosa-associated lymphoid tissue; NK, natural killer; WHO, World Health Organization.

Note: Not all subtypes are listed. **Malignancies in bold occur in at least 1% of patients.**

(Adapted from Swerdlow SH, et al. WHO Classification of Tumours of Haematopoietic and Lymphoid Tissues, 4th ed. World Health Organization; 2008.)

includes CD15⁺, CD30⁺, PAX-5⁺ (weak), CD3⁻, CD20⁻, CD45⁻, and CD79a⁻. NLPHL is separated because of its distinct immunophenotype: CD15⁻, CD20⁺, CD30⁻, and CD45⁺ (the opposite of classical Hodgkin lymphoma). With the use of extensive staging, sophisticated radiotherapy, and effective combination chemotherapy, the prognostic value of these subtypes is becoming less clear. The true value of understanding these subtypes is likely tied to the pathogenesis of the disease and its potential prevention in the future.

Clinical Presentation

Most patients with Hodgkin lymphoma present with a painless, rubbery, enlarged lymph node in the supradiaphragmatic area and commonly have mediastinal nodal involvement. Lymphadenopathy may come and go, but the persistence of lymphadenopathy for more than 2 months warrants evaluation. Hodgkin lymphoma is occasionally diagnosed in an asymptomatic patient who has a mediastinal mass found with chest radiography or another imaging procedure. Asymptomatic adenopathy of the inguinal and axillary regions may be present at diagnosis but is less common (Fig. 155-1).[2,3] Patients can also present with constitutional symptoms (B symptoms) before the discovery of lymph node enlargement, and these symptoms include fever greater than 38°C (100.4°F), drenching night sweats, and weight loss greater than 10% within 6 months of diagnosis. At diagnosis, these symptoms may appear in about 25% of all patients and up to 50% of patients with advanced disease. Patients may also experience other nonspecific symptoms including pruritus, fatigue, and development of pain after alcohol consumption at sites where nodes are involved.[3] Extranodal manifestations, such as bowel or hepatic involvements, are much less common in Hodgkin lymphoma than NHL.[2]

Diagnosis, Staging, and Prognostic Factors

Diagnostic and staging procedures are based on recommendations made at the Ann Arbor and Cotswolds conferences and new scientific advances. The diagnosis and pathologic classification of Hodgkin lymphoma can only be made by review of a biopsy (preferably an excisional biopsy) of the enlarged node by an expert hematopathologist.

In addition to a careful physical examination, routine laboratory tests including a complete blood count, complete metabolic panel to assess renal and hepatic function, lactate dehydrogenase (LDH), and erythrocyte sedimentation rate (ESR) are helpful in treatment planning and aid in prognosis. Pregnancy test and HIV status should be assessed. Computed tomography (CT) scans of the chest, abdomen, and pelvis are routinely performed. Furthermore, positron emission tomography (PET) plays an important role in the initial staging of Hodgkin lymphoma, as it has shown high sensitivity and specificity in the staging of the disease response to treatment.[6] The use of integrated PET-CT has further improved the staging of Hodgkin lymphoma given that it can provide more sensitive and specific imaging as compared with each imaging alone. Bone marrow biopsy is now recommended only in patients with cytopenias and a negative PET.

CLINICAL PRESENTATION Hodgkin Lymphoma

General

- Most patients with Hodgkin lymphoma have lymph node involvement in the supradiaphragmatic and mediastinal areas.

Symptoms

- Fatigue, malaise, and pruritus.
- About 25% of all patients present with fever, night sweats, and weight loss (ie, B symptoms), and up to 50% of patients with advanced disease.

Signs

- Enlarged lymph node, which may present as painless and rubbery.

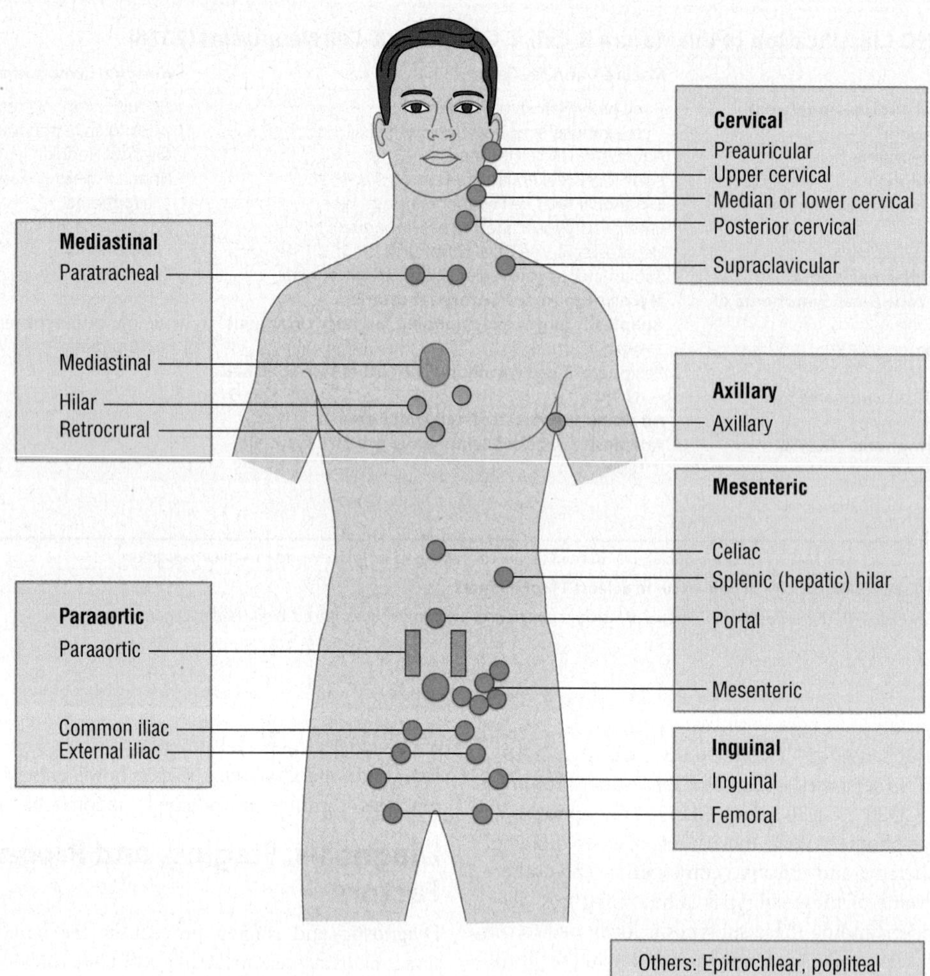

FIGURE 155-1 Areas of lymph nodes used in the staging of Hodgkin and non-Hodgkin lymphoma. Each rectangle corresponds to a nodal area.

Staging can be based on clinical or pathologic findings. The clinical stage is based on all noninvasive procedures (history, physical examination, laboratory tests, and radiologic findings), whereas the pathologic stage is based on the biopsy findings of strategic sites (bone marrow, spleen, and abdominal nodes). Patients with extranodal disease (bone marrow, bone, or Waldeyer ring) contiguous to involved nodes are classified with the subscript "E" in the Cotswolds staging system.

The Ann Arbor staging classification, which was developed at the 1970 Ann Arbor conference, has proven to be a good schema. At the Cotswolds meeting in 1989, the Ann Arbor classification was modified to incorporate new diagnostic techniques (eg, CT and magnetic resonance imaging), and the understanding that prognosis is associated with the bulk of the disease and the number of involved nodal sites (Fig. 155-1, Table 155-2).[3] After careful staging, about one-half of patients have localized disease (stages I, II, and II_E) and the remainder have advanced disease (stage III or IV). About 10% to 15% present with metastatic disease (stage IV). Hodgkin lymphoma follows a predictable pattern of nodal spread that is not seen with the NHLs.[3]

Patient prognosis is predominately driven by age and amount of disease. Patients older than 65 to 70 years have a lower cure rate than younger patients. The difference in cure rates may be related to the higher prevalence of comorbid diseases and decreased organ function in older patients, which impairs their ability to tolerate intensive chemotherapy. Stage is a dominant factor in predicting survival; patients with limited-stage disease (stages I-II) have a 90% to 95% cure rate, while those with advanced disease (stages III-IV) have only a 60% to 80% cure rate.[2,3]

Seven adverse prognostic factors with similar impact on survival (each factor reduced survival by 7%-8% per year) have been identified through an international collaborative effort. These factors can be combined to generate an IPS that can be used to predict progression-free and overall survival (Table 155-3).[7]

TREATMENT: HODGKIN LYMPHOMA

Desired Outcomes

The current goal in the treatment of Hodgkin lymphoma is to maximize curability while minimizing short- and long-term treatment-related complications. According to the Surveillance, Epidemiology, and End Results (SEER) database, the 5-year age-adjusted relative survival is greater than 80%.[1] Therefore, the initial treatment goal for all stages of Hodgkin lymphoma is the cure.

General Approach

Combination chemotherapy is the primary treatment modality for most patients with Hodgkin lymphoma. In general, patients of all stages are initially treated with combination chemotherapy for about

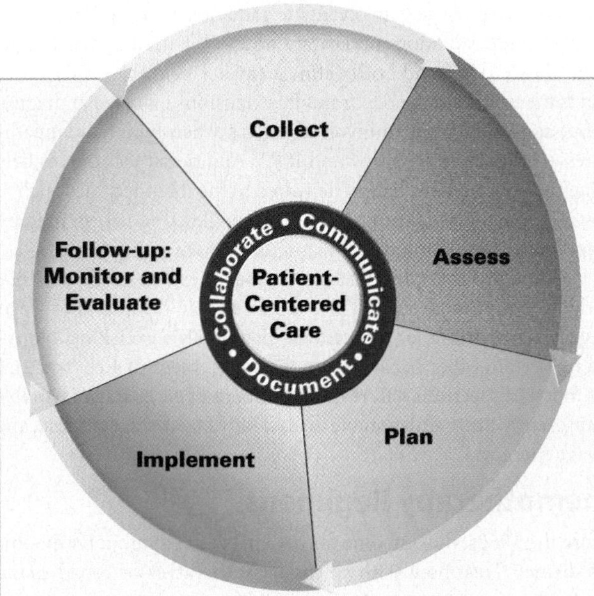

Patient Care Process for Lymphoma

Collect

- Patient characteristics (eg, age, sex, pregnant, smoking history)
- Patient medical history (personal and family)
- Current medications including OTC aspirin/NSAID use, herbal products, dietary supplements
- Objective data
  - Height and weight to calculate body surface area (BSA)
  - Labs include complete blood count (CBC), complete metabolic panel which includes liver function tests, LDH, pregnancy test for women with reproductive potential
  - Baseline assessment of cardiac ejection fraction by ECHO or MUGA if treatment with anthracycline is planned
  - Baseline assessment of pulmonary function (pulmonary function test including diffusing capacity of lungs for carbon monoxide—DLCO) if treatment with bleomycin is planned
  - Lymphoma-specific immunophenotyping, cytogenetics, such as CD20, CD30, t(11:14), t(14;18)
  - Stage and prognostic score (eg, IPS, IPI, FLIPI)

Assess

- Comorbid illnesses that may affect drug therapy selection (baseline neuropathy, CHF, renal or hepatic dysfunction)
- Potential for drug-drug interactions (particularly with oral agents such as idelalisib or ibrutinib)
- Patient's risk of tumor lysis syndrome based on disease, planned therapy, tumor burden, and renal function
- Ability to self-care, family/social support
- Financial challenges—copays, coinsurance, specialty pharmacy medication access
- Birth control and fertility options if the patient is of childbearing age (male and female)
- Emotional status (eg, anxiety, depression)
- Need for central venous access
- Access and availability of eligible clinical trials

Plan*

- Logistics of the treatment plan (inpatient, outpatient, daily oral medication) and monitoring plan
- Patient education (eg, goals and purpose of treatment, treatment schedule, duration/number of treatment cycles, drug-specific information, medication administration)
- Self-monitoring for toxicities, when to seek emergency medical attention
- Referrals to other providers when appropriate (eg, dietician, navigator, behavioral health, integrative health, palliative/supportive care)

Implement*

- Provide patient education regarding all elements of the treatment plan
- Obtain consent for planned treatment
- Use motivational interviewing and coaching strategies to maximize adherence
- Write, order, or review therapy orders to ensure appropriate dosing, supportive care therapies (eg, nausea/vomiting, infection prevention, prevention of hypersensitivity reactions)
- Schedule follow-up (eg, oral therapy medication therapy management, adherence assessment, symptom management)
- Connect patient to resources such as support groups, educational websites, community resources, social worker

Follow-up: Monitor and Evaluate

- Survivorship teaching and follow-up with focus on monitoring for long-term toxicities
- Patient adherence to treatment plan using multiple sources of information
- Imaging studies to be ordered for appropriate follow-up
- Necessary vaccines following stem-cell transplant

**Collaborate with patients, caregivers, and other healthcare professionals.*

8 to 12 weeks (depending on the regimen) and then restaged with PET-CT. Three combination chemotherapy regimens are primarily used for the initial treatment of classical Hodgkin lymphoma: ABVD, BEACOPP (bleomycin, etoposide, doxorubicin [Adriamycin®], cyclophosphamide, vincristine [Oncovin®], procarbazine, and prednisone), and A-AVD (brentuximab vedotin [Adcetris®], doxorubicin [Adriamycin®], vinblastine, and dacarbazine). Depending on the initial radiographic response from the restaging, further chemotherapy with or without radiation is planned. For patients with refractory or recurrent disease, salvage therapy consists of multi-agent chemotherapy with or without high-dose chemotherapy and autologous hematopoietic stem cell transplantation (HSCT).[2,3]

Radiation is often an integral part of the treatment plan. Selected patients with early-stage disease (usually nodular lymphocyte-predominant histology) can receive radiation as the only treatment modality, whereas most other patients with early-stage disease may

TABLE 155-2 The Ann Arbor Staging Classification of Hodgkin Lymphoma

Stage I	Involvement of a single lymph node region or structure (I) or of a single extralymphatic organ or site (I_E)
Stage II	Involvement of two or more lymph node regions on the same side of the diaphragm (II) or localized involvement of an extralymphatic organ or site and one or more lymph node regions on the same side of the diaphragm (II_E). The number of nodal regions involved should be indicated by a subscript (eg, II_2)
Stage III	Involvement of lymph node regions on both sides of the diaphragm (III), which may also be accompanied by localized involvement of an extralymphatic organ or site (III_E) or by involvement of the spleen (IIIS) or both ($IIIS_E$). III_1: with or without splenic, hilar, celiac, or portal node involvement. III_2: with paraaortic, iliac, or mesenteric node involvement
Stage IV	Diffuse or disseminated involvement of one or more extralymphatic organs or tissues with or without associated lymph node enlargement A—No symptoms B—Fever, night sweats, weight loss (>10%) X—Bulky disease >One-third of the width of the mediastinum >10-cm maximal dimension of nodal mass E—Involvement of extralymphatic tissue on one side of the diaphragm by limited direct extension from an adjacent, involved lymph node region S—Involvement of the spleen CS—Clinical stage PS—Pathologic stage

TABLE 155-3 The International Prognostic Factors Project Score for Advanced Hodgkin Lymphoma

Risk Factors

Serum albumin (<4 g/dL [40 g/L])

Hemoglobin (<10.5 g/dL [105 g/L; 6.52 mmol/L])

Male gender

Stage IV disease

Age (≥45 years)

White blood cell (WBC) count (≥15,000 cells/mm^3 [15 × 10^9/L])

Lymphocytopenia (<600 cells/mm^3 [0.6 × 10^9/L] or <8% of WBC count)

Number of Factors	Freedom from Progression*	Overall Survival*
0	84 ± 4	89 ± 2
1	77 ± 3	90 ± 2
2	67 ± 2	81 ± 2
3	60 ± 3	78 ± 3
4	51 ± 4	61 ± 4
≥5	42 ± 5	56 ± 5

*Percentage of patients at 5 years.

Data from Reference 7.

receive chemotherapy and radiation depending on the initial bulk of disease and the response to chemotherapy alone. Although radiation is a local therapy, many patients with advanced disease will also receive radiation therapy to residual or bulky disease sites after chemotherapy. Many different radiation techniques targeting different radiation fields have been used over the last few decades, including involved-field radiation (IFRT), extended-field radiation, subtotal nodal irradiation, and total nodal irradiation. The major concern with radiation therapy is its long-term effects, particularly on organs at risk, such as cardiovascular disease and secondary malignancies that commonly occur in the lung, breast, gastrointestinal tract, and connective tissue.[8] Involved-site radiation therapy (ISRT) and involved-node radiation therapy are now being used as alternatives to the classic IFRT, and both define a smaller field than IFRT. ISRT targets the nodal sites and extranodal extensions involved at diagnosis but spares adjacent uninvolved organs when lymphadenopathy regresses after chemotherapy and ISRT. Additional techniques help refine the volume of radiation delivered to the intended sites such as 4D-CT simulation planning, intensity-modulated radiation therapy, image-guided radiation therapy, and respiratory gating.[9]

Although multiple treatment modalities are used to treat Hodgkin lymphoma, surgery has a limited role regardless of stage. Surgery is important for an accurate diagnosis via excisional biopsy, and on certain other occasions, such as placement of a central line. The following sections will review treatment of early-stage favorable disease, early-stage unfavorable disease, advanced-stage disease, and salvage therapy.

Chemotherapy Regimens

Before the 1960s, the outcome for patients with Hodgkin lymphoma was dismal. Treatment with single-agent therapies or broad radiation fields caused excessive toxicities and few durable responses with advanced disease. The mechlorethamine, vincristine, procarbazine, and prednisone (MOPP) regimen was introduced in the early 1960s and was the initial combination chemotherapy regimen shown to cure advanced Hodgkin lymphoma (Table 155-4). This was a tremendous advance in oncology at that time. MOPP chemotherapy was a mainstay of treatment for patients with stages III and IV advanced Hodgkin lymphoma for many years. However, investigators later learned that MOPP is associated with high rates of sterility and secondary malignancies. The young cohort of Hodgkin survivors would live long enough to endure these consequences. The research focus was then shifted to maintain the high cure rates obtained with MOPP while decreasing the long-term toxicities.

The development of ABVD by Bonadonna et al. at the Milan Cancer Institute about a decade later represents the next important step in the evolution of therapy for Hodgkin lymphoma (see Table 155-4).[10] ABVD was initially shown to be effective in treating MOPP failures and was later compared directly to MOPP in advanced disease, where it produced an 82% complete response rate, as compared to a 67% complete response rate with MOPP. ABVD improved failure-free survival, but no significant differences in 5-year overall survival were noted.[11] Because ABVD was less toxic and provided similar or better outcomes than MOPP, it eventually replaced MOPP as the standard regimen for advanced-stage Hodgkin lymphoma.

In the early 1980s, the Goldie–Coldman hypothesis proposed that chemotherapy resistance was related to spontaneous mutation rates and the development of resistant clones. To test that hypothesis, researchers designed several clinical trials to evaluate the efficacy of alternating non–cross-resistant drug combinations in patients with Hodgkin lymphoma.[12] The initial approach adopted by investigators was to alternate or combine the MOPP and ABVD regimens. When MOPP and ABVD (or doxorubicin [Adriamycin®], bleomycin, vinblastine [ABV]) are combined in a monthly cycle, it is referred to as a hybrid regimen. Besides a potential benefit in efficacy, another potential benefit of alternating or hybrid regimens is the decreased risk of long-term toxicities. In the alternating MOPP/ABVD regimen, the cumulative doses of procarbazine and mechlorethamine are reduced by 50%, and the cumulative doxorubicin dose is reduced by 50%. In the hybrid regimen, the cumulative doxorubicin dose is reduced by 33%, and the cumulative bleomycin dose is reduced by 50%.

Several clinical trials have been performed to evaluate the efficacy of alternating or hybrid MOPP/ABVD regimens. The results of these trials show that alternating and hybrid regimens are superior to MOPP but not to ABVD.[12,13] Another approach evaluated by researchers was the administration of sequential cycles of MOPP and ABVD (MOPP/ABVD). Results of an intergroup trial

TABLE 155-4 Combination Chemotherapy Regimens for Hodgkin Lymphoma

Drug	Dosage (mg/m²)	Route	Days
MOPP			
Mechlorethamine	6	IV	1, 8
Vincristine	1.4	IV	1, 8
Procarbazine	100	Oral	1-14
Prednisone	40	Oral	1-14
Repeat every 21 days			
ABVD			
Doxorubicin (Adriamycin®)	25	IV	1, 15
Bleomycin	10	IV	1, 15
Vinblastine	6	IV	1, 15
Dacarbazine	375	IV	1, 15
Repeat every 28 days			
MOPP/ABVD			
Alternating months of MOPP and ABVD			
MOPP/ABV hybrid			
Mechlorethamine	6	IV	1
Vincristine	1.4	IV	1
Procarbazine	100	Oral	1-7
Prednisone	40	Oral	1-14
Doxorubicin	35	IV	8
Bleomycin	10	IV	8
Vinblastine	6	IV	8
Repeat every 28 days			
Stanford V			
Doxorubicin	25	IV	Weeks 1, 3, 5, 7, 9, 11
Vinblastine	6	IV	Weeks 1, 3, 5, 7, 9, 11
Mechlorethamine	6	IV	Weeks 1, 5, 9
Etoposide	60	IV	Weeks 3, 7, 11
Vincristine	1.4[a]	IV	Weeks 2, 4, 6, 8, 10, 12
Bleomycin	5	IV	Weeks 2, 4, 6, 8
Prednisone	40	Oral	Every other day for 12 weeks; begin tapering at week 10
One course (12 weeks)			
BEACOPP (standard-dose)			
Bleomycin	10	IV	8
Etoposide	100	IV	1-3
Adriamycin (doxorubicin)	25	IV	1
Cyclophosphamide	650	IV	1
Oncovin® (vincristine)	1.4[a]	IV	8
Procarbazine	100	Oral	1-7
Prednisone	40	Oral	1-14
Repeat every 21 days			
BEACOPP (escalated-dose)			
Bleomycin	10	IV	8
Etoposide	200	IV	1-3
Adriamycin (doxorubicin)	35	IV	1
Cyclophosphamide	1250	IV	1
Oncovin® (vincristine)	1.4[a]	IV	8
Procarbazine	100	Oral	1-7
Prednisone	40	Oral	1-14
Granulocyte colony-stimulating factor		Subcutaneously	8+
Repeat every 21 days			
A-AVD			
Adcetris® (brentuximab vedotin)	1.2 mg/kg	IV	1,15
Doxorubicin	25	IV	1,15
Vinblastine	6	IV	1,15
Dacarbazine	375	IV	1,15

[a]Vincristine dose capped at 2 mg.

showed sequential MOPP and ABVD to be inferior to the MOPP/ABV hybrid regimen in terms of response and survival.[13] In another randomized comparison trial of the MOPP/ABV hybrid regimen and ABVD, the complete remission rate, failure-free survival, and overall survival were similar between the two regimens.[14] The latter trial was closed prematurely because of an increased number of treatment-related deaths and secondary malignancies in the patients who received the MOPP/ABV hybrid regimen.

More complex regimens, such as Stanford V and BEACOPP, have been evaluated as alternatives to MOPP or ABVD. Radiation therapy is an integral part of the Stanford V regimen for all patients. The Stanford V regimen generated considerable interest based on the results of phase II trials.[15] Stanford V, ABVD, and an MOPP/ABV hybrid-like regimen (mechlorethamine, vincristine, procarbazine, prednisone, epidoxorubicin, bleomycin, vinblastine, lomustine, doxorubicin, and vindesine [MOPPEBVCAD]) were then compared in a randomized trial to determine the best regimen to support a reduced radiotherapy program.[16] Five-year failure-free and progression-free survival were significantly worse for the Stanford V regimen as compared to the other two regimens. However, no significant differences in overall response rate or 5-year overall or failure-free survival were observed between Stanford V and ABVD in a published randomized trial of patients with advanced Hodgkin lymphoma (E2496).[17] Investigators have speculated that differences in the application of radiotherapy may explain the divergent results in the randomized trials. More pulmonary toxicity occurred in the ABVD group, but other toxicities occurred more frequently in the Stanford V group.

The German Hodgkin Study Group (GHSG) developed the BEACOPP regimens based on the principles of dose density, dose intensity, and mathematical modeling. BEACOPP uses similar drugs as in the cyclophosphamide, vincristine, procarbazine, and prednisone (COPP)/ABVD regimen, but rearranges the drugs in a shorter 3-week cycle. Several different versions of BEACOPP have been developed: standard-dose BEACOPP, escalated-dose BEACOPP, and dose-dense BEACOPP (BEACOPP-14). Granulocyte colony-stimulating factor support is required for the escalated-dose BEACOPP and BEACOPP-14 regimens.

The initial evidence for these regimens focused on patients with advanced or metastatic disease, but subsequent trials have focused on the use of these regimens in early-stage disease.

1 With all stages and risk groups of Hodgkin lymphoma, it is current practice to treat with chemotherapy for 8 to 12 weeks and then obtain a restaging PET-CT.[18] This scan is assessed on a PET 5-point scale, also known as the Deauville Criteria based on visual assessment of radiolabeled glucose uptake in involved sites. Score 1 indicates no uptake and can be called a complete response or no measurable disease.[6] For all stages of Hodgkin lymphoma, further treatment is based on the restaging PET/CT results such that residual uptake at the end of chemotherapy would likely indicate the need for ISRT. If a Deauville score of 5 exists after completion of chemotherapy, then a biopsy of the involved area is indicated. With an interval PET/CT scan, every patient's treatment plan is personalized based on the response to treatment.

Classical Hodgkin Lymphoma

Hodgkin lymphoma can initially be divided into two broad classifications: classical Hodgkin lymphoma and NLPHL. Although classical Hodgkin lymphoma can be further divided into pathologic subtypes, the treatments are based on risk factors and the presence of bulky disease regardless of the subtype of classical Hodgkin lymphoma.

Treatment of Early-Stage Favorable Disease

Patients with early-stage favorable disease have stage IA or IIA disease and no adverse risk factors (B symptoms, extranodal disease, bulky disease, three or more sites of nodal involvement, or an ESR of >50 mm/hr [13.9 μm/s]). Extended-field radiation was previously considered the treatment of choice for stages IA and IIA disease. Although most patients were cured of their disease, the radiation is associated with long-term toxicities due to large radiation fields such as heart disease, pulmonary dysfunction, and secondary malignancies.[3]

Combined modality therapy (chemotherapy and radiation therapy) has replaced radiation therapy alone in patients with early-stage favorable disease. With combined modality therapy, both a shorter duration of chemotherapy and newer, more focused radiation techniques (ISRT, others) are used to decrease the long-term toxicities of both.

Clinical trials comparing radiation alone to radiation plus chemotherapy show lower relapse rates in patients treated with combined modality therapy (radiation and chemotherapy), but no change in overall survival because of the availability of effective salvage therapy. Ongoing trials focus on questions such as the optimal number of chemotherapy cycles, the volume of radiation that must be used to obtain optimal patient outcomes, and the role of PET scanning to individualize therapy. Long-term results of clinical trials also suggest that as few as two cycles of Stanford V or ABVD chemotherapy followed by IFRT is sufficient in favorable, early-stage disease patients.[19,20] Different combination chemotherapy regimens have been used in these studies and no one regimen is superior to another.

Clinical trials have also investigated the use of chemotherapy alone to treat low-risk early-stage Hodgkin lymphoma. Long-term results of clinical trials show a lower rate of disease control versus combined modality therapy. Selected patients can be treated with chemotherapy alone if they achieve a complete response following two cycles of chemotherapy, with a total treatment of four cycles of chemotherapy.

Patients with early-stage favorable disease can be treated with two cycles of ABVD alone or plus ISRT or two to four cycles of the Stanford V regimen (doxorubicin, vinblastine, mechlorethamine, etoposide, vincristine, bleomycin, and prednisone), followed by a restaging PET-CT scan.[19,20] Depending on the response to the initial chemotherapy, consolidative ISRT is recommended if anything less than a complete response is achieved. With this approach, 5-year progression-free and overall survival rates of more than 90% can be achieved in early-stage favorable disease.

Treatment of Early-Stage Unfavorable Disease

Patients with early-stage disease who have certain features associated with a poor prognosis (B symptoms, extranodal disease, bulky disease, three or more sites of nodal involvement, or an ESR >50 mm/hr [13.9 μm/s]) are defined as having unfavorable disease. Different research groups or clinical trials have different definitions for unfavorable disease. Most groups consider an ESR >50 mm/hr (13.9 μm/s), presence of B symptoms, large mediastinal mass, and more than three affected nodal sites to be unfavorable risk factors. Current guidelines recommend combined modality therapy (combination chemotherapy and ISRT) to reduce the relapse rate and avoid the toxicity associated with extended-field radiation.[18]

Randomized trials show that combined modality therapy reduces the relapse rate in patients with early-stage unfavorable disease. Different chemotherapy regimens and the number of chemotherapy cycles have been compared in clinical trials. In most studies involving early-stage unfavorable disease, ABVD is the comparator arm. ABVD plus 30 Gy [3,000 rad] ISRT remains the standard of care for patients with early-stage unfavorable disease, but the Stanford V regimen plus radiation or BEACOPP for two cycles followed by ABVD for two cycles are both alternatives in select patients. The Stanford V regimen has been studied in several single arm trials[15,21] and comparative trials versus ABVD[17,22] report overall response rates in the 90% range and 5-year overall survival from 88% to 94%. All of these trials included radiation therapy as part of the treatment schema. The GHSG studied the use of a more aggressive regimen of escalated-dose BEACOPP for two cycles followed by ABVD for two cycles versus ABVD for four cycles. Both treatment arms received 30 Gy [3,000 rad] of IFRT. Patients treated with BEACOPP had longer progression-free survival but similar 5-year overall survival as compared with ABVD.[23] Stanford V and BEACOPP are associated with more toxicities than ABVD in early-stage unfavorable Hodgkin lymphoma.[17,24]

2 In summary, most patients with early-stage disease will be treated with two to four cycles of ABVD chemotherapy and involved-site radiation. The number of cycles initially administered is based on the classification of favorable versus unfavorable disease. Restaging with a PET-CT after 4 to 12 weeks of chemotherapy further guides the need for more chemotherapy or radiation (ISRT), but most patients with unfavorable disease will require radiation. Clinical trials have demonstrated the utility of PET scans as biomarkers to personalize therapy and minimize the amount of therapy necessary for cure.[6] Despite excellent results from treatment with ABVD and radiation, about 5% of patients do not respond to initial treatment and another 15% of patients will relapse following an initial response.

Treatment of Advanced-Stage Disease

Advanced-stage disease consists of stages III and IV disease. In some studies, stage IIB with a large mediastinal mass or extranodal disease is also considered advanced-stage disease (see Table 155-2). By definition, patients with stages III and IV disease have tumors on both sides of the diaphragm, which almost always precludes the use of radiation alone as a therapeutic modality. Intensive combination chemotherapy is the mainstay of treatment, although some patients will benefit from radiation following chemotherapy. The prognosis of advanced-stage disease is excellent with 5-year overall survival rates ranging from 56% to 90%. Most patients obtain a complete response from their initial treatment. Prognostic factors have been identified and standardized to predict an individual's prognosis, according to the IPS (see Table 155-3).[7]

Patients with advanced-stage Hodgkin lymphoma can be classified into two groups based on the number of prognostic factors present from the IPS (see Table 155-3). Advanced-stage patients with three or fewer poor prognostic factors are considered to have favorable disease and have about a 60% likelihood of being failure-free at 5 years with traditional combination chemotherapy. Advanced-stage patients with four or more poor prognostic factors are considered to have unfavorable disease and a less than 50% likelihood of being failure-free at 5 years with traditional combination chemotherapy. Cures are possible in patients with high-risk disease, but long-term disease control is a more realistic goal for most patients.

Doxorubicin (Adriamycin®), bleomycin, vinblastine, and dacarbazine (ABVD) for decades have continued to be the standard initial regimen for advanced Hodgkin lymphoma in many cancer programs. As discussed in the section "Chemotherapy Regimens," many international randomized large trials have demonstrated ABVD's sustained positive outcomes and lower toxicity profile as compared to other regimens.

The BEACOPP regimens were designed to provide a more aggressive treatment for advanced disease. Several randomized trials have compared BEACOPP to other regimens.[3,25] The GHSG conducted a large randomized comparison of COPP/ABVD (alternating), BEACOPP, or an escalated-dose BEACOPP regimen (HD9 trial).[25] Escalated-dose BEACOPP was the most active regimen in this study, with 10-year freedom from treatment failure at 82% and overall survival at 86%, but this regimen was also associated with more toxicities, including secondary leukemias, and was particularly toxic in older adults.[26] In the HD2000 study, patients with advanced Hodgkin lymphoma were randomized to receive six cycles of ABVD, four cycles of escalated-dose BEACOPP with two cycles of standard-dose BEACOPP, or a third chemotherapy regimen that is not a current standard of care.[27] BEACOPP was superior to ABVD for 5-year progression-free survival (81% vs 68%), but 5-year overall survival was not significantly different between ABVD and BEACOPP. BEACOPP may be superior to ABVD in patients with high-risk advanced Hodgkin lymphoma (IPS ≥3). Higher rates of neutropenia and severe infections were observed with BEACOPP as compared with ABVD. The HD2000 trial also demonstrated a higher risk of secondary malignancy in the BEACOPP versus ABVD arm at 10 years.[28] Finally, GHSG has conducted several trials to evaluate the optimal number and intensity of BEACOPP. The HD12 and HD15 trials are two examples of this research.[29,30] The results of these studies suggest that escalated-dose BEACOPP is superior to ABVD in the treatment of advanced Hodgkin lymphoma, but at the cost of more treatment-related toxicity.

Current treatment options for patients with advanced disease are ABVD or escalated-dose BEACOPP. BEACOPP may be considered in patients less than 60 years old with an IPS of greater than or equal to 4.[30] As with earlier stage disease, combination chemotherapy should be administered for 4 to 18 weeks, depending on the regimen, followed by a restaging PET scan. Based on the residual Deauville score, additional chemotherapy and/or radiation may be administered. The Response-Adapted Therapy in Advanced Hodgkin Lymphoma (RATHL) trial evaluated the use of AVD, ABVD and escalated-dose BEACOPP based on interim PET-CT results after two cycles of ABVD. Those patients with a favorable response on PET-CT received either 4 cycles of ABVD or AVD. There was no difference in 3-year progression-free or overall survival, but there was less pulmonary toxicity in the AVD group due to the omission of bleomycin. Those patients with an unfavorable response on interim PET-CT had treatment intensified to dose-escalated BEACOPP with a 3-year progression-free survival and overall survival of 67.5% and 87.8% respectively.[31]

Brentuximab vedotin is an antibody-drug conjugate (ADC) comprised of an anti-CD30 antibody conjugated by a protease cleavable linker to a potent antimicrotubule agent, monomethyl auristatin E (MMAE). After the ADC binds to CD30 on the cell surface, the ADC-CD30 complex is internalized and then releases MMAE via proteolytic cleavage in the lysosomal compartment. Tubulin binding by MMAE disrupts the microtubule network, which causes apoptotic death of the cancer cells. The A-AVD regimen incorporates brentuximab vedotin instead of bleomycin into the "AVD" backbone (doxorubicin, vinblastine, and dacarbazine). In a large international phase III trial, A-AVD was compared to ABVD in patients with newly diagnosed stage III or IV Hodgkin lymphoma. Toxicities differed in the two arms, where neutropenia, neutropenic fever, and peripheral neuropathy were more common in the A-AVD arm as compared to ABVD. Grade 3 or higher pulmonary toxicity was more common in patients receiving ABVD arm as compared to A-AVD. Of the deaths that occurred in this trial, 11 of the 13 receiving ABVD were associated with pulmonary toxicities, and 7 of the 9 receiving A-AVD were associated with neutropenia. The authors concluded that A-AVD was superior to ABVD, based on the absolute difference of 4.9% in the combined risk of death, progressive disease or incomplete response. Possible candidates for the A-AVD regimen are patients with newly diagnosed disease, no preexisting neuropathy, and a contraindication to bleomycin.[32] The modified 3-year progression-free survival rates were 83.1% in the A-AVD arm and 76% in the ABVD arm.[33]

3 In summary, there are several approaches to the initial treatment of stages III and IV Hodgkin lymphoma. A standard treatment of advanced-stage favorable Hodgkin lymphoma is to administer two cycles of ABVD chemotherapy followed by a restaging PET-CT. If minimal disease is found (Deauville score 1-3), four additional courses of AVD should be given (total of six cycles). If

residual disease is suspected (Deauville score 4-5), a switch to escalated-BEACOPP for four cycles should be considered. Escalated-dose BEACOPP or A-AVD for six cycles should be considered for select patients with unfavorable disease. This risk-adapted approach should result in 70% to more than 90% of patients achieving a complete remission and 60% to 80% of patients being cured of their disease. No further treatment is needed for patients who achieve a complete remission (Deauville 1-2) with chemotherapy alone. Patients who achieve a partial remission (Deauville 3-5) should be considered for consolidative radiation to residual sites of disease. As with all stages and risk-groups of Hodgkin lymphoma, if a Deauville score of 5 remains after completion of initial chemotherapy, a biopsy is recommended to determine if refractory disease is present.

Nodular Lymphocyte-Predominant Hodgkin Lymphoma

Nodular lymphocyte-predominant Hodgkin lymphoma has been described as more indolent in nature, and has a better prognosis as compared with classical Hodgkin lymphoma. The use of radiation alone for stages I and II NLPHL patients who choose to omit chemotherapy or who cannot tolerate chemotherapy does not adversely affect survival.[18] The disadvantage of radiation therapy alone as compared with combination chemotherapy plus radiation is the higher relapse rate. Patients who relapse after radiation alone (20%-25%) can be successfully salvaged with chemotherapy. If the decision is made to use radiation alone, ISRT is the preferred method. Patients with advanced-stage disease can be treated with combined chemotherapy and radiation therapy. Historically, MOPP and MOPP/ABVD have been used, but these regimens have fallen out of favor much like classical Hodgkin lymphoma. ABVD is frequently used in these patients due to the available evidence to support its use for classical Hodgkin lymphoma, although other regimens, such as CHOP (cyclophosphamide, doxorubicin, vincristine, and prednisone), and CVP (cyclophosphamide, vincristine, and prednisone), have been studied. No randomized clinical trials of different chemotherapy regimens have been conducted in NLPHL. NLPHL reliably expresses CD20 and therefore rituximab has demonstrated efficacy in both newly diagnosed and progressive NLPHL. Several phase II trials have reported overall response rates of 90% to 100% with single-agent rituximab.[34,35] Current NCCN guidelines recommend that patients with stage IA or IIA nonbulky disease preferentially be treated with ISRT alone. In select patients with stage IA disease that was completely resected with the excisional biopsy, observation may be an option. Patients with IB, IIB, or advanced disease should receive chemotherapy with or without rituximab and with or without ISRT.[18]

4 Treatment of Refractory or Relapsed Disease

Refractory disease is defined as disease that persists following initial therapy, including any response less than a complete response. Relapsed disease suggests tumor recurrence following attainment of a complete response. Patients who experience relapsed disease less than 12 months after the completion of therapy have a poor prognosis. The goal of second-line or salvage therapy is still cure. With the increasing use of chemotherapy with or without radiation, regardless of disease extent, the rate of primary refractory disease is decreasing. Many therapeutic options are available for treatment of refractory or relapsed disease, so each patient's treatment should be personalized. The highest survival and cure rates are reported for patients with chemosensitive disease who are medically able to undergo high-dose therapy and autologous HSCT.[36] Since most patients are initially treated with ABVD, doxorubicin should be avoided in salvage chemotherapy regimens if the cumulative dose has reached between 300 and 400 mg/m^2, particularly in those patients who have received mediastinal radiotherapy, because of the higher risk of cardiotoxicity.

The response to salvage therapy depends on the extent and site of recurrence, previous therapy, and duration of initial remission. Patients who relapse after radiation therapy alone have a good chance of being cured with combination chemotherapy, although fewer patients are being treated with radiation alone. High response rates (60%-87%) have been reported with salvage chemotherapy regimens.[2,3] Other patient groups who have a favorable prognosis following salvage therapy include patients who experience a local recurrence in a nonirradiated location and those who relapse more than 1 year after completion of their initial chemotherapy. Patients who experience late relapses can be cured with retreatment with the same chemotherapy regimen, treatment with a different, potentially non–cross-resistant regimen, or high-dose chemotherapy and autologous HSCT.

Patients who have an early relapse (<1 year after treatment) generally respond poorly to standard-dose salvage chemotherapy. High-dose chemotherapy and autologous HSCT are more effective, but also produce a higher risk of treatment-related mortality. Therefore, the choice of salvage treatment should consider the patient's tolerance for a particular set of chemotherapeutic agents and treatment approach (standard-dose chemotherapy vs high-dose chemotherapy and autologous HSCT).

High-dose therapy should be considered in patients who relapse within 12 months of initial remission and in those who are refractory to first-line chemotherapy. Although no single preparative regimen is superior to another, most regimens do not include total-body irradiation because of its potential pulmonary toxicity. Most patients are already at higher risk for pulmonary toxicity because of previous exposure to one or more of the following: bleomycin, thoracic radiation, and nitrosoureas.

Brentuximab vedotin is effective in the relapsed or refractory setting. In a pivotal multicenter phase II study of 102 patients with relapsed or refractory Hodgkin lymphoma after HSCT, 75% and 34% of patients treated with brentuximab vedotin had an objective response and complete remission, respectively.[37] End-of-study results showed that response to brentuximab was durable; patients who achieved complete remission had an overall survival rate of 64% at 5 years and 26% remained in remission with no further anticancer therapy after receiving brentuximab.[38] Brentuximab vedotin has also been evaluated as posttransplant consolidation therapy in a phase III trial in 329 patients undergoing autologous HSCT. All patients had a high risk of relapse, defined as disease refractory to initial therapy or relapsed disease less than 12 months from completion of initial therapy with extranodal disease. Patients randomized to receive 16 cycles of brentuximab had significantly longer median progression-free survival (42.9 vs 24.1 months) as compared with placebo.[39] Common toxicities associated with brentuximab vedotin include neuropathy, neutropenia, nausea, and fatigue.[37] Based on these results, brentuximab vedotin received FDA approval for the treatment of classical Hodgkin lymphoma after failure of autologous HSCT or after failure of at least two prior multi-agent chemotherapy regimens in patients who are not candidates for autologous HSCT, and also for patients with classical Hodgkin lymphoma at high risk of relapse or progression as consolidation therapy after autologous HSCT.

Many single-agent and combination regimens can be used as salvage therapy. In this setting, the goal of therapy is disease control and cures are unlikely. Gemcitabine, vinorelbine, and pegylated liposomal doxorubicin (GVD), ifosfamide, carboplatin, and etoposide (ICE) and ifosfamide, gemcitabine, and vinorelbine are examples of chemotherapy regimens that include drugs with different mechanisms of action and toxicity profiles than regimens used earlier in therapy. Bendamustine, lenalidomide, and everolimus have shown activity in patients with refractory or relapsed Hodgkin lymphoma.

Immune checkpoint inhibitors, specifically PD-1 (programmed death 1 pathway) inhibitors, are treatment options in refractory

Hodgkin lymphoma. Promising results have been reported from phase II trials of heavily pretreated patients. One trial with single-agent nivolumab reported an objective response rate of 87%, with some complete responses; progression-free survival at 24 weeks was 86%.[40] In another phase II trial of nivolumab in 80 patients with classical Hodgkin lymphoma after failure to both HSCT and brentuximab (median of 4 previous therapies), objective responses were achieved in two-thirds of patients.[41] Pembrolizumab, another PD-1 inhibitor, has also been studied in patients with relapsed or refractory disease. In a trial of 31 heavily pretreated patients, a complete response rate of 16% and a partial remission rate of 48% were observed, and the 52-week progression-free survival rate was 46%.[42] A large phase II trial of 210 patients treated with pembrolizumab 200 mg IV every 3 weeks also reported an overall response rate of 69% and a complete response rate of 22%.[43] Based on these results, both nivolumab and pembrolizumab received FDA approval for relapsed Hodgkin lymphoma. Potentially severe graft-versus-host disease has been described in patients who received a checkpoint inhibitor following allogeneic HSCT.[44]

Long-Term Complications

A variety of acute and chronic toxicities may occur as a result of treatment for Hodgkin lymphoma. Long-term complications of radiation therapy, chemotherapy, and combined modality therapy have become more evident as the curability and long-term survival of Hodgkin lymphoma patients have improved.[2,3,18,45] Gonadal dysfunction (including sterility and hypothyroidism), secondary malignancies, and cardiopulmonary diseases are important considerations in the treatment of this malignancy. Almost all men and up to 50% of premenopausal women treated with six cycles of regimens containing alkylating agents become sterile. This is a dose-related phenomenon. For men, even a single dose of nitrogen mustard or chlorambucil can cause sterility, so if fertility is a major concern, ABVD is the best alternative.

The risk of secondary malignancies is increased about threefold in long-term survivors of Hodgkin lymphoma. The risk of developing leukemia carries the highest increase in risk and is seen with radiotherapy, chemotherapy, and chemoradiotherapy. Solid tumors, including breast cancers, gastrointestinal cancers, and lung cancers, are also likely to develop more than 10 years after the completion of treatment. A recently published British cohort study suggested that unlike radiotherapy, which may increase the occurrence of cancer at almost all anatomic sites, chemotherapy is associated with an increased risk of leukemia, NHL, and lung cancer. However, studies that evaluate the risk of secondary malignancies (and other complications) must be interpreted cautiously because many factors probably contribute to the development of secondary malignancies. In addition, much of the long-term complication data are derived from patients who were treated with older regimens and extensive field radiotherapy, which are no longer commonly used in clinical practice. As the field of cancer survivorship continues to grow, more specific recommendations for long-term follow-up are developed. Regular mammograms and breast MRI are recommended starting 10 years following the completion of therapy or at age 40 (whichever is earlier) for females. Patients are at increased risk of lung cancer if they have a smoking history, chest irradiation, and/or alkylating agent exposure. These patients should be considered for low-dose screening chest CT. For cardiovascular monitoring, annual blood pressure monitoring and aggressive management of cardiovascular risk factors are strongly encouraged. Hypothyroidism is reported in about 50% of long-term survivors who received irradiation to this area. Thyroid function tests should be performed annually. Monitoring and follow-up should be personalized after assessing a patient's risks for long-term complications.[18]

NON-HODGKIN LYMPHOMA

The NHLs are a heterogeneous group of lymphoproliferative disorders that affect individuals from early childhood to late adulthood. Advances in molecular biology techniques and our understanding of the human immune system have led to major progress in understanding the pathogenesis and treatment of lymphomas. NHLs are classified into distinct clinical entities defined by a combination of morphology, immunophenotype, genetic features, and clinical features. These differences influence the natural history, approach, and response to treatment. The use of extensive combination chemotherapeutic regimens shows dramatic improvement in survival and cure in patients with a disease that was once considered incurable. The 5-year survival rate for patients with NHL has increased from 48% to 73% over the past 30 years, and the mortality rate actually *declined* from 1997 to 2015.[1,4] Further improvement in survival is anticipated with the continued expansion of our therapeutic armamentarium, including high-dose chemotherapy and targeted therapy.

Epidemiology and Etiology

NHL is the fifth most common cause of newly diagnosed cancer in the United States and accounts for about 4% of all cancers. An estimated 80,470 new cases were diagnosed in 2022, and 20,250 people will die from NHL during this same period.[4] Although the average age of patients at the time of diagnosis is about 67 years, NHL can occur at any age. The incidence rate generally increases with age and is higher in men than in women and in white patients than in black patients.[4] The age-adjusted incidence rate of NHL increased by more than 80% in the United States since the early 1970s, from about 11 cases per 100,000 in 1975 to about 20 cases per 100,000 in 2011 and 2012.[1] The incidence of NHL increased by 3% to 4% from 1975 to 1991, but has finally begun to decline since reaching its peak in 1994. The increased incidence of NHL over the past three decades is second only to melanoma and has been referred to as an epidemic of NHL. Although the increase has been noted particularly among older adults and patients with acquired immune deficiency syndrome (AIDS), much of it cannot be explained by known risk factors.

The etiology of NHL is unknown, although several genetic diseases, environmental agents, and infectious agents are associated with the development of NHL. An increased incidence of NHL is seen in many congenital and acquired immunodeficiency states, supporting the role of immune dysregulation in the etiology of NHL. Patients with congenital immunodeficiency disorders such as Wiskott–Aldrich's syndrome and ataxia telangiectasia, acquired immunodeficiency disorders such as AIDS, and those receiving chronic pharmacologic immunosuppression in the setting of solid-organ transplantation are predisposed to the development of NHL. Autoimmune diseases (Hashimoto's thyroiditis and Sjögren's syndrome) cause chronic inflammation in the mucosa-associated lymphoid tissue (MALT), which predisposes patients to subsequent lymphoid malignancies. Other autoimmune diseases, such as systemic lupus erythematosus and rheumatoid arthritis, are also associated with the development of NHL, but the use of immunosuppressive agents in these diseases makes the pathologic cause less clear.

Certain infections are associated with the development of lymphoma. EBV was discovered in cell lines from tumors of patients with African (endemic) Burkitt lymphoma, and EBV DNA is associated with nearly all cases of endemic Burkitt lymphoma. However, EBV is associated with sporadic Burkitt lymphoma in 15% to 85% of cases. EBV is also associated with posttransplant lymphoproliferative disorders and some lymphomas in patients with AIDS or congenital immunodeficiencies. Extranodal NK-T cell lymphoma is also strongly associated with EBV infection. The nasal-type extranodal NK-T cell lymphoma is more common in East Asia, and less common in Central and South America than in other regions. The human T-cell lymphotropic virus type 1 was the first human retrovirus associated with malignancy. Infection with human T-cell lymphotropic virus type 1, especially in early childhood, is strongly associated with an aggressive form of T-cell lymphoma, known as adult T-cell leukemia/lymphoma. Human T-cell lymphotropic virus type 1 is endemic in parts of southern Japan, Africa, South America, and the Caribbean. In endemic areas, more than 50% of all NHL cases are adult T-cell leukemia/lymphoma. A third virus associated with NHL is human herpesvirus 8 (also referred to as Kaposi sarcoma–associated herpesvirus [KSHV]). This virus was originally isolated from Kaposi sarcoma lesions in AIDS patients. Gastric infection with *Helicobacter pylori*, a gram-negative bacteria that leads to chronic gastritis, is associated with gastric MALT lymphomas. Finally, hepatitis C virus has been associated with splenic and nodal marginal zone lymphomas.

Several physical agents are also associated with the development of NHL. Exposure to herbicides, particularly phenoxyl herbicides, is associated with the development of NHL. These observations may explain why certain occupations, such as farmers, forestry workers, and agricultural workers, are associated with a higher risk of NHL. Exposure to lawn-care pesticides is also increasing in the general population. A higher risk of NHL is also associated with exposure to other chemical solvents and dyes, exposure to radiation from nuclear explosions, and high intake of meats and dietary fats. Smoking or alcohol consumption is not strongly associated with an increased risk of NHL.

Molecular Abnormalities

Chromosomal translocations are a hallmark of many lymphoid malignancies.[46] The presence of these specific translocations can be helpful in the diagnosis and classification of lymphoid malignancies. The mechanisms leading to the translocations are unknown, but they usually involve the antigen receptor loci. In contrast to most myeloid and some lymphoid leukemias, NHLs usually place a structurally intact cellular proto-oncogene under the regulatory influence of highly expressed immunoglobulin or T-cell receptor genes, leading to effects on cell growth, cellular differentiation, or apoptosis. The most common chromosomal translocations involve t(8;14), t(14;18), and t(11;14); each translocation involves the immunoglobulin heavy-chain gene locus on chromosome 14 at 14q32. The translocation t(8;14) that involves c-*MYC*, a well-characterized oncogene associated with malignancy, is implicated in nearly all cases of Burkitt lymphoma. The translocation t(14;18) that involves *BCL*-2, one of several putative B-cell lymphoma-associated oncogenes, is found in about 90% of cases of follicular B-cell lymphomas. The translocation t(11;14) that involves *BCL*-1 is found in about 70% of patients with mantle cell lymphoma (MCL). Another putative B-cell lymphoma-associated oncogene, *BCL*-6, is found in about one-third of diffuse large B-cell lymphomas (DLBCLs).

Although mutations in the *p53* tumor suppressor gene are found in many human neoplasms, such mutations have not been consistently found in patients with lymphoma, which suggests that it may occur late in malignant evolution. Because of their role in the pathogenesis of lymphoma, oncogenes are attractive molecular targets for new and novel therapies.

Pathology and Classification

NHLs are neoplasms derived from the monoclonal proliferation of malignant B or T lymphocytes and their precursors. About 85% to 90% of NHLs in the United States are of B-cell origin. Proliferation of malignant cells replaces the normal cells and architecture of lymph nodes or bone marrow with a relatively uniform population of lymphoid cells. The current classification schemes characterize the NHLs according to the cell of origin (B cell vs T cell), clinical features, and morphologic features. Additional immunohistochemical markers, cytogenetic features, and genotypic characteristics may further classify NHL into subtypes.

5 The 2016 WHO classification categorizes lymphoid malignancies into two major categories: B-cell lymphomas and T-cell (and natural killer cell) lymphomas (see Table 155-1).[47] B-cell lymphomas represent about 85% to 90% of all NHLs. Lymphomas within each category can be divided into malignancies of precursor or mature cells. Hodgkin lymphoma and multiple myeloma are recognized as mature B-cell neoplasms. The WHO classification uses the term *grade* to refer to histologic parameters such as cell and nuclear size, density of chromatin, and proliferation fraction, and the term *aggressiveness* to denote clinical behavior of a tumor. This classification scheme includes both lymphomas and lymphoid leukemias, because there is no distinction between the solid and circulating forms of these diseases. The WHO classification includes several previously unrecognized types of lymphomas, and new entities not specifically recognized in the Working Formulation account for about 20% to 25% of the cases.

The WHO classification has broad clinical implications. The WHO Clinical Advisory Committee has agreed that clinical groupings of lymphoid neoplasms into prognostic categories are neither necessary nor desirable because such arbitrary groupings are of no practical value and may be misleading.[48]

Clinical Presentation

6 Patients with NHL present with a wide variety of symptoms, depending on the site of involvement and whether tumor involvement is nodal or extranodal. Sites of involvement and dissemination of the malignant cells can sometimes be predicted based on the cell of origin and the tendency of tumors to frequently disseminate to areas where the normal counterparts of the lymphoma cells are located. For example, B-cell lymphomas involve areas of the lymphoid system normally populated by B-lymphocytes such as lymph nodes, spleen, and bone marrow. T-cell lymphomas commonly disseminate to various extranodal sites such as the skin and lungs.[46]

Most patients present with peripheral lymphadenopathy. The lymphadenopathy may be either localized or generalized, and the involved nodes are often painless, rubbery, and discrete, and usually located in the cervical and supraclavicular regions as in Hodgkin lymphoma (see Fig. 155-1). Rapid and progressive lymphadenopathy is more characteristic of aggressive lymphomas. Waxing and waning of lymph nodes, including their complete disappearance and reappearance, is more characteristic of indolent lymphomas. Massive lymphadenopathy can sometimes lead to organ dysfunction. For example, patients with NHL may present with acute renal failure from retroperitoneal adenopathy causing ureteral obstruction or from metabolic abnormalities such as hyperuricemia with uric acid nephropathy.

About 40% of patients with NHL present with fever (temperature >38°C [100.4°F]), weight loss (unexplained weight loss of 10% of body weight over the past 6 months), or night sweats (drenching night sweats). If one or more of these symptoms are present, the patient is noted to have B symptoms, and a B is added to the stage of disease (discussed in the section "Diagnosis, Staging, and Prognostic Factors" under Hodgkin Lymphoma earlier in this chapter). B symptoms are more commonly observed in patients with aggressive NHLs.

Patients with Hodgkin lymphoma rarely present with extranodal (ie, extralymphatic) disease, but 10% to 35% of patients with NHL have primary extranodal disease at the time of diagnosis. The frequency of extranodal presentation varies dramatically among different subtypes. The most common extranodal sites are the gastrointestinal tract followed by the skin. The liver or spleen may be

CLINICAL PRESENTATION Non-Hodgkin Lymphoma

General

- Patients with NHL present with a wide variety of symptoms, depending on the site of involvement and whether tumor involvement is nodal or extranodal.

Symptoms

- About 40% of patients present with fever, night sweats, and weight loss (ie, B symptoms).
- Fatigue, malaise, and pruritus.

Signs

- More than two-thirds of patients present with peripheral lymphadenopathy.

Laboratory Tests

- A complete blood count, tests of renal and liver function, and serum electrolytes should be obtained.
- Serum β_2-microglobulin and LDH levels may be useful as prognostic factors and for monitoring response to therapy.

Other Diagnostic Tests

- Varies depending on the sites of involvement.

enlarged in patients with generalized adenopathy. Patients with mesenteric or gastrointestinal involvement may present with signs and symptoms of nausea, vomiting, obstruction, abdominal pain, a palpable abdominal mass, or gastrointestinal bleeding. Patients with bone marrow involvement may have symptoms related to anemia, neutropenia, or thrombocytopenia. Other sites of extranodal disease include the testes and bone. The incidence of solitary brain lymphoma is increasing, especially in patients with AIDS.

Diagnosis, Staging, and Prognostic Factors

As with Hodgkin lymphoma, the diagnosis of NHL must be established by pathologic review of tissue obtained by biopsy.[46,49,50] The preferred procedure is an excisional biopsy, where the entire involved lymph node is removed for review by an experienced hematopathologist. This procedure should be done carefully to prevent distortional artifact of the architecture, which could lead to an inaccurate diagnosis. Needle biopsy of the node can sometimes provide adequate tissue for pathologic diagnosis if an excisional biopsy cannot be performed. When adenopathy is not present, diagnosis may be established by biopsy of cutaneous lesions, bone marrow biopsy and aspiration in patients with unexplained myelosuppression, liver biopsy in patients with hepatomegaly or elevated liver function tests, or biopsy of involved extranodal organs such as bone, Waldeyer's ring, lung, and testis.

After the diagnosis is established, further workup is required to determine the extent of involvement.[46,49,50] Clinical staging always begins with a thorough history and physical examination. Patients should be questioned about the presence or absence and extent of fever, night sweats, and weight loss. A detailed history of lymphadenopathy should also be obtained, including when and where the lymph nodes were first noted, and their rate of growth. A complete physical examination is performed to assess the extent of disease involvement, with special attention given to all nodal areas (see Fig. 155-1). All patients should have a complete blood count, serum chemistries including liver and renal profiles. Lumbar puncture to evaluate the cerebrospinal fluid is recommended in patients who have histologic types of lymphoma that often spread to the CNS.

Imaging studies are important in the staging workup. In the most recent recommendations, PET-CT is the gold standard for assessment of essentially all lymphoma histologies, except chronic lymphocytic leukemia/small lymphocytic lymphoma, lymphoplasmacytic lymphoma/Waldenstrom's macroglobulinemia, mycosis fungoides, and marginal zone NHLs, unless there is a suspicion of aggressive transformation.[50] The total metabolic tumor volume at diagnosis may play a prognostic role.[51] Magnetic resonance imaging is of limited usefulness in the staging of NHL. Gallium scans are sometimes used as part of the staging workup. Other tests, such as liver-spleen scan, bone scan, upper gastrointestinal series, and IV pyelogram, are sometimes useful in patients with organ symptomatology or serum chemistry abnormalities.

The likelihood of bone marrow involvement varies among the different histologic types of lymphoma (Table 155-6). In the NCCN guidelines, bone marrow biopsy with or without aspirate is included in the essential workup for all lymphomas. Although PET-CT scans are as sensitive as bone marrow biopsy in the identification of bone marrow involvement in certain subtypes of NHL including DLBCL, bone marrow biopsy remains preferable for identifying bone marrow involvement in indolent lymphomas such as follicular lymphoma.

The Ann Arbor staging classification developed for the clinical staging of Hodgkin lymphoma is also used to stage patients with NHL (see Table 155-2). After completion of the staging workup, most patients will be found to have advanced disease (stages III and IV). The frequency of localized disease at the time of diagnosis varies depending on the histologic type of lymphoma (see Table 155-5). Stage is a more important prognostic factor in Hodgkin lymphoma than in NHL.

7 The Ann Arbor system emphasizes the distribution of nodal disease sites because Hodgkin lymphoma usually spreads through contiguous lymph nodes and does not involve extranodal sites. But NHL is a disease with tremendous heterogeneity that does not spread through contiguous lymph nodes and often involves extranodal sites. As a result of these clinical differences between Hodgkin lymphoma and NHL, Ann Arbor stage correlates poorly with prognosis.

8 This lack of accuracy with the Ann Arbor staging system in NHL has led to several international projects to develop prognostic models for the most common types of NHLs—DLBCLs and follicular lymphomas. The International Non-Hodgkin Lymphoma Prognostic Factors Project was based on more than 2,000 patients with diffuse aggressive lymphomas treated with an anthracycline-containing combination chemotherapy regimen in the United States, Europe, and Canada.[52] The Project identified five risk factors that correlated with low complete response rate to chemotherapy and poor survival, and a subgroup analysis found three specific risk factors correlated with low complete response rate to chemotherapy

TABLE 155-5 Clinical Characteristics of Patients with Common Types of Non-Hodgkin Lymphomas

Disease	Median Age (Years)	Frequency in Children	% Male	Stage I/II vs III/IV (%)	B Symptoms (%)	BM Involvement (%)	GI Tract Involvement (%)	5 Year Survival (%)
B-cell chronic lymphocytic leukemia/small lymphocytic lymphoma	65	Rare	53	9 vs 91	33	72	3	51
Mantle cell lymphoma	63	Rare	74	20 vs 80	28	64	9	27
Extranodal marginal zone B-cell lymphoma of MALT type	60	Rare	48	67 vs 33	19	14	50	74
Follicular lymphoma	59	Rare	42	33 vs 67	28	42	4	72
Diffuse large B-cell lymphoma	64	≈25% of childhood NHL	55	54 vs 46	33	16	18	46
Burkitt lymphoma	31	≈30% of childhood NHL	89	62 vs 38	22	33	11	45
Precursor T-cell lymphoblastic lymphoma	28	≈40% of childhood NHL	64	11 vs 89	21	50	4	26
Anaplastic large T-/null cell lymphoma	34	Common	69	51 vs 49	53	13	9	77
Peripheral T-cell non-Hodgkin lymphoma	61	≈5% of childhood NHL	55	20 vs 80	50	36	15	25

BM, bone marrow; GI, gastrointestinal; MALT, mucosa-associated lymphoid tissue; NHL, non-Hodgkin lymphoma.

Reproduced with permission from Longo DL. Malignancies of lymphoid cells. In: Kasper D, Fauci A, Hauser S, Longo D, Jameson J, Loscalzo J, eds. Harrison's Principles of Internal Medicine. 19th ed. New York, NY: McGraw-Hill; 2015.

TABLE 155-6 Risk Factors According to the International Non-Hodgkin Lymphoma Prognostic Factors Project

All Patients	Patients ≤60 Years of Age
Age >60 years	Abnormal LDH level
Abnormal LDH level	Performance status ≥2
Performance status ≥2	Ann Arbor stage III or IV
Ann Arbor stage III or IV	
Extranodal involvement ≥2 sites	

LDH, lactic dehydrogenase.
Data from Reference 52.

and poor survival in patients 60 years old and above (Table 155-6). It is unclear whether the effect of serum LDH level is related to a tumor or a host event. LDH likely measures cellular catabolism (the enzyme is released from injured cells) or the product of tumor burden and proliferation. Because each of the factors has about the same impact (eg, relative risk) on prognosis, the number of adverse risk factors is summed to provide the IPI. Patients could therefore have a score of 0 to 5. For patients older than or equal to 60 years, a simplified IPI score can be determined based on Ann Arbor stage, serum LDH level, and performance status.

It is important to periodically reevaluate prognostic factors as prognosis improves as a result of more effective therapy. The IPI was based on patients treated from 1982 to 1987 with anthracycline-based combination chemotherapy; none of the patients received rituximab. Therefore, an enhanced IPI (NCCN-IPI) was developed to stratify newly diagnosed DLBCL patients based on their clinical features (age, normalized LDH, sites of involvement, Ann Arbor, and ECOG performance status) in the rituximab era.[53] Through an independent validation, the NCCN-IPI was shown to discriminate patients in the low- and high-risk subgroups better than the IPI.

Although the IPI is often used to predict prognosis in patients with other NHL subtypes, the IPI has several shortcomings when applied to patients with indolent lymphomas. Because only patients with diffuse aggressive lymphomas were used to develop the IPI system, some important prognostic factors may have been missed. Furthermore, the IPI system has limited discriminating power in follicular lymphoma because only about 10% of patients are categorized as high-risk in the IPI system. To address these concerns, an international cooperative study was designed to develop a prognostic model similar to the IPI in patients with follicular lymphoma. The results of that study, which was based on more than 4,000 patients with follicular lymphoma diagnosed between 1985 and 1992, identified five factors that correlated with poor survival (Table 155-8).[54] Analogous to the IPI, the number of adverse risk factors is summed to provide the Follicular Lymphoma International Prognostic Index (FLIPI). FLIPI had higher discriminating power among groups as compared with the IPI system. Table 155-8 shows the number of risk factors stratified with FLIPI. The survival data from FLIPI, however, may not reflect current treatment results because none of the patients in the cohort used to derive the FLIPI were treated with rituximab. In an updated prognostic model (FLIPI-2) derived from patients with newly diagnosed follicular lymphoma treated with rituximab-containing chemoimmunotherapy regimens, age older than 60 years, low hemoglobin level (<12 g/dL [120 g/L; 7.45 mmol/L]), longest diameter of the largest lymph node more than 6 cm, abnormal β_2-microglobulin levels and bone marrow involvement were identified as adverse risk factors. FLIPI-2 was highly predictive of treatment outcomes and separated patients into three distinct risk groups: low-risk (0 factors), intermediate-risk (1 or 2 factors), and high-risk (≥3 factors). Three-year progression-free survival was 91%, 69%, and 51%, and overall survival was 99%, 96%, and 84% in low-, intermediate-, and high-risk patients, respectively.[55]

Although IPI and FLIPI are clinically useful tools to estimate prognosis, the factors used to calculate these scores probably represent clinical surrogates for the biologic heterogeneity among NHLs and many researchers are interested in determining the prognostic importance of certain phenotypic and molecular characteristics of NHLs. For example, molecular markers of apoptosis, cell-cycle regulation, cell lineage, and cell proliferation are being evaluated as potential prognostic factors.[56]

Gene expression profiling with microarrays may also correlate with survival. Using gene expression profiling, investigators identified at least two molecularly distinct types of DLBCLs based on gene expression patterns indicative of different stages of B-cell differentiation: germinal center B-cell–like (GCB) and activated B-cell–like (ABC), with 10% to 15% being unclassifiable.[56,57] The GCB subtype of DLBCL probably arises from normal germinal center B-cells while the ABC subtype may arise from postgerminal center B-cells. Many oncogenic pathways are different for the GCB and ABC subtypes, and these differences may lead to the development of targeted therapies for each subtype.[56] Patients with the germinal center B-cell profile had significantly better overall survival independent of IPI score after treatment with cyclophosphamide, doxorubicin [hydroxydaunorubicin], vincristine (Oncovin®), prednisone (CHOP), or CHOP-like chemotherapy. In a published study of patients with DLBCL treated with either CHOP or rituximab and CHOP (R-CHOP), Lenz et al. identified several gene expressions signatures that predicted survival in both CHOP and R-CHOP cohorts: GCB, stromal-1, and stromal-2.[58] The GCB and stromal-1 signatures were associated with a favorable prognosis while the stromal-2 signature was associated with an unfavorable prognosis. The stromal-1 signature reflects extracellular matrix deposition and histiocytic infiltration, whereas the stromal-2 signature reflects tumor blood vessel density. It is speculated that DLBCLs that express the stromal-2 signature may respond to antiangiogenic agents.

Another important but rare molecular subtype is double-hit NHL, which is now classified by WHO as high-grade B cell lymphoma with MYC gene arrangement and BCL2 or BCL6 translocation. If all three are rearranged, it is referred to as triple-hit NHL. Patients with double-hit or triple-hit NHL have a poor prognosis, with a median overall survival that is 4 to 6 months even with highly aggressive chemotherapy.[59] Some lymphoma experts suggest that patients with double-hit NHL should be treated with more dose-intensive regimens.[56] Besides double-hit NHL, a more common molecular subtype is double-expressor NHL, accounting for 20% to 30% of DLBCL cases. Unlike double-hit NHL, patients with double-expressor lymphoma co-express MYC and BCL2 proteins without underlying chromosomal rearrangements. Double-expressor NHL is associated with a worse prognosis than other DLBCLs, but it has slightly better outcomes than double-hit NHLs. More intensive treatment regimens are also being evaluated in patients with double-expressor NHL.[60]

Two molecularly distinct profiles of follicular lymphoma have been identified. The first includes genes encoding for T-cell markers and genes highly expressed in macrophages, and the second includes genes that are preferentially expressed in macrophages, dendritic cells, or both.[61] Patients with the first molecular signature have a more favorable outcome than those with the second signature. These results suggest that molecular classification of NHL based on gene expression may allow the identification of clinically significant subtypes.

TREATMENT: NON-HODGKIN LYMPHOMA

Desired Outcomes

The primary goals in the treatment of NHL are to relieve symptoms, cure the patient of the disease whenever possible, and minimize the risk of serious toxicities. The treatment strategy depends on many factors, including the patient's age, concomitant disease, disease type, stage of disease, site of disease, and patient preference.

General Approach

9 Historically, the clinical behavior and degree of aggressiveness are used to describe NHLs. Indolent lymphomas, which make up about 25% to 40% of all NHLs, are characterized by their slow-growth behavior. Patients with indolent lymphoma usually have a relatively long survival (measured in years), with or without aggressive chemotherapy. Although these lymphomas respond to a wide range of therapeutic approaches, there is no convincing evidence of a survival plateau, which indicates that patients are rarely cured of their disease. In contrast, aggressive lymphomas, which make up about 60% to 75% of all NHLs, are characterized by rapid growth rate and short survival (measured in weeks to months) if appropriate therapy is not initiated. Despite their more aggressive nature, many patients with aggressive lymphomas who respond to chemotherapy can experience prolonged disease-free survival and some are cured of their disease. Therefore, the terminology for the NHLs represents a paradox, where "indolent" is bad and "aggressive" is good in terms of the likelihood of cure.

Therapeutic approaches to NHL include radiation therapy, chemotherapy, and biologic or targeted agents. The role of radiation therapy in the treatment of NHL differs from its role in the treatment of Hodgkin lymphoma. Although the disease responds to radiation therapy, only a small percentage of patients with NHL present with truly localized disease that can be treated with local or regional radiation therapy. Radiation therapy is used more commonly in advanced disease, primarily as a palliative measure to control local bulky disease.

Effective chemotherapy for NHL ranges from single-agent therapy in indolent lymphomas to aggressive, complex chemotherapy regimens in aggressive lymphomas. The most active agents used in the treatment of NHL include the alkylating agents (eg, cyclophosphamide, chlorambucil), bleomycin, doxorubicin, purine analogs, etoposide, methotrexate, vincristine, and corticosteroids (eg, prednisone, dexamethasone). The most aggressive chemotherapy approaches are dose-dense chemotherapy or high-dose chemotherapy followed by autologous or allogeneic HSCT.

B-cell lymphomas have served as a model for immunotherapy with monoclonal antibodies for more than 20 years, beginning with the successful use of custom-made monoclonal antibodies targeted against the idiotype present on the patient's cancer cells.[62] These encouraging results lead to the development of monoclonal antibodies against a more generic target, a molecule on the surface of B cells that would be present on tumor cells. One potential target, the CD20 molecule, is present only on cells in the B-lymphocyte lineage. It is expressed on the surface of both normal and malignant B cells, but not on other normal tissues. Rituximab (Rituxan®) is a chimeric monoclonal antibody directed at the CD20 molecule. Its antitumor activity is mediated through complement-dependent cytotoxicity, antibody-dependent cytotoxicity, and induction of apoptosis.[62] With the availability of monoclonal antibodies and radioimmunoconjugates for the therapy of lymphoma, nearly all patients with NHL will receive one or more biologic agents during the course of their disease.

Objective response to therapy for NHL should be defined according to the Lugano classification. The Lugano classification

TABLE 155-7 Risk Factors According to the Follicular Lymphoma International Prognostic Index

All Patients	
Age >60 years	
Ann Arbor stage III or IV	
Number of nodal sites ≥5	
Abnormal lactate dehydrogenase level	
Hemoglobin <12 g/dL (120 g/L; 7.45 mmol/L)	
Risk Group (% of Patients)	**Number of Risk Factors**
Low (36)	0-1
Intermediate (37)	2
High (27)	≥3

was established at the 12th International Conference on Malignant Lymphoma 2013. The revised guidelines describe criteria for response (eg, complete response, partial response, and stable disease) and emphasize the role of PET-CT and CT in the assessment of response in lymphoma treatment. PET-CT is recommended in FDG-avid histologies such as Hodgkin lymphoma, DLBCL, and follicular lymphoma while CT is advised for other lymphomas with low or variable FDG-avidity.[50]

Appropriate therapy for NHL depends on the patient's age, histologic type, stage of disease, site of disease, presence of adverse prognostic factors (as measured by IPI or FLIPI score), and patient preferences. In general, treatment of lymphoma can be divided into limited disease and advanced disease. Limited disease includes those patients with localized disease (Ann Arbor stages I and II). Advanced disease is defined as all Ann Arbor stage III or IV patients, and also frequently includes Ann Arbor stage II patients with poor prognostic features (see Tables 155-6 and 155-7).[52,54]

The following section discusses the clinical characteristics and therapy of the most common disease entities.

Follicular Lymphomas

The combined group of follicular lymphomas makes up the second most common histologic type of NHL in the United States, comprising about 20% to 25% of all new NHLs diagnosed in western countries.[61] The WHO classification includes criteria for grading follicular lymphoma based on the number of centroblasts per high-power field: grade 1 to 2 (0-15 centroblasts/high-power field) and grade 3 (>15 centroblasts/high-power field).[5] The clinical behavior and treatment outcome of grades 1 and 2 follicular lymphoma are similar, and they are usually treated as indolent lymphomas. The current WHO classification subdivides grade 3 follicular lymphoma into grades 3A and 3B. The WHO recommends that grade 3A follicular lymphoma should be treated in the same way as low-grade follicular lymphoma, whereas grade 3B should be treated in the same way as an aggressive lymphoma.

Follicular lymphomas tend to occur in older adults, with a slight female predominance (see Table 155-5). Most patients have advanced disease at diagnosis, but about 25% to 33% of patients have localized disease (clinical stage I or II) at diagnosis.[63] Extranodal disease, bulky disease, and B symptoms are uncommon features at diagnosis. Most patients with follicular lymphoma have chromosomal translocation t(14;18) at the time of diagnosis.

The clinical course is generally indolent, with median survivals of 8 to 10 years. But the natural history of follicular lymphoma can be unpredictable. Spontaneous regression of objective disease has been noted in as many as 20% to 30% of patients. There is also a high conversion rate of follicular lymphoma to a more aggressive histology over time that steadily increases after diagnosis and reaches about 30% at 10 years.[64] At autopsy, most patients with follicular lymphoma have some evidence of DLBCL. Patients with transformed indolent lymphoma should be treated in the same way as patients with an aggressive lymphoma.

Most patients have dramatic responses to initial therapy, and their disease course is characterized by multiple relapses, with responses to salvage therapy becoming progressively shorter after every relapse, eventually leading to death from disease-related causes. This pattern of constant relapses over time without evidence of a survival plateau and the failure of randomized controlled trials to show a survival benefit with aggressive chemotherapy led to the conclusion that therapy does not prolong overall survival or cure patients of their disease. However, the use of biologic agents, particularly rituximab, has changed the natural history of follicular lymphoma. In a study of patients enrolled in Southwest Oncology Group (SWOG) trials over more than 20 years, patients treated with CHOP and a monoclonal antibody had a significantly longer 4-year overall survival than those treated with CHOP alone (91% vs 69%).[65] With advances in therapeutics, the life expectancy of patients with follicular lymphoma has correspondingly increased. However, lymphoma is still the leading cause of death among patients diagnosed with follicular lymphoma in the rituximab era, especially among those patients experiencing disease transformation.[66]

Certain subsets of patients with follicular lymphoma have a much better or worse prognosis. The natural history of follicular large cell lymphoma (ie, grade 3 follicular lymphoma) is similar to that of other aggressive lymphomas and that treatment with intensive combination chemotherapy regimens may result in long-term disease-free survival, including a possible plateau in the survival curve.[67] The recent development of the FLIPI prognostic model should help clinicians to identify patients in different prognostic groups based on disease characteristics at the time of diagnosis.[54] Patients who are predicted to have a poor prognosis (ie, high-risk) could then be offered aggressive or experimental therapy, while those who are predicted to have a good prognosis (ie, low-risk) would be treated with standard therapy, avoiding unnecessary toxicity.

Treatment of Localized Disease (Stages I and II)

Radiation therapy is the standard treatment for early-stage follicular lymphoma. Involved-field, extended-field, and total nodal irradiation have been used. Carefully staged patients with either stage I or contiguous stage II disease treated with radiation therapy alone can achieve disease-free survival rates of 40% to 50% and overall survival rates of 60% to 70% at 10 years.[67] Late relapses are uncommon; only 10% of patients who reached 10 years without relapse subsequently experienced a recurrence.

Chemotherapy is not usually given in most patients with localized follicular lymphoma, but it may be helpful in some patients with high-risk stage II disease (eg, multiple sites of involvement or bulky disease).[68]

10 About 40% to 60% of patients with clinical stage I or II follicular lymphoma are cured of their disease with radiation therapy alone.[49] Most centers use radiation at a dose of 30 to 40 Gy (3,000-4,000 rad) to either involved (ie, local) or regional fields, which would consist of irradiation to the involved nodal region plus one additional uninvolved region on each side of the involved nodes. Extended-field irradiation is not usually used because of the absence of a survival benefit and possible increased risk of secondary malignancies. In addition, previous use of extended-field irradiation compromises the ability of that patient to receive subsequent chemotherapy. The current NCCN guideline states that locoregional radiation therapy is preferred for most patients with early-stage follicular lymphoma.[49] Anti-CD20 antibodies, in combination with chemotherapy, are also listed as an option.

Treatment of Advanced Disease (Stages II Bulky, III, and IV)

The management of stages II Bulky, III, and IV indolent lymphomas remains controversial because until recently, no therapeutic approaches had been shown to prolong overall survival despite the high complete remission rates to initial therapy. More than 80% of patients with stage III or IV follicular lymphoma are alive at 5 years, and the median survival ranges between 7 and 10 years.

Although complete remission can be achieved in 50% to 80% of patients with various treatments, the median time to relapse is usually only 18 to 36 months. About 20% of patients who have a complete response remain in remission for longer than 10 years. After relapse, patients are retreated and high remission rates can be achieved. Unfortunately, response rates and duration of response decrease with each retreatment.

Several different approaches can be used to treat follicular lymphoma. Carefully selected patients may receive no initial therapy followed by chemoimmunotherapy or single-agent anti-CD20 therapy, or radiation therapy when treatment is needed. Candidates for the conservative approach are usually older, asymptomatic, and have minimal tumor burden. Patients with symptoms, extensive extranodal involvement, bulky disease, cytopenia due to bone marrow involvement, splenomegaly and steady progression over at least 6 months, or impaired end-organ function at the time of diagnosis are not candidates for conservative treatment. Patients who respond to induction therapy may receive maintenance therapy with single-agent anti-CD20 therapy.

At the time of relapse, many of the same treatment options are available, and the following factors must be considered: age, symptomatic status of the patient, tumor burden, rate of regrowth (based on previous assessment of active disease sites), presence or absence of characteristics suggesting transformation or biologic progression, prior therapy, degree and duration of response to prior therapy, availability of clinical trials, and patient preferences.[49]

Watch-and-Wait Because there are no convincing data that standard treatment approaches have improved survival, some clinicians have adopted a "watch-and-wait" approach for asymptomatic patients where therapy is delayed until the patient experiences systemic symptoms or disease progression such as rapidly progressive or bulky adenopathy, anemia, thrombocytopenia, or disease in threatening sites such as the orbit or spinal cord.[68] In a randomized study of asymptomatic patients with indolent lymphomas (mostly follicular), patients who underwent watchful waiting had similar cause-specific and overall survival as compared with those who received immediate chlorambucil.[69] With a median length of follow-up of 16 years, about 17% of patients who were randomized to the watchful waiting group died of other causes without receiving chemotherapy and an additional 9% are alive and have not yet had chemotherapy. Due to the frequent use of rituximab in current clinical practice, a recent study has evaluated whether the use of the "watch-and-wait" approach is more effective than the use of rituximab to delay the need for chemotherapy or radiotherapy in patients with advanced-stage, low tumor burden follicular lymphoma. Immediate treatment with rituximab significantly delays disease progression and the time until chemotherapy or radiotherapy compared with a watchful waiting approach.[69] However, an overall survival advantage has not been demonstrated with this approach.

As described above, patients with follicular lymphoma who are followed without therapy sometimes have spontaneous regressions that can be complete while the disease in other patients can convert to a more aggressive histology. Current guidelines suggest that "watch and wait" is an acceptable initial management approach for patients with low-grade follicular lymphoma who are asymptomatic; have no threatened end-organ function, cytopenias secondary to lymphoma, or bulky disease; and in whom the disease is not steadily progressing. If the watchful waiting approach is chosen, the patient should be evaluated at least every 3 to 6 months for 5 years and then annually, so that intervention can occur before serious problems occur.[49]

Single-Agent Rituximab The approval of rituximab is arguably the most important development in the treatment of NHL. Its initial approval in 1997 was based on an open-label multicenter study that enrolled 166 patients with relapsed or recurrent indolent lymphoma.[70] Rituximab, given IV at a dose of 375 mg/m^2 weekly for 4 weeks, resulted in an overall response of 48% (complete response: 6%, partial response: 42%). The median time to progression for responders was 13.2 months and the median duration of response was 11.6 months. Other studies of single-agent rituximab in patients with relapsed or refractory indolent NHL have reported overall response rates of 40% to 60% and complete response rates of 5% to 10%.[71]

Based on the activity of rituximab in relapsed or refractory patients, it is currently being used as first-line therapy, either alone or in combination with chemotherapy.[71] When given as a single agent to patients with previously untreated indolent NHL, the overall response rate is 60% to 70% and the complete response rate is 20% to 30%. It is interesting to note that many of these patients remain in molecular remission (ie, polymerase chain reaction—negative) at 12 months. Single-agent rituximab is listed as an acceptable option for first-line therapy of follicular lymphoma, particularly for patients who cannot tolerate more intensive chemotherapy regimens.[49]

In patients who respond to rituximab, either alone or combined with chemotherapy, maintenance therapy with single-agent rituximab is often given to prolong the duration of remission. Rituximab is FDA-approved as single-agent maintenance therapy in patients achieving a complete or partial response following induction chemotherapy. The FDA approval was based on a randomized controlled trial in previously untreated patients with advanced-stage follicular lymphoma treated with maintenance rituximab after CVP chemotherapy.[72] After a median follow-up of 11.5 years in the E1496 study, patients with indolent lymphoma receiving maintenance rituximab had longer median progression-free survival than patients on observation (4.8 vs 1.3 years). However, no significant difference in 10-year overall survival between maintenance rituximab and the observation group was observed (67% vs 59%).[73] Maintenance rituximab is expensive and may be associated with serious adverse drug reactions, including an increased risk of grades 3 or 4 infections. The NCCN guideline lists maintenance therapy with rituximab (one dose every 8 weeks for up to 2 years) as an option following first-line therapy for patients initially presenting with a high tumor burden.[49]

Rituximab maintenance following second-line therapy has also been evaluated in patients with relapsed or refractory disease. Two randomized trials have demonstrated a progression-free survival advantage with rituximab maintenance over observation for patients treated with induction chemotherapy.[74,75] Patients who develop progressive disease during or within 6 months of first-line maintenance rituximab will likely experience little, if any, benefit from maintenance therapy in the second-line setting. The NCCN guideline recommends optional maintenance therapy with rituximab (one dose every 12 weeks for 2 years) for patients who are in remission after second-line therapy.[49]

Most of the adverse drug reactions of rituximab are infusion-related, particularly after the first intravenous infusion, and consist of fever, chills, respiratory symptoms, fatigue, headache, pruritus, and angioedema. Premedication with oral acetaminophen 650 mg and diphenhydramine 50 mg is usually given 30 minutes before rituximab infusion. Duration of infusions may take up to 5 hours. The package insert recommends a step-up infusion rate of rituximab to decrease the risk of infusion-related events. The FDA has approved rapid infusions of rituximab, but they are not recommended in patients with clinically significant cardiovascular disease and high circulating lymphocyte counts (>5,000 cells/mm^3 [5 × 10^9/L]). Reactivation of hepatitis B has been reported in patients receiving chemotherapy, either alone or combined with rituximab. Hepatitis B testing is recommended in patients who are considering rituximab therapy.[49]

In addition to the intravenous formulation of rituximab, a subcutaneous formulation of rituximab was approved. In this formulation, rituximab is combined with recombinant human hyaluronidase, which allows rituximab to be rapidly dispersed and absorbed after subcutaneous administration. Subcutaneous administration shortens the administration time to 5 to 7 minutes as compared to several hours for the intravenous infusion. FDA approval for the subcutaneous rituximab was based on multiple randomized clinical trials that demonstrated non-inferior rituximab blood concentrations and comparable efficacy and safety for the two formulations.[76,77] Premedication with acetaminophen and antihistamine is still required before each dose of subcutaneous rituximab, and subcutaneous administration should only be considered after patients receive at least one full dose of a rituximab product by intravenous infusion with no severe adverse drug reactions.

Chemoimmunotherapy Patients with high tumor burden or with disease-related symptoms are typically treated with chemoimmunotherapy, with or without maintenance therapy with an anti-CD20 monoclonal antibody. The rationale for the use of rituximab in combination with conventional agents is based on the clinical activity of both agents/regimens, non–cross-resistant mechanisms of action, non-overlapping toxicities, and synergistic antitumor activity in vitro. In a meta-analysis of randomized controlled trials, patients with indolent lymphoma treated with rituximab and chemotherapy had a significantly higher overall response rate and reduced risk of treatment failure and death.[78] Currently, the most widely used front-line regimen is R-CHOP or bendamustine plus rituximab (BR). Table 155-8 shows the CHOP regimen that is widely used in the treatment of NHL, and the development of the CHOP regimen is described in more detail later in this chapter.

Bendamustine is an alkylating agent with structural similarities to both alkylating agents and purine analogs. The mechanism of action of bendamustine is different from other alkylating agents and it does not show cross-resistance to other alkylating agents. When used as a single agent, bendamustine shows antitumor activity in relapsed or refractory indolent lymphomas. Overall and complete response rates of 70% to 80% and 30% to 35% have been reported, respectively, in phase II trials.[79] Two randomized, noninferiority studies have reported that BR is noninferior to R-CHOP for indolent lymphomas. In a randomized noninferiority phase III study of patients with advanced indolent lymphoma (with slightly over half follicular lymphoma patients), patients randomized to receive BR had longer median progression-free survival as compared to those in the R-CHOP group. In the subgroup analysis of patients with follicular lymphoma subtype, a significant benefit for progression-free survival was observed with BR versus R-CHOP.[80] In another study, BR was demonstrated to be noninferior to standard therapies (R-CHOP or R-CVP) for overall and complete response rate, with

TABLE 155-8 CHOP Regimen

Drug	Dose	Route	Treatment Days
Cyclophosphamide	750 mg/m^2	IV	1
Doxorubicin[a]	50 mg/m^2	IV	1
Vincristine[b]	1.4 mg/m^2	IV	1
Prednisone	100 mg	Oral	1-5
One cycle is 21 days			

[a]Another name for doxorubicin is hydroxydaunorubicin.

[b]Vincristine dose is typically capped at 2 mg.

significant improvement in 5-year progression-free survival (65.5% vs 55.8%).[81,82] Both studies also reported that BR was associated with fewer infectious episodes and fewer hematological toxicities such as grade 3 to 4 leukopenia and neutropenia. BR was also associated with less peripheral neuropathy and alopecia.[80,81] However, dermatological toxicities, drug-related hypersensitivities, and vomiting were more common with BR. Based on these results, BR, R-CHOP, and R-CVP are all listed as first-line therapy of follicular lymphoma (category 1).[49]

Obinutuzumab-based chemoimmunotherapy regimens are also approved in the treatment of follicular lymphomas. Obinutuzumab is a humanized anti-CD20 monoclonal antibody developed to have lower complement-dependent cytotoxicity, but greater antibody-dependent cellular cytotoxicity, phagocytosis, and direct B-cell killing than rituximab. Obinutuzumab has been evaluated in both first- and second-line settings. In the first-line trial, patients with previously untreated advanced-stage follicular lymphoma were randomized to receive chemotherapy (CHOP, CVP, or bendamustine) combined with either obinutuzumab or rituximab.[83,84] Patients who achieved a complete or partial remission received maintenance therapy with the same antibody. Although progression-free survival at 3 years favored patients receiving obinutuzumab, overall survival was similar in the two groups. Serious adverse drug reactions such as infusion-related events occurred more frequently in patients receiving obinutuzumab. In the second-line setting, patients with indolent lymphoma (majority being follicular lymphoma) refractory to rituximab were randomized to bendamustine, either alone or combined with obinutuzumab for 6 cycles, followed by maintenance obinutuzumab therapy for 2 years.[85,86] Patients in the obinutuzumab arm had increased progression-free and overall survival as compared to bendamustine monotherapy. The NCCN guidelines list obinutuzumab, combined with chemotherapy, as first-line, second-line, and subsequent therapy options for treatment of follicular lymphoma.[49] To reduce the risk of infusion reactions associated with obinutuzumab, patients should receive premedication including glucocorticoids, acetaminophen, and antihistamines, as well as a step-up infusion rate. In addition, patients receiving obinutuzumab and bendamustine should receive prophylaxis for *Pneumocystis jiroveci* pneumonia and varicella zoster virus.

Lenalidomide Lenalidomide is an immunomodulating agent that binds to the cereblon E3 ubiquitin ligase complex, which degrades transcription factors and leads to apoptosis of lymphoma cells.[87] The NCCN guidelines list rituximab-lenalidomide as a treatment option for first-line and second-line therapy for treatment of follicular lymphoma.[49] In the first-line setting, one phase III study compared rituximab and lenalidomide versus rituximab and chemotherapy (R-CHOP, BR, or R-CVP) in advanced-stage follicular lymphoma. Patients received different lenalidomide doses and treatment duration (maximum duration of 18 cycles) depending on their response. Maintenance rituximab was given to all patients. Complete response rates at 120 weeks and 3-year progression-free survival were similar in both arms. Safety profiles, however, differed between the two treatment arms, with more patients in the rituximab and chemotherapy group experiencing grade 3 or 4 neutropenia. Patients receiving lenalidomide and rituximab experienced more grade 3 or 4 cutaneous reactions.[88]

The combination of rituximab and lenalidomide was compared to lenalidomide monotherapy in patients with recurrent follicular lymphoma. Compared to lenalidomide monotherapy, the combination had higher overall and complete response rates. The time-to-progression was also longer in the rituximab and lenalidomide group (2.0 vs 1.1 year). Commonly reported toxicities of lenalidomide include neutropenia, fatigue, and thrombosis.[89]

Radioimmunotherapy ^{90}Y-Ibritumomab tiuxetan (Zevalin®) is an anti-CD20 radioimmunoconjugate used for patients with indolent NHLs.[90] It is a mouse antibody linked to yttrium-90$^{(90Y)}$, a radioisotope. Indolent lymphomas are known to be responsive to radiation therapy (ie, radiosensitive), and the rationale for radioimmunotherapy is that the antibody acts as a guided missile to deliver its payload (ie, radiation) to its target (ie, lymphoma cells that express the CD20 antigen). The specificity of the monoclonal antibody allows delivery of the radiation selectively to the tumor (and adjacent normal tissues).

^{90}Y-Ibritumomab tiuxetan has shown activity in relapsed and refractory patients with indolent or transformed lymphomas.[90] In patients who respond to radioimmunotherapy, the duration of remission can be more than several years. Radioimmunotherapy is generally well-tolerated. The major acute toxicities with both radioimmunoconjugates are infusion-related reactions and myelosuppression. The primary concern with radioimmunotherapy is the development of treatment-related myelodysplastic syndrome or acute myelogenous leukemia.

The decision to use radioimmunotherapy must be made carefully because of the complexity, risks, and costs of the treatment regimen. Because of safety concerns related to delivery of radiation to bone marrow, candidates for radioimmunotherapy usually have limited bone marrow involvement and adequate absolute neutrophil and platelet counts. Although medical oncologists usually select patients for therapy, the radioimmunotherapy regimen must be administered at a radiation oncology or nuclear medicine facility.

Phosphatidylinositol-3-Kinase (PI3K) Inhibitor The B-cell receptor signaling pathway plays an important role in the maintenance and progression of FL. The PI3K pathway is downstream from the B-cell receptor and is essential for the survival of FL. Inhibition of PI3K reduces phosphatidylinositol 3,4,5-triphosphate (PIP_3), which is a messenger that affects pivotal cell function including cell proliferation, survival, and metabolism. Among the four isoforms of PI3K, PI3Kδ mediates B-cell receptor signaling and microenvironment support signals that promote the growth and survival of malignant B lymphocytes. Four PI3K inhibitors (idelalisib, copanlisib, duvelisib, and umbralisib) are currently approved for treatment of relapsed and refractory follicular lymphoma. Idelalisib is an isoform-selective PI3K inhibitor and targets specifically PI3Kδ, whereas copalisinb is a pan-class I PI3K inhibitor, predominantly targeting PI3Kα and PI3Kδ. Duvelisib targets PIK3Kδ and PI3Kγ, and umbralisib inhibits PI3Kδ and casein kinase-1ε (CK1ε). CK1ε is a component of the Wnt signaling pathway which has been shown to drive the pathogenesis of B-cell lymphoproliferative disorders.

The use of PI3K inhibitors for follicular lymphoma is based on three Phase II studies. In one study, patients with relapsed or refractory indolent NHL received oral idelalisib 150 mg twice daily until disease progression. The overall response rate was 57% in patients with follicular lymphoma who had relapsed within 24 months of chemoimmunotherapy, with a median duration of response of 11.8 months.[91,92] Similar results were reported with other PI3K inhibitors.[93-95] All of the PI3K inhibitors can cause severe neutropenia, diarrhea, infection, and pneumonia. Idelalisib is also associated with severe hepatotoxicity, severe diarrhea, colitis, and lung infection. Hypertension and hyperglycemia are more prominent with copanlisib because of its potent inhibition of PI3Kα. Severe skin infections have also been observed with copanlisib while duvelisib is associated with serious adverse drug reactions including infection and death. Umbralisib is associated with neutropenia, diarrhea, and transaminitis. The NCCN guidelines list idealisib, copanlisib, and duvelisib as treatment options for second-line therapy and umbralisib is listed as third-line therapy for patients with relapsed or refractory follicular lymphoma.[49]

Tazemetostat Among patients with follicular lymphoma, 20% to 25% harbor an activating mutation of the epigenetic regulator EZH2. Such mutation allows the escape from the normal B-cell clonal selection process and allows GCB cells to survive and proliferate. Tazemetostat is a first-generation EZH2 inhibitor and is currently approved for EZH2 mutation positive in relapsed or refractory disease after two prior therapies, or EZH2 wild-type or unknown relapsed/refractory disease in patients who have no satisfactory alternative treatment options. In a trial of tazemetostat, patients with relapsed or refractory FL harboring an EZH2 mutation had a 71% overall response rate, whereas patients without this mutation had an overall response rate of 33%.[96]

Axicabtagene Ciloleuce Chimeric antigen receptor (CAR) T-cell therapies have also been explored in relapsed/refractory follicular lymphomas. In a phase 2 trial (ZUMA-5), 84 patients with relapsed/refractory follicular lymphoma after two or more lines of therapy received axicabtagene ciloleuce. The overall response rate was 94%, with 80% having a complete response. The 12-month progression-free and overall survival were 74% and 93%, respectively. However, grade 3 or above adverse drug reactions occurred in 85% of the patients, with cytokine release syndrome and neurologic toxicities occurring in 6% and 15%, respectively.[97]

Hematopoietic Stem Cell Transplantation High-dose chemotherapy, followed by autologous or allogeneic HSCT, is another option for patients with relapsed follicular lymphoma.[98] In patients who are transplanted at the time of initial treatment failure, 5-year event-free survival is about 40% to 50%. Although the rate of recurrence is lower after allogeneic HSCT as compared with autologous HSCT, that benefit is offset by increased treatment-related mortality after allogeneic HSCT. The presence of a survival plateau after allogeneic HSCT suggests that some patients may be cured of their disease.

A recent study has evaluated the role of HSCT in relapsed/refractory follicular lymphoma following disease relapse after prior rituximab-based therapy. Allogeneic HSCT was associated with an increased risk of death on analysis. Autologous HSCT, on the other hand, was associated with a 3-year overall survival rate of 87%.[99] The current NCCN guideline lists autologous HSCT as an appropriate consolidative therapy for patients achieving second or third remission.[49] However, emerging data suggest that patients transplanted after their first or second relapse could achieve better outcomes than those who receive transplants later in their course of illness.[100]

Diffuse Large B-Cell Lymphoma

The DLBCLs are the most common lymphoma in the International NHL Classification Project, accounting for about 30% of all NHLs.[63] DLBCLs are characterized by the presence of large cells, which are similar in size to or larger than tissue macrophages and usually more than twice the size of normal lymphocytes. The median age at the time of diagnosis is in the seventh decade, but DLBCL can affect individuals of all ages, from children to older adults. Patients often present with a rapidly enlarging symptomatic mass, with B symptoms in about 30% to 40% of cases.[49] About 30% to 40% of patients with DLBCL present with extranodal disease; common sites include the head and neck, gastrointestinal tract, skin, bone, testis, and CNS. DLBCL is the most common type of diffuse aggressive lymphomas, which are characterized by an aggressive clinical behavior that leads to death within weeks to months if the tumor is not treated. Diffuse aggressive lymphomas are also sensitive to many chemotherapeutic agents, and some patients treated with chemotherapy can be cured of their disease.

Several factors correlate with response to chemotherapy and survival in patients with aggressive lymphoma. Because the IPI was originally developed based on patients with aggressive lymphoma, the IPI score correlates with prognosis (see Table 155-7).[52] As described above, the revised NCCN-IPI score may more accurately predict prognosis in patients receiving rituximab-containing combination chemotherapy.[53]

Therapy of DLBCL is based on the Ann Arbor stage, IPI (or revised IPI) score, and other prognostic factors.[49] About one-half of patients present with localized (stage I or II) disease. However, many patients present with large bulky masses (ie, larger than 10 cm), and patients with bulky stage II disease are treated with the same approach used for patients with advanced disease (stage III or IV).

Treatment of Localized Disease (Stages I and II)

11 Before 1980, radiation therapy was the primary treatment for patients with localized DLBCL. Five-year disease-free survival with radiation therapy alone was about 50% and 20% in patients with stage I and stage II disease, respectively.[49] Randomized trials in the 1980s showed that radiation therapy followed by chemotherapy resulted in significantly longer disease-free and overall survival as compared with radiation therapy alone. Other studies reported excellent results with a short course of chemotherapy (three cycles) followed by involved-field radiotherapy or six to eight cycles of CHOP chemotherapy, with or without consolidation radiotherapy. With either of these approaches, 5-year progression-free survival was more than 90% for patients with stage I disease and about 70% for patients with stage II disease.[49]

Because the most effective approach was not clear, the SWOG performed a randomized trial that compared three cycles of CHOP and involved-field radiotherapy or six cycles of CHOP in patients with stage I and nonbulky stage II aggressive lymphoma.[101] Patients treated with three cycles of CHOP plus radiotherapy had significantly better 5-year progression-free and overall survival with a lower incidence of life-threatening toxicity than patients treated with CHOP alone. However, with longer follow-up, the differences in progression-free or overall survival were no longer significant between the two arms.

In the rituximab era, most patients with localized disease are treated with either three to four cycles of R-CHOP followed by radiotherapy or six to eight cycles of R-CHOP with no radiotherapy. Although these two treatment options have not been directly compared in a randomized controlled trial, observational data show similar 5-year overall survival in patients with stage I and II DLBCL. Patients who received the abbreviated course of R-CHOP plus radiotherapy experienced less acute toxicity and a lower risk of requiring second-line therapy.[102] Based on these findings, three cycles of R-CHOP followed by locoregional radiation is recommended for patients with localized, nonbulky DLBCL. Alternatively, if the disease presents at sites where radiotherapy may lead to significant morbidity, six cycles of R-CHOP without radiation can be considered.[49]

A recent study has examined the use of interim PET scans to determine the need for radiotherapy. Patients with a negative interim PET scan received four cycles of R-CHOP alone with no radiotherapy while those with a positive PET scan were subsequently treated with radiotherapy and ibritumomab tiuxetan. Patients with both positive and negative interim PET scans demonstrated similarly excellent survival outcomes, suggesting the potential role of interim PET scans to guide treatment of localized DLBCL.[102]

Treatment of Advanced Disease (Bulky Stage II, Stages III, and IV)

It has been known since the late 1970s that intensive combination chemotherapy can cure some patients with disseminated DLBCL.[46] Initial studies with cyclophosphamide, vincristine (Oncovin®), and prednisone or prednisolone (COP; same as CVP) produced a plateau on the survival curve of just 10%, with a median survival of less than 1 year. Based on the activity of single-agent doxorubicin, McKelvey et al. developed the CHOP regimen (see Table 155-8).[103] A few years later, a SWOG study showed that CHOP was more active than COP, and CHOP chemotherapy rapidly became the treatment of choice for patients with aggressive lymphomas.[104] Studies in larger numbers of patients showed that about 50% of patients had a complete remission to CHOP chemotherapy, and 50% to 75% of the patients who had a complete response (about one-third of all patients) experienced long-term disease-free survival and cure of their disease.

To improve these results, many investigators used several approaches to develop second- and third-generation regimens in the 1980s. Results of phase II trials suggested that these second- and third-generation regimens were more active than CHOP, with slightly higher complete response rates and improved disease-free survival rates. However, they were also more difficult to administer, more toxic, and more expensive. Based on these results, many oncologists adopted one of these second- or third-generation combination regimens as their standard regimen for patients with advanced aggressive lymphomas.

Many randomized studies have compared different combination regimens in patients with aggressive lymphoma. Although the results of these studies show that no one regimen is superior to another, they demonstrate the superiority of anthracycline-containing regimens over those that do not contain an anthracycline. In the largest and most widely cited study, the SWOG initiated a randomized trial in 1986 that compared CHOP to three of the most commonly used third-generation regimens in patients with advanced NHL. At the time of the initial publication (median follow-up: 35 months), no differences in disease-free and overall survival were observed between the four groups.[105] Furthermore, no significant differences in disease-free or overall survival were observed in any subgroup of patients. But the risk of treatment-related mortality was higher in patients receiving one of the third-generation regimens. Extended follow-up of that trial shows that about 35% of patients who participated in that trial are probably cured of their disease, regardless of the initial combination chemotherapy regimen. Interestingly, the overall survival is about 10% higher than the disease-free survival, which probably reflects the effectiveness of salvage high-dose chemotherapy with autologous HSCT (see the "Treatment of Refractory or Relapsed Disease" section).

Based on the lack of survival benefit with the newer combination chemotherapy regimens, the less-complicated and less-expensive CHOP regimen was considered as the treatment of choice for most patients with DLBCL and other aggressive NHLs for many years. Even with CHOP chemotherapy, however, less than 50% of patients with DLBCL were cured of their disease and most patients who relapse after an initial response do so in the first 2 years. New treatment approaches were needed.

Based on the encouraging results of R-CHOP in indolent lymphomas, several studies evaluated this combination in aggressive lymphomas. The first randomized controlled trial that established the efficacy of R-CHOP in advanced-stage DLBCL showed that R-CHOP significantly increased complete response rates and overall survival in older adults (≥60 years old) as compared with CHOP alone (discussed in the "Treatment of Older Patients with Advanced Disease" section).[106] Although the results of that study established R-CHOP as standard therapy in older patients, the role of R-CHOP in the treatment of younger patients was not clear. That issue was addressed in the MabThera International Trial, which enrolled younger (18-60 years old) patients with good-prognosis DLBCL.[107] Patients randomized to receive rituximab plus CHOP-like chemotherapy had significantly higher complete response rates (86% vs 68%) and longer 3-year event-free and overall survival (79% vs 59%; HR 0.44 and 93% vs 84%; HR 0.40, respectively). Updates from the study cohort indicate that the survival benefits of adding rituximab are sustained at 6 years with no increase in the incidence of secondary malignancies.[108] Based on these trial results, rituximab received FDA approval for first-line treatment in combination with CHOP or CHOP-like chemotherapy and R-CHOP is recommended for all patients with advanced-stage DLBCL in the current NCCN guideline.[49]

Several studies attempted to improve treatment results by increasing chemotherapy dose (ie, dose-intensity), shortening the interval between chemotherapy cycles (ie, dose-density), or both. Because of the increased risk of severe neutropenia, these treatment approaches require growth factor support. Dose-dense chemotherapy, where the interval between cycles is shortened from 3 to 2 weeks, has been evaluated in randomized trials. Before the rituximab era, event-free, and overall survival rates were longer with biweekly CHOP-14 compared to standard CHOP-21 every 21 days.[109] However, long-term follow-up data show that with the addition of rituximab, the survival benefit associated with a dose-dense schedule is not superior to that of R-CHOP-21.[110,111] In one of the trials conducted in older adults, the incidence of severe neutropenia was significantly higher despite an increased use of granulocyte colony-stimulating factor.[111]

Treatment outcomes for high-risk patients according to the IPI (or revised IPI) score are unsatisfactory. High-risk groups generally include all patients older than 60 years and those with an IPI score of 3 or more (or an age-adjusted IPI score of ≥2). Since progression-free survival is only about 50% in these high-risk patients treated with R-CHOP, other more aggressive treatments, preferably as part of a clinical trial, should be considered in these patients.

One approach is to give high-dose chemotherapy with autologous HSCT as intensive consolidation in high-risk patients with DLBCL who achieve a remission with standard chemotherapy. This approach improves progression-free survival in patients with high-risk disease (age-adjusted IPI score of ≥2) who have a response to CHOP-based chemotherapy.[49]

In summary, all patients with bulky stage II, stage III, or stage IV disease should be treated with R-CHOP or rituximab and CHOP-like chemotherapy until a complete response is achieved (usually four to six cycles).[49] The use of long-term maintenance therapy following a complete response has not been shown to improve overall survival. Treatment outcomes for high-risk patients according to the IPI (or revised IPI) score are unsatisfactory and alternative treatment approaches, preferably as part of a clinical trial, should be considered in these patients. High-dose chemotherapy with autologous HSCT should be considered in high-risk patients who respond to standard chemotherapy and are candidates for autologous HSCT.[49]

Treatment of Older Patients with Advanced Disease

More than one-half of patients with NHL are older than 60 years of age at diagnosis, and about one-third are older than age 70 years. The International Non-Hodgkin Lymphoma Prognostic Factors Project showed that patients older than 60 years had a significantly lower complete response rate and overall survival.[52] The reasons for the poorer outcome in older adults are not clear. Older patients do not tolerate intensive chemotherapy as well as younger patients, and some studies report that older patients have a higher risk of treatment-related mortality. As a result, many clinicians treat older adults with reduced dose or less-aggressive chemotherapy regimens. In general, these less-intensive regimens use anthracyclines with less cardiotoxicity than doxorubicin, substitute mitoxantrone for doxorubicin, or use short-duration weekly therapy.[112]

Over the past few years, several nonrandomized and randomized trials have evaluated different treatment approaches in older patients with aggressive NHL. The results of these studies suggest that carefully selected older adults with good performance status and without significant comorbidities can tolerate aggressive anthracycline-containing regimens as well as younger patients. These patients should be treated initially with full-dose R-CHOP or similar regimens; dosages can be reduced later if severe toxicity occurs. Hematopoietic growth factors may allow older adults to maintain dose intensity.[112]

The combination therapy, R-CHOP, has replaced CHOP as standard treatment for older adults with aggressive lymphoma, based on the results of the Groupe d'Etude des Lymphomes de l'Adulte (GELA) study.[106] In that study of older adults with DLBCL, patients who were randomized to receive R-CHOP had a significantly higher complete response rate and longer event-free and overall survival as compared with those who received CHOP. After 10 years of follow-up, progression-free survival was significantly longer among those who received R-CHOP than CHOP.[106] A higher risk of death or secondary cancer was not observed with the addition of rituximab to CHOP after 10 years of follow-up. In another randomized controlled trial conducted primarily in the United States (Eastern Cooperative Oncology Group 4494), older adults (≥60 years old) who received rituximab, either as induction or maintenance with CHOP chemotherapy, had significantly longer failure-free survival as compared with those not given rituximab during their treatment course.[113] Maintenance therapy with single-agent rituximab did not provide any additional benefit in patients who received R-CHOP as induction therapy. Rituximab is given differently in the two studies. In the GELA study, rituximab is given on day 1 (the same day that cyclophosphamide, doxorubicin, and vincristine are administered) with each cycle of CHOP chemotherapy.[106] In the Eastern Cooperative Oncology Group 4494 study, R-CHOP was modeled after the regimen developed by Czuczman et al.: two doses of rituximab are given before cycle 1, and one dose is given before cycles 3, 5, and 7 (if administered).[114] In most NHL protocols and in clinical practice, rituximab is given on day 1 of each cycle of CHOP chemotherapy.

Previous trials have evaluated different drugs, including rituximab, as maintenance treatment in DLBCL but have failed to show survival benefits. Lenalidomide as maintenance in older adults (60-80 years old) who had responded to R-CHOP was recently evaluated in the REMARC trial. Maintenance lenalidomide for 24 months prolonged progression-free survival but did not improve overall survival and was associated with a higher premature discontinuation rate.[115] Based on these results, lenalidomide is an option if maintenance therapy is considered in older adults who have responded to treatment.[49]

Treatment of Refractory or Relapsed Disease

12 Although many patients with aggressive NHL experience long-term survival and cure with intensive chemotherapy, about 10% to 20% of patients fail to achieve a complete remission and about 20% to 30% of patients who do achieve a complete remission will subsequently relapse. Therefore, about 30% to 40% of all patients with aggressive NHL will require salvage therapy at some point during their disease course. Response to salvage therapy depends on the initial responsiveness of the tumor to chemotherapy. Patients who achieve an initial complete remission and then relapse generally have a better response to salvage therapy than those who are primarily or partially resistant to chemotherapy.[116]

Many conventional-dose salvage chemotherapy regimens have been used in patients with relapsed or refractory NHL. Many patients who respond to salvage therapy (ie, chemosensitive relapse) will then receive high-dose chemotherapy with autologous HSCT. To avoid cross-resistance, most salvage regimens incorporate drugs not used in the initial therapy. Some of the more commonly used salvage regimens include ICE, dexamethasone, cytarabine, cisplatin (DHAP), etoposide, methylprednisolone, cytarabine, cisplatin (ESHAP), mesna, ifosfamide, mitoxantrone, etoposide (MINE), gemcitabine, dexamethasone, and cisplatin (GDP) and no one regimen is superior to any other regimen.[117] With these salvage regimens, about 30% to 50% of patients achieve a complete response, with a median duration of remission of 1 to 2 years. Only about 5% to 10% of patients will have long-term disease-free survival.[116]

Rituximab is sometimes added to these salvage regimens. It is recommended, however, to exclude rituximab in second-line therapy if the patient's disease is refractory or if the duration of remission is less than 6 months. One study (CORAL study) compared two salvage regimens (R-ICE and R-DHAP) in patients with relapsed or refractory DLBCL, followed by autologous HSCT.[118] No significant difference in 3-year event-free survival or overall survival was observed between R-ICE and R-DHAP. However, patients who had received prior rituximab and experienced early relapse (defined as less than 12 months after diagnosis) had a poor prognosis. New treatment strategies are needed to improve the response rates of salvage regimens.

To improve the cure rate, many studies have evaluated high-dose chemotherapy with autologous HSCT as intensive consolidation therapy in patients who respond to salvage therapy. In the PARMA study, patients with relapsed aggressive NHL who had a response to DHAP salvage therapy were randomized to receive either high-dose chemotherapy or continued DHAP therapy.[119] Patients who received high-dose chemotherapy had significantly longer 5-year disease-free survival (46% vs 12%) and overall survival (53% vs 32%) than those treated with conventional salvage therapy. Further analysis of that study showed that patients who relapsed within 12 months of their initial diagnosis were less likely to benefit from high-dose chemotherapy than patients who relapsed after 12 months. Based on a review of the available evidence, including the PARMA study, high-dose chemotherapy with autologous HSCT is considered to be the treatment of choice in younger patients with chemotherapy-sensitive relapse.[49] High-dose chemotherapy with autologous HSCT is not recommended in patients with untested or chemotherapy-refractory relapse.

In patients who have failed multiple lines of treatment, several agents have been studied, including selinexor and chimeric antigen receptor (CAR) T-cell therapy. CAR T-cell therapy is a type of adoptive immunotherapy where the patient's own T-lymphocytes are collected, modified genetically in the laboratory to target antigens on malignant cells, and then administered back to the patient by infusion.[120] In recent years, three CAR T-cell therapies, tisagenlecleucel, axicabtagene ciloleucel, and lisocabtagene maraleucel have been approved by the FDA for relapsed and refractory DLBCL after two or more lines of systemic treatment have failed. The approval of CAR T-cell therapies was based on high response rates reported in phase II trials, which compared favorably to historical data. In the JULIET trial, an overall best response rate of 52% was reported in 93 patients with refractory disease treated with tisagenlecleucel.[121] In the ZUMA-1 trial, a response rate of 82% and 18-month overall survival of 52% was reported in 101 patients with refractory disease.[122] The TRANSCEND trial, with 256 evaluable patients, reported an objective response rate of 73% among those with refractory disease who received lisocabtagene maraleucel.[123] Ongoing randomized trials are investigating the role of CAR T-cell therapy as first-line therapy or in combination with other immunotherapy agents in relapsed and refractory DLBCL[124,125]

CAR T-cell therapies are associated with a high incidence of cytokine release syndrome, which is characterized by fever, hypoxia, and hypotension, and may require the use of vasopressors in severe cases. Severe neurological toxicities such as encephalopathy and seizures can also occur, usually within days of T-cell infusion. While mild episodes can be symptomatically managed, moderate-to-severe grades of cytokine release syndrome and neurological toxicities may require immunosuppressants including tocilizumab and corticosteroids.[49,120,126]

Mantle Cell Lymphoma

Mantle cell lymphoma (MCL) is found in 6% of cases in the International Lymphoma Classification Project.[63] The chromosomal translocation t(11;14) occurs in most cases of MCL. MCL usually occurs in older adults, particularly in men, and most patients have advanced disease at the time of diagnosis (see Table 155-6). Extranodal involvement is found in about 90% of cases. The course of the disease is moderately aggressive; the median overall survival is about 3 years, with no evidence of a survival plateau.

Both aggressive and less-aggressive chemotherapy regimens have been evaluated in patients with disseminated MCL. One widely used aggressive combination regimen is cyclophosphamide, vincristine, doxorubicin, dexamethasone alternating with methotrexate and cytarabine (hyperCVAD) with or without rituximab. Overall response rates to these regimens are about 90%, with long-term progression-free survival rates of 59% and 35% at 5 and 10 years, respectively.[127] Less-aggressive regimens are often used for patients who are not candidates of HSCT. Because MCL usually expresses CD20, rituximab, either alone or combined with CHOP and bendamustine, has been used with some success in patients with newly diagnosed and relapsed MCL.[80,128] In a phase III study, BR was compared to R-CHOP for first-line therapy in patients with advanced follicular, indolent, and MCL. In the MCL subgroup, progression-free survival was higher with BR compared to R-CHOP up to 5 years after treatment completion, and it is associated with less hematologic toxicities.[80-82] However, a higher number of secondary malignancies were observed in the BR group during long-term follow-up.[82] Another less-aggressive option that has been found to yield favorable results was lenalidomide in combination with rituximab, with 5-year progression-free and overall survival rates of 63.9% and 77.4%, respectively.[129] Bortezomib (Velcade®), in combination with rituximab, cyclophosphamide, doxorubicin, and prednisolone, (VR-CAP, similar to R-CHOP regimen but with bortezomib replacing vincristine) is also indicated for newly diagnosed MCL.[130] In a phase III randomized study, patients with newly diagnosed MCL who were ineligible or not considered for HSCT received R-CHOP or VR-CAP. After a median follow-up of 40 months, median progression-free survival was longer in the VR-CAP arm compared to R-CHOP (24.7 vs 14.4 months). Rates of neutropenia and thrombocytopenia were higher in the VR-CAP group.[130]

Despite the high response rates, MCL is not considered curable with standard chemotherapy. Therefore, younger patients who have an initial response to chemotherapy often undergo autologous or allogeneic HSCT as consolidation therapy. The NCCN guidelines recommend that patients with advanced-stage MCL be treated initially with rituximab and combination chemotherapy, followed by autologous HSCT as first-line consolidation therapy.[49] In patients who respond to autologous HSCT, maintenance rituximab or lenalidomide are options that have been demonstrated to prolong progression-free and overall survival.[131-133] Findings from a prospective study suggest that similar survival benefits are also associated with the use of maintenance rituximab after R-CHOP in older patients who are not candidates for autologous HSCT.[134]

Unfortunately, most patients with MCL eventually relapse and are treated with salvage therapy or enrolled in trials of investigational agents, some of which are directed at molecular targets. First-line regimens such as R-CHOP, VR-CAP, and bendamustine can be considered if they have not been previously given.[49] Bortezomib with or without rituximab is also approved for the treatment of MCL that has relapsed after at least one prior therapy.

Novel agents that have been approved for the treatment of relapsed or refractory MCL include the Bruton tyrosine kinase (BTK) inhibitors ibrutinib, acalabrutinib, and zanubrutinib. In a phase III randomized trial, ibrutinib had a higher response rate and longer median duration of response with a more favorable safety profile than temsirolimus.[135] Addition of rituximab to ibrutinib was further evaluated in a phase II trial that reported a response rate of 88%, with a median duration of response of 46 months.[136] Other oral BTK inhibitors, acalabrutinib and zanubrutinib, have demonstrated overall response rates of more than 80% in phase II trials in patients with relapsed and refractory MCL.[137] The most common adverse drug reactions of BTK inhibitors include diarrhea and fatigue. Since cytopenias are also common, complete blood counts should be monitored monthly while patients are on treatment. Bleeding may rarely occur during the first 6 months of BTK inhibitor therapy. Cases of new-onset atrial fibrillation have also been reported. A CAR T-cell therapy, brexucabtagene autoleucel, has also recently been approved for the treatment of relapsed and refractory mantle cell lymphoma in adult patients. Approval was granted based on ZUMA-2, a single-arm trial that demonstrated a response rate of 93% and a 12-month overall survival rate of 83%.[138]

EVALUATION OF THERAPEUTIC OUTCOMES

Hodgkin lymphoma and NHLs tend to respond well to radiation, chemotherapy, and biologic therapy. The goal of therapy for patients with Hodgkin lymphoma and aggressive NHL is long-term survival and cure. The therapeutic goal in patients with indolent NHLs is less clear because of the indolent nature of the disease and the lack of convincing evidence showing that therapy prolongs survival. Therapeutic responses should be evaluated based on physical examination, radiologic evidence, PET/CT scanning, and other positive findings at baseline. The current standard of care to evaluate response to treatment in Hodgkin lymphoma, follicular lymphoma, and DLBCL is PET imaging. As described earlier, the 5-point scale is recommended for PET-CT interpretation where a Deauville score of 1, 2, or 3 (uptake less than or equivalent to liver) indicates complete response, even in the presence of a persistent mass. If salvage treatment is considered based on a metabolically active residual mass, a biopsy or follow-up scan should be considered.[50] CT is advised for other lymphomas with low or variable FDG avidity. The rapidity of response to therapy in patients with indolent NHL depends on the choice of therapy. Early interim PET-CT scans may also possess prognostic value in patients with advanced Hodgkin lymphoma.[18] In NHL, the prognostic value of interim PET-CT scans is less established and they are currently not recommended to guide changes in therapy.[49] Patients should be clinically monitored every 3 months for 2 years, then every 6 to 12 months as appropriate. Surveillance scans after disease remission has been achieved are currently not advised, especially in Hodgkin lymphoma and DLBCL, but they can be considered in the event of equivocal findings at the end of treatment or in indolent lymphomas with residual disease.[50]

CONCLUSION

Hodgkin lymphoma and NHL are the two primary histologic classifications of lymphoma. Hodgkin lymphoma is defined by the presence of Reed–Sternberg cells. Restaging PET-CT serves to guide patient-specific treatment plans primarily comprised of combination chemotherapy with or without radiation therapy. The primary combination chemotherapy utilized is ABVD. NHL is a much more heterogeneous group of malignancies and is classified by a combination of morphology, immunophenotype, genetic features, and clinical features. Treatment response is often based on the aggressiveness of the NHL. Aggressive NHLs, such as DLBCL, can often be cured with combination chemoimmunotherapy with R-CHOP. Indolent NHLs, such as follicular lymphoma, are often uncurable but can be managed long-term with a variety of different treatment approaches. In the relapsed setting, salvage chemoimmunotherapy is used along with high-dose chemotherapy followed by autologous HSCT. Several novel agents, including the CAR T-cell therapy is a new approach for NHL and an area of ongoing research.

ABBREVIATIONS

A-AVD	brentuximab vedotin (Adcetris®), doxorubicin (Adriamycin®), vinblastine, and dacarbazine
ABC	activated B-cell–like
ABV	doxorubicin (Adriamycin®), bleomycin, vinblastine
ABVD	doxorubicin (Adriamycin®), bleomycin, vinblastine, and dacarbazine
ADC	antibody-drug conjugate
AIDS	acquired immune deficiency syndrome
BEACOPP	bleomycin, etoposide, doxorubicin (Adriamycin®), cyclophosphamide, vincristine (Oncovin®), procarbazine, and prednisone
BR	bendamustine and rituximab
BTK	Bruton tyrosine kinase
CAR	chimeric antigen receptor
CHOP	cyclophosphamide, doxorubicin, vincristine (Oncovin®), prednisone
COP	cyclophosphamide, vincristine (Oncovin®), and prednisone or prednisolone
COPP	cyclophosphamide, vincristine, procarbazine, and prednisone
CT	computed tomography
CVP	cyclophosphamide, vincristine, and prednisone
DHAP	dexamethasone, cytarabine, cisplatin
DLBCL	diffuse large B-cell lymphoma
EBV	Epstein-Barr virus
EPOCH	etoposide, prednisone, vincristine, cyclophosphamide, and doxorubicin
ESHAP	etoposide, methylprednisolone, cytarabine, cisplatin
ESR	erythrocyte sedimentation rate
FDA	Food and Drug Administration
FLIPI	Follicular Lymphoma International Prognostic Index
GCB	germinal center B-cell like
GDP	gemcitabine, dexamethasone, cisplatin
GELA	Groupe d'Etude des Lymphomes de l'Adulte
GHSG	German Hodgkin Study Group
GVD	gemcitabine, vinorelbine, and pegylated liposomal doxorubicin
HAART	highly active antiretroviral therapy
HIV	human immunodeficiency virus
HLA	human leukocyte antigen
HR	hazard ratio
HSCT	hematopoietic stem cell transplantation
Hyper CVAD	cyclophosphamide, vincristine, doxorubicin, dexamethasone alternating with methotrexate and cytarabine
ICE	ifosfamide, carboplatin, and etoposide
IFRT	involved-field radiation
IPI	International Prognostic Index
IPS	International Prognostic Score
ISRT	involved-site radiation therapy
JAK–STAT	Janus kinase–signal transduction and transcription
KSHV	Kaposi sarcoma–associated herpesvirus
LDH	lactate dehydrogenase
MALT	mucosa-associated lymphoid tissue
MCL	mantle cell lymphoma
MINE	mesna, ifosfamide, mitoxantrone, etoposide
MMAE	monomethyl auristatin
MOPP	mechlorethamine, vincristine, procarbazine, and prednisone
MOPPEBVCAD	mechlorethamine, vincristine, procarbazine, prednisone, epidoxorubicin, bleomycin, vinblastine, lomustine, doxorubicin, and vindesine
NCCN	National Comprehensive Cancer Network
NHL	non-Hodgkin lymphoma
NLPHL	nodular lymphocyte-predominant Hodgkin lymphoma
PET	positron emission tomography

PI3K	phosphatidylinositol-3-kinase
R-CHOP	rituximab, cyclophosphamide, doxorubicin, vincristine (Oncovin®), prednisone
REAL	Revised European-American Classification of Lymphoid Neoplasms
RICE	rituximab, ifosfamide, carboplatin, and etoposide
SEER	surveillance, epidemiology, and end results
SWOG	Southwest Oncology Group
WHO	World Health Organization

REFERENCES

1. Howlader N, Noone AM, Krapcho M, et al. SEER Cancer Statistics Review, 1975-2018. National Cancer Institute. Updated April 2018. Accessed April 2021. https://seer.cancer.gov/csr/1975_2018/.
2. Diehl V, Re D, Harris NL, Mauch PM. *Hodgkin's Lymphoma*. 10th ed. Devita, Hellman and Rosenberg's Cancer: Principles and Practice of Oncology. Lippincott Williams and Wilkins; 2015.
3. Bartlett NL, Triska G. Hodgkin's Lymphoma. In: Niederhuber JE, Armitage JO, Doroshow JH, Kastan MB, Tepper JE, eds. *Abeloff's Clinical Oncology*. 6th ed. Churchill Livingstone; 2019.
4. Siegel RL, Miller KD, Jemal A. Cancer statistics, 2022. *CA Cancer J Clin.* Jan 2022;72(1):7–33. doi:10.3322/caac.21708.
5. Swerdlow SH, Campo E, Pileri SA, et al. The 2016 revision of the World Health Organization classification of lymphoid neoplasms. *Blood.* 2016;127(20):2375–2390. doi:10.1182/blood-2016-01-643569.
6. Barrington SF, Mikhaeel NG, Kostakoglu L, et al. Role of imaging in the staging and response assessment of lymphoma: Consensus of the International Conference on Malignant Lymphomas Imaging Working Group. *J Clin Oncol.* 2014;32(27):3048–3058. doi:10.1200/jco.2013.53.5229.
7. Hasenclever D, Diehl V. A prognostic score for advanced Hodgkin's disease. International Prognostic Factors Project on Advanced Hodgkin's Disease. *New England J Med.* Nov 19 1998;339(21):1506–1514. doi:10.1056/NEJM199811193392104.
8. Ng AK, van Leeuwen FE. Hodgkin lymphoma: Late effects of treatment and guidelines for surveillance. *Semin Hematol.* Jul 2016;53(3):209–215. doi:10.1053/j.seminhematol.2016.05.008.
9. Specht L, Yahalom J, Illidge T, et al. Modern radiation therapy for Hodgkin lymphoma: Field and dose guidelines from the international lymphoma radiation oncology group (ILROG). *Int J Radiation Oncol, Biol, Phys.* Jul 15 2014;89(4):854–862. doi:10.1016/j.ijrobp.2013.05.005.
10. Bonadonna G, Zucali R, Monfardini S, De Lena M, Uslenghi C. Combination chemotherapy of Hodgkin's disease with adriamycin, bleomycin, vinblastine, and imidazole carboxamide versus MOPP. *Cancer.* Jul 1975;36(1):252–259.
11. Canellos GP, Anderson JR, Propert KJ, et al. Chemotherapy of advanced Hodgkin's disease with MOPP, ABVD, or MOPP alternating with ABVD. *New Eng J Med.* Nov 19 1992;327(21):1478–1484. doi:10.1056/NEJM199211193272102.
12. Goldie JH, Coldman AJ, Gudauskas GA. Rationale for the use of alternating non-cross-resistant chemotherapy. *Cancer Treatment Reports.* Mar 1982;66(3):439–449.
13. Glick JH, Young ML, Harrington D, et al. MOPP/ABV hybrid chemotherapy for advanced Hodgkin's disease significantly improves failure-free and overall survival: The 8-year results of the intergroup trial. *J Clin Oncol.* Jan 1998;16(1):19–26. doi:10.1200/JCO.1998.16.1.19.
14. Duggan DB, Petroni GR, Johnson JL, et al. Randomized comparison of ABVD and MOPP/ABV hybrid for the treatment of advanced Hodgkin's disease: Report of an intergroup trial. *J Clin Oncol.* Feb 15 2003;21(4):607–614. doi:10.1200/JCO.2003.12.086.
15. Horning SJ, Hoppe RT, Breslin S, Bartlett NL, Brown BW, Rosenberg SA. Stanford V and radiotherapy for locally extensive and advanced Hodgkin's disease: Mature results of a prospective clinical trial. *J Clin Oncol.* Feb 1 2002;20(3):630–637. doi:10.1200/JCO.2002.20.3.630.
16. Gobbi PG, Levis A, Chisesi T, et al. ABVD versus modified Stanford V versus MOPPEBVCAD with optional and limited radiotherapy in intermediate- and advanced-stage Hodgkin's lymphoma: Final results of a multicenter randomized trial by the Intergruppo Italiano Linfomi. *J Clin Oncol.* Dec 20 2005;23(36):9198–9207. doi:10.1200/JCO.2005.02.907.
17. Gordon LI, Hong F, Fisher RI, et al. Randomized phase III trial of ABVD versus Stanford V with or without radiation therapy in locally extensive and advanced-stage Hodgkin lymphoma: An intergroup study coordinated by the Eastern Cooperative Oncology Group (E2496). *J Clin Oncol.* Feb 20 2013;31(6):684–691. doi:10.1200/JCO.2012.43.4803.
18. National Comprehensive Cancer Network. Hodgkin's Lymphoma (Version 4.2021). Accessed 30, August 2021, https://www.nccn.org/professionals/physician_gls/pdf/hodgkins.pdf.
19. Engert A, Plutschow A, Eich HT, et al. Reduced treatment intensity in patients with early-stage Hodgkin's lymphoma. *New Eng J Med.* Aug 12 2010;363(7):640–652. doi:10.1056/NEJMoa1000067.
20. Advani RH, Hoppe RT, Baer D, et al. Efficacy of abbreviated Stanford V chemotherapy and involved-field radiotherapy in early-stage Hodgkin lymphoma: Mature results of the G4 trial. *Ann Oncol.* Apr 2013;24(4):1044–1048. doi:10.1093/annonc/mds542.
21. Edwards-Bennett SM, Jacks LM, Moskowitz CH, et al. Stanford V program for locally extensive and advanced Hodgkin lymphoma: The Memorial Sloan-Kettering Cancer Center experience. *Ann Oncol.* Mar 2010;21(3):574–581. doi:10.1093/annonc/mdp337.
22. Hoskin PJ, Lowry L, Horwich A, et al. Randomized comparison of the Stanford V regimen and ABVD in the treatment of advanced Hodgkin's Lymphoma: United Kingdom National Cancer Research Institute Lymphoma Group Study ISRCTN 64141244. *J Clin Oncol.* Nov 10 2009;27(32):5390–5396. doi:10.1200/JCO.2009.23.3239.
23. von Tresckow B, Plutschow A, Fuchs M, et al. Dose-intensification in early unfavorable Hodgkin's lymphoma: Final analysis of the German Hodgkin Study Group HD14 trial. *J Clin Oncol.* Mar 20 2012;30(9):907–913. doi:10.1200/JCO.2011.38.5807.
24. Eich HT, Diehl V, Gorgen H, et al. Intensified chemotherapy and dose-reduced involved-field radiotherapy in patients with early unfavorable Hodgkin's lymphoma: Final analysis of the German Hodgkin Study Group HD11 trial. *J Clin Oncol.* Sep 20 2010;28(27):4199–4206. doi:10.1200/JCO.2010.29.8018.
25. Diehl V, Franklin J, Pfreundschuh M, et al. Standard and increased-dose BEACOPP chemotherapy compared with COPP-ABVD for advanced Hodgkin's disease. *New EngJ Med.* Jun 12 2003;348(24):2386–2395. doi:10.1056/NEJMoa022473.
26. Engert A, Diehl V, Franklin J, et al. Escalated-dose BEACOPP in the treatment of patients with advanced-stage Hodgkin's lymphoma: 10 Years of follow-up of the GHSG HD9 study. *J Clin Oncol.* Sep 20 2009;27(27):4548–4554. doi:10.1200/JCO.2008.19.8820.
27. Federico M, Luminari S, Iannitto E, et al. ABVD compared with BEACOPP compared with CEC for the initial treatment of patients with advanced Hodgkin's lymphoma: Results from the HD2000 Gruppo Italiano per lo Studio dei Linfomi Trial. *J Clin Oncol.* Feb 10 2009;27(5):805–811. doi:10.1200/JCO.2008.17.0910.
28. Merli F, Luminari S, Gobbi PG, et al. Long-Term Results of the HD2000 Trial Comparing ABVD Versus BEACOPP Versus COPP-EBV-CAD in Untreated Patients With Advanced Hodgkin Lymphoma: A Study by Fondazione Italiana Linfomi. *J Clin Oncol.* Apr 10 2016;34(11):1175–1181. doi:10.1200/JCO.2015.62.4817.
29. Borchmann P, Haverkamp H, Diehl V, et al. Eight cycles of escalated-dose BEACOPP compared with four cycles of escalated-dose BEACOPP followed by four cycles of baseline-dose BEACOPP with or without radiotherapy in patients with advanced-stage Hodgkin's lymphoma: Final analysis of the HD12 trial of the German Hodgkin Study Group. *J Clin Oncol.* Nov 10 2011;29(32):4234–4242. doi:10.1200/JCO.2010.33.9549.
30. Engert A, Haverkamp H, Kobe C, et al. Reduced-intensity chemotherapy and PET-guided radiotherapy in patients with advanced stage Hodgkin's lymphoma (HD15 trial): A randomised, open-label, phase 3 non-inferiority trial. *Lancet (London, England).* May 12 2012;379(9828):1791–1799. doi:10.1016/S0140-6736(11)61940-5.
31. Johnson P, Federico M, Kirkwood A, et al. Adapted Treatment Guided by Interim PET-CT Scan in Advanced Hodgkin's Lymphoma. *New Eng J Med.* Jun 23 2016;374(25):2419–2429. doi:10.1056/NEJMoa1510093.
32. Connors JM, Jurczak W, Straus DJ, et al. Brentuximab Vedotin with Chemotherapy for Stage III or IV Hodgkin's Lymphoma. *New Eng J Med.* Jan 25 2018;378(4):331–344. doi:10.1056/NEJMoa1708984.
33. Straus DJ, Dlugosz-Danecka M, Alekseev S, et al. Brentuximab vedotin with chemotherapy for stage III/IV classical Hodgkin lymphoma: 3-year update of the ECHELON-1 study. *Blood.* Mar 5 2020;135(10):735–742. doi:10.1182/blood.2019003127.
34. Advani RH, Horning SJ, Hoppe RT, et al. Mature results of a phase II study of rituximab therapy for nodular lymphocyte-predominant Hodgkin lymphoma. *J Clin Oncol.* Mar 20 2014;32(9):912–918. doi:10.1200/JCO.2013.53.2069.
35. Schulz H, Rehwald U, Morschhauser F, et al. Rituximab in relapsed lymphocyte-predominant Hodgkin lymphoma: Long-term results of a phase 2 trial by the German Hodgkin Lymphoma Study

Group (GHSG). *Blood.* Jan 1 2008;111(1):109–111. doi:10.1182/blood-2007-03-078725.

36. Majhail NS, Weisdorf DJ, Defor TE, et al. Long-term results of autologous stem cell transplantation for primary refractory or relapsed Hodgkin's lymphoma. *Biol Blood Marrow Transplant.* Oct 2006;12(10):1065–1072. doi:10.1016/j.bbmt.2006.06.006.
37. Younes A, Gopal AK, Smith SE, et al. Results of a pivotal phase II study of brentuximab vedotin for patients with relapsed or refractory Hodgkin's lymphoma. *J Clin Oncol.* Jun 20 2012;30(18):2183–2189. doi:10.1200/JCO.2011.38.0410.
38. Chen R, Gopal AK, Smith SE, et al. Five-year survival and durability results of brentuximab vedotin in patients with relapsed or refractory Hodgkin lymphoma. *Blood.* 2016;128(12):1562–1566. doi:10.1182/blood-2016-02-699850.
39. Moskowitz CH, Nademanee A, Masszi T, et al. Brentuximab vedotin as consolidation therapy after autologous stem-cell transplantation in patients with Hodgkin's lymphoma at risk of relapse or progression (AETHERA): A randomised, double-blind, placebo-controlled, phase 3 trial. *Lancet (London, England).* May 9 2015;385(9980):1853–1862. doi:10.1016/s0140-6736(15)60165-9.
40. Ansell SM, Lesokhin AM, Borrello I, et al. PD-1 blockade with nivolumab in relapsed or refractory Hodgkin's lymphoma. *New England J Med.* Jan 22 2015;372(4):311–319. doi:10.1056/NEJMoa1411087.
41. Younes A, Santoro A, Shipp M, et al. Nivolumab for classical Hodgkin's lymphoma after failure of both autologous stem-cell transplantation and brentuximab vedotin: A multicentre, multicohort, single-arm phase 2 trial. *The Lancet Oncology.* Sep 2016;17(9):1283–1294. doi:10.1016/s1470-2045(16)30167-x.
42. Armand P, Shipp MA, Ribrag V, et al. Programmed death-1 blockade with pembrolizumab in patients with classical Hodgkin lymphoma after brentuximab vedotin failure. *J Clin Oncol.* Nov 1 2016;34(31):3733–3739. doi:10.1200/JCO.2016.67.3467.
43. Chen R, Zinzani PL, Fanale MA, et al. Phase II study of the efficacy and safety of pembrolizumab for relapsed/refractory classic Hodgkin lymphoma. *J Clin Oncol.* Jul 1 2017;35(19):2125–2132. doi:10.1200/JCO.2016.72.1316.
44. Herbaux C, Gauthier J, Brice P, et al. Efficacy and tolerability of nivolumab after allogeneic transplantation for relapsed Hodgkin lymphoma. *Blood.* May 4 2017;129(18):2471–2478. doi:10.1182/blood-2016-11-749556.
45. Hodgson DC. Late effects in the era of modern therapy for Hodgkin lymphoma. *Hematology American Society of Hematology Education Program.* 2011;2011:323–329. doi:10.1182/asheducation-2011.1.323.
46. Abramson JS. Non-Hodgkin's Lymphoma. In: Niederhuber JE, Armitage JO, Doroshow JH, Kastan MB, Tepper JE, eds. *Abeloff's Clinical Oncology.* 6th ed. Churchill Livingstone; 2019.
47. *WHO Classification of Tumours of Haematopoietic and Lymphoid Tissues.* 4th ed. Vol. 2. WHO Classification of Tumours. International Agency for Research on Cancer; 2008.
48. Harris NL, Jaffe ES, Diebold J, et al. World Health Organization classification of neoplastic diseases of the hematopoietic and lymphoid tissues: Report of the Clinical Advisory Committee meeting-Airlie House, Virginia, November 1997. *J Clin Oncol.* Dec 1999;17(12):3835–3849. doi:10.1200/JCO.1999.17.12.3835.
49. National Comprehensive Cancer Network. B-Cell Lymphomas (Version 4.2021). Accessed 30 August 2021, https://www.nccn.org/professionals/physician_gls/pdf/b-cell.pdf.
50. Cheson BD, Fisher RI, Barrington SF, et al. Recommendations for initial evaluation, staging, and response assessment of Hodgkin and non-Hodgkin lymphoma: The Lugano Classification. *J Clin Oncol.* 2014;32(27):3059–3067. doi:10.1200/jco.2013.54.8800.
51. Vercellino L, Cottereau AS, Casasnovas O, et al. High total metabolic tumor volume at baseline predicts survival independent of response to therapy. *Blood.* Apr 16 2020;135(16):1396–1405. doi:10.1182/blood.2019003526.
52. International Non-Hodgkin's Lymphoma Prognostic Factors Project. A predictive model for aggressive non-Hodgkin's lymphoma. *New England J Med.* Sep 30 1993;329(14):987–94. doi:10.1056/NEJM199309303291402.
53. Zhou Z, Sehn LH, Rademaker AW, et al. An enhanced International Prognostic Index (NCCN-IPI) for patients with diffuse large B-cell lymphoma treated in the rituximab era. *Blood.* 2013;123(6):837–842. doi:10.1182/blood-2013-09-524108.
54. Solal-Celigny P, Roy P, Colombat P, et al. Follicular lymphoma international prognostic index. *Blood.* Sep 1 2004;104(5):1258–1265. doi:10.1182/blood-2003-12-4434.
55. Federico M, Bellei M, Marcheselli L, et al. Follicular lymphoma international prognostic index 2: A new prognostic index for follicular lymphoma developed by the international follicular lymphoma prognostic factor project. *J Clin Oncol.* Sep 20 2009;27(27):4555–4562. doi:10.1200/JCO.2008.21.3991.
56. Nowakowski GS, Czuczman MS. ABC, GCB, and double-hit diffuse large B-cell lymphoma: Does subtype make a difference in therapy selection? *Am Soc Clin Oncol Educ Book.* 2015;35:e449–e457. doi:10.14694/EdBook_AM.2015.35.e449.
57. Sehn LH, Salles G. Diffuse large B-cell lymphoma. *New England J Med.* Mar 4 2021;384(9):842–858. doi:10.1056/NEJMra2027612.
58. Lenz G, Wright G, Dave SS, et al. Stromal gene signatures in large-B-cell lymphomas. *New England J Med.* Nov 27 2008;359(22):2313–2323. doi:10.1056/NEJMoa0802885.
59. Green TM, Young KH, Visco C, et al. Immunohistochemical double-hit score is a strong predictor of outcome in patients with diffuse large B-cell lymphoma treated with rituximab plus cyclophosphamide, doxorubicin, vincristine, and prednisone. *J Clin Oncol.* Oct 1 2012;30(28):3460–7. doi:10.1200/JCO.2011.41.4342.
60. Riedell PA, Smith SM. Double hit and double expressors in lymphoma: Definition and treatment. *Cancer.* 2018;doi:10.1002/cncr.31646.
61. Carbone A, Roulland S, Gloghini A, et al. Follicular lymphoma. *Nat Rev Dis Primers.* Dec 12 2019;5(1):83. doi:10.1038/s41572-019-0132-x.
62. Maloney DG. Anti-CD20 antibody therapy for B-cell lymphomas. *New England J Med.* May 24 2012;366(21):2008–2016. doi:10.1056/NEJMct1114348.
63. The Non-Hodgkin's Lymphoma Classification Project. A clinical evaluation of the International Lymphoma Study Group Classification of Non-Hodgkin's Lymphoma. *Blood.* 1997;89:3909–3918.
64. Bernstein SH, Burack WR. The incidence, natural history, biology, and treatment of transformed lymphomas. *Hematology Am Soc Hematol Educ Program.* 2009:532–541. doi:10.1182/asheducation-2009.1.532.
65. Fisher RI, LeBlanc M, Press OW, Maloney DG, Unger JM, Miller TP. New treatment options have changed the survival of patients with follicular lymphoma. *J Clin Oncol.* Nov 20 2005;23(33):8447–8452. doi:10.1200/JCO.2005.03.1674.
66. Sarkozy C, Maurer MJ, Link BK, et al. Cause of death in follicular lymphoma in the first decade of the rituximab era: A pooled analysis of French and US Cohorts. *J Clin Oncol.* Jan 10 2019;37(2):144–152. doi:10.1200/JCO.18.00400.
67. Armitage JO, Mauch PM, Harris NL, Coiggier B, Dalla-Favera R. *Non-Hodgkin Lymphomas.* 2nd ed. Wolters Kluwer/Lippincott Williams & Wilkins Health; 2010.
68. Armitage JO, Longo DL. Is watch and wait still acceptable for patients with low-grade follicular lymphoma? *Blood.* Jun 9 2016;127(23):2804–2808. doi:10.1182/blood-2015-11-632745.
69. Ardeshna KM, Qian W, Smith P, et al. Rituximab versus a watch-and-wait approach in patients with advanced-stage, asymptomatic, non-bulky follicular lymphoma: An open-label randomised phase 3 trial. *The Lancet Oncology.* 2014;15(4):424–435. doi:10.1016/s1470-2045(14)70027-0.
70. McLaughlin P, Grillo-López AJ, Link BK, et al. Rituximab chimeric anti-CD20 monoclonal antibody therapy for relapsed indolent lymphoma: Half of patients respond to a four-dose treatment program. *J Clin Oncol.* 1998;16(8):2825–2833. doi:10.1200/jco.1998.16.8.2825.
71. Friedberg JW, Taylor MD, Cerhan JR, et al. Follicular lymphoma in the United States: First report of the national LymphoCare study. *J Clin Oncol.* Mar 10 2009;27(8):1202–1208. doi:10.1200/JCO.2008.18.1495.
72. Hochster H, Weller E, Gascoyne RD, et al. Maintenance rituximab after cyclophosphamide, vincristine, and prednisone prolongs progression-free survival in advanced indolent lymphoma: Results of the randomized phase III ECOG1496 Study. *J Clin Oncol.* Apr 1 2009;27(10):1607–1614. doi:10.1200/JCO.2008.17.1561.
73. Barta SK, Li H, Hochster HS, et al. Randomized phase 3 study in low-grade lymphoma comparing maintenance anti-CD20 antibody with observation after induction therapy: A trial of the ECOG-ACRIN Cancer Research Group (E1496). *Cancer.* Oct 2016;122(19):2996–3004. doi:10.1002/cncr.30137.
74. Forstpointner R, Unterhalt M, Dreyling M, et al. Maintenance therapy with rituximab leads to a significant prolongation of response duration after salvage therapy with a combination of rituximab, fludarabine, cyclophosphamide, and mitoxantrone (R-FCM) in patients with recurring and refractory follicular and mantle cell lymphomas: Results of a prospective randomized study of the German Low Grade Lymphoma Study Group (GLSG). *Blood.* Dec 15 2006;108(13):4003–4008. doi:10.1182/blood-2006-04-016725.
75. van Oers MH, Van Glabbeke M, Giurgea L, et al. Rituximab maintenance treatment of relapsed/resistant follicular non-Hodgkin's lymphoma: Long-term outcome of the EORTC 20981 phase III

randomized intergroup study. *J Clin Oncol.* Jun 10 2010;28(17):2853–2858. doi:10.1200/JCO.2009.26.5827.
76. Davies A, Merli F, Mihaljević B, et al. Efficacy and safety of subcutaneous rituximab versus intravenous rituximab for first-line treatment of follicular lymphoma (SABRINA): A randomised, open-label, phase 3 trial. *Lancet Haematol.* 2017;4(6):e272–e282. doi:10.1016/s2352-3026(17)30078-9.
77. Lugtenburg P, Avivi I, Berenschot H, et al. Efficacy and safety of subcutaneous and intravenous rituximab plus cyclophosphamide, doxorubicin, vincristine, and prednisone in first-line diffuse large B-cell lymphoma: The randomized MabEase study. *Haematologica.* Nov 2017;102(11):1913–1922. doi:10.3324/haematol.2017.173583.
78. Schulz H, Bohlius JF, Trelle S, et al. Immunochemotherapy with rituximab and overall survival in patients with indolent or mantle cell lymphoma: A systematic review and meta-analysis. *J Natl Cancer Inst.* May 2 2007;99(9):706–714. doi:10.1093/jnci/djk152.
79. Rummel MJ, Gregory SA. Bendamustine's emerging role in the management of lymphoid malignancies. *Semin Hematol.* Apr 2011;48(Suppl 1):S24–S36. doi:10.1053/j.seminhematol.2011.03.004.
80. Rummel MJ, Niederle N, Maschmeyer G, et al. Bendamustine plus rituximab versus CHOP plus rituximab as first-line treatment for patients with indolent and mantle-cell lymphomas: An open-label, multicentre, randomised, phase 3 non-inferiority trial. *Lancet (London, England).* 2013;381(9873):1203–1210. doi:10.1016/s0140-6736(12)61763-2.
81. Flinn IW, van der Jagt R, Kahl BS, et al. Randomized trial of bendamustine-rituximab or R-CHOP/R-CVP in first-line treatment of indolent NHL or MCL: The BRIGHT study. *Blood.* 2014;123(19):2944–2952. doi:10.1182/blood-2013-11-531327.
82. Flinn IW, van der Jagt R, Kahl B, et al. First-line treatment of patients with indolent non-Hodgkin lymphoma or mantle-cell lymphoma with bendamustine plus rituximab versus R-CHOP or R-CVP: Results of the BRIGHT 5-year follow-up study. *J Clin Oncol.* Apr 20 2019;37(12):984–991. doi:10.1200/JCO.18.00605.
83. Hiddemann W, Barbui AM, Canales MA, et al. Immunochemotherapy with obinutuzumab or rituximab for previously untreated follicular lymphoma in the GALLIUM Study: Influence of chemotherapy on efficacy and safety. *J Clin Oncol.* Aug 10 2018;36(23):2395–2404. doi:10.1200/JCO.2017.76.8960.
84. Marcus R, Davies A, Ando K, et al. Obinutuzumab for the first-line treatment of follicular lymphoma. *New England J Med.* 2017;377(14):1331–1344. doi:10.1056/NEJMoa1614598.
85. Cheson BD, Chua N, Mayer J, et al. Overall survival benefit in patients with rituximab-refractory indolent non-Hodgkin lymphoma who received obinutuzumab plus bendamustine induction and obinutuzumab maintenance in the GADOLIN study. *J Clin Oncol.* Aug 1 2018;36(22):2259–2266. doi:10.1200/JCO.2017.76.3656.
86. Sehn LH, Chua N, Mayer J, et al. Obinutuzumab plus bendamustine versus bendamustine monotherapy in patients with rituximab-refractory indolent non-Hodgkin lymphoma (GADOLIN): A randomised, controlled, open-label, multicentre, phase 3 trial. *The Lancet Oncology.* 2016;17(8):1081–1093. doi:10.1016/s1470-2045(16)30097-3.
87. Gandhi AK, Kang J, Havens CG, et al. Immunomodulatory agents lenalidomide and pomalidomide co-stimulate T cells by inducing degradation of T cell repressors Ikaros and Aiolos via modulation of the E3 ubiquitin ligase complex CRL4(CRBN.). *Br J Haematol.* Mar 2014;164(6):811–821. doi:10.1111/bjh.12708.
88. Morschhauser F, Fowler NH, Feugier P, et al. Rituximab plus lenalidomide in advanced untreated follicular lymphoma. *New England J Med.* 2018;379(10):934–947. doi:10.1056/NEJMoa1805104.
89. Leonard JP, Jung S-H, Johnson J, et al. Randomized trial of lenalidomide alone versus lenalidomide plus rituximab in patients with recurrent follicular lymphoma: CALGB 50401 (Alliance). *J Clin Oncol.* 2015;33(31):3635–3640. doi:10.1200/jco.2014.59.9258.
90. Hohloch K. Radioimmunotherapy of lymphoma: An underestimated therapy option. *The Lancet Haematology.* 2017;4(1):e6–e7. doi:10.1016/s2352-3026(16)30188-0.
91. Gopal AK, Kahl BS, Flowers CR, et al. Idelalisib is effective in patients with high-risk follicular lymphoma and early relapse after initial chemoimmunotherapy. *Blood.* Jun 1 2017;129(22):3037–3039. doi:10.1182/blood-2016-12-757740.
92. Gopal AK, Kahl BS, de Vos S, et al. PI3Kdelta inhibition by idelalisib in patients with relapsed indolent lymphoma. *New England J Med.* Mar 13 2014;370(11):1008–1018. doi:10.1056/NEJMoa1314583.
93. Dreyling M, Santoro A, Mollica L, et al. Phosphatidylinositol 3-kinase inhibition by copanlisib in relapsed or refractory indolent lymphoma. *J Clin Oncol.* 2017;35(35):3898–3905. doi:10.1200/jco.2017.75.4648.
94. Zinzani P, Wagner-Johnston N, Miller C, et al. DYNAMO: A phase II study demonstrating the clinical activity of duvelisib in patients with double-refractory indolent non-Hodgkin lymphoma. *Hematol Oncol.* 2017;35:69–70. doi:10.1002/hon.2437_57.
95. Fowler NH, Samaniego F, Jurczak W, et al. Umbralisib, a Dual PI3Kdelta/CK1epsilon inhibitor in patients with relapsed or refractory indolent lymphoma. *J Clin Oncol.* May 20 2021;39(15):1609–1618. doi:10.1200/JCO.20.03433.
96. Morschhauser F, Tilly H, Chaidos A, et al. Tazemetostat for patients with relapsed or refractory follicular lymphoma: An open-label, single-arm, multicentre, phase 2 trial. *Lancet Oncol.* 2020;21(11):1433–1442. doi:10.1016/s1470-2045(20)30441-1.
97. Jacobson C, Chavez JC, Sehgal AR, et al. Primary analysis of zuma-5: A phase 2 study of axicabtagene ciloleucel (Axi-Cel) in patients with relapsed/refractory (R/R) indolent non-Hodgkin lymphoma (iNHL). *Blood.* 2020;136(Suppl 1):40–41. doi:10.1182/blood-2020-136834.
98. Kuruvilla J. The role of autologous and allogeneic stem cell transplantation in the management of indolent B-cell lymphoma. *Blood.* 2016;127(17):2093–2100. doi:10.1182/blood-2015-11-624320.
99. Evens AM, Vanderplas A, LaCasce AS, et al. Stem cell transplantation for follicular lymphoma relapsed/refractory after prior rituximab: A comprehensive analysis from the NCCN lymphoma outcomes project. *Cancer.* Oct 15 2013;119(20):3662–3671. doi:10.1002/cncr.28243.
100. Oh DH, Li H, Duan Q, et al. Quantifying benefit of autologous transplantation for relapsed follicular lymphoma patients via instrumental variable analysis. *Biol Blood Marrow Transplant.* 2016;22(5):941–948. doi:10.1016/j.bbmt.2016.01.015.
101. Miller TP, Dahlberg S, Cassady JR, et al. Chemotherapy alone compared with chemotherapy plus radiotherapy for localized intermediate- and high-grade non-Hodgkin's lymphoma. *New England J Med.* Jul 2 1998;339(1):21–26. doi:10.1056/NEJM199807023390104.
102. Odejide OO, Cronin AM, Davidoff AJ, LaCasce AS, Abel GA. Limited stage diffuse large B-cell lymphoma: Comparative effectiveness of treatment strategies in a large cohort of elderly patients. *Leukemia Lymphoma.* 2014;56(3):716–724. doi:10.3109/10428194.2014.930853.
103. McKelvey EM, Gottlieb JA, Wilson HE, et al. Hydroxyldaunomycin (Adriamycin) combination chemotherapy in malignant lymphoma. *Cancer.* 1976;38(4):1484–1493.
104. Jones SE, Grozea PN, Metz EN, et al. Superiority of adriamycin-containing combination chemotherapy in the treatment of diffuse lymphoma: A Southwest Oncology Group study. *Cancer.* 1979;43(2):417–425.
105. Fisher RI, Gaynor ER, Dahlberg S, et al. Comparison of a Standard Regimen (CHOP) with three intensive chemotherapy regimens for advanced non-Hodgkin's lymphoma. *New England J Med.* 1993;328(14):1002–1006. doi:10.1056/nejm199304083281404.
106. Coiffier B, Thieblemont C, Van Den Neste E, et al. Long-term outcome of patients in the LNH-98.5 trial, the first randomized study comparing rituximab-CHOP to standard CHOP chemotherapy in DLBCL patients: A study by the Groupe d'Etudes des Lymphomes de l'Adulte. *Blood.* 2010;116(12):2040–2045. doi:10.1182/blood-2010-03-276246.
107. Pfreundschuh M, Trümper L, Österborg A, et al. CHOP-like chemotherapy plus rituximab versus CHOP-like chemotherapy alone in young patients with good-prognosis diffuse large-B-cell lymphoma: A randomised controlled trial by the MabThera International Trial (MInT) Group. *Lancet Oncol.* 2006;7(5):379–391. doi:10.1016/s1470-2045(06)70664-7.
108. Pfreundschuh M, Kuhnt E, Trümper L, et al. CHOP-like chemotherapy with or without rituximab in young patients with good-prognosis diffuse large-B-cell lymphoma: 6-year results of an open-label randomised study of the MabThera International Trial (MInT) Group. *Lancet Oncol.* 2011;12(11):1013–1022. doi:10.1016/s1470-2045(11)70235-2.
109. Pfreundschuh M. Two-weekly or 3-weekly CHOP chemotherapy with or without etoposide for the treatment of young patients with good-prognosis (normal LDH) aggressive lymphomas: Results of the NHL-B1 trial of the DSHNHL. *Blood.* 2004;104(3):626–633. doi:10.1182/blood-2003-06-2094.
110. Cunningham D, Hawkes EA, Jack A, et al. Rituximab plus cyclophosphamide, doxorubicin, vincristine, and prednisolone in patients with newly diagnosed diffuse large B-cell non-Hodgkin lymphoma: A phase 3 comparison of dose intensification with 14-day versus 21-day cycles. *Lancet (London, England).* 2013;381(9880):1817–1826. doi:10.1016/s0140-6736(13)60313-x.
111. Delarue R, Tilly H, Mounier N, et al. Dose-dense rituximab-CHOP compared with standard rituximab-CHOP in elderly patients with diffuse large B-cell lymphoma (the LNH03-6B study): A randomised

phase 3 trial. *Lancet Oncol.* 2013;14(6):525–533. doi:10.1016/s1470-2045(13)70122-0.

112. Morrison VA, Hamlin P, Soubeyran P, et al. Approach to therapy of diffuse large B-cell lymphoma in the elderly: The International Society of Geriatric Oncology (SIOG) expert position commentary. *Ann Oncol.* Jun 2015;26(6):1058–1068. doi:10.1093/annonc/mdv018.
113. Habermann TM, Weller EA, Morrison VA, et al. Rituximab-CHOP versus CHOP alone or with maintenance rituximab in older patients with diffuse large B-cell lymphoma. *J Clin Oncol.* Jul 1 2006;24(19):3121–7. doi:10.1200/JCO.2005.05.1003.
114. Czuczman MS, Grillo-Lopez AJ, White CA, et al. Treatment of patients with low-grade B-cell lymphoma with the combination of chimeric anti-CD20 monoclonal antibody and CHOP chemotherapy. *J Clin Oncol.* Jan 1999;17(1):268–276. doi:10.1200/JCO.1999.17.1.268.
115. Thieblemont C, Tilly H, Gomes da Silva M, et al. Lenalidomide maintenance compared with placebo in responding elderly patients with diffuse large B-cell lymphoma treated with first-line rituximab plus cyclophosphamide, doxorubicin, vincristine, and prednisone. *J Clin Oncol.* Aug 1 2017;35(22):2473–2481. doi:10.1200/JCO.2017.72.6984.
116. Crump M, Neelapu SS, Farooq U, et al. Outcomes in refractory diffuse large B-cell lymphoma: Results from the international SCHOLAR-1 study. *Blood.* Oct 19 2017;130(16):1800–1808. doi:10.1182/blood-2017-03-769620.
117. Crump M, Kuruvilla J, Couban S, et al. Randomized comparison of gemcitabine, dexamethasone, and cisplatin versus dexamethasone, cytarabine, and cisplatin chemotherapy before autologous stem-cell transplantation for relapsed and refractory aggressive lymphomas: NCIC-CTG LY.12. *J Clin Oncol.* Nov 1 2014;32(31):3490–6. doi:10.1200/JCO.2013.53.9593.
118. Gisselbrecht C, Glass B, Mounier N, et al. Salvage regimens with autologous transplantation for relapsed large B-cell lymphoma in the rituximab era. *J Clin Oncol.* Sep 20 2010;28(27):4184–4190. doi:10.1200/JCO.2010.28.1618.
119. Philip T, Guglielmi C, Hagenbeek A, et al. Autologous bone marrow transplantation as compared with salvage chemotherapy in relapses of chemotherapy-sensitive non-Hodgkin's lymphoma. *New England J Med.* Dec 7 1995;333(23):1540–1545. doi:10.1056/NEJM199512073332305.
120. Dai H, Wang Y, Lu X, Han W. Chimeric antigen receptors modified t-cells for cancer therapy. *J Natl Cancer Inst.* Jul 2016;108(7). doi:10.1093/jnci/djv439.
121. Schuster SJ, Bishop MR, Tam CS, et al. Tisagenlecleucel in adult relapsed or refractory diffuse large B-cell lymphoma. *New England J Med.* Jan 3 2019;380(1):45–56. doi:10.1056/NEJMoa1804980.
122. Locke FL, Ghobadi A, Jacobson CA, et al. Long-term safety and activity of axicabtagene ciloleucel in refractory large B-cell lymphoma (ZUMA-1): A single-arm, multicentre, phase 1–2 trial. *Lancet Oncol.* 2019;20(1):31–42. doi:10.1016/s1470-2045(18)30864-7.
123. Abramson JS, Palomba ML, Gordon LI, et al. Lisocabtagene maraleucel for patients with relapsed or refractory large B-cell lymphomas (TRANSCEND NHL 001): A multicentre seamless design study. *The Lancet.* 2020;396(10254):839–852. doi:10.1016/s0140-6736(20)31366-0.
124. Neelapu SS, Locke FL, Bartlett NL, et al. Axicabtagene ciloleucel CAR T-cell therapy in refractory large B-cell lymphoma. *New England J Med.* Dec 28 2017;377(26):2531–2544. doi:10.1056/NEJMoa1707447.
125. Schuster SJ, Bishop MR, Tam CS, et al. Primary analysis of Juliet: A global, pivotal, phase 2 trial of CTL019 in adult patients with relapsed or refractory diffuse large B-cell lymphoma. Abstract. *Blood.* 2017;130(Suppl 1):577.
126. Neelapu SS, Tummala S, Kebriaei P, et al. Chimeric antigen receptor T-cell therapy: Assessment and management of toxicities. *Nat Rev Clin Oncol.* Jan 2018;15(1):47–62. doi:10.1038/nrclinonc.2017.148.
127. Massaro F, Stepanishyna Y, Manni M, et al. Long-term results of the MCL01 phase II trial of rituximab plus HyperCVAD alternating with high-dose cytarabine and methotrexate for the initial treatment of patients with mantle cell lymphoma. *Br J Haematol.* Mar 2021;192(6):1011–1014. doi:10.1111/bjh.16714.
128. Delarue R, Haioun C, Ribrag V, et al. CHOP and DHAP plus rituximab followed by autologous stem cell transplantation in mantle cell lymphoma: A phase 2 study from the Groupe d'Etude des Lymphomes de l'Adulte. *Blood.* Jan 3 2013;121(1):48–53. doi:10.1182/blood-2011-09-370320.
129. Ruan J, Martin P, Christos P, et al. Five-year follow-up of lenalidomide plus rituximab as initial treatment of mantle cell lymphoma. *Blood.* Nov 8 2018;132(19):2016–2025. doi:10.1182/blood-2018-07-859769.
130. Robak T, Huang H, Jin J, et al. Bortezomib-based therapy for newly diagnosed Mantle-cell lymphoma. *New England J Med.* 2015;372(10):944–953. doi:10.1056/NEJMoa1412096.
131. Graf SA, Stevenson PA, Holmberg LA, et al. Maintenance rituximab after autologous stem cell transplantation in patients with mantle cell lymphoma. *Ann Oncol.* 2015;26(11):2323–2328. doi:10.1093/annonc/mdv364.
132. Le Gouill S, Thieblemont C, Oberic L, et al. Rituximab after autologous stem-cell transplantation in mantle-cell lymphoma. *New England J Med.* Sep 28 2017;377(13):1250–1260. doi:10.1056/NEJMoa1701769.
133. Ladetto M, Cortelazzo S, Ferrero S, et al. Lenalidomide maintenance after autologous haematopoietic stem-cell transplantation in mantle cell lymphoma: Results of a Fondazione Italiana Linfomi (FIL) multicentre, randomised, phase 3 trial. *Lancet Haematol.* 2021;8(1):e34–e44. doi:10.1016/s2352-3026(20)30358-6.
134. Hoster E, Kluin-Nelemans H, Hermine O, et al. Rituximab maintenance after first-line immunochemotherapy in Mantle cell lymphoma: Long-term follow-up of the randomized European MCL Elderly Trial. Abstract. *Blood.* 2017;130(Suppl 1):153.
135. Rule S, Jurczak W, Jerkeman M, et al. Ibrutinib versus temsirolimus: 3-year follow-up of patients with previously treated mantle cell lymphoma from the phase 3, international, randomized, open-label RAY study. *Leukemia.* 2018;32(8):1799–1803. doi:10.1038/s41375-018-0023-2.
136. Jain P, Romaguera J, Srour SA, et al. Four-year follow-up of a single arm, phase II clinical trial of ibrutinib with rituximab (IR) in patients with relapsed/refractory mantle cell lymphoma (MCL). *Br J Haematol.* May 22 2018;doi:10.1111/bjh.15411.
137. Tam CS, Opat S, Simpson D, et al. Zanubrutinib for the treatment of relapsed or refractory mantle cell lymphoma. *Blood Adv.* Jun 22 2021;5(12):2577–2585. doi:10.1182/bloodadvances.2020004074.
138. Wang M, Munoz J, Goy A, et al. KTE-X19 CAR T-cell therapy in relapsed or refractory Mantle-cell lymphoma. *New England J Med.* Apr 2 2020;382(14):1331–1342. doi:10.1056/NEJMoa1914347.

156

Ovarian Cancer

Grace A. Martin and Judith A. Smith

KEY CONCEPTS

1. Ovarian cancer is denoted "the silent killer" because of the nonspecific signs and symptoms that contribute to the delay in diagnosis. The few patients who present with disease still confined to the ovary will have a 5-year survival rate greater than 90%, but most patients present with advanced disease and have a 5-year survival rate around 30%.
2. Ovarian cancer is a sporadic disease with less than 20% of cases of ovarian cancer attributed to heredity. However, a history of two or more first-degree relatives with ovarian cancer increases an individual's risk of developing ovarian cancer by greater than 50%.
3. As there are currently no effective screening tools for early detection of ovarian cancer, considerable education efforts have been made to identify patients with the persistence (ie, greater than 2 weeks) of nonspecific presenting symptoms of ovarian cancer including: abdominal pressure/pain, difficulty eating or feeling full quickly, urinary urgency/frequency, change in bowel habits, or unexplained vaginal bleeding.
4. Serum cancer antigen 125 (CA-125) is a nonspecific antigen used as a tumor marker for diagnosing and monitoring epithelial ovarian carcinoma. If CA-125 is positive at the time of diagnosis, changes in CA-125 levels correlate with disease response and progression.
5. Although most patients will achieve a complete response to initial treatment, more than 50% of patients will have recurrence within the first 2 years. If recurrence occurs less than 6 months after completion of chemotherapy, the tumor is defined to be platinum-resistant. The antitumor activities of second-line chemotherapy regimens are similar, and the choice of treatment for recurrent platinum-resistant ovarian cancer depends on residual toxicities, physician preference, and patient convenience. Participation in a clinical trial is also a reasonable option for these patients.
6. Ovarian cancer is staged surgically with the International Federation of Gynecology and Obstetrics (FIGO) staging algorithm. Tumor-debulking and total abdominal hysterectomy–bilateral oophorectomy surgery are the primary surgical interventions for ovarian cancer. After the completion of the staging and primary surgical treatment, the current standard of care is six cycles of a taxane/platinum-containing chemotherapy regimen.
7. Neoadjuvant chemotherapy is intended to reduce tumor burden in preparation for surgery and should be used in patients who are poor surgical candidates because of comorbidities or bulky tumors. The goal of neoadjuvant chemotherapy is to improve the likelihood of optimal tumor debulking.
8. A platinum-containing doublet chemotherapy regimen is the standard of care for the first recurrence of platinum-sensitive ovarian cancer.
9. Despite recent advances, enrollment in an investigational study is still the primary treatment recommendation for patients with recurrent platinum-resistant ovarian cancer.
10. Poly(adenosine diphosphate [ADP]-ribose) polymerase (PARP) inhibitors cause double-stranded DNA breaks that cannot be repaired in cancer cells with homologous recombination deficiency, such as those with *BRCA1/2* mutations.
11. Patients receiving a platinum or taxane-containing regimen should be monitored for signs of hypersensitivity or infusion-related reactions.

BEYOND THE BOOK

Pair up with a classmate and create flashcards of treatment regimens for ovarian cancer on one side and the appropriate line of therapy (first-line following primary surgery, consolidation/maintenance therapy following a complete response with first-line therapy, treatment for relapse greater than 6 months from last platinum therapy, treatment for relapse less than 6 months from last platinum therapy) and common adverse drug reactions of that treatment on the other side. Present your partner with the treatment and have them recommend a patient scenario when that would be an appropriate therapy based on the line of treatment and describe the adverse drug reactions of that regimen. Discuss supportive care interventions to prevent or minimize common adverse drug reactions from the chemotherapy. Compare and contrast your recommendations and discuss other possible situations when the treatment may be considered or any patient-specific factors that may cause you to consider an alternative therapy or recommend dose modifications (eg, avoid bevacizumab in a patient with recent bowel surgery).

INTRODUCTION

1 Ovarian cancer is a gynecologic cancer that usually arises from the disruption or mutations in the epithelium of the ovary. It is associated with the highest mortality among the gynecologic cancers,

primarily because most patients present with advanced disease. Ovarian cancer is denoted "the silent killer" because of the nonspecific signs and symptoms that often lead to a delayed diagnosis. Ovarian cancers often metastasize via the lymphatic and blood systems to the liver or lungs. Common complications of advanced and progressive ovarian cancer include ascites and small bowel obstruction. Patients who present with disease still confined to the ovary will have a 5-year survival rate greater than 90%, but most patients present with advanced disease and have a 5-year survival rate around 30%.[1] Primary treatment includes tumor-debulking surgery followed by six cycles of a taxane-platinum chemotherapy regimen. Although 70% of patients achieve an initial complete response to chemotherapy, most of these patients will have recurrence within the first 2 years from diagnosis.[2]

EPIDEMIOLOGY

In this chapter, the term "woman" is used to reflect the gender identified in previous research studies and other literature on ovarian cancer and to recognize the biological sex of individuals at birth. In doing so, we recognize that not all patients with ovarian cancer identify as females at the time of diagnosis and treatment of this condition. It is estimated that 19,880 new cases of ovarian cancer were diagnosed and 12,810 women died of the disease in 2022.[1] Unfortunately, despite clinical advances over the past two decades, the overall mortality rate for ovarian cancer is an estimated 60% and has not changed over the past two decades. Ovarian cancer is still associated with the highest mortality rate among the gynecologic cancers and is the fifth leading cause of cancer-related deaths in women. The high mortality rate is related to the insidious onset of nonspecific symptoms and the lack of adequate screening tools, which allows the disease to go undiagnosed until it has progressed beyond the pelvic cavity.

ETIOLOGY

As with many other cancers, the risk of ovarian cancer increases with increasing age. A woman's risk increases from 2.9 to 41.2 per 100,000 as their age advances from less than 40 to 75 years or more, and the median age at diagnosis is 63 years.[3] Most cases of ovarian cancer are diagnosed during the peri- and postmenopausal phase of individual's reproductive life span.

2 Heredity accounts for approximately 20% of ovarian cancer cases.[2] Family history of ovarian or breast cancer is an important risk factor in the development of ovarian cancer. If a first-degree relative has a diagnosis of ovarian cancer, the associated lifetime risk is increased by 50%. An individual's risk of ovarian cancer is increased by 10% if a first-degree relative has a diagnosis of breast cancer.[4] Risk is greatest in individuals with multiple family members with ovarian cancer and in those with family members who were diagnosed at an early age.[5]

Breast cancer activator gene 1 (*BRCA1*) and breast cancer activator gene 2 (*BRCA2*) are tumor suppressor genes thought to be involved in one or more pathways of DNA damage recognition and repair. The *BRCA1* gene is located on chromosome 17q12–21 and the *BRCA2* gene is located on chromosome 13q12–13. Both *BRCA1* and *BRCA2* mutations are associated with ovarian cancer. However, *BRCA1* is more prevalent and is associated with 90% of inherited and 10% of sporadic cases of ovarian cancer.[6] Patients with *BRCA1*-associated ovarian cancer are usually considerably younger than patients with *BRCA2* mutations, with a mean age of 54 years.[6] Patients usually present with advanced stage at diagnosis, and the *BRCA1*-linked ovarian cancers are more aggressive tumors that typically are serous histology, moderate-to-high grade. As *BRCA1* and *BRCA2* are thought to be involved in DNA damage or repair, their mutations may be associated with an increased resistance of ovarian cancer cells to cytotoxic agents.

Hereditary breast and ovarian cancer syndrome is one of the two different forms of hereditary ovarian cancer that are associated with germline mutations in *BRCA1* and *BRCA2*. The hereditary nonpolyposis colorectal cancer or Lynch syndrome is a familial syndrome with germline mutations causing defects in enzymes involved in DNA mismatch repair, which is associated with 10% to 15% of hereditary ovarian cancer cases.[7] This syndrome is associated with mutations in DNA mismatch repair genes such as *MSH2, MLH1, PMS1*, and *PMS2* and leads to microsatellite instability.

Hormone exposure, specifically estrogen, and reproductive history is also associated with the risk of developing ovarian cancer. Conditions that increase the total number of ovulations in individual's reproductive history, such as nulliparity, early menarche, or late menopause, are associated with an increased risk for epithelial ovarian cancers.[7] Conversely, those conditions that limit ovulations are associated with a protective effect. Each time ovulation occurs, the ovarian epithelium is broken, followed by cellular repair. According to *incessant ovulation hypothesis*, the risk of mutations and, ultimately, cancer increases each time the ovarian epithelium undergoes cell repair.

Finally, ovarian cancer is associated with certain dietary, lifestyle, and environmental factors. A diet that is high in galactose, animal fat, and meat may increase the risk of ovarian cancer, whereas a vegetable-rich diet may decrease the risk of ovarian cancer.[5] Although controversial, exogenous factors such as asbestos and talcum powder use in the perineal area are also associated with an increased risk of ovarian cancer.[5] Obesity has also been associated with an increased risk of low-grade ovarian cancer in some studies.[5]

PATHOPHYSIOLOGY

Ovarian carcinomas can be separated into three major entities: epithelial carcinomas, germ cell tumors, and stromal carcinomas. Most ovarian tumors (85%-90%) are derived from the epithelial surface of the ovary.[2] The classification of common epithelial tumors has been developed by the World Health Organization and FIGO.[2] The nomenclature considers cell type, location of the tumor, and the degree of the malignancy, which ranges from benign tumors to tumors of low malignancy to invasive carcinomas. Epithelial tumors classified as low malignancy ("borderline malignancy") are characterized by epithelial papillae with atypical cell clusters, cellular stratification, nuclear atypia, and increased mitotic activity, and have a much better prognosis than those classified as invasive carcinomas. Malignant tumors are characterized by an infiltrative destructive growth pattern with malignant cells growing in a disorganized manner and dissection into stromal planes.

Invasive epithelial adenocarcinomas are characterized by histologic subtype and grade, which measures the degree of cellular differentiation. Although the histologic type of the tumor is not a significant prognostic factor, with the exception of clear cell, the histopathologic grade is an important prognostic factor. Undifferentiated tumors are associated with a poorer prognosis than those lesions that are well or moderately differentiated. A universal grading system for ovarian cancer was developed that combines mitotic score, nuclear atypia score, and architectural score based on the histologic pattern.[8]

The histologic subtypes of ovarian epithelial tumors include serous, mucinous, endometrioid, clear cell, Brenner tumors, mixed epithelial, and undifferentiated carcinomas.[2] High-grade serous carcinoma is the most common type of epithelial ovarian cancer and accounts for about 70% to 80% of cases.[9] The peak age of diagnosis ranges from 55 to 64 years with 63 years as the median age of diagnosis.[3] Endometrioid carcinomas are seen in individuals 40 to 50 years of age and comprise about 8% of ovarian carcinomas, of which about 6% are surface epithelial neoplasms.[10] Endometrioid tumors are usually diagnosed as stage I disease and have a better prognosis than tumors with serous histology. Mucinous carcinomas occur in individuals between 40 and 70 years of age and account for about 36% of all ovarian cancers. The overall prognosis for mucinous carcinoma is better than for serous carcinoma because most patients present with stage I disease. Clear cell carcinoma comprises about 3% of ovarian carcinomas in individuals, with a mean age of 57 years. Although clear cell carcinoma is the least common ovarian neoplasm, it is most commonly associated with paraneoplastic-related hypercalcemia.

Germ cell tumors of the ovary, including malignant teratoma and dysgerminomas, are rare, comprising about 2% to 3% of all ovarian cancers in Western countries with an increased incidence in Black and Asian individuals.[9] These tumors are highly curable and affect primarily young individuals. In contrast to epithelial tumors, about 60% to 70% of germ cell tumors are stage I at diagnosis, which is related to earlier detection and response to symptoms in this younger patient population.[9] Serum markers (human β-chorionic gonadotropin and α-fetoprotein) are helpful to confirm the diagnosis and monitor response to treatment.

Finally, ovarian sex cord-stromal tumors account for 7% of all ovarian cancers and tend to be diagnosed at an early stage.[9] Sex cord-stromal tumors are associated with hormonal effects, such as precocious puberty, amenorrhea, and postmenopausal bleeding. Because these tumors are rare, the optimal treatment of ovarian sex cord-stromal tumors is not clear. The current recommended standard of care is surgery followed by treatment with a platinum-based chemotherapy regimen.

Ovarian cancer is usually confined to the abdominal cavity, but can spread to the lung, liver, and, less commonly, the bone or brain. Direct extension, peritoneal seeding, lymphatic dissemination, or blood borne metastasis spreads disease. Lymphatic seeding is the most common pathway and frequently causes ascites.

SCREENING AND PREVENTION

Screening

3 Ovarian cancer is an uncommon disease with no known preinvasive component, which has made it difficult to detect early disease. In addition, the risk factors for developing ovarian cancer are not well understood, which also makes it difficult to identify a high-risk group of individuals. At the present time, there are no effective screening tools for early detection of ovarian cancer. However, considerable education efforts have been made to identify patients with the persistence of nonspecific presenting symptoms of ovarian cancer including abdominal pressure/pain, difficulty eating or feeling full quickly, urinary urgency/frequency, change in bowel habits, or unexplained vaginal bleeding.

Pelvic examinations are noninvasive and may be able to detect large tumors; however, routine pelvic examinations are not an effective screening tool and do not decrease overall mortality because pelvic examinations cannot detect minimal or microscopic disease.[11]

Transvaginal ultrasound (TVUS) creates an image of the ovary by releasing sound waves. It can be used to evaluate the size and shape and to detect the presence of cystic or solid masses or abdominal fluid. Transvaginal ultrasound can also evaluate blood flow within an ovarian mass. Transvaginal ultrasound is sensitive in identifying ovarian lesions and abnormalities, but its use as a routine screening test is limited by a lack of specificity and an inability to detect peritoneal cancer or cancer in normal-size ovaries.[11]

Serum CA-125 is a nonspecific inflammatory antigen that can be elevated in numerous conditions associated with inflammation in the abdominal cavity. CA-125 has been extensively studied as a potential tumor marker for ovarian cancer based on the observation that CA-125 levels in an individual without ovarian cancer tend to stay the same or decrease over time, whereas levels associated with malignancy tend to gradually increase over time.[11] However, CA-125 is a nonspecific test that can be elevated in a number of benign conditions, including other gynecologic conditions, such as endometriosis, and many nongynecologic conditions, such as diverticulitis and peptic ulcer disease. Because of these limitations, CA-125 levels are not recommended as a routine screening test for detection of ovarian cancer. Numerous other serologic markers such as carcinoembryonic antigen and lipid-associated sialic acid have been evaluated but cannot be recommended for routine screening for ovarian cancer.

The United States Preventive Services Task Force found fair evidence to support screening with CA-125 or TVUS and concluded that earlier detection would likely have a small effect, at best, on mortality from ovarian cancer.[12] Unfortunately, because of the low prevalence of ovarian cancer and the invasive nature of diagnostic testing after a positive screening test, the Task Force also found fair evidence that screening could likely lead to important harms. The United States Preventive Services Task Force concluded that the potential harms outweigh the potential benefits and recommended against any form of routine screening with CA-125 or TVUS for ovarian cancer for asymptomatic individuals who do not have a high-risk hereditary cancer syndrome.

In high-risk individuals, as defined by family history, most clinicians use a multimodality approach for ovarian cancer screening that includes an annual TVUS in combination with a CA-125 blood test every 6 months. Changes in CA-125 are monitored over time, and changes such as a persistent elevation or consistent increases in CA-125 levels in conjunction with TVUS abnormalities are evaluated further.

Prevention

It is difficult to make recommendations for prevention for the general population because ovarian cancer is a sporadic disease with no established risk factors. Noninvasive measures, such as chemoprevention, can decrease the risk of developing ovarian cancer. Ovulation itself is considered a potential insult to the ovarian epithelium, increasing its susceptibility to damage and, ultimately, to cancer. Interventions or reproductive conditions associated with decreasing the number of ovulations, including multiparity, may have a protective effect for the prevention of ovarian cancer. However, the more invasive prevention interventions, such as prophylactic surgery and genetic screening, should be reserved for those individuals identified to be at high risk based on their inherited risk for developing ovarian cancer.

Although a number of agents have been investigated as chemoprevention of ovarian cancer, including oral contraceptives, aspirin, nonsteroidal anti-inflammatory agents, and retinoids, none of these agents is currently accepted as a standard treatment for the prevention of ovarian cancer. Oral contraceptives may be considered for patients at high risk of ovarian cancer as they inhibit ovulation, which reduces the potential for damage to the ovarian epithelium. When taken for longer than 10 years, oral contraceptives decrease the relative risk to less than 0.4.[13] Because oral contraceptive use has been associated with an increased risk of breast cancer, individuals with a family history of breast cancer should carefully consider the use of oral contraceptives as chemoprevention of ovarian cancer, though modern oral contraceptives are far less likely to increase the risk of breast cancer than those used prior to 1975.[13]

Prophylactic Surgery

Prophylactic surgical interventions for the prevention of ovarian cancer are reserved for patients with a significant family history or known genetic mutations such as *BRCA1* and should be postponed until after childbearing is completed, preferably between the ages of 35 to 40 years.[14] The goal is to remove healthy, at-risk organs before any carcinogenic activity is initiated, ultimately reducing the risk of developing cancer. These surgeries include prophylactic oophorectomy or bilateral salpingo-oophorectomy and tubal ligation. These procedures cause surgical menopause, which can be associated with severe hot flashes, vaginal dryness, sexual dysfunction, and increased risk for development of osteoporosis and heart disease.

Because of the potential impact on quality of life and increased health risks, prophylactic surgery is not recommended as a general prevention intervention.

Although prophylactic surgical interventions are the most effective way to reduce the risk of developing ovarian cancer in high-risk populations, patients who choose to have a prophylactic oophorectomy/bilateral salpingo-oophorectomy need to be informed that complete protection is not guaranteed.[13-15] Although a 67% risk reduction has been shown, a potential 2% to 5% risk of primary peritoneal cancer remains.[15] Primary peritoneal cancers have identical histology of ovarian tumors with diffuse involvement of peritoneal surfaces. Primary peritoneal cancers can often result from "seeding" during the prophylactic surgery. It is recommended for peritoneal washings to be completed during the prophylactic surgery to check for the presence of tumor cells on peritoneal surfaces. If positive, then prophylactic surgery would change to staging and treatment surgery to determine extent of disease and remove any other possible lesions.

Tubal ligation is another procedure that can reduce the risk for developing ovarian cancer. In a case-control study, Narod and colleagues[16] reported that tubal ligation in *BRCA*-positive patients was associated with a 63% reduction in risk of developing ovarian cancer. However, it is not recommended as a sole procedure in prophylaxis. The mechanism for its protective effect is not clear, but it has been proposed that tubal ligation may limit exposure of the ovary to environmental carcinogens.

Genetic Screening

Genetic screening should be considered for all individuals who are suspected of carrying a BRCA mutation, based on family history or young age (less than 50 years old) at diagnosis and a high-grade serous tumor. Patients should be evaluated for the presence of genes such as *BRCA1*, *BRCA2*, or other genes such as those associated with hereditary nonpolyposis colorectal cancer or the hereditary breast ovarian cancer (hereditary breast and ovarian cancer syndrome) syndrome.[16] Prior to genetic screening, appropriate patient/family counseling and genetic counseling should be available to help individuals prepare and deal with the health and psychosocial implications of the genetic screening results.

CLINICAL PRESENTATION

Patients with early ovarian cancer are often asymptomatic and the ovarian mass is detected incidentally during an unrelated surgery, procedure, or imaging. Patients with ovarian cancer often present with nonspecific, vague symptoms such as abdominal bloating, pressure or pain, indigestion, or change in bowel movements.[2] These symptoms can easily be confused with symptoms of common benign gastrointestinal disorders. Patients will often not seek medical attention until these symptoms become unrelenting and bothersome, which allows the disease to progress undetected. Patients with advanced disease may report symptoms such as pain, abdominal distension, and ascites.[2]

Several groups have partnered together to educate individuals about early signs and symptoms of ovarian cancer. Goff and colleagues[17] developed a symptom index, based on a comparison of symptoms experienced in patients with ovarian cancer and a matched control group. Symptoms that were correlated with ovarian cancer include persistent or recurrent bloating, pelvic or abdominal pain, difficulty eating or feeling full quickly, and urinary symptoms (either urgency or frequency). The Gynecologic Cancer Foundation, Society of Gynecologic Oncologists, and American Cancer Society recommend that individuals who have any of those problems nearly every day for more than 2 weeks should see a gynecologist, especially if the symptoms are new and quite different from the usual state of health. Furthermore, healthcare professionals should keep ovarian cancer in the differential for patients presenting with these persistent symptoms.

The diagnostic workup for suspected ovarian cancer includes a careful physical examination including a Papanicolaou, or Pap, smear and a pelvic and rectovaginal examination.[18] The presence of a pelvic mass that is unilateral or bilateral, solid, irregular, fixed, or nodular is highly suggestive of ovarian cancer. Unfortunately, by the time a pelvic mass can be palpated on physical exam, the disease would have already advanced beyond the pelvic cavity. A detailed family history should be taken, especially noting the number and pattern of first-degree relatives with malignancies. All patients with suspected ovarian malignancies should be referred to a gynecologic oncologist for evaluation as survival is increased when primary assessment and surgery is performed by a specialist.[19]

4 A complete blood count, chemistry profile (including liver and renal function tests), and CA-125, carcinoembryonic antigen, or CEA, and cancer antigen 19-9, or CA19-9, levels should be performed. Although CA-125 is a nonspecific antigen, it is the best current tumor marker for epithelial ovarian carcinoma.[18] A normal CA-125 value is less than 35 units/mL (kU/L). If the CA-125 is elevated at the time of diagnosis, changes in CA-125 levels correlate with tumor burden. Rising CA-125 levels are often associated with disease progression, but CA-125 can be elevated in various other conditions such as different phases of the menstrual cycle, diverticulitis,

CLINICAL PRESENTATION Ovarian Cancer

General

- Ovarian cancer is sometimes referred to as "the silent killer" because of the vague nonspecific signs and symptoms that contribute to the delay in diagnosis.

Symptoms

- The patient may complain of abdominal discomfort, nausea, dyspepsia, flatulence, bloating, fullness, early satiety, urinary frequency, change in bowel function (diarrhea or constipation), weight change, and digestive disturbances.

Signs

- Abdominal or pelvic mass may be palpable.
- Lymphadenopathy may be present.
- Vaginal bleeding may be irregular.
- Patient may have signs of ascites (abdominal distension, shifting, and dullness to percussion—may present like "pregnant abdomen").

Laboratory Tests

- CA-125 may be elevated (normal level is <35 units/mL [kU/L]).
- Abnormalities in liver function tests may suggest hepatic involvement.
- Abnormalities in renal function tests may suggest compression of the renal system by the tumor.

endometriosis, as well as other nongynecologic cancers. When a patient presents with an abdominal mass, it is important to rule out other cancers in the abdominal cavity. Carcinoembryonic antigen and CA19–9 are markers for other gastrointestinal cancers and may be helpful in the differential diagnosis.

Other diagnostic tests should include a TVUS or abdominal ultrasonography, chest radiography, computed tomography, magnetic resonance imaging, or positron emission tomography scan. An upper gastrointestinal series, intravenous pyelogram, cystoscopy, proctoscopy, or barium enema is sometimes indicated to confirm diagnosis and extent of disease.

TREATMENT

Desired Outcomes

The goals of treatment of ovarian cancer depend upon the FIGO stage at diagnosis. While ideally "treatment for cure" is desired, it is important to set realistic expectations for the patient. Most patients will achieve a complete response to the initial multimodality treatment, but over 75% of these patients will have disease recurrence.[20] Although overall survival has not significantly changed for ovarian cancer patients, progression-free survival has improved, which translates to less time on chemotherapy and overall improvement in quality of life for these patients.

In patients who present with metastatic disease or are not surgical candidates, the goal of treatment is to alleviate symptoms and prolong survival as long as quality of life is acceptable. In the setting of recurrent platinum-resistant ovarian cancer, the treatment goal is also to alleviate symptoms and prolong survival as long as quality of life is acceptable.

General Approach

5 A multimodal approach that includes comprehensive surgery and chemotherapy is used for the initial treatment of ovarian cancer with curative intent. Although most patients will initially achieve a complete response, more than 50% will recur within the first 2 years.[21] A clinical complete response to treatment is defined as no evidence of disease by physical examination or diagnostic tests and a normal CA-125 level.

Chemotherapy regimens for ovarian cancer have evolved over the past several decades to the current standard of care for first-line treatment that includes a taxane- and platinum-based regimen. Certain subgroups of patients have a better or worse response to chemotherapy. The histologic subtype of the tumor is a prognostic factor; clear cell histology is more likely to be poorly differentiated, faster growing, and have intrinsic drug resistance.[2,9] However, the extent of residual disease, size larger than 1 cm, and tumor grade are better predictors of response to chemotherapy and overall survival.[2] In general, younger patients have a better performance status and tolerate chemotherapy better than older adult patients. For unknown reasons, white women tend to have a worse prognosis and response to therapy as compared with women of other ethnic backgrounds.[2]

In patients with recurrent ovarian cancer, the goals of treatment are to relieve symptoms such as pain or discomfort from ascites, slow disease progression, and prevent serious complications such as small bowel obstructions.

Surgery

Surgery is the primary treatment intervention for ovarian cancer.[22-24] Surgery may be curative for selected patients with limited stage IA disease. Primary surgical treatment includes a total abdominal hysterectomy with bilateral salpingo-oophorectomy (TAH/BSO), omentectomy, and lymph node dissection (Fig. 156-1).[22-24]

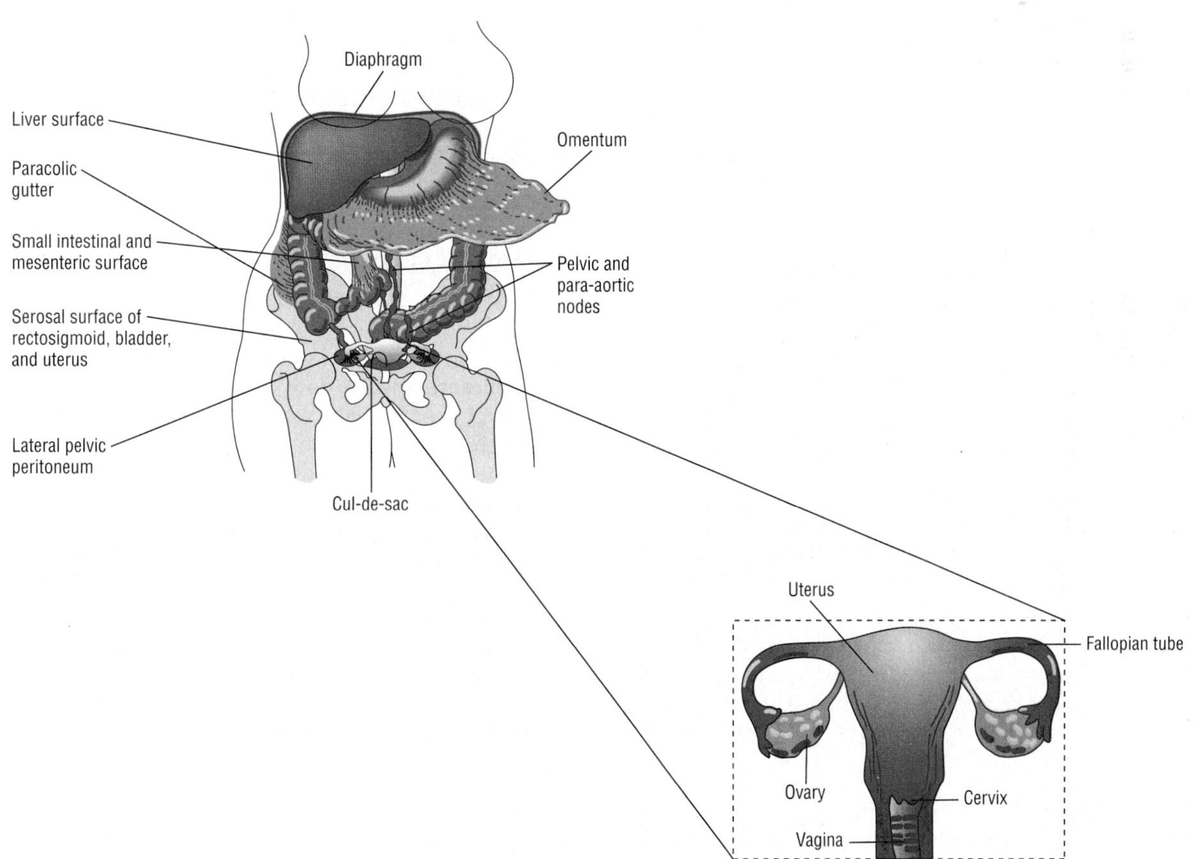

FIGURE 156-1 Staging laparotomy for ovarian cancer with diagram of female reproductive tract (uterus, fallopian tubes, ovaries, and vagina). Dashed line box outlines what is removed during the TAH/BSO. (*Data from References 22-24.*)

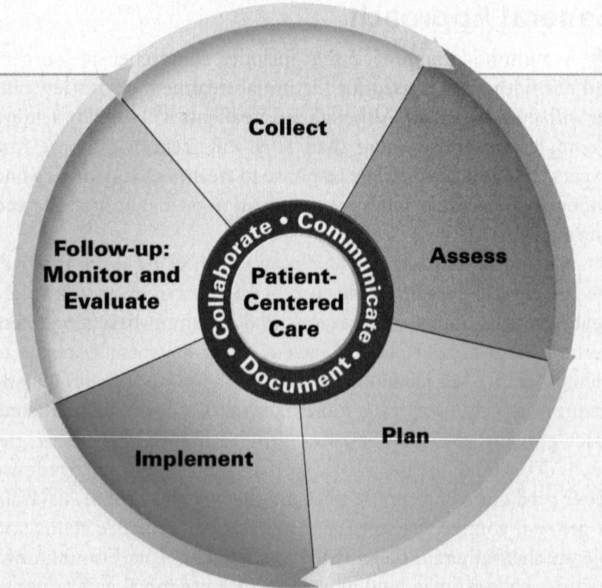

Patient Care Process for Ovarian Cancer

Collect

- Patient characteristics and medication history, including any allergies
- Medical history, family cancer history, and physical assessment findings
- Patient-specific factors, tumor-specific factors, and laboratory information that may influence chemotherapy selection and drug dosing
- Lifestyle habits, preferences and beliefs, health goals, and socioeconomic factors that affect medication access and other aspects of care

Assess

- Goal of therapy defined by prognosis-based stage of disease and patient preferences
- Medication profile to identify agents that may worsen the patient's symptoms, potential interactions, duplicate therapies, or unnecessary medications. Determine need for symptomatic supportive care medications including antiemetics or pain medications
- Medical and family history to determine whether the patient has compelling indications or contraindications for specific chemotherapy and if additional genetic testing is recommended
- Relevant laboratory tests (eg, CBC, electrolytes, complete metabolic panel to determine liver and hepatic function, tumor markers [eg, CA-125, CEA, and CA19-9 as part of differential], tumor genetic profile) that may impact drug selection or dosing
- Potential appropriate chemotherapy regimens and the related toxicities; review chemotherapy history to determine potential for platinum sensitivity/resistance and consider genetic mutation status in selection of treatment options

Plan*

- Recommendations for any medications or supplements that need to be held temporarily before surgery (eg, anticoagulants, nonsteroidal anti-inflammatory agents, omega 3 fatty acids, etc.)
- Anticancer therapy order with dosages based on organ function and patient characteristics (calculate body surface area), list of drug interactions and possible adverse drug reactions from the regimen
- Determine whether patient has insurance coverage for planned anticancer therapy regimen and supportive care medications as indicated; consider institution's formulary if applicable
- Recommendations for lifestyle modifications that may assist in symptom and disease management and supportive care options
- Counseling for potential adverse drug reactions of the regimen and management strategies

Implement

- Patient education treatment plan
  - Patients undergoing surgery: use of low-molecular weight heparin for postoperative clot prevention, list of medication to stop prior to surgery and when to resume, plan for postoperative pain
  - Patients undergoing anticancer treatment: anticancer therapy agents including timing of administration, expected adverse drug reactions and prevention and management of these toxicities (nausea, infection, neuropathy, alopecia, electrolyte disturbances), necessary laboratory monitoring and follow-up visits; help patient set realistic expectations during treatment

Follow-up: Monitor and Evaluate

- Patients undergoing surgery (2-3 weeks postoperative): evaluate symptom management including nausea, pain control, and determine if adjuvant anticancer therapy is required
- Patients undergoing anticancer therapy:
  - CBC with differential should be obtained prior to each anticancer therapy dose
  - Complete laboratory values should be obtained with each cycle
  - Adjust doses based on unacceptable toxicity or organ dysfunction when indicated
  - Tumor markers obtained with each cycle: consider reevaluating therapy if a 50% increase or consistent trend upwards
  - Radiographic scan (CT scan/MRI/PET) once every 3 months: assess tumor response, following current RECIST criteria

Collaborate with patient, caregivers, and other healthcare professionals.

The primary objective of the surgery is to optimally debulk the tumor to remove all gross disease.[18] Long-term follow-up studies confirm that residual disease smaller than 1 cm correlates with higher complete response rates to chemotherapy and longer overall survival as compared to patients with bulky residual disease (>1 cm).[23]

6 A comprehensive exploratory laparotomy is vital for the accurate confirmation of diagnosis and staging of ovarian cancer.[22,23]

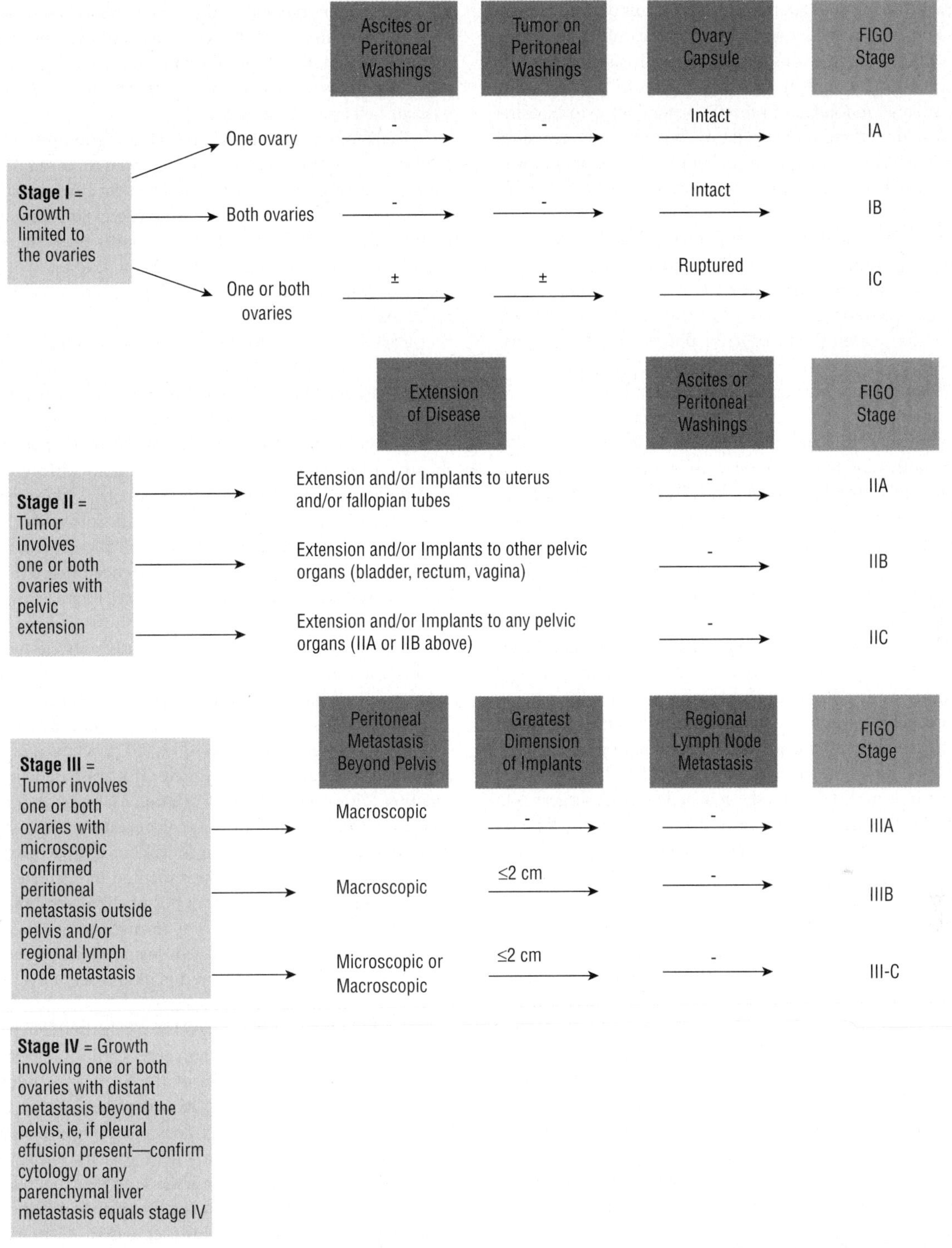

FIGURE 156-2 FIGO staging algorithm.

Unlike other cancers that are typically diagnosed by biopsy or laboratory results and clinically staged by results from imaging tests, gynecologic cancers are surgically diagnosed and then staged according to the FIGO staging algorithm (Fig. 156-2). The FIGO staging system requires an extensive surgery by an experienced gynecologic oncologist. The training and skill of the surgeon has a significant effect on prognosis, with definitive benefit of a trained gynecologic oncologist performing surgery as compared with a gynecologist or general surgeon.[19,25] The reasons for this approach include (a) pelvic tumors cannot be readily biopsied without risk of "tumor seeding," which can increase the risk of recurrence, and (b) surgical staging takes into account the presence of microscopic disease in samples obtained by pelvic washing and lymph node dissection and read by a pathologist during the surgical procedure. It is recommended that the initial surgical staging and tumor-debulking surgery be completed by a trained gynecologic oncology surgeon when ovarian cancer is suspected to prevent understaging and to optimize overall outcome.[18,19,22,26]

Secondary cytoreduction or interval debulking is when surgery is performed after completion of some or all chemotherapy to remove residual disease. Some protocols include additional cycles of chemotherapy after the surgical procedure. The importance of cytoreduction before, during, or after chemotherapy is still controversial, but it has been recommended to facilitate response to chemotherapy and improve overall survival.[18] Randomized trials of secondary surgical cytoreduction have reported conflicting results. In a study of 550 women with stage III or IV disease treated with primary cytoreductive surgery and three cycles of paclitaxel and cisplatin, patients randomized to receive secondary cytoreductive surgery followed by three more cycles of chemotherapy had similar progression-free survival and overall survival as compared with those randomized to receive three more cycles of chemotherapy alone.[27]

The overall effect of interval debulking is influenced by several factors, including initial response to chemotherapy, the amount of residual disease before and after second-look surgery, and the presence of microscopic residual disease. The results of recent trials suggest that secondary surgical cytoreduction does not prolong survival in patients who are treated with maximal primary cytoreductive surgery followed by appropriate postoperative chemotherapy.[28]

"Second-look surgery" is an elective surgical procedure performed in patients who achieve a clinical complete response after primary chemotherapy to determine if any visible or microscopic disease is present in the peritoneal cavity. The benefit of "second-look laparotomy" to evaluate residual disease after completing chemotherapy remains controversial because it has been difficult to establish any impact on overall survival. It has questionable benefit because about 50% of those with a negative second look still relapsed.[27] If visible or microscopic disease is detected during second look, then the clinician may decide to give additional chemotherapy. But if no visible or microscopic disease is detected during second look, the clinician may decide to observe and monitor the patient. Use of laparoscopic surgical techniques is controversial for initial surgery but is sometimes considered in debulking of recurrent or advanced disease when the intent is palliative rather than curative.[24] In patients with recurrent disease, the goal of debulking surgery is to relieve symptoms associated with complications such as small bowel obstructions and to improve the patient's quality of life.

Radiation Therapy

Radiation therapy has a limited role in the management of ovarian cancer. Use of radiation therapy for treatment of early stage disease has no impact on overall survival.[29] Radiation therapy is most beneficial for palliation of symptoms in patients with recurrent pelvic disease, often associated with small bowel obstructions. The two forms of radiation therapy used in ovarian cancer are external beam whole-abdominal irradiation and intraperitoneal isotopes such as phosphorus-32, or ^{32}P. Alleviation of symptoms with external beam whole-abdominal irradiation is associated with a significant improvement in the patient's quality of life. The recommended dose ranges from 35 to 45 Gy (3,500-4,500 rad), depending on the treatment history and ability to tolerate radiation treatments.

First-Line Chemotherapy

The mainstay of ovarian cancer treatment is chemotherapy. It is used as a component of first-line treatment after completion of surgery and is the primary modality of treatment for recurrent ovarian cancer. Systemic chemotherapy with a taxane and platinum regimen following optimal surgical debulking is the standard of care for treatment of epithelial ovarian cancer (Fig. 156-3).[18] Table 156-1 summarizes the chemotherapeutic regimens used as the initial treatment of newly diagnosed epithelial ovarian cancer. More than 60 randomized controlled clinical trials have evaluated combination chemotherapy regimens for the treatment of advanced ovarian cancer, and a meta-analysis of these trials confirms the efficacy of platinum and taxane regimens over other regimens.[30]

Single-agent alkylating agents such as melphalan, and later cyclophosphamide, were used for the treatment of advanced ovarian cancer until cisplatin was introduced in the 1970s. Combination chemotherapy regimens containing cisplatin and cyclophosphamide achieved higher response and overall survival rates than regimens without cisplatin in patients with advanced ovarian cancer.[31] Based on the results of these trials, the combination of cisplatin plus cyclophosphamide remained the standard of care for the treatment of ovarian cancer until the early 1990s.

The combination of paclitaxel (135 mg/m^2 over 24 hours) and cisplatin (75 mg/m^2) has been an accepted standard of care for the treatment of ovarian cancer because of its effectiveness since the early 1990s. It is associated with a median progression-free survival of 18 months and overall survival of 38 months from the Gynecologic Oncology Group (GOG)-11 and OV10 studies.[32,33] Neutropenia, alopecia, and peripheral neuropathy are common adverse drug reactions.

Carboplatin can be substituted for cisplatin, which spares patients from the significant nephrotoxicity and peripheral neuropathy associated with cisplatin. Several prospective randomized comparisons of carboplatin plus paclitaxel versus cisplatin plus paclitaxel in patients with advanced ovarian cancer have shown carboplatin plus paclitaxel is equally efficacious and better tolerated than cisplatin and paclitaxel.[34-37] As expected, the incidence of nausea and vomiting, nephrotoxicity, and peripheral neuropathy is higher in patients in the cisplatin arm, while patients in the carboplatin arm experienced more thrombocytopenia. Based on these results, paclitaxel plus carboplatin is the preferred standard-of-care regimen.

While most chemotherapy drugs used to treat ovarian cancer are dosed according to body surface area, or BSA, carboplatin dosing is personalized based on each individual's renal function with the Calvert formula: carboplatin dose = area under the curve (AUC) × (glomerular filtration rate [GFR] + 25).[38] When it was originally developed and validated, measured GFR was used in the Calvert equation. However, estimated creatinine clearance (CrCl) is now used in clinical practice in place of measured GFR. Despite more than 30 years of clinical use, it is still not clear which equation to use to estimate CrCl and the best method to estimate CrCl in certain patient subgroups. The use of personalized carboplatin dose has reduced potential toxicity such as thrombocytopenia, neuropathy, and nephrotoxicity.[38] Personalized dosing of carboplatin is one of the reasons why it is the preferred platinum agent over cisplatin for primary treatment for ovarian cancer.[36]

Similarly the use of docetaxel as a substitute for paclitaxel has been evaluated as paclitaxel can cause significant peripheral neuropathy over time. The results of the Scottish Randomized Trial in Ovarian Cancer, or SCOTROC, study showed that the substitution of docetaxel for paclitaxel does not compromise efficacy and improves tolerability, particularly neurotoxicity, but patients receiving docetaxel experienced more grade 3 to 4 neutropenia and neutropenic complications.[39] These findings were not confirmed in another randomized controlled trial. However, based on the results of this study, the combination of docetaxel plus carboplatin is considered a reasonable treatment option for patients with advanced ovarian cancer. Docetaxel and paclitaxel both cause alopecia and have a risk of infusion-related reactions or true hypersensitivity reactions, though reactions are more common with paclitaxel. Paclitaxel infusions require premedication with a corticosteroid, diphenhydramine, and an H_2-blocker like famotidine to help prevent severe reactions. Due to the risk of fluid retention with docetaxel, premedication with dexamethasone is recommended to reduce the incidence and severity. Six cycles of paclitaxel plus carboplatin following tumor-debulking surgery remain the current standard of care for treatment of advanced ovarian cancer. Although the choice of taxane or platinum agent does not appear to have a major effect on antitumor activity, the impact of paclitaxel dose and frequency of administration has been controversial.[40-42] Due to less favorable treatment-related toxicities and questionable benefit on progression-free survival, dose-dense weekly paclitaxel regimens are not widely used.

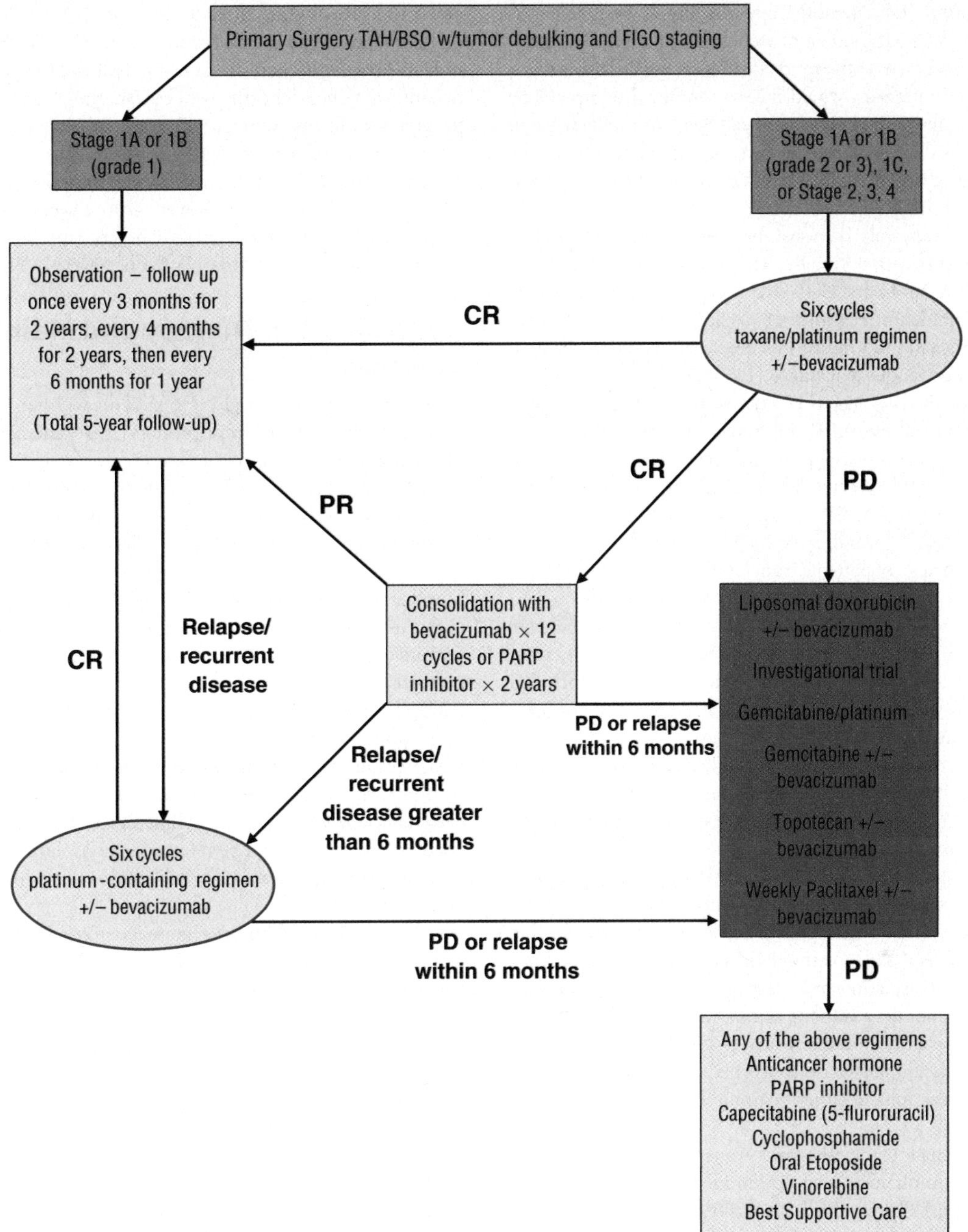

FIGURE 156-3 Management of newly diagnosed, refractory, and progressive epithelial ovarian cancer. (CR, complete response; PD, progression of disease; PR, partial response; TAH/BSO, total abdominal hysterectomy/bilateral salpingo-oophorectomy.)

TABLE 156-1 Initial Chemotherapeutic Regimens of Epithelial Ovarian Cancer

Regimen	Initial Dose(s)/Usual Range	Cycle Frequency
Paclitaxel + carboplatin	Paclitaxel 175 mg/m^2 IV (3-hour infusion) day 1 Carboplatin AUC 5-6 IV day 1	Every 21 days
Paclitaxel + carboplatin + bevacizumab	Paclitaxel 175 mg/m^2 IV (3-hour infusion) day 1 Carboplatin AUC 5-6 IV day 1 Bevacizumab 7.5-15 mg/kg IV on day 1	Every 21 days
Paclitaxel + carboplatin (dose-dense)	Paclitaxel 80 mg/m^2 IV (1-hour infusion) on days 1, 8, 15 Carboplatin AUC 5-6 IV day 1 or AUC 2 on days 1, 8, and 15	Every 21 days
Paclitaxel + cisplatin (IP)	Paclitaxel 135 mg/m^2 IV infused over 24 hours on day 1 Cisplatin 100 mg/m^2 IP infused over 1 hour on day 2 Paclitaxel 60 mg/m^2 IP infused over 1 hour on day 8	Every 21 days
Carboplatin + pegylated liposomal doxorubicin	Carboplatin AUC 5 IV day 1 Pegylated liposomal doxorubicin 30 mg/m^2 IV day 1	Every 28 days
Docetaxel + carboplatin	Docetaxel 75 mg/m^2 IV day 1 Carboplatin AUC 5-6 IV day 1	Every 21 days

Intraperitoneal (IP) chemotherapy was initially employed as palliative care in the management of ascites and uncontrolled intra-abdominal tumors based on the rationale that exposure of the tumor to high drug concentrations would increase tumor drug uptake by passive diffusion and ultimately cancer cell death.[43] The increase in AUC exposure in the peritoneal cavity was demonstrated, but the correlative increase in drug uptake in tumor tissue has yet to be validated in any preclinical or clinical study.

IP chemotherapy has demonstrated benefit in the first-line treatment of patients with optimally debulked advanced-stage ovarian cancer.[44,45] In a landmark GOG-172 study, which evaluated the intravenous combination regimen of paclitaxel (135 mg/m^2 over 24 hours) and cisplatin (75 mg/m^2) or a new combination regimen that included intravenous paclitaxel (135 mg/m^2 over 24 hours) followed by cisplatin 100 mg/m^2 IP infused over 1 hour on day 2, and then paclitaxel 60 mg/m^2 IP infused over 1 hour on day 8.[46] Both treatment regimens were given once every 21 days for a total of six cycles. Patients receiving IP chemotherapy experienced a 5.5-month increase in median progression-free survival and a 15.9-month increase in overall survival.[46] A secondary analysis by Tewari and colleagues[47] of patients from GOG-172 and GOG-114 IP therapy studies reported a 10.4 month improvement in the median overall survival and 23% decreased risk of death in those patients that had received IP chemotherapy compared to IV chemotherapy. Contributing factors that negatively impacted survival included gross residual disease, clear cell or mucinous histology, and not completing all six cycles of IP chemotherapy.

A limitation of IP therapy is significantly more toxicity, including pain, fatigue, myelosuppression, gastrointestinal, metabolic, and neurotoxicity.[18,46,48,49] The significant increase in systemic toxicity, primarily neurotoxicity, has led to the question of whether IP carboplatin could be substituted for IP cisplatin. Although these platinum agents have demonstrated equal efficacy when administered intravenously (IV) to ovarian cancer patients, it is difficult to extrapolate the IP activity of cisplatin to carboplatin because of the difference in molecular size of cisplatin versus carboplatin and the importance of passive diffusion of drug into the tumor. Most clinical trials used platinum agents given IP until the GOG-172 trial that incorporated IP paclitaxel. Many clinicians are concerned about how to manage hypersensitivity reactions to either platinum or taxane agents when administered IP.

In the National Comprehensive Cancer Network (NCCN) guidelines, IP chemotherapy is an option for first-line treatment of stage II to III, optimally debulked, <1 cm residual disease, ovarian cancer but is not without clinical controversy.[18] Because of the significant toxicities associated with IP therapy, only carefully selected patients should receive IP therapy. Ideal candidates for IP therapy are younger patients with good performance status, minimal comorbidities, adequate renal and liver function, and optimally debulked disease without significant bowel resection.[18,49] The IP regimens have recently fallen out of favor due to the results of GOG-252. Bevacizumab was administered in combination with IV/IP paclitaxel and carboplatin compared to IV/IP paclitaxel and cisplatin, or IV paclitaxel and carboplatin.[50] With the addition of bevacizumab to first-line chemotherapy, no progression-free or overall survival benefit with IP administration was observed and the IV regimen was as effective and better tolerated.[50]

Neoadjuvant Chemotherapy

7 Neoadjuvant chemotherapy is first-line treatment for patients who are poor surgical candidates or patients with bulky or significant tumor burden.[51] The neoadjuvant chemotherapy regimen typically includes a combination of taxane with platinum agent and is administered every 21 to 28 days as tolerated with intent to reduce tumor burden to where it potentially could be surgically resected and ideally optimally debulked during surgery.[51] After surgery, patients usually receive another three to six cycles (IV or IP/IV), depending on their response to chemotherapy.[18,52] In patients who are poor candidates for surgery because of comorbidities, the primary intent of neoadjuvant chemotherapy is to relieve symptoms and slow disease progression. In this setting, palliative chemotherapy alone has not been curative for patients with advanced ovarian cancer.[51] If tolerated, these patients will receive the standard taxane plus platinum chemotherapy regimen once every 3 to 4 weeks. Another option for palliative neoadjuvant chemotherapy, especially in older adult patients, is single-agent carboplatin once every 4 weeks.

Consolidation Therapy and Maintenance Therapy

Consolidation therapy is given to patients without "measurable disease" after the completion of primary chemotherapy, with the goal of eliminating any microscopic residual disease that may be present to extend progression-free and overall survival. It will have a set duration to therapy and typically is less toxicity than primary chemotherapy regimens. Patients undergoing consolidation therapy are monitored for signs of recurrent disease. Maintenance therapy, however, is given to patients with measurable disease, with the goal of prevent progression/growth of disease. It is given for an undetermined duration and may alternate or "switch maintenance" between aggressive cytotoxic regimens and less toxic regimens. Patients undergoing maintenance therapy are monitored for clinical response or progression of disease. Both bevacizumab and PARP inhibitors are the only agents approved by the US Food and Drug Administration for use as consolidation in the first-line setting however mislabeled as "first-line maintenance". For the purpose of this chapter, this therapy will be referred to consolidation because there is no measurable disease and it is administered for a defined two-year duration.

Consolidation with bevacizumab and/or PARP inhibitor therapy is recommended by the NCCN guidelines following first-line treatment depending on the agents used as first-line therapy and the patient's mutation status (category 2A recommendation).[18] Single-agent bevacizumab is recommended as consolidation therapy only if it was used with first-line chemotherapy based on GOG-0218 and ICON7.[18] No data exists to support bevacizumab consolidation if it was not used with first-line chemotherapy.

Olaparib, an oral PARP inhibitor, should be considered as consolidation therapy in individuals with a germline mutation in *BRCA1* or *BRCA2* and a response to first-line platinum-based therapy. Continuous twice-daily oral dosing of olaparib provides substantial clinical benefit in progression-free survival when compared to placebo.[53] The use of consolidation therapy with olaparib results in a 70% lower risk of disease progression or death. Niraparib, another PARP inhibitor, should also be considered as consolidation because it improves progression-free survival by 5.6 months (13.8 months compared to 8.2 months with placebo).[54] This effect is more pronounced in patients with *BRCA* or other homologous recombination repair gene mutations. The NCCN guidelines recommend niraparib as an option for those who are *BRCA1/2* wild-type or unknown who did not receive bevacizumab with primary treatment and as an option for patients with a *BRCA1/2* mutation.[18]

Bevacizumab in combination with olaparib was studied as consolidation following frontline chemotherapy with bevacizumab in patients with homologous recombination repair gene mutations, including those without *BRCA* mutations, in the PAOLA-1 study.[55] The addition of olaparib to bevacizumab resulted in a 51% risk reduction in disease progression or death compared to bevacizumab alone.[55] One major limitation of this study is that it did not include an arm with olaparib alone, so the addition of bevacizumab to olaparib compared to single-agent olaparib is unknown.

The clinical challenge with consolidation therapy after first-line treatment is selection of which agent based on molecular profile and cost of therapy. Patients need to be evaluated for tumor molecular status, residual toxicity, renal function, and comorbidities to determine if bevacizumab or PARP inhibitor or perhaps combination of bevacizumab plus PARP inhibitor would be the best option for consolidation. However, from the cost perspective neither bevacizumab nor PARP inhibitors are cost effective for consolidation therapy after completion of primary treatment of ovarian cancer.[56]

Treatment of Recurrent Disease

Although most patients will achieve a complete response to initial treatment, most patients will eventually have recurrence of their disease within the first 2 years. When a patient relapses, the prognostic factors are similar to the factors after initial surgery except that the disease-free interval—defined as the length of time that has lapsed since the completion of chemotherapy—should be considered to determine if the tumor is likely to be drug resistant to agents used in first-line treatment (ie, platinum and taxanes). If recurrence occurs less than 6 months after completion of chemotherapy or if the patient progresses during platinum-based chemotherapy, the tumor is defined as platinum-resistant. Patients with platinum-sensitive disease generally have a better prognosis than platinum-resistant patients.

8 9 If the patient had a clinical complete response to first-line chemotherapy and the recurrence occurred more than 6 months after chemotherapy is completed, the tumor is considered platinum-sensitive. In patients with platinum-sensitive ovarian cancer, the standard of care is to treat the first recurrence with a doublet, platinum-containing chemotherapy regimen (Table 156-2). Because the chemotherapy agents used for second-line treatment of recurrent or refractory platinum-resistant disease have similar response rates that average less than 30%, the selection of the agent depends on the toxicity profile of the agent, physician preference, patient performance status, residual toxicities, and patient convenience (see Fig. 156-3). In this setting, the intent of treatment is to prolong survival and alleviate symptoms, not necessarily and unlikely to achieve another "complete response" to chemotherapy. Because of poor response rates of the available agents, participation in a clinical trial of an investigational agent is recommended if available for patients with recurrent platinum-resistant ovarian cancer.

Platinum-Sensitive Disease

8 Retreatment with a platinum-containing regimen should be considered in patients with platinum-sensitive disease. The 2021 NCCN guidelines recommend the combination of platinum agent with gemcitabine, pegylated liposomal doxorubicin, or paclitaxel for treatment of platinum-sensitive recurrent ovarian cancer (Table 156-3).[18] In addition, the combination of gemcitabine plus cisplatin, gemcitabine plus carboplatin and bevacizumab and carboplatin plus paclitaxel and bevacizumab has demonstrated improvement in progression-free survival.[57-59] Carboplatin alone or any of the second-line agents is recommended for patients with platinum-sensitive disease who are unable to tolerate additional combination chemotherapy regimens because of residual toxicity or poor performance status.

Biologic and targeted agents play an important role in the treatment of recurrent disease. Bevacizumab is a recombinant humanized monoclonal antibody that targets vascular endothelial growth factor (VEGF), a key mediator of angiogenesis. In patients with platinum-sensitive recurrent disease, the addition of bevacizumab to chemotherapy (eg, carboplatin/gemcitabine, carboplatin/paclitaxel) improves disease outcomes.[58,59] Due to the toxicity profile of bevacizumab, patients considered for bevacizumab therapy must be carefully selected. Further details regarding the role of bevacizumab and other targeted and biologic agents in the treatment of ovarian cancer will be discussed in the following section.

TABLE 156-2 Chemotherapy Regimens for Platinum-Sensitive Recurrent Ovarian Cancer

Regimen	Initial Dose(s)/Usual Range	Cycle Frequency
Carboplatin + gemcitabine	Carboplatin AUC 5 IV day 1 Gemcitabine 800 mg/m² IV days 1 and 8	Every 21 days
Carboplatin + gemcitabine + bevacizumab	Carboplatin AUC 5 IV day 1 Gemcitabine 800 mg/m² IV days 1 and 8 Bevacizumab 15 mg/kg IV day 1	Every 21 days
Carboplatin + pegylated liposomal doxorubicin	Carboplatin AUC 5 IV day 1 Pegylated liposomal doxorubicin 30 mg/m² IV day	Every 28 days
Carboplatin + pegylated liposomal doxorubicin + bevacizumab	Carboplatin AUC 5 IV day 1 Pegylated liposomal doxorubicin 30 mg/m² IV day Bevacizumab 15 mg/kg IV days 1 and 15	Every 28 days
Carboplatin + paclitaxel	Carboplatin AUC 5-6 IV day 1 Paclitaxel 175 mg/m² IV day 1	Every 21 days
Carboplatin + paclitaxel + bevacizumab	Carboplatin AUC 5-6 IV day 1 Paclitaxel 175 mg/m² IV day 1 Bevacizumab 15 mg/kg IV day 1	Every 21 days
Cisplatin + gemcitabine	Cisplatin 30 mg/m² IV days 1 and 8 Gemcitabine 600-750 mg/m² IV days 1 and 8	Every 28 days
Bevacizumab	Bevacizumab 10 mg/kg on days 1 and 15 or Bevacizumab 15 mg/kg IV on day 1	Every 28 days Every 21 days
Olaparib	300 mg PO twice daily	
Niraparib	300 mg PO daily	
Rucaparib	600 mg PO twice daily	

PO, by mouth.

TABLE 156-3 Chemotherapy Regimens for Platinum-Resistant Recurrent Ovarian Cancer

Drug(s)	Initial Dose(s)/Usual Range	Cycle Frequency
Paclitaxel + bevacizumab	Paclitaxel 60-80 mg/m² IV days 1, 8, 15, and 22 Bevacizumab 10 mg/m² IV days 1 and 15	Every 28 days
Paclitaxel	60-80 mg/m² IV days 1, 8, 15, and 22	Every 28 days
Pegylated liposomal doxorubicin + bevacizumab	Pegylated liposomal doxorubicin 40 mg/m² IV day 1 Bevacizumab 10 mg/m² IV days 1 and 15	Every 28 days
Pegylated liposomal doxorubicin	40 mg/m² IV day 1	Every 28 days
Topotecan + bevacizumab	Topotecan 3-4 mg/m² IV days 1, 8, and 15 Bevacizumab 10 mg/m² IV days 1 and 15	Every 28 days
Topotecan	3-4 mg/m² IV days 1, 8, and 15	Every 28 days
Gemcitabine	800 mg/m² IV days 1 and 8	Every 21 days
Docetaxel	100 mg/m² IV day 1	Every 21 days
Etoposide (oral)	50 mg/m² PO daily on days 1-21	Every 28 days
Cyclophosphamide (oral) + bevacizumab	Cyclophosphamide 50 mg PO once daily Bevacizumab 10 mg/kg on days 1 and 15	Every 28 days
Bevacizumab	10 mg/kg on days 1 and 15 OR 15 mg/kg IV on day 1	Every 28 days Every 21 days
Olaparib	300 mg PO twice daily	
Niraparib	300 mg PO daily	
Rucaparib	600 mg PO twice daily	

The preferred regimen for platinum-sensitive recurrent disease varies by clinician. Some clinicians will recommend retreatment with a chemotherapy regimen including a platinum agent. Other clinicians suggest that the platinum-free interval for these patients should be extended and recommend that recurrent disease first be treated with a nonplatinum regimen (ie, liposomal doxorubicin) and reserve the platinum agent until the next relapse.

Platinum-Resistant Disease

Patients frequently present with recurrent drug-resistant disease after initial platinum-based therapy and cytoreductive surgery.[2] Patients who progress on a platinum agent or have no response are considered "platinum-refractory," while those patients who have recurrence within 6 months of completing a platinum-containing regimen are considered "platinum-resistant."[18] The NCCN guidelines list many possible treatment options for recurrent platinum-resistant or refractory ovarian carcinoma.[18] The optimal chemotherapeutic agent or regimen in the treatment of platinum-resistant disease is unclear. Ideally, the agent should be active in ovarian cancer and non–cross-resistant with taxanes or platinum agents. Unfortunately, the response rate is low for all agents in platinum-refractory or resistant ovarian cancer.[2] Patients should typically be evaluated for response after treatment with at least three cycles of the chemotherapy agent or regimen. Because partial responses are rare, stable disease with relief of symptoms is considered a treatment success. If no response is observed, then an alternative chemotherapy regimen may be selected. Because all the potential agents have similar efficacy, the selection of agents and sequence used for treatment as the patient progresses will vary based on residual toxicity and the adverse effect profile of the regimen (Table 156-4), dosing schedule, patient convenience, and physician preference.

Topotecan, an analog of the plant alkaloid 20(S)-camptothecin, is active in patients with metastatic ovarian cancer and is non–cross-resistant with platinum-based chemotherapy.[60] It produces an overall response rate of 21%, with a median time-to-progression of 32 weeks.[61] Topotecan is well-tolerated with minimal nonhematologic toxicities.[61,62] The dose-limiting toxicity is myelosuppression with neutropenia as the most common adverse drug reaction but patients may experience fatigue as well. Patients receiving topotecan have often received multiple other lines of chemotherapy, so they may require dose adjustments or treatment delays for their counts to recover between cycles. For patients unable to tolerate conventional topotecan over 5 days, weekly topotecan on days 1, 8, and 15 of a 28-day cycle may be considered as it has been found to be better tolerated.[63]

Pegylated liposomal doxorubicin is one of the primary agents used for second-line therapy of recurrent ovarian cancer.[64-66] The drug tends to be better tolerated than topotecan, which is important for heavily pretreated patients with advanced disease. The overall response rate with pegylated liposomal doxorubicin is 20%.[65] Median overall survival is longer with pegylated liposomal doxorubicin than topotecan, with a median of 108 weeks versus 71 weeks. Palmar–plantar erythrodysesthesia (PPE) occurs with pegylated liposomal doxorubicin. However, the incidence of PPE in current clinical practice has decreased because the standard dose of pegylated liposomal doxorubicin used currently (40 mg/m²) is less than the dose that was used in the initial clinical trials and approved by the FDA.[67] Other adverse drug reactions include cardiotoxicity, mucositis, skin rash or hyperpigmentation, and discoloration of urine or body fluids for a day or two following the infusion due to the red color of the drug.

Gemcitabine, a pyrimidine antimetabolite, is also widely used in the treatment of recurrent platinum-resistant ovarian cancer. Although the overall response rate is only about 13% to 22% with single-agent gemcitabine in patients with platinum-refractory recurrent ovarian cancer, an additional 16% to 50% of patients have stable disease for a median of 7 months.[68] The main toxicities include myelosuppression, fatigue, myalgia, and skin rash.

Other agents that have shown an overall response rate of 10% to 25% in patients with recurrent ovarian cancer include etoposide, capecitabine, tamoxifen, letrozole, vinorelbine, and oxaliplatin.[18] Response rates tend to be higher in the platinum-sensitive subgroups. Most of these agents are available in oral formulations, which allows for outpatient administration in the palliative care setting.

TABLE 156-4 Adverse Drug Reactions of Treatments for Ovarian Cancer

Class	Drug	Common Adverse Drug Reactions
Taxane agents	Paclitaxel	Peripheral neuropathy (DLT), nausea/vomiting, alopecia, hypersensitivity reactions
	Docetaxel	Neutropenia (DLT), fluid retention, nail disorders, myelosuppression, alopecia
Platinum analogues	Carboplatin	Myelosuppression (DLT), nephrotoxicity, nausea/vomiting, electrolyte wasting, hypersensitivity reactions
	Cisplatin	Nephrotoxicity (DLT), nausea/vomiting, ototoxicity, peripheral neuropathy, myelosuppression, electrolyte wasting, diarrhea
Anthracycline	Liposomal doxorubicin	Hand-foot syndrome, mucositis, myelosuppression, discoloration of body fluids, cardiotoxicity
Pyrimidine Antimetabolite	Gemcitabine	Myelosuppression, flu-like symptoms (fever, headache, arthralgias, myalgias), transient skin rash, transient hepatic dysfunction, pneumonitis
Topoisomerase Inhibitor	Topotecan	Myelosuppression (DLT), fatigue
Anti-angiogenesis agent	Bevacizumab	Hypertension, proteinuria, headache, increased risk of thrombosis, surgery and wound healing complications
PARP inhibitors	Olaparib	Fatigue, anemia, nausea
	Niraparib	Fatigue, nausea, thrombocytopenia, neutropenia, elevated liver function tests
	Rucaparib	Nausea, fatigue, anemia, elevations in liver function tests, rash

DLT, dose limiting toxicity; PARP, poly-ADP-ribose polymerase.

The three most commonly used agents in clinical practice are pegylated liposomal doxorubicin, gemcitabine, and topotecan. These agents have demonstrated efficacy when used as a single agent and in combination with other agents. Selection of chemotherapy for treatment of recurrent disease is based on the patient's residual toxicities, scheduling and convenience, and physician preference.

Biologic and Targeted Agents

Although biologic agents as single agents have not demonstrated significant activity for the treatment of ovarian cancer, the results of several clinical trials show that the addition of bevacizumab into first-line and consolidation regimens improves progression-free survival. However, the impact on overall survival is controversial. PARP inhibitors have become a mainstay for ovarian cancer, especially for patients with BRCA mutations, while other targeted therapies, like tyrosine kinase inhibitors, have a limited scope within this malignancy. Though immunotherapy has been found to be effective in many other disease types, ovarian cancer is far more resistant to its effects except in very specific situations like high microsatellite instability.

Anti-Angiogenesis Agents

Bevacizumab is a recombinant humanized monoclonal antibody that targets VEGF, a key mediator of angiogenesis. In the setting of recurrent disease, single-agent bevacizumab produces a response rate similar to other therapies of 16% to 21%.[69,70] Response rates with combinations of bevacizumab range from 15% to 80%.[69-74] However, these phase II trials have also reported a higher risk of bowel perforation in patients treated with bevacizumab-containing regimens.[69,70] Bevacizumab should therefore not be given to patients who have had recent bowel surgery or a history of significant bowel resections. Common adverse drug reactions with bevacizumab include hypertension, proteinuria, and headache, while rare but serious adverse drug reactions include thrombotic events, surgery and wound healing complications, and posterior reversible encephalopathy syndrome. Overall, bevacizumab is typically well-tolerated. In an open-label phase III study (AURELIA Study) that evaluated the combination of bevacizumab in combination with chemotherapy (pegylated liposomal doxorubicin, weekly paclitaxel, or topotecan), the addition of bevacizumab to chemotherapy had no significant impact on overall survival but did improve median progression-free survival (6.4 vs 3.7 months).[75] Based on this study, bevacizumab was approved for use in combination with pegylated liposomal doxorubicin, weekly paclitaxel, or topotecan for treatment of recurrent ovarian cancer.

Recent efforts have focused on the use of bevacizumab in first-line treatment regimens. Although bevacizumab has demonstrated some progression-free survival advantages when used in combination, its effect on overall survival is not clear.[76,77] Furthermore, the benefits do not appear to justify the high cost of bevacizumab (based on pharmacoeconomic studies).[78] As a result, health insurance companies do not consistently reimburse for bevacizumab when used for the primary treatment of ovarian cancer.

Pazopanib, an oral anti-angiogenesis agent, is an alternative treatment regimen for platinum-refractory recurrence.[79] A phase 2 trial assessed oral pazopanib in patients with low-volume recurrent disease who had achieved complete response to initial therapy, with an overall response rate 18%. Single-agent pazopanib is listed as an alternative option for the treatment of platinum-resistant disease in the NCCN guidelines (category 2B recommendation).[18] Adverse drug reactions of pazopanib include diarrhea, hypertension, hair discoloration, hand-foot skin reaction, and a boxed warning for hepatotoxicity.

PARP Inhibitors

10 PARP plays a critical role in the repair of single-strand DNA breaks via the base-excision repair pathway. Specifically, PARP keeps the low-fidelity nonhomologous-end-joining DNA repair machinery functioning. PARP inhibition results in double-stranded DNA breaks that cannot be repaired in cancer cells with homologous recombinant deficiency, such as those with *BRCA1/2* mutations. Three oral PARP inhibitors are commercially approved for treatment of ovarian cancer—olaparib, rucaparib, and niraparib—with similar FDA-labeled approvals for treatment and maintenance therapy for recurrent ovarian cancer. Both olaparib and niraparib also have FDA-approved indications for "first-line maintenance treatment" after achieving a clinical complete response to platinum-based regimen for ovarian cancers.

In the treatment setting, patients with platinum-sensitive disease have a higher response rate to PARP inhibitors compared to those with platinum-resistant disease (66% vs 20%-30%).[80] However, PARP inhibitors are considered a preferred option in this setting because of the lack of active agents in platinum-resistant disease.[18]

While not commonly discussed, creatinine is a substrate of the MATE 1/2 renal transporter and drug interactions that inhibit or induce the MATE 1/2 pathway will alter serum creatinine levels and ultimately cause a change in CrCl. The class of PARP inhibitors are substrates of and inhibit the MATE 1/2 renal transporter that influences CrCl, so caution is needed in patients with renal insufficiency to monitor for cumulative toxicity.[81] Rucaparib is the only PARP inhibitor with known cytochrome P450 drug interactions involving the 1A2 and 2D6 pathways, so drug interactions must be closely evaluated.[82] The common adverse drug reactions associated with PARP inhibitors include nausea and vomiting and significant anemia with associated fatigue. Patients often require antiemetics and some require transfusion support due to drug-induced anemia. Additional serious but infrequent toxicities include thrombocytopenia, neutropenia, and rarely secondary myelodysplastic syndrome or acute myeloid leukemia. The challenge of combining PARP inhibitors with chemotherapy has been the fatigue, nausea, and significant hematological toxicity, primarily anemia, thrombocytopenia, and neutropenia. The three PARP inhibitors have comparable efficacy and toxicity profiles. Selection of PARP inhibitors will dependent upon patient factors, renal function, and potential drug interactions with concomitant medication.

Other Targeted Agents

Tyrosine kinase inhibitors such as sorafenib and pazopanib inhibit angiogenesis by specifically targeting the VEGF receptor, or VEGFR. When given as single agents, tyrosine kinase inhibitors have demonstrated some antitumor activity in ovarian cancer, but these agents are rarely used due to the toxicity profile. Estrogen receptor antagonists and aromatase inhibitors have also been studied in early phase clinical trials with modest responses.[83] Hormone therapy may be considered in patients who cannot tolerate other regimens or who have not responded to chemotherapy.[18,84]

Immunotherapy

Based on changes in chromosomal instability and epigenetic silencing in ovarian cancer, in theory immunotherapy would be a useful treatment option; however, studies to date have not demonstrated benefit in ovarian cancer. Improved survival has been correlated with the increased presence of CD3+ tumor-infiltrating lymphocytes and a high CD8+/regulatory T-cell ratio in ovarian cancer patients provides evidence for the immunogenicity of this tumor.[85,86] Increased tumor-infiltrating lymphocytes are linked to tumors with high chromosomal instability such as those with *BRCA* mutation or epigenetic loss. Immunotherapy with pembrolizumab is currently indicated for those with high microsatellite instability, or MSI-H, tumors, which are only seen in 2% of ovarian cancers, or in patients with high tumor mutational burden with at least 10 mutations/megabase and no satisfactory alternative treatment options.[18] Dostarlimab-gxly was also recently approved in patients with solid tumors and no alternative treatment options who have deficient mismatch repair, or dMMR, or high microsatellite instability.[18]

EVALUATION OF THERAPEUTIC OUTCOMES

11 During chemotherapy, patients may experience numerous adverse drug reactions such as nausea and vomiting, myelosuppression, neuropathy, and changes in organ function. Patients receiving a taxane or platinum chemotherapy regimen should be monitored for signs of hypersensitivity or infusion-related reactions. Patients treated with paclitaxel often experience infusion-related reactions, which have been attributed to the polyethoxylated castor oil (Cremophor) diluent. Premedications including an H_1-blocker, H_2-blocker, and steroid should be administered prior to each chemotherapy administration to prevent hypersensitivity reactions. If a patient has a reaction, increasing the duration of the infusion from 3 to 6 hours may help with infusion-related reactions. For patients with a true taxane allergy, paclitaxel desensitization can be attempted with 24 hours of premedications (H_1-blocker, H_2-blocker, and steroids) followed by paclitaxel given as a titrated infusion (1:1000 → 1:100 → 1:10 → full dose) over 8 hours. With repeated exposure (ie, seven cycles or more) to carboplatin, patients can develop a delayed hypersensitivity reaction. A similar protocol can be used for carboplatin desensitization.

Ovarian cancer patients receive multiple courses of chemotherapy that can have varying effects on kidney and liver function, often with a delayed onset. Appropriate laboratory tests should be ordered to assess organ function so that chemotherapy doses can be adjusted as indicated. Patients on platinum-containing regimens can often experience electrolyte wasting, so patients should be monitored for electrolyte replacement, IV or oral, as indicated. The use of myeloid growth factors should be considered to prevent treatment delays or dose reductions. Prevention of nausea and vomiting, both acute and delayed, is critical for patients receiving emetogenic chemotherapy regimens.

During initial taxane plus platinum chemotherapy, a CA-125 level should be obtained with each cycle and monitored for at least a 50% reduction in CA-125 after completion of four cycles, which is related to an improved prognosis. Patients who achieve a complete response after completion of first-line treatment should have follow-up once every 3 months, including CA-125, physical examination, pelvic examination, and appropriate diagnostic scans (eg, computed tomography, magnetic resonance imaging, or positron emission tomography), which should be evaluated for presence of disease. In addition to routine follow-up examinations, clinicians should monitor for resolution of any residual chemotherapy-related adverse drug reactions, including neuropathies, nephrotoxicity, ototoxicity, myelosuppression, and nausea and vomiting.

In the progressive disease or recurrent setting, CA-125 levels can be used to monitor for response and should be checked with each cycle, although no change in therapy is recommended until after completion of at least three cycles of the second-line chemotherapy. In addition to laboratory monitoring, appropriate diagnostic scans (eg, computed tomography, magnetic resonance imaging, or positron emission tomography) should be done once every three cycles. Patients need to be monitored with each cycle of chemotherapy to evaluate for new or persistent toxicities such as neuropathies, fluid retention, PPE, myelosuppression, and nausea and vomiting. Another precaution to keep in mind for patients with significant ascites, the "dry weight" or an adjusted body weight should be used for dosing chemotherapy.

Most patients with ovarian cancer will eventually progress through all chemotherapy regimens and investigational treatment options, after which the best supportive care measures should be provided to maintain patient comfort and quality of life. A plan to treat common complications of progressive ovarian cancer, including thrombosis, ascites, uncontrollable pain, and small bowel obstruction, should be developed. This plan should include an opioid-based pain regimen with both long-acting agents and short-acting opioids for breakthrough or progressive pain; it should also include a bowel regimen to prevent opioid-induced constipation. Nausea can be a problem in individuals with advanced ovarian cancer when disease progression causes ascites or partial/complete bowel obstruction. Both antiemetic medications and nonpharmacologic interventions with nutrition and hydration can be helpful. Management of partial or complete small bowel obstruction focuses on controlling symptoms of pain and nausea. Bowel rest with best supportive care may lead to spontaneous resolution of the small bowel obstruction but most often it is a complication associated with rapidly progressive disease. Palliative surgery may be considered for selected patients to relieve symptoms.

ABBREVIATIONS

AUC	area under the curve
BRCA1	breast cancer activator gene 1
BRCA2	breast cancer activator gene 2
CA-125	cancer antigen 125
CrCl	creatinine clearance
FDA	Food and Drug Administration
FIGO	International Federation of Gynecology and Obstetrics
GFR	glomerular filtration rate
GOG	Gynecologic Oncology Group
H_1-blocker	histamine receptor 1 blocker
H_2-blocker	histamine receptor 2 blocker
IP	intraperitoneal
IV	intravenous
NCCN	National Comprehensive Cancer Network
PARP	poly-ADP-ribose polymerase
PPE	palmar–plantar erythrodysesthesia
TAH/BSO	total abdominal hysterectomy/bilateral salpingo-oophorectomy
TVUS	transvaginal ultrasound
VEGF	vascular endothelial growth factor

REFERENCES

1. Siegel RL, Miller KD, Fuchs HE, Jemal A. Cancer statistics. *CA Cancer J Clin.* 2022;72(1):7–33. 10.3322/caac.21708.
2. Berek JS, Kehoe ST, Kumar L, Friedlander M. Cancer of the ovary, fallopian tube, and peritoneum. *Int J Gynaecol Obstet.* 2018;143:59–78. doi:10.1002/ijgo.12614.
3. SEER: An interactive website for SEER cancer statistics. Accessed 2021 June 13, https://seer.cancer.gov/explorer/.
4. Torre LA, Trabert B, DeSantis CE, et al. Ovarian cancer statistics. *CA Cancer J Clin* 2018;68(4):284–296. doi:10.3322/caac.21456.
5. Reid BM, Permuth JB, Sellers TA. Epidemiology of ovarian cancer: a review. *Cancer Biol Med.* 2017;14(1):9–32. doi:10.20892/j.issn.2095-3941.2016.0084.
6. Bai H, Cao D, Yang J, Li M, Zhang Z, Shen K. Genetic and epigenetic heterogeneity of epithelial ovarian cancer and the clinical implications for molecular targeted therapy. *J Cell Mol Med.* 2016;20(4):581–593. doi:10.1111/jcmm.12771.
7. Lheureux S, Gourley C, Vergote I, et al. Epithelial ovarian cancer. *Lancet.* 2019;393(10177):1240–1253. doi:10.1016/S0140-6736(18)32552-2.
8. Silverberg SG. Histopathologic grading of ovarian carcinoma: a review and proposal. *IJGC.* 2000;19(1):7–15. doi:10.1097/00004347-200001000-00003.
9. Sundar S, Neal RD, Kehoe S. Diagnosis of ovarian cancer. *BMJ.* 2015;351. doi:10.1136/bmj.h4443.
10. Longuespée R, Boyon C, Desmons A, et al. Ovarian cancer molecular pathology. *Cancer Metastasis Rev.* 2012;31(3):713–732. doi:10.1007/s10555-012-9383-7.
11. USPSTF, Grossman DC, Curry SJ, et al. Screening for Ovarian Cancer: US Preventive Services Task Force Recommendation Statement. *JAMA.* 2018;319(6):588–594. doi:10.1001/jama.2017.21926.
12. USPSTF. Screening for Ovarian Cancer: US Preventive Services Task Force Recommendation Statement. *JAMA.* 2018;319(6):588–594. doi:10.1001/jama.2017.21926.
13. Walker JL, Powell CB, Chen LM, et al. Society of Gynecologic Oncology recommendations for the prevention of ovarian cancer. *Cancer.* 2015;121(13):2108–2120. doi:10.1002/cncr.29321.
14. Lancaster JM, Powell CB, Chen L-M, et al. Society of Gynecologic Oncology statement on risk assessment for inherited gynecologic cancer predispositions. *Gynecol Oncol.* 2015;136(1):3–7. doi:10.1016/j.ygyno.2014.09.009.
15. Hartmann LC, Lindor NM. The role of risk-reducing surgery in hereditary breast and ovarian cancer. *N Engl J Med.* 2016;374(5):454–468. doi:10.1056/NEJMra1503523.
16. Narod SA, Sun P, Ghadirian P, et al. Tubal ligation and risk of ovarian cancer in carriers of BRCA1 or BRCA2 mutations: a case-control study. *Lancet.* 2001;357(9267):1467–1470.
17. Goff BA, Mandel LS, Drescher CW, et al. Development of an ovarian cancer symptom index: possibilities for earlier detection. *Cancer.* 2007;109(2):221–227. doi:10.1002/cncr.22371.
18. National Comprehensive Cancer Network. Ovarian Cancer Including Fallopian Tube Cancer and Primary Peritoneal Cancer (Version 3.2021). Accessed November 13, 2021, https://www.nccn.org/professionals/physician_gls/pdf/ovarian.pdf.
19. Earle CC, Schrag D, Neville BA, et al. Effect of surgeon specialty on processes of care and outcomes for ovarian cancer patients. *J Natl Cancer Inst.* 2006;98(3):172–180. doi:10.1093/jnci/djj019.
20. Hess LM, Rong N, Monahan PO, et al. Continued chemotherapy after complete response to primary therapy among women with advanced ovarian cancer: a meta-analysis. *Cancer.* 2010;116(22):5251–5260. doi:10.1002/cncr.25487.
21. Giornelli GH. Management of relapsed ovarian cancer: a review. *Springerplus.* 2016;5(1):1197. doi:10.1186/s40064-016-2660-0.
22. Chang S-J, Bristow RE, Chi DS, Cliby WA. Role of aggressive surgical cytoreduction in advanced ovarian cancer. *J Gynecol Oncol.* 2015;26(4):336. doi:10.3802/jgo.2015.26.4.336.
23. Schorge JO, McCann C, Del Carmen MG. Surgical debulking of ovarian cancer: what difference does it make? *Rev Obstet Gynecol.* 2010;3(3):111.
24. Ibeanu OA, Bristow RE. Predicting the outcome of cytoreductive surgery for advanced ovarian cancer: a review. *Int J Gynecol Cancer.* 2010;20(S1):1–11. doi:10.1111/IGC.0b013e3181cff38b.
25. Mayer AR, Chambers SK, Graves E, et al. Ovarian cancer staging: does it require a gynecologic oncologist? *Gynecol Oncol.* 1992;47(2):223–227. doi:10.1016/0090-8258(92)90110-5.
26. Nguyen HN, Averette HE, Hoskins W, et al. National survey of ovarian carcinoma part V. The impact of physician's specialty on patients' survival. *Cancer.* 1993;72(12):3663–3670. doi:10.1002/1097-0142(19931215)72:12<3663::aid-cncr2820721218>3.0.co;2-s.
27. Martinek IE, Kehoe S. When should surgical cytoreduction in advanced ovarian cancer take place? *J Oncol.* 2010;2010. doi:10.1155/2010/852028.
28. Coleman RL, Spirtos NM, Enserro D, et al. Secondary surgical cytoreduction for recurrent ovarian cancer. *NEJM.* 2019;381(20):1929–1939. doi:10.1056/NEJMoa1902626.
29. Lorusso D, Mancini M, Di Rocco R, et al. The role of secondary surgery in recurrent ovarian cancer. *Int J Surg Oncol.* 2012;2012. doi:10.1155/2012/613980.
30. Bohra U. Recent advances in management of epithelial ovarian cancer. *Apollo Medicine.* 2012;9(3):212–218. doi:10.1016/j.apme.2012.07.011.
31. Pokhriyal R, Hariprasad R, Kumar L, et al. Chemotherapy resistance in advanced ovarian cancer patients. *Biomark Cancer.* 2019;11:1179299X19860815. doi:10.1177/1179299X19860815.
32. McGuire WP, Hoskins WJ, Brady MF, et al. Cyclophosphamide and cisplatin compared with paclitaxel and cisplatin in patients with stage III and stage IV ovarian cancer. *N Engl J Med.* 1996;334(1):1–6. doi:10.1056/NEJM199601043340101.
33. Piccart MJ, Bertelsen K, Stuart G, et al. Long-term follow-up confirms a survival advantage of the paclitaxel–cisplatin regimen over the cyclophosphamide–cisplatin combination in advanced ovarian cancer. *Int J Gynecol Cancer.* 2003;13(Suppl 2):144–148. doi:10.1111/j.1525-1438.2003.13357.x.
34. Bookman M, Greer B, Ozols RJ. Optimal therapy of advanced ovarian cancer: carboplatin and paclitaxel vs. cisplatin and paclitaxel (GOG 158) and an update on GOG0 182-ICON5. *Int J Gynecol Cancer.* 2003;13(6):735–740. doi:10.1111/j.1525-1438.2003.13602.x.
35. Du Bois A, Lück H-J, Meier W, et al. A randomized clinical trial of cisplatin/paclitaxel versus carboplatin/paclitaxel as first-line treatment of ovarian cancer. *J Natl Cancer Inst.* 2003;95(17):1320–1329. doi:10.1093/jnci/djg036.
36. Neijt JP, Engelholm SA, Tuxen MK, et al. Exploratory phase III study of paclitaxel and cisplatin versus paclitaxel and carboplatin in advanced ovarian cancer. *J Clin Oncol.* 2000;18(17):3084–3092. doi:10.1200/JCO.2000.18.17.3084.
37. Ozols RF, Bundy BN, Greer BE, et al. Phase III trial of carboplatin and paclitaxel compared with cisplatin and paclitaxel in patients with optimally resected stage III ovarian cancer: a Gynecologic Oncology Group study. *J Clin Oncol.* 2003;21(17):3194–3200. doi:10.1200/JCO.2003.02.153.
38. Calvert A, Newell D, Gumbrell L, et al. Carboplatin dosage: prospective evaluation of a simple formula based on renal function. *J Clin Oncol.* 1989;7(11):1748–1756. doi:10.1200/JCO.1989.7.11.1748.
39. Vasey PA, Jayson GC, Gordon A, et al. Phase III randomized trial of docetaxel–carboplatin versus paclitaxel–carboplatin as first-line chemotherapy for ovarian carcinoma. *J Natl Cancer Inst.* 2004;96(22):1682–1691. doi:10.1093/jnci/djh323.

40. Fennelly D, Aghajanian C, Shapiro F, et al. Phase I and pharmacologic study of paclitaxel administered weekly in patients with relapsed ovarian cancer. *J Clin Oncol.* 1997;15(1):187–192. doi:10.1200/JCO.1997.15.1.187.
41. Markman M, Blessing J, Rubin SC, et al. Phase II trial of weekly paclitaxel (80 mg/m^2) in platinum and paclitaxel-resistant ovarian and primary peritoneal cancers: a Gynecologic Oncology Group study. *Gynecol Oncol.* 2006;101(3):436–440. doi:10.1016/j.ygyno.2005.10.036.
42. Katsumata N, Yasuda M, Takahashi F, et al. Dose-dense paclitaxel once a week in combination with carboplatin every 3 weeks for advanced ovarian cancer: a phase 3, open-label, randomised controlled trial. *Lancet.* 2009;374(9698):1331–1338. doi:10.1016/S0140-6736(09)61157-0.
43. Fujiwara K, Armstrong D, Morgan M, et al. Principles and practice of intraperitoneal chemotherapy for ovarian cancer. *Int J Gynecol Cancer.* 2007;17(1):1–20. doi:10.1111/j.1525-1438.2007.00809.x.
44. Jaaback K, Johnson N, Lawrie TA. Intraperitoneal chemotherapy for the initial management of primary epithelial ovarian cancer. *Cochrane Database Syst Rev.* 2016;(1): CD005340. doi:10.1002/14651858.CD005340.pub4.
45. Markman M, Bundy BN, Alberts DS, et al. Phase III trial of standard-dose intravenous cisplatin plus paclitaxel versus moderately high-dose carboplatin followed by intravenous paclitaxel and intraperitoneal cisplatin in small-volume stage III ovarian carcinoma: an intergroup study of the Gynecologic Oncology Group, Southwestern Oncology Group, and Eastern Cooperative Oncology Group. *J Clin Oncol.* 2001;19(4):1001–1007. doi:10.1200/JCO.2001.19.4.1001.
46. Armstrong DK, Bundy B, Wenzel L, et al. Intraperitoneal cisplatin and paclitaxel in ovarian cancer. *N Engl J Med.* 2006;354(1):34–43. doi:10.1056/NEJMoa052985.
47. Tewari D, Java JJ, Salani R, et al. Long-term survival advantage and prognostic factors associated with intraperitoneal chemotherapy treatment in advanced ovarian cancer: a gynecologic oncology group study. *J Clin Oncol.* 2015;33(13):1460. doi:10.1200/JCO.2014.55.9898.
48. Alberts DS, Liu P, Hannigan EV, et al. Intraperitoneal cisplatin plus intravenous cyclophosphamide versus intravenous cisplatin plus intravenous cyclophosphamide for stage III ovarian cancer. *N Engl J Med.* 1996;335(26):1950–1955. doi:10.1056/NEJM199612263352603.
49. Walker JL, Armstrong DK, Huang HQ, et al. Intraperitoneal catheter outcomes in a phase III trial of intravenous versus intraperitoneal chemotherapy in optimal stage III ovarian and primary peritoneal cancer: a Gynecologic Oncology Group Study. *Gynecol Oncol.* 2006;100(1):27–32. doi:10.1016/j.ygyno.2005.11.013.
50. Walker JL, Brady MF, Wenzel L, et al. Randomized Trial of Intravenous Versus Intraperitoneal Chemotherapy Plus Bevacizumab in Advanced Ovarian Carcinoma: An NRG Oncology/Gynecologic Oncology Group Study. *J Clin Oncol.* 2019;37(16):1380–1390. doi:10.1200/JCO.18.01568.
51. Seward SM, Winer I. Primary debulking surgery and neoadjuvant chemotherapy in the treatment of advanced epithelial ovarian carcinoma. *Cancer Metastasis Rev.* 2015;34(1):5–10. doi:10.1007/s10555-014-9536-y.
52. Provencher D, Gallagher C, Parulekar W, et al. OV21/PETROC: a randomized Gynecologic Cancer Intergroup phase II study of intraperitoneal versus intravenous chemotherapy following neoadjuvant chemotherapy and optimal debulking surgery in epithelial ovarian cancer. *Ann Oncol.* 2018;29(2):431–438. doi:10.1093/annonc/mdx754.
53. Moore K, Colombo N, Scambia G, et al. Maintenance olaparib in patients with newly diagnosed advanced ovarian cancer. *N Engl J Med.* 2018;379(26):2495–2505. doi:10.1056/NEJMoa1810858.
54. González-Martín A, Pothuri B, Vergote I, et al. Niraparib in patients with newly diagnosed advanced ovarian cancer. *N Engl J Med.* 2019;381(25):2391–2402. doi:10.1056/NEJMoa1910962.
55. Ray-Coquard I, Pautier P, Pignata S, et al. Olaparib plus bevacizumab as first-line maintenance in ovarian cancer. *N Engl J Med.* 2019;381(25):2416–2428. doi:10.1056/NEJMoa1911361.
56. Penn CA, Wong MS, Walsh CS. Cost-effectiveness of maintenance therapy based on molecular classification following treatment of primary epithelial ovarian cancer in the United States. *JAMA Netw Open.* 2020;3(12):e2028620. doi:10.1001/jamanetworkopen.2020.28620.
57. Bozas G, Bamias A, Koutsoukou V, et al. Biweekly gemcitabine and cisplatin in platinum-resistant/refractory, paclitaxel-pretreated, ovarian and peritoneal carcinoma. *Gynecol Oncol.* 2007;104(3):580–585. doi:10.1016/j.ygyno.2006.09.006.
58. Aghajanian C, Blank SV, Goff BA, et al. OCEANS: a randomized, double-blind, placebo-controlled phase III trial of chemotherapy with or without bevacizumab in patients with platinum-sensitive recurrent epithelial ovarian, primary peritoneal, or fallopian tube cancer. *J Clin Oncol.* 2012;30(17):2039. doi:10.1200/JCO.2012.42.0505.
59. Coleman RL, Brady MF, Herzog TJ, et al. Bevacizumab and paclitaxel–carboplatin chemotherapy and secondary cytoreduction in recurrent, platinum-sensitive ovarian cancer (NRG Oncology/Gynecologic Oncology Group study GOG-0213): a multicentre, open-label, randomised, phase 3 trial. *Lancet Oncol.* 2017;18(6):779–791. doi:10.1016/S1470-2045(17)30279-6.
60. Guichard S, Montazeri A, Chatelut E, et al. Schedule-dependent activity of topotecan in OVCAR-3 ovarian carcinoma xenograft: pharmacokinetic and pharmacodynamic evaluation. *Clin Cancer Res.* 2001;7(10):3222–3228.
61. Creemers G, Bolis G, Gore M, et al. Topotecan, an active drug in the second-line treatment of epithelial ovarian cancer: results of a large European phase II study. *J Clin Oncol.* 1996;14(12):3056–3061. doi:10.1200/JCO.1996.14.12.3056.
62. ten Bokkel Huinink W, Gore M, Carmichael J, et al. Topotecan versus paclitaxel for the treatment of recurrent epithelial ovarian cancer. *J Clin Oncol.* 1997;15(6):2183–2193. doi:10.1200/JCO.1997.15.6.2183.
63. Sehouli J, Stengel D, Harter P, et al. Topotecan Weekly Versus Conventional 5-Day Schedule in Patients with Platinum-Resistant Ovarian Cancer: a randomized multicenter phase II trial of the North-Eastern German Society of Gynecological Oncology Ovarian Cancer Study Group. *J Clin Oncol.* 2011;29(2):242–248. doi:10.1200/JCO.2009.27.8911.
64. Muggia FM, Hainsworth JD, Jeffers S, et al. Phase II study of liposomal doxorubicin in refractory ovarian cancer: antitumor activity and toxicity modification by liposomal encapsulation. *J Clin Oncol.* 1997;15(3):987–993. doi:10.1200/JCO.1997.15.3.987.
65. Gordon AN, Fleagle JT, Guthrie D, et al. Recurrent epithelial ovarian carcinoma: a randomized phase III study of pegylated liposomal doxorubicin versus topotecan. *J Clin Oncol.* 2001;19(14):3312–3322. doi:10.1200/JCO.2001.19.14.3312.
66. Gordon AN, Granai C, Rose PG, et al. Phase II study of liposomal doxorubicin in platinum- and paclitaxel-refractory epithelial ovarian cancer. *J Clin Oncol.* 2000;18(17):3093–3100. doi:10.1200/JCO.2000.18.17.3093.
67. Wilailak S, Linasmita V. A study of pegylated liposomal Doxorubicin in platinum-refractory epithelial ovarian cancer. *Oncology.* 2004;67(3-4):183–186. doi:10.1159/000081315.
68. Lund B, Hansen OP, Theilade K, et al. Phase II study of gemcitabine (2′,2′-difluorodeoxycytidine) in previously treated ovarian cancer patients. *J Natl Cancer Inst.* 1994;86(20):1530–1533. doi:10.1093/jnci/86.20.1530.
69. Cannistra SA, Matulonis UA, Penson RT, et al. Phase II study of bevacizumab in patients with platinum-resistant ovarian cancer or peritoneal serous cancer. *J Clin Oncol.* 2007;25(33):5180–5186. doi:10.1200/JCO.2007.12.0782.
70. Burger RA, Sill MW, Monk BJ, et al. Phase II trial of bevacizumab in persistent or recurrent epithelial ovarian cancer or primary peritoneal cancer: a Gynecologic Oncology Group Study. *J Clin Oncol.* 2007;25(33):5165–5171. doi:10.1200/JCO.2007.11.5345.
71. Garcia AA, Hirte H, Fleming G, et al. Phase II clinical trial of bevacizumab and low-dose metronomic oral cyclophosphamide in recurrent ovarian cancer: a trial of the California, Chicago, and Princess Margaret Hospital phase II consortia. *J Clin Oncol.* 2008;26(1):76–82. doi:10.1200/JCO.2007.12.1939.
72. McGonigle KF, Muntz HG, Vuky J, et al. Combined weekly topotecan and biweekly bevacizumab in women with platinum-resistant ovarian, peritoneal, or fallopian tube cancer: results of a phase 2 study. *Cancer.* 2011;117(16):3731–3740. doi:10.1002/cncr.25967.
73. Penson RT, Dizon DS, Cannistra SA, et al. Phase II study of carboplatin, paclitaxel, and bevacizumab with maintenance bevacizumab as first-line chemotherapy for advanced Müllerian tumors. *J Clin Oncol.* 2010;28(1):154–159. doi:10.1200/JCO.2009.22.7900.
74. Wright AA, Cronin A, Milne DE, et al. Use and effectiveness of intraperitoneal chemotherapy for treatment of ovarian cancer. *J Clin Oncol.* 2015;33(26):2841. doi:10.1200/JCO.2015.61.4776.
75. Pujade-Lauraine E, Hilpert F, Weber B, et al. Bevacizumab combined with chemotherapy for platinum-resistant recurrent ovarian cancer: the AURELIA open-label randomized phase III trial. *J Clin Oncol.* 2014;69(7):402–404. doi:10.1200/JCO.2013.51.4489.
76. Perren TJ, Swart AM, Pfisterer J, et al. A phase 3 trial of bevacizumab in ovarian cancer. *N Engl J Med.* 2011;365(26):2484–2496. doi:10.1056/NEJMoa1103799.
77. Burger RA, Brady MF, Bookman MA, et al. Incorporation of bevacizumab in the primary treatment of ovarian cancer. *N Engl J Med.* 2011;365(26):2473–2483. doi:10.1056/NEJMoa1104390.

78. Cohn DE, Barnett JC, Wenzel L, et al. A cost–utility analysis of NRG Oncology/Gynecologic Oncology Group Protocol 218: incorporating prospectively collected quality-of-life scores in an economic model of treatment of ovarian cancer. *Gynecol Oncol.* 2015;136(2):293–299. doi:10.1016/j.ygyno.2014.10.020.
79. Friedlander M, Hancock KC, Rischin D, et al. A Phase II, open-label study evaluating pazopanib in patients with recurrent ovarian cancer. *Gynecol Oncol.* 2010;119(1):32–37. doi:10.1016/j.ygyno.2010.05.033.
80. Kristeleit R, Shapiro GI, Burris HA, et al. A phase I–II study of the oral PARP inhibitor rucaparib in patients with germline BRCA1/2-mutated ovarian carcinoma or other solid tumors. *Clin Cancer Res.* 2017;23(15):4095–4106. doi:10.1158/1078-0432.CCR-16-2796.
81. Smith JA, Le T, Martin GA, et al. Identifying the need to refine the potential patient risk factors for niraparib-induced thrombocytopenia. *Gynecol Oncol.* 2019;152(2):265–269. doi:10.1016/j.ygyno.2018.11.024.
82. Xiao JJ, Nowak D, Ramlau R, et al. Evaluation of drug–drug interactions of rucaparib and CYP 1A2, CYP 2C9, CYP 2C19, CYP 3A, and P-gp substrates in patients with an advanced solid tumor. *Clin Transl Sci.* 2019;12(1):58–65. doi:10.1111/cts.12600.
83. Langdon SP, Gourley C, Gabra H, et al. Endocrine therapy in epithelial ovarian cancer. *Expert Rev Anticancer Ther.* 2017;17(2):109–117. doi:10.1080/14737140.2017.1272414.
84. Ramirez PT, Schmeler KM, Milam MR, et al. Efficacy of letrozole in the treatment of recurrent platinum- and taxane-resistant high-grade cancer of the ovary or peritoneum. *Gynecol Oncol.* 2008;110(1):56–59. doi:10.1016/j.ygyno.2008.03.014.
85. Zhang L, Conejo-Garcia JR, Katsaros D, et al. Intratumoral T cells, recurrence, and survival in epithelial ovarian cancer. *N Engl J Med.* 2003;348(3):203–213. doi:10.1056/NEJMoa020177.
86. Sato E, Olson SH, Ahn J, et al. Intraepithelial CD8+ tumor-infiltrating lymphocytes and a high CD8+/regulatory T cell ratio are associated with favorable prognosis in ovarian cancer. *Proc Natl Acad Sci USA.* 2005;102(51):18538–18543. doi:10.1073/pnas.0509182102.

157

Acute Leukemias

David DeRemer and Tara A. Higgins

KEY CONCEPTS

1. Acute leukemias are the most common malignancies in children and the leading cause of cancer-related death in patients younger than 20 years.
2. Several risk factors correlate with prognosis for acute lymphoblastic leukemia (ALL). Poor prognostic factors include high white blood cell (WBC) count at presentation, very young or very old age at diagnosis, delayed remission induction, and presence of certain cytogenetic abnormalities (eg, Philadelphia chromosome positive [Ph^+]).
3. For children with ALL, remission induction therapy includes vincristine, a corticosteroid, and asparaginase, with or without an anthracycline. For adults with ALL, vincristine, prednisone, anthracycline, and asparaginase are used.
4. All patients with ALL require prophylactic therapy to prevent CNS disease because of the high risk of central nervous system (CNS) relapse. The choice for therapy includes a combination of cranial irradiation, intrathecal chemotherapy, or high-dose systemic chemotherapy with drugs that cross the blood-brain barrier.
5. Long-term maintenance therapy for 2 to 3 years is essential to eradicate residual leukemia cells and prolong the duration of remission. Maintenance therapy consists of oral methotrexate and mercaptopurine, with or without monthly pulses of vincristine and a corticosteroid.
6. Disease-free survival is lower in adults with ALL and has been attributed to greater drug resistance, poor tolerance with subsequent nonadherence, and possibly less-effective therapy. This population is also more likely to have Ph^+ ALL, which is associated with a worse outcome, but the use of tyrosine kinase inhibitors (TKIs) has improved treatment results.
7. Several poor prognostic factors for adult acute myeloid leukemia (AML) include older age, organ impairment, extramedullary disease, and certain cytogenetic and molecular abnormalities.
8. Treatment of AML usually includes therapy with an anthracycline and cytarabine. Postremission therapy is required in all patients and consists of either consolidation chemotherapy with or without maintenance therapy, or hematopoietic stem cell transplantation (HSCT). Novel oral therapies that inhibit FMS-related tyrosine kinase (FLT-3), isocitrate dehydrogenase (IDH1 and IDH2), and B-cell leukemia/lymphoma (BCL-2) have emerged in the AML treatment landscape.
9. Treatment of acute promyelocytic leukemia (APL) consists of induction therapy, consolidation, and maintenance therapy. Induction includes tretinoin and an anthracycline; consolidation therapy consists of two to three cycles of anthracycline-based therapy; maintenance consists of pulse doses of tretinoin, mercaptopurine, and methotrexate for 2 years.
10. Hematopoietic growth factors can be safely and effectively used with myelosuppressive chemotherapy for acute leukemias. They reduce the risk of serious infections, hospital length of stay, and treatment delays but do not prolong disease-free or overall survival.

BEYOND THE BOOK

Watch the video "Valerie Shares Her Story for AML Awareness Month" (https://www.youtube.com/watch?v=8_CD1Yt1-2k). In this Cancer Care video, patient Valerie shares her journey with AML while she underwent treatment at the MD Anderson Cancer Center. After you watch this video, answer the following questions:

1. What are the signs/symptoms of a newly diagnosed AML patient?
2. What economic challenges does Valerie mention? What are some ongoing initiatives to reduce cancer disparities?
3. Discuss the AML treatment options for induction therapy (pediatric, 18-60, ≥60 years old population).
4. When should an AML patient consider a hematopoietic stem cell transplant?

INTRODUCTION

The leukemias are heterogeneous hematologic malignancies characterized by unregulated proliferation of the blood-forming cells in the bone marrow. These immature proliferating leukemia cells (blasts) physically "crowd out" or inhibit normal cellular maturation in bone marrow, resulting in anemia, granulocytopenia, including neutropenia, and thrombocytopenia. Leukemic blasts may also infiltrate various tissues such as lymph nodes, skin, liver, spleen, kidney, testes, and the central nervous system (CNS).

Leukemia is historically classified based on the cell of origin and cell line, and as acute or chronic based on differences in clinical presentation, rapidity of progression of the untreated disease, and response to therapy. The four major leukemias are acute lymphoblastic (or lymphocytic) leukemia (ALL), acute myeloid (or myelogenous) leukemia (AML), chronic lymphocytic leukemia (CLL), and chronic myeloid (or myelogenous) leukemia (CML). Undifferentiated immature cells that proliferate autonomously characterize acute leukemias. Chronic leukemias also proliferate autonomously, but the cells are more differentiated and mature. If untreated, acute leukemia is fatal within weeks to months.

EPIDEMIOLOGY

1 About 26,710 new cases of acute leukemia—20,050 cases of AML and 6,660 cases of ALL were diagnosed in the United States in 2022, accounting for about 1.5% of the total number of cancers diagnosed. The incidence has been relatively stable for two decades. An estimated 13,100 deaths per year, representing about 2% of all cancer deaths, are caused by acute leukemias.[1]

Leukemia is the leading cause of cancer-related deaths in persons younger than 20 years.[2] It is the leading cause of cancer death for males aged 20 to 39 years, but it is an uncommon cause of cancer-related death for both genders after the age of 40 years. Among adults, acute and chronic leukemias occur at equal rates. More than 90% of the cases of acute and chronic leukemia occur in adults. AML accounts for most cases of acute leukemia in adults and occurs with increasing frequency in older patients.[1]

Despite the low incidence, acute leukemias are the most common malignancy in persons younger than 20 years, accounting for nearly 30% of all childhood malignancies. About 75% of children with leukemia have ALL and most of the remaining cases are AML.[1] Conversely, AML represents about 80% of acute leukemias in adults while only 20% of cases are ALL. Pediatric ALL is about 30% more common in males than in females, peaks at 1 to 4 years of age, and is almost twice as likely to affect Caucasian children than African American children.[2] Geographically, the highest rates of ALL have been identified in the Western portion of the US region.[3] Acute leukemia during the first year of life (infant leukemia) slightly favors ALL over AML.

ETIOLOGY

The exact cause of acute leukemias is unknown. A multifactorial process involving genetics, environmental and socioeconomic factors, toxins, immunologic status, and viral exposures is likely. Infectious and genetic factors have the strongest associations. In pediatric ALL, many environmental factors have been associated with the disease: exposure to ionizing radiation, toxic chemicals, herbicides and pesticides; maternal use of contraceptives, diethylstilbestrol, or cigarettes; parental exposure to drugs, diagnostic radiographs, alcohol consumption, coffee and cola consumption, or chemicals before and during pregnancy; and chemical contamination of groundwater.[4,5] Some studies have reported that high birth weight is a risk factor for ALL. Ionizing radiation and benzene exposure are the only environmental risk factors strongly associated with ALL or AML. Some studies have reported an association between electromagnetic fields of high-voltage power lines and the development of leukemia, but larger studies could not confirm this association. In most patients who develop leukemia, a cause cannot be identified.

PATHOPHYSIOLOGY

Normal hematopoiesis consists of multiple well-orchestrated steps of cellular development. Pluripotent stem cells undergo differentiation, proliferation, and maturation, to form the mature blood cells seen in the peripheral circulation. These pluripotent stem cells initially differentiate into two distinct stem cell pools. The myeloid stem cell gives rise to six types of blood cells (erythrocytes, platelets, monocytes, basophils, neutrophils, and eosinophils). Lymphoid stem cells differentiate into natural killer cells, B-lymphocytes, and T-lymphocytes. Leukemia may develop at any stage and within any cell line.

Two features are common to both AML and ALL. First, both arise from a single leukemic cell that expands and acquires additional mutations, culminating in a monoclonal population of leukemia cells. Second, there is a failure to maintain a relative balance between proliferation and differentiation, so that the cells do not differentiate past a particular stage of hematopoiesis. Cells (lymphoblasts or myeloblasts) then proliferate uncontrollably. Proliferation, differentiation, and apoptosis are under genetic control, and leukemia can occur when the balance between these processes is altered.

AML likely arises from a defect in the pluripotent stem cell or a more committed myeloid precursor, resulting in partial differentiation and proliferation of immature precursors of the myeloid blood-forming cells. In older patients, trilineage leukemia occurs, suggesting that the cell of origin is probably a stem or very early progenitor cell. In younger patients, a more differentiated progenitor becomes malignant, allowing some granulocytic and erythroid populations to mature. These two forms of AML exhibit different patterns of resistance to chemotherapy, with resistance more evident in older adults with AML. ALL is a disease characterized by the proliferation of immature lymphoblasts. In this type of acute leukemia, the defect is probably at the level of the lymphoid stem cell or an early lymphoid precursor.

Leukemic cells have growth and survival advantages over normal cells, leading to a "crowding out" phenomenon in the bone marrow. This growth advantage is not caused by more rapid proliferation than normal cells. It may be caused by factors produced by leukemic cells that either inhibit normal cellular proliferation and differentiation or reduce apoptosis compared with normal blood cells.

Specific genetic alterations that lead to leukemia continue to be elucidated. Genetic defects may include (a) activation of a normally suppressed gene (protooncogene) to create an oncogene that produces a protein product that signals increased proliferation; (b) loss of signals for the blood cell to differentiate; (c) loss of tumor suppressor genes that control normal proliferation; and (d) loss of signals for apoptosis. Most normal cells are programmed to die eventually through apoptosis, but the appropriate programmed signal is often interrupted in cancer cells, leading to continued survival, replication, and drug resistance. Signal transduction, RNA transcription, cell-cycle control factors, cell differentiation, and programmed cell death may all be affected.[6,7]

LEUKEMIA CLASSIFICATION

In 2016, the World Health Organization (WHO) revised the current classification system for myeloid neoplasms (Table 157-1).[8] This classification system incorporates not only morphologic findings, but also genetic, immunophenotypic, cytochemical, and clinical features. With the recent discoveries of mutations involved in AML, the revised classification system expanded the prognostic significance of mutations such as c-KIT, FLT-3, CEBPA, NPM1, IDH, WT1, and TET2 in AML subtypes.

ALL is classified based on lymphoblast analysis. Immunophenotype is determined by flow cytometry that analyzes specific antigens, known as clusters of differentiation (often abbreviated "CD"), present on the cell surface. Although no leukemia-specific antigens have been identified, the pattern of cell-surface antigen expression reliably distinguishes between lymphoid and myeloid leukemia. The immunophenotype defines the cell of origin. The major phenotypes are mature B-cell, precursor B-cell, and T-cell disease, but the WHO classifies ALL as either B lymphoblastic or T lymphoblastic. About 80% of childhood ALL derives from precursor B cells and about 15% from T cells; the remainder is from mixed lineage or mature B cells. T-cell ALL is more common in teenage males. In adults, about 75% of ALL is B-cell lineage and 25% is T-cell lineage ALL.

Leukemias may also be described by cytogenetic abnormalities. Chromosome alterations include numerical (hyperdiploidy and hypodiploidy) and structural abnormalities due to exchanges of genetic information within (inversion) or between (translocation) chromosomes. Unique translocations can identify specific subtypes of acute leukemia. The most common translocation in adult ALL,

TABLE 157-1 World Health Organization Classification of Acute Myeloid Leukemia and Related Neoplasms

Acute myeloid leukemia (AML) with recurrent genetic abnormalities
AML with t(8;21)(q22;q22.1); RUNX1-RUNX1T1
AML with inv(16)(p13.1q22) or t(16;16)(p13.1;q22); CBFB-MYH11
APL with PML-RARA
AML with t(9;11)(p21.3;q23.3); MLLT3-KMT2A
AML with t(6;9)(p23;q34.1); DEK-NUP214
AML with inv(3)(q21.3q26.2) or t(3;3)(q21.3;q26.2); GATA2, MECOM
AML (megakaryoblastic) with t(1;22)(p13.3;q13.3); RBM15-MKL1
AML with BCR-ABL1
AML with biallelic mutations of CEBPA
AML with mutated RUNX1
AML with myelodysplasia-related changes
Therapy-related myeloid neoplasms
AML, not otherwise specified
AML with minimal differentiation
AML without maturation
AML with maturation
Acute myelomonocytic leukemia
Acute monoblastic/monocytic leukemia
Pure erythroid leukemia
Acute megakaryoblastic leukemia
Acute basophilic leukemia
Acute panmyelosis with myelofibrosis
Myeloid sarcoma
Myeloid proliferations related to Down syndrome
Transient abnormal myelopoiesis
Myeloid leukemia associated with Down syndrome

PML, promyelocytic leukemia, RARα, retinoic acid receptor-α.

occurring in 25% of patients, is the t(9;22) or Philadelphia chromosome positive (Ph$^+$), which causes fusion of the BCR signaling protein to the ABL nonreceptor tyrosine kinase, resulting in constitutive tyrosine kinase activity. Acute promyelocytic leukemia (APL) is characterized by a specific translocation between chromosomes 15 and 17: t(15;17). Molecular tests may be used to identify products of specific translocations, such as promyelocytic leukemia (PML) retinoic acid receptor-α (RARα) in APL and *AML1-ETO* and *CBFβ/MYH 11* in other subtypes of AML.

Several factors can affect the cytogenetics of AML in adults. First, in about 5% of patients, simultaneous blood and marrow samples demonstrate normal cytogenetics versus abnormal cytogenetics, respectively. Second, central cytogenetic analysis is done in multicenter trials because of variability in specimen examination. Some patients have a normal karyotype on standard review, but carry fusion genes, which are identical to those of translocations or inversions.[8] These insertions of very small chromosome segments do not alter chromosome morphology but may affect outcome.

CLINICAL PRESENTATION

At presentation, common signs and symptoms result from malignant cells that replace and suppress normal hematopoietic progenitor cells and infiltrate into extramedullary spaces. Patients with acute leukemia often present with symptoms related to complications of pancytopenia (eg, anemia, neutropenia, and thrombocytopenia) which include fatigue, infections, gingival bleeding, ecchymoses, and epistaxis.

In addition to clinical presentation, laboratory and pathology evaluations are required for a definitive diagnosis of leukemia. An abnormal complete blood count (CBC) is usually the diagnostic test that initiates a leukemia workup. Although leukemic blast cells may be present on the peripheral blood smear, they are not diagnostic of leukemia because there are other explanations for why immature blast cells may be present in peripheral blood. The most important diagnostic test is a bone marrow biopsy and aspirate, which is submitted to hematopathology for numerous evaluations, including flow cytometry, cytogenetics, and immunophenotyping. A lumbar puncture is performed to determine if there are blasts in the CNS. Unlike ALL, AML is less commonly associated with CNS involvement. A chest radiograph or computed tomography is performed to screen for a mediastinal mass (most common in T-cell disease). The results of these evaluations help to determine the patient's prognosis and therapeutic plan.[9]

ACUTE LYMPHOBLASTIC LEUKEMIA

Risk Classification

2 Several clinical and biological features at diagnosis are associated with response to treatment, as measured by the complete remission rate, duration of remission, and long-term survival. The patient's response to initial therapy is strongly associated with response to treatment. Identifying these risk factors allows the clinician to better understand the disease and personalize treatment according to the risk of disease recurrence (ie, risk-adapted therapy). For example, if a patient has many clinical and laboratory features that are associated with a favorable response to antineoplastic therapy (standard risk), the clinician may give less-intensive therapy to reduce the risk of long-term adverse effects. Conversely, if a patient is unlikely to respond well to standard therapy (high-risk or very-high-risk disease), the clinician may give more intensive antineoplastic therapy. The factors can be grouped as follows: patient characteristics at diagnosis, leukemic cell features at diagnosis, and patient response to initial therapy.

The National Cancer Institute (NCI) developed an ALL-risk stratification to create a standard for comparison in children.[10] Induction therapy is initially selected based on this classification, which divides children into standard- or high-risk categories based on age and initial WBC count (Table 157-2a). Age remains an independent predictor of outcome with children aged 1 to 9 years having the best event-free survival, possibly due to a more frequent favorable cytogenetics in this age group.[11] Age and WBC count has limited prognostic importance in T-cell ALL.[10] The presence of CNS disease at diagnosis is associated with a higher relapse rate. About 2% of males have testicular disease at diagnosis, but not all cooperative groups classify this as an adverse prognostic factor. Male ALL patients have a slightly worse prognosis.[12]

TABLE 157-2a National Cancer Institute Risk Classification for Pediatric Acute Lymphoblastic Leukemia

Risk Group	Standard Risk	High Risk
Age (years)	1–<10	<1 or ≥10
WBC count (× 10^3 cells/mm^3 or × 10^9/L)	<50	≥50
Karyotype	No t(9;22) or t(4;11)	t(9;22) or t(4;11)

WBC, white blood cell.

Data from Smith M, Arthur D, Camitta B, et al. Uniform approach to risk classification and treatment assignment for children with acute lymphoblastic leukemia. J Clin Oncol. 1996;14:18-24.

CLINICAL PRESENTATION Acute Leukemias

General

- Recent history of vague symptoms such as tiredness, lack of exercise tolerance, weight loss, and "feeling unwell," but in no obvious distress.

Signs and Symptoms

- Common: Patients with anemia present with pallor, malaise, palpitations, and fatigue. Patients with low platelet count present with bruising, ecchymoses, and petechiae. Temperature is often elevated and may be caused by disease or infection. Patients may have bone pain from hyperactive bone marrow.
- Other possible symptoms include epistaxis, dyspnea on exertion, seizures, or headache. Splenomegaly, hepatomegaly, or lymphadenopathy is common in patients presenting with ALL, but painless testicular enlargement and rarely, small, blue-green collections of leukemia cells under the skin (chloromas) may also be present. Patients with AML may present with gum hypertrophy and bleeding.

Laboratory Tests

- Complete blood count with differential. Anemia (<7 g/dL [70 g/L; 4.34 mmol/L]) is normochromic and normocytic (without a compensatory increase in reticulocytes). Thrombocytopenia (severe, <20,000 cells/mm^3 [20 × 10^9/L]) is present in 28% of ALL and 50% of AML cases. Patients can present with leukopenia or leukocytosis; about 20% of patients will present with a WBC count ≥50,000 cells/mm^3 (50 × 10^9/L) and 53% of ALL and 20% of AML cases with a WBC <10,000 cells/mm^3 (10 × 10^9/L). Even patients with elevated counts can be considered functionally neutropenic.
- Uric acid may be elevated because of rapid cell turnover and is more common in patients presenting with elevated WBC count and with ALL.
- Electrolytes: potassium and phosphate may be elevated with a compensatory decrease in calcium, more common with ALL.
- Coagulation (more common with AML): elevated prothrombin time, partial thromboplastin time, D-dimers; hypofibrinogenemia.

Other Diagnostic Tests

- Bone marrow aspirate and biopsy: send for morphologic examination, cytochemical staining, immunophenotyping, and cytogenetic (chromosome) analysis. Molecular testing for FMS-like tyrosine kinase 3 (FLT3), nucleophosmin (NPM1), and CCAAT/enhancer binding-protein α (CEBPA), mutations is warranted for suspected AML.
- All adults with ALL should have a screening lumbar puncture performed to assess CNS involvement. Screening in patients with AML is not routine and depends on multiple factors at presentation including symptoms, WBC count, and morphology that includes monocytic disease.
- All pediatric patients with acute leukemias will receive a diagnostic lumbar puncture and intrathecal chemotherapy at that time (intrathecal is usually performed on day 1 of induction chemotherapy for ALL and within the first week of induction for AML patents).

Cell surface and immunophenotype classify childhood ALL into B-cell (85%) or T-cell (15%). T-cell ALL patients are often male, African American, older, and less likely to be Hispanic than B-cell ALL. T-cell ALL generally presents with higher WBC counts and has mediastinal lymph node and CNS involvement. Historically, survival for T-cell ALL was inferior to B-cell ALL, but this difference has narrowed with more intensive therapy.[10] Several cytogenetic abnormalities are associated with prognosis. Favorable outcomes are associated with the presence of trisomy of chromosomes 4 and 10, high hyperdiploidy (chromosome number >50 and DNA index >1.16), and the *ETV6-RUNX1* cryptic translocation, t(12;21).[13] Unfavorable or poor prognostic genetic factors are hypodiploidy (chromosome number <44), MLL rearrangement, BCR-ABL1, Ph-like ALL, CRLF2 rearrangement, intrachromosomal amplification of chromosome 21, and IKZF1 alterations (common in Ph-positive and Ph-like ALL).[10] Ph-like ALL can have translocations similar to BCR/ABL (ie, fusions including ABL1 [non-BCR], ABL2, CSF1R, and PDGFRB) or defects in the Janus kinase (JAK) pathway. The most common cytogenetic abnormalities in B-cell ALL are hyperdiploidy (25%), ETV6-RUNX1 (25%), MLL (5%), hypodiploidy (1%-5%), and Ph-positive (4%).[13]

The strongest prognostic factor for ALL is response to therapy. Previous predictors for early response to treatment were response to the first week of glucocorticoid therapy and evaluation of marrow blasts following 1 to 2 weeks of induction therapy. Minimal residual disease (MRD) quantification at the end of induction has become the most important prognostic factor. Molecular measurement of subclinical MRD by either flow cytometry or polymerase chain reaction detects leukemic cells not visible on morphologic examination to assess treatment response and detect relapse. This technique detects one leukemia cell per 10^4 to 10^5 normal cells. The goal is to have MRD less than 0.01% at the end of remission induction therapy. Children with higher levels have a 3 to 5 times greater risk of treatment failure and death.[10]

The Children's Oncology Group uses a risk- and response-based classification of childhood ALL (Fig. 157-1). This classification system uses the NCI-risk assignment to initially categorize patients into standard- or high-risk groups (see Table 157-2a). Following induction therapy, the risk is reclassified based on completeness of response to therapy, the presence or absence of cytogenetic abnormalities, and CNS involvement (Table 157-2b). Patients are then reclassified as low risk, standard risk, high risk, or very-high risk (see Fig. 157-1). Patients who are initially high risk do not have their therapy reduced, but may have it intensified to very high risk.

Children are classified as low risk and will have therapy reduced if they have trisomy 4 and 10 or the *ETV6-RUNX1* cryptic translocation with less than 0.01% MRD on day 29 bone marrow samples and do not have CNS or testicular disease. Children with testicular disease, MRD greater than or equal to 0.01% on day 29, or who received steroids before diagnosis have postinduction therapy intensified and are classified as high risk. Childhood precursor B-ALL

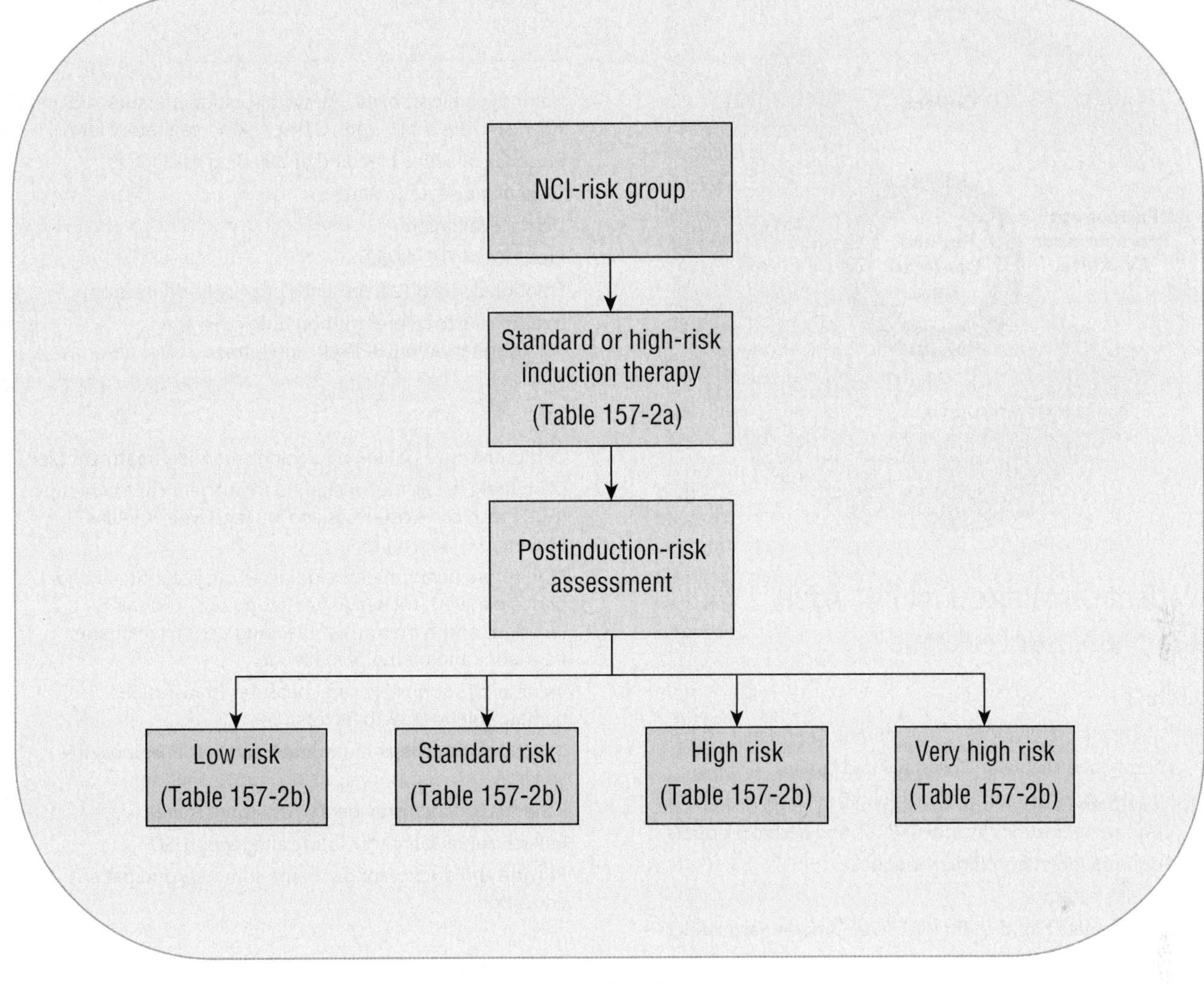

FIGURE 157-1 Risk and response classification of childhood acute lymphoblastic leukemia.

TABLE 157-2b Pediatric Precursor B-Cell Acute Lymphoblastic Leukemia Risk Classification

	Low	Standard			High Risk			Very High Risk		
NCI Risk	**SR**	**SR**	**SR**	**SR**	**SR**	**HR (age <13)**	**SR**	**HR**	**HR (age >13)**	**Any**
Favorable Genetics	Yes	Yes	No	Yes	No	Any	No	Any	Any	Any
Unfavorable Characteristics	None	None	None	None	None	None	None	None	None	Yes
Day 29 Marrow MRD	<0.01%	<0.01%	<0.01%	>0.01%	<0.01%	>0.01%	<0.01%	>0.01%	<0.01%	Any

HR, high risk; MRD, minimal residual disease; NCI, National Cancer Institute; SR, standard risk.

Note: See Table 157-2a for criteria used to categorize patients into initial risk categories.

Data from Schultz KR, Pullen DJ, Sather HN, et al. Blood. 2007;109:926-935.

with more than five WBCs and blasts present in the cerebrospinal fluid (CSF), Ph+ disease, hypodiploidy, $iAMP_{21}$, induction failure, or *MLL* gene rearrangement have therapy intensified and are considered very high risk. Infant ALL, trisomy 21, or childhood T-cell ALL have unique risk classification schemas.[13] Relapse occurs in 15% to 20% of children with ALL. Factors associated with prognosis include time to relapse (ie, shorter time), immunophenotype (ie, T cell), and site of relapse (ie, bone marrow disease). If relapse occurs following the completion of primary treatment, the likelihood of cure is about 50%. If a patient relapses during therapy, only 20% to 30% are cured.[10]

TREATMENT—ACUTE LYMPHOBLASTIC LEUKEMIA

Desired Outcomes

The short-term goal for ALL treatment is to rapidly achieve a complete clinical and hematologic remission (CR), defined as the disappearance of all physical and bone marrow evidence (normal cellularity with less than 5% blasts) of leukemia, with restoration of

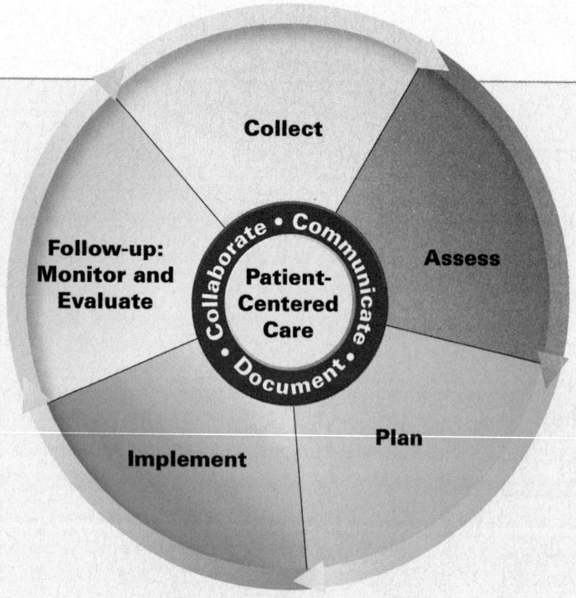

Patient Care Process for Ph+ Adult Lymphoblastic Leukemia

Collect

- Patient characteristics (eg, age, gender, pregnancy status)
- Patient medical history (personal and family)
- Social history (eg, tobacco/marijuana, ethanol use)
- Current medications including OTCs and herbal products
- Confirmation of histological diagnosis
- Objective data
  - Complete blood count (CBC) with differential, platelets
  - Hepatic function tests
  - Basic chemistry panel
  - DIC panel: D-dimer, fibrinogen, PT, PTT
  - Tumor lysis panel (uric acid, potassium, calcium, phosphate)
  - Hepatitis B/C serologies, HIV, CMV status
  - ABO blood typing
  - Human leukocyte antigen (HLA) typing
- Molecular/cytogenetic information

Assess

- Tumor lysis syndrome risk
- Risk for Hepatitis B reactivation (CD20+ monoclonal antibody)
- Central venous access device
- Echocardiogram or MUGA scan (anthracycline component in ALL therapy)
- Chemotherapy consent (willingness for intrathecal chemotherapy)
- Chemotherapy-induced nausea/vomiting risk
- Hemodynamic stability (eg, systolic blood pressure <90 mm Hg, heart rate >110 bpm, O_2 sat <90%, respiratory rate)
- Presence of active bleeding or bleeding risk factors
- Testicular disease (males)
- Dental evaluation
- Presence of Ph+ disease
- Emotional status (eg, presence of anxiety, depression)
- Health insurance/prescription drug coverage (eg, hospitalization, BCR-ABL inhibitor)

Plan

- Comprehensive patient education regarding treatment plan
- Drug therapy regimen including multiagent chemotherapy (IV, IT) with corticosteroids and TKI (eg, Hyper-CVAD + rituximab + dasatinib)
- Monitoring parameters including efficacy (eg, circulating blasts, platelets, trilineage hematopoiesis) and safety (eg, signs and symptoms of bleeding, serum creatinine); frequency and timing of follow-up
- Implement supportive care measures (transfusions, hematopoietic growth factors)
- Infection prophylaxis (antifungal, antiviral, *Pneumocystis jirovecii*)
- Referrals to other providers when appropriate
- Initiate donor search for future allogeneic HSCT
- Provide and document discharge summary and patient education

Implement*

- Provide patient education regarding all elements of the treatment plan
- Use motivational interviewing and coaching strategies to maximize adherence with tyrosine kinase inhibitor (ie, dasatinib)
- Schedule clinic follow-up visits

Follow-up: Monitor and Evaluate

- Response assessment (monitor for minimal residual disease [RT-PCR or next generation sequencing to detect BCR-ABL1]) after completion of induction
- PET scans for extramedullary disease if applicable
- Repeat echocardiogram or MUGA scan if applicable
- Physical examination every 1 to 2 months within the first year following completion of therapy
- Referral to Cancer Survivorship clinic

Collaborate with patient, caregivers, and other healthcare professionals.

normal hematopoiesis. After a CR is achieved, the goal is to maintain the patient in continuous CR. A child is generally considered cured after being in continuous CR for 5 years.

Successful treatment of ALL was first developed in children. Cure rates in children have risen from less than 10% with treatments used in the 1960s to current rates of about 90%.[10] The reason for this improvement lies primarily in improved scheduling of existing drugs, as relatively few new drugs have come to the market since the 1960s. MRD is a strong predictor of relapse in ALL. Children with low-risk disease have a 5-year event-free survival of more than 95%. The 5-year event-free survival for average-risk disease is 90% to 95%. The 5-year event-free survival is nearly 90% for high-risk childhood B-precursor and T-cell ALL. Children with very-high-risk disease have a 5-year event-free survival of less than 80%.[14]

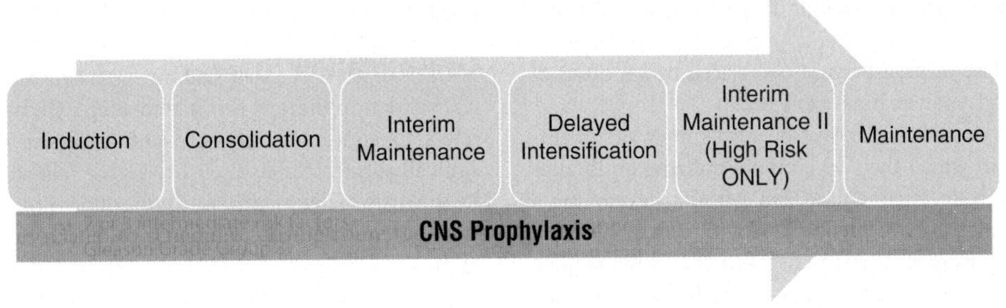

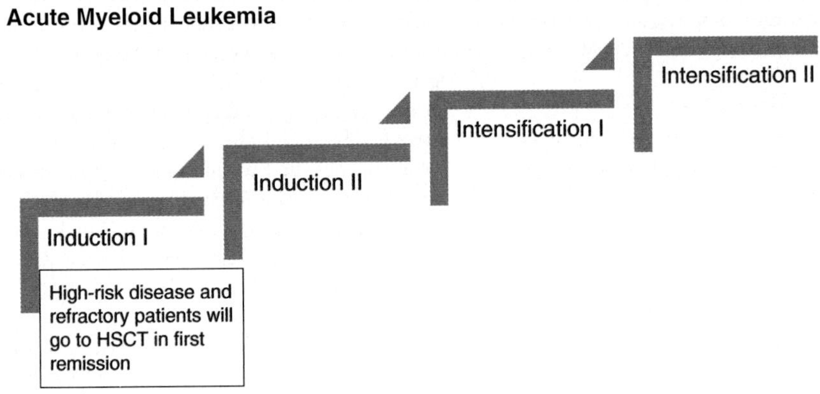

FIGURE 157-2 Treatment phases for acute leukemias.

Response to treatment is determined by intrinsic drug sensitivity and the patient's pharmacogenomics and pharmacodynamics, treatment received, and treatment adherence.

Although treatment response with adult ALL is worse than those with childhood ALL, recent use of aggressive chemotherapy in adult ALL has increased the initial CR rate after induction therapy from 60% to 85%. Long-term event-free survival in this population, however, remains low (between 30% and 40%) because a higher proportion of adults present with high-risk disease. CR rates and event-free survival depend on several poor prognostic factors and certain types of ALL are associated with a very poor outcome.

Treatment Phases

Therapy for childhood ALL is divided into five or six phases: (a) induction, (b) consolidation therapy, (c) interim maintenance, (d) delayed intensification, (e) interim maintenance II, and (f) maintenance therapy (Fig. 157-2). CNS prophylaxis is a mandatory component of ALL treatment regimens and is administered longitudinally during all phases of treatment. The total duration of treatment is 2 to 3 years.[13,15]

Induction

3 The goal of induction is to rapidly induce a CR. The CR rate is about 98% for standard-risk children treated with vincristine, a glucocorticoid (dexamethasone or prednisone), and pegaspargase.[10] Many treatment protocols include daunorubicin in induction (four-drug induction) for high-risk or very-high-risk ALL. Most children achieve a CR in 4 weeks. Those who have positive MRD at day 29 receive intensified therapy. About 2% to 3% of children fail induction therapy and have a 10-year survival rate of 32%.

Prednisone has been the primary glucocorticoid used in pediatric ALL regimens but has been replaced with dexamethasone in most standard-risk protocols due to its longer duration of action and higher CSF penetration.[16] Dexamethasone improves event-free survival and decreases the risk of CNS relapse, but increases the risk of osteonecrosis, mood alteration, steroid myopathy, hyperglycemia, and infections.[16,17] Adolescents (older than 10 years) are particularly prone to osteonecrosis and receive prednisone instead of dexamethasone to minimize this adverse drug reaction.[12] Patients with Down syndrome also receive prednisone because they have increased infections and mortality with dexamethasone.[18]

Asparaginase has historically been available in three forms. L-Asparaginase (no longer manufactured in the United States) and pegaspargase are isolated from *Escherichia coli,* while Erwinia asparaginase is isolated from *Erwinia chrysanthemi.* Erwinia asparaginase is generally utilized in the setting of an allergic reaction to *E. coli* asparaginase. Erwinia asparaginase is given intramuscularly or intravenously. Erwinia asparaginase intravenously may require more frequent administration every 48 hours or the need for nadir serum asparaginase activity if every 72 hour dosing is required (ie, Monday, Wednesday, and Friday administration).[19] Asparaginase erwinia chrysanthemi (recombinant)-rywn is a new asparaginase product on the market. The dose is vastly different from Erwinia asparaginase.[20] An additional novel asparaginase product calaspargase pegol-mknl has also been developed.[21] Pegaspargase is pegylated *E. coli* asparaginase; pegylation prolongs its duration of activity and allows it to be given less frequently. Pegaspargase is used in most protocols and is preferred over L-asparaginase because of fewer intramuscular injections, decreased antibody formation, and superior response rates. Pegaspargase is also approved for IV administration.[22] The addition of asparaginase and an anthracycline to vincristine and prednisone improves remission rates from 85% to 95%.[15]

Asparaginase products are the antineoplastic agents used in ALL which are most likely to cause hypersensitivity reactions. Depending on the type of asparaginase used and the presence of a co-administered steroid, 8% to 42% of patients may develop hypersensitivity reactions to asparaginase.[23] Hypersensitivity reactions to pegaspargase may have a delayed onset (when administered intramuscularly) and prolonged duration, sometimes requiring hospitalization.[24] *Erwinia* asparaginase is only used for patients who are allergic to pegaspargase. Because *Erwinia* asparaginase has a short half-life, it must be administered more frequently. A single dose of pegaspargase is replaced by six doses of *Erwinia* asparaginase, given three times per week.[25]

Patients may develop silent inactivation, also known as subclinical hypersensitivity, in which they develop neutralizing antibodies that can rapidly inactivate asparaginase, but without developing a clinical hypersensitivity reaction. Silent inactivation can be detected by therapeutic monitoring of asparaginase activity. If inadequate asparaginase activity is detected, a therapeutic switch from pegaspargase to *Erwinia* asparaginase can be made to optimize activity and outcomes. The use of therapeutic drug monitoring to optimize the dosing of asparaginase has also been demonstrated in clinical trials.[26]

Central Nervous System Prophylaxis

4 Central nervous system prophylaxis is incorporated throughout all phases of therapy. The rationale for CNS prophylaxis is based on two observations. First, many antineoplastic agents do not readily cross the blood-brain barrier. Second, results from early clinical trials showed that most patients with ALL experienced CNS relapse.[10] These observations indicate that the CNS is a potential sanctuary for leukemic cells and undetectable leukemic cells are present in the CNS in many patients at the time of diagnosis, while only 3% of children have detectable CNS involvement at diagnosis.[11]

The goal of CNS prophylaxis is to eradicate undetectable leukemic cells from the CNS while minimizing neurotoxicity and late effects. Once CNS relapse has occurred, patients are at increased risk of bone marrow relapse and death from refractory leukemia. Initial trials of childhood ALL in the 1960s established craniospinal irradiation as the standard for prevention of CNS relapse. However, this approach is associated with long-term sequelae including neuropsychological deficits, precocious puberty, osteoporosis, decreased intellect, thyroid dysfunction, brain tumors, short stature, and obesity. Subsequent trials showed that irradiation may be replaced by frequent administration of intrathecal chemotherapy in children with ALL. Some centers may treat children with CNS disease at diagnosis or very-high-risk disease with cranial radiation. The use of CNS irradiation and early intensified intrathecal chemotherapy has decreased the rate of CNS relapse to less than 5%.[12]

The CNS prophylaxis regimen is selected based on efficacy, toxicity, and risk of CNS disease. Intrathecal chemotherapy, cranial irradiation, dexamethasone, and high-dose IV methotrexate or cytarabine can be used to treat or prevent CNS disease. At least 80% of children with newly diagnosed ALL are treated without cranial radiation.[10] Risk factors for CNS relapse include male sex, hepatomegaly, T-cell phenotype, CNS2 disease (the presence of leukemic blasts in a CSF sample that contains less than 5 WBC/mm^3 [5×10^6/L]), age younger than 2 years or older than 6 years, and a bloody diagnostic lumbar puncture.[14,27] Intrathecal therapy consists of methotrexate and cytarabine, given either alone or in combination. When given together, hydrocortisone is commonly added (triple intrathecal therapy) to decrease the incidence of arachnoiditis. Triple intrathecal therapy is typically reserved for children with refractory CNS disease. For standard-risk ALL, triple intrathecal therapy decreased CNS relapse rates by 30% as compared to intrathecal methotrexate but had no effect on event-free survival and worsened overall survival.[27] Liposomal cytarabine given intrathecally can induce remission of CNS disease but is associated with arachnoiditis and other CNS-related adverse effects.[28]

Patients with T-cell leukemia have an increased incidence of CNS disease and usually receive systemic therapy that penetrates the CNS such as high-dose methotrexate. Patients with T-cell disease have lower methotrexate polyglutamate accumulation in leukemic blasts and therefore were expected to require higher doses of methotrexate intravenously. The Capizzi methotrexate regimen, which consists of low escalating doses of methotrexate without leucovorin rescue plus pegaspargase, was superior to high-dose methotrexate with leucovorin rescue in 90% of patients receiving cranial radiation therapy.[29]

Consolidation Therapy

Consolidation therapy is initiated after a CR has been achieved and refers to continued intensive antineoplastic therapy to eradicate clinically undetectable disease to secure (consolidate) the remission. Regimens usually incorporate either non–cross-resistant drugs that are different from the induction regimen, or more dose-intensive use of the same drugs.

Randomized trials show that consolidation therapy improves patient outcomes in children, but its benefit in adults is less clear. The relative benefit of individual components of treatment regimens is difficult to demonstrate because of the overall complexity of therapy in ALL. Standard consolidation lasts 4 weeks and usually consists of vincristine, mercaptopurine, and intrathecal methotrexate. In children, the intensity of consolidation therapy is personalized based on the child's initial risk classification and response to induction therapy. Children with high-risk disease receive intensified consolidation that includes the addition of pegaspargase, cyclophosphamide, and low-dose cytarabine to standard therapy.[10,13] Children with testicular disease usually receive radiation during this phase of therapy if a complete clinical response in the testes is not achieved by the end of induction. Patients with T-cell leukemia also receive nelarabine, a prodrug of ara-G that preferentially accumulates in T-lymphoblasts as ara-guanosine triphosphate (GTP), during consolidation and throughout the remainder of their treatment course because it improves event-free survival when it is added to an intensified-therapeutic backbone.[30]

Reinduction (Interim Maintenance and Delayed Intensification)

One or two interim maintenance phases separated by a high-intensity delayed intensification cycle can be added to maintain remission and decrease cumulative toxicity (Fig. 157-2). Interim maintenance is given to all ALL patients. Standard-risk patients receive one interim maintenance cycle that includes IV methotrexate (low dose that escalates over the course of the cycle) and vincristine while high-risk patients receive interim maintenance which includes vincristine, high-dose methotrexate, and mercaptopurine. High-risk patients receive a second interim maintenance after delayed intensification which is similar to standard-risk interim maintenance but adds asparaginase. Delayed intensification is similar for both standard- and high-risk patients and includes vincristine, glucocorticoid, doxorubicin, asparaginase, cyclophosphamide, cytarabine, and thioguanine.[11,12,15] ALL patients previously received one interim maintenance and two delayed intensification cycles. Delayed intensification with dose intensification improved event-free survival and decreased late relapses for high-risk childhood ALL, but there was no additional benefit for the second delayed intensification cycle. Children on the intensified arms of the study received significantly more antimicrobial drugs, blood products, and parenteral nutrition but had no increase in treatment-related mortality.[31] These phases use an augmented schedule and chemotherapy dose that reduces tumor burden and prevents the emergence of drug resistant clones.[12]

Maintenance Therapy

5 Maintenance therapy provides long-term drug exposure to slowly dividing cells, allows the immune system time to eradicate leukemia cells, and promotes apoptosis (programmed cell death). The goal of maintenance therapy is to further eradicate residual leukemic cells and prolong remission duration. Although maintenance therapy is clearly beneficial in childhood ALL, the benefit in adults has only been demonstrated.

Maintenance therapy usually consists of daily mercaptopurine and weekly methotrexate for 12-week courses, at doses that produce mild myelosuppression, with monthly pulses of vincristine and a steroid.[10,31] Since male children treated for 2 years versus 3 years have a slightly higher risk of late relapse (excluding isolated testicular relapse), some centers treat female children for 2 years while males receive maintenance for a total of 3 years of therapy.[11] The most recent Children's Oncology Group trial requires 2 years of therapy for male and female children.

Mercaptopurine and oral methotrexate are available as tablets and as an FDA-approved commercially available oral suspension. It was previously recommended that mercaptopurine be taken at night and administered on an empty stomach without concomitant milk products. It was thought xanthine oxidase in milk products would inactivate the drug and circadian rhythm would affect absorption. However, red cell thioguanine levels are not influenced by coadministration of food or dairy, timing of administration or whether the tablet is swallowed whole, crushed, or chewed. Therefore, previous recommendations may hinder drug adherence.[32] Interpatient variability in the adherence and systemic exposure to oral methotrexate and mercaptopurine is an important determinant of the effectiveness and toxicity of maintenance therapy. Children with an adherence rate less than 95% with mercaptopurine have a 2.7-fold higher risk of suffering a relapse.[33] Factors associated with nonadherence include single-parent household, adolescence, lower socioeconomic status, and Hispanic ethnicity.[34] To account for the interpatient variability, most clinicians will titrate the dose of these agents to achieve adequate myelosuppression.[11] Some clinicians overcome variable bioavailability and poor adherence issues by administering methotrexate IV or intramuscularly. The importance of these pharmacokinetic issues in adults is not well defined.

Genetic polymorphisms may affect drug metabolism, receptor expression, drug transport, drug disposition, and pharmacologic response. Pharmacogenomic polymorphisms are an important determinant of mercaptopurine toxicity. Thiopurine methyltransferase (TPMT) is the predominant inactivating enzyme for thiopurines in hematopoietic tissues. About 10% of the population has intermediate TPMT activity because of heterozygous polymorphisms in the gene encoding for TPMT, and 1 in 300 has extremely low activity because of homozygous presence of this TPMT polymorphism. Patients with low activity (homozygous mutant TPMT genotype) require a tenfold dose reduction and frequency change to three times weekly instead of daily. Heterozygous or intermediate metabolizers will require an initial dose reduction of 30% to 80% if the dose is 75 mg/m^2/day or greater. If the mercaptopurine dose is less than 75 mg/m^2/day, then dose reduction may not be recommended.[35] TPMT testing is now a standard of care at many institutions and treatment dosing is adjusted to minimize toxicity without compromising anti-leukemic outcomes. A coding variant in nudix hydrolase 15 (NUDT15) is another important determinant of thiopurine toxicity. NUDT15 encodes a nucleoside diphosphatase that dephosphorylates active thiopurine metabolites, which prevents them from incorporating into DNA and minimizes their cytotoxicity. If a patient has defective NUDT15 alleles, active thiopurine metabolites can accumulate and cause toxicity.[36]

Philadelphia Chromosome Positive Acute Lymphoblastic Leukemia

Ph$^+$ ALL has historically been treated as very-high-risk disease, which includes the use of a four-drug induction regimen with continuous imatinib mesylate, a tyrosine kinase inhibitor (TKI) that inhibits BCR-ABL kinase, throughout all phases of treatment. This targeted therapeutic approach results in a 5-year overall survival of 70%. The results for patients receiving chemotherapy with imatinib were similar to those receiving hematopoietic stem cell transplantation (HSCT).[37] Imatinib is incorporated into childhood treatment trials for Ph$^+$ ALL in Europe and the United States. Dasatinib shows improved event-free and overall survival compared to imatinib-treated patients with pediatric Ph$^+$ ALL.[38,39] Ph-like ALL is more common in the adolescent and young adult age group (ie, 15-39 years). TKIs (dasatinib), JAK inhibitor (ruxolitinib), and mTOR inhibitors (sirolimus and everolimus) are being investigated for Ph-like ALL.[12,15]

Acute Lymphoblastic Leukemia in Adolescents and Young Adults

Although ALL is relatively uncommon in adolescents and young adults (15-39 years old [AYA]), the outcomes are generally worse than for childhood ALL.[13] The number of AYA patients with ALL has doubled since 1975 and it is estimated to be about 1,200 new diagnoses per year since 2006. In the last decade, about 50% of AYA patients with ALL survived 10 years. ALL in AYA has a higher frequency of T-cell immunophenotype and a lower frequency of the t(12;21)(p13;q22) cryptic translocation responsible for hyperdiploidy and the *ETV6-RUNX1* fusion gene; and increased incidence of Ph$^+$ ALL, intrachromosomal amplification of chromosome 21, and Ph-like ALL which occurs most frequently in the AYA population. Thirteen studies have compared outcomes of AYA patients treated with either pediatric or adult regimens. Pediatric-inspired regimens had better outcomes reported in 12 of the 13 studies. Event-free survival rates ranged from 60% to 77% with pediatric regimens versus 32% to 72% with adult regimens, with an overall survival rate of 27% to 80% versus 10% to 74% for pediatric and adult regimens, respectively. Treatment outcomes for AYA patients undergoing related or unrelated HSCT were compared to similar patients treated with pediatric chemotherapy regimens. Patients treated with chemotherapy alone had a similar relapse rate but significantly less treatment-related mortality. The AYA patients treated with chemotherapy had a significantly higher 4-year survival rate.

The toxicity of chemotherapy regimens is a vital consideration when treating the AYA population. Pediatric regimens do not usually require hospitalization and have a low potential for cardiotoxicity, infertility, and carcinogenesis while adult regimens often require hospitalization for neutropenic fever and other infectious complications. Pediatric chemotherapy regimens are associated with an overall increase in both life years and quality-adjusted life years (QALYs) following the initial stages of treatment. Based on mental health and quality-of-life surveys, depression, anxiety, and posttraumatic stress disorder were present in one-third of AYA patients. Adherence is more problematic in the AYA population due to education, employment, various relationships, and insurance. Oral chemotherapy agents are a large portion of treatment in pediatric regimens while adult regimens often require inpatient therapy, thus affecting school or employment. Both require reliable access to transportation.[40]

Acute Lymphoblastic Leukemia in Adults

6 Risk stratification for adult patients depends on age and Philadelphia chromosome status. The National Comprehensive Cancer Network (NCCN) guidelines recommend different strategies for AYA (15-39 years), adults (40-65 years), and older adults (≥65 years) with substantial comorbidities.[41] The most common treatment regimens use a four-drug induction regimen consisting of an anthracycline, vincristine, an asparaginase, and a corticosteroid. These regimens produce high CR rates (>70%), but the long-term event-free survival is unsatisfactory.[42] Poorer outcomes in adults have been attributed to differences in cytogenetic abnormalities, greater drug resistance, higher risk of treatment-related adverse drug reactions with subsequent nonadherence, and possibly less-effective therapy. Several different regimens are considered appropriate first-line therapies in adults including the Cancer and Leukemia Group B (CALGB) 8811 (Larson regimen), Eastern Cooperative Oncology Group (ECOG) 2903, or Linker regimen.[41] Some studies suggest that high-dose methotrexate and cytarabine alternating with fractionated cyclophosphamide plus vincristine, doxorubicin,

and dexamethasone (hyper-CVAD) may improve response and survival in adults with ALL. Many cases occur in patients older than 65 years, and the response to therapy and durability of response in this subgroup is less than in other populations. Treatment-related mortality rates during remission induction therapy are also higher in this population.[42]

While the overall incidence of Ph$^+$ disease is 25% in adults, the incidence rises to over 40% in adults older than 50 years. Historically, patients with Ph$^+$ ALL had a poor prognosis, with 1-year survival of about 10% without an allogeneic HSCT.[42] As compared with historical control patients treated with standard chemotherapy alone, the addition of BCR-ABL TKI-based therapy to chemotherapy is associated with an increased CR rate and overall survival.[43-46] TKIs should be incorporated early in the Ph$^+$ ALL patient and continuous dosing has demonstrated superior outcomes compared to pulse or intermittent dosing strategies. For patients older than 65 years or those with poor performance status, remission induction regimens may include a BCR-ABL TKI (imatinib, dasatinib, bosutinib, or nilotinib) combined with corticosteroids.[41]

The emergence of resistance to BCR-ABL TKIs provides a challenge in patients relapsing after treatment. Point mutations within the ABL kinase domain and the activation of alternative signaling pathways due to SRC kinase have been identified. A patient's specific mutation analysis should be considered when a specific TKI is selected in the relapsed or refractory setting. Second- and third-generation TKIs have demonstrated activity in patients with imatinib-resistant Ph$^+$ ALL, but ABL mutations such as T315I, V299L, and F317L have demonstrated resistance to dasatinib. Ponatinib is the only BCR-ABL TKI available with known activity against T315I mutations. With the emergence of more potent inhibitors that can induce sustained remissions, studies evaluating the need for intensive chemotherapy are ongoing.[47]

In adults with B-cell ALL, about 50% have leukemic cells that express CD20. CD20 expression is associated with decreased CR rates, higher risk of relapse, and shorter overall survival.[48] The addition of rituximab to hyper-CVAD results in a higher CR rate (70% vs 38%) and longer overall survival (75% vs 47%) as compared with hyper-CVAD alone.[49] Ofatumumab, a more potent second-generation anti-CD20 monoclonal antibody, was also added to hyper-CVAD and produced CR and MRD negativity rates of 98% and 93%, respectively.[50]

HSCT plays an important role in the treatment of adult patients with ALL. For patients with ALL who have a CR after induction therapy, consolidation with allogeneic HSCT should be considered if a human leukocyte antigen (HLA)-matched sibling or matched unrelated donor is available. After HSCT, patients with Ph$^+$ ALL should continue with standard maintenance therapy that includes a TKI. Allogeneic HSCT should be considered for patients with Philadelphia chromosome negative (Ph$^-$) disease who have MRD after induction therapy if a matched donor is available. Allogenic HSCT is preferred over autologous HSCT because of lower disease relapse rates.[51]

Relapsed Acute Lymphoblastic Leukemia

About 20% of children with ALL will relapse, but about 40% will experience long-term overall survival following relapsed treatment regimens.[10] In adults, about 30% to 60% of patients will relapse despite aggressive consolidation and maintenance chemotherapy.[52] The most common site for relapse is the bone marrow, although relapses can occur in the CNS, testicles, or multiple sites. Patients who have completed treatment and remained in remission for longer periods are more likely to achieve remission again.[11,41]

Clofarabine, a purine antimetabolite, is an option for patients with second or later relapses, but the duration of response is short. Single-agent clofarabine is associated with hepatotoxicity, prolonged myelosuppression, and febrile neutropenia.[53] Nelarabine, a T-cell-specific purine nucleoside analog, is approved to treat T-cell ALL who have relapsed disease following at least two prior therapies.[54] The drug is being evaluated in the frontline setting.[55] Adverse drug reactions such as severe peripheral and sensory neurotoxicity, severe somnolence, and seizures have occurred with nelarabine.[54]

Blinatumomab is approved for relapsed or refractory B-cell precursor ALL and in first or second CR with minimal residual disease (MRD) greater than or equal to 0.1%. As a bispecific T-cell engager (BiTE), blinatumomab binds to both CD19, an antigen present throughout B-cell development, and CD3, a T-cell receptor. By linking CD19 and CD3, blinatumomab enables a cascade of events resulting in lysis of CD19 cells.[56] Blinatumomab can induce a CR and achieve MRD negativity in adult and pediatric patients with relapsed or refractory ALL. In a randomized Phase 3 clinical trial, patients receiving blinatumomab had improved overall survival as compared to standard chemotherapy.[57] Blinatumomab has a short half-life and therefore must be administered as a continuous infusion for 28 days of a 6-week cycle. Adverse drug reactions occur in most patients, ranging from mild, reversible symptoms such as fever and rigors to more severe toxicities including neurotoxicity, infections, and cytokine release syndrome.[56]

Inotuzumab ozogamicin, an antibody-drug conjugate targeting CD22, received FDA approval in 2017 for relapsed or refractory B-cell ALL.[58] In a Phase 3 clinical trial, inotuzumab ozogamicin had significantly higher CR rates (80.7% vs 29.4%) compared to a standard chemotherapy group in patients with relapsed or refractory ALL. Positive responses occurred in patients with heavy disease burden and Ph$^+$ disease.[59] In a pediatric study, inotuzumab ozogamicin was evaluated in 51 children who received therapy in a compassionate use program. A CR was achieved in 67% of patients with overt marrow disease with most responders having MRD negativity.[60] Inotuzumab ozogamicin is associated with hepatotoxicity (including veno-occlusive disease [ie, sinusoidal obstruction syndrome]) and increased non-relapse mortality for patients who proceed to HSCT.[59]

Chimeric antigen receptor (CAR) T-cell therapy is a therapeutic option for ALL patients without other curative options. This novel therapeutic modality involves genetically engineered T cells that express CARs directed against CD19, resulting in T cells targeting leukemic cells that express CD19. In August 2017, the FDA-approved tisagenlecleucel, a CD19-directed autologous T-cell immunotherapy, for treatment of patients up to 25 years of age with B-cell ALL that is refractory or in second or later relapse.[61] An impressive 81% of children and young adults had a CR, many of which were durable.[62] The enthusiasm over CAR T-cell therapy based on its activity must be balanced by its significant adverse events and cost. Serious adverse drug reactions of CAR T-cell therapy include hypogammaglobulinemia, encephalopathy, seizures, and cytokine release syndrome (CRS), ranging from mild, flu-like symptoms to multiorgan system failure.[63] A single infusion of tisagenlecleucel is estimated to cost $475,000.[64] In October 2021, the FDA approved brexucabtagene autoleucel, an autologous anti-CD19 CAR T-cell therapy for adult patients with relapsed or refractory B-cell precursor ALL. In the ZUMA-3 trial, 83% of patients achieved a CR following brexucabtagene autoleucel. Adverse drug reactions were frequent with Grade ≥3 CRS and neurologic events occurring in 31% and 38% of patients, respectively.[65]

Allogeneic HSCT has traditionally been the treatment of choice for early bone marrow relapse (continuous CR less than 36 months) while children who relapse more than 36 months after completion of initial therapy have traditionally received chemotherapy alone.[10] The American Society for Transplantation and Cellular Therapy (ASTCT) guidelines recommend allogeneic HSCT for both standard- and high-risk ALL patients in first CR (CR1).[51] This recommendation is based on a meta-analysis of randomized trials that reported significantly reduced all-cause mortality with allogeneic HSCT in CR1 when compared to autologous HSCT.[66] For older patients, reduced-intensity conditioning (RIC) nonmyeloablative transplants may produce similar outcomes with less treatment-related morbidity and mortality.[67]

The decision for pediatric patients with relapsed ALL depends on the time from diagnosis to relapse and MRD at the end of reinduction. Patients who relapse <18 months since diagnosis are considered to have a *very early* relapse; these patients usually relapse while receiving their initial therapy. *Early* relapse occurs 18 months to 3 years; these patients relapse during maintenance or soon after finishing therapy. *Late* relapse occurs greater than 3 years from the start of their initial treatment. Patients are considered low risk if they have a late B-ALL marrow relapse with an end of reinduction marrow MRD <0.1% or late isolated extramedullary relapse with an end of reinduction MRD <0.1%. Intermediate risk patients have a late B-ALL marrow relapse with an end of reinduction MRD greater than or equal to 0.1% or late isolated extramedullary relapse with an end of reinduction RMD greater than or equal to 0.1%. Finally, high-risk patients have an early B-ALL marrow or isolated extramedullary relapse or T-ALL relapse. All patients receive the same four-drug reinduction regimen. Based on the end of reinduction MRD and risk stratification, patients may receive more chemotherapy for a total of 2 years, blinatumomab and HSCT, or continued reinduction cycles and HSCT. If a patient does not achieve MRD less than 0.01%, HSCT is not considered and alternative strategies such as investigational trials should be considered.[14]

TABLE 157-3 AML Risk Status According to Cytogenetics and Molecular Abnormalities

Risk	Cytogenetics	Molecular Abnormalities
Favorable	Inv(16) t(8;21) t(15;17)	NPM1 mutation in the absence of FLT3-ITD or presence of FLT3-ITD^{low} Biallelic CEBPA mutation
Intermediate	Cytogenetics abnormalities not classified as favorable or poor t(9;11)	Core binding factor with KIT mutation Mutated NPM1 and FLT3-ITD^{high} WT-NPM1 without FLT3-ITD^{low}
Poor risk	Complex (≥3 clonal chromosomal abnormalities) Monosomal karyotype -5, 5q, -7, 7q- 11q23 Inv(3) t(6;9) t(9;22)	Normal cytogenetics with FLT3-ITD Mutated TP53 Mutated RUNX1 Mutated ASXL WT-NPM1 and FLT3-ITD^{high}

AML, acute myeloid leukemia; ASXL, additional sex combs; FLT-3-ITD, FMS-like tyrosine kinase 3 internal tandem duplication; NPM1, nucleophosmin; RUNX1, Runt-related transcription factor 1; TP53, tumor protein.

Data from Dohner H, Estey E, Grimwade D, et al. Blood. 2017;129:424-447. National Comprehensive Cancer Network Clinical Practice Guidelines in Oncology. Acute Myeloid Leukemia. Version 3.2021. Accessed November 15, 2021.

ACUTE MYELOID LEUKEMIA

Risk Classification

7 Risk stratification for AML is based on patient-related and disease-related factors that influence a patient's likelihood of responding to drug therapy.[6] Early identification of these risk factors allows clinicians to personalize treatment according to the risk of disease recurrence. A key prognostic factor for AML is age. Patients aged 60 years and older have significantly worse outcomes than their younger counterparts. Older patients have differences in tumor biology which confers resistance and patient characteristics (eg, impaired performance status) that reduce treatment tolerance. Other unfavorable prognostic factors in adult AML include multidrug-resistance gene expression, WBC greater than 100,000 cells/mm^3 (100×10^9/L) and therapy-related AML.[68] Patients who develop "secondary" leukemia after treatment of another malignancy (ie, therapy-related AML) usually have a very poor response to antileukemic chemotherapy. Patient factors such as where patients received treatment, educational level, and cohabitation status may also affect treatment-related mortality.[69,70]

The genetic analysis includes karyotyping and molecular mutational profiling and provides important prognostic information (Table 157-3). For example, patients with core-binding factor with t(8;21)(q22;q22) or inv(16)(p13;q22)/t(16;16)(p13;q22) treated with a cytarabine-based regimen have a relatively favorable prognosis. Adults and children with chromosomal deletions such as 3q[abn(3q)] or 5q[del(5q)], monosomies of chromosome 5 or 7(−5/−7) have a poor prognosis with standard chemotherapy for AML and may be candidates for experimental treatments. About 40% of cases have a normal karyotype.[68] Molecular markers such as FMS-like tyrosine kinase 3 (FLT3), nucleophosmin 1(NPM1), c-KIT, DNA (cytosine-5)-methyltransferase (DNMT3), CEBPA, and isocitrate dehydrogenase 1 and 2 (IDH 1/2) can provide prognostic information and guide postremission therapy.[71]

Two major types of FLT3 mutations have been identified—internal tandem duplications (ITD) and tyrosine kinase domain (TKD) point mutations. Patients with FLT3-ITD mutations have shorter remission durations and worse survival outcomes.[71,72] FLT3-ITD mutations occur in about 15% of older patients and 25% of patients younger than 60 years.[73] *NPM1* mutations occur in about 30% of patients with AML, even in patients with normal karyotype, and commonly coexists with FLT3. They are associated with a higher CR and reduced relapse risk as compared to patients without the mutation. c-KIT mutations have been observed in about 20% of patients with core-binding factor AML and are associated with decreased duration of CR and overall survival.[69,74] CEBPA mutations occur in about 10% of patients with AML. The most common CEBPA mutation, a biallelic (double) mutation, is associated with improved prognosis.[8] IDH1/2 mutations occur in <10% of patients and its effect on prognosis is unclear.[69]

Prognostic factors associated with pediatric AML include response to the first course of remission induction therapy, cytogenetics, and molecular genetics. Poor prognostic factors include monosomy 7, age older than 10 years, black race, internal tandem duplications of FLT3, *MLL* gene rearrangements, and a diagnosis of AML secondary to prior chemotherapy or radiation therapy. Conversely, inversion of chromosome 16, trisomy 21, CBF-AML, *PML-RARA*, *NPM1*, biallelic CEBPA, and *RUNX1-RUNX1T1* fusion transcript t(8;21) are associated with a favorable outcome.[75]

TREATMENT—ACUTE MYELOID LEUKEMIA

Desired Outcomes

The short-term goal of treatment for AML is to rapidly achieve a complete clinical and hematologic remission. In the absence of a CR, a rapid and fatal outcome is inevitable. After a CR is achieved, the goal is to maintain the patient in continuous CR.[72,73] The occurrence of leukemic relapse in the bone marrow significantly reduces the likelihood of cure. Upon relapse, available clinical trials, additional chemotherapy, or best supportive care should be pursued depending on the patient's clinical status.[72] Most patients who will die from acute leukemia die within the first 6 years. Survival curves tend to plateau after that time, and patients alive without disease are considered to be cured of their leukemia.

With recent advances in antineoplastic therapy and supportive care, 20% to 40% become long-term survivors. Overall, the median duration of remission is 1 to 2 years.[74] In contrast to ALL, effective therapies utilized in AML result in severe and often prolonged myelosuppression. As a result, patients with AML, particularly patients older than 60 years, are at greater risk for treatment-related fatal infectious and bleeding complications.

Treatment Phases

Therapy for AML is divided into two phases: (a) induction and (b) postremission therapy (eg, consolidation, intensification) (Fig. 157-2).

Induction

8 As with ALL, the goal of remission induction for AML is to rapidly induce a CR, defined as the disappearance of all clinical and bone marrow evidence (normal cellularity more than 20% with less than 5% blasts) of leukemia, with restoration of normal hematopoiesis (neutrophils more than or equal to 1,000 cells/mm^3 [1 × 10^9/L] and platelets more than 100,000 cells/mm^3 [100 × 10^9/L]). Partial remission is a significant response to treatment (a decrease of at least 50% of blasts). Evidence of residual disease in the bone marrow (5%-25% blasts) is considered a treatment failure requiring additional therapy. The definition of CR has several categories, including CR (morphologic CR with restoration of normal hematopoiesis), CR with incomplete hematological recovery (CRi), cytogenetic CR ([CRc] patient with normal cytogenetics in which cytogenetics were previously abnormal), and molecular CR ([CRm] molecular studies negative). A bone aspirate/biopsy should be obtained 14 to 21 days after the start of induction therapy to assess for response.[72]

A CR is achieved in 60% to 85% of adults aged 60 years or younger. Compared to ALL, however, the CR rate is lower with AML. Because the CR rate in AML is related to the intensity of the remission induction regimen, the drugs used in AML are given at doses that uniformly cause severe myelosuppression (except tretinoin). One reason for the lower CR rate in AML as compared to ALL is the inability to give optimal doses of chemotherapy because of marrow toxicity. With continued improvement of supportive care, more intensive treatment regimens are given to reduce the high rate of leukemic relapse and increase the proportion of long-term survivors. Most patients achieve a CR after one or two courses of chemotherapy. Patients who require additional chemotherapy to achieve a CR have been reported to have a poor prognosis, even if remission is ultimately achieved.

The most active single agents in AML are the anthracycline antibiotics (daunorubicin, doxorubicin, and idarubicin), mitoxantrone, and the antimetabolite cytarabine. The standard therapy for the treatment of adult AML has not changed in several decades. The most common regimen ("7+3") combines daunorubicin administered as a short infusion of 60 to 90 mg/m^2/day on days 1 to 3, along with cytarabine administered as a continuous 24-hour infusion of 100 to 200 mg/m^2/day on days 1 to 7.[6,72] The CR rate with the 7+3 regimen is 65% to 75% in patients aged 18 to 60 years. Several trials have attempted to improve on conventional 7+3 therapy, but have shown no improvement by (a) increasing cytarabine to 10 days, (b) shortening cytarabine to 5 days, (c) substituting doxorubicin, idarubicin, or mitoxantrone for daunorubicin, (d) adding other agents such as etoposide, thioguanine, or topotecan, or (e) increasing cytarabine to higher doses (2 g/m^2 every 12 hours for 8-12 doses).[72] The most recent change to the standard 7+3 regimen is to increase the daunorubicin dose. Adults younger than 60 years with AML who were randomized to receive higher daunorubicin dosages (90 mg/m^2/day on days 1-3) in combination with 7 days of standard-dose cytarabine (100 mg/m^2/day) had a significantly higher CR rate (71% vs 57%) and longer median overall survival (23.7 vs 15.7 months) as compared with those who received the standard 7+3 regimen of daunorubicin (45 mg/m^2/day on days 1-3) and cytarabine. However, on subgroup analysis, the survival benefit with high-dose daunorubicin was restricted to patients with favorable or intermediate-risk cytogenetics and those younger than 50 years.[76]

Idarubicin and mitoxantrone have been evaluated as alternatives to daunorubicin in combination with standard-dose continuous infusion cytarabine. Trials in younger patients reported improved CR rates with these newer anthracyclines (idarubicin) or anthracenediones (mitoxantrone), and one trial reported prolonged survival. Among older adults, the CR rate and overall survival are not different among the different anthracyclines or anthracenediones.[74] Therefore, the anthracycline of choice for the standard 7+3 regimen is daunorubicin or idarubicin (12 mg/m^2) and many centers adopt idarubicin or higher doses of daunorubicin into the induction regimen in younger AML patients.

Based on experimental tumor models that showed a steep dose-response curve for cytarabine, higher cytarabine doses have been evaluated to increase its antileukemic activity. The decision to give high-dose cytarabine during induction depends on the treatment plan for postremission or consolidation therapy. In a study of patients aged 15 through 60 years with AML, the cytarabine dose (conventional dose versus high-dose) in the remission induction regimen (with both cohorts receiving daunorubicin and etoposide) was evaluated in a treatment protocol that did not include high-dose cytarabine as consolidation.[77] Patients who received high-dose cytarabine had higher remission rates and longer overall survival, particularly in patients younger than 46 years. A retrospective study conducted by the European Group for Blood and Marrow Transplantation reported that the cytarabine dose administered during induction and/or consolidation does not influence the outcome in patients who ultimately received allogeneic or autologous HSCT.[78] These data suggest that high doses of cytarabine during induction may not be needed in patients who receive HSCT as postremission therapy. In summary, the role of high-dose cytarabine during induction remains controversial. If used during induction, high-dose cytarabine is more appropriate in younger patients than in older patients because of poor tolerance by older patients. In addition, it may be an option in patients unable to tolerate anthracyclines.

A novel remission induction option has emerged for patients with poor prognosis AML. In August 2017, the FDA granted regular approval to a liposome-encapsulated combination of daunorubicin and cytarabine (CPX-351) to treat adults with newly diagnosed therapy-related AML or AML with myelodysplasia-related changes.[79] Approval was based on an open-label phase 3 trial of newly diagnosed high-risk AML patients aged 60 to 75 years who were randomized to receive the standard 7+3 regimen or CPX-351 for one to two cycles of induction followed by similar consolidation. The CPX-351 induction course consisted of 100 units/m^2 (100 mg/m^2 cytarabine and 44 mg/m^2 daunorubicin) administered as a 90-minute infusion on days 1, 3, and 5. Patients who received CPX-351 had significantly higher CR rates (37.3% vs 25.6%) and overall remission rates (47.7% vs 33.3%) as compared to those receiving the standard 7+3 regimen.[80] Adverse drug reactions associated with CPX-351 include hemorrhagic events, febrile neutropenia, rash, fatigue, and increased risk of infections. Since CPX-351 includes daunorubicin, cardiotoxicity remains a concern and clinicians should monitor cardiac function.[79]

Another recent addition to remission induction therapy is gemtuzumab ozogamicin, which was withdrawn from the US market in 2010 because no survival benefit and increased treatment-related mortality were observed in the pivotal trial. Subsequent trials evaluated lower doses of gemtuzumab ozogamicin.[81] In a Phase 3 trial, patients were randomized to receive daunorubicin (60 mg/m^2 days 1-3) and cytarabine (200 mg/m^2 days 1-7) with or without gemtuzumab ozogamicin (days 1, 4, and 7) for the treatment of adults with newly diagnosed *de novo* AML. Patients in the gemtuzumab ozogamicin group had significantly longer median event-free survival (17.3 vs 9.5 months) as compared with those in the daunorubicin and cytarabine group, but also a higher risk of grade 3 or higher adverse drug reactions (infection, hemorrhage, veno-occlusive disease, and thrombocytopenia).[82]

Several small molecule FLT3 inhibitors have been developed and are changing the AML treatment landscape.[83] Midostaurin is an oral multitargeted TKI that is active against FLT3. In a large phase 3 trial, patients younger than 60 years with AML and an *FLT3* mutation were randomly assigned to receive standard remission induction with daunorubicin and cytarabine plus either midostaurin or placebo. Patients who remained in remission after consolidation therapy received either midostaurin or placebo as maintenance therapy. Patients in the midostaurin arm had a significant improvement in overall survival (74.7 vs 25.6 months).[84] Midostaurin is administered days 8 to 21 of each cycle of induction chemotherapy and during each consolidation cycle.[85]

The NCCN guidelines recommend the standard 7+3 regimen for AML patients younger than 60 years. Younger patients with intermediate-risk disease cytogenetics with *FLT3*-mutant disease should receive 7+3 therapy combined with midostaurin. Patients with therapy-related AML should receive standard 7+3 as remission induction, but CPX-351 administered on days 1, 3, and 5 for one cycle is a recommended alternative option.[72]

Older patients (more than or equal to 60 years) who are not candidates for intensive remission induction therapy should be offered venetoclax, an oral BCL-2 inhibitor, once daily with ramp-up dosing with a hypomethylating agent such as azacitidine or decitabine.[72,86] Azacitidine and decitabine are pyrimidine nucleoside analogs of cytidine that inhibit DNA methylation. While each agent has shown promising results versus conventional chemotherapy and best supportive care, the agents have not been compared to each other in trials.[86,87] Azacitidine is usually given IV or SQ for 7 days while decitabine is given IV for 5 days. Cycles are repeated every 28 days. Median overall survival was increased 4 months with azacitidine compared to standard induction chemotherapy (10.4 vs 6.5 months).[88] These agents are generally well-tolerated with the most significant adverse drug reaction being myelosuppression. Best supportive care includes the use of blood product transfusion support.

Other options for older patients who are not candidates for intensive remission induction therapy include gemtuzumab ozogamicin in CD33-positive patients and IDH inhibitors for patients with IDH1/2 mutations.[72] A single remission induction course of gemtuzumab on days 1 and 8 improves overall survival as compared to best supportive care.[89] Ivosidenib (IDH1 inhibitor) and enasidenib (IDH2 inhibitor) are both FDA-approved for relapsed/refractory AML.[90] These agents are evaluated in combination with hypomethylating agents in the frontline setting. A novel oral hedgehog pathway inhibitor, glasdegib, is approved in combination with low-dose cytarabine for patients ≥75 years who cannot tolerate intensive remission induction therapy.[91]

The NCCN guidelines recommend venetoclax, in combination with decitabine or azacytidine, in AML patients ≥60 years who are not candidates for intensive induction therapies.[72] Venetoclax is associated with tumor lysis syndrome (TLS), and patients should have a WBC <25,000 cells/mm^3 (25 × 10^9/L) prior to initiation.[92] Clinicians should provide prophylactic strategies such as hydration and anti-hyperuricemic therapies and monitor blood chemistries (uric acid, potassium, phosphorus, and calcium).

All adult patients who present with CNS symptoms or asymptomatic monocytic disease should have a diagnostic lumbar puncture and should be treated for disease if it is positive. Methotrexate or cytarabine should be administered intrathecally twice a week until clearance of leukemic blasts from the CSF, and then weekly for 4 to 6 weeks. Continued secondary prophylaxis is recommended following treatment for CNS disease.[72]

Postremission Therapy

8 Although most adults with AML achieve a CR, the duration of remission is short (6-9 months) if no further treatment is given. Relapse is presumably a consequence of the presence of residual, but clinically undetectable, leukemic cells after remission induction therapy. The goal of intensive postremission therapy is to eradicate these residual leukemic cells and prevent the emergence of drug-resistant disease. The need for postremission therapy is based on postmortem analysis and cell kinetic data suggesting that nearly 10^9 residual leukemic cells remain after effective remission induction therapy. Strategies evaluated as postremission therapy include (a) low-dose, prolonged maintenance therapy, (b) short-course intensive chemotherapy-alone regimens, and (c) high-dose chemotherapy followed by allogeneic or autologous HSCT.

In the treatment of AML, intensive postremission therapy is referred to as consolidation therapy. Results of randomized controlled trials in adults clearly show that intensive postremission therapy following remission induction therapy prolongs survival versus no therapy, although the exact duration of postremission therapy is controversial.[6,74]

The intensity of postremission therapy is important. In a large CALGB trial, all patients who achieved a CR after standard 7+3 induction were randomized to receive one of the three cytarabine-based consolidation regimens: 100 mg/m^2/day or 400 mg/m^2/day as a continuous 24-hour infusion, or 3,000 mg/m^2 every 12 hours on days 1, 3, and 5. For adults younger than 60 years, the probability of remaining in CR after 4 years was significantly higher in patients who received high-dose cytarabine (25% vs 29% vs 44%, respectively). Older patients had lower response rates in all arms and did not benefit from the higher cytarabine doses, probably because they could not tolerate the high-dose regimen. Dose-limiting neurotoxicity in the high-dose arm was more common in older patients and those with impaired renal function.[93]

High-dose cytarabine is an essential component of postremission therapy, particularly if it is not used in induction therapy. However, many questions remain, such as the optimal dose (g/m^2), number of doses per cycle, and number of cycles of high-dose cytarabine. Among patients with core-binding factor AML, defined as the presence of either t(8;21) or inv(16), multiple cycles are beneficial. The NCCN guideline recommends three to four cycles of high-dose cytarabine for adults younger than 60 years with favorable cytogenetics. Patients with intermediate-risk cytogenetics should receive three to four cycles of high-dose cytarabine or proceed directly to a matched sibling or alternative donor HSCT.[72] For those patients with FLT3-positive AML, midostaurin on days 8 to 21 should be added to high-dose cytarabine.[83,84] Gemtuzumab ozogamicin, in combination with daunorubicin and cytarabine, is an option for patients with CD33-positive, intermediate-risk cytogenetics AML.

If the patient is 60 years of age or older, standard-dose cytarabine with or without an anthracycline for one to two cycles, a reduced-dose high-dose cytarabine regimen (1-1.5 g/m^2/day for 4-6 doses) for one to two cycles, continuation of low-intensity therapy such as azacitidine or decitabine, or enrollment in a clinical trial is recommended. The reduced dose of high-dose cytarabine in older patients is related to their reduced ability to tolerate cytarabine and the higher risk of neurotoxicity. Patients with high-risk cytogenetics, underlying MDS, or secondary AML should either be enrolled in a clinical trial or be referred for either a matched sibling or alternative donor allogeneic HSCT.[72]

After remission is achieved, maintenance therapy with oral azacitidine (days 1-14 of a 28-day cycle) is recommended for patients <60 years old with intermediate or unfavorable cytogenetics.[72] In a Phase 3 trial of patients >55 years old who were in CR1, oral azacitidine improved overall survival (24.7 vs 14.8 months) as compared to placebo. Common grades 3/4 adverse drug reactions associated with oral azacitidine are neutropenia and thrombocytopenia.[94]

Allogeneic Hematopoietic Stem Cell Transplantation Allogeneic HSCT is the most aggressive postremission therapy in the management of AML. This treatment approach is controversial, specifically the appropriateness, timing, treatment design, and donor selection.

The antileukemic activity of allogeneic HSCT is based on the administration of pretransplant high-dose chemotherapy and the development of a posttransplant immune-based antileukemic response. The immune-based response, referred to as a graft-versus-leukemia (GVL) effect, often accompanies the graft-versus-host disease (GVHD) reaction. Evidence for the immune-based benefit of allogeneic HSCT is based on the observation of consistently lower relapse rates with allogeneic HSCT as compared to autologous or syngeneic HSCT. This potential benefit of allogeneic HSCT can be offset by the risk of posttransplant complications such as GVHD, sinusoidal obstruction syndrome, graft failure, and infections.

Allogeneic HSCT was first evaluated as a treatment modality for AML in refractory patients, but because of initial success in small numbers of patients, it has also been evaluated as intensive-postremission therapy in AML patients in first or subsequent remission.[95] Transplant-related mortality following HLA-matched sibling allogeneic HSCT ranges from 10% to 25%. However, these data are based on studies of HSCT with HLA-identical sibling donors. With increasing use of matched unrelated donors and umbilical cord blood as donor sources, transplant-related mortality of allogeneic transplants continues to be evaluated. With the availability of more effective immunosuppressive and antibiotic regimens, transplant-related mortality has decreased and survival has increased.[96]

Allogeneic HSCT from an HLA-matched sibling donor for AML patients in CR1 results in long-term event-free survival in 43% to 55% of patients. Although the results vary, some of the studies show longer event-free survival and lower relapse rates with allogeneic HSCT in AML in CR1 as compared to chemotherapy-alone postremission regimens. Single center prospective trials have not shown an overall survival advantage for allogeneic HSCT in all patients with AML CR1. Meta-analyses of clinical trials comparing allogeneic HSCT to other consolidation strategies in CR1 show that allogeneic HSCT does provide an overall survival advantage for patients with intermediate- and high-risk AML. The ASTCT recommends allogeneic HSCT for AML patients who are in CR1 with intermediate- or high-risk disease and CR2 patients.[51]

Myeloablative allogeneic HSCT is generally restricted to patients younger than 60 years, which limits the number of patients eligible for treatment of a disease that primarily affects older adults. Non-myeloablative transplantation (NMT) uses RIC preparative regimens and is now being used in AML patients, particularly in older patients and those with comorbid illnesses that would limit their eligibility for conventional allogeneic HSCT.[97] NMT is designed to provide enough immunosuppression in the preparative regimen to allow for engraftment of donor cells and depends primarily on the development of a GVL effect as a means to treat and prevent relapse of AML. The procedure is well tolerated in a wide age range of patients, with low rates of regimen-related toxicity. In a large study of 1,637 patients who received NMT, age was not associated with outcome.[98] Registry data of patients aged 70 years or older (89% received NMT) reported that 2-year overall survival significantly improved between 2000-2007 and 2008-2013 (26% vs 39%).[99]

Given that only 30% of patients have an HLA-matched sibling donor, matched unrelated donor HSCT is also an option for children and younger adults with AML. This approach is associated with improved survival, but the risk of transplant-related mortality is higher than in patients undergoing HLA-matched sibling allogeneic HSCT. A large observational study of matched unrelated donor transplants indicates that overall survival, nonrelapse mortality, and relapse rate have improved over the last two decades.[100]

Autologous Hematopoietic Stem Cell Transplantation Compared to allogeneic HSCT, autologous HSCT has the advantages of a lower risk of posttransplant complications because of lack of immunosuppression and GVHD, and more broad applicability because of a lack of donor limitations and fewer age restrictions. Although the preparative regimen still provides antileukemic activity, autologous HSCT is associated with a higher risk of relapse because of a lack of a GVL effect and potential tumor contamination with autologous stem cells. The ASTCT does not recommend autologous HSCT in pediatric patients.[51] Autologous HSCT is an alternative option in adults, particularly in low-risk patients but should not be pursued in patients with high-risk cytogenetics.[51,101] The NCCN guideline does not recommend autologous HSCT outside the setting of a clinical trial.[72]

Postremission Therapies Several randomized trials in AML patients in CR1 have compared outcomes following allogeneic HSCT, autologous HSCT, or intensive consolidation chemotherapy.[101] In most trials, eligible patients based on age and donor availability received an allogeneic HSCT and the remaining patients were randomized between autologous HSCT and chemotherapy alone. The effect of stem cell source (bone marrow or peripheral blood) on event-free and overall survival has been evaluated in several trials. The ASTCT recommends bone marrow grafts with myeloablative conditioning regimens given comparable survival with a lower risk of chronic GVHD. Peripheral blood may offer improved leukemia-free survival for patients who receive RIC, but additional prospective trials are needed.[96]

The decision to transplant is often based on the cytogenetic risk category.[69] Allogeneic HSCT is the treatment of choice in patients with high-risk cytogenetics because they do poorly with conventional chemotherapy or autologous HSCT. Patients with favorable-risk cytogenetics should not proceed to transplant in CR1, as neither autologous nor allogeneic HSCT is superior to conventional chemotherapy. The optimal treatment of choice in patients with intermediate-risk cytogenetics is not clear and is based on the availability of a matched-related donor and clinician preference. Despite recommendations that patients with intermediate-risk cytogenetics should receive HSCT in CR1, a recent study reported only 27% of patients in a European study proceeded to transplant at CR1.[102]

For patients 60 years and older, additional consolidative chemotherapy or immediately proceeding to HSCT is recommended if the patient has achieved a CR1 and is deemed a suitable transplant candidate. The NCCN guideline recommends NMT rather than a myeloablative transplant in this patient population. For the AML patient who relapses early after induction therapy, if a sibling or matched unrelated donor is available, then allogeneic HSCT is the primary reinduction therapy because conventional chemotherapy offers little benefit. If the relapse occurs late, then HSCT may be used as postremission consolidation after reinduction therapy. In those patients who achieve remission with an intensive regimen but experience significant toxicities, the use of maintenance hypomethylating agents (eg, decitabine or azacitidine) every 4 to 6 weeks until progression is an option.[72]

Acute Myeloid Leukemia in Children

AML comprises about 20% of leukemias in children and adolescents. Most cases of AML in children arise *de novo* but AML is associated with trisomy 21, Fanconi anemia, dyskeratosis congenital, Schwachman-Diamond syndrome, and Kostmann syndrome. Secondary AML is extremely rare in children and is associated with alkylating agents, topoisomerase inhibitors and radiation therapy.[12] AML patients are classified as low risk or high risk based on molecular and cytogenetic markers and response to therapy. Examples of low-risk cytogenetic and molecular markers (ie, favorable prognostic markers) are PML-RARA, inv(16), RUNX1, CEBPα, and NPM1 and examples of high-risk markers (unfavorable prognostic markers) are monosomy 5, monosomy 7, KMT2A (MLL), FLT3/ITD with allelic ratio greater than 0.1%, and rearrangement or loss of ETV6.[103] The CR rate in pediatric AML is high at about 90%, with an event-free and overall survival of 45% and 65%, respectively. Unfortunately, relapse occurs in nearly half of pediatric AML patients. Even in low-risk children, the relapse rate is about 35%. Children with high-risk genetic features are at highest risk of relapse and only one in three are alive at 3 years.

Therapy for AML in children includes one to two cycles of induction therapy followed by two to three cycles of consolidation therapy. The number of cycles varies by protocol. Induction therapy with cytarabine and an anthracycline is standard. Etoposide is often included in induction but its contribution to efficacy is unclear.[104] Gemtuzumab ozogamicin was FDA-approved for newly diagnosed CD33-positive AML patients aged 1 month and older. It has been incorporated into the standard backbone in Children's Oncology Group trials of children with newly diagnosed AML.[105] Consolidation therapy or intensification phases of treatment involve the use of high-dose cytarabine in combination with an anthracycline and etoposide.[13] Maintenance therapy has no role in pediatric AML (see Fig. 157-2). Intrathecal chemotherapy for CNS prophylaxis is routinely used, but the optimal regimen is unknown and varies by protocol.[75] Cranial radiation is only used for patients with refractory CNS disease.

Certain patients may be eligible to receive an HSCT as consolidation therapy instead of continued chemotherapy. The use of HSCT in CR1 rather than waiting until relapse/CR2 is controversial. Most trials recommend consolidation with chemotherapy for favorable-risk patients. The role of HSCT in unfavorable or high-risk patients has been utilized in recent childhood AML studies upfront.[106]

Relapsed or Refractory Acute Myeloid Leukemia

Treatment of relapsed or refractory AML is a therapeutic challenge despite the emergence of novel agents and the increasing number of available donors for HSCT. The most common cause of treatment failure in AML patients receiving chemotherapy alone or undergoing HSCT is relapse. In addition, many patients, particularly older patients, have refractory disease as defined by the inability to achieve a CR after two courses of induction therapy. In most cases, the preferred method of treatment for relapsed or refractory disease is HSCT if patients can tolerate it. Unfortunately, most patients receive salvage chemotherapy because only a small percentage of relapsed or refractory adult patients will be eligible for HSCT, particularly allogeneic HSCT because of age and donor restrictions.

Commonly used salvage chemotherapy regimens include FLAG-IDA (fludarabine, cytarabine, idarubicin, and granulocyte colony stimulating factor), MEC (mitoxantrone, etoposide, cytarabine), and GCLAC (clofarabine, high-dose cytarabine, and priming granulocyte colony stimulating factor). These regimens are associated with CR rates of 40% to 65% in younger patients and significant toxicity.[107] Patients who achieve a CR2 should pursue an allogeneic HSCT since this modality is the only potentially curative therapy. Allogeneic HSCT should be performed when a patient is in CR to allow for a robust GVL effect.

In patients unfit to receive intensive salvage chemotherapy, less-aggressive therapies such as hypomethylating agents (azacitidine, decitabine) are options.[72] In a large multicenter retrospective study of hypomethylating agents in relapsed/refractory AML, 11% of patients achieved a CR with a median overall survival of 6.7 months.[108] Given these poor outcomes with current options, older or unfit patients with relapsed or refractory AML are encouraged to enroll in clinical trials.[72]

Several novel classes of agents are treatment options for relapsed or refractory AML including FLT-3 inhibitors (eg, midostaurin, gilteritinib), IDH (eg, enasidenib, ivosidenib), Hedgehog inhibitors (glasdegib), and BCL-2 inhibitors (venetoclax). Table 157-4 lists novel oral agents for AML. These agents are given either as single agents or combined with other agents such as low-dose cytarabine and hypomethylating agents. Immunotherapy approaches such as CAR T-cells, BiTEs, antibody-drug conjugates, and cell-based vaccines are being investigated in clinical trials.[109]

Acute Promyelocytic Leukemia

Acute promyelocytic leukemia (APL) is a subclass of AML that accounts for about 10% of all cases. APL is the most curable AML subtype, but its clinical presentation is associated with a high early death rate secondary to coagulopathy.[110] Most patients are diagnosed between the ages of 15 and 60 years, and the average age is 44 years.[72] Although the management of APL is complex, remission induction regimens produce CR rates exceeding 90% with 5-year event-free survival rates of 70% to 80%.[111] APL is clinically unique from the other subclasses because of the common occurrence of severe coagulopathy (characterized by disseminated intravascular coagulation) at diagnosis and during induction therapy, which frequently results in intracerebral hemorrhage. In APL, differentiation and maturation arrest are caused by alterations in the retinoic acid receptor (RAR) because of the translocation of chromosomes 15 and 17. The discovery of t(15;17) provides a cytogenetic marker of the disease and is predictive of response to differentiation therapy with tretinoin (commonly referred to as all-*trans* retinoic acid or ATRA). This translocation leads to a fusion protein of the *PML* gene on chromosome 15 and the RARα on chromosome 17.

Before the availability of tretinoin in the late 1980s, treatment of APL consisted of the same combination chemotherapy regimens used in the treatment of other subclasses of AML. Such standard regimens produced CR rates of 50% to 60% but were associated with high treatment-related mortality caused by hemorrhagic complications. The introduction of targeted therapy with tretinoin results in high CR rates with a lower risk of life-threatening bleeding complications. Arsenic trioxide targets the PML moiety, resulting in apoptosis, and is synergistic with tretinoin.[112] The initial WBC count at presentation is the most important prognostic factor in patients with APL. Risk stratification of patients at diagnosis based on WBC count has improved outcomes. Abnormal creatinine, increased peripheral blast count, and coagulopathy are risk factors associated with early death due to hemorrhage.[113]

Treatment Phases

Induction Therapy 9 Tretinoin, an oral vitamin A analog, is given orally in a dose of 45 mg/m²/day, as a single dose or divided into two doses, after a meal. Tretinoin-based regimens achieve CR rates as high as 95% in APL patients within 1 to 3 months. Because tretinoin does not cross the blood-brain barrier, leukemic meningitis should be treated with conventional intrathecal chemotherapy.

Although it is not myelosuppressive, tretinoin therapy is associated with headache, skin and mucous membrane reactions, bone pain, nausea, and retinoic acid syndrome. When tretinoin is started, rapid onset of differentiation of promyelocytes occurs, which can lead to leukocytosis and retinoic acid syndrome. The retinoic acid syndrome (unexplained fever, acute respiratory distress, interstitial pulmonary infiltrates, pleural effusions, and weight gain) is now referred to as APL differentiation syndrome (or APL hyperleukocytosis syndrome) because it is associated with other treatment modalities in the management of APL. The syndrome is fatal in 5% to 29% of cases. A combination of chemotherapy with tretinoin induction decreases the risk of APL differentiation syndrome, and

TABLE 157-4 Novel Oral Therapies for Acute Myeloid Leukemia

Agent	Class	Dosing	FDA Indication	Drug Interactions
Midostaurin	FLT3 inhibitor	50 mg PO twice daily with food	• Newly diagnosed AML that is FLT3 mutation positive as detected by an FDA-approved test, in combination with standard cytarabine and daunorubicin induction and cytarabine consolidation	• Strong CYP3A4 inhibitors; consider alternative therapies • Avoid concomitant CYP3A4 inducers • CYP2B6, BCRP, OATP1B1 substrates; dose adjustment may be necessary
Gilteritinib	FLT3 inhibitor	120 mg PO once daily	• Treatment of adult patients who have relapsed or refractory AML with an FLT3 mutation as detected by an FDA-approved test	• Strong CYP3A inhibitors; consider alternative therapies • Avoid concomitant P-gp and strong CYP3A inducers
Enasidenib	IDH inhibitor	100 mg PO once daily	• Treatment of adult patients with relapsed or refractory AML with an isocitrate dehydrogenase-2 (IDH2) mutation as detected by an FDA-approved test	• Decrease the dose of OATP1B1, OATP1B3, and BCRP substrates
Ivosidenib	IDH inhibitor	500 mg PO once daily with or without food	• Newly diagnosed with IDH1 mutation positive AML who are ≥75 years old or who have comorbidities that preclude use of intensive induction chemotherapy • Relapsed or refractory AML IDH1 mutation positive	• Avoid concomitant CYP3A4 inducers • Avoid concomitant CYP3A4 substrates • Strong or moderate CYP3A4 inhibitors; reduce ivosidenib dose to 250 mg/day if given with strong CYP3A4 inhibitor • QTc prolonging drugs
Glasdegib	Hedgehog inhibitor	100 mg PO once daily	• Treatment of newly diagnosed AML in adult patients who are ≥75 years old or who have comorbidities that preclude use of intensive induction chemotherapy (in combination with low dose cytarabine)	• Avoid concomitant strong and moderate CYP3A4 inducers • Strong CYP3A4 inhibitors; consider alternative therapies • QTc prolonging drugs
Venetoclax	BCL-2 inhibitor	Day 1: 100 mg PO once daily Day 2: 200 mg PO once daily Day 3: 400 mg PO once daily Day 4 and beyond: 400 mg PO once daily of each 28-day cycle in combination with azacitidine or decitabine; 600 mg PO once daily of each 28-day cycle in combination with low-dose cytarabine	• Treatment of newly diagnosed AML in adult patients who are ≥75 years old, or who have comorbidities that preclude use of intensive induction chemotherapy (in combination with azacitidine, or decitabine, or low-dose cytarabine)	• Avoid concomitant strong and moderate CYP3A4 inducers • Strong or moderate CYP3A inhibitors or P-gp inhibitors; adjust dosage of venetoclax • P-gp substrates, take 6 hours prior to venetoclax
Azacitidine	Nucleoside metabolic inhibitor	300 mg PO once daily on days 1 through 14 of each 28-day cycle	• Treatment of adult patients with AML who achieved first complete remission or complete remission with incomplete blood count recovery following intensive induction chemotherapy and are not able to complete intensive curative therapy	• Coadministration with omeprazole increased azacitidine AUC by 19%

BCRP, breast cancer resistance protein; CYP, cytochrome P43550; P-gp, P-glycoprotein; OATP, organic anion-transporting polypeptide.

rapid initiation of dexamethasone 10 mg (0.2 mg/kg per dose in children) twice daily on development of symptoms decreases associated mortality.[113]

For newly diagnosed low-risk APL patients (WBC ≤10,000/mm^3 [10×10^9/L]), induction therapy should consist of tretinoin 45 mg/m^2 in two divided doses daily in addition to arsenic trioxide (ATO) 0.15 mg/kg IV daily until hematologic CR.[72] This "chemotherapy-free" strategy achieved an impressive 100% CR rate in a Phase 3 clinical trial. Furthermore, early mortality and hematological toxicities were significantly less with patients who received tretinoin + ATO compared to those who received tretinoin and chemotherapy.[113] For patients with adequate cardiac function, the combination of daily tretinoin and idarubicin 12 mg/m^2 on days 2, 4, 6, and 8 is also a recommended alternative regimen. Assessment of response to treatment of APL is completed when the bone marrow has recovered after induction therapy. A 28- to 35-day bone marrow biopsy is recommended to document morphologic remission before consolidation.[72] ATO induces clinical remissions in APL through its induction of apoptosis and differentiation.

ATO therapy is associated with two specific adverse drug reactions. First, it can cause the APL differentiation syndrome, similar to tretinoin. Management is similar: corticosteroids at first signs of pulmonary distress or a rapidly rising WBC count. The second adverse drug reaction is prolonged QT_c interval. It is important to obtain a baseline 12-lead electrocardiogram before starting therapy with ATO and correct any electrolyte abnormalities, including potassium, calcium, and magnesium. Other medications known to prolong the QT_c interval should be avoided, if possible, during arsenic trioxide therapy. The QT_c interval should not exceed 500 ms at baseline, and if it increases to more than 500 ms during therapy, the patient should be reevaluated. ATO should not be restarted until the QT_c is less than 460 ms.

High-risk patients (WBC > 10,000/mm^3 [10 × 10^9/L]) represent about 30% of APL patients. They should proceed with induction therapy that consists of tretinoin in addition to an anthracycline. All of these regimens include tretinoin 45 mg/m^2/day until a CR is achieved, in combination with an anthracycline (either daunorubicin or idarubicin) or tretinoin plus ATO for patients unable to tolerate anthracycline therapy. Several induction regimens also contain cytarabine; similar CR rates are observed with daunorubicin or idarubicin.[72] APL cells are more sensitive to anthracyclines, possibly because of decreased P-glycoprotein expression. Gemtuzumab ozogamicin has been added to tretinoin and anthracycline combinations for high-risk patients but does not increase event-free or overall survival.[114]

Consolidation Therapy Due to a high relapse rate, all APL patients should receive consolidation therapy. The NCCN guideline recommends ATO 5 days/week for 4 weeks every 8 weeks for four cycles in addition to tretinoin 45 mg/m^2/day for 2 weeks every 4 weeks for seven cycles in low-risk patients. If ATO is unavailable or contraindicated, low-risk patients should receive tretinoin in combination with an anthracycline in consolidation. In high-risk patients, consolidation therapy consists of multiple cycles of ATO and tretinoin. In patients who have ATO or tretinoin discontinued for toxicity, gemtuzumab ozogamicin may be given once every 4 to 5 weeks until 28 weeks have elapsed from the CR date. Intrathecal chemotherapy (methotrexate alternating with cytarabine) is recommended in high-risk patients during consolidation.[72]

Maintenance Therapy Unlike other subtypes of AML, maintenance therapy is an important but controversial component of therapy for APL. Before the development of tretinoin, nonrandomized trials suggested a benefit of continuous low-dose methotrexate and mercaptopurine as maintenance therapy. Larger prospective randomized trials have demonstrated decreased relapse rates in patients who received maintenance therapy (either tretinoin or combination chemotherapy) and some trials have demonstrated increased event-free and overall survival. However, several large APL study (APL0406, UK AML17, and MD Anderson) protocols do not include maintenance therapy for patients in molecular remission at the end of consolidation.[114] The AIDA 0493 study evaluated four maintenance cohorts (intramuscular methotrexate and mercaptopurine, tretinoin, alternating chemotherapy with tretinoin, and observation) and reported a 12-year event-free survival of 69%, with no significant differences between cohorts. Some experts do not recommend the use of maintenance therapy, particularly in low-risk patients.[113,114] NCCN guidelines recommend that APL patients who achieve molecular remission after consolidation should receive maintenance therapy if indicated by treatment protocol.[72]

Relapsed Acute Promyelocytic Leukemia

The overall incidence of relapsed or refractory APL is 5% to 10%, with rates as high as 20% to 30% in high-risk disease. Most relapses occur in the first 3 years following induction therapy. ATO is the agent of choice for relapsed APL, and this agent serves as a backbone for treatment regimens. Multiple studies have reported CR rates of about 80%.[111]

Several regimens consisting of tretinoin, anthracyclines, ATO, high-dose cytarabine, and gemtuzumab ozogamicin are options for relapsed or refractory APL. For patients in early first relapse (<6 months), an anthracycline-based regimen is recommended for those patients with no prior anthracycline. Similarly, ATO should be integrated into the treatment regimen if the patient has not received prior ATO. For patients who relapse (≥6 months) following an ATO-containing regimen, ATO should be continued with tretinoin plus an anthracycline (or single dose of gemtuzumab ozogamicin).

Patients who achieve a hematologic and molecular remission after ATO therapy should proceed to autologous HSCT.[72] Outcomes with autologous HSCT depend on the patient's disease status at the time of transplant. Autologous HSCT in CR2 (vs CR1) is associated with lower overall survival, leukemia-free survival, and increased treatment-related mortality. Autologous HSCT has shown increased disease-free and overall survival as compared to allogeneic HSCT. In patients who present with bone marrow involvement by cytogenetics or molecular testing before transplant, an allogeneic HSCT should be pursued.[72,115]

Patient Monitoring

In comparison to non-APL AML, molecular and cytogenetic testing at the end of remission induction therapy in APL has no prognostic value. Clinicians should therefore not make decisions based on the presence or absence of any genetic abnormalities. Since terminal differentiation of blasts in APL requires more than 40 days, results of a bone marrow biopsy obtained at the end of remission induction can be misleading because insufficient time has elapsed to determine response. Molecular and cytogenetic response assessment should occur after the completion of consolidation treatment.

Detection of residual PML/RARα transcripts in the bone marrow at the end of consolidation therapy is strongly associated with subsequent hematologic relapse. Achievement of PML/RARα-negative status is associated with a higher probability of cure. This molecular technique allows the clinician to assess response to therapy and detect relapse earlier, which might prevent the development of overt disease recurrence and is associated with improved outcomes as compared with delaying treatment until overt morphologic relapse. Most experts recommend that APL patients be routinely evaluated with polymerase chain reaction for PML/RARα every 3 to 6 months for 2 years, and then every 6 months for 2 years.[72]

ROLE OF HEMATOPOIETIC GROWTH FACTORS IN ACUTE MYELOID LEUKEMIA

10 Hematopoietic growth factors have been evaluated in AML patients to enhance chemotherapy cytotoxicity, shorten the duration of neutropenia, and reduce the incidence and severity of infection following induction and consolidation chemotherapy. Most studies show limited benefit with the use of colony-stimulating factors as "priming" agents administered during remission induction therapy to recruit leukemia cells into the cycle to enhance susceptibility to cell-cycle–specific chemotherapy agents, leading to increased cell kill. The use of hematopoietic growth factors concurrently during chemotherapy administration is discouraged outside the setting of a clinical trial and is not recommended in the American Society of Clinical Oncology (ASCO) guidelines.[116]

Both filgrastim and sargramostim are FDA-approved to prevent neutropenic complications in adult AML patients receiving intensive chemotherapy. Since myeloid blast cells have receptors for granulocyte colony-stimulating factor and granulocyte-macrophage colony-stimulating factor, some experts were initially concerned that the use of these factors would stimulate regrowth of leukemia. Although subsequent studies have addressed these concerns, many clinicians do not initiate filgrastim until an initial remission is achieved. Growth factors are not recommended in APL patients during induction therapy because they can increase the risk of differentiation syndrome.[72]

Several randomized trials, primarily in older patients, show that filgrastim or sargramostim reduces the duration of neutropenia following AML-induction chemotherapy. The ASCO Guidelines for the Use of White Blood Cell Growth Factors consider the use of hematopoietic growth factors after initial induction therapy reasonable, with the understanding that the effects on length of hospitalization and incidence of severe infection are modest. Patients older than 55 years derive the greatest benefit, and use is appropriate in this population where more rapid marrow recovery might decrease the duration of hospitalization.[116] Hematopoietic growth factors have been evaluated in patients with AML, including sargramostim, filgrastim, and pegfilgrastim. Although pegfilgrastim is not FDA-approved for this indication, evidence supports its use in this setting. Multiple biosimilar products are available. Filgrastim-sndz was the first FDA-approved growth factor indicated in patients with AML receiving induction and consolidation therapy.[117] Filgrastim-aafi was approved to reduce the time of neutrophil recovery and duration of fever in AML patients.[118] The use of hematopoietic growth factors can also interfere with the interpretation of the day 14 bone marrow examination. Hematopoietic growth factors should be discontinued at least 7 days before a bone marrow aspirate and biopsy to avoid interfering with the interpretation of the results (ie, may see immature myeloid forms that would suggest residual disease).[72]

SUPPORTIVE CARE

The most common and significant adverse drug reaction of antileukemic agents is marrow suppression. Except for corticosteroids, tretinoin, asparaginase/pegaspargase, and vincristine, antineoplastic agents used to treat acute leukemia cause myelosuppression. During AML remission and postremission therapy, daily monitoring of the complete blood count and the absolute neutrophil count is necessary to determine when red cell and platelet transfusions are needed and when neutropenia occurs and resolves. Marrow hypoplasia from the myelosuppressive regimens usually reaches its lowest point (nadir) after 1 to 2 weeks of therapy and lasts for another 1 to 2 weeks. During this period of hypoplasia, infectious and bleeding complications are major causes of death in leukemic patients.

Since typical signs and symptoms of infection may be absent in the neutropenic host, frequent monitoring of vital signs (particularly fever) and daily assessment are essential. Infection control strategies often include routine handwashing; dietary restrictions; reverse isolation and laminar-air flow rooms; fungal, *Pneumocystis*, and bacterial prophylaxis; and the empiric use of broad-spectrum antibiotics when fever occurs. A joint ASCO/IDSA guideline recommends antibacterial and antifungal prophylaxis in high-risk neutropenic patients (<100 cells/mm^3 [0.1 × 10^9/L] for 7 days). Furthermore, *Pneumocystis jirovecii* prophylaxis is recommended in patients receiving chemotherapy associated with >3.5% risk for pneumonia. Leukemia patients who are herpes simplex virus seropositive undergoing induction therapy should receive antiviral prophylaxis.[119,120] See Chapters 144 and 145 for more detailed discussion of infections in immunocompromised patients.

In children, short-term levofloxacin prophylaxis is recommended during intensive chemotherapy for acute leukemias (ie, *de novo* AML, relapsed AML, secondary AML, ambiguous lineage leukemia treated on AML therapy and relapsed ALL) to reduce the risk of bacteremias. However, pediatric HSCT patients have not shown a significant reduction in bacteremia with levofloxacin prophylaxis. Levofloxacin prophylaxis in pediatric leukemia patients decreases the risk of febrile episodes but does not reduce the risk of severe infection or invasive fungal disease.[121] Infectious complications, especially fungi, are a major cause of morbidity and mortality. Therefore, primary antifungal prophylaxis with a mold active agent is strongly recommended for children with AML, undergoing allogeneic HSCT or receiving systemic treatment for GVHD.[122]

Acute leukemia patients, particularly those with an initial elevated WBC count, are at risk for tumor lysis syndrome (see Chapter 150). Measures to prevent the development of urate nephropathy from the rapid destruction of WBCs include allopurinol or rasburicase, and adequate hydration before and during chemotherapy. Rasburicase, a recombinant urate oxidase enzyme produced by genetic modification of *Saccharomyces cerevisiae*, catalyzes the enzymatic oxidation of uric acid into the inactive soluble metabolite, allantoin. In children, rasburicase more rapidly reduces uric acid levels in patients with aggressive malignancies as compared to allopurinol, and reduces the need for dialysis. Rasburicase has been evaluated in adults, and some studies show that fixed dosing produces equivalent outcomes to a weight-based, milligram per kilogram dosing strategy. Due to its high cost, rasburicase is usually limited to patients with ALL who have a high-WBC count or bulky extramedullary disease, aggressive lymphoma, or patients with AML with a high-presenting WBC. Most institutions also include an elevated uric acid as part of the criteria for use. Rasburicase has a rapid onset of action and long duration of action, so many institutions also limit its use to a single dose and allow repeat doses as needed. Rasburicase is contraindicated in patients with glucose-6-phosphate dehydrogenase (G6PD) deficiency due to an increased risk of methemoglobinemia. Tumor lysis syndrome may result in hyperuricemia, hyperkalemia, hyperphosphatemia, hypocalcemia, and subsequent renal insufficiency.[123]

Hematologic support consists primarily of platelet and packed red blood cell transfusions. Platelet transfusions are often given for peripheral counts below 10,000 cells/mm^3 (10 × 10^9/L) or clinical signs of bleeding. Transfusions of packed red cells may also be indicated for a hemoglobin less than 8 g/dL (80 g/L; 4.96 mmol/L), fatigue, dyspnea, tachycardia, or chest pain. APL can release procoagulants that can cause disseminated intravascular coagulation, necessitating close monitoring and replacement of coagulation factors with cryoprecipitate.

EVALUATION OF THERAPEUTIC OUTCOMES

The development of a pharmaceutical care plan for a acute leukemia patient begins with information about the patient's diagnosis and prognosis. Long-term therapeutic goals for the patient may include long-term event-free survival, although palliative care is possible in some patients. The desired short-term outcome is the achievement of remission. Restoration of normal hematopoiesis and a repeat bone marrow biopsy that demonstrates no evidence of disease serve as documentation that remission has been achieved. After the appropriate postremission therapy has been completed, the patient may return monthly for 1 year, and then every 3 months, to check hematologic values. If no evidence of disease exists after 5 years from the diagnosis and the patient has been in continuous CR, the patient is considered cured.

Frequent monitoring of fevers, hematologic and chemistry laboratory values, microbiology reports, and the patient's physical condition are necessary to identify infection, risk of bleeding, and tumor lysis syndrome early. A coagulation screening panel will identify patients with ongoing disseminated intravascular coagulation, a particular risk with APL.

Clinicians should provide patient education on acute and chronic toxicities of the chemotherapy administered and information regarding antibiotics, antiemetics, nutritional support, hematopoietic growth factors, and other supportive care issues. With the emergence of novel oral agents in the treatment landscape of AML, patients should receive institutional assistance to prevent financial toxicity given potential out-of-pocket expenses that can occur. Financial distress can impact drug therapy adherence, which could potentially impact clinical outcomes. Clinicians need to be actively engaged in assessing drug doses and any dose modifications for organ dysfunction.

Numerous late sequelae from leukemia therapy have been recognized and should be included in the monitoring plan after therapy is completed. Chapter e163 discusses the long-term consequences of HSCT. The Children's Oncology Group Long-Term Follow-Up Guidelines provide an additional resource for assessment and monitoring.[124]

CONCLUSION

Major scientific discoveries, particularly in the elucidation of molecular and genetic alterations, advanced diagnostic methodologies, and the emergence of novel therapeutics, have improved clinical responses and survival in acute leukemias. In ALL, multiagent chemotherapy with vincristine, corticosteroids, and an anthracycline followed by an allogeneic HSCT remains the standard of care for eligible candidates. Second- and third-generation TKIs in combination with chemotherapy have significantly improved survival in patients with Ph^+ ALL. The development of CAR T-cell therapies, in which a patient's T-cells are genetically programmed to recognize leukemic cells, have offered hope to patients with relapsed or refractory ALL. Childhood ALL requires multiple phases of therapy including CNS prophylaxis and most children treated today are cured of their leukemia. In adult AML, the historical induction therapy "7+3" continues to be used, but the FDA has approved nine new agents since 2017. Next-generation sequencing has identified frequently mutated genes including FLT3, NPM1, DNMT3A, IDH1/2, TET2, and others which are associated with prognosis. Novel therapies such as venetoclax, FLT3 inhibitors, IDH inhibitors, Hedgehog inhibitors, and novel anti-CD33 directed agents are changing the AML treatment landscape.

ABBREVIATIONS

ASTCT	American Society for Transplantation and Cellular Therapy
ASCO	American Society of Clinical Oncology
ALL	acute lymphoblastic leukemia
AML	acute myeloid leukemia
APL	acute promyelocytic leukemia
ATRA	all-*trans* retinoic acid
AYA	adolescents and young adults
BCL-2	B-cell lymphoma 2
BCR-ABL	breakpoint cluster region-Abelson protooncogene
BiTE	bi-specific T-cell engager
BMI	body mass index
CALGB	Cancer and Leukemia Group B
CAR	chimeric antigen receptor
CD	cluster of differentiation
CEBPA	CCAAT/enhancer binding-protein α
CNS	central nervous system
CR	complete remission
CR1	first complete remission
CR2	second complete remission
CRi	complete remission with incomplete hematological recovery
CRc	cytogenetic complete remission
CRm	molecular complete remission
CSF	cerebrospinal fluid
ECOG	Eastern Cooperative Oncology Group
FDA	Food and Drug Administration
FLT3	FMS-like tyrosine kinase 3
GTP	guanosine triphosphate
GVHD	graft-versus-host disease
GVL	graft-versus-leukemia
HLA	human leukocyte antigen
HSCT	hematopoietic stem cell transplantation
Hyper-CVAD	high-dose methotrexate and cytarabine alternating with fractionated cyclophosphamide plus vincristine, doxorubicin, and dexamethasone
JAK	Janus kinase
$iAMLP_{21}$	intrachromosomal amplification of chromosome 21
IDH	isocitrate dehydrogenase
ITD	internal tandem duplication
MDS	myelodysplastic syndrome
MLL	mixed lineage leukemia
MRD	minimal residual disease
m-TOR	mammalian target of rapamycin
NCCN	National Comprehensive Cancer Network
NCI	National Cancer Institute
NMT	nonmyeloablative transplant
NPM1	nucleophosmin 1
PETHEMA	Programa para el Estudio de la Terapeutica en Hemopatıa Maligna
Ph-	Philadelphia chromosome negative
Ph^+	Philadelphia chromosome positive
PML	promyelocytic leukemia
QALYs	quality adjusted life years
RARα	retinoic acid receptor-α
RIC	reduced intensity conditioning
TET	ten-eleven translocation methylcytosine dioxygenase
TKD	tyrosine kinase domain
TKI	tyrosine kinase inhibitor
TPMT	thiopurine *S*-methyltransferase
WBC	white blood cell
WHO	World Health Organization
WT1	Wilms tumor 1

REFERENCES

1. Siegel RL, Miller KD, Fuchs HE, Jemal A. Cancer statistics, 2022. *CA Cancer J Clin.* 2022 Jan;72(1):7–33.
2. Howlader N, Noone AM, Krapcho M, et al, eds. SEER Cancer Statistics Review, 1975-2018, National Cancer Institute; 2021.
3. Siegel DA, Henley SJ, Li J, Pollack LA, Van Dyne EA, White A. Rates and trends of pediatric acute lymphoblastic leukemia—United States, 2001-2014. *MMWR Morb Mortal Wkly Rep.* 2017;66:950–954.
4. Wiemels J. New insights into childhood leukemia etiology. *Eur J Epidemiol.* 2015;30:1225–1227.
5. Thomopoulos TP, Ntouvelis E, Diamantaras AA, et al. Maternal and childhood consumption of coffee, tea and cola beverages in association with childhood leukemia: A meta-analysis. *Cancer Epidemiol.* 2015;39:1047–1059.
6. Short NJ, Rytting ME, Cortes JE. Acute myeloid leukaemia. *Lancet.* 2018;392:593–606.
7. Rose-Inman H, Kuehl D. Acute leukemia. *Hematol Oncol Clin North Am.* 2017;31:1011–1028.
8. Arber DA, Orazi A, Hasserjian R, et al. The 2016 revision to the World Health Organization classification of myeloid neoplasms and acute leukemia. *Blood.* 2016;127:2391–2405.
9. Arber DA, Borowitz MJ, Cessna M, et al. Initial diagnostic workup of acute leukemia: Guideline from the College of American Pathologists and the American Society of Hematology. *Arch Pathol Lab Med.* 2017;141:1342–1393.
10. Hunger SP, Mullighan CG. Acute lymphoblastic leukemia in children. *N Engl J Med.* 2015;373:1541–1552.
11. Cooper SL, Brown PA. Treatment of pediatric acute lymphoblastic leukemia. *Pediatr Clin North Am.* 2015;62:61–73.
12. Madhusoodhan PP, Carroll WL, Bhatla T. Progress and prospects in pediatric leukemia. *Curr Probl Pediatr Adolesc Health Care.* 2016;46:229–241.
13. Inaba H, Pui CH. Advances in the diagnosis and treatment of pediatric acute lymphoblastic leukemia. *J Clin Med.* 2021 Apr 29;10(9):1926.
14. Hunger SP, Raetz EA. How I treat relapsed acute lymphoblastic leukemia in the pediatric population. *Blood.* 2020;136(16):1803–1812.
15. National Comprehensive Cancer Center Network Practice Guidelines in Oncology. Pediatric acute lymphoblastic leukemia. Version 1.2022. Accessed January 14, 2022.
16. Inaba H, Pui CH. Glucocorticoid use in acute lymphoblastic leukaemia. *Lancet Oncol.* 2010;11:1096–1106.
17. Mitchell CD, Richards SM, Kinsey SE, et al. Benefit of dexamethasone compared with prednisolone for childhood acute lymphoblastic leukaemia: Results of the UK Medical Research Council ALL97 randomized trial. *Br J Haematol.* 2005;129:734–745.

18. Lee P, Bhansali R, Izraeli S, Hijiya N, Crispino JD. The biology, pathogenesis and clinical aspects of acute lymphoblastic leukemia in children with down syndrome. *Leukemia.* 2016;30(9):1816–1823.
19. Vrooman LM, Kirov II, Dreyer ZE, et al. Activity and toxicity of intravenous Erwinia asparaginase following allergy to *E. coli*-derived asparaginase in children and adolescents with acute lymphoblastic leukemia. *Pediatr Blood Cancer.* 2016;63:228–233.
20. Rylaze (asparaginase erwinia chrysanthemi (recombinant)-rwyn) [package insert]. Palo Alto, CA: Jazz Pharmaceuticals; 2021.
21. Asparlas (calaspargase pegol-mknl) [package insert]. Boston, MA. Servier Pharmaceuticals; 2018.
22. Place AE, Stevenson KE, Vrooman LM, et al. Intravenous pegylated asparaginase versus intramuscular native *Escherichia coli* L-asparaginase in newly diagnosed childhood acute lymphoblastic leukaemia (DFCI 05-001): A randomised, open-label phase 3 trial. *Lancet Oncol.* 2015;16:1677–1690.
23. Hasan H, Shaikh OM, Rassekh SR, et al. Comparison of hypersensitivity rates to intravenous and intramuscular PEG-asparaginase in children with acute lymphoblastic leukemia: A meta-analysis and systematic review. *Pediatr Blood Cancer.* 2017;64:81–88.
24. Petersen WC Jr, Clark D, Senn SL, et al. Comparison of allergic reactions to intravenous and intramuscular pegaspargase in children with acute lymphoblastic leukemia. *Pediatr Hematol Oncol.* 2014;31:311–317.
25. Burke MJ, Devidas M, Maloney K, et al. Severe pegaspargase hypersensitivity reaction rates (grade ≥3) with intravenous infusion vs. intramuscular injection: Analysis of 54,280 doses administered to 16,534 patients on children's oncology group (COG) clinical trials. *Leuk Lymphoma.* 2018 Jul;59(7):1624–1633.
26. Asselin B, Rizzari C. Asparaginase pharmacokinetics and implications of therapeutic drug monitoring. *Leuk Lymphoma.* 2015;56:2273–2280.
27. Matloub Y, Lindemulder S, Gaynon PS, et al. Intrathecal triple therapy decreases central nervous system relapse but fails to improve event-free survival when compared with intrathecal methotrexate: Results of the Children's Cancer Group (CCG) 1952 study for standard-risk acute lymphoblastic leukemia, reported by the Children's Oncology Group. *Blood.* 2006;108:1165–1173.
28. Levinsen M, Harila-Saari A, Grell K, et al. Efficacy and toxicity of intrathecal liposomal cytarabine in first-line therapy of childhood acute lymphoblastic leukemia. *J Pediatr Hematol Oncol.* 2016;38:602–609.
29. Sison EA, Silverman LB. CNS prophylaxis in pediatric acute lymphoblastic leukemia. *Hematol Am Soc Hematol Educ Program.* 2014;2014:198–201.
30. Winter SS, Dunsmore KP, Devidas M, et al. Safe integration of nelarabine into intensive chemotherapy in newly diagnosed T-cell acute lymphoblastic leukemia: Children's Oncology Group Study AALL0434. *Pediatr Blood Cancer.* 2015;62:1176–1183.
31. Seibel NL, Steinherz PG, Sather HN, et al. Early postinduction intensification therapy improves survival for children and adolescents with high-risk acute lymphoblastic leukemia: A report from the Children's Oncology Group. *Blood.* 2008;111:2548–2555.
32. Landier W, Hageman L, Chen Y, et al. Mercaptopurine ingestion habits, red cell thioguanine nucleotide levels, and relapse risk in children with acute lymphoblastic leukemia: A report from the children's oncology group study AALL03N1. *J Clin Oncol.* 2017;35:1730–1736.
33. Bhatia S, Landier W, Hageman L, et al. Systemic exposure to thiopurines and risk of relapse in children with acute lymphoblastic leukemia: A Children's Oncology Group Study. *JAMA Oncol.* 2015;1:287–295.
34. Gupta S, Bhatia S. Optimizing medication adherence in children with cancer. *Curr Opin Pediatr.* 2017;29(1):41–45.
35. Schwab M, Whirl-Carrillo M, Suarez-Kurtz G, et al. Clinical Pharmacogenetics Implementation Consortium (CPIC) guideline for thiopurine dosing based on TPMT and NUDT15 genotypes: 2018 Update. *Clin Pharmacol Ther.* 2019;105(5):1095–1105.
36. Lee SHR, Yang JJ. Pharmacogenomics in acute lymphoblastic leukemia. *Best Pract Res Clin Haematol.* 2017;30:229–236.
37. Schultz KR, Carroll A, Heerema NA, et al. Long-term follow-up of imatinib in pediatric Philadelphia chromosome-positive acute lymphoblastic leukemia: Children's Oncology Group study AALL0031. *Leukemia.* 2014;28:1467–1471.
38. Cerchione C, Locatelli F, Martinelli G, et al. Dasatinib in the management of pediatric patients with Philadelphia chromosome-positive acute lymphoblastic leukemia. *Front Oncol.* 2021 Mar 25;11:632231.
39. Shen S, Chen X, Cai J, et al. Effect of dasatinib vs imatinib in the treatment of pediatric Philadelphia chromosome positive acute lymphoblastic leukemia: A randomized clinical trial. *JAMA Oncol.* 2020;6(3):358–366.
40. McNeer JL, Bleyer A. Acute lymphoblastic leukemia and lymphoblastic lymphoma in adolescents and young adults. *Pediatr Blood Cancer.* 2018;65:e26989.
41. National Comprehensive Cancer Center Network Practice Guidelines in Oncology. Acute lymphoblastic leukemia. Version 2.2021. Accessed November 15, 2021.
42. Paul S, Kantarjian H, Jabbour EJ. Adult acute lymphoblastic leukemia. *Mayo Clin Proc.* 2016;91:1645–1666.
43. Ravandi F, O'Brien SM, Cortes JE, et al. Long-term follow-up of a phase 2 study of chemotherapy plus dasatinib for the initial treatment of patients with Philadelphia chromosome-positive acute lymphoblastic leukemia. *Cancer.* 2015;121:4158–4164.
44. Lim SN, Joo YD, Lee KH, et al. Long-term follow-up of imatinib plus combination chemotherapy in patients with newly diagnosed Philadelphia chromosome-positive acute lymphoblastic leukemia. *Am J Hematol.* 2015;90:1013–1020.
45. Kim DY, Joo YD, Lim SN, et al. Nilotinib combined with multiagent chemotherapy for newly diagnosed Philadelphia-positive acute lymphoblastic leukemia. *Blood.* 2015;126:746–756.
46. Jabbour E, Kantarjian H, Ravandi F, et al. Combination of hyper-CVAD with ponatinib as first-line therapy for patients with Philadelphia chromosome-positive acute lymphoblastic leukaemia: A single-centre, phase 2 study. *Lancet Oncol.* 2015;16:1547–1555.
47. Short NJ, Kantarjian H, Jabbour E, Ravandi F. Which tyrosine kinase inhibitor should we use to treat Philadelphia chromosome-positive acute lymphoblastic leukemia? *Best Pract Res Clin Haematol.* 2017;30:193–200.
48. Esteban RE, Christianne B, Alvaro A, et al. Prognostic effect of CD20 expression in adult B-cell acute lymphoblastic leukemia. *Clin Lymphoma Myeloma Leuk.* 2018 May;18(5):361–367.
49. Thomas DA, OBrien S, Faderl S, et al. Chemoimmunotherapy with a modified hyper-CVAD and rituximab regimen improves outcome in de novo Philadelphia chromosome-negative precursor B-lineage acute lymphoblastic leukemia. *J Clin Oncol.* 2010;28:3880–3889.
50. Bazarbachi A, Yilmaz M, Ravandi F, Thomas D, Khouri M. A phase 2 study of hyper-CVAD plus ofatumumab as frontline therapy in CD20+ acute lymphoblastic leukemia (ALL): Updated results. *J Clin Oncol.* 2018;36:7041.
51. Kanate AS, Majhail NS, Savani BN, et al. Indications for hematopoietic cell transplantation and immune effector cell therapy: Guidelines from the American Society for Transplantation and Cellular Therapy. *Bio Blood Marrow Transplant.* 2020 Jul;26(7):1247–1256.
52. Gokbuget N. How should we treat a patient with relapsed Ph-negative B-ALL and what novel approaches are being investigated? *Best Pract Res Clin Haematol.* 2017 Sep;30(3):261–274.
53. Clolar (clofarabine) [package insert]. Cambridge. MA: Genzyme; 2016.
54. Arranon (nelarabine) [package insert]. East Hanover, NJ: Novartis Pharmaceuticals; 2019.
55. Abaza MY, Kantarjian H, Faderl S, et al. Hyper-CVAD plus nelarabine in newly diagnosed adult T-cell acute lymphoblastic leukemia and T-lymphoblastic lymphoma. *Am J Hematol.* 2018 Jan;93(1):91–99.
56. Blincyto (blinatumomab) [package insert]. Thousand Oaks, CA: Amgen; 2021.
57. Kantarjian H, Stein A, Gokbuget N, et al. Blinatumomab versus chemotherapy for advanced acute lymphoblastic leukemia. *N Engl J Med.* 2017;376:836–847.
58. Besponsa (inotuzumab ozogamicin) [package insert]. Philadelphia, PA: Wyeth Pharmaceuticals; 2017.
59. Kantarjian HM, DeAngelo DJ, Stelljes M, et al. Inotuzumab ozogamicin versus standard therapy for acute lymphoblastic leukemia. *N Engl J Med.* 2016;375:740–753.
60. Bhojwani D, Sposto R, Shah NN, et al. Inotuzumab ozogamicin in pediatric patients with relapsed/refractory acute lymphoblastic leukemia. *Leukemia.* 2019;33(4):884–892.
61. O'Leary MC, Lu X, Huang Y, et al. FDA approval summary: Tisagenlecleucel for treatment of patients with relapsed or refractory B-Cell precursor acute lymphoblastic leukemia. *Clin Cancer Res.* 2019;25:1142–1146.
62. Maude SL, Laetsch TW, Buechner J, et al. Tisagenlecleucel in children and young adults with B-Cell lymphoblastic leukemia. *N Engl J Med.* 2018;378:439–448.
63. Hansen DK, Dam M, Faramand RG. Toxicities associated with adoptive cellular therapies. *Best Pract Res Clin Haematol.* 2021 Sep;34(3):101287.
64. Bach PB, Giralt SA, Saltz LB. FDA approval of tisagenlecleucel: Promise and complexities of a $475000 cancer drug. *JAMA.* 2017;318:1861–1862.
65. Shah BD, Bishop MR, Oluwole O, et al. KTE-X19 anti-CD19 CAR T-cell therapy in adult relapsed/refractory acute lymphoblastic leukemia: ZUMA-3 phase 1 results. *Blood.* 2021 Jul 8;138(1):11–22.

66. Ram R, Gafter-Gvili A, Vidal L, et al. Management of adult patients with acute lymphoblastic leukemia in first complete remission: Systematic review and meta-analysis. *Cancer.* 2010;116:3447–3457.
67. Akahoshi Y, Nishiwaki S, Arai Y, et al. Reduced-intensity conditioning is a reasonable alternative for Philadelphia chromosome-positive acute lymphoblastic leukemia among elderly patients who have achieved negative minimal residual disease: A report from the Adult Acute Lymphoblastic Leukemia Working Group of the JSHCT. *Bone Marrow Transplant.* 2020 Jul;55(7):1317–1325.
68. Cordoba R, Eyre TA, Klepin HD, et al. A comprehensive approach to therapy of haematological malignancies in older patients. *Lancet Haematol.* 2021 Nov;8(11);e840–e852.
69. Estey EH. Acute myeloid leukemia: 2021 Update on risk-stratification and management. *Am J Hematol.* 2020 Nov;95(11):1368–1398.
70. Sorror ML, Storer BE, Fathi AT, et al. Development and validation of a novel acute myeloid leukemia-composite model to estimate risks of mortality. *JAMA Oncol.* 2017;3:1675–1682.
71. Papaemmanuil E, Dohner H, Campbell PJ. Genomic classification in acute myeloid leukemia. *N Engl J Med.* 2016;375:900–901.
72. National Comprehensive Cancer Network Clinical Practice Guidelines in Oncology. Acute Myeloid Leukemia. Version3.2021. Accessed November 18, 2021.
73. Daver N, Schlenk RF, Russell NH, et al. Targeting *FLT3* mutations in AML: Review of current knowledge and evidence. *Leukemia.* 2019;33:299–312.
74. Dohner H, Weisdorf DJ, Bloomfield CD. Acute myeloid leukemia. *N Engl J Med.* 2015;373:1136–1152.
75. Zwaan CM, Kolb EA, Reinhardt D, et al. Collaborative efforts driving progress in pediatric acute myeloid leukemia. *J Clin Oncol.* 2015;33:2949–2962.
76. Pophali P, Litzow M. What is the best daunorubicin dose and schedule for acute myeloid leukemia induction? *Curr Treat Options Oncol.* 2017;18:3.
77. Willemze R, Suciu S, Meloni G, et al. High-dose cytarabine in induction treatment improves the outcome of adult patients younger than age 46 years with acute myeloid leukemia: Results of the EORTC-GIMEMA AML-12 trial. *J Clin Oncol.* 2014;32:219–228.
78. Cahn JY, Labopin M, Sierra J, et al. No impact of high-dose cytarabine on the outcome of patients transplanted for acute myeloblastic leukaemia in first remission. Acute Leukaemia Working Party of the European Group for Blood and Marrow Transplantation (EBMT). *Br J Haematol.* 2000;110:308–314.
79. Vyexos (daunorubicin and cytarabine; liposome) [package insert]. Palo Alto, CA: Jazz Pharmaceuticals; 2021.
80. Lancet JE, Uy GL, Cortes JE, et al. CPX-351 (cytarabine and daunorubicin) liposome for injection versus conventional cytarabine plus daunorubicin in older patients with newly diagnosed secondary acute myeloid leukemia. *J Clin Oncol.* 2018;36:2684–2692.
81. Jen EY, Ko CW, Lee JE, et al. FDA approval: Gemtuzumab ozogamicin for the treatment of adults with newly diagnosed CD33-positive acute myeloid leukemia. *Clin Cancer Res.* 2018;24:3242–3246.
82. Lambert J, Pautas C, Terre C, et al. Gemtuzumab ozogamicin for de novo acute myeloid leukemia: Final efficacy and safety updates from the open-label, phase III ALFA-0701 trial. *Haematologica.* 2019;104:113–119.
83. Assi R, Ravandi F. FLT3 inhibitors in acute myeloid leukemia: Choosing the best when the optimal does not exist. *Am J Hematol.* 2018;93:553–563.
84. Stone RM, Mandrekar SJ, Sanford BL, et al. Midostaurin plus chemotherapy for acute myeloid leukemia with a FLT3 mutation. *N Engl J Med.* 2017;377:454–464.
85. Rydapt (midostaurin) [package insert]. East Hanover, NJ: Novartis Pharmaceuticals; 2021.
86. DiNardo CD, Jonas BA, Pullarkat V, et al. Azacitidine and venetoclax in previously untreated acute myeloid leukemia. *N Eng J Med.* 2020;383:617–629.
87. Kantarjian HM, Thomas XG, Dmoszynska A, et al. Multicenter, randomized, open-label, phase III trial of decitabine versus patient choice, with physician advice, of either supportive care or low-dose cytarabine for the treatment of older patients with newly diagnosed acute myeloid leukemia. *J Clin Oncol.* 2012;30:2670–2677.
88. Dombret H, Seymour JF, Butrym A, et al. International phase 3 study of azacitidine vs conventional care regimens in older patients with newly diagnosed AML with >30% blasts. *Blood.* 2015;126:291–299.
89. Amadori S, Suciu S, Selleslag D, et al. Gemtuzumab ozogamicin versus best supportive care in older patients with newly diagnosed acute myeloid leukemia unsuitable for intensive chemotherapy: Results of the randomized Phase III EORTC-GIMEMA AML-19 Trial. *J Clin Oncol.* 2016;34:972–979.
90. McMurry H, Fletcher L, Traer E. IDH inhibitors in AML-promise and pitfalls. *Curr Hematol Malig Rep.* 2021 Apr;16(2):207–217.
91. Daurismo (glasdegib) [package insert]. New York, NY: Pfizer; 2020.
92. Vencelexta (venetoclax) [package insert]. North Chicago, IL: AbbVie; 2021.
93. Li W, Gong X, Sun M, et al. High-dose cytarabine in acute myeloid leukemia treatment: A systematic review and meta-analysis. *PLoS One.* 2014;9:e110153.
94. Weil AH, Dohner H, Pocock C, et al. Oral azacitidine maintenance therapy for acute myeloid leukemia in first remission. *N Eng J Med.* 2020;383:2526–2537.
95. Cornelissen JJ, Blaise D. Hematopoietic stem cell transplantation for patients with AML in first complete remission. *Blood.* 2016;127:62–70.
96. Penack O, Peczynski C, Mohty M, et al. How much has allogeneic stem cell transplant–related mortality improved since the 1980s? A retrospective analysis from the EBMT. *Blood Adv.* 2020;4(24):6283–6290.
97. Dholoaria B, Savani BN, Hamilton BK, et al. Hematopoietic cell transplantation in the treatment of newly diagnosed adult acute myeloid leukemia: An evidence-based review from the American Society of Transplantation and Cellular Therapy. *Transplant Cell Ther.* 2021 Jan;27(1):6–20.
98. Sorror ML, Sandmaier BM, Storer BE, et al. Allogeneic hematopoietic cell transplantation (HCT) in the eighth decade of life: How much does age matter. *Biol Blood Marrow Transplant.* 2017;23:S98–S99.
99. Muffly L, Pasquini MC, Martens M, et al. Increasing use of allogeneic hematopoietic cell transplantation in patients aged 70 years and older in the United States. *Blood.* 2017;130:1156–1164.
100. Canaani J, Beohou E, Labopin M, et al. Trends in patient outcome over the past two decades following allogeneic stem cell transplantation for acute myeloid leukaemia: An ALWP/EBMT analysis. *J Intern Med.* 2019;(4):407–418.
101. Cornelissen JJ, Blaise D. Hematopoietic stem cell transplantation for patients with AML in first complete remission. *Blood.* 2016;127:62–70.
102. Ostgard LSG, Lund JL, Norgaard JM, et al. Impact of allogeneic stem cell transplantation in first complete remission in acute myeloid leukemia: A national population-based cohort study. *Biol Blood Marrow Transplant.* 2018;24:314–323.
103. Conneely SE, Stevens AM. Acute myeloid leukemia in children: Emerging paradigms in genetic and new approaches to therapy. *Curr Oncol Rep.* 2021;23(2):16.
104. Kim H. Treatments for children and adolescents with AML. *Blood Res.* 2020;55(S1):S5–S13.
105. Mylotarg (gemtuzumab ozogamicin) [package insert]. Philadelphia, PA. Wyeth Pharmaceuticals; 2021.
106. Gibson BES. The EBMT Handbook: Hematopoietic Stem Cell Transplantation and Cellular Therapies [Internet]. 7th edition. Chapter 70 Acute Myeloid Leukemia in Children.
107. Rashidi A, Weisdorf DJ, Bejanyan N. Treatment of relapsed/refractory acute myeloid leukaemia in adults. *Br J Haematol.* 2018;181:27–37.
108. Stahl M, DeVeaux M, Montesinos P, et al. Hypomethylating agents in relapsed and refractory AML: Outcomes and their predictors in a large international patient cohort. *Blood Adv.* 2018;2(8):923–932.
109. Moeinafshar A, Hemmati S, Rezaei N. Immunotherpay in AML: A brief review or emerging strategies. *Clin Transl Oncol.* 2021 Dec;23(12):2431–2447.
110. Sanz MA, Pontesinos P. Advances in the management of coagulopathy in acute promyelocytic leukemia. *Thromb Res.* 2020 Jul;191(Suppl 1):S63–S67.
111. Yilmaz M, Kantarjian H, Ravandi F. Acute promyelocytic leukemia current treatment algorithms. *Blood Cancer J.* 2021 Jun 30;11(6):123.
112. McCulloch D, Brown C, Iland H. Retinoic acid and arsenic trioxide in the treatment of acute promyelocytic leukemia: Current perspectives. *Onco Targets Ther.* 2017;10:1585–1601.
113. Kayser S, Schlenk RF, Platzbecker U. Management of patients with acute promyelocytic leukemia. *Leukemia.* 2018;32:1277–1294.
114. Osman AEG, Anderson J, Churpek JE, et al. Treatment of acute promyelocytic leukemia in adults. *J Oncol Pract.* 2018;14:649–657.
115. Hashmi J, Nishihori T. Role of hematopoietic cell transplantation in relapsed acute promyelocytic leukemia. *Clin Transplant.* 2020 Sep;34(9):e14009.
116. Smith TJ, Bohlke K, Lyman GH, et al. Recommendations for the use of WBC growth factors: American Society of Clinical Oncology Clinical Practice Guideline Update. *J Clin Oncol.* 2015;33:3199–3212.
117. Zarxio (filgrastim-sndz) [package insert]. Princeton, NJ: Sandoz; 2017.
118. Nivestym (filgrastim-aafi) [package insert]. New York, NY: Pfizer; 2021.

119. Taplitz RA, Kennedy EB, Bow EJ, et al. Antimicrobial prophylaxis for adult patients with cancer-related immunosuppression: ASCO and IDSA clinical practice guideline update. *J Clin Oncol.* 2018;36:3043–3054.
120. National Comprehensive Cancer Network Clinical Practice Guidelines in Oncology. Myeloid Growth Factors. Version 4.2021. Accessed November 21, 2021.
121. Alexander S, Fisher BT, Gaur AH, et al. Effect of levofloxacin prophylaxis on bacteremia in children with acute leukemia or undergoing hematopoietic stem cell transplantation: A randomized clinical trial. *JAMA.* 2018;320:995–1004.
122. Lehrnbecher T, Fisher BT, Phillips B, Beauchemin M, Carlesse F, Castagnola E, et al. Clinical practice guideline for systemic antifungal prophylaxis in pediatric patients with cancer and hematopoietic stem-cell transplantation recipients. *J Clin Oncol.* 2020;38(27):3205–3216.
123. Howard SC, Trifilio S, Gregory TK, Baxter N, McBride A. Tumor lysis syndrome in the era of novel and targeted agents in patients with hematologic malignancies: A systematic review. *Ann Hematol.* 2016;95:563–573.
124. Children's Oncology Group. Long-Term Follow-Up Guidelines. V 5.0. 2018. Available at: http://www.survivorshipguidelines.org

158

Chronic Leukemias

Karen M. Fancher and Jill M. Comeau

KEY CONCEPTS

1. Chronic myeloid leukemia (CML) is defined by the presence of the Philadelphia chromosome (Ph), a translocation between chromosomes 9 and 22. The resulting abnormal fusion protein, p210 *BCR-ABL*, phosphorylates tyrosine kinase residues and is constitutively active, resulting in uncontrolled hematopoietic cell proliferation.
2. Without treatment, the disease course of CML is characterized by a progressive increase in white blood cells over a period of years that ultimately transforms into acute leukemia.
3. Allogeneic hematopoietic stem cell transplant (HSCT) is the only known curative treatment option for CML and is reserved for patients with a suitable donor who progress after treatment with tyrosine kinase-based therapy.
4. The commercially available BCR-ABL tyrosine kinase inhibitors, imatinib, dasatinib, nilotinib, bosutinib, and ponatinib, have demonstrated efficacy in the treatment of newly diagnosed CML patients in chronic phase as well as in patients in accelerated phase or blast crisis.
5. CML monitoring requires the assessment of milestones throughout therapy, which includes hematologic, cytogenetic, and most importantly, molecular responses.
6. The management of chronic lymphocytic leukemia (CLL) is highly individualized. It includes observation in patients with early-stage disease and treatment with targeted therapy, chemotherapy, and/or biologic therapy in patients with more advanced disease.
7. Rituximab, obinutuzumab and ofatumumab are monoclonal antibodies indicated for the treatment of CLL.
8. Regimens such as fludarabine, cyclophosphamide, and rituximab are considered first-line therapy for patients with CLL who are younger and have immunoglobulin heavy-chain variable (IGHV) mutation.
9. Novel agents such as ibrutinib, acalabrutinib, zanubrutinib, idelalisib, duvelisib, and venetoclax provide orally administered options for the treatment of CLL. These agents, alone or in combination with anti-CD20 monoclonal antibodies, are now preferred treatment options.

BEYOND THE BOOK

Chronic Myeloid Leukemia (CML)

Watch the video entitled "What Is Chronic Myelogenous Leukemia?" by the Khan Academy. https://www.youtube.com/watch?v=ST6mSB-RvE0

This 10-minute video provides a brief overview of CML, its signs and symptoms, diagnosis, and a basic treatment overview. This video is useful to enhance student understanding regarding COLLECT and ASSESS steps in the patient care process.

Chronic Lymphocytic Leukemia (CLL)

Watch the video: "Understanding Chronic Lymphocytic Leukemia with Lindsey Roeker, MD." https://www.youtube.com/watch?v=cgYuEC69QXg

This 11-minute video by the Lymphoma Research Foundation briefly reviews CLL, diagnosis, and treatment options. This video is designed to aid in the student's patient care process, particularly the COLLECT and ASSESS steps.

INTRODUCTION

Chronic leukemias include chronic myeloid leukemia (CML), chronic lymphocytic leukemia (CLL), hairy cell leukemia, and prolymphocytic leukemia. The typical clinical presentation of chronic leukemias is an indolent course, in contrast to patients with acute leukemia who will die of their diseases within weeks to months if not treated. This chapter focuses on the two most common types of chronic leukemia, CML and CLL.

CHRONIC MYELOID LEUKEMIA

CML is a myeloproliferative disease that results from malignant transformation of a subpopulation of pluripotent hematopoietic stem cells.[1,2] Bone marrow hyperplasia and the accumulation of differentiated myeloid cells in the peripheral blood are the initial presenting features of the disease. The terminal stage of CML is characterized by the rapid accumulation of blast cells in the bone marrow and suppression of normal hematopoiesis that ultimately leads to death. CML was the first malignant disease identified with a consistent cytogenetic abnormality, namely the Philadelphia Chromosome (Ph) that contains the BCR-ABL oncogene. This dominant cytogenetic abnormality has allowed CML to become the template for the development of targeted drug therapies.[2]

Epidemiology and Etiology

It is estimated that 8,860 new cases of CML will be diagnosed in the United States in 2022.[3] The median age at diagnosis is 67 years.[4] The development of CML is not associated with hereditary, familial, geographic, ethnic, or economic status. An increased risk of CML has been noted with ionizing radiation exposure and in atomic bomb survivors from Hiroshima and Nagasaki.[2]

Pathophysiology

CML was first described in 1845, but extensive research into the genetic and molecular characteristics of the disease began with the discovery of the Ph in 1960 by Nowell and Hungerford.[5] Research in the 1980s identified the molecular changes that occur as a result of the Ph when an oncogenic protein was identified and associated with the pathophysiology of CML.[1,5] Ph is the first karyotypic abnormality specifically implicated in the pathogenesis of cancer, and its discovery has resulted in extensive research into the molecular biology of CML. This chromosomal abnormality is characteristic of CML and is present in about 95% of patients with the disease.[1]

1 Ph, identified as a shortened long arm of chromosome 22, is found in granulocyte and erythrocyte progenitors, macrophages, megakaryocytes, and lymphocytes. The Ph is the consequence of breaks in chromosomes 9 and 22, resulting in a transposition that relocates the 3′ end of *ABL* (Abelson proto-oncogene) from its normal site on chromosome 9 at band 34 to the 5′ end of *BCR* (breakpoint cluster region) on chromosome 22 at band 11 (symbolized as *t*[9;22][q34;q11]).[1,6] This results in the formation of the hybrid *BCR-ABL* fusion gene (Fig. 158-1). Through this chromosomal translocation, the *ABL* proto-oncogene escapes normal genetic controls and is activated into a functional oncogene, directing the transcription of messenger ribonucleic acid (mRNA). The mRNA is translated into a 210-kDa protein—p210 BCR-ABL—that is constitutively (ie, constantly) activated compared to the 145-kDa protein translated by the normal *ABL* gene.[1,6]

CML is considered a clonal disease because it begins with the malignant transformation of a single cell. The progeny from this transformed primitive hematopoietic stem cell results in a proliferative advantage over normal hematopoietic cells that displaces normal hematopoiesis. The Ph is found in both myeloid and lymphoid cells, which suggests that the transformed cell of CML is a pluripotent stem cell.[2] Disrupted maturation leads to a number of circulating granulocytes that may be many times higher than normal. In the advanced stages of CML, cytopenias may occur in association with fibrotic changes in the bone marrow.

The *BCR-ABL* fusion gene encodes for a constitutively active tyrosine kinase that is involved in both the increased proliferation of the CML clone and a reduction in apoptosis.[7] Characterization of the adenosine triphosphate binding site on the BCR-ABL tyrosine kinase has provided a target for inhibition of tyrosine kinase activity. The first Food and Drug Administration (FDA)-approved tyrosine kinase inhibitor (TKI), imatinib mesylate (Gleevec®), was indicated for patients in chronic phase who had failed interferon alfa (IFN-α) or for those with advanced disease. Imatinib received additional FDA approval in 2002 for first-line treatment in newly diagnosed CML. Second-generation TKIs with a higher binding affinity and selectivity for BCR-ABL kinase are now approved as both first-line agents and salvage therapy for patients with resistance or intolerance to imatinib.

Clinical Presentation

The diagnosis of CML is often made incidentally during a routine examination or when a complete blood count is obtained for unrelated reasons, as patients are often asymptomatic upon presentation. The differential diagnosis of CML includes infection, myeloproliferative disorders (ie, polycythemia vera, essential thrombocythemia, myelofibrosis), and chronic myelomonocytic leukemia. Initial laboratory workup includes complete blood count with differential and complete metabolic panel. A bone marrow aspiration and biopsy are required to confirm the diagnosis of CML.[6] Bone marrow is markedly hypercellular (75%-90%) with increased erythropoiesis and normal megakaryocytes.[4,6] Karyotyping (ie, cytogenetic analysis) is required for a diagnosis. The bone marrow aspiration is analyzed with fluorescence in situ hybridization (FISH) to determine the presence of the Ph chromosome. Quantitative reverse-transcription polymerase chain reaction (RT-PCR) is also performed to assess the baseline *BCR-ABL* transcript levels in the blood and monitored with the International Scale (IS). In the IS, the standardized baseline, defined as the mean expression of *BCR-ABL1* transcripts observed from previous study patients, is set to 100%. Levels measured by

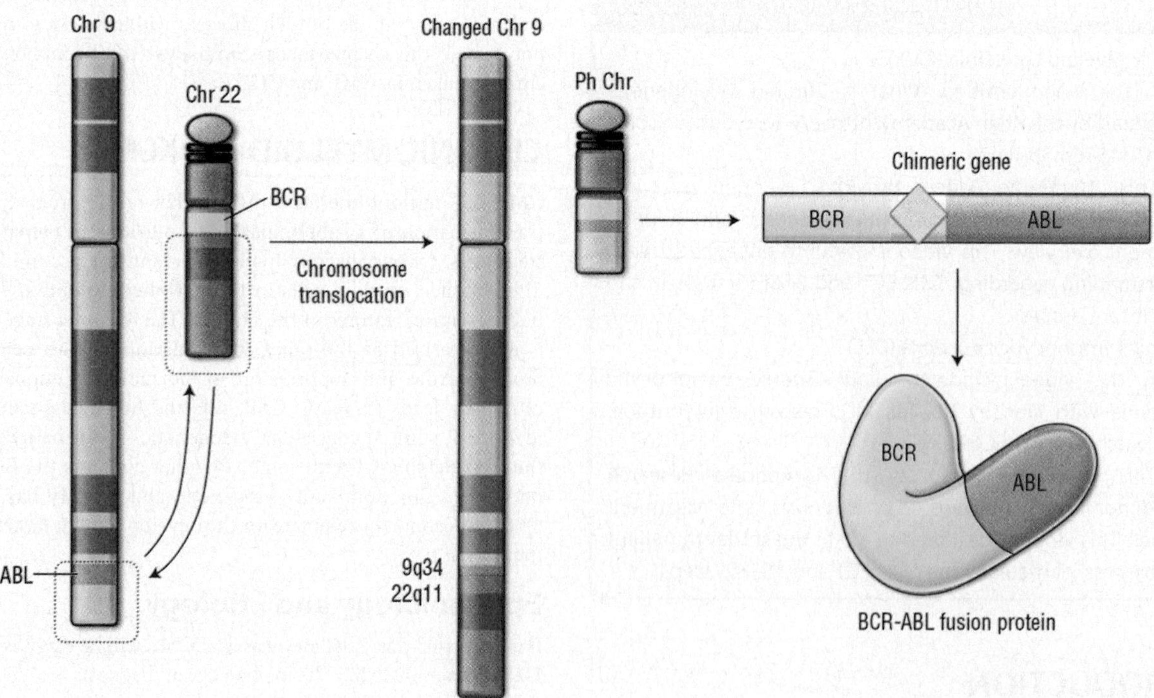

FIGURE 158-1 Specific chromosomal translocation that results in the Philadelphia chromosome. The fusion of these DNA sequences allows the generation of a constitutively activated fusion protein. *(Reproduced, with permission, from Jameson JL, Fauci AS, Kasper DL, Hauser SL, Longo DL, Loscalzo J, eds. Harrison's Principles of Internal Medicine. 20th ed. New York, NY: McGraw Hill; 2019.)*

CLINICAL PRESENTATION Chronic Myeloid Leukemia

General

- 90% of patients are diagnosed in CP
- 50% are asymptomatic in CP and often diagnosed following abnormal complete blood count

Signs and Symptoms

- Fatigue
- Left upper quadrant pain
- Abdominal pain or distension
- Weight loss
- Night sweats

Physical Examination

- Splenomegaly
- Hepatomegaly

Data from References 4 and 6.

Laboratory Tests

Peripheral blood

- Leukocytosis
- Thrombocytosis
- Basophilia
- Low or undetectable leukocyte alkaline phosphatase
- Elevated uric acid and lactate dehydrogenase

Molecular testing

- Presence of *BCR-ABL* by RT-PCR

Bone marrow

- Hypercellular
- Fully mature myeloid cells
- Increased megakaryocytes
- <10% blasts in CP

Cytogenetics

- Presence of Ph
- Additional abnormalities may occur

individual laboratories may need to be converted to the IS by a conversion factor.

2 Historically, the three clinical phases of CML were chronic phase (CP), accelerated phase (AP), and blast crisis (BC) (Table 158-1).[4,6] Newer classification systems now classify CML into two clinical phases: chronic phase and advanced phase (AP).[6] Although many patients in CP-CML are asymptomatic, signs and symptoms may include fatigue, sweating, bone pain, weight loss, abdominal discomfort, and early satiety secondary to splenomegaly.[8] Leukocytosis is the hallmark of CP, and the white blood cell count can be as high as 1,000,000 cells/mm^3 (1,000 × 10^9/L), placing patients at risk for complications of leukostasis. Symptoms secondary to leukostasis include acute abdominal pain resulting from splenic infarctions, priapism, retinal hemorrhage, cerebrovascular accidents, confusion, hyperuricemia, and gouty arthritis.

AP is characterized by a loss of efficacy of drug therapy and the progressive arrest of myeloid maturation. The most commonly observed cytogenetic changes with disease progression are an additional Ph chromosome, trisomy 8, trisomy 19, and isochromosome 17q.[8,11]

BC is the terminal stage of the disease and clinically resembles acute leukemia, in which the leukemic clone overwhelmingly dominates the bone marrow at the expense of normal hematopoiesis. The WHO classification defines BC CML as the presence of one or more of the following: greater than 20% blasts in the peripheral blood or bone marrow, extramedullary disease, or large clusters of blasts in the bone marrow.[6,9] Patients can present occasionally with BC without an apparent AP. One-third of patients present with BC of lymphoid lineage, while two-thirds present with BC of myeloid lineage or undifferentiated phenotype. The transformation to BC CML is the consequence of several factors in addition to *BCR-ABL*, such as the activation of the oncogene signaling pathways and loss of tumor suppressors such as p53.

TABLE 158-1 Criteria for Different Phases of Chronic Myeloid Leukemia

Chronic Phase	Accelerated Phase	Blast Crisis
• <10% blasts in peripheral blood or bone marrow	• 10%-19% blasts in peripheral blood or bone marrow • Platelets <100,000 cells/mm^3 (100 × 10^9/L) unrelated to therapy or >1,000,000 cells/mm^3 (1,000 × 10^9/L) unresponsive to therapy • Persistent or increasing white blood cells >10,000 cells/mm^3 (10 × 10^9/L), unresponsive to therapy • 20% or more basophils in the peripheral blood • Any new clonal chromosomal abnormalities in Ph+ cells that occur during therapy Additional findings • Cytogenetic evolution • Progressive splenomegaly, unresponsive to therapy	• >20% blasts in peripheral blood or bone marrow • Large clusters of blasts on bone marrow biopsy • Presence of extramedullary infiltrates

Data from References 6, 10, and 11.

Prognosis

Several models have been proposed to estimate prognosis in patients with CML, but the model developed by Sokal et al. is the historical standard.[12] The Sokal algorithm uses spleen size, percentage of circulating blasts, platelet count, and age as prognostic factors for patients in CP. However, this scoring system was developed before the advent of TKI therapy and may have limited predictive value in the current treatment landscape. The median overall survival for patients diagnosed with CP, AP, and BC CML was reported to be 47 months, 12 to 24 months, and 3 to 6 months, respectively, in the era before TKIs were introduced.[13]

The European Treatment and Outcome Study (EUTOS) Long Term Survival (ELTS) score is gaining popularity since it is based on data from patients with CML treated with TKIs.[6,14] Factors such as age, spleen size, platelet count, and percentage of circulating blasts are used to stratify patients into low, intermediate, or high risk of disease progression.

TREATMENT: CHRONIC MYELOID LEUKEMIA

Desired Outcomes

Without effective treatment, CML disease progression leads inexorably to a fatal outcome within 5 years. The introduction of TKI therapy has dramatically altered the clinical course of CML, as patients can now expect to maintain disease control for many years.[4] The survival of patients who are newly diagnosed with CML in CP is now nearly equivalent to that of the general population, with the risk of death from other comorbid conditions greater than from CML.[4,6,15]

The overriding treatment goals for CML include the eradication of the leukemic clone from the bone marrow and maintenance of CP with minimal toxicity from treatment.[4,6] The only proven therapy to eradicate the malignant clone from the bone marrow is allogeneic hematopoietic stem cell transplantation (HSCT). Both immunotherapy with IFN-α and TKI-based therapies have demonstrated the ability to extend CP beyond the expected period of several years, with TKIs now being the preferred treatment option.[4,6]

Clinical response in CML is measured by hematologic, cytogenetic, and molecular indices, all of which have standardized criteria.[1,4,16] *Hematologic response* is defined as the normalization of peripheral blood counts and is the earliest type of response observed in CML patients. *Cytogenetic responses* are based on the percentage of cells positive for Ph in a bone marrow biopsy. A *complete*

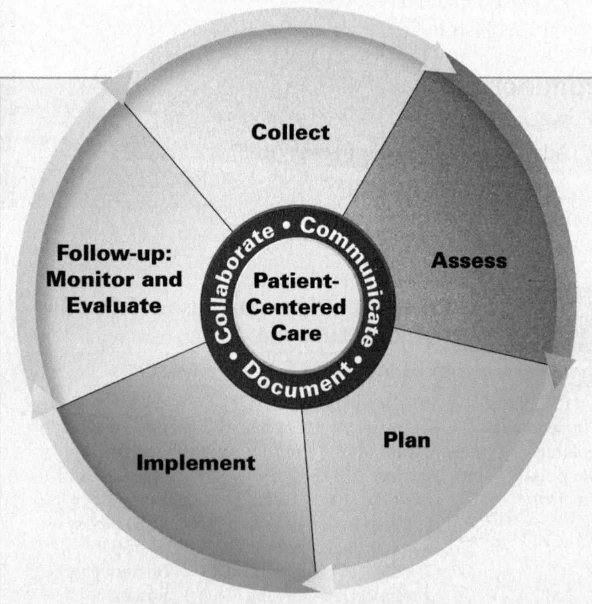

Patient Care Process for Chronic Myeloid Leukemia (CML)

Collect

- Patient characteristics (eg, age, sex)
- Patient medical history (personal and family)
- Social history (eg, tobacco/ethanol use)
- Current medications including acid-suppressing agents, herbal products, dietary supplements, and inhibitors/inducers of CYP3A4
- Objective data
  - Blood pressure (BP), heart rate (HR), respiratory rate (RR), height, weight, O_2-saturation
  - Labs including Complete Blood Counts (CBC) with differential, comprehensive metabolic panel, liver function tests, and uric acid
  - Objective confirmation of CML via bone marrow biopsy with chromosomal and molecular analysis

Assess

- Bone marrow biopsy morphology, cytogenetics, molecular mRNA transcripts
- CBC and presence of active bleeding due to potential thrombocytopenia
- Presence of VTE provoking factors (eg, recent surgery, plaster casting of lower extremity, indwelling catheter)
- Ability/willingness to obtain laboratory monitoring tests (eg, CBC, CMP, BCR-ABL assessments)
- Comorbidities (eg, diabetes, chronic kidney disease, pulmonary arterial hypertension)
- Emotional status (eg, presence of anxiety, depression)

Plan

- Drug therapy regimen including tyrosine kinase inhibitor dose, route, frequency, and duration (see Tables 158-3 and 158-4)
- Monitoring parameters including efficacy (eg, cytogenetic response, BCR-ABL mRNA PCR) and safety (eg, sign and symptoms of bleeding, anemia, fluid retention, ECG); frequency and timing of follow-up
- Patient education (eg, goals of treatment, drug-specific information, oral medication adherence, drug-drug interactions)

Implement*

- Provide patient education regarding all elements of the treatment plan
- Use motivational interviewing and coaching strategies to maximize adherence to oral therapy

Follow-up: Monitor and Evaluate

- Routinely monitor for assessment of hematologic, cytogenetic, and molecular milestones
- Presence of adverse drug reactions
- Patient adherence to treatment plan using multiple sources of information
- Addition of any new medications, including over-the-counter agents and/or herbal supplements

**Collaborate with patient, caregivers, and other healthcare professionals.*

cytogenetic response is defined as the elimination of Ph from all cells in the marrow sample and a *major cytogenetic response* is defined as ≤35% Ph-positive cells. Patients who have a major or complete cytogenetic response have improved survival compared to those who fail to achieve a cytogenetic response.

More sensitive and less invasive tests to monitor disease status are now used because most patients on BCR-ABL TKIs achieve a complete cytogenetic response.[4] *Molecular responses* are determined by RT-PCR (based on IS), which are several logs more sensitive than methods used to measure cytogenetic responses. An early molecular response is the observation of ≤10% *BCR-ABL* (IS) at 3 and 6 months. A *major molecular response* is a ≥3 log reduction in *BCR-ABL* mRNA from the baseline or a BCR-ABL (IS) of <0.1%. A *complete molecular response* is the absence of *BCR-ABL* transcripts by RT-PCR. Clinicians should interpret RT-PCR assays carefully because they have varying sensitivities and may show a complete molecular remission even when low levels of *BCR-ABL* transcripts are present.[17] Quantitative RT-PCR should be performed before initiating therapy and throughout therapy to monitor residual disease. Peripheral blood can often be used for this analysis because bone marrow and peripheral blood *BCR-ABL* mRNA levels are correlated.

Hematopoietic Stem Cell Transplantation

3 The advent of TKI therapy has resulted in fewer transplants for patients with CML. Allogeneic HSCT remains the only proven therapy to cure patients with CML, with many patients alive and disease-free decades after transplant. Patients undergoing allogeneic HSCT from a human leukocyte antigen (HLA)-matched sibling donor have 5-year survival rates ranging from 60% to 80% and long-term survival of about 50%.[17] In most long-term survivors, the *BCR-ABL* translocation is absent in all diagnostic tests including RT-PCR. Prognostic risk factors associated with survival outcomes include age, phase of disease, and disease duration.[4,6] Increased age is associated with a poorer prognosis, with higher transplant-related mortality in patients older than age 50 years. Patients with CP who receive allogeneic HSCT have better outcomes than those in AP or BC at the time of transplant. The time from diagnosis to transplantation also affects outcomes. Patients who undergo matched-sibling allogeneic HSCT within the first year of diagnosis have a better 5-year survival rate than those who undergo transplantation more than 1 year after their diagnosis (70%-80% vs 50%-60%).[17] However, these data were reported prior to the use of imatinib as first-line therapy for CML.

The major limitation for the application of HSCT is that fewer than 30% of transplant-eligible patients will have an HLA-matched sibling donor. The most practical approach is to use an HLA-matched unrelated donor, if an HLA-matched sibling donor is not available. Matched unrelated donor HSCT has an overall 5-year survival reported to be 40% to 70%, which approaches overall survival data results reported for matched-sibling donor HSCT.[17] Imatinib use before transplantation does not appear to adversely affect transplant-related mortality.[18]

Treatment options in patients who relapse after HSCT are limited. Graft-versus-leukemia (GVL) effect, TKIs, omacetaxine, IFN-α, and a clinical trial are reasonable options.[6] The infusion of donor lymphocytes functions as a form of adoptive immunotherapy that can induce a GVL effect. In relapsed CML, donor lymphocytes induce durable responses and these responses strongly correlate with the development of graft-versus-host disease (GVHD).[6,19]

Conventional Chemotherapy

At present, conventional cytotoxic chemotherapy is only used in CML to reduce and temporarily control high peripheral white blood cell (WBC) counts. The agent most often used for cytoreduction is hydroxyurea (Hydrea®).[20] Hydroxyurea rapidly lowers high circulating WBCs in CML by inhibiting ribonucleotide reductase, which inhibits DNA synthesis, eliminating cells in the S phase of the cell cycle, and synchronizing cells in the G_1 or pre-DNA synthesis phase. Hydroxyurea is initiated at 40 to 50 mg/kg/day in divided doses until the WBC count falls to approximately 10,000 cells/mm^3 (10×10^9/L). Hydroxyurea may be discontinued once adequate control of the WBC count is achieved and a TKI has been initiated. Hydroxyurea does not change the natural progression of the disease to BC.

Interferon Alfa

The interferons are a family of glycoproteins involved in many of the functional aspects of the hematopoietic system. Before imatinib was available, IFN-α was the preferred agent in the treatment of CML. The use of IFN-α in the treatment of CP CML was based on reports that 20% to 50% of patients achieved a major cytogenetic response, which led to prolonged survival.[1,21] However, IFN-α use is limited by its toxicity profile, as it is associated with both short-term constitutional toxicities and potentially dose-limiting long-term toxicities.[1,22,23] The most predictable early toxicity is a flu-like syndrome characterized by fever, chills, myalgia, headache, and anorexia. These dose-dependent effects may be a result of IFN-α–induced leukocytosis and the release of inflammatory cytokines. Cardiovascular toxicities (eg, tachycardia, hypotension) are seen in about 15% of patients in the first few weeks. Long-term adverse drug reactions include weight loss, alopecia, neurologic effects (eg, paresthesia, cognitive impairment, and depression), and immune-mediated complications (eg, hemolysis, thrombocytopenia, nephrotic syndrome, systemic lupus erythematosus, and hypothyroidism), which occur in about 5% to 20% of patients. The National Comprehensive Cancer Network (NCCN) guidelines now recommend IFN-α only for CML patients with post-transplant relapse or during pregnancy if the treatment benefit outweighs the risk to the mother and fetus.[6]

Tyrosine Kinase Inhibitors

4 A transformative discovery in cancer therapeutics was the characterization of the adenosine triphosphate binding site on the BCR-ABL tyrosine kinase. This specific receptor established a novel drug discovery platform for molecularly targeted therapy in CML. Numerous TKIs were in development in the 1990s and STI571 (STI stands for *signal transduction inhibitor*), subsequently named imatinib, has high binding affinity for the BCR-ABL tyrosine kinase and emerged as the drug with the best oral bioavailability at that time.[24] Imatinib competitively binds to the adenosine triphosphate (ATP)-binding site on BCR-ABL, which inhibits the phosphorylation of proteins involved with CML clone proliferation. In 2001, imatinib mesylate received FDA approval for patients in CP-CML who had failed IFN-α treatment and in patients with AP- or BC-CML based on phase II studies. In 2002, it received FDA approval for first-line treatment in newly diagnosed CML based on the IRIS phase III trial results.[22] Imatinib inhibits several other tyrosine kinases including BCR-ABL, c-Kit, and platelet-derived growth factor receptor (PDGFR) (Table 158-2).[22]

Table 158-3 summarizes the dosing, food-drug interactions, and drug-drug interactions of imatinib and other TKIs.

Adverse Drug Reactions and Drug Interactions Tables 158-3 and 158-4 summarize drug-drug interactions, adverse drug reactions, and monitoring of BCR-ABL TKIs.

Myelosuppression is one of the most common adverse drug reactions observed during therapy with imatinib.[25] Moderate-to-severe myelosuppression occurs in about 5% to 10% of patients with CP-CML and 50% to 60% of patients in AP or BC. Myelosuppression typically occurs within the first 4 weeks of therapy and is more common in patients with advanced disease (ie, high blastic involvement of the bone marrow), those receiving higher doses and those with low hemoglobin. When imatinib is initiated, patients should have complete blood counts drawn every 1 to 2 weeks to assess for myelosuppression until they have stabilized.[26] Appropriate initial management of myelosuppression is to interrupt imatinib treatment rather than dose reduce because dose reductions below 300 mg daily do not fully inhibit BCR-ABL and may lead to the emergence of imatinib resistance.[4,6]

TABLE 158-2 Cytogenetic and Molecular Response Rate Associated with Tyrosine Kinase Inhibitor Therapy in Chronic Myeloid Leukemia

Drug (Disease Status)	Daily Dose (mg)	CCyR (%)	MMR	Median Follow-up (months)
Imatinib (CP)	400	82	57%	70
	800	90	NR	30
Imatinib (AP)	600	43	NR	12
	400	11	NR	
Imatinib (BC)	400-800	7.40	NR	—
Dasatinib (CP)	100	83	76%	60
Dasatinib (AP)	140	32	NR	15
Nilotinib (CP)	600	87	77%	36
Nilotinib (AP)	800	16	NR	24
Bosutinib (CP–3rd line)	500	24	15%	28.5
Bosutinib (CP–1st line)	500	79	59%	12
Omacetaxine (CP–2nd line, T315I mutation)	2.5	16	NR	19.1
Ponatinib (CP-resistant/intolerant disease)	45	37	NR	10
Ponatinib (CP-T315I mutation)	45	66	NR	10

AP, accelerated phase; BC, blast crisis; CCyR, complete cytogenetic response; CP, chronic phase; MCyR, major cytogenetic response; MMR, major molecular response; NR, no response.

Many other non-hematologic toxicities associated with imatinib have been reported (Table 158-4).[4,6,26] Drug rash frequently occurs but is usually mild and can be managed with antihistamines or topical steroids. Hepatotoxicity can occur with imatinib, and the drug should be withheld if liver function tests exceed five times the upper limits of normal. It is recommended that patients on imatinib limit their use of acetaminophen to 1,300 mg daily.[6] Other medications that are known to be hepatotoxic should be used with caution while patients are treated with imatinib.

Dasatinib can cause edema and pleural effusions, which can be managed by drug holiday, diuretics, thoracentesis, and/or short courses of steroids.[4,6,26,27] Dasatinib may also be associated with an increased risk of bleeding due to its effects on PDGFR.[28] A rare adverse drug reaction of dasatinib is pulmonary arterial hypertension (PAH), which warrants permanent discontinuation.[6,27] Nilotinib can be associated with indirect bilirubin elevations in 10% to 15% of patients.[4,6,26,27] Nilotinib may prolong the QTc interval (Black Box Warning), and patients should have an electrocardiogram at baseline, at 7 days following initiation of therapy, and periodically thereafter. Nilotinib has also been associated with "metabolic syndrome," consisting of hyperglycemia, hypercholesterolemia and hypertriglyceridemia; careful attention should be given to eliminate or reduce risk factors for these conditions. Bosutinib is associated with gastrointestinal adverse drug reactions such as diarrhea, nausea and vomiting, and abdominal discomfort.[4,6,26] These gastrointestinal effects are typically self-limiting and can be managed with over-the-counter medications. Ponatinib can cause hepatotoxicity (including reports of liver failure), vascular occlusion, and heart failure, with some events occurring within 1 week of starting therapy.[4,6,27,29] The ponatinib manufacturer recommends specific dose modifications for myelosuppression, hepatotoxicity, and elevated lipase; monitoring for cardiovascular effects should also be routinely performed.

Similar to imatinib, advanced-generation TKIs are metabolized by cytochrome P450 (CYP) 3A4.[30] Clinicians need to be aware of possible drug interactions with inducers and inhibitors of the CYP3A4 pathway such as phenytoin, azole antifungals, or macrolide antibiotics (Table 158-3).[6,26] Drug interactions with BCR-ABL can

TABLE 158-3 Dosing of Tyrosine Kinase Inhibitors in Chronic Myeloid Leukemia*

Drug	Brand Name	Dose Range	Food-Drug Interactions	Drug-Drug Interactions
Imatinib	Gleevec®	• 400 mg/day (CP) • 600 mg/day (AP/BC)	Take with food and a large glass of water	• CYP3A4 inducers may decrease C_{max} and AUC • CYP3A4 inhibitors may increase C_{max} and AUC • Imatinib inhibits CYP3A4 and 2D6 • Package labeling recommendations against using warfarin concurrently
Dasatinib	Sprycel®	• 100 mg/day (CP) • 140 mg/day (AP/BC)	With or without meals; do not crush tablets	• CYP3A4 inhibitors may increase dasatinib levels • CYP3A4 inducers may decrease dasatinib levels • H_2 antagonists/PPIs decrease dasatinib levels
Nilotinib	Tasigna®	• 300 mg BID (CP) • 400 mg BID (AP/BC)	Take with water; avoid food 2 hours prior to a dose or 1 hour after	• Avoid drugs concurrently known to prolong QT interval • CYP inducers may decrease nilotinib concentrations • CYP inhibitors may increase nilotinib concentrations • H_2 antagonists/PPIs decrease nilotinib levels • Nilotinib is an inhibitor of CYP3A4, CYP2C8, CYP2C9, and CYP2D6 • Nilotinib is an inducer of CYP2B6, CYP2C8, and CYP2C9
Bosutinib	Bosulif®	• 400 mg/day (CP) • 500 mg/day (AP/BC or resistance/intolerance to other TKI therapy)	Take with food; PPIs may decrease absorption	• Concurrent use with CYP3A4 or Pgp inhibitors increase bosutinib concentrations • Concurrent use with CYP3A4 inducers reduces bosutinib concentrations
Ponatinib	Iclusig®	45 mg/day (lower dosing may be required as the optimal dose is not defined)	With or without food	• Concurrent use with CYP3A4 or Pgp inhibitors increase ponatinib concentrations • Concurrent use with CYP3A4 inducers reduces ponatinib concentrations

AP, accelerated phase; AUC, area under the curve; BC, blast crisis; BID, twice daily; C_{max}, maximum concentration; CP, chronic phase; CYP, cytochrome P450; Pgp, P-glycoprotein; PPI, proton pump inhibitor.

Information obtained from each agent's prescribing information.

TABLE 158-4 Monitoring of Tyrosine Kinase Inhibitors in Chronic Myeloid Leukemia*

Drug	Adverse Drug Reactions	Monitoring Parameters	Comments
Imatinib	Common: • Myelosuppression • Fluid retention (pleural/pericardial effusion, ascites, periorbital, and peripheral edema) • Nausea/vomiting • Rash • Fatigue • Hepatotoxicity • Hypothyroidism • Myalgias Rare but serious: • Congestive heart failure/left ventricular dysfunction • Hemorrhage • Bullous dermatologic reactions	• CBC for myelosuppression • CMP for hepatotoxicity • Consider baseline echocardiogram if preexisting cardiac dysfunction or risk factors for cardiac dysfunction, repeat if experiencing symptoms of cardiac dysfunction • Thyroid-stimulating hormone	Nausea and vomiting improved when administered with food
Dasatinib	Common: • Myelosuppression • Myalgia • Fluid retention • Cardiotoxicity • Rash • Gastrointestinal toxicity • Hypophosphatemia • Hepatotoxicity Rare but serious: • Pleural effusion • Pericardial effusion • QT prolongation • Congestive heart failure/left ventricular dysfunction • Pulmonary arterial hypertension • Hemorrhage	• CBC for myelosuppression • CMP for hypophosphatemia and hepatotoxicity • ECG if risk factors for QTc prolongation • Chest radiograph for signs and symptoms of pleural effusion • Evaluate for signs/symptoms of underlying cardiopulmonary disease for pulmonary arterial hypertension	Gastrointestinal hemorrhage reported to be fatal; severe pleural effusions requiring thoracentesis; fatal myocardial infarction are reported
Nilotinib	Common: • Myelosuppression • Rash • Gastrointestinal toxicity • Peripheral edema • Liver function abnormalities • Elevated serum lipase/amylase • Electrolyte abnormalities (hypophosphatemia, hypokalemia, hypocalcemia, and hyponatremia) Rare but serious: • Tumor lysis syndrome • Cardiotoxicity (QTc prolongation/sudden cardiac death/ left ventricular dysfunction)	• CBC for myelosuppression • CMP for hypophosphatemia and hepatotoxicity • Serum amylase/lipase • Lipid panel • ECG if risk factors for QTc prolongation at baseline, 7 days thereafter and then as clinically indicated	Sudden deaths reported with nilotinib; ventricular repolarization abnormalities may have been contributory
Bosutinib	Common: • Myelosuppression • Gastrointestinal toxicity • Fluid retention • Hepatotoxicity • Hypophosphatemia • Rash Rare but serious: • Embryofetal toxicity	• CBC for myelosuppression • CMP for hypophosphatemia and hepatotoxicity • Serum amylase/lipase • ECG if risk factors for QTc prolongation at baseline, 7 days thereafter and then as clinically indicated	Potential for additive risk of hepatotoxicity when given concurrently with letrozole
Ponatinib	Common: • Myelosuppression • Arthralgia • Headache • Fatigue • Fever • Pancreatitis • Elevated lipase • Hypertension • Gastrointestinal toxicity • Dermatologic toxicity • Electrolyte abnormalities • Fluid retention Rare but serious: • Arterial thrombosis • Hepatotoxicity • Cardiotoxicity (arrhythmia/congestive heart failure) • Embryofetal toxicity • Hemorrhage • Tumor lysis syndrome • Impaired wound healing/GI perforation • Ocular toxicity	• CBC for myelosuppression • Serum lipase • CMP for hepatotoxicity, at baseline for tumor lysis syndrome • Blood pressure as clinically indicated • Ocular exam at baseline and then as clinically indicated	Deaths reported from hepatotoxicity, thrombosis including myocardial infarction and hemorrhage

CBC, complete blood count; CMP, comprehensive metabolic panel; ECG, electrocardiogram; GI, gastrointestinal.

Information obtained from each agent's prescribing information.

not only affect toxicity but efficacy outcomes as well. It is recommended to re-evaluate drug-drug and, if applicable, drug-food interactions in patients do not reach their disease response goal.

Similar to other chronic medications, adherence should be reinforced in patients taking BCR-ABL TKIs.[4,6,26,31] Potential barriers to adherence, such as cost, adverse drug reactions, and frequency of dosing, should be identified and routinely assessed. An observational study, ADAGIO, evaluated 169 patients receiving imatinib and found that only 67% of patients were adherent. The percent of imatinib not taken was associated with a lower rate of complete cytogenetic response.[32]

Treatment of Chronic Phase

The IRIS study compared imatinib 400 mg orally daily to IFN-α plus low-dose subcutaneous cytarabine in 1,106 patients with newly diagnosed CP-CML.[22] After a median follow-up of 19 months, patients who received imatinib achieved a complete hematologic response of 95%, major cytogenetic response of 85%, and complete cytogenetic response of 76%. Six percent of patients had progressed to AP or BC, and only four patients discontinued imatinib because of an adverse drug reaction. After 5 years of follow-up, only 3% of patients randomized to receive IFN-α remained on this agent compared to 69% of patients in the imatinib arm.[33] The estimated 10-year overall survival of the 553 patients originally randomized to receive imatinib is 83.3%, with 47% alive and still on initial imatinib treatment. At 10 years, the estimated event-free survival was 79.6%.[34]

Higher doses of imatinib have been evaluated in clinical trials. The German CML IV study randomized 1,551 patients with CP-CML to 400 mg or 800 mg of imatinib daily in a phase III trial.[35,36] Patients who received 800 mg daily were significantly more likely to achieve a major molecular response at 12 months than patients who received 400 mg daily. However, there was no difference between the treatment groups in progression-free or overall survival at 3 or 10 years. Higher doses of imatinib were associated with higher rates of dose interruption, reduction, and discontinuation. The results of this study and others do not justify the routine use of imatinib 800 mg daily as first-line therapy in patients with CML.[6,35-37]

Dasatinib (Sprycel®), nilotinib (Tasigna®), and bosutinib (Bosulif®) are second-generation TKIs originally used for the treatment of CML in patients who are resistant or intolerant to imatinib therapy; all three drugs are also approved for first-line treatment of CP CML. The encouraging results of phase III trials of these agents make them viable alternatives to imatinib for first-line treatment for newly diagnosed CP-CML.[6]

Dasatinib is an oral BCR-ABL TKI that was FDA-approved in 2006 to treat imatinib-resistant CML. Dasatinib is also a TKI of the SRC family, c-KIT, EPHA2, and PDGFR.[28] Preclinical data show that dasatinib is approximately 300 times more potent than imatinib and inhibits the growth of imatinib-resistant clones, except for the T315I mutation. Dasatinib has been evaluated as first-line therapy in the phase III DASISION trial, which included 519 patients with CP-CML.[38] Patients were randomized to dasatinib 100 mg once daily or imatinib 400 mg once daily. A greater percentage of patients achieved a complete cytogenetic response at 12 months with dasatinib compared to imatinib (83% vs 72%). The rate of complete cytogenetic response at 5 years was higher with dasatinib as compared to imatinib (83% vs 78%).[39] The rate of major molecular response was significantly higher in the dasatinib group (76% vs 64%). Five-year progression-free and overall survival were similar in the two groups. A trial evaluating different dosing strategies of dasatinib showed that 100 mg once daily was as efficacious as dasatinib 70 mg twice daily, 50 mg twice daily or 140 mg once daily but with decreased adverse drug reactions such as pleural effusions.[40] The standard dose of dasatinib for patients with CP-CML is now accepted to be 100 mg daily.

Nilotinib has 20 to 30 times the inhibitory activity of the BCR-ABL tyrosine kinase than imatinib, with activity against c-Kit and PDGFR (but not SRC kinases) due to a modification of the methylpiperazinyl structure of imatinib.[28] Nilotinib has inhibitory activity against imatinib-resistant mutants, with the exception of T315I. For first-line treatment of CP-CML, results of the phase III randomized ENESTnd trial comparing nilotinib at two doses (300 or 400 mg twice daily) to imatinib 400 mg once daily in 846 patients has been published.[41] The primary end point of the trial was major molecular response. In the final 5-year analysis, both nilotinib arms had a significantly higher major molecular response rate at 12 months (77% for nilotinib 300 and 400 mg twice daily) as compared to imatinib (60%).[42] The nilotinib arms also had significantly improved time-to-progression to AP or BC, as compared to the imatinib arm. The number of patients who discontinued treatment was similar in the three treatment arms.

Bosutinib has 15 to 100 times the inhibitory activity of the BCR-ABL tyrosine kinase as imatinib, with activity against SRC kinases but minimal activity against c-Kit and PDGFR.[28] Bosutinib has demonstrated clinical activity against many BCR-ABL kinase domain mutations that are resistant to imatinib, dasatinib, and nilotinib, with T315I as the notable exception. The phase III BELA trial of bosutinib 500 mg daily compared to imatinib 400 mg daily in CP-CML did not meet its primary endpoint of complete cytogenetic response at 12 months, likely as a result of a premature discontinuation rate in the bosutinib arm due to gastrointestinal toxicities.[43] A second phase III trial entitled BFORE compared bosutinib at a lower dose of 400 mg daily to imatinib 400 mg daily in 536 CP-CML patients.[44] Patients who received bosutinib had significantly higher rates of both major molecular response and complete cytogenetic response at 12 months compared to patients receiving imatinib. However, more patients in the bosutinib arm had dose interruptions, reductions, or discontinuation of therapy due to adverse drug reactions.

Ponatinib is considered a third-generation TKI, as it contains a novel triple-bond linkage in its chemical structure that avoids the steric hindrance caused by the bulky isoleucine residue at position 315 in T315I BCR-ABL binding site cleft, providing clinical activity against this resistance phenotype. However, off-target inhibition of vascular endothelial growth factor receptor (VEGFR), PDGFR, SRC, c-Kit, and other receptors may occur.[28] The EPIC trial was a phase III randomized trial comparing ponatinib to imatinib in patients with newly diagnosed CP-CML.[45] The study was terminated in October 2013 after events of arterial thrombosis were reported. The FDA subsequently released a Drug Safety Communication reporting an increased risk of life-threatening blood clots and narrowing of vessels within the extremities in patients who received ponatinib.[46] This agent also carries a Black Box Warning for vascular occlusion, heart failure, and hepatotoxicity.

Now, imatinib, dasatinib, nilotinib, and bosutinib are all recommended for patients with CP-CML who are at low risk of progression according to the ELTS model.[6] In patients with intermediate or high risk of progression, recommended first-line treatment includes dasatinib, nilotinib, and bosutinib. Imatinib may also be used in this setting, although it is not preferred. There are no head-to-head comparisons of dasatinib, nilotinib, and bosutinib, and therefore the clinician should personalize the selection of first-line therapy in CP-CML.[4,6,26] Factors such as comorbidities, potential toxicities, drug-drug interactions, dosing schedule, cost, and patient and physician preference should all be considered. Due to the risk of serious toxicities, ponatinib is generally reserved for patients with a documented T315I mutation or for patients in whom no other TKI therapy is indicated.[4,6]

Monitoring for Response 5 Careful monitoring is necessary to guide clinician decision making for modification of therapy. Recommendations for monitoring include baseline molecular and cytogenetic assessment. Patients with CP-CML who have an optimal response have a complete hematologic response within 3 months, partial cytogenetic response within 6 months, complete cytogenetic response within 12 months and major molecular response within 18 months of starting treatment.[4,6] *BCR-ABL* transcripts should be evaluated by RT-PCR every 3 months and bone marrow cytogenetics performed at 3 months if RT-PCR is unavailable or 12 months if neither complete cytogenetic response nor major molecular response is achieved. Bone marrow cytogenetics are repeated at 18 months if the patient is not in major molecular response or did not have a complete cytogenetic response at 12 months. The loss of hematologic or cytogenetic responses or clonal evolution at any time should be considered a treatment failure warranting a change in therapy. *BCR-ABL* kinase domain mutation analysis is performed for patients who have an inadequate initial response at 3, 6, 12, or 18 months, have any sign of loss of response or demonstrate disease progression to AP or BC.

Although most patients attain a complete cytogenetic response on TKIs, very few patients achieve a complete molecular response. In a study of patients enrolled in the IRIS study, Hughes et al. reported that less than 5% of patients on imatinib have undetectable levels of *BCR-ABL* when analyzed by RT-PCR.[47] Recent data suggest that the level of residual disease is predictive of progression-free survival.[48] Cytogenetic and molecular responses secondary to imatinib are associated with event-free survival and risk of progression to AP or BC.[33] Patients who do not achieve a hematologic response by 3 months, cytogenetic response by 6 months or major cytogenetic response by 12 months fare significantly worse as compared to responders. In addition, a complete cytogenetic response and at least a 3-log reduction in *BCR-ABL* levels via RT-PCR correlated with a 100% survival without disease progression at 18 months. The risk of disease progression according to the Sokal scoring system predicted the rates of disease progression to be 3%, 8%, and 17% in low-risk, intermediate-risk, and high-risk patients, respectively.

Discontinuation of TKIs The treatment of CML requires long-term therapy that can have significant adverse drug reactions and financial consequences. Discontinuation of TKI therapy with close monitoring has recently emerged as a possibility in carefully selected patients.[4,6] Candidates for discontinuation include those who achieve and maintain a major molecular response, or what is referred to as a deep molecular response (>4 log decrease in *BCR-ABL* RT-PCR or <0.01% *BCR-ABL* [IS] detection), for at least 3 years. Other criteria include no history of AP or BC, access to reliable response monitoring, and a thorough discussion of the risks and benefits of discontinuing therapy with the patient.

Studies of TKI discontinuation show that about 40% of patients who have achieved a deep molecular response remain in treatment-free remission (TFR) after stopping treatment.[49-51] Most patients who do relapse after stopping TKI do so within the first 6 months after cessation of treatment, and a molecular response is regained in almost all patients when the same TKI is promptly resumed.

An unexpected phenomenon of TKI discontinuation is "TKI withdrawal syndrome."[4,6,52] Pruritis and musculoskeletal pain requiring treatment are seen in up to 30% of patients. However, this phenomenon is reversible, and symptoms often rapidly disappear if TKI therapy is reinitiated.

Careful patient selection for discontinuation of TKI therapy, followed by close monitoring of *BCR-ABL* transcripts and restarting therapy if *BCR-ABL* levels rise may become standard management in the future.

TKI Resistance and Subsequent Treatment Up to 25% of patients with CP-CML will develop intolerance or resistance to first-line BCR-ABL TKI therapy.[53] Dasatinib, nilotinib, and bosutinib have all demonstrated efficacy in imatinib-intolerant and resistant patients.[53,54] Patients who cannot tolerate or do not respond to imatinib in the first-line setting should be treated with dasatinib, nilotinib, or bosutinib.[4,6] Patients who do not respond to a second-generation TKI in the first-line setting should receive an alternate second-generation TKI. There are not enough data at this time to recommend one second-generation TKI over another in second-line therapy. Mutational analysis may be helpful in this setting, as well as consideration of concurrent disease states, prior therapy, and expected adverse drug reactions.

The most prominent mechanism of TKI resistance is the presence of point mutations in one or more areas of the ABL kinase. More than 100 different mutations have been discovered thus far. Many of these mutations can cause a conformational change in the ATP binding site, which greatly decreases the ability of the TKI to bind and inhibit kinase activity.[55] Imatinib binds to BCR-ABL by establishing a series of hydrogen bonds with side chains of amino acids within the kinase domain. Mutations that alter this surface can decrease the affinity of imatinib for BCR-ABL, potentially preventing binding entirely.[56] The T315I mutation, known as the "gatekeeper mutation," occurs directly within the imatinib binding site and completely disrupts imatinib binding.[57-59] This mutation occurs in up to 20% of patients and is important because it confers resistance not only to imatinib but also to all second-generation BCR-ABL kinase inhibitors.

The PACE trial evaluated the use of ponatinib in 449 patients with resistance or intolerance to prior TKI therapy or with the T315I mutation.[59,60] Complete cytogenetic response rate at 12 months and major molecular response rate were 66% and 56%, respectively, in patients with CP-CML and the T315I mutation. Ponatinib is now recommended in patients with the T315I mutation or in patients who have failed 2 or more TKIs.[4,6]

A phase II trial of omacetaxine was conducted in 62 CP-CML patients with a history of the T315I mutation.[61] Complete hematologic response was achieved in 77%, complete cytogenetic response in 16%, and major molecular response in 17% of evaluable patients.

Treatment of Accelerated Phase/Blast Crisis

The goal of therapy in AP or BC is to return the patient to CP.[62] All of the BCR-ABL TKIs can induce responses in AP- and BC-CML, but response rates are lower as compared with those in CP-CML.

Omacetaxine mepesuccinate (Synribo®) was approved by the FDA in October 2012 for the treatment of CP- or AP-CML with resistance or intolerance to two or more TKIs. Omacetaxine is a first-in-class cephalotaxine ester that inhibits protein synthesis independent of direct BCR-ABL binding.[63] It is a semisynthetic form of homoharringtonine derived from the *Cephalotaxus harrintonia* alkaloid. Efficacy with omacetaxine has been demonstrated in two patient groups: CP- or AP-CML resistant to two or more TKIs and patients previously treated with imatinib harboring the T315I mutation. In a combined analysis of two phase II studies for CP- and AP-CML, omacetaxine was administered at 1.25 mg/m^2 subcutaneously twice daily for 14 consecutive days every 28 days then for 7 days every 28 days as maintenance.[64] Of the 41 patients in AP, 14% achieved or maintained a major hematologic response for a median of 4.7 months. The median overall survival of these patients was 14.3 months.

Traditional therapy for BC-CML is cytotoxic chemotherapy in treatment regimens similar to acute leukemia induction.[4,6,62] Etoposide (VP-16), cytarabine (Ara-C), and carboplatin (VAC-regimen) has demonstrated efficacy in patients with BC-CML with a median overall survival of 7 months.[65] The BCR-ABL TKIs have demonstrated modest activity in BC-CML and they may be added to cytotoxic chemotherapy to improve outcomes. Clinical guidelines recommend induction chemotherapy for acute leukemia based on the type of BP-CML, lymphoid or myeloid, along with a BCR-ABL TKI.[4,6] A BCR-ABL TKI can also be used alone in those with myeloid BP-CML or with a steroid in those with lymphoid BP-CML. Evaluation for allogeneic HSCT should be performed in all patients in BP-CML.[4,6,62] Please refer to the HSCT section above for more information regarding the indications and timing of this approach.

Summary of Treatment Options

The current standard of care is for patients with newly diagnosed CP-CML to receive a BCR-ABL TKI.[4,6] Low-risk patients may receive imatinib, dasatinib, nilotinib, or bosutinib based on comorbid conditions, expected adverse drug reactions, and patient or physician preference. Patients with intermediate- or high-risk disease should receive dasatinib, nilotinib, or bosutinib in the front-line setting. The goal of disease monitoring in CML is to differentiate patients who have optimally responded to an initial course of TKI therapy from those at high risk for treatment failure. With imatinib, nilotinib, dasatinib, and bosutinib as appropriate options for initial therapy for newly diagnosed CP-CML, and ponatinib and omacetaxine approved for salvage therapy, clinicians have many treatment options before allogeneic HSCT is warranted. Future research opportunities will focus on how to select second-, third-, and fourth-line therapies and whether combination therapy provides additional long-term benefits.

CHRONIC LYMPHOCYTIC LEUKEMIA

Epidemiology and Etiology

CLL is a lymphoproliferative disorder characterized by the accumulation of functionally incompetent clonal B lymphocytes.[66,67] CLL is the most common form of leukemia in the United States but is rare in other countries, such as Japan and China.[68] It is estimated that 20,160 new cases of CLL will be diagnosed in the United States in 2022.[3] Occasional family clusters of CLL have been recognized, and first-degree relatives of patients with CLL are at three times the risk of developing a lymphoid malignancy as compared with the general population. Male sex, white race, family history, and advanced age are known risk factors for the disease. CLL is a disease of older adults, with a median age of 71 years, although 20% to 30% of CLL occurs in patients who are younger than 55 years of age.[66,67]

Pathophysiology

CLL cells are comprised of a neoplastic clone of $CD5^+$ cells, which express low levels of surface-membrane immunoglobulin M (IgM) and immunoglobulin D (IgD) compared to normal peripheral blood B cells.[66,67] Normal $CD5^+$ B lymphocytes are present in the lymph nodes and blood. Neoplastic $CD5^+$ cells accumulate in the lymph nodes and spleen because of the loss of apoptosis by either the overexpression of an oncogene, such as *BCL-1* or *2*, or loss of a tumor suppressor gene, such as *RB1*.[66] The BCL-2 protein is a major regulator of apoptosis or programmed cell death.

A monoclonal population of B cells with a similar surface antigen phenotype as CLL cells has been recently identified in patients up to several years before diagnosis of the disease.[67] This phenomenon, termed monoclonal B-cell lymphocytosis (MBL), appears to predict whether a patient is at risk for developing CLL over time.

Although CLL lacks a common genetic target as observed in CML, B-cell-receptor signaling is a driver for CLL tumor survival.[66,67] Bruton's tyrosine kinase (BTK), a member of the Tec family of kinases, is essential for the activation of several constitutively active pathways for CLL cell survival. Phosphatidylinositol 3-Kinase (PI3K)-δ is a lipid kinase that plays a critical role in normal B-cell development, function, and transducing signals from receptors. The PI3Kδ signaling pathway is hyperactive in CLL and other B-cell cancers.

Cytogenetic abnormalities correlate with disease progression in CLL.[67] About 80% of patients with CLL have a karyotypic abnormality. The chromosomes that are most frequently involved include chromosomes 11, 12, 13, and 17.[67,69] Additional cytogenetic abnormalities may be acquired during therapy, particularly with deletions of chromosome 17, which have an adverse effect on survival.

About 4% to 10% of patients with CLL will undergo transformation of their disease to an aggressive lymphoma, most commonly non-Hodgkin lymphoma (diffuse large B-cell), which is termed as *Richter's syndrome*.[66,68,70] Richter's syndrome may be triggered by accumulation of additional cytogenetic abnormalities in the malignant clone of lymphocytes or by viral infections, such as Epstein-Barr virus.[70] Patients with Richter's syndrome will typically have a rapidly advancing disease course that mimics diffuse large B-cell non-Hodgkin lymphoma, but a small percentage of patients diagnosed with Richter's syndrome will transform into a Hodgkin lymphoma instead of a non-Hodgkin lymphoma.[68]

Clinical Presentation

Staging and Prognosis

Survival times for patients with CLL are widely variable, with some patients succumbing to the disease within 3 years and others living into a second decade from the time of diagnosis.[66,71]

The Rai and the Binet staging systems are commonly used in CLL, with the Rai being favored in the United States and the Binet in Europe.[67,71] The Rai staging system has been combined into a risk classification scheme: low risk (stage 0), intermediate risk (stages I and II), and high risk (stages III and IV) with median survivals of greater than 10, 7, and 2 to 4 years, respectively.[72] While historically useful, the Rai and Binet staging systems are not predictive for individual patients because they do not include immunohistochemistry, cytogenetic, or molecular markers or abnormalities.

Immunoglobulin heavy-chain variable (IGHV) gene mutation status is an important predictor of survival outcomes.[66,73] Unmutated IGHV (≤2% mutated) is an independent indicator of poor prognosis and significantly decreased survival compared to mutated IGHV, regardless of the patient's disease stage.

Biomarkers, such as CD38 expression and ζ-associated protein 70 (ZAP-70) expression, have been explored as prognostic factors for CLL.[67,71] CD38 is a cell-surface antigen that is associated with early progression, shorter overall survival, and a poor response to fludarabine. ZAP-70 is an intracellular protein with tyrosine kinase activity. Once considered as simply a surrogate marker for unmutated IGHV, elevated ZAP-70 expression appears to predict for rapid CLL disease progression and independently correlates with prognosis.

Cytogenetic changes can be biomarkers of response to therapy. Specific chromosomal abnormalities and their associated survival are listed in Table 158-5. Deletion of the short arm of chromosome 17 (del[17p]), which corresponds to p53 silencing, is associated with the shortest survival times. Mutations in the p53 gene (ie, *TP53*) can also occur separately from del(17p) and are associated with uncontrolled cell proliferation and shorter overall survival.[67,71]

TABLE 158-5 Prognosis Associated with Cytogenetic Changes in CLL

Chromosomal Abnormality	Median Overall Survival (months)
del(13)	133
del(12)	114
del(11q)	79
del(17p)	32

Data from References 71 and 73.

TREATMENT: CHRONIC LYMPHOCYTIC LEUKEMIA

Desired Outcomes

The primary goals of treatment for CLL are to achieve and maintain a prolonged remission with minimal treatment-related toxicity.[67,71] The management of patients with CLL is highly personalized, with

CLINICAL PRESENTATION Chronic Lymphocytic Leukemia

Constitutional Symptoms

- Fever, fatigue, weight loss

Physical Examination

- Lymphadenopathy (87%)
- Splenomegaly (54%)
- Hepatomegaly (14%)

Laboratory Tests

Peripheral blood

- Lymphocytosis
- Coombs-positive autoimmune hemolytic anemia
- Hyper- or hypogammaglobulinemia
- Monoclonal gammopathy
- Anemia
- Thrombocytopenia

Bone marrow

- Hypercellular
- Increased mature lymphocytes
- Increased megakaryocytes

Molecular markers

- Cytogenetics (11q, del(13p), del (17p))
- IGHV status
- CD38+ status
- ZAP-70 status

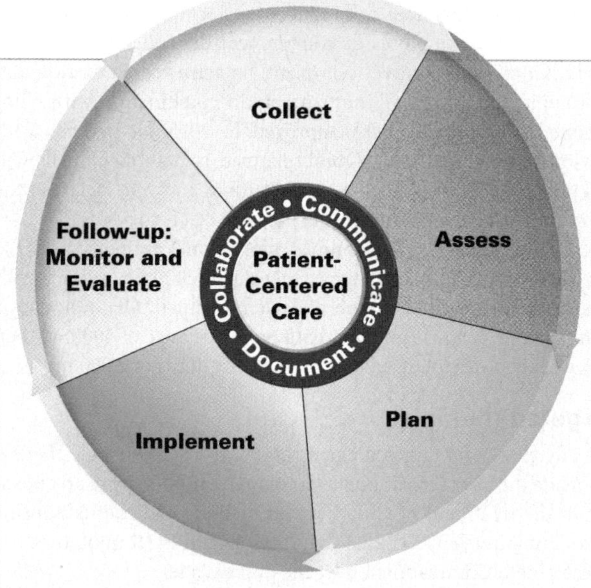

Patient Care Process for Chronic Lymphocytic Leukemia (CLL)

Collect

- Patient characteristics (eg, age, sex)
- Medical history (personal and family), including personal history of infections
- Social history (eg, tobacco, alcohol, chemical exposure)
- Current medications (eg, complementary or alternative medicines, inducers or inhibitors of CYP3A4, QT prolonging medications, warfarin, over-the-counter medications including aspirin/NSAID use)
- Objective data:
  - Vital signs: height, weight, blood pressure, heart rate, respiratory rate, oxygen status
  - Laboratory data: CBC with differential, CMP
  - Flow cytometry (chromosomal and molecular markers of CLL) and bone marrow analysis if performed
  - Imaging studies (PET or CT scan, if performed)

Assess

- Performance status (ie, to determine if the patient is fit enough to receive chemotherapy)
- Comorbidities
- Cytogenetic and molecular markers of CLL (eg, high-risk disease with del(17p) or *TP53* mutation)
- Immunoglobulin heavy-chain variable (IGHV) mutation status
- Infection risk (eg, IgG <500 mg/dL [5 g/L] or absolute neutrophil count <500 cells/mm^3 [0.5 × 10^9/L])
- Symptoms of disease
- Patient and family's goals of care

Plan*

- Observation (also known as "watch and wait") versus treatment
- Drug therapy based on high-risk CLL features, patient age, comorbidities, and schedule and route of therapy
- Monitoring parameters of efficacy (ie, disease response criteria) and safety (eg, myelosuppression, nausea, vomiting)
- Patient education (eg, goals of treatment, drug-specific education, medication adherence, food-drug and drug-drug interactions)

Implement*

- Educate patient on all aspects of the treatment plan
- Patient compliance (intravenous vs oral)

Follow-up: Monitor and Evaluation of Response*

- Evaluate efficacy using disease response criteria
- Assess safety and adverse drug reactions of treatment regimen
- Assess adherence to treatment plan (eg, patient-initiated delays vs toxicity-related delays)

**Collaborate with patient, caregivers, and other healthcare professionals.*

some patients receiving therapy on diagnosis, while other patients, particularly with early-stage disease, are managed expectantly. Indications for initiating treatment include disease-related symptoms (fatigue, night sweats, weight loss, and fever), threatened end-organ function, bulky disease, doubling of lymphocyte doubling time in less than 6 months, progressive anemia, and platelet count less than 100,000/mm^3 (100 × 10^9/L) or steroid-refractory autoimmune cytopenias.[68] Consideration of initial treatment options is based on several factors, including patient age and comorbid conditions, disease stage, and high-risk prognostic factors, such as del(17p) or *TP53* mutation.

Most patients diagnosed with stage 0 CLL do not require treatment and can be managed with observation.[67] In patients with stage I disease, treatment is controversial. A consistent survival benefit from early therapy has not been reported in asymptomatic patients.[71] In stages II through IV disease, treatment is required, with the goal of achieving a partial or complete remission.

Response definition varies based on the sites of involvement: resolution of lymphadenopathy and organomegaly, reduction of blood or marrow lymphocytes, and restoration of normal hematopoiesis.[67,71] An emerging goal of therapy is minimal residual disease (MRD), but this endpoint has only been recently introduced in CLL.[67] The clinical relevance of this assessment is currently undefined, as there is controversy as to whether this is a realistic treatment goal in patients with many comorbid conditions.

Cytotoxic Chemotherapy

Alkylating Agents Historically, orally administered alkylating agents such as chlorambucil, given either alone or with corticosteroids, were used as the primary treatment for CLL.[74] Chlorambucil has been used in older, symptomatic patients as initial treatment for CLL, but its use is based on a small number of studies with no demonstrable survival advantage. Common dosing schedules for chlorambucil are intermittent pulse dosing of 15 to 40 mg/m^2 orally every 28 days or daily doses of 4 to 8 mg/m^2/day.[71] The dose of chlorambucil is often titrated to circumvent myelosuppression.

Bendamustine is an alkylating agent with a purine-derivative benzimidazole ring in its chemical structure that yields a compound that is non–cross-resistant with other alkylating agents. Bendamustine induces cell death via single- and double-stranded cross-links.[75] It is usually combined with an anti-CD20 monoclonal antibody, most often rituximab (eg, BR regimen). The use of bendamustine in the treatment of CLL is declining due to the availability of more targeted agents.[71]

Purine Analogs Purine analogs, including fludarabine, 2-chlorodeoxyadenosine (cladribine) and 2-deoxycoformycin (pentostatin), are highly active in CLL, and fludarabine is the most widely studied.[67,73,74] Fludarabine is particularly useful in younger patients who can tolerate immunosuppressive chemotherapy. Although it was initially studied as a single agent in the treatment of CLL, fludarabine is now exclusively used in combination with other cytotoxic chemotherapy and/or immunotherapy. The most widely studied combination is fludarabine, cyclophosphamide and biologic therapy with rituximab (discussed below) in the FCR regimen.

Biologic Therapy

Monoclonal antibodies are a mainstay in the treatment of CLL. Rituximab is a chimeric monoclonal antibody that targets CD20 antigens expressed on B lymphocytes. Rituximab received FDA approval for the treatment of CD20-positive CLL in 2010. CLL cells have less prominent CD20 expression on their surface as compared to non-Hodgkin lymphoma, which may explain the lower clinical response in this setting. Rituximab as a single agent has moderate activity in CLL, with a 58% overall response rate reported with 9% complete responses.[67,71] Subsequent studies have used higher rituximab doses (up to 500 mg/m^2 per cycle) when given in combination with other agents. There are currently several biosimilar products of intravenous rituximab that are FDA-approved for use in the CLL population. Rituximab-arrx (approved in 2020), rituximab-pvvr (approved in 2019), and rituximab-abbs (approved in 2018) can all be substituted for rituximab. The decision regarding the specific product is usually based on the hospital or infusion center's formulary and the patient's insurance.

The FDA recently approved subcutaneous rituximab and hyaluronidase (1,600 mg/26,800 units) in combination with fludarabine and cyclophosphamide for the treatment of CLL. Subcutaneous administration of rituximab greatly reduces the time patients spend in an infusion center during their therapy by decreasing rituximab infusion from several hours to 15 minutes. Because of the large volume of rituximab, hyaluronidase is a component of the viscous, subcutaneous solution.[76] The hyaluronidase breaks down collagen, increasing the subcutaneous space for rituximab solution and facilitating absorption. Due to concerns over reactions, the intravenous formulation is given for the first treatment or cycle, and then the subcutaneous version is given with cycle 2 and beyond as long as the patient does not have an infusion-related reaction to intravenous rituximab.

Obinutuzumab is a glycoengineered type II anti-CD20 monoclonal antibody that does not induce translocation of CD20 monoclonal antibody complexes or complement-dependent cytotoxicity, but rather stimulates direct cell death via actin reorganization and homotypic adhesion.[77] Obinutuzumab, in combination with chlorambucil, was initially FDA approved in 2013 for patients with previously untreated CLL. Obinutuzumab is now combined with oral targeted therapies, such as acalabrutinib and venetoclax, in the frontline setting depending on the patient's del(17p) status.[71]

Ofatumumab is a fully human monoclonal antibody to CD20 that was approved as single-agent therapy in 2009 for patients with CLL refractory to fludarabine and alemtuzumab. Ofatumumab is administered as an IV infusion with an initial dose of 300 mg, then four weekly doses followed by four monthly doses of 2,000 mg.

Targeted Therapy

The advent of oral targeted agents and anti-CD20 biologic therapy has made the use of traditional cytotoxic chemotherapy nearly obsolete in the treatment of CLL.[67] The availability of Bruton's tyrosine kinase inhibitors (BTKi), BCL-2 inhibitors and PI3K inhibitors, has transformed CLL treatment over the past decade.

Bruton's tyrosine kinase (BTK) plays a key role in B cell survival, proliferation, adhesion, and cell migration. The introduction of BTKi has radically changed the treatment landscape of CLL. BTK is primarily expressed in B cells, but not plasma cells or T cells, making it an ideal target in CLL.[66] Ibrutinib is an orally administered compound that covalently binds to the cysteine-481 amino acid of the BTK enzyme and inhibits signaling of ERK, NF-κB, and cytosine phosphate-guanine–mediated tumor cell proliferation and migration.[67] Ibrutinib was FDA-approved in 2014 for the treatment of CLL after at least 1 prior therapy and in 2016 for patients who are treatment-naïve. Acalabrutinib is an irreversible second-generation BTKi with greater occupancy and improved selectivity compared to ibrutinib.[78] Zanbrutinib is a second-generation BTKi designed to minimize off-target kinase inhibition while achieving maximal exposure; it is more selective than ibrutinib for BTK and has less off-target activity against EGFR, TEC, and other kinases.[79]

Venetoclax is an orally administered selective BCL-2 inhibitor.[80,81] BCL-2 is an antiapoptotic protein that regulates the intrinsic apoptosis pathway. BCL-2 is overexpressed in CLL cells resulting in lymphocyte accumulation. BCL-2 inhibition with venetoclax results in apoptosis. Venetoclax was FDA-approved in 2016 based on a phase I/IIb trial of venetoclax in 116 patients with relapsed CLL.

Idelalisib is a small-molecule inhibitor of PI3Kδ and interferes with the PI3Kδ-AKT signaling pathway leading to increased apoptosis.[67] Duvelisib is a dual small-molecule inhibitor of both PI3Kδ and PI3Kγ.[82] While PI3Kδ is involved in the survival and proliferation of B-cells, PI3Kγ is a mediator in the migration and differentiation of T-cells and macrophages. Inhibition of both the delta and gamma kinases blocks malignant B-cell survival and proliferation and disrupts the malignant microenvironment.

Tables 158-6 and 158-7 summarize dosing, drug interactions, adverse drug reactions, and monitoring of oral targeted agents used to treat CLL.

BTKis have several characteristic adverse drug reactions that require active management and may necessitate pharmacologic treatment.[83] Diarrhea occurs early and often in patients who receive ibrutinib and acalabrutinib, but is usually self-limiting and can be managed with supportive care.[66,71] A common toxicity unique to BTKi is redistribution lymphocytosis secondary to tumor cell mobilization to the peripheral blood.[66] Patient adherence to therapy should be stressed, as this lymphocytosis is *not* an indicator of disease progression and the BTKi should be continued at the standard dose. Resolution of lymphocytosis usually occurs after several weeks.

Minor bleeding or bruising may occur during BTK therapy, and up to 10% of patients may have serious bleeding events.[66] For patients having planned surgical procedures that are considered to be high risk for bleeding, BTKi may be held up to 7 days before and 7 days after the procedure; more minor procedures may warrant holding the BTKi for 3 days before and after the procedure.

BTKis are associated with cardiotoxic adverse effects.[84] Atrial fibrillation (AF) has been noted, most often with ibrutinib but also with acalabrutinib and zanubrutinib. In a phase III trial of acalabrutinib compared to ibrutinib for the treatment of relapsed CLL, the incidence of AF was significantly lower in the acalabrutinib arm.[85] The mechanism of this adverse drug reaction is poorly understood, but off-target inhibition of cardiac phosphoinositide 3-kinase (PI3K-AKT) has been proposed. The advanced age and comorbid conditions of many patients with CLL make this adverse drug reaction particularly troublesome.[86] If possible, modifiable risk factors for AF such as hypertension, heart failure, obesity, and thyroid function should be identified and treated before the BTKi is started.[71,84] Patients with recurrent AF that is not medically controlled should avoid BTKis; AF that occurs during BTKi therapy should be managed according to current national guidelines.[84,86] The selection of drug therapy for AF during BTKi therapy may be problematic, as drug-drug interactions have been reported between BTKi and amiodarone or non-dihydropyridine calcium channel blockers. Further, the addition of anticoagulation may predispose the patient to

TABLE 158-6 Oral Targeted Agents in Chronic Lymphocytic Leukemia*

Drug	Brand Name	Dosing	Food-Drug Interactions	Drug-Drug Interactions
Acalabrutinib	Calquence®	• 100 mg orally twice daily • Avoid with severe hepatic impairment	• Avoid taking with proton pump inhibitors • Take 2 hours prior to taking an H_2-receptor antagonist • Separate from antacids by at least 2 hours • Avoid grapefruit, Seville oranges, star fruit, and pomegranate	• Substrate of CYP 3A4 to an active metabolite (ACP-5862), 50% less potent than the parent compound • Strong CYP 3A4 inhibitors increase C_{max} by 3.9-fold and AUC by 5.1-fold • Strong CYP 3A4 inducers decrease C_{max} by 68% and AUC by 77% • Weak inhibitor of CYP 3A4/5, 2C8, and 2C9 • Weak inducer of CYP1A2, 2B6, and 3A4
Duvelisib	Copiktra®	25 mg orally twice daily	None	• Substrate of CYP 3A4, P-gp, and BCRP • Strong CYP 3A4 inhibitors increase C_{max} 1.7-fold and AUC 4-fold • Strong CYP 3A4 inducers decrease C_{max} by 66% and AUC by 82% • Moderate inhibitor of CYP 3A4
Ibrutinib	Imbruvica®	• 420 mg/day • 140 mg/day with mild hepatic impairment • 70 mg/day with moderate hepatic impairment	Avoid grapefruit, Seville oranges, and pomegranate	• Strong CYP 3A4 inhibitors increase C_{max} 6.7-fold to 29-fold and AUC 5.7-fold to 24-fold • Strong CYP 3A4 inducers decrease C_{max} >13-fold and AUC >10-fold • Minor substrate of CYP2D6
Idelalisib	Zydelig®	• 150 mg twice daily • Moderate or severe hepatic impairment, reduce dose to 150 mg daily	None	• Idelalisib is a CYP 3A4, 2C8, 2C19, UGT1A1, and P-gp inhibitor • Strong CYP 3A4 inducers decrease C_{max} by 58% and AUC by 75% • Strong CYP 3A4 inhibitors increase AUC 1.8-fold (no change in C_{max})
Venetoclax	Venclexa®	• Week 1: 20 mg once daily • Week 2: 50 mg once daily • Week 3: 100 mg once daily • Week 4: 200 mg once daily • Week 5: 400 mg once daily	• Take with a meal and water • Avoid grapefruit, Seville oranges, star fruit, and pomegranate	• Substrate of CYP 3A4, P-gp, and BRCP • Inhibits CYP 2C8, 2C9, UGT1A1, P-gp, BCRP, and OATP1B1 • Concomitant strong 3A4 inhibitors, reduce dose to 100 mg • Concomitant moderate 3A4 inhibitors, reduce dose to 200 mg
Zanubrutinib	Brukinsa®	• 320 mg daily or 160 mg twice daily • 80 mg twice daily for severe hepatic impairment	Can be taken with or without food	• Primarily metabolized by CYP 3A4 • Concomitant strong or moderate CYP 3A4 inhibitors, reduce dose to 80 mg twice daily • Avoid concomitant use with strong CYP 3A4 inducers • Weak inhibitor of CYP 3A4 and CYP 2C19

AUC, area under the curve; C_{max}, maximum concentration; CYP, cytochrome P450; Pgp, P-glycoprotein; UGT, uridine 5′-diphospho-glucuronosyltransferase; BRCP, breast cancer resistance protein; OATP, organic-anion-transporting polypeptide.

Information obtained from each agent's prescribing information.

TABLE 158-7 Monitoring of Oral Targeted Agents in Chronic Lymphocytic Leukemia*

Drug	Adverse Drug Reactions	Monitoring Parameters	Comments
Acalabrutinib	Common • Dermatologic toxicity • Diarrhea • Myalgias • Headaches • Fatigue • Infections • Myelosuppression Rare but Serious • Atrial fibrillation and flutter • Hemorrhage	• CBC for myelosuppression • CMP for renal function and liver function • ECG at baseline if cardiac risk factors	• Acalabrutinib increases the risk of bleeding; therapy may be held from 3 to 7 days prior to and after surgery • Upon initiation, transient increase in lymphocyte count (not progression) • Headaches can usually be managed with acetaminophen and caffeine combination products
Duvelisib	Common • Edema • Skin rash • Fatigue • Dizziness • Electrolyte abnormalities (hypophosphatemia, hyponatremia, hyperkalemia, hypocalcemia) • Colitis • Diarrhea • Hepatotoxicity • Myelosuppression Rare but serious • Pneumonitis • PJP • Cytomegalovirus disease	• CBC for myelosuppression • CMP for liver function • Signs and symptoms of CMV reactivation or PJP • Signs and symptoms of diarrhea/colitis, intestinal perforation • Signs and symptoms of pneumonitis	PJP prophylaxis needed
Ibrutinib	Common • Edema • Hypertension • Fatigue • Dizziness • Dermatologic toxicity • Myalgias and arthralgias • Fever • Myelosuppression • Renal toxicity Rare but Serious • Hemorrhage • Cardiovascular effects: atrial fibrillation, atrial flutter, ventricular tachyarrhythmias • Nonmelanoma skin carcinoma	• CBC for myelosuppression • CMP for renal function and liver function • ECG at baseline if cardiac risk factors	• Ibrutinib increases bleeding risk; hold 3-7 days prior to and after procedures • If anticoagulation is necessary, avoid warfarin • Upon initiation, transient increase in lymphocyte count (not progression)
Idelalisib	Common • Myelosuppression • Hepatotoxicity • Diarrhea/Colitis • Fatigue • Edema Rare but serious • Dermatologic toxicity • Gastrointestinal perforation • PJP • Pneumonitis	• CBC for myelosuppression • CMP for renal function and liver function • Signs and symptoms of diarrhea/colitis, intestinal perforation • Signs and symptoms of pneumonitis • CMV reactivation	• Upon initiation, transient increase in lymphocyte count (not progression) • PJP prophylaxis needed
Venetoclax	Common • Myelosuppression • Tumor lysis syndrome • Edema • Dermatologic toxicity • Fatigue • Dizziness • Electrolyte abnormalities (hypocalcemia, hyperkalemia, hypophosphatemia, hyponatremia) • Diarrhea • Nausea • Hepatotoxicity • Myalgias, arthralgias	• CBC for myelosuppression • CMP and uric acid for tumor lysis syndrome, renal toxicity, hepatoxicity	Risk for tumor lysis is based on patient's disease burden and rate of dose escalation
Zanubrutinib	Common • Myelosuppression • Upper respiratory tract infection • Rash • Bruising • Diarrhea Rare but Serious • Atrial fibrillation and flutter • Hemorrhage	• CBC for myelosuppression • CMP for renal function and liver function • ECG at baseline if cardiac risk factors	• Zanubrutinib may increase the risk of bleeding; therapy may be held from 3-7 days prior to and after surgery • Upon initiation, transient increase in lymphocyte count (not progression)

CBC, complete blood count; CMP, comprehensive metabolic panel; ECG, electrocardiogram; PJP, *Pneumocystis jiroveci* pneumonia.

**Information obtained from each agent's prescribing information.*

bleeding, as noted above. If anticoagulation is necessary, non-warfarin alternatives should be considered since patients taking warfarin were excluded from many BTKi clinical trials.[71,84,86]

BTKis have also been associated with hypertension, with a potential continual rise in risk over time.[87] In retrospective studies, no single anti-hypertensive agent or class of drugs has been associated with the prevention or control of BTKi-related hypertension. The selection of drug therapy should be carefully considered to avoid drug-drug interactions with antihypertensive medications and the patient's current BTKi.[83]

Patients treated with venetoclax can develop tumor lysis syndrome when therapy is initiated.[83] The manufacturer recommends slow dose titration (known as "ramp up") from 20 mg daily to the target dose of 400 mg daily weekly over 5 weeks to minimize the risk of tumor lysis, although faster escalations of dosing may be used in select patient groups. Specific recommendations regarding inpatient versus outpatient initiation, dose escalation, and tumor lysis syndrome prophylaxis are based on disease burden and the patient's clinical status.[71] Drug-drug interactions must also be considered during venetoclax therapy.

Idelalisib, and duvelisib to a lesser extent, has been associated with immune-mediated adverse drug reactions such as colitis, intestinal perforation, elevated liver function tests, and pneumonitis.[66,88] Patients should have complete blood counts and hepatic function monitored before initiation and throughout treatment. Patients receiving idelalisib or duvelisib should receive *Pneumocystis jiroveci* pneumonia prophylaxis and monitoring for CMV reactivation.[71]

Infections are a major cause of morbidity and mortality in patients with CLL, due to both the underlying disease and treatment-related immunosuppression.[66,71,83] Although hypogammaglobulinemia often occurs, intravenous immunoglobulin should only be considered in patients with serum IgG <500 mg/dL (5 g/L) and with recurrent sinopulmonary infections requiring hospitalization or intravenous antibiotics. Prevention of herpes virus infections with acyclovir or an equivalent should be considered, especially if patients are receiving purine analogs, bendamustine or corticosteroids. Hepatitis B reactivation may occur in patients treated with anti-CD20 monoclonal antibodies; screening should be conducted prior to initiation of therapy, and prophylaxis may be required. Finally, vaccination for influenza, pneumococcus and zoster, should be administered as recommended by national guidelines; recombinant forms should be used and live vaccines should be avoided.

Hematopoietic Stem Cell Transplantation

The experience with the use of HSCT in CLL is limited. Although allogeneic HSCT may offer the potential of cure in CLL, the advanced age of most patients, reduced donor availability, and high treatment-related mortality precludes the routine application in the management of this disease.[71] Patients treated with allogeneic HSCT achieve higher remission rates and appear to have longer disease-free survival, but this approach is associated with high treatment-related mortality of about 40%.

Additionally, the new, targeted therapies provide additional options for disease control and overall survival advantages, so the role of allogeneic HSCT is further limited. Older patients who are not candidates for full-intensity allogeneic HSCT may be candidates for non-myeloablative allogeneic HSCT.

Figure 158-2 shows the molecular targets of the various chemotherapy, targeted, and biologic agents used to treat CLL.

Initial Therapy

An evaluation of the patient's fitness for therapy must be conducted before therapy is initiated. Up to 90% of patients with CLL have one or more comorbidities, which may influence the choice of therapy and the patient's treatment goals.[89] There is no standard tool to assess a patient's fitness for therapy at this time, although NCCN Guidelines currently base the choice of initial therapy on age (older or younger than 65 years), the presence of significant comorbidities, and the presence or absence of deletion 17p or *TP53* mutation.[71]

At present, conventional cytotoxic chemotherapy in CLL is only recommended in younger, fit patients with mutated IGHV. This recommendation is based on the CLL10 study, in which bendamustine and rituximab (BR) was compared to FCR in over 500 previously untreated, fit patients with CLL.[90] The FCR arm showed improved progression-free survival, but overall survival was not different between the treatment groups. A progression-free survival benefit was also seen in those who had mutated IGHV CLL with a median

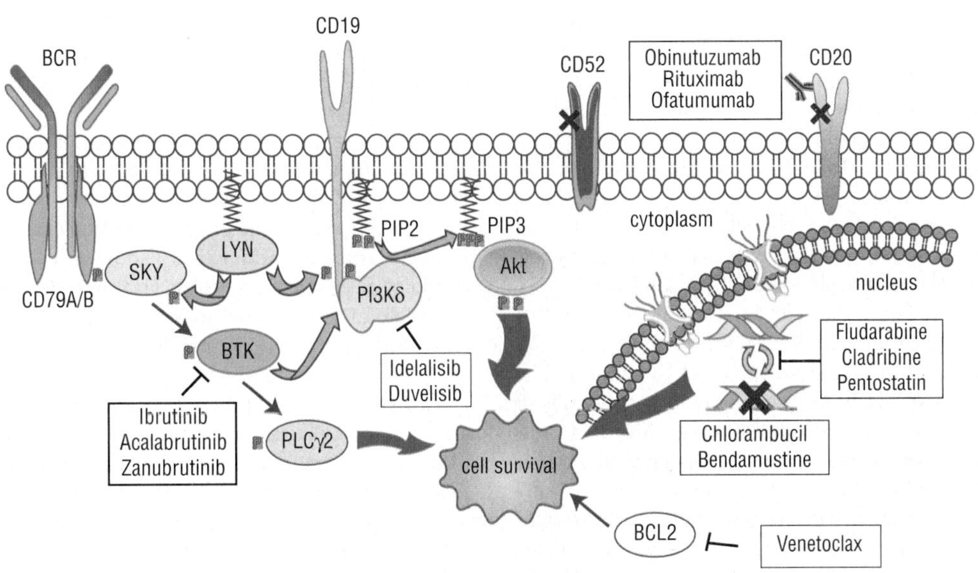

FIGURE 158-2 Current treatments and their molecular targets in chronic lymphocytic leukemia. *(Reprinted, with permission, from Manman W, Wang X, Song Z, et al. Targeting PI3Kδ: Emerging Therapy for Chronic Lymphocytic Leukemia and Beyond. Med Res Rev 2015;35:720-752.)*

of 42.7 months versus a median of 33.6 months in those without an IGHV mutation. However, the benefit of improved progression-free survival with FCR was not observed in patients older than 65 years of age. Patients who received FCR experienced more grade 3 to 4 neutropenia and infections, as well as an increased risk of secondary myelodysplastic syndromes and leukemias. Therefore, FCR is now only recommended for the first-line treatment of younger, fit patients with IGHV-mutated CLL.[71]

Preferred regimens for initial therapy of younger, fit patients include ibrutinib, acalabrutinib with or without obinutuzumab, and venetoclax plus obinutuzumab.[71]

Ibrutinib plus rituximab was compared to FCR in 529 previously untreated patients with CLL who were less than 70 years of age without del(17p).[91] At 45 months, progression-free survival favored ibrutinib and rituximab. Improved progression-free survival was seen across subgroups, but was not observed in patients with mutated IGHV, which strengthens the recommendation for FCR in the first-line treatment of younger, fit patients with IGHV-mutated CLL as discussed above. Although this study examined the use of ibrutinib and rituximab, the true benefit of an anti-CD20 monoclonal antibody in this setting is not clear due to a lack of comparative studies, and therefore ibrutinib alone is recommended in the first-line treatment of CLL.[71,73]

The ELEVATE-TN study was a three-arm phase III trial that randomized 535 patients with untreated CLL to acalabrutinib plus obinutuzumab, acalabrutinib alone, or chlorambucil plus obinutuzumab.[78] Of note, acalabrutinib was continued until disease progression or unacceptable toxicity while chlorambucil was given for a specific period of time. At a follow-up of 24 months, both of the acalabrutinib-containing treatment arms had significantly longer progression-free survival (87% for acalabrutinib alone and 93% for the acalabrutinib plus obinutuzumab compared to 47% for chlorambucil plus obinutuzumab). Overall survival was not different between the three treatment groups.

In June 2019, the combination of venetoclax plus obinutuzumab was approved by the FDA for treatment-naïve patients with CLL. In an open-label, phase III trial comparing venetoclax plus obinutuzumab with chlorambucil plus obinutuzumab, patients treated with venetoclax plus obinutuzumab had a significant improvement in progression-free survival over chlorambucil plus obinutuzumab after a median follow-up of 28.1 months. No benefit in overall survival has been reported in this trial.[80]

Patients who are 65 years of age or older or who have comorbid conditions may also be treated with ibrutinib, acalabrutinib with or without obinutuzumab, and venetoclax plus obinutuzumab in the first-line setting as discussed above.[71] The use of ibrutinib in the first-line treatment of older patients with CLL was explored in a phase III open-label trial in which 269 patients with CLL were randomized to ibrutinib or chlorambucil.[92] Patients who received ibrutinib had significantly longer progression-free and overall survival and higher overall response rates as compared to chlorambucil. Sustained increases in hemoglobin and platelet levels and greater improvements in quality of life were also observed with ibrutinib.

The combination of obinutuzumab plus chlorambucil is also a recommended regimen in the first-line treatment of patients who are 65 years of age or older or who have comorbid conditions.[71] The CLL11 study was a phase III trial that randomized 781 patients with untreated CLL and coexisting conditions to one of three treatment groups: single-agent chlorambucil, obinutuzumab plus chlorambucil, or rituximab plus chlorambucil.[93] Median progression-free survival was longer with obinutuzumab plus chlorambucil as compared to the other treatment arms. Overall survival also favored obinutuzumab plus chlorambucil as compared to rituximab plus chlorambucil. However, this regimen has fallen out of favor because of the data showing better progression-free survival outcomes with acalabrutinib and obinutuzumab.[71]

Preferred regimens for the first-line treatment of patients with del(17p) or TP53 mutation include ibrutinib, acalabrutinib with or without obinutuzumab, or venetoclax plus obinutuzumab, regardless of patient age or comorbidities.[71] Zanbrutinib is also currently recommended as an option for first-line treatment in this setting based on arm C of the SEQUOIA trial, which enrolled 104 patients with newly diagnosed CLL with del(17p).[94] All patients received zanubrutinib as a single agent. After a median of 18.2 months, the overall response rate was 94.5%, progression-free survival was 88.6%, and overall survival was 95.1%.

Treatment of Relapsed or Refractory CLL

Despite impressive results with the use of new agents in the first-line treatment of CLL, the disease remains incurable and nearly all patients will relapse. Selection of therapy for relapsed disease depends on age, performance status, previous therapy, and response and duration of previous therapy.[67,71] Recommended treatment regimens in this setting include BTKis, venetoclax plus rituximab, and PI3K inhibitors.

Patients who did not receive ibrutinib in the first-line setting may be considered for this agent at relapse. In a phase III trial, ibrutinib was compared to ofatumumab in patients with relapsed or refractory CLL with a primary endpoint of progression-free survival.[95] At 4 years of follow-up, the median progression-free survival was still not reached in patients who had received ibrutinib as compared to 8 months with ofatumumab, and 3-year overall survival continued to favor ibrutinib (59% vs 3%).[96] Patient-reported outcomes were significantly greater in patients who received ibrutinib. Acalabrutinib was compared to ibrutinib in patients with previously treated CLL with del(17p) or del (11q) in the phase III ELEVATE-RR trial.[85] Acalabrutinib was determined to be noninferior to ibrutinib, with a median progression-free survival of 38.4 months in both arms as assessed by an independent review committee. Zanubrutinib is currently recommended as second-line or subsequent treatment of CLL in patients who are intolerant or have contraindications to other BTKis.[71] This recommendation is based on a single-arm phase II study of 91 patients with relapsed or refractory CLL. Overall response rate, as assessed by an independent review committee, was 84.6% at a median of 15.1 months.[97]

The combination of venetoclax plus rituximab was compared to bendamustine plus rituximab in 389 patients with relapsed or refractory CLL.[81] Progression-free and overall survival were both significantly higher in the venetoclax plus rituximab arm, and these benefits were maintained across all subgroups. A higher percentage of patients receiving venetoclax plus rituximab also had undetectable MRD at the end of therapy.

Idelalisib and duvelisib may also be considered in the relapsed and refractory setting.[71] In a randomized phase III trial, patients with relapsed CLL who had comorbidities that precluded them from being treated with standard chemotherapy were randomized to receive rituximab with either placebo or idelalisib.[98] The primary endpoint of progression-free survival was 20.3 months in the idelalisib group as compared to 5.5 months in the rituximab monotherapy group. Patients in the idelalisib group had a higher overall response rate and significantly longer overall survival. In an open-label, phase III clinical trial of previously treated patients, duvelisib showed improved progression-free survival over ofatumumab.[82] The improvement in progression-free survival was also observed in patients with high-risk cytogenetic markers.

For patients with relapsed or refractory disease who have del(17p) or *TP53* mutation, preferred treatment options include ibrutinib (if not previously received), acalabrutinib, and venetoclax with rituximab (all Category 1 recommendations in the NCCN Guidelines).[71] Other recommended regimens include duvelisib, idelalisib plus rituximab, and single-agent venetoclax.

Summary of Treatment Options

CLL is an incurable disease, and the goal of therapy is to achieve and maintain disease remission while minimizing the burden of treatment-related adverse drug reactions.[66,67] Therefore, patients should not be initiated on therapy unless symptomatic. The specific treatment depends on cytogenetics, age, and comorbidities. The NCCN guidelines recommend first-line treatment options based on the presence of deletion 17p or *TP53* mutation, age (older or younger than 65) and the presence of significant comorbidities.[71]

Historically, FCR has been the preferred initial therapy for symptomatic CLL in younger patients without significant comorbidities, but this regimen is now limited to younger, fit patients with IGHV mutation.[66,67,71] First-line choices for patients without del(17p) include ibrutinib, acalabrutinib with or without obinutuzumab, or venetoclax plus obinutuzumab. At relapse, therapy options include alternative regimens used in the first-line setting as well as idelalisib plus rituximab, duvelisib or zanubrutinib. Patients with del(17p) or *TP53* mutation may receive ibrutinib, acalabrutinib with or without obinutuzumab, zanubrutinib or venetoclax plus obinutuzumab as initial therapy, with alternative regimens employed at relapse.

Careful attention should be paid to the management of adverse drug reactions, and pharmacologic therapy to treat such effects must be carefully chosen to avoid drug-drug interactions (Tables 158-6 and 158-7). Cost must also be considered because many of the oral therapies are given for long periods of time. Patients with CLL are also at risk for opportunistic infections, and prophylactic therapy may be warranted. Future research in CLL will determine the optimum sequence, length, and goals of therapy in CLL, as well as management strategies for long-term adverse drug reactions of such therapies.

ABBREVIATIONS

ABL	Abelson proto-oncogene
ALL	acute lymphoblastic leukemia
AP	accelerated phase
ATP	adenosine triphosphate
BC	blast crisis
BCR	breakpoint cluster region
BTK	Bruton's tyrosine kinase
BTKi	Bruton's tyrosine kinase inhibitor
CLL	chronic lymphocytic leukemia
CML	chronic myeloid leukemia
CMV	cytomegalovirus
CP	chronic phase
CYP	cytochrome P450
Del(17p)	deletion 17p
ERK	extracellular signal-regulated kinase
FCR	fludarabine, cyclophosphamide, rituximab
FDA	Food and Drug Administration
FISH	fluorescence in situ hybridization
GVHD	graft-versus-host disease
GVL	graft-versus-leukemia (effect)
HLA	human leukocyte antigen
HSCT	hematopoietic stem cell transplantation
Ig	immunoglobulin M
IGHV	immunoglobulin heavy chain gene
IFN-α	interferon alfa
IRIS	International Randomized study of Interferon vs STI571 trial
IS	international scale
MBL	monoclonal B-cell lymphocytosis
mRNA	messenger ribonucleic acid
NCCN	National Comprehensive Cancer Network
NSAID	nonsteroidal anti-inflammatory drug
PDGFR	platelet-derived growth factor receptor
Ph	Philadelphia chromosome
PI3K	phosphatidylinositol 3-kinase
RT-PCR	reverse-transcription polymerase chain reaction
STI	signal transduction inhibitor
TKI	tyrosine kinase inhibitor
VTE	venous thromboembolism
WBC	white blood cell
WHO	World Health Organization
ZAP-70	ζ-associated protein 70

REFERENCES

1. Faderl S, Talpaz M, Estrov Z, et al. Chronic myelogenous leukemia: Biology and therapy. *Ann Intern Med.* 1999;131(3):207–219.
2. Hehlmann R, Hochhaus A, Baccarani M, et al. Chronic myeloid leukaemia. *Lancet.* 2007;370(9584):342–350.
3. Siegel RL, Miller KD, Fuchs HE, Jemal A. Cancer statistics, 2022. *CA Cancer J Clin.* 2022;72(1):7–33.
4. Hochhaus A, Baccarani M, Silver RT, et al. European leukemianet 2020 recommendations for treating chronic myeloid leukemia. *Leukemia.* 2020;34(4):966–984.
5. Borgaonkar DS. Philadelphia-chromosome translocation and chronic myeloid leukaemia. *Lancet.* 1973;1(7814):1250.
6. National comprehensive cancer network clinical practice guidelines in oncology. Chronic myeloid leukemia version 1. 2022. Available at www.NCCN.org. Accessed September 28, 2021.
7. Jabbour E, Fava C, Kantarjian H. Advances in the biology and therapy of patients with chronic myeloid leukaemia. *Best Pract Res Clin Haematol.* 2009;22(3):395–407.
8. Shanmuganathan N, Hughes TP. Early management of CML. *Curr Hematol Malig Rep.* 2019;14(6):480–491.
9. Swerdlow SH, Harris NL, Jaffe ES, et al. *Who Classification of Tumours.* revised 4th ed. Vol 2. Lyon, France: IRAC; 2017.
10. Kantarjian HM, Deisseroth A, Kurzrock R, et al. Chronic myelogenous leukemia: A concise update. *Blood.* 1993;82(3):691–703.
11. Fabarius A, Leitner A, Hochhaus A, et al. Impact of additional cytogenetic aberrations at diagnosis on prognosis of CML: Long-term observation of 1151 patients from the randomized CML study IV. *Blood* 2011;118(26):6760–6768.
12. Sokal JE, Cox EB, Baccarani M, et al. Prognostic discrimination in "good-risk" chronic granulocytic leukemia. *Blood.* 1984;63(4):789–799.
13. Jabbour E, Kantarjian H. Chronic myeloid leukemia: 2012 Update on diagnosis, monitoring, and management. *Am J Hematol.* 2012;87(11):1037–1045.
14. Pfirrmann M, Clark RE, Prejzner W, et al. The eutos long-term survival (ELTS) score is superior to the sokal score for predicting survival in chronic myeloid leukemia. *Leukemia.* 2020;34(8):2138–2149.
15. Jabbour E, Kantarjian H. Chronic myeloid leukemia: 2018 Update on diagnosis, therapy and monitoring. *Am J Hematol.* 2018;93(3):442–459.
16. Radich JP. The biology of chronic myelogenous leukemia progression: Who, what, where, and why? *Hematol Oncol Clin North Am.* 2011;25(5):967–980, v.
17. Gratwohl A, Brand R, Apperley J, et al. Allogeneic hematopoietic stem cell transplantation for chronic myeloid leukemia in Europe 2006: Transplant activity, long-term data and current results. An analysis by the chronic leukemia working party of the European group for blood and marrow transplantation (EBMT). *Haematologica.* 2006;91(4):513–521.
18. Deininger M, Schleuning M, Greinix H, et al. The effect of prior exposure to imatinib on transplant-related mortality. *Haematologica.* 2006;91(4):452–459.
19. Porter D, Levine JE. Graft-versus-host disease and graft-versus-leukemia after donor leukocyte infusion. *Semin Hematol.* 2006;43(1):53–61.
20. Liesveld JL, Lichtmann MA. *Chronic Myelogenous Leukemia and Related Disorders.* McGraw Hill; 2021.
21. Cortes J, Kantarjian H. How I treat newly diagnosed chronic phase CML. *Blood.* 2012;120(7):1390–1397.
22. O'Brien SG, Guilhot F, Larson RA, et al. Imatinib compared with interferon and low-dose cytarabine for newly diagnosed chronic-phase chronic myeloid leukemia. *N Engl J Med.* 2003;348(11):994–1004.
23. Preudhomme C, Guilhot J, Nicolini FE, et al. Imatinib plus peginterferon alfa-2a in chronic myeloid leukemia. *N Engl J Med.* 2010; 363(26):2511–2521.

24. Pasic I, Lipton JH. Current approach to the treatment of chronic myeloid leukaemia. *Leuk Res.* 2017;55:65–78.
25. Steegmann JL, Baccarani M, Breccia M, et al. European leukemianet recommendations for the management and avoidance of adverse events of treatment in chronic myeloid leukaemia. *Leukemia.* 2016;30(8):1648–1671.
26. Reff MJ, Shillingburg A, Shah B, et al. Front-line use of tyrosine kinase inhibitors in chronic phase chronic myeloid leukemia: Practice considerations. *J Oncol Pharm Pract.* 2020;26(1):156–174.
27. Medeiros BC, Possick J, Fradley M. Cardiovascular, pulmonary, and metabolic toxicities complicating tyrosine kinase inhibitor therapy in chronic myeloid leukemia: Strategies for monitoring, detecting, and managing. *Blood Rev.* 2018;32(4):289–299.
28. Green MR, Newton MD, Fancher KM. Off-target effects of BCR-ABL and JAK2 inhibitors. *Am J Clin Oncol.* 2016;39(1):76–84.
29. Luciano L, Annunziata M, Attolico I, et al. The multi-tyrosine kinase inhibitor ponatinib for chronic myeloid leukemia: Real-world data. *Eur J Haematol.* 2020;105(1):3–15.
30. Haouala A, Widmer N, Duchosal MA, et al. Drug interactions with the tyrosine kinase inhibitors imatinib, dasatinib, and nilotinib. *Blood.* 2011;117(8):e75–e87.
31. Marin D, Bazeos A, Mahon FX, et al. Adherence is the critical factor for achieving molecular responses in patients with chronic myeloid leukemia who achieve complete cytogenetic responses on imatinib. *J Clin Oncol.* 2010;28(14):2381–2388.
32. Noens L, van Lierde MA, De Bock R, et al. Prevalence, determinants, and outcomes of nonadherence to imatinib therapy in patients with chronic myeloid leukemia: The adagio study. *Blood.* 2009;113(22):5401–5411.
33. Druker BJ, Guilhot F, O'Brien SG, et al. Five-year follow-up of patients receiving imatinib for chronic myeloid leukemia. *N Engl J Med.* 2006;355(23):2408–2417.
34. Hochhaus A, Larson RA, Guilhot F, et al. Long-term outcomes of imatinib treatment for chronic myeloid leukemia. *N Engl J Med.* 2017;376(10):917–927.
35. Hehlmann R, Muller MC, Lauseker M, et al. Deep molecular response is reached by the majority of patients treated with imatinib, predicts survival, and is achieved more quickly by optimized high-dose imatinib: Results from the randomized CML-study IV. *J Clin Oncol.* 2014;32(5):415–423.
36. Hehlmann R, Lauseker M, Jung-Munkwitz S, et al. Tolerability-adapted imatinib 800 mg/d versus 400 mg/d versus 400 mg/d plus interferon-alpha in newly diagnosed chronic myeloid leukemia. *J Clin Oncol.* 2011;29(12):1634–1642.
37. Cortes JE, Baccarani M, Guilhot F, et al. Phase III, randomized, open-label study of daily imatinib mesylate 400 mg versus 800 mg in patients with newly diagnosed, previously untreated chronic myeloid leukemia in chronic phase using molecular end points: Tyrosine kinase inhibitor optimization and selectivity study. *J Clin Oncol.* 2010;28(3):424–430.
38. Kantarjian H, Shah NP, Hochhaus A, et al. Dasatinib versus imatinib in newly diagnosed chronic-phase chronic myeloid leukemia. *N Engl J Med.* 2010;362(24):2260–2270.
39. Cortes JE, Saglio G, Kantarjian HM, et al. Final 5-year study results of dasision: The dasatinib versus imatinib study in treatment-naive chronic myeloid leukemia patients trial. *J Clin Oncol.* 2016;34(20):2333–2340.
40. Shah NP, Kantarjian HM, Kim DW, et al. Intermittent target inhibition with dasatinib 100 mg once daily preserves efficacy and improves tolerability in imatinib-resistant and -intolerant chronic-phase chronic myeloid leukemia. *J Clin Oncol.* 2008;26(19):3204–3212.
41. Saglio G, Kim DW, Issaragrisil S, et al. Nilotinib versus imatinib for newly diagnosed chronic myeloid leukemia. *N Engl J Med.* 2010;362(24):2251–2259.
42. Hughes TP, Larson RA, Kim DW, et al. Efficacy and safety of niloting vs imatinib in patients with newly diagnosed chronic myelogenous leukemia in chronic phase: 6-year follow-up of enestnd. *Hematologica.* 2015;100:61.
43. Gambacorti-Passerini C, Cortes JE, Lipton JH, et al. Safety of bosutinib versus imatinib in the phase 3 bela trial in newly diagnosed chronic phase chronic myeloid leukemia. *Am J Hematol.* 2014;89(10):947–953.
44. Cortes JE, Gambacorti-Passerini C, Deininger MW, et al. Bosutinib versus imatinib for newly diagnosed chronic myeloid leukemia: Results from the randomized bfore trial. *J Clin Oncol.* 2018;36(3):231–237.
45. Lipton JH, Chuah C, Guerci-Bresler A, et al. Ponatinib versus imatinib for newly diagnosed chronic myeloid leukaemia: An international, randomised, open-label, phase 3 trial. *Lancet Oncol.* 2016;17(5):612–621.
46. FDA drug safety communication: FDA asks manufacturer of the leukemia drug iclusig (ponatinib) to suspend marketing and sales. Available at http://wayback.Archive-it.Org/7993/20170112031621/http://www.Fda.Gov/drugs/drugsafety/ucm373040.Htm. Accessed May 29, 2021.
47. Hughes TP, Kaeda J, Branford S, et al. Frequency of major molecular responses to imatinib or interferon alfa plus cytarabine in newly diagnosed chronic myeloid leukemia. *N Engl J Med.* 2003;349(15):1423–1432.
48. Press RD, Love Z, Tronnes AA, et al. BCR-ABL mRNA levels at and after the time of a complete cytogenetic response (CCR) predict the duration of CCR in imatinib mesylate-treated patients with CML. *Blood.* 2006;107(11):4250–4256.
49. Mahon FX, Rea D, Guilhot J, et al. Discontinuation of imatinib in patients with chronic myeloid leukaemia who have maintained complete molecular remission for at least 2 years: The prospective, multicentre stop imatinib (STIM) trial. *Lancet Oncol.* 2010;11(11):1029–1035.
50. Ross DM, Branford S, Seymour JF, et al. Safety and efficacy of imatinib cessation for CML patients with stable undetectable minimal residual disease: Results from the twister study. *Blood.* 2013;122(4):515–522.
51. Saussele S, Richter J, Hochhaus A, et al. The concept of treatment-free remission in chronic myeloid leukemia. *Leukemia.* 2016;30(8):1638–1647.
52. Clark RE. Tyrosine kinase inhibitor therapy discontinuation for patients with chronic myeloid leukaemia in clinical practice. *Curr Hematol Malig Rep.* 2019;14(6):507–514.
53. Khoury HJ, Bixby DL. Outcomes of chronic-phase chronic myeloid leukemia beyond first-line therapy. *Leuk Lymphoma.* 2015;56(3):568–576.
54. Gambacorti-Passerini C, Aroldi A, Cordani N, et al. Chronic myeloid leukemia: Second-line drugs of choice. *Am J Hematol.* 2016;91(1):67–75.
55. Mathisen MS, Kantarjian HM, Cortes J, et al. Practical issues surrounding the explosion of tyrosine kinase inhibitors for the management of chronic myeloid leukemia. *Blood Rev.* 2014;28(5):179–187.
56. Hughes TP, Saglio G, Quintas-Cardama A, et al. BCR-ABL1 mutation development during first-line treatment with dasatinib or imatinib for chronic myeloid leukemia in chronic phase. *Leukemia.* 2015;29(9):1832–1838.
57. Hochhaus A, Ernst T, Eigendorff E, et al. Causes of resistance and treatment choices of second- and third-line treatment in chronic myelogenous leukemia patients. *Ann Hematol.* 2015;94(Suppl 2):S133–S140.
58. Molica M, Scalzulli E, Colafigli G, et al. Insights into the optimal use of ponatinib in patients with chronic phase chronic myeloid leukaemia. *Ther Adv Hematol.* 2019;10:2040620719826444.
59. Cortes JE, Talpaz M, Kantarjian H. Ponatinib in philadelphia chromosome-positive leukemias. *N Engl J Med.* 2014;370(6):577.
60. Cortes JE, Kim DW, Pinilla-Ibarz J, et al. A phase 2 trial of ponatinib in philadelphia chromosome-positive leukemias. *N Engl J Med.* 2013;369(19):1783–1796.
61. Cortes J, Lipton JH, Rea D, et al. Phase 2 study of subcutaneous omacetaxine mepesuccinate after tki failure in patients with chronic-phase CML with t315i mutation. *Blood.* 2012;120(13):2573–2580.
62. Bonifacio M, Stagno F, Scaffidi L, et al. Management of chronic myeloid leukemia in advanced phase. *Front Oncol.* 2019;9:1132.
63. Al Ustwani O, Griffiths EA, Wang ES, et al. Omacetaxine mepesuccinate in chronic myeloid leukemia. *Expert Opin Pharmacother.* 2014;15(16):2397–2405.
64. Cortes JE, Kantarjian HM, Rea D, et al. Final analysis of the efficacy and safety of omacetaxine mepesuccinate in patients with chronic- or accelerated-phase chronic myeloid leukemia: Results with 24 months of follow-up. *Cancer.* 2015;121(10):1637–1644.
65. Amadori S, Picardi A, Fazi P, et al. A phase II study of VP-16, intermediate-dose Ara-C and carboplatin (VAC) in advanced acute myelogenous leukemia and blastic chronic myelogenous leukemia. *Leukemia.* 1996;10(5):766–768.
66. Burger JA. Treatment of chronic lymphocytic leukemia. *N Engl J Med.* 2020;383(5):460–473.
67. Hallek M. Chronic lymphocytic leukemia: 2020 Update on diagnosis, risk stratification and treatment. *Am J Hematol.* 2019;94(11):1266–1287.
68. Strati P, Jain N, O'Brien S. Chronic lymphocytic leukemia: Diagnosis and treatment. *Mayo Clin Proc.* 2018;93(5):651–664.
69. Kurtin S, McBride A. Risk assessment and risk-adapted treatment selection: A case-based approach for chronic lymphocytic leukemia. *J Adv Pract Oncol.* 2017;8(5):502–520.

70. Jamroziak K, Tadmor T, Robak T, et al. Richter syndrome in chronic lymphocytic leukemia: Updates on biology, clinical features and therapy. *Leuk Lymphoma.* 2015;56(7):1949–1958.
71. National comprehensive cancer network clinical practice guidelines in oncology. Chronic lymphocytic leukemia/small lymphocytic leukemia version 1. 2022. Available at www.Nccn.Org. Accessed September 29, 2021.
72. Hallek M. Chronic lymphocytic leukemia: 2015 Update on diagnosis, risk stratification, and treatment. *Am J Hematol.* 2015;90(5):446–460.
73. Hanna KS. Updates in the management of chronic lymphocytic leukemia/small lymphocytic leukemia. *J Oncol Pharm Pract.* 2020;26(1):146–155.
74. Byrd JC, Jones JJ, Woyach JA, et al. Entering the era of targeted therapy for chronic lymphocytic leukemia: Impact on the practicing clinician. *J Clin Oncol.* 2014;32(27):3039–3047.
75. Cheson BD, Rummel MJ. Bendamustine: Rebirth of an old drug. *J Clin Oncol.* 2009;27(9):1492–1501.
76. Assouline S, Buccheri V, Delmer A, et al. Pharmacokinetics, safety, and efficacy of subcutaneous versus intravenous rituximab plus chemotherapy as treatment for chronic lymphocytic leukaemia (sawyer): A phase 1b, open-label, randomised controlled non-inferiority trial. *Lancet Haematol.* 2016;3(3):e128–e138.
77. Goede V, Fischer K, Busch R, et al. Obinutuzumab plus chlorambucil in patients with CLL and coexisting conditions. *N Engl J Med.* 2014;370(12):1101–1110.
78. Sharman JP, Egyed M, Jurczak W, et al. Acalabrutinib with or without obinutuzumab versus chlorambucil and obinutuzmab for treatment-naive chronic lymphocytic leukaemia (ELEVATE TN): A randomised, controlled, phase 3 trial. *Lancet.* 2020;395(10232):1278–1291.
79. Song Y, Zhou K, Zou D, et al. Treatment of patients with relapsed or refractory mantle-cell lymphoma with zanubrutinib, a selective inhibitor of bruton's tyrosine kinase. *Clin Cancer Res.* 2020;26(16):4216–4224.
80. Fischer K, Al-Sawaf O, Bahlo J, et al. Venetoclax and obinutuzumab in patients with CLL and coexisting conditions. *N Engl J Med.* 2019;380(23):2225–2236.
81. Seymour JF, Kipps TJ, Eichhorst B, et al. Venetoclax-rituximab in relapsed or refractory chronic lymphocytic leukemia. *N Engl J Med.* 2018;378(12):1107–1120.
82. Flinn IW, Hillmen P, Montillo M, et al. The phase 3 duo trial: Duvelisib vs ofatumumab in relapsed and refractory CLL/SLL. *Blood.* 2018;132(23):2446–2455.
83. Chen KY, Brunk KM, Patel BA, et al. Pharmacists' role in managing patients with chronic lymphocytic leukemia. *Pharmacy (Basel).* 2020;8(2).
84. Pineda-Gayoso R, Alomar M, Lee DH, et al. Cardiovascular toxicities of bruton's tyrosine kinase inhibitors. *Curr Treat Options Oncol.* 2020;21(8):67.
85. Byrd JC, Hillmen P, Ghia P, et al. Acalabrutinib versus ibrutinib in previously treated chronic lymphocytic leukemia: Results of the first randomized phase III trial. *J Clin Oncol.* 2021: JCO2101210.
86. Stephens DM, Byrd JC. How I manage ibrutinib intolerance and complications in patients with chronic lymphocytic leukemia. *Blood.* 2019;133(12):1298–1307.
87. Dickerson T, Wiczer T, Waller A, et al. Hypertension and incident cardiovascular events following ibrutinib initiation. *Blood.* 2019;134(22):1919–1928.
88. Cuneo A, Barosi G, Danesi R, et al. Management of adverse events associated with idelalisib treatment in chronic lymphocytic leukemia and follicular lymphoma: A multidisciplinary position paper. *Hematol Oncol.* 2019;37(1):3–14.
89. Strati P, Ferrajoli A. Treating older patients with chronic lymphocytic leukemia: A personalized approach. *Drugs Aging.* 2019;36(9):841–851.
90. Eichhorst B, Fink AM, Bahlo J, et al. First-line chemoimmunotherapy with bendamustine and rituximab versus fludarabine, cyclophosphamide, and rituximab in patients with advanced chronic lymphocytic leukaemia (CLL10): An international, open-label, randomised, phase 3, non-inferiority trial. *Lancet Oncol.* 2016;17(7):928–942.
91. Shanafelt TD, Wang XV, Kay NE, et al. Ibrutinib-rituximab or chemoimmunotherapy for chronic lymphocytic leukemia. *N Engl J Med.* 2019;381(5):432–443.
92. Burger JA, Barr PM, Robak T, et al. Long-term efficacy and safety of first-line ibrutinib treatment for patients with CLL/SLL: 5 years of follow-up from the phase 3 resonate-2 study. *Leukemia.* 2020;34(3):787–798.
93. Goede V, Fischer K, Engelke A, et al. Obinutuzumab as frontline treatment of chronic lymphocytic leukemia: Updated results of the CLL11 study. *Leukemia.* 2015;29(7):1602–1604.
94. Tam CS, Robak T, Ghia P, et al. Zanubrutinib monotherapy for patients with treatment naive chronic lymphocytic leukemia and 17p deletion. *Haematologica.* 2020; Online ahead of print.
95. Byrd JC, Brown JR, O'Brien S, et al. Ibrutinib versus ofatumumab in previously treated chronic lymphoid leukemia. *N Engl J Med.* 2014;371(3):213–223.
96. Munir T, Brown JR, O'Brien S, et al. Final analysis from resonate: Up to six years of follow-up on ibrutinib in patients with previously treated chronic lymphocytic leukemia or small lymphocytic lymphoma. *Am J Hematol.* 2019;94(12):1353–1363.
97. Xu W, Yang S, Zhou K, et al. Treatment of relapsed/refractory chronic lymphocytic leukemia/small lymphocytic lymphoma with the BTK inhibitor zanubrutinib: Phase 2, single-arm, multicenter study. *J Hematol Oncol.* 2020;13(1):48.
98. Sharman JP, Coutre SE, Furman RR, et al. Final results of a randomized, phase III study of rituximab with or without idelalisib followed by open-label idelalisib in patients with relapsed chronic lymphocytic leukemia. *J Clin Oncol.* 2019;37(16):1391–1402.

159

Multiple Myeloma

Amy M. Pick and Jared E. Matya

KEY CONCEPTS

1. Multiple myeloma (MM) is a cancer that develops in plasma cells, leading to excessive production of a monoclonal immunoglobulin.
2. Most patients have skeletal involvement at the time of diagnosis, including bone pain and fractures. The acronym CRAB summarizes common clinical manifestations of MM and stands for hyper**c**alcemia, **r**enal failure, **a**nemia, and **b**one disease.
3. Primary therapy is initiated in patients with symptomatic MM, while patients with asymptomatic disease, such as smoldering myeloma or monoclonal gammopathy of undetermined significance, may be routinely observed.
4. Patients should be assessed for autologous hematopoietic stem cell transplantation (HSCT) eligibility before the initiation of treatment and, if eligible, hematopoietic stem cells should be harvested for transplantation following primary induction therapy. Autologous HSCT maximizes complete remissions and prolongs survival.
5. Initial therapy for patients with newly diagnosed MM should be personalized and based on their disease presentation, cytogenetic risk stratification, and functional status.
6. Initial therapy often consists of drug regimens incorporating a proteasome inhibitor, immunomodulatory drug, and dexamethasone. The regimen VRd (bortezomib, lenalidomide, and dexamethasone) is recommended for transplant eligible and ineligible patients with MM. A bortezomib-based regimen incorporating daratumumab is recommended by the Mayo mSMART guidelines in patients with high-risk cytogenetics.
7. Novel anti-myeloma drugs continue to be approved with encouraging results. Newer therapies include monoclonal antibodies, which are added to combination therapy, and chimeric antigen receptor T-cell therapy.
8. Maintenance therapies with lenalidomide or bortezomib may be used in both transplant-eligible and ineligible patients, with the goal of increasing progression-free survival.
9. There are numerous treatment options for patients with relapsed or refractory MM. Treatment selection depends on the patient's performance status, drug toxicity profile, and prior drugs used for treatment.
10. The bisphosphonates, zoledronic acid and pamidronate, and denosumab are used to manage myeloma bone disease, resulting in decreased pain and skeletal-related events and improved quality of life.

BEYOND THE BOOK

Watch the online YouTube video (https://www.youtube.com/watch?v=jdytgW5wKa4), "What is multiple myeloma" by Khan Academy Medicine. This 10-minute video provides an overview of multiple myeloma, highlighting classic myeloma disease presentation in the patient "Babs the CRAB," and the pathogenesis and diagnosis of myeloma. This video increases the students' understanding regarding the COLLECT and ASSESS steps in the patient care process.

INTRODUCTION

1 Multiple myeloma (MM) is a malignancy of plasma cells (ie, immunoglobulin-producing B lymphocytes).[1] The cancer is characterized by clonal proliferation and accumulation of a monoclonal immunoglobulin secreted from the plasma cell that can be measured in the plasma or urine. Patients with MM often have osteolytic bone lesions at the time of diagnosis, which is probably related to various bone-mobilizing cytokines secreted from the MM clone and bone marrow stromal cells. Other clinical manifestations include end-organ damage such as renal insufficiency, hypercalcemia, and anemia. The treatment of MM often consists of a three-drug combination incorporating a proteasome inhibitor (PI), immunomodulatory drug (IMiD), and dexamethasone. These regimens have improved response rates and outcomes compared to conventional chemotherapeutic agents. Although therapy is not curative, MM continues to be a remarkable example of bench-to-bedside translation in new drug development.

EPIDEMIOLOGY AND ETIOLOGY

The incidence of MM has increased globally, with a 126% increase in cases reported from 1990 to 2016.[2] In the United States, about 34,470 cases of MM were diagnosed in 2022, accounting for 12,640 deaths.[3] MM is a disease that affects older adults, with a median age at diagnosis of 69 years.[1,4] MM occurs more frequently in men than in women. The incidence of MM in Black individuals is twice that of White individuals, with Black patients having poorer survival rates.[5] Socioeconomic factors such as lack of access to care, medications, and clinical trials have been associated with poor outcomes.[5-7]

Risk factors for the development of MM are multifactorial. Inherited, societal, and environmental factors contribute to the incidence and outcomes of MM. Familial clusters of MM and multiple genetic mutations, including immunoglobin gene rearrangements, have been identified in the development and proliferation of MM.[8] Certain environmental influences have also been implicated with MM. Radiation exposure has been historically linked to the development of MM with atomic bomb survivors having a five times higher risk of MM. Even low levels of radiation may be a risk factor.[9] MM has been associated with exposure to various chemicals including pesticides, aromatic hydrocarbons, and petroleum products used in farming, cleaning works, mining, and other occupational groups working with these chemicals.[2]

PATHOPHYSIOLOGY

MM is a genetically heterogeneous disease characterized by abnormal clonal plasma cell infiltration in the bone marrow. Monoclonal gammopathy of undetermined significance (MGUS) and smoldering (ie, asymptomatic) MM may precede active MM. These conditions do not require treatment but do require active monitoring. MGUS is associated with the presence of monoclonal immunoglobulin in the blood (≤3 g/dL [30 g/L]), less than 10% clonal plasma cells in the bone marrow, and the absence of clinical manifestations of MM (eg, end-organ damage).[10,11] The conversion rate of MGUS to MM is about 1% per year. The molecular changes associated with the conversion of MGUS to MM are not clear, but genome-wide studies have identified several candidate genes associated with disease progression.[10,12] Smoldering MM is an advanced premalignant stage that is clinically distinct from MGUS with criteria including high monoclonal immunoglobulin in the blood (≥3 g/dL [30 g/L]) and 10% to 60% plasma cells in bone marrow with no clinical manifestations of MM. Although patients with smoldering MM have asymptomatic disease, the risk of progression to MM is about 10% per year for the first 5 years after diagnosis, about 3% per year for the next 5 years, and about 1% per year for the next 10 years.[13] Certain cytogenetic characteristics are associated with a higher risk of transformation to active MM including translocation of 4 and 14 (t(4;14)) and deletion of 17p (del (17p)).[10,14] Multiple genetic changes may occur over time leading to more symptomatic disease. Understanding the clinical features of the disease may help clinicians identify which patients are at high-risk for progression from MGUS or smoldering MM to active MM.

MM is characterized by the accumulation of malignant plasma cells in the bone marrow. Both MM and normal plasma cells are produced from differentiated B cells after antigen stimulation. Normal plasma cells will die within days to weeks after differentiation, whereas MM plasma cells are long-lived, with low proliferative activity.[1] MM was thought to originate from a single tumor cell, but it is now believed that MM is composed of genetically diverse clones and subclones that originate from one or more stem cells. The malignant plasma cell is involved in the unregulated production of a monoclonal antibody referred to as *M-protein.* MM cells are seldom seen in large quantities in the peripheral blood because of their close interaction with bone marrow stromal cells. MM cells are supported by a supportive bone marrow microenvironment that promotes the further expansion of MM clones. Molecules such as interleukin-6 (IL-6), vascular endothelial growth factor (VEGF), insulin-like growth factor-1 (IGF-1), and the transcriptional regulator nuclear factor kappa B (NF-κB) are part of the microenvironment and stimulate clonal growth, disease progression, and promote resistance to therapy (see Fig. 159-1).[15] Disruption of the microenvironment is an important strategy for therapy.

Figure 159-1 shows the molecules released during cytokine-mediated signaling and adhesion-mediated signaling. In a BMSC cell, NF-kappa B is added to the nucleus. The cell releases cytokines, IL-6, VEGF, IGF-1, and SDF-1 alpha, which result in cytokine-mediated

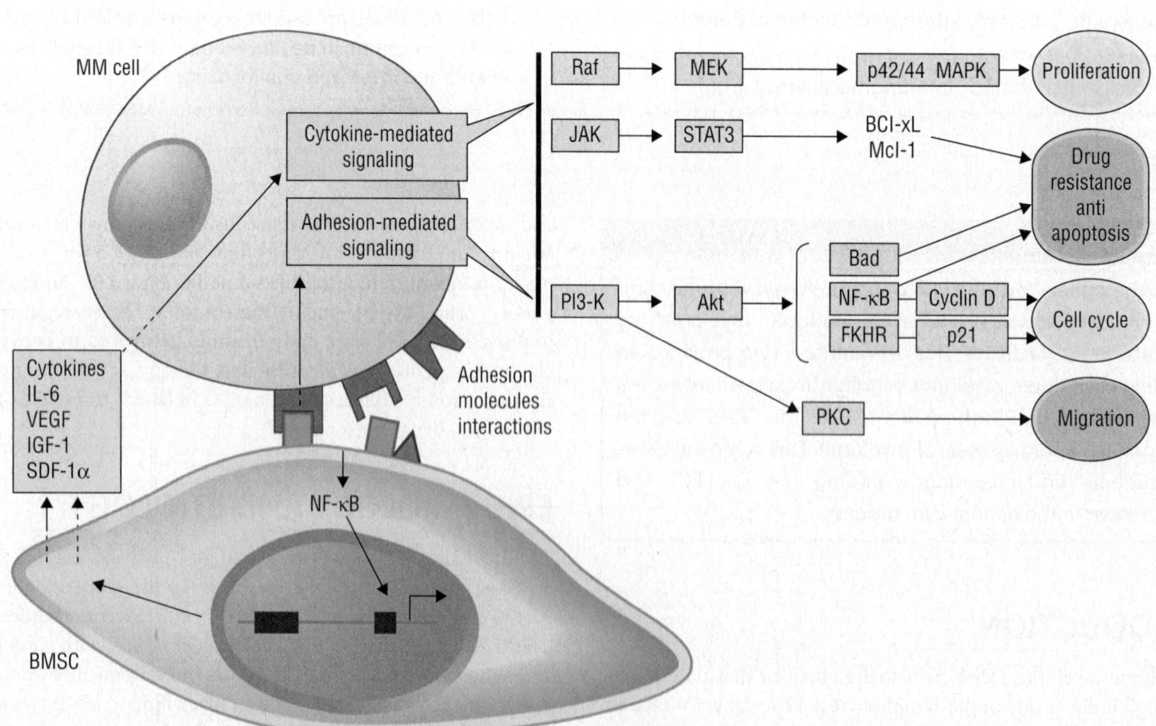

FIGURE 159-1 Pathogenesis of multiple myeloma. Multiple myeloma (MM) cells interact with bone marrow stromal cells (BMSCs) and extracellular matrix proteins via adhesion molecules, triggering adhesion-mediated signaling as well as cytokine production. This triggers cytokine-mediated signaling that provides growth, survival, and antiapoptotic effects as well as development of drug resistance. *(Reproduced, with permission, from Jameson JL, Fauci AS, Kasper DL, Hauser SL, Longo DL, Loscalzo J, eds. Harrison's Principles of Internal Medicine. 20th ed. New York: McGraw Hill; 2019.)*

signaling and adhesion-mediated signaling in the MM cells. During cytokine-mediated signaling, Raf forms MEK, which in turn forms p42/44 MAPK and promotes proliferation. JAK forms STAT3, which produces BCL-xL and Mcl-1 and promotes drug resistance and anti-apoptosis. During adhesion-mediated signaling, P13-K releases Akt and PKC. Akt releases Bad, NF-kappa B, and FKHR. Bad promotes drug resistance and anti-apoptosis. NF-kappa B promotes drug resistance and anti-apoptosis and produces cyclin D which results in cell cycle dysregulation. FKHR produces p21, which results in cell cycle dysregulation. PKC is involved in migration.

CLINICAL PRESENTATION

2 The clinical manifestations are related to the effects of MM cells on the bone microenvironment and the unregulated production of the M protein. Most patients with MM present with complaints of bone pain and fatigue at diagnosis. Initial laboratory evaluation often reveals hypercalcemia, renal insufficiency, anemia, and other abnormalities. Serum β_2-microglobulin is a useful measure of tumor burden. Skeletal evaluation shows gross abnormalities in most patients. Bone scans show abnormalities that often include lytic lesions, osteoporosis, and fractures. This group of findings—hyper**c**alcemia, **r**enal insufficiency, **a**nemia, and **b**one lesions—is often referred to by the acronym ***CRAB*** and is considered myeloma-defining events and suggests end-organ damage.[1,11] A confirmed diagnosis is defined by a bone marrow biopsy with 10% or more plasma cells, one or more myeloma-defining events, or biomarkers of malignancy.[11] The National Comprehensive Cancer Network (NCCN), International Myeloma Working Group (IMWG), and European Society of Medical Oncology (ESCO) have described criteria to diagnose MM.[11,16,17]

Following the diagnosis of MM, further workup analyzes and measures the quantity of the isotype of M-protein present. M-protein is a surrogate marker used to assess treatment response and disease progression. Serum protein and urine electrophoresis and serum and urine immunofixation identify the M-protein isotype secreted.[1] About 60% of patients have intact monoclonal immunoglobulin G (IgG), 20% have monoclonal IgA, and the remaining 20% secrete only monoclonal light chains. Antibodies are composed of two light chains, where antigen binds, and two heavy chains. Light-chain immunoglobulins, called Bence Jones proteins, can be secreted by the MM clone and excreted in the urine due to their low molecular weight, resulting in MM-associated renal failure. Serum-free light chains (SFCs) may also be measured, and these results may provide valuable information on the likelihood of disease progression.

Most patients have bone involvement at the time of diagnosis.[11] The effects of MM on the bone result from the abnormal production of cytokines, including IL-1, IL-6, tumor necrosis factor-α (TNF-α), and the receptor for activation of NF-κB ligand (RANK-L).[2] Bone involvement results from the activation of osteoclasts and inhibition of osteoblastogenesis and leads to bone destruction and resorption predisposing the patient to pathologic fractures and lytic lesions. Patients with MM are frequently anemic due to infiltration of the bone marrow with the MM clone and poor erythropoietin response. Patients can have clinically important hypercalcemia, which results from calcium mobilization due to bone resorption. Renal failure can occur as a result of high protein load from the monoclonal protein secretion and dehydration.

STAGING AND PROGNOSTIC FACTORS

Tumor cell features, tumor burden, and patient characteristics influence MM clinical outcomes. The revised International Staging System (R-ISS) is the primary staging system used to predict clinical outcomes for patients with MM. The R-ISS incorporates serum β_2-microglobulin, albumin, and lactate dehydrogenase levels, and high-risk chromosomal abnormalities to stage patients.[2,18] The R-ISS has largely replaced the older staging system, Durie-Salmon. Table 159-1 shows the R-ISS and median survival times for each stage.

Certain cytogenetic abnormalities are important prognostic factors. High-risk features associated with shortened overall survival include the presence of chromosomal 13 deletion (del 13), translocation of 4 and 14 (t(4;14)), and deletion of 17p (del (17p)).[11] The translocation of 11 and 14 (t(11;14) is the most common translocation, found in 20% of newly diagnosed patients. t(11;14) may be associated with intermediate outcomes and poor response to the novel agents used to treat MM.[19] The Mayo Clinic developed a risk-adapted approach, known as the mSMART (Mayo Stratification for

CLINICAL PRESENTATION Multiple Myeloma

General Criteria

- Most patients present with symptomatic disease

Signs and Symptoms

- Bone pain (fractures, lytic lesions)
- Fatigue (anemia)
- Infection (reduced polyclonal response)
- Neurologic symptoms (nerve compression)
- Polyuria (hypercalcemia)
- Nausea and vomiting (hypercalcemia)

Laboratory Parameters

- Elevated M-protein
  - Plasma electrophoresis
  - Urine electrophoresis
  - Immunofixation
- Elevated serum creatinine
- Hypercalcemia
- Low hemoglobin
- Low albumin
- Elevated β_2-microglobulin
- Elevated C-reactive protein

Bone Marrow

- More than or equal to 10% plasma cells

Imaging

- Skeletal survey with MRI or low-dose CT scan, as indicated

Cytogenetics

- Chromosome 13 deletion
- Translocations of t(4;14), t(11;14), t(14;16), and t(14;20)
- Del (17p)
- Chromosome 1 amplification

TABLE 159-1 Revised-International Staging System (R-ISS) for Multiple Myeloma

Stage	Characteristics	Frequency (% of pts)	5-Year Survival (months)
I	Serum β_2-microglobulin <3.5 µg/mL (mg/L) and Serum albumin ≥3.5 g/dL (35 g/L) No high-risk cytogenetics Normal LDH	28	82
II	Not stage I or stage III	62	62
III	Serum β_2-microglobulin ≥5.5 µg/mL (mg/L) and High-risk cytogenetics [t(4;14), t(14;16), or del(17p)] or elevated LDH	10	40

Reprinted, with permission, from Rajkumar SV. Updated Diagnostic Criteria and Staging System for Multiple Myeloma, American Society of Clinical Oncology Educational Book 36 (October 29, 2018) e418-e423.

Myeloma and Risk-Adapted Therapy), that categorizes patients into risk groups based on cytogenetics and gene expression profiling: high or standard risk.[20,21] Therapeutic options and treatment length are then recommended for each risk group. Additional prognostic factors generally represent the underlying pathologic changes associated with MM, including proinflammatory biomarkers (elevated C-reactive protein), tumor load (increased β_2-microglobulin), and dysregulated cellular growth (labeling index and marrow microvessel density).

TREATMENT

Desired Outcomes

The primary goal in the treatment of MM is to prolong the patient's survival and improve quality of life. This can be achieved by inducing a deep response (ie, MRD). Newly diagnosed MM patients who can tolerate chemotherapy will receive primary therapy where the goal is to achieve at least a major response. In transplant-eligible patients, primary therapy may be followed by transplant and

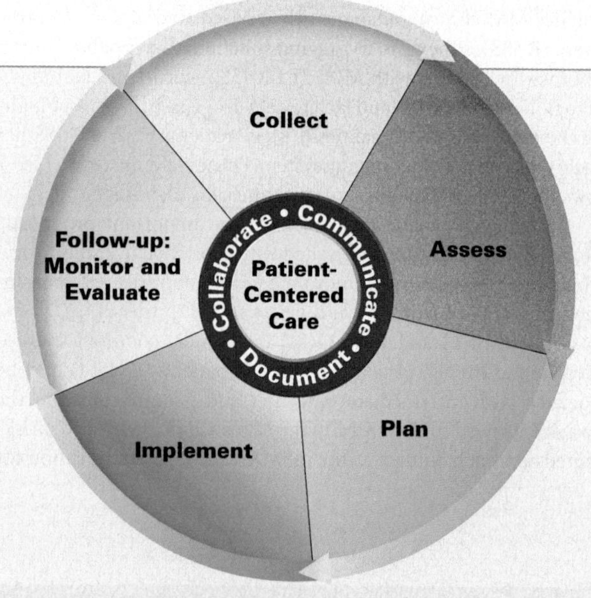

Patient Care Process for Multiple Myeloma

An illustration shows that patient-centered care includes collaboration, communication, and documentation. The actions associated with the care are collect, assess, plan, implement, and follow-up by monitoring and evaluating.

Collect

- Patient characteristics (eg, age at diagnosis)
- Patient medical history (personal and family)
- Patient comorbidities
- Patient organ function
- Current medications including over-the-counter (OTC) agents
- Prior treatment history for myeloma, if any
- Objective data
  - Labs including CBC, comprehensive metabolic panel, β_2-microglobulin
  - Results of bone scan

Assess

- Indication for therapy
- Candidate for autologous HSCT
- Impact of comorbidities on tolerance of therapy (eg, diabetes)
- Health literacy and adherence
- Emotional status (eg, presence of anxiety, depression)
- Ability/willingness to pay for antimyeloma treatment options (PO vs IV therapy)

Plan

- Drug therapy regimen (primary therapy vs relapsed therapy)
- Supportive care regimen (treatment of anemia, renal dysfunction, use of bone modifying agents)
- Monitoring parameters including efficacy and safety; frequency and timing of follow-up
- Patient education (eg, goal of therapy, schedule of treatments, adherence, self-monitoring)

Implement*

- Provide patient education
- Assess steps needed for insurance approval for oral/at home agents
- Ensure follow-up appointments are scheduled for active and supportive therapy

Follow-up: Monitor and Evaluate

- Response (minimum residual disease [MRD], M-protein)
- Safety (skeletal-related events, adverse drug reactions of antimyeloma therapy)
- Address supportive care concerns
- Adherence

**Collaborate with patient, caregivers, and other healthcare professionals.*

maintenance therapy. The goals of these subsequent phases are to further improve response rates. With the integration of novel agents into therapy, progression-free survival and overall survival have steadily improved, and responses have increased in frequency, depth, and duration. Unfortunately, there is no convincing evidence that patients are cured of their disease.

General Approach

3 The decision to initiate treatment depends on whether the patient has symptoms of the disease. Early conventional treatment is not beneficial in patients with MGUS or smoldering MM.[10] Therefore, watchful waiting is the most common practice for patients with asymptomatic disease and is recommended by the NCCN guidelines.[11] However, this treatment paradigm is evolving with the availability of novel agents. Several small published studies, including a phase III randomized trial of 119 patients with high-risk smoldering MM, suggest that early treatment with novel agents may improve overall survival and delay time-to-progression.[10] Clinical trials are highly encouraged and close monitoring every 3 to 6 months should be considered in patients with high-risk smoldering MM.[11]

Pharmacotherapy plays a major role in the management of MM. In the last two decades, the availability of novel drugs such as IMiDs, PIs, and monoclonal antibodies has improved survival in patients with MM. Patients with MM are usually treated initially with combination drug therapy, and most patients will respond to that therapy (see "Initial Therapy" section). Eligible patients will also undergo autologous HSCT. Unfortunately, most patients will eventually relapse and require additional therapies.

The IMWG has developed uniform response criteria to assess response to drug therapy in patients with MM.[22] Clinical response to therapy is generally defined by a reduced serum and urine M-protein by immunofixation and electrophoresis and plasma cells in bone marrow. Numerous response types have been defined, including a stringent complete response (sCR), complete response (CR), very good partial response (VGPR), partial response (PR), and stable disease (SD). The depth-of-response correlates with improved outcomes and a complete response correlates with prolonged overall survival.[17,23] Since the depth of response is important, measurements of MRD with more sensitive assays such as quantitative polymerase chain reaction (Q-PCR) and next generation sequencing are included in the IMWG Response Criteria. Table 159-2 describes the most common types of clinical responses.[17]

TABLE 159-2 IMWG Response Criteria in Multiple Myeloma

Standard IMWG Response Criteria	
Stringent complete response	Complete response as defined below plus normal FLC ratio and absence of clonal cells in bone marrow biopsy by immunohistochemistry
Complete response	Negative immunofixation on the serum and urine and disappearance of any soft tissue plasmacytomas <5% plasma cells in bone marrow aspirates
Very good partial response	Serum and urine M-protein detectable by immunofixation but not on electrophoresis or ≥90% reduction in serum M-protein plus urine M-protein level <100 mg/24 hr
Partial response	≥50% reduction of serum M-protein plus reduction in 24 hours urinary M-protein by ≥90% or to <20 mg/24 hr If the serum and urine M-protein are unmeasurable, a ≥50% decrease in the difference between involved and uninvolved FLC levels is required in place of the M-protein criteria If serum and urine M-protein is unmeasurable, and serum-free light assay is also unmeasurable, ≥50% reduction in plasma cells is required in place of M-protein, provided baseline bone marrow plasma-cell percentage was ≥30%. In addition to these criteria, if present at baseline, a ≥50% reduction in the size of soft tissue plasmacytomas is required
Minimal response	≥25% but ≤49% reduction of serum M-protein and reduction in 24-hour urine M-protein by 50% to 89%. In addition to the above listed criteria, if present at baseline, a ≥50% reduction in the size of soft tissue plasmacytomas is also required
Stable disease	Not recommended for use as an indicator of response; stability of disease is best described by providing the time-to-progression estimates. Not meeting criteria for complete response, very good partial response, partial response, minimal response, or progressive disease
Progressive disease	Any one or more of the following criteria: Increase of 25% from lowest confirmed response value in one or more of the following criteria: Serum M-protein (absolute increase must be ≥0.5 g/dL [5 g/L]); Serum M-protein increase ≥1 g/dL (10 g/L), if the lowest M component was ≥5 g/dL (50 g/L); Urine M-protein (absolute increase must be ≥200 mg/24 hr); In patients without measurable serum and urine M-protein levels, the difference between involved and uninvolved FLC levels (absolute increase must be ≥10 mg/dL [100 mg/L]); In patients without measurable serum and urine M-protein levels and without measurable involved FLC levels, bone marrow plasma cell percentage irrespective of baseline status (absolute increase must be ≥10%); Appearance of a new lesion(s), ≥50% increase from nadir in the size of >1 lesion, or ≥50% increase in the longest diameter of a previous lesion >1 cm in short axis; ≥50% increase in circulating plasma cells (minimum of 200 cells/μL [0.2 × 10^9/L]) if this is the only measure of disease

Data from Reference 17.

Pharmacotherapy

6 Treatment of MM is based on the combination of dexamethasone with novel agents from two classes of drugs, the IMiDs and PIs. A three-drug regimen is preferred for primary treatment based on increased response rates and improved survival in clinical trials when compared to two-drug regimens. Although there is a lack of head-to-head comparative trials, several highly active combination regimens are available. VRd (bortezomib, lenalidomide, and dexamethasone) is a frequently used regimen based on improved outcomes and is considered standard of care.[14] Tables 159-3 and 159-4 show dosing and monitoring parameters for the commonly used agents in the treatment of MM. Dose reductions in elderly patients and patients experiencing adverse drug reactions are often required.

Conventional Chemotherapy

Novel regimens have replaced conventional chemotherapy in the treatment of MM. Conventional drugs such as melphalan and cyclophosphamide may be combined with novel agents to improve overall survival, but their use is limited.[7] High-dose melphalan is commonly used in the conditioning regimen for patients with MM before autologous HSCT.

Corticosteroids

Corticosteroids are the cornerstone of MM therapy. Dexamethasone is incorporated into most treatment regimens, given in higher doses than those used in the treatment of other diseases. High-dose dexamethasone is associated with a higher risk of infection and central nervous system toxicity so it should be used with caution, particularly in older patients.[24] In current regimens, PIs and IMiDs are combined with dexamethasone to maximize initial response rates.

Immunomodulatory Drugs

IMiDs are incorporated into most treatment regimens for MM. Three IMiDs, thalidomide, lenalidomide, and pomalidomide, are

TABLE 159-3 Dosing of Drugs Used in the Treatment of Multiple Myeloma

Drug (Brand Name)	Dosing	Comments/Special Population
Lenalidomide (Revlimid®)	Induction therapy 25 mg/day PO on days 1-21 (28-day cycle) Maintenance therapy 10 mg/day, may be increased to 15 mg/day as tolerated	Adjust dose in renal impairment 30-60 mL/min (0.5-1.0 mL/s): 10 mg every 24 hours <30 mL/min (0.5 mL/s): 15 mg every 48 hours <30 mL/min (0.5 mL/s) (dialysis): 5 mg every 24 hours *Note:* Doses noted above are when used in combination therapy
Pomalidomide (Pomalyst®)	4 mg/day PO for 21 days (28-day cycle)	Mild-to-moderate hepatic impairment (Child-Pugh class A or B): 3 mg/day Severe hepatic impairment (Child-Pugh class C): 2 mg/day
Thalidomide (Thalidomide®)	200 mg/day	Start low in elderly adults; increase dose every 1-3 weeks
Bortezomib (Velcade®)	1.3 mg/m² SQ Days 1, 4, 8, and 11 Every 21 days	Reduce initial dose in hepatic impairment (serum bilirubin >1.5 × ULN) to 0.7 mg/m²
Carfilzomib (Kyprolis®)	20 mg/m² on day 1 of cycle 1 and then 70 mg/m² on day 8; continue with 70 mg/m² for subsequent doses	Dosing for relapsed/refractory disease Alternate dosing schedules are available
Ixazomib (Ninlaro®)	4 mg/day PO Days 1, 8, and 15 Every 28 days	Renal impairment <30 mL/min (0.5 mL/s): 3 mg Hepatic impairment serum bilirubin >3 × ULN: 3 mg
Daratumumab (Darzalex®)	16 mg/kg (actual body weight) IV weekly × 8 weeks then 16 mg/kg IV every other week × 8 weeks, then 16 mg/kg every 4 weeks until disease progression	
Elotuzumab (Emplicit®)	10 mg/kg IV weekly on days 1, 8, 15, 22 for cycles 1 and 2; dosing changes with subsequent cycles	
Isatuximab-irfc (Sarclisa®)	10 mg/kg IV on days 1, 8, 15, 22 of a 28-day cycle for cycle 1; 10 mg/kg IV on days 1 and 15 of a 28-day cycle for subsequent cycles	
Panobinostat (Farydak®)	20 mg PO every other day for 3 doses/week (days 1, 3, 5, 8, 10, 12) of a 21-day cycle	Hepatic impairment serum bilirubin >1-1.5 × ULN: 15 mg serum bilirubin >1.5-3 × ULN: 10 mg serum bilirubin >3 × ULN: Not recommended
Selinexor	60-80 mg PO twice weekly (days 1 and 3) 100 mg PO once weekly	Dosing depends on regimen selected
Belantamab mafodotin	2.5 mg/kg IV every 3 weeks	
Melphalan flufenamide	40 mg IV once every 28 days	

approved for the treatment of MM, with lenalidomide most frequently utilized. Although thalidomide was the initial IMiD studied in MM, it has been largely replaced by lenalidomide due to increased potency and fewer adverse drug reactions. Thus, the discussion below on IMiDs will primarily focus on lenalidomide. IMiDs are often used in combination with a PI and dexamethasone to treat newly diagnosed and previously treated MM.

IMiDs have complex immune effects and block several pathways that are involved in disease progression in MM.[25] While not fully understood, IMiDs have anti-angiogenic and anti-inflammatory properties that directly or indirectly affect MM cells. IMiDs decrease the production of cytokines and growth factors that are believed to have a role in the pathogenesis of the disease, such as IL-6, TNF-α, and VEGF. IMiDs may also inhibit NF-κB activation, either directly or indirectly via TNF, which results in increased apoptosis of the MM clone. Further discussion of NF-κB can be found in the PIs treatment section. IMiDs also induce IL-2 mediated T-cell proliferation including natural killer cell activity. Figure 159-1 shows the proposed involvement of cytokines on MM cells.

A major concern with IMiDs is the rates of VTE. Patients with MM have up to a ninefold increased risk of VTE for the first 6 to 12 months of therapy compared to patients without MM.[26] The risk of VTE is also increased when IMiDs are combined with dexamethasone- or anthracycline-based chemotherapy. The underlying mechanism for thrombosis in these patients is unknown but is likely multifactorial. The IMPEDE VTE score is a VTE risk stratification tool that has been developed and validated to assist clinicians with the identification of high-risk VTE patients and with the appropriate selection of VTE prophylaxis.[27] That tool incorporates IMiD use in addition to other factors. NCCN guidelines have adopted the IMPEDE VTE score in their VTE prevention guidelines because the tool better predicts VTE in MM as compared to previously published guidelines.[27] Prophylactic aspirin may be an option for patients at low risk of VTE. High-risk patients should receive LMWH, warfarin (target INR 2-3) or a direct oral anticoagulant indefinitely while on MM therapy.[11] The use of direct oral anticoagulants is a recent addition to the NCCN guidelines and is based on emerging literature showing them to be safe and effective.[11] Apixaban has the most evidence to support its use in patients with MM.[28,29]

IMiDs are considered teratogenic based on the known teratogenicity of thalidomide. All of the IMiDs have black box warnings for the potential for severe birth defects and embryo-fetal death. The drugs are commercially available through restricted distribution programs and require enrollment into their respective Risk Evaluation and Mitigation Strategy (REMS) programs. The intent is to encourage safe use of the medication and minimize the risk of fetal exposure.

Table 159-4 shows additional adverse drug reactions for IMiDs.

Lenalidomide Lenalidomide is a potent thalidomide analog and shares a similar mechanism of action to other IMiDs by targeting the

TABLE 159-4 Adverse Reactions and Monitoring Parameters for Drugs Used in the Treatment of Multiple Myeloma

Drug	Adverse Drug Reactions	Monitoring Parameters	Comments
Lenalidomide	Myelosuppression, rash, constipation, VTE, teratogenicity	CBC, LFTs, renal function, REMS Program (pregnancy testing), serum electrolytes and uric acid, thyroid function tests	Adjust dose in renal impairment VTE prophylaxis Secondary malignancies
Pomalidomide	Myelosuppression, rash, VTE, teratogenicity, infection	CBC, LFTs, renal function, REMS Program (pregnancy testing), serum electrolytes and uric acid	Adjust dose in hepatic impairment VTE prophylaxis
Thalidomide	Neuropathy, sedation, constipation, VTE, rash, neutropenia, teratogenicity	CBC, REMS Program (pregnancy testing), serum electrolytes and uric acid	Evening dose to decrease sedation Laxatives VTE prophylaxis
Bortezomib	Myelosuppression, neuropathy, infection including herpes zoster, gastrointestinal	CBC, LFTs, serum electrolytes and uric acid, neurologic examination	Antiviral prophylaxis
Carfilzomib	Myelosuppression, infection including herpes zoster, cardiac toxicity, infusion reactions, renal failure, neuropathy	CBC, LFTs, serum electrolytes and uric acid, renal function	Hydration to reduce risk of renal toxicity and TLS Dexamethasone premedication for infusion reactions Antiviral prophylaxis
Ixazomib	Myelosuppression, rash, neuropathy, infection including herpes zoster, gastrointestinal	CBC, LFTs, serum electrolytes and uric acid, renal function	Antiviral prophylaxis
Daratumumab	Severe infusion reactions, myelosuppression, infections, gastrointestinal	CBC	Premedicate with acetaminophen, diphenhydramine, methylprednisolone for infusion reactions Oral corticosteroid for 2 days following infusion Inhaled corticosteroids and bronchodilators may be needed for patients with COPD Antiviral prophylaxis is continued for 3 months after therapy
Elotuzumab	Severe infusion reactions, infections, hepatotoxicity, fatigue	LFTs	Premedicate with acetaminophen, H_1-receptor antagonist (ie, diphenhydramine), H_2-receptor antagonist (ie, ranitidine), dexamethasone for infusion reactions
Isatuximab	Severe infusion reactions, myelosuppression, infections, gastrointestinal, hypertension	CBC	Premedicate with acetaminophen, H_1-receptor antagonist (ie, diphenhydramine), H_2 receptor antagonist (ie, famotidine), dexamethasone for infusion reactions Consider antiviral and antibiotic prophylaxis
Panobinostat	Severe gastrointestinal toxicity (vomiting/diarrhea) resulting in dehydration, cardiac toxicity including QTc prolongation, myelosuppression, infection, hepatotoxicity	CBC, LFTs, serum electrolytes and uric acid, ECG	Anti-diarrheals Anti-emetics
Selinexor	Myelosuppression, infection, gastrointestinal, infection, neurotoxicity, ocular, electrolytes, hepatotoxicity, fatigue	CBC, serum electrolytes, LFTs, serum creatinine, neurologic, vision	Moderate-high emetic risk-administer with 5-HT_3 antagonist Specific dose adjustments for toxicity
Belantamab mafodotin	Infusion reactions, myelosuppression, electrolytes, hepatotoxicity, ocular, including vision loss	CBC, REMS-ophthalmic exam (baseline, before each dose), serum electrolytes	No premedications unless the patient experiences infusion reaction Lubricating eye drops QID while on therapy Avoid contact lenses
Melphalan flufenamide	Myelosuppression, infection, gastrointestinal, secondary malignancies	CBC	Moderate emetic risk-administer with 5-HT_3 antagonist Specific dose interruptions/reductions for toxicity

CBC, complete blood count; REMS, Risk Evaluation and Mitigation Strategy; VTE, venous thromboembolism.

microenvironment. Lenalidomide can be used as primary therapy in transplant-eligible or -ineligible patients, in relapsed/refractory MM and as maintenance therapy following transplant. Lenalidomide is preferred over thalidomide because of its improved toxicity profile.

Lenalidomide is Food and Drug Administration (FDA)-approved for the treatment of newly diagnosed patients with MM. In this setting, the doublet of lenalidomide and dexamethasone was compared with dexamethasone alone. The trial was halted when a planned interim analysis showed the combination to be more active than dexamethasone alone, with increased progression-free survival and overall response rate in the combination arm.[30] Subsequent trials examined the addition of a third agent, bortezomib, to the lenalidomide-dexamethasone regimen. A phase III study reported longer median progression-free and overall survival with the triplet regimen compared to the doublet lenalidomide and dexamethasone.[31] The regimen of bortezomib, lenalidomide, and dexamethasone is a category 1 NCCN recommendation for the primary treatment of MM patients regardless of transplant eligibility.[11] Other PIs and monoclonal antibodies may also be combined with lenalidomide and dexamethasone for primary therapy.

Lenalidomide is also used in the treatment of relapsed or refractory MM. Initial trials randomized patients to receive either lenalidomide (25 mg/day on days 1-21 of a 28-day cycle) and high-dose dexamethasone or high-dose dexamethasone alone. In one trial, patients receiving lenalidomide and dexamethasone had overall response and CR rates of 61% and 14%, respectively, compared with 20% and 0.6% in the dexamethasone alone group.[32] The improved response rates translated into a longer median overall survival in the lenalidomide and dexamethasone groups. Similar results were reported in the second trial.[33] Other trials have evaluated the combination of lenalidomide and dexamethasone with a third agent for relapsed/refractory MM. The triplet regimens of lenalidomide, dexamethasone, and carfilzomib, ixazomib, elotuzumab, or daratumumab show longer progression-free survival, resulting in the approval of these regimens for the treatment of relapsed/refractory disease.[30]

The most appropriate dosing of dexamethasone with lenalidomide has also been evaluated. An open-label noninferiority phase III trial addressed this question in untreated patients with MM.[34] Patients were randomized to lenalidomide and high-dose dexamethasone (40 mg on days 1-4, 9-12, and 17-20 of each 28-day cycle) compared with lenalidomide and low-dose dexamethasone (40 mg/week). Patients who received lenalidomide with low-dose dexamethasone had longer 2-year overall survival and less toxicity than those who received lenalidomide with high-dose dexamethasone. The trial was halted after a second interim analysis and patients were allowed to cross-over to the low-dose arm. Patients in the lenalidomide plus high-dose dexamethasone arm had a 26% incidence of VTE compared to a 12% rate in those randomized to the lenalidomide plus low-dose dexamethasone arm.[34] The improved survival in the low-dose dexamethasone arm is likely related to lower mortality from adverse drug reactions, particularly VTE. Deaths in the high-dose dexamethasone group usually occurred during the first 4 months in older patients.

Lenalidomide is better tolerated than thalidomide. Lenalidomide causes less neurotoxicity, somnolence, and constipation but more myelosuppression than thalidomide. Patients receiving lenalidomide have an increased risk of secondary malignancies, particularly patients >74 years old receiving maintenance lenalidomide.[35] Multiple cycles of lenalidomide can impair stem cell mobilization. The IMWG recommends that transplant-eligible patients receiving lenalidomide have stem cells collected within the first four cycles of therapy.[11,36] Mobilization with chemotherapy or plerixafor may be utilized if stem cell collection is decreased.

Pomalidomide Pomalidomide is a third-generation IMiD used in the treatment of MM. It is FDA-approved in relapsed MM in patients who have received at least two prior therapies, including lenalidomide and a PI. Pomalidomide is not approved for first-line therapy. Its initial approval was in combination with low-dose dexamethasone, where the pomalidomide combination demonstrated a progression-free and overall survival benefit versus high-dose dexamethasone.[37] Following that approval, pomalidomide was evaluated as part of various three-drug combinations. Pomalidomide shows good efficacy in patients who are refractory to lenalidomide and/or PI therapy. In refractory patients or those experiencing early relapse (<60 days after last therapy), the NCCN recommends pomalidomide, dexamethasone, and any of the available PIs as a preferred regimen after at least two lines of prior therapy. Similarly, regimens including pomalidomide and dexamethasone in combination with an anti-CD38 monoclonal antibody or elotuzumab are recommended for patients previously treated with lenalidomide and a PI.[11] Overall, pomalidomide is well tolerated with a toxicity profile similar to that observed with lenalidomide, except for a slightly higher incidence of peripheral neuropathy.

Proteasome Inhibitors

6 PIs are incorporated into most treatment regimens for MM. Three PIs, bortezomib, carfilzomib, and ixazomib, are approved for the treatment of MM. Bortezomib is the backbone of many regimens while the newer generation drugs seek to improve the toxicity profile, specifically lessening the degree of neuropathy. PIs are often used in combination with an IMiD and dexamethasone for the treatment of primary and relapsed/refractory MM.

PIs inhibit the proteasome and NF-κB activation. The proteasome is a protease complex responsible for degrading cytosolic proteins that are conjugated to ubiquitin. Ubiquitin is a 76-amino acid protein that tags various proteins for destruction.[38] By reversibly binding to the chymotrypsin site in the catalytic core of the 26S proteasome, bortezomib inhibits the degradation of these targeted proteins. Ixazomib is a reversible inhibitor while carfilzomib irreversibly binds to the chymotrypsin site, which explains the differences in pharmacokinetics among the drugs in this class.[38]

As discussed earlier, NF-κB activity is increased in MM. In the cytosol, NF-κB is bound to and is inhibited by IκB. The proteasome degrades IκB. When the proteasome is inhibited, cytosolic concentrations of IκB remain high, and NF-κB is retained in the cytosol as an inactive complex. The resulting inhibition of the NF-κB signal leads to a reduction in cytokine production and growth inhibition of the MM clone. Other proteins involved in cell-cycle regulation and apoptotic signaling that may be affected by PIs include p53 and map kinase.[38]

Bortezomib Bortezomib was the first drug in the class of PIs and continues to be the backbone of many regimens used in the treatment of MM. A 2016 Cochrane review concluded that bortezomib treatment improves response rates, progression-free survival, and overall survival and should be considered standard of care for the treatment of MM.[39] Bortezomib has been extensively studied and is approved as primary therapy for newly diagnosed and relapsed/refractory MM. Bortezomib was initially approved in 2003 under the FDA's accelerated approval process for relapsed or refractory MM in patients who had failed at least two prior therapies. The approval was based on a phase II trial in which refractory MM received 1.3 mg/m^2 of bortezomib twice weekly for 2 weeks followed by 1 week of rest. Patients received up to eight cycles. The overall response rate was 35% (includes minor responses) with seven (3.6%) patients achieving a CR.[40] Subsequently, a large phase III study (Assessment of Proteasome Inhibition for Extending Remissions [APEX] trial) demonstrated that bortezomib had superior activity compared with high-dose dexamethasone in relapsed MM. Bortezomib-treated patients had higher CR and PR rates, longer median time-to-progression, and improved 1-year overall survival compared with patients receiving dexamethasone.[41] The differences in each of these end points were statistically significant. The results from this study led to expanded FDA approval in 2005 to include patients who had relapsed after one therapy. Numerous trials have examined bortezomib in combination with monoclonal antibodies, IMiDs, and/or traditional chemotherapy for relapsed and refractory MM. Various triplet combinations include bortezomib and dexamethasone with lenalidomide or daratumumab.[11]

Bortezomib is extensively used in the primary treatment of MM. As discussed earlier, the triple drug regimen of lenalidomide, bortezomib, and dexamethasone is the preferred treatment regimen for primary therapy in patients regardless of transplant eligibility. The inclusion of bortezomib in three- or four-drug combinations improves response rates and increases progression-free and overall survival. Bortezomib-based therapies may also be preferred in patients with high-risk disease, based on data that shows bortezomib may be able to overcome certain cytogenetic abnormalities, including the t(4;14) translocation.[42]

Bortezomib can cause serious adverse drug reactions. The most common adverse drug reactions are mild-to-moderate fatigue and gastrointestinal toxicities. Neuropathy occurs frequently and is the most common cause of discontinuation of therapy. Other important toxicities are listed in Table 159-4. An increased risk of shingles has been reported in bortezomib-treated patients, and the NCCN guidelines recommend herpes zoster prophylaxis.[11] Bortezomib-based therapy is an attractive option for those patients with renal dysfunction since renal dose modifications are not required. In patients with renal dysfunction, the NCCN recommends the combination of bortezomib-cyclophosphamide-dexamethasone, as lenalidomide requires renal dose adjustments. If the patient's renal function improves after initial treatment with bortezomib-cyclophosphamide-dexamethasone, it is reasonable to switch to bortezomib-lenalidomide-dexamethasone.[11] Unlike lenalidomide, bortezomib does not affect stem cell mobilization.

Since neurotoxicity is a concern with bortezomib, investigators have explored modifying the route of administration and dosing schedule of bortezomib. In a phase III trial in relapsed MM, therapeutic equivalence was found between intravenous and subcutaneous routes of administration.[11] In addition, subcutaneous administration offers the potential advantage of administration in patients without IV access, is more convenient, and has a lower risk of peripheral neuropathy. Subcutaneous bortezomib administration is now the preferred route of administration.[11] Dose schedules have also been modified to decrease toxicity-related treatment delays. Once-weekly bortezomib has been compared with twice-weekly dosing with similar overall response rates.[11] The once-weekly schedule was associated with fewer dose reductions, and the risk of neuropathy was similar.

Carfilzomib Carfilzomib is a second-generation, irreversible PI approved for patients with relapsed and refractory disease. Its mechanism, higher selectivity for the chymotryptic site of the 20S proteasome, and toxicity profile are distinct compared to bortezomib.[38] The dosing schedule is also different than bortezomib. Carfilzomib is more potent, yet tolerable with two consecutive daily doses or once weekly dosing. Collectively, clinical trials start with carfilzomib 20 mg/m^2 IV over 10 to 30 minutes on the first cycle/week and increase to 27 to 70 mg/m^2 depending on tolerability and dosing frequency.[43,44]

Numerous trials have examined carfilzomib in the treatment of progressive or relapsed MM. The ASPIRE trial showed the addition of carfilzomib to a lenalidomide-dexamethasone backbone improved progression-free survival, overall survival, and health-related quality of life without any change in adverse drug reactions.[44] The incidence of neuropathy was similar in both arms. Carfilzomib-dexamethasone was compared to bortezomib-dexamethasone in relapsed or refractory MM in the head-to-head Phase III trial (ENDEAVOR). Median progression-free survival was longer with carfilzomib as compared to the bortezomib group.[45] A second interim analysis showed that carfilzomib also improved median overall survival as compared to bortezomib.[46] Based on these data, carfilzomib in combination with lenalidomide-dexamethasone or dexamethasone is an NCCN category 1 recommendation for previously treated MM.[11] Additional studies are evaluating carfilzomib with traditional chemotherapy and other novel drugs.

The activity of carfilzomib in combination regimens as first-line treatment is also impressive. The phase III, open-label, ENDURANCE trial compared bortezomib, lenalidomide and dexamethasone and carfilzomib, lenalidomide and dexamethasone in the first-line setting for standard and intermediate-risk patients with MM.[47] The trial showed similar progression-free survival between the two arms. Carfilzomib was associated with less neuropathy but increased pulmonary and cardiac adverse events.[47] According to the NCCN guidelines, certain carfilzomib-containing regimens may be used for primary therapy, especially in patients with peripheral neuropathy.[11]

The toxicity profile of carfilzomib differs from that of bortezomib. The incidence of peripheral neuropathy is less with the second-generation PIs which should be considered when treatment is selected. The ENDEAVOR trial reported a lower risk of grade 2 or higher peripheral neuropathy in patients who received carfilzomib as compared with bortezomib.[45,46] Carfilzomib is associated with serious cardiac and pulmonary toxicities. The cardiovascular adverse events include congestive heart failure, hypertension, arrhythmias, and ischemia. A meta-analysis of 24 studies reported the rate of cardiovascular events as 18.1%, with higher doses of carfilzomib ($\geq$45 mg/m^2) associated with higher rates of cardiovascular events.[47] The pulmonary adverse events of dyspnea, cough, respiratory tract infections, and pneumonia are also of concern.[48] Clinicians should monitor patients for carfilzomib-related cardiac and pulmonary symptoms and initiate symptom management when necessary.

Ixazomib Ixazomib is the first oral PI approved for the treatment of MM. It is given once-weekly as second-line therapy in combination with lenalidomide and dexamethasone. The approval is based on the TOURMALINE-MM1 phase III trial, which showed the addition of ixazomib to lenalidomide and dexamethasone prolonged progression-free survival in patients with relapsed or refractory MM as compared with lenalidomide and dexamethasone alone.[49] The TOURMALINE-MM2 phase III trial evaluated ixazomib, lenalidomide, and dexamethasone in newly diagnosed patients with MM. The trial showed improved response rates with the addition of ixazomib to lenalidomide and dexamethasone but failed to reach statistical significance in progression-free survival.[50] The results of this study led to an NCCN category 2B recommendation for ixazomib, lenalidomide, dexamethasone in the first-line setting for transplant-eligible patients.[11] Despite this recommendation, the regimen is an attractive option for some patients because it allows for a completely oral triple-drug combination. Similarly, ixazomib can be administered in combination with oral cyclophosphamide and dexamethasone. This may be beneficial in patients with renal dysfunction but lacks the supporting evidence associated with bortezomib-containing regimens. As discussed in a previous section, ixazomib combined with pomalidomide and dexamethasone is highly effective in patients experiencing early progression following two lines of IMiD and PI therapy. Table 159-4 lists the adverse drug reactions of ixazomib. Unlike carfilzomib, cardiac toxicity with ixazomib is minimal.[51]

Monoclonal Antibodies

7 Three monoclonal antibodies and one antibody-drug conjugate are FDA-approved for the treatment of MM. These monoclonal antibodies are often added to a combination drug regimen, with daratumumab incorporated into regimens for high-risk patients with MM.

Daratumumab Daratumumab is an IgG1-κ fully human monoclonal antibody that targets CD38, a glycoprotein highly expressed on MM cells. Accelerated FDA approval for daratumumab in relapsed/refractory MM was granted after two open-label phase II trials of daratumumab showed single-agent activity (overall response rates of 29% and 36%).[52] Subsequent studies confirmed the role of daratumumab in combination therapy. A phase III trial of daratumumab, bortezomib, and dexamethasone reported a higher 12-month progression-free survival as compared to bortezomib and dexamethasone.[52] Similar findings were reported with daratumumab, lenalidomide, and dexamethasone, with a higher 12-month progression-free survival as compared with lenalidomide and dexamethasone.[52] Daratumumab, in combination with bortezomib, carfilzomib, lenalidomide, or pomalidomide and dexamethasone are NCCN category 1 recommendations for patients with relapsed and refractory MM.

Daratumumab combinations are also used in front-line therapy for newly diagnosed MM patients. The combination of daratumumab with bortezomib, melphalan, and prednisone was the first regimen approved for newly diagnosed, transplant-ineligible patients with MM. FDA approval was based on the phase III trial that showed that the addition of daratumumab to the regimen resulted in a higher overall response rate and a lower risk of disease progression and death as compared to bortezomib, melphalan, and prednisone.[53] Additional studies have reported the benefits of daratumumab combination therapy. The three-drug regimen of daratumumab, lenalidomide, and dexamethasone is considered a NCCN category 1 preferred recommendation as primary therapy for transplant-ineligible patients, and the four-drug regimen of daratumumab, bortezomib, thalidomide, and dexamethasone may be used as primary therapy for transplant eligible candidates.[11] Mayo Clinic mSMART guidelines recommend the four-drug regimen—daratumumab, lenalidomide, bortezomib, and dexamethasone—as initial treatment for patients with high-risk cytogenetics.[21]

Daratumumab is well-tolerated (Table 159-4). Infusion-reactions are common, occurring in 48% of patients.[53] Patients should be pre-medicated with a corticosteroid, acetaminophen, and an antihistamine to reduce the risk of a severe infusion reaction. Since daratumumab can interfere with cross-matching and red blood cell antibody screening, blood typing should occur before starting therapy.

Isatuximab-irfc Isatuximab-irfc is a chimeric IgG-derived monoclonal antibody that also targets CD38 but at a different epitope than daratumumab. This leads to enhanced direct apoptosis without the need for effector cells or the complement system.[54] Isatuximab also inhibits the enzymatic activity of CD38 more effectively than daratumumab. This suggests more potent MM activity in vitro, although it is unknown if this will translate into increased clinical efficacy. Isatuximab may be active in patients who were refractory to daratumumab.[54] Isatuximab was initially approved in the third-line setting, following progression after lenalidomide and a PI, in combination with pomalidomide and dexamethasone. The combination with isatuximab showed improved response rates and progression-free survival over pomalidomide and dexamethasone alone.[55] Isatuximab is approved for patients who have received at least one prior line of therapy in combination with carfilzomib and dexamethasone. The adverse drug reaction profile of isatuximab is similar to that of daratumumab.

Elotuzumab Elotuzumab is a monoclonal antibody directed against signaling lymphocyte activation molecule family 7 (SLAMF7), which is expressed on MM cells.[56] The binding of elotuzumab to SLAMF7 results in cytotoxicity through various mechanisms including antibody-dependent cellular cytotoxicity. Elotuzumab was evaluated in a phase III trial in combination with lenalidomide and dexamethasone in patients with relapsed and refractory MM. The elotuzumab combination improved progression-free survival and overall response rate as compared to lenalidomide and dexamethasone. Elotuzumab also improves progression-free survival when combined with either bortezomib or pomalidomide and dexamethasone. The elotuzumab, lenalidomide, and dexamethasone regimen is considered an NCCN category 1 recommendation for previously treated patients with MM.[11] Common adverse effects are listed in Table 159-4. Patients should be premedicated with dexamethasone, diphenhydramine, ranitidine, and acetaminophen to reduce the risk of an infusion reaction. Infusion reactions occurred in 10% of patients despite premedication, and most of the infusion reactions occurred with the first dose.[56] Patients receiving an elotuzumab-containing combination should also be monitored for infections because infections are the most common cause of non-myeloma-related death.

Belantamab mafodotin Belantamab mafodotin is an antibody-drug conjugate targeting B cell maturation antigen (BCMA). Upon binding to BCMA, belantamab mafodotin is internalized and releases its monomethyl auristatin F (MMAF) payload, which inhibits microtubule formation.[57] Belantamab mafodotin is approved for patients who have received at least four prior lines of therapy, including a CD38 antibody, a PI, and an IMiD. The approval was based on the results of a phase II, DREAMM-2 study, in which belantamab mafodotin had an overall response rate of 31%.[57] Of those responders, nearly 75% of patients had a duration of response of 6 months or greater. The most common adverse drug reactions observed during the study were cytopenias, liver function test abnormalities, infusion reactions, and ocular toxicity, including vision loss. Due to the risk of ocular toxicity, belantamab mafodotin is only available through a restricted program under a Risk Evaluation and Mitigation Strategy (REMS). The REMS program requires the patient to undergo a thorough ophthalmic exam prior to each dose. Patients should use lubricating eye drops while on therapy and avoid the use of contact lenses.

Panobinostat

Panobinostat is an oral inhibitor of histone deacetylase enzymes and has shown activity in MM. Panobinostat was evaluated in a phase III trial in patients with refractory or relapsed MM who had received prior therapy with an IMiD and bortezomib.[58] Patients were randomized to receive bortezomib, dexamethasone, and panobinostat or bortezomib, dexamethasone, and placebo. The addition of panobinostat significantly improved progression-free survival.[58] No overall survival data have been reported. Adverse drug reactions are listed in Table 159-4. The regimen is considered an NCCN category 1 option for the treatment of relapsed/refractory MM who have received at least two prior therapies with an IMiD and bortezomib.[11]

Selinexor

Selinexor is the first in a new class of drugs that inhibits the nuclear export of tumor suppressor proteins (TSPs) and exportin 1 (XPO1).[59] The inhibition of XPO1 allows the cell to restore endogenous tumor suppressing proteins resulting in cancer cell apoptosis. Selinexor received accelerated FDA approval in 2019 for use with dexamethasone in patients with relapsed or refractory MM who have received at least four prior therapies, including an anti-CD38 monoclonal antibody (eg, daratumumab).[11] Serious adverse drug reactions are listed in Table 159-4. Following its initial approval, selinexor was combined with bortezomib and dexamethasone in patients progressing after at least one therapy, where the regimen showed an increase in progression-free survival compared to bortezomib and dexamethasone alone.[59] Weekly dosing of selinexor improves the tolerability of the drug, with less grade >3 hematologic toxicity when compared to twice weekly dosing.[59]

Melphalan Flufenamide

Melphalan flufenamide is a first-in-class peptide-drug conjugate, combining melphalan with a modified phenylalanine amino acid. The drug requires cleavage by an aminopeptidase for activation. Aminopeptidases are often overexpressed in malignant cells which allows for more targeted activity in MM cells. The FDA granted melphalan flufenamide, in combination with low-dose dexamethasone, accelerated approval for patients who have received at least four lines of therapy. The approval was based on a single-arm phase II trial that showed an overall response rate of 24%, with a median duration of response of 4.2 months.[60] Adverse drug reactions are listed in Table 159-4. While the phase III confirmatory study comparing melphalan flufenamide to pomalidomide and dexamethasone was being conducted, a significant increase in mortality was observed in patients receiving melphalan flufenamide. This caused the FDA to issue a safety warning in July 2021 and required the manufacturer to suspend all studies involving melphalan flufenamide pending further evaluation.[61]

Chimeric Antigen Receptor T-Cell Therapy

7 Chimeric antigen receptor (CAR) T-cell therapy is a novel form of immunotherapy in which a patient's T-cells are collected

and genetically modified to target malignant cells. Multiple CAR T-cell products, directed at CD19, are FDA-approved for the treatment of B-cell malignancies. In 2021, the FDA-approved idecabtagene vicleucel for the treatment of relapsed or refractory MM after four or more prior lines of therapy, including an IMiD, a PI, and an anti-CD38 monoclonal antibody. The CAR T-cell product targets BCMA found on the surface of mature B lymphocytes and plasma cells. In the phase II trial that led to its approval, idecabtagene vicleucel showed an overall response rate of 73%, with 33% of patients achieving a complete response or better. MRD negative status was reached in 79% of those with a complete response.[62] In many cases, the responses are durable with a median progression-free survival of 19 months in patients achieving a complete response. Patients achieving a VGPR had a lower median progression-free survival of 10.4 months. These results are impressive considering the heavily pretreated patient population (median six lines of prior therapy, 95% prior autologous transplant). The most common adverse events observed were cytopenias, cytokine release syndrome (CRS), and immune effector cell-associated neurotoxicity syndrome (ICANS).[62] CRS is characterized by immune activation and release of inflammatory cytokines secondary to CAR T-cells interacting with target cells. CRS presentation can range from mild, flu-like symptoms to severe life-threatening organ dysfunction. CRS is treated with supportive care, tocilizumab (an interleukin-6 receptor antagonist), and steroids. The pathophysiology of ICANS is less completely understood but may be related to immune activation and vascular dysfunction. Similar to CRS, ICANS can present with a wide variety of symptoms, ranging from mild somnolence to cerebral edema and seizures. ICANS and CRS often present together but can occur independently. ICANS is treated with steroid therapy, antiepileptics, and other supportive care.[63] The NCCN has added idecabtagene vicleucel to its guidelines, but further studies are needed to determine its optimal place in therapy.

Initial Therapy

4 Initial therapy is guided by the NCCN, IMWG, ESMO, and mSMART recommendations and depends on whether the patient is symptomatic and a candidate for autologous HSCT (see Fig. 159-2). Eligibility factors for HSCT include patient age, renal function, performance status, and comorbidities. All patients with symptomatic MM are treated with primary therapy, with the selected regimen depending on transplant eligibility. Patients who are candidates for autologous HSCT will often receive 4 to 6 months of therapy before proceeding to hematopoietic stem cell collection, harvesting enough stem cells for two transplants.[11] Most patients will undergo autologous HSCT immediately following collection, but some patients may decide to delay the transplant until first relapse. Therapies that may compromise stem cell reserve are avoided in transplant-eligible patients. The selected regimen will often be composed of agents from multiple, distinct classes. Triplet combination regimens are commonly used and often include dexamethasone, a PI, and an IMiD. Patients who are not candidates for autologous HSCT usually continue their MM therapy or receive maintenance therapy, although the optimal duration of therapy after the desired response is achieved is unknown. Single-agent maintenance therapy, consisting of lenalidomide or bortezomib, may be given in both transplant-eligible and ineligible patients.

VRd is frequently used for primary therapy in both transplant-eligible and ineligible patients. Daratumumab, carfilzomib, or ixazomib-based therapy are additional treatment options for select patients. Treatment decisions are made based on physician preference, patient characteristics, and transplant eligibility. Some experts recommend a risk-adapted approach that personalizes treatment based on cytogenetics and gene expression profiling. The high cost of medications can pose a financial challenge for patients and clinicians who must consider the financial implications when selecting a regimen.

Some clinicians use a risk-adapted approach to select therapies (eg, mSMART). Bortezomib-containing induction regimens are recommended in patients with high-risk cytogenetics (see Fig. 159-2).[21] In this approach, high-risk patients receive a combination of daratumumab, bortezomib, lenalidomide, and dexamethasone as primary therapy. The combination of VRd is recommended in standard-risk patients. These regimens are continued in transplant-eligible patients for four cycles before transplant, but transplant can be delayed depending on patient preference. Transplant-ineligible patients will receive therapy for about 1 year and then possibly maintenance therapy. Lenalidomide- and bortezomib-based therapies may be used for maintenance therapy depending on risk.

5 A flow diagram shows the management of newly diagnosed myeloma. If the patient is transplant ineligible, there are two pathways. The first pathway is for patients with t(11;14), t(6;14), or trisomies, and is classified as standard risk. These patients should be treated with DVd or VRd for nine cycles, followed by lenalidomide maintenance until disease progression. The second pathway is for patients with t(4;14), t(14;16), t(14;20), or del17p and is classified as high risk. These patients should be treated with DVd or VRd for nine cycles, followed by bortezomib-based maintenance until progression. If the patient is transplant eligible, there are three pathways. The first pathway is for patients with t(11;14), t(6;14), or trisomies, and is classified as standard risk. These patients should be treated with four cycles of VRd, followed by stem cell collection. The patient then either proceeds with autologous transplant (preferred), followed by lenalidomide maintenance for a minimum of 2 years, or proceeds with four cycles of VRd, followed by lenalidomide until disease progression. The second pathway is for patients with Del17p, Gain 1q, t(4;14), or t(14;16) and is classified as high risk. These patients should be treated with four cycles of Dara-VRd followed by autologous transplant, and then bortezomib-based maintenance until progression. The third pathway is for patients with double or triple hit myeloma and is classified as high risk. These patients should be treated with four cycles of Dara-VRd followed by autologous transplant, and then bortezomib-based maintenance until progression.

Autologous Hematopoietic Stem Cell Transplantation

4 Although MM is a chemosensitive tumor with significant response rates after treatment with conventional chemotherapy, the duration of response is usually short. To improve outcomes with chemotherapy, high-dose chemotherapy regimens with autologous stem cell support is used after initial induction therapy. The intent of the induction therapy before transplant is to reduce tumor burden. With newer treatment regimens being used for induction, higher rates of quality responses (CR, VGPR, nCR) can be obtained which may improve the outcomes associated with autologous HSCT.

Randomized, controlled trials have evaluated the role of high-dose chemotherapy followed by autologous HSCT in patients with MM. Studies have confirmed that primary therapy followed by high-dose chemotherapy and autologous HSCT improves overall survival and increases complete response rates.[11,64] The timing of autologous HSCT has also been explored. An induction regimen of lenalidomide and dexamethasone followed by either chemotherapy (melphalan/prednisone/lenalidomide) or tandem melphalan-based autologous transplants was evaluated.[64] Results of this trial showed a progression-free survival and overall survival benefit for the autologous transplant arm. In a separate trial, patients received induction therapy with VRd, with either upfront or delayed consolidation with autologous HSCT, followed by lenalidomide maintenance therapy. Results of this trial showed that upfront transplant followed by maintenance resulted in significant improvements in progression-free survival but no difference in overall survival.[65] Based on available

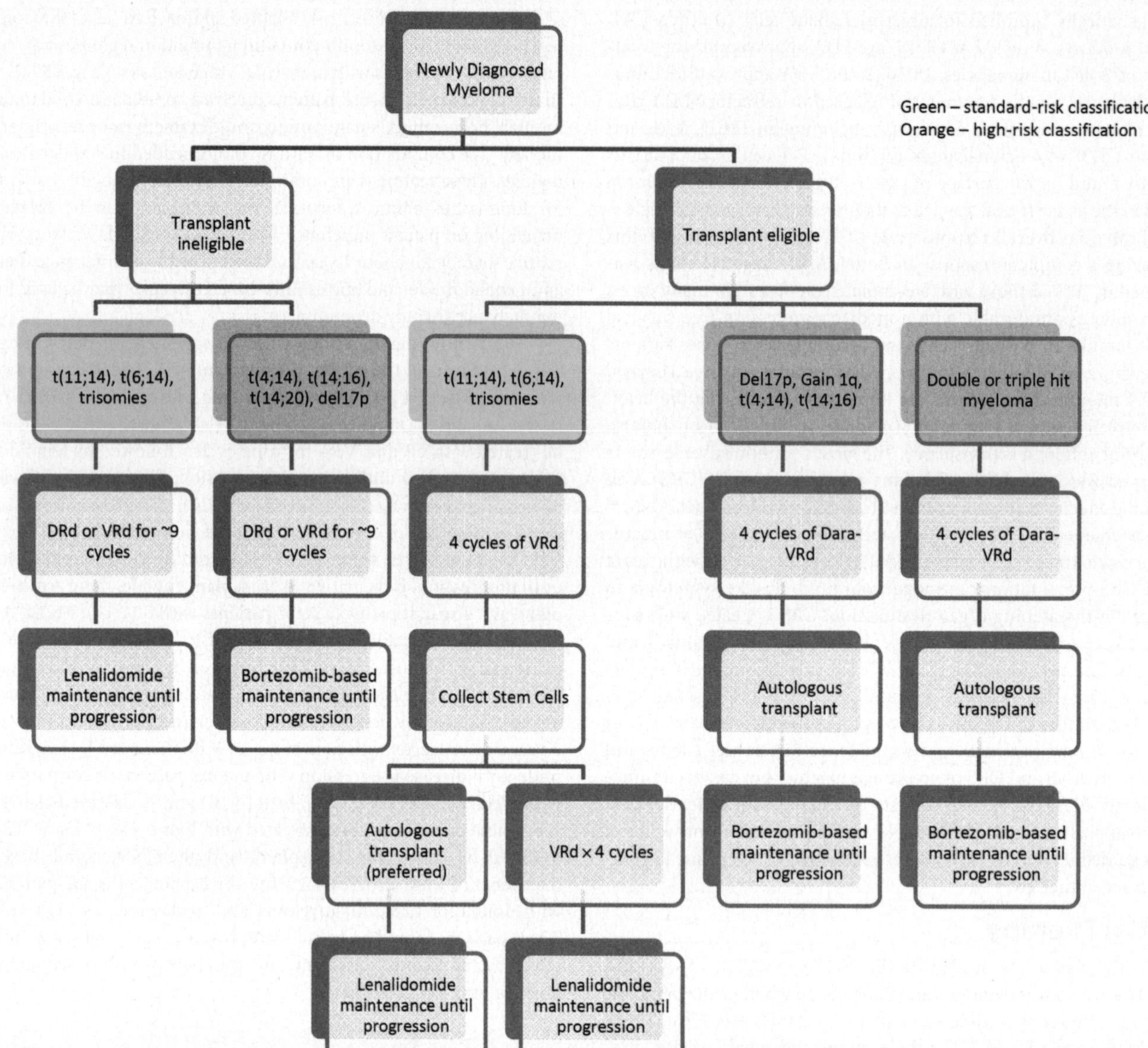

FIGURE 159-2 Risk-adapted treatment of multiple myeloma based on eligibility for hematopoietic stem cell transplantation. (Dara-VRd, daratumumab, bortezomib, lenalidomide, dexamethasone; DRd, daratumumab, lenalidomide, dexamethasone; VRd, bortezomib, lenalidomide, and dexamethasone.) (*Adapted from mSMART.org. http://www.msmart.org/mm-treatment-guidelines. Accessed October 1, 2021.)*

data, autologous HSCT improves response rates, symptom-free and progression-free survival but may not prolong overall survival. The lack of an overall survival advantage is likely due to improved salvage therapy. Despite this, current recommendations support high-dose chemotherapy and autologous HSCT in eligible patients with a first remission after primary therapy.[11,16,21]

The optimal timing of autologous HSCT (early vs late) in MM has also been investigated. In a landmark trial, patients were randomized to early (within 12 months of diagnosis) or late transplantation (>12 months after diagnosis), and no significant difference in 5-year overall survival was observed between the groups.[66] Event-free survival, however, was significantly longer in the early transplantation group (39 vs 13 months). In an analysis that factors in the time without symptoms, treatment, or treatment toxicity (TWiSTT), patients receiving early transplantation had a longer time in a state associated with a good quality of life (27.8 vs 22.3 months). The results of this study supported early autologous HSCT because of its effects on event-free survival and quality of life. Since then, two retrospective studies comparing early versus delayed autologous HSCT have been published.[67,68] These studies included MM patients who received an induction regimen that included either lenalidomide, thalidomide or another novel therapy. Both trials demonstrated similar time-to-progression and overall survival in the early (within 12 months) and delayed transplant groups. While most of the phase III trials have shown improvements in progression-free survival with transplantation, not all trials have shown an improvement in overall survival with transplantation.[69] This has been attributed to variations in primary treatment and study design. The collective results of these trials may support the idea that, in the setting of novel therapies, delaying transplant may be feasible for certain standard-risk patients, but the lack of rigorous, prospective, randomized data prevents the uniform recommendation to delay transplant. For patients with high-risk disease, current data do not support delaying transplant. Enrollment in clinical trials is highly recommended for most patients when evaluating the appropriate timing of HSCT in MM.[11]

A specialized form of autologous HSCT, tandem transplantation, involves the use of two separate autologous HSCT procedures separated by a rest period of several months. It was hypothesized that this more intensive approach would lead to improvements in therapeutic outcomes. Since the initial report of a benefit to the tandem transplant approach, several trials investigated this approach to therapy. Many of these trials were conducted before the availability of novel drugs and were shown to have conflicting results regarding overall survival.[69] Thus, the current data do not support the routine use of tandem transplants. Tandem autologous HSCT may be considered in selected patients with high-risk disease or those failing to achieve a VGPR after the first transplant, but any such decision would be best evaluated in the context of a clinical trial.[11,16,69]

The primary conclusion from the current data on autologous HSCT as consolidation therapy in MM is that it should be used in patients with good performance status. Advanced age and/or renal dysfunction should not be considered contraindications to transplant.[11] Before transplant, all patients should receive primary therapy to reduce tumor burden. Prolonged exposure to drugs such as lenalidomide and daratumumab can decrease the yield of stem cell harvest, so cells should be collected early on in therapy. Similarly, alkylating agents and nitrosoureas should be avoided before stem cell collection. NCCN recommends collecting sufficient hematopoietic stem cells for a second, salvage transplant in younger patients. The Mayo Clinic mSMART guidelines recommend autologous HSCT in transplant-eligible high-risk patients after the bortezomib-based induction therapy.[21] Standard-risk patients are given the option of autologous HSCT followed by maintenance therapy or continued induction followed by maintenance therapy (see Fig. 159-2).

Maintenance Therapy 8 Even with the advances in induction therapy and autologous HSCT, most patients will eventually progress within 3 to 5 years, suggesting that effective maintenance therapy could control or delay disease progression. Lenalidomide is frequently used as maintenance therapy in both transplant-ineligible and post-autologous HSCT patients with MM. Numerous trials have investigated the use of lenalidomide maintenance after autologous HSCT, showing improvements in progression-free and, possibly, overall survival compared to no maintenance therapy.[70] A 2017 meta-analysis examined the use of lenalidomide maintenance in newly diagnosed post-autologous HSCT patients with MM.[70] The analysis found significant benefits with lenalidomide maintenance compared to placebo or observation, extending median progression-free and overall survival.[70] While there are no direct head-to-head comparisons, a 2018 meta-analysis examined all regimens used for maintenance therapy and concluded that lenalidomide was the only maintenance therapy to improve progression-free and overall survival.[71] One unique adverse effect noted in these trials was second primary malignancy, including solid tumors, hematologic malignancies, and nonmelanoma skin cancers. These second malignancies occurred at a significantly higher rate as compared to placebo or control arms. Based on these data, the FDA issued a safety announcement to be added to the warning section of the lenalidomide drug labeling. Some practitioners advocate limiting the duration of maintenance lenalidomide to 2 years after transplant to minimize risk.[11]

Bortezomib may also be used for maintenance therapy in transplant-ineligible and post-autologous HSCT high-risk patients with MM. The 2018 meta-analysis of maintenance therapy showed that bortezomib-based therapies prolonged progression-free survival but did not improve overall survival.[71] Bortezomib is recommended over lenalidomide in the mSMART treatment and ESMO guidelines for maintenance therapy in high-risk patients.[16,21] Additionally, patients who do not achieve at least a VGPR after autologous transplant may benefit from bortezomib maintenance.[11]

Ixazomib has also been studied as maintenance therapy following autologous HSCT. The phase III TOURMALINE-MM3 trial randomized patients to oral ixazomib dosed on days 1, 8, and 15 in 28-day cycles or placebo as maintenance therapy for 2 years.[72] The trial showed that ixazomib maintenance therapy prolonged progression-free survival in newly diagnosed patients who received a single autologous HSCT within 12 months of diagnosis. While lenalidomide is the preferred maintenance medication by the NCCN guidelines, the guidelines added ixazomib as an option.[11] Since ixazomib is administered weekly, the convenient dosing may make it the preferred PI for maintenance therapy. The lack of secondary malignancies and low risk of peripheral neuropathy may make ixazomib a desirable alternative to lenalidomide. Future comparative trials are needed to determine the preferred maintenance therapy, particularly in patients with high-risk MM. The decision to use any of these agents in the maintenance setting must include careful consideration of the benefits and risks.

Allogeneic Hematopoietic Stem Cell Transplantation

Allogeneic HSCT uses a stem cell source other than the patient and is therefore a transplant across immunologic barriers. Unlike autologous HSCT, which is simply a method of increasing the dose intensity of chemotherapy, allogeneic HSCT is a form of immunotherapy. The interest in allogeneic transplantation for MM is based on the use of a stem cell source free of tumor, which may potentially offer longer disease control and possible cure. The major posttransplant complications associated with allogeneic transplants are acute and chronic graft-versus-host disease (GVHD). GVHD may be accompanied by a graft-versus-myeloma effect. The graft-versus-myeloma effect, which is mediated by antitumor effector cells from the GVHD reaction, reduces relapse risk and may offer the patient the best chance for long-term disease-free survival.

Myeloablative allogeneic HSCT has traditionally been associated with high treatment-related mortality, between 20% and 60%.[73] Historically, allogeneic transplant has been used after patients have received and progressed after an autologous HSCT. Several trials have compared tandem autologous transplants to autologous followed by allogeneic stem cell transplant, although there is wide variability in trial design patient selection and protocols for the prevention and treatment of GVHD.[74] In all trials to date, no consistent improvement in overall survival or progression-free survival has been reported. Meta-analyses show that allogeneic HSCT may result in a higher CR rate, including long term remissions, but this comes at the cost of a higher rate of transplant-related mortality.[11]

Allogeneic HSCT may have a role in the management of patients with high-risk disease. Ongoing clinical trials are evaluating the role of allogeneic HSCT in patients with MM who have high-risk cytogenetic characteristics, who are not likely to respond to upfront therapy or who relapse quickly after upfront therapy or autologous HSCT. There is increasing interest in the use of reduced-intensity conditioning regimens. Based on the available data, upfront myeloablative allogeneic HSCT is not routinely recommended.

Relapsed or Refractory Disease

9 The most appropriate therapy for an individual who relapses depends on the type and duration of previous therapies, whether the patient received a transplant, presence or absence of adverse prognostic factors, toxicity of prior therapies (eg, peripheral neuropathy), organ dysfunction (eg, renal impairment), and how much time has elapsed from initial response to relapse.[11] The same drugs used to treat MM initially can also be used as salvage therapy in patients who have relapsed more than 6 months after primary induction therapy.[11] Patients with relapsed or refractory MM can be treated with active agents in combination or single agents used sequentially. With the growing number of highly active agents, combination therapy is more commonly given. There are no direct comparisons of the frequently utilized regimens for relapsed and refractory disease making

it difficult to determine the best treatment option. The NCCN has seventeen category 1 recommendations (13 triplet and 4 doublet regimens) and lists many other additional regimens.[11] Combination therapy continues to incorporate a PI, IMiD, and dexamethasone. Daratumumab, elotuzumab, and isatximab-irfc may also be used in various regimens. A systematic review suggests the combination of daratumumab, lenalidomide, and dexamethasone may be superior in patients with progressive disease.[75] Other meta-analyses have reported triplet-based combinations with monoclonal antibodies are superior (extending progression-free survival) compared to other regimens in patients with relapsed and refractory disease.[76] CAR T-cell therapy with idecabtagene vicleucel has reported encouraging results and may be considered in patients who have progressed after multiple lines of therapy. Despite clear progress, most salvage therapies produce less than a 50% response rate, and new drugs and drug combinations are needed.

Questions remain on the optimal timing for autologous HSCT. For patients who are eligible for autologous HSCT and did not receive a transplant as part of initial therapy, autologous HSCT should be considered at first relapse. Autologous HSCT in first remission trends toward longer progression-free survival compared to those transplanted beyond first remission.[77] Salvage autologous HSCT may be beneficial in patients who were heavily pretreated and refractory to daratumumab.[78] The role of salvage autologous transplant may continue to be minimized with the approval of additional drugs and the use of maintenance therapy.

Supportive Care

Bone-Modifying Agents

10 Along with anti-MM therapy, supportive care measures are aggressively used to stabilize skeletal abnormalities. Patients with MM have a high rate of bone involvement. The mechanism of MM-associated bone disease is thought to be mediated through several pathways, including IL-6, IL-1, and TNF-α, but the most targeted pathway is that involving receptor activator factor kappa B ligand (RANK-L) and osteoprotegerin (OPG).[23] Skeletal homeostasis is complex. In normal bone, RANK-L and OPG are both produced by osteoblasts. RANK-L binds to RANK receptors on osteoclasts, to stimulate bone resorption, and to OPG, a "decoy receptor," to inhibit bone resorption and stimulate bone formation. A balance between RANK-L and OPG is the basis for normal bone remodeling. In MM, an imbalance in normal bone homeostasis leads to increased osteoclast activity and the formation of osteolytic bone lesions which can lead to clinically significant skeletal-related events, including fracture, hypercalcemia, and bone pain. Based on the 2019 ASCO guidelines, clinical indications for bone modifying therapies include hypercalcemia, renal dysfunction, anemia, and bone disease. In the absence of these features, patients with >60% plasma cells in the bone marrow or more than one site of bone disease are now recommended for treatment.[79] The NCCN guidelines recommend bone modifying therapies for all patients regardless of documented bone disease. Preventative therapies are initiated early to delay myeloma bone disease. Myeloma bone modifying therapies should be continued for at least 2 years with discontinuation based on clinical judgment.[11]

The primary therapies for the prevention of myeloma bone disease include antiresorptive bisphosphonates (ie, zoledronic acid and pamidronate) and denosumab. Bisphosphonates bind to hydroxyapatite and are incorporated into the bone matrix, suppressing osteoclast activity.[80] There are two classes of bisphosphonates (ie, nitrogen and non-nitrogen containing) based on their binding affinity with hydroxyapatite. The nitrogen-containing bisphosphonates of zoledronic acid and pamidronate are 100 to 10,000 fold more potent than the non-nitrogen containing bisphosphonates (ie, etidronate).[80] For this reason, zoledronic acid and pamidronate are used in the management of myeloma bone disease. Bisphosphonates may also promote apoptosis in MM cells, modify the cytokine microenvironment, inhibit the adhesion of MM cells to bone marrow matrix cells, and inhibit angiogenesis.[81] A meta-analysis in patients with MM shows bisphosphonates reduce pain, overall fractures, and fractures of the vertebrae.[80]

Pamidronate and zoledronic acid are usually well tolerated. Acute-phase reactions consisting of flu-like symptoms can occur after the administration of bisphosphonates. Acute renal impairment can occur with both agents and is related to both infusion time and dose. Patients with moderate renal impairment (creatinine clearance: 30-60 mL/min [0.5-1.0 mL/s]) require renal dose adjustments of zoledronic acid, and the use of zoledronic acid is not recommended in patients with severe renal impairment.[82] This is important as patients with MM often have renal dysfunction. Osteonecrosis of the jaw (ONJ) is a serious adverse effect of bisphosphonates. ONJ is characterized by an area of exposed necrotic bone and often affects the mandible and the maxilla, but it can also affect the soft palate. The development of ONJ may be related to dental disease and tooth extraction, dependent on the dose and duration, and is more common with IV bisphosphonates (vs oral) and zoledronic acid (vs pamidronate).[79] The incidence of ONJ is unknown but may be as high as 10% in MM patients receiving zoledronic acid for extended periods. A meta-analysis found no difference between the bisphosphonate used and the incidence of ONJ.[83] Patients should be advised to have dental work completed before the initiation of bisphosphonates, if possible.

Denosumab has also been shown to reduce the incidence of myeloma skeletal-related events and is used in the prevention of myeloma bone disease. Denosumab is a monoclonal antibody directed toward RANK-L. By binding to RANK-L, denosumab prevents binding of RANK-L to RANK, reducing osteoclast activity and allowing bone formation and osteoblast function to predominate. A phase III trial evaluated the efficacy and safety of denosumab compared to zoledronic acid in patients with newly diagnosed MM.[84] Results from this study found denosumab to be noninferior to zoledronic acid in delaying time to first skeletal-related event. Rates of overall survival and ONJ were similar between groups. In an exploratory analysis of an international phase III study, denosumab showed an increase in median progression-free survival compared to zoledronic acid, which suggests that denosumab may have antimyeloma activity.[85] The results were most favorable in the subset of patients who had received PI-based triple therapy and were transplant eligible. While the risk of ONJ with denosumab and zoledronic acid is similar, the risk of renal adverse effects is higher with zoledronic acid.[84] The NCCN guidelines recommend denosumab for patients with renal disease because denosumab does not worsen renal function or require dose adjustments with renal impairment.[11]

EVALUATION OF THERAPEUTIC OUTCOMES

The goals of therapy are to prolong survival and improve quality of life. Patients with asymptomatic MM are usually observed and not treated. Asymptomatic patients are assessed every 3 to 6 months for disease progression, which would then warrant therapy. Assessment involves measurement of M protein in blood and urine and laboratory tests that include complete blood count, serum creatinine, and calcium. Patients are treated as the disease produces symptoms. Disease response is defined by a decline in M protein. After completion of the initial course of therapy and once a response is obtained, patients should be monitored every 3 months. NCCN guidelines have been updated to include assessment of MRD status after treatment. Bone surveys are performed yearly or as required because of changes in symptoms. Various other tests, including bone marrow biopsy, magnetic resonance imaging, and positron emission tomography, or computed tomography scan, are performed as needed to evaluate disease status.

CONCLUSION

MM is a cancer that occurs due to the abnormal proliferation of plasma cells. Hallmark symptoms are associated with the acronyms CRAB. While MM is an incurable disease, novel drug classes have improved response rates and overall survival compared to conventional chemotherapeutic agents. Triple regimens are often used and include dexamethasone, a PI, and an IMiD. Autologous HSCT plays a role in patients who are transplant eligible. Unfortunately, most patients will eventually experience refractory/relapsed disease where multiple agents and classes of drugs may be utilized to manage disease progression. To improve quality of life, clinicians should address and manage disease symptoms and adverse effects. Future advances in the treatment of MM depend on a better understanding of the pathophysiology of MM, identification of new drug targets, and development of new drugs.

ABBREVIATIONS

ASCO	American Society of Clinical Oncology
CAR	chimeric antigen receptor
CI	confidence interval
CR	complete remission
CRS	cytokine release syndrome
HSCT	hematopoietic stem cell transplantation
ICANS	immune effector cell-associated neurotoxicity syndrome
IκB	inhibitory factor kappa B
IFN	interferon
IGF-1	insulin-like growth factor
IgG	immunoglobulin G
IL	interleukin
IL-6	interleukin-6
IMiD	immunomodulatory drug
IMWG	International Myeloma Working Group
ISS	International Staging System
LMWH	low-molecular-weight heparin
MGUS	monoclonal gammopathy of undetermined significance
MM	multiple myeloma
MRD	minimal residual disease
mSMART	Mayo Stratification for Myeloma and Risk-Adapted Therapy
NCCN	National Comprehensive Cancer Network
NF-κB	nuclear factor kappa B
ONJ	osteonecrosis of the jaw
OPG	osteoprotegerin
PI	proteasome inhibitor
PR	partial response
RANK	receptor activator of nuclear factor-κB
RANK-L	receptor for activation of NF-κB ligand
SFC	serum-free light chains
TNF-α	tumor necrosis factor-α
VEGF	vascular endothelial growth factor
VGPR	very good partial response
VRd	bortezomib, lenalidomide, dexamethasone
VTE	venous thromboembolism

REFERENCES

1. Röllig C, Knop S, Bornhäuser M. Multiple myeloma. *Lancet.* 2015;385(9983):2197–2208.
2. van de Donk N, Pawlyn C, Yong KL. Multiple myeloma. *Lancet.* 2021;397(10272):410–427.
3. Siegel RL, Miller KD, Fuchs HE, Jemal A. Cancer statistics, 2022. *CA: A Cancer Journal for Clinicians* 2022;72:7–33. https://doi.org/10.3322/caac.21708. Accessed February 20, 2022.
4. Surveillance, epidemiology, and end results (SEER) program. SEER cancer stat facts: Myeloma. https://seer.cancer.gov/statfacts/html/mulmy.html. Accessed September 1, 2021.
5. Kazandjian D. Multiple myeloma epidemiology and survival: A unique malignancy. *Semin Oncol.* 2016;43(6):676–681.
6. Ruan G, Goyal G, Hashmi SK, Kapoor P, Go RS. Trends in multiple myeloma incidence in the united states (US): Demographic and geographic considerations and focus on young adults. *Blood.* 2018;132:5575.
7. Marinac CR, Ghobrial IM, Birmann BM, Soiffer J, Rebbeck TR. Dissecting racial disparities in multiple myeloma. *Blood Cancer J.* 2020;10(2):19.
8. Landgren O, Kristinsson SY, Goldin LR, et al. Risk of plasma cell and lymphoproliferative disorders among 14621 first-degree relatives of 4458 patients with monoclonal gammopathy of undetermined significance in sweden. *Blood.* 2009;114(4):791–795.
9. DeVita VT, Lawrence TS, Rosenberg SA. *DeVita, Hellman, and Rosenberg's Cancer: Principles & Practice of Oncology.* Vol 10th edition. Philadelphia: Wolters Kluwer Health; 2011.
10. Mateos MV, Landgren O. MGUS and smoldering multiple myeloma: Diagnosis and epidemiology. *Cancer Treatment and Research.* 2016;169:3–12. doi:10.1007/978-3-319-40320-5_1. PMID: 27696254.
11. National comprehensive cancer network. The NCCN multiple myeloma clinical practice guidelines in oncology (version 4.2022). https://www.nccn.org/professionals/physician_gls/pdf/myeloma.pdf. Accessed February 20, 2022.
12. Morgan GJ, Walker BA, Davies FE. The genetic architecture of multiple myeloma. *Nat Rev Cancer.* 2012;12(5):335–348.
13. Landgren O. Monoclonal gammopathy of undetermined significance and smoldering multiple myeloma: Biological insights and early treatment strategies. *Hematology Am Soc Hematol Educ Program.* 2013;2013:478–487.
14. Rajkumar SV. Multiple myeloma: 2020 update on diagnosis, risk-stratification and management. *Am J Hematol.* 2020;95(5):548–567.
15. Ahn IE, Mailankody S, Korde N, Landgren O. Dilemmas in treating smoldering multiple myeloma. *J Clin Oncol.* 2015;33(1):115–123.
16. Dimopoulos MA, Moreau P, Terpos E, et al. Multiple myeloma: EHA-ESMO clinical practice guidelines for diagnosis, treatment and follow-up. *Annals of Oncology.* 2021;32(3):309–322.
17. Kumar S, Paiva B, Anderson KC, et al. International myeloma working group consensus criteria for response and minimal residual disease assessment in multiple myeloma. *Lancet Oncol.* 2016 Aug;17(8):e328–e346. doi:10.1016/S1470-2045(16)30206-6. PMID: 27511158.
18. Palumbo A, Avet-Loiseau H, Oliva S, et al. Revised international staging system for multiple myeloma: A report from international myeloma working group. *JCO.* 2015;33(26):2863–2869.
19. Paner A, Patel P, Dhakal B. The evolving role of translocation t(11;14) in the biology, prognosis, and management of multiple myeloma. *Blood Rev.* 2019;41:100643.
20. Mikhael JR, Dingli D, Roy V, et al. Management of newly diagnosed symptomatic multiple myeloma: Updated mayo stratification of myeloma and risk-adapted therapy (mSMART) consensus guidelines 2013. *Mayo Clin Proc.* 2013;88(4):360–376.
21. mSMART. stratification for myeloma & risk-adapted therapy. https://www.msmart.org/mm-treatment-guidelines. Accessed September 21, 2021.
22. Palumbo A, Avet-Loiseau H, Oliva S, et al. Revised international staging system for multiple myeloma: A report from international myeloma working group. *Journal of Clinical Oncology.* 2015 33:26, 2863–2869.
23. Hanbali A, Hassanein M, Rasheed W, Aljurf M, Alsharif F. The evolution of prognostic factors in multiple myeloma. *Advances in Hematology.* 2017;2017:11.
24. Facon T, Mary JY, Pégourie B, et al. Dexamethasone-based regimens versus melphalan-prednisone for elderly multiple myeloma patients ineligible for high-dose therapy. *Blood.* 2006;107(4):1292–1298. doi:10.1182/blood-2005-04-1588.
25. Chang X, Zhu Y, Shi C, Stewart AK. Mechanism of immunomodulatory drugs' action in the treatment of multiple myeloma. *Acta Biochim Biophys Sin (Shanghai).* 2014;46(3):240–253. doi:10.1093/abbs/gmt142.
26. Schoen MW, Carson KR, Luo S, et al. Venous thromboembolism in multiple myeloma is associated with increased mortality. *Res Pract*

Thromb Haemost. 2020;4(7):1203–1210. Published 2020 Sep 25. doi:10.1002/rth2.12411.
27. Sanfilippo KM, Luo S, Wang TF, et al. Predicting venous thromboembolism in multiple myeloma: Development and validation of the IMPEDE VTE score. *Am J Hematol.* 2019;94(11):1176–1184. doi:10.1002/ajh.25603.
28. Cornell RF, Goldhaber SZ, Engelhardt BG, et al. Primary prevention of venous thromboembolism with apixaban for multiple myeloma patients receiving immunomodulatory agents. *Br J Haematol.* 2020;190(4):555–561. doi:10.1111/bjh.16653.
29. Cornell RF, Goldhaber SZ, Engelhardt BG, et al. Apixaban for primary prevention of venous thromboembolism in patients with multiple myeloma receiving immunomodulatory therapy. *Frontiers in Oncology.* 2019;9.
30. Holstein SA, Suman VJ, McCarthy PL. Update on the role of lenalidomide in patients with multiple myeloma. *Ther Adv Hematol.* 2018;9(7):175–190. doi:10.1177/2040620718775629.
31. Durie BG, Hoering A, Abidi MH, et al. Bortezomib with lenalidomide and dexamethasone versus lenalidomide and dexamethasone alone in patients with newly diagnosed myeloma without intent for immediate autologous stem-cell transplant (SWOG S0777): A randomised, open-label, phase 3 trial. *Lancet.* 2017;389(10068):519–527. doi:10.1016/S0140-6736(16)31594-X.
32. Weber DM, Chen C, Niesvizky R, et al. Lenalidomide plus dexamethasone for relapsed multiple myeloma in North America. *N Engl J Med.* 2007;357(21):2133–2142. doi:10.1056/NEJMoa070596.
33. Dimopoulos M, Spencer A, Attal M, et al. Lenalidomide plus dexamethasone for relapsed or refractory multiple myeloma [published correction appears in *N Engl J Med.* 2009 July 30;361(5):544]. *N Engl J Med.* 2007;357(21):2123–2132. 10.1056/NEJMoa070594.
34. Rajkumar SV, Jacobus S, Callander NS, et al. Lenalidomide plus high-dose dexamethasone versus lenalidomide plus low-dose dexamethasone as initial therapy for newly diagnosed multiple myeloma: An open-label randomised controlled trial [published correction appears in *Lancet Oncol.* 2010 January;11(1):14]. *Lancet Oncol.* 2010;11(1):29–37. 10.1016/S1470-2045(09)70284-0.
35. Jones JR, Cairns DA, Gregory WM, et al. Second malignancies in the context of lenalidomide treatment: An analysis of 2732 myeloma patients enrolled to the myeloma XI trial. *Blood.* 2016;6(12):e506.
36. Kumar S, Giralt S, Stadtmauer EA, et al. Mobilization in myeloma revisited: IMWG consensus perspectives on stem cell collection following initial therapy with thalidomide-, lenalidomide-, or bortezomib-containing regimens. *Blood.* 2009;114(9):1729–1735. doi:10.1182/blood-2009-04-205013.
37. Miguel JS, Weisel K, Moreau P, et al. Pomalidomide plus low-dose dexamethasone versus high-dose dexamethasone alone for patients with relapsed and refractory multiple myeloma (MM-003): A randomised, open-label, phase 3 trial. *Lancet Oncol.* 2013;14(11):1055–1066. doi:10.1016/S1470-2045(13)70380-2.
38. Teicher BA, Tomaszewski JE. Proteasome inhibitors. *Biochem Pharmacol.* 2015;96(1):1–9. doi:10.1016/j.bcp.2015.04.008.
39. Scott K, Hayden PJ, Will A, Wheatley K, Coyne I. Bortezomib for the treatment of multiple myeloma. *Cochrane Database of Systematic Reviews.* 2016(4).
40. Richardson PG, Barlogie B, Berenson J, et al. A phase 2 study of bortezomib in relapsed, refractory myeloma. *N Engl J Med.* 2003;348(26):2609–2617. doi:10.1056/NEJMoa030288.
41. Richardson PG, Sonneveld P, Schuster MW, et al. Bortezomib or high-dose dexamethasone for relapsed multiple myeloma. *N Engl J Med.* 2005;352(24):2487–2498. doi:10.1056/NEJMoa043445.
42. Sonneveld P, Avet-Loiseau H, Lonial S, et al. Treatment of multiple myeloma with high-risk cytogenetics: A consensus of the international myeloma working group. *Blood.* 2016;127(24):2955–2962.
43. Moreau P, Mateos MV, Berenson JR, et al. Once weekly versus twice weekly carfilzomib dosing in patients with relapsed and refractory multiple myeloma (A.R.R.O.W.): Interim analysis results of a randomised, phase 3 study [published correction appears in *Lancet Oncol.* 2018 August;19(8):e382]. *Lancet Oncol.* 2018;19(7):953–964. 10.1016/S1470-2045(18)30354-1.
44. Stewart AK, Rajkumar SV, Dimopoulos MA, et al. Carfilzomib, lenalidomide, and dexamethasone for relapsed multiple myeloma. *N Engl J Med.* 2015;372(2):142–152. doi:10.1056/NEJMoa1411321.
45. Dimopoulos MA, Goldschmidt H, Niesvizky R, et al. Carfilzomib or bortezomib in relapsed or refractory multiple myeloma (ENDEAVOR): An interim overall survival analysis of an open-label, randomised, phase 3 trial [published correction appears in *Lancet Oncol.* 2017 October;18(10):e562]. *Lancet Oncol.* 2017;18(10):1327–1337. 10.1016/S1470-2045(17)30578-8.
46. Kumar SK, Jacobus SJ, Cohen AD, et al. Carfilzomib or bortezomib in combination with lenalidomide and dexamethasone for patients with newly diagnosed multiple myeloma without intention for immediate autologous stem-cell transplantation (ENDURANCE): A multicentre, open-label, phase 3, randomised, controlled trial. *Lancet Oncol.* 2020;21(10):1317–1330. doi:10.1016/S1470-2045(20)30452-6.
47. Waxman AJ, Clasen S, Hwang W, et al. Carfilzomib-associated cardiovascular adverse events: A systematic review and meta-analysis. *JAMA Oncology.* 2018;4(3):e174519.
48. Lataifeh AR, Nusair A. Fatal pulmonary toxicity due to carfilzomib (Kyprolis™). *J Oncol Pharm Pract.* 2016;22(5):720–724. doi:10.1177/1078155215588630.
49. Moreau P, Masszi T, Grzasko N, et al. Oral Ixazomib, lenalidomide, and dexamethasone for multiple myeloma. *N Engl J Med.* 2016;374(17):1621–1634. doi:10.1056/NEJMoa1516282.
50. Facon T, Venner CP, Bahlis NJ, et al. MM-347: Ixazomib plus lenalidomide-dexamethasone (IRd) vs. placebo-rd for newly diagnosed multiple myeloma (NDMM) patients not eligible for autologous stem cell transplant: The double-blind, placebo-controlled, phase 3 TOURMALINE-MM2 trial. *Clinical Lymphoma, Myeloma and Leukemia.* 2020(20):S307–S308.
51. Kumar S, Moreau P, Hari P, et al. Management of adverse events associated with ixazomib plus lenalidomide/dexamethasone in relapsed/refractory multiple myeloma. *Br J Haematol.* 2017;178(4):571–582. doi:10.1111/bjh.14733.
52. Blair HA. Daratumumab: A review in relapsed and/or refractory multiple myeloma. *Drugs.* 2017;77(18):2013–2024.
53. Mateos M, Dimopoulos MA, Cavo M, et al. Daratumumab plus bortezomib, melphalan, and prednisone for untreated myeloma. *N Engl J Med.* 2018;378(6):518–528.
54. Mikhael J, Belhadj-Merzoug K, Hulin C, et al. A phase 2 study of isatuximab monotherapy in patients with multiple myeloma who are refractory to daratumumab. *Blood Cancer J.* 2021;11(5):89.
55. Attal M, Richardson PG, Rajkumar SV, et al. Isatuximab plus pomalidomide and low-dose dexamethasone versus pomalidomide and low-dose dexamethasone in patients with relapsed and refractory multiple myeloma (ICARIA-MM): A randomised, multicentre, open-label, phase 3 study. *The Lancet.* 2019;394(10214):2096–2107.
56. Lamb YN. Elotuzumab: A review in relapsed and/or refractory multiple myeloma. *Drugs.* 2018;78(14):1481–1488. doi:10.1007/s40265-018-0969-4.
57. Lonial S, Lee HC, Badros A, et al. Belantamab mafodotin for relapsed or refractory multiple myeloma (DREAMM-2): A two-arm, randomised, open-label, phase 2 study. *Lancet Oncol.* 2020;21(2):207–221. doi:10.1016/S1470-2045(19)30788-0.
58. San-Miguel JF, Hungria VT, Yoon SS, et al. Panobinostat plus bortezomib and dexamethasone versus placebo plus bortezomib and dexamethasone in patients with relapsed or relapsed and refractory multiple myeloma: A multicentre, randomised, double-blind phase 3 trial. *Lancet Oncol.* 2014;15(11):1195–1206. doi:10.1016/S1470-2045(14)70440-1.
59. Grosicki S, Simonova M, Spicka I, et al. Once-per-week selinexor, bortezomib, and dexamethasone versus twice-per-week bortezomib and dexamethasone in patients with multiple myeloma (BOSTON): A randomised, open-label, phase 3 trial. *The Lancet.* 2020;396(10262):1563–1573.
60. Richardson PG, Oriol A, Larocca A, et al. Melflufen and dexamethasone in heavily pretreated relapsed and refractory multiple myeloma. *J Clin Oncol.* 2021;39(7):757–767. doi:10.1200/JCO.20.02259.
61. US Food and Drug Administration. FDA alerts patients and health care professionals about clinical trial results showing an increased risk of death associated with Pepaxto (melphalan flufenamide). FDA. July 28, 2021. https://www.fda.gov/drugs/drug-safety-and-availability/fda-alerts-patients-and-health-care-professionals-about-clinical-trial-results-showing-increased. Accessed September 27, 2021.
62. Munshi NC, Anderson LDJr, Shah N, et al. Idecabtagene vicleucel in relapsed and refractory multiple myeloma. *N Engl J Med.* 2021;384(8):705–716. doi:10.1056/NEJMoa2024850.
63. Neelapu SS, Tummala S, Kebriaei P, et al. Chimeric antigen receptor T-cell therapy - assessment and management of toxicities. *Nat Rev Clin Oncol.* 2018;15(1):47–62. doi:10.1038/nrclinonc.2017.148.
64. Palumbo A, Cavallo F, Gay F, et al. Autologous transplantation and maintenance therapy in multiple myeloma. *N Engl J Med.* 2014;371(10):895–905. doi:10.1056/NEJMoa1402888.
65. Attal M, Lauwers-Cances V, Hulin C, et al. Lenalidomide, bortezomib, and dexamethasone with transplantation for myeloma. *N Engl J Med.* 2017;376(14):1311–1320.

66. Fermand JP, Ravaud P, Chevret S, et al. High-dose therapy and autologous peripheral blood stem cell transplantation in multiple myeloma: Up-front or rescue treatment? Results of a multicenter sequential randomized clinical trial. *Blood.* 1998;92(9):3131–3136.
67. Kumar SK, Lacy MQ, Dispenzieri A, et al. Early versus delayed autologous transplantation after immunomodulatory agents-based induction therapy in patients with newly diagnosed multiple myeloma. *Cancer.* 2012;118(6):1585–1592. doi:10.1002/cncr.26422.
68. Dunavin NC, Wei L, Elder P, et al. Early versus delayed autologous stem cell transplant in patients receiving novel therapies for multiple myeloma. *Leuk Lymphoma.* 2013;54(8):1658–1664.
69. Voorhees PM, Usmani SZ. The role of high-dose melphalan and autologous stem cell transplant in the rapidly evolving era of modern multiple myeloma therapy. *Clin Adv Hematol Oncol.* 2016;14(9):719–728.
70. McCarthy PL, Holstein SA, Petrucci MT, et al. Lenalidomide maintenance after autologous stem-cell transplantation in newly diagnosed multiple myeloma: A meta-analysis. *J Clin Oncol.* 2017;35(29):3279–3289. doi:10.1200/JCO.2017.72.6679.
71. Gay F, Jackson G, Rosiñol L, et al. Maintenance treatment and survival in patients with myeloma: A systematic review and network meta-analysis. *JAMA Oncol.* 2018;4(10):1389–1397.
72. Dimopoulos MA, Gay F, Schjesvold F, et al. Oral ixazomib maintenance following autologous stem cell transplantation (TOURMALINE-MM3): A double-blind, randomised, placebo-controlled phase 3 trial. *Lancet.* 2019;393(10168):253–264. doi:10.1016/S0140-6736(18)33003-4.
73. Barlogie B, Kyle RA, Anderson KC, et al. Standard chemotherapy compared with high-dose chemoradiotherapy for multiple myeloma: Final results of phase III US intergroup trial S9321. *J Clin Oncol.* 2006;24(6):929–936.
74. Shah N, Callander N, Ganguly S, et al. Hematopoietic stem cell transplantation for multiple myeloma: Guidelines from the American Society for Blood and Marrow Transplantation. *Biol Blood Marrow Transplant.* 2015;21(7):1155–1166. doi:10.1016/j.bbmt.2015.03.002.
75. van Beurden-Tan CHY, Franken MG, Blommestein HM, Uyl-de Groot CA, Sonneveld P. Systematic literature review and network meta-analysis of treatment outcomes in relapsed and/or refractory multiple myeloma. *J Clin Oncol.* 2017;35(12):1312–1319. doi:10.1200/JCO.2016.71.1663.
76. Botta C, Ciliberto D, Rossi M, et al. Network meta-analysis of randomized trials in multiple myeloma: Efficacy and safety in relapsed/refractory patients. *Blood Adv.* 2017;1(7):455–466. 10.1182/bloodadvances.2016003905 2017 February 27.
77. Aggarwal M, Agrawal N, Yadav N, et al. Autologous stem cell transplantation in first remission is associated with better progression-free survival in multiple myeloma. *Ann Hematol.* 2018;97(10):1869–1877. doi:10.1007/s00277-018-3370-1
78. Yarlagadda L, Gundarlapalli S, Parikh R, et al. Salvage autologous stem cell transplantation in daratumumab-refractory multiple myeloma. *Cancers (Basel).* 2021;13(16):4019. doi:10.3390/cancers13164019
79. Anderson K, Ismaila N, Flynn PJ, et al. Role of Bone-modifying agents in multiple myeloma: American Society of Clinical Oncology Clinical Practice Guideline Update. *J Clin Oncol.* 2018;36(8):812–818. doi:10.1200/JCO.2017.76.6402
80. Mhaskar R, Kumar A, Miladinovic B, Djulbegovic B. Bisphosphonates in multiple myeloma: An updated network meta-analysis. *Cochrane Database Syst Rev.* 2017;12(12):CD003188.
81. Lu H, Pundole X, Lee HC. The role of bone-modifying agents in myeloma bone disease. *JBMR Plus* 2021;5(8):e10518. Published 2021 June 15. doi:10.1002/jbm4.10518.
82. Zometa [package insert].East Hanover, NJ: Novartis Pharmaceutical Corporation; December 2016. https://www.accessdata.fda.gov/drugsatfda_docs/label/2016/021223s035lbl.pdf. Accessed September 27, 2021.
83. Clézardin P. Bisphosphonates' antitumor activity: An unravelled side of a multifaceted drug class. *Bone.* 2011;48(1):71–79. doi:10.1016/j.bone.2010.07.01
84. Raje N, Terpos E, Willenbacher W, et al. Denosumab versus zoledronic acid in bone disease treatment of newly diagnosed multiple myeloma: An international, double-blind, double-dummy, randomised, controlled, phase 3 study. *Lancet Oncol.* 2018;19(3):370–381. doi:10.1016/S1470-2045(18)30072-X
85. Terpos E, Raje N, Croucher P, et al. Denosumab compared with zoledronic acid on PFS in multiple myeloma: Exploratory results of an international phase 3 study. *Blood Advances.* 2021;5(3):725–736.

Myelodysplastic Syndromes

e160

Jill S. Bates and Jolynn Knoche Sessions

KEY CONCEPTS

1. Myelodysplastic syndromes (MDS) primarily affect older adults.
2. The exact cause of MDS is unknown and is probably multifactorial. MDS have been associated with host-specific characteristics, environmental, lifestyle, and therapeutic exposures.
3. Genomic instability drives MDS development and progression. The clonal population of cells manifested as MDS results from enhanced self-renewal of a hematopoietic stem cell or acquisition of self-renewal in a progenitor cell, increased proliferative capacity in the abnormal clone, impaired cell differentiation, evasion of immune regulation, and antiapoptotic mechanisms in the disease-sustaining cell.
4. Most patients with MDS present with fatigue, infection, bleeding/bruising, lethargy, or other symptoms related to cytopenias.
5. The prognosis of patients with MDS depends on the biology of the MDS and host characteristics. Overall survival time ranges from a few months to several years and is most accurately estimated with the International Prognostic Scoring System—Revised (IPSS-R).
6. The goals of therapy for MDS are to change the natural history of the disease, reduce the number of red blood cell transfusions, and improve quality of life.
7. Lenalidomide should be considered for patients with MDS that harbor a del(5q) clone and is particularly beneficial in those with symptomatic anemia.
8. Patients with lower-risk MDS and symptomatic anemia who have a serum erythropoietin level ≤500 mU/mL (U/L) are suitable candidates for an erythropoiesis stimulating agent with or without growth factor support.
9. A subset of lower-risk MDS patients respond well to antithymocyte globulin (ie, immunosuppressive therapy), which is most effective in patients who have a hypocellular marrow, MDS that expresses HLA DR15 with trisomy 8 as the sole cytogenetic abnormality, refractory anemia, and younger than 60 years.
10. Further evaluation is required to determine the optimal hypomethylating agent treatment regimen.
11. Allogeneic hematopoietic stem cell transplantation offers potentially curative therapy to patients with MDS who have a donor and are healthy enough for the procedure.

BEYOND THE BOOK

Name of drug	Target	Dosing	Top 3 counseling points
Lenalidomide			
Antithymocyte globulin (equine)			
Cyclosporine			
Azacitidine			
Decitabine			
Decitabine + Cedazuridine			
Venetoclax			

INTRODUCTION

Myelodysplastic syndromes (MDS) are a heterogeneous group of myeloid stem cell disorders that are clonal in nature and characterized by ineffective hematopoiesis with morphologic dysplasia in hematopoietic cells and peripheral cytopenias.[1] About one-third of patients with MDS will have a disease course that progresses to acute myeloid leukemia (AML). The diagnostic criteria for MDS is the presence of bone marrow dysplasia in at least 10% of cells in one or more of three major bone marrow lineages. Additionally, a diagnosis of MDS can be achieved if 5% to 19% blasts or an MDS-associated karyotype is noted in the bone marrow.[1-3] The clinical course of patients with MDS varies from a slowly progressing, indolent disease, to more aggressive disease characterized by excess bone marrow blasts and rapid progression to AML.[2,3]

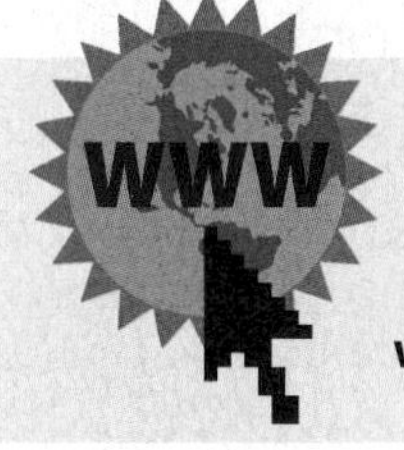

The complete chapter, learning objectives, and other resources can be found at **www.pharmacotherapyonline.com.**

e161

Renal Cell Carcinoma

Erin B. Bailey and David D. Stenehjem

KEY CONCEPTS

1. Renal cell carcinoma (RCC) predominantly occurs later in life, with about 70% of all cases diagnosed between the ages of 55 and 84 years.
2. Established risk factors for RCC include smoking, obesity, hypertension, and inherited susceptibility.
3. Inactivation of the von Hippel-Lindau tumor suppressor gene (*VHL*) is the hallmark of the most common type of RCC, the clear cell histologic subtype.
4. More than 50% of RCC cases are diagnosed by incidental findings on routine imaging for unrelated reasons.
5. The Memorial Sloan-Kettering Cancer Center (MSKCC) Prognostic Factors Model for Survival and International Metastatic Renal Cell Carcinoma Database Consortium (IMDC) Criteria classifies patients into favorable-, intermediate-, and poor-risk groups based on clinical factors, and can predict survival among both untreated patients and those treated with immunotherapy and/or targeted agents.
6. Surgical excision of the primary tumor, either by radical or partial nephrectomy, is the preferred treatment modality for patients with stage I-III RCC, but some patients with stage IV disease may also benefit from surgery.
7. Immunotherapy (programmed cell death protein-1 [PD-1], PD-ligand 1 [PD-L1] and cytotoxic T lymphocyte-associated antigen-4 [CTLA-4] inhibitors) and targeted therapy (multikinase inhibitors, mammalian target of rapamycin [mTOR] inhibitors, and vascular endothelial growth factor [VEGF] inhibitors) are integral components of the management of advanced or metastatic RCC with unique mechanisms of action and adverse drug reaction profiles.
8. First-line treatment options for metastatic RCC (mRCC) are chosen based on patient-specific factors and include small molecule tyrosine kinase inhibitors (sunitinib, pazopanib, axitinib, cabozantinib), an mTOR inhibitor (temsirolimus), and immune checkpoint inhibitor combinations (ipilimumab plus nivolumab, nivolumab plus cabozantinib, pembrolizumab plus axitinib, and pembrolizumab plus lenvatinib).
9. In patients who progress after first-line treatment, multikinase inhibitors cabozantinib, axitinib, and lenvatinib (in combination with everolimus) or immunotherapy with nivolumab may be considered. Combination of nivolumab and ipilimumab and combination immunotherapy with a multikinase inhibitor (eg, pembrolizumab plus axitinib) are also options. A multikinase inhibitor, tivozanib, is an option for patients who have received two or more prior therapies.

BEYOND THE BOOK

Develop a study table showing appropriate first-line treatment options for advanced and metastatic clear cell RCC in different patient groups. This summary table should include factors included in the MSKCC and IMDC Criteria prognostic scoring tools. The summary table should also include how these prognostic tools stratify patients into favorable/low-, intermediate-, and poor-risk categories. This summary table should include both orally and intravenously administered pharmacotherapeutic options. The intent of this activity is to help students practice their skills in the Collect and Assess steps of the patient care process and apply them to patients with advanced and metastatic RCC.

INTRODUCTION

Renal cell carcinoma (RCC) represents about 2% to 4% of all adult malignancies and is the most common type of malignancy of the kidney and renal pelvis. Few treatment options existed, and those that were available had modest activity and were poorly tolerated by patients. However, treatment for the disease has been revolutionized by targeted agents and immunotherapies that were developed based on an increased understanding of RCC pathophysiology. Clear cell is the predominant histologic subtype of RCC (about 80% of all cases) and is characterized by the inactivation of the von Hippel-Lindau (*VHL*) tumor suppressor gene located on chromosome 3p25. *VHL* inactivation leads to increased production of growth factors, such as vascular endothelial growth factor (VEGF), transforming growth factor (TGF), platelet-derived growth factor (PDGF), and others responsible for angiogenesis and cell growth.[1]

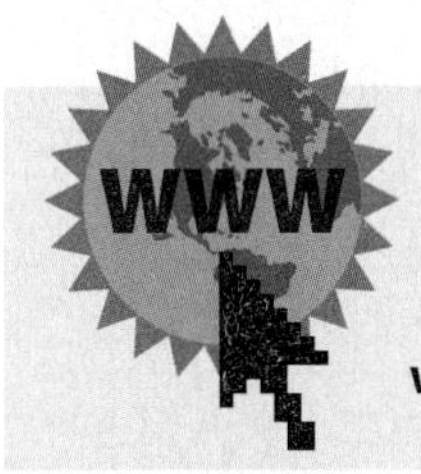

The complete chapter, learning objectives, and other resources can be found at **www.pharmacotherapyonline.com.**

162

Melanoma

Cindy L. O'Bryant and Christina M. Davis

KEY CONCEPTS

1. Cutaneous melanoma is an increasingly common malignancy that can be cured if detected early. Public education about screening and early detection is one strategy to reduce the mortality associated with cutaneous melanoma.
2. Surgical resection can cure patients with early-stage melanoma.
3. Adjuvant therapy should be considered in patients with locally advanced disease; recommended options include ipilimumab, nivolumab, pembrolizumab, BRAF and MEK inhibitors, and clinical trial.
4. Chemotherapy and biochemotherapy offer limited benefit in the treatment of metastatic melanoma.
5. Immunotherapy with ipilimumab, nivolumab, the combination of ipilimumab/nivolumab and pembrolizumab have led to durable responses and significantly prolonged overall survival in patients with metastatic melanoma.
6. Immune-related toxicities associated with immunotherapy can be severe and life-threatening. Consequently, the use of these agents warrants appropriate patient selection, close monitoring, and toxicity management by an experienced healthcare team.
7. As the biology of melanoma has been further delineated, a growing number of potential targets for drug therapy have been identified. *BRAF* mutations occur in up to 70% of melanoma patients. The combination of BRAF and MEK inhibitors improves overall survival in patients with this mutation.
8. Treatment of melanoma is determined by many factors. As the number of treatment options for patients with metastatic melanoma grows, disease- and patient-related factors should be considered to determine appropriate therapy.

BEYOND THE BOOK

Review educational materials regarding skin self-examinations created by the American Cancer Society (https://www.cancer.org/healthy/be-safe-in-sun/skin-exams.html) and the American Academy of Dermatology Association (https://www.aad.org/public/diseases/skin-cancer/find/check-skin). Assess the level of understanding and ease of use from a patient perspective for each. Then perform your own skin self-examination based on the ABCDE rule to identify any new or suspicious spots on your skin. This activity will enhance student understanding regarding the COLLECT and ASSESS steps in the patient care process.

INTRODUCTION

Skin cancer is the most common malignancy worldwide and is associated with chronic ultraviolet (UV) exposure. The two types of skin cancer are nonmelanoma skin cancers (NMSCs) and melanoma. Although NMSCs are the most common malignancy of the skin, cutaneous melanoma accounts for up to 80% of all skin cancer-related deaths.[1] Melanoma cases are increasing globally with the highest rates found in Australia, New Zealand, North America, and Northern Europe.[2] Melanoma is the fifth most common cancer in the United States.[1] The incidence of melanoma has rapidly increased in the United States over the last 30 years, and has increased an average of 1.4% each year over the last decade.[3] When detected early, patients generally have a good prognosis. Skin cancer prevention and screening have a major impact on public health and the success of treatment for those individuals diagnosed with NMSC and melanoma. Skin cancers tend to occur more frequently in older individuals with a median age of diagnosis of 65 years.[3] Therefore, as the population continues to age, effective strategies to prevent, detect, and treat individuals with these cancers are necessary. An understanding of the biology of melanoma has led to the development of therapies targeted toward somatic mutations and the immune response, which have shown improved outcomes in patients with advanced melanoma.

EPIDEMIOLOGY

In the United States, it is estimated that 99,780 cases of melanoma will be diagnosed in 2022, accounting for 7,650 deaths.[4] The overall incidence is greater in men than women, but rates are higher in women before the age of 50. Risk also varies with ethnicity, with most melanoma cases occurring among White individuals.[4] Childhood and adolescent melanoma account for only 1% and 3%, respectively, of new melanoma cases each year but is the most common skin cancer in individuals younger than 20 years.[5] The majority of childhood and adolescent melanoma occurs in females and non-Hispanic White patients.[6] From the 1970s to the early 2000s, the incidence of melanoma in those younger than 20 years increased by 2% to 3% per year, but data from 2004 to 2010 show a decrease of 11.6% per year.[6]

Survival rates for patients with melanoma have gradually increased over the past four decades. Due to recent advances in treatment, the 5-year relative survival rate is 93.3% for all stages of melanoma, but survival declines to 29.8% in patients with more

TABLE 162-1 Risk Factors for Melanoma

Patient-Specific Risk Factors
Adulthood (older than 15 years)
History of cutaneous melanoma
Dysplastic nevi
High density of common nevi and atypical nevi
Cutaneous melanoma in first-degree relative
Immunodeficiency or immunosuppression
High degree of freckling
Sunburns easily or tans rarely
Blonde or red hair
Blue, green, or gray eyes
Socioeconomic status (higher > lower)
Race (Caucasians > Hispanics > African Americans)
External Risk Factors
Intense, intermittent sun exposures
History of sunburn
More than four painful sunburns before the age of 15 years
Recreational sun exposure

advanced disease.[3] Over the last decade, the death rate from melanoma has declined around 1% per year in adults older than 50 years and 3% per year in adults younger than 50 years.[3]

Several patient-specific and environmental risk factors have been identified (see Table 162-1), and it is likely these factors alone, or in combination, increase the risk of cutaneous melanoma.

Both UVB and UVA are known carcinogens and are related to the development of melanoma. Caucasian individuals with fair-colored hair (red or blond), light-colored eyes (blue or green), high degrees of freckling, and those who tend to burn and rarely tan with sun exposure, are especially at risk. Clinical and epidemiologic research shows a higher rate of melanoma in those who have extensive or repeated intense UV and sun exposure.[1] Intermittent, intense sun exposure, blistering sunburns, tanning bed use, and the time of life when exposed to the sun are critical factors for the development of cutaneous melanoma.[7,8] The risk of melanoma seems to be greater during childhood and adolescence due to sunlight and UV radiation exposure and lower in adults who have had chronic sun exposure, are without a history of burning, and those with occupational exposure.

A significant risk factor for melanoma is the number and size of melanocytic nevi (pigmented lesions or moles) on the body. The formation of these nevi is directly related to cumulative sun exposure. The relative risk of developing melanoma increases with the number of typical nevi on an individual. A second risk factor is the presence of atypical melanocytic nevi. Atypical nevi may progress from a normal nevus or be dysplastic from the onset. Up to 20% of melanomas develop from atypical nevi. Congenital melanocytic nevi may be present at birth or within the first few months of life, and the associated risk of melanoma increases with size.[1,6]

Other risk factors in the development of melanoma include immunodeficiency (either inherited or acquired), a personal history of NMSC or melanoma skin cancer, and a diagnosis of xeroderma pigmentosum, a rare skin disorder. Patients with these risk factors often have more aggressive disease and have been shown to have a poor prognosis.[1,6]

Family history is associated with up to 10% of cases of melanoma. Familial atypical multiple mole syndrome (FAMMM) or dysplastic nevus syndrome is an autosomal dominant hereditary disease that accounts for about 1% of melanoma cases. It is characterized by the presence of numerous common and atypical moles and a family history of melanoma in multiple first-degree relatives and younger age at diagnosis.[9,10] Patients with FAMMM syndrome are at considerable risk for developing melanoma which increases with age. FAMMM syndrome is associated with mutations in the *CDKN2A* gene. *CDKN2A* encodes two distinct proteins: p16, an inhibitor of cyclin-dependent kinase 4 and 6, and p14ARF, which inhibits p53 degradation. Mutations in *CDKN2A* result in increased proliferation and decreased apoptosis.[9,10]

ETIOLOGY

Melanoma arises from the melanocytes in the basal layer of the epidermis. DNA damage, most commonly a result of UV radiation, leads to cellular mutations that transform the cell and result in uncontrolled proliferation and the formation of tumors. The identification of these genetic alterations has led to the recognition of molecular subgroups of melanoma and more focused drug development for treatment.

A major signaling pathway associated with the development of melanoma is the mitogen-activated protein kinase pathway (MAPK), which mediates receptor tyrosine kinases, resulting in activation of RAS and downstream BRAF. Activating *BRAF* mutations are the most common somatic genetic event in human melanoma, occurring in about 50% of melanoma patients and primarily noted by a single point mutation at residue V600. The V600E mutation, in which valine is substituted for glutamic acid at codon 600, is the most common point mutation. The V600K mutation may also occur at this residue. *BRAF* mutations are associated with younger age at diagnosis, intermittent sun exposure, and superficial spreading melanoma.[10]

Upstream of BRAF, mutations in *NRAS,* and *KIT* can act as molecular drivers in the development of melanoma. Mutations in *NRAS* are found in up to 20% of patients. These tumors are associated with chronic sun exposure and high growth rates.[7] *KIT* is a transmembrane receptor tyrosine kinase that, when activated, signals the MAPK and phosphatidyl-inositol-3-OH kinase (PI3K) pathways, resulting in transcription and cell proliferation. Mutations in *KIT* are commonly found in acral and mucosal melanomas as well as those with chronic sun exposure.[10]

Other genetic alterations involved in the development of melanoma include *MITF* (microphthalmia-associated transcription factor) and *MCIR* (melanocortin 1 receptor gene). *MITF* is a gene important to the survival of melanocytes and, when mutated, acts as an oncogene. *MCIR* is prevalent in individuals with melanoma and signals through the MITF pathway. It is involved in melanin synthesis and is associated with the red hair and fair skin phenotype.[10]

PATHOPHYSIOLOGY

Melanomas most often arise within epidermal melanocytes of the skin, although they can also arise from noncutaneous melanocytes. During fetal development, melanocytes migrate over a predictable route to multiple sites within the body, including the skin, uveal tract, meninges, and ectodermal mucosa. Melanocytes synthesize melanin to protect various tissues, such as the skin, from UV damage and reach the keratinocytes in the upper layers of the epidermis via dendrites. Primary melanoma can arise in any area of the body with melanocytes. Cutaneous melanoma is the most frequent site constituting 90% of all melanomas. Other sites of primary melanoma include the eye (uveal melanoma), the mucosa, and in some cases, as metastatic disease with an unknown primary site.[10]

The pathogenesis of human melanoma involves a series of morphologic stages: melanocytic atypia, atypical melanocytic hyperplasia, radial growth phase, vertical growth phase with or without in-transit metastasis, regional lymph node metastatic melanoma, and distant metastatic melanoma. Melanoma gains the potential for metastasis with the onset of a vertical growth phase. Therefore, the thickness of a primary melanoma is an important prognostic factor and is used in the staging classification of cutaneous melanoma. As the disease progresses, melanoma cells increase the production of certain growth factors and cytokines which, in turn, activate cellular growth and survival pathways, including the MAPK, PI3K/AKT, and mammalian target of rapamycin (mTOR). Understanding the biology of melanoma has provided targets for innovative drug therapy.

The role of the immune system in the development of melanoma is well documented and spontaneous cancer regressions associated with host immunity have been reported.[11] Melanoma cells evade the immune system by exploiting immune checkpoints. Immune checkpoint receptors such as cytotoxic T-lymphocyte antigen 4 (CTLA-4) and programmed death-1 (PD-1) are found on the surface of activated T cells and, when bound to a ligand, inhibit the function of the T cell. In the case of PD-1, when interferon is released by T-cell recognition of the melanoma cell, janus-kinase (JAK) and signal-transducer-and-activator-of-transcription (STAT) are upregulated, leading to increased expression of programmed cell death ligand 1 (PD-L1) on the melanoma cell surface. When PD-L1 binds to PD-1, the T cell becomes inactivated and the antitumor immune response is inhibited.[7]

MELANOMA SUBTYPES

Histologic

Cutaneous melanomas are categorized by growth patterns. Four major histologic subtypes, or growth patterns of primary cutaneous melanoma, have been identified: superficial spreading melanoma (SSM), nodular melanoma (NM), lentigo maligna melanoma (LMM), and acral lentiginous melanoma (ALM). While these subtypes do not directly correlate with clinical outcomes, certain subtypes have been shown to demonstrate a higher frequency of genetic mutations.

SSM is the most common type of cutaneous melanoma, accounting for up to 70% of all melanomas and is associated with intense, intermittent sun exposure. Early in lesion development, SSM is flat, growing radially before vertically. SSM evolves slowly, typically over 1 to 5 years. As the lesion progresses, it may become raised or ulcerated. The borders are often irregular and asymmetrical as the lesion progresses and may vary in color (blue, black, brown, pink, or other colors). SSMs may occur at any anatomic site on the body but are more commonly found on the trunk and extremities. The average age of a diagnosis of SSM is 50 years. These lesions can be linked to mutations in *BRAF*.

Nodular melanoma is the second most common histological type of melanoma, occurring in 15% to 30% of patients. Since nodular melanoma is a pure vertical growth phase disease, it is more aggressive and develops more rapidly than other subtypes.[10] Nodular melanomas are often dark blue–black and uniform in color with a shiny surface, although a small percentage of nodular melanomas are amelanotic and have a fleshy appearance. Nodular melanomas are raised, often symmetric, and can occur at any site. *LMM* represents 10% to 20% of melanomas and is commonly found on the head and neck. It is unique from other histologic subtypes; it does not have the same propensity to metastasize because of a prolonged radial growth phase. LMM arises on chronically sun-exposed sites in older individuals and presents as a freckle-like lesion. LMMs are generally large flat, tan-colored lesions with shades of brown and black that gradually grow, develop, and begin to change in color.[10] Evolution into invasive melanoma is characterized by nodular development within the flat lesion. These lesions can be linked to mutations in *KIT*.

ALM makes up about 5% of melanomas and is not related to UV exposure. It presents commonly as melanoma on the palms of the hands or soles of the feet but may present as subungual melanoma and mucosal melanoma. ALMs located on the soles of the feet appear as a large tan or brown stain. The lesions often have irregular convoluted borders and may be masked by thick skin on the feet. Subungual melanoma arises in the nail matrix or nail bed. The most common presentation is a brown or black line in the great toe or the thumbnail. Mucosal melanoma is rare and can occur on any mucosal surface. Most commonly is seen in the oropharyngeal mucosa followed by the anal and rectal, genital, and urinary mucosa. Unfortunately, mucosal melanoma often does not become clinically apparent until the mass is large or the lesion bleeds. ALM is the most common type of melanoma reported in individuals with a dark complexion.[10] Similar to LMMs, this subtype is characterized by a protracted radial growth phase and is associated with mutations in *KIT*.

Uveal melanoma arises from the pigmented epithelium of the choroid. It is the most common primary intraocular malignancy seen in adults but is an uncommon tumor. Unlike cutaneous melanoma, the frequency and mortality rates of uveal melanoma have remained steady.[12] The risk of metastasis varies with the histologic type and size of the tumor and the location in the eye. The liver is the most frequent site of metastasis but uveal melanoma can spread to a variety of tissues.[10]

Clinical

Based on our understanding of the role of genetic alterations in the treatment and outcomes of patients with melanoma, four distinctive clinical subtypes have emerged based on UV exposure and anatomic site. The four subtypes are divided into (1) nonchronic sun damage (non-CSD): melanomas on the skin without chronic sun-induced damage; (2) chronic sun damage (CSD): melanomas on the skin with chronic sun-induced damage characterized by the presence of solar elastosis; (3) acral; and (4) mucosal.[8] The primary genetic differences of these subtypes are based on the activation of the MAPK and PI3K pathways. *BRAF* mutations predominantly occur in non-CSD (56%) and less commonly in the other groups. About 5% to 20% of all the subtypes contain *NRAS* mutations and these mutations occur independent of *BRAF*. Further studies showed *KIT* mutations are found in almost 40% of acral and mucosal subtypes, in almost one-third of CSD melanomas and not at all in non-CSD melanomas.[8] Guidelines recommend uveal and mucosal melanoma be treated differently than CSD and non-CSD melanoma because of their differences in presentation and outcomes.[8] This further emphasizes the need for continued refinement of tumor classifications in melanoma based on genetic and biological features, which will lead to more personalized treatment options and improved outcomes for patients.

PREVENTION AND DETECTION

1 Skin cancer is a major health problem in the United States. In 2014, the US Surgeon General released a Call to Action to Prevent Skin Cancer that addressed the following goals to support skin cancer prevention: increase opportunities for sun protection in outdoor settings; provide individuals with the information they need to make informed, healthy choices about UV radiation exposure; promote policies to advance the national goal of preventing skin cancer; reduce harms from indoor tanning; and strengthen research, surveillance, monitoring, and evaluation related to skin cancer prevention.[13]

Both UVA and UVB exposure plays a major role in melanoma development and is the most preventable cause of melanoma. The incidence of melanoma has been associated with latitude and the intensity of solar exposure among susceptible populations. As such, the mainstay of melanoma prevention remains strategies to protect individuals from the harmful effects of the sun (see Table 162-2).

Strategies such as sun avoidance, especially during peak hours of sun intensity (10 AM–4 PM), seeking the shade when outdoors, and use of protective clothing are important education concepts for individuals who are in the sun for prolonged periods or who are at high risk for burning. In addition, the use of sunglasses, with both UVA and UVB protection, is important. Due to its correlation with the development of melanoma, the World Health Organization

TABLE 162-2 Options for Sun Protection

Behavioral	Sunscreens: Physical Blockers (Reflectants)	Sunscreens: Chemical Absorbers
Protective clothing and accessories	Zinc oxide	Ultraviolet B absorbers
Seek shade (avoid peak sun hours)	Talc	Salicylates
Avoid tanning equipment	Titanium dioxide	Cinnamates
	Red petrolatum	Camphor derivatives
		Aminobenzoates
		Ultraviolet A absorbers
		Benzophenone-6
		Dibenzoylmethanes

TABLE 162-3 Self-Examination of Suspicious Moles

1. Examine your body front and back in the mirror and then the right and left sides with the arms raised
2. Bend the elbows and look carefully at the forearms and upper arms and palms
3. Look at the backs of the legs and feet. Look specifically in the spaces between toes and at the soles of the feet
4. Examine the back of the neck and scalp with the help of a hand-held mirror; part the hair (or use a blow dryer) to lift the hair and give yourself a closer look
5. Check the back and buttocks with a handheld mirror

Data from the American Academy of Dermatology (www.aad.org).

International Agency for Research on Cancer has declared UV light emitted from tanning beds a human carcinogen and the United States Food and Drug Administration (FDA) reclassified UV tanning devices to class II (moderate-to-high risk) devices.[14] As a result, 44 states have regulations in place to restrict minors' access to indoor tanning, including 23 that prohibit the use of indoor tanning for anyone younger than 18 years.

Sunscreens are another strategy to decrease UV exposure. A broad-spectrum sunscreen with both UVA and UVB protection and an SPF of 15 or higher used regularly as directed is recommended with other sun protective measures to prevent sunburn and reduce the risk of skin cancer. Of note, current regulations limit the SPF value on sunscreen labels to 50+ because of the lack of evidence to show that products with SPF values greater than 50 provide greater protection.[15] However, the FDA proposed several changes regarding labeling requirements and reducing the number of active ingredients to be generally recognized as safe and effective for over-the-counter sunscreen products. It is important to counsel patients about the appropriate use of sunscreen. Sunscreen should be applied 30 minutes before going into the sun and reapplied every 2 hours, after swimming or after perspiring heavily. About one ounce (30 mL) of sunscreen (a "palmful") should be used to cover the arms, legs, neck, and face of the average adult. Sun protection must be used regularly and not merely limited to times of recreation or anticipated "prolonged" exposure.

There are no consistent recommendations for the screening and early detection of melanoma. Early detection can play a large part in preventing a premalignant precursor from becoming melanoma or preventing a melanoma recurrence. About 50% of initial melanoma lesions are discovered by self-skin examination (SSE). Improved survival rates for melanoma have been attributed to the identification and treatment of disease at an early stage when the disease is limited and has not yet metastasized. High-risk patients with a strong family history should have additional clinical examinations, and in some cases, screening photography to document the size, shape, and location of moles. The entire cutaneous surface, including the scalp, should be examined. Both patients and clinicians need to be properly educated in the clinical features of the disease to ensure a more appropriate diagnosis.

In some cases, an individual may need the help of a partner or caregiver to perform an SSE. This is especially important for older adults as they are more likely to develop and die from melanoma. Barriers to successful SSEs in older adults, such as failing eyesight, lack of partners, and poor memory impact older adults in detecting new or changing lesions. These barriers, coupled with the higher incidence of melanoma in older adults, present challenges and opportunities for healthcare professionals to target education on this growing segment of our population.

Healthcare professionals who routinely work with the public have an opportunity to increase public awareness concerning the benefits and appropriate methods for SSE. Educational pamphlets describing SSE (see Table 162-3) for the public are widely available through the American Cancer Society, American Academy of Dermatology, and Skin Cancer Foundation. If a newly discovered pigmented lesion is identified on SSE, or if a preexisting pigmented lesion changes, the individual should be immediately evaluated by a clinician.

Benign nevi often occur in sun-exposed areas and are typically 4 to 6 mm in diameter (about the size of a pencil eraser), raised or flat, uniform in color and round in shape. Dysplastic nevi, an intermediate between benign nevi and melanoma, tend to be larger than common nevi (>5 mm), appear as flat macules with asymmetry, have a fuzzy or ill-defined shape, and vary in color.

CLINICAL PRESENTATION

The initial clinical presentation of melanoma is often a cutaneous pigmented skin lesion that changes over time. Any changes in the skin surrounding a nevus, including redness or swelling, are important clinical signs. Uncommonly, the lesion may become itchy or tender and painful. Friability of the lesion, resulting in bleeding or oozing, is a danger sign. Perhaps the most important warning sign of danger is the evolution of any characteristic of a lesion. A biopsy of the lesion is critical to establish the diagnosis of melanoma. Subsequent pathologic interpretation of the biopsy will provide information on prognosis and treatment options. An excisional biopsy, with a 1- to 3-mm margin of normal appearing skin, is recommended for a suspicious lesion and should include a portion of underlying subcutaneous fat for microstaging. For larger lesions, an incisional or punch biopsy can be performed and should include a core of full-thickness skin and subcutaneous tissue. When excisional biopsies are not appropriate, as with the face or palmar surface of the hands, a full-thickness incisional or punch biopsy is preferred. A shave biopsy is rarely appropriate because it can underestimate the thickness of the lesion, and may not fully remove it. A broad shave biopsy could be considered for melanoma in site or LMM. Evaluation of any individual with a suspected melanoma includes a complete history and total-body skin examination. The focus of the patient history is to identify potential risk factors including family history of melanoma, personal history of skin cancer or nevus excisions, immunosuppression or an immunosuppressive condition, sun exposure, tanning bed use, and phenotype. A total dermatologic examination is necessary to determine melanoma risk factors (eg, mole pattern, mole type, or freckling) and for staging. Since melanoma commonly spreads to the lymph nodes, individuals suspicious for advanced disease should be examined for lymphadenopathy. Lactate dehydrogenase (LDH) should be measured because elevated serum levels are an independent predictor of decreased survival.[8,16] In addition, any other signs or symptoms suggestive of metastatic disease should be completely evaluated.

STAGING AND PROGNOSTIC FACTORS

The size of a primary melanoma lesion is associated with the likelihood of metastasis. The Breslow tumor thickness of the lesion

CLINICAL PRESENTATION Melanoma

General

- Any lesion that changes in appearance over time

Local Signs and Symptoms

- The clinical features used to describe suspicious lesions are highlighted with the mnemonic "ABCDE"
  - Asymmetry: Melanoma lesions are often asymmetric
  - Border: Melanoma lesions have irregular borders
  - Color: Color is often variegated in a melanoma ranging from tan, blue-black, red, purple, or white
  - Diameter: Melanoma lesions are frequently greater than 6 mm
  - Enlargement or evolution: A sudden enlargement or change in the lesion is concerning for melanoma
- Other signs of melanoma include a lesion that swells, bleeds, or oozes

Systemic Signs and Symptoms

- Palpable lymph nodes
- Depending on the site of metastasis, shortness of breath, abdominal pain, bone pain, headache, and mental status changes

Laboratory Tests

- In addition to a comprehensive metabolic panel, LDH should be evaluated

Other Diagnostic Tests

- Biopsy and pathology review for staging with molecular testing for *BRAF*, *NRAS*, and *KIT*
- When applicable, SLNB
- Systemic staging should include chest, abdomen, and pelvic CT scan or CT/PET bone scan, and brain MRI

CT, computed tomography; LDH, lactate dehydrogenase; MRI, magnetic resonance imaging; PET, positron emission tomography; SLNB, sentinel lymph node biopsy.

is commonly used as a prognostic factor to predict outcomes.[6] Tumor thickness is quantified to the nearest 0.1 mm with an ocular micrometer, measuring from the top of the granular layer of the overlying epidermis to the deepest contiguous invasive melanoma cell. The correlation between tumor thickness and the risk of tumor metastasis is strong but does not include aspects such as tumor satellites, defined rather arbitrarily, as skin involvement within 2 cm of the primary lesion, and vascular invasion. Patients with satellitosis have a worse prognosis than patients with thick primary lesions (tumor thickness > 4 mm), and the prognosis is more similar to that of patients with nodal metastasis. The American Joint Committee on Cancer (AJCC) developed an early-staging system for melanoma that divides patients with localized melanoma into four stages according to the microstaging criteria of Breslow. Additionally, ulceration of the melanoma, satellite lesions of the primary tumor, and location of distant metastases must be considered for accurate staging. As a result, the revised AJCC staging system for cutaneous melanoma was implemented in 2018.[16] Carefully examine older clinical trials to determine which staging system was used to determine patient inclusion and exclusion criteria, as results may differ based on these patient criteria. Clinical staging includes microstaging the primary melanoma with clinical, laboratory, and radiologic evaluation. It is used after complete excision of the primary melanoma and clinical assessment to determine regional and distant metastasis. Pathologic staging includes microstaging of the primary melanoma and pathologic information about the regional nodes after partial or complete lymphadenectomy. Patients with limited disease (in situ, stage 0 or stage 1A) do not require pathologic evaluation of lymph nodes (see Tables 162-4 and 162-5).[8]

As with other solid tumors, regional lymph node involvement is a powerful predictor of tumor burden and patient outcome. Sentinel lymph node biopsy (SLNB) is a minimally invasive procedure that determines if a patient is a candidate for a complete lymph node dissection. The rationale for lymphatic mapping and subsequent SLNB is based on the observation that skin regions have patterns of lymphatic drainage to specific lymph nodes in the regional lymphatic basin. The sentinel lymph node is the first node in the lymphatic basin into which the primary melanoma drains. Unlike other solid tumors, melanoma progresses in an orderly nodal distribution. SLNB allows for the detection of micrometastases with a more thorough examination of a single sentinel node than is possible when examining multiple lymph nodes with a lymph node dissection. SLNB is associated with low false-negative rates and low complication rates.[18] SLNB may be most useful for melanomas located in ambiguous drainage sites such as the head and neck. Detection of clinically undetectable disease in a lymph node basin not directly adjacent to the primary lesion may allow for upstaging of patients who initially are believed to have node-negative disease. The American Society of Clinical Oncology and Society of Surgical Oncology joint clinical practice guidelines recommend SLNB for patients with any intermediate-thickness melanoma and may be considered for a thinner melanoma.[18]

Tumor thickness, ulceration, and mitotic rate, in addition to age and gender, are the primary indicators of the natural history of the disease and correlate with prognosis. Mitotic rate, defined as the number of mitosis per square millimeter, is an important prognostic factor for developing metastatic disease. Increasing mitotic rate, characterized as greater than ≥ 1 mitosis/mm^2, represents a more aggressive lesion and is associated with a poorer survival rate. Other factors such as tumor growth pattern, vertical growth phase, histological subtype, density of tumor-infiltrating lymphocytes (TILs) in the tumor tissue, elevated LDH level, satellite lesions, and angiolymphatic invasion may be associated with survival.[19] The location of the primary tumor on the skin is also important as tumors of the extremities have increased survival compared with those with axial, neck, head, and trunk tumors. In addition, several additional prognostic factors have been identified in patients with advanced disease. The number of metastatic sites, involvement of the central nervous system, gastrointestinal tract, liver, pleura, or lung, Eastern Cooperative Oncology Group (ECOG) performance status of 1 or greater, male sex, and prior immunotherapy have all been associated with poor prognosis.[8]

TABLE 162-4 Melanoma Tumor (T), Node (N), Metastasis (M) Classification

T Classification	Thickness	Ulcerative Status
T_X	Primary tumor cannot be addressed (eg, shave biopsy)	
T_0	No evidence of primary tumor	
T_{is}	Melanoma in situ	
T_1	≤1 mm	Unknown or unspecified
	0.8-1 mm	With or without ulceration
	<0.8 mm	A: Without ulceration B: With ulceration
T_2	>1-2 mm	Unknown or unspecified A: Without ulceration B: With ulceration
T_3	>2-4 mm	Unknown or unspecified A: Without ulceration B: With ulceration
T_4	>4 mm	Unknown or unspecified A: Without ulceration B: With ulceration
N Classification	**No. of Tumor Involved Nodes**	**Presence of In-Transit, Satellite, and/or Microsatellite Metastases**
N_X	Regional lymph nodes cannot be assessed	No
N_0	No regional lymph nodes	No
N_1	1 node	
N_{1a}	1 clinically occult node[a]	No
N_{1b}	1 clinically detected node	No
N_{1c}	No regional lymph node disease	Yes
N_2	2-3 nodes	
N_{2a}	2-3 clinically occult nodes	No
N_{2b}	2-3, with 1 clinically detected node	No
N_{2c}	1 clinically occult or detected node	Yes
N_3	≥4 nodes	
N_{3a}	≥4 clinically occult nodes	No
N_{3b}	≥4, with 1 clinically detected, or presence of any matted nodes	No
N_{3c}	≥2 clinically occult or detected and/or any matted nodes	Yes
M Classification	**Site**	**Serum Lactate Dehydrogenase**
M_0	No detectable distant metastasis	
M_{1a}	Distant skin, soft tissue, and/or nonregional lymph nodes	Not elevated Elevated: $M_{1a(1)}$
M_{1b}	Lung metastases	Not elevated Elevated: $M_{1b(1)}$
M_{1c}	Any distant metastasis visceral metastases	Not elevated Elevated: $M_{1c(1)}$
M_{1d}	Distant metastases to the CNS	Not elevated Elevated: $M_{1d(1)}$

M, metastasis; N, node; T, tumor.

[a]Clinically occult node detected by sentinel lymph node biopsy.

Data from Reference 17.

TREATMENT

Desired Outcomes

Treatment of cutaneous melanoma depends on the stage of disease. Localized disease is managed, and often cured, with surgical ablation. Regional disease is treated with surgical resection of the primary lesion and, depending on the risk of recurrence, adjuvant therapy to eradicate any residual disease and cure the patient. The role of ipilimumab as adjuvant therapy after surgical resection is limited with combination BRAF and MEK inhibitors and PD-1 inhibitors now favored in this setting based on recent FDA approvals. Historically, metastatic melanoma has been a difficult disease to treat. The goals of treatment for metastatic disease are to slow tumor progression, prolong survival, relieve acute symptoms, and improve quality of life. After decades of poor treatment options, several effective treatment options are now available, including targeted agents (BRAF and MEK inhibitors) and immunotherapy (CTLA-4 and PD-1 inhibitors) approved to treat metastatic melanoma. Targeted agents offer rapid and high-response rates with prolonged time-to-disease progression, while immunotherapy can induce durable responses. These new treatment options have increased survival expectations to an all-time high in the history of melanoma treatment. As a result of the differences in the underlying pathophysiology and treatment of uveal melanoma, the NCCN developed disease-specific guidelines.[20]

Surgery

Patients who present with a suspicious pigmented lesion should undergo a full-thickness excisional biopsy, if possible. A full-thickness incisional or punch biopsy is preferred in cases where an excisional biopsy is not possible, to provide microstaging and ultimately determine therapy.

2 Localized cutaneous melanoma can often be cured with surgical excision. The cure rates for melanomas smaller than 1 mm are as high as 98%.[21] The extent of the excision margin determines the risk of local recurrence and ultimately survival. For melanoma in situ, excision of the visible lesion or biopsy site with a 0.5- to 1 cm border of clinically normal skin and a layer of subcutaneous tissue along with confirmation of histologically negative peripheral margins is recommended. The recommended clinical margin for invasive melanoma depends on tumor thickness. Excision with a 1-cm margin of clinically normal skin and underlying subcutaneous tissue is recommended for invasive melanomas 1 mm thick or smaller. Current guidelines recommend a 1 to 2 cm margin for melanoma with a tumor thickness of 1.01 to 2 mm.[8] Lesions that are 2 to 4 mm thick should be excised with a 2 cm margin and primary tumors more than 4 mm thick require at least a 2 cm margin. Surgical management of lentigo maligna melanoma is problematic as subclinical extension of atypical junctional melanocytic hyperplasia may extend beyond the visible margins. Complete excision of these lesions is important.

When isolated regional lymph nodes in the absence of distant disease are detected via physical examination, a therapeutic lymphadenectomy is recommended. Neoadjuvant therapy should also be considered in patients at high risk of perioperative morbidity or if gross complete resection of nodal disease may not be achieved. The extent of the therapeutic lymph node dissection is often modified according to the anatomic area of the lymphadenopathy. Selective regional lymphadenectomy performed after scintigraphic and dye lymphographic identification of the affected draining sentinel lymph node(s) is the standard of care for melanomas more than 1 mm thick. If the lesion is less than 0.8 mm in thickness with ulceration, 0.8 to 1 mm in thickness with or without ulceration, or <0.8 mm with other adverse features (very high mitotic index >2/mm^2 or lymphovascular invasion), lymphatic mapping with

TABLE 162-5 American Joint Committee on Cancer Tumor (T), Node (N), Metastasis (M) Stage Grouping for Cutaneous Melanoma

Pathologic Stage	T	N	M	Clinical Stage	T	N	M
0	T_{is}	N_0	M_0	0	T_{is}	N_0	M_0
IA	T_{1a}	N_0	M_0	IA	T_{1a}	N_0	M_0
	T_{1b}	N_0	M_0	IB	T_{1b} T_{2a}	N_0 N_0	M_0 M_0
IB	T_{2a}	N_0	M_0				
IIA	T_{2b}	N_0	M_0				
	T_{3a}	N_0	M_0	IIA	T_{2b}	N_0	M_0
IIB	T_{3b}	N_0	M_0		T_{3a}	N_0	M_0
	T_{4a}	N_0	M_0	IIB	T_{3b}	N_0	M_0
	T_{4a}	N_0	M_0		T_{4a}	N_0	M_0
IIC	T_{4b}	N_0	M_0	IIC	T_{4b}	N_0	M_0
IIIA	$T_{1a/b}$, T_{2a}	N_{1a}, N_{2a}	M_0	III	Any T, T_{is}	$>N_1$	M_0
IIIB	T_0	N_{1b}, N_{1c}	M_0				
	$T_{1a/b}$, T_{2a}	$N_{2b/c}$, N_{2b}	M_0				
	T_{2b}, T_{3a}	N_{1a-c}, $N_{2a/b}$					
IIIC	T_0	$N_{2b/c}$, $N_{3b/c}$	M_0				
	T_{1a}-T_{3a}	N_{2c}, N_{3a-c}	M_0				
	T_{3b}, T_{4a}	Any $N \geq N_1$	M_0				
	T_{4b}	N_{1a-c}-N_{2a-c}	M_0				
IIID	T_{4b}	N_{3a-c}	M_0				
IV	Any T, T_{is}	Any N	M_1	IV	Any T	Any N	M_1

SLNB should be discussed and considered. If the sentinel node is found to have micrometastatic melanoma, regional dissection of the involved nodal basin is performed. The likelihood of detecting metastatic disease in the sentinel lymph node is <5% in thin melanomas that are less than 0.8 mm, but increases to more than 30% in tumors 4 mm thick.[22] The Multicenter Selective Lymphadenectomy Trial (MSLT-1) investigated the use of SLNB and immediate complete lymph node dissection (CLND) compared to nodal observation in patients with melanoma undergoing a wide local excision. Results showed a significant improvement in disease-free survival but not melanoma-specific survival, supporting the staging value of SLNB.[23] The Multicenter Selective Lymphadenectomy Trial II (MSLT-II) then randomized sentinel lymph node-positive patients to either CLND or nodal observation. No difference in melanoma-specific survival was observed despite an increased rate of regional disease control.[24] As a result, the value of CLND in routine practice remains unclear, with nodal basin ultrasound surveillance preferred for patients without clinically positive nodes.[8] However, SLNB results are important for accurate staging and aid in the decision to offer adjuvant treatment.[22]

One of the most important aspects of surgical management for cutaneous melanoma is patient follow-up. Postsurgical follow-up of patients who have had a melanoma excised is essential to monitor for undetected metastatic disease and the development of a second primary cutaneous melanoma or nonmelanoma malignancy. Scheduled screening, in addition to routine surgical follow-up, is required for any patient with a melanoma; the recommended frequency and duration depend on the stage of melanoma. The optimal duration of follow-up remains controversial. Most patients who develop recurrent disease do so within the first 5 years after treatment but late recurrences (more than 10 years after surgery) have been observed. The increased lifetime risk of developing a second primary melanoma supports lifetime dermatologic surveillance for all patients.[8]

A patient with stage III melanoma typically has lymph node involvement but intralymphatic metastases, including satellite metastases and in-transit metastases, may also occur. Satellite metastases are either clinically (visible) or pathologically (microscopic) detectable and occur within 2 cm of the primary site. In-transit metastases are defined as regional metastases that occur more than 2 cm from the original lesion and are more common in individuals with thick, ulcerated lesions.[8] Surgery may be used to manage in-transit lesions with the goal of complete resection with clear margins. Unfortunately, surgery is not always feasible and subsequent recurrence in the same extremity often occurs after initial resection of an in-transit metastasis.

The role of surgery beyond that of cure is less clear, although surgery may offer palliation for patients with isolated metastasis.[22] Brain metastases occur in up to 50% of patients with metastatic melanoma. Surgical resection, with or without radiation, has been used in select individuals. High control rates of brain metastasis have been achieved with focal radiation therapy such as linear accelerator–based stereotactic radiosurgery or gamma-knife technologies.[8] Surgical resection or bypass may also offer significant symptom relief to patients with a bowel obstruction due to metastasis. Despite the lack of controlled clinical trials, the impact of palliative surgery should be evaluated in the context of a patient's comfort and quality of life. Surgery may improve quality of life, result in long-term disease control, and extend survival in select patients with metastatic disease.[22]

Adjuvant Therapy

3 The risk of relapse and death after resection of a local or regional cutaneous melanoma is the primary determinant for the use of adjuvant therapy. Adjuvant trials have focused on patients at intermediate or high risk for recurrence.

Historically, melanoma has shown resistance to traditional treatment modalities such as radiation and chemotherapy. However,

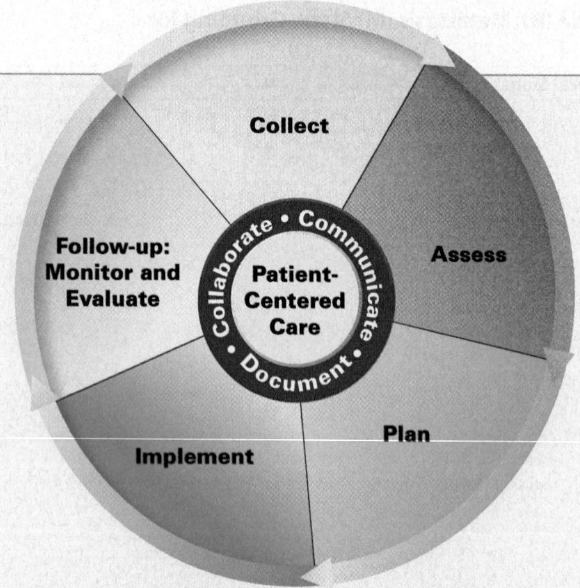

Patient Care Process for Melanoma

An illustration shows that patient centered care includes collaboration, communication, and documentation. The actions associated with the care are collect, assess, plan, implement, and follow up by monitoring and evaluating.

Collect

- Patient characteristics (eg, age, sex, physical features)
- Patient medical history (personal/family) including autoimmune diseases
- Social history (eg, history of blistering sunburns; intermittent, intense sun exposure; tanning bed use)
- Current medications including OTC products, herbal products, dietary supplements, current or past use of immunosuppressants
- Objective data
    - o Type of biopsy performed
    - o Pathology report: Breslow thickness, presence or absence of ulceration, mitotic rate
    - o Routine imaging and labs not recommended for early stage/localized disease; perform for baseline staging in stage IIIB or higher (can be considered for stage IIIA)
    - o Labs: serum creatinine (SCr), liver function (AST, ALT, total bilirubin), lactate dehydrogenase (LDH), complete blood count (CBC), thyroid function (TSH, free T4) for regional/metastatic disease

Assess

- Appropriate primary treatment (wide excision, need for sentinel lymph node biopsy)
- Status of sentinel lymph node biopsy (if performed); if positive sentinel lymph node, appropriateness of nodal basin ultrasound surveillance versus complete lymph node dissection
- Mutational analysis, if appropriate
- Presence of active autoimmune disease
- Ability/willingness to complete 1 year of adjuvant treatment, if recommended
- Ability/willingness to pay for treatment options
- Ability/willingness to obtain laboratory monitoring tests and imaging to evaluate signs and symptoms
- Emotional status (eg, presence of anxiety, depression)

Plan

- Wide excision for all stages; consider sentinel lymph node biopsy for stage IB; offer to stage II
- Adjuvant treatment with either PD-1 inhibitor or BRAF and MEK inhibitor combination for patients with fully resected stage III or stage IV disease that are appropriate for therapy
- Drug therapy regimen including specific drug(s) dose, route, frequency, and duration (see Tables 162-7 and 162-8)
- Referral to neurosurgery for treatment of brain metastases (Gamma Knife stereotactic radiosurgery; resection by craniotomy)
- Monitoring parameters including efficacy (eg, CT and brain MRI as indicated) and safety (eg, signs and symptoms of immune-related adverse events [irAEs]); frequency and timing of follow-up
- Patient education (eg, purpose of treatment, drug-specific information, proper administration/storage/handling for targeted therapies, when to seek emergency medical attention; see Tables 162-7 to 162-10)
- Referrals to other specialists when appropriate (eg, endocrinology, GI)

Implement*

- Provide patient education regarding all elements of the treatment plan
- Use motivational interviewing and coaching strategies to maximize adherence
- Schedule follow-up

Follow-up: Monitor and Evaluate

- At least annual skin examination; self-examination of skin and lymph node
- Imaging to assess signs/symptoms and/or every 3 to 12 months to screen for recurrence
- Presence of adverse drug reactions
- Patient adherence to treatment plan using multiple sources of information

**Collaborate with patient, caregivers, and other healthcare professionals.*

melanoma is considered one of the most immunogenic solid tumors and lymphocyte infiltration in the tumor suggests that immunomodulation may impact the biology of the disease. Early work with nonspecific immunomodulators, such as levamisole and Bacillus Calmette-Guérin (BCG), resulted in tumor regression but many of these responses were limited and short-lived. The use of adjuvant immunotherapy to treat these patients has been investigated to prevent distant recurrence and improve long-term survival.

CTLA-4 Inhibitor

It is well known that T cells play a crucial role in cell-mediated immunity. They are activated when the T-cell receptor (TCR) binds to its antigen in conjunction with the binding of CD28 on the T cell to the costimulatory molecule B7 on antigen-presenting cells (APCs). To prevent over activation of T cells, immune checkpoints such as CTLA-4 function as inhibitory receptors for the costimulatory molecule B7. Crosslinking of CTLA-4 by B7 inhibits T-cell activation, transcription, translation, and transduction. CTLA-4 blockade overcomes this inhibition and results in the activation and proliferation of T cells.[11] Ipilimumab, a monoclonal antibody against CTLA-4, has efficacy in both the adjuvant and metastatic setting in the treatment of melanoma. The EORTC 18071 trial evaluated 475 patients treated with high-dose ipilimumab as compared to placebo in the adjuvant setting. Median recurrence-free survival was longer in patients treated with high-dose ipilimumab as compared with placebo (26.1 vs 17.1 months). Long-term data demonstrated significantly higher 5-year recurrence-free and overall survival with adjuvant ipilimumab as compared to placebo.[25]

However, these results did not come without toxicity. CTLA-4 inhibitors produce immune-related adverse events (irAEs) that are distinct and different from adverse drug reactions associated with conventional cancer treatments (see Table 162-6). irAEs are the result of the activation of self-reactive T cells. The incidence of irAEs with the high-dose ipilimumab in EORTC 18071 was 90% and up to 55% of patients experienced grade 3 or 4 irAEs.[25] The most common serious irAEs observed in the EORTC 18071 adjuvant trial were autoimmune colitis and autoimmune hepatitis. Autoimmune endocrinopathies occurred at a higher frequency than in the metastatic disease trials. irAEs led to treatment discontinuation in 52% of patients treated with ipilimumab. Of concern, five deaths were attributed to adverse drug reactions.[25]

TABLE 162-6 Management of Immune-Related Adverse Effects (irAEs)

Organ Toxicity	Signs/Symptoms	Management	Comments
Skin and Mucosa	Pruritus, rash, desquamation, mucositis	Grade 1 Topical corticosteroids (betamethasone 0.1%) Urea-based creams Oral antipruritic as needed (diphenhydramine or hydroxyzine) Grade 2 Moderate-high potency topical corticosteroids If unresponsive to topical, consider prednisone 0.5 mg/kg/day Oral antipruritic as needed (diphenhydramine or hydroxyzine) Grade 3 or 4 Hold therapy High-potency topical corticosteroids to affected areas Prednisone 0.5-1 mg/kg/day or equivalent (increase up to 2 mg/kg/day if no improvement) Consider inpatient care	Rare cases of toxic epidermal necrosis and Stevens–Johnson syndrome have been reported. Permanent discontinuation of immunotherapy is warranted in these cases.
Gastrointestinal	Diarrhea, hematochezia, abdominal cramping, nausea, and vomiting	Grade 1 Consider holding treatment Oral hydration/electrolyte repletion Close monitoring Loperamide or diphenoxylate hydrochloride Grade 2 Hold immunotherapy Prednisone/methylprednisolone 1-2 mg/kg/day No response in 2-3 days, consider adding infliximab or vedolizumab Grade 3 or 4 Consider inpatient care Methylprednisolone 1-2 mg/kg/day No response in 1-2 days, add infliximab or vedolizumab	Infliximab 5 mg/kg IV may be given if symptoms do not improve with 48-72 hours of high-dose steroids. Bowel perforation and obstruction may occur in cases of severe colitis.
Hepatic	Transaminitis, jaundice, sclera icterus	Grade 1 Consider holding therapy Increase lab monitoring Grade 2 Hold therapy Monitor liver function tests every 3-5 days Consider prednisone 0.5-1 mg/kg/day Grade 3 Hold treatment Prednisone 1-2 mg/kg/day or equivalent No response in 1-2 days, consider adding mycophenolate Grade 4 Permanently discontinue treatment Prednisone/methylprednisolone 1-2 mg/kg/day or equivalent Inpatient care Monitor liver enzymes daily	Mycophenolate mofetil 500 mg IV/PO every 12 hours can be used in patients who do not respond to steroids within 48 hours. Avoid infliximab in hepatitis.

(continued)

TABLE 162-6 Management of Immune-Related Adverse Effects (irAEs) (*Continued*)

Organ Toxicity	Signs/Symptoms	Management	Comments
Neurologic	Muscle weakness, motor neuropathies, sensory neuropathies	Grade 1-2 Consider holding treatment Monitor Grade 3 or 4 Inpatient care Permanently discontinue treatment Methylprednisolone 1-2 mg/kg/day Prednisone if severe or progressing symptoms, consider pulse steroids methylprednisolone 1 g IV daily × 3-5 days plus IVIG or plasmapheresis	Rare case reports of Guillain–Barre' syndrome and myasthenia gravis have been reported with ipilimumab.
Endocrine	Headache, weakness, visual changes, behavioral changes, electrolyte imbalances	Grade 1 or 2 Appropriate hormone replacement therapy Endocrine consultation Grade 3 or 4 Hold therapy until acute symptoms resolve Carefully consider high-dose steroids for acute severe symptoms	Potential endocrinopathies include Addison's disease, pan-hypopituitarism, adrenal crisis, and hypophysitis. These effects may be permanent.
Ocular	Photophobia, eye dryness, blurred vision	Grade 1 or 2 Consider holding treatment Prednisolone acetate 1% topical Grade 3 or 4 Hold treatment Ophthalmic and systemic prednisone/methylprednisolone	Rare cases of episcleritis and uveitis have been reported.
Pulmonary	Dyspnea, new or worsened cough, chest pain, hemoptysis	Grade 1 Consider holding treatment Consider chest CT with contrast Grade 2 Hold treatment Consider infectious workup Prednisone 1-2 mg/kg/day or equivalent If no improvement after 2-3 days, treat as Grade 3 Grade 3 or 4 Permanently discontinue treatment Methylprednisolone 1-2 mg/kg IV then 1-2 mg/kg/day of oral prednisone or equivalent If no improvement after 2 days, consider adding infliximab, IVIG, or mycophenolate	Pneumonitis is more common with pembrolizumab and nivolumab than ipilimumab.

Data from Reference 26.

The incidence of irAEs with ipilimumab are dose related and tend to follow a pattern: skin-related toxicities typically occur after the first dose; colitis tends to occur after the second dose; and hepatitis and endocrinopathies often occur after the third or fourth dose.[27] However, irAEs can occur at any time during treatment and even after the treatment is discontinued. Their development cannot be predicted because they result from the individual's immune system and not the treatment itself. Most irAEs are reversible with treatment and resolve after 6 to 8 weeks; the exception being endocrinopathies which may require lifelong hormonal treatment. Close monitoring and early intervention are necessary for effective management of irAEs while on therapy.[8] It is recommended that patients obtain a comprehensive metabolic panel (with liver function tests), complete blood count, and thyroid function tests at baseline, throughout treatment and for up to 6 months after treatment.[26,27]

Ipilimumab therapy should be held and high-dose systemic corticosteroids initiated for grade 2 irAEs that do not improve from withholding therapy or for any grade 3 or 4 irAE. Consideration may be given to restart ipilimumab after an irAE improves to grade 0 or 1 and systemic corticosteroid dose is less than or equal to prednisone 10 mg per day. In early studies, corticosteroids were discouraged due to the theoretical risk of blunting the desired immune response. However, the efficacy of ipilimumab is not compromised when corticosteroids are given for toxicity management.[26] For patients who develop steroid-refractory irAEs, defined as no response to high-dose steroids within 48 to 72 hours of initiation, other immunosuppressive agents have been used in addition to corticosteroids. For example, infliximab and mycophenolate have been used as secondary immunosuppressants for patients who develop steroid-refractory colitis and hepatitis, respectively. Due to case reports of hepatotoxicity with infliximab, this agent should be avoided in patients with autoimmune hepatitis. Published guidelines for the treatment of irAEs are available.[26] In cases of severe or life-threatening irAEs, permanent discontinuation of ipilimumab therapy is recommended. In clinical studies reported to date, patients who experienced grade 3 or 4 autoimmune toxicities were also the most likely to exhibit tumor regression and increased time to relapse in the metastatic setting.[26]

PD-1 Inhibitors

Physiologically, the binding of PD-1 to its ligand (PD-L1 or PD-L2) results in an inhibitory signal to suppress T-cell activation, therefore preventing autoimmunity and recognition of self. However, melanoma cells can overexpress PD-L1, leading to T-cell exhaustion and the inability to mount an immune response against a tumor. Monoclonal antibodies directed against PD-1 block the binding of PD-L1, thus allowing T cells to remain stimulated.[7] PD-1 inhibitors have exhibited improved efficacy and reduced toxicity compared to ipilimumab.

Pembrolizumab and nivolumab are PD-1 inhibitors initially approved for the treatment of metastatic melanoma that have been evaluated in the adjuvant setting. Checkmate-238 was the first in a series of published adjuvant studies that changed the treatment landscape of early-stage melanoma. A total of 906 patients with high-risk stage III or stage IV melanoma who underwent complete resection were randomized to receive either ipilimumab 10 mg/kg IV every 3 weeks for four doses then every 12 weeks or nivolumab 3 mg/kg IV every 2 weeks for up to 1 year. Results showed 1-year recurrence-free survival of 70.5% with nivolumab as compared to 60.8% with ipilimumab.[28] The risk of grade 3 to 4 toxicities was significantly lower in the patients receiving nivolumab (14.4%) versus ipilimumab (45.9%). Treatment discontinuation due to an adverse drug reaction occurred in 9.7% of patients treated with nivolumab versus 42.6% of patients treated with ipilimumab.[28] With longer follow-up, nivolumab has demonstrated a sustained recurrence-free survival benefit over ipilimumab. However, fewer deaths than anticipated occurred and 4-year overall survival was similar in both groups.[29] Based on these results, nivolumab is an efficacious adjuvant treatment with less toxicity than ipilimumab.

A similar study of adjuvant pembrolizumab, Keynote-054, was conducted in patients with stage III melanoma undergoing complete resection. Patients were randomized to receive pembrolizumab 200 mg IV every 3 weeks or placebo for up to 1 year. The 1-year recurrence-free survival rate was 75.4% with pembrolizumab compared to 61.0% with placebo. Grade 3 to 4 adverse drug reactions were reported in 14.7% of patients who received pembrolizumab.[30] Based on these two studies, PD-1 inhibitors are now considered the standard of care for the adjuvant treatment of melanoma in patients with stage III disease who have undergone complete resection.[8]

With significant benefit seen in stage III melanoma, adjuvant treatment with PD-1 inhibitors has been studied in patients with high-risk stage II disease. KEYNOTE-716 was a multicenter, randomized, double-blind, placebo-controlled trial that randomized patients with fully resected stage IIB or IIC melanoma to receive either pembrolizumab 200 mg every 3 weeks or placebo for up to 1 year. At a median follow-up of 14.4 months, this study showed a significant improvement in recurrence-free survival, with a 35% reduction in risk in those who received pembrolizumab compared to placebo.[31] Although further follow-up is needed to evaluate if there is an overall survival benefit, the FDA approved pembrolizumab for the adjuvant treatment of patients with stage IIB or IIC melanoma following complete resection based on this data. This approval supports the introduction of immunotherapy, specifically PD-1 inhibitors, in the adjuvant setting due to their ability to reduce the risk of melanoma recurrence and their favorable toxicity profile.

Targeted Therapy

Mutations in BRAF, found in up to 50% of melanomas, lead to the constitutive activation of the MAPK pathway and uncontrolled cell growth/differentiation.[7] BRAF-targeted therapies have shown an improvement in survival in patients with metastatic melanoma. However, resistance eventually develops, potentially caused by mutations in MEK. The use of MEK inhibitors in combination with BRAF inhibitors delays the development of acquired resistance and increases efficacy in the metastatic setting.

For patients with early-stage melanoma and molecular mutations identified in BRAF, the combination of BRAF and MEK inhibitors has been studied in the adjuvant setting. The COMBI-AD trial investigated the use of adjuvant dabrafenib and trametinib in patients with completely resected, stage III melanoma, and the presence of a *BRAF* V600E or V600K mutation. Patients were randomized to receive dabrafenib 150 mg twice daily plus trametinib 2 mg daily or placebo for up to 1 year. The 3-year relapse-free survival rate was 58% in the dabrafenib/trametinib group and 39% in the placebo group, with a 53% lower risk of relapse at 2.8 years.[32] Overall survival was also increased in the combination arm but this did not reach statistical significance in the first interim analysis. No new or unexpected adverse drug reactions were observed in the adjuvant setting. Relapse-free survival at 5 years was 52% in patients treated with dabrafenib and trametinib versus 36% with placebo and no long-term adverse drug reactions were seen.[33] The major toxicities of BRAF and MEK inhibitor therapy will be discussed in the Treatment of Metastatic Melanoma section. Based on this data, the combination of dabrafenib and trametinib received FDA approval for adjuvant treatment in patients with stage III melanoma and the presence of a *BRAF* V600E or V600K mutation following complete resection.

Summary of Adjuvant Therapy

High-dose ipilimumab is a treatment option for patients with high-risk disease, but it has fallen out of favor because of its toxicities and has been removed from the list of recommended adjuvant treatment options in the NCCN guidelines. The treatment of choice in this setting is PD-1 inhibitors (nivolumab or pembrolizumab) or dabrafenib and trametinib for patients with BRAF V600-activating mutation due to improved efficacy and reduced toxicity.[8]

Treatment of Metastatic Melanoma

Chemotherapy and Biochemotherapy

4 Although many chemotherapy drugs show in vitro activity against melanoma, only a few have consistently shown a response rate greater than 10% in individuals with metastatic melanoma. Dacarbazine and temozolomide, the oral prodrug of the active metabolite of dacarbazine, are alkylating agents that have been studied in the treatment of metastatic melanoma. Dacarbazine is the only FDA-approved chemotherapeutic agent for treatment in this setting and once was considered the standard of care. Reported response rates with these two cytotoxic drugs are 10% to 25%, with an average duration of response of 5 to 7 months.[8] Common adverse drug reactions include myelosuppression and severe nausea and vomiting. Carboplatin in combination with paclitaxel demonstrated activity in the second-line setting.[34] Response rates of 15% to 17% were seen in trials with single-agent paclitaxel.[8] A phase III trial comparing albumin-bound paclitaxel with dacarbazine in chemotherapy-naïve melanoma patients reported an increase in progression-free survival and a trend in overall survival in patients receiving albumin-bound paclitaxel. Neuropathy and neutropenia were more common in the albumin-bound paclitaxel arm.[35] The NCCN guidelines state that these chemotherapy agents should not be routinely used because of their lack of overall survival benefit and toxicity and should only be considered for patients who are not candidates for immunotherapy or targeted therapy.[8]

To improve the low response rates with chemotherapy, the strategy of combining chemotherapy (dacarbazine, platinum agents, or vinca alkaloids) and cytokines (aldesleukin or interferon), often termed biochemotherapy, has been evaluated for the management of metastatic melanoma as well as the adjuvant setting. The primary rationale for this combination is to increase overall activity and response rates based on preclinical work suggesting potential synergistic interactions between cytokines and some chemotherapy agents. Results of clinical studies with biochemotherapy have not demonstrated a clear survival advantage and toxicities are additive and can be severe. The NCCN guidelines do not recommend biochemotherapy in the adjuvant or metastatic setting.[8]

Immunotherapy

Significant attention has been given to immunotherapy as a treatment option in metastatic melanoma due to its general resistance to traditional treatment modalities. Over the past decade, advances in immunotherapy for the treatment of melanoma have improved survival in patients with metastatic disease.

Interleukin-2 *Interleukin-2* is a glycoprotein produced by activated lymphocytes. IL-2 was first identified as a T-cell growth factor, but IL-2 is also a growth factor for various cells, including lymphocytes and natural killer (NK) cells. The precise mechanism of cytotoxicity of IL-2 is unknown. In vitro and in vivo, IL-2 stimulates the production and release of many secondary monocyte-derived and T-cell–derived cytokines, including IL-4, IL-5, IL-6, IL-8, tumor necrosis factor (TNF)-α, granulocyte-macrophage colony-stimulating factor, and IFN-γ, which may have direct or indirect antitumor activity. In addition, IL-2 stimulates the cytotoxic activities of NK cells, monocytes, lymphokine-activated killer (LAK) cells, and cytotoxic T lymphocytes (CTLs). IL-2 also activates endothelial cells, which results in increased expression of adhesion molecules.[36]

High-dose IL-2, as known as aldesleukin, was evaluated in a series of trials with objective response rates around 16%. Of significance, 6% of those patients exhibited durable complete responses (median response, 70 months).[36] Responses were seen in various metastatic sites such as the lung, liver, bone, lymph nodes, and subcutaneous tissue. The FDA-approved high-dose aldesleukin regimen for the treatment of metastatic melanoma is 600,000 IU/kg/dose every 8 hours for a maximum of 14 doses in a 5-day period given for two cycles, with a 10- to 14-day rest period between cycles. At these doses, cytokine-induced capillary leak syndrome is a common problem and often is accompanied by significant hypotension, visceral edema, dyspnea, tachycardia, and arrhythmias. Increased permeability of capillary walls allows for a fluid shift from the intravascular space into tissues. Hypotension may occur as the patient becomes intravascularly dehydrated, resulting in reflex tachycardia and arrhythmias. In addition, the decrease in blood volume may result in decreased renal blood flow, manifesting as increases in blood urea nitrogen, serum creatinine, edema, and weight gain, and a decrease in urine output (input greater than output). Visceral edema may result in pulmonary congestion, pleural effusions, and edema. The management of patients receiving high-dose aldesleukin requires extensive supportive care medications, careful monitoring, and staff trained in aspects of critical care such as hypotension management. Constitutional symptoms are a frequent complication of aldesleukin therapy and become more intense as therapy progresses. Additional adverse drug reactions of aldesleukin include pruritus, eosinophilia, bone marrow suppression, increased liver function tests, neurologic disturbances, diarrhea, and nausea.[8]

Careful patient selection for aldesleukin therapy is important. Pretreatment factors such as performance status, site of metastasis, and LDH may predict who will respond. Based on reports of long-term responses (>10 years) experienced by some patients, the benefit certainly exceeds the risk for those individuals. Unfortunately, it is difficult to determine which individuals will respond to aldesleukin therapy because no biologic or immunologic biomarkers have been found to correlate with response. The decision to treat an individual with high-dose aldesleukin should be based on an analysis of an individual patient's risk versus potential benefit. With newer agents now available on the market, and its complexity of administration, the role of aldesleukin has diminished.[8]

CTLA-4 Inhibitors (5) CTLA-4 was the first immune checkpoint identified as a target for immunotherapy and ipilimumab was the first drug in this class to demonstrate efficacy in metastatic melanoma. Results from phase I and II trials with ipilimumab demonstrate up to 20% response rates in advanced disease.[8] In a phase III trial of 676 HLA-A*0201-positive patients with refractory metastatic melanoma, ipilimumab (3 mg/kg) plus a glycoprotein 100 (gp100) peptide vaccine was compared with ipilimumab (3 mg/kg) alone or gp100 alone.[8] The median overall survival time was significantly longer in patients treated with ipilimumab, alone or combined with gp100, as compared with patients treated with gp100 alone. Another phase III trial compared a higher dose of ipilimumab (10 mg/kg) plus dacarbazine with dacarbazine alone in patients previously untreated for metastatic melanoma. Ipilimumab plus dacarbazine demonstrated significantly longer median overall survival and higher survival rates at 1 year (47.3% vs 36.3%), 2 years (28.5% vs 17.9%), and 3 years (20.8% vs 12.2%) than dacarbazine alone.[8] Based on these results, ipilimumab, dosed at 3 mg/kg IV every 3 weeks for four doses became the first FDA-approved drug for the treatment of unresectable or metastatic melanoma with a survival benefit. With longer follow-up, the survival benefit was maintained in patients who had an initial response to ipilimumab. Five-year follow-up data demonstrate survival rates of 13% to 23% with survival durations of 13 to 16 months.[37] It is also important to note that the 3-year survival mark is noteworthy for patients treated with ipilimumab. Up to 85% of the patients who were alive at 3 years were alive at 4 years, suggesting that the 3-year survival mark may be a useful surrogate endpoint.[38] After a period of time, it is felt that the balance between immune response and tumor growth can shift leading to disease relapse after an extended duration of response. Retreatment can be an option for patients who had an initial clinical benefit and has been shown to re-induce a response; no additional toxicities have been observed with re-induction.[34]

One of the greatest lessons learned from early clinical trials with ipilimumab was the difference in the kinetics of response seen with immunotherapies and how to evaluate response to treatment. Patients have no regression of disease for many weeks after treatment initiation. Even more alarming was around 10% of patients initially experienced a significant increase in tumor burden which suggested disease progression. This pseudoprogression was then followed by a delayed response to the drug after about 12 weeks of therapy; some patients continued to have a steady reduction in tumor burden over time which eventually produced a durable clinical benefit. It is hypothesized that the delayed response is related to the time needed to stimulate the immune system.[37] Due to this phenomenon, the Response Evaluation Criteria in Solid Tumors (RECIST) has developed immune-related response criteria (irRECIST) to evaluate response to immunotherapies.[39]

(6) The greatest challenge with the use of ipilimumab is the management of irAEs. Patients must be thoroughly educated on signs and symptoms of irAEs and when to seek medical attention. Clinicians should be familiar with the different types, timing, and appropriate management of irAEs (see Table 162-6). As previously discussed, management of irAEs should follow established treatment guidelines.[26]

PD-1 Inhibitors (5) As the next generation of immune checkpoint inhibitors, these agents have demonstrated response rates of up to 40% in metastatic melanoma with long-term clinical benefit seen in early phase I trials.[40] It became clear that PD-1 inhibitors have a more favorable safety profile with significantly fewer irAEs compared to ipilimumab. Additionally, clinical benefit was seen in patients who had previously been treated with ipilimumab. The KEYNOTE-001 trial evaluated the efficacy of pembrolizumab in patients who were previously treated with ipilimumab. The trial reported an overall response rate of 26%, progression-free survival of 45% at 24 weeks, and 1-year overall survival of 58%.[41] Treatment was well tolerated with grade 3 or 4 adverse events occurring in 12% of patients. In the CheckMate 037 randomized controlled trial of patients previously treated with ipilimumab, nivolumab produced higher response rates (32% vs 11%) with fewer irAEs when compared to chemotherapy.[42] An important observation from these studies is the lack of cross-resistance between ipilimumab and PD-1 inhibitors. As with ipilimumab, if patients are able to achieve a response to these agents, that response can be maintained for an extended duration. Both pembrolizumab 2 mg/kg IV every 3 weeks and nivolumab 3 mg/kg IV every 2 weeks were approved to treat patients with advanced or unresectable melanoma who progressed on previous ipilimumab therapy and, if applicable, a BRAF inhibitor. Each agent has received FDA approval for flat dosing (pembrolizumab 200 mg every 3 weeks or 400 mg every 6 weeks; nivolumab 240 mg every 2 weeks or 480 mg every 4 weeks) based on dose/exposure, efficacy, and safety data.

6 Like ipilimumab, the response to PD-1 inhibitors is delayed but the response to PD-1 inhibitors may be slightly faster than with ipilimumab. The irAE profile with PD-1 inhibitors is different, with the most common adverse drug reactions with pembrolizumab and nivolumab being fatigue, cough, nausea, pruritus, rash, decreased appetite, constipation, arthralgias, and diarrhea.[41,42] The risk of grade 3 or 4 irAEs is significantly lower as compared to ipilimumab. Specifically, the incidence of grade 3 or 4 diarrhea/colitis with PD-1 inhibitors is dramatically lower and occurs in only 1% to 2% of patients. However, a higher incidence of autoimmune pneumonitis (1%-2%) is seen with nivolumab and pembrolizumab as compared to ipilimumab.[27] Patients should be counseled to notify a clinician if they notice new or worsening cough, chest pain, or shortness of breath. Treatment of irAEs follows the same established treatment algorithms as ipilimumab (Table 162-6).

First-line therapy with PD-1 inhibitors has been evaluated to treat unresectable or metastatic melanoma. In the KEYNOTE-006 trial, pembrolizumab was compared directly to ipilimumab for first-line treatment. In this trial, 834 patients with unresectable or metastatic melanoma were randomized to receive pembrolizumab 10 mg/kg every 2 weeks or every 3 weeks or ipilimumab 3 mg/kg every 3 weeks for four doses. One-year overall survival rates were 75% for the pembrolizumab every 2 weeks, 68.4% for the pembrolizumab every 3 weeks, and 58.2% for ipilimumab.[43] Treatment-related grade 3 or 4 adverse effects were lower in both pembrolizumab arms. With better efficacy and less toxicity compared to ipilimumab, the FDA-approved pembrolizumab 2 mg/kg IV every 3 weeks as a first-line treatment option for metastatic melanoma. Similarly, in a randomized controlled trial comparing nivolumab with dacarbazine for first-line treatment of BRAF wild-type metastatic melanoma, nivolumab produced significantly better 1-year overall survival rates, median progression-free survival, and overall response rates.[44] The NCCN Guidelines recommend both pembrolizumab and nivolumab as preferred first-line treatment options for patients with unresectable or metastatic disease.[8]

Combination CTLA-4 and PD-1 Inhibitors 5 6 The combination of a CTLA-4 inhibitor, which stimulates the immune system at the central level in the priming phase of T-cell activation and proliferation, and a PD-1 inhibitor, which acts in the peripheral phase within the tumor microenvironment, can result in synergistic activity. Survival rates of 90% at 1 year and >80% at 2 years were unprecedented in the treatment of metastatic melanoma in early trials.[8] This combination was studied in the landmark Checkmate-067 trial, which included 945 previously untreated patients with unresectable stage III or IV melanoma. Patients were randomized to receive either nivolumab 3 mg/kg alone, nivolumab 1 mg/kg plus ipilimumab 3 mg/kg, or ipilimumab 3 mg/kg alone. The median progression-free survival was 11.5 months with nivolumab plus ipilimumab, compared with 6.9 months with nivolumab alone and 2.9 months with ipilimumab alone.[45] After 6.5 years of follow-up, the median overall survival with the combination is 72.1 months, 36.9 months with nivolumab alone, and 19.9 months with ipilimumab alone.[46] Of particular importance, 81% of patients who received the combination were off treatment and never received subsequent systemic therapy, highlighting the durability of treatment responses. A second trial, CheckMate-069, confirmed the benefits of this combination. In this double-blind, randomized, controlled trial, 142 untreated melanoma patients were randomized to receive ipilimumab 3 mg/kg plus nivolumab 1 mg/kg or the same dose of ipilimumab with placebo once every 3 weeks for four doses. Patients then received nivolumab (ipilimumab arm) or placebo at the same dose every 2 weeks until disease progression or unacceptable toxicity.[47] The objective response rate was 61% for patients receiving the combination versus 11% for patients receiving ipilimumab alone. Complete responses were seen in 22% of the combination arm with none in the ipilimumab arm and responses were seen regardless of *BRAF* mutational status. Median progression-free survival was significantly longer in the combination arm. As with previous studies, the responses were durable, with 82% of responding patients in the combination arm maintaining their response.[47]

One of the most significant concerns with a combination of two immune checkpoint inhibitors is the safety profile. In Checkmate-067, grade 3 or 4 treatment-related adverse drug reactions were significantly higher with the combination arm than nivolumab or ipilimumab alone.[45] Similar safety results were observed in Checkmate-069, with grade 3 or 4 drug-related adverse reactions occurring more frequently in the combination arm than ipilimumab alone.[47] As a result of the data from these two trials, the FDA granted approval for combination therapy with nivolumab 1 mg/kg plus ipilimumab 3 mg/kg every 3 weeks for four doses followed by nivolumab maintenance (240 mg every 2 weeks or 480 mg every 4 weeks) in patients with unresectable or metastatic melanoma. While this combination offers higher response rates with the potential for durable responses, judicious monitoring and aggressive management of toxicities are important.

Summary of Immune Checkpoint Inhibitors Over the last decade, advances in immunotherapy have provided new treatment options and offered new hope regarding survival for patients with metastatic melanoma. These benefits are realized with single-agent or combination immune checkpoint inhibitors. Despite advances in the treatment of melanoma, several questions still surround the use of immunotherapy. First, how do we identify which patients will benefit from immunotherapy treatment? Some clinicians are hesitant to treat older patients or those with autoimmune conditions with ipilimumab because of toxicity concerns. These unique patient populations require further investigation. Second, what are the biomarkers of response to immunotherapy? Immunologic markers and other biomarkers have been investigated without success.[48] Tumors that express PD-L1, regardless of the type of cancer, have demonstrated higher responses to PD-1/PD-L1 blockade. However, patients with tumors that do not express PD-1/PD-L1 may also benefit and should not be excluded from this treatment option. In addition, it remains unclear as to the best approach for assessing PD-L1 expression, definition of positivity in the assay, and clinical application.[40] Lastly, what is the optimal sequencing of systemic therapy with immunotherapy and targeted therapy? A recent study (DREAMseq) evaluated the sequencing of initial treatment with combination immunotherapy versus combination targeted therapy. Patients with untreated *BRAF* V600-mutant metastatic melanoma were randomized to receive initial therapy with nivolumab and ipilimumab or dabrafenib and trametinib; patients were crossed over to the alternate combination at progression. Initial overall response rates were similar at 46% with nivolumab and ipilimumab versus 43% with dabrafenib and trametinib. However, 88% of patients who responded to nivolumab and ipilimumab remained in response compared to 49% of those who responded to dabrafenib and trametinib. In addition, response rates to nivolumab and ipilimumab were lower in the second-line setting, which suggests that combination immunotherapy is less effective after progression on dabrafenib and trametinib. A meaningful difference in overall survival was observed. At a median follow-up of 27.7 months, overall survival for the nivolumab and ipilimumab group was 72% compared to 52% for dabrafenib and trametinib, a 20% absolute difference in survival.[49] These results suggest that the combination of nivolumab and ipilimumab is preferred as initial therapy over BRAF and MEK inhibitor combination therapy.

Other Immunotherapy Approaches Vaccine therapy has been investigated for over a decade in metastatic melanoma. The rationale for vaccination is that antigens expressed on the surface of tumor cells differ from normal cells and a vaccine has the ability to induce effective tumor-specific immune responses with less toxicity than conventional chemotherapy or other immunotherapies.

A variety of melanoma vaccines, based on whole tumor cells, peptides, and proteins have been evaluated to treat patients with metastatic disease or intermediate-risk and high-risk patients following surgical resection. To date, no vaccine has shown a survival advantage.[11] Occasional clinical responses have been observed in trials of melanoma vaccines. Vaccines in combination with other biologic therapies have been evaluated. Although early efficacy signals have been seen with some combination approaches, none have improved survival.[11] Clinical trials that incorporate vaccines into approved immunotherapeutic treatments are ongoing.

Oncolytic immunotherapy has been investigated for the treatment of metastatic melanoma. Talimogene laherparepvec (T-VEC) is a genetically modified oncolytic virus derived from herpes simplex-1. T-VEC works by two distinct mechanisms: (1) modification of attenuated HSV-1 to selectively replicate within tumor cells causing death while sparing other cells and (2) secretion of GM-CSF to attract dendritic cells to the site for antigen presentation and T-cell activation. Activated T cells can then target the cancer cells systemically. In a phase III study, T-VEC demonstrated better response rates (including complete responses) and a trend toward improved survival compared to GM-CSF alone.[50] It was well tolerated with fatigue, chills, and fever being the most common adverse drug reactions with few severe events reported. T-VEC is FDA-approved for the local treatment of unresectable cutaneous, subcutaneous, and nodal lesions in patients with recurrent melanoma after initial surgery. T-VEC is administered intratumorally (injected directly into the tumor) and therefore patients with internal visceral disease are not appropriate candidates for treatment. With its favorable toxicity profile, T-VEC has been studied in combination with other immunotherapies. Masterkey-265 was a phase III, randomized, double-blind study evaluating the use of TVEC plus pembrolizumab versus pembrolizumab alone in unresectable or metastatic melanoma. Unfortunately, the combination did not significantly improve progression-free or overall survival, indicating that TVEC did not add any additional benefit to PD-1 inhibitor monotherapy.[51]

Targeted Therapy

7 Oral kinase inhibitors have emerged as standard therapy for malignancies such as renal cell carcinoma, chronic myelogenous leukemia, subsets of lung cancer, and gastrointestinal stromal tumors. As our understanding of the biology of melanoma grows, there is increasing interest in developing therapies against molecular targets involved in the development and progression of melanoma. Several orally administered targeted therapies are FDA-approved to treat melanoma (see Tables 162-7 and 162-8).

Vemurafenib was the first BRAF inhibitor developed to treat patients with metastatic melanoma who harbor a V600E mutation. In a phase III trial comparing vemurafenib with dacarbazine in patients with unresectable, previously untreated stage IIIC or IV melanoma with a *BRAF* V600E mutation, vemurafenib significantly improved response rate and overall survival. Patients treated with vemurafenib had longer median progression-free survival and a higher overall survival rate at 6 months. The median time-to-response was also shorter with vemurafenib than dacarbazine.[8]

Dabrafenib, another oral selective BRAF inhibitor, demonstrated similar activity to vemurafenib in early-stage clinical trials in patients with previously untreated *BRAF* V6000E mutated melanoma. In a phase III study, dabrafenib was compared to dacarbazine in patients with untreated stage IV or unresectable stage III melanoma. Patients in the dabrafenib arm had longer median progression-free survival. A follow-up analysis showed that overall survival at 12 months was 70% with dabrafenib as compared to 63% with dacarbazine.[8] Both vemurafenib and dabrafenib have been studied in melanoma patients with CNS metastasis with some activity. Other targeted agents, such as the pan-RAF inhibitor sorafenib, have historically been studied in this setting without encouraging results.[8]

BRAF inhibitors are generally well tolerated (see Table 162-9). Skin complications, comprising of cutaneous squamous cell carcinoma or keratoacanthoma and photosensitivity reactions, are a major concern with the use of these agents. In clinical trials, the incidence of cutaneous squamous cell carcinoma or keratoacanthoma with vemurafenib was 18% and 6% with dabrafenib. The development of these lesions result from the activation of the MAPK pathway in healthy skin cells lacking *BRAF* alterations. As a result, patients receiving a BRAF inhibitor should have dermatologic evaluations prior to starting therapy, every 2 months while on therapy and for up to 6 months following discontinuation of therapy. Cutaneous complications can be effectively managed by surgical resection and treatment with the BRAF inhibitor can continue without dose adjustment.[52]

Resistance to BRAF inhibitors is potentially caused by mutations in *MEK*, dependency on MEK/ERK antiapoptotic signaling, PI3K/AKT pathway involvement, *NRAS* mutation, or MAPK pathway reactivation. Concurrent treatment with an MEK inhibitor in combination with a BRAF inhibitor can delay the onset of acquired resistance.

7 MEK inhibitors have been studied in the treatment of metastatic melanoma and have shown modest activity as monotherapy. Trametinib is an oral small-molecule inhibitor of MEK1/2 that was studied in a phase III trial that compared trametinib to chemotherapy (dacarbazine or paclitaxel). In this trial, median progression-free survival was 4.8 versus 1.5 months in the trametinib and chemotherapy arms, respectively. Overall survival at 6 months was 81% for trametinib and 67% for chemotherapy, even with crossover at progression. Common adverse drug reactions seen with trametinib were rash, diarrhea, and peripheral edema (see Table 162-10). Interestingly, secondary skin neoplasms were not observed in this trial.[8]

In addition to delaying drug resistance, the combination of BRAF and MEK inhibitors shows additive efficacy in the treatment of melanoma. The combination of trametinib 2 mg orally once daily and dabrafenib 150 mg orally twice daily received accelerated approval for treatment in patients with unresectable or metastatic melanoma with *BRAF* V600 mutations based on higher objective response rates compared to either agent alone. Additional trials with this combination compared to BRAF inhibitors in the same patient population confirmed early findings and led to a full FDA approval. In a clinical trial that compared the combination to dabrafenib alone, patients randomized to the combination had longer median progression-free survival, overall survival at 6 months and higher overall response rates as compared with dabrafenib alone.[53] In another phase III trial, the combination of dabrafenib and trametinib showed significantly longer median overall survival and higher overall survival at 12 months. Median progression-free survival was also significantly longer and the overall response rate was higher in patients treated with the combination.[54] The safety profile with the combination was similar to that observed with either drug given alone, with the notable exception of decreased incidence of skin complications in the combination arms.

Cobimetinib is another inhibitor of MEK1/2 approved in combination with vemurafenib to treat patients with unresectable or metastatic melanoma with a *BRAF* V600E or V600K mutation. The recommended dosing with this regimen is vemurafenib 960 mg orally twice daily on days 1 to 28 and cobimetinib 60 mg orally once daily on days 1 to 21 of a 28-day cycle. In a phase III trial, median

TABLE 162-7 Dosing of BRAF Inhibitors in Melanoma

Drug	Brand Name	Dose	Dose Reductions for Adverse Drug Reactions	Food-Drug Interaction	Drug-Drug Interactions
Dabrafenib	Tafinlar	• 150 mg BID • Missed dose may be taken up to 6 hours prior to next dose	• First: 100 mg BID • Second: 75 mg BID • Third: 50 mg BID • Subsequent: permanently discontinue if unable to tolerate 50 mg BID	• Take at least 1 hour before or 2 hours after a meal • High-fat meals decrease C_{max} and AUC	• Dabrafenib may decrease drug levels of CYP2B6, CYP2C19, CYP2C8, CYP2C9, and CYP3A4 substrates • Strong CYP2C8 and CYP3A4 inhibitors may increase dabrafenib concentrations • Concurrent use with antacids, H2-antagonists, and proton pump inhibitors may decrease dabrafenib concentrations • Concurrent use with St. John's wort may decrease dabrafenib concentrations • Monitor closely if dabrafenib is used concurrently with other drugs known to prolong QT interval
Encorafenib	Braftovi	• 450 mg daily • Missed dose may be taken up to 12 hours prior to next dose	• First: 300 mg daily • Second: 200 mg daily • Subsequent: permanently discontinue if unable to tolerate 200 mg daily	• Take with or without food • Avoid grapefruit juice	• Strong and moderate CYP3A4 inhibitors may increase encorafenib concentrations • Reduce encorafenib dose to one-third original dose if used concurrently with strong CYP3A4 inhibitor • Reduce encorafenib dose to one-half original dose is used concurrently with moderate CYP3A4 inhibitor • Strong or moderate CYP3A4 inducers may decrease encorafenib concentrations • Encorafenib may increase toxicity or decrease efficacy of sensitive CYP3A4 substrates • Coadministration with hormonal contraceptives can result in decreased concentrations and loss of efficacy • Avoid coadministration of encorafenib with other drugs known to prolong QTc interval
Vemurafenib	Zelboraf	• 960 mg BID • Missed dose may be taken up to 4 hours prior to next dose	• First: 720 mg BID • Second: 480 mg BID • Subsequent: permanently discontinue if unable to tolerate 480 mg BID	• Take with or without food • Avoid grapefruit juice	• Avoid concomitant administration with CYP1A2 substrates with a narrow therapeutic window • Strong CYP3A4 inhibitors/inducers may increase/decrease vemurafenib concentrations and should be avoided • Vemurafenib may increase concentrations of CYP2D6 substrates • Avoid concurrent use with P-gp substrates known to have narrow therapeutic indices • Monitor closely if vemurafenib is used concurrently with other drugs known to prolong QT interval

AUC, area under the curve; CYP, cytochrome P450.

TABLE 162-8 Dosing of MEK Inhibitors in Melanoma

Drug	Brand Name	Dose	Dose Reductions for Adverse Drug Reactions	Food-Drug Interactions	Drug-Drug Interactions
Binimetinib	Mektovi	• 45 mg BID • Missed dose may be taken up to 6 hours prior to the next dose	• First: 30 mg BID • Subsequent: permanently discontinue if unable to tolerate 30 mg BID	• Take with or without food	• No known significant interactions
Cobimetinib	Cotellic	• 60 mg daily on days 1-21 of 28-day cycle	• First: 40 mg daily • Second: 20 mg daily • Subsequent: permanently discontinue if unable to tolerate 20 mg daily	• Take with or without food	• CYP3A4 inducers may decrease cobimetenib concentrations • CYP3A4 inhibitors may increase cobimetenib concentrations
Trametinib	Mekinist	• 2 mg daily • Store in the refrigerator (36-46°F [2-8°C]) • Missed dose may be taken up to 12 hours prior to the next dose	• First: 1.5 mg daily • Second: 1 mg daily • Permanently discontinue if unable to tolerate 1 mg daily	• Take at least 1 hour before or 2 hours after a meal • High-fat meals may decrease AUC	• May enhance the adverse effects of dabrafenib

AUC, area under the curve; CYP, cytochrome P450.

TABLE 162-9 Monitoring of BRAF Inhibitors in Melanoma

Drug	Adverse Drug Reactions: Common	Adverse Drug Reactions: Rare but Serious	Monitoring Parameters	Comments
Dabrafenib	• Pyrexia • Rash • Chills • Headache • Arthralgia • Fatigue • Hyperkeratosis • Nausea/vomiting/diarrhea • Alopecia • Palmar-plantar erythrodysesthesia • Increased LFTs • Hyperglycemia • Hypophosphatemia	• New primary malignancies (cutaneous and noncutaneous) • Hemorrhage • Uveitis • Pancreatitis • Interstitial nephritis	• CMP including serum phosphorus, albumin, glucose, and LFTs • CBC for myelosuppression • Dermatologic examinations at baseline, every 2 months during treatment, then 6 months after discontinuation for secondary skin malignancies • ECG for QT prolongation • Signs/symptoms of uveitis (vision changes, photophobia, eye pain)	• Risk of secondary skin malignancies decreases when used in combination with MEK inhibitor • ECHO to assess LVEF when used in combination with MEK inhibitor • Patients with G6PD deficiency are at risk for hemolytic anemia
Encorafenib	• Fatigue • Nausea/vomiting • Abdominal pain • Arthralgia • Rash • Myopathy • Hyperkeratosis • Headache • Anemia • Increased LFTs • Pyrexia	• New primary malignancies (cutaneous and noncutaneous) • Hemorrhage • Uveitis • QTc prolongation	• Dermatologic evaluation prior to, while on therapy, and following discontinuation of treatment • CMP including serum phosphorus, magnesium, glucose, and LFTs • ECG for QT prolongation; electrolytes before and during treatment • Signs/symptoms of uveitis (vision changes, photophobia, eye pain)	• Only FDA-approved in combination with binimetinib • If binimetinib is held, the encorafenib dose must be reduced to 300 mg daily
Vemurafenib	• Arthralgia • Rash • Alopecia • Fatigue • Nausea • Photosensitivity • Pruritus • Skin papilloma	• New primary malignancies (cutaneous and noncutaneous) • Uveitis • QTc prolongation • Severe dermatologic reactions (SJS, TEN) • Hypersensitivity reactions (including DRESS) • Renal failure	• LFTs at baseline and monthly or as clinically indicated • Serum creatinine at baseline and periodically during treatment • ECG and electrolytes (including potassium, magnesium, and calcium) at baseline, after 15 days, monthly for the first 3 months, then every 3 months or as clinically indicated • Dermatologic examinations at baseline, every 2 months during treatment. Consider monitoring for 6 months following discontinuation • Signs/symptoms of uveitis (vision changes, photophobia, eye pain) • Monitor closely if administered concomitantly or sequentially with radiation treatment	• Off-label indication for *BRAF* V600K mutation • Associated with rare cases of pancreatitis; evaluate unexplained abdominal pain • Due to photosensitivity, patients should avoid the sun, wear protective clothing, and wear sunscreen

CMP, comprehensive metabolic panel; CBC, complete blood count; CPK, creatine phosphokinase; DVT, deep vein thrombosis; DRESS, drug reaction with eosinophilia and systemic symptoms; LFTs, liver function tests; LVEF, left ventricular function; PE, pulmonary embolism.

TABLE 162-10 Monitoring of MEK Inhibitors in Melanoma

Drug	Adverse Drug Reactions: Common	Adverse Drug Reactions: Rare but Serious	Monitoring Parameters	Comments
Binimetinib	• Fatigue • Nausea/vomiting • Abdominal pain • Diarrhea • Constipation • Rash • Increased LFTs • Anemia • Increased creatinine • Increased CPK • Hyponatremia	• VTE • Cardiomyopathy • Ocular toxicity (serous retinopathy/retinal pigment epithelial detachments, retinal vein occlusion) • Interstitial lung disease/pneumonitis • New primary malignancies (cutaneous and noncutaneous) • Hemorrhage • Rhabdomyolysis	• LFTs at baseline, monthly during treatment, and as clinically indicated • CPK and serum creatinine at baseline, periodically during treatment, and as clinically indicated • Assess for visual symptoms at each visit. Perform ophthalmologic examination at regular intervals and for any new/worsening visual disturbances • Signs and symptoms of bleeding • LVEF at baseline, 1 month after therapy initiation, then at 2- to 3-month intervals for cardiomyopathy • Evaluate for signs/symptoms of pulmonary toxicity (cough, dyspnea, hypoxia, pleural effusions, infiltrates)	• If encorafenib is permanently discontinued, discontinue binimetinib • Serous retinopathy occurred in 20% of patients treated with binimetinib in combination with encorafenib • Elevation in LFTs can occur with combination; monitor prior to beginning treatment and monthly during treatment

(continued)

TABLE 162-10 Monitoring of MEK Inhibitors in Melanoma (*Continued*)

Drug	Adverse Drug Reactions: Common	Adverse Drug Reactions: Rare but Serious	Monitoring Parameters	Comments
Cobimetinib	• Nausea/vomiting • Diarrhea • Hypertension • Photosensitivity • Pyrexia • Hypophosphatemia • Electrolyte disturbances • Hypoalbuminemia • Lymphopenia • Anemia • Increased LFTs • Increased CPK • Increase in serum creatinine • Hyponatremia	• Cardiomyopathy • Hemorrhage • New primary malignancies (cutaneous and noncutaneous) • Ocular toxicity (serous retinopathy, retinal vein occlusion • Hepatotoxicity • Rhabdomyolysis	• CMP at baseline and monthly during treatment for hepatotoxicity, renal failure, and electrolyte replacement • CPK at baseline, periodically during treatment, and as clinically indicated • LVEF at baseline, 1 month after initiation of therapy, and every 3 months until discontinuation • Dermatologic examinations at baseline, every 2 months during treatment, then 6 months after discontinuation for secondary skin malignancies • Ophthalmological evaluation at regular intervals and at any sign of new or worsening visual disturbances • Signs and symptoms of hemorrhage and rhabdomyolysis	• Due to photosensitivity, patients should avoid the sun, wear protective clothing, and wear sunscreen • Hypertension has been seen in combination with vemurafenib
Trametinib	• Dermatologic toxicity (rash, acneiform dermatitis, palmar-plantar erythrodysesthesia, erythema) • Diarrhea • Lymphedema (including edema, peripheral edema) • Pyrexia • Hypertension • Fatigue • Nausea/vomiting • Hyperglycemia • Increased LFTs • Anemia • Hypoalbuminemia	• VTE • Cardiomyopathy • Ocular toxicity (retinal pigment epithelial detachments, retinal vein occlusion) • Interstitial lung disease/pneumonitis • New primary malignancies (cutaneous and noncutaneous) • Hemorrhage • Colitis/GI perforation • Rhabdomyolysis	• CBC and CMP at baseline and as clinically indicated • LVEF at baseline, 1 month after therapy initiation, then at 2- to 3-month intervals • Ophthalmological evaluation periodically and at any sign of visual disturbance • Evaluate for signs/symptoms of pulmonary toxicity (cough, dyspnea, hypoxia, pleural effusions, infiltrates) • Blood pressure • Signs and symptoms of bleeding • Dermatologic examinations at baseline, every 2 months during treatment, then 6 months after discontinuation • Monitor closely for colitis and GI perforation	• Severe skin toxicities can require hospitalization • Intracranial hemorrhage can be fatal • Many adverse effects are increased when trametinib is used in combination with dabrafenib • Increased incidence of DVT/PE when used in combination with dabrafenib • Increase in serious febrile reactions when used in combination with dabrafenib

CMP, comprehensive metabolic panel; CBC, complete blood count; CPK, creatine phosphokinase; DVT, deep vein thrombosis; DRESS, drug reaction with eosinophilia and systemic symptoms; LFTs, liver function tests; LVEF, left ventricular function; PE, pulmonary embolism; VTE, venous thromboembolism.

progression-free survival was significantly improved with the combined regimen of cobimetinib and vemurafenib versus vemurafenib alone. The difference in median overall survival was also statistically significant in favor of the combination. Overall response rates were 70% and 50% for the combination and single-agent arms, respectively. Adverse drug reactions were similar across the two groups and similar to the other MEK and BRAF combination, the number of secondary cutaneous cancer was decreased.[55]

The safety and efficacy of encorafenib and binimetinib, a BRAF and MEK inhibitor combination, were established in the COLUMBUS trial, a phase III study where 577 patients were randomized to receive encorafenib 450 mg daily plus binimetinib 45 mg twice daily, encorafenib 300 mg daily, or vemurafenib 960 mg twice daily. Median progression-free survival was significantly longer with the combination as compared with vemurafenib alone. The overall response rate was higher with encorafenib and binimetinib as compared to BRAF inhibitor monotherapy. The median overall survival was 33.6 months for the combination of encorafenib and binimetinib as compared to 16.9 months with vemurafenib. This is the longest overall survival observed of all studies conducted with combination BRAF and MEK inhibitors. The adverse drug reactions seen with encorafenib and binimetinib are similar to those of other BRAF and MEK inhibitor combinations.[56]

Another agent of interest in the treatment of metastatic melanoma is imatinib mesylate, an oral agent that inhibits *KIT* and platelet-derived growth factor receptor. *KIT* is expressed primarily in acral and mucosal melanomas and treatment with imatinib showed activity against melanoma cell growth in preclinical studies. In clinical trials with unselected patients, imatinib did not show benefit in metastatic melanoma despite downregulation of phosphorylated *KIT*.[8] However, a phase II trial of imatinib in patients with *KIT* mutations reported that 23% had a partial response, 30% had stable disease, and progression-free survival was 3.5 months.[8] Responses in these patients were short, similar to what is seen with BRAF inhibitor monotherapy. Other potential molecular targets in the treatment of melanoma include vascular endothelial growth factor and cyclin-dependent kinases. Studies with drugs that inhibit these pathways are ongoing.

Combination Targeted Therapy Plus Immunotherapy

With the success of both immunotherapy and targeted therapy, combining agents from both classes is another area of great interest and ongoing research interest. Studies combining ipilimumab with BRAF inhibitors have been conducted but are associated with significant toxicity. A phase I trial combining vemurafenib and ipilimumab showed high rates of hepatotoxicity while case reports of dabrafenib/trametinib plus ipilimumab resulted in severe gastrointestinal toxicity, specifically perforation. Based on these results, the use of targeted therapy in combination with ipilimumab is not recommended.[8]

The combination of BRAF and MEK inhibitors plus other immune checkpoint inhibitors has shown promising results in the treatment of metastatic melanoma. IMspire150, a Phase III, double-blind study, randomized 514 patients with untreated *BRAF* V600-mutated metastatic melanoma to receive combination BRAF and MEK inhibitors (vemurafenib and cobimetinib) and either atezolizumab or placebo. At a median follow-up of 18.9 months, the median progression-free survival was significantly longer in patients treated with combination BRAF and MEK inhibitors and atezolizumab versus combination BRAF and MEK inhibitors alone (15.1 vs 10.6 months). Common treatment-related adverse drug reactions that occurred more frequently in the atezolizumab arm were increased blood creatinine phosphokinase, pyrexia, arthralgia, myalgia, increased liver enzymes and bilirubin, hyper/hypothyroidism, pneumonitis, pruritus, and peripheral edema.[57] Based on this study, the combination of vemurafenib, cobimetinib, and atezolizumab was FDA-approved for the treatment of patients with *BRAF* V600 mutation-positive unresectable or metastatic melanoma and is also recommended per the NCCN guidelines in this treatment setting.[8] The dosing for this regimen includes a run-in period with vemurafenib 960 mg by mouth twice daily for 21 days then 720 mg twice daily thereafter plus cobimetinib 60 mg daily days 1 to 21 every 28 days in addition to atezolizumab 840 mg IV every 2 weeks. Another BRAF and MEK inhibitor combination (dabrafenib and trametinib) has also been studied in combination with immunotherapy. Keynote-022 was a double-blind, phase II study evaluating the use of dabrafenib and trametinib and either pembrolizumab or placebo for patients with untreated *BRAF* V600-mutated advanced melanoma. This study showed that at 36.6 months of follow-up, the addition of immunotherapy to combination BRAF and MEK inhibitor therapy substantially improved progression-free survival, duration of response, and overall survival but with a higher incidence of treatment-related adverse drug reactions. These results show the importance of careful patient selection to identify the best candidates for combined modality therapy.[58]

Radiation

The role of radiation in the adjuvant treatment of melanoma has been investigated. Recent data from a prospective study suggest patients treated with therapeutic lymphadenectomy for lymph node relapse benefit from postoperative radiation to the nodal basins as compared to observation. Lymph node recurrence was significantly less in the adjuvant radiation arm, but increased toxicity was noted. No difference in overall survival or relapse-free survival was observed between the groups.[59] Adjuvant radiation may be an acceptable option for selected patients. Radiation can also be used in patients with in-transit metastasis, satellite metastasis, or for extranodal tumor extension. For patients with metastatic melanoma, radiation is palliative to symptomatic areas of disease progression. Stereotactic radiosurgery (SRS), or stereotactic radiotherapy (SRT), is the preferred type of treatment for brain metastases. Adjuvant radiation, given after resection of brain metastases, can help with disease control. Whole brain radiation is associated with worse cognitive decline compared to SRS/SRT, and therefore should be used in situations when SRS/SRT is not achievable.[60] Whole brain radiation may be needed in situations that involve numerous brain metastasis or leptomeningeal disease.

Limb Perfusion and Limb Infusion

Isolated limb perfusion is a surgical procedure involving regional intravascular delivery of chemotherapy or biotherapy (or both) into an extremity with cutaneous melanoma. When in-transit metastases occurs in extremities, local therapy with isolated limb perfusion or isolated limb infusion has been used.[8] Isolated limb perfusion is a method for escalating the dose of chemotherapeutic drugs to a specific region of the body while limiting the systemic toxicities of the agent. Most perfusions can be performed with drug exposures of less than 2%. The most significant adverse drug reaction of isolated limb perfusion is regional toxicity because the skin, subcutaneous tissue, and tissue of the extremity receives the same dose and is subjected to the same perfusion conditions as the tumor located within the extremity. After regional perfusions, objective response rates greater than 50% in treated limbs have been reported, with overall response rates possibly as high as 80%. Although most clinical trials have used melphalan, it is not known whether the combination of melphalan with other agents may improve results.[8] This is also a technically complex procedure that should only be performed at centers with the proper clinical expertise. A simplified form of isolated limb perfusion, called isolated limb infusion, is a low-flow isolated limb perfusion performed under hypoxic conditions via small-caliber arterial and venous catheters. It has been proposed that the hypoxia which develops during isolated limb infusion may be beneficial with certain cytotoxic agents such as melphalan.[8]

EVALUATION OF THERAPEUTIC OUTCOMES

The outcome of patients treated with melanoma depends on the stage of disease at presentation. The prognosis of patients with thin tumors (less than 1 mm in thickness) and localized disease is good with long-term survival in more than 90% of patients. The risk of regional nodal involvement rises with increasing tumor thickness and survival rates decrease in patients with nodal involvement. Long-term survival in patients with distant metastasis is even lower. Therefore, early diagnosis and appropriate treatment of early disease are essential. Patients with suspicious pigmented lesions should be evaluated and the lesion excised whenever possible. Treatment is determined by patient factors and stage of disease.

Clinical practice guidelines published by the NCCN and European Society of Clinical Oncology (ESMO) provide guidance for treatment and follow-up of patients with melanoma.[8,61] Intensive surveillance has the benefit of early detection of recurrent disease, which may lead to better options for surgical resection. Emphasis on the evaluation of locoregional areas is important. For patients with in situ melanoma, periodic skin examinations for life are recommended, with frequency determined based on patient risk factors. Local recurrence is associated with aggressive tumor biology and frequently is a manifestation of an aggressive primary tumor. If a local recurrence occurs after inadequate primary disease management, the patient should undergo a workup based on the lesion thickness of the original melanoma. Patients with nodal recurrence should be evaluated for lymph node metastasis. Patients with systemic recurrence should be evaluated and treated similarly to patients presenting with systemic disease.

CONCLUSION

Treatment of cutaneous melanoma is determined by both disease-related and patient-related issues. Treatment recommendations are based on stage of disease. Treatment of localized disease is surgical excision, with the extent of excision based on the tumor size. Wide excision is recommended for in situ melanoma and wide excision with SLNB for stage IA, IB, and II disease.

The addition of new immunotherapy and targeted agents has increased the number of adjuvant treatment options for patients with melanoma who are at high risk of recurrence. Identifying which patients are appropriate candidates for treatment after resection of the primary tumor remains a challenge. When choosing an adjuvant treatment, the clinician should consider patient preference, age, comorbidities, and risk of recurrence.[8]

(8) Due to the rapid influx of effective therapies, the management of metastatic melanoma has become complex. The NCCN guidelines list a variety of preferred systemic therapies for advanced or metastatic melanoma, including ipilimumab/nivolumab, pembrolizumab, nivolumab, combination BRAF and MEK inhibitors, triple therapy with BRAF and MEK inhibitors plus PD-1 (or PD-L1) inhibitor, ipilimumab, high-dose aldesleukin, and in certain cases chemotherapy or other targeted agents.[8] The choice of drug therapy should be based on *BRAF* mutational status, the aggressiveness of the disease, and disease-related symptoms. Patients with a more indolent clinical picture may respond better to immunotherapy. Patients with a documented *BRAF* mutation are candidates for treatment with a BRAF and MEK inhibitor combination regimen. Best supportive care is also an option for some individuals. Surgical treatment of metastatic melanoma should be considered in select individuals based on the extent and location of disease and performance status.

ABBREVIATIONS

AJCC	American Joint Committee on Cancer
ALM	acral lentiginous melanoma
ARF	alternative reading frame
CSD	chronic sun damage
CTL	cytotoxic T lymphocyte
CTLA-4	cytotoxic T lymphocyte antigen 4
ECOG	Eastern Cooperative Oncology Group
EORTC	The European Organization for Research and Treatment of Cancer
ESMO	European Society of Clinical Oncology
FAMMM	familial atypical multiple mole syndrome
FDA	Food and Drug Administration
HLA	human leukocyte antigen
IL-2	interleukin-2
irAE	immune-related adverse effect
JAK	janus-kinase
LAK	lymphokine-activated killer
LDH	lactate dehydrogenase
LMM	lentigo maligna melanoma
MAPK	mitogen-activated protein kinase pathway
mTOR	mammalian target of rapamycin
NCCN	National Comprehensive Cancer Network
NK	natural killer
NMSC	nonmelanoma skin cancer
NSAID	nonsteroidal anti-inflammatory drug
PD-1	programmed death receptor 1
PD-L1	programmed death receptor 1 ligand
PET	positron emission tomography
PI3K	phosphatidylinositol-3 kinase
SLNB	sentinel lymph node biopsy
SPF	sun protection factor
SRS	stereotactic radiosurgery
SRT	stereotactic radiotherapy
SSE	skin self-examination
SSM	superficial spreading melanoma
STAT	signal-transducer-and-activator-of-transcription
TNF	tumor necrosis factor
TIL	tumor-infiltrating lymphocyte
UV	ultraviolet
UVA	ultraviolet A
UVB	ultraviolet B
VEGF	vascular endothelial growth factor

REFERENCES

1. Saginala K, Barsouk A, Aluru JS, et al. Epidemiology of melanoma. *Med Sci (Basel).* 2021;9(4):63. 10.3390/medsci9040063
2. Sung H, Ferlay J, Siegel R, et al. Global cancer statistics 2020: GLOBOCAN estimates of incidence and mortality worldwide for 36 cancers in 185 countries. *CA Cancer J Clin.* 2021;71:209–249. 10.3322/caac.21660
3. SEER Cancer Statistics Factsheets: Melanoma of the Skin. Bethesda, MD: National Cancer Institute. Available at: https://seer.cancer.gov/statfacts/html/melan.html. Accessed February 21, 2022.
4. American Cancer Society. *Cancer Facts & Figures 2022.* Atlanta, GA: American Cancer Society; 2022.
5. Siegel RL, Miller KD, Fuchs HE, Jemal A. Cancer statistics, 2022. *CA Cancer J Clin.* 2022;72;7–33. 10.3322/caac.21708
6. Saiyed FK, Hamilton EC, Austin MT. Pediatric melanoma: Incidence, treatment, and prognosis. *Pediatric Health Med Ther.* 2017;8:39–45. 10.2147/PHMT.S115534
7. Schadendof D, van Akkool ACJ, Berking C, et al. Melanoma. *Lancet.* 2018;392:971–984. 10.1016/S0140-6736(18)31559-9
8. National Comprehensive Cancer Network. NCCN Clinical Practice Guidelines in Oncology: Cutaneous Melanoma version 2.2022. Available at: http://www.nccn.org. Accessed February 21, 2022.
9. Soura S, Eliades PJ, Shannon K, et al. Hereditary melanoma: Update on syndromes and management: Emerging melanoma cancer complexes and genetic counseling. *J Am Acad Dermatol.* 2016;74:411–420. 10.1016/j.jaad.2015.08.037
10. Mitchell TC, Karakousis G, Schuchter L. Melanoma. *Ableoff's Clinical Oncology.* 6th ed. Philadelphia, PA: Elsevier, Inc.; 2020;1034–1051 e2.
11. Zhu Z, Liu W, Gotlieb V. The rapidly evolving therapies for advanced melanoma: Towards immunotherapy, molecular targeted therapy, and beyond. *Crit Rev Oncol Hematol.* 2016;99:91–99. 10.1016/j.critrevonc.2015.12.002
12. Lane AM, Kim IK, Gragoudas ES. Survival rates in patients after treatment for metastasis from uveal melanoma. *JAMA Ophthalmol.* 2018;136:981–986. 10.1001/jamaophthalmol.2018.2466
13. U.S. Department of Health and Human Services. *The Surgeon General's Call to Action to Prevent Skin Cancer.* Washington, DC: U.S. Dept of Health and Human Services, Office of the Surgeon General; 2014.
14. Ogden N. General and plastic surgery devices: Reclassification of ultraviolet lamps for tanning, henceforth to be known as sunlamp products and ultraviolet lamps intended for use in sunlamp products. Available at: https://www.federalregister.gov/articles/2014/06/02/2014-12546/general-and-plastic-surgery-devices-reclassification-of-ultraviolet-lamps-for-tanning-henceforth-to. Accessed February 21, 2022.
15. Department of Health and Human Services, Food and Drug Administration 21 CFR Parts 201 and 310, labeling and effectiveness testing; sunscreen drug products for over-the-counter human use. Available at: https://www.gpo.gov/fdsys/pkg/FR-2011-06-17/pdf/2011-14766.pdf. Accessed February 21, 2022.
16. Gershenwald JE, Scolyer RA. Melanoma staging: American Joint Committee on Cancer (AJCC) 8th edition and beyond. *Ann Surg Oncol.* 2018;25:2105–2010. 10.1245/s10434-018-6513-7
17. Gershenwald JE, Scolyer RA, Hess KR. Melanoma Staging: Evidence-Based Changes in the American Joint Committee on Cancer Eighth Edition Cancer Staging Manual. *CA Cancer J Clin.* 2017;67:472–492.
18. Wong SL, Farles MB, Kennedy EB, et al. Sentinel lymph node biopsy and management of regional lymph nodes in melanoma: American Society of Clinical Oncology and Society of Surgical Oncology clinical practice guideline update. *J Clin Oncol.* 2018;36:399–413. 10.1200/JCO.2017.75.7724
19. Cherobin ACFP, Wainstein AJA, Colosimo EA, Goulart EMA, Bittencourt FV. Prognostic factors for metastasis in cutaneous melanoma. *An Bras Dermatol.* 2018;93(1):19–26. 10.1590/abd1806-4841.20184779
20. National Comprehensive Cancer Network. NCCN Clinical Practice Guidelines in Oncology: Uveal Melanoma version 2.2021. Available at: http://www.nccn.org. Accessed February 21, 2022.
21. Keung EZ, Gershenwald JE. The eighth edition American Joint Committee on Cancer (AJCC) melanoma staging system: Implications for melanoma treatment and care. *Expert Rev Anticancer Ther.* 2018;18(8):775–784. 10.1080/14737140.2018.1489246
22. Joyce KM. Chapter 7: Surgical management of melanoma. In: Ward WH, Farma JM, eds. *Cutaneous Melanoma: Etiology and Therapy* [Internet]. Brisbane (AU): Codon Publications; 2017.
23. Morton DL, Thompson JF, Cochran AJ, et al. Final trial report of sentinel-node biopsy versus nodal observation in melanoma. *N Engl J Med.* 2014;370:599–609. 10.1056/NEJMoa1310460

24. Faries MB, Thompson JF, Cochran AJ, et al. Completion dissection or observation for sentinel-node metastasis in melanoma. *N Engl J Med.* 2017;376:2211–2222. 10.1056/NEJMoa1613210
25. Eggermont AMM, Chiarion-Sileni V, Grob JJ, et al. Adjuvant ipilimumab versus placebo after complete resection of high-risk stage III melanoma (EORTC 18071): A randomised, double-blind, phase 3 trial. *Lancet Oncol.* 2015;16:522–530. 10.1016/S1470-2045(15)70122-1
26. National Comprehensive Cancer Network. NCCN Clinical Practice Guidelines in Oncology: Management of Immunotherapy-Related Toxicities version 4.2021. Available at: http://www.nccn.org. Accessed February 21, 2022.
27. Weber JS, Yang JC, Atkins MB, Disis ML. Toxicities of immunotherapy for the practitioner. *J Clin Oncol.* 2015:2092–2099. 10.1200/JCO.2014.60.0379
28. Weber J, Mandala M, Del Vecchio M, et al. Adjuvant nivolumab versus ipilimumab in resected stage III or IV melanoma. *N Engl J Med.* 2017;377:1824–1835. 10.1056/NEJMoa1709030
29. Ascierto PA, Del Vecchio M, Mandalá M, et al. Adjuvant nivolumab versus ipilimumab in resected stage IIIB-C and stage IV melanoma (CheckMate 238): 4-year results from a multicentre, double-blind, randomised, controlled, phase 3 trial [published correction appears in *Lancet Oncol.* 2021 Oct;22(10):e428]. *Lancet Oncol.* 2020;21(11):1465–1477. 10.1016/S1470-2045(20)30494-0
30. Eggermont AMM, Blank CU, Mandala M, et al. Adjuvant pembrolizumab versus placebo in resected stage III melanoma. *N Engl J Med.* 2018;378:1789–1801. 10.1056/NEJMoa1802357
31. Luke JJ, Ascierto PA, Carlino MS, et al. KEYNOTE-716: Phase III study of adjuvant pembrolizumab versus placebo in resected high-risk stage II melanoma. *Future Oncol.* 2020;16(3):4429–4438. 10.2217/fon-2019-0666
32. Long GV, Hauschild A, Santinami M, et al. Adjuvant dabrafenib plus trametinib in stage III BRAF-mutated melanoma. *N Engl J Med.* 2017;377:1813–1823. 10.1056/NEJMoa1708539
33. Dummer R, Hauschild A, Santinami M, et al. Five-year analysis of adjuvant dabrafenib plus trametinib in stage III melanoma. *N Engl J Med.* 2020;383(12):1139–1148. 10.1056/NEJMoa2005493
34. Chiarion-Sileni V, Pigozzo J, Ascietro PA, et al. Ipilimumab retreatment in patients with pretreated advanced melanoma: The expanded access programme in Italy. *Br J Can.* 2014;110:1721–1726. 10.1038/bjc.2014.126
35. Hersh E, Del Vecchio M, Brown M, et al. A randomized, controlled phase III trial of nab-paclitaxel versus dacarbazine in chemotherapy-naïve patients with metastatic melanoma. *Ann Oncol.* 2015;26:2267–2274. 10.1093/annonc/mdv324
36. Sim GC, Radvanyi L. The IL-2 cytokine family in cancer immunotherapy. *Cytokine Growth Factor Rev.* 2014;25:377–390. 10.1016/j.cytogfr.2014.07.018
37. Delyon J, Maio M, Lebbé C. The ipilimumab lesson in melanoma: Achieving long-term survival. *Semin Oncol.* 2015;42:387–401. 10.1053/j.seminoncol.2015.02.005
38. McDermott D, Lebbe C, Hodi FS, et al. Durable benefit and the potential for long-term survival with immunotherapy in advanced melanoma. *Can Treat Review.* 2014;40:1056–1064. 10.1016/j.ctrv.2014.06.012
39. Seymour L, Bogaerts J, Perrone A, et al. iRECIST: Guidelines for response criteria for use in trials testing immunotherapeutics. *Lancet Oncol.* 2017;18:e143–e152. 10.1016/S1470-2045(17)30074-8
40. Postow MA, Callahan MK, Wolchok JD. Immune checkpoint blockade in cancer. *J Clin Oncol.* 2015;33:1974–1982. 10.1200/JCO.2014.59.4358
41. Ribas A, Hodi FS, Kefford R, et al. Efficacy and safety of the anti-PD-1 monoclonal antibody MK-3475 in 411 patients with melanoma. *J Clin Oncol.* 2014;32:5s.
42. Weber JS, D'Angelo SP, Minor D, et al. Nivolumab versus chemotherapy in patients with advanced melanoma who progressed after anti-CTLA-4 treatment (CheckMate 037): A randomised controlled, open-label, phase 3trial. *Lancet Oncol.* 2015;16:375–384. 10.1016/S1470-2045(15)70076-8
43. Robert C, Schachter J, Long GV, et al. Pembrolizumab versus ipilimumab in advanced melanoma. *N Engl J Med.* 2015;372:2521–2532. 10.1056/NEJMoa1503093
44. Roberts C, Long GV, Brady B, et al. Nivolumab in previously untreated melanoma without BRAF mutation. *N Engl J Med.* 2015;372:320–330. 10.1056/NEJMoa1412082
45. Larkin J, Chiarion-Sileni V, Gonzalez R, et al. Combined nivolumab and ipilimumab or monotherapy in untreated melanoma. *N Engl J Med.* 2015;373:23–34. 10.1056/NEJMoa1504030
46. Wolchok JD, Chiarion-Sileni V, Gonzalez R, et al. Long-term outcomes with nivolumab plus ipilimumab or nivolumab alone versus ipilimumab in patients with advanced melanoma. *J Clin Oncol.* 2022;40(2):127–137. 10.1200/JCO.21.02229
47. Postow MA, Chesney J, Pavlick AC, et al. Nivolumab and ipilimumab versus ipilimumab in untreated melanoma. *N Engl J Med.* 2015;372:2006–2017. 10.1056/NEJMoa1414428
48. Eggermont AMM, Maio M, Robert C. Immune checkpoint inhibitors in melanoma provide the cornerstones for curative therapies. *Semin Oncol.* 2015;42:429–435. 10.1053/j.seminoncol.2015.02.010
49. Atkins MB, Lee SJ, Chmielowski B, et al. DREAMseq: A phase III trial—ECOG-ACRIN EA6134. *ASCO Plenary Series.* Abstract 356154. Presented November 16, 2021.
50. Andtbacka RHI, Collichio FA, Amatruda T, et al. OPTiM: A randomized phase III trial of talimogene laherparepvec versus subcutaneous granulocyte-macrophage colony-stimulating factor for the treatment of unresected stage IIIB/C and IV melanoma. *J Clin Oncol.* 2015;58:3377.
51. Long G, Dummer R, Andtbacka R, et al. Follow-up analysis of MASTERKEY-265 Phase 1b (ph1b) trial of talimogene laherparepvec (T-VEC) in combination (combo) with pembrolizumab (pembro) in patients (pts) with unresectable stage IIIB–IVM1c melanoma (MEL). *Pigment Cell Melanoma Res.* 2019;32:133–134.
52. Welsh SJ, Corrie PG. Management of BRAF and MEK inhibitor toxicities in patients with metastatic melanoma. *Ther Adv Med Oncol.* 2015;7(2):122–136. 10.1177/1758834014566428
53. Long GV, Stroyakovskiy D, Gogas H, et al. Combined BRAF and MEK inhibition versus BRAF inhibition alone in melanoma. *N Engl J Med.* 2014;371:1877–1888. 10.1056/NEJMoa1406037
54. Robert C, Karaszewska B, Schachter J, et al. Improved overall survival in melanoma with combined dabrafenib and trametinib. *N Engl J Med.* 2015;372:30–39. 10.1056/NEJMoa1412690
55. Larkin J, Ascierto B, Dreno V, et al. Combined vemurafenib and cobimetinib in BRAF-mutated melanoma. *N Engl J Med.* 2014;371:1867–1876. 10.1056/NEJMoa1408868
56. Dummer R, Ascierto PA, Gogas HJ, et al. Overall survival in patients with BRAF-mutant melanoma receiving encorafenib plus binimetinib versus vemurafenib or encorafenib (COLUMBUS): A multicentre, open-label, randomised, phase 3 trial. *Lancet Oncol.* 2018;19:1315–1327. 10.1016/S1470-2045(18)30497-2
57. Gutzmer R, Stroyakovskiy D, Gogas H, et al. Atezolizumab, vemurafenib, and cobimetinib as first-line treatment for unresectable advanced BRAFV600 mutation-positive melanoma (IMspire150): Primary analysis of the randomised, double-blind, placebo-controlled, phase 3 trial [published correction appears in *Lancet.* 2020 August 15;396(10249):466]. *Lancet.* 2020;395(10240):1835–1844. 10.1016/S0140-6736(20)30934-X
58. Ferrucci PF, Di Giacomo AM, Del Vecchio M, et al. KEYNOTE-022 part 3: A randomized, double-blind, phase 2 study of pembrolizumab, dabrafenib, and trametinib in BRAF-mutant melanoma [published correction appears in *J Immunother Cancer.* 2021 Nov;9(11):]. *J Immunother Cancer.* 2020;8(2):e001806. 10.1136/jitc-2020-001806
59. Burmeister BH, Ainslie J, et al. Adjuvant lymph-node field radiotherapy versus observation only in patients with melanoma at high risk for further lymph-node filed relapse after lymphadenectomy (ANZMTG 01.02/TROG02.01): 6-Year follow-up of a phase 3, randomised controlled trial. *Lancet Oncol.* 2015;16:1049–1060. 10.1016/S1470-2045(15)00187-4
60. Brown PD, Ballman KV, Cerhan JH, et al. Postoperative stereotactic radiosurgery compared to whole brain radio-therapy for resected metastatic brain disease: A multicenter, randomized, controlled, phase 3 trial. *Lancet Oncol.* 2017;18:1049–1060. 10.1016/S1470-2045(17)30441-2
61. Michieli O, van Akkooi ACJ, Ascierto PA, Dummer R, Keilholz U. Cutaneous melanoma: ESMO Clinical Practice Guidelines for diagnosis, treatment and follow-up. *Ann Oncol.* 2019;30:1884–1901. 10.1093/annonc/mdz411

Hematopoietic Cell Transplantation

e163

Elizabeth Dimaggio and Janelle Perkins

KEY CONCEPTS

1. Hematopoietic cell transplantation (HCT) is a procedure that involves intravenous infusion of hematopoietic stem cells from a donor into a recipient, after the administration of chemotherapy with or without radiation. The rationale is to increase tumor cell kill by increasing the dose of myelotoxic therapies and giving donor hematopoietic stem cells to "rescue" the recipient from the hematologic toxicity. Immune-mediated effects also contribute to the tumor cell kill observed after allogeneic HCT.
2. Hematopoietic stem cells used for transplantation can come from the recipient (autologous) or from a related or unrelated donor (allogeneic). If the related donor is a twin, the transplant is referred to as a syngeneic transplant.
3. Human leukocyte antigen (HLA) mismatching of allogeneic donor-recipient pairs at either class I or class II loci increases the risk of graft failure, graft-versus-host disease (GVHD), and worsens survival in the absence of effective GVHD prophylaxis. The ideal donor is one that is matched at HLA-A, B, C, and DRB1.
4. Hematopoietic stem cells are found in the bone marrow, peripheral blood, and umbilical cord blood. These stem cells express the CD34 antigen, and the number of $CD34^+$ cells is a clinically useful measure of the number of hematopoietic stem cells. Infusion of a minimum number of $CD34^+$ cells is necessary to ensure posttransplant engraftment. Due to the rarity of these cells in the peripheral blood, mobilization strategies are used to increase the number of $CD34^+$ cells prior to collection procedures.
5. Because of clinical and economic advantages, peripheral blood has replaced bone marrow as the most common source of hematopoietic stem cells in the autologous and adult allogeneic HCT setting.
6. The purpose of the preparative (or conditioning) regimen in traditional myeloablative transplants is twofold: (a) maximal tumor cell kill and (b) immunosuppression of the recipient to reduce the risk of graft rejection (allogeneic HCT only).
7. Reduced-intensity conditioning regimens (including those that are nonmyeloablative) have been developed to reduce early posttransplant morbidity and mortality while maximizing the graft-versus-malignancy (GVM) effect. The advantage of this approach is that patients who would otherwise not be eligible for allogeneic HCT can be offered a potentially curative therapy.
8. Transplant-related mortality associated with allogeneic HCT depends on recipient age, recipient performance status, donor source and degree of HLA matching, and disease status. Major causes of death include relapse, infection, organ toxicity, and GVHD. The most common cause of death after autologous HCT is disease relapse; transplant-related mortality is lower than after allogeneic HCT and depends on the conditioning regimen, age, underlying comorbidities, and disease status.
9. Patients undergoing allogeneic HCT receive immunosuppressive therapy to prevent GVHD, which inhibits T-cell activation, proliferation, or both. Commonly used GVHD prophylaxis regimens include combinations of tacrolimus, methotrexate, sirolimus, mycophenolate mofetil, or posttransplant cyclophosphamide.
10. Initial treatment of acute and chronic GVHD consists of prednisone, either alone or combined with other immunosuppressants. New agents are available for the treatment of steroid-refractory GVHD.

BEYOND THE BOOK

Watch the "What is GVHD?" video available on YouTube and visit the "Hematopoietic Cell Transplantation (HCT)—Clinicians Resource" (select posttransplant care, then chronic GVHD) on bethematchclinical.org. The video gives a brief overview of GVHD for the purposes of patient education. The Website provides more detail about the clinical manifestations of chronic GVHD. Both will help students to learn the basics about GVHD in preparation for a more in-depth discussion provided by the chapter.

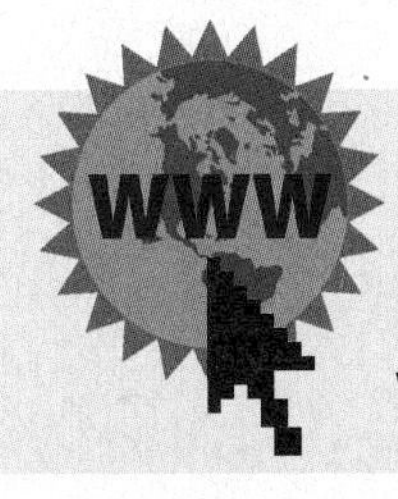

The complete chapter, learning objectives, and other resources can be found at **www.pharmacotherapyonline.com.**

Assessment of Nutrition Status and Nutrition Requirements

164

Katherine H. Chessman and Angela L. Bingham

KEY CONCEPTS

1. Malnutrition encompasses both undernutrition and overnutrition (obesity); although, the term is most often used to refer to undernutrition.
2. Nutrition screening is distinct from nutrition assessment; an effective screening process should be designed to identify quickly and consistently those with pre-existing malnutrition or those at risk for malnutrition.
3. A comprehensive medical, surgical, and dietary history; a nutrition-focused physical examination (NFPE); and anthropometric and laboratory measurements are essential components of a comprehensive nutrition assessment.
4. Anthropometrics, physical measurements of the size, weight, and proportions of the human body, are important parameters used to assess nutrition status.
5. Laboratory assessment of nutrition status must be interpreted in the context of clinical status and acute and chronic inflammation.
6. Macronutrient or micronutrient deficiencies or toxicities or risk factors for these deficiencies or toxicities can be identified by a comprehensive nutrition assessment.
7. Evidence-based patient-specific goals should be established considering the patient's clinical condition and the need for maintenance or repletion in adults and continued growth and development in children.
8. Validated predictive equations and population estimates are most often used to determine energy requirements; however, if available, indirect calorimetry is the most accurate bedside method to determine energy requirements.
9. Daily protein needs are based on age, sex, nutrition status, disease state, and clinical condition.
10. Drug–nutrient interactions can affect response to medication therapy and nutrition status.

BEYOND THE BOOK

Watch these videos from the American Society for Parenteral and Enteral Nutrition to enhance understanding of malnutrition, the etiology of malnutrition, and identification of malnourished patients. These videos will aid in the COLLECT and ASSESS steps in the patient care process:

- "Malnutrition Matters: A Call to Action for Providers Caring for Adult Patients" (15 minutes): https://youtu.be/JORLgsyri5U
- "GLIM Educational Series Part 1: What is GLIM?" (11 minutes): https://youtu.be/XIgB7eobGRY

INTRODUCTION

Nutrition care is an essential component of quality patient care. Nutrition screening and assessment are integral components of the nutrition care process. No single clinical or laboratory parameter is an absolute indicator of nutrition status, so information must be collected and analyzed from a number of sources. This chapter reviews tools most commonly used for accurate, relevant, and cost-effective nutrition screening and assessment, including various methods used to determine patient-specific macro- and micronutrient requirements and potential drug–nutrient interactions (DNI).

CLASSIFICATION OF NUTRITION STATUS

1 *Malnutrition* encompasses both undernutrition and overnutrition (obesity); although, the term is most often used to refer to undernutrition. Malnutrition is a consequence of nutrient imbalance. In general, deficiency states can be classified as those involving protein, energy, or single nutrients such as individual vitamins or trace elements. Many terms have been used to define malnutrition leading international nutrition experts to propose standardization of nomenclature and diagnosis for both adults and children.[1-3] Starvation-associated malnutrition, *marasmus*, results from prolonged inadequate intake, absorption, or utilization of protein and energy. It can occur in patients with an inadequate food supply, anorexia nervosa, major depression, and malabsorption syndromes (Fig. 164-1). Somatic protein (skeletal muscle) and adipose tissue (subcutaneous fat) wasting occurs, but visceral protein (albumin [ALB] and transferrin [TFN]) production is usually preserved. Moderate weight loss of 10% of usual body weight (UBW; typical weight) over a 6-month period is prognostic of poor clinical outcomes. A severe weight loss (30% or more of UBW) is life-threatening.[4] Patients with starvation-associated malnutrition commonly have a prototypical wasted appearance. When starvation-associated malnutrition develops as a consequence of primarily inadequate protein intake as is seen in areas of famine or limited food supply, affected individuals may not appear malnourished because of

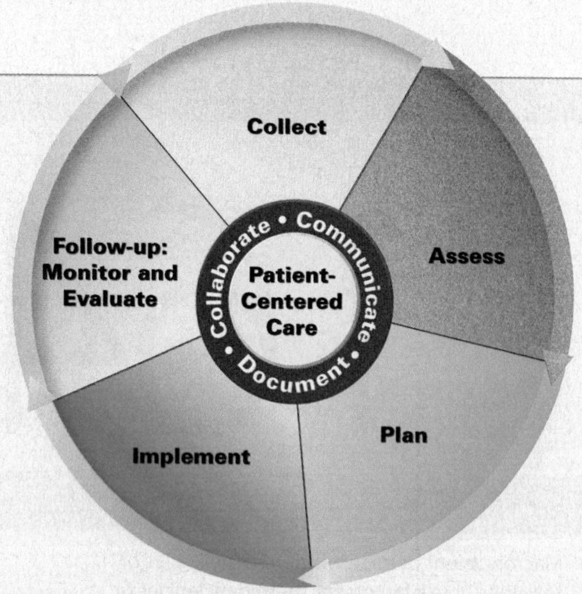

Patient Care Process for Nutrition Screening and Assessment

Collect

- Patient characteristics (eg, age, sex, diagnosis)
- Patient history (eg, medical, surgical, diet, recent GI losses, environmental exposures, alcohol use; see Tables 164-1, 164-2)
- Current medications, including nutrition supplements
- Objective data
  - o Body weight (current and usual)
  - o Stature, body mass index (BMI), head circumference
  - o Recent dietary and fluid intake
  - o Nutrition-focused physical exam (see Table 164-3)
  - o Labs (eg, serum electrolytes; glucose; blood urea nitrogen; serum creatinine [SCr]; albumin, prealbumin; C-reactive protein [CRP]; liver function tests; vitamin, mineral, and trace element concentrations)

Assess

- Nutrition status: presence of malnutrition, obesity (see Table 164-4)
- Risk of refeeding syndrome (eg, unintentional weight loss of more than 5% to 10% of usual body weight, prolonged period with poor caloric intake, BMI less than 18.5 kg/m^2, loss of subcutaneous fat, loss of muscle mass, electrolyte abnormalities)
- Signs and symptoms of micronutrient deficiencies or toxicities (see Tables 164-7, 164-8)
- Determine nutrition requirements based on current clinical condition (see Tables 164-9, 164-10, 164-11, 164-12, 164-13, 164-14, 164-15)

Plan*

- Conduct indirect calorimetry to estimate energy needs, if appropriate
- Develop a nutrition care plan to ensure delivery of estimated nutrition needs (energy, protein, fluid, vitamins, trace elements)
- Develop a plan to avoid or manage potential drug-nutrient interactions (see Table 164-16)
- Develop a plan to monitor nutritional recovery
- Make referrals to other providers, when appropriate (eg, dietitian, speech therapist, wound care nurse, lactation specialist)

Implement*

- Provide nutrition support using estimated goals
- Provide nutrient supplements to correct deficiencies
- Restrict nutrients to avoid toxicities
- Provide patient education regarding all elements of the nutrition care plan

Follow-up: Monitor and Evaluate

- Appropriate weight gain, loss, or maintenance
- Appropriate gains in length and head circumference in children
- Maintenance or return of function, including muscle strength
- Laboratory parameters, as indicated
- Monitor for side effects of nutrition care
- Monitor for patient adherence to nutrition care plan

**Collaborate with patient, caregivers, and other healthcare professionals*

relative adipose tissue sparing, especially with mild undernutrition, but visceral (and to some degree somatic) protein stores are depleted, resulting in severe hypoalbuminemia and edema in more advanced cases. In patients with starvation-related malnutrition, enhancing nutritional intake or bypassing impaired absorption with nutrition support can reverse the condition. Careful nutritional resuscitation is required to avoid complications related to refeeding.[5]

Malnutrition (undernutrition) may also develop as the result of an acute or chronic condition or disease, especially those associated with mild-to-severe inflammation (see Fig. 164-1).[1,2,4,6] Patients with severe acute disease or injury (major infections, burns, trauma) or with chronic inflammatory diseases (Crohn's disease), organ failure, or cancer can develop disease-related malnutrition because of increased metabolic demands despite seemingly adequate nutrition intake. Individuals with pre-existing starvation-related malnutrition can develop pronounced malnutrition if they experience a severe injury or inflammatory process. In patients with disease-related, acute or chronic, malnutrition, simply providing nutrients in usual or even increased amounts may not be sufficient to reverse the nutrient imbalance due to the chronic inflammatory process. As a patient's clinical course progresses, they may change from one malnutrition classification to another.[4] Regardless of the cause, malnutrition (undernutrition and overnutrition) can result in changes in subcellular, cellular, or organ function that increase morbidity and mortality.

Nutrition screening is also used to identify overnutrition: overweight and obese individuals and those at risk of becoming overweight or obese. Obesity is a major global healthcare concern; during 2017 to 2018, the age-adjusted prevalence of obesity (defined as a BMI $\geq$ 30 kg/m^2) was 42.4% and severe obesity (defined as a BMI $\geq$ 40 kg/m^2) was 9.2% of US adults.[7] In all states, more than 20% of adults were obese. Obesity prevalence in 2020 was 20% to 24.99% only in Colorado, Hawaii, Massachusetts, and the District

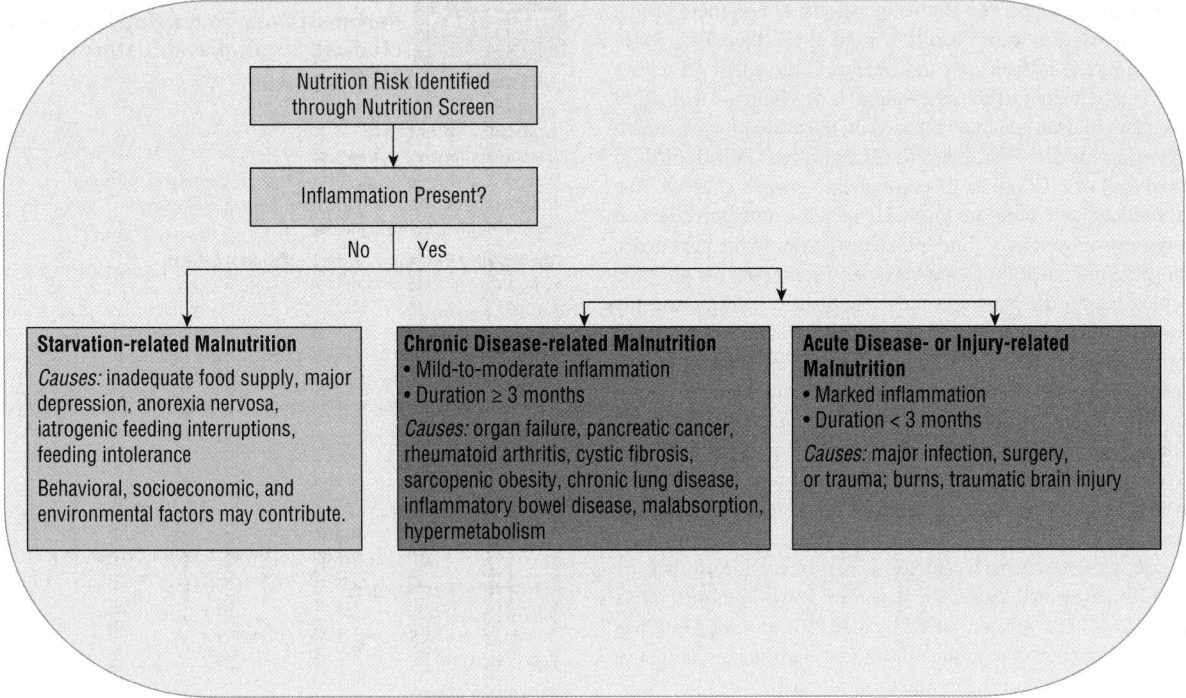

FIGURE 164-1 Etiologic basis for malnutrition diagnosis. (*Data from References* 1 and 2.)

of Columbia; and 35% or more in 16 states (Alabama, Arkansas, Delaware, Indiana, Iowa, Kansas, Kentucky, Louisiana, Michigan, Mississippi, Ohio, Oklahoma, South Carolina, Tennessee, Texas, and West Virginia).[8] In fact, US obesity and severe obesity prevalence has increased from 1999-2000 to 2017-2018, 30.5% to 42.4% and 4.7% to 9.2%, respectively.[8] Additionally, 19.3% (14.4 million) of all US children and adolescents, aged 2 to 19 years, were obese (BMI $\geq$ 95th percentile-for-age on the gender-appropriate BMI-for-age Centers for Disease Control and Prevention's [CDC] 2000 growth chart).[7,9] The prevalence of obesity in children varied by age group: 2 to 5 years, 13.4%; 6 to 11 years, 20.3%; and, 12 to 19 years, 21.2%.[7] The consequences of obesity are numerous and include type 2 diabetes mellitus, cardiovascular disease, hypertension, and stroke. Obesity contributes significantly to all-cause mortality and decreased life expectancy.[10]

Because malnutrition is associated with higher morbidity and mortality rates in many settings, an effective nutrition screening program is essential to identify patients at nutrition-related risk, alerting clinicians to perform a comprehensive nutrition assessment to accurately characterize baseline nutrition status, estimate nutrition needs, and develop a patient-specific nutrition care plan. Diligent monitoring of ongoing nutrition status can ensure that nutrition-related goals are being met and improve patient outcomes.

NUTRITION SCREENING

2 Nutrition screening is distinct from nutrition assessment; an effective screening process should be designed to identify quickly and consistently those with pre-existing malnutrition or those at risk for malnutrition.[11] It is not practical, expedient, cost-effective, nor clinically warranted to conduct a comprehensive nutrition assessment on every individual; thus, nutrition screening provides a reliable, systematic method to identify persons for whom a detailed nutrition assessment is warranted. A validated nutrition screening tool can be used to detect those who are overweight, obese, malnourished, or at risk for malnutrition; predict their health outcomes based on nutrition-related factors; and identify individuals who would benefit from nutritional intervention.[11,12]

The ideal nutrition screening tool is quick, simple, and noninvasive and can be done by lay and healthcare providers in homes, long-term care facilities, ambulatory care clinics, and hospitals. In 1995, The Joint Commission implemented a standard for accredited healthcare institutions requiring a nutrition screen be completed within 24 hours of inpatient admission on all applicable patients.[13] Because nutrition assessment has been routinely adopted in the United States, this standard was deleted in 2016. Periodic rescreening should occur at regular intervals determined by the institution and the patient population, usually every 3 to 7 days. For outpatients, nutrition screening should occur at the first visit with a new provider and thereafter as warranted by the patient's condition.

Risk factor identification is the foundation of appropriate nutrition screening. Risk factors for malnutrition include recent unintended weight loss; presence and severity of acute and chronic disease states; medications and or other treatments; socioeconomic factors that may result in a decreased nutrient intake; and, altered nutrient absorption, metabolism, or utilization. Risk factors for obesity include a family history of obesity, certain medical diagnoses (eg, polycystic ovary syndrome, Prader-Willi syndrome, Cushing's syndrome), poor dietary habits, inadequate exercise, and some medication therapies. Various rating and classification systems have been proposed to screen for nutrition risk and guide subsequent interventions.[11] In general, checklists of varying complexity are used to quantify a person's food and alcohol consumption habits; ability to buy, prepare, and eat food; weight history; diagnoses; medical and surgical procedures; medication and supplement therapies; and, history of nutrition support (enteral nutrition [EN] or parenteral nutrition [PN]). Although no tool is 100% sensitive and specific for detecting malnutrition, the Mini Nutritional Assessment – Short Form and the Malnutrition Screening Tool (MST) have high sensitivity and specificity.[12] The Mini Nutritional Assessment – Short Form is used extensively in older adults and found to be useful in several care settings.[12] The Nutrition Risk Screening 2002 (NRS 2002) and the Nutrition Risk in the Critically Ill (NUTRIC) may be used as nutrition assessment tools in critically ill adults, but supporting literature is limited.[14–16] Given the drawbacks with use of these tools, a more simple approach is to ask two simple questions: 1) Has there been a recent weight loss of at least 5% to 10%?; and 2) Has there been inadequate food intake for at least 1 to 2 weeks? If the answer to either question is *Yes*, then further assessment is warranted.[11] Nutrition screening for children generally is based on the evaluation of growth parameters against the World Health Organization (WHO; birth to 2 years of age) or CDC (2 to 19 years of age) growth charts,[9,17] the presence of medical conditions known to increase nutrition risk, and recent changes in weight or food intake. Estimates of the prevalence of in-hospital malnutrition for pediatric and adult patients are variable depending on the patient population, disease severity, and the criteria used. According to data from the 2018 Healthcare Cost and Utilization Project, 8.9% of all US nonmaternal, nonneonatal hospital discharges included a coded diagnosis of malnutrition.[18]

In any setting, patients screened to be nutritionally-at-risk should receive a timely comprehensive nutrition assessment to verify nutrition-related risk and to formulate a complete nutrition care plan which includes monitoring parameters to ensure that desired outcomes are met. For patients who are screened to be *nutritionally-at-risk*, a comprehensive nutrition assessment ideally will be completed by a trained professional within 48 to 72 hours. Most nutrition assessments are completed by dietitians or nurses but may be completed by others including pharmacists, physicians, and physician assistants with training in nutrition support.

NUTRITION ASSESSMENT

3 A comprehensive medical, surgical, and dietary history; a nutrition-focused physical examination (NFPE); and anthropometric and laboratory measurements are essential components of a comprehensive nutrition assessment. Goals of nutrition assessment include identification of risk factors associated with malnutrition, including disorders resulting from macro- or micronutrient deficiencies (undernutrition), obesity (overnutrition), or impaired nutrient absorption, metabolism, or utilization; determination of the risk of nutrition-related complications; estimation of nutrition needs; and establishment of baseline nutrition parameters against which to measure nutrition therapy outcomes.[11]

Nutrition-Focused History and Physical Examination

The nutrition-focused medical, surgical, and dietary history serves to identify factors that predispose to malnutrition (eg, prematurity, chronic disease, gastrointestinal [GI] dysfunction, alcohol misuse, acute or chronic inflammation [eg, cancer, surgery, trauma]), and overnutrition (eg, poor dietary habits, limited exercise, chronic disease, family history) (Table 164-1). The clinician should clarify any history of weight gain or loss (intended or unintended), anorexia, vomiting, diarrhea, decreased or restrictive food intake, and EN or PN. Any conditions that suggest ongoing inflammation, including fever, hyperthermia, tachycardia, or infection should be documented (Table 164-2).[6]

The NFPE uses a systematic approach to assess for abnormal nutrition-related clinical and physical findings in each region of the body. Components of the NFPE include: general inspection; vital signs; skin; nails; head/hair; eyes/nose; mouth; neck/chest; abdomen; and, musculoskeletal.[15] The clinician completing a NFPE assesses for muscle and fat loss; fluid status; micronutrient deficiency/toxicity; functional status/hand grip strength; and, for children, mid-arm muscle circumference (MUMC).[19,20] Findings commonly associated with malnutrition (eg, muscle wasting, alopecia, dermatitis, glossitis, cheilosis, jaundice) are noted (Table 164-3).

The Subjective Global Assessment (SGA) and the tool described in the Academy of Nutrition and Dietetics (AND) and the American Society for Parenteral and Enteral Nutrition (ASPEN) consensus statement on the identification and documentation of adult malnutrition are representative examples of a relatively simple, reproducible, cost-effective, bedside approach to nutrition assessment.[1,11] The SGA assesses five aspects of the medical and dietary history: weight change in the previous 6 months, dietary changes, GI symptoms, functional capacity, and disease states known to affect nutrition status. Weight loss of less than 5% of UBW is considered a "small" loss, 5% to 10% loss is "potentially significant," and more than a 10% loss is "definitely significant." Dietary intake is characterized as normal or abnormal, and the duration and degree of abnormal intake are noted. The presence of daily GI symptoms (anorexia, nausea, vomiting, diarrhea) for longer than 2 weeks is significant. Functional capacity assesses the patient's energy level and whether the patient is active or bedridden. Finally, disease state impact on metabolic demands (no, low, moderate, or high stress) is documented. Four physical examination findings are rated as normal, mild, moderate,

TABLE 164-1 Pertinent Data from a Nutrition-Focused Medical, Surgical, and Dietary History

Nutrition Intake and Dietary Habits
Anorexia
Unusual or absent taste
Diet, including vegetarian, vegan
Specialized nutrition support (enteral or parenteral nutrition)
Supplemental vitamin, mineral, or herbal intake
Food allergies or intolerances
Underlying Pathology with Nutritional Effects
Chronic infection or inflammatory state
Cancer
Endocrine disorders
Chronic illness (lung disease, cirrhosis, kidney failure)
Hypermetabolic states (trauma, burns, sepsis)
Digestive/absorptive disease, nausea, vomiting, diarrhea, constipation
Hyperlipidemia
End-organ Effects
Weight changes
Skin or hair changes
Exercise intolerance or fatigue
Gastrointestinal tract symptoms (diarrhea, vomiting, constipation)
Gastrointestinal Surgery
Bariatric surgery
Small bowel or colon resection or diversion
Gastrectomy
Miscellaneous
Catabolic medications or therapies (corticosteroids, immunosuppressive agents, radiation, chemotherapy)
Other medications (diuretics, laxatives, antipsychotics, anabolic steroids)
Genetics (body habitus of parents, siblings, family)
Alcohol or drug misuse
Pregnancy or lactation

TABLE 164-2 Assessment of Inflammation

Laboratory Assessment	Clinical Findings	Acute/Chronic Disease States
Decreased	Fever	Cancer
Albumin	Hyperthermia	Celiac disease
Transferrin	Infection	Cystic fibrosis
Prealbumin	Urinary tract	Inflammatory bowel disease
Nitrogen balance	Pneumonia	Organ failure (ARDS)
Elevated	Bacteremia	Pancreatitis
CRP	Wound/incision	Rheumatologic disorders (RA, SLE)
Serum glucose	Abscess	Trauma (burns, major surgery, TBI)
% neutrophils		
Decreased or increased WBC		

ARDS, acute respiratory distress syndrome; CRP, C-reactive protein; RA, rheumatoid arthritis; SLE, systemic lupus erythematosus; TBI, traumatic brain injury; WBC, white blood cell count.

TABLE 164-3 Nutrition Focused Physical Examination (NFPE) Findings Suggestive of Malnutrition

General Inspection	**Eyes/Nose**
Edema	Dull dry appearance to sclerae or inner lids
Cachexia or obesity	Dull milky appearance of cornea
Signs/symptoms of dehydration (poor skin turgor, sunken eyes, orthostasis, dry mucous membranes)	Bitot's spots[a]
Muscle wasting or loss of subcutaneous fat	Icteric sclerae
Vital Signs	Pale conjunctiva
Fever	Cracked red corners of eyes
Tachycardia	**Mouth**
Skin	Pale, red, or bleeding gums
Thin, shiny, dry, or scaly skin	Dry, cracked, red lips
Dermatitis, rash	Fissures at corners (angular stomatitis)
Decubitus ulcers, poorly healing wounds	Vertical cracks of the lips (cheilosis)
Bruising, petechiae	Magenta or beefy red tongue (glossitis)
Follicular hyperkeratosis	Atrophied papillae
Pallor, cyanosis, jaundice	Excessive dental caries
Nails	**Neck/Chest**
Spoon shape, clubbing	Enlarged thyroid
Transverse ridging/banding	Distended neck veins
Mottled, pale, poor capillary refill	Prominent bony chest, visible ribs (muscle and fat wasting)
Head/Hair	**Abdomen**
Dry, dull, brittle, sparse, easily pluckable hair	Scaphoid, concave, or protuberant abdomen
Corkscrew, coiled, or depigmented hair	Hepatomegaly, ascites
Alopecia	**Musculoskeletal**
Scaly, flaky scalp	Ataxia (poor muscle control)
Moon face	Numbness, tingling
Bilateral temporal wasting	Swollen or painful joints
	Rickets, knock knees, bowleg

[a]Bitot's spots are foamy spots on the surface of the eye.

or severe: loss of subcutaneous fat (triceps and chest), muscle wasting (quadriceps and deltoids), edema (ankle and sacral), and ascites. The patient's nutrition status is then rated as adequately nourished, moderately malnourished or suspected of being malnourished, or severely malnourished. Critics of the SGA find it time-consuming and complex. The AND/ASPEN consensus tool assesses six characteristics: insufficient energy intake, weight loss, loss of muscle mass, loss of subcutaneous fat, localized or generalized fluid accumulation, and diminished functional status measured by hand grip strength. The presence of two or more of these characteristics identifies malnutrition in an adult.

Given variability in diagnostic criteria for malnutrition, the Global Leadership Initiative on Malnutrition (GLIM) was convened to reach global consensus.[3] GLIM established a two-step model that includes malnutrition risk screening of at-risk individuals with a validated tool and assessment for diagnosis and severity grading. Patients who are identified at-risk undergo diagnostic assessment that incorporates phenotypic criteria (nonvolitional weight loss, low BMI, reduced muscle mass) and etiologic criteria (reduced food intake or assimilation, disease burden/inflammatory condition). Malnutrition is diagnosed in patients with at least one phenotypic and one etiologic criterion with further severity grading based on phenotypic metrics.

Anthropometric Measurements

4 Anthropometrics, physical measurements of the size, weight, and proportions of the human body, are important parameters used to assess nutrition status. Common measurements are weight, stature (standing height or recumbent length), waist circumference, and head circumference (occipital frontal circumference) for children younger than 3 years of age. Measurement of limb size, such as skinfold thickness, MUMC, and wrist circumference, may be useful in selected individuals. Accurate measurement of anthropometrics rather than the use of self-reported values is critical for accurate assessment. Measurement can be difficult in injured and critically ill patients but should be conducted as soon as feasible.

Bioelectrical impedance analysis (BIA) is also an anthropometric assessment tool. Body measurements can be compared with normative population standards to identify clinical concerns and may be repeated at various intervals to monitor response to a nutrition care plan. In adults, nutrition-related changes in anthropometric measurements tend to occur slowly; several weeks or more may be required before detectable changes are noted. In infants and young children, changes occur more quickly. Significant acute changes in weight and skinfold thickness usually reflect changes in hydration status, which must be considered when interpreting these parameters.

Weight, Stature, and Head Circumference

Body weight is a nonspecific measure of body cell mass, representing skeletal mass, body fat, and the energy-using component, lean body mass (LBM). Fat-free mass includes skeletal muscle, bone, connective tissue, organs, and water while fat mass includes the subcutaneous fat beneath the skin and the visceral (internal) fat. Change in weight over time, particularly in the absence of edema, ascites, or voluntary losses, is an important indicator of altered LBM. Actual body weight (ABW) interpretation should include consideration of ideal weight-for-height, referred to as ideal body weight (IBW), UBW (typical weight), fluid status, and age (Table 164-4). Both acute and chronic changes in fluid status can affect the ABW; these changes often can be detected by monitoring the patient's daily fluid intake and output. Patients who are dehydrated will have a decreased ABW but not a loss of LBM. Once rehydrated, these patients must be reweighed to establish an appropriate baseline weight for nutrition evaluation. Edema and ascites increase total body water (TBW), thus increasing ABW but not LBM. The ABW of patients with severe edema and ascites should not be used for nutrition assessment, and practitioners often use an estimated "*dry weight*" to account for this TBW increase.

The IBW is a population reference standard against which the ABW can be compared. IBW-for-height reference tables are available, and IBW can be calculated using mathematical equations based on sex and height. The most commonly used equations for calculating IBW for adults are the Devine equations where IBW is calculated as follows:[21]

$$\text{Adult men: IBW} = 50\text{ kg} + (2.3 \times \text{inches over 6 feet})$$
$$\text{Adult women: IBW} = 45.5\text{ kg} + (2.3 \times \text{inches over 6 feet})$$

Adjusted body weight (AdjBW) has been suggested as a logical means to account for the percentage of the obese weight that is LBM (22% to 38%). For obese adults, use of an AdjBW has been recommended for nutrition-related calculations, as follows:

$$\text{AdjBW} = ([\text{ABW} - \text{IBW}] \times 0.25) + \text{IBW}$$

However, the use of AdjBW is generally not recommended; its use is not evidence-based because most of the metabolic rate equations were formulated using ABW in a mix of obese and nonobese individuals.[22]

Multiple methods are available for estimating the IBW of children.[23] The Traub equation can be used for a child younger than 18 years of age and 60 inches or shorter:

$$\text{IBW} = ([\text{height(cm)}]^2 \times 1.65)/1{,}000$$

The McLaren method uses the WHO or CDC growth chart to compare height and weight relative to the child's age. A vertical line is

TABLE 164-4 Evaluation of Body Weight and Waist Circumference

Parameter	Interpretation	NHLBI Obesity Classification	Waist Circumference	
ABW compared with IBW				
ABW <69% IBW	Severe malnutrition			
ABW 70%-79% IBW	Moderate malnutrition			
ABW 80%-89% IBW	Mild malnutrition			
ABW 90%-120% IBW	Normal			
ABW >120% IBW	Overweight			
ABW ≥150% IBW	Obese			
ABW ≥200% IBW	Morbidly obese			
ABW compared with UBW				
ABW 85%-95% UBW	Mild malnutrition			
ABW 75%-84% UBW	Moderate malnutrition			
ABW <75% UBW	Severe malnutrition			
BMI (kg/m²)				
Adults				
<16	Severe malnutrition			
16-16.9	Moderate malnutrition			
17-18.9	Mild malnutrition			
19-24.9	Healthy		Disease risk above BMI-related risk[a]	
22-30 (Older adults)	Healthy		Women ≤89 cm (35 in) Men ≤102 cm (40 in)	Women >89 cm (35 in) Men >102 cm (40 in)
25-29.9	Overweight		Increased	High
30-40	Moderate obesity			
30-34.9		I	High	Very high
35-39.9		II	Very high	Very high
>40	Severe or morbid obesity	III	Extremely high	Extremely high
Children				
BMI for age <5th percentile	Underweight			
BMI for age 5th-84th percentile	Healthy			
BMI for age 85th-94th percentile	Overweight			
BMI for age ≥95th percentile	Obese			

[a]Increased risk for Type 2 diabetes mellitus, hypertension, and cardiovascular disease.
NHLBI, National Heart, Lung, and Blood Institute.

graphed between the child's height-for-age measurement and the corresponding 50th percentile weight-for-age to determine the IBW. This approach becomes less accurate as the child's height deviates from the 50th percentile.[23]

Change in weight over time can be calculated as a percentage of UBW. Use of UBW as a reference point provides a more accurate reflection of clinically significant weight change over time (Table 164-4). The use of UBW avoids the inherent problems with normative tables and documents comparative changes in body weight. However, unless documented in the medical record, determining UBW depends on patient or family recall, which is often inaccurate. All weight changes should be interpreted relative to time because unintentional weight loss, especially rapid weight loss (5% of UBW in 1 month or 10% of UBW in 6 months), increases the risk of nutrition-related poor clinical outcomes.[12]

Stature is determined by both genetics and nutrition. Accurate measurement of stature is critical to appropriate interpretation. In older children and adults, a standing height should be obtained. If a standing height cannot be measured using a wall-mounted stadiometer, recumbent length, knee height, and arm spam have been used. Each of these methods yields different results.[24] In infants and young children who are unable to stand, a recumbent length is measured using a *length board* which requires two people to obtain an accurate measurement.

Demispan is determined in a seated patient by measuring the distance from the sternal notch to the web between the middle and ring fingers along a horizontally outstretched arm with the wrist in neutral rotation and zero extension or flexion. Demispan may more accurately assess stature in elderly adults, especially those with kyphosis or vertebral collapse. After the demispan is measured, height is estimated using the following equations:[25]

$$\text{Women: Height (cm)} = (1.35 \times \text{demispan [cm]}) + 60.1$$
$$\text{Men: Height (cm)} = (1.4 \times \text{demispan [cm]}) + 57.8$$

Knee height may also be used to estimate stature and is helpful in patients with limb contractures, such as patients with cerebral palsy and the elderly. Knee height is measured from just under the heel to the anterior surface of the thigh just proximal to the patella. Using the average of two measurements rounded to the nearest 0.1 cm, height can be estimated using the following equations:[12]

$$\text{Women: Height(cm)} = [1.83 \times \text{knee height(cm)}] - [0.24 \times \text{age(yr)}] + 84.8$$

$$\text{Men: Height(cm)} = [2.02 \times \text{knee height(cm)}] - [0.04 \times \text{age(yr)}] + 64.9$$

Appropriate growth is predictable and the best indicator of adequate nutrition in a child. At each medical encounter, weight, stature, head circumference (until 3 years), and BMI (after 2 years) should be plotted on the WHO (younger than 2 years) or CDC gender- and age-specific growth curves.[9,17] The CDC charts were revised in 2000 from US data only and indicate how US children grow. The WHO charts developed in 2006 are preferred in those younger than 2 years because they include data from infants from six industrialized countries including the United States who were predominantly breastfed for the first 4 months of life and who were receiving some breast milk at 12 months, conditions felt to ensure optimal growth.[17] Specialized charts are also available for assessment of growth of premature infants.[26,27] For premature infants with corrected postnatal age of 40 weeks or more, the WHO growth charts can be used; however, weight-for-age, length-for-age, and head circumference-for-age should be plotted according to corrected postnatal age until 2 years, 1.5 to 3 years, and 3 years of age, respectively.

Recommended intervals between measurements in young children are weight, 7 days; length, 4 weeks; height, 8 weeks; and head circumference, 7 days in infants and 4 weeks in children until 3 years of age. Daily weight fluctuations can occur with changes in fluid status. Growth velocity can be used to assess growth at intervals too close to plot accurately on a growth chart (Table 164-5). In newborns, average weight gain is 10 to 20 g/kg/day (24-35 g/day in term infants; 10-25 g/day in preterm infants depending on gestational age). The rate of weight gain declines considerably after 3 months of age; children 6 to 10 years of age gain about 2 to 3 kg/yr. The adolescent "growth spurt" typically begins at 9 to 10 years in girls and 11 to 12 years in boys. During the 11 to 13 year-old-interval of maximum growth in height, girls will gain about 10 kg (22 lb) while boys gain 15.5 kg (33 lb). Length increases rapidly in infancy (see Table 164-5). In children 6 to 10 years of age, height increases by 2 to 3 in/yr (approximately 5-7.5 cm/yr) and continues until about 16 to 18 years of age in girls and 18 to 20 years of age in boys. Head growth (measured by head circumference), usually 0.5 cm/wk (0.2 in/wk) during the first year of life, can be compromised during periods of critical illness or malnutrition. Rapid head growth, at a rate faster than expected, suggests hydrocephalus which may be benign but must be further evaluated.

In the International Classification of Disease-10 (ICD-10), failure-to-thrive (growth faltering) in a child is defined as *lack of expected normal physical growth, failure to gain weight,* or *lack of growth.* Not all children with low weight have failure-to-thrive, but it has been defined as weight-for-age, length-for-age, BMI-for-age, or weight velocity below the 2nd percentile or a weight deceleration crossing two or more major percentiles (major percentiles are defined as 97th, 95th, 90th, 75th, 50th, 25th, 10th, 5th, and 3rd), or if an infant is not gaining the expected daily weight.[28] In children, a significant weight loss is defined as: greater than 2% in 1 week; greater than 5% in 1 month; greater than 7.5% in 3 months; and, greater than 10% in 6 months. Growth faltering is best defined by using z-scores for weight-for-length, BMI-for-age, or length- or height-for age: a z-score of -1 indicates mild malnutrition; -2 moderate malnutrition; and, -3 severe malnutrition.[2] Weight-for-height evaluation is age independent and helps differentiate a stunted child (chronic malnutrition) from a wasted child (acute malnutrition). Short stature can be associated with chronic undernutrition, but short stature in the absence of poor weight gain suggests another etiology, such as growth hormone deficiency or constitutional growth delay.[29]

TABLE 164-5 Expected Growth Velocities in Term Infants and Children

Age	Weight (g/day)	Height (cm/mo)[a]
0-3 mo	24-35	2.8-3.4
4-6 mo	15-21	1.7-2.4
7-12 mo	10-13	1.3-1.6
1-3 yr	5-9	0.6-1
4-6 yr	5-6	0.5-0.6
7-10 yr	7-11	0.4-0.5

Example of growth assessment

Age: 2 mo; weight: 3.2 kg; weight at 1 mo of age, 3.1 kg; time since last weight was obtained: 30 days.

Growth velocity = ([3.2 kg−3.1 kg] × 1,000 g/kg)/30 days = 3.3 g/day.

Interpretation: suboptimal growth; comprehensive nutrition assessment needed.

[a]Growth velocity of 1 cm/mo is equivalent to 0.4 in/mo.

Body Mass Index

BMI can be calculated as either body weight in kilograms divided by height in meters squared (kg/m^2) or body weight in pounds multiplied by 703 divided by height in inches squared (lb/in^2). The assessment of BMI is the first step but not the sole criterion to judge potential health risk.[30] A BMI of 25 kg/m^2 or higher is a risk factor for premature death and disability. Health risks increase with increasing BMI; however, individual variation, especially in very muscular persons, can lead to erroneous nutrition status classification when BMI alone is used. Thus, BMI must be interpreted based on characteristics such as sex, frame size, race/ethnicity, and age. For example, at the same BMI, a woman tends to have more body fat than a man, and an older adult will have more body fat than a younger one.

The National Institutes of Health obesity expert panel report classifies a BMI between 18.5 and 24.9 kg/m^2 as a healthy or normal weight, between 25 kg/m^2 and 29.9 kg/m^2 as overweight, between 30 kg/m^2 and 39.9 kg/m^2 as obese; and, 40 kg/m^2 or higher as extreme obesity (see Table 164-4).[31] These BMI classifications may not be appropriate for adults older than 60 to 65 years. The Centers for Medicaid and Medicare Services defines normal BMI for adults older than 65 years to be between 23 kg/m^2 and 30 kg/m^2; the National Screening Initiative defined normal BMI for this age as 22 to 27 kg/m^2. The NIH classifies a BMI of less than 18.5 kg/m^2 as undernutrition, but this relationship is not as well established.[31] BMI values below 18.5 kg/m^2 have been associated with higher mortality rates in patients with cancer.[32] Children 2 years of age and older whose BMI is at or above the 85th percentile or at or above the 95th percentile on the age- and gender-specific CDC BMI chart are classified as overweight and obese, respectively.[9,17] Use of these charts at each medical encounter helps to heighten awareness of children whose BMI and family history put them at risk for adult obesity and its associated complications.

Waist Circumference

Body fat distribution is associated with health risk. Waist circumference is a simple measurement used to assess abdominal (visceral) fat. Waist circumference is determined by measuring the distance around the waist just above the iliac crest after exhaling. Extra weight around the waist rather than peripheral (subcutaneous) fat confers a greater health risk than extra weight around the hips and thighs. The larger the waist circumference, the greater the risk of obesity-related complications, especially diabetes mellitus, cardiovascular disease, and all-cause mortality.[30,33] Men and women are considered to have abdominal obesity and at increased risk (beyond their BMI-related risk) when the waist circumference is greater than 40 inches (102 cm) and greater than 35 inches (89 cm), respectively (Table 164-4). Children have abdominal obesity if the waist circumference is at or above the 90th percentile according to CDC age- and sex-specific standards.[34]

Waist-to-Hip and Waist-to-Height Ratios

The waist-to-hip ratio is determined by dividing the waist circumference by the hip circumference (maximal posterior extension of the buttocks). In adults, a waist-to-hip ratio of greater than 0.9 in men and 0.85 in women is considered an independent risk factor for adverse health consequences.[33] Waist-to-height ratio (both measured in centimeters) has been used to evaluate children at risk for the metabolic syndrome because, unlike waist circumference, it is independent of age and sex. A child (aged 6 to 18 years) with a waist-to-height ratio of more than 0.5 is considered to have abdominal obesity and at risk for developing the metabolic syndrome. This cutoff may overestimate abdominal obesity in younger children (aged 2 to 5 years).[34]

Skinfold Thickness and Mid-Arm Muscle Circumference

More than 50% of the body's fat is subcutaneous; thus, changes in subcutaneous fat reflect changes in total body fat. Skinfold thickness measurement provides an estimate of subcutaneous fat, and MUMC, which is calculated using the skinfold thickness and mid-arm circumference, estimates skeletal muscle mass. Although simple and noninvasive, these anthropometric measurements are used most commonly in population analysis and long-term monitoring of individuals. Triceps skinfold thickness measurement is used most often, but reference standards also exist for subscapular and suprailiac measurements.[35] Consistent technique in the use of pressure-regulated calipers is essential for reproducibility and reliability in measuring skinfold thickness. Published standards do not account for variation in bone size, muscle mass, hydration, or skin compressibility, and they do not consider obesity, ethnicity, illness, and increased age. Results should be interpreted cautiously as these parameters change slowly in adults, often requiring weeks before significant alterations from baseline can be detected. These parameters will change more rapidly in young children.

Bioelectrical Impedance

BIA is a portable, simple, quick, noninvasive, and relatively inexpensive technique used to measure body composition.[36,37] When a weak, alternating electric current is applied to two appendages (wrist and ankle or both feet), impedance (resistance) to flow is measured as it passes through the body. Different body tissues have varying amounts of water and will conduct the electrical current differently. Water and electrolyte-rich tissues such as blood and muscle are highly conductive, but fat and bone are poor conductors. Assessment of LBM, TBW, and water distribution can be determined with BIA. Increased TBW decreases impedance; thus, it is important to evaluate hydration status when performing BIA. Other potential limitations of BIA include variability with electrolyte imbalance and interference by large fat masses, environment, ethnicity, menstrual cycle phase, and underlying medical conditions.[37] Although BIA equations have high validity when used in the population in which they were developed (mostly young healthy adults), BIA calculations are subject to considerable errors if applied to other populations or when conditions are not identical (eg, electrode placement).[37] The use of BIA in clinical practice may be limited by the lack of reference standards that reflect variations in individual age, body size, and clinical conditions.[36] Due to the proprietary nature of manufacture-specific BIA regression models and inability to compare studies using different devices, current guidelines do not provide recommendations regarding the use of BIA in clinical practice.[38]

OTHER NUTRITION ASSESSMENT TOOLS

Functional status is dependent on nutrition, but the specific tools to assess it are not well defined. Muscle function is an end-organ response; thus, diminished skeletal muscle function can be a useful indicator of malnutrition. Muscle function may also recover more quickly in response to adequate nutrition support than anthropometric measurements. Simple functional assessments include the ability to perform activities of daily living, participate in physical and occupational therapy, and wean from the ventilator. Hand-grip strength (forearm muscle dynamometry), respiratory muscle strength, and muscle response to electrical stimulation also have been used. Measuring hand-grip strength is part of a NFPE and is a relatively simple, noninvasive, and inexpensive procedure that correlates well with patient outcome.[39–41] Normative standards supplied by the manufacturer of the specific dynamometer must be used for assessment. Hand grip strength is an indirect measurement of LBM making it a good parameter for assessment of undernutrition. However, some conditions will limit hand grip strength, such as rheumatoid arthritis, stroke, neuromuscular disease, dementia, and heavy sedation. Ulnar nerve stimulation causes measurable muscle contraction and is used in most intensive care units to monitor neuromuscular blockade. In malnourished patients, increased fatigue and a slowed muscle relaxation rate are noted, and these indices may return to normal with refeeding.

Other methods used to determine body composition include bioimpedance spectroscopy, dual energy x-ray absorptiometry (DXA), quantitative computed tomography (CT), air displacement plethysmography (BodPod®), three-dimensional photonic scanning, quantitative magnetic resonance imaging (MRI), ultrasonography, and positron emission tomography.[14,37,38,42] These methods are often complex and expensive to perform. DXA, best known for its use in measuring bone density, is a promising method for routine clinical practice because it can quantify mineral, fat, and LBM compartments and is available in most hospitals and many outpatient facilities. Current guidelines recommend the use of DXA for assessing fat mass in patients with a variety of disease states, but the validity for lean mass assessment is unknown.[38] A central body DXA scanner requires a fair amount of space, and the cost depends on the scanner's complexity. Portable (or peripheral) DXA devices can be used to measure bone density in peripheral bones, such as the wrist, fingers, or heel, and have also been used to assess subcutaneous fat. Portable DXA scanners are much less expensive than central scanners and can be used in community screenings. Further research is needed to determine how DXA can be used clinically in nutrition assessment. MRI and CT can measure subcutaneous, intra-abdominal, and regional fat distribution and thus also have the potential to be useful clinically. Ultrasound uses high-frequency sound waves to image soft tissue structures in an inexpensive and noninvasive manner. Current guidelines do not recommend ultrasound to assess body composition due to the lack of evidence for supporting its validity in clinical practice.[38]

Laboratory Assessment

5 Laboratory assessment of nutrition status must be interpreted in the context of clinical status and acute and chronic inflammation. Biochemically, serum visceral proteins (ALB, TFN, and prealbumin [also known as transthyretin]) have traditionally been used to assess LBM. C-reactive protein (CRP) can be useful as a marker of inflammation.

Serum Visceral Proteins

Visceral proteins synthesized by the liver have historically been considered useful parameters for nutrition assessment, but newer literature challenges this premise.[43] It is assumed that in undernutrition states, a low serum protein concentration reflects diminished hepatic protein synthetic mass and indirectly reflects the functional protein mass of other organs (heart, lung, kidney, and intestines). However, visceral proteins are not valid proxy measures of total body mass.[43] Many factors other than nutrition can affect the serum concentrations of these proteins including age; abnormal kidney (nephrotic syndrome), GI tract (protein-losing enteropathy) or skin (burns) losses; hydration (dehydration results in hemoconcentration, overhydration in hemodilution); liver function (synthesis); and metabolic stress and inflammation (chronic disease, sepsis, trauma, surgery, infection). Thus, visceral protein concentrations must be interpreted relative to the individual's overall clinical condition and inflammatory state (Table 164-6).

The significant influence of inflammation on visceral protein concentrations is now well established; thus, these *negative acute phase reactants* may be considered to reflect the extent of physiologic stress or inflammation rather than the presence of undernutrition (Table 164-3).[43,44] During severe acute stress (eg, trauma, burns, sepsis), these proteins are decreased because the resultant increased vascular permeability can lead to dramatic fluid shifts and the reprioritizing of liver protein synthesis increases the production of acute-phase reactants such as CRP, ferritin, fibrinogen, and haptoglobin.[11,44] CRP is a true acute-phase protein rising within 10 hours after major surgery or acute sepsis; it can be used to assess the degree of inflammation present.[44] If CRP is elevated, then inflammation is likely contributing to decreased visceral protein concentrations making visceral proteins inflammatory markers associated with nutrition risk rather than markers of malnutrition or protein and energy intake inadequacy.[43] The role of visceral protein monitoring in nutrition support remains unclear; however, normalizing values may indicate resolving stress and inflammation, decreased nutrition risk, shift to anabolism, and/or decreasing nutritional requirements.[43] Thus, assessing individual patient trends, not comparison to normative standards, may be useful in monitoring recovery.

ALB is the most abundant serum protein and is critical for the maintenance of colloid oncotic pressure and binding and transport of numerous hormones, anions, medications, and fatty acids. As an insensitive index of protein malnutrition, ALB is not a component of currently accepted definitions for malnutrition.[43] Factors that lead to ALBs insensitivity include the large amount normally in the body (4-5 g/kg of body weight), extensive distribution in the extravascular compartment (60%), and long half-life (18-20 days). As discussed, ALB is a negative acute-phase reactant, and serum concentrations decrease with inflammation, infection, trauma, stress, and burns. Serum ALB concentrations less than 2.5 g/dL (25 g/L) can be expected to exacerbate ascites and peripheral, pulmonary, and GI mucosal edema because of decreased colloid oncotic pressure. Hypoalbuminemia also affects the interpretation of serum concentrations of calcium and highly protein bound medications (eg, phenytoin, valproic acid).

TFN is a glycoprotein that binds and transports ferric iron to the liver and reticuloendothelial system for storage. TFN is also a negative acute-phase reactant, and its concentration is decreased in the presence of critical illness and inflammation.[12] Because it has a shorter half-life (8-9 days) and there is less of it in the body (less than 100 mg/kg of body weight), TFN concentration decreases in response to various factors before the serum ALB concentration. If a direct measure of serum TFN is not available, TFN concentration can be estimated indirectly from measurement of total iron-binding capacity, as follows:

$$\text{TFN(mg/dL)} = (\text{total iron} - \text{binding capacity[mcg/dL]} \times 0.8) - 43$$

Alternatively, TFN (mg/dL) = 0.7 × total iron-binding capacity (mcg/dL) and TFN (g/L) = 0.039 × total iron-binding capacity (μmol/L). Iron stores affect serum TFN concentrations: in iron deficiency, hepatic TFN synthesis is increased, resulting in increased serum TFN concentrations.

Prealbumin (transthyretin) is the transport protein for thyroxine and a carrier for retinol-binding protein. While prealbumin was historically used to monitor the short-term, acute effects of nutrition support or deficits, it is now recognized as an inflammatory marker that may be associated with risk of developing malnutrition or poor clinical outcomes.[43] Prealbumin stores are low (10 mg/kg of body weight), and it has a very short half-life (2-3 days); thus, the serum prealbumin concentration will decrease rapidly with severe metabolic stress (trauma, burns, sepsis). As with ALB and TFN, prealbumin synthesis is decreased in liver disease. Prealbumin is renally excreted, so falsely elevated prealbumin concentrations may be seen in patients with kidney dysfunction.

Nitrogen Balance Study

Nitrogen is found only in protein and at a relatively constant ratio of 1 g nitrogen per 6.25 g of protein. This ratio may vary somewhat for EN and PN formulations, depending on the biologic value of the protein source. The adequacy of protein intake can be assessed clinically by a nitrogen balance study—measuring urinary nitrogen excretion and comparing it with nitrogen intake. Nitrogen balance indirectly reflects protein utilization and/or the protein catabolic rate. As the stress level increases, a concomitant increase in protein catabolism (hypercatabolism) results in an increase in urinary nitrogen excretion. The amount of urine urea nitrogen (UUN) measured in a 24-hour urine collection in healthy individuals, accounts for 80% to 90% of the total urine nitrogen (TUN) excreted. Nitrogen output (g/day) can be approximated as 24-hour UUN + 4, where 4 is a factor representing usual skin, fecal, and respiratory nitrogen losses.[12]

TABLE 164-6 Serum Proteins Associated with Nutrition Risk

Serum Protein	Half-Life (Days)	Functions	Factors Resulting in Increased Values	Factors Resulting in Decreased Values
Albumin	18-20	Maintains plasma oncotic pressure; transports small molecules	Dehydration, anabolic steroids, insulin, infection	Fluid overload; edema; kidney dysfunction; nephrotic syndrome; poor dietary intake; impaired digestion; burns; heart failure; cirrhosis; thyroid, adrenal, or pituitary hormones; trauma; sepsis
Transferrin	8-9	Binds Fe in plasma; transports Fe to bone	Fe deficiency, pregnancy, hypoxia, chronic blood loss, estrogens	Chronic infection, cirrhosis, burns, enteropathies, nephrotic syndrome, cortisone, testosterone
Prealbumin (transthyretin)	2-3	Binds T_3 and, to a lesser extent, T_4; retinol-binding protein carrier	Impaired kidney function	Cirrhosis, hepatitis, stress, surgery, inflammation, hyperthyroidism, cystic fibrosis, burns, zinc deficiency

Fe, iron; T_3, triiodothyronine; T_4, thyroxine.

Alternatively, nitrogen output can be estimated using the equation: 24-hour UUN + 2 + 20% of urinary urea losses.[45] At higher UUN values (30 g nitrogen or more), then the use of a factor of + 6 may yield a more accurate measure of nitrogen output.[46] Alternatively, if available, TUN can be measured and may be more accurate, especially in critically ill patients who excrete more nitrogen-containing substances such as 3-methylhistidine. If TUN is used, then the best estimate of nitrogen output is TUN + 1.05, where 1.05 is the average extraurinary nitrogen losses.[46] In patients with decreased kidney function, in which case neither UUN nor TUN accurately represents net protein degradation, nitrogen output can be approximated with equations based on urea nitrogen appearance.[47]

Immune Function Tests

Nutrition status affects immune function either directly, via actions on the lymphoid system, or indirectly by altering cellular metabolism or organs that are involved with immune system regulation. Immune function tests most often used in nutrition assessment are the total lymphocyte count and delayed cutaneous hypersensitivity (DCH) reactions. Both tests are simple, readily available, and inexpensive. A lack of specificity, however, limits the usefulness of these tests as nutrition status markers.

Total lymphocyte count reflects the number of circulating T and B lymphocytes. Tissues that generate T cells are very sensitive to malnutrition, undergoing involution resulting in decreased T-cell production and eventually lymphocytopenia. A total lymphocyte count less than 1200 cells/mm^3 (1.2 × 10^9 cells/L) is a nonspecific marker for nutrition depletion.[12] Total lymphocyte count is reduced in the presence of infection (eg, human immunodeficiency virus [HIV], other viruses, tuberculosis), immunosuppressive drugs (eg, corticosteroids, cyclosporine, tacrolimus, sirolimus, chemotherapy, antilymphocyte globulin), leukemia, and lymphoma.

DCH is commonly assessed using recall antigens to which the patient was likely previously sensitized, such as mumps and *Candida albicans*. Although not specific for nutrition status, anergy is associated with severe malnutrition, and response can be restored with nutrition repletion.[12] Factors affecting DCH include fever, viral illness, recent live-virus vaccination, critical illness, irradiation, immunosuppressive drugs, diabetes mellitus, HIV, cancer, and surgery. Other immune function tests used in nutrition research include lymphocyte surface antigens (eg, CD4, CD8, CD4:CD8 ratio), T-lymphocyte responsiveness, and various serum interleukin concentrations.

Nutrients such as arginine, omega-3 fatty acids, and nucleic acids given in pharmacologic doses may improve immune function. Monitoring efficacy of a nutrition care plan that includes these potentially immune-modulating nutrients may include these immune function assessments.

NUTRIENT DEFICIENCIES AND TOXICITIES

6 Macronutrient or micronutrient deficiencies or toxicities or risk factors for these deficiencies or toxicities may be identified by a comprehensive nutrition assessment. A comprehensive nutrition assessment should include an evaluation for possible essential fatty acid deficiency (EFAD) or vitamin or trace element toxicities. Because of their key role in metabolic processes (coenzymes and cofactors), a deficiency of any of these nutrients may result in altered metabolism and cell dysfunction. An accurate history to identify symptoms and risk factors for a specific nutrient deficiency or toxicity is critical. A NFPE and biochemical assessment to confirm a suspected deficiency or toxicity should be done in all nutritionally-at-risk patients. Ideally, biochemical assessment would be based on the nutrient's function (eg, metalloenzyme activity) rather than simply measuring the serum concentration. Unfortunately, few practical methods to assess micronutrient function are available; thus, the serum concentration is most often measured (Table 164-7).

Trace Elements

Trace elements considered essential in humans (at least one important role and a range of intakes within which homeostasis is maintained) are iron, zinc, selenium, copper, chromium, manganese, molybdenum, and iodine. A complete discussion of each of these elements is beyond the scope of this chapter.[48-52] Each trace element is involved in a variety of biologic functions and is necessary for normal metabolism, acting as a coenzyme or in other roles in hormonal metabolism or erythropoiesis. Toxicities can occur with excess intake of some trace elements. With the current interest in complementary medicine, clinicians must ask patients about their use of all dietary supplements.

Iron

Iron is the most abundant trace element and is an important component of hemoglobin, myoglobin, and cytochrome enzymes; it is also involved in oxygen transport and cellular energy production. Patients with iron-deficiency anemia typically present with fatigue, weakness, and pallor. Inadequate iron intake, malabsorption, and chronic blood loss are the principal causes of iron-deficiency anemia. Iron toxicity (overload) with possible organ damage can occur when chronic iron intake exceeds requirements, such as in patients receiving multiple blood transfusions over an extended period (1 unit of packed red blood cells provides 200-250 mg elemental iron). Iron deficiency or overload is confirmed by assessment of iron stores, as reflected indirectly by measurement of hemoglobin, serum iron, total iron-binding capacity, and serum ferritin or directly by bone marrow staining or liver biopsy. Direct methods are most accurate but invasive and rarely necessary. Because indirect parameters such as ferritin are altered by acute or chronic inflammation independent of iron stores, concomitant illness must be considered in their interpretation. As with visceral protein assessment, CRP measurement simultaneously with iron assessments will help to determine the degree to which inflammation influences these parameters.[50]

Zinc

Zinc, the second-most abundant trace element, is a cofactor in many enzymatic reactions involved in protein, fat, and carbohydrate metabolism and is involved in the regulation of gene expression, immunity, growth, wound healing, and liver regeneration.[49,50,53] Most of the body's zinc (85%) is found in muscle and bone; less than 1% is found in the serum. Zinc is eliminated through the urine and the GI tract. Zinc deficiency develops with decreased intake or absorption, increased loss, or increased demand. Risk factors for zinc deficiency include bariatric surgery, anorexia/bulimia, alcohol misuse, excessive fluid losses (bile, intestinal, urine), and increased metabolic demands (sepsis, burns).[53] Urinary zinc losses are increased by thiazide diuretics, angiotensin converting enzyme inhibitors, angiotensin receptor blockers, and hemofiltration.[51] Zinc deficiency can develop in 14 days to 3 months with insufficient intake and is characterized by skin lesions (acrodermatitis enteropathica), a moist eczematous dermatitis that is most apparent in the nasolabial folds and around orifices, and other symptoms (Table 164-7).[49] Recovery is rapid with zinc supplementation; severe dermatitis can improve in as little as 4 to 5 days. Zinc deficiency can be documented by the presence of low serum zinc concentrations. However, serum zinc concentrations decrease during acute stress states and generally remain depressed until the stress resolves. Hair zinc analysis and urinary zinc excretion can be used as biomarkers of zinc status.[53] Excess zinc intake is eliminated by the kidneys and GI tract; thus, zinc toxicity is uncommon except in overdoses or with excessive, prolonged parenteral supplementation.

TABLE 164-7 Assessment of Trace Element Status

Trace Element	Signs of Deficiency	Signs of Toxicity	Factors Associated with Altered Plasma Concentrations	Monitoring
Chromium	Impaired glucose/protein utilization, peripheral neuropathy, weight loss, increased LDL-C, increased free fatty acid concentrations	Industrial exposure: skin or nasal septum lesions, allergic dermatitis, increased incidence of lung cancer	**Decreased**: long-term inadequate intake **Increased**: kidney failure	Serum glucose, plasma chromium (unreliable)
Copper	Menkes' syndrome: progressive mental deterioration, vomiting, diarrhea, protein-losing enteropathy, hypopigmentation, bone and hair changes Deficiency: neutropenia, hypochromic anemia, pallor, dermatitis, neurological dysfunction, osteoporosis, myopathy, thrombocytopenia, decreased bone mineralization (children)	Wilson's disease: cirrhosis, Kayser-Fleischer rings[a], kidney dysfunction, neurologic or psychiatric symptoms (tremors, slow speech, inappropriate behavior, personality changes) Mild chronic toxicity: fatigue, anemia, thrombocytopenia Acute toxicity: nausea, vomiting, diarrhea	**Decreased**: high zinc, iron, or vitamin C intake; corticosteroid use **Increased**: infection, rheumatoid arthritis, pregnancy, oral contraceptives, decreased biliary excretion	Serum copper and ceruloplasmin with CRP[b], CBC
Iodine	Hypothyroid goiter, neuromuscular impairment, deaf-mutism, increased embryonic and postnatal mortality, cognitive impairment, impaired fertility, congenital hypothyroidism (severe cases)	Thyrotoxicosis: nodular goiter, weight loss, tachycardia, muscle weakness, warm skin	**Decreased**: long-term inadequate intake	Serum T_3, T_4, TSH
Iron	Microcytic, hypochromic anemia (weakness, pallor, fatigue), glossitis, headache, dysphasia, nail changes, gastric atrophy, paresthesia, decreased cognitive function	Cirrhosis, cardiomyopathy, pancreatic damage, skin pigmentation changes	**Increased**: blood transfusion **Decreased**: blood loss; long-term iron-free PN	Serum ferritin[c], iron, percent iron saturation, iron binding capacity; CBC
Manganese	Nausea; vomiting; dermatitis; hair color changes; hypocholesterolemia; growth retardation; defective carbohydrate, lipid, and protein metabolism	Parkinsonian-like symptoms, hyperirritability, hallucinations, libido disturbances, ataxia, mental confusion, lack of attention, memory loss, weakness, seizures, facial nerve abnormalities, headache, dizziness, dystonia, peripheral neuropathy	**Increased**: decreased biliary excretion, high iron or vitamin C intake	Whole blood manganese, brain MRI
Molybdenum	Tachycardia, tachypnea, altered mental status, visual changes, headache, nausea, vomiting	Gout-like syndrome, increased urinary copper	**Decreased**: low birth weight, excessive GI losses	Urinary hypoxanthine, xanthine, and sulfite oxidase
Selenium	Muscle weakness or pain, cardiomyopathy, skin and hair pigmentation changes, macrocytosis, alopecia and growth retardation in infants	Nausea, vomiting, hair or nail loss, tooth decay, skin lesions, irritability, fatigue, peripheral neuropathy	**Decreased**: malignancy, liver failure, pregnancy, stress, infection **Increased**: reticuloendothelial-neoplasia	Plasma, serum, or whole blood selenium: RBC glutathione peroxidase; CBC
Zinc	Dermatitis (scaly, hyperpigmented skin lesions), stomatitis, glossitis, perioral and periungual ulceration, altered taste and smell, alopecia, diarrhea, apathy, depression, growth retardation, impaired wound healing, anorexia, confusion, immunosuppression, delayed sexual maturation, hypogonadism (decreased sperm count and function)	Acute: diarrhea, vomiting, nausea, dizziness, garlic-smelling breath; death with large IV doses Chronic: immunosuppression, decreased HDL-C, copper deficiency	**Decreased**: infection, burns, stress, hypoalbuminemia, corticosteroids, pregnancy, inflammation **Increased**: tissue injury, hemolysis, contaminated collection tube	Plasma or serum zinc with albumin and CRP, stool or ostomy output, serum copper

CBC, complete blood count; CRP, C-reactive protein; GI, gastrointestinal; HDL-C, high-density-lipoprotein cholesterol; IV, intravenous LDL-C, low-density-lipoprotein cholesterol; MRI, magnetic resonance imaging; PN, parenteral nutrition; RBC, red blood cell; RQ, respiratory quotient; T_3, triiodothyronine; T_4, thyroxine TSH, thyroid stimulating hormone.

[a]Kayser-Fleischer rings are dark rings that appear to encircle the iris of the eye.

[b]If CRP > 4 mg/dL (40 mg/L), serum copper concentration will be falsely elevated. Ceruloplasmin increased with inflammation, pregnancy, liver disease, malignancy, and myocardial infarction.

[c]If ferritin low, iron deficiency; if high, inflammation or iron overload.

Selenium

Selenium is not an antioxidant itself but an integral part of selenoproteins. There are 25 genes coding for these selenoproteins, about half of which have a defined metabolic function. Important selenoproteins include selenoprotein P (antioxidant activity), glutathione peroxidase (antioxidant activity), iodothyronine deiodinase (thyroid hormone regulation), thioredoxin reductase (vitamin C), selenoprotein V (spermatogenesis), and selenoprotein S (inflammation, immune response).[50,54] A key metabolic function of selenium is its role in the enzymatic cofactor selenocysteine, the 21st proteinogenic amino acid.[54] Selenoprotein P is the major (60%) circulating form of selenium in serum.

Prematurity, critical illness, burns, chronic GI losses, and long-term selenium-free PN are associated with low serum selenium concentrations and decreased glutathione peroxidase activity.[49] The clinical significance of reduced serum selenium concentrations is unclear, but low selenium concentrations may increase susceptibility to physiologic stressors. Low serum selenium concentrations in critically ill patients correlate with low triiodothyronine (T_3) concentrations.[55] Serum selenium concentrations reflect acute distribution between tissues rather than selenium stores. Selenium deficiency is associated with muscle pain, wasting, and weakness (see Table 164-7), but severe biochemical deficiency is not always accompanied by these symptoms. Statins inhibit 3-hydroxy-3-methylglutaryl coenzyme A reductase and can induce myopathy by interfering with synthesis of selenoproteins.[50] Fatal cardiomyopathy may occur. Although critically ill patients may require higher selenium intakes than normal, optimal intake is unknown; current recommendations range from 20 to 1,000 mcg/day.[55]

Serum, erythrocyte, and whole-blood selenium; serum selenoprotein P; and serum, platelet, and whole-blood glutathione peroxidase activity respond to changes in selenium intake, but the response is heterogeneous.[56] Decreased serum selenium concentrations may indicate selenium deficiency, but reductions have also been observed in patients with malignancies, liver failure, pregnancy, alcohol misuse, and HIV; in patients receiving statins or corticosteroids; and in patients who smoke. Selenium toxicity (selenosis) generally occurs only in those with long-term exposure to foods grown in selenium-rich soil (eg, US Great Plains area) but may occur when intake exceeds 200 mcg/day or 5 mcg/kg/day for prolonged periods.[50] Selenium toxicity results in hair and nail brittleness and loss, GI disturbance, skin rash, garlic breath odor, fatigue, irritability, nervous system abnormalities, and has been linked to type 2 diabetes mellitus.[54]

Copper

Copper is a cofactor in oxidative enzymes vital to the function of hematopoietic, vascular, and skeletal tissue, as well as structure and function of the nervous system.[47,48,57] It is a component of ceruloplasmin and key metalloenzymes involved in iron and manganese metabolism (ceruloplasmin), electron transfer and oxidation-reduction reactions (cytochrome c oxidase), connective tissue and collagen cross-linking (lysyl oxidase), dopamine conversion to norepinephrine (dopamine monooxygenase), free radical scavenging (superoxide dismutase), and many others.[49,50] Copper is absorbed in the duodenum and excreted through the bile bound to bile salts. Most copper (67%) is found in bone and muscle, and 60% to 95% of serum copper is bound to ceruloplasmin.[58] Signs and symptoms of copper deficiency are listed in Table 164-7 and include anemia, neutropenia, thrombocytopenia, and neurologic dysfunction. In severe cases, such as in Menkes' syndrome, copper deficiency is further manifested as hypothermia, hair and skin depigmentation, progressive mental deterioration, and growth retardation. Factors predisposing to copper deficiency include generalized malabsorption, protein-losing enteropathy, nephrotic syndrome, prematurity, and copper-free PN.[57–59] Long-term PN supplemented with copper may increase the risk of copper toxicity in patients who develop cholestasis; however, copper deficiency has been reported with copper-free PN after copper removal from the PN solution due to a rising direct bilirubin concentration (cholestasis).[58] Patients undergoing bariatric surgery are at risk for copper deficiency as early as 2 months after surgery. Typically 1 to 3 weeks of oral copper supplementation or 5 days of IV supplementation (1 mg/day) is sufficient to correct the deficiency.[49,57]

Copper deficiency is assessed using serum copper concentrations along with CRP and ceruloplasmin, which appear to reflect changes in copper status in both copper-depleted and copper-replete individuals.[59] While reliable indicators of severe copper deficiency, serum copper and ceruloplasmin concentrations may not detect marginal copper deficiency because serum concentrations may be altered by a variety of conditions including inflammation (Table 164-7). Copper concentrations should be monitored every 2 to 6 months in patients receiving long-term PN. The chronic ingestion of excessive copper or inadequate elimination can result in cirrhosis as seen in Wilson's disease, an autosomal-recessive genetic disorder.

Chromium

Historically, trivalent chromium was thought to be essential for insulin function and maintenance of normal blood glucose concentrations. A low-molecular-weight chromium binding substance, *the glucose tolerance factor*, that may enhance insulin receptor response has been discussed. In 2014, the European Food Safety Authority (EFSA) determined that chromium is not an essential element in humans.[60] Chromium is stored in the heart, muscle, kidney, and liver and excreted in the urine.[49,52] Chromium deficiency may occur in patients receiving long-term chromium-free PN; symptoms include hyperglycemia, weight loss, and neuropathy.[49] Urine and serum chromium concentrations reflect chromium absorption not stores.[60] Chromium toxicity varies depending on the valence; trivalent chromium used in PN solutions is generally not toxic. No chromium toxicity has been reported in patients receiving PN, even though intake may be 30 to 60 times higher than estimated requirements through chromium contamination, primarily Dextrose 70%,; additional supplementation is rarely needed.[52] Chromium toxicity has only been reported with contaminated drinking water or industrial exposure. Chromium supplementation as an adjunct to aerobic exercise for weight loss or diabetes mellitus management is ineffective.[60,61]

Manganese

Manganese is needed as a cofactor for several metalloenzymes, including isocitrate dehydrogenase (Krebs cycle), superoxide dismutase (mitochondrial antioxidant), glutamine synthetase (astrocytes), arginase (urea cycle), pyruvate carboxylase (carbohydrate metabolism), glycosyltransferases (bone formation), and prolidase (wound healing).[50,62] Excess manganese is rapidly and efficiently eliminated in bile in the absence of significant cholestasis. Excretion may be compromised in newborns due to immature liver function. Manganese deficiency is only associated with the ingestion of chemically defined manganese-deficient oral diets. Table 164-7 lists symptoms associated with manganese deficiency.

Manganese toxicity is more concerning and has been described in industrial exposures via inhaled manganese (welding) and in patients receiving long-term manganese-supplemented PN in the setting of chronic cholestasis. Toxicity may occur in adults receiving more than 500 mcg/day and in children receiving more than 40 mcg/kg/day.[62] Manganese can accumulate in brain tissue; an intravenous dosage of 1.1 mg/day has been associated with brain deposition.[50] Because of its paramagnetic properties, manganese is detectable using MRI with increased signal intensity on T1-weighted images of the basal ganglia, especially in the striatum, globus pallidus, and substantia nigra. Manganese appears to target the dopaminergic

(DAergic) neurons but may affect other neurotransmitters.[62] Whole-blood manganese concentrations are used to assess manganese status; serum concentrations do not correlate with either whole blood concentrations or MRI findings.[62] The neurodegenerative process induced by manganese is termed *manganism*. Symptoms mimicking Parkinson's disease, including psychiatric symptoms, cognitive deficits, motor impairment, extrapyramidal symptoms, headache, dizziness, rigidity, tremors, ataxia, and facial muscle spasms.[49,62] Lewy bodies, the hallmark of Parkinson's disease, are not seen in manganism.[62] Removing manganese from the PN solution results in resolution of neurologic symptoms with partial or total MRI normalization within 1 year.[62] The newborn brain may be more susceptible to the effects of manganese toxicity which has implications for manganese supplementation in premature neonates receiving PN.[62]

Molybdenum

Molybdenum is a cofactor for enzymes involved in catabolism of sulfur-containing amino acids, purines, and pyrimidines (xanthine, aldehyde, sulfite oxidases).[49,50,63] Molybdenum deficiency is uncommon, but a rare genetic defect that prevents sulfite oxidase synthesis resulting in molybdenum deficiency has been identified. A continuous supply of sulfated compounds is needed during brain development; thus, young infants are at risk if an adequate molybdenum supply is not provided.[63] Molybdenum deficiency may occur in patients receiving long-term molybdenum-free PN; although significant molybdenum contamination is present in all PN solutions. Currently, there is no IV molybdenum product marketed in the United States, and no marketed trace element combination product contains molybdenum. Molybdenum deficiency symptoms include tachycardia, tachypnea, headache, night blindness, nausea, vomiting, central scotomas, lethargy, disorientation, and coma (Table 164-7).[49,50,63] Symptoms reverse with molybdenum supplementation. Plasma and serum molybdenum are very low and difficult to measure, and plasma concentrations do not reflect molybdenum status.[52] Biochemical abnormalities expected in molybdenum deficiency include very low serum and urine uric acid concentrations (low xanthine oxidase activity) and low urine inorganic sulfate concentrations with high urine inorganic sulfite concentrations (low sulfate oxidase activity).[49,50] Molybdenum toxicity has not been described.

Iodine

Iodine, found primarily in the thyroid gland (70%-80%) incorporated into thyroid hormones, is required for normal thyroid function which affects resting energy expenditure and growth. In iodine deficiency, there is a constant release of thyroid stimulating hormone (TSH), resulting in thyroid gland hyperplasia and goiter formation. However, not everyone with an iodine-deficient diet will develop a goiter. The most serious effects of iodine deficiency are during pregnancy and in childhood, including fetal death, cretinism, abnormal growth, and mental retardation.[49] Measurement of thyroxine (T_4), T_3, and thyroid stimulating hormone (TSH) can be used to assess iodine status (Table 164-7). Iodine needs may be met by consumption of iodized salt or cutaneous iodine absorption from povidone–iodine, a topical antiseptic, used in catheter care.[50] Use of povidone–iodine for this indication has virtually been eliminated with the increased use of chlorhexidine for catheter site care, putting patients requiring long-term PN at risk. An IV iodine product is no longer available, and no trace element combination product marketed in the United States contains iodine. Iodine excess is rarely a clinical concern when thyroid and kidney function are normal except in overdoses or too rapid correction of iodine deficiency.[50]

Vitamins

Vitamins act as both catalysts (cofactors) and substrates in essential metabolic reactions. They are needed for normal growth, metabolism, and cellular integrity. They facilitate energy-yielding chemical reactions; they do not contribute energy. A thorough review of vitamins and their complex effects on nutrition and metabolism is beyond the scope of this chapter.[50,52,64] A comprehensive nutrition-focused history and NFPE are valuable means of assessing patients for vitamin deficiency or toxicity (Table 164-8). Generalized malnutrition is often associated with multiple vitamin deficiencies or increased needs; however, single vitamin deficiencies do occur. Thiamine (B_1) deficiency can result in early symptoms (dry or wet beriberi, GI symptoms) or advanced symptoms (lactic acidosis, Wernicke's encephalopathy, polyneuropathy, ataxia, mental confusion) due to impaired oxidative and energy metabolism often leading to serious and potentially irreversible neurological damage or death.[50,65] Macrocytic anemia, peripheral neuropathy, and neuropsychiatric sequelae may be caused by vitamin B12 (cyanocobalamin) deficiency which can occur after gastric or ileal resection due to the loss of intrinsic factor or absorption sites of the intrinsic factor-B_{12} complex, respectively. Vitamin B12 deficiency has been reported with increasing frequency in older adults, especially with prolonged gastric acid suppression with proton pump inhibitors.[66] There is a high prevalence of subclinical vitamin K deficiency in patients with chronic kidney disease, including those on hemodialysis or peritoneal dialysis. Vitamin K deficiency is a modifiable risk factor for cardiovascular disease and bone fracture in this patient population.[67]

Patients with steatorrhea have an increased risk of fat-soluble vitamin (A, D, E, K) deficiencies. However, the increasing prevalence of vitamin D deficiency is a worldwide concern, including all ages, genders, and racial/ethnic groups. Risk for deficiency is higher in children and older adults, pregnant women, individuals with dark skin, patients receiving long-term PN, those living in temperate and higher latitudes, and those with disabilities or who are obese.[68] Laboratory assessment can confirm the clinical suspicion of a deficiency state. Vitamin D2 (ergocalciferol from plant-based sources) and vitamin D3 (cholecalciferol from conversion of cholesterol in the skin by ultraviolet light) are quickly converted to 25(OH)D via hydroxylation in the liver. The best marker for vitamin D deficiency is the serum concentration of 25(OH)D. Reference ranges for US laboratories are typically 20-100 ng/mL (50-250 nmol/L), but the optimal range is likely above 30 ng/mL (75 nmol/L) based on the concentration associated with parathyroid hormone (PTH) stimulation and calcium absorption efficiency.[68] The first indication of a deficiency is usually a decrease in circulating serum 25(OH)D. Subsequently, there is a decrease in urinary vitamin D excretion, which is followed by diminished tissue concentrations. Because the active form of vitamin D, $1,25(OH)_2D$, is produced only when needed, not stored, and dependent on kidney function, intact PTH concentration, and calcium and phosphorus supply, it is not a useful marker of vitamin D stores but may be helpful if assessing the kidney's ability to hydroxylate to the active form.

Vitamin toxicity can occur, especially with fat-soluble vitamins, which are stored in the body. Vitamin D toxicity can cause significant hypercalcemia, hypercalciuria, and soft tissue calcifications leading to kidney and cardiovascular damage.[50] Vitamin A toxicity is associated with many signs and symptoms including effects on bone.[50] Water-soluble vitamins, except cyanocobalamin (vitamin B_{12}), are not stored; consequently, the toxicity risk is minimal unless ingested in very high doses. However, evidence suggests that even water-soluble vitamins may be associated with adverse medication reactions when taken chronically in high doses. Preconception folic acid supplementation is definitively associated with a reduction in neural tube defects.[69] Multivitamin supplementation containing folic acid does not prevent cardiovascular disease despite its effects on homocysteine concentrations.[70] With North Americans consuming large amounts of nutrition supplements, spending more than $15.5B (2020 USD) for them each year, clinicians should be alert for signs of inappropriate vitamin use and hypervitaminosis (see Table 164-8) and be prepared to discuss rational supplement use with all patients.[71]

TABLE 164-8 Assessment of Vitamin Status

Vitamin	Signs of Deficiency	Laboratory Assay	Comments
Water-Soluble Vitamins			
Thiamine (B1)	Early: anorexia, fatigue, depression, impaired memory or concentration Late: paresthesia, nystagmus, GI beriberi (nausea, vomiting, abdominal pain, lactic acidosis), beriberi (heart failure, edema), Wernicke's encephalopathy, Korsakoff's psychosis, peripheral neuropathy	Whole blood or erythrocyte transketolase activation test Blood thiamine pyrophosphate Erythrocyte glutathione reductase activity coefficient	Increased need with hemo- and peritoneal dialysis, alcohol misuse, malabsorption, hypermetabolism
Riboflavin (B2)	Mucositis, dermatitis, cheilosis, glossitis, photophobia, corneal vascularization, lacrimation, decreased vision, impaired wound healing and growth, normocytic anemia	Urine riboflavin	
Pantothenic acid	Fatigue, malaise, headache, insomnia, vomiting, abdominal cramps	Serum pantothenic acid	
Niacin	Pellagra: dermatitis, dementia, glossitis, diarrhea, memory loss, headaches	Urine niacin and N1-methylnicotinamide Erythrocyte NAD and NADP concentrations to determine "niacin number"	Flushing, nausea, and vomiting seen with hyperlipidemia treatment; increased need with hemo- and peritoneal dialysis
Pyridoxine (B6)	Pellagra, dermatitis, glossitis, cheilosis, distal limb numbness or paresthesia, convulsions, microcytic anemia	Plasma pyridoxal 5-phosphate Urine 4-pyridoxic acid	Sensory neuropathy and seizures with very high doses (>2 g/day)
Folic acid	Macrocytic anemia, diarrhea, glossitis, cheilosis, angular stomatitis, fatigue, difficulty concentrating, irritability, headache, palpitations, shortness of breath, heart failure, tachycardia, postural hypotension, lactic acidosis, neural tube defects, impaired cellular immunity, paranoid behavior	Serum or plasma folate (acute) Red blood cell folate (chronic) Serum homocysteine	Decreased with increased cellular/tissue turnover (pregnancy, malignancy, hemolytic anemia); masks diagnosis of vitamin B12 deficiency; decreases risks of neural tube defects
Cyanocobalamin (B12)	Pernicious (megaloblastic) anemia, glossitis, spinal cord degeneration, peripheral neuropathy, paresthesias, pancytopenia, personality changes, dementia, depression, psychosis	Serum cobalamin Plasma homocysteine Urine or plasma methylmalonic acid[a] CBC	Decreased absorption in older adults, distal ileal resection, loss of gastric intrinsic factor due to gastrectomy or long-term gastric acid suppression
Biotin	Dermatitis, depression, lassitude, somnolence	Urine biotin	
Ascorbic acid (C)	Enlargement or keratosis of hair follicles, impaired wound healing, anemia, lethargy, depression, bleeding, ecchymosis, scurvy	Plasma ascorbic acid Leukocyte ascorbate	GI disturbances, hyperoxaluria and kidney stones, excess iron absorption with excess intake; individuals who smoke need 35 mg/day more than nonsmokers; rebound scurvy with abrupt discontinuation after long-term high doses
Fat-Soluble Vitamins			
Vitamin A (includes retinol, retinal, retinoic acid, and retinyl esters)	Dermatitis, night blindness, xerophthalmia, Bitot spots[b], pruritus, follicular hyperkeratosis, excessive deposition of periosteal bone, hair changes, poor growth and wound healing, impaired resistance to infection Irreversible: punctate keratopathy, keratomalacia, corneal perforation	Serum retinol Serum retinol-binding protein Serum retinyl esters (toxicity)	Teratogenic, liver toxicity with excessive intake; alcohol use, liver disease, hyperlipidemia, and severe protein malnutrition increase susceptibility to adverse effects of high intake; β-carotene supplements recommended only for those at risk of deficiency (fat malabsorption); may reverse corticosteroid-induced poor wound healing
D	Rickets, osteomalacia, osteoporosis, muscle weakness, poor growth, hypocalcemia, immune dysfunction, cardiomyopathy	Serum 25-hydroxy-vitamin D (storage form); 1,25-dihydroxyvitamin D (active form)	Elevated intake causes hypercalcemia, nephrocalcinosis, azotemia, poor growth; decreased concentration in uremia, older adults (especially in winter), and fat malabsorption
α-Tocopherol (E)	Hemolysis	Serum α-tocopherol Ratios of serum α-tocopherol to total lipids	Excess intake: hemorrhagic toxicity; increased risk of bleeding with anticoagulants; impaired leukocyte function
K	Bleeding (ecchymosis, petechiae, hematoma)	Prothrombin time INR	Anticoagulant therapy can be affected by supplements or diet

CBC, complete blood count; GI, gastrointestinal; INR, international normalized ratio; NAD, nicotinamide adenine dinucleotide; NADP, nicotinamide adenine dinucleotide phosphate.

[a]Plasma methylmalonic acid concentrations increase with vitamin B12 deficiency.

[b]Bitot spots are spots which are oval, triangular, or irregular in shape and located superficially in the conjunctiva.

Essential Fatty Acids

The human body can synthesize all fatty acids except the essential fatty acids, linoleic acid (an omega-6 fatty acid) and α-linolenic acid (an omega-3 fatty acid). EFAD can be prevented if approximately 5% (linoleic acid) and 0.6% (linolenic acid) of total energy is ingested as these fatty acids.[72,73] EFAD is rare in adults and children but can occur with prolonged lipid-free PN, severe fat malabsorption, very low-fat enteral feeding formulations or diets, high medium chain triglyceride-containing diets, and severe malnutrition, especially in stressed patients.[74] Although the time needed to develop EFAD is variable, symptomatic EFAD has occurred after only 4 weeks of lipid-free PN, and biochemical evidence can occur within 1 week.[74] The brain grows rapidly during the last trimester of gestation and the first 2 years of life. Large amounts of essential fatty acids are needed for central nervous system myelin synthesis. Newborns, especially those born prematurely, who have limited to no fat stores, may develop EFAD more rapidly than adults and should generally receive a source of essential fatty acids within 72 hours after birth.[74] Symptoms reported with EFAD include dermatitis (dry, scaly skin), increased susceptibility to infection, impaired wound healing, poor growth and brain development, and immune dysfunction.[73,74]

Linoleic acid is converted to arachidonic acid (20:4ω-6; a tetraene fatty acid). When linoleic acid is unavailable, oleic acid (18:1ω-9) is the preferred substrate, resulting in production of eicosatrienoic acid (20:3ω-9; a triene fatty acid). Thus, EFAD is associated with decreased tetraene and increased triene production. Different methods to measure fatty acids have resulted in variable proposed threshold triene-to-tetraene (T:T) values to diagnose EFAD.[75] The usual T:T ratio is approximately 0.01 to 0.05 depending on the assay; thus a T:T ratio greater than 0.05 generally suggests early EFAD. The T:T ratio will be abnormal before there are overt clinical symptoms. Clinical symptoms of EFAD will be present in patients with higher T:T ratios. EFAD diagnosis is generally made based on risk assessment and/or clinical findings with confirmation by measuring serum fatty acid concentrations.

Carnitine

Carnitine is a quaternary amine required for transport of long-chain fatty acids into the mitochondria for β-oxidation and energy production. Additionally, acyl compounds that are trapped within cells due to cell membrane impermeability can be esterified with carnitine, forming acylcarnitine derivatives, which are transported out of the cell, preventing the acyl compounds from accumulating to toxic concentrations (detoxification). Carnitine is also important in the metabolism of intracellular acetyl coenzyme A.[76,77] The L isomer is the physiologic active form.

Carnitine is available from a wide variety of dietary sources (especially dairy products and meats) and can be synthesized when intake is low from lysine and methionine.[78] Carnitine is filtered by the kidney and reabsorbed in the proximal tubule.[79] Hepatic synthesis is decreased in premature infants, and low serum carnitine concentrations and overt carnitine deficiency have been documented in premature infants receiving carnitine-free PN or diets (secondary deficiency), as well as in those with primary deficiency due to carnitine inborn errors of metabolism (eg, defect in the OCTN2 transporter; biosynthetic defects).[78,79] Other predisposing factors for secondary carnitine deficiency include pregnancy, malabsorption (cystic fibrosis, short bowel syndrome), chronic disease (HIV, kidney, liver), chronic medication therapy (valproic acid, verapamil, zidovudine), and a vegetarian diet.[79,80]

The clinical presentation of carnitine deficiency varies by type but may include generalized skeletal muscle weakness, hypotonia, lethargy, gross motor delay, poor feeding, growth failure, hypoglycemia, seizures, encephalopathy, hepatomegaly, hyperammonemia, recurrent infections, cardiomyopathy, and coma.[78,79] Symptoms are typically more severe in patients with primary deficiency. In clinical practice, carnitine status is assessed by measuring the serum total and free carnitine concentrations along with acylcarnitine; although, carnitine is distributed primarily in the muscle. When only total and free concentrations are available, the free is subtracted from the total to give the acylcarnitine concentration. Serum and urine carnitine concentrations are most helpful in primary carnitine deficiency; acylcarnitine concentrations are more helpful in secondary deficiency.[79]

Daily supplementation of neonatal PN solutions with 2 to 5 mg/kg carnitine is recommended when no enteral source is provided.[52] Higher doses (100-200 mg/kg/day) may be required for treatment of primary deficiency.[77]

NUTRIENT REQUIREMENTS

7 Evidence-based patient-specific goals should be established considering the patient's clinical condition and the need for maintenance or repletion in adults and continued growth and development in children. Individual nutrient requirements vary with age, sex, size, and clinical condition. Nutrition status, physical activity, and the need for continued maintenance of adequate nutrition or repletion in those with ongoing metabolic stress or malnutrition dictate the nutrient requirements for an individual. For obese patients, usual nutrition requirements may be altered because of desired weight loss and after bariatric surgery. In children, sustaining or reestablishing normal growth and development is critical. Organ function (intestine, kidney, liver, pancreas) may affect nutrient utilization. Nutrient requirements can be estimated using various methods interpreted in the context of patient-specific factors.

Recommended Dietary Allowances

The Recommended Dietary Allowances (RDAs) were first established in 1941. In 1997, the Food and Nutrition Board introduced a new designation for nutrition reference values, the Dietary Reference Intakes (DRIs). The four DRI categories are estimated average requirements (EARs), RDAs, adequate intakes (AIs), and tolerable upper intake levels (ULs). The nutrient intake that meets the needs of half of the healthy persons in a group (EAR) can be used for planning nutrient intakes for groups. The RDA, the nutrient intake that meets the needs of almost all persons in a designated group, is approximately two standard deviations above the EAR for nutrients for which the requirement is well defined and 1.2 times the EAR for other nutrients. To evaluate an individual's daily intake, the RDA is the most appropriate comparator. The AI, defined as the average intake for the designated group that appears to sustain growth or other indicator of health, is reserved for nutrients for which no EAR or RDA has been determined. The UL is the maximum nutrient intake unlikely to pose adverse effects in almost all persons in a designated group.[81] A new DRI category, Chronic Disease Risk Reduction level (CDRR), was recently added and defined as the nutrient intake that is expected to reduce the risk of developing chronic disease.[82] This new category has been applied to sodium and potassium guidelines.[83]

Dietary reference intakes have been established for six nutrient groups: calcium, phosphorus, magnesium, vitamin D, and fluoride; folate and other B vitamins; antioxidants (eg, selenium, vitamin C, vitamin E); trace elements; macronutrients (eg, protein, fat, carbohydrates, fiber); and electrolytes and water. An online Interactive DRI for Healthcare Professionals is available to calculate DRI-based nutrition needs for a generally healthy individual.[84]

In general, healthy adults and children older than 2 year of age should consume 45% to 65% of their total calories as carbohydrates. Protein recommendations also vary by age: 2 to 3 years, 5% to 20%; 4 to 18 years, 10% to 30%; and, adults, 10% to 35% of total calories. Recommended fat intakes vary by age: 2 to 3 years, 30% to 40%;

4 to 18 years, 25% to 35%; and, adults, 20% to 35% of total calories. Infants, especially premature infants, require a higher proportion of calories from fat (approximately 40%-50% of total calories) to ensure normal neurological development.

Energy

8 Validated predictive equations or population estimates are most often used to determine energy requirements; however, if available, indirect calorimetry is the most accurate bedside method to determine energy requirements. The method used will be determined by a variety of factors, including illness severity, resource availability, and clinician preference.

Estimating Energy Expenditure

Daily energy expenditure consists of the basal energy expenditure (BEE), diet-induced thermogenesis (10%), and energy used for physical activity. In sick or injured patients, the BEE is increased because of stress-related hypermetabolism, but the physical activity is usually greatly reduced. Continuous infusion EN, often used in critically ill patients, results in minimal diet-induced thermogenesis (not more than 5%) unless overfeeding. Failure to account for these changes can result in overfeeding.[22]

Numerous methods for determining an individual's daily energy requirement in a variety of settings have been published. These methods use population estimates of calories per kilogram of body weight (kcal/kg), equations that estimate energy expenditure (kcal/day or kJ/day; 1 kcal is equivalent to 4.184 kJ), or indirect calorimetry. The simplest and most convenient method to determine energy requirements is to use population estimates of calories required per kilogram of body weight. This method assumes standard values for health or the energy requirements associated with various disease states or clinical conditions, as well as the additional requirements for repletion of a malnourished individual. Most do not take into consideration age- or sex-related differences in energy needs. No stress or activity modifiers are used with these equations because the effect of the clinical condition (hypermetabolism) has been captured in the calculation. Daily adult requirements by this method can be estimated as shown below:[15,16,85]

Healthy, normal nutrition status, minimal illness severity:

20-25 kcal ABW/kg/day (84-105 kJ ABW/kg/day)

Illness, metabolic stress (first 7-10 days of intensive care unit stay):

12-25 kcal ABW/kg/day (50-105 kJ ABW/kg/day)

Illness, metabolic stress (BMI < 30 kg/m^2):

25-30 kcal ABW/kg/day (105-126 kJ ABW/kg/day)

Illness, metabolic stress (BMI ≥ 30 kg/m^2):

11-14 kcal ABW/kg/day (46-59 kJ ABW/kg/day) or
22 to 25 kcal IBW/kg/day (92-105 kJ ABW/kg/day)

Major burn [$\geq$ 50% total body surface area (TBSA)]:

25 kcal/kg ABW(kg) + 40 kcal per % TBSA burned (adult) or 25-35 kcal/kg/day in non obese patients and 21 kcal/kg/day in obese patients

When using the equations for individuals with a BMI over 30 kg/m^2, as the BMI increases, the number derived using ABW compared to IBW becomes quite disparate. Accuracy is improved by using the ABW recommendation for patients with BMI 30 to 50 kg/m^2 and the IBW recommendation when the BMI is greater than 50 kg/m^2. When these recommendations are used for patients with a BMI of 30 kg/m^2 or more, the calories provided allow for permissive underfeeding (provision of approximately 65% to 75% of usual estimated energy needs), which decreases infection rates and hospital lengths of stay.[22] DRIs for energy for healthy infants and children are shown in Table 164-9.[72] These maintenance energy requirements are approximately 130% to 150% of the basal metabolic rate, with the additional calories provided to support usual activity and growth. For all ages, energy requirements may increase with fever, sepsis, major surgery, trauma, burns, and long-term growth failure and in the presence of chronic conditions such as bronchopulmonary dysplasia, congenital heart disease, and cystic fibrosis.

There are many equations available to estimate energy expenditure in adults and children with an accuracy of approximately 40% to 77% when compared to indirect calorimetry (Tables 164-10 and 164-11,

TABLE 164-9 Dietary Reference Intakes for Energy and Protein in Healthy Children

Age (Reference age/weight)	Estimated Energy Requirement (kcal/day)[a] Boys	Girls	Protein RDA (g/kg/day)[b]
0-6 mo (3 mo/6 kg)	570	520	1.52[c]
7-12 months (9 mo/9 kg)	743	676	1.5
1-2 yr (24 mo/12 kg)	1,046	992	
1-3 yr (24 mo/12 kg)			1.1
3-8 yr (6 yr/20 kg)	1,742	1,642	
4-8 yr (6 yr/20 kg)			0.95
9-13 yr (11 yr/M: 36 kg; F: 37 kg)	2,279	2,071	0.95
14-18 yr (16 yr/M: 61 kg; F: 54 kg)	3,152	2,368	0.85

F, female; M, male; RDA, recommended dietary allowance.

[a]1 kcal is equal to approximately 4.18 kJ.

[b]Protein requirements in children with moderate to severe stress increase by 50% or more.

[c]Adequate intake.

TABLE 164-10 Equations to Estimate Energy Expenditure in Adults[a]

Healthy Adults

Harris-Benedict[b] Equations (kcal/day)

Men: BEE = 66 + (13.75W + 5H [cm]) – (6.8A)

Women: BEE = 655 + (9.6W + 1.8H [cm]) – (4.7A)

DRI Equations (kcal/day)[c]

Men: EER = 662 – 9.53A + (PA × 15.91W) + 539.6H (m)

Women: EER = 354 – 6.91A + (PA × 9.36W) + 726H (m)

PA = 1 if sedentary; 1.12 if low active; 1.27 if active; and 1.45 if very active

Mifflin-St. Jeor Equations (kcal/day)

Men: 10W + 6.25H (cm) – 5A + 5

Women: 10W + 6.25H (cm) – 5A – 161

Critically Ill Adults

Penn State Equation (kcal/day): Mifflin(0.96) + Tmax(167) + Ve(31) – 6212

Penn State Equation, modified (kcal/day) for age ≥60 yr with BMI ≥30 kg/m²: Mifflin(0.71) + Tmax(85) + Ve(64) – 3085

A, age in years; BEE, basal energy expenditure; BMI, body mass index; DRI, dietary reference intakes; EER, estimated energy requirement; H, height in centimeters or meters, as indicated; PA, physical activity factor; Tmax, maximum body temperature in the previous 24 hours in degrees centigrade; Ve, minute ventilation in L/min; W, actual body weight in kilograms; yr, years.

[a]No real consensus exists as to which formula is best in all situations. Many clinicians use more than one equation and calculate a range of acceptable intakes.

[b]The common practice of using an adjusted body weight for obesity in these calculations is not supported by the original data that used actual body weight in all cases up to a BMI of 56 kg/m^2 in men and 40 kg/m^2 in women.

[c]1 kcal is equal to approximately 4.18 kJ.

respectively).[15,22,72,85-89] The Harris-Benedict equations, derived in 1919 from a study of 239 individuals, are still used by some clinicians for assessing energy requirements in adults. They have the advantage of incorporating the patient's age, height, weight, and sex. These equations were derived from oxygen consumption measurements made in normally nourished healthy individuals who were in a fasting and resting state. Although they are commonly referred to as the "BEE equations," they estimate resting energy expenditure (REE), the amount of energy expended at rest by a fasting, awake individual in a temperature-controlled environment performing only basal functions such as breathing, circulation, and metabolic processes.

Because these equations approximate REE, the results have been modified by an activity or stress factor that adjusts for the individual's clinical condition. For example, an individual who is confined to bed may require a calorie intake that is only 20% to 30% above the REE, while a person who has sustained a severe burn injury may require 150% to 200% of the calculated REE. Multiplying the calculated REE by both a stress factor and an activity factor will overestimate needs because these equations overestimate REE by at least 6% to 15%. Stress factors used in adults and children are shown in Table 164-12 and Table 164-13, respectively.[88] ABW (up to a BMI of 56 kg/m^2 in men and 40 kg/m^2 in women), not IBW or adjusted body weight, was used to generate the original data with these equations and thus should be used for these calculations.[22,86]

TABLE 164-11 Equations to Estimate Energy Expenditure in Children[a,b]

FAO/WHO/UNU 2001 (kcal/day)[b]

0-12 Months

Breastfed

TEE (kcal/day) = −152 + 92.8W

TEE (MJ[c]/day) = −0.635 + 0.388W

Formula fed

TEE (kcal/day) = −29 + 82.6W

TEE (MJ[c]/day) = −0.122 + 0.346W

Boys 1-17 Years

TEE (kcal/day) = 310.2 + 63.3W - 0.263W2

TEE (MJ[c]/day) = 1,298 + 0.265W - 0.0011W2

Girls 1-17 Years

TEE (kcal/day) = 263.4 + 65.3W - 0.454W2

TEE (MJ[c]/day) = 1,102 + 0.273W - 0.0019W2

DRI Equations (kcal/day)

Birth through 2 years of age

EER = (89W - 100) + GF

GF = 175 kcal if 0-3 months; 56 kcal if 4-6 months; 22 kcal if 7-12 months; 20 kcal if 13-35 months

3-18 years of age

Boys: EER = 88.5 - (61.9A) + PA (26.7W + 903H) + GF

Girls: EER = 135.3 - (30.8A) + PA (10W + 934H) + GF

GF = 20 kcal if 3-8 years; 25 kcal if 9-18 years

PA = 1 if sedentary; 1.13-1.16 if low activity; 1.26-1.31 if normal activity; and 1.42-1.56 if very active

A, age in years; DRI, dietary reference intakes; EER, estimated energy requirement; FAO/WHO/UNU, Food and Agriculture Organization/World Health Organization/United Nations University; GF, growth factor; H, height in meters; PA, physical activity factor; TEE, total energy expenditure; W, actual body weight in kilograms.

[a]No real consensus exists as to which formula is best in all situations. Many clinicians use more than one equation and calculate a range of acceptable intakes.

[b]Additional daily calories are needed for growth; about 2 kcal/g of weight gain desired.

[c]1 kcal is equivalent to approximately 4.18 kJ; 1 MJ = 1,000 kJ.

TABLE 164-12 Stress Factors for Use in Adults

Condition	Factor
No Stress	
Confined to bed	1.2
Out of bed: normal activity	1.3
Mild Stress[a]	
Postoperative recovery: uncomplicated surgery	1-1.15
Trauma: mild (eg, long-bone fracture)	1.2
Moderate Stress[a]	
Sepsis (moderate)	1.2-1.4
Trauma: CNS (sedated)	1.3
Trauma: moderate to severe	1.3-1.4
Severe Stress[a]	
Sepsis (severe)	1.3
Trauma: CNS (severe)	Up to 1.3
Burns (proportionate to TBSA burned)[b]	Up to 2.0

CNS, central nervous system; TBSA, total body surface area.

[a]Assumes decreased activity during periods of stress.

[b]Formulas specifically for estimating energy needs in burned children and adults have been published and are likely to be more accurate.

TABLE 164-13 Stress Factors for Use in Children

Condition	Factor
Well-nourished child at bedrest with mild-moderate stress	REE × 1.3
Normally active child with mild-moderate stress OR inactive child with severe stress (eg, trauma, cancer) OR child with minimal activity and malnutrition requiring catch-up	REE × 1.5
Active child requiring catch-up growth OR an active child with severe stress	REE × 1.7

There is no individual method proven to accurately determine the energy needs of all critically ill patients (see Table 164-10). The Penn State equations appear to be most accurate in critically ill adults receiving mechanical ventilation. However, when compared to indirect calorimetry in mechanically ventilated patients, the accuracy of these equations has been shown to be only 34%.[90] The Penn State equations were found to have an accuracy rate of 77%, 70%, and 53% in older nonobese, younger obese (BMI ≥ 30 kg/m^2) and nonobese, and older obese patients, respectively. In older obese patients, use of the modified Penn State equation increased accuracy to 74%.[22,90] There is no consensus as to the best equation for critically ill adults who are not mechanically ventilated.

Measuring Energy Expenditure

The most accurate method to determine energy expenditure in clinical practice is to measure it using indirect calorimetry (metabolic gas monitoring), but capital and operational costs may limit its availability in many settings. Handheld calorimeters have been shown to be more accurate than predictive equations and may be a viable alternative to the more expensive equipment in both inpatient and outpatient settings.[91,92]

Indirect calorimetry methodology is based on pulmonary gas exchange: when a substrate (carbohydrate, fat, protein) is oxidized, heat is produced, oxygen is consumed, and carbon dioxide is expired in a constant amount depending on the substrate being oxidized. More carbon dioxide is produced when a gram of glucose is metabolized than either a gram of protein or a gram of fat. Indirect calorimetry is a noninvasive procedure in which oxygen consumption (VO_2, mL/min) and carbon dioxide production (VCO_2, mL/min) are measured, and the measured resting energy expenditure (MREE; kcal/day) is calculated using the modified Weir equation, as follows:[91-93]

$$MREE = ([3.94\ VO_2 + 1.11\ VCO_2] + [2.17\ uN_2]) \times 1.44$$

The urinary nitrogen component (uN_2) is often omitted when calculating energy expenditure because it accounts for less than 4% of the energy expenditure, and its omission results in an insignificant measurement error.[86,91] Excluding the nitrogen component eliminates the need for a 24-hour urine collection, which can be difficult and delay the measurement.

The MREE represents the total energy expended during the period over which the measurements were taken extrapolated to a 24-hour period to approximate daily energy requirements. MREE reflects changes in energy requirements resulting from diseases or clinical conditions, but it does not include energy required for repletion of a malnourished individual or growth. No multiplier (activity/stress factor) should be used in critically ill adults.[82] Modifiers may be used in other settings (eg, weight loss clinics). In children, the MREE should be multiplied by a factor for physical activity or stress (Table 164-13).[88]

Indirect calorimetry can be used to determine the patient's respiratory quotient (RQ), calculated as VCO_2/VO_2, which reflects substrate utilization. RQ values for nutrient substrates are fat, 0.71; carbohydrate, 1; protein, 0.82; and mixed substrate (fat, carbohydrate, and protein), 0.85. An RQ value greater than 1 denotes either lipogenesis or hyperventilation; less than 0.7 may indicate a ketogenic diet, fat gluconeogenesis, or ethanol oxidation. Values outside the physiologic range of 0.67 to 1.3 suggest an invalid test. Clinically, the RQ is used to determine if a patient is being overfed, which is likely if the RQ value is greater than 1.[86] Increased carbon dioxide production with overfeeding leads to increased respiratory demand which can be decreased by reducing overall energy and carbohydrate administration.

Indirect calorimetry should be considered in any patient in whom uncertainty in estimating energy requirements needs to be minimized, such as adults and children who are severely malnourished (BMI < 18.5 kg/m^2) or obese (BMI ≥ 30 kg/m^2), who have unexplained high partial arterial pressure of carbon dioxide ($PaCO_2$) concentrations or minute ventilation, spinal cord injuries, who experience weight loss despite apparently receiving adequate protein and energy intakes, critically ill surgery patients receiving PN, patients with large total body surface area burns, and patients unable to be weaned from the ventilator.[20,92]

Indirect calorimetry may not be accurate in all clinical situations. Indirect calorimetry overestimates REE for patients with hyperventilation, metabolic acidosis, overfeeding, and if there is an air leak anywhere in the ventilator circuit. Underestimation of REE is likely with hypoventilation, metabolic alkalosis, underfeeding, and gluconeogenesis. Mechanically ventilated patients are technically easier to study because the indirect calorimeter can be integrated directly into the ventilator circuit. However, the patient must be at complete rest for 1 hour, must not receive bolus feedings either by enteral feeding tube or orally for 4 hours, should have no changes in substrate delivery for 12 hours, and must be on a fraction of inspired O_2 (FiO_2) of less than 0.6 with a positive end-expiratory pressure (PEEP) less than 10 cm H_2O (approximately 1.0 kPa) and peak airway pressure of less than 30 cm H_2O [2.9 kPa]) to ensure an accurate steady-state reading.[86,88] Newer indirect calorimeters may have less restrictions on ventilator settings, but many of the patients who would benefit most from indirect calorimetry often will not meet qualifications for the measurement.

Protein

9 Daily protein requirements are based on age, sex, nutrition status, disease state, and clinical condition. For adults, the RDA for protein is 0.8 g/kg/day, which is significantly less than most Americans typically consume.[72] In adults older than 60 years of age, protein needs are increased to 1.5 g/kg/day to reduce the loss of LBM that occurs with aging, and 1.5 to 2 g/kg/day or more may be needed in states of metabolic stress.[15,72,94] Protein requirements increase in pregnant and lactating women (1.1 g/kg/day or 6-10 g protein per day above the usual RDA). Table 164-9 lists the RDAs for protein for children.[72]

Protein metabolism depends on both kidney and liver function. Critical illness results in a hypercatabolic state in which there is both increased protein synthesis and degradation. The goal of protein administration is to minimize catabolism by maximizing protein synthesis. Consequently, protein requirements are increased to 1.2 to 2 g/kg/day in critically ill patients.[15,16] For obese critically ill patients, protein needs are 2 g/kg IBW if the BMI is between 30 and 40 kg/m^2 and 2.5 g/kg IBW or more if the BMI is greater than 40 kg/m^2.[15] Adults with significant burns have protein requirements of 2.5 to 3 g/kg ABW/day or more; children with burns required between 20% and 25% of their energy needs as protein.[89] Large stool or ileostomy losses increase protein requirements. Liver failure typically results in the need for protein restriction (0.5 g/kg/day) unless a hypercatabolic state is also present, which will increase requirements to 1.5 g/kg/day. Protein needs in patients with kidney failure are variable and affected by the various renal replacement therapies. The application of these protein intake guidelines requires both clinical judgment and frequent monitoring of kidney and liver function, serum chemistries, clinical condition, and nutrition outcomes.

Fat

The daily AI for men and women for α-linolenic acid is 1.6 and 1.1 g, respectively; for linoleic acid, it is 14 to 17 g/day for men and 11 to 12 g/day for women.[72] For adults, fat should represent no more than 10% to 35% of total calories, with the recommendation that saturated fatty acids, *trans* fatty acids, and dietary cholesterol intake be kept as low as possible while a nutritionally adequate diet is consumed. Fat should constitute 30% to 40% of energy in children 1 to 3 years of age and 25% to 35% of energy in children 4 to 18 years of age.[72] Fat intake in children younger than 3 years of age is critical for proper central nervous system growth and development; generally, fat-restricted diets (skim milk) should not be imposed until after the age of 2 to 3 years except under medical supervision.

Fiber

Decreased serum cholesterol, improved glycemic control in patients with metabolic syndrome and type 2 diabetes mellitus, and maintenance of normal laxation have been attributed to dietary fiber intake, but only 5% of Americans consume the recommended amount of fiber daily.[95] Men and women 50 years of age and younger should ingest 38 g/day and 25 to 26 g/day of total fiber, respectively. For men and women older than 50 years of age, the AI is 30 g/day and 21 g/day, respectively.[72] The AI for fiber has not been set for children younger than 1 year of age. Breast milk and infant formulas are essentially fiber-free. For older children, the recommended fiber intake is 19 g/day for children 1 to 3 years of age, 24 g/day for children 4 to 8 years of age, and 26 to 31 g/day for children 9 to 13 years of age.[72]

Fluid

The daily fluid requirement for an adult depends on many factors but is generally estimated to be 30-40 mL/kg.[96] Fluid requirements per kilogram of body weight are higher for children and even higher for preterm infants because of their higher percentage of TBW and basal energy needs. Additionally, premature neonates have increased fluid requirements because of greater insensible losses and decreased concentrating ability of the kidneys. The Holliday-Segar method is a commonly used, quick, and simple method for estimating minimum daily fluid needs of children and adults. Children weighing

TABLE 164-14 Factors That Alter Fluid Requirements

Increased Requirements	Decreased Requirements
Fever	Fluid overload
Radiant warmers	Heart failure
Diuretics	Decreased urine output
Vomiting	Heat shields
Nasogastric suction	Relatively high humidity
Ostomy or fistula drainage	Humidified air via endotracheal tube
Diarrhea	Kidney failure
Glycosuria	Hypoalbuminemia with starvation
Phototherapy	Syndrome of inappropriate secretion of antidiuretic hormone (SIADH)
Diabetes insipidus	
Increased ambient temperatures	
Hyperventilation	
Prematurity	
Excessive sweating	
Increased metabolism (eg, hyperthyroidism)	

less than 10 kg should receive at least 100 mL/kg/day. An additional 50 mL/kg/day should be provided for each kilogram of body weight between 11 kg and 20 kg and 20 mL/kg/day for each kilogram above 20 kg.[97] Thus, the minimum fluid required for a child weighing 8-kg would be 800 mL/day, a 17-kg child would need 1,350 mL/day; and a 50-kg individual would need 2,000 mL/day.

Factors that may alter fluid needs in both adults and children are listed in Table 164-14. All sources of fluid (and sodium) intake should be considered (eg, vehicles for IV medications, IV or feeding tube flushes) when determining fluid requirements. Urine output, sodium, and specific gravity as well as serum electrolytes and weight changes can be used to assess fluid status. A urine output of at least 1 mL/kg/h (in children) and approximately 0.5 mL/kg/h or 40 to 50 mL/h (in adults) is considered adequate to ensure tissue perfusion. Urine output should be higher if large fluid volumes or high renal solute loads (eg, concentrated PN or EN formulations) are being administered. Urine sodium will be low (≤30 mmol/L) if the patient has volume and/or sodium deficits. Urine specific gravity depends on the kidneys' concentrating and diluting capabilities. Concomitant diuretic therapy, resulting in increased solute or water excretion, may limit the use of urine specific gravity and sodium as assessments of fluid status.

Micronutrients

Requirements for micronutrients (electrolytes, minerals, trace elements, vitamins) vary with age, sex, and route of ingestion (Table 164-15).[48–52,64,98,99] Enteral and parenteral requirements vary due to bioavailability considerations. Micronutrients poorly absorbed via the GI tract usually are required in greater amounts when given by the enteral than parenteral route. However, many water-soluble micronutrients are excreted more rapidly via the kidneys when administered intravenously. In these situations, the IV dose is greater than the enteral dose. Other factors that affect micronutrient requirements include GI losses through diarrhea, vomiting, or high-output fistula or ostomies; wound healing; and hypermetabolism or hypercatabolism. Cutaneous micronutrient losses (eg, zinc, copper, selenium) also may be significant after major burn injury. Sodium, potassium, magnesium, and phosphorus excretion are particularly dependent on kidney function, and in the setting of acute kidney injury or chronic kidney disease, intake will likely need to be restricted. Calcium needs, on the other hand, may be increased in these patients. Patients with moderate-to-severe malnutrition will have increased requirements during early refeeding owing to pre-existing deficiencies and rapid intracellular uptake with anabolism. Failure to provide adequate electrolyte replacement, especially potassium and phosphorus, and vitamin supplementation (thiamine) before advancing caloric provision can result in significant morbidity and even death from refeeding syndrome.[5,100,101]

DRUG–NUTRIENT INTERACTIONS

10 DNIs can affect response to medication therapy and nutrition status. A comprehensive discussion of DNIs is beyond the scope of this chapter.[102–105] Medication-induced nutrient deficiency, poor therapeutic response, enhanced toxicity, and failure to achieve desired nutrition outcomes can occur if either nutrition support or medication therapy is stopped because of adverse effects. Patient outcomes may be enhanced when an effective method to identify significant DNIs is coupled with a patient counseling program. An important part of the assessment process is to recognize risk factors that influence DNIs. The potential for significant DNIs is greatest in children and older adults. Other risk factors include critical illness, multiple medications, and EN.

Mineral and electrolyte serum concentrations may change because of medication therapy. For example, with loop diuretics, urine sodium, potassium, calcium, and magnesium wasting may occur, causing a reduction in their respective serum concentrations. Alternatively, calcium excretion is reduced with thiazide diuretics. Serum electrolyte concentrations also may increase as a direct result of the medication's mechanism (potassium-sparing diuretics) or because of the medication's salt form (sodium piperacillin/tazobactam). Corticosteroids and cyclosporine are known to cause hyperglycemia; other medications are prescribed to pharmacologically lower blood glucose concentrations (insulin, oral hypoglycemics).

Vitamin and trace element status also may be affected by medications (Table 164-16). For example, sulfasalazine therapy causes a decrease in folic acid, isoniazid therapy causes pyridoxine deficiency, and furosemide therapy may result in decreased thiamine concentrations. Medication therapy outcomes also may be affected by vitamin intake. For instance, the ingestion of high folic acid doses may decrease the therapeutic effect of methotrexate, and changes in an individual's usual vitamin K or vitamin E intake may cause variability in warfarin's anticoagulant effects.

Vehicles for medication delivery also may contain nutrients. Most IV therapies (maintenance IV fluids, medications, electrolyte replacements) are delivered using solutions of either dextrose (dextrose 5% or 10% in water) or sodium (0.9% NaCl). Lipid emulsion is used as the vehicle for the anesthetic agent propofol (10% lipid) and the IV calcium channel blocker clevidipine (20% lipid), and both contribute fat calories (1.1 kcal/mL or 4.6 kJ/mL for 10% and 2.0 kcal/mL or 8.4 kJ/mL for 20%) when these medications are used. Nutrition support regimens must be adjusted to accommodate calories, sodium, and other nutrients delivered through these therapies to avoid overfeeding, sodium overload, and other complications.

PRACTICAL GUIDELINES

The value of any marker used for nutrition screening is only as good as its ability to accurately identify malnourished patients and to correlate with nutrition-related complications. The response of the various nutrition status markers to nutrition therapy and the correlation between improvement in these markers and decreased morbidity and mortality support their validity. However, when applied to an individual, most of these markers lack specificity and sensitivity, which makes the development of a clinically useful, cost-effective approach to nutrition screening challenging.

The importance of the nutrition-focused history and NFPE in both nutrition screening and assessment cannot be overemphasized. Objective data such as weight can further substantiate the clinical impression and provide a baseline for subsequent monitoring. The cost effectiveness of many biochemical parameters is unknown. The assessment of other anthropometric measures is most useful in the

TABLE 164-15 Recommended Daily Electrolyte, Trace Element, and Vitamin Intake in Healthy Individuals[a]

	Adult (≥19 yr of age)[b]		Pediatric (≥6 mo of age)[c]	
Nutrient	**Enteral**	**Parenteral**	**Enteral**	**Parenteral**
Electrolytes and Minerals				
Acetate[d]	—	—	—	—
Calcium	1,000 mg F (> 50 yr): 1,200 mg Lactating: 1,300[e]	0-15 mEq (0-7.5 mmol)	6-11 mo: 260 mg 12-36 mo: 700 mg 4-8 yr: 1,000 mg 9-18 yr: 1,300 mg	Premature: 2-4 mEq/kg (1-2 mmol/kg) Other: 1-2.5 mEq/kg (0.5-1.25 mmol/kg)
Chloride[d]		—	—	2-6 mEq/kg (mmol/kg)
Magnesium	M: 400-420 mg F: 310-320 mg Pregnant: 350-400 mg[e] Lactating: 310-360 mg	10-20 mEq (5-10 mmol)	6-11 mo: 75 mg 12-36 mo: 80 mg 4-8 yr: 130 mg 9-13 yr: 240 mg 14-18 yr: 360-410 mg	0.25-1 mEq/kg (0.12-0.5 mmol/kg)
Phosphorus	700 mg Pregnant, lactating (14-18 yr): 1,250 mg	20-45 mmol	6-12 mo: 275 mg 12-36 mo: 460 mg 4-8 yr: 500 mg 9-18 yr: 1,250 mg	Premature: 1-2 mmol/kg Others: 0.5-1 mmol/kg
Potassium	M: 3,400 mg F: 2,600 mg Pregnant, lactating (14-18 yr): 2,500-2,600 mg Pregnant, lactating (>18 yr): 2,800-2,900 mg	60-100 mEq (60-100 mmol) (1-2 mEq/kg [1-2 mmol/kg])	6-12 mo: 860 mg 12-36 mo: 2,000 mg F: 4-18 yr: 2,300 mg M (4-8 yr): 2,300 M (9-13 yr): 2,500 mg M (14-18 yr): 3,000 mg	2-5 mEq/kg (mmol/kg)
Sodium	2,300 mg	60-100 mEq (60-100 mmol) (1-2 mEq/kg [1-2 mmol/kg])	6-12 mo: 370 mg 12-36 mo: 1,200 mg 4-8 yr: 1,500 mg 9-13 yr: 1,800 mg 14-18 yr: 2,300 mg	2-6 mEq/kg (mmol/kg)
Trace Elements				
Chromium (mcg)	20-45 (varies with age and sex)	10-15 0.14-0.87[f]	0-6 mo: 0.2 7-12 mo: 5.5 1-8 yr: 11-15 9-18 yr: 21-35	0-6 mo: 0.0006 mcg/kg[f] 7-12 mo: 0.012 mcg/kg[f] 1-3 yr: 0.22 mcg[f] 4-8 yr: 0.3 mcg[f] 9-13 yr: M 0.5 mcg; F 0.42 mcg[f] 14-18 yr: M 0.7 mcg; F 0.48 mcg[f]
Copper[g] (mcg)	900 1,000 (pregnancy) 1,300 (lactation)	0.3-1.5 (increased with GI loss)	0-12 mo: 200-220 1-8 yr: 340-440 9-18 yr: 700-890	20 mcg/kg (maximum, 300 mcg)
Fluoride (mg)	M: 4 F: 3	NA[h]	0-6 mo: 0.01 mg 7-12 mo: 0.5 mg 1-8 yr: 0.7-1 mg 9-18 yr: 2-3 mg	NA[h]
Iodine (mcg)	150 Pregnant: 220 Lactating: 290	70-140[h]	0-12 mo: 110-130 1-8 yr: 90 9-18 yr: 120-150	1 mcg/kg[h]
Iron (mg)	M: 8 F (≤50 yr): 18 F (>50 yr): 8 Pregnant: 27 Lactating: 9-10	1 1.5 (blood loss)	6-12 mo: 11 12-36 mo: 7 4-8 yr: 10 9-13 yr: 8 M (14-18 yr): 11 F (14-18 yr): 15	Varies
Manganese[g] (mg)	M: 2.3 F: 1.8 Pregnant: 2 Lactating: 6	0.15-1	0-6 mo: 0.003 7-12 mo: 0.6 1-8 yr: 1.2-1.5 9-18 yr: 1.6-2.2	1 mcg/kg (maximum, 50 mcg)
Molybdenum (mcg)	45 Pregnant, lactating: 50	100-200[h]	0-12 mo: 2-3 1-8 yr: 17-22 9-18 yr: 34-43	0.25 mcg/kg (maximum, 5 mcg)[h]
Selenium (mcg)	55 Pregnant: 60 Lactating: 70	20-60	0-12 mo: 15-20 1-8 yr: 20-30 9-18 yr: 40-55	1.5-3 mcg/kg (maximum, 30 mcg)
Zinc[i] (mg)	M: 11 F: 8 Pregnant: 11-12 Lactating: 12-13	2.5-5	6-36 mo: 3 4-8 yr: 5 9-13 yr: 8 M (14-18 yr): 11 F (14-18 yr): 8	Premature: 300-400 mcg/kg Other: 50-250 mcg/kg

(Continued)

TABLE 164-15 Recommended Daily Electrolyte, Trace Element, and Vitamin Intake in Healthy Individuals[a] (*Continued*)

Nutrient	Adult (≥19 yr of age)[b]		Pediatric (≥6 mo of age)[c]	
	Enteral	**Parenteral**	**Enteral**	**Parenteral**
Vitamins				
Ascorbic acid (mg) (vitamin C)	M: 90 F: 75 Pregnant: 80-85 Lactating: 115-120	100	6-12 mo: 50 12-36 mo: 15 4-8 yr: 25 9-13 yr: 45 M (14-18 yr): 75 F (14-18 yr): 65	80
Biotin (mcg)	30	60	0-12 mo: 5-6 1-8 yr: 8-12 9-18 yr: 20-25	20
Choline (mg)	M: 550 F: 425 Pregnant: 450 Lactating: 550	NA[h]	6-12 mo: 150 12-36 mo: 200 4-8 yr: 250 9-13 yr: 375 M (14-18 yr): 550 F (14-18 yr): 400	NA[h]
Cobalamin (mcg) (vitamin B12)	2.4 Pregnant: 2.6 Lactating: 2.8	5	6-12 mo: 0.5 12-36 mo: 0.9 4-8 yr: 1.2 9-13 yr: 1.8 14-18 yr: 2.4	1
Folate (mcg DFE)	400 Pregnant: 600 Lactating: 500	400	6-12 mo: 80 12-36 mo: 150 4-8 yr: 200 9-13 yr: 300 14-18 yr: 400	140
Niacin (mg)	M: 16 F: 14 Pregnant: 18 Lactating: 17	40	6-12 mo: 4 12-36 mo: 6 4-8 yr: 8 9-13 yr: 12 M (14-18 yr): 16 F (14-18 yr): 14	17
Pantothenic acid (mg)	5	15	0-12 mo: 1.7-1.8 1-8 yr: 2-3 9-18 yr: 4-5	5
Pyridoxine (mg) (vitamin B6)	1.3 M (>50 yr): 1.7 F (<50 yr): 1.5 Pregnant: 1.9 Lactating: 2	4	6-12 mo: 0.3 12-36 mo: 0.5 4-8 yr: 0.6 9-13 yr: 1 M (14-18 yr): 1.3 F (14-18 yr): 1.2	1
Riboflavin (mg)	M: 1.3 F: 1.1 Pregnant: 1.4 Lactating: 1.6	3.6	6-12 mo: 0.3 12-23 mo: 0.5 1-8 yr: 0.5-0.6 M (9-18 yr): 1.3 F (9-18 yr): 1.0	1.4
Thiamine (mg) (vitamin B1)	M: 1.2 F: 1.1 Pregnant, lactating: 1.4	3	6-12 mo: 0.3 12-36 mo: 0.5 4-8 yr: 0.6 9-13 yr: 0.9 M (14-18 yr): 1.2 F (14-18 yr): 1.0	1.2
Vitamin A (mcg RAE)[j]	M: 900 F: 700 Pregnant: 750-770 Lactating: 1200-1300	600-1,000	6-12 mo: 500 12-23 mo: 300 4-8 yr: 400 9-13 yr: 600 M (9-18 yr): 900 F (9-18 yr): 700	700
Vitamin D (IU)[k]	≤70 yr: 600 IU >70 yr: 800 IU	200 IU	6-12 mo: 400 IU 1-18 yr: 600 IU	200-400 IU
Vitamin E (mg AT)	15 Pregnant, lactating: 19	10	6-12 mo: 5 12-23 mo: 6 4-8 yr: 7 9-13 yr: 11 14-18 yr: 15	7

(*Continued*)

TABLE 164-15 Recommended Daily Electrolyte, Trace Element, and Vitamin Intake in Healthy Individuals[a]

	Adult (≥19 yr of age)[b]		Pediatric (≥6 mo of age)[c]	
Nutrient	**Enteral**	**Parenteral**	**Enteral**	**Parenteral**
Vitamin K (mcg)	M: 120 F: 90	0.7-2.5 mg	6-12 mo: 2.5 12-36 mo: 30 4-8 yr: 55 9-13 yr: 60 14-18 yr: 75	200

AT, alpha-tocopherol; DFE, dietary folate equivalent; F, female; IU, international units M, male; NA, not applicable; NE, niacin equivalents; RAE, retinol activity equivalents; TE, tocopherol equivalent

[a]Data represent either the Recommended Dietary Allowance (RDA), the Adequate Intake (AI), or the CDRR (Chronic Disease Risk Reduction level) for each nutrient.

[b]Intake in nonhealthy adults must be individualized.

[c]Term newborns, low-birthweight, and very-low-birthweight infants or older infants and children may have higher or lower requirements. Intake in nonhealthy children must be individualized.

[d]Not established; as needed to maintain acid–base balance.

[e]Pregnancy and lactation recommendations provided if different than age-specific recommendations; recommendations include pregnant or lactating females aged 14 to 50 yr unless otherwise specified.

[f]American Society for Parenteral and Enteral Nutrition recommendations

[g]May accumulate in cholestasis.

[h]No IV product available in the United States

[i]Additional intake needed with small bowel losses, which can be 12 mg zinc/L or 17 mg zinc/kg of stool or ileostomy output; an additional 2 mg/day needed for acute catabolic stress.

[j]1 mcg RAE = 3.3 international units

[k]40 international units = 1 mcg

TABLE 164-16 Drug–Nutrient Interactions

Medication	Effect
Angiotensin converting enzyme inhibitors	Increased urinary zinc losses
Angiotensin receptor blockers	Increased urinary zinc losses
Antacids	Thiamine deficiency
Antibiotics	Vitamin K deficiency
Aspirin	Folic acid deficiency; increased vitamin C excretion
Cathartics	Increased requirements for vitamins D, C, and B6
Cholestyramine	Vitamins A, D, E, and K and β-carotene malabsorption
Colestipol	Vitamins A, D, E, and K and β-carotene malabsorption
Corticosteroids	Decreased vitamins A, D, and C
Diuretics (loop)	Thiamine deficiency
Diuretics (thiazides)	Increased urinary zinc losses
Efavirenz	Vitamin D deficiency caused by increased metabolism of 25(OH)-vitamin D and 1,25-(OH)2-vitamin D
Histamine2 antagonists	Vitamin B12 malabsorption (reduced acid results in impaired release of B12 from food)
Isoniazid	Vitamin B6 and niacin deficiency
Isotretinoin	Vitamin A increases toxicity
Mercaptopurine	Niacin deficiency
Methotrexate	Folic acid inhibits effect
Orlistat	Vitamins A, D, E, and K malabsorption caused by fat malabsorption
Pentamidine	Folic acid deficiency
Phenobarbital	Increased vitamin D metabolism
Phenytoin	Increased vitamin D metabolism; decreased folic acid concentrations
Primidone	Folic acid deficiency
Protease inhibitors	Vitamin D deficiency (impaired renal hydroxylation)
Proton pump inhibitors	Decreased iron and vitamin B12 absorption (reduced acid results in impaired release of B12 from food)
Sulfasalazine	Folic acid malabsorption
Trimethoprim	Folic acid depletion
Warfarin	Vitamin K inhibits effect; vitamins A, C, and E may affect prothrombin time
Valproic acid	Zinc, carnitine
Zidovudine	Folic acid and B12 deficiencies increase myelosuppression

setting of anticipated long-term nutrition support in which these measurements will serve as longitudinal markers of response to the nutrition care plan.

Better markers of nutrition status and methods for determining patient-specific nutrition requirements are needed to allow further refinement of estimates of an individual's nutrition needs. Functional tests and simple, noninvasive tests for body composition analysis hold promise for the future. However, until better methods of assessment become available and are demonstrated to be cost effective, the currently available battery of tests will continue to be the mainstay of nutrition assessment.

Initially, nutrition requirements are determined based on assumptions made about the patient's clinical condition and the nutrition needs associated with repletion or growth, if needed. After a nutrition intervention has been initiated, periodic reassessment of nutrition status is critical to determine the accuracy of the initial estimate. Nutrition requirements are dynamic in the setting of acute or critical illness—as the patient's clinical status changes, so will protein and energy requirements, further emphasizing the need for continued reassessment.

ABBREVIATIONS

ABW	actual body weight (kg)
AdjBW	adjusted body weight (kg)
AI	Adequate Intake
ALB	albumin
AND	Academy of Nutrition and Dietetics
ASPEN	American Society for Parenteral and Enteral Nutrition
BEE	basal energy expenditure
BIA	bioelectrical impedance analysis
BMI	body mass index
CDC	Centers for Disease Control and Prevention
CDRR	Chronic Disease Reduction Risk level
CRP	C-reactive protein
CT	computed tomography
DCH	delayed cutaneous hypersensitivity
DNI	drug-nutrient interaction
DRI	Dietary Reference Intake
DXA	dual-energy x-ray absorptiometry
EAR	Estimated Average Requirement
EFAD	essential fatty acid deficiency
EN	enteral nutrition
GI	gastrointestinal
HIV	human immunodeficiency virus
IBW	ideal body weight
IV	intravenous
LBM	lean body mass
MREE	measured resting energy expenditure
MRI	magnetic resonance imaging
MST	Malnutrition Screening Tool
MUMC	mid-arm muscle circumference
NFPE	nutrition-focused physical examination
PN	parenteral nutrition
RDA	Recommended Dietary Allowance
REE	resting energy expenditure
RQ	respiratory quotient
SCr	serum creatinine
SGA	Subjective Global Assessment
TBSA	total body surface area
TBW	total body water
TFN	transferrin
TUN	total urine nitrogen
UBW	usual body weight
UL	tolerable upper intake level
UUN	urine urea nitrogen
VCO_2	carbon dioxide production
VO_2	oxygen consumption
WHO	World Health Organization

REFERENCES

1. JV White, P Guenter, G Jensen, et al. Consensus statement: Academy of Nutrition and Dietetics and American Society for Parenteral and Enteral Nutrition: characteristics recommended for the identification and documentation of adult malnutrition (undernutrition). *JPEN J Parenter Enteral Nutr.* 2012;36(3):275–283. doi:10.1177/0148607112440285..
2. Mehta NM, Corkins MR, Lyman B, et al. Defining pediatric malnutrition: A paradigm shift toward etiology-related definitions. *JPEN J Parenter Enteral Nutr.* 2013;37(4):460–481. doi: 10.1177/0148607113479972.
3. GL Jensen, T Cederholm, MITD Correia, et al. GLIM criteria for the diagnosis of malnutrition: A consensus report from the global clinical nutrition community. *JPEN J Parenter Enteral Nutr.* 2019;43(1):32–40. doi:https://doi.org/10.1002/jpen.1440.
4. Jensen GL, Hsiao PY, Wheeler D. Adult nutrition assessment tutorial. *JPEN J Parenter Enteral Nutr.* 2012;36(3):267–274. doi: 10.1177/0148607112440284.
5. da Silva JSV, Seres DS, Sabino K, et al. ASPEN consensus recommendations for refeeding syndrome. *Nutr Clin Pract.* 2020;35(2):178–195. doi: https://doi.org/10.1002/ncp.10474.
6. Malone A, Hamilton C. The Academy of Nutrition and Dietetics/ the American Society for Parenteral and Enteral Nutrition consensus malnutrition characteristics: Application in practice. *Nutr Clin Pract.* 2013;28(6):639–650. doi: 10.1177/0884533613508435.
7. Hales CM, Carroll MD, Fryar CD, et al., Prevalence of obesity among adults and youth: United States, 2017-2018 Hyattsville, MD: National Center for Health Statistics; 2020. Available at: https://www.cdc.gov/nchs/products/databriefs/db360.htm. Accessed January 15, 2022.
8. Centers for Disease Control and Prevention. Overweight and obesity: Adult obesity facts 2021. Available at: https://www.cdc.gov/obesity/data/adult.html. Accessed January 15, 2022.
9. Centers for Disease Control and Prevention. Growth chart 2016. Available at: https://www.cdc.gov/growthcharts/cdc_charts.htm. Accessed January 15, 2022.
10. Bhaskaran K, Dos-Santos-Silva I, Leon DA, et al. Association of BMI with overall and cause-specific mortality: a population-based cohort study of 3.6 million adults in the UK. *Lancet Diabetes Endocrinol.* 2018;6(12):944–953. doi: 10.1016/S2213-8587(18)30288-2.
11. Correia MITD. Nutrition screening vs nutrition assessment: What's the difference? *Nutr Clin Pract.* 2018;33(1):62–72. doi:10.1177/0884533617719669.
12. AK JeVenn, M Galang, P Hipskind, C Bury. Malnutrition screening and assessment. In: CM Mueller ed. *The ASPEN Adult Nutrition Support Core Curriculum.* 3rd ed. Silver Spring, MD: American Society for Parenteral and Enteral Nutrition; 2017.
13. The Joint Commission. Standards. Available at: https://www.jointcommission.org/standards/. Accessed January 15, 2022.
14. Lee ZY, Heyland DK. Determination of nutrition risk and status in critically ill patients: What are our considerations? *Nutr Clin Pract.* 2019;34(1):96–111. doi:10.1002/ncp.10214.
15. SA McClave, BE Taylor, RG Martindale, et al. Guidelines for the provision and assessment of nutrition support therapy in the adult critically ill patient: Society of Critical Care Medicine (SCCM) and American Society for Parenteral and Enteral Nutrition (ASPEN). *JPEN J Parenter Enteral Nutr.* 2016;40(2):159–211. doi:10.1177/0148607115621863.
16. Compher C, Bingham AL, McCall M, et al. Guidelines for the provision of nutrition support therapy in the adult critically ill patient: The American Society for Parenteral and Enteral Nutrition. *JPEN J Parenter Enteral Nutr.* 2022. doi:https://doi.org/10.1002/jpen.2267.
17. Grummer-Strawn LM, Reinold C, Krebs NF, et al. Use of World Health Organization and CDC growth charts for children aged 0-59 months in the United States. *MMWR Recomm Rep.* 2010;59(RR-9):1–15.
18. Guenter P, Abdelhadi R, Anthony P, et al. Malnutrition diagnoses and associated outcomes in hospitalized patients: United States, 2018. *Nutr Clin Pract.* 2021;36(5):957–969. https://doi.org/10.1002/ncp.10771.
19. Esper DH. Utilization of nutrition-focused physical assessment in identifying micronutrient deficiencies. *Nutr Clin Pract.* 2015;30(2):194–202. doi:10.1177/0884533615573054.
20. Corkins KG. Nutrition-focused physical examination in pediatric patients. *Nutr Clin Pract.* 2015;30(2):203–209. 10.1177/0884533615572654.
21. Devine BJ. Gentamicin therapy. *Drug Intell Clin Pharm.* 1974;8:650–655.
22. Frankenfield DC, Ashcraft CM. Estimating energy needs in nutrition support patients. *JPEN J Parenter Enteral Nutr.* 2011;35(5):563–570. doi: 10.1177/0148607111415859.
23. Kang K, Absher R, Farrington E, et al. Evaluation of different methods used to calculate ideal body weight in the pediatric population. *J Pediatr Pharmacol Ther.* 2019;24(5):421–430. doi: 10.5863/1551-6776-24.5.421.
24. Froehlich-Grobe K, Nary DE, Van Sciver A, et al. Measuring height without a stadiometer: empirical investigation of four height estimates among wheelchair users. *Am J Phys Med Rehabil.* 2011;90(8):658–666. doi: 10.1097/PHM.0b013e31821f6eb2.
25. Hickson M, Frost G. A comparison of three methods for estimating height in the acutely ill elderly population. *J Hum Nutr Diet.* 2003;16(1):13–20. doi:10.1046/j.1365-277x.2003.00416.x.
26. Fenton TR, Kim JH. A systematic review and meta-analysis to revise the Fenton growth chart for preterm infants. *BMC Pediatr.* 2013;13:59. doi:10.1186/1471-2431-13-59.
27. Olsen IE, Groveman SA, Lawson ML, et al. New intrauterine growth curves based on United States data. *Pediatrics* 2010;125(2):e214–e224. doi: 10.1542/peds.2009-0913.

28. Cole SZ, Lanham JS. Failure to thrive: An update. *Am Fam Physician* 2011;83(7):829–834.
29. Braun LR, Marino R. Disorders of growth and stature. *Pediatr Rev.* 2017;38(7):293–304. doi:10.1542/pir.2016-0178.
30. Jensen MD, Ryan DH, Apovian CM, et al. 2013 AHA/ACC/TOS guideline for the management of overweight and obesity in adults: a report of the American College of Cardiology/American Heart Association Task Force on Practice Guidelines and The Obesity Society. *J Am Coll Cardiol.* 2014;63(25 Pt B):2985–3023. doi:10.1016/j.jacc.2013.11.004.
31. National Institutes of Health. Managing overweight and obesity in adults: Systematic evidence review from obesity expert panel 2013. Available at: https://www.nhlbi.nih.gov/health-topics/managing-overweight-obesity-in-adults. Accessed January 15, 2022.
32. Martin L, Senesse P, Gioulbasanis I, et al. Diagnostic criteria for the classification of cancer-associated weight loss. *J Clin Oncol.* 2015;33(1):90–99. doi: 10.1200/JCO.2014.56.1894.
33. Ness-Abramof R, Apovian CM. Waist circumference measurement in clinical practice. *Nutr Clin Pract.* 2008;23(4):397–404. doi:10.1177/0884533608321700.
34. Xi B, Mi J, Zhao M, et al. Trends in abdominal obesity among U.S. children and adolescents. *Pediatrics* 2014;134(2):e334–e339. doi: 10.1542/peds.2014-0970.
35. Fryar CD, Carroll MD, Gu Q, et al. Anthropometric reference data for children and adults: United States, 2015-2018. *Vital Health Stat.* 3 2021(36):1–44.
36. Mulasi U, Kuchnia AJ, Cole AJ, et al. Bioimpedance at the bedside: Current applications, limitations, and opportunities. *Nutr Clin Pract.* 2015;30(2):180–193. doi: 10.1177/0884533614568155.
37. Earthman CP. Body composition tools for assessment of adult malnutrition at the bedside: A tutorial on research considerations and clinical applications. *JPEN J Parenter Enteral Nutr.* 2015;39(7):787–822. doi:10.1177/0148607115595227.
38. Sheean P, Gonzalez MC, Prado CM, et al. American Society for Parenteral and Enteral Nutrition clinical guidelines: The validity of body composition assessment in clinical populations. *JPEN J Parenter Enteral Nutr.* 2020;44(1):12–43. doi:https://doi.org/10.1002/jpen.1669.
39. Guerra RS, Fonseca I, Pichel F, et al. Handgrip strength and associated factors in hospitalized patients. *JPEN J Parenter Enteral Nutr.* 2015;39(3):322–330. doi: 10.1177/0148607113514113.
40. Flood A, Chung A, Parker H, et al. The use of hand grip strength as a predictor of nutrition status in hospital patients. *Clin Nutr.* 2014;33(1):106–114. doi: 10.1016/j.clnu.2013.03.003.
41. Whiting SJ, Cheng PC, Thorpe L, Viveky N, Alcorn J, Hadjistavropoulous T. Hand grip strength as a potential nutritional assessment tool in long-term care homes. *J. Aging Res. Healthcare* 2016;1(2):1–11.
42. Fields DA, Gunatilake R, Kalaitzoglou E. Air displacement plethysmography: Cradle to grave. *Nutr Clin Pract.* 2015;30(2):219–226. doi: 10.1177/0884533615572443.
43. Evans DC, Corkins MR, Malone A, et al. The use of visceral proteins as nutrition markers: An ASPEN position paper. *Nutr Clin Pract.* 2021;36(1):22–28. doi: https://doi.org/10.1002/ncp.10588.
44. Soeters PB, Wolfe RR, Shenkin A. Hypoalbumi nemia: Pathogenesis and clinical significance. *JPEN J Parenter Enteral Nutr.* 2019;43(2):181–193. doi: 10.1002/jpen.1451.
45. Young LS, Kim DW. Protein. In: Mueller CM, ed. *The ASPEN Adult Nutrition Support Core Curriculum.* 3rd ed. Silver Springs, MD: American Society for Parenteral and Enteral Nutrition; 2017.
46. Velasco N, Long CL, Otto DA, et al. Comparison of three methods for the estimation of total nitrogen losses in hospitalized patients. *JPEN J Parenter Enteral Nutr.* 1990;14(5):517–522. doi: 10.1177/0148607190014005517.
47. Sarav M, Kovesdy CP. Renal disease. In: Mueller CM, ed. *The ASPEN Adult Nutrition Support Core Curriculum.* 3rd ed. Silver Springs, MD: American Society for Parenteral and Enteral Nutrition; 2017.
48. Food and Nutrition Board National Academies. Dietary Reference Intakes: Recommended dietary allowances and adequate intakes, elements 2019. Available at: https://www.ncbi.nlm.nih.gov/books/NBK545442/table/appJ_tab3/?report=objectonly. Accessed January 15, 2022.
49. Fessler TA. Trace elements in parenteral nutrition: A practical guide for dosage and monitoring for adult patients. *Nutr Clin Pract.* 2013;28(6):722–729. doi: 10.1177/0884533613506596.
50. McKeever L. Vitamins and trace elements. In: Mueller CM, ed. *The ASPEN Adult Nutrition Support Core Curriculum.* 3rd ed. Silver Springs, MD: American Society for Parenteral and Enteral Nutrition; 2017.
51. Jin J, Mulesa L, Carrilero Rouillet M. Trace elements in parenteral nutrition: Considerations for the prescribing clinician. *Nutrients.* 2017;9(5). doi:10.3390/nu9050440.
52. Vanek VW, Borum P, Buchman A, et al. ASPEN position paper: Recommendations for changes in commercially available parenteral multivitamin and multi-trace element products. *Nutr Clin Pract.* 2012;27(4):440–491. doi: 10.1177/0884533612446706.
53. Livingstone C. Zinc: physiology, deficiency, and parenteral nutrition. *Nutr Clin Pract.* 2015;30(3):371–382. doi: 10.1177/0884533615570376.
54. Steinbrenner H, Speckmann B, Klotz LO. Selenoproteins: Antioxidant selenoenzymes and beyond. *Arch Biochem Biophys.* 2016;595:113–119. doi: 10.1016/j.abb.2015.06.024.
55. Manzanares W, Langlois PL, Heyland DK. Pharmaconutrition with selenium in critically ill patients: What do we know? *Nutr Clin Pract.* 2015;30(1):34–43. doi:10.1177/0884533614561794.
56. Ashton K, Hooper L, Harvey LJ, et al. Methods of assessment of selenium status in humans: A systematic review. *Am J Clin Nutr.* 2009;89(6):2025S–39S. doi:10.3945/ajcn.2009.27230F.
57. Moon N, Aryan M, Westerveld D, et al. Clinical manifestations of copper deficiency: A case report and review of the literature. *Nutr Clin Pract.* 2021;36(5):1080–1085. doi: 10.1002/ncp.10582.
58. MacKay M, Mulroy CW, Street J, et al. Assessing copper status in pediatric patients receiving parenteral nutrition. *Nutr Clin Pract.* 2015;30(1):117–121. doi: 10.1177/0884533614538457.
59. Harvey LJ, Ashton K, Hooper L, et al. Methods of assessment of copper status in humans: a systematic review. *Am J Clin Nutr.* 2009;89(6):2009S–24S. doi:10.3945/ajcn.2009.27230E.
60. Vincent JB. New evidence against chromium as an essential trace element. *J Nutr.* 2017;147(12):2212–2219. doi: 10.3945/jn.117.255901.
61. Tian H, Guo X, Wang X, et al. Chromium picolinate supplementation for overweight or obese adults. *Cochrane Database Syst Rev.* 2013(11):CD010063. doi:10.1002/14651858.CD010063.pub2.
62. Peres TV, Schettinger MR, Chen P, et al. Manganese-induced neurotoxicity: A review of its behavioral consequences and neuroprotective strategies. *BMC Pharmacol Toxicol.* 2016;17(1):57. doi:10.1186/s40360-016-0099-0.
63. Sardesai VM. Molybdenum: An essential trace element. *Nutr Clin Pract.* 1993;8(6):277–281. doi: 10.1177/0115426593008006277.
64. Food and Nutrition Board National Academies. Dietary Reference Intakes: Recommended allowances and adequate intakes, vitamins 2011. Available at: https://www.ncbi.nlm.nih.gov/books/NBK56068/table/summarytables.t2/?report=objectonly. Accessed January 15, 2022.
65. Frank LL. Thiamin in clinical practice. *JPEN J Parenter Enteral Nutr.* 2015;39(5):503–520. doi: 10.1177/0148607114565245.
66. Lam JR, Schneider JL, Zhao W, et al. Proton pump inhibitor and histamine 2 receptor antagonist use and vitamin B12 deficiency. *JAMA.* 2013;310(22):2435–2442. doi: 10.1001/jama.2013.280490.
67. McCabe KM, Adams MA, Holden RM. Vitamin K status in chronic kidney disease. *Nutrients* 2013;5(11):4390–4398. doi: 10.3390/nu5114390.
68. Holick MF. The vitamin D deficiency pandemic: Approaches for diagnosis, treatment and prevention. *Rev Endocr Metab Disord.* 2017;18(2):153–165. doi: 10.1007/s11154-017-9424-1.
69. De-Regil LM, Pena-Rosas JP, Fernandez-Gaxiola AC, et al. Effects and safety of periconceptional oral folate supplementation for preventing birth defects. *Cochrane Database Syst Rev.* 2015(12):CD007950. doi:10.1002/14651858.CD007950.pub3.
70. Kim J, Choi J, Kwon SY, et al. Association of multivitamin and mineral supplementation and risk of cardiovascular disease: A systematic review and meta-analysis. *Circ Cardiovasc Qual Outcomes.* 2018;11(7):e004224. doi:10.1161/CIRCOUTCOMES.117.004224.
71. Dietary supplements market size, share & COVID-19 impact analysis, by type (vitamins, minerals, enzymes, fatty acids, proteins, and other), form (tablets, capsules, liquids, and powders), and regional forecasts, 2021-2028. Available at: www.fortunebusinessinsights.com/dietary-supplements-market-102082. Accessed February 13, 2022.
72. Food and Nutrition Board National Academies. Dietary Reference Intakes: Recommended dietary allowances and adequate intakes, Total water and macronutrients 2011. Available at: https://www.ncbi.nlm.nih.gov/books/NBK56068/table/summarytables.t4/?report=objectonly. Accessed January 15, 2022.
73. Hise M, Brown JC. Lipids. In: Mueller CM, ed. *The ASPEN Adult Nutrition Support Core Curriculum.* 3rd ed. Silver Springs, MD: American Society for Parenteral and Enteral Nutrition; 2017.
74. Borum P. Fats. In: Corkins MR, ed. *The ASPEN Pediatric Nutrition Support Core Curriculum.* 2nd ed. Silver Springs, MD: American Society for Parenteral and Enteral Nutrition; 2015: 31–40.

75. Gramlich L, Ireton-Jones C, Miles JM, et al. Essential fatty acid requirements and intravenous lipid emulsions. *JPEN J Parenter Enteral Nutr.* 2019;43(6):697–707. doi:https://doi.org/10.1002/jpen.1537.
76. Gramlich L, Meddings L, Alberda C, et al. Essential fatty acid deficiency in 2015: The impact of novel intravenous lipid emulsions. *JPEN J Parenter Enteral Nutr.* 2015;39(1 Suppl):61S–66S. 10.1177/0148607115595977.
77. Almannai M, Alfadhel M, El-Hattab AW. Carnitine inborn errors of metabolism. *Molecules (Basel, Switzerland).* 2019;24(18):3251. doi:10.3390/molecules24183251.
78. Buist NR. Historical perspective on clinical trials of carnitine in children and adults. *Ann Nutr Metab.* 2016;68 (Suppl 3):1–4. doi:10.1159/000448320.
79. Reuter SE, Evans AM. Carnitine and acylcarnitines: Pharmacokinetic, pharmacological and clinical aspects. *Clin Pharmacokinet* 2012;51(9):553–72. doi: 10.1007/BF03261931.
80. Scruggs ER, Dirks Naylor AJ. Mechanisms of zidovudine-induced mitochondrial toxicity and myopathy. *Pharmacology* 2008;82(2):83–88. doi: 10.1159/000134943.
81. Institute of Medicine. *The development of DRIs 1994-2004: Lessons learned and new challenges.* Washington, DC: The National Academies Press; 2008.
82. U.S. Department of Agriculture and U.S. Department of Health and Human Services. Dietary guidelines for Americans, 2020-2025 2020. Available at: https://www.dietaryguidelines.gov/. Accessed February 12, 2022.
83. National Academies of Sciences, Engineering, and Medicine. VA Stallings, M Harrison, M Oria, eds. *Dietary Reference Intakes for Sodium and Potassium.* Washington, DC: The National Academies Press; 2019.
84. United States Department of Agriculture National Agricultural Library. DRI Calculator for Healthcare Professionals. Available at: https://www.nal.usda.gov/legacy/fnic/dri-calculator/. Accessed January 15, 2022.
85. Frankenfield DC. Factors related to the assessment of resting metabolic rate in critically ill patients. *JPEN J Parenter Enteral Nutr.* 2019;43(2):234–244. doi: 10.1002/jpen.1484.
86. Frankenfield DC. Energy. In: Mueller CM, ed. *The ASPEN Adult Nutrition Support Core Curriculum.* 3rd ed. Silver Springs, MD: American Society for Parenteral and Enteral Nutrition; 2017.
87. Mehta NM, Skillman HE, Irving SY, et al. Guidelines for the provision and assessment of nutrition support therapy in the pediatric critically ill patient: Society of Critical Care Medicine and American Society for Parenteral and Enteral Nutrition. *JPEN J Parenter Enteral Nutr.* 2017;41(5):706–42. doi:10.1177/0148607117711387.
88. Sentongo T. Assessment of nutrition status by age and determining nutrient needs. In: Corkins MR, ed. *The ASPEN Pediatric Nutrition Support Core Curriculum* 2nd ed. Silver Springs, MD: American Society for Parenteral and Enteral Nutrition; 2015:531–565.
89. Rollins C, Huettner F, Neumeister MW. Clinician's guide to nutritional therapy following major burn injury. *Clin Plast Surg.* 2017;44(3):555–566. doi: 10.1016/j.cps.2017.02.014.
90. Cooney RN, Frankenfield DC. Determining energy needs in critically ill patients: Equations or indirect calorimeters. *Curr Opin Crit Care* 2012;18(2):174–177. doi: 10.1097/MCC.0b013e3283514bbc.
91. Hipskind P, Glass C, Charlton D, et al. Do handheld calorimeters have a role in assessment of nutrition needs in hospitalized patients? A systematic review of literature. *Nutr Clin Pract.* 2011;26(4):426–433. doi: 10.1177/0884533611411272.
92. Oshima T, Berger MM, De Waele E, et al. Indirect calorimetry in nutritional therapy. A position paper by the ICALIC study group. *Clin Nutr.* 2017;36(3):651–662. doi: 10.1016/j.clnu.2016.06.010.
93. McClave SA, Martindale RG, Kiraly L. The use of indirect calorimetry in the intensive care unit. *Curr Opin Clin Nutr Metab Care* 2013;16(2):202–208. doi: 10.1097/MCO.0b013e32835dbc54.
94. Wolfe RR, Miller SL, Miller KB. Optimal protein intake in the elderly. *Clin Nutr.* 2008;27(5):675–684. doi: 10.1016/j.clnu.2008.06.008.
95. Lambeau KV, McRorie JW Jr. Fiber supplements and clinically proven health benefits: How to recognize and recommend an effective fiber therapy. *J Am Assoc Nurse Pract.* 2017;29(4):216–223. doi: 10.1002/2327-6924.12447.
96. Canada TW, Lord LM. Fluids, electrolytes, and acid-base disorders. In: Mueller CM, ed. *The ASPEN Adult Nutrition Support Core Curriculum.* Silver Springs, MD: American Society for Parenteral and Enteral Nutrition; 2017.
97. Schmidt GL. Fluids and electrolytes. In: Corkins MR, ed. *The ASPEN Pediatric Nutrition Support Core Curriculum.* 2nd ed. Silver Springs, MD: American Society for Parenteral and Enteral Nutrition; 2015.
98. Food and Nutrition Board. Dietary reference intakes for calcium and vitamin D 2011. Available at: https://www.nap.edu/read/13050/chapter/1. Accessed January 15, 2022.
99. Greene HL, Hambidge KM, Schanler R, et al. Guidelines for the use of vitamins, trace elements, calcium, magnesium, and phosphorus in infants and children receiving total parenteral nutrition: report of the Subcommittee on Pediatric Parenteral Nutrient Requirements from the Committee on Clinical Practice Issues of the American Society for Clinical Nutrition. *Am J Clin Nutr.* 1988;48(5):1324–1342. doi: 10.1093/ajcn/48.5.1324.
100. Friedli N, Stanga Z, Sobotka L, et al. Revisiting the refeeding syndrome: Results of a systematic review. *Nutrition* 2017;35:151–160. doi: 10.1016/j.nut.2016.05.016.
101. Pulcini CD, Zettle S, Srinath A. Refeeding syndrome. *Pediatr Rev.* 2016;37(12):516–23. doi:10.1542/pir.2015-0152.
102. Robien K, Oppeneer SJ, Kelly JA, et al. Drug-vitamin D interactions: A systematic review of the literature. *Nutr Clin Pract.* 2013;28(2):194–208. doi:10.1177/0884533612467824.
103. Chan LN. Drug-nutrient interactions. *JPEN J Parenter Enteral Nutr.* 2013;37(4):450–459. doi: 10.1177/0148607113488799.
104. Boullata JI. *Guidebook on enteral medication administration.* Silver Springs, MD: American Society for Parenteral and Enteral Nutrition; 2019.
105. Deng J, Zhu X, Chen Z, et al. A review of food-drug interactions on oral drug absorption. *Drugs* 2017;77(17):1833–1855. doi: 10.1007/s40265-017-0832-z.

165

Parenteral Nutrition

Todd W. Mattox and Catherine M. Crill

KEY CONCEPTS

1. Development and implementation of an appropriate, individualized nutrition care plan requires definition of nutrition goals, determination of nutrition requirements and appropriate route of nutrient delivery, and design of a monitoring plan to evaluate suitability of the nutrition regimen as a patient's clinical condition changes.
2. The appropriate route of nutrition support depends on the functional condition of the patient's gastrointestinal (GI) tract, risk of aspiration, expected duration of nutrition therapy, and clinical condition.
3. Suitable candidates for parenteral nutrition (PN) therapy can be identified on the basis of their age, nutrition status, expected duration of GI dysfunction, and potential risks of PN therapy.
4. PN formulations include injectable amino acids, dextrose, water, electrolytes, vitamins, trace elements, and other additives. Some formulations may include lipid injectable emulsion (ILE).
5. PN solutions may be appropriately formulated for administration by peripheral or central venous access.
6. PN formulations are available as standardized commercial multichamber bag products or they may be compounded with an automated compounding device (ACD).
7. PN solutions may be infused continuously or intermittently.
8. Biochemical and clinical measurements for effective monitoring of patients receiving PN include serum chemistries, vital signs, body weight, total daily fluid intake and losses, and nutritional intake.
9. Non-catheter–related complications of PN therapy can be minimized by using age-appropriate nutrient dosing guidelines, frequent monitoring, and implementing rational adjustments to the PN regimen when metabolic abnormalities occur.
10. Individualized PN therapy should be based on nutrition therapy goals determined from a patient-specific nutrition assessment, type of available intravenous (IV) access, and macronutrient and micronutrient requirements.
11. A patient's nutrient requirements are affected by age, degree of metabolic demand, organ function, medication therapy, exogenous losses, acid-base status, and enteral intake in patients with recovering GI function.

BEYOND THE BOOK

These audiovisual materials are useful to enhance student understanding regarding the COLLECT and ASSESS steps (video) as well as the PLAN, IMPLEMENT, and FOLLOW-UP: MONITOR AND EVALUATE steps (podcast) in the patient care process.

Video: Watch the video entitled "PN Appropriateness: The General Approach" at the American Society for Parenteral and Enteral Nutrition (ASPEN) Website <http://www.nutritioncare.org/smartpn/>. This 13.5-minute video provides a brief overview regarding selection of appropriate PN candidates.

Podcast: Listen to the podcast entitled "When Times are Short: Managing Drug Shortages in PN" <https://soundcloud.com/user-67457490/when-times-are-short-managing-drug-shortages-mixdown?in=user-67457490/sets/parenteral-nutrition>. This podcast is just 14 minutes in length and discusses the approach to manage product shortages in PN support.

INTRODUCTION

Maintenance of adequate nutrition status during illness has been recognized for more than 50 years as an integral part of the treatment plan for patients who are unable to attain and sustain oral nourishment. Successful techniques for providing IV nutrition support were introduced to clinical practice in adults and subsequently, infants in the late 1960s.[1] Use of central venous access was investigated to reduce risk of metabolic complications associated with IV fluid overload and electrolyte imbalances. The use of large central vessels permitted infusion of concentrated formulas, which decreased the fluid volume required and avoided the phlebitis that commonly occurred when hypertonic infusions were given peripherally.

Clinical experience and research fostered development of protocols that promoted better patient care and resulted in a decline in complications and costs associated with parenteral nutrition (PN) therapy.[2] The scope of practice for nutrition support clinicians has broadened as a result of increasing knowledge regarding the metabolic consequences associated with acute injury and chronic disease states. The pharmacist's role in providing safe and effective nutrition-support care requires knowledge of the principles of patient selection, initial therapy design, outcome monitoring, and strategies for providing therapy during PN product shortages.[3-5] In addition, the pharmacist is uniquely prepared to take on the responsibility for PN order verification as well as compounding and dispensing of the PN admixture. The PN order must be verified by a pharmacist to ensure the order is clear, complete, and correctly transcribed. A clinical review should be performed to confirm appropriate indication, nutrient dosing, and non-nutrient medication dosing. A pharmaceutical review should be performed to confirm compatibility of ordered nutrients and any non-nutrient medications in addition to the expected stability of the formulation.[4,5] Other responsibilities of the nutrition support pharmacist may include development of policy and procedures as well as quality improvement activities for patient care and operational processes associated with providing PN and enteral nutrition (EN).[4,5] The clinical role of other healthcare professionals may be similar because of the evolving interprofessional approach to nutritional support.[6-10] This chapter reviews indications for PN, components of PN formulations, routes of IV administration, practical aspects of regimen design, solution admixture, outcome monitoring, and management of complications for both adult and pediatric (neonates, infants, and children) patients.

DESIRED OUTCOMES

1 The primary objective of nutrition support therapy is to promote positive clinical outcomes of an illness and improve a patient's quality of life. Four fundamental steps are key to providing optimal care for patients who require nutrition support. They are establishing patient-specific nutrition goals, determining nutrient requirements to achieve the nutrition goals, assuring delivery of the required nutrients, and subsequently assessing the nutrition regimen.[5-7]

A patient's nutrition goals can be established after a thorough nutritional assessment (see Chapter 164). Nutrient requirements and an appropriate route for delivery of the required nutrients can then be determined. Nutrition support goals include correction of the patient's caloric and nitrogen imbalances and any fluid, electrolyte, vitamin, or trace element abnormalities. An additional goal is to lessen the metabolic response to injury by minimizing oxidant stress and favorably modulating immune response. These interventions should not cause or worsen other metabolic complications.

2 The gastrointestinal (GI) tract is the optimal route for providing nutrients unless obstruction or other GI complications are present (see Chapter 166).[11] Two other considerations that may impact selection of the optimal route for delivery of nutrition support include expected duration of nutrition therapy and risk of aspiration. Patients who have nonfunctional GI tracts or are otherwise not candidates for EN may benefit from PN.

INDICATIONS FOR PARENTERAL NUTRITION SUPPORT

The association between malnutrition and development of complications and mortality is well documented for adult and pediatric patients.[7,11-13] Although various clinical nutrition markers are improved for patients who receive PN, the impact on clinical outcomes has been difficult to demonstrate in many adult populations. The effect of PN on complications and mortality is unclear.[11] Consensus guidelines for PN use for adults and pediatric patients are based on clinical experience and investigations in specific patient populations.[11-18] Unfortunately, a lack of consistency in published guidelines from different sources complicates identification of the patient who is most likely to benefit from PN.

3 PN use should not be determined by medical diagnosis or disease state.[11] However, there are more detailed considerations for specific disease states.[11-18] The decision to initiate PN is based on the findings of an assessment performed after a patient demonstrates an inability to meet nutritional needs enterally for an extended time period (Tables 165-1 and 165-2). This assessment must include an evaluation of the patient's nutrition status, clinical status, age, and potential risks of initiating therapy (eg, infection, metabolic abnormalities). The appropriate length of time to wait before starting PN therapy depends on patient's age and clinical status.[11-18] PN therapy is not an emergent intervention and should not be initiated until the patient is hemodynamically and metabolically stable.[11]

TABLE 165-1 Time Frame for Initiating Parenteral Nutrition

1. Adults
   a. Previously well-nourished patients: Initiate PN after 7 days of oral intake or EN less than 50% of estimated requirements
   b. Nutritionally at-risk patients (ie, involuntary loss of 10% or more of usual body weight within 6 months; involuntary loss of greater than or 5% or more of usual body weight in 1 month; involuntary loss or gain of 10 pounds within 6 months; BMI less than 18.5 kg/m^2; inadequate nutrition intake, including inadequate food or nutrition products for greater than 7 days): Initiate PN after 3 to 5 days of oral intake or EN less than 50% of estimated requirements.
   c. Moderate or severely malnourished patients: Initiate PN as soon as feasible for those in whom oral intake or EN is not possible or sufficient.
   d. Delay PN in metabolically unstable patients until improvement in clinical condition.
2. Neonates
   a. Very low birth weight infant (birth weight less than 1,500 g): Begin PN promptly.
   b. Critically ill: Initiate PN when EN is unable to meet energy requirements for energy expenditure and growth.
3. Pediatrics
   a. Infant, child, or adolescent with self-limited illness: Delay PN for up to 7 days.
   b. Infants: Initiate PN within 1 to 3 days when EN is unable to provide sufficient nutrients to support growth for an extended period.
   c. Older children and adolescents: Initiate PN within 4 to 5 days when EN is unable to provide sufficient nutrients to support growth for an extended period.

BMI, body mass index; EN, enteral nutrition; PN, parenteral nutrition.

Data from Reference 11.

COMPONENTS OF PARENTERAL NUTRITION

4 PN formulations include IV sources of protein, dextrose, fat or lipid, water, electrolytes, vitamins, trace elements, and other additives. PN solutions should provide the optimal combination of macro- and micronutrients to provide a patient's specific nutritional requirements. Macronutrients include water, protein, dextrose, and lipid (Table 165-3). Micronutrients include vitamins, trace elements, and electrolytes. Both macronutrients and micronutrients are necessary for maintenance of normal metabolism. In general, macronutrients are used for energy (dextrose and lipid) and as structural substrates (protein and lipid). Micronutrients on the other hand support a variety of metabolic activities necessary for cellular homeostasis such as enzymatic reactions, fluid balance, and regulation of electrophysiologic processes.

Over the past 5 to 10 years, there have been shortages of all PN components.[3] The unavailability of these products has resulted in delays in PN therapy initiation, restricted or limited nutrient dosing, and negative effects on all steps of the PN process that have compromised patient health and safety. Providing safe therapy during PN product shortages can be challenging for PN patients and practitioners.[3,5] Conservation recommendations and alternative therapy measures may need to be employed to optimize quality of care and avoid patient harm.[3,5] In addition, the Food and Drug Administration (FDA) may permit the temporary importation of PN products from foreign manufacturers that have been used safely and successfully in the foreign market. However, the products may have not received official FDA approval for routine use and distribution in the United States because the manufacturer has not sought FDA approval. Imported products have included PN components such as sodium glycerophosphate, multitrace element products, and amino acids.[3] If such products are imported and used in the United States, practitioners should thoroughly familiarize themselves with the prescribing information located in the product's package insert because

TABLE 165-2 Indications for Parenteral Nutrition

1. Impaired absorption or loss of nutrients via the GI tract because of one or more of the following:
   a. Massive small bowel resection: Adult patients with less than 120 cm of small bowel distal to the ligament of Treitz without a colon or less than 60 cm of small bowel with an intact colon; neonates, infants, and pediatric patients who are unable to meet nutrient, electrolyte, and fluid requirements regardless of intestinal length
   b. High output GI fistulae: Greater than 500 mL/day; location precludes enteral access
   c. High volume fistula output with EN
   d. Neutropenic colitis: Typhlitis or opportunistic infection in an immunocompromised patient
   e. Small bowel mucosal disease: Radiation or chemotherapy-related enteritis, autoimmune enteropathy, intractable diarrhea of infancy
   f. Intestinal atresia
   g. Gastroschisis
   h. Volvulus
   i. Meconium ileus
   j. Necrotizing enterocolitis
   k. Mesenteric thrombosis
2. Mechanical bowel obstruction: Intrinsic or extrinsic blockage of intestinal lumen
   a. Stenosis or stricture
   b. Inflammatory disease
   c. Peritoneal carcinomatosis
   d. Severe adhesive disease
   e. Severe superior mesenteric artery syndrome
3. Restricted oral intake or EN necessary for bowel rest
   a. Ischemic bowel
      - Mesenteric artery stenosis
      - Abdominal compartment syndrome
      - Low flow states
   b. Severe pancreatitis
      - EN exacerbated pain
      - Worsening serum lipase levels
      - Infected pancreatic phlegmon/pseudocyst
      - Complex pancreatic fistula
      - Abdominal compartment syndrome
   c. Chylous fistula: High output with low-fat diet or elemental formula
   d. Preoperative status: Severely malnourished patient with non-functional GI tract for 7 to 10 days prior to surgery
4. Motility disorders
   a. Prolonged ileus
      - Diffuse peritonitis
      - Medical treatment-induced
      - Other disease states
   b. Pseudo-obstruction
   c. Scleroderma
   d. Visceral organ myopathy
   e. Very long segment Hirschsprung's disease
   f. Severe adhesive disease
5. Inability to achieve or maintain enteral access or EN
   a. Hemodynamic instability
   b. Active GI bleeding
   c. Severe neutropenic fever
   d. Low birth weight infant

EN, enteral nutrition; GI, gastrointestinal.

Data from Reference 11.

TABLE 165-3 Macronutrient Components of PN Solutions

Nutritional Substrate	IV Source	Description
Fluid	Sterile water for injection USP	
Nitrogen	Crystalline amino acids	
	Standard solutions	Contain a balanced profile of essential, semi-essential, and nonessential L-amino acids
	Pediatrics	Amino acid profile includes standard essential, semi-essential, and nonessential amino acids with lower methionine, phenylalanine, and glycine concentrations; these solutions also contain taurine, glutamate, and aspartate
Energy		
Carbohydrate	Dextrose	
Fat	Lipid injectable emulsion	Fatty acid source
	LCT emulsions	Soybean
	Fish oil emulsions	Fish oil
	Mixed lipid emulsions	Soybean-olive oil SMOF (soybean oil, MCT, olive, and fish oils)

LCT, long-chain triglycerides; MCT, medium-chain triglycerides; PN, parenteral nutrition; SMOF, soybean oil, MCT, olive, and fish oils; USP, United States Pharmacopeia.

of potential differences in product ingredients and concentration that may affect dosing. In addition, potential interactions resulting in stability or compatibility problems should be considered.

Amino Acids

Protein in PN solutions is provided in the form of crystalline amino acids (CAAs), which when oxidized for energy yield 4 cal or approximately 17 J/g of protein. However, including the caloric contribution from protein when calculating calories provided by the PN regimen is controversial.[19] While sufficient energy substrate should be provided to allow utilization of amino acids for protein synthesis rather than an energy source, oxidation of amino acids for energy has been demonstrated in critically ill patients and is thought to occur because of metabolic derangements seen during severe metabolic stress. Hence, some practice settings may differ in expressing calories provided by a PN regimen as total calories (protein, carbohydrate, and lipid calories) or non-protein calories (carbohydrate and lipid calories).

Commercially available CAA solutions may be categorized as standard amino acid solutions or modified amino acid solutions. Standard CAA solutions are designed for patients with "normal" organ function and nutritional requirements (see Table 165-3). Although standard CAA solutions differ in the proportion of specific amino acids, they contain a balanced profile of essential, semi-essential, and nonessential L-amino acids. Despite these differences, there are similar effects on markers of protein metabolism.[20] The protein concentration, total nitrogen, and electrolyte content may also differ among products. Because the nitrogen concentration of dietary protein is approximately 16%, 6.25 (100 g protein/16 g nitrogen) is commonly accepted as the conversion figure for calculating the nitrogen amount provided by CAA protein. Differences in nitrogen content per gram of amino acids among CAA products may affect calculation of nitrogen amounts infused when determining nitrogen balance.[20,21] The clinical significance of these differences in determining nitrogen balance for routine clinical use is unknown.[21]

Standard CAA solutions may also include obligatory electrolyte concentrations that may affect PN compounding as well as the total clinical dose provided to the patient.[22] CAAs are available in several different concentrations, which facilitate compounding of patient-specific PN regimens. Use of highly concentrated products (15%-20% amino acids) is attractive for critically ill patients who typically require fluid restriction but have large protein needs. Modified amino acid solutions are designed for patients who have altered protein requirements, such as neonates and pediatric patients (see Table 165-3). For example, several commercially available CAA solutions are designed to provide conditionally essential amino acids, which are considered nonessential during health because

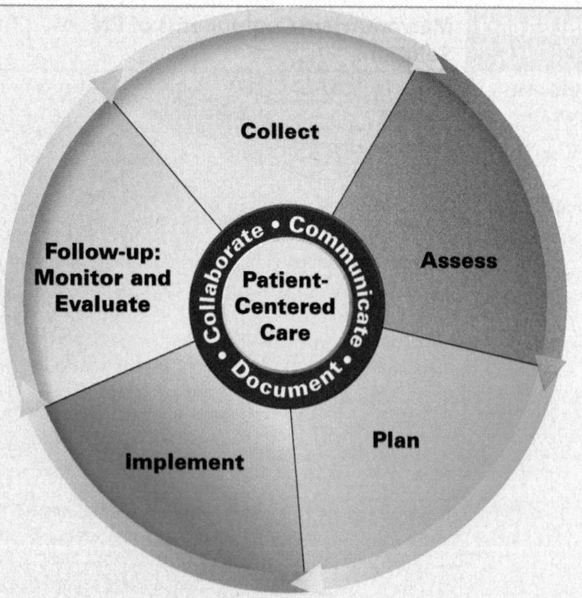

Patient Care Process for Use of Parenteral Nutrition

Collect

- Patient characteristics (eg, age, race, sex)
- Patient history (past medical, surgical, family, social, alcohol use)
- Nutrition history (dietary history, weight history)
- Current medications (including nutritional supplements)
- Age appropriate objective data (Fig. 165-3)
  - Height/length, weight, body mass index (BMI), head circumference
  - Fluid balance (intake and output)
  - Labs (eg, serum electrolytes, SCr, BUN, glucose, albumin, AST, ALT, alkaline phosphatase)
  - Vital signs (eg, temperature, pulse rate, respiration rate, blood pressure)

Assess

- Current nutrition status and time period of insufficient nutrient intake
- Clinical condition(s) preventing adequate oral nutrient intake
- Clinical condition(s) preventing use of enteral tube feeding to determine if an indication for PN therapy exists (Tables 165-1 and 165-2)
- Vascular access
- Current degree of metabolic instability (eg, hemodynamics, organ function, fluid/electrolyte status)
- Appropriate route of PN (central or peripheral)

Plan*

- Design an age-appropriate PN regimen that provides estimated nutrient requirements and minimizes risk of adverse medication reactions or worsening current metabolic conditions (see Designing a PN Regimen; Figs. 165-1 and 165-2)
- Monitoring parameters for efficacy (Fig. 165-3)

Implement*

- Provide education regarding all elements of treatment plan to patient/caregivers and other members of the healthcare team
- Use a standardized PN order form for ordering PN prescription to minimize risk of errors
- Verify the order to ensure that it is clear, complete, and correctly transcribed
- Confirm stability of formulation and compatibility of ordered nutrients and any non-nutrient medications
- Determine if PN solution will be provided as compounded sterile preparation according to United States Pharmacopoeia Chapter 797 standards or provided as a standardized, commercially available PN product
- Determine appropriate plan for patient-specific monitoring based on the patient's clinical condition to anticipate, prevent or treat mechanical/technical, metabolic/nutritional or infectious complications (Fig. 165-3)

Follow-up: Monitor and Evaluate

- Evaluate patient for mechanical, metabolic, and infectious complications (Fig. 165-3)
- Re-evaluate clinical condition(s) preventing adequate oral intake or precluding use of enteral tube feeding to anticipate either transition off of PN support or need for continuing PN therapy (Fig. 165-3)

**Collaborate with patient, caregivers, and other healthcare professionals.*

they are produced from other amino acids. However, under certain physiologic conditions, such as prematurity or sepsis, these amino acids cannot be synthesized in sufficient quantities.[20,22] CAA solutions specifically designed for neonates and pediatric patients contain increased amounts of taurine, aspartic acid, and glutamic acid. Other conditionally essential amino acids, such as cysteine, carnitine, and glutamine, are not available in commercial CAA solutions in pharmacologic amounts because they are relatively unstable or poorly soluble.[20,22]

Consequently, PN solutions may need to be modified to provide the desired amount of supplemental conditionally essential amino acids. For example, cysteine is a conditionally essential amino acid for preterm and term infants because of their enzymatic immaturity of the trans-sulfuration pathway. Cysteine may be added to PN solutions at the time of compounding as a supplement to CAA solutions and to enhance calcium and phosphate solubility by decreasing solution pH.[22] Carnitine is a quaternary amine required for long-chain fatty acid transport into the mitochondria for β-oxidation and energy production. Newborns are at risk for carnitine deficiency because of their immature biosynthetic capacity. Decreased plasma carnitine concentrations occur in infants and children receiving PN without carnitine.[16] Supplemental carnitine may be added to the PN solution at the time of compounding. Although the benefit of carnitine supplementation in PN has not been clearly identified, positive effects on nutritional markers, including improved fatty acid oxidation, weight gain, and nitrogen balance, have been documented. In general, carnitine supplementation is reserved for neonates expected to receive PN support for 7 days or longer.[16]

Glutamine is the most abundant free amino acid in the body and is an important intermediate for many metabolic processes. Glutamine has an important role in maintaining intestinal integrity, immune function, and protein synthesis during conditions of metabolic stress.[23] Positive effects on nutritional markers (eg, improved nitrogen balance) as well as outcome markers (eg, decreased length of hospitalization, incidence of infections, GI toxicities associated with chemotherapy or radiation) are associated with glutamine.[23] Unfortunately, the best candidate for response to glutamine therapy has not been clearly identified.[23,24] Use of both IV and enteral glutamine in combination with a variety of antioxidant supplements in critically ill adult patients has been associated with increased mortality.[24] Despite an association between increased brain volume and head circumference in school-aged children, who were premature at birth and received glutamine during the first year of life, the clinical usefulness of glutamine in neonates and infants is unclear.[23,25,26] Plasma glutamine concentrations increase with supplementation, but there is no beneficial effect on sepsis incidence or outcome, enteral feeding tolerance, necrotizing enterocolitis, growth, or mortality.[23,26,27] The clinical use of glutamine is further complicated because there is no parenteral glutamine formulation commercially available in the United States. Available CAA solutions do not contain glutamine because of poor solubility and instability.[22] Use of parenteral glutamine requires special manufacturing techniques not readily available in many institutional pharmacies.[23] However, parenteral glutamine has been made available from several licensed pharmacies that extemporaneously compound glutamine crystalline powder under sterile conditions either as a separate parenteral solution or as a part of a CAA solution.

Dextrose

The primary energy source in PN solutions is carbohydrate, usually in the form of dextrose monohydrate, hereafter referred to as dextrose which is available in concentrations ranging from 5% to 70%. When oxidized, each gram of dextrose provides 3.4 kcal (14.2 kJ). The appropriate IV dextrose dose depends on the patient's age, estimated caloric requirements, and clinical condition. For example, minimum dextrose requirements for neonates are estimated to be approximately 6 to 8 mg/kg/min and infusion rates should not exceed 14 to 18 mg/kg/min for infants or 4 to 7 mg/kg/min for adults.[16,28,29] The recommended dextrose dose for routine clinical care rarely exceeds 5 mg/kg/min for adolescents and adults.[16,28,29] Maintaining an age-appropriate dextrose infusion rate is necessary to minimize risk of adverse medication reactions. If the dextrose infusion rate exceeds the glucose oxidation rate, metabolically expensive pathways, such as glycogen repletion and lipid synthesis, are favored, resulting in increased energy expenditure, increased oxygen consumption, and increased carbon dioxide production. Excessive dextrose infusion rates also may contribute to the development of hyperglycemia and an increase in the concentration of biochemical markers indicative of fatty infiltration of the liver.[29,30]

Lipid Injectable Emulsion

Lipid injectable emulsion (ILE) is used as a concentrated source of calories and essential fatty acids.[31-35] Commercially available ILE products have traditionally contained soybean oil (SO) or a combination of SO and safflower oil. However, SO-based ILE may have negative effects on immune function and hepatic function, and this has led to approval of alternative mixed oil ILE for clinical use.[35,36] These products contain combinations of SO and olive oil, as well as SO, olive oil, medium chain triglyceride oil (MCT), and fish oil (FO), collectively known as SMOF.[32,33] An additional ILE alternative containing 100% FO is also approved for clinical use (Table 165-3).[34]

As a caloric source, ILE use may facilitate provision of adequate calories and minimize complications of nutrition therapy such as hyperglycemia, hepatotoxicity, or increased carbon dioxide production.[35] In the past, SO-based ILE has been used for treatment or prevention of essential fatty acid deficiency (EFAD) in both adult and pediatric patients because of the higher linoleic and linolenic FA composition.[35,36] EFAD is the result of a biochemical deficiency of linoleic acid and arachidonic acid, which are considered essential for humans.[28,35,36] Linoleic acid, an omega-3 FA, and linolenic acid, an omega-6 FA, are important for a variety of functions such as cellular integrity, platelet function, postnatal brain development, and wound healing.[36] Both are polyunsaturated long chain triglycerides (LCT). Normally, linoleic acid is converted to the tetraene arachidonic acid. When linoleic acid is not present in sufficient amounts, oleic acid is converted to the tetraene 5,8,11-eicosatrienoic acid, an FA of lesser physiologic integrity, and as a result, EFAD develops. EFAD may be prevented by providing 2% to 4% of total calories as linoleic acid and 0.25% to 0.5% of total calories as linolenic acid. This may be achieved for most adult patients by giving approximately 100 g SO ILE weekly and approximately 200 g mixed oil ILE weekly (based on approximately 2,000 calories/day [~8,400 J/day]).[35,36] Neonates and infants require a minimum of 0.5 to 1 g/kg SO ILE daily.[16] The SO-olive oil product is not approved for use in pediatric patients because of the lower linoleic and linolenic acid content and inadequate provision of essential fatty acids to prevent or treat EFAD when used in recommended doses.[32] In general, the 100% FO product is not indicated for treating EFAD because of the relatively lower essential FA content.[34,35] This product is indicated for use in pediatric patients with PN associated cholestasis.[34] However, EFAD may be prevented in PN-dependent infants who received FO ILE as the sole source of fat calories for at least 1 month.[37]

ILEs with SO as the lipid source may have negative effects on immune function as the result of omega-6 PUFA influence on proinflammatory eicosanoid production through arachidonic acid metabolic pathways.[35,36] Mixed oil ILE may promote lower production of proinflammatory cytokines by providing lower amounts of omega-6 FA. Olive oil–based ILEs provide essential fatty acids, are a rich source of vitamin E, and have a neutral effect on immune function because of the decreased amount of omega-6 PUFA linoleic acid.[35] MCTs may offer several advantages, especially for critically ill patients. MCTs are hydrolyzed and cleared more rapidly than LCTs, and they do not accumulate in the liver. In addition, MCTs do not require carnitine for entrance into mitochondria for oxidation. However, MCTs are not a source of essential fatty acids. IV MCT-LCT mixtures demonstrate safety and efficacy comparable with standard LCT emulsions.[35,36] FO–based ILE contain predominantly omega-3 PUFAs, which are metabolized to cytokine mediators that may be less inflammatory and immunosuppressive than those derived from omega-6 PUFAs. The clinical effect of FO-containing ILE administration on immune function, as well as on patient morbidity and mortality, is not clear.[35,36,38]

Phytosterols are sterols that are a natural component of plant-based oils used in ILE formulations.[39] SO-based ILE and phytosterol intake are associated with cholestasis of PN-associated liver disease (PNALD). SO-based ILE have a higher phytosterol content relative to the other mixed oil ILE products.[39] Use of mixed oil or 100% FO ILE in PN-dependent patients who developed cholestasis while receiving SO-based ILE may improve in or reverse of PNALD.[39]

Commercially available products are reviewed in Table 165-3. All commercially available ILE formulations contain egg phospholipids as an emulsifying agent and glycerol to make the emulsion isotonic.[22] Although the caloric contribution of fat is 9 kcal/g (38 kJ/g), the caloric content of 10% ILE is 1.1 kcal/mL (4.6 kJ/mL), 2 kcal/mL (8.4 kJ/mL) for 20% ILE, and 3 kcal/mL (12.6 kJ/mL) for 30% ILE because of the caloric contribution of the egg phospholipid and glycerol.

Commercially available ILE products may be administered by either the central or the peripheral route. They may be added directly to the PN solution as a total nutrient admixture (TNA), also referred to as a three-in-one system (lipids, protein, glucose, and additives), or they may be co-infused with the CAA-dextrose solution, commonly referred to as a two-in-one admixture.[5,31-34,40] However, 30% ILEs are only approved for use in the preparation of TNA and are not intended for direct IV administration.

Plasma ILE clearance is directly related to gestational age of infants and is influenced by the infusion rate and the patient's clinical status.[16] Rapid SO-ILE infusions contribute to decreased oxygenation for neonates.[41] Adverse pulmonary effects are thought to be caused by polyunsaturated fatty acid (PUFA)–driven prostaglandin production, which results in altered vascular tone. Although the association between ILE and pulmonary dysfunction is not clear, a boxed warning appears in the FDA product labeling for both SO and SO-olive oil ILE that acknowledges deaths in preterm infants associated with pulmonary fat accumulation thought to be related to ILE infusions.[31,32] In addition, rapid infusion of long-chain fatty acid formulations may have a negative impact on immunocompetence by saturating the reticuloendothelial system.[28,35,42]

Although the frequency of acute adverse medication reactions is less than 1% with current formulations, patients receiving their first ILE dose should be monitored for dyspnea, chest tightness, palpitations, and chills. Headache, nausea, and fever may also occur, especially with a rapid infusion rate. In general, ILE use is contraindicated for patients with an impaired ability to clear fat emulsion, such as patients with pathologic hyperlipidemia, lipoid nephrosis, and hypertriglyceridemia associated with pancreatitis.[31-35] Patients should be evaluated for hypersensitivity to any of the product-dependent ingredients such as fish, egg, soybean, or peanut protein prior to initiating ILE.[31-34,43]

ILE products remain the most common source of parenteral fat, but a number of medications have been introduced that contain lipid either as a vehicle for delivery or as a portion of the medication formulation. Propofol, an IV anesthetic, is delivered in a soybean-oil-in-water emulsion that has essentially the same composition and caloric concentration as 10% SO-ILE. This agent is used commonly for continuous sedation of mechanically ventilated patients and should be considered a potential source of calories that may require adjustment of a patient's nutrition regimen.[35,44] Clevidipine is an injectable calcium channel blocker that contains 20% ILE as a vehicle that may also be a potential source of IV fat when used as a continuous infusion for multiple days of therapy.[45] The antifungal amphotericin B is available in several lipid-containing combinations such as liposomal and lipid complex formulations. The caloric contribution from amphotericin B is generally small and not clinically relevant when used in standard doses.

Vitamins

The Nutrition Advisory Group of the American Medical Association (NAG-AMA) recommended in 1975 the daily parenteral supplementation of 13 essential (four fat-soluble and nine water-soluble) vitamins for pediatric and adult patients based on requirements for healthy people.[46]

Since these original recommendations, the NAG-AMA has revised the guidelines for children to primarily reflect changes for preterm infants requiring PN.[46] The FDA also mandated in 2000 changes in adult parenteral vitamin formulations (inclusion of vitamin K and higher doses of vitamins B_1, B_6, and C).[46] Vitamin K was not included in early multivitamin formulations due to the potential for drug-nutrient interactions in patients receiving anticoagulants. Although the NAG-AMA recommendation for vitamin K for adults is 2 to 4 mg weekly, only 150 μg/day was mandated to be included in newer formulations by the FDA.[47] However, in adult patients receiving long-term SO-ILE-containing PN with vitamin K–free parenteral multivitamins at home, supplemental vitamin K may not be necessary to maintain normal prothrombin times and plasma vitamin K concentrations.[48] Indeed, SO used in ILEs is a natural source of phylloquinone (vitamin K1). However, the other commercially available mixed-oil ILE formulations contain phylloquinone as well.[49] SO-ILE formulations contain the highest amount of vitamin K and the concentration is generally dependent on the SO concentration in the ILE.[35,47-49] Although current vitamin K-containing multiple-vitamin products should provide sufficient amounts to prevent adverse effects associated with vitamin K deficiency, supplemental vitamin K may be given intramuscularly or subcutaneously or added to the PN solution if needed.[47]

The 2012 ASPEN recommendations advocate for the continued availability of multivitamin products with and without vitamin K so that clinicians have the ability to withhold vitamin K supplementation in patients receiving warfarin therapy. Most adult parenteral multiple-vitamin products which are available commercially contain vitamin K. MVI-12, multivitamin infusion without vitamin K is available from Hospira, Inc. Lake Forest, IL. Two parenteral multiple-vitamin products are commercially available for use for pediatric patients. MVI-Pediatric (Hospira Inc.) and Infuvite Pediatric (Baxter Healthcare Corporation) are formulated to meet the revised NAG-AMA guidelines for infants weighing less than 1 kg (2.2 lb) and children up to 11 years. However, there are no commercially available injectable multivitamin products designed to specifically meet the unique requirements of premature infants, including higher vitamin A and lower doses of vitamins B_1, B_2, B_6, and B_{12}.

Vitamin requirements may be altered in malnutrition and other specific disease states or with certain medication therapies. Individual and combination products are available to provide additional or tailored supplementation, which may be necessary to prevent development of vitamin toxicities or deficiencies caused by altered metabolism or medication therapy.

The 2012 ASPEN recommendations question whether the vitamin D content of parenteral multivitamins is adequate to meet current Recommended Dietary Allowances (RDA) and advocate for the addition of a parenteral vitamin D product for PN-dependent patients who are unresponsive to additional enteral vitamin D supplementation.[46] In addition, the recommendations support the continued production of adult-injectable multivitamin products with and without vitamin K and for the supplementation of carnitine (2-5 mg/kg/day) in neonatal PN and choline in all patients receiving PN.[46]

Trace Elements

Many trace elements are an important part of metalloenzymes and function as cofactors in a variety of regulatory metabolic pathways.[50] Although 17 trace elements have demonstrated biologic importance, clear deficiency syndromes in humans have been described only for cobalt (as vitamin B_{12}), copper, iodine, iron, and zinc.[50-52] In 1979, the NAG-AMA recommended chromium, copper, manganese, and zinc supplementation for patients receiving PN.[46,50] Recommendations followed in 1984 to also supplement with selenium.[46,50] Although there is not a clear deficiency syndrome for manganese, the NAG-AMA considered manganese essential based on case reports of patients receiving PN with metabolic complications that corrected after manganese supplementation. Reports of deficiency syndromes associated with selenium and molybdenum suggest that they may also be essential.[46,50,51] Although iodine deficiency does not occur for patients receiving short-term PN, it has been observed in patients receiving long-term PN and may be related to the use of chlorhexidine for central-line care instead of povidone-iodine.[46,50,52]

Injectable trace elements are available as single-trace element solutions and as multiple-trace element combinations.[22] The use of single-entity injectable products allows for individualization of trace mineral supplementation of chromium, copper, iodine, manganese, selenium, and zinc. Requirements for trace elements vary on the basis of the patient's clinical condition. For example, higher doses of supplemental zinc are likely necessary for patients with high-output ostomies or diarrhea because the GI tract is the predominant excretion route for zinc. Whereas manganese and copper are excreted through the biliary tract, chromium, molybdenum, and selenium are excreted renally. Hence, these trace elements should be restricted or withheld from PN solutions for patients with cholestatic liver disease and kidney disease, respectively. ASPEN recommended formulation changes to the available injectable multiple-trace element preparations for PN patients.[46] In general, the recommendations support overall decreased trace element contamination in large- and small-volume PN products.[46] The recommendations advocate for decreased copper and manganese, no (or decreased) chromium, and inclusion and increased dose of selenium in all injectable adult multiple-trace products.[46] The recommendations also support products with no chromium, decreased manganese, and the inclusion of selenium in all injectable pediatric multiple-trace products.[46] These recommendations were recognized by injectable trace element manufacturers and reformulated products for adults and pediatric patients are now available.[22] The trace element combination product for adults provides the daily requirements for the trace elements considered essential by the NAG-AMA except chromium (ie, copper, manganese, selenium, zinc).[53] Chromium amounts provided as a contaminate in PN injectable products are considered adequate to meet daily requirements.[46] The combination product approved for use in the United States for neonates and pediatric patients contains zinc, copper, manganese, and selenium.[54] The addition of single-entity zinc, copper, and selenium is required in many pediatric weight ranges to meet recommended needs when using these combination products.

Electrolytes

Electrolytes such as sodium, potassium, calcium, magnesium, phosphorus, chloride, and acetate are necessary PN components for the maintenance of many cellular functions. Electrolytes may be given to maintain normal serum concentrations or to correct deficits. Patients who have "normal" organ function and relatively normal serum concentrations of any electrolyte should receive "normal" maintenance electrolyte doses when PN is initiated and daily thereafter. Specific electrolyte requirements vary according to the patient's age, disease state, organ function, previous and current medication therapy, nutrition status, and extrarenal losses. Electrolytes are available commercially as single- and multiple-nutrient solutions.[22] Multiple-electrolyte solutions are useful for stable patients with normal organ function who are receiving PN. Concentrated multiple-electrolyte solutions designed for addition to PN solutions generally contain only sodium, potassium, calcium, and magnesium. Phosphorus must be added as a separate additive. Further information regarding metabolism and requirements of vitamins, trace elements, and electrolytes is given elsewhere.[55]

DESIGNING A PARENTERAL NUTRITION REGIMEN

5 Several factors, including the patient's venous access, fluid status, and macronutrient and micronutrient requirements, are important considerations when designing the PN regimen. A patient's venous access and fluid status determines the maximum PN osmolar concentration, which will impact the nutrient amount that may be provided. PN solutions may be administered by central or peripheral venous access. The patient's clinical condition determines which route is most appropriate.

PN formulations may be provided as a two-in-one admixture that contains dextrose, CAA, and other necessary micronutrients or as a three-in-one admixture or TNA that contains dextrose, CAA, and ILE, as well as other necessary micronutrients. Use of TNA solutions offers several potential advantages, including reduced inventory (infusion pumps, tubing, and other related supplies), decreased time for compounding and administration, a potential decrease in manipulations of the infusion line (which should correspond with a decreased risk of catheter contamination), and ease of delivery and storage for patients receiving home PN.[40] Potential disadvantages include increased risk of infections and stability and compatibility concerns. For example, the stability of TNA admixtures is less predictable than that of two-in-one admixtures, which makes their use less desirable in some patient populations such as neonates and infants.[41,56]

Routes of Parenteral Nutrition Administration

Peripheral Route

Peripheral parenteral nutrition (PPN) is an option for mild-to-moderately stressed patients in whom adequate GI tract function is expected to return within 10 to 14 days.[11] PPN may also be used as a temporary source of PN, or as a bridge therapy during transition periods where oral intake or EN is suboptimal or clinical circumstances do not justify placing a central venous catheter (CVC) access.[11] In general, potential PPN candidates should not be fluid-restricted or require large nutrient amounts. Lower concentrations of amino acids (3%-5% final concentration), dextrose (5%-10% final concentration), and micronutrients compared with central parenteral nutrition (CPN) must be used for peripheral administration. Because PPN solutions are relatively dilute, larger volumes are usually necessary to provide nutrient requirements. Additionally, many patients who receive PPN likely will require ILE to achieve the desired caloric intake at levels consistent with CPN regimens. The primary advantages of PPN include a potentially lower risk of infectious and technical complications associated with CVC access.[11] Patients who are likely to be poor candidates for PPN include those with poor venous access as the result of multiple courses of chemotherapy, malnutrition, illness of long duration that has required multiple venous accesses for fluid and medication administration, premature infants, and the elderly. PPN use is also limited by relatively poor peripheral vein tolerance to hypertonic solutions. Thrombophlebitis is a common complication for patients receiving PPN.[56] Although the risk of phlebitis is greater with solution osmolarities greater than 600 to 900 mOsm/L, peripherally administered TNA with much higher osmolarities to adults has been associated with low infusion-site complications in some centers.[56,57] Efforts to minimize development of phlebitis or infiltration sequelae for patients receiving PPN include addition of ILE as a possible venous lumen protectant, subtherapeutic heparin doses (0.5-1 unit/mL) to prevent thrombus formation, or small doses of hydrocortisone (5 mg/L) to minimize access site inflammation.[56,57] However, the co-infusion of ILE with PPN (ie, not provided as a TNA) does not reduce phlebitis. In addition, heparin does not reduce catheter-related thrombosis and is not compatible for use in TNAs.[56] Midline catheter use may offer some advantage and has been associated with a reduced risk of thrombophlebitis.[11,58] Although these catheters are not central venous access devices, they are longer and infuse into larger venous vessels that may dilute the PPN solution to a more tolerable osmolarity. The osmolarity of a PN solution may be estimated by using the guidelines for osmolarities of selected PN components listed in Table 165-4.

Central Route

CPN is the preferred route for PN delivery and is used predominantly for patients who require PN for periods of more than 7 to 14 days during hospitalization or indefinitely at home.[11,59,60] These patients may have large nutrient requirements; poor peripheral venous access; or fluctuating fluid requirements, such as metabolically stressed patients with extensive surgery, trauma, sepsis, multiple-organ failure, or malignancy. CPN solutions are highly

TABLE 165-4 Osmolarities of Selected Parenteral Nutrients

Nutrient	Osmolarity
Amino acid	100 mOsm/%
Dextrose	50 mOsm/%
Lipid emulsion (20%)	1.3-1.5 mOsm/g
Sodium (acetate, chloride)	2 mOsm/mEq
Sodium phosphate	3 mOsm/mEq sodium
Potassium (acetate, chloride)	2 mOsm/mEq
Potassium phosphate	1.7-2.7 mOsm/mEq potassium
Magnesium sulfate	1 mOsm/mEq
Calcium gluconate	1.4 mOsm/mEq

concentrated hypertonic solutions that must be administered through a large central vein. Unlike peripheral veins, central veins have a higher blood flow, which quickly dilutes the hypertonic solutions. Disadvantages of CPN include risks associated with catheter insertion, routine catheter use, and care of the access site. Relative to peripheral venous access, CVC access is associated with a greater potential for infection. In addition, the risk of more serious catheter-induced trauma and related sequelae and other serious technical or mechanical problems is greater than that with peripheral access.

The choice of central venous access site depends on a number of factors, including the patient's age and anatomy. CVCs vary in composition, lumen size, number of injection ports, and other features that affect ease or convenience of care and maintenance. CVCs for short-term use for adults are commonly inserted percutaneously into the subclavian vein and advanced so that the tip is at the superior vena cava.[58] If this approach is not possible, the internal jugular vein can be used. Frequently, short-term central venous access is obtained for critically ill neonates via a catheter placed in the umbilical vein. Other sites for central venous access in infants and older children are similar to those in adults. When therapy is expected to last longer than 4 weeks, the catheter is tunneled subcutaneously before entering the central vessel, secured initially with retaining sutures, and anchored in place with a felt cuff that promotes subcutaneous fibrotic tissue growth around the catheter. The injection port may remain external or may be concealed entirely beneath the skin. Implanted CVCs have a larger port or reservoir that is surgically placed beneath the skin surface and anchored in the chest wall muscle. Peripherally inserted central catheters (PICCs) are venous access devices that are inserted into a peripheral vein (basilic, cephalic, or brachial) and advanced so that the tip is at the superior vena cava.[58] PICCs are increasingly used for both short- and long-term central venous access in acute or home care settings because of ease and economy of bedside placement.[11,58,60]

Constructing a Parenteral Nutrition Regimen

After the route of delivery is chosen, the components of the PN regimen are determined based on the patient's nutritional assessment. Although not recommended due to increased potential for errors, some healthcare systems may require the entire PN order to be written in individual components and additives on traditional paper order forms without the use of a standard order form. Standardized electronic PN orders suitable for computerized prescriber order entry (CPOE) are recommended for all patients to minimize risk of errors associated with the ordering process.[5,61] Standardized order forms or clinical decision support within electronic PN ordering systems promote education of practitioners by providing brief guidelines for initiating PN and foster cost-efficient nutrition support by minimizing errors in ordering, compounding, and administration.[5,56,61] Standardized order forms also may include options for ordering certain related procedures, laboratory tests, protocols for patient management, or consultations with other medical services related to the patient's nutrition support.

Adult Parenteral Nutrition Solutions

6 In general, there are two methods for ordering adult PN. The "standard formula approach" offers a variety of admixtures with a fixed nonprotein-calorie-to-nitrogen ratio. This method usually includes different formulas for mild-to-moderately stressed patients, and those who have kidney or liver failure or are fluid-restricted. Because the nonprotein-calorie-to-nitrogen ratio is fixed, the daily amount of nutrient delivered depends solely on the volume infused. Standard institutional PN formulations may be compounded; however, standardized commercial PN products or multichamber bag PN solutions are available from several manufacturers.[62] A standard institutional formula may promote clinician prescribing of a complete, balanced formulation and promote consistent provision of stable and compatible admixtures. However, efficiencies associated with use of the standard formula approach may be hindered if there is a frequent need to modify the PN formulation. Finally, standard PN formulations may be difficult to use in complicated patients, such as neonatal or pediatric patients, and those with severe malnutrition, organ failure, glucose intolerance, large GI losses, or critical illness.[62]

The "individualized formula approach" permits compounding of patient-specific admixtures. Compounding of the PN admixture is limited only by the concentrations of stock solutions and stability of the additives. The nutrient amount delivered depends on the daily volume of the PN solution infused and the nutrient amounts in the PN solution. The total daily amount of PN solution may be prepared in multiple bags or more cost-effectively in a single container.[40]

Historically, adult PN formulations were ordered by expressing the final concentrations of each component in the solution. However, this inconsistency may promote confusion and misinterpretation of PN admixture contents that may result in harm, especially when patients are transferred between health system environments. To ensure that PN labels in all health system environments clearly and accurately reflect the PN admixture contents, guidelines for standardized adult PN labeling have been recommended.[5,61] In addition to including a variety of other information on the label such as dosing weight and administration route, the guidelines recommend expressing PN ingredients in amounts per daily volume, which minimizes the need for pharmaceutical calculations to determine the nutrient value of the admixture. For example, macronutrients ordered in grams per day and electrolytes in milliequivalents or millimoles per day in an adult patient. Commercially available computer software for calculating PN formulations include the recommended ASPEN labeling guidelines (Baxter Healthcare, Deerfield, Il.; B. Braun Medical Inc., Bethlehem, PA).[5,61] Pharmaceutical calculations of an adult TNA PN regimen are briefly reviewed in Fig. 165-1.

Several guidelines are available to help simplify calculation of a PN regimen after a patient's nutritional requirements have been decided. For example, adult patients receiving only PN therapy may need larger volumes of fluid to provide maintenance requirements and replace extrarenal losses. However, patients requiring other IV medication therapy may receive adequate fluid from an additional IV maintenance solution (eg, 0.45% NaCl in 5% dextrose) or co-infused medications (or both). Depending on individual institutional practices, maximally concentrating the PN admixture and using an inexpensive maintenance fluid to manage hydration may provide a cost-effective regimen that requires fewer adjustments. Another guideline that may be helpful in designing a PN regimen is to allow a volume of approximately 100 to 150 mL/L of base solution (~200-300 mL/day) for electrolytes and other additives.

Calculation of an Adult PN Regimen

Patient case: A patient's daily nutritional requirements have been estimated to be 105 g protein and 2,200 total kcal. The patient has central venous access and reports no history of diabetes, hyperlipidemia, or egg allergy. The patient is not fluid-restricted. The PN formulation will be compounded as an individualized regimen using a single-bag, 24-hour infusion of a TNA. Determine the total PN volume and administration rate by calculating the macronutrient solution volumes required to provide the desired daily nutrients. The PN products used for this regimen are 10% CAA, 70% dextrose, and 30% ILE.

1. Determine the daily ILE calories and volume.
   - 2,200 kcal/day × 30%-40% of total calories as fat = 660-880 kcal/day
   - Choose 660 kcal to minimize ILE calories; calculate 30% ILE volume

     660 kcal ÷ 3 cal/mL 30% ILE = X mL   X = 220 mL 30% ILE

   - Calculate ILE gram amount
     30 g/100 mL = X g/220 mL 30% ILE   X = 66 g ILE
2. Determine the appropriate volume of 70% dextrose to deliver the desired dextrose calories
   - Dextrose calories = Total kcal – ILE kcal – Protein kcal
     = 2,200 kcal – 660 kcal ILE – (4 kcal × 105 g CAA) = 1,120 kcal
   - Calculate required dextrose (grams):

     1,120 kcal ÷ 3.4 kcal/g dextrose = 329 g dextrose

   - Determine 70% dextrose volume
     70 g/100 mL = 329 g/X mL 70% dextrose;   X = 470 mL 70% dextrose
3. Determine the appropriate volume of 10% CAA
   10 g/100 mL = 105 g/X mL 10% CAA   X = 1,050 mL 10% CAA
4. Determine the TNA PN volume and administration rate
   - Calculate CAA/dextrose/ILE volume:
     470 mL 70% dextrose + 1,050 mL 10% CAA + 220 mL 30% ILE = 1,740 mL
   - Add 100-200 mL for additives:
     Total TNA volume = approximately 1,840-1,940 mL/day
   - Calculate the administration rate:
     1,840 to 1,940 mL/day ÷ 24 h = 77 to 81 mL/h; round up to 80 to 85 mL/h
5. Choose final TNA regimen and determine final concentrations of CAA, dextrose, and ILE
   - Final TNA regimen
     105 g CAA/329 g dextrose/66 g ILE in 1,920 mL/d to infuse at 80 mL/h
   - Calculate final concentrations of CAA, dextrose, and ILE
     - 105 g CAA/1,920 mL = X g/100 mL   X = 5.5% CAA
     - 329 g dextrose/1,920 mL = X g/100 mL   X = 17.1% dextrose
     - 66 g ILE/1,920 mL = X g/100 mL   X = 3.4% ILE

FIGURE 165-1 Calculation of an adult PN regimen. To convert to energy units of kilojoules (kJ) multiply values with kilocalories as the numerator (kcal, kcal/mL, kcal/kg, kcal/g) by 4.18 to give the corresponding value in kilojoules (kJ, kJ/mL, kJ/kg, kJ/g). (CAA, crystalline amino acids; ILE, lipid injectable emulsion; PN, parenteral nutrition; TNA, total nutrient admixture.)

PN regimens for patients who require small amounts of additives, such as patients with kidney failure, may need further concentration.

Pediatric Parenteral Nutrition Solutions

Pediatric PN admixtures are typically ordered using an individualized approach because current safe clinical practice guidelines recommend nutrient intakes based on the patient's weight.[5] To simplify pediatric PN ordering, many institutions use a pediatric-specific PN order form that expresses daily nutrient amount based on weight. For example, protein and fat are ordered as grams per kilogram per day, dextrose as milligrams per kilogram per minute, and electrolytes as milliequivalents per kilogram per day. However, some institutions may order macronutrients by expressing the final concentration of each component in the solution. Current safe practice guidelines recommend ordering all PN ingredients based on weight as "amount per kilogram per day."[5] The PN bag label should accurately reflect the weight-based order as well. Calculations for determining a pediatric PN admixture are reviewed to illustrate fundamental concepts for ordering pediatric PN formulations (Fig. 165-2). Additional features of the pediatric PN label include the dosing weight, administration date and time, expiration date, infusion rate, and duration of infusion. Because infants and children generally receive daily maintenance fluid from the PN regimen, supplemental IV solutions are rarely needed. Pediatric PN may be provided as a two-in-one

Calculation of a Pediatric PN Regimen

The nutrition requirements for a 2-week-old preterm neonate (28 weeks gestation; weight 1.2 kg) have been estimated to be 3.5 g/kg/day protein, 3 g/kg/day ILE, 100 nonprotein kcal/kg/day, and 150 mL/kg/day fluid. The neonate has central access and no prior history of hyperlipidemia or egg allergy. The PN regimen will be compounded as an individualized regimen using a single-bag, 24-hour infusion of a 2-in-1 solution with 20% ILE co-infused into the PN infusion line. Determine the macronutrient calculations to deliver this neonate's nutrition goals; 10% pediatric CAA and 70% dextrose stock solutions will be used to compound the solution.

1. Determine the goal daily ILE amount, volume, and administration rate
   - 3 g/kg/day ILE × 1.2 kg = 3.6 g
   - Calculate 20% ILE volume
     - 20 g/100 mL = 3.6 g/X mL
     - X = 18 mL/day of 20% ILE (15 mL/kg/day)
   - Calculate the ILE administration rate:
     - 18 mL 20% ILE ÷ 24 hours = 0.75 mL/h (rate may need to be rounded up to 0.8 mL/h or down to 0.7 mL/h depending on precision capability of infusion pump)

2. Determine the goal 2-in-1 PN volume and administration rate
   - Total volume based on maintenance fluid requirements
     - 150 mL/kg/day (estimated fluid goal) – 15 mL/kg/day (20% ILE) = 135 mL/kg/day for PN volume
     - 135 mL/kg/day × 1.2 kg = 162 mL/day
   - PN infusion rate is 162 mL/day ÷ 24 hours = 6.75 mL/h (rate may need to be rounded up to 6.8 mL/h or down to 6.7 mL/h depending on precision capability of infusion pump)

3. Determine the daily protein amount and the corresponding 10% CAA volume
   - Calculate the goal protein amount
     - 3.5 g/kg/day × 1.2 kg = 4.2 g/day
   - Calculate the 10% pediatric CAA stock solution volume
     - 10 g/100 mL = 4.2 g/X mL 10% pediatric CAA
     - X = 42 mL 10% pediatric CAA

4. Determine the daily dextrose amount, corresponding 70% dextrose volume, and final dextrose concentration in the 2-in-1 PN solution
   - Goal is to provide approximately 14 mg/kg/min dextrose
     - 14 mg x 1.2 kg × 1,440 min/day ÷ 1,000 mg/g = 24.2 g dextrose
   - Calculate the 70% dextrose volume
     - 70 g/100 mL = 24.2 g/X mL 70% dextrose
     - X = 34.6 mL 70% dextrose
   - Calculate the final dextrose concentration of the PN solution
     - 24.2 g dextrose/162 mL = X g/100 mL
     - X = 14.9% dextrose (round up to 15% dextrose final concentration)
     - 162 mL × 15% dextrose = 162 × 15 g/100 mL = 24.3 g dextrose

5. Determine the available volume for additives
   - 162 mL – 42 mL (10% pediatric CAA) – 34.6 mL (70% dextrose) = 85.4 mL
   - Depending on volume needed for additives, sterile water may be necessary to add to formulation to make final total volume of 162 mL

6. Determine the final PN regimen and provided nutrient amounts
   - Final PN regimen
     - 3.5 g/kg/day pediatric CAA and 15% dextrose to infuse at 6.75 mL/h
     - 3 g/kg/day (or 18 mL) 20% ILE to infuse at 0.75 mL/h
   - Macronutrient calories

Dextrose:	24.3 g × 3.4 kcal/g	=	82.6 kcal
Protein:	4.2 g × 4 kcal/g	=	16.8 kcal
20% ILE	18 mL × 2 kcal/mL	=	36 kcal
Total kcal (kcal/kg):			135.4 kcal (113 kcal/kg)
Nonprotein kcal (kcal/kg):			118.6 kcal (99 kcal/kg)

FIGURE 165-2 Calculation of a pediatric PN regimen. To convert to energy units of kilojoules, multiply values with kilocalories as the numerator (kcal, kcal/mL, kcal/kg, kcal/g) by 4.18 to give the corresponding value in kilojoules (kJ, kJ/mL, kJ/kg, kJ/g). (CAA, crystalline amino acids; ILE, lipid injectable emulsion.)

admixture or TNA. However, the TNA system is not recommended for compounding neonatal and infant PN because of ILE instability with the often needed higher calcium and phosphorus concentrations.[41,56] The ILE labeling guidelines for pediatric PN are similar to adult ILE labeling recommendations.

Administration Techniques

PN admixtures should be administered with an infusion pump. The IV administration line for CAA-dextrose solutions should include a 1.2 μm inline filter to remove any particulate matter that may be present in the solution.[63] This filter size also removes *Candida albicans.*

ILE's may be administered separately from the CAA-dextrose solution by co-infusion into the PN line. However, co-infused ILE should also be filtered with a 1.2 μm filter.[31-35,41,63] A single 1.2 μm filter may be placed below the Y-site of the IV administration line where the dextrose-amino acid admixture and the ILE co-infuse to simplify PN filtering practices.[63] TNA solutions should be filtered with a 1.2 μm filter placed as close to the IV catheter hub as possible.

INITIATING AND ADVANCING THE PARENTERAL NUTRITION INFUSION

Adult Parenteral Nutrition

The patient's nutrition status, current clinical status, history of glucose tolerance, and dextrose concentration in the formula will dictate the infusion rate at which the adult PN solution should be initiated. Stable patients with normal organ function and stable baseline serum glucose concentrations have demonstrated minimal effect on serum glucose concentrations when PN is abruptly initiated or discontinued.[5,64] However, another approach is to begin the PN infusion and increase the rate gradually over 12 to 24 hours to the desired rate. The infusion rate may likewise be reduced in a stepwise fashion, such as decreasing the rate by 50% for 1 hour before discontinuation.[5,64] This approach should prevent development of hyperglycemia and rebound hypoglycemia, respectively. Alternatively, the PN regimen may be initiated at the goal infusion rate but with a hypocaloric dextrose dose. The dextrose dose can be increased daily to the goal based on patient response. Tapered initiation and cessation should be considered for patients receiving intermittent subcutaneous regular insulin; patients with severe kidney or liver disease; and patients with other disease states who have an increased risk for development of hyperglycemia or hypoglycemia, such as severe diabetes mellitus or pancreatic malignancy.

The SO-ILE dose should not exceed 2.5 g/kg/day or 60% of total daily calories, lower doses of 1 g/kg/day not to exceed 30% of calories have been recommended to minimize negative effects associated with long-chain fatty acids.[12,31,35] Higher doses of mixed-oil ILE up to 2.5 g/day may be necessary to prevent EFAD in patients with larger energy requirements. Manufacturer's dosing and administration recommendations differ depending on the product.[31-35] However, co-infusion over 12 hours as a separate infusion with two-in-one admixtures and infusion over no longer than 24 hours in a TNA formulation is the best clinical strategy to promote ILE clearance and minimize risk of negative effects on infection control and pulmonary and immune function.[5]

The manufacturer's guidelines recommend initiating SO-ILE and SMOF ILE with a test dose of 0.5 to 1 mL/min for the first 15 to 30 minutes because of the potential for an immediate hypersensitivity reaction.[31,37] For most adult patients, this is probably not necessary because of the relatively low incidence and benign nature of acute adverse reactions. In addition, infusion over 12 to 24 hours eliminates the need for a test dose because the infusion rate is within the range of the recommended test dose rates. Appropriate electrolytes should be provided to patients with normal organ function based on standard nutrient ranges Adjustments may be necessary depending on the patient's clinical condition. Adults and children older than 11 years should receive daily amounts of trace elements and an adult vitamin formulation.

Pediatric Parenteral Nutrition

Pediatric PN solutions are typically initiated with a volume calculated to provide the patient's daily maintenance fluid requirements on the first day of therapy. Individual nutrient substrates are then advanced daily as tolerated with the goal PN regimen generally being achieved by day 3 of therapy. However, the PN formulation should be initiated with the goal of achieving the desired protein dose on day 1. The initial dextrose dose for older infants and children is based on their previous glucose tolerance. Although practices may vary, one approach is to start with 10% dextrose and advance the concentration in 5% increments daily, as tolerated, to goals of 10 to 14 mg/kg/min in infants, 8 to 10 mg/kg/min in children, or 5 to 6 mg/kg/min in adolescents.[16] Initial dextrose doses for premature infants should approximate fetal nutrient delivery rates of 5 to 6 mg/kg/min. Frequently, this results in a final PN dextrose concentration of 5% to 10%. The dextrose concentration for the neonatal PN should be advanced daily by 1% to 2.5% or by 2 to 4 mg/kg/min increments to a goal of 10 to 14 mg/kg/min (maximum, 14-18 mg/kg/min).[16] SO-ILE is usually initiated at 0.5 g/kg/day for neonates and 0.5 to 1 g/kg/day for infants and children and increased daily by 0.5 to 1 g/kg/day. Incremental increases of SO-ILE dose allow daily serum triglyceride evaluation and early detection of those with impaired fat clearance. The SO-ILE dose should not exceed 60% of total daily calories for neonates and 30% of total calories for children, and the maximum SO-ILE dose should not exceed 3 g/kg/day (approximately 30 kcal/kg/day [126 kJ/kg/day]) for infants and 2.5 g/kg/day for children.[16] The maximum dose for FO-ILE is 1 g/kg/day.[34] The best clinical strategy for minimizing the risk of adverse medication reactions associated with SO-ILE administration and promoting ILE clearance is to infuse SO-ILE over 20 to 24 hours, not exceeding 1 g/kg in 4 hours. FO-ILE may be infused over 8 to 12 hours.[34,41]

IV electrolytes, vitamins, and trace elements should be initiated on the first day of therapy and continued as a daily component of the PN solution.[5,16] Children younger than 11 years should receive a vitamin product formulated for pediatric patients. Two multivitamin dosing schemas may be used for infants and children.[16] One method recommends 2 mL/kg/day for infants weighing less than 2.5 kg (15.5 lb) and 5 mL/day for infants and children weighing 2.5 kg (5.5 lb) or greater. The other suggests 30% of a vial (1.5 mL/day) for infants weighing less than 1 kg (2.2 lb), 65% of a vial (3.25 mL/day) for infants weighing 1 to 3 kg (2.2-6.6 lb), and 100% of the vial (5 mL/day) for children weighing more than 3 kg (6.6 lb) (up to 11 years of age). Adult injectable vitamin products should not be used for infants because of potential neurotoxicity from accumulation of polysorbate and propylene glycol preservatives. Dosage recommendations for the reformulated multiple trace element products approved for use in pediatric patients are 0.2 mL every other day for neonates weighing less than 0.6 kg and 0.3 mL/kg/day for neonates and infants at least 0.6 kg and less than 10 kg (maximum daily dose of 1 mL) using the product approved for pediatric patients less than 10 kg. The daily dose for the product approved for pediatric patients 10 kg and greater is 0.2 mL, 0.4 mL, 0.6 mL, or 0.8 mL (based on weight range). Children weighing 50 kg (110 lb) or greater should receive the adult dose of 1 mL daily. Weight-based doses of the multiple trace element products do not provide the recommended daily intake for all trace elements, so additional supplementation or individual dosing with single-entity products is necessary. Individualized dosing allows for dose adjustment based on serum trace element assessment, individual patient characteristics (eg, cholestasis, stool losses, wounds), and the provision of the recommended intake across the pediatric age spectrum from a single source for each trace element supplemented. And while the amounts of chromium and manganese are lower in the reformulated multiple trace element products, individualized dosing allows for the need to minimize or remove these trace elements in patients with evidence of accumulation. Pediatric patients receiving PN commonly transition from PN support to EN gradually, over a period of days to weeks, by decreasing the PN infusion rate while increasing the enteral intake. The PN infusion rate should be reduced for 1 to 2 hours before stopping the infusion for neonates and infants because of their immature counter-regulatory mechanisms that contribute to an increased risk for developing rebound hypoglycemia.[5] Blood glucose concentrations should be measured within 15 to 60 minutes after the PN infusion ends.

Continuous Versus Cyclic Infusions

7 Continuous infusions are attractive for patients with unstable fluid balance or glucose homeostasis. The intermittent or cyclic infusion of PN over less than 24 hours, usually for 12 to 18 hours each day, is useful for hospitalized patients with limited venous access in whom administration of multiple other medications requires interruption of the PN infusion.[64] Cyclic PN may also minimize the incidence or reverse the liver injury associated with continuous PN therapy. In addition, this delivery mode allows patients receiving PN at home the ability to resume a relatively normal lifestyle.[16,60,64] Various protocols suggest incremental increases to the maximum infusion rate for a desired period of time followed by a gradual taper to discontinue the solution.[64] However, metabolically stable adults and children older than 2 years receiving ILE-based PN regimens are likely candidates for abrupt initiation and discontinuation of their intermittent PN regimen.[5,64,65] Cyclic PN should be used with caution for those with severe glucose intolerance, diabetes mellitus, or unstable fluid balance.

EVALUATION OF THERAPEUTIC OUTCOMES

8 Thorough and consistent monitoring of patients who are receiving PN is necessary to ensure that the desired nutritional outcomes are achieved and to prevent the occurrence of adverse effects or complications. Routine evaluation should include the assessment of the patient's clinical condition with a focus on nutritional and metabolic effects of the PN regimen. Serial documentation of a patient's response to their PN regimen is a helpful guide for determining appropriate adjustments in fluid, electrolyte, and nutrient therapies.

Serum concentrations of electrolytes, hematologic indices, and biochemical markers for kidney and liver function, and nutrition status should be measured before PN initiation and periodically thereafter depending on the patient's age, nutrition status, and clinical condition. The frequency of blood laboratory measurements for neonates and infants tends to be more conservative because of their smaller blood volumes and, in some cases, lack of central vascular access. Other important clinical measurements include vital signs, weight, total fluid intake and output, and nutritional intakes. Weekly measurements of height, length, and head circumference are helpful for monitoring nutritional changes in neonates. Monitoring parameters considered important for patients receiving PN and the suggested frequency of measurement for each are outlined in Fig. 165-3. Appropriate assessment and evaluation of patient data can identify potential complications that may be avoided or treated early. Monitoring protocols should be developed and tailored for the patient population, medical practices, and resources of individual practice settings.

COMPOUNDING, STORAGE, AND INFECTION CONTROL

The USP Chapter 797 details the procedures and requirements for compounding sterile preparations, including PN admixtures.[66] These standards apply to all healthcare settings in which sterile preparations are compounded and are used by boards of pharmacy, the FDA, and accreditation organizations such as The Joint Commission. Compounded sterile preparations are defined by risk level (immediate use, low, low with 12-hour beyond-use date, medium, and high) based on the probability of microbial, chemical, or physical contamination. PN solutions are classified as a medium-risk compounded sterile preparation. In general, PN solutions should be prepared using aseptic technique in a device or room that meets International Organization for Standardization (ISO) class 5 standards that is located in an ISO class 7 buffer area with an ISO class 8 ante area.[66] Preparation of PN formulations should be supervised by a pharmacist experienced in compounding IV solutions and knowledgeable about the stability, compatibility, and storage of PN admixtures. Quality assurance procedures should be developed to maintain safe and accurate admixture preparation. A standardized process for PN ordering, labeling, determining nutrient requirements, screening of the PN order, PN administration, and monitoring has been recommended to minimize risk of potentially life-threatening compounding errors.[5,62] The potential risk of infectious complications associated with PN solution contamination can be decreased greatly when pharmacy-based admixture programs follow specific guidelines developed to ensure proper compounding of PN solutions.[5,66] USP Chapter 797 is under revision.[67] However, the published version of the chapter, which became official on June 1, 2008, is enforceable.

In general, the type of solution being prepared dictates the compounding, storage, and infusion methods. The two most commonly used types of PN solutions are two-in-one admixtures with or without ILE co-infused into the PN administration line and TNAs. Methods for compounding PN admixtures vary based on a healthcare system's patient population and medical practices and the number of PN admixtures that need to be prepared. PN base admixtures may be prepared by using gravity-driven transfer of CAA stock solutions to partially filled bags of concentrated dextrose stock solutions.[5,68] Other practice settings may use standardized commercial PN products with CAA and dextrose, and ILE separated within a single bag that must be mixed before use.[5,44,62] Advances in compounding technology have facilitated the use of ACDs for preparing PN solutions. ACD systems usually include computer software that communicates calculated volumes of nutrient stock solutions directly to a transfer pump device that delivers fluid from the source container to the final container by either a volumetric or gravimetric fluid pumping system.[5,68] Advantages of ACDs include reduced personnel time and compounding materials and improved compounding accuracy. Disadvantages include the potential for equipment failure. Because of their acidic pH and hypertonicity, two-in-one PN admixtures are poor media for microbial growth.[5,40] However, several characteristics of ILE, such as isoosmotic tonicity, near neutral to alkaline pH, glycerol content, and preservative-free formulations favor microbial growth, particularly at room temperature.[35,41,56] Other factors contributing to the potential for compromised ILE stability or sterility include the container material, length of ILE co-infusion with PN, length of time between administration set change, effect of infusion from the source container such as the original container, and infusion of ILE transferred to a secondary container. When ILEs are added to dextrose-CAA solutions to make TNAs, the growth potential is decreased, presumably because of the protective effects of the hypertonic dextrose-CAA solution and decreased pH.[35,41,56]

Because of the risk for microbial contamination, manufacturers recommend storage of PN solutions for as little time as possible after preparation. The USP 797 standards recommend storage times of not more than 30 hours at controlled room temperature (20°C-25°C [68°F-77°F]) and not more than 9 days at refrigerated temperatures (2°C-8°C [36°F-46°F]) for all medium-risk compounded sterile preparations, including PN admixtures.[66]

When co-infusing ILE with PN (ie, not as a TNA), the appropriate ILE dosage form (original packaging or re-packaged doses) and administration time to minimize risk of contamination is controversial. Unfortunately, the Centers for Disease Control and Prevention (CDC) guidelines offer no guidance for administration times.[58] Instead, the guidelines recommend administration tubing replacement every 24 hours for both ILE infused separately or when given as part of a TNA. The guidelines also recommend administration tubing replacement no more frequently than at 96-hour intervals but at least every 7 days for tubing used continuously for infusion of IV

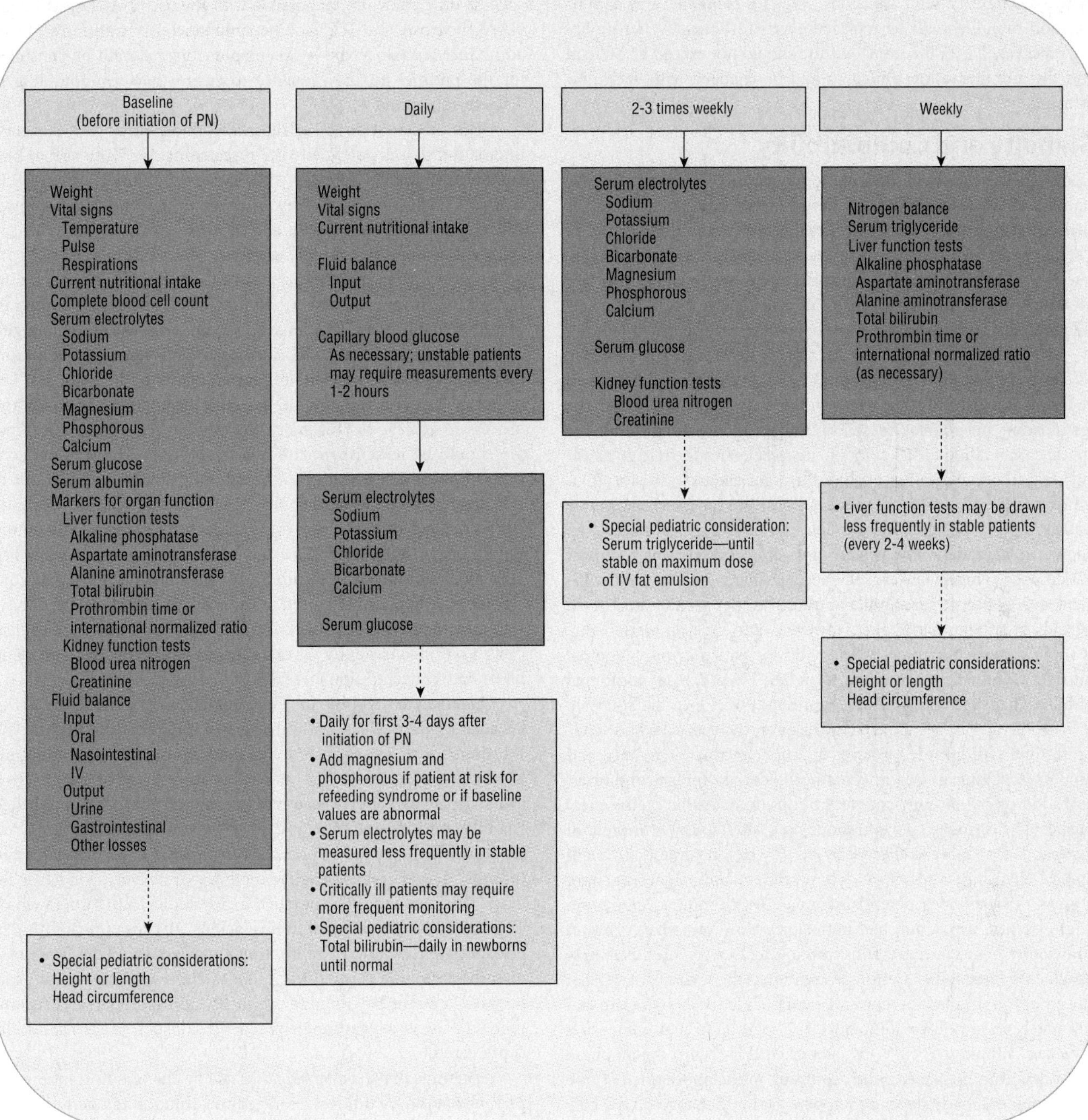

FIGURE 165-3 Monitoring strategy for patients receiving parenteral nutrition (PN).

solutions other than blood, blood products, or ILE. More conservative recommendations have been presented.[5,56] The ASPEN 2013 PN Safety Consensus suggests a 24-hour infusion time and administration tubing replacement every 24 hours for TNAs and two-in-one PN formulations and a 12-hour infusion time and administration tubing replacement every 12 hours for ILE co-infused separately.[5]

Compliance with ASPEN recommendations in pediatric patients is problematic. For example, an infant receiving 3 g/kg/day ILE at the recommended infusion rate of 0.15 g/kg/hr to promote lipid clearance and minimize metabolic complications, would require at least a 20-hour infusion.[16,69] To accommodate prolonged ILE infusions, many institutions routinely infuse ILE separately over 24 hours and change administration tubing for the ILE and PN solution with each new bag because the use of TNA formulations is not recommended in neonates and infants. In addition, since commercially available ILE products are not manufactured in unit volumes suitable for safe use in neonates and infants, institutions commonly transfer ILE from the original container into another container to accommodate the smaller patient-specific volume to decrease risk of adverse events from infusion-related errors. A variety of methods have been utilized for repackaging ILE. Syringe repackaging and aseptic transfer into sterile bags with the use of an ACD are not recommended because of higher contamination rates. Other methodologies, such as aseptic withdrawal of an appropriate ILE volume resulting in a patient-specific dose in the original manufacturer's container (drawing-down) has been recommended as a potential option.[41,56,69] These multifactorial concerns with providing ILE to pediatric patients have been addressed by the ASPEN Safety Consensus Recommendations.[5] When prolonged ILE infusions are required in neonates and infants, the daily dose should be divided in two separate 12-hour infusions. The ILE container and administration tubing should be replaced every 12 hours.[5] When utilizing repackaged ILE, the infusion time should not exceed 12 hr/Unit and the administration tubing should be changed with each new infusion.[5,41,56,69]

Stability and Compatibility

Comprehensive current information regarding compatibility and stability of PN solutions can be found in several reference sources such as *ASHP Injectable Drug Information*[70] and *King Guide to Parenteral Admixtures*.[71] In many cases, the answer to a compatibility question may not be readily available, and a review of the primary literature may be necessary. When information is not available, clinical judgment and experience must be used to resolve the situation.

The stability of a PN formulation is determined by the rate or degree of component degradation and any resulting changes in chemical integrity or pharmacologic activity that may render the formulation unsuitable for safe administration.[22] In general, the sterile combination of PN components accelerates the rate of physicochemical destabilization of all of the components in the formulation; certain amino acids, vitamins, and ILE are the most susceptible nutrients.[5,22,28,46] When compounded and stored appropriately, the degree of degradation is usually not clinically relevant for most patients receiving short-term PN because many patients have sufficient stores of those susceptible nutrients to support any short-term periods of suboptimal intake. However, nutrient degradation that is more extensive may be problematic for patients with marginal nutrient stores who receive long-term PN. TNAs present additional stability challenges because of the presence of ILE in the solution. ILE stability in TNAs is affected by the amino acid and dextrose concentration, solution pH, order of mixing, electrolyte amounts, and final TNA volume as well as container material, storage conditions, and addition of non-nutrient medications. Information on the effect of specific electrolyte concentrations on TNA stability is limited. In general, ILE stability is affected by the PN cation content. Divalent and trivalent cation additives such as calcium and magnesium have a greater destabilizing potential compared with monovalent cation additives such as sodium and potassium. However, when given in sufficiently high concentrations, monovalent cation additives may also increase instability. Cations act to reduce the surface potential of the emulsion droplet, thereby enhancing tendency to aggregate and ultimately, in some cases, destabilize the solution to coalescence or a "cracked" admixture.[5,22,40] When a cracked ILE occurs, the oil phase separates from the water phase, resulting in the appearance of free oil fat globules. Early stages may appear as subtle changes in the uniformly white appearance of the TNA, which may progress to yellow oil streaks throughout the bag or development of an amber oil layer at the top of the admixture bag. TNA formulations with any visible free oil should be considered unsafe for parenteral administration because infusion of circulating fat globules may be of sufficient size to accumulate in the pulmonary vasculature and potentially compromise respiratory function. In general, the likelihood of preparing an unstable TNA formulation can be minimized by maintaining the final concentrations of CAA greater than 4%, dextrose greater than 10%, and ILE greater than 2%.[5] Specific guidelines for compounding TNAs are reviewed elsewhere.[2,5,31-35,56]

Because of differences in pH among various CAA products and phospholipid content among ILE products, the manufacturer of each product should be consulted for compatibility and stability information before routinely admixing components. One approach to compounding TNAs manually is to combine CAA, dextrose, and sterile water (if necessary) followed by the addition of electrolytes, vitamins, and trace elements. Then the solution should be visually inspected for precipitate or other particulates. Finally, ILE may be added and the solution should then be visually inspected again to ensure a uniform emulsion exists.[31-34] Mixing components in this specific order may not be possible with the use of ACDs. Although CAA, dextrose, and ILE may be simultaneously transferred to an admixture container, the ACDs manufacturer should be consulted for the optimal mixing sequence to ensure safe compounding of TNA formulations.

The precipitation of calcium and phosphorus is a common interaction that is potentially life-threatening.[16,22,72] The risk of precipitate formation is greater with increased solution temperature and pH, higher concentrations of calcium and phosphorus, lower concentrations of amino acids and dextrose, use of the chloride salt of calcium, improper mixing sequence when adding calcium and phosphorus salts, and the presence of other additives (including ILEs).[16,22,72] In general, steps to minimize risk of calcium and phosphate precipitation in PN admixtures include the use of calcium gluconate instead of calcium chloride because it is less reactive, adding phosphate salts early in the mixing sequence, adding calcium last or nearly last, and agitating the mixture throughout the admixture process to achieve homogeneity. PN admixtures with a lower final pH should be used when clinically appropriate. Higher final concentrations of dextrose and CAA and lower final concentrations of ILE favor a lower admixture pH. CAA product-specific solubility curves that are available from the manufacturer or primary literature should be consulted to project calcium and phosphorous solubility. The calculation of a sum or product of calcium and phosphate concentrations should not be used as the sole criterion for determining solubility because the product of calcium and phosphate concentrations vary inconsistently as calcium concentration decreases and phosphate concentration increases.[72]

Electrolyte stability in TNA solutions is difficult to assess because of poor visualization of a precipitate if one occurs. PN solutions for neonates and infants tend to contain larger amounts of calcium and phosphorus, as well as other divalent cations, that limit the use of TNAs. Because of the limited amount of published stability information, the use of a two-in-one admixture with separate administration of ILEs is recommended for neonates and infants.[56] In general, alternative methods of delivering electrolytes or medications should be pursued in any clinical situation in which TNA compatibility information is lacking. Because the addition of bicarbonate to acidic PN admixtures may result in the formation of carbon dioxide gas and insoluble calcium and magnesium carbonates, sodium bicarbonate use in PN admixtures is not recommended. Use of a bicarbonate precursor salt such as acetate usually is preferred.[22]

Vitamins may be affected adversely by changes in solution pH, presence of other additives, storage time, solution temperature, and exposure to light.[22,28] Because of variable stabilities of individual vitamins, IV vitamin solutions should be added to the PN solution as near to the time of administration as is clinically feasible and should not be in the PN solution longer than 24 hours.

Peroxide concentrations are increased in ILE and dextrose-amino acid solutions after addition of injectable multivitamins or exposure to air or light.[73] Peroxides and associated metabolites have negative effects on organ and immune function. Specifically, peroxides are associated with neonatal hypoxic-ischemic encephalopathy, intraventricular hemorrhage, periventricular leukomalacia, chronic lung disease, retinopathy of prematurity, and necrotizing enterocolitis.[73] Neonates and infants are at increased risk for harmful effects of peroxides because they receive a higher daily peroxide load from PN solutions compared to adults and they have lower endogenous antioxidant levels. However, premature infants are more vulnerable to consequences of peroxide formation in PN admixtures.[73] Complete PN photoprotection from light (admixture and administration line) beginning as soon as possible during the PN compounding process and continued until the entire PN admixture and ILE infusion is complete is recommended to minimize risk of peroxides formation and by-products of lipid peroxidation.[73]

Many patients receiving PN also receive other IV medications. The compatibility of these medications with the PN solution is an important consideration for safe and effective medication delivery. Although some medications may be added directly to the PN solution and administered at the same rate as the PN infusion, most are administered as a separate admixture co-infused in the PN line. Several criteria should be considered before medications are added directly to the PN solution because of the potential for ineffective medication therapy or other complications associated with physiochemical incompatibility and stability of the PN solution.[22,56] First, the medication should be stable for at least 24 hours and should have pharmacokinetic properties appropriate for continuous infusion. Second, the chemical and physical compatibility of the medication with PN admixture components and other medications that may be co-infused concomitantly into the PN line should be verified. Advantages of using PN admixtures as medication vehicles include consolidation of dosage units, improved pharmacodynamics for certain medications, conservation of fluid in volume-restricted patients, fewer venous catheter violations, and decreased compounding and administration times. However, a major disadvantage to the use of PN solutions as medication-delivery vehicles is the lack of compatibility and stability data. Medications frequently added to PN solutions include regular insulin and histamine-2 receptor antagonists.[22,56]

COMPLICATIONS OF PARENTERAL NUTRITION

Mechanical and Technical Complications

Mechanical and technical complications include malfunctions in the system used for IV delivery of the solution, such as infusion pump failure, problems with administration sets or tubing, or the CVC. Although problems associated with infusion pumps and administration sets can be decreased by appropriate equipment selection and routine care and monitoring, CVC-related complications are potentially life-threatening. Pneumothorax, catheter misdirection or migration into the wrong vein or improper positioning within the cardiac chambers, arterial puncture, bleeding, and hematoma formation may occur during surgical placement of the catheter. Many of these complications, in addition to venous thrombosis and air embolism, can occur after insertion. CVCs occasionally occlude or break during use and if these problems cannot be rectified easily, the catheter may need to be surgically replaced.

Infectious Complications

Infectious complications can be a major hazard for patients receiving CPN because of the increased risk associated with the presence of an indwelling CVC. The source of a CVC infection may be skin organisms from the catheter insertion site, contamination of the catheter hub, or hematogenous seeding of the catheter from a distant site. In addition, patients receiving PN therapy are often predisposed to infection because of compromised immunity or concomitant infection. Frequent use of broad-spectrum antibiotic therapy and malnutrition are also predisposing factors for development of infection. The risk of catheter infection is increased for those who require multiple manipulations of the line used for PN administration as well as those who experience, poor catheter placement technique, and poor CVC and insertion site care.[58]

Infection rarely develops secondary to solution contamination.[58,63] Strict adherence to protocols for preparation of PN admixtures should minimize this occurrence.[66,74] Catheter-related bloodstream infections (CRBSIs), defined as the presence of clinical manifestations of infection (eg, fever, chills, hypotension) associated with bacteremia or fungemia resulting from no apparent source other than the catheter, are common sources of systemic infection.[74] Before this diagnosis can be made, there should be evidence of more than one positive blood culture result obtained from the peripheral vein with growth of the same organism from a blood culture obtained from the catheter or catheter segment. When a CRBSI is suspected or confirmed, appropriate antimicrobial therapy should be initiated. Retention or removal of the CVC depends on the patient's severity of illness, the suspected or identified pathogen, and the type of catheter involved. The catheter may be removed and replaced in the same site, the catheter may be removed and replaced at a different anatomic location, or it may not be replaced.[74] Filling the catheter with antimicrobials such as vancomycin or antiseptics such as 70% alcohol and allowing the solution to dwell for a period of time while the catheter is not in use is referred to as a catheter lock.[58] Antimicrobial catheter locks have been used to prevent and treat CRBSI in patients with long-term catheters such as those receiving home PN.[58,59]

Metabolic and Nutritional Complications

9 Metabolic and nutritional complications associated with PN therapy are numerous, frequently multifactorial in origin, and potentially fatal if left untreated. Metabolic abnormalities related to substrate intolerance, fluid and electrolyte disorders, and acid-base disorders are summarized in multiple recent review articles and their management is briefly summarized in the following sections.[28-30,39,55,75-82]

Liver Disease

PNALD presents as elevations in total bilirubin, aspartate aminotransferase, alanine aminotransferase, and alkaline phosphatase. Both adult and pediatric patients who receive PN are at risk for developing PNALD; it occurs in approximately 50% to 60% of children who receive long-term PN, with a higher incidence in premature infants.[28,29,75] No single etiology has been identified, although several risk factors have been described, such as degree of prematurity, sepsis, hypoxia, lack of EN, small bowel bacterial overgrowth, GI conditions requiring surgical intervention, duration of PN therapy, and long-term administration of excessive calories.[29,39,75] PNALD in infants is characterized clinically by a serum direct bilirubin concentration greater than 2 mg/dL (more than 34.2 μmol/L).[29] Taurine deficiency has been proposed as an etiology of cholestasis for preterm infants and neonates.[29,39] Taurine is a conditionally essential amino acid that is not present in standard CAA solutions but is important for neonatal and infant bile metabolism. However, the preventative or therapeutic benefit of PN regimens with CAA solutions containing supplemental taurine is unclear. SO-based ILEs contain large concentrations of plant sterols or phytosterols, which are inefficiently metabolized to bile acids by the liver and may impair bile flow. Improvement or reversal of PNALD may occur for patients who receive FO-ILE.[37,39] Other PNALD treatments that have been investigated include providing reduced doses of SO-based ILE and use of enteral fish oil in patients with limited oral intake.[39,76]

Risk factors for PNALD in adults include preexisting liver disease, sepsis, preexisting malnutrition, extensive bowel resection, prolonged duration of PN therapy, lack of enteral intake, nutrient deficiencies such as choline deficiency, and long-term administration of excessive calories.[28,29,39,75] PNALD in adults typically presents as steatosis and steatohepatitis on biopsy. Clinically, PNALD is characterized by mild elevations in serum liver enzymes, usually less than three times the upper limit of normal, with peak enzyme levels usually occurring between 1 and 4 weeks after initiating PN. In many cases, the liver abnormalities improve or resolve with manipulation of substrate intake or discontinuation of PN therapy. However, in severe cases, liver dysfunction may progress to overt failure and death despite use of traditional therapies such as using cyclic PN, ursodiol, and oral antibiotics for bacterial overgrowth; maximizing enteral feeding; and avoiding sepsis and parenteral overfeeding.[28,29,75]

Intestinal transplant with or without liver transplantation has become a treatment option for PN-dependent patients who have progressive PNALD.

Hypertriglyceridemia

Hypertriglyceridemia, defined as serum triglyceride concentrations greater than 400 mg/dL (4.52 mmol/L) for adults and 150 mg/dL (1.70 mmol/L) to 200 mg/dL (2.26 mmol/L) for preterm infants, neonates, and older pediatric patients, may occur in patients receiving ILE-based PN. Risk factors include preexisting liver or pancreatic dysfunction, sepsis, multiple-organ failure, degree of prematurity, ILE infusion rate, and dose.

ILE-associated hypertriglyceridemia is generally caused by defective lipid clearance or an excessive rate of ILE administration.[28] Premature infants and neonates have relatively slower lipid clearance than do adults because of immature metabolic pathways, including decreased lipoprotein lipase activity.[16,41] Reducing the ILE infusion rate or dose or withholding ILE therapy should be considered when patients present with hypertriglyceridemia or lipemic serum.[28] Use of low-dose heparin (1 unit/mL of two-in-one PN formulation) to stimulate lipoprotein lipase activity may be a potential therapeutic intervention to treat ILE-associated hypertriglyceridemia in neonates.[16] However, the risk associated with heparin delivery via PN may outweigh the clinical benefits because of the potential for compounding errors associated with confusion between heparin and insulin doses.[77] Carnitine does not have a defined role for treatment of ILE-associated hypertriglyceridemia.[16,28]

Hyperglycemia

Hyperglycemia is one of the most common complications of PN administration and is associated with a history of diabetes mellitus, metabolic stress, adverse medications reactions to agents such as glucocorticoids, and excessive carbohydrate administration. In the pediatric population, additional risks for hyperglycemia include prematurity and surgery. The optimal blood glucose concentration for acutely ill hospitalized patients receiving PN is not known. However, a target range of 140 to 180 mg/dL (7.8-10 mmol/L) has been suggested for adults, and less than 150 mg/dL (8.3 mmol/L) has been suggested for neonates.[78,79] Clinical management of PN patients with hyperglycemia has not been well studied and is largely empiric.[80,81] Blood glucose concentrations can be controlled with regular insulin, which may be given subcutaneously or added to the PN formulation. One approach for adult PN patients requiring insulin or oral hypoglycemic agents before starting PN therapy is to initiate PN with approximately 100 to 200 g of dextrose and add 0.05 to 0.1 Units of regular insulin per gram of dextrose in the PN solution for those patients with mild hyperglycemia (140-180 mg/dL [7.8-10 mmol/L]). The insulin dose may be increased to 0.15 to 0.2 Units/g of dextrose for patients with moderate hyperglycemia (181-200 mg/dL [10-11.1 mmol/L]).[28,80,81] Others have suggested continuing preadmission basal insulin with long-acting insulin (detemir or glargine). Response to blood glucose monitoring prior to initiating PN therapy can be useful in determining initial insulin dosing. Blood glucose concentrations should be monitored every 4 to 6 hours. Blood glucose measurements above the goal range should be treated with short-acting insulin administered subcutaneously according to an appropriate sliding scale (see Chapter 94). The insulin dose is modified daily by adding 60% to 100% of the sliding-scale insulin given over the previous 24 hours to the PN formulation daily until blood glucose concentrations are stable and within the target range. When blood glucose measurements are stable, the dextrose dose may be advanced to achieve the therapeutic goal and the frequency of monitoring blood glucose concentrations may be decreased after blood glucose concentrations are stable within the target range at the goal dextrose dose. Use of a separate IV insulin infusion is most commonly used for pediatric patients, but it may also provide better and safer glycemic control for patients with large insulin requirements or those with unstable marked fluctuations in their blood glucose concentrations.

Refeeding Syndrome

Severe and rapid declines in serum phosphate, potassium, and magnesium concentrations; fluid retention; and other micronutrient deficiencies are common features of the refeeding syndrome.[82] Individuals at greatest risk for refeeding syndrome are severely malnourished patients with considerable weight loss who receive aggressive nutritional supplementation. In addition, those who are unfed for 7 to 10 days with evidence of stress or nutritional depletion; those with chronic diseases causing undernutrition such as cancer, cardiac cachexia, chronic obstructive pulmonary disease, or cirrhosis; and individuals who were previously morbidly obese and have experienced massive weight loss are at heightened risk for this syndrome.[82] Electrolyte abnormalities are related to acute provision of macronutrient substrates that promote anabolism in an environment of depleted total body stores of phosphorus, potassium, and magnesium. Recommendations for initiating PN in adults at risk for refeeding syndrome include providing 100 to 150 g of dextrose or 10 to 20 kcal/kg (42-84 kJ/kg) for the first 24 hours and advancing calories by 33% of goal every 1 to 2 days. Recommendations for initiating PN in pediatric patients include providing a maximum of 40% to 50% goal, and initiating the glucose infusion rate at approximately 4 to 6 mg/kg/min. The dextrose dose should be advanced by 1 to 2 mg/kg/min daily to a maximum dose of 14 to 18 mg/kg/min depending on blood glucose response. Other non-PN sources such as IV fluids or EN should be considered as well. Supplemental thiamine 100 mg/day for adults and 2 mg/kg/day to a maximum of 100 to 200 mg/day for pediatric patients should be considered before feeding or before initiating dextrose-containing IV fluids in patients at risk.

Because the metabolic abnormalities described with refeeding syndrome are related primarily to acute provision of large amounts of dextrose, the goal protein dose may usually be provided with the initial PN infusion. Pediatric PN regimens are usually advanced over several days as a general practice for all pediatric patients.

Complications Associated with Long-Term Parenteral Nutrition

Other nutritional complications of PN therapy may develop over a prolonged course of therapy (weeks to months) as a result of inappropriate intake of a particular nutrient. Certain conditions, such as metabolic stress in a previously malnourished patient, may elicit symptoms of deficiency much earlier if a nutrient is not appropriately provided. For example, lactic acidosis and other life-threatening complications associated with severe thiamine deficiency may occur in patients who received PN solutions without multivitamin supplementation.[46] Maintenance doses of vitamins, trace elements, and essential fatty acids should be provided to all patients with normal age-related organ function receiving PN.

Essential Fatty Acid Deficiency

Patients receiving PN regimens without ILEs for weeks to months are at risk for development of EFAD. Clinical signs of EFAD include hair loss, desquamative dermatitis, thrombocytopenia, malabsorption, and diarrhea resulting from changes in intestinal mucosa.[28,36] EFAD may also be diagnosed by evaluating plasma fatty acid profiles. Although this assessment is not routinely available, it can be provided by several larger regional laboratories. Historically, a triene-to-tetraene ratio more than 0.4 was considered biochemical evidence for EFAD; however, individual laboratory reference ranges should be used when evaluating patients for EFAD.[16,36] Although the time in which EFAD may develop depends on the patient's nutrition status, disease state, and age, these manifestations may occur

2 to 4 weeks after initiation of lipid-free PN in adults and within 48 hours in newborn infants.[36,37]

Metabolic Bone Disease

Metabolic bone disease may occur in adults and children receiving long-term home PN.[28,29] This disorder in adults is characterized by osteomalacia with or without osteoporosis that may present without associated clinical, radiologic, or biochemical abnormalities. The diagnosis may not be made for premature infants until after the development of bone fractures or overt rickets. The etiology is poorly understood and likely multifactorial. Treatment options include pharmacologic intervention, calcium and vitamin D supplementation, and exercise. Because excessive vitamin D has also been implicated in the development of metabolic bone disease, others have recommended removal of vitamin D from the PN for patients with a normal 25-hydroxyvitamin D concentration and low serum parathyroid hormone and 1,25-hydroxyvitamin D concentrations.[28,29]

Trace Element and Vitamin Complications

Clinical symptoms of trace element deficiencies, although rare, may occur for patients receiving long-term PN. More commonly, decreased serum trace element concentrations are seen in a variety of patient populations. However, the clinical significance of abnormally low concentrations of many trace elements is unknown because serum concentrations often do not correlate with total body stores.[46] Occasionally, patients may develop clinical toxicities from elevated vitamin or trace element concentrations as the result of increased intake or decreased metabolism. These abnormalities are frequently associated with an underlying disease state such as severe kidney or hepatic failure and may necessitate reduction in vitamin and trace element intake.

Many trace elements are present in PN components as contaminants.[46,56] In patients with normal organ function who receive PN supplemented with commercially available parenteral multiple trace element solutions, elevated serum concentrations of trace elements such as chromium and manganese may develop.[46,56] Aluminum is a common contaminant of many sterile IV solutions, including those used for compounding PN. Calcium and phosphorus solutions are among those components with the highest levels of aluminum contamination.[83,84] Aluminum accumulation may occur during long-term PN therapy, especially for patients with reduced kidney function, and is associated with abnormal neurologic and hematologic function and metabolic bone disease in adults and premature infants.[28,83,84] Preterm infants are at higher risk of aluminum toxicities because they receive larger doses (μg/kg) from PN solutions than adults.[84] Preterm infants are also more likely to retain aluminum because of immature kidney function. Although the maximum safe level of IV aluminum intake is unknown, parenteral doses of 4 to 5 μg/kg/day may be associated with central nervous system and bone toxicity.[85] Even smaller amounts may result in tissue accumulation but no documented toxicity.

The FDA implemented a mandate in 2004 to restrict aluminum content in large-volume PN stock solutions (CAA, dextrose, sterile water for injection, ILE) to a maximum of 25 μg/L and for manufacturers to indicate the maximum aluminum concentration at expiration for both large- and small-volume parenteral products used for PN.[85] Actual aluminum concentrations in parenteral products should be lower than the amounts described on the manufacturer's label; however, aluminum amounts in PN solutions still exceed FDA guidelines.[83,84] In addition, the aluminum content of parenteral products varies considerably during the shelf life of the products and increases with time because of leaching from glass containers. The amount of aluminum contamination delivered to patients receiving long-term parenteral therapy such as chronic PN patients or dialysis patients, can be substantially reduced if newer stock solutions are used to prepare their PN.[83,84]

HOME PARENTERAL NUTRITION

Advances in technology for the delivery of IV solutions have allowed medically stable patients who require extended PN therapy to be maintained indefinitely on IV nutrition. An increasing concern for cost containment of healthcare services has fostered use of sophisticated infusion devices to provide PN at home. Numerous programs are now available outside the traditional healthcare setting to support patients who require long-term or permanent PN. Standards have been developed to promote safe and effective care.[60] Home PN services may be coordinated and administered through a hospital or by a commercial home care company.[59]

Many factors are considered in selecting candidates for home PN therapy. Meaningful benefit must be expected from the therapy. Examples of patients who have been maintained successfully with home PN include those with severe GI dysfunction secondary to Crohn's disease, ischemic bowel disease, severe GI motility disorders, extensive intestinal obstruction, and congenital bowel dysfunction.[59] The patient and the patient's caregiver must be willing to complete training and assume numerous responsibilities for managing the new daily routine. Other logistics such as funding, procurement of solutions and supplies, and clinical management and follow-up must be individualized for each patient in order to achieve the desired outcomes.[59]

Patients commonly receive PN solutions from their home care provider. IV vitamins or other additives may be added daily by the patient or caregiver, depending on the arrangement with the home care provider. The solution is administered through the night by infusion pump over 8 to 20 hours.[59,64] A cycled regimen allows the patient time away from the pump during daylight hours and provides many patients with the freedom to have a reasonably normal daily routine. Clinical management and follow-up are performed periodically according to the needs of the patient and the protocol of the home care provider or the managing healthcare team. A coordinated effort among several healthcare professionals, including physicians, pharmacists, nurses, dietitians, social workers, and the patient and the patient's caregiver, as well as the suppliers, is paramount to providing safe and effective management. Home PN affords some patients the potential for an ambulatory lifestyle while maintaining an IV feeding regimen that was previously only available in the hospital setting. For others, home PN may contribute to a better quality of life in the comfort of their homes.[59]

PHARMACOECONOMIC CONSIDERATIONS

Determining the true cost of PN support is difficult because numerous variables affect the provision of PN and the clinical response to therapy. PN therapy cost variables include the underlying indication for treatment, the administration setting (home or acute care), timing of PN initiation, therapy associated complications, and the type of PN formulation provided (compounded or standardized commercial PN product).[59,86-91] Expenses associated with PN therapy may be categorized as direct and indirect costs.[89] Direct costs may be further categorized as fixed or variable costs. Fixed costs do not depend on the volume of patients receiving therapy. For example, an ACD and the tubing sets required to transfer volumes of stock solutions to the administration bag would be considered fixed costs in many practice settings. These costs per patient tend to be highest in low-volume environments. Variable costs such as PN administration bags or standard commercial PN products depend directly on the number of patients receiving PN. Other direct costs include ancillary services required by patients receiving PN and costs related to the management of PN associated complications.

Clinical benefits and other clinical effects of PN (ie, reduction in hospital length of stay and frequency of complications) in specific patient populations have been evaluated but few investigations include a comprehensive economic assessment of PN therapy. Attempting to measure the cost or cost savings associated with the benefits of PN therapy and other clinical effects is difficult.[87,88] Clinical outcome measurements and hence economic outcomes are influenced by multiple factors, including experimental design, sample size, and specific health system practices.[87,89-93] More recent cost analyses for PN therapy have focused on timing of initiating therapy in critically ill patients and choice of PN formulation (compounded or standard commercial PN product). The cost advantage of supplemental PN in critically ill patients unable to meet nutritional goals within 24 to 48 hours of intensive care unit (ICU) admission is unclear.[91] Similarly, the cost advantage of using standard commercial PN products compared to PNs compounded with an ACD is uncertain.[93,94]

Although the results of economic analyses of PN remain controversial, similarities among several reports provide a basis for minimizing the costs of PN therapy:

1. Use PN only for the most appropriate patients as described by institution-specific criteria based on current consensus statements. EN should be used whenever feasible because the associated costs and complications are demonstrated to be less than those associated with PN.[90,92,95]
2. Reassess the need for routine laboratory monitoring measurements used for PN therapy. In general, the level of laboratory monitoring should decrease as a patient's clinical condition stabilizes.
3. Minimize the direct cost of PN by using efficient purchasing practices for PN solutions and compounding supplies through contract purchasing, streamlined compounding procedures, standardized administration times, single-bag PN solutions, and optimized monitoring plans. Some institutions may realize direct cost savings with use of standardized, commercial PN products depending on the usual daily PN census and patient population.[94,96] Others may reduce direct costs by outsourcing PN compounding to a third-party compounding pharmacy facility.

PHARMACOTHERAPY CONSIDERATIONS

10 11 Considerations for individualizing a patient's PN regimen include goals determination based on a patient-specific nutrition assessment, selection of the optimal type of available vascular access, and macronutrient and micronutrient requirements. In general, both macronutrient and micronutrient doses are age and weights based but are also affected by the patient's degree of metabolic demand, organ function, other medication therapy, exogenous losses, and acid-base status. Nutrient amounts provided by the PN may also require adjustment based on enteral intake either orally or by feeding tube in patients with recovering GI tract function.

Patient-specific caloric goals include (a) adequate energy intake to promote normal growth and development in neonates, infants, and children; (b) energy equilibrium and preservation of fat calorie stores in well-nourished adults; and (c) positive energy balance in malnourished patients with depleted endogenous fat stores. Overweight patients with a BMI above 30 kg/m^2 may require less caloric support than nonobese patients with the same clinical condition.[12] Critically ill adults may also benefit from a hypocaloric regimen.[12] Specific nitrogen goals are positive nitrogen balance or nitrogen equilibrium and improvement in the serum concentration of visceral protein markers such as transferrin or prealbumin in patients without systemic inflammation. Routine monitoring is necessary to ensure that the nutrition regimen is suitable for a given patient as the patient's clinical condition changes and to minimize or treat complications. The PN component doses usually require individualized adjustments as the patient's clinical condition affects further changes in metabolic stress, organ function, fluid and electrolyte balance, and acid-base status.

Appropriate patient selection, assessment, and monitoring are key to successful PN therapy and the prevention of unnecessary complications. Because pharmacists are actively involved in the provision of PN at many levels, including order verification, PN compounding and dispensing, direct patient care, education, and research, nutrition support is recognized as a pharmacy practice specialty.[97] In addition, as the interprofessional team-based approach to specialized nutrition support has evolved, standards of practice have been defined for pharmacists as well as for other healthcare professionals.[4,8-10] Standardized order forms and monitoring protocols are useful tools to ensure safe administration and monitoring of PN therapy. The future of PN therapy and the role of nutrition-support clinicians will be affected primarily by new insights from clinical research and economic challenges in the evolving healthcare environment.

ABBREVIATIONS

AAP	American Academy of Pediatrics
ASPEN	American Society for Parenteral and Enteral Nutrition
BMI	body mass index
CAA	crystalline amino acid
CDC	Centers for Disease Control and Prevention
CPN	central parenteral nutrition
CRBSI	catheter-related bloodstream infection
CVC	central venous catheter
EN	enteral nutrition
EFAD	essential fatty acid deficiency
FO	fish oil
FDA	Food and Drug Administration
GI	gastrointestinal
ICU	intensive care unit
ILE	lipid injectable emulsion
IV	intravenous
LCT	long-chain triglyceride
MCT	medium-chain triglyceride
NAG-AMA	Nutrition Advisory Group of the American Medical Association
NF	National Formulary
PICC	peripherally inserted central catheter
PN	parenteral nutrition
PNALD	parenteral nutrition-associated liver disease
PPN	peripheral parenteral nutrition
PUFA	polyunsaturated fatty acid
SO	soybean oil
SMOF	soybean oil, medium chain triglyceride oil, olive oil, fish oil
TNA	total nutrient admixture
USP	United States Pharmacopeia

REFERENCES

1. Dudrick SJ, Palesty JA. Historical highlights of the development of total parenteral nutrition. *Surg Clin N Am.* 2011;91(3):693–717. doi:10.1016/j.suc.2011.02.009.
2. Mistiaen P, Van den Heede K. Nutrition support teams: A systematic review. *JPEN J Parenter Enteral Nutr.* 2020;44(6):1004–1020. doi:10.1002/jpen.1811.
3. Holcombe B, Mattox TW, Plogsted S. Drug shortages: Effect on parenteral nutrition therapy. *Nutr Clin Pract.* 2018;33(1):53–61. doi:10.1002/ncp.10052.

4. Tucker A, Ybarra J, Bingham A, et al. American Society for Parenteral and Enteral Nutrition (ASPEN) standards of practice for nutrition support pharmacists. *Nutr Clin Pract.* 2015;30(1):139–146. doi:10.1177/0884533614550318.
5. Ayers P, Adams S, Boullata J, et al. ASPEN parenteral nutrition safety consensus recommendations. *JPEN J Parenter Enteral Nutr.* 2014;38(3):296–333. doi:10.1177/0148607113511992.
6. Ukleja A, Gilbert K, Mogensen KM, et al. Standards for nutrition support: Adult hospitalized patients. *Nutr Clin Pract.* 2018;33(6): 906–920. doi:10.1002/ncp.10204.
7. Corkins MR, Griggs KC, Groh-Wargo S, et al. Standards for nutrition support: Pediatric hospitalized patients. *Nutr Clin Pract.* 2013;28(2):263–276. doi:10.1177/0884533613475822.
8. Corrigan ML, Bobo E, Rollins C, et al. Academy of Nutrition and Dietetics and American Society for Parenteral and Enteral Nutrition: Revised 2021 standards of practice and standards of professional performance for registered dietitian nutritionists (competent, proficient, and expert) in nutrition support. *Nutr Clin Pract.* 2021;36(6):1126–1143. doi:10.1002/ncp.10774.
9. DiMaria-Ghalili RA, Gilbert K, Lord L, et al. Standards of nutrition care practice and professional performance for nutrition support and generalist nurses. *Nutr Clin Pract.* 2016;31(4):527–547. doi:10.1177/0884533616653835.
10. Mascarenhas MR, August DA, DeLegge MH, et al. Standards of practice for nutrition support physicians. *Nutr Clin Pract.* 2012;27(2):295–299. doi:10.1177/0884533612438286.
11. Worthington P, Balint J, Bechtold M, et al. When is parenteral nutrition appropriate? *JPEN J Parenter Enteral Nutr.* 2017;41(3):324–377. doi:10.1177/0148607117695251.
12. McClave SA, Taylor BE, Martindale RG, et al. Guidelines for the provision and assessment of nutrition support therapy in the adult critically ill patient: Society of Critical Care Medicine (SCCM) and American Society for Parenteral and Enteral Nutrition (ASPEN). *JPEN J Parenter Enteral Nutr.* 2016;40(2):159–211. doi:10.1177/0148607115621863.
13. Mehta NM, Skillman HE, Irving SY, et al. Guidelines for the provision and assessment of nutrition support therapy in the pediatric critically ill patient: Society of Critical Care Medicine and American Society for Parenteral and Enteral Nutrition. *JPEN J Parenter Enteral Nutr.* 2017;41(5):706–742. doi:10.1177/0148607117711387.
14. Arends J, Bachman P, Baracos V, et al. ESPEN guidelines on nutrition in cancer patients. *Clin Nutr.* 2017;36(1):11–48. doi:10.1016/j.clnu.2016.07.015.
15. Plauth M, Bernal W, Dasarathy S, et al. ESPEN guideline on clinical nutrition in liver disease. *Clin Nutr.* 2019;38(2):485–521. doi:10.1016/j.clnu.2018.12.022.
16. Crill CM, Gura KM. Parenteral nutrition support: In: Corkins MR, ed. *The ASPEN Pediatric Nutrition Support Core Curriculum.* 2nd ed. Silver Spring, MD: American Society for Parenteral and Enteral Nutrition (ASPEN); 2015:593–614.
17. Fiaccadori E, Sabatino A, Barazzoni R, et al. ESPEN guideline on clinical nutrition in hospitalized patients with acute or chronic kidney disease. *Clin Nutr.* 2021;40(4):1644–1668. doi:10.1016/j.clnu.2021.01.028.
18. Moyses HE, Johnson MJ, Leaf AA, et al. Early parenteral nutrition and growth outcomes in preterm infants: As systematic review and meta-analysis. *Am J Clin Nutr.* 2013;97(4):816–826. doi:10.3945/ajcn.112.042028.
19. Skipper A, Tupesis N. Is there a role for nonprotein calories in developing and evaluating the nutrient prescription? *Nutr Clin Pract.* 2005;20(3):321–324. doi:10.1177/0115426505020003321.
20. Furst P, Stehle P. Are intravenous amino acid solutions unbalanced? *New Horiz.* 1994;2(2):215–223.
21. Dickerson RN. Using nitrogen balance in clinical practice. *Hosp Pharm.* 2005;40:1081–1085.
22. Boullata JI, Mirtallo JM, Sacks GS, et al. Parenteral nutrition compatibility and stability: A comprehensive review. *JPEN J Parenter Enteral Nutr.* 2021 Nov 17 Epub. doi:10.1002/jpen.2306.
23. Vaek VW, Matarese LE, Robinson M, et al. ASPEN position paper: Parenteral nutrition glutamine supplementation. *Nutr Clin Pract.* 2011;26(4):479–494. doi:10.1177/0884533611410975.
24. Mulherin DW, Sacks GS. Uncertainty about the safety of supplemental glutamine: An editorial on "A randomized trial of glutamine and antioxidants in critically ill patients." *Hepatobiliary Surg Nutr.* 2015;4(1):76–79. doi:10.3978/j.
25. de Kieviet JF, Vuijk PJ, van den Berg A, et al. Glutamine effects on brain growth in very preterm children in the first year of life. *Clin Nutr.* 2014;33(1):69–74. doi:10.1016/j.clnu.2013.03.019.
26. Moe-Byrne T, Wagner JV, McGuire W. Glutamine supplementation to prevent morbidity and mortality in preterm infants. *Cochrane Database Syst Rev.* 2012;(3):CD001457. doi:10.1002/14651858.CD001457.pub4.
27. Brown JV, Moe-Byrne T, McGuire W. Glutamine supplementation for young infants with severe gastrointestinal disease. *Cochrane Database Syst Rev.* 2014;(12):CD005947. doi:10.1002/14651858.CD005947.pub4.
28. Kumpf VJ, Gervasio J. Complications of parenteral nutrition. In: Mueller CM, ed. *The ASPEN Adult Nutrition Core Curriculum.* 3rd ed. Silver Spring, MD: American Society for Parenteral and Enteral Nutrition (ASPEN);2017:345–358.
29. Btaiche IF, Khalidi N. Metabolic complications of parenteral nutrition in adults, part 2. *Am J Health Syst Pharm.* 2004;61(19):2050–2057. doi:10.1093/ajhp/61.19.2050.
30. Btaiche IF, Khalidi N. Metabolic complications of parenteral nutrition in adults, part 1. *Am J Health Syst Pharm.* 2004;61(18):1938–1949. doi:10.1093/ajhp/61.18.1938.
31. Intralipid. Package insert. Baxter Healthcare Corporation; 2016.
32. Clinolipid. Package insert. Baxter Healthcare Corporation; 2021.
33. Smoflipid. Package insert. Fresenius Kabi; 2022.
34. Omegaven. Package insert. Fresenius Kabi; 2020.
35. Mirtallo JM, Ayers P, Boullata J, et al. ASPEN Lipid injectable emulsion safety recommendations, part 1: Background and adult considerations. *Nutr Clin Pract.* 2020;35(5):769–782. doi:10.1002/ncp.10496.
36. Gramlich L, Ireton-Jones C, Miles JM, et al. Essential fatty acid requirements and intravenous lipid emulsions. *JPEN J Parenter Enteral Nutr.* 2019;43(6):697–707. doi:10.1002/jpen.1537.
37. de Meijer VE, Le HD, Meisel JA, et al. Parenteral fish oil as monotherapy prevents essential fatty acid deficiency in parenteral nutrition-dependent patients. *J Pediatr Gastroenterol Nutr.* 2010;50(2):212–218. doi:10.1097/MPG.0b013e3181bbf51e.
38. Kreymann KG, Heyland DK, de Heer G, et al. Intravenous fish oil in critically ill and surgical patients-historical remarks and critical appraisal. *Clin Nutr.* 2018;37(3):1075–1081. doi:10.1016/j.clnu.2017.07.006.
39. Zaloga GP. Phytosterols, lipid administration, and liver disease during parenteral nutrition. *JPEN J Parenter Enteral Nutr.* 2015;39(suppl 1):39S–60S. doi:10.1177/0148607115595978.
40. Gervasio J. Total nutrient admixtures (3-in-1): Pros and cons for adults. *Nutr Clin Pract.* 2015;30(3):331–335. doi:10.1177/0884533615578458.
41. Cober MP, Gura KM, Mirtallo JM, et al. ASPEN lipid injectable emulsion safety recommendations part 2: Neonate and pediatric considerations. *Nutr Clin Pract.* 2021;36(3):1106–1125. doi:10.1002/ncp.10778.
42. Raman M, Almutairdi A, Mulesa L, et al. Parenteral nutrition and lipids. *Nutrients.* 2017; 9(4): 388. doi:10.3390/nu9040388.
43. Franz N, Pleva M, Nordbeck S. Lipid emulsion therapies and type 1 hypersensitivity reactions: Risk assessment and management. *Nutr Clin Pract.* 2021;36(2):398–405. doi:10.1002/ncp.10443.
44. Diprivan. Package insert. Fresenius Kabi USA LLC; 2014.
45. Cleviprex (clevidipine) injectable emulsion. Package insert. Fresenius Kabi Austria GmbH; 2021.
46. Vanek VW, Borum P, Buchman A, et al. ASPEN Position paper: Recommendations for changes in commercially available parenteral multivitamin and multi-trace element products. *Nutr Clin Pract.* 2012;27(4):440–491. doi:10.1177/0884533612446706.
47. Helphingstine CJ, Bistrian BR. New food and drug administration requirements for inclusion of vitamin K in adult parenteral multivitamins. *JPEN J Parenter Enteral Nutr.* 2003;27(3):220–224. doi:10.1177/0148607103027003220.
48. Chambrier C, Lellerq M, Saudin F, et al. Is vitamin K1 supplementation necessary in long-term parenteral nutrition? *JPEN J Parenter Enteral Nutr.* 1998;22(2):87–90. doi:10.1177/014860719802200287.
49. Forchielli ML, Conti M, Motta R, et al. Phytonadione content in branded intravenous fat emulsions. *JPEN J Parenter Enteral Nutr.* 2017;41(3):489–495. doi:10.1177/0148607115589989.
50. Greene HL, Hambidge KM, Schanler R, et al. Guidelines for the use of vitamins, trace elements, calcium, magnesium, and phosphorus in infants and children receiving total parenteral nutrition: Report of the Subcommittee on Pediatric Parenteral Nutrient Requirements from the Committee on Clinical Practice Issues of the American Society for Clinical Nutrition. *Am J Clin Nutr.* 1988;48(5):1324–1342. doi:10.1093/ajcn/48.5.1324.
51. Stehle P, Stoffel-Wagner B, Kuhn KS. Parenteral trace element provision: Recent clinical research and practical conclusions. *Eur J Clin Nutr.* 2016;70(8):886–893. doi:10.1038/ejcn.2016.53.
52. Zimmermann MB, Crill CM. Iodine in enteral and parenteral nutrition. *Best Pract Res Clin Endocrinol Metab.* 2010;24(1):143–158. doi:10.1016/j.beem.2009.09.003.

53. TRALEMENT (trace elements injection 4). Package insert. American Regent, Inc; 2020.
54. MULTRYSTM (trace elements injection 4). Package insert. American Regent, Inc; 2021.
55. Bruno J, Canada N, Canada T, et al., eds. *ASPEN Fluids, Electrolytes, and Acid-Base Disorders Handbook*. 2nd ed. Silver Spring, MD: American Society for Parenteral and Enteral Nutrition; 2020.
56. Boullata JI, Gilbert K, Sacks G, et al. ASPEN clinical guidelines: Parenteral nutrition ordering, order review, compounding, labeling, and dispensing. *JPEN J Parenter Enteral Nutr.* 2014;38(3):334–377. doi:10.1177/0148607114521833.
57. Anderson ADG, Palmer D, MacFie J. Peripheral parenteral nutrition. *Br J Surg.* 2003;90(9):1048–1054. doi:10.1002/bjs.4328.
58. O'Grady NP, Alexander M, Burns LA, et al. Guidelines for the prevention of intravascular catheter-related infections. *Clin Infect Dis.* 2011;52(9):e162–e193. doi:10.1093/cid/cir257.
59. Kirby DF, Corrigan ML, Hendrickson E, et al. Overview of home parenteral nutrition: An update. *Nutr Clin Pract.* 2017;32(6):739–752. doi:10.1177/088453361773452.
60. Kovacevich DS, Corrigan M, Ross VM, et al. Guidelines for the selection and care of central venous access devices for adult home parenteral nutrition administration. *JPEN J Parenter Enteral Nutr.* 2019;43(1):15–31. doi:10.1002/jpen.1455.
61. Ayers P, Foster J, Kanorwala A, et al. Electronic health record and parenteral nutrition functionality: A gap analysis. *Nutr Clin Pract.* 2021;36(2):433–439. doi:10.1002/ncp.10463.
62. Kochevar M, Guenter P, Holcombe B, et al. ASPEN statement on parenteral nutrition standardization. *JPEN J Parenter Enteral Nutr.* 2007;31(5):441–448. doi:10.1177/014860710703100544l.
63. Worthington P, Gura KM, Kraft MD, et al. Update on the use of filters for parenteral nutrition: An ASPEN position paper. *Nutr Clin Pract.* 2021;36(1):29–39. doi:10.1002/ncp.10587.
64. Speerhas R, Wang J, Seidner D, et al. Maintaining normal blood glucose concentrations with total parenteral nutrition: Is it necessary to taper total parenteral nutrition? *Nutr Clin Pract.* 2003;18(5):414–416. doi:10.1177/0115426503018005414.
65. Stout ST, Cober MP. Metabolic effects of cyclic parenteral nutrition infusion in adults and children. *Nutr Clin Pract.* 2010;25(3):277–281. doi:10.1177/0884533610368701.
66. USP <797> Guidebook to Pharmaceutical Compounding—Sterile Preparations. Rockville, MD: United States Pharmacopeia Convention; 2008.
67. General Chapter <797> Pharmaceutical Compounding—Sterile Preparations. Available at: http://www.usp.org/compounding/general-chapter-797. Accessed September 26, 2021.
68. American Society for Health-System Pharmacists. ASHP guidelines on the safe use of automated compounding devices for the preparation of parenteral nutrition admixtures. *Am J Health Syst Pharm.* 2000;57(14):1343–1348. doi:10.1093/ajhp/57.14.1343.
69. Cober MP. Repackaging of intravenous fat emulsions: A clinical conundrum. *Nutr Clin Pract.* 2016;31(5):642–646. doi:10.1177/0884533616662994.
70. *ASHP Injectable Drug Information: A Comprehensive Guide to Compatibility and Stability*. Bethesda, MD: American Society of Health-System Pharmacists, 2021.
71. King JC, Catania PN, ed. *King Guide to Parenteral Admixtures*. Napa, CA: King Guide Publications, Inc. https://kingguide.com. Accessed September 26, 2021.
72. Newton DW, Driscoll DF. Calcium and phosphate compatibility: Revisited again. *Am J Health-Syst Pharm.* 2008;65:73–80.
73. Robinson DT, Ayers P, Fleming B, et al. Recommendations for photoprotection of parenteral nutrition for premature infants: An ASPEN position paper. *Nutr Clin Pract.* 2021;36(5):927–941. doi:10.1002/ncp.10747.
74. Mermel LA, Allon M, Bouza E, et al. Clinical practice guidelines for the diagnosis and management of intravascular catheter-related infection: 2009 Update by the Infectious Diseases Society of America. *Clin Infect Dis.* 2009;49(1):1–45. doi:10.1086/599376.
75. Tillman EM. Review and clinical update on parenteral nutrition-associated liver disease. *Nutr Clin Pract.* 2013;28(1):30–39. doi:10.1177/0884533612462900.
76. Tillman EM, Helms RA. Omega-3 long chain polyunsaturated fatty acids for treatment of parenteral nutrition-associated liver disease: A review of the literature. *J Pediatr Pharmacol Ther.* 2011;16(1):31–38.
77. ISMP Medication Safety Alert!® Acute Care. Action needed to prevent dangerous heparin-insulin confusion. May 3, 2007. Available at: https://www.ismp.org/resources/action-needed-prevent-dangerous-heparin-insulin-confusion. Accessed September 26, 2021.
78. McMahon MM, Nystrom E, Braunschweig C, et al. ASPEN clinical guidelines: Nutrition support of adult patients with hyperglycemia. *JPEN J Parenter Enteral Nutr.* 2012;37(1):23–36. doi:10.1177/0148607112452001.
79. Arsenault D, Brenn M, Kim S, et al. ASPEN clinical guidelines: Hyperglycemia and hypoglycemia in the neonate receiving parenteral nutrition. *JPEN J Parenter Enteral Nutr.* 2012;36(1):81–95. doi:10.1177/0148607111418980.
80. Vennard KC, Selen DJ, Gilbert MP. The management of hyperglycemia in noncritically ill hospitalized patients treated with continuous enteral or parenteral nutrition. *Endocr Pract.* 2018;24(10):900–906. doi:10.4158/EP-2018-0150.
81. Drincic AT, Knezevich JT, Akkireddy P. Nutrition and hyperglycemia management in the inpatient setting (meals on demand, parenteral, or enteral nutrition). *Curr Diab Rep.* 2017;17(8):59–71. doi:10.1007/s11892-017-0882-3.
82. da Silva JSV, Seres DS, Sabino K, et al. ASPEN consensus recommendations for refeeding syndrome. *Nutr Clin Pract.* 2020;35(2):178–195. doi:10.1002/ncp.10474.
83. Gura KM. Aluminum contamination in products used in parenteral nutrition: Has anything changed? *Nutrition.* 2010;26(6):585–594. doi:10.1016/j.nut.2009.10.015.
84. Gura KM. Aluminum contamination in parenteral products. *Curr Opin Clin Nutr Metab Care.* 2014;17(6):551–557. doi:10.1097/MCO.0000000000000091.
85. Food and Drug Administration. Aluminum in large and small volume parenterals used in total parenteral nutrition. *Fed Regist.* 2000;65:4103–4111.
86. Howard L. Home parenteral nutrition: Survival, cost, and quality of life. *Gastroenterology.* 2006;130(2 Suppl 1):S52–S59. doi:10.1053/j.gastro.2005.09.065.
87. Lipman TO. The cost of TPN: Is the price right? *JPEN J Parenter Enteral Nutr.* 1993;17(3):199–200. doi:10.1177/0148607193017003199.
88. Eisenberg JM, Glick HA, Buzby GP, et al. Does perioperative total parenteral nutrition reduce medical care costs? *JPEN J Parenter Enteral Nutr.* 1993;17(3):201–209. doi:10.1177/0148607193017003201.
89. Eisenberg JM, Glick H, Hillman AL, et al. Measuring the economic impact of perioperative total parenteral nutrition: Principles and design. *Am J Clin Nutr.* 1988;47(2 Suppl):382–391. doi:10.1093/ajcn/47.2.382.
90. Pimiento JM, Evans DC, Tyler R, et al. Value of nutrition support therapy in patients with gastrointestinal malignancies: A narrative review and health economic analysis of impact on clinical outcomes in the United States. *J Gastrointest Oncol.* 2021;12(2):864–873. doi:10.21037/jgo-20-326.
91. Bost RBC, Tjan DHT, Van Zanten ARH. Timing of (supplemental) parenteral nutrition in critically ill patients: A systematic review. *Ann Intensive Care.* 2014;4:31. doi:10.1186/s13613-014-0031-y.
92. DeLegge MH, Base MD, Bannister C, et al. Parenteral nutrition (PN) use for adult hospitalized patients: A study of usage in a tertiary medical center. *Nutr Clin Pract.* 2007;22(2):246–249. doi:10.1177/0115426507022002246.
93. Busch RA, Curtis CS, Leverson GA, et al. Use of piggyback electrolytes for patients receiving individually prescribed vs premixed parenteral nutrition. *JPEN J Parenter Enteral Nutr.* 2015;39(5):586–590. doi:10.1177/0148607113518583.
94. Alfonso JE, Berlana D, Ukleja A, et al. Clinical, ergonomic, and economic outcomes with multichamber bags compared with (hospital) pharmacy compounded bags and multibottle systems: A systematic literature review. *JPEN J Parenter Enteral Nutr.* 2017;41(7):1162–1177. doi:10.1177/0148607116657541.
95. Zaloga GP. Parenteral nutrition in adult inpatients with functioning gastrointestinal tracts: Assessment of outcomes. *Lancet.* 2006;367:1101–1111. doi:10.1016/S0140-6736(06)68307-4.
96. Bozat E, Korubuk G, Abbasoglu O. Cost analysis of premixed multichamber bags versus compounded parenteral nutrition: Breakeven point. *Hosp Pharm.* 2014;49(2):170–176. doi:10.1310/hpj4902-170.
97. Mirtallo JM. Advancement of nutrition support in clinical pharmacy. *Ann Pharmacother.* 2007;41(5):869–872. doi:10.1345/aph.1K164.

166

Enteral Nutrition

Diana W. Mulherin

KEY CONCEPTS

1 The gastrointestinal (GI) tract defends the host from toxins and antigens by both immunologic and nonimmunologic mechanisms, collectively referred to as the gut barrier function. Whenever possible, enteral nutrition (EN) is preferred over parenteral nutrition (PN) because it is associated with a lower risk of metabolic and infectious complications and is less expensive and invasive.

2 Candidates for EN are those with a sufficiently functioning GI tract to allow adequate nutrient absorption who cannot or will not eat and in whom enteral access can be safely obtained.

3 Critically ill patients benefit from early initiation of EN. It is acceptable to deliver EN at low rates (eg, trophic feeds) for the first week in most ICU patients. However, this method may not be appropriate for severely malnourished patients who should have their EN advanced to goal as quickly as tolerated.

4 The most common route for both short- and long-term EN access is directly into the stomach. The method of delivery may be continuous via an infusion pump, intermittently via a pump or gravity drip, or bolus administration via gravity or syringe.

5 Patients unable to tolerate tube feeding into the stomach because of impaired gastric motility may benefit from feeding tube placement into the duodenum or jejunum. When feeding into the small bowel, the continuous method of delivery via an infusion pump is required to enhance tolerance.

6 Selection of the enteral feeding formulation depends on nutritional requirements, the patient's primary disease state and related complications, and nutrient digestibility and absorption. A standard polymeric formulation is appropriate for the majority of adults.

7 Management of diarrhea in patients receiving EN should focus on identification and correction of the most likely cause(s). Tube feeding-related causes include too rapid delivery or advancement, intolerance to the formula composition, and occasionally formula contamination.

8 Medication administration through a feeding tube requires selection of an appropriate dosage form and verification of appropriate enteral access. Medications that should not be crushed and administered through a tube include enteric-coated or sustained-release capsules or tablets and sublingual or buccal tablets.

9 The coadministration of medications with EN can result in alterations in bioavailability and/or changes in the desired pharmacologic effects. Numerous medications are known to interact with EN including phenytoin, warfarin, levothyroxine, select antimicrobials, antacids, and proton-pump inhibitors.

BEYOND THE BOOK

Visit the "Feeding Tube Awareness Foundation" Website <https://www.feedingtubeawareness.org> and navigate to "Tube Feeding Basics." The webpage contains information on each type of feeding tube. The information is presented in a patient education format and is useful to enhance student understanding of the types of feeding tubes available, how these appear when inserted into a patient, and general clinical and patient considerations for each tube. This will aid in the COLLECT and ASSESS steps in the patient care process.

INTRODUCTION

Enteral nutrition (EN) is defined as the delivery of nutrients by tube or by mouth into the gastrointestinal (GI) tract. This chapter focuses on nutrient delivery through a feeding tube rather than oral food ingestion. The terms *enteral nutrition* and *tube feeding* are thus used interchangeably in this context. The goal of EN is to provide calories, macronutrients, and micronutrients to those patients who are unable to achieve these requirements from an oral diet. Increased recognition of malnutrition, along with improvements in enteral access techniques, feeding formulations, and methods to prevent and manage complications, have resulted in an increased use of EN across all healthcare settings. In this chapter, principles and practices related to the safe and successful use of EN therapy are described.

GASTROINTESTINAL TRACT PHYSIOLOGY

The GI tract plays a key role in the processing of ingested foods. Many of the processes involved in digestion, absorption, and utilization of nutrients are modifiable by the presence of acute and chronic illnesses.

Digestion and Absorption

Digestion and absorption are GI processes that generate the body's usable fuels.[1,2] Ingested nutrients are primarily large polymers that cannot be absorbed across the intestinal cell membrane unless they

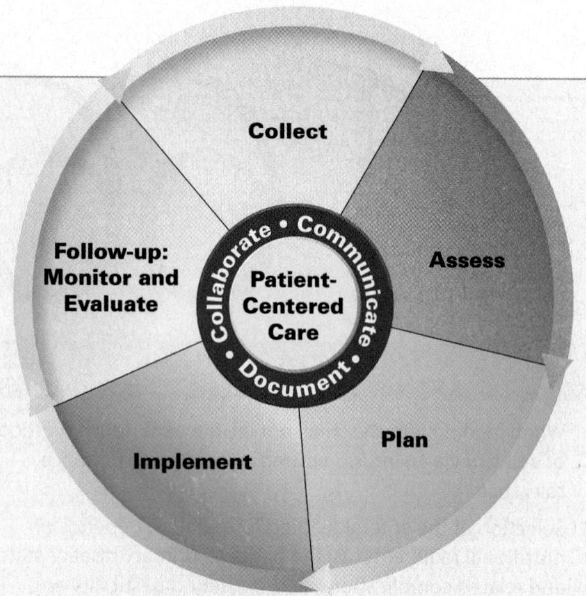

Patient Care Process for the Use of Enteral Nutrition

Collect

- Patient characteristics (eg, age, sex)
- Patient history (past medical, surgical, family, social—alcohol use)
- Nutrition history (dietary history, weight history, dietary intolerance, prior enteral, or parenteral nutrition therapy)
- Current medications (including nutritional supplements)
- Current diet and current nutrition support regimen
- Procedures related to enteral access placement
- Objective data
  - Height, weight, body mass index (BMI)
  - Fluid balance (intake and output)
  - Labs (eg, serum electrolytes, SCr, blood urea nitrogen [BUN], glucose, albumin)
  - Other diagnostic tests when indicated (eg, abdominal imaging, gastric emptying study, swallow study)

Assess

- Appropriate time to initiate EN
- Presence of altered GI anatomy or function (eg, intestinal surgeries, delayed gastric emptying, pancreatic insufficiency)
- Nutritional status and risk of refeeding syndrome (eg, unintentional weight loss, prolonged-time period with poor nutritional intake, BMI <18 kg/m^2, low visceral proteins, muscle wasting)
- Nutrition requirements (goal protein, calories, fluid, and micronutrient intake)
- Appropriate enteral access (see Table 166-3)

Plan

- EN regimen includes specific enteral feeding formulation, method of administration (continuous, bolus), and initiation and advancement guidelines (see Table 166-5).
- Monitoring parameters for efficacy (weight, enteral intake), GI tolerance (stool output, nausea, vomiting, abdominal distension), and metabolic complications (serum electrolytes, SCr, BUN, glucose, liver function tests [LFTs]; see Table 166-6).

Implement

- Initiate EN when the oral route fails or is not possible, the GI tract is functional, and enteral access can be safely achieved
- Patient education when home EN is indicated

Follow-up: Monitor and Evaluate*

- Determine nutrition goal attainment
- Provide adjustments to the EN regimen when nutrition goals are not achieved and consider transition to PN if repeated adjustments fail or intolerance develops
- Transition off EN when nutrition needs are safely met by oral dietary intake
- Presence of adverse medication reactions and GI intolerance
- Plan for transitioning off EN

**Collaborate with patient, caregivers, and other health professionals.*

are transformed into an absorbable molecular form. Digestion consists of the stepwise conversion of a complex chemical and physical nutrient into a molecular form that is absorbable by the intestinal mucosa.[1] Absorption from the GI tract is a multistep process that includes the transfer of a nutrient across the intestinal cell membrane. The nutrient ultimately reaches the systemic circulation through the portal venous or splanchnic lymphatic systems, provided that the GI or biliary tract does not excrete it. In addition, a coordinated interplay of GI motility and neurohormonal secretion is required to facilitate adequate digestion and absorption.

Nutrient digestion involves the complex coordination of multiple mechanical, enzymatic, and physiochemical processes.[1,2] Mechanical dissolution of food occurs by chewing, then mixing and grinding the stomach contents. Food stimulates the secretion of numerous hormones and enzymes from the salivary glands, stomach, liver and biliary system, pancreas, and intestines (Table 166-1). As food traverses the gut lumen, these hormones modulate GI motility and the secretions from other organs of the digestive system. Nutrient absorption occurs within the gut lumen and is a specific function of the intestinal cell membrane, which is comprised of fingerlike projections called villi. Each individual villus is made up of epithelial cells called enterocytes. The enterocyte surface contains special luminal projections called microvilli, which provide an increased surface area that is referred to as the brush-border membrane.

The digestion and absorption of carbohydrates, fat, and protein within the small intestine are illustrated in Fig. 166-1. Carbohydrates are presented to the small intestine in either a digestible or a nondigestible form. Polysaccharides (starches) and oligosaccharides (sucrose and lactose) undergo enzymatic digestion to simple sugars. The simple sugars are absorbed via active and passive transport mechanisms and are eventually released into the portal vein. Polysaccharides, such as cellulose complexes and other fiber components, pass undigested to the colon, where they are digested by bacteria and enzymes to short-chain fatty acids. Colonic absorption of short-chain fatty acids stimulates sodium and water reabsorption.

TABLE 166-1 Gastrointestinal Enzymes and Hormones

Enzyme/Hormone	Site of Secretion	Main Actions
Amylase	Salivary glands, pancreas	Converts carbohydrates, starch, and glycogen to simple disaccharides
Cholecystokinin	Duodenum, jejunum	Stimulates pancreatic enzyme secretion and gallbladder contraction
Chymotrypsinogen	Pancreas	Breaks down proteins into peptides
Enteroglucagon	Duodenum, small intestine	Inhibits pancreatic enzyme secretion and bowel motility
Gastric inhibitory peptide	Small intestine	Decreases gastric motility and stimulates insulin secretion
Gastrin	Stomach, duodenum	Stimulates gastric acid secretion and mucosal growth
Glucagon	Pancreas	Stimulates hepatic glycogenolysis and inhibits motility
Lipase	Pancreas	Hydrolyzes dietary fat to release fatty acids
Pancreatic polypeptide	Pancreas	Inhibits gallbladder contraction and pancreatic and biliary secretion
Pepsinogen	Stomach	Converts large proteins into polypeptides
Secretin	Small intestine	Stimulates hepatic and pancreatic water and bicarbonate release
Trypsinogen	Pancreas	Breaks down proteins into peptides
Vasoactive inhibitory peptide	Small intestine, pancreas	Vasodilator; stimulates water and bicarbonate secretion, insulin and glucagon release, and small bowel secretions

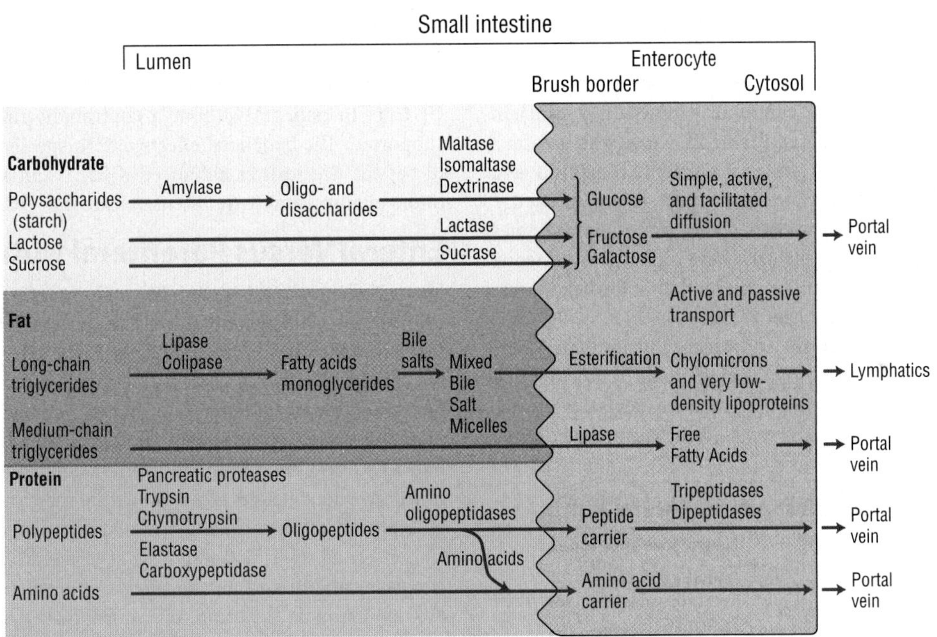

FIGURE 166-1 Schematic of carbohydrate, fat, and protein digestion.

The short-chain fatty acids serve as a systemic energy source and provide nourishment for the colonic mucosa cells.

Fat is most often presented to the small intestine as long-chain triglycerides. Fat digestion requires pancreatic lipase release and formation of mixed bile salt micelles, which are then absorbed across the intestinal enterocyte. Within the enterocyte, triglycerides are reesterified and packaged into chylomicrons that are then transported into the lymphatic system. Medium-chain triglycerides (MCTs) can be absorbed intact by the mucosal membrane and are acted on by intracellular lipase within the enterocyte to release free fatty acids that pass directly into the portal vein.[3]

Protein is presented to the small intestine primarily as large polypeptides and to a lesser extent as free amino acids because of protein denaturation in the stomach. Polypeptide digestion generates oligopeptides, which are further hydrolyzed to dipeptides and tripeptides. Peptide absorption occurs via a peptide transport system while free amino acids are absorbed via specific amino acid transporters. These peptide carriers are efficient, whereas free amino acid absorption is free amino acid absorption is less efficient.[2]

Understanding the mechanisms involved in digestion and absorption can greatly enhance the rational use of EN in patients with normal or altered GI anatomy and/or function. Various circumstances may alter the efficacy of nutrient digestion and absorption. For example, pancreatic insufficiency may result in malnutrition associated with inadequate absorption of fat and fat-soluble vitamins.

Gut Host Defense Mechanisms

1 Besides digesting and absorbing nutrients to maintain nutritional health, the GI tract is actively involved in defending the host from toxins and antigens by both immunologic and nonimmunologic mechanisms.[4] These gut host defense mechanisms are collectively referred to as the gut barrier function. The gut barrier acts to prevent the systemic spread of intraluminal bacteria and endotoxins to other organs and tissues. Hydrochloric acid secreted by

the stomach kills most of the bacteria ingested with food. Under normal circumstances, a mucus layer coats the intestinal epithelium and thereby alters the adherence of bacteria to the cells of the GI tract but provides a favorable environment for anaerobic bacteria. Anaerobic bacteria, which normally colonize the mucus layer, aid in preventing tissue colonization by potential pathogens. Small bowel peristalsis further prevents bacterial stasis and overgrowth. The gut barrier function is also maintained by the intestinal immune system, known as the gut-associated lymphoid tissue (GALT). GALT regulates the local immune response to antigens within the GI tract. Specific immunoglobulins are secreted to kill the remaining organisms and neutralize any toxins they produce. The liver Kupffer cells help to maintain gut barrier function by clearing the portal blood of gut-derived bacteria and endotoxins. Gut barrier integrity may be affected negatively by numerous pathogenic insults, such as physiologic stress and ischemia, and a variety of medications, including chemotherapeutic agents. The administration of certain probiotics can modify intestinal flora and may have beneficial effects in various disease states and patient populations by positively affecting the maintenance of gut barrier function and intestinal immune function.[5,6]

INDICATIONS FOR ENTERAL NUTRITION

2 The decision to initiate EN is based on a variety of factors. Suitable candidates are those who cannot or will not eat a sufficient amount to meet their nutritional requirements, those who exhibit a sufficient functioning GI tract to allow for nutrient absorption, and those in whom a method of enteral access can be safely initiated.[7,8] Thus, EN may be indicated in a variety of conditions or disease states (Table 166-2). For example, patients who have difficulty swallowing due to stroke, altered mental status, or obstruction in the head, neck, or esophagus due to cancer may benefit from EN.

Critically ill patients who are endotracheally intubated represent a large percentage of hospitalized patients requiring EN. Traditionally, EN in the critically ill population was regarded as supportive care designed to provide nutrients during the period of time the patient was unable to maintain adequate oral dietary intake. EN may also be used as a tool to modulate the stress response to critical illness and improve patient outcomes. Nutrition guidelines support the initiation of EN in critically ill adults who are unable to maintain volitional intake, and this can usually be achieved by feeding directly into the stomach.[9-11] Some of these patients may have reduced gastric emptying caused by sepsis, GI surgery, anesthetic agents, opioid analgesics, and underlying pathology, such as diabetic gastroparesis and burns. However, successful EN can often still be achieved by advancing the tip of the feeding tube beyond the pylorus into the duodenum, or preferably into the jejunum. Small bowel feeding may also be appropriate for patients with gastric outlet obstruction, those with pancreatitis, those with moderate-to-severe gastroesophageal reflux, or those with high aspiration risk.

Contraindications to EN use are distal mechanical intestinal obstruction, bowel ischemia, and necrotizing enterocolitis. Contraindications to tube placement include active peritonitis and uncorrectable coagulopathy.[1,12] Conditions that may result in challenges to EN use include severe diarrhea, protracted vomiting, enteric fistulas, severe GI hemorrhage, hemodynamic instability, and intestinal dysmotility.

TABLE 166-2 Potential Indications for Enteral Nutrition

Neoplastic disease	**Neurologic impairment**
Chemotherapy	Comatose state
Radiation therapy	Cerebrovascular accident
Upper GI tumors	Demyelinating disease
Cancer cachexia	Severe depression
Organ dysfunction	Cerebral palsy
Liver disease/failure	**Other indications**
Kidney disease/failure	AIDS
Cardiac cachexia	Anorexia nervosa
ARDS/ALI	Complications during pregnancy
Bronchopulmonary dysplasia	Failure-to-thrive
Congenital heart disease	Geriatric patients with multiple chronic diseases
Organ transplantation	Inborn errors of metabolism
Hypermetabolic states	Cystic fibrosis
Closed head injury	
Burns	
Trauma	
Postoperative major surgery	
Sepsis	
GI disease	
Inflammatory bowel disease	
Short bowel syndrome	
Esophageal motility disorder	
Pancreatitis	
Fistulas	
Gastroesophageal reflux disease (severe)	
Esophageal or intestinal atresia	

AIDS, acquired immune deficiency syndrome; ALI, acute lung injury; ARDS, acute respiratory distress syndrome.

BENEFITS OF ENTERAL NUTRITION

The importance of maintaining nutrient delivery through the GI tract in patients without a contraindication to its use is well supported. The beneficial effects of EN, specifically in the critically ill patient, are further enhanced if EN is initiated within 24 to 48 hours of admission to an intensive care unit (ICU).[9-11]

Enteral Versus Parenteral Nutrition

Historically, comparisons of EN and parenteral nutrition (PN) in critically ill adult patients have demonstrated a decrease in infectious complications with the use of EN.[13] Infectious complications are thought to be less common with EN in part because EN supports functional gut integrity by stimulating bile flow and the release of endogenous trophic agents, such as cholecystokinin, gastrin, and bile salts. Provision of enteral nutrients help maintain the intestinal mucosal villous height and support the mass of secretory immunoglobulin A (IgA)-producing immunocytes that comprise the GALT. In the setting of critical illness or severe injury, adverse changes in gut permeability and gut barrier function that result in increased risk for systemic infection and multiorgan dysfunction syndrome have been noted. By supporting gut integrity, the enteral feeding route is thought to lower infection risk and minimize organ failure.[9]

The use of EN in patients with abdominal trauma, burns, severe head injury, major surgery, and acute pancreatitis is generally thought to lower infectious complications compared to PN. This reduction in infectious complications is primarily associated with a lower incidence of pneumonia and catheter-related bloodstream infections and a decrease in abdominal abscess in trauma patients.[13] However, the use of EN as the preferred route for early nutritional support in critically ill patients has been challenged.[14-16] EN is more physiologic than PN in terms of nutrient utilization and therefore is generally associated with fewer metabolic complications, such as glucose intolerance and elevated insulin requirements.[17] Enteral formulations contain both complex and simple carbohydrates, which results in slower carbohydrate absorption compared with the simple carbohydrate, dextrose, used in PN. In addition, enteral formulations that contain fiber and/or a high-fat content will further slow carbohydrate absorption and reduce blood glucose elevations by delaying gastric emptying, accounting for better blood glucose control when carbohydrates are given via the enteral route. An additional physiologic benefit of enteral feeding is that it stimulates bile flow through the biliary tract and thus reduces the risk of developing cholestasis, gallbladder sludge, and gallstones, conditions that have

TABLE 166-3 Options and Considerations in the Selection of Enteral Access

Access	EN Duration/Patient Characteristics	Tube Placement Options	Advantages	Disadvantages
Nasogastric or orogastric	Short-term Intact gag reflex Normal gastric emptying	Manually at bedside	Ease of placement Allows for all methods of administration Inexpensive Multiple commercially available tubes and sizes	Potential tube displacement Potential increased aspiration risk
Nasojejunal	Short-term Impaired gastric motility or emptying High risk of GER or aspiration	Manually at bedside Fluoroscopically Endoscopically	Potential reduced aspiration risk Allows for early postinjury or postoperative feeding Multiple commercially available tubes and sizes	Manual transpyloric passage requires greater skill Potential tube displacement or clogging Bolus or intermittent feeding not tolerated
Gastrostomy	Long-term Normal gastric emptying	Surgically Endoscopically Radiologically Laparoscopically	Allows for all methods of administration Low-profile buttons available Large-bore tubes less likely to clog Multiple commercially available tubes and sizes	Attendant risks associated with each type of procedure Potential increased aspiration risk Risk of stoma site complications
Jejunostomy	Long-term Impaired gastric motility or gastric emptying High risk of GER or aspiration	Surgically Endoscopically Radiologically Laparoscopically	Allows for early postinjury or postoperative feeding Potential reduced aspiration risk Multiple commercially available tubes and sizes Low-profile buttons available	Attendant risks associated with each type of procedure Bolus or intermittent feeding not tolerated Risk of stoma site complications

EN, enteral nutrition; GER, gastroesophageal reflux

been associated with long-term PN and bowel rest.[18] EN avoids the potential infectious and technical complications associated with the placement and the use of a central venous access device required for PN. Finally, EN is less costly than PN when all factors associated with the therapy are considered.

Timing of Initiation

The timing of initiation of EN in the critically ill patient is of clinical significance. Initiating EN in the first 24 to 48 hours following admission to the ICU is associated with decreased disease severity and infectious complications when compared with the initiation of feedings after 48 hours.[9-11] Early EN has also been associated with a decrease in the release of inflammatory cytokines and fewer effects on gut permeability.[9] In addition, a trend toward reduction in mortality associated with early EN has been noted.[9-11]

In critically ill patients who are hemodynamically unstable, there is concern that EN may result in bowel necrosis because of poor gastric perfusion and increased oxygen demand. It is recommended that initiation of EN be delayed until the patient is fluid resuscitated and vasopressors are being withdrawn or are infusing at low, stable doses.[9] EN is well-tolerated in patients receiving lower doses of vasopressors, and early EN has been associated with decreased mortality in patients receiving vasopressors.[19,20] Therefore, early EN (within 24-48 hours after hospital admission) can safely be initiated in most critically ill adult patients.[9-11] Early EN initiation is not warranted for previously well-nourished, mild-to-moderately stressed adult patients who are not critically ill. When oral intake is inadequate, it is reasonable to delay the initiation of EN for 5 to 7 days in these patients.[7] In the mild-to-moderately stressed adult patient who is moderately to severely malnourished, most clinicians would initiate EN sooner.

ENTERAL ACCESS

Advances in enteral access techniques have contributed to the expanded use of EN for conditions in which PN had previously been used. In particular, improved methods of achieving jejunal access for feeding have allowed the use of EN during the early postoperative and postinjury period when gastric motility is typically impaired. As outlined in Table 166-3, various factors influence the selection of enteral access site and device, including anticipated duration of use and whether to feed into the stomach or small bowel. Figure 166-2 illustrates the predominant enteral access options.

Short-Term Access

3 Short-term enteral access is easier to initiate, less invasive, and less costly than the establishment of long-term access.[21] The most frequently used routes for short-term enteral access are established by inserting a tube through the nose or mouth and passing the tip into the stomach (nasogastric [NG], orogastric [OG]), or jejunum (nasojejunal [NJ], orojejunal [OJ]). In general, these tubes are used in the hospitalized patient when the anticipated tube feeding duration is less than 4 to 6 weeks. The orogastric route is generally reserved for patients in whom the nasopharyngeal area is inaccessible. Because these routes do not require surgical intervention, they are the least invasive options. The most common technique for placement is blind passage at the bedside by trained medical personnel. Several techniques have been described in the literature to help facilitate bedside placement, and greater skill is required to advance the tip of the feeding tube beyond the pylorus and into the small bowel.[12] Metoclopramide, a prokinetic agent, has been used with variable success to aid passage of the tube beyond the pylorus. A bedside electromagnetic tube placement device has also been used to guide tip position into the small bowel by attracting a metal tip on the end of the tube.[22,23] Alternatively, a variety of endoscopic and fluoroscopic techniques have been described to insert tubes into the small bowel.[12,21] Radiographic confirmation of appropriate tip placement should be obtained prior to use for all bedside placed feeding tubes.[12,24]

NG tubes vary in diameter and stiffness. Large-bore (greater than or equal to 14F) rigid NG tubes are used primarily to decompress the stomach (eg, removal of gas and fluid in the setting of an ileus or obstruction) but can also be used for feeding. There is a low incidence of clogging with these tubes, and they provide a reliable

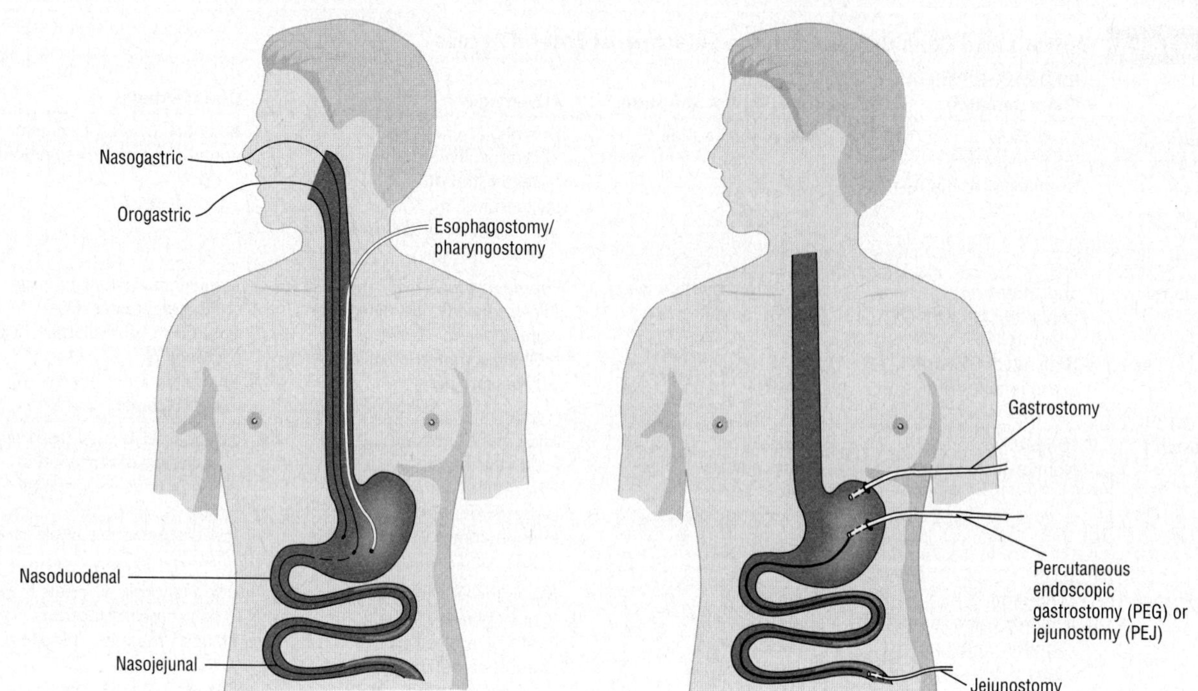

FIGURE 166-2 Access sites for tube feeding.

way to measure gastric residual volumes (GRVs). The major disadvantages associated with the use of these tubes are patient discomfort and the risk of irritation or trauma to the gastric mucosa. Small-bore nasal tubes designed solely for feeding are available in varying lengths (12-60 inches [30-152 cm]) and diameters (3.5F-12F) to accommodate both pediatric (including neonates) and adult patients. The tip of the tube can be placed into the stomach or into the duodenum or jejunum (also referred to as transpyloric placement). These tubes consist of a lightweight, pliable silicone or polyurethane material that is designed for patient comfort. A disadvantage of small-bore tubes is that they more easily occlude, often as a result of improper medication administration or flushing technique. The feeding tube is frequently held in place only by a piece of tape on the nose or face; therefore, it can be inadvertently dislodged relatively easily. Nasal bridles have been used with variable results to secure the nasoenteric tube in place.[12] A bridle involves passing a piece of thin tubing or suture into one nostril, then around the bony portion of the nose, and out the other nostril, and finally tying the tubing around the feeding tube.

4 In general, gastric feeding is the least expensive and the least labor-intensive method for enteral feeding; however, feeding into the stomach is not always tolerated. Patients with impaired gastric motility may be predisposed to aspiration and pneumonia when fed into the stomach. Many critically ill, injured, and postoperative patients exhibit delayed gastric emptying, which limits their ability to tolerate gastric feeding. In addition, patients with diabetic gastroparesis or patients with severe gastroesophageal reflux disease or intractable vomiting are at a higher risk for aspiration of gastric contents, which can result in pneumonia. In these patients, placing the tip of the tube into the duodenum or jejunum may be used as a method to decrease aspiration risk.[12] Transpyloric feeding has been associated with a lower rate of vomiting and ventilator-associated pneumonia when compared to NG feeding. However, the difference in aspiration and aspiration pneumonia risk associated with gastric and small bowel feeding is inconclusive.[9] In general, small bowel feeding may be beneficial in patients who do not tolerate gastric feeding and offers an alternative option for EN prior to resorting to PN.[9-11]

Long-Term Access

Feeding tubes used for short-term enteral access are usually not optimal for long-term use because of patient discomfort, complications, and mechanical failures that develop over time. Long-term access should generally be considered when the need for EN is anticipated to be longer than 4 to 6 weeks. Many techniques can be used to establish long-term enteral access, including laparotomy, laparoscopy, endoscopic and image guidance (eg, fluoroscopy and ultrasound).[12] The ability to perform the various techniques is somewhat dependent on the expertise and facilities available within each institution. Long-term enteral access options include gastrostomy and jejunostomy tubes.

A gastrostomy is the most common type of long-term enteral access. It eliminates the nasal irritation and discomfort associated with nasoenteric feeding tubes and inadvertent removal is uncommon. In addition, because feeding gastrostomies use large-bore tubes, clogging is less of a problem. The most commonly placed is the percutaneous endoscopic gastrostomy (PEG). The technique is minimally invasive and can be performed safely and cost-effectively in an endoscopy suite or at the bedside using conscious sedation and local anesthesia in adult patients. Gastrostomy tubes are available in various sizes (12F-28F; 0.8-5 cm shaft lengths) and materials (eg, silicone and polyurethane) and have different retention mechanisms. Since smaller-diameter tubes are prone to more frequent occlusion and dysfunction, the largest diameter size possible is preferred. For patient convenience, comfort, and cosmetic appearance, a low-profile skin-level gastrostomy device may be used. It is typically placed as an exchange tube for a preexisting gastrostomy or jejunostomy once the tract has matured but can also be used at the time of initial tube placement. This "gastric button" consists of a short, silicone, self-retaining conduit with either a mushroom-type or a balloon-type tip at the internal end and a one-way valve and small flange at the skin surface. Because this averts the external tube presence, it tends to be preferred in children or ambulatory adults who are receiving intermittent feedings. The exit site of all gastrostomies requires general stoma care to prevent inflammation and infection. Routine replacement of the gastrostomy tube at defined intervals (usually 3-6 months) is a standard of practice of many clinicians to prevent failure of the retention mechanism that can occur over time.[12]

In patients with a functional bowel but impaired gastric motility, pancreatitis, or who otherwise do not tolerate gastric feeding and require long-term enteral access, a jejunostomy may be an appropriate option.[21] Various endoscopic and fluoroscopic techniques are available for direct jejunostomy placement. A surgically placed jejunostomy may also be an option. For patients who require small bowel feeding with simultaneous gastric decompression, a gastrojejunal (GJ) tube may be placed utilizing various endoscopic, fluoroscopic, and surgical techniques.[21] Because jejunostomies use smaller-bore tubes, occlusion occurs more commonly than with gastrostomy tubes. GJ tubes are often replaced every 3 to 6 months to prevent occlusion.

There are ethical implications regarding the determination of appropriate candidates for long-term feeding tube placement.[12,25-27] Because a gastrostomy is relatively easy to place and many patients, families, and clinicians overestimate the benefits of EN, it is prone to inappropriate use. In certain patient populations, such as those with advanced dementia or other near end-of-life conditions, the placement of a gastrostomy is not recommended. Artificial nutrition and hydration (ANH) do not promote the healing of pressure ulcers, increase patient comfort or functional status, or prolong survival when compared to hand feeding in patients with advanced dementia.[25] From a clinical standpoint, ANH does not increase a patient's comfort or improve the nutrition parameters of most terminally ill individuals and can result in medical complications.[25] Survival rates are not improved in older adults with advanced dementia who receive tube feedings, and it is associated with substantial burden, including agitation, greater use of physical and chemical restraints, recurrent aspiration, and tube-related complications.[26,27] Evaluation by a multidisciplinary team is warranted for all patients near the end of life to establish whether the benefit of EN outweighs the risks of feeding tube placement.[25-27]

ADMINISTRATION METHODS

EN may be administered by continuous, cyclic (continuous rate over a portion of the day), intermittent (infused over 20-60 minutes), or bolus (generally given in 5-10 minutes) methods and may be accomplished by syringe, gravity, or pump-controlled techniques. The delivery method depends on the location of the tip of the feeding tube, the patient's clinical condition and intestinal function, and the patient's tolerance to the tube feeding.

Continuous

Pump-assisted continuous administration of EN is generally the method of choice for most hospitalized patients, especially when initiating therapy. They may be candidates for transitioning to intermittent or bolus feeding for long-term use as their medical condition stabilizes, as described below. However, when EN is to be delivered into the small intestine, the continuous method is always preferred because it is associated with enhanced tolerance. The rapid delivery of feeding into the small intestine may contribute to abdominal distension, cramping, hyperperistalsis, and diarrhea. Therefore, conversion to intermittent or bolus administration is not recommended for those with jejunostomies.

The delivery system for continuous administration generally includes a feeding set with an attached reservoir bag or spike set that connects to a feeding container. The feeding set is attached to a pump and then connected to the patient's enteral access tube with an adaptor. Continuous administration may increase nursing time because routine checks are needed, but this disadvantage is usually offset by the improved tolerance. For adults, target EN administration rates generally range from 50 to 125 mL/hr, although this varies considerably based on the EN formula and specific needs of the patient. The primary disadvantage to this method of administration is the cost and inconvenience associated with the pump and administration sets. In the home care setting, battery-operated ambulatory enteral pumps that fit into a backpack with the feeding bag are available to allow the patient greater mobility.

Cyclic

A patient who is not eating well during the day because of complaints of fullness and lack of appetite or who is not able to consume enough calories during the day to meet increased needs (eg, trauma and burns) may benefit from cyclic EN, in which the enteral feeding is administered by pump during part of the day—this typically occurs at night. In addition, nocturnal EN administration will free the patient from the pump during the day and allow for greater mobility. This increased mobility may be particularly useful for the home patient or patient requiring therapy for physical rehabilitation during the day. This method may be used in patients with either gastric or small bowel access.

Bolus

The bolus administration of EN is commonly used for patients in the home or long-term care setting who have a gastrostomy. This administration technique involves the delivery of the enteral feeding formulation over 5 to 10 minutes. Essentially, the only equipment needed is a syringe to instill the feeding volume into the tube. Depending on the patient's nutritional requirements, a feeding volume of 240 to 500 mL is generally used and repeated four to six times daily. From a convenience standpoint, it is generally preferable to adjust the bolus volume in increments of the feeding formulation container size (usually 240-250 mL). Bolus delivery is not appropriate for patients with duodenal or jejunal access, as it may result in cramping, nausea, vomiting, aspiration, and diarrhea. Bolus administration should also be avoided in patients with delayed gastric emptying and in patients who are at high risk of aspiration.

Intermittent

The intermittent method is used in patients with a gastric feeding tube who may be experiencing intolerance to bolus administration over 5 to 10 minutes. In this scenario, the prescribed volume is administered over a longer duration, generally 20 to 60 minutes every 4 to 6 hours. For this method, the desired volume of feeding formulation is emptied into a reservoir bag or container with attached tubing and administered by an enteral pump or via gravity drip using a roller clamp. The bolus and intermittent methods of administration are more consistent physiologically with normal eating patterns compared to the continuous method.

INITIATION AND ADVANCEMENT PROTOCOL

Guidelines for the initiation and advancement of enteral feeding formulations vary greatly and are primarily tailored to patient tolerance. The typical recommendation for continuous EN administration for adults is to start at 20 to 50 mL/hr and advance by 10 to 25 mL/hr every 4 to 8 hours until the desired goal is achieved. For intermittent administration, the typical recommendation is to start with 120 mL every 4 hours and advance by 30 to 60 mL every 8 to 12 hours.[7] Schedules for progression of tube feeding from initial to target rates are important and may influence tolerance. If the protocol is too conservative, it may take an excessively long period of time to reach nutrient goals. The development of an EN protocol within an institution that outlines initiation and advancement criteria is recommended to optimize achievement of nutrient goals.[9,11] Due to frequent interruptions of EN, some institutions have implemented volume-based feeding protocols to improve success in meeting targeted goals. Such a protocol shifts the focus from an hourly rate target goal to a 24-hour volume goal and provides guidance on how to adjust the rate of administration when EN is interrupted for reasons unrelated to GI tolerance such as surgeries or procedures.[28,29]

The optimal dose of EN in critically ill adult patients is a subject of debate. The intentional use of permissive underfeeding (50%-80% of goal) or trophic EN (10-20 mL/hr) in critically ill adult patients requiring short ICU lengths of stay may result in improved GI tolerance and similar short-term outcomes when compared to full feeding.[9] However, the strategy of intentional underfeeding may not be appropriate for patients at high nutrition risk as defined by validated scores accounting for nutrition status, disease severity, preexisting malnutrition, and comorbidities. Patients who are severely malnourished or at high nutrition risk should have their EN advanced toward their energy goal over 24 to 48 hours while monitoring for refeeding syndrome. This is due to an association with lower mortality in critically ill patients at high nutrition risk who receive adequate nutrition.[9,30]

WATER FLUSHES

All feeding tubes require routine flushing with water before and after administration of EN and medications.[24] Flushing may be done manually with a syringe or via the tube feeding pump. Feeding tubes should be flushed immediately before and after bolus or intermittent feedings and at standard intervals (eg, a minimum of 30 mL every 4 hours) with continuous feedings. Safe drinking water is an appropriate flushing source for most patients. Purified water is the preferred flushing source for immunocompromised or critically ill patients. Any fluid needs unmet by the tube feeding formula itself can be achieved via tube feeding water flushes.[24]

ENTERAL FEEDING FORMULATION SELECTION

Historically, enteral formulas were designed primarily to provide essential nutrients. Over the years, enhancements have been made to meet specific patient needs and improve tolerance. For example, nutrient composition has been enhanced by changing the content of the amino acids (eg, glutamine and arginine), increasing the omega-3 polyunsaturated fatty acid content, and adding ribonucleic acid (RNA) to enhance immune function and improve therapeutic outcomes. These specific nutrients have been called pharmaconutrients or immunonutrients because of the intent to use them to modify the activity of the immune system and improve clinical outcomes.[31] Enteral feeding formulations are categorized by the Food and Drug Administration (FDA) as medical foods.[32] They are considered components of supportive care and are simply regulated to ensure sanitary manufacture. Unfortunately, they are not subject to rules governing health claims, and the promotion of medical foods for therapeutic intent is not regulated by the FDA.[32]

The macronutrient content of enteral formulas (namely, protein, carbohydrate, and fat) varies in nutrient complexity (Table 166-4). Nutrient complexity refers to the amount of hydrolysis and digestion a substrate requires prior to intestinal absorption. Polymeric or intact substrates are of similar molecular form as the foods we eat. Enteral formulas that contain partially hydrolyzed or elemental substrates are characterized as elemental or defined-formula diets. The caloric contribution of each of the macronutrients is as follows: carbohydrates, 4 kcal/g (17 kJ/g); protein, 4 kcal/g (17 kJ/g); and fat, 9 kcal/g (38 kJ/g).

TABLE 166-4 Enteral Formula Nutrient Complexity

Nutrient	Polymeric or Intact	Partially Hydrolyzed or Elemental
Carbohydrate	Starches Fruit, vegetable, cereal solids Glucose polymers Corn syrup solids Polysaccharides	Oligosaccharides Maltodextrins Disaccharides Maltose, sucrose, lactose Monosaccharides Glucose Galactose
Fat	Long-chain triglycerides Polyunsaturated fatty acids Corn oil Safflower oil Soybean oil Canola oil Marine oils	Medium-chain triglycerides Coconut oil Palm kernel oil Free fatty acids Linoleic
Protein	Whole Egg, milk, wheat, whey Isolates Caseinate salts Lactalbumin	Oligopeptides Dipeptides Tripeptides L-Amino acids

Protein Composition

The essential amino acid content of the protein source determines the quality of the protein, and most commercially available enteral feeding formulations contain proteins of high quality. The form of the protein source in enteral formulas will determine the amount of digestion that is required for absorption. Polymeric or intact protein sources require digestion to smaller peptides and free amino acids before absorption. Protein sources, such as meat, milk, eggs, and caseinates, require digestion by hydrochloric acid, specific protein enzymes, and pancreatic proteases. Enteral formulations may also contain protein sources that are partially hydrolyzed to peptides or L-amino acids. As the molecular form of protein is reduced in size, the osmotic load of the enteral formulation is increased. Many commercially available enteral feeding formulations contain combinations of intact and partially hydrolyzed protein sources. Most enteral formulations are gluten-free.

Conditionally Essential Amino Acids

Glutamine and arginine are generally considered nonessential amino acids. However, during periods of high physiologic stress, the need for these nutrients may be increased beyond the body's synthetic ability; consequently, these amino acids are characterized as conditionally essential. Because they are usually present in low amounts in most enteral feeding formulations, formulations targeted for the critically ill may be supplemented with glutamine and/or arginine.

Glutamine serves as a key fuel for rapidly dividing cells, including enterocytes, endothelial cells, lymphocytes, and fibroblasts. The primary site of glutamine production is skeletal muscle. During critical illness, skeletal muscle catabolism provides an increased glutamine supply, but this may not be enough to meet the high rate of glutamine used by cells of the immune system and other cells involved in recovery and repair. Glutamine depletion may develop, particularly during prolonged periods of metabolic stress. Favorable outcomes have been documented in subtypes of critically ill patients when enteral formulations have been supplemented with glutamine.[9] Immune-modulating EN formulas containing glutamine are specifically recommended in patients with traumatic brain injury due to their association with decreased infections.[9] However, high dose glutamine supplementation in critically ill patients with shock and multisystem organ failure should be avoided.[9,33]

Arginine has been added to some immune-modulating enteral formulations in concentrations that range from 4.5 to 14 g/L.

Immune-modulating EN formulas containing arginine in combination with fish oil in perioperative patients in the surgical ICU is associated with decreased infections and decreased length of stay.[9] However, arginine supplementation remains controversial, especially in patients with sepsis.[31] Many of arginine's physiologic effects are mediated by its conversion to nitric oxide, which, in turn, modulates immune function, inflammation, and vasodilation. Some of these effects may be potentially harmful in the patient with sepsis, especially when higher arginine intakes are used.[9] Unfortunately, the effects of individual immunonutrients have not been extensively evaluated.

Carbohydrate Composition

The carbohydrate component of enteral feeding formulations usually provides the major source of calories. Polymeric or intact enteral formulations contain starches and numerous types of glucose polymers, which require digestion to monosaccharides prior to intestinal absorption (see Fig. 166-1). As the extent of hydrolysis of carbohydrates increases within an enteral formulation, the osmolality of the formulation increases. Simple sugars, such as glucose and galactose, contribute significantly to the osmolality of enteral formulations. Consequently, polymeric entities, rather than elemental sugars, are preferred. Glucose polymers provide a useful carbohydrate source that is tolerated by most individuals (see Table 166-4). The polymers are large chains that provide minimal osmotic load, yet are absorbed easily in the intestine. The one shortcoming of glucose polymers and oligosaccharides is that they are not as sweet as simple glucose and thus may decrease the palatability of orally consumed products. Finally, almost all commercially available enteral feeding formulations used in adults and older children are lactose-free because disaccharidase production within the gut lumen is reduced during illness and periods of prolonged bowel rest and because lactose intolerance is relatively common in the general adult population.

Fat and Fatty Acid Composition

Fat is an important constituent in the diet because it provides a concentrated calorie source and serves as a carrier for fat-soluble vitamins. Sufficient linoleic acid is required to prevent essential fatty acid deficiency and should approximate at least 1% to 3% of total daily calories. The most common fat sources in enteral feeding formulations are vegetable oils (soy or corn) that are rich in polyunsaturated fatty acids. The fat concentration varies between less than 2% and 45% of total calories. High dietary fat content is associated with delayed gastric emptying. Enteral feeding formulations can also contain fat in the form of MCTs derived from palm kernel or coconut oils. Because MCTs do not contain linoleic acid, enteral formulations that contain MCTs will also have a source of long-chain triglycerides to provide essential fatty acids. Potential advantages of MCTs compared to long-chain triglycerides are that they are more water soluble, undergo rapid hydrolysis, require no pancreatic lipase or bile salts for absorption, and do not require carnitine for transport into the mitochondria, where they are converted to energy. They also do not require chylomicron formation for small bowel enterocyte absorption and are not transported via the lymphatic system.

The source of long-chain fat within some enteral formulations has been modified from omega-6 to omega-3 fatty acids in an effort to modulate the inflammatory response in critically ill patients.[9] The omega-6 fatty acids are high in linoleic acid and are derived from vegetable oil, whereas the omega-3 fatty acids, derived from cold-water fish oils, are high in linolenic acid. Omega-6 fatty acids serve as precursors to certain arachidonic acid-derived cytokines that are potent inflammatory mediators and also decrease cell-mediated immune response, whereas omega-3 fatty acids are precursors for eicosapentanoic acid-derived cytokines which are less inflammatory. It has been proposed that if the dietary proportion of omega-3 fatty acids is increased and omega-6 fatty acids is decreased, less inflammation and immunosuppression may occur during metabolic stress. However, use of enteral formulas containing omega-3 fatty acids in patients with acute respiratory distress syndromes (ARDS) and acute lung injury (ALI) has fallen out of favor, specifically in the medical ICU population with ARDS or ALI. Thus, immune-modulating formulas containing fish oil (in combination with arginine) are reserved for patients requiring EN in the perioperative setting in the surgical ICU.[9]

Fiber Content

Fiber, in both soluble and insoluble forms, is added to several enteral feeding formulations in amounts ranging from 5.9 to 24 g/L. Fiber supplementation is common in clinical practice, primarily because fiber-free enteral formulations are implicated as a contributing factor to both diarrhea and constipation. Soluble fiber stimulates the growth of "healthy" bacteria such as *Bifidobacterium* and *Lactobacillus* species. It undergoes bacterial degradation within the colon to produce short-chain fatty acids, which in turn provide an energy source for colonocytes and trophic effects on the colonic mucosa by promoting sodium and water absorption. Insoluble fiber is undigested and may help decrease GI transit time by increasing fecal weight. Fiber may play an integral role in regulating bowel function with minimal associated risk.[34] Fiber supplementation may be beneficial when long-term EN is required or in patients who experience diarrhea or constipation while receiving a fiber-free enteral formulation. Supplementation with a fermentable soluble fiber is recommended for routine use in all medical and surgical ICU patients who are on a fiber-free EN formula, particularly in the setting of diarrhea, due to possible benefits in maintaining a healthy gut microbiome. Both insoluble and soluble fiber should be avoided in critically ill patients who are at risk for bowel ischemia or severe dysmotility due to potential for bowel obstruction in surgical and trauma ICU patients.[9]

Osmolality and Renal Solute Load

The unit of measure of osmolality is milliosmoles per kilogram (mOsm/kg) or millimoles per kilogram (mmol/kg); iso-osmolar is considered to be approximately 300 mOsm/kg (mmol/kg). Osmolality and renal solute load can affect tolerance to enteral feeding formulations. The osmolality of a given enteral formulation is a function of the size and quantity of ionic and molecular particles, primarily related to the protein, carbohydrate, electrolyte, and mineral content within a given volume. Enteral formulations with greater amounts of partially hydrolyzed or elemental substrates have a higher osmolality than formulations containing polymeric or intact substrates. Therefore, formulations that contain sucrose or glucose, dipeptides and tripeptides, and amino acids are generally hyperosmolar. Increased caloric density also increases the osmolality of an enteral formulation. In general, the osmolality of commercially available enteral feeding formulations ranges from 280 to 875 mOsm/kg (mmol/kg).[32]

Symptoms of gastric retention, diarrhea, abdominal distension, nausea, and vomiting have been attributed to enteral formulations with a high osmolality based on the assumption that higher osmolality draws water into the gut lumen. However, clinical evidence to support this relationship between osmolality and GI tolerance is lacking. The practice of diluting hyperosmolar formulations does not enhance tolerance and is not recommended due to the increased risk of microbial contamination.[17,24] Factors, such as concurrent antibiotic therapy, method of enteral feeding administration, and the formulation's composition, are likely to play a greater role in GI tolerance than the osmolality.

The renal solute load is determined by the protein, sodium, potassium, and chloride content of the enteral formulation. Formulations that contain a greater solute load increase the obligatory water loss via the kidney. It is estimated that 40 to 60 mL of water is the minimal amount necessary to excrete 1 g of nitrogen. Those receiving high-protein enteral formulations unable to ingest or tolerate supplemental water may be at risk for developing dehydration.

CLASSIFICATION OF ENTERAL FEEDING FORMULATIONS

5 Most patients' nutritional needs can be met using a standard enteral feeding formulation; however, certain disease states or clinical conditions may warrant the use of a specialty feeding formulation. Development of an evidence-based, enteral formulary should focus on clinically significant characteristics of available formulations and avoid duplication. Categorizing enteral feeding formulations according to therapeutic class is necessary for developing a formulary system for adults (Table 166-5).

Standard Polymeric

A large number of commercially available enteral feeding formulations fall into the standard polymeric formulation category. These formulations are approximately isotonic (300 mOsm/L), provide 1 to 1.2 kcal/mL (4.2-5 kJ/mL), and are composed of intact nutrients in a nutritionally balanced mix of carbohydrates, fat, and protein. They may contain dietary fiber. The nonprotein calorie-to-nitrogen ratio of these products is approximately 125:1 to 150:1. This ratio is a useful parameter for assessing protein density in relation to calories provided (see Chapter 164). Certain feeding formulations in this category may be promoted as high nitrogen but actually fall within standard protein amounts. To maintain isotonicity, many products within this category are not sweetened, making them unpalatable and generally suited only for tube feeding; however, flavored products are available for oral supplementation. The nutrient requirements of the majority of adults receiving EN can generally be met using feeding formulations in this category.

High Protein

Enteral feeding formulations with a nonprotein calorie-to-nitrogen ratio less than 125:1 can be categorized as high protein. The lower the ratio, the higher the protein density in relation to calories provided. In patients with high protein requirements, it is generally unacceptable to use a feeding formulation with standard protein amounts because the volume necessary to meet protein requirements will result in excessive calorie intake. Patients who may be candidates for a high-protein feeding formulation are critically ill patients and those with pressure sores, surgical wounds, and high output enterocutaneous fistulas. In general, adult patients with estimated protein requirements exceeding 1.5 g/kg/day may benefit from a high-protein formulation. High-protein formulations may also be beneficial in mechanically ventilated patients who are receiving propofol for sedation. The vehicle for propofol is a soybean fat emulsion that contains 1.1 kcal/mL (4.6 kJ/mL). At therapeutic dosages, propofol intake can contribute to caloric intake, and a high protein formulation

TABLE 166-5 Adult Enteral Feeding Formulation Classification System

Category	Features	Indications
Standard polymeric	Isotonic 1-1.2 kcal/mL (4.2-5 kJ/mL) NPC:N 125:1-150:1 May contain fiber	Designed to meet the needs of the majority of patients Patients with functional GI tract Not suitable for oral use
High protein	NPC:N <125:1 May contain fiber	Patients with protein requirements >1.5 g/kg/day, such as trauma patients and those with burns, pressure sores, or wounds Patients receiving propofol
High caloric density	1.5-2 kcal/mL (6.3-8.4 kJ/mL) Lower electrolyte content per calorie Hypertonic	Patients requiring fluid and/or electrolyte restriction, such as kidney insufficiency
Elemental	High proportion of free amino acids Low in fat	Patients who require low fat Use has generally been replaced by peptide-based formulations
Peptide-based	Contains dipeptides and tripeptides Contains MCTs	Indications/benefits not clearly established Trial may be warranted in patients who do not tolerate intact protein due to malabsorption
Disease-specific		
Kidney	Caloric dense Protein content varies Low electrolyte content	Alternative to high caloric density formulations, but generally more expensive
Liver	Increased branched-chain and decreased aromatic amino acids	Patients with hepatic encephalopathy
Lung	High fat, low carbohydrate Anti-inflammatory lipid profile and antioxidants	Patients with ARDS and severe ALI
Diabetes mellitus	High fat, low carbohydrate	Alternative to standard, fiber-containing formulation in patients with uncontrolled hyperglycemia
Immune-modulating	Supplemented with glutamine, arginine, nucleotides, and/or omega-3 fatty acids	Patients undergoing major elective GI surgery, trauma, burns, head and neck cancer, and critically ill patients on mechanical ventilation Use with caution in patients with sepsis Select nutrients may be beneficial or harmful in subgroups of critically ill patients
Oral supplement	Sweetened for taste Hypertonic	Patients who require supplementation to an oral diet

ALI, acute lung injury; ARDS, acute respiratory distress syndrome; MCT, medium-chain triglyceride; NPC, N, nonprotein calorie-to-nitrogen ratio.

may be beneficial in allowing for the provision of protein requirements while minimizing overfeeding.

High Caloric Density

High caloric density formulations are concentrated to provide less fluid and electrolyte intake in comparison to a standard polymeric formulation. They provide approximately 1.5 to 2 kcal/mL (6.3-8.4 kJ/mL) and similar calorie and protein intake can be achieved as a standard polymeric formulation, using less volume. High caloric density formulations are often necessary for patients who require fluid and/or electrolyte restriction, such as those with heart, kidney, liver, or respiratory failure. Although specialty enteral formulations targeted for acute kidney injury and chronic kidney disease are available, many patients with kidney failure can be managed using a product in this category.

Elemental/Peptide-Based

Formulations in this category contain protein and/or fat components that are hydrolyzed into smaller, predigested forms. Traditionally, enteral formulations in this category were referred to as elemental and contained a high proportion of protein in the form of free amino acids and a low amount of fat. Many of these formulations have been reformulated to provide a portion of the protein in the form of dipeptides and tripeptides and fewer free amino acids because dipeptides and tripeptides are more readily absorbed than an equivalent intake of free amino acids.[35] These peptide-based formulations may be beneficial in patients with impaired digestion or absorption. Peptide-based formulations are generally higher in fat than the more elemental formulations and use MCTs in varying proportions as the fat source.

Evidence to support the use of elemental or peptide-based formulations is limited, and their routine use is generally not recommended. Patients who do not tolerate standard, intact nutrient formulations as a result of malabsorption or short bowel syndrome might be candidates for a trial of a peptide-based formulation. In addition, elemental or peptide-based products that have higher percentages of MCTs and small amounts of long-chain triglycerides may be beneficial for patients with severe pancreatic insufficiency, such as chronic pancreatitis and cystic fibrosis; severe abnormalities of the intestinal mucosa, such as untreated celiac disease; biliary tract disease, such as biliary atresia or severe cholestasis; or chylothorax or chylous ascites.

Disease-Specific

Enteral feeding formulations have also been designed to meet unique nutrient requirements and manage metabolic abnormalities associated with specific disease states. Specialized enteral feeding formulations are marketed for use in adult patients with kidney and liver failure; lung disease, including ARDS; diabetes mellitus; wound healing; and metabolic stress (see Table 166-5).

Specialized enteral formulations designed to modulate the inflammatory response in adult patients with severe metabolic stress have been referred to as immune-modulating formulations or immunonutrition. These formulations are supplemented with nutrients such as glutamine, arginine, antioxidants, nucleotides, and omega-3 polyunsaturated fatty acids, because of their potential role in regulating immune function. However, nutrition guidelines recommend against the routine use of immune-modulating enteral formulations in the medical ICU population due to the lack of benefit and potential harm. These formulas should be reserved for patients in the surgical ICU and in patients with traumatic brain injury where beneficial effects have been demonstrated.[9,36,37]

Diabetes-specific formulas are lower in carbohydrate and higher in fat and fiber compared to standard formulas.[38] They contain slowly digestible carbohydrates and their primary fat sources are omega-3 fatty acids and monounsaturated fatty acids. The rationale for this combination of ingredients is to slow gastric emptying and improve glycemic control. Use of diabetes-specific formulas in hospitalized patients may lead to an improvement in glycemic control and a decrease in total insulin requirements, but to date the supporting evidence is limited. Therefore, in hospitalized patients with diabetes mellitus or stress-induced hyperglycemia, a standard enteral formula in combination with pharmacologic management of hyperglycemia is appropriate.[38]

Enteral formulas with lower protein, higher amounts of branched-chain amino acids (BCAAs) (leucine, valine, and isoleucine), and lower amounts of aromatic amino acids (AAAs) have been marketed for use in patients with hepatic encephalopathy. However, these formulations may result in under-dosing protein in a population with a high prevalence of malnutrition. Additionally, they do not improve outcomes in patients with hepatic encephalopathy and are therefore not recommended for routine use in this patient population.[32]

Oral Supplements

In general, oral supplements are not intended for tube feeding but are taken by mouth to enhance an oral diet. They are sweetened to improve taste and therefore are hypertonic (~450-700 mOsm/kg [mmol/kg]), but osmolality is rarely a problem in the patient with a functioning GI tract. However, in the tube-fed patient, a sweetened product is unnecessary and may contribute to GI intolerance, particularly diarrhea. Powder supplements that are mixed with milk should be avoided in lactose-intolerant patients. In addition to liquid supplements, puddings, gelatins, bars, and milkshake-like supplements are available.

Modular Products

A module is a powder or liquid form of a single nutrient (eg, protein, carbohydrate, fat, and dietary fiber) that is used to supplement nutrition intake when the diet or commercially available enteral formulation does not fully meet a patient's needs.[32] Alternatively, formulations available in powder or concentrate can be mixed with less water than needed for the standard dilution to deliver more nutrients in less volume. The mixing process required for modular components increases the potential for bacterial contamination and incorrect preparation. Contamination is a particular concern with the use of blenders and reconstitution of powders.[24] Modular products used to supplement tube feedings should not be mixed with the EN formula but administered separately via a feeding tube similar to the process required for medication administration.

Rehydration

Oral rehydration formulations are useful in maintaining hydration or treating dehydration in patients with high GI output (eg, frequent vomiting, diarrhea, ostomy output). Such formulations are available commercially in powder or liquid form or can be extemporaneously compounded. They can be administered orally or given via a feeding tube. The glucose content of oral rehydration solutions is essential to the absorption of sodium, because it stimulates active transport systems, which, in turn, stimulate passive glucose-coupled sodium and water uptake for rehydration. Therefore, oral or enteral administration of rehydration solutions may decrease fecal water loss and generate a positive fluid and electrolyte balance.[39]

FORMULARY AND DELIVERY SYSTEM CONSIDERATIONS

For an institution's enteral formulary, generally no more than one product per category is necessary, and it may be possible to omit certain categories based on the specific patient population cared for within a given institution. Additional selection criteria include container size and type, liquid or powder form, shelf life, ease of use, and cost.

Most enteral products are available as ready-to-use, prepackaged liquids, but a few are available in the powdered state and require reconstitution prior to use. Advantages of ready-to-use liquid formulations are convenience and reduced susceptibility to microbiologic contamination. One disadvantage is that more storage space may be required. The ease or convenience of a ready-to-use liquid is especially important for self-care patients, those with disabilities, and those who have difficulty reading or following printed instructions. Ready-to-use liquid enteral formulations are generally available in ready-to-hang rigid plastic containers or bags (*closed systems*), cans, or bottles. Bolus administration of EN is usually achieved using formulas available in cans or bottles. However, when formula from a can/bottle is used for continuous or cyclic administration, it must first be poured into a feeding bag and attached to an administration set to allow for administration via a pump. This "open system" has a higher risk of microbial contamination than the ready-to-hang containers. The use of a powder formula is also considered an open delivery system.

Contamination of enteral feeding formulations is a potential cause of diarrhea.[7,24] Contamination is caused by a lack of attention to proper handling techniques, inadequate cleaning and disinfection of preparation equipment, and the use of nonsterile or contaminated tube-feeding additives. Unlike liquid formulations, powdered products are not guaranteed by the manufacturer to be sterile because it is not possible to sterilize the powder without destruction of some of its components. Closed-system containers supply a ready-to-hang, prefilled, sterile supply of formula in volumes of 1 to 1.5 L. Most but not all enteral formulations intended for use in adults are available in the closed-administration system. The closed-administration system also offers the advantage of not requiring refrigeration and allowing hang times of 24 to 48 hours, whereas the conventional open-delivery system necessitates hang times of generally 4 to 8 hours.[24]

New enteral connectors are being integrated into the EN marketplace to prevent enteral misconnections and improve patient safety. An enteral misconnection occurs when a component of the enteral feeding system is inadvertently connected to a non-enteral site, such as a tracheostomy tube, peritoneal dialysis catheter, or other medical device or intravenous (IV) tubing. Misconnections are commonly attributed to the use of universal connectors that allow for misconnections between incompatible systems. Due to potential serious patient harm, including death, an international standard (ISO 80369) has been developed to guide the redesign of all small-bore connectors and the new enteral connectors, referred to as the ENFit™ system.[40] The ENFit™ connector provides a unique connection that is not compatible with any other device and has been specifically designed for all nutrition sources, enteral administration sets, enteral syringes, and all feeding tubes.[40] Thus, filling and administration instructions for syringes used to deliver medications via feeding tubes should differ from oral syringes with the implementation of the ENFit™ system. Information about these processes and other resources is available at the Global Enteral Device Supplier Association (GEDSA) Website (www.stayconnected.org).[41]

COMPLICATIONS AND MONITORING

The majority of complications associated with EN are metabolic, GI, or mechanical. The early detection and management of potential complications is necessary to allow for the safe and successful use of EN. In addition, measures to avoid complications should be incorporated into the management of all patients receiving EN (Table 166-6).

Metabolic Complications

Metabolic complications associated with EN are similar to those associated with PN, but the incidence tends to be lower.[17] Critically ill patients, especially those with underlying organ dysfunction, are at the risk of developing complications related to hydration and electrolyte imbalance and altered glucose control. Patients who present with a history of minimal dietary intake for an extended period of time and have experienced significant weight loss are at risk of developing refeeding syndrome, which can be evidenced by hypophosphatemia, hypokalemia, hypomagnesemia, thiamine deficiency, and sodium retention.[42] The frequency of clinical and laboratory assessment to monitor hydration, electrolytes, organ function, and glucose adequately for a patient who is critically ill or at risk of developing refeeding syndrome is greater than for a stable hospitalized patient or patients residing in rehabilitation units or at home (see Table 166-6). Patients receiving long-term EN at home may require laboratory monitoring only every 2 to 3 months, depending on their clinical status. It is also important to evaluate the actual water and micronutrient content provided by the enteral formulation, especially in critically ill patients. Supplemental fluid, electrolytes, and minerals may be required in some patients. Conversely, for patients who have fluid retention or elevated serum electrolytes, the enteral formulation may need to be changed to one that is more concentrated or provides less of a particular nutrient, if available.

TABLE 166-6 Suggested Monitoring for Adult Patients on Enteral Nutrition

Parameter	During Initiation of EN Therapy	During Stable EN Therapy
Vital signs	Every 4-6 hours	As needed with suspected change (ie, fever)
Clinical assessment		
Weight	Daily	Weekly
Total intake/output	Daily	As needed with suspected change in intake/output
Tube-feeding intake	Daily	Daily
Enterostomy tube site assessment	Daily	Daily
GI tolerance		
Stool frequency/volume	Daily	Daily
Abdomen assessment	Daily	Daily
Nausea or vomiting	Daily	Daily
Tube placement	Prior to starting, then ongoing	Ongoing
Laboratory		
Electrolytes, blood urea nitrogen/serum creatinine, glucose	Daily until stable, then 2-3 times/week	Every 1-3 months
Calcium, magnesium, phosphorus	Daily until stable, then 2-3 times/week	Every 1-3 months
Liver function tests	Weekly	Every 1-3 months
Trace elements, vitamins	If deficiency/toxicity suspected	If deficiency/toxicity suspected

EN, enteral nutrition.

Gastrointestinal Complications

6 The GI complications associated with tube feeding include nausea, vomiting, abdominal distension, cramping, aspiration, diarrhea, and constipation. GRV refers to the volume of contents in the stomach and is measured by using a syringe and aspirating from a large-bore NG or gastrostomy tube. Historically, GRV has been used to identify patients at risk of vomiting, aspiration, and/or ventilator-associated pneumonia. However, when GRV alone is used to assess

tolerance to EN, it can lead to unnecessary holding of EN and prevent patients from meeting their EN goal.[43] Further, introducing stomach acid into feeding tubes may contribute to clogging. Current guidelines recommend against the use of GRV as part of routine monitoring for ICU patients receiving EN.[9,44] However, some argue that GRV monitoring remains a useful tool in patients at high risk for EN intolerance, and it continues to be used in some practice settings.[44] For ICUs that continue to utilize GRV, avoid holding EN in response to any GRV less than 500 mL in the absence of other symptoms suggesting intolerance (eg, nausea, abdominal pain, distension).[9]

If symptoms of intolerance are present, and GRVs are greater than 500 mL, a decrease in the tube feeding rate or discontinuation may be warranted. Unless GRVs are excessive (greater than 500 mL in adults), they are generally reinstilled through the tube to minimize nutrient, fluid, and electrolyte losses. In patients at high risk for aspiration, clinicians should implement other measures to reduce aspiration risk, including elevating the head of the patient's bed to a 30° to 45° angle, advancement of the feeding tube into the small bowel, and initiation of a prokinetic agent such as metoclopramide or erythromycin.[17,24] Other potential interventions include minimizing the use of narcotics, sedatives, or other agents that may slow gastric emptying and correcting underlying fluid and electrolyte imbalances that can impair GI motility.[24] Aspiration pneumonia is considered the most serious complication associated with tube feeding. Although aspiration is a fairly common event for critically ill patients receiving tube feeding, progression to aspiration pneumonia is difficult to predict. Risk factors for aspiration include a previous aspiration episode, decreased consciousness, neuromuscular disease, structural airway or GI tract abnormalities, endotracheal intubation, vomiting, persistently high GRVs, and prolonged supine positioning.[44] Historically, blue food coloring had been added to enteral formulations in an attempt to detect aspiration. However, because of its low sensitivity for detection and association with several serious adverse medication reactions, including death associated with mitochondrial toxicity, the addition of blue food dye to enteral formulations is not advised. There are no reliable methods available to detect aspiration in enterally fed patients.[9]

Diarrhea is the most common GI complication in patients receiving EN, but the actual incidence is unclear due to the lack of a standard definition and the large number of contributing factors.[7,17] When monitoring for diarrhea, stool frequency, consistency, and volume should be evaluated, and previous bowel habits should be considered. Diarrhea has been defined as more than three liquid stools daily or a stool volume of more than 250 to 500 mL/day for at least 2 consecutive days.[17] Therefore, the intermittent occurrence of one or two loose stools does not constitute diarrhea or require intervention.

7 Diarrhea in patients receiving tube feeding may be caused by a number of factors, and the management should be directed at identifying and correcting the most likely cause(s).[17] Tube feeding-related factors that may contribute to diarrhea include too rapid delivery or advancement of formula, intolerance to the formula composition, administration of large volumes of feeding into the small bowel, and formula contamination. Thus, measures to prevent or manage diarrhea-related directly to the tube feeding should address these potential causes.[17] If diarrhea occurs when using a fiber-free formulation, a fiber-containing formulation or supplement may be considered in hemodynamically stable patients. If using a high-fat formulation, it may be beneficial to switch to a formulation lower in fat or having a higher proportion of the fat supplied as MCTs; although, a high MCT concentration has also been associated with diarrhea. Finally, it is important to assess the risk of bacterial contamination of the formula and take steps to minimize any potential risk factors. If infectious etiologies have been excluded, severe diarrhea may require pharmacologic treatment with loperamide, diphenoxylate/atropine, or opioids (see Chapter 54).

Medication therapy, particularly the use of broad-spectrum antibiotics, is a common cause of diarrhea that is unrelated to tube feeding. Sorbitol, used as a sweetening agent in many liquid formulations to enhance palatability, is an osmotic laxative that can cause diarrhea. In addition, many medications available in a liquid form are hyperosmolar, which may contribute to diarrhea, especially when these medications are not diluted properly before administration. Because many patients receiving tube feeding also receive medications in a liquid form, all medications should be evaluated for their potential contribution. Malabsorption, secondary to the underlying disease state or condition, may also cause diarrhea. Infectious causes, such as antibiotic-induced bacterial overgrowth by *Clostridioides difficile* or other intestinal flora, need to be considered when diarrhea develops. Certain probiotic strains may have a role in the prevention and treatment of infectious and antibiotic-associated diarrhea.[45] However, the value of adding probiotics to patients on EN in the ICU setting is unclear. The makeup of intestinal flora becomes disrupted in response to antimicrobial treatment and stress response of ICU patients. The use of probiotics has been associated with the reduction of ventilator-associated pneumonia, antibiotic-associated diarrhea, and overall infections in critically ill patients.[5,9] However, the existing evidence is limited. Further, the use of probiotics concomitantly with fiber and jejunal feeding in patients with severe acute pancreatitis increases risk of mortality. Therefore, the use of studied probiotic strains should be considered only for select ICU patient populations such as trauma, pancreatectomy, and liver transplantation.[9]

Mechanical Complications

Mechanical complications of EN are those associated with the feeding tube, including tube occlusion or malposition, and inadvertent nasopulmonary intubation. Feeding tube occlusion usually results from improper medication administration and/or flushing. Kinking of the tube may also cause occlusion. Adult feeding tubes should be flushed with at least 15 to 30 mL of water before and after administering any medication. If more than one medication is scheduled for a given time, each should be administered separately, and the tube should be flushed with 5 to 15 mL of water between medications.[24,46] The frequency of flushing should be at least every 8 hours during continuous feeding and before and after each intermittent feeding. If tube occlusion occurs, the tube should be irrigated with warm water. Other fluids such as carbonated beverages and cranberry juice have been used to irrigate occluded tubes but are likely not any more effective than warm water. Because the acid in these liquids may actually precipitate with protein in the enteral formula and lead to new or worsening of occlusions, this practice should be avoided.[24] Pancreatic enzymes mixed with sodium bicarbonate may be used to reestablish patency in this situation.[46] Declogging devices that are specifically designed to unclog feeding tubes are available. They have been designed to either mechanically break through or remove the occlusion or provide an applicator and syringe prefilled with pancreatic enzymes and various powders targeted to restore patency.[7,46]

Inadvertent nasoenteric tube removal or displacement has been reported in approximately 40% of patients receiving EN.[47] An agitated or confused patient may pull at the feeding tube and cause its removal or malposition. Measures to decrease agitation and confusion should be attempted. Securing the tube with tape may be helpful, as well as marking the tube with permanent ink at the exit site to assess for position change. A nasal bridle that uses a magnetic retrieval system has proven to be a simple and effective method for securing nasoenteric feeding tubes and preventing accidental removal.[48]

When a feeding tube is inserted nasally or orally, there is a risk that the tube may inadvertently enter the tracheobronchial tree. The risk may be higher in patients who have an impaired cough or gag reflex and when a stylet is used for tube insertion. Proper positioning of the tube should always be confirmed by radiography prior to feeding initiation and routinely reassessed to avoid inadvertent administration of enteral formula into the lung.[24]

Other Complications

Infectious complications of feeding tube placement include sinusitis (with nasoenteric placement), exit site-related infections (eg, cellulitis, subcutaneous abscess, necrotizing fasciitis), and intraabdominal infections (eg, peritonitis, abscess). Leaking and bleeding around the exit site can also occur.[12] Formation of excessive granulation tissue around the exit site is often the cause of leaking and bleeding and can be managed by applying silver nitrate and topical corticosteroids.[49]

NUTRITION CARE PLAN

A nutrition care plan that incorporates nutrition assessment and therapy goals should be developed for all patients who require EN (see Chapter 164). Desired outcomes of EN are to promote an adequate nutritional state while minimizing any associated metabolic complications. The EN goals are individualized and based on meeting estimated fluid, calorie, protein, and micronutrient requirements. The desired end point should be included in the care plan. The end point may be resolution of a disease or condition that impairs ability to eat, such as in a critically ill patient who is expected to transition back to an oral diet. EN may be considered a lifelong therapy for those with a permanent impairment that restricts or limits eating, such as gastroparesis.

Assessing the outcome of EN requires monitoring objective measures of body composition, protein and energy balance, and muscle function and wound healing. In addition to optimizing nutrition, the goal of EN is to reduce disease-related morbidity and mortality. Measures of disease-related morbidity include length of hospital stay, infectious complications, and the patient's functional status and sense of well-being. A target weight should be established for each patient and energy content from the EN regimen adjusted as needed to safely achieve or maintain the target weight. Adult patients should generally gain or lose no more than 1 to 2 pounds (~0.45-0.9 kg) per week. EN may be used to supplement an oral diet when oral intake is inadequate and should be modified as needed based on changes in tolerance.

MEDICATION DELIVERY VIA FEEDING TUBE

Using enteral feeding tubes to deliver medications is a common practice and offers an alternative for patients unable to take medications by the oral route. However, in addition to tube occlusion, effects on medication bioavailability and other potential interactions need to be considered when using this route. Medications have been given as a concomitant bolus administration via the feeding tube or admixed with the enteral feeding formulation.

Concomitant Medication Administration

8 Concomitant administration of medications with enteral feedings can be extremely complicated and potentially deleterious. Depending on the indication for enteral nutrition (eg, inadequate oral intake), oral administration may still be the most appropriate route for medication administration.[24] Therefore, if it is feasible and appropriate, oral medications should be continued to be delivered orally whenever possible. If medication must be delivered through a feeding tube, then larger bore feeding tubes (eg, nasogastric or gastrostomy tubes) are preferred over small bore tubes. Delivering medications directly into the stomach allows for the normal process of drug dissolution. Medication delivery directly into the small bowel, however, may result in alterations in drug dissolution because the stomach is bypassed. In addition, therapeutic effects designed to occur within the stomach, such as with antacids and sucralfate, may not be achieved. Because many medications are best absorbed in the fasting state, care should be taken to ensure proper timing of drug administration relative to EN administration when clinically appropriate. Patients on bolus gastric feeding must receive these medications appropriately spaced between feedings, and patients on continuous feeding may require feeding interruptions for drug administration.

Selecting the proper medication dosage form for coadministration with the tube feeding is another important consideration. If crushing a given solid dosage form results in changes to medication absorption, then it should be avoided. Medications in sublingual form, sustained-release capsules or tablets, and enteric-coated tablets should not be crushed and therefore should not be administered via enteral feeding tubes.[24,46] Solid dosage forms that are appropriate to crush should be prepared as a fine powder and mixed with 15 to 30 mL of purified water or other appropriate solvents before administering through the tube. In addition, many capsules may be opened and the contents administered in the same manner. Pellets contained inside microencapsulated dosage forms should generally not be crushed. It may be acceptable to administer intact pellets through larger bore feeding tubes, provided that the pellets are small enough and drug absorption is not compromised.[50] To avoid the need to crush a solid dosage form, liquid dosage forms are commonly preferred for administration through feeding tubes. However, the risk of GI intolerance should be considered because of the hyperosmolality of many liquid formulations and possible sorbitol content.[46,51] Although the use of a liquid dosage preparation may be more convenient than a solid dosage form, it may not be the best choice if GI intolerance is an issue.

Admixture of Medications with Enteral Feeding

Mixing liquid medications with certain enteral feeding formulations is associated with several types of physical incompatibilities, including granulation, gel formation, separation, and precipitation.[46,51] Not only can these physical incompatibilities inhibit drug absorption, but gel formation may clog small-bore feeding tubes. Physical incompatibility with medications is more common in formulations that contain intact protein than in those with hydrolyzed protein. Also, medication and enteral formula incompatibilities are more common with the use of acidic pharmaceutical syrups. The most prudent recommendation is to avoid the routine admixture whenever possible, especially for nonaqueous preparations and syrups. In the clinical setting, exceptions do exist, such as adding sodium or magnesium to enteral formulas to assist in maintaining or repleting electrolytes. However, this practice has fallen out of favor, and a closed EN delivery system should be used whenever possible to minimize the risk of contamination.[24]

Drug-Nutrient Interactions

9 The most significant drug-nutrient interactions that can occur during continuous enteral feeding are those in which the drug's bioavailability is reduced, and the desired pharmacologic effect is not achieved (Table 166-7).[52] One of the well-documented interactions is between phenytoin and enteral feeding. Phenytoin serum concentrations may decrease by 50% to 75% when phenytoin is given concomitantly with EN, possibly as a result of the binding of phenytoin to calcium caseinates or protein hydrolysates in the enteral formulation. Management options include holding EN for 1 to 2 hours before and after drug administration in addition to flushing the tube with water before and after medication delivery. The dosing of phenytoin should be divided into two doses per day rather than three divided doses to minimize interruption of EN. If EN cannot be held around the administration of phenytoin

TABLE 166-7 Select Medications with Special Considerations for Enteral Feeding Tube Administration

Drug	Interaction	Comments
Phenytoin	Reduced bioavailability in the presence of tube feedings Possible phenytoin binding to calcium caseinates or protein hydrolysates in enteral feeding	To minimize interaction, holding tube feedings 1-2 hours before and after phenytoin has been suggested Adjust tube-feeding rate to account for time held for phenytoin administration Monitor phenytoin serum concentration and clinical response closely Consider switching to IV phenytoin or an alternative treatment option if unable to reach therapeutic serum concentration
Fluoroquinolones Tetracyclines	Potential for reduced bioavailability because of complexation of drug with divalent and trivalent cations found in enteral feeding	Consider holding tube feeding 1 hour before and after administration Avoid jejunal administration of ciprofloxacin Monitor clinical response
Warfarin	Decreased absorption of warfarin because of enteral feeding; therapeutic effect antagonized by vitamin K in enteral formulations	Adjust warfarin dose based on INR Anticipate need to increase warfarin dose when enteral feedings are started and decrease dose when enteral feedings are stopped Consider holding tube feeding 1 hour before and after administration
Omeprazole Lansoprazole	Administration via feeding tube complicated by acid-labile medication within delayed-release, base-labile granules	Granules become sticky when moistened with water and may occlude small-bore tubes Granules should be mixed with acidic liquid when given via a gastric feeding tube An oral liquid suspension can be extemporaneously prepared for administration via a feeding tube

INR, International normalized ratio.

suspension per tube, then patients will typically require higher than normal phenytoin doses.[46] The patient's clinical response and phenytoin serum concentrations should be monitored to assure that the desired therapeutic effects are achieved.

Decreased bioavailability of certain antibiotics, particularly quinolones, has been documented when coadministered with enteral feeding due to complexation with multivalent cations such as calcium, magnesium, and iron contained in the feeding.[46,50] Although the practice of holding tube feeding for 30 minutes before and 30 minutes after quinolone administration has been recommended, it does not improve drug absorption. Another option is to increase the quinolone dose when given concurrently with EN. Oral ciprofloxacin is absorbed primarily in the duodenum and early jejunum. Ciprofloxacin bioavailability is significantly decreased when given via a jejunostomy tube due to bypassing the site of absorption, so this practice should be avoided.[46]

Warfarin resistance has been documented during enteral feeding, possibly as a consequence of decreased absorption, binding to protein in EN, or the antagonist effects of vitamin K in the feeding formulation. Before 1980, it was thought that the content of vitamin K (up to 1,330 μg/1,000 kcal [or 317 μg/1,000 kJ] of enteral feeding formula) was contributing to the pharmacologic interaction with warfarin. Subsequently, the vitamin K content within formulas intended for use in adults was reduced to less than 200 μg/1,000 kcal (or 48 μg/1,000 kJ). However, warfarin resistance continues to be reported in patients on EN. Holding EN for one hour before and after warfarin administration along with close monitoring of the International Normalized Ratio is warranted to ensure therapeutic drug concentrations are maintained.[53] Conversely, when EN is discontinued, a reduction in warfarin dosage may be required.

Decreased absorption of levothyroxine has been described in patients receiving continuous EN.[50,54] This is thought to be due to the binding of the medication to the tube feeding formula and/or the binding of thyroid hormones to enteral nutrition during enterohepatic recirculation. Several recommendations have been described, including holding tube feedings for 1 hour before and after medication administration and increasing the dose of levothyroxine while continuous tube feedings are required. Thyroid function tests should be monitored closely (eg, every 7 days) during this time.[54]

CONCLUSION

Identifying appropriate candidates for EN and designing a personalized EN regimen and monitoring plan is a complex process that is often under-appreciated. The successful use of EN can minimize the need for PN in patients unable to meet nutrient requirements with an oral diet. Ultimately, no disease process can improve with prolonged starvation and malnutrition. The American Society for Parenteral and Enteral Nutrition (ASPEN) has identified safety issues related to the administration and management of EN and created practice recommendations based on evidence-based research and expert opinion. These guidelines address the provision and assessment of nutrition support therapy, including EN for adult critically ill patients.[9,24] A multidisciplinary team approach, either as a formal nutrition support service or as a team of caregivers within the practice setting, is recommended to optimize patient outcomes.

ABBREVIATIONS

ALI	acute lung injury
ASPEN	American Society for Parenteral and Enteral Nutrition
ANH	artificial nutrition and hydration
ARDS	acute respiratory distress syndrome
EN	enteral nutrition
FDA	Food and Drug Administration
GALT	gut-associated lymphoid tissue
GI	gastrointestinal
GJ	gastrojejunal
GRV	gastric residual volume
ICU	intensive care unit
IV	intravenous
IgA	immunoglobulin A
MCT	medium-chain triglyceride
NG	nasogastric
NJ	nasojejunal
NPO	nothing by mouth
OG	orogastric
OJ	orojejunal
PEG	percutaneous endoscopic gastrostomy
PN	parenteral nutrition
RNA	ribonucleic acid

REFERENCES

1. Colaizzo-Anas T. Nutrient intake, digestion, absorption, and excretion. In: Mueller CM, ed. *The ASPEN Adult Nutrition Support Core Curriculum*. 3rd ed. Silver Spring, MD: American Society for Parenteral and Enteral Nutrition; 2017:3–25.

2. Abumrad NA, Nassir F, Marcus A. Digestion and absorption of dietary fat, carbohydrate, and protein. In: Feldman M, Friedman LS, Brandt LJ, eds. *Sleisenger & Fordtran's Gastrointestinal and Liver Disease: Pathophysiology/Diagnosis/Management*. 10th ed. Philadelphia, PA: Saunders Elsevier; 2016:1736–1764.
3. Hise M, Brown JC. Lipids. In: Mueller CM, ed. *The ASPEN Adult Nutrition Support Core Curriculum*. 3rd ed. Silver Spring, MD: American Society for Parenteral and Enteral Nutrition; 2017:71–95.
4. Dotan I, Mayer L. Mucosal immunology and inflammation. In: Feldman M, Friedman LS, Brandt LJ, eds. *Sleisenger & Fordtran's Gastrointestinal and Liver Disease: Pathophysiology/Diagnosis/Management*. 10th ed. Philadelphia, PA: Saunders Elsevier; 2016:16–27.
5. Manzanares W, Langlois PL, Wischmeyer PE. Restoring the microbiome in critically ill patients: Are probiotics our true friends when we are seriously ill? *JPEN J Parenter Enteral Nutr.* 2017;41(4):530–533. doi:10.1177/0148607117700572
6. Sanders ME, Merenstein DJ, Reid G, et al. Probiotics and prebiotics in intestinal health and disease: From biology to the clinic. *Nat Rev Gastroenterol Hepatol.* 2019;16(10):605–616. doi:10.1038/s41575-019-0173-3
7. Kozeniecki M, Fritzshall R. Enteral nutrition for adults in the hospital setting. *Nutr Clin Pract.* 2015;30(5):634–651. doi:10.1177/0884533615594012
8. Doley J, Phillips W. Overview of enteral nutrition. In: Mueller CM, ed. *The ASPEN Adult Nutrition Support Core Curriculum*. 3rd ed. Silver Spring, MD: American Society for Parenteral and Enteral Nutrition; 2017:213–225.
9. McClave SA, Taylor BE, Martindale RG. Guidelines for the provision and assessment of nutrition support therapy in the adult critically ill patient: Society of Critical Care Medicine (SCCM) and American Society for Parenteral and Enteral Nutrition (A.S.P.E.N.). *JPEN J Parenter Enteral Nutr.* 2016;40(2):159–211. doi:10.1177/0148607115621863
10. Singer P, Blaser AR, Berger MM, et al. ESPEN guideline on clinical nutrition in the intensive care unit. *Clin Nutr.* 2019;38(1):48–79. doi:10.1016/j.clnu.2018.08.037
11. Dhaliwal R, Cahill N, Lemieux M, et al. The Canadian critical care nutrition guidelines in 2013: An update on current recommendations and implementation strategies. *Nutr Clin Pract.* 2014;29(1):29–43. doi:10.1177/0884533613510948
12. Itkin M, DeLegge MH, Fang JC, et al. Multidisciplinary practical guidelines for gastrointestinal access for enteral nutrition and decompression from the Society of Interventional Radiology and American Gastroenterological Association (AGA) Institute, with endorsement by Canadian Interventional Radiological Association (CIRA) and Cardiovascular and Interventional Radiological Society of Europe (CIRSE). *Gastroenterol.* 2011;141(2):742–65. doi:10.1053/j.gastro.2011.06.001
13. McCleary EJ, Tajchman S. Parenteral nutrition and infection risk in the intensive care unit: A practical guide for the bedside clinician. *Nutr Clin Pract.* 2016;31(4):476–489. doi:10.1177/0884533616653808
14. Doig GS, Simpson F, Sweetman EA, et al. Early parenteral nutrition in critically ill patients with short-term relative contraindications to early enteral nutrition: A randomized controlled trial. *JAMA.* 2013;309(20):2130–2138. doi:10.1001/jama.2013.5124
15. Harvey SE, Parrott F, Harrison DA, et al. Trial of the route of early nutritional support in critically ill adults. *N Engl J Med.* 2014;371(18):1673–1684. doi:10.1056/NEJMoa1409860
16. Reignier J, Boisrame-Helms J, Brisard L, et al. Enteral versus parenteral early nutrition in ventilated adults with shock: A randomised, controlled, multicentre, open-label, parallel-group study (NUTRIREA-2). *Lancet.* 2018;391(10116):133–143. doi:10.1016/S0140-6736(17)32146-3
17. Malone AM, Seres DS, Lord LM. Complications of enteral nutrition. In: Mueller CM, ed. *The ASPEN Adult Nutrition Support Core Curriculum*. 3rd ed. Silver Spring, MD: American Society for Parenteral and Enteral Nutrition; 2017:265–283.
18. Lal S, Pironi L, Wanten G, et al. Clinical approach to the management of Intestinal Failure Associated Liver Disease (IFALD) in adults: A position paper from the Home Artificial Nutrition and Chronic Intestinal Failure Special Interest Group of ESPEN. *Clin Nutr.* 2018;37(6):1794–1797. doi:10.1016/j.clnu.2018.07.006
19. Sabino KM, Fuller J, May S, et al. Safety and tolerance of enteral nutrition in the medical and surgical intensive care unit patient receiving vasopressors. *Nutr Clin Pract.* 2021;36(1):192–200. doi:10.1002/ncp.10548
20. Wischmeyer PE. Enteral nutrition can be given to patients on vasopressors. *Crit Care Med.* 2020;48(1):122–125. doi:10.1097/CCM.0000000000003965
21. Fang JC, Kinikini M. Enteral access devices. In: Mueller CM, ed. *The ASPEN Adult Nutrition Support Core Curriculum*. 3rd ed. Silver Spring, MD: American Society for Parenteral and Enteral Nutrition; 2017:251–264.
22. McCutcheon KP, Whittet WL, Kirsten JL, et al. Feeding tube insertion and placement confirmation using electromagnetic guidance: A team review. *JPEN J Parenter Enteral Nutr.* 2018;42(1):247–254. doi:10.1002/jpen.1015
23. Powers J, Luebbehusen M, Aguirre L, et al. Improved safety and efficacy of small-bore feeding tube confirmation using an electromagnetic placement device. *Nutr Clin Pract.* 2018;33(2):268–273. doi:10.1002/ncp.10062
24. Boullata JI, Carrera AL, Harvey L, et al. ASPEN safe practices for enteral nutrition therapy. *JPEN J Parenter Enteral Nutr.* 2017;41(1):15–103. doi:10.1177/0148607116673053
25. Schwartz DB, Barrocas A, Annetta MG, et al. Ethical aspects of artificially administered nutrition and hydration: An ASPEN position paper. *Nutr Clin Pract.* 2021;36(2):254–267. doi:10.1002/ncp.10633
26. American Geriatrics Society Ethics Committee and Clinical Practice and Models of Care Committee. American Geriatrics Society feeding tubes in advanced dementia position statement. *J Am Geriatr Soc.* 2014;62(8):1590–1593. doi:10.1111/jgs.12924
27. Schwartz DB, Barrocas A, Wesley JR, et al. Gastrostomy tube placement in patients with advanced dementia or near end of life. *Nutr Clin Pract.* 2014;29(6):829–840. doi:10.1177/0884533614546890
28. McClave SA, Saad MA, Esterle M, et al. Volume-based feeding in the critically ill patient. *JPEN J Parenter Enteral Nutr.* 2015;39(6):707–712. doi:10.1177/0148607114540004
29. Taylor B, Brody R, Denmark R, et al. Improving enteral delivery through the adoption of the "Feed Early Enteral Diet Adequately for Maximum Effect (FEED ME)" protocol in a surgical trauma ICU: A quality improvement review. *Nutr Clin Pract.* 2014;29(5):639–648. doi:10.1177/0884533614539705
30. Rahman A, Hasan RM, Agarwala R, et al. Identifying critically-ill patients who will benefit most from nutritional therapy: Further validation of the "modified NUTRIC" nutritional risk assessment tool. *Clin Nutr.* 2016;35(1):158–162. doi:10.1016/j.clnu.2015.01.015
31. McCarthy MS, Martindale RG. Immunonutrition in critical illness: What is the role? *Nutr Clin Pract.* 2018;33(3):348–358. doi:10.1002/ncp.10102
32. Roberts S, Kirsch R. Enteral nutrition formulations. In: Mueller CM, ed. *The ASPEN Adult Nutrition Support Core Curriculum*. 3rd ed. Silver Spring, MD: American Society for Parenteral and Enteral Nutrition; 2017:227–249.
33. Heyland D, Muscedere J, Wischmeyer PE, et al. A randomized trial of glutamine and antioxidants in critically ill patients. *N Eng J Med.* 2013;368(16):1489–1497. doi:10.1056/NEJMoa1212722
34. Zaman MK, Chin KF, Rai V, et al. Fiber and prebiotic supplementation in enteral nutrition: A systematic review and meta-analysis. *World J Gastroenterol.* 2015;21(17):5372–5381. doi:10.3748/wjg.v21.i17.5372
35. Young LS, Kim DW. Protein. In: Mueller CM, ed. *The ASPEN Adult Nutrition Support Core Curriculum*. 3rd ed. Silver Spring, MD: American Society for Parenteral and Enteral Nutrition; 2017:97–112.
36. van Zanten ARH, Sztark F, Kaisers UX, et al. High-protein enteral nutrition enriched with immune-modulating nutrients vs standard high-protein enteral nutrition and nosocomial infections in the ICU: A randomized clinical trial. *JAMA.* 2014;312(5):514–524. doi:10.1001/jama.2014.7698
37. Rice TW, Wheeler AP, Thompson BT, et al. Enteral omega-3 fatty acid, gamma-linolenic acid, and antioxidant supplementation in acute lung injury. *JAMA.* 2011;306(14):1574–1581. doi:10.1001/jama.2011.1435
38. Walker R, Tucker AM, Birtcher KK. Diabetes mellitus. In: Mueller CM, ed. *The ASPEN Adult Nutrition Support Core Curriculum*. 3rd ed. Silver Spring, MD: American Society for Parenteral and Enteral Nutrition; 2017:675–700.
39. Limketkai BN, Hurt RT, Palmer LB. Short bowel syndrome. In: Mueller CM, ed. *The ASPEN Adult Nutrition Support Core Curriculum*. 3rd ed. Silver Spring, MD: American Society for Parenteral and Enteral Nutrition; 2017:587–601.
40. Guenter P. New enteral connectors: Raising awareness. *Nutr Clin Pract.* 2014;29(5):612–614. doi:10.1177/0884533614543330
41. Global Enteral Device Supply Associate (GEDSA). Stay Connected. Available at: www.stayconnected.org. Accessed July 19, 2021.
42. da Silva JSV, Seres DS, Sabino K, Adams SC, et al. ASPEN consensus recommendations for refeeding syndrome. *Nutr Clin Pract.* 2020;35(2):178–195. doi:10.1002/ncp.10474
43. Marik PE. Enteral nutrition in the critically ill: Myths and misconceptions. *Crit Care Med.* 2014;42(4):962–969. doi:10.1097/Ccm.0000000000000051

44. Elke G, Felbinger TW, Heyland DK. Gastric residual volume in critically ill patients: A dead marker or still alive? *Nutr Clin Pract.* 2015;30(1):59–71. doi:10.1177/0884533614562841
45. Guarino A, Guandalini S, Lo Vecchio A. Probiotics for prevention and treatment of diarrhea. *J Clin Gastroenterol.* 2015;49:S37–S45. doi:10.1097/MCG.0000000000000349
46. Williams NT. Medication administration through enteral feeding tubes. *Am J Health Syst Pharm.* 2008;65(24):2347–2357. doi:10.2146/ajhp080155
47. Gunn SR, Early BJ, Zenati MS, et al. Use of a nasal bridle prevents accidental nasoenteral feeding tube removal. *JPEN J Parenter Enteral Nutr.* 2009;33(1):50–54. doi:10.1177/0148607108321704
48. Bechtold ML, Nguyen DL, Palmer LB, et al. Nasal bridles for securing nasoenteric tubes: A meta-analysis. *Nutr Clin Pract.* 2014;29(5):667–671. doi:10.1177/0884533614536737
49. Warriner L, Spruce P. Managing overgranulation tissue around gastrostomy sites. *Br J Nurs.* 2012;21(5):S14–S16, S8, S20 passim. doi:10.12968/bjon.2012.21.Sup5.S14
50. Wohlt PD, Zheng L, Gunderson S, et al. Recommendations for the use of medications with continuous enteral nutrition. *Am J Health Syst Pharm.* 2009;66(16):1458–1467. doi:10.2146/ajhp080632
51. Klang M, McLymont V, Ng N. Osmolality, pH, and compatibility of selected oral liquid medications with an enteral nutrition product. *JPEN J Parenter Enteral Nutr.* 2013;37(5):689–694. doi:10.1177/0148607112471560
52. Chan LN. Drug-nutrient interactions. *JPEN J Parenter Enteral Nutr.* 2013;37(4):450–459. doi:10.1177/0148607113488799
53. Dickerson RN, Garmon WM, Kuhl DA, et al. Vitamin K-independent warfarin resistance after concurrent administration of warfarin and continuous enteral nutrition. *Pharmacotherapy.* 2008;28(3):308–313. doi:10.1592/phco.28.3.308
54. Dickerson RN, Maish GO, Minard G, et al. Clinical relevancy of the levothyroxine-continuous enteral nutrition interaction. *Nutr Clin Pract.* 2010;25(6):646–652. doi:10.1177/0884533610385701

167

Obesity

Amy Heck Sheehan, Judy T. Chen, and Jack A. Yanovski

KEY CONCEPTS

1. Two clinical measures of excess body fat, regardless of sex, are the body mass index (BMI) and the waist circumference (WC). BMI and WC provide a better assessment of total body fat than weight alone and are independent predictors of obesity-related disease risk.
2. Excessive central adiposity increases risk for development of type 2 diabetes mellitus, hypertension, and dyslipidemia.
3. Weight loss goals should be determined based on severity of obesity-related complications. Treatment selection and intensity of obesity intervention varies depending on the phase of prevention and treatment in which the patient resides. Sustained, large weight losses (ie, after bariatric surgery) are associated with a lower risk of cardiovascular events and death and with long-term improvements in many of the complications associated with obesity.
4. Clinicians should consider the weight-altering effects of medications used to treat comorbid conditions (eg, antidepressants, antipsychotics, antiepileptics, and antidiabetics) and select medications that promote weight loss or are weight-neutral.
5. Bariatric surgery is reserved for adolescents with extreme obesity (BMI more than or equal 35 kg/m^2 or more than or equal 120% of the 95th percentile for age, whichever is lower, with a severe comorbidity, or in youth with BMI more than or equal 40 kg/m^2 or more than or equal 140% of the 95th percentile for BMI, whichever is lower, with any obesity-related comorbidity) and adults with extreme obesity (BMI more than or equal 40 kg/m^2 or BMI more than or equal to 35 kg/m^2 with a major comorbidity).
6. Pharmacotherapy may be considered an adjunctive treatment in adolescents age 12 years and older with BMI corresponding to 30 kg/m^2 or greater for adults (more than or equal to the 95th percentile for age) and adults with a BMI more than or equal to 30 kg/m^2 or BMI of 27 to 30 kg/m^2 with a comorbidity if comprehensive lifestyle modifications (eg, diet, exercise, behavioral modification) fail to achieve or sustain weight loss.
7. Weight regain occurs with a high probability when pharmacotherapy for obesity is discontinued.
8. Pharmacotherapy should be discontinued if weight loss of at least 5% is not achieved after 12 weeks of maximum-dose therapy with phentermine-topiramate, bupropion-naltrexone, or setmelanotide because significant weight loss is unlikely to be achieved despite continued therapy. Liraglutide should be discontinued if weight loss of at least 4% is not achieved after 16 weeks of therapy. There is no recommendation for early discontinuation of semaglutide.
9. The Food and Drug Administration (FDA) does not regulate labeling of herbal and food supplement diet agents, and content is not guaranteed.

BEYOND THE BOOK

Access the Centers for Disease Control and Prevention (CDC) Overweight & Obesity website found at https://www.cdc.gov/obesity/index.html. Review the latest obesity statistics and recommended strategies to prevent and manage obesity. This Website is useful to enhance student awareness of the significant public health impact of overweight and obesity and provides tools to assist in the IMPLEMENT step of the patient care process.

INTRODUCTION

Since 1975, the prevalence of obesity worldwide has nearly tripled.[1] It is now estimated that at seven out of every ten adult women and three of every four adult men have overweight or obesity in the United States, and the number of women with obesity outnumbers those who are overweight.[2] While the rise in obesity among young children ages 2 to 5 years appears to have reached a plateau,[3] the prevalence of obesity persistently increased among 6 to 11 year-olds, 12 to 17 year-olds, and adults over the most recent decade between 1999 and 2000 and 2017 and 2018.[2] The presence of obesity and overweight is associated with a dramatically increased risk for the development of many diseases (Table 167-1), poorer outcomes of comorbid disease states, compromise quality of life, and increased healthcare costs.[4-24] As of 2013, it was estimated that obesity accounted for 28.2% of total healthcare spending in non-institutionalized adults in the United States, and the total medical costs of obesity were $342.2 billion annually in 2013.[25] National and global initiatives to stem the obesity epidemic have been established through prevention strategies, consensus guidelines, and best practices.[4-6,22,26-34] This chapter reviews the epidemiology, pathophysiology, and therapeutic approaches for the management of obesity. Although nonpharmacologic treatment modalities are discussed, the pharmacotherapy of obesity is highlighted, and the role of pharmacotherapy relative to the other therapeutic options is critically reviewed.

TABLE 167-1 Conditions More Prevalent Among Patients with Obesity

Cancer	**Genitourinary**
Biliary tract system cancer	Chronic kidney disease
Breast cancer (postmenopausal)	End-stage renal disease
Colorectal cancer	Increased serum urate
Cervical cancer	Nephrolithiasis (kidney stones)
Endometrial cancer (premenopausal)	Obesity-related glomerulopathy
Esophageal cancer	Urinary stress incontinence
Gallbladder cancer	**Immune System**
Gastric cardia cancer	Chronic inflammatory reaction
Leukemia	Immune dysfunction
Liver cancer	**Metabolic**
Multiple myeloma	Diabetes mellitus
Meningioma	Gestational diabetes mellitus
Melanoma	Hyperlipidemia
Non-Hodgkin's lymphoma	Hyperinsulinemia
Ovarian cancer	Hypertriglyceridemia
Pancreatic cancer	Impaired glucose tolerance
Prostate cancer	Low high-density lipoprotein
Rectal cancer	Metabolic syndrome
Renal cell cancer	**Musculoskeletal**
Thyroid cancer	Degenerative joint disease
Cardiovascular	Diffuse idiopathic skeletal hyperostosis
Atrial fibrillation	Disc disease
Cerebral vascular accidents	Fibromyalgia
Chronic heart failure	Flat feet
Coronary artery disease	Gait disturbance
Cor pulmonale	Gout and hyperuricemia
Hypertension	Immobility
Left ventricular hypertrophy	Low back pain/back strain
Myocardial infarction	Osteoarthritis (knee, hips, ankles, feet)
Peripheral vascular disease	Osteoporosis
Peripheral venous insufficiency	Plantar fasciitis
Pulmonary embolism	Sarcopenic obesity
Sudden cardiac death	Total knee arthroplasty (total knee replacement)
Thrombophlebitis	Tendinopathy
Varicose veins	**Neurologic**
Venous thromboembolism	Carpal tunnel syndrome
Ventricular arrhythmias	Idiopathic intracranial hypertension
Dermatologic	Migraines
Acanthosis nigricans	Meralgia paresthetica
Acrochordons (skin tags)	Pseudotumor cerebri
Acne	Stroke
Atopic dermatitis	**Oral Health**
Cellulitis	Dental caries
Hidradenitis suppurativa	Loss of teeth
Intertrigo, carbuncles	Periodontitis
Lymphedema	Xerostomia
Keratosis pilaris	**Psychological**
Panniculitis	Affective disorders
Plantar hyperkeratosis	Anxiety
Psoriasis (women)	Body image disturbance
Status pigmentation of legs	Cognitive dysfunction
Striae distensae (stretch marks)	Depression
Xerosis	Eating disorders
Endocrine and Reproductive	Low self-esteem
Amenorrhea and other menstrual disorders	Social stigmatization
	Social isolation
Congenital anomalies	
Fetal abnormalities	**Respiratory**
Hirsutism	Asthma
Hyperandrogenism	Chronic obstructive pulmonary disease
Hypogonadism (male)	Dyspnea
Infertility	Hypoventilation syndrome
Precocious thelarche	Obstructive sleep apnea
Polycystic ovary syndrome	Pickwickian syndrome
Pregnancy complications	Pneumonia
Sexual dysfunction	Pulmonary hypertension
Gastrointestinal	Respiratory viral infections (coronavirus, influenza, parainfluenza, metapneumovirus, and rhinovirus)
Altered gut microbiome	
Cholelithiasis	
Gastroesophageal reflux disease	
Hepatic cirrhosis	
Hernias	
Nonalcoholic fatty liver disease	
Pancreatitis	
Nonalcoholic steatohepatitis	
Vitamin deficiencies (fat-soluble and water-soluble vitamins)	

Data from References 4-24.

EPIDEMIOLOGY

One of the global health targets set by the World Health Organization (WHO) is to halt the rise of diabetes mellitus and obesity.[27,35] Obesity in the United States has climbed since the 1960s.[2] The National Health and Nutrition Examination Survey (NHANES) II estimated the prevalence of obesity among adults in the United States was at 15% in 1976 to 1980.[2] By 2017 to 2018, the prevalence of obesity had increased almost threefold and affected 42.4% of the adult population and severe obesity affected 9.2% of the adult population.[2] While the speed with which the prevalence of obesity has increased appears to have somewhat leveled off in recent years, prevention of obesity remains a public health priority due to its high prevalence. If the current trend continues, new projection indicates that by 2030, 78% of the adults in the United States projected will have overweight or obesity and one in every two adults will have obesity.[36] In children, 1 in every 3 children aged 6 to 11 years and 1 in every 2 adolescents aged 12 to 19 years will have overweight or obesity by 2030.[36] Children who are overweight are likely to remain overweight as adults.[37] Furthermore, children and adolescents with overweight or obesity have a higher risk of premature mortality and morbidity as adults.[37] Therefore, childhood and early adulthood are critical intervention periods for prevention of obesity in the next generation and require long-term commitment and investment from all stakeholders.[35] The prevalence of obesity using the 30 kg/m^2 cut point varies by sex and race/ethnicity within the United States. Non-Hispanic Asian men (17.5%) and women (17.2%) have the lowest prevalence of obesity compared to other ethnic groups, though they develop obesity-linked complications at lower BMI than other races/ethnicities.[2] The highest prevalence of obesity is observed among non-Hispanic Black women (56.9%) compared with non-Hispanic Black men (41.1%).[2] This disparity is also associated with the level of education. Black women without a college degree are at greater risk of obesity compared with Black men.[38]

Educational achievement, which is linked to socioeconomic status, is also correlated with the fraction of people who have obesity. The prevalence of obesity is greatest in those with high school education or less among non-Hispanic White women and men, non-Hispanic Black women, and Hispanic Women.[38]

ETIOLOGY

Obesity occurs when there is increased energy storage resulting from an imbalance between energy intake and energy expenditure over time. The specific etiology for this imbalance in the vast majority of individuals is multifactorial, with genetic and environmental factors contributing to various degrees. In a small minority of individuals, excess weight may be attributed to an underlying medical condition or an unintended effect of a medication.

Genetic Influences

Genetics plays an important role in determining both obesity and distribution of body fat. In some individuals, genetic factors are the primary determinants of obesity, whereas in others, obesity may be caused primarily by environmental factors. The genetic contribution to the actual variance in BMI and body fat distribution is estimated to be up between 40% and 50%.[39] A number of single-gene mutations producing extreme obesity have been identified, but such mutations are rare and account for a relatively small number of the total cases of obesity.[39] The total number and identity of contributing genes are still being determined, as is the means by which the many potential so-called obesity genes interact with each other and with the environment to produce the obese phenotype.

Environmental Factors

Many of the societal changes associated with economic development over the past 50 years have been implicated as potential causes for the increase in the prevalence of obesity.[40] These include an abundant and easily accessible food supply and the material comforts of modern life in Western civilizations, which have contributed to a reduction in physical activity. Advances in technology and automation have resulted in more sedentary lifestyles during both work and leisure time for most individuals. At the same time, there has been a substantial increase in the availability and portion size of high-fat foods, which are aggressively marketed and are often more convenient and less expensive than healthier alternatives. This modern environment has been described by some as "obesogenic" because it is likely to result in a state of positive energy balance in many individuals (Fig. 167-1).[41] Obesity is observed more frequently among individuals within close social networks (eg, siblings, spouses, and friends), with a person's risk of developing obesity increasing dramatically if a friend in their social network has obesity.[42] Cultural factors such as socioeconomic status, and religious beliefs may influence eating habits and body weights. Obesity has also been linked to changes in gut microorganisms and lack of sleep.[40]

Medical Conditions

Occasionally, patients present with obesity secondary to an identifiable medical condition. Conditions associated with weight gain include iatrogenic and idiopathic Cushing syndrome, growth hormone deficiency, insulinoma, leptin deficiency, and various psychiatric disorders, such as depression, binge-eating disorder, and schizophrenia. Hypothyroidism is often included in this list, but it mostly causes fluid retention (myxedema) and is generally not a cause of obesity. Genetic syndromes that have obesity as a major component are extremely rare and include Prader-Willi, Wilms' tumor, aniridia, genitourinary abnormalities or gonadoblastoma, mental retardation (WAGR), Simpson-Golabi-Behmel, Cohen, Bardet-Biedl, Carpenter, Börjeson, and Wilson-Turner syndromes. The clinician evaluating a patient for obesity needs to be aware of these potential conditions. The physical examination of patients with obesity patients always should include an assessment for secondary causes of obesity, including genetic syndromes.

Medications

An increasing number of medications are associated with unintended weight gain. These include several antiseizure medications (eg, carbamazepine, gabapentin, pregabalin, valproic acid), antidepressants (eg, mirtazapine, tricyclic antidepressants), atypical antipsychotics (eg, clozapine, olanzapine, quetiapine, risperidone), conventional antipsychotics (eg, haloperidol), lithium, hormones (eg, corticosteroids, insulin, medroxyprogesterone), beta adrenergic

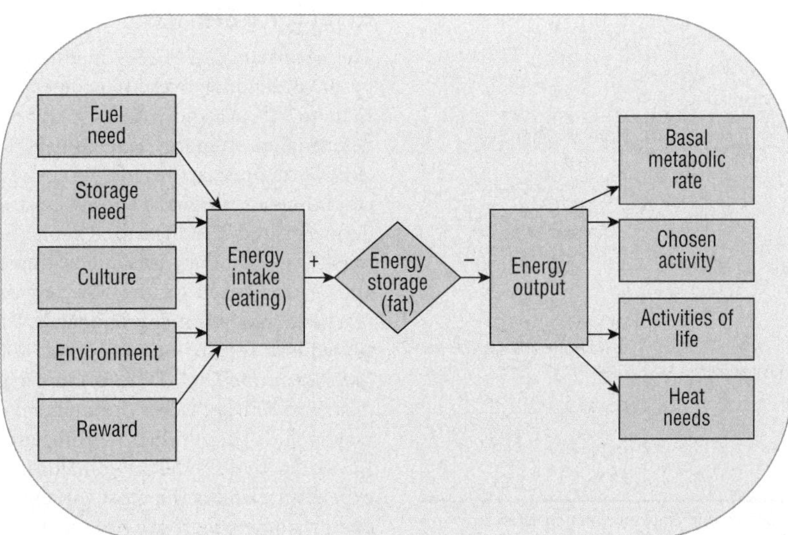

FIGURE 167-1 Net energy stores are determined by various inputs and outputs. Simply stated, obesity occurs when there is an imbalance between energy intake and expenditure.

blockers, sulfonylureas, thiazolidinediones, and antiretrovirals.[43] Although the pharmacologic mechanism responsible for weight gain is usually medication-specific, in most cases the precise mechanism is unknown.

PATHOPHYSIOLOGY

The pathophysiology of obesity involves numerous factors that regulate appetite and energy balance.[29,44,45] Disturbance of these homeostatic functions results in an imbalance between energy intake and energy expenditure.

Appetite

Human appetite is a complex process that is the net result of many inputs within a neural network involving principally the hypothalamus, limbic system, brainstem, hippocampus, and elements of the cortex.[29,44,45] Within this neural network, many neurotransmitters and neuropeptides have been identified that can stimulate or inhibit the brain's appetite network and thereby affect total caloric intake. The first receptor systems found to alter food intake in animals and humans were the biogenic amines. Serotonin, also known as 5-hydroxytryptamine (5-HT), and cells known to respond to 5-HT are found throughout the central nervous system (CNS) and the periphery. Currently, two major noradrenergic receptor subtypes are recognized (α and β), each with multiple subtypes. Histamine and dopamine also demonstrate multiple receptor subtypes, but their role in the regulation of human eating behaviors and food intake is less well documented. Table 167-2 summarizes the major effects of direct receptor stimulation, inhibition, and changes in synaptic cleft amine concentrations on food intake.

Many neuropeptides also influence appetite within the hypothalamus. Most research has focused on the neural projection between parts of the hypothalamus and the arcuate nucleus with signals to the paraventricular nucleus. The key peptides in this projection are thought to include neuropeptide Y and α-melanocyte–stimulating hormone. Neuropeptide Y is the most potent known stimulator of eating, and α-melanocyte–stimulating hormone action at the melanocortin 3 and 4 receptors is one of the crucial inhibitors of eating.[44] The lateral hypothalamus has been referred to as the "hunger" center within the brain. The most prominent of the lateral hypothalamic peptides, orexin, increases food intake stimuli within the lateral hypothalamus.[40] Another important neuropeptide stimulator of eating that principally originates in the lateral hypothalamus is melanocyte-concentrating hormone. Neurons in the lateral hypothalamus use orexin and melanocyte-concentrating hormone to communicate with other neurons throughout the brain and thereby affect a number of functions beyond appetite.[44] Table 167-2 summarizes the major effects of various neuropeptides on food intake.[44,45] Although hunger and satiety functions are thought to be primarily regulated by the hypothalamus, humans eat in response to a broad set of stimuli, including reward, pleasure, learning, and memory.

TABLE 167-2 Effects of Various Neurotransmitters, Receptors, and Peptides on Food Intake

Anatomic Region	Increased Eating	Decreased Eating
Arcuate nucleus of hypothalamus	NPY AgRP	α-MSH CART Leptin Insulin GLP-1 PYY
Paraventricular nucleus of hypothalamus	NPY AgRP	α-MSH, melanocortin CRH CCK
Lateral hypothalamus	Orexin MCH	
Hypothalamus	Norepinephrine α_2 Serotonin 5-HT_{1A}	Norepinephrine α_1 and β_2 Serotonin 5-HT_{1B} and 5-HT_{2C} Histamine H_1 and H_3
Nucleus accumbens	Dopamine	
Brainstem (hindbrain)	NPY AgRP Opioids (especially μ)	Leptin α-MSH, melanocortin CCK
Vagus nerve	Ghrelin	Leptin CCK GLP-1 PYY

AgRP, agouti-related protein; CART, cocaine-and-amphetamine-regulated transcript; CCK, cholecystokinin; CRH, corticotropin-releasing hormone; GLP-1, glucagon-like peptide-1; MCH, melanocyte concentration hormone; α-MSH, α-melanocyte-stimulating hormone; NPY, neuropeptide Y; PYY, peptide YY.

Data from References 44 and 45.

Peripheral appetite signals also dramatically affect food intake.[45] Leptin, a hormone that is secreted by adipose cells, acts on the arcuate nucleus of the hypothalamus and elsewhere in the brain to decrease appetite and increase energy expenditure.[45] Exogenous leptin administration produces considerable weight loss in leptin-deficient patients; however, recombinant leptin replacement therapy in patients with obesity who are not leptin-deficient has not proved successful because most with obesity appear to be leptin resistant.[44] Figure 167-2 shows the peripheral link that leptin appears to provide in signaling the CNS about the status of fat cell mass.

Other peripheral signals important to the brain's processing of appetite include several gut hormones, notably those released by the intestine in response to passage of digesting food such as glucagon-like peptide-1 (GLP-1), oxyntomodulin, and peptide YY.[45] Each of these hormonal signals suppresses eating. GLP-1 has other effects, most importantly as an incretin, which facilitates release of insulin by pancreatic β cells in response to meal-related glucose. Ghrelin, another important gut hormone that is released from the distal stomach and duodenum, stimulates appetite. An understanding of the relationships among the brain, its many neurotransmitters and neuropeptides, environmental stimulation of brain activities, and other hormones is still evolving.

Energy Balance

The net balance of energy ingested relative to energy expended by an individual over time determines the degree of obesity (Fig. 167-1). An individual's metabolic rate is the single largest determinant of energy expenditure. Resting energy expenditure (REE) is defined as the energy expended by a person at rest under conditions of thermal neutrality. Basal metabolic rate (BMR) is defined as the REE measured soon after awakening in the morning at least 12 hours after the last meal. Metabolic rate increases after eating based on the size and composition of the meal. It reaches a maximum approximately 1 hour after the meal is consumed and returns to basal levels 4 hours after the meal. This increase in metabolic rate is known as the *thermogenic effect of food*. The REE measures the energy costs of the wakeful state and may include the residual thermogenic effect of a previous meal. Physical activity is the other major factor that affects total energy expenditure and is the most variable component. With regard to energy storage, there are two major types of adipose tissue, white adipose tissue (WAT) and brown adipose tissue (BAT). The primary function of WAT is energy storage, whereas BAT is brown because it has much greater mitochondrial density along with

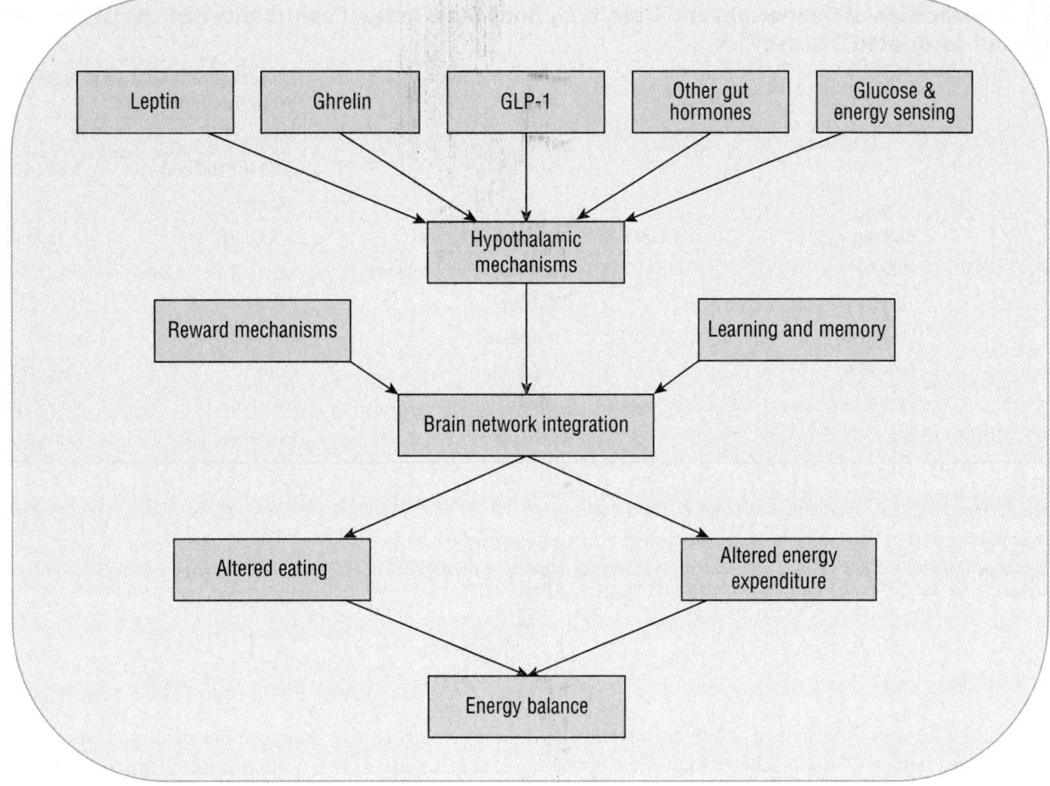

FIGURE 167-2 Intrinsic hypothalamic hunger and satiety mechanisms are modified by input from fat tissue via leptin, and from the gut via ghrelin, glucagon-like peptide-1 (GLP-1), and other hormones. Additional input is derived by direct sensing of prevailing glucose and other energy signals. The hypothalamus generates signals that are integrated within brain networks, which also receive additional signals. The brain network effects change in energy balance by modifying food intake and energy expenditure.

high expression of uncoupling proteins that give it the capacity to uncouple oxidative phosphorylation to produce heat and maintain body temperature.[46] BAT is more commonly identified in those who are lean than those with obesity, but its importance for human obesity remains unclear. Both white and brown adipose tissues are highly innervated by the sympathetic nervous system, and adrenergic stimulation via β-adrenergic receptors (β_1, β_2, and β_3) is known to activate lipolysis in fat cells as well as increase energy expenditure in adipose tissue and skeletal muscle.

CLINICAL PRESENTATION

Although obesity is often readily apparent, most patients with obesity seek healthcare only when obesity-associated comorbidities become problematic. The National Institutes of Health (NIH) has established a stratification of weight excess based on associated medical risks.[4,7] These levels of excess weight are defined on the basis of BMI, a measure of total body weight relative to height. Using metric units, BMI (kg/m^2) is defined as weight in kilograms divided by height in meters squared (kg/m^2). Using pounds and inches, BMI (kg/m^2) is estimated as (weight [lb]/height [inches^2]) × 703. Adults with a BMI of 25 to 29.9 kg/m^2 are considered "*overweight*"; the terms *obesity* and *extreme obesity* are reserved for those with a BMI of 30 to 39.9 kg/m^2 and 40 kg/m^2 and over, respectively. The Endocrine Society clinical practice guideline currently classifies children and adolescents older than 2 years of age with a BMI at 120% or above of the 95th percentile or BMI at 35 kg/m^2 or above as having extreme obesity, BMI at the 95th percentile or above as obesity, and those with a BMI between the 85th and 94th percentiles as overweight.[34] Because BMI may overestimate the degree of excess body fat in some clinical situations (eg, edematous states, extreme muscularity, muscle wasting, hydration status, large tumor, short stature), the assessment of body composition in such cases often requires clinical judgment.

1 BMI measurement is the practical method of defining obesity in the clinic and in epidemiologic studies; however, it does not always correspond to excess fat. There are well-established differences in the relationship between BMI and obesity-related risks among disparate racial, sex, and ethnic groups. For example, the standard cut points for BMI underestimates risks among Asian patients and utilizing a lower BMI value of 23 kg/m^2 or above to confirm excess body adiposity in this population is recommended.[6,26,47] Across all ethnic groups, men tend to have higher visceral adipose tissues.[48] Central obesity reflects high levels of intra-abdominal or visceral fat, and this pattern of obesity is associated with an increased propensity for the development of hypertension, dyslipidemia, type 2 diabetes mellitus, and cardiovascular disease (sometimes referred to as the "metabolic syndrome") and have an increased cardiometabolic disease risk.[5] Thus, in addition to the absolute excess fat mass, the distribution of this fat regionally in the body has important clinical effects. Intra-abdominal fat is best estimated by imaging techniques such as computed tomography (CT) and magnetic resonance imaging (MRI) but can be approximated through measurement of waist circumference (WC). Clinically, WC is the narrowest circumference measured in the area between the last rib and the top of the iliac crest. Currently in the United States, Canada, and Europe, the definition for high-risk WC is greater than 40 inches (102 cm) in men and greater than 35 inches (89 cm) in women.[7] Specific region- and ethnicity-specific waist circumference thresholds should be used to assess abdominal obesity and disease risks in other populations.[6] Routine determination of WC should be implemented in those with

TABLE 167-3 Classification of Overweight and Obesity by Body Mass Index, Comorbidity Risk, Waist Circumference, and Associated Disease Risk

				Disease Risk[a] (Relative to Normal Weight and Waist Circumference)	
				Men	
				≤40 in (102 cm)	>40 in (102 cm)
				Women	
	BMI (kg/m²)	Obesity Class	Comorbidity Risk	≤35 in (89 cm)	>35 in (89 cm)
Underweight	<18.5		Low but other problems	—	—
Normal weight[b]	18.5-24.9		Average	—	High
Overweight	25.0-29.9		Increased	Increased	High
Obesity	30.0-34.9	I	Moderate	High	Very high
	35.0-39.9	II	Severe	Very high	Very high
Extreme obesity	≥40	III	Very severe	Extremely high	Extremely high

BMI, body mass index.

[a]Disease risk for type 2 diabetes mellitus, hypertension, and cardiovascular disease.

[b]Increased waist circumference can also be a marker for increased risk even in persons of normal weight.

Data from WHO Consultation on Obesity (1999: Geneva, Switzerland) & World Health Organization. (2000). Obesity: preventing and managing the global epidemic: report of a WHO consultation. World Health Organization. Available at: https://apps.who.int/iris/handle/10665/42330.

BMIs between 25 and 34.9 kg/m² to assess additional metabolic risk.[5,31-33] However, after a patient's BMI reaches 35 kg/m², it is not necessary to measure WC because it will likely be elevated and adds little in terms of risk prediction.[32]

(2) Although BMI and WC are related, each measure independently predicts disease risk. Both measurements should be assessed and monitored during therapy for obesity.[5-7] The risks for development of type 2 diabetes mellitus, hypertension, or cardiovascular disease at various stages of obesity based on BMI or WC are outlined in Table 167-3. Note that increased WC confers increased risk even in normal-weight individuals. A higher prevalence of cardiometabolic abnormalities among normal weight individuals is particularly evident in racial/ethnic minority populations.[49]

Comorbidities

Obesity and overweight are associated with an increased risk of all-cause mortality and contributed to approximately 7.1% of total death globally.[50] A U-shaped association is noted between BMI and all-cause mortality for patients with diabetes mellitus, hypertension, coronary artery disease, and peripheral artery disease because underweight, obesity, and morbid obesity are all associated with increased risk of cardiovascular diseases (CVD) and mortality.[51] For each standard deviation higher BMI the risk of type 2 diabetes mellitus increases by 67% and coronary artery disease by 20%.[52] While substantial reduction in life expectancy has been predicted in adults with BMIs greater than 35 kg/m²,[53,54] healthy life-years lost due to obesity is estimated to be two to four times greater than total years of life lost.[53] Excessive body fat affects virtually all organ systems. A plethora of evidence continue to link obesity with numerous disease states and health conditions (Table 167-1).[4-24] Therefore, current clinical practice guidelines recommend a "complication-centric approach" for management of obesity.[6,29] It is important for clinicians to assess presence and severity of weight-related complications to determine the appropriate treatment and intensity of weight loss therapy in all individuals with overweight and obesity (Fig. 167-3).[6] Because individuals with obesity are also at risk for developing many malignancies, adherence to routine age- and risk-appropriate cancer screening guidelines is recommended.[29] Furthermore, hypertension, hyperlipidemia, coronary heart disease, cerebrovascular accidents, insulin resistance, glucose intolerance, and diabetes mellitus are all known cardiac risk factors that tend to cluster in individuals with obesity. Aggressive management of these comorbid cardiovascular risk factors and other weight-related complications (eg, sleep apnea, major depression, osteoarthritis, nonalcoholic fatty liver disease) is warranted in an individual with obesity regardless of an individual's weight loss efforts.[6,7,29]

TREATMENT

Available treatment options for the chronic management of obesity include reduced caloric intake, comprehensive lifestyle intervention, pharmacotherapy, medical devices, and bariatric surgery.

Desired Outcomes

Weight management is commonly considered successful when a predefined amount of weight has been lost such that a final goal is achieved. However, in the current "complication-centric approach" in obesity management, the primary goal is to ameliorate weight-related complications and ultimately improve patient's health and quality of life rather than a preset decline in body weight.[6] In 2016, comprehensive clinical practice guidelines published by the American Association of Clinical Endocrinologists (AACE) and American College of Endocrinology (ACE) outlined intervention and weight loss goals from at least 5% to 40% based on severity of obesity-related complications (see Table 167-4).[6] The AACE/ACE guideline further outlines the three-phase paradigm of chronic disease prevention and treatment: primary, secondary, and tertiary. The goal of primary phase is to prevent overweight and obesity; the goal of secondary phase is to prevent progressive weight gain or achieve weight loss to prevent complications; the goal of tertiary phase is to achieve sufficient weight loss to improve obesity-related complications and prevent further deterioration. Treatment selection and intensity of obesity intervention varies depending on the phase of prevention and treatment in which the patient resides. If improvement in type 2 diabetes mellitus, dyslipidemia, hypertension, and polycystic ovary syndrome are primary goals, then the recommended weight loss goals is at least 5% to 15% or more.[6] For patient with steatohepatitis, the recommended weight loss goal is 10% to 40% in order to reduce inflammation and fibrosis of the liver.[6] Success may also include end points of decreasing the rate of weight

DIAGNOSIS AND MEDICAL MANAGEMENT OF OBESITY

DIAGNOSIS		COMPLICATION-SPECIFIC STAGING AND TREATMENT		
Anthropometric Component (BMI kg/m²)	**Clinical Component**	**Disease Stage**	**Chronic Disease Phase of Prevention**	**Suggested Therapy (based on clinical judgment)**
<25 <23 in certain ethnicities waist circumference below regional/ ethnic cutoffs		**Normal weight** (no obesity)	**Primary**	• **Healthy lifestyle:** healthy meal plan/ physical activity
25-29.9 **23-24.9 in certain ethnicities**	Evaluate for presence or absence of adiposity-related complications and severity of complications • Metabolic syndrome • Prediabetes • Type 2 diabetes • Dyslipidemia • Hypertension • Cardiovascular disease • Nonalcoholic fatty liver disease • Polycystic ovary syndrome • Female infertility • Male hypogonadism • Obstructive sleep apnea • Asthma/reactive airway disease • Osteoarthritis • Urinary stress incontinence • Gastroesophageal reflux disease • Depression	**Overweight stage 0** (no complications)	**Secondary**	• **Lifestyle therapy:** Reduced-calorie healthy meal plan/physical activity/ behavioral interventions
≥30 **≥25 in certain ethnicities**		**Obesity stage 0** (no complications)	**Secondary**	• **Lifestyle therapy:** Reduced-calorie healthy meal plan/physical activity/ behavioral interventions • **Weight-loss medications:** Consider if lifestyle therapy fails to prevent progressive weight gain (BMI ≥27)
≥25 **≥23 in certain ethnicities**		**Obesity stage 1** (1 or more mild-to-moderate complications)	**Tertiary**	• **Lifestyle therapy:** Reduced-calorie healthy meal plan/physical activity/ behavioral interventions • **Weight-loss medications:** Consider if lifestyle therapy fails to achieve therapeutic target or initiate concurrently with lifestyle therapy (BMI ≥27)
≥25 **≥23 in certain ethnicities**		**Obesity stage 2** (at least 1 severe complication)	**Tertiary**	• **Lifestyle therapy:** Reduced-calorie healthy meal plan/physical activity/ behavioral interventions • **Add weight-loss medication:** Initiate concurrently with lifestyle therapy (BMI ≥27) • **Consider bariatric surgery:** (BMI ≥35)

a. All patients with BMI ≥25 have either overweight or obesity stage 0 or higher, depending on the initial clinical evaluation for presence and severity of complications. These patients should be followed over time and evaluated for changes in both anthropometric and clinical diagnostic components. The diagnoses of overweight/obesity stage 0, obesity stage 1, and obesity stage 2 are not static, and disease progression may warrant more aggressive weight-loss therapy in the future. BMI values ≥25 have been clinically confirmed to represent excess adiposity after evaluation for muscularity, edema, sarcopenia, etc.

b. Stages are determined using criteria specific to each obesity-related complication; stage 0 = no complication; stage 1 = mild to moderate; stage 2 = severe.

c. Treatment plans should be individualized; suggested interventions are appropriate for obtaining the sufficient degree of weight loss generally required to treat the obesity-related complication(s) at the specified stage of severity.

d. BMI ≥27 is consistent with the recommendations established by the US Food and Drug Administration for weight-loss medications.

FIGURE 167-3 Diagnosis and Medical Management of Obesity. *(Reprinted from Garvey WT, Mechanick JI, Brett EM, et al. American Association of Clinical Endocrinologist and American College of Endocrinology Comprehensive Clinical Practice Guidelines for medical care of patients with obesity. Endocr Pract. 2016;3:1–203.)*

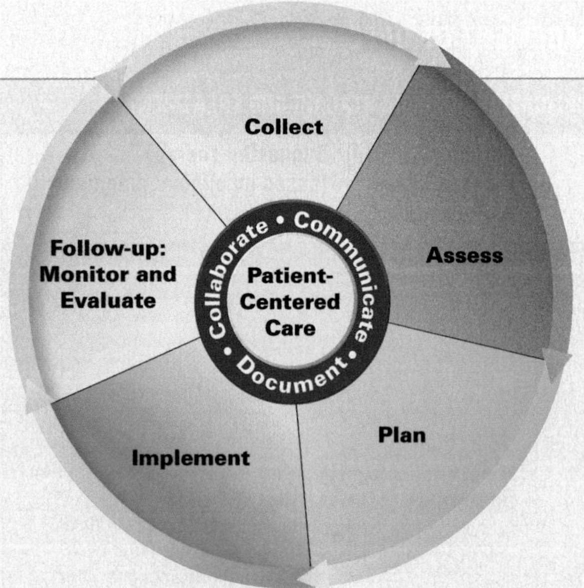

Patient Care Process for Management of Obesity

Collect

- Patient characteristics (eg, age, race, sex)
- Patient history (past medical, family, social—dietary habits, tobacco use)
- Obesity-related conditions (see Table 167-1)
- Current medications including prescription, non-prescription, and herbal product use
- Weight loss history and prior attempts to lose weight
- Objective data
    - Height, weight, BMI, waist circumference, and blood pressure
    - Labs (eg, fasting glucose, hemoglobin A1c, lipid panel)

Assess

- Causes of secondary obesity (eg, insulinoma, Cushing syndrome)
- Current medications that may contribute to weight gain
- Presence of obesity-related comorbidities (eg, hypertension, dyslipidemia, coronary artery disease, type 2 diabetes mellitus, sleep apnea, increased waist circumference; see Fig. 167-3)
- Class of overweight and obesity determined by BMI, waist circumference, and obesity-related comorbidities (see Table 167-3)
- Readiness to engage in weight loss efforts and potential barriers to success
- Candidacy for treatment with pharmacotherapy, medical devices, or bariatric surgery

Plan*

- Nonpharmacologic lifestyle intervention including low-calorie diet, physical activity, and behavioral modifications
- Determine appropriate weight loss goals based on severity of existing obesity-related complications (see Table 167-4)
- Pharmacotherapy (if appropriate) including specific medication, dose, route, frequency, and duration; specify the continuation and discontinuation of existing therapies (see Tables 167-6 and 167-8)
- Medical devices (if appropriate) including specific instruction for use, dose, route, duration, and adverse medication reactions (see Table 167-5)
- Monitoring parameters including efficacy (weight loss) and tolerability (medication and/or medical device–specific adverse effects) (see TableS 167-5 and 167-8)
- Bariatric surgery (if appropriate) ensuring specific pre- and post-operative criteria are met
- Patient education (eg, purpose of dietary and lifestyle modification, medication therapy)
- Self-monitoring of weight—when and how to record results
- Referrals to other providers when appropriate (eg, physician, dietitian, psychologist)

Implement*

- Educate patient regarding health risks associated with overweight and obesity
- Provide patient education regarding all elements of treatment plan
- Use motivational interviewing and coaching strategies to maximize adherence
- Schedule appropriate follow-up (eg, monthly for first 3 months and every 3 months thereafter) based on treatment selected

Follow-up: Monitor and Evaluate

- Determine weight loss goal attainment
- Presence of adverse medication reactions
- Patient adherence to treatment plan using multiple sources of information

** Collaborate with patient, caregivers, and other healthcare professionals.*

gain or maintaining a weight-neutral status. All too often patients expect to lose weight overnight, only to be disappointed. Thus, it is important to set a time course for the plan. Numerous web-based resources for supporting both patient and practitioner weight-management activities are available.[7,55-58]

General Approach to Treatment

To achieve meaningful weight loss goals, successful obesity treatment plans require incorporation of comprehensive lifestyle interventions such as healthy diet, adequate physical activity, and behavioral modifications as the cornerstone of weight management.[5,6,26,28,29,31-33] Psychological interventions such as cognitive therapy or stress management to address the emotional relationship with food may help further promote adherence, intrinsic motivation, and treatment success.[32,33] Once the need for weight loss has been determined, the clinician needs to assess a patient's readiness to engage in weight loss efforts and identify any potential barriers to success. They need to initiate a dialogue with each patient who has overweight or obesity

TABLE 167-4 Tertiary Prevention Treatment Goals Based on Diagnosis in the Medical Management of Patients with Overweight or Obesity[a]

Diagnosis	Weight Loss Goals	Clinical Goals
Urinary stress incontinence	5% to 10% or more	Reduced frequency of incontinence episodes
Metabolic syndrome	10%	Prevention of type 2 diabetes mellitus
Prediabetes	10%	Prevention of type 2 diabetes mellitus
Gastroesophageal reflux disease	10% or more	Reduced symptoms frequency and severity
Female infertility	10% or more	Ovulation, pregnancy, and live birth
Asthma/reactive air way disease	7% to 8% or more	Improved in forced expiratory volume at 1 second (FEV1), improved symptoms
Obstructive sleep apnea	7% to 11% or more	Improved symptoms, decreased apnea-hyponea index
Osteoarthritis	≥10% (5%-10% or more when coupled with exercise)	Improved symptoms, increased function
Type 2 diabetes mellitus	5% to ≥15%	Reduced A1c, reduced number and/or doses of diabetes medications, diabetes remission (if diabetes duration is short)
Dyslipidemia	5% to ≥15%	Lowered triglycerides, raised HDL-C, lowered non-HDL-C
Hypertension	5% to ≥15%	Lowered blood pressure, reduced number and/or doses of antihypertensive medications
Polycystic ovary syndrome	5% to ≥15%	Ovulation, regularization of menses, reduced hirsuitism, enhanced insulin sensitivity, reduced serum androgen levels
Nonalcoholic fatty liver disease		
Steatosis	5% or more	Reduced intrahepatocellular lipid
Steatohepatitis	10% to 40%	Reduced inflammation and fibrosis
Depression	Uncertain	Improved depressive symptoms and depression scores

A1c, glycated hemoglobin A1c; HDL-C, high density lipoprotein cholesterol.

[a]Patients with BMI ≥25 kg/m² (≥23 kg/m² in certain ethnicities).

Adapted from Garvey WT, Mechanick JI, Brett EM, et al. American Association of Clinical Endocrinologist and American College of Endocrinology Comprehensive Clinical Practice Guidelines for medical care of patients with obesity. Endocr Pract. 2016;3:1–203.

to ensure they understand the potential health consequences of excess body weight and benefits of appropriate weight management. Specific weight goals should be established that are consistent with medical needs, weight-related complications, and the patient's personal desire.[6] Patients should not be allowed to attain an abnormally low body weight (ie, less than their estimated ideal body weight).

(3) Patients seeking help for obesity do so for many reasons, including improvement in their quality of life, a reduction in associated morbidity, and increased life expectancy. Because weight stigma is prevalent in the western culture, numerous individuals seek therapy for obesity primarily for cosmetic purposes and often have unrealistic goals and expectations. Aggressive marketing of weight loss programs, therapies, and diets—parallel to the fashion industry's standards of desirable body profiles—has led many individuals to set impossible goals and expectations. Often, these individuals will go to extreme measures to achieve weight loss. Consequently, clinicians must be careful to fully discuss the risks of therapies and to clearly define the achievable benefits and magnitude of weight loss. Patients with obesity should be redirected away from trying to achieve an "ideal weight" to the more realistic goal of modest (eg, loss of 5%-10% of body weight) but sustained, medically relevant weight loss. In practice, goals should be set based on many factors, including initial body weight, patient motivation and desire, presence of obesity-related comorbid conditions, and age. The Look Action for Health in Diabetes (AHEAD) study found that patients with diabetes mellitus who maintained weight loss of at least 7% with intensive lifestyle modifications for a period of almost 10 years did not experience a reduced incidence of cardiovascular events, but they did have a reduced need for diabetes mellitus medications and improvement in physical function, lipids, blood pressure, kidney disease, sleep apnea, fitness, and depression.[59] When behavioral-based weight loss intervention is incorporated, with or without medication therapy, patients are able to achieve more weight loss and have a lower risk of developing diabetes mellitus.[60] In patients with overweight and obesity with diabetes mellitus, lifestyle modification with sustained weight loss of greater than 5% improves HbA1c level and ameliorates hyperglycemia, hyperlipidemia, and hypertension within a year.[61] For individuals with obesity who have gastroesophageal reflux disease, a 10% or more weight reduction may be required to improve symptoms.[6] This highlights the importance of defining end points and measures of success in any weight-loss plan.

(4) Weight-loss interventions must be founded on lifestyle changes, such as a modification in eating practices; complemented by medication therapy, if indicated; and in some cases, surgery. Before recommending any therapy, the clinician must evaluate the patient for the presence of secondary causes of obesity.[62] If a secondary cause is suspected, then a more complete diagnostic workup and the initiation of appropriate therapy may be warranted. The next step in patient evaluation is to determine the presence and severity of other medical conditions that are either directly associated with obesity (eg, diabetes mellitus, cardiovascular diseases, uncontrolled hypertension) or that have an impact on therapeutic decision making (eg, history of pancreatitis, cardiac arrhythmia, seizure disorders, concurrent medications).[6,29] The Endocrine Society Clinical Practice Guideline for the Pharmacological Management of Obesity emphasizes that clinicians should always consider the potential weight-altering effects of all medications a patient is receiving for the management of comorbid conditions and select medications that are weight-neutral or promote weight loss (strong recommendation with moderate quality evidence).[29] For example, in patients with type 2 diabetes mellitus, antidiabetic agents that promote weight loss (eg, metformin, glucagon-like peptide-1 analogs, sodium-glucose-linked transporter-2 inhibitors) are preferred. Appropriate laboratory tests to exclude or quantify the degree of specific conditions such as diabetes mellitus, liver dysfunction, and nephropathy should be performed as indicated by the history and physical examination. Based on the outcome of this medical evaluation, the patient should be counseled on treatment options, benefits, and risks. Ultimately,

lifelong therapeutic goals should consist of maintenance of reduced body weight and prevention of weight gain.

Nonpharmacologic Therapy

Nonpharmacologic therapy, including reduced caloric intake, increased physical activity, and behavioral modification, is the mainstay of obesity management. This combination, also known as lifestyle therapy, is recommended for all patients with overweight and obesity by the ACC/AHA Guideline on the Primary Prevention of Cardiovascular Disease,[5] the Endocrine Society Clinical Practice Guidelines for the Pharmacological Management of Obesity (graded as strong recommendation with high quality evidence),[29] and the AACE/ACE Guidelines for the Medical Care of Patients with Obesity (grade A recommendation with the best level of evidence).[6] Weight loss will require major effort on the part of the patient to change their lifestyle and comply with the management plan. If the patient is not ready to meet these expectations, then early counseling will reduce the chance of frustration for the patient, clinician, and possibly other family members. Providing basic education can lead to a substantial change in motivation and desire to lose weight and improved compliance.

Reduced Caloric Intake

Current adult guidelines recommend reduced energy intake through adherence to a low-calorie diet (LCD).[5,6] The LCD should provide a daily energy deficit of 500 to 750 kcal (2,100-3,150 kJ), which generally correlates to a total intake of 1,200 to 1,500 kcal/day (5,000-6,300 kJ/day) for women and 1,500 to 1,800 kcal/day (6,300-7,550 kJ/day) for men. Individuals with severe obesity will require more energy, at least at the start of dietary restriction. Adherence to the LCD results in an average weight loss of 8% after 6 months.[7]

Numerous diet and nutrition plans are available to aid patients in their pursuit of weight loss, and current guidelines allow for choice among many potential evidence-based diet plans.[6,7,63] Popular diets include moderate energy-deficient plans (eg, DASH [Dietary approaches to Stop Hypertension], Mediterranean, Weight Watchers, LEARN [Lifestyle, Exercise, Attitude, Relationships, Nutrition], Jenny Craig), vegetarian-based plans (eg, Ornish), and low carbohydrate plans (eg, Zone, Atkins). Short-term weight loss is considerable for almost all diet plans. However, long-term weight loss and maintenance of weight loss are less promising, primarily because of difficulty with adherence. Therefore, the choice of diet plan should be determined based on patient-specific preferences, health status, and ability to consistently adhere to the specific recommendations of the diet.[6] A meta-analysis of 121 clinical trials assessing the efficacy of various diets concluded that differences in weight loss among popular named diets are not clinically significant,[64] highlighting the general consensus that macronutrient composition of the diet may not be as important as consistent adherence to reduced energy consumption. Time restricted eating (TRE), defined as consuming all calories within a restricted time window (eg, 6-8 hours) and fasting during the rest of the day, has recently become a popular diet intervention for weight loss and other health benefits. Although short-term weight loss data are promising, long-term data on the sustained efficacy, ability for patients to adhere to the required lifestyle changes, and safety in patients with obesity-related comorbidities are limited.[65]

Very-low-calorie diets, providing less than 800 kcal/day (3,350 kJ/day), are generally not recommended.[7] Although very-low-calorie diets can often result in substantial early weight loss, long-term results have been disappointing because it is difficult for individuals to maintain compliance. Additionally, very-low-calorie diets require intensive medical monitoring and should only be used in certain situations under the supervision of an experienced clinician. Regardless of the diet program, it is clear that energy consumption must be less than energy expenditure to achieve weight loss (see Fig. 167-1). The challenge is to develop a diet plan that leads to consistent adherence by the patient and sustained weight loss and maintenance.

Comprehensive Lifestyle Intervention

Comprehensive lifestyle intervention encompasses the combination of reduced energy intake, increased physical activity, and behavioral modification. Increased physical activity is an important component in achieving the state of greater energy expenditure than energy intake that is necessary to lose weight and maintain weight loss. Weight loss is modest when increased physical activity is attempted as monotherapy. However, when it is combined with reduced energy intake and behavior modification, it can augment weight loss and improve obesity-related comorbidities and cardiovascular risk factors.[5,7] Aerobic physical activity for at least 150 minutes per week, completed over 3 to 5 days is recommended for adults.[6,66] Greater levels (ie, 200-300 min/wk) may be required to augment weight loss and maintain lost weight. Patients should be advised to start slowly and gradually increase intensity. All patients with obesity should receive a medical examination before embarking on a physical activity program.

Current adult guidelines recommend initiation of a comprehensive lifestyle program to help patients with overweight and obesity adhere to the prescribed LDC and increased physical activity per week (NHLBI Grade A; strong recommendation).[5,6] For patients who have successfully lost weight during the first 6 months, long-term participation in a comprehensive lifestyle program is recommended. The primary aim is to help patients choose lifestyles that are conducive to safe and sustained weight loss. Most such programs use self-monitoring of diet and exercise to increase patient awareness of behavior and as a tool for the clinician to determine patient compliance as well as patient motivation. High-intensity comprehensive lifestyle interventions that include a reduced-calorie diet, increased exercise, and in-person behavioral counseling sessions result in an average weight loss of 8 kg (17.6 lb) after 6 months.[7]

Bariatric Surgery

5 Consistent with the growing obesity epidemic, the demand for bariatric surgery has increased drastically over the past two decades. Surgery currently remains the most powerful and effective intervention for the treatment of obesity.[67,68] Current clinical practice guidelines recommend that surgical intervention be reserved for adults with extreme obesity (BMI ≥40 kg/m^2 or BMI >37.5 kg/m^2 in Asian Americans) without other comorbidity, or BMI at 35 kg/m^2 or above (BMI 32.5-37.4 kg/m^2 in Asian Americans) with at least one or more major comorbidity such as hypertension, type 2 diabetes mellitus, or obstructive sleep apnea (NHLBI Grade A; strong recommendation).[6,26,29,68] Surgery may also be advocated to adults with BMI between 30 kg/m^2 and 34.9 kg/m^2 (27.5-32.4 kg/m^2 in Asian Americans) with diabetes mellitus or metabolic syndrome, as a similar efficacy and safety profile for improving type 2 diabetes mellitus and metabolic disorders is observed among bariatric patients with a BMI below or above 35 kg/m^2.[26,69] This has led to use of the term "metabolic surgery" with focus on treating metabolic diseases independent of body weight.[68] Bariatric surgery is also endorsed by the American Academy of Pediatrics for severe obesity. For adolescents, the American Society for Metabolic and Bariatric Surgery recommends bariatric surgery can be considered in youth (ages 13 to 18) with BMI ≥35 kg/m^2 or ≥120% of the 95th percentile for age, whichever is lower, with a severe comorbidity, or in youth with BMI ≥40 kg/m^2 or ≥140% of the 95th percentile for BMI, whichever is lower, with any obesity-related comorbidity.[69]

Surgical weight loss options should only be considered in patients who have met the eligibility criteria and have failed other recommended methods for weight loss. It is critical for bariatric surgical candidates to fully understand the surgical risks and be able to commit fully to the extensive postoperative care plan, follow-ups, and necessary lifelong vitamin supplementation, medical monitoring (including costs required), dietary, lifestyle, and behavioral adjustments to ensure the long-term success of the procedure.[68]

Appropriate selection of a bariatric procedure should be individualized based on goals of therapies, available expertise, patient preferences, and inherent risks. The four available surgical procedures currently endorsed by the American Society of Metabolic and Bariatric Surgery are (1) adjustable gastric banding, (2) sleeve gastrectomy, (3) biliopancreatic diversion with duodenal switch, and (4) conventional Roux-en-Y gastric bypass. The adjustable gastric banding and sleeve gastrectomy are designed to reduce the volume of the stomach and thus restrict the rate of nutrient intake. The biliopancreatic diversion with duodenal switch is primarily malabsorptive in nature, and the length of the diversion determines the extent of nutrient malabsorption. This hybrid procedure combines a restrictive approach with a degree of malabsorption induced by reducing the size of the stomach pouch and causing food to bypass parts of the small intestine. Techniques that involve redirection of the flow of nutrients so as to have humoral and malabsorptive effects generally yield greater and longer lasting weight loss than the purely restrictive methods.[67] The sleeve gastrectomy has increased in its popularity worldwide and is currently the most common procedure performed in the United States.[68] Resection of the gastric segment from sleeve gastrectomy also removes the endocrine cells, which alters neuro-humoral activity and results in earlier satiety and improvements in glucose metabolism. The amount of total body weight loss and remission of comorbidities is proportional to intestinal bypass, which is expected from the metabolic effect of the surgery [eg, adjustable gastric banding (20%-25%) < sleeve gastrectomy (25%-30%) < Roux-en-Y gastric bypass (30%-35%) < duodenal switch (35%-45%)].[68] Patients usually achieve the lowest post-bariatric weight from 1 to 2 years after bariatric surgery.

After 5 years, patients with type 2 diabetes mellitus with BMI of 27 to 43 kg/m^2 who undergo gastric bypass surgery lose more (23%) of their initial body weight compared to patients who receive sleeve gastrectomy (19%) and patients who receive intensive medical therapy (5%).[70] Results from gastric bypass appear at least as promising among adolescents, for whom the likelihood for, and durability of remission from comorbid conditions is often greater than observed in adults.[71,72] The extent of weight loss and the potential for weight regain after bariatric surgery is multifactorial as metabolic, anatomic, and lifestyle changes can all impact the outcome of the procedure. Bariatric surgeries are now considered among the safest abdominal surgical procedures performed in the United States today; the operative 30-day mortality rates for gastric bypass and sleeve gastrectomy are 0.2% and 0.1%, respectively.[67] Some of the most common early surgical complications are gastric and anastomotic leaks, bleeding, wound infections, and pulmonary emboli. Due to the disruption of the normal gastric anatomy and physiology, postsurgical patients are often at risk for severe micronutrient deficiencies (eg, vitamin B_{12}, vitamin B_1, vitamin K, zinc, copper, folate, iron, calcium) as well as deficiencies in fat soluble vitamins such as vitamins A, D, E, and K due to fat malabsorption.[68] Therefore, empiric supplementation with daily adult multivitamin plus minerals, elemental calcium, vitamin D, folic acid, thiamine, elemental iron, and vitamin B_{12} is essential to prevent nutritional deficiencies in bariatric patients.[68] Because many commercial dietary supplements products are adulterated with compounds that are not included in the original manufacturer's label, use of supplements verified by the US Pharmacopeia (https://www.quality-supplements.org/verified-products), or other brands that have been safely and effectively tested in clinical trials are recommended.[68] All bariatric surgical patients should undergo life-long monitoring of nutritional deficiencies after the procedure. Profound weight loss resulting from bariatric surgery provide multitude of health benefits, which are often accompanied by dramatic improvements, and sometimes complete resolution, of many obesity-related complications.[67,68]

Significant reduction in risks of myocardial infarction, cardiovascular deaths, as well as the incidence of type 2 diabetes mellitus, hypertension, dyslipidemia, and cancer occur after adult's bariatric surgery.[14,67,70,73,74] It has long been known that bariatric surgery improves microvascular diseases,[75] and substantially reduces macrovascular disease and mortality in patients with type 2 diabetes mellitus and severe obesity.[73] Patients who undergo Roux-en-Y gastric bypass surgery are expected to have a 40% decrease in all-cause mortality, 60% decrease in mortality due to cancer, 92% decrease in mortality due to diabetes mellitus, and 56% decrease in mortality due to coronary artery disease at 12 years.[74] An increase in life expectancy is also expected after bariatric surgery, regardless of the type of bariatric procedure.[76] Metabolic surgery can prolong median life expectancy by 6.1 years and substantial survival benefit is seen in patients with preexisting diabetes mellitus than those without after surgery (9.3 years vs 5.1 years gain in median life expectancy).[76] Every 1% increase in metabolic surgery utilization rate is estimated to yield 5.1 million to 6.6 million potential life-years saved.[76] Despite the expenses of the bariatric procedure, bariatric surgery is a cost-saving alternative to conventional management over the lifetime for patients who suffer from severe obesity.[77]

After experiencing weight loss, many gastric surgery patients are able to discontinue pharmacotherapy for glucose lowering, dyslipidemia, hypertension, and reduce medication costs.[67,68,70] However, the need for use of proton-pump inhibitors are often increased as a prophylactic therapy for anastomotic ulcers.[68,78] It is imperative for clinicians to recognize that bariatric interventions not only alter nutrient absorption but also may impede medication absorption and can cause potential serious consequences.[78] Achlorhydria, reduced contact time with digestive enzymes, reduced surface area for intestinal and gastric absorption, reduced bile acid exposure after bariatric surgery can lead to altered absorption, distribution, metabolism, and/or elimination of many medications.[78] Use of direct oral anticoagulant (eg, apixaban, rivaroxaban) and nonsteroidal anti-inflammatory drugs (eg, ibuprofen) should be avoided after surgery.[78] Reduced serum concentrations may be observed for some antimicrobials, antidepressants, selective serotonin reuptake inhibitors (SSRIs), antipsychotics, and tamoxifene.[78] Furthermore, concurrent administration of proton-pump inhibitors may also alter bioavailability of weak basic medications such as antifungals (eg, posaconzale),[78] certain antibiotics and some cardiovascular medications (eg, digoxin) as well as hinder the absorption of micronutrients.[78] Therefore, clinicians need to recognize that the standard dosage regimens recommended for presurgical patients may need to be adjusted. Switching from solid medications to opened capsules or liquid formulations (without high sugar loads) for post-surgical patients may be beneficial when inadequate clinical response is observed.[78] Long-term close therapeutic monitoring of all orally administered medications after surgery, particularly those with narrow therapeutic ranges (eg, warfarin, levothyroxine, lithium) is highly recommended because dosage form selection, dose conversion, or therapeutic interchange may be necessary to avoid or minimize absorption problems and ensure optimal patient outcomes.[68,78] Controlled-release formulations may be used after surgery but close monitoring is needed.[78] With increased fertility rate and decreased absorption of oral contraceptives after bariatric surgery, alternative non-oral contraceptive is recommended for all reproductive-aged women who have undergone surgery.[68,78] Women who desire to conceive should wait at least 12 to 18 months after bariatric surgery to ensure stable weight and balance nutrition is achieved.[68]

Implantable Medical Devices

Despite meeting the medical necessity for bariatric surgery, some individuals may not qualify as surgical candidates or may choose to not undergo the procedure. Medical devices may fill the existing treatment gap in obesity management and may address the unmet needs in these individuals. Currently, there are six FDA-approved medical devices for weight reduction involving electrical stimulation, gastric emptying, gastric balloon systems, or superabsorbent hydrogel (Table 167-5).[79-84] Each of these devices is fully

TABLE 167-5 FDA-Approved Medical Devices for Weight Loss

Device	Mechanism of Action	BMI Indication	Contraindications	Weight Loss Outcomes	Adverse Medication Reactions	Comments
Gastric Emptying System						
AspireAssist®[79,80]	An implanted percutaneous gastrostomy aspiration tube removes approximately 25%-30% of the meal from stomach 20-30 minutes after ingestion	Adult age ≥22 with BMI 35-55 kg/m²	- Uncontrolled hypertension - Bulimia - Binge eating disorder - Night-eating syndrome - Previous abdominal surgery - Esophageal stricture, gastric obstruction, gastroparesis - Inflammatory bowel disease - Stomach ulcer - History of serious pulmonary or cardiovascular disease - Coagulation disorders - Anemia - Chronic abdominal pain - Pregnancy or lactation, or desire to become pregnant	%TBWL across trials demonstrated 17.8%, 18.3%, 19.1%, and 18.6% after 1 year, 2 years, 3 years, and 4 years, respectively/[80]	- Abdominal pain - Indigestion - Nausea - Vomiting - Constipation - Diarrhea - Peristomal granulation tissue - Peristomal irritation and inflammation	Patient must take extra time to chew thoroughly and drink sufficient liquid with each meal to ensure proper aspiration Frequent medical visits are also necessary to monitor device use and weight loss and to provide counseling on lifestyle therapies The device contains a safety feature to keep track the number of times the drain tube is connected to the port and automatically stops working after 115 cycles (approximately 5-6 weeks of therapy) to ensure proper use
Electrical Stimulation System						
Maestro® Rechargeable System[79]	A neurometabolic therapy, deliver via a pacemaker-like device that is implanted on the vagal trunk. The device is designed to intermittently block the communication with the vagus nerve (vBloc) through the delivery of electrical impulse to increase satiety and improve food-related cognitive restraints	Age ≥18 with BMI 40-45 kg/m² OR Age ≥18 with BMI 35-39.9 kg/m² with at least 1 comorbidity	- Liver cirrhosis - Portal hypertension - Esophageal varices - Hiatal hernia - Planned MRI or diathermy - Permanently implanted, electrical-powered medical device (ie, pacemaker, defibrillator, neurostimulator)	%TBWL after 1 year of therapy is 9.2% and excess body weight is 24.4%.	- Neuroregulator site pain - Nausea - Abdominal pain - Heartburn - Dyspepsia	The implanted neuroregulatory is controlled by the clinician with an external programming device to deliver 12 to 15 hours of intermittent nerve block. Battery is recharged daily for 30 minutes Once the device is turn-off, patient often will regain the weight lost
Gastric Balloon System						
Orbera Intragastric Balloon[79,81-83]	Endoscopically placed intragastric balloon device designed to occupy space in the stomach to reduce hunger and improve appetite control	Orbera® Adult age ≥22 with BMI 30-40 kg/m² Orbera365™ Adults with BMI >40 kg/m² OR Adult with BMI ≥35 kg/m² with comorbidities OR Adults with BMI between 27 and 50 kg/m² who failed to achieve and maintain weight loss with a supervised weight-controlled program	- Previous gastric surgery - Hiatal hernia - Coagulation disorder - A potential bleeding lesion of the upper gastrointestinal tract - Alcohol or drug misuse - Severe liver disease - Pregnancy or lactation, or desire to become pregnant - Any contraindication to endoscopy	%TBWL after 1 year of therapy is 11.3%.[81]	- Abdominal pain - Nausea - Vomiting - Dysphagia - Heartburn - Early explantation - Gastric ulcer - Deflation - Migration - Perforation - Hyperinflation of balloon - Acute pancreatitis	The device placement is intended to be temporarily. After 6 months (Orbera®) or 12 months (Orbera365™), the balloon is punctured and removed through the mouth via a grasping device Patients who fail to remove the device after 6 months (Orbera®) or 12 months (Orbera365™), will be at increased risk of intestinal obstruction due to migration of the deflated balloon Aggressive symptoms control with triple antiemetic medications in the early period after insertion Use of proton pump inhibitor and avoidance of nonsteroidal anti-inflammatory agents during treatment **Weight regain occurs after device removal**

TABLE 167-5 FDA-Approved Medical Devices for Weight Loss

Device	Mechanism of Action	BMI Indication	Contraindications	Weight Loss Outcomes	Adverse Medication Reactions	Comments
[a]The ReShape Integrated Dual Balloon System[79,82,83]	Endoscopically placed intragastric balloon device designed to occupy space in the stomach to reduce hunger and improve appetite control	Adult age 22-60 with BMI 30-40 kg/m^2 with at least 1 comorbidity	- Prior gastrointestinal or bariatric surgery - Inflammatory intestinal or bowel disease - Large hiatal hernia - Delayed gastric emptying - Upper gastrointestinal bleed - Coagulation disorder - Severe liver disease - Active *Helicobacter pylori* infection - A structural abnormality in the esophagus or pharynx - Use of anticoagulants or anti-inflammatory agents - Pregnancy or lactation, or desire to become pregnant - Any contraindication to endoscopy	%TBWL after 6 months of therapy is 15.4%	- Abdominal pain - Nausea - Vomiting - Heartburn - Gastric ulcer - Deflation - Perforation - Dysphagia - Gastric bleeding - Hyperinflation of balloon - Acute pancreatitis	The device placement is intended to be temporarily and should be removed 6 months after insertion as the device will deflate over time Patients who fail to remove the device after 6 months will be at increased risk of intestinal obstruction due to migration of the deflated balloon Aggressive symptoms control with triple antiemetic medications in the early period after insertion Use of proton pump inhibitor and avoidance of nonsteroidal anti-inflammatory agents during treatment Patients currently taking selective serotonin reuptake inhibitors (SSRIs), serotonin-norepinephrine reuptake inhibitors (SNRIs), and monoamine oxidase inhibitors (MAOIs) should use this device with caution due to the potential for balloon rupture and release of methylene blue which with these concurrent therapies can increase risk of developing serotonin syndrome Weight regain occurs after device removal
Obalon Balloon System™[79,83]	Sequentially swallowed balloon device designed to occupy space in the stomach to reduce hunger and improve appetite control. A total of 3 balloons are placed over 3 months	Adult age ≥22 with BMI 30-40 kg/m^2	- Any structural or functional abnormality in the esophagus, pharynx, stomach, intestines, or any portion of the gastrointestinal tract - Prior bariatric surgery - Inflammatory and other conditions of the gastrointestinal tract - Active *Heliocobacter pylori* infection - Bulimia, binge eating or other eating disorders - Use of gastric irritants such as NSAIDs and aspirin - Use of anti-platelets or anticoagulants - Irritable bowel syndrome or other inflammatory bowel disease - Taking medications on specified hourly intervals that may be affected by changes in gastric emptying (eg, anti-seizure or anti-arrhythmic medications) - Alcohol or drug misuse - Pregnancy or lactation, or desire to become pregnant	%TBWL after 6 months of therapy is 6.8%	- Abdominal pain - Nausea - Vomiting - Heartburn - Bloating - Deflation - Gastric ulcer - Hyperinflation of balloon	The only intragastric balloon that does not require endoscopic placement. The balloon is encapsulated, attached to a tube, and swallowed under provider supervision The device placement is intended to be temporarily and should be endoscopically removed after 3 to 6 months Aggressive symptoms control with triple antiemetic medications in the early period after insertion Use of proton pump inhibitor and avoidance of nonsteroidal anti-inflammatory agents during treatment Weight regain occurs after device removal

(*Continued*)

TABLE 167-5 FDA-Approved Medical Devices for Weight Loss (*Continued*)

Device	Mechanism of Action	BMI Indication	Contraindications	Weight Loss Outcomes	Adverse Medication Reactions	Comments
Nonsystemic Oral Superabsorbent Hydrogel						
Plenity[a84]	Oral capsule releases carboxymethylcellulose and citric acid hydrogel when taken with water. The particles rapidly absorb water and mix with ingested food, which expands to ¼ of the stomach volume, to create a sensation of satiety to reduce hunger and improve appetite control.	Adult with BMI 25-40 kg/m^2	- Allergic reaction to cellulose, citric acid, sodium stearyl fumarate, gelatin, or titanium dioxide - Pregnancy	%TBWL demonstrated 6.4% and 9.5% after 6 months and 48 weeks, respectively	- Abdominal pain - Diarrhea - Abdominal distension - Infrequent bowel movements - Flatulence - Constipation	Take three capsules (2.25 g total) orally twice daily, administer 20 to 30 minutes before lunch and dinner

BMI: Body Mass Index; TBWL: Total Body Weight Loss.
[a]As of January 2019, ReShape has been voluntary withdrawn from the market due to marketing reasons.

reversible and are designed to work in conjunction with prescribed diet and exercises programs. A patient's ability to provide appropriate follow-up is essential to enhance the safety and to avoid complications related to the devices. Unfortunately, once the device is removed, patients will often regain the lost weight.

Pharmacologic Therapy

6 7 According to current guidelines, pharmacotherapy is an adjunct to comprehensive lifestyle intervention in adults who are motivated to lose weight, have failed to achieve or sustain weight loss with lifestyle changes alone, and have a BMI more than or equal to 30 kg/m^2 or a BMI more than or equal to 27 kg/m^2 with at least one weight-related comorbidity (Graded as a strong recommendation with high quality evidence).[6,29] Furthermore, patients who meet the BMI requirements and have a history of failed attempts to lose weight or maintain weight loss with comprehensive lifestyle intervention alone may also be candidates for pharmacotherapy.[29] Long-term pharmacotherapy may have a place in the treatment of obesity for patients who have no obvious contraindications to approved medication therapy, as the likelihood of weight regain after treatment discontinuation is quite high. Table 167-6 lists FDA-approved pharmacotherapeutic agents currently available for management of overweight and obesity.

A multidisciplinary team approach to the management of obesity is necessary to ensure long-term success. It is common for

TABLE 167-6 FDA-Approved Pharmacotherapeutic Agents for Weight Loss

Medication	Brand Name	Initial Dose	Usual Range	Special Population Dose	Comments
Gastrointestinal Lipase Inhibitor					
Orlistat	Xenical®	120 mg three times daily with each main meal containing fat	120 mg three times daily with each main meal containing fat	120 mg three times daily is approved for adolescents ages 12 or greater with BMI for age equivalent to 30 kg/m^2 in adults	Approved for long-term use Take during or up to 1 hour after the meal Omit dose if meal is occasionally missed or contains no fat
Orlistat	Alli®[a]	60 mg three times daily with each main meal containing fat	60 mg three times daily with each main meal containing fat		Same as Xenical®
Phentermine–Topiramate Combination					
Phentermine and topiramate extended release	Qsymia®	3.75 mg of phentermine and 23 mg of topiramate once daily for 14 days; then increase to 7.5 mg of phentermine and 46 mg of topiramate once daily	7.5 mg of phentermine and 46 mg of topiramate once daily to a maximum dose of phentermine 15 mg and topiramate 92 mg once daily	Maximum dose for patients with moderate or severe kidney impairment or patients with moderate hepatic impairment is 7.5 mg of phentermine and 46 mg of topiramate	Approved for long-term use Take dose in the morning to avoid insomnia Controlled substance: C–IV
Naltrexone-Bupropion Combination					
Bupropion and naltrexone extended release	Contrave®	8 mg naltrexone/90 mg bupropion (1 tablet) once daily in the morning for 1 week; then 8 mg naltrexone/90 mg bupropion twice daily (morning and evening) for 1 week; then 16 mg naltrexone/180 mg bupropion in the morning and 8 mg naltrexone/ 90 mg bupropion in the evening for 1 week; then 16 mg naltrexone/180 mg bupropion twice daily (morning and evening)	16 mg naltrexone and 180 mg bupropion (2 tablets) twice daily	Maximum dose for patients with moderate or severe kidney impairment is 8 mg naltrexone/90 mg bupropion (1 tablet) twice daily Maximum dose for patients with hepatic impairment is 8 mg naltrexone/90 mg bupropion (1 tablet) once daily in the morning	Approved for long-term use Do not take dose with high-fat meal
Glucagon-Like Peptide-1 Agonists					
Liraglutide	Saxenda®	0.6 mg once daily for 1 week 1.2 mg once daily for 1 week 1.8 mg once daily for 1 week 2.4 mg once daily for 1 week 3.0 mg once daily for 1 week	3 mg once daily	Use with caution in mild, moderate, and severe kidney and hepatic impairment. Dose escalation to 3.0 mg once daily is approved for adolescents ages 12 or greater with weight 60 kg (132 lb) or greater and BMI for age equivalent to 30 kg/m^2 in adults	Approved for long-term use Inject subcutaneously in the abdomen, thigh, or upper arm
		Administered by subcutaneous injection			Administer at any time of day without regard to the timing of meals

(continued)

TABLE 167-6 FDA-Approved Pharmacotherapeutic Agents for Weight Loss (*Continued*)

Medication	Brand Name	Initial Dose	Usual Range	Special Population Dose	Comments
Semaglutide	Wegovy™	0.25 mg once weekly for 4 weeks 0.5 mg once weekly for 4 weeks 1 mg once weekly for 4 weeks 1.7 mg once weekly for 4 weeks 2.4 mg once weekly Administered by subcutaneous injection	2.4 mg once weekly		Approved for long-term use Inject subcutaneously in the abdomen, thigh, or upper arm Administer at any time of day without regard to the timing of meals
Melanocortin 4 (MC4) Receptor Agonist					
Setmelanotide	Imcivree™	Adults and adolescents >12 years: 2 mg once daily for 2 weeks, then increase to 3 mg once daily if tolerated and additional weight loss is desired (or decrease to 1 mg once daily based on tolerability) Children aged 6 to <12 years: 1 mg once daily for 2 weeks, then increase to 2 mg once daily if tolerated (or decrease to 0.5 mg once daily based on tolerability), then increase to 3 mg once daily if tolerated and additional weight loss is desired Administered by subcutaneous injection	2-3 mg once daily	Not recommended for patients with moderate to severe kidney impairment	Approved for long-term use in patients aged 6 years and above with genetically confirmed or suspected deficiency of POMC, PCSK1, or LEPR. Inject subcutaneously in the abdomen, thigh, or upper arm rotating sites each day Administer at the beginning of the day without regard to timing of meals
Noradrenergic Agents					
Phendimetrazine	Bontril® PDM; Bontril® Slow-Release	Conventional tablet: start at 17.5 mg two or three times daily, given 1 hour before meals Extended-release capsule: 105 mg once daily 30-60 minutes before morning meal	70-105 mg/day	Use caution in patients with kidney impairment	Approved for short-term monotherapy Controlled substance: C–III Prescriptions should be written for the smallest quantity to minimize possibility of overdose
Phentermine	Lomaira™ Adipex-P®	8 mg three times daily, given ½ hour before meal Orally disintegrating tablet: 15 or 30 mg once every morning Phentermine hydrochloride: 15-37.5 mg/day given in one or two divided doses; administer before breakfast or 1-2 hours after breakfast	8 mg three times daily, given ½ hour before meal Orally disintegrating tablet: 15 or 30 mg once every morning Phentermine hydrochloride: 15-37.5 mg/day given in one or two divided doses; administer before breakfast or 1-2 hours after breakfast	Use with caution in patients with kidney impairment	Approved for short-term monotherapy Controlled substance: C–IV Prescriptions should be written for the smallest quantity to minimize possibility of overdose Individualize to achieve adequate response with lowest effective dose
Diethylpropion	Tenuate®, Tenuate Dospan	Immediate release: 25 mg three times daily administered 1 hour before meals Controlled release: 75 mg once daily administered at midmorning	75 mg/day	Use with caution in patients with kidney impairment	Approved for short-term monotherapy Dose should not be administered in the evening or at bedtime Controlled substance: C–IV

[a]Available without a prescription.

patients to use a combination of nonprescription, prescription, and other complementary and alternative therapies to attain the desired weight loss goal. Therefore, clinicians should maintain a high degree of sensitivity toward the potential polypharmacy practices of patients with obesity. Finally, it is prudent to consider specific patient factors and characteristics along with the efficacy and safety profiles of individual therapies when determining if use of a pharmacologic intervention is warranted.

Agents Approved for Long-Term Use

8 There are currently six products approved in the United States for the chronic management of obesity. These include the lipase inhibitor

orlistat (Xenical®, Genentech USA, South San Francisco, CA; Alli®, GlaxoSmithKline, Middlesex, UK), the combination product phentermine–topiramate extended release (Qsymia®, Vivus, Inc, Mountain View, CA), the combination product naltrexone-bupropion extended-release tablets (Contrave®, Takeda Pharmaceuticals America Inc, Cambridge, MA), the GLP-1 receptor agonists liraglutide (Saxenda®, Novo Nordisk Inc, Plainsboro, NJ) and semaglutide (Wegovy™, Novo Nordisk Inc, Plainsboro, NJ), and the melanocortin 4 (MC4) receptor agonist, setmelanotide (Imcivree™, Rhythm Pharmaceuticals Inc, Boston, MA). Pharmacotherapy management guidelines recommend discontinuation of medication therapy in patients who fail to lose sufficient amounts of body weight after 3 months and in patients who experience significant adverse medication reactions, with consideration given to potential alternative weight loss agents (strong recommendation with high-quality evidence).[29] Table 167-7 lists clinical and economic considerations for use of the products approved for long-term use.

Lipase Inhibitor: Orlistat Excessive intake of dietary fat is one of the contributing factors in the development of obesity. GI (gastric, pancreatic, and carboxyl ester) lipases are essential in the absorption of the long-chain triglycerides. Additionally, lipase is known to play a role in facilitating gastric emptying and secretion of other pancreaticobiliary substances. Orlistat (Xenical®) is a synthetic derivative of lipstatin, a natural lipase inhibitor produced by *Streptomyces toxytricini*. The medication is minimally absorbed and induces weight loss by persistent lowering of dietary fat absorption through selective inhibition of the GI lipase. Furthermore, lower luminal free fatty acid concentrations result in malabsorption of cholesterol. Up to 30% reduction in fat absorption occurs with daily doses of 120 mg three times daily with meals.[89] A nonprescription formulation of orlistat (Alli®) is approved in the United States at a reduced daily dose of 60 mg three times daily.[89] The medication must be taken within 1 hour of consuming foods that contain fat in order to exert its effect. If a meal is skipped or contains no fat, the dose of orlistat can be omitted.

As an adjunct to diet therapy, orlistat results in dose-dependent reductions in fat absorption. Orlistat modestly increases the amount of weight lost and decreases the amount of weight regained during medically supervised weight loss programs.[89] Improved glycemic control can be attained in patients with type 2 diabetes mellitus by inducing or increasing weight loss with orlistat in addition to diet management.[89] In some cases, dosages or the number of antidiabetic medications may be reduced or discontinued. Improvements in the lipid profile (reduction in total and low-density lipoprotein [LDL] cholesterol), glucose control, and other markers of metabolism are seen when using orlistat in addition to the diet.[89,90] Orlistat is approved for the chronic treatment of obesity in adults and adolescents between ages 12 and 16 years. The recommended dose is 120 mg three times daily taken within 1 hour of consuming a fat-containing meal.

At least one GI complaint (soft stools, abdominal pain or colic, flatulence, fecal urgency, or incontinence) has been reported in up to 80% of individuals using prescription-strength orlistat. These complaints are most common in the first 1 to 2 months of therapy, are mild to moderate in severity, and tend to improve with continued orlistat use. Limiting dietary fat before initiation of orlistat therapy may be beneficial in decreasing initial GI complaints. Severe diarrhea secondary to orlistat use can affect the absorption of orally administered medications, such as oral contraceptives, fat-soluble vitamins (A, D, E, and K), and β-carotene. Therefore, supplementation with a multivitamin should be considered during therapy. In the presence of severe diarrhea, women receiving oral contraceptives should be advised of the need to use alternative backup methods because absorption of oral contraceptive may be reduced.

TABLE 167-7 Clinical and Economic Considerations for Long-Term Pharmacotherapy Options

Medication	Brand Name	Weight Loss Above Diet and Exercise Alone (1 year)[85-88]	Cost for 30 Days of Therapy[a]	Comments
Orlistat	Xenical®	2.9-3.4 kg (6.5-7.5 lb)	$685.81	- Use may be limited by GI intolerance
Phentermine and topiramate extended release	Qsymia®	6.6-8.6 kg (14.5-18.9 lb)	$186.00, 7.5 mg-46 mg $199.50, 15 mg-92 mg	- Limited distribution under FDA Risk Evaluation Mitigation Strategy (REMS)
Bupropion and naltrexone extended release	Contrave®	4.9 kg (10.8 lb)	$303.60	- Lowers seizure threshold (bupropion) - Rare reports of hepatotoxicity (naltrexone) - Drug interactions with opioids, CYP2B6 inducers and CYP2D6 substrates
Liraglutide	Saxenda®	5.2 kg (11.4 lb)	$1,349.00	- Injectable (daily dosing) - Available as pre-filled dosing pen - Reduces HbA1c and fasting glucose - Risk of medullary thyroid carcinoma and multiple endocrine neoplasia syndrome type 2 - Rare reports of pancreatitis, gallbladder disease, and suicidal ideation
Semaglutide	Wegovy™	15.5 kg (34.1 lb)[b]	$1,349.00	- Injectable (weekly dosing) - Available as pre-filled dosing pen - Reduces HbA1c and fasting glucose - Risk of medullary thyroid carcinoma and multiple endocrine neoplasia syndrome type 2 - Rare reports of pancreatitis, gallbladder disease, and suicidal ideation
Setmelanotide	Imcivree™	23.1% (patients with POMC or PCSK1 deficiency) 9.7% (patients with LEPR deficiency)	$19,800	- Injectable (daily dosing) - Available as multiple-dose vial (10 mg/mL) - Indicated for genetically confirmed or suspected deficiency POMC, PCSK1, or LEPR

[a]Cost of therapy based on maintenance dose using wholesaler acquisition cost (WAC) as of September 29, 2021.

[b]Data from 68-week trial.

Reduced fat absorption can potentially affect the absorption of lipophilic medications, such as lamotrigine, valproic acid, gabapentin, and amiodarone.[91,92] Decreased vitamin K absorption has also been noted and can alter the patient's warfarin dosage needs. Clinicians should also be aware that orlistat may directly interfere with the absorption of other narrow therapeutic range medications, such as cyclosporine, levothyroxine, and antiretrovirals.[92] In patients requiring concomitant therapies with orlistat, close monitoring is warranted to ensure an adequate therapeutic response. Separation of the administration times of the medications may minimize these potential drug interactions. Finally, there have been rare postmarketing reports of liver damage with the use of orlistat.[92] Although causality has not been definitively linked to orlistat, patients are advised to notify their healthcare providers if they notice signs and symptoms of liver injury, such as development of itching, yellow eyes or skin, dark urine, loss of appetite, or light-colored stools.

Phentermine–Topiramate Extended Release A combination product containing phentermine and topiramate extended release (Qsymia®) is approved for chronic weight management in patients who have obesity (BMI of greater than or equal to 30 kg/m^2) or overweight (BMI of greater than 27 kg/m^2) with at least one weight-related comorbidity.[93] Phentermine is structurally similar to amphetamine, but it has less severe CNS stimulation and a lower misuse potential. Its mechanism of action centers on its ability to enhance norepinephrine (NE) and dopamine neurotransmission, resulting in appetite suppressing effects. Topiramate is an antiseizure medication. Although the exact mechanism for its efficacy in weight management is unknown, it may decrease appetite and increase satiety through multiple pathways, including effects on γ-aminobutyrate, voltage-gated ion channels, excitatory glutamate receptors, or carbonic anhydrase.[93] The doses of phentermine (3.75-15 mg) and topiramate (23-92 mg) in this combination are lower than the therapeutic doses of each separate product when used as monotherapy for obesity (37.5 mg) and seizures (400 mg), respectively. The recommended dosing strategy for phentermine–topiramate extended release involves gradual titration, staring with 3.75 mg of phentermine and 23 mg of topiramate once daily for 14 days and then increasing the dose to 7.5 mg of phentermine and 46 mg of topiramate once daily.[93] After 12 weeks of therapy, the dose may be increased again to 11.25 mg of phentermine and 69 mg of topiramate for 14 days and then to a maximum dose of 15 mg of phentermine and 92 mg of topiramate daily. Likewise, when discontinuing therapy, the dose should be gradually decreased by taking a dose every other day for at least 1 week to prevent the possible precipitation of seizures.

When used as an adjunct to a reduced-calorie diet and lifestyle changes, phentermine–topiramate leads to dose-dependent weight loss and reductions in blood pressure, total cholesterol, LDL cholesterol, triglycerides, fasting glucose, and HbA_{1c}.[85] Mean weight loss after 1 year of treatment is 8.1 kg (17.8 lb) for the 7.5-mg phentermine and 46-mg topiramate dose and 10.2 kg (22.4 lb) for the 15-mg phentermine and 92-mg topiramate group. The efficacy of phentermine–topiramate has also been documented in patients with class II and class III obesity (mean BMI, 42 kg/m^2), with a mean weight loss of 10.9% after 1 year of treatment.[85]

The most common adverse medication reactions associated with the use of phentermine–topiramate are constipation, dry mouth, paraesthesia, dysgeusia, and insomnia.[85,93] Because topiramate is a known teratogen, this medication is contraindicated in pregnancy because fetal exposure in the first trimester increases the risk of cleft lip or cleft palate. To manage the potential risk of teratogenicity, the medication is only available through a limited distribution process under a risk evaluation and mitigation strategy (REMS).[93] All women of childbearing age must have a documented negative pregnancy test result before beginning treatment and then monthly to continue therapy. Topiramate has been associated with acute myopia associated with secondary angle-closure glaucoma, and phentermine can cause mydriasis from adrenergic stimulation. Therefore, this product is also contraindicated in patients with glaucoma. The potential for hypertensive crisis with coadministration of phentermine and monoamine oxidase inhibitors (MAOIs) exists; therefore, patients should have stopped an MAOI for at least 14 days before use of any adrenergic agent. Phentermine–topiramate is also contraindicated in patients with untreated hyperthyroidism.

Monitoring parameters and drug interactions that clinicians should be aware of include known issues related to both components of the formulation. Of note, increases in heart rate greater than 10 beats/min are observed in approximately 50% of patients receiving phentermine–topiramate.[93] In patients receiving the highest dose, 19% experience increases in heart rate that are greater than 20 beats/min. Therefore, heart rate should be monitored in all patients, particularly those with preexisting CVD. Decreases in serum bicarbonate are generally mild, but peak after 4 weeks of therapy. Decreases in serum potassium and increases in serum creatinine are also seen. Therefore, monitoring of serum electrolytes and creatinine is recommended at baseline and during therapy. Clinicians should be aware that concomitant use of non–potassium-sparing diuretics may potentiate the risk for hypokalemia. Although pregnancy risk is not expected, use of phentermine–topiramate concomitantly with oral contraceptives may result in breakthrough bleeding because of increased exposure to progestin and decreases exposure to estrogen. Phentermine–topiramate is classified as a controlled substance in schedule IV because of the misuse potential of phentermine. Therapy should be discontinued if 5% weight loss is not achieved after 12 weeks with the 7.5-mg phentermine and 46-mg topiramate dose.[93]

Naltrexone–Bupropion Extended Release A combination product containing naltrexone and bupropion extended release (Contrave®) is approved for chronic weight management in patients who have obesity (BMI of more than or equal to 30 kg/m^2) or overweight (of more than or equal to 27 kg/m^2) with at least one weight-related comorbidity.[94] Naltrexone and bupropion are both approved separately for treatment of alcohol and opioid physical dependence, and depression and smoking cessation, respectively.[95] Bupropion is a dopamine and norepinephrine reuptake inhibitor, and naltrexone is an opioid antagonist. Although the exact weight-loss mechanism of action is not known for this medication combination, stimulation of release of α-MSH in hypothalamus by bupropion and inhibition of endogenous opioids by naltrexone are thought to contribute to a decrease in appetite.[95] The recommended dosing strategy for naltrexone-bupropion extended-release involves gradual titration, starting with one tablet (8-mg naltrexone/90-mg bupropion) per day and slowly increasing the dose over a period of 4 weeks to a maintenance dose of two tablets twice daily. Doses greater than 32 mg of naltrexone and 360 mg of bupropion (ie, 4 tablets) per day are not recommended. Patients should be advised to not take their dose with a high-fat meal as this would result in increased systemic exposure to both naltrexone and bupropion.

When used in combination with a reduced-calorie diet and lifestyle changes, naltrexone/bupropion is associated with improvements in high-density lipoprotein (HDL) cholesterol, triglycerides, glucose, and insulin.[85,95] Average total weight loss is 7.3 kg (16.1 lb) following 1 year of treatment,[95] with the greatest weight loss (9.7 kg [21.3 lb]) seen in patients without diabetes mellitus also receiving intensive behavior modification therapy.[85]

The most common adverse medication reactions associated with the use of naltrexone/bupropion are nausea, constipation, headache, vomiting, dizziness, insomnia, dry mouth, and diarrhea.[94] Approximately 24% of patients who receive naltrexone-bupropion discontinue treatment due to adverse medication reactions, with nausea being the most frequent reason.[94] Statistically significant increases in heart rate (2.1 beats/min) and blood pressure (1.8-2.3 mm Hg systolic and 1.7-2.1 mm Hg diastolic) occur in patients receiving naltrexone-bupropion during the first 3 months of therapy, but the clinical significance of these increases is unknown. Blood pressure and pulse should be monitored at baseline and at regular intervals following initiation of therapy. Naltrexone-bupropion should not be used in patients with uncontrolled hypertension.[94] Naltrexone monotherapy is associated with rare reports of hepatotoxicity, and patients receiving naltrexone-bupropion should be advised of the signs and symptoms of acute hepatitis. Bupropion lowers the seizure threshold in a dose-dependent manner and has been associated with serious neuropsychiatric reactions and an increased risk of suicidal thoughts and behavior when used for smoking cessation and treatment of depression. Bupropion may also be associated with activation of mania, serious allergic reaction, and angle-closure glaucoma.

Clinicians should also be aware of potential drug interactions with naltrexone-bupropion. Because of the opioid antagonist effects of naltrexone, naltrexone-bupropion is contraindicated in patients receiving chronic opioid or opiate agonist therapy, and also in patients undergoing abrupt withdrawal of chronic alcohol, benzodiazepine, barbiturate or antiseizure medications. Bupropion is metabolized by cytochrome P450 2B6 (CYP2B6) and inhibits cytochrome P450 2D6 (CYP2D6). Therefore, any medication that induces CYP2B6 (eg, rifampin, carbamazepine) could potentially reduce the effects of bupropion, and bupropion could increase the effects of medications that are CYP2D6 substrates (eg, SSRIs, tricyclic antidepressants, antipsychotics). Bupropion is also contraindicated with concomitant use of MAOIs. As with other long-term pharmacologic treatments for obesity, weight loss may increase the risk of hypoglycemia in patients with type 2 diabetes mellitus receiving antidiabetic medications. Finally, treatment with naltrexone-bupropion should be discontinued if 5% weight loss is not achieved after 12 weeks.[94]

Glucagon-Like Peptide-1 Receptor Agonists

Liraglutide Liraglutide (Saxenda®), an analog of GLP-1, is approved in the United States for chronic weight management in adult patients who have obesity (BMI of more than or equal to 30 kg/m^2) or overweight (BMI of more than 27 kg/m^2) with at least one weight-related comorbidity and in adolescents age 12 years and older with body weight above 60 kg (132 lb) and an initial BMI corresponding to obesity according to international cut-offs for age and sex.[96] Endogenous GLP-1 is released in response to food digestion and stimulates GLP-1 receptors in the brain to reduce appetite. GLP-1 also stimulates insulin secretion and reduces glucagon secretion. For that reason, several GLP-1 receptor agonists, including liraglutide, are currently approved for the treatment of type 2 diabetes mellitus at recommended doses of 1.2 mg or 1.8 mg daily far less than the maintenance dose for weight loss of 3 mg daily. Liraglutide is administered subcutaneously and is available in prefilled, multidose pens. When used for weight loss, a 5-week dose escalation schedule is recommended to improve tolerability of GI adverse medication reactions. It should be initiated at a dose of 0.6 mg daily, and increased weekly by 0.6-mg increments to a final maintenance dose of 3 mg daily. If the patient cannot tolerate the GI adverse medication reactions at any point during the dose escalation phase, a dose increase may be delayed by a week. Patients should be instructed on the proper technique for subcutaneous injection into the abdomen, thigh, or upper arm.

The efficacy of liraglutide for the management of overweight and obesity has been studied in patients with and without diabetes mellitus. A mean weight loss of 5.2 kg (11.4 lb) more than placebo is observed after 1 year of treatment with liraglutide[86]; slightly less weight loss is reported for adolescents.[97] As expected, patients who receive liraglutide also experience improvements in HbA_{1c}, fasting glucose and insulin, and had a lower prevalence of prediabetes. Similarly, patients with diabetes mellitus experience a 6% average weight loss after 1 year of treatment.[93] Improvements in fasting glucose and the number of subjects achieving HbA_{1c} targets are also observed. The most common adverse medication reactions associated with the use of liraglutide are nausea, diarrhea, constipation, vomiting, dyspepsia, hypoglycemia, and abdominal pain.[96] GI complaints are the most common reason for premature discontinuation of therapy, underscoring the importance of the slow dose-escalation schedule with initiation of therapy. Rare cases of acute pancreatitis (0.3%), potentially leading to fatal hemorrhagic or necrotizing pancreatitis, may occur with the use of liraglutide.[93] Resting heart rate increases an average of 2 to 3 beats/min with liraglutide; however, increases as high as 20 beats/min may be seen. Although the clinical significance of these increases is unknown, heart rate should be regularly monitored in all patients receiving liraglutide. Cholelithiasis (1.5%), cholecystitis (0.6%), and suicidal ideation (0.2%) are also observed.[96] Liraglutide carries a boxed-warning about the risk of thyroid C-cell tumors, including medullary thyroid carcinoma (MTC), and is contraindicated in patients with a personal or family history of MTC or multiple endocrine neoplasia syndrome type 2 (MEN2). Hypoglycemia may occur when liraglutide is used in combination with other antidiabetic agents (particularly sulfonylureas and insulin) in patients with type 2 diabetes mellitus. Therefore, dose adjustments of antidiabetic medications may be necessary. Because liraglutide increases gastric emptying time, clinicians also should be aware that absorption of concomitantly administered oral medications may be altered. Liraglutide should be discontinued if weight loss of at least 4% is not achieved after 16 weeks of therapy.

Semaglutide Semaglutide (Wegovy™) is the most recent medication approved in the United States for chronic weight management in patients who have obesity (BMI of more than or equal to 30 kg/m^2) or overweight (BMI of more than 27 kg/m^2) with at least one weight-related comorbidity.[98] Similar to liraglutide, semaglutide stimulates GLP-1 receptors in the brain to reduce appetite. Semaglutide (Ozempic®) is also approved for the treatment of type 2 diabetes mellitus and to reduce the risk of major cardiovascular events in adults with type 2 diabetes mellitus and cardiovascular disease as a subcutaneous injection at a dose of 1 mg once weekly.[99] When used for weight loss, the starting of semaglutide is 0.25 mg once weekly for 4 weeks, followed by monthly dose escalation to improve tolerability of GI adverse medication reactions, to a maintenance dose of 2.4 mg weekly. If the patient cannot tolerate the GI adverse medication reactions at any point during the dose escalation phase, a dose increase may be delayed by a month. If a patient cannot tolerate the 2.4 mg weekly dose, the dose may be decreased to 1.7 mg weekly for 1 month before increasing the dose back to 2.4 mg weekly. Patients should be instructed on the proper technique for subcutaneous injection into the abdomen, thigh, or upper arm.

The efficacy of semaglutide for the management of overweight and obesity has been studied in patients with and without diabetes mellitus and has been associated with the greatest amount of weight loss when compared to all other approved weight loss medications.[87,100] Patients receiving semaglutide 2.4 mg weekly lose an average of 14.9% of their original body weight (15.5 kg [34.1 lb]) after 68 weeks of treatment and experience considerable improvements in systolic blood pressure, LDL cholesterol, and HbA1C measurements.[87] Notably, 50% of subjects receiving semaglutide achieve >15% reduction in body weight. In patients with type 2 diabetes mellitus, average weight loss is 9.6% after 68 weeks of therapy.[100]

Adverse medication reactions associated with the use of semaglutide are similar to those observed with liraglutide and include nausea, diarrhea, constipation, vomiting, dyspepsia, and abdominal pain.[87,98,100] Semaglutide is also associated with rare cases of acute pancreatitis, acute gall bladder disease, acute kidney injury, diabetic retinopathy, and small increases in resting heart rate.[98] Semaglutide carries a boxed-warning about the risk of thyroid C-cell tumors, including MTC, and is contraindicated in patients with a personal or family history of MTC or multiple endocrine neoplasia syndrome type 2 (MEN2). As with liraglutide, hypoglycemia may occur when semaglutide is used in combination with other antidiabetic agents in patients with type 2 diabetes mellitus. Therefore, dose adjustments of antidiabetic medications may be necessary.

Melanocortin 4 (MC4) Receptor Agonist

Setmelanotide Setmelanotide (Imcivree™) is a peptide analog of endogenous alpha-melanocyte stimulating hormone (α-MSH) approved for chronic weight management in patients with genetically confirmed or suspected proopiomelanocortin (POMC), proprotein convertase subtilisin/kexin type 1 (PCSK1) or leptin receptor (LEPR) deficiency.[101] Patients with variants in POMC, PCSK1, or LEPR genes are thought to have obesity due to insufficient activation of MC4 receptors in the brain. Setmelanotide is an MC4 receptor agonist that results in reduced hunger and promotes weight loss through decreased energy intake and slightly increased energy expenditure. Setmelanotide is indicated in adults and children aged 6 years and older. It is administered once daily as a subcutaneous injection with a starting dose of 2 mg daily for those 12 years and older and 1 mg daily for children aged 6 to less than 12 years.[101] Depending on tolerability the dose can be gradually increased to a maximum of 3 mg daily. In patients with LEPR or POMC deficiency, setmelanotide is associated with >10% weight loss after 1 year of treatment in 45% and 80% of subjects, respectively.[88] The most common adverse medication reactions associated with setmelanotide include injection site reactions (96%), skin hyperpigmentation (78%), nausea (56%), headache (41%), diarrhea (37%), and abdominal pain (33%).[101] Sexual adverse medication reactions such as spontaneous penile erections may occur. Male patients should be advised to seek medical treatment for an erection lasting longer than 4 hours. It is also advised to monitor for the potential of new or worsening depression and suicidal ideation. According to the manufacturer, if a patient fails to lose at least 5% of baseline body weight (or 5% of baseline BMI) after 12 to 16 weeks of treatment, it is recommended to discontinue setmelanotide due to a low potential for a meaningful weight loss with continued treatment.[101]

Agents Approved for Short-Term Use Several noradrenergic agents are currently approved by the FDA for short-term weight loss. Because short-term therapy is not consistent with current national guidelines for the chronic management of obesity, these agents have limited clinical utility in practice.[6,7]

Phentermine Phentermine is available in both immediate-release and sustained-release formulations. However, the value of sustained-release formulations is questionable based on the phentermine plasma half-life of 12 to 24 hours. Phentermine is an effective adjunct to diet, exercise, and behavior modification for producing weight loss.[102] Intermittent phentermine therapy appears to elicit comparable weight loss as that seen with continuous use. However, most individuals experience weight regains during therapy and generally always after discontinuing use.[102] A single dose of 30 mg once daily in the morning provides effective appetite suppression throughout the day. Divided doses of 8 mg immediately before meals, however, are common.[103] Evening or nighttime dosing should be avoided because of insomnia. Large increases in blood pressure, palpitations, and arrhythmias can occur with phentermine administration. Use is not advisable in hypertensive patients. Pharmacotherapy management guidelines recommend against the use of sympathomimetic agents in patients with uncontrolled hypertension or a history of CVD (strong recommendation with high-quality evidence).[29]

The potential for hypertensive crisis with coadministration of phentermine and MAOIs is noted in the product labeling of each agent; therefore, patients should be off an MAOI for at least 14 days before use of any adrenergic agent to avoid excessive adrenergic stimulation syndromes.[104] Phentermine use is contraindicated in patients with hyperthyroidism or agitated states and in those who misuse substances such as cocaine, phencyclidine, and methamphetamine, again because of the potential for excessive adrenergic stimulation syndromes and misuse potential. Mydriasis from adrenergic stimulation can worsen glaucoma, and patients diagnosed with glaucoma should not receive phentermine. Patients with diabetes mellitus may experience altered insulin or oral hypoglycemic dosage requirements soon after beginning therapy and before any substantial weight loss. Phentermine remains the most widely prescribed weight management medication by obesity specialists despite product labeling that indicates short-term (a few weeks), monotherapy use only.[102] This usage pattern deviates from the current national recommendations that promote only long-term medication intervention when obesity pharmacotherapy is appropriate.[7] Some clinicians consider use of long-term phentermine to be reasonable in select patients given the low cost and a lack of serious long-term adverse medication reactions reported over the past 20 years. Select patients include those without CVD, psychiatric disease, or substance misuse; without clinically significant increases in blood pressure or heart rate while receiving phentermine; and documentation of weight loss while receiving phentermine.

Diethylpropion Diethylpropion stimulates NE release from presynaptic storage granules. Increased adrenergic neurotransmitter concentrations activate hypothalamic centers, which result in decreased appetite and food intake. Diethylpropion can be taken in divided daily doses, generally 25 mg three times daily before meals. An extended-release formulation is also used by some clinicians, usually as 75 mg taken once daily in the morning or midmorning.[102] Both dosing regimens are effective in achieving short-term weight loss. Complaints of insomnia increase if late afternoon dosing is used. Diethylpropion causes less stimulation of the CNS than mazindol and generally causes less insomnia than phentermine. Patients with severe hypertension or CVD should not receive diethylpropion. Patients with diabetes mellitus may experience decreased insulin or oral hypoglycemic dosage requirements soon after beginning therapy and before any substantial weight loss. In patients with diabetes mellitus, more frequent blood glucose self-monitoring and medical follow-up are warranted when treating patients with diethylpropion.

Amphetamines Appetite suppressant effects of the amphetamines were well recognized in the 1930s. Amphetamines activate central noradrenergic receptor systems as well as dopaminergic pathways at higher doses by stimulating neurotransmitter release. Increases in blood pressure and mild bronchodilation are attributed to peripheral α- and β-receptor activation. Amphetamines are no longer widely used for the treatment of obesity because of their powerful stimulant effects and addictive potential.

Complementary and Alternative Therapies 9 Many complementary and alternative therapy products are currently promoted for weight loss. A nationwide survey of US consumers reported that about 15.2% of adults had used "dietary supplements" specifically for the purposes of weight loss.[105] It is important for clinicians to be aware that the regulation of dietary supplements is less rigorous than that of prescription and over-the-counter medications. As such, a manufacturer of a dietary supplement does not have to prove the safety or effectiveness of the product before it is marketed. Of concern, some herbal and food supplement diet agents contain pharmacologically active substances that should be used with caution or avoided in patients who have obesity who also have conditions such as diabetes mellitus, hypertension, and CVD. In addition, many marketed products lack consistency in labeling versus actual product content, and a number of dietary supplements have been found to contain undeclared prescription medications. Common herbal and natural products that have been used for weight loss include hoodia, green tea, citrus aurantium, forskolin, caffeine, glucomannan, yohimbine, chitosan, guar gum, hydroxycitric acid, and garcinia cambogia.[105,106]

EVALUATION OF THERAPEUTIC OUTCOMES

The evaluation and management of a patient with obesity requires careful clinical; biochemical; and, if necessary, psychological evaluation. This evaluation should include an assessment of the patient's current medical condition and medication regimen. A multidisciplinary team including, but not limited to, a physician, dietitian, psychologist, behavioral expert, and pharmacist should ideally be involved in the care of individuals with obesity.

Monitoring the Pharmaceutical Care Plan

Assessment of patient progress should be documented frequently.[6] Each encounter should document weight, WC, BMI, blood pressure, medical history, and patient assessment of obesity medication tolerability.[6] Chronic use of obesity medications should be consistent with the approved product labeling. According to current pharmacologic management guidelines, efficacy and tolerability of the medication should be assessed monthly for the first 3 months, followed by visits every 3 months thereafter (weak recommendation with low quality evidence).[29] If the patient has failed to demonstrate weight loss or maintenance of prior weight, medication therapy should be discontinued after 3 months (strong recommendation with high quality evidence).[29]

To achieve optimal weight loss, patients should be instructed about the importance of adherence to prescribed medication and lifestyle changes. The Short Form 36 (SF-36) is used as a quality-of-life evaluation tool for patients with obesity undergoing programmatic weight loss. Quarterly assessments of well-being and quality of life using validated assessment tools can be helpful in objectively quantifying the effectiveness of therapy. Table 167-8 provides monitoring parameters and potential adverse medication reactions of agents used for long-term management of overweight and obesity.

Patients with diabetes mellitus receiving weight loss medication require more intense medical monitoring and self-monitoring of blood glucose to minimize the risk for hypoglycemia. Insulin therapy may need to be reduced with the start of obesity medication

TABLE 167-8 Adverse Medication Reactions and Monitoring Parameters

Medication	Brand Name	Adverse Medication Reactions	Monitoring Parameters	Comments
Gastrointestinal Lipase Inhibitor				
Orlistat	Xenical®, Alli®[a]	Soft stools, diarrhea, abdominal pain or colic, flatulence, fecal urgency, incontinence, liver damage (rare)	BMI; calorie and fat intake; serum glucose in patients with diabetes; thyroid function in patients with thyroid disease; liver function tests in patients exhibiting symptoms of hepatic dysfunction	Supplement with a multivitamin during therapy to prevent vitamin deficiency
Phentermine–Topiramate Combination				
Phentermine and topiramate extended release	Qsymia®	Constipation, dry mouth, paresthesia, dysgeusia, insomnia, hypoglycemia in patients with diabetes	BMI; calorie and fat intake; serum glucose in patients with diabetes; pregnancy; depression or suicidal thoughts; mood or sleep disorders; heart rate; serum electrolytes and creatinine at baseline and during treatment	Discontinue or escalate dose if 3% weight loss not achieved by week 12 on phentermine 7.5 mg and topiramate 46 mg Discontinue if 5% weight loss not achieved by week 12 on phentermine 15 mg and topiramate 92 mg Gradually discontinue phentermine 15 mg and topiramate 92 mg to prevent possible seizure
Bupropion-Naltrexone Combination				
Bupropion and naltrexone extended release	Contrave®	Nausea, constipation, headache, vomiting, dizziness, insomnia, dry mouth, and diarrhea	BMI; calorie and fat intake; serum glucose in patients with diabetes; heart rate and blood pressure; signs and symptoms of hepatotoxicity, neuropsychiatric reactions, and suicidal thoughts or behavior	Discontinue if 5% weight loss not achieved by week 12
Glucagon-Like Peptide-1 Antagonists				
Liraglutide Semaglutide	Saxenda® Wegovi™	Nausea, diarrhea, constipation, vomiting, dyspepsia, hypoglycemia, and abdominal pain	BMI; calorie and fat intake; serum glucose in patients with diabetes; signs and symptoms of pancreatitis; heart rate; signs and symptoms of gallbladder disease and suicidal ideation	Discontinue liraglutide if 4% weight loss not achieved by week 16. At present, there is no recommendation to discontinue semaglutide therapy for inadequate weight loss at week 16.

(continued)

TABLE 167-8 Adverse Medication Reactions and Monitoring Parameters (*Continued*)

Medication	Brand Name	Adverse Medication Reactions	Monitoring Parameters	Comments
Melanocortin 4 Receptor Agonist				
Setmelanotide	Imcivree™	Injection site reactions, skin hyperpigmentation, nausea, headache, diarrhea, and abdominal pain	BMI; calorie and fat intake; serum glucose in patients with diabetes, sexual adverse medication reactions, new or worsening depression, and suicidal ideation	Approved for patients with genetically confirmed or suspected deficiency of POMC, PCSK1, or LEPR Discontinue if 5% weight loss (or 5% decrease in BMI) not achieved after 12 to 16 weeks
Noradrenergic Agents				
Phendimetrazine Phentermine Diethylpropion	Bontril® PDM; Bontril® Slow-Release Adipex-P®, Suprenza™ Tenuate®, Tenuate Dospan	Increased blood pressure, ischemic events, palpitations, tachycardia, valvular disease, urticaria, agitation, dizziness, headache, insomnia, overstimulation, psychosis, restlessness, dry mouth, constipation, thirst, diarrhea	Baseline cardiac evaluation (for preexisting valvular heart disease, pulmonary hypertension); echocardiogram during therapy; weight, waist circumference; blood pressure	Approved as monotherapies only for short-term use (a few weeks) Discontinue if satisfactory weight loss has not occurred within the first 4 weeks of treatment or if tolerance develops Abrupt discontinuation after prolonged high doses may be associated with extreme fatigue and depression

BMI, body mass index.

[a]Available without a prescription.

therapy. Some patients with diabetes mellitus may require daily telephone contact with a healthcare provider to assist in adjusting their hypoglycemic therapy. Weekly patient visits to a healthcare setting may be necessary for 1 to 2 months until the effects of diet, exercise, and weight loss medication become more predictable. As frequent as quarterly assessment of HbA_{1c} may be appropriate in patients with type 2 diabetes mellitus who lose weight to aid in adjustment of hypoglycemic therapy. Lipid profiles can normalize or improve with weight loss. Lipid status should be assessed semiannually or annually in patients with hyperlipidemia to determine the need for continued hyperlipidemia therapies. Weight loss also can result in normalization of blood pressure in hypertensive patients who have obesity. Assessment of appropriateness of antihypertensive therapy should occur with each follow-up visit.

CONCLUSION

Obesity is a complex chronic disease with a prevalence that has increased dramatically over the past 50 years. Increased body weight is a consequence of increased energy storage resulting from an imbalance between energy intake and energy expenditure over time, which is influenced by many factors, including genetics and the environment. Nonpharmacologic therapy, including reduced caloric intake, increased physical activity, and behavioral modification, is currently the mainstay of obesity management. Medication therapy may be considered as an adjunct for patients who fail to achieve adequate weight loss with comprehensive lifestyle modifications. Currently, six products—orlistat, phentermine–topiramate extended release, naltrexone-bupropion extended release, liraglutide, semaglutide, and setmelanotide—are approved by the FDA for the long-term treatment of overweight and obesity. Bariatric procedures have long-term efficacy for weight reduction, but they also introduce surgical comorbidities and, for the most efficacious procedures, may cause nutritional deficiencies. For patients who are not able to undergo bariatric surgery, medical devices may also be considered. Treatment of obesity should be individualized, considering factors such as patient desires, age, degree and duration of obesity, and the presence and severity of medical conditions both directly related to obesity and those that may have an impact on the therapeutic decisions. Regardless of the chosen treatment plan, the management of obesity is a lifelong process requiring patient support and careful monitoring for safety and efficacy.

ABBREVIATIONS

5-HT	5-hydroxytryptamine (serotonin)
α-MSH	alpha-melanocyte stimulating hormone
AACE	American Association of Clinical Endocrinologists
ACE	American College of Endocrinology
AHEAD	Action for Health in Diabetes
BAT	brown adipose tissue
BMI	body mass index
BMR	basal metabolic rate
CDC	Centers for Disease Control and Prevention
CNS	central nervous system
CT	computed tomography
CVD	cardiovascular disease
DASH	Dietary Approaches to Stop Hypertension
FDA	Food and Drug Administration
GI	gastrointestinal
GLP-1	glucagon-like peptide-1
HbA_{1c}	hemoglobin A_{1c}
HDL	high-density lipoprotein
LCD	low-calorie diet
LDL	low-density lipoprotein
LEPR	leptin receptor
MAOI	monoamine oxidase inhibitor
MC4	melanocortin 4
MEN2	multiple endocrine neoplasia syndrome type 2
MRI	magnetic resonance imaging
MTC	medullary thyroid carcinoma
NE	norepinephrine
NHANES	National Health and Nutrition Examination Survey
NIH	National Institutes of Health
REE	resting energy expenditure
REMS	risk evaluation and mitigation strategy
POMC	proopiomelanocortin
PCSK1	proprotein convertase subtilisin/kexin type 1

SF-36	Short Form 36
SNRI	serotonin-norepinephrine reuptake inhibitor
SSRI	selective serotonin reuptake inhibitor
TRE	time-restricted eating
WAT	white adipose tissue
WAGR	Wilms' tumor, aniridia, genitourinary abnormalities or gonadoblastoma, and mental retardation
WC	waist circumference

REFERENCES

1. World Health Organization. Obesity and overweight. Fact sheet, June 2021. https://www.who.int/news-room/fact-sheets/detail/obesity-and-overweight. Accessed August 18, 2021.
2. Fryar CD, Carroll MD, Afful J. Prevalence of overweight, obesity, and severe obesity among adults aged 20 and over: United States, 1960-1962 through 2017-2018. NCHS Health E-Stats. 2020. https://www.cdc.gov/nchs/data/hestat/obesity-adult-17-18/overweight-obesity-adults-H.pdf. Accessed August 18, 2021.
3. Fryar CD, Carroll MD, Afful J. Prevalence of overweight, obesity, and severe obesity among children and adolescents aged 2-19 years: United States, 1963-1965 through 2017-2018. NCHS Health E-Stats. 2020. https://www.cdc.gov/nchs/data/hestat/obesity-child-17-18/overweight-obesity-child-H.pdf. Accessed August 17, 2021.
4. U.S. Department of Health and Human Services. National Heart Lung and Blood Institute. Obesity Initiative Expert Panel on the Identification, Evaluation, and Treatment of Overweight and Obesity in Adults. Washington, DC: U.S. Public Health Service, 1998.
5. Arnett DK, Blumenthal RS, Albert MA et al. 2019 ACC/AHA Guideline on the Primary Prevention of Cardiovascular Disease: A Report of the American College of Cardiology/American Heart Association Task Force on Clinical Practice Guidelines. *Circulation.* 2019;140(11):e596–e646. doi:10.1161/CIR.0000000000000678.
6. Garvey WT, Mechanick JI, Brett EM, et al. American Association of Clinical Endocrinologist and American College of Endocrinology Comprehensive Clinical Practice Guidelines for medical care of patients with obesity. *Endocr Pract.* 2016;3:1–203. doi:10.4158/EP161365.GL.jnjnmoil8i.
7. Managing Overweight and Obesity in Adults: Systemic Review from the Obesity Expert Panel, 2013. Content last reviewed August 2018. Agency for Healthcare Research and Quality, Rockville, MD. https://www.ahrq.gov/evidencenow/heart-health/overall/obesity.html. Accessed August 18, 2021.
8. Upadhyay J, Farr O, Perakakis N, et al. Obesity as a disease. *Med Clin North Am.* 2018;102(1):13–33. doi:10.1016/j.mcna.2017.08.004.
9. Chughtai M, Khlopas A, Newman JM, et al. What is the impact of body mass index on cardiovascular and musculoskeletal health? *Surg Technol Int.* 2017;30:379–392.
10. Collins KH, Herzog W, MacDonald GZ, et al. Obesity, metabolic syndrome, and musculoskeletal disease: Common inflammatory pathways suggest a central role for loss of muscle integrity. *Front Physiol.* 2018 Feb 23;9:112. doi:10.3389/fphys.2018.00112.
11. Kwok S, Adam S, Ho JH, et al. Obesity: A critical risk factor in the COVID-19 pandemic. *Clin Obes.* 2020;10(6):e12403. doi:10.1111/cob.12403.
12. Rubino F, Puhl RM, Cummings DE, et al. Joint international consensus statement for ending stigma of obesity. *Nat Med.* 2020;26(4):485–497. doi:10.1038/s41591-020-0803-x.
13. Thomas-Valdés S, Tostes MDGV, Anunciação PC, et al. Association between vitamin deficiency and metabolic disorders related to obesity. *Crit Rev Food Sci Nutr.* 2017;57(15):3332–3343. doi:10.1080/10408398.2015.1117413.
14. Ghiassi S, El Chaar M, Aleassa EM, et al. ASMBS position statement on the relationship between obesity and cancer, and the role of bariatric surgery: Risk, timing of treatment, effects on disease biology, and qualification for surgery. *Surg Obes Relat Dis.* 2020;16(6):713–724. doi:10.1016/j.soard.2020.03.019.
15. Sarwer DB, Hanson AJ, Voeller J, et al. Obesity and sexual functioning. *Curr Obes Rep.* 2018;7(4):301–307. doi:10.1007/s13679-018-0319-6.
16. Avgerinos KI, Spyrou N, Mantzoros CS, et al. Obesity and cancer risk: Emerging biological mechanisms and perspectives. *Metabolism.* 2019;92:121–135. doi:10.1016/j.metabol.2018.11.001.
17. Kushner RF, Roth JL. Assessment of the obese patient. *Endocrinol Metab Clin North Am.* 2003;32(4):915–933. doi:10.1016/s0889-8529(03)00068-9.
18. Roa I, Del Sol M. Obesity salivary glands and oral pathology. *Colomb Med (Cali).* 2018;49(4):280–287. 10.25100/cm.v49i3.3919.
19. Robinson PD. Obesity and its impact on the respiratory system. *Paediatr Respir Rev.* 2014;15(3):219–26. doi:10.1016/j.prrv.2014.06.003.
20. Lakkis JI, Weir MR. Obesity and kidney disease. *Prog Cardiovasc Dis.* 2018;61(2):157–167. 10.1016/j.pcad.2018.07.005.
21. Hirt PA, Castillo DE, Yosipovitch G, et al. Skin changes in the obese patient. *J Am Acad Dermatol.* 2019;81(5):1037–1057. doi:10.1016/j.jaad.2018.12.070.
22. McAuliffe FM, Killeen SL, Jacob CM, et al. Management of prepregnancy, pregnancy, and postpartum obesity from the FIGO Pregnancy and Non-Communicable Diseases Committee: A FIGO (International Federation of Gynecology and Obstetrics) guideline. *Int J Gynaecol Obstet.* 2020;151(Suppl 1):16–36. doi:10.1002/ijgo.13334.
23. Kinlen D, Cody D, O'Shea D. Complications of obesity. *QJM.* 2018;111(7):437–443. doi:10.1093/qjmed/hcx152.
24. Bhaskaran K, Santos-Silva I, Leon DA, et al. Association of BMI with overall and cause-specific mortality: A population-based cohort study of 3.6 million adults in the UK. *Lancet Diabetes Endocrinol.* 2018;(12):944–953. doi:10.1016/S2213-8587(18)30288-2.
25. Biener A, Cawley J, Meyerhoefer CJ. The high and rising costs of obesity to the US Health Care System. *Gen Intern Med.* 2017;32(Suppl 1):6–8. doi:10.1007/s11606-016-3968-8.
26. American Diabetes Association. Obesity management for the treatment of type 2 diabetes: Standards of Medical Care in Diabetes-2021. *Diabetes Care.* 2021;44(Suppl 1):S100–S110. 10.2337/dc21-S008.
27. World Health Organization. Reducing the burden of noncommunicable diseases through strengthening prevention and control of diabetes. The Seventy-fourth World Health Assembly, May 31, 2021. WHA74.4. Geneva: World Health Organization; 2021. https://apps.who.int/gb/ebwha/pdf_files/WHA74/A74_R4-en.pdf. Accessed August 18, 2021.
28. US Preventative Services Task Force. Behavioral weight loss interventions to prevent obesity-related morbidity and mortality in adults: US Preventative Services Task Force Recommendation Statement. *JAMA.* 2018;320(11):1163–1171.
29. Apovian CM, Aronne LJ, Bessesen DH, et al. Pharmacological management of obesity: An Endocrine Society Clinical Practice Guideline. *J Clin Endocrinol Metab.* 2015;100:342–362. doi:10.1210/jc.2014-3415.
30. Rubino F, Puhl RM, Cummings DE, et al. Joint international consensus statement for ending stigma of obesity. *Nat Med.* 2020;26(4):485–497. doi:10.1038/s41591-020-0803-x.
31. Semlitsch T, Stigler FL, Jeitler K, et al. Management of overweight and obesity in primary care: A systematic overview of international evidence-based guidelines. *Obes Rev.* 2019;20(9):1218–1230. doi:10.1111/obr.12889.
32. Durrer Schutz D, Busetto L, Dicker D, et al. European practical and patient-centered guidelines for adult obesity management in primary care. *Obes Facts.* 2019;12(1):40–66. doi:10.1159/000496183.
33. Wharton S, Lau DCW, Vallis M, et al. Obesity in adults: A clinical practice guideline. *CMAJ.* 2020;192(31):E875–E891. doi:10.1503/cmaj.191707.
34. Styne, DM, Arslanian SA, Conner EL, et al. Pediatric obesity—Assessment, treatment, and prevention: An endocrine society clinical practice guideline. *Clin Endocrinol Metab.* 2017;102(3):709–757. doi:10.1210/jc.2016-2573.
35. World Health Organization. Report of the Commission on Ending Childhood Obesity: Implementation plan. Seventieth World Health Assembly, March 2017. http://apps.who.int/gb/ebwha/pdf_files/WHA70/A70_31-en.pdf. Accessed August 18, 2021.
36. Wang Y, Beydoun MA, Min J, et al. Has the prevalence of overweight, obesity and central obesity levelled off in the United States? Trends, patterns, disparities, and future projections for the obesity epidemic. *Int J Epidemiol.* 2020;49(3):810–823. doi:10.1093/ije/dyz273.
37. Kelsey MM, Zaepfel A, Bjornstad P, et al. Age-related consequences of childhood obesity. *Gerontology.* 2014;60(3):222–28. doi:10.1159/000356023.
38. Ogden CL, Fakhouri TH, Carroll MD, et al. Prevalence of obesity among adults, by household income and education—United States, 2011-2014. Center for Disease Control and Prevention. *Morbidity and Mortality Weekly Report: MMWR.* 2017;66(50):1369–1371. https://www.cdc.gov/mmwr/volumes/66/wr/mm6650a1.htm?s_cid=mm6650a1_w. Accessed December 27, 2018.
39. Bouchard C. Genetics of obesity: What we have learned over decades of research. *Obesity.* 2021;29:802–820. doi:10.1002/oby.23116.

40. Apovian CM. Obesity: definition comorbidities, causes and burden. *Am J Manag Care.* 2016;22(Suppl):s176–s185.
41. Berthoud HR. The neurobiology of food intake in an obesogenic environment. *Proc Nutr Soc.* 2012;71(4):478–487. doi:10.1017/S0029665112000602.
42. Powell K, Wilcox J, Clonan A, et al. The role of social networks in the development of overweight and obesity among adults: Scoping review. *BMC Public Health.* 2015;15:996.
43. Verhaegen AA, Van Gall LF. Drugs affecting body weight, body fat distribution, and metabolic function—Mechanisms and possible therapeutic or preventive measures: An update. *Curr Obes Rep.* 2021;10:1–13. doi:10.1007/s13679-020-00419-5.
44. Schneeberger M, Gomis R, Claret M. Hypothalamic and brainstem neuronal circuits controlling homeostatic energy balance. *J Endocrinol.* 2014;220:T25–T46. doi:10.1530/JOE-13-0398.
45. Theilade S, Christensen MB, Vilsboll T, et al. An overview of obesity mechanisms in humans: Endocrine regulation of food intake, eating behavior and common determinants of body weight. *Diabetes Obes Metab.* 2021;23(1):17–35. doi:10.1111/dom.14270.
46. Suchacki KJ, Stimson RH. Nutritional regulation of human brown adipose tissue. *Nutrients.* 2021;13(6): 1748. doi:10.3390/nu13061748.
47. Fang J, Zhang Z, Ayala C, et al. Cardiovascular health among non-Hispanic Asian Americans: NHANES, 2011-2016. *J Am Heart Assoc.* 2019 Jul 2;8(13):e011324. doi:10.1161/JAHA.118.011324.
48. Rønn PF, Andersen GS, Lauritzen T, et al. Abdominal visceral and subcutaneous adipose tissue and associations with cardiometabolic risk in Inuit, Africans and Europeans: A cross-sectional study. *BMJ Open.* 2020;10(9):e038071. doi:10.1136/bmjopen-2020-038071.
49. Gujral UP, Vittinghoff E, Mongraw-Chaffin M, et al. Cardiometabolic abnormalities among normal-weight persons from five racial/ethnic groups in the United States: A cross-sectional analysis of two cohort studies. *Ann Intern Med.* 2017;166(9):628–636. doi:10.7326/M16-1895.
50. The GBD 2015 Obesity Collaborators. Health effects of overweight and obesity in 195 countries over 25 years. *N Engl J Med.* 2017;377:13–27. doi:10.1056/NEJMoa1614362.
51. Dwivedi AK, Dubey P, Cistola DP, et al. Association between obesity and cardiovascular outcomes: Updated evidence from meta-analysis studies. *Curr Cardiol Rep.* 2020;22(4):25. doi:10.1007/s11886-020-1273-y.
52. Riaz H, Khan MS, Siddiqi TJ, et al. Association between obesity and cardiovascular outcomes: A systemic review and meta-analysis of mendelian randomization studies. *JAMA Netw Open.* 2018;1(7):e183788.
53. Grover SA, Kaouache M, Rempel P, et al. Years of life lost and healthy life-years lost from diabetes and cardiovascular disease in overweight and obese people: A modeling study. *Lancet Diabetes Endocrinol.* 2015;3(2):114–122.
54. Bjørnelv GMW, Halsteinli V, Kulseng BE, et al. Modeling Obesity in Norway (The MOON Study): A decision-analytic approach—prevalence, costs, and years of life lost. *Med Decis Making.* 2021;41(1):21–36. doi:10.1177/0272989X20971589.
55. Center for Disease Control and Prevention. Overweight and obesity: strategies to prevent obesity. https://www.cdc.gov/obesity/strategies/index.html. Accessed August 20, 2021.
56. Community Preventative Services Task Force (CPSTF). CPSTF findings for obesity. https://www.thecommunityguide.org/content/task-force-findings-obesity. Accessed August 31, 2021.
57. World Obesity. Global Obesity Observatory. United States: Policies, interventions, and actions. World Obesity Federation website. https://data.worldobesity.org/country/united-states-227/#data_policies. Accessed August 31, 2021.
58. Bays HE, McCarthy W, Burridge K, et al. Obesity Algorithm eBook. Obesity Medicine Association. www.obesityalgorithm.org. 2021. https://obesitymedicine.org/obesity-algorithm/. Accessed September 3, 2021.
59. Salvia MG. The Look AHEAD Trial: Translating lessons learned into clinical practice and further study. *Diabetes Spectr.* 2017;30(3):166–170. doi:10.2337/ds17-0016.
60. LeBlanc ES, Patnode CD, Webber EM, et al. Behavioral and pharmacotherapy weight loss interventions to prevent obesity-related morbidity and mortality in adults: Updated evidence report and systematic review for the US Preventive Services Task Force. *JAMA.* 2018;320(11):1172–1191. doi:10.1001/jama.2018.7777.
61. Franz MJ, Boucher JL, Rutten-Ramos S, et al. Lifestyle weight-loss intervention outcomes in overweight and obese adults with type 2 diabetes: A systematic review and meta-analysis of randomized clinical trials. *J Acad Nutr Diet.* 2015;S2212-2672(15):00259-2. doi:10.1016/j.jand.2015.02.031.
62. Pasquali R, Casanueva F, Haluzik M, et al. European Society of Endocrinology Clinical Practice Guideline: Endocrine work-up in obesity. *Eur J Endocrinol.* 2020;182(1):G1–G32. doi:10.1530/EJE-19-0893.
63. Laudenslager M, Chaudhry ZW, Rajagopal S, et al. Commercial weight loss programs in the management of obesity: An update. *Curr Obes Rep.* 2021;10:90–99. doi:10.1007/s13679-021-00428-y.
64. Ge L, Sadeghirad B, Ball GDC. Comparison of dietary macronutrient patterns of 14 popular named dietary programs for weight and cardiovascular risk factor reduction in adults: Systematic review and network meta-analysis of randomized trials. *BMJ.* 2020;3679:m696. doi:10.1136/bmj.m696.
65. Fanti M, Mishr A, Longo VD, et al. Time-restricted eating, intermittent fasting, and fasting-mimicking diets in weight loss. *Curr Obes Rep.* 2021;10:70–80. doi:10.1007/s13679-021-00424-2.
66. Piercy KL, Troiano RP, Ballard RM, et al. The physical activity guidelines for Americans. *JAMA.* 2018;320:2020–2028. doi:10.1001/jama.2018.14854.
67. English WJ, Williams DB. Metabolic and bariatric surgery: An effective treatment option for obesity and cardiovascular Disease. *Prog Cardiovasc Dis.* 2018;61(2):253–269. doi:10.1016/j.pcad.2018.06.003.
68. Mechanick JI, Apovian C, Brethauer S, et al. Clinical Practice Guidelines for the Perioperative Nutrition, Metabolic, and Nonsurgical Support of Patients Undergoing Bariatric Procedures—2019 Update: Cosponsored by American Association of Clinical Endocrinologists/American College of Endocrinology, The Obesity Society, American Society for Metabolic and Bariatric Surgery, Obesity Medicine Association, and American Society of Anesthesiologists. *Obesity (Silver Spring).* 2020;28(4):O1–O58. doi:10.1002/oby.22719.
69. Armstrong SC, Bolling CF, Michalsky MP, et al. Pediatric metabolic and bariatric surgery: Evidence, barriers, and best practices. *Pediatrics.* 2019;144(6):e20193223. doi:10.1542/peds.2019-3223.
70. Schauer PR, Bhatt DL, Kirwan JP, et al. Bariatric surgery versus intensive medical therapy for diabetes: 5-Year outcomes. *N Engl J Med.* 2017;376(7):641–651. doi:10.1056/NEJMoa1600869.
71. Inge TH, Courcoulas AP, Jenkins TM, et al. Five-year outcomes of gastric bypass in adolescents as compared with adults. *N Engl J Med.* 2019;380(22):2136–45. doi:10.1056/NEJMoa1813909.
72. Inge TH, Jenkins TM, Xanthakos SA, et al. Long-term outcomes of bariatric surgery in adolescents with severe obesity (FABS-5+): A prospective follow-up analysis. *Lancet Diabetes Endocrinol.* 2017;5(3):165–173. doi:10.1016/S2213-8587(16)30315-1.
73. Billeter AT, Eichel S, Scheurlen KM, et al. Meta-analysis of metabolic surgery versus medical treatment for macrovascular complications and mortality in patients with type 2 diabetes. *Surg Obes Relat Dis.* 2019;15(7):1197–1210. doi:10.1016/j.soard.2019.04.029.
74. Adams TD, Davidson LE, Litwin SE, et al. Weight and metabolic outcomes 12 years after gastric bypass. *N Engl J Med.* 2017;377:1143–1155. doi:10.1056/NEJMoa1700459.
75. Billeter AT, Scheurlen KM, Probst P, et al. Meta-analysis of metabolic surgery versus medical treatment for microvascular complications in patients with type 2 diabetes mellitus. *Br J Surg.* 2018;105(3):168–181. doi:10.1002/bjs.10724.
76. Syn NL, Cummings DE, Wang LZ, et al. Association of metabolic-bariatric surgery with long-term survival in adults with and without diabetes: A one-stage meta-analysis of matched cohort and prospective controlled studies with 174 772 participants. *Lancet.* 2021;397(10287):1830–1841. doi:10.1016/S0140-6736(21)00591-2.
77. Xia Q, Campbell JA, Ahmad H, Si L, et al. Bariatric surgery is a cost-saving treatment for obesity: A comprehensive meta-analysis and updated systematic review of health economic evaluations of bariatric surgery. *Obes Rev.* 2020;21(1):e12932. doi:10.1111/obr.12932.
78. Kingma JS, Burgers DMT, Monpellier VM, et al. Oral drug dosing following bariatric surgery: General concepts and specific dosing advice. *Br J Clin Pharmacol.* 2021. doi:10.1111/bcp.14913.
79. Saunders KH, Igel LI, Saumoy M, et al. Devices and endoscopic bariatric therapies for obesity. *Curr Obes Rep.* 2018;7:162–171. doi:10.1007/s13679-018-0307-x.
80. Jirapinyo P, Kumar N, Saumoy M, et al. Association for Bariatric Endoscopy systematic review and meta-analysis assessing the American Society for Gastrointestinal Endoscopy Preservation and Incorporation of Valuable Endoscopic Innovations thresholds for aspiration therapy. *Gastrointest Endosc.* 2021;93(2):334–342.e1. doi:10.1016/j.gie.2020.09.021.
81. Bariatric Endoscopy Task Force ASGE. Technology Committee ASGE, Abu Dayeh BK, Kumar N, et al. ASGE Bariatric Endoscopy Task Force systemic review and meta-analysis assessing the ASGE PIVI thresholds

for adopting endoscopic bariatric therapies. *Gastrointest Endosc.* 2015;82(3)425–438. doi:10.1016/j.gie.2015.03.1964.

82. Ali MR, Moustarah F, Kim JJ. American Society for Metabolic and Bariatric Surgery Clinical Issues Committee. American Society for Metabolic and Bariatric Surgery position statement on intragastric balloon therapy endorsed by the Society of American Gastrointestinal and Endoscopic Surgeons. *Surg Obes Relat Dis.* 2016;12(3):462–467. doi:10.1016/j.soard.2015.12.026.
83. Bazerbachi F, Vargas EJ, Abu Dayyeh BK. Endoscopic bariatric therapy: A guide to the intragastric balloon. *Am J Gastroenterol.* 2019;114(9):1421–1431. doi:10.14309/ajg.0000000000000239.
84. Pass A, Bialonczyk D, Chiquette E, et al. Oral superabsorbent hydrogel (plenity) for weight management. *Ann Pharmacother.* 2021;55(9):1146–1152. doi:10.1177/1060028020983046.
85. Tak YJ, Lee SY. Long-term efficacy and safety of anti-obesity treatment: Where do we stand? *Curr Obes Rep.* 2021;10:14–30. doi:10.1007/s13679-020-00422-w.
86. Khera R, Murad MH, Chandar AK, et al. Association of pharmacological treatments for obesity with weight loss and adverse events: A systematic review and meta-analysis. *JAMA.* 2016;315(22):2424–2434. doi:10.1001/jama.2016.7602.
87. Wilding JPH, Batterham RL, Calanna S, et al. Once-weekly semaglutide in adults with overweight or obesity. *N Engl J Med.* 2021;384:989–1002. doi:10.1056/NEJMoa2032183.
88. Clément K, van den Akker E, Argente J, et al. Efficacy and safety of setmelanotide, an MC4R agonist, in individuals with severe obesity due to LEPR or POMC deficiency: Single-arm, open-label, multicentre, phase 3 trials. *Lancet Diabetes Endocrinol.* 2020;8(12):960–970. doi:10.1016/S2213-8587(20)30364-8.
89. Yanovski SZ, Yanovski JA. Long-term drug treatment for obesity: A systematic and clinical review. *JAMA.* 2014;311(1):74–86. doi:10.1001/jama.2013.281361.
90. Sahebkar A, Simental-Mendia LE, Reiner Z, et al. Effect of orlistat on plasma lipids and body weight: A systematic review and meta-analysis of 33 randomized controlled trials. *Pharmacol Res.* 2017;122:53–65. doi:10.1016/j.phrs.2017.05.022.
91. Halpern B, Halpern A. Safety assessment of FDA-approved (orlistat and lorcaserin) antiobesity medications. *Expert Opin Drug Saf.* 2015;14(2):185–189. doi:10.1517/14740338.2015.994502.
92. Xenical.® Package insert. Greifswald, Germany: Cheplapharm Arzneimittel GmbH; 2020.
93. Qsymia.™ Package insert. Mountain View, CA: Vivus Inc; 2020.
94. Contrave.® Package insert. San Diego, CA: Nalpropion Pharmaceuticals Inc; 2020.
95. Yanovski SZ, Yanovski JA. Naltrexone extended-release plus bupropion extended-release for treatment of obesity. *JAMA.* 2015;313(12):1213–1214. doi:10.1001/jama.2015.1617.
96. Saxenda.® Package insert. Plainsboro, NJ: Novo Nordisk Inc; 2020.
97. Kelly AS, Auerbach P, Barrientos-Perez M, et al. NN8022-4180 Trial Investigators. A randomized, controlled trial of liraglutide for adolescents with obesity. *N Engl J Med.* 2020;382(22):2117–2128. doi:10.1056/NEJMoa1916038.
98. Wegovy.™ Package insert. Plainsboro, NJ: Novo Nordisk Inc; 2021.
99. Ozempic.™ Package insert. Plainsboro, NJ: Novo Nordisk Inc; 2020.
100. Davis M, Faerch L, Jeppesen OK, et al. Semaglutide 2.4 mg once a week in adults with overweight or obesity, and type 2 diabetes (STEP 2): A randomized, double-blind, double-dummy, placebo-controlled, phase 3 trial. *Lancet.* 2021;397:971–984. doi:10.1016/S0140-6736(21)00213-0.
101. Imcivree.™ Package insert. Boston MA: Rhythm Pharmaceuticals, Inc; 2021.
102. Velazquez A, Apovian CM. Update on obesity pharmacotherapy. *Ann N Y Acad Sci.* 2018;1411:106–119.
103. Saunders KH, Umashanker D, Igel L, et al. Obesity pharmacotherapy. *Med Clin N Am.* 2018;102:135–148.
104. Adipex-P.® Package insert. Horsham, PA: Teva Select Brands; 2020.
105. Bray GA, Heisel WE, Afshin A, et al. The science of obesity management: An Endocrine Society Scientific Statement. *Endocr Rev* 2018;39:79–132. doi:10.1210/er.2017-00253.
106. Rios-Hoyo A, Gitierrez-Salmean G. New dietary supplements for obesity: What we currently know. *Curr Obes Rep.* 2016;5:262–270. doi:10.1007/s13679-016-0214-y.

Index

Page numbers followed by *f*, *t*, or *b* indicate figures, tables, or clinical presentation boxes, respectively.

INDEX

INDEX

D

E

H

I

M

O

INDEX

Q

R

INDEX

V

W

X

Y

Z